Clarke's Analysis of Drugs and Poisons

Clarke's Analysis of Drugs and Poisons

in pharmaceuticals, body fluids and postmortem material

THIRD EDITION

Consulting Editors

Anthony C Moffat M David Osselton Brian Widdop

Managing Editor

Laurent Y Galichet

London • Chicago Pharmaceutical Press

Published by the Pharmaceutical Press
Publications division of the Royal Pharmaceutical Society of Great Britain

1 Lambeth High Street, London SE1 7JN, UK
100 South Atkinson Road, Suite 206, Grayslake, IL 60030-7820, USA

First edition, edited by E G C Clarke, published 1969 (Vol. 1) and 1975 (Vol. 2)
Second edition (in one volume) published 1986
Third edition published 2004

Text design by Barker/Hilsdon, Lyme Regis, Dorset
Typeset by Bibliocraft Ltd, Dundee
Printed in Great Britain by The Bath Press, Bath

ISBN 0 85369 473 7

A catalogue record for this book is available from the British Library

Contents

Abbreviations

A_1^1	specific absorbance (abbreviation of $A_{1cm}^{1\%}$)
AC	acetylated
AFID	alkali flame ionisation detector
agg.	aggregate (in botanical names), including 2 or more species which resemble each other closely
AIDS	acquired immunodeficiency syndrome
API	atmospheric pressure ionisation
APCI	atmospheric pressure chemical ionisation
Art	artefact
AUC	area under the curve
AV	atrioventricular
B.P.	British Pharmacopoeia
b.p.	boiling point
CAS	Chemical Abstracts Service
CFTB	5-chloro-2′-fluoro-2-(2,2,2-trifluoroethylamino)-benzophenone
CHF	congestive heart failure
-CHNO	descarbamoyl artefact
CI	chemical ionisation
CIn	colour index
Cl	clearance
CNS	central nervous system
$-CO_2$	artefact formed by decarboxylation
CSF	cerebrospinal fluid
CT	computed tomography
DMES	dimethylethylsilyl
DMF	dimethylformamide
DMSO	dimethylsulfoxide
ECD	electron capture detection
ECG	electrocardiogram
EDTA	ethylene diamine tetra-acetate
EI	electron impact
ELISA	enzyme-linked immunosorbent assay
ELS	evaporative light-scattering
ET	ethylated
eV	electron volts
FAB	fast atom bombardment
fg	femtograms
FID	flame ionisation detection
f.p.	freezing point
FPD	flame photometric detector
ft	foot (feet)
FTIR	Fourier transform infra-red
G-CSF	granulocyte colony-stimulating factor
GC	gas chromatography
GI	gastro-intestinal
h	hour (s)
-HCl	artefact formed by the elimination of hydrochloric acid
-HCN	artefact formed by the elimination of hydrogen cyanide
HIV	human immunodeficiency virus
$-H_2O$	artefact formed by dehydration of an alcohol or by rearrangement of an amino oxo compound
HPLC	high performance liquid chromatography
-HY	acid-hydrolysed/acid hydrolysis
i.d.	internal diameter
IM	intramuscular
IR	infra-red
IV	intravenous
I.S.	internal standard
k	column capacity ratio
λ	wavelength
log	logarithm to the base 10
ln	logarithm to the base e (natural logarithm)
M	molar (moles per litre)
M (OH-)	hydroxy metabolite
M (COOH-)	carboxy metabolite
M (nor-)	*N*-desmethyl metabolite
M (ring)	ring compound as metabolite
MAO	monoamine oxidase
mEq	milliequivalent(s)
μg	microgram(s)
μm	micrometer(s)
MID	multiple ion detector
min	minute
mol	mole
m.p.	melting point
MRM	multiple reaction monitoring
MS	mass spectrometry
m/z	mass to charge ratio
Me or ME	methylated
ng	nanogram(s)
$-NH_3$	artefact formed by elimination of ammonia
NIAPCI	negative ion atmospheric pressure chemical ionisation
NICI	negative ion chemical ionisation
nm	nanometer(s)
NPD	nitrogen-phosphorus detection
NSD	nitrogen-specific detector
P	apparent partition coefficient
PAD	peripheral arterial disease
PDHID	pulsed discharge helium ionisation detector
PEEK	polyether etherketone
PFB	pentafluorobenzoyl
-PFP	pentafluoropropionylated
pg	picogram(s)
PIAPCI	positive ion atmospheric pressure chemical ionisation
PICI	positive ion chemical ionisation
PID	photoionisation detector
PIFAB	positive ion fast atom bombardment
pK_a	negative logarithm of the dissociation constant
ppb	part(s) per billion
ppm	part(s) per million
PTFE	polytetrafluoroethylene
r.d.	relative density
RI	retention index
RRT	relative retention time
s	second(s)
SDS	sodium dodecyl sulfate
SIM	selected ion monitoring
$-SO_2NH$	artefact formed by elimination of the sulfonamide group
sp.	species (plural spp.)
sp.gr.	specific gravity

$t_{1/2}$	half-life
TBA	tetrabutyl ammonium hydrogen sulfate
TBAF	tetrabutyl ammonium fluoride
TBSA	total body surface area
TCD	thermal conductivity detector
TEA	triethylamine
-TFA	trifluoroacetylated
TIC	total ion current
TLC	thin-layer chromatography
TMS	trimethylsilyl
TMSTFA	trimethylsilyltrifluoroacetyl
TOF	time of flight
TSD	thermionic specific detection
UV	ultraviolet
V	volt(s)
var.	variety
V_D	volume of distribution
Vet.	veterinary
Vol	volume(s)
v/v	volume in volume
Wt	weight
w/v	weight in volume
w/w	weight in weight

Part Two

Monographs

Analytical and toxicological data

Ultraviolet absorption data

In the reproductions of ultraviolet spectra, the following notation has been used:

———————— acid solution

.... alkaline solution

– – – – – – – – neutral solution

The A_1^1 values are divided into three categories in order to provide an indication of reliability:

- The letter 'a' after a figure indicates that the value is a mean value based on several reported figures all of which lie within a range of ±10% of the mean.
- The letter 'b' after a figure indicates that the value is a single reported value of unknown reliability.
- The letter 'c' after a figure indicates that the value is a mean value based on several reported figures some of which lie outside ±10% of the mean.

Infra-red absorption data

The data have been selected from recorded spectra over the range 2000 to 650 cm^{-1} (5 to 15 μm). The selected peaks are the six most intense peaks, except that peaks in the region where Nujol absorbs (1490 to 1320 cm^{-1}, 6.7 to 7.6 μm) have been omitted. The spectra show transmittance plotted against wavelength (μm) and wavenumber (cm^{-1}).

Mass spectral data

The *m*/*z* values of the eight most intense ions are listed in descending order of intensity for drugs and other compounds of forensic interest. The spectra show percentage abundance of ions plotted against mass:charge ratio. Note that the x axis has not been titled '*m*/*z*' as this is assumed.

Abacavir

Antiretroviral

Synonym. 1592
(1*S*,4*R*)-4-[2-Amino-6-(cyclopropylamino)-9*H*-purin-9-yl]-2-cyclopentene-1-methanol
$C_{14}H_{18}N_6O$=286.3
CAS—136470-78-5

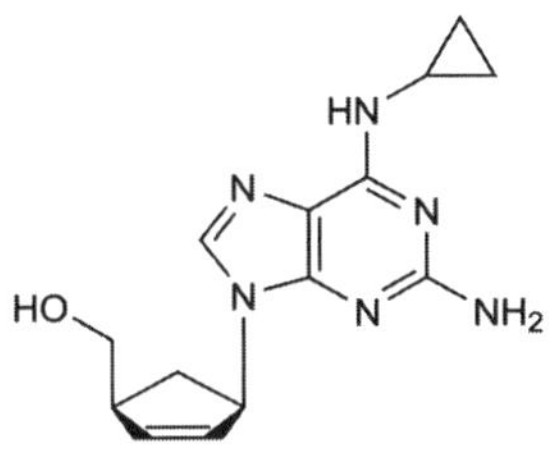

Abacavir Succinate
Synonym. 1592U89
$C_{18}H_{24}N_6O_5$=404.4
CAS—168146-84-7

Abacavir Sulfate
Proprietary name. Ziagen
$(C_{14}H_{18}N_6O)_2,H_2SO_4$=670.8
A white to off-white solid which is soluble in water (0.077 mg/L at 25°).

Dissociation Constant. pK_a 5.01.

Partition Coefficient. (Sulfate) Log *P* (octanol/water, pH 7.1 to 7.3), 1.20 (25°).

High Performance Liquid Chromatography. System HAB—retention time 1.0 min; system HAD—k 8.1.

Column: (analytical) Symmetry C_{18} (100 × 4.6 mm i.d, 3.5 μm), (guard) (20 × 3.8 mm i.d.). Column temperature: 41°. Mobile phase: phosphate buffer (25 mM, pH 7.0):acetonitrile (85:15), 1.0 mL/min flow rate. UV detection (λ=285 nm). Retention time: 4.8 min. [A. I. Veldkamp *et al.*, *J. Chromatogr. Biomed. Sci. Appl.*, 1999, *736*, 123–128].

Ultraviolet Spectrum. Aqueous base—217, 260, 285 nm.

Mass Spectrum. Principal ions at *m*/*z* 175, 189, 190, 286, 173, 162, 271, 163.

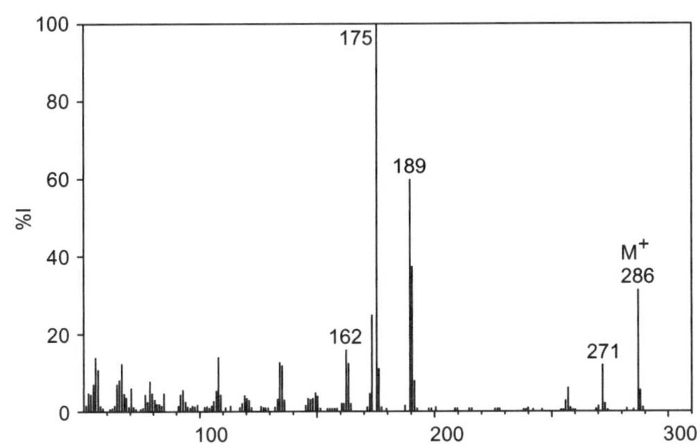

Quantification

High performance liquid chromatography. In plasma: limit of quantification 0.02 mg/L. UV detection (λ=285 nm)—A. I. Veldkamp *et al.*, *J. Chromatogr. Biomed. Sci. Appl.*, 1999, *736*, 123–128. In plasma: limit of quantification 0.02 mg/L. UV detection (λ=260 nm)—G. Aymard *et al.*, *J. Chromatogr. Biomed. Sci. Appl.*, 2000, *744*, 227–240.

Disposition in the Body. Abacavir is extensively and rapidly absorbed after oral administration. It is metabolised by alcohol dehydrogenase to 5′-carboxylic acid and by glucuronyl transferase to 5′-glucuronide. 1.2% of a dose is excreted unchanged in urine, 30% as the two metabolites and 15% as an unidentified metabolite. 16% of the dose can also be detected in faeces.

Therapeutic concentration

12 HIV-infected adult patients were administered with single oral doses of 100, 300, 600, 900 and 1200 mg abacavir. Peak plasma concentrations of 0.6, 3.0, 4.7 and 9.6 mg/L were reached for 100, 300, 600 and 1200 mg doses, respectively, and within 1.0 to 1.7 h. [P. N. Kumer *et al.*, *Antimicrob. Agents Chemother.*, 1999, *43(3)*, 603–608].

22 HIV-infected children, aged between 3 months and 13 years, were administered with either a 4 or 8 mg/kg body weight dose of abacavir. Peak plasma concentrations of 1.69 and 3.94 mg/L, respectively, were reached within 1.5 h. [W. Hughes *et al.*, *Antimicrob. Agents Chemother.*, 1999, *43(3)*, 609–615].

Toxicity. Life-threatening hypersensitivity reactions have been reported, as well as life-threatening lactic acidosis and severe hepatomegaly with steatosis.

Bioavailability. Between 83 and 96% depending on formulation.

Half-life. Elimination half-life is 0.9 to 1.7 h.

Volume of distribution. Apparent volume of distribution is 0.65 to 0.95 L/kg.

Clearance. In adults: mean apparent clearance is 0.56 (single 1200 mg dose) to 1.94 (100 mg dose) L/h/kg. In children (2 to 5 years): 0.08 (8 mg/kg body weight dose) to 0.12 (4 mg/kg dose) L/h/kg, (6 to 13 years): 0.03 to 0.05 L/h/kg, respectively.

Protein binding. Around 50%.

Dose. Adults: 300 mg twice daily. Children aged between 3 months and 16 years: 8 mg/kg body weight twice daily.

Acamprosate Calcium

Alcohol Deterrent

Synonyms. Ca-AOTA; calcium acetylhomotaurinate; calcium bisacetyl homotaurine.
Proprietary names. Aotal; Campral.
Calcium 3-acetamido-1-propanesulfonate
$Ca(C_5H_{10}NO_4S)_2$=400.5
CAS—77337-76-9 (acamprosate); *77337-73-6* (acamprosate calcium)

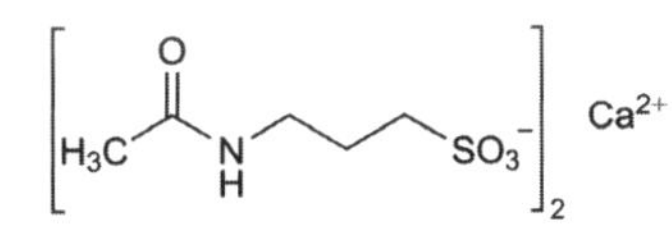

A colourless crystalline powder. M.p. 270°.

Gas Chromatography. Column: fused-silica capillary coated with OV-1701 liquid phase (25 m × 0.35 mm i.d., 0.2 μm film thickness). Column temperature: 240° to 310° at 10°/min, held 2 min. MS detection (NICI, SIM at *m*/*z* 424). Retention time: 5.5 min. [J. Girault *et al.*, *J. Chromatogr.*, 1990, *530*; Biomed. Appl., 7, 295–305].

High Performance Liquid Chromatography. System HAA—retention time 3.0 min.

Ultraviolet Spectrum. Water—192 nm.

Quantification.

Gas chromatography–mass spectrometry. In plasma: limit of detection 0.001 mg/L—J. Girault *et al.*, *J. Chromatogr.*, 1990, *530*; *Biomed. Appl.*, *7*, 295–305.

High performance liquid chromatography. In plasma: limit of detection 0.01 mg/L, fluorescence detection—C. Chabenat *et al.*, *J. Chromatogr.*, 1987, *414*; *Biomed. Appl.*, *58*, 417–422.

Disposition in the Body. Absorption is slow after oral administration but sustained and shows large intersubject variability. Steady state concentrations are observed 7 days after administration. The drug crosses the blood–brain barrier. It is not significantly metabolised and is excreted unchanged in urine.

Therapeutic concentration

Following single oral doses of 666 mg to 24 healthy subjects, aged 19 to 35 years, the mean maximum plasma concentration was 0.180 mg/L. Most of the dose was absorbed within 4 h. [J. Girault *et al.*, *J. Chromatogr.*, 1990, *530*; *Biomed. Appl.*, *58*, 295-305].

6 healthy volunteers and 12 patients with moderate or severe chronic renal impairment were administered with a single dose of 666 mg. Maximum peak plasma concentrations were 0.198 mg/L for the healthy individuals and 0.813 mg/L for those with severe impairment. These were observed at 6 and 23 h, respectively. [J. Sennesael, *Lipha, France*, 1994, *Data on file]*.

Half-life. Plasma, 13–18 h (healthy individuals); 47 h (patients with severe renal impairment).

Clearance. Plasma, 184 L/h (healthy volunteers); 16 L/h (patients with moderate renal impairment); 66.5 L/h (severe impairment).

Protein binding. In plasma, not bound.

Note. For a review of acamprosate calcium, see M. I. Wilde and A. J. Wagstaff, *Drugs*, 1997, *53*, 1038–1053.

Dose. Patients with a body weight <60 kg: 1.3 g daily. Patients with body weight >60 kg: 2 g daily.

Acarbose

Antidiabetic

Synonym. Bay-g-5421
Proprietary names. Glicobase; Glucobay; Glucor; Glumide; Prandase; Precose.
O-4,6-Dideoxy-4-[[(1*S*,4*R*,5*S*,6*S*)-4,5,6-trihydroxy-3-(hydroxymethyl)-2-cyclohexen-1-yl] amino]-α-D-glucopyranosyl-(1→4)-*O*-α-D-glucopyranosyl-(1→4)-D-glucose
$C_{25}H_{43}NO_{18}$=645.6
CAS—56180-94-0

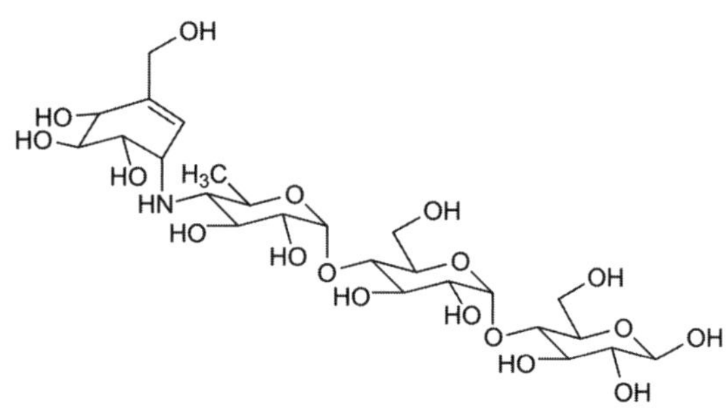

A white to off-white amorphous powder, which is soluble in water.

Dissociation Constant. pK_a 5.1.

Partition Coefficient. Log *P* (octanol/water), −8.08.

High Performance Liquid Chromatography. Column: aminopropyl-bonded (Nucleosil, 5 µm, 250 × 4.6 mm i.d.). Mobile phase: methanol: dichloromethane (65:35). Detection: ELS. Retention time: 4.3 min. [S. Cherkaoui *et al.*, *J. Pharm. Biomed. Anal.*, 1998, *18*, 729–735].

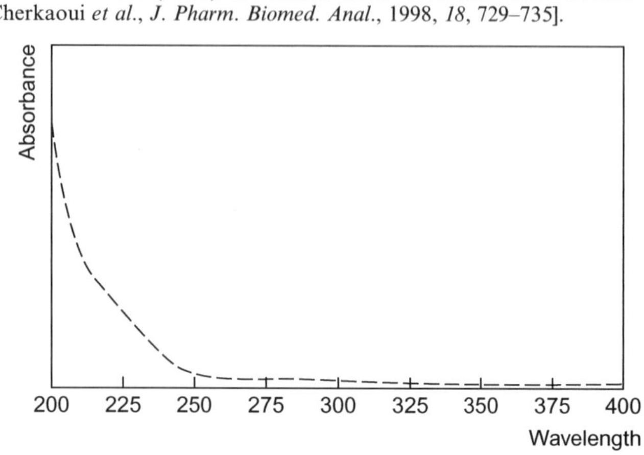

Infra-red Spectrum. Principal peaks at wavenumber 1033, 1153, 1458 cm^{-1} (KBr disk).

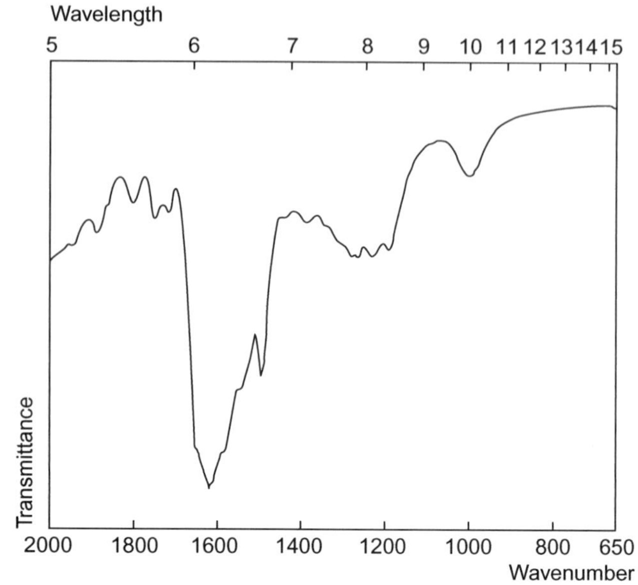

Quantification

High performance liquid chromatography. In pharmaceuticals: limit of detection <5 mg/L and limit of quantification >15 mg/L. ELS detection—S. Cherkaoui *et al.*, *J. Pharm. Biomed. Anal.*, 1998, *18*, 729–735.

Bioassay. In plasma and urine: limit of detection 5 µg/L and 150 µg/L, respectively—H. J. Ahr *et al.*, *Arzneimittelforschung*, 1989, *39*, 1254–1260.

Disposition in the Body. Acarbose is metabolised by intestinal digestive enzymes and by the microbial flora of the gastro-intestinal tract, where the majority of the active unchanged drug remains. The major metabolites are the 4-methylpyrogallol derivatives (sulfate, methyl and glucuronide conjugates) produced by biotransformation (mainly reduction and conjugation). 35% of an oral dose is absorbed as the metabolites and only 1 to 2% absorbed as the active drug. After intravenous administration, approximately 90% of a dose is excreted in urine, within 48 h, as the active drug (parent drug or active metabolite). After oral administration, <2% of the dose is recovered in urine as the active drug and 34% as metabolites, and approximately 50% as the unabsorbed drug in faeces (within 96 h post ingestion).

Therapeutic concentration
Patients with severe renal impairment, creatinine clearance <25 mL/min/1.73 m^2, have a peak plasma concentration of acarbose five times greater than those with normal renal function.

6 healthy volunteers were administered with a single oral 200 mg dose of acarbose. Peak plasma concentrations of 49.5 ± 27.0 µg/L were reached approx. 2 h after administration. [H. J. Ahr *et al.*, *Arzneimittelforschung*, 1989, *39*, 1254–1260].

Toxicity. Acarbose is associated with hepatotoxicity and has low toxicity by ingestion, subcutaneous and intravenous routes. A 360 mg/kg body weight dose in women over a 60-day period and given intermittently in a number of separate and discrete doses can cause non-fatal toxic effects. Acarbose competitively and reversibly inhibits the α-glucosidase enzymes; glucoamylase, sucrase, maltase and isomaltase, found in the small intestine, and this delays hydrolysis of complex carbohydrates. It is unlikely to produce hypoglycaemia in overdose, but abdominal discomfort and diarrhoea may occur.

Bioavailability. Systemic bioavailability is 0.5 to 1.7%.

Half-life. Elimination half-life is 3.2 ± 0.9 h.

Volume of distribution. Steady state volume of distribution is 0.32 L/kg.

Clearance. Total body clearance, 600 L/h.

Protein binding. Minimal protein binding with plasma concentrations of more than 1 µg/L and up to 98% with 0.008 µg/L.

Dose. An initial dose of 25 mg three times a day is administered and can be increased to a maintenance dose of 50 to 100 mg three times daily. Doses up to 200 mg three times daily have been reported. Patients with a body weight ≤60 kg have a maximum dose of 50 mg three times a day.

Acebutolol

Beta-blocker

N-[3-Acetyl-4-[2-hydroxy-3-[(1-methylethyl)amino]propoxy]-butanamide
$C_{18}H_{28}N_2O_4$=336.4
CAS—3751-730-9

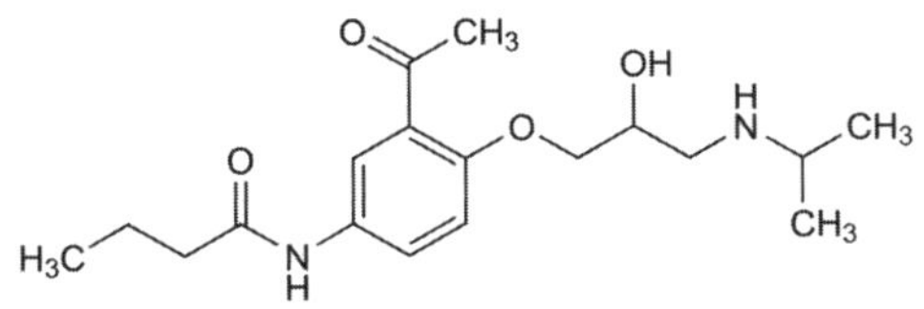

Crystals. M.p. 119° to 123°.

Acebutolol Hydrochloride

Proprietary names. Acecor; Acetanol; Neptal; Prent; Sectral. It is an ingredient of Secadrex.
$C_{18}H_{28}N_2O_4$,HCl=372.9
CAS—34381-68-5
A white or slightly cream-coloured powder. M.p. 141° to 143°.

Dissociation Constant. pK_a 9.4.

Colour Tests. Methanolic potassium hydroxide—yellow; Nessler's reagent—orange (slow); Sulfuric acid—yellow.

Thin-layer Chromatography. System TA—Rf 47; system TB—Rf 00; system TC—Rf 03; system TE—Rf 33; system TL—Rf 06; system TAE—Rf 13; system TAF—Rf 71.

Gas Chromatography. System GA—RI 2811; RI 2850 Art (-H_2O); RI 2450 M (phenol-); system GB—RI 2926; RI 2569 Art (-H_2O); RI 2056 M (phenol-); RI 2089 Art (desacetyl-).

High Performance Liquid Chromatography.

System HA—*k* 1.4; system HX—RI 325; system HX—RI 264; system HZ—Retention time(s) 2.3 min; system HAA—Retention time(s) 10.2 min.

Ultraviolet Spectrum. Aqueous acid—234 (A^1_1=655b), 320 nm (A^1_1=75b); methanol—235 (A^1_1=866a), 328 nm.

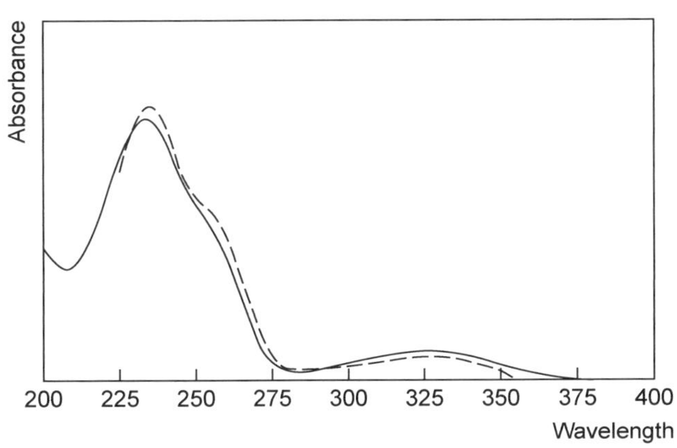

Infra-red Spectrum. Principal peaks at wavenumbers 1665, 1245, 1525, 1495, 1217, 1285 cm^{-1} (acebutolol hydrochloride, KBr disk).

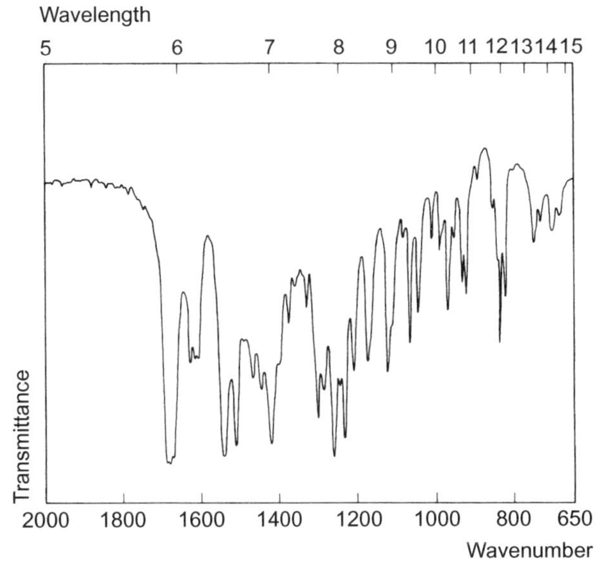

Mass Spectrum. Principal ions at *m/z* 72, 43, 30, 56, 151, 221, 41, 98.

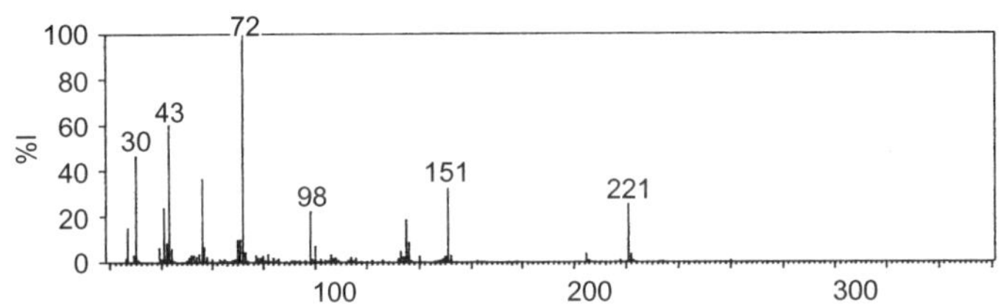

Quantification

High performance liquid chromatography. In plasma or urine: acebutolol and metabolites, limit of detection 20 µg/L, UV detection—J. N. Buskin *et al.*, *J. Chromatogr.*, 1982, *230*; *Biomed. Appl.*, *19*, 438–442.

Disposition in the Body. Absorbed after oral administration; bioavailability about 40%. The major metabolite is the acetyl derivative, diacetalol, which is active. After an oral dose, about 20 to 40% of the dose is excreted in the urine in 24 h, about 9 to 12% of the dose as unchanged drug and about 12 to 24% as diacetalol. Up to about 60% of the dose is eliminated in the faeces as unchanged drug and diacetalol. After an intravenous dose, relatively more is excreted in the urine than in the faeces, and the proportion of unchanged drug in the urine is greater than after an oral dose.

Therapeutic concentration

After a single oral dose of 400 mg, administered to 8 subjects, a mean peak plasma concentration of 0.7 mg/L was attained in 2 h; a mean peak concentration of diacetalol of 0.8 mg/L was attained in 4 h [A. A. Gulaid *et al.*, *Biopharm. Drug Disp.*, 1981, *2*, 103–114].

Steady-state concentrations of 0.51 to 1.23 (mean 0.7) mg/L were reported during chronic oral administration of 300 mg every 6 to 8 h to 6 subjects; the concentration of diacetalol was 0.63 to 4.43 (mean 2.2) mg/L. [R. A. Winkle *et al.*, *Br. J. Clin. Pharmacol.*, 1977, *4*, 519–522].

Toxicity

A fatal case of self-poisoning with acebutolol was reported with a blood concentration of 34.7 µg/mL. [A. Tracqui *et al.*, *J. Anal. Toxicol.*, 1992, *16(6)*, 398–400].

Half-life. Plasma half-life, acebutolol about 7 to 11 h, diacetalol about 12 h.

Volume of distribution. About 1 to 3 L/kg.

Distribution in blood. Plasma:whole blood ratio, about 0.8.

Protein binding. In plasma, about 20%.

Dose. The equivalent of 0.2 to 1.2 g of acebutolol daily.

Acecainide

Anti-arrhythmic

Synonyms. *N*-Acetylprocainamide; NAPA.
4-(Acetylamino)-*N*-[2-(diethylamino)ethyl]benzamide
$C_{15}H_{23}N_3O_2$=277.4
CAS—32795-44-1

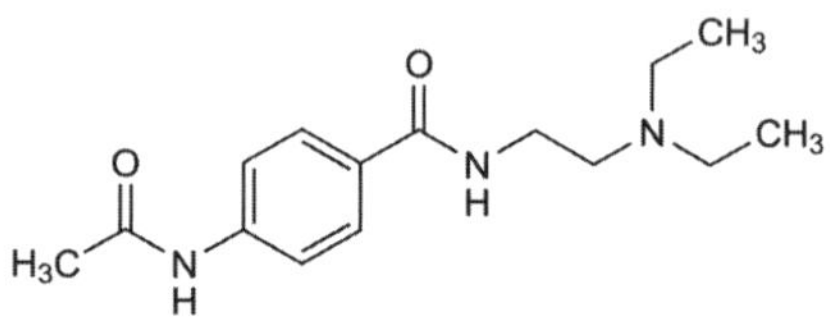

Acecainide Hydrochloride

$C_{15}H_{23}N_3O_2$,HCl=313.8
CAS—34118-92-8
Crystals. M.p. 190° to 193°.

Gas Chromatography. System GA—RI 2550; system GB—RI 2724.

Ultraviolet Spectrum. Aqueous acid or alkali—266 nm.

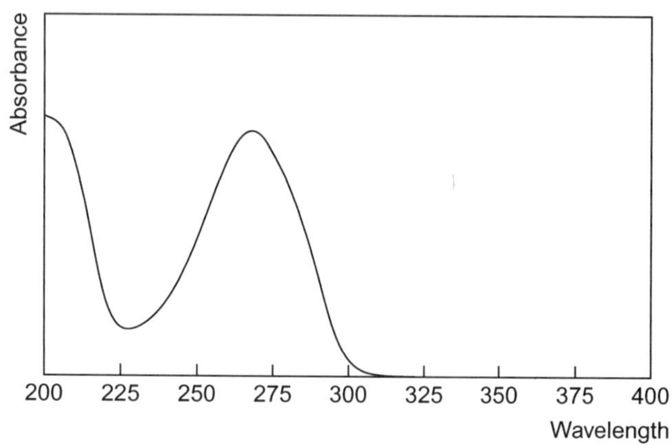

Infra-red Spectrum. Principal peaks at wavenumbers 1639, 1509, 1527, 1696, 1600, 1259 cm^{-1} (acecainide hydrochloride, KBr disk).

Mass Spectrum. Principal ions at *m/z* 86, 58, 99, 56, 162, 132, 149, 205.

Quantification. See also under Procainamide.

Gas chromatography–mass spectrometry. In plasma: limit of detection 500 µg/L—J. M. Strong *et al., J. Pharmacokinet. Biopharm.*, 1975, *3*, 223–235.

High performance liquid chromatography. In plasma: limit of detection 2 µg/L and limit of quantification 4 µg/L (UV detection, λ=280 nm)—E.Lessard *et al., J. Chromatogr. Sci.*, 1998, *36(1)*, 49–54.

Disposition in the Body. Readily absorbed after oral administration. Up to 85% of a dose is excreted in the urine as unchanged drug in 48 h, with only 2 to 3% excreted as procainamide and less than 1% as the mono-desethyl metabolite. Acecainide is the principal active metabolite of procainamide.

Therapeutic concentration. In plasma, usually in the range 10 to 30 mg/L.

After a single oral dose of 1.5 g to 9 subjects, peak plasma concentrations of 7.4 to 17.2 (mean 12) mg/L, were attained in 1.5 to 4 h. [W. K. Lee *et al., Clin. Pharmacol. Ther.*, 1976, *19*, 508–514].

Following oral administration of 1 g four times a day to 8 subjects, steady-state plasma concentrations of 9.3 to 25.5 (mean 18) mg/L were reported. [A. J. Atkinson *et al., Clin. Pharmacol. Ther.*, 1977, *21*, 575–587].

Toxicity. Toxic effects may occur at plasma concentrations within the therapeutic range.

Bioavailability. About 85%.

Half-life. Plasma half-life, about 6 to 9 h in normal subjects; increased in subjects with heart disease or renal impairment.

Volume of distribution. About 1.5 L/kg.

Clearance. Plasma clearance, about 3 mL/min/kg.

Protein binding. In plasma, about 10%.

Note. For a review of the pharmacokinetics of acecainide, see S. J. Connolly and R. E. Kates, *Clin. Pharmacokinet.*, 1982, *7*, 206–220.

Dose. Acecainide has been given in doses of 2 to 6 g daily.

Acecarbromal

Sedative/Hypnotic

Synonym. Acetylcarbromal
Proprietary names. Abasin; Sedamyl.
N-[(Acetylamino)carbonyl]-2-bromo-2-ethylbutanamide
$C_9H_{15}BrN_2O_3$=279.1
CAS—77-66-7

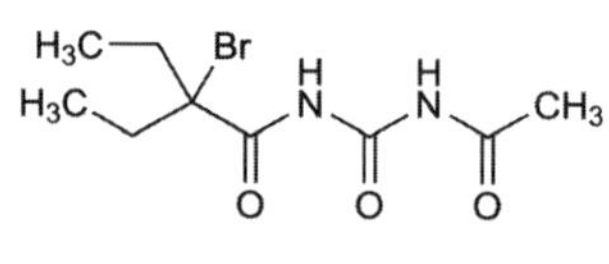

Colourless crystals or white crystalline powder. M.p. 109°.
Soluble 1 in 1000 of water; soluble in ethanol, chloroform, and ether.

Colour Test. Nessler's Reagent—brown-orange (slow).

Thin-layer Chromatography. System TD—Rf 49; system TE—Rf 57; system TF—Rf 48; system TAD—Rf 60; system TAE—Rf 84; system TAF—Rf 84; system TAJ—Rf 61; system TAK—Rf 58; system TAL—Rf 90.

Gas Chromatography. System GA—acecarbromal RI 1720, M (carbromal) RI 1513, M (desbromocarbromal) RI 1380.

High Performance Liquid Chromatography. System HX—RI 429; system HY—RI 374.

Infra-red Spectrum. Principal peaks at wavenumbers 1776, 1730, 1183, 1267, 1149, 1236 cm^{-1} (Nujol mull).

Mass Spectrum. Principal ions at *m/z* 43, 129, 69, 41, 86, 97, 55, 44.

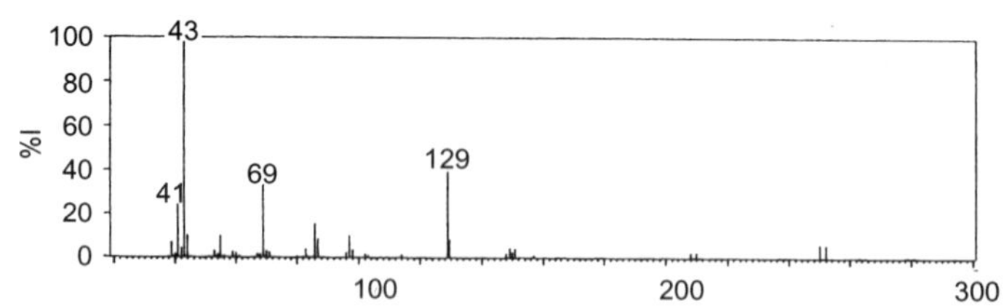

Quantification.
High Performance Liquid Chromatography. In plasma and urine—M. Höbel and G. Bender, *Arch Toxicol.*, 1977, *37*, 307.

Dose. 0.75 to 1.5 g daily.

Aceclofenac

Anti-inflammatory

Synonyms. Aceclofenacum; PR-82/3.
Proprietary names. Airtal; Barcan; Biofenac; Difucrem; Falcol; Gerbin; Preservex; Sanein; Tresquim.
2-[(2,6-Dichlorophenylamino)phenyl]acetoxyacetic acid
$C_{16}H_{13}Cl_2NO_4$=354.2
CAS—89796-99-6

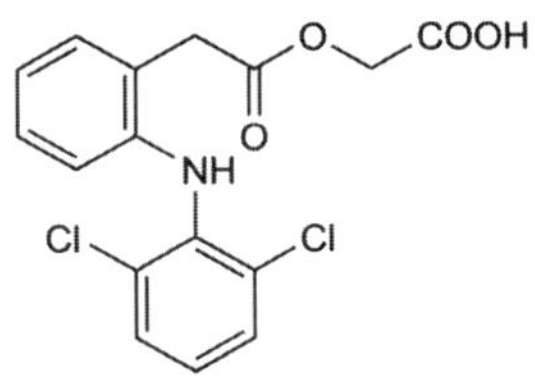

A white to almost white crystalline powder. M.p. 149° to 150°. It is practically insoluble in water; soluble in alcohol and methyl alcohol; freely soluble in acetone and dimethylformamide.

Thin-layer Chromatography. Plate: silica gel. Mobile phase: chloroform:methanol:acetic acid (90:10:1). Aceclofenac, Rf 0.44; 4′-OH aceclofenac, Rf 0.25. [R. Bort *et al.*, *Drug Metab. Dispos.*, 1996, *24*(8), 834–841].

High Performance Liquid Chromatography. System HZ—retention time 10.7 min.

Column: C_{18} (Spherisorb ODS–2, 5 µm, 200 × 4.6 mm). Mobile phase: triethanolamine (0.02% in 100 mM phosphate buffer, pH 7.4):acetonitrile (75:25), flow rate 1.0 mL/min. UV Detection (λ = 282 nm). Retention time: aceclofenac, 23.4 min; 4′-hydroxyaceclofenac, 7.6 min. [R. Bort *et al.*, *Drug Metab. Dispos.*, 1996, *24(8)*, 834–841].

Ultraviolet Spectrum. Ethanol—275 nm.

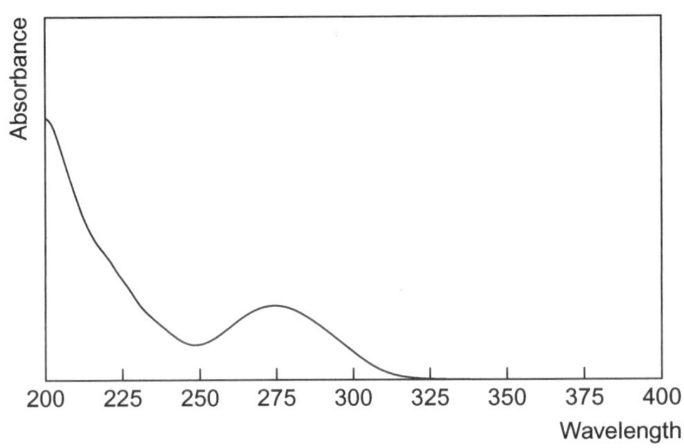

Quantification

High performance liquid chromatography. In urine and plasma: limit of detection, 6.5 mg/L. UV detection (λ = 282 nm)—R. Bort *et al.*, *Drug Metab. Dispos.*, 1996, *24(8)*, 834–841. In plasma: limit of detection, 0.010 mg/L. UV detection (λ = 278 nm)—H. S. Lee *et al.*, *J. Pharm. Biomed. Anal.* 2000, *23*, 775–781.

Disposition in the Body. Aceclofenac is well absorbed after oral administration and circulates mainly as the unchanged drug. It is metabolised in hepatocytes and microsomes to 4′-hydroxyaceclofenac, which can undergo further conjugation. Other metabolites also identified include diclofenac and 4-hydroxydiclofenac, and their hydroxylated derivatives. Aceclofenac penetrates into synovial fluid and concentrations here reach approximately 57% of those in plasma. 70% of an administered dose is excreted in urine as glucuronides of aceclofenac and diclofenac.

Therapeutic concentration

8 healthy, male, Caucasian volunteers, aged between 26 and 68 years, were orally administered a 100 mg dose of aceclofenac. Peak plasma concentrations of 7.6 ± 1.3 mg/L were reached within 2.6 ± 1.8 h. [R. Bort *et al.*, *Drug Metab. Dispos.*, 1996, *24(8)*, 834–841].

Toxicity. Type III hypersensitivity reactions have been reported.

Half-life. Elimination half-life is approx. 4 h.

Volume of distribution. Apparent volume of distribution is approx. 25 L.

Protein binding. >99% plasma protein bound.

Dose. A usual dose of 100 mg twice daily is administered with a reduction to 100 mg daily for patients with hepatic impairment.

Acefylline Piperazine

Xanthine Bronchodilator

Synonyms. Acepifylline; Piperazine Theophylline Ethanoate.
Proprietary names. Dynaphylline; Etaphylline; Etophylate.
Piperazine bis(theophyllin-7-ylacetate)
$(C_9H_{10}N_4O_4)_2,C_4H_{10}N_2 = 562.5$
CAS—18833-13-1

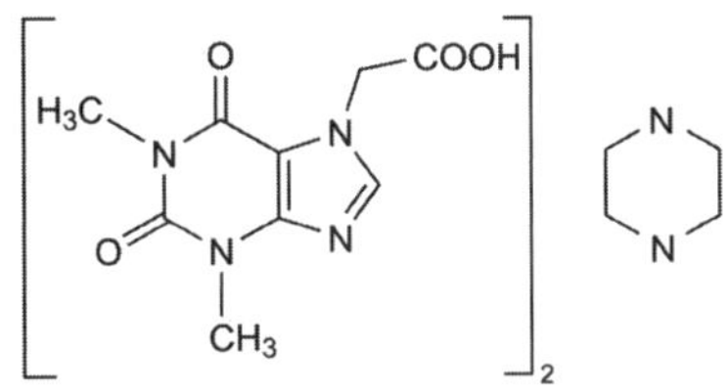

A white crystalline powder. M.p. 260°.
Freely soluble in water; slightly soluble in ethanol.

Colour Test. Amalic Acid Test—orange/violet.

Thin-layer Chromatography. System TA—Rf 04; system TB—Rf 01; system TC—Rf 01; system TL—Rf 01. (Acidified iodoplatinate solution, positive.)

Gas Chromatography. System GA—RI 1000.

Ultraviolet Spectrum. Aqueous acid—274 nm ($A^1_1 = 317a$).

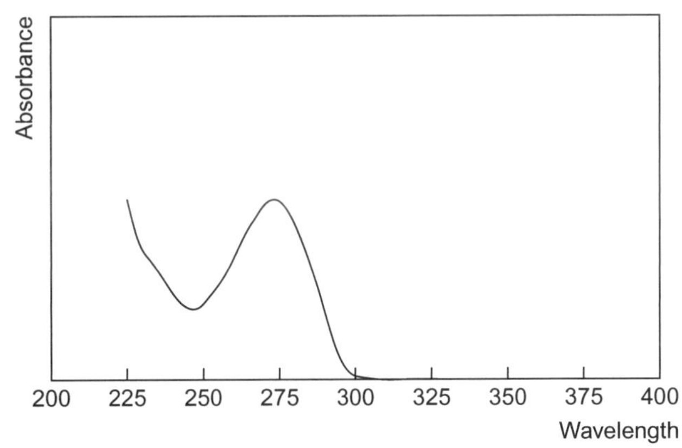

Infra-red Spectrum. Principal peaks at wavenumbers 1700, 1660, 1612, 1538, 1298, 1219 cm^{-1} (KBr disk).

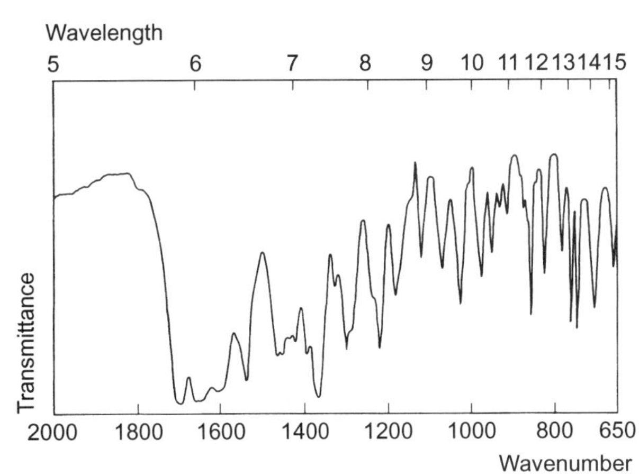

Mass Spectrum. Principal peaks at *m/z* 44, 194, 109, 67, 86, 238, 56, 85.

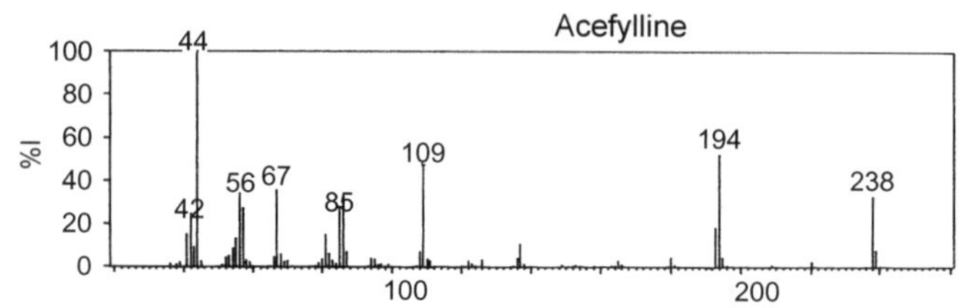

Quantification

Gas chromatography. In urine: FID—J. Zuidema and H. Hilbers, *J. Chromatogr.* 1980, *182* (8); *B Biomed. Appl.*, 445–447.

High pressure liquid chromatography. In plasma: theophylline-7-acetic acid, limit of detection 25 µg/L, UV detection—S. Sved *et al.*, *Biopharm. Drug Disp.*, 1981, *2*, 177–184.

Disposition in the Body. Very poorly absorbed after oral administration. It is metabolised to theophylline-7-acetic acid but does not appear to be converted to theophylline.

Therapeutic concentration Following a single oral dose of 1 g to 2 subjects, peak plasma concentrations of 0.28 and 0.14 µg/mL of theophylline-7-acetic acid were attained in 1.5 and 2 h, respectively. [S. Sved *et al.*, *Biopharm. Drug Disp.*, 1981, *2*, 177–184.]

Half-life. Plasma half-life, theophylline-7-acetic acid about 1 to 2 h.

Volume of distribution. Theophylline-7-acetic acid 0.5 L/kg (single subject).

Clearance. Plasma clearance, theophylline-7-acetic acid 7 mL/min/kg (single subject).

Dose. 1.5 to 3 g daily.

Acemetacin

NSAID

Synonyms. TV-1322, TVX-1322.
Proprietary names. Acemix; Altren; Emflex; Espledol; Oldan; Peran; Rantudil; Rheumibis; Rheutrop; Solart; Tilur.
1-(4-Chlorobenzoyl)-5-methoxy-2-methyl-1*H*-indole-3-acetic acid carboxymethyl ester
$C_{21}H_{18}ClNO_6$=415.8
CAS—53164-05-9

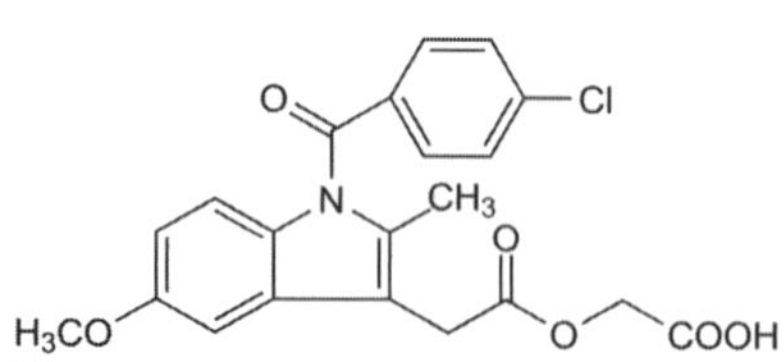

Very fine, pale yellow crystals from petroleum ether. M.p. 150° to 153°.

Dissociation Constant. pK_a 2.9.

Partition Coefficient. Log *P* (octanol/water), 4.13.

Gas Chromatography. System GA—acemetacin RI 0, acemetacin-ME RI 3150, acemetacin-ET RI 3220, acemetacin art-ME_2 RI 2390.

High Performance Liquid Chromatography. Column: ODS (Hypersil, 150 × 4.5 mm i.d., 5 µm). Mobile phase: methanol:0.02 M potassium dihydrogen phosphate (57:43), adjusted to pH 4.5 with 88% phosphoric acid, 1.25 mL/min flow rate. UV detection (λ=245 nm). Retention time: acemetacin, 5.58 min; indometacin, 9.03 min. [L. J. Notarianni and A. J. Collins, *J. Chromatogr.*, 1987, *413*; *Biomed. Appl.*, *57*, 305–308].

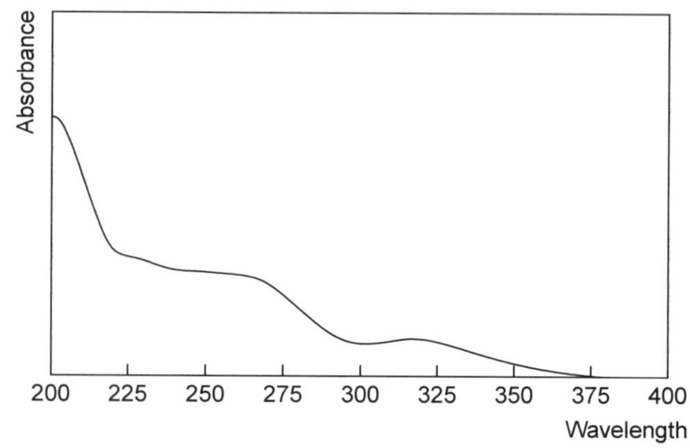

Mass Spectrum. Principal peaks at *m/z* 355, 139, 113, 371, 341, 415.

Quantification

High performance liquid chromatography. In blood or plasma: acemetacin and indometacin, limit of detection 25 µg/L, UV detection—G. Schöllnhammer *et al.*, *J. Chromatogr.*, 1986, *375*; *Biomed. Appl.*, *48*, 331–338. In plasma: acemetacin and metabolites, limit of detection 10 µg/L for acemetacin and indometacin and 20 µg/l for *p*-chlorobenzoic acid, UV detection (λ=245 nm)—L. J. Notarianni and A. J. Collins, *J. Chromatogr.*, 1987, *413*; *Biomed. Appl.*, *57*, 305–308.

Disposition in the Body. Acemetacin is rapidly and well absorbed after oral administration. It is metabolised to indometacin (major metabolite) and *p*-chlorobenzoic acid (PCBA, minor metabolite and degradation product) by hydrolysis in the liver. The drug is eliminated by both hepatic and renal routes; the pharmacokinetics are unaffected by moderate renal or hepatic impairment.

Therapeutic concentration

Following administration of 60 mg orally twice a day for 8 days to 10 young (mean age of 30.9 years, between 22 and 44) and 10 elderly subjects (75.9 years, ranging between 68 and 80 years), mean peak plasma concentrations of 187 µg/L and 277 µg/L were reached after 2.6 and 2.5 h in the two groups, respectively, on day 8 of the study. The peak concentrations for the metabolite, indometacin, were 705 µg/L for the young and 804 µg/L for the elderly. These were observed at 3.1 and 2.9 h, respectively. Each individual suffered with osteoarthiritis and was fasted overnight before administration of the drug with a standard breakfast. [R. W. Jones *et al.*, *Br. J. Clin. Pharmacol.*, 1991, *31*, 543–545].

Half-life. Plasma, 1 h.

Dose. 120 to 180 mg daily.

Acenocoumarol

Anticoagulant

Synonyms. Acenocumarin; Nicoumalone; G-23350.
Proprietary names. Sinthrome; Sintrom.
4-Hydroxy-3-[1-(4-nitrophenyl)-3-oxobutyl]-2*H*-1-benzopyran-2-one
$C_{19}H_{15}NO_6$=353.3
CAS—152-72-7

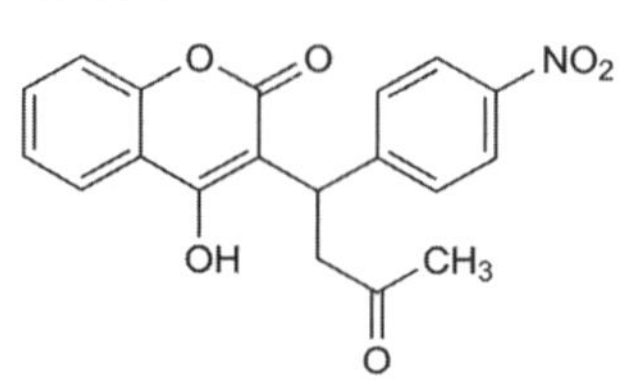

An almost white to buff-coloured powder. M.p. 196° to 199°.
Sparingly soluble in water; soluble 1 in 400 of ethanol and 1 in 200 of chloroform; soluble in solutions of alkali hydroxides.

Dissociation Constant. pK_a 4.7.

Partition Coefficient. Log *P* (octanol/water), 2.0.

Thin-layer Chromatography. System TB—Rf 00; system TD—Rf 52; system TE—Rf 16; system TF—Rf 48; system TAD—Rf 60; system

TAE—Rf 92; system TAF—Rf 92; system TAJ—Rf 68; system TAK—Rf 51; system TAL—Rf 92. (Acidified iodoplatinate solution, positive; acidified potassium permanganate solution, positive.)

Gas Chromatography. System GA—acenocoumarol-Me RI 3035; M(amino-)-Me_3 RI 2985; M(acetamido-)-Me_2 RI 3265; M(OH-) isomer 1-Me_2 RI 3350; M(OH-) isomer 2-Me_2 RI 3500.

High Performance Liquid Chromatography. System HX—RI 563; system HZ—Retention time(s), 9.1 min; system HAA—Retention time(s), 20.1 min.

Ultraviolet Spectrum. Methanol—283 (A_1^1=640a), 306 nm.

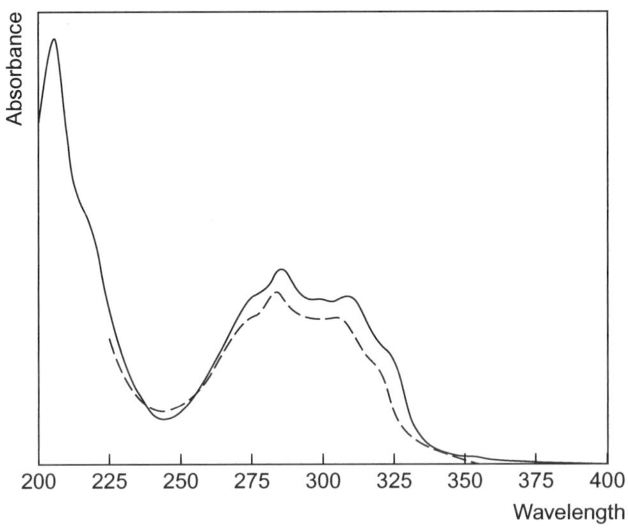

Infra-red Spectrum. Principal peaks at wavenumbers 1686, 1616, 1508, 1070, 762, 1570 cm^{-1} (KBr disk).

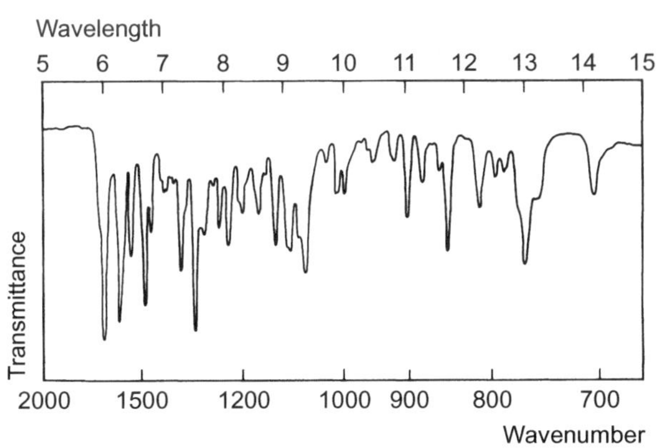

Mass Spectrum. Principal ions at *m/z* 310, 121, 353, 311, 43, 120, 92, 296.

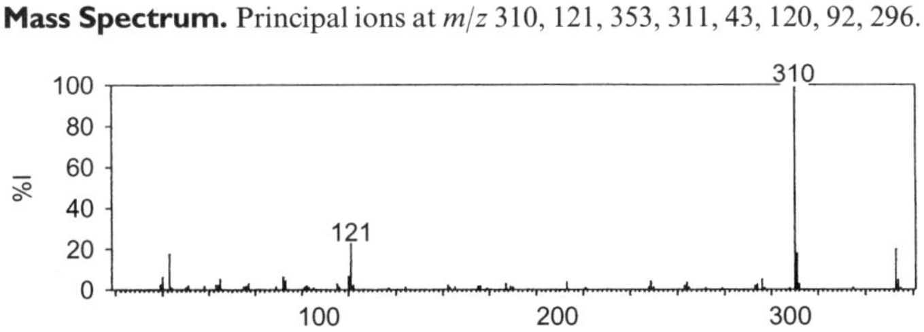

Quantification

Gas chromatography. In plasma: limit of detection 500 pg, ECD—G. Bianchetti *et al., J. Chromatogr.*, 1976, *124*, 331–335.

Gas chromatography–mass spectrometry. In plasma: limit of detection 0.8 µg/L—F. Pommier *et al., J. Chromatogr.*, 1994, *654*; *Biomed. Appl.*, 35–41.

High performance liquid chromatography. In serum: limit of detection 15 µg/L, UV detection—F. A. de Wolff *et al., J. Anal. Toxicol.*, 1980, *4*, 156–159. In plasma: acenocoumarol enantiomers—T. S. Gill *et al., Br. J. Clin. Pharmacol.*, 1988, *25*, 591–598.

High performance liquid chromatography–mass spectrometry. In plasma: acenocoumarol and other coumarins, limit of detection for acenocoumarol 10 µg/L—M. Kollroser and C. Schober, *Clin. Chem.*, 2002, *48*, 84–91 and 1372.

Thin-layer chromatography. In plasma: limit of detection 10 µg/L, fluorescence detection—G. M. J. van Kempen *et al., J. Chromatogr.*, 1978, *145*; *Biomed. Appl.*, *2*, 332–335.

Disposition in the Body. Acenocoumarol is readily absorbed after oral administration. It is extensively metabolised by reduction to a number of metabolites including the amino derivative, and the two diastereoisomers of 4-hydroxy-3-[1-(4-nitrophenyl)-3-hydroxybutyl]coumarin. Two further inactive metabolites, the 6-hydroxy- and 7-hydroxycoumarin derivatives have been identified in urine. About 50 to 60% of a dose is excreted in the urine in 48 h, mostly as metabolites, with less than 1% as unchanged drug; about 30% of a dose is eliminated in the faeces.

Therapeutic concentration

After a single oral dose of 12 mg to 2 subjects, peak plasma acenocoumarol concentrations of 0.17 and 0.41 mg/L were attained in 3 h; peak concentrations of the amino metabolite of 0.28 and 0.16 mg/L were reported after 6 to 10 h. [W. Dieterle *et al., Eur. J. Clin. Pharmacol.*, 1977, *11*, 367–375].

Following a single oral dose of 10 mg to 3 subjects, peak plasma concentrations of about 0.3 mg/L were attained in 2 to 3 h; the amino metabolite was not detected in plasma. [H. H. W. Thijssen and L. G. Baars, *Br. J. Clin. Pharmacol.*, 1983, *16*, 491–496].

Following oral administration of 2.5 mg twice daily to 2 subjects, steady-state plasma concentrations of 0.02 to 0.07 mg/L were reported. [G. Bianchetti *et al., J. Chromatogr.*, 1976, *124*, 331–335].

Half-life. Plasma half-life, about 8 h.

Volume of distribution. About 0.3 L/kg.

Clearance. Plasma clearance, about 0.5 mL/min/kg.

Protein binding. In plasma, about 98%.

Dose. Maintenance, 1 to 8 mg daily.

Acepromazine

Tranquilliser

Synonyms. 1522-CB; Acetazine; Acetylpromazine; Acetylpromazine.
Proprietary name. Plégicil
1-[10-[3-(Dimethylamino)propyl]-10*H*-phenothiazin-2-yl]ethanone
$C_{19}H_{22}N_2OS$=326.5
CAS—61-00-7

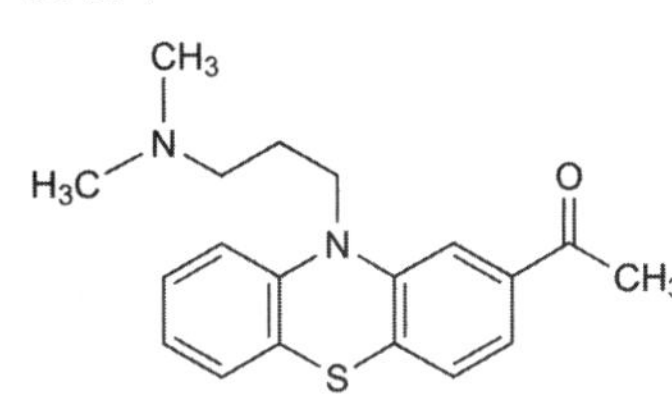

An orange-coloured oil, b.p. 220° to 240°.

Acepromazine Maleate

Proprietary names. Atravet; Calmivet; Plégicil; PromAce; Sedalin; Vetranquil. It is an ingredient of Immobilon (for large animals).
$C_{19}H_{22}N_2OS,C_4H_4O_4$=442.5
CAS—3598-37-6
A yellow crystalline powder. M.p. 135° to 136°.
Soluble 1 in 27 of water, 1 in 13 of ethanol, and 1 in 3 of chloroform; slightly soluble in ether and light petroleum.

Dissociation Constant. pK_a 9.3.

Partition Coefficient. Log *P* (octanol/pH 7.4), 2.3.

Colour Tests. Formaldehyde–Sulfuric acid—blue-violet; Forrest reagent—red; FPN reagent—brown-orange; Liebermann's test—brown; Mandelin's test—green→red; Marquis test—yellow-green→red.

Thin-layer Chromatography. System TA—Rf 48; system TB—Rf 26; system TC—Rf 24; system TE—Rf 63; system TL—Rf 12; system TAE—Rf 28; system TAJ—Rf 04; system TAK—Rf 00; system TAL—Rf 39. (Acidified iodoplatinate solution, positive.)

Gas Chromatography. System GA—RI 2735 acepromazine; RI 2720 M (dihydro-)-H_2O; system GB—RI 2844 acepromazine; RI 2824 M (dihydro-)-H_2O; RI 3160 M (7-OH-); system GF—RI 3230.

Column: Fused silica capillary (1) J&W DB-1 (0.25 µm film thickness, 15 m x 0.32 mm); (2) J&W DB-1301 (0.25 µm, 15 m x 0.25 mm); (3) J&W DB-1 capillary (0.4 µm, 10 m x 0.18 mm). Column temperature: (1&2) 120° increased to 280° at 20°/min; (3) 80° to 300° at 20°/min. Injector temperature: (1&2) 250°; (3) 280°. Carrier gas: helium. Detection: (1&2) NPD; (3) MS (*m/z* 41 to 550). Retention time(s): (1) 8.1 min; (2) 9.4 min; (3) 12.19 min. [L. I. Stowell, *J. Anal. Toxicol.*, 1998, *22*, 166–168].

High Performance Liquid Chromatography. System HA—*k* 4.1; system HY—RI 350; system HAA—Retention time(s) 10.8 min.

Column: (analytical) Spherisorb S_5OD/CN (150 x 4.6 mm); (pre-column) Spherisorb S_5ODS_2 (10 × 4 mm). Mobile phase: 0 to 70% MeCN in 15 min, held at 70% MeCN for 3 min, flow rate 2 mL/min. UV detection (λ=200 to 595 nm). Retention time(s): 10.5 min. [S. P. Elliott and K. A. Hale, *J. Anal. Toxicol.*, 1999, *23*, 367–371].

Ultraviolet Spectrum. Aqueous acid—243 (A^1_1=765a), 279; aqueous alkali—245, 283 nm.

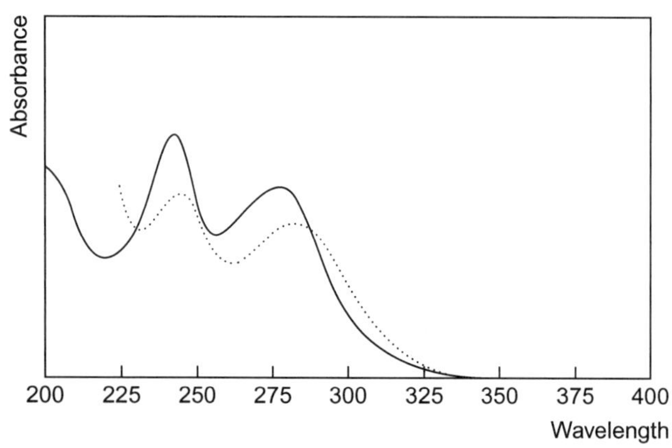

Infra-red Spectrum. Principal peaks at wavenumbers 1675, 1220, 1265, 1587, 746, 1562 cm^{-1} (KBr disk).

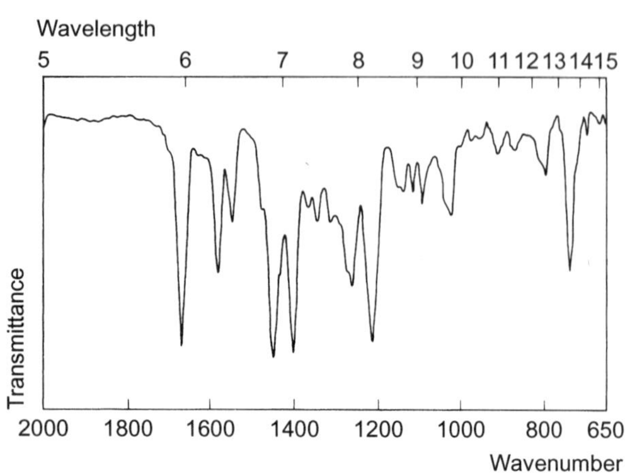

Mass Spectrum. Principal ions at *m/z* 100, 72, 240, 340, 44, 197, 254, 43 (acepromazine maleate).

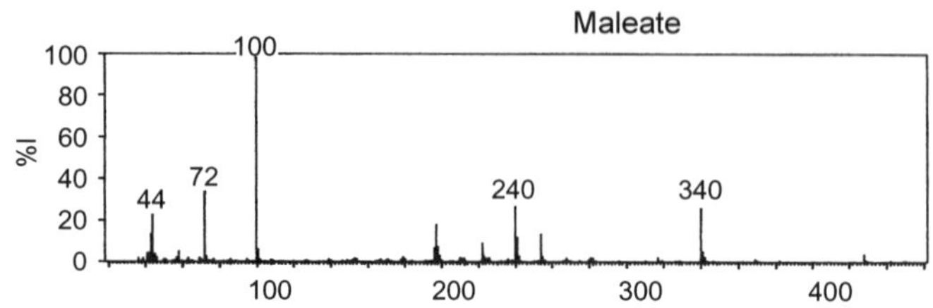

Quantification

High performance liquid chromatography. In blood: limit of detection 5 µg/L, UV detection—S. P. Elliott and K. A. Hale, *J. Anal. Toxicol.*, 1999, *23*, 367–371.

Disposition in the Body. Acepromazine is converted to 2-(1-hydroxyethyl)promazine, by red blood cells, and 2-(1-hydroxyethyl)promazine which may be the major unconjugated metabolite of acepromazine in humans.

Toxicity

A 43-year-old woman was found dead where acepromazine was found in chest-cavity blood, the liver, brain and bile at concentrations of 0.6, 3.0, 0.4, and 6.5 mg/L, respectively. The stomach contents contained a total of 2.5 mg acepromazine. [L. I. Stowell, *J. Anal. Toxicol.*, 1998, *22(2)*, 166–168].

A 28-year-old woman was found dead and toxicological analysis showed a blood concentration of 2.4 mg/L acepromazine and 3.29 mg/L zolpidem, urine concentration of 0.37 mg/L and 2.54 mg/L, respectively, and gastric contents concentration of 20.05 mg/L and 34.27 mg/L, respectively. [A. Tracqui *et al.*, *Am. J. Forensic Med. Pathol.*, 1993, *14(4)*, 309–312].

Dose. Acepromazine has been given in doses of 6 to 60 mg daily.

Acetaldehyde

Synonyms. Acetic Aldehyde; Aldehyde; Ethanal; Ethyl Aldehyde.
C_2H_4O=44.1
CAS—75-07-0

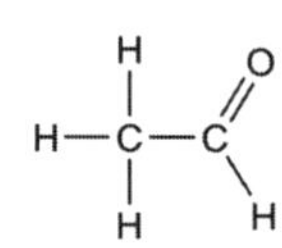

A colourless inflammable liquid. M.p. −123.5°. B.p. 21.0°. Refractive index, at 20°, 1.3316. Miscible with water, ethanol, and ether.

Colour Tests. Potassium dichromate (Method 2)—green; Schiff's reagent—violet; Sodium nitroprusside (Method 2)—red.

Gas Chromatography. System GA—RI 372; system GI—Retention time(s) 0.7 min.

Column: Carbowax megabore capillary (Alltech, 1.2 µm film thickness, 30 m × 0.54 mm). Carrier gas: helium, 7.9 mL/min flow rate. Internal standard: 1-propanol. Detection: FID. Retention time(s): 1.44 min. [D. Gail McCarver-May and L. Durisin, *J. Anal. Toxicol.*, 1997, *21*, 134–141].

Mass Spectrum. Principal ions at *m/z* 29, 44, 43, 42, 26, 41, 28, 27.

Quantification

Gas chromatography. In blood: head-space analysis, limit of detection 18 µg/L, FID—J. M. Christensen *et al.*, *Clinica Chim. Acta*, 1981, *116*, 389–395.

Disposition in the Body. Acetaldehyde is a major intermediate metabolite of ethanol and is also a metabolite of metaldehyde, paraldehyde and phenacetin. It undergoes further metabolism by oxidation to acetic acid and, eventually, to carbon dioxide and water. A minor pathway involves condensation with pyruvic acid to form acetoin.

Toxicity. Acetaldehyde is more toxic than ethanol or acetic acid. The maximum permissible atmospheric concentration is 100 ppm.

Acetanilide

Analgesic

Synonyms. Acetylaniline, Acetylaminobenzene, Antifebrin.
N-Phenylacetamide
C_8H_9NO=135.2
CAS—103-84-4

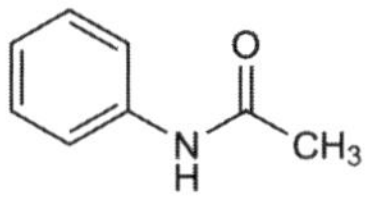

Colourless shining lamellar crystals or white crystalline powder. M.p. 113° to 115°. Soluble 1 in 200 of water, 1 in 20 of boiling water, 1 in 3.5 of ethanol, 1 in 8 of chloroform, and 1 in 50 of ether; soluble in acetone.

Dissociation Constant. pK_a 0.6 (25°).

Partition Coefficient. Log *P* (octanol/water), 1.2.

Colour Test. Liebermann's Test—red→orange.

Thin-layer Chromatography. System TD—Rf 45; system TE—Rf 70; system TF—Rf 45; system TAD—Rf 52; system TAE—Rf 80; system TAF—Rf 84. (Acidified potassium permanganate solution, positive.)

Gas Chromatography. System GA—acetanilide RI 1368, paracetamol RI 1665; system GB—RI 1400.

High Performance Liquid Chromatography. System HA—*k* 0.1; system HD—acetanilide *k* 0.5, paracetamol *k* 0.1; system HW—acetanilide *k* 2.3, paracetamol *k* 0.32; system HY—RI 281.

Ultraviolet Spectrum. Aqueous acid—239 nm (A_1^1=815 a). No alkaline shift.

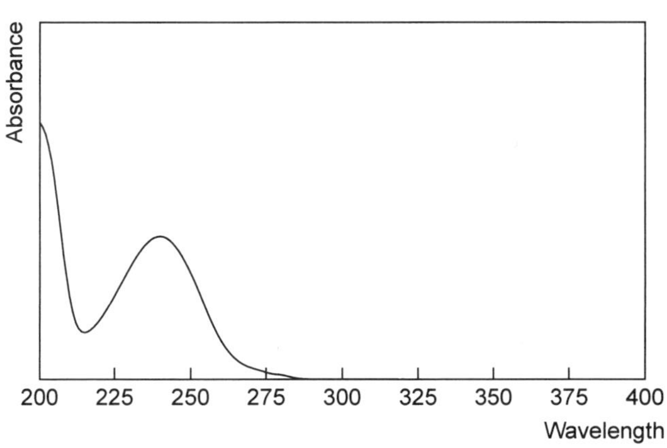

Infra-red Spectrum. Principal peaks at wavenumbers 1660, 1598, 752, 1538, 1315, 1500 cm^{-1} (KBr disk).

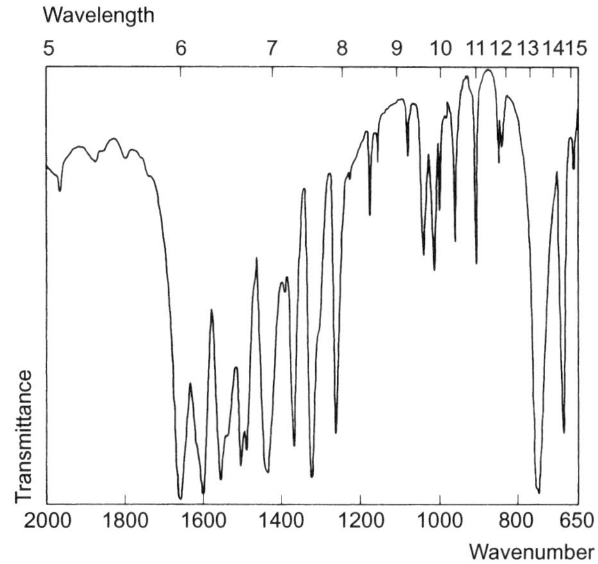

Mass Spectrum. Principal ions at *m/z* 93, 135, 43, 66, 65, 39, 94, 92; paracetamol 109, 151, 43, 80, 108, 81, 53, 52.

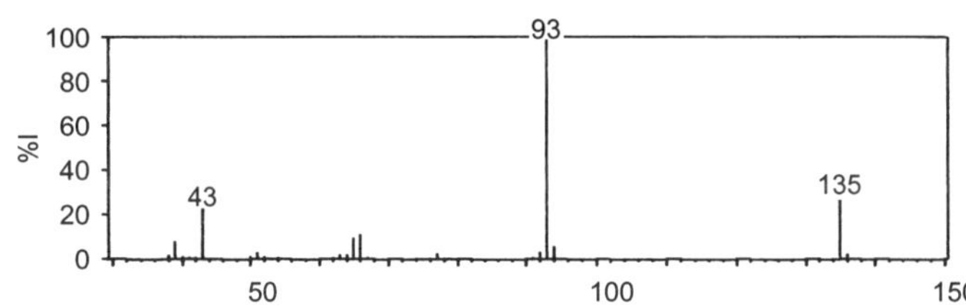

Quantification

Gas chromatography. In plasma: FID—N. Buchanan *et al.*, *Br. J. Clin. Pharmacol.*, 1980, *9*, 525–526.

Disposition in the Body. Rapidly and completely absorbed after oral administration, with maximum plasma concentrations achieved after 1 to 2 h. It is distributed throughout the body. The main metabolic reaction is oxidation to paracetamol through which the analgesic and antipyretic effects of the drug are chiefly exerted; paracetamol is then conjugated with glucuronic acid or sulfate. A minor reaction is deacetylation of acetanilide to aniline. About 0.1% of an oral dose is excreted unchanged in the urine in 24 h, about 4% as free paracetamol, 80% as paracetamol conjugates, and 0.05% as aniline. About 0.1% of an oral dose may be eliminated in the faeces.

Toxicity. The main toxic effect is the formation of methaemoglobin due to the production of aniline or other toxic metabolites.

Half-life. Plasma half-life, about 1.5 h.

Volume of distribution. About 0.7 L/kg.

Clearance. Plasma clearance, about 6 mL/min/kg.

Protein binding. In plasma, not significantly bound.

Dose. Acetanilide was formerly given in doses of 0.36 to 1.2 g daily.

Acetarsone

Antiprotozoal

Synonyms. Acetarsol; Acetphenarsine; Acetphenarsinum; Osarsolum.
Proprietary names. Ehrlich 594; Fourneau 190; F—190; Gynoplix; Orarsan; Spirocid; Stovarsol; SVC.
[3-(Acetylamino)-4-hydroxyphenyl]arsonic acid
$C_8H_{10}AsNO_5$=275.1
CAS—97-44-9

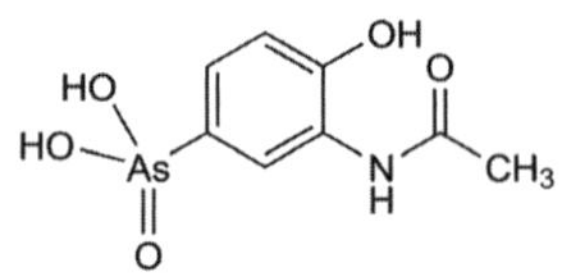

A white crystalline powder. M.p. about 240°, with decomposition. Practically insoluble in cold water, moderately soluble in boiling water; practically insoluble in ethanol; soluble in dilute alkalis.

Acetarsone Sodium
$C_8H_9AsNNaO_5,5H_2O$=387.2
CAS—5892-48-8 (anhydrous)
White crystals or crystalline powder. Soluble 1 in 7 of water; practically insoluble in ethanol, chloroform and ether.

Dissociation Constant. pK_a 3.7, 7.9, 9.3.

Ultraviolet Spectrum. Aqueous acid—281 nm (A_1^1=94 b); aqueous alkali—250 nm (A_1^1=567 b), 299 nm (A_1^1=177 b).

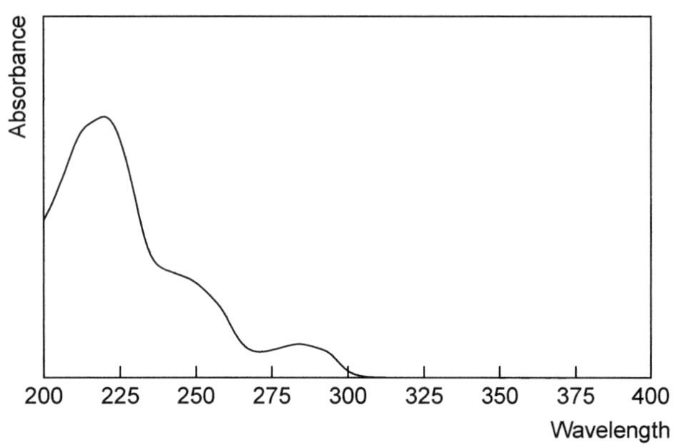

Infra-red Spectrum. Principal peaks at wavenumbers 887, 1538, 784, 823, 1297, 1584 cm^{-1} (KBr disk).

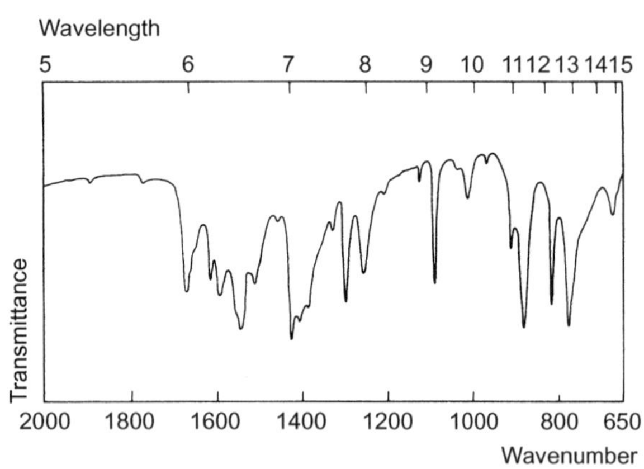

Dose. Up to 500 mg daily for 10 days.

Acetazolamide

Antiglaucoma/Diuretic/Carbonic Anhydrase Inhibitor

Synonyms. 6063; Acetazolam; Acetazoleamide.
Proprietary names. Acetamox; Atenezol; Défiltran; Diamox; Didoc; Diuriwas; Donmox; Edemox; Fonurit; Glaucomide; Glaupax; Inidrase.
N-[5-(Aminosulfonyl)-1,3,4-thiadiazol-2-yl]acetamide
$C_4H_6N_4O_3S_2$=222.3
CAS—59-66-5

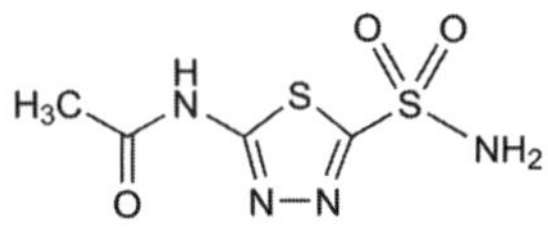

A fine, white to yellowish-white, crystalline powder. M.p. about 260°, with decomposition. Soluble 1 in 1400 of water, 1 in 400 of ethanol, and 1 in 100 of acetone; practically insoluble in carbon tetrachloride, chloroform and ether.

Acetazolamide Sodium
Proprietary names. Diamox Sodium; Vetamox.
$C_4H_5N_4NaO_3S_2$=244.2
CAS—1424-27-7
Soluble in water.

Dissociation Constant. pK_a 7.2, 9.0 (25°).

Colour Test. Koppanyi–Zwikker test—red-violet (transient).

Thin-layer Chromatography. System TA—Rf 85; system TD—Rf 04; system TE—Rf 03; system TF—Rf 31; system TAD—Rf 18; system TAE—Rf 84; system TAJ—Rf 18; system TAK—Rf 01; system TAL—Rf 60.

Gas Chromatography. Column: fused silica capillary cross-linked 5% phenylmethylsilicone (0.33 µm film thickness, 25 m × 0.2 mm). Column temperature: 230° increased to 320° at 35°/min. Injector: 280°. Detector: 300°. Carrier gas: helium, 1 mL/min flow rate. Internal standard (IS): mefruside. MS detection: (SIM at *m/z* 249 and *m/z* 85 for IS). Retention time(s): acetazolamide, 3.62 min (*k* 0.684); IS, 7.43 min (*k* 2.46). [D. Carreras *et al.*, *J. Chromatogr. A*, 1994, *683*, 195–202].

High Performance Liquid Chromatography. System HA—*k* 0.1; system HX—RI 268; system HY—RI 226; system HZ—Retention time(s) 1.9 min; system HAA—Retention time(s) 6.9 min.

Ultraviolet Spectrum. Aqueous acid—265 (A_1^1=475a); aqueous alkali—240, 291 nm.

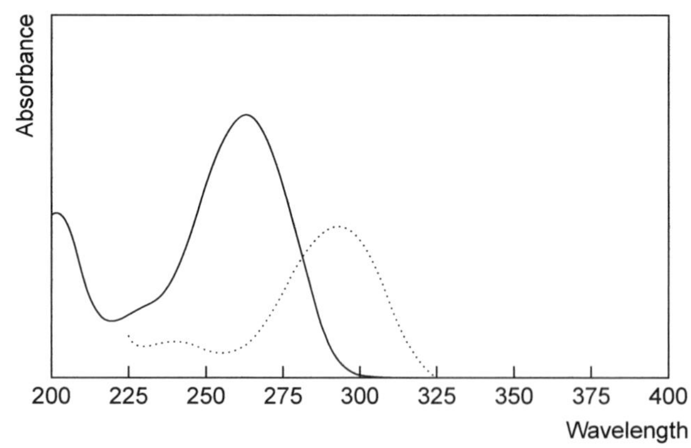

Infra-red Spectrum. Principal peaks at wavenumbers 1167, 1548, 1316, 1665, 671, 1115 cm^{-1} (KBr disk).

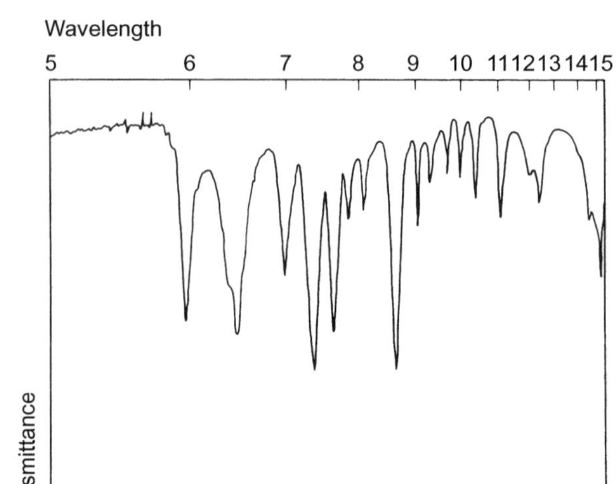

Mass Spectrum. Principal ions at *m/z* 43, 180, 42, 45, 44, 64, 100, 222.

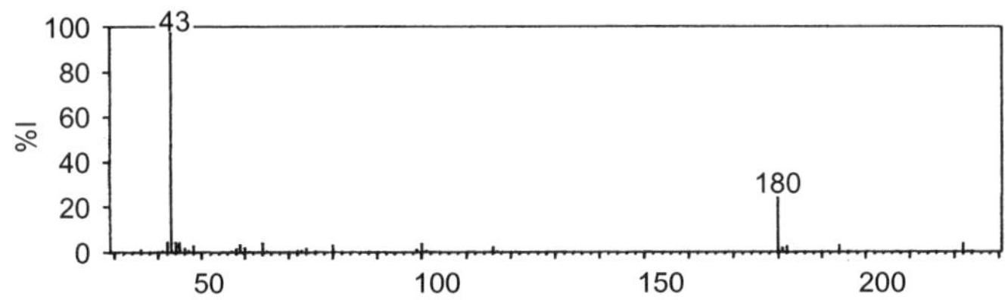

Quantification

Gas chromatography. In blood, plasma or saliva: limit of detection 10 ng, ECD—S. M. Wallace *et al.*, *J. Pharm. Sci.*, 1977, *66*, 527–530.

Gas chromatography–mass spectrometry. In blood or saliva: limit of detection 25 pg—K. Kishida *et al.*, *Anal. Lett. (Part B)*, 1981, *14*, 335–347.

High performance liquid chromatography. In plasma: limit of detection 5 µg/L, UV detection (λ=254 nm)—A Zarghi and A. Shafaati, *J. Pharm. Biomed. Anal.*, 2002, *28*, 169–172. In blood, plasma, or urine: limit of detection 50 µg/L, UV detection—D. J. Chapron and L. B. White, *J. Pharm. Sci.*, 1984, *73*, 985–989.

Disposition in the Body. Acetazolamide is readily absorbed after oral administration. It binds tightly to carbonic anhydrase and will accumulate in tissues in which this enzyme is present, particularly in red blood cells and the renal cortex. About 70 to 90% of a dose is excreted in the urine as unchanged drug in 24 h but the renal clearance is increased if the urine is alkaline; small amounts of unchanged drug are excreted in the bile. The plasma:saliva ratio is about 100.

Therapeutic concentration. In plasma, usually in the range 10 to 15 mg/L.

Following a single oral dose of 250 mg to 5 subjects, peak plasma concentrations of 10 to 18 (mean 14) mg/L were attained in 1 to 3 h; peak erythrocyte concentrations of 13 to 29 mg/L were reached about 1 h after the peak plasma concentrations. [S. M. Wallace *et al.*, *J. Pharm. Sci.*, 1977, *66*, 527–530].

A patient with type I diabetes and end-stage renal disease (ESRD) undergoing continuous ambulatory peritoneal dialysis (CAPD) was administered a 250 mg oral dose of acetazolamide after surgery for a detached retina. The concentration of acetazolamide in serum was measured prior to the dose and 12 additional times over a 24-hour dosing period. The serum concentration at the beginning of the dosing period was 18 µg/mL and at the end 17 µg/mL with a maximum concentration of 27 µg/mL at 6.5 h. The therapeutic range was 5 to 10 µg/mL. [M. H. Schwenk *et al.*, *Adv. Perit. Dial.*, 1994, *10*, 44–46].

Toxicity. Fatal cases of agranulocytosis, aplastic anaemia and thrombocytopenia have been reported.

Half-life. Plasma half-life, about 13 h; blood and erythrocyte concentrations decrease more slowly.

Volume of distribution. About 0.2 L/kg.

Protein binding. In plasma, about 90 to 95%.

Dose. In the treatment of glaucoma 0.25 to 1 g daily.

Acetic Acid Glacial

Synonyms. Acetic Acid; Acide Acetique Cristallisable; Concentrated Acetic Acid
$CH_3{\cdot}COOH$=60.1
CAS—64-19-7

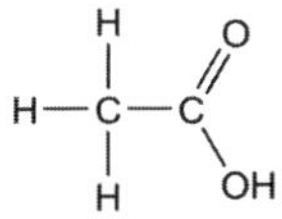

A translucent crystalline mass or a clear colourless liquid. M.p. 15°. B.p. about 117°. Refractive index, at 20°, 1.3718. Miscible with water, ethanol, chloroform and ether.

Dissociation Constant. pK_a 4.8 (25°).

Colour Test. Ferric Chloride—red.

Mass Spectrum. Principal ions at *m/z* 45, 29, 43, 60, 42, 28, 44, 41.

Quantification

Gas chromatography. In blood: limit of detection 1 µg/mL, FID—D. Lester, *Anal. Chem.*, 1964, *36*, 1810–1812.

Disposition in the Body. Acetic acid occurs as a metabolite of ethanol and also of paraldehyde after its depolymerisation to acetaldehyde. It is further oxidised to carbon dioxide and water.

Toxicity. The estimated minimum lethal dose is 5 mL and the maximum permissible atmospheric concentration is 10 ppm.

Acetohexamide

Antidiabetic

Synonyms. Cyclamide; Tsiklamid
Proprietary names. Dimelor; Dimeline; Dymelor; Ordimel.
4-Acetyl-*N*-[(cyclohexylamino)carbonyl]benzenesulfonamide
$C_{15}H_{20}N_2O_4S$=324.4
CAS—968-81-0

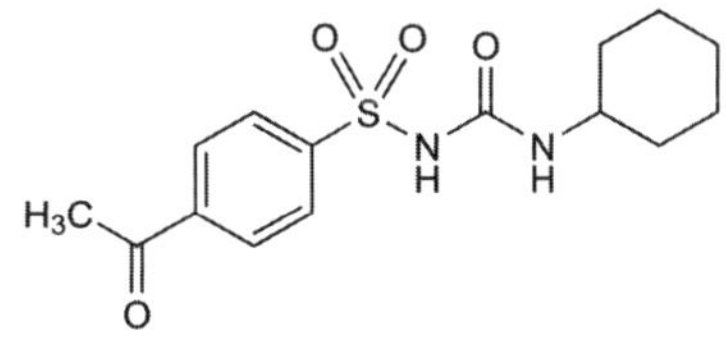

A white crystalline powder. M.p. 182° to 187°. Practically insoluble in water and ether; soluble 1 in 230 of ethanol and 1 in 210 of chloroform; soluble in pyridine and in dilute solutions of alkali hydroxides.

Colour Test. Koppanyi–Zwikker Test—violet.

Thin-layer Chromatography. System TD—Rf 39; system TE—Rf 12; system TF—Rf 43; system TAD—Rf 53; system TAJ—Rf 60; system TAK—Rf 66; system TAL—Rf 91.

High Performance Liquid Chromatography. System HY—RI 438.

Ultraviolet Spectrum. Aqueous acid—247 nm (A_1^1=508 b); aqueous alkali—249 nm (A_1^1=427 a).

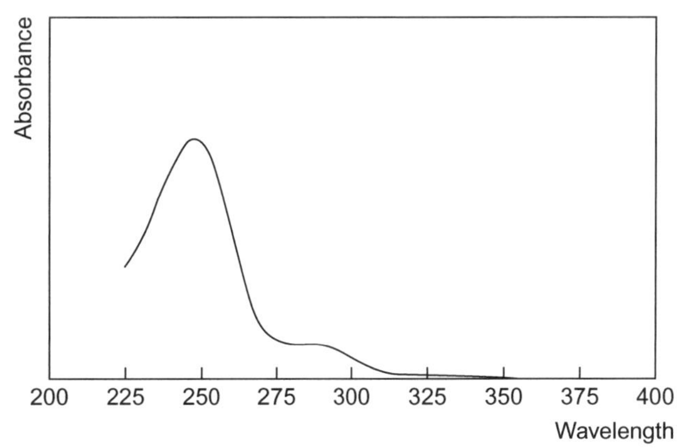

Infra-red Spectrum. Principal peaks at wavenumbers 1165, 1031, 1681, 1531, 905, 1264 cm^{-1} (Nujol mull).

Mass Spectrum. Principal ions at *m/z* 210, 56, 43, 184, 211, 75, 99, 76.

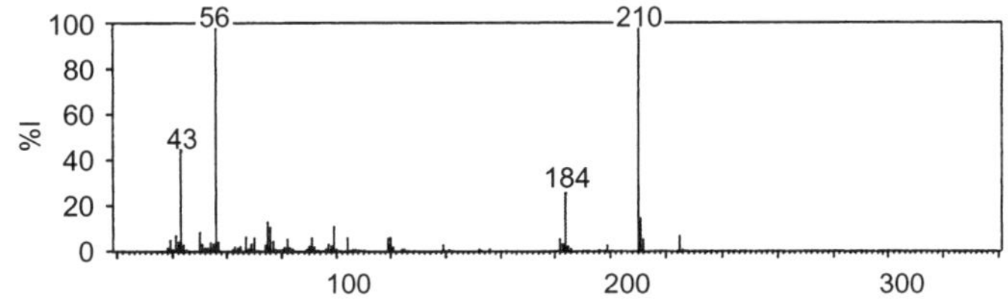

Quantification

Spectrofluorimetry. In plasma: limit of detection 200 ng—P. Girgis-Takla and I. Chroneos, *Analyst*, 1979, *104*, 117–123.

Gas chromatography. In biological fluids: FID—J. W. Kleber *et al.*, *J. Pharm. Sci.*, 1977, *66*, 635–638.

Disposition in the Body. Readily absorbed after oral administration and rapidly metabolised to (–)-1-hydroxyhexamide which has about 2.5 times the hypoglycaemic activity of the unchanged drug. Minor metabolites include 4′-*trans*-hydroxyacetohexamide, 4′-*trans*-hydroxy-1-hydroxyhexamide and, to a lesser extent, the 4′-*cis*-, 3′-*cis*-, and 3′-*trans*-isomers. About 80% of a dose is excreted in the urine in 24 h, mainly as metabolites.

Therapeutic concentration. In plasma, usually in the range 20 to 60 μg/mL.

Following oral administration of 750 mg of three different tablet formulations to 8 subjects, mean peak plasma-acetohexamide concentrations of about 28, 40, and 44 μg/mL were attained 2 h after a dose; mean peak plasma concentrations of (–)-1-hydroxyhexamide averaged about 30 μg/mL. [J. W. Kleber *et al.*, *J. Pharm. Sci.*, 1977, *66*, 635–638].

After daily oral doses of 0.5 g to 18 subjects, an average serum concentration of 42 μg/mL was reported 3 to 5 h after the dose. [J. Sheldon *et al.*, *Diabetes*, 1965, *14*, 362–367].

Toxicity. Prolonged hypoglycaemia has been reported.

Half-life. Plasma half-life, acetohexamide about 1.3 h, (–)-1-hydroxyhexamide about 5 h.

Protein binding. In plasma, about 96%.

Note. For a review of the pharmacokinetics of oral hypoglycaemic agents see L. Balant, *Clin. Pharmacokinet.*, 1981, *6*, 215–241.
For a review of the relationship between the pharmacokinetics and pharmacodynamic effects of oral hypoglycaemic drugs see R. E. Ferner and S. Chaplin, *Clin. Pharmacokinet.*, 1987, *12*, 379–401.

Dose. 0.25 to 1.5 g daily.

Acetomenaphthone

Vitamin K Activity

Synonyms. Acetomenadione; Dihydrovitamin K_3, Menadiol Diacetate, Vitamin-K_4.
Proprietary names. Kapilin; Prokayvit Oral; Vitavel K; It is an ingredient of Pernivit.
1,4-Diacetoxy-2-methylnaphthalene
$C_{15}H_{14}O_4$=258.3
CAS—573-20-6

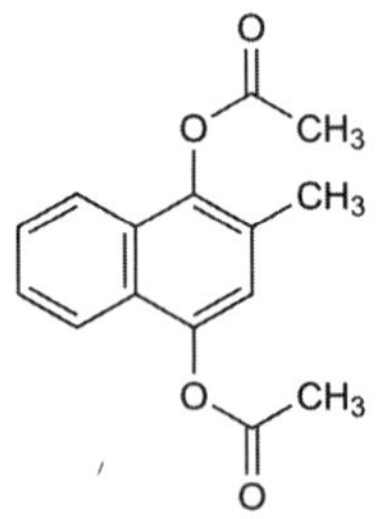

A white crystalline powder. M.p. 112° to 115°. Practically insoluble in water; slightly soluble in cold ethanol; soluble 1 in 3.3 of boiling ethanol; soluble in acetic acid.

Colour Test. Liebermann's Test—black.

Ultraviolet Spectrum. Dehydrated alcohol—285 nm (A^1_1=245 b), 322 nm (A^1_1=37 b).

Infra-red Spectrum. Principal peaks at wavenumbers 1210, 1760, 1163, 1070, 775, 1030 cm^{-1} (KBr disk).

Dose. 5 to 20 mg daily.

Acetone

Solvent

Synonyms. Cetona; Dimethylformaldehyde; Dimethyl Ketone; β-Ketopropane; Pyroacetic Ether.
2-Propanone
C_3H_6O=58.08
CAS—67-64-1

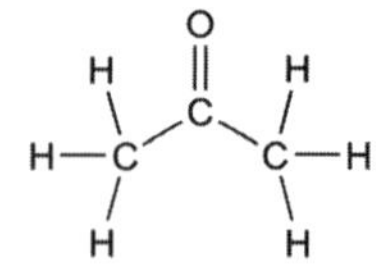

A clear, colourless, volatile, mobile, inflammable liquid. M.p. –94°. B.p. about 56°. Refractive index 1.3591. Miscible with water, ethanol, chloroform, and ether.

Partition Coefficient. Log *P* (octanol/water), –0.2.

Colour Test. Sodium nitroprusside (method 1)—red.

Gas Chromatography. System GA—RI 469; system GI—Retention time(s) 2.5 min.

Column: Trifluoropropylmethylpolysiloxane Crossbond Rtx-200 (3 μm film thickness, 30 m × 0.53 mm). Column temperature: 40° for 1 min increasing to 260° at 70°/min. Injector and detector temperature: 250°. Carrier gas: helium, 80.1 mL/min flow rate. Internal standard (IS): *n*-propanol. Detection: FID. Retention time(s): acetone, 1.8 min; IS, 1.5 min [R. H. Williams *et al.*, *J. Anal. Toxicol.*, 2000, *24*, 621–626].

High Pressure Liquid Chromatography. Column: RP C_{18} Pecosphere (3 × 3). Mobile phase: acetonitrile:water (45:55, v/v), flow-rate 1 mL/min. UV detection (λ=365 nm). Retention time(s): 3 min [A. Brega *et al.*, *J. Chromatogr.*, 1991, *553(1–2)*, 249–254].

Ultraviolet Spectrum. Aqueous acid—265 nm.

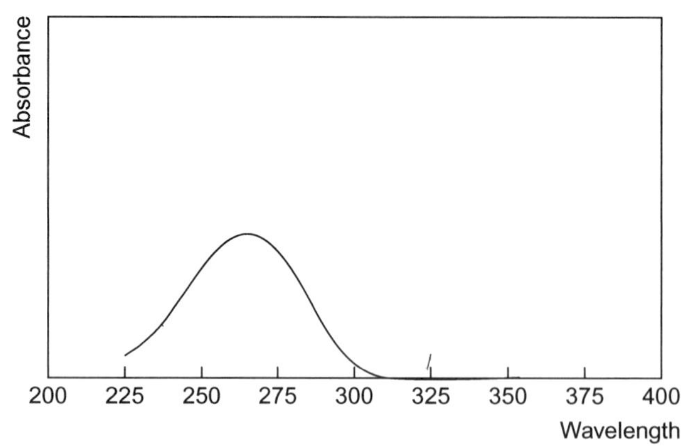

Mass Spectrum. Principal ions at *m*/*z* 43, 58, 59, 27, 42, 26, 39, 29.

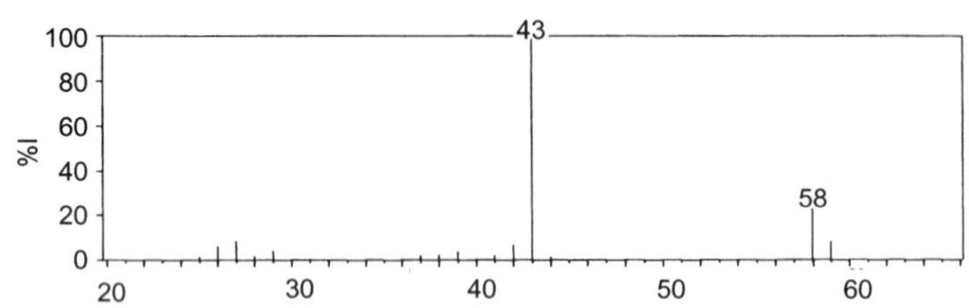

Quantification

Gas chromatography. In serum: limit of detection 10 mg/L and limit of quantification 25 mg/L, FID—R. H. Williams *et al.*, *J. Anal. Toxicol.*, 2000, *24*, 621–626. In plasma or breath: FID—M. D. Trotter *et al.*, *Clinica Chim. Acta*, 1971, *35*, 137–143.

High pressure liquid chromatography. In or urine: limit of detection 0.034 mmol/L—A. Brega *et al.*, *J. Chromatogr.*, 1991, *553(1–2)*, 249–254.

Disposition in the Body. Acetone is absorbed through the lungs and skin. It is excreted in the urine and through the lungs; large amounts are mainly excreted unchanged but small doses may be oxidised to carbon dioxide or utilised in the body as acetate or formate. Acetone is the main metabolite of isopropyl alcohol; it occurs naturally in the blood and urine of diabetics.

Therapeutic concentration

89 non-occupationally exposed subjects and 3 groups of workers exposed to acetone or isopropanol on a daily basis were observed. Acetone was

detected in all samples from the non-exposed subjects at mean concentrations of 840 µg/L in blood (C_b), 842 µg/L in urine (C_u), 715 mg/L in alveolar air (C_a) and 154 ng/L in environmental air (C_i). The morning after a shift, the workers had C_b 3.5 mg/L and C_u 13 mg/L of acetone. This was after mean acetone exposure of 336 µg/L. [G. Wang *et al.*, *Int. Arch. Occup. Environ. Health*, 1994, *65(5)*, 285–289].

Toxicity. Acetone is one of the solvents abused in 'glue-sniffing'. Severe toxic effects have been associated with blood concentrations of 200 to 300 mg/L; a blood concentration of 550 mg/L has been reported in a fatality. The maximum permissible atmospheric concentration is 1000 ppm. Exposure to 1600 ppm for about 15 min causes irritation to the eyes and nose. Up to 20 mL has been ingested without ill-effect.

Acetophenazine

Tranquilliser/Antipsychotic

Synonym. Acephenazine

1-[10-[3-[4-(2-Hydroxyethyl)-1-piperazinyl]propyl]-10*H*-phenothiazin-2-yl]ethanone

$C_{23}H_{29}N_3O_2S = 411.6$

CAS—2751-68-0

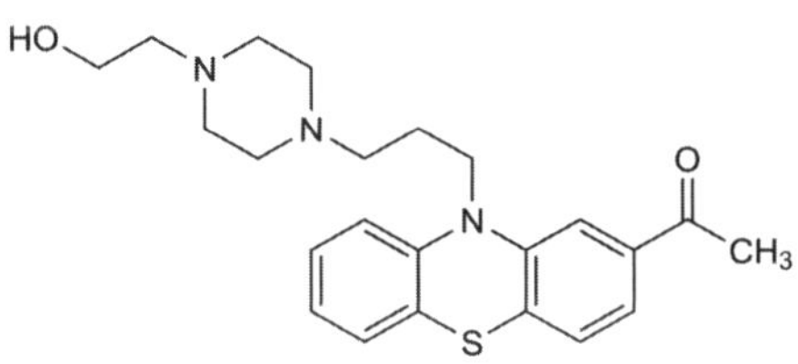

Acetophenazine Dimaleate

Proprietary name. Tindal

$C_{23}H_{29}N_3O_2S,2C_4H_4O_4 = 643.7$

CAS—5714-00-1

A fine yellow powder. M.p. about 165°, with decomposition. Soluble 1 in 10 of water, 1 in 260 of ethanol, 1 in 370 of acetone, 1 in 2850 of chloroform, 1 in 6000 of ether, and 1 in 11 of propylene glycol.

Colour Tests. Formaldehyde–Sulfuric acid—blue-violet; Forrest reagent—pink-orange; FPN reagent—orange; Liebermann's test—brown; Marquis test—red-violet.

Thin-layer Chromatography. System TA—Rf 53; system TB—Rf 03; system TC—Rf 25; system TE—Rf 38; system TL—Rf 03; system TAE—Rf 34; system TAF—Rf 32; system TAJ—Rf 05; system TAK—Rf 00; system TAL—Rf 33. (Dragendorff spray, positive; FPN reagent, pink; acidified iodoplatinate solution, positive; Marquis reagent, orange.)

Gas Chromatography. System GA—not eluted.

High Performance Liquid Chromatography. System HA—*k* 1.9.

Ultraviolet Spectrum. Aqueous acid—243 (A_1^1 = 500a), 278 nm.

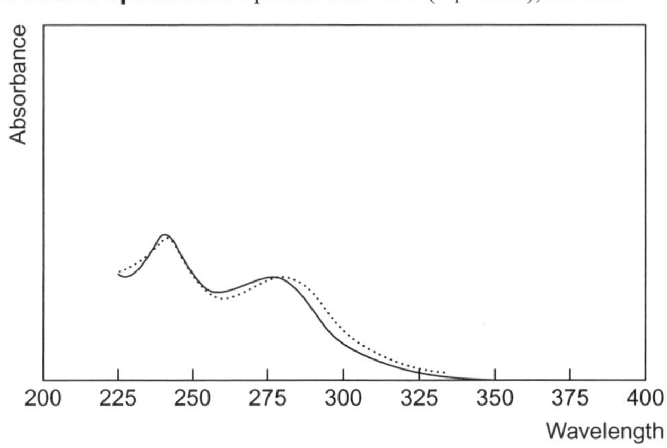

Infra-red Spectrum. Principal peaks at wavenumbers 1670, 1220, 1265, 1587, 746, 1149 cm^{-1} (KBr disk).

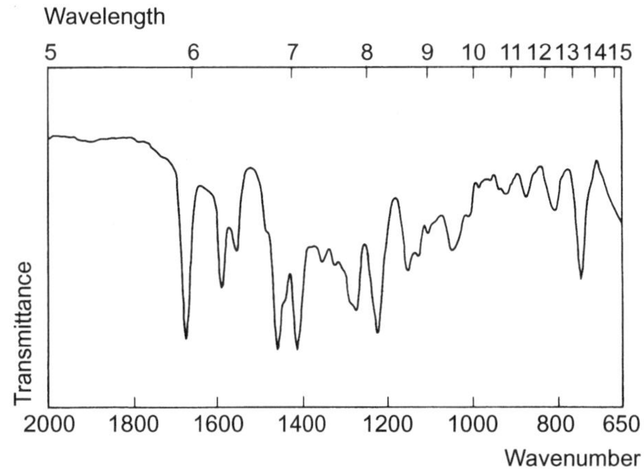

Mass Spectrum. Principal ions at *m/z* 254, 143, 42, 70, 411, 113, 56, 157.

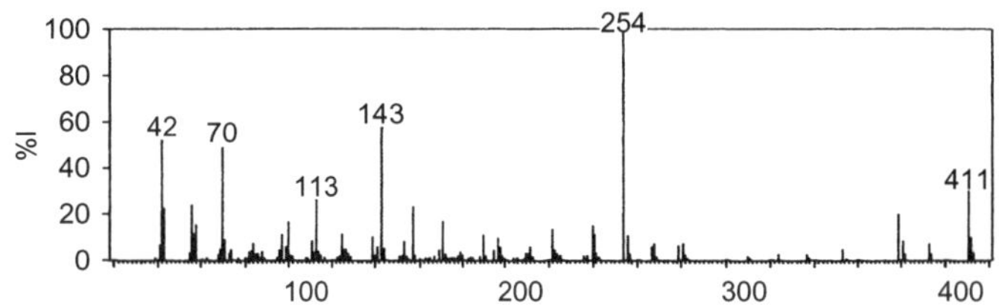

Dose. 40 to 120 mg of acetophenazine maleate daily; up to 600 mg daily has been given.

Acetorphine

Narcotic Analgesic (Veterinary)

O^3-Acetyl-7,8-dihydro-7α-[1(*R*)-hydroxy-1-methylbutyl]-O^6-methyl-6,14-*endo*-ethenomorphine

$C_{27}H_{35}NO_5 = 453.6$

CAS—25333-77-1

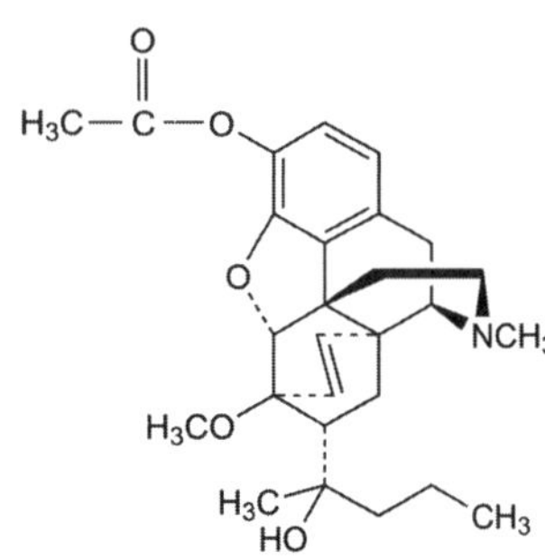

M.p. 193°.

Soluble 1 in 4000 of water; freely soluble in ethanol, chloroform, and ether.

Caution. It is dangerous to smell or taste this substance.

Acetorphine Hydrochloride

Synonym. M183

$C_{27}H_{35}NO_5,HCl = 490.0$

CAS—25333-78-2

A white, crystalline, hygroscopic powder. M.p. 204°. It is hydrolysed in solution to etorphine and acetic acid.

Soluble 1 in 50 of water and 1 in 10 of ethanol.

Colour Test. Marquis Test—blue-grey→yellow-brown.

Thin-layer Chromatography. System TA—Rf 72. (Acidified iodoplatinate solution, positive; Marquis reagent, grey; acidified potassium permanganate solution, positive.)

High Pressure Liquid Chromatography. System HA—*k* 0.4.

Ultraviolet Spectrum. Aqueous acid—284 nm (A_1^1 = 45b).

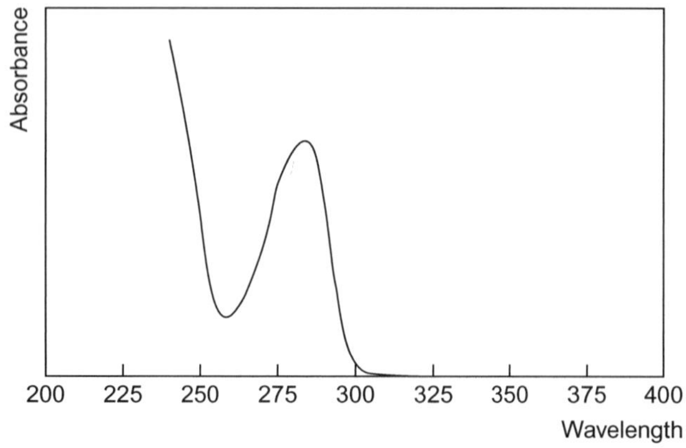

Infra-red Spectrum. Principal peaks at wavenumbers 1200, 1218, 1168, 1760, 1150, 1122 cm^{-1} (acetorphine hydrochloride, KBr disk).

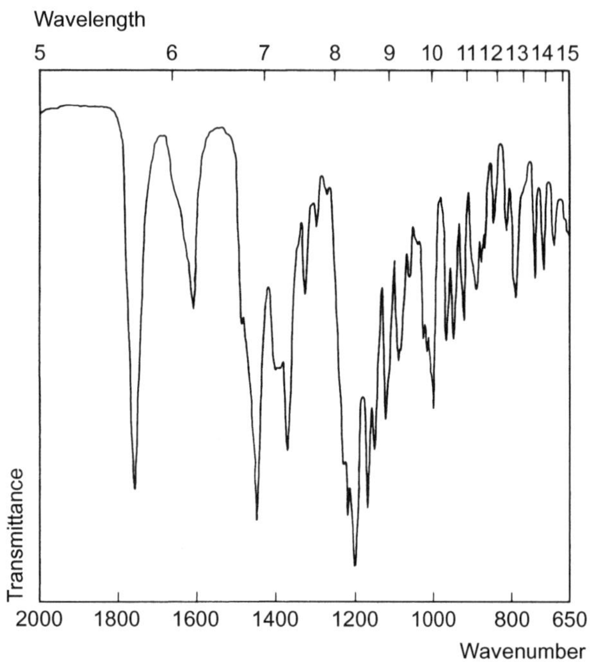

Acetylcholine Chloride

Parasympathomimetic

Proprietary names. Acecoline; Arterocoline; Miochol; Ovisot
2-(Acetyloxy)-*N*,*N*,*N*-trimethylethanaminium chloride
$C_7H_{16}ClNO_2$=181.7
CAS—60-31-1
A white, very hygroscopic, crystalline powder. M.p. about 150°. Very soluble in water yielding unstable solutions; very soluble in ethanol and propylene glycol; freely soluble in chloroform; practically insoluble in ether.

Acetylcholine Bromide

$C_7H_{16}BrNO_2$=226.1
CAS—66-23-9
Deliquescent colourless crystals or white crystalline powder. Hydrolysed by hot water and alkalis. M.p. 143°. Freely soluble in water; soluble in ethanol; practically insoluble in ether.

Thin-layer Chromatography. System TA—Rf 02; system TN—Rf 70; system TO—Rf 60. (Acidified iodoplatinate solution, positive.)

Infra-red Spectrum. Principal peaks at wavenumbers 949, 1089, 869, 1231, 1000, 1740 cm^{-1} (KBr disk).

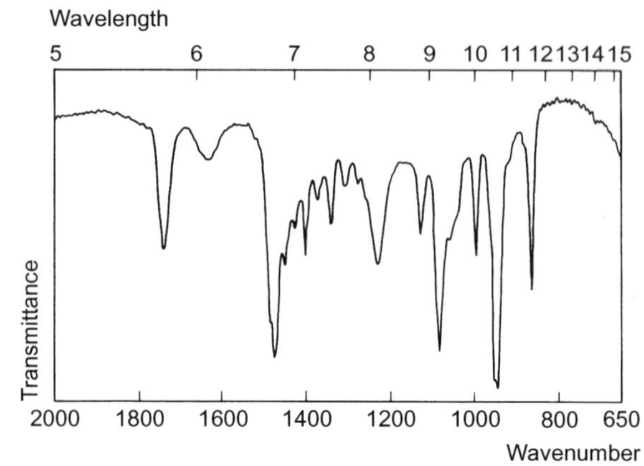

Mass Spectrum. Principal ions at *m/z* 58, 43, 57, 149, 71, 42, 41, 55.

Dose. Acetylcholine chloride is used as a 1% ophthalmic solution; it was formerly given parenterally in doses of 20 to 200 mg.

Acetylcodeine

3-*O*-Methyl-6-*O*-acetylmorphine
$C_{20}H_{23}NO_4$=341.4
CAS—6703-27-1

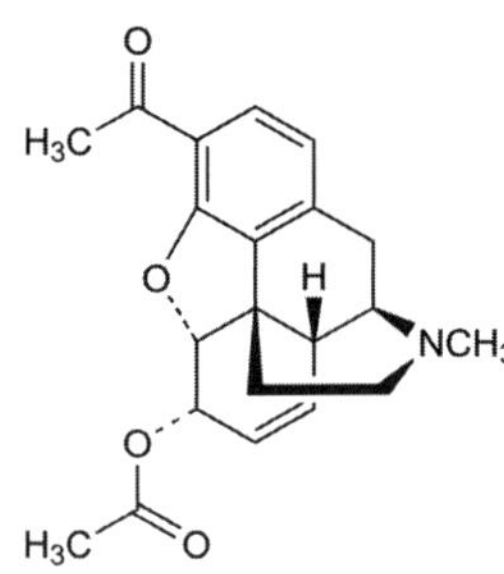

M.p. 134° to 135°.
It is a contaminant of codeine and up to 12% may be found in illicit heroin.

Thin-layer Chromatography. System TA—Rf 44; system TB—Rf 23; system TC—Rf 43; system TE—Rf 54; system TL—Rf 12; system TAE—Rf 26; system TAF—Rf 25; system TAJ—Rf 32; system TAK—Rf 05; system TAL—Rf 61.

Gas Chromatography. System GA—RI 2503; system GB—RI 2645; system GM—RRT 1.449 (relative to iprindole).

High Pressure Liquid Chromatography. System HC—*k* 0.78; system HS—*k* 0.50; system HX—RI 336.

Ultraviolet Spectrum. Aqueous acid—284 nm (A^1_1=37b).

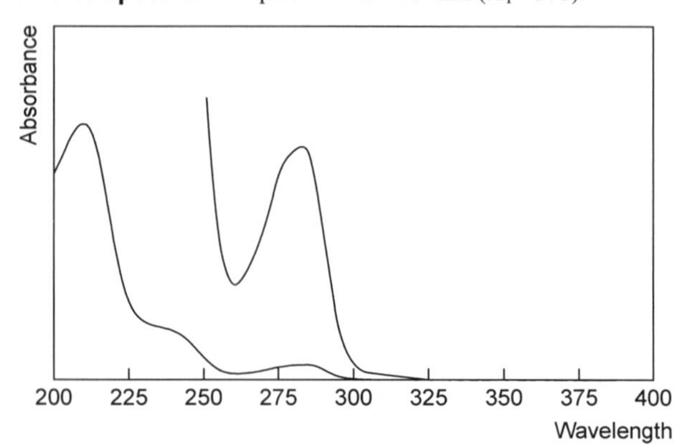

Infra-red Spectrum. Principal peaks at wavenumbers 1233, 1731, 1272, 1042, 1055, 1501 cm^{-1}.

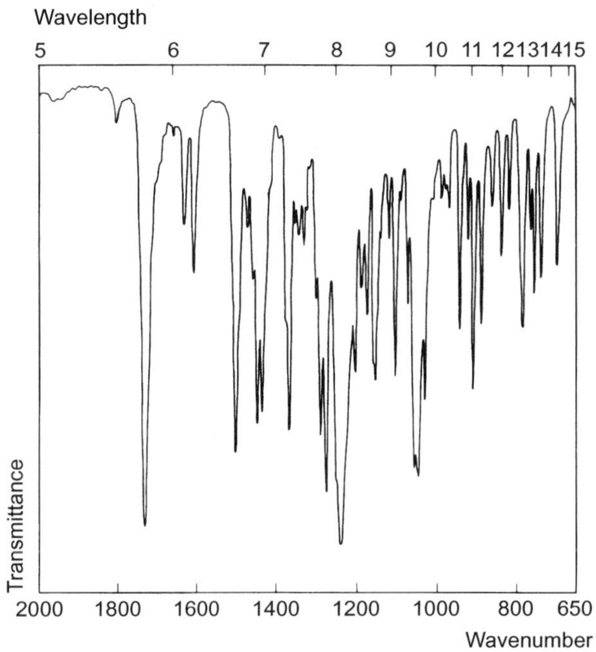

Mass Spectrum. Principal peaks at *m*/*z* 341, 282, 229, 42, 43, 59, 342, 204.

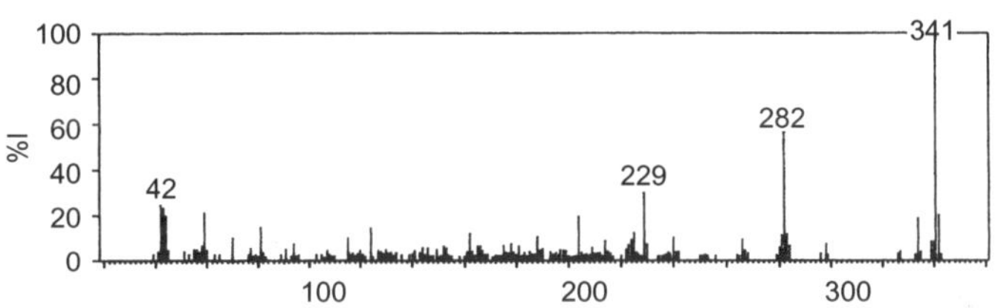

Quantification

Gas chromatography–mass spectrometry. In hair: limit of quantification 0.1 ng/mg—P. Kintz *et al.*, *J. Anal. Toxicol.*, 1998, *22*, 425–429. In hair: —A. Polettini *et al.*, *Forensic Sci. Int.*, 1997, *84*, 259–269. In urine: limit of quantification 0.2 µg/L—R. Brenneisen *et al.*, J. Anal. Toxicol., 2002, *26*, 561–566. In hair—C. Girod and C. Staub, *J. Anal. Toxicol.*, 2001, *25*, 106–111.

High performance liquid chromatography. In illicit diamorphine samples —P. B. Baker and T. A. Gough, *J. Chromatogr. Sci.*, 1981, *19*, 483–489.

Acetylcysteine

Mucolytic/Paracetamol Antidote

Synonyms. *N*-Acetylcysteine; L-α-Acetamido-*β*-mercaptopropionic Acid.
Proprietary names. Airbron; Brunac; Fabrol; Fluimucil; Fluprowit; Mucocedyl; Mucolyticum; Mucolator; Mucomyst; Muco Sanigen; Mucosil; Mucret; Neo-Flumucil; Nac; Parvolex; Tixair.
N-Acetyl-L-cysteine
$C_5H_9NO_3S$=163.2
CAS—616-91-1

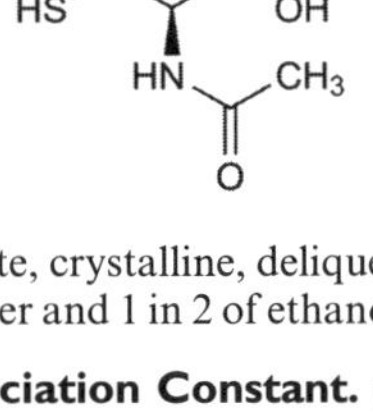

A white, crystalline, deliquescent powder. M.p. 104° to 110°. Soluble 1 in 8 of water and 1 in 2 of ethanol; practically insoluble in chloroform and ether.

Dissociation Constant. pK_a 9.5 (30°).

Thin-layer Chromatography. System TE—Rf 00; system TF—Rf 00; system TAJ—Rf 00; system TAK—Rf 10; system TAL—Rf 26.

Gas Chromatography. System GA—RI 1547.

High Performance Liquid Chromatography. System HX—RI 149; system HY—RI 176; system HZ—Retention time(s) 1.6 min.

Ultraviolet Spectrum. No significant absorption, 230 to 360 nm.

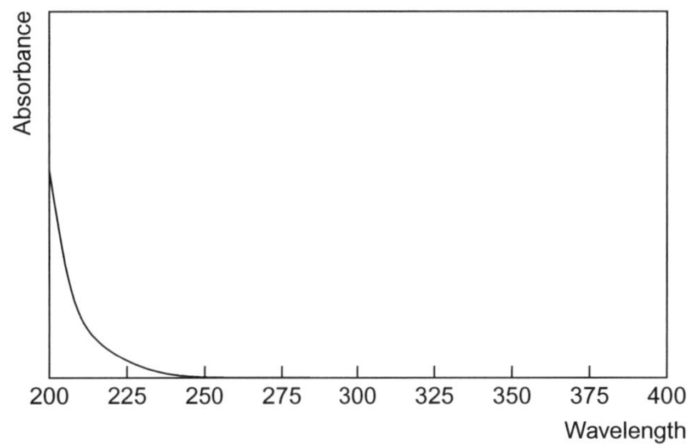

Infra-red Spectrum. Principal peaks at wavenumbers 1530, 1300, 1230, 1275, 1580, 1715 cm^{-1} (Nujol mull).

Quantification

High performance liquid chromatography. In plasma: limit of detection *N*-acetylcysteine 0.17 µg/L and cysteine 0.35 µg/L, UV detection (λ=333 nm)—D. Tsikas *et al.*, *J. Chromatogr. B, Biomed. Sci. Appl.*, 1998, *708*, 55–60. In plasma or urine: limit of detection 50 µg/L, UV detection—P. A. Lewis *et al.*, *J. Pharm. Sci.*, 1984, *73*, 996–998.

Disposition in the Body. Acetylcysteine is readily absorbed after oral administration, peak plasma concentrations being attained in 2 to 3 h; concentrations in the lung are similar to those in plasma. About 20% of a dose is excreted in the urine in 24 h. Acetylcysteine is primarily metabolised to cysteine.

Therapeutic concentration

5 healthy male and female subjects with a mean age of 28.8 years were fasted overnight for 12 h and administered 600 mg Acetylcysteine orally. Acetylcysteine was observed in plasma at a mean concentration of 4.6 µg/L after 60 min and 2.5 µg/L after 90 min. Cysteine was observed at a mean maximum concentration of 18.6 µg/L. [D. Tsikas *et al.*, *J. Chromatogr. B, Biomed. Sci. Appl.*, 1998, *708*, 55–60].

9 patients with cirrhosis, mean age 51.1 years (40 to 74 years), male and female, and 6 healthy subjects with mean age 39.8 years (28 to 61 years) were administered 600 mg acetylcysteine intravenously over 3 min. After 30 min, the peak plasma concentration was 60 mg/L for both groups and after 10 h, the plasma concentration was 4.5 mg/L for the patients and 1.5 mg/L for the healthy subjects. [A. L. Jones *et al.*, *Aliment. Pharmacol. Ther.*, 1997, *11(4)*, 787–791].

Half-life. 2.6 h (healthy subjects); 4.9 h (patients with cirrhosis).

Volume of distribution. 25.5 L (healthy subjects); 17.4 L (patients with cirrhosis).

Clearance. Body, 6.5 L/h (healthy subjects); 4.5 L/h (patients with cirrhosis).

Protein binding. In plasma, about 78%.

Note. D. Rodenstein *et al.*, *Clin. Pharmacokinet.*, 1978, *3*, 247–254.

Dose. As a mucolytic, 600 mg daily by mouth. In the treatment of paracetamol overdosage, initially 150 mg/kg by rapid intravenous infusion.

Acetyldigitoxin

Cardiac Glycoside

Synonyms. Acetyldigitoxoside; β-Digitoxin monoacetate.
Proprietary name. Acylanid(e)
3β-[(*O*–3-*O*-Acetyl-2,6-dideoxy-β-D-*ribo*-hexopyranosyl-(1→4)-*O*-2,6-dideoxy-β-D-*ribo*-hexopyranosyl(1→4)-2,6-dideoxy-β-D-*ribo*-hexopyranosyl)oxy]-14-hydroxy-5β,14β-card-20(22)-enolide

$C_{43}H_{66}O_{14}$=807.0
CAS—1111-393

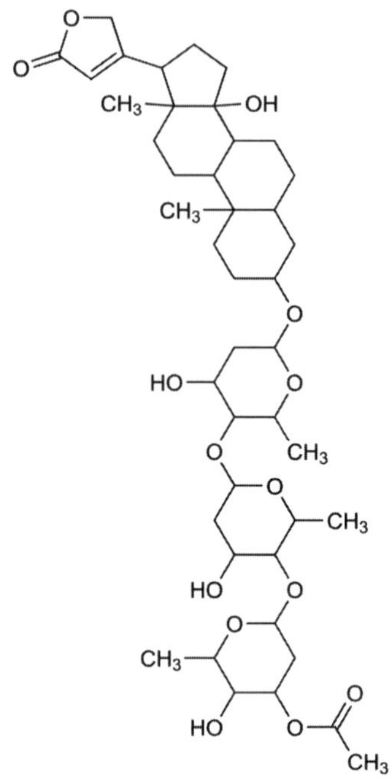

A white hygroscopic crystalline powder. M.p. 217° to 221°. Soluble 1 in 6100 of water, 1 in 63 of ethanol, and 1 in 12 of chloroform; practically insoluble in ether and light petroleum; soluble in methanol.

Ultraviolet Spectrum. No significant absorption, 230 to 360 nm.

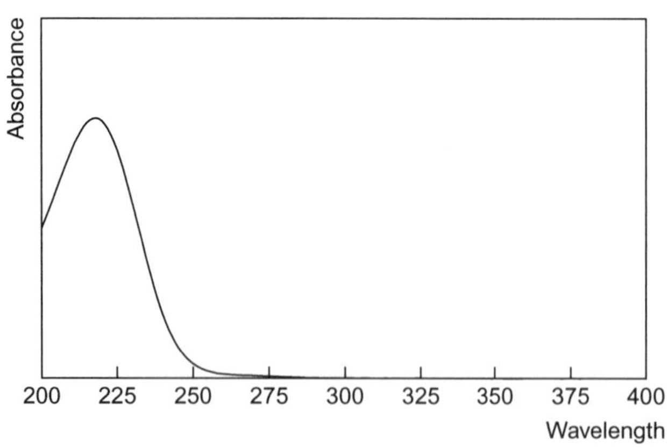

Quantification
High performance liquid chromatography. In plasma: limit of detection 0.15 µg/L. MS detection—A. Tracqui *et al.*, *J. Chromatogr. B Biomed. Sci. Appl.*, 1997, *692*, 101–109.

Disposition in the Body. About 65% of a dose is absorbed after oral administration. It is slowly excreted in the urine, about 20% of a dose being excreted in 6 days; digitoxin accounts for about 60% of the urinary material. About 15 to 20% of a dose is eliminated in the faeces over a period of 18 days.

Half-life. Plasma half-life, about 8 to 9 days.

Protein binding. In plasma, about 80%.

Dose. Maintenance, 100 to 200 µg daily.

Aciclovir

Antiviral

Synonyms. Acycloguanosine; Acyclovir; BW-248U.
Proprietary names. Aciviran; Activir; Acyvir; Alovir; Avirase; Avyclor; Clovix; Cusiviral; Cycloviran; Dravyr; Efriviral; Esavir; Geavir; Maynar; Milavir; Neviran; Rexan; Sifiviral; Viclovir; Vipral; Virherpes; Virmen; Zovir; Zovirax; Zyclir.
2-Amino-1,9-dihydro-9-(2-hydroxyethoxymethyl)-6*H*-purin-6-one
$C_8H_{11}N_5O_3$=225.2
CAS—59277-89-3

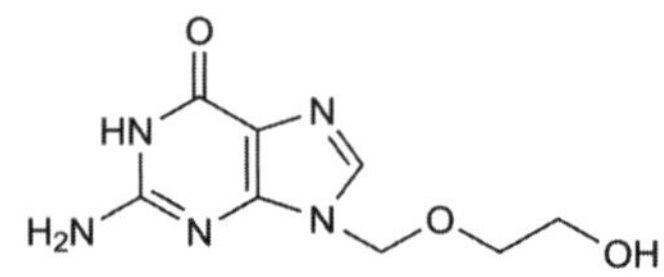

A white to almost white crystalline powder. M.p. 255°, with decomposition. It is sparingly to slightly soluble in water; practically insoluble or very slightly soluble in ethanol; dissolves in dilute solutions of mineral acids and alkali hydroxides; and is freely soluble in dimethyl sulfoxide.

Aciclovir Sodium

Proprietary names. Cusiviral; Geavir; Herpotern; Maynar; Viclovir; Virherpes; Virmen; Zovirax; Zyclir.
$C_8H_{10}N_5NaO_3$=247.2
CAS—69657-51-8
A white crystalline powder. It is soluble 1 in 10 of water.

Dissociation Constant. pK_a 2.3, 9.2.

Partition Coefficient. Log *P* (octanol/water), −1.56.

High Performance Liquid Chromatography. System HAA—retention time 3.1 min.

Column: (analytical) LiChrosorb RP-8 (250 × 4 mm i.d., 7 µm); (guard) Perisorb RP-18 (30–40 µm, pellicular). Mobile phase: 1% acetonitrile in 0.02 M disodium hydrogen orthophosphate, adjusted to pH 2.5 with 60–62% perchloric acid, 1.2 mL/min flow rate. Fluorescence detection (λ_{ex}=270 nm, λ_{em}=380 nm). Retention time: 9.6 min. [K.-K. Peh and K.-H. Yuen, *J. Chromatogr. Biomed. Sci. Appl.*, 1997, *693*, 241–244].

Column: ODS R-P (Ultrasphere, 75 × 4.6 mm, 3 µm). Mobile phase: 30 mM phosphate buffer, pH 2.1 containing 5 mM dodecyl sulfate and 18% acetonitrile, 1.5 mL/min flow rate. Fluorescence detection (λ_{ex}=285 nm, λ_{em}=380 nm). Retention time: aciclovir, 1.7 min; 9-carboxy-methoxymethylguanine, 1.5 min. [J.-O. Svensson *et al.*, *J. Chromatogr. Biomed. Sci. Appl.*, 1997, *690*, 363–366].

Column: C_8 (Symmetry, 150 × 4.6 mm, 5 µm) with 1 cm pre-column (same material). Mobile phase: acetate citrate buffer (0.1 M) containing 3.7 mM octane sulfonic acid:methanol (92:8), adjusted to pH 3.0 with 14.8 M orthophosphoric acid, 1 mL/min flow rate. UV detection (λ=250 nm). Retention time: 5.3 min. [J-M. Poirier *et al.*, *Ther. Drug Monit.*, 1999, *21*, 129-133].

Column: (analytical) RP-8 (SymmetryShield, 6 mm i.d., 5 µm); (guard) RP-8 (20 × 3.9 mm). Mobile phase: acetonitrile:monoammonium phosphate buffer (0.025 M) adjusted to pH 4.0 with 10% diluted phosphoric acid (2:98), 1.0 mL/min flow rate. UV detection. Retention time: 9.7 min. [C. Pham-Huy *et al.*, *J. Chromatogr. Biomed. Sci. Appl.*, 1999, *732*, 47–3].

Ultraviolet Spectrum. Aqueous acid (0.2 M H_2SO_4)—255 nm: basic—261 nm.

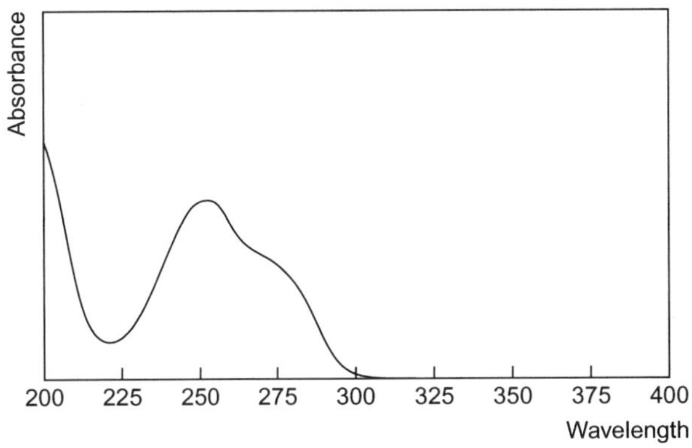

Infra-red Spectrum. Principal peaks at wavenumber 1717, 1632, 1485, 1104 cm^{-1}.

Mass Spectrum. Principal peaks at *m/z* 151, 164, 45, 43, 165, 109, 110, 108.

Quantification

High performance liquid chromatography. In serum: limit of detection 50 µg/L, UV detection—P. Nebinger and M. Koel, *J. Chromatogr.*, 1993, *619*; *Biomed. Appl.*, *130*, 342–344. In plasma: limit of detection, 10 µg/L, UV detection—K. J. Swart *et al.*, *J. Chromatogr. A*, 1994, *663*, 65–69. In plasma: limit of detection 30 µg/L, fluorescence detection (λ_{ex}=270 nm, λ_{em}=380 nm)—K.-K. Peh and K.-H. Yuen, *J. Chromatogr. Biomed. Sci. Appl.*, 1997, *693*, 241–244. In plasma or urine: limit of detection 0.12 µg/L and 0.60 µg/L, respectively, fluorescence detection (λ_{ex}=285 nm, λ_{em}=380 nm)—J.-O. Svensson *et al.*, *J. Chromatogr. Biomed. Sci. Appl.*, 1997, *690*, 363–366. In serum: limit of detection 50 g/L and limit of quantification 200 µg/L, UV detection—C. Pham-Huy *et al.*, *J. Chromatogr. Biomed. Sci. Appl.*, 1999, *732*, 47–53. In plasma: limit of detection 62.5 µg/L. UV detection (λ=250 nm)—J-M. Poirier *et al.*, *Ther. Drug Monit.*, 1999, *21*, 129–133.

Enzyme-linked immunosorbent assay. In plasma or urine: limit of detection 0.2 ng/L—S. M. Tadepalli *et al.*, *Antimicrob. Agents Chemother.*, 1986, *29*, 93–98.

Disposition in the Body. Aciclovir is poorly absorbed after oral administration. Peak plasma concentrations occur about 1.5 to 2.5 h after administration. It is excreted mostly unchanged through the kidney both by glomerular filtration and tubular secretion. 30 to 70% of an administered dose can be detected in urine. About 14% is excreted as the inactive metabolite 9-carboxymethoxymethylguanine (the main metabolite), and also 8-hydroxy-9-(2-hydroxyethoxymethyl)guanine has been detected (<0.2% of the dose). Faecal excretion accounts for about 2% of a dose. It is widely distributed into various tissues, including CSF where concentrations reach about 50% those of plasma. It crosses the placenta and is distributed into breast milk. Aciclovir is removed by haemodialysis but not by peritoneal dialysis.

Therapeutic concentration. The trough serum therapeutic concentration range is 0.5 to 1.5 mg/L and the peak, 5 to 15 mg/L.

Single dose and multiple dosing studies were carried out on adult volunteers aged 45 to 60 years old. Single dose studies involved administering intravenous doses of 0.5, 1.0, 2.5, 5.0, 10.0 and 15.0 mg/kg over a 1 h infusion period and mean peak plasma concentrations were 1.0, 2.1, 4.2, 8.8, 14.6 and 22.7 mg/L, respectively. All concentrations were observed by the end of infusion. The mean peak and trough plasma concentrations measured after administration of 2.5 mg/kg intravenously over 1 h every 8 h were 5.1 and 0.5 mg/L, respectively. Following doses of 5.0, 10.0, and 15.0 mg/kg administered similarly, the mean peak and trough concentrations were: 9.8 and 0.7, 20.7 and 2.3, 23.6 and 2.0 mg/L, respectively. A study was also carried out on children, from birth up to 17 years old, and they were administered with a 250 or 500 mg/m^2 dose. The mean peak concentrations were 4 to 18 mg/L and 14 to 30 mg/L, respectively. [M. R. Blum *et al.*, *Am. J. Med.*, 1982, *73*, *Suppl. 1A*, 186–192].

Bioavailability. Oral bioavailability, 20%.

Toxicity. Nephrotoxicity may occur occasionally. The risk may be increased if large doses are given or if it is administered very rapidly or as a bolus. Neurotoxicity may also occur. Patients have ingested up to 20 g with no unexpected effects. If the solubility of aciclovir in intratubular fluid is exceeded (2.5 g/L), aciclovir may precipitate in the renal tubules and therefore urine flow must be maintained in cases of overdosage.

Severe neurological impairment and nonoliguric renal failure developed in a 68-year-old man a week after starting treatment with aciclovir 600 mg four times daily by mouth. On presentation the blood-aciclovir concentration was 18 mg/L. Intravascular volume depletion secondary to profuse diarrhoea and a history of chronic renal failure were contributory factors. Symptoms resolved on discontinuation of aciclovir and haemodialysis. [J. Bradley *et al.*, *Chest*, 1997, *112*, 538–540].

7 of 8 subjects treated with high-dose aciclovir (400 to 1200 mg/m^2/day) by intravenous infusion for cytomegalovirus pneumonia following bone-marrow transplant died. Plasma-aciclovir concentrations at autopsy for 4 of the subjects were 0.018 to 0.2 mg/L. The following corresponding concentrations in various organs were reported: lung 0.023 to 0.28 mg/L, heart 0.027 to 0.25 mg/L, liver 0.022 to 0.31 mg/L, renal medulla 0.16 to 2.68 mg/L, renal cortex 0.13 to 2.62 mg/L, brain 0.142 mg/L, spinal cord 0.0063 to 0.118 mg/L. [A. Wade *et al.*, *Am. J. Med.*, 1982, *73*, *Suppl. 1A*, 249–255].

Half-life. Plasma, 2 to 3 h.

Volume of distribution. 4L to 55 L/1.73 m^2.

Clearance. Plasma, 327 mL/min/1.73 m^2.

Protein binding. In plasma, 9 to 33%.

Dose. Up to 30 mg/kg body weight daily intravenously; up to 4 g daily by mouth.

Acitretin

Dermatological

Synonyms. Etretin; Ro-10-1670.
Proprietary names. Neotigason; Soriatane.
(2*E*,4*E*,6*E*,8*E*)-9-(4-Methoxy-2,3,6-trimethylphenyl)-3,7-dimethyl-nona-2,4,6,8-tetraenoic acid
$C_{21}H_{26}O_3$=326.4
CAS—55079-83-9

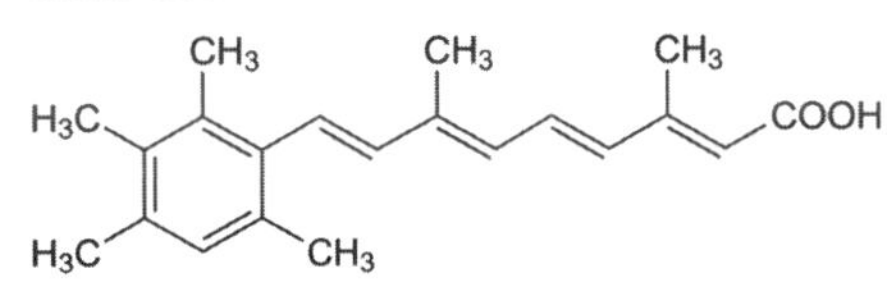

A yellow to greenish-yellow powder. M.p. 228° to 230°. Protect from light.

Dissociation Constant. pK_a 3.7.

Partition Coefficient. Log *P* (octanol/water), 6.4.

Thin-layer Chromatography. System TE—Rf 4; system TF—Rf 43.

High Performance Liquid Chromatography. Column: RP C_{18} (Nucleosil, 250 × 4.2 mm i.d., 5 µm). Mobile phase: methanol–acetonitrile (7:3):purified water with 1.5% acetate acid (85:15), 1.2 mL/min flow rate. UV detection (λ=350 nm). Retention times: 13-*cis*-acitretin, 6.0 min; all-*trans*-acitretin, 6.9 min—J. P. Laugier *et al.*, *J. Pharm. Sci.*, 1994, *83(5)*, 623–628].

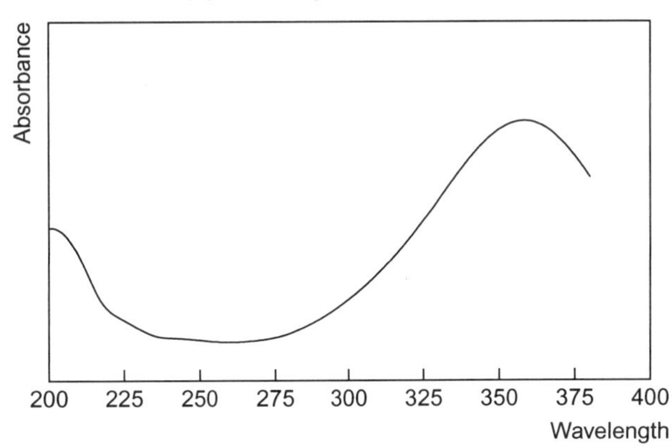

Mass Spectrum. Principal peaks at *m/z* 150, 326, 163, 203, 251, 281, 41, 311.

Quantification

High performance liquid chromatography. In plasma or subcutaneous tissue: limit of detection 0.1 μg/L and 8 ng/g (50 mg tissue sample), respectively—M. C. Sturkenboom *et al.*, *Br. J. Clin. Pharmacol.* 1994, *38*, 229–235. In plasma: acitretin and metabolites, limit of detection 0.1 μg/L, UV detection ($\lambda=360$ nm)—R. Wyss and F. Bucheli, *J. Chromatogr.*, 1988, *431*, 297–307. In plasma: acitretin and metabolites, limit of detection 3 μg/L, UV detection—A. P. De Leenheer *et al.*, *J. Chromatogr.* 1990, *500*, 637–642. In plasma: acitretin and metabolites, limit of quantification 0.3 μg/L, UV detection ($\lambda=360$ nm)—R. Wyss and F. Bucheli, *J. Chromatogr.*, 1992, *593*, 55–62. In blood, plasma, or urine: limit of detection 2 μg/L (plasma) —N. R. Al-Mallah *et al.*, *J. Chromatogr.*, 1987, *421*; *Biomed. Appl.*, *65*, 177–186. In plasma: acitretin and metabolites, limit of detection 1 μg/L, UV detection—P. Jakobsen *et al.*, *J. Chromatogr.*, 1987, *415*; *Biomed. Appl.*, *59*, 413–418. In skin, suction blister or plasma: limit of detection 1 ng/g, UV detection ($\lambda=350$ nm)—J. P. Laugier *et al.*, *J. Pharm. Sci.*, 1994, *83*, 623–628. In plasma: limit of detection 2 μg/L, UV detection—J. Klein *et al.*, *Ther. Drug Monit.*, 1992, *14*, 197–202.

Disposition in the Body. Acitretin is absorbed after oral administration and peak plasma concentrations occur after about 1 to 6 h. Administration with food increases bioavailability. The drug is widely distributed in the body. It undergoes extensive metabolism and interconversion by simple isomerisation to 13-*cis*-acitretin. Both acitretin and 13-*cis*-acitretin may be conjugated. An additional three metabolites have been identified. Etretinate has been detected following administration of acitretin; this may be a route of metabolism if there is concomitant alcohol consumption. It is excreted in urine and bile. Neither acitretin nor its 13-*cis* metabolite are removed by dialysis.

Therapeutic concentration

Following administration of a single dose of acitretin (40 mg) to 6 subjects, aged between 23 and 76 years (mean, 52), with psoriasis, peak plasma concentrations of 98 to 526 μg/L (mean, 241 μg/L) occurred after 0.6 to 3.0 h. The dose was administered after an overnight fast. [F. G. Larsen *et al.*, *Pharmacol. Toxicol.*, 1987, *61*, 85–88].

Following administration of 50 mg acitretin to 18 healthy male subjects (18 to 40 years old) with or without food, peak plasma concentrations of 87 to 480 μg/L and 196 to 728 μg/L were measured, respectively. A mean concentration of 245 and 416 μg/L was observed for the doses administered with food and without, respectively. Peak concentrations were reached between 2 and 5 h. [P. J. McNamara *et al.*, *J. Clin. Pharmacol.*, 1988, *28*, 1051–1055].

Peak plasma concentrations of 229 to 408 μg/L occurred after 1.0 to 2.8 h in 4 subjects who were administered with 40 mg acitretin daily for 3 months. This dose was ingested after an overnight fast followed by a 3 h additional fast post-administration. The individuals used in the study were aged 23 to 59 years (mean, 55) and suffered from severe psoriasis (healthy otherwise). [F. G. Larsen *et al.*, *Pharmacol. Toxicol.*, 1988, *62*, 159–165].

Toxicity. Acitretin is teratogenic. Although acitretin has a relatively short half-life, etretinate has also been detected in the plasma of some patients taking acitretin and since etretinate is also teratogenic and has a much longer half-life than acitretin, pregnancy must be avoided for at least 3 years after stopping acitretin therapy. Plasma concentrations may be a poor guide to presence of etretinate in the body since etretinate concentrates in fatty tissues. The minimum plasma concentrations associated with teratogenicity are unknown.

In a woman who had taken a cumulative dose of acitretin of 9900 mg and who had stopped taking acitretin 52 months previously, concentrations of etretinate of 0.30 μg/L and 128.5 ng/g were found in plasma and subcutaneous fat, respectively. Another woman who was still taking acitretin (cumulative dose, 1075 mg) had plasma and fat concentrations of etretinate of 0.48 μg/L and 18.7 ng/g, respectively. [H. Maier and H. Hönigsmann, *Lancet*, 1996, *348*, 1107].

Bioavailability. Approximately, 60%.

Half-life. Plasma, acitretin, 50 h; 13-*cis*-acitretin, 63 h.

Volume of distribution. 2.3 to 4.5 L/kg; mean, 3.47 L/kg.

Clearance. Plasma, 175.9 ± 81.4 mL/kg/h.

Protein binding. In plasma, >99.9%.

Note. For general references, see C. K. Brindley, *Dermatologica*, 1989, *178*, 79–87 and T. Pilkington and R. N. Brogden, *Drugs*, 1992, *43*, 597–627.

Dose. Usually 25 to 50 mg daily.

Aclarubicin

Antineoplastic

Synonym. Aclacinomycin A

[1*R*-(1α,2β,4β)]-2-Ethyl-1,2,3,4,6,11-hexahydro-2,5,7-trihydroxy-6,11-dioxo-4-[[2,3,6-trideoxy-4-*O*-[2,6-dideoxy-4-*O*-[(2*R*-*trans*)-tetrahydro-6-methyl-5-oxo-2*H*-pyran-2-yl]-α-L-*lyxo*-hexopyranosyl]-3-(dimethylamino)-α-L-*lyxo*-hexopyranosyl]oxy]-1-naphthacenecarboxylic acid methyl ester

$C_{42}H_{53}NO_{15}=811.8$

CAS—57576-44-0

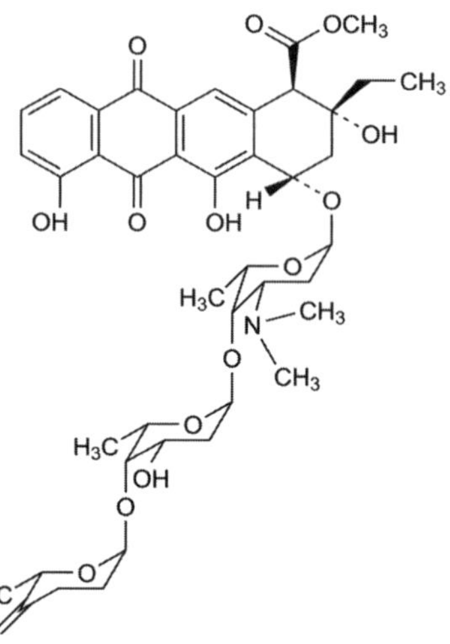

It is soluble in chloroform and in ethyl acetate; insoluble in ether, in *n*-hexane and in light petroleum.

Aclarubicin Hydrochloride

Proprietary names. Aclacin; Aclacinomycine; Aclaplastin.

$C_{42}H_{53}NO_{15}$,HCl=848.3

High Performance Liquid Chromatography. Column: C_{18} (μBondapak, 300 × 4 mm i.d., 10 μm). Mobile phase: acetonitrile:methanol:water (40:90:70) acidified with orthophosphoric acid 85% (1.5 mL per 100 ml), 2 mL/min flow rate. UV detection ($\lambda=254$ nm). Retention time: 5.9 min. [R. Erttmann, *J. Chromatogr.*, 1983, *277*; *Biomed. Appl.*, *28*, 433–435].

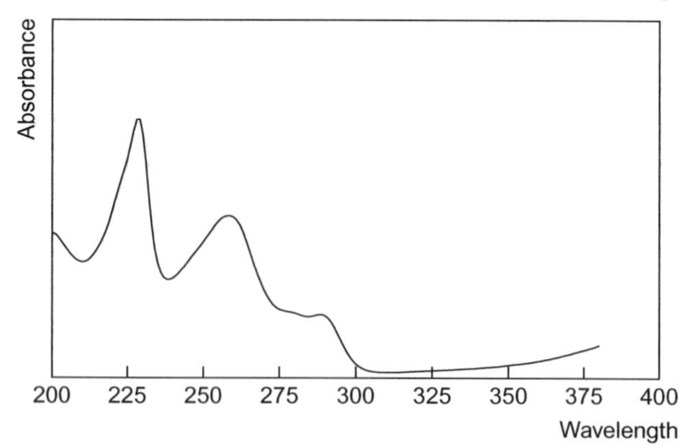

Mass Spectrum. Principal peaks at *m/z* 113, 100, 71, 43, 73, 81, 96, 376.

Quantification

High performance liquid chromatography. In serum: limit of detection 10.8 μg/L, UV detection ($\lambda=254$ nm)—R. Erttmann, *J. Chromatogr.*, 1983, *277*; *Biomed. Appl.*, *28*, 433–435.

Disposition in the Body. Aclarubicin is rapidly distributed following intravenous administration. It is rapidly and highly metabolised to biologically active glycosides and inactive aglycones. The metabolites are excreted mainly in urine, and small amounts may be excreted in faeces.

Therapeutic concentration. The mean peak concentration of the principal active metabolite is 130 μg/L and occurs at a mean time of 191 min after dosing.

Half-life. Plasma, aclarubicin, 3 h; principal metabolite, 13 h.

Clearance. Plasma, 1.6 to 8.8 L/min/m^2.

Volume of distribution. Apparent volume of distribution is 600 to 1900 L/m^2.

Dose. 25 to 100 mg/m^2 as a single infusion every 3 to 4 weeks (maintenance therapy). Usual maximum total dose is 400 mg/m^2.

Aconitine

Alkaloid

Synonym. Acetylbenzoylaconine
(1α,3α,6α,14α,15α,16β)-20-Ethyl-1,6,16-trimethoxy-4-(methoxymethyl)aconitane-3,8,13,14,15-pentol 8-acetate 14-benzoate
$C_{34}H_{47}NO_{11}$=645.7
CAS—302-27-2

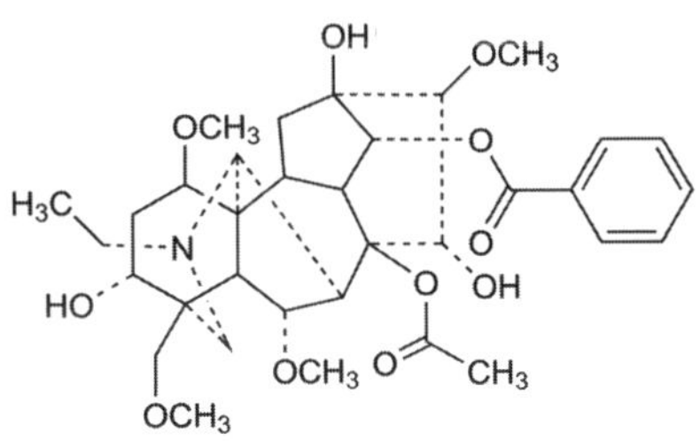

An alkaloid present in species of *Aconitum*, including *A. napellus* agg. (Ranunculaceae).
Colourless crystals or white crystalline powder. M.p. 204°, with decomposition.
Solubility (g/mL): 1 in 3300 of water, 1 in 28 abs. alcohol, 1 in 2 of chloroform, 1 in 50 of ether, and 1 in 7 benzene; slightly soluble in petroleum ether.

Aconitine Nitrate

Proprietary names. Aconitysat; Bromofotyl; Herbadon.
$C_{34}H_{47}NO_{11},HNO_3$=708.8
CAS—6509-18-8
Colourless crystals or white crystalline powder. M.p. about 200°, with decomposition.
Soluble 1 in 10 in boiling water; less soluble in cold water; soluble in alcohol.

Dissociation Constant. pK_a 8.1 (25°).

Partition Coefficient. Log *P* (octanol/water), 0.13.

Thin-layer Chromatography. System TA—Rf 68; system TB—Rf 11; system TC—Rf 39; system TE—Rf 75; system TL—Rf 58; system TAE—Rf 42; system TAF—Rf 68; system TAJ—Rf 06; system TAK—Rf 00; system TAL—Rf 24. (Acidified iodoplatinate solution, positive.)

Gas Chromatography. System GA—not eluted.

Column: Fused silica cross-linked with 5% phenylsilicone (15 m × 0.25 mm i.d.). Injector and transfer line temperature: 320°. Column temperature: 250° for 1 min, to 320° at 16°/min. Carrier gas: helium, flow rate 25 cm/s. Detection: MS (SIM mode). [M. Mizugaki *et al.*, *Planta. Med.*, 1997, *63(1)*, 75–79.]

High Performance Liquid Chomatography. System HX—RI 432.

Column: L-column ODS (150 × 4.6 mm i.d.) at 40°. Mobile phase: tetrahydrofuran:trifluoroacetic acid (0.2%) (14:86), flow rate 1 mL/min. UV detection (λ = 235 nm). [H. Ohta *et al.*, *J. Chromatogr. B Biomed. Sci. Appl.*, 1995, *669*, 408–412.]

Ultraviolet Spectrum. Aqueous acid—234 (A_1^1=233a), 275 nm.

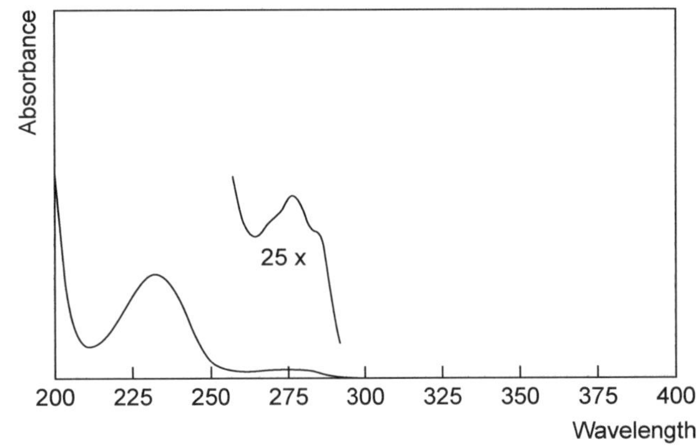

Infra-red Spectrum. Principal peaks at wavenumbers 1092, 1273, 1713, 1235, 710, 1020 cm^{-1} (KBr disk).

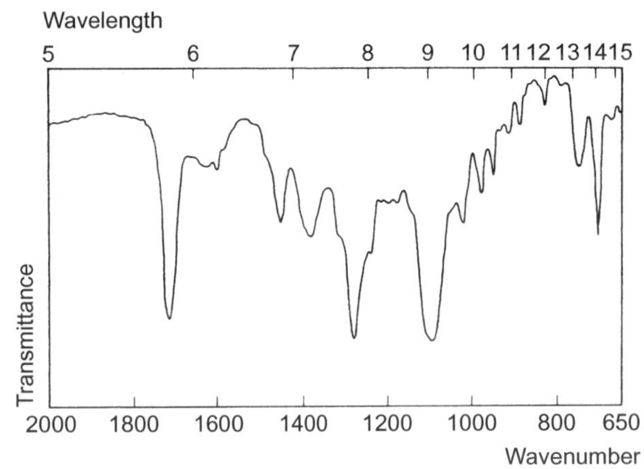

Mass Spectrum. Principal ions at *m/z* 105, 554, 540, 43, 45, 77, 31, 29.

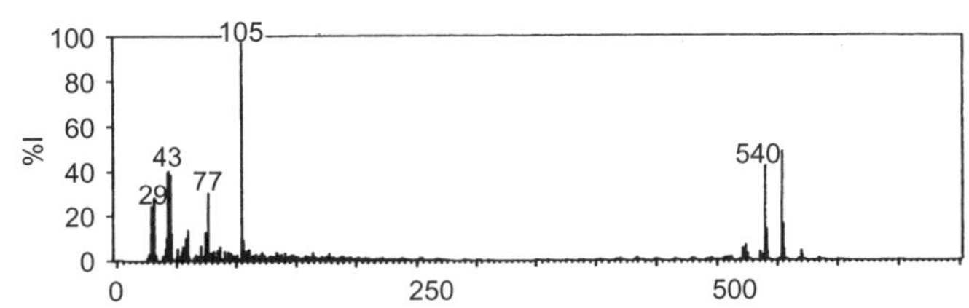

Quantification

Gas chromatography–mass spectrometry. In serum: limit of detection 10 pg—K. Ito *et al.*, *Planta. Med.*, 1997, *63*, 75–79. In body fluids: aconitine and mesaconitine, limit of detection 10 pg, SIM—K. Ito *et al.*, *J. Chromatogr. B Biomed. Sci. Appl.*, 1998, *714*, 197–203.

High Performance Liquid Chromatography. In blood: limit of detection 50 μg/L—H. Ohta *et al.*, *J. Chromatogr.* 1995, *669*, *B Biomed. Sci. Appl.*, 408–412. In blood or urine: aconitine and other aconite alkaloids, limit of detection 1 ng, UV detection—H. Ohta *et al.*, *J. Chromatogr. B Biomed. Sci. Appl.*, 1997, *691*, 351–356.

High performance liquid chromatography–mass spectrometry. In blood and urine: 1 μg/L and 0.5 μg/L, respectively—H. Ohta *et al.*, *J. Chromatogr. B Biomed. Sci. Appl.*, 1998, *714*, 215–221.

Disposition in the Body

Toxicity. Aconitine affects both the heart and the CNS and is one of the most potent and quick-acting poisons. It is well absorbed from the gastro-intestinal tract and death may occur within a few minutes. The estimated minimum lethal dose is 2 mg of aconitine, 5 mL of aconite tincture (25%v/v), or 1 g of aconite root, although recovery after ingestion of 10 mg of aconitine has been reported.

In a fatality resulting from the deliberate ingestion of *Aconitum napellus* extract, the following postmortem tissue concentrations of aconitine were reported: femoral blood 10.8 μg/L, urine 264< μg/L. The antemortem concentrations were 6 μg/L in the serum (estimate) and 334 μg/L in the urine. [S. P. Elliott, *Sci. Justice*, 2002, *42*, 111–115.]

A 61-year-old man developed nausea and diarrhoea 2 h after ingesting aconite, mistaken for edible grass. Resuscitation and antiarrhythmic drugs did not work. Ventricular tachycardia and fibrillation developed and lasted for 6 h. The man fell into a coma and died of brain oedema on the sixth day. No aconitine was detected in serum after 24 h. Urine was tested after 9, 13, and 18 h and aconitine levels were 14.9, 20.2, and 2.8 μg/L respectively. [N. Yoshioka *et al.*, *Forensic Sci. Int.*, 1996, *81(2–3)*, 117–123.]

Acriflavinium Chloride

Antiseptic

Synonyms. Acid trypaflavine; Acriflavinium chloride hydrochloride.
Proprietary names. Diacrid; Panflavin.
A mixture of 3,6-diamino-10-methylacridinium chloride hydrochloride and 3,6-diaminoacridine dihydrochloride, the latter being present to the extent of approximately one-third.
$C_{14}H_{14}ClN_3,HCl$=296.2; $C_{13}H_{11}N_3,2HCl$=282.2
CAS—8063-24-9

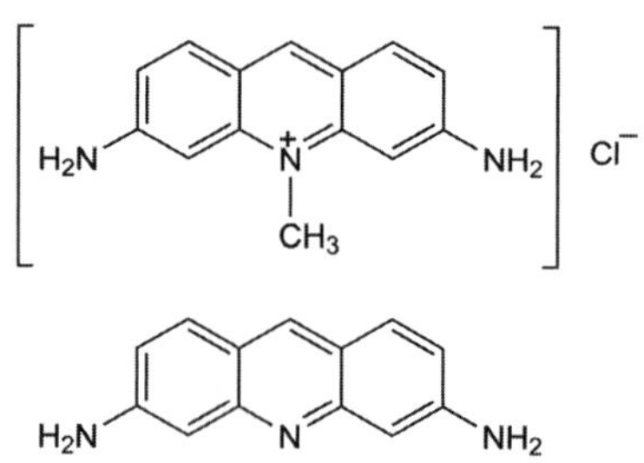

An orange-red to red crystalline powder. A precipitate may form in aqueous solutions on dilution or on standing. Soluble 1 in about 3 of water and 1 in 40 of ethanol; practically insoluble in chloroform and ether.

Dissociation Constant. pK_a 9.1 (25°).

Colour Test. Marquis Test—yellow→red.

Thin-layer Chromatography. System TA—four spots at Rf 07, 22, 28, and 62. (Location under ultraviolet light, yellow-green fluorescence.)

Ultraviolet Spectrum. Aqueous acid—262 nm (A_1^1=1515 a). No alkaline shift.

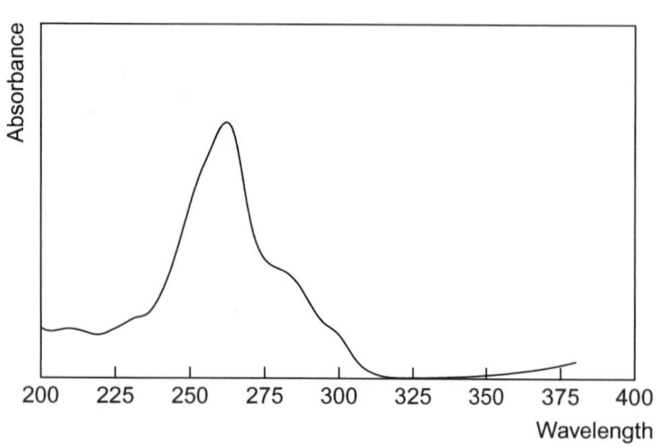

Infra-red Spectrum. Principal peaks at wavenumbers 1631, 1590, 1171, 1181, 1316, 1242 cm^{-1}.

Acrivastine

Antihistamine

Synonyms. BW-270C; BW-825C; BW-A825C.
Proprietary names. Benadryl; Semprex.
(*E*)-3-{6-[(*E*)-3-Pyrrolidin-1-yl-1-*p*-tolylprop-1-enyl]-2-pyridyl}acrylic acid
$C_{22}H_{24}N_2O_2$=348.4
CAS—87848-99-5

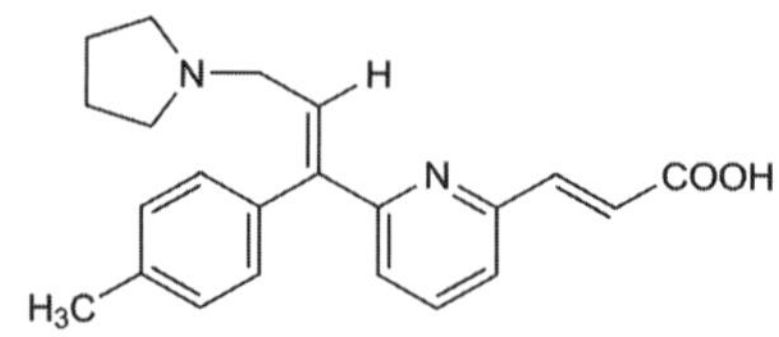

An odourless, white to pale cream crystalline powder. It is slightly soluble in water; soluble in chloroform and ethanol. M.p. 222°.

Partition Coefficient. Log *P* (octanol/water), 2.83.

High Performance Liquid Chromatography. Column: RP-C_{18} (LiChrosorb, 200 × 4.6 mm i.d., 5 μm). Mobile phase: water:acetonitrile: methanol:perchloric acid:*n*-octylamine (500:130:25:13:0.3), 3 mL/min flow rate. UV detection (λ=260 nm). Retention time: 6.6 min. [T. G. Altuntas *et al.*, *J. Pharm. Biomed. Anal.*, 1998, *17*, 103–109].

Mass Spectrum. Principal ions at *m/z* 351, 420, 73, 232, 233, 260, 405, 200 (TMS derivative).

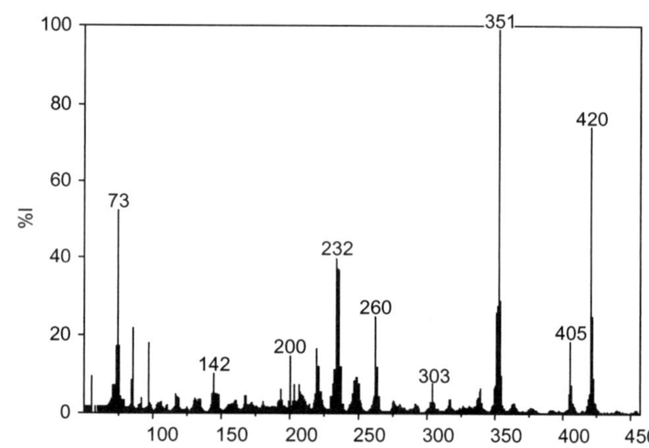

Quantification
Gas chromatography–mass spectrometry. In plasma: acrivastine and propionic acid metabolite, limit of detection about 2 μg/L—S. Y. Chang *et al.*, *J. Chromatogr.*, 1989, *497*; *Biomed. Appl.*, *89*, 288–295.

Disposition in the Body. Acrivastine is well absorbed after oral administration. Peak plasma concentrations are reached in about 1.5 h. It is does not cross the blood–brain barrier to a significant extent. The drug undergoes some metabolism to form a propionic acid analogue that has pharmacological activity and makes up approximately, 10% of the total plasma drug concentration. About 60% of an administered dose is excreted unchanged in urine and 15 to 17% of this is detected as the metabolite.

Therapeutic concentration
A mean peak plasma concentration of 73.1 (range, 48.1 to 101.0) μg/L was obtained 1.42 h (range, 0.75 to 2 h) after oral administration of a single dose of 4 mg to 12 healthy male subjects, aged between 20 and 42 years. [A. F. Cohen *et al.*, *Eur. J. Clin. Pharmacol.*, 1985, *28*, 197–204].

Bioavailability. 18%.

Half-life. Plasma, 1.4 to 2.1 h (acrivastine); 2.3 h (metabolite).

Volume of distribution. 0.64 L/kg (single dose); 0.75 L/kg (multiple).

Clearance. Total body, 4.41 ± 0.63 mL/min/kg.

Protein binding. In plasma, 50%.

Note. For a review of acrivastine see R. N. Brogden and D. McTavish, *Drugs*, 1991, *41*, 927–940 (correction R. N. Brogden and D. McTavish, *Drugs*, 1991, *42*, 639).

Dose. 8 mg three times daily (in Europe and UK) or four times daily (USA).

Adenosine

Anti-arrhythmic

Synonyms. Adenine nucleoside; adenine riboside.
Proprietary names. Adenocard; Adenocor; Adenoscan; Adenosin; Adrekar; Krenosin.
6-Amino-9-β-D-ribofuranosyl-9*H*-purine
$C_{10}H_{13}N_5O_4$=267.2
CAS—58-61-7

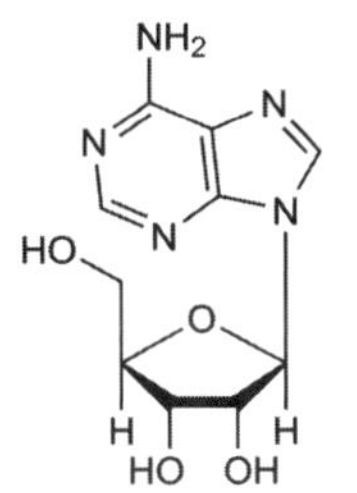

Adenosine is a white crystalline powder. M.p. 234°. Melts with decomposition >300°. Adenosine is soluble in water (approx. 8 g/L) and practically insoluble in alcohol.

Adenosine Triphosphate

Synonyms. Adenosine 5′-triphosphate; 5′-adenyldiphosphoric acid; adenylpyrophosphoric acid; ATP; adenosine 5′-(tetrahydrogen triphosphate).
Proprietary names. Atepadene; Atepodin; Bio-Regenerat; Striadyne.
$C_{10}H_{16}N_5O_{13}P_3$=507.2
CAS—56-65-5

Dissociation Constant. pK_a 3.5.

Partition Coefficient. Log *P* (octanol/water), −1.05.

Thin-layer Chromatography.

Plate: Octadecyl-modified silica treated with copper acetate and (2*S*,4*R*,2′*RS*)-4-hydroxyl-1-(2-hydroxydodecyl)proline (Chiral). Mobile phase: methanol:water:acetonitrile (50:50:50). Rf 0.8. [R. S. Feldburg and L. M. Reppuci, *J. Chromatogr*., 1987, *410*, 226].

Plate: Whatman LK5DF. Mobile phase: IPA:water:ammonia (7:2:1). Rf 0.6.

Plate: Whatman LHPKDF. Mobile phase: IPA:water:ammonia (7:2:1). Rf 0.7.

Plate: Whatman LKC18DF. Mobile phase: IPA:water:DMSO (16:4:1). Rf 0.6.

Plate: Whatman C2. Mobile phase: IPA:water:DMSO (16:4:1). Rf 0.8.

Plate: Whatman SCX. Mobile phase: ammonium hydrogen phosphate (0.1 M) and sodium chloride (1 M). Rf 0.7. [B. P. Sherma *et al*., *Techniques and Application of Thin Layer Chromatography*, John Wiley & Sons, New York, 1982].

Plate: silanised aminopropyl. Mobile phase: methanol:water (46:60), and sodium chloride (0.18 mol/L). Rf 0.8. [H. E. Hauck and W. Jost, *J. Chromatogr*., 1983, *261*, 235].

High Performance Liquid Chromatography. System HAA—retention time 2.7 min.

Ultraviolet Spectrum. Aqueous acid (0.1 M hydrochloric acid), alkali (0.1 M sodium hydroxide) and water—209, 259 nm.

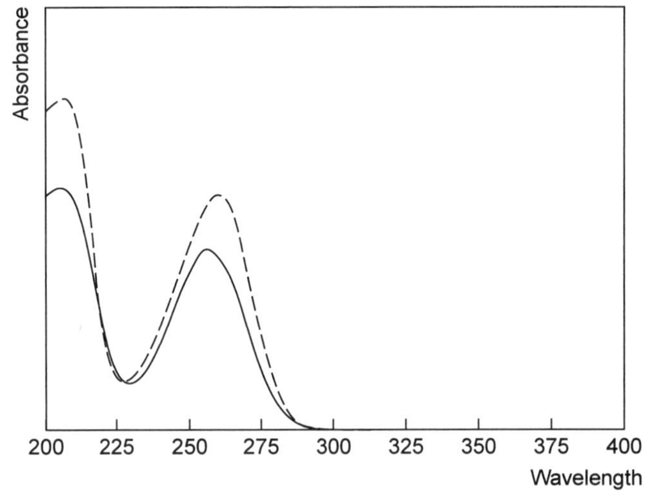

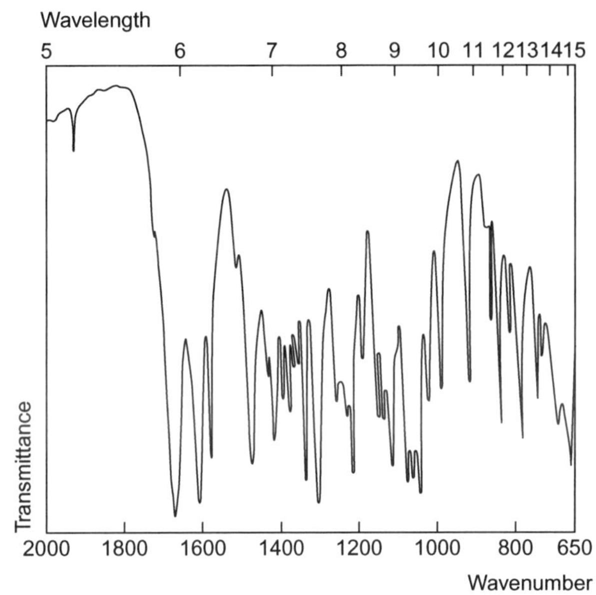

Mass Spectrum. Principal peaks at *m*/*z* 135, 136, 164, 29, 31, 108, 178, 237.

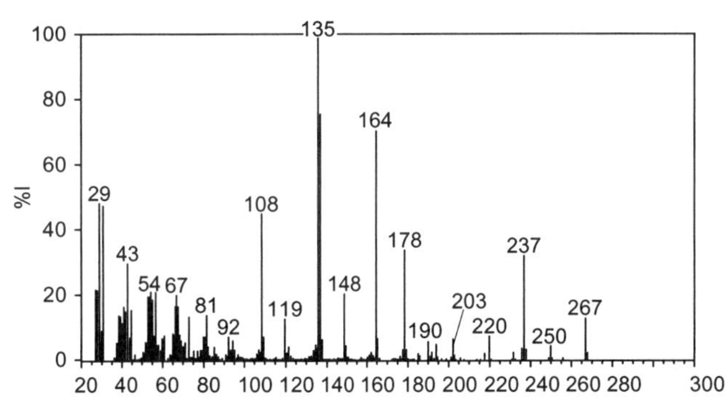

Disposition in the Body. Extremely efficient re-uptake of adenosine from plasma by red blood cells and blood vessel endothelial cells. Once inside the blood cells, adenosine is phosphorylated, by adenosine kinase, to adenosine monophosphate (AMP). Alternatively, it is deaminated, by adenosine deaminase, to inactive inosine, which can be further degraded to hypoxanthine and then uric acid. Adenosine is almost completely eliminated after a single pass through the coronary circulation. It is naturally found in various forms in all cells of the body.

Therapeutic concentration. Administrated dose is minute in comparison with adenosine concentrations already in the body and due to the efficient re-uptake, classic ADME (absorption, distribution, metabolism and excretion) studies are not possible.

Half-life. 0.6 to 10 s.

Distribution in blood. Erythrocytes transport adenosine from the liver to tissues which cannot synthesise it.

Dose. Initial dose is 6 mg (rapid intravenous bolus injection, administered over 1 to 2 s), followed by a saline flush. Up to two additional 12 mg boluses, within 1 to 2 min after initial dose, if necessary. A dose of 0.05 to 0.1 mg/kg body weight is effective in children with a maximum of 0.3 mg/kg.

Adiphenine

Anticholinergic

Synonyms. Diphacil; Diphenylacetyldiethylaminoethanol
α-Phenylbenzeneacetic acid 2-(diethylamino)ethyl ester
$C_{20}H_{25}NO_2$=311.4
CAS—64-95-9

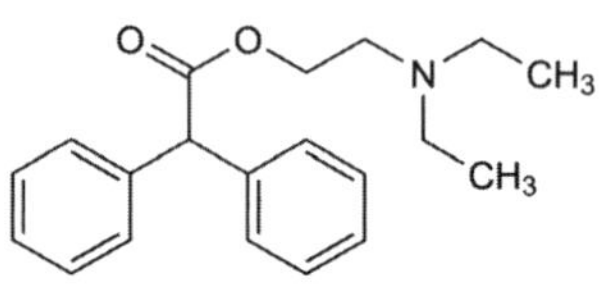

Adiphenine Hydrochloride

Synonym. Spasmolytine
Proprietary name. Trasentine
$C_{20}H_{25}NO_2$,HCl=347.9
CAS—50-42-0
A white crystalline powder. M.p. 112° to 115°.
Soluble in water, ethanol and chloroform; practically insoluble in ether.

Colour Tests. Liebermann's Test—brown; Mandelin's Test—green→blue.

Thin-layer Chromatography. System TA—Rf 64; system TB—Rf 56; system TC—Rf 60; system TE—Rf 83; system TAE—Rf 49; system TL—Rf 51. (Acidified iodoplatinate solution, positive.)

Gas Chromatography. System GA—RI 2186.

High Performance Liquid Chromatography. System HA—*k* 1.8; system HX—RI 422.

Ultraviolet Spectrum. Aqueous acid—253, 258 (A^1_1=14.5a), 264 nm.

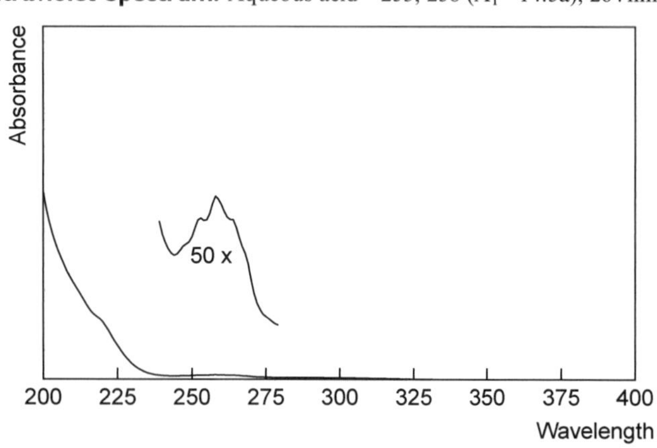

Infra-red Spectrum. Principal peaks at wavenumbers 1736, 1145, 700, 1190, 1500, 746 (KBr disk) cm^{-1}.

Mass Spectrum. Principal ions at *m*/*z* 86, 30, 167, 99, 87, 58, 165, 29.

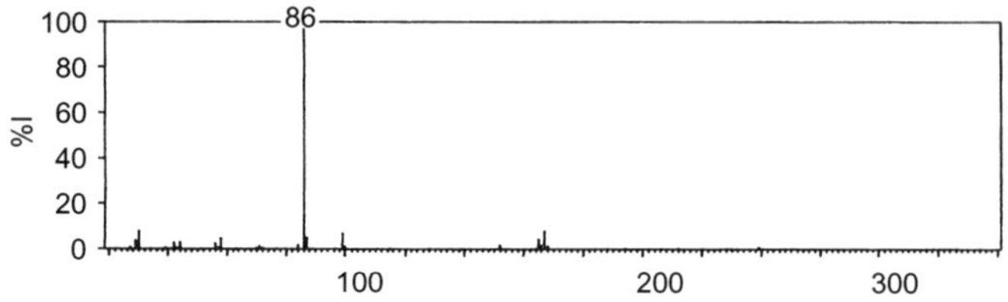

Dose. Adiphenine hydrochloride has been given in doses of 225 to 450 mg daily.

Adrafinil

Alpha-adrenergic Agonist

Synonym. Adrafinilum
Proprietary name. Olmifon
2-[(Diphenylmethyl)sulfinyl]-*N*-hydroxyacetamide
$C_{15}H_{15}NO_3S$=289.4
CAS—63547-13-7

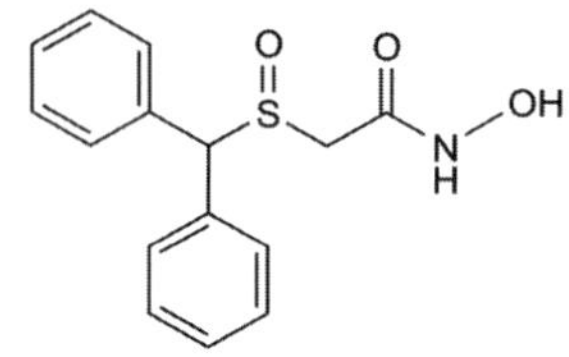

White to off-white crystalline powder with m.p. 154° to 160°. Slightly soluble in water (< 1 g/L), more soluble in ethanol and soluble in methanol.

High Performance Liquid Chromatography. System HAA—retention time 13.8 min.

Disposition in the Body. After oral administration, adrafinil is partly metabolised to its amide, 2-(benzhydrylsulfinyl)acetamide/2-[(diphenylmethyl)sulfinyl]acetamide (modafinil), which is also metabolised into its inactive acid and sulfone forms.

Toxicity. Low toxicity.

Half-life. Elimination half-life, adrafinil 1 h; modafinil 3 h.

Protein binding. 80% (albumin).

Dose. Between 600 mg and 1.2 g daily by mouth (to the elderly).

Adrenaline

Sympathomimetic

Synonyms. Epinephrine; Epirenamine; Levorenin; Suprarenin.
Proprietary names. Bronkaid Mistometer; Dyspné-Inhal; Epi-glaufrin; Epinal; Eppy; Glauposine; Primatene Mist; Simplene; Sus-Phrine; Suprarenaline; Vaponefrin. It is an ingredient of Asma-Vydrin, Brovon, Ganda, Isopto Epinal, Riddovydrin Inhalant and Rybarvin.
4-[(1*R*)-1-Hydroxy-2-(methylamino)ethyl]-1,2-benzenediol
$C_9H_{13}NO_3$=183.2
CAS—51-43-4

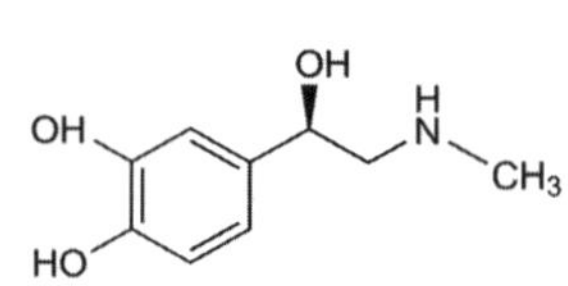

A white or creamy-white crystalline powder or granules. It darkens in colour on exposure to air and light. It is unstable in neutral or alkaline solution. M.p. about 212°, with decomposition. Sparingly soluble in water; practically insoluble in ethanol, chloroform, ether and light petroleum; freely soluble in solutions of mineral acids and boric acid solution, and in solutions of sodium or potassium hydroxide.

Adrenaline Acid Tartrate

Synonyms. Adrenaline [Epinephrine] Tartrate; Epinephrine Bitartrate.
Proprietary Names. E1; E2; Epitrate; Liadren; Lyophrin; Medihaler Epi. It is an ingredient of E-Pilo, Mydricaine, PE and Welder's Flash Drops.
$C_9H_{13}NO_3,C_4H_6O_6$=333.3
CAS—51-42-3
A white to greyish-white or light brownish-grey, crystalline powder. It slowly darkens on exposure to air and light. Incompatible with alkalis. M.p. 147° to 152°, with decomposition. Soluble 1 in 3 of water and 1 in 520 of ethanol; practically insoluble in chloroform and ether.

Adrenaline Hydrochloride

Proprietary names. Epifrin; Glaucon; Glycirenan. It is an ingredient of Riddobron Inhalant and Riddofan.
$C_9H_{13}NO_3,HCl$=219.7
CAS—55-312

Dissociation Constant. pK_a 8.7, 10.2, 12.0 (20°).

Colour Tests. Ammoniacal silver nitrate—red-brown/red-brown; Ferric chloride—green; Folin–Ciocalteu reagent—blue; Marquis test—orange→violet; Methanolic potassium hydroxide—pink-orange→brown; Nessler's reagent—black; Palladium chloride—orange→brown; Potassium dichromate (Method 1)—green→brown.

Thin-layer Chromatography. System TA—Rf 00; system TB—Rf 00; system TC—Rf 01; system TE—Rf 13; system TL—Rf 00; system TAE—Rf 03. (Acidified potassium permanganate solution, positive.)

High Performance Liquid Chromatography. System HC—*k* 0.63; system HX—RI 30.

Column: (analytical) RP C_{18} Ultrasphere-ODS (5 mm, 250 × 4.6 mm i.d., 5 µm); (guard) RP C_{18} Licrocart (5 mm, 4 × 4.0 mm i.d., 5 µm). Mobile phase: 0.1 M citrate buffer, 0.3 M disodium ethylenediaminetetraacetic acid (EDTA) and 0.5 mM sodium 1-octanesulfonic acid in methanol:water (7:93), final pH adjusted to 2.5 with 20% sodium hydroxide solution, 1.2 mL/min flow rate, ECD. Internal standard (IS): isoproterenol. Retention time(s): noradrenaline [norepinephrine], 3.5 min; adrenaline [epinephrine], 4.1 min; IS, 9.6 min [Y. Wang *et al.*, *J. Pharm. Biomed. Anal.*, 1999, *21*, 519–525].

Ultraviolet Spectrum. Aqueous acid—280 (A_1^1=155a); aqueous alkali—242, 297 nm.

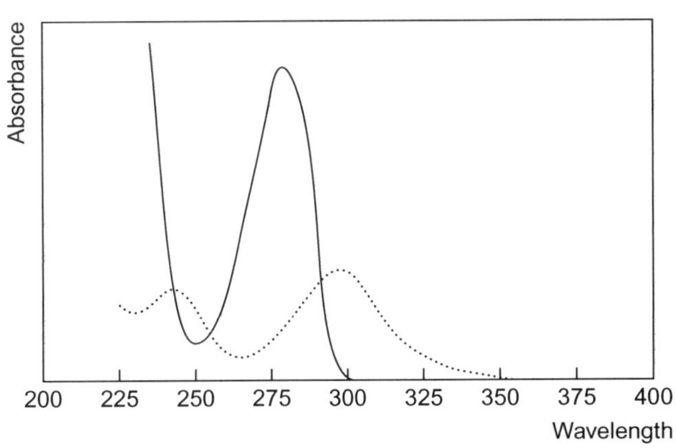

Infra-red Spectrum. Principal peaks at wavenumbers 1253, 1274, 1500, 945, 1224, 871 cm^{-1} (KBr disk).

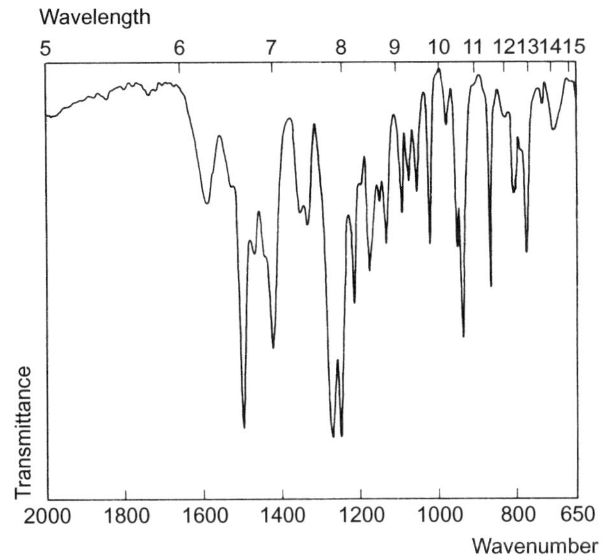

Mass Spectrum. Principal ions at *m/z* 44, 42, 124, 165, 163, 123, 93, 65.

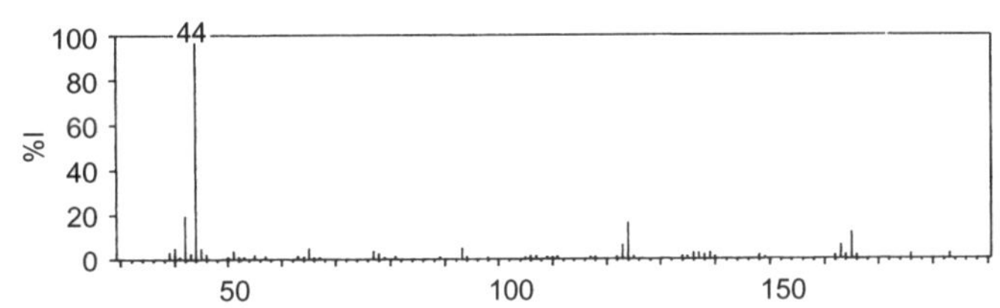

Quantification

Spectrofluorimetry. In plasma: adrenaline [epinephrine] and noradrenaline [norepinephrine]—J. F. O'Hanlon *et al.*, *Anal. Biochem.*, 1970, *34*, 568–581.

Gas chromatography. In plasma, erythrocytes, serum or urine: adrenaline [epinephrine] and noradrenaline [norepinephrine], limit of detection 10^{-7} µg, FID—H. G. Lovelady and L. L. Foster, *J. Chromatogr.*, 1975, *108*, 43–52.

High performance liquid chromatography. In plasma: limit of detection <10 pg, ECD—Y. Wang *et al.*, *J. Pharm. Biomed. Anal.*, 1999, *21*, 519–525.

Disposition in the Body. Adrenaline [epinephrine] is rapidly destroyed in the gastro-intestinal tract after oral administration; the effects of the drug after subcutaneous injection are produced within 5 min and appear more slowly than after intramuscular injection. It is rapidly taken up by the heart, spleen, several glandular tissues and adrenergic nerves; only metabolites are detectable in the cerebrospinal fluid. The major metabolic reactions are oxidative deamination and *O*-methylation followed by reduction or by glucuronic acid or sulfate conjugation. About 70 to 95% of an intravenous dose is excreted in the urine; of the excreted material about 80% is *O*-methyl metabolites, 2% is catechol metabolites, and only 1% is unchanged drug. The major urinary metabolite is 4-hydroxy-3-methoxymandelic acid (HMMA); other metabolites include 4-hydroxy-3-methoxyphenylacetic acid (homovanillic acid, HVA), conjugated metanephrine, and 4-hydroxy-3-methoxyphenylglycol, together with minor amounts of 3,4-dihydroxymandelic acid in free or conjugated form and *N*-methyladrenaline. Endogenous plasma concentrations of adrenaline [epinephrine] in normal subjects are in the range 30 to 160 pg/mL.

Toxicity. The minimum subcutaneous lethal dose is about 4 mg, but recoveries have occurred after accidental overdosage with 16 mg subcutaneously and 30 mg intravenously, followed by immediate supportive treatment.

Protein binding. In plasma, about 50%.

Dose. 200 to 500 µg, subcutaneously or intramuscularly, as a single dose which may be repeated.

Ajmaline

Anti-arrhythmic

Synonym. Rauwolfine
Proprietary names. Aritmina; Cardiorythmine; Gilurytmal; Ritmos; Tachmalin.
Ajmalan-17,21-diol
$C_{20}H_{26}N_2O_2$=326.4
CAS—4360-12-7

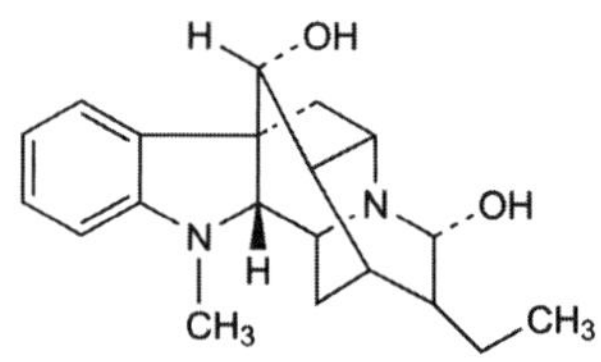

An alkaloid obtained from the root of *Rauwolfia serpentina* (*Apocynaceae*). A white or slightly yellowish crystalline powder. M.p. about 195°, with decomposition. Practically insoluble in water; freely soluble in ethanol, chloroform and glacial acetic acid; sparingly soluble in ether and methanol; soluble in dilute hydrochloric acid.

Ajmaline Hydrochloride

Proprietary name. Cardiorythmine
$C_{20}H_{26}N_2O_2,2HCl,2H_2O$=435.4
Crystals. M.p. 140°. Soluble 1 in 40 of water.

Ajmaline Monoethanolate

$C_{20}H_{26}N_2O_2,C_2H_6O$=372.5
CAS—60991-48-2
A white or slightly yellowish crystalline powder.
Practically insoluble in water; freely soluble in ethanol, chloroform, and glacial acetic acid; sparingly soluble in ether and methanol.

Dissociation Constant. pK_a 8.2.

Colour Tests. Liebermann's test—red; Mandelin's test—red; Marquis test—violet.

Thin-layer Chromatography. System TA—Rf 62; system TB—Rf 7; system TE—Rf 56; system TAE—Rf 22. (Acidified potassium permanganate solution, positive.)

Gas Chromatography. System GA—RI 2880.

High Performance Liquid Chromatography. System HA—*k* 2.8 (tailing peak); system HY—RI 277.

Column: RP_{18} (5 µm, 125 × 4 mm). Column temperature: 40°. Mobile phase: methanol: phosphate buffer (0.1 mol/L) adjusted to pH 3.5 with H_3PO_4 (26:74), 1 mL/min flow rate. Internal standard (IS): detajmium. Fluorescence detection (λ_{ex}=247 nm; λ_{em}=353 nm). Retention time(s): ajmaline, 3.5 min; IS, 7.0 min. [R. Oertel *et al.*, *J. Chromatogr. A*, 1998, *797*, 203–209].

Column: Nucleosil C_{18} (5 µm, 12 cm × 4 mm) with pre-column (2 cm × 4 mm). Mobile phase: (1) acetontrile:0.07% orthophosphoric acid (22:78 v/v), flow rate 1.5 mL/min; (2) aqueous 0.2 M trifluoroacetic acid: acetonitrile (80:20 v/v), flow rate 1.1 mL/min. UV detection (λ=254 nm). Retention time(s): ajmaline, 5.9 min; isoajmaline, 5.1 min; ajmaline *N*-oxide, 4.4 min; dihydroajmaline, 7.1 min. [C. Koppel *et al.*, *J. Chromatogr.*, 1992, *575(1)*, 87–91].

Ultraviolet Spectrum. Aqueous acid—204, 245 (A_1^1=223a), 289 nm. No alkaline shift.

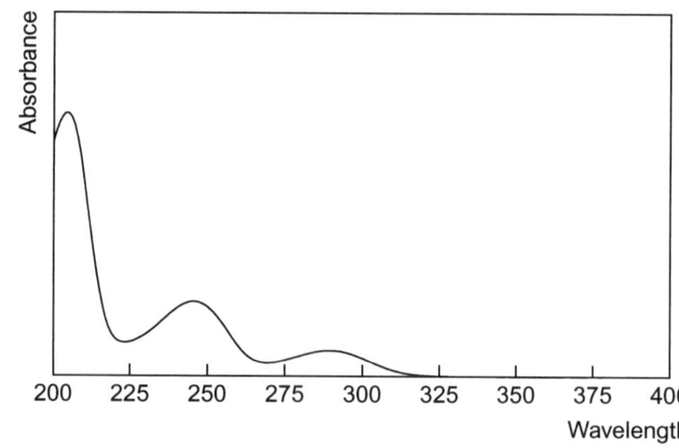

Infra-red Spectrum. Principal peaks at wavenumbers 756, 741, 1103, 1092, 1046, 1280 cm^{-1}.

Quantification

Spectrofluorimetry. In plasma—E. Welman *et al.*, *Br. J. Clin. Pharmacol.*, 1977, *4*, 549–551.

Thin-layer chromatography. In plasma—L. J. Drombowski *et al.*, *J. Pharm. Sci.*, 1975, *64*, 643–645.

Gas chromatography–mass spectrometry. In blood—D. St. Clemans *et al.*, *Arzneimittelforschung*, 1977, *27*, 1128–1130.

High performance liquid chromatography. In plasma—limit of detection 1 µg/L with extraction and 50 µg/L without. Fluorescence detection (λ_{ex}=296 nm; λ_{em}=358 nm)—C. Koppel *et al.*, *J. Chromatogr.*, 1992, *575(1)*, 87–91.

Disposition in the Body. Variably absorbed after oral administration, and mainly metabolised by the liver.

Therapeutic concentration

6 patients with acute myocardial infarction and ventricular arrhythmia were intravenously administered 20 mg/h ajmaline for 24 h. After 24 h, the plasma concentrations ranged from 0.25 to 0.95 mg/L. [C. Koppel *et al.*, *J. Chromatogr.*, 1992, *575(1)*, 87–91].

After intravenous injection of 50 mg to 1 subject, a plasma concentration of about 1.7 mg/L was reported at 1 min. [E. Welman *et al.*, *Br. J. Clin. Pharmacol.*, 1977, *4*, 549–551].

Toxicity

A 4-year-old girl died 3 h after ingestion of her mother's ajmaline tablets: 17 50-mg tablets were found to be missing. The ajmaline concentrations were determined to be 5.5 mg/L in her blood and 178.2 µg/g in her stomach contents (46.3 mg in total was found in the stomach). The lethal dose was estimated to be 500 mg/kg. [N. Ikeda *et al.*, *J. Forensic Sci.*, 1988, *33(2)*, 558–561].

In a fatality due to the ingestion of 2.5 g of ajmaline and 300 mg of diazepam the following postmortem tissue concentrations of ajmaline were reported: blood 10 mg/L, liver 50 µg/g, urine 44 mg/L; a blood-alcohol concentration of 1590 mg/L was also reported [A. R. Alha 1966, personal communication].

Dose. Maintenance, 200 to 300 mg daily.

Alachlor

Herbicide

Synonyms. Alachlore; CP-50144; Metachlor.
Proprietary names. Alanex; Lasso.
2-Chloro-*N*-(2,6-diethylphenyl)-*N*-(methoxymethyl)acetamide
$C_{14}H_{20}ClNO_2$=269.8
CAS—15972-60-8

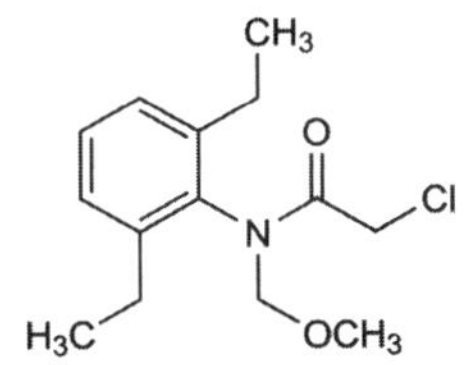

A colourless to yellow crystalline solid. M.p. 40° to 41°.
It is soluble in water (240 mg/L at 25°), acetone, benzene, ethanol, ethyl acetate, diethyl ether, and chloroform; sparingly soluble in heptane.

Partition Coefficient. Log *P* (octanol/water), 2.64, 2.92, and 3.52.

Thin-layer Chromatography. System TX—Rf 40; system TY—Rf 45.

Gas Chromatography. System GA—RI 1876.

Column: DB-1 (2 m × 0.25 mm i.d., 0.25 μm film thickness). Column temperature: 120°, held for 0.3 min and increased to 180° at 15°/min. Carrier gas: hydrogen, 1.9 mL/min. FID. Reference compounds: pentachlorophenol, heptadecanoic acid. Retention time: 2.75 min. [Z. Liu *et al.*, *Anal. Chem.*, 1994, *66*, 3086–3092.]

Ultraviolet Spectrum. Aqueous acid—265, 273 nm.

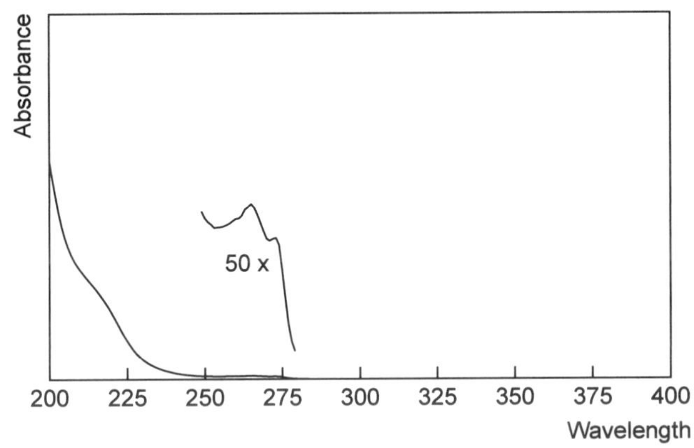

Infra-red Spectrum. Principal peaks at 1106, 1702, 1365, 1458 cm^{-1}.

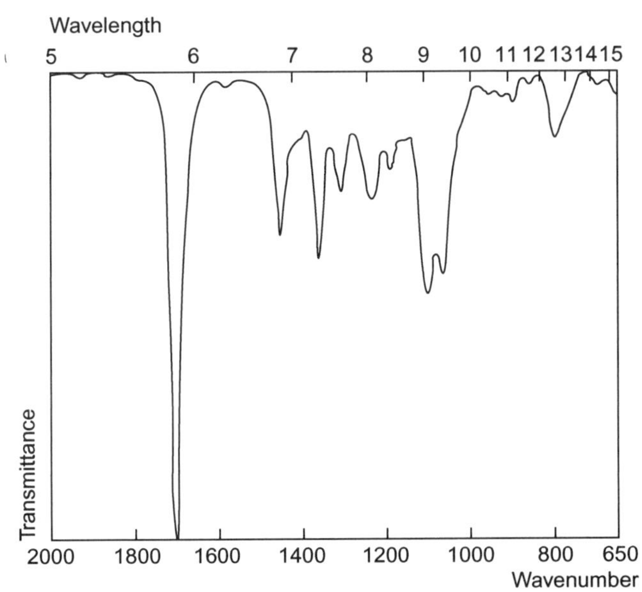

Mass Spectrum. Principal ions at *m/z* 45, 160, 188, 146, 237, 132, 117, 77.

Quantification

Gas chromatography. In serum: limit of detection 11.5 μg/L— Z. Liu *et al.*, *Anal. Chem.*, 1994, *66*, 3086–3092.

High performance liquid chromatography. In serum: limit of detection <50 mg/L—R. Galati *et al.*, *Anticancer Res.*, 1998, *18*, 979–982.

Enzyme-linked immunoassay. In plasma: limit of detection 0.001 μg/L—R. E. Biagini *et al.*, *Bull. Envir. Contam. Toxicol.*, 1995, *54(2)*, 245–250.

Disposition in the Body. Alachlor is absorbed through the skin and can be metabolised to 2,6-diethylbenzoquinoneimine (DEBQI) which is a carcinogenic metabolite and 2-chloro-*N*-(2,6-diethylphenyl)acetamide (CDEPA) which can subsequently be converted into DEBQI. Additionally, 2,6-diethylaniline (DEA), alachlor mercapturate and conjugated metabolites have been detected in urine. No free alachlor has been detected in urine.

Toxicity. Alachlor may cause mild eye and skin irritations after exposure.

Albendazole

Anthelmintic (Veterinary)

Proprietary names. Albenza; Eskazole; Proftril; Valbazen; Zental.
[5-(Propylthio)-1*H*-benzimidazol-2-yl]carbamic acid methyl ester
$C_{12}H_{15}N_3O_2S$=265.3
CAS—54965-21-8

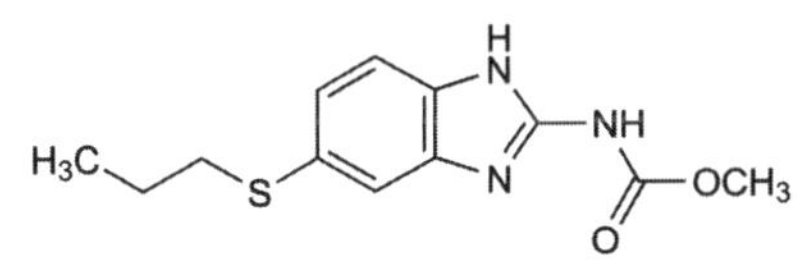

Colourless crystals. M.p. 208° to 210°.

Ultraviolet Spectrum. Aqueous acid—292 nm (A^1_1=370b); aqueous alkali—309 nm (A^1_1=742b).

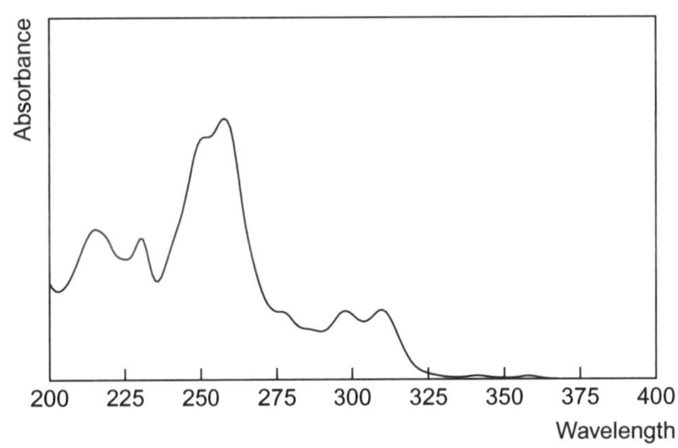

High Performance Liquid Chromatography. Column: amylose tris(3-dimethylphenyl carbamate) coated on silica gel substrate (Chiralpak AD, 10 μm, 250 × 4.6 mm). Mobile phase: hexane: isopropanol:ethanol (81:14.25:4.74 v/v/v), flow rate 1.2 mL/min. Fluorescence detection (λ_{ex}=280 nm; λ_{em}=320 nm). Retention time(s): albendazole, 8.5 min; albendazole sulfoxide, 13.7 (+) 21.6 (−) min; albendazole sulfone, 25.7 min [V. L. Lanchote *et al.*, *J. Chromatogr. B, Biomed. Sci. Appl.*, 1998, *709*, 273–279].

Column: RP C_{18} Lichrocart (5 μm, 125 × 4 mm). Mobile phase: acetonitrile:0.25 N sodium acetate buffer (3:7 v/v), 1.5 mL/min flow rate. Internal standard (IS): mebendazole. UV detection (λ=290 nm). Retention time(s): albendazole sulfoxide, 1.2 min; albendazole sulfone, 1.9 min; IS, 5.6 min; albendazole, 11.7 min [M. E. C. Valois *et al.*, *J. Anal. Toxicol.*, 1994, *18*, 86–89].

Quantification

High performance liquid chromatography. In plasma: limit of quantification of albendazole and metabolites, 10 μg/L and 7.5 μg/L, respectively—P. Chiap *et al.*, *J. Chromatogr. A.*, 2000, *870(1–2)*, 121–134. In plasma: limit of quantification albendazole sulfoxide 40 μg/L and sulfone 10 μg/L, UV detection (λ=290 nm)—M. E. C. Valois *et al.*, *J. Anal. Toxicol.*, 1994, *18*, 86–89. In plasma: limit of detection, albendazole sulfoxide 14 μg/L and albendazole sulfone 30 μg/L, UV detection (λ=290 nm)—T. Zeugin *et al.*, *Ther. Drug Monit.*, 1990, *12*, 187–190.

Therapeutic concentration

13 subjects, male and female, with a mean age of 38.9 (15 to 64) years were administered a mean daily dose of 18.3 mg/kg albendazole (range 16.0 to

22.2 mg/kg). The mean peak plasma concentration of albendazole sulfoxide was 0.71 mg/L (range 0.36 to 1.52 mg/L) and albendazole sulfone was 0.06 (range 0.02 to 0.14) mg/L. [M. E. C. Valois *et al.*, *J. Anal. Toxicol.*, 1994, *18*, 86–89]

A patient with echinococcosis was administered 200 mg albendazole orally and a peak plasma concentration of 1.57 µmol/L was observed at 0.9 h. [T. Zeugin *et al.*, *Ther. Drug Monit.*, 1990, *12*, 187–190].

Alclofenac

Analgesic

Proprietary names. Allopydin; Epinal; Mervan; Reufenac; Zumaril.
3-Chloro-4-(2-propenyloxy)benzeneacetic acid
$C_{11}H_{11}ClO_3$=226.7
CAS—22131-79-9

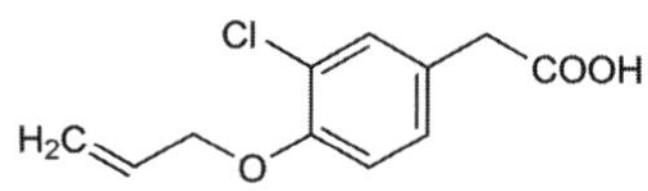

A white or slightly yellowish-white crystalline powder. M.p. about 91°. Slightly soluble in water; soluble 1 in 3 of ethanol, 1 in 4 of chloroform, and 1 in 6 of ether.

Dissociation Constant. pK_a 4.6.

Thin-layer Chromatography. System TD—Rf 18; system TE—Rf 04; system TF—Rf 28; system TG—Rf 12; system TAD—Rf 33; system TAJ—Rf 17; system TAK—Rf 70; system TAL—Rf 90. (Ludy Tenger reagent, orange.)

Gas Chromatography. System GD—Retention time of methyl derivative 1.13 relative to n-$C_{16}H_{34}$.

High Performance Liquid Chromatography. System HD—*k* 2.6; system HV—RRT 0.61 relative to meclofenamic acid.

Ultraviolet Spectrum. Aqueous acid—277 (A^1_1=77b); dehydrated alcohol—282 (A^1_1=88a), 290 nm (A^1_1=78a).

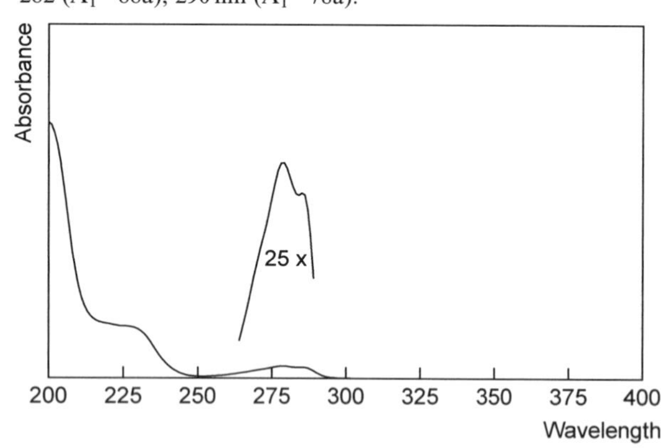

Infra-red Spectrum. Principal peaks at wavenumbers 1258, 1689, 1235, 933, 1016, 1500 cm^{-1} (KBr disk).

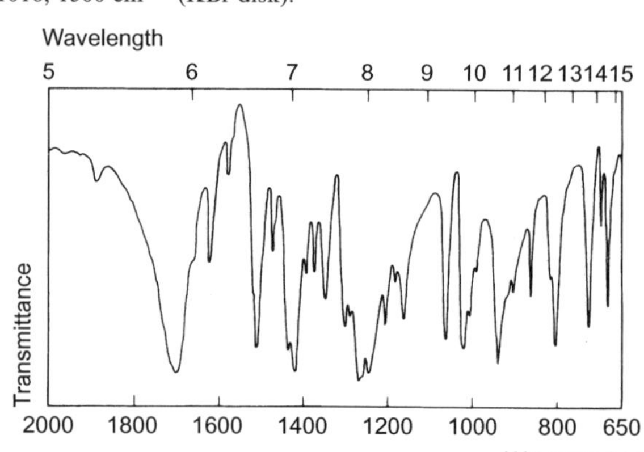

Mass Spectrum. Principal ions at m/z 41, 226, 77, 143, 181, 141, 39, 145.

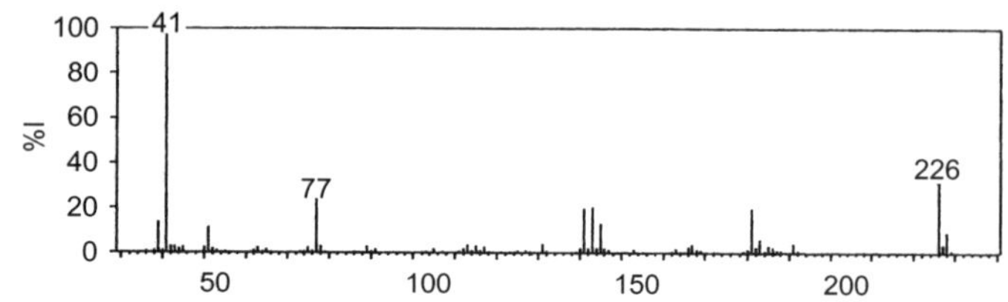

Quantification
Gas chromatography. In plasma or urine: alclofenac and two metabolites, FID—R. Roncucci *et al.*, *J. Chromatogr.*, 1971, *62*, 135–137.

High performance liquid chromatography. In urine: limit of quantification 1 mg/L—F. T. Delbeke *et al.*, *J. Chromatogr.*, 1993, *621(2)*, 209–214.

Disposition in the Body. Alcofenac is variably absorbed after oral or rectal administration and distributed into the synovial fluid. It is metabolised by glucuronic acid conjugation; there is some conjugation with glycine, deallylation to form 3-chloro-4-hydroxyphenylacetic acid, and hydroxylation to form 3-chloro-4-(2,3-dihydroxypropyloxy)phenylacetic acid which may be methylated; an epoxide metabolite has also been identified. Up to about 90% of an oral dose is excreted in the urine in 24 h, mostly as unchanged drug and the glucuronide conjugate.

Therapeutic concentration
After an oral dose of 1 g to 10 subjects, a mean peak plasma concentration of 136 mg/L was attained in about 1 h; concentrations in the synovial fluid reached a mean peak of 32 mg/L in 2 h. [G. M. Thomas *et al.*, *Curr. Med. Res. Opinion*, 1975, *3*, 264–267].

Half-life. Plasma half-life, 1.5 to 5.5 h (mean 2.5 h).

Volume of distribution. About 0.1 L/kg.

Protein binding. In plasma, about 99%.

Note. For a review of the pharmacokinetics of alclofenac, see R. N. Brogden *et al.*, *Drugs*, 1977, *14*, 241–259.

Dose. Alclofenac has been given in doses of 1.5 to 3 g daily.

Alcuronium Chloride

Muscle Relaxant

Synonyms. Allnortoxiferin Chloride; Diallylnortoxiferine Dichloride; Diallyltoxiferine Chloride.
Proprietary name. Alloferin
4,4′-Didemethyl-4,4′-di-2-propenyltoxiferine dichloride
$C_{44}H_{50}Cl_2N_4O_2,5H_2O$=827.9
CAS—23214-96-2 (alcuronium); 15180-03-7 (chloride)

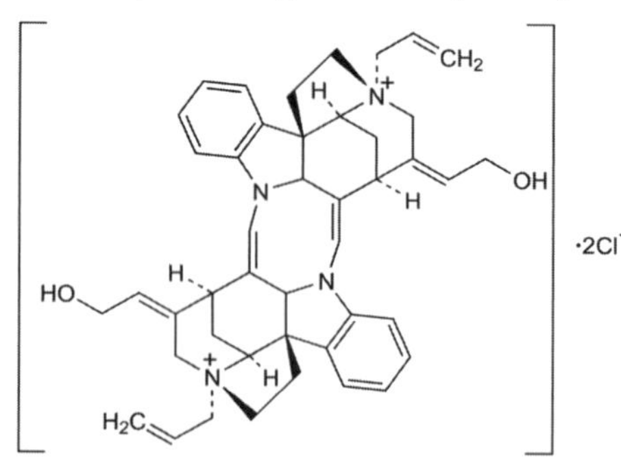

A colourless crystalline powder. No characteristic melting-point; a brown colour appears at 220°; still not melted at 350°. Soluble in water and ethanol; soluble 1 in 5 of methanol.

Colour Tests. Mandelin's test—blue-violet; Marquis test—green-brown.

Thin-layer Chromatography. System TA—Rf 01; system TB—Rf 00 (alcuronium); system TE—Rf 00; system TAE—Rf 00. (Acidified potassium permanganate solution, positive.)

High Performance Liquid Chromatography. System HX—RI 354.

Column: Spherisorb 5-CN. (250 × 4 mm) Mobile phase: acetonitrile:aqueous solution of 60 mM Na_2SO_4 and 5 mM H_2SO_4 (46:54 v/v), flow-rate 1 mL/min. Internal standard (IS): laudanosine. UV detection

(λ=294 nm). Retention time(s): IS 3.2 min; alcuronium, 5.4 min. [T. Kunzer *et al.*, *J. Chromatogr. B, Biomed. Appl.*, 1994, *653(1)*, 63–68].

Ultraviolet Spectrum. Aqueous acid—255, 291 nm (A_1^1=185b).

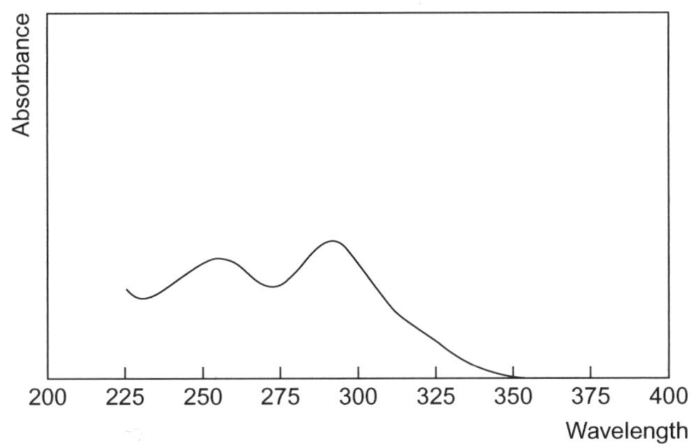

Infra-red Spectrum. Principal peaks at wavenumbers 1495, 1592, 1283, 1650, 1030, 757 cm^{-1} (KBr disk).

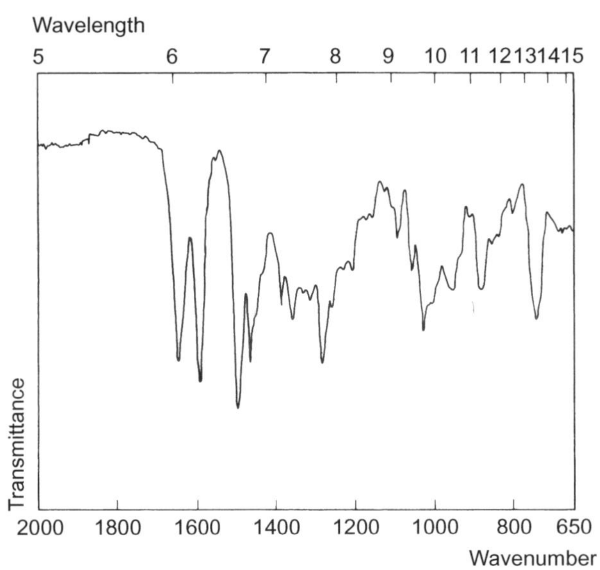

Quantification

Spectrofluorimetry. In plasma—J. Walker *et al.*, *Eur. J. Clin. Pharmacol.*, 1980, 17, 449–457.

High performance liquid chromatography. In plasma and urine: limit of detection 25 µg/L—T. Kunzer *et al.*, *J. Chromatogr. B, Biomed. Appl.*, 1994, *653(1)*, 63–68. In plasma: limit of detection 100 µg/L, ECD—C. Tovey *et al.*, *J. Chromatogr.*, 1983, *278*; *Biomed. Appl.*, *29*, 216–219.

Disposition in the Body. After intravenous administration it is widely distributed throughout the tissues. About 80 to 85% of a dose is excreted in the urine as unchanged drug and about 10 to 15% is secreted in the bile and eliminated in the faeces.

Therapeutic concentration

Following intravenous administration of 0.25 mg/kg to 17 subjects, plasma concentrations of 0.74 to 2.25 mg/L (mean 1.4 mg/L) were reported after 3 to 30 min [J. Walker *et al.*, *Eur. J. Clin. Pharmacol.*, 1980, 17, 449–457].

Half-life. Plasma half-life, about 3 h; increased in subjects with renal failure.

Volume of distribution. About 0.4 L/kg.

Clearance. Plasma clearance, about 1.3 mL/min/kg.

Protein binding. In plasma, about 40%.

Note. For a review of the pharmacokinetics of alcuronium chloride and other muscle relaxants, see M. I. Ramzan *et al.*, *Clin. Pharmacokinet.*, 1981, *6*, 25–60.

Dose. Initially 200 to 300 µg/kg intravenously.

Aldesleukin

Antineoplastic/Immunomodulator/Biological Response Modifier

Synonyms. DRG-0021; recombinant human interleukin-2; rIL-2; r-ser-HuIL-2.
Proprietary name. Proleukin
Serine-125 human interleukin-2
$C_{690}H_{1115}N_{177}O_{203}S_6$=15330.7
CAS—110942-02-4

A human recombinant interleukin-2 product, approximate molecular weight 15 300 daltons.

Quantification

Immunobioassay. In serum: limit of quantification 0.1 µg/L—R. W. Nadeau *et al.*, *Anal. Chem.*, 1989, *61*, 1732–1736.

Disposition in the Body. The pharmacokinetics of aldesleukin show considerable inter- and intra-subject variation. Following intravenous administration it undergoes rapid distribution into extravascular space. Distribution may be related to the method of administration and may therefore affect its efficacy. It is eliminated by the kidneys by both glomerular filtration and peritubular secretion.

Therapeutic concentration

12 patients with either metastatic renal cell carcinoma or melanoma were administered with aldesleukin at a dose of 1.1 mg/m^2 daily (18 × 10^6 IU/m^2 daily) as a continuous intravenous infusion for 5 days. The maximum serum concentration was 2.2 ± 1.1 µg/L (40 IU/L) after 24 or 48 h. After that time, the serum concentrations decreased to 0.59 ± 0.43 µg/L (10.6 IU/L) by the end of the 5-day treatment. [Fish *et al.*, *Br. J. Cancer*, 1991, *64* (*Suppl.15*), 4].

Toxicity. Capillary leak syndrome leading to pulmonary oedema and hypertension is a major adverse effect.

Half-life. Plasma, 85 min to 4 h (intravenous bolus); 12 h (1-h infusion).

Volume of distribution. 6.3 to 7.9 L (following intravenous bolus or 2-h infusion) which increases with repeated doses.

Clearance. Plasma, 140 to 300 mL/min (mean clearance 268 mL/min); 8.4 to 18 L/h.

Note. For a review of aldesleukin see R. Whittington and D. Faulds, *Drugs*, 1993, *46*, 446–514.

Dose. 600 000 units/kg every 8 h by intravenous infusion over 15 min for a maximum of 14 doses repeated after 9 days. Alternatively, a dose of up to 18 million international units may be given subcutaneously.

Aldicarb

Acaricide, Insecticide, Nematicide

Synonyms. Aldicarbe; carbanolate; ENT 27093; NCI-CO8640; OMS 771; UC 21149.
Proprietary names. Sentry; Temic; Temik.
2-Methyl-2-(methylthio)propanal *O*-[(methylamino)carbonyl]oxime
$C_7H_{14}N_2O_2S$=190.3
CAS—116-06-3

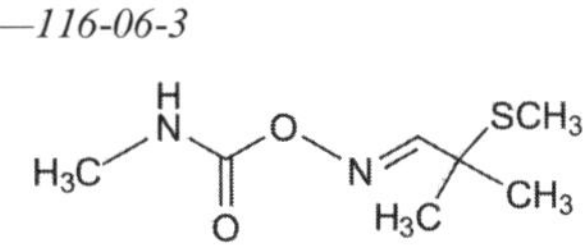

A white crystalline powder. M.p. 90° to 100°.
It is soluble in water (0.1 to 1.0 mg/mL at 22°), DMSO (>100 mg/mL at 21°), 95% ethanol (>100 mg/mL at 21°), acetone (>100 mg/mL at 21°), chloroform, isopropane, toluene, and most organic solvents; insoluble in heptane and mineral oils.

Partition Coefficient. Log P (octanol/water), 1.13 (25°).

Thin-layer Chromatography. System TX—Rf 18; system TY—Rf 12; system TZ—Rf 65; system TAA—Rf 12; system TAB—Rf 04; system TAC—Rf 03.

Plate: silica gel G. Mobile phase: *n*-hexane:acetone (4:1). Developed with zinc chloride–diphenylamine spray reagent. Rf 0.4. [T. Murlidhar *et al.*, *J. Assoc. Off. Anal. Chem.*, 1991, *74*, 545–546.]

Gas Chromatography. System GA—RI 1320; system GKA—RI 866; system GKB—RI 966; system GKC—RI 1088.

High Performance Liquid Chromatography. System HZ—retention time 3.6 min; system HAA—retention time 15.1 min; system HAO—k 7.63; system HAP—k 0.69.

Column: RP-C_{18} (250 × 4.6 mm i.d., 5 μm). Mobile phase: acetonitrile: water (35:65), flow rate 1.5 mL/min. Retention time 7.2 min. [A. Covaci *et al.*, *J. Anal. Toxicol.*, 1999, *23*, 290–293.]

Ultraviolet Spectrum. Aqueous solution—201 nm; acetonitrile—249 nm.

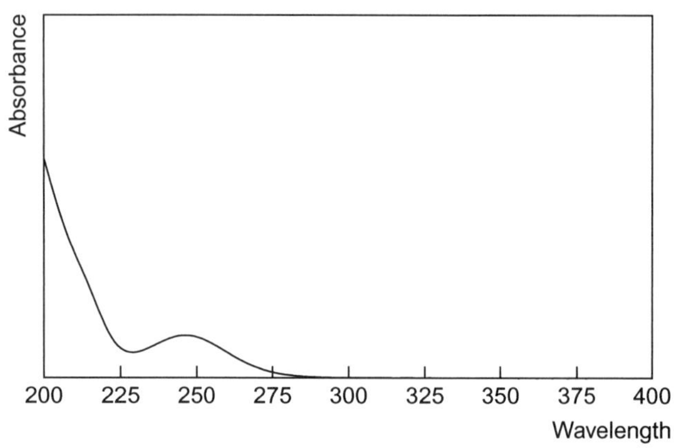

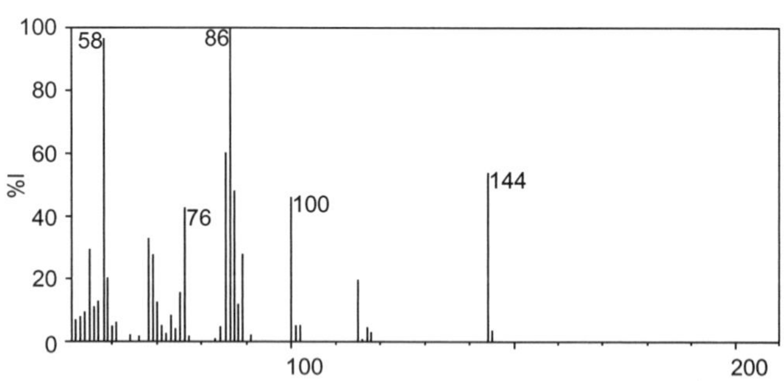

Quantification

Gas chromatography. In urine: limit of detection 2.4 μg/L, FPD—D. X. Lian *et al.*, *J. Chromatogr.*, 1991, *542(2)*, 526–530.

High performance liquid chromatography. In urine: limit of detection between 4 and 10 μg/L, UV detection, and 0.1 to 0.5 μg/L, electrospray MS detection—F. J. Martinez *et al.*, *Anal. Chim. Acta*, 2000, *412 (1–2)*, 131–139. In serum and urine: 0.05 μg/L—A. Covaci *et al.*, *J. Anal. Toxicol.*, 1999, *23*, 290–293.

Disposition in the Body. Aldicarb is efficiently absorbed from the gastrointestinal tract and at a lesser extent through the skin. It is distributed to all tissues, but it does not significantly cross the blood–brain barrier, and is metabolised to aldicarb sulfoxide and aldicarb sulfone metabolites which are both toxic. Both metabolites can be detoxified by hydrolysis to oximes and nitriles. The drug and metabolites are excreted primarily in urine but also a small amount through biliary elimination. Aldicarb does not accumulate in the body during long-term exposure.

Toxicity. Aldicarb features prominently in accidental pesticide poisonings because of the way it is misused. Aldicarb exposure may be fatal and may occur by ingestion, inhalation, or when absorbed through the skin. Very high doses may result in paralysis of the respiratory system and the nervous system. Toxicity can occur between 15 min and 3 h post-exposure but effects can disappear quite quickly within 4 to 12 h. The allowed daily intake is 5 μg/kg bodyweight.

A 40-year-old woman was found unconscious and later pronounced dead. It was believed that she had ingested a black granular substance known as Temic. Postmortem analysis revealed the following aldicarb levels: blood concentration 11 mg/L, total stomach contents 213 mg, and more than 1 mg/kg in her liver. [S. Hoai Ngo, *TIAFT Bulletin Case Notes*, 1991, *21 (2)*].

Aldosterone

Corticosteroid

Synonym. Electrocortin
Proprietary name. Aldocorten
(11β)-11,21-Dihydroxy-3,20-dioxopregn-4-en-18-al
$C_{21}H_{28}O_5$=360.4
CAS—52-39-1

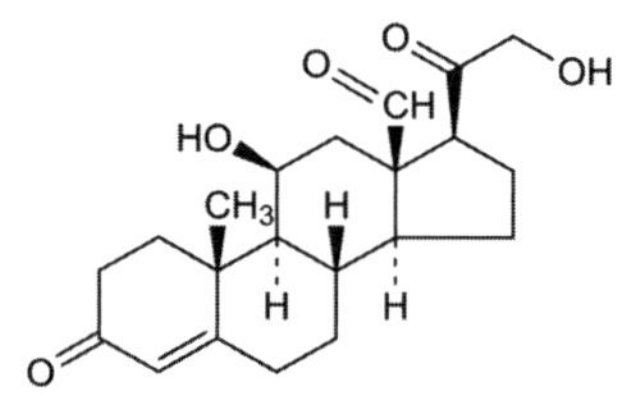

M.p. 164° (anhydrous).

Ultraviolet Spectrum. Methanol—241 nm (A^1_1=437b).

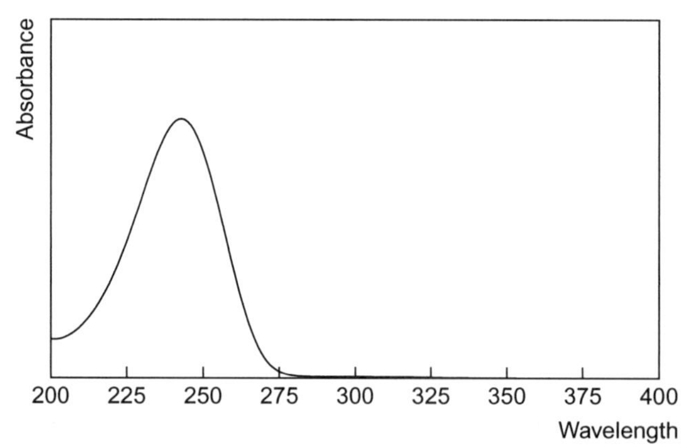

Infra-red Spectrum. Principal peaks at wavenumbers 1650, 986, 1020, 999, 1062, 1075 cm^{-1} (KBr disk).

Quantification

High performance liquid chromatography–mass spectrometry. In serum and plasma: limit of detection 10 ng/L and limit of quantification 15 ng/L, MS detection (m/z 359.2 to 331.2)—V. F. Fredline *et al.*, *Anal. Biochem.*, 1997, *252*, 308–313.

Dose. Aldosterone has been given in doses of 500 μg intravenously, repeated several times a day.

Aldrin

Insecticide

Synonyms. Compd 118; HHDN.
Proprietary names. Alderstan; Aldrex; Octalene.
Aldrin usually contains 95% w/w of 1,2,3,4,10,10-hexachloro-1,4,4a,5,8,8a-hexahydro-1,4:5,8-dimethanonaphthalene (HHDN) together with 5% w/w of active related compounds.
$C_{12}H_8Cl_6$=364.9
CAS—309-00-2

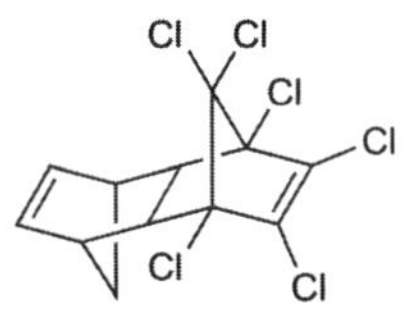

White crystals. When heated to decomposition it evolves highly toxic fumes of phosgene and hydrogen chloride. The technical grade is a tan to dark brown solid containing 85% or more of HHDN. M.p. 104° (pure grade), 49° to 60° (technical grade).
Practically insoluble in water; soluble 1 in 20 of ethanol, 1 in 1 of acetone, 1 in 0.55 of benzene, and 1 in 0.33 of carbon tetrachloride; soluble in ether.

Partition Coefficient. Log *P* (octanol), 3.0.

Colour Tests. Nitric–Sulfuric Acid—pink; Sulfuric Acid–Fuming Sulfuric Acid—red (slow).

Thin Layer Chromatography. System TX—aldrin Rf 89, dieldrin Rf 65; system TY—aldrin Rf 98, dieldrin Rf 87; system TAB—aldrin Rf 67, dieldrin Rf 51; system TAC—aldrin Rf 52; dieldrin Rf 27.

Gas Chromatography. System GA—aldrin RI 1943, dieldrin RI 2110; system GK—aldrin RRT 0.88, dieldrin RRT 1.13 (both relative to caffeine); system GKA—aldrin RI 2008, dieldrin RI 2170; system GKB—aldrin RI 2096, dieldrin RI 2304; system GKC—aldrin RI 2226, dieldrin RI 2528.

Column: fused silica capillary (30 m x 0.25 mm i.d., 0.25 μm film thickness). Column temperature: 250°. Carrier gas: helium. IS: endosulfan-I-d_4. MS detection. Retention time: aldrin, 21.9 min; dieldrin, 31.4 min. [Siming Liu and J. D. Pleil, *J. Chromatogr. B Analyt. Technol. Biomed. Life Sci.*, 2002, *769*, 155–167].

High Performance Liquid Chromatography. System HAO—*k* 0; system HAP—*k* 33.86.

Ultraviolet Spectrum. No significant absorption, 230 to 360 nm.

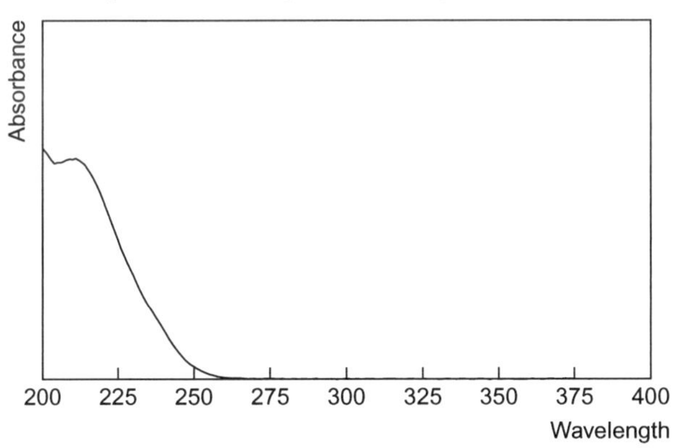

Infra-red Spectrum. Principal peaks at wavenumbers 696, 1036, 835, 723, 1255, 893 cm^{-1} (KBr disk).

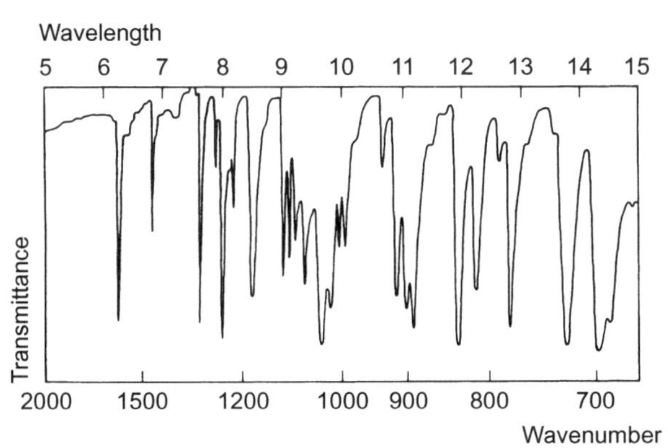

Mass Spectrum. Principal ions at *m/z* 66, 91, 79, 263, 65, 101, 261, 265; dieldrin 79, 82, 81, 263, 77, 108, 265, 80.

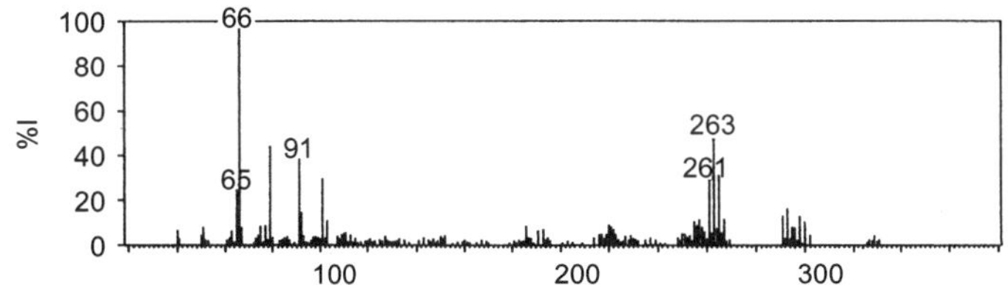

Quantification

Gas chromatography. In blood: limit of detection 0.1 μg/L, ECD—M. G. Rosell *et al.*, *J. Chromatogr.*, 1993, *655(1)*, 151–154.

Gas chromatography–mass spectrometry. In blood: limit of quantification 25–50 pg (*m/z* 263, 378)—Siming Liu and J. D. Pleil, *J. Chromatogr. B Analyt. Technol. Biomed. Life Sci.*, 2002, *769*, 155–167.

Disposition in the Body. Poorly absorbed after oral ingestion but when dissolved in oils or other lipids it is readily absorbed by the skin and gastrointestinal tract. It is rapidly metabolised in the body by epoxidation to dieldrin; dieldrin is stored in the body fat and persists for several weeks after the cessation of exposure. It is slowly eliminated in the faeces, mainly as unknown hydrophilic metabolites; a small amount is excreted in the urine as metabolites.

Blood concentration. Blood concentrations of dieldrin averaging 1 μg/L have been reported in 10 subjects with no occupational exposure to insecticides. Serum concentrations in subjects with low to high occupational exposure averaged 1 to 2 μg/L for aldrin and 9 to 27 μg/L for dieldrin.

Toxicity. Severe symptoms may follow absorption of 1 to 3 g; the estimated minimum lethal dose is 5 g. The maximum permissible atmospheric concentration is 0.25 mg/m^3 and the maximum permissible concentration in food is 0.1 ppm.

The body fat of a 23-year-old man poisoned by aldrin, while working in a formulating plant, contained 60 μg/g of dieldrin 15 days after the last exposure; a blood concentration of 0.1 mg/L was reported 4 months later. The blood concentrations of two men exposed to aldrin in the same plant and showing symptoms of poisoning were 0.28 and 0.13 mg/L of dieldrin 1 month after the last exposure. In 2 further cases of poisoning, the concentrations of dieldrin in the body fat 3 and 5 weeks after exposure were 149 and 44 μg/g respectively; the corresponding blood concentrations were 0.53 and 0.13 mg/L. [G. Kazantzis *et al.*, *Br. J. Ind. Med.*, 1964, *21*, 46–51].

Half-life. Blood half-life, dieldrin 50 to 170 days (mean 97).

Distribution in blood. Plasma:whole blood ratio, dieldrin about 1.5.

Alendronic Acid

Bone Modulator

Synonyms. Alendronate; aminohydroxybutylidene diphosphonic acid.
(4-Amino-1-hydroxybutylidene)bisphosphonic acid
$C_4H_{13}NO_7P_2$=249.1
CAS—66376-36-1

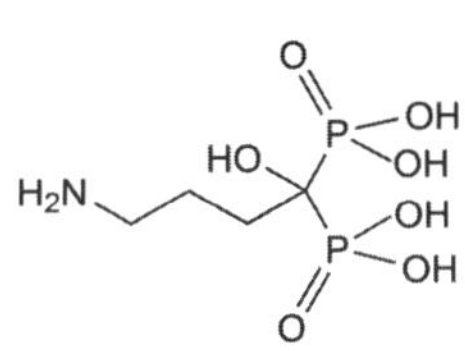

A fine white powder. M.p. 233° to 235°, with decomposition.

Alendronate Sodium

Proprietary names. Adronat; Alendros; Dronal; Fosamax.
$C_4H_{12}NNaO_7P_2,3H_2O$=325.1
CAS—121268-17-5
A white crystalline nonhygroscopic powder. It is soluble in water; very slightly soluble in ethanol; practically insoluble in chloroform.

Dissociation Constant. pK_a (25°) 2.7, 8.7, 10.5, 11.6.

Partition Coefficient. Log *P* (octanol/water), −1.30.

Quantification

High performance liquid chromatography. In urine: limit of quantification is 5 μg/L, fluorescence detection—W. F. Kline *et al.*, *J. Chromatogr.*, 1990, *534*; *Biomed. Appl.*, *99*, 139–149. In urine and plasma: limit of quantification is 1 μg/L and 5 μg/L, respectively, fluorescence detection; in urine: 2.5 μg/L, electrochemical detection—W. F. Kline and B. K. Matuszewski, *J. Chromatogr.*, 1992, *583*; *Biomed. Appl.*, *121*, 183–193.

Disposition in the Body. Alendronate is poorly absorbed after oral administration and absorption is decreased by food, especially products containing calcium or other polyvalent cations. The drug is rapidly cleared from plasma and about half of the absorbed dose is excreted in urine with the remainder being sequestered to bone for a prolonged period. It does not appear to be metabolised and is slowly released from skeletal deposits. Approximately, 45% is excreted in urine in the first 8 h after an intravenous dose and then 5% is excreted much more slowly between 8 and 72 h. The drug is probably bound to the mineral phase of the skeleton and of that retained, approximately one-third is excreted over the first 6 months.

Half-life. 10.5 years.

Volume of distribution. Steady state (estimated), greater than 28 L.

Clearance. Systemic clearance (estimated), no more than 11.94 L/h.

Protein binding. In plasma, 78%.

Dose. For Paget's disease of bone the equivalent of 40 mg of alendronic acid daily; for treatment of postmenopausal osteoporosis 10 mg daily.

Aletamine

Analgesic

Synonym. Alfetamine
α-Allylphenethylamine
$C_{11}H_{15}N = 161.2$
CAS—4255-23-6

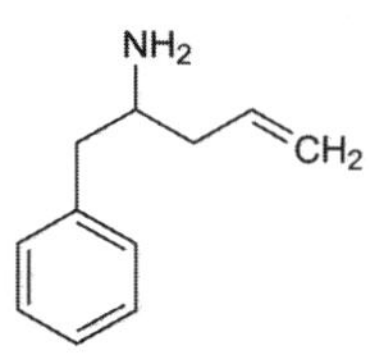

Aletamine Hydrochloride

$C_{11}H_{15}N,HCl = 197.7$
CAS—4255-24-7
White crystals.
Soluble in water.

Colour Tests. Liebermann's Test—orange; Marquis Test—orange.

Thin-layer Chromatography. System TA—Rf 59; system TB—Rf 37; system TC—Rf 40; system TL—Rf 42. (Acidified iodoplatinate solution, positive; acidified potassium permanganate solution, positive.)

Gas Chromatography. System GA—RI 1293.

Ultraviolet Spectrum. Aqueous acid—251, 257 ($A^1_1 = 10b$), 263 nm.

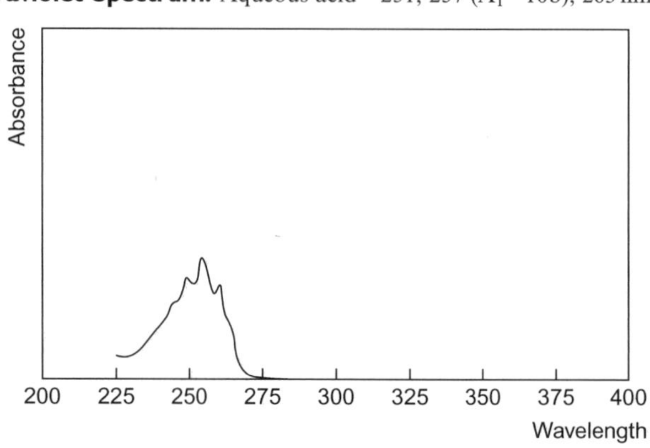

Mass Spectrum. Principal peaks at *m/z* 70, 120, 43, 91, 39, 103, 71, 65.

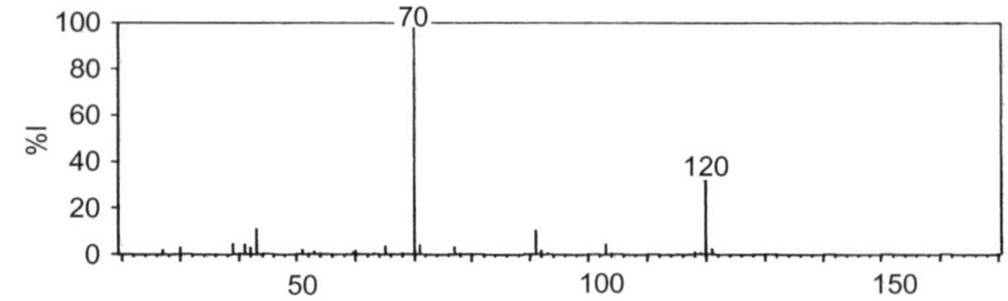

Dose. Aletamine hydrochloride has been given in doses of 375 to 750 mg daily.

Alfacalcidol

Vitamin

Synonyms. 1α-Hydroxycholecalciferol; 1α-hydroxyvitamin D_3.
Proprietary names. Alfa D; AlfaD; Alfadelta; Alfarol; Bondiol; Dediol; Diseon; Doss; EinsAlpha; Etalpha; One-Alpha; Un-Alfa.
(5*Z*,7*E*)-9,10-Secocholesta-5,7,10(19)-triene-1α,3β-diol
$C_{27}H_{44}O_2 = 400.6$
CAS—41294-56-8

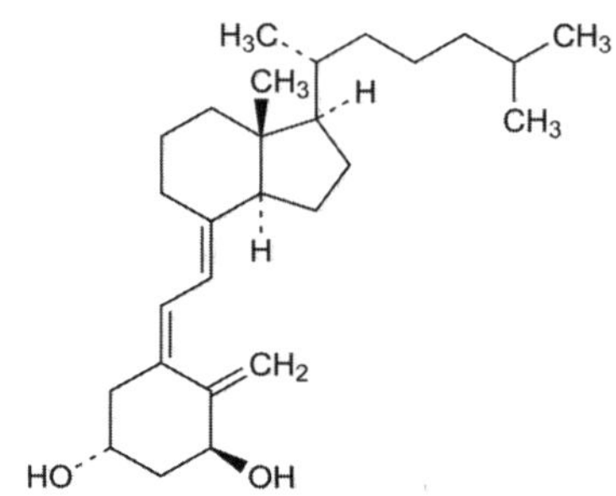

White or almost white crystals that are sensitive to air, heat, and light. M.p. 134° to 136°. It is practically insoluble in water; freely soluble in ethanol; soluble in fatty oils. Reversible isomerisation to pre-alfacalcidol may take place in solution.

Partition Coefficient. Log *P* (octanol/water), 9.11.

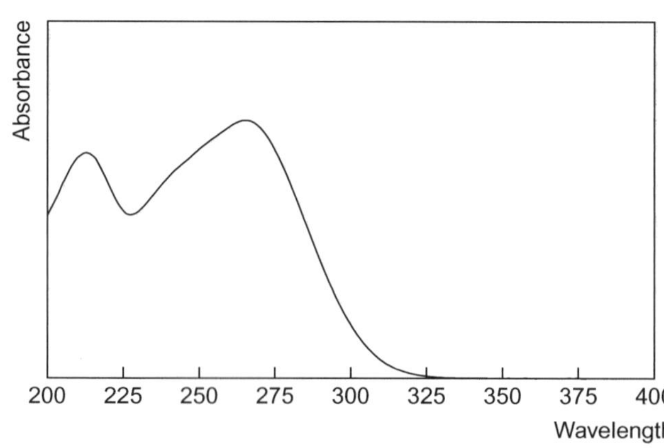

Disposition in the Body. Alfacalcidol is well absorbed after oral administration. Bile is essential for intestinal absorption. It is converted rapidly in the liver to calcitriol and eliminated via bile and kidneys.

Therapeutic concentration. Peak serum concentrations occur about 12 h after a single dose.

Half-life. Plasma, calcitriol 3 to 6 h.

Protein binding. Bound to specific α-globulins for transport.

Dose. Initially 1 μg daily, usual maintenance 0.25 to 1 μg daily.

Alfadolone

General Anaesthetic

Synonym. Alphadolone
3α,21-Dihydroxy-5α-pregnane-11,20-dione
$C_{21}H_{32}O_4$=348.5
CAS—14107-37-0

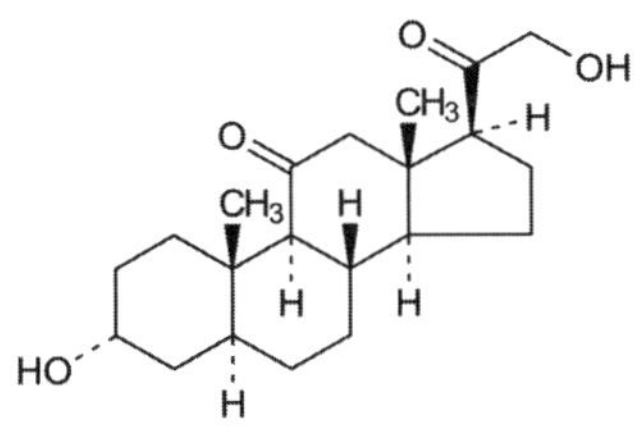

M.p. 167° to 170°.

Alfadolone Acetate
Synonym. It is an ingredient of Alphadione (with alfaxalone)
Proprietary names. It is an ingredient of Alfatesin(e), Alfathesin, Althesin, and Saffan (vet.).
$C_{23}H_{34}O_5$=390.5
CAS—23930-37-2
A white to creamy-white powder. M.p. 175° to 177°.
Practically insoluble in water; soluble 1 in 15 of ethanol and 1 in 2 of chloroform.

Partition Coefficient. Log *P* (octanol/water), 2.67 (alfadolone acetate).

Colour Tests. Antimony Pentachloride—yellow; Naphthol–Sulfuric Acid—orange-brown/orange; Sulfuric Acid—yellow

Thin-layer Chromatography. Alfadolone acetate: system TD—Rf 35; system TE—Rf 71; system TF—Rf 40; system TP—Rf 59; system TQ—Rf 22; system TR—Rf 80; system TS—Rf 45, streaking may occur; system TAD—Rf 62. (*p*-Toluenesulfonic acid solution, positive.)

Ultraviolet Spectrum. Alfadolone acetate: methanol—290 nm (A^1_1=about 2).

Infra-red Spectrum. Principal peaks at wavenumbers 1228, 1758, 1710, 1278, 1010, 1043 cm^{-1} (alfadolone acetate, KBr disk).

Mass Spectrum. Principal peaks at *m/z* 317, 43, 271, 147, 289, 390, 95, 81 (alfadolone acetate).

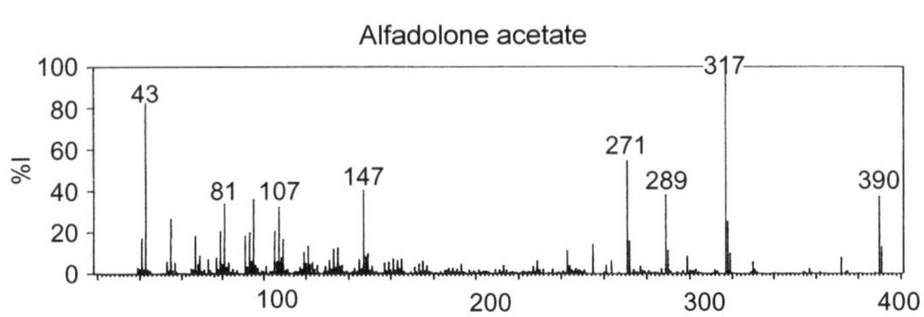

Quantification
Gas chromatography. In plasma: limit of detection 10 μg/L, ECD—A. J. Pateman, *J. Chromatogr.* 1981, *226(15) B Biomed. Appl.*, 213–218. In biological material—H. Heusler, *J. Chromatogr.*, 1985, *340*, 273–319.

Disposition in the Body. Rapidly and widely distributed after injection. Alfadolone acetate is metabolised in the liver to alfadolone and alfadolone glucuronide which are excreted in the urine. Alfadolone is considered to be about 50% as potent an anaesthetic as alfaxalone.

Protein binding. In plasma, 20 to 40%.

Dose. See under Alfaxalone.

Alfaxalone

General Anaesthetic

Synonyms. Alphaxalone. It is an ingredient of Alphadione (with alfadolone acetate).

Proprietary names. It is an ingredient of Alfatesin(e), Alfathesin, Althesin and Saffan (vet.).
(3α,5α)-3-Hydroxypregnane-11,20-dione
$C_{21}H_{32}O_3$=332.5
CAS—23930-19-0

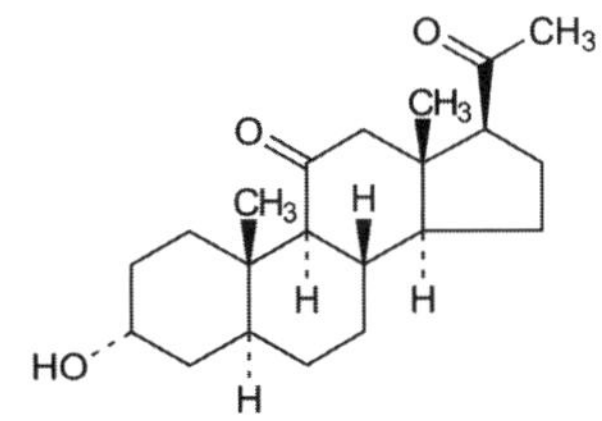

A white to creamy-white powder. M.p. 165° to 171°. Practically insoluble in water; soluble 1 in 10 of ethanol and 1 in 2 of chloroform.

Thin-layer Chromatography. System TP—Rf 60; system TQ—Rf 22; system TR—Rf 90; system TS—Rf 72, streaking may occur. (*p*-Toluenesulfonic acid solution, positive.)

Ultraviolet Spectrum. Methanol—290 nm (A^1_1=about 2).

Infra-red Spectrum. Principal peaks at wavenumbers 1695, 1148, 1220, 1267, 1000, 1252 cm^{-1} (KBr disk).

Quantification.
Gas chromatography. In plasma: limit of detection 10 μg/L, AFID—J. W. Sear *et al.*, *J. Pharm. Pharmacol.*, 1980, *32*, 349–352.

Disposition in the Body. Alfaxalone is rapidly and widely distributed following injection. It undergoes almost 100% first-pass metabolism by reduction of the 20-oxo group and conjugation with glucuronic acid, and is excreted in the urine. About 60% of a dose is excreted in the urine in 24 h and 80% in 5 days.

Therapeutic concentration
During constant intravenous infusion of 18, 52 and 90 μg/min/kg, to 22 subjects, mean steady-state plasma concentrations of 1.9, 2.9 and 3.9 mg/L, respectively, were reported. [J. W. Sear and C. Prys-Roberts, *Br. J. Anaesth.*, 1979, *51*, 861–865].

Half-life. Plasma half-life, about 0.5 h.

Volume of distribution. About 0.8 L/kg.

Clearance. Plasma clearance, about 20 mL/min/kg.

Protein binding In plasma, 20 to 50%.

Note. For a review of the pharmacokinetics of intravenous anaesthetic agents, see P. Duvaldestin, *Clin. Pharmacokinet.*, 1981, *6*, 61–82.

Dose. A solution containing alfaxalone 9 mg and alfadolone acetate 3 mg/mL has been administered intravenously; doses of 0.05 to 0.075 mL/kg and 10 to 20 mL/h have been given to induce and maintain anaesthesia, respectively.

Alfentanil

Narcotic Analgesic

N-[1-[2-(4-Ethyl-4,5-dihydro-5-oxo-1*H*-tetrazol-1-yl)ethyl]-4-(methoxymethyl)-4-piperidinyl]-*N*-phenylpropanamide
$C_{21}H_{32}N_6O_3$=416.5
CAS—71195-58-9

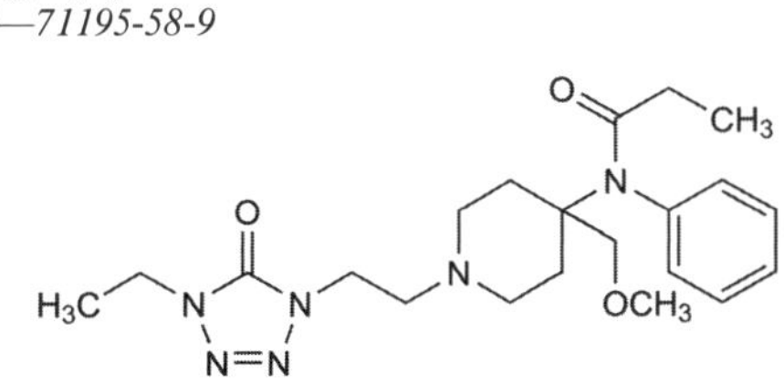

Alfentanil Hydrochloride
Proprietary name. Alfenta; R-39209; Rapifen
$C_{21}H_{32}N_6O_3,HCl,H_2O$=471.0
CAS—69049-06-5 (anhydrous); 70879-28-6 (monohydrate)
A white powder. M.p. 135° to 140°.

Readily soluble in water; soluble 1 in 5 of ethanol, 1 in less than 2 of chloroform, and 1 in less than 2 of methanol; practically insoluble in ether.

Dissociation Constant. pK_a 6.5.

Thin Layer Chromatography. System TB—Rf 16; system TE—Rf 72; system TF—Rf 08; system TAE—Rf 78.

Gas Chromatography. System GA—RI 2970; system GB—RI 3108; system GM—not eluted.

High Performance Liquid Chromatography. System HX—RI 378.

Column: (analytical) Econosphere CN (250 × 4.6 mm i.d., 5 μm); (guard) Newguard Cyano (15 × 3.2 mm i.d., 7 μm). Mobile phase: potassium dihydrogen phosphate (0.01 M) pH 2.8, adjusted with 85% orthophosphoric acid: acetonitrile (65:35 v/v), flow rate 1.4 mL/min. Internal standard: papaverine. Detection: UV (λ = 195 nm). Retention time(s): IS, 4.8 min; alfentanil, 5.3 min. (K. Kumar *et al.*, *J. Pharm. Biomed. Anal.*, 1996, *14*, 667–673).

Ultraviolet Spectrum. Isopropyl alcohol—258 (A_1^1 = 6.3b), 264 (A_1^1 = 4.5b), 268 nm (A_1^1 = 3.1b).

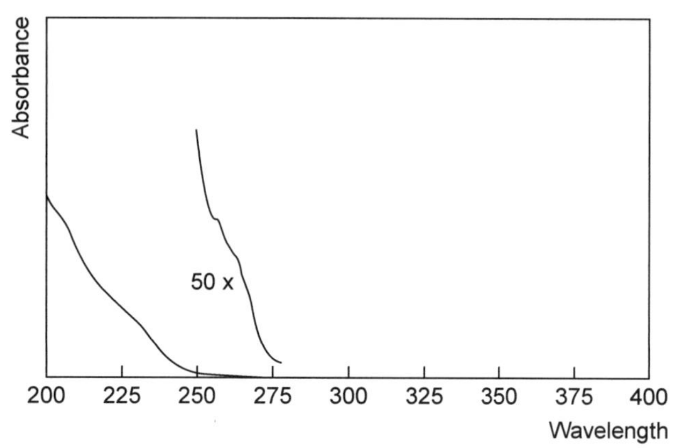

Infra-red Spectrum. Principal peaks at wavenumbers 1722, 1654, 1252, 1109, 715, 967 cm^{-1} (alfentanil hydrochloride, KBr disk).

Quantification

Gas chromatography. In plasma: limit of detection 1 μg/L, AFID—R. Woestenborghs *et al.*, *J. Chromatogr.*, 1981, *224*; *Biomed. Appl.*, *13*, 122–127.

Gas chromatography–mass spectrometry. In urine: limit of detection of metabolites 0.3 μg/L—A. K. Valaer *et al.*, *J. Chromatogr. Sci.*, 1997, *35(10)*, 461–466. In plasma: limit of quantification 0.4 μg/L noralfentanil and 5 μg/L alfentanil (*m/z* 321 and 326)—D. S. Mautz *et al.*, *J. Chromatogr.*, 1994, *658(1)*; *Biomed. Sci. Appl.*, 149–153.

High performance liquid chromatography. In plasma: limit of quantification 2 μg/L and limit of detection 0.25 μg/L, UV detection—K. Kumar *et al.*, *J. Pharm. Biomed. Anal.*, 1996, *14*, 667–673.

Disposition in the Body

Therapeutic concentration

8 patients undergoing lower abdominal surgery were anaesthetised and 1 mg alfentanil was administered epidurally before induction of the general anaesthesia. The mean peak plasma concentration was 9.7 μg/L observed between 30 and 120 min. [F. van der Lely Haak *et al.*, *Anaesthesia*, 1994, *49(10)*, 850–852].

Following an IV injection of 50 μg/kg to 2 subjects, a mean plasma concentration of 0.54 mg/L was reported at 1 min, decreasing to 0.038 mg/L at 1 h. [M. Michiels *et al.*, *J. Pharm. Pharmacol.*, 1983, *35*, 86–93].

Half-life. Plasma half-life, about 1.5 h.

Volume of distribution. About 0.5 to 1.0 L/kg.

Clearance. Plasma clearance, about 3 to 8 mL/min/kg.

Distribution in blood. Plasma : whole blood ratio, 1.6.

Protein binding. In plasma, about 90% (concentration-dependent; decreases at plasma concentrations greater than 0.1 μg/mL).

Note. For a review of alfentanil, see L. E. Mather, *Clin. Pharmacokinet.*, 1983, *8*, 422–446.

Dose. Initially the equivalent of up to 500 μg of alfentanil intravenously, followed by supplementary doses of 250 μg. With assisted ventilation, an initial dose of 30 to 50 μg/kg intravenously may be given.

Alfuzosin

Alpha₁-adrenoceptor Blocker

Synonym. SL-77.499

N-[(3-[(4-Amino-6,7-dimethoxy-2-quinazolinyl)(methyl amino]propyl]tetrahydro-2-furancarboxamide

$C_{19}H_{27}N_5O_4$ = 389.5

CAS—81403-80-7

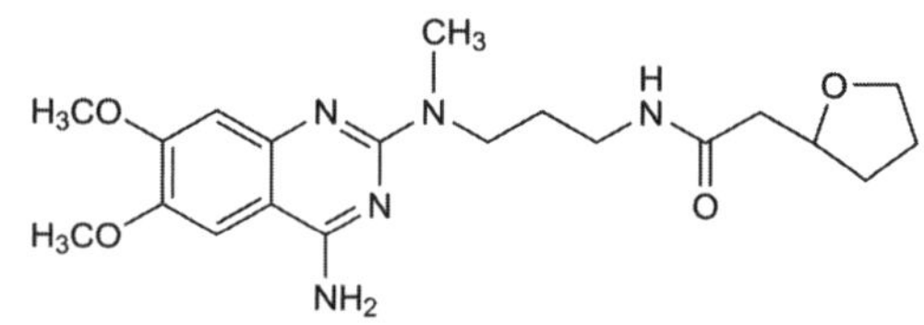

Alfuzosin Hydrochloride

Synonym. SL-77.499-10

Proprietary names. Alfoten; Benestan; Dalfaz; Mittoval; Urion; UroXatral; Xatral.

$C_{19}H_{27}N_5O_4$,HCl = 425.9

CAS—81403-68-1

A white or almost white slightly hygroscopic crystalline powder. M.p. 225°, also reported as 235°. It is freely soluble in water; sparingly soluble in ethanol; practically insoluble in dichloromethane.

Dissociation Constant. pK_a 8.1.

High Performance Liquid Chromatography. System HZ—retention time 2.4 min; system HAA—retention time 10.4 min.

Ultraviolet Spectrum. Neutral (water)—245, 210, 331 nm (hydrochloride).

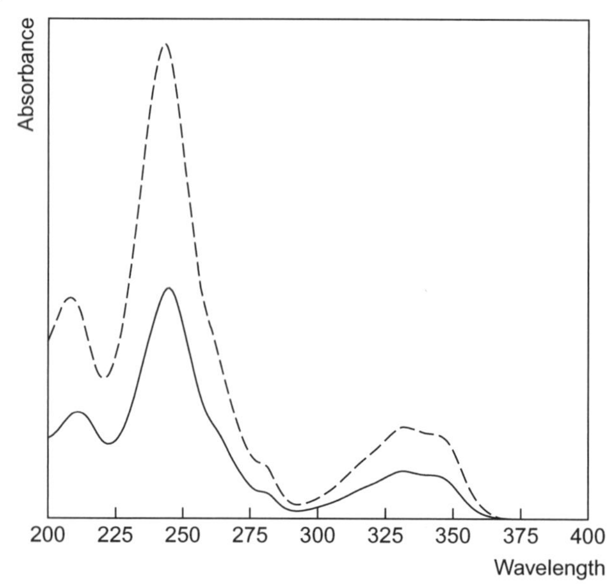

Infra-red Spectrum. Principal peaks at wavenumber 1598, 1492, 1238, 3366, 873 cm^{-1} (hydrochloride).

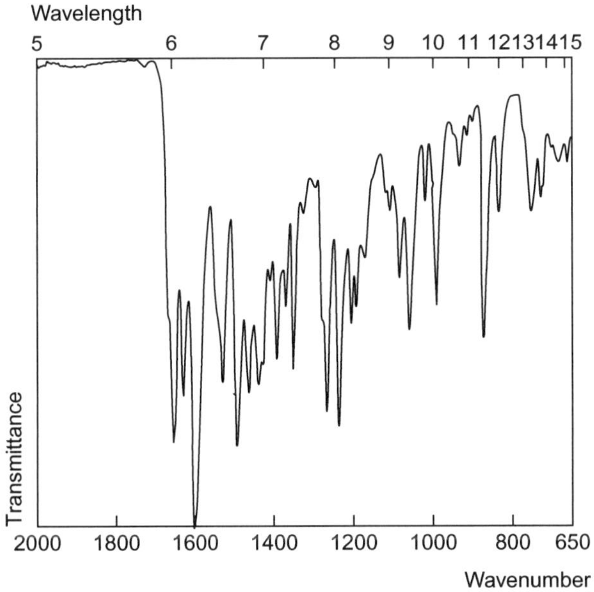

Mass Spectrum. Principal ions at *m/z* 248, 261, 219, 233, 247, 205, 318, 389.

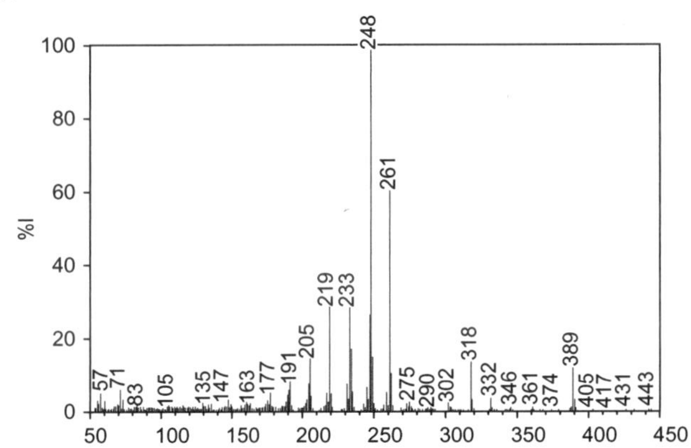

Quantification

High performance liquid chromatography. In blood, plasma, or urine: limit of detection 0.5 to 1.0 µg/L in plasma, fluorescence detection—P. Guinebault *et al.*, *J. Chromatogr.*, 1986, *353*, 361–369. In plasma: limit of detection 1 µg/L for each enantiomer—A. Rouchouse *et al.*, *J. Chromatogr.*, 1990, *506*, 601–610.

Disposition in the Body. Alfuzosin is readily absorbed after oral administration. Peak plasma concentrations occur about 0.5 to 3 h after a dose. It is extensively metabolised in the liver to inactive metabolites and excreted primarily in faeces via bile. About 11% of a dose is excreted unchanged in urine.

Therapeutic concentration

Following oral administration of 1, 2.5, 5 and 10 mg twice daily for 3 days to 6 subjects and 10 mg twice daily to 3 subjects, peak plasma concentrations measured after a dose on the fourth day were 4.1, 11.8, 20.8 and 46.0 µg/L, respectively. These concentrations were observed after 1.8, 1.3, 1.0 and 2.0 h for the doses 1, 2.5, 5 and 10 mg, respectively. All subjects were healthy males, aged between 21 and 32 years with a mean of 23.8 years. [M. G. Scott *et al.*, *Eur. J. Clin. Pharmacol.*, 1989, *37*, 53–58].

Bioavailability. About 64%.

Half-life. Plasma, 3 to 5 h.

Protein binding. In plasma, 90%.

Dose. Up to 10 mg daily.

Alimemazine

Antihistamine/Sedative

Synonym. Trimeprazine

N,N,β-Trimethyl-10*H*-phenothiazine-10-propanamine

$C_{18}H_{22}N_2S=298.4$

CAS—84-96-8

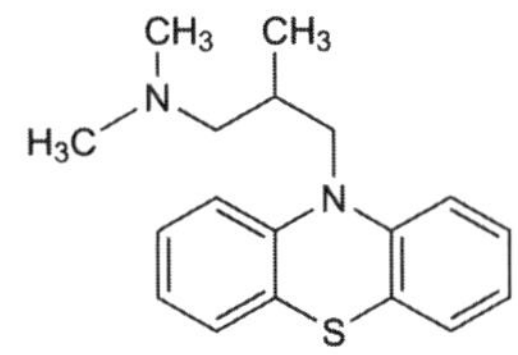

Crystals. M.p. 68°. Its solubility in water is 0.9415 mg/L at 25°.

Alimemazine Tartrate

Proprietary names. Nedeltran; Panectyl; Repeltin; Theralen(e); Vallergan; Variargil.

$(C_{18}H_{22}N_2S)_2,C_4H_6O_6=747.0$

CAS—4330-99-8

A white or slightly cream-coloured crystalline powder which darkens in colour on exposure to light. M.p. 159° to 163°.

Soluble 1 in 4 of water, 1 in 30 of ethanol and 1 in 5 of chloroform; very slightly soluble in ether.

Partition Coefficient. Log *P* (octanol/pH 7.4), 2.9; (octanol/water), 4.71.

Colour Tests. Formaldehyde–Sulfuric Acid—red-violet; Forrest Reagent—brown-red; FPN Reagent—brown-red; Mandelin's Test—violet; Marquis Test—violet

Thin-layer Chromatography. System TA—Rf 58; system TB—Rf 54; system TC—Rf 39; system TE—Rf 77; system TL—Rf 31; system TAE—Rf 32; system TAF—Rf 46. (Dragendorff spray, positive; FPN reagent, pink; acidified iodoplatinate solution, positive; Marquis reagent, pink; ninhydrin spray, positive.)

Gas Chromatography. System GA—alimemazine RI 2305, M (OH-) RI 2650, M (OH-)-AC RI 2600, M (bis-nor-)-AC RI 2765, M (nor-) RI 2335, M (nor-OH-)-AC_2 RI 2930, M (ring) (phenothiazine) RI 2020, M (sulfoxide) RI 2665; system GB—alimemazine RI 2402, M (nor-) RI 2432, M (sulfoxide) RI 2805, M (OH-) RI 2829, M (norsulfoxide) RI 2817, M (nor-OH-) RI 2845; system GC—RI 2646; system GF—RI 2715; system GW—Retention time 20.3 min.

High Performance Liquid Chromatography. System HA—*k* 3.1; system HX—RI 420; system HAX—Retention time 14.9 min; system HAY—Retention time 7.1 min.

Ultraviolet Spectrum. Aqueous acid—251 nm ($A^1_1=926a$), 300 nm; aqueous alkali—256, 310 nm.

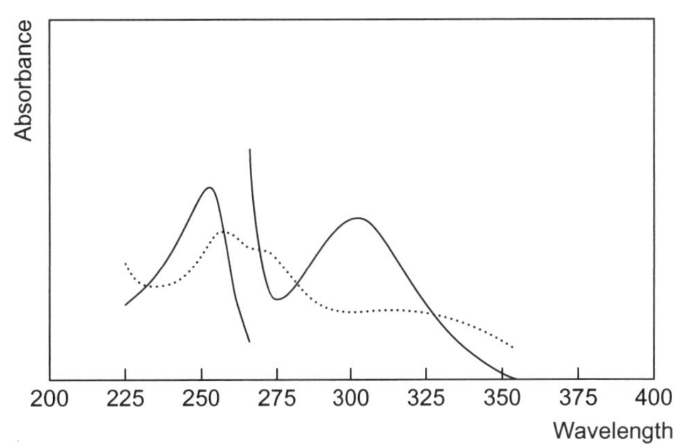

Infra-red Spectrum. Principal peaks at wavenumbers 748, 1248, 1260, 1305, 1590, 1275 cm^{-1} (alimemazine tartrate, KBr disk).

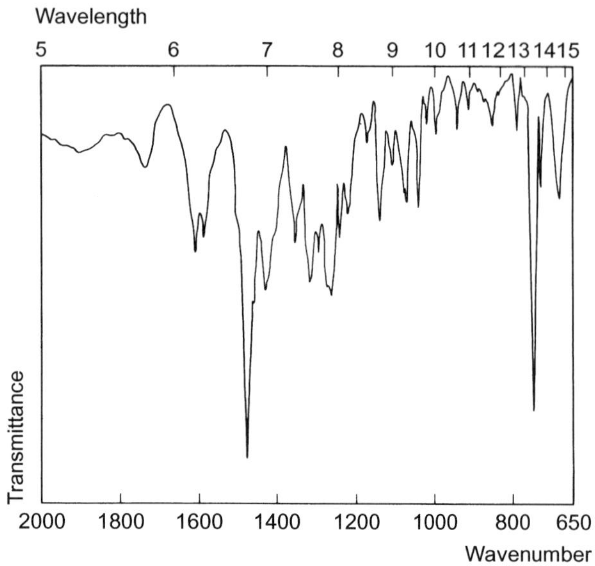

Mass Spectrum. Principal ions at *m/z* 58, 298, 212, 198, 100, 299, 252, 199.

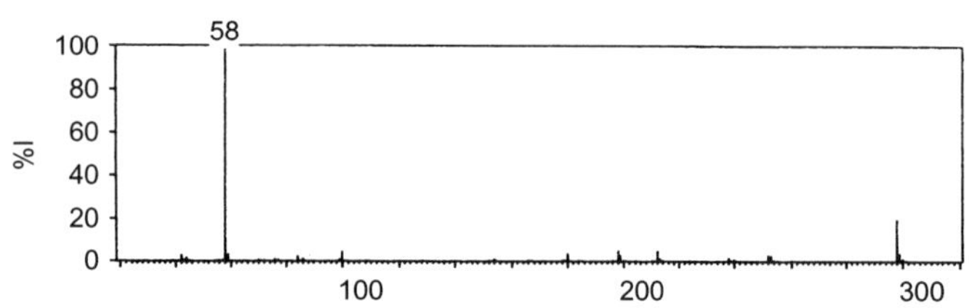

Quantification

Gas chromatography. In body fluid: limit of detection 0.25 to 0.5 μg/L, SID—H. Hattori *et al.*, *J. Chromatogr.*, 1992, *579(2)*, 247–252.

High performance liquid chromatography. In plasma: limit of detection 0.1 μg/L, electrochemical detection—J. E. Holt *et al.*, *Br. J. Clin. Pharmacol.*, 1983, *15*, 604P–605P. Limit of detection 0.004 μg/L, fluorescence detection—G. Diehl and U. Karst, *J. Chromatogr. A.*, 2000, *890(2)*, 281–287.

Disposition in the Body. Readily absorbed after oral administration and widely distributed throughout the body. About 70% of an oral dose is excreted in the urine in 48 h mostly as sulfoxides and glucuronides.

Therapeutic concentration

Following single oral doses of 5 mg to 2 subjects, peak plasma concentrations of 0.8 and 1.8 μg/L were reported at 4 h [G. McKay *et al.*, *J. Chromatogr.*, 1982, *233*; *Biomed. Appl.*, *22*, 417–422].

6 healthy males, aged 20 to 40 years, were administered with 5 mg alimemazine as a syrup and in tablet form, after an overnight fast. The mean peak blood concentrations were 2.34 μg/L after the syrup and 0.95 μg/L with the tablet. These concentrations were observed at 3.5 and 4.5 h, respectively [O. Y.-P. Hu *et al.*, *J. Pharm. Pharmacol.*, 1986, *38*, 172–176].

6 children, aged 1.5 to 9.5 years, were orally administered with 3 mg/kg body weight for 30 to 85 min (median 65 min). The mean peak blood alimemazine concentration was 0.357 μmol/L (range 0.27 to 0.51) observed at 55 to 105 min [S. Sponheim *et al.*, *Pharmacol. Toxicol.*, 1990, *67(3)*, 243–245].

Toxicity

A 50-year-old male was found dead at his home with a suicide note. Toxicological analysis showed that he had a alimemazine concentration of 1.91 mg/L in his blood and 25.05 mg/L in his urine. Noralimemazine was detected in his urine at 13.59 mg/L and alimemazine sulfoxide at 7.84 mg/L. In this case the blood alimemazine concentration was 1000 times greater than reported therapeutic concentrations [P. Kintz and P. Mangin, *TIAFT Bulletin Case Notes*, 1995, *25(3)*].

A 58-year-old man who had a history of clinical depression was found dead at his home. Several empty containers of alimemazine were found near his bed. Alimemazine was detected in his femoral blood at a concentration of 6.52 mg/L; in urine at 6.22 mg/L; bile, 4.44 mg/L; gastric contents, 80.19 mg/L; brain, 19.9 μg/g (the major site of drug disposition); liver, 18.69 μg/g; kidney, 19.13 μg/g; heart, 16.62 μg/g, and in muscle a concentration of 1.43 μg/g. The postmortem blood concentration was 10 000 times that observed at therapeutic levels [P. Kintz *et al.*, *J. Anal. Toxicol.*, 1995, *19(7)*, 591–594].

Half-life. Mean, 6.8 h (children).

Clearance. Blood, 3.7 L/kg/h (children).

Blood distribution. Plasma:red blood cell ratio, 1.17.

Dose. Usually 10 to 40 mg of alimemazine tartrate daily; up to 100 mg daily has been given. Elderly, 10 to 20 mg daily. Children >2 years old, 2.5 to 5 mg three or four times daily.

Allobarbital

Sedative/Barbiturate

Synonyms. Allobarbitone; Diallylbarbitone; Diallylmalonylurea; Diallymalum.

Proprietary name. It is an ingredient of Dialog.

5,5-Di-2-propenyl-2,4,6(1*H*,3*H*,5*H*)pyrimidinetrione

$C_{10}H_{12}N_2O_3$=208.2

CAS—52-43-7

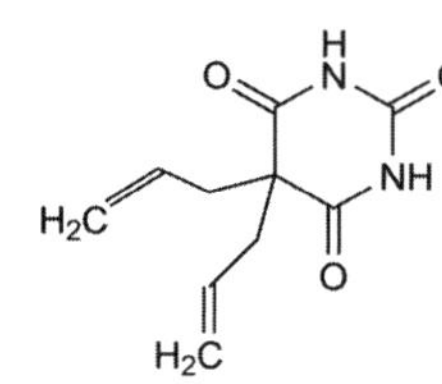

A white crystalline powder. M.p. about 173°.

Soluble 1 in 700 of water, 1 in 15 of ethanol and 1 in 20 of ether; soluble in solutions of alkalis.

Dissociation Constant. pK_a 7.8 (25°).

Colour Tests. Koppanyi–Zwikker Test—violet; Mercurous Nitrate—black; Vanillin Reagent—brown-orange/violet (transient).

Thin-layer Chromatography. System TD—Rf 50; system TE—Rf 34; system TF—Rf 66; system TH—Rf 53; system TAD—Rf 56; system TAE—Rf 87. (Mercurous nitrate spray, black; acidified potassium permanganate solution, yellow-brown.)

Gas Chromatography. System GA—allobarbital RI 1600, allobarbital-Me_2 RI 1636; system GB—allobarbital-Me_2 RI 1505; system GF—allobarbital RI 2340.

High Performance Liquid Chromatography. System HG—*k* 2.46; system HH—*k* 1.33; system HX—RI 346; system HZ—Retention time(s) 2.7 min.

Column: (1) C_{18} RP TSK gel Super-ODS (100 × 4.6 mm i.d., 2 μm); (2) C_{18} RP Hypersil ODS-C_{18} (100 × 4.6 mm i.d., 5 μm). Mobile phase: acetonitrile: 8 mM KH_2PO_4 (30:70 v/v), flow rate 0.4 mL/min. Internal standard: 5-(4-methylphenyl)-5-phenylhydantoin. UV detection (λ=215 nm). Retention time(s): (1) 5.1 min; (2) 5.7 min. (E. Tanaka *et al.*, *Forens. Sci. Int.*, 1997, *85*, 73–82).

Ultraviolet Spectrum. Borax buffer 0.05 M (pH 9.2)—241 (A_1^1=460a); 1 M sodium hydroxide (pH 13)—256 nm (A_1^1=356b).

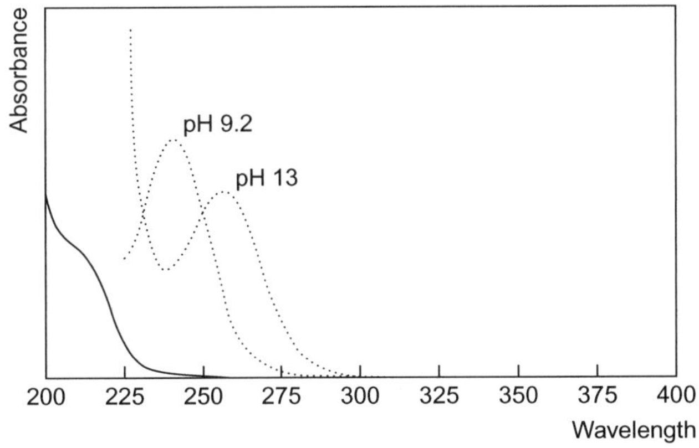

Infra-red Spectrum. Principal peaks at wavenumbers 1687, 1315, 925, 1219, 847, 1640 cm^{-1} (KBr disk).

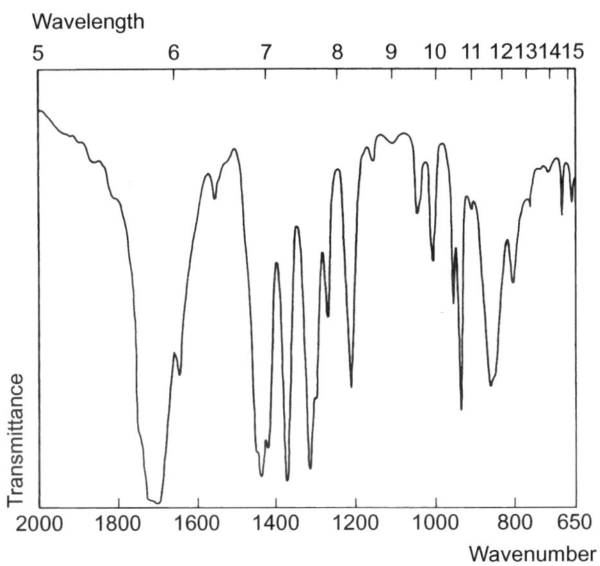

Mass Spectrum. Principal ions at *m/z* 41, 167, 124, 39, 80, 53, 68, 141.

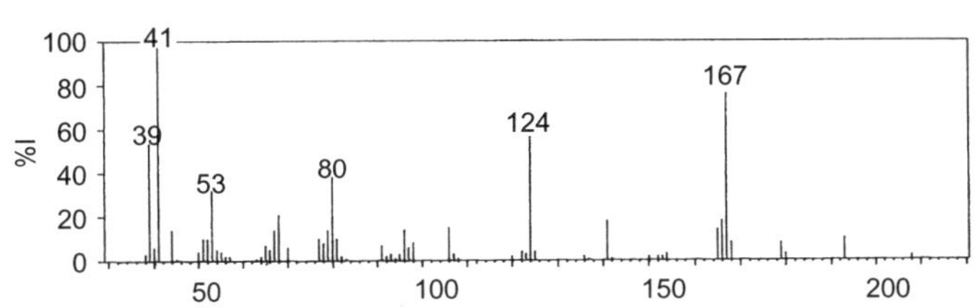

Quantification See under Amylobarbital.

High performance liquid chromatography. In blood, urine, brain and liver: limit of quantification 50 µg/L, UV detection (λ=215 nm)—E. Tanaka *et al.*, *Forens. Sci. Int.*, 1997, *85*, 73–82.

Disposition in the Body. Allobarbital is absorbed after oral administration. It may persist unchanged in the body for up to one week; about 10 to 35% of a dose is slowly excreted unchanged in the urine.

Therapeutic concentration. In plasma, usually in the range 15 to 40 mg/L.

Toxicity. The estimated minimum lethal dose is 2 g. Plasma concentrations of 50 mg/L or more are usually toxic.

Dose. Allobarbital has been given in doses of 90 to 200 mg daily.

Allopurinol

Xanthine-oxidase Inhibitor

Synonyms. HPP; Isopurinol; BW-56158.
Proprietary names. Adenock; Alloprin; Allopur; Aloral; Alositol; Aluline; Anoprolin; Blemimol; Bloxanth; Caplenal; Cosuric; Dabroson; Embarin; Epidropal; Foligan; Gichtex; Hexanurat; Ledopor; Lysuron; Miniplanor; Monarch; Progout; Remin; Sigapural; Takanarumin; Uriscel; Urobenyl; Urtias; Xanturat; Zyloprim; Zyloric.
1,5-Dihydro-4*H*-pyrazolo[3,4-*d*]pyrimidin-4-one
$C_5H_4N_4O$=136.1
CAS—315-30-0

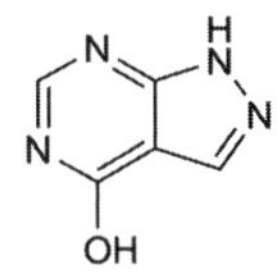

A white microcrystalline powder. No characteristic melting point; it is unchanged up to 300°, after which it begins to darken and at an indefinite high temperature it chars and decomposes. Very slightly soluble in water and ethanol; practically insoluble in chloroform and ether; soluble in dimethylformamide and in dilute solutions of alkali hydroxides.

Dissociation Constant. pK_a 9.4.

Colour Test. Folin–Ciocalteu reagent—grey-blue.

Thin-layer Chromatography. System TE—Rf 21; system TAE—Rf 75.

Gas Chromatography. System GA—RI 882.

High Performance Liquid Chromatography. System HY—RI 128; system HZ—Retention time(s) 1.55 min.

Ultraviolet Spectrum. Aqueous acid (prepared by dissolving in alkali and diluting with acid)—250 (A^1_1=563a); aqueous alkali—257 nm (A^1_1=523a).

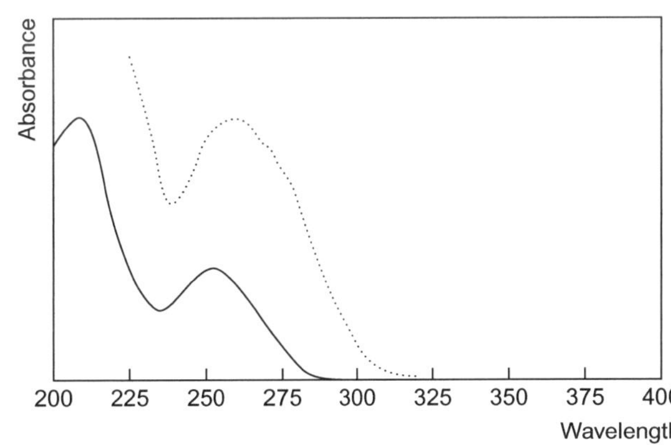

Infra-red Spectrum. Principal peaks at wavenumbers 1692, 1587, 916, 1224, 1235, 956 cm^{-1} (KBr disk).

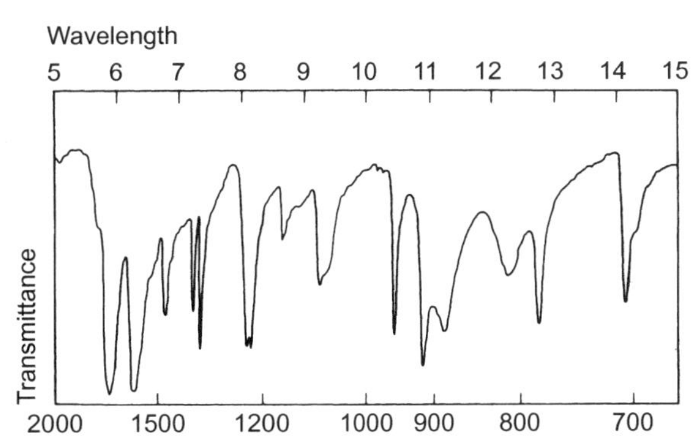

Mass Spectrum. Principal ions at *m/z* 136, 135, 52, 28, 137, 109, 29, 18.

Quantification

Gas chromatography–mass spectrometry. In serum or urine: limit of detection 25 µg/L for allopurinol—C. Lartigue-Mattei *et al.*, *J. Chromatogr.*, 1982, *229*; *Biomed. Appl.*, *18*, 211–216.

High performance liquid chromatography. In plasma and urine: limit of detection 0.1 mg/L and 0.2 mg/L, respectively. UV detection—J. X. de Vries *et al.*, *Arzneimittelforschung*, 1993, *43(1)*, 1072–1075. In plasma or urine: allopurinol and oxipurinol, limit of detection 100 µg/L, UV detection—H. Breithaupt and G. Goebel, *J. Chromatogr.*, 1981, *226*; *Biomed. Appl.*, *15*, 237–242.

Disposition in the Body. Allopurinol is rapidly absorbed after oral administration. The major metabolite, oxipurinol (alloxanthine), is active but less potent than allopurinol. Subjects with a genetic deficiency of xanthine oxidase are unable to metabolise allopurinol to oxipurinol. The excretion of unchanged drug appears to vary with acute or chronic administration, less than 10% of a single dose being excreted unchanged in the urine whereas about 30% is excreted in the urine as unchanged drug after chronic administration. Most of the remainder of a dose is slowly excreted in the urine as oxipurinol; about 20% of a dose is eliminated in the faeces in 72 h.

Therapeutic concentration. Oxipurinol accumulates during chronic administration and may contribute significantly to the therapeutic effect.

10 elderly patients with bronchitis, angina and degenerative bone/joint disease (mean age 76.5 years; range 71 to 93 years) and 9 young volunteers (30.3; 24 to 35 years) were administered 200 mg allopurinol orally and 200 mg intravenously after a standard breakfast. The peak allopurinol concentrations were 1.24 mg/L at 0.8 h and 0.64 mg/L at 1.2 h for the young and elderly subjects, respectively. The peak oxipurinol concentrations were 3.75 mg/L at 4.2 h and 5.63 mg/L at 4.5 h, respectively. [J. X. de Vries *et al.*, *Arzneimittelforschung*, 1993, *43(1)*, 1072–1075].

18 healthy volunteers, aged 22 to 27 years, were administered a single dose of two different tablet formulations of allopurinol with an interval between of 2 weeks. The mean peak concentrations were 1.91 and 1.93 mg/L for allopurinol at 1.17 and 1.53 h, respectively, and for the metabolite, oxipurinol, 4.59 and 4.78 mg/L at 5.22 and 4.94 h, respectively. [W. Barthel *et al.*, *Int. J. Clin. Pharmacol. Ther.*, 1999, *37(3)*, 148–152].

Following a single oral dose of 300 mg given to 6 subjects, peak plasma concentrations of 1.4 to 2.6 mg/L (mean 2) of allopurinol and 4.4 to 7.8 mg/L (mean 6.3) of oxipurinol were attained in about 0.5 to 2 h and 2 to 5 h, respectively. [H. Breithaupt and M. Tittel, *Eur. J. Clin. Pharmacol.*, 1982, *22*, 77–84].

Following daily oral administration of 300 mg to 7 subjects, steady-state serum concentrations of oxipurinol, determined immediately prior to a dose, were reported to range from 3.4 to 19.4 mg/L (mean 9.7). [G. P. Rodnan *et al.*, *J. Am. Med. Assoc.*, 1975, *231*, 1143–1147].

Bioavailability. About 90%

Half-life. Plasma half-life, allopurinol about 0.5 to 2 h, oxipurinol 12 to 40 h.

Volume of distribution. About 0.6 L/kg.

Clearance. Plasma clearance, about 11 mL/min/kg.

Protein binding. In plasma, allopurinol less than 5%, oxipurinol about 17%.

Dose. 100 to 600 mg daily.

Allylestrenol

Progestogen

Synonym. Allyloestrenol
Proprietary names. Gestanin; Gestanon; Gestanyn; Orageston; Turinal.
(17β)-17-(2-Propenyl)-estr-4-en-17-ol
$C_{21}H_{32}O = 300.5$
CAS—432-60-0

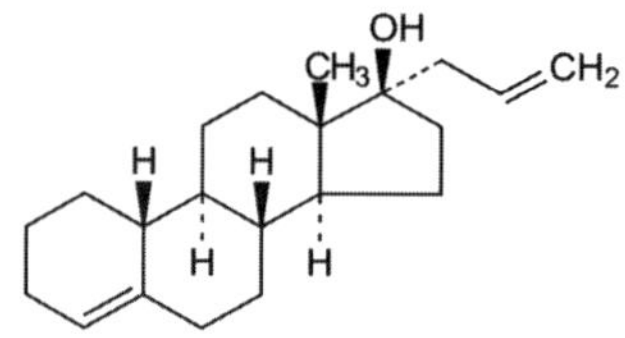

Crystals. M.p. 80°. Practically insoluble in water; soluble in ethanol, chloroform and ether.

Ultraviolet Spectrum. No significant absorption, 230 to 360 nm.

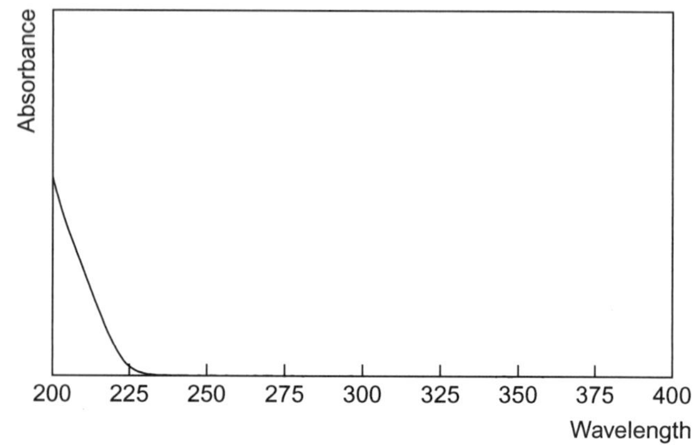

Infra-red Spectrum. Principal peaks at wavenumbers 905, 1008, 999, 1020, 1101, 985 cm^{-1} (Nujol mull).

Dose. Allylestrenol has been given in doses of 5 to 20 mg daily.

Almotriptan

Anti-migraine

Synonym. LAS-31416
1-[[[3-[2-(Dimethylamino)ethyl-1H-indol-5-yl]methyl]sulfonyl]pyrrolidine
$C_{17}H_{25}N_3O_2S = 335.5$
CAS—154323-57-6

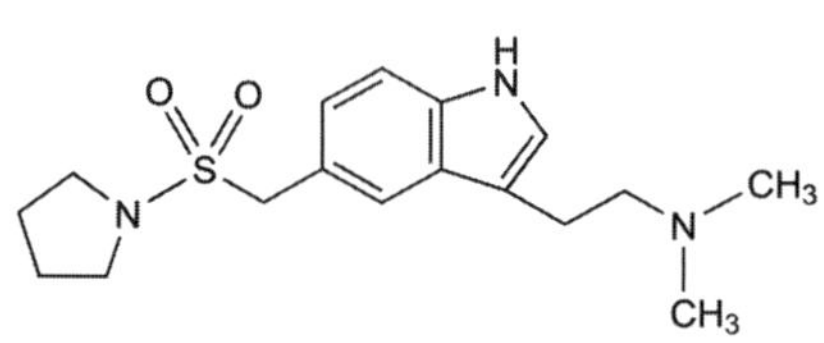

Almotriptan Maleate
Synonym. PNU-180638E
Proprietary names. Almogran; Axert.
$C_{19}H_{25}N_3O_2S,C_4H_6O_5 = 469.6$
CAS—181183-52-8

Quantification

High performance liquid chromatography–mass spectrometry. In plasma and urine: lower limit of quantification 0.5 µg/L in plasma and 50 µg/L in urine, tandem MS detection—J. C. Fleishaker *et al.*, *Br. J. Clin. Pharmacol.*, 2001, *51*, 437–441.

Disposition in the Body. Almotriptan is well absorbed after oral administration and metabolised in the liver by monoamine oxidase and cytochrome P450 isoenzymes (CYP3A4 and CYP2D6). Metabolites are inactive. It is eliminated by a number of pathways and 40 to 50% of a dose is recovered unchanged in urine.

Therapeutic concentration

12 healthy male and female volunteers aged 18 to 51 years (mean, 31 years) were treated with 12.5 mg almotriptan with 1 week wash-out periods in-between. The peak plasma concentration was 39.6 µg/L at 2.67 h. [J. C. Fleishaker *et al.*, *Clin. Pharmacol. Ther.*, 2000, *67(5)*, 498–503].

11 healthy women and 3 men, aged 18 to 55 years (mean, 35.3 years), were administered with a single 12.5 mg dose of almotriptan after a 10 h fast. The same dose was also administered on day 8 of treatment after 20 mg three

times daily of fluoxetine for days 1 to 8. The peak plasma concentration of almotriptan was 44.3 µg/L for the single dose and 52.5 µg/L for the dose administered with fluoxetine. The time to reach these concentrations was 2.46 and 1.86 h, respectively. [J. C. Fleishaker *et al.*, *J. Clin. Pharmacol.*, 2001, *41(2)*, 217–223].

Bioavailability. 69 to 80%.

Half-life. 3.1 to 3.6 h.

Volume of distribution. 249 L.

Clearance. 26.6 L/h.

Dose. 12.5 mg repeated after 2 h if migraine recurs with a maximum of 25 mg in 24 h.

Aloin

Purgative

A crystalline substance extracted from aloes and consisting almost entirely of barbaloin.
10-Glucopyranosyl-1,8-dihydroxy-3-(hydroxymethyl)-9(10*H*)-anthracenone
$C_{21}H_{22}O_9$=418.4
CAS—8015-61-0; 1415-73-2 (barbaloin)

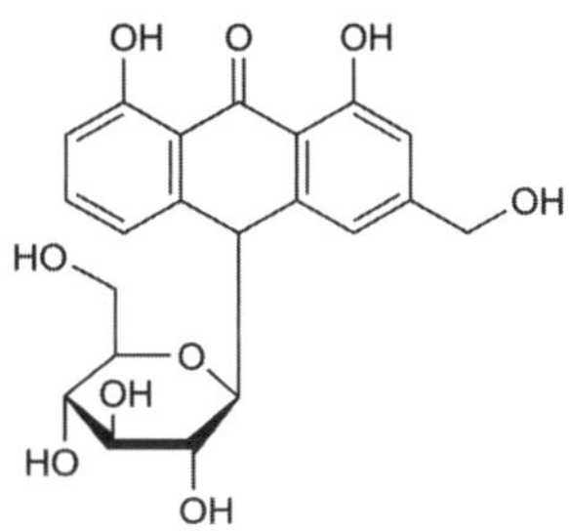

A pale or dull yellow crystalline powder. It darkens on exposure to light. M.p. of barbaloin about 148°. It quickly forms a monohydrate, m.p. 70° to 80°. Almost completely soluble 1 in 130 of water; soluble 1 in 20 of ethanol; soluble in acetone; very slightly soluble in chloroform and ether.

Colour Tests. Ferric chloride—brown; Folin–Ciocalteu reagent—blue; Liebermann's test—black; Millon's reagent—pink→red.

Ultraviolet Spectrum. Aqueous acid—245, 253, 300 nm; aqueous alkali—268 nm.

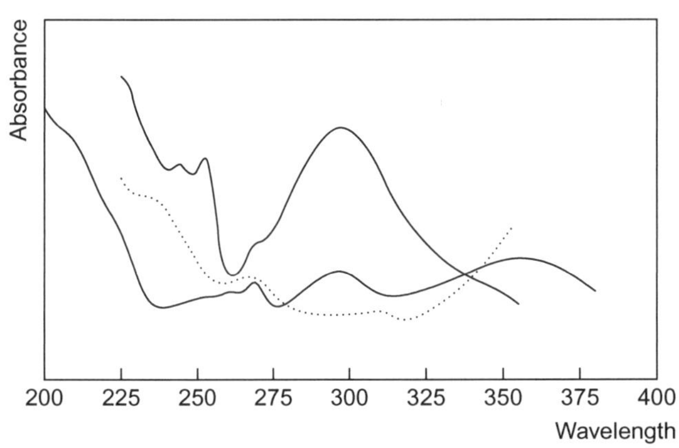

Thin-layer Chromatography. Plate: silica gel (Merck). Mobile phase: methyl-isobutylketone:*m*-xylene:hexane:glacial acetic acid (60:20:12:0.5 v/v). Detection: sprayed with potassium hydroxide (3 M) and examined at 254 nm (yellow/red) and 366 nm (orange/red). Rf 0.75. [S. L. Perkins and J. F. Livesey, *Clin. Biochem.*, 1993, *26*, 179–181].

Dose. Aloin has been given in doses of 13 to 60 mg.

Aloxiprin

Analgesic

Proprietary names. Lyman; Palaprin Forte; Rumatral.
A polymeric condensation product of aluminium oxide and aspirin which contains about 83% of total salicylates. Approx. formula:
$Al_3O_2[C_6H_4(OOCCH_3)COO]_5$
CAS—9014-67-9

A fine white or slightly pink powder.
Practically insoluble in water, ethanol, and ether; soluble 1 in 200 of chloroform.

Thin-layer Chromatography. System TD—Rf 04; system TE—Rf 09; system TF—Rf 10; system TAD—Rf 22.

Ultraviolet Spectrum. Aqueous acid—231 nm; aqueous alkali—298 nm.

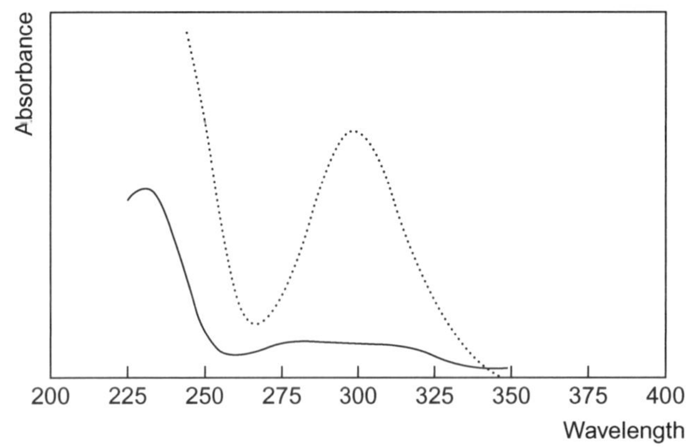

Infra-red Spectrum. Principal peaks at wavenumbers 1597, 1198, 1562, 1220, 1745, 760 cm^{-1} (KBr disk).

Mass Spectrum. Principal ions at *m/z* 43, 45, 60, 120, 42, 92, 138, 44.

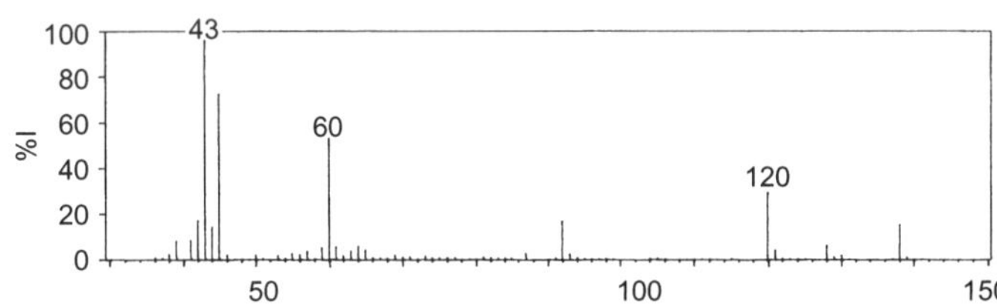

Disposition in the Body. Aloxiprin is hydrolysed to aspirin in the gastro-intestinal tract.

Dose. Up to 100 mg/kg daily, by mouth.

Alpha Tocoferil Acetate

Vitamin E Activity

Synonyms. α-Tocopherol Acetate; *dl*-α-Tocopherol Acetate; α-Tocoferil Acetate; Vitamin E Acetate.
Proprietary names. Aquasol E; Ephynal; Evion; Tocomine; Tokols (*d*= +); Vita-E (*d*= +); Detulin; Eusovit.
(±)-α-Tocopheryl acetate
$C_{31}H_{52}O_3$=472.8
CAS—52225-20-4

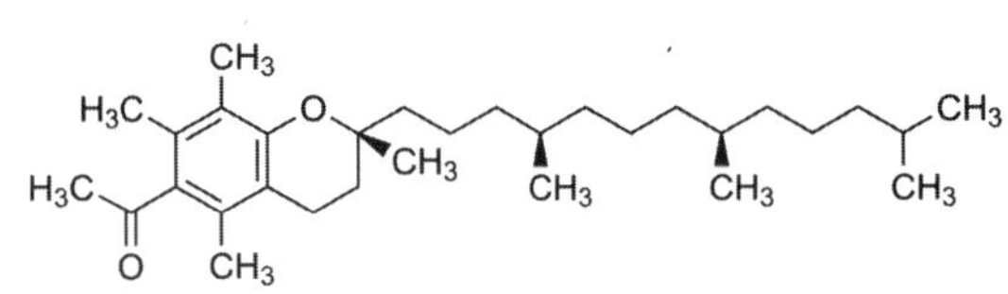

A clear, slightly greenish-yellow, viscous, oily liquid. Relative density 0.952 to 0.966.

Practically insoluble in water; soluble in ethanol; freely soluble in dehydrated alcohol, chloroform, and ether.

Ultraviolet Spectrum. Methanol—284 nm (A_1^1=43a).

Infra-red Spectrum. Principal peaks at wavenumbers 1210, 1755, 1075, 1105, 1160, 1250 cm^{-1} (thin film).

Alphachloralose

Rodenticide

Synonyms. α-Chloralosane; Chloralose; Glucochloral; Glucochloralose.
Proprietary names. Alfamat; Alphabird; Alphakil; Alphamouse; Aphosal; Dulcidor; Murex; Somi.
(*R*)-1,2-*O*-(2,2,2-trichloroethylidene)-α-D-glucofuranose
$C_8H_{11}Cl_3O_6$=309.5
CAS—15879-93-3

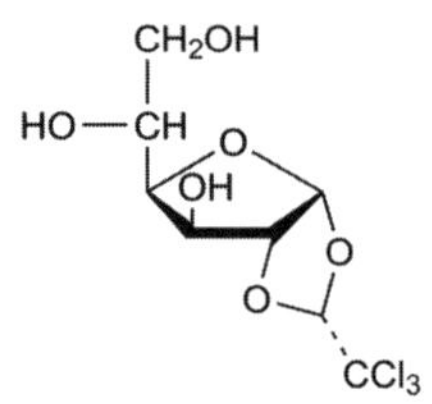

M.p. 182° to 184°.
It is soluble in water 4.44 g/L at 15°.

Partition Coefficient. Log *P* (octanol/water), 1.02.

Quantification

Gas chromatography–mass spectrometry. In blood, bile, and tissue: limit of detection 0.5 mg/L (mg/kg)—P. Kintz *et al.*, *Forens. Sci. Int.*, 1999, *104*, 59–63.

Disposition in the Body. Alphachloralose is detected in urine as the parent compound and also as the *β*-isomer.

Toxicity. The toxic dose of alphachloralose is approximately 1 g in adults and 20 mg/kg in infants.

> An 18-year-old man was found dead at home with 3 bags, which had contained 5 g 100% alphachloralose. Postmortem toxicological analysis showed that the man had a peripheral blood alphachloralose concentration of 175.7 mg/L, cardiac blood concentration of 282.2 mg/L, and bile concentration of 279.6 mg/L. No other drugs or ethanol was detected. [P. Kintz *et al.*, *Forens. Sci. Int.*, 1999, *104*, 59–63].

Alphaprodine

Narcotic Analgesic

Synonyms. Prisilidene; (±)-α-Prodine.
(*cis*)-1,3-Dimethyl-4-phenyl-4-piperidinol propanoate
$C_{16}H_{23}NO_2$=261.4
CAS—77-20-3; 15867-21-7 (±)

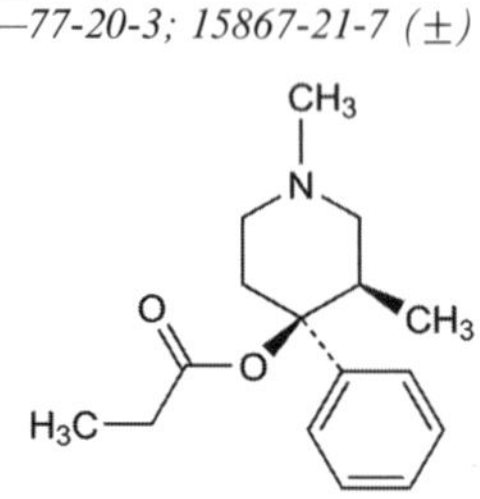

(+)-form

Practically insoluble in water; soluble in chloroform.

Alphaprodine Hydrochloride

Proprietary name. Nisentil
$C_{16}H_{23}NO_2$,HCl=297.8
CAS—*561-78-4 (±)*
A white crystalline powder. M.p. 218° to 220°.
Soluble 1 in 2 of water, 1 in 7 of ethanol, 1 in 47 of acetone and 1 in 3 of chloroform; very slightly soluble in ether.

Dissociation Constant. pK_a 8.7 (20°).

Colour Tests. Mandelin's test—blue-grey; Marquis test—brown-red.

Thin-layer Chromatography. System TA—Rf 50; system TB—Rf 30; system TC—Rf 35; system TE—Rf 62; system TF—Rf 01; system TL—Rf 11; system TAE—Rf 28; system TAJ—Rf 23; system TAK—Rf 05; system TAL—Rf 60. (Dragendorff spray, positive; Acidified iodoplatinate solution, positive; Marquis reagent, red-brown.)

Gas Chromatography. System GA—RI 1792; system GB—RI 1862.

High Performance Liquid Chromatography. System HA—*k* 2.8 (tailing peak); system HX—RI 363; system HY—RI 317.

Ultraviolet Spectrum. Aqueous acid—251, 257 (A_1^1=9a), 263 nm. No alkaline shift.

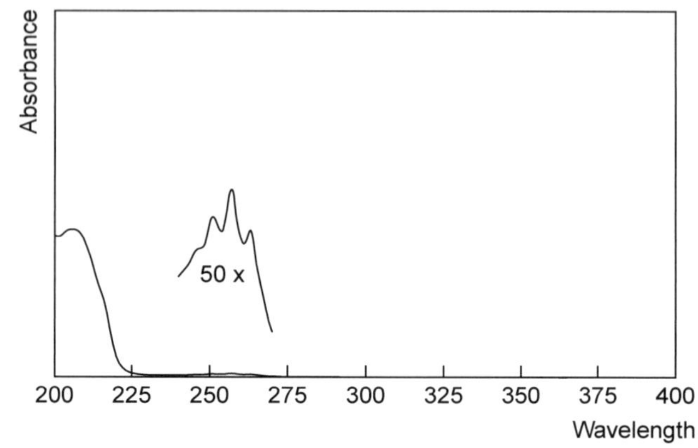

Infra-red Spectrum. Principal peaks at wavenumbers 1740, 1178, 1134, 694, 1030, 1055 cm^{-1} (KBr disk).

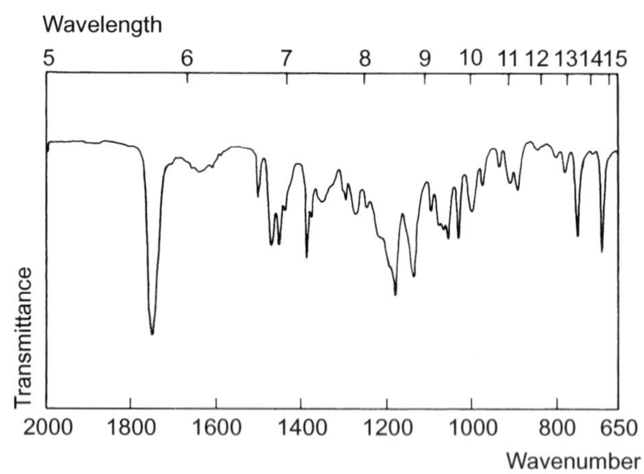

Mass Spectrum. Principal ions at *m/z* 172, 187, 84, 57, 42, 188, 44, 43.

Quantification

Gas chromatography. In plasma: limit of detection 30 µg/L, FID—D. L. Fung *et al.*, *J. Clin. Pharmacol.*, 1980, *20*, 37–41.

Disposition in the Body. Alphaprodine is a homologue of pethidine but its action is more rapid in onset and of shorter duration.

Therapeutic concentration

> After a rapid IV injection of 0.5 mg/kg to 6 subjects, plasma concentrations of about 0.8 mg/L were measured after 5 min, declining to 0.07 mg/L at 5 h. [D. L. Fung *et al.*, *J. Clin. Pharmacol.*, 1980, *20*, 37–41].

Toxicity. The estimated minimum lethal dose is 0.1 g. Prolonged use of alphaprodine is liable to produce dependence of the morphine type.

> The following post-mortem tissue concentrations were reported in an accidental fatality caused by the IV administration of 40 mg of alphaprodine: blood 0.62 mg/L, liver 0.97 µg/g, urine 0.30 mg/L; a blood-alcohol concentration of 1.7 mg/L was also reported. [E. Griesemer and G. R. Nakamura, *Bull. Int. Ass. Forens. Toxicol.*, 1973, *9(1–2)*, 5].

Half-life. Plasma half-life, about 2 h.

Volume of distribution. About 2 L/kg.

Clearance. Plasma clearance, about 10 mL/min/kg.

Dose. 20 to 60 mg of alphaprodine hydrochloride by subcutaneous injection, or 10 to 30 mg intravenously.

Alprazolam

Anxiolytic

Proprietary names. Alpralid; Alpraz; Alprox; Alzam; Anxirid; Apo-Alpraz; Apox; Azor; Calmax; Cassadan; Drimpam; Esparon; Gerax; Kalmor; Mialin; Novo-Alprazol; Nu-Alpraz; Panix; Ralozam; Valeans; Xanagis; Xanax; Xanolam; Xanor; Zopax.

8-Chloro-1-methyl-6-phenyl-4*H*-[1,2,4]triazolo[4,3-*a*][1,4]-benzodiazepine

$C_{17}H_{13}ClN_4$=308.8

CAS—28981-97-7

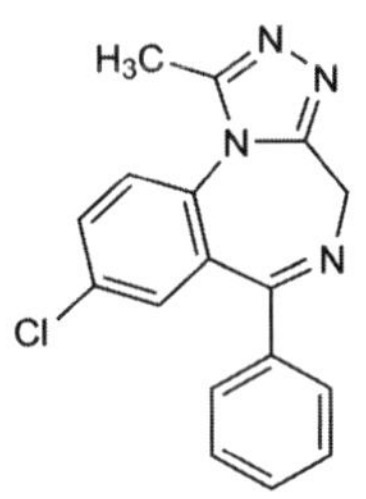

A white crystalline powder. M.p. 228° to 228.5° (from ethyl acetate). Practically insoluble in water; sparingly soluble in alcohol and in acetone; freely soluble in chloroform and dichloromethane.

Dissociation Constant. pK_a 2.4.

Partition Coefficient. Log *P*, 2.12.

Thin-layer Chromatography. System TA—Rf 67; system TB—Rf 01; system TC—Rf 57; system TD—Rf 07; system TE—Rf 47; system TF—Rf 02; system TL—Rf 14; system TAD—Rf 40; system TAE—Rf 67; system TAF—Rf 66.

Gas Chromatography. System GA—alprazolam RI 3100, M (α-OH-) RI 3045, M (OH-) RI 3245, M (4-OH-) not eluted; system GB—alprazolam RI 3108, M (OH-) not eluted.

Column: Hydroguard (5 m × 0.32 mm i.d.) guard column coupled to BP1 polydimethylsiloxane (30 m × 0.25 mm i.d., 0.25 μm film thickness) column. Carrier gas: helium, flow rate 1.2 mL/min. Injector temperature: 70°. Column temperature: 65° for 1 min, to 250° at 15°/min, held for 8 min, to 300° at 10°/min and held for 2 min. MS detection. Retention time: 21.49 min. [D. Borrey *et al.*, *J. Chromatogr. A*, 2001, *910(1)*, 105–118.]

High Performance Liquid Chromatography. System HI—*k* 4.70; system HK—*k* 2.79; system HX—RI 470; system HY—RI 379; system HZ—retention time 4.0 min; system HAA—retention time 17.0 min; system HAL—retention time 6.3 min; system HAM—not detected; system HAX—retention time 6.4 min; system HAY—retention time 6. 4 min; system HBH—*k* 3.35; system HBI—*k* 1.28.

Column: C_{18} Hypersil (100 × 4.6 mm i.d., 3 μm). Mobile phase: acetonitrile:phosphate buffer (0.04 M, pH 4.5 with 0.4 % octylamine) (35:65), flow rate, 1 mL/min. UV detection (λ = 240 nm). Retention time: 3.5 and 5.0 min for α-hydroxyalprazolam and alprazolam, respectively. [M. Segura *et al.*, *J. Anal. Toxicol.*, 2001, *25(2)*, 130–136.]

Column: C_{18} ODS (150 × 4.6 mm i.d., 5 μm) at 30°. Mobile phase: methanol:water with 1% diethylamine (pH 6) (60:40), flow rate, 1.5 mL/min. UV detection (λ = 240 nm). [A. J. Jenkins *et al.*, *J. Anal. Toxicol.*, 1997, *21(3)*, 218–220.]

Ultraviolet Spectrum. Aqueous acid—260 nm.

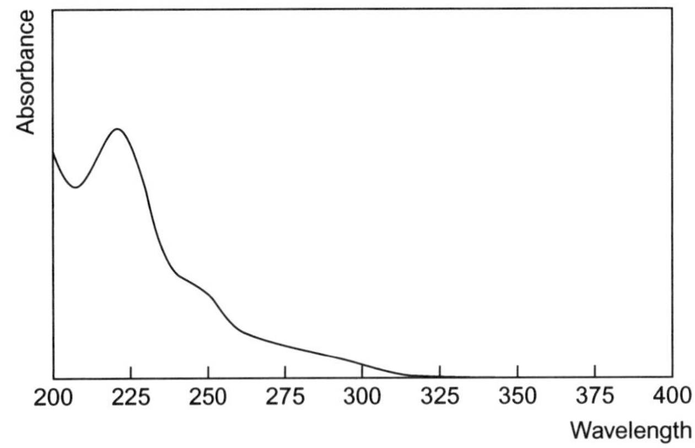

Infra-red Spectrum. Principal peaks at wavenumbers 1490, 1610, 697, 1316, 1540, 827 cm^{-1} (KBr disk). Three polymorphic forms may occur.

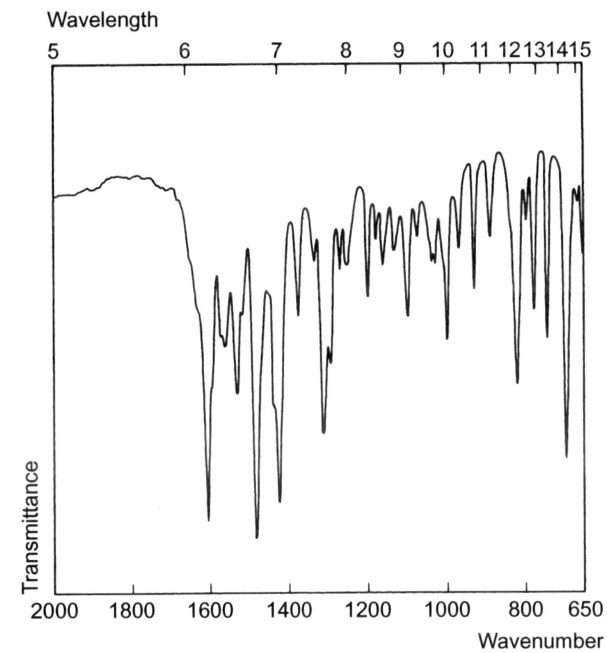

Mass Spectrum. Principal ions at *m/z* 308, 279, 204, 273, 77, 307, 310, 309.

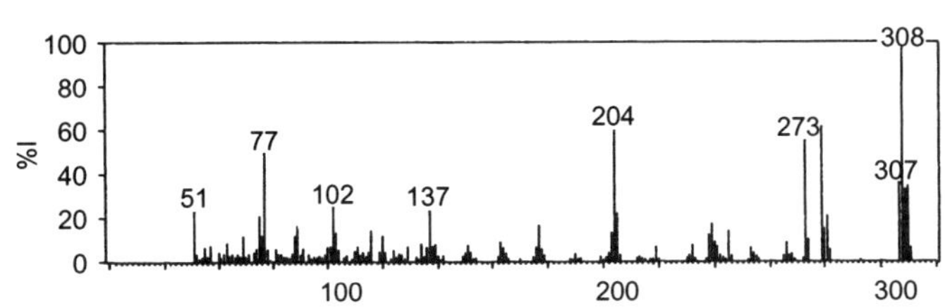

Quantification

Gas chromatography. In plasma or whole blood: alprazolam and other benzodiazepines, NPD and ECD—P. Lillsunde and T. Seppala, *J. Chromatogr.*, 1990, *533*, 97–110. In plasma: alprazolam and other anxiolytics, NPD and ECD—Y. Gaillard *et al.*, *J. Chromatogr.*, 1993, *622*, 197–208. In plasma or urine: alprazolam and other benzodiazepines, limits of detection 0.01 to 0.45 μmol/L in urine and 0.01 to 0.48 μmol/L in plasma—K. J. Reubsaet *et al.*, *J. Pharm. Biomed. Anal.*, 1998, *18*, 667–680.

Gas chromatography–mass spectrometry. In urine: alprazolam and other benzodiazepines, limits of quantification 13 to 25 μg/L—W. A. Joern, *J. Anal. Toxicol.*, 1992, *16*, 363–367. In plasma: alprazolam and triazolam, limit of quantification for alprazolam 4 μg/L, NICI—E. R. Cairns *et al.*, *J. Anal. Toxicol.*, 1994, *18*, 1–6. In urine: alprazolam and other benzodiazepines, limit of quantification 0.16 mg/L—D. A. Black *et al.*, *J. Anal. Toxicol.*, 1994, *18*, 185–188 and D. A. Black *et al.*, *J. Anal. Toxicol.*, 1995, *19*, 58–59. In plasma: alprazolam and α-hydroxyalprazolam, limit of quantification 0.25 μg/L—K. M. Hold *et al.*, *J. Mass Spectrom.*, 1996, *31*, 1033–1038. In urine: alprazolam, α-hydroxyalprazolam, 4-hydroxyalprazolam and other benzodiazepines, limits of detection 13 to 30 μg/L—D. Borrey *et al.*, *J. Chromatogr. B. Biomed. Sci. Appl.*, 2001, *765*, 187–197. Limit of quantification 2.5 to 5 μg/L (full scan) and 0.1 to 0.5 μg/L (SIM, *m/z* 279)—D. Borrey *et al.*, *J. Chromatogr. A*, 2001, *910*, 105–118.

High performance liquid chromatography. In serum: alprazolam and its active metabolites—V. D. Schmith *et al.*, *J. Chromatogr.*, 1991, *568*, 253–260. In plasma: alprazolam, limit of quantification 1 μg/L—W. Rieck and D. Platt, *J. Chromatogr.*, 1992, *578*, 259–263. In serum: alprazolam and estazolam—A. Goldnik *et al.*, *Acta Pol. Pharm.*, 1994, *51*, 311–312. In postmortem blood: limit of quantification 18 μg/L—M. A. Hall *et al.*, *J. Anal. Toxicol.*, 1995, *19*, 511–513. In serum or plasma: limit of detection 5 nmol/L, UV detection—K. K. Akerman *et al.*, *Clin. Chem.*, 1996, *42*, 1412–1416. In plasma and tissue: limit of detection 200 μg/L for alprazolam—A. J. Jenkins *et al.*, *J. Anal. Toxicol.*, 1997, *21*, 218–220. In urine: limits of detection, 9.2 μg/L and 8.5 μg/L for alprazolam and α-hydroxyalprazolam, respectively—M. Segura *et al.*, *J. Anal. Toxicol.*, 2001, *25*, 130–136.

High performance liquid chromatography–mass spectrometry. In plasma: alprazolam and α-hydroxyalprazolam, limit of detection 0.05 μg/L—D. J. Crouch *et al.*, *J. Anal. Toxicol.*, 1999, *23*, 479–485.

Disposition in the Body. Readily absorbed after oral administration and undergoes extensive metabolism. The major metabolites are α-hydroxyalprazolam, 4-hydroxyalprazolam (both active), and a benzophenone derivative of alprazolam. About 80% of a dose is excreted in the urine in 72 h of which 11% is unchanged drug, 15% is α-hydroxyalprazolam, and 9% is the benzophenone metabolite. Small amounts of desmethylalprazolam and 4-hydroxyalprazolam are also excreted in the urine. About 7% of a dose is eliminated in the faeces.

Therapeutic concentration. The serum therapeutic concentration range is 0.005 to 0.05 mg/L and has also been reported as 0.025 to 0.102 mg/L.

After a single oral dose of 1 mg given to 10 subjects, peak plasma concentrations of 0.011 to 0.020 mg/L (mean 0.015) were attained in about 1.75 h. Following daily oral doses of 0.5 mg three times a day to the same subjects, minimum steady-state plasma concentrations of 0.006 to 0.017 mg/L (mean 0.011) and a mean maximum steady-state plasma concentration of 0.018 mg/L were reported. [R. B. Smith *et al.*, *Clin. Pharm.*, 1983, *2*, 139–143.]

In 227 patients treated for panic disorder with alprazolam (dosage titrated up to 6 mg daily), after 3 weeks of treatment, alprazolam plasma levels were significantly correlated with daily dosage—70% of those with levels greater than 0.02 mg/L achieved complete remission of attacks compared with 30% of those with levels below 0.02 mg/L. At week 8, plasma alprazolam levels no longer correlated with efficacy. [D. J. Greenblatt *et al.*, *Arch. Gen. Psychiatry*, 1993, *50*, 715–722.]

Toxicity. The serum toxic concentration range is 0.1 to 0.4 mg/L.

In a fatality attributed to acute alprazolam toxicity, the following postmortem tissue concentrations were reported for alprazolam and α-hydroxyalprazolam, respectively: heart blood 2.1 mg/L and not detected, subclavian blood 2.3 and 0.12 mg/L, urine 1.0 and 1.4 mg/L, bile 2.8 and 1.3 mg/L, vitreous humour 0.58 mg/L and not detected, liver 9.2 and 0.83 μg/g, kidney 3.8 μg/g and not detected, stomach contents 13 mg in 110 mL and not detected; the alprazolam concentration in the heart blood (2.1 mg/L) was the highest reported thus far in the literature. [A. J. Jenkins *et al.*, *J. Anal. Toxicol.*, 1997, *21*, 218–220.]

The following postmortem concentrations were reported in a 30-year-old female who ingested an unknown quantity of alprazolam and tramadol, respectively: peripheral blood 0.21, not detected and 38.3 mg/L alprazolam, α-hydroxyalprazolam, and tramadol, respectively, bile 0.27, 0.12, and 44.0 mg/L, liver 0.23, <0.005, and 27.6 μg/g, gastric contents (100 mL) 2.73, not detected and 130 mg. [K. Michaud *et al.*, *Forensic Sci. Int.*, 1999, *105*, 185–189.]

Half-life. Plasma half-life, 11 to 15 h (mean 12).

Volume of distribution. About 0.7 L/kg.

Clearance. Plasma clearance, about 0.7 mL/min/kg.

Protein binding. In plasma, about 70 to 80%.

Note. For a review of alprazolam, see G. W. Dawson *et al.*, *Drugs*, 1984, *27*, 132–147 and for its pharmacokinetics, see D. J. Greenblatt and C. E. Wright, *Clin. Pharmacokinet.*, 1993, *24*, 453–471 and D. G. Greenblatt *et al.*, *J. Clin. Psychiatry*, 1993, *54(Suppl.)*, 4–11.

Dose. 1 to 3 mg daily; up to 10 mg in the treatment of panic attacks.

Alprenolol

Beta-blocker

1-[(1-Methylethyl)amino]-3-[2-2-propenyl)phenoxy]-2-propanol
$C_{15}H_{23}NO_2$=249.4
CAS—13655-52-2; 23846-70-0 (±)

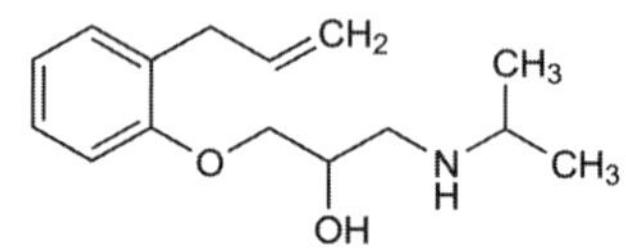

M.p. 57° to 59°.

Alprenolol Hydrochloride

Proprietary names. Apllobal; Aptin(e); Betacard; Duriles; Gubernal; Regletin; Yobir.
$C_{15}H_{23}NO_2$,HCl=285.8
CAS—13707-88-5; 13678-97-2 (±)
Colourless crystals or a white crystalline powder. M.p. 108° to 111°. Soluble 1 in less than 1 of water, 1 in 2 of ethanol and 1 in 3 of chloroform; soluble in acetone and dilute acetic acid; practically insoluble in ether.

Dissociation Constant pK_a 9.5 (20°).

Partition Coefficient. Log *P* (octanol/pH 7.0), 0.5.

Colour Tests. Liebermann's test—red; Mandelin's test—brown-violet; Marquis test—red; Sulfuric acid—orange.

Thin-layer Chromatography. System TA—Rf 52; system TB—Rf 11; system TC—Rf 12; system TE—Rf 49; system TL—Rf 11; system TAE—Rf 22; system TAJ—Rf 06; system TAK—Rf 17; system TAL—Rf 70. (Acidified iodoplatinate solution, positive.)

Gas Chromatography. System GA—RI 1820.

High Performance Liquid Chromatography. System HA—*k* 1.2; system HY—RI 323; system HZ—Retention time 3.9 min.

Column: (analytical) C_{18} μBondapack (300 × 3.9 mm, 10 μm); (guard) C_{18} μBondapack. Column temperature: 30°. Mobile phase: acetonitrile:water (40:60) containing 5 mM potassium dihydrogenphosphate/dipotassium hydrogenphosphate, pH adjusted with phosphoric acid or 1 M potassium hydroxide, flow rate 1.3 mL/min. Electrochemical detection. Retention time(s): 11.42 min (*k* 4.71). [M. J. Maguregui *et al.*, *J. Chromatogr. B, Biomed. Appl.*, 1995, *674*, 85–91].

Ultraviolet Spectrum. Aqueous acid—270 (A_1^1=69b), 276 nm. No alkaline shift.

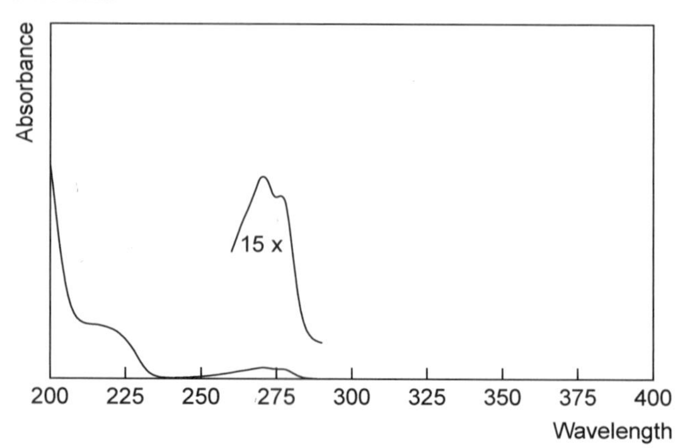

Infra-red Spectrum. Principal peaks at wavenumbers 1242, 746, 1031, 1492, 1079, 916 cm^{-1} (KBr disk).

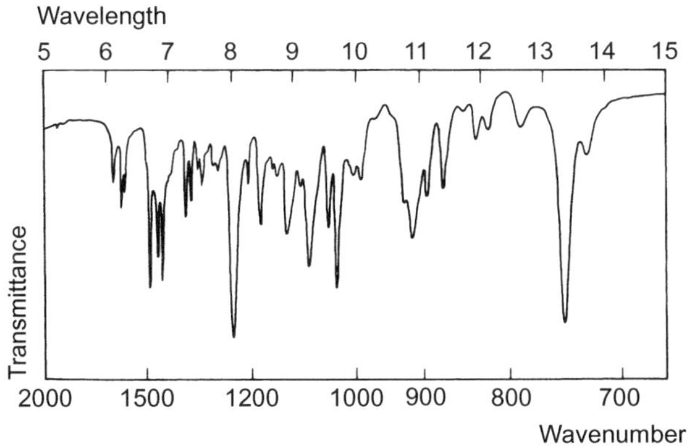

Mass Spectrum. Principal ions at *m/z* 72, 30, 56, 73, 249, 98, 234, 102.

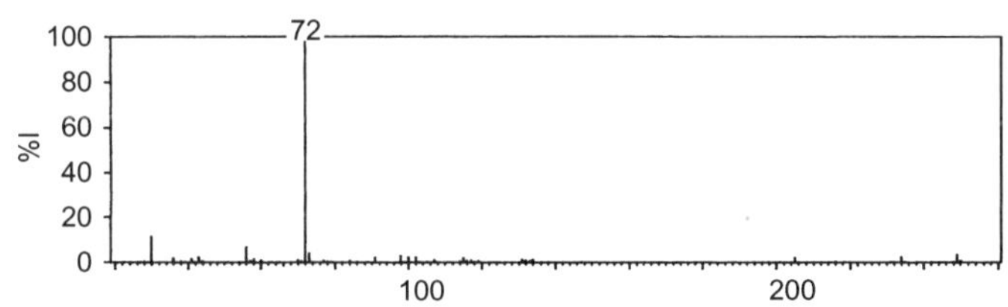

Quantification

Gas chromatography. In plasma: limit of detection 2.5 µg/L, ECD—C. F. Poole *et al.*, *J. Chromatogr.*, 1980, *194*, 365–377. In serum: limit of detection 2 pg, ECD—D. DeBruyne *et al.*, *J. Pharm. Sci.*, 1979, *68*, 511–512.

High performance liquid chromatography. In urine: limit of quantification 500 µg/L, ECD—M. J. Maguregui *et al.*, *J. Chromatogr. B, Biomed. Sci. Appl.*, 1995, *674*, 85–91.

Disposition in the Body. Alprenolol is rapidly and almost completely absorbed after oral administration but undergoes extensive first-pass metabolism. About 90% of an oral dose is excreted in the urine in 24 h with about 40% as the glucuronide conjugate of the active metabolite 4-hydroxyalprenolol, 5% as free 4-hydroxyalprenolol, 20 to 30% as alprenolol glucuronide, 1% as desisopropylalprenolol, and less than 1% as unchanged drug; unknown metabolites account for the remainder of the dose.

Therapeutic concentration. There is considerable intersubject variation in plasma concentrations and in the ratio of 4-hydroxyalprenolol to alprenolol.

After oral administration of 200 mg to 2 subjects, peak plasma alprenolol concentrations of 0.07 and 0.22 mg/L were reported; peak plasma concentrations of the 4-hydroxy metabolite were 0.04 and 0.06 mg/L. [G. Alvan *et al.*, *J. Pharmacokinet. Biopharm.*, 1977, *5*, 193–205].

Following oral administration of 200 mg three times a day to 16 subjects, average steady-state plasma-alprenolol concentrations of 0.01 to 0.14 mg/L (mean 0.04 mg/L) were reported. [P. Collste *et al.*, *Eur. J. Clin. Pharmacol.*, 1976, *10*, 85–88].

Toxicity

In 2 fatalities due to the ingestion of about 4 g and 20 g, respectively, the following postmortem tissue-alprenolol concentrations were reported: blood 40 and 43 mg/L, liver 72 and 91 µg/g. [S. J. Dickson *et al.*, *J. Anal. Toxicol.*, 1978, *2*, 242–244].

Bioavailability. About 5 to 10%.

Half-life. Plasma half-life, alprenolol and 4-hydroxyalprenolol about 2 to 3 h.

Volume of distribution. About 3 L/kg.

Clearance. Plasma clearance, about 15 mL/min/kg.

Distribution in blood. Plasma:whole blood ratio, about 1.6.

Protein binding. In plasma, 80 to 90%.

Dose. 200 to 800 mg of alprenolol hydrochloride daily.

Alprostadil

Prostaglandin/ Vasodilator

Synonyms. Prostaglandin E_1; PGE_1.
Proprietary names. Alprostar (alprostadil alfadex); Caverject; Edex; Liple; Minprog; Muse; Prostandin (alprostadil alfadex); Prostavasin (alprostadil alfadex); Prostin VR; Prostine VR; Prostivas; Sugiran (alprostadil alfadex); Viridal (alprostadil alfadex).
(*E*)-(8*R*,11*R*,12*R*,15*S*)-11,15-Dihydroxy-9-oxoprost-13-en-1-oic acid
$C_{20}H_{34}O_5$=354.5
CAS—745-65-3

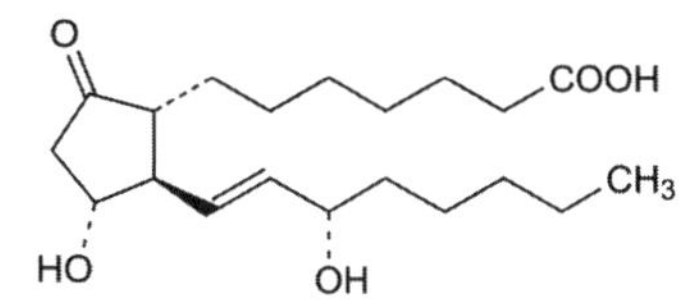

A white to off-white crystalline powder. M.p. about 110°. It is soluble in water and in acetone; freely soluble in ethanol; very slightly soluble in chloroform and in ether; slightly soluble in ethyl acetate.

Dissociation Constant. pK_a 4.85.

Partition Coefficient. Log *P* (octanol/water), 3.20.

Thin-layer Chromatography. Plate: silica LK6D (5 × 20 cm). Mobile phase: ethyl acetate:acetic acid (99.5:0.5). PGE_0, Rf 0.50; PGE_2 Rf 0.31. [H. Scweer *et al.*, *Biol. Mass Spectrom.*, 1994, *23*, 165–170].

Quantification

Gas chromatography–mass spectrometry. In plasma: limit of quantification is 1 ng/L for alprostadil and 5 ng/L for its metabolite—H. Scweer *et al.*, *Biol. Mass Spectrom.*, 1994, *23*, 165–170.

Disposition in the Body. Alprostadil is rapidly distributed throughout the body (except the CNS) following intravenous administration. Between 60 and 90% (depending on dose) is rapidly metabolised by oxidation during passage through pulmonary circulation. It is also metabolised by the liver and kidneys to prostaglandin E_0 (PGE_0) and 15-hydroxy-PGE_0. The drug is excreted principally in urine (88% of a dose) as metabolites and a small amount is excreted in faeces via bile (12%).

Therapeutic concentration

Following intravenous infusion of 20 µg over 30 min in 24 subjects, mean peak plasma concentrations of 8.2 ng/L were observed. Following intracavernous injection of 20 µg, mean peak plasma concentrations of 17.6 ng/L were reached after a mean of 4.8 min. [W. Cawello *et al.*, *J. Urol.*, 1997, *158*, 1403–1407].

Mean peak plasma concentrations of 4.8 (range, 3.4 to 6.3), 7.7 (6.7 to 10.8), and 12.9 (10.2 to 14.6) ng/L were measured in 12 healthy male subjects (aged between 20 and 35 years) after intravenous infusion over 2 h of 30, 60 and 120 µg, respectively. These levels were observed by the end of the infusion. The mean peak plasma PGE_0 concentrations were 8.3, 15.1 and 29.2 ng/L for the 30, 60 and 120 µg doses and the 15-hydroxy-PGE_0 metabolite, 108.6, 203.6 and 395.6 ng/L, respectively. [W. Cawello *et al.*, *Br. J. Clin. Pharmacol.*, 1995, *40*, 273–276].

Bioavailability. 15%.

Half-life. Plasma, 0.2 to 8 min (after single dose).

Volume of distribution. 0.8 L/kg.

Clearance. Plasma, 115 L/min; also reported as 20 mL/min/kg.

Protein binding. In plasma, 81% to 93% (to albumin).

Note. For a review of the pharmacokinetics of alprostadil see R. Kirsten *et al.*, *Clin. Pharmacokinet.*, 1998, *35*, 9–36.

Dose. Usually, 5 to 20 µg by intracavernous injection; 250 µg by transurethral delivery (initial dose); 50 to 100 ng/kg/min by intravenous infusion (reduced to lowest dose).

Alteplase

Antithrombotic

Synonyms. G-11044; G-11021; recombinant tissue-type plasminogen activator; rt-PA.

Proprietary names. Actilyse; Actiplas; Activase; Besospartin; Lysatec-rt-PA.
$C_{2569}H_{3894}N_{746}O_{781}S_{40}$=59007.6
CAS—105857-23-6

A white to off-white powder.

Quantification
Enzyme immunoassay. In plasma: limit of detection 0.2 µg/L—O. Matsuo *et al*., *Anal. Biochem*., 1983, *135*, 58–63.

Disposition in the Body. Alteplase is rapidly cleared from plasma and metabolised mainly in the liver to low molecular weight compounds and amino acids. After intravenous infusion, 50% of the dose is cleared from plasma within 5 min and 80% within 10 min. 80% of a dose of alteplase is excreted within 18 h, via the kidneys.

Therapeutic concentration
6 healthy volunteers were administered with a 0.25 mg/kg dose of alteplase and 6 with 0.5 mg/kg. Peak plasma concentrations of 0.96 mg/L and 1.83 mg/L, respectively, were reached by the end of infusion. [P. Tanswell *et al*., *Clin. Pharmacol. Ther*., 1989, *46*, 1310–1319].

Patients with acute myocardial infarction show increased peak plasma concentrations with similar doses.

Toxicity. Acute overdosing (over 150 mg) can lead to internal bleeding including, intracranial, gastro-intestinal and peripheral and ocular haemorrhaging.

Half-life. Plasma half-life (α-phase) is 4 to 5 min, (β-phase) approximately 40 min.

Volume of distribution Initial volume of distribution approximates plasma volume, 2–5 L.

Clearance. Plasma clearance, 550 to 650 L/min.

Dose. Adult: dose ranges between 0.02 to 0.04 mg/kg body weight and 1.5 mg/kg body weight, depending on symptoms. Maximum dose of 100 mg. Children: 0.01 to 0.05 mg/kg body weight.

Altretamine

Antineoplastic

Synonyms. ENT-50852; hexamethylmelamine; HMM; NSC-13875.
Proprietary names. Hexalen; Hexastat; Hexinawas.
2,4,6-Tris(dimethylamino)-1,3,5-triazine
$C_9H_{18}N_6$=210.3
CAS—645-05-6

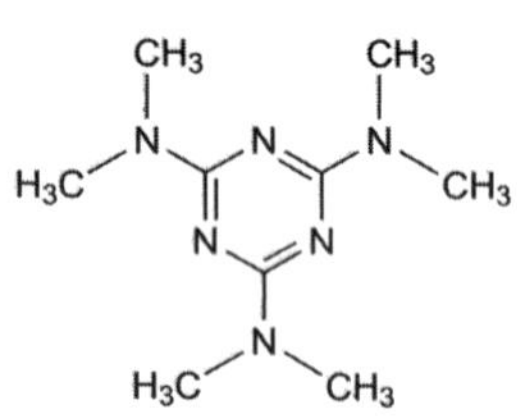

A white crystalline powder. M.p. about 172°. It is practically insoluble in water and physiological solvents; soluble in chloroform, DMSO, ethanol and acetone.
Caution. Altretamine is an irritant; avoid contact with skin and mucous membranes.

Partition Coefficient. Log *P* (octanol/water), 2.73.

High Performance Liquid Chromatography. System HAA—retention time 17.8 min.
Column: ODS Hypersil (100 × 4.6 mm i.d., 5 µm). Mobile phase: methanol, 0.5 mL/min flow rate. UV diode array detection. Retention time: 3.2 min. [T. Mills and J. C. Roberson, *Instrumental Data for Drug Analysis*, 1993, CRC Press, Boca Raton, US. 2nd Edn, Vol. 4–5].

Ultraviolet Spectrum. Aqueous acid (0.2 M NH_2SO_4)—240 nm; (ethanol)—226 nm; basic—241 nm.

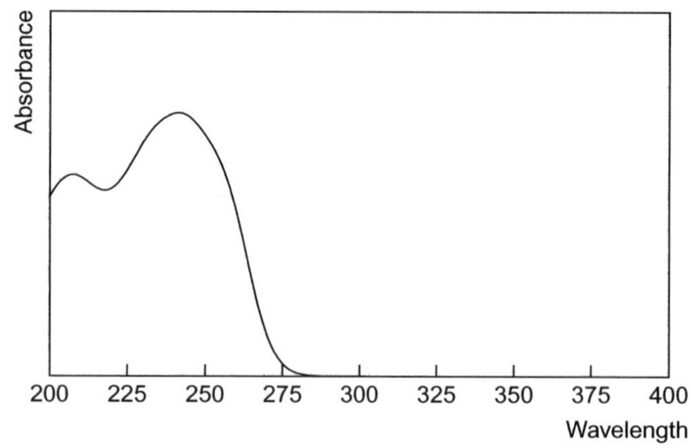

Infra-red Spectrum. Principal peaks at wavenumber 1527, 1387, 1051 cm^{-1} (KBr pellet).

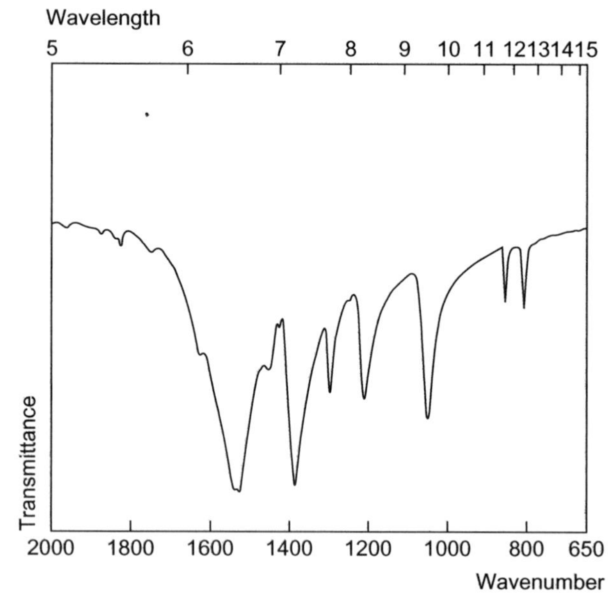

Mass Spectrum. Principal peaks at *m*/*z* 96, 42, 195, 210, 71, 69, 44, 152.

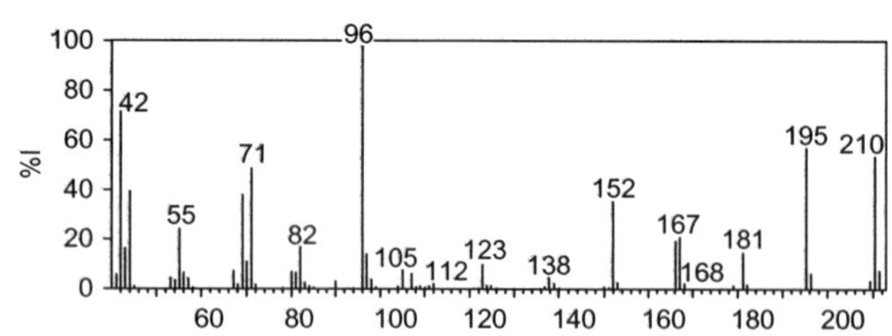

Quantification
Gas chromatography. In plasma or serum: limit of detection 0.005 mg/L, AFID—A. Hulshoff *et al*., *J. Chromatogr*., 1980, *181*; *Biomed. Appl*., *7*, 363–371. In plasma or urine: limit of detection altretamine, 0.2 mg/L and pentamethylmelamine, 0.025 mg/L, AFID—M. M. Ames and G. Powis, *J. Chromatogr*., 1979, *174*, 245–249.

High performance liquid chromatography. In plasma: limit of quantification 0.15 mg/L, UV detection—I. K. Barker *et al*., *J. Chromatogr. Biomed. Sci. Appl*., 1994, *660*, 121–126.

Disposition in the Body. Altretamine is rapidly and well absorbed after oral administration and quickly distributed to tissues with a high lipid component. It is rapidly demethylated in the liver to pentamethylmelamine and other metabolites that are excreted in urine. Formaldehyde is also produced which is subsequently oxidised to carbon dioxide and expired. Other metabolites include dimethylmelamine, monomethylmelamine, trimethylmelamine and melamine, and these have been detected in urine. No parent drug has been detected in urine. Metabolism is catalysed by cytochrome P450 enzymes. Accumulation in plasma has not been observed with multiple dosing.

Therapeutic concentration

20 patients with gynaecological malignancies were administered with 200 to 300 mg/m^2 doses and peak plasma concentrations of 0.32 to 4.28 mg/L were observed after 0.5 to 3 h. 12 patients administered with a 200 mg dose reached peak concentrations of 0.3 to 0.9 mg/L at approximately 1 h. Peak plasma concentrations vary widely among patients because of the rapid hepatic metabolism. [G. Damia and M. D'Incalci, *Clin. Pharmacokinet.*, 1995, *28*, 439–448].

Half-life. Plasma, 4 to 13 h.

Protein binding. In plasma, altretamine 94%; pentamethylmelamine 75%.

Dose. 260 mg/m^2 daily for 14 consecutive days in a 28-day cycle.

Alverine

Antispasmodic

Synonyms. Dipropyline; Phenpropamine.
N-Ethyl-*N*-(3-phenylpropyl)-benzenepropanamine
$C_{20}H_{27}N$=281.4
CAS—150-59-4

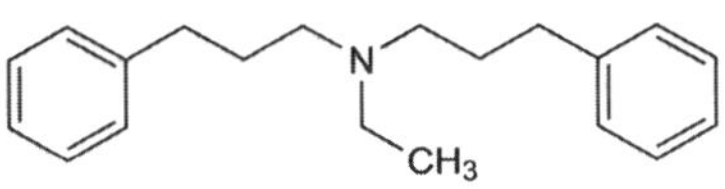

Alverine Citrate

Proprietary names. Profenil; Spasmavérine; Spasmonal.
$C_{20}H_{27}N,C_6H_8O_7$=473.6
CAS—5560-59-8
A white powder. M.p. 100° to 103°.
Slightly soluble in water and chloroform; sparingly soluble in ethanol; very slightly soluble in ether.

Colour Tests. Liebermann's Test—orange; Mandelin's Test—grey–green; Marquis Test—orange–red.

Thin-layer Chromatography. System TA—Rf 66; system TB—Rf 65; system TC—Rf 39; system TL—Rf 38. (Acidified potassium permanganate solution, positive.)

Gas Chromatography. System GA—RI 2142.

High Performance Liquid Chromatography. System HA—*k* 1.8.

Ultraviolet Spectrum. Aqueous acid—253, 259 nm (A^1_1=14.4 b), 264, 268 nm.

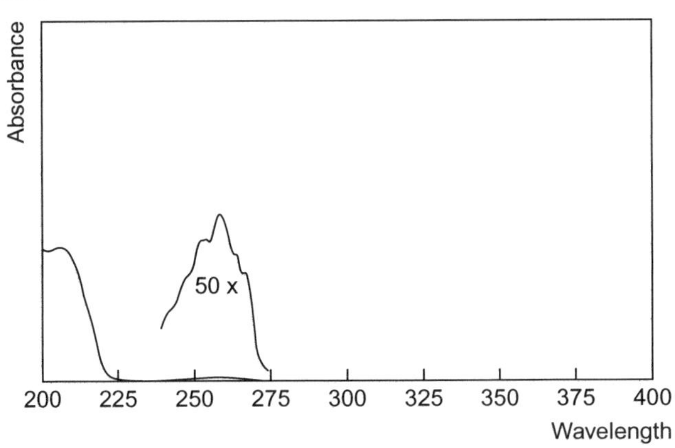

Infra-red Spectrum. Principal peaks at wavenumbers 694, 1190, 740, 1075, 1020, 1694 cm^{-1} (KBr disk).

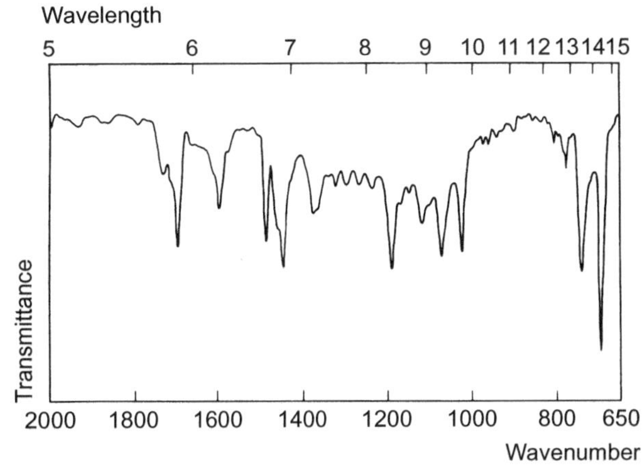

Mass Spectrum. Principal ions at *m/z* 72, 176, 91, 58, 177, 41, 42, 30.

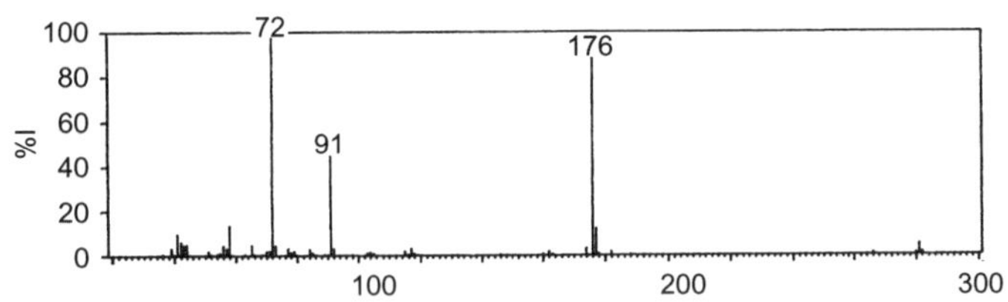

Dose. The equivalent of 40 to 240 mg of alverine daily.

Amantadine

Antiviral/Antiparkinsonian

Synonym. 1-Adamantanamine
Tricyclo[3.3.1.1^{3,7}]decan-1-amine
$C_{10}H_{17}N$=151.3
CAS—768-94-5

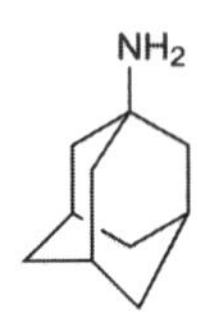

Crystals. M.p. 160° to 190°, also reported as M.p. 180° to 192°.
Sparingly soluble in water; soluble in chloroform.

Amantadine Hydrochloride

Synonyms. EXP-105-1; NSC-83653.
Proprietary names. Amazolon; Antadine; Mantandan; Mantadine; Mantadix; Symmetrel; Virofral.
$C_{10}H_{17}N,HCl$=187.7
CAS—665-66-7
A white crystalline powder. M.p. 360°, with decomposition.
Soluble 1 in 2.5 of water, 1 in about 5 of ethanol, and 1 in 18 of chloroform; practically insoluble in ether.

Amantadine Sulfate

Proprietary names. Contenton; PK-Merz; Trivaline.
$C_{10}H_{17}N,\frac{1}{2}H_2SO_4$=200.3
CAS—31377-23-8

Dissociation Constant. pK_a 10.1.

Partition Coefficient. Log *P* (octanol/pH 7.4), −0.4.

Colour Test. Ninhydrin—pink-violet.

Thin-layer Chromatography. System TA—Rf 23; system TB—Rf 19; system TC—Rf 07; system TE—Rf 35; system TL—Rf 04; system TAE—Rf 07; system TAF—Rf 77. (Acidified iodoplatinate solution, positive.)

Gas Chromatography. System GA—amantadine RI 1240, amantadine-AC RI 1640.

Ultraviolet Spectrum. No significant absorption, 230 to 360 nm.

Infra-red Spectrum. Principal peaks at wavenumbers 1503, 1497, 1316, 1603, 1089, 1517 cm^{-1} (amantadine hydrochloride, KBr disk).

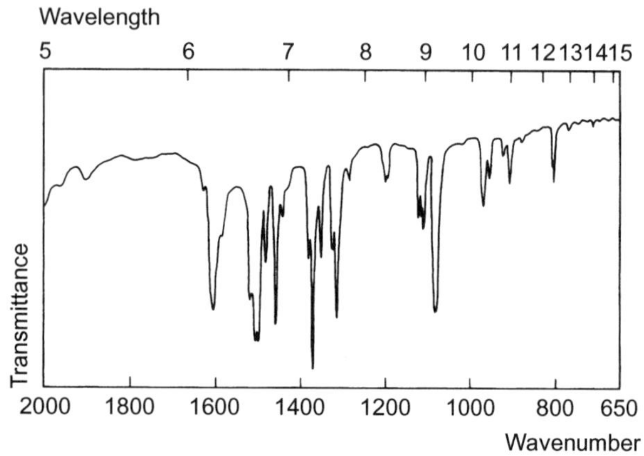

Mass Spectrum. Principal peaks at m/z 94, 151, 57, 95, 40, 41, 58, 108.

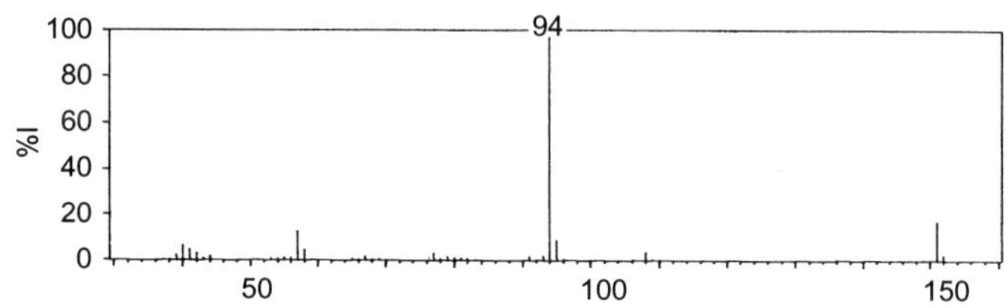

Quantification

Gas chromatography. In plasma: limit of quantification 2.3 µg/L, ECD—D. Rakestraw, *J. Pharm. Biomed. Anal.*, 1993, *11*, 699–703. In plasma or urine: limit of detection 100 µg/L in plasma and 4 mg/L in urine, FID—P. M. Bélanger and O. Grech-Bélanger, *J. Chromatogr.* 1982, *228*(17) *B Biomed. Appl.*, 327–332. In plasma or urine: limit of detection 10 µg/L, ECD—A. Sioufi and F. Pommier, *J. Chromatogr.* 1980, *183*(9) *B Biomed. Appl.*, 33–39.

High performance liquid chromatography. In plasma and urine: fluorescence detection—F. X. Zhou *et al.*, *J. Chromatogr.*, 1993, *619*, 93–101. In urine: limit of detection 2.0 mg/L, fluorescence detection (λ_{ex}=355 nm, λ_{em}=405 nm)—H. Fujino *et al.*, *Yakugaku Zasshi*, 1993, *113*, 391–395. In urine: limit of detection 75 µg/L, fluorescence detection—F. A. van der Horst *et al.*, *J. Pharm. Biomed. Anal.*, 1990, *8*, 799–804.

Disposition in the Body. Slowly but almost completely absorbed after oral administration. It is mainly excreted unchanged in the urine (about 56% of a dose being excreted unchanged in 24 h and about 86% in 4 days) although small amounts of metabolites have also been detected. The major metabolic pathway is *N*-acetylation but several unusual routes (*N*-methylation, formation of Schiff bases and *N*-formates) have also been observed. Amantadine crosses the placenta and the blood–brain barrier. It is also distributed into breast milk.

Therapeutic concentration

Following a single oral dose of 150 mg given to 6 subjects, peak plasma concentrations of 0.32 to 0.56 mg/L (mean 0.4) were attained in about 3 to 4 h. [F. Y. Aoki *et al.*, *Clin. Pharmacol. Ther.*, 1979, *26*, 729–736.]

After oral administration of 100 mg twice daily, steady-state plasma concentrations of 0.1 to 1.1 mg/L (mean 0.5) were observed in 22 patients. [D. J. Greenblatt *et al.*, *J. Clin. Pharmacol.*, 1977, *17*, 704–708.]

Toxicity

An adolescent who ingested 1.3 g of amantadine developed complex ventricular arrhythmias and altered mental status. The arrhythmias were completely suppressed with intravenous lidocaine. [L. Pimentel and B. Hughes, *Pediatr. Emerg. Care*, 1991, *7*, 89–92.]

In a fatality involving the ingestion of amantadine, the following postmortem tissue concentrations were reported: blood 21 mg/L, bile 418.6 mg/L, liver 135.4 µg/g, urine 1330 mg/L. [P. C. Reynolds and S. Van Meter, *J. Anal. Toxicol.*, 1984, *8*, 100.]

Half-life. Plasma half-life, 10 to 15 h in patients with normal renal function but significantly prolonged in the elderly and in patients with renal impairment.

Protein binding. About 67%.

Note. For studies on the use of amantadine as a medication for cocaine dependence, see S. Shoptaw *et al.*, *Drug Alcohol Depend.*, 2002, *66*, 217–224.

Dose. Usually 100 to 200 mg of amantadine hydrochloride daily. Doses up to 400 mg daily have occasionally been used, but this dose should not be exceeded.

Ambazone

Bacteriostat

Proprietary names. Bridal; Iversal; Primal(s).

2-[4-[(Aminoiminomethyl)hydrazono]-2,5-cyclohexadien-1-ylidene]-hydrazinecarbothioamide monohydrate

$C_8H_{11}N_7S,H_2O$=255.3

CAS—6011-12-7; 539-21-9

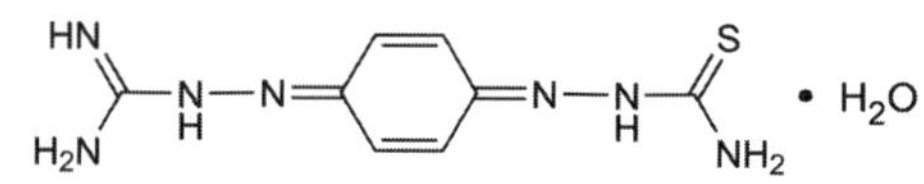

A brown microcrystalline powder. M.p. 192° to 194°, with decomposition. Practically insoluble in water; very slightly soluble in ethanol; soluble in DMF and in solutions of acids and of alkali hydroxides.

Colour Test. Palladium Chloride—brown.

Thin-layer Chromatography. System TA—Rf 55; system TB—Rf 00; system TC—Rf 04; system TE—Rf 38; system TL—Rf 08; system TAD—Rf 00; system TAE—Rf 70. (Acidified potassium permanganate solution, positive.)

Ultraviolet Spectrum. No significant absorption, 230 to 360 nm.

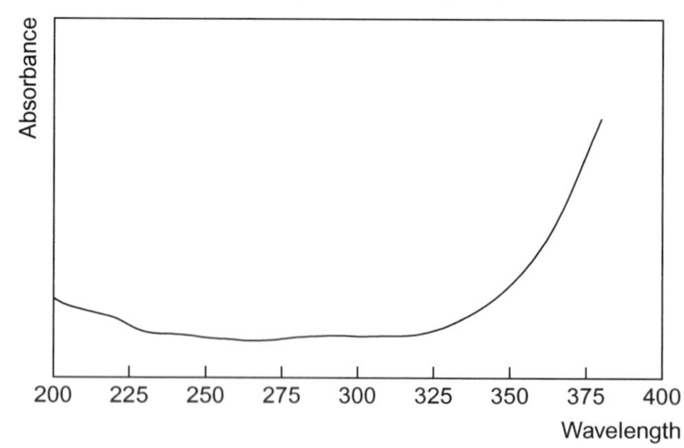

Infra-red Spectrum. Principal peaks at wavenumbers 1130, 1515, 1587, 1612, 1639, 1315 cm^{-1}.

Note. For the chemical and analytical characterisation of ambazone, see N. Miosga *et al.*, *Pharmazie*, 1988, *43*, 541–543.

Dose. Ambazone is given as 10-mg lozenges in doses of 30 to 50 mg daily.

Ambenonium Chloride

Anticholinesterase

Synonyms. Ambestigmini Chloridum; Oxazyl.

Proprietary names. Mysuran; Mytelase.

N,N'-[(1,2-Dioxo-1,2-ethanediyl)bis(imino-2,1-ethanediyl)]bis[2-chloro-*N,N*-diethylbezenemethanaminium] dichloride

$C_{28}H_{42}Cl_4N_4O_2$=608.5

CAS—7648-98-8 (ambenonium); 115-79-7 (chloride, anhydrous); 52022-31-8 (chloride, tetrahydrate)

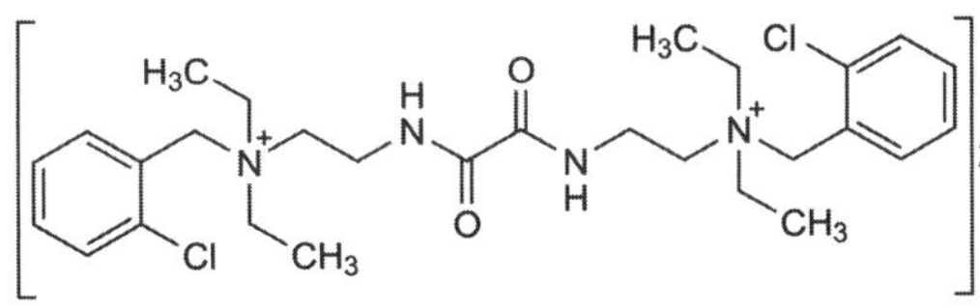

A white powder. M.p. about 200°. Soluble 1 in 5 of water and 1 in 20 of ethanol; slightly soluble in chloroform; practically insoluble in acetone and ether.

Thin-layer Chromatography. System TA—Rf 02. (Acidified iodoplatinate solution, positive.)

Ultraviolet Spectrum. Aqueous acid—271 (A_1^1=30c), 277 nm (A_1^1=29c). No alkaline shift.

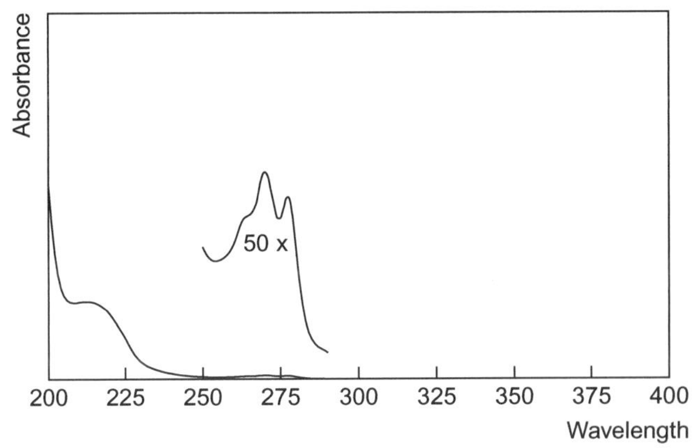

Infra-red Spectrum. Principal peaks at wavenumbers 1675, 1505, 767, 806, 1136, 1190 cm^{-1} (KBr disk).

Therapeutic concentration

6 patients with myasthenia gravis with mean age, 47.8 years (34 to 56 years) were administered 10 mg ambenonium chloride (group A) and 7 patients with mean age, 48.1 years (25 to 68 years) administered 5 mg (group B) after an overnight fast of 12 h or 30 min after a standard meal. The mean peak concentrations were 9.12 μg/L observed at 85 min for group A when fasting and 2.50 μg/L at 120 min after a meal. For group B, mean concentrations were 5.61 μg/L at 55.7 min when fasting and 1.29 μg/L at 72.9 min after a meal. [K. Ohtsubo *et al.*, *Eur. J. Clin. Pharmacol.*, 1992, *42(4)*, 371–374].

Dose. 15 to 100 mg daily; doses of over 200 mg daily have been given.

Ambucetamide

Antispasmodic

Proprietary name. It is an ingredient of Femerital.

2-Dibutylamino-2-(4-methoxyphenyl)acetamide

$C_{17}H_{28}N_2O_2$=292.4

CAS—519-88-0

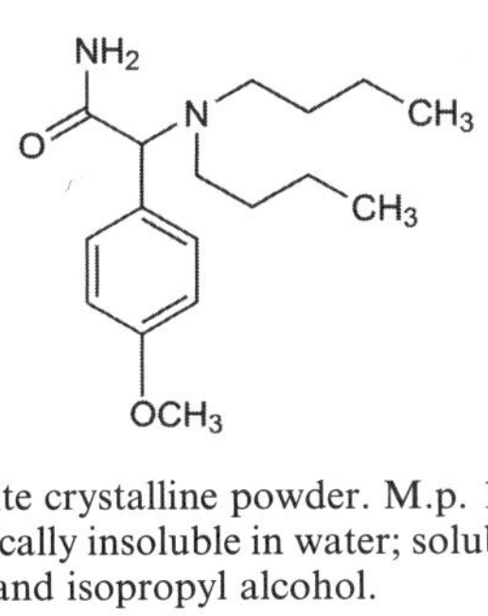

A white crystalline powder. M.p. 134°.

Practically insoluble in water; soluble in ethanol, chloroform, glacial acetic acid, and isopropyl alcohol.

Thin-layer Chromatography. System TA—Rf 73; system TB—Rf 05; system TC—Rf 68; system TE—Rf 76; system TL—Rf 61; system TAE—Rf 76; system TAF—Rf 88. (Acidified iodoplatinate solution, positive.)

Gas Chromatography. System GA—RI 2330.

Ultraviolet Spectrum. Aqueous acid—235; aqueous alkali—279, 286 nm.

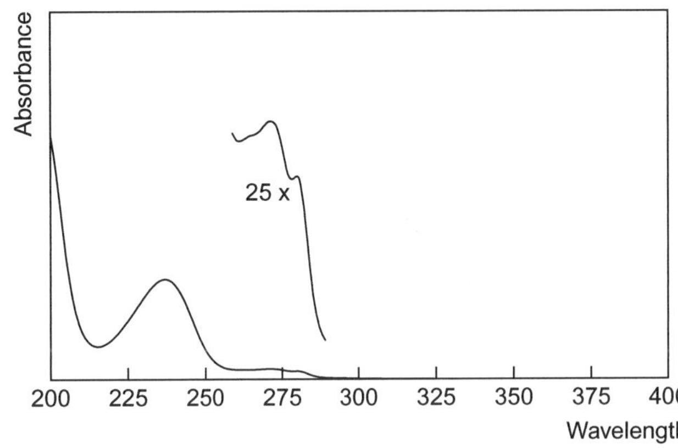

Infra-red Spectrum. Principal peaks at wavenumbers 1656, 1513, 1176, 1250, 1026, 820 cm^{-1} (KBr disk).

Mass Spectrum. Principal peaks at *m/z* 248, 44, 249, 121, 136, 29, 164, 192.

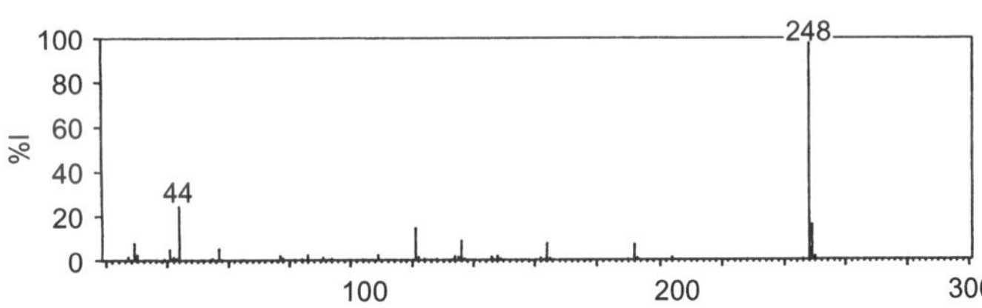

Dose. 300 to 600 mg daily.

Ambutonium Bromide

Anticholinergic

Proprietary name. It is an ingredient of Aludrox SA and Praxiten SP.

γ-(Aminocarbonyl)-*N*-ethyl-*N,N*-dimethyl-γphenylbenzenepropanaminium bromide

$C_{20}H_{27}BrN_2O$=391.4

CAS—14007-49-9 (ambutonium); 115-51-5 (bromide)

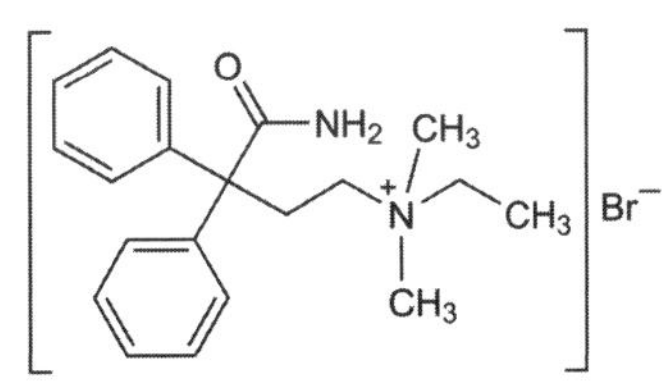

White crystals. M.p. 228° to 229°, with decomposition. Soluble 1 in 1.4 of water, 1 in 27 of ethanol, 1 in 500 of acetone and 1 in 3.5 of chloroform.

Colour Test. Liebermann's test—brown-orange.

Thin-layer Chromatography. System TA—Rf 03. (Acidified iodoplatinate solution, positive.)

Ultraviolet Spectrum. Aqueous acid—253, 259 (A_1^1=11.5b), 265 nm.

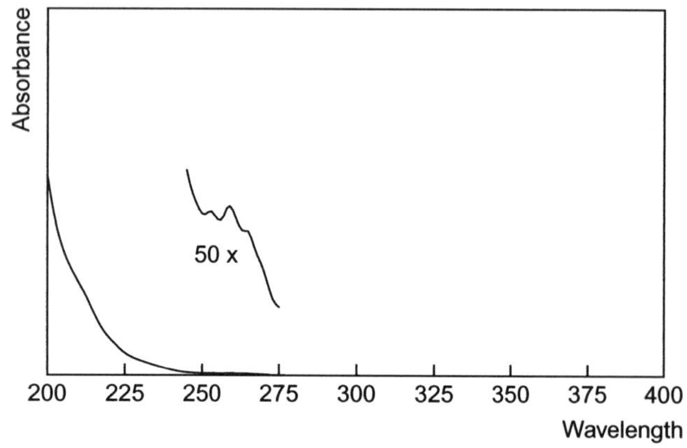

Infra-red Spectrum. Principal peaks at wavenumbers 700, 1664, 764, 1590, 1315, 979 cm^{-1}.

Dose. 7.5 to 20 mg daily.

Ametazole

Diagnostic Agent (Gastric Secretion)

Synonyms. Betazole; Gastramine.
1*H*-Pyrazole-3-ethanamine
$C_5H_9N_3$=111.1
CAS—105-20-4

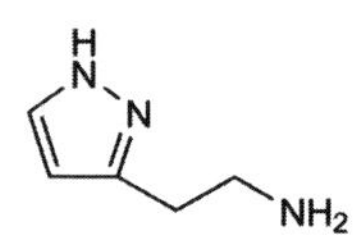

A viscous liquid. B.p. 118° to 123°.

Ametazole Hydrochloride

Proprietary names. Betazol; Histalog.
$C_5H_9N_3$,2HCl=184.1
CAS—138-92-1
A white, hygroscopic, crystalline powder. M.p. about 240° after softening at about 215°. Soluble 1 in 3 of water and 1 in 50 of ethanol; practically insoluble in chloroform; very slightly soluble in ether.

Dissociation Constant. pK_a 2.2, 9.6 (20°).

Thin-layer Chromatography. System TA—Rf 26; system TB—Rf 11; system TC—Rf 00. (Dragendorff spray, positive; acidified iodoplatinate solution, positive; Marquis reagent, brown; ninhydrin spray, positive; acidified potassium permanganate solution, positive.)

Gas Chromatography. System GA—RI 1390.

Ultraviolet Spectrum. No significant absorption, 230 to 360 nm.

Infra-red Spectrum. Principal peaks at wavenumbers 1563, 1316, 1647, 775, 928, 1044 cm^{-1}.

Mass Spectrum. Principal ions at *m/z* 82, 30, 81, 83, 55, 54, 42, 27.

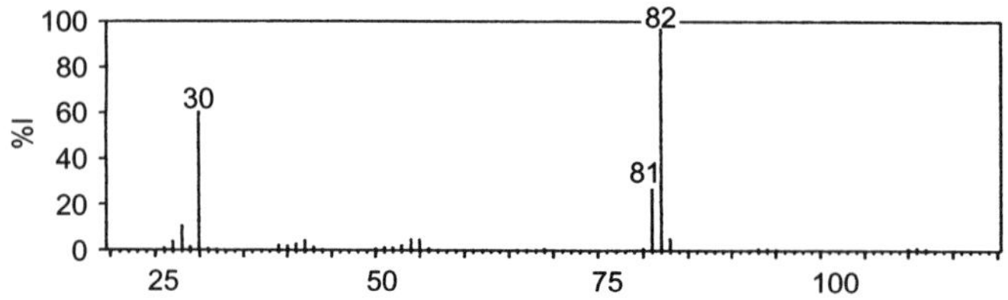

Dose. 500 µg/kg of ametazole hydrochloride by subcutaneous or intramuscular injection.

Ametryne

Herbicide

Synonym. Ametryn
Proprietary names. Ametrex; Evik; Gesapax; G-34162.
N-Ethyl-*N*′-(1-methylethyl)-6-(methylthio)-1,3,5-triazine-2,4-diamine
$C_9H_{17}N_5S$=227.3
CAS—834-12-8

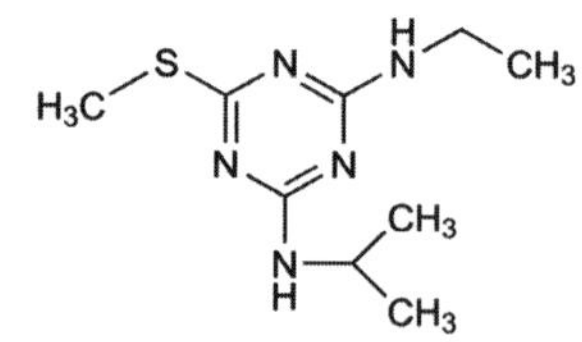

Colourless crystals. M.p. 84° to 86°.
Very slightly soluble in water; soluble in chloroform and methanol.

Thin-layer Chromatography. System TA—Rf 76; system TX—Rf 26; system TY—Rf 23. (Dragendorff spray, positive.)

Gas Chromatography. System GA—RI 1879.

Infra-red Spectrum. Principal peaks at wavenumbers 1515, 1595, 1294, 1166, 806, 1140 cm^{-1} (KBr disk).

Amfetamine

Central Stimulant

Synonyms. Amphetamine; Anfetamina; Racemic Desoxynorephedrine.
Proprietary names. It is an ingredient of Biphetamine and Durophet.
α-Methylbenzeneethanamine
$C_9H_{13}N$=135.2
CAS—300-62-9

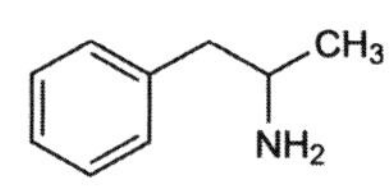

A colourless, mobile, slowly volatile liquid. It absorbs carbon dioxide from the air forming a volatile carbonate. B.p. 200° to 203°.
Soluble 1 in 50 of water; soluble in ethanol chloroform and ether; readily soluble in acids.

Amfetamine Phosphate

Synonyms. Amphetamine Phosphate; Benzpropaminum Phosphoricum; Monobasic Racemic Amphetamine Phosphate.
$C_9H_{13}N,H_3PO_4$=233.2
CAS—139-10-6
A white crystalline powder with no characteristic melting point; it sinters at about 150° and decomposes at about 300°.
Freely soluble in water; slightly soluble in ethanol; practically insoluble in benzene, chloroform, and ether.

Amfetamine Sulfate

Synonyms. Amphetamine Sulfate; Phenaminum; Phenopromini Sulfas; Phenylaminopropanum Racemicum Sulfuricum; Psychedrinum.
Proprietary names. Benzedrine; Centramina. It is an ingredient of Adderall, Epipropane, and Ortenal.
$(C_9H_{13}N)_2,H_2SO_4$=368.5
CAS—60-13-9
A white crystalline powder. M.p. above 300°, with decomposition.
Soluble 1 in 9 of water and 1 in 515 of ethanol; practically insoluble in chloroform and ether.

Dissociation Constant. pK_a 10.1.

Partition Coefficient. Log *P* (octanol/water), 1.8.

Colour Tests. Liebermann's Test—red-orange; Marquis Test—orange→brown; Ninhydrin—pink-orange.

Thin-layer Chromatography. System TA—Rf 43; system TB—Rf 20; system TC—Rf 09; system TE—Rf 43; system TL—Rf 18; system TAE—Rf 12; system TAF—Rf 75. (Dragendorff spray, positive; FPN reagent, pink; acidified iodoplatinate solution, positive; Marquis reagent, brown; ninhydrin spray, positive; acidified potassium permanganate solution, positive.)

Gas Chromatography. System GA—amfetamine RI 1125, amfetamine-TFA RI 1095, amfetamine-PFP RI 1330, amfetamine-TMS RI 1190, amfetamine-AC RI 1501, art (formyl) RI 1100, M (3-OH-)-PFP$_2$ RI 1520, M (3-OH-)-TMS$_2$ RI 1850, M (3-OH-)-AC$_2$ RI 1930, M (4-OH-) RI 1480, M (4-OH-)-AC$_2$ RI 1900, M (3,4-di-OH-)-AC$_3$ RI 2150, M (OH-methoxy-) RI 1465, M (OH-methoxy-)-AC$_2$ RI 2065, M (desamino-oxo-OH-)-AC RI 1520, M (desamino-oxo-OH-methoxy-) RI 1510, M (desamino-oxo-OH-methoxy-)-AC RI 1600, M (desamino-oxo-di-OH-)-AC$_2$ RI 1735; system GB—amfetamine RI 1150; art (formyl) RI 1142; system GC—RI 1536; system GF—RI 1315; system GAK—retention time 4.9 min.

Column: DB-5 fused silica (30 m × 0.25 mm i.d., 0.25 µm film thickness). Column temperature: 70° for 1 min, ramp to 100° at 30°/min, and to 270° at 10°/min. Injector temperature: 280°. Carrier gas: helium, flow rate 0.8 mL/min. MS detection. Retention time: 6.5 min. [E. Meyer *et al.*, *J. Anal. Toxicol.*, 1997, *21*, 236–239.]

High Performance Liquid Chromatography. System HA—*k* 0.9; system HB—*k* 8.48; system HC—*k* 0.98; system HX—RI 244; system HAA—retention time, 3.7 min; system HBC—retention time 2.1 min; system HBD—retention time 3.7 min.

Column: Chiralcel OD-RH (150 × 2 mm i.d., 5 µm) at 35°. Mobile phase: phosphate–citrate buffer (pH 4.0) with sodium hexafluorophosphate (0.3 M):acetonitrile (43:57), flow rate 0.1 mL/min. Fluorescence detection (λ_{ex} = 330 nm, λ_{em} = 440 nm). Retention time: 24.6 min. [O. Y. Al-Dirbashi *et al.*, *Biomed. Chromatogr.*, 2000, *14(5)*, 293–300.]

Ultraviolet Spectrum. Aqueous acid—251, 257 nm (A_1^1 = 14a), 263 nm.

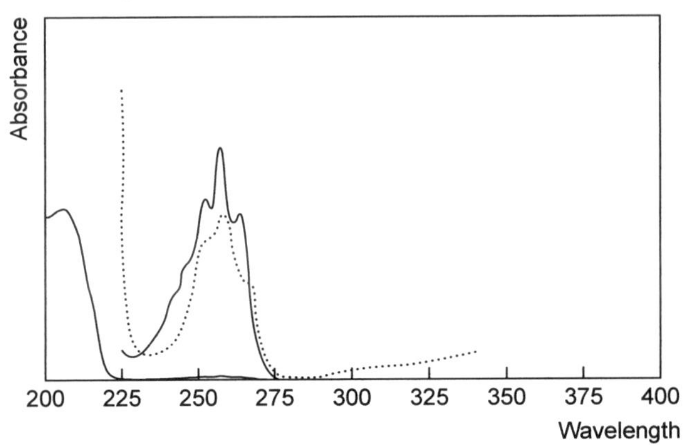

Infra-red Spectrum. Principal peaks at wavenumbers 700, 740, 1495, 1090, 1605, 825 cm^{-1} (thin film). (See below)

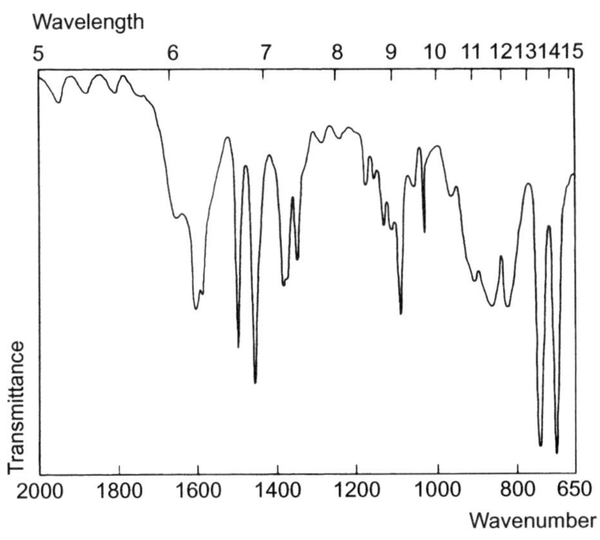

Mass Spectrum. Principal ions at *m/z* 44, 91, 40, 42, 65, 45, 39, 43; phenylacetone 43, 91, 134, 92, 65, 39, 63, 135.

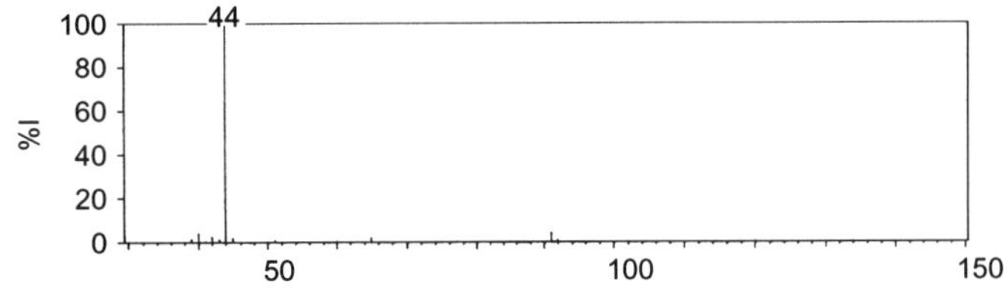

Quantification

Gas chromatography. In urine: amfetamine and metamfetamine, limit of detection <10 µg/L, FTIR—K. S. Kalasinsky *et al.*, *J. Anal. Toxicol.*, 1993, *17*, 359–364. In urine: amfetamine and related drugs, limit of quantification for amfetamine 50 µg/L, NPD—J. Jonsson *et al.*, *J. Forensic Sci.*, 1996, *41*, 148–151. In urine: amfetamine and α-phenethylamine enantiomers, FID or FTIR—J. F. Van Bocxlaer *et al.*, *J. Anal. Toxicol.*, 1997, *21*, 5–11. In plasma or urine: amfetamine, metamfetamine, and *p*-hydroxylated metabolites, limit of detection 1 µg/L, NPD—S. Cheung *et al.*, *J. Chromatogr. B Biomed. Sci. Appl.*, 1997, *690*, 77–87. In urine: amfetamine and metamfetamine, limit of detection 50 µg/L, NPD or MS—H. G. Ugland *et al.*, *J. Chromatogr. B Biomed. Sci. Appl.*, 1997, *701*, 29–38. In hair: amfetamine and metamfetamine, limits of detection 0.1 µg/g and 0.4 µg/g, respectively, NPD—I. Koide *et al.*, *J. Chromatogr. B Biomed. Sci. Appl.*, 1998, *707*, 99–104. In urine: amfetamine and related drugs, limit of detection for amfetamine 15 µg/L, NPD—H. G. Ugland *et al.*, *J. Pharm. Biomed. Anal.*, 1999, *19*, 463–475. In urine: amfetamine and related drugs, limit of detection for amfetamine 500 µg/L, PDHID—C. Casari and A. R. Andrews, *Forensic Sci. Int.*, 2001, *120*, 165–171. In plasma: limit of detection <1 µg/L, ECD—S. J. Asghar *et al.*, *J. Pharmacol. Toxicol. Methods*, 2001, *46*, 111–115.

Gas chromatography–mass spectrometry. In plasma—H. J. Leis *et al.*, *Biol. Mass Spectrom.*, 1994, *23*, 637–641. In fingernails and hair: limits of detection, 12.0 µg/g and 10.2 µg/g, respectively—V. Cirimele *et al.*, *Arch. Toxicol.*, 1995, *70*, 68–69. In hair: amfetamine and related drugs, limit of detection for amfetamine 0.05 µg/g—P. Kintz *et al.*, *J. Chromatogr.* 1995, *670 B Biomed. Appl.* 162–166. In urine: amfetamine and metamfetamine—J. L. Valentine *et al.*, *J. Anal. Toxicol.*, 1995, *19*, 581–590. In urine: amfetamine and metamfetamine—M. Yashiki *et al.*, *Forensic Sci. Int.*, 1995, *76*, 169–177. In blood: amfetamine and metamfetamine—N. Nagasawa *et al.*, *Forensic Sci. Int.*, 1996, *78*, 95–102. In urine: amfetamine and metamfetamine, limits of detection 2.1 mg/L and 0.9 mg/L, respectively—P. Dallakian *et al.*, *J. Anal. Toxicol.*, 1996, *20*, 255–261. In urine: amfetamine and related drugs—F. Centini *et al.*, *Forensic Sci. Int.*, 1996, *83*, 161–166. In hair: amfetamine and derivatives, limit of detection 0.01 µg/g—J. Rohrich and G. Kauert, *Forensic Sci. Int.*, 1997, *84*, 179–188. In urine: amfetamine and related drugs—K. McCambly *et al.*, *J. Anal. Toxicol.*, 1997, *21*, 438–444. In whole blood: amfetamine and related drugs, limits of detection 0.5 to 8 µg/L—P. Marquet *et al.*, *J. Chromatogr. B. Biomed. Sci. Appl.*, 1997, *700*, 77–82. In blood: amfetamine and metamfetamine—M. Sato and T. Mitsui, *J. Pharm. Biomed. Anal.*, 1997, *16*, 139–145. In urine: amfetamine and metamfetamine, limit of detection 100 µg/L—A. Dasgupta and J. Spies, *Am. J. Clin. Path.*, 1998, *109*, 527–532. In urine: amfetamine, metamfetamine, and dimethylamfetamine, limits of detection 1 to 10 µg/L—S. W. Myung *et al.*, *J. Chromatogr. B Biomed. Sci. Appl.*, 1998, *716*, 359–365. In plasma: limit of detection, 0.43 µg/L—N. Pizarro *et al.*, *J. Pharm. Biomed. Anal.*, 1999, *21*, 739–747. In meconium: amfetamine and other drugs of abuse—M. A. ElSohly *et al.*, *J. Anal. Toxicol.*, 1999, *23*, 436–445. In urine: amfetamine enantiomers and related drugs, limit of quantification for amfetamine 10 µg/L—D. Hensley and J. T. Cody, *J. Anal. Toxicol.*, 1999, *23*, 518–523. In urine: amfetamine and related drugs, limit of quantification for amfetamine 10 µg/L—C. Jurado *et al.*, *J. Anal. Toxicol.*, 2000, *24*, 11–16. In whole blood: amfetamine, metamfetamine, and fenfluramine, limit of detection for amfetamine 10 ng/g—A. Namera *et al.*, *Forensic Sci. Int.*, 2000, *109*, 215–223. In serum: amfetamine and other drugs of abuse—W. Weinmann *et al.*, *Int. J. Legal Med.*, 2000, *113*, 229–235. In serum: amfetamine and metamfetamine—M. R. Lee *et al.*, *J. Chromatogr. A*, 2000, *896*, 265–273. In urine: amfetamine and other drugs of abuse, limits of detection 3 to 12 µg/L—V. Karacic and L. Skender, *Arh. Hig. Rada. Toksikol.*, 2000, *51*, 389–400. In whole blood: amfetamine and metamfetamine, limit of quantification 0.5 ng/g—K. Okajima *et al.*, *Forensic Sci. Int.*, 2001, *116*, 15–22. In hair: amfetamine and metamfetamine, limit of quantification 0.1 µg/g—J. Liu *et al.*, *J. Chromatogr. B. Biomed. Sci. Appl.*, 2001, *758*, 95–101. In urine: amfetamine and metamfetamine, limits of detection 19 to 50 µg/L—S. M. Wang *et al.*, *J. Chromatogr. B. Biomed. Sci. Appl.*, 2001, *759*, 17–26. In urine: amfetamine and related drugs, limit of quantification for amfetamine 2 µg/L—A. Namera *et al.*, *J. Chromatogr. Sci.*, 2002, *40*, 19–25. In hair: amfetamine and other drugs of abuse, limits of detection 0.05 to 0.3 µg/g—L. Skender *et al.*, *Forensic Sci. Int.*, 2002, *125*, 120–126. In urine: amfetamine and related 'designer' drugs, limit of detection 5 to 10 µg/L—M. Pellegrini *et al.*, *J. Chromatogr. B Anal. Technol. Biomed. Life Sci.*, 2002, *769*, 243–251. In hair: amfetamine and related 'designer' drugs, limits of detection 0.01 to 0.19 µg/g—F. Musshoff *et al.*, *J. Chromatogr. A*, 2002, *958*, 231–238; F. Musshoff *et al.*, *J. Chromatogr. Sci.*, 2002, *40*, 359–364. In urine: amfetamine and related drugs, limit of detection for amfetamine 62.5 µg/L—P. R. Stout *et al.*, *J. Anal. Toxicol.*, 2002, *26*, 253–261. In plasma or serum: amfetamine and metamfetamine—F. T. Peters *et al.*, *Clin. Chem.*, 2002, *48*, 1472–1485. In urine: amfetamine and metamfetamine, limit of detection 0.3 µg/L—M. K. Huang *et al.*, *Analyst*, 2002, *127*, 1203–1206. In plasma: amfetamine enantiomers, limit of quantification 6 ng/L—H. J. Leis *et al.*, *Rapid Commun. Mass Spectrom.*, 2003, *17*, 569–575.

High performance liquid chromatography. In urine: limit of detection 14 µg/L, UV detection—D. H. Fisher and A. J. Bourque, *J. Chromatogr.*, 1993, *614*, 142–147. In urine: amfetamine and metamfetamine—P. Campins Falco *et al.*, *J. Chromatogr.* 1995, *663 B Biomed. Appl.*, 235–245. In urine: amfetamine and metamfetamine, limits of detection 4 µg/L and 2 µg/L, respectively, UV–Vis detection—C. Molins Legua *et al.*, *J. Chromatogr.* 1995, *672 B Biomed. Appl.*, 81–88. In urine: fluorescence detection—T. K. Wang and M. S. Fuh, *J. Chromatogr.* 1996, *686 B Biomed. Appl.*, 285–290. In urine: amfetamine and metamfetamine, limits of detection 100 µg/L and 400 µg/L, respectively—P. Campins-Falco *et al.*, *J. Chromatogr.* 1996, *687 B Biomed. Appl.*, 239–246. In serum or urine: amfetamine and its analogues, limits of detection 10 to 30 µg/L (UV detection) or 50 to 100 µg/L (diode-array detection), also MS—M. J. Bogusz *et al.*, *J. Anal. Toxicol.*, 1997, *21*, 59–69. In hair: amfetamine and metamfetamine, limit of detection about 0.1 µg/L chemiluminescence detection—N. Takayama *et al.*, *Biomed. Chromatogr.*, 1997, *11*, 25–28. In urine: amfetamine, metamfetamine, and related compounds, limits of detection 0.2 to 0.3 µg/L, fluorescence detection—O. Al-Dirbashi *et al.*, *J. Chromatogr. B Biomed. Sci. Appl.*, 1997, *695*, 251–258. In urine: amfetamine and metamfetamine enantiomers, limit of detection 160 µg/L, fluorescence detection—B. S. Foster *et al.*, *J. Anal. Toxicol.*, 1998, *22*, 265–269. In urine: amfetamine and metamfetamine enantiomers, limits of detection 75 ng/L to 238 ng/L, fluorescence detection—O. al-Dirbashi *et al.*, *Analyst*, 1998, *123*, 2333–2337. In hair: amfetamine and metamfetamine, limits of detection 51.4 ng/g and 74.6 ng/g, respectively, fluorescence detection—O. al-Dirbashi *et al.*, *Analyst*, 1999, *124*, 493–497. In urine: amfetamine and related drugs, UV detection—D. Talwar *et al.*, *J. Chromatogr. B Biomed. Sci. Appl.*, 1999, *735*, 229–241. In urine: amfetamine and metamfetamine, fluorescence detection—O. Y. Al-Dirbashi *et al.*, *J. Forensic Sci.*, 2000, *45*, 708–714. Limit of detection, 10 µg/L—T. Veress, *J. Forensic Sci.*, 2000, *45*, 161–166. In hair: amfetamine and metamfetamine enantiomers, limit of detection, >27 ng/L injection, fluorescence detection—O. Y. Al-Dirbashi *et al.*, *Biomed. Chromatogr.*, 2000, *14*, 293–300.

High performance liquid chromatography–mass spectrometry. In urine: amfetamine and metamfetamine enantiomers, limits of detection for amfetamine 0.5 µg/L (SIM) and 10 µg/L (scan mode)—M. Katagi *et al.*, *J. Chromatogr.* 1996, *676 B Biomed. Appl.*, 35–43. In serum: amfetamine and other drugs of abuse, limits of detection 1 to 5 µg/L—M. J. Bogusz *et al.*, *J. Anal. Toxicol.*, 2000, *24*, 77–84.

Reviews. In blood: methods for the analysis of amfetamine and other drugs of abuse—M. R. Moeller *et al.*, *J. Chromatogr. B. Biomed. Sci. Appl.*, 1998, *713*, 91–109. In blood or urine: methods for analysis of amfetamine, metafetamine and derivatives—T. Kraemer and H. H. Maurer, *J. Chromatogr. B Biomed. Sci. Appl.*, 1998, *713*, 163–187.

Disposition in the Body. Readily absorbed after oral or rectal administration; rapidly distributed extravascularly and taken up, to some extent, by red blood cells. The main metabolic reaction is oxidative deamination to form phenylacetone, which is then oxidised to benzoic acid and conjugated with glycine to form hippuric acid; minor reactions include aromatic hydroxylation to form 4-hydroxyamfetamine (an active metabolite), β-hydroxylation which is stereoselective for the (+)-isomer of amfetamine, to form norephedrine (phenylpropanolamine), and *N*-oxidation to form a hydroxylamine derivative. The products of aromatic hydroxylation and *N*-oxidation may be conjugated with sulfate or glucuronic acid.

Excretion of amfetamine is markedly dependent on urinary pH, being greatly increased in acid urine. After large doses, amfetamine may be detected in urine for several days. Under uncontrolled urinary pH conditions, about 30% of the dose is excreted unchanged in the urine in 24 h and a total of about 90% of the dose is excreted in 3 to 4 days. The amount excreted unchanged in 24 h may increase to 74% of the dose in acid urine and decrease to 1 to 4% in alkaline urine; under alkaline conditions, hippuric acid and benzoic acid account for about 50% of the urinary material. Under normal conditions 16 to 28% is excreted as hippuric acid, about 4% as benzoylglucuronide, 2 to 4% as 4-hydroxyamfetamine, and about 2% as norephedrine in 24 h; small amounts of conjugated 4-hydroxynorephedrine and phenylacetone are also excreted. No elimination in the faeces has been detected.
Amfetamine is a metabolite of benzfetamine, metamfetamine, and selegiline.

Therapeutic concentration. After normal therapeutic doses the plasma concentration is usually below 0.1 mg/L. However, continued use of amfetamine may cause addiction, and ingestion of 10 times the usual therapeutic dose is common among addicts; in such cases the plasma concentration may be up to 3 mg/L.

After a single oral dose containing 10 mg of amfetamine to 4 subjects, peak plasma concentrations of about 0.02 mg/L were attained. [S. H. Wan *et al.*, *Clin. Pharmacol. Ther.*, 1978, *23*, 585–590.]

Steady-state blood concentrations of 2 to 3 mg/L were observed in a regular user who ingested about 1 g a day. [R. H. Cravey and N. C. Jain, *Trauma*, 1973, *15*, 49–94.]

The intravenous administration of 160 mg of amfetamine to a regular user resulted in a plasma concentration of 0.59 mg/L after 1 h. [E. Anggard *et al.*, *Scand. J. Clin. Lab. Invest.*, 1970, *26*, 137–143.]

Toxicity. The estimated minimum lethal dose in non-addicted adults is 200 mg. Toxic effects may be produced with blood concentrations of 0.2 to 3 mg/L, and fatalities with concentrations greater than 0.5 mg/L. Death from overdosage is comparatively rare.

In a fatality caused by intravenous administration of amfetamine, the following postmortem tissue concentrations were reported: blood 41 mg/L, liver 23 µg/g, urine 39 mg/L. [G. Adjutantis *et al.*, *Med., Sci. Law*, 1975, *15*, 62–63.]

Urine concentrations of <0.5 to 320 mg/L (mean 76) were reported in 11 fatalities caused by amfetamine. [P. Holmgren and O. Lindquist, *Z. Rechtsmed.*, 1975, *75*, 265–273.]

In a 22-year-old man who died of cardiorespiratory arrest following amfetamine ingestion, the following postmortem tissue concentrations were reported for racemic, (*R*)- and (*S*)-amfetamine, respectively: blood 2.44, 1.26, and 1.18 mg/L, urine 33.4, 16.7, and 16.7 mg/L, liver 11.7, 6.07, and 5.64 µg/g, kidney 3.85, 2.00, and 1.85 µg/g, brain 5.50, 2.95, and 2.55 µg/g. [E. Meyer *et al.*, *J. Anal. Toxicol.*, 1997, *21*, 236–239.]

Half-life. Plasma half-life, 4 to 8 h when the urine is acidic and about 12 h in subjects whose urinary pH values are uncontrolled.

Volume of distribution. About 3 to 4 L/kg.

Saliva. Plasma:saliva ratio, about 0.35.

Protein binding. In plasma, 15 to 40%.
For a review of the toxicokinetics of amfetamines see T. Kraemer and H. H. Maurer, *Ther. Drug Monit.*, 2002, *24*, 277–289. For a study of the pharmacokinetic and pharmacodynamic drug interactions in the treatment of attention-deficit hyperactivity disorder, see J. S. Markowitz and K. S. Patrick, *Clin. Pharmacokinet.*, 2001, *40*, 753–772.

Dose. 20 to 100 mg of amfetamine sulfate daily has been used in the treatment of narcolepsy.

Amicarbalide

Antiprotozoal (Veterinary)

3,3′-(Carbonyldiimino)bisbenzenecarboximidamide
$C_{15}H_{16}N_6O$=296.3
CAS—3459-96-9

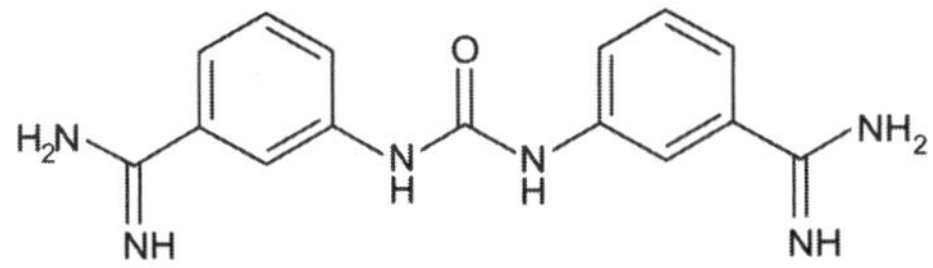

Amicarbalide Isetionate
Synonym. M&B 5062A
Proprietary name. Diampron
$C_{19}H_{28}N_6O_9S_2$=548.6
CAS—3671-72-5
A white or slightly cream-coloured powder. M.p. 200° to 204°.
Soluble 1 in less than 1 of water and 1 in 250 of ethanol; practically insoluble in chloroform and ether.

Colour Tests. Aromaticity (Method 2)—yellow/orange; Liebermann's test (100°)—yellow.

Thin-layer Chromatography. System TA—Rf 05, streaking. (Acidified iodoplatinate solution, positive.)

Ultraviolet Spectrum. Aqueous acid—231 (A_1^1=1236a), inflexion at 256 nm.

Infra-red Spectrum. Principal peaks at wavenumbers 1195, 1590, 1672, 1250, 1562, 1052 cm^{-1} (KBr disk).

Amidefrine

Sympathomimetic

Synonyms. Amidephrine; MJ-1996.
N-[3-[1-Hydroxy-2-(methylamino)ethyl]phenyl]methanesulfonamide
$C_{10}H_{16}N_2O_3S$=244.3
CAS—3354-67-4

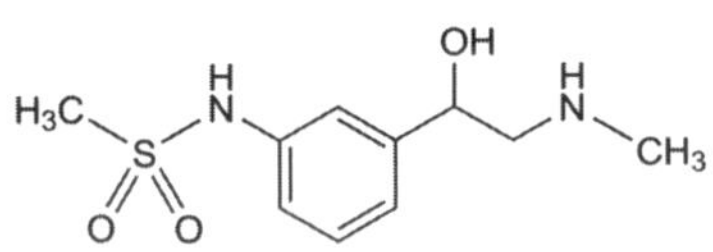

Crystals. M.p. 159° to 161°.

Amidefrine Mesilate
$C_{10}H_{16}N_2O_3S,CH_3SO_3H$=340.4
CAS—1421-68-7
A white crystalline solid. M.p. 207° to 209°.
Soluble 1 in about 5 of water; very slightly soluble in chloroform.

Dissociation Constant. pK_a 9.1.

Colour Test. Mandelin's Test—violet.

Thin-layer Chromatography. System TA—Rf 15; system TB—Rf 00; system TC—Rf 01; system TE—Rf 00; system TL—Rf 02; system TAE—Rf 01. (Acidified potassium permanganate solution, positive.)

Gas Chromatography. System GA—not eluted.

Ultraviolet Spectrum. Aqueous acid—272 nm (A_1^1=22a).

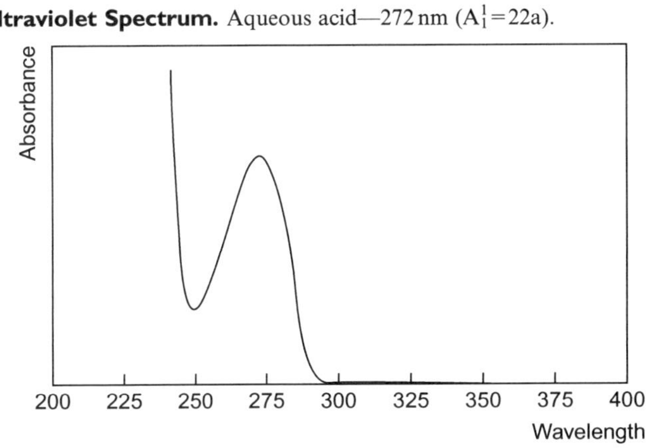

Infra-red Spectrum. Principal peaks at wavenumbers 1101, 1153, 1270, 799, 1207, 1316 cm^{-1}.

Mass Spectrum. Principal ions at *m/z* 44, 42, 147, 120, 65, 43, 45, 39.

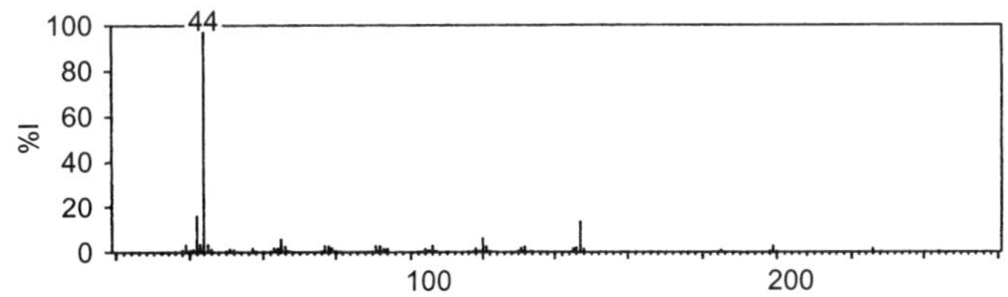

Use. A 0.1% solution of amidefrine mesilate has been used as a nasal decongestant.

Amifostine

Cytoprotective

Synonyms. Ethiofos; Gammaphos; NSC-296961; WR-2721; YM-08310.
Proprietary name. Ethyol
Phosphorothioic acid *S*-[2-[(3-aminopropyl)amino]ethyl] ester
$C_5H_{15}N_2O_3PS$=214.2
CAS—20537-88-6

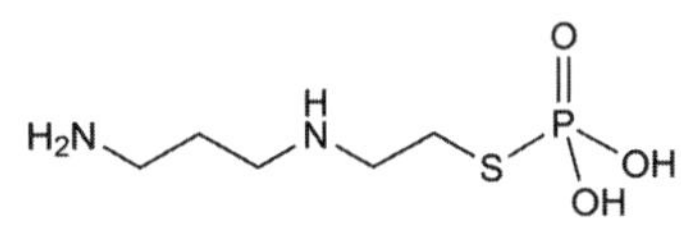

A white to off-white crystalline powder. M.p. 160°. It is freely soluble in water, >9 g/100 ml.

Dissociation Constant. pK_a (water), 10.14, 7.26.

Partition Coefficient. Log *P* (octanol/water), −1.07.

Thin-layer Chromatography. (All systems are for the *S*-2-(3-aminopropylamino)-ethanethiol, WR-1065, metabolite.)
Plate 1: silica 60 (0.25 mm particles). Mobile phase: sodium acetate buffer (pH 5.5, 0.50 M):methanol (50 to 90%). Rf 0.03.

Plate 2: alumina 60 (0.25 mm particles). Mobile phase 1: sodium acetate buffer (pH 5.5, 0.50 M):methanol (50 to 90%). Rf 0.70 (50% methanol), Rf 0.45 (60%) and Rf 0.03 (70 to 90%). Mobile phase 2: phosphate buffer (pH 5.5, 0.1 M):methanol (50 to 90%). Rf 0.03. [A. J. G. Mank *et al.*, *J. Pharm. Biomed. Anal.*, 1995, *13*(3), 255–263].

High Performance Liquid Chromatography. Column: LC-ABZ (Supelcosil, 15 cm × 4.6 mm i.d., 5 μm). Mobile phase: methanol:ethylamine (10 mM) in monochloroacetic acid (0.1 mol/l, pH 2.8) (10:90), 1.0 mL/min flow rate. Fluorescence detection (λ_{ex}=385 nm, λ_{em}=515 nm). Retention time: amifostine metabolite, WR-1065, 4.0 min. [H. S. Bonner and L. M. Shaw, *J. Chromatogr. Biomed. Sci. Appl.*, 2000, *739*, 357–362].

Quantification

High performance liquid chromatography. In whole blood: limit of detection 0.25 mg/L. Fluorescence detection (λ_{ex}=385 nm, λ_{em}=515 nm)—H. S. Bonner and L. M. Shaw, *J. Chromatogr. Biomed. Sci. Appl.*, 2000, *739*, 357–362.

Disposition in the Body. Amifostine is rapidly cleared from plasma with <10% remaining in plasma 6 min after administration. It is metabolised in the liver, by alkaline phosphatase, to the active free thiol metabolite, *S*-2-(3-aminopropylamino)-ethanethiol, WR-1065, and the inactive WR-33278 metabolite. <4% of the parent drug and metabolites are excreted in urine, WR-1065 is found in bone marrow.

Therapeutic concentration
5 cancer patients were administered with a 740 mg/m^2 dose of amifostine and 7 patients with 910 mg/m^2. Peak plasma levels of 0.10 and 0.24 nmol/L were reached. [L. Shaw *et al.*, *Proc. Am. Soc. Cancer Res.*, 1994, *13*, 144].

Toxicity. Hypotension is the main toxic effect.

Half-life. Elimination half-life is approx. 9 min.

Volume of distribution. Steady state, between 3.5 and 7 L.

Clearance. Plasma clearance, 2.17 L/min.

Protein binding. Approx 4% amifostine is bound to plasma proteins.

Dose. Usual dose given is 910 mg/m^2 body surface but can be reduced to 740 mg/m^2, if necessary.

Amikacin

Antibacterial

O-3-Amino-3-deoxy-α-D-glucopyranosyl-(1→6)-*O*-[6-amino-6-deoxy-α-D-glucopyranosyl-(1→4)]-N^1-[(2*S*)-4-amino-2-hydroxy-1-oxobutyl]-2-deoxy-D-streptamine
$C_{22}H_{43}N_5O_{13}$=585.6
CAS—37517-28-5

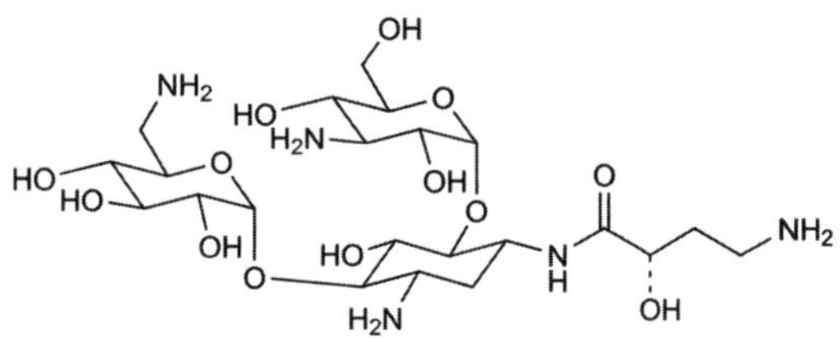

A white crystalline powder. M.p. 201° to 204°, with decomposition. Sparingly soluble in water.

Amikacin Sulfate

Proprietary names. Amiglyde-V; Amikin; BB-K8; Biklin; Lukadin; Mikavir; Novamin; Pierami.
$C_{22}H_{43}N_5O_{13},2H_2SO_4$=781.8
CAS—39831-55-5
Freely soluble in water.

Thin-layer Chromatography. System TAE—Rf 00.

High Performance Liquid Chromatography. Column: (analytical) C_{18} μBondapak (10 μm, 300 × 3.9 mm); (pre-column) C_{18}/Corasil (37 to 50 μm, 25 × 4 mm). Column temperature: 58°. Mobile phase: acetonitrile:2-methoxyethanol:tetrahydrofuran:glacial acetic acid:tris(hydroxymethyl):aminoethane (1% aqueous solution) (41:4:52:4:0.21:50). Elution programme: 0 to 8.5 min at 1.0 mL/min; 8.5 to 19 min at 0.5 mL/min; 19 to 25 min at 3.0 mL/min; 25 to 30 min at 1.0 mL/min. Internal standard (IS): Cefepine. UV detection. Retention time(s): 16.5 min. [E. A. Papp *et al.*, *J. Chromatogr.*, 1992, *574*; *B Biomed. Appl.*, 93–99].

Ultraviolet Spectrum. No significant absorption, 230 to 360 nm.

Infra-red Spectrum. Principal peaks at wavenumbers 1050, 1630, 1120, 1145, 1545, 940 cm^{-1} (KBr disk).

Quantification

Gas chromatography. In serum: amikacin, gentamicin and tobramycin, limit of detection 600 μg/L, ECD—J. W. Mayhew and S. L. Gorbach, *J. Chromatogr.*, 1978, *151*, 133–146.

High performance liquid chromatography. In plasma and urine: limit of quantification 0.5 mg/L, UV detection—E. A. Papp *et al.*, *J. Chromatogr.*, 1992, *574*; *B Biomed. Appl.*, 93–99. In plasma: limit of quantification 25 μg/L, fluorescence detection (λ_{ex}=340 nm; λ_{em}=418 nm)—B. Wichert *et al.*, *J. Pharm. Biomed. Anal.*, 1991, *9(3)*, 251–254. In serum: amikacin, gentamicin and tobramycin, limit of detection 1 mg/L, fluorescence detection—J. P. Anhalt and S. D. Brown, *Clin. Chem.*, 1978, *24*, 1940–1947.

Immunoassay. In serum: fluoroimmunoassay—S. G. Thompson and J. F. Burd, *Antimicrob. Agents Chemother.*, 1980, *18*, 264–268.

Bioassay. Aminoglycoside antibiotics in biological fluids—J. M. Broughall, Aminoglycosides, in *Laboratory Methods in Antimicrobial Chemotherapy*, D. S. Reeves *et al.* (Ed.), 1978, Churchill Livingstone, Edinburgh, pp. 194–207.

Review. For a review of methods for the determination of aminoglycoside antibiotics in biological fluids, see S. K. Maitra *et al.*, *Clin. Chem.*, 1979, *25*, 1361–1367.

Disposition in the Body. Poorly absorbed after oral administration but rapidly absorbed after intramuscular injection. About 90% of a dose is excreted in the urine unchanged in 24 h.

Therapeutic concentration. During treatment, the serum concentration should be in the range 15 to 25 mg/L and should be monitored regularly, especially in patients who have renal insufficiency. During multiple dosing, the trough concentration immediately preceding a dose should not exceed 10 mg/L.

A male patient, aged 36 years, with multi-drug resistant tuberculosis was administered 750 mg amikacin intravenously for 5 days. The mean peak concentration was 39.27 mg/L observed between 0.5 and 1.5 h. [W. W. Yew *et al.*, *Int. J. Clin. Pharmacol. Res.*, 1999, *19(3)*, 65–71].

18 patients with cystic fibrosis, aged 1.7 to 22.2 years, were administered a daily intravenous dose of 35 mg/kg amikacin over 30 min. The mean peak serum concentration was 121.4 mg/L (range 42.7 to 176 mg/L) after the 30 min and the trough concentration was 0.88 (0.2 to 1.9) mg/L. The peak concentration in sputum was 10.95 mg/L observed at 2 h which decreased slowly to a mean concentration of 2.14 mg/L just before the next infusion. [F. Canis *et al.*, *J. Antimicrob. Chemother.*, 1997, *39(3)*, 431–433].

A patient received 300 mg only of amikacin intravenously over a 30-min infusion or in combination with 2000 mg cefepime. The mean plasma amikacin concentration was 27.4 mg/L when the drug was administered alone and 24.6 mg/L when in combination with cefepime. The peak concentrations were observed at the end of the infusion [E. A. Papp *et al.*, *J. Chromatogr.*, 1992, *574*; *B Biomed. Appl.*, 93–99].

A single intramuscular dose of 500 mg given to 6 subjects, produced a mean peak serum concentration of 20 mg/L in 1.5 h. [R. A. Yates *et al.*, *J. Antimicrob. Chemother.*, 1978, *4*, 335–341].

Toxicity. Toxic effects may be produced at serum concentrations of 30 mg/L or more or, during chronic treatment, if the trough serum concentration exceeds 10 mg/L.

The following postmortem tissue concentrations were reported in a patient who died 5 days after discontinuation of amikacin treatment: serum 2.2 mg/L, heart 20 μg/g, kidney 794 μg/g, liver 30 μg/g, lungs 48 μg/g, muscle 11 μg/g. [M. A. French *et al.*, *Antimicrob. Agents Chemother.*, 1981, *19*, 147–152].

Half-life. Plasma half-life, 2 to 3 h.

Volume of distribution. About 0.2 L/kg.

Clearance. Plasma clearance, about 1 mL/min/kg.

Protein binding. In plasma, less than 10%.

Note. For a review of the pharmacokinetics of amikacin, see D. Andrews, *Can. J. Hosp. Pharm.*, 1977, *30*, 146–148.

Dose. The equivalent of 15 mg of amikacin/kg daily, given parenterally; maximum of 1.5 g daily. The total dose should not exceed 15 g.

Amiloride

Diuretic

Synonyms. Amipramidin; Amipramizide; Guanamprazine
3,5-Diamino-*N*-(aminoiminomethyl)-6-chloropyrazinecarboxamide
$C_6H_8ClN_7O$=229.6
CAS—2609-46-3

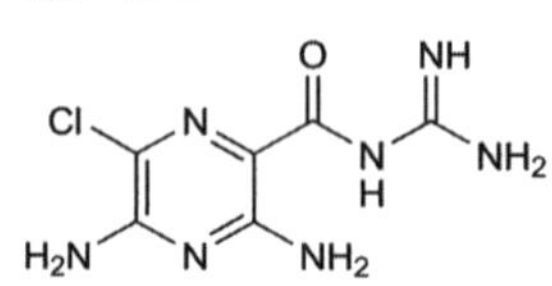

M.p. 240° to 242°.

Amiloride Hydrochloride

Synonym. Amipramizide
Proprietary names. Arumil; Midamor; Modamide. It is an ingredient of Amilco, Frumil, Moducren and Moduretic.
$C_6H_8ClN_7O,HCl,2H_2O$=302.1
CAS—2016-88-8 (anhydrous)
A pale yellow to greenish-yellow powder. M.p. 285° to 288°, with decomposition. Soluble in water and ethyl acetate; soluble 1 in 350 of ethanol; practically insoluble in chloroform and ether.

Dissociation Constant. pK_a 8.7.

Colour Tests. Marquis test—yellow; Sulfuric acid—yellow.

Thin-layer Chromatography. System TA—Rf 24; system TB—Rf 00; system TC—Rf 01; system TE—Rf 24; system TL—Rf 02; system TAD—Rf 00; system TAE—Rf 06; system TAF—Rf 74; system TAJ—Rf 00; system TAK—Rf 00; system TAL—Rf 29. (Acidified iodoplatinate solution, strong reaction.)

High Performance Liquid Chromatography. System HY—RI 190; system HX—RI 257; system HAA—Retention time(s) 3.6 min.

Ultraviolet Spectrum. Aqueous acid—285 (A^1_1=731a), 361 nm (A^1_1=802a).

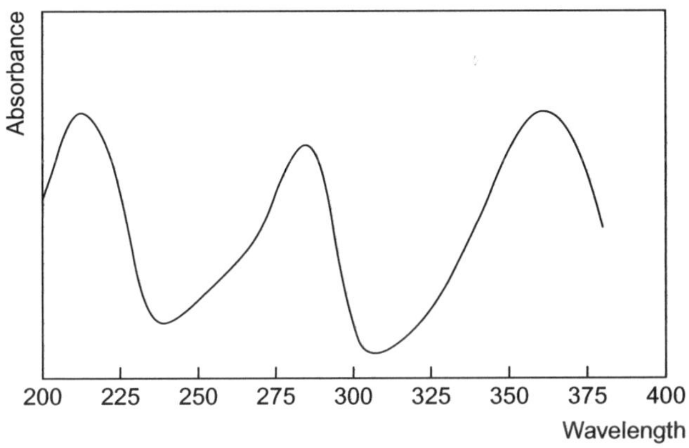

Infra-red Spectrum. Principal peaks at wavenumbers 1634, 1602, 1504, 1686, 1238, 1538 cm^{-1} (amiloride hydrochloride, KBr disk).

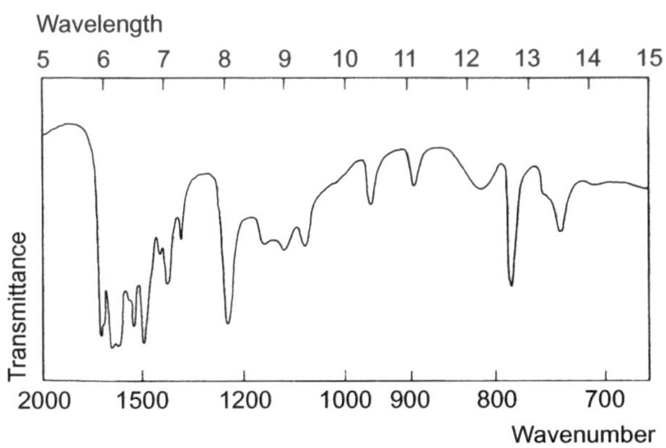

Mass Spectrum. Principal ions at *m/z* 43, 187, 42, 171, 229, 86, 144, 170.

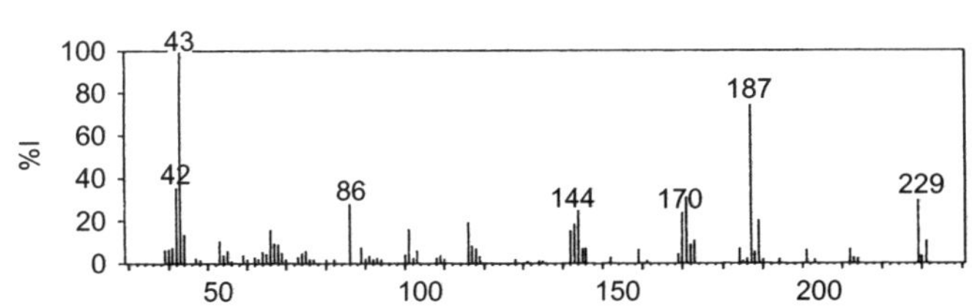

Quantification

Spectrofluorimetry. In plasma, serum or urine—J. E. Baer *et al.*, *J. Pharmacol Exp. Ther.*, 1967, *157*, 472–485.

Thin-layer chromatography–spectrofluorimetry. In plasma—K. Reuter *et al.*, *J. Chromatogr.*, 1982, *233*; *Biomed. Appl.*, *22*, 432–436.

Gas chromatography–mass spectrometry. In urine: limit of detection 4 mg/L—H. Bi *et al.*, *J. Chromatogr.*, 1992, *582(1–2)*, 93–101.

High performance liquid chromatography. In urine: limit of detection 0.12 mg/L, UV detection (λ=363, 213 and 285 nm)—H. Bi *et al.*, *J. Chromatogr.*, 1992, *582(1–2)*, 93–101. In plasma: limit of detection 0.03 μg/L, fluorescence detection (λ_{ex}=360 nm; λ_{em}=413 nm)—H. J. Reeuwijk *et al.*, *J. Chromatogr.*, 1992, *575(2)*, 269–274. In plasma and urine: limit of detection 0.5 μg/L, fluorescence detection (λ_{ex}=286 nm; λ_{em}=418 nm)—Dan-Ke Xu *et al.*, *J. Chromatogr.*, 1991, *567*; B Biomed. Appl., 451–458. In urine: limit of detection 1.0 mg/L, diode-array detection—S. J. Park *et al.*, *J. Anal. Toxicol.*, 1990, *14(2)*, 84–90.

Disposition in the Body. Incompletely absorbed after oral administration; it does not appear to be metabolised. About 50% of an oral dose is excreted unchanged in the urine and 40% is eliminated in the faeces in 72 h.

Therapeutic concentration

8 healthy subjects aged 22 to 33 years (mean 25 years) inhaled 1 mg/mL (a volume of 4.5 mL in container) amiloride for 12 min. The mean volume aerolised was 3.5 mL in the 12 min. The peak plasma concentrations of amiloride were 3.36 μg/L after 30 min. [P. G. Noone *et al.*, *Chest*, 1997, *112(5)*, 1283–1290].

6 adult subjects were administered 10 mg amiloride as a Chinese formulation and an imported formulation. After 4 h, the peak plasma amiloride concentration was 27.76 μg/L for the Chinese and 23.17 μg/L for the imported formulations, respectively. After 24 h, the plasma concentrations had decreased to 5.76 μg/L and 3.57 μg/L, respectively. [Dan-Ke Xu *et al.*, *J. Chromatogr.*, 1991, *567*; *B Biomed. Appl.*, 451–458].

After a single oral dose of 20 mg to 6 subjects, peak serum concentrations of about 0.05 mg/L were attained in 4 h. [A. J. Smith and R. N. Smith, *Br. J. Pharmacol.*, 1973, *48*, 646–649].

Half-life. Plasma half-life, 6 to 10 h.

Volume of distribution. About 5 L/kg.

Protein binding. In plasma, not significantly bound.

Dose. 5 to 20 mg of amiloride hydrochloride daily.

Amineptine

CNS Stimulant

7-[(10,11-dihydro-5*H*-dibenzo[*a*,*d*]-cyclohepten-5-yl)amino]heptanoic acid

$C_{22}H_{27}NO_2$=337.5

CAS—57574-09-1

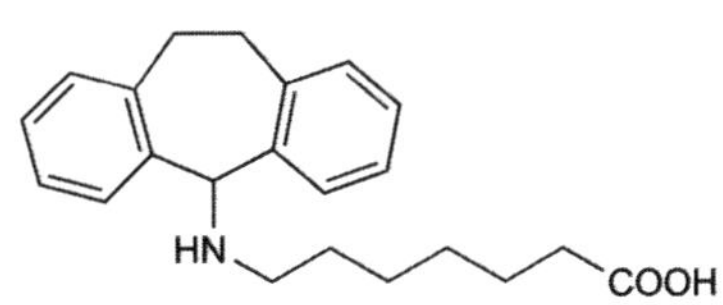

Amineptine Hydrochloride

Synonym. S-1694

Proprietary names. Maneon; Survector.

$C_{22}H_{28}ClNO_2$=373.9

CAS—30272-08-3

Crystals from distilled water. M.p. 226° to 230°.

Partition Coefficient. Log *P* (octanol/water), 2.66.

High Performance Liquid Chromatography. System HAA—retention time 14.0 min.

Column: (analytical) C_{18} (μBondapak, 300 × 3.9 mm i.d., 10 μm), (guard) C_{18} (μBondapak, 5 × 6 mm i.d., fitted with 2-μm filters at either end). Mobile phase: acetonitrile:potassium dihydrogen phosphate (0.025 M) (45:55), flow rate 0.8 mL/min. UV detection (λ=210 nm). *k* values: amineptine, 1.47; metabolite, 0.93. [P. P. Rop *et al.*, *J. Chromatogr. B Biomed. Sci. Appl.*, 1990, *532*, 351–361].

Ultraviolet Spectrum. Aqueous acid—266 nm.

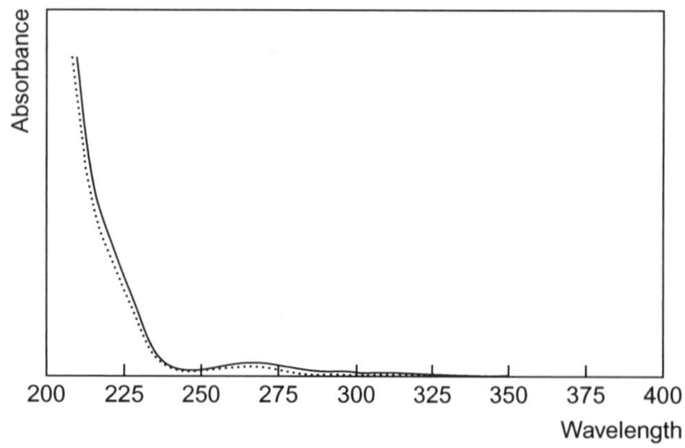

Mass Spectrum. Principal peaks at *m/z* 191, 192, 207, 208, 209.

Quantification

High perfomance liquid chromatography. In plasma: limit of quantification <0.05 mg/L, UV detection (λ=210 nm)— P. P. Rop *et al.*, *J. Chromatogr. B Biomed. Sci. Appl.*, 1990, *532*, 351–361. Limit of detection ⩾0.01 mg/L— G. Lachatre *et al.*, *Fundam. Clin. Pharmacol.*, 1989, *3*, 19–26.

Disposition in the Body. Amineptine is rapidly absorbed and metabolised to produce seven metabolites. Metabolism is mainly via *β*-oxidation of the heptanoic side chain, resulting in pentanoic and propanoic side chain metabolites, and hydroxylation of the dibenzocycloheptyl ring to produce two diastereoisomers. *N*-Dealkylation of the lateral alkyl chain can, also, occur to produce dibenzosuberamine (DBZ), which is only found as a trace. Elimination is mainly via urine and complete within about 12 h.

Therapeutic concentration

6 healthy males and 6 females, aged between 23 and 46 years, were administered with a single dose of 100 mg of amineptine hydrchloride. Mean peak plasma concentrations of 0.28 to 2.22 mg/L amineptine were reached within 0.36 to 1.40 h. Peak plasma concentrations of the metabolites reached 0.14 to 1.07 mg/L within 0.44 to 2.32 h. No significant differences were observed between the male and female data. [G. Lachatre *et al.*, *Fundam. Clin. Pharmacol.*, 1989, *3*, 19–26].

Toxicity. Severe acne-type lesions are associated with chronic self-administration of high doses (200 to 1000 mg). They occur mainly on the face, back, and thorax but, also, on the extremities and in the perineal region.

Half-life. Elimination half-life of amineptine is 0.8 h and, for its metabolite, 2.5 h.

Volume of distribution. Apparent volume of distribution is 2.4 L/kg.

Clearance. Plasma clearance, 124.8 L/h.

Dose. A usual dose of 100 to 200 mg is administered daily.

Aminitrozole

Antiprotozoal

Synonyms. Acinitrazole; Nithiamide.
Proprietary names. Enheptin-A; Trichorad; Tricosil; Trigamma; Tritheon.
N-(5-Nitro-2-thiazolyl)acetamide
$C_5H_5N_3O_3S$=187.2
CAS—140-40-9

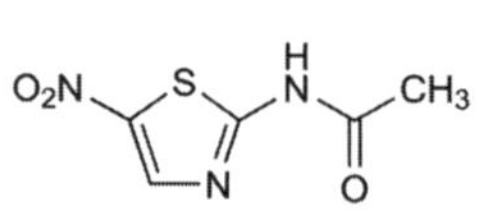

A buff or yellowish-buff powder. M.p. 264° to 265°; slight decomposition may occur. Very slightly soluble in water; soluble 1 in 300 of ethanol and 1 in 900 of chloroform; slightly soluble in ether; soluble in aqueous solutions of sodium hydroxide and ammonia.

Colour Test. Methanolic potassium hydroxide—orange.

Thin-layer Chromatography. System TA—Rf 80. (Acidified potassium permanganate solution, positive.)

Ultraviolet Spectrum. Aqueous acid—237, 345 nm (A_1^1=435b).

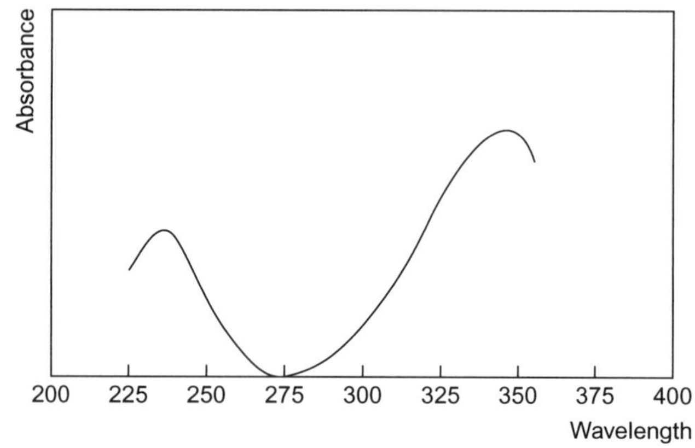

Infra-red Spectrum. Principal peaks at wavenumbers 1314, 1176, 1709, 1215, 818, 740 cm^{-1}.

Dose. Aminitrozole has been given in doses of 200 to 400 mg daily.

Aminoacridine

Antiseptic

Synonym. Aminacrine
9-Acridinamine
$C_{13}H_{10}N_2$=194.2
CAS—90-45-9

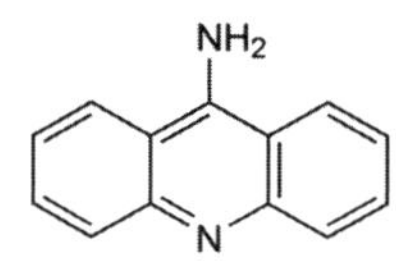

Yellow needles. M.p. 241°. Freely soluble in ethanol; soluble in acetone; slightly soluble in chloroform.

Aminoacridine Hexylresorcinate

Synonyms. Acrisorcin; Aminoacridine 4-Hexylresorcinate.
$C_{13}H_{10}N_2,C_{12}H_{18}O_2$=388.5
CAS—7527-91-5
A yellow crystalline powder. Slightly soluble in water and ethanol.

Aminoacridine Hydrochloride

Synonym. Acramine Yellow
Proprietary names. Aminopt; Monacrin.
$C_{13}H_{10}N_2,HCl,H_2O$=248.7
CAS—134-50-9 (anhydrous)
A yellow crystalline powder. M.p. about 235°. Soluble 1 in 300 of water; a saturated solution in water is pale yellow with a greenish-blue fluorescence, becoming blue when freely diluted. Soluble 1 in 150 of ethanol; practically insoluble in chloroform and ether.

Dissociation Constant. pK_a 9.5 (25°).

Colour Tests. Aromaticity (Method 2)—yellow/red; Liebermann's test (100°)—red. Cold nitric acid gives a red colour in 15 s.

Thin-layer Chromatography. System TA—Rf 54; system TB—Rf 00; system TE—Rf 57; system TAE—Rf 09. (Acidified iodoplatinate solution, positive.)

Gas Chromatography. System GA—RI 2240.

High Performance Liquid Chromatography. System HX—RI 320.

Ultraviolet Spectrum. Aqueous acid—260 (A_1^1=4442a), 313 (A_1^1=74b), 326 (A_1^1=81b) nm; methanol—260 (A_1^1=4480 b), 311, 325 nm.

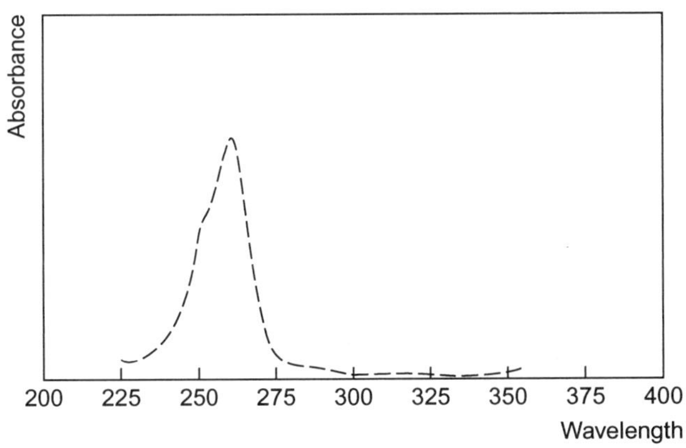

Infra-red Spectrum. Principal peaks at wavenumbers 760, 1556, 1645, 1655, 750, 1612 cm^{-1} (KBr disk).

Aminobenzoic Acid

Sunscreen Agent

Synonyms. Amben; PAB; PABA; Pabacidum; Para-aminobenzoic Acid; Vitamin H′.
Proprietary names. Hill-Shade; Pabagel; Pabanol; Paraminan; Presun 8; RVPaba.
4-Aminobenzoic acid
$C_7H_7NO_2$=137.1
CAS—150-13-0

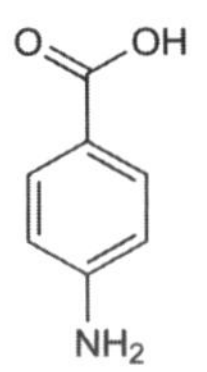

White or slightly yellow crystals or crystalline powder. It gradually darkens on exposure to air and light. M.p. 186° to 189°. Soluble 1 in 200 of water, 1 in 10 of boiling water, 1 in 8 of ethanol, and 1 in 50 of ether; slightly soluble in chloroform; freely soluble in solutions of alkali hydroxides and carbonates.

Potassium Aminobenzoate
Proprietary name. Potaba
$C_7H_6KNO_2$=175.2
CAS—138-84-1
A crystalline powder. Very soluble in water; less soluble in ethanol; practically insoluble in ether.

Dissociation Constant. pK_a 2.4, 4.9 (25°).

Colour Tests. Coniferyl alcohol—orange; Diazotisation—red.

Thin-layer Chromatography. System TA—Rf 58; system TD—Rf 19; system TE—Rf 01; system TF—Rf 43; system TAD—Rf 31; system TAJ—Rf 44; system TAK—Rf 44; system TAL—Rf 83 (*p*-aminobenzoic acid). (Acidified potassium permanganate solution, positive; Van Urk reagent, yellow.)

Gas Chromatography. System GA—RI 1547.

High Performance Liquid Chromatography. System HY—RI 66 (*m*-aminobenzoic acid), RI 235 (*o*-aminobenzoic acid), RI 212 (*p*-aminobenzoic acid).
Column: C_{18} Separon-6 RP (150 × 3.2 mm i.d., 5 μm). Mobile phase: methanol: 0.02 M ammonium acetate (20:80 v/v), pH 4, flow rate 0.5 mL/min. UV detection (λ=280 nm). *k* values: *p*-aminobenzoic acid, 1.86; *m*-hydroxybenzoic acid, 2.74; *N*-acetyl-*p*-aminobenzoic acid, 3.89 [R. Kastel *et al.*, *Biomed. Chromatogr.*, 1994, *8*, 294–296].

Ultraviolet Spectrum. Aqueous acid—270 nm (A^1_1=95b); aqueous alkali—265 nm (A^1_1=1063a).

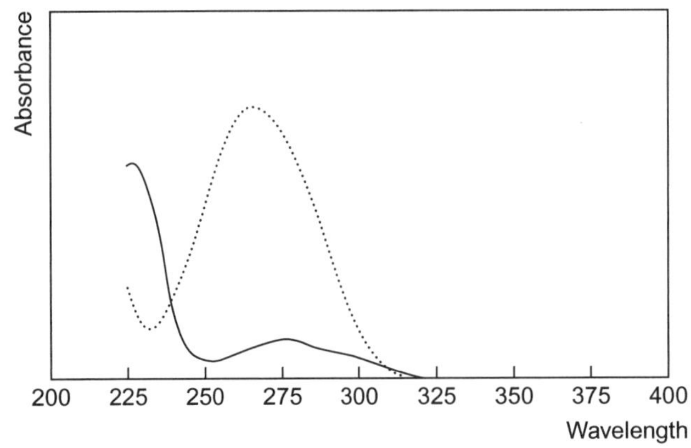

Infra-red Spectrum. Principal peaks at wavenumbers 1597, 1168, 1290, 1665, 1305, 1625 cm^{-1} (KBr disk).

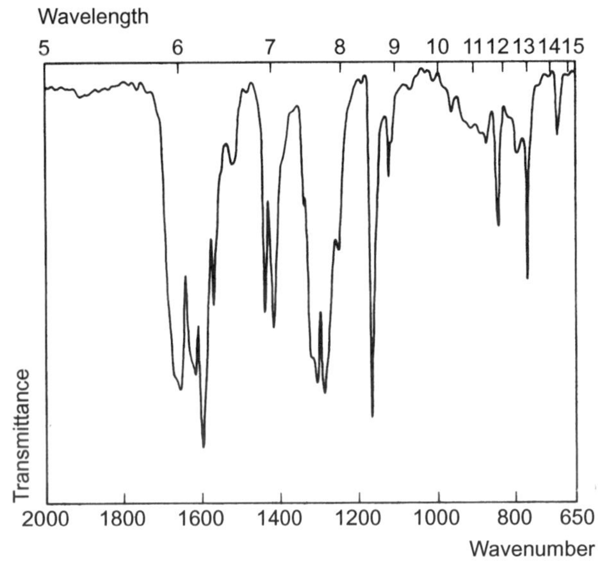

Mass Spectrum. Principal ions at *m/z* 137, 120, 92, 65, 39, 138, 121, 63.

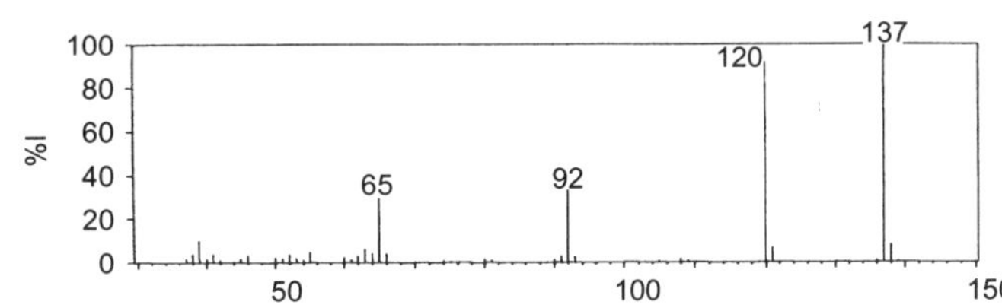

Quantification

High performance liquid chromatography. In urine: limit of detection 12.5 mg/L, UV detection (λ=280 nm)—R. Kastel *et al.*, *Biomed. Chromatogr.*, 1994, *8*, 294–296. In serum or urine: aminobenzoic acid and metabolites, UV detection—N. D. Brown and E. J. Michalski, *J. Chromatogr.*, 1976, *121*, 76–78.

Disposition in the Body. Aminobenzoic acid is readily absorbed after oral administration. It is conjugated with aminoacetic acid to form *p*-aminohippuric acid which is excreted in the urine together with a small amount of *p*-aminobenzoyl glucuronide, *p*-acetamidobenzoyl glucuronide, and traces of *p*-acetamidohippuric acid, *p*-acetamidobenzoic acid and unchanged aminobenzoic acid.
Aminobenzoic acid may be detected in the urine as a metabolite of tetracaine, benzocaine and procaine.

Toxicity. Toxic effects are infrequent and are usually associated with plasma concentrations greater than about 600 mg/L.

Uses. Aminobenzoic acid is used topically as a 5% solution; potassium aminobenzoate has been given orally, in doses of 12 g daily.

Aminocaproic Acid

Haemostatic

Synonyms. CY-116; EACA; Epsilcapramin; Epsilon Aminocaproic Acid.
Proprietary names. Amicar; Capracid; Capralense; Capramol; Ekaprol; Epsikapron; Hemocaprol; Ipsilon.
6-Aminohexanoic acid
$C_6H_{13}NO_2$=131.2
CAS—60-32-2

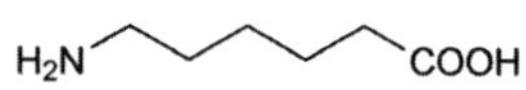

Colourless crystals or white crystalline powder. M.p. about 204°, with decomposition. Soluble 1 in 1.5 of water; slightly soluble in ethanol; practically insoluble in chloroform and ether; freely soluble in solutions of acids and alkalis.

Dissociation Constant. pK_a 4.4, 10.8 (25°).

Thin-layer Chromatography. System TAJ—Rf 01; system TAL—Rf 45.

Infra-red Spectrum. Principal peaks at wavenumbers 1538, 1613, 1098, 1319, 1258, 1203 cm^{-1} (KBr disk).

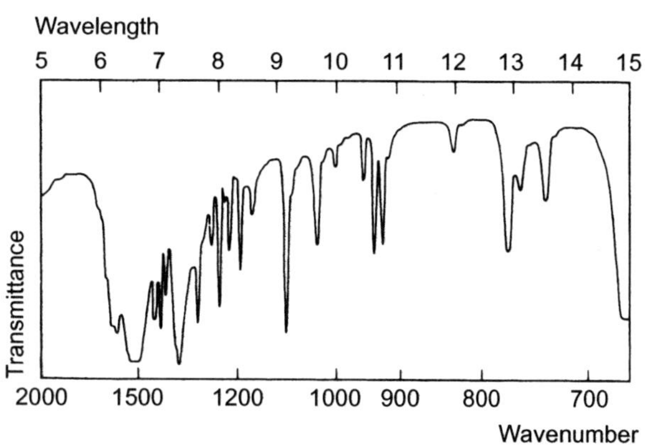

Quantification

High performance liquid chromatography. In plasma and urine: limit of detection 50 µg/L, fluorescence detection—S. Lam, *Biomed. Chromatogr.*, 1990, *4(4)*, 175–177. In serum: limits of detection 0.01 ng and 3 ng for fluorescence or UV detection, respectively—N. A. Farid, *J. Pharm. Sci.*, 1979, *68*, 249–252.

Disposition in the Body. Aminocaproic acid is readily absorbed after oral administration and widely distributed throughout the body fluids. About 70 to 80% of a dose is excreted in the urine unchanged in 12 h.

Therapeutic concentration. In plasma, usually in the range 100 to 400 mg/L.

Half-life. Plasma half-life, about 2 to 5 h.

Volume of distribution. About 0.4 L/kg.

Note. For a review of aminocaproic acid, see *Aust. J. Pharm.*, 1981, *62*, 403–407.

Dose. 3 to 6 g may be given 4 to 6 times daily.

Aminoglutethimide

Antineoplastic

Proprietary names. Cytadren; Elipten; Orimeten.
3-(4-Aminophenyl)-3-ethyl-2,6-piperidinedione
$C_{13}H_{16}N_2O_2$=232.3
CAS—125-84-8

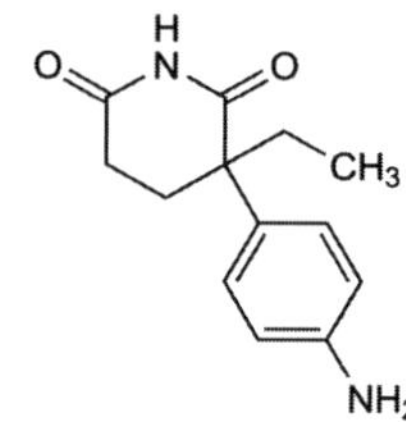

A white crystalline powder. M.p. about 151°. Very slightly soluble in water; freely soluble in organic solvents.

Colour Tests. Coniferyl alcohol—yellow; Koppanyi–Zwikker test—violet; Mercurous nitrate—black.

Thin-layer Chromatography. System TD—Rf 32; system TE—Rf 65; system TF—Rf 47; system TAD—Rf 53.

Gas Chromatography. System GA—RI 2227.

High Performance Liquid Chromatography. System HZ—Retention time(s) 2.5 min.

Column: cellulose tris(3,5-dimethylphenyl carbamate) (Chiralcel OD). Mobile phase: hexane:methanol:isopropyl alcohol (65:17.5:17.5), flow rate 0.7 mL/min. UV detection. Retention time(s): *R-N*-acetylaminoglutethimide 17.7 min (*k* 1.2); *S-N*-acetylaminoglutethimide 21.5 min (*k* 1.5); (*R*-aminoglutethimide) 32.7 min (*k* 2.6); (*S*-aminoglutethimide) 37.7 min (*k* 3.3). [I. A. Alshowaier *et al.*, *Ther. Drug Monit.*, 1995, *17*, 538–543].

Ultraviolet Spectrum. Aqueous acid—251 (A_1^1=18b), 257 nm (A_1^1=18b).

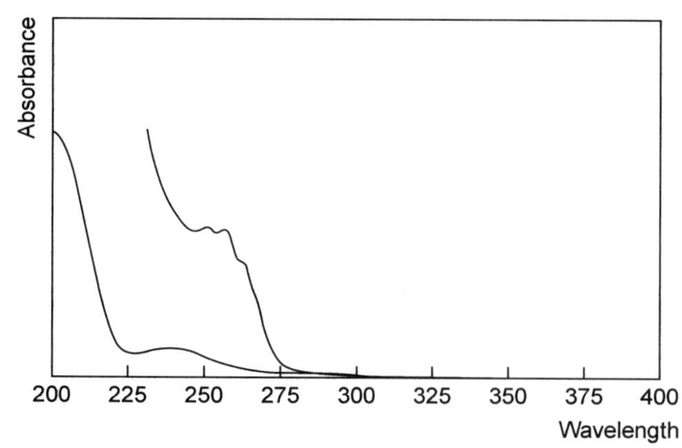

Infra-red Spectrum. Principal peaks at wavenumbers 1695, 1185, 1200, 1515, 1623, 1267 cm^{-1} (KCl disk).

Mass Spectrum. Principal ions at *m/z* 203, 232, 132, 175, 204, 233, 160, 118.

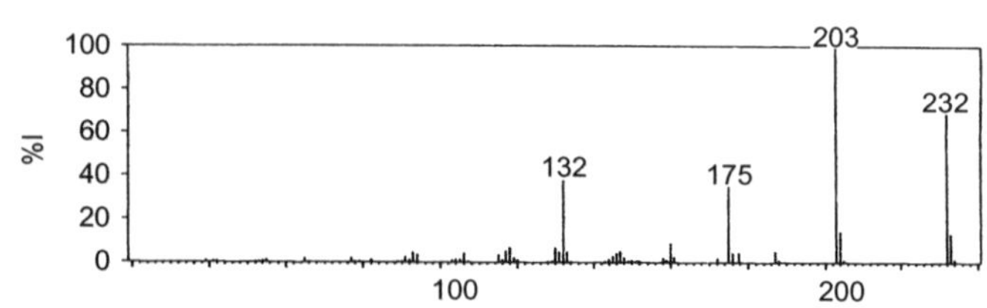

Quantification

High performance liquid chromatography. In plasma, saliva and urine: limit of detection of *N*-acetylaminoglutethimide 0.24 mg/L and aminoglutethimide 0.32 mg/L, UV detection—I. A. Alshowaier *et al.*, *Ther. Drug Monit.*, 1995, *17*, 538–543. In plasma: limit of detection <230 µg/L, UV detection—B. A. Robinson and F. N. Cornell, *Clin. Chem.*, 1983, *29*, 1104–1105.

Disposition in the Body. Aminoglutethimide is readily absorbed after oral administration. About 10% of an oral dose is excreted in the urine as unchanged drug in 48 h; acetamidoglutethimide has been identified as a metabolite. Aminoglutethimide appears to induce its own metabolism.

Therapeutic concentration

Postmenopausal women with advanced metastatic breast carcinoma, mean age 53 years, were administered 500 mg aminoglutethimide after an overnight fast. The mean peak concentration of *R*-aminoglutethimide was 3.8 (range 2.5 to 4.3) g/L observed at 1.4 (0.5 to 2.0) h and for *S*-aminoglutethimide 3.3 (2.4 to 4.3) g/L at 1.3 (1 to 2) h. [*J. Clin. Pharmacol.*, 1999, *39(11)*, 1136–1142].

After a single oral dose of 500 mg given to 6 subjects, peak plasma concentrations of 5.8 to 6.3 (mean 5.9) mg/L were attained in 1.3 h. [T. A. Thompson *et al.*, *J. Pharm. Sci.*, 1981, *70*, 1040–1043].

Steady-state serum concentrations of 4.7 to 32.4 (mean 11.5) mg/L were reported in 7 subjects receiving chronic treatment with oral doses of 1 g daily. [F. T. Murray *et al.*, *J. Clin. Pharmacol.*, 1979, *19*, 704–711].

Toxicity. The estimated minimum lethal dose is 5 g.

Half-life. Plasma half-life, about 13 h following a single dose but appears to decrease during chronic treatment.

Volume of distribution. About 1.4 L/kg.

Clearance. Plasma clearance, about 1.3 mL/min/kg.

Distribution in blood. Plasma:whole blood ratio, about 0.7.

Protein binding. In plasma, about 25%.

Dose. 0.5 to 1 g daily.

Aminohippuric Acid

Diagnostic Agent (Renal Function)

Synonyms. *p*-Aminobenzoylglycine; PAHA; Para-aminohippuric Acid.
N-(4-Aminobenzoyl)glycine
$C_9H_{10}N_2O_3$=194.2
CAS—61-78-9

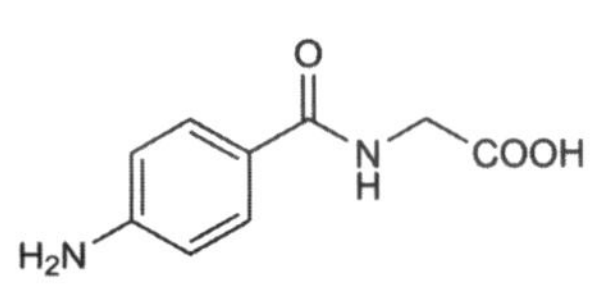

A white crystalline powder, which discolours on exposure to light. M.p. about 195°, with decomposition. Soluble 1 in 45 of water, 1 in 50 of ethanol and 1 in 5 of dilute hydrochloric acid; very slightly soluble in carbon tetrachloride, chloroform and ether; freely soluble, with decomposition, in solutions of alkali hydroxides and carbonates.

Sodium Aminohippurate

Proprietary name. Nephrotest
$C_9H_9N_2NaO_3$=216.2
CAS—94-16-6
Soluble in water.

Dissociation Constant. pK_a 3.6.

Colour Test. Diazotisation—red.

Thin-layer Chromatography. System TA—Rf 55. (Van Urk reagent, yellow.)

High Performance Liquid Chromatography. Column: Ultracarb ODS 30 (150 × 4.6 mm i.d., 5 μm). Mobile phase: 7 mmol/L 1-decanesulfonic acid adjusted to pH 3.7 with orthophosphoric acid (89%):acetonitrile (82:18 v/v), flow rate 1.0 mL/min. Internal standard (IS): *p*-aminobenzoic acid. UV detection (λ=280 nm). Retention time(s): 2.4 min. [A. Pastore *et al.*, *J. Chromatogr. B, Biomed. Sci. Appl.*, 2001, *751*, 187–191].

Ultraviolet Spectrum. Methanol—280 nm (A_1^1=880b).

Quantification

High performance liquid chromatography. In plasma and urine: limit of detection 1 mg/L, UV detection (λ=280 nm)—A. Pastore *et al.*, *J. Chromatogr. B Biomed. Sci. Appl.*, 2001, *751*, 187–191. In plasma and urine: limit of quantification 6.25 mg/L, UV detection (λ=285 nm)—T. C. Dowling *et al.*, *J. Chromatogr. B Biomed. Sci. Appl.*, 1999, *124(6)*, 833–836. In serum and urine: limit of detection 0.18 mg/L, UV detection (λ=275 nm)—R. Marsilio *et al.*, *J. Chromatogr. B Biomed. Sci. Appl.*, 1997, *704*, 359–364. In plasma or urine: limit of detection 1 mg/L, UV detection—T. Prueksaritanont *et al.*, *J. Chromatogr.*, 1984, *306*; *B Biomed. Appl.*, *31*, 89–97.

Disposition in the Body. Aminohippuric acid is a major metabolite of aminobenzoic acid. After intravenous administration it is rapidly excreted in the urine in subjects with normal renal function.

Half-life. Biological half-life, about 0.2 h.

Dose. 2 to 30 g of sodium aminohippurate intravenously, to measure renal function.

Aminonitrothiazole

Antiprotozoal (Veterinary)

5-Nitro-2-thiazolamine
$C_3H_3N_3O_2S$=145.1
CAS—1320-42-9

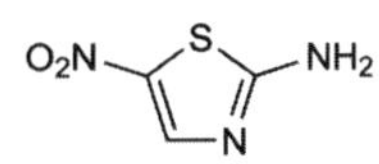

A greenish-yellow to orange-yellow light powder. M.p. 200°, with decomposition.
Slightly soluble in water; soluble 1 in 250 of ethanol and ether; practically insoluble in chloroform; soluble in dilute mineral acids and propylene glycol.

Colour Test. Diazotisation—violet.

Thin-layer Chromatography. System TA—Rf 75. (Visible yellow spot; acidified iodoplatinate solution, strong reaction.)

Gas Chromatography. System GA—not eluted.

Ultraviolet Spectrum. Water—386 nm (A_1^1=1060a).

Infra-red Spectrum. Principal peaks at wavenumbers 1200, 1623, 1176, 1504, 1515, 1252 cm^{-1} (KBr disk).

Aminophenazone

Analgesic

Synonyms. Amidazofen; Amidopyrine; Amidopyrine-Pyramidon; Aminopyrine; Dimethylaminoantipyrine; Dimethylaminophenazone.
Proprietary names. It is an ingredient of Gineburno; Thermocutan; Virdex.
4-(Dimethylamino)-1,2-dihydro-1,5-dimethyl-2-phenyl-3*H*-pyrazol-3-one
$C_{13}H_{17}N_3O$=231.3
CAS—58-15-1

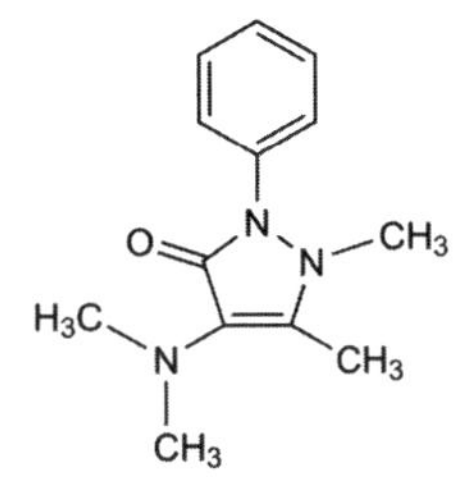

Small colourless crystals or white crystalline powder. M.p. 107° to 109°. Soluble 1 in 18 of water, 1 in 12 of benzene, 1 in 1.5 of ethanol, 1 in 1 of chloroform, and 1 in 13 of ether.
A number of salts of aminophenazone have been used including the ascorbate, gentisate, hydroxyisophthalate, and salicylate.

Dissociation Constant. pK_a 5.0 (20°).

Partition Coefficient. Log *P* (octanol/water), 1.0.

Colour Tests. Ferric Chloride—blue-violet; Liebermann's Test (100°)—blue; Nitrous Acid—violet (transient).

Thin-layer Chromatography. System TA—Rf 66; system TB—Rf 21; system TD—Rf 25; system TE—Rf 62; system TF—Rf 10; system TAD—Rf 58; system TAE—Rf 70; system TAF—Rf 68; system TAJ—Rf 53;

system TAK—Rf 00; system TAL—Rf 76. (Acidified iodoplatinate solution, positive.)

Gas Chromatography. System GA—aminophenazone RI 1895, M (nor-) RI 1980, M (bis-nor-) RI 1955, M (desamino-OH-) RI 1855; system GB—RI 1992; system GC—RI 2370; system GF—RI 2265.

High Performance Liquid Chromatography. System HA—*k* 0.3; system HD—*k* 0.2; system HW—*k* 0.32; system HX—RI 262; system HY—RI 204; system HZ—retention time 2.1 min.

Column: Spherisorb ODS (250 × 4.6 mm i.d., 5 μm). Mobile phase: water:methanol:triethylamine:acetic acid (70.9:27.7:0.9:0.5), flow rate 1 mL/min. UV detection (λ = 254 nm). Retention time 29 min. [J. A. Agundez *et al.*, *Ther. Drug Monit.*, 1994, *16*, 316–322.]

Ultraviolet Spectrum. Aqueous acid—257 (A^1_1=443c); aqueous alkali—264 nm (A^1_1=353b).

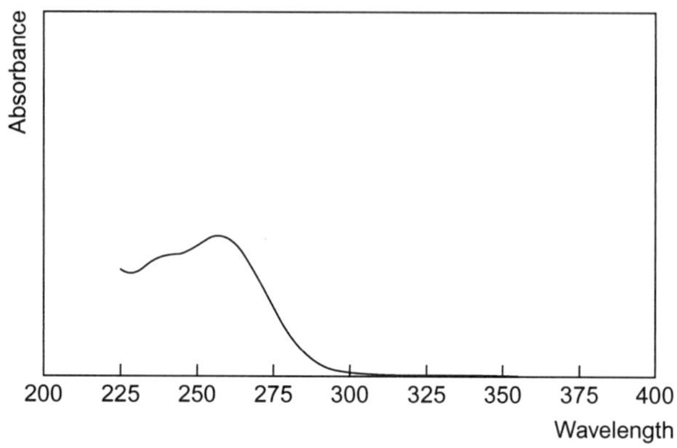

Infra-red Spectrum. Principal peaks at wavenumbers 1660, 1315, 1126, 750, 700, 1620 cm^{-1} (KBr disk).

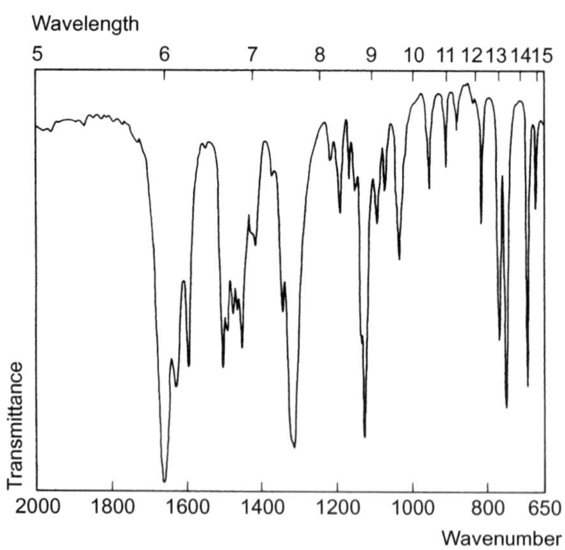

Mass Spectrum. Principal ions at *m/z* 56, 231, 97, 111, 112, 42, 77, 71.

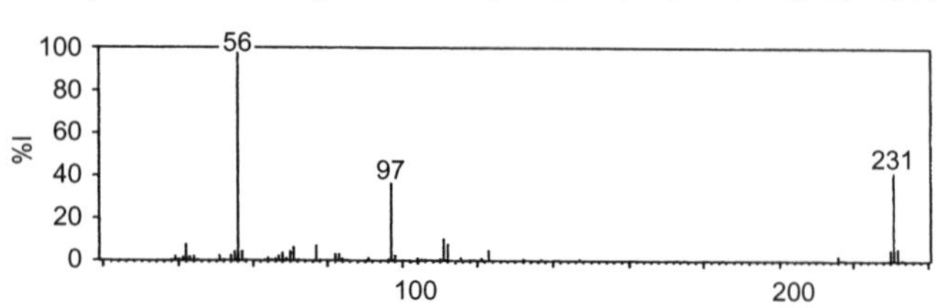

Quantification

Gas chromatography. In plasma: limit of detection 100 μg/L, FID—A. Sioufi and D. Colussi, *J. Chromatogr.* 1978, *146*(3) *B Biomed. Appl.*, 503–507.

High performance liquid chromatography. In urine: aminophenazone and related compounds, limits of detection 120 ng for aminophenazone and 25 ng for 4-acetamidophenazone, UV detection—K. Shimada and Y. Nagase, *J. Chromatogr.* 1980, *181*(7) *B Biomed. Appl.*, 51–57. In urine: aminophenazone, and dipyrone and metabolites, limit of detection 0.10 mg/L, limit of quantification 1 mg/L for aminophenazone, UV detection—J. A. Agundez *et al.*, *Ther. Drug Monit.*, 1994, *16*, 316–322.

Disposition in the Body. Absorbed after oral administration. It is rapidly and extensively metabolised. About 30 to 50% of a dose is excreted in the urine in 3 days as 4-aminophenazone and its acetyl derivative 4-acetamidophenazone which is the major urinary metabolite; other metabolites found in the urine include two red pigments, rubazonic acid and methylrubazonic acid; dimethylnitrosamine may be formed in the stomach. Less than 5% of a dose is excreted in the urine unchanged.

Toxicity. The use of aminophenazone is discouraged due to the risk of fatal agranulocytosis. The estimated minimum lethal dose is 5 g.

Half-life. Plasma half-life, about 2 to 3 h.

Protein binding. In plasma, 25 to 30%.

Dose. Aminophenazone was formerly given in doses of up to 1.5 g in 24 h.

4-Aminophenol

Synonyms. *p*-Aminophenol; *p*-Hydroxyaniline.
C_6H_7NO = 109.1
CAS—123-30-8

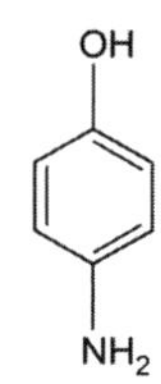

Crystals. M.p. about 190°. The commercial product is usually pink; M.p. 186°.
Slightly soluble in water; soluble in dehydrated alcohol; practically insoluble in chloroform.

Colour Test. Liebermann's Test—black

Thin-layer Chromatography. System TB—Rf 03; system TD—Rf 21; system TE—Rf 59; system TF—Rf 40; system TAD—Rf 30; system TAE—Rf 75. (Ferric chloride solution, violet; acidified potassium permanganate solution, positive; Van Urk reagent, yellow.)

Gas Chromatography. System GA—4-aminophenol RI 1253, 4-aminophenol-AC$_2$ RI 1765, 4-aminophenol-AC$_3$ RI 2085, 4-aminophenol-Me RI 1100; system GB—4-aminophenol RI 1280.

Ultraviolet Spectrum. Aqueous acid—271 nm (A^1_1 = 133b); aqueous alkali—266 nm (broad) (A^1_1=731b); methanol—233 nm (A^1_1=587b), 303 nm (A^1_1=177b).

Mass Spectrum. Principal peaks at *m/z* 109, 80, 53, 81, 108, 52, 54, 110.

Quantification

High performance liquid chromatography. In urine: limit of detection 1 mg/L, UV detection (λ=215 nm)—A. Brega *et al.*, *J. Chromatogr.*, 1990, *535*, 311–316.

Disposition in the Body. 4-Aminophenol is a metabolite of aniline, nitrobenzene, paracetamol and phenazopyridine.

Toxicity

Following paracetamol overdose, three patients were observed to have urine discoloration. Investigation by chromatographic and colorimetric methods revealed the presence of 4-aminophenol, responsible for the dark brown discoloration [P. M. Clark *et al.*, *Clin. Chem.*, 1986, *32*, 1777–1778].

Aminopromazine

Antispasmodic (Veterinary)

Synonyms. Proquamezine; Tetrameprozine; RP-3828.
N,N,N′,N′-Tetramethyl-3-(10*H*-phenothiazin-10-yl)-1,2-propanediamine
$C_{19}H_{25}N_3S$=327.5
CAS—58-37-7

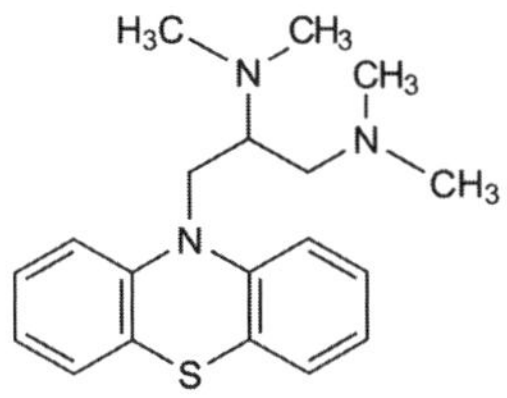

Aminopromazine Fumarate

Synonym. Proquamezine Fumarate
Proprietary names. Lispamol; Sedofarmolo.
$(C_{19}H_{25}N_3S)_2,C_4H_4O_4$=771.1
CAS—3688-62-8
A white powder. M.p. about 166° to 170°, with decomposition.
Soluble 1 in 11 of water, 1 in 200 of ethanol, and 1 in 20 of methanol; practically insoluble in ether.

Dissociation Constant. pK_a 9.8.

Partition Coefficient. Log *P* (octanol/water), 4.8.

Colour Tests. Forrest Reagent—violet→red→orange; FPN Reagent—violet-red→red→orange; Mandelin's Test—orange→violet; Marquis Test—violet.

Thin-layer Chromatography. System TA—Rf 50; system TB—Rf 42; system TC—Rf 19; system TE—Rf 60; system TL—Rf 08; system TAE—Rf 12; system TAJ—Rf 00; system TAK—Rf 00; system TAL—Rf 22. (Acidified iodoplatinate solution, positive.)

Gas Chromatography. System GA—RI 2434.

High Performance Liquid Chromatography. System HX—RI 427.

Ultraviolet Spectrum. Aqueous acid—248 (A^1_1=965a), 297 nm (broad) (A^1_1=106a).

Infra-red Spectrum. Principal peaks at wavenumbers 1584, 745, 660, 1278, 1190, 765 cm^{-1} (aminopromazine fumarate, KBr disk).

Mass Spectrum. Principal ions at *m/z* 198, 58, 115, 70, 269, 199, 72, 71.

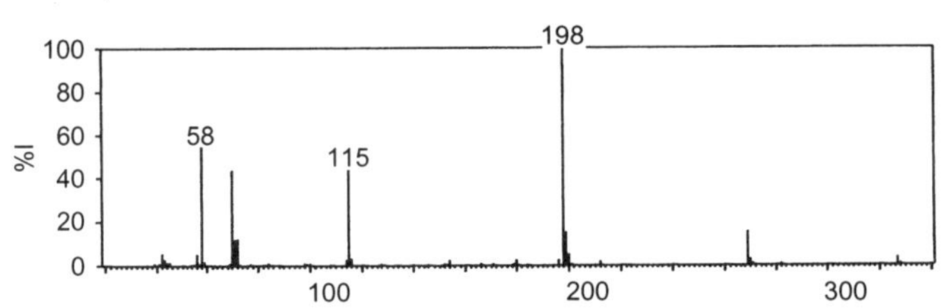

Aminosalicylic Acid

Antituberculous

Synonyms. Aminosalylum; Para-aminosalicylic Acid; PAS; Pasalicylum.
Proprietary names. Nemasol; Parasal; Rezipas; Teebacin Acid.
4-Amino-2-hydroxybenzoic acid
$C_7H_7NO_3$=153.1
CAS—65-49-6

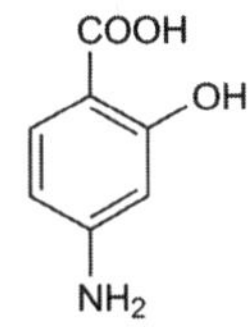

A white bulky powder, which darkens on exposure to air and light. Aqueous solutions are unstable. M.p. 150° to 151°, with effervescence. Soluble 1 in about 600 of water, 1 in about 20 of ethanol, 1 in 6 of acetone, 1 in 4000 of chloroform, and 1 in 50 of ether.

Calcium Aminosalicylate

Synonym. Aminosalicylate Calcium
$(C_7H_6NO_3)_2Ca,3H_2O$=398.4
CAS—133-15-3 (anhydrous)
A white or slightly yellow, hygroscopic, crystalline powder. Aqueous solutions are unstable and darken in colour. Soluble 1 in 7 to 1 in 10 of water; slightly soluble in ethanol.

Phenyl Aminosalicylate

Synonym. Fenamisal
$C_{13}H_{11}NO_3$=229.2
CAS—133-11-9
A white crystalline solid. M.p. 153°. Practically insoluble in water.

Potassium Aminosalicylate

Synonym. Aminosalicylate Potassium
Proprietary name. Teebacin Kalium
$C_7H_6KNO_3$=191.2
CAS—133-09-5
A white to cream-coloured crystalline powder. Aqueous solutions are unstable. Freely soluble in water; sparingly soluble in ethanol; very slightly soluble in chloroform and ether.

Sodium Aminosalicylate

Synonyms. Aminosalicylate Sodium; Pasalicylum Solubile.
Proprietary names. Eupasal Sodico; Italpas Sodico; Parasal Sodium; Pasalba; Teebacin.
$C_7H_6NNaO_3,2H_2O$=211.1
CAS—133-10-8 (anhydrous); 6018-19-5 (dihydrate)
White or cream-coloured crystals or crystalline powder. Aqueous solutions are unstable. Soluble 1 in 2 of water; sparingly soluble in ethanol; practically insoluble in chloroform and ether.

Dissociation Constant. pK_a 1.8 ($-NH_2$), 3.6 (-COOH).

Partition Coefficient. Log *P* (octanol/water), 0.87.

Colour Tests. Coniferyl alcohol—orange; Ferric chloride—violet; Folin–Ciocalteu reagent—blue; McNally's test—brown precipitate.

Thin-layer Chromatography. System TA—Rf 70; system TD—Rf 05; system TE—Rf 07; system TF—Rf 24; system TAD—Rf 15. (Location under UV light, blue fluorescence; ferric chloride solution, violet; acidified potassium permanganate solution, positive; Van Urk reagent, yellow.)

Gas Chromatography. System GA—RI 1309.

High Performance Liquid Chromatography. System HZ—Retention time(s) 1.5 min.

Column: (analytical) LiChrospher 60 RP-select B (250 × 4.6 mm i.d., 5 μm); (pre-column) LiChroCARetention time(s) 4-4 (4 × 4 mm i.d., 5 μm). Mobile phase: deionised water (adjusted to pH 3 with perchloric acid):methanol:acetonitrile (60:20:20 v/v), flow rate 1.2 mL/min. Internal standard (IS): *N*-acetyl-anthranilic acid. Fluorescence detection (λ_{ex}=311 nm; λ_{em}=449 nm). Retention time(s): acetyl-5-aminosalicylic acid 4 min. [B. Bystrowska *et al.*, *J. Pharm. Biomed. Anal.*, 2000, *22*, 341–347].

Column: (analytical) C_{18} Erbasil S (250 × 4.6 mm i.d., 10 μm); (pre-column) Pelliguard (50 × 4.6 mm i.d., 40 μm). Mobile phase: 0.01 M Na_2HPO_4 containing 0.1 mM EDTA, 0.1 M citric acid and 0.1 mM heptanesulfonic acid:methanol (85:15 v/v), pH adjusted to 3 with 0.1 M NaOH, flow rate 1.0 mL/min. IS: 3,4-dihydroxybenzylamine. Electrochemical detection. Retention time(s): (5-aminosalicylic acid) 3.2 min; (acetyl-5-aminosalicylic acid) 8.3 min; (2,5-dihydroxybenzoic acid) 6.5 min. [G. Palumbo *et al.*, *J. Pharm. Biomed. Anal.*, 1995, *14*, 175–180]

Ultraviolet Spectrum. Aqueous acid—234 (A^1_1=496a), 300 (A^1_1=330a); aqueous alkali—265 (A^1_1=846a), 300 nm (A^1_1=532a).

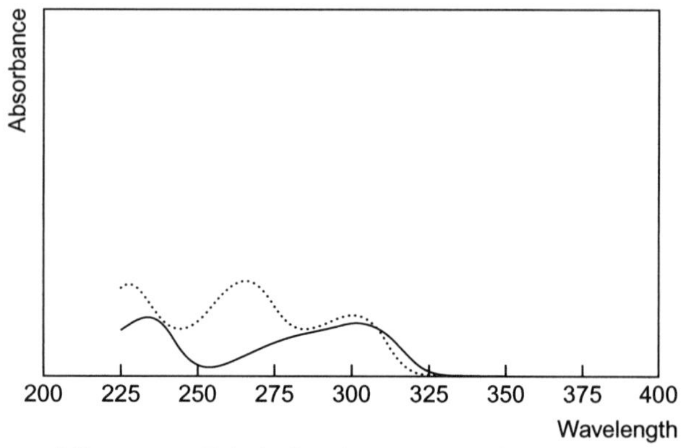

Infra-red Spectrum. Principal peaks at wavenumbers 1301, 1638, 1595, 1510, 805, 1180 cm^{-1} (KBr disk).

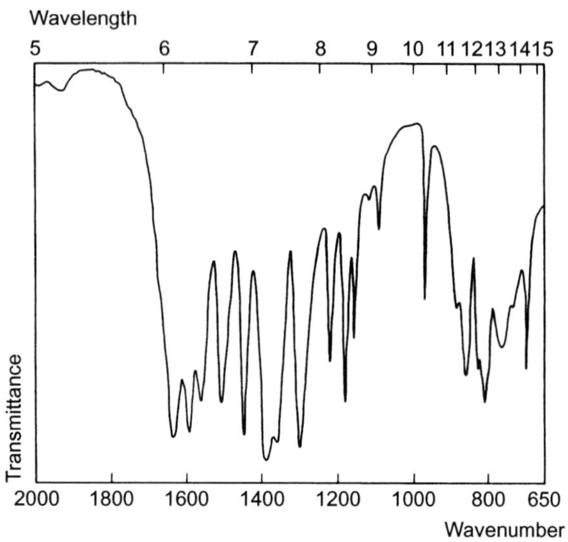

Mass Spectrum. Principal ions at *m/z* 109, 80, 44, 81, 53, 39, 52, 54.

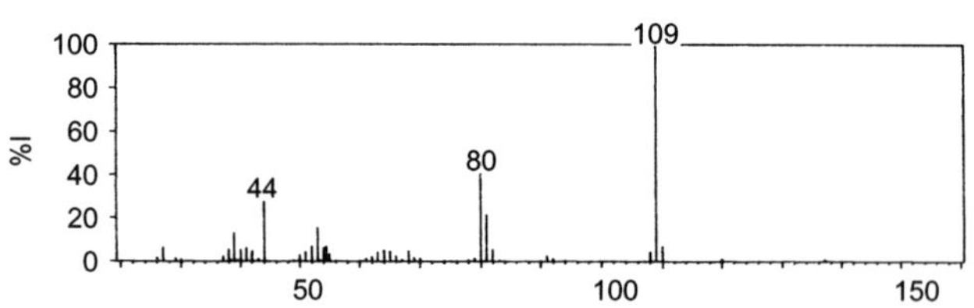

Quantification

High performance liquid chromatography. In plasma and urine: limit of detection 20 µg/L and limit of quantification 100 µg/L, fluorescence detection (λ_{ex}=311 nm; λ_{em}=449 nm)—B. Bystrowska *et al., J. Pharm. Biomed. Anal.*, 2000, *22*, 341–347. In intestinal biopsy samples: limit of detection 1 µg/L for 5-aminosalicylic acid and acetyl-5-aminosalicylic acid, and 0.1 µg/L for 2,5-dihydroxybenzoic acid, electrochemical detection— G. Palumbo *et al., J. Pharm. Biomed. Anal.*, 1995, *14*, 175–180. In plasma or urine: aminosalicylic acid and *p*-acetamidosalicylic acid, limit of detection 500 µg/L, fluorescence detection—R. G. Stoll *et al., Res. Commun. Chem. Path. Pharmacol.*, 1972, *4*, 327–338. In plasma: limit of detection 0.5 ng, fluorescence detection—I. L. Honigberg *et al., J. Chromatogr.*, 1980, *181; B Biomed. Appl.*, *7*, 266–271.

Disposition in the Body. Aminosalicylic acid is readily absorbed after oral administration and widely distributed throughout the body, with high concentrations in the kidneys, lungs and liver. It is metabolised by acetylation to *p*-acetamidosalicylic acid and by conjugation with glycine, producing *p*-aminosalicyluric acid; both metabolites are inactive. More than 80% of a dose is excreted in the urine in 24 h with about 50% of the dose consisting of *p*-acetamidosalicylic acid; up to 25% of the dose may be excreted as free and acetylated *p*-aminosalicyluric acid, and the remainder is mostly unchanged drug with small amounts of 2,4-dihydroxybenzoic acid.

Therapeutic concentration

Following a single oral dose of 4 g of aminosalicylic acid to 12 subjects, a mean peak plasma concentration of 50 mg/L was attained in 3.5 h; after oral administration of 4 g of sodium aminosalicylate to the same subjects, a mean peak plasma concentration of 155 mg/L was attained in about 0.8 h. [S. H. Wan *et al., J. Pharm. Sci.*, 1974, *63*, 708–711].

Toxicity. Prolonged administration may give rise to toxic symptoms characteristic of the salicylates.

Half-life. Plasma half-life, aminosalicylic acid about 0.5 to 1 h, *p*-acetamidosalicylic acid about 1.5 h.

Protein binding. In plasma, 60 to 70%.

Dose. 12 g of sodium aminosalicylate daily; up to 20 g daily has been given.

Aminotriazole

Herbicide

Synonyms. Amitrole; ATA; ENT-25445.
Proprietary names. Amizol; Cytrol; Weedazol. It is an ingredient of a number of proprietary weed-killers.
1*H*-1,2,4-Triazol-3-amine
$C_2H_4N_4$=84.1
CAS—61-82-5

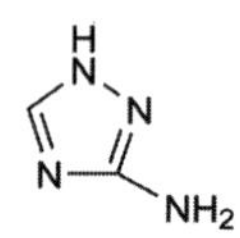

A white crystalline powder. M.p. 159°.
Soluble 1 in 3.5 of water and 1 in 4 of ethanol; practically insoluble in acetone, ether, and non-polar solvents; sparingly soluble in ethyl acetate.

Colour Test. Add sodium hypobromite solution to the sample—orange-red.

Thin-layer Chromatography. System TA—Rf 68. (Acidified iodoplatinate solution, positive.)

Gas Chromatography. System GA—aminotriazole RI 1312, aminotriazole-Me_2 RI 1050, aminotriazole-AC RI 1010; system GK—not eluted.

Ultraviolet Spectrum. No significant absorption, 230 to 360 nm.

Infra-red Spectrum. Principal peaks at wavenumbers 1639, 1047, 1534, 1595, 1211, 971 cm^{-1} (KBr disk).

Mass Spectrum. Principal peaks at *m/z* 84, 58, 43, 44, 42, 53, 55, 86.

Toxicity

A 54-year-old man was hospitalised following poisoning with Radoxone TL, a weed-killer containing ammonium thiocyanate and aminotriazole. The patient was in a coma with myoclonic jerks and vascular collapse. Thiocyanate and aminotriazole blood levels were 750 mg/L and 138 mg/L, respectively, more than 12 h after ingestion. The patient died 48 h later of potanoxic coma. [A. Legras *et al., J. Toxicol. Clin. Toxicol.*, 1996, 34, 441–446.]

Amiodarone

Anti-arrhythmic

(2-Butyl-3-benzofuranyl)[4-[2-(diethylamino)ethoxy]-3,5-diiodophenyl]methanone
$C_{25}H_{29}I_2NO_3$=645.3
CAS—1951-25-3

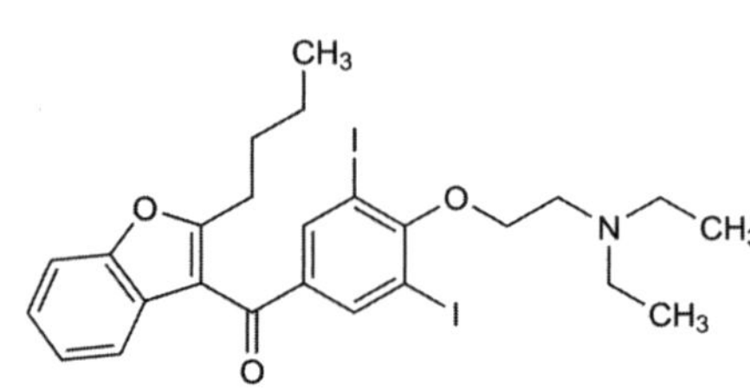

Amiodarone Hydrochloride
Proprietary names. Amiodar; Ancaron; Cordarex; Cordarone; Cordarone X; Ortacrone; Tachydaron; Trangorex.
$C_{25}H_{29}I_2NO_3,HCl=681.8$
CAS—19774-82-4
A white crystalline powder. M.p. about 161°. Very slightly soluble in water; soluble in ethanol; freely soluble in chloroform.

Dissociation Constant. pK_a 5.6.

Colour Tests. Iodine test (omitting MnO_2)—positive; Liebermann's test—brown-yellow; Sulfuric acid—yellow.

Thin-layer Chromatography. System TA—Rf 72; system TB—Rf 62; system TC—Rf 68; system TE—Rf 82; system TL—Rf 55; system TAE—Rf 54; system TAF—Rf 64. (Dragendorff spray, positive; acidified iodoplatinate solution, positive; Marquis reagent, yellow.)

Gas Chromatography. System GA—RI 3335 amiodarone; RI 2800 Art (*O*-desalkyl).

High Performance Liquid Chromatography. System HA—amiodarone k 2.4, monodesethylamiodarone k 1.8; system HX—RI 683; system HY—RI 476; system HZ—Retention time(s) 90.4 min.

Ultraviolet Spectrum. Aqueous acid—241 nm; aqueous alkali—251 nm.

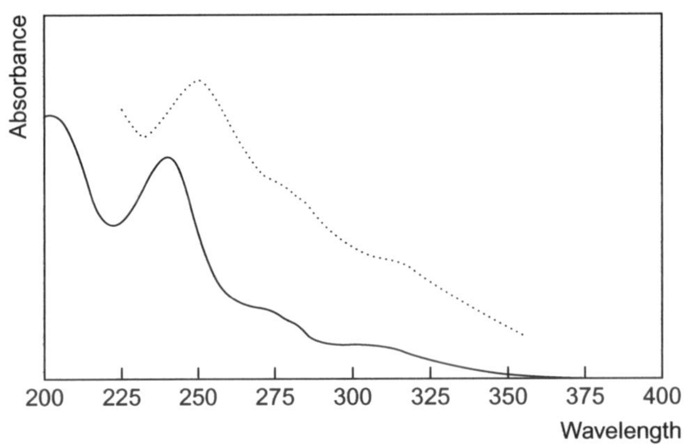

Infra-red Spectrum. Principal peaks at wavenumbers 1630, 748, 1245, 1558, 1170, 998 cm^{-1} (amiodarone hydrochloride, KBr disk).

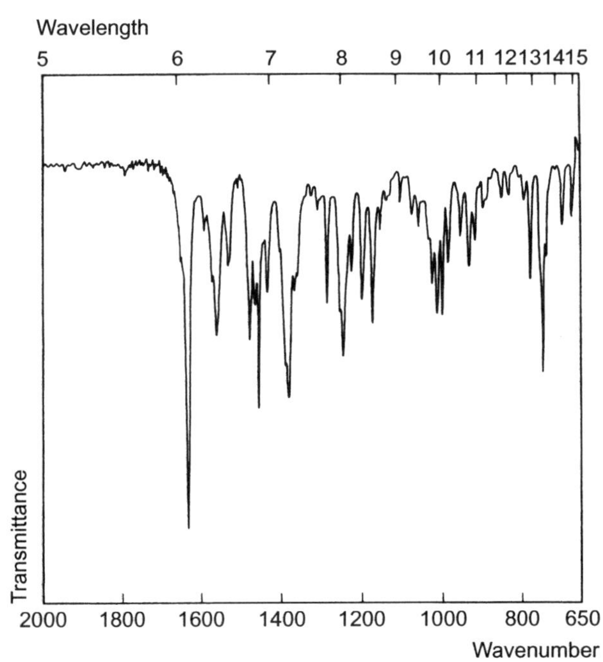

Mass Spectrum. Principal ions at *m*/*z* 86, 36, 87, 84, 58, 56, 44, 38.

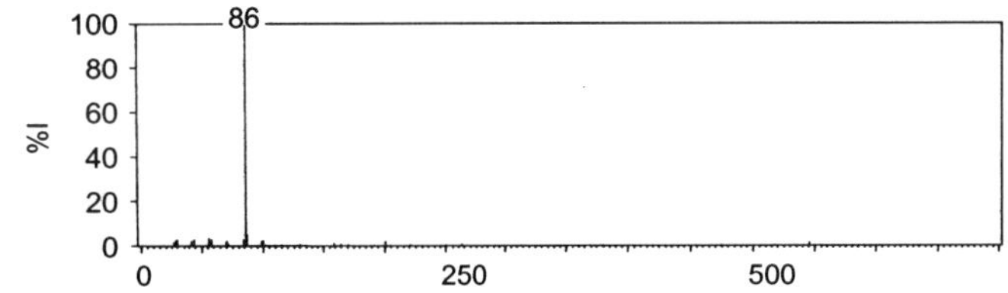

Quantification
High performance liquid chromatography. In plasma: limit of detection 1 µg/L for amiodarone and 0.5 µg/L for desethylamiodarone, and limit of quantification 50 µg/L for drug and metabolite, UV detection—M. Kollroser and C. Schober, *J. Chromatogr. B Biomed. Sci. Appl.*, 2002, *766*, 219–226. In plasma: amiodarone and monodesethylamiodarone, limit of detection 100 µg/L, UV detection—G. C. A. Storey *et al.*, *Ther. Drug Monit.*, 1982, *4*, 385–388. In plasma, urine or tissues: amiodarone and monodesethylamiodarone, limit of detection 25 µg/L, UV detection—T. A. Plomp *et al.*, *J. Chromatogr.*, 1983, *273*; *B Biomed. Appl.*, *24*, 379–392.

Disposition in the Body. Amiodarone is slowly and incompletely absorbed after oral administration; it is distributed to the tissues where it is strongly bound. It is metabolised by *N*-dealkylation to monodesethylamiodarone which is the major plasma metabolite during chronic dosing. High concentrations of amiodarone and monodesethylamiodarone are found in the liver, lungs and adipose tissue. Enterohepatic circulation may occur. Only a small amount is excreted in the urine as unchanged drug.

Therapeutic concentration. Accumulates on chronic administration; steady-state plasma concentrations are attained in about 1 month.

15 patients were administered 400 mg amiodarone three times daily and peak plasma concentrations of the drug were 1.478 to 1.983 mg/L. Peak plasma concentrations of the metabolite, desethylamiodarone, were 0.522 to 1.008 mg/L. [M. Kollroser and C. Schober, *J. Chromatogr. B Biomed. Sci. Appl.*, 2002, *766*, 219–226].

Following oral administration of 400 mg to 7 subjects, peak plasma concentrations of about 0.5 to 1 mg/L were attained in about 7 h. After administration of 200 mg 8-hourly to 6 subjects for 1 month, plasma concentrations determined immediately before the morning dose ranged from 0.75 to 2.8 mg/L (mean 1.5 mg/L). [F. Andreasen *et al.*, *Eur. J. Clin. Pharmacol.*, 1981, *19*, 293–299].

During chronic treatment with 400 mg daily to 33 subjects, mean steady-state plasma concentrations of 2.2 mg/L of amiodarone and 2.0 mg/L of monodesethylamiodarone were reported. [R. J. Flanagan *et al.*, *J. Pharm. Pharmacol.*, 1982, *34*, 638–643].

Half-life. Plasma half-life during chronic dosing, 14 to 107 days (mean 50).

Distribution in blood. Plasma:whole blood ratio, 1.3.

Protein binding. In plasma, extensively bound.

Note. For a review of the pharmacokinetics of amiodarone, see R. Latini *et al.*, *Clin. Pharmacokinet.*, 1984, *9*, 136–156.

Dose. Initially 600 mg of amiodarone hydrochloride daily; maintenance, 200 to 400 mg daily.

Amiphenazole

Narcotic Antagonist/ Respiratory Stimulant

Synonyms. DAPT; Phenamizole
Proprietary names. Dizol; Daptazole; Daptazile; Fenamizol.
5-Phenyl-2,4-thiazolediamine
$C_9H_9N_3S=191.3$
CAS—490-55-1

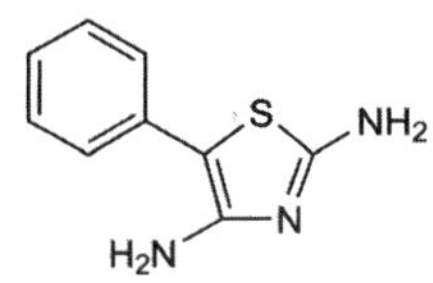

Flakes which turn brown on exposure to light and air. M.p. 163° to 164°, with decomposition.

Amiphenazole Hydrochloride
Synonym. Amiphenazole Chloride
Proprietary names. Daptazile; Daptazole.
$C_9H_9N_3S,HCl=227.7$
CAS—942-31-4
A white, fine crystalline or granular, mobile powder. Aqueous solutions hydrolyse slowly. M.p. 236°. Soluble 1 in 16 of water and 1 in 50 of ethanol; slightly soluble in acetone, chloroform and ether.

Colour Test. Liebermann's test (100°)—green-blue.

Thin-layer Chromatography. System TA—Rf 61; system TB—Rf 02; system TC—Rf 33.; system TE—Rf 62; system TL—Rf 57. (Acidified iodoplatinate solution, positive.)

Gas Chromatography. System GB—RI 1150; system GC—RI 2563.

Ultraviolet Spectrum. Aqueous acid—230 (A_1^1=998 a), 261 nm.

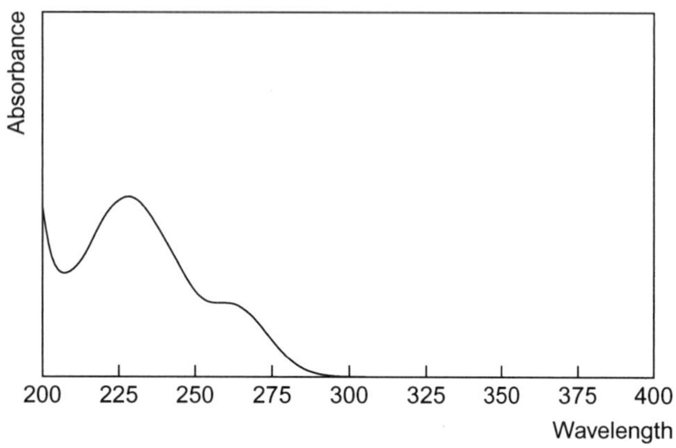

Infra-red Spectrum. Principal peaks at wavenumbers 1495, 1637, 688, 750, 1665, 1050 cm^{-1} (KBr disk).

Mass Spectrum. Principal ions at *m/z* 191, 121, 77, 104, 122, 43, 51, 192.

Dose. Amiphenazole hydrochloride has been given parenterally in doses of 100 to 150 mg.

Amisulpride

Antipsychotic

Synonyms. Aminosultopride; DAN-2163.
Proprietary names. Deniban; Solian; Sulamid.
4-Amino-*N*-[(1-ethyl-2-pyrrolidinyl)methyl]-5-(ethylsulfonyl)-2-methoxybenzamide
$C_{17}H_{27}N_3O_4S=369.5$
CAS—71675-85-9

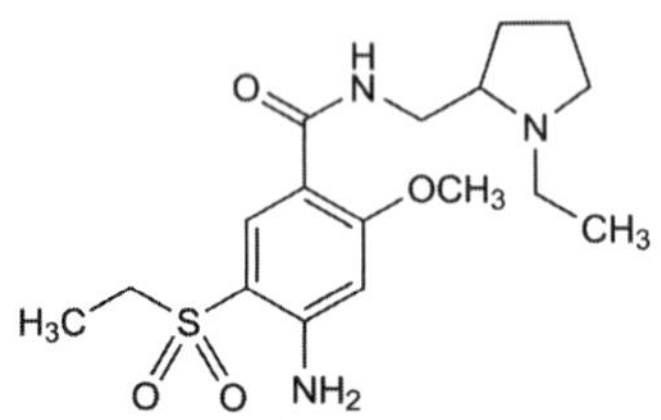

Crystals from acetone with m.p. 126° to 127°.

Dissociation Constant. pK_a 9.37.

Partition Coefficient. Log *P* (octanol/water), 1.10.

High Performance Liquid Chromatography. System HAA—retention time amisulpride, 8.9 min; metabolite-1, 7.1 min; metabolite-2, 10.9 min.

Column: (analytical) Hypersil C_{18} BDS (150 × 4.6 mm i.d., 5 µm); (guard) Pelliguard LC_8 (20 × 4.6 mm, 40 µm). Mobile phase: solution A: water:triethylamine:potassium dihydrogen phosphate (1 M) (974:1:25), pH 3 with phosphoric acid; 1 mL/min flow rate. Fluorescence detection (λ_{ex}=280 nm, λ_{em}=370 nm). Retention time: 4 min. [B. Malavasi *et al.*, *J. Chromatogr. Biomed. Sci. Appl.*, 1996, *676*, 107–115].

Ultraviolet Spectrum. Aqueous acid—230, 285 nm.

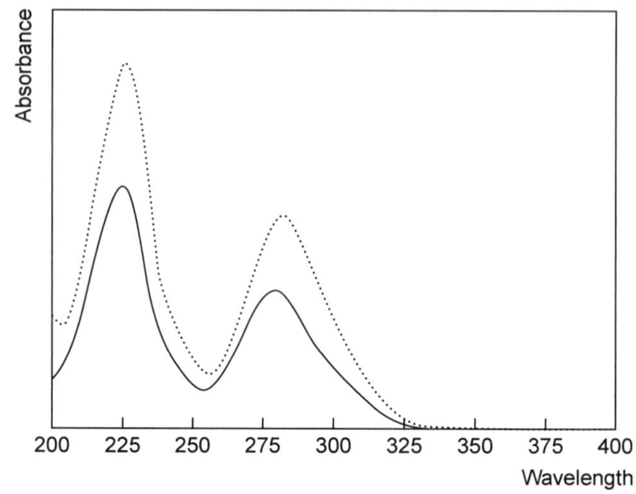

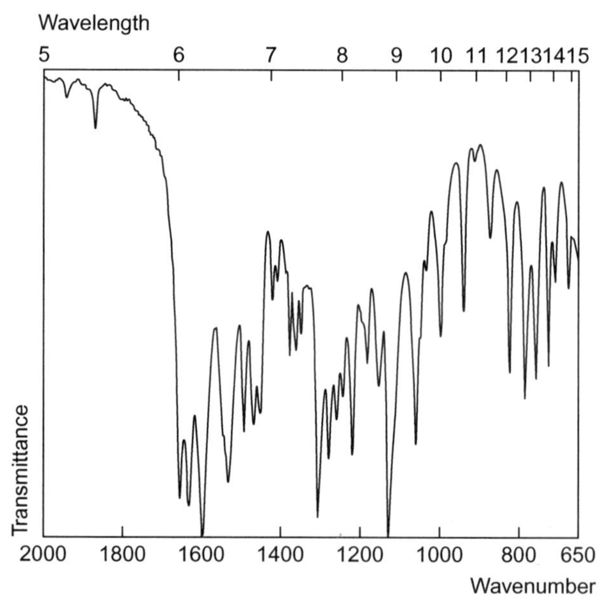

Mass Spectrum. Principal ions at *m/z* 98, 99, 44, 242, 70, 28, 111, 149.

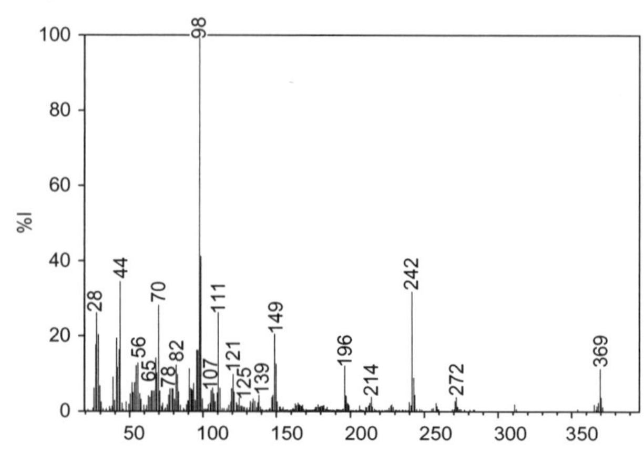

Quantification

High performance liquid chromatography. In plasma or urine: limit of detection (both enantiomers) 0.5 µg/L in plasma and 50 µg/L in urine,

UV or fluorescence detection—V. Ascalone *et al*., *J. Chromatogr. Biomed. Sci. Appl*., 1996, *676*, 95–105. In plasma or urine: limit of detection 0.5 µg/L in plasma and 100 µg/L in urine, fluorescence detection—B. Malavasi *et al*., *J. Chromatogr. Biomed. Sci. Appl*., 1996, *676*, 107–115. In plasma: limit of detection 5 µg/L, UV detection—M. Bohbot *et al*., *J. Chromatogr*., 1987, *416*; *Biomed. Appl*., *60*, 414–419.

Disposition in the Body. Following oral administration of amisulpride, this drug is readily absorbed with two absorption peaks being observed, the first after about 1 h and the second between 3 and 4 h after administration. It is only weakly metabolised; metabolites account for only about 4% of the dose and are inactive. It is excreted largely unchanged in urine (70%) and a small amount in faeces as the unchanged drug. Amisulpride is widely distributed throughout the body and is only very weakly dialysed.

Therapeutic concentration

Following administration of a single oral dose of 50 mg of amisulpride to 18 healthy subjects the following mean plasma concentrations were measured at 2, 4 and 6.5 h; 18.8, 17.9 and 17.2 µg/L, respectively. Following administration of a single 200-mg dose, the plasma concentrations were; 76.2, 83.0 and 92.1 µg/L, respectively. [M. J. Mattila *et al*., *Eur. J. Clin. Pharmacol*., 1996, *51*, 161–166].

Toxicity

In a non-fatal overdosage case, a 30-year-old Caucasian woman who had taken about 3 g of amisulpride and an unknown amount of dothiepin had a blood-amisulpride concentration of 9.63 mg/L. Her gastric fluid concentration was 14.25 mg/L. The patient experienced generalised convulsions which resolved spontaneously followed by coma, motor restlessness, tachycardia, and slight prolongation of the QT interval. The subject was treated with gastric lavage and recovered within 48 h. The drug blood concentration was 10 to 50 times higher than that observed at therapeutic levels. A second subject who had been found dead had a blood-amisulpride concentration of 41.7 mg/L. This was 40 to 200 times the observed therapeutic concentration. [A. Tracqui *et al*., *Human Exp. Toxicol*., 1995, *14*, 294–298].

Half-life. Plasma, 12 h.

Volume of distribution. 5.8 L/kg.

Clearance. 20 L/h

Protein binding. In plasma, 16%.

Dose. Up to 1200 mg daily by mouth; up to 400 mg daily has been given intramuscularly.

Amitriptyline

Antidepressant

3-(10,11-Dihydro-5*H*-dibenzo[*a*,*d*]cyclohepten-5-ylidene)-*N*,*N*-dimethyl-1-propanamine

$C_{20}H_{23}N = 277.4$

CAS—50-48-6

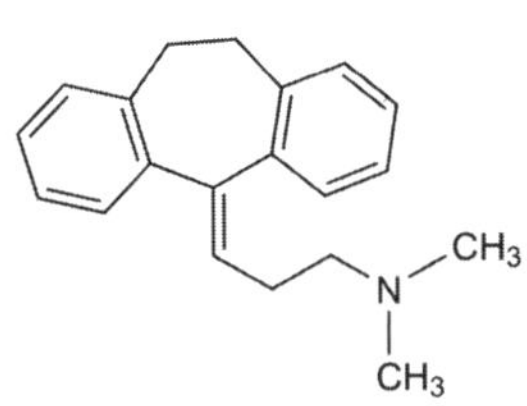

A colourless oil, which becomes yellow on standing due to oxidation to a ketonic product.

Amitriptyline Embonate

Proprietary name. Tryptizol (syrup)

$(C_{20}H_{23}N)_2,C_{23}H_{16}O_6 = 943.2$

CAS—17086-03-2

A pale yellow to brownish-yellow powder. M.p. about 140°.

Practically insoluble in water; soluble 1 in 120 of ethanol, 1 in 6 of acetone, and 1 in 8 of chloroform.

Amitriptyline Hydrochloride

Proprietary names. Adepril; Amavil; Amiline; Amineurin; Amioxid; Amitid; Amitril; Amitrip; Amitrol; Domical; Elatrol; Elavil; Endep; Equilibrin; Klotriptyl; Laroxyl; Lentizol; Levate; Meravil; Novoprotect; Novotriptyn; Redomex; Saroten; Sarotex; Syneudon; Triptyl; Tryptanol; Tryptil; Tryptizol. It is an ingredient of Etrafon, Limbatril, Limbitrol, Triavil, and Triptafen.

$C_{20}H_{23}N,HCl = 313.9$

CAS—549-18-8

Colourless crystals or white powder. M.p. 196° to 197°.

Soluble 1 in 1 of water, 1 in 1.5 of ethanol, 1 in 56 of acetone, 1 in 1.2 of chloroform, and 1 in 1 of methanol; practically insoluble in ether.

Dissociation Constant. pK_a 9.4 (25°).

Partition Coefficient. Log *P* (octanol/water), 4.94.

Colour Tests. Mandelin's Test—brown→green; Marquis Test—brown-orange; Sulfuric Acid—orange.

Thin-layer Chromatography. System TA—Rf 51; system TB—Rf 50; system TC—Rf 32; system TE—Rf 69; system TL—Rf 15; system TAE—Rf 27; system TAF—Rf 51; system TAJ—Rf 13; system TAK—Rf 05; system TAL—Rf 56. (Dragendorff spray, positive; acidified iodoplatinate solution, positive; Marquis reagent, brown.)

Gas Chromatography. System GA—amitriptyline RI 2194, M (*cis*-10-OH-) RI 2348, M (*trans*-10-OH-) RI 2348, M (*N*-oxide) RI 1975, M (nor-) RI 2215, M (cyclobenzaprine) RI 2235, M (OH-) RI 2380, M (nor-OH-) RI 2390; system GB—amitriptyline RI 2284, M (*cis*-10-OH-) RI 2454, M (*cis*-10-OH-*N*-oxide) RI 2215, M (*trans*-10-OH-) RI 2466, M (*trans*-10-OH-*N*-oxide) RI 2239, M (cyclobenzaprine) RI 2330, M (*N*-oxide) RI 2051; system GF—amitriptyline RI 2510, M (10-OH-) RI 2830 or 2880 (stereoisomers); system GM—amitriptyline RRT 0.723, M (*cis*-10-OH-) RRT 1.149, M (*trans*-10-OH-) RRT 1.168, M (cyclobenzaprine) RRT 0.850 (all relative to iprindole); system GS—retention time 16.1 min.

High Performance Liquid Chromatography. System HA—amitriptyline *k* 3.3, 10-hydroxyamitriptyline *k* 2.9, 10-hydroxynortriptyline *k* 1.8, nortriptyline *k* 2.0; system HF—amitriptyline *k* 5.42, nortriptyline *k* 4.58; system HX—RI 440; system HY—RI 375; system HZ—retention time 7.5 min; system HAA—retention time 15.9 min; system HAX—retention time 15.8 min; system HAY—retention time 7.3 min; system HAZ—amitriptyline *k* 1.76, nortriptyline *k* 1.71.

Column: RP C_{18} (Nova-Pak, 150 × 4.6 mm i.d., 4 µm). Mobile phase: potassium dihydrogen phosphate (5 mM):acetonitrile:diethylamine (500:500:2) adjusted to pH 8 with phosphoric acid. Flow rate 0.9 mL/min. UV detection (λ=242 nm). Retention time 17.0 min. [R. Theurillat and W. Thormann, *J. Pharm. Biomed. Anal*., 1998, *18*, 751–760.]

Column: RP C_{18} ODS (150 × 4.6 mm i.d., 5 µm) at 25°. Mobile phase: acetonitrile:tetramethylethylene diamine (12 mM) (40:60), adjusted to pH 5.5 with acetic acid. Flow rate, 1.5 mL. UV detection (λ=242 nm). Retention time 8.9 min. [Y. Shu *et al*., *Zhongguo Yao Li Xue Bao*, 1998, *19*, 343–346.]

Column: RP C_{18} (Symmetry, 250 × 4.6 mm i.d., 5 µm). Mobile phase: potassium dihydrogen phosphate (0.067 M, adjusted to pH 3 with phosphoric acid):acetonitrile (65:35) Flow rate 1.2 mL/min. UV detection (diode array: 200 to 450 nm). Retention time 11.3 min. [G. Aymard *et al*., *J. Chromatogr. B Biomed. Sci. Appl*., 1997, *700*, 183–189.]

Ultraviolet Spectrum. Aqueous acid—239 nm (A_1^1 = 504a).

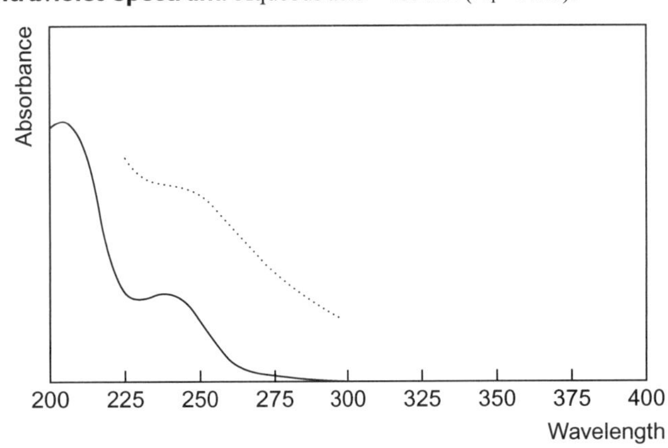

Infra-red Spectrum. Principal peaks at wavenumbers 756, 770, 746, 969, 1014, 1258 cm^{-1} (amitriptyline hydrochloride, KBr disk).

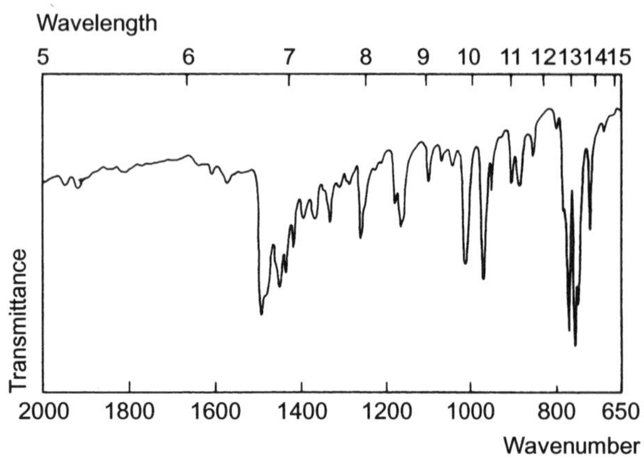

Mass Spectrum. Principal ions at *m/z* 58, 59, 202, 42, 203, 214, 217, –; 10-hydroxyamitriptyline 58, 42, 69, 41, 30, 215, 202, 59; 10-hydroxynortriptyline 44, 45, 26, 218, 215, 203, 202, 42; nortriptyline 44, 202, 45, 220, 218, 215, 91, –.

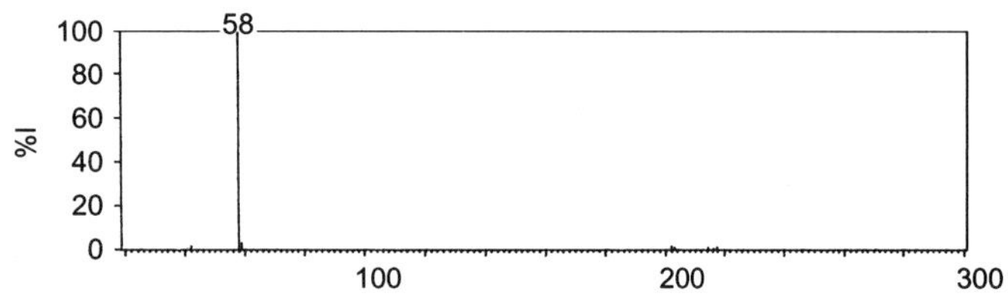

Quantification

Gas chromatography. In plasma: amitriptyline and nortriptyline, limit of detection 10 µg/L, AFID—S. Dawling and R. A. Braithwaite, *J. Chromatogr.* 1978, *146*(3) *B Biomed. Appl.*, 449–456. In plasma: amitriptyline and nortriptyline, comparison with enzyme immunoassay—S. Vandel *et al.*, *Therapie*, 1992, *47*, 41–45. In serum: amitriptyline, nortriptyline, and metabolites, limit of detection for amitriptyline 1.5 µg/L, NPD—S. Ulrich *et al.*, *J. Chromatogr.* 1996, *685 B Biomed. Appl.*, 81–89. In plasma: amitriptyline and other antidepressants and their metabolites, limit of quantification for amitriptyline 125 µg/L, NPD—S. Ulrich and J. Martens, *J. Chromatogr. B Biomed. Sci. Appl.*, 1997, *696*, 217–234. In whole blood: amitriptyline and other tricyclic antidepressants, limits of detection 32 to 50 µg/L, FID—X. P. Lee, *J. Chromatogr. Sci.*, 1997, *35*, 302–308. In plasma: amitriptyline and other tricyclics and their metabolites, limits of detection 1.2 to 5.8 µg/L, NPD—R. de la Torre *et al.*, *Ther. Drug Monit.*, 1998, *20*, 340–346.

Gas chromatography–mass spectrometry. In hair—A. Tracqui *et al.*, *Hum. Exp. Toxicol.*, 1992, *11*, 363–367; F. J. Couper *et al.*, *J. Forensic Sci.*, 1995, *40*, 87–90. In plasma: amitriptyline and nortriptyline, limits of detection 2 ng/g and 5 ng/g, respectively—K. Kudo *et al.*, *J. Anal. Toxicol.*, 1997, *21*, 185–189.

High performance liquid chromatography. In serum: amitriptyline and other tricyclics, UV detection—M. P. Segatti *et al.*, *J. Chromatogr.*, 1991, *536*, 319–325. In plasma or serum: amitriptyline, nortriptyline, and their hydroxylated metabolites, limit of quantification 5 µg/L, UV detection—S. Hartter and C. Hiemke, *J. Chromatogr.*, 1992, *578*, 273–282. In serum: amitriptyline and nortriptyline, UV detection—M. Dolezalova, *J. Chromatogr.*, 1992, *579*, 291–297. In postmortem and clinical samples: amitriptyline and other antidepressants and metabolites, limit of detection 50 µg/L, UV detection—I. M. McIntyre *et al.*, *J. Chromatogr.*, 1993, *621*, 215–223. In urine: amitriptyline and drugs of abuse, diode-array detection—S. Li *et al.*, *J. Chromatogr.* 1994, *655 B Biomed. Appl.*, 213–223. In urine: glucuronides of amitriptyline and diphenhydramine—D. Fischer and U. Breyer-Pfaff, *J. Pharm. Pharmacol.*, 1995, *47*, 534–538. In plasma: amitriptyline and other tricyclics and metabolites, UV detection—R. H. Queiroz *et al.*, *Pharm. Acta Helv.*, 1995, *70*, 181–186. In plasma or liver microsomes: amitriptyline and nortriptyline, limit of detection 2 µg/L—P. Ghahramani and M. S. Lennard, *J. Chromatogr.* 1996, *685 B Biomed. Appl.*, 307–313. In plasma: amitriptyline and nortriptyline, limits of detection 5 ng/g and 10 ng/g, respectively, UV detection—K. Kudo *et al.*, *J. Anal. Toxicol.*, 1997, *21*, 185–189. In biological samples: amitriptyline and other antidepressants, UV detection—E. Tanaka *et al.*, *J. Chromatogr. B Biomed. Sci. Appl.*, 1997, *692*, 405–412. In plasma: amitriptyline and other antidepressants, 5 µg/L, UV detection (λ = 226 nm or 400 nm)—G. Aymard *et al.*, *J. Chromatogr. B Biomed. Sci. Appl.*, 1997, *700*, 183–189. In liver microsomes: limit of detection for amitriptyline and nortriptyline, 10 µg/L—Y. Shu *et al.*, *Zhongguo Yao Li Xue Bao*, 1998, *19*, 343–346. In serum or plasma: amitriptyline and other tricyclic antidepressants, limit of detection for amitriptyline, 0.06 µg/L, UV detection—R. Theurillat and W. Thormann, *J. Pharm. Biomed. Anal.*, 1998, *18*, 751–760. In plasma: amitriptyline and other tricyclic antidepressants, UV detection—K. Johansen and K. E. Rasmussen, *J. Pharm. Biomed. Anal.*, 1998, *16*, 1159–1169. In plasma: limit of detection 5 µg/L, UV detection—A. Zarghi *et al.*, *Boll. Chim. Farm.*, 2001, *140*, 458–461.

High performance liquid chromatography–mass spectrometry. In plasma: amitriptyline and other tricyclic antidepressants, limit of detection 5 µg/L—H. Zang *et al.*, *J. Mass Spectrom.*, 2000, *35*, 423–431. In plasma: amitriptyline and other antidepressants—M. Kollroser and C. Schober, *Ther. Drug Monit.*, 2002, *24*, 537–544.

Fluorescence polarisation immunoassay. In serum: amitripyline and other tricyclic antidepressants, limit of detection about 20 µg/L, comparison with GC and HPLC—M. L. Rao *et al.*, *Clin. Chem.*, 1994, *40*, 929–933. In plasma: amitriptyline and other tricyclic antidepressants, comparison with HPLC—L. P. Hackett *et al.*, *Ther. Drug Monit.*, 1998, *20*, 30–34.

Disposition in the Body. Readily absorbed after oral administration and rapidly taken up by the tissues. The main metabolic reaction, demethylation to form the major active metabolite, nortriptyline, is catalysed by CYP2C19 and CYP3A4 isoenzymes; hydroxylation is catalysed by CYP2D6; *N*-oxidation and conjugation also occur; other metabolites include didesmethylamitriptyline, 10-hydroxy- derivatives, conjugates, and amitriptyline *N*-oxide; the 10-hydroxy- metabolites may also have some activity. It is mainly excreted in the urine as free and conjugated metabolites, up to about 35% of a single dose being excreted in 24 h. About 50% of the excreted material is 10-hydroxynortriptyline and its glucuronide conjugate; up to 27% is 10-hydroxyamitriptyline (mainly conjugated); unchanged drug and nortriptyline each account for less than 5% of the excreted material. About 8% of a dose may be eliminated in the faeces as unchanged drug. There appears to be polymorphic variation in the metabolite pattern. Amitriptyline and nortriptyline are widely distributed; they cross the placenta and are excreted in breast milk.

Therapeutic concentration. In plasma, usually in the range 0.1 to 0.2 mg/L (combined amitriptyline and nortriptyline).

After a single oral dose of 50 mg to 3 subjects, peak plasma concentrations for amitriptyline of 0.02 to 0.04 mg/L (mean 0.025) and for nortriptyline of about 0.01 mg/Lwere attained in 2 to 4 h. [W. A. Garland, *J. Pharm. Sci.*, 1977, *66*, 77–81.]

Following daily oral doses of 150 mg to 14 subjects for 3 weeks, steady-state serum concentrations of 0.05 to 0.24 mg/L (mean 0.13) of amitriptyline, 0.04 to 0.26 mg/L (mean 0.11) of nortriptyline, 0.05 to 0.25 mg/L (mean 0.13) of *E*-10-hydroxynortriptyline, and 0.005 to 0.04 mg/L (mean 0.02) of 10-hydroxyamitriptyline were reported. [P. M. Edelbroek *et al.*, *Clin. Pharmacol. Ther.*, 1984, *35*, 467–473.]

Toxicity. Moderate intoxication is associated with plasma concentrations of 0.05 to 0.43 mg/L (mean 0.17) and severe toxic symptoms with concentrations greater than 0.3 mg/L. The fatal blood concentration range is 0.55 to 16.1 mg/L (mean 3.3). Corresponding toxic doses are greater than 1 g (moderate intoxication) and greater than 2 g (severe or fatal).

In 7 fatalities attributed to amitriptyline overdose, postmortem concentrations, mg/L or mg/kg (mean), were:

	Amitriptyline	Nortriptyline
Blood	0.43–8.30 (3.4)	0.29–6.50 (1.6)
Liver	10.4–243 (92)	4.2–456 (94)

[D. N. Bailey and R. F. Shaw, *J. Anal. Toxicol.*, 1980, *4*, 232–236.]

In a fatality involving the suicidal ingestion of amitriptyline, 10 blood samples taken 21 h after discovery of the body and approximately 28.5 h after the ingestion revealed concentrations of 2.5 to 12 mg/L of amitriptyline, 0.7 to 3.1 mg/L of nortriptyline, and 81 to 244 mg/L of salicylate; 10 h later, the concentrations were 1 to 39 mg/L, 0.6 to 7.0 mg/L, and 86 to 310 mg/L, respectively. Of tissue samples, drug concentrations were highest in the liver (amitriptyline 301 mg/kg, salicylates 670 mg/kg). [D. J. Pounder *et al.*, *Am. J. Forensic Med. Pathol.*, 1994, *15*, 224–230.]

Bioavailability. 30 to 60%.

Half-life. Plasma half-life, 9 to 36 h, increased in overdosage.

Volume of distribution. About 15 L/kg.

Clearance. Plasma clearance, 11.5 mL/min/kg.

Distribution in blood. Plasma:whole blood ratio, 1.2.

Saliva. Plasma:saliva ratio, 3.

Protein binding. In plasma, 91 to 97%.

Note. For a review of the pharmacokinetics of tricyclic antidepressants, see G. Molnar and R. N. Gupta, *Biopharm. Drug Dispos.*, 1980, *1*, 283–305.

Dose. For depression, 50 to 150 mg of amitriptyline hydrochloride daily; up to 300 mg daily has been given.

Amlodipine

Calcium-channel Blocker

Synonym. UK-48340

2-[(2-Aminoethoxy)methyl]-4-(2-chlorophenyl)-1,4-dihydro-6-methyl-3,5-pyridinedicarboxylic acid 3-ethyl 5-methyl ester

$C_{20}H_{25}ClN_2O_5$=408.9

CAS—88150-42-9

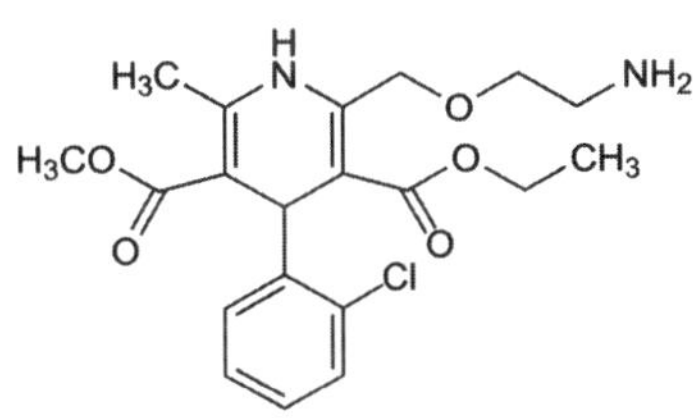

Amlodipine Maleate

Synonyms. UK-48340-11

$C_{20}H_{25}ClN_2O_5,C_4H_4O_4$=525.0

CAS—88150-47-4

A white crystalline powder with m.p. 178° to 179°.

Amlodipine Besilate

Synonyms. Amlodipine Besylate; Amlodipine Monobenzenesulfonate.

Proprietary name. Amlodin; Amlor; Antacal; Astudal; Istin; Monopina; Norvas; Norvasc.

$C_{20}H_{25}ClN_2O_5,C_6H_5SO_3H$=567.1

CAS—111470-99-6

A white crystalline powder. It is slightly soluble in water; sparingly soluble in ethanol.

Dissociation Constant. pK_a 8.6.

Partition Coefficient. Log *P* (octanol/water), 3.00.

Thin-layer Liquid Chromatography. System TE—Rf 36; system TB—Rf 2; system TAE—Rf 11.

Gas Chromatography. System GB—RI 2982; system GP—M (dehydro-2-HOOC$^-$)-ME, RI 2430, M (dehydro-desamino-HOOC$^-$)-ME, RI 2635.

Column: fused-silica coated with cross-linked 5% phenylmethyl silicone gum (25 m × 0.31 mm i.d., 0.17 µm film thickness). Column temperature: 280° to 320° at 20°/min, held 9 min. Carrier gas: nitrogen, 1 mL/min flow rate. Detection: electron capture. Retention time: 4.4 min. [J. K. Faulkner *et al.*, *Br. J. Clin. Pharmacol.*, 1986, *22*, 21–25].

Column: (analytical) fused-silica (DB1, 40 m × 0.25 mm i.d. × 0.25 mm); (pre-column) fused-silica (DB1, 7 m × 0.56 mm × 0.15 m). Column temperature: 250°. Carrier gas: hydrogen, 32 cm/s. Detection: ^{63}Ni electron-capture. Retention time: 9.9 min. [S. C. Monkman *et al.*, *J. Chromatogr. Biomed. Sci. Appl.*, 1996, *678*, 360–364].

High Performance Liquid Chromatography. System HX—RI 428; system HZ—retention time 4.9 min; system HAA—retention time 15.1 min.

Column: octadecyl-bonded silica (Cosmosil 5 C_{18}-P, 150 × 4.6 mm, 5 µm). Mobile phase: phosphate buffer solution (0.05 M, pH 3.1):acetonitrile (65:35) containing sodium octane sulfonate (0.005 M) and EDTA (5 mg/L), 1 mL/min flow rate. Amperometric detection. Retention time 10.1 min. [K. Shimooka *et al.*, *J. Pharm. Biomed. Anal.*, 1989, 7, 1267–1272].

Ultraviolet Spectrum. Aqueous acid (0.2 M NH_2SO_4)—239 nm; basic—238 nm (besilate).

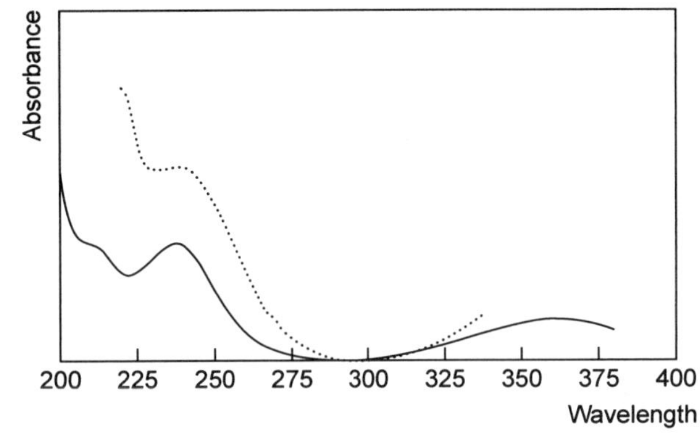

Infra-red Spectrum. Principal peaks at wavenumber 1208, 1182, 1094 cm^{-1} (KBr pellet).

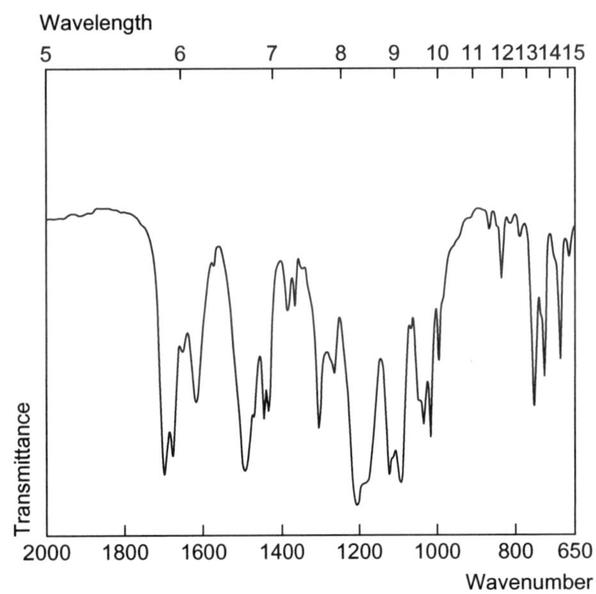

Mass Spectrum. Principal ions at *m*/*z* 297, 208, 44, 254, 298, 347, 236, 165.

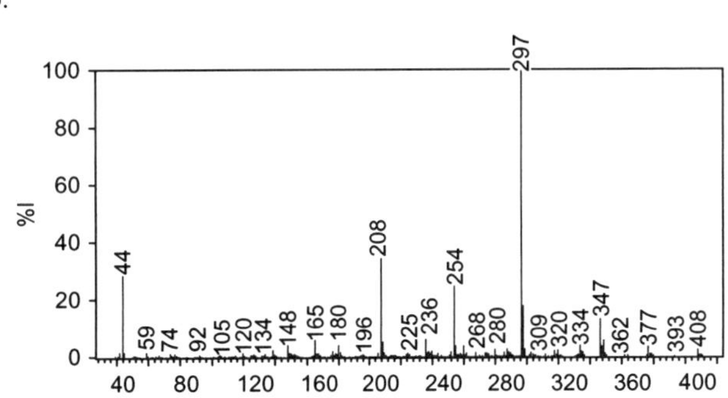

Quantification

Gas chromatography. In plasma: limit of detection 0.2 µg/L, ECD—J. K. Faulkner *et al.*, *Br. J. Clin. Pharmacol.*, 1986, *22*, 21–25. In plasma: limit of detection 0.2 µg/L, ECD—A. P. Beresford *et al.*, *J. Chromatogr.*, 1987, *420*; *Biomed. Appl.*, *64*, 178–183. In plasma or tissue: limit of detection 0.02 µg/L for each enantiomer in plasma and 0.5 ng/g for each enantiomer in tissue, ECD—F. Scharpf *et al.*, *J. Chromatogr. Biomed. Sci. Appl.*, 1994, *655*,

225–233. In plasma or gingival crevicular fluid: limit of detection 0.5 μg/L, ECD—S. C. Monkman *et al.*, *J. Chromatogr. Biomed. Sci. Appl.*, 1996, *678*, 360–364.

Gas chromatography–mass spectrometry.
A. P. Beresford *et al.*, *Xenobiotica*, 1988, *18*, 245–254.

High performance liquid chromatography. In serum: limit of detection 0.1 μg/L, electrochemical detection—K. Shimooka *et al.*, *J. Pharm. Biomed. Anal.*, 1989, *7*, 1267–1272. In plasma: limit of detection about 0.2 μg/L for each enantiomer, electrochemical detection—M. Josefsson and B. Norlander, *J. Pharm. Biomed. Anal*, 1996, *15*, 267–277.

Disposition in the Body. Amlodipine is slowly and almost completely absorbed after oral administration; peak plasma concentrations occur after 6 to 12 h. Absorption is not affected by food. It undergoes minimal presystemic metabolism; bioavailability is about 60 to 65% and it undergoes extensive but slow metabolism in the liver. Metabolites lack significant pharmacological activity and are excreted predominantly in urine (about 60% of a dose); less than 10% of a dose is excreted as the unchanged drug. About 20 to 25% of a dose is eliminated via bile. It is not removed by haemodialysis.

Therapeutic concentration
The mean peak plasma concentration 7.6 h after administration of a 10 mg single oral dose in 12 healthy male subjects (with a mean age of 25.8 years) was 5.9 μg/L. The drug was administered after an overnight fast. Following oral administration of 15 mg daily for 14 days in 56 subjects mean peak plasma concentration was 18.1 μg/L after 8.7 h. [J. K. Faulkner *et al.*, *Br. J. Clin. Pharmacol.*, 1986, *22*, 21–25].

Toxicity
A 42-year-old female ingested 50 to 100 mg of amlodipine besylate together with alcohol in a suicide attempt. Symptoms included hypotension and sinus tachycardia. Serum-amlodipine concentration measured 2.5 h after ingestion was 88 μg/L; this had reduced to 79 μg/L 37.5 h after ingestion. Treatment included activated charcoal, whole bowel irrigation and intravenous sodium chloride 0.9%; the woman was discharged on day 2. [E. J. Stanek *et al.*, *Ann Pharmacother.*, 1997, *31*, 853–856].

Bioavailability. 60 to 65%.

Half-life. Plasma, 35 to 50 h; 65 h in elderly subjects; 56 h in patients with hepatic impairment.

Volume of distribution. 21 L/kg.

Clearance. Plasma, 18.5 L/h (elderly); 24.6 L/h (young); also, stated as 7 mL/min/kg.

Protein binding. In plasma, 95 to 98%.

Dose. Up to 10 mg (of the base) daily.

Amobarbital

Barbiturate

Synonyms. Amylobarbital; Amylobarbitone; Pentymalum.
Proprietary names. Amal; Amytal; Eunoctal; Neur-Amyl; Stadadorm.
5-Ethyl-5-(3-methylbutyl)-2,4,6-(1*H*,3*H*,5*H*)-pyrimidinetrione
$C_{11}H_{18}N_2O_3$=226.3
CAS—57-43-2

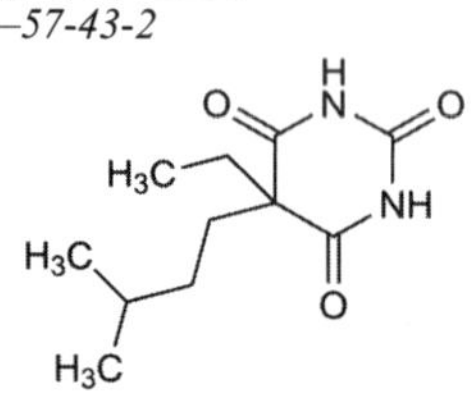

A white crystalline powder. M.p. 156° to 158°.
Soluble 1 in 1300 of water, 1 in 5 of ethanol, 1 in 17 of chloroform, and 1 in 6 of ether; freely soluble in benzene; soluble in aqueous solutions of alkali hydroxides and carbonates; insoluble in petroleum ether and aliphatic hydrocarbons.

Amobarbital Sodium

Synonyms. Amylobarbitone Sodium; Barbamylum; Soluble Amylobarbital.
Proprietary names. Amylbarb Sodium; Amylobeta; Neur-Amyl Sodium; Sodium Amytal. It is an ingredient of Tuinal.
$C_{11}H_{17}N_2NaO_3$=248.3
CAS—64-43-7
A white, hygroscopic, granular powder. M.p. about 156°.
Soluble 1 in less than 1 of water and 1 in 1 of ethanol; practically insoluble in chloroform and ether. Solutions in water decompose on standing.

Dissociation Constant. pK_a 7.9 (25°).

Partition Coefficient. Log *P* (octanol/pH 7.4), 1.6.

Colour Tests. Koppanyi–Zwikker Test—violet; Mercurous Nitrate—black

Thin-layer Chromatography. System TD—Rf 52; system TE—Rf 44; system TF—Rf 66; system TH—Rf 74; system TAD—Rf 58; system TAE—Rf 88. (Mercuric chloride–diphenylcarbazone reagent, positive; mercurous nitrate spray, black; Zwikker's reagent, pink.)

Gas Chromatography. System GA—amobarbital RI 1710; amobarbital-Me_2 RI 1593, M (3-OH-) RI 1915, M (3-OH-)-Me_2 RI 1750, M (COOH-) RI 1960; system GB—amobarbital RI 1742; M (3-OH-) RI 2015; system GF—RI 2430; system GAJ—amobarbital RRT 0.794, M (3-OH-) RRT 1.138, M (COOH-) RRT 0.775 (relative to methylphenobarbital).

High Performance Liquid Chromatography. System HG—*k* 10.91; system HH—*k* 7.05; system HX—RI 424; system HY—RI 374; system HZ—retention time 4.0 min; system HAA—retention time 16.6 min.

Ultraviolet Spectrum. Borax buffer 0.05 M (pH 9.2)—240 nm (A_1^1=445a); 1 M sodium hydroxide (pH 13)—255 nm (A_1^1=364b). (See below)

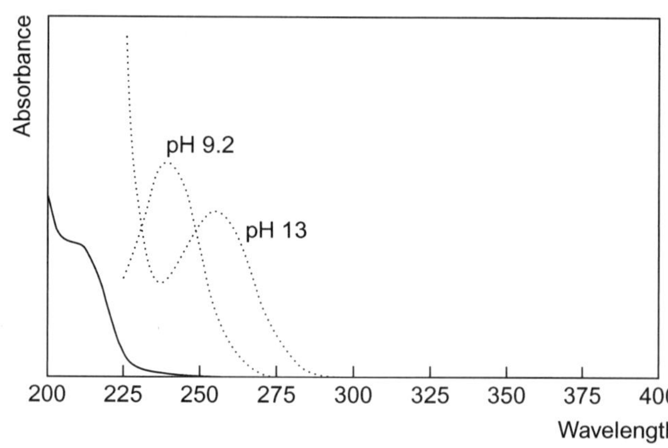

Infra-red Spectrum. Principal peaks at wavenumbers 1725, 1696, 1758, 1317, 1240, 850 cm^{-1} (KBr disk). (See below.)

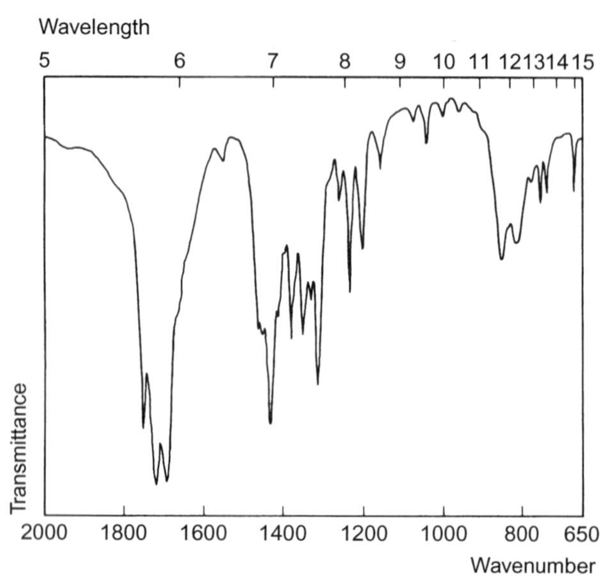

Mass Spectrum. Principal ions at *m/z* 156, 141, 157, 41, 55, 142, 98, 39; 3′-hydroxyamylobarbital 59, 157, 156, 141, 43, 41, 71, 69.

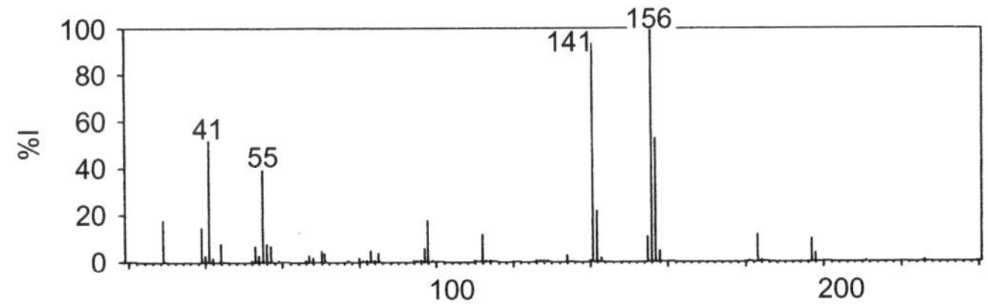

Quantification. The following are general methods for most barbiturates. **Gas chromatography.** In plasma or urine: limit of detection <500 ng/L, AFID—T. Villén and I. Petters, *J. Chromatogr.*, 1983, *258*, 267–270. In plasma: limit of detection <500 µg/L, AFID—A. Turcant *et al.*, *J. Chromatogr.* 1982, *229(18) Biomed. Appl. B* 222–226. For a review of gas chromatographic methods see D. N. Pillai and S. Dilli, *J. Chromatogr.*, 1981, *220*; *Chromatogr. Rev.*, *25*, 253–274. In serum: limit of detection 500 µg/L, nitrogen–phosphorus detection—V. A. Soo *et al.*, *Clin. Chem.*, 1986, *32*, 325–328.

Gas chromatography–mass spectrometry. In urine: limit of detection about 20 µg/L—R. H. Lui *et al.*, *J. Forensic Sci.*, 1994, *39*, 1504–1514.

High performance liquid chromatography. In blood: limit of detection <1 mg/L, UV detection—R. Gill *et al.*, *J. Chromatogr.* 1981, *226(25)*; *Biomed. Appl. B* 117–123. In saliva: limits of detection 0.5 to 2.5 ng, UV detection—J. Haginaka and J. Wakai, *J. Chromatogr.*, 1987, *390*, 421–428. In urine: amobarbital *N*-glycosides, UV detection—V. Nandi and W. H. Soine, *J. Pharm. Biomed. Anal.*, 1997, *15*, 1187–1195.

Immunoassay. In urine: barbiturates and metabolites, limit of detection 2 mg/L for quinalbarbital using EMIT and 10 µg/L using RIA—B. Law and A. C. Moffat, *J. Forensic Sci. Soc.*, 1981, *21*, 55–66. In plasma or serum: FPIA on COBAS INTEGRA, comparison with GC–MS—R. D. Cannon *et al.*, *Ther. Drug Monit.*, 1999, *21*, 553–558. In serum or urine: FPIA on COBAS INTEGRA, comparison with EMIT and GC–MS—K. S. Schwenzer *et al.*, *J. Anal. Toxicol.*, 2000, *24*, 726–732.

Disposition in the Body. Readily and almost completely absorbed after oral administration.. It is metabolised by hydroxylation to give the major metabolite 3′-hydroxyamobarbital, which has about one-third of the activity of the parent substance. About 80 to 90% of a dose is excreted in the urine in 6 days, of which 30 to 50% is 3′-hydroxyamobarbital, up to 30% is *N*-*β*-D-glucopyranosylamobarbital, and about 1% is unchanged drug. The metabolite pattern appears to be genetically determined. 5-(3′-Carboxybutyl)-5-ethylbarbituric acid has also been identified as a metabolite in urine. About 5% of a dose is eliminated in the faeces in 6 days.

Therapeutic concentration. In plasma, usually in the range 2 to 12 mg/L.

Toxicity. The estimated minimum lethal dose is 1.5 g. Toxic effects are associated with plasma concentrations greater than 9 mg/L and fatalities with postmortem blood concentrations of 9 to 26 to 72 mg/L.

In a review of 55 cases of fatal overdosage, postmortem blood concentrations were in the range 13 to 96 mg/L. [R. C. Gupta and J. Kofed, *Can. Med. Assoc. J.*, 1966, *94*, 863–865.]

In 3 fatalities attributed to amobarbital overdose, the following post-mortem tissue concentrations, mg/L or µg/g, were reported:

	Amobarbital	3′-Hydroxyamobarbital
Blood	36, 35, 25	2, –, 2
Bile	198, 178, –	6, –, –
Kidney	32, 59, 87	–, 2, 4
Liver	71, 79, 224	1, 2, 2
Lung	43, 40, 84	–, 2, 4
Spleen	77, 63, 104	–, 1, –
Urine	12, 12, –	9, –, –

[A. E. Robinson and R. D. McDowall, *J. Pharm. Pharmacol.*, 1979, *31*, 357–365.]

Bioavailability. About 95%

Half-life. Plasma half-life, 8 to 40 h (mean 24).

Volume of distribution. About 1 L/kg.

Clearance. Plasma clearance, about 0.5 mL/min/kg.

Saliva. Plasma:saliva ratio, about 2.8.

Protein binding. In plasma, 40 to 60%.

Note. For a review of the clinical pharmacokinetics of barbiturates, see D. D. Breimer, *Clin. Pharmacokinet.*, 1977, *2*, 93–109.

Dose. 30 to 240 mg daily; up to 600 mg daily has been given.

Amodiaquine

Antimalarial

Synonym. Amodiachin
Proprietary name. Basoquin
4-[(7-Chloro-4-quinolinyl)amino]-2-[(diethylamino)methyl]phenol
$C_{20}H_{22}ClN_3O = 355.9$
CAS—86-42-0

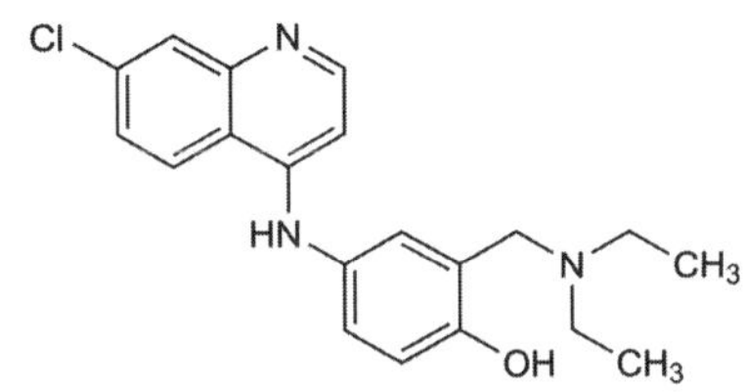

White crystals. M.p. 208°.

Amodiaquine Hydrochloride

Proprietary names. Camoquin; Flavoquine.
$C_{20}H_{22}ClN_3O,2HCl,2H_2O = 464.8$
CAS—69-44-3 (anhydrous); 6398-98-7 (dihydrate)
A yellow crystalline powder. M.p. about 158°. Soluble 1 in about 22 of water and 1 in about 70 of ethanol; practically insoluble in chloroform and ether.

Colour Tests. Folin–Ciocalteu reagent—blue; Liebermann's test—black; Millon's reagent—orange.

Thin-layer Chromatography. System TA—Rf 62; system TB—Rf 08; system TC—Rf 40; system TE—Rf 74; system TL—Rf 37; system TAE—Rf 38; system TAJ—Rf 15; system TAK—Rf 00; system TAL—Rf 09. (Acidified iodoplatinate solution, positive.)

Gas Chromatography. System GA—not eluted.

Ultraviolet Spectrum. Aqueous acid—237 ($A_1^1 = 600$b), 343; aqueous alkali—273, 287 nm.

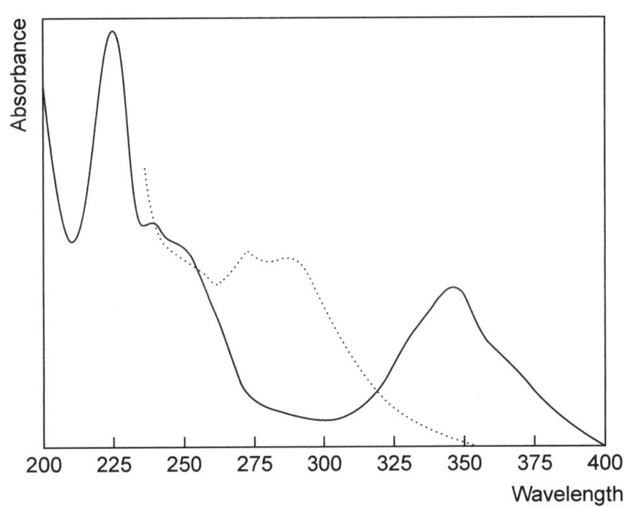

Infra-red Spectrum. Principal peaks at wavenumbers 1565, 815, 1535, 1255, 869, 847 cm^{-1} (KBr disk).

Mass Spectrum. Principal ions at *m*/*z* 58, 282, 30, 284, 355, 73, 283, 44.

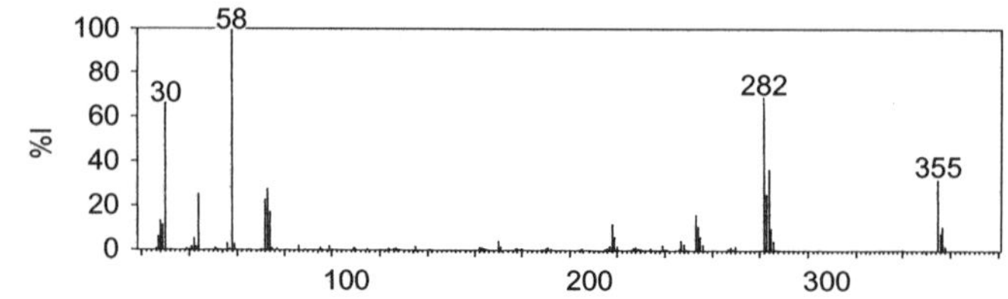

Quantification

Spectrofluorimetry. In plasma or serum: limit of detection 50 µg/L—G. M. Trenholme *et al.*, *Bull. WHO*, 1974, *51*, 431–434.

Disposition in the Body. Amodiaquine is readily absorbed after oral administration and widely distributed throughout the tissues. After absorption it is slowly released into the blood and excreted in the urine for at least 7 days after a single dose; the rate of excretion is increased in acid urine.

Therapeutic concentration

Following a single oral dose of 10 mg/kg to 5 subjects, serum concentrations of 0.30 to 0.68 (mean 0.5) mg/L were reported after 4 h; the ratio of erythrocyte to serum concentration varied with time and between individuals, but erythrocyte concentrations were generally higher than serum concentrations after 48 h. [G. M. Trenholme *et al.*, *Bull. WHO*, 1974, *51*, 431–434].

Dose. For an acute attack, the equivalent of 1.5 g of amodiaquine in 48 h (1.2 g in the first 24 h); for suppression, the equivalent of 300 to 600 mg every 7 days.

Amosulalol

Antihypertensive

5-[1-Hydroxy-2-[[2-(2-methoxy-phenoxy)ethyl]amino]ethyl]-2-methylbenzene sulfonamide

$C_{18}H_{24}N_2O_5S$=380.5

CAS—85320-68-9

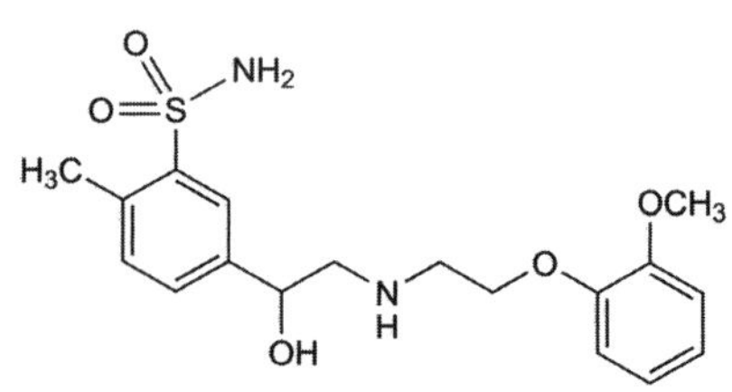

Amosulalol Monohydrochloride

Synonym. YM-09538

Proprietary name. Lowgan

$C_{18}H_{25}ClN_2O_5S$=416.9

CAS—70958-86-0; 93633-92-2

Colourless crystals with m.p. 158° to 160°.

Dissociation Constant. pK_a 7.72; 10.04.

Partition Coefficient. Log *D* (octanol/pH 7.5), 0.82.

High Performance Liquid Chromatography. Column: C_{18} (µBondapak, 300 × 7.8 mm i.d., 8 to 10 µm) with RP-18 (LiChrosorb, 15 cm × 4 mm i.d., 5 µm), stainless steel. Mobile phase: acetonitrile:methanol:acetic acid (0.6 M):ammonium acetate (0.02 M) (20:5:30:50). UV detection (λ=271 nm). Retention time: amosulalol, 7.2 min; 5-hydroxylated amosulalol, 3.3 min. [H. Kamimura *et al.*, *Xenobiotica*, 1985, *15(5)*, 413–420].

Ultraviolet Spectrum. Aqueous acid—272 nm; aqueous alkali—272 nm.

Infra-red Spectrum. Principal peaks at wavenumber 1330, 1260, 1165, 755 cm^{-1}.

Mass Spectrum. (5-hydroxylated amosulalol) Principal peaks at *m/z* 196, 239, 208, 200, 225, 397, 396, 257.

Quantification

Gas chromatography. In urine: limit of detection 0.2 mg/L—H. Kamimura *et al.*, *J. Chromatogr. Biomed. Sci. Appl.*, 1983, *275*, 81–87.

High performance liquid chromatography. In plasma: limit of detection 0.02 mg/L. UV detection (λ=271 nm)—H. Kamimura *et al.*, *J. Chromatogr. Biomed. Sci. Appl.*, 1981, *255*, 115–121.

Disposition in the Body. Amosulalol is metabolised to at least six metabolites (free and conjugated forms), the main metabolite in humans being the sulfate conjugate of 5-hydroxyl amosulalol. 25 to 35% of an administered dose is excreted in urine unchanged within the first 6 h.

Therapeutic concentration

25 healthy men, aged between 24 and 45 years, were administered with single oral doses of 12.5, 25, 50, 100 and 150 mg amosulalol after a fast. Mean peak plasma concentrations of 0.2, 0.49, 1.11, 1.87 and 4.09 mg/L were reached, respectively within 2.5 to 4 h. [M. Nakashima *et al.*, *Clin. Pharmacol. Ther.*, 1984, *36*, 436–443].

Toxicity. Toxic by subcutaneous and intravenous routes.

Bioavailability. Approx. 100%.

Half-life. Approximately, 2.8 h (intravenous administration) or 5.7 h (oral).

Volume of distribution. 0.75 L/kg.

Clearance. Approx. 8.09 L/h (intravenous); 7.28 L/h (oral).

Protein binding. 97 to 98%.

Dose. Starting oral dose of 10 mg twice daily, up to a maximum daily dose of 60 mg.

Amoxapine

Antidepressant

Synonym. CL-67772

Proprietary names. Asendin; Asendis; Defanyl; Demolox; Moxadil.

2-Chloro-11-(1-piperazinyl)dibenz[*b,f*][1,4]oxazepine

$C_{17}H_{16}ClN_3O$=313.8

CAS—14028-44-5

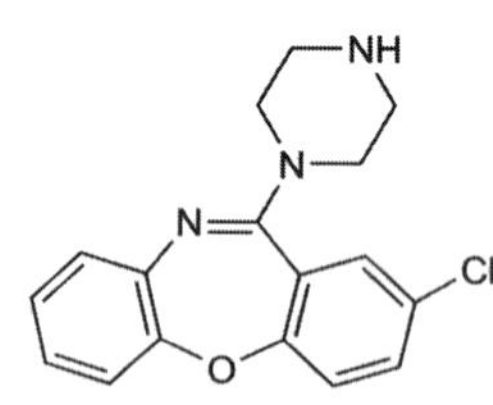

Crystals. M.p. 175° to 176°.

Gas Chromatography. System GA—RI 2638 amoxapine; RI 2951 M ($7\text{-}OH^-$); RI 2959 M (8-OH); system GB—RI 2746 amoxapine; RI 3525 M ($7\text{-}OH^-$); RI 3546 M ($\text{-}OH^-$); system GM—RRT 2.831 amoxapine (relative to iprindole).

High Performance Liquid Chromatography. System HX—RI 398; system HAA—Retention time(s) 14.2 min.

Column: (1) C_8 RP TSK gel Super-Octyl (100 × 4.6 mm i.d., 2 µm); (2) Hypersil MOS-C_8 (100 × 4.6 mm i.d., 5 µm). Mobile phase: methanol:20 mM KH_2PO_4 (pH 7) (60:40 v/v), flow rate 0.6 mL/min. Internal standard (IS): diazepam. UV detection (λ=254 nm). Retention time(s): column (1): 5.6 min; column (2): 7.8 min. [E. Tanaka *et al.*, *J. Chromatogr. B Biomed. Sci. Appl.*, 1997, *692*, 405–412].

Ultraviolet Spectrum. Aqueous acid—210, 252 (A_1^1=362 a), 297 (A_1^1=315 a); aqueous alkali—250, 299 nm.

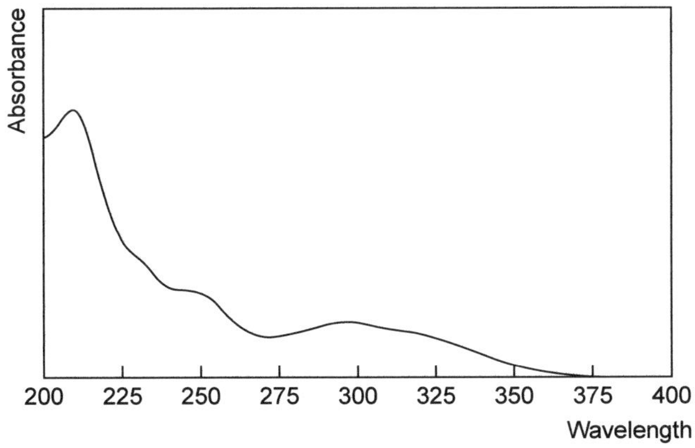

Infra-red Spectrum. Principal peaks at wavenumbers 1604, 1592, 752, 1181, 1246, 1107 cm^{-1}.

Mass Spectrum. Principal ions at *m/z* 245, 257, 247, 193, 56, 246, 228, 259.

Quantification

Gas chromatography. In blood: limit of detection 42 to 62 µg/L and limit of quantification 140 to 204 µg/L depending on column, NPD—M. A. Martinez *et al.*, *J. Anal. Toxicol.*, 2002, *26(5)*, 296–302. In serum or urine: amoxapine and metabolites, ECD for serum and FID for urine—T. B. Cooper and R. G. Kelly, *J. Pharm. Sci.*, 1979, *68*, 216–219.

High performance liquid chromatography. In serum and urine: limit of quantification 0.05 mg/L, UV detection (λ=254 nm)—E. Tanaka *et al.*, *J. Chromatogr. B Biomed. Sci. Appl.*, 1997, *692*, 405–412. In serum: amoxapine and 8-hydroxyamoxapine, limit of detection 50 µg/L, UV detection—J. J. Tasset and F. M. Hassan, *Clin. Chem.*, 1982, *28*, 2154–2157. In plasma: amoxapine and metabolites, limit of detection 25 µg/L, UV detection—S. M. Johnson *et al.*, *J. Pharm. Sci.*, 1984, *73*, 696–699.

Disposition in the Body. Amoxapine is rapidly and almost completely absorbed after oral administration. It is metabolised by hydroxylation to 7-hydroxyamoxapine and 8-hydroxyamoxapine which are both active. The hydroxylated metabolites are excreted in the urine as glucuronide conjugates and are also eliminated in the faeces in unconjugated form. Less than 5% of a dose is excreted in the urine as unchanged drug.
Amoxapine is a metabolite of loxapine.

Therapeutic concentration

After a single oral dose of 50 mg to 26 subjects, a mean peak serum-amoxapine concentration of 0.03 mg/L was attained in 1 to 2 h; the peak concentration of 8-hydroxyamoxapine was of a similar order. [T. B. Cooper and R. G. Kelly, *J. Pharm. Sci.*, 1979, *68*, 216–219].

Following oral administration of 300 mg daily in divided doses to 10 subjects, steady-state serum concentrations of 0.02 to 0.09 mg/L of amoxapine and 0.16 to 0.51 mg/L of 8-hydroxyamoxapine were reported. [W. E. Boutelle, *Neuropharmacology*, 1980, *19*, 1229–1231].

Toxicity

The following postmortem concentrations were reported in 3 fatalities due to amoxapine overdose: blood 11.5, 2.8, 0.89 mg/L, bile 1264.5, 69.1, 14.3 mg/L, liver 112.2, 40.1, 16.8 µg/g; in the first case brain and urine concentrations of 2.5 µg/g and 28.3 mg/L, respectively, were also reported. [C. L. Winek *et al.*, *Forensic Sci. Int.*, 1984, *26*, 33–38].

In a review of 33 cases of amoxapine overdose, 3 subjects had no toxic symptoms, 10 suffered mild toxic reactions, 15 developed severe toxicity and 5 died. Postmortem blood concentrations of 0.26 to 6.70 (mean 2.8) mg/L of amoxapine plus 8-hydroxyamoxapine were reported in 4 of the 5 fatalities. [T. L. Litovitz and K. G. Troutman, *J. Am. Med. Assoc.*, 1983, *250*, 1069–1071].

The following postmortem tissue concentrations were reported in a fatality due to ingestion of 2 grams of amoxapine: blood 7.2 mg/L, bile 823 mg/L, liver 36 µg/g; a blood-alcohol concentration of 280 mg/L was also reported. In a further 2 cases where amoxapine was a contributory cause of death, postmortem concentrations were: blood 1.66 and 2.95 mg/L; bile 75 mg/L; liver 23.2 µg/g; urine 22 mg/L. [N.B. Wu Chen *et al.*, *J. Forensic Sci.*, 1983, *28*, 116–121].

Half-life. Plasma half-life, amoxapine about 8 h, 7-hydroxyamoxapine about 6 h, 8-hydroxyamoxapine about 30 h.

Protein binding. In plasma, about 90%.

Note. For a review of the pharmacokinetics of amoxapine, see S. G. Jue *et al.*, *Drugs*, 1982, *24*, 1–23.

Dose. 150 to 600 mg daily.

Amoxicillin

Antibacterial

Synonyms. D(−)-α-Amino-*p*-hydroxybenzylpenicillin; Amoxycillin; Amoxicilline.

Proprietary names. AMPC; Amolin; Amopenixin; Helvamox; Moxal; Pasetocin; Penimox; Zamocilline.

(2*S*,5*R*,6*R*)-6-[[(2*R*)-Amino(4-hydroxyphenyl)acetyl]amino]-3,3-dimethyl-7-oxo-4-thia-1-azabicyclo[3.2.0]heptane-2-carboxylic acid

$C_{16}H_{19}N_3O_5S$=365.4

CAS—26787-78-0

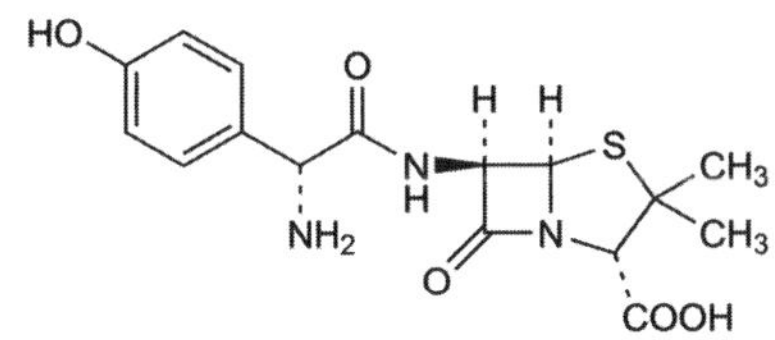

Amoxicillin Sodium

Proprietary names. Amoxil (injection); Clamoxyl (injection).

$C_{16}H_{18}N_3NaO_5S$=387.4

CAS—34642-77-8

A white powder. Soluble 1 in less than 1 of water.

Amoxicillin Trihydrate

Synonym. Amoxicillin

Proprietary names. Amoxican; Amoxil; Amoxypen; Clamoxyl; Imacillin; Larotid; Moxacin; Moxilean; Novamoxin; Penamox; Polymox; Robamox; Trimox; Utimox; Wymox. It is an ingredient of Augmentin.

$C_{16}H_{19}N_3O_5S,3H_2O$=419.4

CAS—61336-70-7

A white crystalline powder. Soluble 1 in 400 of water, 1 in 1000 of ethanol, and 1 in 200 of methanol; practically insoluble in chloroform and ether.

Dissociation Constant. pK_a 2.4, 7.4, 9.6.

Partition Coefficient Log *P* (octanol/water), 0.87.

High Performance Liquid Chromatography. System HY—RI 226; system HAA—Retention time(s) 3.1 min.

Ultraviolet Spectrum. Amoxicillin trihydrate: aqueous acid—230 (A^1_1=225a), 272 (A^1_1=26a); aqueous alkali—247 (A^1_1=286b), 291 nm (A^1_1=62a).

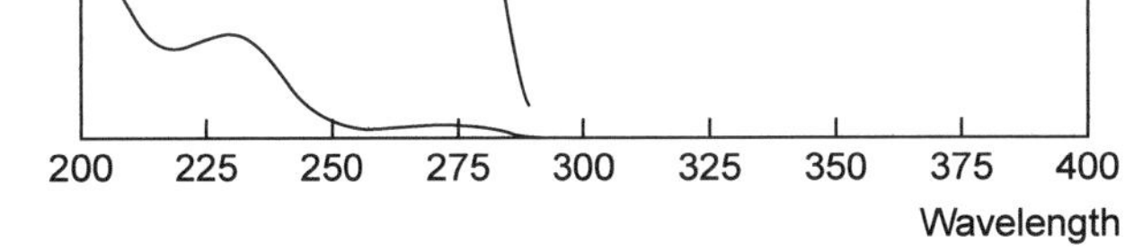

Infra-red Spectrum. Principal peaks at wavenumbers 1775, 1583, 1684, 1248, 1613, 1313 cm^{-1} (amoxicillin trihydrate, KBr disk).

Quantification

High performance liquid chromatography. In plasma: limit of quantification 1.0 mg/L, photodiode array detection—A. Menelaou *et al.*, *J. Chromatogr. B, Biomed. Sci. Appl.*, 1999, *731*, 261–266. In serum and plasma: limit of quantification 0.1 mg/L, fluorescence detection (λ_{ex}=395 nm; λ_{em}=485 nm)—H. J. Mascher and C. Kikuta, *J. Chromatogr. A*, 1998, *812(1–2)*, 221–226. In blood, plasma and ear fluid: limit of quantification 1.0 mg/L in whole blood and 0.25 mg/L in plasma and ear fluid, UV detection (λ=210 nm)—Z. Yuan *et al.*, *J. Chromatogr. B Biomed. Sci. Appl.*, 1997, *692(2)*, 361–366. In urine: amoxicillin and penicilloic acid, limit of detection 2.5 mg/L, fluorescence detection—T. L. Lee, *J. Pharm. Sci.*, 1979, *68*, 454–458. In plasma: limit of detection 500 μg/L, UV detection—T. L. Lee and M. A. Brooks, *J. Chromatogr.*, 1984, *306*; *B Biomed. Appl.*, *31*, 429–435.

Disposition in the Body. Amoxicillin is rapidly absorbed after oral administration. About 60% of an oral dose is excreted in the urine as unchanged drug in 6 h and 20% as the inactive metabolite, penicilloic acid, in the same period. After parenteral administration, up to 75% of a dose is excreted in the urine unchanged in 6 h.

Therapeutic concentration

12 healthy male and female subjects with a mean age of 33.7 years (range 18 to 47 years) were fasted overnight and after administration of 1 g standard reference formulation amoxicillin (A), dispersible tablet (B) and 1 g dispersible tablet in suspension (C) the mean peak serum concentrations observed were 14.1 mg/L at 2.3 h for A, 15.1 mg/L at 2.0 h for B and 15.1 mg/L at 1.5 h for C. [M. H. Prevot *et al.*, *Eur. J. Drug Metab. Pharmacokinet.*, 1997, *22(1)*, 47–52].

Following an oral dose of 500 mg to 8 subjects, peak plasma concentrations of 6.0 to 15.3 (mean 10) mg/L were attained in 1 to 2 h. [A. Arancibia *et al.*, *Antimicrob. Agents Chemother.*, 1980, 17, 199–202].

Half-life. Plasma half-life, about 1 h, increased in renal failure.

Volume of distribution. About 0.2 to 0.4 L/kg.

Clearance. Plasma clearance, 3 to 5 mL/min/kg.

Protein binding. In plasma, about 20%.

Note. For reviews of the pharmacokinetics of amoxicillin, see R. N. Brogden *et al.*, *Drugs*, 1975, *9*, 88–140 and R. N. Brogden *et al.*, *Drugs*, 1979, *18*, 169–184 (amoxicillin injectable).

Dose. The equivalent of 0.75 to 1.5 g of amoxicillin daily. One-day courses of 3 to 6 g are also given.

Amphotericin B

Antifungal

Synonyms. Amphotericin; Anfotericina B.

Proprietary names. Ampho-Moronal; Fungilin; Fungizone. It is an ingredient of Mysteclin (syrup).

A mixture of antifungal polyenes produced by the growth of certain strains of *Streptomyces nodosus* or by any other means.

$C_{47}H_{73}NO_{17}$=924.1

CAS—1397-89-3

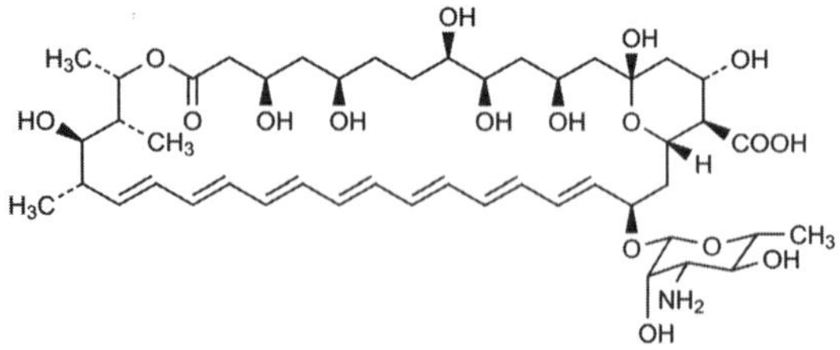

A yellow to orange powder. It gradually decomposes above 170°. Practically insoluble in water, ethanol, chloroform and ether; soluble 1 in 200 of dimethylformamide and 1 in 20 of dimethylsulfoxide; soluble in propylene glycol.

Dissociation Constant. pK_a 5.5, 10.0.

High Performance Liquid Chromatography. System HAA—Retention time(s) 15.7 min.

Column: RP-C_{18} μBondapak (300 × 3.9 mm i.d., 10 μm). Mobile phase: acetonitrile:acetate buffer 10 mM, pH 4 (37:63 v/v). Elution: flow rate 1 mL/min for first 6 min and 2 mL/min until completion. Internal standard (IS): natamycin. UV detection (λ=383 nm). Retention time(s): 15 min. [M. Polikandritou *et al.*, *J. Chromatogr.*, 1996, *685*; *B Biomed. Appl.*, 135–140].

Column: RP-C_{18} μBondapak (300 × 4.6 mm i.d., 5 μm). Mobile phase: acetonitrile:disodium edetate 20 mM, pH 5 (45:55 v/v), flow rate 1 mL/min. IS: 1-amino-4-nitronaphthalene. UV detection (λ=407 nm). Retention time(s): 6.3 min [T. Eldem and N. Arica-Cellat, *J. Pharm. Biomed. Anal.*, 2001, *25*, 53–64].

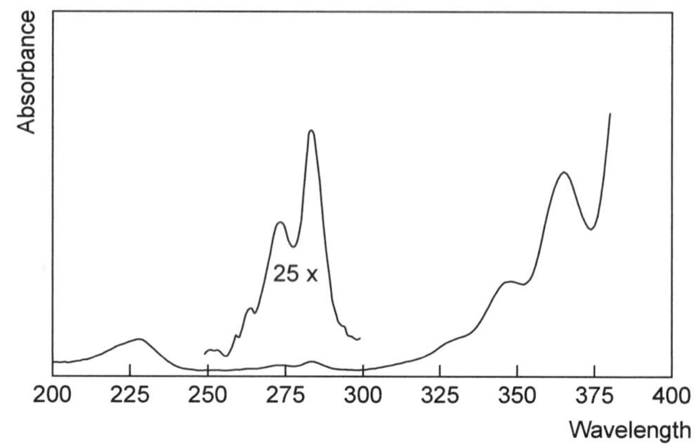

Infra-red Spectrum. Principal peaks at wavenumbers 1010, 1065, 1038, 1103, 1183, 1126 cm^{-1} (KBr disk).

Quantification

High performance liquid chromatography. In plasma, urine and faecal homogenate: limit of quantification 2 mg/L, 0.05 mg/L and 0.4 mg/L, respectively, MS/MS detection—J. W. Lee *et al.*, *Ther. Drug Monit.*, 2001, *23(3)*, 268–276. In plasma: limit of detection 5 μg/L, UV detection (λ=407 nm)—T. Eldem and N. Arica-Cellat, *J. Pharm. Biomed. Anal.*, 2001, *25*, 53–64. In serum, lung and liver: limit of detection 0.1 mg/L, UV detection (λ=383 nm)—M. Polikandritou *et al.*, *J. Chromatogr.*, 1996, *685*; *B Biomed. Appl.*, 135–140. In serum: limit of quantification 0.05 mg/L, UV detection—A. Alak *et al.*, *Ther. Drug Monit.*, 1996, *18(5)*, 604–609. In serum or cerebrospinal fluid: limit of detection 20 μg/L, UV detection—I. Nilsson-Ehle *et al.*, *J. Infect. Dis.*, 1977, *135*, 414–422.

Immunoassay. In plasma and tissue: limit of quantification 0.1 μg/L and 1.0 ng/g, respectively—S. Machard *et al.*, *Antimicrob. Agents Chemother.*, 2000, *44(3)*, 546–550.

Disposition in the Body. Amphotericin B is poorly absorbed after oral, intramuscular or subcutaneous administration. It is slowly excreted in the urine, less than 10% of a dose being excreted unchanged in 24 h; up to 40% of a dose is excreted in the urine in 7 days and traces are still detectable in urine 2 months after cessation of treatment.

Therapeutic concentration

10 critically ill patients, aged 20 to 67 years, were intravenously administered liposomal amphotericin B at a dose of 1.2 to 4.2 mg/kg over 1 h, and 6 male and female patients, aged 49 to 76 years, were administered amphotericin B deoxycholate at a standard dose of 1.0 mg/kg over 1 h. The median peak concentration of amphotericin B was 14.4 (range 6.4 to 89.0) mg/L after the infusion and for amphotericin B deoxycholate, 1.7 (1.5 to 2.1) mg/L. [V. Heinemann *et al.*, *Antimicrob. Agents Chemother.*, 1997, *41(6)*, 1275–1280].

Adult patients, children (aged 1 to 12 years) and neonates (aged 14 to 30 days) all with invasive fungal infection were administered 1.0 mg/kg liposomal amphotericin B as a 60-min infusion. Mean peak plasma concentrations 1.02 mg/L were detected at 0.83 to 1.22 h on day 1 which increased to 1.66 mg/L on day 28 for the adults. In the children, the peak concentrations were 0.63 mg/L at 0.36 to 0.95 h on day 1 and 1.1 mg/L on day 28. For the neonates, the peak plasma concentration was 0.54 mg/L at 0.34 to 1.0 h on day 1 and 0.73 mg/L on day 28. [R. N. Kotwami *et al.*, *Int. J. Pharm.*, 2002, *238(1–2)*, 11–15].

A mean serum concentration of 1.2 mg/L was reported in 20 subjects 1 h after an intravenous infusion of 50 mg. [B. T. Fields *et al.*, *Appl. Microbiol.*, 1970, *19*, 955–959].

Half-life. Plasma half-life, about 24 to 48 h; a longer terminal elimination phase of about 15 days has also been reported.

Volume of distribution. About 4 L/kg.

Clearance. Plasma clearance, about 0.4 mL/min/kg.

Protein binding. In plasma, 90 to 97%.

Note. For a review of amphotericin B, see T. K. Daneshead and D. W. Warnock, *Clin. Pharmacokinet.*, 1983, *8*, 19–23.

Dose. Up to 800 mg daily by mouth. Doses of 0.25 to 1 mg/kg daily are given intravenously.

Ampicillin

Antibiotic

Synonyms. AY-6108; BRL-1341; P-50; Aminobenzylpenicillin; Anhydrous Ampicillin.
Proprietary names. A-Cillin; Albipen; Alpen; Amblosin; Amcill; Amfipen; Amipenix; Ampipenin; Amperil; Ampilar; Ampilean; Ampitab; Binotal; Biosan; Bonapicillin; Britacil; Britcin; D-Amp; Doktacillin; Domicillin; Dumopen; Grampenil; Nuvapen; Omnipen; Pen A; Penbritin(e); Penicicline; Pensyn; Pentrexyl; Polycillin; Principen; Robamox; Supen; Tokiocillin; Totacillin; Vidopen.
(2*S*,5*R*,6*R*)-6-[[(2*R*)-Aminophenylacetyl]amino]-3,3-dimethyl-7-oxo-4-thia-1-azabicyclo[3.2.0]heptane-2-carboxylic acid
$C_{16}H_{19}N_3O_4S$=349.4
CAS—69-53-4

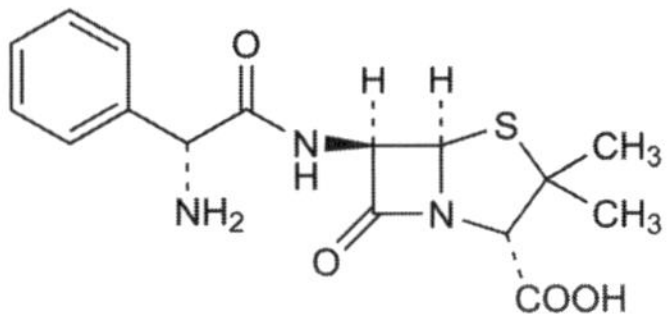

A white crystalline powder. M.p. about 200°. Soluble 1 in 170 of water; practically insoluble in ethanol, acetone, carbon tetrachloride, chloroform and ether.

Ampicillin Sodium

$C_{16}H_{18}N_3NaO_4S$=371.4
CAS—69-52-3
A white, hygroscopic, crystalline or amorphous powder. Aqueous solutions containing 10% or more deteriorate rapidly on storage. M.p. about 205°, with decomposition. Soluble 1 in 2 of water and 1 in 50 of acetone; slightly soluble in chloroform; practically insoluble in ether. With ethanol, ampicillin sodium forms a colloidal dispersion which gels on standing.

Ampicillin Trihydrate

$C_{16}H_{19}N_3O_4S,3H_2O$=403.4
CAS—7177-48-2
A white crystalline powder. Soluble 1 in 150 of water; practically insoluble in ethanol, acetone, carbon tetrachloride, chloroform and ether.

Dissociation Constant. pK_a 2.5 (-COOH), 7.3 ($-NH_2$) (25°).

Colour Tests. Liebermann's test—orange. Suspend 10 mg in 1 mL of water and add 2 mL of a mixture of 2 mL of potassium cupritartrate solution and 6 mL of water—red-violet.

High Performance Liquid Chromatography. System HY—RI 250; system HAA—Retention time(s) 3.8 min.

Ultraviolet Spectrum. Aqueous acid—257 (A^1_1=9.2a), 262, 268 nm.

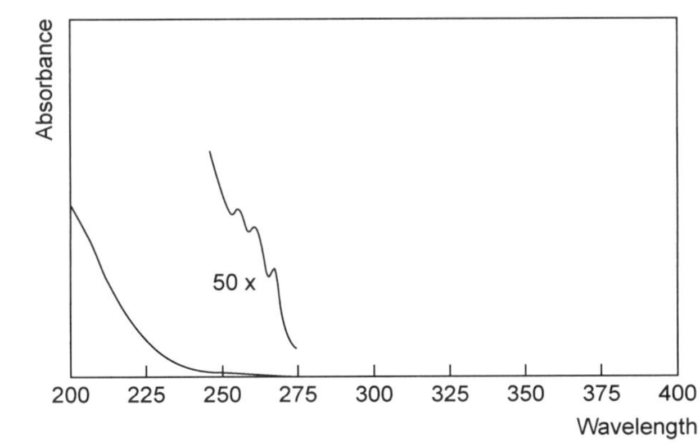

Infra-red Spectrum. Principal peaks at wavenumbers 1775, 1693, 1526, 1308, 1497, 1583 cm^{-1} (KBr disk).

Quantification

Spectrofluorimetry. In serum: limit of detection 50 µg/L—H. J. H. Keshavan *et al.*, *Clin. Chem.*, 1979, *25*, 1674–1675.

High performance liquid chromatography. In serum: limit of detection 2 µg/L, fluorescence detection (λ_{ex}=364 nm; λ_{em}=422 nm)—J. Lal *et al.*, *J. Chromatogr.*, 1994, *655*; *B Biomed. Appl.*, *1*, 142–146. In plasma, saliva or urine: limit of detection 500 µg/L, UV detection—T. B. Vree *et al.*, *J. Chromatogr.*, 1978, *145*; *B Biomed. Appl.*, *2*, 496–501.

Polarography. In serum or urine—S. Schroeder *et al.*, *Pharmazie*, 1978, *33*, 432–434.

Disposition in the Body. Ampicillin is readily but incompletely absorbed after oral administration. About 30% of an oral dose is excreted in the urine in 6 h as unchanged drug and about 10% as penicilloic acid; after parenteral administration about 75% is excreted unchanged in 6 h. High concentrations of ampicillin are attained in the bile.

Therapeutic concentration

After an oral dose of 500 mg given to 6 young subjects, peak plasma concentrations of 2.65 to 4.0 (mean 3.4) mg/L were attained in about 2 h; higher concentrations were reported when a similar dose was given to 6 elderly subjects. [E. J. Triggs *et al.*, *Eur. J. Clin. Pharmacol.*, 1980, *18*, 195–198].

Half-life. Plasma half-life, about 1 to 2 h.

Volume of distribution. About 0.2 to 0.5 L/kg.

Clearance. Plasma clearance, about 3 to 4 mL/min/kg.

Distribution in blood. Plasma:whole blood ratio, 1.8.

Protein binding. In plasma, about 20%.

Note. For a review of the pharmacokinetics of penicillins, see M. Barza and L. Weinstein, *Clin. Pharmacokinet.*, 1976, *1*, 297–308.

Dose. 1 to 8 g daily.

Amprenavir

Antiviral

Synonyms. KVX-478; VX-478; 141-W94.
Proprietary names. Agenerase; Vertex.
[(1*S*,2*R*)-3-[[(4-Aminophenyl)sulfonyl]-(2-methylpropyl)amino]-2-hydroxy-1-(phenylmethyl)propyl]carbamic acid (3*S*)-tetrahydro-3-furanyl ester
$C_{25}H_{35}N_3O_6S$=505.6
CAS—161814-49-9

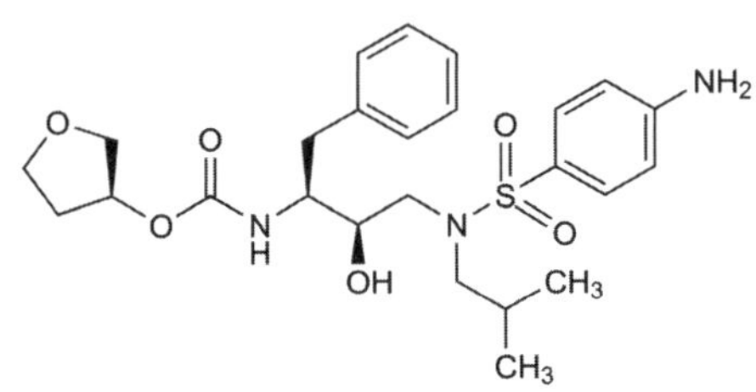

A white to cream coloured solid with a solubility of 0.04 g/l in water, 86 g/l in alcohol at 25°.

Dissociation Constant. pK_a 1.97 at 25°.

High Performance Liquid Chromatography. System HAB—retention time, 4.0 min; system HAC—*k* 2.5; system HAE—retention time, 9.4 min.

Column: C_{18} AB (Nucleosil 100, 5 µm). Mobile phase: (gradient elution) acetonitrile:phosphate buffer, adjusted to pH 5.15, and containing sodium heptanesulfonate (0.02%). 15:85 at 0 min, increased to 30:70 at 2 min, 32:68 (8 min), 42:58 (18 min), 46:54 (34 min). UV detection (λ=201 nm). Retention time: 16.3 min. [C. Marzolini *et al.*, *J. Chromatogr. Biomed. Sci. Appl.*, 2000, *740(1)*, 43–58].

Column: C_{18} (Novapak, 4 µm, 150 × 2.1 mm i.d.). Mobile phases: (A)-orthophosphoric acid (0.5%, 5.8 M) and triethylamine (0.02%) adjusted to pH 5.0 with sodium hydroxide (10 M); (B)-acetonitrile; (C)-methanol. 40% A, 35% B and 25% C (first 10 min), 25% A and 75% B (next 15 min), 0.4

mL/min flow rate. UV detection (λ=265 nm). Retention time: 3.1 min. [J-M. Poirier *et al.*, *Ther. Drug Monit.*, 2000, *22*, 465–473].

Ultraviolet Spectrum. Aqueous alkali—265 nm.

Quantification

High performance liquid chromatography. In plasma: limit of quantification 10 μg/L—L. Veronese *et al.*, *Antimicrob. Agents Chemother.*, 2000, *44(4)*, 821–826. In plasma and semen: limit of quantification 1 μg/L—R. W. Sparidans *et al.*, *J. Chromatogr. Biomed. Sci. Appl.*, 2000, *742(1)*, 185–192. In plasma: limit of quantification is 25 μg/L. UV detection (λ =261 nm)—G. Aymard *et al.*, *J. Chromatogr. Biomed. Sci. Appl.*, 2000, *744*, 227–240. In plasma: limit of quantification 5 μg/L. UV detection (λ =265 nm)—J-M. Poirer *et al.*, *Ther. Drug Monit.*, 2000, *22*, 465–473. In plasma: limit of quantification is 50 μg/L. UV detection (λ =260 nm)—V. Proust *et al.*, *J. Chromatogr. Biomed. Sci. Appl.*, 2000, *742*, 453–458.

Disposition in the Body. Amprenavir is rapidly absorbed and metabolised in the liver to two major metabolites by oxidation, and minor metabolites which are glucuronide conjugates of these oxidised metabolites. In total there are 24 detected metabolites. <2% of the drug is recovered unchanged with the majority as metabolites in urine (14%) and faeces (75%).

Therapeutic concentration

10 healthy volunteers, 10 patients with moderate cirrhosis and 10 with severe cirrhosis, male and female, aged between 18 and 65 years, were administered with a 600 mg dose of amprenavir. Peak plasma concentrations of 4.9, 6.5 and 9.4 mg/L were observed for the three groups of people, respectively. These levels were reached within 1 h. [L. Veronese *et al.*, *Antimicrob. Agents Chemother.*, 2000, *44(4)*, 821–826].

12 HIV infected patients, 18 to 55 years old, were administered with single oral doses of 150, 300, 600, 900 and 1200 mg. Peak plasma concentrations reached 2.00, 3.51, 6.27, 7.76 and 9.11 mg/L, respectively, within 1 to 2 h. [B. M. Sadler *et al.*, *Antimicrob. Agents Chemother.*, 1999, *43(7)*, 1686–1692].

Toxicity. A severe or life-threatening rash including Stevens–Johnson syndrome has been observed.

Half-life. Approximately, 8 h (range, 5.6 to 10.6 h).

Volume of distribution. 430 L.

Clearance. 946 mL/min (healthy volunteers); 564 mL/min (patients with moderate cirrhosis); 295 mL/min (severe cirrhosis).

Distribution in blood. Partitioning into erythrocytes is low.

Protein binding. 90%.

Note. For a review of the pharmacokinetics of amprenavir see L. Veronese *et al.*, *Antimicrob. Agents Chemother.*, 2000, *44(4)*, 821–826 and B. M. Sadler *et al.*, *Antimicrob. Agents Chemother.*, 1999, *43(7)*, 1686–1692.

Dose. The usual dose administered is 1200 mg twice daily. Children aged between 4 and 12 years or those weighing below 50 kg: 40 to 45 mg/kg body weight is administered. The maximum dose is 2400 mg daily. The dose is reduced in patients with hepatic impairment.

Amprolium Hydrochloride

Coccidiostat (Veterinary)

Proprietary names. It is an ingredient of Amprolmix-UK, Amprol-Plus, Pancoxin, and Supacox.

1-[(4-Amino-2-propyl-5-pyrimidinyl)methyl]-2-methylpyridinium chloride hydrochloride

$C_{14}H_{19}ClN_4,HCl$=315.2

CAS—121-25-5 (amprolium); 137-88-2 (hydrochloride)

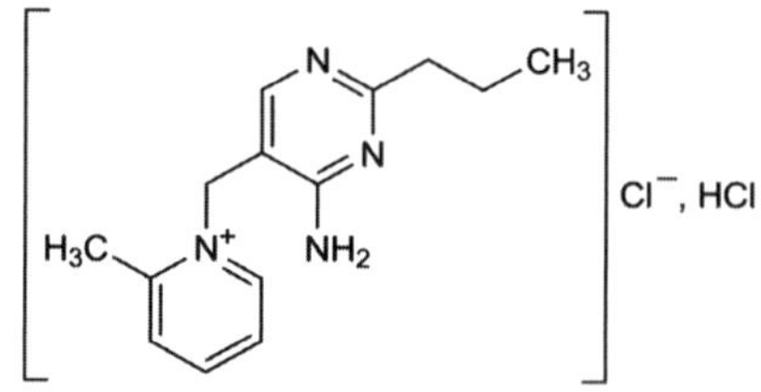

A white powder. M.p. 247°, with decomposition. Soluble 1 in 2 of water and 1 in 170 of ethanol; practically insoluble in chloroform; very slightly soluble in ether.

Colour Test. Aromaticity (Method 2)—colourless/yellow.

Thin-layer Chromatography. System TA—Rf 02. (Acidified iodoplatinate solution, positive.)

Ultraviolet Spectrum. Aqueous acid—246 (A^1_1=420b), 262 nm.

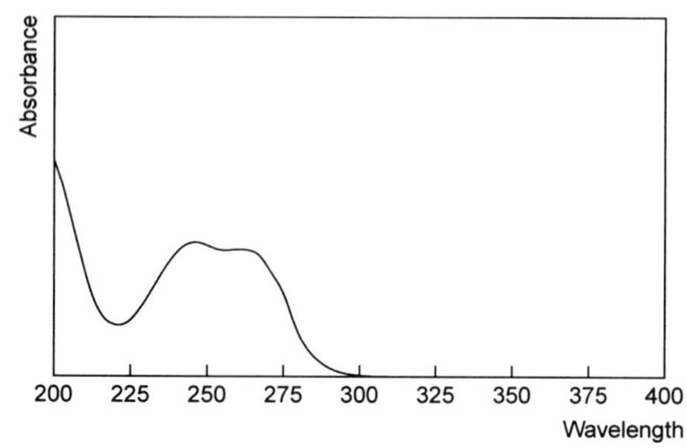

Infra-red Spectrum. Principal peaks at wavenumbers 1638, 1522, 1593, 787, 1562, 1149 cm^{-1} (amprolium, KBr disk).

Amsacrine

Antineoplastic

Synonyms. Acridinyl anisidide; *m*-AMSA; CI-880; NSC-249992; SN-11841

Proprietary names. Amekrin; Amsa P-D; Amsidine; Amsidyl.

N-[4-(9-Acridinylamino)-3-methoxyphenyl]methanesulfonamide

$C_{21}H_{19}N_3O_3S$=393.5

CAS—51264-14-3

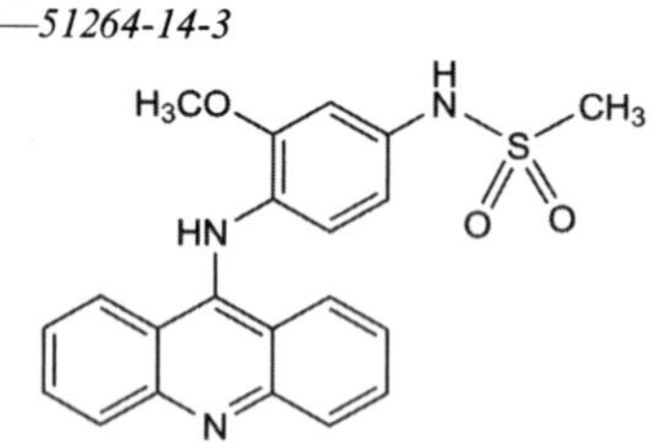

Partition Coefficient. Log *P* (octanol/water), 3.89.

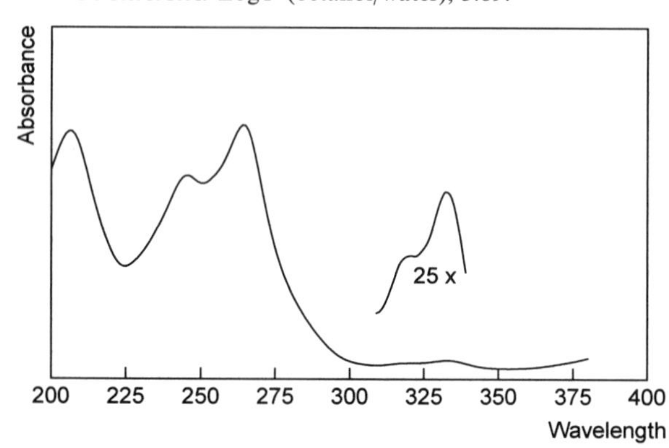

Mass Spectrum. Principal peaks at *m/z* 314, 315, 393, 270, 283, 79, 271, 394.

Quantification

Gas chromatography. In plasma: limit of detection 0.05 mg/L (NPD), 0.125 mg/L (FID)—S. Eksborg and H. Ehrsson, *J. Chromatogr.*, 1985, *340*; *Biomed. Appl.*, *41*, 31–72.

High performance liquid chromatography. In plasma: limit of detection 50 nmol/L, UV detection (λ=254 nm)—J. L. Jurlina and J. W. Paxton, *J. Chromatogr.*, 1983, *276*, 367–374.

Disposition in the Body. Amsacrine is poorly absorbed after oral administration. Following intravenous administration it is well distributed, except to the brain and CSF (cerebrospinal fluid). It is metabolised in the liver mostly as amasacrine–glutathione metabolites. It is excreted primarily in the bile by an active transport mechanism. >20% of the drug is recovered unchanged in urine.

Therapeutic concentration. The trough serum therapeutic concentration is 0.03 mg/L and the peak, 0.15 to 5.5 mg/L.

Half-life. Plasma, 7 h.

Volume of distribution. 1.67 L/kg; 87.1 L/m^2.

Clearance. 150 $mL/min/m^2$.

Protein binding. In plasma, 98%.

Dose. For induction therapy up to 120 mg/m^2 intravenously daily for 5 to 8 days.

Amygdalin

Synonym. Amygdaloside
Note. The name 'laetrile' is frequently used to describe amygdalin but it has also been used to describe L-mandelonitrile-β-glucuronide, a substance that may be derived from amygdalin.
[(6-*O*-β-D-Glucopyranosyl-β-D-glucopyranosyl)oxy]benzeneacetonitrile
$C_{20}H_{27}NO_{11}$=457.4
CAS—29883-15-6

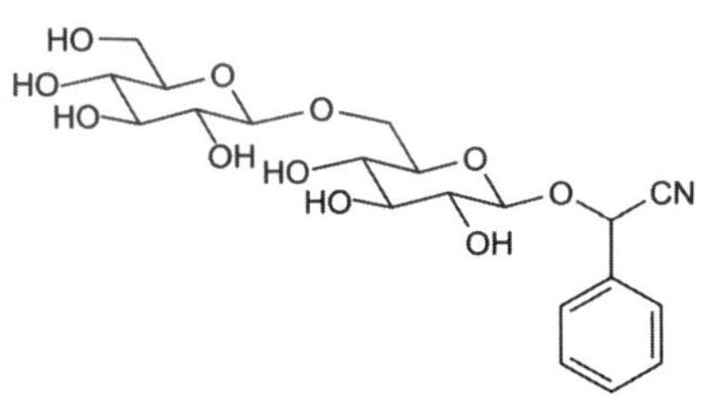

A colourless, crystalline, cyanogenic glycoside present in bitter almond seeds, *Prunus amygdalus* var. *amara*, apricot kernels and other seeds of the Rosaceae. M.p. about 220°; after solidifying the substance remelts at 125° to 130°.
Soluble 1 in 12 of water and 1 in 900 of ethanol; almost insoluble in ether.

Thin-layer Chromatography. System TA—Rf 87; system TE—Rf 56; system TAJ—Rf 54; system TAK—Rf 62; system TAL—Rf 92.

Partition Coefficient. Log *P* (octanol/water), −4.3.

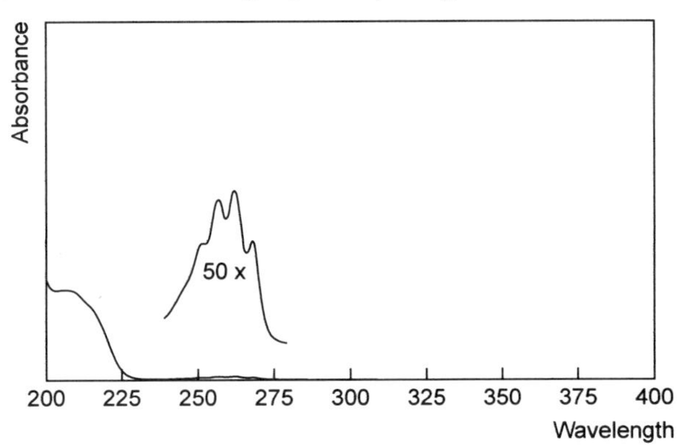

Infra-red Spectrum. Principal peaks at wavenumbers 1065, 1025, 695, 758, 1272, 890 cm^{-1} (KCl disk).

Mass Spectrum. Principal ions at *m/z* 43, 31, 57, 73, 60, 29, 55, 44.

Quantification.

Gas chromatography. In plasma: limit of detection 2 mg/L, FID—J. F. Stobaugh, *Anal. Lett. (Part B)*, 1978, *11*, 753–764.

High performance liquid chromatography. In plasma or urine: amygdalin and prunasin, limit of detection 1 mg/L, UV detection—A. G. Rauws *et al.*, *Pharm. Weekbl. (Sci.)*, 1982, *4*, 172–175.

Review. In body fluids or tissues: methods including GC–MS, HPLC, or TLC—J. Balkon, *J. Anal. Toxicol.*, 1982, *6*, 244–246.

Disposition in the Body. Poorly absorbed after ingestion and slowly hydrolysed in the gastro-intestinal tract to mandelonitrile-β-glucoside (prunasin), mandelonitrile, and glucose, and finally to benzaldehyde and hydrogen cyanide. After ingestion, about 8 to 32% of a dose is excreted unchanged in the urine; after parenteral administration, only small amounts are hydrolysed and most of a dose is excreted unchanged in the urine. Urinary cyanide and thiocyanate concentrations are not significantly elevated after oral or intravenous administration.

Blood concentration

In 6 subjects ingesting 500 mg of amygdalin three times a day, peak plasma concentrations of <1 mg/L of amygdalin were attained in 30 to 60 min; peak plasma-cyanide concentrations of 0.4 to 2.1 mg/L (mean 1.0) were reported 1.5 to 2 h after a dose on the second day; plasma-thiocyanate concentrations accumulated on repeated administration of amygdalin to about 25 mg/L on the last day of ingestion. [C. G. Moertel *et al.*, *JAMA*, 1981, *245*, 591–594.]

Following an intramuscular injection of 6 g to 1 subject, a peak plasma concentration of 180 mg/L was attained in 1.25 h. [M. M. Ames *et al.*, *Res. Commun. Chem. Pathol. Pharmacol.*, 1978, *22*, 175–185.]

Toxicity. Several reports of cyanide poisoning following administration of amygdalin have been recorded, mostly involving the ingestion of apricot or other fruit kernels. Cyanide release from amygdalin is known to occur in the presence of β-glucosidase enzymes that are present in some raw fruits and vegetables. Toxic effects or fatalities have been associated with blood-cyanide concentrations greater than 2 mg/L.

A blood-cyanide concentration of 10 mg/L was reported in one subject with toxic effects following daily ingestion of 1500 mg of amygdalin. [F. P. Smith *et al.*, *JAMA*, 1977, *238*, 1361.]

In a fatality involving amygdalin ingestion, a postmortem blood-cyanide concentration of 2.18 mg/L was reported. [S. N. Vogel *et al.*, *Clin. Toxicol.*, 1981, *18*, 367–383.]

Note. For a review of the literature on amygdalin, see R. F. Chandler *et al.*, *Pharm. J.*, 1984, *232*, 330–332.

Amyl Acetate

Solvent

A mixture of isomers, principally isoamyl acetate (3-methylbutyl acetate), *sec*-amyl acetate (2-methylbutyl acetate), and *n*-amyl acetate.
$C_7H_{14}O_2$=130.2
*CAS—123-92-2 (iso); 53496-15-4 (*sec*); 628-63-7 (n)*
A colourless, mobile, flammable liquid. B.p. about 140°. Refractive index 1.1400.
Slightly soluble in water; miscible with ethanol and ether.

Partition Coefficient. Log *P* (octanol/water), 2.3.

Mass Spectrum. Principal ions at *m/z* 43, 70, 55, 42, 41, 73, 61, 87.

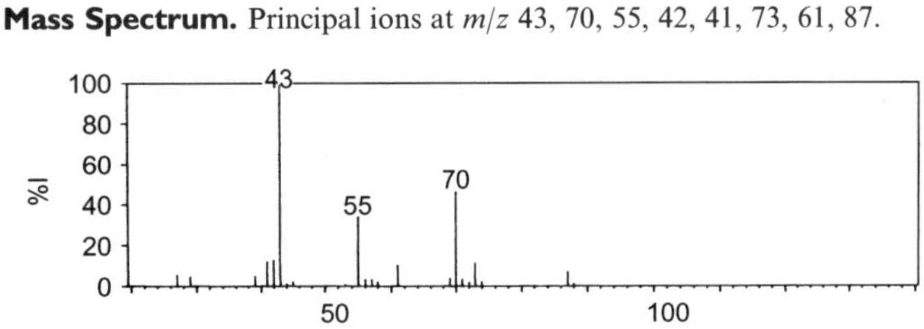

Disposition in the Body.

Toxicity. The estimated minimum lethal dose is 50 g and the maximum permissible atmospheric concentration is 100 ppm for isoamyl acetate or *n*-amyl acetate and 125 ppm for *sec*-amyl acetate.

Amyl Alcohol

Solvent

Synonym. Amylic Alcohol

A mixture of mainly 3-methyl-1-butanol (primary isoamyl alcohol) [$(CH_3)_2CHCH_2CH_2OH$] with some 2-methyl-1-butanol (primary amyl alcohol) [$CH_3CH_2CH(CH_3)CH_2OH$].

$C_5H_{12}O$=88.15

CAS—123-51-3 (3-methyl-1-butanol); 137-32-6 (2-methyl-1-butanol)

A colourless liquid obtained by purifying fusel oil. B.p. 128° to 132°. Refractive index 1.4075.

Slightly soluble in water; miscible with ethanol, chloroform, and ether.

Partition Coefficient. Log *P* (octanol/water), 1.2 (3-methyl-1-butanol), 1.3 (2-methyl-1-butanol).

Mass Spectrum. Principal ions at *m/z* 55, 41, 42, 43, 70, 57, 29, 31.

Disposition in the Body.

Toxicity. It is toxic after ingestion. The estimated minimum lethal dose is 30 g and the maximum permissible atmospheric concentration is 100 ppm.

Amyl Nitrite

Anti-anginal Vasodilator

Synonyms. Isoamyl Nitrite; Isopentyl Nitrite.

It consists of the nitrites of 3-methylbutan-1-ol [$(CH_3)_2CHCH_2CH_2OH$] and 2-methylbutan-1-ol [$CH_3CH_2CH(CH_3)CH_2OH$], with other nitrites of the homologous series.

$C_5H_{11}NO_2$=117.1

CAS—8017-89-8; 110-46-3

A clear, yellow, volatile, flammable liquid with a fragrant odour. Incompatible with ethanol. Store in a cool place in airtight containers; protect from light. Mass per mL 0.868 to 0.878 g. B.p. 96°. Refractive index 1.3871.

Practically insoluble in water; miscible with ethanol, chloroform, and ether.

Caution. Amyl nitrite forms an explosive mixture with air or oxygen. It is very inflammable and must not be used where it may be ignited.

Partition Coefficient. Log *P* (octanol/water), 2.8.

Colour Tests. To 0.2 mL add 2 mL of a 2% ferrous sulfate solution and 5 mL of dilute hydrochloric acid—green-brown; to 0.2 mL add 0.5 mL of aniline and 5 mL of acetic acid—orange-red.

Gas Chromatography. System GA—RI 680; system GI—retention time 20.3 min.

Mass Spectrum. Principal ions at *m/z* 70, 43, 55, 41, 57, 42, 71, –.

Disposition in the Body. Absorbed from the mucous membranes after inhalation but rapidly inactivated by hydrolysis. Inactive after ingestion owing to hydrolysis in the gastro-intestinal tract.

Toxicity. Recovery has occurred after the ingestion of 12 mL.

Dose. 0.12 to 0.3 mL, by inhalation.

Amylmetacresol

Antiseptic

Synonym. 6-Pentyl-*m*-cresol

Proprietary name. It is an ingredient of Strepsils.

5-Methyl-2-pentylphenol

$C_{12}H_{18}O$=178.3

CAS—1300-94-3; 53043-14-4

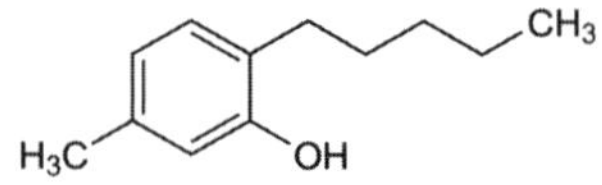

A colourless or slightly yellow, clear liquid or solid crystalline mass, which darkens on keeping. M.p. 24°.

Practically insoluble in water; soluble in ethanol and ether.

Partition Coefficient. Log *P* (octanol/water), 4.6.

Ultraviolet Spectrum. Acidified dehydrated alcohol—278 nm (A^1_1=132a), 286 nm.

Infra-red Spectrum. Principal peaks at wavenumbers 1120, 1225, 1272, 805, 1584, 938 cm^{-1} (thin film).

Anagrelide

Antithrombotic

6,7-Dichloro-1,5-dihydroimidazo-[2,1-*b*]quinazolin-2-(3*H*)-one

$C_{10}H_7Cl_2N_3O$=256.1

CAS—68475-42-3

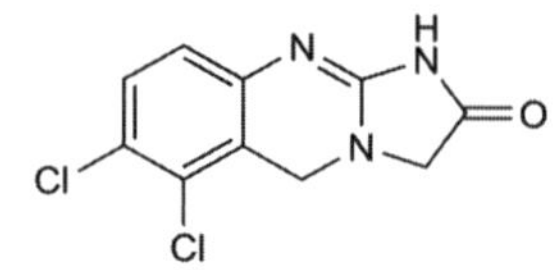

Anagrelide Hydrochloride

Synonyms. BL-4162A; BMY-26538-01.

Proprietary names. Agrelin; Agrylin.

$C_{10}H_8Cl_3N_3O$=292.5

CAS—58579-51-4

It is an off white powder with m.p. >280°. It is very slightly soluble in water; sparingly soluble in dimethylsulfoxide and dimethylformamide.

High Performance Liquid Chromatography. Column: (analytical) phenyl (μBondapak, 300 × 3.9 mm i.d.); (guard) phenyl/corasil (μBondapak, 40 mm). Mobile phases: (A)-acetonitrile:sodium acetate (0.01 M) adjusted to pH 4 with glacial acetic acid (25:75), 2.5 mL/min flow rate for first 10 min. (B)-dimethylsulfoxide, flow rate 2.5 mL/min, reduced to 1 mL/min at 13 min. Mobile phase A re-used at minute 18, flow rate 2.5 mL/min. UV detection (λ=254 nm). Retention time: 6 to 8 min. [R. C. Gaver *et al., Clin. Pharmacol. Ther.*, 1981, *29(3)*, 381–386].

Quantification

High performance liquid chromatography. In plasma: limit of detection, 5 μg/L. UV detection (λ=254 nm)—R. C. Gaver *et al., Clin. Pharmacol. Ther.*, 1981, *29(3)*, 381–386.

Disposition in the Body. Anagrelide is rapidly absorbed after oral administration (minimum 75%) and is extensively metabolised. A minimum of four metabolites have been identified, none of which are glucuronide or sulfate conjugates. It is excreted mainly in urine (70 to 75% over 5 days) and in faeces (10%). Less than 1% of the dose is excreted unchanged. It is extensively distributed.

Therapeutic concentration

5 healthy men, aged 19 to 26 years, were administered with a 1.2 mg anagrelide hydrochloride (1 mg free base) dose after an overnight fast. Mean peak plasma concentrations were 4.5 ± 0.9 μg/L and reached within 0.9 ± 0.4 h, rapidly declining in the first 6 to 8 h. [R. C Gaver *et al., Clin. Pharmacol. Ther.*, 1981, *29(3)*, 381–386].

Toxicity. Cardiac and CNS toxicity can be expected with overdose. It may also cause fetotoxicity and renal failure. Doses greater than 5 mg daily can lead to hypotension.

Bioavailability. 13.8% after administration with food.

Half-life. 1.3 h (fasting state); 1.8 h (dose administered with food).

Volume of distribution. 12 L/kg.

Clearance. 9 L/h.

Dose. An initial dose of 2 mg daily is administered which can be increased to a maximum of 10 mg daily.

Anastrozole

Antineoplastic

Synonyms. ZD1033; ICI-D-1033.

Proprietary name. Arimidex

α,α,α′,α′-Tetramethyl-5-(1*H*-1,2,4-triazol-1-ylmethyl)-1,3-benzenediacetonitrile

$C_{17}H_{19}N_5$=293.4

CAS—120511-73-1

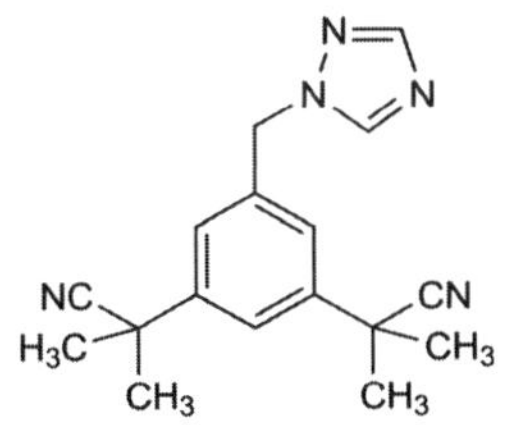

An off-white powder. M.p. 81 to 82°. It is soluble in water 0.5 mg/ml at 25°; freely soluble in acetone, ethanol, methanol and tetrahydrofuran; very soluble in acetonitrile.

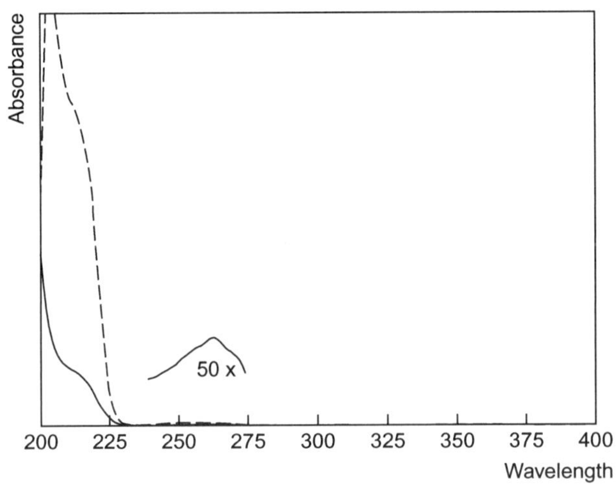

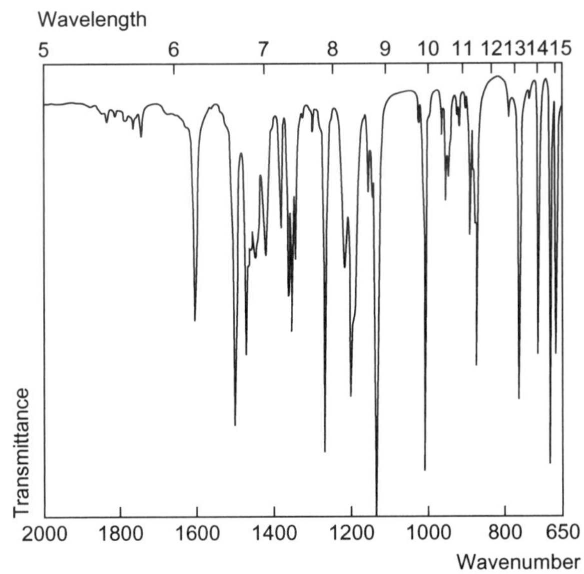

Mass Spectrum. Principal ions at m/z 209, 70, 224, 293, 115, 41, 156, 266.

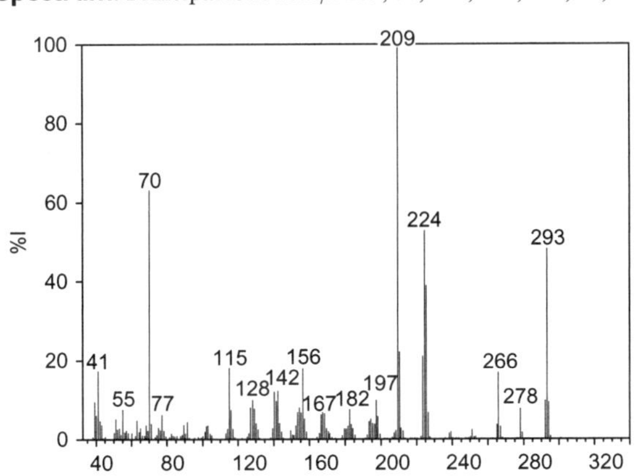

Quantification

Gas chromatography. In plasma: limit of detection is 0.5 μg/L and limit of quantification 3 μg/L, ECD—M. J. H. Bock *et al.*, *J. Chromatogr. Biomed. Sci. Appl.*, 1997, *700*, 131–138.

Disposition in the Body. Anastrozole is rapidly and almost completely absorbed after oral administration; peak plasma concentrations occur within about 2 h. The drug undergoes metabolism in the liver by *N*-dealkylation, hydroxylation and glucuronidation. The main inactive metabolite is triazole. The metabolites are excreted mainly in urine; less than 11% is excreted unchanged. It is removed by dialysis.

Half-life. Plasma, 50 h.

Protein binding. In plasma, 40%.

Dose. 1 mg daily.

Androstanolone

Anabolic Steroid

Synonyms. Dihydrotestosterone; Stanolone.
Proprietary names. Anabolex; Andractim; Androlone.
(5α,17β)-17-Hydroxyandrostan-3-one
$C_{19}H_{30}O_2$=290.4
CAS—521-18-6

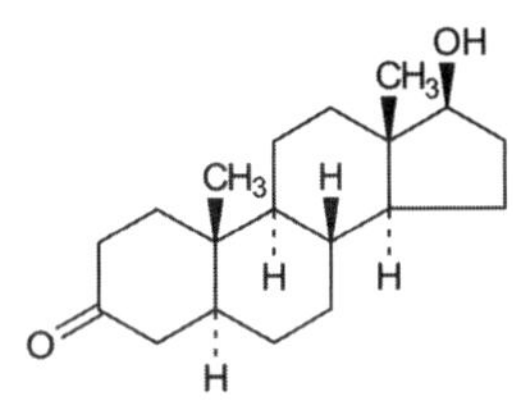

A white crystalline powder. M.p. 181°.
Practically insoluble in water; soluble 1 in 20 of ethanol and 1 in 70 of ether; soluble in acetone.

Partition Coefficient. Log *P* (octanol/water), 3.6.

Thin-layer Chromatography. System TP—Rf 78; system TQ—Rf 11; system TR—Rf 90; system TS—Rf 72.

Gas Chromatography. System GA—dihydrotestosterone RI 2510, dihydrotestosterone-AC RI 2630, dihydrotestosterone-TMS RI 2485, dihydrotestosterone enol-TMS_2 RI 2450; system GAI—urinary metabolite: 5α-dihydrotestosterone RRT 0.95 (relative to 17α-methyl-5α-androstan-3β,17β-diol).

Infra-red Spectrum. Principal peaks at wavenumbers 1698, 1046, 1277, 1027, 1064, 1079 cm^{-1} (KBr disk).

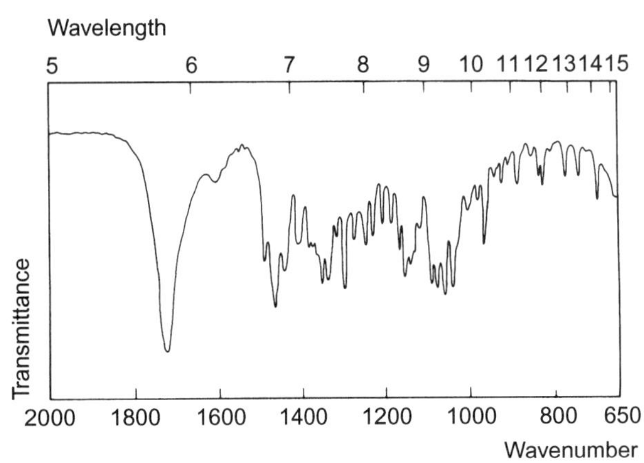

Dose. Androstanolone has been given sublingually or sublabially in doses of 50 to 75 mg daily.

Androstenediol

Anabolic steroid

Proprietary name. Hermaphrodiol
(3β,17β)-Androst-5-ene-3,17-diol
$C_{19}H_{30}O_2$=290.4
CAS—521-17-5

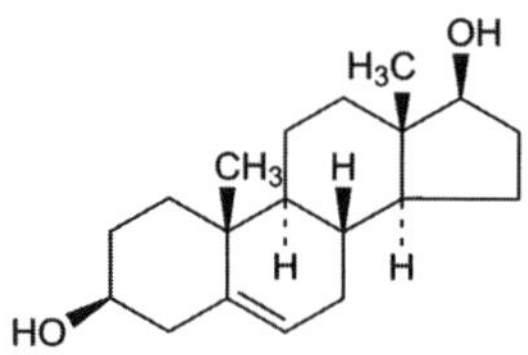

Leaflets. M.p. 179° to 182° (sublimes in high vacuum).
It is insoluble in water.

Androstenediol Diacetate

$C_{23}H_{34}O_4$=374.5
CAS—2099-26-5

Androstenediol Dipropionate

Proprietary names. Bisexovis; Disexovister; Ginandrin; Stenandiol.
$C_{25}H_{38}O_4$=402.6
CAS—2297-30-5
Solid. M.p. 115° to 116°.

Partition Coefficient. Log *P* (octanol/water), 4.58.

Gas Chromatography. Column: 5% phenyl, methyl silicone (HP Ultra-2, 25 m × 0.2 mm i.d., 0.33 μm film thickness). Column temperature: 100° for 1 min, 16°/min to 220°, 3.8°/min to 300°, held for 10 min. Carrier gas: helium, flow rate 0.6 to 0.8 mL/min. IS: 5α-androstane-17-one. MS detection. Retention time: androstenediol 24.0 min; androstenedione 24.5 min. [R. Masse *et al.*, *J. Chromatogr.* 1989, *489 B Biomed. Sci. Appl.*, 23–50.]

Column: methyl silicone (HP1, 0.2 mm i.d., 0.33 μm). Column temperature: 280°. Carrier gas: helium, 0.9 mL/min flow rate. MS detection. RI: androstenediol, 2613; androstenediol diacetate, 2816; androstenediol dipropionate, 3013. [T. Mills and J. C. Roberson, *Instrumental data for drug analysis*, 2nd Edn, CRC Press, Boca Raton, 1993, *5*, 20–21.]

High Pressure Liquid Chromatography. Column: ODS Hypersil (100 × 4.6 mm i.d., 5 μm). Mobile phase: methanol:aqueous 0.01 M dihydrogen potassium phosphate buffer, adjusted to pH 3.5 with 85% phosphoric acid (90:10), 1 mL/min flow rate. UV diode array detection. Retention time: (androstenediol diacetate), 4.1 min; (dipropionate), 6.7 min. [T. Mills and J. C. Roberson, *Instrumental data for drug analysis*, 2nd Edn, CRC Press, Boca Raton, 1993, *5*, 20–21, 28–32.]

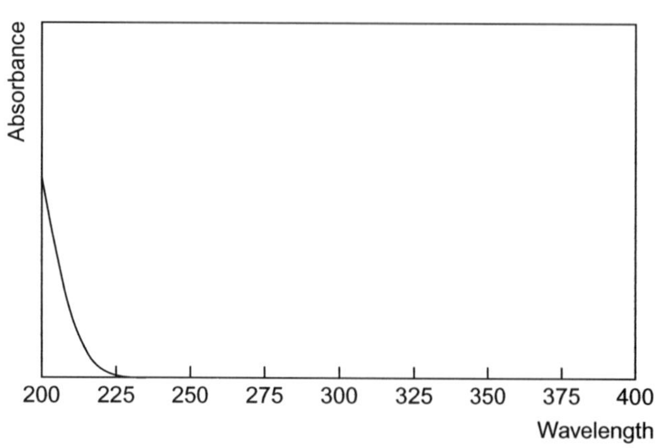

Infra-red Spectrum. Principal peaks at wavenumber 1429, 1048, 583 cm^{-1}; (androstenediol diacetate) 1725, 1238, 1041 cm^{-1}; (dipropionate) 1724, 1351, 1182 cm^{-1} (KBr pellets).

Mass Spectrum. Principal peaks at *m/z* 57, 328, 121, 145, 91, 105, 79, 239; (diacetate) 43, 314, 121, 133, 91, 107, 57, 239; (dipropionate) 57, 328, 121, 146, 91, 105, 79, 159.

Toxicity. Moderately toxic by ingestion (dipropionate form).

Androstenedione

Anabolic Steroid

Proprietary name. Androtex
Androst-4-ene-3,17-dione
$C_{19}H_{26}O_2$=286.4
CAS—63-05-8

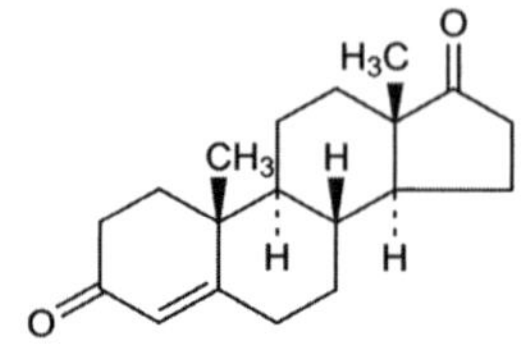

Appears as needles or crystals. M.p. 158°.
Soluble in water (57.82 mg/L at 25°).

Partition Coefficient. Log *P* (octanol/water), 2.75.

Gas Chromatography. System GA—RI 2600.

Column: 5% phenyl, methyl silicone (HP Ultra-2, 25 m × 0.2 mm i.d., 0.33 μm film thickness). Column temperature: 100° for 1 min, 16°/min to 220°, 3.8°/min to 300°, held for 10 min. Carrier gas: helium, flow rate 0.6 to 0.8 mL/min. IS: 5α-androstane-17-one. MS detection (EI, SIM). Retention time: androstenediol 24 min; androstenedione 24.5 min. [R. Masse *et al.*, *J. Chromatogr. B Biomed. Sci. Appl.*, 1989, *489*, 23–50.]

Ultraviolet Spectrum. Water—235 nm.

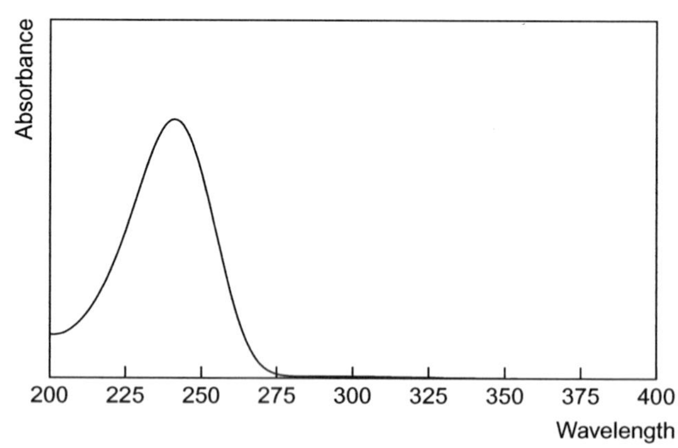

Mass Spectrum. Principal peaks at *m/z* 286, 124, 244, 148, 109, 107, 287, 147.

Quantification

High pressure liquid chromatography. In serum or plasma: limit of detection 5 pg—V. R. Walker *et al.*, *Anal. Biochem.*, 1996, *234*, 194–203.

Disposition in the Body. After oral administration, androstenedione is metabolised in the liver to testosterone. Blood testosterone levels increase approx. 15 min after oral administration and remain elevated for up to 3 h. Blood testosterone peaks at approx. 1 to 1.5 h after ingestion.

Therapeutic concentration. In young males, a single oral dose of 100 mg can increase endogenous androstenedione serum concentrations by 175% within the first 60 min after administration and 325 to 350% between 90 and 270 min after administration.

Dose. The recommended dosage is between 50 and 300 mg daily.

Androsterone

Androgen

(3α,5α)-3-Hydroxyandrostan-17-one
$C_{19}H_{30}O_2$=290.4
CAS—53-41-8

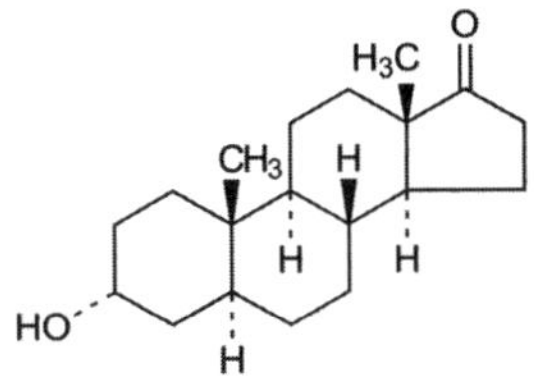

A white crystalline powder. M.p. about 185°.
Practically insoluble in water; soluble in ethanol, ether, and most organic solvents.

Partition Coefficient. Log *P* (octanol/water), 3.7.

Colour Tests. Antimony Pentachloride—yellow→brown; Naphthol–Sulfuric Acid—orange-brown/orange; Sulfuric Acid—yellow

Thin-layer Chromatography. System TB—Rf 16; system TE—Rf 72; system TF—Rf 52; system TAE—Rf 90.

Gas Chromatography. System GA—androsterone RI 2475, androsterone-AC RI 2580, androsterone enol-TMS_2 RI 2500; system GAR—retention time 11.9 min.

Ultraviolet Spectrum. No significant absorption, 230 to 360 nm.

Infra-red Spectrum. Principal peaks at wavenumbers 1724, 1000, 1031, 1062, 1242, 1282 cm^{-1} (Nujol mull).

Mass Spectrum. Principal ions at *m/z* 290, 67, 108, 107, 79, 55, 41, 93.

Quantification.
Gas chromatography–mass spectrometry. In urine: androsterone glucuronide and other androgen glucuronides, limits of detection 15 to 20 pg—M. H. Choi *et al.*, *Steroids*, 2000, *65*, 54–59.

Disposition in the Body. Androsterone is a naturally occurring androgen which may be isolated from male urine. It is a major metabolite of testosterone.

Anileridine

Narcotic Analgesic

Ethyl-1-[2-(4-aminophenyl)ethyl]-4-phenyl-4-piperidinecarboxylate
$C_{22}H_{28}N_2O_2$=352.5
CAS—144-14-9

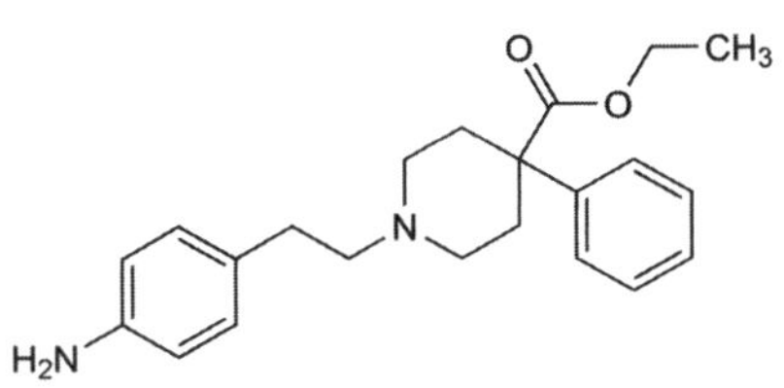

A white to yellowish-white crystalline powder. When exposed to light and air it oxidises and darkens in colour. There are 2 crystalline forms which melt at about 80° and about 89°.
Very slightly soluble in water; soluble 1 in 2 of ethanol and 1 in 1 of chloroform; soluble in ether but solutions may be turbid.

Anileridine Hydrochloride

Proprietary name. Leritine (tablets)
$C_{22}H_{28}N_2O_2$,2HCl=425.4
CAS—126-12-5
A white crystalline powder. M.p. about 270°, with decomposition.
Soluble 1 in 5 of water and 1 in 80 of ethanol; practically insoluble in chloroform and ether.

Anileridine Phosphate

Proprietary name. Leritine (injection)
$C_{22}H_{28}N_2O_2,H_3PO_4$=450.5
CAS—4268-37-5
A white crystalline powder.
Very soluble in water. Solutions are unstable above pH 4.

Dissociation Constant. pK_a 3.7, 7.5.

Partition Coefficient. Log *P* (octanol/water), 4.1.

Colour Tests. Diazotisation—red; Marquis Test—orange (slow).

Thin-layer Chromatography. System TA—Rf 73; system TB—Rf 12; system TC—Rf 56; system TE—Rf 79; system TL—Rf 51; system TAE—Rf 60; system TAF—Rf 66; system TAJ—Rf 20; system TAK—Rf 00; system TAL—Rf 68. (Acidified iodoplatinate solution, positive).

Gas Chromatography. System GA—RI 2850; system GC—RI 3469.

High Performance Liquid Chromatography. System HA—*k* 1.1; System HAX—retention time 11.7 min; System HAY—retention time 5.9 min.

Ultraviolet Spectrum. Aqueous acid—252, 258, 264 nm.

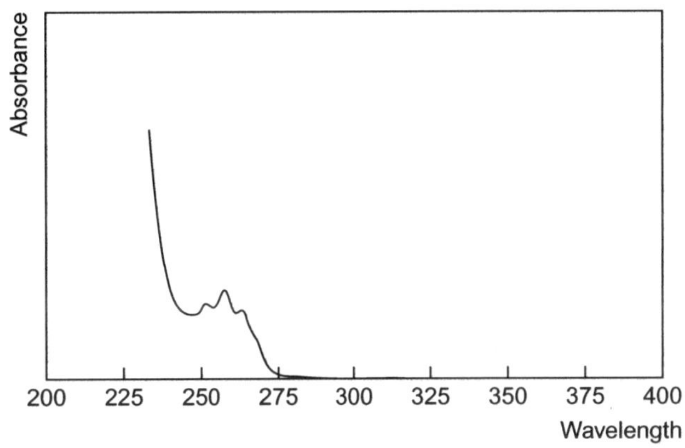

Infra-red Spectrum. Principal peaks at wavenumbers 1700, 1120, 1179, 1512, 1219, 1620 cm^{-1} (KCl disk).

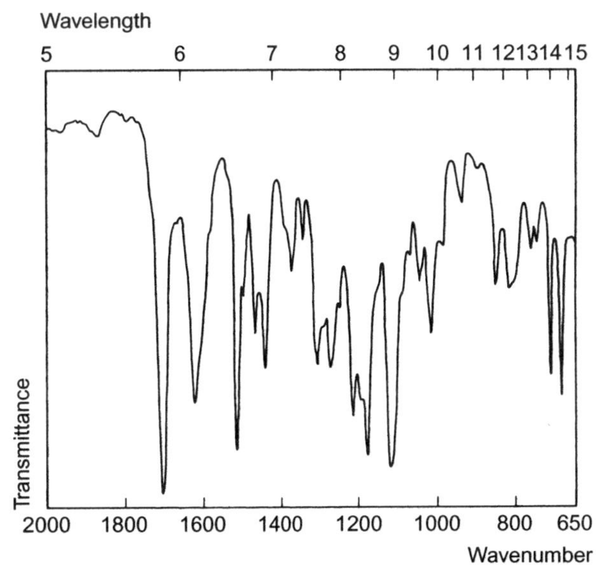

Mass Spectrum. Principal ions at *m/z* 246, 247, 42, 120, 218, 172, 106, 91.

Disposition in the Body. Readily absorbed after oral administration. Metabolised by hydrolysis to anileridinic acid followed by acetylation to acetylanileridinic acid; conjugation with acetic acid followed by partial de-esterification to acetylanileridinic acid also occurs. After oral administration, 5% of the dose is excreted in the urine as unchanged drug, with 7 to 14% as free anileridinic acid, 1 to 2% as acetylanileridinic acid, 0.5 to 2% as acetylanileridine, and 15 to 35% as diazotisable metabolites, tentatively identified as *p*-acetylaminophenylacetic acid; norpethidine has also been detected in urine.

Toxicity. The estimated minimum lethal dose is 0.5 g but it may be up to 5 g in addicts.

The following postmortem concentrations were reported in a fatality attributed to oral overdosage of anileridine: blood 0.9 mg/L, bile 2.4 mg/L, urine 11.4 mg/L, vitreous humour 0.07 mg/L; diazepam was also detected. [M. A. Peat and L. Kopjak, *Bull. Int. Assoc. Forensic Toxicol.*, 1979, *14*(3), 19.]

Dose. Up to the equivalent of 200 mg of anileridine daily.

Aniline

Synonym. Phenylamine
$C_6H_5NH_2$=93.1
CAS—62-53-3

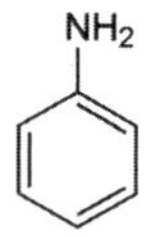

A colourless or pale yellow, oily liquid, with a characteristic odour. It readily darkens to brown on exposure to air and light. F.p. −6°. B.p. about 183°. Refractive index 1.5863.
Soluble 1 in about 29 of water; miscible with ethanol, benzene, chloroform, and ether.

Dissociation Constant. pK_a 4.6 (25°).

Partition Coefficient. Log *P* (octanol/water), 0.9.

Colour Tests. Coniferyl Alcohol—orange; Diazotisation—red; Liebermann's Test—red-orange; Potassium Dichromate—blue-green (2 min).

Thin-layer Chromatography. System TA—Rf 72; system TE—Rf 00; system TAJ—Rf 64; system TAK—Rf 00; system TAL—Rf 96. (Acidified potassium permanganate solution, positive; Van Urk reagent, bright yellow.)

Gas Chromatography. System GA—aniline RI 1158, 4-aminophenol RI 1253.

Ultraviolet Spectrum. Aqueous acid—229 nm (A^1_1=13b), 255 nm (A^1_1=16b), 261 nm (A^1_1=12.5b); ethanol—235 nm (A^1_1=1007b), 286 nm (A^1_1=179b).

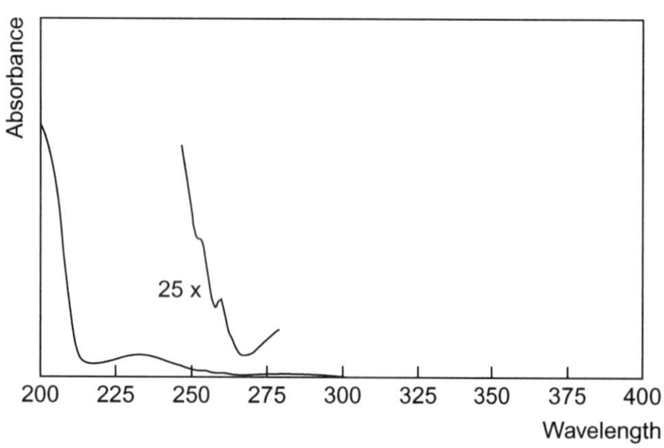

Mass Spectrum. 4-Aminophenol: principal ions at *m/z* 109, 80, 53, 81, 108, 52, 54, 110.

Quantification.
Gas chromatography. In postmortem tissues: AFID—J. S. Oliver and D. J. Williams, *Bull. Int. Assoc. Forensic Toxicol.*, 1974, *10*, 6–7.

Gas chromatography–mass spectrometry. In serum: limit of detection 0.1 mg/L—A. Dasgupta, *J. Chromatogr. B. Biomed. Sci. Appl.*, 1998, *716*, 354–358; A. Dasgupta and C. Jagannath, *Ther. Drug Monit.*, 1999, *21*, 238–242. In urine: aniline and other aromatic amines and aromatic nitro metabolites, limits of detection 0.05 to 2 μg/L—T. Weiss and J. Angerer, *J. Chromatogr. B. Anal. Technol. Biomed. Life Sci.*, 2002, *778*, 179–192.

Disposition in the Body. Readily absorbed from the skin and mucous membranes. Metabolised to 4-aminophenol and 4-acetamidophenol which are excreted in the urine as glucuronide and sulfate conjugates. *N*-Phenylsulfamic acid (aniline *N*-sulfate) is also a metabolite. The main toxic effect of aniline, the formation of methaemoglobin, is thought to be due to an oxidation product of aniline, phenylhydroxylamine.
Aniline is a metabolite of phenazopyridine.

Toxicity. The minimum lethal dose may be as low as 1 g although recovery has followed the ingestion of 30 g. Serious toxic effects may occur after exposure for about 1 h to atmospheric concentrations of 100 to 160 ppm. The maximum permissible atmospheric concentration is 2 ppm. Urinary concentrations of greater than 10 mg/L of 4-aminophenol may indicate toxic exposure to aniline.

The following postmortem tissue concentrations were reported in a fatality attributed to ingestion of an aniline-based ink: blood 6.3 mg/L, liver 20 μg/g, urine 40 mg/L. [J. S. Oliver and D. J. Williams, *Bull. Int. Assoc. Forensic Toxicol.*, 1974, *10*, 6–7.]

Aniracetam

Cognition Enhancer/Nootropic

Synonym. Aniracetamum
Proprietary names. Ampamet; Draganon; Reset; Sarpul.
1-(4-Methoxybenzoyl)-2-pyrrolidinone; 1-*p*-Anisoyl-2-pyrrolidinone
$C_{12}H_{13}NO_3$=219.2
CAS—72432-10-1

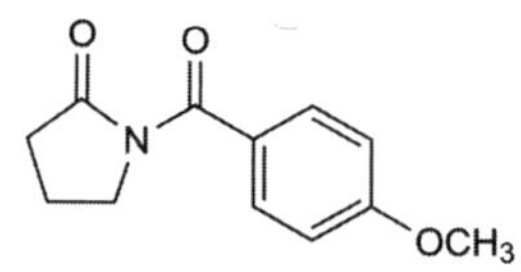

Odourless and colourless crystals, with m.p. 121° to 122°. It has limited aqueous solubility (approximately, 1.5 g/L) which is not affected by pH (1.47 g/L at pH 1.2 and 1.38 g/L at pH 7.5). It is essentially a neutral molecule with moderate lipophilicity.

Partition Coefficient. Log *P* (octanol/buffer pH 7.4), 10 (22°).

High Performance Liquid Chromatography. Column: (analytical) ODS-silica (Hypersil ODS, 3 μm, 60 × 4.0 mm i.d.), (guard) (RP-2, 10 μm, 30 × 4.6 mm i.d.). Mobile phase: water:methanol:acetonitrile (70:30:10), 1.0 mL/min flow rate. UV detection (λ=282 nm). Retention time: 4.3 min.

Column: (analytical) C_{18} (μBondapak, 10 μm, 300 × 3.9 mm i.d.), (guard) (RP-8 Spheri, 5 μm, 30 × 4.6 mm i.d.). Mobile phase: methanol:triethylamine:phosphate buffer (0.1 M, pH 3.0) (530:0.05:470). 1.0 mL/min flow rate. UV detection (diode array). Retention time: *N*-anisoyl-GABA, 5.3 min. [A. Guenzi and M. Zanetti, *J. Chromatogr.*, 1990, *530*, 397–406].

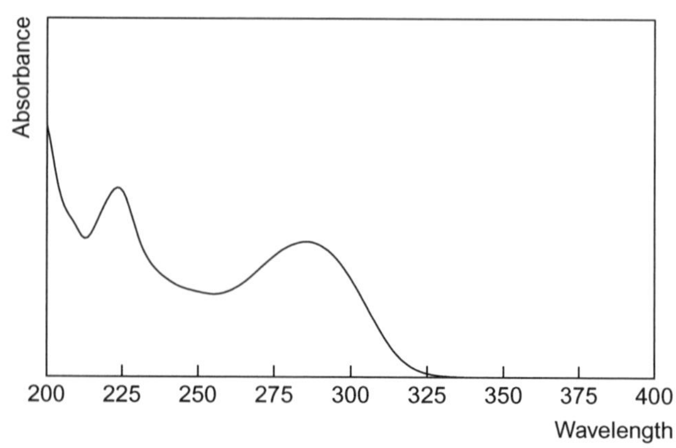

Quantification
High performance liquid chromatography. In plasma: limits of quantification for aniracetam and *N*-anisoyl-GABA, 5 μg/L and 50 μg/L, respectively, and detection limits 2 μg/L and 5 μg/L, respectively. UV

detection—A. Guenzi and M. Zanetti, *J. Chromatogr. Biomed. Sci. Appl.*, 1990, *530*, 397–406.

Disposition in the Body. Aniracetam is rapidly absorbed from the gastro-intestinal tract and essentially absorption is complete. Aniracetam undergoes extensive biodegradation and therefore bioavailability is very low at approximately 0.2% (only 0.2% reaches the systemic circulation as the parent drug). Aniracetam is metabolised in the body and the main metabolite produced is *N*-anisoyl-GABA (approx. 70%) but 2-pyrrolidinone, 5-hydroxy-2-pyrrolidinone and anisic acid are also produced. Rapid and complete elimination occurs via urine (84%), faeces (0.8%) and expired air (11%) as CO_2. Elimination is biphasic. *N*-Anisoyl-GABA and anisic acid are secreted in breast milk. All can traverse the placenta from blood and/or metabolites formed before reaching fetus.

Therapeutic concentration

After oral administration, 1000 mg, peak plasma concentrations varied greatly between 42 and 246 µg/L for 6 subjects and were detected at 5 min. Peak plasma concentrations for a 2 g dose varied between 55 and 116 µg/L, and between 42 and 1087 µg/L for a 4 g dose. [Roncari *et al.*, 1984, F. Hoffman-La Roche data on file B-104′488.]

Toxicity. Toxicity testing in several animal species, including mouse, rat, rabbit and dog shows that aniracetam has extremely low toxicity.

Half-life. For the parent drug, aniracetam, the half-life is 30 min and for its metabolites, 12.8 to 15.7 h.

Volume of distribution. Steady state, 2.5 L/kg (ranging between 1.9 and 4.1 L/kg).

Clearance. Total clearance, approximately, 9.9 L/min (range between 6.4 and 14.9 L/min).

Distribution in blood. Aniracetam is equally distributed between red blood cells and plasma (blood:plasma concentration ratio range 0.92 to 0.95). Distribution outside the vascular space and probable binding with tissue components also occurs.

Protein binding. Aniracetam has a protein-binding rate of 66%.

Dose. Recommended dose of 1500 mg daily by mouth, either as a single dose (as sugar-free sachets) or as 750 mg doses in the form of a tablet.

Anisindione

Anticoagulant

Proprietary names. Miradon; Unidone.
2-(4-Methoxyphenyl)-1*H*-indene-1,3(2*H*)-dione
$C_{16}H_{12}O_3$=252.3
CAS—117-37-3

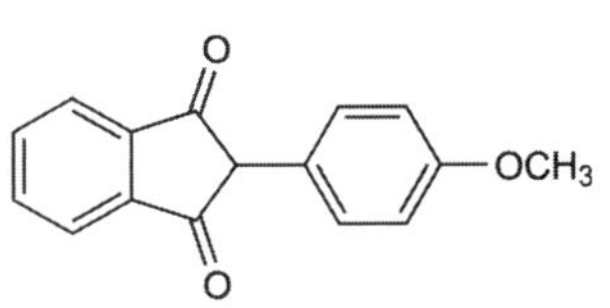

A white or creamy-white powder. M.p. 152° to 158°.
Practically insoluble in water; soluble in ether and methanol.

Dissociation Constant. pK_a 4.1.

Partition Coefficient. Log *P* (octanol/water), 2.9.

Thin-layer Chromatography. System TA—Rf 98; system TE—Rf 15; system TAJ—Rf 82; system TAK—Rf 70; system TAL—Rf 95.

Gas Chromatography. System GA—RI 2273.

Ultraviolet Spectrum. Aqueous acid—273 nm; ethanol—286 nm (A^1_1=1400b), 340 nm.

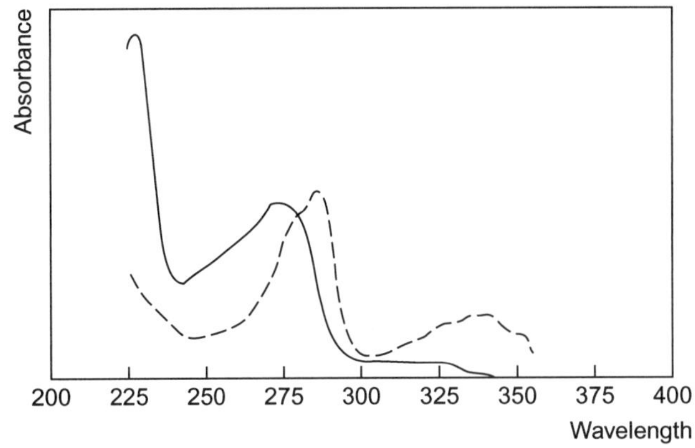

Mass Spectrum. Principal ions at *m/z* 252, 237, 253, 181, 238, 77, 76, 209.

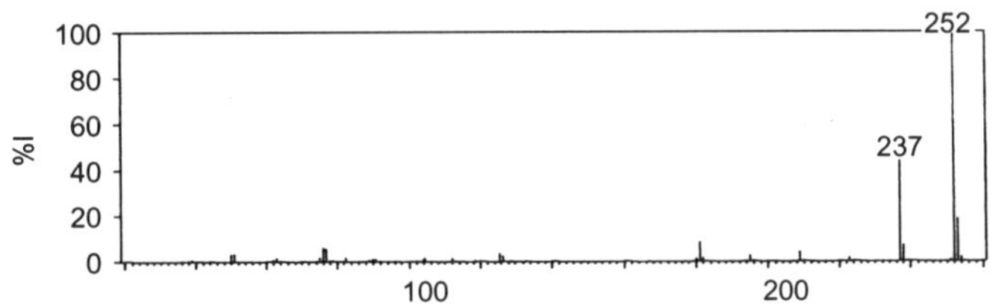

Dose. Maintenance, 25 to 250 mg daily.

Antazoline

Antihistamine

Synonyms. Imidamine; Phenazoline.
4,5-Dihydro-*N*-phenyl-*N*-(phenylmethyl)-1*H*-imidazole-2-methanamine
$C_{17}H_{19}N_3$=265.4
CAS—91-75-8

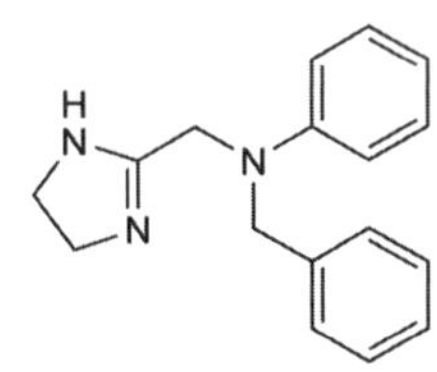

Crystals. M.p. 120° to 122°.

Antazoline Hydrochloride

Synonyms. Imidamine Hydrochloride; Phenazolinum.
Proprietary names. Wasp-Eze (ointment). It is an ingredient of Modantis and RBC.
$C_{17}H_{19}N_3$,HCl=301.8
CAS—2508-72-7
A white crystalline powder. M.p. 237° to 241°.
Soluble 1 in 40 of water and 1 in 25 of ethanol; practically insoluble in ether, benzene, and chloroform.

Antazoline Mesilate

Synonyms. Antazoline Mesylate; Antazoline Methanesulphonate; Imidamine Mesilate.
$C_{17}H_{19}N_3$,CH_3SO_3H=361.5
CAS—3131-32-6
A white, slightly hygroscopic powder. M.p. 165° to 168°.
Soluble 1 in 6 of water, 1 in 7 of ethanol, and 1 in 12 of chloroform; practically insoluble in ether.

Antazoline Phosphate

Synonym. Imidamine Phosphate
Proprietary names. It is an ingredient of Albalon-A, Antazoline-V, and Vasocon A.
$C_{17}H_{19}N_3$,H_3PO_4=363.4
CAS—154-68-7
A white crystalline powder. M.p. 194° to 198°.

Soluble in water; sparingly soluble in methanol; practically insoluble in benzene and ether.

Antazoline Sulfate
Synonym. Imidamine Sulphate
Proprietary names. It is an ingredient of Antistin(e)-Privin(e) and Otrivine-Antistin.
$(C_{17}H_{19}N_3)_2,H_2SO_4,2H_2O$=664.8
CAS—24359-81-7 (anhydrous antazoline sulfate)

Dissociation Constant. pK_a 2.5, 10.1 (25°).

Partition Coefficient. Log *P* (octanol/water), 3.4.

Colour Tests. Liebermann's Test—red; Mandelin's Test—red-violet.

Thin-layer Chromatography. System TA—Rf 31; system TB—Rf 06; system TC—Rf 07; system TE—Rf 47; system TL—Rf 03; system TAE—Rf 05; system TAF—Rf 66; system TAJ—Rf 00; system TAK—Rf 00; system TAL—Rf 15. (Dragendorff spray, positive; FPN reagent, pink; acidified iodoplatinate solution, positive.)

Gas Chromatography. System GA—RI 2318; system GB—RI 2421; system GC—RI 2749.

High Performance Liquid Chromatography. System HA—*k* 1.8; system HX—RI 383; system HY—RI 294.

Ultraviolet Spectrum. Aqueous acid—241 nm (A_1^1=578a), 291 nm; aqueous alkali—247, 295 nm.

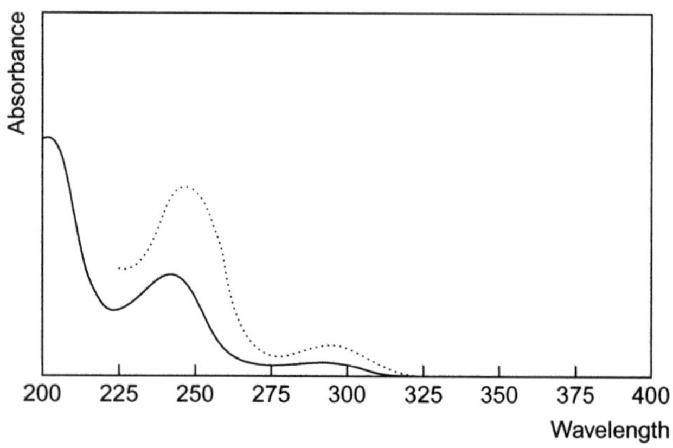

Infra-red Spectrum. Principal peaks at wavenumbers 1164, 1599, 1042, 1508, 750, 700 cm^{-1} (antazoline mesilate, KBr disk).

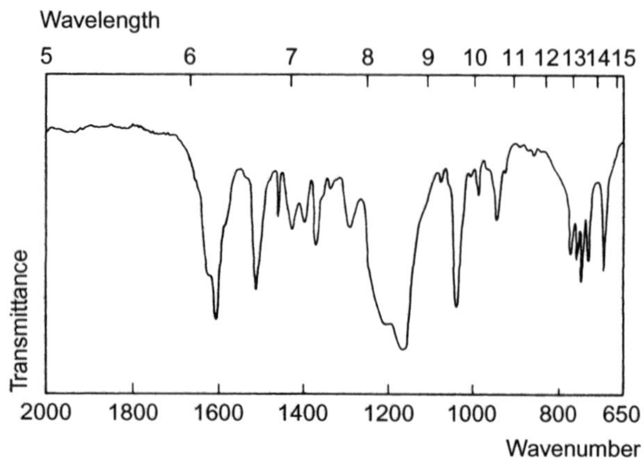

Mass Spectrum. Principal ions at *m/z* 84, 91, 77, 55, 182, 85, 65, 104.

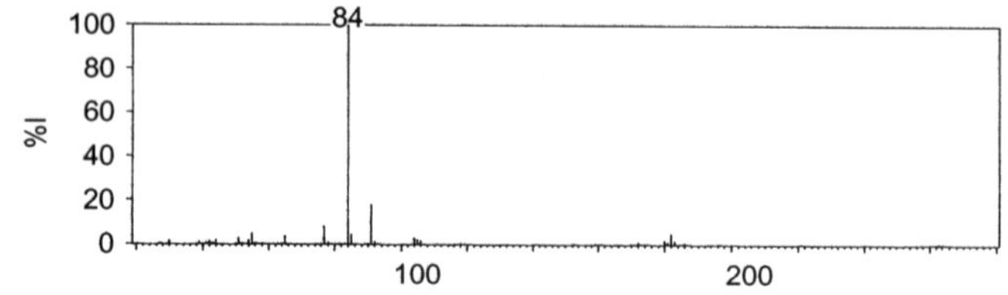

Quantification
Colorimetry. In urine—N. Wahba *et al.*, *Pharmazie*, 1974, *29*, 790–791.

Disposition in the Body. Readily absorbed after oral or parenteral administration. About 2% of an oral dose is excreted unchanged in the urine in 24 h.

Dose. Antazoline hydrochloride has been given in doses of 100 to 600 mg daily.

Apomorphine

Antoparkinsonian/Emetic

(6a*R*)-5,6,6a,7-Tetrahydro-6-methyl-4*H*-dibenzo[*de*,*g*]quinoline-10,11-diol
$C_{17}H_{17}NO_2$=267.3
CAS—58-00-4

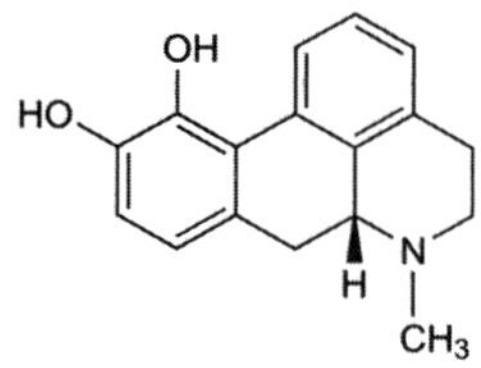

Crystals. M.p. about 195°, with decomposition. The crystals and aqueous solutions oxidise rapidly in light and air, turning green.
Slightly soluble in water, benzene, ether, and petroleum ether; soluble in ethanol and chloroform.

Apomorphine Hydrochloride
Proprietary names. Apofin; APO-go; Apokinon; Apomine; Britaject; Uprima.
$C_{17}H_{17}NO_2$,HCl,½H_2O=312.8
CAS—314-19-2 (anhydrous); 41372-20-7 (hemihydrate)
White or greyish-white glistening crystals or microcrystalline powder. Decomposes between 225° and 236°.
Soluble 1 in 50 of water and 1 in 17 of water at 80°; soluble 1 in 50 of ethanol; very slightly soluble in chloroform and ether.

Dissociation Constant. pK_a 7.2, 8.9 (15°).

Partition Coefficient. Log *P* (octanol/water), 2.3.

Colour Tests. Ferric Chloride—blue; Liebermann's Test—black; Marquis Test—violet→black; Methanolic Potassium Hydroxide—green→red; Nessler's Reagent—black

Thin-layer Chromatography. System TA—Rf 83; system TB—Rf 00; system TC—Rf 21; system TE—Rf 58; system TL—Rf 27; system TAE—Rf 54; system TAJ—Rf 06; system TAK—Rf 00; system TAL—Rf 22. (Acidified iodoplatinate solution, positive.)

Gas Chromatography. System GA—apomorphine RI 2530; apomorphine-AC_2 RI 2830.

High Performance Liquid Chromatography. System HA—*k* 3.7 (tailing peak); system HX—RI 348; system HY—RI 256; system HAA—retention time 9.0 min.

Ultraviolet Spectrum. Aqueous acid—272 nm (A_1^1=626a); aqueous alkali—253 nm. (See below)

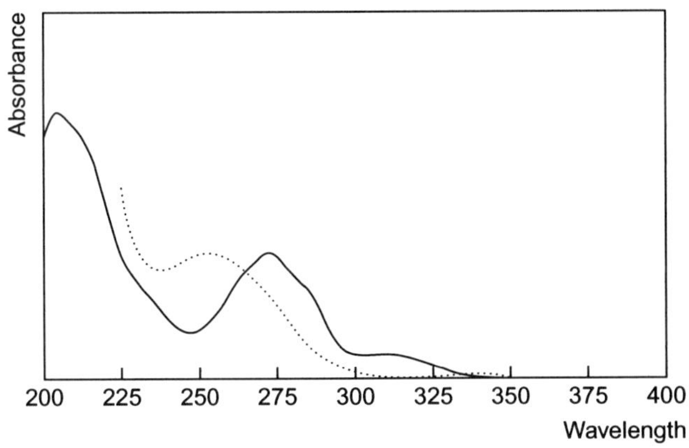

Infra-red Spectrum. Principal peaks at wavenumbers 1265, 1298, 1204, 752, 985, 790 cm^{-1} (KBr disk).

Mass Spectrum. Principal ions at *m/z* 266, 267, 224, 220, 268, 44, 250, 248.

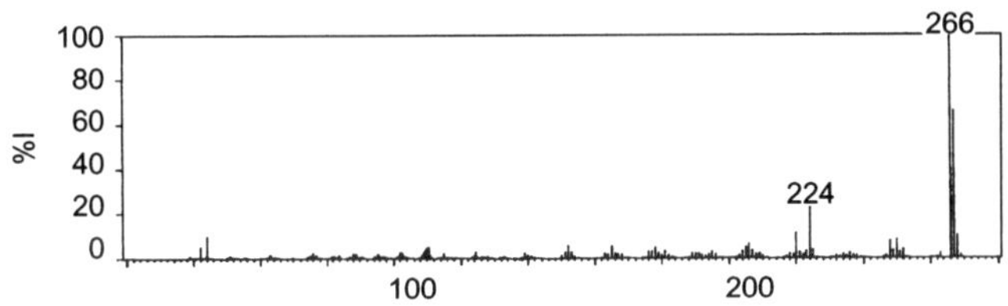

Quantification

Gas chromatography. In plasma: limit of detection 1 mg/L, FID—D. M. Baaske *et al.*, *J. Chromatogr.*, 1977, *140*, 57–64.

High performance liquid chromatography. In plasma: limit of detection 100 µg/L, fluorescence detection—R. V. Smith and M. R. De Moreno, *J. Chromatogr.* 1983, *274(25) Biomed. Appl. B* 376–380. In plasma: limit of detection 0.5 µg/L, electrochemical detection—A. W. Essink *et al.*, *J. Chromatogr.* 1991, *570*, 419–424. In plasma: electrochemical detection—E. Sam *et al.*, *J. Chromatogr.* 1994, *658 Biomed. Appl. B* 311–317. In plasma: fluorescence detection—M. J. Priston and G. J. Sewell, *J. Chromatogr.* 1996, *681 Biomed. Appl. B* 161–167. In plasma: limit of detection 20 pg, electrochemical detection—A. Bolner *et al.*, *Forensic Sci. Int.*, 1997, *89*, 81–91. In plasma or urine: *R*- and *S*-apomorphine, apocodeine, isoapocodeine, and conjugated metabolites, limits of detection 0.3 µg/L and 0.6 µg/L for *R*- and *S*-apomorphine respectively, electrochemical detection—R. van der Geest *et al.*, *J. Chromatogr. B. Biomed. Sci. Appl.*, 1997, *702*, 131–141.

Disposition in the Body

Therapeutic concentration

Apomorphine was administered by intravenous infusion (the rate was increased by 10 µg/kg every 20 min up to 100 µg/kg/h or until adverse effects occurred) to 10 subjects with parkinsonism, 8 of whom responded. Clinical efficacy occurred at a minimum concentration of 1.4 to 10.7 µg/L (mean 4.7) and dyskinesia occurred at 2.7 to 20 µg/L (mean 8.5); the minimal toxic concentration was 6.5 to24.5 µg/L (mean 16.7). [T. van Laar *et al.*, *Clin. Neuropharmacol.*, 1998, *21*, 152–158.]

After a single sublingual dose of apomorphine 0.21 to 0.91 mg/kg to 5 patients (2 received 18 mg, 3 received 39 mg), peak plasma concentrations of 11.3 to 144.0 µg/L were attained at 45 to 90 min. [F. Durif *et al.*, *Eur. J. Clin. Pharmacol.*, 1991, *41*, 493–494.]

Dose. 100 µg/kg of apomorphine hydrochloride subcutaneously, as a single dose.

Aprindine

Anti-arrhythmic

N-(2,3-Dihydro-1*H*-inden-2-yl)-*N'*,*N'*-diethyl-*N*-phenyl-1,3-propanediamine
$C_{22}H_{30}N_2$=322.5
CAS—37640-71-4

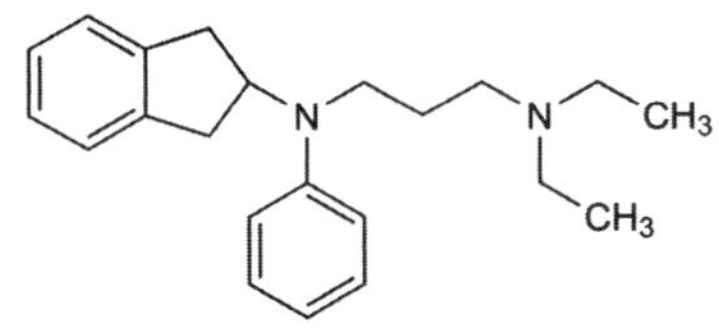

Aprindine Hydrochloride
Proprietary names. Amidonal; Fiboran.
$C_{22}H_{30}N_2$,HCl=359.0
CAS—33237-74-0
A white to yellowish-white microcrystalline powder. M.p. 127° to 130°.
Very soluble in water; freely soluble in ethanol and chloroform; practically insoluble in ether.

Dissociation Constant. pK_a 10.1.

Partition Coefficient. Log *P* (octanol/water), 4.9.

Thin-layer Chromatography. System TB—Rf 63; system TE—Rf 76; system TAE—Rf 20.

Gas Chromatography. System GA—aprindine RI 2462; M (*N*-desalkyl-) RI 1920, M (*p*-aminophenol) RI 1253, M (OH-)-AC RI 2850, M (OH-methoxy-)-AC RI 2995, M (desindane)-AC RI 1880, M (desphenyl-)-AC RI 2300.

High Performance Liquid Chromatography. System HX—RI 433; system HAA—retention time 17.0 min.

Ultraviolet Spectrum. Aqueous acid—260, 266 nm(A^1_1=38a), 272 nm; ethanol—258 nm (A^1_1=389a), 296 nm (A^1_1=47a).

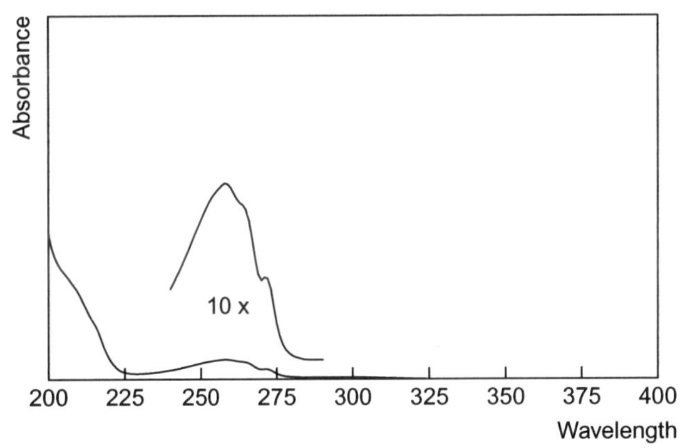

Infra-red Spectrum. Principal peaks at wavenumbers 745, 1510, 1602, 1187, 1258, 1035 cm^{-1} (aprindine hydrochloride, KBr disk).

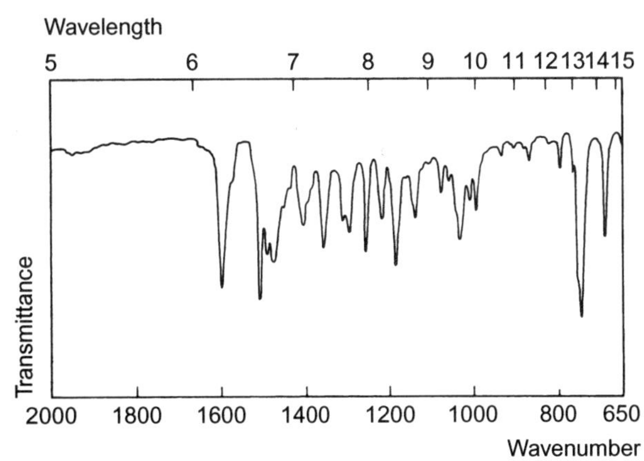

Mass Spectrum. Principal ions at *m/z* 113, 86, 116, 98, 117, 115, 58, 84; M (*N*-desalkyl-) *m/z* 104, 209, 77, 116, 115, 94.

Quantification

Gas chromatography. In plasma: limit of detection 20 µg/L, AFID—J. F. Nash and R. H. Carmichael, *J. Pharm. Sci.*, 1980, *69*, 1094–1096. In serum:

limit of detection 16 pg, surface ionization detection—H. Kawano *et al.*, *J. Chromatogr.*, 1989, *493*, 71–78.

High performance liquid chromatography. In plasma: aprindine and monodesethylaprindine, limits of detection 20 µg/L and 50 µg/L, respectively, UV detection—T. Kobari *et al.*, *J. Chromatogr.* 1983, *278 (29) Biomed. Appl.* 220–224. In plasma: aprindine and other antiarrhythmic drugs, UV or fluorescence detection—R. Verbesselt *et al.*, *Ther. Drug Monit.*, 1991, *13*, 157–165. In plasma: UV detection—G. Misztal and L. Przyborowski, *Pharmazie*, 1995, *50*, 187–188.

Disposition in the Body. Almost completely absorbed after oral administration. Extensively metabolised by aromatic hydroxylation and N-dealkylation followed by glucuronic acid conjugation; the monodesethyl metabolite, which can be detected in plasma after chronic administration, is active. Less than 1% of a dose is excreted in the urine as unchanged drug and about 40 to 65% as conjugated metabolites; 35 to 60% of the dose is eliminated in the faeces over a period of 5 days.

Therapeutic concentration. In plasma, usually in the range 0.7 to 2 mg/L.

After a single oral dose of 200 mg to 12 subjects, peak plasma concentrations of 0.6 to 2 mg/L (mean 0.9) were attained in 2 h. [A. F. Fasola and R. Carmichael, *Acta Cardiol.*, 1974, Suppl., *18*, 317–333.]

Following daily oral doses of 100 to 150 mg, plasma concentrations in 28 patients ranged from 0.73 to 2.55 mg/L. [J. P. Van Durme *et al.*, *Eur. J. Clin. Pharmacol.*, 1974, *7*, 343–346.]

In 38 patients given a single oral dose of 100 to 150 mg aprindine hydrochloride, mean peak plasma concentrations of 0.33 to 1.40 mg/L (mean 0.77) were achieved in 1.5 to 4.0 h (mean 2.9). With repeated administration of 10 or 20 mg doses every 8 h, steady-state plasma concentrations of 0.155 to 0.455 mg/L and 0.39 to 1.53 mg/L, respectively, were attained in 7 to 19 days. [M. Yokota *et al.*, *Arzneimittelforschung.*, 1987, *37*, 184–188.]

Toxicity. Toxic effects are usually associated with plasma concentrations greater than 2 mg/L.

Toxic effects were found in 9 patients whose plasma concentrations ranged from 1.2 to 4.9 mg/L (mean 2.6). [J. P. Van Durme *et al.*, *Eur. J. Clin. Pharmacol.*, 1974, *7*, 343–346.]

Bioavailability. About 75%.

Half-life. Plasma half-life, 12 to 66 h (mean 30) in normal subjects but the half-life is apparently longer in patients with chronic ventricular arrhythmias and myocardial infarction (average, about 50 h).

Volume of distribution. About 4 L/kg.

Clearance. Plasma clearance, about 2.5 mL/min/kg in normal subjects; decreased to about 1 mL/min/kg in patients with cardiac disease.

Protein binding. In plasma, more than 95% at therapeutic concentrations, decreasing at higher concentrations.

Note. For a review of the pharmacokinetics of anti-arrhythmic agents see R. A. Ronfeld, *Am. Heart J.*, 1980, *100*, 978–983.

Dose. 50 to 100 mg of aprindine hydrochloride daily; initial doses of up to 200 mg daily may be given.

Aprobarbital

Sedative/Barbiturate

Synonyms. Allylisopropylmalonylurea; Allypropymal; Aprobarbitone.
Proprietary name. Alurate
5-(1-Methylethyl)-5-(2-propenyl)-2,4,6(1*H*,3*H*,5*H*)-pyrimidinetrione
$C_{10}H_{14}N_2O_3$=210.2
CAS—77-02-1

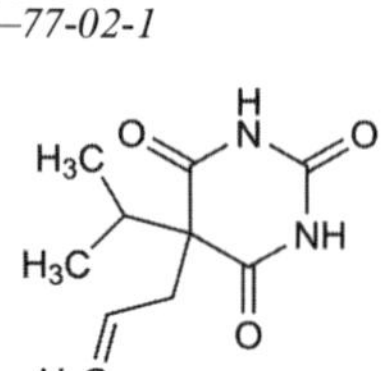

A white crystalline powder. M.p. 140° to 141.5°.

Soluble 1 in 350 of water, 1 in 30 of boiling water, 1 in 2.5 of ethanol, 1 in 40 of chloroform, and 1 in 5 of ether; soluble in acetone, glacial acetic acid, and aqueous solutions of alkali hydroxides and carbonates; almost insoluble in petroleum ether and aliphatic hydrocarbons.

Aprobarbital Sodium

Synonym. Aprobarbitone Sodium
$C_{10}H_{13}N_2NaO_3$=232.2
CAS—125-88-2
A white, hygroscopic, microcrystalline powder.
Very soluble in water; slightly soluble in ethanol; practically insoluble in ether.

Dissociation Constant. pK_a 8.0 (25°).

Partition Coefficient. Log *P* (octanol/water), 1.2.

Colour Test. Koppanyi–Zwikker Test—violet.

Thin-layer Chromatography. System TD—Rf 48; system TE—Rf 40; system TF—Rf 65; system TH—Rf 66; system TAD—Rf 57; system TAE—Rf 86. (Mercurous nitrate spray, black; acidified potassium permanganate solution, yellow-brown; Zwikker's reagent, pink.)

Gas Chromatography. System GA—aprobarbital RI 1618, M (OH-) RI 1815, aprobarbital-Me_2 RI 1540.

High Performance Liquid Chromatography. System HG—*k* 3.42; system HH—*k* 2.22; system HX—RI 357; system HY—RI 319; system HZ—retention time 2.8 min; system HAL—retention time 2.0 min.

Ultraviolet Spectrum. Borax buffer 0.05 M (pH 9.2)—241 nm (A^1_1=451a); 1 M sodium hydroxide (pH 13)—257 nm (A^1_1=331b).

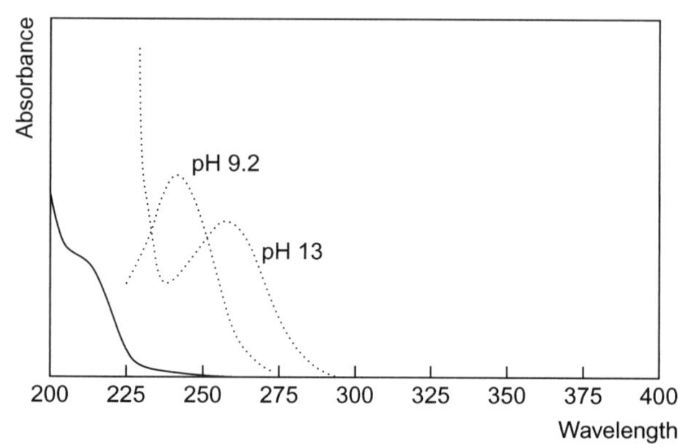

Infra-red Spectrum. Principal peaks at wavenumbers 1693, 1720, 1745, 1316, 1255, 860 cm^{-1}(KBr disk).

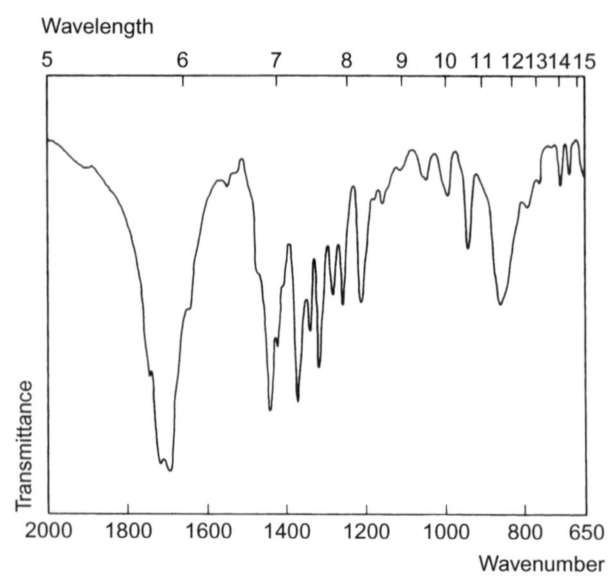

Mass Spectrum. Principal ions at *m/z* 167, 41, 124, 168, 97, 39, 169, 45; *N*-hydroxyaprobarbital 41, 43, 183, 167, 140, 184, 124, 109.

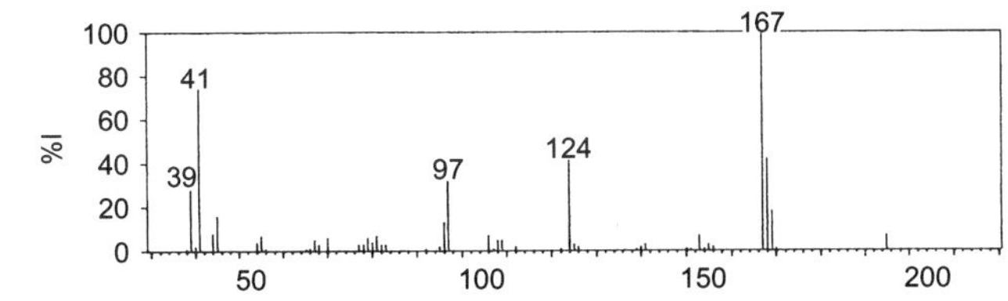

Quantification. See also under Amobarbital.

Gas chromatography–mass spectrometry. In urine: aprobarbital, *N*-hydroxyaprobarbital and aprobarbital diol—J. N. T. Gilbert *et al.*, *J. Pharm. Pharmacol.*, 1978, *30*, 173–175.

Disposition in the Body. Absorbed after oral administration and slowly excreted in the urine, mainly as metabolites, less than 3% of a dose being excreted as unchanged drug in 24 h. About 12% of a dose is excreted in the urine as the diol derivative and 4% as *N*-hydroxyaprobarbital in 3 days, together with 9% as unchanged drug.

Therapeutic concentration. In plasma, usually in the range 10 to 40 mg/L.

Toxicity. The estimated minimum lethal dose is 2 g. Plasma concentrations greater than 40 mg/L are usually associated with toxic effects; concentrations greater than 50 mg/L may be fatal.

In 4 cases of death attributed to overdoses ranging from 2.5 to 7.7 g, antemortem serum concentrations ranged from 120 to 150 mg/L. In 44 cases of overdose in which the patients subsequently recovered, the serum concentrations 24 h after ingestion were in the range 40 to 130 mg/L. [P. Lous, *Acta Pharmacol.Toxicol.*, 1954, *10*, 261–280.]

In a number of fatalities attributed to aprobarbital, a mean postmortem blood concentration of 50 mg/L in 9 cases and a mean postmortem liver concentration of 83 μg/g in 12 cases were reported. [R. Bonnichen *et al.*, *J. Forensic Sci.*, 1961, *6*, 411–443.]

Half-life. Plasma half-life, 0.5 to 1.5 days.

Protein binding. In plasma, 55 to 70%.

Dose. 40 to 160 mg daily.

Apronal

Hypnotic/Sedative

Synonyms. Allylisopropylacetylurea; Apronalide.
Proprietary name. Sedormid
N-(Aminocarbonyl)-2-(1-methylethyl)-4-pentenamide
$C_9H_{16}N_2O_2$=184.2
CAS—528-92-7

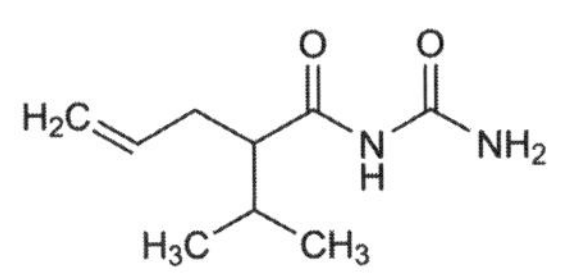

Colourless crystals or white crystalline powder. M.p. 194°.
Soluble 1 in 3000 of cold water, 1 in 210 of boiling water, 1 in 10 of ethanol, 1 in 45 of chloroform, and 1 in 75 of ether.

Partition Coefficient. Log *P* (octanol/water), 1.7.

Thin-layer Chromatography. System TD—Rf 33; system TE—Rf 67; system TF—Rf 52. (Acidified potassium permanganate solution, positive.)

Gas Chromatography. System GA—RI 1331.

High Performance Liquid Chromatography. System HX—RI 396.

Ultraviolet Spectrum. No significant absorption, 230 to 360 nm.

Infra-red Spectrum. Principal peaks at wavenumbers 1676, 1704, 1092, 1620, 1185, 750 cm^{-1} (KBr disk).

Mass Spectrum. Principal ions at *m/z* 55, 44, 142, 141, 41, 61, 81, 82.

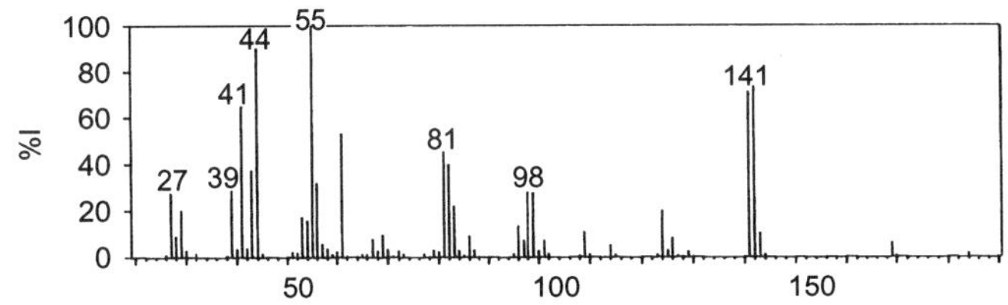

Dose. Apronal was formerly given in doses of 250 to 750 mg daily.

Arecoline

Purgative/Taenifuge (Veterinary)

Methyl-1,2,5,6-tetrahydro-1-methyl-3-pyridinecarboxylate
$C_8H_{13}NO_2$=155.2
CAS—63-75-2

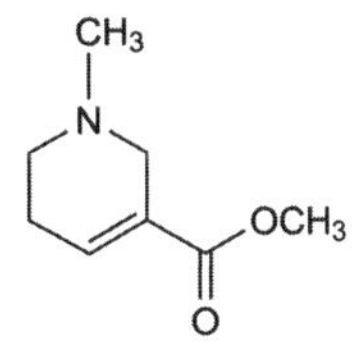

Arecoline is an alkaloid which is obtained from the seeds of *Areca catechu* (Palmae).
An oily liquid which is a strong base. B.p. 209°.
Miscible with water, ethanol, and ether; soluble in chloroform.

Arecoline Hydrobromide

$C_8H_{13}NO_2$,HBr=236.1
CAS—300-08-3
A white crystalline powder. Unstable in light. M.p. 169° to 171°.
Soluble 1 in 1 of water and 1 in 10 of ethanol; slightly soluble in chloroform and ether.

Dissociation Constant. pK_a 7.4 (20°).

Partition Coefficient. Log *P* (octanol/water), 0.4.

Thin-layer Chromatography. System TA—Rf 53; system TB—Rf 39; system TE—Rf 59; system TAE—Rf 41; system TAJ—Rf 28; system TAK—Rf 00; system TAL—Rf 28. (Acidified potassium permanganate solution, positive.)

Gas Chromatography. System GA—RI 1195.

High Performance Liquid Chromatography. System HX—RI 79; system HAA—Retention time 3.1 min.

Ultraviolet Spectrum. No significant absorption, 230 to 360 nm.

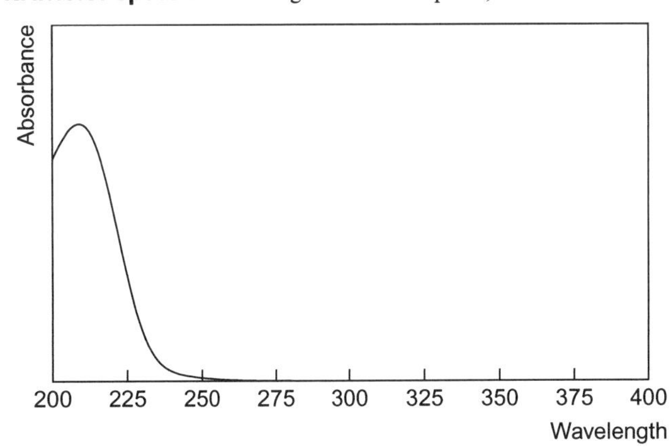

Infra-red Spectrum. Principal peaks at wavenumbers 1712, 1262, 1135, 1282, 1020, 1650 cm^{-1} (KCl disk).

Mass Spectrum. Principal ions at *m/z* 155, 96, 140, 43, 42, 81, 94, 53.

Quantification

Gas chromatography–mass spectrometry. In plasma: limit of detection <1 µg/L—M. J. Hayes *et al.*, *Biomed. Environ. Mass Spectrom.*, 1989, *18*, 1005–1009. In biological tissue: arecoline, acetylcholine, and choline, limit of detection <25 pmol—T. A. Patterson and J. W. Kosh, *Biol. Mass Spectrom.*, 1992, *21*, 299–304.

Arsenic Trioxide

Antineoplastic

Synonyms. Arsenic oxide; arsenic (III) oxide; arsenious acid; arsenious acid anhydride; arsenious oxide; arsenite; arsenous acid; arsenous acid anhydride; arsenous oxide; arsenic sesquioxide; white arsenic.
Proprietary name. Trisenox
As_2O_3=197.8
CAS—1327-53-3

White or transparent, glassy, amorphous lumps or crystalline powder. Two crystalline modifications: claudetite, m.p. 313°; arsenolite, m.p. 275°. B.p. 465°. It is intensely poisonous. It is sparingly and extremely slowly soluble in cold water; soluble in boiling water, dilute hydrochloric acid, alkali hydroxide and carbonate solutions; practically insoluble in alcohol, chloroform and ether.

Partition Coefficient. Log *P* (octanol/water), −0.13.

Disposition in the Body. The extent of arsenic trioxide absorption depends on the physical form of the compound; for example, a coarse powder may be eliminated in faeces before significant dissolution and absorption can occur. Arsenic trioxide is partly methylated (detoxification) to monomethylarsonic acid (MMA) and dimethylarsinic acid (DMA) in the liver. Both of these metabolites are relatively non-toxic and are excreted mostly in urine along with other inorganic arsenic compounds. During treatment with arsenic trioxide, the arsenic content of urine over a 24-h period accounted for 1% to 8% of the administered daily dose. Smaller amounts of arsenic are also excreted in faeces, sweat and via the lungs and skin. It has also been detected in breast milk and is known to cross the placenta. After ingestion of large doses, arsenic is widely distributed throughout the body to all organs with the highest concentrations in liver and kidneys with 10-fold and 3-fold higher concentrations, respectively.

Therapeutic concentration

Arsenic trioxide was administered to 8 patients with relapsed acute promyelocytic leukaemia at a dose of 10 mg daily. The peak plasma concentration reached 0.94 mg/L 4 h after dosing. [J. Ni *et al.*, *Chin. Med. J. (Engl.)*, 1998, *111(12)*, 1107–1110].

Toxicity. In severe arsenic poisoning, the major toxic effect is haemorrhagic gastro-enteritis which may lead to severe dehydration, collapse, shock and even death. Cardiac arrhythmias and convulsions have also been reported. A dose of 70 to 300 mg arsenic trioxide has been associated with fatalities depending on the physical form of the compound and the extent of its absorption. In the absence of adequate treatment, death may occur within 1 h but can be prolonged to 12 to 48 h.

A 28-year-old man died 3 days after committing suicide by ingesting approximately 8 g of arsenic trioxide. Major intoxication symptoms observed were hepatic and renal failure and cardiovascular and neurological effects. After toxicological analysis of his organs, the highest arsenic concentrations were found in the liver (147 µg/g) and kidneys (26.6 µg/g). Other organs contained lower but very similar concentrations: muscle, 12.3 µg/g; heart, 11.75 µg/g; spleen, 11.72 µg/g; pancreas, 11.2 µg/g; lungs, 11.13 µg/g; cerebellum, 10.95 µg/g; and brain, 8.33 µg/g. Skin had the lowest concentration at 2.9 µg/g. These concentrations were made up of arsenic (III) and the two metabolites, MMA and DMA. [L. Benramdane *et al.*, *Clin. Chem.*, 1999, *45(2)*, 301–306].

Half-life. Plasma, 12 h.

Clearance. Systemic, 1.43 L/h.

Artemether

Antimalarial

Synonyms. Dihydroartemisinin methyl ether; dihydroqinghaosu methyl ether; *o*-methyl-dihydroartemisinin; SM-224.

Proprietary names. Artemos; Qing Hao.
(3*R*,5a*S*,6*R*,8a*S*,9*R*,10*S*,12*R*,12a*R*)-Decahydro-10-methoxy-3,6,9-trimethyl-3,12-epoxy-12*H*-pyrano[4,3-j]-1,2-benzodioxepin
$C_{16}H_{26}O_5$=298.4
CAS—71963-77-4

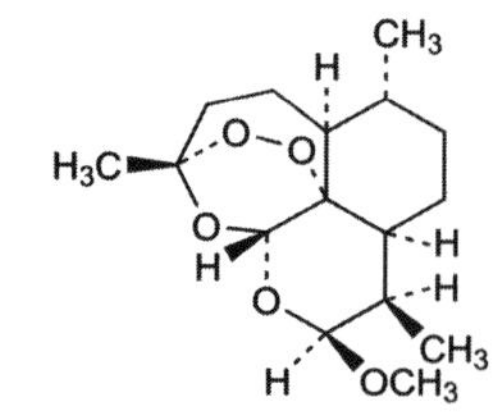

White crystalline powder. M.p. 86° to 88°.

Quantification

Gas chromatography–mass spectrometry. In plasma: limit of quantification 5 µg/L—S. S. Mohamed *et al.*, *J. Chromatogr. Biomed. Sci. Appl.*, 1999, *731*, 251–260.

High performance liquid chromatography. In plasma: limit of quantification for artemether and metabolite, DHA, 26 µg/L. Electrochemical detection—P. Teja-Isavadharm *et al.*, *Br. J. Clin. Pharmacol.*, 1996, *42*, 599–604.

Bioassay. In plasma: limit of quantification for DHA, 60 µg/L—P. Teja-Isavadharm *et al.*, *Br. J. Clin. Pharmacol.*, 1996, *42*, 599–604.

Disposition in the Body. Artemether is rapidly but incompletely absorbed after oral administration and is metabolised in the liver to the demethylated derivative dihydroartemisinin (DHA). It is rapidly eliminated. Oral bioavailability, after intramuscular injection, is approx. 43%.

Therapeutic concentration

6 healthy Malaysian males were administered with a single oral dose of 200 mg artemether. Peak plasma concentrations of 310 ± 153 µg/L were reached within 1.88 ± 0.21 h. The peak concentration of the metabolite, DHA, was 273 ± 64 µg/L which was reached within 1.92 ± 0.13 h. [M. N. Mordi *et al.*, *Br. J. Clin. Pharmacol.*, 1997, *43*, 363–365].

6 patients with severe falciparum malaria and acute renal failure and 11 patients without renal failure were intramuscularly administered with a total dose of 640 mg (over 7 days) artemether. Patients with renal failure had a slightly higher peak plasma concentration compared with those without failure (1.89 to 3.95 µg/L/mg dose versus 1.05 to 3.38 µg/L/mg dose). [J. Karbwang *et al.*, *Br. J. Clin. Pharmacol.*, 1998, *45*, 597–600].

Toxicity. Neurotoxicity.

Half-life. Elimination half-life for artemether is 1.5 to 3.5 h and for DHA is 1.4 to 2.4 h.

Volume of distribution. Apparent volume of distribution is 3.2 to 6.9 L/kg for patients with acute renal failure and 4.2 to 12.3 L/kg for those without.

Clearance. Plasma clearance is 5.4 to 13.8 mL/min/kg for patients with acute renal failure and 8.5 to 25.1 mL/min/kg for those without.

Protein binding. Binding to plasma proteins is about 50%.

Dose. An intramuscular dose of 3.2 mg/kg is administered initially followed by 1.6 mg/kg daily for a maximum of 7 days, then changed to oral administration. Capsule formulation: 160 mg on the first day followed by 80 mg daily for the next 4 days.

Artesunate

Antimalarial

Synonyms. Artesunic acid; dihydroartemisinin hemisuccinate; dihydroqinghaosu hemisuccinate.
Butanedioic acid mono[(3*R*,5a*S*,6*R*,8a*S*,9*R*,10*R*,12*R*,12a*R*)-decahydro-3,6,9-trimethyl-3,12-epoxy-12*H*-pyrano[4,3-*j*]-1,2-benzodioxepin-10-yl] ester
$C_{19}H_{28}O_8$=384.4
CAS—88495-63-0

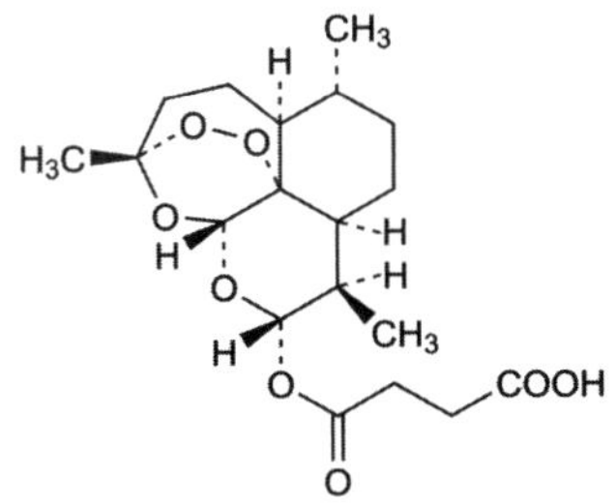

A fine white crystalline powder.

Artesunate Sodium
Synonyms. Dihydroartemisinin hemisuccinate sodium; dihydroqinghaosu hemisuccinate sodium; SM-804.
Proprietary name. Arsumex
$C_{19}H_{27}NaO_8$=406.4
Poor stability in aqueous solutions.

Gas Chromatography. Column: 3% OV-3 on 100-120 Supelcocort (silanised glass, 2 m × 2 mm i.d.). Column temperature: 160° to 24° at 10°/min. Carrier gas: methane, flow rate 20 mL/min. MS detection (EI, SIM at *m/z* 221). Internal standard: cedrol. Retention time: dihydroqinghaosu (cyclohexane pyrolysis product) 5.5 min. [A. D. Theoharides *et al.*, *Anal. Chem.*, 1988, *60*, 115–120].

High Performance Liquid Chromatography. Column: C_{18} (Nova-Pak, 5 µm, 150 × 3.9 mm i.d.), column and detector oven set at 20°. Mobile phase (kept at 35°): acetonitrile:dilute acetic acid (0.1 M, pH 4.80) (45:55). Flow rate 1.5 mL/min. Electrochemical detection. Retention time: α-dihydroartemisinin (DHA), 2.9 min; β-DHA, 4.2 min; artesunate, 4.5 min. [K. Na-Bangchang *et al.*, *J. Chromatogr. Biomed. Sci. Appl.*, 1998, *708*, 201–207].

Column: C_8 (Econosil, 10 µm, 250 × 4.6 mm). Mobile phase: acetonitrile:acetic acid (0.05 M) (42:58), adjusted to pH 5.0 with sodium hydroxide (1.0 M), 1.5 mL/min flow rate. Electrochemical detection. Retention time: artesunate, 6.6 min; DHA, 8.7 min. [V. Navaratnam *et al.*, *J. Chromatogr. Biomed. Sci. Appl.*, 1997, *692*, 157–162].

Mass Spectrum. (Cyclohexane pyrolysis product of dihydroqinghaosu), principal ions at *m/z* 43, 55, 69, 81, 152, 210, 95, 180.

Quantification
Gas chromatography–mass spectrometry. In blood: limit of detection of DQHS 2 µg/L—A. D. Theoharides *et al.*, *Anal. Chem.*, 1988, *60*, 11–120.

High performance liquid chromatography. In plasma: limit of detection is 4.0 µg/L for artesunate and the metabolite, DHA. Electrochemical detection—V. Navaratnam *et al.*, *J. Chromatogr. Biomed. Sci. Appl.*, 1997, *692*, 157–162. In plasma: limit of quantification for artesunate is 5 µg/L and 3 µg/L DHA. Electrochemical detection—K. Na-Bangchang *et al.*, *J. Chromatogr. Biomed. Sci. Appl.*, 1998, *708*, 207–207.

Disposition in the Body. Artesunate is rapidly metabolised to its active metabolite dihydroartemisinin (DHA) (dihydroqinghaosu, DQHS). After oral administration, bioavailability of DHA is 82%.

Therapeutic concentration
26 Vietnamese patients with falciparum malaria were administered with either a 120 mg intravenous dose or 100 mg oral dose of artesunate. With the intravenous dose, peak plasma concentrations of 11 mg/L artesunate and 2.64 mg/L DHA were reached. With the oral dose of artesunate, peak concentrations of 0.74 mg/L DHA were observed. [K. T. Barry *et al.*, *Br. J. Clin. Pharmacol.*, 1998, *45*, 123–129].

11 Thai patients, aged between 15 and 37 years, with acute uncomplicated falciparum malaria were administered with an initial, oral dose of 200 mg, followed by 100 mg daily (total of 700 mg). After the initial dose, peak plasma concentrations of artesunate at 0.5 to 1.9 µg/L were reached within 0.5 to 1 h and 1.2 to 4.1 µg/L for the metabolite, DHA (1.5 to 2.5 h). After the first 100 mg dose, peak concentrations reached 0.62 to 2.9 µg/L and 1.3 to 4.2 µg/L, respectively, within 2 h. [J. Karbwang *et al.*, *Clin. Drug Invest.*, 1998, *15*, 37–43].

Bioavailability. Bioavailability of DHA is 82%.

Half-life. Elimination half-life of artesunate is 2.7 min and 40 min for DHA (intravenous administration) and 21.6 and 38.4 min, respectively, for oral administration.

Volume of distribution. Artesunate, 0.14 L/kg; DHA, 0.76 L/kg (intravenous administration). (Oral administration) 6.8 L/kg for artesunate and DHA.

Clearance. Clearance of artesunate is 2.33 L/h/kg and of DHA is 0.75 L/kg/h (intravenous administration). (Oral administration) 0.005 and 0.003 L/kg/h, respectively.

Distribution in blood. Blood cells:plasma concentration ratio 5.5.

Note. Refer to J. Karbwang *et al.*, *Clin. Drug Invest.*, 1998, *15*, 37–43 and K. T. Barry *et al.*, *Br. J. Clin. Pharmacol.*, 1998, *45*, 123–129 for a review of the pharmacokinetics.

Dose. A dose of 10 mg/kg body weight daily (intravenously) is administered for a minimum of 5 days (3 days if in combination). Lowest dose of 2 mg/kg body weight daily. Total oral dose of 600 mg over 5 days.

Ascorbic Acid

Vitamin

Synonyms. L-Ascorbic Acid; Cevitamic Acid; Vitamin C.
Proprietary names Alba CE; Ascorbicap; Ascorbicin; Ascorvit; Buffered C; Cantan; Cebid; Cebion; Cecon; Celaskon; Celin; Cenolate; Cetebe; Cevi-Bid; Cevilan; Ce-Vi-Sol; Cevitan; Cewin; Dull-C; Favorcee; Halib-orange Halibonbons; Hybrin; N'ice Vitamin C; RedoxonVitacin; Vitascorbol includes proprietary names of Sodium Ascorbate.
Ascorbic acid and ascorbates are ingredients of many proprietary preparations—see *Martindale, The complete drug reference*, 33rd Edn., Pharmaceutical Press, London, 2002.
The enolic form of 3-oxo-L-gulofuranolactone
$C_6H_8O_6$=176.1
CAS—50-81-7

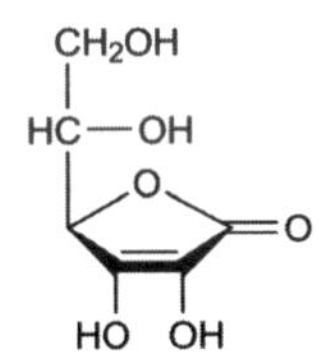

Colourless crystals or white or very pale yellow crystalline powder. Solutions, especially when made alkaline, deteriorate rapidly in air. M.p. 190° to 192°, with some decomposition.
Soluble 1 in about 3 of water, 1 in 30 of ethanol, 1 in 10 of methanol, and 1 in 20 of propylene glycol; soluble in acetone; insoluble in benzene, chloroform, ether, petroleum ether, oils, fats, and fat solvents.

Sodium Ascorbate
$C_6H_7NaO_6$=198.1
CAS—134-03-2
White or very faintly yellow crystals or crystalline powder. It gradually darkens on exposure to light. M.p. 218° with decomposition.
Soluble 1 in 1.3 of water; very slightly soluble in ethanol; practically insoluble in chloroform and ether.

Dissociation Constant. pK_a 4.2, 11.6 (25°).

Partition Coefficient. Log *P* (octanol/water), −1.8.

Colour Tests. Ammoniacal Silver Nitrate—black; Benedict's Reagent—red; Nessler's Reagent—black; Palladium Chloride—black

Gas Chromatography. System GA—ascorbic acid RI 2120; ascorbic acid—AC_2 RI 2065; ascorbic acid—Me_2 RI 1700.

High Performance Liquid Chromatography. System HY—RI 52; system HZ—retention time 1.5 min (ascorbate).

Ultraviolet Spectrum. Aqueous acid—243 nm (A_1^1=556a).

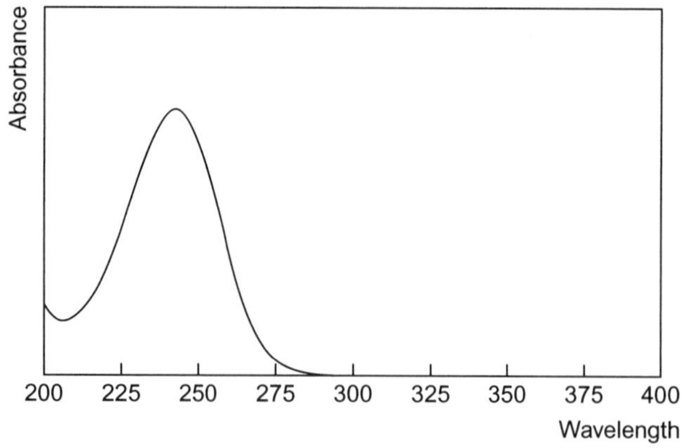

Infra-red Spectrum. Principal peaks at wavenumbers 1026, 1111, 1312, 1136, 1653, 990 cm^{-1} (Nujol mull).

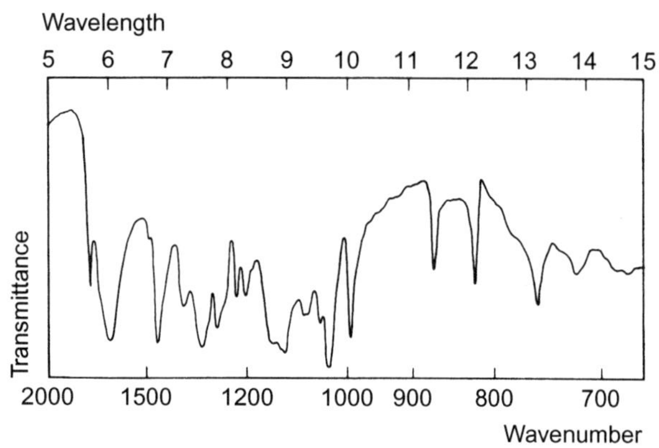

Mass Spectrum. Principal ions at *m*/*z* 29, 41, 39, 42, 69, 116, 167, 168.

Quantification

Colorimetry. In plasma: comparison with HPLC—W. Y. Chung *et al.*, *Clin. Biochem.*, 2001, *34*, 623–627.

Gas chromatography–mass spectrometry. In plasma: ascorbic and dehydroascorbic acids—J. C. Deutsch and J. F. Kolhouse, *Anal. Chem.*, 1993, *65*, 321–326.

High performance liquid chromatography. In serum or urine: electrochemical detection—L. A. Pachla and P. T. Kissinger, *Anal. Chem.*, 1976, *48*, 364–367. In urine: UV detection—E. S. Wagner *et al.*, *J. Chromatogr.* 1979, *163(5) Biomed. Appl. B* 225–229. In postmortem tissues: UV detection—W. J. Allender, *J. Anal. Toxicol.*, 1982, *6*, 202–204. In urine: fluorescence detection—T. Seki *et al.*, *J. Chromatogr.*, 1987, *385*, 287–291. In blood cells—S. T. Omaye *et al.*, *Ann. N. Y. Acad. Sci.*, 1987, *498*, 389–401. In plasma or blood cells: ascorbate-2-phosphate—G. L. Moore and R. M. Fishman, *J. Chromatogr.*, 1987, *419*, 95–102. In plasma or blood cells—M. A. Kutnink *et al.*, *Anal. Biochem.*, 1987, *166*, 424–430. In plasma or serum: ascorbic acid and dehydroascorbic acid, electrochemical detection—K. R. Dhariwal *et al.*, *Am. J. Clin. Nutr.*, 1991, *54*, 712–716. In plasma: limit of detection 120 µg/L, UV detection (comparison with electrochemical detection)—L. S. Liau *et al.*, *J. Chromatogr.*, 1993, *612*, 63–70. In plasma or aqueous humour: electrochemical detection—D. G. Watson *et al.*, *J. Pharm. Biomed. Anal.*, 1993, *11*, 389–392. In plasma: UV detection—K. Tanishima and M. Kita, *J. Chromatogr.*, 1993, *613*, 275–280. In plasma: electrochemical detection—K. Umegaki *et al.*, *J. Nutr. Sci. Vitaminol. (Tokyo)*, 1994, *40*, 73–79. In plasma or urine: limits of detection 0.4 mg/L and 0.1 mg/L respectively, UV detection—M. Manoharan and P. O. Schwille, *J. Chromatogr.* 1994, *654*, *Biomed. Appl. B* 134–139. In plasma: limit of detection 240 µg/L, electrochemical detection—H. Iwase and I. Ono, *J. Chromatogr.* 1994, *655*, *Biomed. Appl. B* 195–200. In plasma: ascorbic acid and uric acid, UV detection—M. A. Ross, *J. Chromatogr.* 1994, *657 B Biomed. Appl.*, 197–200. In plasma: ascorbic acid and dehydroascorbic acid, coulometric detection—J. Lykkesfeldt *et al.*, *Anal. Biochem.*, 1995, *229*, 329–335. In plasma: ascorbic acid and dehydroascorbic acid, fluorescence detection (comparison with coulometric detection)—F. Tessier *et al.*, *Int. J. Vitam. Nutr. Res.*, 1996, *66*, 166–170. In plasma or urine: ascorbate and dehydroascorbate—I. Koshiishi and T. Imanari, *Anal. Chem.*, 1997, *69*, 216–220. In plasma or serum: ascorbic and dehydroascorbic acids, UV detection—M. J. Esteve *et al.*, *J. Chromatogr. B Biomed. Sci. Appl.*, 1997, *688*, 345–349. In vitreous humour: UV detection—S. Takano *et al.*, *Curr. Eye Res.*, 1997, *16*, 589–594. In plasma or urine: UV detection—A. Rumelin *et al.*, *Clin. Chem. Lab. Med.*, 1999, *37*, 533–536. In plasma: ascorbic and dehydroascorbic acids, fluorescence detection—M. A. Kall and C. Andersen, *J. Chromatogr. B Biomed. Sci. Appl.*, 1999, *730*, 101–111.

Review. In biological samples, pharmaceuticals and food: analysis methods—L. A. Pachla *et al.*, *J. AOAC*, 1985, *68*, 1–12.

Disposition in the Body. Readily absorbed after oral administration; the proportion of a dose absorbed tends to decrease with increasing dose; it is widely distributed in the body tissues. The concentration of ascorbic acid is higher in leucocytes and platelets than in erythrocytes and plasma. Ascorbic acid is metabolised to dehydroascorbic acid, 2,3-diketogulonic acid, oxalate and carbon dioxide; some conjugation with sulfate occurs to form ascorbate-3-sulfate. Ascorbic acid in excess of the body's requirements is rapidly eliminated in the urine. About 85% of an intravenous dose, given to subjects previously saturated with the vitamin, is excreted in the urine in 24 h, with about 70% of the dose excreted unchanged and 15% as dehydroascorbic acid and diketogulonic acid. The amount normally present in the body is in excess of 1.5 g.

Blood concentration. Concentrations in plasma and in leucocytes are normally about 5 to 12 mg/L and 25 to 30 µg/10^8 cells respectively; these concentrations exhibit circadian and seasonal rhythms.

Protein binding. In plasma, about 25%.

Dose. 0.2 to 3 g daily.

Asparaginase

Antineoplastic

Synonyms. L-Asnase; L-Asparaginase; L-Asparagine Amidohydrolase; Colaspase; E.C.3.5.1.1; Mk-965; NSC-109229.
Proprietary names. Crasnitin; Crasnitine; Elspar; Erwinase (Crisantaspase-recombinant); Kidrolase; Laspar; Leucogen; Leunase; Oncaspar (Pegaspargase-recombinant); Paronal.
CAS—9015-68-3
Commonly obtained from *E. coli* and *Erwinia* sp. Asparaginase from *E.coli* has a molecular weight of about 136 000.
A white crystalline powder. It is freely soluble in water where it appears to be global in shape; practically insoluble in methanol, in acetone and in chloroform.

Quantification

Thin-layer chromatography. In serum: limit of detection 0.05 U/mL, reaction with ^{14}C-asparagine and detection with scintillation counter—N. Clausen and E. Christensen, *Clin. Chim. Acta*, 1986, *161*, 111–116.

Disposition in the Body. It is sequestered slowly by the reticuloendothelial system. It is found in the lymph at about 20% of the concentration in plasma. There is virtually no diffusion into the CSF. Little is excreted in the urine. Preparations derived from *E. coli* and *Erwinia* differ in their pharmacokinetic and pharmacodynamic properties.

Toxicity. Allergic reactions are frequent and can lead to death.

Half-life. Plasma, 8 to 30 h (intravenous administration); up to 49 h (intramuscular administration).

Protein binding. In plasma, 30%.

Dose. Up to 1000 units/kg intravenously daily for 10 days.

Aspirin

Analgesic

Synonyms. Acetylsalicylic Acid; Salicylic Acid Acetate.
Proprietary names. Adprin-B; Angettes; Ascriptin; Aspergum; Asprimox; Aspro; Beechams Lemon Tablets; Bufferin; Buffex; Caprin; Disprin; Easprin; Empirin; Enprin; Gencardia; Genprin; Halfprin; Micropirin; Magnaprin; Nu-Seals; Platet; PostMI; Solprin; ZORprin.
Aspirin is an ingredient of many proprietary preparations—see *Martindale, The complete drug reference*, 33rd Edn, London, Pharmaceutical Press, 2002.
2-(Acetyloxy)benzoic acid
$C_9H_8O_4$=180.2
CAS—50-78-2

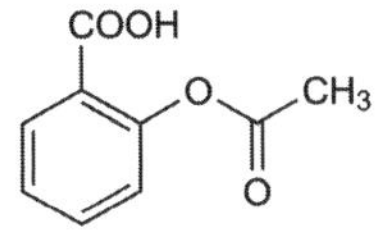

Colourless or white crystals or white crystalline powder or granules. It is stable in dry air but gradually hydrolyses in contact with moisture to acetic and salicylic acids. M.p. 135°.
Soluble 1 in 300 of water, 1 in 5 of ethanol, 1 in 17 of chloroform, and 1 in 10 to 15 of ether; soluble in solutions of acetates and citrates and, with decomposition, in solutions of alkali hydroxides and carbonates.

Dissociation Constant. pK_a 3.5 (25°).

Partition Coefficient. Log *P* (octanol/buffer pH 7.4), –1.1.

Colour Test. McNally's Test—red (after hydrolysis).

Thin-layer Chromatography. System TA—Rf 90; system TD—aspirin Rf 18, salicylic acid Rf 07, salicyluric acid Rf 00; system TE—aspirin Rf 09, salicylic acid Rf 10, salicyluric acid Rf 00; system TF—aspirin Rf 30, salicylic acid Rf 01, salicyluric acid Rf 00; system TAD—aspirin Rf 31, salicylic acid Rf 24; system TAE—aspirin Rf 78, salicylic acid Rf 86; system TAJ—Rf 40; system TAK—Rf 65; system TAL—Rf 90.

Gas Chromatography. System GA—aspirin RI 1545, salicylic acid RI 1307, aspirin-Me RI 1394, salicylic acid-Me RI 1195; system GB—salicylic acid RI 1340, salicylic acid-Me RI 1228.

High Performance Liquid Chromatography. System HD—aspirin *k* 0.5, salicylic acid *k* 0.7; system HW—aspirin *k* 2.7, salicylic acid *k* 4.6; system HX—aspirin RI 350; system HY—aspirin RI 318; system HZ—aspirin retention time 2.7 min; system HAX—salicylic acid retention time 5.2 min; system HAY—salicylic acid retention time 4.4 min.

Ultraviolet Spectrum. Aqueous acid—230 (A_1^1=466a), 278 (A_1^1=68a); aqueous alkali—231 (A_1^1=409b), 298 nm (A_1^1=190b).

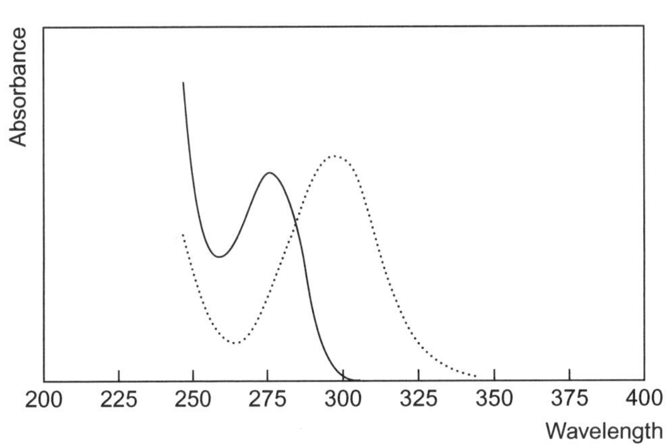

Infra-red Spectrum. Principal peaks at wavenumbers 1183, 1688, 1305, 1755, 925, 1219 cm^{-1} (KBr disk).

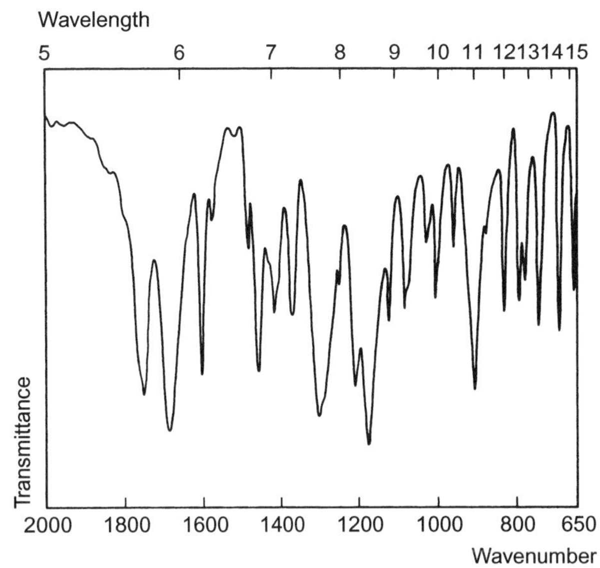

Mass Spectrum. Principal ions at *m/z* 120, 43, 138, 92, 121, 39, 64, 63; salicylic acid 120, 92, 138, 64, 39, 63, 121, 65; salicyluric acid 121, 120, 69, 92, 195, 39, 93, 45.

Quantification

Gas chromatography. In plasma: aspirin, salicylic acid, and salicylamide, limit of detection 200 to 500 µg/L for all three compounds, FID—M. J. Rance *et al.*, *J. Pharm. Pharmacol.*, 1975, *27*, 425–429.

Gas chromatography–mass spectrometry. In plasma—D. Tsikas *et al.*, *J. Chromatogr. B Biomed. Sci. Appl.*, 1998, *709*, 79–88.

High performance liquid chromatography. In plasma: aspirin, salicylic acid, and salicyluric acid, limit of detection 50 µg/L for aspirin in plasma; also aspirin metabolites in urine, UV detection—J. N. Buskin *et al.*, *Clin. Chem.*, 1982, *28*, 1200–1203. In plasma or urine: aspirin and its major metabolites, limits of detection in plasma 100 µg/L for aspirin and salicyluric acid, 500 µg/L for salicylic acid, and 200 µg/L for gentisic acid, UV detection—R. H. Rumble *et al.*, *J. Chromatogr.* 1981, *225*(14) *B Biomed. Appl.*, 252–260. In plasma: aspirin and NSAIDs, UV detection—S. G. Owen *et al.*, *J. Chromatogr.*, 1987, *416*, 293–302. In plasma: aspirin and salicylic acid, limit of detection 0.1 mg/L, UV detection—F. Gaspari and M. Locatelli, *Ther. Drug Monit.*, 1987, *9*, 243–247. In urine: salicylate glucuronide conjugates—J. J. Shen *et al.*, *J. Chromatogr.*, 1991, *565*, 309–320. In plasma or saliva: UV detection—M. E. Legaz *et al.*, *Tokai J. Exp. Clin. Med.*, 1992, *17*, 229–237. In plasma: aspirin and salicylic acid, limit of detection 100 µg/L, UV detection—F. Kees *et al.*, *J. Chromatogr.* 1996, *677 B Biomed. Appl.*, 172–177. In plasma: salicylic acid, limit of detection 5 µmol/L—C. Coudray *et al.*, *J. Chromatogr. Sci.*, 1996, *34*, 166–173. In plasma or urine: aspirin, salicylic acid, and salicyluric acid, UV detection—Z. Krivosikova *et al.*, *Methods Find. Exp. Clin. Pharmacol.*, 1996, *18*, 527–532. In plasma: aspirin and salicylic acid, limit of detection 40 µg/L, UV detection—G. P. McMahon and M. T. Kelly, *Anal. Chem.*, 1998, *70*, 409–414. In plasma or skin: aspirin and salicylic acid, limits of detection 0.1 µg/mL and 0.1 µg/cm^2 respectively—R. Pirola *et al.*, *J. Chromatogr. B Biomed. Sci. Appl.*, 1998, *705*, 309–315.

Disposition in the Body. Readily absorbed after oral administration and rapidly hydrolysed to salicylic acid which is the active agent. Salicylic acid is conjugated with glucuronic acid and glycine to form acyl and ether glucuronides and salicyluric acid; some hydroxylation also occurs to give dihydroxy and trihydroxy derivatives of salicylic acid. Aspirin is excreted almost entirely in the urine with about 50 to 80% of a dose as salicyluric acid, 10 to 30% as salicyl *O*-glucuronide, 5% as salicyl ester glucuronide, and 5 to 10% as free salicylic acid, together with small amounts of gentisic acid, gentisuric acid, and unchanged drug; salicylates are reabsorbed by the renal tubules from acid urine and thus alkaline diuresis increases the rate of salicylate elimination; about 85% of a dose is excreted as free salicylic acid if the urine is made alkaline.

Aspirin is a metabolite of aloxiprin and benorilate.

Therapeutic concentration. In plasma, salicylic acid usually in the range 20 to 100 mg/L for analgesia and 150 to 300 mg/L for anti-inflammatory effect.

After a single oral dose of 900 mg given to 5 subjects, peak plasma-aspirin concentrations of 16 to 50 mg/L (mean 37) were attained in about 14 min, and peak plasma-salicylic acid concentrations of 47 to 113 mg/L (mean 78) were reported at 0.5 to 1 h. [B. E. Cham *et al.*, *Ther. Drug Monit.*, 1980, *2*, 365–372.]

Following daily oral doses of 3.9 g to 8 subjects for 8 days, steady-state plasma-salicylic acid concentrations of 105 to 227 mg/L (mean 173) were reported; by the 36th day of treatment the steady-state plasma concentrations had declined to 45 to 208 mg/L (mean 129). [R. H. Rumble *et al.*, *Br. J. Clin. Pharmacol.*, 1980, *9*, 41–45.]

Toxicity. The estimated minimum lethal dose is 15 g. Plasma concentrations of salicylic acid greater than 300 mg/L are likely to produce toxic reactions and concentrations greater than 500 mg/L are associated with moderate to severe intoxication. The maximum permissible atmospheric concentration is 5 mg/m^3.

A 43-year-old female attempted suicide by self-administration, in the form of an enema, of approximately 700 aspirin tablets dissolved in water. The initial salicylate concentration in the serum was 590 mg/L and rose to 900 mg/L 12 h later; after haemodialysis, serum salicylate concentration fell to 160 mg/L but the patient remained in a coma for more than a year. The patient's poor outcome was attributed to retention of aspirin products in the rectal vault plus poor recognition of the delayed absorption properties of rectally administered aspirin. [J. E. Watson and E. T. Tagupa, *Ann. Pharmacother.*, 1994, *28*, 467–469.]

Half-life. Plasma half-life, aspirin about 17 min, salicylic acid dose-dependent (2 to 4 h after doses of less than 3 g, increasing to about 19 h after large doses).

Volume of distribution. Aspirin about 0.15 L/kg, salicylic acid about 0.1 to 0.2 L/kg (dose-dependent).

Protein binding. In plasma, salicylic acid about 90% at concentrations below 100 μg/mL, decreasing to 50% at concentrations above 400 μg/mL.

Note. For reviews of the pharmacokinetics of salicylates, see M. Mandelli and G. Tognoni, *Clin. Pharmacokinet.*, 1980, *5*, 424–440, and G. Levy, *Pediatrics*, 1978, *62*, Suppl., 865–872.

Dose. Usually 1.2 to 4 g daily; doses of up to 8 g daily are given in acute rheumatic disorders.

Astemizole

Antihistamine

Synonym. R-43512

Proprietary names. Alermizol; Esmacen; Hismacap; Hismanal; Histamen; Histaminos; Hubermizol; Laridal; Paralergin; Pollon-eze; Pollonis; Retolen; Rifedot; Rimbol; Romadin; Simprox; Urdrim.

1-[(4-Fluorophenyl)methyl]-*N*-[1-[2-(4-methoxyphenyl)ethyl]-4-piperidinyl]-1*H*-benzimidazol-2-amine

$C_{28}H_{31}FN_4O = 458.6$

CAS—68844-77-9

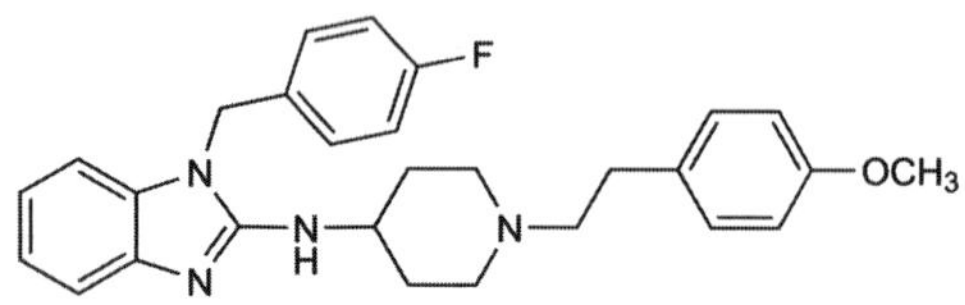

A white or almost white powder with m.p. 175° to 178°. Also described as white, odourless crystals with m.p. 149.1°. It is practically insoluble in water; soluble in ethanol; freely soluble in dichloromethane, methanol and other organic solvents.

Partition Coefficient. Log *P* (octanol/water), 6.43.

Thin-layer Chromatography. System TB—Rf 1 (astemizole) ; Rf 0 (M-nor) ; system TE—Rf 64 (astemizole) ; Rf 51 (M-nor) ; system TAE—Rf 56 (astemizole) ; Rf 55 (M-nor).

Plate: silica gel 60 F_{254}. Mobile phase: *n*-butanol:acetic acid:twice distilled water (12:5:2). UV detection (280 nm). Rf 0.45. [S. Mangalan *et al.*, *J. Chromatogr. Biomed. Sci. Appl.*, 1991, *567*, 498–503].

Plate: silica gel 60 F_{254} (20 × 20 cm, 0.25 mm thin layer). Mobile phase: chloroform:methanol (85:15). UV detection (254 nm). Rf 0.67 (astemizole); 0.36 (demethylated derivative). Relative Rf value of drug to its metabolite, 1.86. [O. A. Al-Deeb *et al.*, *Eur. J. Drug Metab. Pharmacokinet.*, 1992, *17(4)*, 251–255].

Gas Chromatography. System GA—RI 3150 (astemizole) ; RI 2470 (*M-N*-desalkyl).

High Performance Liquid Chromatography. System HX—RI 383 (astemizole), RI 361 (M-nor); system HY—RI 286; system HZ—3.9 min; system HAA—retention time 13.2 min.

Column: ODS Hypersil (100 × 4.6 mm i.d., 5 μm). Mobile phase: methanol:aqueous 0.01 M dihydrogen potassium phosphate buffer, adjusted to pH 3.5 with 85% phosphoric acid (70:30), 1 mL/min flow rate. UV diode array detection. Retention time: 3.2 min. [T. Mills and J. C. Roberson, *Instrumental Data for Drug Analysis*, 1993, CRC Press, Boca Raton, US. 2nd Edn, Vol. 34–35].

Ultraviolet Spectrum. Aqueous acid (ethanol)—219, 249, 286 (A = 306.5) nm; (0.1 M hydrochloric acid)—209, 277 nm.

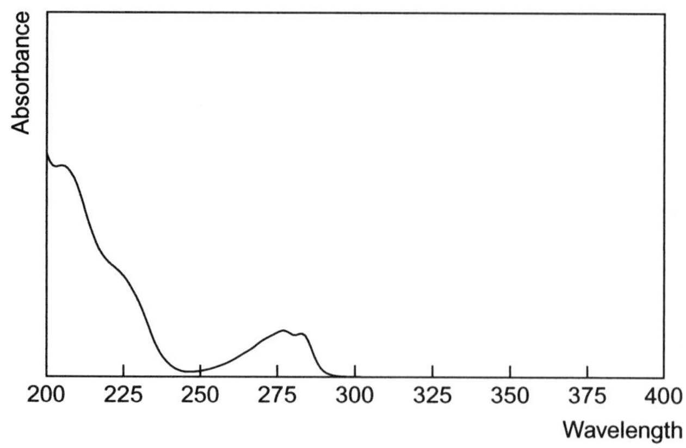

Infra-red Spectrum. Principal peaks at wavenumber 1506, 1217, 738 cm^{-1} (KBr pellets).

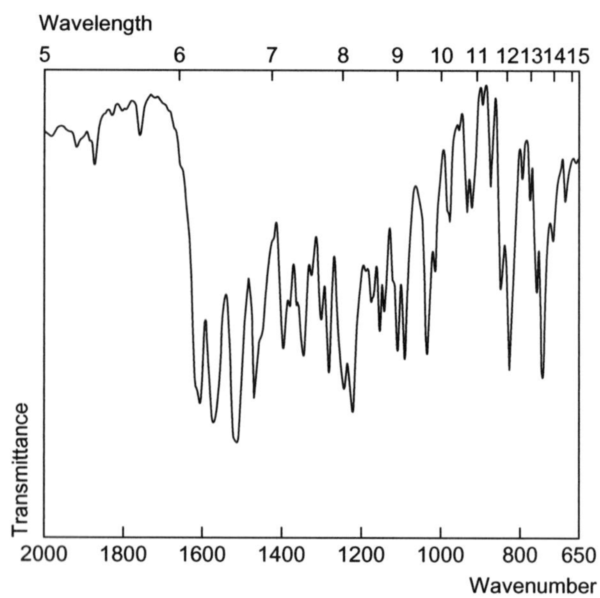

Mass Spectrum. Principal peaks at *m/z* 96, 109, 97, 294, 95, 135, 121, 242 (astemizole); 109, 241, 132, 83, 242, 111 (*M-N*-desalkyl).

Quantification

High performance liquid chromatography. In plasma or tissues: astemizole and desmethylastemizole, limit of detection 1 μg/L in plasma and 5 ng/g in tissue, UV detection—R. Woestenborghs *et al.*, *J. Chromatogr.*, 1983, *278*; *Biomed. Appl.*, *29*, 359–366.

Disposition in the Body. Astemizole is rapidly absorbed after oral administration. It is widely distributed although does not cross the blood–brain barrier to a significant extent. It is distributed into breast milk. The drug undergoes extensive first-pass metabolism mediated by the cytochrome P450 enzyme system (mainly by isoenzyme CYP 3A4 and to a lesser extent by CYP2D6 and CYP2A6). Desmethylastemizole is the major metabolite and has histamine-H_1 blocking activity. Other metabolites include norastemizole and 6-hydroxydesmethylastemizole. The metabolites are slowly excreted primarily in faeces via bile and undergo enterohepatic recycling. No unchanged drug has been detected and it is not known to accumulate once steady state levels have been reached.

Therapeutic concentration. Peak plasma concentrations are reached within 1 to 2 h. At steady state, the average peak plasma concentration of astemizole plus desmethylastemizole is 3 to 5 μg/L.

Toxicity. Elevated plasma-astemizole concentrations are associated with QT interval prolongation and serious cardiotoxicity. Arrhythmias, including *torsade de pointes*, have occurred rarely at doses as low as 20 to 30 mg daily.

Plasma-astemizole concentrations following accidental overdose in a 28-month old child who had taken 16.7 mg/kg and in a 24-month old child who had taken 2.5 to 3.3 mg/kg were 250 and 15.9 μg/L, respectively (time after ingestion not stated). The child who had ingested 16.7 mg/kg developed ventricular fibrillation requiring DC cardioversion 46 h after ingestion. Both children made a full recovery. [K. Hoppu *et al.*, *Lancet*, 1991, *338*, 538–540].

A 4-year-old boy who ingested 1.7 mg/kg of astemizole became lethargic 4 h later. Serum-astemizole concentration measured 4.5 h after ingestion was 14 μg/L. Four other children aged 1.5 to 11 years who had ingested 2.2 to 12.2 mg/kg all had prolonged QT intervals on ECG recordings that took 1 to 3 days to resolve. [J. F. Wiley *et al.*, *J. Pediatr.*, 1992, *120*, 799–802].

A 16-year-old girl who had taken an overdose of 200 mg of astemizole became unconscious with no cardiac output 7 h later. After another hour she developed ventricular tachyarrhythmia requiring DC cardioversion. [T. M. Craft, *BMJ*, 1986, *292*, 660].

Half-life. Plasma: astemizole, 1 to 2 days; desmethylastemizole, 9 to 13 days. The half-life of the drug and metabolites may increase after long-term administration to 18 to 20 days.

Volume of distribution. 250 L/kg.

Clearance. Plasma, 11 mL/min/kg.

Protein binding. In plasma, 96%.

Note. For reviews of astemizole see D. M. Richards *et al.*, *Drugs*, 1984, *28*, 38–61 and D. M. Paton and D. R. Webster, *Clin. Pharmacokinet.*, 1985, *10*, 477–497.

Dose. 10 mg daily (maximum).

Atenolol

Beta-adrenoceptor Blocking Agent

Proprietary names. Anselol; Antipressan; Ate; Atebeta; Atehexal; Atendol; Atenix; Ateno; Betatop; Blocotenol; Cuxanorm; Duratenol; Evitocor; Falitonsin; Jenatenol; Juvental; Noten; Tenlol; Teno; Tenormin(e); Tensig; Tonoprotect; Totamol; Xaten. It is an ingredient of AtenixCo, Beta-Adalat, Kalten, Tenben, Tenchlor, Tenif, Tenoret(ic) and Totaretic.

4-[2-Hydroxy-3-[(1-methylethyl)amino]propoxy]benzeneacetamide

$C_{14}H_{22}N_2O_3$=266.3

CAS—29122-68-7

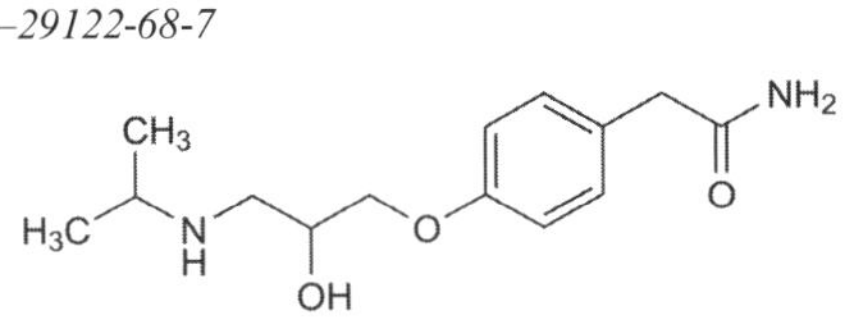

Crystals. M.p. 146° to 148°.

Slightly soluble in water and isopropanol; freely soluble in methanol; soluble in acetic acid and dimethylsulfoxide; very slightly soluble in acetone and dioxane; practically insoluble in acetonitrile, ethylacetate, and chloroform.

Dissociation Constant. pK_a 9.6 (24°).

Partition Coefficient. Log *P* (octanol/water), 0.23.

Colour Tests. Liebermann's Test—black; Nessler's Reagent—yellow-brown (slow).

Thin-layer Chromatography. System TA—Rf 45; system TB—Rf 00; system TC—Rf 02; system TE—Rf 22; system TL—Rf 02; system TAE—Rf 14.

Gas Chromatography. System GA—atenolol RI 2385, Art (-H_2O) RI 2150, Art (HOOC-)-Me RI 2140 and 2175; system GB—atenolol RI 2469, Art (-H_2O) RI 2090.

High Performance Liquid Chromatography. System HA—*k* 1.3; system HX—RI 243; system HY—RI 194; system HZ—retention time 1.7 min; system HAA—retention time 3.6 min; system HAX—retention time 5.3 min; system HAY—retention time 3.1 min.

Ultraviolet Spectrum. Aqueous acid—274 nm (A^1_1=48b), 280 nm. No alkaline shift.

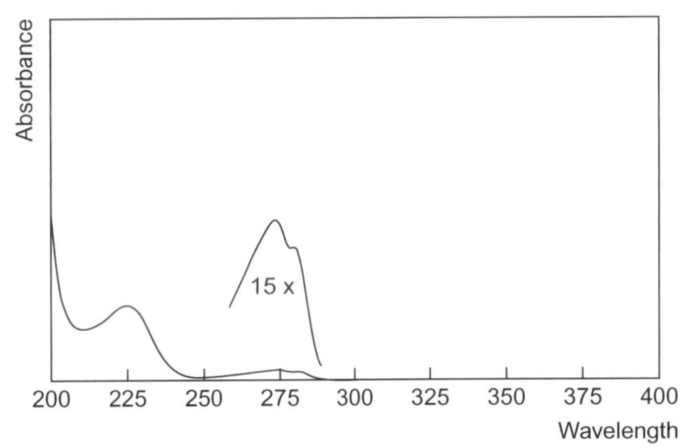

Infra-red Spectrum. Principal peaks at wavenumbers 1633, 1245, 1510, 1184, 805, 820 cm^{-1}.

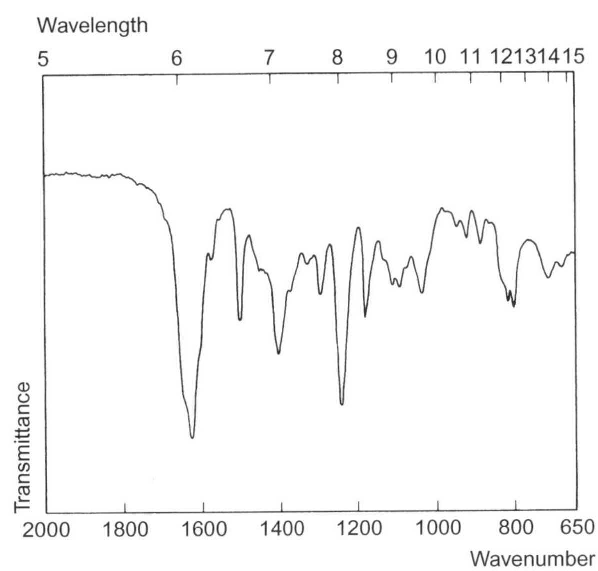

Mass Spectrum. Principal ions at *m/z* 72, 30, 56, 98, 43, 107, 41, 73.

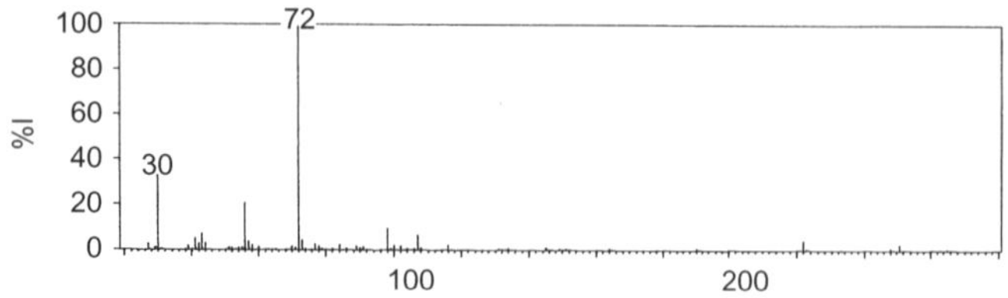

Quantification

Gas chromatography. In plasma or urine: limit of detection 5 μg/L, ECD—M. Ervik *et al.*, *J. Chromatogr.* 1980, *182(8) B Biomed. Appl.*, 341–347.

High performance liquid chromatography. In plasma or whole blood: limit of detection 2 μg/L, fluorescence detection—Y. G. Yee *et al.*, *J. Chromatogr.*, 1979, *171*, 357–362. In plasma, urine, or breast-milk: limit of detection <50 μg/L, fluorescence detection—D. W. Holt *et al.*, *Br. J. Clin. Pharmacol.*, 1982, *14*, 148P–149P. In plasma or urine: atenolol and other beta-blockers, limits of detection for atenolol 5 μg/L in plasma and 50 μg/L in urine, fluorescence detection—K. U. Buhring and A. Garbe, *J. Chromatogr.*, 1986, *383*, 215–224. In serum: fluorescence detection—T. Alebic-Kolbah *et al.*, *J. Pharm. Biomed. Anal.*, 1989, *7*, 1777–1781. In plasma or urine: atenolol enantiomers, fluorescence detection—R. Mehvar, *J. Pharm. Sci.*, 1989, *78*, 1035–1039. In plasma or urine: *R*- and *S*-atenolol, limits of detection <6 μg/L, fluorescence detection—M. Enquist and J. Hermansson, *Chirality*, 1989, *1*, 209–215. In blood: limit of detection <10 μg/L, fluorescence detection—R. B. Miller, *J. Pharm. Biomed. Anal.*, 1991, *9*, 849–853. In plasma or urine: limit of detection 0.5 μg/L, fluorescence detection—R. G. Morris *et al.*, *Ther. Drug Monit.*, 1991, *13*, 345–349. In plasma: *R*- and *S*-atenolol, limits of detection 0.5 μg and 0.6 μg respectively, fluorescence detection—G. Egginger *et al.*, *Chirality*, 1993, *5*, 505–512. In plasma: atenolol enantiomers—J. He *et al.*, *Chem. Pharm. Bull (Tokyo)*, 1993, *41*, 544–548. In plasma or urine: limit of detection 1 μg/L, fluorescence detection—F. C. Chiu *et al.*, *J. Chromatogr. B Biomed. Sci. Appl.*, 1997, *691*, 473–477. In plasma: atenolol and chlorthalidone, fluorescence detection for atenolol—C. Giachetti *et al.*, *J. Chromatogr. B Biomed. Sci. Appl.*, 1997, *698*, 187–194. In urine: atenolol enantiomers, fluorescence detection—G. Lamprecht *et al.*, *J. Chromatogr. B Biomed. Sci. Appl.*, 2000, *740*, 219–226. In plasma or urine: atenolol enantiomers, limit of detection <10 μg/L—M. H. Iha *et al.*, *J. Chromatogr. B Anal. Technol. Biomed. Life Sci.*, 2002, *767*, 1–9.

Thin-layer chromatography. In plasma or urine: limits of detection 5 μg/L in plasma and 500 μg/L in urine, fluorescence detection—M. Schaefer and E. Mutschler, *J. Chromatogr.*, 1979, *169*, 477–481.

Review. In biological fluids: HPLC methods for enantiomers of atenolol and other beta-blockers—G. Egginger *et al.*, *Biomed. Chromatogr.*, 1993, *7*, 277–295.

Disposition in the Body. Rapidly but incompletely absorbed after oral administration. It is excreted almost entirely as unchanged drug, 35 to 50% of an oral dose being excreted in the urine and 30 to 50% in the faeces in 24 h; small amounts of 2-hydroxyatenolol and atenolol glucuronide are excreted in the urine.

Therapeutic concentration

After a single oral dose of 100 mg given to 12 subjects, peak plasma concentrations of 0.41 to 0.87 mg/L (mean 0.6) were attained in about 3 h. [J. McAinsh *et al.*, *Biopharm. Drug Dispos.*, 1980, *1*, 323–332.]

Following daily oral doses of 25, 50, and 100 mg to 7, 7, and 6 subjects respectively, mean maximum steady-state plasma concentrations of 0.12, 0.22, and 0.39 mg/L were reported 4 h after a dose; the corresponding mean trough concentrations were 0.02, 0.04, and 0.07 mg/L. [T. Ishizaki et al., *Br. J. Clin. Pharmacol.*, 1983, *16*, 17–25.]

Toxicity. Atenolol is relatively non-toxic; a case of ingestion of 1.2 g with subsequent recovery has been reported.

A 44-year-old obese female survived after ingesting 200 mg diazepam and 1000 mg atenolol in a suicide attempt. Upon admission to hospital 24 h later she was in deep coma with a blood atenolol level of 250 mg/L. [K. Hagemann, *Dtsch. Med. Wochenschr.*, 1986, *111*, 1523–1525].

A man survived after ingesting a massive overdose of atenolol and diazepam despite having an atenolol level of 35 mg/L. [C. P. Snook *et al*, *J. Toxicol. Clin. Toxicol.*, 2000, *38*, 661–665.]

A 28-year-old patient with end-stage renal failure suffered cardiac arrest and cardiogenic shock after receiving an overdose of atenolol. During haemodialysis with charcoal haemoperfusion (4 dialyses carried out over 72 h), plasma atenolol levels declined from 7.4 to 2.1 mg/L. [S. D. Salhanick and P. M. Wax, *Vet. Hum. Toxicol.*, 2000, *42*, 224–225.]

Bioavailability. About 50%.

Half-life. Plasma half-life, 4 to 14 h (mean 7).

Volume of distribution. About 0.5 to 1.5 L/kg.

Clearance. Plasma clearance, about 2 mL/min/kg.

Distribution in blood. Plasma:whole blood ratio, about 0.8 to 0.9.

Protein binding. In plasma, less than 5%.

Note. For reviews of the pharmacokinetics of atenolol, see R. C. Heel *et al.*, *Drugs*, 1979, *17*, 425–460 and W. Kirch and K. G. Görg, *Eur. J. Drug Metab. Pharmacokinet.*, 1982, *7*, 81–91.

Dose. 50 to 100 mg daily.

Atorvastatin

HMG-CoA Reductase Inhibitor

Synonym. CI-981

[*R*-(R^*,R^*)]-2-(4-Fluorophenyl)-β,δ-dihydroxy-5-(1-methylethyl)-3-phenyl-4-[(phenylamino)carbonyl]-1*H*-pyrrole-1-heptanoic acid

$C_{33}H_{35}FN_2O_5$=558.7

CAS—134523-00-5

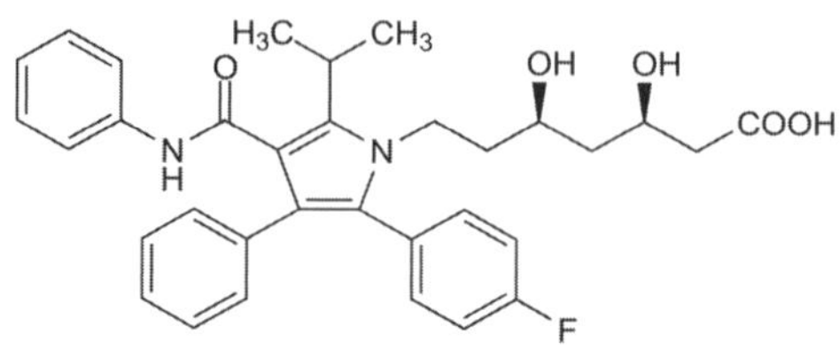

Atorvastatin Calcium

Proprietary names. Lipitor; Sortis; Torvast; Totalip; Xarator.

$C_{66}H_{68}CaF_2N_4O_{10}$,$3H_2O$=1209.4

CAS—134523-03-8

A white to off-white crystalline powder, which is insoluble in aqueous solutions with pH ⩽4.0. It is very slightly soluble in distilled water, phosphate buffer (pH 7.4) and acetonitrile; slightly soluble in ethanol; freely soluble in methanol.

Atorvastatin Lactone

$C_{33}H_{33}FN_2O_4$=540.6

M.p. 159.2° to 160.7°. Solubility, 1.34 ± 0.53 mg/L (pH 2.3 to 7.7 at 30°).

Atorvastatin Sodium

$C_{33}H_{34}FN_2NaO_5$=580.6

Soluble in water at 30°, with a solubility of 20.4 mg/L at pH 2.1 and 1.23 g/L at pH 6.0.

Dissociation Constant. pK_a 4.46.

Partition Coefficient. Log *P* (octanol/water), 6.36.

High Performance Liquid Chromatography. Column: C_{18} (YMC J'Sphere H80, 4 μm, 150 × 2 mm i.d.). Mobile phase: acetonitrile:acetic acid (0.1%) (70:30). Flow rate: 0.2 mL/min. MS–MS detection. Retention times: *para*-hydroxyatorvastatin, 2.27 min; *ortho*-hydroxyatorvastatin, 3.36 min; atorvastatin, 4.12 min. [W. W. Bullen *et al.*, *J. Am. Soc. Mass Spectrom.*, 1999, *10*, 55–66].

Column: ODS (Ultrasphere, 5 μm, 250 × 4.6 mm). Mobile phase: acetonitrile:sodium acetate in water, pH adjusted to 4.0 with glacial acetic acid (50 mM) (60:40), 1.0 mL/min flow rate. UV detection (λ=246 nm). Retention time: atorvastatin sodium, 4 min; atorvastatin lactone, 7 min. [A. S. Kearney *et al.*, *Pharm. Res.*, 1993, *10*, 1461–1465].

Column: YMC basic (5 μm, 2 × 50 mm) (at 40°). Mobile phases: (gradient elution) A—water:methanol:formic acid (88%) (950 mL:50 mL:43 μL), B—acetonitrile:methanol:formic acid (950 mL:50 mL:43 μL). 70% A and 30% B to 45% A and 55% B, 0 to 1 min; hold 0.5 min; to 70% A and 30% B, 0.1 min; hold, 0.3 mL/min flow rate. MS–MS detection. Retention time: atorvastatin, 2.78 min; 2-hydroxyatorvastatin, 2.69 min; 4-hydroxyatorvastatin, 2.31 min. [M. Jemal *et al.*, *Rapid Commun. Mass Spectrom.*, 1999, *13*, 1003–1015].

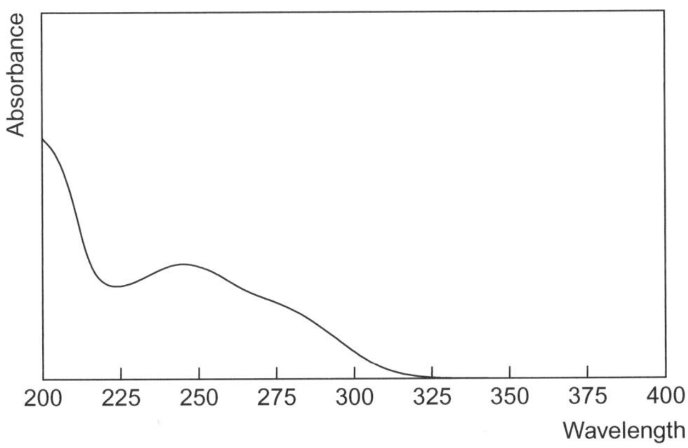

Quantification

High performance liquid chromatography. In plasma: limit of quantification is 0.25 μg/L. MS–MS detection—W. W. Bullen *et al.*, *J. Am. Soc. Mass Spectrom.*, 1999, *10*, 55–66. In serum: 0.5 μg/L. MS–MS detection—M. Jemal *et al.*, *Rapid Commun. Mass Spectrom.*, 1999, *13*, 1003–1015.

Bioassay. In plasma: limit of quantification is 0.36 μg/L—Y. Y. Shum *et al.*, *Ther. Drug Monit.*, 1998, *20*, 41–49. In plasma: limit of quantification 0.3 μg/L—D. M. Gibsa *et al.*, *J. Clin. Pharmacol.*, 1996, *36*, 242–246.

Disposition in the Body. Atorvastatin is rapidly absorbed after oral administration, which increases in proportion to the dose administered. Absolute bioavailability is approximately 12% due to presystemic clearance in the gastro-intestinal mucosa and metabolism by cytochrome P450 3A4 in the liver. A number of metabolites have been identified, all with inhibitory activity, including 2- and 4-hydroxyatorvastatin, *ortho-* and *para*-hydroxylated derivatives and various β-oxidation products. Atorvastatin is excreted as metabolites, primarily in bile, with less than 2% of the dose present in urine.

Therapeutic concentration

16 young, healthy men and women, aged between 19 and 35 years, and 16 healthy, elderly men and women, 66 to 92 years old, were administered with a 20-mg dose of atorvastatin, after fasting for 8 h. Maximum plasma concentrations for the young volunteers reached 12.7 μg/L within 1 to 2 h and 18.1 μg/L for the elderly. Differences were also observed between the men and women with 14.2 μg/L (within 2.3 h) and 16.7 μg/L (1.4 h), respectively. [D. M. Gibsa *et al.*, *J. Clin. Pharmacol.*, 1996, *36*, 242–246].

Toxicity

A 73-year-old, moderately obese woman with type II diabetes and hypertension was admitted to hospital. She had been receiving a number of medications with no other problems and was prescribed a 10 mg daily dose of atorvastatin. 4 days later, she developed a red, itchy, painful rash (potentially life-threatening dermatosis). Treatment with atorvastatin was stopped but she still developed severe stomatitis, diffuse erythema, oedema of face, trunk and extremities, and other symptoms. Supportive care including intravenous fluids, morphine, corticosteroids and a liquid diet were required. She eventually recovered after being seriously ill for 4 months. [C. M. Pfeiffer *et al.*, *J. Am. Med. Ass.*, 1998, *279*, 1613–1614].

Half-life. Elimination half-life, approximately 14 h.

Volume of distribution. Mean, approximately 565 L.

Distribution in blood. Blood cells:plasma, 0.25.

Protein binding. 98% plasma protein bound.

Dose. An initial dose of 10 mg daily is administered with a maximum of 80 mg daily.

Atovaquone

Antiprotozoal

Synonyms. 566C80; BW-566C; BW-566C-80.
Proprietary names. Acuvel; Mepron; Wellvone.
trans-2-[4-(4-Chlorophenyl)cyclohexyl]-3-hydroxy-1,4-naphthalenedione
$C_{22}H_{19}O_3Cl = 366.8$
CAS—95233-18-4

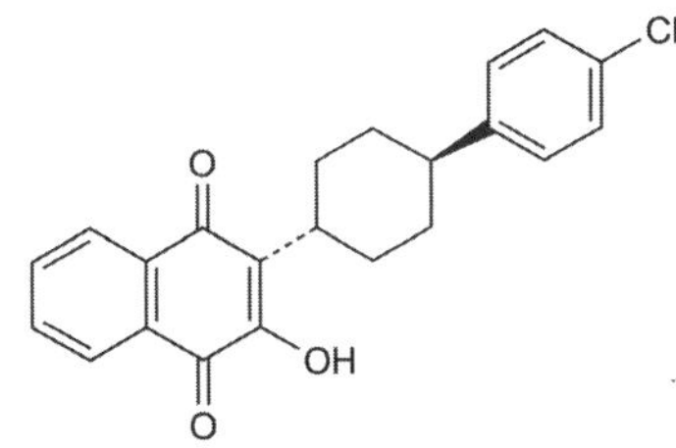

A yellow crystalline solid. Also, reported as crystals from acetonitrile with m.p. 216° to 219°. It is practically insoluble in water (>0.2 mg/L); poorly soluble in a variety of organic solvents.

High Performance Liquid Chromatography. Column: C_6 (Spherisorb, 250 × 4.6 mm i.d., 5 μm). Mobile phase: methanol:10 mM triethylamine in 0.2% aqueous trifluoroacetic acid, pH 2 (76:24), 1 mL/min flow rate. UV detection (λ = 254 nm). Retention time: 8.8 min. [A. G. Hansson *et al.*, *J. Chromatogr. Biomed. Sci. Appl.*, 1996, *675*, 180–182].

Ultraviolet Spectrum. Basic—252, 276 nm.

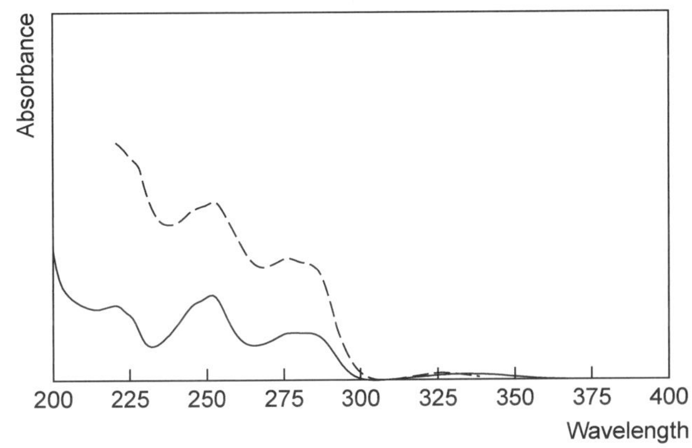

Infra-red Spectrum. Principal peaks at wavenumber 1659, 1278, 1370 cm^{-1} (KBr pellet).

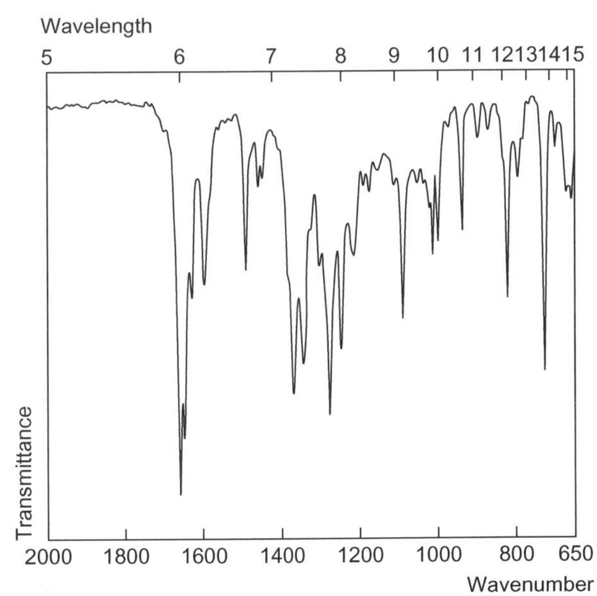

Mass Spectrum. Principal peaks at *m/z* 202, 366, 115, 77, 368, 125, 105, 213.

Quantification

Gas chromatography. In plasma: sensitivity 0.01 mg/L, ECD—P. E. Rolan *et al.*, *Br. J. Clin. Pharmacol.*, 1994, *37*, 13–20.

High performance liquid chromatography. In plasma: limit of detection 0.05 mg/L, UV detection—P. E. Rolan *et al.*, *Br. J. Clin. Pharmacol.*, 1994,

37, 13–20. In plasma: limit of quantification 0.25 mg/L, UV detection (λ=254 nm)—D. V. DeAngelis *et al.*, *J. Chromatogr. Biomed. Sci. Appl.*, 1994, *652*, 211–219. In plasma: limit of detection 0.25 mg/L, UV detection—S. D. Studenberg *et al.*, *J. Pharm. Biomed. Anal.*, 1995, *13*, 1383–1393. In plasma: limit of detection 0.5 mg/L, UV detection—A. G. Hansson *et al.*, *J. Chromatogr. Biomed. Sci. Appl.*, 1996, *675*, 180–182. In plasma: limit of quantification 0.1 mg/L, UV detection (λ=254 nm)—S. L. Hannan *et al.*, *J. Chromatogr. Biomed. Sci. Appl.*, 1996, *678*, 297–302.

Disposition in the Body. Atovaquone is rapidly but poorly absorbed after oral administration; bioavailability shows considerable inter-individual variation and is increased by concomitant administration with food, especially food with high fat content. The drug is excreted almost entirely in faeces (94% of an administered dose over 21 days) as the unchanged drug, with little present in urine. There is no evidence that atovaquone is metabolised in the body. It may undergo enterohepatic recycling. Plasma concentrations do not increase proportionally with dose.

Therapeutic concentration

6 male individuals, HIV-sero-positive, with CD4 counts >200 cells/mm^3 were administered with single 500, 1000 and 1500 mg doses after an overnight fast. Peak plasma concentrations reached 2.7, 5.6 and 4.3 mg/L, respectively, between 1.5 and 2.5 h. Following administration of 1000 mg daily with a high-fat meal and 1000 mg twice daily with or without a high-fat meal, for 14 days, the mean concentrations were 24.2, 41.3 and 34.4 mg/L, respectively. These levels were detected at 9.1, 3.7 and 2.1 h. [R. Dixon *et al.*, *Antimicrob. Agents Chemother.*, 1996, *40*, 556–560].

The mean peak plasma concentration occurring 6 h after administration of 750 mg three times a day for 5 days followed by 750 mg twice a day for 16 days, with a standard breakfast, was 51 mg/L in 4 male subjects, aged over 18 years, with CD4 counts ⩾250 cells/mm^3. Single doses of 100, 250, 750, 1500 and 3000 mg administered to the same group produced peak concentrations of 4.5, 14.3, 37.9, 33.4 and 39.0 mg/L, respectively, observed between 4 and 8 h. [W. T. Hughes *et al.*, *J. Infect. Dis.*, 1991, *163*, 843–848].

Toxicity. It is safe to give doses of up to 3000 mg daily.

Half-life. Plasma, between 60 and 70 h.

Volume of distribution 0.6 L/kg.

Clearance. Plasma, 0.15 mL/min/kg; also, reported as 1.56 L/h.

Protein binding. In plasma, more than 99%.

Note. For reviews of atovaquone see L. G. Haile and J. F. Flaherty, *Ann. Pharmacother.*, 1993, *27*, 1488–1494 and C. M. Spencer and K. L. Goa, *Drugs*, 1995, *50*, 176–196.

Dose. 750 mg as an oral suspension twice a day or 750 mg as tablets three times a day.

Atracurium

Skeletal Muscle Relaxant

2,2′-[1,5-Pentanediylbis[oxy(3-oxo-3,1-propanediyl)]]bis[1-[(3,4-dimethoxyphenyl)-methyl]-1,2,3,4-tetrahydro-6,7-dimethoxy-2-methylisoquinolinium]
$C_{53}H_{72}N_2O_{12}$=929.2
CAS—64228-79-1

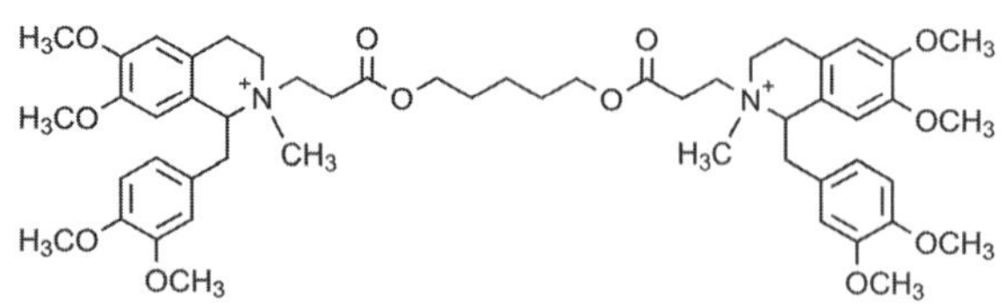

Atracurium Besilate

Synonyms. Atracurium besylate; BW-33A.
Proprietary name. Tracrium
$C_{53}H_{72}N_2O_{12},2C_6H_5O_3S$=1243.5
CAS—64228-81-5
An off-white powder. M.p. 85° to 90°. Softens at 60°.

High Performance Liquid Chromatography. Column: (analytical) µPorasil (150 × 3.9 mm i.d.); (pre-column) (0.002 mm). Mobile phase: acetonitrile:0.002 M sulfuric acid (50:50), 2 mL/min flow rate. UV detection (λ=210 nm). Retention time: 3.5 min. [A. R. Bjorksten *et al.*, *J. Chromatogr.*, 1990, *533*; *Biomed. Appl.*, *98*, 241–247].

Column: Spherisorb C_8 (100 × 4.9 mm, 5 µm). Mobile phase: (A)—acetonitrile:methanol:0.03 M dibasic potassium phosphate buffer (37.5:5:57.5); (B)—acetonitrile:methanol:0.1 M dibasic potassium phosphate buffer (37.5:15:47.5), final pH 5. Elution program: 0 to 100% (B) over 8 min, 1.7 mL/min flow rate. Fluorescence detection (λ_{ex}=240 nm, λ_{em}=320 nm). Retention time: 6.2 min. [F. Varin *et al.*, *J. Chromatogr.*, 1990, *529*; *Biomed. Appl.*, *94*, 319–327].

Ultraviolet Spectrum. Ethanol—231, 280 nm; basic—281 nm.

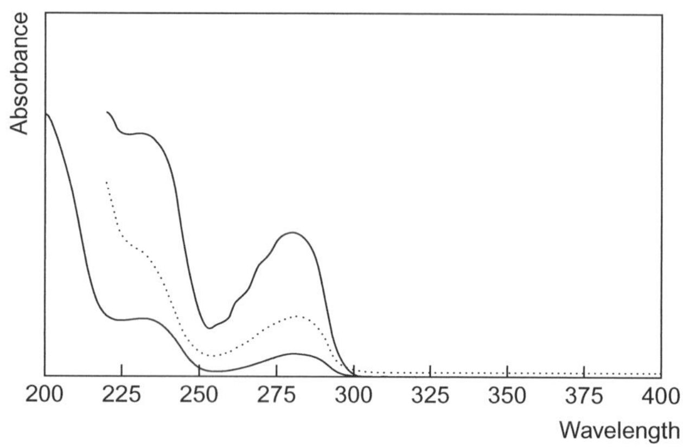

Infra-red Spectrum. Principal peaks at wavenumber 1725, 1513, 1189 cm^{-1} (KBr pellets).

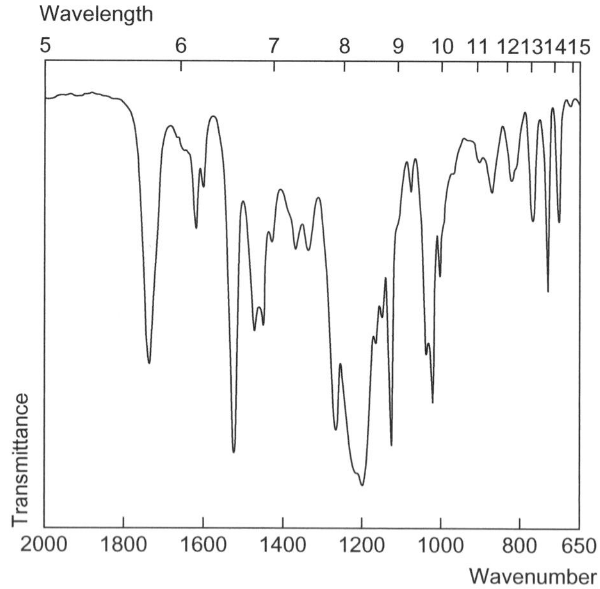

Quantification

High performance liquid chromatography. In plasma: atracurium and laudanosine, limit of detection 0.025 mg/L, UV detection (λ=210 nm)—A. R. Bjorksten *et al.*, *J. Chromatogr.*, 1990, *533*; *Biomed. Appl.*, *98*, 241–247. In plasma: atracurium and laudanosine, limit of detection 0.02 mg/L and 0.01 mg/L respectively, fluorescence detection (λ_{ex}=240 nm, λ_{em}=320 nm)—F. Varin *et al.*, *J. Chromatogr.*, 1990, *529*; *Biomed. Appl.*, *94*, 319–327. In plasma: atracurium and laudanosine, limit of detection about 0.01 mg/L atracurium and 0.005 mg/L laudanosine, fluorescence detection—R. J. Simmonds, *J. Chromatogr.*, 1985, *343*; *Biomed. Appl.*, *44*, 431–436.

Disposition in the Body. After intravenous administration, it is inactivated in plasma by Hofmann elimination, a non-enzymatic breakdown process occurring at physiological pH and temperature, to produce laudanosine and other metabolites. It also undergoes ester hydrolysis by non-specific plasma esterases. The metabolites have no neuromuscular blocking activity although laudanosine may have some stimulatory action on the CNS. Excreted in urine and bile, mostly as metabolites. It crosses the placenta.

Therapeutic concentration. The serum therapeutic concentration range is 0.1 to 1.0 mg/L.

A study in 20 male and female subjects undergoing major surgery, with a mean age of 59.4 years, found that 90% paralysis was maintained by a mean infusion rate of 4.25 µg/kg/min of atracurium (mean plasma concentration 1.13 mg/L). [G. H. Beemer *et al.*, *Br. J. Anaesth.*, 1990, *65*, 668–674].

A study in 20 subjects on mechanical ventilation receiving atracurium infusion found that stable neuromuscular blockade was associated with a plasma-atracurium concentration of 1.5 mg/L, but this had increased to 5.3 mg/L at 38 h. Plasma-laudanosine concentrations were measured in 6 of the subjects and the maximum concentrations measured ranged from 1.9 to 5.1 mg/L. [P. M. Yate *et al.*, *Br. J. Anaesth.*, 1987, *59*, 211–217].

An atracurium infusion was given for 71 days to a 35-year-old intravenous drug abuser who contracted tetanus. The mean rate of infusion over the period was 1.3 mg/kg/h. There was no evidence of accumulation of laudanosine as plasma concentration at the end of the infusion was 0.985 mg/L. The plasma-atracurium concentration was 1.5 mg/L. [S. J. Peat *et al.*, *Anaesthesia*, 1988, *43*, 962–963].

Toxicity

A 59-day-old infant weighing 2.75 kg received 37 mg of atracurium over 75 min when the syringe driver was set up incorrectly. The infant made a full recovery by 135 min after the infusion was stopped. It was estimated that the plasma-laudanosine concentration at the time neuromuscular function recovered was about 19 mg/L. No atracurium was detectable in the plasma sample taken. [A. J. Charlton *et al.*, *Anaesthesia*, 1989, *44*, 485–486].

A 3-week-old ventilated neonate weighing 3.9 kg received a bolus overdose of atracurium of 5.1 mg/kg in error. Intense bronchospasm occurred, systolic blood pressure fell to 28 mmHg and pulse rate increased from 140/min to 180/min. The neonate recovered within 3 h following treatment with adrenaline and ventilatory support. [J. Durcan and J. A. Carter, *Anaesthesia*, 1986, *41*, 767].

Half-life. Plasma, atracurium 20 min; laudanosine 3 h.

Volume of distribution. 0.16 L/kg.

Clearance. Plasma, 4.4 to 6.5 mL/min/kg.

Protein binding. In plasma, 80%.

Dose. Initially 300 to 600 µg/kg of atracurium besilate intravenously with subsequent doses of 100 to 200 µg/kg as necessary; 5 to 10 µg/kg/min has been given as a continuous intravenous infusion.

Atrazine

Herbicide

6-Chloro-*N*-ethyl-*N*′-(1-methylethyl)-1,3,5-triazine-2,4-diamine
$C_8H_{14}ClN_5$=215.7
CAS—1912-24-9

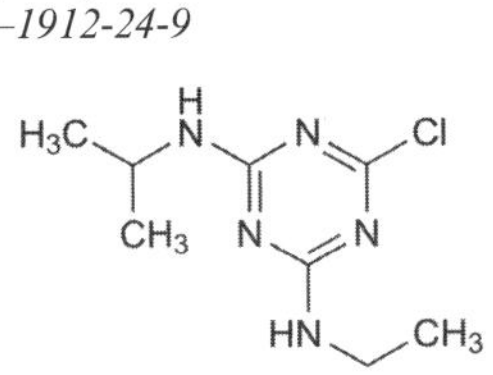

Colourless crystals. M.p. 171° to 174°.
Practically insoluble in water; soluble 1 in 20 of chloroform, 1 in 80 of ether, and 1 in 55 of methanol.

Dissociation Constant. pK_a 1.7.

Partition Coefficient. Log *P* (octanol/water), 2.6.

Thin-layer Chromatography. System TA—Rf 77; system TAB—Rf 04; system TAC—Rf 08.

Gas Chromatography. System GA—atrazine RI 1714, M (desethyl-) RI 1680, M (desethyl-deschloro-methoxy-) RI 1670; system GK—RRT 0.79 (relative to caffeine).

High Performance Liquid Chromatography. System HY—RI 401; system HAA—retention time 18.2 min; system HAO—*k* 10.75; system HAP—*k* 1.24.

Ultraviolet Spectrum. Ethanol—263 nm (A^1_1=195b).

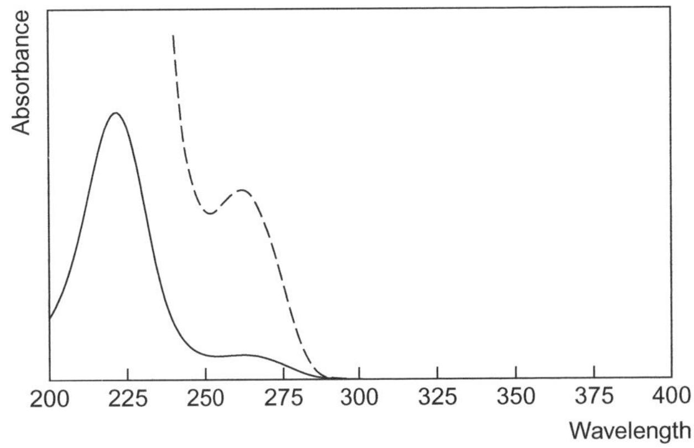

Infra-red Spectrum. Principal peaks at wavenumbers 1539, 1612, 1295, 804, 1161, 1121 cm^{-1} (KBr disk).

Mass Spectrum. Principal ions at *m/z* 43, 58, 44, 200, 68, 215, 41, 42.

Quantification

High performance liquid chromatography–mass spectrometry. In urine: atrazine metabolites—B. A. Buchholz *et al.*, *Anal. Chem.*, 1999, *71*, 3519–3525. In urine: atrazine metabolites, limit of detection 0.5 µg/L—M. D. Beeson *et al.*, *Anal. Chem.*, 1999, *71*, 3526–3530. In urine: atrazine and other pesticide metabolites, limits of detection 0.2 to 0.5 µg/L—S. E. Baker *et al.*, *J. Exp. Anal. Environ. Epidemiol.*, 2000, *10*, 789–798.

Immunoassay. In urine: atrazine and its major metabolite, ELISA—A. D. Lucas *et al.*, *Chem. Res. Toxicol.*, 1993, *6*, 107–116.

Toxicity.

In a fatality involving the ingestion of 500 mL of a herbicide mix containing atrazine (100 g), aminotriazole (25 g), ethylene glycol (25 g), and formaldehyde (0.15 g), the postmortem tissue concentrations of atrazine were reported to be: liver 32.04 µg/g, pancreas 30.99 µg/g, small intestine µg/g, kidney 97.62 µg/g, lung 79.53 µg/g, heart 15.27 µg/g, muscle 19.93 µg/g. At the time of death, about 3 days after ingestion, the plasma atrazine concentration was 1.49 mg/L. [J. Pommery *et al.*, *Clin Toxicol.*, 1993, *31*, 323–331.]

Atropine

Anticholinergic

Synonym. (±)-Hyoscyamine
Proprietary name. Atropinol
Atropine and its salts are ingredients in and also used as adjuncts in many proprietary preparations—see *Martindale, The complete drug reference*, 33rd Edn., Pharmaceutical Press, London, 2002.
(3-*endo*)-8-Methyl-8-azabicyclo[3.2.1]oct-3-yl-α-(hydroxymethyl)-benzeneacetate
$C_{17}H_{23}NO_3$=289.4
CAS—51-55-8

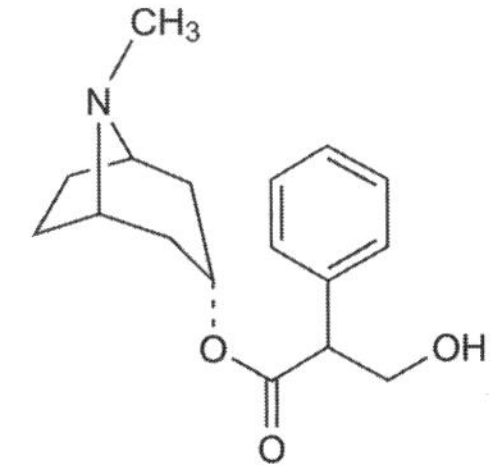

An alkaloid obtained from *Duboisia* spp. and other solanaceous plants, or prepared by synthesis.
Colourless crystals or white crystalline powder. M.p. 114° to 118°.
Soluble 1 in 455 of water, 1 in 50 of boiling water, 1 in 2 of ethanol, 1 in 1 of chloroform, 1 in 25 of ether, and 1 in 27 of glycerol.

Atropine Sulfate

Proprietary names. AtroPen; Atropisol; Atropocil; Atropt; Atrospan; Liotropina; Ocu-Tropine; Sal-Tropine.

$(C_{17}H_{23}NO_3)_2,H_2SO_4,H_2O$=694.8

CAS—55-48-1 (anhydrous); 5908-99-6 (monohydrate)

Colourless crystals or white crystalline powder. It effloresces in dry air. M.p. about 190°, with decomposition, after drying at 135° for 15 min.

Soluble 1 in 0.4 of water and 1 in 5 of ethanol; practically insoluble in chloroform and ether.

Dissociation Constant. pK_a 9.9 (20°).

Partition Coefficient. Log *P* (octanol/water), 1.8.

Colour Test. Liebermann's Test—red-orange.

Thin-layer Chromatography. System TA—Rf 18; system TB—Rf 05; system TC—Rf 03; system TE—Rf 24; system TL—Rf 01; system TAE—Rf 05; system TAF—Rf 28; system TAJ—Rf 00; system TAK—Rf 00; system TAL—Rf 14. (Dragendorff spray, positive; acidified iodoplatinate solution, positive; Marquis reagent, pink.)

Gas Chromatography. System GA—atropine RI 2190, Art (-CH_2O) RI 1980, Art (-H_2O) RI 2085, atropine-AC RI 2275; system GB—atropine RI 2293, Art (-CH_2O) RI 2051, Art (-H_2O) RI 2250; system GF—RI 2660.

High Performance Liquid Chromatography. System HA—*k* 3.9 (tailing peak); system HX—RI 306; system HY—RI 251; system HZ—retention time 2.2 min; system HAA—retention time 10.4 min; system HAX—retention time 7.0 min; system HAY—retention time 3.8 min.

Ultraviolet Spectrum. Aqueous acid—252, 258 nm (A^1_1=6.3c), 264 nm. No alkaline shift.

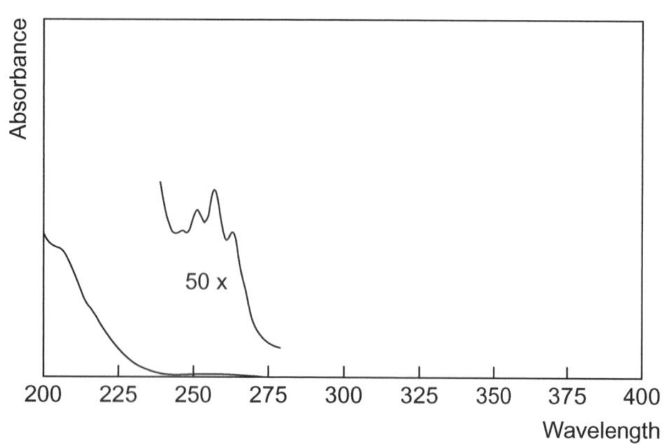

Infra-red Spectrum. Principal peaks at wavenumbers 1720, 1035, 1153, 1163, 1063, 1204 cm^{-1} (KBr disk).

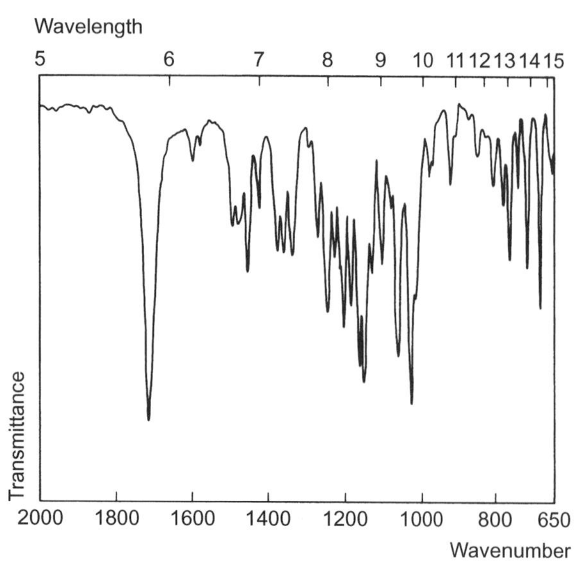

Mass Spectrum. Principal ions at *m/z* 124, 82, 94, 83, 42, 96, 103, 67.

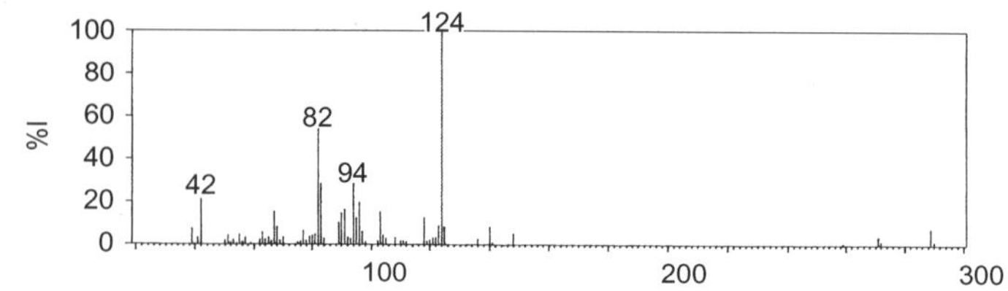

Quantification

Gas chromatography–mass spectrometry. In blood: limit of detection <10 μg/L—J. J. Saady and A. Poklis, *J. Anal. Toxicol.*, 1989, *13*, 296–299.

High performance liquid chromatography. In biological samples: UV detection—T. Okuda *et al.*, *J. Chromatogr.*, 1991, *567*, 141–149.

Radioimmunoassay. In plasma or serum: atropine and hyoscyamine, limit of detection 2.5 μg/L for both compounds—R. Virtanen *et al.*, *Acta Pharmacol. Toxicol.*, 1980, 47, 208–212.

Disposition in the Body. Readily absorbed from the mucous membranes, skin and gastro-intestinal tract but not from the stomach. About 80 to 90% of a dose is excreted in the urine in 24 h, 50% of the dose as unchanged drug, less than 2% as tropic acid and tropine, and about 30% as unknown metabolites. Traces of the dose are eliminated in the faeces.

Therapeutic concentration

Following an intravenous dose of 1 mg to 6 subjects, plasma concentrations of about 0.25 mg/L were observed at 2 min decreasing to 0.005 mg/L at 20 min; following an intramuscular dose of 1 mg to 4 subjects, peak plasma concentrations of about 0.003 mg/L were attained in 30 min. [L. Berghem *et al.*, *Br. J. Anaesth.*, 1980, *52*, 597–601.]

Toxicity. The amount of a toxic dose appears to vary considerably with individuals. Fatalities are reported to have occurred with doses of 50 to 100 mg but recovery has occurred after administration of 1 g; doses of 10 mg or less may be lethal in children or in susceptible individuals.

A man was found dead after having ingested an unknown amount of atropine sulfate tablets. The blood contained 0.2 mg/L and the urine 1.5 mg/L of atropine. [B. W. Corbett and A. J. McBay, *Bull. Int. Assoc. Forensic Toxicol.*, 1978, *14*(1), 36–37.]

Of 240 children accidentally injected with automatic atropine injectors, which had been distributed in Israel during the Persian Gulf Crisis as an antidote to chemical warfare agents, 20 (8%) showed signs of severe atropinization; no fatalities occurred. High serum atropine levels of 6.2 to 61 μg/L were noted approximately 1 h after injection in 6 of the children. [Y. Amitai *et al.*, *JAMA*, 1992, *268*, 630–632.]

Half-life. Plasma half-life, about 2 to 4 h; a longer terminal phase of 13 to 38 h has also been reported.

Volume of distribution. About 2 to 3 L/kg.

Clearance. Plasma clearance, about 8 mL/min/kg.

Protein binding. In plasma, about 50%.

Dose. Usually 0.25 to 2 mg of atropine sulfate daily.

Atropine Methobromide

Anticholinergic

Synonyms. Atropine Methylbromide; Methylatropine Bromide; Mydriasine.

$C_{18}H_{26}BrNO_3$=384.3

CAS—2870-71-5

Colourless crystals or a white crystalline powder. M.p. 222° to 223°.

Soluble 1 in 1 of water and 1 in 20 of ethanol; very slightly soluble in dehydrated alcohol; almost insoluble in chloroform and ether.

Partition Coefficient. Log *P* (octanol/water), −1.6.

Colour Tests. Aromaticity (Method 2)—colourless/yellow; Liebermann's Test—orange.

Atropine Methonitrate

Anticholinergic

Synonym. Methylatropine Nitrate
$C_{18}H_{26}N_2O_6$=366.4
CAS—52-88-0
Colourless crystals or a white crystalline powder. M.p. 163°.
Soluble 1 in less than 1 of water and 1 in 13 of ethanol; very slightly soluble in chloroform and ether. Aqueous solutions are unstable.

Partition Coefficient. Log *P* (octanol/water), −2.2.

Colour Tests. Aromaticity (Method 2)—colourless/violet (transient); Liebermann's Test—orange

Thin-layer Chromatography. System TA—Rf 02; system TB—Rf 00; system TE—Rf 00; system TN—Rf 95; system TO—Rf 35; system TAE—Rf 00. (Acidified iodoplatinate solution, positive.)

High Performance Liquid Chromatography. System HX—RI 299.

Ultraviolet Spectrum. Aqueous acid—252 nm (A_1^1=about 5), 258 nm (A_1^1=about 5), 264 nm (A_1^1=about 4).

Infra-red Spectrum. Principal peaks at wavenumbers 1159, 1045, 1718, 1176, 700, 1212 cm^{-1} (Nujol mull).

Atropine Oxide

Anticholinergic

Synonyms. Aminoxytropine Tropate; Atropine Aminoxide; Atropine *N*-oxide.
(3-*endo*)-8-Methyl-8-azabicyclo[3.2.1]oct-3-yl-α-(hydroxymethyl)-benzeneacetate *N*-oxide
$C_{17}H_{23}NO_4$=305.4
CAS—4438-22-6
A very hygroscopic, crystalline powder. M.p. 127° to 128°; it decomposes at 135°.
Soluble in ethanol and chloroform; practically insoluble in ether.

Atropine Oxide Hydrochloride
Proprietary name. Génatropine
$C_{17}H_{23}NO_4$,HCl=341.8
CAS—4574-60-1
Crystals. M.p. 192° to 193°.

Thin-layer Chromatography. System TA—Rf 21. (Acidified iodoplatinate solution, positive.)

Infra-red Spectrum. Principal peaks at wavenumbers 1164, 1730, 1118, 1026, 1056, 1195 cm^{-1}.

Azacyclonol

Tranquilliser

α,α-Diphenyl-4-piperidinemethanol
$C_{18}H_{21}NO$=267.4
CAS—115-46-8

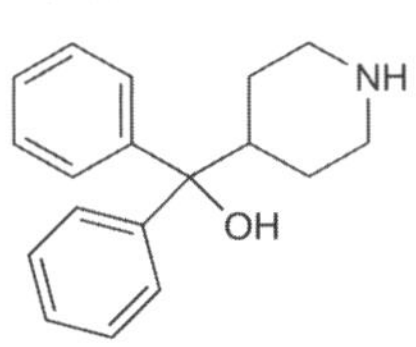

Crystals. M.p. 160° to 161°.

Azacyclonol Hydrochloride
Synonym. Azacyclonolium Chloride
Proprietary names. Frenoton; Frenquel.
$C_{18}H_{21}NO$,HCl=303.8
CAS—1798-50-1
Small white crystals or crystalline powder. M.p. 270° to 281°.
Soluble 1 in 200 of water and 1 in 1000 of ethanol; practically insoluble in acetone, chloroform, ether, and light petroleum.

Partition Coefficient. Log *P* (octanol/water), 3.4.

Colour Tests. Liebermann's Test—brown; Mandelin's Test—red; Marquis Test—yellow

Thin-layer Chromatography. System TA—Rf 10; system TB—Rf 00; system TC—Rf 03; system TE—Rf 14; system TL—Rf 01; system TAE—Rf 03; system TAL—Rf 40. (Acidified iodoplatinate solution, positive.)

Gas Chromatography. System GA—RI 2243; system GB—RI 2361.

High Performance Liquid Chromatography. System HA—*k* 1.2; system HAX—retention time 8.7 min; system HAY—retention time 4.5 min.

Ultraviolet Spectrum. Aqueous acid—253, 259 nm (A_1^1=17.4a).

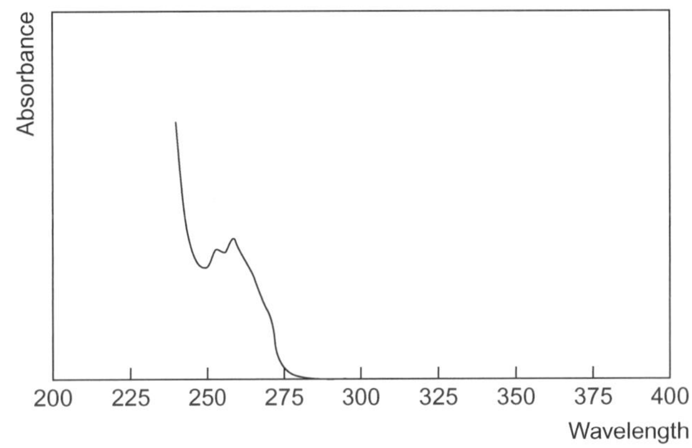

Infra-red Spectrum. Principal peaks at wavenumbers 702, 745, 1316, 1063, 971, 1155 cm^{-1} (KBr disk).

Mass Spectrum. Principal ions at *m/z* 85, 84, 183, 105, 56, 77, 55, 30.

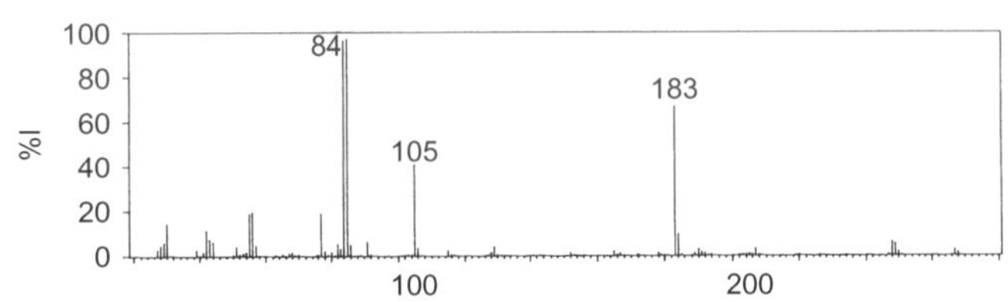

Dose. Azacyclonol hydrochloride has been given in doses of 100 to 800 mg daily.

Azaperone

Tranquilliser (Veterinary)

Proprietary names. Stresnil; Suicalm. It is an ingredient of Fentazin. (All veterinary.)
1-(4-Fluorophenyl)-4-[4-(2-pyridinyl)-1-piperazinyl]-1-butanone
$C_{19}H_{22}FN_3O$=327.4
CAS—1649-18-9

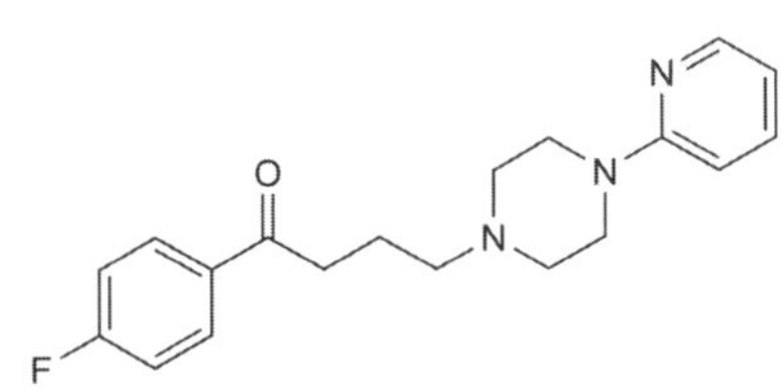

A white to yellowish-white microcrystalline powder. M.p. 73° to 75°.
Practically insoluble in water; soluble 1 in 29 of ethanol, 1 in 4 of chloroform, and 1 in 31 of ether; soluble in dilute organic acids.

Partition Coefficient. Log *P* (octanol/water), 3.3.

Colour Tests. Cyanogen Bromide—orange; Mandelin's Test—yellow

Thin-layer Chromatography. System TA—Rf 66; system TB—Rf 30; system TE—Rf 72; system TL—Rf 09; system TAE—Rf 65; system TAJ—Rf 54; system TAK—Rf 00; system TAL—Rf 67. (Acidified iodoplatinate solution, positive.)

Gas Chromatography. System GA—RI 2705; system GV—retention time 19.0 min.

High Performance Liquid Chromatography. System HX—RI 319.

Ultraviolet Spectrum. Aqueous acid—242 nm (A_1^1=800a), 312 nm; methanol—247 nm (A_1^1=1260b), 300 nm (A_1^1=200b).

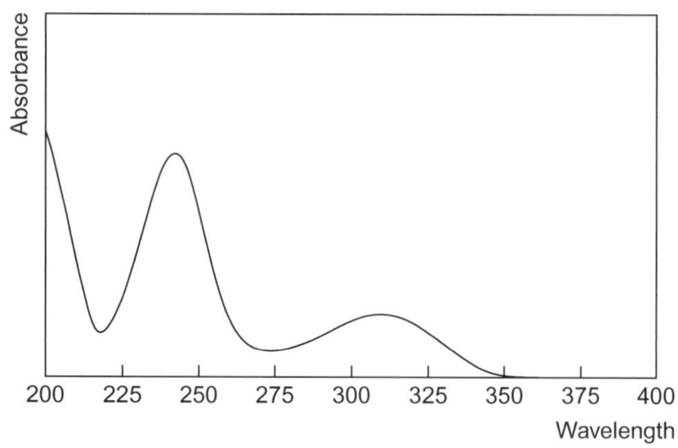

Infra-red Spectrum. Principal peaks at wavenumbers 1587, 1669, 775, 1236, 1222, 1152 cm^{-1} (KBr disk).

Mass Spectrum. Principal ions at *m/z* 107, 165, 123, 95, 121, -, -, -.

Quantification

Gas chromatography–mass spectrometry. In urine (animal): azaperone and other tranquillisers, limit of detection for azaperone 5 µg/L—M. L. Olmos-Carmona and M. Hernandez-Carrasquilla, *J. Chromatogr. B Biomed. Sci. Appl.*, 1999, *734*, 113–120. In muscle and kidney (swine): azaperone, azaperol, and carazolol—D. Fluchard *et al.*, *J. Chromatogr. B Biomed. Sci. Appl.*, 2000, *744*, 139–147.

Azapetine

Vasodilator

Synonym. Azepine

6-Allyl-6,7-dihydro-5*H*-dibenz[*c*,*E*]azepine

$C_{17}H_{17}N$=235.3

CAS—146-36-1

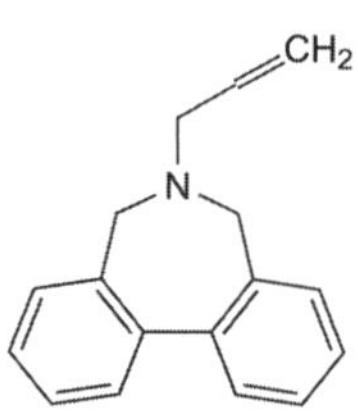

Azapetine Phosphate

$C_{17}H_{17}N,H_3PO_4$=333.3

CAS—130-83-6

Crystals. M.p. 211° to 215°, with decomposition.

Soluble at least 1 in 100 of water.

Colour Test. Mandelin's Test—brown

Thin-layer Chromatography. System TA—Rf 70; system TB—Rf 57; system TC—Rf 67; system TE—Rf 78; system TL—Rf 56; system TAE—Rf 14; system TAJ—Rf 59; system TAK—Rf 26; system TAL—Rf 90. (Acidified iodoplatinate solution, positive.)

Gas Chromatography. System GA—RI 1939.

Ultraviolet Spectrum. Aqueous acid—248 nm.

Infra-red Spectrum. Principal peaks at wavenumbers 748, 918, 1063, 990, 1111, 1639 cm^{-1} (KBr disk).

Mass Spectrum. Principal ions at *m/z* 165, 234, 194, 235, 193, 196, 166, 179.

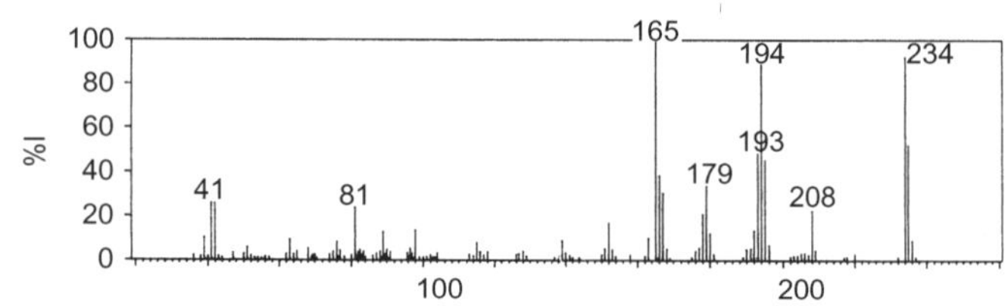

Dose. The equivalent of 75 to 225 mg of azapetine has been given daily.

Azapropazone

Analgesic

Synonym. Apazone

Proprietary names. Prolixan(a); Rheumox; Tolyprin.

5-(Dimethylamino)-9-methyl-2-propyl-1*H*-pyrazolo[1,2-*a*][1,2,4]-benzotriazine-1,3(2*H*)-dione dihydrate

$C_{16}H_{20}N_4O_2,2H_2O$=336.4

CAS—13539-59-8 (anhydrous)

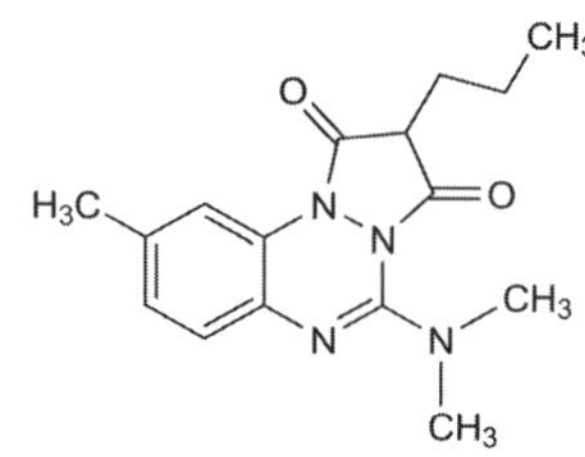

Almost colourless crystals. M.p. 228° (anhydrous); 247° to 248° (dihydrate).

Partition Coefficient. Log *P* (octanol/pH 7.4), 1.0.

Colour Tests. Liebermann's Test—grey-green; Mandelin's Test—grey-green.

Thin-layer Chromatography. System TA—Rf 68; system TB—Rf 53; system TC—Rf 05; system TE—Rf 08; system TL—Rf 67; system TAE—Rf 88; system TAJ—Rf 11; system TAK—Rf 06; system TAL—Rf 61.

Gas Chromatography. System GA—RI 2461; system GF—RI 3010.

High Performance Liquid Chromatography. System HZ—retention time 2.0 min.

Ultraviolet Spectrum. Azapropazone dihydrate: aqueous acid—250 nm (A_1^1=1040b); aqueous alkali—255 nm (A_1^1=1080b), 325 nm.

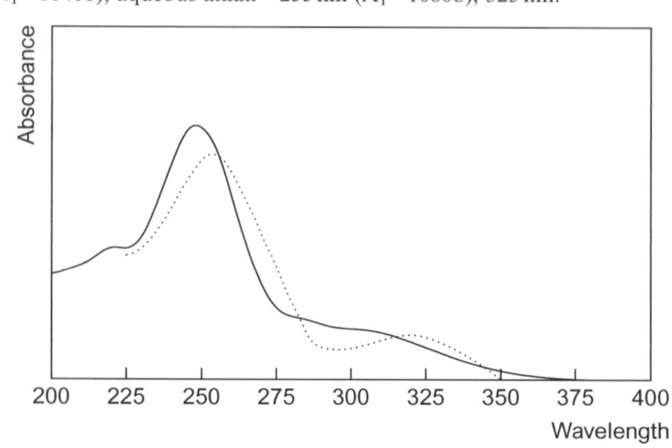

Infra-red Spectrum. Principal peaks at wavenumbers 1590, 1640, 1500, 1133, 1270, 1695 cm^{-1}.

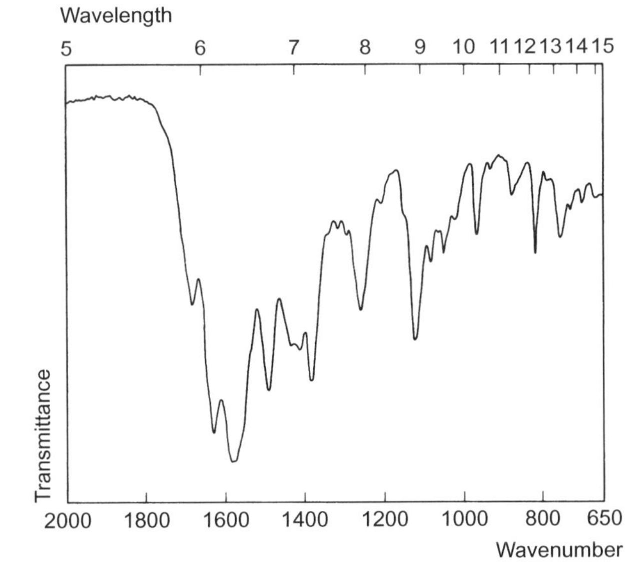

Mass Spectrum. Principal ions at m/z 160, 300, 189, 145, 188, 301, 161, 42.

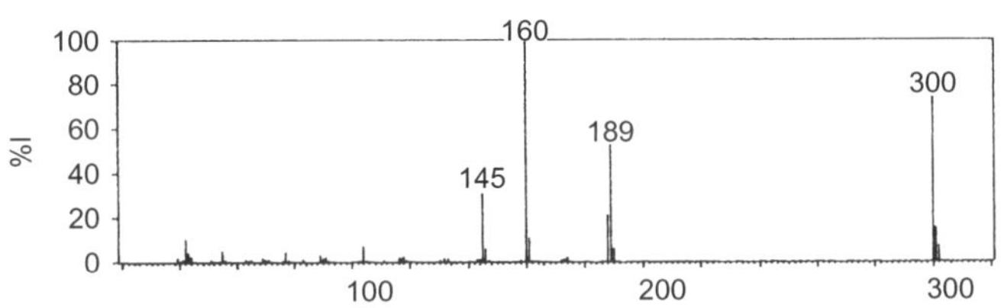

Quantification

Colorimetry. In serum: limit of detection 10 mg/L—D. S. Farrier, *Arzneimittelforschung*, 1974, *24*, 747–751.

Ultraviolet spectrophotometry. In plasma: comparison with gas chromatographic and colorimetric methods—H. Leach, *Curr. Med. Res. Opin.*, 1976, *4*, 35–43.

High performance liquid chromatography. In plasma or urine: limits of detection 400 µg/L for azapropazone and 1.5 to 3 mg/L for 6-hydroxyazapropazone, UV detection—B. J. Kline *et al.*, *Arzneimittelforschung*, 1983, *33*, 504–506.

Disposition in the Body. Readily absorbed after oral administration. About 95% of a dose is excreted in the urine, of which about 60% is unchanged drug and about 20% is the inactive metabolite, 6-hydroxyazapropazone.

Therapeutic concentration

After a single oral dose of 600 mg, administered to 6 subjects, plasma concentrations of 34 to 54 mg/L (mean 43) were attained in 4 h. [A. E. S. Ritch *et al.*, *Br. J. Clin. Pharmacol.*, 1982, *14*, 116–119.]

Steady-state plasma concentrations of 32 to 89 mg/L (mean 57) were reported during the daily administration of 800 mg to 10 subjects. [S. Thune, *Curr. Med. Res. Opin.*, 1976, *4*, 70–75.]

Half-life. Plasma half-life, 8 to 24 h (mean 15), increased in elderly subjects and in subjects with impaired renal or liver function.

Volume of distribution. About 0.2 L/kg.

Clearance. Plasma clearance, 0.1 to 0.2 mL/min/kg.

Protein binding. In plasma, about 99%.

Dose. 0.6 to 1.2 g daily.

Azatadine

Antihistamine

6,11-Dihydro-11-(1-methyl-4-piperidinylidene)-5*H*-benzo[5,6]cyclohepta-[1,2-*b*]pyridine
$C_{20}H_{22}N_2$=290.4
CAS—3964-81-6

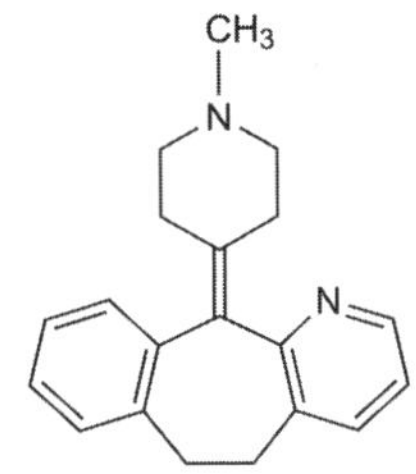

Azatadine Maleate

Proprietary names. Idulamine; Idulian; Lergocil; Optimine; Zadine.
$C_{20}H_{22}N_2,2C_4H_4O_4$=522.6
CAS—3978-86-7
A white crystalline powder.
M.p. 145° to 154°.
Soluble in water, ethanol, chloroform, dimethylformamide, and methanol; practically insoluble in ether.

Partition Coefficient. Log *P* (octanol/water), 3.6.

Colour Tests. Cyanogen Bromide—pink; Marquis Test—violet

Thin-layer Chromatography. System TA—Rf 39. (Acidified potassium permanganate solution, strong reaction.)

Gas Chromatography. System GA—azatadine RI 2377, M (OH-alkyl-)-H_2O RI 2410, M (OH-alkyl-)-AC RI 2520, M (OH-aryl-)-AC RI 2540, M (nor-)-AC RI 2720; system GB—azatadine RI 2499.

High Performance Liquid Chromatography. System HAX—retention time 10.7 min; System HAY—retention time 4.6 min.

Ultraviolet Spectrum. Aqueous acid—283 nm (A_1^1=330b).

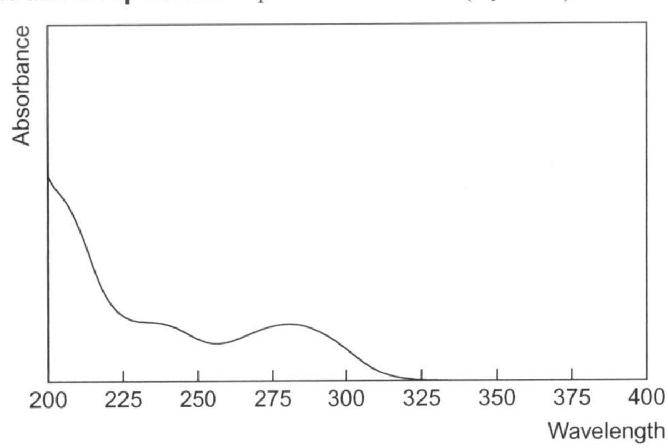

Infra-red Spectrum. Principal peaks at wavenumbers 752, 1271, 1124, 803, 984, 795 cm^{-1} (KBr disk).

Quantification

High performance liquid chromatography. In urine: UV detection—K. B. Alton *et al.*, *J. Chromatogr.*, 1987, *385*, 249–259.

Dose. 2 to 4 mg of azatadine maleate daily.

Azathioprine

Immunosuppressant

Proprietary names. Aseroprim; Azahexal; Azamun(e); Azatrilem; Azopi; Azopine; Berkaprine; Immunoprin; Imuprin; Imuran; Imurek; Imurel; Oprisine; Satedon; Thioprine; Tiosalprin; Zytrim.
6-[(1-Methyl-4-nitro-1*H*-imidazol-5-yl)thio]-1*H*-purine
$C_9H_7N_7O_2S$=277.3

CAS—446-86-6

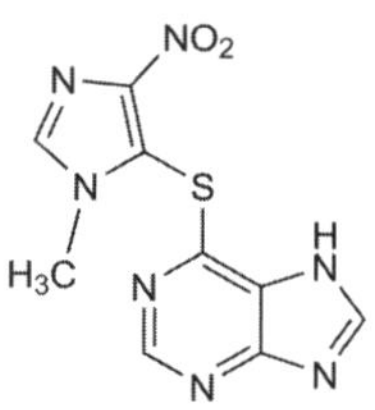

A pale yellow powder. M.p. about 238°, with decomposition.
Practically insoluble in water; very slightly soluble in ethanol and chloroform; sparingly soluble in dilute mineral acids; soluble in dilute solutions of alkali hydroxides but decomposes in stronger solutions.

Dissociation Constant. pK_a 8.2 (25°).

Partition Coefficient. Log *P* (octanol/water), 0.1.

Thin-layer Chromatography. System TA—Rf 53; system TB—Rf 03; system TC—Rf 08; system TE—Rf 06; system TL—Rf 04; system TAD—Rf 71; system TAE—Rf 80.

High Performance Liquid Chromatography. System HX—RI 323.

Ultraviolet Spectrum. Aqueous acid—280 nm (A^1_1=600a); aqueous alkali—285 nm.

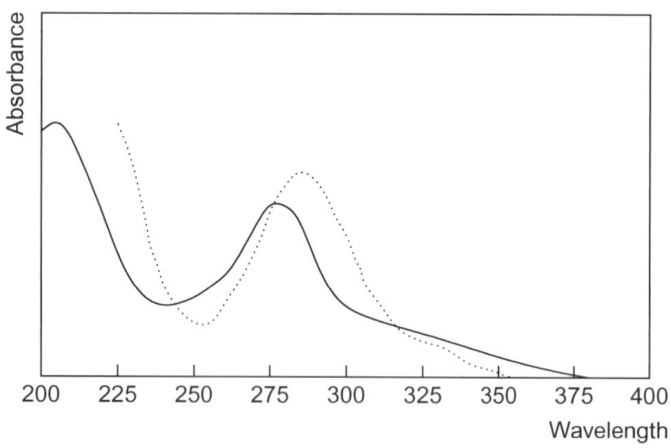

Infra-red Spectrum. Principal peaks at wavenumbers 1237, 1306, 1580, 832, 1500, 1531 cm^{-1} (KBr disk).

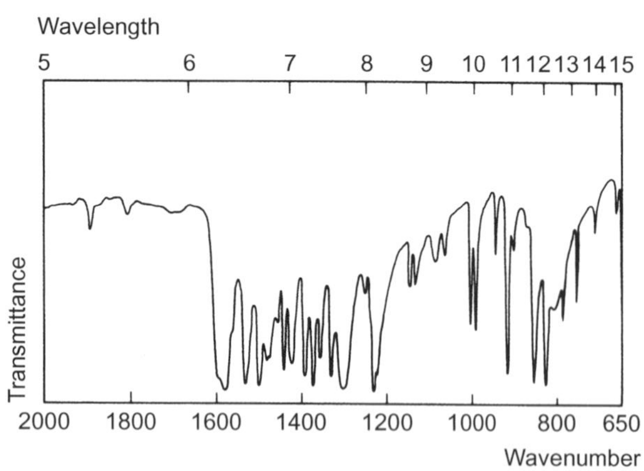

Mass Spectrum. Principal ions at *m/z* 231, 42, 119, 232, 92, 65, 67, 74.

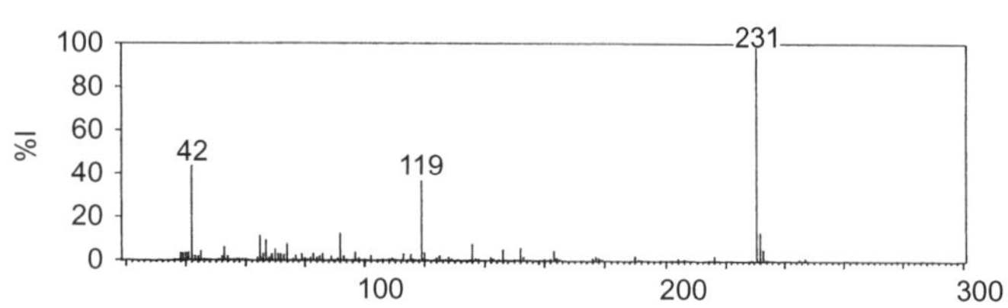

Quantification

Spectrofluorimetry. In plasma: azathioprine and mercaptopurine, limit of detection 10 µg/L—J. L. Maddocks, *Br. J. Clin. Pharmacol.*, 1979, *8*, 273–278.

High performance liquid chromatography. In plasma: azathioprine and mercaptopurine, limit of detection 40 µg/L for azathioprine and 5 µg/L for mercaptopurine, UV detection—T. L. Ding and L. Z. Benet, *J. Chromatogr.* 1979, *163(5) B Biomed. Appl.*, 281–288. In biological fluids: thiopurine metabolites of azathioprine—R. Boulieu *et al.*, *J. Chromatogr.*, 1993, *615*, 352–356. In red blood cells, plasma or urine: azathioprine metabolites, limit of detection in plasma 5 µg/L—S. Weller *et al.*, *Int. J. Clin. Pharmacol. Ther.*, 1995, *33*, 639–645. In serum: limit of detection <2.5 ng, UV detection—T. Binscheck *et al.*, *J. Chromatogr.* 1996, *675 B Biomed. Appl.*, 287–294. In plasma: azathioprine and 6-mercaptopurine, limit of detection for azathioprine <5 µg/L—E. C. Van Os *et al.*, *J. Chromatogr.* 1996, *679 B Biomed. Appl.*, 147–154. In red blood cells: azathioprine metabolites—T. Dervieux and R. Boulieu, *Clin. Chem.*, 1998, *44*, 551–55.

Disposition in the Body. Absorbed after oral administration and distributed throughout the body. It is readily metabolised to mercaptopurine, which is the major active metabolite, and to 1-methyl-4-nitro-5-(*S*-glutathionyl)-imidazole; other metabolites include 1-methyl-4-nitroimidazole, 1-methyl-4-nitro-5-thioimidazole, and 6-thiouric acid; mercaptopurine is further metabolised to its ribonucleotide, thioinosinic acid, which is the active moiety. About 50% of a dose is excreted in the urine in 24 h, mainly as thiouric acid and other metabolites, with about 10% consisting of unchanged drug; about 12% of a dose is eliminated in the faeces in 48 h.

Therapeutic concentration

After daily oral doses of 50 to 100 mg to 3 renal transplant patients, peak steady-state plasma concentrations of 0.05 to 0.08 mg/L of mercaptopurine were reported 1 h after a dose. [T. L. Ding and L. Z. Benet, *J. Chromatogr.*, 1979, *163*; *Biomed. Appl.*, *5*, 281–288.]

Half-life. Plasma half-life, azathioprine about 3 h, mercaptopurine about 0.5 to 1.5 h.

Protein binding. In plasma, about 30%.

Dose. 1 to 5 mg/kg daily, by mouth.

Azinphos-ethyl

Acaricide, Insecticide

Synonyms. Bayer 16259; ENT-22014; Ethyl Guthion; Gusathion A; R-1513.
Proprietary names. Azinos; Azinugec E; Bionex; Contrion-Ethyl; Gutex; Sepizin L; Triazotion.
Phosphorodithioic acid *O,O*-diethyl *S*-[(4-oxo-1,2,3-benzotriazin-3(4*H*)-yl)methyl] ester
$C_{12}H_{16}N_3O_3PS_2$=345.4
CAS—2642-71-9

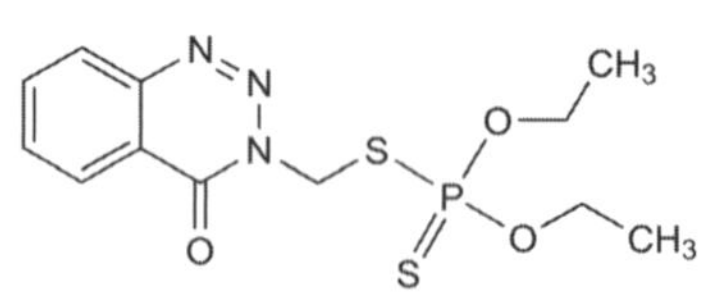

Colourless crystals. M.p. 53°. B.p. 111° at 0.001 mmHg.
It is soluble in water (4 to 5 mg/L at 20°); readily soluble in most organic solvents except aliphatic hydrocarbons.

Partition Coefficient. Log *P* (octanol/water), 3.40.

Thin-layer Chromatography. System TX—Rf 24; system TY—Rf 48; system TAE—Rf 81.

Gas Chromatography. System GA—RI 2560.

Column: 3% OV-1 on 100–120 mesh Gas-Chrom Q (1.8 m × 0.25 mm i.d.). Column temperature: 245°. Detector temperature: 300°. Carrier gas: 5% methane in argon, flow rate 50 mL/min. Detection: electron capture ^{63}Ni. Retention time: azinphos-ethyl, 1.5 min. [V. B. Stein and K. A. Pittman, *J. Ass. Off. Anal. Chem.*, 1976, *59(5)*, 1094–1096.]

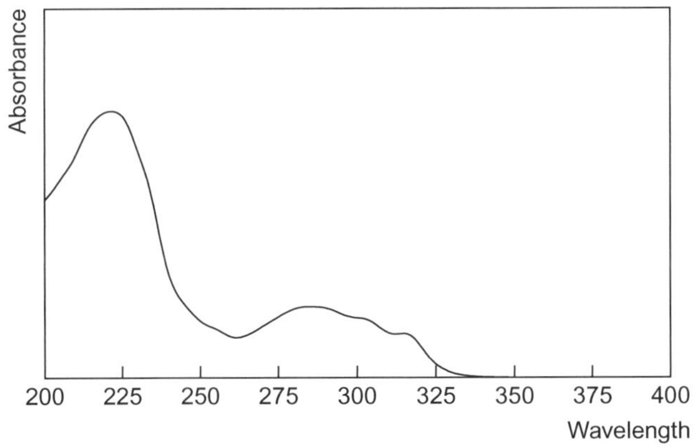

Mass Spectrum. Principal ions at *m/z* 132, 77, 160, 105, 29, 65, 76, 97.

Quantification
Gas chromatography. In plasma: limit of detection 1 μg/L. ECD—V. B. Stein and K. A. Pittman, *J. Ass. Off. Anal. Chem.*, 1976, *59(5)*, 1094–1096. In blood: limit of detection 1 μg/L, FPD—E. G. Pinto Marques, *J. Anal. Toxicol.*, 1990, *14(4)*, 243–246.

Disposition in the Body. Azinphos is rapidly absorbed from the gastro-intestinal tract after ingestion. It is excreted in urine.

Toxicity
In a series of azinphos-ethyl poisoning cases, fatal cases were found to have blood levels of 1.112 mg/L and above, serious cases of intoxication with levels of 494 μg/L and above, and less serious cases with levels above 57 μg/L. Serious intoxication was always observed with concentrations above 370 μg/L. [E. G. Pinto Marques, *J. Anal. Toxicol.*, 1990, *14*, 243–246.]

Azinphos-methyl

Pesticide

Synonym. DBD
Proprietary names. Gusathion M; Guthion.
Phosphorodithioic acid *O,O*-dimethyl-*S*-[(4-Oxo-1,2,3-benzotriazin-3(4*H*)-yl)methyl] ester
$C_{10}H_{12}N_3O_3PS_2$ = 317.3
CAS—86-50-0

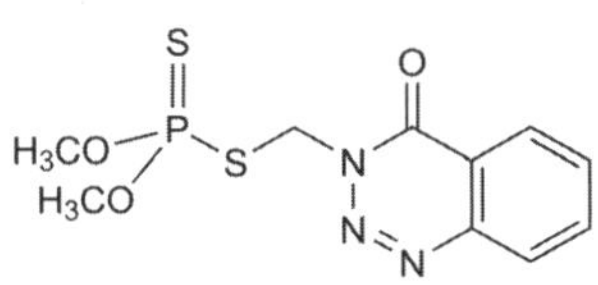

Colourless crystals. It is rapidly hydrolysed in alkaline or acid media. M.p. 73° to 74°.
Soluble 1 in 30 000 of water; soluble in ethanol, methanol, and propylene glycol.

Partition Coefficient. Log *P* (octanol/water), 2.8.

Colour Tests. Palladium Chloride—brown; Phosphorus Test—yellow

Thin-layer Chromatography. System TA—Rf 84; system TB—Rf 40; system TC—Rf 99; system TD—Rf 91; system TE—Rf 99; system TF—Rf 93; system TL—Rf 99; system TW—Rf 68; system TX—Rf 20; system TY—Rf 42; system TAD—Rf 94; system TAE—Rf 81; system TAF—Rf 87.

Gas Chromatography. System GA—RI 2473; system GK—RRT 1.60 (relative to caffeine).

High Performance Liquid Chromatography. System HY—RI 513.

Ultraviolet Spectrum. Hexane—285 nm (A^1_1 = 280b), 302, 315 nm.

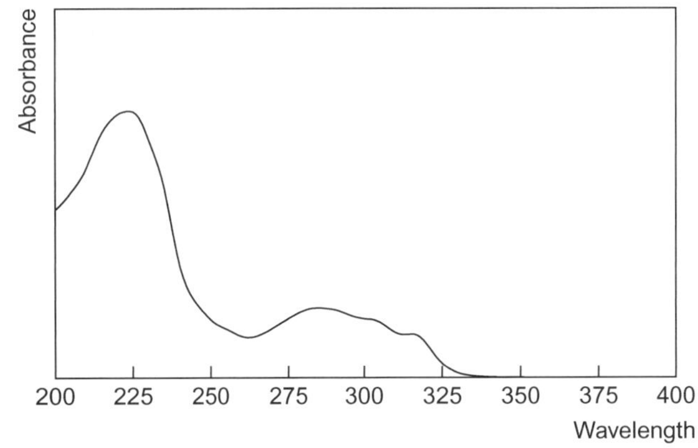

Infra-red Spectrum. Principal peaks at wavenumbers 1000, 1666, 833, 781, 1041, 775 cm^{-1}.

Mass Spectrum. Principal ions at *m/z* 77, 160, 132, 44, 105, 104, 93, 76.

Disposition in the Body.
Toxicity. Azinphos-methyl is less toxic than mevinphos or parathion. The maximum permissible atmospheric concentration is 0.2 mg/m^3.

Azithromycin

Antibacterial

Synonyms. 9-Deoxo-9a-aza-9a-methyl-9a-homoerythromycin A; CP-62993; XZ-450.
Proprietary names. Azitrocin; Azitromax; Goxil; Ribotrex; Sumamed; Toraseptol; Trozocina; Vinzam; Zentavion; Zithromax; Zitromax.
[2*R*-(2*R**,3*S**,4*R**,5*R**,8*R**,10*R**,11*R**,12*S**,13*S**,14*R**)]-13-[2,6-Di-deoxy-3-*C*-methyl-3*O*-methyl-α-L-*ribo*-hexopyranosyl)oxy]-2-ethyl-3,4,10-trihydroxy-3,5,6,8,10,12,14-heptamethyl-11-[[3,4,6-trideoxy-3-(dimethylamino)-β-D-*xylo*-hexopyranosyl]oxy]-1-oxa-6-azacyclopent-adecan-15-one
$C_{38}H_{72}N_2O_{12}$ = 749.0
CAS—83905-01-5 (anhydrous); 117772-70-0 (dihydrate)

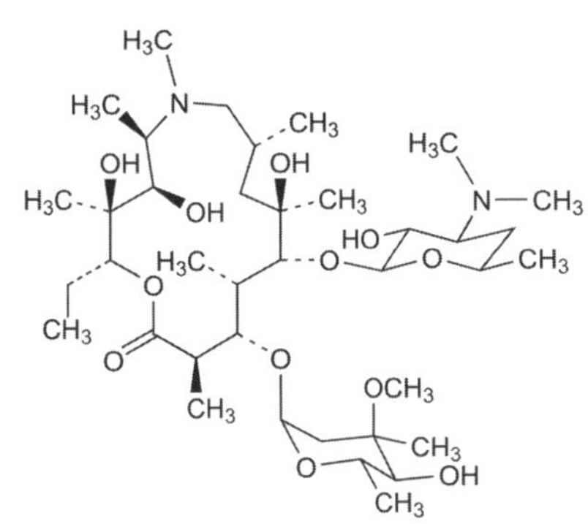

M.p. 113° to 115°.

Dissociation Constant. pK_a 8.1 and 8.8.

Partition Coefficient. Log *P* (octanol/water), 4.02.

High Performance Liquid Chromatography. System HBA—retention time 20.7 min; system HBB—retention time 9.6 min.

Infra-red Spectrum. Principal peaks at wavenumber 1721, 1188, 1052 cm^{-1} (KBr pellet).

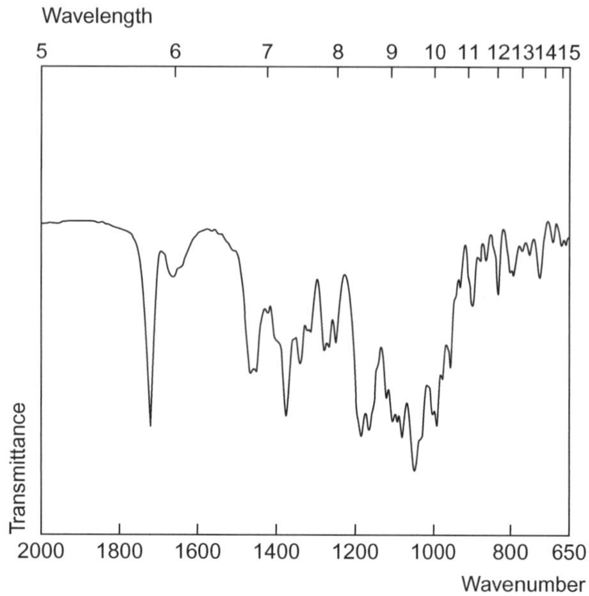

Quantification

High performance liquid chromatography. In plasma: limit of quantification 0.03 mg/L. Electrochemical detection—C. Taninaka *et al.*, *J. Chromatogr. Biomed. Sci. Appl.*, 2000, *738*, 405–411. In serum: limit of detection 0.09 mg/L, fluorescence detection (λ_{ex}=255 nm, λ_{em}=315 nm)—J. Sastre Toraño and H.-J. Guchelaar, *J. Chromatogr. Biomed. Sci. Appl.*, 1998, *720*, 89–97. In serum or tissues: limit of detection 0.01 mg/L in serum and 100 mg/g in tissue, amperometric or electrochemical detection—R. M. Shepard *et al., J. Chromatogr. Biomed. Sci. Appl.*, 1991, *565*, 321–337.

Note. For a comparison of microbiological assay and high performance liquid chromatography methods for the determination of azithromycin see K.-D. Riedel *et al., J. Chromatogr. Biomed. Sci. Appl.*, 1992, *576*, 358–362.

Disposition in the Body. Azithromycin is rapidly absorbed after oral administration with a bioavailability of about 40%. Absorption from the capsule formulation, but not the tablet formulation, is reduced by food. It is extensively distributed to the tissues; tissue concentrations are much higher than those in blood and high concentrations are taken up into white blood cells. There is little diffusion into CSF unless meninges are inflamed. Some demethylation of the drug occurs in the liver and it is excreted in bile as the unchanged drug and its metabolites (approx. 10 with no microbial activity); more than 50% of a dose is excreted in faeces as the unchanged drug. About 12% of an oral dose is excreted in urine over the course of about a week.

Therapeutic concentration

Peak plasma concentrations of 0.165 to 0.623 mg/L (mean, 0.383 mg/L) were reported following oral administration of 10 mg/kg on day 1 followed by 5 mg/kg on days 2 to 5 in 14 children aged 6 to 15 years, both boys and girls. Peak concentrations were reached after 1 to 4 h (mean 2.4 h). [M. C. Nahata *et al., Antimicrob. Agents Chemother.*, 1993, *37*, 314–316].

Following administration of a 1-g oral dose to 14 male subjects, mean peak serum concentrations at 1.7 h were 0.82 mg/L and mean peak lymph concentrations after 3.1 h were 0.22 mg/L. [T. Bergan *et al., Scand. J. Infect. Dis.*, 1992, *24*, *Suppl. 83*, 15–21].

Bioavailability. 37%.

Half-life. Plasma half-life, 14 to >40 h.

Volume of distribution. 23 to 31 L/kg.

Clearance. Plasma clearance, 630 mL/min.

Protein binding. In plasma, decreasing from 51% at 0.02 to 0.05 mg/L to 7% at 1 mg/L.

Note. For reviews of azithromycin see S. Hopkins, *Am. J. Med.*, 1991, *91*, *Suppl. 3A*, 40S–45S, D. H. Peters *et al., Drugs*, 1992, *44*, 750–799, and N. J. Lalak and D. L. Morris, *Clin. Pharmacokinet.*, 1993, *25*, 370–374.

Dose. Usually 500 mg daily.

Azlocillin

Antibacterial

Synonym. Bay e 6905
(6*R*)-6-[D-2-(2-oxoimidazolidine-1-carboxamido)-2-phenylacetamido]penicillin
$C_{20}H_{23}N_5O_6S$=461.5
CAS—37091-66-0

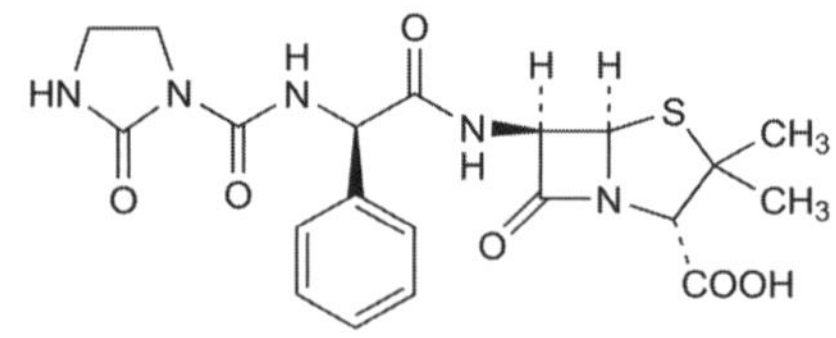

Azlocillin Sodium

Proprietary names. Azlin; Securopen.
$C_{20}H_{22}N_5NaO_6S$=483.5
CAS—*37091-65-9*

A white to pale yellow hygroscopic powder. It is freely soluble in water; soluble in dimethyl formamide and methanol; slightly soluble in ethanol and isopropanol; practically insoluble in acetone, chloroform, and ether.

Ultraviolet Spectrum. Water—257, 320 nm (sodium salt).

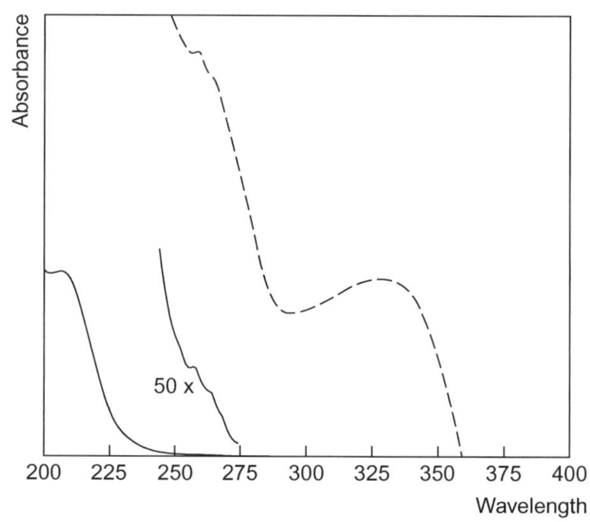

Infra-red Spectrum. Principal peaks at wavenumber 1722, 1606, 1532, 1772, 1272, 3295 cm^{-1} (sodium salt) (KBr disk).

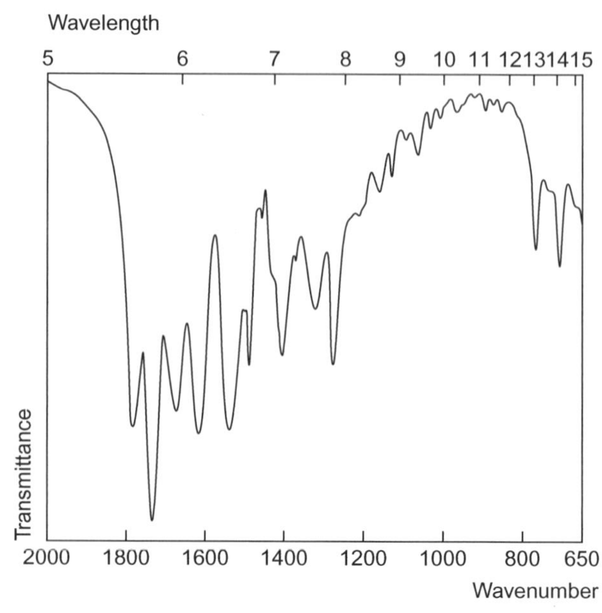

Quantification

High performance liquid chromatography. In urine: azlocillin and penicilloic acid metabolite, limit of detection 1 to 2 mg/L for azlocillin and 5 to 7 mg/L for the penicilloic acid metabolite, UV detection—Von W. Gau and F. A. Horster, *Arzneimittelforschung*, 1979, *29*, 1941–1943. In plasma: limit of detection 0.7 mg/L, UV detection—U. Gundert-Remy and J. X. De Vries, *Br. J. Clin. Pharmacol.*, 1979, *8*, 589–592. In plasma: limit of detection 1.3 μg/mL, limit of quantification 5 μg/mL. UV detection (λ=220 nm)—R. Hildebrandt and U. Gundert-Remy, *J. Chromatogr.*, 1982, *228*; *Biomed. Appl.*, *17*, 409–412. In serum: limit of detection 0.4 mg/L, UV detection—A. Weber *et al.*, *Antimicrob. Agents. Chemother.*, 1983, *24*, 750–753. In bile, serum, or urine: limit of detection 0.1 mg/L, UV detection (λ=214 nm)—F. Jehl *et al.*, *J. Chromatogr.*, 1987, *413*; *Biomed. Appl.*, *57*, 109–119. In plasma, serum, tissues, or urine: limit of detection 0.1 mg/L, UV detection (λ=220 nm)—J. Knöller *et al.*, *J. Chromatogr.*, 1988, *427*; *Biomed. Appl.*, *71*, 257–267.

Disposition in the Body. Azlocillin is poorly absorbed from the gastrointestinal tract but is widely distributed following intravenous administration in body tissues and fluids. It crosses the placenta and small amounts are distributed into breast milk. There is little diffusion into CSF unless meninges are inflamed. It is metabolised to a limited extent and about 50 to 70% of a dose is excreted unchanged in the urine by glomerular filtration and tubular secretion. This occurs within 24 h of administration, therefore, producing high urinary concentrations. It is partly excreted in bile. Concomitant administration of probenecid increases plasma concentrations. It can be removed by haemodialysis.

Therapeutic concentration

Following administration of 4 g as an IV infusion over 20 min to 12 healthy male and female subjects, the mean peak plasma concentration was 451 mg/L. This decreased to 223 mg/L after 30 min and 33 mg/L 4 h from the beginning of infusion. [P. A. Colaizzi *et al.*, *Antimicrob. Agents Chemother.*, 1986, *29*, 938–940].

Half-life. Plasma half-life, 1 h; 2 to 6 h in renal impairment.

Volume of distribution. 0.22 L/kg.

Clearance. Serum clearance, 153 mL/min/1.73 m^2.

Protein binding. In plasma, between 20 and 46%.

Note. For a review of the pharmacokinetics of azlocillin see T. Bergan, *J. Antimicrob. Chemother.*, 1983, *11*, *Suppl.* B, 101–114.

Dose. Up to 5 g (of the base) intravenously every 8 h; reduced in patients with renal dysfunction.

Aztreonam

Antibacterial

Synonyms. Azthreonam; SQ-26776.
Proprietary names. Azactam; Azonam; Aztreon; Nebactam; Primbactam; Urobactam.
[2*S*-[2α,3β(*Z*)]]-2-[[[1-(2-Amino-4-thiazolyl)-2-[(2-methyl-4-oxo-1-sulfo-3-azetidinyl)amino]-2-oxoethylidene]amino]oxy]-2-methylpropanoic acid
$C_{13}H_{17}N_5O_8S_2$=435.4
CAS—78110-38-0

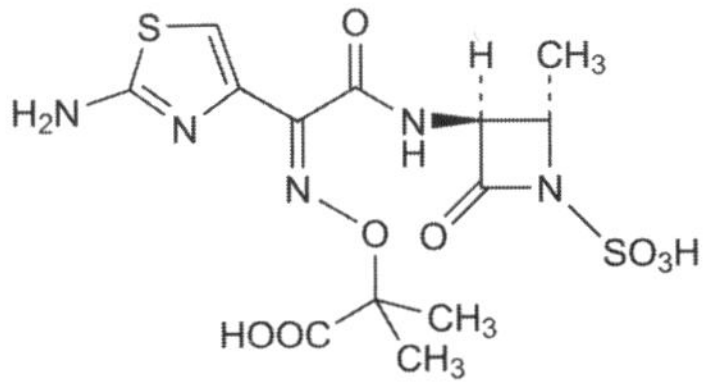

A white crystalline odourless powder. Decomposes at 227°. It is very slightly soluble in dehydrated alcohol; slightly soluble in methanol; soluble in dimethylformamide and dimethylsulfoxide; practically insoluble in chloroform, ethyl acetate and toluene.

Aztreonam Disodium
$C_{13}H_{15}N_5Na_2O_8S_2$=479.4

Dissociation Constant. pK_a, less than 2.0.

Ultraviolet Spectrum. Aqueous acid (ethanol)—268, 281 nm; basic—289 nm.

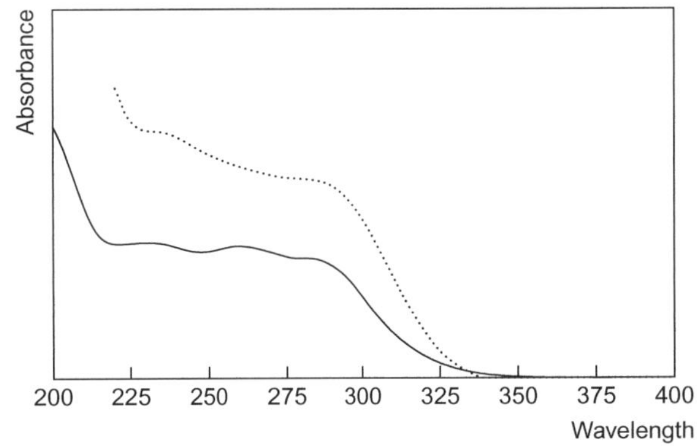

Infra-red Spectrum. Principal peaks at wavenumber 1640, 1041, 633 cm^{-1} (KBr disk).

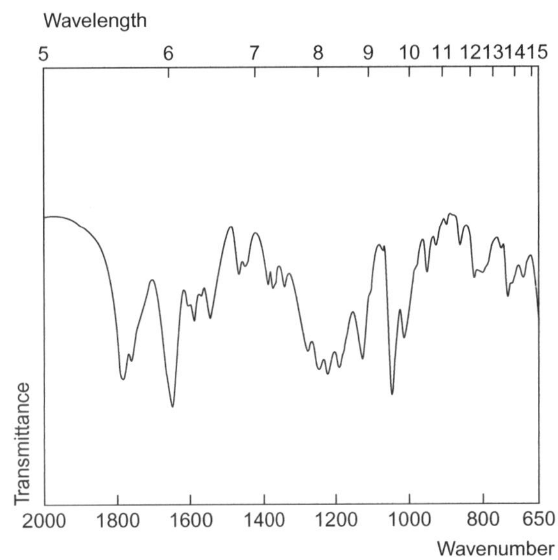

Quantification

High pressure liquid chromatography. In serum or urine: limit of detection 1 mg/L in serum and 5 mg/L in urine, UV detection—E. A. Swabb *et al.*, *J. Antimicrob. Chemother.*, 1981, *8*, *Suppl.* E, 131–140. In serum or urine: limit of detection 1 mg/L in serum and 5 mg/L in urine, UV detection (λ=293 nm)—F. G. Pilkiewicz *et al.*, *Antimicrob. Agents Chemother.*, 1983, *23*, 852–856. In serum or urine: limit of detection 1 mg/L in serum and urine, UV detection—J. C. L. Mihindu *et al.*, *Antimicrob. Agents Chemother.*, 1983, *24*, 252–261. In bile, serum, or urine: limit of detection 0.5 mg/L, UV detection—F. Jehl *et al.*, *J. Chromatogr.*, 1987, *413*; *Biomed. Appl.*, *57*, 109–119. In faeces: limit of detection about 2 μg/g, UV detection—W. Ehret *et al.*, *J. Antimicrob. Chemother.*, 1987, *19*, 541–549.

Bioassay. In faeces: limit of detection, 0.03 mg/L—W. Ehret *et al.*, *J. Antimicrob. Chemother.*, 1987, *19*, 541–549.

Disposition in the Body. Aztreonam is completely absorbed after intramuscular administration with peak concentrations reached within 1 h. It takes 1 to 3 h for equilibrium to be reached between tissues and plasma. It is widely distributed in body tissues and fluids, including bile, but diffusion into CSF is poor unless meninges are inflamed. It crosses the placenta and small amounts are distributed into breast milk. Only about 6 to 16% is metabolised to inactive metabolites by hydrolysis. The drug is excreted predominantly in urine by renal tubular secretion and glomerular filtration; about 60 to 75% of a dose appears within 8 h as the unchanged drug with only small quantities of metabolites. Only small amounts of the unchanged drug and metabolites are excreted in faeces. It is removed by haemodialysis and to a lesser extent by peritoneal dialysis.

Therapeutic concentration. The trough serum therapeutic concentration range is 1 to 10 mg/L and the peak, 50 to 250 mg/L.

24 male volunteers were divided into 4 groups according to the degree of creatinine clearance. Group 1 (mean age, 27 years): creatinine clearance, ⩾80 mL/min, group 2 (mean age, 43): 30 to 79 mL/min, group 3 (mean age, 44): 10 to 29 mL/min, group 4 (mean, 40 years old): <10 mL/min. Each group was administered with an intravenous dose of 1 g aztreonam over 2 min, after an overnight fast followed by a 2-h fast after administration. The mean peak serum concentrations for the groups were 78, 98, 98 and 145 mg/L, respectively, observed after 10 min. [J. C. L. Mihindu *et al.*, *Antimicrob. Agents. Chemother.*, 1983, *24*, 252–261].

Half-life. Plasma half-life, 1.4 to 2.2 h; prolonged to 4.7 to 6 h in renal impairment and to some extent in hepatic impairment.

Volume of distribution. 0.11 to 0.21 L/kg; increased in neonates and paediatric patients (from 1 week to 12 years old) to 0.3 to 1 L/kg.

Clearance. Plasma clearance, 93 mL/min; reduced in neonates.

Protein binding. In plasma, about 56%.

Note. For reviews of aztreonam see R. N. Brogden and R. C. Heel, *Drugs*, 1986, *31*, 91–130 and H. C. Neu, *Am. J. Med.*, 1990, *88*, *Suppl.* 3c, 2S–6S. For reviews of the pharmacokinetics of aztreonam see H. Mattie, *Clin. Pharmacokinet.*, 1988, *14*, 148–155 and H. Mattie, *Clin. Pharmacokinet.*, 1994, *26*, 99–106.

Dose. Up to 8 g daily by intravenous or intramuscular injection. Dose may need to be reduced in patients with severe renal impairment.

Bacampicillin

Antibacterial

Synonym. Carampicillin

(2*S*,5*R*,6*R*)-6-[[(2*R*)-Aminophenylacetyl]amino]-3,3-dimethyl-7-oxo-4-thia-1-azabicyclo[3.2.0]heptane-2-carboxylic acid 1-[(ethoxycarbonyl)oxy]ethyl ester

$C_{21}H_{27}N_3O_7S = 465.5$

CAS—50972-17-3

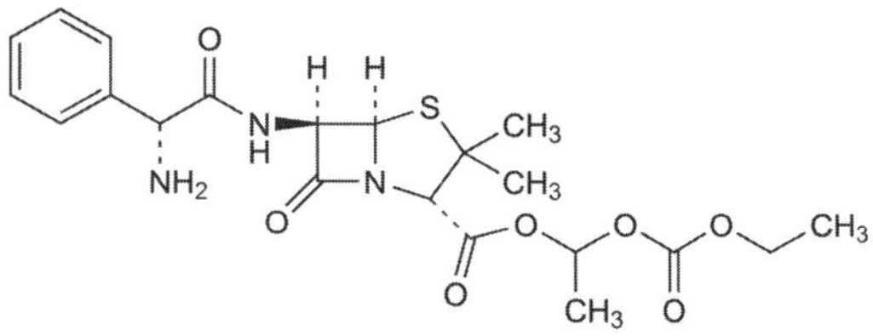

Bacampicillin Hydrochloride

Proprietary names. Ambaxin; Penglobe; Spectrobid.

$C_{21}H_{27}N_3O_7S,HCl = 502.0$

CAS—37661-08-8

A white crystalline powder. M.p. 171° to176°. Soluble 1 in 15 of water, 1 in 7 of ethanol, and 1 in 10 of chloroform; practically insoluble in ether.

High Performance Liquid Chromatography. System HAA—Retention time(s) 14.7 min.

Ultraviolet Spectrum. Water—258, 263 (A_1^1 = 13b), 269; aqueous alkali—310 nm.

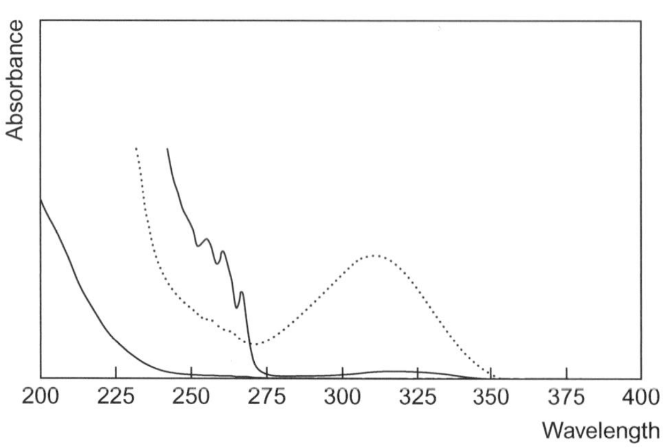

Infra-red Spectrum. Principal peaks at wavenumbers 1770, 1075, 1788, 1263, 1687, 1744 cm^{-1} (bacampicillin hydrochloride, KBr disk).

Dose. 0.8 to 2.4 g of bacampicillin hydrochloride daily.

Bacitracin

Antibacterial

Proprietary names. Baciguent; Bacitin. It is an ingredient of Ototrips and Polybactrin Soluble GU.

CAS—1405-87-4

Bacitracin is a polypeptide produced by the growth of an organism of the licheniformis group of *Bacillus subtilis*.

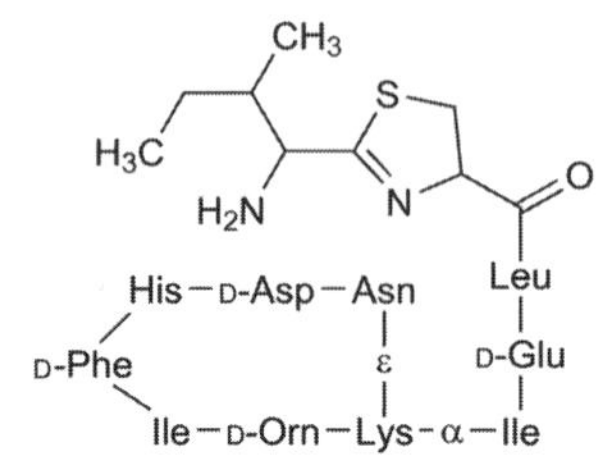

Bacitracin A

A white to pale buff hygroscopic powder. Freely soluble in water; soluble in ethanol; practically insoluble in acetone, chloroform, and ether.

Bacitracin Zinc

Synonyms. Bacitracins Zinc Complex; Zinc Bacitracin.

Proprietary names. It is an ingredient of Cicatrene, Cicatrex, Cicatrin, Dispray Antibiotic, Polyfax and Tribiotic.

CAS-1405-89-6

A white, pale buff or tan, hygroscopic powder. Soluble 1 in 900 of water and 1 in 500 of ethanol; very slightly soluble in ether; practically insoluble in chloroform.

Ultraviolet Spectrum. Bacitracin zinc: aqueous acid—252 nm (A_1^1 = 18b).

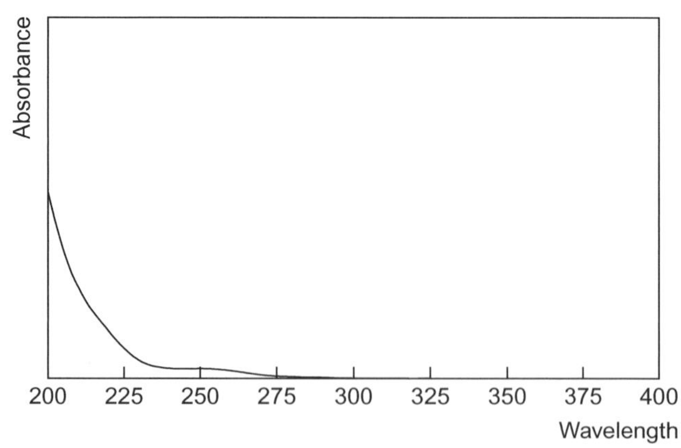

Baclofen

Muscle Relaxant

Synonym. Aminomethyl Chlorohydrocinnamic Acid

Proprietary Name. Lioresal

β-(Aminomethyl)-4-chlorobenzenepropanoic acid

$C_{10}H_{12}ClNO_2 = 213.7$

CAS—1134-47-0

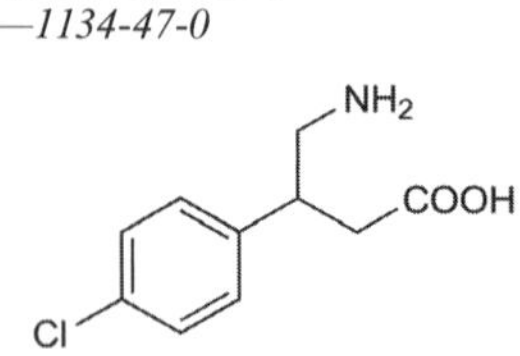

A white crystalline solid. M.p. about 207°. Slightly soluble in water; poorly soluble in organic solvents.

Dissociation Constant. pK_a 3.9, 9.6.

Partition Coefficient. Log *P* (octanol/water), −1.0.

Colour Test. Liebermann's test—orange.

Thin-layer Chromatography. System TD—Rf 01; system TE—Rf 00; system TF—Rf 00; system TAD—Rf 00.

Gas Chromatography. System GA—RI 2010.

High Performance Liquid Chromatography. System HZ—Retention time(s) 2.0 min.
Column: C_{18} Bondapak (300 × 3.9 mm i.d., 10 μm). Mobile phase: methanol:water (45:55 v/v), flow rate 0.4 mL/min. Fluorescence detection (λ_{ex}=463 nm; λ_{em}=524 nm). Retention time(s): 4.0 min. [S. Tosunoglu and L. Ersoy, *Analyst*, 1995, *120*, 373–375].

Ultraviolet Spectrum. Aqueous acid—259, 266 (A_1^1=11.3a), 274 nm. No alkaline shift.

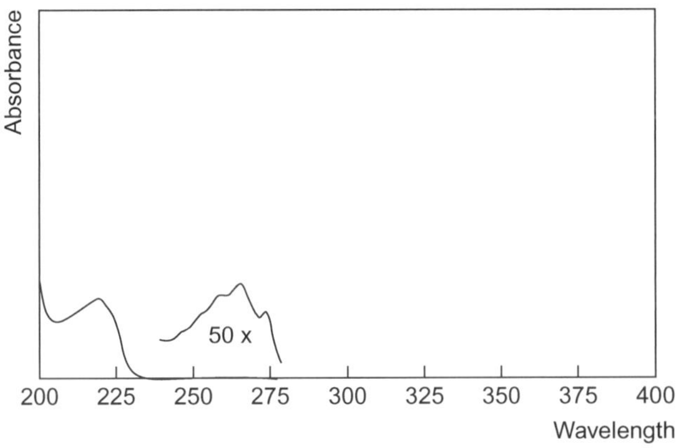

Infra-red Spectrum. Principal peaks at wavenumbers 1527, 835, 1574, 1495, 1624, 1095 cm^{-1} (KBr disk).

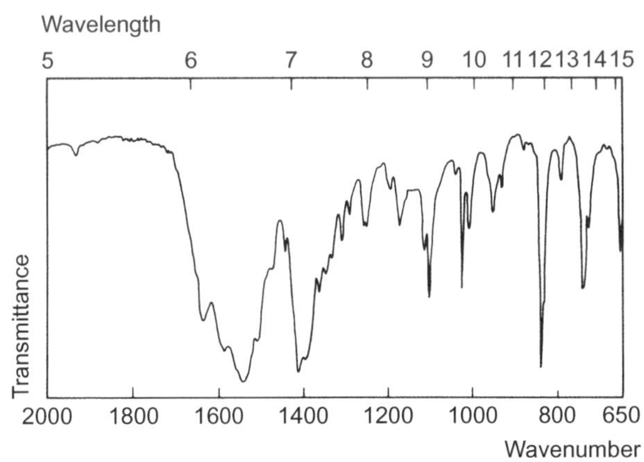

Mass Spectrum. Principal ions at *m/z* 30, 138, 195, 140, 103, 197, 77, 196.

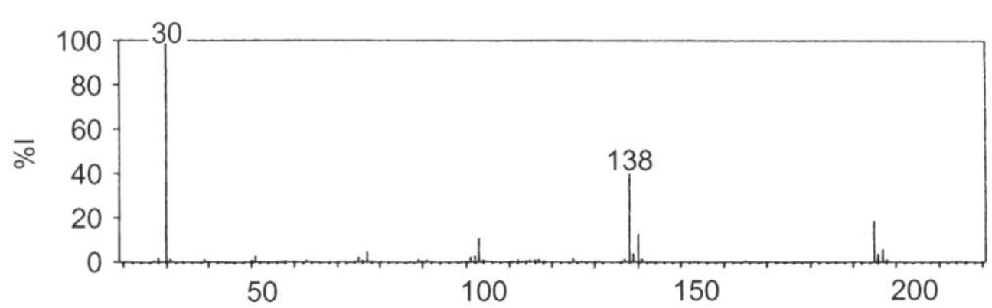

Quantification

Gas chromatography. In plasma or urine: limit of detection 50 μg/L, ECD—P. H. Degen and W. Riess, *J. Chromatogr.*, 1976, *117*, 399–405.

Gas chromatography–mass spectrometry. In serum or cerebrospinal fluid: limit of detection 5 μg/L—C. G. Swahn *et al.*, *J. Chromatogr.*, 1979, *162*; *B Biomed Appl.*, *4*, 433–438.

High performance liquid chromatography. In plasma: limit of detection 2.5 μg/L and limit of quantification 10 μg/L, ECD—L. Millerioux *et al.*, *J. Chromatogr. A*, 1996, *729*, 309–314.

Disposition in the Body. Baclofen is rapidly absorbed after oral administration. About 80% of a dose is excreted in the urine in 24 h, mostly as unchanged drug. About 15% of a dose is metabolised, mainly to the deaminated derivative; about 20% of a dose may be eliminated in the faeces as unchanged drug and metabolites.

Therapeutic concentration

A 45-year-old, healthy, woman administered 20 mg baclofen orally produced a peak plasma concentration of 270 μg/L after 2.5 h. [S. Tosunoglu and L. Ersoy, *Analyst*, 1995, *120*, 373–375].

After an oral dose of 40 mg to 1 subject, a peak plasma concentration of unchanged drug of about 0.6 mg/L was attained in 2 h; a peak concentration of metabolites of about 0.1 mg/L was attained in about 4 h. [J. W. Faigle and H. Keberle, *Postgrad. Med. J.*, 1972, *48* (Oct.), Suppl., 9–13].

Toxicity. Recovery has occurred after the ingestion of 1.5 g.

A fatality occurred after ingestion of baclofen. Baclofen was detected in serum at a concentration of 17 mg/L and in urine at 760 mg/L which was collected 12 h after ingestion of the drug. [A. D. Fraser *et al.*, *J. Forensic Sci.*, 1991, *36(5)*, 1596–1602].

Coma, respiratory failure and severe seizures occurred in a 39-year-old female subject after ingestion of 450 mg of baclofen; following treatment, the patient regained consciousness within 36 h, at which time a plasma concentration of 0.2 mg/L was reported; the plasma half-life was found to be 35 h. [K. Ghose *et al.*, *Postgrad. Med. J.*, 1980, *56*, 865–867].

Half-life. Plasma half-life, about 2 to 4 h.

Protein binding. In plasma, about 30%.

Dose. 15 to 60 mg daily; maximum of 100 mg daily.

Balsalazide

Anti-ulcer

5-[(1*E*)-[4-[[(2-Carboxyethyl)amino]carbonyl]phenyl]azo]-2-hydroxybenzoic acid
$C_{17}H_{15}N_3O_6$=357.3
CAS—80573-04-2

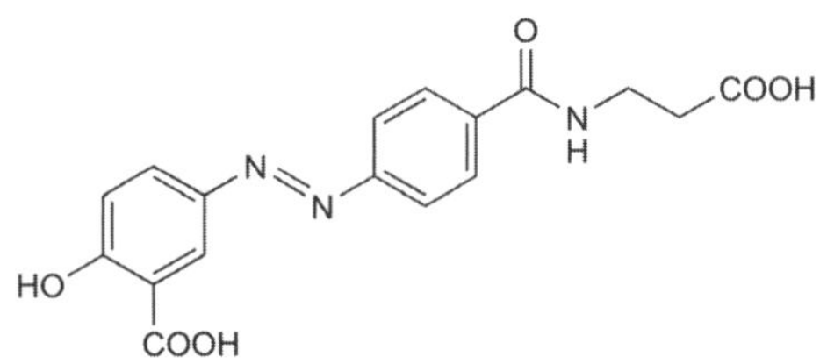

Balsalazide Disodium
Synonyms. Balsalazide sodium; BX-661A.
Proprietary name. Colazide
$C_{17}H_{17}N_3Na_2O_8$=437.3
CAS—150399-21-6

Disposition in the Body. Balsalazide is metabolised in the colon, by bacterial azoreductases, to 5-aminosalicyclic acid (5-ASA) which is responsible for the anti-inflammatory action, and 4-aminobenzoyl-β-alanine (4-ABA), an inert carrier. 25% of the released 5-ASA is inactivated in the colonic mucosa and liver to the *N*-acetylated metabolite, NASA. Likewise, 4-ABA becomes converted to its *N*-acetylated metabolite, NABA. It is only NASA and NABA which are detected in urine; the parent drug is excreted mainly in faeces.

Therapeutic concentration.

54 adult patients with ulcerative colitis (in remission) were administered with 3 to 6 g daily for at least a year. Peak plasma concentrations of 0.324 mg/L were reached within 2 h. [J. R. B. Green *et al.*, Glycyx Pharmaceuticals Ltd., GLY01/93, 1998 (data on file)].

Peak plasma concentrations of the metabolite, 4-ABA, were less than 0.096 mg/L within 9 to 10 h after administration of a 2.25 g dose of balsalazide. [J. G. Riddel *et al.*, Glycyx Pharmaceuticals Ltd., Harris Project no. 20060, 1998 (data on file)].

Toxicity.
Hypersensitivity reaction: a 59-year-old woman was administered with 2.25 g balsalazide 3 times a day and after 8 days, was admitted into hospital with central chest pain, shortness of breath and back pain, which worsened over the next 3 days. Examination showed a pyrexial, splinter haemorrhages in her fingernails, raised jugular venous pressure, a loud pericardial rub and a soft, tender liver. Balsalazide treatment was stopped and all symptoms were resolved within a month. [V. Adhiyaman *et al.*, *BMJ*, 2000, *320*, 613].

Half-life. Elimination half-life of NASA is 6 to 9 h, and of 5-ASA is approx. 1 h.

Clearance. 4.5 L/h.

Protein binding. 5-ASA, approximately 40% and NASA, 80%.

Dose. An initial dose of 2.25 g three times a day is administered for up to 12 weeks. Maintenance dose of 1.5 g twice daily with a maximum of 6 g daily.

Bambuterol

Bronchodilator/Beta$_2$-agonist

Dimethylcarbamic acid 5-[2-[(1,1-dimethylethyl)amino]-1-hydroxyethyl]-1,3-phenylene ester
$C_{18}H_{29}N_3O_5$=367.5
CAS—81732-65-2

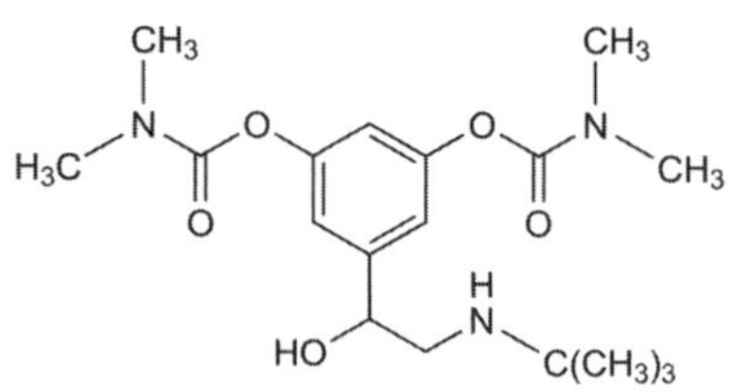

Bambuterol Hydrochloride
Synonym. KWD-2183
Proprietary name. Bambec
$C_{18}H_{29}N_3O_5$,HCl=403.9
CAS—81732-46-9
A white or almost white crystalline powder. Exhibits polymorphism. It is freely soluble in water; soluble in ethanol.

Thin-layer Chromatography. System TB—Rf 02 (bambuterol); Rf 00 (bambuterol monocarbamate); system TE—Rf 37 (bambuterol); Rf 21 (bambuterol monocarbamate); system TAE—Rf 18 (bambuterol); Rf 19 (bambuterol monocarbamate).

High Performance Liquid Chromatography. System HX—RI 353 (bambuterol); RI 304 (bambuterol monocarbamate).

Column: LC-18-DB (Supelcosil, 150 × 4.6 mm i.d., 5 μm). Mobile phase: 6.0 mM sodium octane sulfonate and methanol:acetonitrile:50 mM phosphate buffer pH 3.0 (34:11:55), 1.0 mL/min flow rate. UV detection (λ=214 nm). Retention time: 10 min. [O. Wannerberg and B. Persson, *J. Chromatogr.*, 1988, *435*, 199–203].

Ultraviolet Spectrum. Water—264 nm.

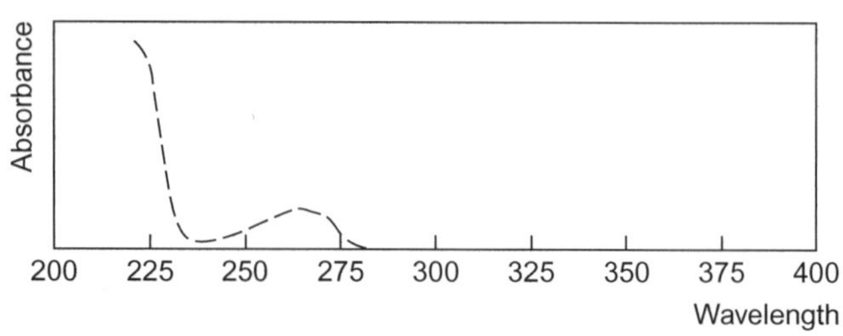

Infra-red Spectrum. Principal peaks at wavenumber 1695, 1720, 1190, 1200, 1390, 1350 cm^{-1}.

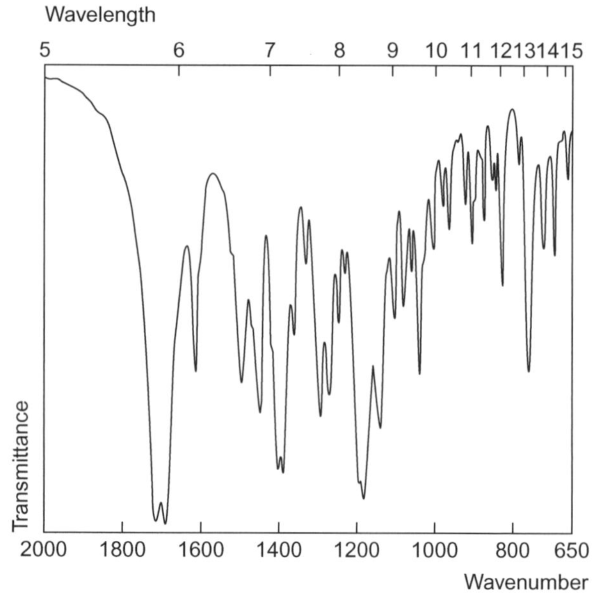

Mass Spectrum. Principal ions at *m/z* 72, 86, 57, 70, 367, 282, 352, 334.

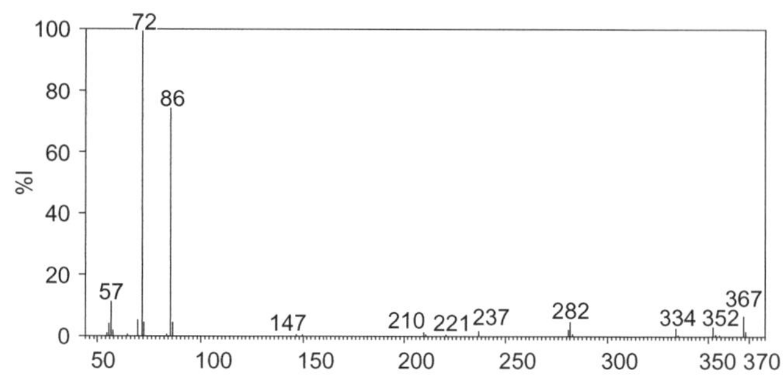

Quantification
Gas chromatography–mass spectrometry. In plasma and urine: limit of quantification is 0.2 μg/L and 1.5 μg/L, respectively—C. Lindberg *et al.*, *Biomed. Env. Mass Spectrom.*, 1990, *19*, 218–224.

Disposition in the Body. About 20% of a dose is absorbed after oral administration. It concentrates in lung tissue where it is hydrolysed primarily by a plasma cholinesterase to its active metabolite terbutaline (β_2 adrenergic receptor agonist). It is also metabolised by oxidative enzymes in the liver. Approximately one-third of an intravenous dose is converted to terbutaline. It also undergoes oxidative metabolism to products that are then metabolised to terbutaline. Very little bambuterol is excreted unchanged in urine.

Therapeutic concentration
12 healthy volunteers, male and female, aged between 23 and 62 years, were administered with intravenous doses of 30 g/kg over 5 min and oral doses of 7 g/kg as an aqueous solution. Peak plasma concentrations after the intravenous dose ranged between 72.5 and 184 nmol/L with a mean of 129 nmol/L. The mean peak plasma concentration, after a single oral dose, was 6.9 nmol/L (2.3 to 24.3 nmol/L) and was reached within 2.3 h (ranging between 1 and 4 h). [L. Nyberg *et al.*, *Br. J. Clin. Pharmacol.*, 1998, *45(5)*, 471–478].

23 healthy Caucasian volunteers (12 women), aged between 20 and 56 years, were administered with oral tablets: 10, 20 and 30 mg, and a 20 mg solution as an open, crossover, random study. After the first dose, the mean peak plasma concentration was 3.69 nmol/L (1.0 to 8.8 nmol/L) for the 10 mg tablet, 8.56 nmol/L (ranging between 3.5 and 16.9 nmol/L) for the 20 mg tablet, 14.23 nmol/L (range, 5.3 to 30.4 nmol/L) for 30 mg and 6.13 nmol/L (1.7 to 13.6 nmol/L) for the 20 mg solution. The mean time to the peak concentration was 1.4 to 1.8 h. [J. Rosenborg *et al.*, *Br. J. Clin. Pharmacol.*, 2000, *49*, 199–206].

Bioavailability. Less than 15%.

Half-life. Plasma, 12 h (oral administration); 2.6 h (intravenous administration).

Volume of distribution. Women, between 1.6 and 2.1 L/kg; men, 1.2 to 1.4 L/kg.

Clearance. Plasma, 1250 mL/min.

Protein binding. Plasma, 40 to 50%.

Distribution in blood. Distributes extensively outside the plasma component.

Note. For a review of the pharmacokinetics of bambuterol see D. S. Sitar, *Clin. Pharmacokinet.*, 1996, *31*, 246–256.

Dose. Usually 20 mg daily.

Bamethan

Vasodilator

α-[(Butylamino)methyl]-4-hydroxybenzenemethanol
$C_{12}H_{19}NO_2$=209.3
CAS-3703-79-5

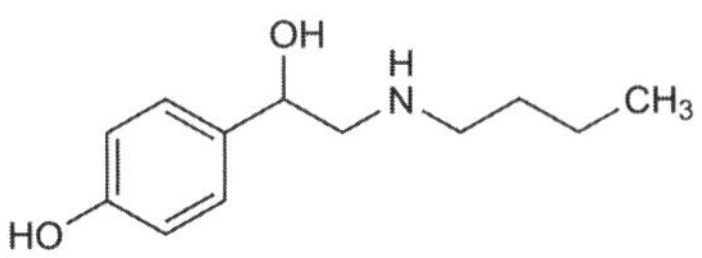

Crystals. M.p. 123.5° to 125°.

Bamethan Sulfate
Proprietary names. Vasculat; Vasculit.
$(C_{12}H_{19}NO_2)_2,H_2SO_4$=516.7
CAS—5716-20-1
Soluble in water.

Dissociation Constant. pK_a 9.0, 10.2 (25°).

Partition Coefficient. Log *P* (octanol/water), 1.3.

Colour Tests. Folin–Ciocalteu reagent—blue; Liebermann's test—violet-brown; Mandelin's test—blue→green.

Thin-layer Chromatography. System TA—Rf 55; system TB—Rf 04; system TC—Rf 06; system TL—Rf 00; system TAE—Rf 23. (Acidified potassium permanganate solution, positive.)

Gas Chromatography. System GA—RI 1920.

High Performance Liquid Chromatography. System HA—*k* 0.9; system HX—RI 250; system HAA—Retention time(s) 5.9 min.

Ultraviolet Spectrum. Aqueous acid—275 (A_1^1=64a); aqueous alkali—242, 290 nm.

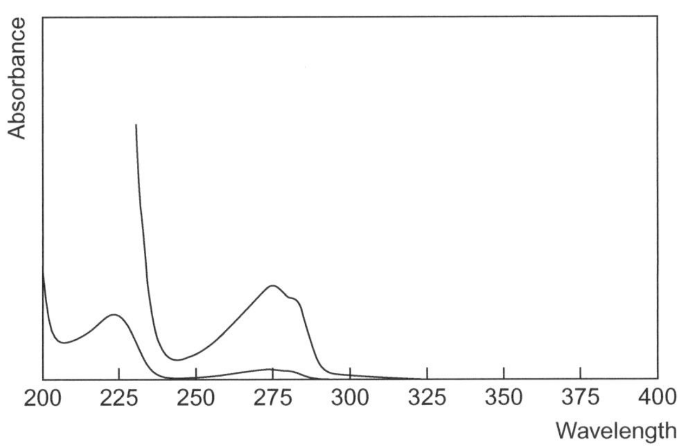

Infra-red Spectrum. Principal peaks at wavenumbers 832, 1228, 1066, 1264, 1494, 1108 cm^{-1} (KBr disk).

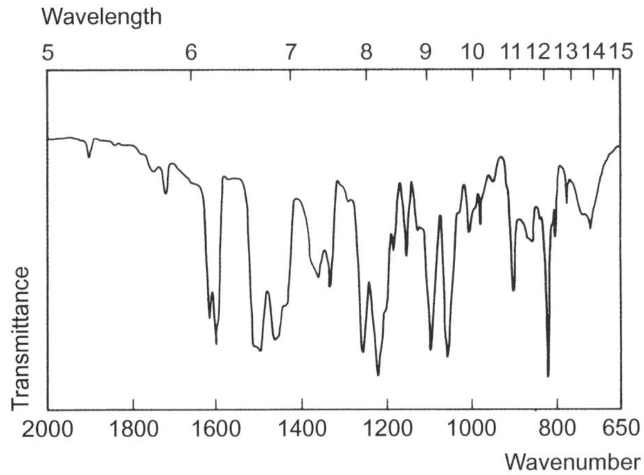

Mass Spectrum. Principal ions at *m/z* 86, 30, 57, 108, 44, 29, 84, 41.

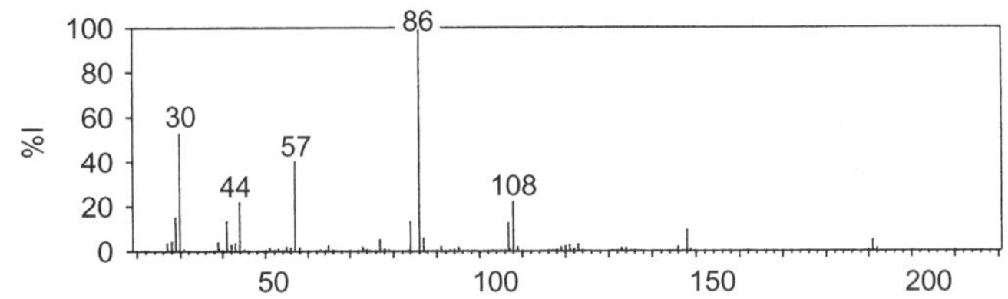

Disposition in the Body. Bamethan is rapidly absorbed after oral administration. About 80% of a dose is excreted in the urine in 24 h, with about 30% of the dose as unchanged drug.

Therapeutic concentration

After a single oral dose of 25 mg given to 5 subjects, peak serum concentrations of 0.04 to 0.11 mg/L (mean 0.07) were attained in 0.5 to 1 h. [J. H. Hengstmann and B. Steinkamp, *Arzneimittelforschung*, 1981, *31*, 843–848].

Half-life. Plasma half-life, about 2.5 h.

Volume of distribution. 2.5 to 5 L/kg (mean 3.7).

Clearance. Plasma clearance, 12 to 20 (mean 16) mL/min/kg.

Dose. 100 mg of bamethan sulfate daily.

Bamifylline

Bronchodilator

7-[2-[Ethyl(2-hydroxyethyl)amino]ethyl]-3,7-dihydro-1,3-dimethyl-8-(phenylmethyl)-1*H*-purine-2,6-dione
$C_{20}H_{27}N_5O_3$=385.5
CAS-2016-63-9

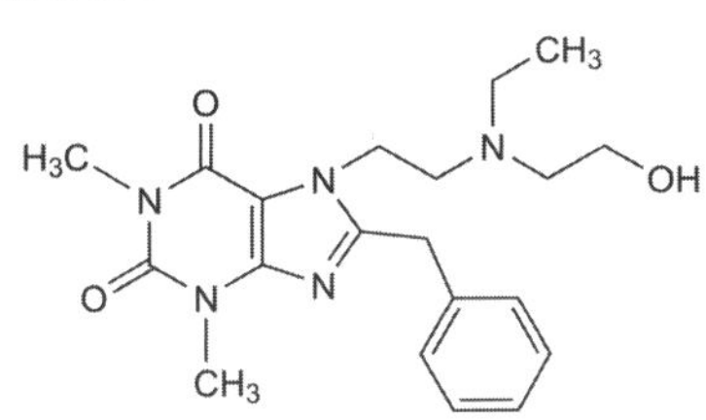

Crystals. M.p. 80° to 80.5°.

Bamifylline Hydrochloride
Proprietary name. Trentadil
$C_{20}H_{27}N_5O_3$,HCl=421.9
CAS-20684-06-4
A crystalline solid. M.p. 185° to 186°. Soluble in water.

Partition Coefficient. Log *P* (octanol), 1.6.

Colour Test. Amalic acid test—orange/violet.

Thin-layer Chromatography. System TA—Rf 65; system TB—Rf 00; system TC—Rf 54; system TL—Rf 34; system TAE—Rf 71. (Acidified iodoplatinate solution, positive.)

High Performance Liquid Chromatography. System HAA—Retention time(s) 10.3 min.

Ultraviolet Spectrum. Aqueous acid—278(A^1_1=310a); methanol—277 nm (A^1_1=280b).

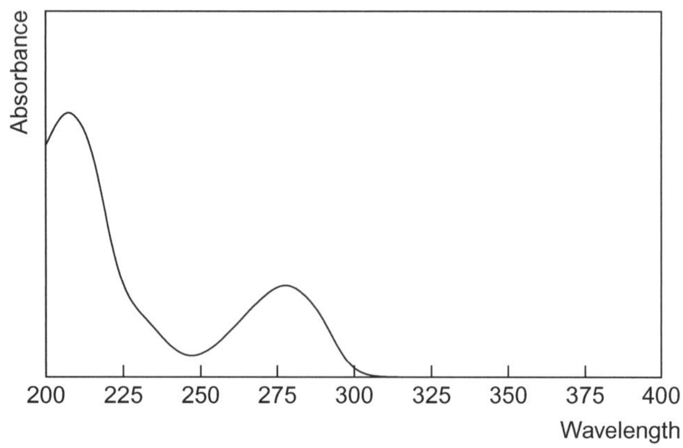

Infra-red Spectrum. Principal peaks at wavenumbers 1650, 1698, 1538, 729, 1041, 1205 cm^{-1} (KBr disk).

Mass Spectrum. Principal ions at *m/z* 102, 84, 58, 56, 42, 30, 103, 91.

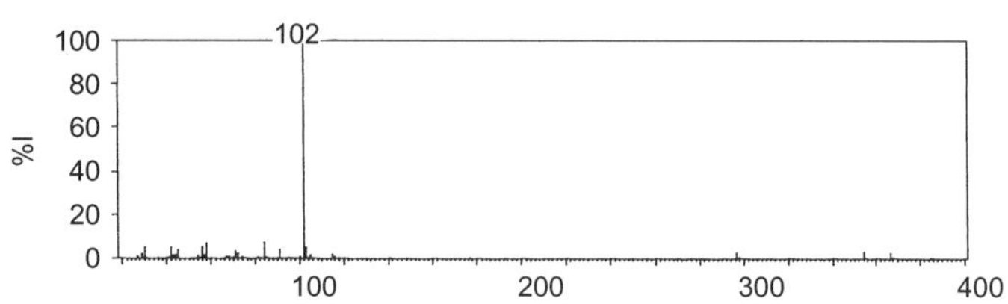

Quantification

High performance liquid chromatography. In plasma: limit of detection 20 µg/L, UV detection (λ=280 nm)—G. Segre *et al., Arzneimittelforschung*, 1990, *40(4)*, 450–452. In plasma: bamifylline and desalkyl metabolites, limit of detection 10 µg/L, UV detection—G. Nicot *et al., J. Chromatogr.*, 1983, *277; B Biomed. Appl., 28*, 239–249.

Therapeutic concentration

6 male and female healthy subjects, mean age 33.3 years, were administered 600 mg bamifylline every 12 h for 7 days. The mean peak plasma concentration after the first dose was 1165 µg/L (range 463 to 1708 µg/L) observed 1 h after dosing and 1038 (777 to 1238) µg/L for the last dose administered. [G. Segre *et al., Arzneimittelforschung*, 1990, *40(4)*, 450–452].

Toxicity

A 21-year-old woman, suffering from asthma, was found dead with a blood concentration of 205 mg/L. [C. Offidani *et al., Am. J. Forensic Med. Pathol.*, 1993, *14(3)*, 244–245].

Dose. Bamifylline hydrochloride has been given in doses of 0.9 to 1.8 g daily.

Bamipine

Antihistamine

1-Methyl-*N*-phenyl-*N*-(phenylmethyl)-4-piperidinamine
$C_{19}H_{24}N_2$=280.4
CAS-4945-47-5

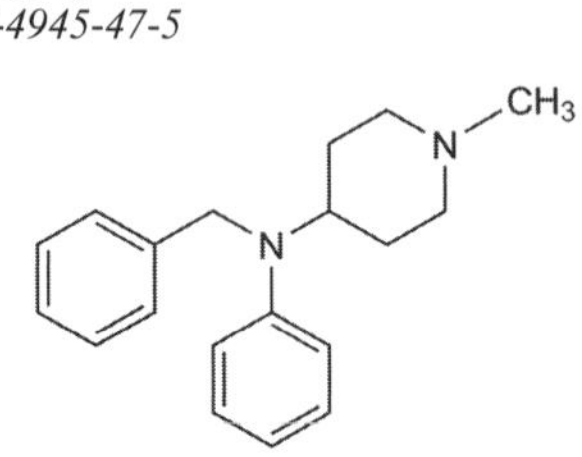

Crystals. M.p. about 115°. Soluble 1 in 75 of water.

Bamipine Hydrochloride

Proprietary names. Soventol; Taumidrine.
$C_{19}H_{24}N_2$,HCl=316.9
CAS-1229-69-2

Partition Coefficient. Log *P* (octanol), 4.1.

Colour Tests. Liebermann's test—red-orange; Mandelin's test—brown.

Thin-layer Chromatography. System TA—Rf 49; system TB—Rf 40; system TC—Rf 43; system TL—Rf 13; system TAE—Rf 24. (Acidified iodoplatinate solution, positive.)

Gas Chromatography. System GA—RI 2250; RI 2580 M (OH^-).

High Performance Liquid Chromatography. System HX—RI 468.

Ultraviolet Spectrum. Aqueous acid—251, 298 nm; methanol—251 (A^1_1=439b), 298 nm (A^1_1=62b).

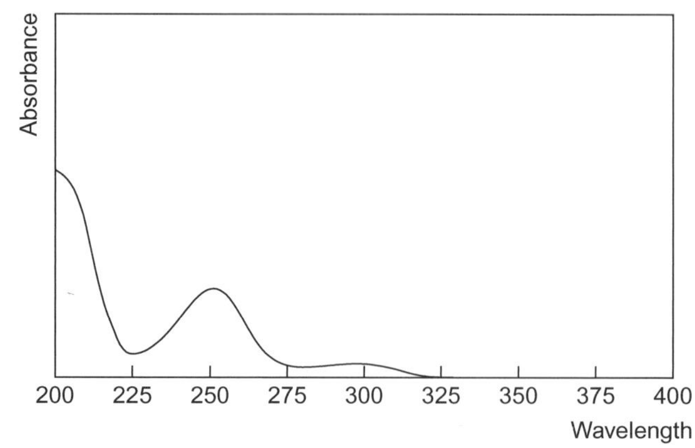

Infra-red Spectrum. Principal peaks at wavenumbers 745, 1593, 725, 1495, 690, 1275 cm^{-1} (KBr disk).

Mass Spectrum. Principal ions at *m/z* 97, 43, 71, 70, 96, 91, 98, 42.

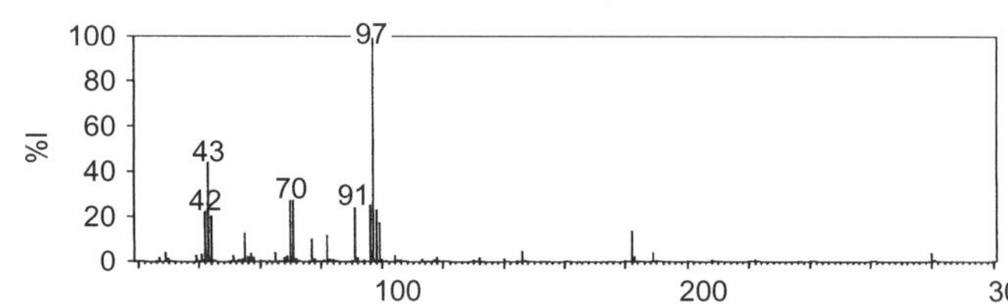

Dose. Bamipine hydrochloride has been given in doses of 75 to 400 mg daily.

Barbital

Sedative/Barbiturate

Synonyms. Barb; Barbitalum; Barbitone; Diemalum; Diethylmalonylurea; Malonal.
5,5-Diethyl-2,4,6(1*H*,3*H*,5*H*)-pyrimidinetrione
$C_8H_{12}N_2O_3$=184.2
CAS—57-44-3

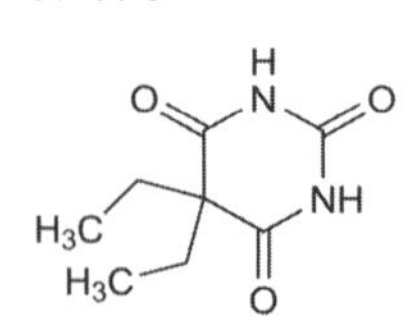

Colourless crystals or white crystalline powder. M.p. 188° to 192°. Soluble 1 in about 130 of water, 1 in 13 of boiling water, 1 in 14 of ethanol, 1 in 75 of chloroform, and 1 in 35 of ether; soluble in acetone, ethyl acetate, petroleum ether, acetic acid, amyl alcohol, pyridine, aniline, and nitrobenzene, and in solutions of alkalis.

Barbital Sodium

Synonyms. Barbitalum Natricum; Barbitone Sodium; Diemalnatrium; Soluble Barbitone.
Proprietary name. Neurinase
$C_8H_{11}N_2NaO_3$=206.2
CAS—144-02-5
A white crystalline powder. A solution in water slowly decomposes. M.p. about 190°.
Soluble 1 in 5 of water (1 in 2.5 of boiling water) and 1 in 400 of ethanol; practically insoluble in chloroform and ether.

Dissociation Constant. pK_a 8.0 (25°).

Partition Coefficient. Log *P* (octanol/water), 0.7.

Colour Tests. Koppanyi–Zwikker Test—violet; Mercurous Nitrate—black.

Thin-layer Chromatography. System TD—Rf 41; system TE—Rf 32; system TF—Rf 61; system TH—Rf 51; system TAD—Rf 57; system TAE—Rf 84. (Mercuric chloride–diphenylcarbazone reagent, positive; mercurous nitrate spray, black; Zwikker's reagent, pink.)

Gas Chromatography. System GA—barbital RI 1489, barbital-Me_2 RI 1420, barbital-Me (metharbital) RI 1470, barbituric acid-Me_3 RI 1645; system GF—RI 2230; system GAJ—RRT 0.612 (relative to methylphenobarbital).

High Performance Liquid Chromatography. System HG—*k* 1.11; system HH—*k* 0.63; system HX—RI 308; system HY—RI 258; system HZ—retention time 2.2 min; system HAA—retention time 10.4 min; system HAL—retention time 1.4 min.

Ultraviolet Spectrum. Borax buffer 0.05 M (pH 9.2)—239 nm (A^1_1=549a); M sodium hydroxide (pH 13)—254 nm (A^1_1=427b).

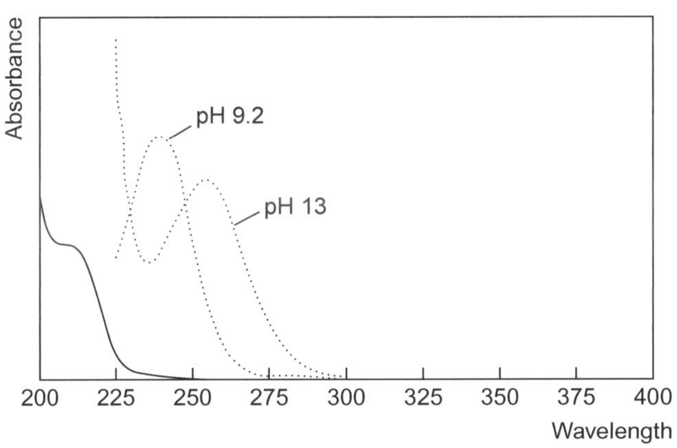

Infra-red Spectrum. Principal peaks at wavenumbers 1680, 1720, 1767, 1320, 1245, 875 cm^{-1} (KBr disk).

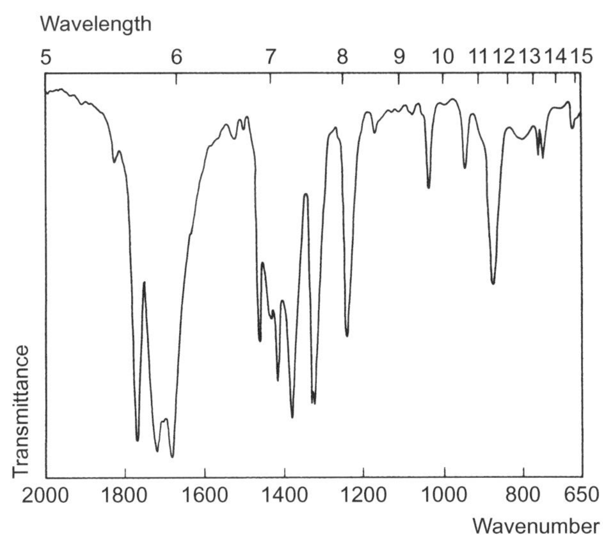

Mass Spectrum. Principal ions at *m*/*z* 156, 141, 55, 155, 98, 39, 82, 43.

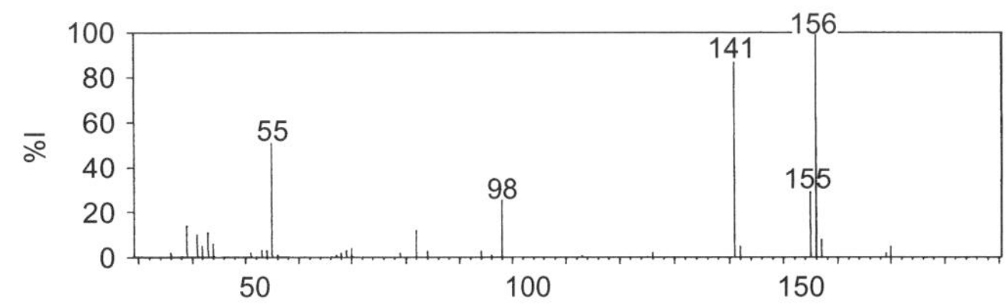

Quantification. See also under Amylobarbital.

Gas chromatography–mass spectrometry. In plasma: limit of detection 0.5 mg/L—F. Varin *et al.*, *J. Pharm. Sci.*, 1980, *69(6)*, 640–643.

Disposition in the Body. Readily absorbed after oral administration. It is excreted slowly in the urine almost entirely as unchanged drug; about 2% of a dose is excreted in 8 h, about 16% in 32 h, and detectable amounts may still be present in the urine after 16 days.
Barbital is a metabolite of metharbital.

Therapeutic concentration. In plasma, usually in the range 5 to 30 mg/L.

Toxicity. The estimated minimum lethal dose is 2 g. Toxic effects may be produced with blood concentrations of about 20 mg/L or more, and concentrations greater than 90 mg/L may be lethal.

In 6 cases of acute poisoning, the amounts ingested ranged from 5 to about 25 g. In 2 cases, death ensued after 150 and 160 h when the serum concentrations were about 100 and 170 mg/L respectively. In the other 4 cases, the serum concentrations on awakening from coma were 70 to 150 μg/L. [P. Lous, *Acta Pharmacol. Toxicol.*, 1954, *10*, 147–165 and P. Lous, *Acta Pharmacol. Toxicol.*, 1954, *10*, 261–280.]

Half-life. Plasma half-life, about 2 days.

Volume of distribution. About 0.5 L/kg.

Saliva. Plasma:saliva ratio, about 1.

Protein binding. In plasma, less than 20%.

Dose. Barbital has been given in a dose of 300 to 600 mg.

Barbituric Acid

Synonym. Malonylurea
2,4,6-(1*H*,3*H*,5*H*)-pyrimidinetrione
$C_4H_4N_2O_3$=128.1
CAS—67-52-7

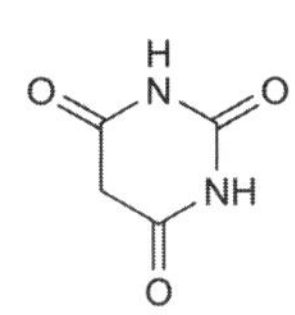

Crystals. M.p. about 248°, with some decomposition.

Dissociation Constant. pK_a 4.0 (25°).

Partition Coefficient. Log *P* (octanol/water), −1.5.

Thin-layer Chromatography. System TD—Rf 00; system TE—Rf 00; system TF—Rf 00; system TH—Rf 03; system TAD—Rf 00; system TAE—Rf 84.

Ultraviolet Spectrum. Borax buffer 0.05 M (pH 9.2)—257 nm; 1 M sodium hydroxide (pH 13) —259 nm.

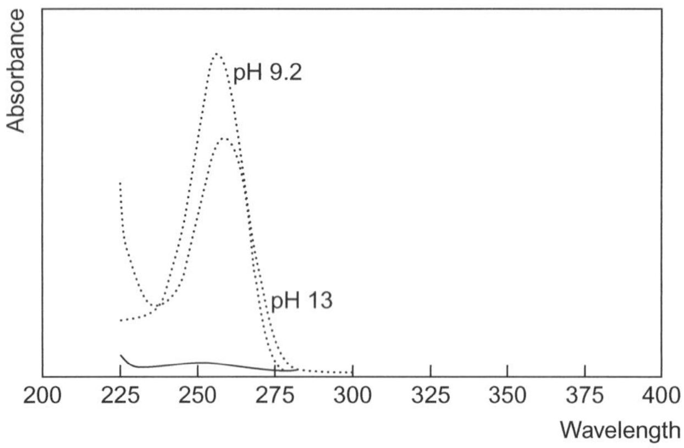

Infra-red Spectrum. Principal peaks at wavenumbers 1710, 1734, 1750, 1225, 775, 1190 cm^{-1} (KBr disk).

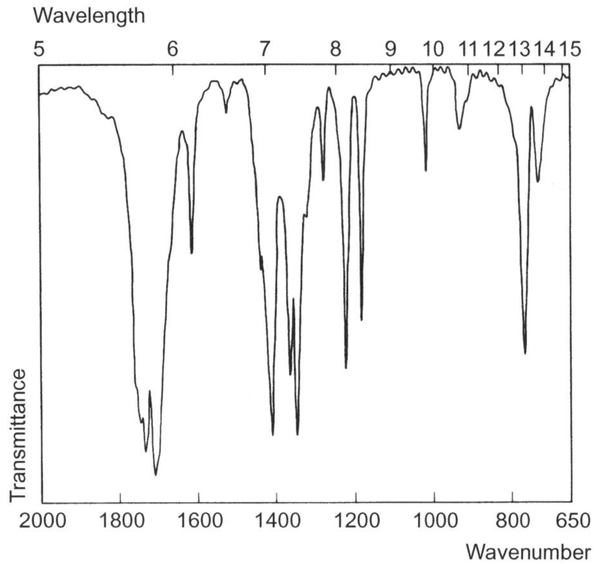

Mass Spectrum. Principal ions at *m/z* 42, 128, 85, 43, 44, 41, 70, 69.

Beclamide

Anticonvulsant

Synonyms. Benzchlorpropamide; Chloroethylphenamide.
Proprietary names. Neuracen; Nydrane; Posedrine.
3-Chloro-*N*-(phenylmethyl)propanamide
$C_{10}H_{12}ClNO = 197.7$
CAS—501-68-8

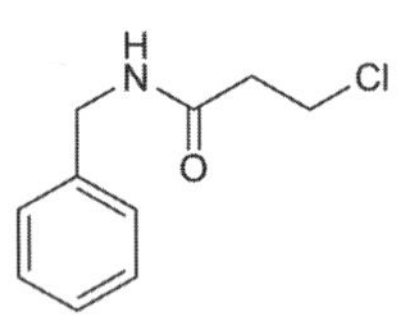

Colourless crystals. M.p. 91° to 94°.
Slightly soluble in water; soluble 1 in 14 of ethanol, 1 in 5 of chloroform, and 1 in less than 100 of ether.

Partition Coefficient. Log *P* (octanol/water), 1.8.

Colour Test. Liebermann's Test—red-orange.

Thin-layer Chromatography. System TA—Rf 65; system TB—Rf 08; system TC—Rf 65; system TL—Rf 64; system TAE—Rf 90. (Acidified potassium permanganate solution, positive, developing slowly.)

Gas Chromatography. System GA—beclamide RI 1720, beclamide-Art RI 1680; system GB—beclamide RI 1778, beclamide-Art RI 1539.

High Performance Liquid Chromatography. Column: Apex ODS (250 × 4.5 mm i.d., 5 μm). Mobile phase: acetonitrile:water (22.5:77.5): potassium dihydrogen phosphate (1.4 g/L), flow rate 2 mL/min. Internal standard: hexobarbital. UV detection (λ = 215 nm). Retention time(s): beclamide 8.8 min; 4-hydroxybeclamide 3.0 min; 3-hydroxybeclamide 3.5 min. (M. Ahmadi *et al.*, *J. Pharm. Pharmacol.*, 1995, *47*, 876–878).

Ultraviolet Spectrum. Aqueous acid—252, 258, 264; methanol—252, 258 (A_1^1 = 9.6b), 264, 268 nm.

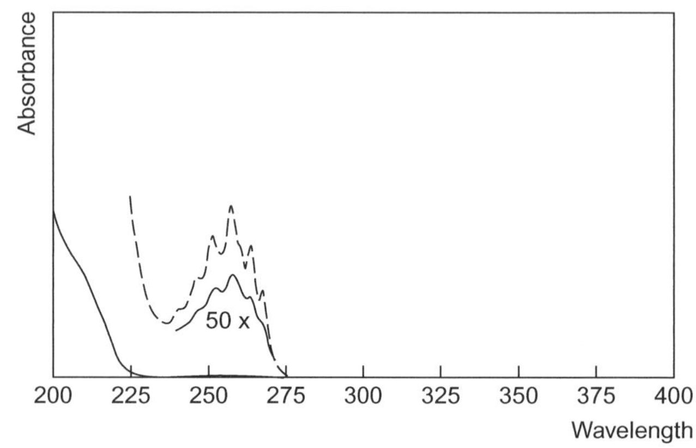

Infra-red Spectrum. Principal peaks at wavenumbers 1640, 696, 736, 1558, 1275, 1290 cm^{-1} (KBr disk).

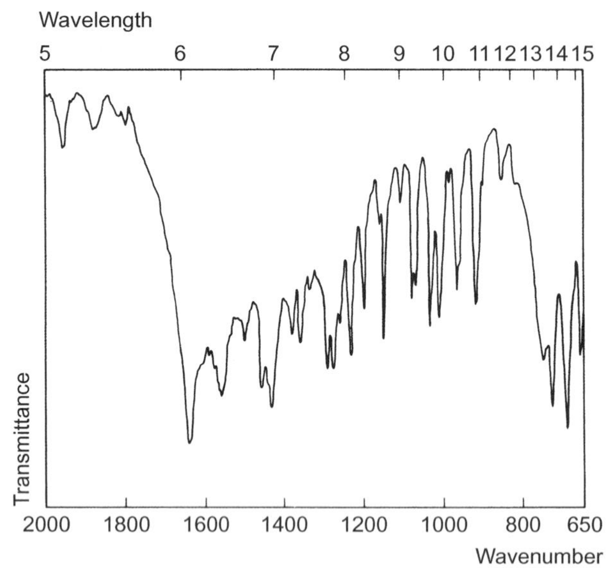

Mass Spectrum. Principal ions at *m/z* 91, 106, 197, 162, 107, 148, 27, 63.

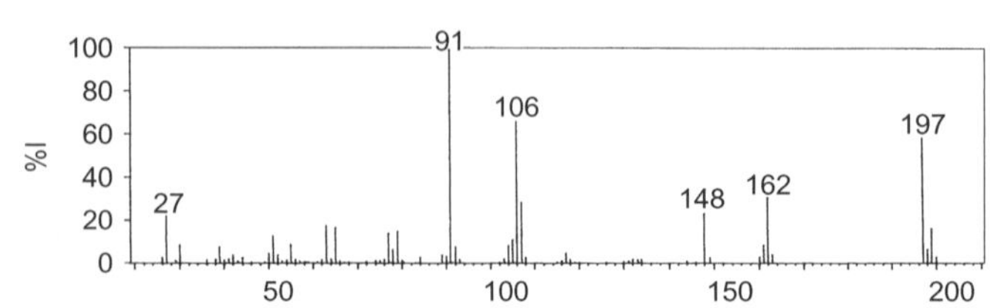

Quantification

Gas chromatography. In plasma: limit of detection 200 μg/L, FID—O. P. Jones *et al.*, *Br. J. Clin. Pharmacol.*, 1975, *2*, 364–365.

High performance liquid chromatography. In urine: limit of detection of beclamide and metabolites 0.2 mg/L—M. Ahmadi *et al.*, *J. Pharm. Pharmacol.*, 1995, *47*, 876–878.

Disposition in the Body. Beclamide is absorbed after oral administration. Less than 0.5% of a dose is excreted in the urine as unchanged drug in 24 h; a metabolite, tentatively identified as an *N*-hydroxybenzyl-3-chloropropionamide, has been detected in the urine as a glucuronide conjugate. Its 3-hydroxyphenyl (7% excreted over 24 h) and 4-hydroxyphenyl (24% over 24 h) metabolites are detected as both glucuronide (majority) and sulfate conjugates in urine. Approx. 22% of an administered dose is excreted as hippuric acid.

Therapeutic concentration

Following a single oral dose of 1 g to 6 subjects, peak plasma concentrations of 8.7 to 18.9 (mean 13) mg/L were attained in 1 to 4 h. [H. Leach *et al.*, *Br. J. Clin. Pharmacol.*, 1975, *2*, 377P–378P].

Dose. 1.5 to 4 g daily.

Beclometasone

Corticosteroid

Synonyms. Beclomethasone; 9α-Chloro-16β-methylprednisolone.
(11β,16β)-9-Chloro-11,17,21-trihydroxy-16-methylpregna-1,4-diene-3,20-dione
$C_{22}H_{29}ClO_5$=408.9
CAS—4419-39-0

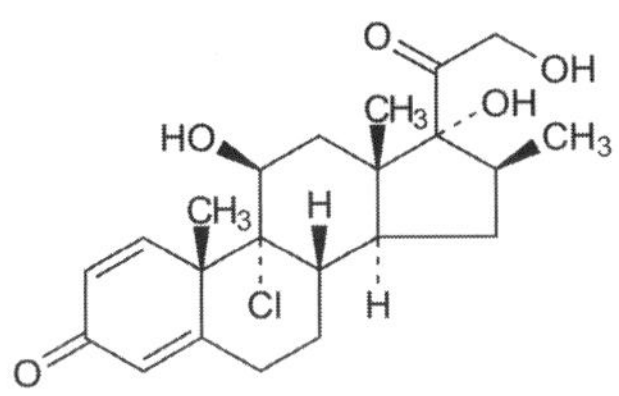

Beclometasone Dipropionate

Proprietary names. Aldecin; Becloforte; Beclovent; Beconase; Becotide; Clenil; Propaderm; Sanasthmyl; Turbinal; Vancenase; Vanceril; Viarox. It is an ingredient of Ventide.
$C_{28}H_{37}ClO_7$=521.0
CAS—5534-09-8
A white to creamy-white powder. M.p. about 212°, with decomposition. Practically insoluble in water; soluble 1 in 60 of ethanol and 1 in 8 of chloroform; freely soluble in acetone.

Partition Coefficient. Log *P* (octanol/water), 2.0.

Colour Tests. Naphthol–Sulfuric acid—green/brown-yellow; Sulfuric acid—orange (slow).

Thin-layer Chromatography. Beclometasone dipropionate: system TP—Rf 75; system TQ—Rf 38; system TR—Rf 89; system TS—Rf 42, streaking may occur. (*p*-Toluenesulfonic acid solution, positive.)

High Performance Liquid Chromatography. System HT—*k* 4.2; system HX—RI 444; system HY—RI 711 (dipropionate).

Column: C_{18} Alltima (250 × 4.6 mm i.d.). Mobile phase: methanol:water:acetonitrile:glacial acetic acid (650:262:88:1.75), flow rate 1.3 mL/min. Internal standard (IS): dexamethasone-21-acetate. UV detection (λ=242 nm). Retention time(s): beclometasone, 3.9 min; beclometasone propionate, 15.4 min [K. Foe *et al.*, *Biopharm. Drug Dispos.*, 1998, *19*, 1–8].

Column: (1) C_{18} Alltima 16% carbon load (250 × 4.6 mm i.d., 5 μm); (2) C_{18} Econosphere 10% carbon load (250 × 4.6 mm i.d., 5 μm); (3) C_8 Ultrasphere (150 × 4.6 mm i.d., 5 μm). Mobile phase: (1) methanol:water:acetonitrile:acetic acid (309:146:44:1), flow rate 1.3 mL/min; (2) (250:205:44:1), 1.2 mL/min; (3) (275:180:44:1), 1.3 mL/min. UV detection (λ=242 nm). Retention time(s): beclometasone, (1) 4.9 min (2) 5.5 min (3) 3.3 min; beclometasone propionate, (1) 23.0 min (2) 25.9 min (3) 17.6 min [K. Foe *et al.*, *Drug Metab. Dispos.*, 1998, *26(2)*, 132–136].

Ultraviolet Spectrum. Beclometasone dipropionate: dehydrated alcohol—239 nm (A_1^1=292a).

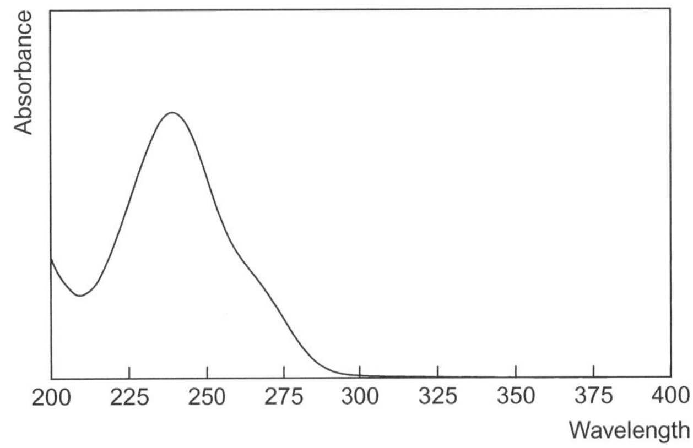

Infra-red Spectrum. Principal peaks at wavenumbers 1190, 1658, 1730, 1608, 890, 1053 cm^{-1} (beclometasone dipropionate, KBr disk).

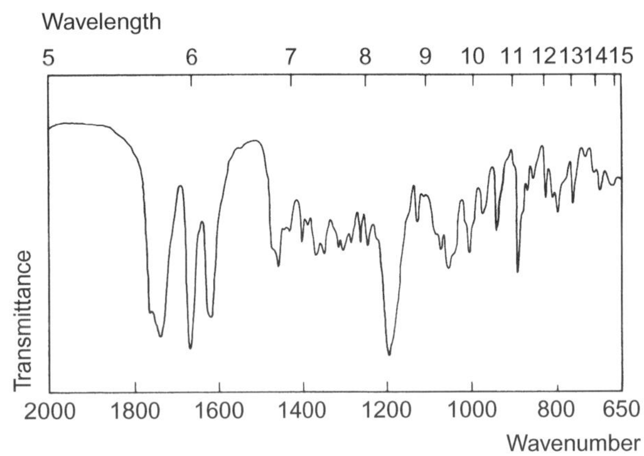

Quantification

High performance liquid chromatography–mass spectrometry. In hair: limit of detection 0.17 ng/g, MS detection (*m/z* 411)—V. Cirimele *et al.*, *Forensic Sci. Int.*, 2000, *107(1–3)*, 381–383.

Disposition in the Body. Beclometasone dipropionate is rapidly converted to the metabolite beclometasone-17-monopropionate.

Therapeutic concentration

12 healthy males, aged 22 to 39 years, were administered a single IV dose of 1.0 mg over a 10-min infusion, a single intranasal dose of 1.344 mg, a single inhaled dose of 1.0 mg and a single oral dose of 4.0 mg as an aqueous solution. Subjects were fasted 12 h before dosing and for 2 h afterwards. The median peak plasma beclometasone dipropionate concentrations for the above doses were 35.356 μg/L (range 20.2 to 61.7 μg/L) observed at 0.2 to 0.3 h, 0.31 (0.256 to 0.375) μg/L at 4 to 8 h, 0.319 (0.184 to 0.553) μg/L at 0.2 to 0.5 h and 0.703 (0.563 to 0.879) μg/L at 1.5 to 6.0 h, respectively [P. T. Daley-Yates *et al.*, *Br. J. Clin. Pharmacol.*, 2001, *51(5)*, 400–409].

Half-life. Beclometasone dipropionate, 0.3 to 0.7 h; beclometasone 17-monopropionate, 1.3 to 5.3 h.

Volume of distribution. Beclometasone dipropionate, median, 20 (range 10.6 to 39.4) L; beclometasone 17-monopropionate, 424 (362 to 496) L.

Clearance. Plasma, beclometasone dipropionate, median, 150 (98.8 to 228) L/h; beclometasone 17-monopropionate, 120 (104 to 139) L/h.

Dose. Usually 300 to 400 μg of beclometasone dipropionate daily, by aerosol inhalation; maximum of 2 mg daily.

Bemegride

CNS Stimulant/Antidote (Barbiturate Poisoning)

Synonym. Methetharimide
Proprietary names. Eukraton; Megimide.
4-Ethyl-4-methyl-2,6-piperidinedione

$C_8H_{13}NO_2$=155.2
CAS—64-65-3

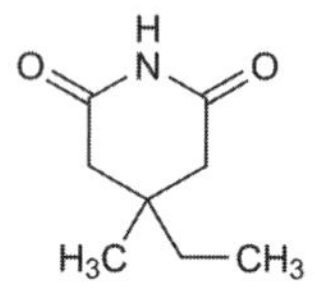

White flakes or crystalline powder. M.p. 126° to 128°. Soluble 1 in 170 of water, 1 in 30 of ethanol, 1 in 12 of acetone, 1 in 4 of chloroform, and 1 in 100 of ether; soluble in aqueous solutions of alkali hydroxides.

Bemegride Sodium
$C_8H_{12}NNaO_2$=177.2
CAS—25334-00-3
A fine white powder. Soluble 1 in 11 of water and 1 in 20 of ethanol; practically insoluble in acetone and ether.

Dissociation Constant. pK_a 11.6.

Partition Coefficient. Log *P* (octanol/water), 0.5.

Colour Tests. Koppanyi–Zwikker test—violet; Mercurous nitrate—black.

Thin-layer Chromatography. System TD—Rf 52; system TE—Rf 68; system TF—Rf 53; system TAD—Rf 64; system TAF—Rf 88. (Mercuric chloride–diphenylcarbazone reagent, positive; mercurous nitrate spray, black.)

Gas Chromatography. System GA—RI 1373; system GC—RI 1253.

Ultraviolet Spectrum. No significant absorption, 230 to 360 nm.

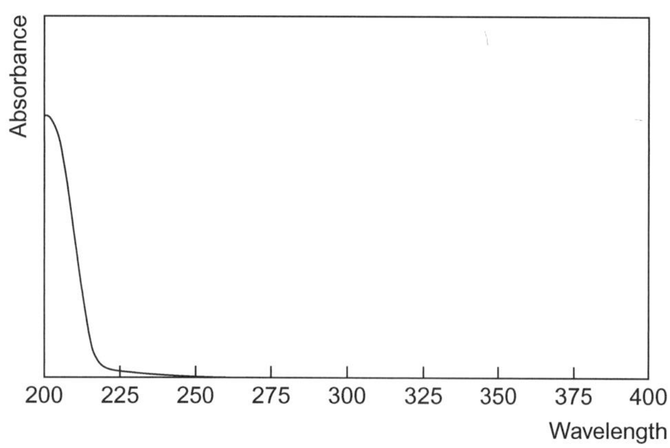

Infra-red Spectrum. Principal peaks at wavenumbers 1680, 1277, 1730, 860, 1160, 1145 cm^{-1} (KBr disk).

Mass Spectrum. Principal ions at *m/z* 55, 83, 82, 41, 113, 70, 29, 69.

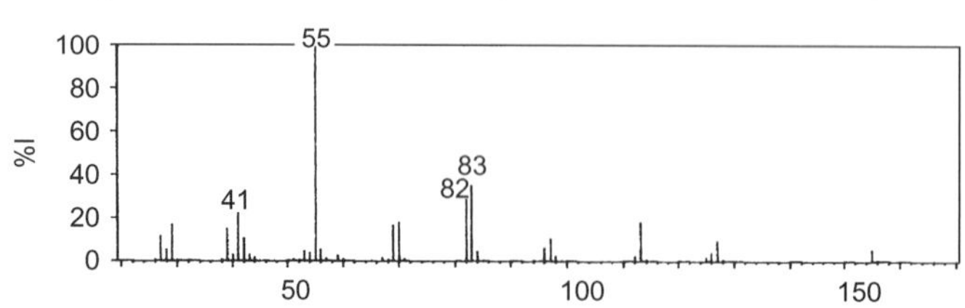

Disposition in the Body. Metabolised by hydroxylation of the ethyl side-chain and excreted in the urine as unchanged drug and as the hydroxy metabolite.

Dose. Bemegride has been given in doses of 25 to 50 mg intravenously, repeated as necessary.

Benactyzine

Antispasmodic

α-Hydroxy-α-phenylbenzeneacetic acid 2-(diethylamino)ethyl ester
$C_{20}H_{25}NO_3$=327.4
CAS—302-40-9

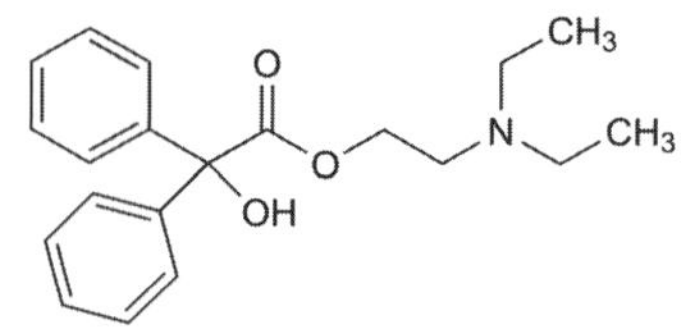

Crystals. M.p. 51°.

Benactyzine Hydrochloride
Proprietary name. It is an ingredient of Deprol.
$C_{20}H_{25}NO_3,HCl$=363.9
CAS—57-37-4
A white crystalline powder. M.p. 177° to 181°. Soluble 1 in 14 of water and 1 in 22 of ethanol; very slightly soluble in ether.

Dissociation Constant. pK_a 6.6.

Partition Coefficient. Log *P* (octanol/water), 2.9.

Colour Tests. Liebermann's test—orange→brown; Marquis test—orange→green→blue; Sulfuric acid—orange.

Thin-layer Chromatography. System TA—Rf 66; system TB—Rf 40; system TC—Rf 53; system TL—Rf 53; system TAE—Rf 52; system TAF—Rf 57; system TAJ—Rf 34; system TAK—Rf 03; system TAL—Rf 48. (Acidified iodoplatinate solution, positive.)

Gas Chromatography. System GA—RI 2255.

High Performance Liquid Chromatography. System HA—*k* 1.7; system HX—RI 382.

Ultraviolet Spectrum. Aqueous acid—252, 258 (A^1_1=14a), 262, 264 nm.

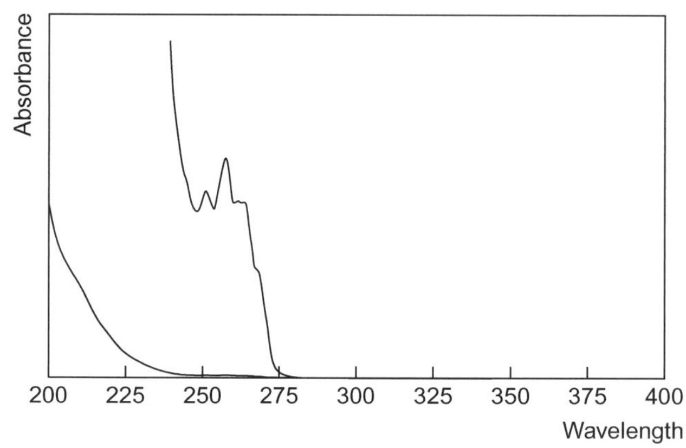

Infra-red Spectrum. Principal peaks at wavenumbers 695, 1723, 1231, 1054, 1162, 751 cm^{-1} (KBr disk).

Mass Spectrum. Principal ions at *m/z* 86, 105, 77, 87, 182, 99, 183, 58.

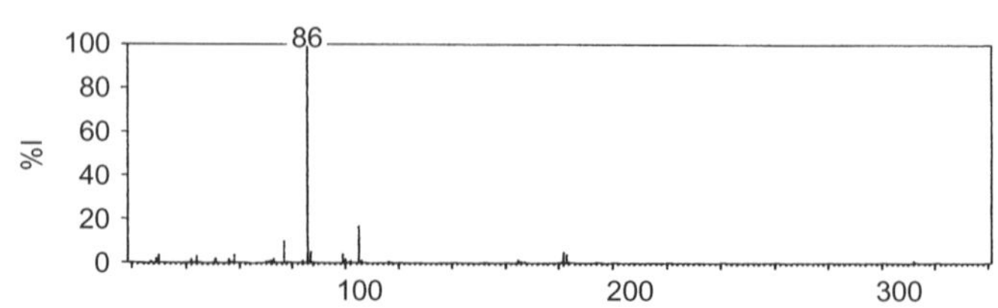

Disposition in the Body. Rapidly metabolised and excreted.

Dose. 3 to 9 mg of benactyzine hydrochloride daily.

Benaprizine

Anticholinergic

Synonym. Benapryzine
2-(*N*-Ethylpropylamino)ethyl benzilate
$C_{21}H_{27}NO_3$=341.4

CAS—22487-42-9

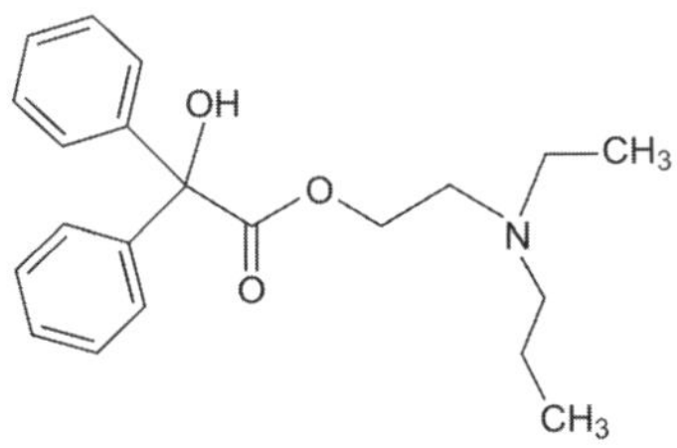

Benaprizine Hydrochloride
$C_{21}H_{27}NO_3$,HCl=377.9
CAS—32702-55-9
A white crystalline powder. M.p. about 166°. Soluble 1 in 35 of water, 1 in 56 of dehydrated alcohol, 1 in 120 of acetone and 1 in 8 of chloroform.

Thin-layer Chromatography. System TAJ—Rf 48; system TAK—Rf 05; system TAL—Rf 58.

Ultraviolet Spectrum. Aqueous acid—251, 257, 261, 264 nm.

Infra-red Spectrum. Principal peaks at wavenumbers 1753, 1215, 700, 690, 1180, 1020 cm^{-1} (benaprizine hydrochloride, KCl disk).

Dose. 150 to 200 mg of benaprizine hydrochloride daily.

Benazepril

Antihypertensive/ACE Inhibitor

(3*S*)-3-[[1-(Ethoxycarbonyl)-3-phenylpropyl]amino]-2,3,4,5-tetrahydro-2-oxo-1*H*-1-benzazepine-1-acetic acid
$C_{24}H_{28}N_2O_5$=424.5
CAS—86541-75-5

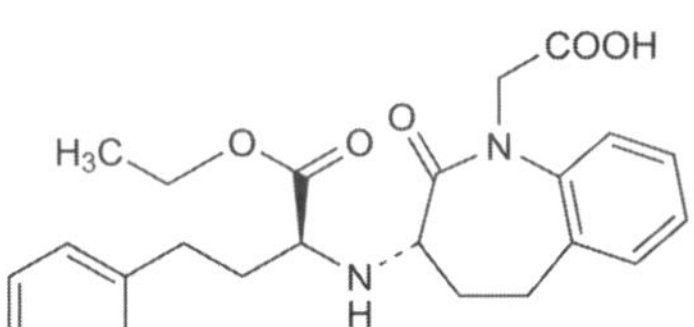

M.p. 148.5°.

Benazepril Hydrochloride
Synonym. CGS 14824A
Proprietary names. Briem; Cibace; Cibacen; Cibacene; Labopal; Lotensin; Tensanil; Zinandril.
$C_{24}H_{28}N_2O_5$,HCl=461.0
CAS—86541-74-4
A white to off-white crystalline powder. It is soluble in water, ethanol and methanol.

Partition Coefficient. Log *P* (octanol/water), 3.50.

Gas Chromatography. System GP—RI 3030 (benazepril-ME); RI 2985 (M (benazeprilate)-ME3).

Column: 3% OV-101 on Gaschrom Q, 80-100 mesh (Ciba-Geigy), pyrex glass (1.5 m × 2 mm i.d.). Column and injector port temperature: 275°. Carrier gas: helium, flow rate 30 mL/min. MS detection (EI, SIM). Retention times: benazepril (methyl ester derivative) 2.55 min; benazeprilat (derivative) 2.3 min. [G. Kaiser *et al.*, *J. Chromatogr.*, 1987, 419, 123–133].

High Performance Liquid Chromatography. System HAA—retention time 17.0 min.

Column: C_{18} (RP-BDS, 5 µm packing, 250 × 3 mm i.d.). Mobile phase: sodium dihydrogen phosphate (0.025 M, pH 4.8):acetonitrile (55:45). 0.4 mL/min flow rate. UV detection (λ=250 nm). Retention time: benazepril hydrochloride, 4.95 min. [I. E. Panderi and M. Parissi-Polou, *J. Pharm. Biomed. Anal.*, 1999, *21*, 1017–1024].

Column: Hypersil ODS (5 µm, 250 × 4.5 mm). Mobile phase: sodium heptanesulfonate (20 mM, pH 2.5):acetonitrile (5% THF) (52:48 v/v), 1.0 mL/min flow rate. UV detection (λ=215 nm). Retention time: 15 min. [D. Bonazzi *et al.*, *J. Pharm. Biomed. Anal.*, 1997, *16*, 431–438].

Ultraviolet Spectrum. Aqueous acid (0.2 M NH_2SO_4)—237 nm; basic—241 nm; aqueous acid (0.1 M hydrochloric acid)—237.2 nm (hydrochloride salt).

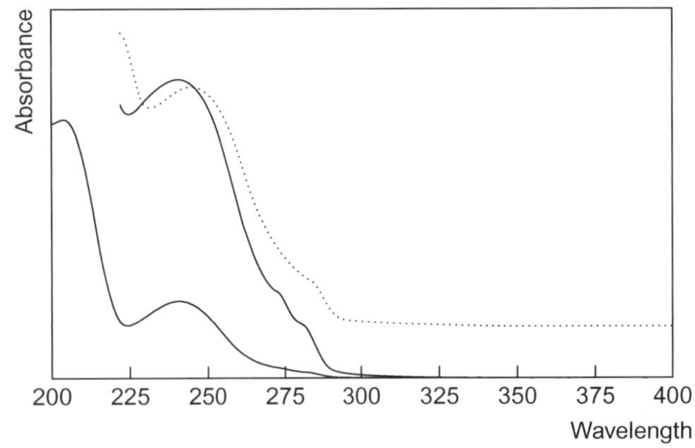

Infra-red Spectrum. Principal peaks at wavenumber 1739, 1674, 1211 cm^{-1} (hydrochloride salt) (KBr pellet).

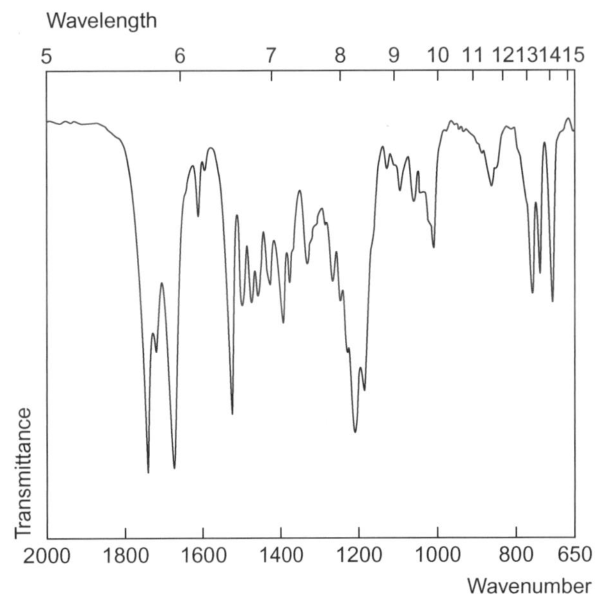

Mass Spectrum. Benazepril (methyl ester derivative): principal ions at *m/z* 91, 204, 365, 144, 118, 117, 120, 122.

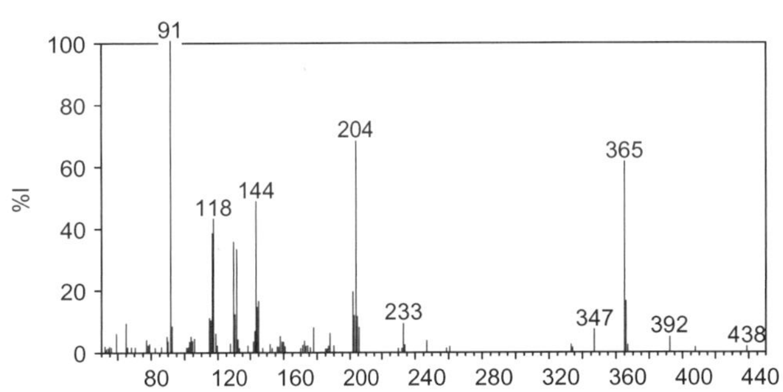

Quantification

Gas chromatography–mass spectrometry. In plasma: limit of quantification, for benazepril, 26 µg/L and limit of detection 3.4 µg/L, for benazeprilat 23 µg/L and 2.3 µg/L, respectively. In urine: for benazepril, limit of quantification 34 µg/L and limit of detection 6.4 µg/L; for benazeprilat

64.5 μg/L and 7.6 μg/L, respectively—K. Gaiser *et al.*, *J. Chromatogr.*, 1987, *419*, 123–133.

High performance liquid chromatography. In pharmaceutical tablets: limit of detection for benazeprilat hydrochloride is 0.88 mg/L and limit of quantification is 2.92 mg/L. UV detection (λ=250 nm)—I. E. Panderi and M. Parissi-Polou, *J. Pharm. Biomed. Anal.*, 1999, *21*, 1017–1024.

Bioassay. In plasma: limit of detection 8.5 μg/L. In urine: 4.25 μg/L—P. Graf *et al.*, *J. Chromatogr.*, 1988, *425*, 353–361.

Disposition in the Body. A minimum of 37% of an oral dose of benazepril is absorbed (fasting) and is rapidly converted to its active carboxylic metabolite, benazeprilat by enzymatic hydrolysis in the liver. Benazepril is cleared mainly by metabolic transformation with < 1% being excreted unchanged in urine along with its acyl glucuronide metabolite. Approximately 18% of an oral dose is recovered in urine as the diacid, benazeprilat. Peak plasma concentrations of benazeprilat occur 1 to 2 h after administration, if fasting, and 2 to 4 h in the non-fasting state. 11 to 12% of benazeprilat is excreted in bile and the majority in urine. Elimination is slow with renal impairment. Very small amounts of benazepril and benazeprilat are secreted into breast milk.

Therapeutic concentration

A daily (oral) dose of 10 mg benazepril was administered to 9 young subjects (male; between 21 and 39 years) and 9 elderly subjects (6 male, 3 female; between 66 and 76 years), over 8 consecutive days. After repeated administration, benazeprilat was detected in plasma immediately before the last dose with mean values of 0.015 μg/L for the young subjects and 0.037 μg/L for the elderly. These values, and those obtained 24 h later, are consistent with steady-state disposition of benazeprilat. Time to peak concentrations was 1.5 h for both groups, after acute and chronic administration. [N. J. MacDonald *et al.*, *Br. J. Clin. Pharmacol.*, 1993, *36*, 201–204]

Toxicity. Severe hypotension with acute overdose.

Half-life. Apparent elimination half-life for benazepril is 0.6 h and it is eliminated from plasma completely within 4 h.
Benazeprilat is eliminated in a biphasic manner with an initial half-life of 3 h and a terminal half-life of 17 h.

Volume of distribution. Steady state, approximately, 0.7 L/kg (metabolite).

Distribution in blood. Benazeprilat is not extensively distributed into extravascular sites with minimum passage across the blood/brain barrier.

Protein binding. Benazepril and benazeprilat both bind serum proteins, approx. 94% and 93%, respectively.

Dose. An initial dose of 10 mg once daily is recommended in patients with creatinine clearance ⩾30 mL/min and those not receiving diuretics. Hypertensive patients with heart failure and those with a creatinine clearance > 30 mL/min are recommended an initial daily dose of 5 mg. A usual daily dose is between 20 and 40 mg with a maximum of 80 mg.

Bendroflumethiazide

Diuretic

Synonyms. Bendrofluazide; Benzydroflumethiazide.
Proprietary names. Aprinox; Berkozide; Centyl; Naturetin; Neo-NaClex; Pluryl; Polidiuril; Salural; Sinesalin; Urizide. It is an ingredient of Abicol, Corgaretic, Inderetic, Inderex, Prestim, Rauzide and Tenavoid.
3,4-Dihydro-3-(phenylmethyl)-6-(trifluoromethyl)-2*H*-1,2,4-benzothiadiazine-7-sulfonamide 1,1-dioxide
$C_{15}H_{14}F_3N_3O_4S_2$=421.4
CAS—73-48-3

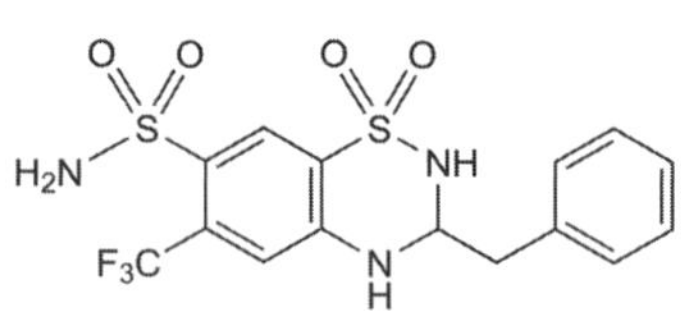

A white or cream-coloured crystalline powder. M.p. about 220°, with decomposition. Practically insoluble in water and chloroform; soluble 1 in 17 of ethanol, 1 in 1.5 of acetone, and 1 in 500 of ether.

Dissociation Constant. pK_a 8.5 (25°).

Partition Coefficient. Log *P* (octanol/water), 1.9.

Colour Tests. Koppanyi–Zwikker test—violet; Liebermann's test—blue; Sulfuric acid—violet.

Thin-layer Chromatography. System TD—Rf 25; system TE—Rf 52; system TF—Rf 71; system TAD—Rf 30; system TAJ—Rf 38; system TAK—Rf 11; system TAL—Rf 72. (Location under UV light, violet fluorescence.)

Gas Chromatography. System GX—Retention time(s) 10.7 min, bendrofluazide-ME4; system GY—Retention time(s) 5.6 min, bendrofluazide-ME4.

High Performance Liquid Chromatography. System HN—*k* 15.35; system HX—RI 508; system HAA—Retention time(s) 18.6 min.

Ultraviolet Spectrum. Aqueous acid—207, 273 (A^1_1=585a), 325; aqueous alkali—273 (A^1_1=410a), 330 nm.

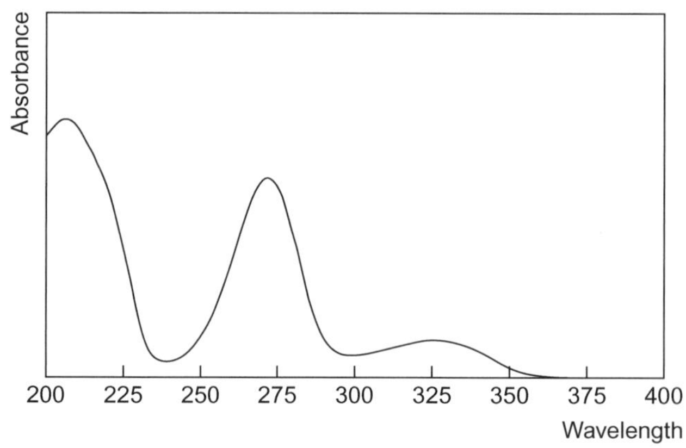

Infra-red Spectrum. Principal peaks at wavenumbers 1170, 1155, 1306, 1518, 1621, 750 cm^{-1} (KBr disk). There are 2 polymorphic forms.

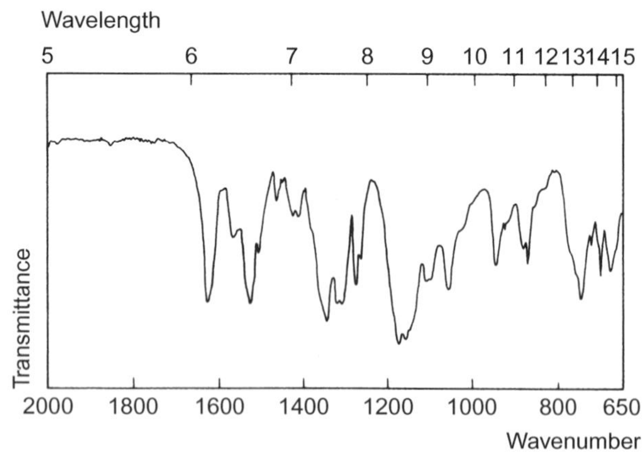

Mass Spectrum. Principal ions at *m/z* 330, 118, 91, 319, 219, 64, 92, 421.

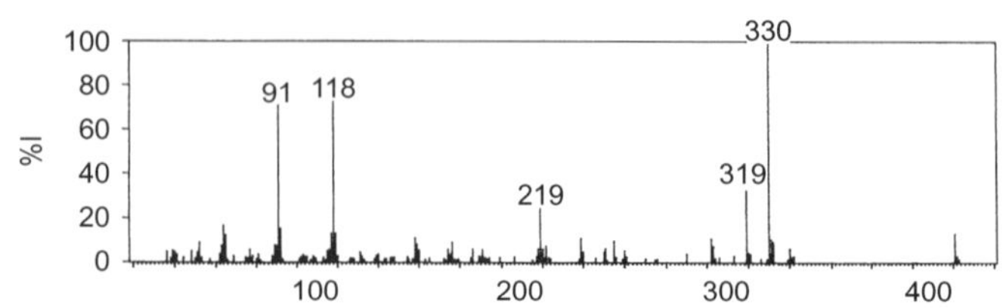

Quantification

Gas chromatography. In plasma: limit of detection 5 μg/L, ECD—B. Beerman *et al.*, *Eur. J. Clin. Pharmacol.*, 1976, *10*, 293–295.

Disposition in the Body. Readily and almost completely absorbed after oral administration. Up to about 30% of a dose is excreted unchanged in the urine in 48 h; the remainder is excreted as unidentified metabolites.

Therapeutic concentration

A single oral dose of 10 mg given to 9 subjects, produced peak plasma concentrations of 0.07 to 0.10 mg/L in 1.6 to 2.4 h. [B. Beerman *et al.*, *Clin. Pharmacol. Ther.*, 1977, *22*, 385–388].

Peak plasma concentrations of 0.04 to 0.06 (mean 0.05) mg/L were reported 2 h after a dose, following administration of 5 mg daily to 8 hypertensive patients. [B. Beerman *et al.*, *Eur. J. Clin. Pharmacol.*, 1978, *13*, 119–124].

Half-life. Plasma half-life, about 9 h.

Volume of distribution. About 1.5 L/kg.

Protein binding. In plasma, about 94%.

Note. For a review of the clinical pharmacokinetics of diuretics see B. Beerman and M. Groschinsky-Grind, *Clin. Pharmacokinet.*, 1980, *5*, 221–245.

Dose. 2.5 to 10 mg daily.

Benethamine

Pharmaceutical Adjuvant

N-Benzylphenethylamine
$C_{15}H_{17}N = 211.3$

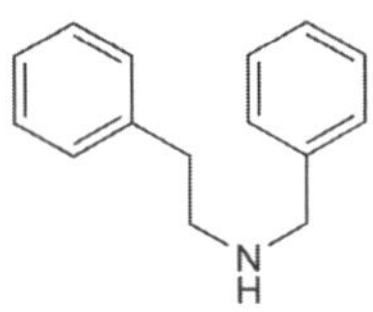

Soluble in chloroform.

Colour Tests. Liebermann's test—red-orange; Marquis test—orange-brown→brown.

Thin-layer Chromatography. System TA—Rf 64; system TB—Rf 48; system TC—Rf 59; system TL—Rf 43. (Acidified iodoplatinate solution, positive.)

Gas Chromatography. System GA—RI 1798.

Ultraviolet Spectrum. Water—258 nm ($A_1^1 = 12b$).

Infra-red Spectrum. Principal peaks at wavenumbers 696, 745, 1111, 1022, 1592, 1067 cm^{-1} (KBr disk).

Mass Spectrum. Principal ions at *m/z* 91, 120, 65, 121, 92, 105, 77, 118.

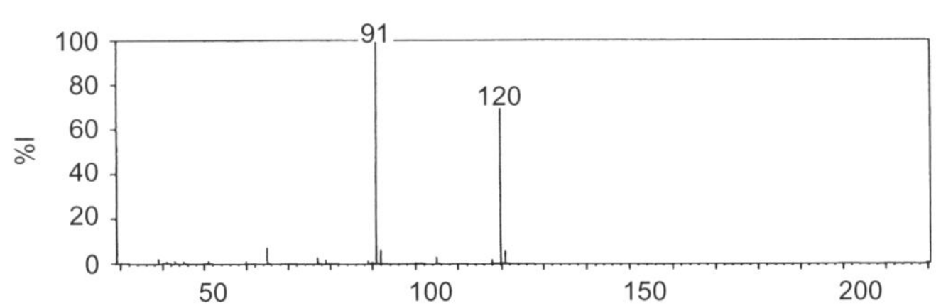

Benorilate

Analgesic

Synonyms. Benorylate; Fenasprate.
Proprietary names. Benoral; Benortan; Salipran.
2-(Acetyloxy)benzoic acid 4-(acetylamino)phenyl ester
$C_{17}H_{15}NO_5 = 313.3$
CAS—5003-48-5

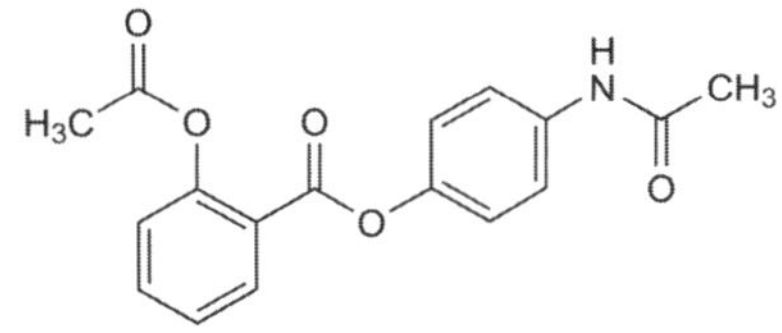

A white crystalline powder. M.p. 178° to 181°. Practically insoluble in water; soluble 1 in 88 of ethanol, 1 in 22 of acetone, 1 in 18 of chloroform, and 1 in 900 of ether.

Partition Coefficient. Log *P* (octanol/water), 2.2.

Colour Tests. Liebermann's test—black; Mandelin's test—green; Marquis test—violet.

Thin-layer Chromatography. System TA—Rf 67; system TB—Rf 00; system TC—Rf 51; system TL—Rf 62; system TAE—Rf 86. (Marquis reagent, positive.)

Gas Chromatography. System GA—benorilate RI 1840, aspirin RI 1309, paracetamol RI 1687.

High Performance Liquid Chromatography. System HD—benorilate *k* 0.7, aspirin *k* 0.5, paracetamol *k* 0.1; system HW—benorilate *k* 22.4, aspirin *k* 2.7, paracetamol *k* 0.32.

Ultraviolet Spectrum. Dehydrated alcohol—240 nm ($A_1^1 = 740a$).

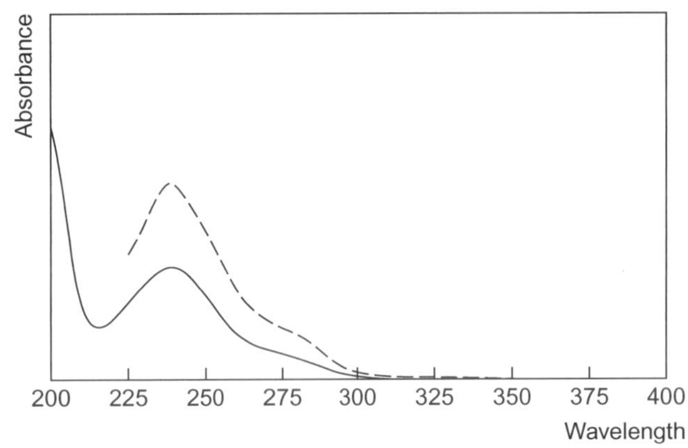

Infra-red Spectrum. Principal peaks at wavenumbers 1182, 1050, 1661, 1730, 1248, 1194 cm^{-1} (KBr disk).

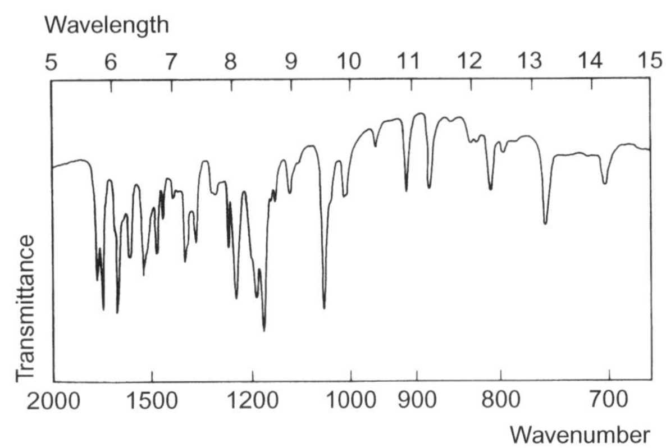

Mass Spectrum. Principal ions at *m/z* 121, 163, 151, 109, 43, 122, 108, 65; aspirin 120, 43, 138, 92, 121, 39, 64, 63; paracetamol 109, 151, 43, 80, 108, 81, 53, 52.

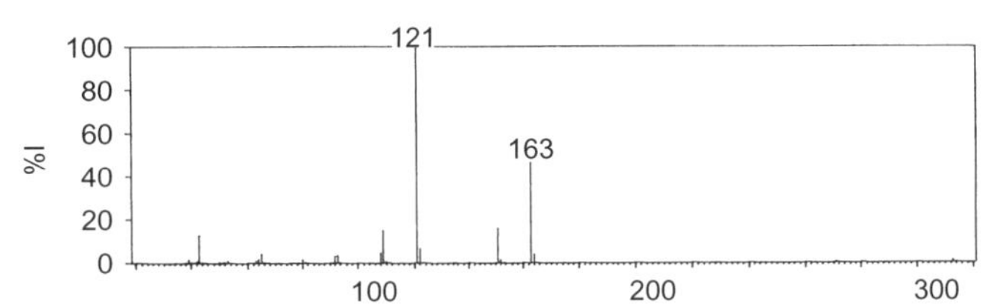

Quantification. See also under Aspirin and Paracetamol.

Gas chromatography. In plasma: aspirin and salicylic acid, limit of detection 2 mg/L for aspirin, FID—A. Cailleux *et al.*, *Therapie*, 1979, *34*, 73–79.

High performance liquid chromatography. In plasma: benorilate and paracetamol, limit of detection 200 μg/L for benorilate and 400 μg/L for paracetamol, UV detection—A. Cailleux *et al.*, *Therapie*, 1979, *34*, 73–79.

Disposition in the Body. Benorilate is readily absorbed after oral administration. It is hydrolysed in the blood to aspirin and paracetamol, and about 85% of a dose is excreted in the urine in 72 h by the normal metabolic routes for these substances. About 15% of a dose is eliminated in the faeces.

Therapeutic concentration

Following oral administration of 4 g as a suspension to 20 subjects, mean peak plasma concentrations of 2.2 mg/L of benorilate and about 120 mg/L of salicylate were attained in 0.5 and 3 h, respectively. [M. Aylward *et al.*, *Scand. J. Rheumatol.*, 1976, Suppl. *13*, 9–12].

Half-life. Plasma half-life, about 1 h.

Dose. 4.5 to 8 g daily.

Benoxaprofen

Analgesic

Proprietary names. Opren; Oraflex.

2-(4-Chlorophenyl)-α-methyl-5-benzoxazoleacetic acid

$C_{16}H_{12}ClNO_3 = 301.7$

CAS—67434-14-4

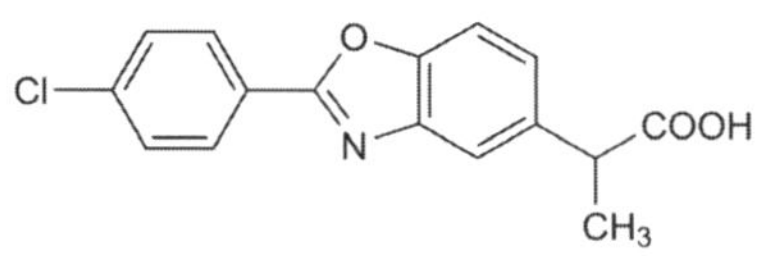

A cream-coloured solid. M.p. 189° to 190°.

Dissociation Constant. pK_a 3.5.

Partition Coefficient. Log *P* (octanol/water), 3.2.

Thin-layer Chromatography. System TG—Rf 14; system TAJ—Rf 56; system TAK—Rf 80; system TAL—Rf 99. (Ludy Tenger reagent, orange.)

Gas Chromatography. System GA—RI 2550; RI 2485 benoxaprofen-ME; system GB—not eluted; system GD—Retention time of methyl derivative 1.98 relative to $n\text{-}C_{16}H_{34}$.

High Performance Liquid Chromatography. System HD—*k* 11.3; system HV—RRT 0.98 relative to meclofenamic acid.

Ultraviolet Spectrum. Aqueous alkali—244 (A^1_1=295b), 309 nm (A^1_1=900b).

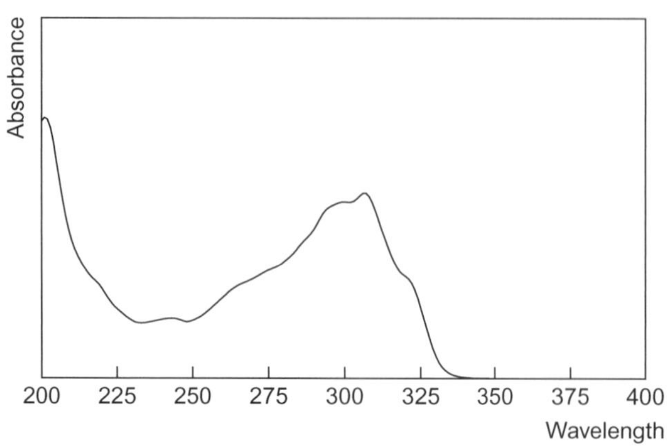

Infra-red Spectrum. Principal peaks at wavenumbers 728, 1695, 833, 1086, 1050, 1010 cm^{-1} (KBr disk).

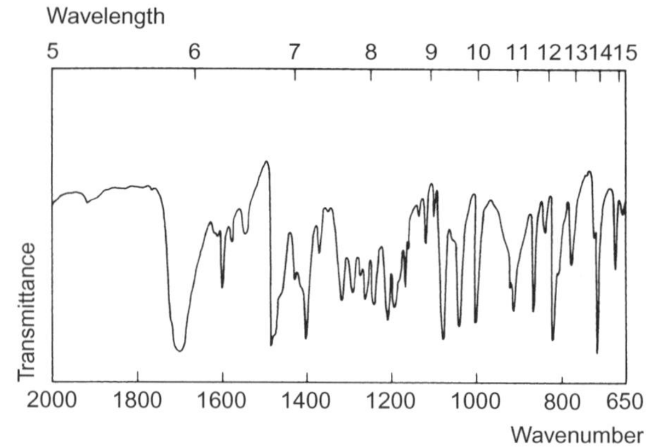

Mass Spectrum. Principal ions at *m/z* 256, 301, 91, 258, 119, 65, 257, 303.

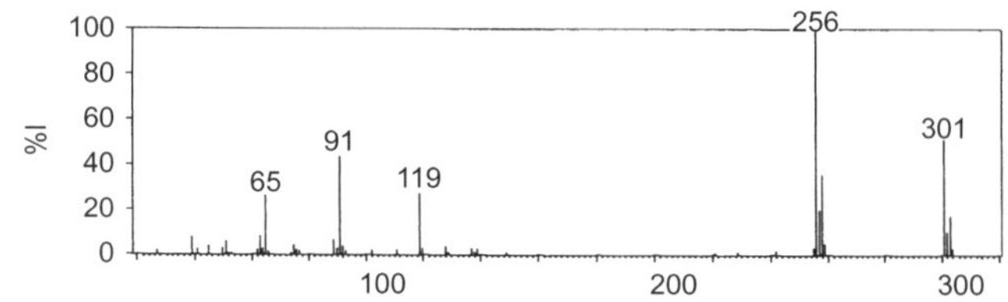

Quantification

Gas chromatography. In plasma or urine: limit of detection 10 μg/L, ECD—D. H. Chatfield and T. J. Woodage, *J. Chromatogr.*, 1978, *153*, 101–106.

High performance liquid chromatography. In plasma or urine: limit of detection 25 μg/L, UV detection—L. Ekman *et al.*, *J. Chromatogr.*, 1980, *182*; *B Biomed. Appl.*, *8*, 478–481.

Disposition in the Body. Benoxaprofen is readily absorbed after oral administration. About 15% of a dose is excreted in the urine in 24 h, mainly as the glucuronic acid conjugate, together with small amounts of unchanged drug. In 5 days about 60% of a dose is excreted in the urine and 40% is eliminated in the faeces.

Therapeutic concentration

After a single oral dose of 400 mg, administered to 4 subjects, a mean peak plasma concentration of 45 mg/L was attained in 2 to 4 h. [G. L. Smith *et al.*, *Br. J. Clin. Pharmacol.*, 1977, *4*, 585–590].

Toxicity. Because of reports of adverse reactions and fatalities, benoxaprofen was withdrawn worldwide in 1982.

Half-life. Plasma half-life, about 30 to 35 h; increased in renal impairment.

Protein binding. In plasma, more than 99%.

Dose. Benoxaprofen has been given in doses of 600 mg daily.

Benperidol

Antipsychotic

Synonym. Benzperidol

Proprietary names. Anquil; Frenactil; Glianimon.

1-[1-[4-(4-Fluorophenyl)-4-oxobutyl]-4-piperidinyl]-1,3-dihydro-2*H*-benzimidazol-2-one

$C_{22}H_{24}FN_3O_2 = 381.4$

CAS—2062-84-2

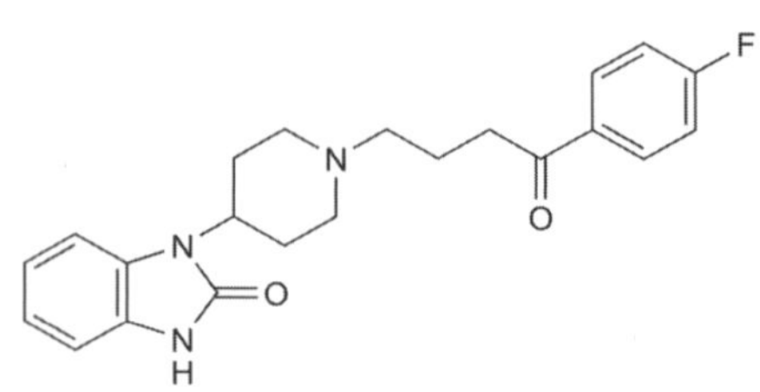

An off-white amorphous powder or crystals. It darkens slowly on exposure to light. M.p. 170° to 171.8°. Practically insoluble in water; soluble 1 in

1000 of ethanol, 1 in 4 of chloroform, and 1 in 625 of ether; sparingly soluble in dilute mineral acids.

Partition Coefficient. Log *P* (octanol/water), 3.9.

Colour Tests. Koppanyi–Zwikker test—violet; Mandelin's test—violet; Mercurous nitrate—black.

Thin-layer Chromatography. System TF—Rf 3; system TL—Rf 32; system TAE—Rf 62; system TAF—Rf 69.

Gas Chromatography. System GA—RI 3433; M (*N*-desalkyl-) RI 2415; system GB—RI 3667.

High Performance Liquid Chromatography. System HA—*k* 1.1; system HX—RI 393; system HY—RI 324; system HZ—Retention time 3.6 min.

Ultraviolet Spectrum. Aqueous acid—231, 249 (A^1_1=348b), 279; aqueous alkali—248 (A^1_1=445b), 288 nm.

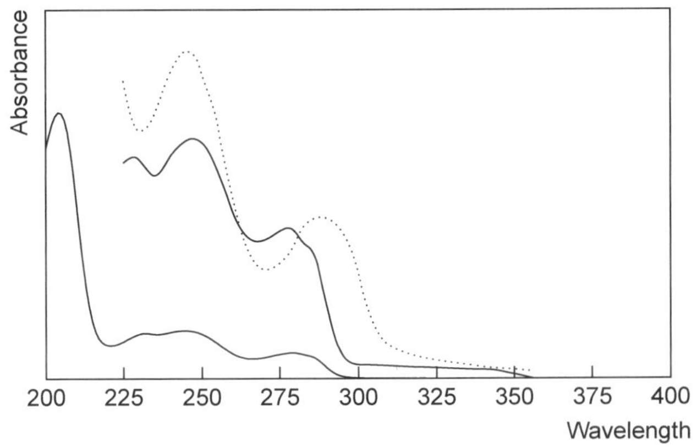

Infra-red Spectrum. Principal peaks at wavenumbers 1694, 757, 1587, 1162, 1204, 1219 cm^{-1}.

Mass Spectrum. Principal ions at *m/z* 230, 109, 82, 187, 243, 363, 42, 123.

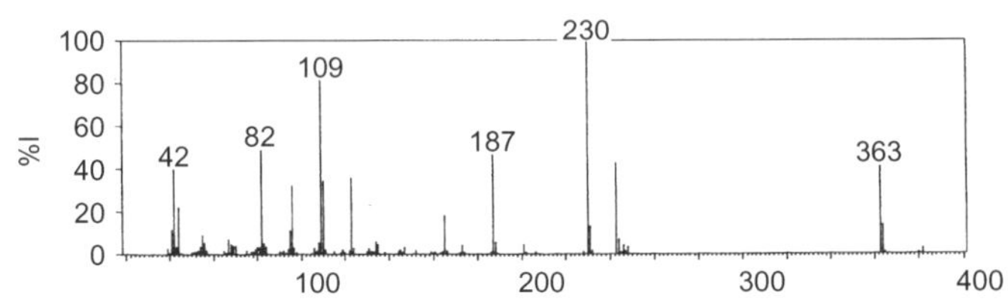

Quantification

Gas chromatography. In plasma: limit of detection 30 μg/L, FID—M. P. Quaglio *et al.*, *Boll. Chim. Farm.*, 1982, *121*, 276–284.

High performance liquid chromatography. In plasma: limit of detection 0.5 μg/L, ECD—S. Suss *et al.*, *J. Chromatogr.*, 1991, *565(1–2)*, 363–373. In serum: limit of detection 0.2 μg/L, ECD—M. Furlanut *et al.*, *Ther. Drug Monit.*, 1987, *9(3)*, 343–346.

Therapeutic concentration

13 schizophrenic patients were orally administered 6 mg benperidol as liquid and 6 mg as tablets. The mean peak plasma concentration were 10.2 μg/L at 1.0 h for the liquid and 7.3 μg/L at 2.7 h for the tablet formulation. [W. Seiler *et al.*, *Psychopharm.*, 1994, *116(4)*, 457–463].

Dose. 0.25 to 1.5 mg daily.

Benserazide

Dopa-decarboxylase Inhibitor/ Antiparkinsonian

Synonym. Serazide
DL-Serine 2-[(2,3,4-trihydroxyphenyl)methyl] hydrazide
$C_{10}H_{15}N_3O_5$=257.2
CAS—322-35-0

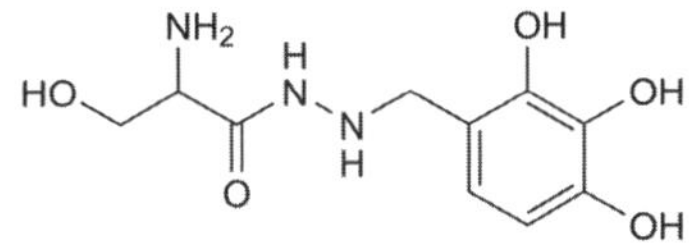

Benserazide Hydrochloride
Proprietary names. It is an ingredient of Madopar and Prolopa.
$C_{10}H_{15}N_3O_5$,HCl=293.7
CAS—14919-77-8; *14046-64-1*
An off-white crystalline powder. M.p. 146° to 148°. Soluble 1 in 3 of water, 1 in 118 of ethanol, 1 in 66 of acetone, 1 in 180 of chloroform and 1 in 455 of ether.

Colour Tests. Ammoniacal silver nitrate—black; *p*-Dimethyl-aminobenzaldehyde—red/-; Ferric chloride—green-brown; Folin–Ciocalteu reagent—blue; Methanolic potassium hydroxide—red; Millon's reagent—red-orange; Nessler's reagent—black; Palladium chloride—orange→brown; Potassium dichromate—brown.

Thin-layer Chromatography. System TA—Rf 01; system TB—Rf 00; system TC—Rf 01; system TL—Rf 03; system TAE—Rf 7.

High Performance Liquid Chromatography. System HX—RI 35.

Ultraviolet Spectrum. Aqueous acid—203, 269 nm.

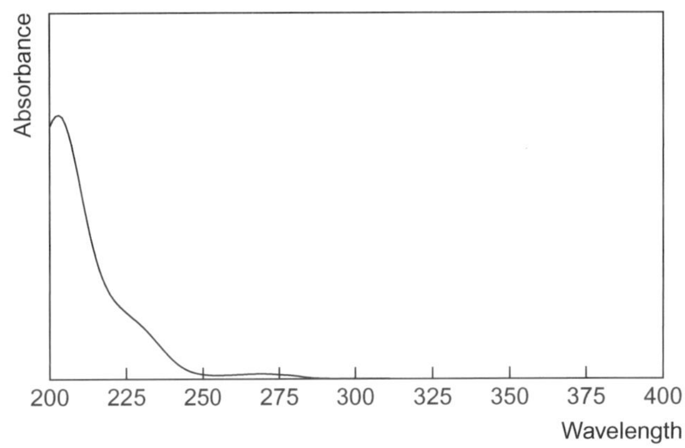

Infra-red Spectrum. Principal peaks at wavenumbers 1500, 1665, 1593, 1195, 1570, 1265 cm^{-1} (KBr disk).

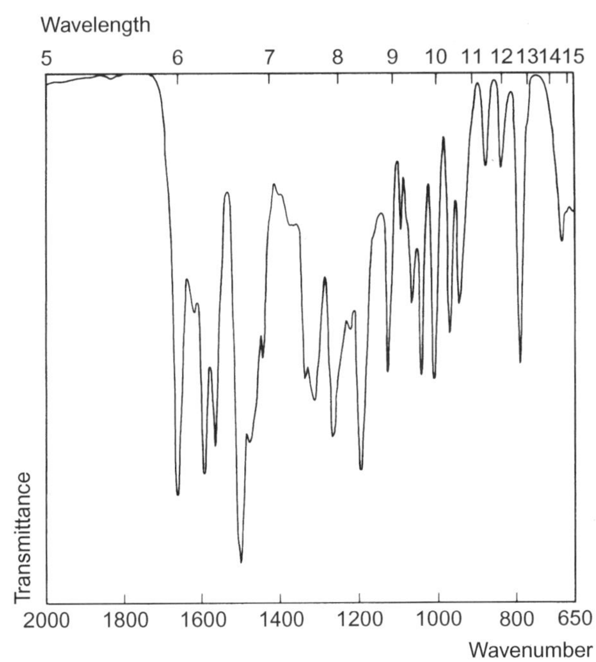

Mass Spectrum. Principal ions at *m/z* 60, 42, 88, 30, 31, 43, 29, 70.

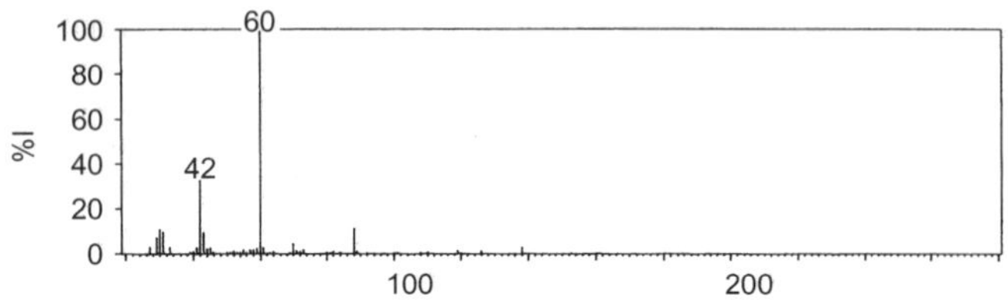

Disposition in the Body. Rapidly absorbed after oral administration and appears to be rapidly metabolised. About 50 to 60% of an oral dose and 80% of an IV dose is excreted in the urine in 24 h, and about 30% and 10% of the respective doses are eliminated in the faeces in 7 days.

Therapeutic concentration

After an oral dose of 50 mg of ^{14}C-benserazide hydrochloride, peak plasma concentrations of about 1 mg/L were attained in 1 h. [D. E. Schwartz *et al.*, *Eur. J. Clin. Pharmacol.*, 1974, *7*, 39–45].

Dose. Usually the equivalent of 50 mg of benserazide daily, increasing to 100 to 250 mg daily (given in combination with levodopa in the treatment of parkinsonism).

Benzaldehyde

Flavouring Agent

Synonym. Artificial Essential Oil of Almond
C_6H_5CHO = 106.1
CAS—100-52-7

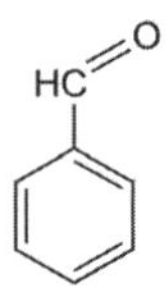

A clear, colourless, strongly refractive liquid, with a characteristic odour of bitter almonds. It becomes yellowish on storage and oxidises in air to benzoic acid. B.p. about 179°. Refractive index, at 20°, 1.544 to 1.5465. Soluble 1 in 350 of water; miscible with ethanol and ether.

Partition Coefficient. Log *P* (octanol/water), 1.5.

Gas Chromatography. System GA—RI 947; system GI—Retention time(s) 34.2 min.

Ultraviolet Spectrum. Ethanol—245 (A_1^1 = 1294b), 279 (A_1^1 = 126b), 289 nm (A_1^1 = 105b).

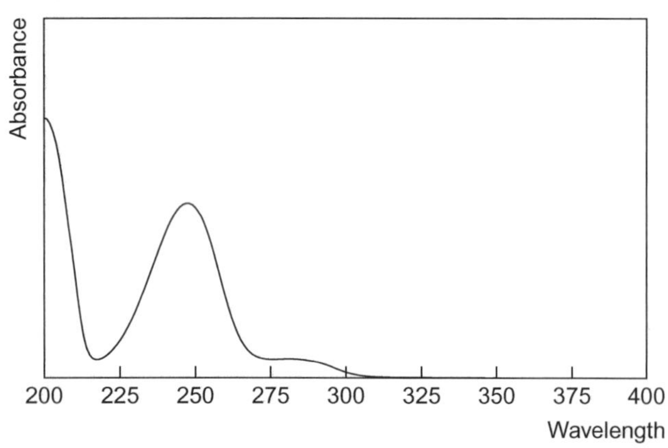

Infra-red Spectrum. Principal peaks at wavenumbers 1700, 1210, 1601, 1175, 1318, 753 cm^{-1} (thin film).

Mass Spectrum. Principal ions at *m/z* 77, 106, 105, 51, 50, 78, 52, 39.

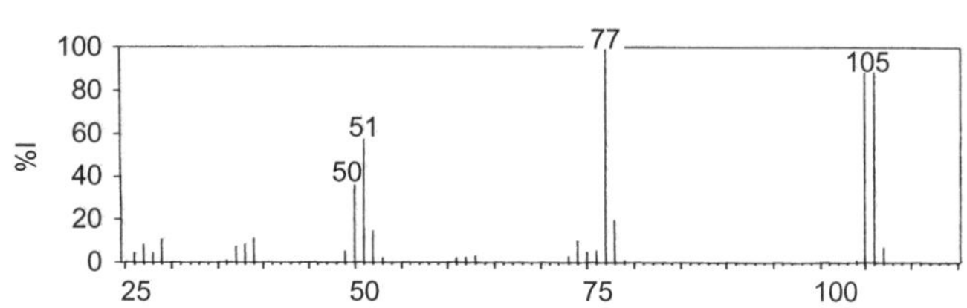

Quantification

Gas chromatography. In blood: detection and identification of volatile compounds using head-space analysis and FID—J. D. Ramsey and R. J. Flanagan, *J. Chromatogr.*, 1982, *240*, 423–444.

Gas chromatography–mass spectrometry. In serum: head-space analysis—A. Zlatkis *et al.*, *J. Chromatogr.*, 1974, *91*, 379–383.

Benzalkonium Chloride

Cationic Disinfectant/Antiseptic

Proprietary names. Benzalchlor-50; Cetal Conc. A and B; Empigen BAC; Hyamine 3500; Laudamonium; Morpan BC; Ovules Pharmatex; Quartamon; Roccal; Sabol; Silquat B10; Silquat B50; Vantoc CL; Zephiran. It is an ingredient of Polycide, Stomosol and Timodine.

A mixture of alkylbenzyldimethylammonium chlorides of the general formula $[C_6H_5{\cdot}CH_2{\cdot}N(CH_3)_2{\cdot}R]Cl$, in which R represents a mixture of the alkyls from C_8H_{17} to $C_{18}H_{37}$.
CAS—8001-54-5

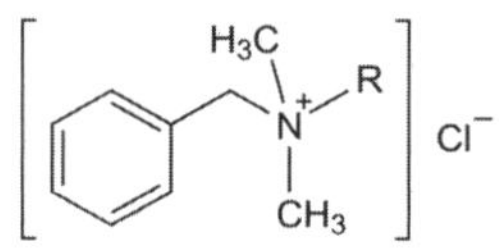

R = C_8H_{17} to $C_{18}H_{37}$

A white or yellowish-white amorphous powder, thick gel, or gelatinous pieces. A solution in water gives a clear, colourless or pale yellow, syrupy liquid, which foams strongly when shaken. Very soluble in water, ethanol and acetone; practically insoluble in ether.

Thin-layer Chromatography. System TL—Rf 00; system TAE—Rf 04; system TAF—Rf 66.

Ultraviolet Spectrum. Water—256 (A_1^1 = 4.9b), 262 (A_1^1 = 5.8b), 268 nm (A_1^1 = 4.6b).

Infra-red Spectrum. Principal peaks at wavenumbers 702, 726, 780, 875, 1618, 1211 cm^{-1} (thin film).

Benzatropine

Anticholinergic

Synonym. Benztropine
3-(Diphenylmethoxy)-8-methyl-8-azabicyclo[3.2.1]octane
$C_{21}H_{25}NO$ = 307.4
CAS—86-13-5

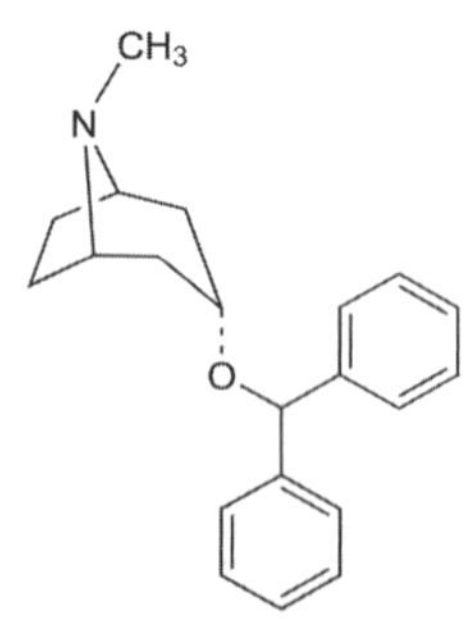

Soluble in chloroform.

Benzatropine Mesilate

Synonyms. Benzatropine Methanesulfonate; Tropine Diphenylmethyl Ether.
Proprietary names. Bensylate; Cogentin.
$C_{21}H_{25}NO,CH_4O_3S$ = 403.5
CAS—132-17-2
A white, slightly hygroscopic, crystalline powder. M.p. 141° to 145°. Soluble 1 in 0.7 of water, 1 in 1.5 of ethanol, and 1 in 2 of chloroform; practically insoluble in ether.

Dissociation Constant. pK_a 10.0 (20°).

Partition Coefficient. Log *P* (heptane), 0.4.

Colour Tests. Mandelin's Test—yellow; Marquis Test—yellow.

Thin-layer Chromatography. System TA—Rf 13; system TB—Rf 26; system TC—Rf 06; system TL—Rf 02; system TAE—Rf 06. (Acidified iodoplatinate solution, positive.)

Gas Chromatography. System GA—RI 2302; system GB—RI 2423.

High Performance Liquid Chromatography. System HA—*k* 3.7 (tailing peak).

Ultraviolet Spectrum. Aqueous acid—253, 259 nm (A^1_1=14.5a).

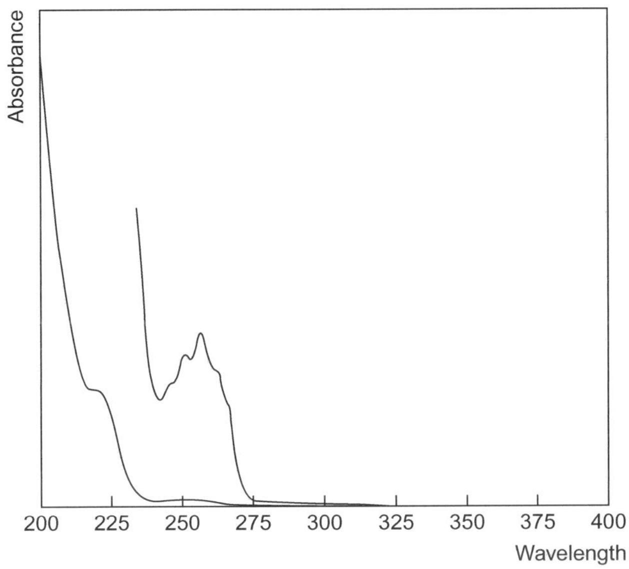

Infra-red Spectrum. Principal peaks at wavenumbers 1054, 700, 742, 1191, 1204, 1075 cm^{-1} (KBr disk).

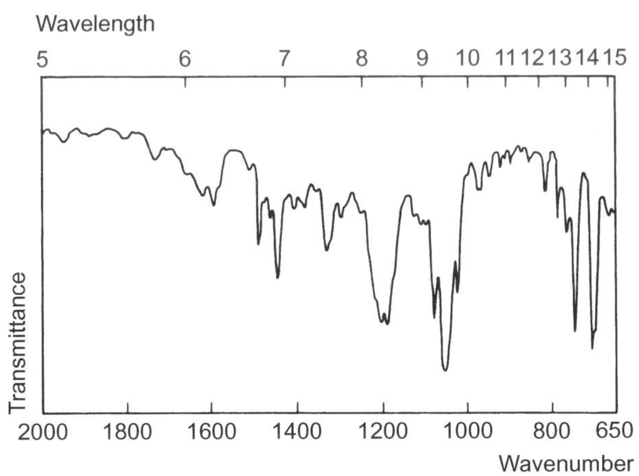

Mass Spectrum. Principal ions at *m*/*z* 83, 140, 82, 124, 96, 97, 42, 125.

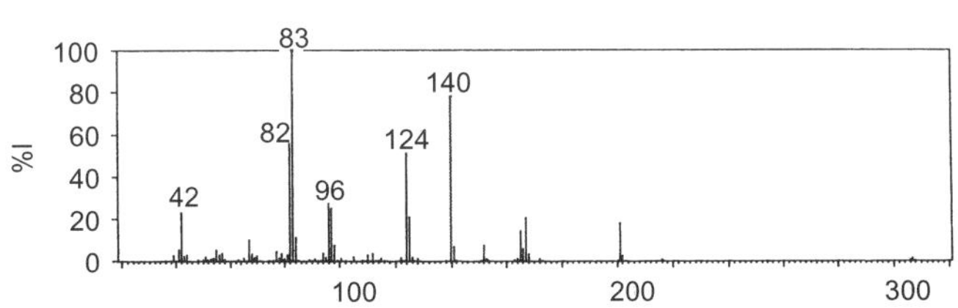

Quantification

High performance liquid chromatography. In plasma—K. Selinger *et al.*, *J. Chromatogr.*, 1989, *491(11)*, 248–252.

Disposition in the Body. Absorbed after oral administration.

Toxicity

In a fatality attributed to the ingestion of an unknown quantity of benzatropine tablets, the following postmortem concentrations were reported: blood 0.7 mg/L, liver 1.6 µg/g, urine 0.8 mg/L. In a second case a liver concentration of 2.3 µg/g was found. [G. del Villar and M. Liddy, *Bull. Int. Assoc. Forensic Toxicol.*, 1976, *12(2)*, 11–12.]

A 41-year-old male with a history of schizophrenia and drug abuse was found dead. Benzatropine was found at a concentration of 0.183 mg/L in his blood and 7.12 mg/L in his urine. [T. G. Rosano *et al.*, *J. Anal. Toxicol.*, 1994, *18(6)*, 348–353.]

Dose. 0.5 to 6 mg of benzatropine mesilate daily.

Benzbromarone

Uricosuric

Proprietary names. Desuric; Narcaricin; Normurat; Uricovac M.
(3,5-Dibromo-4-hydroxyphenyl)(2-ethyl-3-benzofuranyl)methanone
$C_{17}H_{12}Br_2O_3$=424.1
CAS—3562-84-3

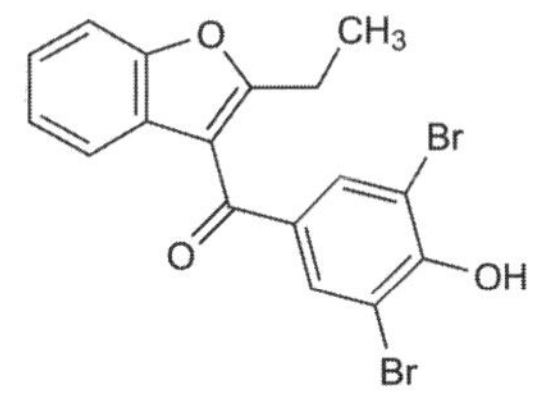

Yellowish crystals. M.p. 151°.

Partition Coefficient. Log *P* (octanol/water), 6.0.

Thin-layer Chromatography. System TF—Rf 49; system TAE—Rf 94.

High Performance Liquid Chromatography. System HX—RI 860; system HAA—Retention time(s) 26.1 min.

Ultraviolet Spectrum. Methanolic acid—237 (A^1_1=666b), 274 (inflexion), 281 (A^1_1=314b); aqueous alkali—240 (A^1_1=440b), 281 (inflexion), 355 nm (A^1_1=513b).

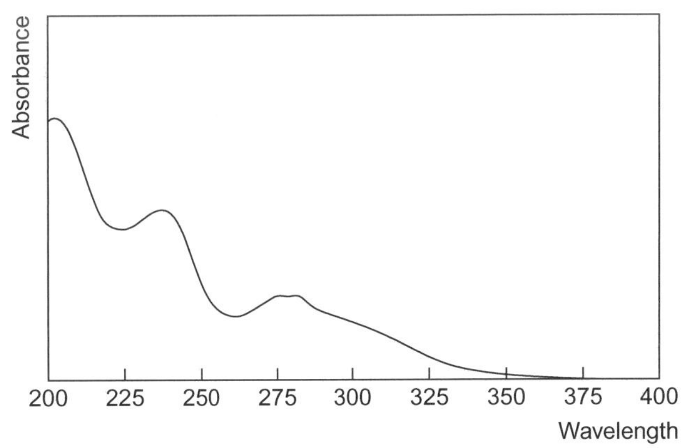

Quantification

High performance liquid chromatography. In plasma and urine: benzarone limit of detection 0.01 mg/L, UV detection—J. X. de Vries *et al.*, *J. Chromatogr.*, 1986, *382*, 167–174. In serum: benzbromarone and benzarone, limits of detection 140 and 90 µg/L, respectively, UV detection—H. Vergin and G. Bishop, *J. Chromatogr.*, 1980, *183*; *Biomed. Appl.*, *9*, 383–386.

Disposition in the Body. Benzbromarone is incompletely absorbed after oral administration. It is metabolised by debromination to bromobenzarone and benzarone which are both active metabolites. About 50% of a dose is excreted in the bile as free and conjugated (glucuronide) metabolites and less than 10% of a dose is excreted in the urine.

Therapeutic concentration

Following a single oral dose of 100 mg to 7 subjects, peak plasma concentrations of 1.4 to 2.9 (mean 2.2) mg/L of benzbromarone and 0.6 to 1.2 (mean 0.8) mg/L of benzarone were attained in about 3 and 6 h, respectively. [H. Ferber *et al.*, *Eur. J. Clin. Pharmacol.*, 1981, *19*, 431–435].

Half-life. Plasma half-life, benzbromarone about 3 h, benzarone about 13 h.

Note. For a review of benzbromarone, see R. C. Heel *et al.*, *Drugs*, 1977, *14*, 349–366.

Dose. Usually 100 mg daily; up to 300 mg daily has been given.

Benzene

Solvent

Synonyms. Cyclohexatriene; Phenyl Hydride
C_6H_6=78.11
CAS—71-43-2

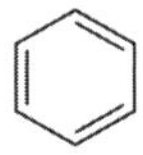

A clear, colourless, mobile, inflammable liquid, with a characteristic aromatic odour, which burns with a smoky flame. B.p. 80.1°. It solidifies when cooled to 0°.
Practically immiscible with water; miscible with dehydrated alcohol, acetone, chloroform, ether, and glacial acetic acid.

Partition Coefficient. Log *P* (octanol/water), 2.1.

Gas Chromatography. System GA—RI 1000; system GI—retention time 14.8 min.

High Performance Liquid Chromatography. System HAA—retention time 19.5 min.

Ultraviolet Spectrum. Ethanol—255 nm (A_1^1=28b).

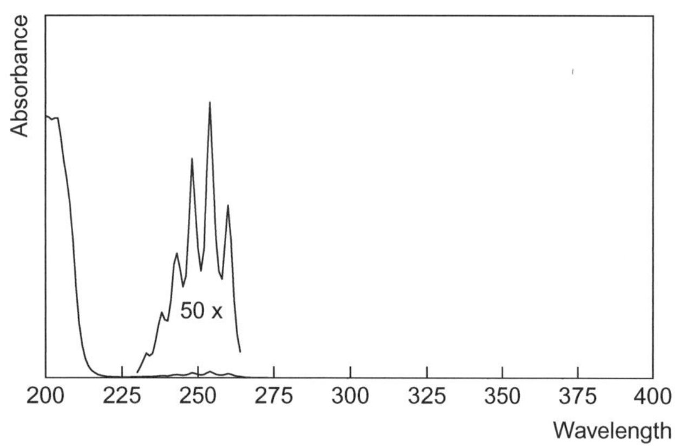

Mass Spectrum. Principal ions at *m/z* 78, 77, 52, 51, 50, 39, 79, 74.

Quantification
Gas chromatography. In blood or tissues: head-space analysis, FID—W. D. Collom and C. L. Winek, *Clin. Toxicol.*, 1970, *3*, 125–130. In tissues—C. A. Snyder *et al.*, *Am. Ind. Hyg. Assoc. J.*, 1977, *38*, 272–276. In urine: phenol, limit of detection 10 μg/L, FID—D. L. Rick *et al.*, *J. Anal. Toxicol.*, 1982, *6*, 297–300. In urine: limit of detection 7 μg/L and limit of quantification 23 μg/L, FID—G. Ljungkvist *et al.*, *Analyst*, 2001, *126(1)*, 41–45.

High performance liquid chromatography. In urine: limit of detection 125 ng, UV detection (λ = 265 nm)—B. L. Lee *et al.*, *Clin. Chem.*, 1993, *39(9)*, 1788–1792. In urine: limit of detection 1 μg/L, fluorescence detection (λ_{ex}=395 nm; λ_{em}=470 nm)—T. Einig and W. Dehnen, *J. Chromatogr. A*, 1995, *697(1–2)*, 371–375. In urine: limit of detection 0.01 mg/L *trans, trans*-muconic acid (metabolite), SIM—T. Ruppert *et al.*, *J. Chromatogr. B Biomed. Sci. Appl.*, 1995, *666(1)*, 71–76.

Disposition in the Body. Benzene is absorbed from the gastro-intestinal tract, through the skin, and from the lungs. About 50% of inhaled benzene is retained in the body; eventually up to 50% of the retained benzene may be eliminated via the lungs, only very small amounts (approximately 0.1%) appearing unchanged in the urine. The remainder of the retained benzene is excreted in the urine, mainly as phenol together with small amounts of catechol and quinol. The excretion of phenol is highest in the first 24 h and is complete within 48 h of exposure. The phenolic metabolites are excreted mainly in the conjugated form as ethereal sulfates and glucuronides.

Toxicity. The maximum permissible atmospheric concentration is 10 ppm or 30 mg/m^3. The maximum exposure limit is 1 ppm. Chronic poisoning may result from exposure to low concentrations over a period of time; 1500 ppm for an hour causes marked depression of the CNS and 7500 ppm for half an hour or 20 000 ppm for a few minutes may cause death; chronic inhalation of as little as 100 ppm is likely to cause severe bone marrow depression. The ingestion of 10 mL has caused death.

In a death attributed to inhalation of benzene vapours (glue sniffing), the postmortem concentration of benzene in the blood was 0.94 mg/L and in the kidney 5.5 μg/g. [W. D. Collom and C. L. Winek, *Clin. Toxicol.*, 1970, *3*, 125–130.]

The following postmortem tissue concentrations were reported in a fatality due to the ingestion of benzene: blood 38 mg/L, brain 253 μg/g, kidney 21 μg/g, liver 105 μg/g, urine 20 mg/L. [A. Alha *et al.*, *Bull. Int. Assoc. Forensic Toxicol.*, 1975, *11(3)*, 9.]

A 3-year-old child drank some benzene and died 2 h later; postmortem concentrations were: brain 250 μg/g, kidney 20 μg/g, liver 800 μg/g. [A. Heyndrickx *et al.*, *J. Pharm. Belg.*, 1966, *21*, 406–408.]

Half-life. Plasma half-life, 9 to 24 h.

Note. For a review of the effects on health of benzene inhalation see T. J. Haley, *Clin. Toxicol.*, 1977, *11*, 531–548.

Benzene Hexachloride

Pesticide

Synonyms. BHC; HCH; Hexachlorocyclohexane; Technical Benzene Hexachloride.
$C_6H_6Cl_6$=290.8
CAS—319-84-6 (α); 319-85-7 (β); 58-89-9 (γ); 319-86-8 (δ); 6108-10-7 (ε)

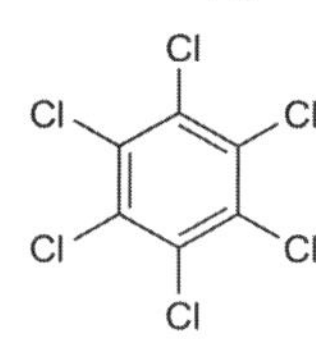

A mixture of the several isomers of 1,2,3,4,5,6-hexachlorocyclohexane; it contains not less than 12% of the gamma isomer. Benzene hexachloride has five known isomers designated alpha, beta, gamma, delta, and epsilon; of these only the gamma isomer (see Lindane) is outstandingly active as an insecticide.
White to light brown granules, flakes or powder, with a characteristic musty odour. M.p. α 159°, β 312°, γ 112°, δ 138°, ε 219°.
Practically insoluble in water; its solubility in organic solvents depends on the proportions of the various isomers present.

Gas Chromatography. System GA—α-isomer RI 1690, β-isomer RI 1710, δ-isomer RI 1755, γ-isomer RI 1745.

Infra-red Spectrum. Principal peaks at wavenumbers 688, 855, 704, 781, 917, 957 cm^{-1} (Nujol mull).

Quantification See under Lindane.

Disposition in the Body. Absorbed after ingestion, inhalation, or through the skin. It is stored in the body fat and adrenal glands. The β-isomer accumulates on chronic exposure (see under Lindane).

Toxicity. Benzene hexachloride has a greater chronic toxicity than lindane. Ingestion of 20 to 30 g may produce serious toxic effects but death is unlikely unless it is dissolved in an organic solvent.

Benzethonium Chloride

Cationic Disinfectant/ Antiseptic

Proprietary names. Hyamine 1622; Phemerol Chloride.
N,N-Dimethyl-*N*-[2-[2-[4-(1,1,3,3-tetramethylbutyl)phenoxy]ethoxy]-ethyl]-benzenemethanaminium chloride

$C_{27}H_{42}ClNO_2$=448.1
CAS—121-54-0

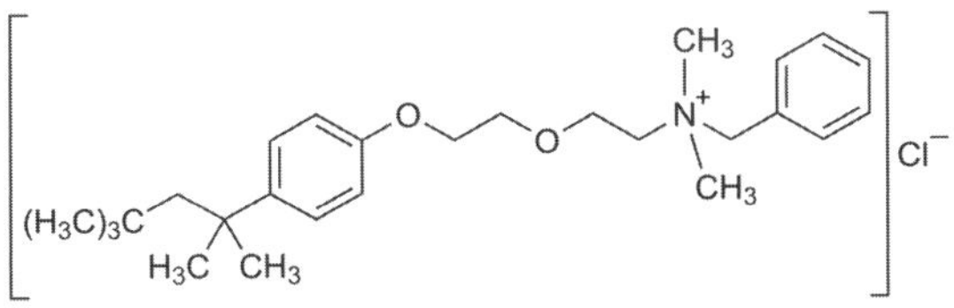

White crystals. A solution in water foams strongly when shaken. M.p. 160° to 165°. Soluble 1 in 0.6 of water, 1 in 0.6 of ethanol and 1 in 1 of chloroform; slightly soluble in ether; practically insoluble in light petroleum.

Partition Coefficient. Log *P* (octanol/water), 4.0.

Colour Test. Marquis test—orange.

Thin-layer Chromatography. System TA—Rf 03. (Acidified iodoplatinate solution, positive.)

Ultraviolet Spectrum. Aqueous acid—263, 269 (A^1_1=29c), 274 nm (A^1_1=28c). No alkaline shift.

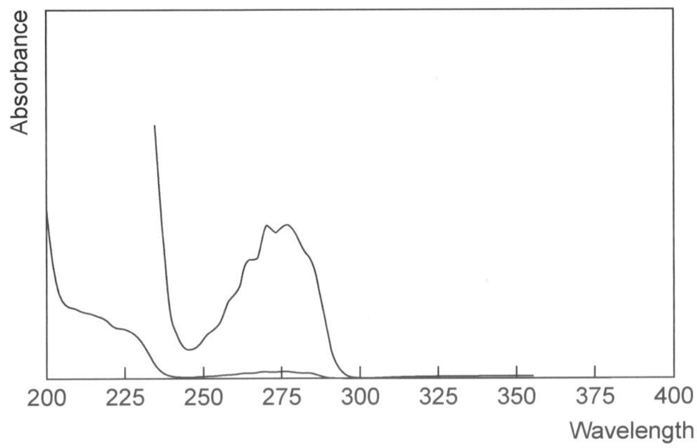

Infra-red Spectrum. Principal peaks at wavenumbers 1240, 1505, 1120, 826, 1063, 769 cm^{-1} (KBr disk).

Use. Used as 0.1 to 0.2% solutions.

Benzfetamine

Anorectic

Synonym. Benzphetamine
Proprietary name. Didrex
(αS)-*N*,α-Dimethyl-*N*-(phenylmethyl)benzeneethanamine
$C_{17}H_{21}N$=239.4
CAS—156-08-1

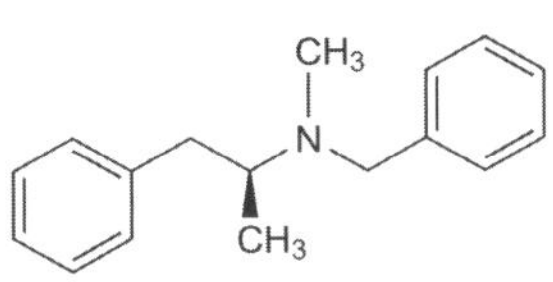

A liquid. B.p. 127°
Practically insoluble in water; soluble in methanol, ethanol, chloroform, acetone, benzene, and ether.

Benzfetamine Hydrochloride

Proprietary names. Didrex; Inapetyl.
$C_{17}H_{21}N,HCl$=275.8
CAS—5411-22-3
A white crystalline powder. M.p. about 131°.
Freely soluble in water, ethanol, and chloroform; slightly soluble in ether.

Dissociation Constant. pK_a 6.6.

Partition Coefficient. Log *P* (octanol/water), 4.1.

Colour Test. Marquis Test—orange

Thin-layer Chromatography. System TA—Rf 73; system TB—Rf 67; system TC—Rf 70; system TE—Rf 87; system TL—Rf 70; system TAE—Rf 60. (Dragendorff spray, positive; acidified iodoplatinate solution, positive; Marquis reagent, brown.)

Gas Chromatography. System GA—benzfetamine RI 1855, amfetamine RI 1125, metamfetamine RI 1175; system GB—benzfetamine RI 1899, amfetamine RI 1150, metamfetamine RI 1200; system GC—benzfetamine RI 2172, amfetamine RI 1536, metamfetamine RI 1722; system GF—benzfetamine RI 2050, amfetamine RI 1315, metamfetamine RI 1335.

Column: HP-1 (12 m × 0.2 mm i.d., 0.33 µm film thickness). Column temperature: 80° held 1 min, ramp to 210° at 20°/min, held for 2 min. Injector temperature: 270°. Carrier gas: helium, flow rate 1 mL/min. MS detection. Retention time(s): amfetamine, 4.2 min; metamfetamine, 5.1 min; benzfetamine, 8.2 min. [J.T Cody and S. Valtier, *J. Anal. Toxicol.*, 1998, *22*, 299–309.]

Column: TC-1 cross-linked methylsilicone (20 m × 0.25 mm i.d., 0.25 µm film thickness). Column temperature: 60° for 0.5 min, ramp to 280° at 20°/min. Injector temperature: 200°. Carrier gas: helium, 1 mL/min flow rate. Detection: MS (SIM). Retention time(s): amfetamine, 4.6 min; metamfetamine, 5.4 min; benzfetamine, 8.2 min. [R. Kikura and Y. Nakahara, *Biol. Pharm. Bull.*, 1995, *18*, 1694–1699.]

High Performance Liquid Chromatography. System HA—benzfetamine *k* 1.2, amfetamine *k* 0.9, metamfetamine *k* 2.0; system HC—benzfetamine *k* 0.15, amfetamine *k* 0.98, metamfetamine *k* 2.07.

Ultraviolet Spectrum. Aqueous acid—252, 258 nm (A^1_1=19c), 262, 268 nm.

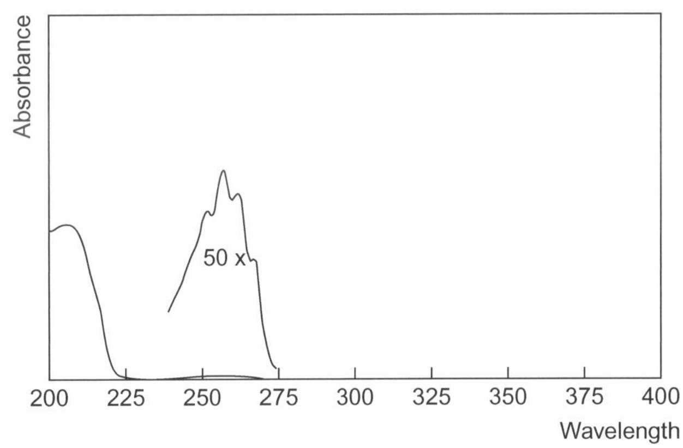

Infra-red Spectrum. Principal peaks at wavenumbers 1497, 740, 698, 1028, 1125, 1220 cm^{-1} (KBr disk).

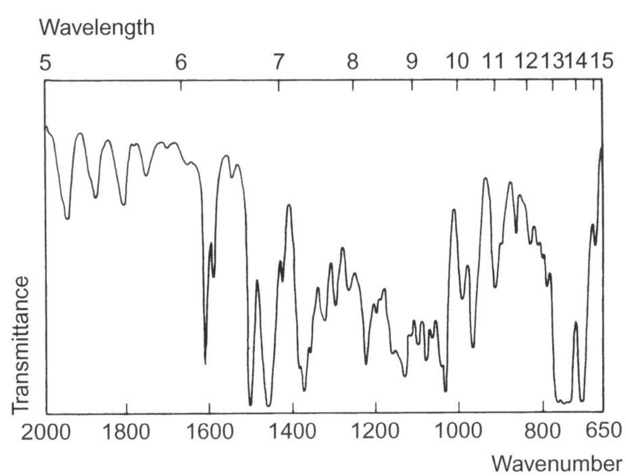

Mass Spectrum. Principal ions at *m*/*z* 91, 148, 149, 65, 92, 42, 56, 39.

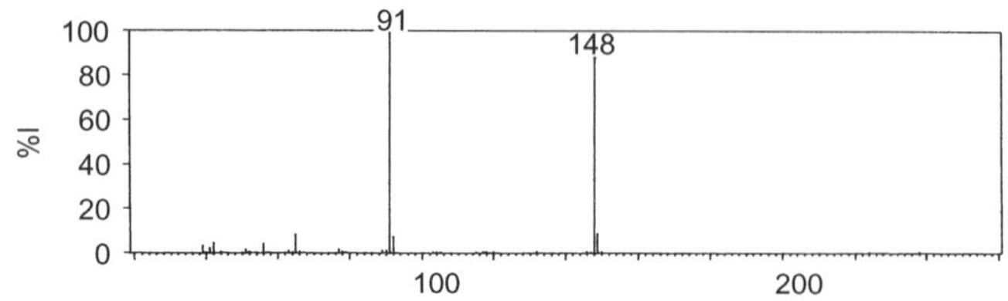

Quantification

Gas chromatography. In hair: benzfetamine, limit of detection 0.5 ng/mg hair, MS—Y. Nakahara, *Forensic Sci. Int.*, 1995, *70*, 135–153.

Gas chromatography–mass spectrometry. In urine: amfetamine and metamfetamine, limit of detection 5 µg/L; benzfetamine 2 µg/L—J. T Cody and S. Valtier, *J. Anal. Toxicol.*, 1998, *22*, 299–309.

High performance liquid chromatography. In urine: benzfetamine metabolites—A. Fujinami *et al.*, *Ann. Clin. Biochem.*, 1998, *35*, 775–779.

Disposition in the Body. Readily absorbed after oral administration and mainly excreted in the urine as amfetamine and metamfetamine; the metabolism of benzfetamine to desmethylbenzfetamine may be a major pathway in its metabolism. It is also excreted in the urine as conjugated metabolites, *p*-hydroxy-*N*-benzylamfetamine glucuronide and *p*-hydroxybenzfetamine glucuronide; very little is excreted as unchanged drug.

Therapeutic concentration

Urinary concentrations of *p*-hydroxy-*N*-benzylamfetamine glucuronide (pHBAG) and *p*-hydroxybenzfetamine glucuronide (pHBZG) were determined in 2 healthy volunteers after the administration of 10 mg benzfetamine hydrochloride. After 6 h, pHBAG concentrations were 450 nM (subject 1) and 800 nM (subject 2), and pHBZG 800 nM (subject 1) and 1900 nM (subject 2). After 24 h, pHBAG levels dropped to 50 nM for both subjects and pHBZG concentrations were negligible. [A. Fujinami *et al.*, *Ann. Clin. Biochem.*, 1998, *35*, 775–779.]

Toxicity

A 16-year-old male was found dead with several medicine bottles in the room. Postmortem examination and toxicological analysis revealed the following benzfetamine concentrations: blood 13.9 mg/L, urine 8.0 mg/L, liver 106.3 mg/kg, brain 30.5 mg/kg, and gastric contents (total) 53.1 mg. [J. P. Brooks *et al.*, *Am. J. Forensic Med. Pathol.*, 1982, *3*, 245–247.]

Dose. 25 to 150 mg of benzfetamine hydrochloride daily.

Benzilonium Bromide

Anticholinergic

Proprietary names. Portyn; Ulcoban.
1,1-Diethyl-3-[(hydroxydiphenylacetyl)oxy]pyrrolidinium bromide
$C_{22}H_{28}BrNO_3$=434.4
CAS—1050-48-2

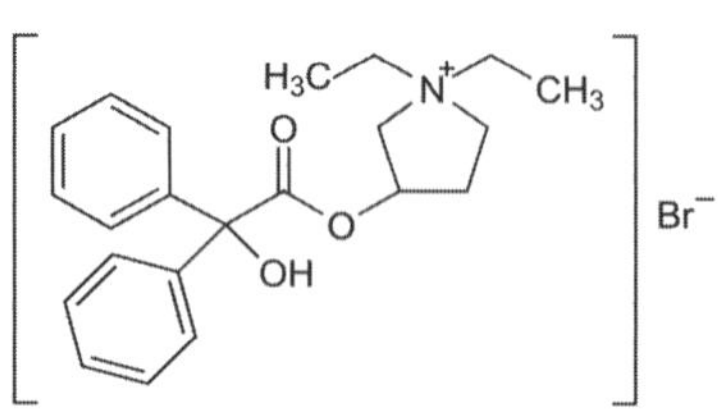

A white crystalline powder. M.p. 203° to 204°. Soluble in water.

Partition Coefficient. Log *P* (octanol/water), −0.3.

Colour Tests. The following tests are performed on benzilonium nitrate (see Chapter 20): Liebermann's test—brown; Marquis test—orange→green→blue; Sulfuric acid—orange.

Thin-layer Chromatography. System TA—Rf 03; system TAJ—Rf 00; system TAK—Rf 00; system TAL—Rf 05. (Acidified iodoplatinate solution, positive.)

Ultraviolet Spectrum. Aqueous acid—252, 258 (A_1^1=11a), 264 nm.

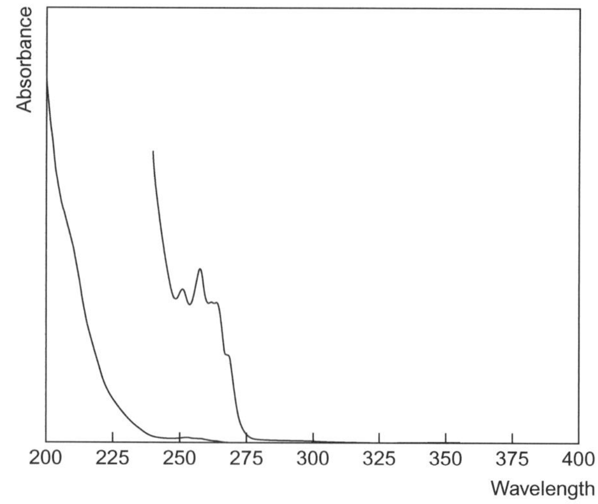

Infra-red Spectrum. Principal peaks at wavenumbers 1728, 1220, 1190, 1162, 690, 1052 cm^{-1} (KBr disk).

Quantification

Gas chromatography–mass spectrometry. In plasma: limit of detection 5 µg/L—H. Dahlström *et al.*, *J. Chromatogr.*, 1980, *183*; *B Biomed. Appl.*, *9*, 511–513.

Dose. 30 to 70 mg daily.

Benziodarone

Uricosuric/Vasodilator

Proprietary name. Amplivix
2-Ethyl-3-benzofuranyl 4-hydroxy-3,5-diiodophenyl methanone
$C_{17}H_{12}I_2O_3$=518.1
CAS-68-90-6

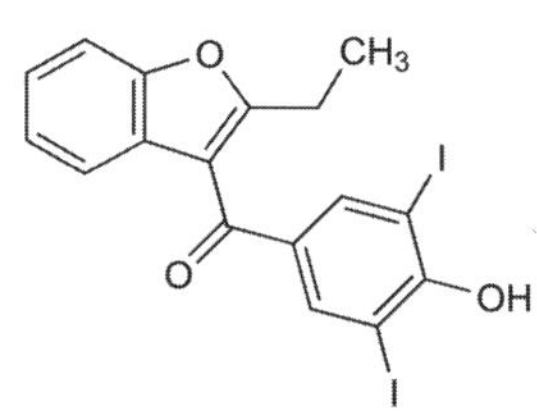

A yellowish powder. M.p. 167°.
Soluble 1 in about 500 of water at 25°, and 1 in about 100 of water at 45°; soluble in acetone and chloroform.

Partition Coefficient. Log *P* (octanol/water) 6.6.

Thin-layer Chromatography. System TD—Rf 62; system TE—Rf 23; system TF—Rf 58; system TAD—Rf 65.

Ultraviolet Spectrum. Methanol—240 nm (A_1^1=1280b), 275, 357 nm.

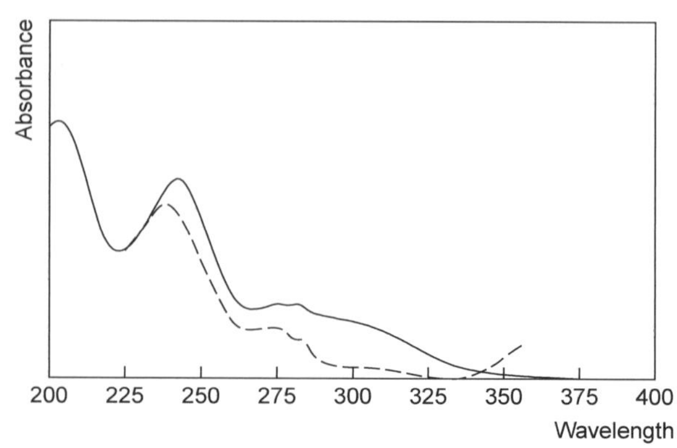

Infra-red Spectrum. Principal peaks at wavenumbers 1618, 756, 1577, 1135, 1293, 1176 cm^{-1} (Nujol mull).

Mass Spectrum. Principal ions at *m/z* 518, 173, 264, 519, 373, 376, 520, 249.

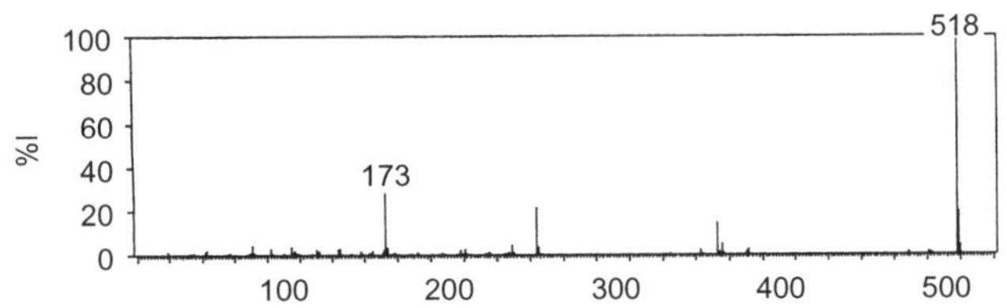

Dose. Benziodarone has been given in initial doses of 600 mg daily and maintenance doses of 300 to 400 mg daily.

Benzocaine

Anaesthetic (local)

Synonyms. Anaesthesinum; Anesthamine; Éthoforme; Ethyl Aminobenzoate.
Proprietary names. Americaine; Anaesthesin; Flavamed; Subcutin. It is an ingredient of AAA, Audicort, Auralgan, Auralgicin, Auraltone, Merocaine, Transvasin, Tyrosolven, and Tyrozets.
4-Aminobenzoic acid ethyl ester
$C_9H_{11}NO_2$=165.2
CAS—94-09-7

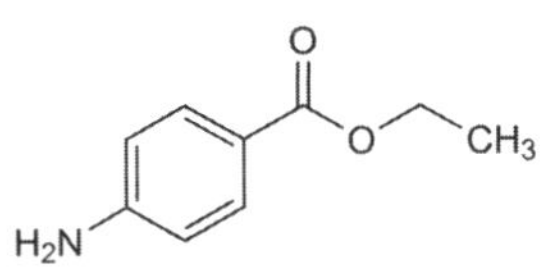

Colourless crystals or white crystalline powder. M.p. 88° to 92°.
Soluble 1 in 2500 of water, 1 in 8 of ethanol, 1 in 2 of chloroform, and 1 in 4 of ether; soluble in dilute acids.

Dissociation Constant. pK_a 2.5 (25°).

Partition Coefficient. Log *P* (octanol/water), 1.9.

Colour Test. Diazotisation—red.

Thin-layer Chromatography. System TA—Rf 67; system TB—Rf 06; system TC—Rf 57; system TD—Rf 56; system TE—Rf 77; system TF—Rf 62; system TL—Rf 66; system TAD—Rf 63; system TAE—Rf 84; system TAF—Rf 87. (Ninhydrin spray, positive; acidified potassium permanganate solution, positive; Van Urk reagent, bright yellow.)

Gas Chromatography. System GA—benzocaine RI 1555, 4-aminobenzoic acid RI 1547; system GF—RI 2100.

High Performance Liquid Chromatography. System HA—*k* 0.1; system HQ—*k* 20.06; system HR—*k* 1.61; system HX—RI 404; system HY—RI 358; system HZ—Retention time(s) 4.3 min.

Ultraviolet Spectrum. Aqueous acid—272 (A_1^1=90c), 278; aqueous alkali—285 (A_1^1=930a); ethanol—293 nm (A_1^1=1238a).

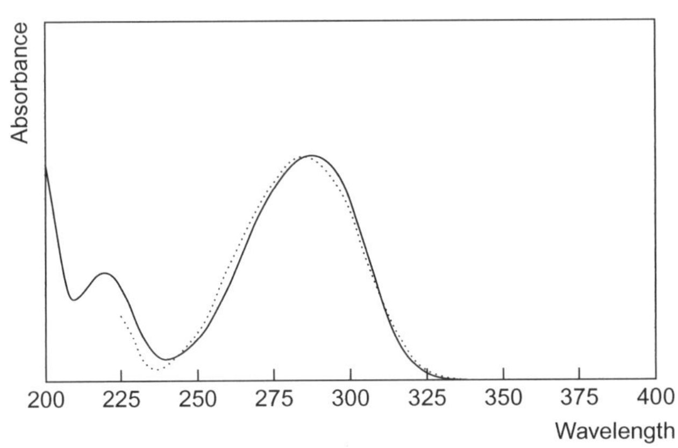

Infra-red Spectrum. Principal peaks at wavenumbers 1280, 1680, 1598, 1170, 1315, 1634 cm^{-1} (KBr disk).

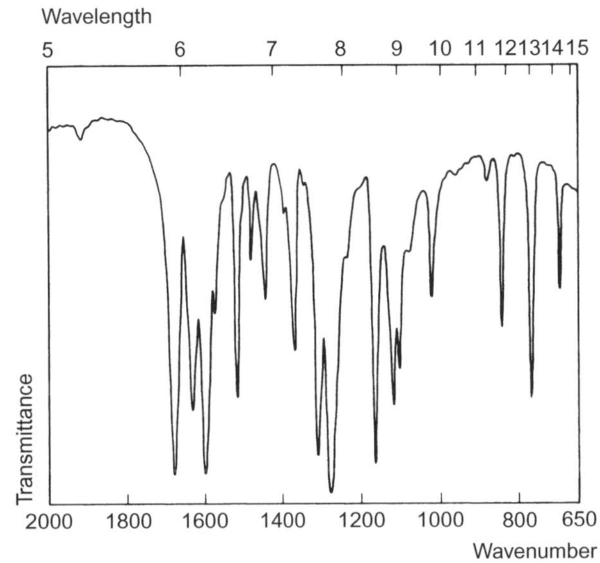

Mass Spectrum. Principal ions at *m/z* 120, 165, 92, 65, 137, 39, 121, 93; 4-aminobenzoic acid 137, 120, 92, 65, 39, 138, 121, 63.

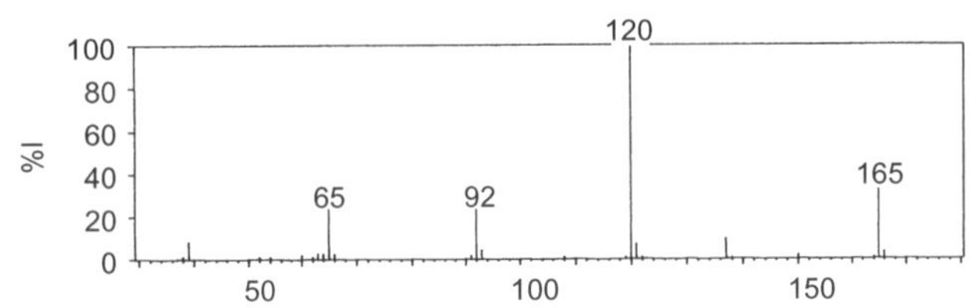

Disposition in the Body. Benzocaine is metabolised by hydrolysis to 4-aminobenzoic acid. At the concentrations normally used (2 to 10%) it is comparatively non-irritant and non-toxic, having only about one-tenth the toxicity of cocaine. The maximum safe amount for topical use is 5000 mg (25 mL of a 20% solution).

Benzoctamine

Tranquilliser

N-Methyl-9,10-ethanoanthracene-9(10*H*)-methenamine
$C_{18}H_{19}N$=249.4
CAS—17243-39-9

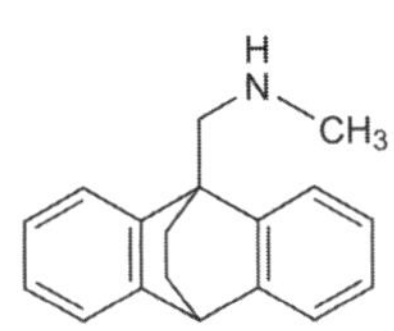

Benzoctamine Hydrochloride

Synonym. Ba-30803
Proprietary name. Tacitin(e)
$C_{18}H_{19}N,HCl$=285.8
CAS—10085-81-1
A white crystalline powder. M.p. 320° to 322°.
Soluble in water, ethanol and chloroform; sparingly soluble in acetone and ether.

Dissociation Constant. pK_a 7.6.

Partition Coefficient. Log *P* (octanol/water), 3.5.

Colour Tests. Mandelin's test—blue-green; Marquis test—red-violet.

Thin-layer Chromatography. System TA—Rf 59; system TB—Rf 57; system TC—Rf 52; system TL—Rf 43; system TAE—Rf 38; system TAJ—Rf 31; system TAK—Rf 14; system TAL—Rf 65. (Acidified iodoplatinate solution, positive.)

Gas Chromatography. System GA—RI 2078; system GB—RI 2172; system GF—RI 2445.

High Performance Liquid Chromatography. System HA—*k* 1.7; system HX—RI 380; system HY—RI 322.

Ultraviolet Spectrum. Aqueous acid—264, 271 nm (A_1^1=57a).

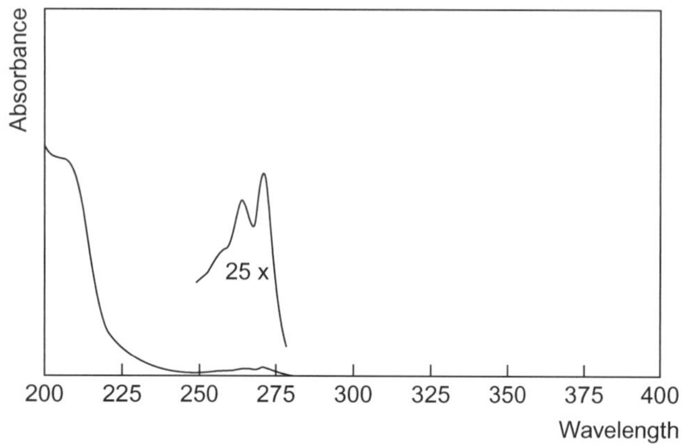

Infra-red Spectrum. Principal peaks at wavenumbers 757, 743, 732, 1134, 1060, 1020 cm^{-1} (KBr disk).

Mass Spectrum. Principal ions at *m/z* 218, 44, 191, 221, 219, 178, 42, 180.

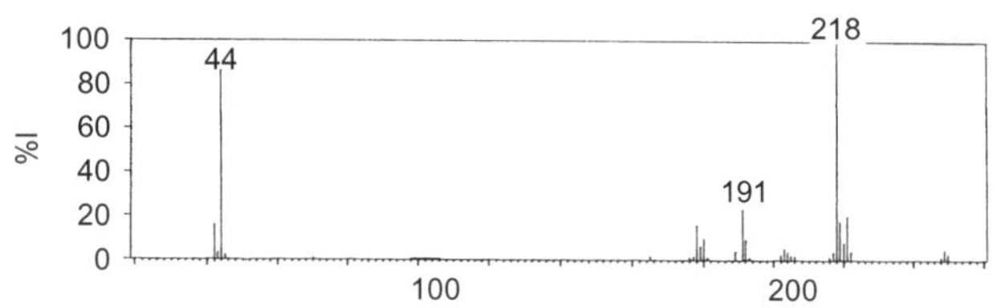

Dose. 30 to 60 mg of benzoctamine hydrochloride daily.

Benzoic Acid

Preservative

Synonyms. Benzenecarboxylic Acid; Phenylformic Acid.
Proprietary names. It is an ingredient of Aserbine and Malatex.
$C_7H_6O_2$=122.1
CAS—65-85-0

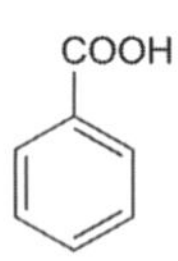

Colourless, light feathery crystals or white scales or powder. M.p. 122.4°. It sublimes on heating.
Soluble 1 in about 350 of water, 1 in 20 of boiling water, 1 in 3 of ethanol, 1 in 5 of chloroform, and 1 in 3 of ether; freely soluble in acetone.

Sodium Benzoate

$C_7H_5O_2Na$=144.1
CAS—532-32-1
A white, amorphous, granular, flaky, or crystalline powder.
Soluble 1 in 2 of water and 1 in 90 of ethanol.

Dissociation Constant. pK_a 4.2 (25°).

Partition Coefficient. Log *P* (octanol/water), 1.9.

Thin-layer Chromatography. System TD—Rf 26; system TE—Rf 07; system TF—Rf 28; system TAD—Rf 35; system TAJ—Rf 55; system TAK—Rf 81; system TAL—Rf 92.

Gas Chromatography. System GA—RI 1180.

High Performance Liquid Chromatography. System HX—RI 360; system HY—RI 327; system HZ—retention time 3.0 min (benzoate).

Ultraviolet Spectrum. Aqueous acid—230 (A_1^1=923a), 273 (A_1^1=85a); methanol—227 (A_1^1=895a), 272 (A_1^1=73a), 280 nm (A_1^1=61b).

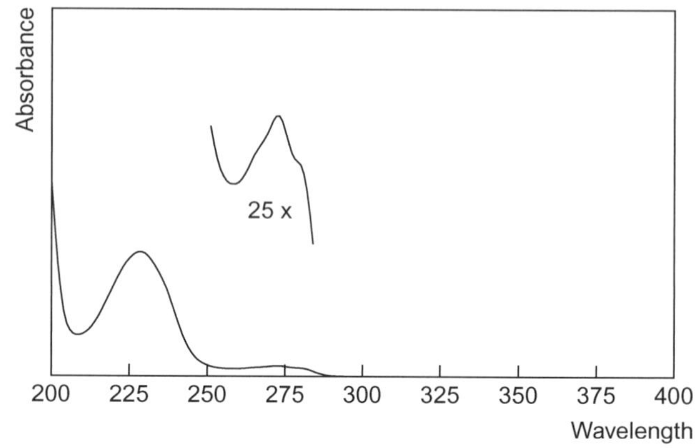

Infra-red Spectrum. Principal peaks at wavenumbers 709, 1689, 1296, 667, 935, 685 cm^{-1} (KBr disk).

Mass Spectrum. Principal ions at *m/z* 105, 77, 51, 122, 50, 39, 74, 76; hippuric acid 105, 135, 51, 134, 77, 106, 50, 78.

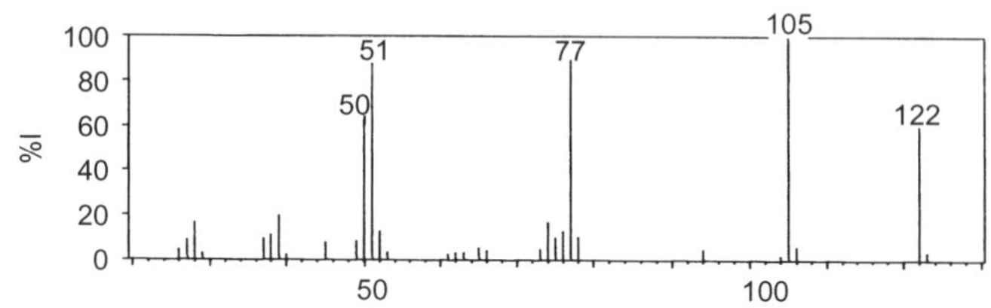

Quantification

Gas chromatography. In plasma or urine: limit of detection 10 μg/L, ECD—A. Sioufi and F. Pommier, *J. Chromatogr.* 1980, *181(7); B Biomed. Appl.*, 161–168. In urine: limit of detection 0.5 μg/L, ECD—C. Aprea *et al.*, *J. Chromatogr. B Biomed. Sci. Appl.*, 1997, *695(2)*, 227–236. In plasma and urine: limit of detection 0.1 mg/L and 0.2 mg/L, respectively, FID—A. Q. Li and X. L. Zhao, *Biomed. Chromatogr.*, 2001, *15(2)*, 75–78.

High performance liquid chromatography. In plasma: limit of quantification 0.05 mg/L, UV detection (λ = 283 nm)—A. A. Nomier *et al.*, *J. Pharm. Biomed. Anal.*, 1994, *12(5)*, 693–698.

Disposition in the Body. Benzoic acid is metabolised in the liver by conjugation with glycine and is rapidly and completely excreted in the urine as hippuric acid. Normal urinary excretion of hippuric acid is 1 to 2.5 g daily, equivalent to 0.7 to 1.7 g of benzoic acid. When taken in large doses, a proportion may be excreted as benzoylglucuronic acid.
Benzoic acid may be found in the urine as a metabolite of benzaldehyde, and is also a metabolite of numerous other compounds.

Uses. Benzoic acid is used as a preservative in a concentration of 0.1%. Sodium benzoate is given by mouth in a dose of 6 g, to test liver function.

Benzonatate

Antitussive

Synonyms. Benzonatine; Benzononatine.
Proprietary name. Tessalon
4-(Butylamino)benzoic acid 3,6,9,12,15,18,21,24,27-nonaoxaoctacos-1-yl ester
$C_{30}H_{53}NO_{17}$=603.7
CAS-104-31-4

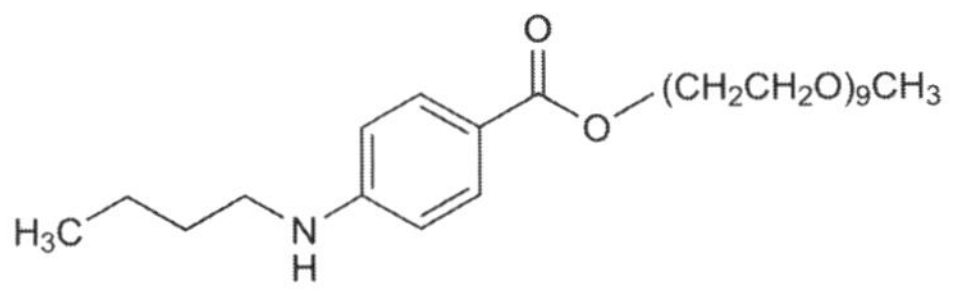

A clear, pale yellow, viscous liquid.
Miscible with water, ethanol, chloroform and ether.

Partition Coefficient. Log *P* (octanol/water) 2.4.

Colour Tests. Aromaticity (Method 2)—yellow/red; Liebermann's Test (at 100°)—blue.

Thin-layer Chromatography. System TA—Rf 61; system TAJ—Rf 56; system TAK—Rf 23; system TAL—Rf 90. (Acidified iodoplatinate solution, positive.)

Gas Chromatography. System GA—not eluted.

Ultraviolet Spectrum. Ethanol—308 nm (A_1^1=473c).

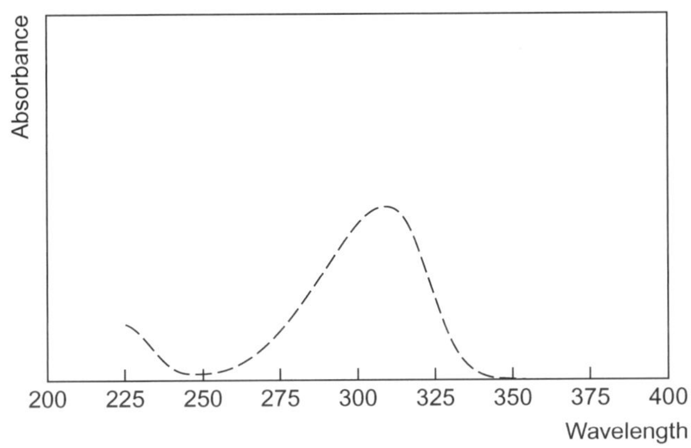

Infra-red Spectrum. Principal peaks at wavenumbers 1095, 1605, 1266, 1172, 1698, 1527 cm^{-1} (KBr disk).

Mass Spectrum. Principal ions at *m/z* 176, 59, 132, 150, 45, 193, 105, 29.

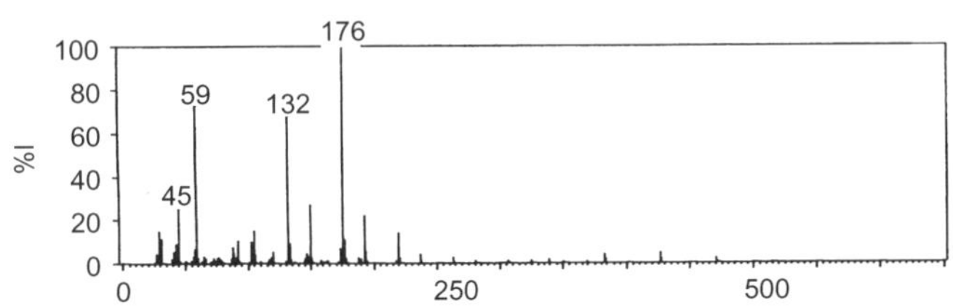

Dose. 300 to 600 mg daily.

Benzoylecgonine

Alkaloid

Synonym. Ecgonine Benzoate
3-(Benzoyloxy)-8-methyl-8-azabicyclo[3.2.1]octane-2-carboxylic acid
$C_{16}H_{19}NO_4$=289.3
CAS—519-09-5

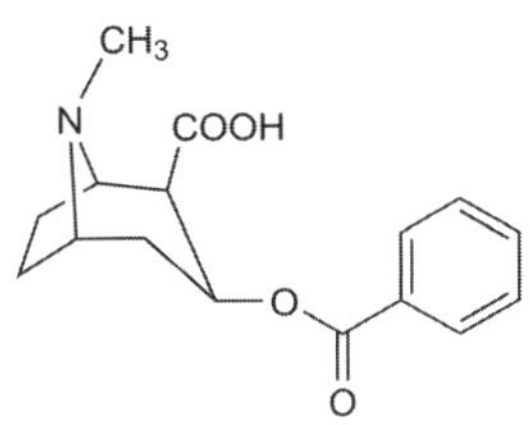

An alkaloid obtained from coca leaves, *Erythroxylum coca* (Erythroxylaceae) and its varieties.
The hydrated form occurs as crystals and melts at 86° to 92°. The anhydrous form melts at 195°, with decomposition.

Very soluble in hot water; soluble in ethanol; practically insoluble in ether; soluble in dilute acids and alkalis.

Partition Coefficient. Log *P* (octanol/water), −1.3.

Thin-layer Chromatography. System TA—Rf 21; system TB—Rf 00; system TC—Rf 01. (Acidified iodoplatinate solution, positive.)
Plate: silica 60 F_{254} (10 × 10 cm). Mobile phase: hexane:toluene: diethylamine (65:20:5). UV detection. Rf 0.02. [L. Antonilli *et al.*, *J. Chromatogr. B Biomed. Sci. Appl.*, 2001, *751*, 19–27.]

Gas Chromatography. System GA—benzoylecgonine RI 2570, cocaine RI 2187; system GB—benzoylecgonine RI 2663, cocaine RI 2289.

High Performance Liquid Chromatography. System HA—*k* 0.9 (tailing peak); system HQ—*k* 5.68; system HY—RI 236; system HZ—retention time 1.7 min; system HAA—retention time 9.7 min.

Column: LiChrocart-LiCrospher 100 RP-18 (250 × 4 mm i.d., 5 μm) pre-column, 100 RP-18 (4 × 4 mm i.d., 5 μm). Mobile phase: (A)-0.045 M ammonium acetate solution:methanol:acetonitrile (80:10:10); (B)-0.045 M ammonium acetate solution:methanol:acetonitrile (20:40:40). Linear gradient: 100 to 47.2% (A) in 20 min, flow rate 1 mL/min. UV detection (λ=235 nm). Retention time: 8.48 min. [L. Antonilli *et al.*, *J. Chromatogr. B Biomed. Sci. Appl.*, 2001, *751*, 19-27.]

Ultraviolet Spectrum. Aqueous acid—234 nm (A_1^1=376a), 274 nm.

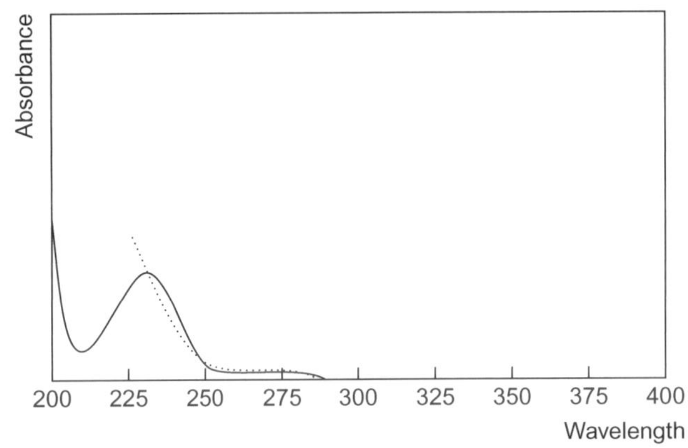

Infra-red Spectrum. Principal peaks at wavenumbers 1275, 1720, 1618, 717, 1116, 1316 cm^{-1}.

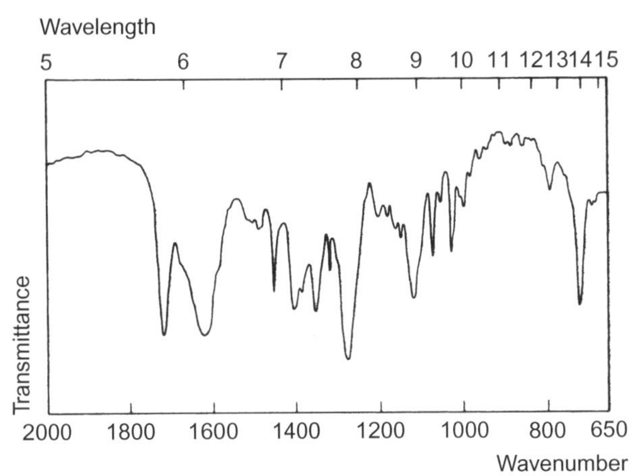

Mass Spectrum. Principal ions at *m/z* 124, 82, 168, 77, 105, 42, 94, 83.

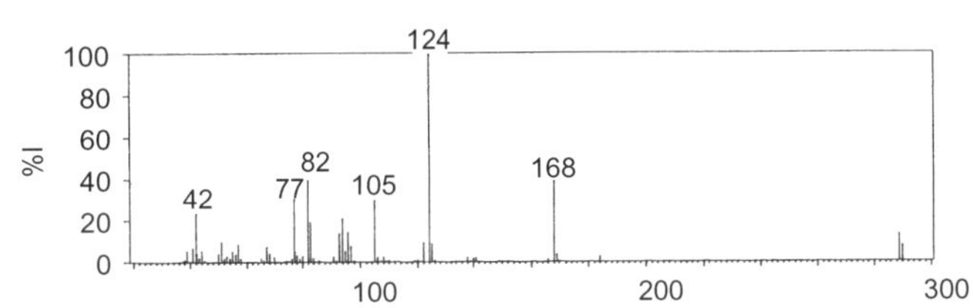

Quantification. See also under Cocaine.

Gas chromatography–mass spectrometry. In hair: limit of detection 0.2 μg/g using a 30 mg sample—P. Kintz and P. Mangin, *Forensic Sci. Int.*, 1995, *73*, 93–100. In hair, plasma, saliva, and urine: limit of detection 0.5 μg/g in hair and 5 μg/L in plasma, saliva, and urine—W. L. Wang *et al.*, *J. Chromatogr.* 1994, *660 B Biomed. Appl.*, 279–290. In urine: limit of detection 1 μg/L—R. de la Torre *et al.*, *J. Pharm. Biomed. Anal.*, 1995, *13(3)*, 305–312.

High performance liquid chromatography. In urine: limit of detection is 25 μg/L and limit of quantification 200 μg/L, UV detection (λ = 235 nm)—L. Antonilli *et al.*, *J. Chromatogr. B Biomed. Sci. Appl.*, 2001, *751*, 19–27.

High performance liquid chromatography–mass spectrometry. In blood: limit of detection is 2 μg/L, tandem MS detection (chemical ionisation)—C. S. Sosnoff *et al.*, *J. Anal. Toxicol.*, 1996, *20*, 179–184. In urine: limit of detection 0.5 μg/L, tandem MS—P. M. Jeanville *et al.*, *J. Anal. Toxicol.*, 2001, *25*, 69–75.

Disposition in the Body. Benzoylecgonine is the first hydrolysis product formed in the metabolism of cocaine; it is then further hydrolysed to ecgonine.

Half-life. About 4.5 hours (based on urinary excretion data).

Note. See under Cocaine for further information on disposition in the body.

Benzquinamide

Anti-emetic

2-(Acetyloxy)-*N*,*N*-diethyl-1,3,4,6,7,11b-hexahydro-9,10-dimethoxy-2*H*-benzo[*a*]-quinolizine-3-carboxamide
$C_{22}H_{32}N_2O_5$=404.5
CAS-63-12-7

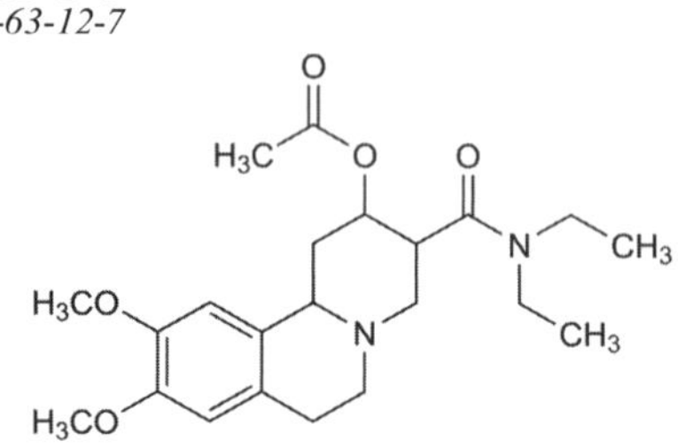

A yellowish crystalline powder. M.p. 130° to 131.5°.
Soluble in dilute acetic acid.

Benzquinamide Hydrochloride
Proprietary name. Emete-con
$C_{22}H_{32}N_2O_5$,HCl=441.0
CAS-113-69-9

Dissociation Constant. pK_a 5.9.

Partition Coefficient. Log *P* (octanol/water) 1.9.

Colour Tests. Liebermann's Test—black; Marquis Test—yellow; Sulfuric Acid—orange.

Thin-layer Chromatography. System TA—Rf 65; system TB—Rf 07; system TC—Rf 69; system TL—Rf 36; system TAJ—Rf 53; system TAK—Rf 06; system TAL—Rf 91. (Acidified iodoplatinate solution, positive.)

High Performance Liquid Chromatography. System HA—*k* 0.3.

Ultraviolet Spectrum. Aqueous acid—282 nm (A_1^1=95b). No alkaline shift.

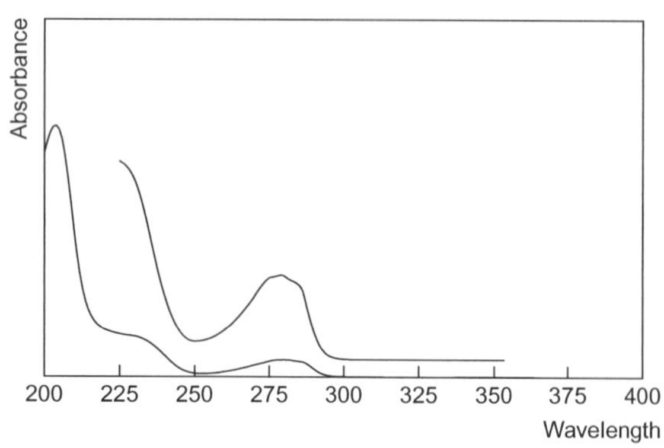

Infra-red Spectrum. Principal peaks at wavenumbers 1244, 1733, 1633, 1204, 1515, 1123 cm^{-1} (KBr disk).

Mass Spectrum. Principal ions at *m/z* 205, 244, 191, 345, 206, 72, 272, 246.

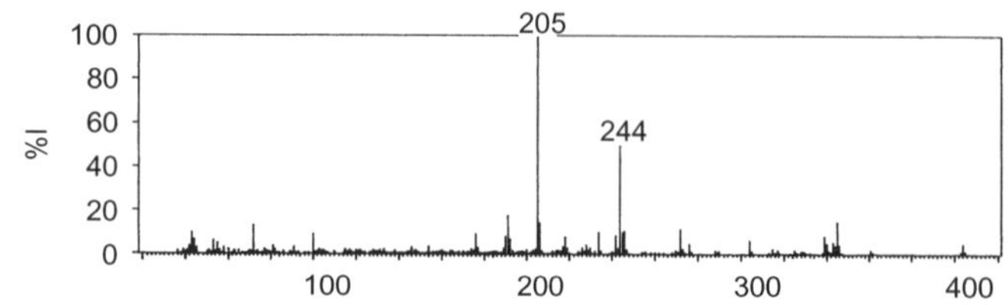

Quantification
Gas chromatography–mass spectrometry. In plasma: limit of detection 10 μg/L—D. C. Hobbs and A. G. Connolly, *J. Pharmacokinet. Biopharm.*, 1978, *6*, 477–485.

Disposition in the Body. Readily absorbed after oral administration; bioavailability about 35%. Metabolised by *O*-demethylation, deacetylation and *N*-dealkylation. After an oral dose, up to about 7% is excreted unchanged in the urine in 24 h.

Therapeutic concentration
Following oral administration of 200 mg to 20 subjects, a mean peak plasma concentration of 0.6 mg/L was attained in 1.2 h. Following intramuscular injection of 50 mg to 20 subjects, a mean peak plasma concentration of 0.7 mg/L was attained in 0.26 h [D. C. Hobbs and A. G. Connolly, *J. Pharmacokinet. Biopharm.*, 1978, *6*, 477–485].

Half-life. Plasma half-life, about 1 h.

Volume of distribution. About 1 L/kg.

Dose. The equivalent of 50 mg of benzquinamide by intramuscular injection, repeated as necessary.

Benzthiazide

Diuretic/Antihypertensive

Proprietary names. Aquatag; Exna; Hydrex. It is an ingredient of Decaserpyl Plus and Dytide.
6-Chloro-3-[[(phenylmethyl)thio]methyl]-2*H*-1,2,4-benzothiadiazine-7-sulfonamide 1,1-dioxide
$C_{15}H_{14}ClN_3O_4S_3$=431.9
CAS-91-33-8

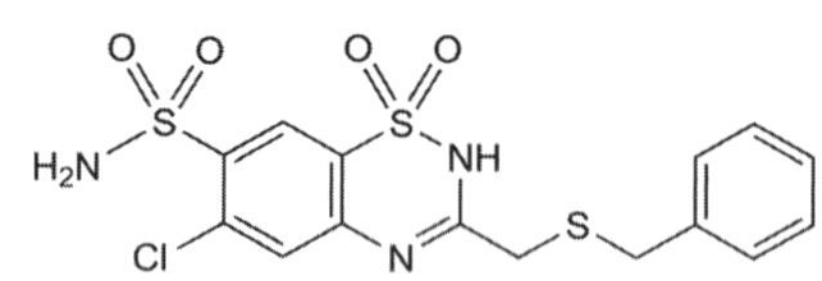

A white crystalline powder. M.p. 231° to 232°.
Practically insoluble in water, chloroform and ether; slightly soluble in ethanol; soluble 1 in 100 of acetone; freely soluble in dimethylformamide and in solutions of alkalis.

Dissociation Constant. pK_a 6.0.

Partition Coefficient. Log *P* (octanol/water) 1.7.

Colour Tests. Koppanyi–Zwikker Test—violet; Liebermann's Test—red-brown; Sulfuric Acid—yellow.

Thin-layer Chromatography. System TD—Rf 14; system TE—Rf 09; system TF—Rf 51; system TAD—Rf 30; system TAJ—Rf 31; system TAK—Rf 06; system TAL—Rf 71.

Gas Chromatography. System GA—RI 2680.

High Performance Liquid Chromatography. System HN—*k* 9.32; system HY—RI 415.

Ultraviolet Spectrum. Aqueous acid—283 nm (A_1^1=292a); aqueous alkali—297 nm (A_1^1=310b).

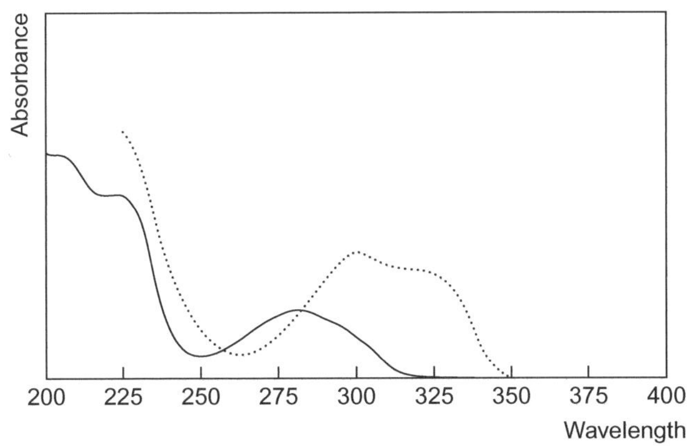

Infra-red Spectrum. Principal peaks at wavenumbers 1180, 1160, 1310, 1502, 1620, 1590 cm^{-1} (KBr disk).

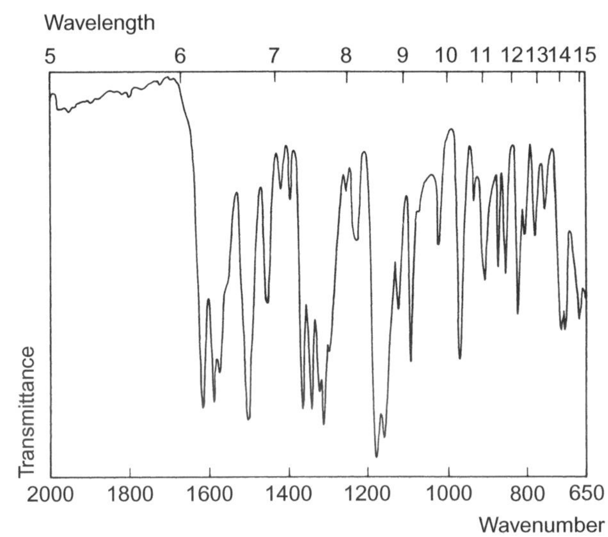

Mass Spectrum. Principal ions at *m/z* 91, 121, 65, 122, 309, 64, 230, 123.

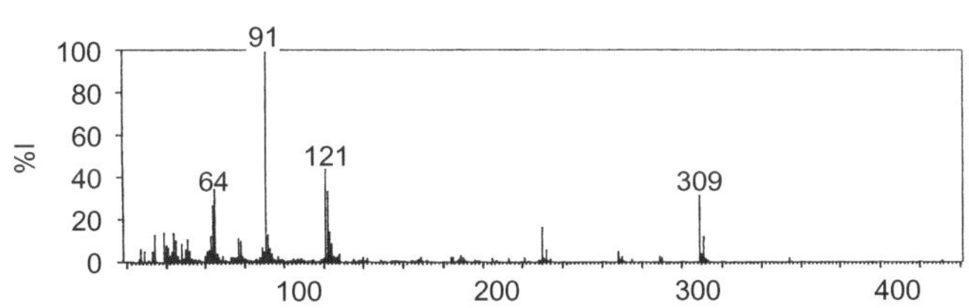

Quantification

High performance liquid chromatography. In plasma, urine or faeces: limit of detection 10 μg/L in plasma and 50 μg/L in urine, UV detection—M. C. Meyer *et al.*, *Biopharm. Drug Dispos.*, 1982, *3*, 1–9.

Disposition in the Body. Poorly absorbed after oral administration. Less than 10% of a dose is excreted in the urine as unchanged drug in 48 h, and about 80% of a dose is eliminated in the faeces.

Therapeutic concentration

Following an oral dose of 50 mg to 4 subjects, peak plasma concentrations of about 0.008 and 0.02 mg/L were attained in 3 h in 2 subjects; in the remaining 2 subjects benzthiazide was not detectable in the plasma [M. C. Meyer *et al.*, *Biopharm. Drug Dispos.*, 1982, *3*, 1–9].

Half-life. Derived from urinary excretion data, about 10 to 15 h.

Dose. 50 to 200 mg daily.

Benzydamine

Analgesic

Synonym. Benzindamine

N,N-Dimethyl-3-[[1-(phenylmethyl)-1*H*-indazol-3-yl]oxy]-1-propanamine

$C_{19}H_{23}N_3O = 309.4$

CAS—642-72-8

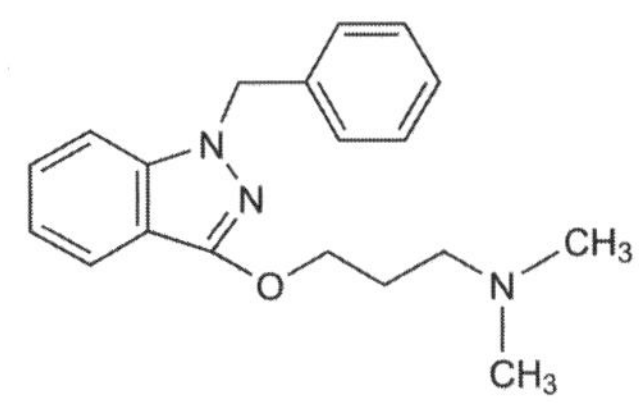

B.p. 160°.

Benzydamine Hydrochloride

Proprietary names. Afloben; A-Termadol; Difflam; Imotryl; Multum; Tantum; Verax.

$C_{19}H_{23}N_3O,HCl = 345.9$

CAS—132-69-4

A white crystalline powder. M.p. 160°.

Soluble 1 in 1 of water, 1 in 8 of ethanol, and 1 in 4 of chloroform; practically insoluble in ether.

Partition Coefficient. Log *P* (octanol/water), 4.2.

Colour Test. Mandelin's Test—brown-green.

Thin-layer Chromatography. System TA—Rf 44; system TB—Rf 36; system TC—Rf 22; system TL—Rf 09; system TAE—Rf 16. (Acidified iodoplatinate solution, positive.)

Gas Chromatography. System GA—RI 2380.

High Performance Liquid Chromatography. System HAA—retention time 15.0 min.

Ultraviolet Spectrum. Aqueous acid—307 nm ($A^1_1 = 144c$). No alkaline shift.

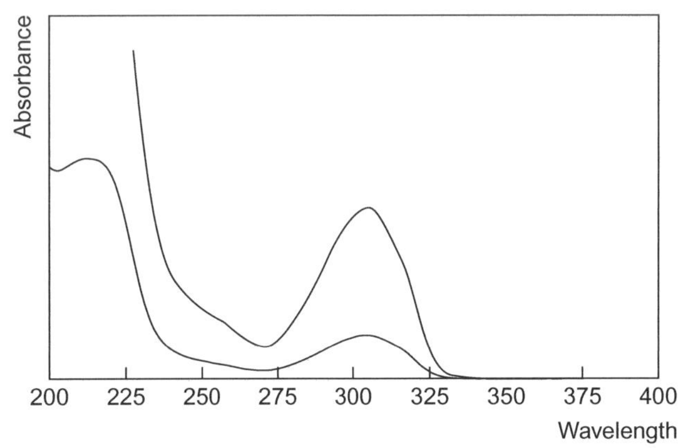

Infra-red Spectrum. Principal peaks at wavenumbers 1529, 740, 1491, 1613, 1182, 1141 cm^{-1} (KBr disk).

Mass Spectrum. Principal ions at *m/z* 85, 58, 86, 91, 84, 70, 42, 225.

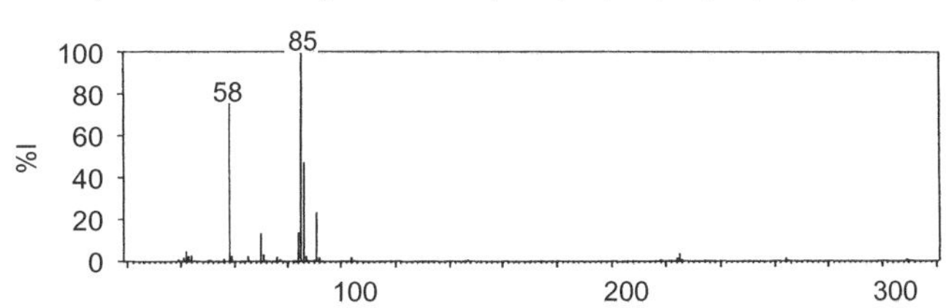

Quantification

High performance liquid chromatography. In plasma and urine: limit of quantification 0.5 μg/L and 1.0 μg/L, respectively—G. A. Baldock *et al.*, *J. Chromatogr.*, 1990, *529(1)*, 113–123.

Disposition in the Body. Absorbed after oral administration. About 50% of a dose is excreted unchanged in the urine.

Therapeutic concentration

An oral dose of 1 mg/kg produced a blood concentration of about 0.8 mg/L within 2 h and a significant concentration was maintained for several hours. [B. Catanese *et al.*, *Arzneimittelforschung*, 1966, *16*, 1354–1357.]

Protein binding. A fraction of benzydamine is bound to proteins in the blood.

Dose. 150 to 200 mg of benzydamine hydrochloride daily.

Benzyl Alcohol

Local Anaesthetic/Disinfectant

Synonyms. Phenylcarbinol; Phenylmethanol.
$C_7H_8O = 108.1$
CAS—100-51-6

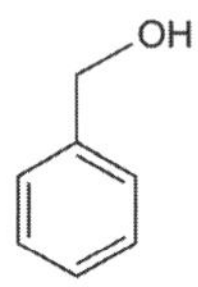

A colourless liquid with a faint aromatic odour. Mass per mL 1.043 to 1.046 g. B.p. 203° to 208°.
Soluble 1 in 25 of water; miscible with ethanol, chloroform, and ether.

Dissociation Constant. pK_a 15.4.

Partition Coefficient. Log *P* (octanol/water), 1.1.

Thin-layer Chromatography. System TAE—Rf 86.

Gas Chromatography. System GA—RI 1040.

Ultraviolet Spectrum. Methanol—252 ($A^1_1 = 14b$), 258 ($A^1_1 = 17b$), 264 nm ($A^1_1 = 13b$).

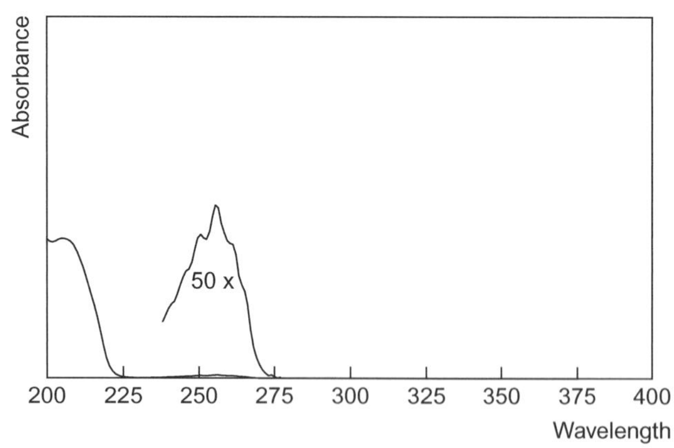

Mass Spectrum. Principal ions at *m/z* 79, 77, 108, 101, 51, 50, 39, 40.

Quantification

Gas chromatography–mass spectrometry. In serum and postmortem blood: limit of detection 1 mg/L—A. Dasgupta and G. Steinagel, *J. Forensic Sci.*, 1997, *42(4)*, 697–700. In serum: limit of detection 0.1 mg/L, SIM (*m/z* 69, 77, 91, 105, 121, 504 and 518)—A. Dasgupta and P. E. Humphrey, *J. Chromatogr. B Biomed. Sci. Appl.*, 1998, *708(1–2)*, 299–303.

High performance liquid chromatography. In plasma—H. S. Tan *et al.*, *J. Chromatogr.*, 1991, *568(1)*, 145–155.

Use. Topically in concentrations of up to 10%.

Benzyl Benzoate

Acaricide

Proprietary names. Antiscabiosum Mago; Ascabiol; Benzemul; Scabanca.

$C_{14}H_{12}O_2 = 212.2$
CAS—120-51-4

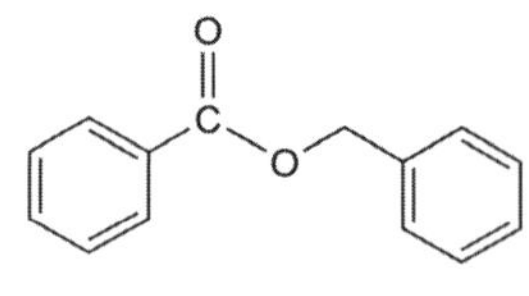

Colourless crystals or a clear, colourless, oily liquid. B.p. 323° to 324°. Practically insoluble in water; miscible with ethanol, acetone, carbon disulfide, chloroform, and ether.

Partition Coefficient. Log *P* (octanol/water), 4.0.

Thin-layer Chromatography. System TF—Rf 73; system TAD—Rf 09.

Gas Chromatography. System GA—RI 1738.

Ultraviolet Spectrum. Ethanol—230 nm ($A^1_1 = 843b$).

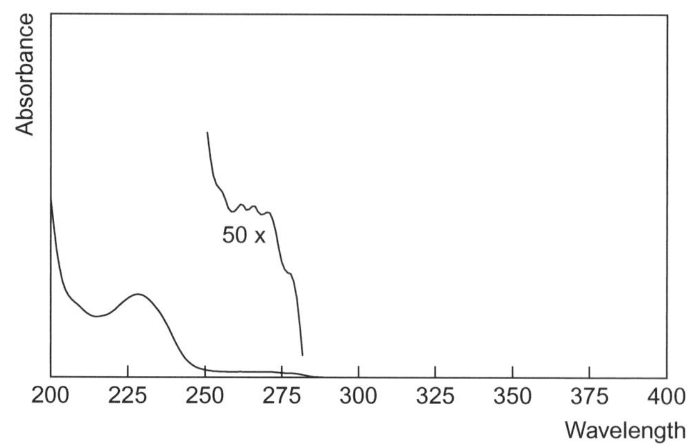

Infra-red Spectrum. Principal peaks at wavenumbers 1263, 1706, 1106, 713, 698, 1067 cm^{-1} (thin film).

Mass Spectrum. Principal ions at *m/z* 77, 105, 91, 51, 65, 212, 50, 78.

Disposition in the Body. Rapidly hydrolysed to benzoic acid and benzyl alcohol; benzyl alcohol then undergoes further oxidation to benzoic acid followed by conjugation with glycine to form hippuric acid. Excreted in the urine mainly as hippuric acid.

Uses. Topically as a 25% application; a 5% solution is used as an insect repellent.

Benzyl Nicotinate

Rubefacient (Topical)

Proprietary names. Rubriment. It is an ingredient of Bayolin.
$C_{13}H_{11}NO_2 = 213.2$
CAS—94-44-0

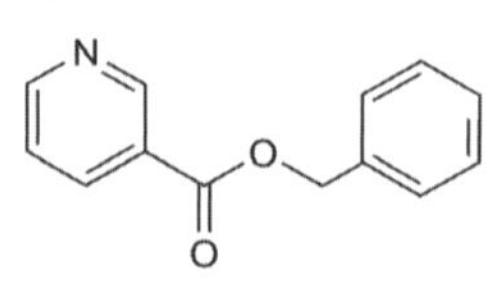

A liquid.

Partition Coefficient. Log *P* (octanol/water), 2.4.

Colour Tests. Cyanogen bromide—red-orange; Liebermann's test—brown; Sulfuric acid—orange.

Thin-layer Chromatography. System TA—Rf 63; system TB—Rf 42; system TC—Rf 71; system TL—Rf 60. (Acidified potassium permanganate solution, positive.)

Ultraviolet Spectrum. Methanol—262 nm ($A^1_1 = 152b$).

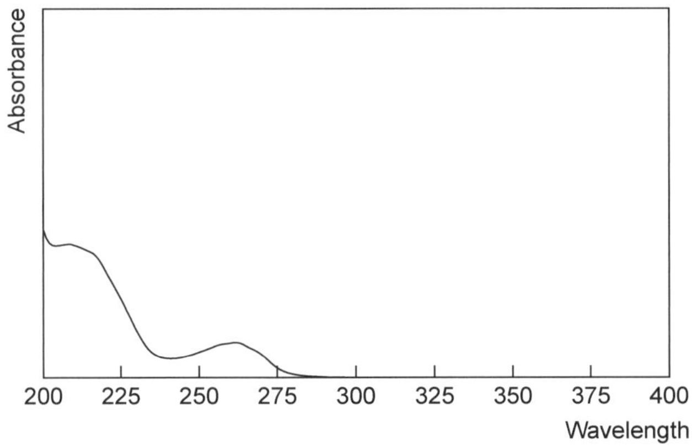

Infra-red Spectrum. Principal peaks at wavenumbers 1278, 1724, 1108, 740, 699, 1587 cm^{-1} (KCl disk).

Use. Topically in a concentration of 2.5%.

Benzylmorphine

Narcotic Analgesic/Antitussive

7,8-Didehydro-4,5-epoxy-17-methyl-3-(phenylmethoxy)morphinan-6-ol
$C_{24}H_{25}NO_3$=375.5
CAS—14297-87-1

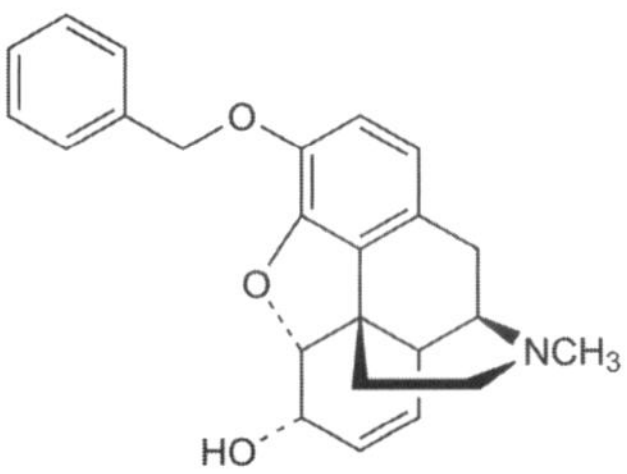

A colourless crystalline powder. M.p. 132°.
Soluble 1 in 2500 of cold water; 1.6 parts dissolves in 100 parts ether; readily soluble in 50% ethanol and in benzene.

Benzylmorphine Hydrochloride

Proprietary name. Peronine
$C_{24}H_{25}NO_3$,HCl=411.9
CAS—630-86-4
A colourless microcrystalline powder.
Soluble 1 in 200 of water and 1 in 160 of ethanol; practically insoluble in chloroform and ether.

Dissociation Constant. pK_a 8.1 (20°).

Partition Coefficient. Log P (octanol/water), 3.0.

Colour Test. Marquis Test—red→violet.

Thin-layer Chromatography. System TA—Rf 41; system TB—Rf 06; system TC—Rf 23; system TL—Rf 08; system TAE—Rf 20; system TAF—Rf 23. (Acidified iodoplatinate solution, positive.)

Gas Chromatography. System GA—RI 3015.

High Performance Liquid Chromatography. System HA—*k* 4.4 (tailing peak); system HC—*k* 1.03.

Ultraviolet Spectrum. Aqueous acid—284 nm (A^1_1=48b).

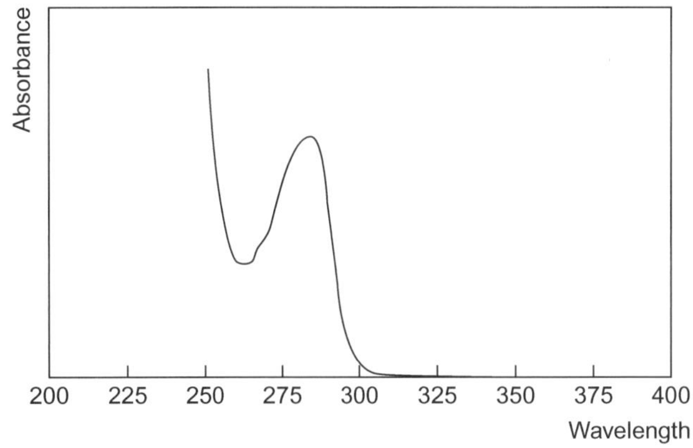

Infra-red Spectrum. Principal peaks at wavenumbers 1274, 1040, 1502, 1017, 763, 1056 cm^{-1}.

Mass Spectrum. Principal ions at m/z 284, 91, 375, 81, 42, 36, 285, 175.

Dose. Benzylmorphine hydrochloride was formerly given in doses of 8 to 30 mg.

Benzylpenicillin

Antibiotic

Synonyms. Crystalline Penicillin G; Penicillin; Penicillin G; Penicillin II.
Note. The name 'benzylpenicillin' and its synonyms are commonly used to describe either benzylpenicillin potassium or benzylpenicillin sodium.
(2*S*,5*R*,6*R*)-3,3-Dimethyl-7-oxo-6-[(phenylacetyl)amino]-4-thia-1-azabicyclo[3.2.0]heptane-2-carboxylic acid
$C_{16}H_{18}N_2O_4S$=334.4
CAS—61-33-6

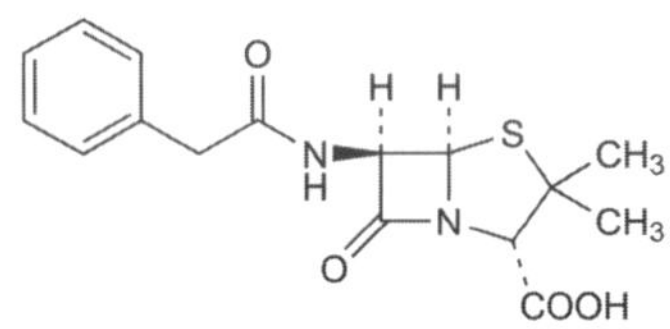

An antimicrobial acid produced by the growth of certain strains of *Penicillium notatum*.

Benzylpenicillin Potassium

Proprietary names. Abbocillin-G; Crystapen G; Falapen; Hyasorb; M-Cillin B; Megacillin; Novopen; P-50; Paclin G; Pentids; Pfizerpen; Sugracillin.
Note. Megacillin is also used as a proprietary name for clemizole penicillin, phenoxymethylpenicillin, and procaine penicillin (procaine benzylpenicillin).
$C_{16}H_{17}KN_2O_4S$=372.5
CAS—113-98-4
A white, finely crystalline powder. M.p. 214° to 217°, with decomposition.
Very soluble in water; soluble in ethanol; practically insoluble in chloroform and ether.

Benzylpenicillin Sodium

Proprietary names. Crystapen; Gonopen; Spécilline G. It is an ingredient of Bicillin and Triplopen.
Note. Bicillin is also used as a proprietary name for benzathine benzylpenicillin.
$C_{16}H_{17}N_2NaO_4S$=356.4
CAS—69-57-8
A white to slightly yellow, finely crystalline powder.
Very soluble in water; soluble in ethanol; practically insoluble in chloroform and ether.

Dissociation Constant. pK_a 2.8 (25°).

Partition Coefficient. Log P (octanol/water), 1.8.

High Performance Liquid Chromatography. System HY—RI 376.

Ultraviolet Spectrum. Benzylpenicillin sodium: water—257 (A^1_1=7b), 264, 325 nm.

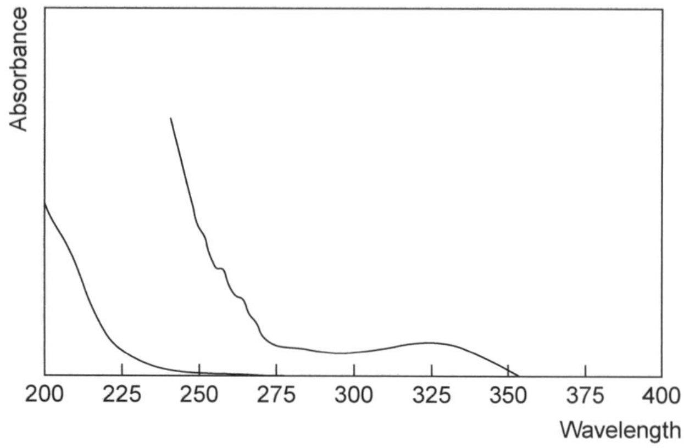

Infra-red Spectrum. Principal peaks at wavenumbers 1620, 1777, 1500, 1310, 1700, 703 cm^{-1} (benzylpenicillin sodium, KBr disk).

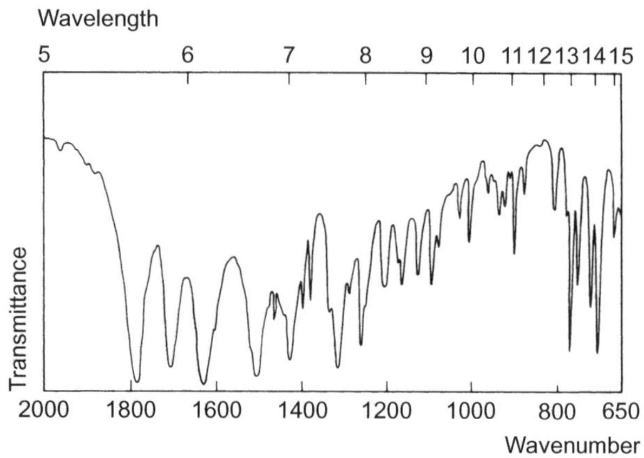

Quantification

High performance liquid chromatography. In serum: limit of quantification 0.5 to 50 mg/L, UV detection (λ=208 nm)—E. Mendez-Alvarez *et al., Biomed. Chromatogr.*, 1991, *5(2)*, 78–82.

Disposition in the Body. About 30% of an oral dose is absorbed, the remainder being inactivated by gastric acid; maximum concentrations are attained about 1 h after oral administration. After IM injection it is rapidly absorbed, peak concentrations being attained in 15 to 30 min. About 60 to 90% of an IM dose is excreted in the urine, mainly in the first few hours; the urinary material consists of unchanged drug and penicilloic acid (about 20% of the dose). Biliary excretion also occurs.

Therapeutic concentration. In plasma, minimum inhibitory concentration 0.006 to 2 mg/L.

Half-life. Plasma half-life, about 0.5 to 1 h; increased in infants and elderly subjects, and in renal impairment.

Distribution in blood. Plasma : whole blood ratio, 1.6.

Protein binding. In plasma, 45 to 65%.

Note. For a review of the pharmacokinetics of penicillin antibiotics see M. Barza and L. Weinstein, *Clin. Pharmacokinet.*, 1976, *1*, 297–308. For a review of clinical pharmacology and therapeutic use of penicillins, see D. Nathwani and M. J. Wood, *Drugs*, 1993, *45*, 866–894.

Dose. 0.6 to 2.4 g daily, given parenterally; up to 24 g daily in severe infections.

Bephenium Hydroxynaphthoate

Anthelmintic

Synonym. Naphthammonum
Proprietary name. Alcopar(a)
N,N-Dimethyl-*N*-(2-phenoxyethyl)benzenemethanaminium 3-hydroxy-2-naphthoate
$C_{28}H_{29}NO_4$=443.5
CAS—7181-73-9 (bephenium); 3818-50-6 (hydroxynaphthoate)

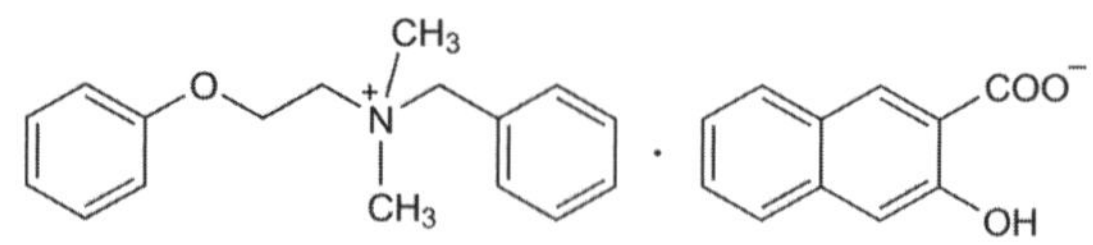

A yellow to greenish-yellow crystalline powder, which gives a green fluorescence when examined under ultraviolet light. M.p. 170° to 171°. Practically insoluble in water; soluble 1 in 50 of ethanol.

Partition Coefficient. Log *P* (octanol/water), 0.5.

Colour Tests. Mandelin's test—green; Marquis test—red-violet.

Thin-layer Chromatography. System TA—Rf 77. (Acidified potassium permanganate solution, positive.)

Ultraviolet Spectrum. Methanol—234 (A_1^1=1300b), 263, 270, 283, 295, 352 nm.

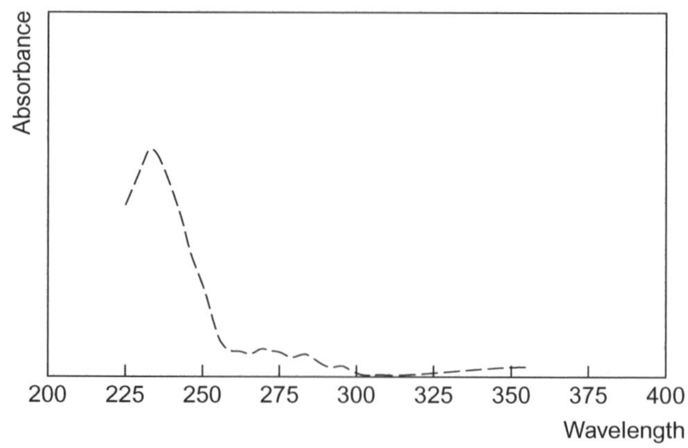

Infra-red Spectrum. Principal peaks at wavenumbers 1233, 768, 1653, 1590, 858, 726 cm^{-1} (KBr disk).

Quantification

Colorimetry. In urine—E. W. Rogers, *BMJ*, 1958, *2*, 1576–1577.

Disposition in the Body. Bephenium hydroxynaphthoate is poorly absorbed after oral administration; less than 1% of a dose is excreted in the urine in 24 h.

Dose. The equivalent of 2.5 g of bephenium, as a single dose.

Berberine

Alkaloid

5,6-Dihydro-9,10-dimethoxybenzo[*g*]-1,3-benzodioxolo[5,6-*a*]quinolizinium
$[C_{20}H_{18}NO_4]^+$=336.4
CAS—2086-83-1 ($C_{20}H_{18}NO_4^+$); 117-74-8 ($C_{20}H_{18}NO_4{\cdot}OH$)

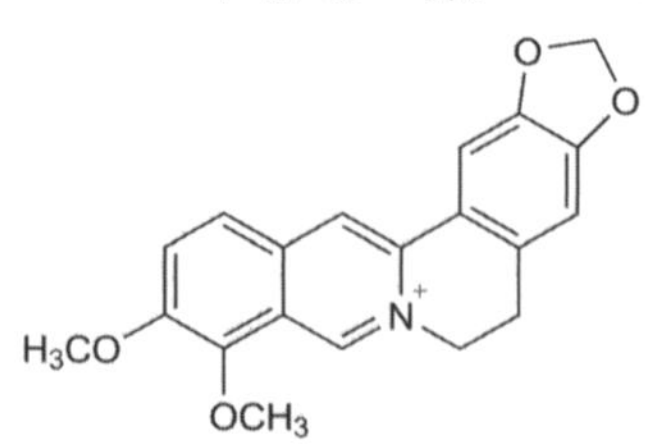

A quaternary alkaloid present in *Hydrastis*, in various species of *Berberis*, and in many other plants.
Yellow crystals. M.p. 145°.
Soluble 1 in 4.5 of water and 1 in 100 of ethanol; very slightly soluble in ether.

Berberine Hydrochloride
Synonym. Berberine Chloride
$C_{20}H_{18}ClNO_4,2H_2O$=407.8
CAS—633-65-8 (anhydrous); 5956-60-5 (dihydrate)
Bright yellow acicular crystals or powder.

Soluble 1 in 400 of water; freely soluble in boiling water; soluble in ethanol; practically insoluble in chloroform and ether.

Berberine Sulfate
Synonyms. Berberine Acid Sulfate; Berberine Bisulfate.
$C_{20}H_{18}NO_4,HSO_4$=433.4
CAS—633-66-9
Bright yellow acicular crystals or dark yellow powder.
Soluble 1 in about 100 of water; slightly soluble in ethanol.

Partition Coefficient. Log *P* (octanol/water), 2.1.

Colour Tests. Mandelin's Test—blue-green→brown; Marquis Test—green.

Thin-layer Chromatography. System TA—Rf 07; system TL—Rf 00; system TAE—Rf 04; system TAF—Rf 56; system TAJ—Rf 00; system TAK—Rf 00; system TAL—Rf 20. (Acidified iodoplatinate solution, positive.)

Gas Chromatography. System GA—RI 2070.

High Performance Liquid Chromatography. System HY—RI 327.

Ultraviolet Spectrum. Aqueous acid—264 (A^1_1=554b), 345 nm.

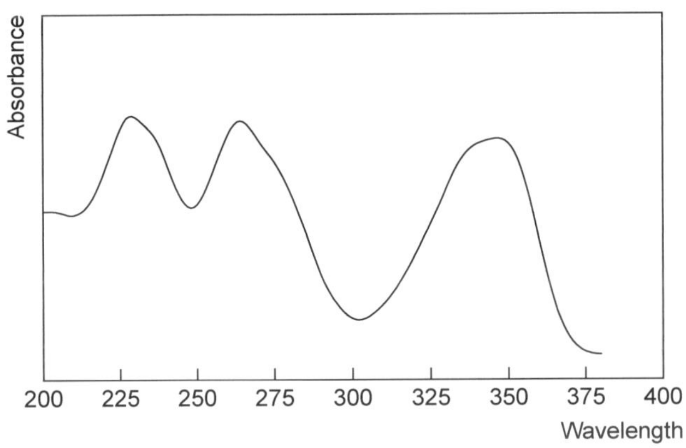

Infra-red Spectrum. Principal peaks at wavenumbers 1505, 1271, 1234, 1030, 1587, 1098 cm^{-1} (KBr disk).

Mass Spectrum. Principal ions at *m/z* 321, 278, 320, 292, 306, 191, 322, 304.

Quantification
Gas chromatography–mass spectrometry. In urine: limit of detection 1 μg/L—H. Miyazaki *et al.*, *J. Chromatogr.*, 1978, *152*, 79–86.

High performance liquid chromatography. In plasma, urine and bile: limit of detection 18.1, 2.3 and 90.4 μg/L—C. M. Chen and H. C. Chang, *J. Chromatogr. B Biomed. Sci. Appl.*, 1995, *665(1)*, 117–123. In plasma: limit of detection 0.4 ng, UV detection (λ=346 nm)—X. Zeng, *Biomed. Chromatogr.*, 1999, *13(7)*, 442–444.

Disposition in the Body. After oral administration, less than 0.1% of a dose is excreted in the urine unchanged in 24 h.

Dose. Berberine sulfate has been given in doses of 150 mg daily.

Betahistine

Vasodilator

N-Methyl-2-pyridine-ethanamine
$C_8H_{12}N_2$=136.2
CAS—5638-76-6

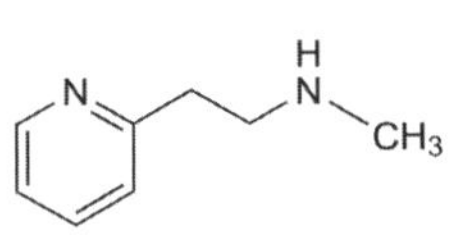

A liquid. B.p. 113° to 114°.
Miscible with water, ethanol, chloroform and ether.

Betahistine Hydrochloride
Proprietary names. Betaserc; Microser; Serc; Vasomotal.
$C_8H_{12}N_2,2HCl$=209.1
CAS—5579-84-0
A white or creamy-white, hygroscopic, crystalline powder. M.p. about 152°.
Freely soluble in water; soluble in ethanol and methanol; practically insoluble in carbon tetrachloride, chloroform and ether.

Dissociation Constant. pK_a 3.5, 9.7.

Partition Coefficient. Log *P* (octanol/water), 0.7.

Thin-layer Chromatography. System TA—Rf 10. (Acidified iodoplatinate solution, strong reaction.)

Gas Chromatography. System GA—RI 1235.

High Performance Liquid Chromatography. System HA—*k* 3.1; system HAA—Retention time(s) 3.2 min.

Ultraviolet Spectrum. Aqueous acid—261 nm (A^1_1=358b).

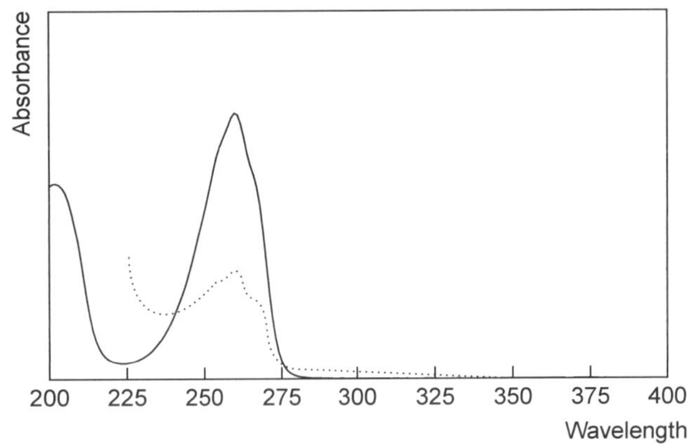

Infra-red Spectrum. Principal peaks at wavenumbers 1585, 1560, 1290, 762, 1238, 1145 cm^{-1} (KBr disk).

Mass Spectrum. Principal ions at *m/z* 79, 105, 104, 51, 78, 52, 50, 77.

Quantification
Gas chromatography. In serum: limit of detection 600 μg/L, FID—J. F. Douglas and T. L. Hohing, *Experientia*, 1978, *34*, 499–500.

Disposition in the Body. Betahistine is readily absorbed after oral administration; peak plasma concentrations of the metabolites are attained in 3 to 5 h. Most of a dose is excreted in the urine as metabolites.

Dose. 24 to 48 mg of betahistine hydrochloride daily.

Betaine

Treatment of Hypochlorhydria

Synonyms. Glycine Betaine; Glycocoll Betaine; Lycine; Oxyneurine; Trimethylglycine.
1-Carboxy-*N*,*N*,*N*-trimethylmethanaminium inner salt
$C_5H_{11}NO_2$=117.2
CAS—107-43-7

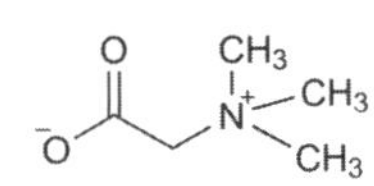

Deliquescent crystals. M.p. about 310°, with decomposition.
Soluble 1 in 0.6 of water and 1 in 11 of ethanol; sparingly soluble in ether; soluble 1 in 2 of methanol.

Betaine Hydrochloride
Proprietary names. It is an ingredient of Acidol-Pepsin and Kloref.
$C_5H_{11}NO_2,HCl$=153.6
CAS—590-46-5
Colourless crystals or white crystalline powder. When dissolved in water betaine hydrochloride hydrolyses and almost 25% of its weight of hydrochloric acid is formed. M.p. about 230°, with decomposition.
Soluble 1 in 2 of water and 1 in 20 of ethanol (90%); practically insoluble in chloroform and ether.

Dissociation Constant. pK_a 1.8 (25°).

Partition Coefficient. Log *P* (octanol/water), −4.9.

Colour Test. To an aqueous solution add iodine solution—red precipitate.

Thin-layer Chromatography. System TA—Rf 23; system TAE—Rf 16; system TAF—Rf 11. (Acidified iodoplatinate solution, positive.)

Gas Chromatography. System GA—not eluted.

Ultraviolet Spectrum. No significant absorption, 230 to 360 nm.

Infra-red Spectrum. Principal peaks at wavenumbers 1731, 1206, 885, 994, 902, 1250 cm^{-1} (KBr disk).

Quantification

High performance liquid chromatography. In urine: limit of detection 0.9 μg, UV detection—M. D. Laryea *et al.*, *Clin. Chim. Acta.*, 1994, *230(2)*, 169–175. In blood and urine: limit of detection 5 μmol/L (=0.6 mg/L), UV detection (λ=254 nm)—M. D. Laryea *et al.*, *Clin. Chem.*, 1998, *44(9)*, 1937–1941.

Dose. 0.18 to 3.5 g of betaine hydrochloride daily.

Betamethasone

Corticosteroid

Synonyms. Flubenisolonum; 9α-Fluoro-16β-methylprednisolone; NSC-39470; Sch-4831.
Proprietary names. Betnelan; Betnesol; Celeston(e); Desacort-Beta; Minisone; No-Reumar; Pertene.
(11β,16β)-9-Fluoro-11,17,21-trihydroxy-16-methylpregna-1,4-diene-3,20-dione
$C_{22}H_{29}FO_5$=392.5
CAS—378-44-9

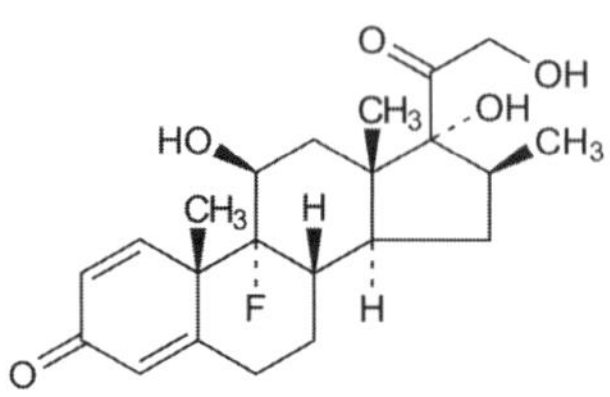

Betamethasone is a synthetic glucocorticoid and an isomer of dexamethasone.
A white to creamy-white crystalline powder. M.p. about 240°, with decomposition. A solution in dioxan is dextrorotatory.
Practically insoluble in water; soluble 1 in 75 of ethanol, 1 in 15 of warm ethanol, and 1 in 1100 of chloroform; very slightly soluble in ether; sparingly soluble in acetone and methanol.

Betamethasone Acetate

$C_{24}H_{31}FO_6$=434.5
CAS—987-24-6
A white to creamy-white powder. M.p. about 165° and, with decomposition, 200° to 220°.
Practically insoluble in water; soluble 1 in 9 of ethanol and 1 in 16 of chloroform; freely soluble in acetone.

Betamethasone Benzoate

Proprietary names. Beben; Benisone; Uticort.
$C_{29}H_{33}FO_6$=496.6
CAS—22298-29-9
A white powder. M.p. about 220°, with decomposition.
Practically insoluble in water; soluble in ethanol, chloroform, and methanol.

Betamethasone Dipropionate

Proprietary name. Diprosone
$C_{28}H_{37}FO_7$=504.6
CAS—5593-20-4
A white or creamy-white powder. M.p. 170° to 179°, with decomposition.
Practically insoluble in water; sparingly soluble in ethanol; freely soluble in acetone and chloroform.

Betamethasone Sodium Phosphate

Synonym. Betamethasone Disodium Phosphate
Proprietary names. Bentelan; Betameson; Betnesol; Celeston(e); Emilan; Paucisone; Vista-Methasone.
$C_{22}H_{28}FNa_2O_8P$=516.4
CAS—151-73-5
A white hygroscopic powder.
Soluble 1 in 2 of water and 1 in 350 of dehydrated alcohol; freely soluble in methanol; practically insoluble in acetone, chloroform, and ether.

Betamethasone Valerate

Synonym. 9α-Fluoro-16β-methylprednisolone 17-Valerate
Proprietary names. Bedermin; Betacort; Betaderm; Betnelan-V; Betnesol-V; Betneval; Betnovat(e); Bextasol; Celestoderm(-V); Celestone-V; Dermovaleas; Ecoval; Valisone.
$C_{27}H_{37}FO_6$=476.6
CAS—2152-44-5
A white to creamy-white powder. M.p. about 190°, with decomposition.
Practically insoluble in water; soluble 1 in 12 to 1 in 16 of ethanol, 1 in 2 of chloroform, and 1 in 50 of isopropyl alcohol; freely soluble in acetone; slightly soluble in ether.
Note. In alkaline media betamethasone 17-valerate undergoes a rearrangement to betamethasone 21-valerate.

Partition Coefficient. Log *P* (octanol/water), 1.9.

Colour Tests. Antimony Pentachloride—green→brown; Naphthol–Sulfuric Acid—green-brown/orange-brown; Sulfuric Acid—pink-orange.

Thin-layer Chromatography. Betamethasone: system TP—Rf 30; system TQ—Rf 00; system TR—Rf 00; system TS—Rf 00; system TAJ—Rf 38; system TAK—Rf 08; system TAL—Rf 80; system TAM—Rf 70. (DPST solution.) Betamethasone valerate: system TP—Rf 58; system TQ—Rf 27; system TR—Rf 20; system TS—Rf 02, streaking may occur. (DPST solution.) Betamethasone sodium phosphate remains on the baseline in all systems.

High Performance Liquid Chromatography. System HY—RI 584 (betamethasone valerate); system HZ—retention time 14.2 min; system HAA—retention time 13.3 min.

Ultraviolet Spectrum. Betamethasone: ethanol—240 nm (A_1^1=390a). Betamethasone sodium phosphate: water—241 nm (A_1^1=296a).

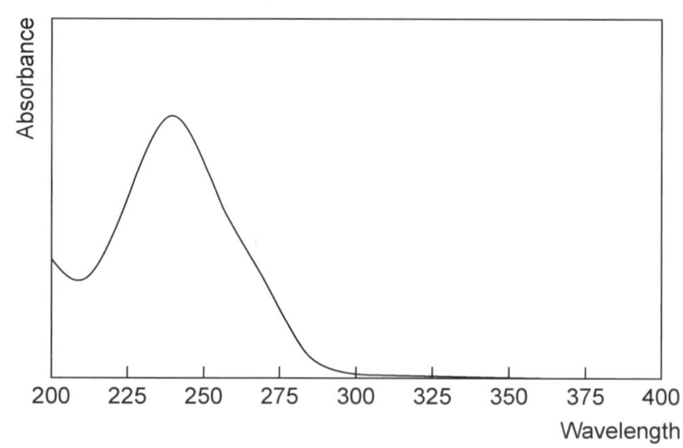

Infra-red Spectrum. Principal peaks at wavenumbers 1660, 1617, 1606, 1710, 1056, 907 cm^{-1} (KBr disk).

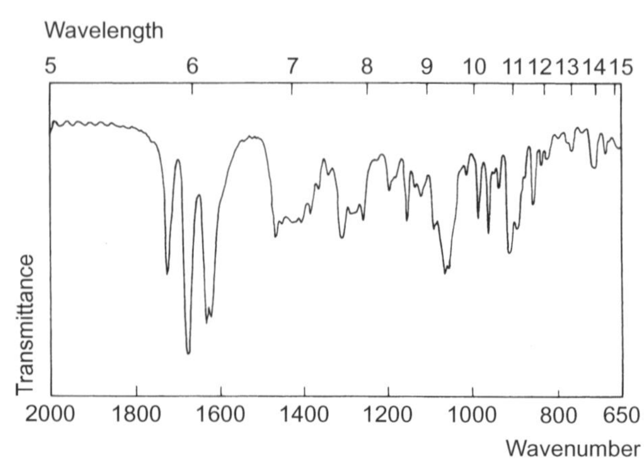

Mass Spectrum. Principal ions at *m/z* 121, 43, 122, 223, 147, 91, 41, 135.

Quantification

High performance liquid chromatography. In urine: limit of detection 10 mg/L (LC/MS/MS), 10 mg/L (LC/LC/MS), 0.2 mg/L (LC/LC/MS/MS) and limit of quantification 1 mg/L (LC/LC/MS/MS)—A. Polettini *et al.*, *J. Chromatogr. B Biomed. Sci. Appl.*, 1998, *713*, 339–352.

Disposition in the Body

Therapeutic concentration

5 healthy volunteers were administered 0.6 mg betamethasone orally and betamethasone 17-valerate as a topical application prepared as a suspension and applied to a 100-cm^2 area on the back for 28 h. The mean peak plasma concentrations were 5.0 and 0.24 mg/L, respectively. (K. Kubota *et al.*, *Br. J. Clin. Pharmacol.*, 1994, *37(1)*, 86–88.)

Dose. 0.5 to 9 mg daily.

Betanaphthol

Parasiticide

Synonyms. *β*-Naftol; Naphthol.

2-Naphthalenol

$C_{10}H_8O = 144.2$

CAS—135-19-3

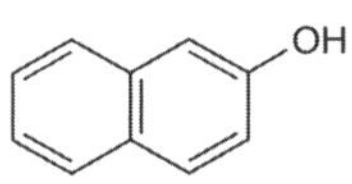

White crystalline leaflets or powder; stable in air but darkens on exposure to light. M.p. 121° to 123°. B.p. 285° to 286°.

Soluble 1 in 1000 of cold water, 1 in 80 of boiling water, 1 in 0.8 of ethanol, and 1 in 1.3 of ether; soluble in chloroform and in solutions of alkali hydroxides.

Dissociation Constant. pK_a 9.5 (25°).

Partition Coefficient. Log *P* (octanol/water), 2.7.

Colour Tests. Ferric Chloride—green; Liebermann's Test—green.

To 200 mg add 2 mL of an 8% sodium hydroxide solution and 1 drop of chloroform, then warm—blue.

Ultraviolet Spectrum. Ethanol—274 (A^1_1=326b), 285 (A^1_1=230b), 322 (A^1_1=120b), 330 nm (A^1_1=140b).

Disposition in the Body. Rapidly absorbed from the gastro-intestinal tract and may be absorbed through intact skin. It is excreted mainly as the glucuronide and gives a reddish tint to the urine.

Toxicity. The estimated minimum lethal dose is 2 g. Severe nephritis and fatalities have occurred following its absorption through intact skin.

Betaxolol

Beta-blocker

1-[4-[2-(Cyclopropylmethoxy)ethyl]phenoxy]-3-[(1-methylethyl)amino]-2-propanol

$C_{18}H_{29}NO_3 = 307.4$

CAS—63659-18-7

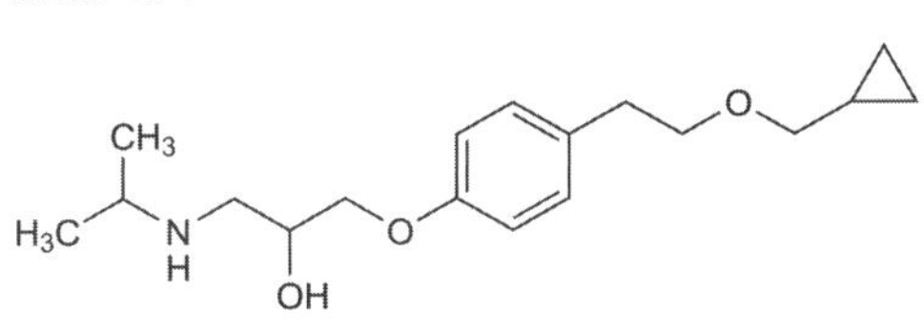

Crystals from petroleum ether. M.p. 70° to 72°.

Betaxolol Hydrochloride

Synonyms. SLD-212; SL-75.212.

Proprietary names. Betoptic; Betoptima; Betoquin; Kerlon; Kerlone; Oxodal.

$C_{18}H_{29}NO_3,HCl = 343.9$

CAS—63659-19-8

A white or almost white crystalline powder. M.p. 113° to 117° . It is very soluble to freely soluble in water; freely soluble in chloroform, ethanol and methanol; soluble in dichloromethane; practically insoluble in ether.

Dissociation Constant. pK_a 9.4.

Partition Coefficient. Log *P* (octanol/water), 2.81.

Thin-layer Chromatography. System TB—Rf 11; system TE—Rf 51; system TF—Rf 00; system TAE—Rf 22.

Gas Chromatography. System GA—RI 2370 (betaxolol); RI 2410 (Art); RI 2400 (Art-H_2O); system GB—RI 2420 (betaxolol); RI 2508 (Art); RI 2519 (Art-H_2O).

Column: 5% phenyl-methyl silicone RTx-5 fused-silica capillary (30 m × 0.25 mm i.d.). Column temperature: 110°, held 1 min; increased to 170° at 20°/min; increased to 225°at 7°/min; 290° at 24°/min, held 10 min. Carrier gas: helium. MS detection. Retention time (relative to isoproteronol, internal standard): 1.32. [G. D. Branum *et al.*, *J. Anal. Toxicol.*, 1998, *22*, 135–141].

High Performance Liquid Chromatography. System HX—RI 386; system HY—RI 301; system HZ—3.8 min; system HAA—retention time 13.4 min.

Column: C_{18} (Ultrasphere, 75 × 4.5 mm i.d., 3 μm). Mobile phase: acetonitrile:0.05 M DMOA, pH 3:water (8:10:82), 1 mL/min. Fluorescence detection (λ_{ex}=200 nm). Retention times: betaxolol, 9.9 min; α-hydroxy-betaxolol, 2.3 min.

Column: C_{18} (Nova-Pak, 150 × 3.9 mm, 5 μm). Mobile phase: acetonitrile:glacial acetic acid:distilled water (29:1:70), 0.9 mL/min flow rate. Fluorescence detection (λ_{ex}=200 nm). Retention times: acid metabolites, 7.4 min. [Y. W. J. Wong and T. M. Ludden, *J. Chromatogr.*, 1990, *534*; *Biomed. Appl.*, *99*, 161–172].

Ultraviolet Spectrum. Ethanol—224, 280 nm.

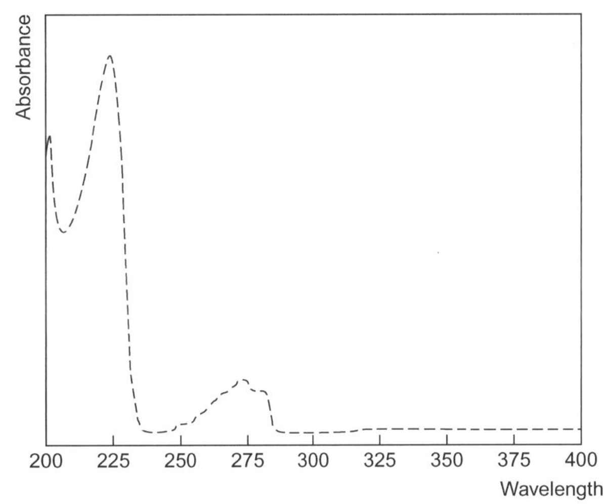

Infra-red Spectrum. Principal peaks at wavenumber 1515, 1249, 1091, 1053, 3250, 830 cm^{-1}.

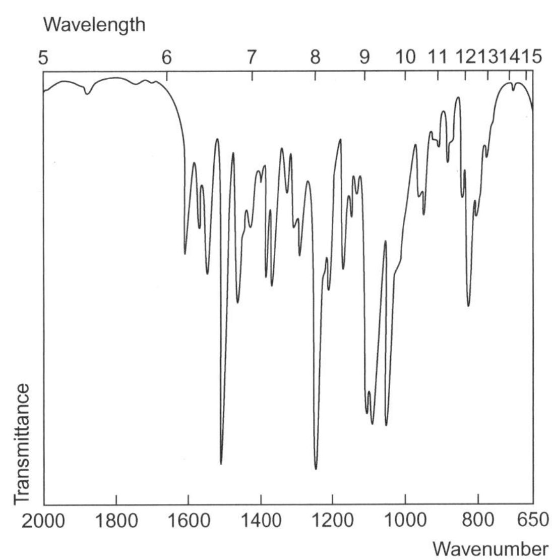

Mass Spectrum. Principal ions at *m/z* 72, 263, 292, 307, 55, 107, 192, 219

(betaxolol); m/z 55, 91, 316, 140, 125, 98, 43, 331 (betaxolol methaneboronate).

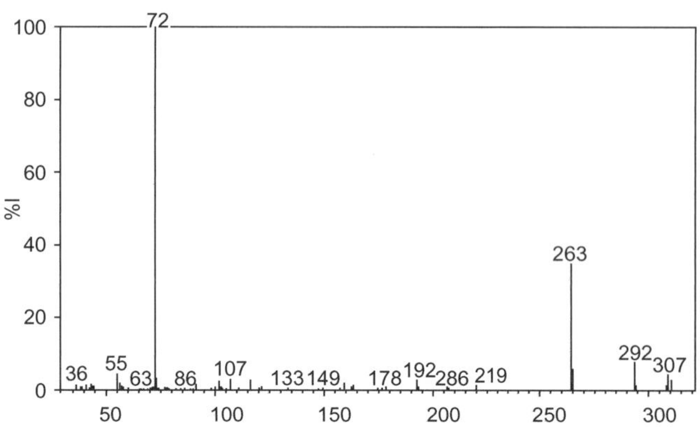

Quantification

Gas chromatography. In blood, urine, or tissues: limit of detection 0.5 µg/L—J. Ganansia *et al.*, *J. Chromatogr.*, 1983, *275*; *Biomed. Appl.*, *26*, 183–188.

High performance liquid chromatography. In blood or urine: limit of detection 5 µg/L, fluorescence detection (λ_{ex}=275 nm, λ_{em}=305 nm)—H. Caqueret and G. Bianchetti., *J. Chromatogr.*, 1984, *311*; *Biomed. Appl.*, *36*, 199–205. In plasma: limit of detection 4 µg/L, fluorescence detection (λ_{ex}=270 nm, λ_{em}=320 nm—M. Canal and B. Flouvat, *J. Chromatogr.*, 1985, *342*; *Biomed. Appl.*, *43*, 212–215. In blood: limit of detection 0.5 µg/L (separate enantiomers), fluorescence detection—A. Darmon and J. P. Thenot, *J. Chromatogr.*, 1986, *374*; *Biomed. Appl.*, *47*, 321–328. In plasma or serum: limit of detection 5 µg/L, fluorescence detection—R. K. Bhamra *et al.*, *J. Chromatogr.*, 1987, *417*; *Biomed. Appl.*, *61*, 229–232. In blood or urine: betaxolol and metabolites, limit of detection 1 to 5 µg/L and 5 to 20 µg/L, respectively, fluorescence detection—Y. W. J. Wong and T. M. Ludden, *J. Chromatogr.*, 1990, *534*; *Biomed. Appl.*, *99*, 161–172.

Disposition in the Body. Betaxolol is completely absorbed after oral administration. Administration with food does not affect the rate or extent of absorption. The primary route of elimination is hepatic metabolism and urinary excretion. About 15% of a dose is excreted in urine as the unchanged drug but the majority is oxidatively metabolised to inactive and weakly active metabolites, including α-hydroxybetaxolol. There are no active metabolites of clinical importance. It has high lipid solubility and crosses the placenta. It is distributed into breast milk where higher concentrations have been achieved than in maternal blood. It is not removed by dialysis.

Therapeutic concentration. The serum therapeutic concentration range is 5 to 50 µg/L.

6 healthy male and female volunteers, aged between 20 and 25 years, were administered with a 20-mg oral dose of betaxolol after a light breakfast and moderate exercise. The peak plasma concentrations were between 48 and 75 µg/L 2 to 4 h after administration. The drug could be measured up to 25 h after administration in all the subjects. [J. F. Giudicelli *et al.*, *Br. J. Clin. Pharmacol.*, 1980, *10*, 41–49].

Bioavailability. Oral, 80 to 90%.

Half-life. Plasma, 14 to 22 h.

Volume of distribution. 8 L/kg; reported as 4.9, 6.0 and 9.8 L/kg for single doses and 7.7 to 8.8 L/kg for repeated doses.

Clearance. Plasma, 0.28 L/h/kg.

Protein binding. In plasma, 55%.

Note. For a review of betaxolol see R. Beresford and R. C. Heel, *Drugs*, 1986, *31*, 6–28.

Dose. Usually 10 to 20 mg daily.

Bethanechol Chloride

Parasympathomimetic

Synonym. Carbamylmethylcholine Chloride
Proprietary names. Duvoid; Mechothane; Myotonachol; Myotonine Chloride; Urecholine; Urocarb; Vesicholine.
2-[(Aminocarbonyl)oxy]-*N*,*N*,*N*-trimethyl-1-propanaminium chloride
$C_7H_{17}ClN_2O_2$=196.7
CAS—674-38-4 (bethanechol); 590-63-6 (chloride)

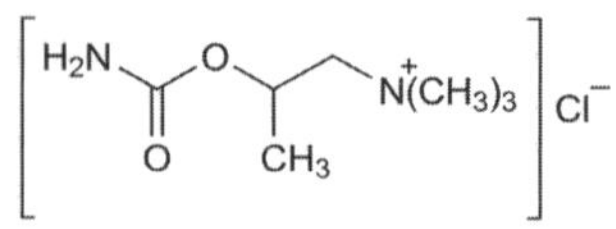

Colourless or white hygroscopic crystals, or white crystalline powder. There are two crystalline forms, one melts at about 211° and the other at about 219°.
Soluble 1 in 0.6 of water and 1 in 10 of ethanol, less soluble in dehydrated alcohol; practically insoluble in chloroform and ether.

Partition Coefficient. Log *P* (octanol/water), −3.4.

Thin-layer Chromatography. System TA—Rf 02. (Acidified iodoplatinate solution, positive.)

Ultraviolet Spectrum. No significant absorption, 230 to 360 nm.

Infra-red Spectrum. Principal peaks at wavenumbers 1712, 1014, 1300, 1062, 1094, 946 cm^{-1} (KBr disk).

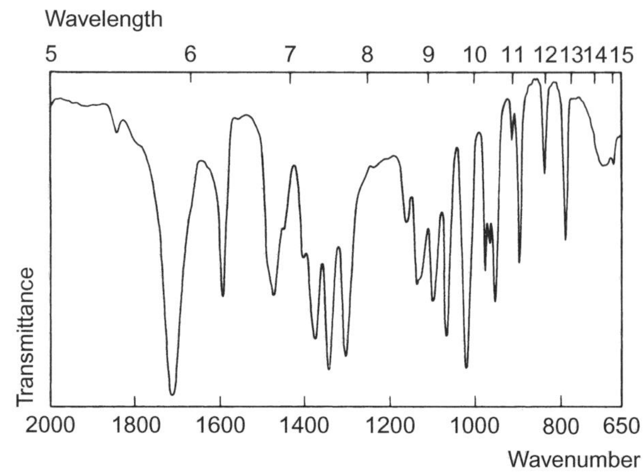

Mass Spectrum. Principal ions at m/z 43, 58, 42, 143, 85, 171, 157, 102.

Dose. 15 to 200 mg daily.

Bethanidine

Antihypertensive

Synonym. Betanidine
N,*N*′-Dimethyl-*N*″-(phenylmethyl)guanidine
$C_{10}H_{15}N_3$=177.2
CAS—55-73-2

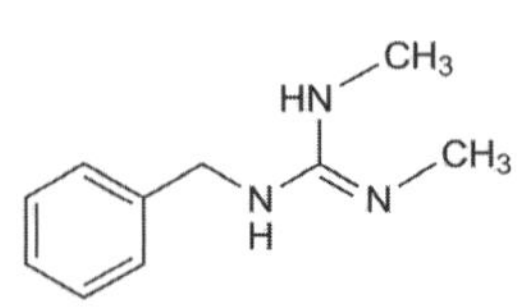

Crystals. M.p. 195° to 197°.

Bethanidine Sulfate

Proprietary names. Esbaloid; Esbatal; Regulin.
$(C_{10}H_{15}N_3)_2,H_2SO_4$=452.6
CAS—114-85-2
A white crystalline powder. M.p. about 280°.
Soluble 1 in 1 of water and 1 in 30 of ethanol; practically insoluble in ether.

Dissociation Constant. pK_a 12 (20°).

Partition Coefficient. Log *P* (octanol/water), 1.6.

Colour Tests. Liebermann's test—orange→brown; Marquis test—orange-red.

Thin-layer Chromatography. System TA—Rf 01; system TB—Rf 00; system TC—Rf 00. (Dragendorff spray, positive.)

Gas Chromatography. System GA—RI 1925.

Ultraviolet Spectrum. Aqueous acid—252, 258 (A_1^1=11a), 264 nm. No alkaline shift.

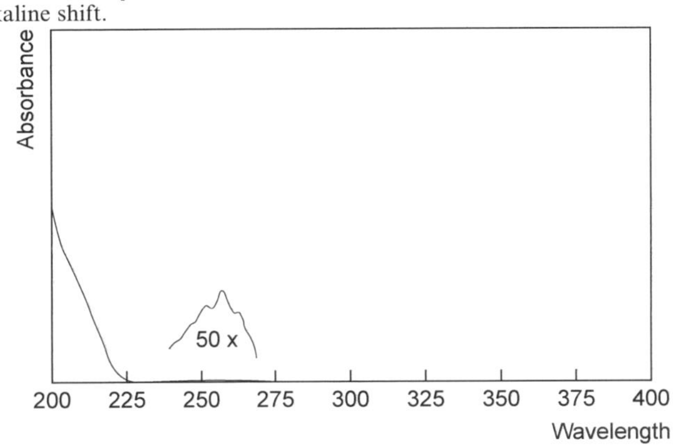

Infra-red Spectrum. Principal peaks at wavenumbers 1630, 1111, 1174, 701, 1192, 1066 cm^{-1} (bethanidine sulfate, KBr disk).

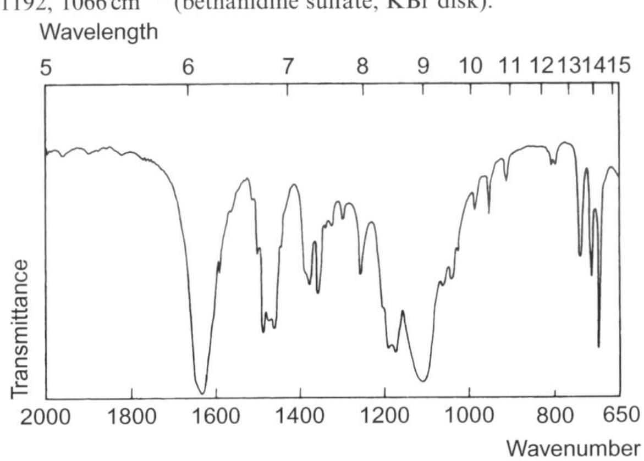

Mass Spectrum. Principal ions at *m/z* 71, 91, 106, 177, 57, 72, 65, 30.

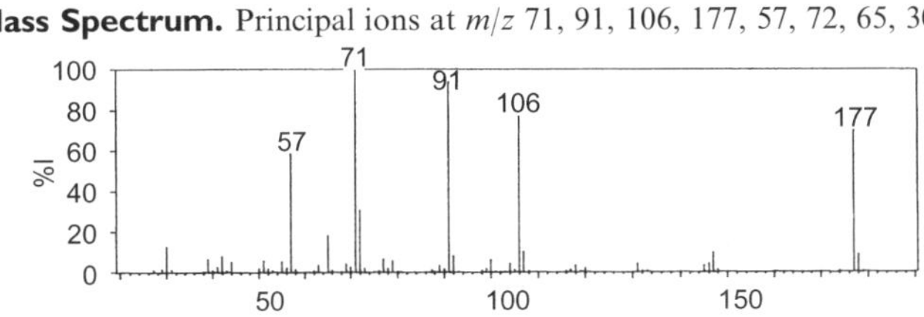

Quantification

Spectrofluorimetry. In plasma: limit of detection 4 µg/L—C. N. Corder *et al.*, *J. Pharm. Sci.*, 1975, *64*, 785–788.

Gas chromatography–mass spectrometry. In plasma or urine: guanethidine and other guanido-containing drugs, limit of detection 1 µg/L—J. H. Hengstmann *et al.*, *Anal. Chem.*, 1974, *46*, 34–39.

High performance liquid chromatography. In plasma: limit of detection 20 µg/L, UV detection—J. R. Shipe *et al.*, *Clin. Chem.*, 1983, *29*, 1793–1795.

Disposition in the Body. Bethanidine is readily but incompletely absorbed after oral administration. It does not appear to be metabolised. After an IV dose, about 90% is excreted unchanged in the urine in 3 to 4 days; after an oral dose, 50 to 85% is excreted in the urine and up to about 50% is eliminated in the faeces.

Therapeutic concentration. In plasma, usually in the range 0.02 to 0.5 mg/L.

After a single oral dose of 10 mg to 3 subjects, peak plasma concentrations of about 0.02 to 0.15 mg/L were attained in 2 h. [C. N. Corder *et al.*, *J. Pharm. Sci.*, 1975, *64*, 785–788].

After daily oral administration of 30 to 150 mg in divided doses to 12 subjects, steady-state plasma concentrations of 0.02 to 0.5 (mean 0.12) mg/L were reported. [C. N. Corder *et al.*, *J. Clin. Pharmacol.*, 1978, *18*, 249–258].

Half-life. The plasma half-life is multiphasic and there is considerable intersubject variation; after intravenous administration, plasma half-lives of about 2 to 6 h and terminal half-lives of several days have been reported.

Protein binding. In plasma, not significantly bound.

Dose. 20 to 200 mg of bethanidine sulfate daily.

Bevantolol

Beta-blocker

1-[[2-(3,4-Dimethoxyphenyl)ethyl]-amino]-3-(3-methylphenoxy)-2-propanol
$C_{20}H_{27}NO_4$=345.4
CAS—59170-23-9

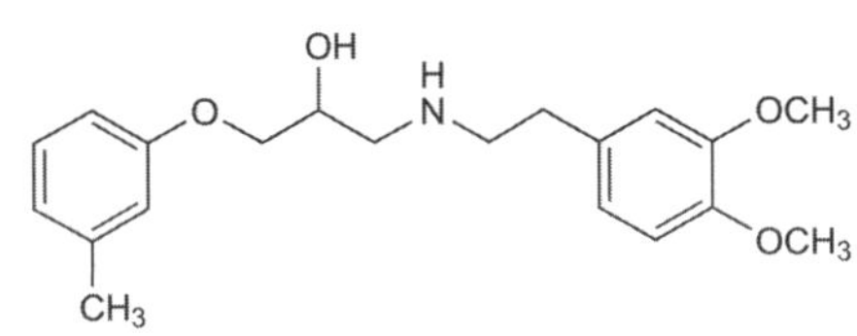

Bevantolol Hydrochloride
Synonyms. CI-775; NC-1400.
Proprietary names. Ranestol; Sentiloc; Vantol.
$C_{20}H_{28}ClNO_4$=381.9
CAS—42864-78-8
M.p. 137° to 138°. Water solubility is 184.3 mg/L at 25°.

Dissociation Constant. pK_a 8.1.

Partition Coefficient. Log *P* (octanol/water), 3.0; (pH 7), 13.0.

High Performance Liquid Chromatography. System HZ—retention time 4.2 min.

Column: LC-CN (Supelcosil, 5 µm, 250 × 4.6 mm i.d.). Mobile phase: ammonium acetate buffer (0.01 M, pH 3.5):acetonitrile:methanol (70:20:10), 1.0 mL/min flow rate. UV detection (λ=205 nm). Retention time: 9.6 min. [A. Selen *et al.*, *Eur. J. Clin. Pharmacol.*, 1986, *30*, 699–704].

Column: ODS-2 (Spherisorb, 5 µm). Mobile phase: phosphate buffer (0.5 M, pH 3.5):acetonitrile:methanol (50:30:20). Fluorescence detection. Retention time: 3.0 min. [S. Nattel *et al.*, *J. Clin. Pharmacol.*, 1987, *27*, 962–966].

Column: Partisil RAC II (5 µm, 100 × 4.6 mm). Mobile phase: dibasic ammonium phosphate buffer (75 mM, adjusted to pH 3.5 with phosphoric acid):acetonitrile (50:50), 2.0 mL/min flow rate. UV detection (λ=220 nm). Retention time: (+)-bevantolol, 7.4 min; (–)-bevantolol, 6.4 min. [S. E. Rose and E. J. Randinitis, *Pharm. Res.*, 1991, *8(6)*, 758–762].

Quantification

High performance liquid chromatography. In plasma: limit of detection is 0.026 mg/L. UV detection (λ=205 nm)—A. Selen *et al.*, *Eur. J. Clin. Pharmacol.*, 1986, *30*, 699–704. In plasma: limit of detection 0.05 mg/L. Fluorescence detection—S. Nattel *et al.*, *J. Clin. Pharmacol.*, 1987, *27*, 962–966.

Disposition in the Body. Bevantolol is virtually completely absorbed (>85%) and undergoes moderate first pass metabolism. It is extensively metabolised to 4 metabolites; the principal metabolite makes up 16% of the dose and 3 minor metabolites in trace amounts. It is excreted in urine (72%) mostly as metabolites and small amounts of the unchanged drug (<10%). It is also excreted in faeces (approx. 12%).

Therapeutic concentration

12 healthy volunteers (11 women and 1 man) with a mean age of 37 years, were administered with a single 100-mg dose of bevantolol in a fasting

state, 15 min before a meal or after a meal. The mean peak plasma concentrations observed were 1.05, 1.06 and 0.92 mg/L, respectively, and these levels were reached at approximately 1.0, 0.9 and 1.8 h. [R. D. Toothaker *et al.*, *J. Clin. Pharmacol.*, 1987, *27*, 297–299].

Bioavailability. 60%.

Half-life. 1.5 to 2 h.

Volume of distribution. Approximately, 1.5 L/kg.

Protein binding. 95 to 98% bound especially to plasma glycoproteins.

Dose. The usual dose of 150 to 400 mg is administered daily.

Bezafibrate

Lipid-regulating Agent

Synonym. BM-15075
Proprietary names. Bezalip; Cedur.
2-[4-[2-[(4-Chlorobenzoyl)amino]ethyl]phenoxy]-2-methylpropanoic acid
$C_{19}H_{20}ClNO_4$=361.8
CAS—41859-67-0

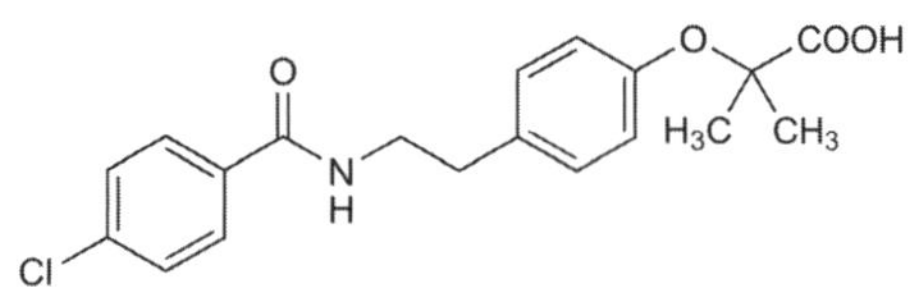

An off-white crystalline powder. M.p. 183° to 186°.
Practically insoluble in water; slightly soluble in ethanol, acetone, and methanol; soluble in dimethylformamide.

Partition Coefficient. Log *P* (octanol/water), 4.2.

Thin-layer Chromatography. System TF—Rf 00; system TAE—Rf 89.

Gas Chromatography. System GA—RI 3100.

High Performance Liquid Chromatography. System HX—RI 513; system HAA—retention time 18.3 min.

Ultraviolet Spectrum. Methanol—230 nm (A_1^1=644b).

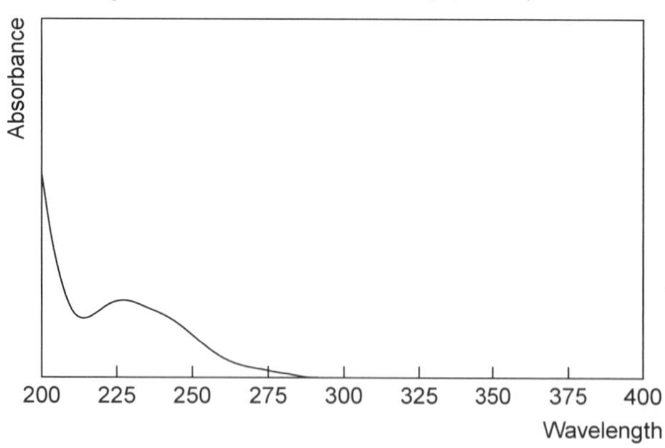

Infra-red Spectrum. Principal peaks at wavenumbers 1715, 1540, 1610, 1140, 1500, 1220 cm^{-1} (KBr disk).

Quantification

High performance liquid chromatography. In plasma: limit of quantification 0.25 mg/L, UV detection (λ=232 nm)—L. D. Masnatta *et al.*, *J. Chromatogr. B Biomed. Sci. Appl.*, 1996, *687(2)*, 437–442.

Dose. 400 to 600 mg daily.

Bezitramide

Narcotic Analgesic

Synonyms. Benzitramide; R-4845.
Proprietary name. Burgodin
1-[1-(3-Cyano-3,3-diphenylpropyl)-4-piperidinyl]-1,3-dihydro-3-(1-oxopropyl)-2*H*-benzimidazol-2-one
$C_{31}H_{32}N_4O_2$=492.6
CAS—15301-48-1

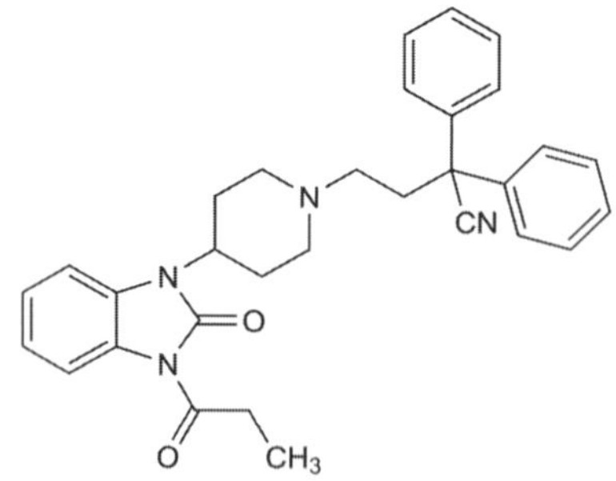

A white, amorphous or crystalline powder. M.p. 145° to 149°.
Practically insoluble in water and ethanol; soluble 1 in 45 of acetone, 1 in 2 of chloroform, and 1 in 400 of ether.

Partition Coefficient. Log *P* (octanol/water), 4.8.

Colour Test. Mandelin's Test—violet→orange.

Thin-layer Chromatography. System TA—Rf 71; system TB—Rf 41; system TC—Rf 79; system TL—Rf 70; system TAE—Rf 92; system TAF—Rf 96. (Acidified iodoplatinate solution, positive.)

Gas Chromatography. System GA—not eluted.

High Performance Liquid Chromatography. System HA—*k* 0.2; system HX—RI 564; system HZ—retention time 22.5 min.

Ultraviolet Spectrum. After solution in chloroform and dilution with acid isopropyl alcohol—251 nm (A_1^1=118b), inflexion at 274 nm.

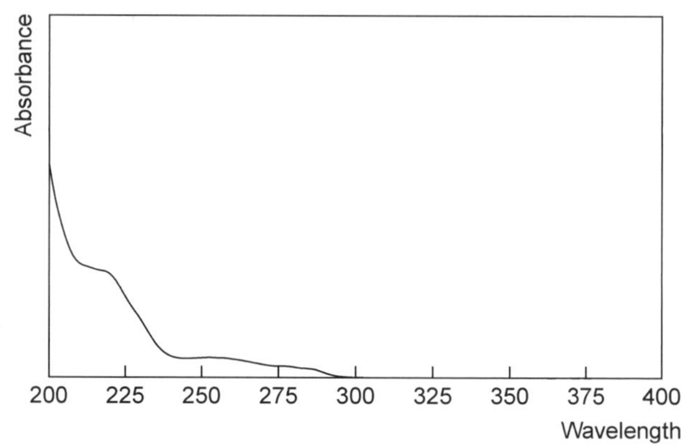

Infra-red Spectrum. Principal peaks at wavenumbers 1733, 755, 1708, 700, 1286, 1054 cm^{-1} (KBr disk).

Mass Spectrum. Principal ions at *m/z* 286, 300, 96, 42, 244, 230, 301, 82.

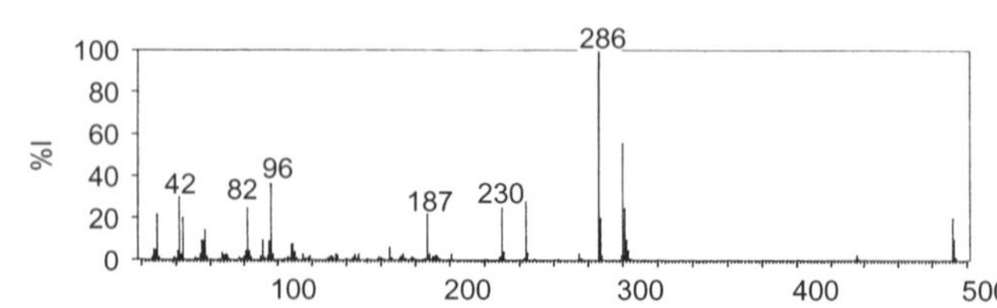

Quantification

Gas chromatography. In urine: 3-cyano-3,3-diphenylpropionic acid, limit of detection 600 µg/L, AFID—H. H. van Rooy *et al.*, *J. Chromatogr.*, 1978, *148*, 447–452. In urine: limit of quantification 10 µg/L acidic metabolite, NPD—S. M. De Baere *et al.*, *J. Anal. Toxicol.*, 1996, *20(3)*, 159–164. In urine: limit of quantification 10 µg/L, NPD—S. M. De Baere *et al.*, *J. Anal. Toxicol.*, 1998, *22(1)*, 18–26.

High performance liquid chromatography. In urine: 1,3-dihydro-1-(piperidin-4-yl)benzimidazol-2-one, limit of detection 150 µg/L, UV detection—H. H. van Rooy and C. Soe-Agnie, *J. Chromatogr.*, 1978, *156*, 189–195. In blood and urine: limit of detection 1 µg/L, fluorescence detection—S. M. De Baere *et al.*, *Anal. Chem.*, 1997, *69(24)*, 5186–5192. In blood, urine, stomach contents, bile, liver, and kidney—S. M. De Baere *et al.*, *Anal. Chem.*, 1999, *71(14)*, 2908–2914.

Disposition in the Body. Absorbed after oral administration. It is metabolised by hydrolysis to 3-cyano-3,3-diphenylpropionic acid and 1,3-dihydro-1-(piperidin-4-yl)benzimidazol-2-one which are excreted in the urine.

Therapeutic concentration

Following a single oral dose of 5 mg to 7 subjects, peak plasma concentrations (bezitramide plus major metabolite) of about 5 µg/L were attained in about 3 h; in 3 of the subjects, plasma concentrations remained fairly constant over a period of 7 h; in a further 2 subjects, distinct secondary peak plasma concentrations were observed. [D. K. F. Meijer *et al.*, *Eur. J. Clin. Pharmacol.*, 1984, *27*, 615–618.]

Dose. Bezitramide has been given in doses of 5 mg; maximum of 30 mg in 24 h.

Bialamicol

Anti-amoebic

Synonyms. Biallylamicol; Biethylamicol.
3,3′-Bis[(diethylamino)methyl]-5,5′-di-2-propenyl-[1,1′-biphenyl]-4,4′-diol
$C_{28}H_{40}N_2O_2$=436.6
CAS—493-75-4

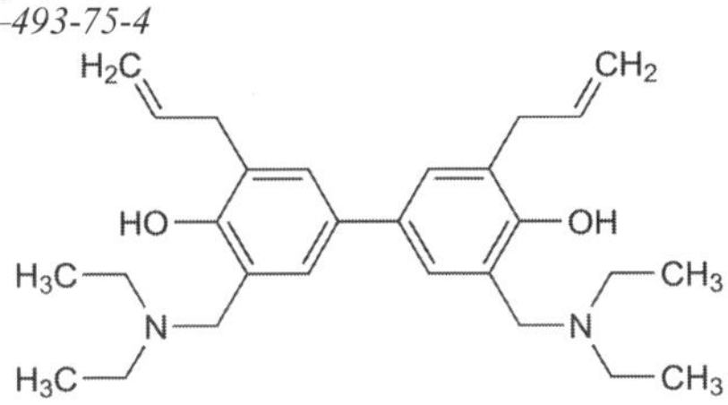

Bialamicol Hydrochloride
Proprietary name. Camoform
$C_{28}H_{40}N_2O_2$,2HCl=509.6
CAS—3624-96-2
A white crystalline powder. M.p. 209° to 210°.
Soluble 1 in 5 of water, 1 in 40 of ethanol and 1 in 150 of chloroform; slightly soluble in ether.

Partition Coefficient. Log *P* (octanol/water), 7.0.

Colour Tests. Folin–Ciocalteu reagent—blue; Liebermann's test—green. Dissolve 100 mg in 2 mL of water and add 2 mL of nitric acid—intense orange-red.

Thin-layer Chromatography. System TA—Rf 74; system TB—Rf 62; system TC—Rf 80; system TL—Rf 73.

Ultraviolet Spectrum. Aqueous acid—266 nm (A^1_1=440a).

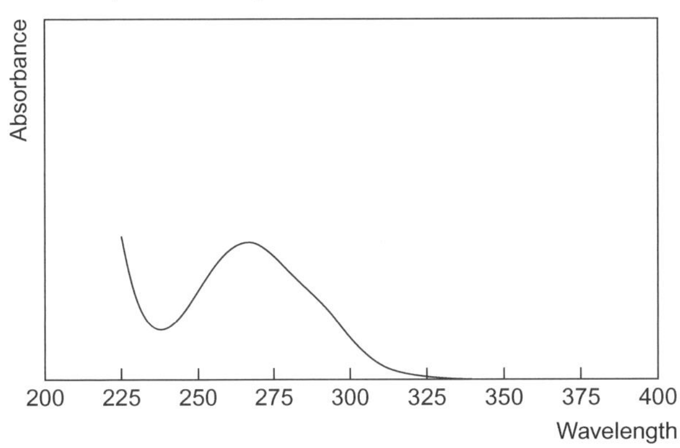

Mass Spectrum. Principal ions at *m/z* 58, 30, 363, 44, 72, 29, 27, 364.

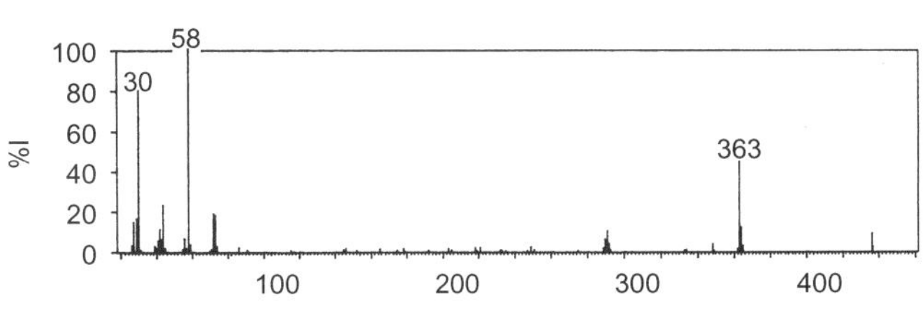

Disposition in the Body. Bialamicol is rapidly absorbed from the gastro-intestinal tract and stored in high concentrations in the liver, lungs and tissues. Slowly excreted in the bile and eliminated in the faeces.

Dose. Bialamicol hydrochloride has been given in doses of 0.75 to 1.5 g daily.

Bibenzonium Bromide

Antitussive

Synonym. Diphenetholine Bromide
Proprietary name. Lysobex, Medipectol, Thoragol.
2-(1,2-Diphenylethoxy)-*N*,*N*,*N*-trimethylethanaminium bromide
$C_{19}H_{26}BrNO$=364.3
CAS—59866-76-1 (bibenzonium); 15585-70-3 (bromide)

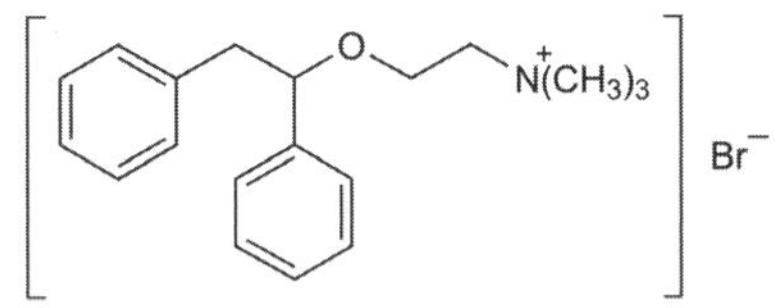

Crystals. M.p. 142° to 144°.
Very soluble in water and ethanol; practically insoluble in benzene and in ether.

Partition Coefficient. Log *P* (octanol/water), 0.6.

Colour Tests. The following tests are performed on bibenzonium nitrate (see Chapter 20): Mandelin's test—green; Marquis test—brown.

Thin-layer Chromatography. System TA—Rf 02. (Acidified iodoplatinate solution, positive.)

Gas Chromatography. System GA—RI 1923.

Ultraviolet Spectrum. Aqueous acid—253, 258 (A^1_1=11.4b), 264, 268 nm.

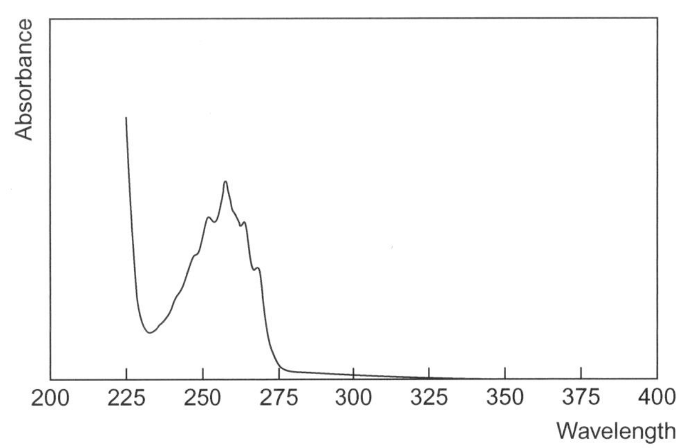

Infra-red Spectrum. Principal peaks at wavenumbers 705, 1095, 749, 759, 1020, 952 cm^{-1} (KBr disk).

Dose. 40 to 120 mg daily.

Bicalutamide

Anti-androgen/ Antineoplastic

Synonym. ICI-176334
Proprietary names. Casodex; Cosudex.
(*RS*)-*N*-[4-Cyano-3-(trifluoromethyl)phenyl]-3-[(4-fluorophenyl) sulfonyl]-2-hydroxy-2-methylpropanamide
$C_{18}H_{14}F_4N_2O_4S$=430.4
CAS—90357-06-5

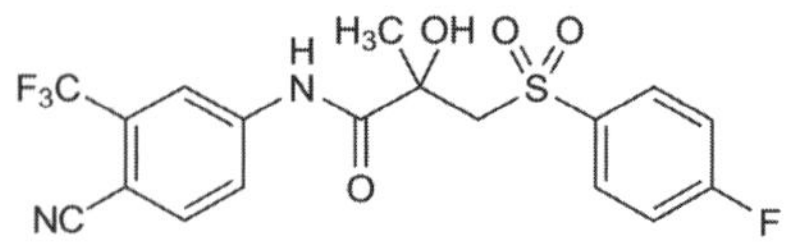

A fine white to off-white powder. M.p. 191° to 193°. It is practically insoluble in water (solubility in aqueous solution is 5 mg/L); slightly soluble in chloroform and anhydrous ethanol; sparingly soluble in methanol; soluble in acetone and in tetrahydrofuran.

Dissociation Constant. pK_a12.

Ultraviolet Spectrum. Aqueous acid (pH 4.0)—217, 272 nm.

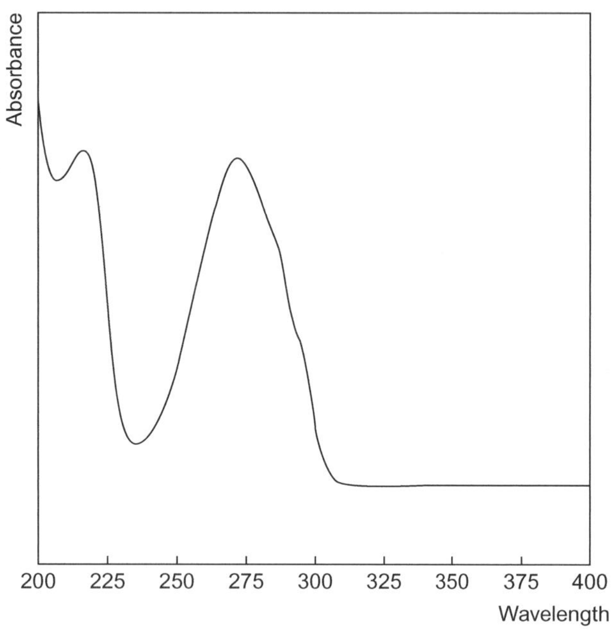

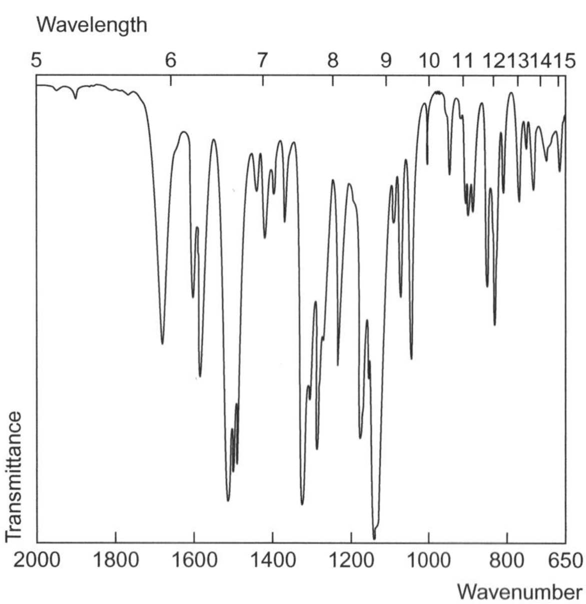

Mass Spectrum. Principal peaks at *m/z* 217, 159, 95, 43, 186, 143, 160, 218.

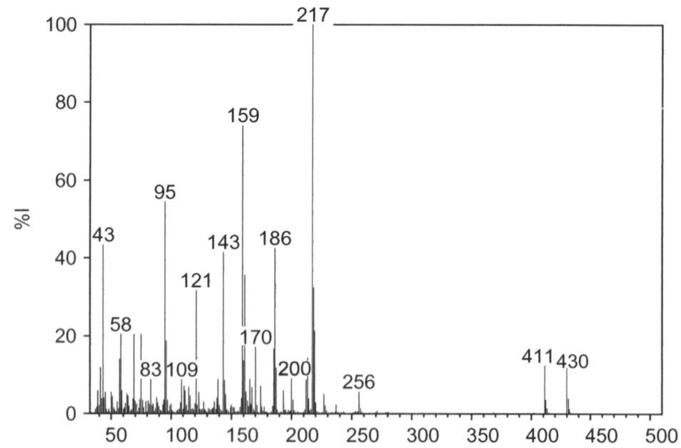

Quantification

High performance liquid chromatography. In plasma: limit of detection is 5 µg/L for (*R*)-bicalutamide and 3.8 µg/L for (*S*)-bicalutamide—I. D. Cockshott *et al.*, *Biopharm. Drug Dispos.*, 1997, *18(6)*, 499–507. In plasma: limit of quantification 7.9 µg/L for (*R*)-bicalutamide and 7.6 µg/L for (*S*)-bicalutamide. UV detection (λ=270 nm)—D. McKillop *et al.*, *Xenobiotica*, 1993, *23(11)*, 1241–1253.

Disposition in the Body. Bicalutamide is extensively absorbed after oral administration and undergoes extensive metabolism in the liver; the active *R*-enantiomer is metabolised predominantly by oxidation, the inactive *S*-enantiomer primarily by glucuronidation. The drug is rapidly cleared and the metabolites are excreted in approximately equal amounts in urine and faeces. Approximately half of an administered dose is excreted in urine as the glucuronide conjugates of the drug and its metabolite, hydroxy-bicalutamide. The remainder is detected in faeces as the drug and metabolite. Bicalutamide is not removed in significant amounts by dialysis.

Therapeutic concentration

15 healthy males, aged 36 to 54 years (mean, 44 years), were administered with a 50 mg single dose after an overnight fast and a standard high-fat cooked breakfast. The mean peak plasma (*R*)-enantiomer concentrations were 836 µg/L for those administered the drug with food and 734 µg/L for those in the fasting state. These concentrations were observed at 15.8 and 23.4 h, respectively. For the (*S*)-enantiomer, the peak concentrations were 100.2 µg/L at 20.8 h for the fed individuals and 84 µg/L for those who were being fasted, observed at 20.7 h. [I. D. Cockshott *et al.*, *Biopharm. Drug Dispos.*, 1997, *18(6)*, 499–507].

Toxicity. Hepatic failure has occurred rarely and consideration should be given to periodic liver function monitoring.

Half-life. Plasma, *R*-enantiomer, 5.8 days to 1 week; the *S*-enantiomer is cleared more rapidly.

Clearance. Plasma, 0.32 L/h (*R*-enantiomer).

Protein binding. In plasma, racemate, 96%; *R*-enantiomer, >99%.

Note. For a review of the pharmacokinetics of bicalutamide see C. Mahler *et al.*, *Clin. Pharmacokinet.*, 1998, *34*, 405–417.

Dose. Up to 150 mg daily.

Biperiden

Anticholinergic

Proprietary name. Roloken

α-Bicyclo[2.2.1]hept-5-en-2-yl-α-phenyl-1-piperidinepropanol

$C_{21}H_{29}NO$=311.5

CAS—514-65-8

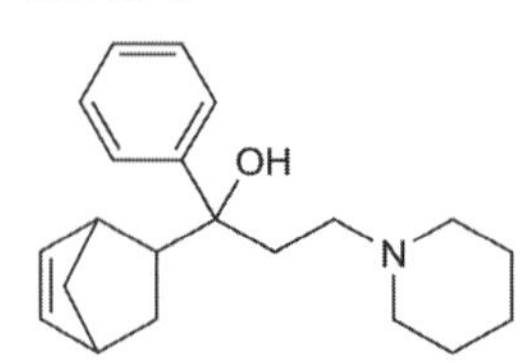

A white crystalline powder. M.p. 101°.

Practically insoluble in water; slightly soluble in ethanol; readily soluble in methanol.

Biperiden Hydrochloride
Proprietary names. Akineton (tablets); Akinophyl; Dekinet; Ipsatol; Norakin N.
$C_{21}H_{29}NO,HCl=347.9$
CAS—1235-82-1
A white crystalline powder. M.p. 238°.
Slightly soluble in water, ethanol, chloroform, and ether; sparingly soluble in methanol.

Biperiden Lactate
Proprietary names. Akineton (injection); Dekinet; Ipsatol.
$C_{21}H_{29}NO,C_3H_6O_3=401.5$
CAS—7085-45-2

Partition Coefficient. Log *P* (octanol/water), 4.25.

Colour Tests. Liebermann's Test—brown; Marquis Test—red-brown; Sulfuric Acid—orange-brown.

Thin-layer Chromatography. System TA—Rf 64; system TB—Rf 68; system TC—Rf 64; system TE—Rf 83; system TL—Rf 64; system TAE—Rf 45; system TAJ—Rf 37; system TAK—Rf 12; system TAL—Rf 73. (Acidified iodoplatinate solution, positive.)

Gas Chromatography. System GA—biperiden RI 2276, M (OH-) RI 2645.

High Performance Liquid Chromatography. System HZ—retention time 6.4 min; system HAA—retention time 14.8 min.

Ultraviolet Spectrum. Aqueous acid—252, 259 ($A_1^1=5.6b$), 264 nm.

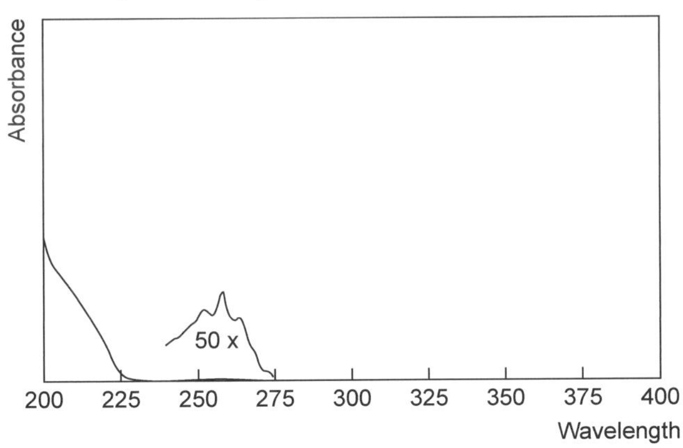

Infra-red Spectrum. Principal peaks at wavenumbers 702, 735, 1121, 997, 760, 1153 cm^{-1} (Nujol mull).

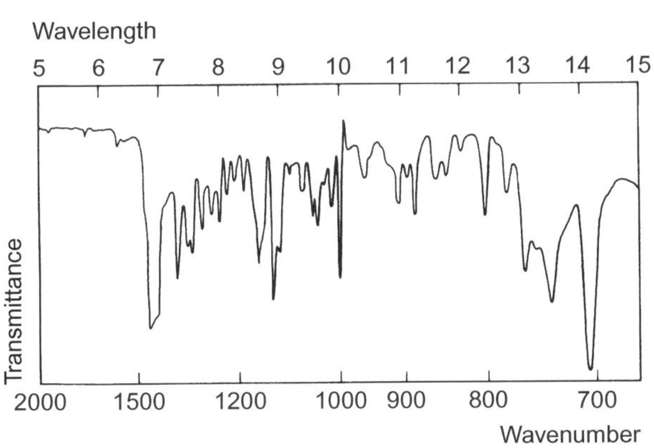

Mass Spectrum. Principal ions at *m/z* 98, 218, 99, 55, 41, 42, 77, 84.

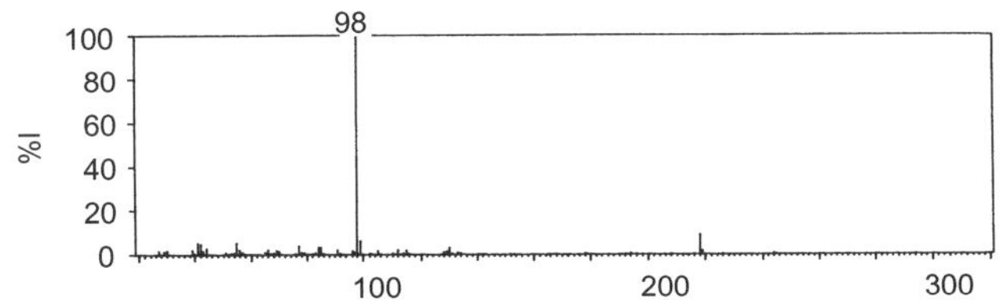

Quantification
Gas chromatography. In plasma: limit of quantification 250 ng/L, AFID—T. Le Bris and E. Brode, *Arzneimittelforschung*, 1985, *35*, 149–151.

Disposition in the Body. Rapidly absorbed after oral administration.

Therapeutic concentration
Following a single oral dose of 4 mg to 6 subjects, peak plasma concentrations of 4 to 6 µg/L were attained in 1.5 h. [M. Hollman *et al.*, *Eur. J. Clin. Pharmacol.*, 1984, *27*, 619–621.]

Toxicity. For a summary of fatalities caused by anticholinergics in Norway, see P. Gjerden *et al.*, *Tidsskr Nor Laegeforen*, 1998, *118*, 42–44.

Bioavailability. About 30%.

Half-life. Plasma half-life, about 18 h.

Clearance. 146 L/h (oral).

Dose. 2 to 12 mg of biperiden hydrochloride daily, by mouth. Biperiden lactate is given parenterally in doses of 5 to 20 mg daily.

Biriperone

Antipsychotic

Synonym. Centbutindole.
Proprietary names. Biriperona; biriperonum.
2-γ-[(*p*-Fluorobenzoyl)propyl]-1,2,3,4,6,7,12,12a-octahydropyrazino[2′,1′:6,1]pyrido[3,4-*b*]indole.
$C_{24}H_{26}FN_3O=381.49$
CAS—41510-23-0

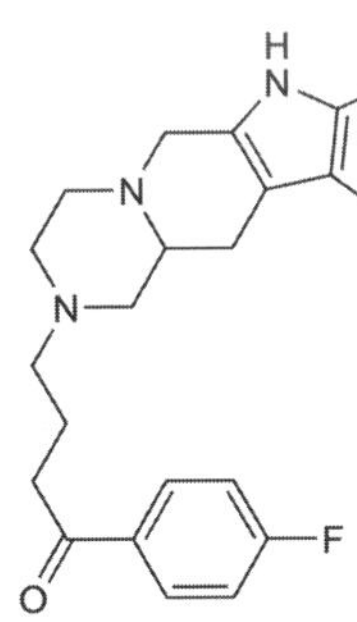

Biriperone is a faint yellow, odourless powder with m.p. 184° to 186°. It is soluble in methanol, ethanol, isopropanol, *n*-butanol, acetone and dilute acids; practically insoluble in *n*-hexane, cyclohexane, propylene glycol and glycerol.

Thin-layer Chromatography. Plate: Neutral alumina (20% gypsum) (6 g) on 5 × 20 cm plate. Mobile phase: Chloroform:methanol (99:1). Detection by exposure to iodine vapour or by spraying with Dragendorff reagent. Rf 48.
Plates: Silica gel GF_{254} (4G) on 10 × 20 cm plate. Mobile phase: Chloroform:methanol (19:1). Detection as above. Rf 25. [R. K. Seth and J. P. S. Sarin, *Indian J. Pharm. Sci.*, 1989, *51(6)*, 244–247].

High Performance Liquid Chromatography. Column: (Analytical) cyano (Nucleosil, 5 µm, 200 × 8 × 4 mm i.d.); Guard: cyano (40 µm, 5 × 4.6 mm). Mobile phase (pH 2.3): Acetonitrile:potassium dihydrogen phosphate (20 mM):orthophosphoric acid (0.3 mM) (20:70:10). 1.0 mL/min flow rate. UV detection (λ=220 nm). Retention time: 6.6 min. [J. K. Paliwal *et al.*, *Indian J. Pharm. Sci.*, 1990, *52(1)*, 22–25].

Column: Cyano (5 µm, 100 × 4.6 mm) with a pre-column (20 mm). Mobile phase: Acetonitrile:potassium dihydrogen phosphate (0.01 M) (60:40), adjusted to pH 3 with orthophosphoric acid. 1.0 mL/min flow rate. Fluorescence detection ($\lambda_{ex}=280$ nm, $\lambda_{em}=350$ nm). Retention time:

biriperone, 10 min and hydroxy-metabolite, 8.6 min. [J. K. Paliwal *et al.*, *J. Chromatogr.*, 1991, *572*, 219–225].

Column: cyano (100 × 4.6 mm i.d., 5 μm); preceded by a 20 mm pre-column. Mobile phase: acetonitrile:potassium dihydrogen phosphate (60:40). Fluorescence detection (λ_{ex}=280 nm, λ_{em}=350 nm). Retention time: 10 min. [J. K. Paliwal *et al.*, *Drug Invest.*, 1992, *4(3)*, 246–251].

Ultraviolet Spectrum. Aqueous acid (0.1 M HCl)—215, 250, 286 nm.

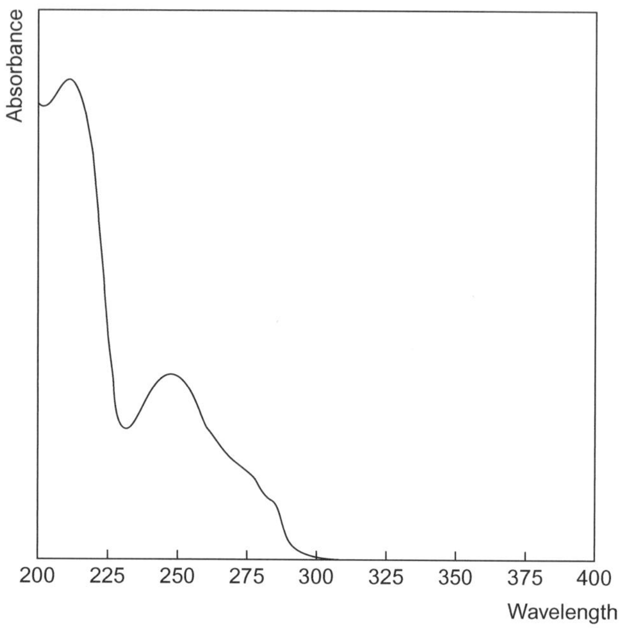

Infra-red Spectrum. Principal peaks at wavenumber 1170, 770, 1290, 1620, 1700, 2850 cm^{-1}.

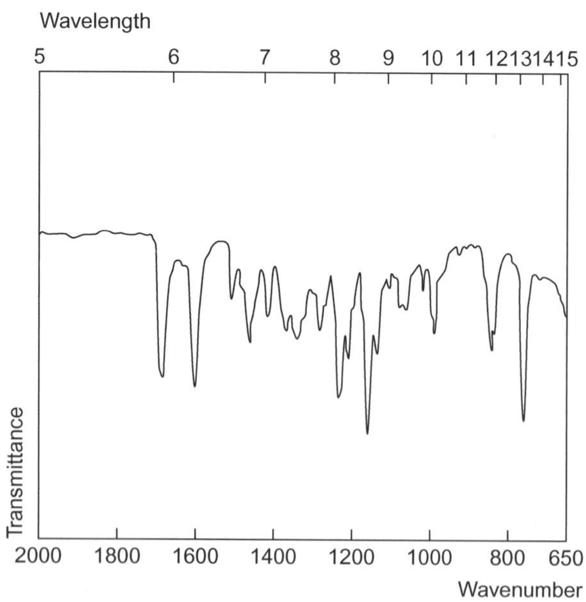

Quantification

High performance liquid chromatography. In serum: limit of detection 0.1 μg/L and 0.02 μg/L for biriperone and its hydroxy-metabolite, respectively, with lower limits of quantification 0.25 and 0.05 μg/L—J. K. Paliwal *et al.*, *J. Chromatogr. Biomed. Sci. Appl.*, 1991, *572*, 219–225.

Disposition in the Body. Large intersubject variation for absorption and bioavailability of biriperone has been observed and extensive tissue distribution has been shown. Biriperone is metabolised to its hydroxy-metabolite, 2-γ-[hydroxy-δ-(4-fluorophenyl)butyl]-1,2,3,4,6,7,12,12a-octahydropyrazino[2′,1′:6,1]pyrido[3,4-b]indole.

Therapeutic concentration

A single 3-mg oral dose of biriperone was administered to five healthy males aged between 24 and 36 years old. The mean peak serum level was 3.48 mg/L (range, 2.24 to 6.13 mg/L), which was achieved within 4.0 h (range, 1.41 to 5.87 h). [J. K. Paliwal *et al.*, *Drug Invest.*, 1992, *4(3)*, 246–251].

Half-life. The absorption half-life for biriperone varies between 0.23 and 2 h and the terminal phase elimination half-life is approximately 12.45 h.

Volume of distribution. 765 L.

Clearance. Systemic clearance is approximately 44.2 h (range between 23.4 and 64.1 h).

Bisacodyl

Purgative

Proprietary names. Bisacolax; Biscolax; Contlax; Deficol; Delco-Lax; Dulcolax; Laco; Laxbene; Perilax; Theralax; Toilax. It is an ingredient of Dulcodos.

4,4′-(2-Pyridylmethylene)bisphenol diacetate

$C_{22}H_{19}NO_4$=361.4

CAS—603-50-9

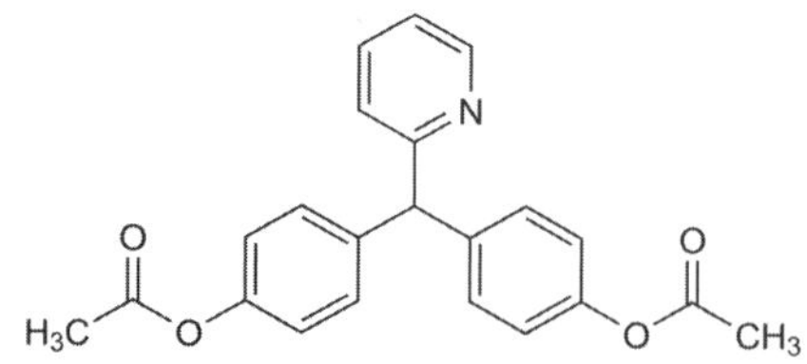

A white crystalline powder. M.p. 138°.

Practically insoluble in water and in alkaline solutions; soluble 1 in 100 of ethanol, 1 in 35 of chloroform, and 1 in 170 of ether; sparingly soluble in methanol; soluble in dilute acids, in acetone, and in propylene glycol.

Partition Coefficient. Log *P* (octanol/water), 3.4.

Colour Tests. Liebermann's Test—red-brown; Mandelin's Test—violet; Marquis Test—violet.

Thin-layer Chromatography. System TA—Rf 74; system TB—Rf 15; system TC—Rf 76; system TL—Rf 66; system TAE—Rf 82; system TAF—Rf 87. (Acidified iodoplatinate solution, positive.)

Gas Chromatography. System GA—bisacodyl RI 2818, M (bismethoxybisdesacetyl) RI 2820, M (bismethoxydesacetyl) RI 2890, M (desacetyl) RI 2750, M (bisdesacetyl) RI 2655, M (methoxybisdesacetyl) RI 2680, M (methoxydesacetyl) RI 2810; system GB—bisacodyl RI 2956, M (desacetyl) RI 2876, M (bisdesacetyl) RI 2793.

High Performance Liquid Chromatography. System HX—RI 531; system HY—RI 431; system HZ—retention time 9.6 min.

Ultraviolet Spectrum. Aqueous acid—264 (A^1_1=270a); methanolic potassium hydroxide—248 nm (A^1_1=650a).

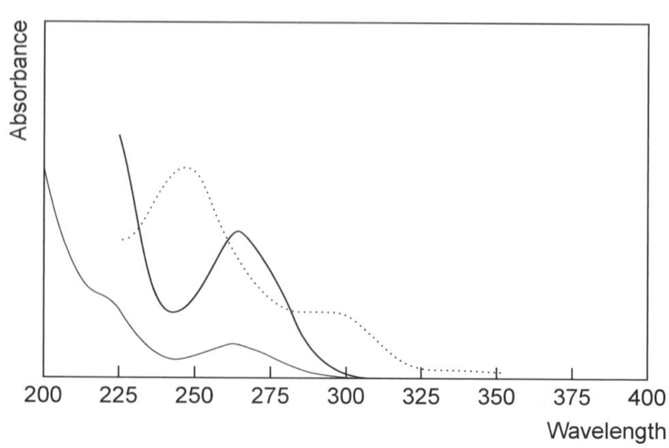

Infra-red Spectrum. Principal peaks at wavenumbers 1212, 1198, 1754, 1162, 1500, 909 cm^{-1} (KBr disk). (See below)

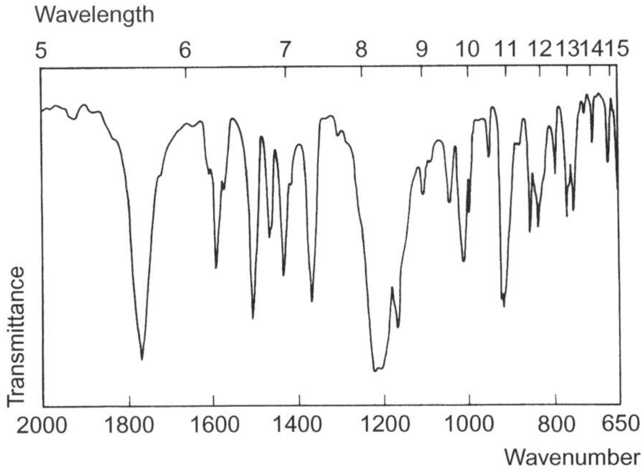

Mass Spectrum. Principal ions at *m/z* 361, 277, 319, 276, 199, 318, 362, 43.

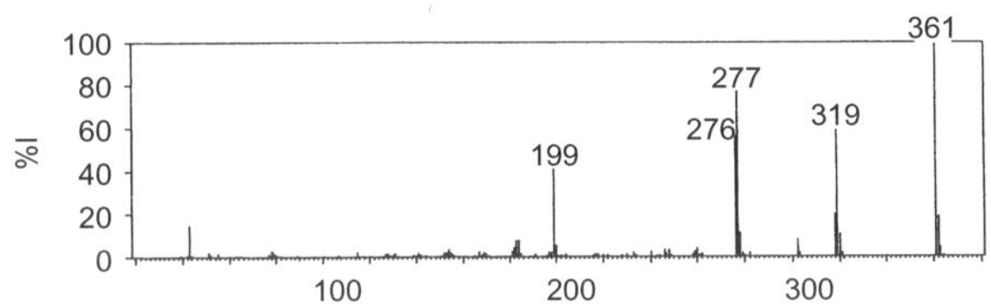

Quantification

Gas chromatography–mass spectrometry. In urine and serum: limit of detection 5 µg/L and 10 µg/L, respectively, SIM *m/z* 305—K. Kudo *et al.*, *J. Anal. Toxicol.*, 1998, *22(4)*, 274–278.

High performance liquid chromatography. In urine: bisacodyl diphenol, limit of detection 1 mg/L, UV detection—L. Loof *et al.*, *Ther. Drug Monit.*, 1980, *2*, 345–349. In urine—S. L. Perkins and J. F. Livesey, *Clin. Biochem.*, 1993, *26(3)*, 179–181.

Thin-layer chromatography–colorimetry. In urine: bisacodyl diphenol—R. Jauch *et al.*, *Arzneimittelforschung*, 1975, *25*, 1796–1800.

Disposition in the Body. Variably absorbed after oral administration and metabolised by deacetylation to the active metabolite, bis(4-hydroxyphenyl)-2-pyridylmethane (bisacodyl diphenol). Up to about 30% of a dose is excreted in the urine in 48 h as bisacodyl diphenol glucuronide; about 50% of a dose is eliminated in the faeces as unconjugated bisacodyl diphenol.

Dose. 5 to 10 mg daily.

Bisoprolol

Beta-blocker

Synonym. EMD-33512

1-[4-[[2-(1-Methylethoxy)ethoxy]methyl]phenoxy]-3-[(1-methylethyl) amino]-2-propanol

$C_{18}H_{31}NO_4$=325.5

CAS—66722-44-9

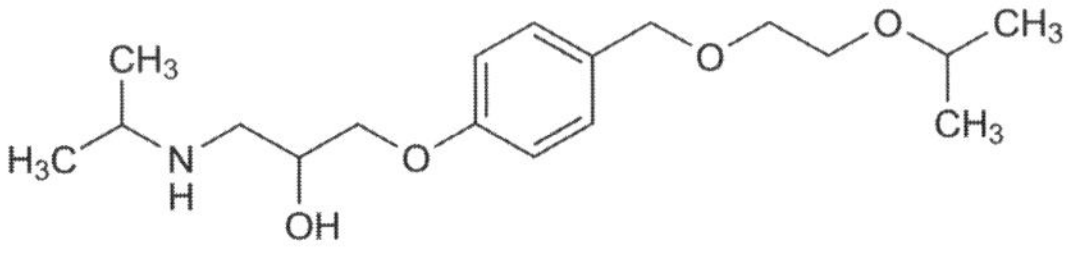

Bisoprolol Fumarate (hemifumerate)

Proprietary names. Bisobloc; Bisomerck; Concor; Cordalin; Detensiel; Emconcor; Emcor; Euradal; Fondril; Godal; Isoten; Monocor; Soprol; Zebeta.

$(C_{18}H_{31}NO_4)_2,C_4H_4O_4$=767.0

CAS—104344-23-2; 66722-45-0

A white crystalline powder. M.p. 100°. It is readily soluble in water, chloroform, ethanol and methanol.

Dissociation Constant. pK_a 9.57.

Partition Coefficient. Log *P* (octanol/water), 2.15; (dodecane/water), −0.24.

Thin-layer Chromatography. System TB—Rf 08; system TE—Rf 48; system TF—Rf 00; system TAE—Rf 22.

Gas Chromatography. System GA—RI 2378 (bisoprolol); RI 2595 (Art); RI 2400 (Art(-H_2O)); RI 1690 (M (phenol)); system GB—RI 2427 (bisoprolol); RI 2680 (Art); RI 2480 (Art(-H_2O)).

Column: 5% phenylmethyl silicone RTx-5 fused-silica capillary (30 m × 0.25 mm i.d.). Injector port: 250°, splitless conditions. Column temperature: 110°, held 1 min; increased to 170° at 20°/min; increased to 225° at 7°/min; 290° at 24°/min, held 10 min. Carrier gas: helium. MS detection. Retention time (relative to isoproteronol, internal standard): 1.31. [G. D. Branum *et al.*, *J. Anal. Toxicol.*, 1998, *22*, 135–141].

High Performance Liquid Chromatography. System HX—RI 358; system HZ—retention time 3.1 min; system HAA—retention time 12.3 min.

Column: (analytical) Chiralcel OD (250 × 4.6 mm i.d., 10 µm); (pre-column) Chiralcel OD (50 × 4.6 mm, 10 µm), at 25°. Mobile phase: hexane:2-propanol (10:0.9) containing 0.01% diethylamine, flow rate 0.5 mL/min. Fluorescence detection (λ_{ex}=228 nm, λ_{em}=298 nm). Retention times: *R*(+)-bisoprolol, 20 min; *S*(−)-bisoprolol, 30 min. [T. Suzuki *et al.*, *J. Chromatogr.*, 1993, *619*; *Biomed. Appl.*, *130*, 267–273].

Ultraviolet Spectrum. Aqueous acid (pH 4)—225, 273 nm.

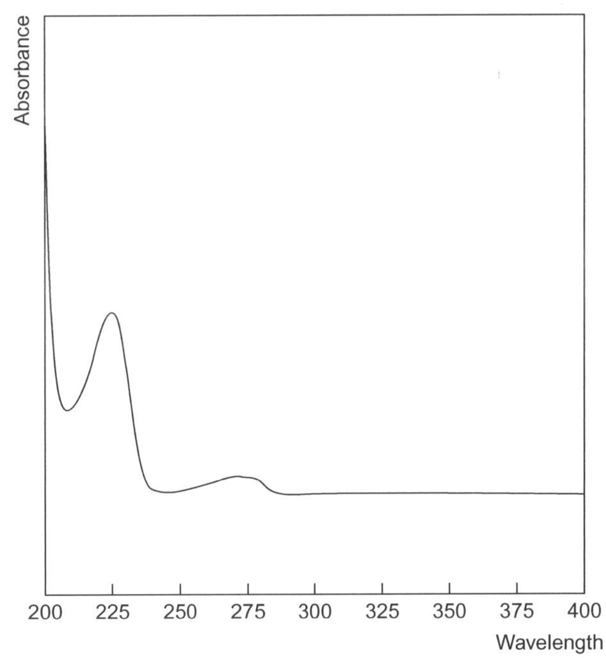

Mass Spectrum. Principal peaks at *m/z* 72, 116, 107, 100, 281, 73, 43, 325.

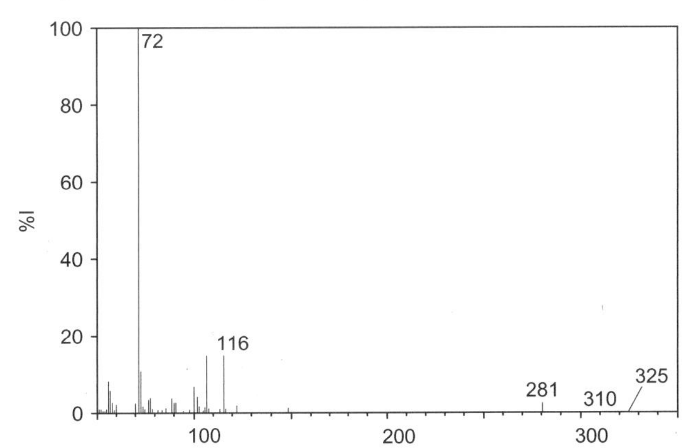

Quantification
High performance liquid chromatography. In plasma or urine: limit of detection 1 to 2 µg/L in plasma and 10 µg/L in urine, fluorescence detection—K. U. Bühring and A. Garbe, *J. Chromatogr.*, 1986, *382*; *Biomed. Appl.*, *55*, 215–224. In plasma or urine: limit of detection 1 µg/L in plasma and 10 µg/L in urine, fluorescence detection—J.-M. Poirier *et al.*, *J.Chromatogr.*, 1988, *426*; *Biomed. Appl.*, *70*, 431–437. In plasma or urine: limit of detection 2 µg/L in plasma for each enantiomer, fluorescence detection—T. Suzuki *et al.*, *J. Chromatogr.*, 1993, *619*; *Biomed. Appl.*, *130*, 267–273.

Disposition in the Body. Bisoprolol is almost completely absorbed after oral administration and undergoes only minimal first-pass metabolism. Peak plasma concentrations are reached 2 to 4 h after oral administration. It is moderately lipid-soluble and rapidly and widely distributed in the body. Approximately 50% of a dose is metabolised in the liver to pharmacologically inactive polar metabolites that are then excreted by the kidneys; the remaining 50% is excreted unchanged by the kidneys. Less than 2% of a dose is excreted in faeces.

Therapeutic concentration. The serum therapeutic concentration range is 0.01 to 0.06 mg/L.

Group 1: 8 healthy subjects (with a mean age of 23 years), group 2: 11 patients with impaired renal function (mean age, 59 years), group 3: 5 patients with acute hepatitis (mean age, 38 years) and group 4: 13 patients with liver cirrhosis (mean age, 52 years). Each group was administered with 10 mg bisoprolol daily for 7 days. The mean peak plasma concentrations were 52, 74, 54 and 62 µg/L for the groups, respectively, and the mean trough concentrations 11, 32, 19 and 22 µg/L. All peak concentrations were observed 1.7 to 3 h after administration. [W. Kirch *et al.*, *Clin. Pharmacokinet.*, 1987, *13*, 110–117].

Bioavailability. 90%.

Half-life. Plasma, 10 to 12 h; increased in patients with renal or liver impairment.

Volume of distribution. 2.9 L/kg for healthy individuals; 3.1 L/kg for patients with impaired renal function; 3.9 L/kg for patients with acute hepatitis; 2.9 L/kg for those with liver cirrhosis.

Clearance. Total, 14.2 L/h for healthy individuals; 7.8 L/h for patients with impaired renal function; 11.9 L/h for patients with acute hepatitis; 10.8 L/h for those with liver cirrhosis.

Protein binding. In plasma, 30 to 35%.

Note. For reviews of bisoprolol see S. G. Lancaster and E. M. Sorkin, *Drugs*, 1988, *36*, 256–285 and T. E. Johns and L. M. Lopez, *Ann. Pharmacother.*, 1995, *29*, 403–414.

Dose. Up to 20 mg of bisoprolol fumarate daily.

Bitoscanate

Anthelmintic

1,4-Di-isothiocyanatobenzene
$C_8H_4N_2S_2$ = 192.3
CAS-4044-65-9

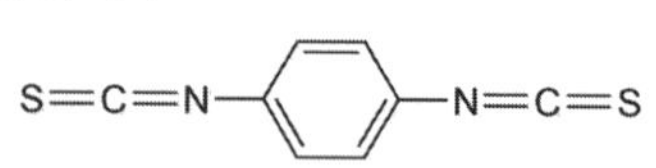

A yellowish-white crystalline powder. M.p. 130° to 132°.
Practically insoluble in water; soluble in ethanol, chloroform and ether.

Partition Coefficient. Log *P* (octanol/water) 4.7.

Colour Tests. Mandelin's Test—brown-violet; Palladium Chloride—orange.

Thin-layer Chromatography. System TA—Rf 65. (Acidified potassium permanganate solution, positive.)

Ultraviolet Spectrum. Ethanol—296, 311 nm (A_1^1 = 1795a).

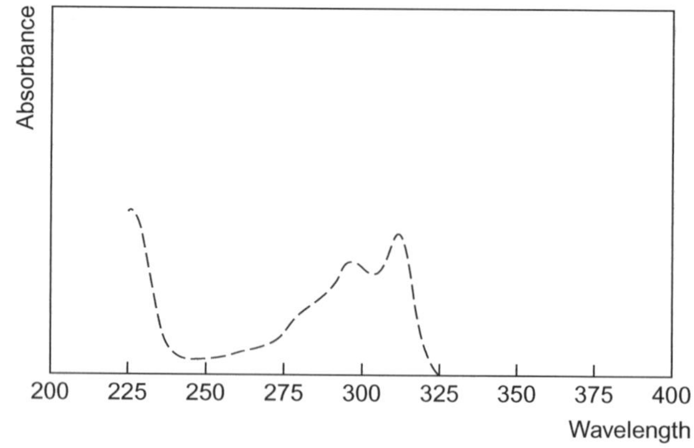

Disposition in the Body. Partly absorbed after oral administration. About 28% of a dose is excreted in the urine in 30 days and 55% is eliminated in the faeces, mainly in the first week.

Therapeutic concentration
Following a single oral dose of 100 mg of ^{14}C-labelled bitoscanate to 6 subjects, peak blood concentrations of total radioactivity equivalent to 0.58 to 2.1 mg/L (mean 1.4) of bitoscanate were reported at about 24 h [O. E. Christ *et al.*, *Arzneimittelforschung*, 1970, *20*, 756–762].

Half-life. Plasma half-life (total radioactivity), about 26 h.

Dose. 100 mg at 12-hourly intervals for 3 doses.

Bleomycin

Antineoplastic

Synonyms. NSC-125066; Bleo.
Bleomycins are a group of related glycopeptide antineoplastic antibiotics isolated from *Streptomyces verticillus*. The main component of bleomycin used clinically is bleomycin A_2 (*N*[1]-[3-(Dimethylsulfonio)propyl]bleomycinamide).
$C_{55}H_{84}N_{17}O_{21}S_3$ = 1415.6
CAS—11056-06-7

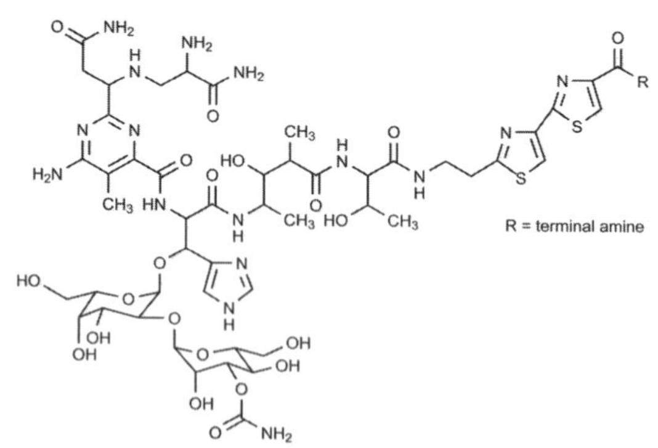

A colourless or yellowish powder which becomes blueish depending on copper content. It is very soluble in water and in methanol; slightly soluble in ethanol; practically insoluble in acetone, in ethyl acetate, in butyl acetate and in ether.

Bleomycin Sulfate
Proprietary names. Blenoxane; Bleo-S; Oil Bleo.
CAS—9041-93-4
A white or yellowish white or cream-coloured amorphous very hygroscopic powder. It is very soluble in water; slightly soluble in ethanol; practically insoluble in acetone and in ether.

Ultraviolet Spectrum. Aqueous acid (0.2 M H_2SO_4)—290 nm: basic—290 nm.

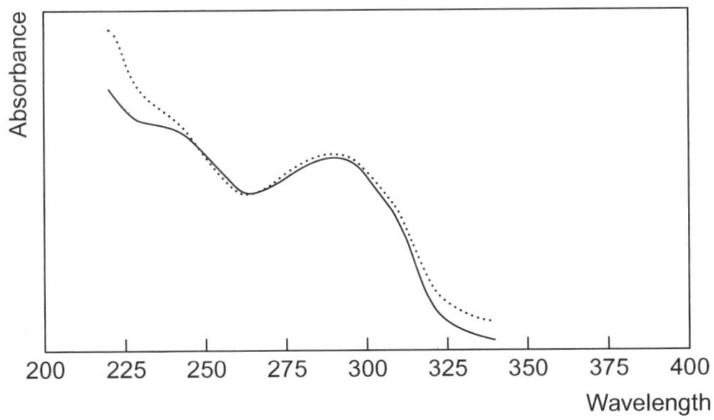

Infra-red Spectrum. Principal peaks at wavenumber 1653, 1548, 1118, 618 cm^{-1} (sulfate salt).

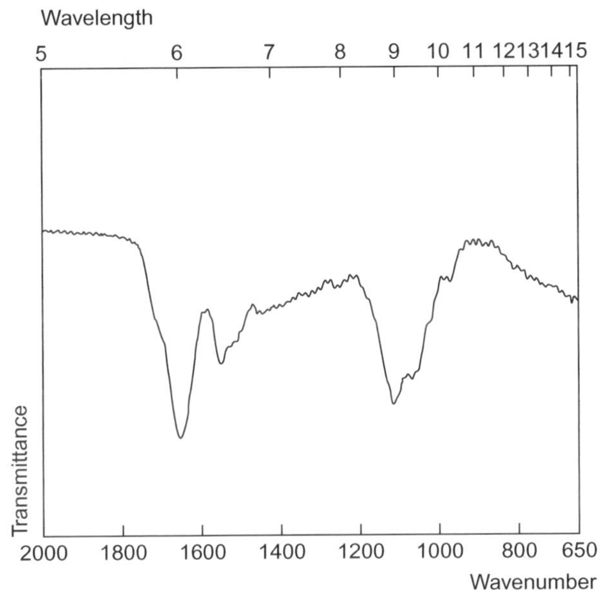

Quantification

High performance liquid chromatography. In plasma: limit of detection 0.5 mg/L, UV detection—G. K. Shiu *et al.*, *J. Pharm. Sci.*, 1979, *68*, 232–234.

Disposition in the Body. It is poorly absorbed after oral administration. After parenteral administration 60 to 70% is excreted in urine as the active drug. Most tissues, except skin and lung, can degrade bleomycin enzymically. About 45% of a dose is absorbed into the systemic circulation following intrapleural or intraperitoneal administration. It does not cross the blood–brain barrier.

Therapeutic concentration

Following intraperitoneal administration of 150 units of bleomycin in 2 L of peritoneal dialysis fluid to 3 subjects, mean peak peritoneal concentration at 15 min was 38 milli-units/L. The corresponding mean plasma concentration was 0.075 milli-units/L. [J. D. Bitran, *Cancer*, 1985, *56*, 2420–2423].

Toxicity. Pulmonary toxicity is the most serious adverse effect and is more likely in those given total cumulative doses greater than 400 units.

Half-life. Plasma, 2 to 4 h.

Volume of distribution. 0.35 to 0.45 L/kg.

Clearance. Plasma, 119 to 128 mL/min/m^2.

Protein binding. In plasma, 1%.

Note. For review of bleomycin, see R. T. Dorr, *Semin. Oncol.*, 1992, *19*, *Suppl. 5*, 3–8.

Dose. Usually 15 to 60 units weekly intravenously. The maximum total cumulative dose is 400 or 500 units.

Boldenone

Anabolic Steroid

Synonym. Dehydrotestosterone

(17β)-17-Hydroxyandrosta-1,4-dien-3-one

$C_{19}H_{26}O_2$=286.4

CAS—846-48-0

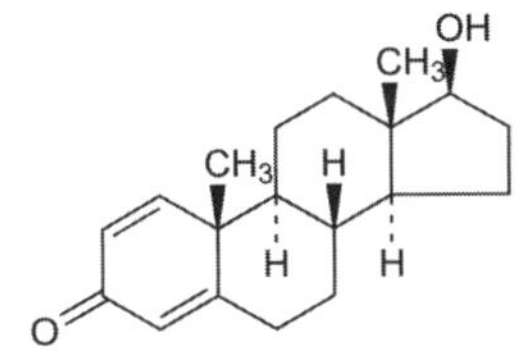

Crystals. M.p. 164° to 166°.

Boldenone Acetate

$C_{21}H_{28}O_3$=328.5

Crystals. M.p. 151° to 153°.

Boldenone Benzoate

$C_{26}H_{30}O_5$=422.5

Boldenone Undecylenate

Synonyms. Ba-29038; 10-Undecenoate.

Proprietary names. Parenabol; Vebonol.

$C_{30}H_{44}O_3$=452.7

CAS—13103-34-9

Partition Coefficient. Log *P* (octanol/water), 3.05.

Thin-layer chromatography. System TA—Rf 98; system TE—Rf 98; system TAJ—Rf 90; system TAK—Rf 88; system TAL—Rf 98; system TAM—Rf 99.

Gas Chromatography. System GAG—boldenone RRT 1.05, boldenone undecylenate RRT 2.62 (both relative to testosterone); system GAI—boldenone RRT 0.961, 5β-androst-1-en-17β-ol-3-one metabolite RRT 0.96 (both relative to 17α-methyl-5α-androstan-3β, 17β-diol); system GAR—retention time: boldenone 12.8 min, boldenone acetate 13.6 min, boldenone benzoate 18.7 min, boldenone undecylenate 22.4 min.

Column: 5% phenylmethylpolysiloxane (Ultra-2, 30 m × 0.2 mm i.d., 0.33 μm film thickness), cross-linked capillary. Column temperature: 150° held for 2 min, step rate of 20°/min to 300°, held for 2 min. MS detection negative chemical ionisation (NCI): Internal standard: 1,2-d_2-testosterone. Retention time: boldenone metabolite, 9.17 min. [Man Ho Choi *et al.*, *Rapid Commun. Mass Spectrom.*, 1998, 12, 1749–1755.]

Column: silica (SE54, cross-linked 5% phenyl, 1% vinyl methyl silicone, 17 m × 0.2 mm i.d., 0.33 μm film thickness). Carrier gas: helium, 1 mL/min flow rate. Split 1:10. MS detection (EI), SIM. Internal standard: 5α-androstane-3,17-dione,bis-TMS. RI: boldenone (TMS derivative) 2685.

Column: silica (OV1, cross-linked methyl silicone, 20 m × 0.25 mm i.d., 0.33 μm film thickness). Carrier gas: helium, flow rate 1 mL/min. MS detection (EI), SIM. Internal standard: 5α-androstane-3,17-dione,bis-TMS. RI: boldenone (TMS derivative) 2672. [W. Schanzer and M. Donike, *Biol. Mass Spectrom.*, 1992, 21, 3–16.]

High Performance Liquid Chromatography. System HAR—RRT 0.74 (relative to testosterone); system HATa—boldenone undecylenate RRT 1.94 (relative to testosterone); system HATb—boldenone RRT 0.76 (relative to testosterone).

Column: C_{18} (Nucleosil, 250 × 10 mm i.d., 7 μm). Mobile phase (A): water, (B) acetonitrile:water (90:10). Elution programme: (A:B) (70:30) to (20:80) over 25 min, flow rate 6 mL/min. Retention time: 13.1 min. [W. Schanzer and M. Donike, *Biol. Mass Spectrom.*, 1992, *21*, 3–16.]

Ultraviolet Spectrum. Aqueous acid—248 nm; aqueous base—250 nm; ethanol—243 nm.

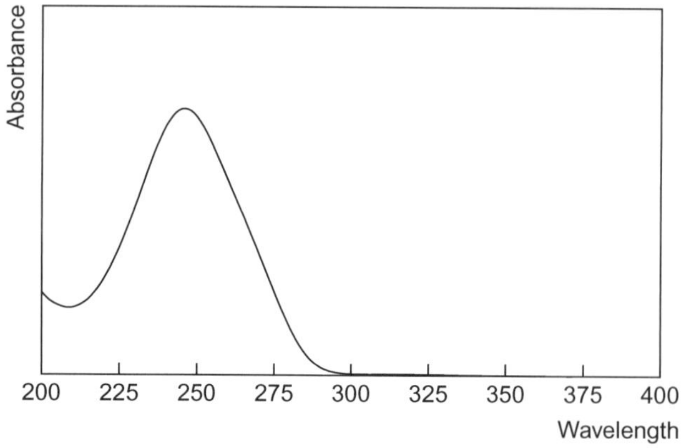

Infra-red Spectrum. Principal peaks at wavenumbers 1654, 1400, 1055 cm^{-1}; (acetate) 1725, 1231, 1034 cm^{-1}; (benzoate) 1658, 1276, 716 cm^{-1}; (undecylenate) 1725, 1654, 1175 cm^{-1} (KBr disks).

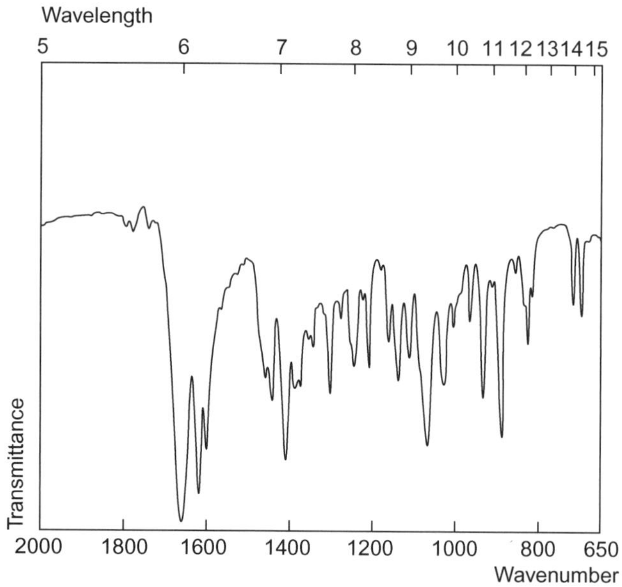

Mass Spectrum. Principal ions at *m/z* 122, 121, 91, 123, 147, 77, 107, 93.

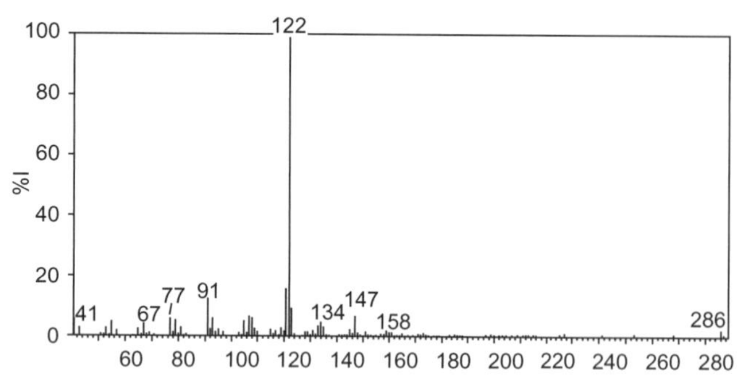

Quantification.

Gas chromatography–mass spectrometry. In urine: limit of detection 2 ppb—Man Ho Choi *et al., Rapid Commun. Mass Spectrom.*, 1998, 12, 1749–1755.

Disposition in the Body. Boldenone is metabolised to 5β-androst-1-en-17β-ol-3-one, 5β-androst-1-ene-3α,17β-diol, 5β-androst-1-en-3α-ol-17-one, 5β-androst-1-ene-3,17-dione, androsta-1,4-diene-6β,17β-diol-3-one, androsta-1,4-dien-6β-ol-3,17β-dione and 5β-androstan-3α-ol-17-one, by 5β-reduction. Excreted, via the kidneys, to a large extent as a conjugate.

Bopindolol

Antihypertensive

1-[(1,1-Dimethylethyl)amino]-3-[(2-methyl-1*H*-indol-4-yl)oxy]-2-propanol benzoate ester

$C_{23}H_{28}N_2O_3$=380.5

CAS—62658-63-3

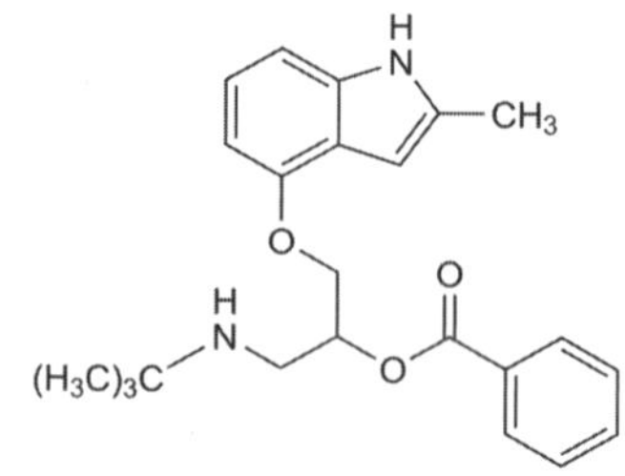

It is soluble in ether and methylene chloride.

Bopindolol Maleate

Proprietary name. Sandonorm

$C_{27}H_{32}N_2O_7$=496.6

Bopindolol Malonate

Synonyms. Bopindolol hydrogen malonate; LT-31-200.

Proprietary name. Wandonorm

$C_{26}H_{32}N_2O_7$=484.5

CAS—82857-38-3

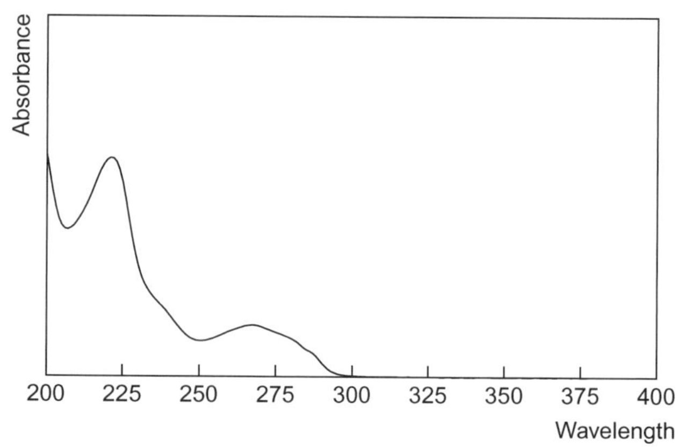

Quantification

High performance liquid chromatography. In plasma: limit of detection is 0.025 µg/L. Electrochemical detection—H. Humbert *et al., J. Chromatogr.*,1987, *422*, 205–215.

Disposition in the Body. Bopindolol is rapidly hydrolysed in plasma and no measurable amounts of the parent drug can be detected after oral administration. The two main metabolites identified are benzoic acid and an active hydrolysed metabolite.

Therapeutic concentration

20 young male volunteers, aged between 18 and 42 years, and 20 elderly males, 62 to 83 years old, were administered with a single 1-mg dose of bopindolol once daily for 7 days. Mean peak plasma concentrations of 4.5 and 5.2 µg/L were reached for the young and elderly volunteers, respectively. All peak concentrations were observed approximately 1.5 h after administration. No significant differences were observed between the young and elderly. [D. Holmes *et al., Eur. J. Clin. Pharmacol.*, 1991, *41*, 175–178].

14 patients with cirrhosis (male and female, aged between 40 and 66 years) and 15 healthy volunteers (21 to 28 years old) were administered with a 1.2-g dose antipyrine on day 1 and 2-mg bopindolol on day 3. The patients with cirrhosis reached a mean peak plasma concentration of 5.8 µg/L at 1.6 h and the healthy volunteers 6.9 µg/L within 1.5 h. No significant difference was observed. [G. Wensing *et al., Eur. J. Clin. Pharmacol.*, 1990, *39*, 569–572].

Half-life. Mean, 4.4 h (range 3.1 to 6.0 h).

Volume of distribution. Mean, 202 L (range, 102 to 504 L) after oral administration; 148 L intravenously.

Clearance. After single dose administration, plasma clearance is 30.9 L/h and for multiple dosing, 38.0 L/h.

Dose. Between 0.5 and 4 mg.

Brallobarbital

Sedative/Barbiturate

Synonym. Brallobarbitone
Proprietary name. It is an ingredient of Vesparax.
5-(2-Bromo-2-propenyl)-5-(2-propenyl)-2,4,6(1*H*,3*H*,5*H*)-pyrimidinetrione
$C_{10}H_{11}BrN_2O_3$=287.1
CAS—561-86-4

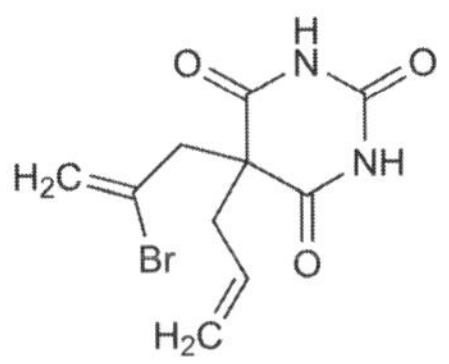

M.p. 168° to 169°.

Partition Coefficient. Log *P* (octanol/water), 1.4.

Colour Test. Vanillin Reagent—brown-orange/brown-orange.

Thin-layer Chromatography. System TD—Rf 52; system TE—Rf 30; system TF—Rf 68; system TH—Rf 47; system TAD—Rf 57; system TAE—Rf 87.

Gas Chromatography. System GA—brallobarbital RI 1853, brallobarbital-Me_2 RI 1725, M(2-OH-) RI 2040, M(desbromo-OH-) RI 1795; system GF—brallobarbital RI 2765; system GM—brallobarbital RRT (relative to methylphenobarbital) 1.000.

High Performance Liquid Chromatography. System HG—*k* 3.09; system HH—*k* 1.72; system HX—RI 371; system HY—RI 336; system HZ—Retention time(s) 3.0 min.

Ultraviolet Spectrum. Borax buffer 0.05 M (pH 9.2)—240 (A^1_1=304b); 1 M sodium hydroxide (pH 13) —256 nm (A^1_1=236b).

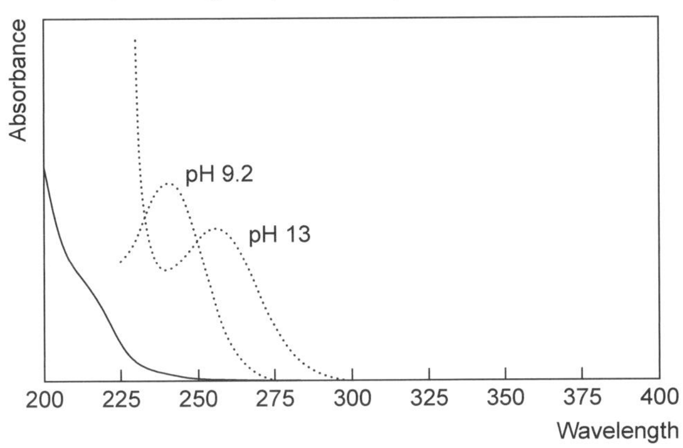

Mass Spectrum. Principal ions at *m/z* 207, 41, 39, 124, 91, 165, 122, 44.

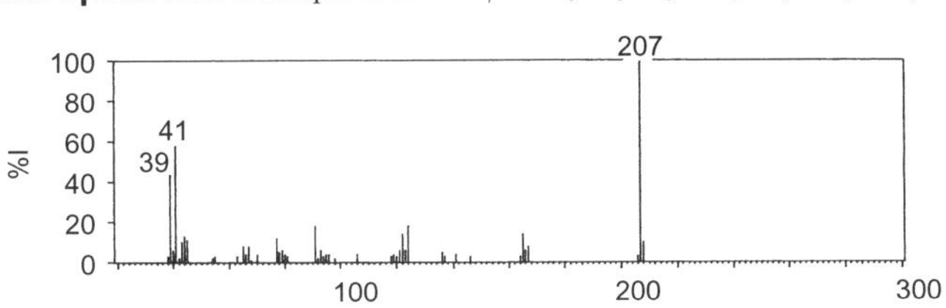

Quantification See under Amylobarbital.

Gas chromatography. In plasma: limit of detection 0.5 mg/L, NPD—F. Coudore *et al., J. Anal. Toxicol.*, 1993, *17(2)*, 109–113.

Disposition in the Body. Brallobarbital is absorbed after oral administration. About 5% of a dose is excreted in the urine as unchanged drug, 9% as 5-acetonyl-5-allylbarbituric acid and less than 1% each as 5-acetonyl-5-(2-bromoallyl)barbituric acid and 5-allyl-5-(2-hydroxypropyl)barbituric acid.

Toxicity
In 10 fatalities involving the ingestion of a preparation containing brallobarbital, quinalbarbital and hydroxyzine, the following post-mortem concentrations, μg/g (mean, *N*) were reported:

	Brallobarbital	Quinalbarbital
Blood	9.8–25 (16.3, 9)	10–33.4 (17.7, 9)
Brain	1.9–24.1 (12.7, 10)	8.6–50 (29.3, 10)
Kidney	8.9–28.1 (20.4, 10)	14.5–83.4 (30.6, 10)
Liver	14.9–241 (50.2, 10)	23.1–231 (95.7, 10)
Urine	1.8–201 (40.8, 6)	1.0–7.1 (4.0, 6)

[G. Sticht and H. Kaferstein, *Z. Rechtsmed.*, 1980, *85*, 169–175].

In an overdose involving the ingestion of more than 3 g of brallobarbital (in combination with quinalbarbital), plasma concentrations of 106 mg/L of brallobarbital and 57 mg/L of quinalbarbital were reported 6 h and 4 h, respectively, after ingestion; the subject slowly recovered after treatment by haemoperfusion. [G. de Groot *et al., Vet. Hum. Toxicol.*, 1979, *21*, 8–11].

Bretylium Tosilate

Anti-arrhythmic/Antihypertensive

Synonym. Bretylium Tosylate
Proprietary names. Bretylate; Bretylol.
2-Bromo-*N*-ethyl-*N*,*N*-dimethylbenzenemethanaminium 4-methylbenzenesulfonate
$C_{11}H_{17}BrN,C_7H_7O_3S$=414.4
CAS—59-41-6 (bretylium); 61-75-6 (tosilate)

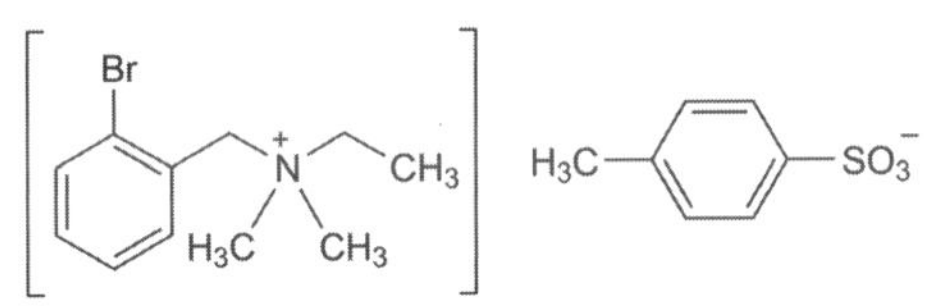

A white crystalline powder. M.p. 97° to 99°.
Soluble 1 in 1 of water and 1 in 0.4 of ethanol; practically insoluble in ether, ethyl acetate and hexane.

Thin-layer Chromatography. System TA—Rf 01; system TN—Rf 94; system TO—Rf 40. (Acidified iodoplatinate solution, positive.)

High Performance Liquid Chromatography. System HA—*k* 4.3 (tailing peak); system HY—RI 275.

Ultraviolet Spectrum. Aqueous acid—263, 272 (A^1_1=22a), 278 nm. No alkaline shift.

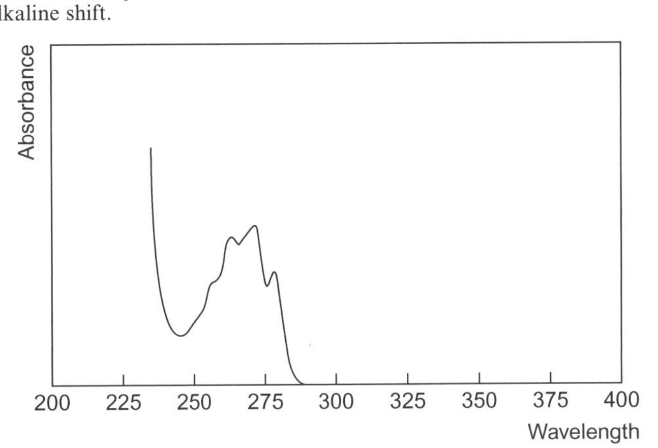

Infra-red Spectrum. Principal peaks at wavenumbers 1188, 1012, 1032, 1120, 680, 815 cm^{-1} (KBr disk).

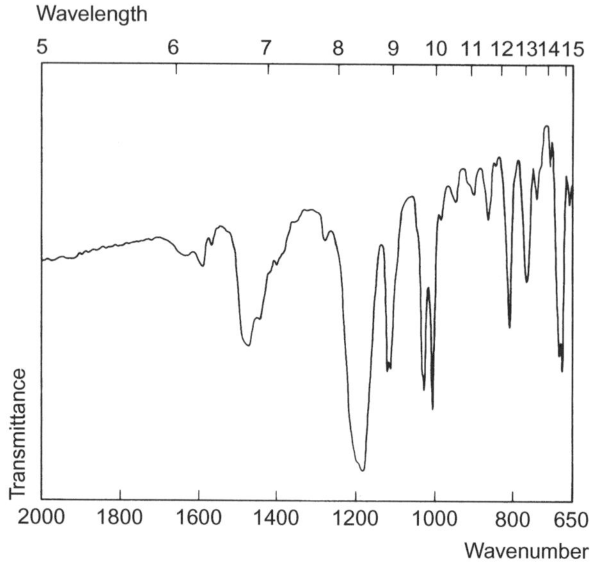

Quantification

Gas chromatography. In plasma or urine: limit of detection 5 µg/L, ECD—C.-M. Lai *et al.*, *J. Pharm. Sci.*, 1980, *69*, 681–683. In plasma, urine or myocardial tissue: limit of detection 1 µg/L, ECD—E. Patterson *et al.*, *J. Chromatogr.*, 1980, *181*; *Biomed. Appl.*, *7*, 33–39.

Disposition in the Body. Bretylium tosilate is poorly absorbed after oral administration. Excreted mainly in the urine as unchanged drug but a high proportion of bretylium is also excreted into the bile. After IV infusion about 70% of the dose is excreted in the urine in 24 h and 90% in 48 h. After chronic oral dosing about 20% of a dose is excreted in the 24-hour urine.

Therapeutic concentration

After a single oral dose of 5 mg/kg to 10 subjects, peak serum concentrations of 0.04 to 0.14 (mean 0.08) mg/L were attained in 1 to 8 h; following IV infusion of 5 mg/kg over 30 min to the same subjects, serum concentrations at the end of the infusion were reported to be in the range 1.1 to 2.4 (mean 1.9) mg/L. [J. L. Anderson *et al.*, *Clin. Pharmacol. Ther.*, 1980, *28*, 468–478].

Bioavailability. About 25%.

Half-life. Plasma half-life, about 7 to 10 h, increased in renal impairment.

Volume of distribution. About 8 L/kg.

Clearance. Plasma clearance, about 11 mL/min/kg.

Protein binding. In plasma, not significantly bound.

Note. For further information on bretylium tosilate, see E. R. Garrett *et al.*, *Biopharm. Drug Disp.*, 1982, *3*, 129–164.

Dose. 5 to 10 mg/kg by IM injection. Bretylium tosilate has been given by mouth in doses of 0.3 to 1.2 g daily.

Bromantane

Psychostimulant

Synonym. Bromantan
N-(4-Bromophenyl)tricyclo[3.3.1.1^{3,7}]decan-2-amine
$C_{16}H_{20}BrN$=306.2
CAS—87913-26-6

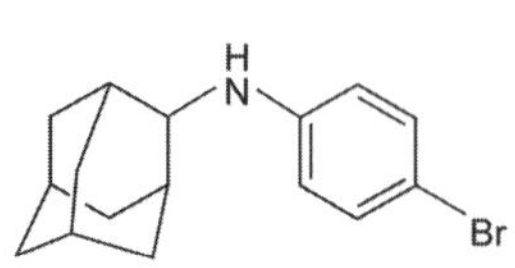

Use. Bromantane is used as a muscle performance-enhancing agent for athletes and as an immunostimulant.

Bromazepam

Tranquilliser

Synonyms. Bromazepamum; Ro-5-3350.
Proprietary names. Anxyrex; Brazepam; Bromam; Bromaze; Bromidem; Brozam; Brozepax; Calmex; Compendium; Creosedin; Deptran; Durazanil; Gityl 6; Lectopam; Lexatin; Lexomil; Lexotan; Lexotanil; neo OPT; Nervium; Normoc; Quietiline; Somalium.
7-Bromo-1,3-dihydro-5-(2-pyridinyl)-2*H*-1,4-benzodiazepin-2-one
$C_{14}H_{10}BrN_3O$=316.2
CAS—1812-30-2

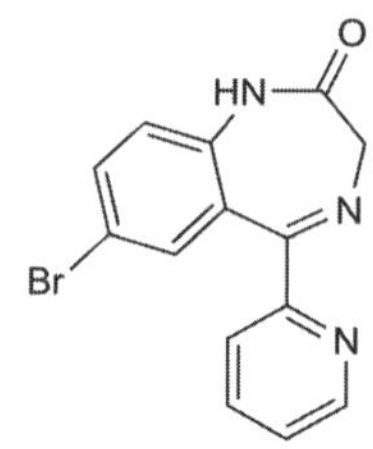

A white or yellowish crystalline powder. M.p. 237° to 238.5° with decomposition.
Practically insoluble in water, sparingly soluble in alcohol and in dichloromethane.

Dissociation Constant. pK_a 2.9, 11.0.

Partition Coefficient. Log *P* (octanol/water), 2.05.

Colour Test. Formaldehyde–Sulfuric Acid—yellow.

Thin-layer Chromatography. System TA—Rf 61; system TB—Rf 6; system TC—Rf 41; system TD—Rf 13; system TE—Rf 63; system TF—Rf 18; system TL—Rf 53; system TAD—Rf 47; system TAE—Rf 73; system TAF—Rf 69; system TAJ—Rf 34; system TAK—Rf 04; system TAL—Rf 63.

Gas Chromatography. System GA—bromazepam RI 2665, M (3-OH-) RI 2470; system GB—bromazepam RI 2760, bromazepam-TMS RI 2702; M (3-OH-)-TMS_2 RI 2650; system GG—RI 3280.

Column: DB-17 (30 m × 0.32 mm i.d., 0.25 µm film thickness). Column temperature: 150°, held for 1 min, ramp to 230°, held for 5 min, ramp to 300° held for 9 min at 10°/min. Injector and detector temperatures: 270° and 300°, respectively. Carrier gas: helium (pre-column pressure, 80 kPa). Detection: ECD. Retention time: 18.0 min. [F. Guan *et al.*, *J. Anal. Toxicol.*, 1999, *23*, 54–61.]

Column: HP5-MS (5% phenyl:95% siloxane, 30 m × 0.25 mm, 0.25 µm film thickness). Column temperature: 60° held for 1 min, ramp to 295° at 30°/min, held for 6 min. Injector temperature: 250°. Carrier gas: helium, flow rate 1 mL/min. MS detection (NCI mode). Retention time: 9.7 min. [P. Kintz *et al.*, *J. Chromatogr. B Biomed. Sci. Appl.*, 1997, *700*, 119–129.]

High Performance Liquid Chromatography. System HI—*k* 2.32; system HK—*k* 2.99; system HX—RI 397; system HY—RI 331; system HZ—retention time 3.0 min; system HAA—retention time 14.7 min; system HAF—retention time 6.6 min (tailing peak); system HAX—retention time 5.8 min; system HAY—retention time 5.1 min; system HBH—*k* 1.63; system HBI—*k* 0.80; system HAL—retention time 8.1 min; system HAM—not detected.

Column: RP C_{18} (150 × 3.9 mm i.d., 5 µm). Mobile phase: water:acetonitrile:triethylamine (700:300:4), adjusted to pH 7.4 with phosphoric acid, flow rate 2 mL/min. UV detection (λ = 240 nm). Retention time: bromazepam, 2.1 min, α-hydroxytriazolam (IS), 3.2 min. [Le Solleu *et al.*, *J. Pharm. Biomed. Anal.*, 1993, *11*, 771–775.]

Ultraviolet Spectrum. Aqueous acid—239, 345 nm; aqueous alkali—237 nm (A^1_1=920b), 348 nm; methanol—233 nm (A^1_1=1050b), 320 nm (A^1_1=61b).

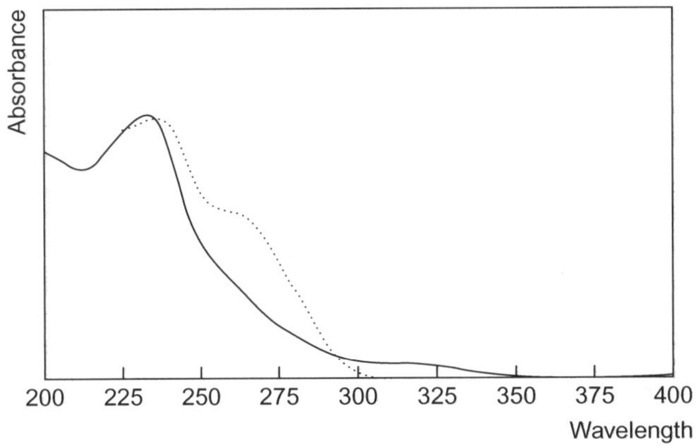

Infra-red Spectrum. Principal peaks at wavenumbers 1685, 825, 750, 802, 1315, 1230 cm^{-1}.

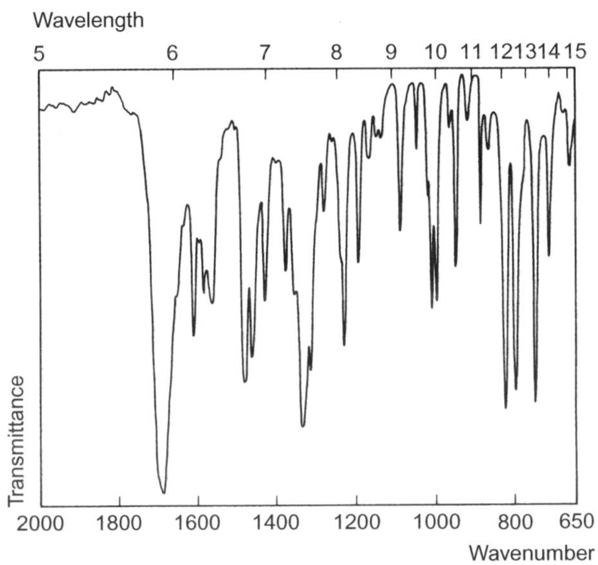

Mass Spectrum. Principal ions at *m/z* 236, 317, 315, 288, 316, 286, 208, 78; 3-hydroxybromazepam 79, 78, 52, 105, 304, 314, 316, 51.

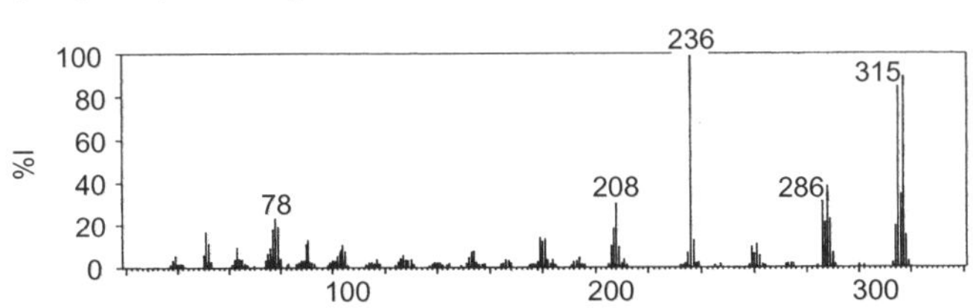

Quantification.

Gas chromatography. In plasma: limit of detection 5 μg/L, ECD—U. Klotz, *J. Chromatogr.* 1981, *222*(21) *B Biomed. Appl.*, 501–506. In plasma or blood: bromazepam and other benzodiazepines, ECD and NPD—P. Lillsunde and T. Seppala, *J. Chromatogr.*, 1990, *533*, 97–110. In hair: limit of detection, 20 pg/mg hair, MS (NCI mode)—P. Kintz *et al.*, *J. Chromatogr. B Biomed. Sci. Appl.*, 1997, *700*, 119–129. In urine: bromazepam and other benzodiazepines, limit of detection for bromazepam 160 μg/L, ECD—F. Guan *et al.*, *J. Anal. Toxicol.*, 1999, *23*, 54–61.

Gas chromatography–mass spectrometry. In tissue: limit of quantification, 50 ng/g tissue, SIM—X.X. Zhang *et al.*, *J. Chromatogr.* 1996, *677 B Biomed. Appl.*, 111–116. In urine: bromazepam, diazepam, and nordazepam, TOF-MS, comparison with MS and ECD—B. Aebi *et al.*, *Forensic Sci. Int.*, 2002, *128*, 84–89.

High performance liquid chromatography. In plasma: limit of detection 5 μg/L, UV detection—H. Hirayama *et al.*, *J. Chromatogr.* 1983, *277*(28) *B Biomed. Appl.*, 414–418. In plasma: limit of detection 3 μg/L, UV detection—A. Boukhabza *et al.*, *Analyst*, 1989, *114*, 639–641. In plasma: limit of detection, 50 μg/L, UV detection—H. Le Solleu *et al.*, *J. Pharm. Biomed. Anal.*, 1993, *11*, 771–775. In serum: bromazepam and other benzodiazepines, UV detection—E. Tanaka *et al.*, *J. Chromatogr.* 1996, *682 B Biomed Appl.*, 173–178 and E. Tanaka *et al.*, *J. Chromatogr. B Biomed. Sci. Appl.*, 1998, *709*, 324.

Disposition in the Body. Well absorbed after oral administration and peak plasma concentrations are usually achieved within 2 h. About 70% of a dose is excreted in the urine in 72 h, including about 2% of the dose as unchanged bromazepam, about 27% as the glucuronide of 3-hydroxybromazepam, about 40% as the glucuronide of 2-amino-5-bromo-3-hydroxybenzoylpyridine, and less than 1% as 2-(2-amino-5-bromobenz-oyl)-pyridine.

Therapeutic concentration

After a single oral dose of 12 mg, administered to 10 subjects, peak plasma concentrations of 0.11 to 0.17 mg/L (mean 0.13) were attained in 1 to 4 h. Steady-state concentrations of 0.08 to 0.15 mg/L (mean 0.12) were measured during dosing of 6 subjects with 9 mg daily. [S. A. Kaplan *et al.*, *J. Pharmacokinet. Biopharm.*, 1976, *4*, 1–16.]

Administration of bromazepam as a slow-release formulation to 24 healthy subjects after an overnight fast resulted in peak plasma concentrations of 9.09 to 13.00 μg/L (mean 11.05 μg/L) attained in 4 to 16 h (mean 8 h); the corresponding values for a conventional-release preparation administered as 2 separate 1.5 mg doses, 12 h apart, were 8.91 to 11.50 μg/L (mean 10.21 μg/L) in 2 to 8 h (mean 8 h). [F. E. Lerner *et al.*, *Arzneimittelforschung*, 2001, *51*, 955–958.]

Toxicity

In a 68-year-old woman who was found unconscious and barely breathing, bromazepam intoxication was discovered to be the cause (a serum level of 6 mg/L was detected); normal functions were restored 12 days after the ingestion. [J. Rudolf *et al.*, *Dtsch. Med. Wochenschr.*, 1998, *123*, 832–834.]

A 42-year-old woman ingested 420 mg bromazepam in a suicide attempt and survived despite being found unconscious outdoors in a state of semi-undress and suffering from hypothermia. About 12 h after the ingestion the blood concentration of bromazepam was 7.7 mg/L. [K. Michaud *et al.*, *Forensic Sci. Int.*, 2001, *124*, 112–114.]

Half-life. Plasma half-life, 8 to 19 h (mean 12).

Volume of distribution. About 0.9 L/kg.

Protein binding. In plasma, 70%.

Dose. Usually 3 to 18 mg daily; up to a maximum of 60 mg daily in divided doses has been given to hospitalised patients.

Bromazine

Antihistamine

Synonyms. Bromodiphenhydramine; Bromdiphenhydramine; Histabromamine.

2-[(4-Bromophenyl)phenylmethoxy]-*N,N*-dimethylethanamine

$C_{17}H_{20}BrNO = 334.3$

CAS-118-23-0

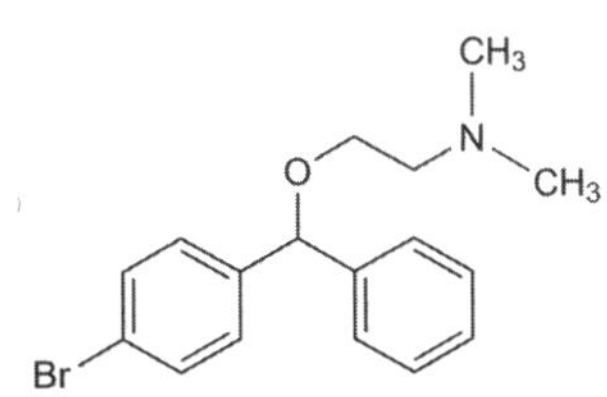

Bromazine Hydrochloride

Proprietary name. Ambodryl

$C_{17}H_{20}BrNO,HCl = 370.7$

CAS-1808-12-4

A white to pale buff-coloured crystalline powder. M.p. 148° to 152°.

Soluble 1 in less than 1 of water, 1 in 2 of ethanol, 1 in 2 of chloroform and 1 in 31 of isopropyl alcohol; practically insoluble in ether.

Dissociation Constant. pK_a 8.6 (25°).

Colour Test. Marquis Test—yellow.

Thin-layer Chromatography. System TA—Rf 54; system TB—Rf 44; system TC—Rf 43; system TL—Rf 13; system TAE—Rf 27; system TAF—Rf 48. (Dragendorff spray, positive; acidified iodoplatinate solution, positive; Marquis reagent, yellow.)

Gas Chromatography. System GA—RI 2155; system GF—RI 2480.

High Performance Liquid Chromatography. System HA—*k* 2.7; system HX—RI 444.

Ultraviolet Spectrum. Aqueous acid—230 nm (A_1^1=465a).

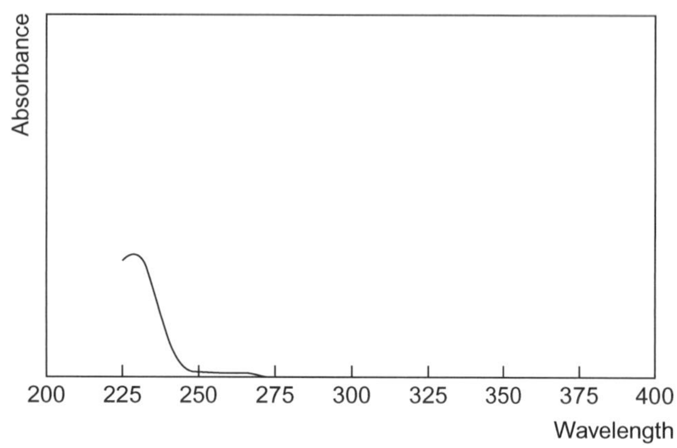

Infra-red Spectrum. Principal peaks at wavenumbers 1067, 1094, 1007, 696, 1041, 746 cm^{-1} (KBr disk).

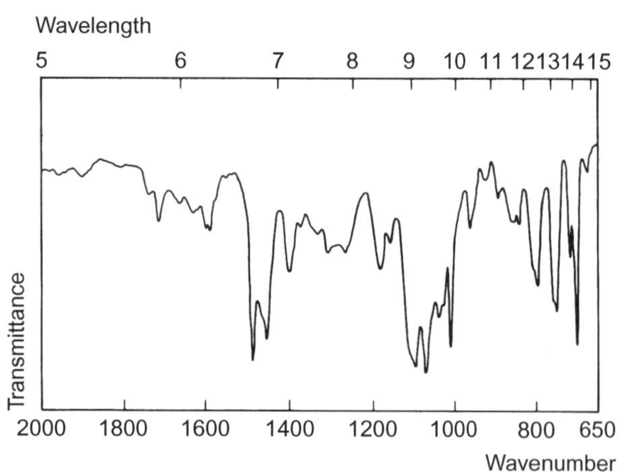

Mass Spectrum. Principal ions at *m/z* 58, 73, 45, 165, 59, 42, 166, 149.

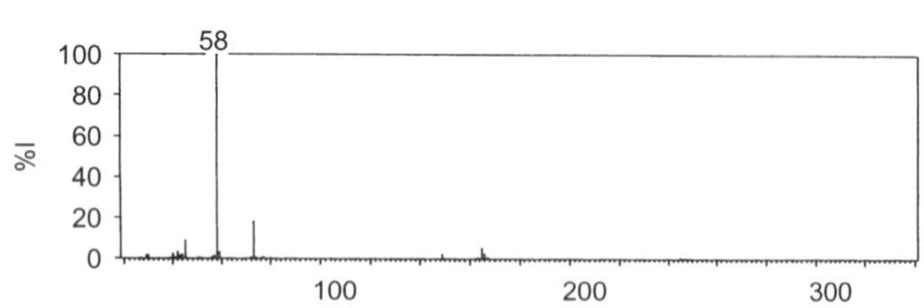

Disposition in the Body. Absorbed after oral administration. A number of metabolites have been identified in the urine including the *N*-oxide, monodesmethyl and didesmethyl derivatives, 4-bromobenzhydrol, 4-bromobenzophenone and 4-hydroxybenzophenone; glucuronide conjugates of some of these metabolites have also been reported. Unchanged drug is also excreted in the urine.

Dose. 75 to 100 mg of bromazine hydrochloride daily.

Bromhexine

Mucolytic Expectorant

2-Amino-3,5-dibromo-*N*-cyclohexyl-*N*-methylbenzenemethanamine
$C_{14}H_{20}Br_2N_2$=376.1
CAS—3572-43-8

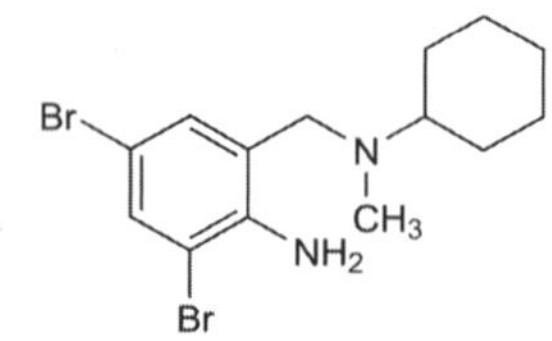

Bromhexine Hydrochloride
Synonym. NA-274.
Proprietary names. Auxit; Bisolvon; Broncokin; Dakryo Biciron; Ophtosol; Quentan. It is an ingredient of Alupent Expectorant and Bisolvomycin.
$C_{14}H_{20}Br_2N_2,HCl$=412.6
CAS—611-75-6
A white crystalline powder. M.p. about 235°.
Soluble 1 in 250 of water, 1 in 100 of ethanol, 1 in 300 of chloroform and 1 in 50 of methanol; practically insoluble in acetone; soluble in glacial acetic acid.

Partition Coefficient. Log *P* (octanol/water), 4.9.

Thin-layer Chromatography. System TA—Rf 75; system TB—Rf 67; system TC—Rf 79; system TL—Rf 71; system TAE—Rf 84; system TAJ—Rf 98; system TAK—Rf 28; system TAL—Rf 78. (Acidified iodoplatinate solution, positive.)

Gas Chromatography. System GA—RI 2337.

High Performance Liquid Chromatography. System HA—*k* 0.4; system HX—RI 417; system HY—RI 334; system HZ—Retention time(s) 7.5 min.

Ultraviolet Spectrum. Aqueous acid—245 (A_1^1=259a), 310; aqueous alkali—262, 317 nm.

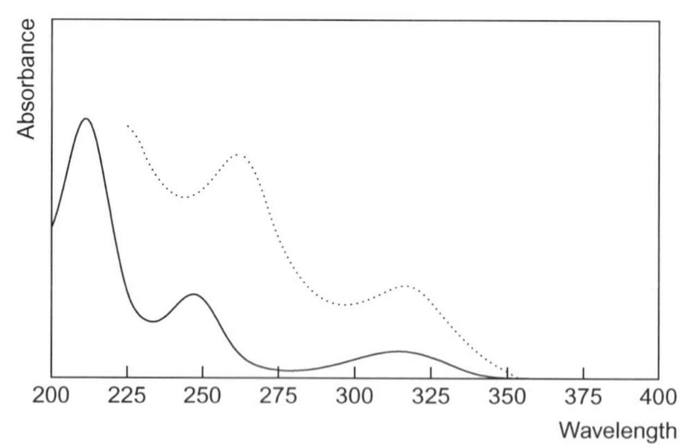

Infra-red Spectrum. Principal peaks at wavenumbers 1602, 1031, 1074, 1548, 1122, 857 cm^{-1} (KBr disk).

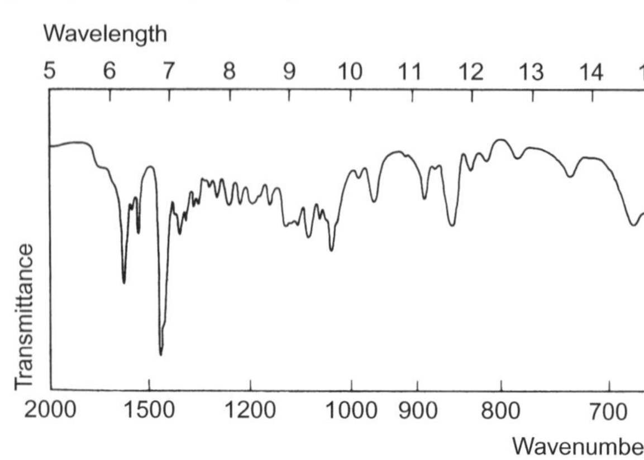

Mass Spectrum. Principal ions at m/z 70, 112, 293, 264, 44, 42, 305, 41.

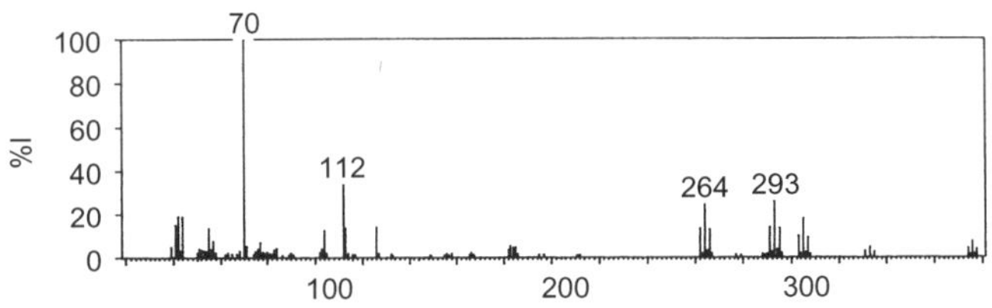

Quantification

Gas chromatography. In plasma: limit of detection 1 µg/L, ECD—A. P. DeLeenheer and L. M. R. Vandecasteele-Thienpont, *J. Pharm. Sci.*, 1980, *69*, 99–100.

High performance liquid chromatography. In plasma or urine: limits of detection 4 µg/L and 2 µg/L, respectively, UV detection—E. Bechgaard and A. Nielsen, *J. Chromatogr.*, 1982, *228*; *B Biomed. Appl.*, *17*, 392–397.

Disposition in the Body. Bromhexine is well absorbed after oral administration but undergoes considerable first-pass metabolism including conjugation with glucuronic acid or sulfate; ambroxol, *trans*-4-(2-amino-3,5-dibromobenzylamino)cyclohexanol, is an active metabolite of bromhexine. About 70% of an oral dose is excreted in the urine in 24 h as metabolites with less than 1% as unchanged drug.

Therapeutic concentration

Following single oral doses of 32 mg to 10 subjects, peak plasma concentrations of 0.01 to 0.14 (mean 0.04) mg/L were attained in 0.5 to 2.5 h. [E. Bechgaard and A. Nielsen, *Biopharm. Drug Disp.*, 1982, *3*, 337–344].

Half-life. Derived from plasma and urinary data, about 6 h.

Dose. 24 to 64 mg of bromhexine hydrochloride daily.

Bromisoval

Hypnotic/Sedative

Synonyms. Bromvaletone; Bromisovalerylurea; Bromisovalum; Bromvalerylurea; Bromylum.
Proprietary names. Bromural. Bromisoval is an ingredient of Seduan, Sekundal, and Steno-Valocordin.
N-(Aminocarbonyl)-2-bromo-3-methylbutanamide
$C_6H_{11}BrN_2O_2 = 223.1$
CAS—496-67-3

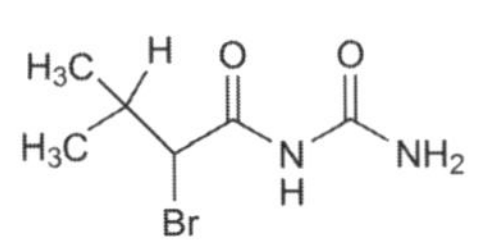

Small, white, acicular or scale-like crystals, which sublime on heating. M.p. 147° to 149°.
Soluble 1 in 500 of water, 1 in 15 of ethanol, 1 in 6 of chloroform, and 1 in 25 of ether; soluble in solutions of alkali hydroxides.

Dissociation Constant. pK_a 10.8.

Partition Coefficient. Log *P* (octanol/water), 1.14.

Colour Test. Nessler's Reagent—brown-orange.

Thin-layer Liquid Chromatography. System TB—Rf 6; system TD—Rf 35; system TE—Rf 68; system TF—Rf 51; system TAD—Rf 52; system TAE—bromisoval Rf 84, α-(*N*-acetylcysteine-*S*-yl)-isovalerylurea (M1) Rf 87, *dl*-isovalthine (M2) Rf 77.

Gas Chromatography. System GA—bromisoval RI 1540, M (Br-isovalerianic acid) RI 1190, M (OH-isovalerianic acid) RI 1140, M (isovalerianic acid carbamide) RI 1850.

High Performance Liquid Chromatography. System HX—bromisoval RI 365, M1 RI 312, M2 RI 211, α-(cystein-*S*-yl)isovalerylurea (M3) 237; system HY—RI 307; system HZ—retention time 2.9 min.

Ultraviolet Spectrum. Aqueous alkali—233 nm ($A^1_1 = 160$b).

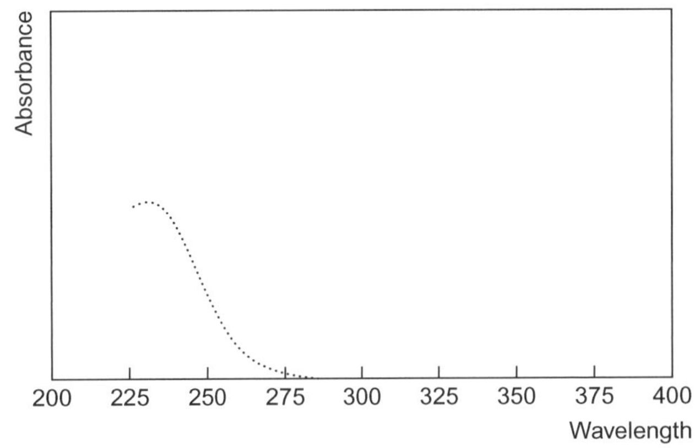

Infra-red Spectrum. Principal peaks at wavenumbers 1720, 1700, 1581, 1210, 1170, 1300 cm^{-1} (KBr disk). Polymorphism may occur.

Mass Spectrum. Principal ions at m/z 44, 83, 180, 182, 137, 143, 139, 41.

Quantification

Gas chromatography. In biological fluids and tissues: limit of detection 200 mg/L, FID—L. R. Goldbaum and T. J. Domanski, *J. Forensic. Sci.*, 1966, *11*, 233–242.

Dose. Bromisoval has been given in doses of 300 to 900 mg.

Bromocriptine

Dopaminergic Agent

Synonyms. 2-Bromo-α-ergocryptine; Bromocryptine; 2-Bromoergocryptine.
(5′α)-2-Bromo-12′-hydroxy-2′-(1-methylethyl)-5′-(2-methylpropyl)-ergotaman-3′,6′,18-trione
$C_{32}H_{40}BrN_5O_5 = 654.6$
CAS—25614-03-3

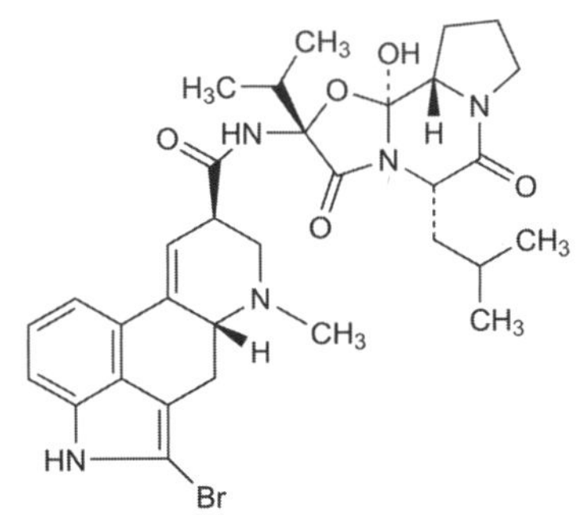

Crystals. M.p. 215° to 218°, with decomposition.

Bromocriptine Mesilate
Synonym. Bromocriptine Methanesulfonate
Proprietary names. Parlodel; Pravidel.
$C_{32}H_{40}BrN_5O_5,CH_4O_3S = 750.7$
CAS—22260-51-1
A yellowish-white crystalline powder. M.p. 192° to 196°, with decomposition.

Thin-layer Chromatography. System TA—Rf 72; system TB—Rf 00; system TC—Rf 69; system TL—Rf 61; system TAE—Rf 84; system TAF—Rf 88.

Gas Chromatography. System GA—RI 2156.

High Performance Liquid Chromatography. System HP—*k* 44.3; system HX—RI 456; system HZ—retention time 5.7 min; system HAA—retention time 16.7 min.

Ultraviolet Spectrum. Aqueous acid—306 ($A^1_1 = 138$b); aqueous alkali—239 ($A^1_1 = 373$b), 300 nm ($A^1_1 = 144$b).

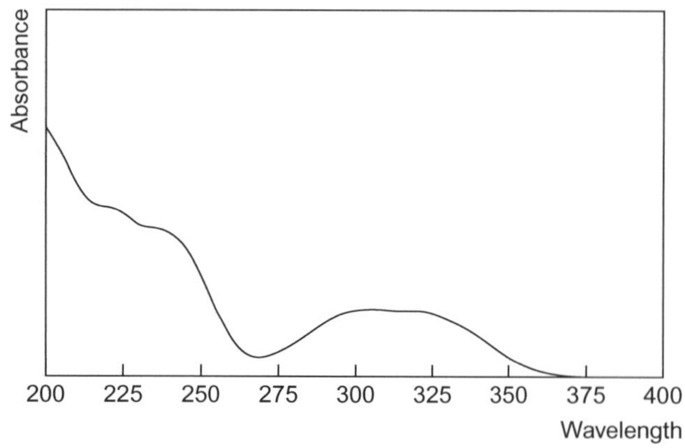

Infra-red Spectrum. Principal peaks at wavenumbers 1170, 1633, 1217, 1660, 1715, 1045 cm^{-1} (bromocriptine mesilate).

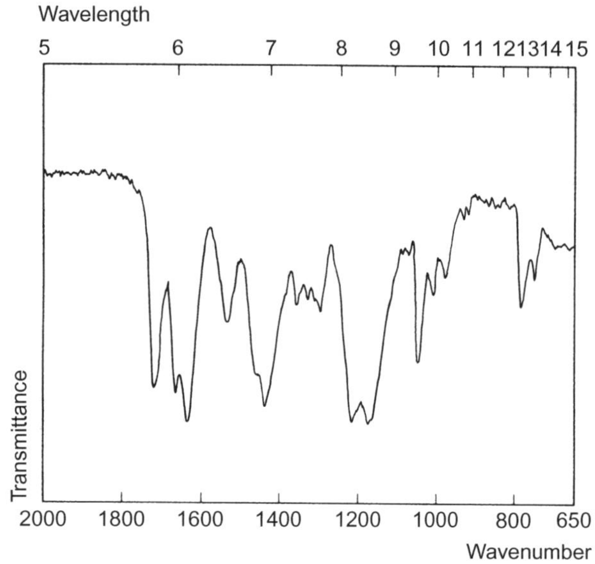

Mass Spectrum. Principal ions at *m/z* 70, 43, 154, 71, 41, 209, 86, 195.

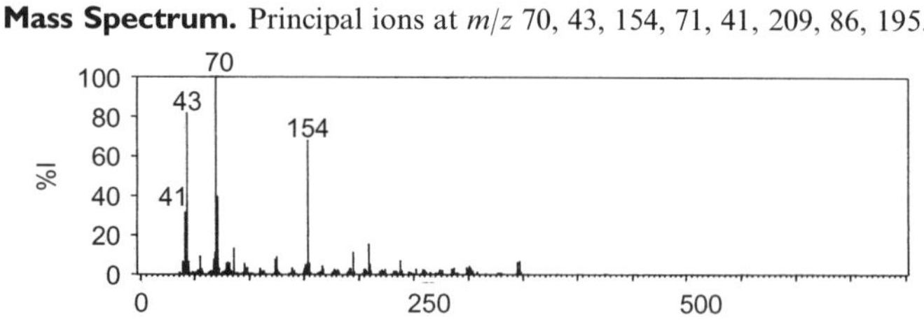

Quantification

Gas chromatography. In plasma: comparison with GC-MS and HPLC, limit of detection 0.5 μg/L for GC and 1 μg/L for GC-MS and HPLC—N. E. Larsen *et al.*, *J. Chromatogr.*, 1979, *174*, 341–349.

Disposition in the Body. Rapidly absorbed after oral administration. It undergoes extensive first-pass metabolism by hydrolysis and isomerisation to 2-bromolysergic acid and 2-bromoisolysergic acid, and, by hydroxylation, further oxidation and conjugation to produce a large number of metabolites. About 7% of a dose is excreted in the urine as metabolites together with a small fraction as unchanged drug. About 70% of a dose is eliminated in the faeces via the bile within 5 days of a single oral dose.

Therapeutic concentration

Following a single oral dose of 25 mg to 9 subjects, peak plasma concentrations of 1 to 4 μg/L were attained in about 90 min; after single doses of 50 and 100 mg to 7 and 5 subjects, respectively, peak plasma concentrations of 3 to 20 μg/L (mean 10) and 6 to 25 μg/L (mean 10) were attained in about 90 to 120 min. [P. Price *et al.*, *Br. J. Clin. Pharmacol.*, 1978, *6*, 303–309.]

Following daily oral administration of 60 to 150 mg in divided doses to 4 subjects, minimum steady-state plasma concentrations of 9 to 54 μg/L (mean 30) and saliva concentrations of 0.1 to 0.4 μg/L were reported. [M. L. Friis *et al.*, *Eur. J. Clin. Pharmacol.*, 1980, *18*, 171–174.]

Half-life. Plasma half-life, about 3 h.

Volume of distribution. About 3 L/kg.

Protein binding. In plasma, 90 to 96%.

Dose. The equivalent of 1.25 to 30 mg of bromocriptine daily. In parkinsonism, the usual maintenance dose is the equivalent of 40 to 100 mg daily, but up to 300 mg daily has been given.

Brompheniramine

Antihistamine

Synonym. Parabromdylamine

γ-(4-Bromophenyl)-*N,N*-dimethyl-2-pyridinepropanamine

$C_{16}H_{19}BrN_2$=319.2

CAS—86-22-6

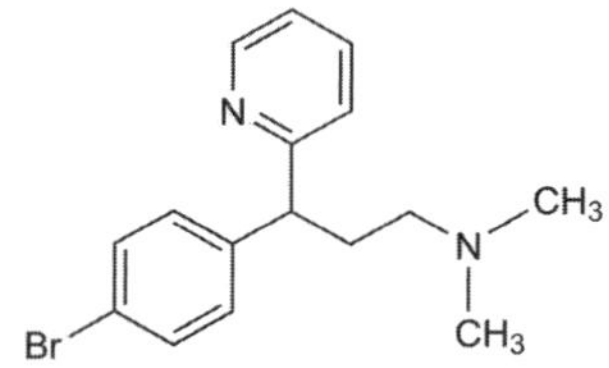

A slightly yellow, oily liquid.
Miscible with dilute acids.

Brompheniramine Maleate

Proprietary names. Antial; Dimegan; Dimetane; Dimotane; Drauxin; Ebalin; Gammistin; Ilvin; Veltane. It is an ingredient of Dimotapp and Exyphen.

$C_{16}H_{19}BrN_2,C_4H_4O_4$=435.3

CAS—980-71-2; 32865-01-3 (±)

A white crystalline powder. M.p. 132° to 134°.

Soluble 1 in 5 of water, 1 in 15 of ethanol, and 1 in 15 of chloroform; slightly soluble in ether.

Dissociation Constant. pK_a 3.9, 9.2.

Partition Coefficient. Log *P* (octanol/water), 4.1.

Colour Test. Cyanogen Bromide—orange.

Thin-layer Chromatography. System TA—Rf 45; system TB—Rf 33; system TC—Rf 16; system TL—Rf 06; system TAE—Rf 12; system TAJ—Rf 01; system TAK—Rf 00; system TAL—Rf 28. (Acidified iodoplatinate solution, positive.)

Gas Chromatography. System GA—RI 2092; system GB—brompheniramine RI 2184, M (nor-) RI 2219, M (bis-nor-) RI 2203; system GC—RI 2457; system GF—RI 2470.

High Performance Liquid Chromatography. System HA—*k* 4.1; system HY—RI 267; system HAA—retention time 13.9 min.

Ultraviolet Spectrum. Aqueous acid—265 (A_1^1=272a); aqueous alkali—262 (A_1^1=177a), 269 nm.

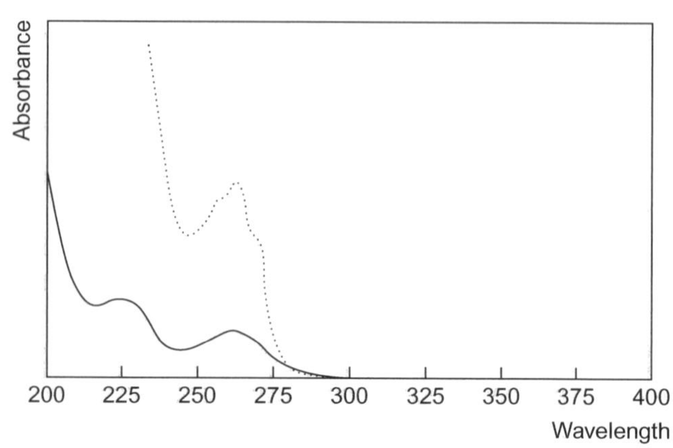

Infra-red Spectrum. Principal peaks at wavenumbers 1585, 750, 1003, 1067, 1565, 1040 cm^{-1} (KBr disk).

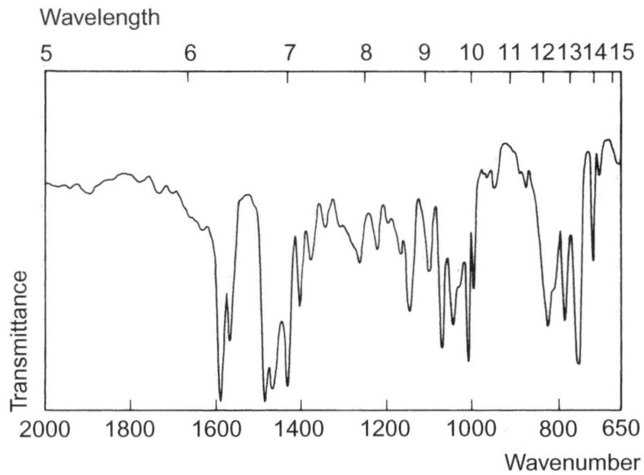

Mass Spectrum. Principal ions at *m/z* 247, 249, 58, 72, 248, 167, 250, 168.

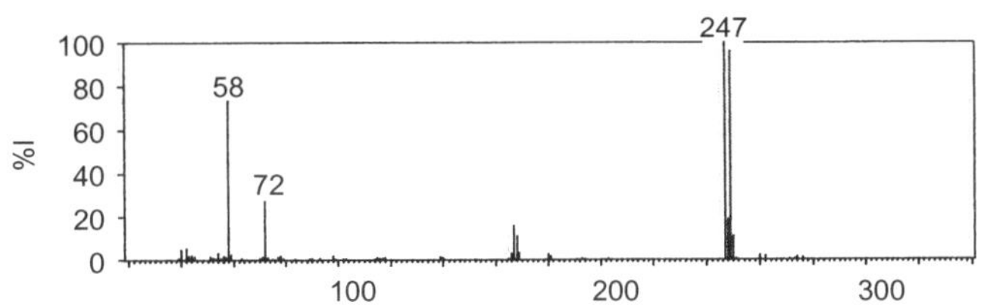

Quantification

Gas chromatography. In blood or urine: limit of detection 10 µg/L in blood, ECD—R. B. Bruce *et al.*, *Anal. Chem.*, 1968, *40*, 1246–1250.

Disposition in the Body. Absorbed after oral administration; accumulates in the body during chronic daily dosing. The main metabolic reactions are *N*-demethylation and deamination. About 50% of a ^{14}C-labelled dose is excreted in the urine in 5 days, with 10% of the dose as unchanged brompheniramine, 11% as monodesmethylbrompheniramine, 10% as didesmethylbrompheniramine, 4% as 3-(4-bromophenyl)-3-(2-pyridyl)-propionic acid, and 2% as its glycine conjugate; other unidentified polar metabolites are also present. Less than 3% of the dose is eliminated in the faeces. Under steady-state conditions the daily excretion rate appears to be dependent on urinary pH and volume.

Therapeutic concentration

After a single oral dose of 8 mg administered to 2 subjects, peak blood concentrations of 12 and 17 µg/L were attained in 3 h. [R. B. Bruce *et al.*, *Anal. Chem.*, 1968, *40*, 1246–1250.]

14 children with a mean age of 9.5 years were administered 4 mg brompheniramine. Mean peak drug concentrations of 7.7 µg/L at 3.2 h. [F. E. Simons *et al.*, *J. Allerg. Clin. Immunol.*, 1999, *103(2)*, 223–226.]

Half-life. Plasma half-life, about 15 h.

Dose. 12 to 32 mg of brompheniramine maleate daily.

Brotizolam

Sedative/Hypnotic

Synonym. WE-941-BS

Proprietary names. Dormex; Landormin; Lendorm; Lendormin; Lindormin; Mederantil; Nimbisan; Noctilen; Sintonal.

2-Bromo-4-(2-chlorophenyl)-9-methyl-6*H*-thieno[3,2-*f*][1,2,4]triazolo[4,3-*a*][1,4]diazepine

$C_{15}H_{10}BrClN_4S = 393.7$

CAS—57801-81-7

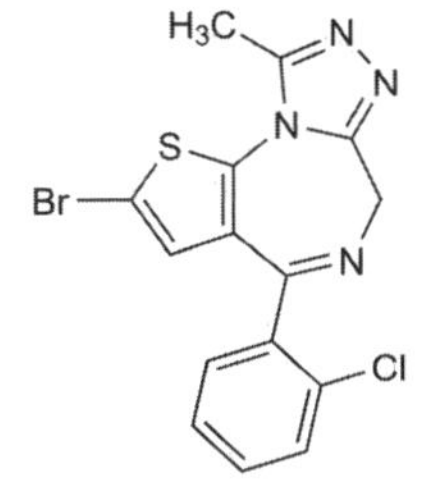

Colourless crystalline powder with m.p. 212° to 214° . Water solubility of 1.078 mg/L at 25°.

Partition Coefficient. Log *P* (octanol/water), 2.79.

Thin-layer Chromatography. System TA—Rf 72 (brotizolam); Rf 68 (M-6-hydroxy); Rf 72 (M-α-hydroxy); system TB—Rf 5 (brotizolam); Rf 1 (M-6-hydroxy); Rf 2 (M-α-hydroxy); TC—Rf 52 (brotizolam); Rf 35 (M-6-hydroxy); Rf 46 (M-α-hydroxy); TD—Rf 15 (brotizolam); Rf 5 (M-6-hydroxy); Rf 7 (M-α-hydroxy); system TE—Rf 52 (brotizolam); Rf 28 (M-6-hydroxy); Rf 45 (M-α-hydroxy); system TF—Rf 5 (brotizolam); Rf 4 (M-6-hydroxy); Rf 6 (M-α-hydroxy); system TL—Rf 27 (brotizolam); Rf 13 (M-6-hydroxy); Rf 31 (M-α-hydroxy); system TAD—Rf 53 (brotizolam); Rf 37 (M-6-hydroxy); Rf 41 (M-α-hydroxy); system TAE—Rf 72 (brotizolam); Rf 76 (M-6-hydroxy); Rf 78 (M-α-hydroxy); system TAF—Rf 71 (brotizolam); Rf 76 (M-6-hydroxy); Rf 78 (M-α-hydroxy).

Plate: silica gel 60 F_{254}. Mobile phase: toluene:isopropanol:NH_3 (25%) (5:4:1). Detection at 254 nm. We 964 Rf 59–62; We 1061 Rf 37–40. [W. D. Bechtel *et al.*, *Arzneimittelforschung*, 1986, *36(1)*, 578–586].

Plate: silica gel 60 F_{254} (10 × 10 cm). Mobile phase 1: cyclohexane:toluene:diethylamine (75:15:10); mobile phase 2: chloroform:methanol (90:10); mobile phase 3: chloroform:acetone (80:20). Dragendorff reagent was used to visualise the spots. Rf 6 (mobile phase 1); Rf 52 (mobile phase 2); Rf 13 (mobile phase 3). [K. Otsubo *et al.*, *J. Chromatogr. Biomed. Sci. Appl.*, 1995, *669*, 408–412].

Gas Chromatography. System GA—RI 3070 (brotizolam); RI 3050 (M(OH) Art(-CH_2O)).

High Performance Liquid Chromatography. System HX—RI 484; system HZ—retention time 4.6 min; system HAX—retention time 7.4 min; system HAY—retention time 7.9 min.

Column: C_{18} (Nucleosil, 5 µm, 200 × 4.5 mm i.d.). Mobile phase: acetonitrile:NH_4CO_3 (0.01 mol/L):diethylamine (35:65:0.1), 1 mL/min flow rate. UV detection (λ = 254 nm). Retention time(s): (metabolites) We 964, 10 to 11 min; We 1061, 12 to 13 min. [W. D. Bechtel *et al.*, *Arzneimittelforschung*, 1986, *36(1)*, 578–586].

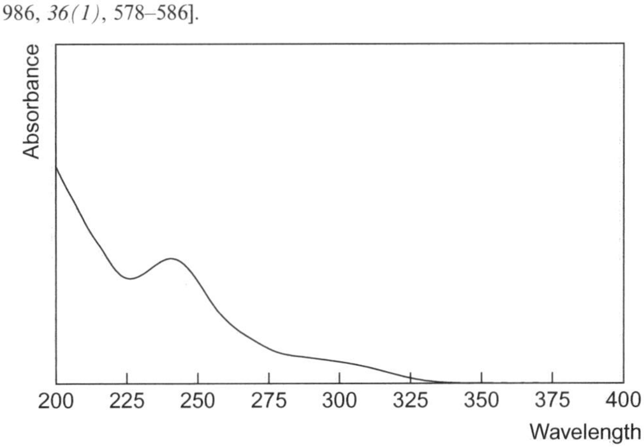

Mass Spectrum. Principal ions at *m/z* 394, 245, 316, 210, 291, 176, 365, 313.

Quantification

High performance liquid chromatography. In serum: limit of detection 2 µg/L—F. Musshoff and T. Daldrup, *Int. J. Legal Med.*, 1992, *105(2)*, 105–109.

Disposition in the Body. Brotizolam is rapidly absorbed after oral administration and is completely metabolised to two major hydroxylated metabolites including 6-hydroxylated brotizolam. The drug is more slowly absorbed in the elderly and metabolic clearance is impaired. The metabolites are excreted in urine as glucuronide and sulfate conjugates, approximately 65%, and in faeces (22%). 2 to 3% of the dose is excreted unchanged. Brotizolam is rapidly distributed throughout the body.

Therapeutic concentration. The serum therapeutic concentration range is 1 to 20 μg/L.

20 elderly patients; 10 males and 10 females aged between 71 and 93 years, and 8 young, healthy volunteers; 5 males and 3 females, 21 to 26 years old, were administered with a 0.25 mg dose of brotizolam in the fasting state. Peak plasma concentrations ranged between 3.8 and 13.6 μg/L for the elderly patients and 5.0 to 6.6 μg/L for the young. These were reached within 1.1 and 1.7 h, respectively. [R. Jochemsen *et al.*, *Br. J. Clin. Pharmacol.*, 1983, *16*, 299S–307S].

Toxicity

A 42-year-old man was found dead and a toxicological screening carried out on his blood, urine and stomach contents. In his blood, 10.4 μg/L brotizolam, 3000 μg/L ibuprofen and 130 μg/L dihydrocodeine were found. In his urine, the brotizolam metabolite We 964, α-OH-triazolam, ibuprofen, dihydrocodeine and phenylpropanolamine were found at varying concentrations. Brotizolam and ibuprofen were both detected in stomach contents. It was determined that death occurred due to a combination of these drugs and alcohol poisoning. [T. Saito *et al.*, *J. Anal. Toxicol.*, 1997, *21*, 584–586].

Bioavailability. 70%.

Half-life. The mean elimination half-life is 4.4 h for the unchanged drug and 9.5 h for the metabolites. In the elderly, the half-life increases to approx. 9.8 h for the parent drug.

Volume of distribution. 0.40 to 0.77 L/kg.

Clearance. For the elderly: 109 mL/min and the young: 40 mL/min.

Protein binding. Approximately 81 to 91% with serum albumin and 89 to 95% plasma proteins.

Dose. The usual dose is 250 μg daily; this is reduced to 125 μg in the elderly and debilitated patients.

Broxaldine

Antiprotozoal

Synonym. Brobenzoxaldine
Proprietary name. It is an ingredient of Intestopan.
5,7-Dibromo-2-methyl-8-quinolyl benzoate
$C_{17}H_{11}Br_2NO_2$=421.1
CAS-3684-46-6

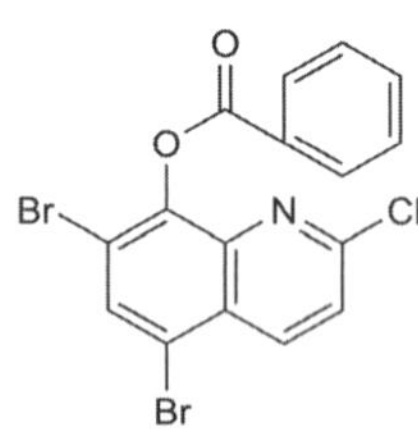

An off-white powder.
Practically insoluble in water; soluble in ether.

Colour Tests. Mandelin's Test—yellow; Marquis Test—yellow; Sulfuric Acid—yellow.

Thin-layer Chromatography. System TA—Rf 74; system TB—Rf 52; system TC—Rf 79; system TL—Rf 71; system TAE—Rf 78. (Acidified iodoplatinate solution, strong reaction.)

Gas Chromatography. System GA—RI 2686.

Mass Spectrum. Principal ions at *m/z* 105, 77, 106, 44, 51, 128, 78, 40.

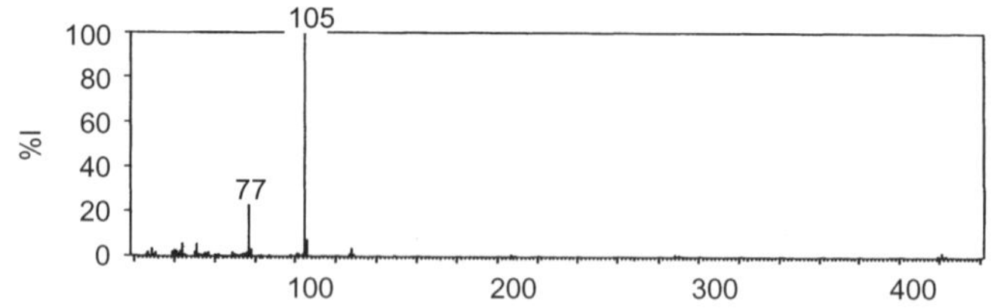

Dose. 120 to 300 mg daily, usually in combination with broxyquinoline.

Broxyquinoline

Antiprotozoal

Synonym. Broxichinolinum
Proprietary name. It is an ingredient of Intestopan.
5,7-Dibromo-8-quinolinol
$C_9H_5Br_2NO$=303.0
CAS-521-74-4

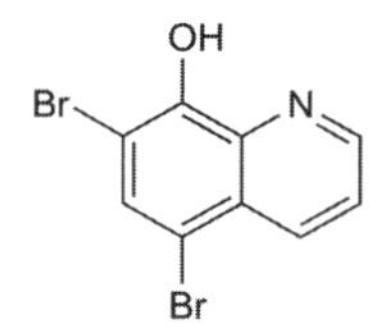

A cream-coloured powder. M.p. 196°.
Practically insoluble in water; freely soluble in acetic acid, benzene, chloroform and ethanol; slightly soluble in ether.

Partition Coefficient. Log *P* (octanol/water) 3.4.

Colour Tests. Liebermann's Test—orange; Marquis Test—yellow; Millon's Reagent—red; Sulfuric Acid—yellow.

Thin-layer Chromatography. System TA—Rf 51; system TL—Rf 03; system TB—Rf 00; system TC—Rf 06. (Acidified potassium permanganate solution, positive.)

Ultraviolet Spectrum. Aqueous acid—263 nm (A_1^1=800b); ethanol—249 nm (A_1^1=1525b), 325 nm (A_1^1=125b).

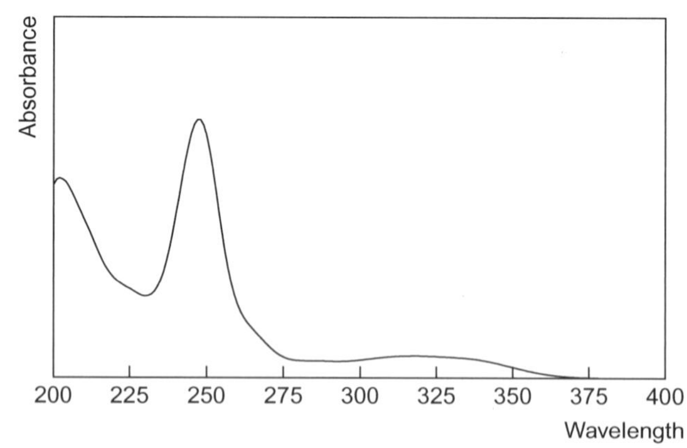

Infra-red Spectrum. Principal peaks at wavenumbers 1316, 1190, 930, 806, 1258, 782 cm^{-1} (KBr disk).

Mass Spectrum. Principal ions at *m/z* 303, 301, 305, 115, 194, 196, 114, 87.

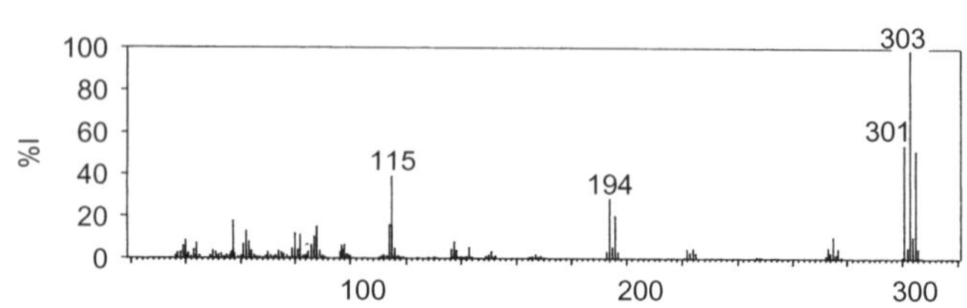

Quantification

Colorimetry. In urine—L. Berggren and O. Hansson, *Clin. Pharmacol. Ther.*, 1968, *9*, 67–70. In urine—L. A. M. Rodriguez and J. A. Close, *Biochem. Pharmacol.*, 1968, *17*, 1647–1653.

Disposition in the Body. Absorbed after oral administration. About 36% of a dose is excreted in the urine in 24 h, mainly as the glucuronide conjugate; very little unchanged drug is excreted and 8-hydroxyquinoline accounts for less than 2% of the dose.

Dose. 0.6 to 1.5 g daily, usually in combination with broxaldine.

Brucine

CNS Stimulant

Synonym. Dimethoxystrychnine
2,3-Dimethoxystrychnidin-10-one
$C_{23}H_{26}N_2O_4$=394.5
CAS—357-57-3 (anhydrous)

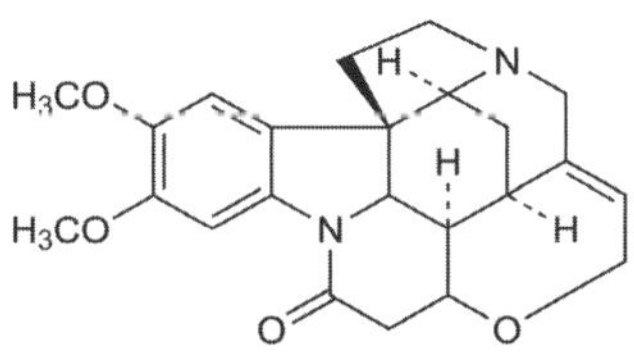

An alkaloid present in the seeds of *Strychnos nux-vomica* and other species of *Strychnos (Loganiaceae)*.
Small white crystals. M.p. 178°.

Brucine Sulfate

$(C_{23}H_{26}N_2O_4)_2,H_2SO_4,7H_2O$=1013
CAS—4845-99-2 (anhydrous); 60583-39-3 (heptahydrate)
Small white crystals or powder.
Soluble 1 in 75 of cold water, 1 in about 10 of boiling water, 1 in 105 of ethanol and 1 in 170 of chloroform.

Brucine tetrahydrate

$C_{23}H_{26}N_2O_4,4H_2O$=466.5
Becomes anhydrous at 100°.
Soluble 1 in 1320 of water, 1 in 100 of benzene, 1 in 1.3 of ethanol, 1 in 5 of chloroform, 1 in 187 of ether, 1 in 25 of ethyl acetate and 1 in 36 of glycerol.

Dissociation Constant. pK_a 2.3, 8.3 (25°).

Partition Coefficient. Log *P* (octanol/water), 1.0.

Colour Test. Liebermann's test—red.

Thin-layer Chromatography. System TA—Rf 16; system TB—Rf 00; system TC—Rf 17; system TL—Rf 01; system TAE—Rf 05; system TAF—Rf 07; system TAJ—Rf 04; system TAK—Rf 00; system TAL—Rf 64. (Acidified iodoplatinate solution, positive.)

Gas Chromatography. System GA—RI 3280.

High Performance Liquid Chromatography. System HA—*k* 11.1 (tailing peak); system HX—RI 312; system HY—RI 267.

Ultraviolet Spectrum. Aqueous acid—265 (A^1_1=330a), 300; aqueous alkali—266 (A^1_1=320a), 304 nm.

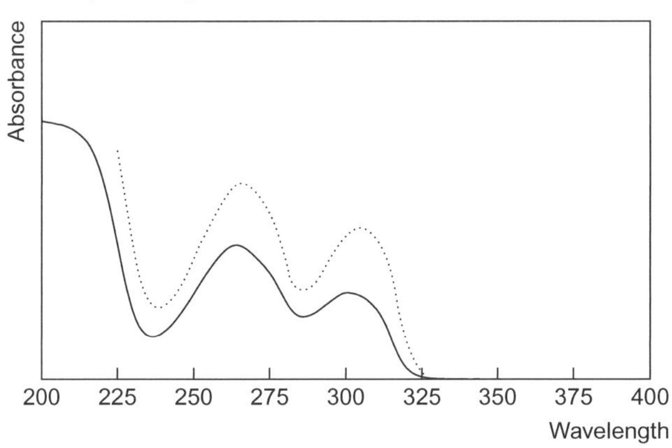

Infra-red Spectrum. Principal peaks at wavenumbers 1500, 1660, 1280, 1195, 1120, 1212 cm^{-1} (KBr disk).

Mass Spectrum. Principal ions at *m/z* 394, 395, 379, 392, 120, 197, 203, 393.

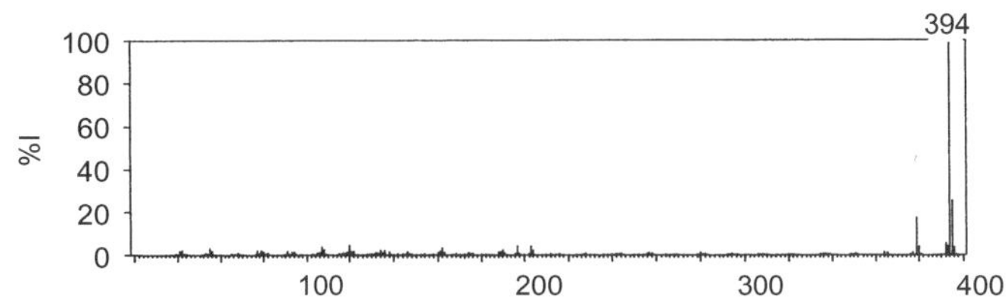

Buclizine

Antihistamine

1-[(4-Chlorophenyl)phenylmethyl]-4-[[4-(1,1-dimethylethyl)phenyl]-methyl]piperazine
$C_{28}H_{33}ClN_2$=433.0
CAS-82-95-1

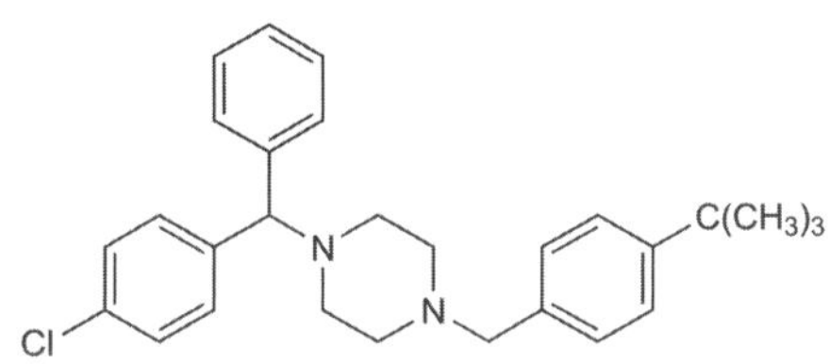

Buclizine Hydrochloride

Proprietary names. Aphilan R; Bucladin-S; Longifene. It is an ingredient of Equivert and Migraleve (pink tablets).
$C_{28}H_{33}ClN_2,2HCl$=506.0
CAS-129-74-8
A white crystalline powder. M.p. 230° to 240°.
Slightly soluble in water.

Thin-layer Chromatography. System TA—Rf 75; system TB—Rf 61; system TC—Rf 83; system TL—Rf 72. (Acidified iodoplatinate solution, positive.)

Gas Chromatography. System GA—buclizine RI 3360; M (desalkyl-) (norchlorcyclizine) RI 2520; M (chlorobenzophenone (ClBP)) RI 1850; M (OH-ClBP) RI 2300; M (carbinol) RI 1750; system GB—buclizine RI 3461; M (4-chloromethylbiphenyl) RI 1688; M (4-chlorobiphenylmethanone) RI 1862.

High Performance Liquid Chromatography. System HA—*k* 0.7; system HY—RI 454.

Ultraviolet Spectrum. Methanol—255, 260 nm (A^1_1=19b).

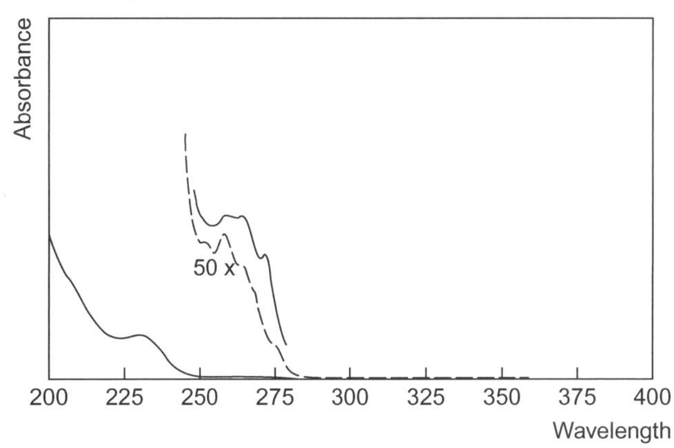

Infra-red Spectrum. Principal peaks at wavenumbers 1002, 1131, 754, 800, 1075, 694 cm^{-1} (KBr disk).

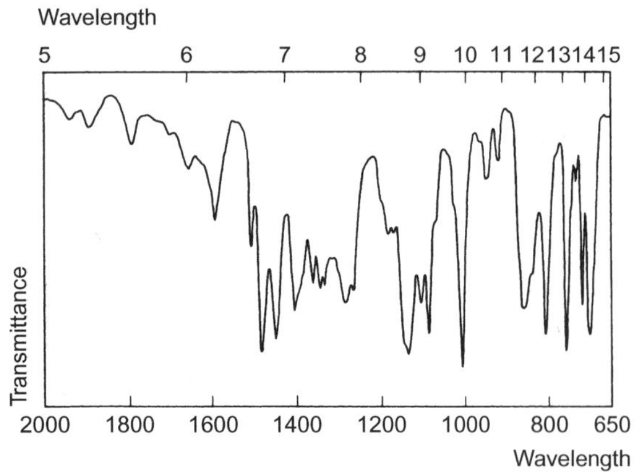

Mass Spectrum. Principal ions at *m/z* 231, 147, 285, 232, 201, 132, 165, 166.

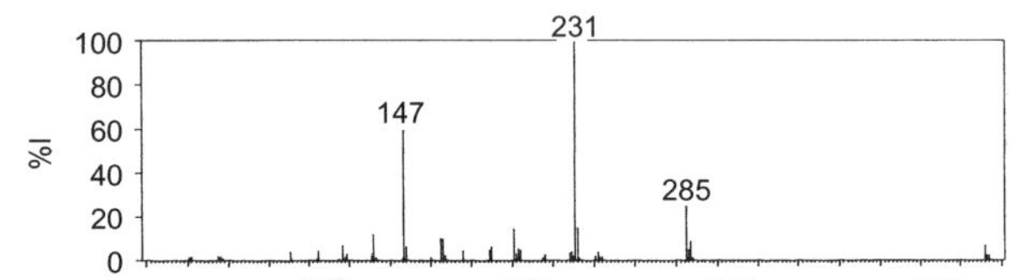

Dose. 25 to 150 mg of buclizine hydrochloride daily.

Buclosamide

Antifungal

N-Butyl-4-chloro-2-hydroxybenzamide
$C_{11}H_{14}ClNO_2$=227.7
CAS-575-74-6

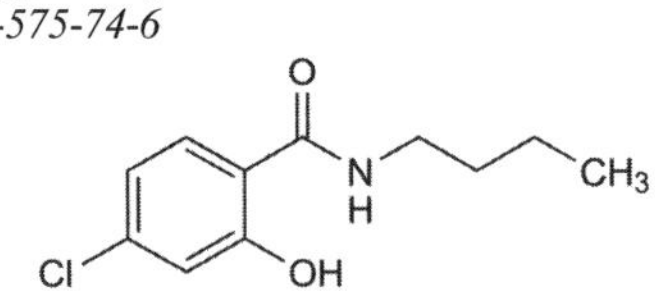

A white crystalline powder. M.p. about 91°.
Practically insoluble in water; soluble 1 in 3 of ethanol, and 1 in 3 of ether.

Partition Coefficient. Log *P* (octanol/water) 3.6.

Colour Tests. Folin–Ciocalteu Reagent—blue; Mandelin's Test—green→blue rim; Millon's Reagent—red.

Thin-layer Chromatography. System TA—Rf 90; system TB—Rf 02; system TC—Rf 67; system TL—Rf 70; system TAE—Rf 90. (Location under ultraviolet light, blue fluorescence; acidified potassium permanganate solution, positive.)

Ultraviolet Spectrum. Aqueous acid—245 nm (A^1_1=532b), 297 nm (A^1_1=204b); aqueous alkali—247 nm (A^1_1=391b), 325 nm (A^1_1=323a); ethanol—243 nm (A^1_1=497a), 301 nm.

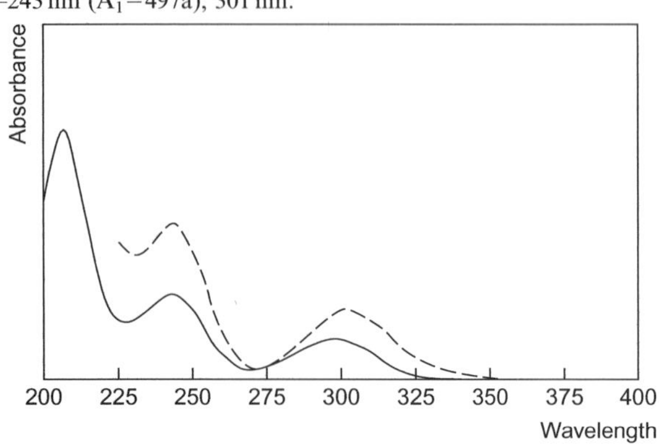

Infra-red Spectrum. Principal peaks at wavenumbers 1543, 898, 1190, 1590, 1201, 1506 cm^{-1} (KBr disk).

Mass Spectrum. Principal ions at *m/z* 155, 157, 227, 154, 185, 44, 30, 156.

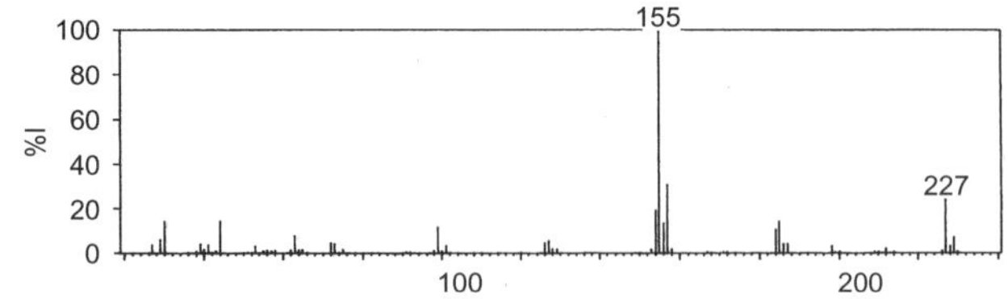

Use. Buclosamide has been applied topically in a concentration of 10%.

Budipine

Dopaminergic

Synonyms. Budipina; BY 701
1-(1,1-Dimethylethyl)-4,4-diphenylpiperidine
$C_{21}H_{27}N$=293.4
CAS—57982-78-2

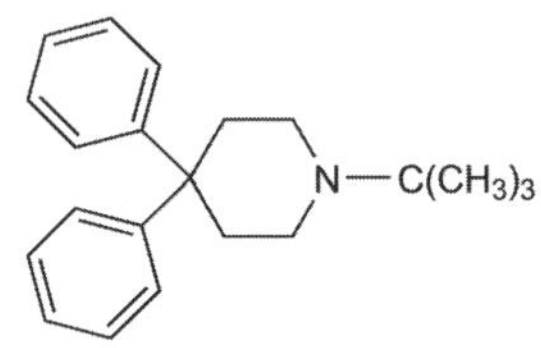

Crystals. M.p. 73° to 75°. B.p. 160° to 165°.

Budipine Hydrochloride
Proprietary name. Parkinsan
$C_{21}H_{28}ClN$=329.9
CAS—63661-61-0
Crystals.

Dissociation Constant. pK_a 10.55.

Partition Coefficient. Log *P* (octanol/water), 5.10; −0.55 (pH 4.5); 1.49 (pH 7.4).

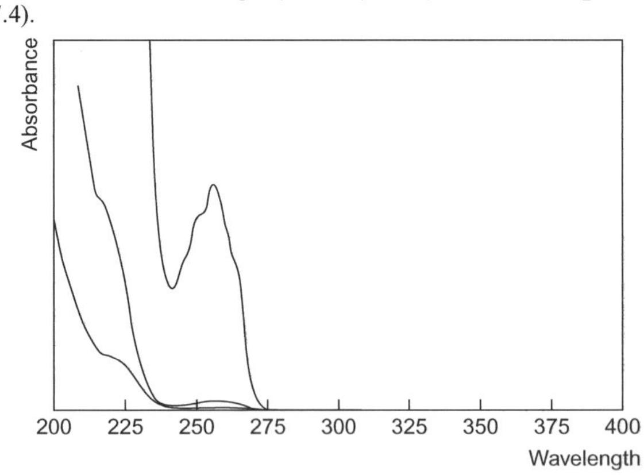

Infra-red Spectrum. Principal peaks at wavenumbers 767, 698, 1446, 1496, 1383, 1242 cm^{-1}.

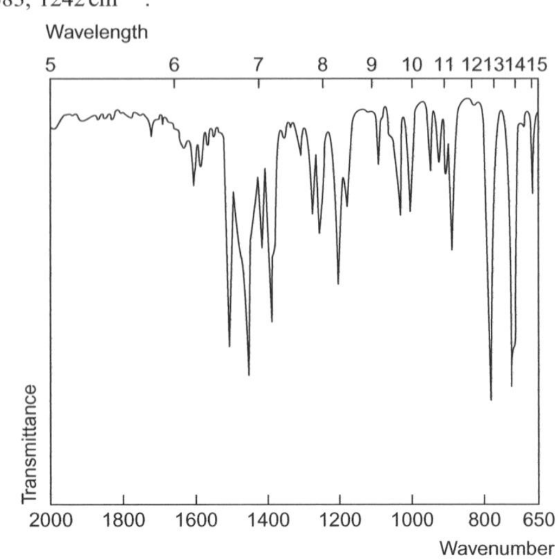

Mass Spectrum. Principal ions at m/z 278, 70, 56, 41, 42, 91, 115, 178.

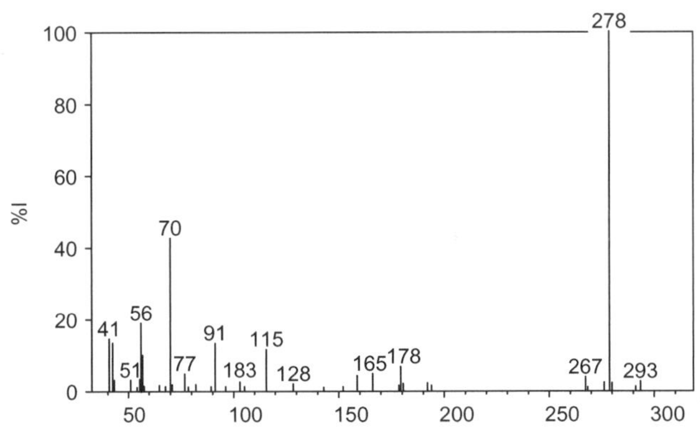

Disposition in the Body. It is well absorbed after oral administration (about 80%). It mainly metabolises to mono-*p*-hydroxybudipine which is significantly less active than budipine. About 80% of a dose is excreted via the kidneys, partly as unchanged budipine and to a greater extent as the hydroxymetabolite.

Toxicity. Can be poisonous intravenously.

Bioavailability. Approx. 47%.

Half-life. About 30 h.

Volume of distribution. 2.7 L/kg.

Protein binding. About 96%.

Dose. Initially, 10 mg three times daily. Maximum dose of 60 mg. In patients with severe impairment of renal function or liver damage, the dose should not exceed 30 mg.

Bufexamac

Analgesic

Synonym. CP-1044-J3
Proprietary names. Droxaryl; Feximac; Malipuran; Mofenar; Norfemac; Paraderm; Parfenac; Parfenal.
4-Butoxy-*N*-hydroxybenzeneacetamide
$C_{12}H_{17}NO_3$=223.3
CAS—2438-72-4

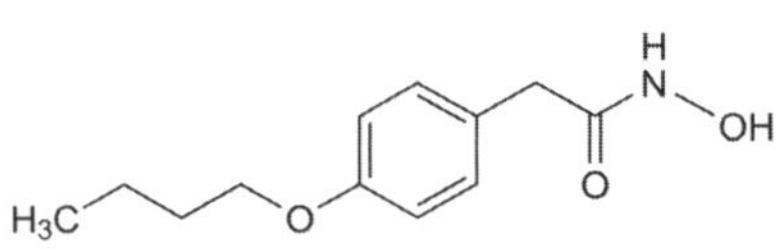

Almost colourless pearly flakes. M.p. 153° to 155°, with decomposition. Practically insoluble in water.

Partition Coefficient. Log *P* (octanol/water), 2.1.

Thin-layer Chromatography. System TD—Rf 11; system TE—Rf 18; system TF—Rf 19; system TG—Rf 36; system TAD—Rf 31.

Gas Chromatography. System GD—RRT of methyl derivative 1.12 relative to *n*-$C_{16}H_{34}$.

High Performance Liquid Chromatography. System HD—*k* 1.95.

Ultraviolet Spectrum. Aqueous alkali—275 nm (A_1^1=72b).

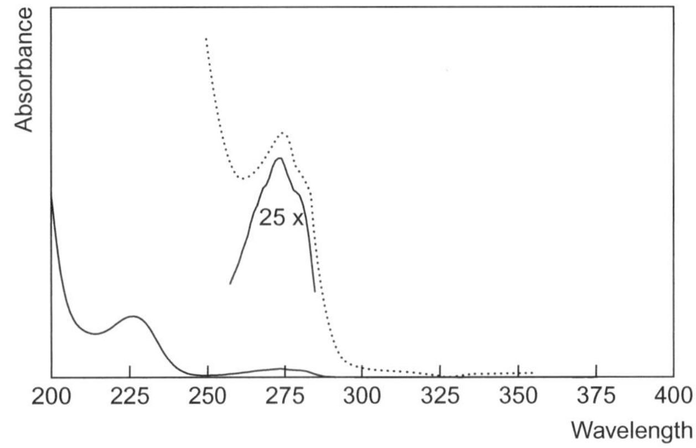

Infra-red Spectrum. Principal peaks at wavenumbers 1612, 1234, 1515, 980, 1052, 1176 cm^{-1}.

Mass Spectrum. Principal ions at m/z 107, 163, 223, 108, 29, 164, 41, 57.

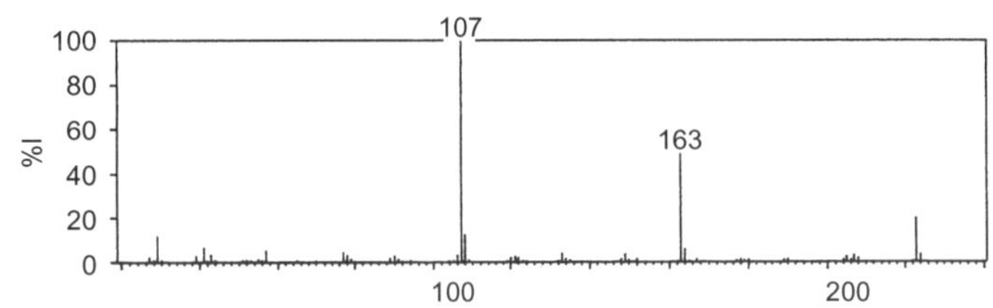

Dose. 0.75 to 1.5 g daily.

Buformin

Antidiabetic

N-Butylimidodicarbonimidic diamide
$C_6H_{15}N_5$=157.2
CAS—692-13-7

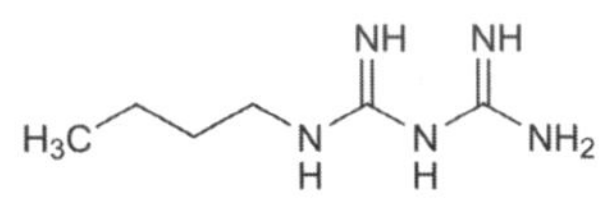

Buformin Hydrochloride
Proprietary names. Silubin; Sindiatil.
$C_6H_{15}N_5$,HCl=193.7
CAS—1190-53-0
A fine white crystalline powder. M.p. 174° to 177°.
Freely soluble in water and ethanol.

Partition Coefficient. Log *P* (octanol), −1.2.

Thin-layer Chromatography. System TA—Rf 02; system TB—Rf 00; system TC—Rf 00; system TL—Rf 00.

Gas Chromatography. System GB—not eluted.

Ultraviolet Spectrum. Aqueous alkali—230 nm (A_1^1=919b).

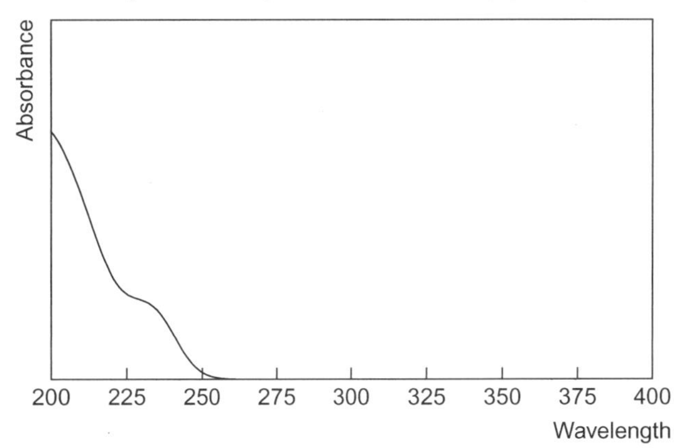

Infra-red Spectrum. Principal peaks at wavenumbers 1530, 1634, 1666, 1562, 1587, 1149 cm^{-1} (KBr disk).

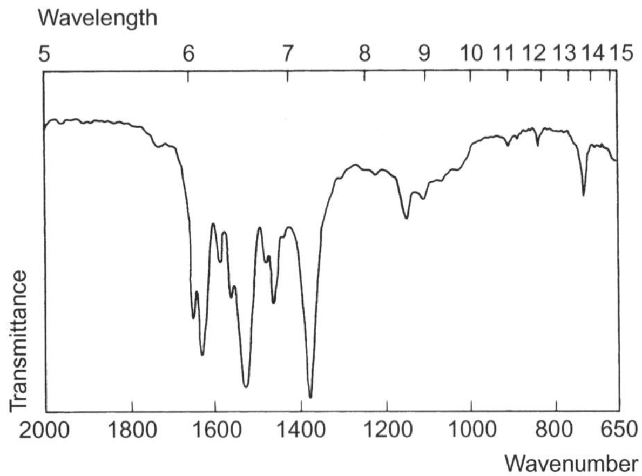

Mass Spectrum. Principal ions at *m/z* 43, 114, 85, 30, 101, 86, 44, 72.

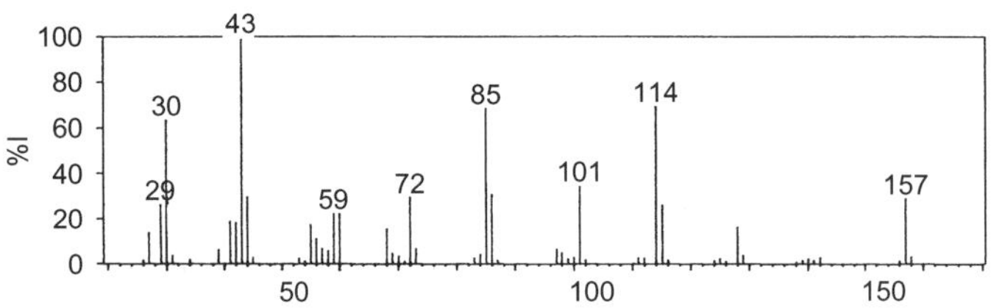

Quantification

Ultraviolet spectrophotometry. In urine—E. R. Garrett and J. Tsau, *J. Pharm. Sci.*, 1972, *61*, 1404–1410. In plasma or whole blood—E. R. Garrett *et al.*, *J. Pharm. Sci.*, 1972, *61*, 1411–1418.

Gas chromatography. In biological fluids or tissues: AFID—G. de Groot *et al.*, *J. Anal. Toxicol.*, 1980, *4*, 281–285. In plasma or urine: limit of detection 1 μg/L, ECD—S. B. Matin *et al.*, *Anal. Chem.*, 1975, *47*, 545–548.

Disposition in the Body. Absorbed after oral administration. About 35% of an oral dose is excreted in the urine as unchanged drug in 24 h and up to 30% is eliminated in the faeces; after intravenous administration about 90% is excreted unchanged in the urine in 12 h.

Therapeutic concentration. In plasma, usually in the range 0.2 to 0.6 mg/L.

Following a single oral dose of 100 mg to 6 subjects, a mean peak plasma concentration of 0.4 mg/L was reported after 2.5 h; plasma concentrations greater than 0.2 mg/L were maintained up to 8 h after the dose. [H. Gutsche *et al.*, *Arzneimittelforschung*, 1976, *26*, 1227–1229.]

Toxicity. Lactic acidosis is associated with plasma concentrations greater than 1 mg/L.

An 84-year-old diabetic died 6 h after admission to hospital with severe lactic acidosis caused by buformin. The plasma concentration on admission was 5.5 mg/L. Postmortem tissue concentrations were: plasma 3.2 mg/L, bile 6.3 mg/L, heart 3.0 μg/g, kidney 98 μg/g, liver 5.2 μg/g, lung 2.8 μg/g. [G. de Groot *et al.*, *J. Anal. Toxicol.*, 1980, *4*, 281–285.]

Half-life. Plasma half-life, about 2 to 6 h.

Volume of distribution. About 2 L/kg.

Protein binding. In plasma, about 10%.

Dose. 100 to 300 mg of buformin hydrochloride daily.

Bufotenine

Hallucinogen

Synonyms. *N,N*-Dimethylserotonin; 5-Hydroxy-*N,N*-dimethyltryptamine; Mappine.

3-[2-(Dimethylamino)ethyl]-1*H*-indol-5-ol

$C_{12}H_{16}N_2O = 204.3$

CAS—487-93-4

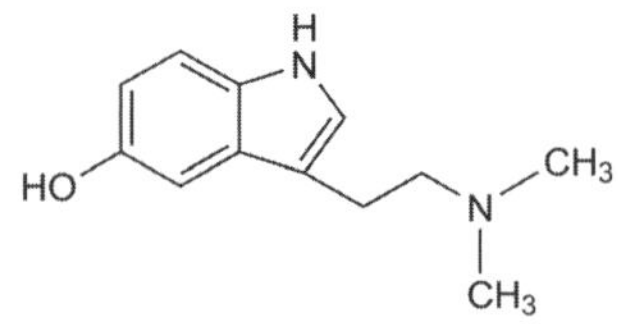

An indole alkaloid obtained from the seeds and leaves of *Piptadenia peregrina* and *P. macrocarpa* (Mimosaceae). It has also been isolated from species of *Amanita* (Agaricaceae) and from the skin glands of toads (*Bufo* spp.; Bufonidae).

A white crystalline powder. M.p. 138° to 140°.

Almost insoluble in water; freely soluble in ethanol; slightly soluble in ether; soluble in dilute acids and alkalis.

Partition Coefficient. Log *P* (octanol/water), 1.5.

Colour Test. Marquis Test—green-brown.

Thin-layer Chromatography. System TA—Rf 35; system TB—Rf 00; system TC—Rf 01; system TE—Rf 33; system TL—Rf 01; system TAE—Rf 10; system TAF—Rf 34. (Van Urk reagent, violet.)

Gas Chromatography. System GA—RI 2057.

High Performance Liquid Chromatography. System HA—*k* 3.1; system HY—RI 181.

Ultraviolet Spectrum. Aqueous acid—278 (A^1_1=269b), 297 nm.

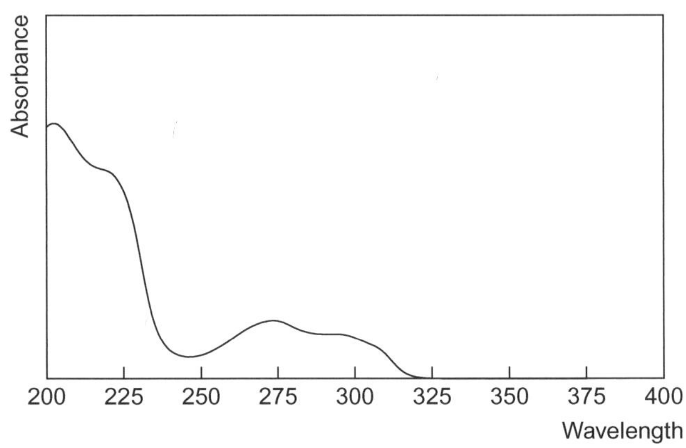

Infra-red Spectrum. Principal peaks at wavenumbers 1232, 824, 1493, 1615, 792, 1052 cm^{-1} (KBr disk).

Mass Spectrum. Principal ions at *m/z* 58, 204, 146, 59, 42, 160, 43, 159.

Quantification

Gas chromatography–mass spectrometry. In urine: limit of detection 300 ng/L—M. Räisänen and J. Kärrkkäinen, *J. Chromatogr.* 1979, *162*(4) *B Biomed. Appl.*, 579–584.

High performance liquid chromatography. In urine: electrochemical detection—N. Takeda *et al.*, *Neuroreport*, 1995, *27*, 2378–2380.

High performance liquid chromatography–mass spectrometry. In urine: —T. Forsstrom *et al.*, *Scand. J. Clin. Lab. Invest.*, 2001, *61*, 547–556.

Note. For reviews of bufotenine, see T. Lyttle *et al.*, *J. Psychoactive Drugs*, 1996, *28*, 267–290 and M. C. McBride, *J. Psychoactive Drugs*, 2000, *32*, 321–331.

Bufotenine and other bufadienolides derived from toad venom or secretions have been used for their aphrodisiac properties, see T.L. Barry *et al.*, *J. Forensic Sci.*, 1996, *41*, 1068–1073.

Bufylline

Xanthine Bronchodilator

Synonyms. Ambuphylline; Theophylline-aminoisobutanol.

Proprietary names. Butaphyllamine; Buthoid. It is an ingredient of Nethaprin and Nethaprin Dospan.

3,7-Dihydro-1,3-dimethyl-1*H*-purine-2,6-dione compound with 2-amino-2-methyl-1-propanol (1:1)
$C_{11}H_{19}N_5O_3$=269.3
CAS—5634-34-4

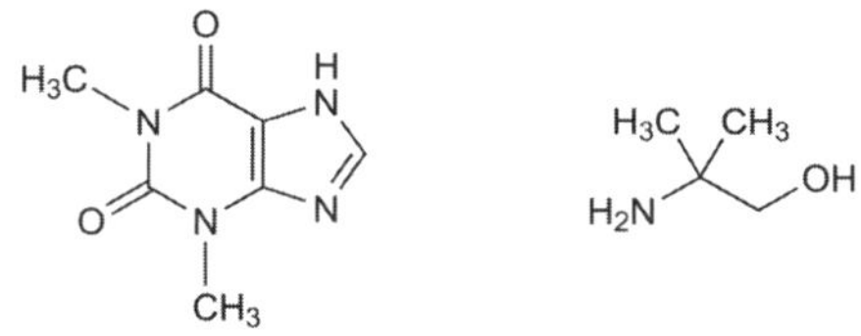

A white crystalline powder. M.p. 254° to 256°.
Slightly soluble in water.

Colour Test. Amalic Acid Test—red/violet.

Gas Chromatography. System GA—RI 2301.

Ultraviolet Spectrum. Aqueous acid—271 nm (A_1^1=350b).

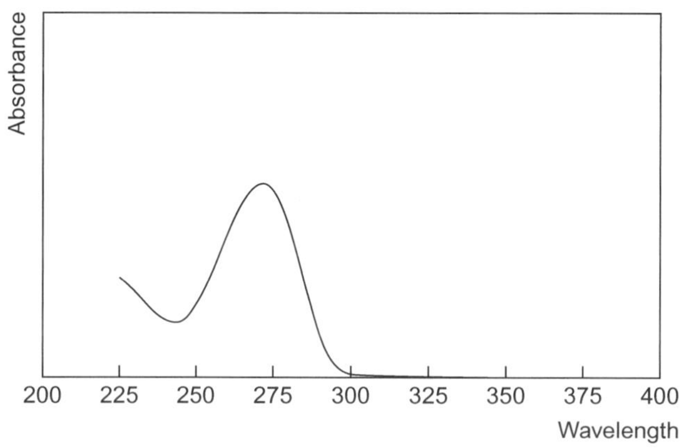

Infra-red Spectrum. Principal peaks at wavenumbers 1665, 1712, 1636, 1562, 740, 1180 cm^{-1} (KBr disk).

Mass Spectrum. Principal ions at *m/z* 180, 95, 68, 41, 58, 53, 123, 96.

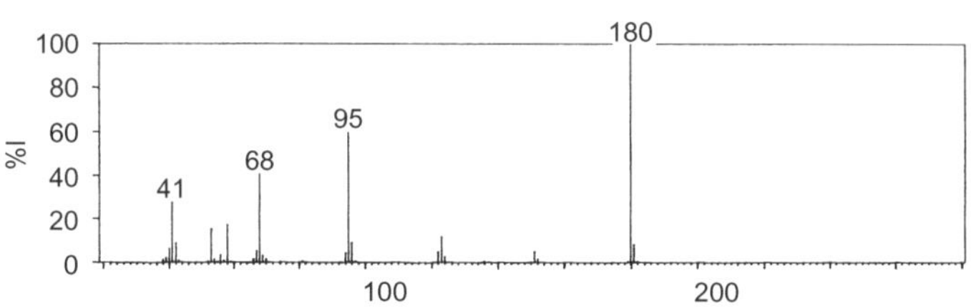

Dose. 60 to 120 mg every 3 to 4 h.

Bumetanide

Diuretic

Synonyms. PF-1593; Ro-10-6338.
Proprietary names. Burinex; Fordiuran.
3-(Aminosulfonyl)-5-(butylamino)-4-phenoxybenzoic acid
$C_{17}H_{20}N_2O_5S$=364.4
CAS—28395-03-1

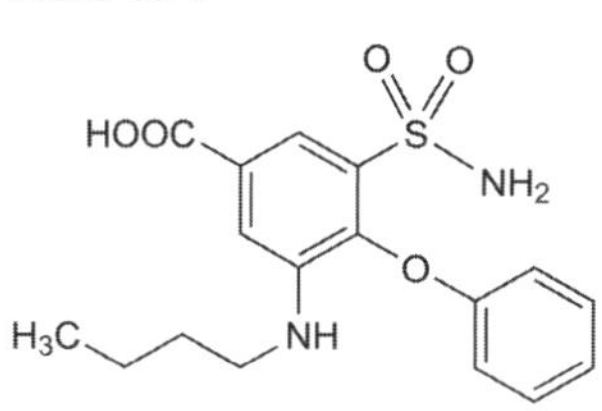

A white crystalline powder. M.p. about 230°.
Soluble 0.1 mg/mL water; 30.6 mg/mL ethanol; 18.7 mg/mL propylene glycol; >500 mg/mL dimethylacetamide; 76.5 mg/mL methanol; 0.4 mg/mL benzene; 21.6 mg/mL benzyl alcohol; 50.2 mg/mL acetone. Soluble in alkaline solutions.

Partition Coefficient. Log *P* (octanol/water), 2.6.

Colour Tests. Koppanyi–Zwikker Test—violet; Liebermann's Test—brown-orange; Mercurous Nitrate—black.

Thin-layer Chromatography. System TD—Rf 01; system TE—Rf 04; system TF—Rf 10; system TAD—Rf 06; system TAE—Rf 87; system TAJ—Rf 18; system TAK—Rf 42; system TAL—Rf 80.

Gas Chromatography. System GA—bumetanide-Me$_3$ RI 2970; system GX—bumetanide-Me$_3$ retention time 7.7 min; system GY—bumetanide-Me$_3$ retention time 4.9 min.

High Performance Liquid Chromatography. System HAA—retention time, 19.1 min.

Ultraviolet Spectrum. Aqueous acid—340 (A_1^1=80b); aqueous alkali—317 nm (A_1^1=87b).

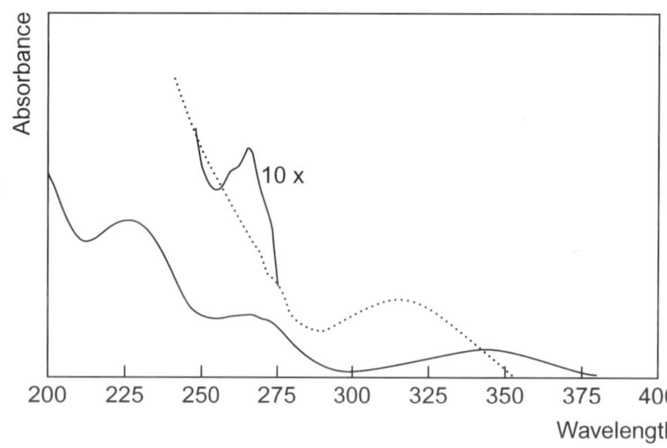

Infra-red Spectrum. Principal peaks at wavenumbers 1695, 1215, 1199, 1153, 1587, 1280 cm^{-1} (KBr disk).

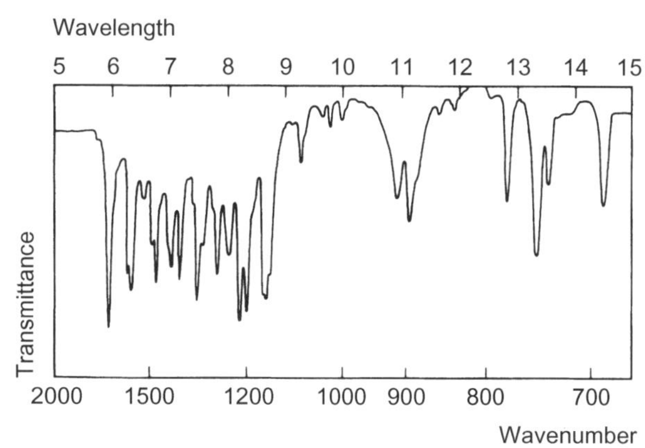

Mass Spectrum. Principal ions at *m/z* 321, 364, 304, 240, 168, 91, 322, 365.

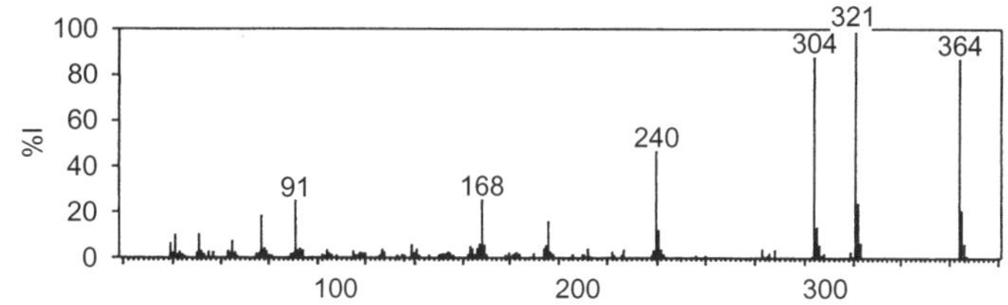

Quantification

Gas chromatography. In serum or urine: limit of detection 1 μg/L, FID—D. L. Davies *et al.*, *Clin. Pharmacol. Ther.*, 1974, *15*, 141–155.

Gas chromatography–mass spectrometry. In urine: limit of detection 10 to 50 µg/L—A. M. Lisi *et al.*, *J. Chromatogr.*, 1992, *581(1)*, 57–63.

High performance liquid chromatography. In plasma: limit of detection 5 µg/L, fluorescence detection—D. E. Smith, *J. Pharm. Sci.*, 1982, *71*, 520–523. In urine: limit of detection <10 µg/L, fluorescence detection—C. Y. Graaden *et al.*, *J. Anal. Toxicol.*, 1990, *14(2)*, 123–126. In plasma and urine: limit of detection 5 µg/L, fluorescence detection (λ_{em}=418 nm; λ_{ex}=228 nm)—T. G. Wells *et al.*, *J. Chromatogr.*, 1991, *570(1)*, 235–242. In urine: limit of detection 0.25 µg/L, amperometric detection—M. J. Legoburu *et al.*, *J. Chromatogr. Sci.*, 2001, *39(10)*, 425–430.

Disposition in the Body. Rapidly and completely absorbed after oral administration. Metabolised to some extent by hydroxylation of the butyl side-chain to give the 2′-, 3′-, and 4′-alcohols; the 3′-carboxylic acid and desbutyl metabolites have also been reported. About 50% of a dose is excreted in the urine as unchanged drug in 24 h together with 4 to 6% as the 3′-alcohol. A total of about 80% of a dose is excreted in the urine and 10% to 15% is eliminated in the faeces in 48 h.

Therapeutic concentration
After a single dose of 1 mg given to 12 subjects, a mean peak plasma concentration of 0.03 mg/L was attained in 1 to 8 h. [A. A. Holazo *et al.*, *J. Pharm. Sci.*, 1984, *73*, 1108–1113.]

Half-life. Plasma half-life, about 1 h.

Volume of distribution. About 0.2 L/kg.

Clearance. Plasma clearance about 3 mL/min/kg.

Protein binding. In plasma, about 96%.

Note. For a review of bumetanide see A. Ward and R. C. Heel, *Drugs*, 1984, *28*, 426–464.

Dose. Usually 1 to 2 mg daily; doses of 20 mg or more daily have been given.

Bunamidine

Anthelmintic (Veterinary)

N,*N*-Dibutyl-4-(hexyloxy)-1-naphthalenecarboximidamide
$C_{25}H_{38}N_2O$=382.6
CAS—3748-77-4

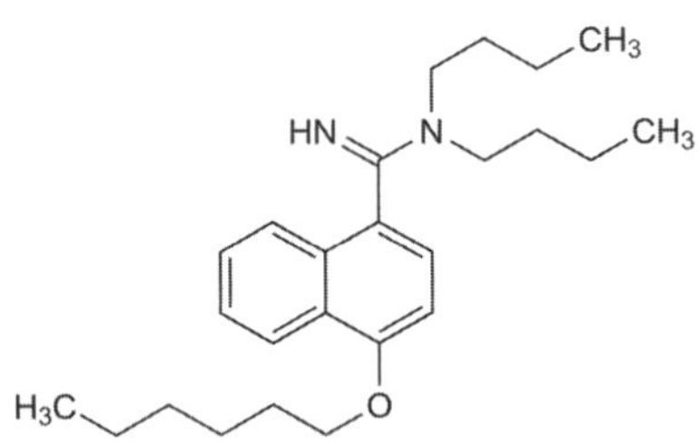

Bunamidine Hydrochloride

Proprietary name. Scolaban
$C_{25}H_{38}N_2O,HCl$=419.0
CAS—1055-55-6
A white crystalline powder. M.p. about 210°.
Soluble 1 in 200 of water, 1 in 2 of ethanol and 1 in 2 of chloroform; practically insoluble in ether.
Caution. Bunamidine hydrochloride is irritant, especially to the eyes, and should be handled with care.

Bunamidine Hydroxynaphthoate

Proprietary name. Buban
$C_{36}H_{46}N_2O_4$=570.8
CAS—13501-04-7
A pale yellow crystalline powder. M.p. 169° to 170°.
Practically insoluble in water; soluble 1 in 35 of ethanol, 1 in 3 of chloroform and 1 in 300 of ether.

Colour Tests. Mandelin's Test—green; Marquis Test—orange→red.

Thin-layer Chromatography. System TA—Rf 64. (Acidified iodoplatinate solution, positive.)

Gas Chromatography. System GA—not eluted.

Ultraviolet Spectrum. Aqueous acid—298 nm (A^1_1=240a).

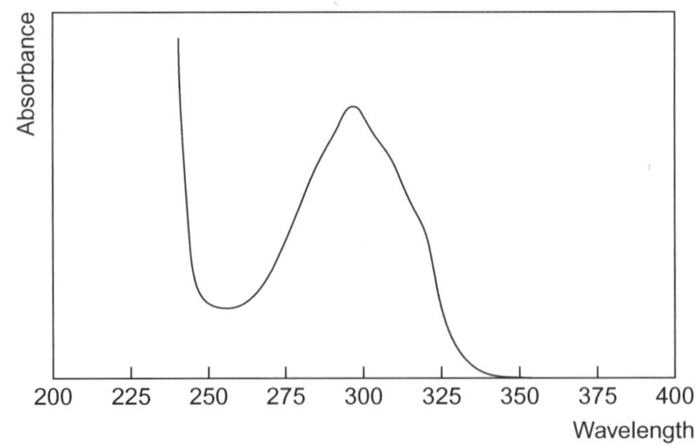

Infra-red Spectrum. Principal peaks at wavenumbers 1572, 1079, 1263, 1234, 763, 1511 cm^{-1} (KBr disk).

Bunazosin

Antihypertensive

Synonyms. Bunazocine; Bunazosine; DDQ
1-(4-Amino-6,7-dimethoxy-2-quinazolinyl)-hexahydro-4-(1-oxobutyl)-1H-1,4-diazepine
$C_{19}H_{27}N_5O_3$=373.5
CAS—80755-51-7

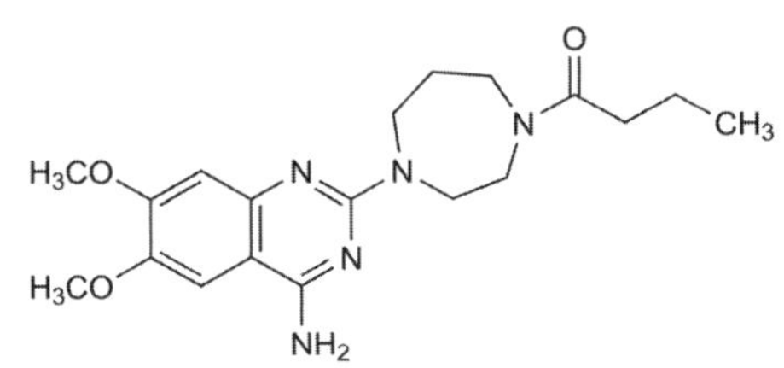

Bunazosin Hydrochloride

Synonym. E643.
Proprietary names. Andante; Bunazosin Retard; Detantol.
$C_{19}H_{28}ClN_5O_3$=409.9
CAS—52712-76-2
A white crystalline powder. M.p. 273°. It is very soluble in formic acid; slightly soluble in water and methanol; very slightly soluble in dehydrated ethanol; practically insoluble in ether.

Partition Coefficient. Log *P* (octanol/water), 0.215.

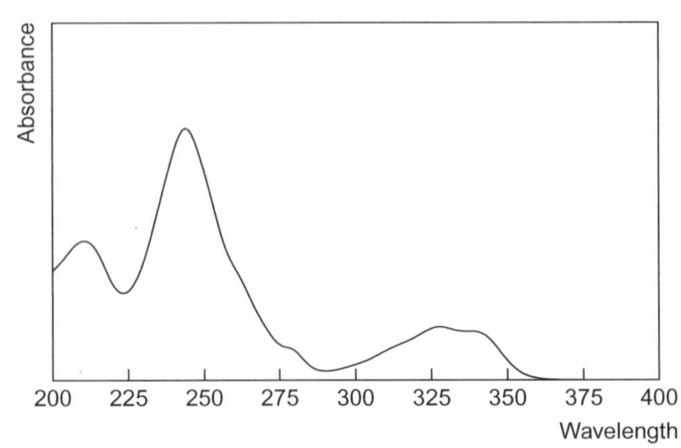

Infra-red Spectrum. Principal peaks at wavenumbers 1598, 1648, 1628, 2953, 3144, 864 cm^{-1} (hydrochloride salt).

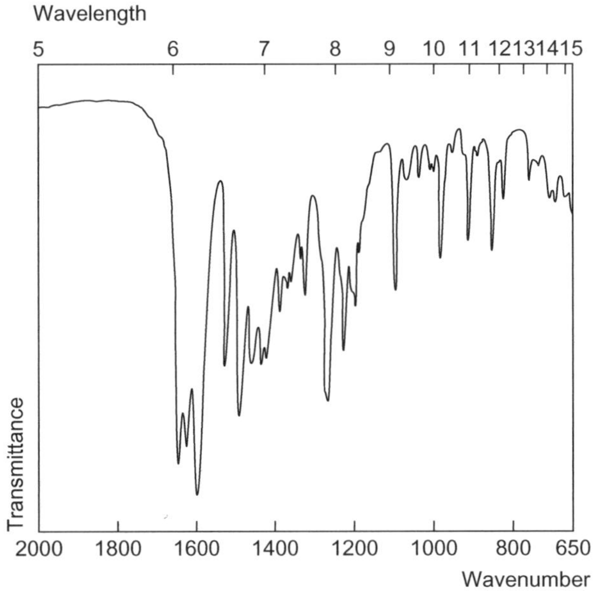

Mass Spectrum. Principal ions at *m/z* 247, 260, 233, 373, 234, 221, 245, 259.

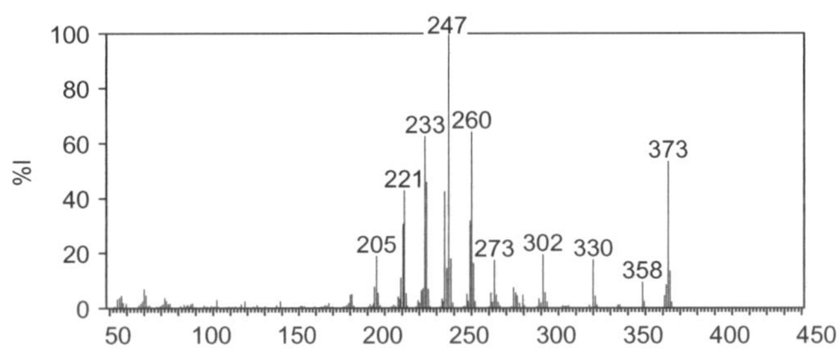

Quantification

High performance liquid chromatography. In plasma and urine: limits of detection 0.1 µg/L and 0.5 µg/L, respectively. Fluorescence detection (λ_{ex}=254 nm; λ_{em}=370 nm)—N. M. Nobumichi *et al.*, *Drug Invest.*, 1993, *6*, 5–9.

Disposition in the Body. Bunazosin is rapidly absorbed after oral administration and undergoes metabolism in the liver. It is eliminated mainly in faeces (60%) and the rest in urine as the unchanged drug (0.7%) and its metabolites. Bunazosin can pass through the placenta to the fetus and is secreted in milk.

Therapeutic concentration

12 healthy, adult males were administered with a 2 mg dose of bunazosin hydrochloride after a meal. The peak plasma concentration of the unchanged drug was 22.5 µg/L which was observed 1 h after administration. [Eisai Product Information Sheets].

12 healthy volunteers, aged between 65 and 75 years (2 males and 10 females), were administered with a single dose of 6 mg bunazosin (sustained release formulation). Peak plasma concentrations of 9.0 ± 4.0 µg/L were reached within 5 to 7 h. 12 healthy young volunteers, 22 to 39 years old (6 males and 6 females), were administered with the same dose. Peak plasma concentrations were lower, reaching 6.1 ± 2.6 µg/L for the males and 5.4 ± 1.5 µg/L for females within 3.5 to 6 h. [N. M. Nobumichi *et al.*, *Drug Invest.*, 1993, *6*, 62–69].

Toxicity. Acute overdose, over 12 mg/day, can result in tachycardia, hypotension, miosis and oliguria. Poison by subcutaneous, intramuscular, intravenous and intraperitoneal routes. Moderate toxicity by ingestion.

Bioavailability. Approx. 45%.

Half-life. Elimination half-life is approx. 2 h.

Volume of distribution. Apparent volume of distribution is approx. 3 to 6 L/kg.

Clearance. Body clearance, approx. 0.25 to 0.35 L/h/kg.

Protein binding. Bunazosin binds plasma proteins up to 97%.

Dose. An initial dose of 1.5 mg bunazosin (as the hydrochloride) is administered, which may be increased to 3 to 6 mg daily (sustained release formulation). The maximum dose is 12 mg/day. The usual adult daily dose for the sustained release preparation is 3 to 9 mg.

Bunitrolol

Beta-blocker

Synonym. Ko-1366
2-[3-[(1,1-Dimethylethyl)amino]-2-hydroxypropoxy]benzonitrile
$C_{14}H_{20}N_2O_2$=248.3
CAS—34915-68-9

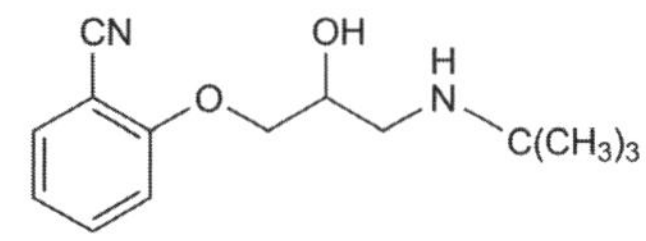

Bunitrolol Hydrochloride

Proprietary name. Stresson
$C_{14}H_{20}N_2O_2$,HCl=284.8
CAS—*23093-74-5*
A crystalline solid. M.p. about 164°.

Partition Coefficient. Log *P* (octanol/water), 1.6.

Thin-layer Chromatography. System TE—Rf 40; system TAE—Rf 16.

Gas Chromatography. System GA—bunitrolol RI 1948, bunitrolol-Art RI 1980.

Ultraviolet Spectrum. Aqueous acid—232 (A^1_1=332b), 292 nm (A^1_1=142b).

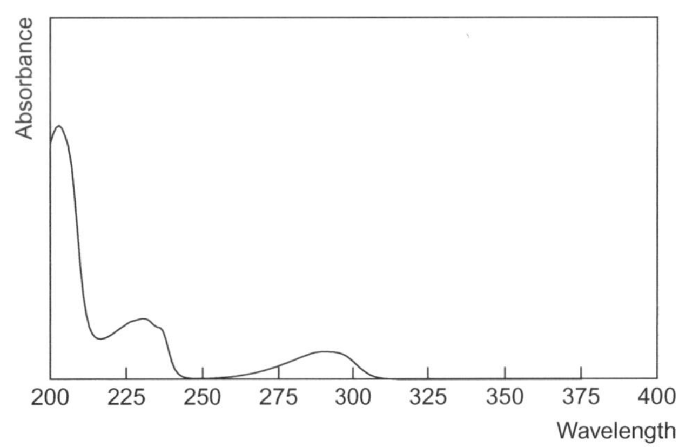

Quantification

High performance liquid chromatography. In plasma or urine: bunitrolol and 4-hydroxybunitrolol, limit of detection 2.5 µg/L in plasma and 250 ng/L in urine, fluorescence detection—A. Nagakura and H. Kohei, *J. Chromatogr.*, 1982, 232; *Biomed. Appl.*, *21*, 137–143.

Disposition in the Body. Bunitrolol is absorbed after oral administration and metabolised by *p*-hydroxylation followed by conjugation with glucuronic acid. About 1% of a dose is excreted in the urine as unchanged drug and 5% as the *p*-hydroxy metabolite, in 6 h.

Dose. Bunitrolol hydrochloride has been given in doses of 20 to 40 mg daily.

Buphenine

Vasodilator

Synonym. Nylidrin
4-Hydroxy-α-[1-[(1-methyl-3-phenylpropyl)amino]ethyl]benzenemethanol
$C_{19}H_{25}NO_2$=299.4
CAS—447-41-6

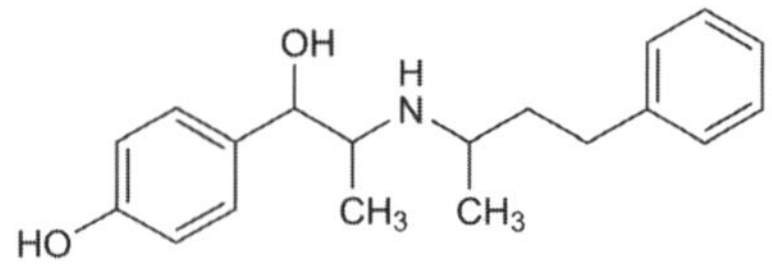

M.p. 111° to 112°.

Buphenine Hydrochloride
Proprietary names. Arlidin; Dilatol; Opino; Penitardon; Pervadil.
$C_{19}H_{25}NO_2,HCl = 335.9$
CAS—849-55-8
A white crystalline powder. M.p. 223° to 226°.
Soluble 1 in 65 of water and 1 in 40 of ethanol; practically insoluble in benzene, chloroform and ether.

Partition Coefficient. Log *P* (octanol/water), 3.3.

Colour Test. Marquis Test—red.

Thin-layer Chromatography. System TA—Rf 74; system TB—Rf 03; system TC—Rf 14; system TE—Rf 62; system TL—Rf 50; system TAE—Rf 33; system TAF—Rf 83. (Dragendorff spray, positive; Acidified iodoplatinate solution, positive; Marquis reagent, brown; Acidified potassium permanganate solution, positive.)

Gas Chromatography. System GA—RI 2314.

High Performance Liquid Chromatography. System HA—*k* 0.9; system HX—RI 370.

Ultraviolet Spectrum. Aqueous acid—273 (A^1_1=40a); aqueous alkali—242 (A^1_1=390b), 291 nm.

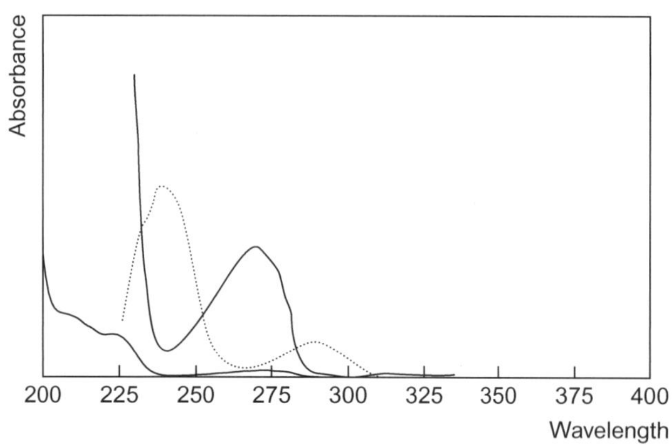

Infra-red Spectrum. Principal peaks at wavenumbers 1512, 1220, 750, 695, 1182, 837 cm^{-1} (KBr disk).

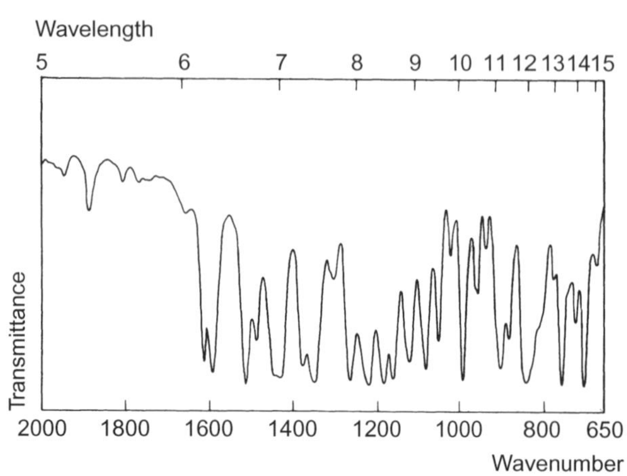

Mass Spectrum. Principal ions at *m/z* 91, 133, 176, 174, 44, 107, 92, 177.

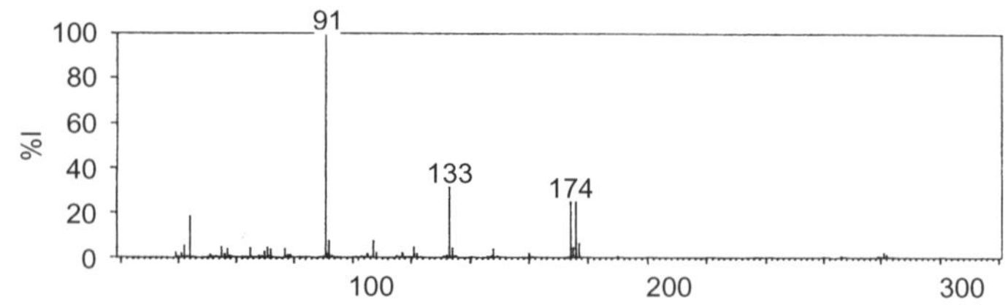

Quantification
Gas chromatography. In urine: FID—H. Li and P. Cervoni, *J. Pharm. Sci.*, 1976, *65*, 1352–1356.

Disposition in the Body. Buphenine is readily absorbed after oral administration. About 5% of a single dose is excreted in the urine as unchanged drug in 24 h.

Toxicity. The estimated minimum lethal dose in adults is 2 g and in children 200 mg.

Dose. 18 to 48 mg of buphenine hydrochloride daily.

Bupivacaine

Local Anaesthetic

1-Butyl-*N*-(2,6-dimethylphenyl)-2-piperidinecarboxamide
$C_{18}H_{28}N_2O = 288.4$
CAS—2180-92-9

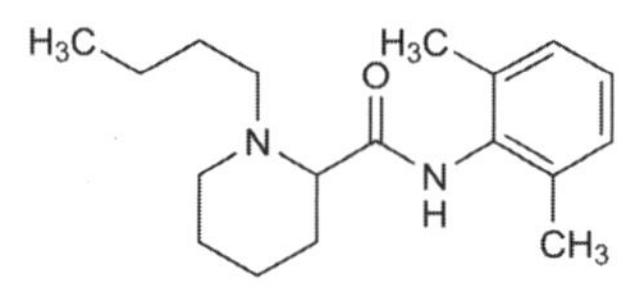

M.p. 107.5° to 108°.

Bupivacaine Hydrochloride
Proprietary names. Carbostesin; Marcain(e).
$C_{18}H_{28}N_2O,HCl,H_2O = 342.9$
CAS—18010-40-7 (anhydrous); 14252-80-3 (monohydrate)
A white crystalline powder. M.p. 258.5°.
Soluble 1 in 25 of water and 1 in 8 of ethanol; slightly soluble in acetone, chloroform, and ether.

Dissociation Constant. pK_a 8.1.

Partition Coefficient. Log *P* (octanol/water), 3.4.

Thin-layer Chromatography. System TA—Rf 69; system TB—Rf 42; system TC—Rf 73; system TE—Rf 80; system TL—Rf 65; system TAE—Rf 69; system TAF—Rf 79; system TAJ—Rf 59; system TAK—Rf 05; system TAL—Rf 40. (Acidified iodoplatinate solution, positive.)

Gas Chromatography. System GA—RI 2269.

High Performance Liquid Chromatography. System HA—*k* 0.9; system HQ—*k* 7.19; system HR—*k* 0.86; system HX—RI 366; system HY—RI 310; system HZ—retention time, 4.1 min.

Ultraviolet Spectrum. Aqueous acid—263 (A^1_1=16a), 271 nm.

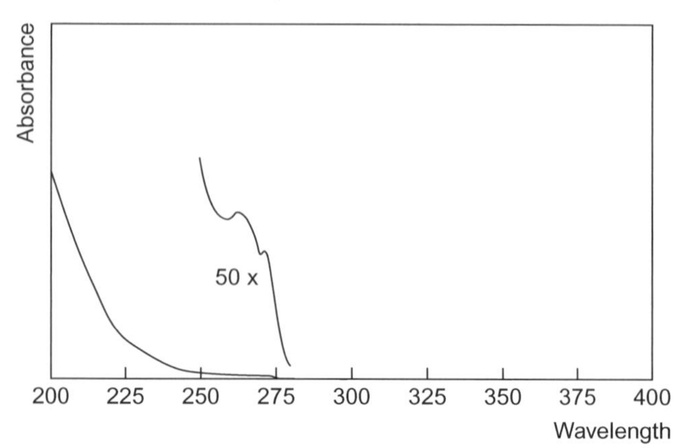

Infra-red Spectrum. Principal peaks at wavenumbers 1667, 1522, 1279, 1222, 787, 944 cm^{-1} (bupivacaine hydrochloride, KBr disk).

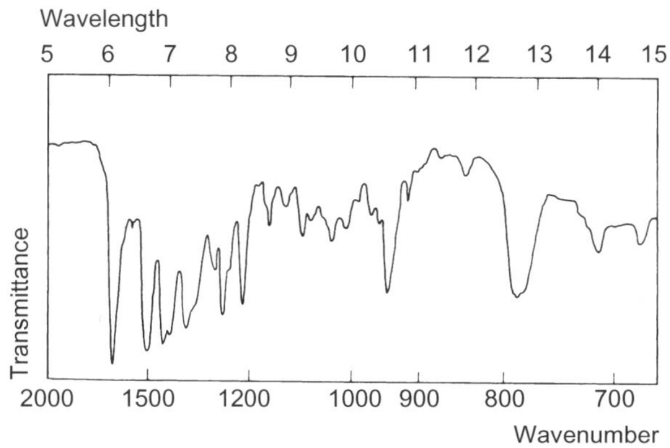

Mass Spectrum. Principal ions at *m/z* 140, 141, 84, 41, 29, 96, 56, 55.

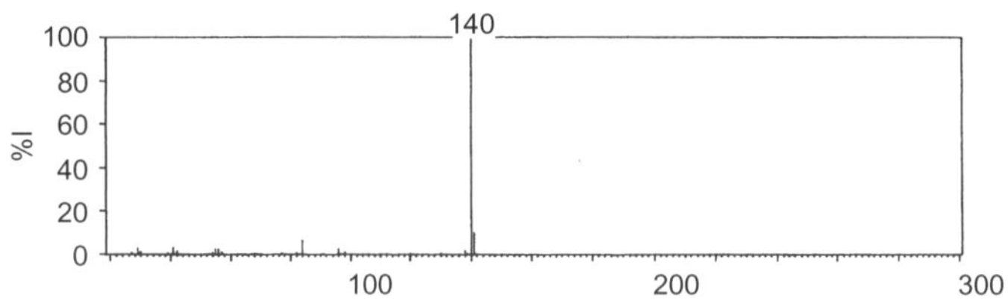

Quantification

Gas chromatography. In serum: bupivacaine and 2′,6′-pipecoloxylidide, limit of detection 50 µg/L for both compounds, AFID—L. J. Lesko *et al.*, *J. Chromatogr.* 1980, *182 B Biomed. Appl.*, *8*, 226–231. In blood: limit of detection 15 µg/L, FID—A. Berlin *et al.*, *J. Pharm. Pharmacol.*, 1973, *25*, 466–469.

Gas chromatography–mass spectrometry. In urine: limit of detection 5 µg/L, SIM (*m/z* 140)—A. Q. Zhang *et al.*, *J. Pharm. Biomed. Anal.*, 1998, *17(6–7)*, 1139–1142.

High performance liquid chromatography. In plasma: limit of quantification 125 µg/L and limit of detection 0.8 ng/70 µL injection, UV (λ=215 nm)—A. S. Gross *et al.*, *J. Chromatogr. B Biomed. Sci. Appl.*, 1999, *728(1)*, 107–115. In plasma: limit of quantification 2.5 µg/L and limit of detection 0.5 µg/L, MS detection—M. Stumpe *et al.*, *J. Chromatogr. B Biomed. Sci. Appl.*, 2000, *748(2)*, 321–330. In plasma: limit of detection 5 µg/L, UV detection—N. Rifai *et al.*, *Ther. Drug Monit.*, 2001, *23(2)*, 182–186.

Disposition in the Body. Bupivacaine is metabolised in the liver by oxidative dealkylation to 2′,6′-pipecoloxylidide (PPX); 3′- and 4′-hydroxylation also occur. Less than 10% of a dose is excreted in the urine as unchanged drug in 24 h.

Therapeutic concentration

15 infants, aged less than 5 months, undergoing minor lower abdominal procedures under a standard general anaesthesia were administered 0.25% bupivacaine at a dose of 2.5 mg/kg or 0.25% bupivacaine with adrenaline. The total plasma drug concentration was 114 to 446 µg/L (median, 400.5 µg/L) for those receiving the drug only compared with 372 to 1423 (median, 742) µg/L for those receiving the drug with adrenaline. [T. G. Hansen *et al.*, *Acta Anaesthesiol. Scand.*, 2001, *45(1)*, 42–47.]

A healthy female patient undergoing tubal ligation was induced with anaesthesia and maintained with propofol, droperidol and fentanyl. Lidocaine (4 mL at 1%) was also administered prior to incision followed by 2 mL *RS*-bupivacaine (0.5%). Peak plasma concentrations of 144 µg/L *R*-bupivacaine and 212 µg/L *S*-bupivacaine were reached 5.4 min after infiltration with the drug. [I. Abraham *et al.*, *J. Chromatogr. B Biomed. Sci. Appl.*, 1997, *703(1–2)*, 203–208.]

After slow IV infusion of 1.35 mg/kg to 3 subjects, peak venous-plasma concentrations of 2.6 to 4.5 mg/L were reported 3 to 17 min after completion of the infusion. [L. E. Mather *et al.*, *Clin Pharmacol. Ther.*, 1971, *12*, 935–943.]

After epidural administration of 150 mg with adrenaline to 12 subjects, mean peak plasma concentrations of 1.1 mg/L were reported at 0.3 h and peak cerebrospinal fluid concentrations averaged 30 mg/L at 0.5 h. [G. R. Wilkinson and P. C. Lund, *Anesthesiology*, 1970, *2*, 482–486.]

Toxicity. Bupivacaine is several times more toxic than lidocaine. Muscular rigidity has been reported in 2 subjects having blood concentrations of 9 and 12 mg/L following the administration of approximately 210 mg, and convulsions have been reported at plasma concentrations greater than 4 mg/L.

Half-life. Plasma half-life, about 1 to 3 h, increased in neonates.

Volume of distribution. About 1 L/kg.

Clearance. Plasma clearance, about 8 mL/min/kg.

Distribution in blood. Plasma : whole blood ratio, about 1.4.

Protein binding. In plasma, about 90%.

Note. For a review of the pharmacokinetics and pharmacodynamics of local anaesthetics, see M. B. Bachmann *et al.*, *Anaesthesiol. Reanim.*, 1991, *16*, 359–373. For a review of pharmacokinetic drug interactions in anaesthetic practice, see M. Wood, *Clin. Pharmacokinet.*, 1991, *21*, 285–307.

Dose. Bupivacaine hydrochloride is given by injection as a 0.25 or 0.5% solution (calculated as the anhydrous hydrochloride); maximum recommended dose is 2 mg/kg in any 4-h period.

Buprenorphine

Narcotic Analgesic

Synonyms. Buprenorphinum; RX-6029-M.
Proprietary name. Nopan
[5α,7α(*S*)]-17-(Cyclopropylmethyl)-α-(1,1-dimethylethyl)-4,5-epoxy-18,19-dihydro-3-hydroxy-6-methoxy-α-methyl-6,14-ethenomorphinan-7-methanol
$C_{29}H_{41}NO_4$=467.6
CAS—52485-79-7

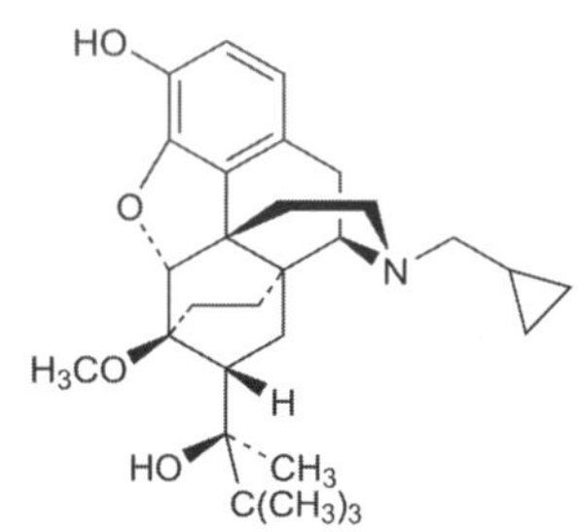

A white or almost white crystalline powder. M.p. 209°.
Very slightly soluble in water; freely soluble in acetone; soluble in methyl alcohol; slightly soluble in cyclohexane. Also dissolves in dilute solutions of acids.

Buprenorphine Hydrochloride

Synonyms. CL-112302; NIH-8805; UM-952.
Proprietary names. Anorfin; Buprenex; Buprex; Buprine; Finibron; Lepetan; Nopan; Prefin; Subutex; Temgesic.
$C_{29}H_{41}NO_4$,HCl=504.1
CAS—53152-21-9
A white or almost white crystalline powder.
Sparingly soluble in water; soluble in alcohol; freely soluble in methyl alcohol; practically insoluble in cyclohexane.

Dissociation Constant. pK_a 8.5, 10.0.

Partition Coefficient. Log *P* (octanol/water), 4.98.

Colour Tests. Liebermann's Test—black; Marquis Test—violet

Thin-layer Chromatography. System TA—Rf 76; system TB—Rf 09; system TC—Rf 68; system TE—Rf 80; system TL—Rf 69; system TAE—Rf 80; system TAJ—Rf 62; system TAK—Rf 04; system TAL—Rf 77.

Gas Chromatography. System GA—buprenorphine RI 3360, buprenorphine-AC RI 3410, art (-H_2O) RI 3240, art (-H_2O)-AC RI 3320; system GB—buprenorphine RI 3610; system GM—not eluted.

High Performance Liquid Chromatography. System HA—*k* 0.4; system HC—*k* 0.05; system HX—RI 397; system HY—RI 339; system HZ—retention time 5.0 min; system HAA—retention time 14.0 min.

Ultraviolet Spectrum. Aqueous acid—286 nm (A_1^1=33b); aqueous alkali—300 nm.

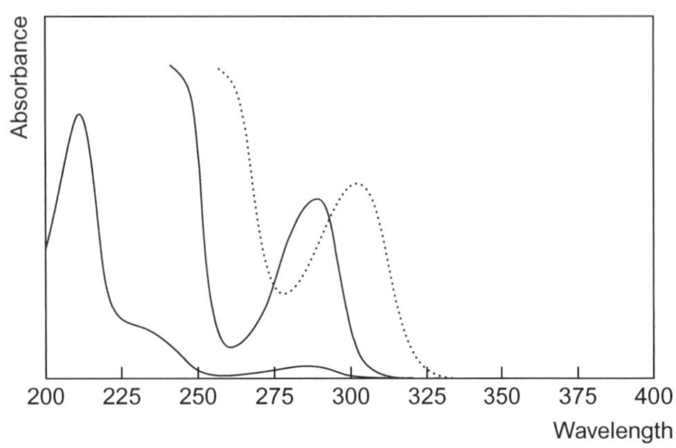

Infra-red Spectrum. Principal peaks at wavenumbers 1320, 1077, 1503, 1155, 1120, 947 cm^{-1} (buprenorphine hydrochloride, KCl disk).

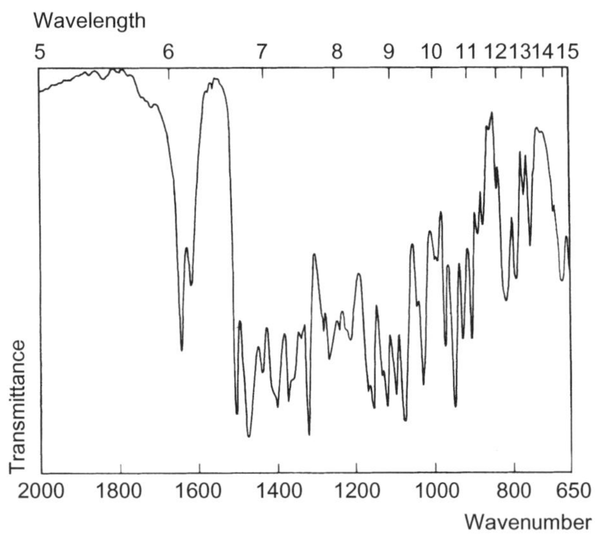

Mass Spectrum. Principal ions at *m/z* 55, 378, 43, 29, 57, 410, 379, 84.

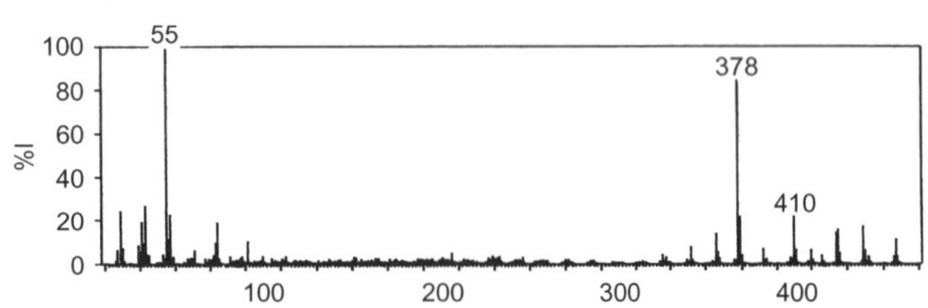

Quantification

Gas chromatography. In plasma: limit of quantification 0.1 µg/L, ECD—E. T. Everhart *et al.*, *Clin. Chem.*, 1997, *43*, 2292—2302.

Gas chromatography–mass spectrometry. In urine: buprenorphine and norbuprenorphine, limit of quantification 1 µg/L—A. M. Lisi *et al.*, *J. Chromatogr. B. Biomed. Sci. Appl.*, 1997, *692*, 67–77. In plasma: limits of quantification 0.1 to 0.5 µg/L—D. E. Moody *et al.*, *J. Anal. Toxicol.*, 1997, *21*, 406–414. In urine or hair: buprenorphine and norbuprenorphine, limits of quantification in urine 0.25 µg/L and 0.2 µg/L, respectively and 0.005 ng/mg for both compounds in hair—F. Vincent *et al.*, *J. Anal. Toxicol.*, 1999, *23*, 270–279. In plasma: buprenorphine and norbupreorphine, limits of quantification 0.05 µg/L and 0.1 µg/L, respectively—S. Gopal *et al.*, *Eur. J. Pharm. Biopharm.*, 2001, *51*, 147–151.

High performance liquid chromatography. In urine: buprenorphine and norbuprenorphine, limits of detection 250 ng/L and 100 ng/L, respectively, electrochemical detection—L. Debrabandere *et al.*, *J. Chromatogr.*, 1991, *564*, 557–566. In plasma: limit of detection 1 µg/L, fluorescence detection—S. T. Ho *et al.*, *J. Chromatogr.*, 1991, *570*, 339–350. In urine: buprenorphine and *N*-dealkylbuprenorphine, limits of detection 0.2 µg/L and 0.15 µg/L, electrochemical detection, comparison with RIA—L. Debrabandere *et al.*, *J. Forensic Sci.*, 1992, *37*, 82–89. In plasma or urine: buprenorphine and norbuprenorphine, limit of detection 40 ng/L, electrochemical detection—E. Schleyer *et al.*, *J. Chromatogr.*, 1993, *614*, 275–283. In hair: buprenorphine and *N*-dealkylbuprenorphine, limits of detection about 0.02 ng/mg and 0.01 ng/mg, respectively, ECD—P. Kintz *et al.*, *J. Forensic Sci.*, 1994, *39*, 1497–1503. In plasma: UV detection—F. Lagrange *et al.*, *J. Pharm. Biomed. Anal.*, 1998, *16*, 1295–1300.

High performance liquid chromatography–mass spectrometry. In biological fluids or hair: buprenorphine and norbuprenorphine, limits of detection 0.1 µg/L and 0.05 µg/L in blood and 4 pg/mg and 2 pg/mg in hair, respectively—A. Traqui *et al.*, *J. Forensic Sci.*, 1997, *42*, 111–114.

Fluoroimmunoassay. In urine: limit of detection 20 µg/L—L. Debradandere *et al.*, *J. Forensic Sci.*, 1995, *40*, 250–253.

Disposition in the Body. Following intramuscular injection, buprenorphine rapidly reaches peak plasma concentration. Absorption also takes place through the buccal mucosa following sublingual administration. It is metabolised mainly by *N*-dealkylation via cytochrome P450 CYP3A4 to *N*-dealkylbuprenorphine (norbuprenorphine) and conjugation. It is eliminated mainly in the faeces with a small proportion excreted in the urine, as metabolites. Buprenorphine is subject to considerable first-pass metabolism following oral administration. Small amounts of buprenorphine are distributed into breast milk.

Therapeutic concentration

After sublingual administration of buprenorphine solution at a dose of 16 mg/70 kg daily to 10 subjects, mean plasma concentrations of 0.67 µg/L were attained 24 h after each dose. Different thrice-weekly dosing schedules with doses of 16 to 44 mg/70 kg resulted in plasma concentrations varying from 0.9 to 1.69 µg/L at 24 h and 0.41 to 0.96 µg/L at 48 h. [M. C. Charwarski *et al.*, *Drug Alcohol Depend.*, 1999, *55*, 157–163.]

In 6 subjects each receiving a 7.7 mg dose of buprenorphine in liquid form (sublingually) and 8 mg in tablet form, 1 week apart, peak plasma levels were 7.1 µg/L at 0.9 h and 2.9 µg/L at 1.2 h for the liquid and tablet dosages, respectively. [R. P. Nath *et al.*, *J. Clin. Pharmacol.*, 1999, *39*, 619–623.]

In 11 patients receiving maintenance doses of 8 mg buprenorphine sublingually, those receiving the dose daily had a mean steady-state plasma concentration (at 24 h) of 0.80 µg/L and those receiving the dose on alternate days had a level of 0.77 µg/L at 24 h. Daily and alternate-day steady-state norbuprenorphine plasma concentrations were 1.0 and 0.9 pg/L, respectively. [J. J. Kuhlman *et al.*, *Addiction*, 1998, *93*, 549–559.]

Toxicity

A 25-year-old male who apparently had committed suicide (drug packages including high-dose sublingual tablets of buprenorphine were found next to his body) had the following postmortem tissue concentrations of buprenorphine and norbuprenorphine: blood 3.3 and 0.4 mg/L, urine 3.4 and 0.6 mg/L, bile 2035 and 536 mg/L, brain 6.4 and 3.9 µg/g; high concentrations of amino-7-flunitrazepam, the main metabolite of flunitrazepam, were also detected in the blood, urine and gastric fluid. [J. M. Gaulier *et al.*, *J. Forensic Sci.*, 2000, *45*, 226–228.]

In 2 series of 39 and 78 fatalities involving buprenorphine, postmortem blood levels were 0.0005 to 0.0510 mg/L (mean 0.0102) and 0.0001 to 0.0760 mg/L (mean 0.0126); norbuprenorphine levels were 0.0002 to 0.0471 mg/L (mean 0.0082) and <0.0001 to 0.0650 mg/L (mean 0.0106), respectively. Two of the deaths were suicides, with blood buprenorphine concentrations of 0.1440 and 3.276 mg/L. [P. Kintz, *Forensic Sci. Int.*, 2001, *121*, 65–69.]

Half-life. Plasma half-life, 1.2 to 7.2 h.

Volume of distribution. About 1.4 L/kg.

Clearance. Plasma, about 13 mL/min/kg.

Protein binding. In plasma, about 96%.

Dose. In the treatment of pain, equivalent of 300 to 600 µg of buprenorphine given parenterally, or 200 to 400 µg by the sublingual route, every 6 to 8 h. In the treatment of opioid dependence, initially 0.8 to 4 mg sublingually once daily; maintenance, up to maximum of 32 mg daily.

Bupropion

Antidepressant

Synonym. Amfebutamone
1-(3-Chlorophenyl)-2-[(1,1-dimethylethyl)-amino]-1-propanone
$C_{13}H_{18}ClNO$=239.7
CAS—34911-55-2

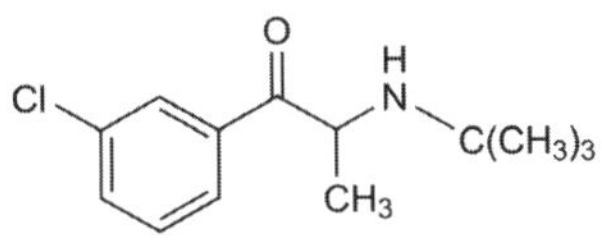

A pale yellow oil. B.p. 52°. It is soluble in methanol, ethanol, acetone, ether and benzene.

Bupropion Hydrochloride

Synonyms. Amfebutamone hydrochloride; BW-323.
Proprietary names. Wellbutrin; Zyban.
$C_{13}H_{19}Cl_2NO$=276.2
CAS—31677-93-7
A white crystalline powder. M.p. 233° to 234°. It is soluble in water, alcohol and hydrochloric acid.

Gas Chromatography. System GB—RI 1645 (bupropion); RI 1898 (M (OH^-)).

Column: silica (DB-5, 12 m) and HP-1 (10 m). Column temperature: 100° to 300° at 10°/min with a 10-min final hold. Detection: nitrogen–phosphorous. Reference compound: *n*-propylamphetamine. Retention time: 8.62 min. [T. P. Rohrig and N. G. Ray, *J. Anal. Toxicol.*, 1992, 16, 343–345].

High Performance Liquid Chromatography. Column: trimethylsilyl (5 µm, 250 × 4.6 mm i.d.). Mobile phase: monobasic potassium phosphate buffer (0.05 M):acetonitrile (80:20) with sodium heptanesulfonate (0.007 M) and triethylamine (0.01 M), pH adjusted to 3.0 with phosphoric acid, 2.3 mL/min flow rate. UV detection (λ=254 nm). Retention time: 11.5 min. [T. B. Cooper *et al.*, *J. Pharm. Sci.*, 1984, *73*, 1104–1107].

Column: silica (Econosphere, 3 µm, 100 × 4.6 mm). Mobile phase: methanol:$(NH_4)H_2PO_4$ (50 mM, adjusted to pH 3.2 with phosphoric acid (50 mM)) (95:5), flow rate 0.9 mL/min. UV detection (λ=248 nm). Retention time: 4.29 min. [T. A. Jennison *et al.*, *J. Anal. Toxicol.*, 1995, *19*, 69–72].

Ultraviolet Spectrum. Methanol—249, 296 nm.

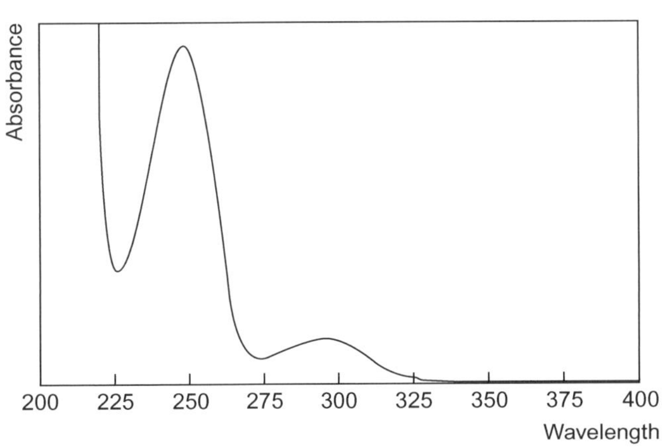

Infra-red Spectrum. Principal peaks at wavenumbers 1560, 1691, 2676, 2982, 1458, 739 cm^{-1}.

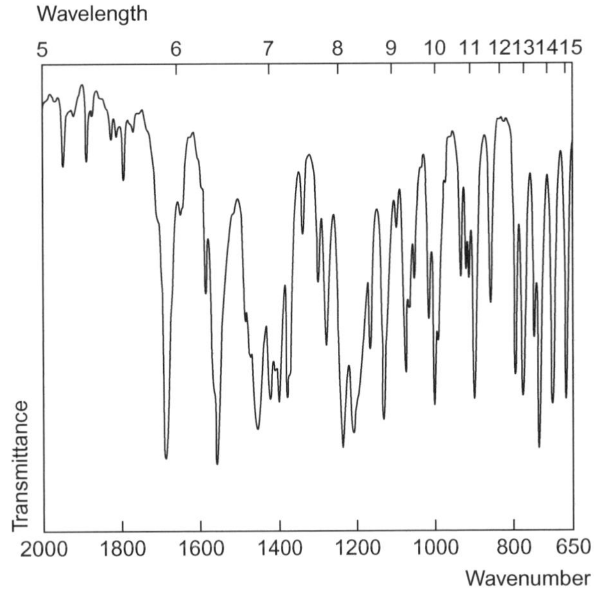

Mass Spectrum. Principal ions at *m/z* 44, 100, 57, 111, 139, 75, 84, 224.

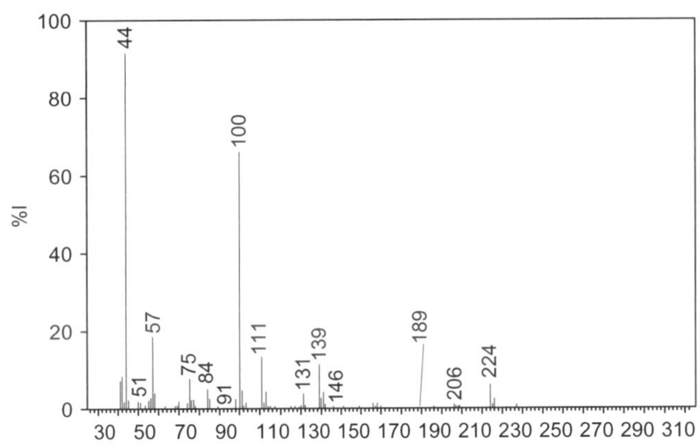

Quantification

Gas chromatography–mass spectrometry. In blood: limit of detection 0.1 mg/L—N. Wohlenberg *et al.*, *TIAFT Bull. Case Notes*, 1992, *22*.

High performance liquid chromatography. In plasma: limit of detection of bupropion is 5.0 µg/L and for its metabolites 0.1 mg/L. UV detection (λ 254 nm)—T. B. Cooper *et al.*, *J. Pharm. Sci.*, 1984, *73*, 1104–1107. In plasma/serum: limit of detection 5.0 µg/L. UV detection (λ 248 nm)—T. A. Jennison *et al.*, *J. Anal. Toxicol.*, 1995, *19*, 69–72.

Disposition in the Body. Bupropion is well absorbed and undergoes hepatic metabolism, via oxidation, hydroxylation and reduction. Peak plasma concentrations are reached within 3 h for sustained release preparations and 2 h for immediate release. Several metabolites are produced which are pharmacologically active. The three active metabolites are hydroxybupropion, the major metabolite, threohydrobupropion and erythrohydrobupropion. More than 60% of a dose is excreted in urine within 24 h, 87% over 96 h and 10% in faeces, with less than 1% being the parent drug. Bupropion crosses the placenta and is secreted in milk.

Therapeutic concentration. The serum therapeutic concentration range is 0.025 to 0.1 mg/L.

Toxicity. Blood levels above 0.17 mg/L are associated with seizures and those above 0.45 mg/L can be fatal. Other toxic effects include tachycardia, hallucinations and loss of consciousness.

A 45-year-old woman with a history of psychological problems took two bottles of bupropion (100 to 150 tablets, up to 22.5 g). She was admitted to hospital semiconscious and died after failing to respond to resuscitation. [J. E. Meeker *et al.*, *TIAFT Bull. Case Notes*, 1992, *22*].

Half-life. Terminal half-life is approx. 14 h (regular release formulation) and 21 h (sustained release).

Volume of distribution. Apparent volume of distribution is 27 to 63 L/kg.

Clearance. Approx. 160 L/h.

Protein binding. Approx. 84%.

Dose. Initial dose of 100 mg twice daily, after 3 days increased to 100 mg three times a day. Maximum dose 450 mg/day. With modified release preparations, initial dose is 150 mg daily, increased to 150 mg twice daily. Maximum dose 200 mg twice daily. Patients with renal or hepatic failure: dose is reduced.

Buserelin

Antineoplastic/Gonadorelin Analogue

6-[*O*-(1,1-Dimethylethyl)-D-serine]-9-(*N*-ethyl-L-prolinamide)-10-deglycinamide-luteinising hormone-releasing factor (pig)
$C_{60}H_{86}N_{16}O_{13}$=1239.4
CAS—57982-77-1

5-oxoPro—His—Trp—Ser—Tyr—D-Ser(t-Bu)—Leu—Arg—ProNHCH$_2$CH$_3$

A white or slightly yellowish hygroscopic powder. It is sparingly soluble in water and in dilute mineral acids.

Buserelin Acetate

Synonym. HOE-766
Proprietary names. Bigonist; Profact; Receptal; Suprecur; Suprefact.
$C_{60}H_{86}N_{16}O_{13},C_2H_4O_2$=1299.5
CAS—68630-75-1

Disposition in the Body. Buserelin is completely absorbed after subcutaneous injection, with peak plasma concentrations occurring after about 1 h. It accumulates in the liver and kidneys as well as in the anterior pituitary. A high degree of inactivation of the drug occurs by the gastrointestinal enzymes (peptidases), and the proportion of active compound reaching systemic circulation is very low. The main serum metabolite is inactive buserelin (5–9) pentapeptide. Buserelin is excreted in urine and bile as the unchanged drug (66% dose) and its metabolites (28% in 24 h). 17 to 32% of a dose is detected in urine after intravenous or subcutaneous administration. Very small amounts are distributed into breast milk.

Therapeutic concentration

A mean peak plasma concentration of 54.2 µg/L was reached 30 min after administration of 30 µg/kg subcutaneously to 11 children being treated for central precocious puberty. Following administration of 200 µg intranasally to 10 children, a mean peak plasma concentration of 0.65 µg/L was obtained after 30 min. [F. J. Holland *et al.*, *J. Clin. Endocrinol. Metab.*, 1986, *63*, 1065–1070].

Following administration of 1000 µg subcutaneously every 12 h for 7 days to 3 women (aged between 18 and 30 years, with laparoscopically diagnosed endometriosis), the mean plasma concentration was 41.7 µg/L at 15 min. Concentrations were also 23.7, 7.3 and 0.97 µg/L after 2, 4 and 8 h, respectively. Mean plasma concentrations of 1.39 µg/L were measured 15 min after the third dose of 300 µg intranasally every 8 h to 5 women. [L. Kiesel *et al.*, *J. Clin. Endocrinol. Metab.*, 1989, *68*, 1167–1173].

Half-life. Plasma, 80 min.

Protein binding. In plasma, 15%.

Note. For a review of buserelin see R. N. Brogden *et al.*, *Drugs*, 1990, *39*, 399–437.

Dose. In prostatic carcinoma, 500 µg (of the base) subcutaneously every 8 h for 7 days, then 200 µg into each nostril every 8 h.

Buspirone

Anxiolytic

8-[4-[4-(2-Pyrimidinyl)-1-piperazinyl]butyl]-8-azaspiro[4.5]decane-7,9-dione
$C_{21}H_{31}N_5O_2$=385.5
CAS—36505-84-7

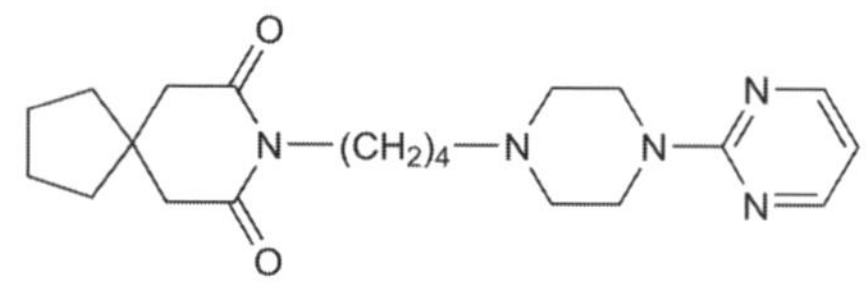

Buspirone Hydrochloride

Proprietary names. Ansial; Ansiced; Axoren; Bespar; Buspar; Buspimen; Buspinol; Buspisal; Censpar; Lucelan; Narol; Travin.
$C_{21}H_{31}N_5O_2,HCl$=422.0
CAS—33386-08-2

A white crystalline powder. M.p. 201.5° to 202.5°. It is very soluble in water; sparingly soluble in ethanol and in acetonitrile; very slightly soluble in ethyl acetate; freely soluble in methanol and in methylene chloride; practically insoluble in hexanes.

Thin-Layer Chromatography. System TB—Rf 30; system TE—Rf 71; system TF—Rf 05; system TAE—Rf 64.

Gas Chromatography. Column: (analytical) fused-silica capillary coated with Ultra 2.5% phenyl methyl silicone (25 m × 0.32 mm i.d., 0.52 µm film thickness); (pre-column) deactivated fused-silica tubing (5 m × 0.53 mm). Column temperature: 210° to 285° at 2.5°/min. Carrier gas: helium, 2.1 mL/min flow rate. Detection: electron-capture/nitrogen–phosphorous. Relative retention time (to prazepam, internal standard): 2.03. [Y. Gaillard *et al.*, *J. Chromatogr.* 1993, *622*; *Biomed. Appl.*, *133*, 197–208].

Column: methyl silicone (HP1, 0.2 mm i.d., 0.33 µm film thickness). Column temperature: 280°. Carrier gas: helium, 0.9 mL/min flow rate. MS detection. Retention index: 3299. [T. Mills and J. C. Roberson, *Instrumental Data for Drug Analysis*, 1993, CRC Press, Boca Raton, US. 2nd Edn, Vol. 5, pp. 76–77].

High Performance Liquid Chromatography. System HX—RI 369; system HY—RI 310; system HZ—3.5 min; system HAA—retention time 12.5 min; system HAX—9.1 min; system HAY—5.0 min.

Column: ODS Hypersil (100 × 4.6 mm i.d., 5 µm). Mobile phase: methanol:aqueous 0.01 M dihydrogen potassium phosphate buffer, adjusted to pH 3.5 with 85% phosphoric acid (70:30), 1 mL/min flow rate. UV diode array detection. Retention time: 2.1 min. [T. Mills and J. C. Roberson, *Instrumental Data for Drug Analysis*, 1993, CRC Press, Boca Raton, US. 2nd Edn, Vol. 5, pp. 76–77].

Ultraviolet Spectrum. Aqueous acid (0.2 M H_2SO_4)—312 nm; basic—307 nm.

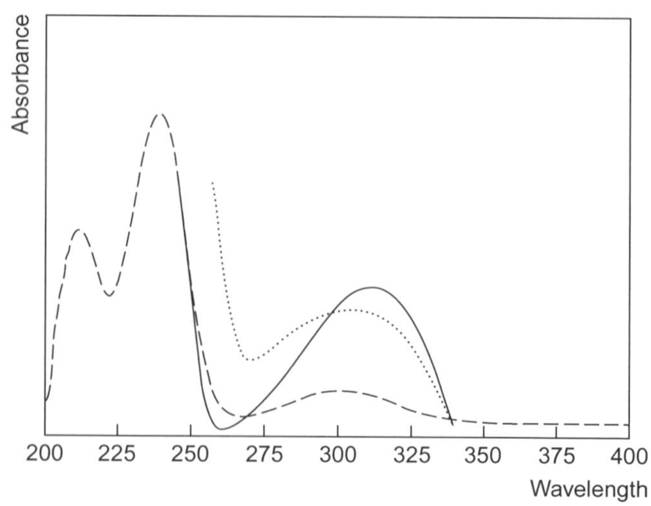

Infra-red Spectrum. Principal peaks at wavenumbers 1668, 1436, 1351 cm^{-1} (KBr pellets).

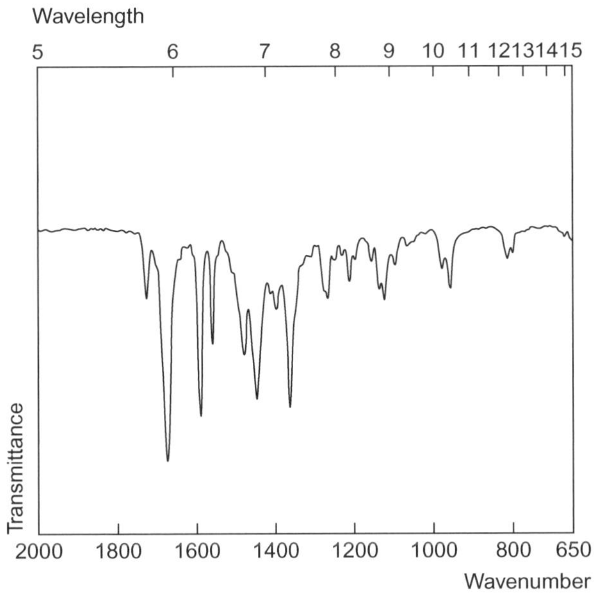

Mass Spectrum. Principal peaks at m/z 177, 277, 265, 122, 148, 108, 56, 70.

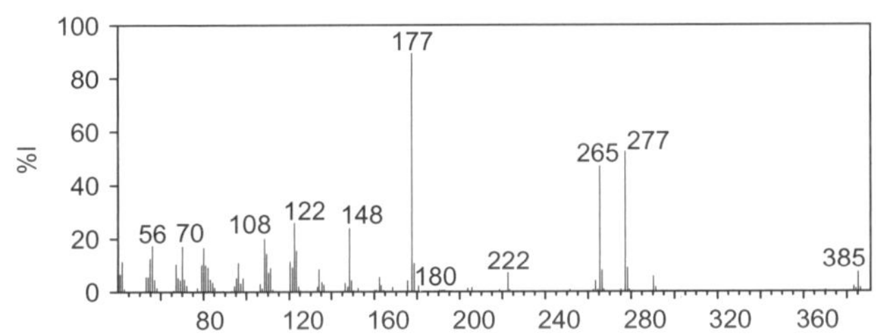

Quantification

Gas chromatography. In plasma: limit of detection 5 µg/L, ECD (electron capture detection) and NPD (nitrogen–phosphorus detection)—Y. Gaillard *et al.*, *J. Chromatogr.*, 1993, *622*; *Biomed. Appl.*, *133*, 197–208.

Gas chromatography–mass spectrometry. In plasma or urine: limit of detection 0.1 µg/L and 0.2 µg/L, respectively—M. A. Sciacca *et al.*, *J. Chromatogr.*, 1988, *428*; *Biomed. Appl.*, *72*, 265–274. In plasma: limit of detection 0.05 µg/L—R. E. Gammans, *J. Chromatogr.*1985, *345*, 285–297.

High performance liquid chromatography. In serum: limit of detection 0.2 µg/L, UV detection—F. Kristjánsson, *J. Chromatogr.*, 1991, *566*; *Biomed. Appl.*, *104*, 250–256. In plasma: limit of detection 0.5 µg/L, electrochemical detection—M. Franklin, *J. Chromatogr.*, 1990, *526*; *Biomed. Appl.*, *91*, 590–596. In plasma: limit of detection 2.5 µg/L, electrochemical detection—P. Betto *et al.*, *J. Chromatogr.*, 1992, *575*; *Biomed. Appl.*, *113*, 117–121. In plasma: limit of detection 0.1 µg/L, electrochemical detection—K. Ary *et al.*, *J. Chromatogr. A*, 1998, *797*, 221–226.

Disposition in the Body. It is rapidly absorbed after oral administration; peak plasma concentrations occur after about 40 to 90 min. It undergoes extensive first-pass metabolism primarily by oxidation and bioavailability is therefore low. Metabolism is probably mediated by CYP3A4. Most metabolites are inactive, although oxidative dealkylation produces 1-(2-pyrimidinyl)-piperazine which is about 20 to 25% as potent as the parent drug. The major metabolite is 5-hydroxybuspirone which may be oxidised further to many more metabolites and its glucuronide conjugate. The metabolites are excreted mainly in urine (65%); some are also excreted in faeces (35%). Less than 1% of a dose is excreted as the unchanged drug. It is not removed by haemodialysis.

Therapeutic concentration. The serum therapeutic concentration range is 0.9 to 5 mg/L.
Plasma concentrations of buspirone are usually very low and variable between subjects. Studies suggest that buspirone has nonlinear pharmacokinetics.

Bioavailability. 4%.

Half-life. Plasma, 2 to 11 h; mean, 2.4 h.

Volume of distribution. 5.3 L/kg after a 20 mg intravenous dose.

Clearance. Plasma, 2.0 to 3.5 L/h/kg, also reported as 1.70 L/h/kg.

Protein binding. In plasma, 95%.

Note. For a review of buspirone, see R. E. Gammans *et al.*, *Am. J. Med.*, 1986, *80*, *Suppl. 3B*, 41–51.

Dose. Usually 15 to 30 mg of buspirone hydrochloride daily.

Busulfan

Antineoplastic

Synonyms. Busulphan; CB-2041; GT-41.
Proprietary names. Misulban; Myleran.
1,4-Butanediol dimethanesulfonate esters
$C_6H_{14}O_6S_2$=246.3
CAS—55-98-1

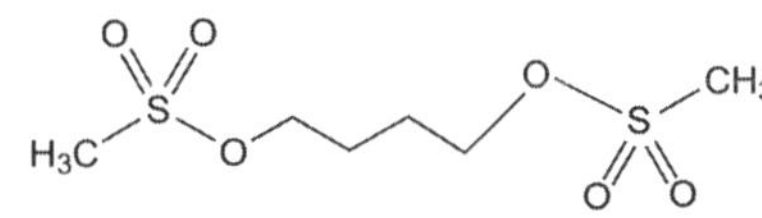

A white crystalline powder. M.p. 114° to 118°.
Soluble 1 in 750 of water and 1 in 25 of acetone; slightly soluble in ethanol.
Caution. Busulfan is irritant; avoid contact with skin and mucous membranes.

Partition Coefficient. Log P (octanol/water), −0.5.

Thin-layer Chromatography. System TAE—Rf 00.

High Performance Liquid Chromatography. System HX—RI 368.

Ultraviolet Spectrum. Methanol—256 nm (A^1_1=20b).

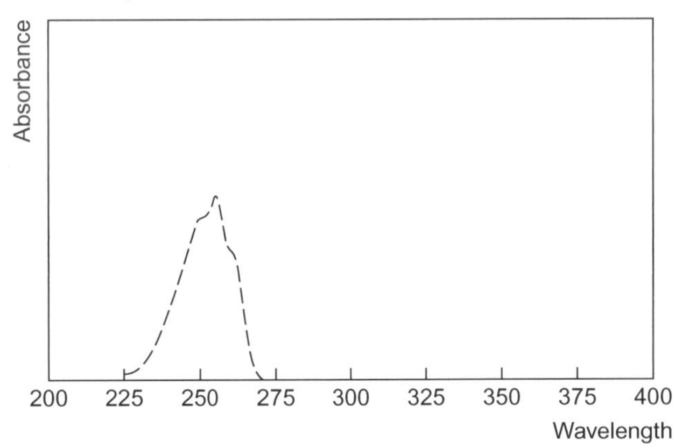

Infra-red Spectrum. Principal peaks at wavenumbers 1178, 934, 861, 980, 962, 773 cm^{-1} (KBr disk).

Quantification

Gas chromatography. In plasma: limit of detection 0.06 mg/L and limit of quantification 0.1 mg/L, ECD—L. Embree *et al.*, *Cancer Chemother. Pharmacol.*, 1993, *32(2)*, 137–142. In plasma: limit of quantification 0.01 mg/L, ECD—R. B. Burns *et al.*, *J. Pharm. Biomed. Anal.*, 1995, *13(9)*, 1073–1078.

Gas chromatography–mass spectrometry. In plasma: limit of detection 10 mg/L—H. Ehrsson and M. Hassan, *J. Pharm. Sci.*, 1983, *72*, 1203–1205. In plasma: limit of quantification 0.04 mg/L, SIM (m/z 183 and 197)—W. K. Lai *et al.*, *Clin. Chem.*, 1998, *44(12)*, 2506–2510.

High performance liquid chromatography. In serum: limit of quantification 10 mg/L, UV detection (λ=278 nm)—K. Funakoshi *et al.*, *J. Chromatogr. B Biomed. Sci. Appl.*, 1994, *660(1)*, 200–204. In plasma: limit of detection 0.02 mg/L and limit of quantification 0.06 mg/L, UV detection (λ=251 nm)—J. R. Heggie *et al.*, *J. Chromatogr. B Biomed. Sci. Appl.*, 1997, *692(2)*, 437–444. In plasma: limit of detection 9 µg/L and limit of quantification 20 µg/L, fluorescence detection (λ_{ex}=360 nm;

λ_{em}=425 nm)—J. E. Peris *et al.*, *J. Chromatogr. B Biomed. Sci. Appl.*, 1999, *730(1)*, 33–40.

Disposition in the Body. Readily absorbed after oral administration. It is mainly excreted in the urine as metabolites; about 1% of a dose is excreted in the urine unchanged in 24 h.

Therapeutic concentration

Following single oral doses of 6 mg to 5 subjects, peak plasma concentrations of 0.05 to 0.13 mg/L (mean 0.08) were reported. [H. Ehrsson *et al.*, *Clin. Pharmacol. Ther.*, 1983, 34, 86–89.]

A patient was administered a 1 mg/kg dose of busulfan on two consecutive days. The maximum plasma concentrations reached were 1.2 mg/L 20 min after dosing on the first day and 1.6 mg/L after approx. 60 min on the following day. [J. E. Peris *et al.*, *J. Chromatogr. B Biomed. Sci. Appl.*, 1999, *730(1)*, 33–40.]

6 adult patients, aged 31.8 to 56.9 years, were administered a single low dose of busulfan of 4.87 to 8.2 mg, and six children, aged 0.9 to 15.8 years were administered 2.29 to 7.72 mg. A mean maximum concentration of 0.504 mg/L was reached by the children and 0.352 mg/L by the adults less than 2 h after dosing. [Z. Hassan *et al.*, *Bone Marrow Transplant.*, 2001, *27(5)*, 479–485.]

Half-life. Plasma half-life, about 2 to 3 h.

Dose. Usually 2 to 4 mg daily; maintenance, 0.5 to 2 mg daily.

Butacaine

Local Anaesthetic

3-(Dibutylamino)-1-propanol 4-aminobenzoate
$C_{18}H_{30}N_2O_2$=306.4
CAS—149-16-6

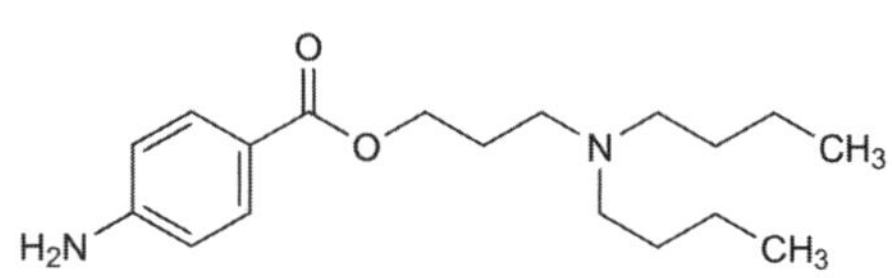

A liquid.

Butacaine Sulfate

Proprietary name. It is an ingredient of Rhinamid.
$(C_{18}H_{30}N_2O_2)_2,H_2SO_4$=711.0
CAS—149-15-5
A white, very hygroscopic, crystalline powder. Unstable to light and moisture. M.p. 100° to 103°.
Soluble 1 in 1.5 of water, 1 in 2 of ethanol, 1 in 2.5 of chloroform and 1 in 2000 of ether; quite soluble in acetone.

Dissociation Constant. pK_a 9.0.

Partition Coefficient. Log *P* (octanol/water), 4.4.

Colour Test. Diazotisation—red.

Thin-layer Chromatography. System TA—Rf 71; system TB—Rf 07; system TC—Rf 30; system TE—Rf 83; system TL—Rf 64; system TAE—Rf 44; system TAF—Rf 76; system TAJ—Rf 27; system TAK—Rf 05; system TAL—Rf 20. (Dragendorff spray, positive; Acidified iodoplatinate solution, positive; Ninhydrin spray, positive; Van Urk reagent, bright yellow.)

Gas Chromatography. System GA—RI 2457.

High Performance Liquid Chromatography. System HA—*k* 1.2; system HQ—*k* 8.97; system HX—RI 392; system HY—RI 331.

Ultraviolet Spectrum. Aqueous acid—272, 278 (A^1_1=72b); aqueous alkali—282 nm.

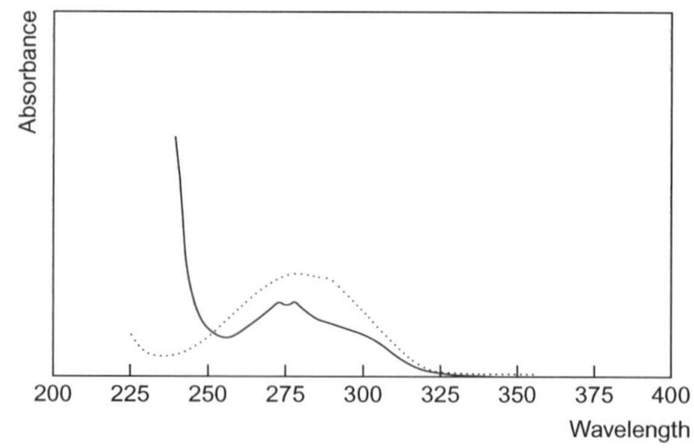

Infra-red Spectrum. Principal peaks at wavenumbers 1275, 1165, 1598, 1694, 1639, 1111 cm^{-1} (KBr disk).

Mass Spectrum. Principal ions at *m/z* 120, 263, 142, 178, 100, 264, 41, 29.

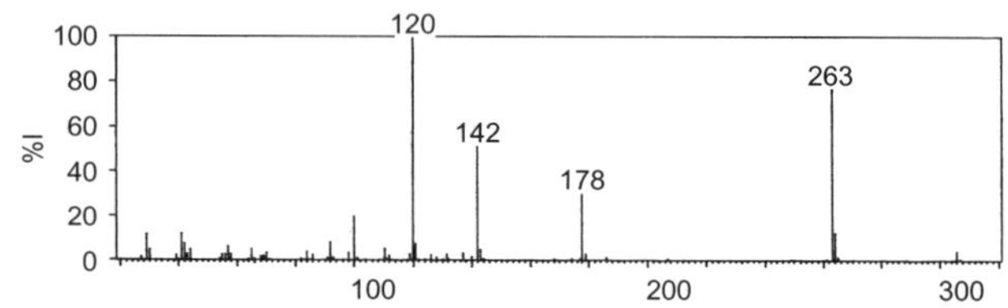

Use. A 2% solution of butacaine sulfate has been used for surface anaesthesia.

Butalamine

Vasodilator

N,N-Dibutyl-*N′*-(3-phenyl-1,2,4-oxadiazol-5-yl)-1,2-ethanediamine
$C_{18}H_{28}N_4O$=316.4
CAS—22131-35-7

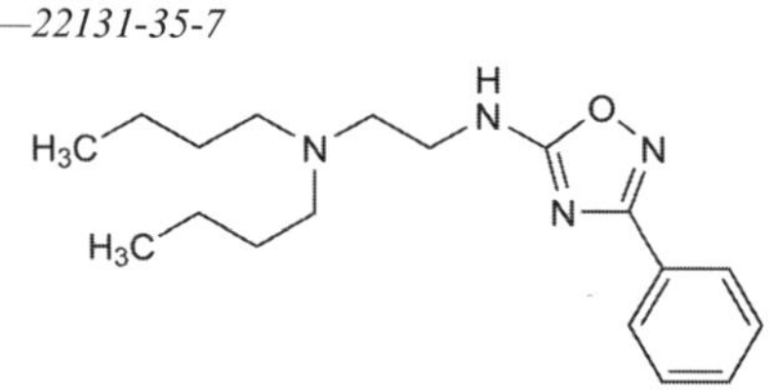

Butalamine Hydrochloride

Proprietary names. Adrevil; Surheme.
$C_{18}H_{28}N_4O,HCl$=352.9
CAS—56974-46-0
A white crystalline powder. M.p. 145°.
Soluble 1 in 7 of water, 1 in 10 of ethanol and 1 in 2.5 of chloroform.

Partition Coefficient. Log *P* (octanol/water), 4.4.

Thin-layer Chromatography. System TA—Rf 68; system TD—Rf 11; system TE—Rf 86; system TF—Rf 29; system TAD—Rf 46. (Acidified iodoplatinate solution, positive.)

Gas Chromatography. System GA—RI 2490.

Ultraviolet Spectrum. Aqueous acid—228 nm (A^1_1=812a).

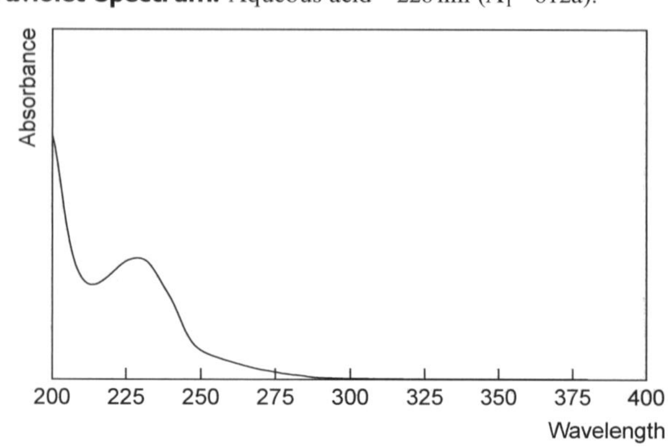

Infra-red Spectrum. Principal peaks at wavenumbers 1639, 751, 1603, 694, 1492, 1170 cm^{-1}.

Mass Spectrum. Principal ions at m/z 142, 143, 100, 155, 44, 112, 57, 29.

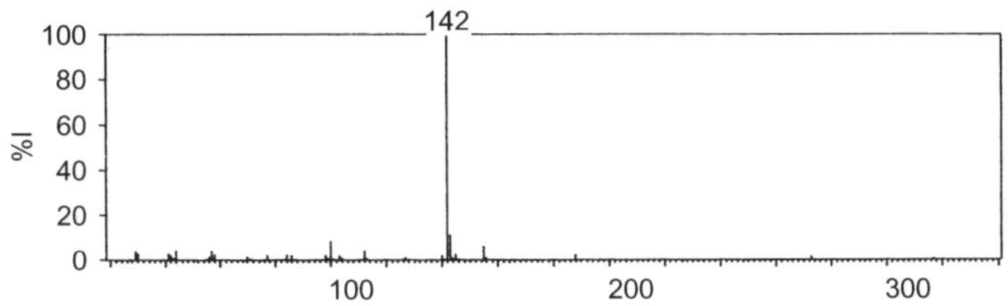

Dose. Butalamine hydrochloride has been given in doses of 160 to 320 mg daily.

Butalbital

Sedative/Barbiturate

Synonyms. Alisobumalum; Allylbarbituric Acid; Itobarbital; Tetrallobarbital.
Proprietary names. Sandoptal. It is an ingredient of Fiorinal.
Note. The name Butalbital has also been applied to talbutal, the *sec*-butyl analogue.
5-(2-Methylpropyl)-5-(2-propenyl)-2,4,6(1*H*,3*H*,5*H*)-pyrimidinetrione
$C_{11}H_{16}N_2O_3$=224.3
CAS—77-26-9

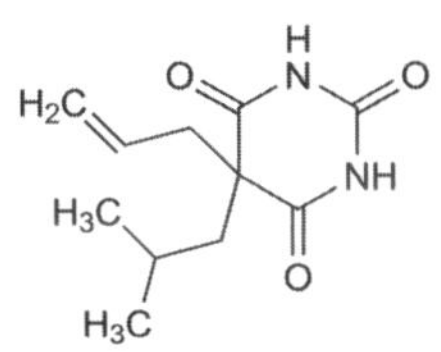

A white crystalline powder. M.p. 138° to 139°.
Slightly soluble in cold water; soluble in boiling water; soluble in acetone, ethanol, chloroform, ether, and glacial acetic acid; soluble in aqueous solutions of alkali hydroxides and carbonates.

Dissociation Constant. pK_a 7.6 (20°).

Partition Coefficient. Log P (octanol/water), 1.9.

Colour Tests. Koppanyi–Zwikker Test—violet; Vanillin Reagent—orange/colourless.

Thin-layer Chromatography. System TB—Rf 01; system TD—Rf 54; system TE—Rf 44; system TF—Rf 67; system TH—Rf 67; system TAD—Rf 57; system TAE—Rf 87. (Mercurous nitrate spray, black; acidified potassium permanganate solution, yellow-brown.)

Gas Chromatography. System GA—butalbital RI 1665, butalbital-Me_2 RI 1655, M (OH-) RI 1940; system GB—butalbital RI 1698, M (OH-) RI 2016; system GF—RI 2395; system GAJ—butalbital RRT 0.778 (relative to methylphenobarbital).

High Performance Liquid Chromatography. System HG—k 6.17; system HH—k 3.48; system HX—RI 394; system HY—RI 342; system HZ—retention time, 3.4 min.

Ultraviolet Spectrum. Borax buffer 0.05 M (pH 9.2)—240 (A_1^1=439a); 1 M sodium hydroxide (pH 13)—255 nm (A_1^1=329b).

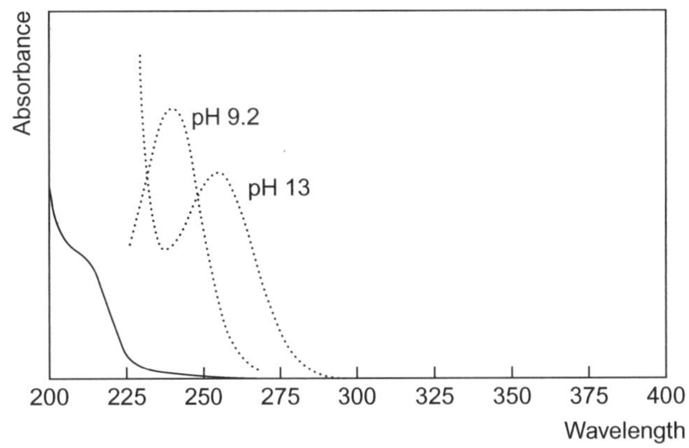

Infra-red Spectrum. Principal peaks at wavenumbers 1690, 1720, 1740, 1310, 1290, 1200 cm^{-1} (KBr disk).

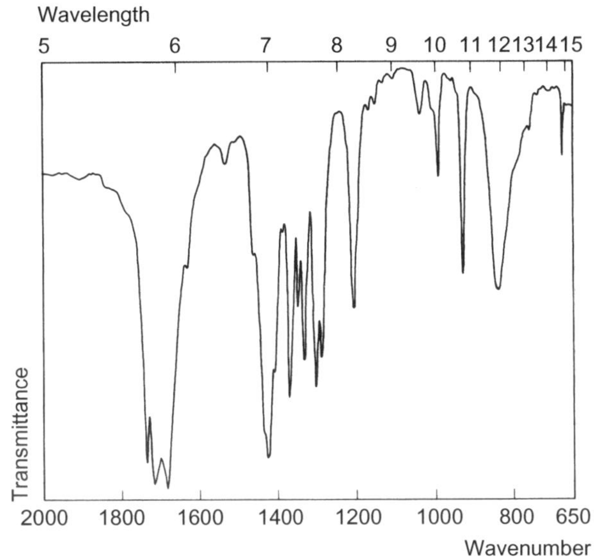

Mass Spectrum. Principal ions at m/z 41, 167, 168, 39, 124, 97, 141, 181.

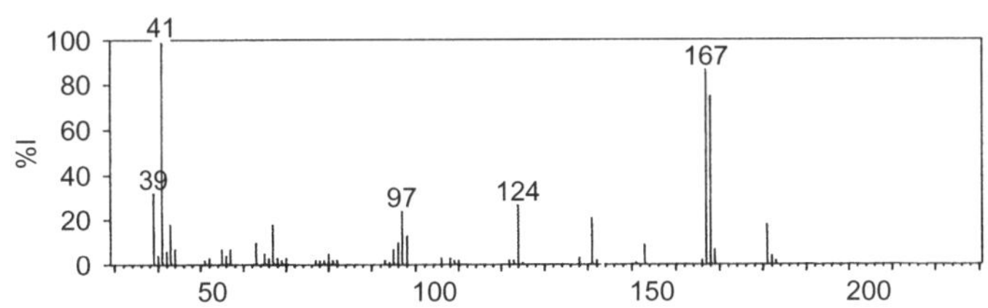

Quantification See under Amylobarbital.

Gas chromatography–mass spectrometry. In blood and urine: limit of detection 5 mg/L and limit of quantification 50 mg/L (blood) and 20 mg/L (urine)—R. Meatherall, *J. Forensic Sci.*, 1997, *42(6)*, 1160–1170.

Disposition in the Body. Absorbed after oral administration. About 5% of a dose is excreted in the urine as unchanged drug in 96 h and 20 to 60% as 5-(2,3-dihydroxypropyl)-5-isobutylbarbituric acid.

Therapeutic concentration. In plasma, usually in the range 1 to 10 mg/L.

A small group of healthy volunteers was administered 100 mg butalbital orally. Peak blood concentrations reached 2.1 mg/L and fell to 1.5 mg/L after 24 h. [M. L. Drost and L. Walter, *J. Anal. Toxicol.*, 1988, *12(6)*, 322–324.]

Toxicity. Plasma concentrations of 10 to 25 mg/L are usually associated with toxic effects.

The following concentrations were reported in one fatality attributed to butalbital overdose: blood 26 mg/L, liver 50 µg/g. [R. C. Baselt and R. H. Cravey, *J. Anal. Toxicol.*, 1977, *1*, 81–103.]

Half-life. Derived from urinary excretion data, about 30 to 40 h.

Dose. 200 mg as a hypnotic; 150 to 400 mg daily as a sedative.

Butanilicaine *Local Anaesthetic*

2-(Butylamino)-*N*-(2-chloro-6-methylphenyl)acetamide
$C_{13}H_{19}ClN_2O = 254.8$
CAS—3785-21-5

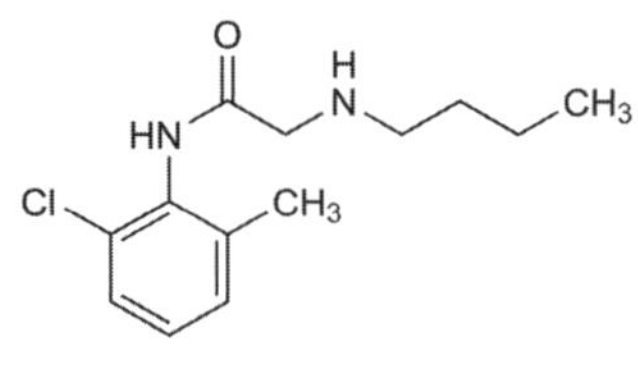

Crystals. M.p. 45° to 46°.

Butanilicaine Phosphate
Proprietary name. Hostacain (also as hydrochloride).
$C_{13}H_{19}ClN_2O,H_3PO_4 = 352.8$
CAS—2081-65-4
Crystals. M.p. 126° to 127°.

Partition Coefficient. Log *P* (octanol/water), 2.0.

Colour Tests. Aromaticity (Method 2)—colourless/orange; Koppanyi–Zwikker Test—violet; Liebermann's Test—orange.

Thin-layer Chromatography. System TA—Rf 76; system TB—Rf 14; system TC—Rf 54; system TE—Rf 75; system TL—Rf 61; system TAE—Rf 65. (Acidified iodoplatinate solution, positive.)

Gas Chromatography. System GA—RI 2025.

High Performance Liquid Chromatography. System HQ—*k* 4.42; system HY—RI 280.

Ultraviolet Spectrum. Aqueous acid—267 ($A_1^1 = 15b$), 275 nm.

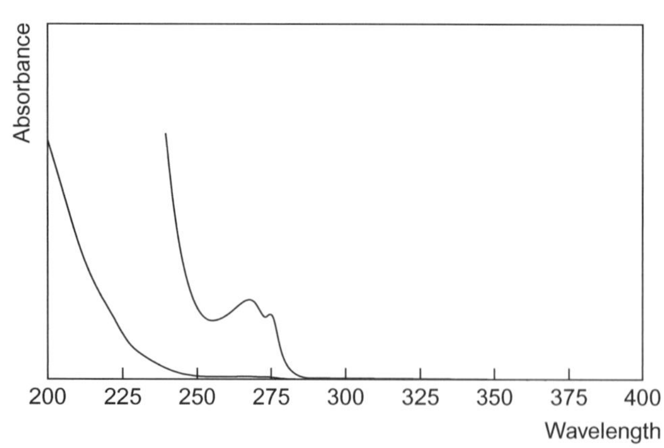

Infra-red Spectrum. Principal peaks at wavenumbers 1495, 1694, 770, 1136, 1562, 1587 cm^{-1}.

Mass Spectrum. Principal ions at *m/z* 86, 30, 72, 44, 141, 42, 29, 57.

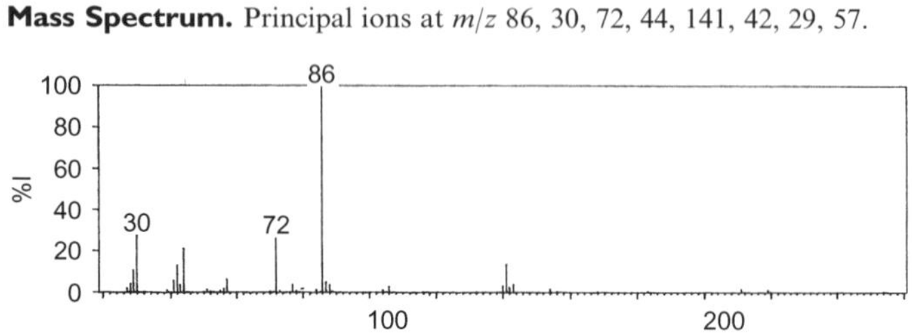

Quantification
Gas chromatography. In horse plasma or urine: limit of detection 5 µg/L, AFID—F. T. Delbeke and M. Debackere, *J. Chromatogr.*, 1982, *237*, 344–349.

Dose. Butanilicaine phosphate has been administered by injection, as a 0.5 to 3% solution.

Butaperazine *Tranquilliser*

Synonym. Butyrylperazine
1-[10-[3-(4-Methyl-1-piperazinyl)propyl]-10*H*-phenothiazin-2-yl]-1-butanone
$C_{24}H_{31}N_3OS = 409.6$
CAS—653-03-2

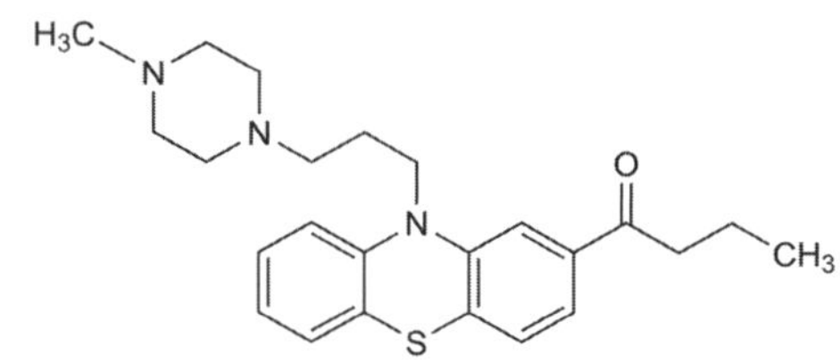

A yellow oil. B.p. 195° to 210°.

Butaperazine Maleate
Synonym. Butaperazine Dimaleate
Proprietary name. Repoise
$C_{24}H_{31}N_3OS,2C_4H_4O_4 = 641.7$
CAS—1063-55-4
A yellow crystalline powder. M.p. about 195°.
Soluble in water; practically insoluble in chloroform and ether.

Butaperazine Phosphate
Synonym. Butaperazine Diphosphate
$C_{24}H_{31}N_3OS,2H_3PO_4 = 605.6$
CAS—7389-45-9
A yellow crystalline powder. M.p. 161° to 162°.
Soluble in water; practically insoluble in chloroform and ether.

Partition Coefficient. Log *P* (octanol/water), 4.8.

Colour Tests. Mandelin's Test—brown-violet; Marquis Test—brown-violet.

Thin-layer Chromatography. System TA—Rf 53; system TB—Rf 28; system TC—Rf 37; system TE—Rf 52; ; system TL—Rf 05; system TAE—Rf 26; system TAJ—Rf 10; system TAK—Rf 00; system TAL—Rf 42. (Acidified potassium permanganate solution, positive.)

Gas Chromatography. System GA—RI 3190.

High Performance Liquid Chromatography. System HA—*k* 3.4; system HX—RI 464; system HY—RI 406.

Ultraviolet Spectrum. Aqueous acid—242 ($A_1^1 = 609a$), 277 nm.

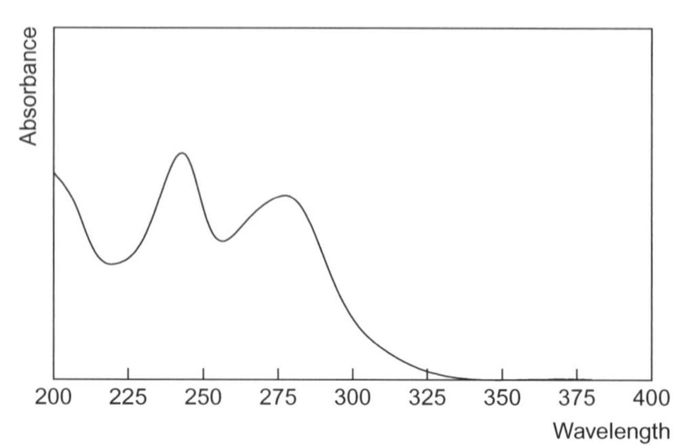

Infra-red Spectrum. Principal peaks at wavenumbers 1675, 749, 1279, 1193, 1163, 1143 cm^{-1}.

Mass Spectrum. Principal ions at *m/z* 113, 70, 409, 43, 141, 283, 42, 127.

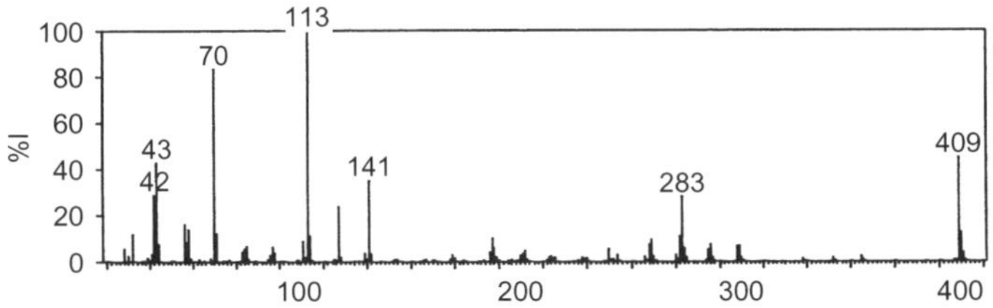

Quantification

Spectrofluorimetry. In plasma—D. H. Manier *et al.*, *Clin. Chim. Acta*, 1974, *57*, 225–230.

Gas chromatography. In biological fluids: limit of detection 5 µg/L, AFID—J. I. Javaid *et al.*, *J. Chromatogr. Sci.*, 1979, *17*, 666–670.

Disposition in the Body. Butaperazine is readily absorbed after oral administration. It is metabolised to the sulfoxide and sulfone; other unidentified metabolites have been detected in plasma.

Therapeutic concentration

Following oral administration of 40 mg as a single dose to 13 subjects, peak plasma concentrations of 0.07 to 0.69 (mean 0.28) mg/L were attained in 2 to 4 h; peak erythrocyte concentrations of 0.01 to 0.52 (mean 0.11) mg/L were also reported. [D. L. Garver *et al.*, *Archs Gen. Psychiat.*, 1976, *33*, 862–866].

Following oral administration of 20 mg twice a day to 9 subjects, minimum steady-state plasma concentrations of 0.02 to 0.20 (mean 0.09) mg/L, and erythrocyte concentrations of 0.01 to 0.06 (mean 0.03) mg/L were reported; therapeutic effect appeared to correlate with erythrocyte concentrations in the range 0.03 to 0.06 mg/L. [R. Casper *et al.*, *Archs Gen. Psychiat.*, 1980, *37*, 301–305].

Half-life. Plasma half-life, 5 to 30 (mean 12) h.

Dose. Usually the equivalent of 15 to 30 mg of butaperazine daily; maximum of 100 mg daily.

Butetamate

Antispasmodic/Bronchodilator

Synonym. Butethamate

Benzeneacetic acid α-ethyl-2-(diethylamino)ethyl ester

$C_{16}H_{25}NO_2$=263.4

CAS—14007-64-8

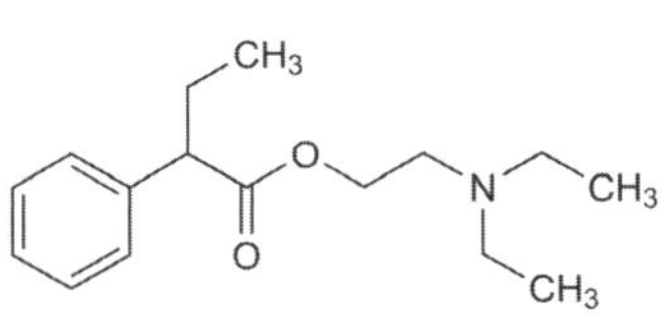

Butetamate Citrate

Proprietary name. It is an ingredient of CAM.

$C_{16}H_{25}NO_2,C_6H_8O_7$=455.5

CAS—3639-12-1

Colourless crystals. M.p. 107° to 110°.

Soluble 1 in 10 of water and 1 in 40 of ethanol.

Partition Coefficient. Log *P* (octanol/water), 3.7.

Thin-layer Chromatography. System TA—Rf 69; system TB—Rf 59; system TC—Rf 57; system TE—Rf 81; system TL—Rf 47; system TAE—Rf 48; system TAF—Rf 56. (Acidified iodoplatinate solution, positive.)

Gas Chromatography. System GA—RI 1754.

High Performance Liquid Chromatography. System HA—*k* 1.7; system HX—RI 390.

Ultraviolet Spectrum. Aqueous acid—253, 258 (A^1_1=7.6b), 264 nm.

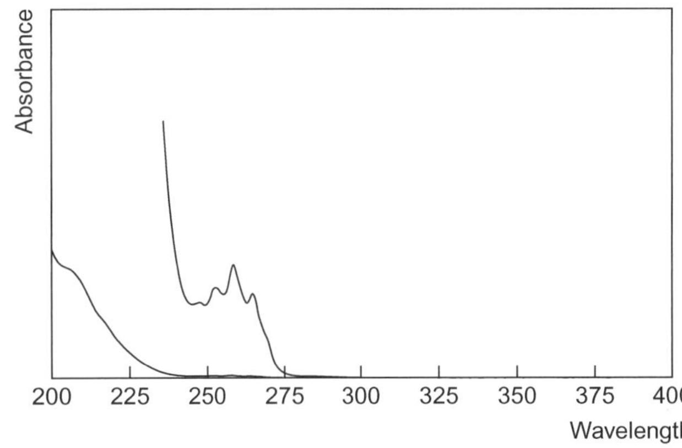

Infra-red Spectrum. Principal peaks at wavenumbers 1730, 1158, 1194, 694, 1265, 1219 cm^{-1} (KBr disk).

Mass Spectrum. Principal ions at *m/z* 86, 99, 91, 191, 87, 119, 58, 248.

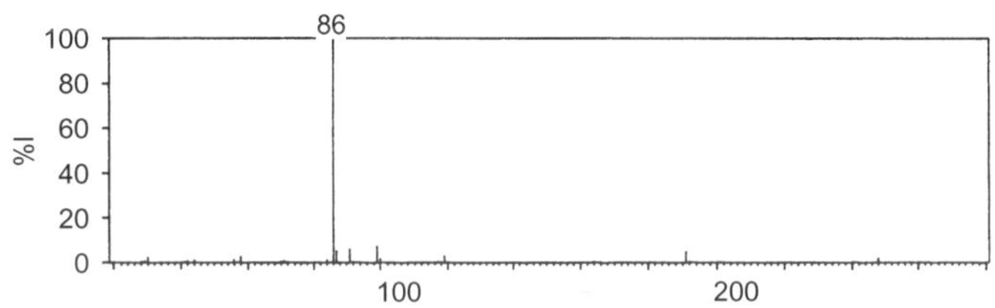

Dose. Butetamate citrate has been given in doses of 18 to 90 mg daily.

Butobarbital

Hypnotic/Barbiturate

Synonyms. Butethal; Butobarbitalum; Butobarbitone. To be distinguished from Butabarbital.

Proprietary names. Sonabarb; Soneryl. It is an ingredient of Belloid and Hypnasmine.

5-Butyl-5-ethyl-2,4,6(1*H*,3*H*,5*H*)-pyrimidinetrione

$C_{10}H_{16}N_2O_3$=212.3

CAS—77-28-1

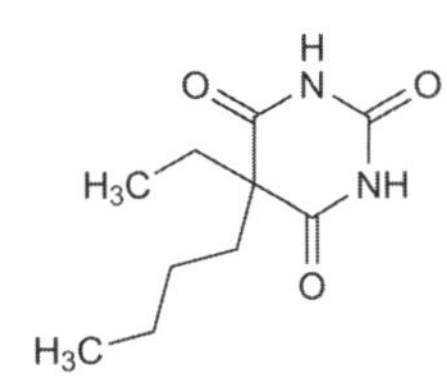

Colourless crystals or white crystalline powder. M.p. 124° to 127°.

Soluble 1 in 5 alcohol and 1 in 10 ether; practically insoluble in water, insoluble in petroleum ether and aliphatic hydrocarbons.

Dissociation Constant. pK_a 8.0 (25°).

Partition Coefficient. Log *P* (octanol/water), 1.73.

Colour Tests. Koppanyi–Zwikker Test—violet; Mercurous Nitrate—black.

Thin-layer Chromatography. System TD—Rf 50; system TE—Rf 41; system TF—Rf 65; system TH—Rf 68; system TAD—Rf 58; system TAE—Rf 86. (Mercuric chloride–diphenylcarbazone reagent, positive; mercurous nitrate spray, black; Zwikker's reagent, pink.)

Gas Chromatography. System GA—butobarbital RI 1660, butobarbital-Me_2 RI 1565, M (3′-OH-) RI 1920, M (3′-OH-)-AC RI 1940, M (3′-oxo-) RI 1880; system GF—RI 2390; system GAJ—butobarbital RRT 0.732, M (3′-OH-) RRT 1.053 (both relative to methylphenobarbital).

High Performance Liquid Chromatography. System HG—*k* 5.43; system HH—*k* 3.42; system HX—RI 384; system HY—RI 355; system HZ—retention time 3.2 min; system HAA—retention time 14.9 min.

Ultraviolet Spectrum. Borax buffer 0.05 M (pH 9.2)—239 (A_1^1=477a); M sodium hydroxide (pH 13)—254 nm (A_1^1=388b).

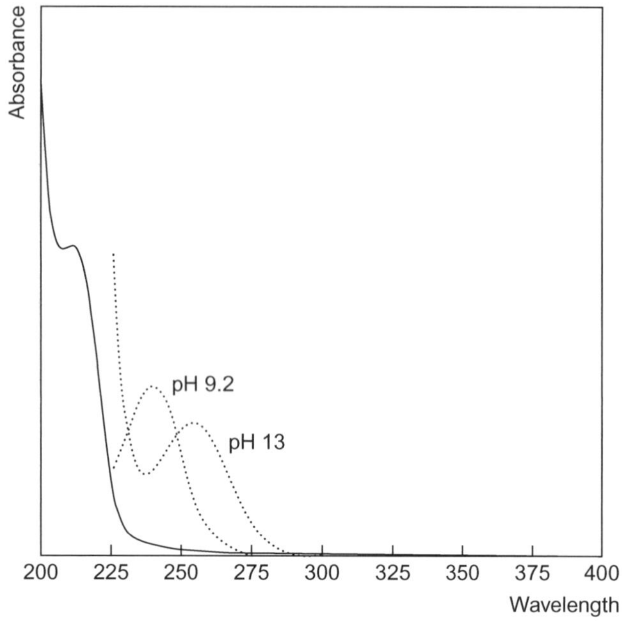

Infra-red Spectrum. Principal peaks at wavenumbers 1696, 1727, 1760, 1242, 850, 1215 cm^{-1} (KBr disk).

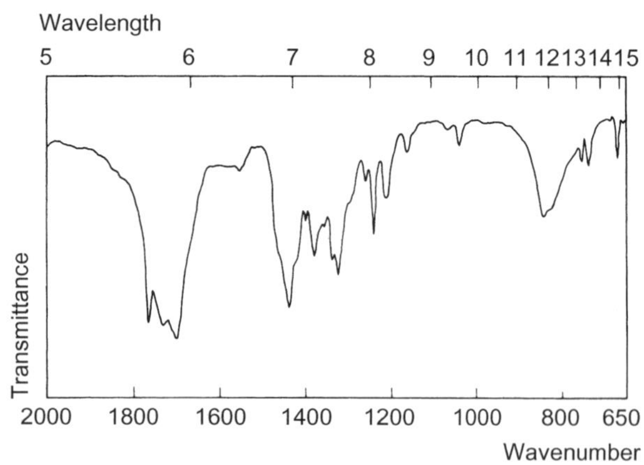

Mass Spectrum. Principal ions at *m/z* 141, 156, 41, 55, 98, 39, 142, 155; 3′-hydroxybutobarbitone 156, 141, 45, 157, 41, 29, 55, 27.

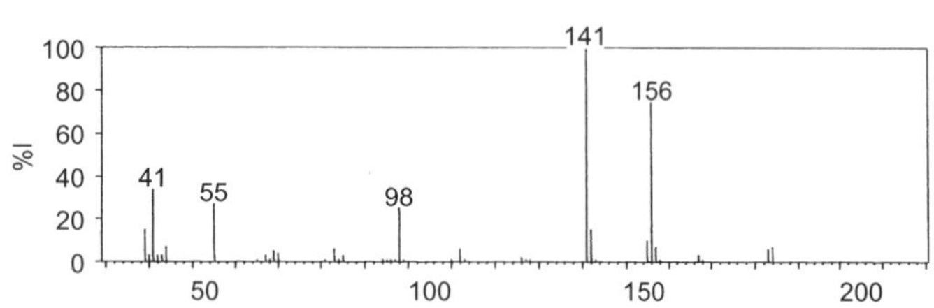

Quantification. See also under Amylobarbital.

Gas chromatography–mass spectrometry. In urine: butobarbital and metabolites—J. N. T. Gilbert and J. W. Powell, *Eur. J. Drug Metab. Pharmacokinet.*, 1976, *1*, 188–193.

Disposition in the Body. Readily absorbed after oral administration. Metabolic reactions include side-chain oxidation to form the 3′-hydroxy, 3′-oxo, and 3′-carboxypropyl metabolites. About 5 to 9% of an oral dose is excreted in the urine unchanged, 22 to 28% as 3′-hydroxybutobarbital, 14 to 18% as 3′-oxobutobarbital, and 4 to 8% as 5-(3′-carboxypropyl)-5-ethylbarbituric acid.

Therapeutic concentration. In plasma, usually in the range 2 to 15 mg/L.

A single oral dose of 200 mg, given to 5 subjects, produced peak plasma concentrations of 2.9 to 4.1 mg/L (mean 3.6) in 0.6 to 2 h; following oral doses of 200 mg daily for 3 days to 2 subjects, plasma concentrations of 6.5 and 6.4 mg/L were observed 9 h after the last dose. [D. D. Breimer, *Eur. J. Clin. Pharmacol.*, 1976, *10*, 263–271.]

Toxicity. The estimated minimum lethal dose is 2 g. Toxic effects are associated with plasma concentrations of 14 to 32 to 98 mg/L and fatalities with blood concentrations of 11 to 30 to 75 mg/L.

In 3 fatalities attributed to butobarbital overdose, the following postmortem tissue concentrations, mg/L or µg/g, were reported:

	Butobarbital	3′-Hydroxybutobarbital
Blood	18, 22, 49	—, 3, —
Bile	49, 27, 131	204, 4, 312
Kidney	31, 23, 72	—, 8, 12
Liver	47, 58, 83	2, 10, 17
Lung	26, 19, 52	—, 8, 19
Urine	4, 26, 38	259, —, 5

[A. E. Robinson and R. D. McDowall, *J. Pharm. Pharmacol.*, 1979, *31*, 357–365.]

Half-life. Plasma half-life, about 40 h following single doses, but may be reduced to about 30 h after multiple dosing.

Volume of distribution. About 0.8 L/kg.

Protein binding. In plasma, about 26%.

Dose. 100 to 200 mg, as a hypnotic.

Butorphanol

Narcotic Analgesic

Synonym. *Levo*-BC-2627
17-(Cyclobutylmethyl)morphinan-3,14-diol
$C_{21}H_{29}NO_2$=327.5
CAS—42408-82-2

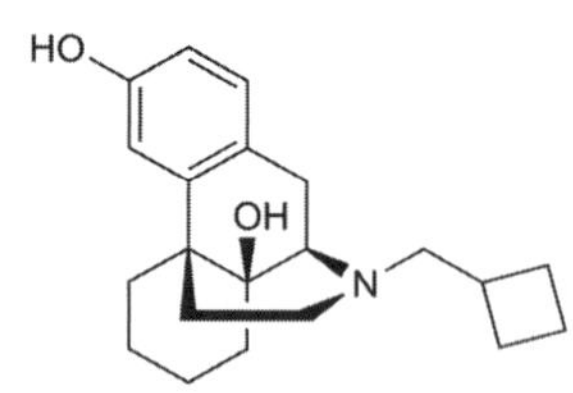

Solid. M.p. 215° to 217°.

Butorphanol Tartrate

Proprietary name. Stadol
$C_{21}H_{29}NO_2,C_4H_6O_6$=477.6
CAS—58786-99-5
A white crystalline powder. M.p. 217° to 219°, with decomposition. Sparingly soluble in water; slightly soluble in methanol; practically insoluble in ethanol, chloroform, and ether; soluble in dilute acids.

Partition Coefficient. Log *P* (octanol/water), 3.7.

Colour Tests. Liebermann's Test—black; Marquis Test—grey.

Thin-layer Chromatography. System TAJ—Rf 16; system TAK—Rf 00; system TAL—Rf 36.

Gas Chromatography. System GA—RI 2761; system GB—RI 2902.

High Performance Liquid Chromatography. System HY—RI 300.

Ultraviolet Spectrum. Aqueous acid—278 (A_1^1=62b); aqueous alkali—299 nm.

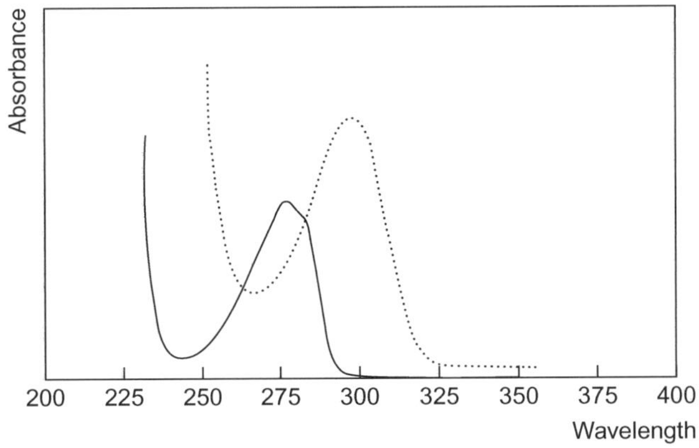

Infra-red Spectrum. Principal peaks at wavenumbers 1269, 1130, 1233, 1575, 1249, 1303 cm^{-1} (butorphanol tartrate, KBr disk). (See below.)

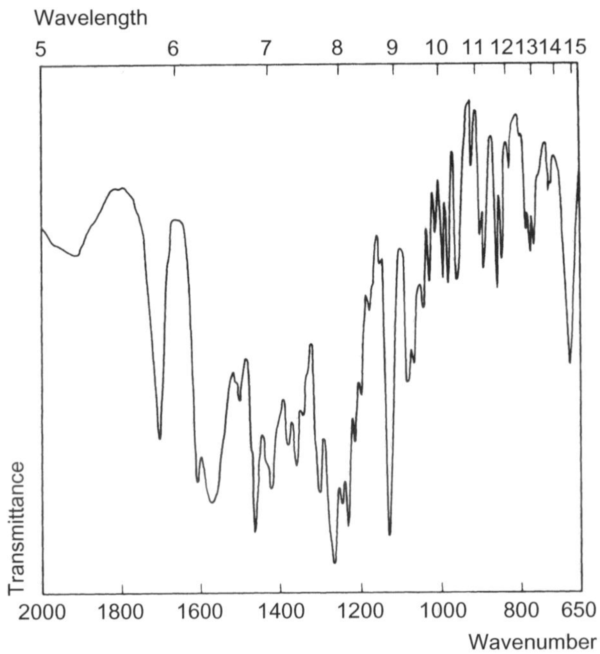

Mass Spectrum. Principal ions at *m/z* 272, 273, 41, 327, 145, 76, 42, 29.

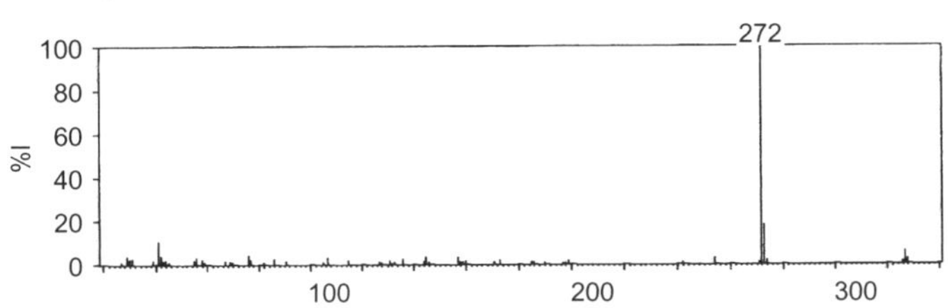

Quantification

Gas chromatography. In serum: limit of detection 2 mg/L, ECD—M. Pfeffer *et al., J. Pharm. Sci.*, 1980, *69*, 801–803. In plasma: MS detection, SIM—D. E. Mulvana *et al., J. Chromatogr. B Biomed. Sci. Appl.*, 1996, *682(2)*, 289–300.

High performance liquid chromatography. In plasma: lower limit of quantification 13.7 ng/L, MS/MS detection—D. W. Boulton *et al., J. Chromatogr. B Biomed. Sci. Appl.*, 2002, *775(1)*, 57–62. In urine: limit of quantification 2 mg/L for drug and metabolites, fluorescence detection—T. A. Willey *et al., J. Chromatogr.*, 1994, *652(2)*, 171–178.

Disposition in the Body. Well absorbed after oral or IM administration. It undergoes extensive first-pass metabolism, mainly by hydroxylation, dealkylation, and conjugation. The major metabolite is 3′-hydroxybutorphanol. About 70% of a dose is excreted in the urine and 13% eliminated in the faeces in 5 days. In 24 h, 5 to 10% of a dose is excreted in the urine as unchanged drug, 5 to 10% as free and conjugated norbutorphanol, and about 50% as 3′-hydroxybutorphanol.

Therapeutic concentration

A single IM dose of 2 mg, administered to 6 subjects, produced a mean peak plasma concentration of 2 µg/L of butorphanol in 0.5 to 1 h, and a mean peak plasma concentration of 1 µg/L of 3′-hydroxybutorphanol in 4 to 6 h. [R. C. Gaver *et al., Drug Met. Disp.*, 1980, *8*, 230–235.]

Following oral administration of 16 mg of butorphanol tartrate to 4 subjects, peak serum concentrations of 0.3 to 3 µg/L (mean 1) were attained in 2 to 4 h. [K. A. Pittman *et al., J. Pharm. Sci.*, 1980, *69*, 160–163.]

Two healthy male volunteers were administered 1 mg butorphanol tartrate as an intranasal dose for 24 h. The maximum plasma concentrations were 1.5 µg/L 0.25 h after the dose and 1.3 µg/L 0.5 h after. [D. W. Boulton *et al., J. Chromatogr. B Biomed. Sci. Appl.*, 2002, *775(1)*, 57–62.]

Bioavailability. About 17%.

Half-life. Plasma half-life, 2 to 4 h.

Volume of distribution. About 5 L/kg.

Protein binding. In plasma, about 80%.

Note. For a review of butorphanol see J. C. Gillis *et al., Drugs*, 1995, *50*, 157–175.

Dose. 1 to 4 mg of butorphanol tartrate every 4 h by IM injection; doses of 4 to 16 mg have been given by mouth.

Butoxyethyl Nicotinate

Topical Vasodilator

Proprietary names. It is an ingredient of Actinac and Finalgon.

2-Butoxyethyl nicotinate

$C_{12}H_{17}NO_3$=223.3

CAS—13912-80-6

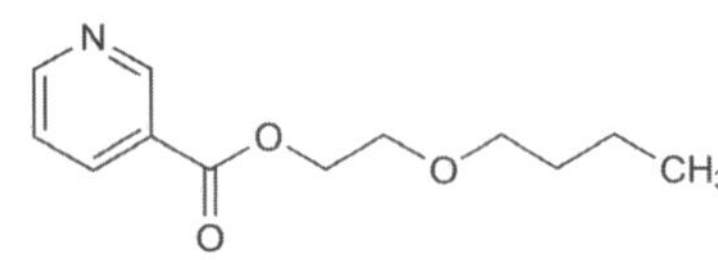

Soluble in ether; slightly soluble in dilute acetic acid.

Thin-layer Chromatography. System TA—Rf 63; system TB—Rf 45; system TC—Rf 69; system TL—Rf 62. (Acidified iodoplatinate solution, positive.)

Gas Chromatography. System GA—RI 1640.

Ultraviolet Spectrum. Methanol—279 nm (A_1^1=152b).

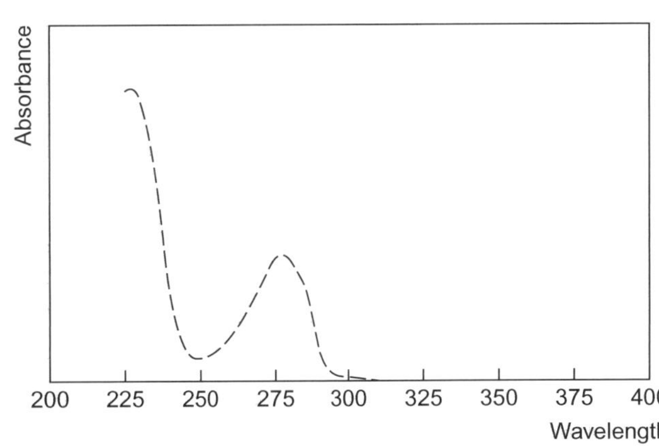

Infra-red Spectrum. Principal peaks at wavenumbers 1282, 1724, 1111, 740, 1020, 1587 cm^{-1}.

Use. Topically in a concentration of 2.5%.

Butriptyline

Antidepressant

10,11-Dihydro-*N*,*N*,*β*-trimethyl-5*H*-dibenzo[*a*,*d*]cycloheptene-5-propanamine
$C_{21}H_{27}N$=293.5
CAS—35941-65-2

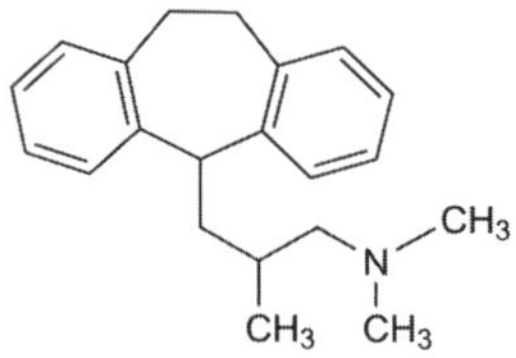

An oil. B.p. 180° to 185°.

Butriptyline Hydrochloride
Proprietary name. Evadyne
$C_{21}H_{27}N,HCl$=329.9
CAS—5585-73-9
A white crystalline powder. M.p. about 186°.
Freely soluble in water; moderately soluble in aliphatic alcohols and chloroform; insoluble in ether.

Colour Test. Marquis Test—violet.

Thin-layer Chromatography. System TA—Rf 59; system TB—Rf 61; system TC—Rf 48; system TL—Rf 38; system TAJ—Rf 22; system TAK—Rf 08; system TAL—Rf 61. (Acidified iodoplatinate solution, positive.)

Gas Chromatography. System GA—RI 2181; system GB—butriptyline RI 2288, M (nor-) RI 2330; system GF—RI 2465; system GM—butriptyline RRT 0.683, M (nor-) RRT 0.761 (relative to iprindole).

High Performance Liquid Chromatography. System HA—butriptyline *k* 2.7, norbutriptyline *k* 1.7; system HF—*k* 7.33; system HY—RI 369.

Ultraviolet Spectrum. Aqueous acid—265 nm.

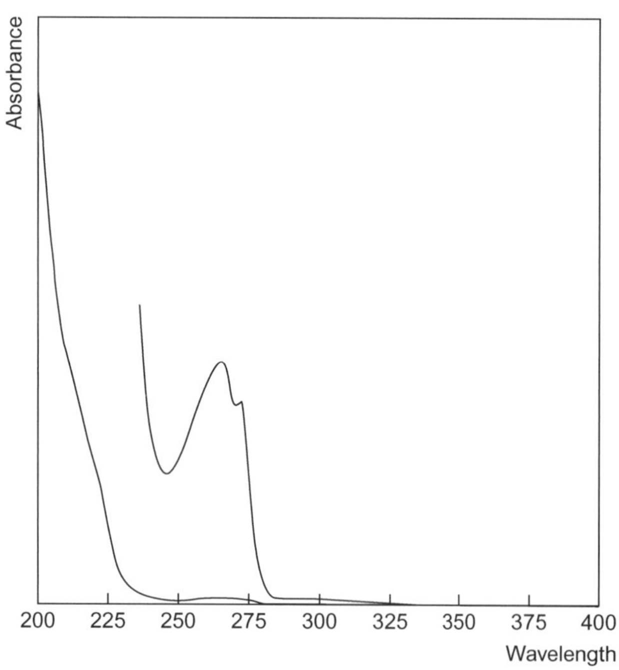

Infra-red Spectrum. Principal peaks at wavenumbers 757, 1033, 1265, 740, 1098, 1149 cm^{-1} (KCl disk).

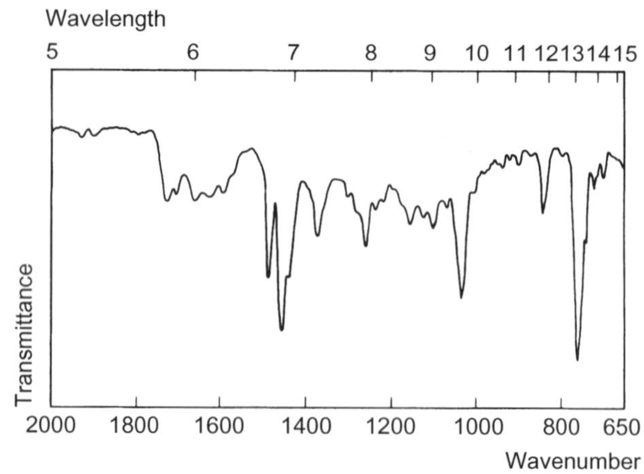

Mass Spectrum. Principal ions at *m/z* 58, 293, 45, 59, 193, 100, 178, 294.

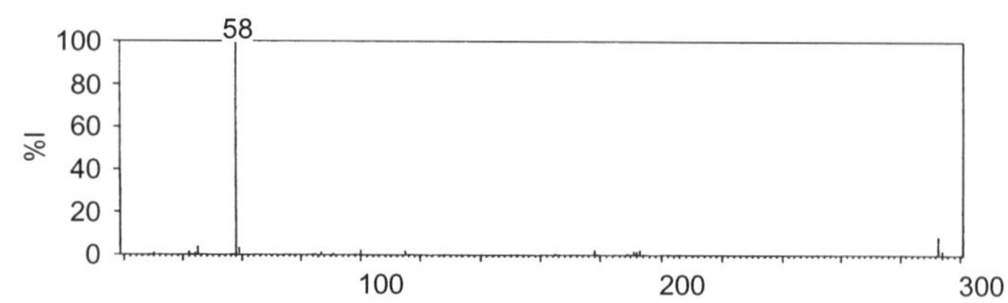

Quantification
Gas chromatography. In plasma: limit of detection 10 mg/L, FID—T. R. Norman *et al.*, *J. Chromatogr.*, 1977, *134*, 524–528.

Disposition in the Body. Readily absorbed after oral administration. It is rapidly metabolised, and the metabolites are thought to undergo enterohepatic circulation; the major metabolite is norbutriptyline. Butriptyline is slowly excreted in the urine mainly as metabolites; up to 25% of a dose is excreted in the urine in 24 h with less than 2% of the dose as unchanged drug, and about 4% as glucuronide conjugates; about 1 to 2% of a dose is eliminated in the faeces in 24 h.

Therapeutic concentration
After a single oral dose of 75 mg to 14 subjects, peak plasma concentrations of 0.024 to 0.11 mg/L (mean 0.05) were attained in about 3 h. [J. Bourgouin *et al.*, *Biopharm. Drug Disp.*, 1981, *2*, 123–130.]

Following oral administration of 50 mg three times a day to 9 subjects, steady-state plasma butriptyline concentrations of 0.06 to 0.28 mg/L (mean 0.15) were reported 6 h after the final dose; plasma concentrations of norbutriptyline were of a similar order. [G. D. Burrows *et al.*, *Med. J. Aust.*, 1977, *2*, 604–606.]

Toxicity
A 16-year-old female was found dead with a number of medication bottles in the vicinity. It was estimated that she had taken approximately 137 butriptyline tablets (25 mg each). The drug was detected in her blood at a concentration of 14.9 mg/L and in her urine at 2.96 mg/L. Salicylate and paracetamol (acetaminophen) were also detected in her blood. [J. D. Hutchison *et al.*, *J. Anal. Toxicol.*, 1994, *18(4)*, 220–224.]

Half-life. Plasma half-life, about 20 h.

Protein binding. In plasma, more than 90%.

Dose. The equivalent of 75 to 150 mg of butriptyline daily.

Butyl Aminobenzoate

Local Anaesthetic

Synonyms. Butamben; Butoforme; Scuroforme.
Butyl 4-aminobenzoate
$C_{11}H_{15}NO_2$=193.2
CAS—94-25-7

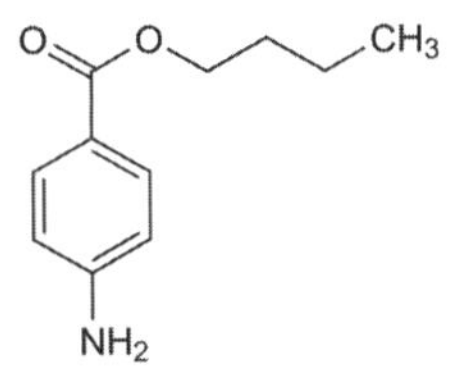

A white crystalline powder. It slowly hydrolyses when boiled with water. M.p. 57° to 59°.
Very slightly soluble in water; soluble 1 in 3 of ethanol, and 1 in 2 of ether; soluble in chloroform and in dilute mineral acids.

Butyl Aminobenzoate Picrate
Proprietary name. Butesin Picrate
$(C_{11}H_{15}NO_2)_2,C_6H_3N_3O_7=615.6$
CAS—577-48-0
A yellow powder. M.p. 109° to 110°.
Very slightly soluble in water; soluble in ethanol, chloroform, and ether.

Dissociation Constant. pK_a 2.5 (25°).

Partition Coefficient. Log *P* (octanol/water), 2.9.

Colour Test. Diazotisation—red.

Thin-layer Chromatography. System TA—Rf 75; system TB—Rf 06; system TC—Rf 63; system TL—Rf 70; system TAE—Rf 83; system TAF—Rf 90.

Gas Chromatography. System GA—RI 1742.

High Performance Liquid Chromatography. System HY—RI 483.

Ultraviolet Spectrum. Aqueous acid—279; aqueous alkali—285; ethanol—294 nm (A_1^1=1065a).

Infra-red Spectrum. Principal peaks at wavenumbers 1273, 1595, 1681, 1630, 1111, 1163 cm^{-1}.

Mass Spectrum. Principal ions at *m/z* 120, 137, 193, 92, 65, 121, 138, 41.

Quantification
Gas chromatography. In plasma, limit of detection 3 mg/L and limit of quantification 6 mg/L, nitrogen selective detection—R. J. Grouls *et al.*, *J. Chromatogr. B Biomed. Sci. Appl.*, 1995, *673(1)*, 51–57.

Note. For a review of the toxicology of topical local anaesthetics, see E. Bangha *et al.*, *Skin Pharmacol.*, 1996, *9*, 376–380.

Dose. The maximum safe dose for topical use is estimated to be 5 g.

Butylated Hydroxyanisole

Antoxidant

Synonym. BHA
Proprietary names. Embanox BHA; Nipantiox 1-F; Tenox BHA.
(1,1-Dimethylethyl)-4-methoxyphenol
$C_{11}H_{16}O_2=180.2$
CAS—25013-16-5

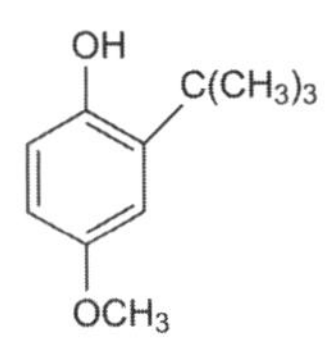

A white crystalline powder or a yellowish-white waxy solid. M.p. 48° to 55°.
It contains a variable proportion of 3-*tert*-butyl-4-methoxyphenol.
Practically insoluble in water; soluble 1 in 4 of ethanol, 1 in 2 of chloroform, 1 in 1.2 of ether and 1 in 2 of propylene glycol; soluble in solutions of alkali hydroxides.

Partition Coefficient. Log *P* (octanol/water), 3.5.

Colour Tests. Dissolve 0.1 g in 10 mL of ethanol, add 2 mL of a 2% solution of borax and a few crystals of 2,6-dichloroquinone-chloroimide—blue (compare blue colour produced by butylated hydroxytoluene).
Dissolve a few crystals in 10 mL of ethanol and add 0.5 mL of a 0.2% solution of ferric ammonium sulfate in 0.5 M sulfuric acid—green-blue.

Gas Chromatography. System GA—RI 1462.

Ultraviolet Spectrum. Acid ethanol—228 (A_1^1=340a), 292 nm (A_1^1=205a).

Infra-red Spectrum. Principal peaks at wavenumbers 1202, 1220, 1050, 805, 1185, 1294 cm^{-1} (KBr disk).

Quantification
Gas chromatography. In plasma or urine: limit of detection <100 µg/L, FID—R. El-Rashidy and S. Niazi, *J. Pharm. Sci.*, 1979, *68*, 103–104.

High performance liquid chromatography. In plasma—H. Verhagen *et al.*, *J. Chromatogr.*, 1987, *413*, 282–286.

Disposition in the Body. Butylated hydroxyanisole is absorbed after oral administration and may be stored in body fat after large doses. It is metabolised by *O*-demethylation and conjugation with glucuronic acid and sulfate. Less than 1% of a dose is excreted in the urine unchanged in 24 h together with 44% as the glucuronide, 26% as the sulfate and about 22% each as the glucuronide and sulfate conjugates of the desmethyl metabolite.

Protein binding. In plasma, highly bound.

Butylated Hydroxytoluene

Antoxidant

Synonyms. BHT; DBPC.
Proprietary names. Anullex BHT; Embanox BHT.
2,6-Bis-(1,1-dimethylethyl)-4-methylphenol
$C_{15}H_{24}O=220.4$
CAS—128-37-0

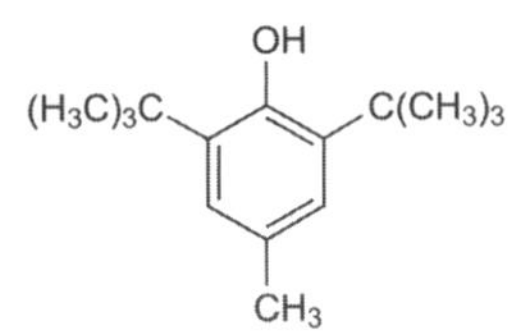

Colourless crystals or white crystalline powder. M.p. 70°.
Insoluble in water; freely soluble in toluene; soluble in acetone; soluble 1 in 4 of ethanol, 1 in 1.1 of chloroform, and 1 in 0.5 of ether; practically insoluble in propylene glycol and in solutions of alkali hydroxides.

Dissociation Constant. pK_a 12.2.

Partition Coefficient. Log *P* (octanol/water), 5.1.

Colour Test. Dissolve 0.1 g in 10 mL of ethanol, add 2 mL of a 2% solution of borax and a few crystals of 2,6-dichloroquinonechloroimide—faint blue (compare blue colour produced by butylated hydroxyanisole).

Gas Chromatography. System GA—RI 1490.

Ultraviolet Spectrum. Dehydrated alcohol—278 nm (A_1^1=85a).

Quantification
High performance liquid chromatography. In plasma and tissue: limit of detection 0.4 mg/L, ECD—L. Bianchi *et al.*, *J. Chromatogr. B Biomed. Sci. Appl.*, 1997, *694(2)*, 359–365.

Disposition in the Body. Readily absorbed after oral administration. About 50% of a dose is excreted in the urine in 24 h mainly as glucuronide conjugates of oxidation products.

Butylchloral Hydrate

Hypnotic

Synonyms. Croton-Cloral Hydrate; Trichlorobutylidene Glycol.
2,2,3-Trichlorobutane-1,1-diol
$C_4H_7Cl_3O_2=193.5$
CAS—76-40-4

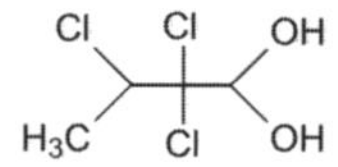

Pearly-white crystalline scales. M.p. about 78°.
Soluble 1 in 40 of water, 1 in 0.6 of ethanol (forming an ethanolate), 1 in 20 of chloroform and 1 in 2 of ether.

Partition Coefficient. Log *P* (octanol/water), 1.9.

Ultraviolet Spectrum. No significant absorption, 230 to 360 nm.

Infra-red Spectrum. Principal peaks at wavenumbers 830, 1090, 1051, 1020, 690, 1300 cm^{-1} (KBr disk).

Dose. Butylchloral hydrate has been given in a dose of 0.3 to 1.2 g.

Cabergoline

Dopamine D_2-agonist

Synonym. FCE-21336.
Proprietary names. Cabaser; Dostinex.
(8β)-*N*-[3-(Dimethylamino)propyl]-*N*-[(ethylamino)carbonyl]-6-(2-propenyl)ergoline-8-carboxamide
$C_{26}H_{37}N_5O_2$=451.6
CAS—81409-90-7

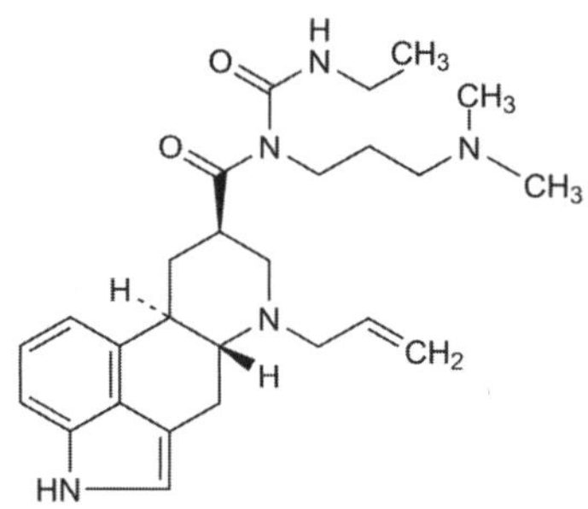

A white powder. It is insoluble in water; soluble in chloroform, ethanol, and dimethylformamide; slightly soluble in 0.1 M hydrochloric acid; very slightly soluble in hexane.

Cabergoline Diphosphate
$C_{26}H_{37}N_5O_2,2H_3PO_4$=647.6
CAS—85329-89-1
M.p. 153° to 155°.

High Performance Liquid Chromatography. Column: C_{18} (Nucleosil, 250 × 4 mm i.d., 5 μm). Mobile phase: acetonitrile:75 mM phosphate buffer pH 3 (20:80), 0.6 mL/min. Electrochemical detection. Retention time: 14 min. [E. Pianezzola *et al.*, *J. Chromatogr.*, 1992, *574*; *Biomed. Appl.*, *112*, 170–174].

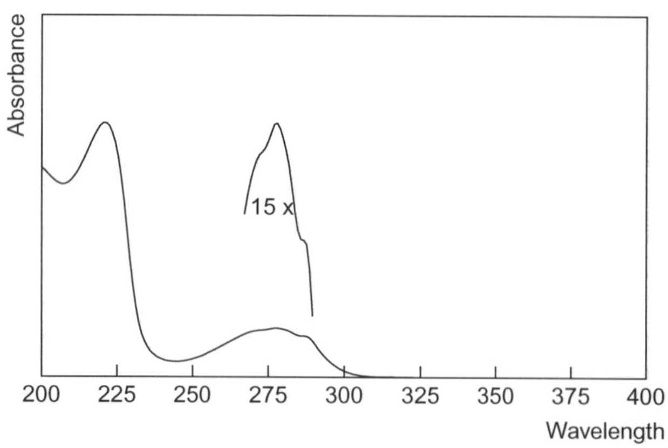

Quantification
High performance liquid chromatography. In plasma or urine: limit of detection 0.25 μg/L and 0.30 μg/L, respectively; electrochemical detection—E. Pianezzola *et al.*, *J. Chromatogr.*, 1992, *574*; *Biomed. Appl.*, *112*, 170–174.

Disposition in the Body. Cabergoline is absorbed after oral administration and undergoes significant first-pass metabolism. It is widely distributed and extensively metabolised, mainly by hydrolysis, to several inactive metabolites. The drug is mainly eliminated via faeces with a small proportion excreted in urine. Less than 4% is excreted unchanged; 1% as the parent drug.

Therapeutic concentration
12 healthy males, aged 21 to 31 years (mean 26 years), were administered with single doses of 0.5, 1.0 and 1.5 mg cabergoline. Mean maximum plasma concentrations were 33.3, 40.3 and 67.0 ng/L, respectively, for the three doses and all were observed at approx. 2 h. [A. C. Andreotti *et al.*, *J. Clin. Endocrinol. Metab.*, 1995, *80(3)*, 841–845].

Half-life. Plasma half-life, 63 to 68 h (in healthy subjects); 79 to 115 h (in hyperprolactinaemic subjects).

Protein binding. In plasma, 40%.

Note. For reviews of cabergoline see C. P. Rains *et al.*, *Drugs*, 1995, *49*, 255–279 and R. G. Fariello, *Drugs*, 1998, *55*, *Suppl.* 1, 10–16.

Dose. Usually 1 mg weekly for hyperprolactinaemia, up to 6 mg daily for Parkinson's disease.

Cadaverine

Putrefactive Base

Synonym. Pentamethylenediamine
1,5-Pentanediamine
$C_5H_{14}N_2$=102.2
CAS—462-94-2

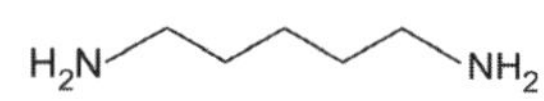

A colourless syrupy basic liquid, which fumes and absorbs carbon dioxide on exposure to air. F.p. 9°. B.p. 178° to 180°.
Soluble in water and ethanol; slightly soluble in ether.

Partition Coefficient. Log *P* (octanol/water), −0.2.

Thin-layer Chromatography. System TA—Rf 02. (Acidified iodoplatinate solution, positive.)

Gas Chromatography. System GA—RI 1035.

Ultraviolet Spectrum. No significant absorption, 230 to 360 nm.

Infra-red Spectrum. Principal peaks at wavenumbers 1565, 1508, 1600, 1120, 1173, 923 cm^{-1} (KBr disk).

Mass Spectrum. Principal ions at *m/z* 56, 55, 41, 43, 45, 85, 42, 84.

Quantification
Gas chromatography. In serum: limit of detection 0.5 mg/L, FID—M. Y. Khuhawar *et al.*, *J. Chromatogr. B Biomed. Sci. Appl.*, 1999, *723(1–2)*, 17–24.

Gas chromatography–mass spectrometry. In hair—M. H. Choi *et al.*, *J. Chromatogr. A*, 2000, *897(1–2)*, 295–305.

Disposition in the Body. Cadaverine is formed during putrefaction by bacterial decarboxylation of lysine in the gastro-intestinal tract. It may be deaminated to yield ammonia and an aldehyde, and it may undergo cyclisation to piperidine. The piperidine normally excreted in the urine is from cadaverine.

Caffeine

Xanthine Stimulant

Synonyms. Anhydrous Caffeine; Coffeinum; Guaranine; Methyltheobromine; Théine.
Proprietary names. Autonic; Cafcit; Caffedrine; Coffee Break; Doxypol; Durvitan; Enerjets; Keep Alert; Percoffedrinol N; Percutafeine; NoDoz; Prolert; Pro-Plus; Quick Pep; Spray-n-Wake; Stay Alert; Tirend; Universal Concentration Tablets; Vivarin; Wake-Up Tablets; Xeramax.

Caffeine is an ingredient of many proprietary preparations—see *Martindale, The complete drug reference*, 33rd Edn., Pharmaceutical Press, London, 2002.
3,7-Dihydro-1,3,7-trimethyl-1*H*-purine-2,6-dione
$C_8H_{10}N_4O_2$=194.2
CAS—58-08-2

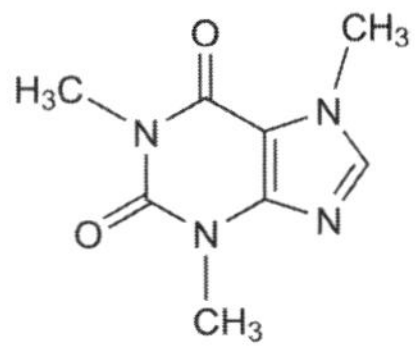

An alkaloid obtained from tea waste, or coffee, or from the dried leaves of *Camellia sinensis* (Theaceae), or prepared synthetically; it is also present in guarana, maté, and kola.
Silky white crystals, usually matted together, or a white crystalline powder. It sublimes at 178°. M.p. 238°. When crystallised from water, caffeine contains 1 molecule of water of crystallisation, but it is anhydrous when crystallised from ethanol, chloroform, or ether. It is decomposed by strong solutions of caustic alkalis.
Soluble 1 in 46 of water, 1 in 5.5 water at 80°, 1 in 1.5 of boiling water, 1 in 66 alcohol, 1 in 22 alcohol at 60°, 1 in 50 acetone, 1 in 5.5 of chloroform, 1 in 530 ether, 1 in 100 benzene, and 1 in 22 boiling benzene. Freely soluble in pyrrole and in tetrahydrofuran containing about 4% water; soluble in ethyl acetate; slightly soluble in petroleum ether. Solubility in water is increased by alkali benzoates, cinnamates, citrates, or salicylates.

Caffeine Citrate

Synonyms. Citrated Caffeine; Coffeinum Citricum.
Proprietary names. It is an ingredient of Antoin, Cojene, and Myolgin.
$C_8H_{10}N_4O_2,C_6H_8O_7$=386.3
CAS—69-22-7
A mixture of caffeine and citric acid containing 47 to 50% of anhydrous caffeine.
A white powder which is decomposed by water.
Soluble 1 in 4 of hot water, dissociating on further dilution with the separation of caffeine on cooling which redissolves in about 32 of water; soluble 1 in 25 of ethanol.

Caffeine Hydrate

Synonyms. Caffeine Monohydrate; Coffeinum Monohydricum.
Proprietary names. It is an ingredient of Migril and Pardale.
$C_8H_{10}N_4O_2,H_2O$=212.2
CAS—5743-12-4
Silky white crystals, usually matted together, or a white crystalline powder. It effloresces in dry air and loses its water of crystallisation when heated, becoming anhydrous at 80°. It sublimes at about 180°. M.p. 234° to 239°.
Soluble 1 in 60 of water and 1 in 110 of ethanol; soluble in chloroform with the separation of water; slightly soluble in ether.

Dissociation Constant. pK_a 14.0 (25°), 10.4 (40°).

Partition Coefficient. Log *P* (octanol/water), −0.07.

Colour Test. Amalic Acid Test—orange/violet.

Thin-layer Chromatography. System TA—Rf 52; system TB—Rf 03; system TC—Rf 58; system TD—Rf 15; system TE—Rf 52; system TF—Rf 10; system TL—Rf 25; system TAD—Rf 55; system TAE—Rf 59; system TAF—Rf 55; system TAJ—Rf 54; system TAK—Rf 18; system TAL—Rf 81. (Dragendorff spray, positive; acidified iodoplatinate solution, positive.)

Gas Chromatography. System GA—caffeine RI 1800, theobromine RI 1807, theophylline RI 2005; system GB—caffeine RI 1904, theobromine RI 1920, theophylline RI 1990; system GC—RI 2376; system GF—RI 2340.

High Performance Liquid Chromatography. System HA—*k* 0.2; system HC—*k* 0.26; system HS—*k* 0.21; system HX—RI 305; system HY—RI 259; system HZ—retention time 1.9 min; system HAA—retention time 6.7 min; system HAM—retention time 1.98 min; system HAX—retention time 4.8 min; system HAY—retention time 3.8 min; system HAZ—*k* 0.18.

Ultraviolet Spectrum. Aqueous acid—273 nm (A^1_1=504a). No alkaline shift.

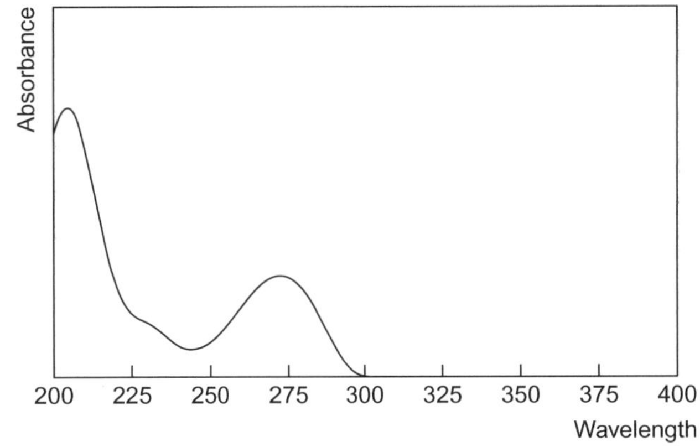

Infra-red Spectrum. Principal peaks at wavenumbers 1658, 1698, 747, 1548, 1242, 760 cm^{-1} (KBr disk).

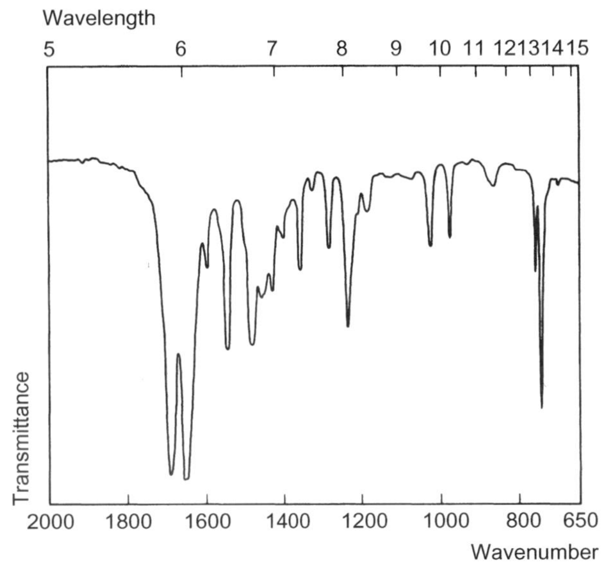

Mass Spectrum. Principal ions at *m/z* 194, 109, 55, 67, 82, 195, 42, 110.

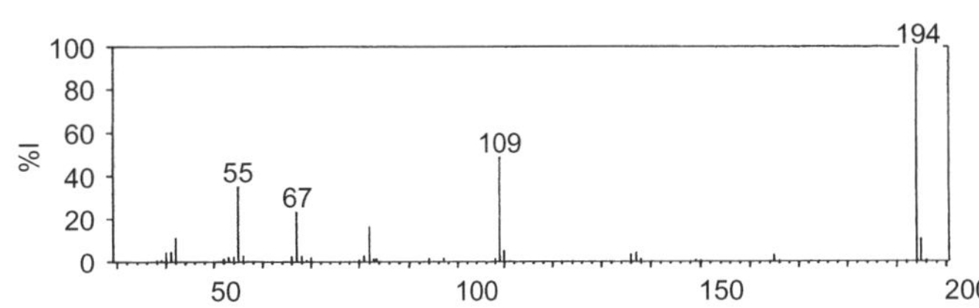

Quantification

Gas chromatography. In plasma: limit of detection 50 µg/L, AFID—I.D. Bradbrook *et al.*, *J. Chromatogr.* 1979, *163*(5) *Biomed. Appl.*, 118–122. In blood , plasma, or saliva: limit of detection in plasma 1 µg/L, nitrogen-sensitive detection—H. W. Teeuwen *et al.*, *Mol. Biol. Rep.*, 1991, *15*, 1–7. In plasma: NPD, comparison with ELISA—A. B. Carregaro *et al.*, *Braz. J. Med. Biol. Res.*, 2001, *34*, 821–824.

Gas chromatography–mass spectrometry. In sweat—T. Tsuda *et al.*, *Biomed. Chromatogr.*, 2000, *14*, 505–510.

High performance liquid chromatography. In plasma, serum or saliva: limit of detection 100 µg/L, UV detection—D. B. Haughey *et al.*, *J. Chromatogr.* 1982, *229*(18) *Biomed. Appl.*, 387–395. In plasma: limit of detection 100 µg/L, UV detection—S. E. O'Connell and F. J. Zurzola, *J. Pharm. Sci.*, 1984, *73*, 1009–1011. In plasma: caffeine and its metabolites, limit of detection for caffeine 5 µg/L, UV detection—E. Tanaka, *J. Chromatogr.*, 1992, *575*, 311–314. In plasma or urine: caffeine and its metabolites—P. Dobrocky *et al.*, *J. Chromatogr.*, 1994, *652*, 104–108. In urine: caffeine and its metabolites, limits of detection 2 to 5 µmol/L, CE—N. Rodopoulos and A.

Norman, *Scand. J. Clin. Lab. Invest.*, 1994, *54*, 305–315. In plasma: caffeine and theophylline, limit of detection 0.1 mg/L, UV detection—E. Schreiber-Deturmeny and B. Bruguerolle, *J. Chromatogr.* 1996, *677 B Biomed. Appl.*, 305–312. In urine: caffeine metabolites, limits of detection 1 to 2 µmol, UV detection—B. B. Rasmussen and K. Brosen, *Ther. Drug Monit.*, 1996, 18, 254–262. In serum: caffeine and paraxanthine, limit of quantification 50 µg/L, UV detection—D. T. Holden *et al.*, *J. Chromatogr. B Biomed. Sci. Appl.*, 1998, *707*, 105–110. In serum: caffeine and theophylline, limit of detection for caffeine 0.5 mg/L, UV detection—T. Umemura *et al.*, *Analyst*, 1998, *123*, 1767–1770. In serum: caffeine and paraxanthine, limit of detection for caffeine 0.3 mg/L, UV detection—J. P. Koch *et al.*, *Biomed. Chromatogr.*, 1999, 13, 309–314. In plasma: caffeine, cotinine, and 3′-hydroxycotinine, limit of detection for caffeine 10 µg/L, UV detection—O. A. Ghosheh *et al.*, *J. Pharm. Biomed. Anal.*, 2000, *23*, 543–549. In urine: caffeine and its metabolites, UV detection—E. K. Bendriss *et al.*, *J. Chromatogr. B Biomed. Sci. Appl.*, 2000, *746*, 331–338; A. Nyeki *et al.*, *J. Chromatogr. B Biomed. Sci. Appl.*, 2001, *755*, 73–84. In serum or urine: caffeine and its metabolites, limit of detection for caffeine 20 µg/L, UV detection—K. A. Georgia *et al.*, *J. Chromatogr. B Biomed. Sci. Appl.*, 2001, *759*, 209–218. In urine: caffeine metabolites, diode-array detection—M. S. Caubet *et al.*, *J. Pharm. Biomed. Anal.*, 2002, *27*, 261–270. In urine: caffeine, theobromine, and theophylline, limit of detection < 1 ng/L, UV detection—M. S. Bispo *et al.*, *J. Chromatogr. Sci.*, 2002, *40*, 45–48.

High performance liquid chromatography–mass spectrometry. In plasma or urine: limit of detection about 5 µg/L—Y. Hieda *et al.*, *J. Chromatogr. 1995, 667 B Biomed. Appl., 241–246.*

Disposition in the Body. Rapidly absorbed after oral administration. It is widely distributed; it crosses the placenta and also enters the CNS and saliva; small amounts are excreted in breast milk. Metabolic reactions include *N*-demethylation, acetylation, and oxidation to uric acid derivatives. About 85% of a dose is excreted in the urine in 48 h with up to 40% of the dose as 1-methyluric acid, 10 to 15% as 1-methylxanthine, and up to 35% as 5-acetylamino-6-formylamino-3-methyluracil and 5-acetylamino-6-amino-3-methyluracil; other metabolites excreted in the urine include theophylline, 1,7-dimethylxanthine (paraxanthine), 7-methylxanthine, and 1,3-dimethyluric acid. About 1% is excreted in the urine as unchanged drug. The extent of *N*-acetylation is genetically determined. In neonates, caffeine is largely excreted unchanged in the urine, because, until about 6 months of age, the capacity to metabolise the drug is reduced. Caffeine, theophylline, theobromine, and paraxanthine are found in plasma from dietary sources especially coffee, tea, and cocoa. An average cup of coffee or tea contains approximately 100 mg of caffeine.

Therapeutic concentration

Following a single dose of 130 mg to 36 subjects, peak plasma concentrations of 2.5 to 6.8 mg/L (mean 4.0) were attained in 20 to 40 min. [S. E. O'Connell and F. J. Zurzola, *J. Pharm. Sci.*, 1984, *73*, 1009–1011.]

Following a single oral dose of 5 mg/kg to 10 subjects, peak plasma concentrations of 6.9 to 16.1 mg/L (mean 10) were attained in about 0.5 h. [J. Blanchard and S. J. A. Sawers, *Eur. J. Clin. Pharmacol.*, 1983, *24*, 93–98.]

Toxicity. Fatalities have occurred after the ingestion of 5 to 50 g of caffeine, but recovery following the ingestion of 30 g has been reported. Toxic effects are associated with blood concentrations greater than 15 mg/L and fatalities with blood concentrations greater than 80 mg/L.

A 1-year-old girl survived after ingesting 2 to 3 g of caffeine (200 to 300 mg/kg) despite having a maximum serum concentration of 385 mg/L 4 h post-ingestion. Symptoms of toxicity included arrhythmias, seizures, metabolic disturbances, and severe pulmonary oedema. [A. M. Dietrich and M. E. Mortensen, *Pediatr. Emerg. Care*, 1990, *6*, 296–298.]

In a fatality due to the ingestion of mail order diet pills containing caffeine as their only active ingredient, a 1560 mg/L postmortem serum concentration was reported in a 22-year-old female. [R. M. Mrvos *et al.*, *Vet. Hum. Toxicol.*, 1989, *31*, 571–572.]

The following postmortem tissue concentrations were reported in a fatality due to the ingestion of 5.3 g of caffeine by a 5-year-old child: blood 159 mg/L, kidney 230 µg/g, liver 198 µg/g, urine 114 mg/L. [V. J. M. DiMaio and J. G. Garriott, *Forensic Sci.*, 1974, *3*, 275–278.]

In a fatality due to the ingestion of 50 g of caffeine, the following postmortem tissue concentrations were reported: blood 79 mg/L, brain 105 µg/g, kidney 145 µg/g, liver 214 µg/g, urine 280 mg/L. [E. Grusz-Harday, *Bull. Int. Assoc. Forensic Toxicol.*, 1973, *9(1–2)*, 6–7.]

Bioavailability. Almost 100%.

Half-life. Plasma half-life, 2 to 10 h (mean 4).

Volume of distribution. About 0.5 L/kg.

Clearance. Plasma clearance, 1 to 2 mL/min/kg.

Distribution in blood. Plasma:whole blood ratio, 0.93.

Saliva. Plasma:saliva ratio, about 1.3.

Protein binding. In plasma, about 35%.

Dose. 50 to 200 mg as a mild stimulant; maximum 1 g daily

Calfactant

Pulmonary Surfactant

Synonyms. CLSE; CLL.
Proprietary name. Infasurf
Chloroform/methanol extract of calf lung lavage fluid consisting of 35 mg/mL phospholipid (of which 55 to 70% is dipalmitoylphosphatidylcholine), 0.9 mg/mL fatty acids, 1.8 mg/mL neutral lipids, and low-molecular-weight surfactant proteins (SP-B and SP-C).
CAS—183325-78-2

Protein binding. Approximately 50%.

Note. For the separation of subfractions of the hydrophobic components of calfactant, see S. B. Hall *et al.*, *J. Lipid Res.*, 1994, *35*, 1386–1394; for a review of calfactant, see D. Willson, *Expert Opin. Pharmacother.*, 2001, *2*, 1479–1493.

Dose. In prophylaxis of respiratory distress syndrome at birth, 3 mL/kg of birth weight in two doses. In treatment of respiratory distress syndrome within 72 h of birth, 3 mL/kg of birth weight, in two doses. Repeat doses of 3 mL/kg of birth weight to a maximum of 3 doses 12 h apart.

Camazepam

Tranquilliser

Proprietary names. Albego; Limpidon.
7-Chloro-2,3-dihydro-1-methyl-2-oxo-5-phenyl-1*H*-1,4-benzodiazepin-3-yl dimethylcarbamate
$C_{19}H_{18}ClN_3O_3 = 371.8$
CAS—36104-80-0

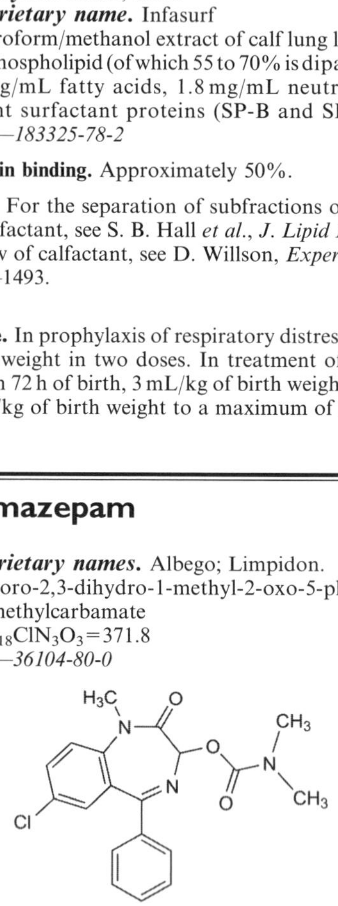

A white crystalline powder. M.p. 173° to 174°.
Moderately soluble in water; soluble in ethanol.

Partition Coefficient. Log *P* (octanol/water), 2.7.

Thin-layer Chromatography. System TA—Rf 76; system TB—Rf 12; system TC—Rf 73; system TD—Rf 55; system TE—Rf 75; system TF—Rf 32; system TL—Rf 65; system TAD—Rf 69; system TAE—Rf 82; system TAF—Rf 83.

Gas Chromatography. System GA—RI 2945; system GB—RI 3162.

High Performance Liquid Chromatography. System HY—RI 506; system HZ—retention time, 9.6 min.

Ultraviolet Spectrum. Methanol—231 (A^1_1 = 937b), 315 nm (A^1_1 = 67b).

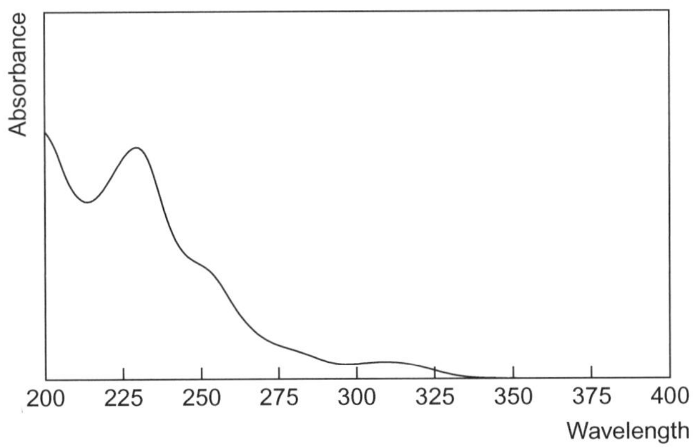

Infra-red Spectrum. Principal peaks at wavenumbers 1680, 1718, 1193, 1318, 1110, 703 cm^{-1}.

Mass Spectrum. Principal ions at *m/z* 58, 72, 43, 78, 271, 57, 44, 77.

Quantification
Gas chromatography. In plasma: limit of detection 1 mg/L, ECD—G. Cuisinaud *et al.*, *J. Chromatogr.*, 1979, *178*, 314–319.

Disposition in the Body. Metabolises to oxazepam and temazepam.

Dose. 20 to 60 mg daily.

Cambendazole

Anthelmintic

Synonym. MK-905
Proprietary names. Bovicam (vet.). It is an ingredient of Porcam (vet.).
[2-(4-Thiazolyl)-1*H*-benzimidazol-5-yl]carbamic acid 1-methylethyl ester
$C_{14}H_{14}N_4O_2S$=302.4
CAS—26097-80-3

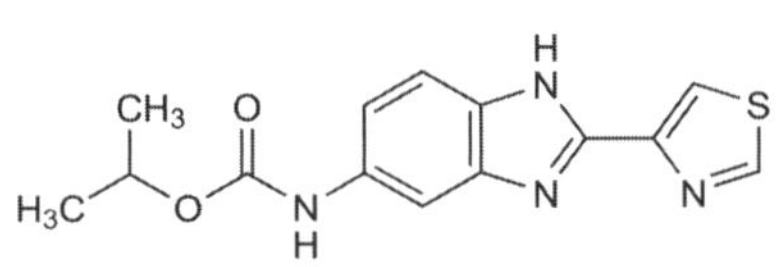

A white crystalline powder. M.p. 238° to 240°, with decomposition.
Practically insoluble in water; soluble in ethanol and dimethylformamide; sparingly soluble in acetone; slightly soluble in benzene; very slightly soluble in 0.1 M HCl.

Partition Coefficient. Log *P* (octanol/water), 2.7.

Ultraviolet Spectrum. Aqueous acid—235 (A^1_1=620b), 319 nm (A^1_1=689b); aqueous alkali—237 (A^1_1=936b), 314 nm (A^1_1=649b).

Mass Spectrum. Principal ions at *m/z* 260, 302, 216, 215, 243, 189, 242, 188.

Camphor

Rubefacient

Synonyms. Alcanfor; 2-Camphanone; Camphre Droit (natural); Camphre du Japon (natural); Cânfora.
Proprietary name. It is an ingredient of Pernomol.
1,7,7-Trimethylbicyclo[2.2.1]heptan-2-one
$C_{10}H_{16}O$=152.2
CAS—76-22-2; 464-49-3 (+)

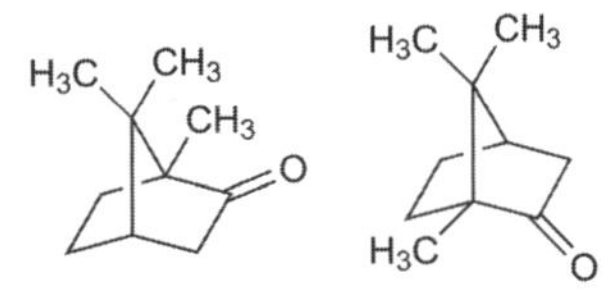

l-form d-form

Camphor is obtained by distillation from the wood of *Cinnamomum camphora* (Lauraceae) and purified by sublimation, or it may be prepared synthetically. Natural camphor is dextrorotatory; the synthetic product is optically inactive.
Colourless transparent or white crystals, crystalline masses, blocks, or powdery masses known as 'flowers of camphor'. M.p. 179°.
Soluble 1 in 700 to 1 in 800 of water, 1 in 1 of ethanol, 1 in 0.5 of chloroform, and 1 in 1 of ether.

Partition Coefficient. Log *P* (octanol/water), 2.4.

Thin-layer Chromatography. System TAF—Rf 93; system TAJ—Rf 98; system TAK—Rf 95; system TAL—Rf 98.

Gas Chromatography. System GA—RI 1143; system GI—retention time 38.2 min.

Ultraviolet Spectrum. Methanol—289 nm (A^1_1=about 2b).

Infra-red Spectrum. Principal peaks at wavenumbers 1730, 1047, 1025, 1277, 1095, 755 cm^{-1} (KCl disk).

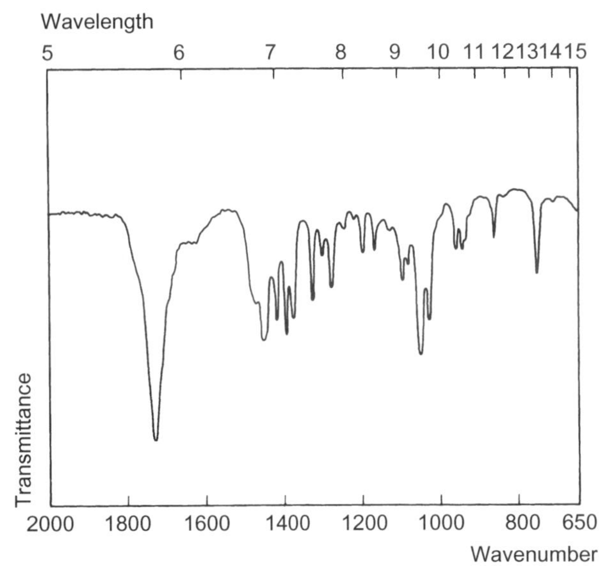

Mass Spectrum. Principal ions at *m/z* 95, 81, 41, 69, 55, 83, 67, 137.

Quantification
Gas chromatography. In plasma: limit of detection 100 mg/L, FID—R. C. Kelly *et al.*, *J. Anal. Toxicol.*, 1979, *3*, 76–77. In plasma: limit of detection 1 mg/L and limit of quantification 5 mg/L, FID—J. S. Valdez *et al.*, *J. Chromatogr. B Biomed. Sci. Appl.*, 1999, *729(1–2)*, 163–171.

Disposition in the Body. Absorbed after ingestion, through the mucous membranes and through the skin. Metabolised by hydroxylation and excreted in the urine mainly as the glucuronides of 2-hydroxy- and 3-hydroxycamphor. Oxidation also occurs at the 7-position yielding a small amount of a carboxylic acid.

Toxicity. Poisoning by camphor has usually been due to ingestion of camphorated oil. The fatal dose in a one-year-old child is stated to be about 1 g of camphor although some children have survived the ingestion of 5 g. In adults, doses in the region of 2 g are likely to produce toxic symptoms and a dose of 4 g or more may be lethal, although a man has survived after ingestion of as much as 30 g in the form of 150 mL of camphorated oil. The maximum permissible atmospheric concentration is 2 ppm.

A plasma concentration of 1.7 mg/L was reported in a severely intoxicated subject, 12 h after the ingestion of about 18 g of camphor; the patient recovered after treatment by resin haemoperfusion. [R. Kopelman *et al.*, *JAMA*, 1979, *241*, 727–728.]

A serum concentration of 19.5 mg/L was observed 7 h after the ingestion of 0.7 g of camphor in a moderately intoxicated 3-year-old child. [W. J. Phelan, *Pediatrics*, 1976, *57*, 428–431.]

Dose. Camphor was formerly given by mouth in doses of 120 to 300 mg.

Candesartan

Angiotensin II Receptor Antagonist

Synonym. CV-11974
2-Ethoxy-1-[[2′-(1H-tetrazol-5-yl)[1,1′-biphenyl]-4-yl]methyl]-1H-benzimidazole-7-carboxylic acid
$C_{24}H_{20}N_6O_3 = 440.5$
CAS—139481-59-7
Colourless crystals., M.p. 183° to 185°.

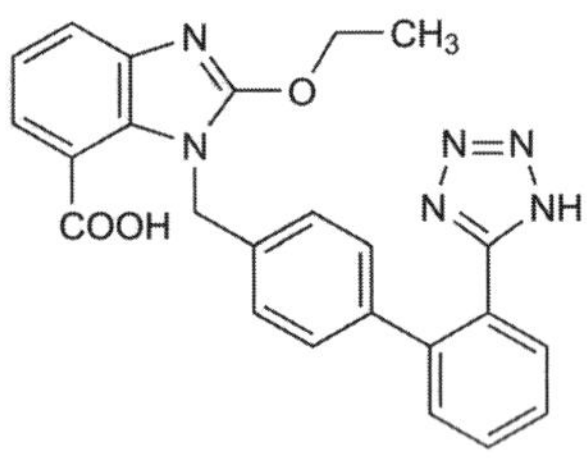

Candesartan Cilexetil

Synonym. TCV-116
Proprietary names. Amias; Atacand.
$C_{33}H_{34}N_6O_6 = 610.7$
CAS—145040-37-5
A white to off-white powder. M.p. 163°. It is practically insoluble in water; sparingly soluble in methanol.

Ultraviolet Spectrum. Aqueous acid (0.2 M H_2SO_4)—246, 281 nm; (ethanol)—253 nm; aqueous base (0.5 M NaOH)—251 nm.

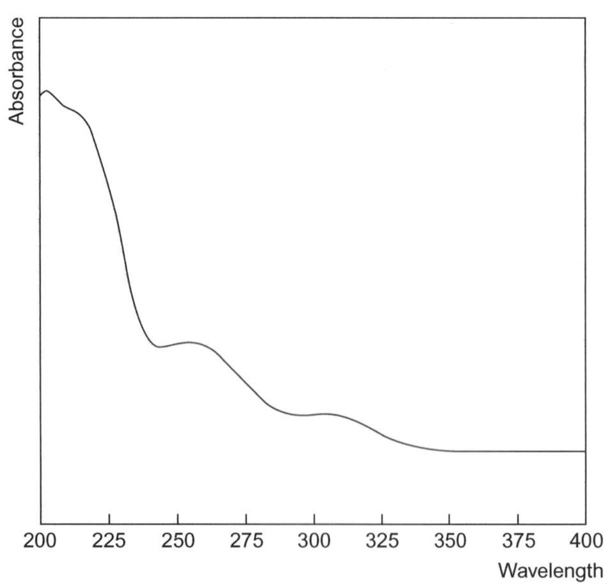

Quantification

High performance liquid chromatography. In serum or urine: limit of detection for candesartan and candesartan cilexetil 2 µg/L in serum and for candesartan cilexetil 10 µg/L in urine, UV detection—J. W. Lee *et al.*, *J. Chromatogr.* 1995, *670*; *Biomed. Appl.*, 287–298. In serum: candesartan, limit of detection 0.8 µg/L—E. Delacrétaz *et al.*, *Hypertension*, 1995, *25*, 14–21.

Disposition in the Body. Candesartan cilexetil is absorbed after oral administration with an absolute bioavailability for candesartan of about 40% following administration of a solution or 14% following administration of tablets. Candesartan is the active metabolite. Peak plasma concentrations occur after about 3 to 4 h. It is excreted in urine and bile mainly as unchanged drug and a small amount of inactive metabolites. Hydrolysed during absorption to form candesartan. Not removed by haemodialysis.

Therapeutic concentration

27 male, healthy volunteers, aged 20 to 36 years (mean age, 26 years), were administered with doses of 1, 2, 4 or 8 g candesartan cilexetil on 8 consecutive days, after an overnight fast. Plasma concentrations of the parent drug were not detected but the active metabolite was detected at peak concentrations between 3.5 and 6.0 h. The mean concentrations on day 1 were 5.5, 12.7, 34.3 and 47.7 µg/L for the 1, 2, 4 and 8 mg doses, respectively. On day 8, the concentrations were 8.8, 17.6, 42.8 and 48.2 µg/L, respectively. [E. Delacrétaz *et al.*, *Hypertension*, 1995, *25*, 14–21].

Half-life. Plasma half-life, 9 h.

Protein binding. In plasma, more than 99%.

Dose. Usually 8 mg of candesartan cilexetil daily, with a maximum dose of 16 mg.

Cannabis

Psychomimetic

Synonyms. Bhang; Cannabis Indica; Chanvre; Charas; Dagga; Ganja; Guaza; Hashish; Hanfkraut; Indian Hemp; Kif; Maconha; Marijuana; Marihuana.
Marijuana usually refers to a mixture of the leaves and flowering tops. Bhang, dagga, ganja, kif, and maconha are commonly used in various countries to describe similar preparations. Hashish and charas are names often applied to the resin, although in some countries hashish is applied to any cannabis preparation.
Note. Many other synonyms, approximate synonyms, and street names for cannabis and cannabis resin have been used—see *Martindale, The complete drug reference*, 33rd Edn., Pharmaceutical Press. London, 2002.
CAS—8063-14-7
The dried flowering or fruiting tops of the pistillate plant of *Cannabis sativa* (Cannabinaceae). In some countries, the legal definition includes the leaves and roots. Cannabis contains over 60 derivatives of 2-(2-isopropyl-5-methylphenyl)-5-pentylresorcinol, known as cannabinoids.
Considerable confusion exists in the nomenclature, depending on whether they are numbered as substituted monoterpenes or dibenzopyrans. To avoid confusion the dibenzofuran system is used in this volume.
Dibenzofuran numbering.

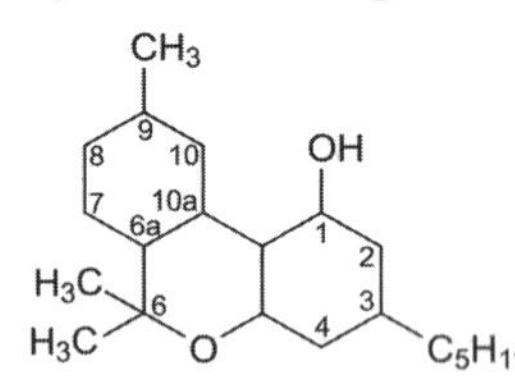

Where appropriate, the alternative numbering system based on a substituted monoterpene structure is given in parentheses.
Monoterpenoid numbering.

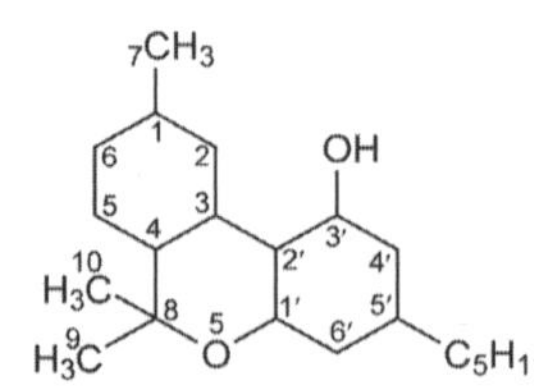

The most important cannabinoids are cannabidiol (CBD), cannabinol (CBN), (−)-*trans*-Δ^9-tetrahydrocannabinol [Δ^9-THC (Δ^1-THC)], (−)-*trans*-Δ^8-tetrahydrocannabinol [Δ^8-THC (Δ^{1-6}-THC)], and Δ^9-tetrahydrocannabinolic acid.

Cannabidiol

Synonym. CBD
2-[3-Methyl-6-(1-methylethenyl)-2-cyclohexen-1-yl]-5-pentyl-1,3-benzenediol
$C_{21}H_{30}O_2 = 314.5$
CAS—13956-29-1

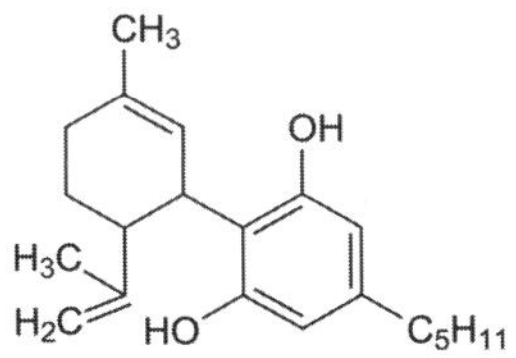

Pale yellow resin or crystal. M.p. 66° to 67°.

Practically insoluble in water or 10% NaOH; readily soluble in ethanol, methanol, ether, benzene, chloroform, and light petroleum.

Cannabinol

Synonym. CBN

6,6,9-Trimethyl-3-pentyl-6*H*-dibenzo[*b*,*d*]pyran-1-ol

$C_{21}H_{26}O_2$=310.4

CAS—521-35-7

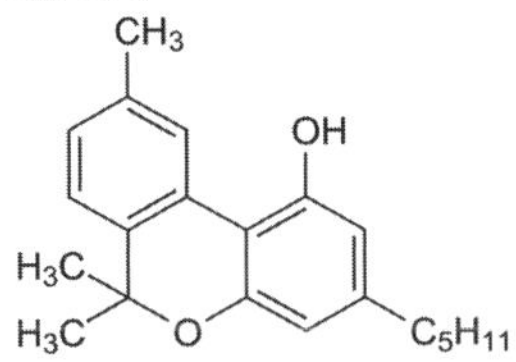

Leaflets from petroleum ether. M.p. 76° to 77°.

Insoluble in water; readily soluble in methanol, ethanol, and aqueous alkaline solutions.

Δ^9-Tetrahydrocannabinol

Synonyms. (−)-*trans*-Δ^9-Tetrahydrocannabinol; Δ^1-THC; Δ^9-THC.

$C_{21}H_{30}O_2$=314.5

CAS—1972-08-3

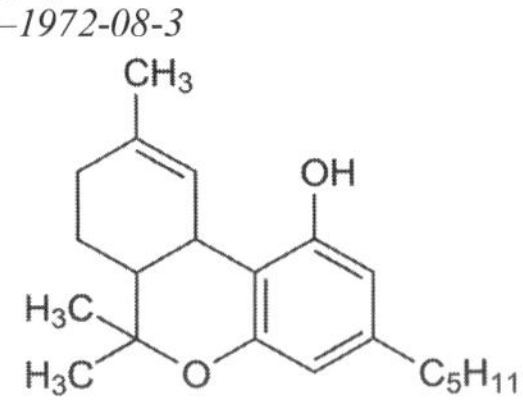

A viscous oil.

Practically insoluble in water; soluble 1 in 1 of ethanol and 1 in 1 of acetone; readily soluble in chloroform and light petroleum.

Δ^8-Tetrahydrocannabinol

Synonyms. (−)-*trans*-Δ^8-Tetrahydrocannabinol; Δ^{1-6}-THC; Δ^8-THC.

$C_{21}H_{30}O_2$=314.5

CAS—5957-75-5

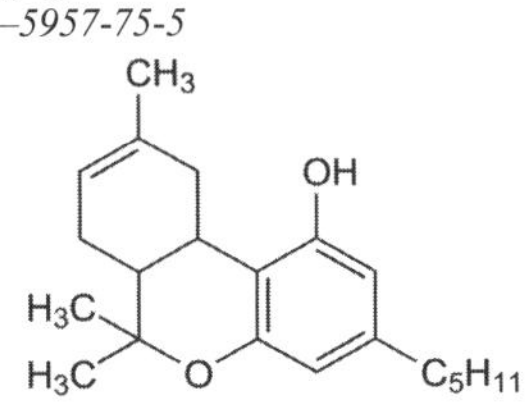

Practically insoluble in water; readily soluble in chloroform and light petroleum.

Δ^9-Tetrahydrocannabinolic Acid

$C_{22}H_{30}O_4$=358.5

CAS—23978-85-0

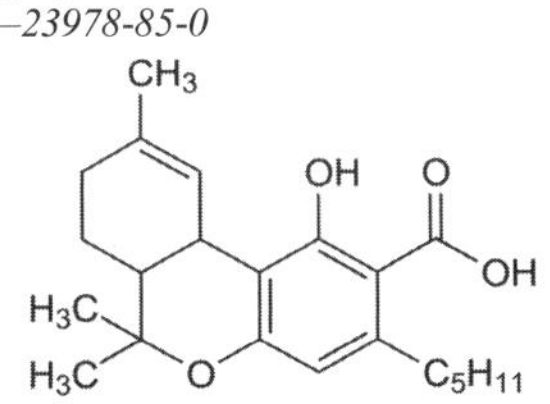

The amount of the major constituents in various samples of cannabis varies between about 5% and zero, depending on climatic and genetic factors. Almost all the psychomimetic activity of the plant is associated with the Δ^9-THC content, which is usually 20 times as great as that of Δ^8-THC. The Δ^9-THC content may average 1, 3, and 5% in marihuana, ganja, and hashish, respectively. However, newer plant strains (e.g. 'skunk weed') can contain much larger Δ^9-THC percentages. The potency of confiscated marijuana samples rose from less than 1.5% Δ^9-THC in 1980 to 4.2% Δ^9-THC in 1997. Δ^9-Tetrahydrocannabinolic acid, which is present in abundance in some cannabis samples, is itself inactive but it is converted by smoking into active Δ^9-THC. Cannabinol and cannabidiol may be present in large amounts but have little activity.

Note. Δ^9-THC binds readily to glass and plastic, reducing recoveries during analytical procedures. Δ^9-THC adsorption can be minimised with storage of solutions in amber silylated glassware and by maintenance of the compound in a basic solution or organic solvent.

Dissociation Constant. Δ^9-THC, pK_a 10.6.

Partition Coefficient. Δ^9-THC, Log *P* (octanol/water), 7.6.

Colour Tests. *p*-Dimethylaminobenzaldehyde—red/violet (cannabinols); Duquenois Test—violet-blue/violet.

Thin-layer Chromatography. System TA—Δ^9-THC Rf 11, CBN Rf 94, CBD Rf 94; system TE—Δ^9-THC Rf 31, CBN Rf 95, CBD Rf 95; system TI—Δ^9-THC Rf 30, CBN Rf 52, CBD Rf 05; system TJ—Δ^9-THC Rf 29, CBN Rf 20, CBD Rf 36; system TAJ—Δ^9-THC Rf 00, CBN Rf 90, CBD Rf 88; system TAK—Δ^9-THC Rf 01, CBN Rf 77, CBD Rf 76; system TAL—Δ^9-THC Rf 31, CBN Rf 97, CBD Rf 97; system TAH—Δ^9-THC Rf 50, CBN Rf 45, CBD Rf 60 (Fast blue B solution—Δ^9-THC red colour, CBD orange colour and CBN purple colour; Duquenois reagent—after spraying reagent, overspray with hydrochloric acid, cannabinoids give blue to violet colours).

Gas Chromatography. System GA—Δ^9-THC RI 2473, CBD RI 2390, CBN RI 2535, cannabigerol RI 2500, M (11-hydroxy-Δ^9-THC) RI 2775; system GB—Δ^9-THC RI 2578, CBN Rf 2644, CBD Rf 2480, M (11-hydroxy-Δ^9-THC) RI 2975; system GH—Δ^9-THC RI 2350, CBD RI 2270, CBN RI 2430, cannabicyclol RI 2280, cannabigerol RI 2440, propylcannabidiol RI 2110, propyl-Δ^9-THC RI 2170, M (8α,11-dihydroxy-Δ^9-THC) RI 2710, M (8α-hydroxy-Δ^9-THC) RI 2580, M (11-hydroxy-Δ^9-THC) RI 2620, M (11-nor-Δ^9-THC-9-carboxylic acid) RI 2756; system GAK—CBN retention time 13.9 min, CBD retention time 13.3 min.

High Performance Liquid Chromatography. System HL—Δ^9-THC *k* 13.35, Δ^8-THC *k* 14.07, CBN *k* 11.77, CBD *k* 7.47, cannabicyclol *k* 14.78, cannabichromene *k* 19.09, cannabidiolic acid *k* 8.76, cannabigerol *k* 8.18, cannabivarin *k* 7.47; tetrahydrocannabinolic acid *k* 25.83; tetrahydrocannabivaric acid *k* 14.64, tetrahydrocannabivarin *k* 8.18; system HX—cannabidiol, RI 990, cannabinol, RI 1080; system HY—cannabidiol, RI 902, cannabinol, RI 1028, M (9-carboxy-11-nor-9-tetrahydrocannabinol) RI 680.

Ultraviolet Spectrum. Ethanol—cannabidiol 278 nm, cannabinol 285 nm, Δ^9-THC 278 nm, and Δ^9-tetrahydrocannabinolic acid 278 nm and 283 nm.

Cannabidiol

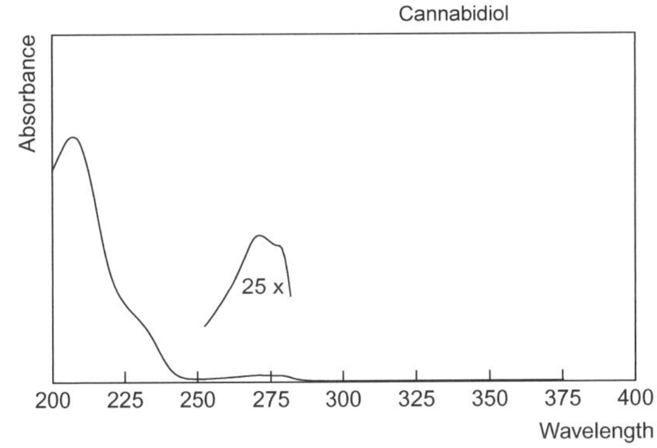

Δ^9-Tetrahydrocannabinol

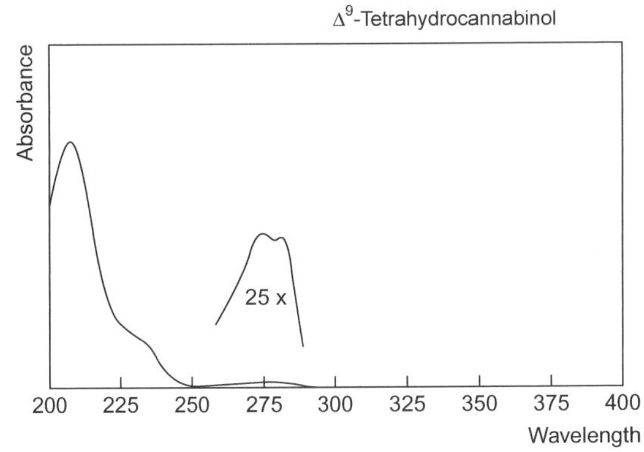

Infra-red Spectrum. Main components have principal peaks at the following wavenumbers (all thin films):
Cannabidiol—1585, 1630, 1020, 1210, 1240, 1050 cm^{-1}
Cannabinol—1620, 1050, 1580, 1030, 1120, 1228 cm^{-1}
Δ^8-THC—1580, 1030, 1620, 1180, 1080, 1260 cm^{-1}
Δ^9-THC—1580, 1040, 1620, 1180, 1130, 1050 cm^{-1}

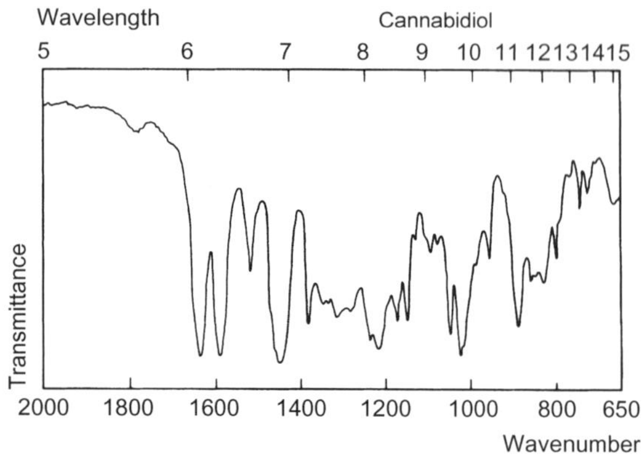

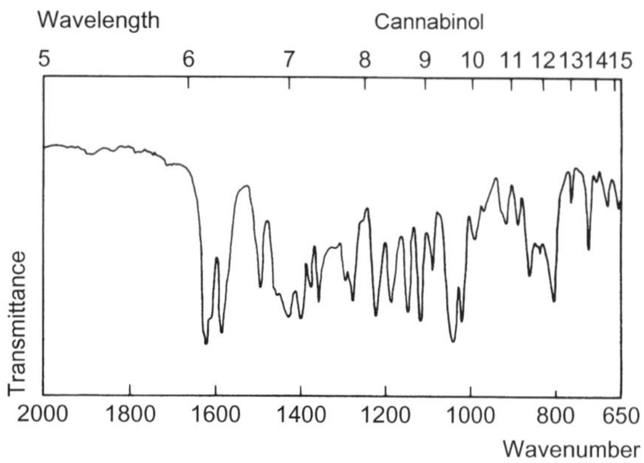

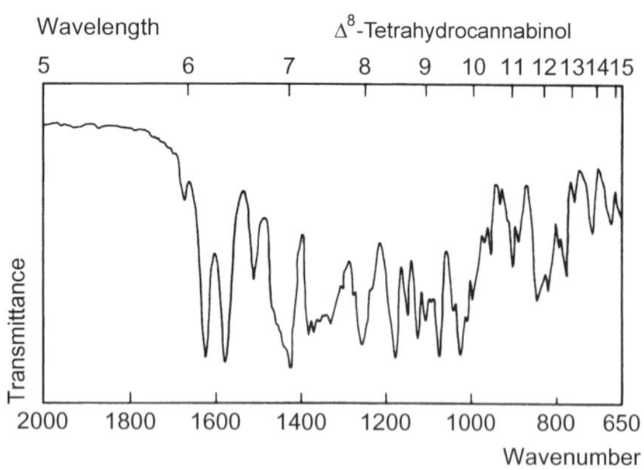

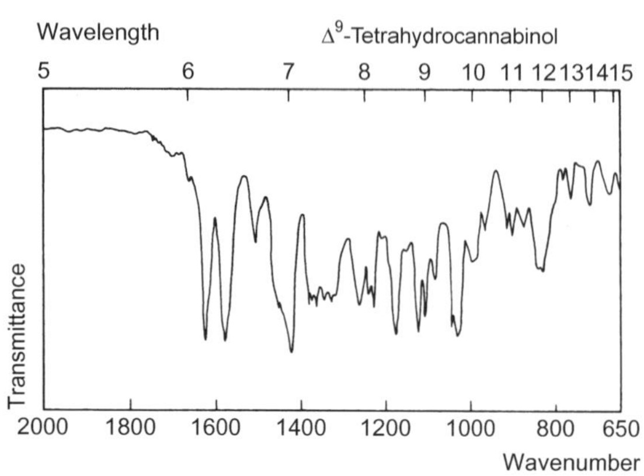

Mass Spectrum. Main components and metabolites have principal peaks at the following *m/z*:
Cannabidiol—231, 246, 314, 232, 121, 193, 74, 174
Cannabinol—295, 296, 238, 310, 119, 43, 251, 239
Δ^8-THC—221, 314, 248, 261, 193, 236, 222, 315
Δ^9-THC—299, 231, 314, 43, 41, 295, 55, 271
8α-Hydroxy-Δ^9-THC—271, 43, 41, 311, 295, 312, 297, 91
8β-Hydroxy-Δ^9-THC—271, 43, 295, 41, 297, 29, 330, 272
11-Hydroxy-Δ^9-THC—299, 43, 41, 67, 300, 69, 231, 29
Δ^9-THC-11-oic acid—41, 229, 43, 329, 69, 344, 29, 283

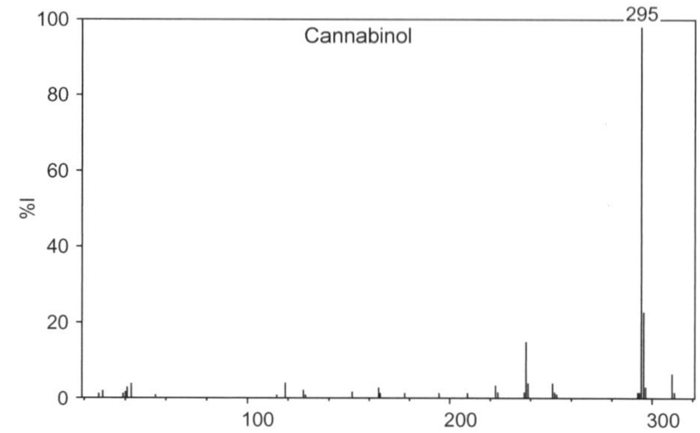

Quantification

Gas chromatography. In blood or brain tissues: Δ^9-THC, limit of detection 200 to 300 ng/L in blood and 2.5 ng/g in brain samples, FID—N. K. McCallum and S. M. Shaw, *J. Anal. Toxicol.*, 1981, *5*, 148–149.

Gas chromatography–mass spectrometry. In urine: 11-nor-Δ^9-THC-9-carboxylic acid, comparison with immunoassays—P. Kintz *et al.*, *J. Anal. Toxicol.*, 1995, *19*, 304–306. In whole blood: Δ^9-THC and 11-nor-9-carboxy-Δ^9-THC, limits of detection 1 µg/L and 0.5 µg/L, respectively—P. Kintz and V. Cirimele, *Biomed. Chromatogr.*, 1997, *11*, 371–373. In hair: cannabinoids, limits of detection 0.1 ng/mg for cannabinol and Δ^9-THC and 0.2 ng/mg for cannabidiol—S. Strano-Rossi and M. Chiarotti, *J. Anal. Toxicol.*, 1999, *23*, 7–10. In fingernails: cannabinoids—N. P. Lemos *et al.*, *J. Anal. Toxicol.*, 1999, *23*, 147–152. In biological samples: Δ^9-THC and 11-nor-carboxy-Δ^9-THC—M. Chiarotti and L. Costamagna, *Forensic Sci. Int.*, 2000, *114*, 1–6. In hair: cannabinoids, limit of detection 0.3 ng/g—H. Sach and U. Dressler, *Forensic Sci. Int.*, 2000, *107*, 239–247. In hair: cannabinoids, limits of quantification for Δ^9-THC, cannabinol and cannabidiol 0.1 µg/g, and 0.01 µg/g for Δ^9-THC carboxylic acid—M. J. Baptista *et al.*, *Forensic Sci. Int.*, 2002, *128*, 66–78. In blood: Δ^9-THC, initial screening by radioimmunoassay, limit of detection 1 µg/L—R. A. Bergman *et al.*, *J. Anal. Toxicol.*, 1981, *5*, 85–89.

High performance liquid chromatography. In plasma or urine: Δ^9-THC and its metabolites, limit of detection 0.5 µg/L, electrochemical detection—Y. Nakahara *et al.*, *J. Anal. Toxicol.*, 1989, *12*, 22–24. In urine: 11-nor-Δ^9-THC-9-carboxylic acid, limit of quantification 10 µg/L, UV detection—V. Bianchi and G. Donzelli, *J. Chromatogr.* 1996, *675 Biomed. Appl.* 162–167. In saliva: Δ^9-THC, limit of quantification 20 µg/L, UV detection—V. Kircher and H. Parlar, *J. Chromatogr.*, 1996, *677 Biomed. Appl.* 245–255.

High performance liquid chromatography–mass spectrometry. In urine: 11-nor-Δ^9-THC-carboxylic acid and its glucuronide conjugate—W. Weinmann *et al.*, *Forensic Sci. Int.*, 2000, *113*, 381–387.

High performance liquid chromatography–radioimmunoassay. In blood, plasma, serum, or urine: Δ^9-THC and metabolites, limit of detection 6.5 µg/L for plasma and 3.3 µg/L for urine—B. Law *et al.*, *J. Anal. Toxicol.*, 1984, *8*, 19–22.

Radioimmunoassay. In body fluids: cannabinoid metabolites, limit of detection 10 µg/L for blood and 2 µg/L for urine—B. Law *et al.*, *J. Anal. Toxicol.*, 1984, *8*, 14–18.

Note. For a study of the detection of cannabis in oral fluid and forehead wipes from impaired drivers see P. Kintz *et al.*, *J. Anal. Toxicol.*, 2000, *24*, 557–561.

Disposition in the Body. Δ^9-THC is absorbed from the gastro-intestinal tract but absorption is slow and irregular. However, Δ^9-THC can be measured in plasma within seconds after inhalation of the first puff of marijuana smoke. Δ^9-THC is lipophilic and is widely distributed in the body. It is oxidised to the active metabolites 11-hydroxy-Δ^9-THC and 8β-hydroxy-Δ^9-THC by the hepatic cytochrome P450 enzyme. The inactive substances 8α-hydroxy-Δ^9-THC and 8α,11-dihydroxy-Δ^9-THC are also formed. 11-Hydroxy-Δ^9-THC is further oxidised to 11-nor-Δ^9-THC-9-carboxylic acid (Δ^9-THC-11-oic acid), and many other polar mono- and dicarboxylic acids are formed; these are conjugated with glucuronic acid to a variable extent. Enterohepatic circulation of metabolites may occur. Up to about 25% of a dose is excreted in the urine in 3 days, mainly as 11-nor-Δ^9-THC-9-carboxylic acid glucuronide, together with the other carboxylic acids in free and conjugated form. Δ^9-THC-*O*-glucuronide has also been detected in urine. The major excretion route is via the faeces, up to about 65% of a dose being excreted in 5 days, mainly as 11-hydroxy-Δ^9-THC and the carboxylic acids in conjugated form. Δ^9-THC metabolites have been detected in urine for up to 12 days following a single oral dose. It crosses the placenta and is distributed into breast milk.

Blood concentration

6 healthy males with histories of marijuana use smoked a single marijuana cigarette (placebo or 1.75% or 3.55% Δ^9-THC). The smoking protocol consisted of a 2 s inhalation, a 10 s hold period and a 72 s exhalation and rest period. A total of 8 puffs were inhaled in 11.2 min. Mean plasma levels of 7.0 and 18.1 µg/L Δ^9-THC were observed after the first inhalation of the 1.75% and 3.55% Δ^9-THC cigarettes, respectively. Levels continued to increase rapidly to mean peak plasma concentrations of 79.0 and 152.0 µg/L for the 1.75% and 3.55% Δ^9-THC cigarettes, respectively, and were reached after 9 min (before initiation of the last puff sequence at 9.8 min). [M. A. Huestis *et al.*, *Clin. Pharmacol. Ther.*, 1992, *52*, 31–41.]

After 11 subjects had smoked 11.6 to 15.6 mg (mean 13.0) of Δ^9-THC from a cigarette over a period of 5 to 7 min, peak plasma concentrations of 0.03 to 0.12 mg/L (mean 0.08) of Δ^9-THC were observed within 3 min after termination of smoking; the concentration fell rapidly to 0.003 to 0.01 mg/L (mean 0.007) at 1 h and to 0.0006 to 0.003 mg/L (mean 0.0016) at 4 h, after smoking. When 20 mg of Δ^9-THC was given orally to the same subjects, peak plasma concentrations of 0.004 to 0.01 mg/L of Δ^9-THC were produced between 60 and 300 min after ingestion. [A. Ohlsson *et al.*, *Clin. Pharmacol. Ther.*, 1980, *28*, 409–416.]

Toxicity. Cannabis or Δ^9-THC intoxication may result in loss of consciousness or even death, but reports of fatalities are rare.

In 6 cardiovascular fatalities following cannabis use, the following tetrahycrocannabinol levels were found in the blood: 22 µg/L, 4 µg/L, 2 µg/L, 5 µg/L, 3 µg/L, and 7 µg/L; no other drugs were detected except for 400 mg/L ethanol in the fourth case [L. Bach and H. Morland, *Forensic Sci. Int.*, 2001, *124*, 200–203.]

In 1 case of fatal poisoning by Δ^9-THC, the following postmortem concentrations of Δ^9-THC in tissues were reported: liver 37.5 µg/g, kidney 42 µg/g, and spleen 12 µg/g [S. N. Tewari and J. D. Sharma, *Toxicol. Lett.*, 1980, *5*, 279–281.]

Bioavailability. After ingestion, about 6 to 20%. During smoking, about 18% to 50%.

Half-life. Plasma half-life, in frequent users Δ^9-THC about 2 h, Δ^9-THC-11-oic acid about 120 h; in infrequent users, 1.5 h and 144 h, respectively.

Volume of distribution. Δ^9-THC about 10 L/kg.

Distribution in blood. Plasma:whole blood ratio, Δ^9-THC 1.8.

Protein binding. In plasma, Δ^9-THC and 11-hydroxy-Δ^9-THC 94 to 99%.

Note. For a general review of cannabis and its effects on human behaviour and performance, see M. A. Huestis, *Forensic Sci. Rev.*, 2002, *14*, 15–60. For a review of the therapeutic aspects of cannabis and cannabinoids, see P. Robson, *Br. J. Psychiatry*, 2001, *178*, 107–115. For a review of Δ^9-THC metabolism and disposition see M. E. Wall and M. Perez-Reyes, *J. Clin. Pharmacol.*, 1981, *21*, 178s–189s. See also M. E. Wall *et al.*, *Clin. Pharmacol. Ther.*, 1983, *34*, 352–363 and B. Law *et al.*, *J. Pharm. Pharmacol.*, 1984, *36*, 289–294. For a review of the clinical pharmacokinetics of non-opiate abused drugs see U. Busto *et al.*, *Clin. Pharmacokinet.*, 1989, *16*, 1–26.

Further references. Relating blood concentrations of tetrahydrocannabinol and metabolites to pharmacological effects and time of marijuana use—E. J. Cone and M. A. Huestis, *Ther. Drug Monit.*, 1993, *15*, 527–532 and M.A. Huestis *et al.*, *J. Anal.Toxicol.*, 1992, *16*, 276–290. Detection and persistence of cannabis DNA on skin—M Wilkinson and A. M. Linacre, *Sci. Justice*, 2000, *40*, 11–14. Determination of the distribution of cannabinoids in cannabis resin—P. B. Baker *et al.*, *J. Anal. Toxicol.*, 1980, *4*, 145–152. The Δ^9-THC and Δ^9-tetrahydrocannabinolic acid content of cannabis products—P. B. Baker *et al.*, *J. Pharm. Pharmacol.*, 1981, *33*, 369–372. Swabbing the hands for traces of marihuana—R. Thibault *et al.*, *J. Forensic Sci.*, 1983, *28*, 15–17. Role of cannabis in motor vehicle crashes—M. N. Bates and T. A. Blakely, *Epidemiol. Rev.*, 1999, *21*, 222–232.

Cantharidin

Vesicant

Proprietary name. Cantharone

Hexahydro-3a,7a-dimethyl-4,7-epoxyisobenzofuran-1,3-dione

$C_{10}H_{12}O_4$=196.2

CAS—56-25-7

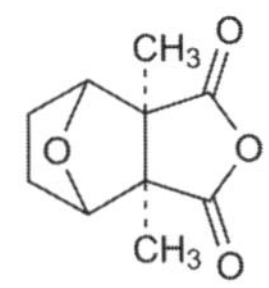

Cantharidin is obtained from cantharides, the dried beetle *Cantharis vesicatoria* (=*Lytta vesicatoria*) (Meloidae) or other species, containing not less than 0.6%, or from mylabris, the dried beetles *Mylabris sidae* (=*M. phalerata*), *M. cichorii* and *M. pustulata* (Meloidae), containing not less than 1%.

Colourless, glistening crystals, which sublime at about 120°. M.p. 218°.

Insoluble in cold water, somewhat soluble in hot water; soluble 1 in about 1100 of ethanol, 1 in 40 of acetone, 1 in 65 of chloroform, 1 in 560 of ether, and 1 in 150 of ethyl acetate. Soluble in oils.

Partition Coefficient. Log *P* (octanol/water), 1.2.

Gas Chromatography. System GA—RI 1492.

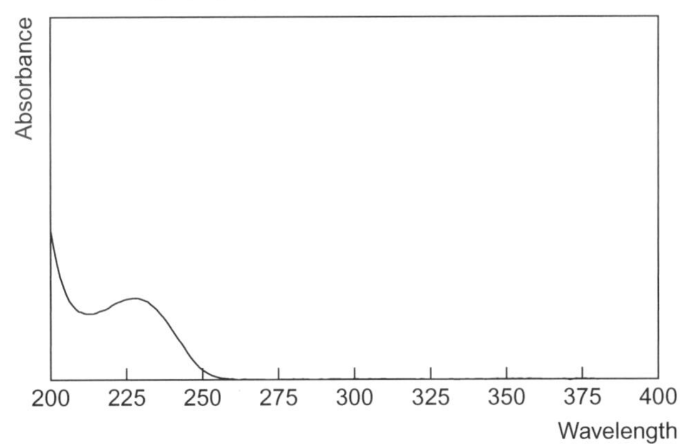

Infra-red Spectrum. Principal peaks at wavenumbers 1242, 962, 900, 1786, 1852, 1002 cm^{-1} (Nujol mull).

Mass Spectrum. Principal ions at *m*/*z* 128, 96, 70, 39, 41, 27, 42, 29.

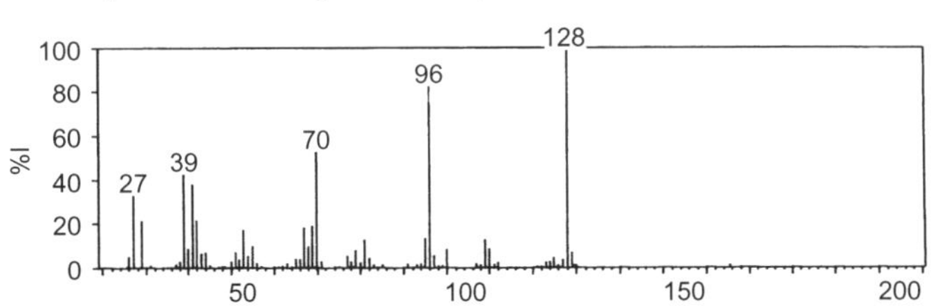

Quantification

Gas chromatography–mass spectrometry. In serum—J. M Steyn and H. K. Hundt, *J. Chromatogr.*, 1988, *432*, 177–184.

Disposition in the Body. Readily absorbed from the skin and mucous membranes. It does not appear to be metabolised.

Toxicity. When taken orally it causes great pain as well as blistering and gross inflammation of the gastro-intestinal tract, the kidneys and the bladder. The lethal dose is between 10 and 60 mg although a crystal weighing not more than 0.5 mg lodged in the mucosa might produce a blister which could be fatal.

A 27-year-old woman died about 17 h after she had eaten coconut ice into which a small quantity of cantharidin had been introduced by a fellow employee. The postmortem findings revealed that between 65 and 130 mg of cantharidin was circulating in the organs. At the same time as the above incident a 19-year-old girl also ate a piece of the cantharidin-impregnated coconut ice. She died 26 h later. The postmortem level of cantharidin in the organs was somewhat less than in the former case. [L. C. Nickolls and D. Teare, *BMJ*, 1954, *2*, 1384.]

Cantharidin was detected at a concentration of 0.11 mg/L in postmortem blood after ingestion of a crude extract of cantharides (over 200 dried beetles). [K. C. Cheng *et al.*, *Med. Sci. Law*, 1990, *30(4)*, 336–340.]

Cantharidin was detected at a concentration of 72.3 mg/L in postmortem serum after ingestion of cantharide powder containing 0.87% cantharidin. [H. K. Hundt *et al.*, *Human Exp. Toxicol.*, 1990, *9(1)*, 35–40.]

Capecitabine

Antineoplastic

Synonym. Ro-09-1978/000
Proprietary name. Xeloda
[1-(5-Deoxy-β-D-ribofuranosyl)-5-fluoro-1,2-dihydro-2-oxo-4-pyrimidinyl]carbamic acid pentyl ester
$C_{15}H_{22}FN_3O_6$=359.4
CAS—154361-50-9

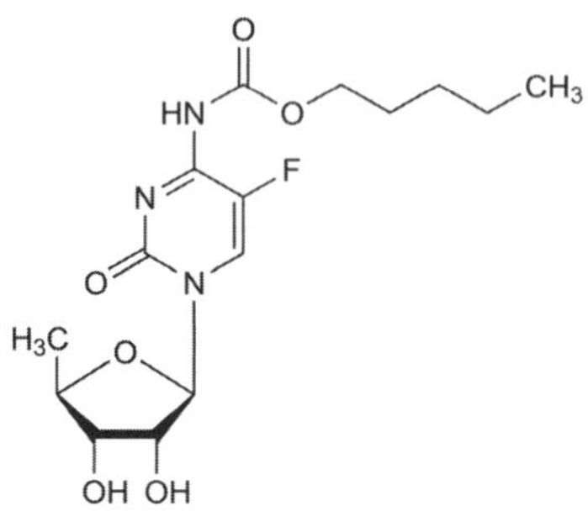

A white to off-white crystalline powder. Aqueous solubility approx. 26 g/L at 20°.

Disposition in the Body. Capecitabine is extensively absorbed after oral administration and hydrolysed first to 5′-deoxy-5-fluorocytidine (5′-DFCR) by a carboxylesterase. 5′-DFCR is then converted to 5′-deoxy-5-fluorouridine (5′-DFUR) by cytadine deaminase to 5′-fluorouracil by thymidine phosphorylase to 5-fluoro-5,6-dihydrofluorouracil (FUH_2) to 5-fluoro-ureidopropionic acid (FUPA) and to α-fluoro-β-alanine (FBAL) by β-ureidopropionase. More than 95% of an administered dose is excreted in urine, with approx. 3% unchanged and 5% as FBAL, the major metabolite. 2.5% of the dose is recovered in faeces.

Therapeutic concentration

A single oral dose of 892 to 2510 mg/m^2 was administered and taken within 30 min of the end of a meal. Mean peak plasma concentrations of the drug ranged from 2.4 to 3.9 mg/L and were reached within approx. 1.5 h. [Roche Laboratories Inc., Xeloda (Capecitabine) prescribing information, USA, 1998].

Toxicity. In patients treated with doses of up to 3514 mg/m^2 daily, i.e. cases of acute overdose, nausea, vomiting, diarrhoea and bleeding were observed.

Half-life. 0.5 to 1 h.

Protein binding. <60% for both the drug and metabolites.

Dose. A usual dose of 2.5 g/m^2 body surface is administered daily.

Capreomycin

Antibacterial

Synonyms. Capromycin; Caprolin; Capostatin.
A mixture of the polypeptide antimicrobial substances produced by certain strains of *Streptomyces capreolus*. Capreomycin I consists of capreomycin IA ($C_{25}H_{44}N_{14}O_8$=668.7), M.p. 246° to 248°; and capreomycin IB ($C_{25}H_{44}N_{14}O_7$=652.7), M.p. 253° to 255°, which predominates. Capreomycin II that makes up about 10% of the mixture consists of capreomycin IIA and capreomycin IIB.
CAS—11003-38-6

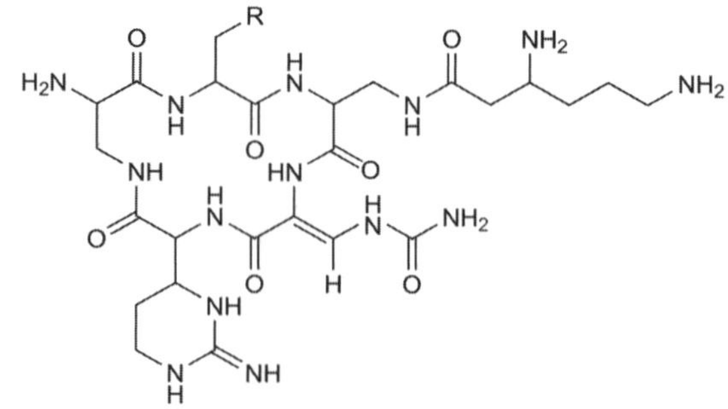

Capreomycin IA R = OH
Capreomycin IB R = H

Capreomycin Sulfate

Proprietary names. Capastat; Caprocin; Ogostal.
CAS—1405-37-4
A white or almost white solid or amorphous powder. It is very soluble in water: practically insoluble in chloroform, ethanol, ether, and most other organic solvents.

Ultraviolet Spectrum. (Capreomycin sulfate) Aqueous acid (0.2 M H_2SO_4)—268 nm; basic—289 nm.

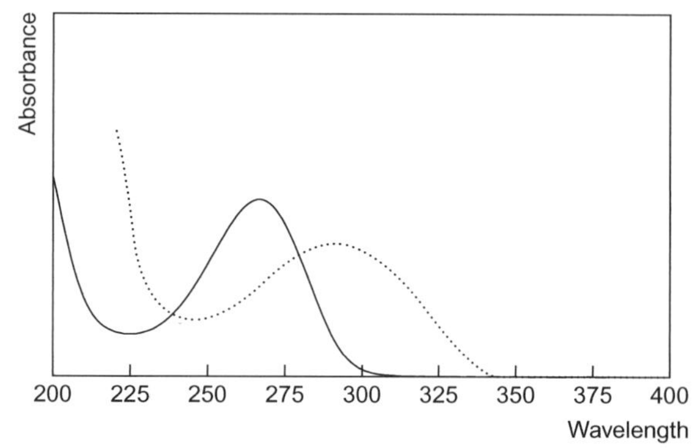

Infra-red Spectrum. Principal peaks at wavenumbers 1668, 1498, 1231, 1118 m^{-1} (sulfate salt).

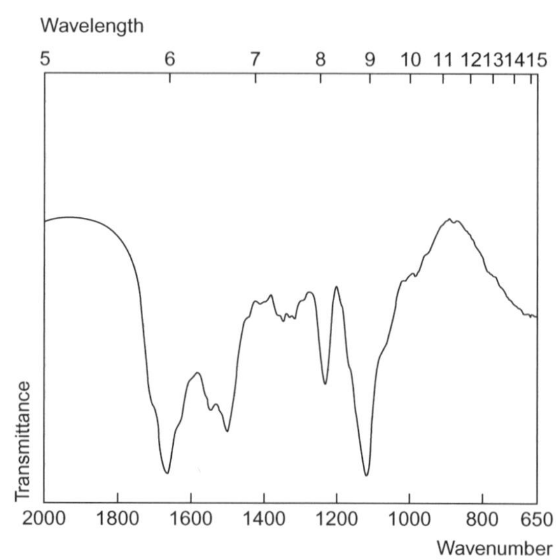

Quantification

Electrophoresis. In urine: limit of detection 0.15 mg/L, UV detection—S. S. Zhang *et al.*, *J. Pharm. Biomed. Anal.*, 1998, *17*, 617–622.

Disposition in the Body. Capreomycin is poorly absorbed after oral administration (less than 1%). It is not distributed into CSF (cerebrospinal fluid), but it does cross the placenta. About 50% of a dose is excreted unchanged in urine by glomerular filtration within 12 h. Small amounts are excreted in bile. It is removed by haemodialysis.

Therapeutic concentration. A 1 g intramuscular dose produces peak serum concentrations of about 30 mg/L (range 20 to 47 mg/L) after 1 to 2 h.

Toxicity

Nephrotoxicity, including acute tubular necrosis, and ototoxicity, including dizziness and vertigo, have been reported. Neuromuscular blockage or respiratory paralysis may also occur after rapid intravenous administration. [Data as supplied by Eli Lilly & Company Ltd.]

Half-life. Plasma half-life, 4 to 6 h.

Clearance. Plasma clearance, 57 mL/h/kg.

Dose. The equivalent of 1 g of capreomycin daily is administered intramuscularly for 60 to 120 days, followed by 1 g two or three times a week. 20 mg/kg daily should not be exceeded. The dose should be reduced in patients with reduced renal function.

Captodiame

Tranquilliser

Synonyms. Captodiamine; Captodramin.
2-[[[4-(Butylthio)phenyl]phenylmethyl]thio]-*N*,*N*-dimethylethanamine
$C_{21}H_{29}NS_2$=359.6
CAS—486-17-9

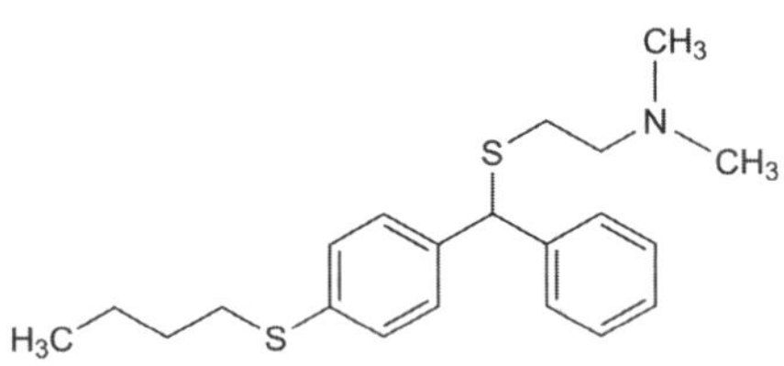

Captodiame Hydrochloride

Proprietary names. Covatine; Covatix; Suvren.
$C_{21}H_{29}NS_2$,HCl=396.1
CAS—904-04-1
Crystals. M.p. 131° to 132°.

Colour Tests. Mandelin's Test—violet; Marquis Test—violet.

Thin-layer Chromatography. System TA—Rf 66; system TB—Rf 49; system TE—Rf 77; system TAE—Rf 47. (Acidified iodoplatinate solution, positive.)

Gas Chromatography. System GA—RI 2774.

High Performance Liquid Chromatography. System HX—RI 561; system HAA—Retention time(s), 20.2 min.

Ultraviolet Spectrum. Aqueous acid—266 nm (A_1^1=370b); aqueous alkali—273 nm.

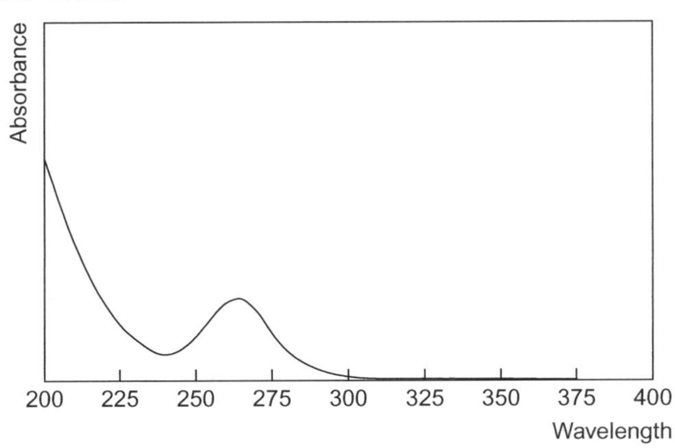

Infra-red Spectrum. Principal peaks at wavenumbers 694, 751, 1086, 1041, 1010, 714 cm^{-1} (KBr disk).

Mass Spectrum. Principal ions at *m/z* 58, 165, 255, 359, 166, 73, 199, 45.

Dose. Captodiame hydrochloride has been given in doses of 150 mg daily.

Captopril

Antihypertensive

Synonyms. SQ-14225; Captoprilum.
Proprietary names. Acediur; Aceomel; Acepril; Aceplus; Alopresin; Acepress; Capoten; Captolane; Captoril; Cesplon; Dilabar; Ecopace; Garranil; Hipertil; Kaplon; Lopirin; Lopril; Tensiomin-Cor; Tensobon; Tensoprel; Tensopril. It is an ingredient of Acezide, Capozid(e), Captea, Capto-Co, and Ecazide.
1-[(2*S*)3-Mercapto-2-methyl-1-oxopropyl]-L-proline
$C_9H_{15}NO_3S$=217.3
CAS—62571-86-2

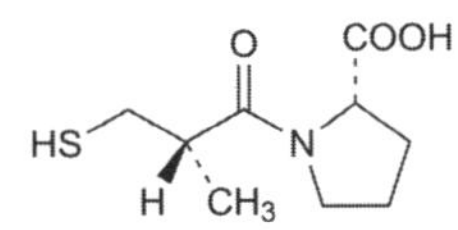

Polymorphic white to off-white crystals. M.p. 106°.
Freely soluble in water, ethanol, chloroform, methylene chloride, and methanol. It dissolves in dilute solutions of alkali hydroxides.

Dissociation Constant. pK_a 3.7, 9.8.

Partition Coefficient. Log *P* (octanol/water), 0.34.

Colour Tests. Palladium Chloride—orange; Sodium Nitroprusside (Method 2)—violet.

Thin-layer Chromatography. System TD—Rf 01; system TE—Rf 00; system TF—Rf 01; system TAD—Rf 06. (Ferric chloride solution, yellow; mercuric chloride–diphenylcarbazone reagent, violet, turns pink on heating; acidified potassium permanganate solution, yellow; Van Urk reagent, yellow, fades on heating.)

Gas Chromatography. System GA—captopril, not eluted captopril-Me RI 1730; system GB—captopril, not eluted.

High Performance Liquid Chromatography. System HZ—retention time 2.1 min; system HY—RI 283; system HX—RI 316; system HAA—retention time 9.7 min.

Column: RP C_{18} (Nova Pak, 150 × 3.9 mm i.d., 4 µm). Mobile phase: acetonitrile:1% acetic acid (pH 2.8) (42:58), flow rate 1.5 mL/min. IS: *N*-acetyl-L-cysteine. Fluorescence detection (λ_{ex}=340 nm; λ_{em}=389 nm). Retention time: captopril, 3.7 min; IS, 2.2 min. [C. Arroyo *et al.*, *J. Chromatogr. B Biomed. Sci. Appl.*, 1997, *688*, 339–344.]

Column: RP C_{18} (250 × 4.6 mm i.d., 5 µm). Mobile phase: acetonitrile:1% acetic acid (60:40), flow rate 1.3 mL/min. IS: nitrazepam. UV detection (λ=260 nm). Retention time: captopril, 4.1 min; IS, 4.6 min. [A. Jankowski *et al.*, *J. Pharm. Biomed. Anal.*, 1995, *13*, 655–660.]

Ultraviolet Spectrum. Aqueous acid—no significant absorption, 230 to 360 nm; aqueous alkali—238 nm (A_1^1=235c).

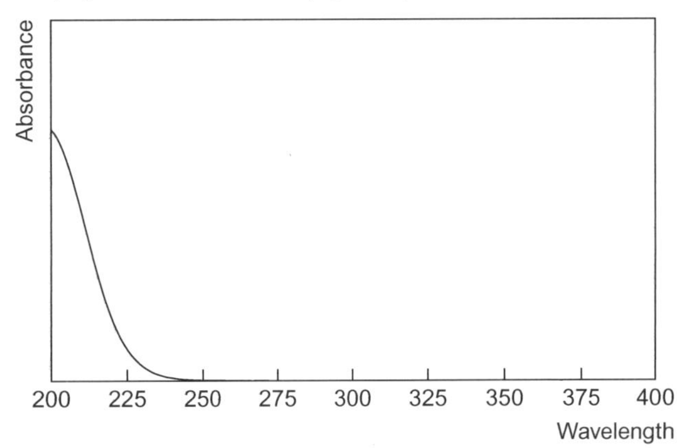

Infra-red Spectrum. Principal peaks at wavenumbers 1589, 1742, 1202, 1192, 1229, 1245 cm^{-1} (KBr disk). Polymorphism may occur.

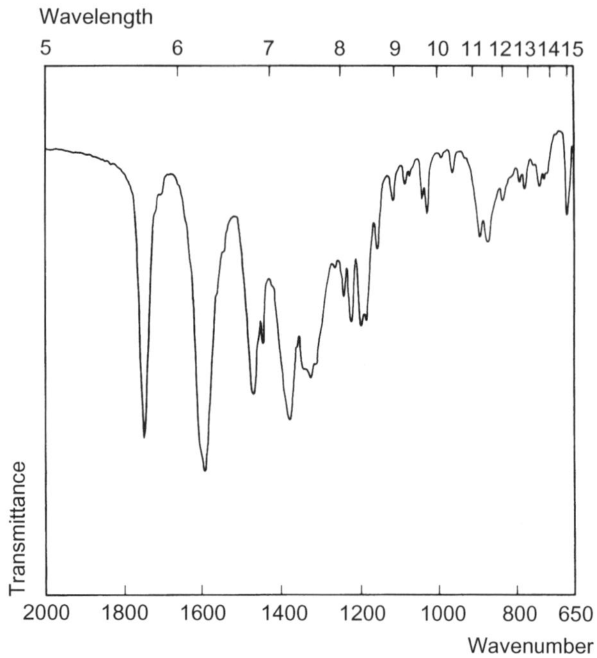

Mass Spectrum. Principal ions at *m/z* 70, 41, 69, 75, 114, 42, 217, 68.

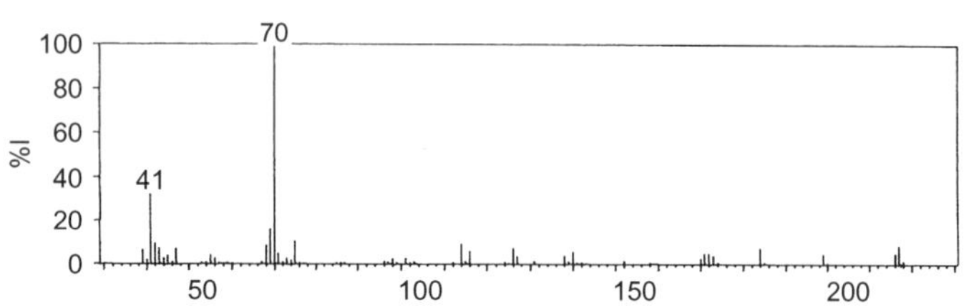

Quantification

Gas chromatography. In plasma or blood: limit of detection 20 µg/L for captopril in blood, 50 µg/L for captopril and metabolites in plasma, ECD—M. S. Bathala *et al.*, *J. Pharm. Sci.*, 1984, *73*, 340–344.

Gas chromatography–mass spectrometry. In plasma or urine: limits of detection 1 µg/L for captopril, 25 µg/L for captopril disulfide—O. H. Drummer *et al.*, *J. Chromatogr.* 1984, *305*(30) *B Biomed. Appl.*, 83–93. In plasma—H. J. Leis *et al.*, *J. Chromatogr.*, 1990, *529*, 299–308. In plasma: limit of quantification 10 µg/L—M. E. Franklin *et al.*, *J. Chromatogr. B Biomed. Sci. Appl.*, 1998, *705*, 47–54.

High performance liquid chromatography. In plasma and urine: limit of quantification 20 µg/L and 10 µg/L, respectively. UV detection (λ=260 nm)—S. Gao *et al.*, *J. Chromatogr.*, 1992, *582*, 258–262. In plasma: limit of detection, 15 µg/L, UV detection (λ=260 nm)—A. Jankowski *et al.*, *J. Pharm. Biomed. Anal.*, 1995, *13*, 655–660. In blood and urine: limit of detection, 0.3 µg/L, UV detection (λ=314 nm)—S. Sypniewski and E. Bald, *J. Chromatogr. A*, 1996, *729*, 335–340. In plasma: limit of detection, 2 µg/L, UV detection (λ=258 nm)—K. Li *et al.*, *Biomed. Chromatogr.*, 1996, *10*, 237–239. In plasma: limit of quantification, 25 µg/L, fluorescence detection (λ_{ex}=340 nm; λ_{em}=389 nm)—C. Arroyo *et al.*, *J. Chromatogr. B Biomed. Sci. Appl.*, 1997, *688*, 339–344. In serum: limit of quantification 50 µg/L, UV detection—M. Bahmaei *et al.*, *J. Pharm. Biomed. Anal.*, 1997, *15*, 1181–1186. In plasma or urine: limits of quantification in plasma 12.5 to 25 µg/L and in urine 250 µg/L, fluorescence detection—R. J. Kok *et al.*, *J. Chromatogr. B Biomed. Sci. Appl.*, 1997, *693*, 181–189. In urine: captopril and hydrochlorothiazide, UV detection—A. Khedr and H. el-Sherief, *Biomed. Chromatogr.*, 1998, *12*, 57–60. In plasma: captopril and its disulfide metabolites, limit of quantification 5 µg/L, fluorescence detection—D. Zhong *et al.*, *Yao Xue Xue Bao*, 1998, *33*, 605–609. In plasma: limit of quantification 10 µg/L. UV detection (λ=246 nm)—M. Amini *et al.*, *Pharm. Acta Helv.*, 1999, *73*, 303–306. In plasma: limit of detection 4 ppb, fluorescence detection—F. Tache *et al.*, *J. Pharm. Biomed. Anal.*, 2002, *28*, 549–557.

Radioimmunoassay. In plasma: limit of detection 2 µg/L—F. M. Duncan *et al.*, *Clinica Chim. Acta*, 1983, *131*, 295–303.

Disposition in the Body. Readily absorbed after oral administration; about 60 to 75% of the dose is absorbed and peak plasma concentrations are achieved within about an hour. It crosses the placenta and is found in breast milk at about 1% of maternal blood concentrations. 40 to 50% of an oral dose is excreted in the urine as unchanged drug, about 3% as captopril disulfide and about 30% as polar metabolites. Excretion in the urine is rapid, about half the dose being excreted within the first 4 h. An *S*-methyl metabolite has been identified in plasma and urine. Captopril is removed by haemodialysis.

Therapeutic concentration

Analysis of captopril concentrations in plasma samples from 20 volunteers following oral administration of 100 mg of captopril resulted in a mean peak concentration of 1.47 mg/L after 0.75 h. [M. E. Franklin *et al.*, *J. Chromatogr. B Biomed. Sci. Appl.*, 1998, *705*, 47–54.]

After a single oral dose of 100 mg of ^{35}S-labelled captopril to 10 subjects, peak blood concentrations of 0.51 to 1.31 mg/L (mean 0.8) of captopril, and 0.11 to 0.49 mg/L (mean 0.23) of captopril disulfide, were attained in 0.5 to 1.5 h. [K. J. Kripalani *et al.*, *Clin. Pharmacol. Ther.*, 1980, *27*, 636–641.]

Following oral administration of 25 mg, three times a day to 12 subjects, a mean maximum steady-state blood concentration of 0.14 mg/L of captopril was reported 0.9 h after a dose. [R. J. Cody *et al.*, *Clin. Pharmacol. Ther.*, 1982, *32*, 721–726.]

Toxicity

A 75-year-old male committed suicide by taking an overdose of captopril. He took approx. 90 12.5-mg captopril tablets. The postmortem plasma concentration of captopril was 60.4 mg/L. This was the first case report of fatal captopril overdose with the measurement of plasma concentration of the drug. [H. Park *et al.*, *J. Toxicol. Clin. Toxicol.*, 1990, *28*, 379–382.]

Serum levels of captopril reached 20 mg/L in a 43 year old who had attempted suicide by ingesting 5 to 7.5 g of captopril 7 hours earlier. The patient survived and displayed minimal symptoms. [P. Lechleitner *et al.*, *Toxicology*, 1990, *64*, 325–329.]

Half-life. Blood half-life, about 1 to 2 h.

Volume of Distribution. In blood, about 0.7 L/kg.

Clearance. Blood clearance, about 13 mL/min/kg.

Protein binding. In plasma, about 30%.

Note. For a review of captopril see J. A. Romankiewicz *et al.*, *Drugs*, 1983, *25*, 6–40.

Dose. 75 to 150 mg daily; maximum of 450 mg daily in divided doses.

Caramiphen

Anticholinergic/Antitussive

2-(Diethylamino)ethyl 1-phenylcyclopentanecarboxylate
$C_{18}H_{27}NO_2$=289.4
CAS—77-22-5

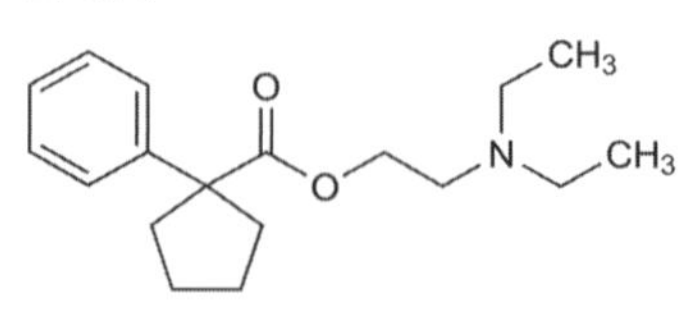

A liquid.

Caramiphen Edisilate

Synonym. Caramiphen Ethanedisulfonate
$C_{18}H_{27}NO_2,\frac{1}{2}C_2H_6O_6S_2$=384.5
CAS—125-86-0
Crystals. M.p. 115° to 116°.
Soluble in water and ethanol.

Caramiphen Hydrochloride

$C_{18}H_{27}NO_2$,HCl=325.9
CAS—125-85-9
White crystals or crystalline powder. M.p. 145° to 146°.

Soluble 1 in 4 of water and 1 in 8 of ethanol; practically insoluble in ether.

Partition Coefficient. Log *P* (octanol/water), 4.5.

Colour Tests. Liebermann's Test—red-orange; Marquis Test—yellow; Sulfuric Acid (when warmed)—red.

Thin-layer Chromatography. System TA—Rf 66. (Acidified iodoplatinate solution, positive.)

Gas Chromatography. System GA—RI 1971.

Ultraviolet Spectrum. Aqueous acid—252 (A_1^1=7.9b), 259 (A_1^1=7.9b), 265 nm.

Infra-red Spectrum. Principal peaks at wavenumbers 1718, 1154, 694, 1173, 1220, 1060 cm^{-1} (KBr disk).

Mass Spectrum. Principal ions at *m/z* 86, 99, 91, 144, 58, 56, 41, 87.

Quantification

Gas chromatography. In blood: limit of detection <2.5 μg/L, AFID—P. Levandoski and T. Flanagan, *J. Pharm. Sci.*, 1980, *69*, 1353–1354.

Disposition in the Body

Therapeutic concentration

Following daily oral administration of 20 mg of caramiphen edisilate at 0, 4, and 8 h to 11 subjects for 4 days, peak blood concentrations of 0.018 to 0.078 (mean 0.046) mg/L were reported 1 to 2 h after a dose. [P. Levandoski and T. Flanagan, *J. Pharm. Sci.*, 1980, *69*, 1353–1354].

Dose. Caramiphen hydrochloride has been given in doses of 50 to 600 mg daily.

Carbachol

Parasympathomimetic

Synonyms. Carbacholine; Carbamoylcholine Chloride; Carbamylcholine Chloride; Choline Chloride Carbamate.
Proprietary names. Carbyl; Doryl; Miostat.
2-[(Aminocarbonyl)oxy]-*N*,*N*,*N*-trimethylethanaminium chloride
$C_6H_{15}ClN_2O_2$=182.6
CAS—51-83-2

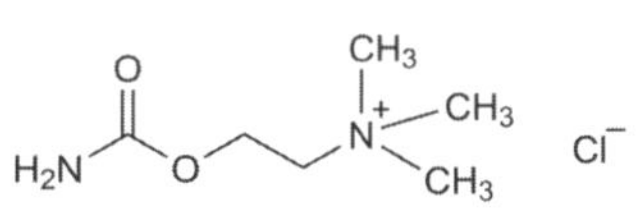

White or faintly yellow, hygroscopic, crystals or crystalline powder. M.p. 200° to 204°, with decomposition.
Soluble 1 in 1 of water and 1 in 50 of ethanol; very slightly soluble in dehydrated alcohol, more readily soluble on boiling; practically insoluble in acetone, chloroform and ether.

Dissociation Constant. pK_a 4.8.

Partition Coefficient. Log *P* (octanol/water), −3.8.

Thin-layer Chromatography. System TA—Rf 00; system TB—Rf 00; system TC—Rf 00; system TE—Rf 00; system TL—Rf 00; system TAE—Rf 04; system TAF—Rf 23. (Acidified iodoplatinate solution, positive.)

Ultraviolet Spectrum. No significant absorption, 230 to 360 nm.

Infra-red Spectrum. Principal peaks at wavenumbers 1730, 1083, 1056, 930, 1102, 1200 cm^{-1} (KBr disk).

Mass Spectrum. Principal ions at *m/z* 43, 58, 42, 44, 30, 129, 36, 143.

Dose. 6 mg daily by mouth. For acute symptoms, 250 μg by subcutaneous injection, repeated if necessary.

Carbamazepine

Anticonvulsant

Synonyms. G-32883; Carbamazepinum.
Proprietary names. Atretol; Biston; Calepsin; Carbagen; Carbatrol; Carbium; Carpaz; Convuline; Epimaz; Epitol; Finlepsin; Fokalepsin; Gericarb; Hermolepsin; Neurotop; Prozine; Sirtal; Stazepin; Tegretol; Telesmin; Teril; Timonil.
5*H*-Dibenz[*b*,*f*]azepine-5-carboxamide
$C_{15}H_{12}N_2O$=236.3
CAS—298-46-4

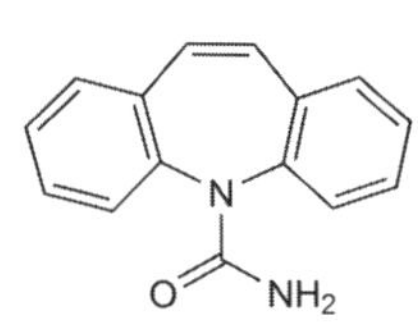

A white or yellowish-white crystalline powder. M.p. 189° to 193°.
Practically insoluble in water and ether; soluble in alcohol, acetone chloroform, and propylene glycol.

Dissociation Constant. pKa 7.0.

Partition Coefficient. Log *P* (octanol/water), 2.45.

Colour Test. Dissolve the sample in 1 mL of chloroform, add 0.2 mL of sodium hypobromite solution and mix for 1 min—blue-violet (detection limit 250 μg/mL).

Thin-layer Chromatography. System TA—Rf 60; system TB—Rf 02; system TC—Rf 56; system TE—carbamazepine Rf 56, M (OH-) Rf 36; system TL—Rf 47; system TAE—carbamazepine Rf 79, M (OH-) Rf 79; system TAF—Rf 75; system TAJ—Rf 44; system TAK—Rf 64; system TAL—Rf 94. (Acidified potassium permanganate solution, positive.)

Gas Chromatography. System GA—carbamazepine RI 2285, carbamazepine-Me RI 1905, M (OH-methoxy-ring) RI 2340, M (OH-ring) RI 2240, M (epoxide) RI 2220, M (iminostilbene) RI 1998, M (acridine) RI 1800, M (formyl-acridine) RI 2025; system GB—carbamazepine RI 2435, M (iminostilbene) RI 2064, M (acridine) RI 1880, M (formyl-acridine) RI 2158, M (methylacridine) RI 2054, M (10,11-di-OH-) RI 2738; system GE—carbamazepine RRT 0.83 (relative to phenytoin); system GF—carbamazepine RI 2610, M (epoxide) RI 2560, M (iminostilbene) RI 2620; system GAJ—carbamazepine RRT 1.716, M (epoxide) RRT 1.188, M (iminostilbene) RRT 1.065 (all relative to methylphenobarbital).

High Performance Liquid Chromatography. System HE—*k* 8.30; system HX—carbamazepine RI 418, M (10,11-di-OH-) RI 355; system HY—carbamazepine RI 368, M (epoxide) RI 336; system HZ—retention time carbamazepine 3.5 min, M (epoxide) 1.9 min, M (10, 11-di-OH-) 2.6 min; system HAA—carbamazepine retention time 15.8 min; system HAK—carbamazepine retention time 4.7 min; system HAX—carbamazepine retention time 6.2 min; system HAY—carbamazepine retention time 5.5 min; system HAZ—carbamazepine *k* 0.82, M (epoxide) *k* 0.38.

Ultraviolet Spectrum. Methanol—237, 285 nm (A_1^1=490a).

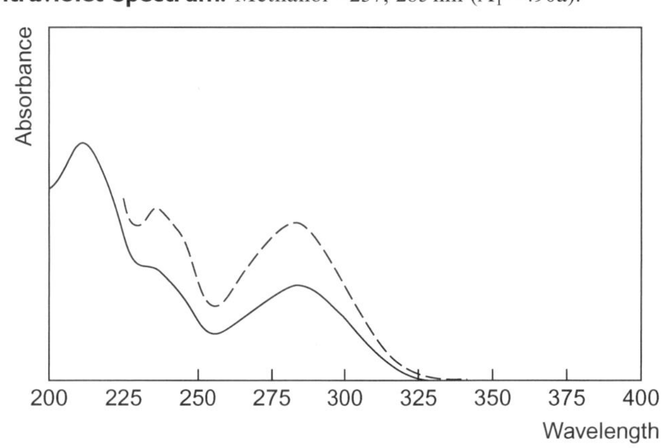

Infra-red Spectrum. Principal peaks at wavenumbers 1678, 1594, 800, 769, 787, 1298 cm^{-1} (KBr disk).

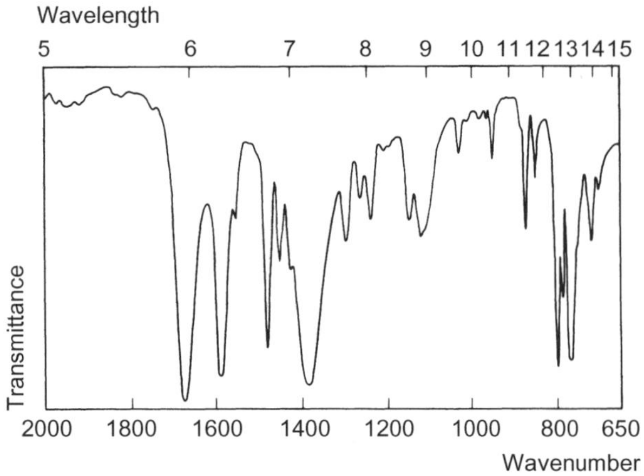

Mass Spectrum. Principal ions at *m/z* 193, 192, 236, 191, 194, 165, 190, 237; carbamazepine-10,11-epoxide 180, 179, 178, 152, 44, 181, 223, 51; *trans*-10,11-dihydro-10,11-dihydroxycarbamazepine 180, 77, 181, 44, 179, 51, 209, 167.

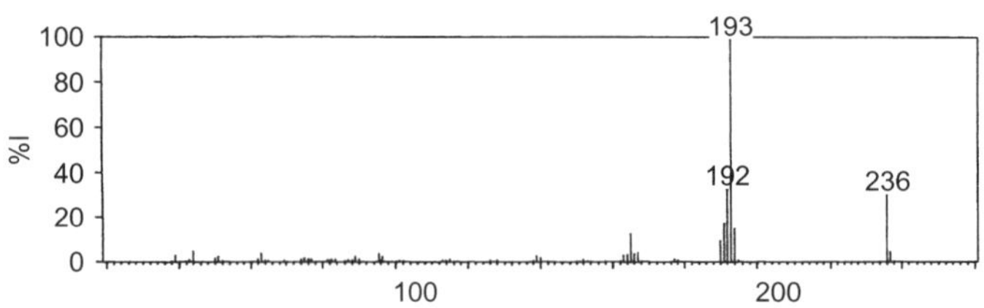

Quantification

Gas chromatography. In plasma or urine: carbamazepine and other anticonvulsants, limit of detection 1000 μg/L, FID—R. Riva *et al.*, *J. Chromatogr.* 1980, *221*(10) *B Biomed. Appl.*, 75–84. In plasma: carbamazepine and carbamazepine-10,11-epoxide, FID—A. Ranise *et al.*, *J. Chromatogr.* 1981, *222*(11) *B Biomed. Appl.*, 120–124. In plasma: carbamazepine, its epoxide, and other anticonvulsants, limits of quantification 50 to 200 μg/L, thermionic detection—E. Queiroz *et al.*, *J. Chromatogr. Sci.*, 2002, *40*, 219–223.

Gas chromatography–mass spectrometry. In serum: carbamazepine, its epoxide, and lamotrigine—J. Hallbach *et al.*, *Eur. J. Clin. Chem. Clin. Biochem.*, 1997, *35*, 755–759. In whole blood and liver tissue: carbamazepine and other anticonvulsants—D. J. Speed *et al.*, *J. Anal. Toxicol.*, 2000, *24*, 685–690. In serum: carbamazepine and its epoxide metabolite, limit of detection 10 μg/L—G. Minkova and D. Getova, *Methods Find. Exp. Clin. Pharmacol.*, 2001, *23*, 481–485.

High performance liquid chromatography. In plasma: carbamazepine and its metabolites, limits of quantification 320 to 640 μg/L, UV detection—P. S. Bonato *et al.*, *J. Anal. Toxicol.*, 1992, *16*, 88–92. In plasma: carbamazepine and its epoxide, limits of detection 80 μg/L and 7 μg/L respectively, comparisons with GC and enzyme immunoassay—J. Martens and P. Banditt, *J. Chromatogr.*, 1993, *620*, 169–173. In serum, saliva, or urine: carbamazepine and other convulsants and their metabolites, photodiode-array detection—H. Liu *et al.*, *J. Chromatogr.*, 1993, *616*, 105–115. In serum: carbamazepine and its metabolites, photodiode-array detection—H. Liu *et al.*, *Ther. Drug Monit.*, 1993, *15*, 317–327. In serum: carbamazepine and other anticonvulsants, limit of quantification for carbamazepine 1000 μg/L, UV detection—Y. Kouno *et al.*, *J. Chromatogr.*, 1993, *622*, 47–52. In plasma: carbamazepine, its metabolites, and other anticonvulsants, UV detection—L. A. Romanyshyn *et al.*, *Ther. Drug Monit.*, 1994, *16*, 90–99. In serum: carbamazepine and phenytoin, comparison with immunoassays—B. Rambeck *et al.*, *Ther. Drug Monit.*, 1994, *16*, 608–612. In plasma: carbamazepine and other anticonvulsants, UV detection—K. Johansen *et al.*, *J. Chromatogr.* 1995, *669 B Biomed. Appl.*, 281–288. In biological fluids: carbamazepine and oxcarbazepine and their metabolites, limits of detection 8 to 12 μg/L—P. Pienimaki *et al.*, *J. Chromatogr.* 1995, *673 B Biomed. Appl.*, 97–105. In plasma: carbamazepine and its epoxide metabolite—D. Chollet *et al.*, *J. Chromatogr.* 1996, *683 B Biomed. Appl.*, 237–243. In serum or saliva: carbamazepine and its epoxide metabolite—M. M. Alexishvili *et al.*, *Biomed. Chromatogr.*, 1997, *11*, 36–41. In hair: carbamazepine and phenytoin, limit of detection for carbamazepine 1.33 μg/g, UV detection—Z. Mei and J Williams, *Ther. Drug Monit.*, 1997, *19*, 92–94. In hair: carbamazepine and its metabolites, UV detection—L. A. Saris *et al.*, *J. Chromatogr. B Biomed. Sci. Appl.*, 1997, *691*, 409–415. In serum: carbamazepine and its epoxide, phenytoin, and lamotrigine, limits of detection 150 to 350 μg/L, UV detection—G. L. Lensmeyer *et al.*, *Ther. Drug Monit.*, 1997, *19*, 292–300. In serum: carbamazepine and other anticonvulsants, UV detection—Y. Kouno *et al.*, *J. Chromatogr. B Biomed. Sci. Appl.*, 1997, *695*, 349–353. In plasma: limit of detection 50 μg/L for carbamazepine and 10,11-carbamazepine epoxide, UV detection (λ=210 nm)—M. M. Bhatti *et al.*, *J. Pharm. Biomed. Anal.*, 1998, *16*, 1233–1240. In plasma: carbamazepine, its metabolites, and other anticonvulsants—K. M. Matar *et al.*, *Ther. Drug Monit.*, 1999, *21*, 559–566. In plasma or breast milk: carbamazepine and its epoxide, limits of quantification 10 μg/L in milk and 20 μg/L in plasma, UV detection—R. Shimoyama *et al.*, *Ann. Clin. Biochem.*, 2000, *37*, 210–215. In plasma or saliva—M. D. Rukhadze *et al.*, *Anal. Biochem.*, 2000, *287*, 279–283. In plasma: carbamazepine and its metabolites, UV detection—R. Mandrioli *et al.*, *J. Chromatogr. B Biomed. Sci. Appl.*, 2001, *762*, 109–116. In serum: carbamazepine and other anticonvulsants, limit of quantification for carbamazepine 660 μg/L, UV detection—H. Levert *et al.*, *Biomed. Chromatogr.*, 2002, *16*, 19–24. In serum or plasma: comparison with immunoassays—J. Hermida *et al.*, *Clin. Biochem.*, 2002, *35*, 251–254 and J. Ma *et al.*, *Acta Pharmacol. Sin.*, 2002, *23*, 87–91. In serum: carbamazepine and other anticonvulsants, UV detection—A. Martinavarro-Dominguez *et al.*, *Clin. Chem.*, 2002, *48*, 1696–1702.

High performance liquid chromatography–mass spectrometry. In urine: carbamazepine metabolites—J. L. Maggs *et al.*, *Drug Metab. Dispos.*, 1997, *25*, 275–280.

Thin-layer chromatography–spectrofluorimetry. In serum: carbamazepine and 2 metabolites, limits of detection 100 μg/L for carbamazepine and 50 μg/L for its metabolites—H. K. L. Hundt and E. C. Clark, *J. Chromatogr.*, 1975, *107*, 149–154.

Fluorescence polarisation immunoassay. In serum: carbamazepine and other anticonvulsants—L. S. Steijns *et al.*, *Ther. Drug Monit.*, 2002, *24*, 432–435.

Disposition in the Body. Slowly but almost completely absorbed after oral administration. Metabolic reactions, catalysed by cytochrome isoenzymes CYP3A4 and CYP2C8, include epoxidation to form the 10,11-epoxide, which is active, followed by hydroxylation to *trans*-10,11-dihydro-10,11-dihydroxycarbamazepine; glucuronic acid conjugation also occurs. The rate of metabolism is higher in children than in adults and levels of the epoxide may be higher in children than in adults. About 25% of a dose is excreted in the urine as the dihydroxy metabolite, together with 2% as the 10,11-epoxide and less than 10% as unchanged drug; other metabolites identified in the urine include carbamazepine-*N*-glucuronide, iminostilbene, and several monohydroxy- and trihydroxycarbamazepine isomers. About 30% of a dose is eliminated in the faeces. Carbamazepine crosses the placental barrier and is distributed into breast milk.

Therapeutic concentration. In plasma, usually in the range 4 to 12 mg/L.

Steady-state plasma concentrations of 3 to 13 mg/L (mean 8) for carbamazepine and 0.6 to 5.7 mg/L (mean 3) for the epoxide metabolite, were reported in 24 subjects receiving daily oral doses of 8 to 30 mg/kg. [J. J. MacKichan *et al.*, *Br. J. Clin. Pharmacol.*, 1981, *12*, 31–37.]

22 children receiving long-term therapy with slow-release carbamazepine tablets (300 to 800 mg daily in 2 divided doses) had their treatment replaced with carbamazepine suppositories for 7 days (at an equivalent dosage—375 to 1000 mg daily in 2 to 4 divided doses). Minimum to maximum plasma concentrations over 24 h were reported as follows: carbamazepine 20.4 to 33.1 μmol/L after slow-release tablets and 18.9 to 31.2 μmol/L after suppositories; 10,11-epoxy-carbamazepine 3.33 to 5.49 μmol/L after slow-release tablets and 3.11 to 4.90 μmol/L after suppositories. [J. Arvidsson *et al.*, *J. Child. Neurol.*, 1995, *10*, 114–117.]

In a study involving 435 blood samples taken from 248 patients receiving carbamazepine therapy (dose: 2.86 to 37.50 mg/kg daily), steady-state plasma concentrations of 2.5 to 82.9 μmol/L (mean 22.3) carbamazepine, 0.85 to 16.9 μmol/L (mean 5.17) carbamazepine-epoxide, and 0.77 to 36.4 μmol/L (mean 11.3) carbamazepine-diol were found. [D. A. Svinarov and C. E. Pippenger, *Ther. Drug Monit.*, 1996, *18*, 660–665.]

Toxicity. The estimated minimum lethal dose is 5 g. Plasma concentrations of 2.4 to 6.0 to 10.5 mg/L have been associated with slight toxic effects and concentrations of 3.2 to 10 to 21 mg/L with severe toxicity.

A 15-year-old girl was admitted having taken at least 23 tablets of Tegretol (4.6 g) 6 h earlier. The carbamazepine level was 44.8 mg/L. Orogastric lavage was followed by activated charcoal. Within 20 h of admission there was no improvement in her neurological status, so it was decided to perform plasmapheresis. The carbamazepine level immediately after the procedure was 23.9 mg/L, and at the 36th, 60th and 84th hours was 72, 33 and 4.7 mg/L, respectively. The patient was discharged on the 4th day. [A. Duzova *et al.*, *Hum. Exp. Toxicol.*, 2001, *20*, 175–177.]

In a massive overdose with controlled-release carbamazepine by a 31-year-old female, serum levels were 17.7 mg/L on admission, fell to 15.6 mg/L 22 h later (39 h post-ingestion), and rose to 46.3 mg/L on day 4 despite treatment with activated charcoal and whole bowel irrigation. Benzodiazepines were also detected. At this time coma and intermittent general seizures developed, so charcoal haemoperfusion was started and serum carbamazepine levels fell from 41.6 to 25.1 mg/L after 1 h. Upon recovery the patient admitted ingesting 300 controlled-release carbamazepine (200 mg) tablets as well as diazepam, nitrazepam, and alcohol. [A. Graudins *et al.*, *Emerg. Med.*, 2002, *14*, 89–94.]

In a fatality involving overdose with carbamazepine, blood concentrations were reported as 47.7 mg/L 2 h antemortem and 53 mg/L 9 h postmortem. [H. A. Spiller and R. D. Carlisle, *J. Forensic Sci.*, 2001, *46*, 1510–1512.]

In 28 cases of massive carbamazepine overdose, peak concentrations ranged from 78 to 285 μmol/L (18.4 to 67.4 mg/L). Serum levels of at least 170 μmol/L (40 mg/L) were associated with serious complications such as coma, seizures, respiratory failure, and cardiac conduction defects. Two of the cases were fatalities. [J. Hojer *et al.*, *J. Toxicol. Clin. Toxicol.*, 1993, *31*, 449–458.]

In a fatality due to carbamazepine and alcohol, postmortem kidney and liver concentrations of 306 mg/kg and 173 mg/kg, respectively, of carbamazepine were reported: the blood-alcohol concentration was 1600 mg/L. [T. Borkowski and E. Janowska, *Bull. Int. Assoc. Forensic Toxicol.*, 1983, *17(2)*, 16–17.]

Bioavailability. More than 70%.

Half-life. Plasma half-life, 18 to 65 h (mean 35) after single doses; reduced during chronic treatment to about 10 to 30 h for adults and 8 to 19 h for children.

Volume of distribution. About 1.4 L/kg.

Clearance. Plasma clearance, about 1.3 mL/min/kg.

Distribution in blood. Plasma:whole blood ratio, about 1.6.

Saliva Plasma:saliva ratio, about 3 to 5.

Protein binding. In plasma, carbamazepine about 75% and 10,11-epoxycarbamazepine about 50%.

Note. For reviews of the pharmacokinetics of carbamazepine, see L. Bertilsson, *Clin. Pharmacokinet.*, 1978, *3*, 128–143 and L. Bertilsson and T. Tomson, *Clin. Pharmacokinet.*, 1986, *11*, 177–198.

Dose. Initially 100 to 400 mg daily, increasing to 0.4 to 1.2 g daily; occasionally up to 2 g daily in epilepsy; in trigeminal neuralgia and bipolar disorder, up to 1.6 g daily.

Carbarsone

Anti-amoebic

Synonym. Aminarsonum
Proprietary names. Amabevan; Ameban; Carb-O-Sep; Fenarsone; Histocarb; Leucarsone.
[4-[(Aminocarbonyl)amino]phenyl]arsonic acid
$C_7H_9AsN_2O_4$=260.1
CAS—121-59-5

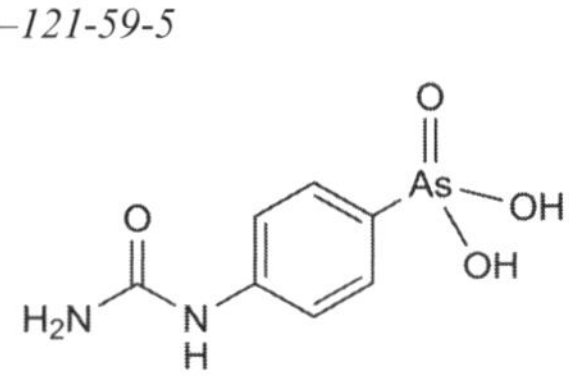

A white powder. M.p. 174°.

Soluble 1 in 330 of water and 1 in 400 of ethanol; nearly insoluble in chloroform and ether; soluble in solutions of alkali hydroxides and carbonates.

Partition Coefficient. Log *P* (octanol/water), −1.2.

Ultraviolet Spectrum. Aqueous acid—257; aqueous alkali—248 nm.

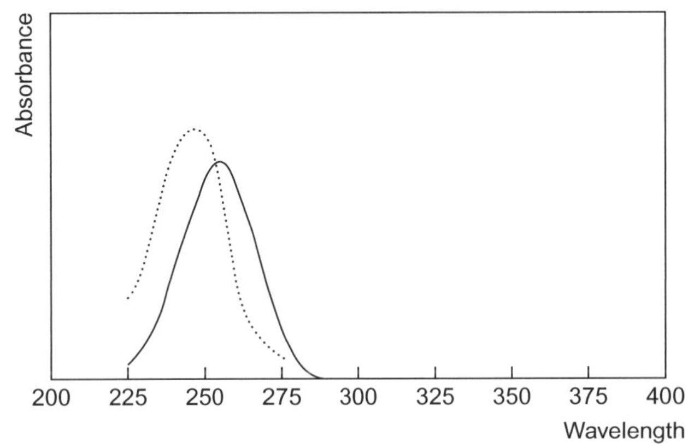

Infra-red Spectrum. Principal peaks at wavenumbers 1508, 1580, 1101, 903, 1681, 1248 cm^{-1}.

Dose. 500 to 750 mg daily, for 10 days.

Carbaryl

Insecticide

Synonym. Carbaril
Proprietary names. Carylderm; Derbac (shampoo); Murvin; Sevin; Suleo-C.
1-Naphthalenol methylcarbamate
$C_{12}H_{11}NO_2$=201.2
CAS—63-25-2

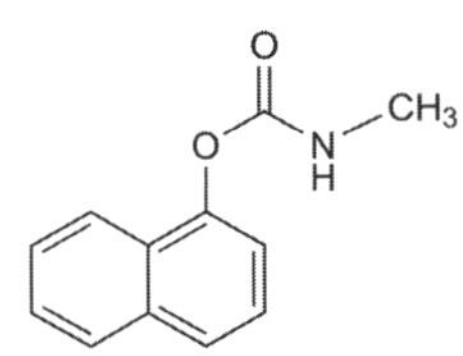

A white crystalline solid. M.p. 142°.
Practically insoluble in water; soluble in most polar organic solvents.

Partition Coefficient. Log *P* (octanol), 2.4.

Colour Tests. Liebermann's Test—black→green; Marquis Test—green.

Thin-layer Chromatography. System TX—Rf 18; system TY—Rf 25; system TZ—Rf 68; system TAA—Rf 17; system TAB—Rf 12; system TAC—Rf 04.

Gas Chromatography. System GA—carbaryl RI 1865, carbaryl-TFA RI 1785, M (1-naphthol) RI 1490, M (1-naphthol)-AC RI 1555; system GK—M (1-naphthol) RRT 0.47 (relative to caffeine).

High Performance Liquid Chromatography. System HY—RI 402; system HAA—retention time 18.0 min.

Ultraviolet Spectrum. Ethanol—279 nm (A_1^1=310b).

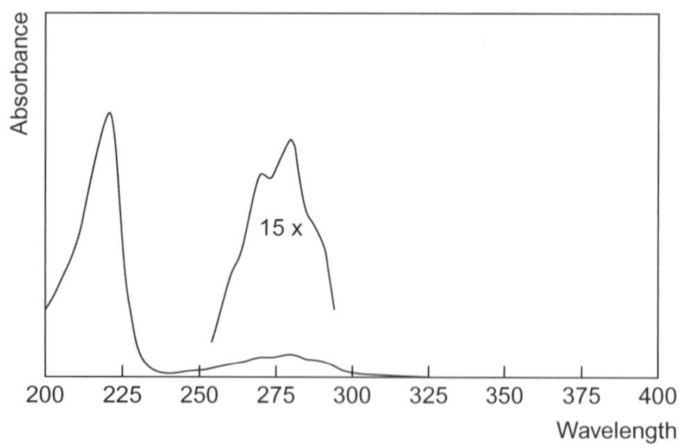

Infra-red Spectrum. Principal peaks at wavenumbers 1724, 1219, 1250, 1111, 781, 1265 cm^{-1}.

Mass Spectrum. Principal ions at *m/z* 144, 115, 116, 57, 58, 63, 145, 89.

Quantification

Gas chromatography. In animal blood or tissues: limit of detection 20 mg/L for blood, 100 mg/L for tissues, ECD—M. E. Mount and F. W. Oehme, *J. Anal. Toxicol.*, 1980, *4*, 286–292.

High performance liquid chromatography. In biological samples: limit of detection 100 ng—V. K. Sharma *et al.*, *Forensic Sci. Int.*, 1990, *48(1)*, 21–25.

Disposition in the Body

Toxicity

A 47-year-old man died due to a possible pesticide poisoning. Carbaryl was found in gastric contents at a concentration of 1.27 g/L and in serum at 8.1 mg/L. Propanil, ethylbenzene, and xylene were also detected. [M. Yamazaki *et al.*, *J. Forensic Sci.*, 2001, *46(1)*, 165–170.]

Carbazochrome

Haemostatic

Synonym. Adrenochrome Monosemicarbazone

Proprietary names. Adrenoxyl; Cromosil.

5,6-Dihydro-3-hydroxy-1-methylindoline-5,6-dione 5-semicarbazone

$C_{10}H_{12}N_4O_3$=236.2

CAS—69-81-8

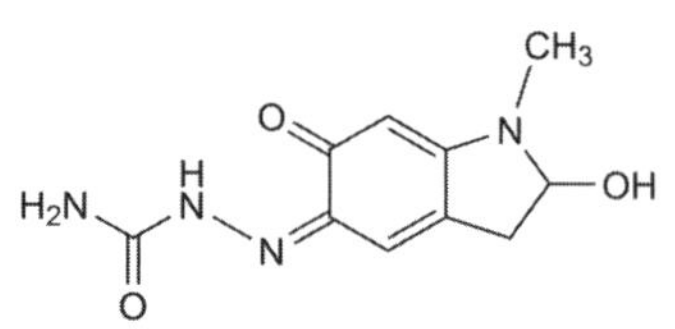

An oxidation product of adrenaline.

Yellowish-red or red crystals or crystalline powder. M.p. about 222°, with decomposition.

Very slightly soluble in water and ethanol; practically insoluble in ether.

Carbazochrome Salicylate

Proprietary name. Adrenosem Salicylate

A complex of carbazochrome with sodium salicylate.

CAS—13051-01-9

A fine, orange-red, crystalline powder. M.p. 196° to 197.5°, with decomposition.

Soluble in water and ethanol; practically insoluble in ether and chloroform.

Carbazochrome Sodium Sulfonate

Proprietary names. Adona; Emex.

$C_{10}H_{11}N_4NaO_5S$=322.3

CAS—51460-26-5

Orange to yellow, fine needle-like crystals. M.p. 227° to 228°, with decomposition.

Soluble 1 in 67 of cold water; slightly soluble in ethanol; practically insoluble in chloroform and ether.

Thin-layer Chromatography. System TD—Rf 00; system TE—Rf 16; system TF—Rf 00; system TAD—Rf 10.

Ultraviolet Spectrum. Methanol—356 nm (A_1^1=960b).

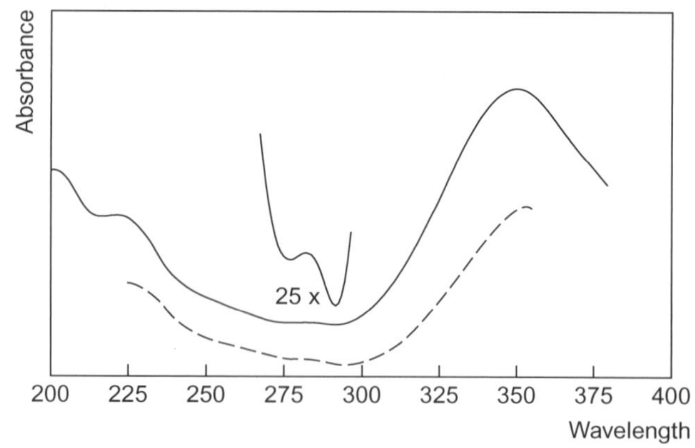

Mass Spectrum. Principal ions at *m/z* 147, 43, 146, 42, 193, 118, 164, 44.

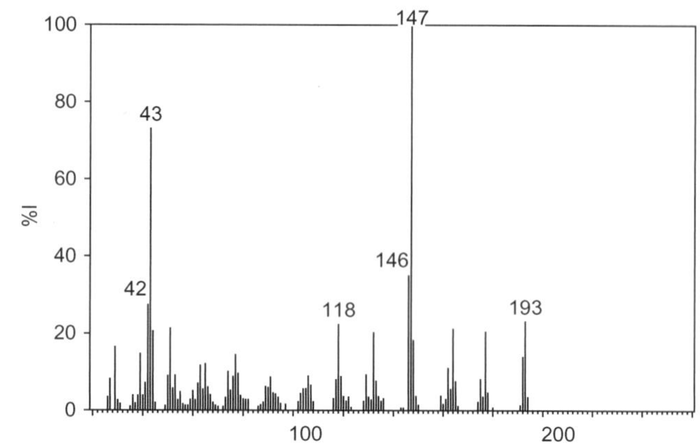

Dose. The equivalent of 5 to 10 mg of carbazochrome has been given intramuscularly or by mouth.

Carbenicillin

Antibiotic

Synonym. α-Carboxybenzylpenicillin

(2*S*,5*R*,6*R*)-6-[(Carboxyphenylacetyl)amino]-3,3-dimethyl-7-oxo-4-thia-1-azabicyclo[3.2.0]heptane-2-carboxylic acid

$C_{17}H_{18}N_2O_6S$=378.4

CAS—4697-36-3

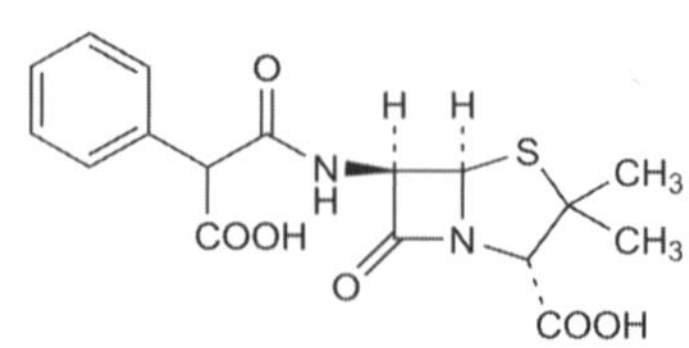

Carbenicillin Sodium

Proprietary names. Anabactyl; Carbapen; Fugacillin; Geopen; Microcillin; Pyopen.

$C_{17}H_{16}N_2Na_2O_6S$=422.4

CAS—4800-94-6

A white, hygroscopic, crystalline powder.

Soluble 1 in 1.2 of water and 1 in 25 of ethanol; practically insoluble in chloroform and ether.

Dissociation Constant. pK_a 2.6, 2.7.

Partition Coefficient. Log *P* (octanol/water), 1.1.

Ultraviolet Spectrum. Aqueous acid—259, 265, 327 nm.

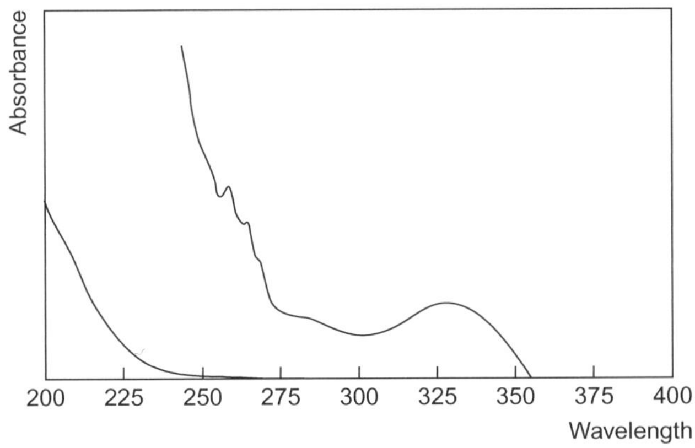

Infra-red Spectrum. Principal peaks at wavenumbers 1612, 1754, 1315, 1123, 1030, 1000 cm^{-1}.

Quantification

High performance liquid chromatography. In serum: limit of quantification 0.25 mg/L, UV detection (λ = 208 nm)—W. Naidong *et al.*, *J Pharm. Biomed. Anal.*, 1994, *12(6)*, 845–850. In plasma and urine: limit of detection 10 mg/L—M. Ishida *et al.*, *J. Chromatogr. B Biomed. Sci. Appl.*, 1994, *652(1)*, 43–49

Disposition in the Body

Therapeutic concentration

Four healthy male volunteers aged 20 to 23 years old were fasted overnight and administered 2 g of carbenicillin intravenously. The peak plasma concentrations of the drug were 88 mg/L for *R*-carbenicillin and 83 mg/L for *S*-carbenicillin approximately 30 min after dosing. [M. Ishida *et al.*, *J. Chromatogr. B Biomed. Sci. Appl.*, 1994, *652(1)*, 43–49.]

Dose. The equivalent of 20 to 30 g of carbenicillin daily, intravenously.

Carbenoxolone

Treatment of Peptic Ulcer

Synonyms. Glycerrhetic Acid Hydrogen Succinate; Glycyrrhetinic Acid Hydrogen Succinate.

(3*β*,20*β*)-3-(3-Carboxy-1-oxopropoxy)-11-oxoolean-12-en-29-oic acid

$C_{34}H_{50}O_7 = 570.8$

CAS—5697-56-3

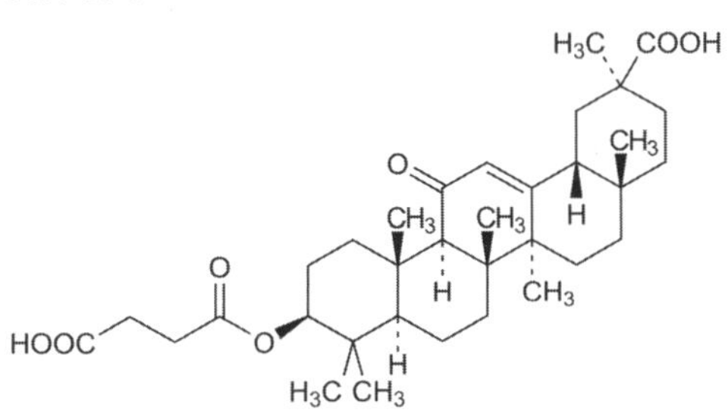

Cream-coloured crystals. M.p. 291° to 294°.

Carbenoxolone Sodium

Synonym. Disodium Enoxolone Succinate

Proprietary names. Biogastrone; Duogastrone; Gastrausil; Neogel; Ulcus-Tablinen. It is an ingredient of Pyrogastrone.

$C_{34}H_{48}Na_2O_7 = 614.7$

CAS—7421-40-1

A white or pale cream-coloured hygroscopic powder.

Soluble 1 in 6 of water and 1 in 30 of ethanol; insoluble in chloroform and ether.

Caution. Carbenoxolone sodium powder is irritating to nasal membranes.

Dissociation Constant. pK_a 6.7, 7.1.

Partition Coefficient. Log *P* (octanol/water), 7.1.

Colour Tests. Antimony Pentachloride—brown; Naphthol–Sulfuric Acid—yellow-brown/orange; Sulfuric Acid—yellow.

Mix 5 mg with 50 mg of resorcinol and 2 mL of 80% v/v sulfuric acid, heat at 200° for 10 min, cool, and add to 200 mL of water; make just alkaline with sodium hydroxide solution—an intense green fluorescence is produced.

Thin-layer Chromatography. System TD—Rf 07; system TE—Rf 00; system TF—Rf 17; system TAD—Rf 28. (Acidified potassium permanganate solution, positive, faint.)

High Performance Liquid Chromatography. System HY—RI 824.

Ultraviolet Spectrum. Carbenoxolone sodium: aqueous acid—248 nm; aqueous alkali—257 nm ($A_1^1 = 172b$).

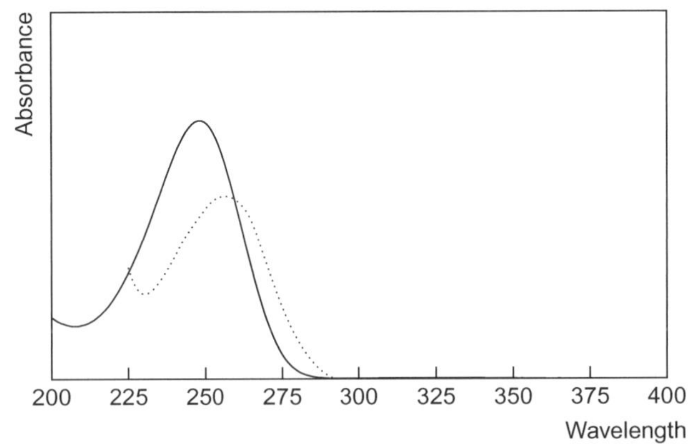

Infra-red Spectrum. Principal peaks at wavenumbers 1562, 1642, 1715, 1289, 1261, 1210 cm^{-1} (carbenoxolone sodium, KBr disk).

Quantification

Gas Chromatography. In serum: limit of detection 5 mg/L, FID—C. Rhodes and P. A. Wright, *J. Pharm. Pharmacol.*, 1974, *26*, 894–898.

Radioimmunoassay. In serum: limit of detection 1 μg/L—B. M. Peskar *et al.*, *J. Pharm. Pharmacol.*, 1976, *28*, 720–721.

Disposition in the Body. Carbenoxolone is rapidly and almost completely absorbed after oral administration; absorption is reduced at gastric pH levels above 2 and delayed after food. It is almost entirely eliminated in the faeces via the bile, less than 5% being excreted in the urine. Carbenoxolone is excreted mainly as the glucuronide conjugate together with small amounts as the sulfate conjugate of β-glycyrrhetic acid (enoxolone).

Therapeutic concentration

After a single oral dose of 200 mg to 10 subjects, peak blood concentrations of 13 to 35 (mean 24) mg/L were attained in 1 to 2 h, followed by a second peak of 3 to 32 (mean 20) mg/L at 3 to 6 h; in some subjects, the second peak was higher than the first. [H. D. Downer *et al.*, *J. Pharm. Pharmacol.*, 1970, *22*, 479–487].

Following oral administration of 100 mg to 3 fasting subjects, peak serum concentrations of 15 to 20 mg/L were attained in 1 to 2 h; following administration of 100 mg to 2 subjects after meals, peak serum concentrations of 8 to 9 mg/L were reported at 5 to 6 h.

After oral doses of 100 mg three times a day to 9 subjects, serum concentrations of 20 to 98 (mean 49) mg/L were reported on the eighth day [J. H. Baron *et al.*, Factors affecting the Absorption of Carbenoxolone in Patients with Peptic Ulcer, in *4th Symposium on Carbenoxolone*, F. A. Jones and D. V. Parke (Ed.), London, Butterworths, 1975, pp. 115–124].

Half-life. Plasma half-life 8 to 20 (mean 13) h, increased in elderly subjects.

Volume of distribution. About 0.1 L/kg.

Protein binding. In plasma, more than 99%.

Note. For a review of carbenoxolone, see R. M. Pinder *et al.*, *Drugs*, 1976, *11*, 245–307.

Dose. 150 to 300 mg of carbenoxolone sodium daily.

Carbetapentane

Antitussive

Synonym. Pentoxyverine

2-(Diethylaminoethoxy)ethyl 1-phenylcyclopentanecarboxylate

$C_{20}H_{31}NO_3 = 333.5$

CAS—77-23-6

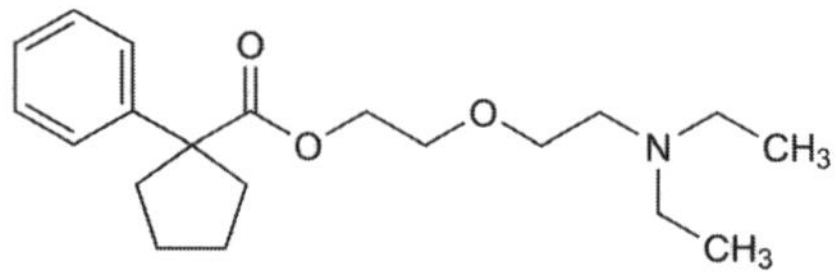

Carbetapentane Citrate

Proprietary names. Atussil; Germapect; Sedotussin; Toclase; Tuclase; Tussa-Tablinen.

$C_{20}H_{31}NO_3,C_6H_8O_7$=525.6

CAS—23142-01-0

A white crystalline powder. M.p. 93°.

Freely soluble in water and chloroform; soluble in ethanol, acetone and ethyl acetate; practically insoluble in ether and in benzene.

Partition Coefficient. Log *P* (octanol/water), 4.2.

Colour Tests. Liebermann's Test—red-orange; Mandelin's Test—brown (slow); Marquis Test—orange (slow).

Thin-layer Chromatography. System TA—Rf 48; system TB—Rf 48; system TC—Rf 22. (Dragendorff spray, positive; Acidified iodoplatinate solution, positive; Marquis reagent, brown.)

Gas Chromatography. System GA—RI 2232; system GF—RI 2455.

Ultraviolet Spectrum. Aqueous acid—252, 258 (A^1_1=6.1a), 264 nm. No alkaline shift.

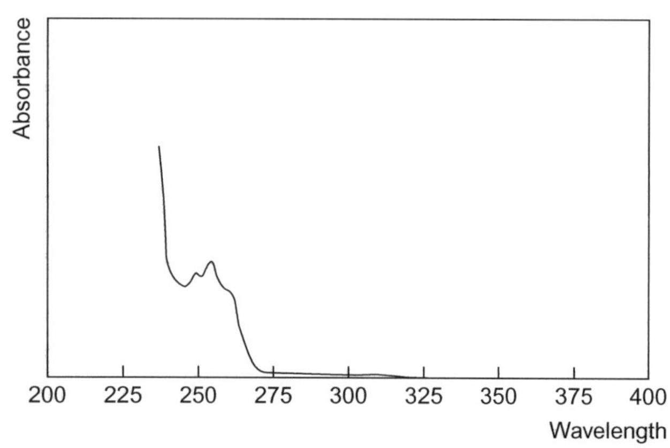

Infra-red Spectrum. Principal peaks at wavenumbers 1725, 1120, 1158, 1176, 694, 1234 cm^{-1} (KBr disk).

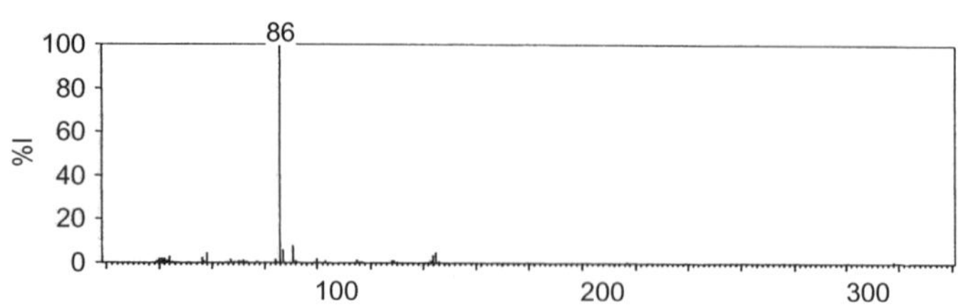

Mass Spectrum. Principal ions at *m/z* 86, 91, 87, 145, 58, 144, 30, 44.

Dose. 25 to 150 mg of carbetapentane citrate daily.

Carbidopa

Dopa-decarboxylase Inhibitor

Synonyms. HMD; (−)-L-α-Methyldopa Hydrazine; Mk-486.

Proprietary name. It is an ingredient of Sinemet.

(α*S*)-α-Hydrazino-3,4-dihydroxy-α-methylbenzenepropanoic acid monohydrate

$C_{10}H_{14}N_2O_4,H_2O$=244.2

CAS—28860-95-9 (anhydrous); 38821-49-7 (monohydrate)

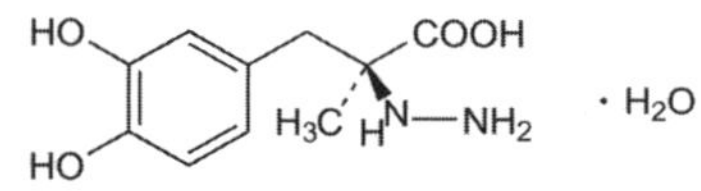

A white or creamy-white powder. M.p. 203° to 205°, with decomposition. Soluble 1 in 500 of water; practically insoluble in ethanol, chloroform, and ether; freely soluble in 3 M hydrochloric acid.

Partition Coefficient. Log *P* (octanol/water), −0.1.

Colour Tests. Ammoniacal Silver Nitrate (on warming) —silver mirror; Ferric Chloride—brown; Folin–Ciocalteu Reagent—blue; Liebermann's Test—black; Marquis Test—brown; Methanolic Potassium Hydroxide—orange; Millon's Reagent (cold)—orange; Nessler's Reagent—orange→black; Palladium Chloride—orange→brown; Potassium Dichromate (Method 1)—red.

Thin-layer Chromatography. System TD—Rf 00; system TE—Rf 00; system TF—Rf 02; system TAD—Rf 04.

Gas Chromatography. System GA—carbidopa, not eluted; carbidopa-Me_2 RI 1660.

High Performance Liquid Chromatography. System HY—RI 190.

Ultraviolet Spectrum. Methanolic acid—282 (A^1_1=130a); aqueous alkali—291 nm.

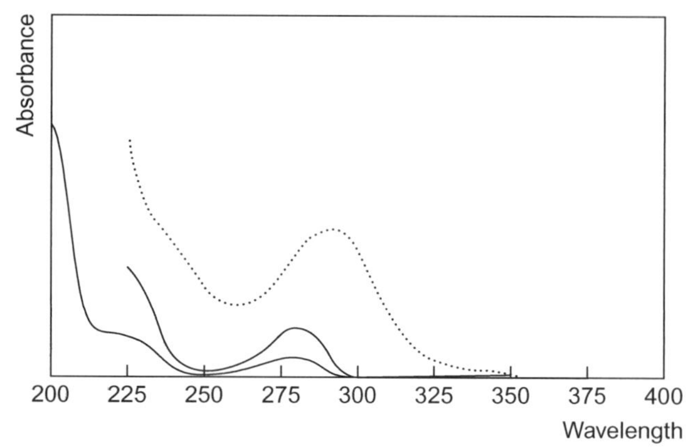

Infra-red Spectrum. Principal peaks at wavenumbers 1625, 1121, 1260, 1525, 1290, 875 cm^{-1} (KBr disk).

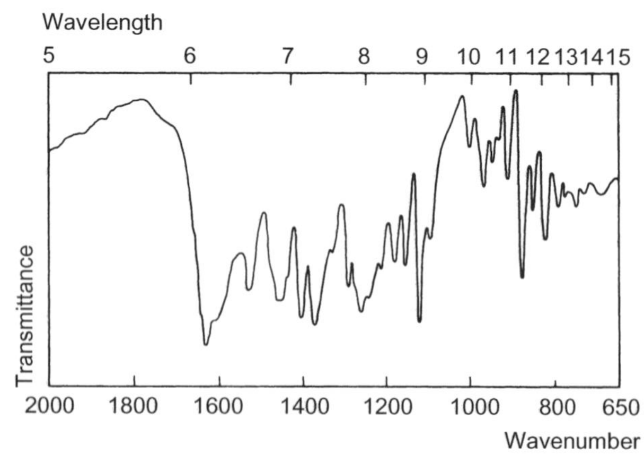

Mass Spectrum. Principal ions at *m/z* 123, 57, 42, 103, 44, 85, 124, 51.

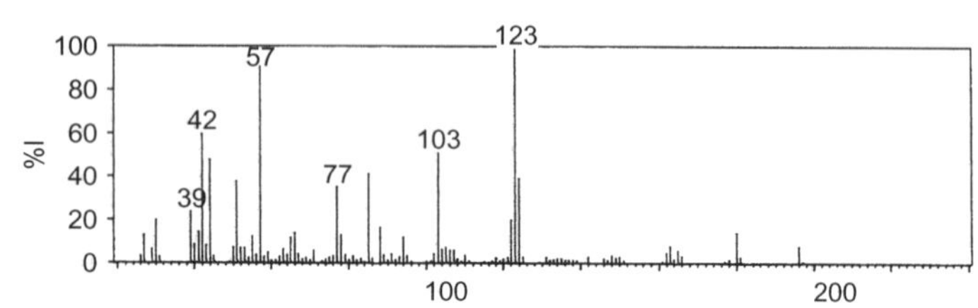

Quantification

High performance liquid chromatography. In plasma: limit of detection 15 µg/L, electrochemical detection—E. Nissinen and J. Taskinen, *J. Chromatogr.* 1982, *231 B Biomed. Appl.*, *20*, 459–462. In plasma: limit of detection 8 µg/L, amperometric detection—K. A. Sagar and M. R. Smyth, *J. Pharm. Biomed. Anal.*, 2000, *22(3)*, 613–624. In plasma, electrochemical detection—C. Lucarelli *et al.*, *J. Chromatogr.*, 1990, *511*, 167–176. In plasma and urine, electrochemical detection—D. C. Titus *et al.*, *J. Chromatogr.*, 1990, *534*, 87–100.

Disposition in the Body. Readily but incompletely absorbed after oral administration. About 50% of an oral dose is excreted in the urine in 48 h and 47% is eliminated in the faeces. Of the urinary material, about 30% is unchanged drug, 10 to 14% is 2-(4-hydroxy-3-methoxybenzyl)propionic acid, 10% is 2-(3,4-dihydroxybenzyl)propionic acid, 5% is 3,4-dihydroxyphenylacetone and 10% is 2-(3-hydroxybenzyl)propionic acid. The metabolites are excreted mainly as glucuronide conjugates.

Therapeutic concentration

Following an oral dose of 50 mg to 10 subjects, a mean peak plasma concentration of 0.2 mg/L was attained in 2 to 4 h. [S. Vickers *et al.*, *Drug Met. Disp.*, 1974, *2*, 9–22.]

Half-life. Plasma half-life, about 2 h.

Protein binding. In plasma, about 36%.

Note. For a review of the pharmacokinetics of carbidopa see R. M. Pinder *et al.*, *Drugs*, 1976, *11*, 329–377.

Dose. Usually the equivalent of 75 to 150 mg of anhydrous carbidopa daily, given in combination with levodopa.

Carbimazole

Antithyroid Agent

Proprietary names. Carbazole; Carbotiroid; Neo-Mercazole; Neo-Morphazole; Neo-Thyreostat; Neo-Tireol.

2,3-Dihydro-3-methyl-2-thioxo-1*H*-imidazole-1-carboxylic acid ethyl ester

$C_7H_{10}N_2O_2S = 186.2$

CAS—22232-54-8

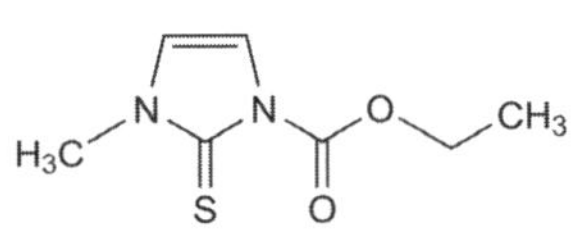

A white or creamy-white crystalline powder. M.p. 122° to 125°.

Soluble 1 in 500 of water, 1 in 50 of ethanol, 1 in 17 of acetone, 1 in 3 of chloroform and 1 in 330 of ether.

Partition Coefficient. Log *P* (octanol/water), 0.5.

Colour Tests. Palladium Chloride—orange.

To a small quantity add 1 drop of iodobismuthous acid solution—red.

Thin-layer Chromatography. System TA—Rf 72; system TB—Rf 01; system TD—Rf 63; system TE—Rf 42; system TF—Rf 47; system TAD—Rf 68; system TAE—Rf 75; system TAF—Rf 75. (Acidified iodoplatinate solution, positive; Acidified potassium permanganate solution, positive.)

Gas Chromatography. System GA—carbimazole RI 1678, thiamazole RI 1550.

High Performance Liquid Chromatography. System HX—RI 318; system HAA—Retention time(s), 11.1 min.

Ultraviolet Spectrum. Aqueous acid—291 nm ($A_1^1 = 557a$); aqueous alkali—244 nm.

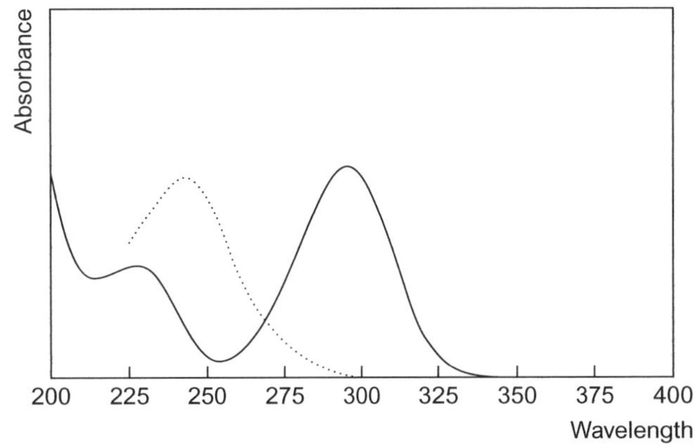

Infra-red Spectrum. Principal peaks at wavenumbers 1574, 1275, 740, 1246, 1150, 767 cm^{-1} (KBr disk).

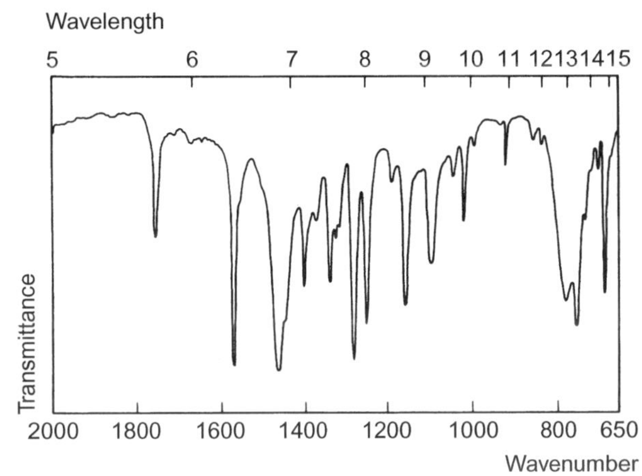

Mass Spectrum. Principal ions at *m/z* 186, 114, 29, 72, 42, 113, 27, 109; thiamazole 114, 42, 72, 113, 69, 81, 54, 115.

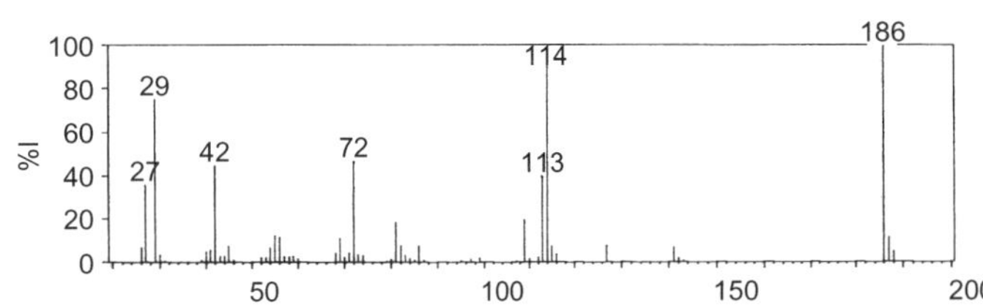

Quantification

Gas chromatography. In plasma: thiamazole, limit of detection 30 µg/L, AFID—M. R. Bending and D. Stevenson, *J. Chromatogr.*, 1978, *154*, 267–271.

Gas chromatography–mass spectrometry. In plasma: thiamazole, limit of detection 2 µg/L—S. Floberg *et al.*, *J. Chromatogr.*, 1980, *182*; *Biomed. Appl.*, *8*, 63–70.

High performance liquid chromatography. In plasma: thiamazole, limit of detection 5 µg/L, absorbance detection at 405 nm—A. Meulemans *et al.*, *J. Liq. Chromatogr.*, 1980, *3*, 287–298.

Disposition in the Body. Carbimazole is rapidly and almost completely absorbed after oral administration and converted to the active metabolite thiamazole. It is almost completely excreted in the urine in 24 h as metabolites; 3-methyl-2-thiohydantoin has been identified as a minor metabolite in urine and plasma. About 3% of a dose is eliminated in the faeces.

Therapeutic concentration

After an oral dose of 60 mg, given to 11 subjects, peak serum concentrations of thiamazole of 0.5 to 3.4 (mean 0.9) mg/L were attained in about 0.7 to 3 h. [A. Melander *et al.*, *Eur. J. Clin. Pharmacol.*, 1980, *17*, 295–299].

Half-life. Plasma half-life, thiamazole about 3 to 5 h.

Volume of distribution. Thiamazole, about 0.5 L/kg.

Protein binding. In plasma, thiamazole, not significantly bound.

Note. For a review of the pharmacokinetics of antithyroid drugs, see J. P. Kampmann and J. M. Hansen, *Clin. Pharmacokinet.*, 1981, *6*, 401–428.

Dose. Initially 30 to 60 mg daily; maintenance, 5 to 20 mg daily.

Carbinoxamine

Antihistamine

Synonym. Paracarbinoxamine
2-[(4-Chlorophenyl)-2-pyridinylmethoxy]-*N*,*N*-dimethylethanamine
$C_{16}H_{19}ClN_2O$=290.8
CAS—486-16-8

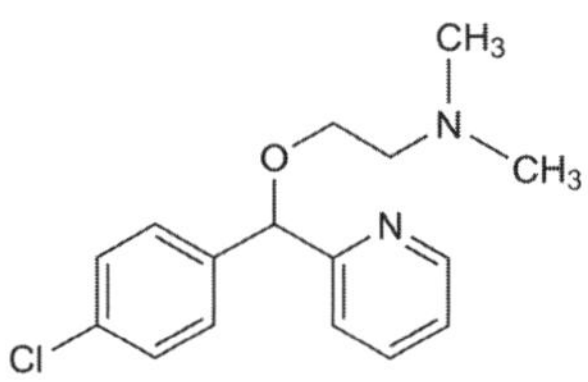

A liquid.

Carbinoxamine Maleate

Proprietary names. Allergefon; Clistin; Histex; Ziriton. It is an ingredient of Davenol, Extil, and Rondec.
$C_{16}H_{19}ClN_2O,C_4H_4O_4$=406.9
CAS—3505-38-2
A white crystalline powder. M.p. 117° to 119°.
Soluble 1 in less than 1 of water, 1 in 1.5 of ethanol, and 1 in 1.5 of chloroform; very slightly soluble in ether.

Dissociation Constant. pK_a 8.1 (25°).

Partition Coefficient. Log *P* (octanol/water), 2.6.

Colour Test. Cyanogen Bromide—orange-pink.

Thin-layer Chromatography. System TA—Rf 48; system TB—Rf 26; system TC—Rf 19; system TE—Rf 50; system TL—Rf 04; system TAE—Rf 13; system TAF—Rf 16; system TAJ—Rf 04; system TAK—Rf 00; system TAL—Rf 27. (Dragendorff spray, positive; acidified iodoplatinate solution, positive; Marquis reagent, pink.)

Gas Chromatography. System GA—carbinoxamine RI 2080, M (chlorobenzoylpyridine) RI 1645, M (carbinol) RI 1670, M (nor-) RI 2150; system GB—RI 2147; system GC—RI 2430.

High Performance Liquid Chromatography. System HA—*k* 4.7 (tailing peak); system HX—RI 359; system HAA—retention time, 12.8 min.

Ultraviolet Spectrum. Aqueous acid—263 (A^1_1=323a); aqueous alkali—261 nm (A^1_1=181a) (see below).

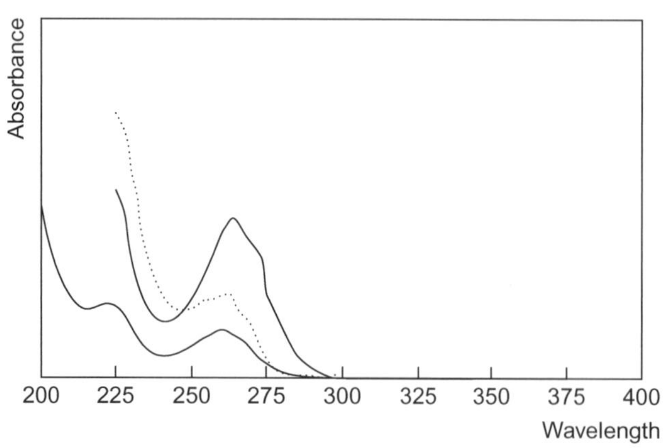

Infra-red Spectrum. Principal peaks at wavenumbers 1084, 1110, 1584, 1041, 763, 1010 cm^{-1} (KBr disk).

Mass Spectrum. Principal ions at *m/z* 58, 71, 26, 54, 167, 72, 42, 44.

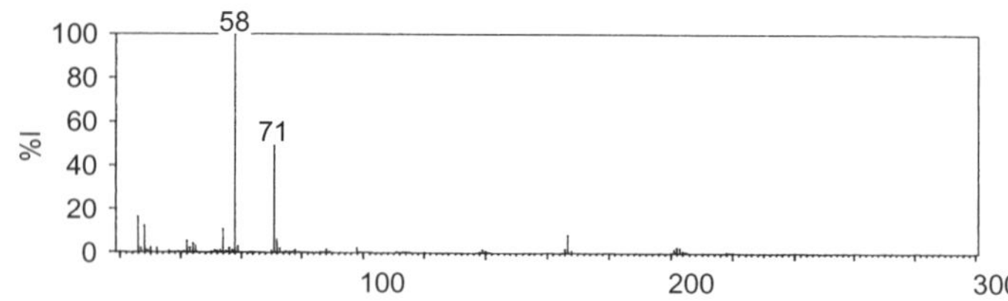

Quantification

Gas chromatography. In plasma: limit of detection 200 ng/L, AFID—D. J. Hoffman *et al.*, *J. Pharm. Sci.*, 1983, *72*, 1342–1344.

High performance liquid chromatography. In plasma, limit of quantification 2 µg/L and limit of detection 0.5 µg/L, coulometric detection—A. Stockis *et al.*, *Arzneimittelforschung*, 1995, *45(9)*, 1009–1112. In plasma, coulometric detection—A. Stockis *et al.*, *Arzneimittelforschung*, 1992, *42(12)*, 1478–1481.

Disposition in the Body

Therapeutic concentration. 20 healthy males and females (20 to 42 years old) were administered a single medication containing 20 mg phenylephrine and 4 mg carbinoxamine maleate. The peak plasma carbinoxamine concentration was 6.5 µg/L, 2 to 6 h after dosing for a single dose and a steady state concentration of 13.5 µg/L, approximately 4.8 h after dosing was observed over a 4-day dosing period. [A. Stockis *et al.*, *Arzneimittelforschung*, 1995, *45(9)*, 1009–1112.]

Dose. 12 to 32 mg of carbinoxamine maleate daily.

Carbocromen

Anti-anginal Vasodilator

Synonym. Chromonar
[[3-[2-(Diethylamino)ethyl]-4-methyl-2-oxo-2*H*-1-benzopyran-7-yl]oxy]-acetic acid ethyl ester
$C_{20}H_{27}NO_5$=361.4
CAS—804-10-4

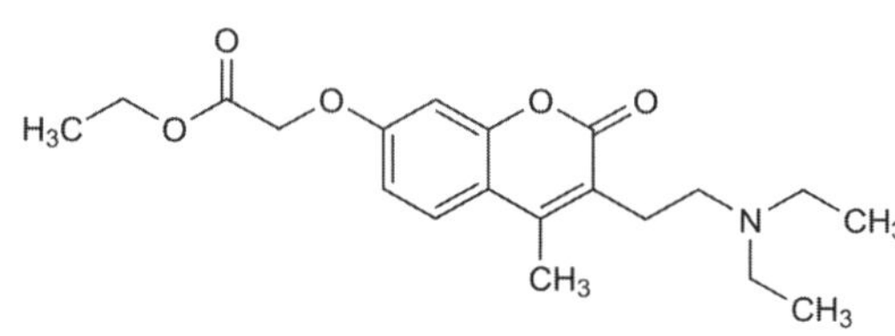

Practically insoluble in water; soluble in chloroform and ether.

Carbocromen Hydrochloride

Synonym. Cassella 4489
Proprietary name. Intensain
$C_{20}H_{27}NO_5,HCl$=397.9
CAS—655-35-6
A white crystalline powder. M.p. 159° to 160°.
Freely soluble in water, ethanol, methylene chloride, and chloroform; sparingly soluble in acetone, benzene, and ether.

Partition Coefficient. Log *P* (octanol/water), 3.4.

Colour Tests. Aromaticity (Method 2)—yellow/orange; Liebermann's Test (100°)—blue (3 min); Sulfuric Acid—violet (blue fluorescence at 350 nm).

Thin-layer Chromatography. System TA—Rf 48; system TB—Rf 17; system TC—Rf 24; system TE—Rf 62; system TL—Rf 12; system TAE—Rf 18. (Acidified iodoplatinate solution, positive.)

Gas Chromatography. System GA—RI 2835.

Ultraviolet Spectrum. Aqueous acid—202, 216, 321 nm (A^1_1=527a).

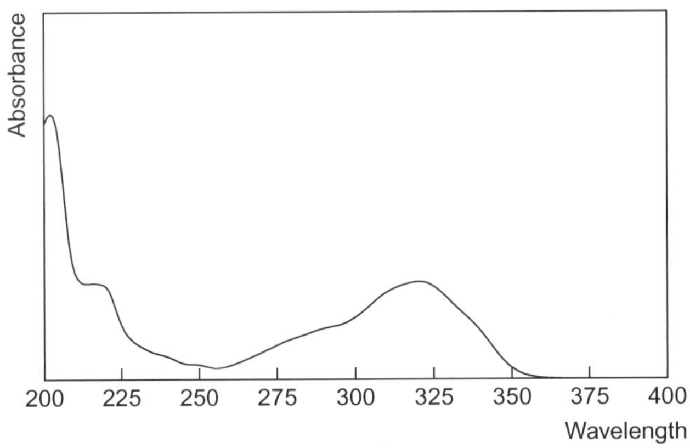

Infra-red Spectrum. Principal peaks at wavenumbers 1708, 1608, 1210, 1755, 1178, 1085 cm^{-1} (KBr disk).

Mass Spectrum. Principal ions at *m/z* 86, 87, 58, 30, 29, 84, 56, 42.

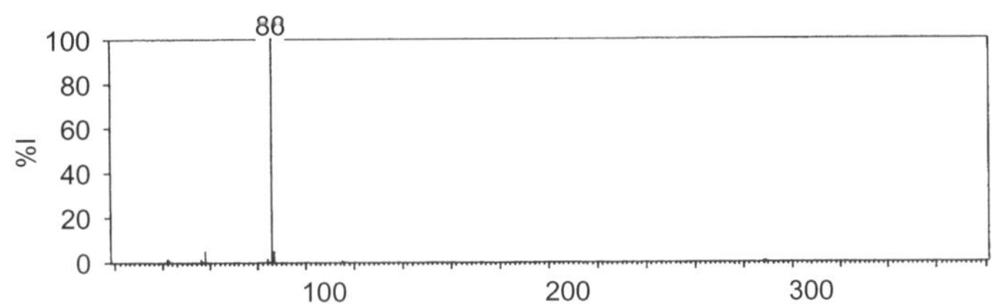

Quantification

Spectrofluorimetry. In plasma or urine: limit of detection 40 µg/L—Y. C. Martin and R. G. Wiegand, *J. Pharm. Sci.*, 1970, *59*, 1313–1318.

Disposition in the Body. Incompletely absorbed after oral administration (about 35%); rapidly hydrolysed to the corresponding carboxylic acid. About 70% of an intravenous dose and 20% of an oral dose are excreted in the 24-h urine as the carboxylic acid metabolite.

Therapeutic concentration

Following oral administration of 150 mg three times a day to 6 subjects, a peak plasma concentration of 0.9 mg/L of the carboxylic acid metabolite was reported, declining to 0.06 mg/L, 10 h after the last dose. [Y. C. Martin and R. G. Wiegand, *J. Pharm. Sci.*, 1970, *59*, 1313–1318.]

Half-life. Plasma half-life, carboxylic acid metabolite about 0.8 h.

Volume of distribution. Carboxylic acid metabolite, about 0.4 L/kg.

Dose. Carbocromen hydrochloride has been given in doses of 225 to 675 mg daily.

Carbon Tetrachloride

Anthelmintic (Veterinary)/Solvent

Synonym. Carboneum Tetrachloratum Medicinale

Tetrachloromethane

CCl_4=153.8

CAS—56-23-5

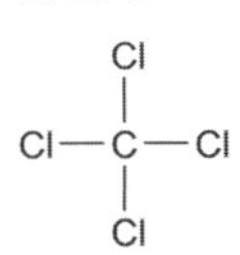

A heavy, clear, colourless, volatile liquid, with a chloroform-like odour. It is non-inflammable but in contact with a flame it decomposes and gives rise to toxic products, which have an acrid odour. Mass per mL 1.592 to 1.595 g. B.p. 76° to 78°. Refractive index 1.4607.

Soluble 1 in 2000 of water; miscible with dehydrated alcohol, benzene, chloroform, and ether.

Partition Coefficient. Log *P* (octanol/water), 2.8.

Colour Test. Fujiwara Test—red.

Gas Chromatography. System GA—RI 1000; system GI—retention time 8.6 min.

Mass Spectrum. Principal ions at *m/z* 117, 119, 47, 35, 121, 82, 84, 49.

Quantification

Gas chromatography. In biological material and expired air: simultaneous determination of carbon tetrachloride and chloroform, limit of detection 5 µg by FID, 15 ng by ECD—C. J. Reddrop *et al.*, *J. Chromatogr.*, 1980, *193*, 71–82.

Disposition in the Body. Readily absorbed after inhalation and also absorbed after ingestion or through the skin; the rate of absorption is increased by the concomitant ingestion of alcohol. It is excreted mainly from the lungs as carbon tetrachloride and carbon dioxide; excretion in the urine, as urea and an unidentified metabolite, and elimination in the faeces also occur.

Toxicity. The minimum lethal dose is 3 to 5 mL but recoveries have occurred following ingestion of 30 to 40 mL. Carbon tetrachloride injures almost all cells of the body including those of the blood, CNS, liver, and kidney; the kidneys and liver of fatal cases often show marked fatty degeneration. The maximum permissible atmospheric concentration is 10 ppm. Inhalation of concentrations of 1000 ppm, even for short periods, may cause acute toxic reactions. Continued exposure to concentrations of about 100 ppm may give rise to chronic poisoning. When carbon tetrachloride is ingested together or immediately after alcohol, its toxicity, particularly nephrotoxicity, is greatly increased. Toxic effects are associated with blood concentrations of 20 to 50 mg/L and a postmortem blood concentration of 260 mg/L has been reported in one fatality.

A 75-year-old man died in hospital after ingesting an unknown amount of carbon tetrachloride. Concentrations were 328.5 mg/L in urine, 169.8 mg/L in bile, 143.4 mg/L in systemic venous blood, 57.5 mg/L in arterial blood, and 170.5 mg/L in vitreous humor. In tissues, the concentrations were 657.9 mg/kg in the pancreas, 243 mg/kg in the brain, 237.3 mg/kg in testes, 127.3 mg/kg in lungs, 150.5 mg/kg in kidneys, 71.1 mg/kg in muscle, 78.5 mg/kg in myocardium, 68.3 mg/kg in spleen, and 58.6 mg/kg in the liver. [A. Tombolini and M. Cingolani, *J. Forensic Sci.*, 1996, *41(1)*, 166–168.]

The following postmortem tissue concentrations were reported in a fatality due to the inhalation of carbon tetrachloride: kidney 32 µg/g, liver 142 µg/g, lung 39 µg/g, muscle 46 µg/g. [H. D. Korenke, O. Pribilla, *Arch. Toxicol.*, 1969, *25*, 109–126.]

The following postmortem tissue concentrations were reported in a fatality due to inhalation of carbon tetrachloride: blood 18 mg/L, brain 175 µg/g, lung 12.5 µg/g. [A. Franc, *Bull. Int. Assoc. Forensic Toxicol.*, 1983, *17(2)*, 22–25.]

Carbromal

Hypnotic

Synonyms. Bromadal; Bromodiethylacetylurea; Karbromal; Uradal.

Proprietary names. Adalin; Mirfudorm.

N-(Aminocarbonyl)-2-bromo-2-ethylbutanamide

$C_7H_{13}BrN_2O_2$=237.1

CAS—77-65-6

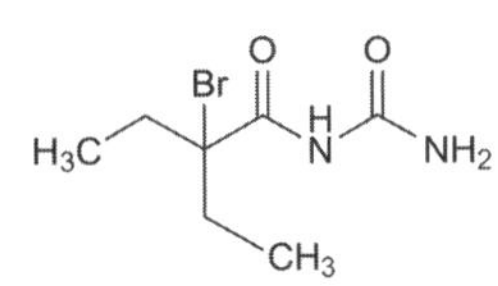

A white crystalline powder. M.p. 116° to 119°.

Soluble 1 in 3000 of water, 1 in 18 of ethanol, 1 in 3 of chloroform and 1 in 14 of ether.

Partition Coefficient. Log *P* (octanol/water), 1.5.

Colour Test. Nessler's Reagent—brown-orange.

Thin-layer Chromatography. System TB—Rf 12; system TD—Rf 53; system TE—Rf 75; system TF—Rf 55; system TAD—Rf 64; system TAE—Rf 85; system TAF—Rf 87. (Fluorescein solution, pink.)

Gas Chromatography. System GA—carbromal RI 1513, M(carbromide) RI 1215, M(OH-carbromide) RI 1340, M(desbromo-) RI 1380, carbromal-Art RI 1450 and 1470.

High Performance Liquid Chromatography. System HX—RI 410; system HY—RI 377; system HZ—Retention time(s), 3.9 min.

Ultraviolet Spectrum. No significant absorption, 230 to 360 nm.

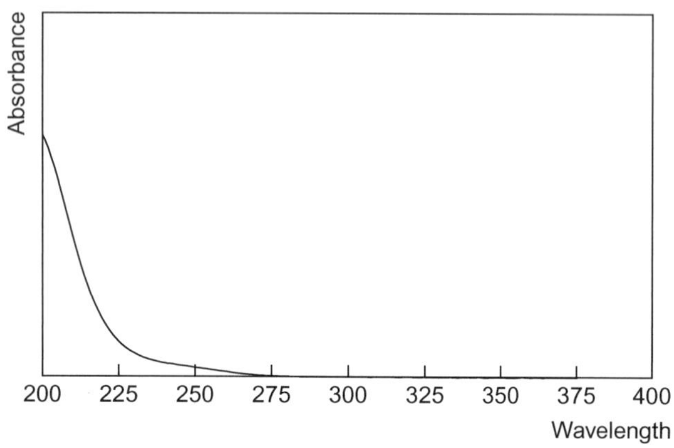

Infra-red Spectrum. Principal peaks at wavenumbers 1694, 660, 1600, 1094, 1212, 834 cm^{-1} (KBr disk).

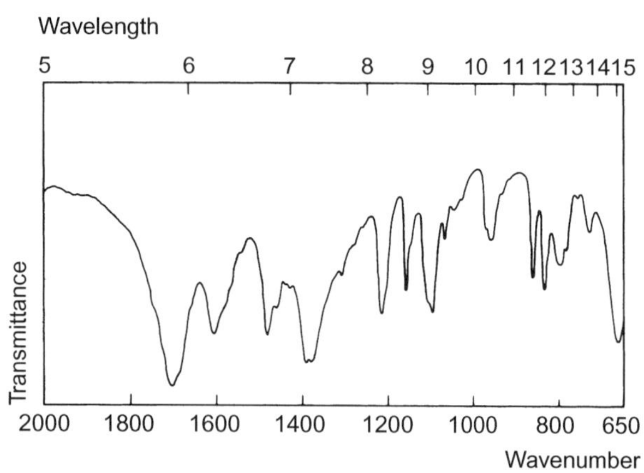

Mass Spectrum. Principal ions at m/z 44, 69, 41, 208, 210, 55, 71, 43; 2-bromo-2-ethylbutyramide 69, 43, 41, 44, 71, 167, 165, 55; 2-bromo-2-ethyl-3-hydroxybutyramide 150, 152, 165, 41, 167, 43, 44, 130; 2-ethylbutyrylurea 45, 130, 44, 71, 42, 61, 115, 55.

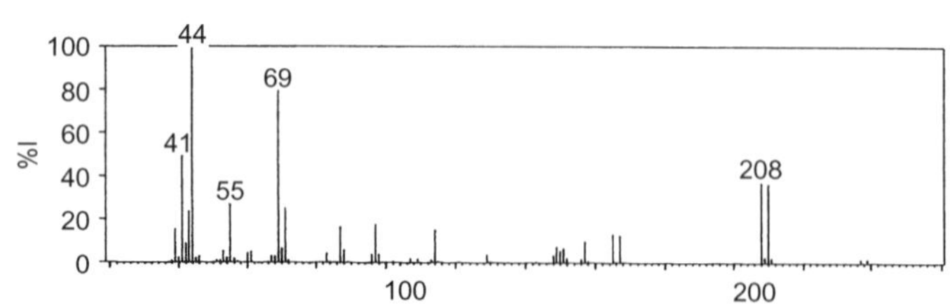

Quantification

Gas chromatography. In blood: determined as inorganic bromide, FID—J. Wells and G. Cimbura, *J. Forensic Sci.*, 1973, i, 437–440.

High performance liquid chromatography. In plasma: carbromal, 2-bromo-2-ethylbutyramide and 2-ethylbutyrylurea, limit of detection 200 μg/L for carbromal, UV detection—M. Eichelbaum *et al.*, *Arch. Toxicol.*, 1978, *41*, 187–193.

Disposition in the Body. Carbromal is readily absorbed after oral administration. The major metabolite is free bromide ion; hydrolysis to an active metabolite, 2-bromo-2-ethylbutyramide, also occurs followed by oxidation to 2-bromo-2-ethyl-3-hydroxybutyramide; other metabolites include 2-ethylbutyrylurea and 2-ethyl-2-hydroxybutyric acid. Carbromal is excreted in the urine mainly as bromide ion and partly as 2-ethyl-2-hydroxybutyric acid, with very little as unchanged drug. Peak bromide excretion is attained after about 48 h.

Therapeutic concentration

Following a single oral dose of 1 g given to 4 subjects, mean peak serum concentrations of about 6 mg/L of carbromal and 3 mg/L of 2-bromo-2-ethylbutyramide were attained in 0.5 and 4 h respectively; the total bromide concentration reached about 12 mg/L in 9 h and was still increasing. [H. W. Vohland *et al.*, *Arch. Toxicol.*, 1976, *36*, 31–42].

Toxicity. Fatalities have occurred in adults following the ingestion of 10 to 25 g but they are rare. Long-term use of carbromal may give rise to symptoms of chronic toxicity resembling bromism. Toxic effects are associated with serum-bromide concentrations of 300 to **1200** to 3200 mg/L.

In 11 fatalities attributed to carbromal overdose, the following post-mortem tissue concentrations, mg/L or μg/g (mean, *N*), were reported

	Carbromal	Bromoethylbutyramide
Blood	19.9–26.1 (23, 3)	0.2–27.2 (15, 10)
Brain	0.6–120.9 (45, 8)	23.3–118.4 (66, 11)
Kidney	0.4–13 (6, 4)	16.1–79.6 (45, 9)
Liver	1.1–2.8 (2.3, 4)	1.75–50.5 (14, 9)
Urine	0.85–47.4 (24, 5)	2.5–36.9 (23, 8)

Total bromide concentrations in the blood ranged from 145 to 1898 (mean 536) mg/L. [H. Kaferstein and G. Sticht, *Z. Rechtsmed.*, 1978, *81*, 269–283].

Post-mortem serum-carbromal concentrations of 158 and 71 mg/L were found in 2 fatalities resulting from acute intoxication. [H. Gruska *et al.*, *Arch. Toxicol.*, 1970, *26*, 149–160 and H. Gruska *et al.*, *Arch. Toxicol.*, 1971, *28*, 149–158].

Half-life. Plasma half-life, carbromal 7 to 15 h, bromide about 15 days.

Dose. 0.3 to 1 g, as a hypnotic.

Carbutamide

Antidiabetic

Synonyms. BZ-55; Glybutamide; U-6987.
Proprietary names. Diabetoplex; Dia-Tablinen; Glucidoral; Insoral; Invenol; Nadisan.
Note. Insoral is also used as a proprietary name for phenformin hydrochloride.
4-Amino-*N*-[(butylamino)carbonyl]benzenesulfonamide
$C_{11}H_{17}N_3O_3S$=271.3
CAS—339-43-5

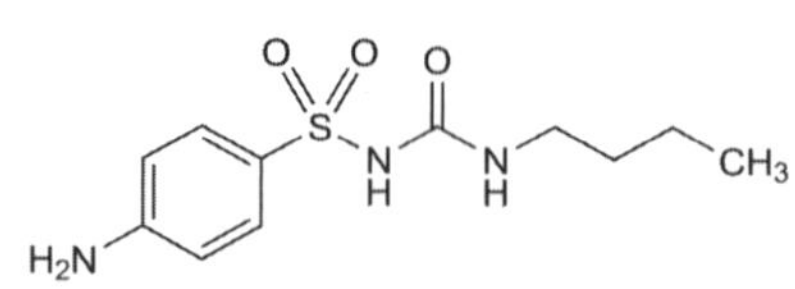

A white finely crystalline powder. M.p. 144° to 145°.
Soluble in water at pH 5 to 8. Practically insoluble in chloroform, and ether; soluble in ethanol and acetone.

Dissociation Constant. pK_a 6.0 (20°).

Partition Coefficient. Log *P* (octanol/water), 1.0.

Thin-layer Chromatography. System TA—Rf 78; system TT—Rf 90; system TU—Rf 27; system TV—Rf 07; system TAE—Rf 87.

High Performance Liquid Chromatography. System HY—RI 321; system HAA—retention time, 14.5 min.

Ultraviolet Spectrum. Aqueous acid—266 (A^1_1=149a); aqueous alkali—255 nm (A^1_1=616a).

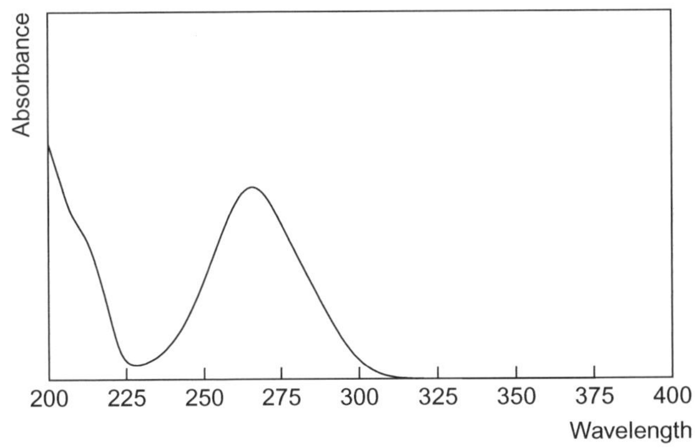

Infra-red Spectrum. Principal peaks at wavenumbers 1661, 1147, 1599, 1089, 1635, 1310 cm^{-1} (KBr disk).

Quantification
High performance liquid chromatography. In serum: UV detection—F. Saffar *et al., Chem. Pharm. Bull.*, 1982, *30*, 679–683.

Disposition in the Body. Absorbed after oral administration. It is excreted in the urine mainly as the acetyl derivative.

Therapeutic concentration
Following an oral dose of 250 mg to 5 subjects, a mean peak serum concentration of 48.8 mg/L was reported at 2.6 h. [F. Saffar *et al., Chem. Pharm. Bull.*, 1982, *30*, 679–683.]

Half-life. Plasma half-life, about 24 h.

Dose. Carbutamide has been given in doses of 0.5 to 1 g daily.

Carfenazine

Antipsychotic/Tranquilliser

Synonym. Carphenazine
1-(10-[3-[4-(2-Hydroxyethyl)-1-piperazinyl]propyl]-10*H*-phenothiazin-2-yl)-1-propanone
$C_{24}H_{31}N_3O_2S=425.6$
CAS—2622-30-2

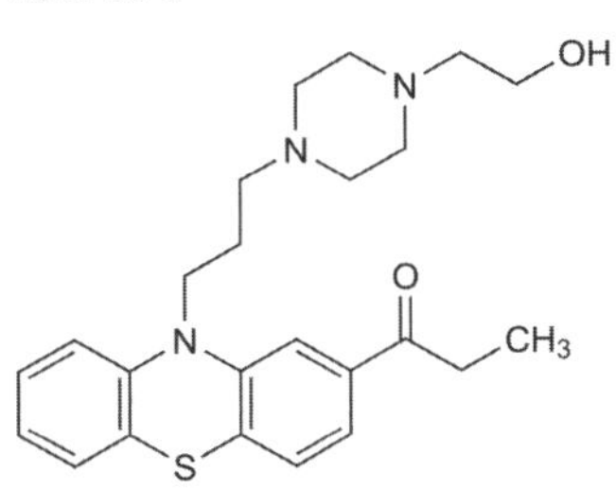

Carfenazine Maleate
Proprietary name. Proketazine
$C_{24}H_{31}N_3O_2S,2C_4H_4O_4=657.7$
CAS—2975-34-0
A fine yellow powder. M.p. 176° to 185°, with decomposition.
Soluble 1 in 600 of water and 1 in 400 of ethanol; practically insoluble in chloroform and ether.

Partition Coefficient. Log *P* (octanol/water), 3.3.

Colour Tests. Formaldehyde–Sulfuric Acid—blue; Forrest Reagent—red; FPN Reagent—red-orange; Liebermann's Test—red-brown; Mandelin's Test—red-violet; Marquis Test—orange→red-violet.

Thin-layer Chromatography. System TA—Rf 54; system TB—Rf 05; system TC—Rf 27; system TE—Rf 39; system TL—Rf 07; system TAE—Rf 39; system TAJ—Rf 08; system TAK—Rf 00; system TAL—Rf 51. (Acidified iodoplatinate solution, positive.)

Gas Chromatography. System GA—RI 3590.

High Performance Liquid Chromatography. System HA—*k* 1.7; system HX—RI 419.

Ultraviolet Spectrum. Aqueous acid—243 ($A_1^1=606a$), 277 nm. No alkaline shift.

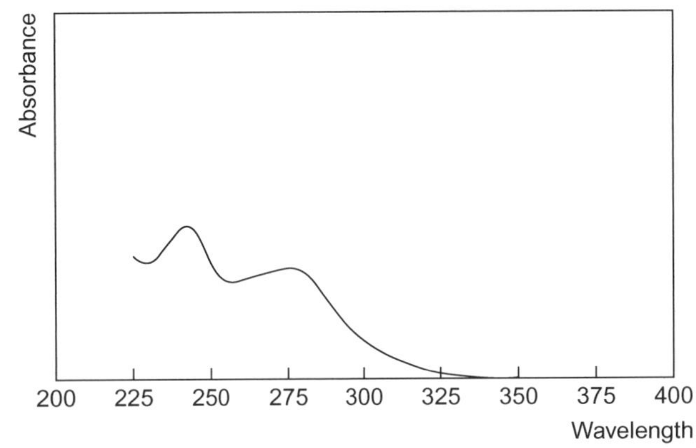

Infra-red Spectrum. Principal peaks at wavenumbers 1585, 1557, 1666, 1204, 751, 1298 cm^{-1} (KBr disk).

Mass Spectrum. Principal ions at *m/z* 268, 143, 425, 70, 269, 42, 394, 157.

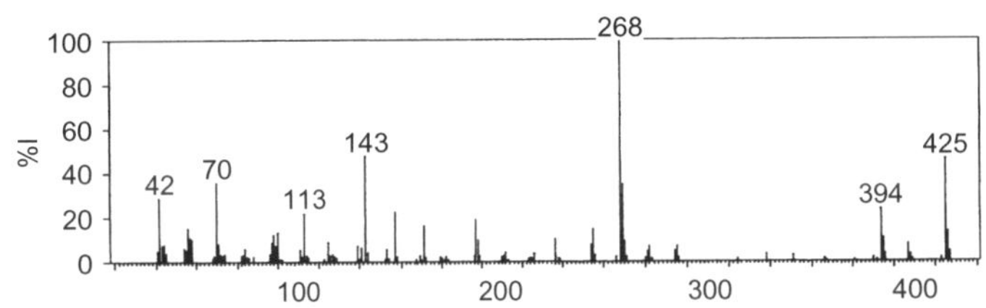

Dose. 75 to 400 mg of carfenazine maleate daily.

Carisoprodol

Muscle Relaxant

Synonyms. Carisoprodate; Carisoprodolum; Isobamate; *N*-Isopropylmeprobamate.
Proprietary names. Artifar; Caridolin; Carisoma; Chinchen; Dolaren; Flexartal; Mio Relax; Mioxom; Muslax; Myolax; Neotica; Rela; Rotalin; Sanoma; Scutamil-C; Soma; Somadril; Somalgit. It is also an ingredient of Flectomas, Flexidone, Lagaflex, Relaxibys, Sodol Compound, Soma Compound, Teknadone.
Note. The name Soma has also been applied to a hallucinogenic fungus.
2-[[(Aminocarbonyl)oxy]methyl]-2-methylpentyl (1-methylethyl)carbamate
$C_{12}H_{24}N_2O_4=260.3$
CAS—78-44-4

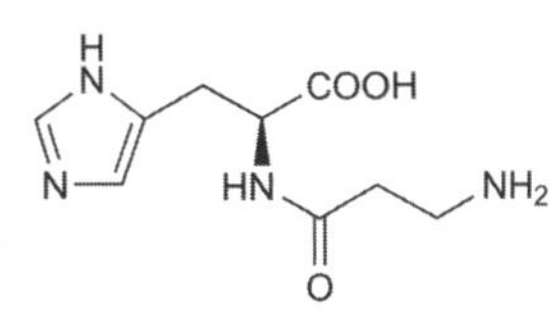

A white crystalline powder. M.p. 92° to 93°.
Soluble in water (30 mg/100 mL at 25°, 140 mg/100 mL at 50°); soluble in most common organic solvents; practically insoluble in vegetable oils. Stable in dilute acids and alkalis.

Partition Coefficient. Log *P* (octanol/water), 2.36.

Thin-layer Chromatography. System TB—Rf 4; system TD—Rf 36; system TE—Rf 75; system TF—Rf 53; system TAD—Rf 59; system TAE—Rf 85; system TAF—Rf 79. (Furfuraldehyde reagent, positive.)

Gas Chromatography. System GA—carisoprodol RI 1830, meprobamate RI 1785.

Ultraviolet Spectrum. No significant absorption, 230 to 360 nm.

Infra-red Spectrum. Principal peaks at wavenumbers 1695, 1527, 1075, 1246, 1101, 1319 cm^{-1} (Nujol mull).

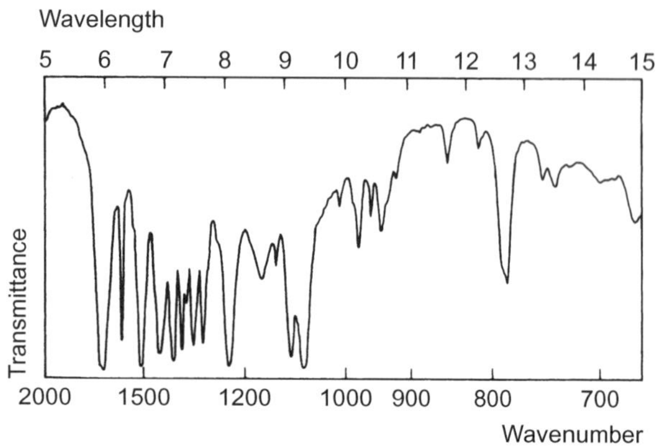

Mass Spectrum. Principal ions at *m/z* 55, 57, 43, 97, 41, 56, 158, 44; meprobamate 83, 84, 55, 56, 43, 71, 41, 62 (no peaks above 160).

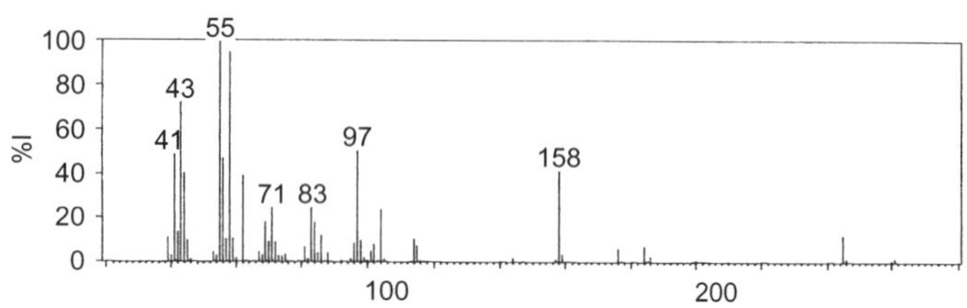

Quantification

Gas chromatography. In serum or urine: carisoprodol and meprobamate, FID—H. R. Adams *et al., J. Forensic Sci.*, 1975, *20*, 200–202. In biological fluids and tissues—R. Maes *et al., Eur. J. Toxicol.*, 1970, *3*, 140–143. In plasma: carisoprodol and meprobamate, FID—P. Kintz *et al., J. Anal. Toxicol.*, 1988, *12*, 73–74.

Disposition in the Body. Absorbed after oral administration. It is metabolised principally to meprobamate, which is active, and to hydroxymeprobamate and their glucuronide conjugates. Less than 1% of a dose is excreted in the urine as unchanged drug in 24 h and about 5% is excreted as meprobamate in the same period. It is distributed in substantial amounts into breast milk.

Therapeutic concentration

Following administration of a 700 mg oral dose of carisoprodol to 9 healthy adults, the mean peak plasma carisoprodol concentration was 3.5 mg/L at 0.8 h and the mean peak meprobamate concentration was 4.0 mg/L at 3.7 h. [H. Olsen *et al., Ther. Drug Monit.*, 1994, *16*, 337–340.]

Toxicity

A 39-year-old man ingested 35 g carisoprodol. He developed agitation, tachycardia, myoclonus, and coma. The blood carisoprodol concentration was 71 mg/L, the meprobamate was 26 mg/L. Carisoprodol overdose is thought to induce simple central nervous system depression. [B. A. Roth *et al., J. Toxicol. Clin. Toxicol*, 1998, *36*, 609–612.]

In 3 cases involving overdose with carisoprodol, the following tissue concentrations were reported in the respective cases: heart blood 39.4, 14.0, and 8.1 mg/L, femoral blood 39.3, 6.5, and 7.9 mg/L, urine 12.6, –, and –, vitreous humour 18.9, 8.7, and 8.1 mg/L. The concentrations of meprobamate in the respective cases were: 40.1, 18.9, and 20.9 mg/L, femoral blood 51.9, 20.5, and 34.3 mg/L, urine 61.0, –, and –, vitreous humour 45.9, 50.2, and 102.0 mg/L. Verapamil was also detected in case 2 and propoxyphene was detected in case 3 in addition to carisoprodol. [R. C. Backer *et al., J. Anal. Toxicol.*, 1990, *14*, 332–334.]

In 21 cases of driving impairment where carisoprodol was the sole drug involved, it was found that most overt symptoms of intoxication were noted when the combined blood concentration of carisoprodol and meprobamate was over 10 mg/L. [B. K. Logan *et al., J. Forensic Sci.*, 2000, *45*, 619–623.]

The following concentrations were reported 4.5 h after the ingestion of 3.5 g by a young child: blood, carisoprodol 36.4 mg/L, meprobamate 15 mg/L; urine, carisoprodol 24.4 mg/L, meprobamate 166.4 mg/L; the child's condition deteriorated and death occurred within 36 h. [H.R. Adams *et al., J. Forensic Sci.*, 1975, *20*, 200–202.]

Half-life. Reported as 0.9 to 2.4 h.

Protein binding. Approx. 58%.

Dose. Usual dose is 350 mg given 3 to 4 times daily by mouth. Half the usual dose or less is recommended in elderly patients.

Carmustine

Antineoplastic

Synonym. BCNU

Proprietary names. Becenun; BiCNU; Carmubris; Gliadel; Nitrourean; Nitrumon.

N,N′-Bis(2-chloroethyl)-*N*-nitrosourea

$C_5H_9Cl_2N_3O_2$=214.0

CAS—154-93-8

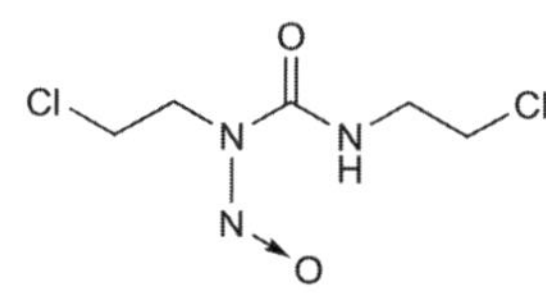

A yellowish granular powder that melts to an oily liquid. M.p. 31°, with decomposition. It is slightly soluble in water; freely soluble in ethanol; very soluble in dichloromethane and ether.

Partition Coefficient. Log *P* (octanol/water), 1.53.

Gas Chromatography. Column: SPB1 fused-silica capillary (60 m × 0.25 mm i.d., 0.25 µm coating) with pre-column (1 m). Column temperature: 50°, 5 min; increased to 100° at 10°/min; increased to 105.5° at 0.1°/min. Detection: ^{63}Ni electron capture. Retention time: 30 min. [S. J. Hassenbusch *et al., J. Pharm. Sci.*, 1995, *84(7)*, 840–842].

High Performance Liquid Chromatography. Column: ODS RP (Ultrasphere, 250 × 4.6 mm i.d., 5 µm) with a Co:Pell ODS guard column (70 × 2 mm, 30 to 38 µm). Mobile phase: 35% acetonitrile:0.1% glacial acetic acid in water, 1.2 mL/min flow rate. UV detection (λ=230 nm). Retention time: 13.8 min. [R. L. Yeager *et al., J. Chromatogr.*, 1984, *305*; Biomed. Appl., *30*, 496–501].

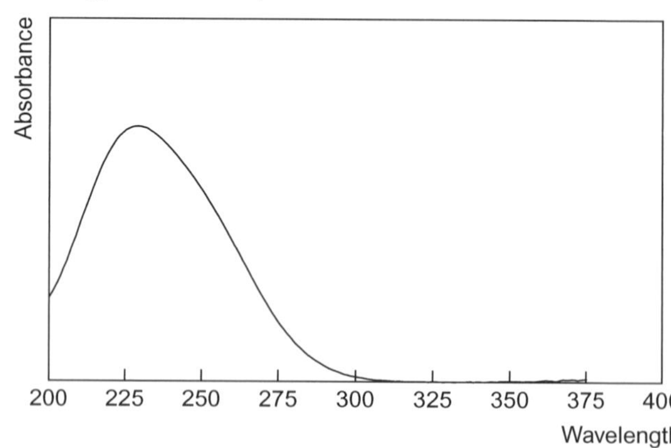

Mass Spectrum. Principal ions at *m/z* 56, 62, 42, 77, 69, 49, 105, 64.

Quantification

Gas chromatography. In brain tissue: limit of detection 0.02 µg, ECD—S. J. Hassenbusch *et al., J. Pharm. Sci.*, 1995, *84(7)*, 840–842.

High performance liquid chromatography. In plasma: limit of detection 50 µg/L, UV detection (λ=230 nm)—R. L. Yeager *et al., J. Chromatogr.*, 1984, *305*; *Biomed. Appl.*, *30*, 496–501.

Disposition in the Body. Rapidly metabolised after intravenous administration. Readily crosses the blood–brain barrier. Alkylates DNA/RNA and has also been shown to inhibit several enzymes by carbamoylation of amino acids in proteins. Metabolites have a longer half-life and are presumed to be responsible for its activity. Some enterohepatic circulation is believed to occur. Excreted primarily in the urine; about 10% is excreted as carbon dioxide via the lungs. Very small amounts (1%) are detected in the faeces.

Therapeutic concentration

10 patients with advanced neoplasms were being treated with a high-dose combination of chemotherapy, cyclophosphamide, cisplatin and carmustine. Each patient received 300 to 750 mg/m^2 carmustine over a 2 h infusion period, but this was increased to 1 g/m^2 for maximum results. Peak plasma concentrations reached 7.8 μg/L at the end of the infusion for the corrected dose. [W. D. Henner *et al.*, *Cancer Treat. Rep.*, 1986, *70(7)*, 877–880].

Toxicity. Hypotension was the most prominent feature with high dose carmustine administration.

Half-life. Plasma half-life, 22 min.

Volume of distribution. 3.25 L/kg; 5.1 L/kg (patients with advanced neoplasms).

Clearance. Plasma clearance, 56 mL/min/kg; 77.6 mL/min/kg (patients with advanced neoplasms).

Protein binding. 77%.

Dose. 150 to 200 mg/m^2 intravenously as a single dose or divided into two doses given on successive days. Implants are also available (containing 7.7 mg/implant).

Carphedon

Psychostimulant/Treatment of Amnesia

Synonyms. BRN-5030440; 4-Phenylpiracetam.

(2-Oxo-4-phenylpyrrolidine)acetamide

$C_{12}H_{14}N_2O_2$=218.3

CAS—77472-70-9

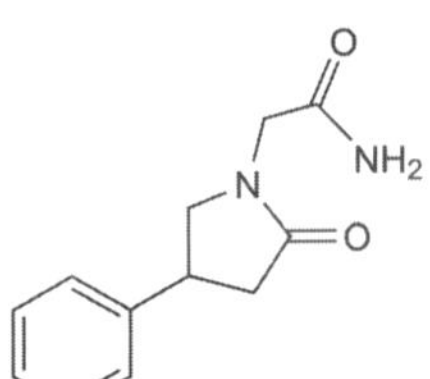

Gas Chromatography. Column: DB-17 (30 m × 0.25 mm i.d., 0.25 μm film thickness). Column temperature: 100° to 280° at 25°/min, held 280° for 8 min. Carrier gas: helium, flow rate 0.9 mL/min. Detection: nitrogen–phosphorous. Retention time: 11.5 min. [S. Kim *et al.*, *Analyst*, 1999, *124*, 1559–1562.]

Mass Spectrum. Principal ions at *m/z* 174, 160, 104, 145, 117, 77, 91, 129.

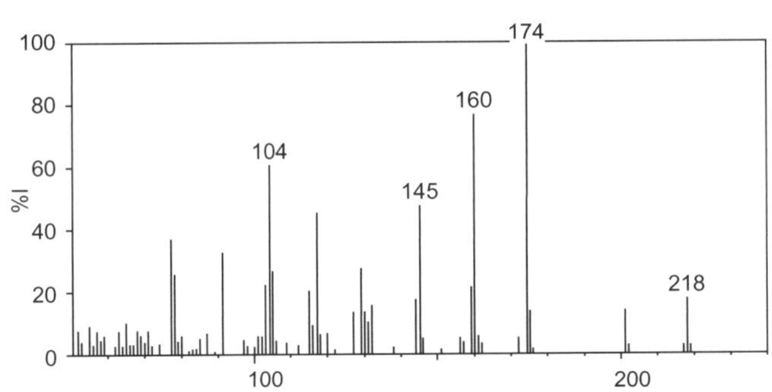

Quantification

Gas chromatography. In urine: limit of detection 0.01 mg/L, NPD—S. Kim *et al.*, *Analyst*, 1999, *124*, 1559–1562.

Disposition in the Body

Therapeutic concentration

A healthy man was administered with a 0.38 mg/kg dose of carphedon. A concentration of 6.34 mg/L was detected in urine after 18 h. [S. Kim *et al.*, *Analyst*, 1999, *124*, 1559–1562.]

Carteolol

Beta-blocker

5-[3-[(1,1-Dimethylethyl)amino]-2-hydroxypropoxy]-3,4-dihydro-2(1*H*)-quinolinone

$C_{16}H_{24}N_2O_3$=292.4

CAS—51781-06-7

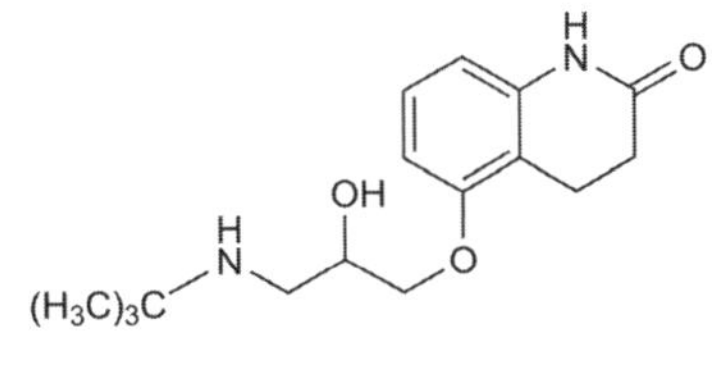

Carteolol Hydrochloride

Synonyms. Abbott-43326, OPC-1085.

Proprietary names. Arteolol; Arteoptic; Carteol; Cartrol; Dispersa; Elebloc; Endak; Mikelan; Ocupress; Teoptic.

$C_{16}H_{24}N_2O_3$,HCl =328.8

CAS—51781-21-6

White crystals or a white crystalline powder., M.p. 278°. It is soluble in water; very slightly soluble in ethanol and glacial acetic acid; sparingly soluble in methanol; practically insoluble in ether.

Dissociation Constant. pK_a 9.74.

Partition Coefficient. Log *P* (octanol/water), 1.42.

Thin-layer Chromatography. System TE—Rf 33; system TAE—Rf 14.

Gas Chromatography. System GA—RI 2588 (carteolol); RI 2690 (Art).

Column: fused-silica capillary coated with dimethylpolysiloxane (15 m × 0.25 mm i.d., 0.25 μm film thickness). Column temperature: 50°, held 0.7 min after injection, 55°/min to 320°, held 3 min. Carrier gas: helium. MS detection, SIM. Retention time: PFB amide–DMES ether derivative, 6.7 min. [M. Nagasawa *et al.*, *J. Chromatogr.*, 1995, *673(2); Biomed. Appl.*, 294–298].

Column: 5% phenyl methyl silicone RTx–5 fused-silica capillary (30 m × 0.25 mm). Column temperature: 110°, held 1 min; increased to 170° at 20°/min; increased to 225° at 7°/min; 290° at 24°/min, held 10 min. Carrier gas: helium. MS detection. Retention time (relative to isoproterenol, internal standard): 1.20. [G. D. Branum *et al.*, *J. Anal. Toxicol.*, 1998, *22*, 135–141].

High Performance Liquid Chromatography. System HAA—retention time 5.9 min.

Ultraviolet Spectrum. Aqueous acid (pH 4)—219, 252, 288 nm.

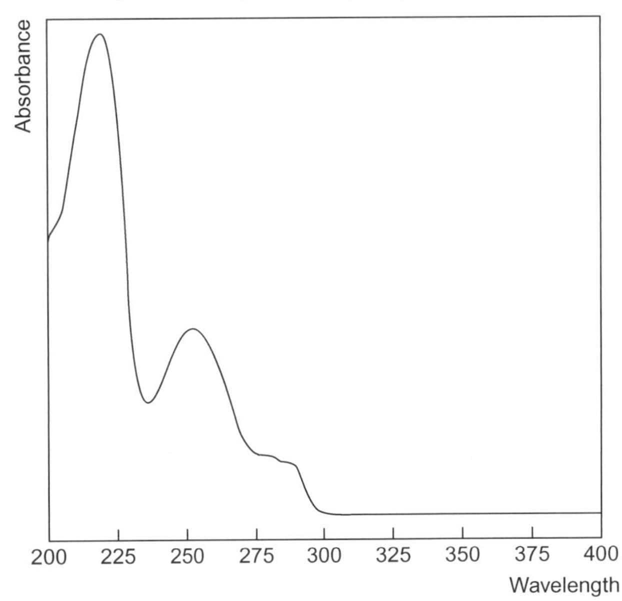

Mass Spectrum. Principal ions at *m/z* 86, 57, 277, 70, 292, 87, 114, 60

(carteolol); *m/z* 301, 138, 41, 70, 96, 84, 316, 153 (carteolol methaneboronate).

Quantification

Gas chromatography–mass spectrometry. In plasma: quantification limit is <0.03 µg/L—M. Nagasawa *et al.*, *J. Chromatogr.* 1995, *673(2); Biomed. Appl.*, 294–298.

High performance liquid chromatography. In plasma or urine: 8-hydroxycarteolol, limit of detection 5 µg/L and 25 µg/L, respectively, electrochemical detection—S.-Y. Chu, *J. Pharm. Sci.*, 1978, *67*, 1623–1625. In plasma or urine: limit of detection 5 µg/L and 100 µg/L, respectively, UV detection—T. Ishizaki *et al.*, *Eur. J. Clin. Pharmacol.*, 1983, *25*, 95–101.

Disposition in the Body. Carteolol is well absorbed after oral administration with peak plasma concentrations being reached within 1 to 3 h. It has low lipid solubility. It is distributed into breast milk. Carteolol undergoes minimal hepatic metabolism to form the active metabolite, 8-hydroxycarteolol and glucuronic acid conjugates of carteolol and 8-hydroxycarteolol. The major route of elimination is renal with 50 to 70% being excreted unchanged in urine.

Bioavailability. Absolute bioavailability, 85%.

Half-life. Plasma, carteolol, 5 to 6 h; 8-hydroxycarteolol, 8 to 12 h.

Volume of distribution. 4 L/kg.

Clearance. Plasma clearance, 10 mL/min/kg.

Protein binding. In plasma, 20 to 30%.

Dose. Usually 2.5 or 5 mg of carteolol hydrochloride daily.

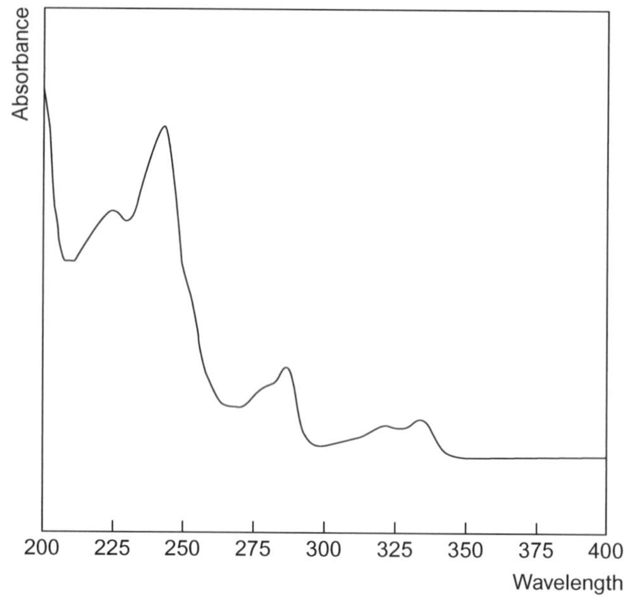

Mass Spectrum. Principal ions at *m/z* 392, 73, 183, 154, 129, 222, 451, 309 (TMSTFA derivative).

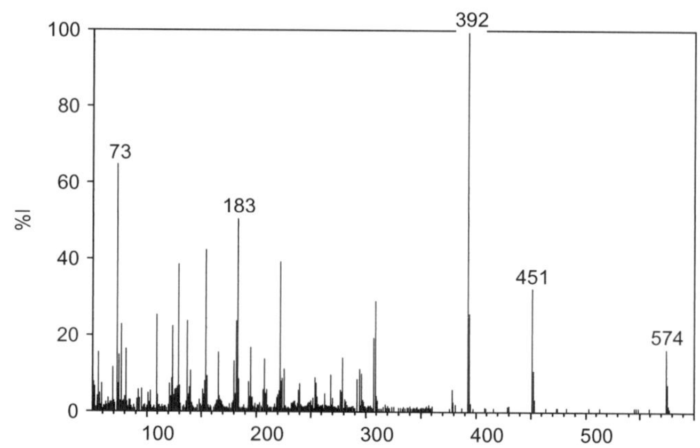

Quantification

High performance liquid chromatography. In serum: limit of detection 0.1 µg/L, fluorescence detection (λ_{ex}=240 nm, λ_{em}=340 nm)—F. Varin *et al.*, *J. Pharm. Sci.*, 1986, *75*, 1195–1197. In plasma: limit of detection 1.55 µg/L, fluorescence detection—M. Fujimaki *et al.*, *J. Pharm. Sci.*, 1990, *79*, 568–572. In plasma: limit of detection 1.1 µg/L (*S*(−)-enantiomer), 0.6 µg/L (*R*(+)-enantiomer), fluorescence detection (λ_{ex}=285 nm, λ_{em}=360 nm)—E. J. Eisenberg *et al.*, *J. Chromatogr.*, 1989, *493*; *Biomed. Appl.*, *85*, 105–115. In plasma or urine: limit of detection 0.38 µg/L and 0.82 µg/L, respectively, fluorescence detection (λ_{ex}=285 nm, λ_{em}=340 nm)—K. Reiff, *J. Chromatogr.*, 1987, *413*; *Biomed. Appl.*, *57*, 355–362. In plasma: limit of quantification 1 µg/L for the *S*(−)-enantiomer and 2 µg/L for the *R*(+)-enantiomer—G. Neugebauer *et al.*, *Eur. J. Clin. Pharmacol.*, 1990, *38*, S108–S111.

Disposition in the Body. Carvedilol is rapidly and well absorbed after oral administration, but is subject to considerable first-pass metabolism in the liver. The rate of absorption is impaired by the co-administration with food but the bioavailability is not affected. The drug is widely distributed and extensively metabolised, primarily by aromatic ring oxidation and glucuronidation. The oxidative metabolites undergo further metabolism by glucuronidation and sulfation. The metabolites are excreted mainly via bile into faeces. Approximately 16% of a dose is detected in urine with less than 2% as the unchanged drug. Some of the metabolites have beta-blocking and vasodilating activity; one metabolite has greater beta-blocking activity than carvedilol but all have weaker vasodilating effects than carvedilol. The *o*-demethyl-*p*-hydroxyl and *m*-hydroxyl metabolites possess beta-blocking activity. Its metabolism is stereoselective and plasma concentrations of *R*(+)-carvedilol are about 2 to 3 times higher than *S*(−)-carvedilol. The

Carvedilol

Beta-blocker

Synonyms. BM-14190; DQ-2466.
Proprietary names. Carvipress; Dilatrend; Dimitone; Eucardic; Kredex; Querto.
1-(9*H*-Carbazol-4-yloxy)-3-[[2-(2-methoxyphenoxy)ethyl]amino]-2-propanol
$C_{24}H_{26}N_2O_4$=406.5
CAS—72956-09-3

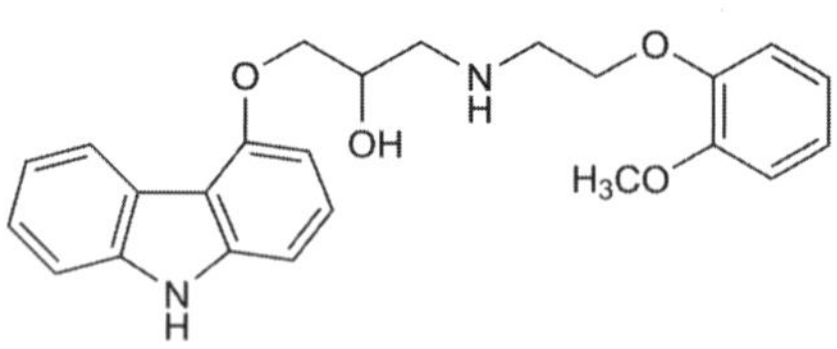

A white to off-white powder. M.p. 114° to 115°. It is practically insoluble in water; freely soluble in dimethyl sulfoxide; soluble in methylene chloride and in methanol; sparingly soluble in ethanol and in isopropyl alcohol; slightly soluble in ethyl ether.

Partition Coefficient. Log *P* (octanol/water), 4.19.

High Performance Liquid Chromatography. System HZ—retention time carvedilol, 5.2 min; desmethylcarvedilol, 4.4 min.

Column: Spherisorb octyl (125 × 5 mm i.d., 5 µm). Mobile phase: acetonitrile:water (45:55) containing dibutylamine (5 mM), 2 mL/min flow rate. Fluorescence detection (λ_{ex}=40 nm, λ_{em}=340 nm). Retention time: 3.8 min. [F. Varin *et al.*, *J. Pharm. Sci.*, 1986, *75(12)*, 1195–1197].

Ultraviolet Spectrum. Aqueous acid (2.0 M HCl)—241, 285, 320, 332 nm; (methanol)—224, 243, 286, 319, 332 nm.

principal enzymes involved are CYP2D6 and CYP2C9. The metabolism of carvedilol is subject to genetic polymorphism with poor metabolisers of debrisoquine having plasma-*R*(+)-carvedilol concentrations 2- to 3-fold higher than extensive metabolisers. It is not significantly cleared by haemodialysis. No accumulation of the drug has been observed.

Therapeutic concentration. In plasma, concentrations are linearly related to the administered dose.

The mean maximum plasma concentration after a 20 mg dose, administered by mouth after an overnight fast, to 5 Japanese healthy males was 0.025 (range, 0.0065 to 0.044) mg/L for the (*R*)-enantiomer and 0.0098 (0.0023 to 0.0187) mg/L, (*S*)-enantiomer. These concentrations were observed 0.5 to 1.0 h after administration. [M. Fujimaki *et al.*, *J. Pharm. Sci.*, 1990, *79*, 568–572].

Following oral administration of a 50 mg tablet to 20 healthy males, aged between 19 and 45 years, maximum plasma concentrations ranged from 34 to 130 mg/L (mean 66 mg/L) after 0.65 to 2.25 h (mean 1.20 h). Peak concentrations of 128 mg/L (range, 55 to 237 mg/L), 0.66 (range, 0.24 to 1.29 h after administration were observed, however, for a 50 mg suspension. Following administration of a 25 mg tablet, maximum plasma concentrations were 5 to 99 mg/L (mean 21 mg/L) seen after 1.46 h (range, 0.68 to 3.10 h). After intravenous administration of 12.5 mg over a 1-h period, the peak concentration was 173 mg/L (range, 109 to 234) by the end of infusion. [E. von Möllendorff *et al.*, *Eur. J. Clin. Pharmacol.*, 1987, *33*, 511–513].

Bioavailability. Absolute bioavailability, 25 to 35%; *S*(−)-enantiomer, 15%; *R*(+)-enatiomer, 31%.

Half-life. Plasma, 4 to 7 h (values outside this range have also been noted).

Volume of distribution. 1.5 to 2.0 L/kg.

Clearance. Plasma clearance, 0.52 L/h/kg.

Protein binding. In plasma, more than 98% with *R*(+)-enantiomer being more tightly bound.

Note. For reviews of carvedilol, see D. McTavish *et al.*, *Drugs*, 1993, *45*, 232–258 and T. Morgan, *Clin. Pharmacokinet.*, 1994, *26*, 335–346.

Dose. It is recommended that all receive 12.5 mg for the first 2 days and then increase if necessary up to 50 mg daily.

Cathine

Anorectic

Synonyms. Katine; (+)-Norpseudoephedrine; Pseudonorephedrine.
(αS)-α-[(1*S*)-1-Aminoethyl]benzenemethanol
$C_9H_{13}NO = 151.2$
CAS—492-39-7; 36393-56-3

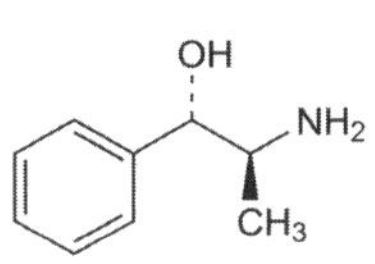

An alkaloid obtained from catha, the fresh or dried leaves of *Catha edulis* (Celastraceae). Catha (also known as Abyssinian, African, or Arabian Tea; Kat; Kath; Khat; Miraa) is used in northern and eastern Africa as a stimulant, the leaves being either chewed or used as an infusion.
Crystals. M.p. 77° to 78°.
Soluble in ethanol, chloroform, ether, and dilute acids.

Cathine Hydrochloride

Proprietary names. Adiposetten N; Amorphan Depot; Fasupond; Minusin.
$C_9H_{13}NO,HCl = 187.7$
CAS—2153-98-2
Crystals. M.p. 180° to 181°.
Soluble in water.

Dissociation Constant. pK_a 9.4 (20°).

Partition Coefficient. Log *P* (octanol/water), 0.8.

Thin-layer Chromatography. System TA—Rf 42; system TB—Rf 25; system TC—Rf 05. (Acidified potassium permanganate solution, positive.)

Gas Chromatography. System GA—RI 1360; system GB—RI 1352; system GC—RI 1383; system GAN—retention time 4.06 min.

High Performance Liquid Chromatography. System HA—*k* 1.0; system HB—*k* 4.39; system HC—*k* 0.83.

Ultraviolet Spectrum. Aqueous acid—252, 258 ($A_1^1 = 10a$), 263 nm. No alkaline shift.

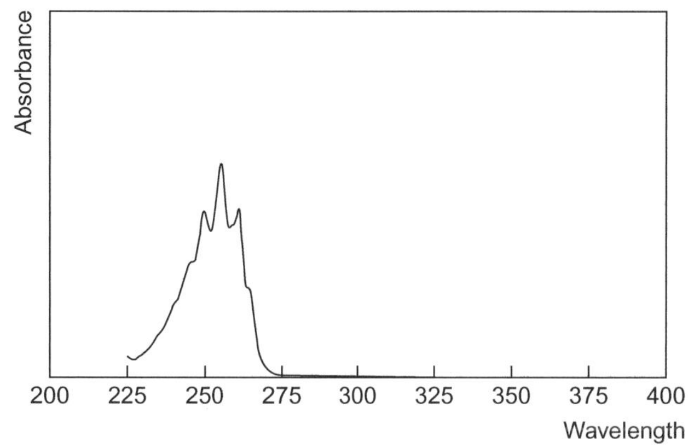

Infra-red Spectrum. Principal peaks at wavenumbers 1045, 695, 754, 704, 1091, 976 cm^{-1} (KBr disk).

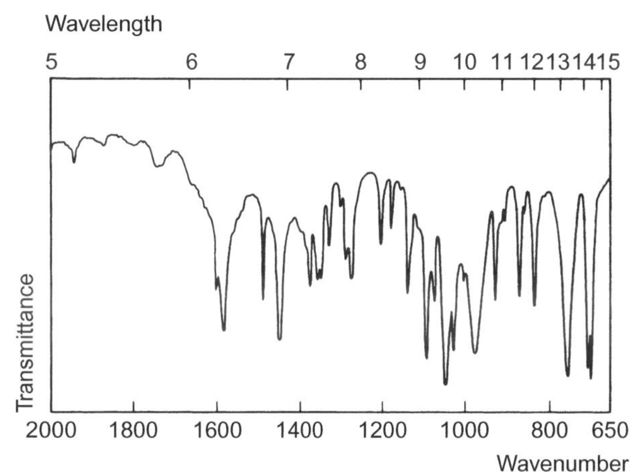

Mass Spectrum. Principal ions at *m/z* 44, 57, 43, 40, 55, 41, 79, 77.

Disposition in the Body. About 40% of an ingested dose is excreted unchanged in the urine in 6 h. Cathine is a metabolite of pseudoephedrine.

Therapeutic concentration
Following a single oral dose of 60 mg to 6 subjects, a mean peak plasma concentration of 0.2 mg/L was attained in 1.3 h; cathine could not be detected in the plasma after 24 h. [F. Frosch, *Arzneimittelforschung*, 1977, *27*, 665–668.]

Toxicity. Addiction to catha has been reported.

Half-life. Plasma half-life, about 3 h.

Dose. Cathine hydrochloride has been given in doses of 20 to 60 mg daily.

Cefaclor

Antibacterial

Proprietary names. Alfatil; Cec; Ceclor; Ceclorbeta; Cefabiocin; Cefallone; Cefa-Wolff; Cef-diolan; Distaclor; Infectocef; Keflor; Kefolor; Keftid; Kloclor; Panacef; Panoral; Sigacefal; Vercef.
(6*R*,7*R*)-7-[[(2*R*)-Aminophenylacetyl]amino]-3-chloro-8-oxo-5-thia-1-azabicyclo[4.2.0]oct-2-ene-2-carboxylic acid monohydrate
$C_{15}H_{14}ClN_3O_4S,H_2O = 385.8$
CAS—53994-73-3 (anhydrous); 70356-03-5 (monohydrate)

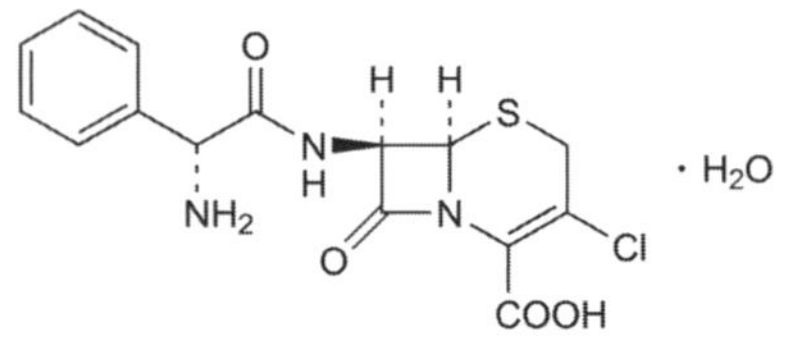

A white to off-white, or slightly yellow, crystalline powder. It is soluble to slightly soluble in water (10 g/L); practically insoluble in benzene, chloroform, dichloromethane, and methanol (all <0.5 g/L).

Dissociation Constant. pK_a 1.5, 7.2 (water); 4.33, 7.34 (66% DMF).

Partition Coefficient. Log *P* (octanol/water), 0.35.

Thin-layer Chromatography. System TE—Rf 0; system TF—Rf 0.

High Performance Liquid Chromatography. System HX—RI 268.

Ultraviolet Spectrum. Aqueous acid (0.1 M hydrochloric acid)—265 nm.

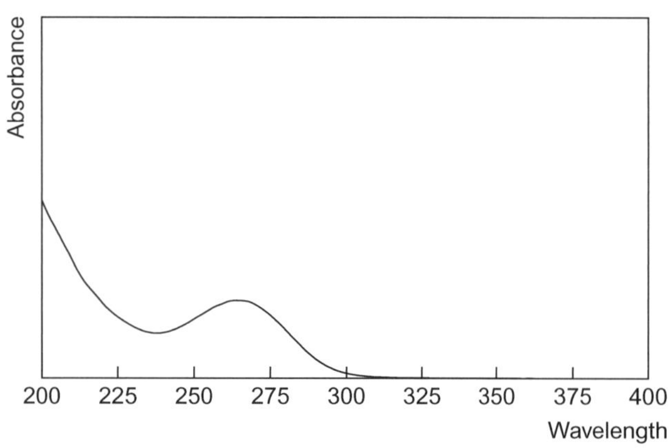

Infra-red Spectrum. Principal peaks at wavenumbers 1775, 1693, 1600, 1365, 1500, 1560 cm^{-1}.

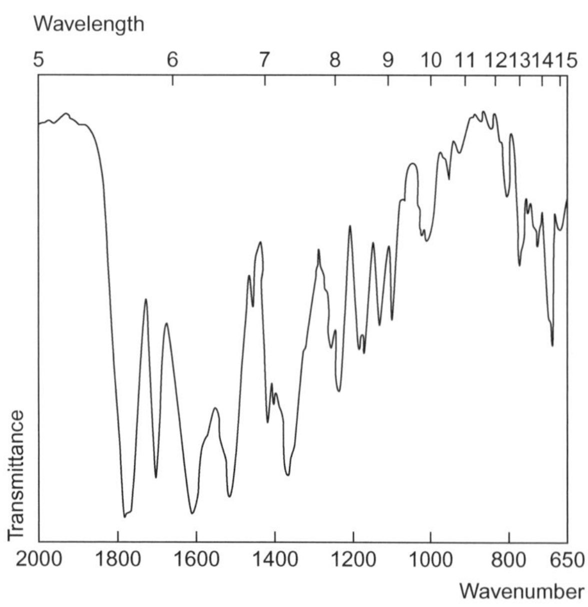

Quantification

High performance liquid chromatography. In serum: limit of detection 1 mg/L, UV detection (λ=240 nm)—J. A. McAteer *et al.*, *Clin. Chem.*, 1987, *33*, 1788–1790. In serum: limit of detection about 1 mg/L, UV detection—K. Lindgren, *J. Chromatogr.*, 1987, *413*; *Biomed. Appl.*, *57*, 351–354. In plasma, serum or urine: limit of detection 0.5 mg/L, UV detection (λ=265 nm)—P. M. Kovach and R. J. Lantz, *J. Chromatogr.*, 1991, *567*; *Biomed. Appl.*, *105*, 129–139. In plasma: limit of detection 0.5 mg/L. UV detection (λ=254 nm)—S. A. Signs *et al.*, *Antimicrob. Agents Chemother.*, 1984, *26(5)*, 652–655.

Disposition in the Body. Cefaclor is well absorbed after oral administration; food may delay absorption but the total amount absorbed is unchanged. The peak concentration, however, with food is 50 to 75% of that observed for the drug when administered in the fasting state. It is widely distributed in the body and crosses the placenta and low concentrations appear in breast milk. Cefaclor is rapidly excreted by the kidneys; up to 85% of a dose appears unchanged in urine within 8 h, with the greater proportion appearing in the first 2 h. Probenecid delays excretion. Some cefaclor is removed by haemodialysis.

Therapeutic concentration. The serum therapeutic concentration range is 13 to 35 mg/L for an oral dose and up to 900 mg/L for an intravenous dose.

Oral doses of 250, 500 and 1000 mg administered to fasting individuals, produce peak plasma concentrations of about 7, 13 and 23 mg/L, respectively at 0.5 to 1 h. [Data as supplied by Eli Lilly & Company Ltd.]

Half-life. Plasma half-life, 0.5 to 1 h; 2.3 to 2.8 h in patients with the complete absence of renal function. Serum, 0.6 to 0.9 h; slightly prolonged in patients with renal impairment.

Protein binding. In plasma, 25%.

Dose. Adults: usually 250 to 500 mg of anhydrous cefaclor every 8 h. Total daily dose should not exceed 4 g. Children: usual recommended daily dose is 20 mg/kg every 8 h.

Cefalexin

Antibiotic

Synonym. Cephalexin
Proprietary names. Ceporex; Ceporexin(e); Keflex; Keforal; Oracef.
(6*R*,7*R*)-7-[[(2*R*)-Aminophenylacetyl]amino]-3-methyl-8-oxo-5-thia-1-azabicyclo[4.2.0]oct-2-ene-2-carboxylic acid monohydrate
$C_{16}H_{17}N_3O_4S,H_2O$=365.4
CAS—15686-71-2 (anhydrous); 23325-78-2 (monohydrate)

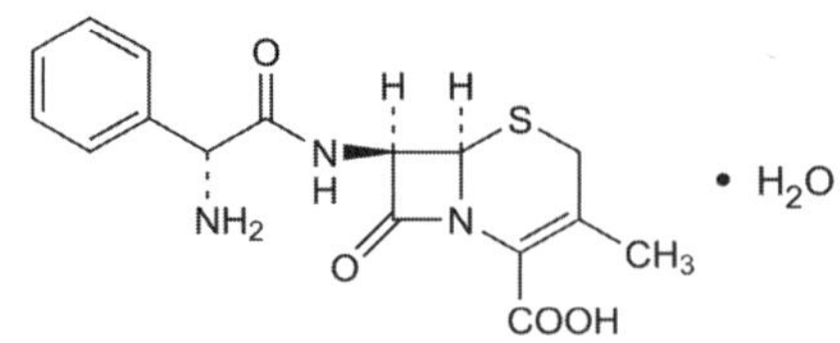

A white to cream-coloured, slightly hygroscopic, crystalline powder. Soluble 1 in 100 of water and 1 in 30 of 0.2% hydrochloric acid; practically insoluble in ethanol, chloroform, and ether; soluble in solutions of dilute alkalis.

Dissociation Constant. pK_a 2.5, 5.2, 7.3.

Partition Coefficient. Log *P* (octanol/water), 0.6.

High Performance Liquid Chromatography. System HAA—retention time, 3.9 min (peak 1).

Ultraviolet Spectrum. Aqueous acid—258; water—260 nm (A_1^1=232a).

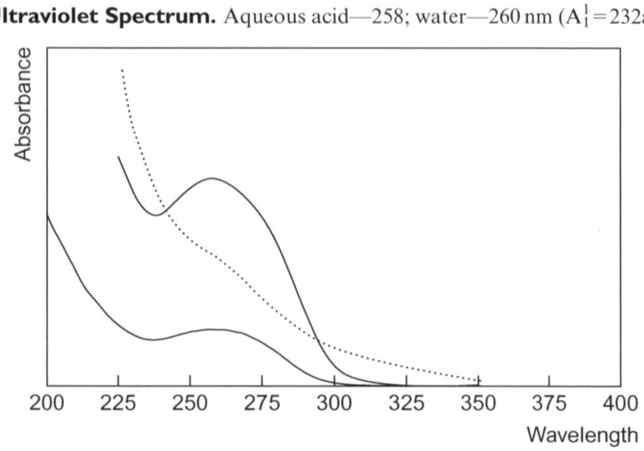

Infra-red Spectrum. Principal peaks at wavenumbers 1754, 1582, 1681, 1271, 695, 1186 cm^{-1} (KBr disk).

Quantification

High performance liquid chromatography. Review of methods for the analysis of antibiotics in biological fluids—I. Nilsson-Ehle, *J. Liq. Chromatogr.*, 1983, *6*, 251–293. In plasma, serum and urine: limit of quantification 0.5 mg/L, UV detection (λ=265 nm)—Eli Lilly and Company, *J. Chromatogr.*, 1991, *567(1)*, 129–139.

Disposition in the Body

Therapeutic concentration

Non-fasting and fasting patients were administered a single oral dose of 250 mg or 500 mg cephalexin. The highest concentration of the drug in radicular granuloma was observed 2 h after dosing at a concentration of 1.65 mg/g after the 250 mg dose in the non-fasting patients. The highest concentration for the 500 mg dose was observed to be 3.35 mg/g after 2 h for the non-fasting and 3.42 mg/g after 1.5 h for the fasting patients. [Y. Akimoto *et al.*, *Gen. Pharmacol.*, 1994, *25(8)*, 1563–1566.]

Dose. 1 to 6 g daily.

Cefaloridine

Antibiotic

Synonym. Cephaloridine

Proprietary names. Cepaloridin; Cepalorin; Ceporan; Ceporin(e); Keflodin; Loridine.

1-[[(6*R*,7*R*)-2-Carboxy-8-oxo-7-[(2-thienylacetyl)amino]-5-thia-1-azabicyclo[4.2.0]oct-2-en-3-yl]methyl]pyridinium inner salt

$C_{19}H_{17}N_3O_4S_2$=415.5

CAS—50-59-9

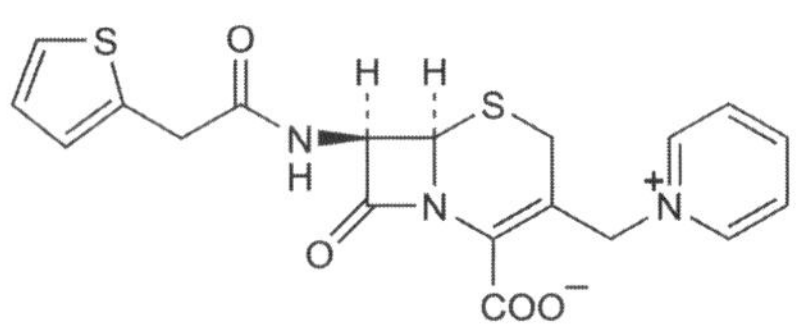

A white crystalline powder, which discolours on exposure to light.

Soluble 1 in 5 of water and 1 in 1000 of ethanol; practically insoluble in chloroform and ether.

Dissociation Constant. pK_a 3.2.

Partition Coefficient. Log *P* (octanol/water), −1.6.

Colour Tests. Mandelin's Test—violet; Marquis Test—red-violet.

Thin-layer Chromatography. System TA—Rf 73. (Acidified potassium permanganate solution, positive.)

Ultraviolet Spectrum. Aqueous acid—241 (A^1_1=350a), 254 (A^1_1=341a); aqueous alkali—261 (A^1_1=88b); methanol—234 nm (A^1_1=372a).

Infra-red Spectrum. Principal peaks at wavenumbers 1600, 1764, 1656, 1538, 715, 1143 cm^{-1} (KBr disk).

Dose. 1 to 3 g daily, intramuscularly; maximum of 6 g daily.

Cefalothin

Antibiotic

Synonym. Cefalotin; Cephalothin

(6*R*,7*R*)-3-[(Acetyloxy)methyl]-8-oxo-7-[(2-thienylacetyl)amino]-5-thia-1-azabicyclo[4.2.0]oct-2-ene-2-carboxylic acid

$C_{16}H_{16}N_2O_6S_2$=396.4

CAS—153-61-7

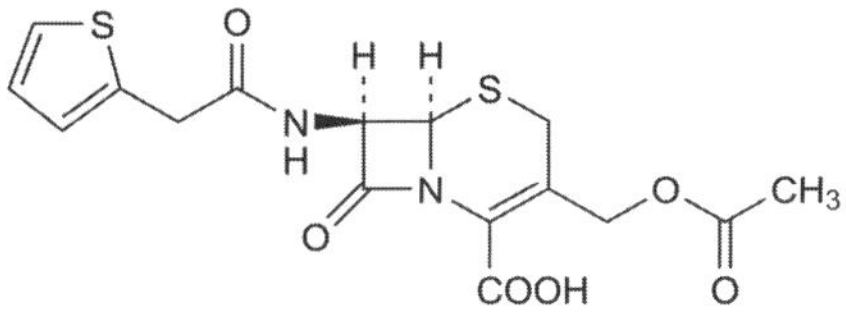

M.p. 160° to160.5°.

Cefalothin Sodium

Proprietary names. Ceporacin; Cepovenin; Keflin.

$C_{16}H_{15}N_2NaO_6S_2$=418.4

CAS—58-71-9

A white crystalline powder. M.p. 204° to 205°.

Soluble 1 in 3.5 of water and 1 in 700 of ethanol; practically insoluble in chloroform and ether.

Dissociation Constant. pK_a 2.2 (35°).

Partition Coefficient. Log *P* (octanol/water), 0.0.

Thin-layer Chromatography. System TAJ—Rf 00; system TAK—Rf 06; system TAL—Rf 41.

Ultraviolet Spectrum. Cefalothin sodium: water—237 (A^1_1=335a), 265 nm (A^1_1=204b).

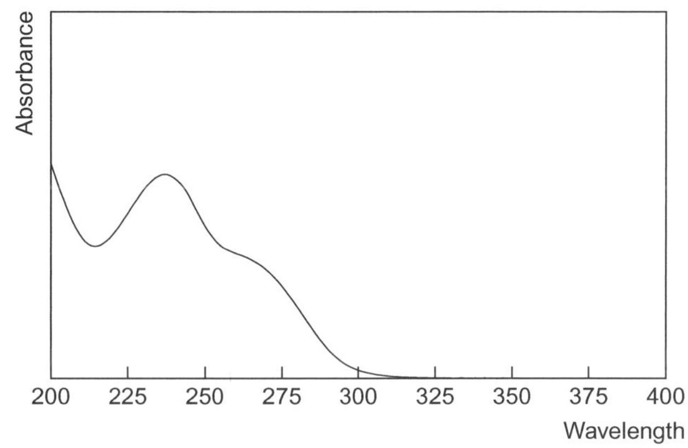

Infra-red Spectrum. Principal peaks at wavenumbers 1704, 1724, 1637, 1600, 1227, 1510 cm^{-1} (cefalothin sodium, KBr disk).

Dose. The equivalent of 4 to 12 g of cefalothin daily, intravenously.

Cefixime

Antibacterial

Synonyms. Cefiximum; CL-284635; FK-027; FR-17027.

Proprietary names. Aerocef; Cefixoral; Cefspan; Cephoral; Denvar; Fixim(e); Oroken; Necopen; Suprax; Tricef; Unixine.

(6*R*,7*R*)-7-[[(2*Z*)-(2-Amino-4-thiazolyl)[(carboxymethoxy)imino]acetyl]amino]-3-ethenyl-8-oxo-5-thia-1-azabicyclo[4.2.0]oct-2-ene-2-carboxylic acid

$C_{16}H_{15}N_5O_7S_2$=453.5

CAS—79350-37-1

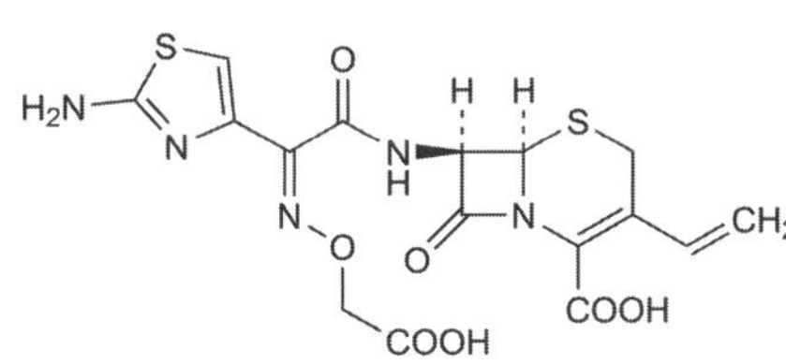

A white/almost white to light yellow crystalline powder. It is slightly soluble in water and alcohol; sparingly soluble in dehydrated alcohol and acetone; freely soluble in methyl alcohol, glycerol and propylene glycol; very slightly soluble in 70% sorbitol and octanol; practically insoluble in ether, ethyl acetate and hexane.

Cefixime Trihydrate

$C_{16}H_{21}N_5O_{10}S_2$=507.5

Pale yellow solid. M.p. 218° to 225°.

Cefixime Disodium Salt

$C_{16}H_{13}N_5Na_2O_7S$=465.4

M.p. >250°.

Dissociation Constant. pK_a, 3.73.

Thin-layer Chromatography. Plate: silica gel with (2.5 × 10 cm). Mobile phase: ethylacetate: acetone:methanol:water (5:2.5:2.5:1.5). Rf

66.9. [S. Eric-Jovanovic *et al.*, *J. Pharm. Biomed. Anal.*, 1998, *18(4–5)*, 893–898].

High Performance Liquid Chromatography. System HAA—retention time 4.8 min.

Quantification

High performance liquid chromatography. In serum: limit of detection 0.1 mg/L (λ=240 nm)—J. A. McAteer *et al.*, *Clin. Chem.*, 1987, *33(10)*, 1788–1790.

Bioassay. In serum and urine: limit of detection 0.1 mg/L and 2.0 mg/L, respectively—D. C. Britain *et al.*, *Clin. Pharmacol. Ther.*, 1985, *38*, 590–594.

Disposition in the Body. 40 to 50% of an orally administered dose of cefixime (tablet form or as a suspension) is slowly absorbed. 20% of a dose (or 50% of the absorbed dose) is excreted unchanged in the urine within 24 h. Possibly up to 60% is eliminated by non-renal pathways, with some excretion in faeces as bile. There is no evidence of metabolism. Cefixime crosses the placenta.

Therapeutic concentration An oral suspension dose provides on average a peak concentration 25 to 50% higher than that for the tablet form.

12 healthy subjects, aged between 24 and 31 years, were administered with a 50, 100, 200 and 400 mg dose of cefixime, after fasting. Peak serum concentrations of 1.02 ± 0.12, 1.46 ± 0.09, 2.63 ± 0.2 and 3.85 ± 0.23 mg/L were reached, respectively, within 2.5 to 4.5 h. [D. C. Britain *et al.*, *Clin. Pharmacol. Ther.*, 1985, *38*, 590–594].

Toxicity. Diarrhoea and pseudomembranous colitis can be mild to life-threatening. Doses up to 2 g have been administered and no other serious toxic effects observed.

Bioavailability. 22 to 54% (oral).

Half-life. Elimination half-life is between 3 and 4 h.

Volume of distribution. 0.1 L/kg.

Clearance. Serum, 0.4 mL/min/kg.

Protein binding. Cefixime is approx. 65% bound to plasma proteins.

Dose. Adults: 200 to 400 mg daily. Children with a body weight <50 kg: 8 mg/kg body weight daily. Patients with a creatinine clearance <20 mL/min: maximum 200 mg daily.

Cefradine

Antibiotic

Synonyms. Cephradine; SQ-11436.
Proprietary names. Anspor; Eskacef; Maxisporin; Megacef; Sefril; Velosef.
(6*R*,7*R*)-7-[[(2*R*)-Amino-1,4-cyclohexadien-1-ylacetyl]amino]-3-methyl-8-oxo-5-thia-1-azabicyclo[4.2.0]oct-2-ene-2-carboxylic acid
$C_{16}H_{19}N_3O_4S$=349.4
CAS—38821-53-3 (anhydrous); 75975-70-1 (monohydrate); 31828-50-9 (dihydrate)

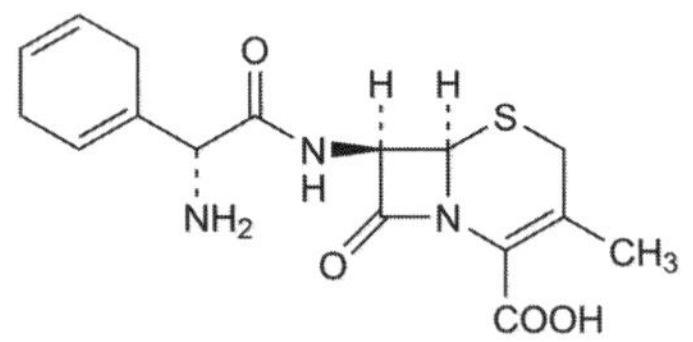

A white to cream-coloured crystalline powder.
Soluble 1 in 100 of water and 1 in 70 of methanol; practically insoluble in ethanol, chloroform, and ether.

Dissociation Constant. pK_a 2.5, 7.3 (35°).

Partition Coefficient. Log *P* (octanol/water), 0.4.

Ultraviolet Spectrum. Aqueous acid—257 nm.

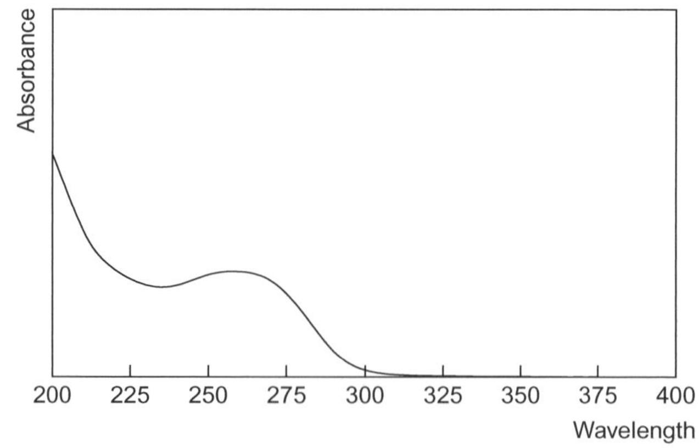

Infra-red Spectrum. Principal peaks at wavenumbers 1754, 1582, 1678, 1271, 1235, 1190 cm^{-1} (KBr disk).

Quantification

High performance liquid chromatography. In plasma: limit of quantification 0.2 mg/L, UV detection (λ=260 nm)—V. M. Johnson *et al.*, *J. Chromatogr. B Biomed. Sci. Appl.*, 2000, *740(1)*, 71–80.

Disposition in the Body

Therapeutic concentration

Ten healthy, young male and female volunteers (aged 19 to 25 years) and nine elderly volunteers (aged 65 to 81 years) were administered 1 g cephradine as a 5-min IV infusion followed by 1 g oral dose the next day. The mean serum drug concentration was 1.52 mg/L 6 h after dosing and 0.73 mg/L after 8 h for the elderly volunteers compared with 0.43 mg/L at 6 h for the younger volunteers. [T. L. Schwinghammer *et al.*, *J. Clin. Pharmacol.*, 1990, *30(10)*, 893–899.]

Dose. 1 to 4 g daily.

Ceftazidime

Antibacterial

Synonym. GR-20263
1-[[(6*R*,7*R*)-7-[[(2*Z*)-(2-Amino-4-thiazolyl)[(1-carboxy-1-methylethoxy)imino]acetyl]amino]-2-carboxy-8-oxo-5-thia-1-azabicyclo[4.2.0]oct-2-en-3-yl]methyl]-pyridinium inner salt
$C_{22}H_{22}N_6O_7S_2$=546.6
CAS—72558-82-8

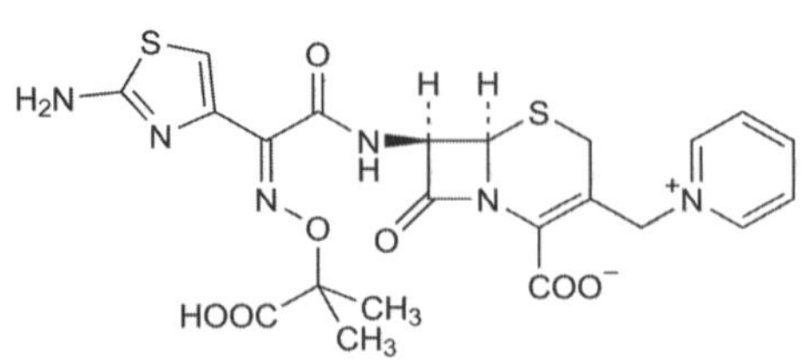

Ceftazidime Pentahydrate

Proprietary names. Ceftim; Ceptaz; Fortam; Fortaz; Fortum; Glazidim; Kefadim; Kefamin; Kefazim; Kefzim; Panzid; Potendal; Spectrum; Starcef; Tazicef; Tazidime.
$C_{22}H_{22}N_6O_7S_2,5H_2O$=636.7
CAS—78439-06-2
A white to cream coloured crystalline powder. M.p. 135° to 137°, with decomposition (dark brown).
It is slightly soluble in water (5 g/L); soluble in dimethylsulfoxide and in alkali; slightly soluble in dimethyl formamide and in methanol; practically insoluble in acetone, in chloroform, in dioxan, in ethanol (<1 g/L), in ether, in ethyl acetate, and in toluene; soluble in alkali.

Dissociation Constant. pK_a 1.9, 2.7, 4.1.

High Performance Liquid Chromatography. Column: (analytical) C_{18} (μBondapak, 300 × 3.9 mm i.d.); (pre-column) C_{18} (μBondapak)/

Corasil 37 to 50 µm. Mobile phase for serum analysis: potassium dihydrogen phosphate buffer (150 mM, pH 6.5):methanol (82:18), 1.2 mL/min flow rate. For urine analysis: potassium dihydrogen phosphate buffer (50 mM, pH 6.5):methanol (88:12). UV detection (λ=255 nm). Retention time in serum and urine: 5.0 min. [J. S. Leeder *et al.*, *Antimicrob. Agents Chemother.*, 1983, *24*, 720–724].

Column: (analytical) RP MCH 10 (Micropak, 300 × 4.0 mm); (guard column) pellicular RP (Vydac, 40 × 4 mm, 40 µm). Column temperature: 50°. Mobile phase: (method A) 20% methanol:80% aqueous ammonium dihydrogen phosphate (50 mM) and perchloric acid (117 µM), 1.0 mL/min flow rate. (Method B) 9% acetonitrile:91% phosphate–perchloric acid solution (as method A), 0.5 mL/min flow rate increased to 1.5 mL/min over first 4 min. UV detection (λ=257 nm). *k* value: 0.3. [C. M. Myers and J. L. Blumer, *Antimicrob. Agents Chemother.*, 1983, *24*, 343–346].

Column: C_{18} (LiChrosorb, 250 × 4.6 mm, 10 µm). Mobile phase: methanol (6%):sodium phosphate buffer (100 mM, pH 6.0), 2.5 mL/min flow rate. UV detection (λ=254 nm). Retention time: 9.6 min. [D. E. Holt *et al.*, *J. Antimicrob. Chemother.*, 1990, *26*, 107–115].

Ultraviolet Spectrum. Aqueous acid (0.2 M NH_2SO_4)—259 nm; (methanol)—257 nm; (0.1 M sulfuric acid)—260 nm (A=2.514); basic—257 nm.

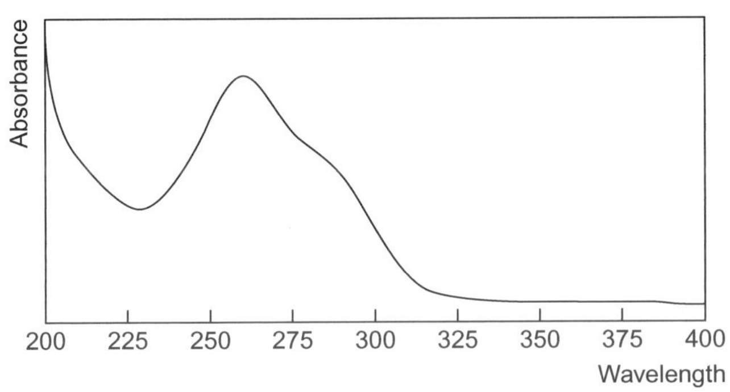

Infra-red Spectrum. Principal peaks at wavenumbers 1621, 1757, 1537, 1157, 3000–3600 cm^{-1} (pentahydrate salt) (KBr pellet).

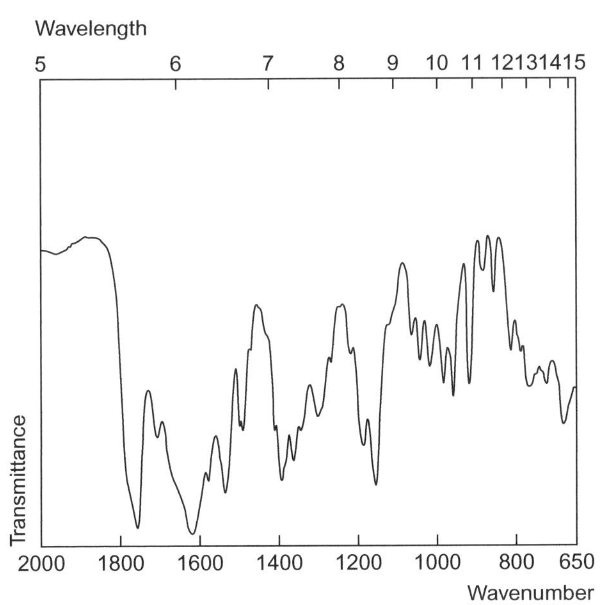

Mass Spectrum. Principal ions at *m/z* 168, 167, 514, 548, 40, 166, 51.

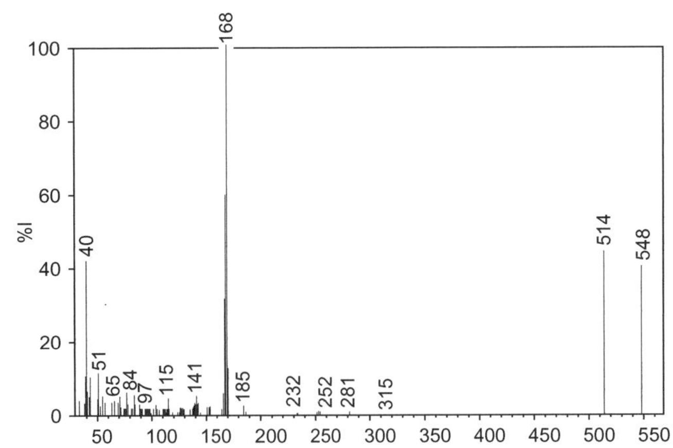

Quantification

High performance liquid chromatography. In serum, urine, or bile: limit of detection 0.2 mg/L (conventional HPLC), 0.05 mg/L (high-speed HPLC), UV detection—F. Jehl *et al.*, *J. Chromatogr.*, 1987, *413*; *Biomed. Appl.*, *57*, 109–119. In serum or urine: limit of detection 1 mg/L, UV detection (λ=255 nm)—J. S. Leeder *et al.*, *Antimicrob. Agents Chemother.*, 1983, *24*, 720–724. In serum or urine: limit of detection 0.3 mg/L, UV detection (λ=257 nm)—C. M. Myers and J. L. Blumer, *Antimicrob. Agents Chemother.*, 1983, *24*, 343–346. In serum, CSF (cerebrospinal fluid) or urine: limit of detection 1 mg/L, UV detection (λ=254 nm)—D. E. Holt *et al.*, *J. Antimicrob. Chemother.*, 1990, *26*, 107–115.

Disposition in the Body. Ceftazidime is not absorbed by oral administration but is given by injection as its sodium salt or in solution with arginine. It is widely distributed in body tissues and fluids including bone, synovial fluid, heart and bile; therapeutic concentrations are achieved in the CSF when the meninges are inflamed. The drug crosses the placenta and is distributed into breast milk. It is passively excreted in bile, although only a small proportion is eliminated by this route. The drug is mainly excreted by the kidneys, almost exclusively by glomerular filtration. About 80 to 90% of a dose is recovered unchanged in urine in 24 h as it does not undergo metabolism. It is removed by haemodialysis and peritoneal dialysis. There is no evidence of accumulation of the drug in serum after multiple dosing.

Therapeutic concentration. The trough serum therapeutic concentration range is 20 to 40 mg/L and peak, 50 to 200 mg/L.

In healthy adults, mean peak serum concentrations of 45 and 90 mg/L have been reported after intravenous administration of 500 mg and 1 g, respectively, over 5 min. Mean peak serum concentrations of 42, 69 and 170 mg/L have been reported after intravenous infusion of 500 mg, 1 g and 2 g, respectively, over 20 to 30 min. These concentrations were observed up to 30 min after the end of infusion. After intramuscular injection of 500 mg and 1 g ceftazidine, mean peak serum concentrations were 17 and 39 mg/L, respectively, at approximately, 1 h. Serum concentrations stayed above 4 mg/L for 6 to 8 h after these doses. [Data as supplied by Eli Lilly & Company Ltd.]

Toxicity

Ceftazidime overdosage may lead to neurological effects including encephalopathy, neuromuscular excitability, convulsions and coma. Seizures may occur in patients with renal impairment. [Data as supplied by Eli Lilly & Company Ltd.]

Half-life. Plasma half-life, approx. 2 h.

Volume of distribution. Steady state, 0.2 to 0.3 L/kg.

Clearance. Plasma clearance, 115 mL/min; serum, 98 to 122 mL/min (healthy individuals); 142 to 376 mL/min/1.73m^2 for patients suffering with cystic fibrosis; 79 mL/min for geriatric patients aged between 63 and 83 years.

Protein binding. In plasma, less than 10%.

Note. For a review of ceftazidime, see C. P. Rains *et al.*, *Drugs*, 1995, *49*, 577–617.

Dose. Adults: usual dose is 500 mg to 2 g every 8 to 12 h. In patients >80 years old, daily dose should not exceed 2 g. Infants and children over 2 months old: between 50 and 150 mg/kg daily intravenously. Maximum is 6 g daily. Neonates and children up to 2 months: 25 to 60 mg/kg daily. Dose should be reduced in patients with impaired renal function.

Ceftriaxone

Antibacterial

Synonyms. Cefatriaxone, Ro-13-9904/000
(6*R*,7*R*)-7-[[(2*Z*)-(2-Amino-4-thiazolyl)(methoxyimino)acetyl]amino]-8-oxo-3-[[(1,2,5,6-tetrahydro-2-methyl-5,6-dioxo-1,2,4-triazin-3-yl)thio]-methyl]-5-thia-1-azabicyclo[4.2.0]oct-2-ene-2-carboxylic acid
$C_{18}H_{18}N_8O_7S_3$=554.6
CAS—73384-59-5

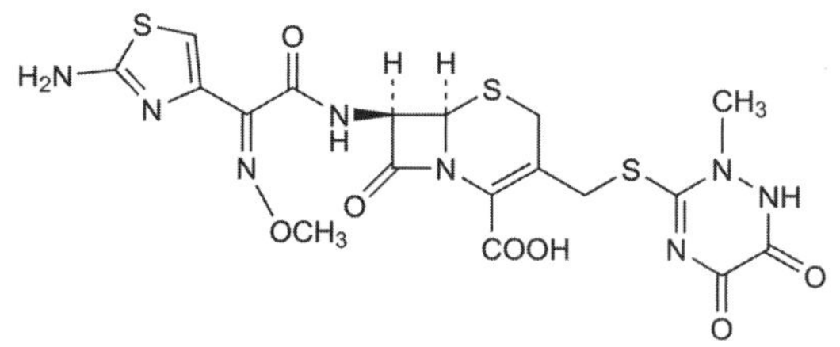

Ceftriaxone Sodium

Synonym. Cefatriaxone sodium
Proprietary names. Hosbocin; Rocefalin; Rocefin; Rocephalin; Rocephin; Rocephine.
$C_{18}H_{16}N_8Na_2O_7S_3,3\frac{1}{2}H_2O$=661.6
CAS—74578-69-1 (anhydrous); 104376-79-6 (hemiheptahydrate)
An almost white to yellowish-orange, slightly hygroscopic, crystalline powder. M.p. >155°, with decomposition. It is freely or very soluble in water (40 g/100 mL at 25°); very slightly soluble in ethanol; sparingly soluble in methanol.

Dissociation Constant. pK_a 3, 3.2, 4.1. (disodium salt, hemiheptahydrate)

Thin-layer Chromatography. System TB—Rf 00; system TE—Rf 00; system TF—Rf 00; system TAE—Rf 88.

High Performance Liquid Chromatography. System HX—RI 239; system HAA—retention time 5.3 min.

Column: (analytical) C_{18} RP (μBondapak, 300 × 4.0 mm i.d.); (pre-column) silica (300 × 4.0 mm, 18 μm). Mobile phase: acetonitrile:potassium phosphate buffer (10 mM, pH 9) containing 10 mM hexadecyltrimethylammonium bromide (46:54), 1.5 mL/min flow rate. UV detection (λ=274 nm). Retention time: 4.6 min. [G. G. Granich and D. J. Krogstad, *Antimicrob. Agents Chemother.*, 1987, *31*, 385–388].

Ultraviolet Spectrum. Aqueous acid (0.2 M NH_2SO_4)—261 nm; basic—242, 269 nm.

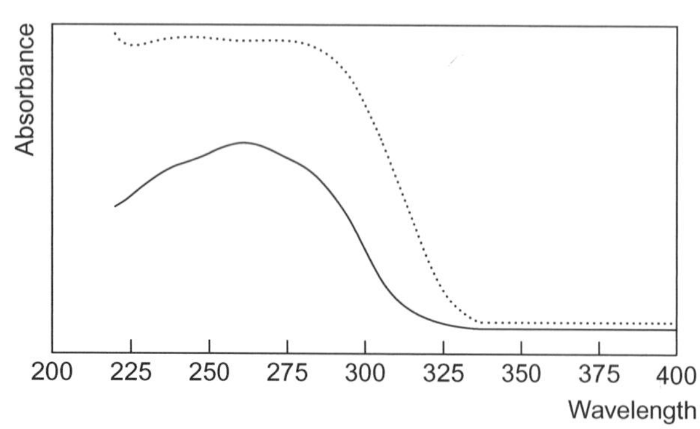

Infra-red Spectrum. Principal peaks at wavenumber 1739, 1598, 1527, 1393 cm^{-1} (KBr pellets).

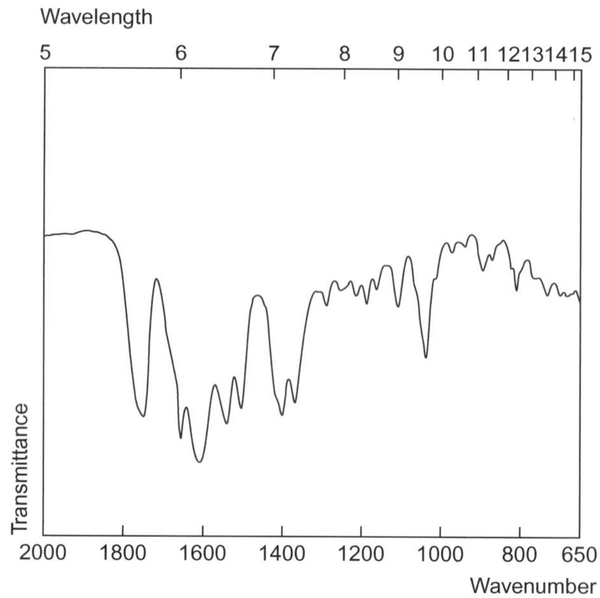

Quantification

High performance liquid chromatography. In plasma, urine or saliva: limits of detection 0.4, 3.0 and 0.03 mg/L, respectively, UV detection—V. Ascalone and L. Dal Bò, *J. Chromatogr.*, 1983, *273*, 357–366. In serum, urine or bile: limits of detection 0.2 mg/L (conventional HPLC), 0.05 mg/L (high-speed HPLC), UV detection—F. Jehl *et al.*, *J. Chromatogr.*, 1987, *413*; *Biomed. Appl.*, *57*, 109–119. In serum, urine or CSF (cerebrospinal fluid): limit of detection 1 mg/L, UV detection (λ=274 nm)—G. G. Granich and D. J. Krogstad, *Antimicrob. Agents Chemother.*, 1987, *31*, 385–388.

Disposition in the Body. Following intramuscular administration of ceftriaxone, peak plasma concentrations occur after about 2 to 3 h. It is widely distributed in body tissues and fluids; therapeutic concentrations may occur in the CSF when the meninges are inflamed. It crosses the placenta and is distributed into breast milk. High concentrations are found in bile. About 40 to 65% of a dose is excreted unchanged in urine, mainly by glomerular filtration; the remainder is excreted in bile and is found in faeces as the unchanged drug and inactive metabolites.

Therapeutic concentration. The serum therapeutic concentration range is 15 to 75 mg/L.

Peak plasma concentrations of 46.2 to 66.5 mg/L (mean, 54.9 mg/L) occurred 1 to 2 h after an intramuscular injection of 500 mg administered to 6 subjects. Those participating in the study were males, mean age 25.7 years (range 19 to 43 years) with maturity-induced diabetes controlled by diet alone. Doses were repeated every 12 h for a total of 5 doses. At steady state, the plasma concentrations ranged from 64.8 to 86.5 mg/L (mean 74.1 mg/L). [M. E. Pickup *et al.*, *Br. J. Clin. Pharmacol.*, 1981, *12*, 111–115].

Half-life. Plasma, 6 to 9 h.

Volume of distribution. 5.8 to 13.5 L.

Clearance. Plasma, 0.58 to 1.45 L/h.

Protein binding. In plasma, 85 to 95% depending on plasma concentration of ceftriaxone.

Note. For reviews of the pharmacokinetics of ceftriaxone, see J. H. Yuk *et al.*, *Clin. Pharmacokinet.*, 1989, *17*, 223–235, I. H. Patel and S. A. Kaplan, *Am. J. Med.*, 1984, *77*, *Suppl. 4C*, 17–25, and R. N. Brogden and A. Ward, *Drugs*, 1987, *35*, 604–645.

Dose. 1 g daily or for severe infections, the equivalent of up to 4 g of ceftriaxone intravenously or intramuscularly daily.

Celecoxib

NSAID

Synonyms. SC-58635; YM-177.
Proprietary name. Celebrex
p-[5-*p*-Methylphenyl-3-(trifluoromethyl)-*1H*-pyrazol-1-yl] benzenesulfonamide
$C_{17}H_{14}F_3N_3O_2S$=381.4
CAS—169590-42-5

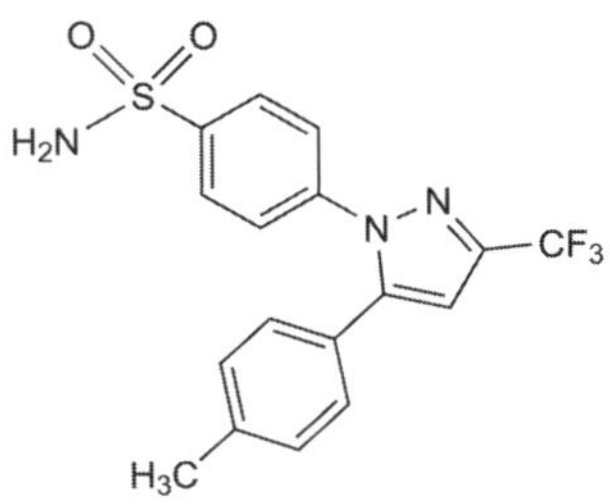

Pale yellow solid. M.p. 157° to 159°.

Dissociation Constant. pK_a 11.1.

Ultraviolet Spectrum. Aqueous acid (ethanol)—254 nm.

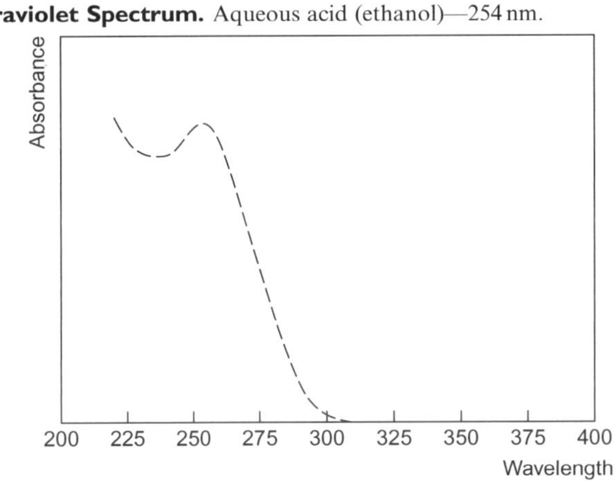

Mass Spectrum. Principal ions at *m/z* 381, 300, 382, 301, 281, 140, 115, 362.

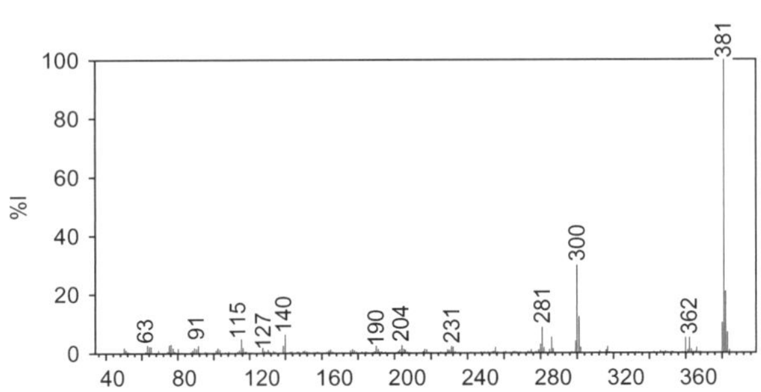

Quantification
High performance liquid chromatography. In plasma: limit of quantification is 0.025 mg/L. UV detection (λ=260 nm)—M. J. Rose *et al.*, *J. Chromatogr. B Biomed. Sci. Appl.*, 2000, *738(2)*, 377–385.

Disposition in the Body. Celecoxib is well and rapidly absorbed and metabolised in the liver to primary alcohol, the corresponding carboxylic acid (the primary metabolite) and its glucuronide conjugate. The drug is widely distributed throughout the body. It is eliminated predominantly by hepatic metabolism (>97%), with approx. 57% of the dose excreted in faeces and 27% urine.

Therapeutic concentration
4 healthy young volunteers were administered with a single 200 mg dose of celecoxib. Peak plasma concentrations of 0.797 mg/L were reached within 1.8 h for those who had not had celecoxib administered with food, and 0.877 mg/L within 6.3 h for the volunteers who had the drug administered with a high fat breakfast. [N. M. Danes *et al.*, *Clin. Pharmacokinet.*, 2000, *38(3)*, 225–242].

Toxicity. Acute overdose: coma, hypertension, acute renal failure and respiratory depression.

Half-life. 11.2 to 15.6 h.

Volume of distribution. 5.7 to 7.1 L/kg; also reported as 455 ± 166 L.

Clearance. 27.7 L/h.

Distribution in blood. Red blood cells:plasma ratio is 0.89.

Protein binding. 97%, albumin.

Dose. 200 mg daily and increased if necessary to 400 mg.

Celiprolol

Beta-blocker

Synonym. ST-1396
N′-[3-Acetyl-4-[3-[(1,1-dimethylethyl)-amino]-2-hydroxypropoxy] phenyl]-*N*,*N*-diethylurea
$C_{20}H_{33}N_3O_4$=379.5
CAS—56980-93-9

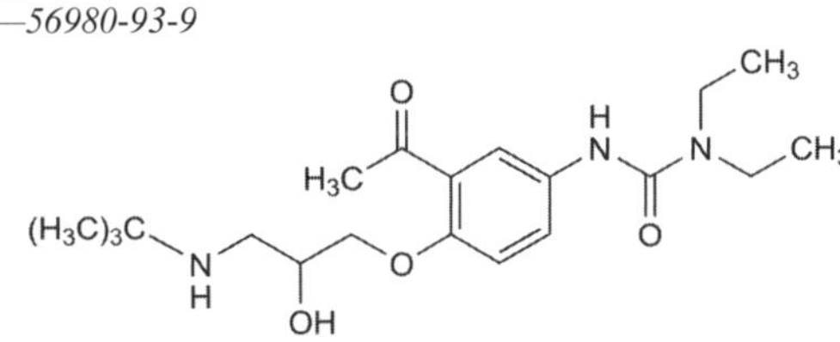

Crystals. M.p. 110° to 112°.

Celiprolol Hydrochloride
Synonyms. REV-5320A; RG-5320A; RHC-5320A; ST-1236.
Proprietary names. Cardem; Celectol; Celipro; Corliprol; Dilanorm; Jofurol; Moderator; Selectol.
$C_{20}H_{33}N_3O_4$,HCl=416.0
CAS—57470-78-7
White odourless crystals. M.p. 197° to 200°, with decomposition. Solubility at 25° in water, 15.1 g/100 mL; methanol, 18.2 g/100 mL; ethanol, 1.61 g/100 mL; chloroform, 0.42 g/100 mL.

Dissociation Constant. pK_a 9.68 (25°).

Partition Coefficient. Log *P* (octanol/aqueous phosphate buffer, pH 7.4), 0.8 (37°); log *P* (chloroform/water), 0.14; log *P* (chloroform/pH 7.1 aqueous phosphate buffer), 2.42; log *P* (octanol/water), 1.92.

Thin-layer Chromatography. System TAE—Rf 15; system TE—Rf 33.

Gas Chromatography. System GA— RI 2610.

High Performance Liquid Chromatography. System HAV—*k* 2.2; system HAA—retention time 11.5 min; system HZ—RI 2.5 min.

Ultraviolet Spectrum. Aqueous acid (0.01 M hydrochloric acid)—231 (A^1_1=660) and 324 (A^1_1=60) nm; aqueous alkali (0.01 M sodium hydroxide)—231 (A^1_1=640) and 324 (A^1_1=60); methanol—232 (A^1_1=775) and 329 (A^1_1=58) nm.

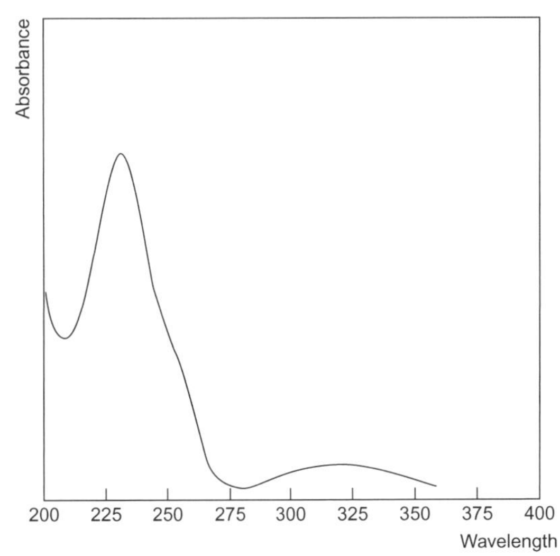

Infra-red Spectrum. Principal peaks at wavenumbers 1674, 1636, 823, 591 cm^{-1}.

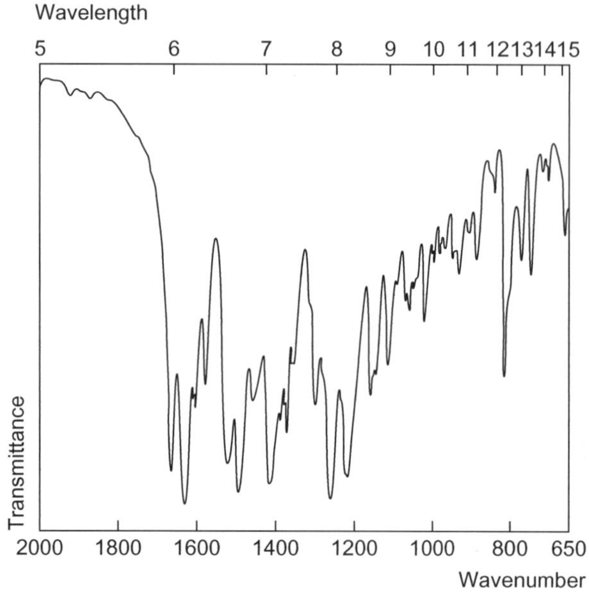

Mass Spectrum. Principal ions at *m/z* 86, 58, 250, 44, 57, 72, 291, 71.

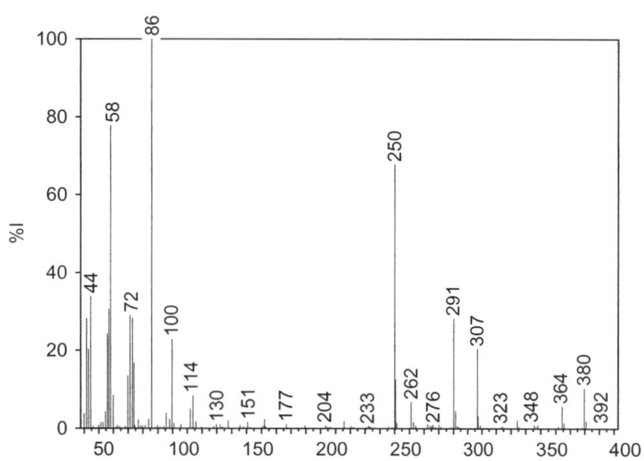

Quantification

High performance liquid chromatography. In blood, plasma or urine: limit of detection 10 µg/L in plasma with UV detection or 5 µg/L in plasma with fluorescence detection—J. N. Buskin *et al.*, *J. Chromatogr.*, 1982, *230*; *Biomed. Appl.*, *19*, 454–460. In plasma or urine: limit of detection 10 µg/L, fluorescence detection—Von D. Hippmann and F. Takacs, *Arzneimittel-forschung*, 1983, *33*, 8–12. In plasma or urine: limit of detection 1.5 µg/L (each enantiomer) in plasma and 2.5 µg/L (each enantiomer) in urine, fluorescence detection—C. Hartmann *et al.*, *J. Chromatogr.*, 1989, *496*; *Biomed. Appl.*, *88*, 387–396. In plasma: limit of detection 4 µg/L, UV detection—D. R. Rutledge *et al.*, *J. Chromatogr. Sci.*, 1994, *32*, 153–156. In plasma: limit of detection 25.7 µg/L, UV detection—D. R. Rutledge *et al.*, *J. Pharm. Biomed. Anal.*, 1994, *12*, 135–140. In plasma: limit of detection 5 µg/L (total celiprolol), 2.5 µg/L (each enantiomer), UV and fluorescence detection—R. Verbesselt *et al.*, *J. Chromatogr. B Biomed. Sci. Appl.*, 1996, *683*, 231–236. In plasma: limit of detection 5 µg/L, fluorescence detection—F. C. K. Chiu and K. Raymond, *J. Chromatogr. B Biomed. Sci. Appl.*, 1996, *687*, 462–465. In plasma: limit of detection about 16 µg/L, UV detection—A. J. Braza *et al.*, *J. Chromatogr. B Biomed. Sci. Appl.*, 1998, *718*, 267–272.

Disposition in the Body. Absorbed after oral administration in a non-linear fashion; the percentage of dose absorbed increases with increasing dose. The extent of absorption is reduced in the presence of food. Peak plasma concentrations are reached after 2 to 3 h. Crosses the placenta. Low lipid solubility. Undergoes only minimal metabolism and is excreted unchanged in the urine (approx. 11%) and faeces (84% in 24 h after an oral dose). After an intravenous dose, approx. 50% is excreted in urine and 31% in faeces. A very low percentage of the drug is excreted as three metabolites.

Bioavailability. 30 to 70%, which is reduced in the presence of food.

Therapeutic concentration. Considerable inter-individual variation in peak plasma concentrations.

Mean peak plasma concentration measured after administration of a 200 mg single oral dose to 12 subjects was 687 µg/L after 3.71 h. Following administration of 200 mg and 400 mg daily for 7 days to 12 subjects, the mean peak plasma concentration was 597 µg/L and 1676 µg/L, respectively. [R. J. Norris *et al.*, *J. Cardiovasc. Pharmacol.*, 1986, *8*, *Suppl. 4*, S91–S92].

Half-life. Plasma, 5 to 6 h.

Protein binding. In plasma, 25%.

Note. For reviews of celiprolol see J. G. Riddell *et al.*, *Drugs*, 1987, *34*, 438–458 and R. J. Milne and M. M.-T. Buckley, *Drugs*, 1991, *41*, 941–969.

Dose. 200 mg of the hydrochloride daily, increased to 400 mg daily if necessary.

Cephaëline

Emetic/Expectorant

Synonyms. Desmethylemetine; Dihydropsychotrine.
7′,10,11-Trimethoxyemetan-6′-ol
$C_{28}H_{38}N_2O_4$=466.6
CAS—483-17-0

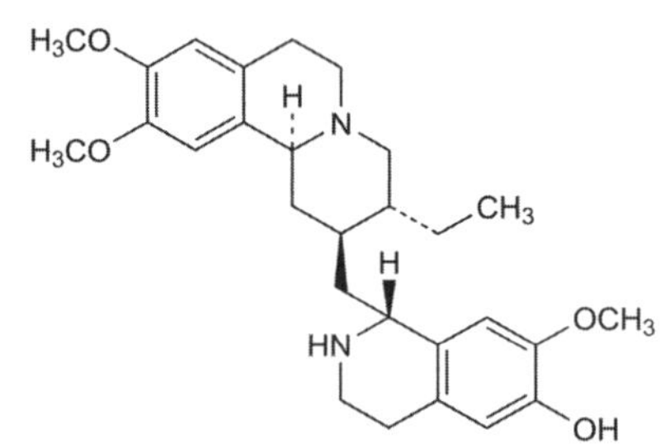

An alkaloid present in ipecacuanha, the dried root, or rhizome and root, of *Cephaëlis ipecacuanha* (=*Uragoga ipecacuanha*) (Rubiaceae) or *C. acuminata*.
Needles. M.p. 115° to 116°.
Practically insoluble in water; freely soluble in acetic acid, acetone, ethanol, and chloroform; slightly soluble in ether.

Cephaëline Hydrochloride

$C_{28}H_{38}N_2O_4$,2HCl=539.5
CAS—5853-29-2
White crystals or crystalline powder. Solutions turn yellow.
Soluble in water; less soluble in alcohol, acetone, and chloroform. Practically insoluble in benzene.

Partition Coefficient. Log *P* (octanol/water), 4.9.

Colour Test. Liebermann's Test—black.

Thin-layer Chromatography. System TA—Rf 53; system TB—Rf 01; system TC—Rf 19; system TL—Rf 08. (Acidified iodoplatinate solution, positive.)

High Performance Liquid Chromatography. System HA—*k* 7.7 (tailing peak).

Ultraviolet Spectrum. Aqueous acid—283 (A_1^1=127b); ethanol—235, 276 nm (A_1^1=144b).

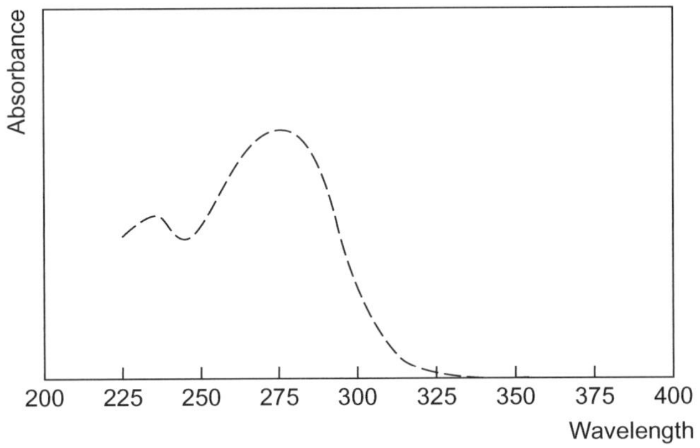

Infra-red Spectrum. Principal peaks at wavenumbers 1264, 1515, 1116, 1229, 1213, 1616 cm^{-1} (cephaëline hydrochloride, KBr disk).

Mass Spectrum. Principal ions at *m/z* 178, 192, 272, 466, 244, 288, 191, 273.

Quantification See under Emetine.

High performance liquid chromatography. In plasma and urine: limit of quantification 1.0 mg/L and 5 mg/L, respectively, fluorescence detection—T. Asano *et al.*, *J. Chromatogr. B Biomed. Sci. Appl.*, 2001, *757(2)*, 197–206.

Disposition in the Body

Therapeutic concentration

Six healthy male volunteers were administered Ipecac syrup containing 0.843 g/L cephaëline and 0.503 g/L emetine at doses of 5, 10, 15, 20, 25, and 30 mL. Cephaëline was found in plasma at a concentration of 1.7, 3.0, 3.1, 3.6, 5.6, and 3.1 mg/L respective to the dosings at times of 2.1, 1.7, 0.8, 1.1, 2.4, and 1.5 h, respectively. [T. Asano *et al.*, *J. Chromatogr. B Biomed. Sci. Appl.*, 2001, *757(2)*, 197–206.]

Dose. Cephaëline hydrochloride has been given in doses of 5 to 10 mg.

Cerivastatin

Lipid Regulator

(3*R*,5*S*,6*E*)-7-[4-(4-Fluorophenyl)-5-(methoxymethyl)-2,6-bis(1-methylethyl)-3-pyridinyl]-3,5-dihydroxy-6-heptenoic acid

$C_{26}H_{34}FNO_5$=459.6

CAS—145599-86-6

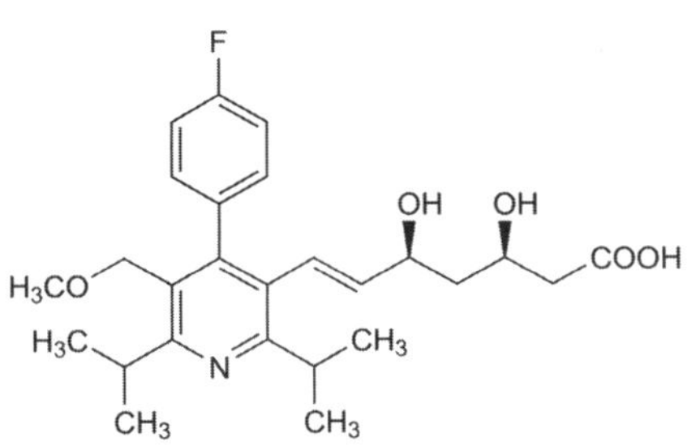

Cerivastatin Sodium

Synonym. Bay-W-6228

Proprietary names. Baycol; Lipobay.

$C_{26}H_{33}FNNaO_5$=481.5

CAS—143201-11-0

A white to off-white hygroscopic amorphous powder. It is soluble in water, ethanol, and methanol; very slightly soluble in acetone.

Ultraviolet Spectrum. Methanol—228, 263 nm.

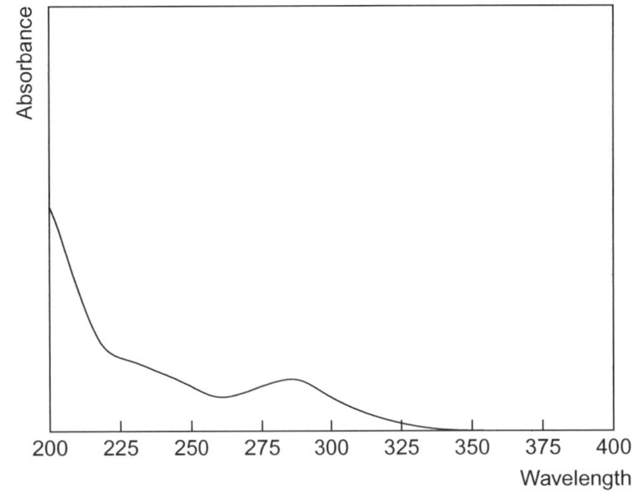

Infra-red Spectrum. Principal peaks at wavenumbers 1603, 1098, 1381, 1222 cm^{-1} (KBr disc).

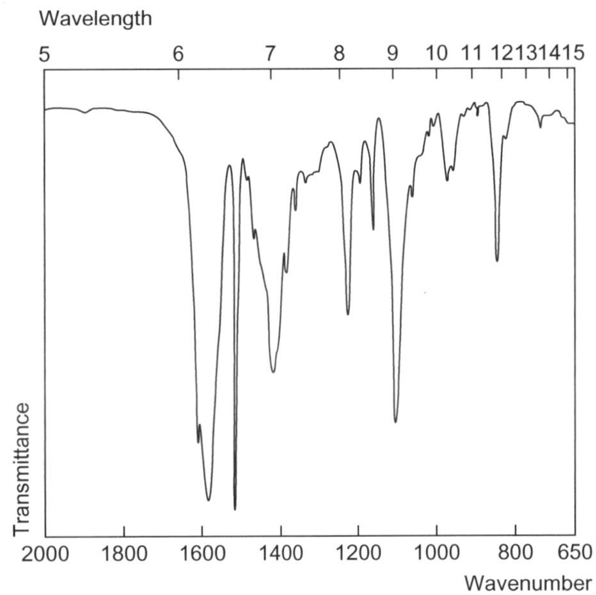

Quantification

High performance liquid chromatography. In serum: limit of quantification 0.01 µg/L for cerivastatin and the lactone form, and 0.05 to 0.5 µg/L for its biotransformation products. MS detection—M. Jemal *et al.*, *J. Chromatogr. B, Biomed. Sci. Appl.*, 1999, *736(1–2)*, 19–41. In plasma: limit of quantification 0.025 µg/L. Fluorescence detection—G. J. Krol *et al.*, *J. Pharm. Biomed. Anal.*, 1993, *11*, 1269–1275.

Disposition in the Body. Cerivastatin is readily and almost completely absorbed after oral administration. It undergoes metabolism in the liver and is catalysed by at least two cytochrome P450 isoenzymes, CYP2C8 and CYP3A4. Three active metabolites are formed. The demethylated metabolite (about 50% as potent as the parent drug) and the hydroxylated metabolite (about 80% as potent) are the major metabolites formed; the product of both demethylation and hydroxylation also has activity, but it is only a minor metabolite. The metabolites are excreted in urine (about 30%) and in faeces (about 70%). There is no unchanged drug found in urine. There is no significant clearance by haemodialysis.

Therapeutic concentration

24 healthy, Caucasian males, aged between 21 and 44 years, were administered with a single dose of 0.8 mg after an overnight fast (group 1), with breakfast (group 2), in the evening with dinner (group 3) or 4 h after dinner (group 4). The peak plasma concentrations were 7.7, 8.7, 7.1 and 7.1 µg/L for the four groups, respectively. These concentrations were reached within 1.5, 2.3 and 2.5 h, respectively. The mean concentration

detected for the demethylated metabolite, M1, was 0.6 μg/L for the four groups and this was observed approx. 4 h after administration. The hydroxylated metabolite, M23, showed a concentration of 1.6 μg/L at approx. 4 to 6 h. [W. Muck *et al.*, *Int. J. Clin. Pharmacol. Ther.*, 2000, *38(6)*, 298–303].

Bioavailability. Absolute bioavailability, 60%.

Half-life. Plasma, 2 to 3 h.

Volume of distribution. 0.3 L/kg.

Clearance. Plasma, 0.2 L/h/kg.

Protein binding. In plasma, 99%; 80% to albumin.

Dose. Initially 0.1 mg of cerivastatin sodium daily, increasing to 0.3 mg daily.

Cetalkonium Chloride

Cationic Disinfectant

Proprietary names. Baktonium. It is an ingredient of AAA, Bonjela, and Teejel.

N-Hexadecyl-*N*,*N*-dimethylbenzenemethanaminium chloride
$C_{25}H_{46}ClN$=396.1
CAS—122-18-9

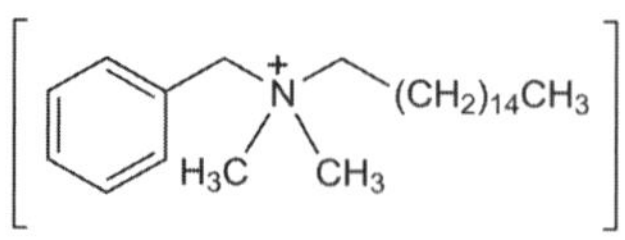

A white crystalline powder. M.p. 58° to 60°.
Sparingly soluble in cold water, soluble in hot water; soluble in acetone, ethanol, chloroform, ether, ethyl acetate, propylene glycol, and glycerol.

Partition Coefficient. Log *P* (octanol/water), 4.9.

Thin-layer Chromatography. System TA—Rf 12, streaking. (Acidified iodoplatinate solution, positive.)

Ultraviolet Spectrum. Aqueous acid—258 (A_1^1=8b), 264 (A_1^1=10b), 270 (A_1^1=8b); methanol—253, 258, 263 (A_1^1=11b), 270 nm.

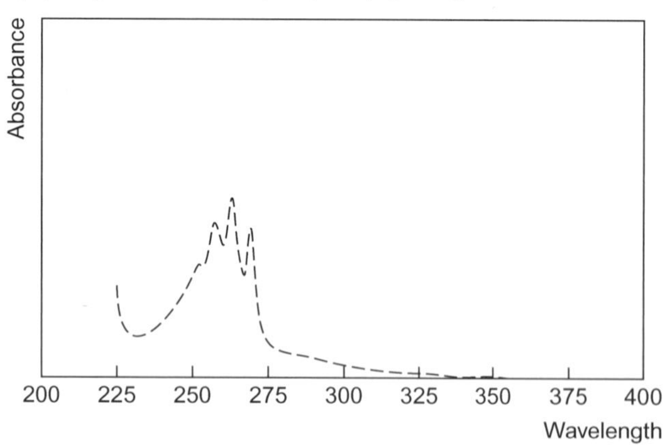

Infra-red Spectrum. Principal peaks at wavenumbers 722, 698, 1612, 1204, 875, 790 cm^{-1} (KBr disk).

Use. In a concentration of 0.01% in preparations applied to the mouth or throat.

Cetirizine

Antihistamine

[2-[4-[(4-Chlorophenyl)phenylmethyl]-1-piperazinyl]ethoxy] acetic acid
$C_{21}H_{25}ClN_2O_3$=388.9
CAS—83881-51-0

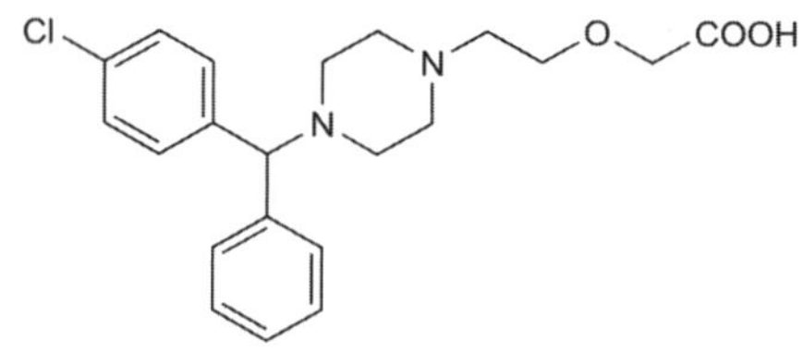

Crystals from ethanol. M.p. 110° to 115°.

Cetirizine Dihydrochloride

Synonyms. P-071; UCB-P071.
Proprietary names. Alerlisin; Formistin; Reactine; Virlix; Voltric; Zirtek; Zyrlex; Zyrtec.
$C_{21}H_{27}Cl_3N_2O_3$=461.8
CAS—83881-52-1
A white to almost white crystalline powder. M.p. 225°. It is freely soluble in water; practically insoluble in acetone and dichloromethane.

Partition Coefficient. Log *P* (octanol/water), −0.61.

Thin-layer Chromatography. Plate: silica 60 F_{254}. Mobile phase: first development with chloroform and second development, chloroform:methanol (85:15). Rf 0.31. [K. K. Pandya *et al.*, *J. Pharm. Pharmacol.*, 1996, *48*, 510–513].

Gas Chromatography. Column: fused-silica methylsilicone (25 m × 0.31 mm i.d., 0.17 μm film thickness). Column temperature: 260°. Carrier gas: helium, 35 cm/s velocity. Detection: nitrogen–phosphorous flame ionisation. Retention time: 8.5 min. [E. Baltes *et al.*, *J. Chromatogr.*, 1988, *430, Biomed. Appl.*, 149–155].

High Performance Liquid Chromatography. System HZ—retention time 3.6 min; system HAA—retention time 15.7 min; system HAX—retention time 8.89 min; system HAY—retention time 5.29 min.

Column: (analytical) C_{18} (Nucleosil 100-3, 150 × 3.2 mm, 3 μm), (pre-column) C_{18} (Nucleosil 120-5, 10 × 4 mm, 5 μm) at 40°. Mobile phase: potassium dihydrogen phosphate (30 mM), pH adjusted to 6.8 with potassium hydroxide. UV detection: λ 232 nm. Retention time: 8.25 min. [J. Macek *et al.*, *J. Chromatogr. B, Biomed. Sci. Appl.*, 1999, *736*, 231–235].

Column: C_{18} (150 × 3.9 mm i.d., 4 μm). Mobile phase: acetonitrile:water (39:61) containing 13 mM phosphate buffer, adjusted to pH 2.8 with 5 M sodium hydroxide. UV detection (λ 230 nm). Retention time: 1.69 min. [M. F. Zaater *et al.*, *J. Pharm. Biomed. Anal.*, 2000, *22*, 739–744].

Ultraviolet Spectrum. Aqueous acid (pH 2.38)—192, 258 nm.

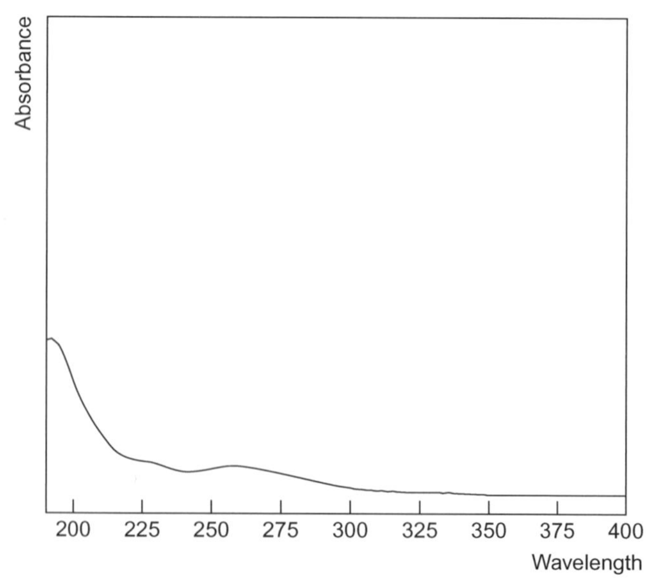

Mass Spectrum. Principal ions at *m/z* 201, 165, 203, 56, 187, 242, 299, 388.

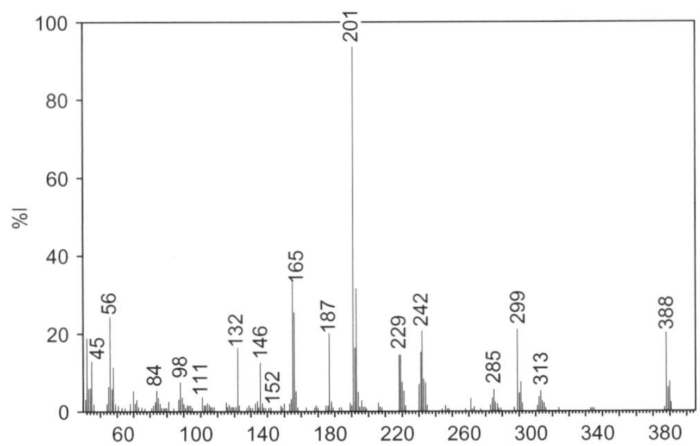

Quantification

Gas chromatography. In plasma: limit of detection 0.02 mg/L, nitrogen–phosphorous detection—E. Baltes *et al.*, *J. Chromatogr.*, 1988, *430, Biomed.; Appl.*, 149–155.

High performance liquid chromatography. In serum: limit of detection is 0.005 mg/L, UV detection (λ=230 nm)—M. F. Zaater *et al.*, *J. Pharm. Biomed. Anal.*, 2000, *22(5)*, 739–744. In plasma: limit of quantification is 0.01 mg/L. UV detection (λ=232 nm)—J. Macek *et al.*, *J. Chromatogr. B, Biomed. Sci. Appl.*, 1999, *736*, 231–235. In serum: limit of detection 0.02 mg/L. UV detection (λ=211 nm)—J. Moncrieff, *J. Chromatogr.* 1992, *583*; *Biomed. Appl.*, 128–130.

Disposition in the Body. Cetirizine is rapidly absorbed after oral administration and undergoes metabolism in the liver, to a very limited extent by *O*-dealkylation. The metabolite produced has negligible antihistaminic activity. Cetirizine is primarily excreted in urine (70%) and in faeces (10%), as the unchanged drug. It is secreted in breast milk.

Therapeutic concentration

15 infants and toddlers, with a mean age of 12.3 months, were admitted to hospital for reoccurring respiratory infections or other hypersensitivity-related diseases and treated with a single dose of 0.25 mg/kg cetirizine solution. A mean peak plasma concentration of 0.39 mg/L was observed at 2.0 h. [V. Spicak *et al.*, *Clin. Pharmacol. Ther.*, 1997, *61(3)*, 325–330].

10 elderly volunteers (aged between 60 and 90 years) and 10 healthy, young volunteers (21 to 29 years old) were administered with a single oral dose of 10 mg. Mean plasma concentrations were 0.362 mg/L for the elderly individuals and 0.337 mg/L for the young. These concentrations were observed at 1.30 and 1.12 h, respectively. [R. A. Lefebvre *et al.*, *Int. J. Clin. Pharmacol. Res.*, 1988, *8(6)*, 463–470].

Toxicity. Two cases of overdose have been reported: an adult took a 150 mg dose of cetirizine and was admitted to hospital with somnolence but no other clinical signs or blood chemistry/haematology. An 18-month-old child overdosed on 180 mg and became restless, irritable and drowsy. Multiple dose toxicity targets the liver and single dose the central nervous system.

Half-life. Elimination half-life is 7 to 11 h in adults; 6 to 7 h in children; 3.1 h in infants.

Volume of distribution. In adults, volume of distribution is 0.6 to 0.8 L/kg; children, 0.44 L/kg.

Clearance. Body clearance, 53 mL/min; 2.13 mL/min/kg (infants).

Protein binding. Cetirizine is approx. 93% bound to plasma proteins.

Dose. Adults and children >6 years: a usual dose of 10 mg is administered daily. Children (2 to 6 years) and patients with renal impairment: usual dose 5 mg daily.

Cetrimide

Cationic Disinfectant

Proprietary names. Cetavlon; Morpan CHSA; Silquat C100. It is an ingredient of Ceanel, Cetal (liquid), Savloclens, Savlodil, Savlon (liquid), and Travasept.

Consists chiefly of tetradecyltrimethylammonium bromide together with smaller amounts of dodecyl- and hexadecyltrimethylammonium bromides.

CAS—8044-71-1

A white to creamy-white, voluminous, free-flowing, hygroscopic powder. A solution in water foams on shaking. M.p. 232° to 247°.

Soluble 1 in 2 of water; freely soluble in ethanol; soluble in ether.

Thin-layer Chromatography. System TA—Rf 00; system TB—Rf 00; system TC—Rf 01; system TE—Rf 00; system TL—Rf 00; system TN—Rf 100; system TO—Rf 50; system TAE—Rf 00; system TAF—Rf 29. (Acidified iodoplatinate solution, positive.)

Gas Chromatography. System GA—RI 1699.

High Performance Liquid Chromatography. System HX—RI 56.

Infra-red Spectrum. Principal peaks at wavenumbers 961, 909, 952, 719, 970, 724 cm^{-1} (KCl disk).

Cetylpyridinium Chloride

Cationic Disinfectant

Proprietary names. Ceepryn; Cepacol; Dobendan; Merocet(s). It is an ingredient of Merocaine and Tyrosolven.

1-Hexadecylpyridinium chloride monohydrate

$C_{21}H_{38}ClN,H_2O$=358.0

CAS—7773-52-6 (cetylpyridinium); 123-03-5 (chloride, anhydrous); 6004-24-6 (chloride, monohydrate)

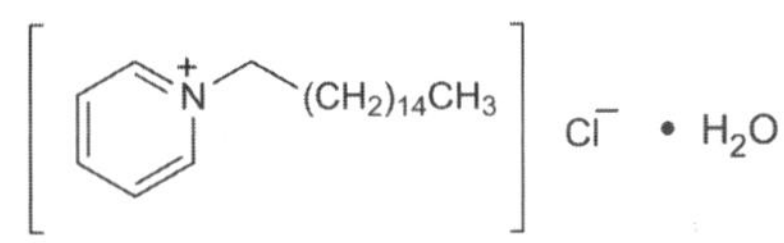

A white powder. A solution in water foams strongly when shaken. M.p. 77° to 83°.

Soluble 1 in 20 of water; freely soluble in ethanol and chloroform; very slightly soluble in ether and in benzene.

Partition Coefficient. Log *P* (octanol), 1.7.

Thin-layer Chromatography. System TA—Rf 20; system TL—Rf 00; system TAE—Rf 00; system TAF—Rf 29. (Acidified iodoplatinate solution, positive.)

Gas Chromatography. System GA—not eluted.

Ultraviolet Spectrum. Aqueous acid—280 nm. No alkaline shift.

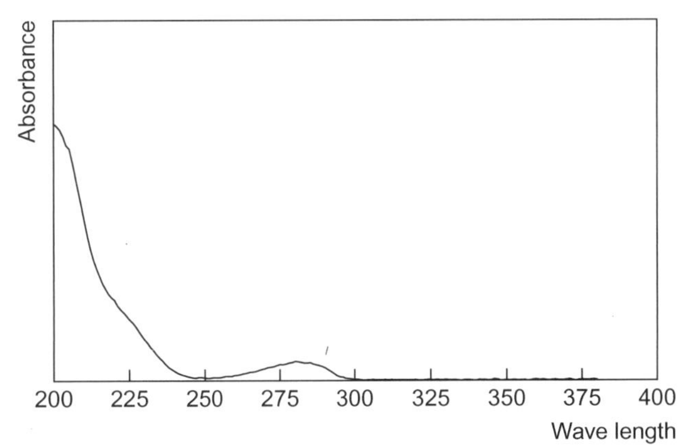

Infra-red Spectrum. Principal peaks at wavenumbers 685, 1629, 776, 1174, 715, 1205 cm^{-1}.

Use. In concentrations of 0.01 to 1%.

Chelidonine

Alkaloid

Synonym. Stylophorin
[5bR-(5bα,6β,12bα)]-5b,6,7,12b,13,14-Hexahydro-13-methyl[1,3]-benzodioxolo[5,6-c]-1,3-dioxolo[4,5-i]phenanthridin-6-ol
$C_{20}H_{19}NO_5$=353.4
CAS—476-32-4

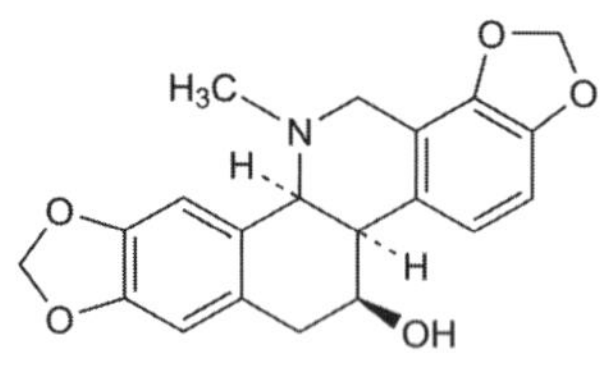

(+)-form

An alkaloid obtained from the greater celandine, *Chelidonium majus* (Papaveraceae).
A white crystalline powder. M.p. 135° to 136°.
Practically insoluble in water; soluble in ethanol, chloroform, and ether.

Partition Coefficient. Log *P* (octanol/water), 2.9.

Colour Tests. Mandelin's Test—yellow→green; Marquis Test—green; Sulfuric Acid—brown.

Thin-layer Chromatography. System TA—Rf 72. (Acidified iodoplatinate solution, positive.)

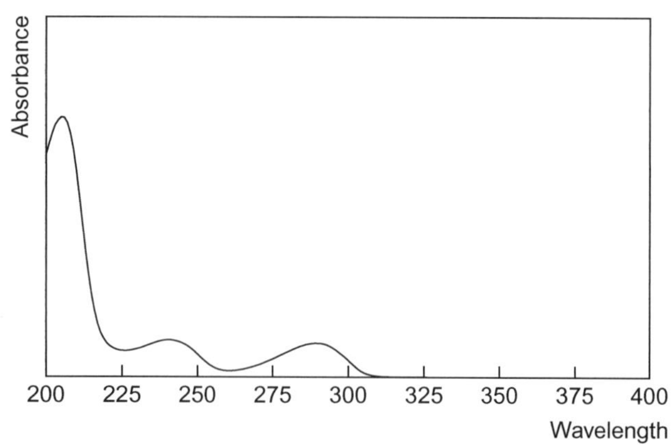

Infra-red Spectrum. Principal peaks at wavenumbers 1035, 1257, 1222, 1497, 748, 1070 cm^{-1} (KBr disk).

Mass Spectrum. Principal ions at *m/z* 332, 333, 304, 335, 176, 303, 334, 162.

Chlorambucil

Antineoplastic

Synonyms. CB-1348; Chlorbutinum.
Proprietary names. Chloraminophène; Leukeran.
4-[Bis(2-chloroethyl)amino]benzenebutanoic acid
$C_{14}H_{19}Cl_2NO_2$=304.2
CAS—305-03-3

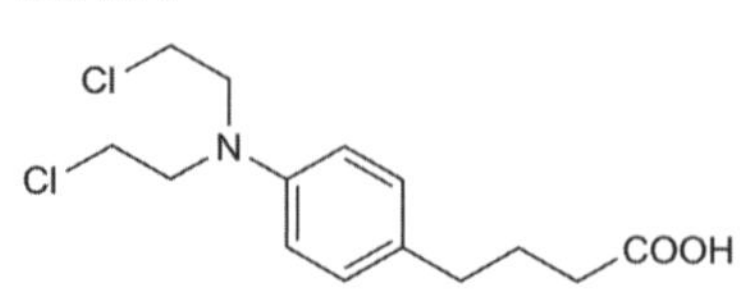

A white crystalline or granular powder. M.p. 66°.
Practically insoluble in water; soluble 1 in 1.5 of ethanol, 1 in 2 of acetone, and 1 in 2.5 of chloroform; soluble in ether.
Caution. Chlorambucil is irritant; avoid contact with skin and mucous membranes.

Dissociation Constant. pK_a 5.8.

Partition Coefficient. Log *P* (octanol/pH 7.4), 1.7.

Thin-layer Chromatography. system TD—Rf 33; system TE—Rf 06; system TF—Rf 40; System TAD—Rf 50; system TAE—Rf 84.

Gas Chromatography. System GA—chlorambucil RI 2420, chlorambucil-Me RI 2340.

High Performance Liquid Chromatography. System HAA—retention time, 22.4 min.

Ultraviolet Spectrum. Methanol—258 (A^1_1=642a), 303 nm. No alkaline shift.

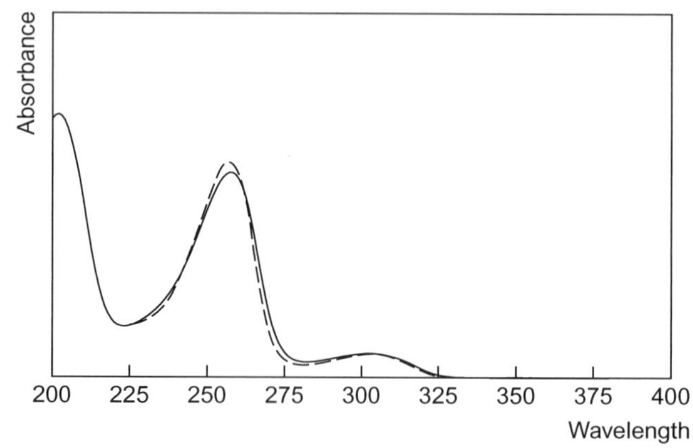

Infra-red Spectrum. Principal peaks at wavenumbers 1695, 1520, 1229, 1610, 1175, 1270 cm^{-1} (KBr disk).

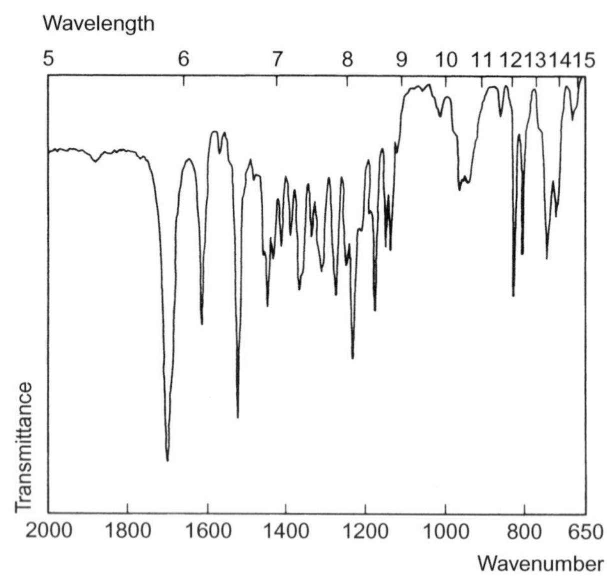

Mass Spectrum. Principal ions at *m/z* 254, 256, 118, 255, 303, 305, 63, 45.

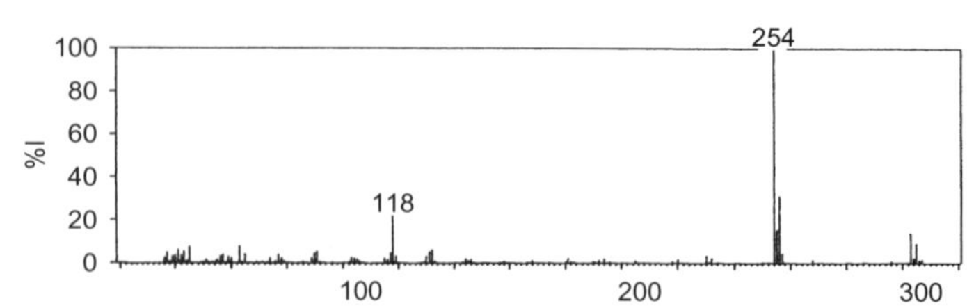

Quantification

Gas chromatography–mass spectrometry. In plasma: limit of detection <10 mg/L—H. Ehrsson *et al.*, *J. Pharm. Sci.*, 1980, *69*, 710–712.

High performance liquid chromatography. In plasma: limit of detection 100 mg/L, UV detection—A. E. Ahmed *et al.*, *J. Chromatogr.* 1982, *233(22) B Biomed. Appl.*, 392–397. In serum and plasma: limit of detection 4 to 800 mg/L for drug and metabolites, MS/MS—I.D. Davies *et al.*, *J. Chromatogr. B Biomed. Sci. Appl.*, 1999, *732(1)*, 173–184.

Disposition in the Body. Rapidly absorbed after oral administration with peak plasma concentrations being attained in 0.5 to 2 h. It is extensively metabolised; less than 1% of a dose is excreted in the urine unchanged. Phenylacetic acid mustard is a major metabolite.

Therapeutic concentration

A single oral dose of 0.2 mg/kg (three different formulations tested: UK, US, and worldwide) was administered to healthy volunteers. Mean peak plasma drug concentrations of 475, 575, and 534 mg/L were observed for the three different formulations, respectively, and 340, 381, and 338 mg/L for the major metabolite, respectively. [I.D. Davies *et al.*, *J. Chromatogr. B Biomed. Sci. Appl.*, 1999, *732(1)*, 173–184.]

Half-life. Plasma half-life, about 1 to 2 h.

Dose. Initially 200 µg/kg daily, by mouth; maintenance, 30 to 100 µg/kg daily.

Chloramphenicol

Antibiotic

Synonyms. Chloranfenicol; Cloranfenicol; Laevomycetinum.
Proprietary names. Amphicol; Chloromycetin; Chloroptic; Econochlor; Fenicol; Kemicetine; Novochlorocap; Sno Phenicol.
2,2-Dichloro-*N*-[(1*R*,2*R*)-2-hydroxy-1-(hydroxymethyl)-2-(4-nitrophenyl)ethyl]acetamide
$C_{11}H_{12}Cl_2N_2O_5$=323.1
CAS—56-75-7

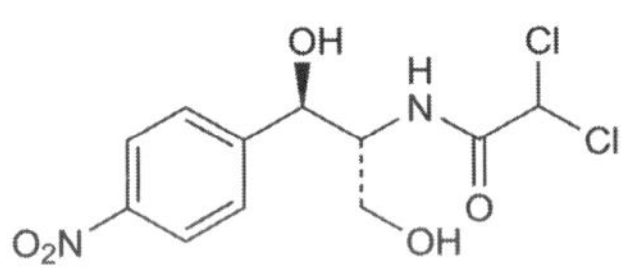

Fine, white to greyish-white or yellowish-white crystals. M.p. 149° to 153°. A solution in dehydrated alcohol is dextrorotatory and a solution in ethyl acetate is laevorotatory.
Soluble 1 in 400 of water and 1 in 2.5 of ethanol; very soluble in acetone and ethyl acetate; slightly soluble in chloroform and ether.

Chloramphenicol Cinnamate

$C_{20}H_{18}Cl_2N_2O_6$=453.3
CAS—14399-14-5
A white or yellowish-white crystalline powder. M.p. about 119°.
Very slightly soluble in water; soluble 1 in 25 of ethanol, 1 in 50 of chloroform, and 1 in 500 of ether.

Chloramphenicol Palmitate

Synonyms. Chloramphenicol α-Palmitate; Palmitylchloramphenicol.
Proprietary names. Chloromycetin Palmitate Suspension; Globenicol.
$C_{27}H_{42}Cl_2N_2O_6$=561.5
CAS—530-43-8
A fine, white, unctuous, crystalline powder. M.p. 87° to 95°.
Very slightly soluble in water; soluble 1 in 45 of ethanol, 1 in 6 of chloroform, and 1 in 14 of ether; freely soluble in acetone; soluble in ethyl acetate.

Chloramphenicol Sodium Succinate

Synonym. Chloramphenicol α-Sodium Succinate
Proprietary names. Chloromycetin Succinate; Globenicol; Kemicetine Succinate; Mychel-S.
$C_{15}H_{15}Cl_2N_2NaO_8$=445.2
CAS—982-57-0
A white or yellowish-white hygroscopic powder.
Soluble 1 in less than 1 of water and 1 in 1 of ethanol; practically insoluble in chloroform and ether.

Dissociation Constant. pK_a 5.5.

Partition Coefficient. Log *P* (octanol/water), 1.1.

Colour Tests. Fujiwara Test—red; Nessler's Reagent—brown-orange.

Thin-layer Chromatography. System TA—Rf 69; system TB—Rf 00; system TC—Rf 31; system TD—Rf 11; system TE—Rf 36; system TF—Rf 31; system TL—Rf 48; system TAD—Rf 34; system TAE—Rf 86; system TAF—Rf 90; system TAJ—Rf 32; system TAK—Rf 08; system TAL—Rf 71.

Gas Chromatography. System GA—RI 2310.

High Performance Liquid Chromatography. System HX—RI 390; system HY—RI 336; system HAA—retention time, 14.1 min.

Ultraviolet Spectrum. Water—278 (A_1^1=298a). Chloramphenicol palmitate: dehydrated alcohol—271 (A_1^1=178a).

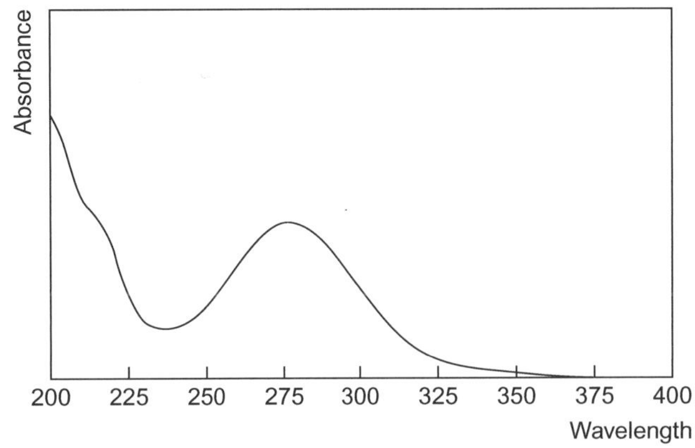

Infra-red Spectrum. Principal peaks at wavenumbers 1681, 847, 1072, 1515, 816, 1562 cm^{-1} (Nujol mull).

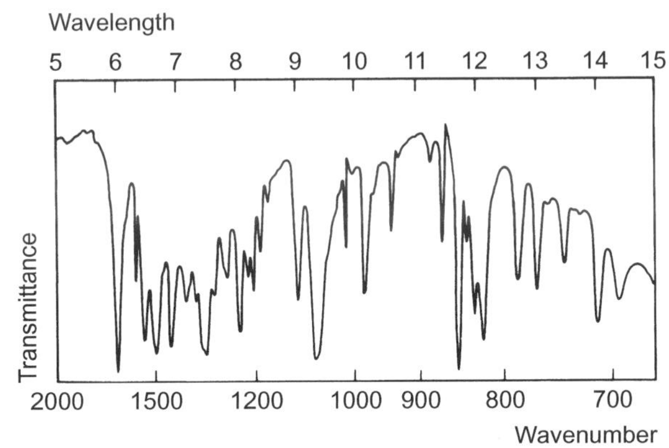

Mass Spectrum. Principal ions at *m/z* 70, 150, 151, 153, 77, 51, 118, 60.

Quantification

Gas chromatography. In cerebrospinal fluid, plasma, or urine: ECD—L. K. Pickering *et al.*, *Clin. Chem.*, 1979, *25*, 300–305. In urine: chloramphenicol or thiamphenicol and their metabolites, FID—T. Nakagawa *et al.*, *J. Chromatogr.*, 1975, *111*, 355–364.

High Performance Liquid Chromatography. In plasma: chloramphenicol and chloramphenicol succinate, limits of detection 500 µg/L for chloramphenicol and 1 mg/L for the succinate, UV detection—R. Velagapudi *et al.*, *J. Chromatogr.* 1982, *228(17) B Biomed. Appl.*, 423–428. In cerebrospinal fluid, plasma, or serum: limit of detection 100 to 200 µg/L, UV detection—R. H. B. Sample *et al.*, *Antimicrob. Agents Chemother.*, 1979, *15*, 491–493.

Disposition in the Body. Readily absorbed after oral administration. The inactive palmitate ester is hydrolysed to free drug in the gastrointestinal tract before absorption and the inactive sodium succinate ester, given parenterally, is similarly hydrolysed *in vivo*. It is widely distributed in the body, giving a concentration in the CSF about 50% of that in the blood. The main metabolic pathway is conjugation with glucuronic acid; chloramphenicol is also hydrolysed to 1-(4-nitrophenyl)-2-aminopropane-1,3-diol. Both metabolites are inactive. Up to about 90% of a dose is excreted in the urine in 24 h, mainly as the glucuronide, with about 5 to 10% of the dose in unchanged form. About 3% of the dose is excreted in the bile but this is mainly reabsorbed to give about 1% eliminated in the faeces.

Therapeutic concentration. In plasma, usually in the range 10 to 20 mg/L.

Following oral administration of chloramphenicol palmitate, equivalent to 15 to 27 mg/kg of chloramphenicol, four times a day to 18 children, plasma concentrations of 15.2 to 38.9 mg/L (mean 27.5) were reported 1.5 h after a dose. [R. E. Kauffman *et al.*, *J. Pediatr.*, 1981, *99*, 963–967.]

29 adults with uncomplicated enteric fever were administered 30 mg/kg chloramphenicol succinate ester intravenously or intramuscularly. The mean peak plasma concentrations of chloramphenicol were 16.2 and 7.8 mg/L, respectively. [G. P. Acharya *et al.*, *J. Antimicrob. Chemother.*, 1997, *40(1)*, 91–98.]

Toxicity. There is an increased incidence of reversible bone marrow depression when plasma concentrations exceed 25 mg/L. The 'grey' syndrome (cardiovascular collapse, respiratory depression, and coma) has been reported in patients with plasma concentrations in the range 40 to 200 mg/L.

A 26-year-old woman received an initial 1-g dose followed in 7 and 12 h by two 10-g doses. A plasma concentration of 201 mg/L was measured 5½ h after the last dose while she was in severe shock, but she recovered. [W. L. Thompson *et al.*, *JAMA*, 1975, *234*, 149–150.]

In a fatality involving ingestion of an unknown quantity of chloramphenicol (probably 2.5 to 4 g) by a 5-year-old boy, postmortem liver and urine concentrations of 10.7 µg/g and 2.09 g/L, respectively, were reported; death occurred about 18 h after ingestion. [E. Grusz-Harday, *Bull. Int. Assoc. Forensic Toxicol.*, 1973, *9(3 and 4)*, 10–11.]

Half-life. Plasma half-life, about 2 to 5 h.

Volume of distribution. About 0.5 to 1 L/kg.

Clearance. Plasma clearance, about 4 mL/min/kg.

Protein binding. In plasma, about 40 to 60%.

Note. For a review of the pharmacokinetics of chloramphenicol see P. J. Ambrose, *Clin. Pharmacokinet.*, 1984, *9*, 222–238.

Dose. Usually 2 g daily.

Chlorcyclizine

Antihistamine

Synonym. Histachlorazine
1-[(4-Chlorophenyl)phenylmethyl]-4-methylpiperazine
$C_{18}H_{21}ClN_2$=300.8
CAS—82-93-9

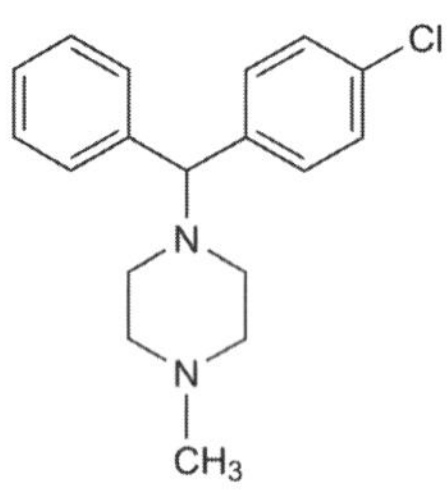

A liquid.

Chlorcyclizine Hydrochloride

Synonym. Chlorcyclizinium Chloride
Proprietary names. Di-Paralene; Trihistan. It is an ingredient of Fedrazil.
$C_{18}H_{21}ClN_2$,HCl=337.3
CAS—1620-21-9; 14362-31-3
A white crystalline powder. M.p. 226° to 227°.
Soluble 1 in 2 of water, 1 in 11 of ethanol, and 1 in 4 of chloroform; practically insoluble in ether and benzene.

Dissociation Constant. pK_a 2.4, 7.8 (25°).

Colour Test. Liebermann's Test—red-orange.

Thin-layer Chromatography. System TA—Rf 57; system TB—Rf 42; system TC—Rf 46; system TE—Rf 67; system TL—Rf 14; system TAE—Rf 35; system TAF—Rf 52; system TAJ—Rf 21; system TAK—Rf 10; system TAL—Rf 70. (Dragendorff spray, positive; acidified iodoplatinate solution, positive.)

Gas Chromatography. System GA—chlorcyclizine RI 2220, M (nor-) RI 2520; system GB—chlorcyclizine RI 2316, M (nor-) RI 2355; system GF—RI 2560.

High Performance Liquid Chromatography. System HA—*k* 2.3; system HY—RI 340.

Ultraviolet Spectrum. Aqueous acid—232 nm (A_1^1=581a).

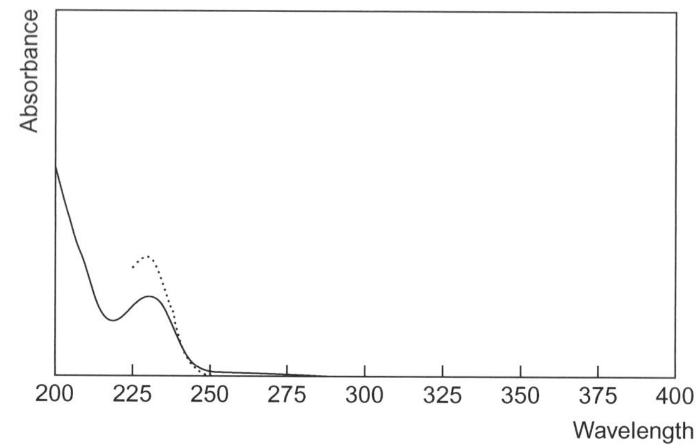

Infra-red Spectrum. Principal peaks at wavenumbers 988, 725, 760, 706, 1087, 870 cm^{-1} (chlorcyclizine hydrochloride, Nujol mull).

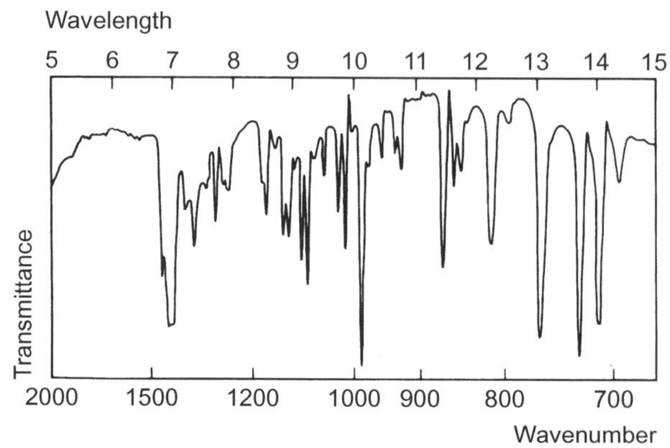

Mass Spectrum. Principal ions at *m/z* 99, 56, 72, 165, 300, 228, 229, 242.

Quantification

Colorimetry. In animal plasma or tissues: chlorcyclizine, cyclizine, and their metabolites—R. Kuntzman *et al.*, *J. Pharmacol. Exp. Ther.*, 1965, *149*, 29–35.

Disposition in the Body. Readily absorbed after oral administration and widely distributed throughout the body. Metabolised by *N*-demethylation to form norchlorcyclizine and by *N*-oxidation. High concentrations of the *N*-desmethyl metabolite are found in the liver, lungs, kidney, and spleen. Slowly excreted in the urine; measurable amounts of norchlorcyclizine have been detected in the urine for up to 3 weeks after the cessation of chronic oral administration. About 0.5% of a dose is excreted in the urine as the *N*-oxide.

Therapeutic concentration

After a single oral dose of 2 mg/kg to 4 subjects, average peak plasma concentrations of about 0.05 mg/L and 0.03 mg/L were attained in 5 h for unchanged drug and norchlorcyclizine, respectively. After oral administration of 50 mg 3 times a day for 6 days, plasma concentrations of norchlorcyclizine of 0.05 to 0.11 mg/L were reported on the first day after the cessation of treatment and plasma concentrations of 0.02 to 0.04 mg/L were found on the 10th day after cessation of treatment. [R. Kuntzman *et al.*, *Ann. N.Y. Acad. Sci.*, 1973, *226*, 131–147.]

Half-life. Plasma half-life, chlorcyclizine about 12 h, norchlorcyclizine 6 to 9 days.

Protein binding. In plasma, norchlorcyclizine, about 85 to 90%.

Dose. 50 to 200 mg of chlorcyclizine hydrochloride daily.

Chlordane

Pesticide

Synonym. Chlordan
Proprietary names. Corodane; Murphy Ant Killer; Nippon Ant Powder; Nizran; Sydane; Toxichlor. It is an ingredient of Cooper Ant Killer.
1,2,4,5,6,7,8,8-Octachloro-2,3,3a,4,7,7a-hexahydro-4,7-methano-1*H*-indene
$C_{10}H_6Cl_8$=409.8
CAS—57-74-9; 12789-03-6 (technical grade); 22212-52-8 (cis); 5103-74-2 (trans)

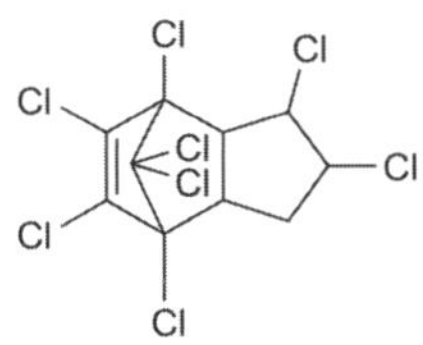

Technical chlordane is a mixture of chlorinated methano-indenes, the major components being the two stereoisomers *cis*-chlordane and *trans*-chlordane.
The technical grade is an amber viscous liquid which is decomposed by alkalis.
Insoluble in water; miscible with ethanol, chloroform, and ether.

Partition Coefficient. Log *P* (octanol/water), 6.3.

Thin-layer Chromatography. System TB—Rf 72; system TE—Rf 87; system TF—Rf 72; system TAB—Rf 64; system TAC—Rf 44; system TAE—Rf 91.

Gas Chromatography. System GA—RI 2020; system GK—*cis*-chlordane and *trans*-chlordane RRT 1.08 and 1.06, respectively (relative to caffeine).

High Performance Liquid Chromatography. system HX—RI 1017; system HAO—*k* 0; system HAP—*k* 99.9.

Infra-red Spectrum. Principal peaks at wavenumbers 704, 1265, 1020, 1075, 1612, 826 cm^{-1}.

Mass Spectrum. Principal ions at *m/z* 373, 375, 377, 371, 44, 109, 75, 272 (*cis*-chlordane); 373, 375, 377, 371, 272, 237, 75, 65 (*trans*-chlordane).

Quantification

Gas chromatography. In blood—W. E. Dale *et al.*, *Life Sci.*, 1966, *5*, 46–54.

Disposition in the Body. Readily absorbed from the gastro-intestinal tract, lungs, and the skin. It is stored in adipose tissue. Oxychlordane has been detected in adipose tissue and breast milk.

Toxicity. Severe toxicity may result after ingestion or skin contamination with greater than 1 g, and fatalities have occurred after the ingestion of more than 2 g and after excessive skin contamination. The maximum permissible atmospheric concentration is 0.5 mg/m^3.

In a non-fatal poisoning case, a 4-year-old child who ingested an unknown amount of chlordane and developed intermittent convulsions had an initial serum concentration of 3.4 mg/L which decreased to 0.14 mg/L after 72 h; the rate of decline of the serum concentration was non-linear with a terminal half-life of 88 days. Urine samples obtained during the first 3 days after ingestion showed a decrease from 1.9 mg/L to 0.05 mg/L, but increased to 0.13 mg/L on the 35th day. [F. D. Aldrich and J. M. Holmes, *Arch. Environ. Health*, 1969, *19*, 129–132.]

The following postmortem concentrations were reported in a fatality due to the ingestion of chlordane: blood 4.4 mg/L, urine 0.24 mg/L. [R. O. Bost, I. Sunshine, *Bull. Int. Assoc. Forensic Toxicol.* 1978, *14(1)*, 30.]

A 66-year-old man who ingested about 400 mL of a 70% commercial solution and died after 40 h had the following postmortem tissue concentrations: blood 1.7 mg/L, fat 378 µg/g, kidney 14 µg/g, liver 43 µg/g, urine 0.6 mg/L. [R. Morano per *Disposition of Toxic Drugs and Chemicals in Man*, 5th Edn, R. C. Baselt (Ed.), Davis, California, Biomedical Publications, 2000, pp. 150–152.]

Chlordiazepoxide

Tranquilliser

Synonyms. Chlordiazepoxidum; Clopoxide; Methaminodiazepoxide.
Proprietary names. Helogaphen; Libritabs; Librium (tablets); Multum; Omnalio; Reposans; Risolid; Silibrin; Tropium. It is an ingredient of Libraxin, Limbatril, Limbitrol and Menrium.
7-Chloro-*N*-methyl-5-phenyl-3*H*-1,4-benzodiazepin-2-amine 4-oxide
$C_{16}H_{14}ClN_3O$=299.8
CAS—58-25-3

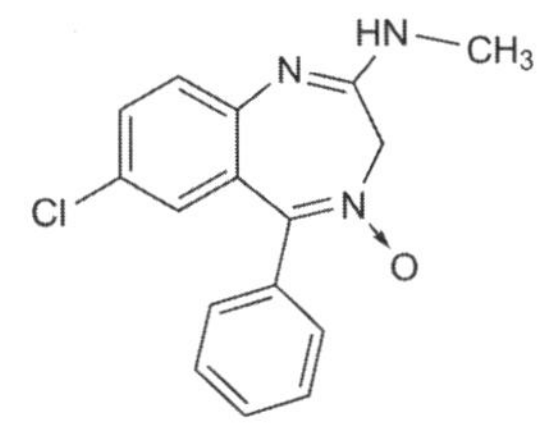

A yellow crystalline powder, sensitive to sunlight. M.p. 236° to 236.5° (from ethanol).
Practically insoluble in water; soluble 1 in 50 of ethanol and 1 in 130 of ether; slightly soluble in chloroform.

Chlordiazepoxide Hydrochloride

Proprietary names. Ansiacal; A-Poxide; Balance; Benzodiapin; Cebrum; Corax; C-Tran; Disarim; Elenium; Equibral; Labican; Librium; Medilium; Mitran; Nack; Novopoxide; O.C.M.; Psichial; Psicoterina; Relaxil; Reliberan; Reposans; Seren Vita; SK-Lygen; Solium; Trilium; Tropium; Viansin. It is an ingredient of Clindex, Librax, Limbitrol, and Menrium.
$C_{16}H_{14}ClN_3O,HCl$=336.2
CAS—438-41-5
A white or slightly yellowish crystalline powder. M.p. 213°, with decomposition. Soluble 1 in 10 of water and 1 in 40 of ethanol; practically insoluble in chloroform and ether.

Dissociation Constant. pK_a 4.8.

Partition Coefficient. Log *P* (octanol/water), 2.44.

Colour Test. Marquis Test—yellow

Thin-layer Chromatography. System TA—Rf 62; system TB—Rf 02; system TC—Rf 50; system TD—Rf 10; system TE—Rf 52; system TF—Rf 11; system TL—Rf 22; system TAD—Rf 53; system TAE—Rf 76; system TAF—Rf 77; system TAJ—Rf 48; system TAK—Rf 02; system TAL—Rf 79. (Dragendorff spray, positive; FPN reagent, yellow; acidified iodoplatinate solution, positive; Marquis reagent, yellow.)

Gas Chromatography. System GA—chlordiazepoxide RI 2795, M (nor-) RI 2452, M (demoxepam) RI 2529, nordazepam RI 2490, oxazepam RI 2325; system GB—chlordiazepoxide RI 2981, M (nor-) RI 2679, M (demoxepam) RI 2806; system GG—chlordiazepoxide RI 3065, nordazepam RI 3041, oxazepam RI 2803.

High Performance Liquid Chromatography. System HI—chlordiazepoxide *k* 6.41, demoxepam *k* 2.42, M (nor-) *k* 4.47, nordazepam *k* 8.00, oxazepam *k* 4.62; system HK—chlordiazepoxide *k* 2.87, demoxepam *k* 0.03, M (nor-) *k* 2.39, nordazepam *k* 1.99, oxazepam *k* 0.73; system HX—RI 363; system HY—RI 285; system HZ—retention time 3.2 min; system HAA—retention time 15.2 min; system HAF—retention time 21.0 min; system HAL—retention time 7.7 min; system HAM—retention time 3.1 min; system HAX—retention time 6.9 min; system HAY—retention time 5.3 min; system HAZ—*k* 1.68; system HBH—*k* 6.68; system HBI—*k* 1.65.

Ultraviolet Spectrum. Aqueous acid—246 nm (A_1^1=1112a), 308 nm; aqueous alkali—262 nm.

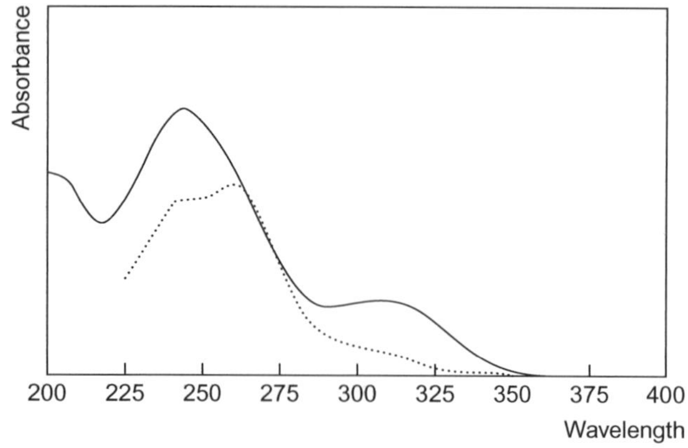

Infra-red Spectrum. Principal peaks at wavenumbers 1625, 760, 1260, 690, 1590, 850 cm^{-1} (KBr disk).

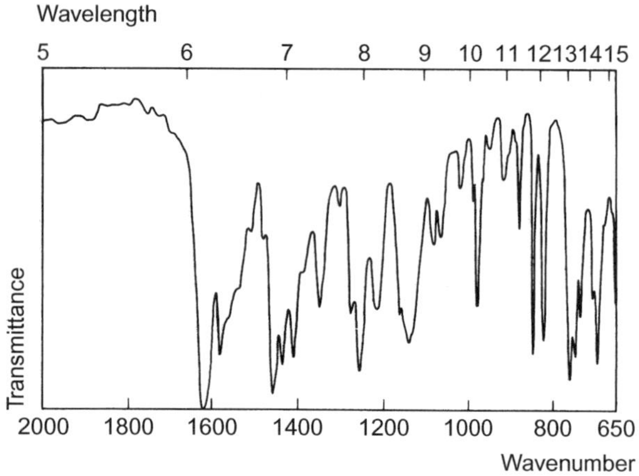

Mass Spectrum. Principal ions at *m/z* 282, 299, 284, 283, 241, 56, 301, 253; demoxepam 285, 286, 269, 287, 241, 242, 77, 270; desmethylchlordiazepoxide 285, 268, 284, 77, 286, 42, 287, 233; desmethyldiazepam (nordazepam) 242, 269, 270, 241, 243, 271, 244, 272; oxazepam 257, 77, 268, 239, 205, 267, 233, 259.

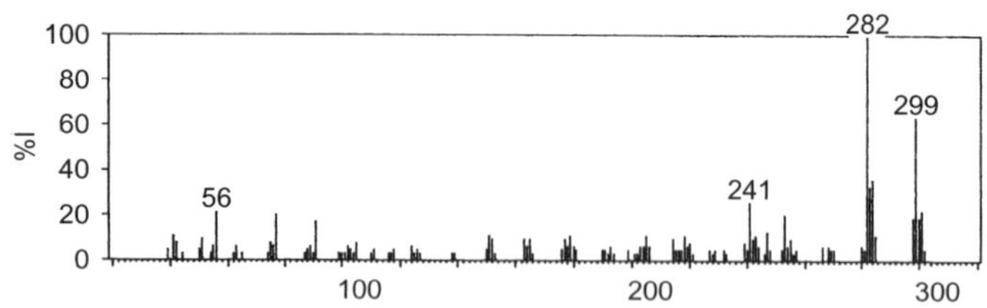

Quantification

Gas chromatography. In serum: chlordiazepoxide and demoxepam, limit of detection 45 µg/L for chlordiazepoxide, ECD—S. R. Sun and D. J. Hoffman, *J. Pharm. Sci.*, 1978, *67*, 1647–1648. In plasma or whole blood: chlordiazepoxide and other benzodiazepines, NPD and ECD—P. Lillsunde and T. Seppala, *J. Chromatogr.*, 1990, *533*, 97–110. In plasma: chlordiazepoxide and other anxiolytics, NPD and ECD—Y. Gaillard *et al.*, *J. Chromatogr.*, 1993, *622*, 197–208.

High performance liquid chromatography. In plasma or urine: chlordiazepoxide and four metabolites, limit of detection 20 µg/L for all compounds, UV detection—T. B. Vree *et al.*, *J. Chromatogr.* 1981, *224*(13) *B Biomed. Appl.*, 519–525. In serum: chlordiazepoxide and other benzodiazepines, UV detection—E. Tanaka *et al.*, *J. Chromatogr.* 1996, *682 B Biomed. Appl.*, 173–178 and E. Tanaka *et al.*, *J. Chromatogr. B Biomed. Appl.*, 1998, *709*, 324.

Radioimmunoassay. In blood, plasma, or saliva: limit of detection 50 µg/L in blood or plasma and 500 ng/L in saliva—R. Dixon *et al.*, *J. Pharm. Sci.*, 1979, *68*, 261.

Disposition in the Body. Readily absorbed after oral administration;. Peak plasma levels are found after 1 to 2 h. Metabolised by demethylation and subsequent deamination to the active metabolites desmethylchlordiazepoxide and demoxepam. Demoxepam is further metabolised by hydrolysis with cleavage of the lactam ring and by reduction to desmethyldiazepam (nordazepam) followed by hydroxylation to oxazepam (desmethyldiazepam and oxazepam are also pharmacologically active). About 60% of a dose is excreted in the urine and 10 to 20% is eliminated in the faeces; less than 1% of a dose is excreted in the urine unchanged, about 6% is excreted as demoxepam, and the remainder as ring-opened derivatives and glucuronide conjugates of oxazepam and other hydroxylated metabolites. Chlordiazepoxide passes into the cerebrospinal fluid and breast milk and crosses the placenta.

Therapeutic concentration. In plasma, usually in the range 0.4 to 4 mg/L. Demoxepam and desmethyldiazepam may accumulate in the plasma of patients on chronic therapy; demoxepam is not normally detectable in plasma after a single dose of chlordiazepoxide.

Following a single oral dose of 20 mg to 6 subjects, peak plasma concentrations of 0.78 to 1.24 mg/L (mean 1.0) of chlordiazepoxide were attained in 2 to 6 h; desmethylchlordiazepoxide was detectable 5 h after the dose and peak plasma concentrations of 0.14 to 0.46 mg/L (mean 0.3) were attained in 8 to 24 h. [M. A. Schwartz *et al.*, *J. Pharm. Sci.*, 1971, *60*, 1500–1503.]

Following daily oral administration of 10 mg 3 times a day to 8 subjects, mean steady-state plasma concentrations were: chlordiazepoxide 0.5 to 1.0 mg/L (mean 0.8), desmethylchlordiazepoxide 0.3 to 0.8 mg/L (mean 0.5), demoxepam 0.24 to 0.44 mg/L (mean 0.36). [H. G. Boxenbaum *et al.*, *J. Pharmacokinet. Biopharm.*, 1977, *5*, 25–39.]

Toxicity. Toxic reactions may be produced by plasma concentrations greater than 3 mg/L; plasma concentrations in the region of 20 mg/L may produce coma or death, but fatalities caused by chlordiazepoxide alone are rare. Recoveries have occurred after the ingestion of single doses of about 2 g.

The following postmortem chlordiazepoxide tissue concentrations were reported in a fatality in which death occurred 18 to 20 h after the ingestion of an unknown quantity of chlordiazepoxide: blood 26.4 mg/L, bile 39 mg/L, kidney 11 µg/g, liver 10 µg/g, spleen 9 µg/g, urine 7.8 mg/L. [H. Moheni, *Bull. Int. Assoc. Forensic Toxicol.*, 1975, *11(2)*, 17–18.]

The following peak plasma concentrations were observed in a comatose adult subject who had ingested 1 g: chlordiazepoxide 20 mg/L after 6 h, desmethylchlordiazepoxide 12 mg/L after 21 h, demoxepam 9 mg/L after 51 h. [J. A. F. de Silva and L. D'Arconte, *J. Forensic Sci.*, 1969, *14*, 184–202.]

Bioavailability. Almost 100%.

Half-life. Plasma half-life, chlordiazepoxide 5 to 30 h (mean 15), demoxepam 14 to 95 h (mean 40), desmethyldiazepam about 40 to 100 h, but there is considerable intersubject variation—see under Nordazepam.

Volume of distribution. 0.3 to 0.6 L/kg.

Clearance. Plasma clearance, about 0.5 mL/min/kg.

Saliva. Plasma:saliva ratio, about 33.

Protein binding. In plasma, about 96%.

Note. For a review of the pharmacokinetics of chlordiazepoxide see D. J. Greenblatt *et al.*, *Clin. Pharmacokinet.*, 1978, *3*, 381–394. For a general review of benzodiazepines see N. S. Miller and M. S. Gold, *Adv. Alcohol Subst. Abuse*, 1990, *8*, 67–84.

Dose. In the treatment of anxiety 30 to 100 mg daily. For symptoms of alcohol withdrawal up to a maximum of 300 mg daily.

Chlorhexidine

Cationic Disinfectant

Proprietary names. Hexol. It is an ingredient of Cetal (liquid).

N,N''-Bis(4-chlorophenyl)-3,12-diimino-2,4,11,13-tetraazatetradecanediimidamide

$C_{22}H_{30}Cl_2N_{10}$=505.5
CAS—55-56-1

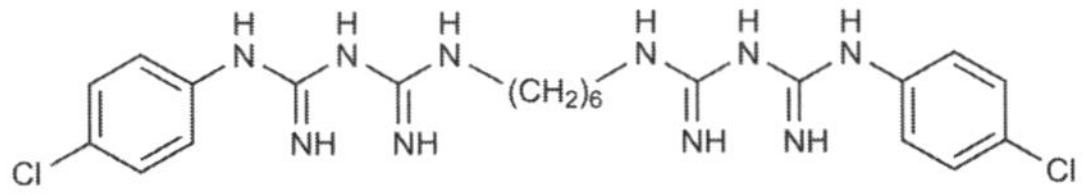

Crystals. M.p. 134°.

Chlorhexidine Acetate
Proprietary names. Chlorasept 2000; Hibitane (powder); Nolvasan.
$C_{22}H_{30}Cl_2N_{10},2C_2H_4O_2$=625.6
CAS—56-95-1
A white to pale cream microcrystalline powder. M.p. 154° to 155°. When heated it decomposes with the production of trace amounts of 4-chloroaniline. Aqueous solutions slowly decompose.
Soluble 1 in 55 of water and 1 in 15 of ethanol; soluble in glycerol and propylene glycol.

Chlorhexidine Gluconate Solution
Proprietary names. Corsodyl; Dispray; Hibicare; Hibiclens; Hibidil; Hibiscrub; Hibisol; Hibitane (solution); pHiso-MED; Rotersept. It is an ingredient of Cyteal, Eludril, Savloclens, Savlodil, Savlon (liquid), and Stomosol.
An aqueous solution containing 19 to 21% of $C_{22}H_{30}Cl_2N_{10}$, $2C_6H_{12}O_7$(=897.8).
CAS—18472-51-0 (chlorhexidine gluconate)
A colourless to pale straw-coloured liquid which is affected by light. Mass per mL 1.06 to 1.07 g.
Miscible with water, with up to 5 parts of ethanol, and with up to 3 parts of acetone.

Chlorhexidine Hydrochloride
Proprietary names. Hibitane (powder); Lisium; Sterilon (powder).
$C_{22}H_{30}Cl_2N_{10},2HCl$=578.4
CAS—3697-42-5
A white crystalline powder, affected by light. M.p. 260° to 262°, with decomposition.
Soluble 1 in 1700 of water, 1 in 450 of ethanol, and 1 in 50 of propylene glycol; slightly soluble in methanol.

Dissociation Constant. pK_a 10.8 (25°).

Partition Coefficient. Log *P* (octanol/water), 0.1.

Colour Test. Stir a small quantity on a white tile with a drop of bromine solution followed by a drop of sodium hydroxide solution—red.

Thin-layer Chromatography. System TA—Rf 33; system TB—Rf 00; system TE—Rf 13; system TAE—Rf 01. (Acidified iodoplatinate solution, positive.)

High Performance Liquid Chromatography. System HX—RI 398; system HY—RI 305; system HAA—retention time, 13.5 min.

Ultraviolet Spectrum. Aqueous acid—245 nm; aqueous alkali (pH 10)—232, 253 nm. (See below)

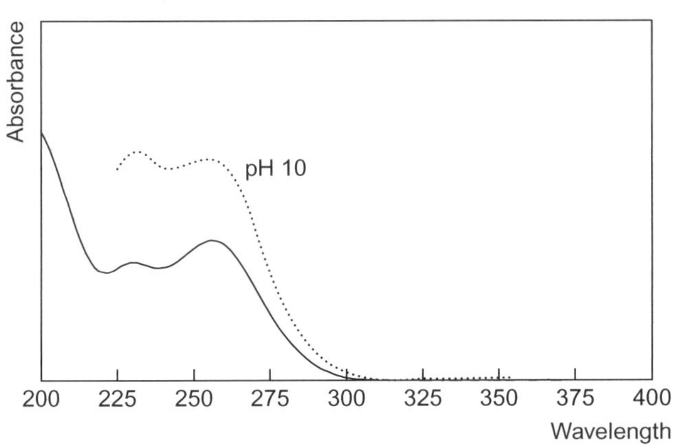

Infra-red Spectrum. Principal peaks at wavenumbers 1527, 1628, 1575, 1235, 820, 1080 cm^{-1} (KBr disk). (See below)

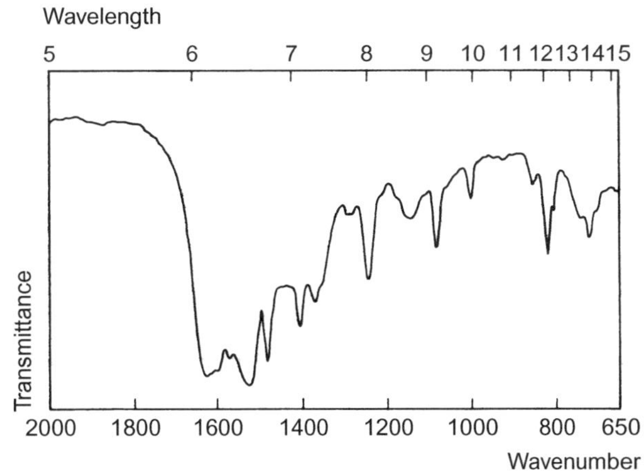

Quantification
High performance liquid chromatography. In blood, serum, or urine: limit of detection 1 mg/L, UV detection—C. E. Huston *et al.*, *J. Chromatogr.*, 1982, *237*, 457–464. In saliva: limit of quantification 50 μg/L, UV detection—H. Tsuchiya *et al.*, *Caries Res.*, 1999, *33(2)*, 156–163. In saliva—T. Pesonen *et al.*, *J. Chromatogr.* 1995, *665(1) B Biomed. Appl.*, 222–225. In serum: limit of detection 0.05 mg/L, UV detection (λ=260 nm)—K. Kudo *et al.*, *J. Anal. Toxicol.*, 2002, *26(2)*, 119–122.

Disposition in the Body
Toxicity
A 58-year-old Japanese woman suffering from articular rheumatism underwent synovectomy on her finger. While in hospital she received an injection of antibiotics. 20 min later she went into cardiac arrest and after 100 min she died. A concentration of chlorhexidine was detected in the serum taken from the right side of her heart at a level of 39.5 mg/L only 27 h after death. [K. Kudo *et al.*, *J. Anal. Toxicol.*, 2002, *26(2)*, 119–122.]

Use. Chlorhexidine gluconate is used in solutions containing 0.01 to 0.5%.

Chlormadinone Acetate
Progestational Steroid

Proprietary names. Chronosym; Cormin; Cyclonorm; Fertiletren; Gestafortin; Lutéran; Matrol; Traslan.
17-(Acetyloxy)-6-chloropregna-4,6-diene-3,20-dione
$C_{23}H_{29}ClO_4$=404.9
CAS—1961-77-9 (chlormadinone); 302-22-7 (acetate)

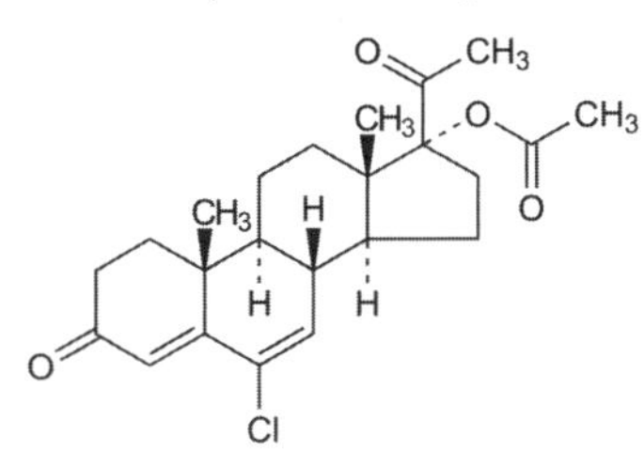

A white to creamy-white, fluffy, crystalline powder. M.p. 208° to 212°.
Practically insoluble in water; soluble 1 in 160 of ethanol, 1 in 1.5 of chloroform, and 1 in 210 of ether.

Partition Coefficient. Log *P* (octanol/water), 4.0.

Gas Chromatography. System GA—chlormadinone-H_2O RI 3340, chlormadinone acetate RI 3360.

High Performance Liquid Chromatography. System HAA—retention time, 24.1 min (chlormadinone).

Ultraviolet Spectrum. Methanol—285 nm (A_1^1=575b).

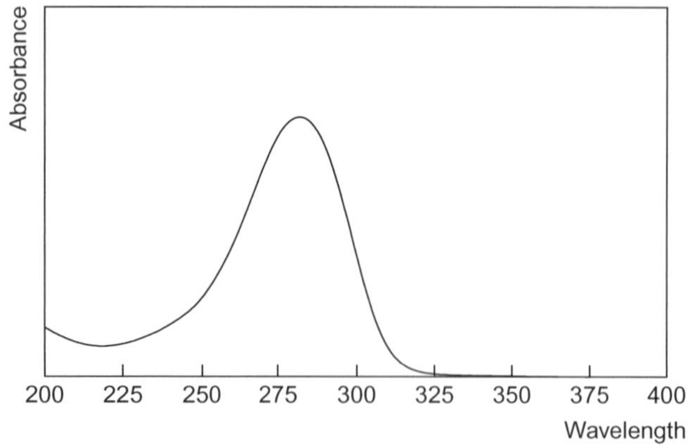

Infra-red Spectrum. Principal peaks at wavenumbers 1238, 1724, 1646, 1219, 881, 1597 cm^{-1} (KBr disk).

Dose. Chlormadinone acetate has been given in doses of 2 to 10 mg daily.

Chlormezanone

Tranquilliser

Synonyms. Chlormethazanone; Chlormezanonum; Dichloromethazanone.
Proprietary names. Trancopal. It is an ingredient of Arcanaflex; Besaprin; Beserol; Clormetadone; Lobak; Trancogesic and Trancoprin.
2-(4-Chlorophenyl)tetrahydro-3-methyl-4*H*-1,3-thiazin-4-one 1,1-dioxide
$C_{11}H_{12}ClNO_3S$=273.7
CAS—80-77-3

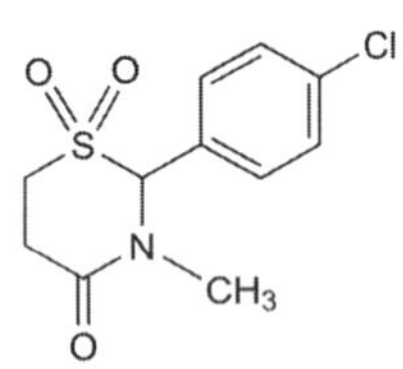

A white crystalline powder. M.p. 116.2° to 118.2°.
Very slightly soluble in water; sparingly soluble in ethanol; freely soluble in acetone and chloroform.

Partition Coefficient. Log *P* (octanol/water), -0.26.

Thin-layer Chromatography. System TA—Rf 66; system TB—Rf 01; system TC—Rf 63; system TE—Rf 68; system TL—Rf 57; system TAE—Rf 84; system TAF—Rf 80; system TAJ—Rf 55; system TAK—Rf 45; system TAL—Rf 94.

Gas Chromatography. System GA—chlormezazone RI 2199, M (4-chlorobenzoic acid) RI 1400, M (*N*-methyl-4-chlorobenzamide) RI 1555, art RI 1235; system GB—chlormezazone RI 2346, M (*N*-methyl-4-chlorobenzamide) RI 1596, art RI 1245.

High Performance Liquid Chromatography. System HY—RI 334; system HAA—Retention time 15.5 min; system HAX—Retention time 6.0 min; system HAY—Retention time 5.3 min.

Column: (analytical) RP C_{18} (Nucleosil, 120 × 4.0 mm i.d., 5 µm), (guard) RP C_{18} (20 × 4.0 mm, 5 µm). Mobile phase: acetonitrile:water: orthophosphoric acid (85%) (35:65:0.1), flow rate 1.5 mL/min. Retention time: not specified [C. Koppel *et al.*, *Eur. J. Drug Metab. Pharmacokinet.*, 1991, *16*, 43–47.]

Ultraviolet Spectrum. Aqueous acid—258, 265 (A^1_1=23b), 272; aqueous alkali—259 nm.

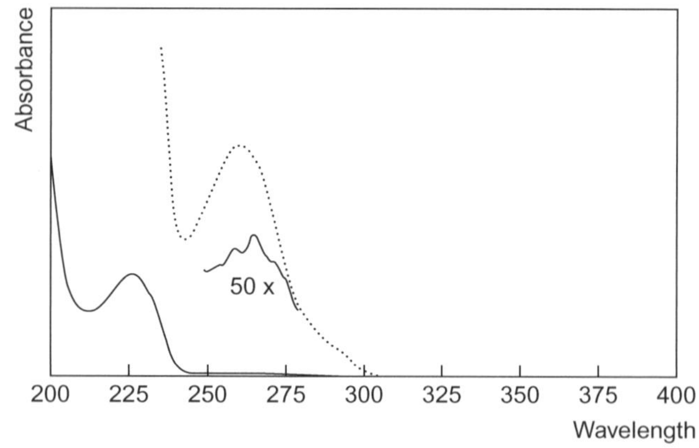

Infra-red Spectrum. Principal peaks at wavenumbers 1650, 1150, 1130, 1315, 880, 1090 cm^{-1} (KBr disk).

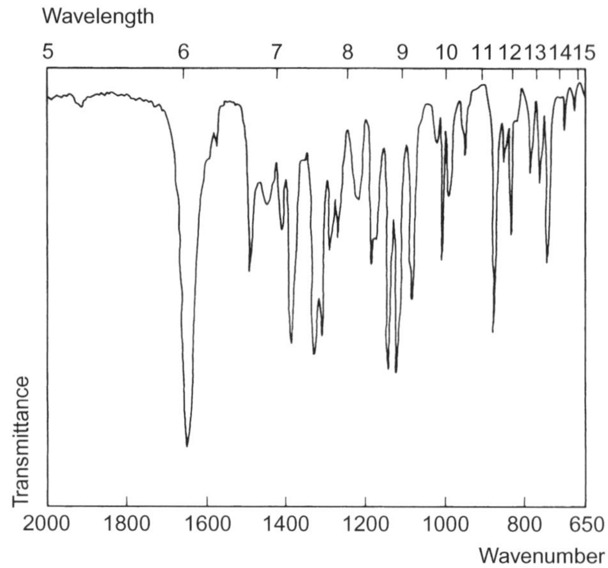

Mass Spectrum. Principal ions at *m/z* 98, 152, 154, 42, 69, 174, 208, 153.

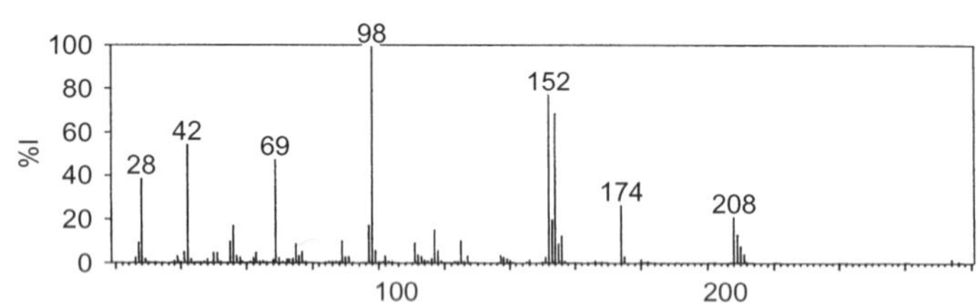

Quantification

Gas chromatography. In plasma: limit of detection 100 µg/L, ECD—K. Ohya *et al.*, *J. Chromatogr.*, 1980, *221*; *B Biomed. Appl.*, *10*, 67–74. In blood: FID—D. S. Lo *et al.*, *Forensic Sci. Int.*, 1997, *90*, 205–214.

High performance liquid chromatography. In blood: DAD—D. S. Lo *et al.*, *Forensic Sci. Int.*, 1997, *90*, 205–214.

High performance liquid chromatography–mass spectrometry. In plasma—S. L. Ali and H. Blume, *Arzneimittelforschung*, 1987, *37*, 1396–1399.

Disposition in the Body. Rapidly absorbed after oral administration, with peak plasma concentrations reached after 1 to 2 h. It appears to be metabolised by hydrolysis then oxidation to chlorobenzaldehyde and conjugation. Less than 5% of a dose is excreted in the urine as unchanged drug in 48 h; about 40% of a dose is excreted in the urine in 72 h as acidic metabolites, mainly 4-chlorohippuric acid.

Therapeutic concentration

After a single oral dose of 200 mg to 5 subjects, peak plasma concentrations of 2.5 to 3.4 mg/L (mean 2.8) were attained in about 4 h. [K. Ohya *et al.*, *J. Chromatogr.*, 1980, *221*; *B Biomed. Appl.*, *10*, 67–74.]

After a single oral dose of 200 mg to 5 subjects a mean peak plasma concentration of 1.86 mg/L was attained in 1 h. Repeated oral doses of 3 × 200 mg (12 subjects) or 4 × 400 mg (10 subjects) produced pre-dose chlormezanone plasma levels of 12.0 and 22.7 mg/L, respectively, after 5 days; levels were comparable after 10 days in 3 patients from each group. After a loading dose of 800 mg and repeated doses of 3 × 200 mg chlormezanone to 5 patients, plasma levels of 6.5, 8.9, 12.7, and 10.4 mg/L were determined after 2, 8, 16, and 36 h, respectively. [C. Koppel *et al.*, *Eur. J. Drug Metab. Pharmacokinet.*, 1991, *16*, 43–47.]

Toxicity. Chlormezanone has been withdrawn from the market in many countries because of reports of serious skin reactions.

A 39-year-old woman was found in a comatose state 6 h after ingesting chlormezanone (possibly up to 12 g). A liver biopsy revealed diffuse hydropic degeneration and necrosis of hepatocytes. Chlormezanone levels 7 to 8 h post ingestion and then every other day were as follows: 78.0, 45.9, 21.6 and 7.8 mg/L in serum and 3.8, 1.1, 0.5 mg/L then untraceable, in urine. [B. S. Sheu *et al.*, *Am. J. Gastroenterol.*, 1995, *90*, 833–835.]

In a fatality due to the combined ingestion of chlormezanone (possibly up to 11 g), diazepam (up to 200 mg) and nitrazepam (up to 80 mg), the following postmortem concentrations of chlormezanone were reported: femoral blood, 53 mg/L; brain 109 μg/g; liver, 88 μg/g and urine, 31 mg/L. [C. Koppel *et al.*, *Eur. J. Drug Metab. Pharmacokinet.*, 1991, *16*, 43–47.]

A 36-year-old woman was admitted to hospital comatose following the ingestion of 7 g of chlormezanone; an initial plasma concentration of 60 mg/L was reported, which declined with a half-life of 29 h; the patient regained consciousness after 15 h. [D. Armstrong *et al.*, *BMJ*, 1983, *286*, 845–846.]

Half-life. Plasma half-life, about 20 to 30 h.

Protein binding. In plasma, about 50%.

Note. For a review of the pharmacokinetics of chlormezanone, see V. Gautier *et al.*, *Therapie*, 1990, *45*, 315–319.

Dose. 300 to 800 mg daily in divided doses.

Chloroaniline

Insecticide

Synonym. NSC-174207
Chlorobenzenamine
$C_6H_6ClN = 127.6$
CAS—27134-26-5

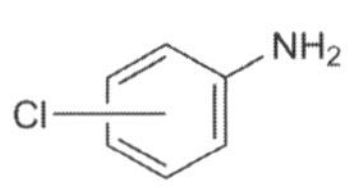

2-Chloroaniline

Synonyms. *o*-Chloroaniline; OCA.
$C_6H_6ClN = 127.6$
CAS—95-51-2
A pale amber liquid. M.p. −1.9°. B.p. 208.8°.
It is practically insoluble in water (<0.1 g/100 mL at 20°) but soluble in acid and most organic solvents.

3-Chloroaniline

Synonyms. *m*-Chloroaniline; MCA.
$C_6H_6ClN = 127.6$
CAS—108-42-9
A colourless to light amber liquid. M.p. −10.3°. B.p. 230.5°.
It is practically insoluble in water (<0.1 g/100 mL at 18°) but soluble in most common organic solvents (completely miscible in methanol and diethyl ether).

4-Chloroaniline

Synonyms. *p*-Chloroaniline; *p*-Chlorophenylamine
$C_6H_6ClN = 127.6$
CAS—106-47-8
A white to pale yellow solid. M.p. 72.5°. B.p. 232.0°.
It is practically insoluble in cold water (39 mg/100 mL) but soluble in hot water and freely soluble in alcohol, ether, acetone, and carbon disulphide.

Gas Chromatography. System GA—4-chloroaniline RI 1210.

Quantification

High performance liquid chromatography. Limit of detection of 3-chloroaniline <6 μg/L and 4-chloroaniline <14 μg/L—E. Marengo *et al.*, *J. Chromatogr. A*, 1999, *863(1)*, 1–11.

Disposition in the Body. Chloroaniline is metabolised primarily to conjugated *p*-chloroaniline (*p*-CA) and 2-amino-5-chlorophenol (2-A-5-CP). Small amounts of 2,4-dichloroaniline (2,4-DCA) and *p*-chloroformanilide (*p*-CFA) have also been detected. All metabolites and the parent chemical are excreted mainly in urine with <1% present in faeces. Accumulation can occur in the liver.

Toxicity. Hepatotoxicity, splenotoxicity, hematotoxicity, and nephrotoxicity.

Half-life. Elimination half-lives of the metabolites: *p*-CA 2.4 h, 2-A-5-CP 1.7 h, and 2,4-DCA 1.7 h.

Chlorobutanol

Preservative

Synonyms. Acetone-Chloroforme; Alcohol Trichlorisobutylicus; Chlorbutanol; Chlorbutanolum Hydratum; Chlorbutol; Chloretone; Trichlorbutanolum.
Proprietary names. Chloretone; Coliquifilm; Methaform; Sedaform.
1,1,1-Trichloro-2-methyl-2-propanol
$C_4H_7Cl_3O = 177.5$
CAS—57-15-8 (anhydrous); 6001-64-5 (hemihydrate)

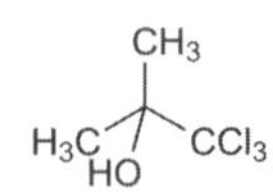

Colourless or white crystals which are volatile at ordinary temperatures.
M.p. 78°; anhydrous chlorobutanol, 97°. B.p. about 167°.
Soluble 1 in 130 of water, 1 in 1 of ethanol and 1 in 3 of chloroform; soluble in ether, acetone, and glacial acetic acid.

Partition Coefficient. Log *P* (octanol/water), 2.0.

Colour Test. Fujiwara Test—red.

Gas Chromatography. System GA—RI 949; system GI—retention time 29.8 min.

Ultraviolet Spectrum. No significant absorption, 230 to 360 nm.

Infra-red Spectrum. Principal peaks at wavenumbers 790, 833, 1145, 1186, 917, 980 cm^{-1} (Nujol mull).

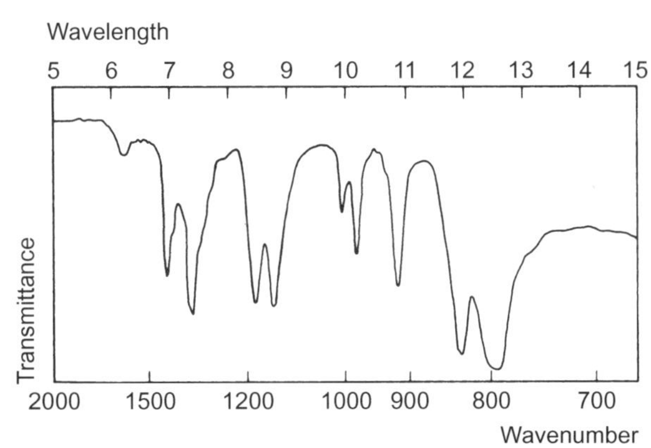

Quantification

Gas chromatography. In blood, urine, or tissues: limit of detection about 100 μg/L, ECD—J. C. Valentour and I. Sunshine, *Z. Rechtsmed.*, 1975, *77*, 61–63.

Disposition in the Body. Rapidly absorbed after oral administration, peak plasma concentrations being attained within 0.25 to 1 h. About 10% of a dose is excreted in the urine in 17 days mostly as the glucuronide and sulfate conjugates.

Toxicity.

In a non-fatal case of chlorobutanol toxicity, a man who had been taking 1 to 1.5 g daily was admitted to hospital. An initial plasma concentration of about 100 mg/L was reported and the plasma half-life was found to be about 13 days. [T. Borody *et al.*, *Med. J. Aust.*, 1979, *1*, 288.]

In a fatality caused by chlorobutanol overdose, the following postmortem tissue concentrations were found: blood 64 mg/L, bile 123 mg/L, brain 161 μg/g, kidney 87 μg/g, liver 141 μg/g, spleen 120 μg/g, urine 31 mg/L. [J. C. Valentour and I. Sunshine, *Z. Rechtsmed.*, 1975, *77*, 61–63.]

Half-life. Plasma half-life, about 10 days.

Volume of distribution. About 3 L/kg.

Protein binding. In plasma, about 50 to 60%.

Note. For a report on the pharmacokinetics of chlorobutanol see C. Tung *et al.*, *Biopharm. Drug Dispos.*, 1982, *3*, 371–378.

Uses. Chlorobutanol is used in a concentration of 0.5%. It was formerly given as a sedative in doses of 0.3 to 1.2 g.

Chlorocresol

Disinfectant

Synonyms. Chlorkresolum; Parachlorometacresol; PCMC.
Proprietary name. Wright's Vaporizing Fluid
4-Chloro-3-methylphenol
$C_7H_7ClO = 142.6$
CAS—59-50-7

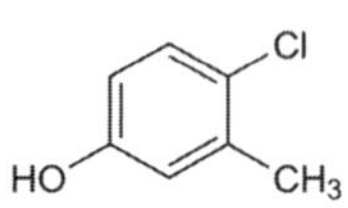

Colourless crystals or crystalline powder. It is volatile in steam. M.p. 55.5° and 66°.
Soluble 1 in 260 of water, 1 in 50 of boiling water, and 1 in 0.4 of ethanol; freely soluble in acetone, benzene, chloroform, aqueous alkaline solutions, and ether. Solutions in water acquire a yellowish colour on exposure to light and air.

Dissociation Constant. pK_a 9.6 (25°).

Partition Coefficient. Log *P* (octanol/water), 3.1.

Gas Chromatography. System GA—RI 1400.

High Performance Liquid Chromatography. System HY—RI 455.

Ultraviolet Spectrum. Aqueous acid—227, 279 nm ($A^1_1 = 105a$); aqueous alkali—244, 299 nm.

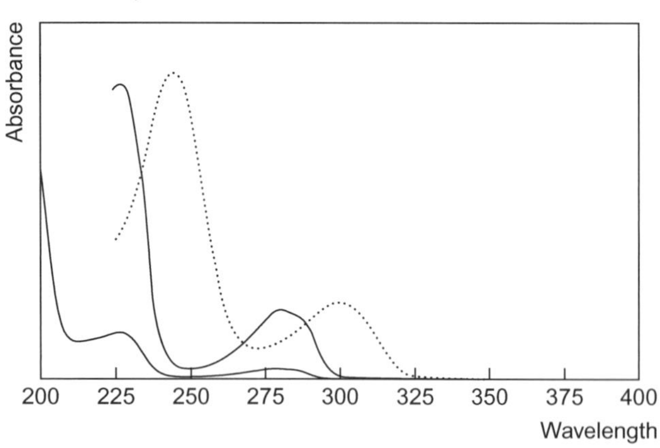

Use. In concentrations of 0.1 to 0.2%.

Chloroform

General Anaesthetic

Synonyms. Chloroformium Anaesthesicum; Chloroformum pro Narcosi. Trichloromethane
$CHCl_3 = 119.4$
CAS—67-66-3
A colourless, mobile, volatile liquid. Mass per mL 1.474 to 1.479 g. B.p. 61° to 62°. Refractive index 1.4464.
Chloroform (B.P.) contains 1 to 2% v/v of ethanol.
Soluble 1 in 200 of water; miscible with dehydrated alcohol, benzene, and ether.

Partition Coefficient. Log *P* (octanol/water), 2.0.

Colour Tests. Fujiwara Test—red; Palladium Chloride—black. Heat with a small amount of resorcinol in 2 M sodium hydroxide—red. Heat with a small amount of either alpha- or beta-naphthol—blue.

Gas Chromatography. System GA—RI 605; system GI—retention time 6.2 min.

Infra-red Spectrum. Principal peaks at wavenumbers 714, 787, 1205, 1220, 928, 1515 cm^{-1} (thin film).

Mass Spectrum. Principal ions at *m/z* 83, 85, 47, 87, 48, 49, 35, 82.

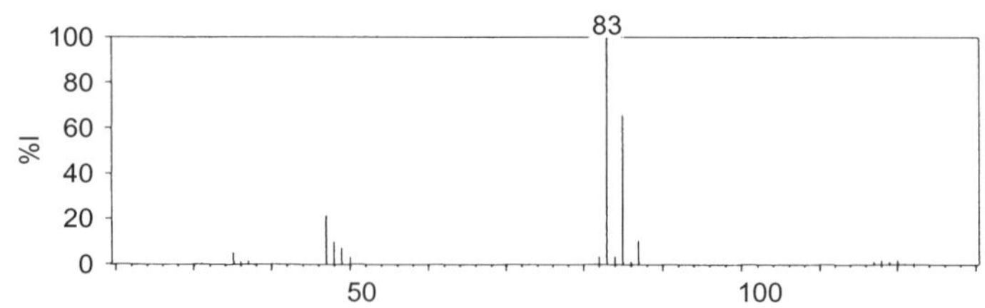

Quantification

Gas chromatography. In blood: FID—N. Poobalasingham, *Br. J. Anaesth.*, 1976, *48*, 953–956. In expired air, blood or urine: ECD—B. J. Fry *et al.*, *Arch. Int. Pharmacodyn. Ther.*, 1972, *196*, 98–111.

Disposition in the Body. Almost completely absorbed after oral administration, rapidly absorbed after inhalation and subject to first-pass metabolism in the liver and lungs. It is rapidly distributed throughout the body and is taken up by adipose tissue. Between 20 and 70% of a dose is exhaled unchanged in 8 h and up to about 50% is exhaled as carbon dioxide in the same period; less than 0.01% of a dose is excreted in the urine.

Blood concentration

After a single oral dose of 500 mg to 2 subjects, peak blood concentrations of about 1 and 5 mg/L were attained in 1 h. [B. J. Fry *et al.*, *Arch. Int. Pharmacodyn. Ther.*, 1972, *196*, 98–111.]

A mean chloroform concentration in arterial blood of 173 mg/L was reported in spontaneously breathing subjects during surgical anaesthesia. [N. Poobalasingham and J. P. Payne, *Br. J. Anaesth.*, 1978, *50*, 325–329.]

Toxicity. The minimum lethal dose is 10 mL by ingestion and the maximum permissible atmospheric concentration is 10 ppm. Exposure to air concentrations of 100 to 1000 ppm for short periods may cause discomfort and dizziness and concentrations of 7000 ppm or more will produce rapid loss of consciousness.

The following postmortem tissue concentrations were reported in 7 fatalities: blood 10 to 48 mg/L (mean 32, 7 cases); brain 50.4 to 156 μg/g (mean 101, 4 cases); kidney 16 to 27 μg/g (mean 20, 3 cases); liver 6 to 86.2 μg/g (mean 43.4, 6 cases); urine 0 to 60 mg/L (mean 15, 5 cases). [R. Bonnichsen, A. C. Maehly, *J. Forensic Sci.*, 1966, *11*, 414–427 and G. V. Giusti, M. Chiarotti, *Med. Sci. Law*, 1981, *21*, 2–3.]

A case of chloroform poisoning was reported with a blood concentration of 60 mg/kg and 14 mg/kg in the lungs in a 30-year-old male. [N. Y. Kim *et al.*, *J. Forensic Sci.*, 1996, *41(3)*, 527–529.]

Half-life. Blood half-life, about 1.5 h.

Volume of distribution. In blood, about 2 to 3 L/kg.

Clearance. Blood clearance, about 20 mL/min/kg.

Dose. Concentrations of 2 to 4% of the vapour have been used for induction and 1 to 2% for maintenance of anaesthesia.

Chloromethylaniline

Insecticide

Synonyms. Chlorotoluidine; 2-Chloro-5-methylaniline; 6-Chloro-*m*-toluidine.
2-Chloro-5-methylbenzeneamine
C_7H_8ClN=141.6
CAS—95-81-8

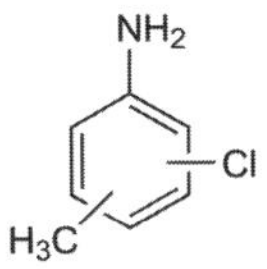

M.p. 29.5°. B.p. 228° to 229°.
It is soluble in water.

Partition Coefficient. Log *P* (octanol/water), 2.27.

Mass Spectrum. Principal ions at *m/z* 106, 141, 77, 143, 140, 142, 52, 79.

Chloronitroaniline

Insecticide

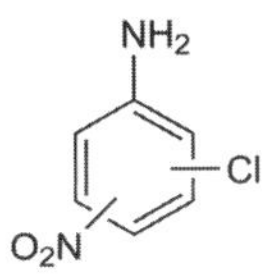

$C_6H_5ClN_2O_2$=172.6
CAS—41587-36-4

Chloronitrotoluene

Pesticide

Synonyms. α-Chloro-*p*-nitrotoluene; *p*-Nitrobenzylchloride.
1-(Chloromethyl)-4-nitrobenzene
$C_7H_6ClNO_2$=171.6
CAS—25567-68-4

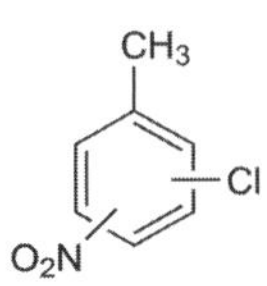

A solid. M.p. 71°.
It is insoluble in water.

Ultraviolet Spectrum. Aqueous solution—260 nm.

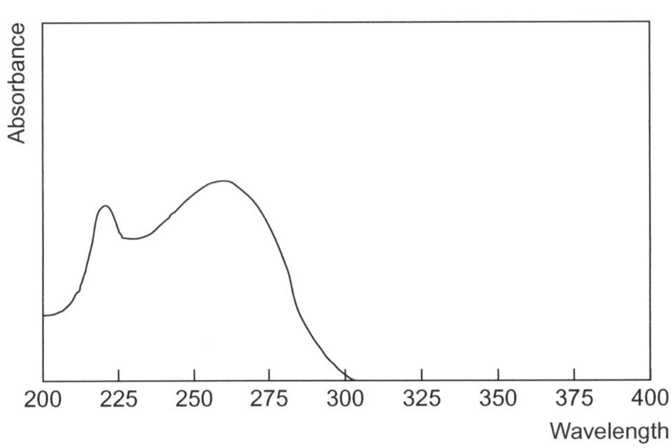

Infra-red Spectrum. Principal peaks at wavenumber 1353, 1541, 809, 719, 1263, 1609 cm^{-1}.

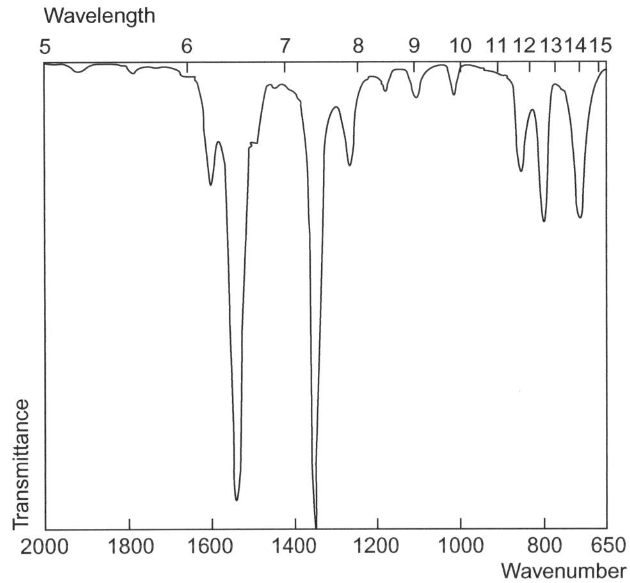

Mass Spectrum. Principal ions at *m/z* 136, 89, 171, 125, 63, 90, 78, 77.

Chloroprocaine

Local Anaesthetic

4-Amino-2-chlorobenzoic acid 2-(diethylamino)ethyl ester
$C_{13}H_{19}ClN_2O_2$=270.8
CAS—133-16-4

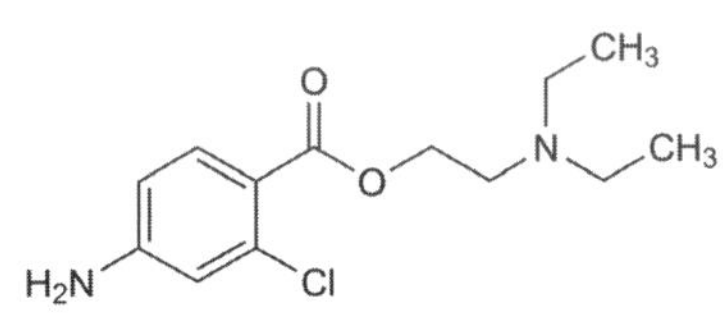

Chloroprocaine Hydrochloride
Proprietary name. Nesacaine
$C_{13}H_{19}ClN_2O_2$,HCl=307.2
CAS—3858-89-7
A white crystalline powder. M.p. 176° to 178°.
Soluble 1 in 20 of water and 1 in 100 of ethanol; very slightly soluble in chloroform; practically insoluble in ether.

Dissociation Constant. pK_a 8.7.

Partition Coefficient. Log *P* (octanol/water), 2.9.

Colour Test. Diazotisation—red.

Thin-layer Chromatography. System TA—Rf 59; system TB—Rf 05; system TC—Rf 23; system TL—Rf 37; system TAJ—Rf 09; system TAK—Rf 00; system TAL—Rf 32. (Acidified iodoplatinate solution, positive; Van Urk reagent, yellow.)

Gas Chromatography. System GA—RI 2241.

High Performance Liquid Chromatography. System HQ—*k* 0.24; system HY—RI 250.

Ultraviolet Spectrum. Aqueous acid—230 nm (A^1_1=330b), 288 nm (A^1_1=311b).

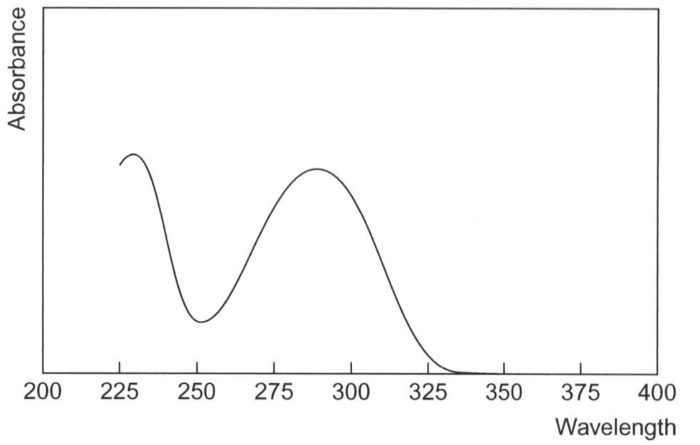

Infra-red Spectrum. Principal peaks at wavenumbers 1595, 1698, 1240, 1625, 1111, 1315 cm^{-1} (KBr disk).

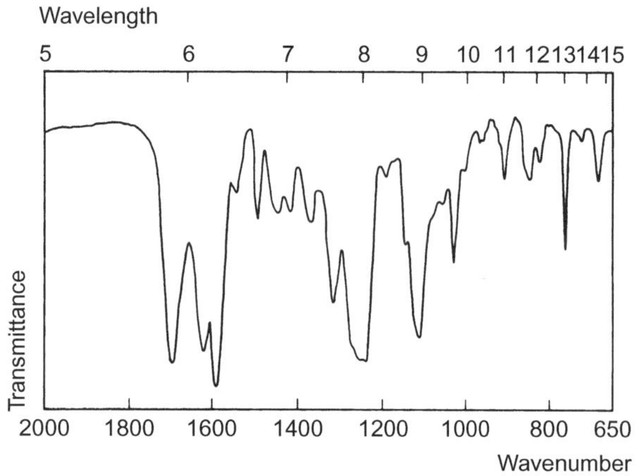

Mass Spectrum. Principal ions at *m/z* 86, 99, 154, 30, 87, 58, 29, 156.

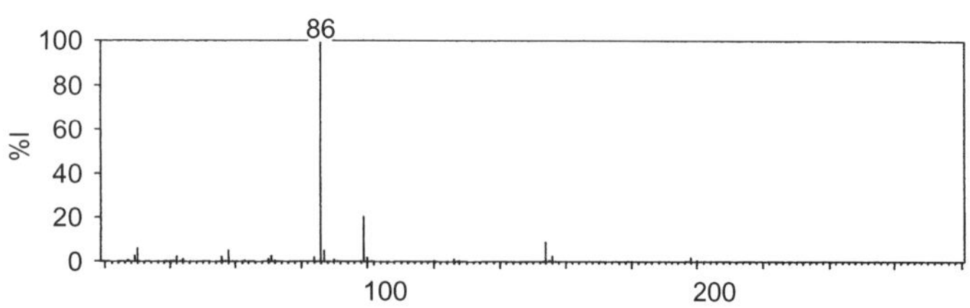

Quantification.

Gas chromatography. In plasma: limit of detection 10 µg/L, FID—J. E. O'Brien *et al.*, *J. Pharm. Sci.*, 1979, *68*, 75–78.

Gas chromatography–mass spectrometry. In plasma: limit of detection <2 µg/L—B. R. Kuhnert *et al.*, *J. Chromatogr.*, 1981, *224(13)*, *B Biomed. Appl.*, 488–491.

High performance liquid chromatography. In blood and serum: limit of detection for diethylaminoethanol 5 µg/L—Q. C. Meng *et al.*, *Reg. Anesth. Pain Med.*, 1999, *24(3)*, 242–245.

Thin-layer chromatography. In plasma, whole blood or urine: 4-amino-2-chlorobenzoic acid—J. E. O'Brien *et al.*, *J.Pharm. Sci.*, 1979, *68*, 75–78.

Disposition in the Body. Rapidly hydrolysed in the plasma to 4-amino-2-chlorobenzoic acid and 2-diethylaminoethanol. About 50% of an intravenous dose is excreted in the urine in 90 min, mainly as an unidentified conjugate (possibly the glycine conjugate) of 4-amino-2-chlorobenzoic acid.

Therapeutic concentration

After intravenous infusion of 250 mg over a period of 30 min to 3 subjects, peak plasma concentrations of 3.5 to 4.3 mg/L of 4-amino-2-chlorobenzoic acid were attained at the end of the infusion; chloroprocaine was not detectable in the plasma. [J. E. O'Brien *et al.*, *J.Pharm. Sci.*, 1979, *68*, 75–78.]

Toxicity. The maximum safe intravenous or topical dose is 750 mg.

Dose. Chloroprocaine hydrochloride is injected as a 0.5 to 3% solution.

Chloropyramine

Antihistamine

Synonyms. Chlortripelennamine; Halopyramine.
N-[(4-Chlorophenyl)methyl]-*N'*,*N'*-dimethyl-*N*-2-pyridinyl-1,2-ethanediamine
$C_{16}H_{20}ClN_3$ = 289.8
CAS—59-32-5

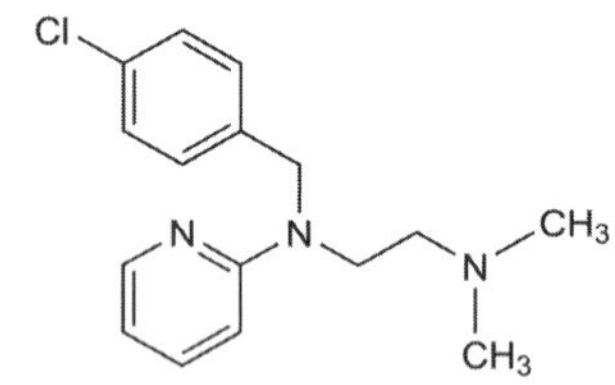

A yellow oil.

Chloropyramine Hydrochloride

Proprietary names. Alegan S; Avapena; Suprastin; Synopen; Synpen.
$C_{16}H_{20}ClN_3,HCl$ = 326.3
CAS—6170-42-9
A white powder. M.p. 172°.
Freely soluble in water, ethanol, and chloroform; practically insoluble in ether.

Partition Coefficient. Log *P* (octanol/water), 3.4.

Colour Test. Cyanogen Bromide—yellow.

Thin-layer Chromatography. System TA—Rf 52; system TB—Rf 41; system TC—Rf 28; system TE—Rf 63; system TL—Rf 17; system TAD—Rf 00; system TAE—Rf 22. (Acidified iodoplatinate solution, positive.)

Gas Chromatography. System GA—chloropyramine RI 2190; M (*N*-desalkyl-) RI 1900; M (nor-) RI 2210; M (OH-)-AC RI 2440; M (*N*-desalkyl-)-AC RI 2160; M (nor-)-AC RI 2470; M (bis-nor-)-AC RI 2420.

High Performance Liquid Chromatography. System HA—*k* 4.2.

Ultraviolet Spectrum. Aqueous acid—239 (A_1^1 = 515a), 315; aqueous alkali—248, 313 nm.

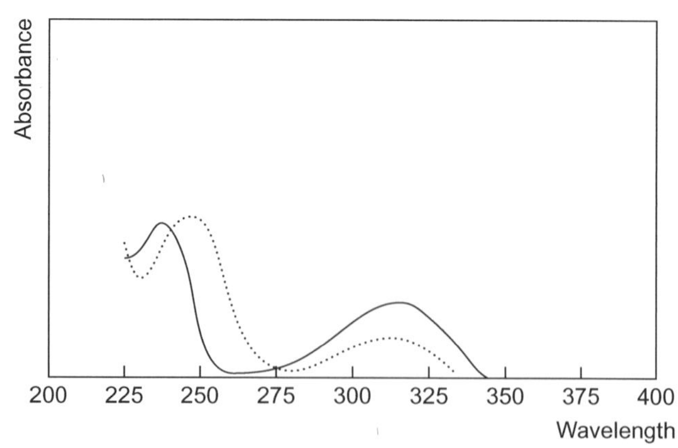

Infra-red Spectrum. Principal peaks at wavenumbers 1494, 1598, 769, 1562, 1010, 1098 cm^{-1} (KBr disk).

Mass Spectrum. Principal ions at *m/z* 58, 125, 71, 72, 36, 127, 79, 219.

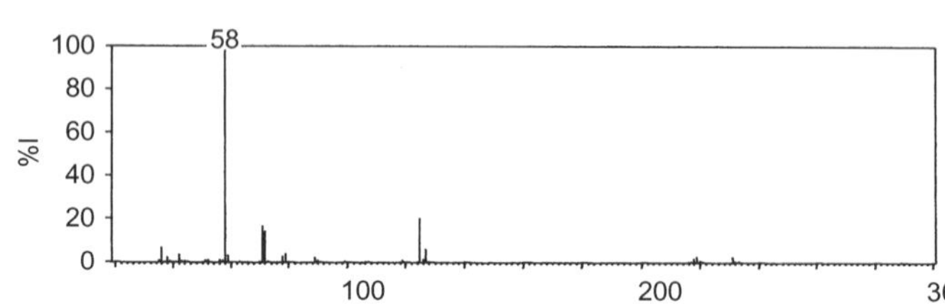

Dose. Chloropyramine hydrochloride has been given in doses of up to 150 mg daily.

Chloropyrilene

Antihistamine

Synonyms. Chloromethapyrilene; Chlorothen; Chlorpyrilen; Histachlorylene.
N-[(5-Chloro-2-thienyl)-methyl]-*N′*,*N′*-dimethyl-*N*-2-pyridinyl-1,2-ethanediamine
$C_{14}H_{18}ClN_3S$=295.8
CAS—148-65-2

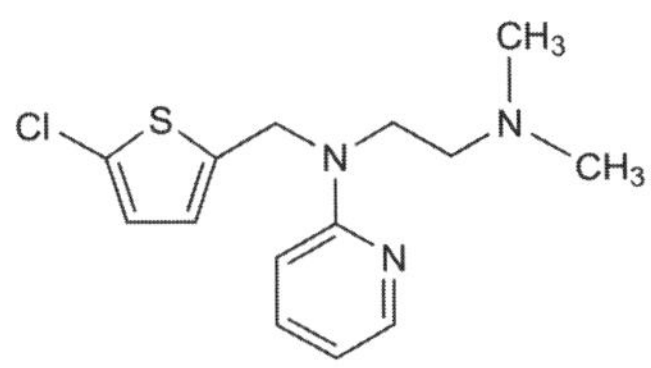

A liquid.

Chloropyrilene Citrate
Proprietary names. Panta; Tagathen.
$C_{14}H_{18}ClN_3S,C_6H_8O_7$=488.0
CAS—148-64-1
A white crystalline powder. M.p. 112° to 116°; on further heating it gradually solidifies and remelts at 125° to 140°, with decomposition.
Soluble 1 in 35 of water and 1 in about 65 of alcohol; practically insoluble in benzene, chloroform, and ether.

Dissociation Constant. pK_a 8.4 (25°).

Partition Coefficient. Log *P* (octanol/water), 3.2.

Colour Tests. Mandelin's Test—violet→orange; Marquis Test—violet.

Thin-layer Chromatography. System TA—Rf 53. (Acidified iodoplatinate solution, positive.)

Gas Chromatography. System GA—RI 2133.

High Performance Liquid Chromatography. System HA—*k* 4.0.

Ultraviolet Spectrum. Aqueous acid—237 nm (A^1_1=520c), 312 nm; aqueous alkali—243 nm (A^1_1=676b), 308 nm (A^1_1=148b).

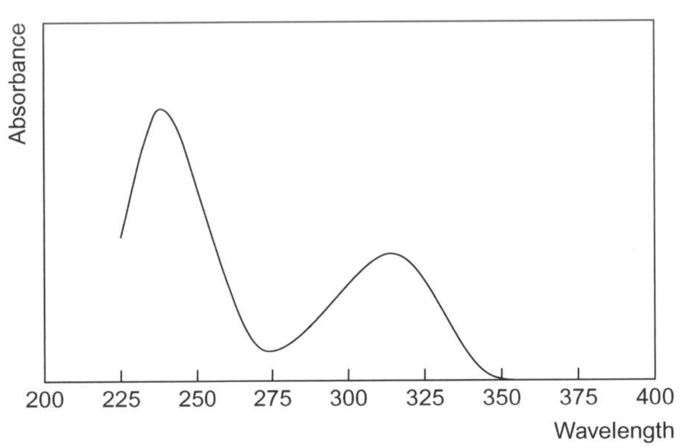

Infra-red Spectrum. Principal peaks at wavenumbers 1595, 767, 990, 1562, 1149, 1234 cm^{-1} (KBr disk).

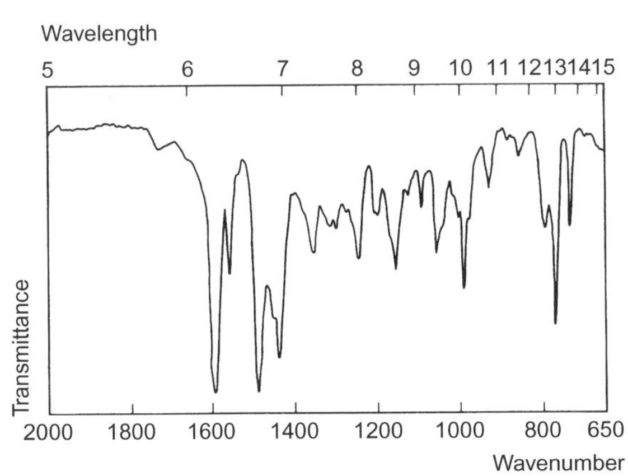

Mass Spectrum. Principal ions at *m/z* 58, 131, 72, 71, 79, 42, 30, 78.

Dose. Up to 150 mg of chloropyrilene citrate daily.

Chloroquine

Antimalarial

Synonyms. RP-3377; Cloroquina
Proprietary names. Aralen; Artrichin; Bemaphate; Capquin; Nivaquine B; Paluken; Resoquine; Reumachlor; Sanoquin.
N^4-(7-Chloro-4-quinolinyl)-N^1,N^1-diethyl-1,4-pentanediamine
$C_{18}H_{26}ClN_3$=319.9
CAS—54-05-7

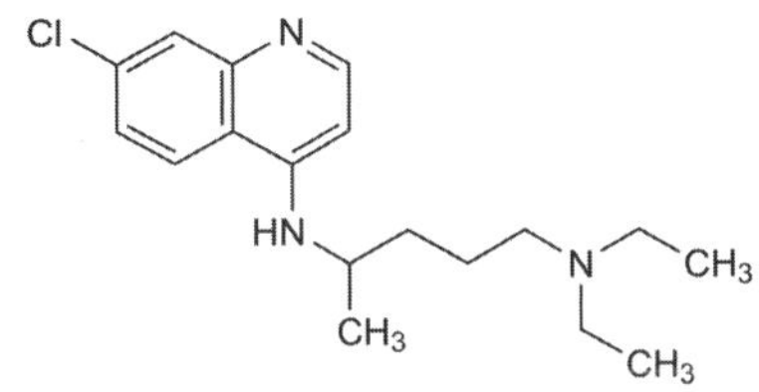

A white or slightly yellow crystalline powder. M.p. 87° to 92°.
Very slightly soluble in water; soluble in chloroform and ether.

Chloroquine Phosphate
Synonyms. SN-7618; Chingaminum; Chlorochinum Diphosphoricum; Quingamine.
Proprietary names. Anoclor; Aralen (tablets); Arechin; Avloclor; Chlorquin; Diroquine; Genocin; Heliopar; Imagon; Klorokin; Malaquin; Malarex; Malarivon; P-Roquine; Palux; Resochin(e); Tresochin; Weimerquin. It is an ingredient of Aralis; Clopirim; Savarine.
$C_{18}H_{26}ClN_3,2H_3PO_4$=515.9
CAS—50-63-5
A white powder. It discolours on exposure to light. There are 2 polymorphic forms which melt at 193° to 195° and at 215° to 218°.
Freely soluble in water, very slightly soluble or practically insoluble in alcohol, in chloroform and in ether; very slightly soluble in methyl alcohol.

Chloroquine Hydrochloride
$C_{18}H_{26}ClN_3$, 2HCl=392.8
CAS—3545-67-3

Chloroquine Sulfate
Synonyms. RP-3377; Chloroquini Sulfas; Chloroquine Sulphate; Sulfato de Cloroquina
Proprietary names. Daramal; Nivaquine; Plasmoquine. It is an ingredient of Daramal-Paludrine.
$C_{18}H_{26}ClN_3,H_2SO_4,H_2O$=436.0
CAS—132-73-0 (anhydrous)
A white or almost white crystalline powder. M.p. 205° to 210°. Protect from light.
Freely soluble in water and methyl alcohol, very slightly soluble in alcohol, practically insoluble in ether.

Dissociation Constant. pK_a 8.4, 10.8 (20°).

Partition Coefficient. Log *P* (octanol/water), 4.63.

Colour Test. Liebermann's Test (100°)—orange.

Thin-layer Chromatography. System TA—Rf 38; system TB—Rf 14; system TC—Rf 04; system TE—Rf 46; system TL—Rf 02; system TAD—Rf 00; system TAE—Rf 04; system TAF—Rf 14; system TAJ—Rf 00; system TAK—Rf 00; system TAL—Rf 04. (Acidified iodoplatinate solution, positive.)

Gas Chromatography. System GA—chloroquine RI 2605, M (desethyl-) RI 2555, M (desethyl-)-AC RI 3010; system GF—RI 3245.

High Performance Liquid Chromatography. System HA—*k* 15.2 (tailing peak); system HX—RI 282; system HY—RI 246; system HZ—Retention time 2.1 min; system HAA—Retention time 5.4 min; system HAX—Retention time 12.7 min; system HAY—Retention time 3.6 min.

Ultraviolet Spectrum. Aqueous acid—257, 329 (A^1_1=600b), 343 (A^1_1=625b); aqueous alkali—254 (A^1_1=555b), 330 nm.

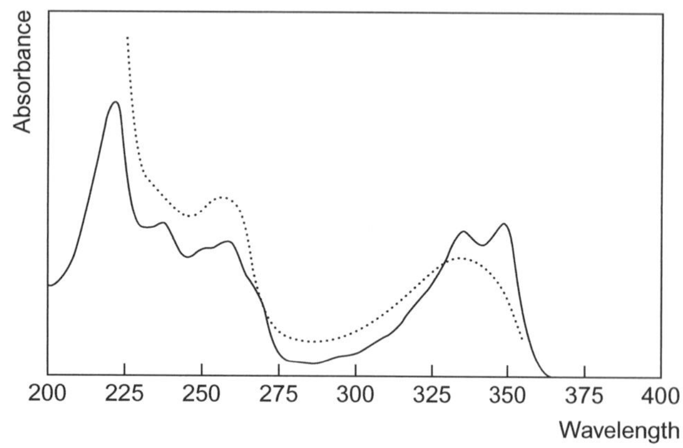

Infra-red Spectrum. Principal peaks at wavenumbers 1573, 1538, 1612, 1155, 800, 870 cm^{-1} (KBr disk).

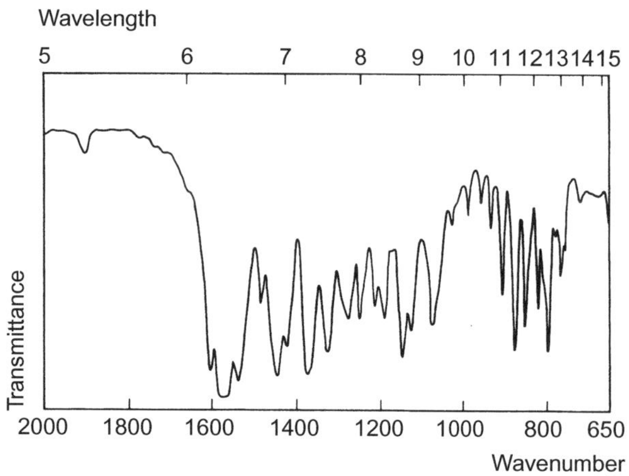

Mass Spectrum. Principal ions at *m/z* 86, 58, 319, 87, 73, 247, 245, 112.

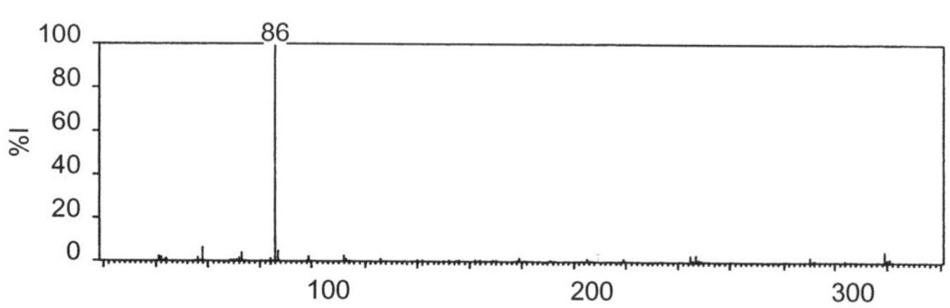

Quantification.

Spectrofluorimetry. In plasma, erythrocytes or urine: limit of detection 5 μg/L—S. A. Adelusi and L. A. Salako, *J. Pharm. Pharmacol.*, 1980, *32*, 711–712.

Gas chromatography. In plasma or blood: limit of detection 3 μg/L for chloroquine and monodesethyl-chloroquine, 10 μg/L for didesethylchloroquine, AFID—Y. Bergqvist and S. Eckerbom, *J. Chromatogr.*, 1984, *306 B Biomed. Appl.*, *31*, 147–153.

High performance liquid chromatography. In plasma: chloroquine, monodesethylchloroquine and didesethylchloroquine, limit of detection 5 ng for all compounds, UV detection—N. D. Brown *et al.*, *J. Chromatogr.*, 1982, *229 B Biomed. Appl.*, *18*, 248–254. In plasma, erythrocytes or urine: chloroquine and monodesethylchloroquine, limits of detection 1 μg/L for chloroquine and 500 ng/L for monodesethylchloroquine in plasma, fluorescence detection—G. Alvan *et al.*, *J. Chromatogr.*, 1982, *229 B Biomed. Appl.*, *18*, 241–247. In plasma, whole blood, or urine: chloroquine and its metabolites, limits of detection 1 to 2 μg/L, UV detection—P. Houze *et al.*, *J. Chromatogr.*, 1992, *574*, 305–312. In plasma: chloroquine and quinine, limit of detection 5 μg/L for chloroquine, fluorescence detection (λ_{ex}=325 nm; λ_{em}=375 nm)—J. F. Chaulet *et al.*, *J. Chromatogr.*, 1993, *613*, 303–310. In plasma: limit of quantification 2.5 μg/L, UV detection—D. Zhong *et al.*, *Pharmazie*, 1993, *48*, 349–352. In plasma: limit of quantification 6 μg/L for chloroquine, UV detection (λ=254 nm)—J. F. Chaulet *et al.*, *J. Pharm. Biomed. Anal.*, 1994, *12*, 111–117. In serum, whole blood and filter paper adsorbed dry blood: limits of quantification, 0.005 mg/L for chloroquine and hydroxychloroquine, 0.05 mg/L for quinine, fluorescence detection (λ_{ex}=215 nm, no emission filter)—K. Croes *et al.*, *J. Anal. Toxicol.*, 1994, *18*, 255–260. In serum: chloroquine and hydroxychloroquine, photodiode-array detection—P. Violin, *J. Chromatogr. B Biomed. Appl.*, 1995, *666*, 347–353. In plasma or urine: chloroquine and desethylchloroquine—O. Walker and O. G. Ademowo, *Ther. Drug Monit.*, 1996, *18*, 92–96. In liver microsomes: limit of detection for chloroquine, monodesethylchloroquine and bisdesethylchloroquine, 25 μg/L, fluorescence detection (λ_{ex}=250 nm; λ_{em}=380 nm)—J. Ducharme and R. Farinotti, *J. Chromatogr. B Biomed. Sci. Appl.*, 1997, *698*, 243–250. In plasma or blood cells—V. K. Dua *et al.*, *J. Pharm. Bimed. Anal.*, 1999, *21*, 199–205.

Disposition in the Body. Rapidly absorbed after oral administration and widely distributed into body tissues. It accumulates in high concentrations in the kidneys, liver, lungs, spleen and is strongly bound in melanin-containing cells (eyes and skin). It also crosses the placenta. Metabolic reactions include *N*-dealkylation and deamination followed by conjugation, possibly with glucuronic acid, of the carboxylic acid metabolites; the metabolites include monodesethyl- and didesethylchloroquine, 4-(7-chloroquinol-4-ylamino)pentan-1-ol, and 4-(7-chloroquinol-4-ylamino)pentanoic acid and its conjugate. Chloroquine is excreted slowly and may persist in the tissues for prolonged periods; about 55% is excreted in the urine and about 10% is eliminated in the faeces in 90 days following therapy with 310 mg of the phosphate daily for 14 days; the urinary excretion of unchanged drug is dependent upon urinary pH and larger amounts are excreted in acid urine than in alkaline urine; of the material excreted in the urine, about 70% is unchanged, 23% is monodesethylchloroquine, 1 to 2% is didesethylchloroquine and an unidentified metabolite, and 1 to 2% is conjugated carboxylic acid metabolites. Chloroquine and its monodesethyl metabolite are both distributed into breast milk.

Therapeutic concentration. In plasma, usually in the range 0.02 to 0.2 mg/L.

Following a single oral dose of 300 mg to 11 subjects, peak plasma concentrations of 0.056 to 0.10 mg/L (mean 0.08) of chloroquine and 0.01 to 0.02 mg/L of monodesethylchloroquine were attained in 1 to 6 h [L. L. Gustafsson *et al.*, *Br. J. Clin. Pharmacol.*, 1983, *15*, 471–479].

In healthy subjects receiving three different chloroquine regimens for 3 weeks (once weekly 300 mg (5 subjects), twice weekly 200 mg (4 subjects), once daily 50 mg (5 subjects)), all regimens produced peak and trough chloroquine concentrations above 16 μg/L after the first week, sufficient to suppress chloroquine-sensitive *Plasmodium falciparum* strains [J. C. Wetsteyn *et al.*, *Br. J. Clin. Pharmacol.*, 1995, *39*, 696–699].

In 29 patients undergoing long-term chloroquine treatment for rheumatoid arthritis, steady-state blood concentrations varied considerably (0.0366 to 3.895 mg/L); concentrations of the 2 main metabolites also varied (bisdesethylchloroquine 0 to 0.267 mg/L, desethylchloroquine 0.0247 to 1.506 mg/L) [P. Augustijns *et al.*, *Eur. J. Clin. Pharmacol.*, 1993, *42*, 429–433].

Toxicity. Doses as low as 1 g have caused deaths in children and fatalities have occurred in adults after the ingestion of 3 to 44 g. Plasma concentrations greater than 0.6 mg/L may produce toxic effects and concentrations greater than 3 mg/L may be fatal.

Plasma concentrations in a 52-year-old woman who ingested 10 g chloroquine in a suicide attempt were 13.1 mg/L 3 h after ingestion, and fell to 0.5 mg/L after 335 h. The chloroquine concentration in the whole blood was 18.4 mg/L at 3 h and rose to a peak of 28.4 mg/L 6 to 6.5 h after ingestion and then fell to 3.1 mg/L at 335 h. Maximum plasma and whole blood concentrations of desethylchloroquine were 1.48 mg/L and 3.7 mg/L, respectively, at 3 h and 6 h [F. T. Boereboom *et al.*, *Crit. Care Med.*, 2000, *28*, 3346–3350].

A 32-year-old man died 3 days after ingesting an unknown quantity of chloroquine in a suicide attempt, despite receiving treatment. The chloroquine concentration on admittance to hospital was 6.5 mg/L in the serum and 683.0 mg/L in the urine. Postmortem concentrations were as follows: peripheral blood 9.2 mg/L, heart blood 26.4 mg/L, vitreous humour 5.3 mg/L, stomach content 2.7 mg/L, bile 18.2 mg/L [T. Keller *et al.*, *Forensic Sci. Int.*, 1998, *96*, 21–28].

In a 27-year-old man whose death was attributed to heart failure caused by chloroquine overdosage, the following tissue concentrations were reported: femoral blood 16.71 mg/L, urine 516.0 mg/L, bile 8410 mg/L, stomach contents 82 020 mg/L, duodenal contents 7550 mg/L, tracheal foam 50

370 mg/L, left lung 1170 µg/g, right lung 1270 µg/g, left kidney 1690 µg/g, right kidney 1690 µg/g, heart 520 µg/g, liver 1110 µg/g, pancreas 5510 µg/g, spleen 1000 µg/g, cerebral hemispheres 100 µg/g, cerebellum 80 µg/g, hair not detected. The blood ethanol concentration was 350 mg/L, which could not have enhanced the effect of chloroquine [P. Kintz *et al.*, *Hum. Toxicol.*, 1988, *7*, 541–543].

Bioavailability. About 80 to 90%.

Half-life. Plasma half-life, about 25 to 60 days.

Volume of distribution. Reported as 116 to 285 L/kg.

Clearance. Plasma, about 3.7 mL/min/kg (after IV administration)

Distribution in blood. Plasma: whole blood ratio, about 0.3.

Protein binding. In plasma, about 50 to 70%.

Note: For reviews of the pharmacokinetics of chloroquine see S. Krishna and N. J. White, *Clin. Pharmacokinet*, 1996, *30*, 263–299 and J. Ducharme and R. Farinotti, *Clin. Pharmacokinet.*, 1996, *31*, 257–274.

Dose. For an acute attack, the equivalent of 1.5 g of chloroquine base over three days (900 mg on the first day); for prophylaxis, 300 mg once every 7 days.
Chloroquine base 300 mg ≅ chloroquine phosphate 500 mg or chloroquine sulfate 400 mg; chloroquine base 40 mg ≅ chloroquine hydrochloride 50 mg.

Chlorothiazide

Diuretic

Synonym. Clorotiazida
Proprietary names. Azide; Chlotride; Diubram; Diuret; Diuril; Diurilix; Diurone; Saluric. It is an ingredient of Aldoclor and Diupres.
6-Chloro-2*H*-1,2,4-benzothiadiazine-7-sulfonamide 1,1-dioxide
$C_7H_6ClN_3O_4S_2$=295.7
CAS—58-94-6

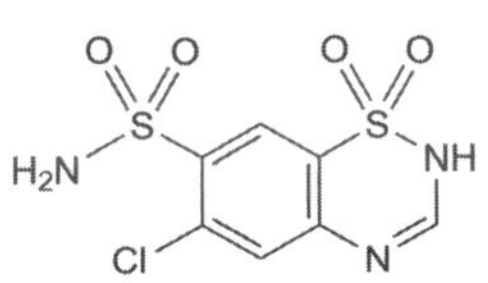

A white crystalline powder. M.p. about 340°, with decomposition.
Very slightly soluble in water; practically insoluble in benzene, chloroform, and ether; soluble 1 in 650 of ethanol and 1 in 100 of acetone; freely soluble in dimethylformamide and dimethyl sulfoxide.

Chlorothiazide Sodium

Synonym. Sodium Chlorothiazide
Proprietary name. Diuril (injection)
$C_7H_5ClN_3NaO_4S_2$=317.7
CAS—7085-44-1
A crystalline solid.
Soluble in water.

Dissociation Constant. pK_a 6.7, 9.5 (20°).

Partition Coefficient. Log *P* (ether/pH 7.4), −1.9.

Colour Tests. Koppanyi–Zwikker Test—blue; Mercurous Nitrate—black.

Thin-layer Chromatography. System TD—Rf 02; system TE—Rf 02; system TF—Rf 16; system TAD—Rf 11; system TAJ—Rf 11; system TAK—Rf 00; system TAL—Rf 41; system TAM—Rf 13. (Mercuric chloride–diphenylcarbazone reagent, positive.)

Gas Chromatography. System GA—RI 1720; system GX—chlorothiazide-Me_3 RT 6.6 min; system GY—chlorothiazide-Me_3 retention time 4.3 min.

High Performance Liquid Chromatography. System HN—*k* 0.54; system HY—RI 239; system HZ—retention time, 2.1 min.

Ultraviolet Spectrum. Aqueous acid—278 nm (A_1^1=400a); aqueous alkali—292 nm (A_1^1=430a).

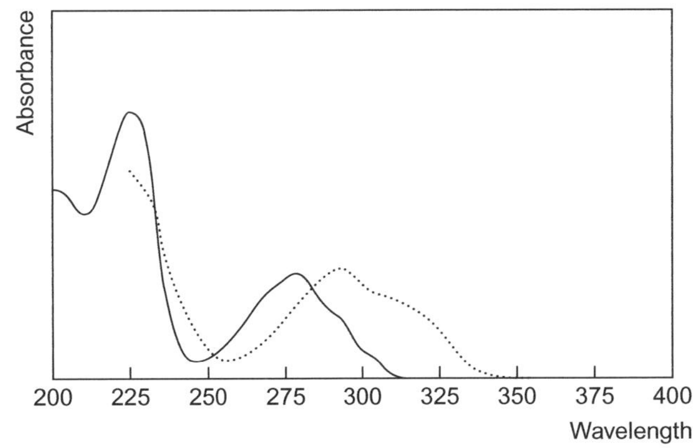

Infra-red Spectrum. Principal peaks at wavenumbers 1157, 1305, 1595, 1090, 1123, 1620 cm^{-1} (KBr disk).

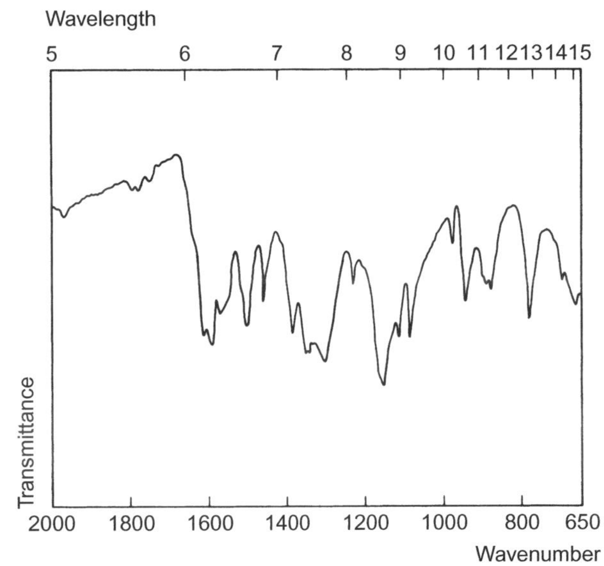

Quantification

High performance liquid chromatography. In plasma or urine: chlorothiazide or hydrochlorothiazide, limit of detection 10 µg/L in plasma and 2 mg/L in urine, UV detection—R. H. Barbhaiya *et al.*, *J.Pharm. Sci.*, 1981, *70*, 291–295. In urine: limit of detection 1 mg/L, UV detection—D. Farthing *et al.*, *J. Pharm. Biomed. Anal.*, 1998, *17(8)*, 1455–1459. In serum: limit of quantification 5 µg/L, electrochemical detection—K. Richter *et al.*, *J. Chromatogr. A*, 1996, *729(1–2)*, 293–296. In plasma and urine: limit of detection 0.01 mg/L and 0.2 mg/L, UV detection—J. X. de Vries and A. Voss, *Biomed. Chromatogr.*, 1993, *7(1)*, 12–14.

Disposition in the Body. Poorly and erratically absorbed after oral administration; bioavailability, about 20 to 30% after doses of 250 mg, decreasing with increasing dose. Chlorothiazide is not significantly metabolised and is excreted in the urine to a variable extent depending on the extent of absorption.

Therapeutic concentration

Following single oral doses of 125, 250, and 500 mg to 12 subjects, mean peak plasma concentrations of 0.64, 0.92, and 1.3 mg/L were attained in about 1 h. [P. G. Welling *et al.*, *Curr. Ther. Res.*, 1982, *31*, 379–385.]

20 healthy males were administered 25 mg of hydrochlorothiazide daily for 11 days. The mean steady-state plasma concentration was 288 µg/L observed at 2 h. [S. J. Weir *et al.*, *Biopharm. Drug Dispos.*, 1998, *19(6)*, 365–371.]

Half-life. Plasma half-life, about 1.5 h.

Protein binding. In plasma, about 95%.

Dose. 0.5 to 2 g daily.

Chlorotrianisene

Oestrogen

Synonym. Tri-*p*-anisylchloroethylene
Proprietary names. Anisene; Chlorotrisin; Merbentul; Tace; Triagen.
1,1′,1″-(1-Chloro-1-ethenyl-2-ylidene)tris[4-methoxybenzene]
$C_{23}H_{21}ClO_3$=380.9
CAS—569-57-3

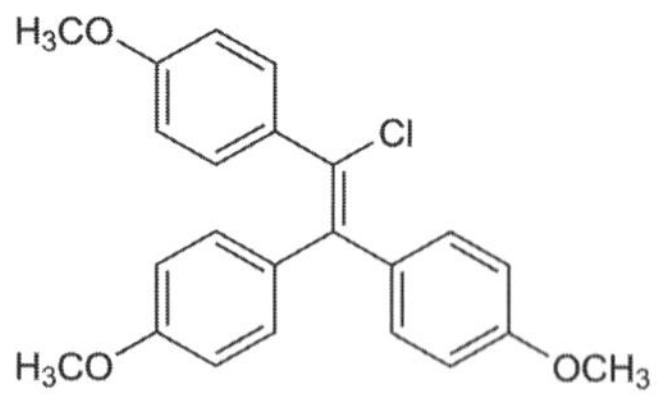

Small white crystals or crystalline powder. M.p. about 118°.
Soluble 1 in 4200 of water, 1 in 360 of ethanol, 1 in 7 of acetone, 1 in 1.5 of chloroform, and 1 in 28 of ether.
Caution. Chlorotrianisene is a powerful oestrogen. Contact with the skin or inhalation should be avoided.

Partition Coefficient. Log *P* (octanol/water), 6.2.

Colour Tests. Liebermann's Test—green; Sulfuric Acid—violet.

Thin-layer Chromatography. System TP—Rf 88; system TQ—Rf 77; system TR—Rf 98; system TS—Rf 92.

Gas Chromatography. System GA—RI 2917.

Ultraviolet Spectrum. Ethanol—247 nm (A^1_1=635a), 307 nm (A^1_1=410a).

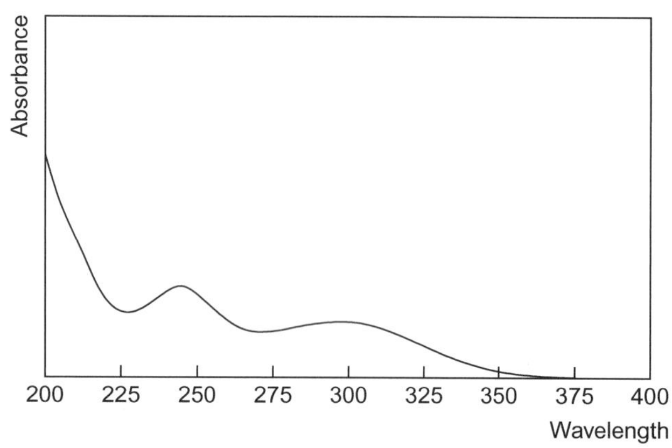

Infra-red Spectrum. Principal peaks at wavenumbers 1250, 1510, 1606, 1174, 813, 1184 cm^{-1} (KBr disk).

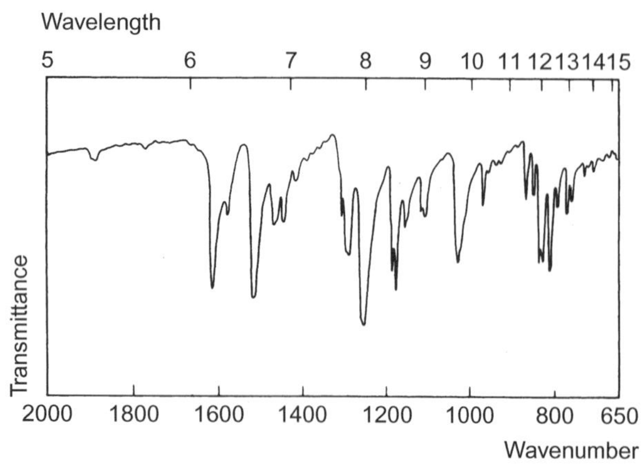

Mass Spectrum. Principal ions at *m/z* 380, 223, 382, 238, 152, 345, 215, 113.

Dose. 12 to 24 mg daily.

Chloroxylenol

Disinfectant

Synonyms. Parachlorometaxylenol; PCMX.
Proprietary names. Dettol; Metasep.
4-Chloro-3,5-dimethylphenol
C_8H_9ClO=156.6
CAS—88-04-0

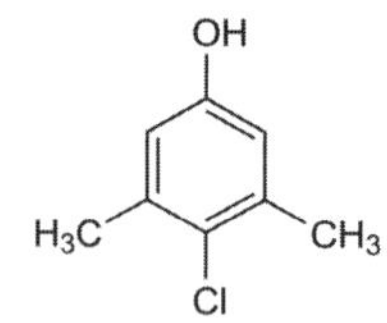

White or cream-coloured crystals or crystalline powder. Volatile in steam. M.p. 114° to 116°.
Soluble 1 in 3000 of water, 1 in 200 of boiling water, and 1 in 1 of ethanol; soluble in benzene and in ether.

Dissociation Constant. pK_a 9.7 (25°).

Partition Coefficient. Log *P* (octanol/water), 3.3.

Colour Test. Liebermann's Test—black.

Gas Chromatography. System GA—RI 1420.

High Performance Liquid Chromatography. System HY—RI 511.

Ultraviolet Spectrum. Aqueous acid—279 nm (A^1_1=83a); aqueous alkali—242 nm (A^1_1=650a), 296 nm.

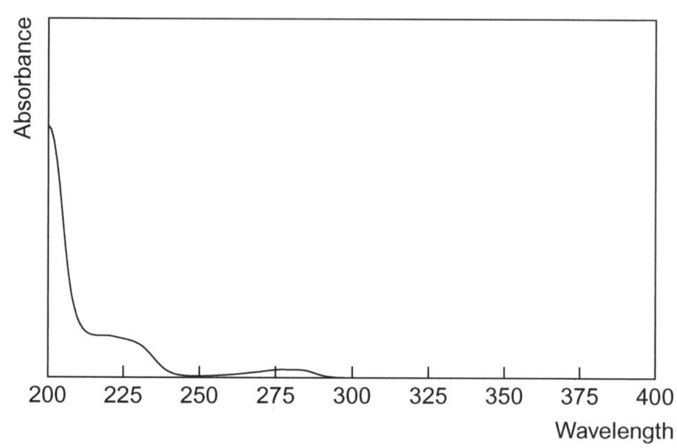

Infra-red Spectrum. Principal peaks at wavenumbers 1158, 1317, 1590, 1020, 858, 848 cm^{-1} (KCl disk).

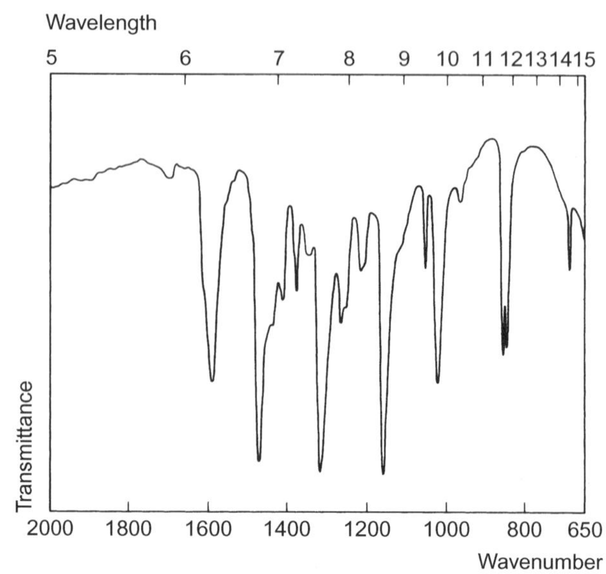

Disposition in the Body. About 14% of ingested chloroxylenol is excreted in the urine as a glucuronide conjugate and 17% as the sulfate, together with traces of unchanged chloroxylenol; the amount of unchanged chloroxylenol excreted is increased if the urine is alkaline.

Toxicity

In a fatality caused by the ingestion of at least 100 mL of a solution containing 4.8% of chloroxylenol, postmortem chloroxylenol concentrations were as follows: blood 23 mg/L, liver 8 μg/g. [A. Coutselinis and D. Boukis, *Med. Sci. Law*, 1976, *16*, 180.]

A subject who had ingested about 17 g of chloroxylenol in solution was admitted to hospital 30 min afterwards and recovered after intensive treatment. [P. Joubert *et al.*, *BMJ*, 1978, *1*, 890.]

Use. Chloroxylenol is available in concentrations of about 5%; it is further diluted before use.

Chlorphenamine

Antihistamine

Synonyms. Chlorpheniramine; Chlorprophenpyridamine.
Proprietary names. Alerdil; Bioflusin; Blendox; Cronal; Pollenase Antihistamine; Rimarin.
γ-(4-Chlorophenyl)-*N*,*N*-dimethyl-2-pyridinepropanamine
$C_{16}H_{19}ClN_2$=274.8
CAS—132-22-9; 42882-96-2 (±)

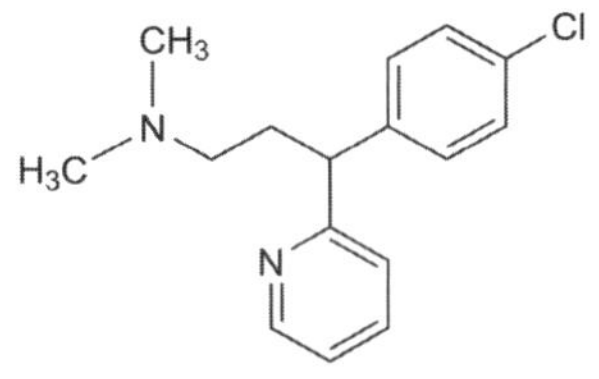

An oily liquid. B.p. 142°.

Chlorphenamine maleate

Synonyms. Chlorphenamini Maleas; Chlorpheniramine maleate.
Proprietary names. Aller-Chlor; Allergex; Allergin; Allerphen; Allergy; Allergy Relief; Calimal; Chlo-Amine; Chlorhist; Chlor-Pro; Chlorpyrimine; Chlorspan; Chlor-Trimeton; Chlor-Tripolon; Histafen; Histalon; Piriject; Piriton; Teldrin; Trimeton. It is an ingredient of many proprietary preparations—see *Martindale, The Complete Drug Reference*, 33rd edn, London, Pharmaceutical Press, 2002.
Note. The name Chloramin has been applied to tosylchloramide sodium.
$C_{16}H_{19}ClN_2,C_4H_4O_4$=390.9
CAS—113-92-8
A white crystalline powder. M.p. 130° to 135°.
Solubility in g/L at 25°: ethanol 330; chloroform 240; water 160; methanol 130. Slightly soluble in benzene and ether.

Dexchlorphenamine Maleate

Synonyms. Dexchlorpheniramine Maleate; Dexchlorphenamini Maleas.
Proprietary names. Phenamin; Polamin; Polaronil; Polaramin(e); Rhiniramine; Trenelone.
CAS—25523-97-1 (dexchlorphenamine); *2438-32-6* (maleate)
A white odourless crystalline powder. Protect from light. Soluble 1 in 1.1 water; 1 in 2 of alcohol; 1 in 1.7 chloroform and 1 in 2500 of ether; freely soluble in methyl alcohol and dichloromethane.

Dissociation Constant. pK_a 9.13 (25°).

Partition Coefficient. Log *P* (octanol/water), 3.38.

Colour Test. Cyanogen Bromide—orange.

Thin-layer Chromatography. System TA—Rf 45; system TB—Rf 35; system TC—Rf 18; system TE—Rf 46; system TL—Rf 02; system TAE—Rf 12; system TAF—Rf 21; system TAJ—Rf 00; system TAK—Rf 00; system TAL—Rf 25. (Dragendorff spray, positive; FPN reagent, blue; acidified iodoplatinate solution, positive; Marquis reagent, violet; ninhydrin spray, positive.)

Gas Chromatography. System GA—chlorphenamine RI 1996, M (nor-) RI 2014, M (OH-)-AC RI 2405, M (bis-nor-)-AC RI 2535, M (desamino-OH-)-AC RI 2130, M (nor-)-AC RI 2530; system GB—chlorphenamine RI 2079, M (nor-) RI 2115, M (bis-nor-) RI 2065, M (nor-)-AC RI 2563; system GC—RI 2586; system GF—RI 2335.

High Performance Liquid Chromatography. System HA—*k* 3.9; system HX—RI 356; system HY—RI 264; system HZ—Retention time 3.5 min; system HAA—Retention time 12.9 min; system HAX—Retention time 10.8 min; system HAY—Retention time 5.3 min.

Ultraviolet Spectrum. Aqueous acid—265 (A_1^1=302a); aqueous alkali—262 nm (A_1^1=205a).

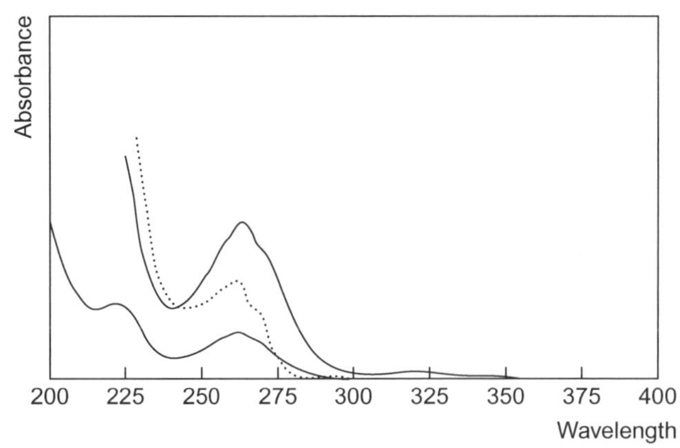

Infra-red Spectrum. Principal peaks at wavenumbers 1585, 1086, 746, 1010, 830, 1562 cm^{-1} (KBr disk).

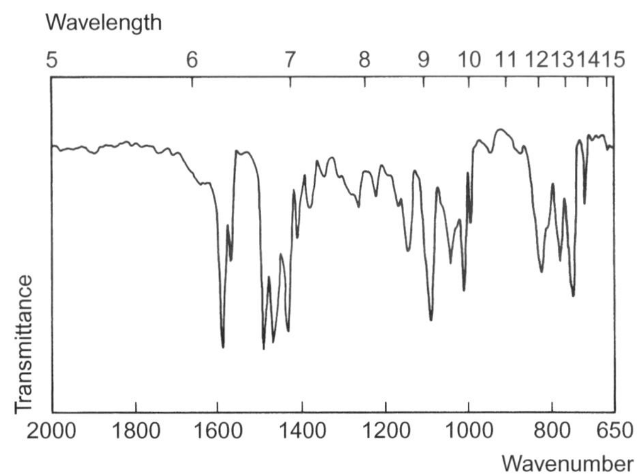

Mass Spectrum. Principal ions at *m/z* 203, 58, 44, 205, 54, 204, 72, 202.

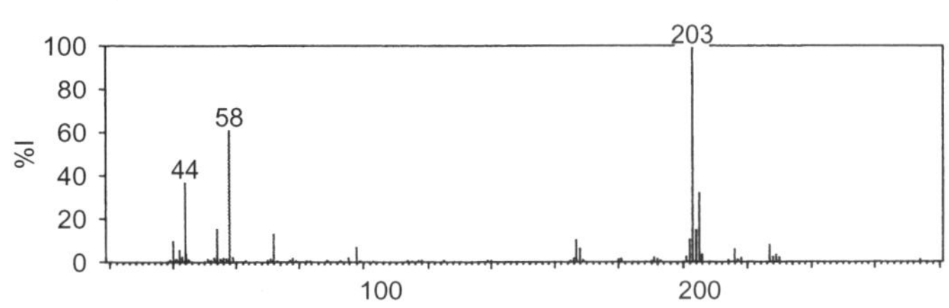

Quantification

Gas chromatography. In urine: limit of detection <60 ng, FID—H. M. Ali and A. H. Beckett, *J. Chromatogr.*, 1981, *223 B Biomed. Appl.*, *12*, 208–212. In serum: limit of detection 0.5 to 1 μg/L, ECD—J. W. Barnhart and J. D. Johnson, *Anal. Chem.*, 1977, *49*, 1085–1086. In plasma: chlorphenamine and codeine, limit of quantification for chlorphenamine 0.4 μg/L, flame thermionic detection—K. Masumoto *et al.*, *J. Chromatogr.*, 1986, *381*, 323–329.

High performance liquid chromatography. In plasma, saliva or urine: chlorphenamine and two metabolites, limit of detection 2 μg/L in plasma for chlorphenamine, UV detection—N. K. Athanikar *et al.*, *J. Chromatogr.*, 1979, *162 B Biomed. Appl.*, *4*, 367–376. In serum: limit of quantification 0.5 μg/L, UV detection—M. Yamaguchi *et al.*, *J. Chromatogr. B Biomed. Appl.*, 1994, *661*, 168–172.

High performance liquid chromatography–mass spectrometry. In plasma: chlorphenamine enantiomers and metabolites, limits of detection for enantiomers, 125 ng/L—K. M. Fried *et al.*, *J. Pharm. Biomed. Anal.*, 2002, *27*, 479–488.

Radioimmunoassay. In plasma: limit of detection 156 ng/L—K. K. Midha *et al.*, *J. Pharm. Sci.*, 1984, *73*, 1144–1147.

Disposition in the Body. Chlorphenamine maleate is readily and almost completely absorbed after oral administration; peak plasma concentrations reached after 2.5 to 6 h. It is widely distributed in the body, including passage into the CNS. The major metabolites are monodesmethyl- and didesmethylchlorphenamine. About 35% of a single dose is excreted in the urine in 48 h; the 24-h excretion of unchanged drug accounts for about 3 to 10% of the dose but this is increased by acidification of the urine and increased urinary flow, and decreased when the urine is alkaline; more non-polar metabolites appear to be excreted after IV than after oral administration. After daily oral administration, about 20% of a dose is excreted in the 24-h urine as unchanged drug, 20% as monodesmethylchlorphenamine, and 5% as didesmethylchlorphenamine. Less than 1% of a dose is eliminated in the faeces.

Therapeutic concentration

Following a single oral dose of 8 mg to 5 subjects, peak plasma concentrations of 0.01 to 0.04 mg/L (mean 0.02) were attained in 2 to 3 h; after repeated oral administration of 6 mg twice a day to 2 subjects, mean plasma steady-state concentrations of 0.02 and 0.03 mg/L were reported; the plasma concentration of monodesmethylchlorphenamine averaged 0.008 mg/L and plasma concentrations of didesmethylchlorphenamine were less than 0.003 mg/L [S. M. Huang *et al.*, *Eur. J. Clin. Pharmacol.*, 1982, *22*, 359–365].

In 13 subjects who received a single oral dose of 8 mg (either as test formulation tablets or as reference tablets), the maximum plasma concentrations were 0.022 and 0.0205 mg/L at 2.5 and 2.08 h for the test and reference preparations, respectively [T. A. Najjar *et al.*, *Int. J. Clin. Pharmacol. Ther.*, 1995, *33*, 619–622].

Toxicity. Toxic effects may be produced by plasma concentrations greater than 20 mg/L.

The following postmortem heart blood concentrations were reported in a fatality due to the ingestion of chlorphenamine, diphenhydramine, and guaifenesin: 0.2 mg/L, 8.8 mg/L and 27.4 mg/L. The cause of death was determined to be acute intoxication by the combined effects of the three drugs [H. Wogoman *et al.*, *Am. J. Forensic Med. Pathol.*, 1999, *20*, 199–202].

Postmortem results from 47 pilot fatalities involving chlorphenamine revealed that where chlorphenamine was the sole agent present, tissue concentrations were as follows: blood 0.109 mg/L, liver 1.412 mg/L, lung 1.160 to 3.260 μg/g. In the remaining 31 cases, in which other drugs were also involved, the chlorphenamine concentration was reported as follows: blood 0.093 mg/L, liver 0.747 mg/L, lung 0.731 to 6.483 μg/g [J. W. Soper *et al.*, *Aviat. Space Environ. Med.*, 2000, *71*, 1206–1209].

The following postmortem tissue concentrations were reported in a fatality due to the ingestion of chlorphenamine and alcohol in mg/L: blood 1.1, bile 1.5, brain 2.5, kidney 1.4, liver 6.6, lung 5.2; a blood-alcohol concentration of 1200 mg/L was also reported [D. Reed, *Clin. Toxicol.*, 1981, *18*, 941–943].

Bioavailability. Between 25 and 50%.

Half-life. Values from 2 to 43 h have been reported; shorter half-life in children.

Volume of distribution. Approximately 3 to 5.9 L/kg.

Clearance. Plasma clearance, about 1.7 mL/min/kg.

Distribution in blood. Plasma:whole blood ratio, about 0.83.

Protein binding. In plasma, about 70%.

Note. For a review of the pharmacokinetics of chlorphenamine, see M.M. Rumore, *Drug Intell. Clin. Pharm.*, 1984, *18*, 701–707. For a review of the pharmacokinetics of general H1-receptor antagonists, see D. M. Paton and D. R. Webster, *Clin. Pharmacokinet.*, 1985, *10*, 477–497.

Dose. 12 to 24 mg of chlorphenamine maleate daily in divided doses; single doses of 8 to 12 mg have been given in sustained-release preparations. Up to 12 mg daily of dexchlorphenamine maleate is given in divided doses.

Chlorphenesin

Antifungal

Synonym. *p*-Chlorophenyl α-Glyceryl Ether
Proprietary names. Adermykon; Mycil; Soorphenesin.
3-(4-Chlorophenoxy)-1,2-propanediol
$C_9H_{11}ClO_3$=202.6
CAS—104-29-0

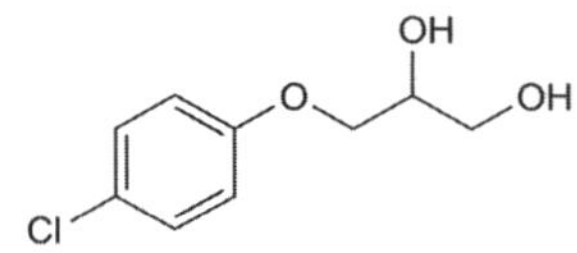

White or pale cream-coloured crystals or crystalline aggregates. M.p. 77° to 79°.
Soluble 1 in 200 of water and 1 in 5 of ethanol; soluble in ether.

Partition Coefficient. Log *P* (octanol/water), 1.5.

Colour Tests. Liebermann's Test—black; Mandelin's Test—brown-green.

Thin-layer Chromatography. System TA—Rf 82; system TE—Rf 62; system TAJ—Rf 38; system TAK—Rf 32; system TAL—Rf 86. (Acidified iodoplatinate solution, positive.)

Gas Chromatography. System GA—chlorphenesin RI 1680, chlorphenesin-AC_2 RI 2070, chlorphenesin-AC RI 2030.

Ultraviolet Spectrum. Methanol—281 (A_1^1=79b), 289 nm.

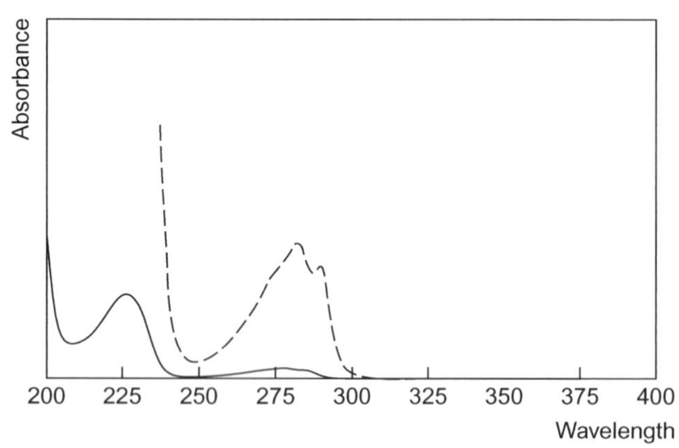

Infra-red Spectrum. Principal peaks at wavenumbers 1232, 1043, 818, 1109, 1490, 710 cm^{-1} (KBr disk).

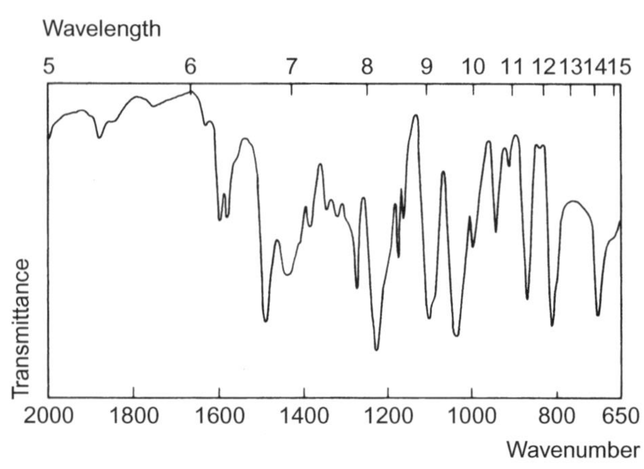

Mass Spectrum. Principal ions at *m/z* 128, 130, 202, 31, 29, 65, 43, 111.

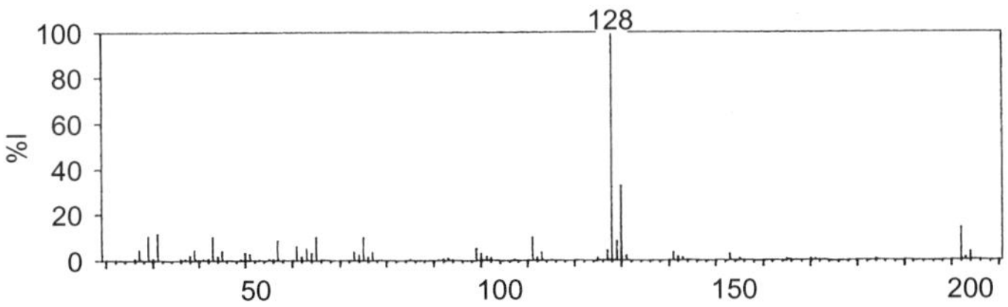

Use. Topically in concentrations of 0.5 to 1%.

Chlorphenesin Carbamate

Muscle Relaxant

Proprietary names. Maolate; Rinlaxer.
3-(4-Chlorophenoxy)-1,2-propanediol-1-carbamate
$C_{10}H_{12}ClNO_4$=245.7
CAS—886-74-8

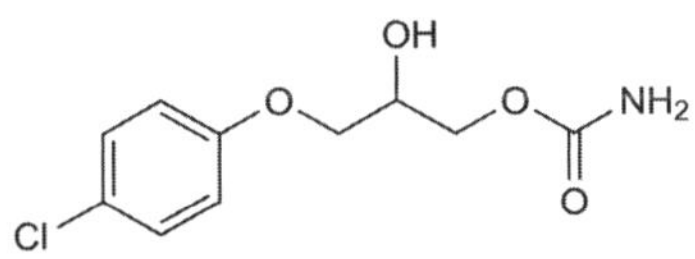

A white crystalline powder. M.p. about 90°.
Practically insoluble in water, benzene, and cyclohexane; readily soluble in ethanol, acetone, and ethyl acetate; soluble in chloroform.

Partition Coefficient. Log *P* (octanol/water), 0.8.

Thin-layer Chromatography. System TA—Rf 82; system TB—Rf 00; system TD—Rf 11; system TE—Rf 52; system TF—Rf 34; system TAD—Rf 32; system TAE—Rf 87; system TAJ—Rf 31; system TAK—Rf 18; system TAL—Rf 80. (Furfuraldehyde reagent, positive.)

Gas Chromatography. System GA—chlorphenesin RI 1680.

High Performance Liquid Chromatography. System HX—RI 387; system HY—RI 348.

Ultraviolet Spectrum. Ethanol—280 nm (A_1^1=75b), 288 nm(A_1^1=62b).

Infra-red Spectrum. Principal peaks at wavenumbers 1724, 1234, 1028, 1692, 1111, 824 cm^{-1} (KBr disk).

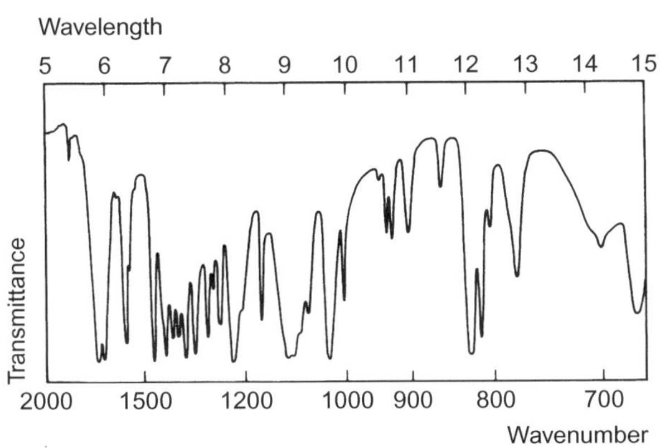

Mass Spectrum. Principal ions at *m/z* 128, 130, 202, 43, 129, 111, 75, 204.

Quantification

Colorimetry. In serum—A. A. Forist and R. W. Judy, *J. Pharm. Sci.*, 1971, *60*, 1686–1688.

Gas chromatography. In serum: limit of detection 500 μg/L, FID—D. G. Kaiser and S. R. Shaw, *J. Pharm. Sci.*, 1974, *63*, 1094–1097.

Disposition in the Body. Readily absorbed after oral administration. About 85% of a dose is excreted in the urine as a glucuronide conjugate in 24 h together with small amounts of unchanged drug, and the oxidised metabolites, 4-chlorophenoxylactic acid, 4-chlorophenoxyacetic acid, and 4-chlorophenol.

Therapeutic concentration
Following a single oral dose of 800 mg to 10 subjects, peak serum concentrations of 3.9 to 17.0 mg/L (mean 10) were attained in about 2 h; after daily oral dosing with 800 mg three times a day for 11 weeks to the same subjects, a mean peak serum concentration of 14.4 mg/L was reported about 2 h after the last dose. [R. G. Stoll *et al.*, *J. Clin. Pharmacol.*, 1974, *14*, 520–524.]

Half-life. Plasma half-life, about 2 to 5 h.

Volume of distribution. About 1 L/kg.

Dose. Initially 2.4 g daily, reduced to 1.6 g daily or less.

Chlorphenoxamine

Anticholinergic

2-[1-(4-Chlorophenyl)-1-phenylethoxy]-*N*,*N*-dimethylethanamine
$C_{18}H_{22}ClNO$=303.8
CAS—77-38-3

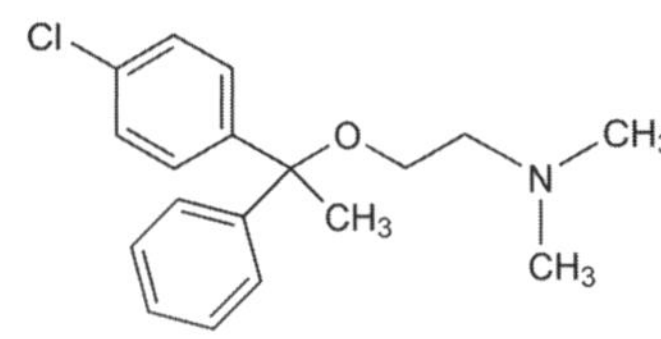

An oil.

Chlorphenoxamine Hydrochloride

Proprietary names. Clorevan; Phenoxene; Systral.
$C_{18}H_{22}ClNO,HCl$=340.3
CAS—562-09-4
A white crystalline powder. M.p. 128°.
Soluble 1 in 2 of water, 1 in 1.8 of ethanol, and 1 in 1.5 of chloroform; practically insoluble in ether.

Colour Test. Marquis Test—yellow→green.

Thin-layer Chromatography. System TA—Rf 53; system TB—Rf 47; system TC—Rf 36; system TE—Rf 70; system TL—Rf 17; system TAE—Rf 29; system TAJ—Rf 11; system TAK—Rf 05; system TAL—Rf 54. (Acidified iodoplatinate solution, positive.)

Gas Chromatography. System GA—chlorphenoxamine RI 2080, M (OH-) RI 2470, M (OH-methoxy-carbinol)-H_2O RI 2220; system GB—chlorphenoxamine RI 2190, M (nor-) RI 2205; system GF—RI 2365.

High Performance Liquid Chromatography. System HA—*k* 2.9; system HY—RI 346.

Ultraviolet Spectrum. Aqueous acid—259 nm (A_1^1=16b).

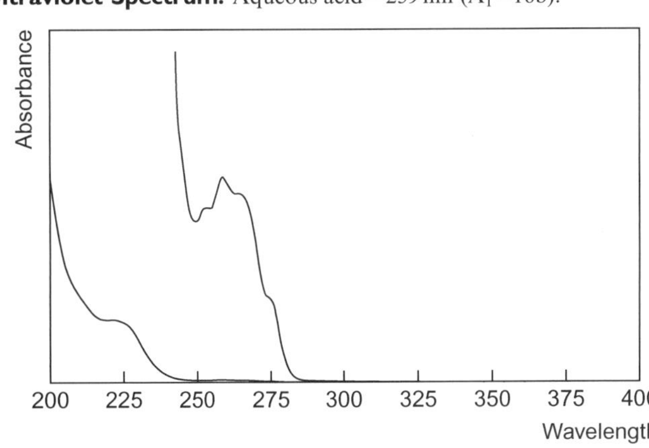

Infra-red Spectrum. Principal peaks at wavenumbers 1088, 1490, 1010, 760, 700, 990 cm^{-1} (chlorphenoxamine hydrochloride, KBr disk).

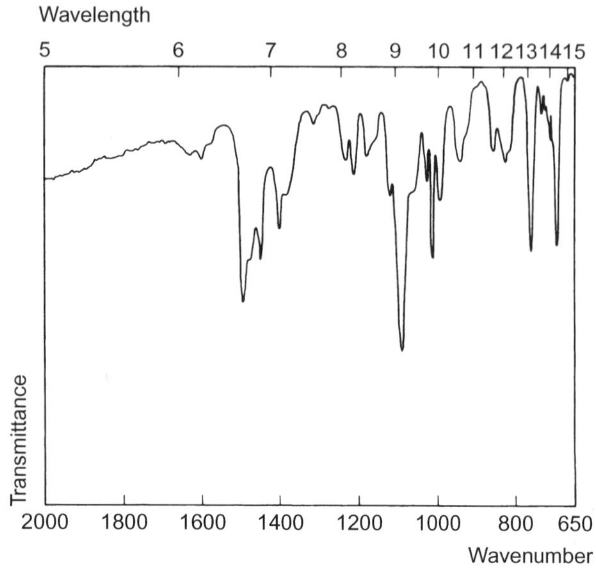

Mass Spectrum. Principal ions at m/z 58, 59, 179, 42, 178, 72, 77, 30.

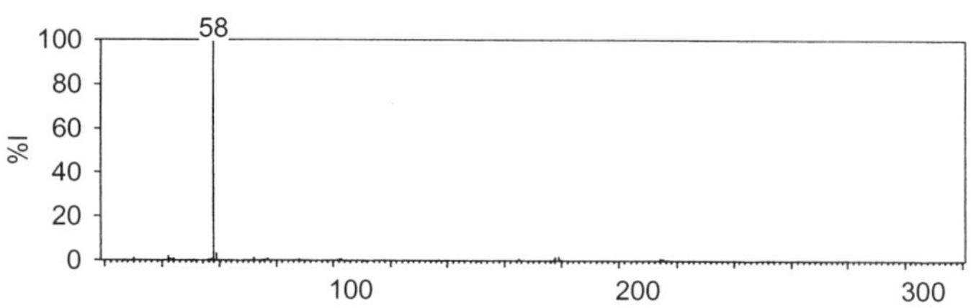

Dose. 150 to 400 mg of chlorphenoxamine hydrochloride daily.

Chlorphentermine

Anorectic

Proprietary names. Lucofen; Teramine.
4-Chloro-α,α-dimethylbenzeneethanamine
$C_{10}H_{14}ClN$=183.7
CAS—461-78-9

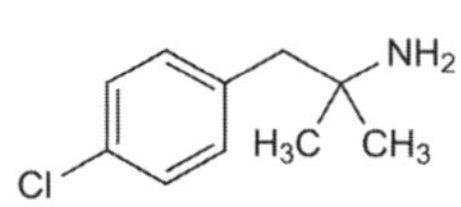

A liquid.

Chlorphentermine Hydrochloride
Proprietary name. Pre-Sate
$C_{10}H_{14}ClN,HCl$=220.1
CAS—151-06-4
A white or off-white crystalline powder. M.p. about 234°.
Soluble in water and ethanol; sparingly soluble in chloroform; practically insoluble in ether.

Dissociation Constant. pK_a 9.6.

Partition Coefficient. Log *P* (octanol/water), 2.6.

Thin-layer Chromatography. System TA—Rf 44; system TB—Rf 18; system TC—Rf 17; system TE—Rf 48; system TL—Rf 08; system TAE—Rf 14; system TAF—Rf 77. (Dragendorff spray, positive; acidified iodoplatinate solution, positive.)

Gas Chromatography. System GA—RI 1344; system GB—RI 1393; system GC—RI 1725.

High Performance Liquid Chromatography. System HA—*k* 0.9; system HC—*k* 0.82.

Ultraviolet Spectrum. Aqueous acid—220, 259, 267 (A^1_1=11.6c), 274 nm. No alkaline shift.

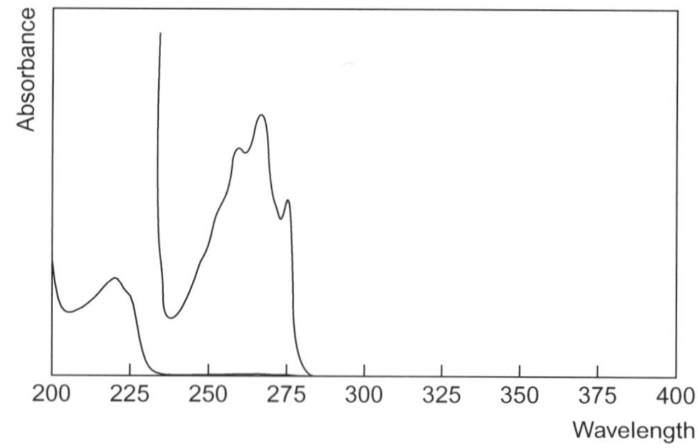

Infra-red Spectrum. Principal peaks at wavenumbers 818, 1493, 1092, 1020, 848, 754 cm^{-1} (chlorphentermine hydrochloride, KBr disk).

Mass Spectrum. Principal ions at m/z 58, 42, 41, 125, 59, 30, 89, 168.

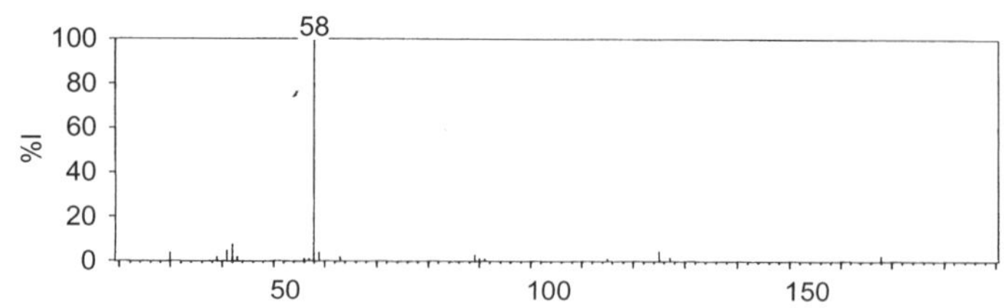

Quantification

Gas chromatography. In urine: chlorphentermine and metabolites, FID—A. H. Beckett and P. M. Bélanger, *Br. J. Clin. Pharmacol.*, 1977, *4*, 193–200. In blood: limit of detection 25 μg/L, FID—H. W. Jun and E. J. Triggs, *J. Pharm. Sci.*, 1970, *59*, 306–309.

Disposition in the Body. Absorbed after oral administration and metabolised mainly by *N*-oxidation and *N*-hydroxylation to nitro, nitroso and hydroxylamine derivatives. Excretion in the urine is dependent upon urinary pH, a much greater proportion of unchanged drug being excreted when the urine is acidic than when it is alkaline. In normal urine, about 17% of a dose is excreted unchanged and about 50% as *N*-oxidised metabolites in 48 h. If the urine is maintained at an acid pH, these proportions are approximately reversed, about 70% of a dose being excreted in 24 h. In alkaline urine less than 12% of a dose is excreted unchanged in 48 h.

Therapeutic concentration

A single oral dose of 100 mg given to 4 subjects produced a mean peak blood concentration of about 0.32 mg/L in 4 h. [H. W. Jun and E. J. Triggs, *J. Pharm. Sci.*, 1970, *59*, 306–309.]

Half-life. Plasma half-life, about 40 h.

Volume of distribution. About 2 to 3 L/kg.

Dose. Usually the equivalent of 65 mg of chlorphentermine daily.

Chlorproguanil

Antimalarial

Synonym. M-5943
N-(3,4-Dichlorophenyl)-*N*′-(1-methylethyl)imidodicarbonimidic diamide
$C_{11}H_{15}Cl_2N_5$=288.2
CAS—537-21-3

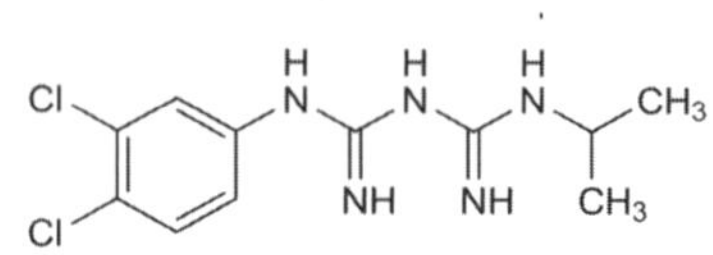

Chlorproguanil Hydrochloride

Proprietary name. Lapudrine
$C_{11}H_{15}Cl_2N_5,HCl=324.6$
CAS—15537-76-5
A white crystalline powder. M.p. 246° to 247°.
Soluble 1 in 100 of water and 1 in 50 of ethanol; practically insoluble in chloroform and ether.

Partition Coefficient. Log *P* (octanol/water), 3.2.

Colour Tests. To 10 mL of a saturated aqueous solution add 1 drop of 10% copper sulfate solution and 2.5 mL of dilute ammonia solution and shake well; add 5 mL of toluene and shake again—toluene layer is violet-red. Dissolve 5 mg in 5 mL of a warm 1% solution of cetrimide in water, add 1 mL of sodium hydroxide solution and 1 mL of bromine solution—red.

Thin-layer Chromatography. System TA—Rf 03; system TB—Rf 00; system TC—Rf 01; system TL—Rf 01. (Acidified potassium permanganate solution, positive.)

Gas Chromatography. System GA—RI 1621.

Ultraviolet Spectrum. Aqueous acid—250 nm (A_1^1=293c); methanol—260 nm (A_1^1=755b).

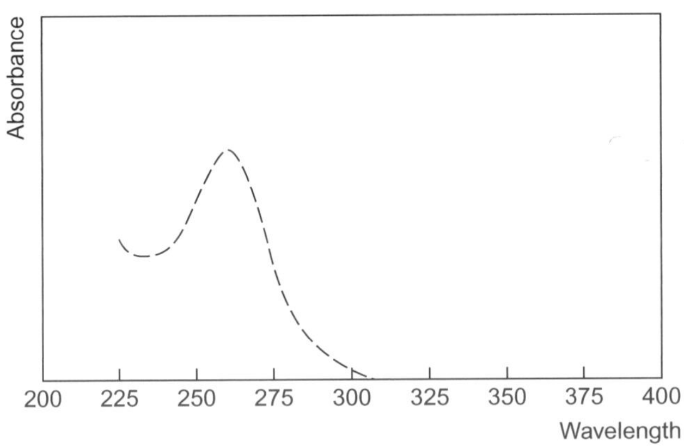

Infra-red Spectrum. Principal peaks at wavenumbers 1520, 1562, 1620, 1600, 1128, 1290 cm^{-1} (chlorproguanil hydrochloride, KBr disk). (See below)

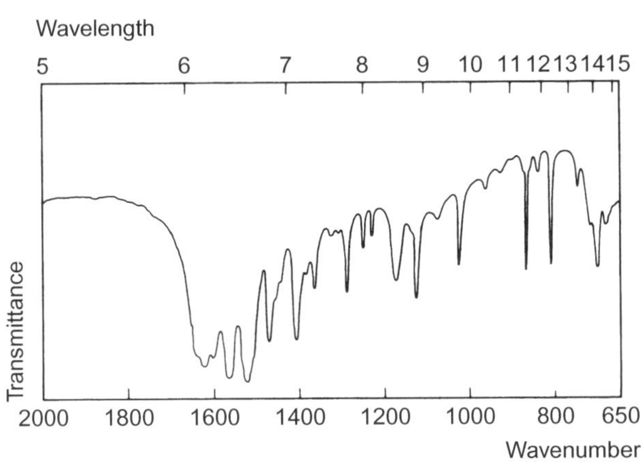

Mass Spectrum. Principal ions at *m/z* 127, 43, 229, 44, 161, 231, 85, 186.

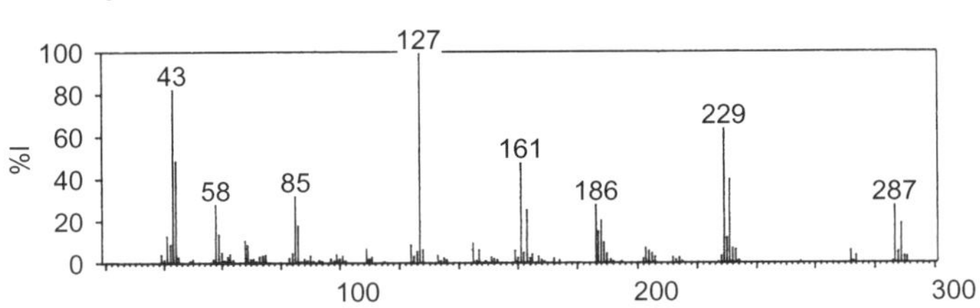

Dose. 20 mg of chlorproguanil hydrochloride every 7 days.

Chlorpromazine

Tranquilliser

Synonyms. 2601-A, HL-5746, RP-4560, SKF-2601-A.
Proprietary names. Amplictil; Largactil (suppositories); Thorazine (suppositories); Aminazine; Chlorderazin; Chlorpromados; Contomin; Esmind; Fenactil; Novomazina; Promactil; Prozil; Plegomazin; Wintermin.
2-Chloro-*N,N*-dimethyl-10*H*-phenothiazine-10-propanamine
$C_{17}H_{19}ClN_2S=318.9$
CAS—50-53-3

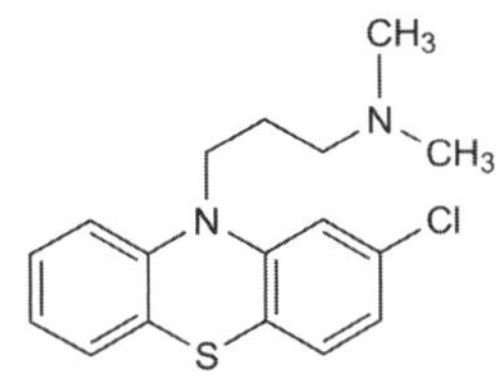

An oily liquid or waxy solid. It darkens on prolonged exposure to light. M.p. 56° to 60°.
Practically insoluble in water; soluble 1 in 2 of ethanol, 1 in less than 1 of chloroform, and 1 in 1 of ether.
Caution. Chlorpromazine may cause severe dermatitis in sensitised persons.

Chlorpromazine Embonate

Synonym. Chlorpromazine Pamoate
Proprietary name. Largactil (suspension)
$(C_{17}H_{19}ClN_2S)_2,C_{23}H_{16}O_6=1026.0$
A pale yellow powder.
Very slightly soluble in water; soluble in acetone.

Chlorpromazine Hydrochloride

Synonym. Aminazine
Proprietary names. Chloractil; Chlorazin; Chlorpromed; Chlor-Promanyl; Clonazine; Hebanil; Hibanil; Hibernal; Klorproman; Klorpromex; Largactil; Lagarktyl; Largatrex; Megaphen; Marazine; Matcine; Propaphenin; Prozin(e); Taroctyl; Thorazine; Torazina.
$C_{17}H_{19}ClN_2S,HCl=355.3$
CAS—69-09-0
A white or creamy-white crystalline powder. It decomposes on exposure to air and light becoming yellow, pink, and finally violet. M.p. with decomposition 179° to 180° (capillary), 194° to 196° (microblock).
Soluble 1 in 2.5 of water; soluble in methanol, ethanol, and chloroform; practically insoluble in ether and benzene.

Dissociation Constant. pK_a 9.3 (20°).

Partition Coefficient. Log *P* (octanol/buffer pH 7.4), 3.4.

Colour Tests. Formaldehyde–Sulfuric Acid—red-violet; Forrest Reagent—red; FPN Reagent—red; Liebermann's Test—red-brown; Mandelin's Test—green→violet; Marquis Test—violet.

Thin-layer Chromatography. System TA—Rf 49; system TB—Rf 45; system TC—Rf 35; system TE—Rf 70; system TL—Rf 17; system TAE—Rf 25; system TAF—Rf 45; system TAJ—Rf 11; system TAK—Rf 02; system TAL—Rf 47. (Dragendorff spray, positive; FPN reagent, pink; acidified iodoplatinate solution, positive; Marquis reagent, pink.)

Gas Chromatography. System GA—chlorpromazine RI 2495; M (nor-) RI 2480; M (didesmethyl-) RI 2480; M (sulfoxide) RI 2809; M (norsulfoxide) RI 2900; M (*N*-oxide) RI 2100; M (ring) RI 2100; M (OH-)-Me RI 2590; M (bis-nor-)-AC RI 2990; M (nor-)-AC RI 3070; system GB—chlorpromazine RI 2618; M (nor-) RI 2656; M (didesmethyl-) RI 2646; M (sulfoxide) RI 3003; M (norsulfoxide) RI 3046; M (7-OH-) RI 2939; M (*N*-oxide) RI 2355; system GF—RI 2940; system GV—Retention time 16.6 min; system GW—Retention time 23.0 min.

High Performance Liquid Chromatography. System HA—chlorpromazine *k* 4.1, M (nor-) *k* 2.2; system HX—chlorpromazine RI 456; system HY—chlorpromazine RI 350; system HZ—chlorpromazine Retention time 9.1 min; system HAA—chlorpromazine Retention time 16.0 min; system HAX—chlorpromazine Retention time 17.0 min; M (sulfoxide) 8.4 min; system HAY—chlorpromazine Retention time 7.8 min; M (sulfoxide) 4.3 min; system HAZ—chlorpromazine *k* 2.64; M (sulfoxide) *k* 0.62.

Ultraviolet Spectrum. Aqueous acid—255 (A^{1}_{1}=1025a). Chlorpromazine sulfoxide: aqueous acid—239 (A^{1}_{1}=1107b), 274 (A^{1}_{1}=343b), 300 (A^{1}_{1}=232b), 341 nm (A^{1}_{1}=168b).

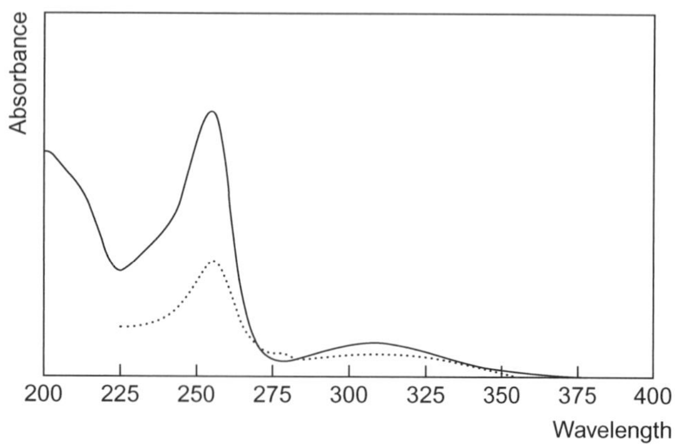

Infra-red Spectrum. Principal peaks at wavenumbers 747, 1240, 1561, 1125, 1095, 1220 cm^{-1} (KBr disk).

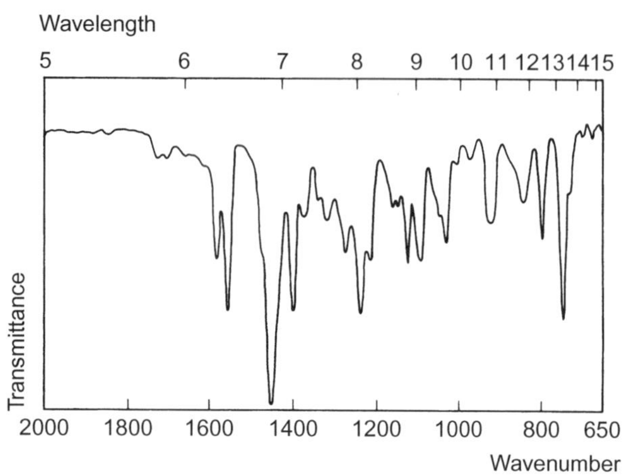

Mass Spectrum. Principal ions at *m/z* 58, 86, 318, 85, 320, 272, 319, 273.

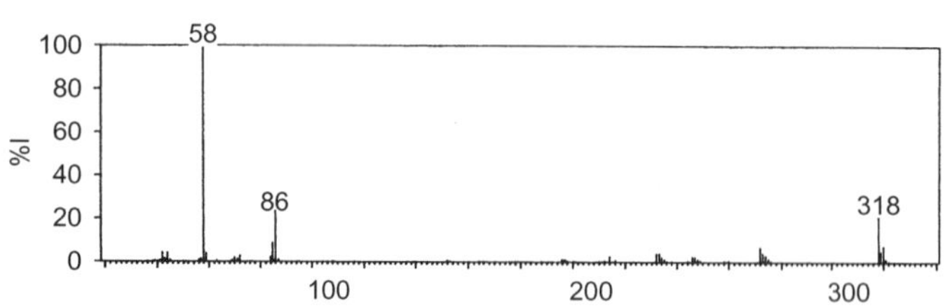

Quantification

Gas chromatography. In serum: limit of detection 5 µg/L for chlorpromazine and chlorpromazine sulfoxide, 20 µg/L for monodesmethylchlorpromazine and 10 µg/L for didesmethylchlorpromazine, AFID—D. N. Bailey and J. J. Guba, *Clin. Chem.*, 1979, *25*, 1211–1215. In whole blood or urine: chlorpromazine and other phenothiazines, limits of detection 250 to 500 ng/L, SID—H. Hattori *et al.*, *J. Chromatogr.*, 1992, *579*, 247–252.

Gas chromatography–mass spectrometry. In urine: limit of detection 5 µg/L (*m/z* 247, 232, 272, 318)—M. L. Olmos-Carmona and M. Hernandez-Carrazquilla, *J. Chromatogr. B Biomed. Sci. Appl.*, 1999, *734(1)*, 113–120. In hair: chlorpromazine and other antipsychotics and antidepressants—M. Shen *et al.*, *Forensic Sci. Int.*, 2002, *126*, 153–161.

High performance liquid chromatography. In plasma: limit of detection 1 µg/L, UV detection—K. K. Midha *et al.*, *J. Pharm. Sci.*, 1981, *70*, 1043–1046. In plasma: limit of detection 0.25 µg/L, electrochemical detection—J. K. Cooper *et al.*, *J. Pharm. Sci.*, 1983, *72*, 1259–1262. In postmortem samples: chlorpromazine and metabolites, UV detection—W. J. Allender *et al.*, *J. Anal. Toxicol.*, 1983, *7*, 203–206. In serum or breast milk: limit of quantification 10 µg/L, UV detection—T. Ohkubo *et al.*, *J. Chromatogr.*, 1993, *614*, 328–332.

Disposition in the Body. Readily absorbed after oral administration with peak plasma levels occurring after 2 to 4 h; it undergoes first-pass metabolism in the gut wall and is extensively metabolised in the liver and excreted in the bile and urine. Metabolism is catalysed by the P450 isoenzyme CYP2D6 and includes sulfoxidation, *N*-demethylation, hydroxylation, *N*-oxidation; glucuronic acid conjugation and possibly ring fission also occur. There is some evidence that chlorpromazine may stimulate its own metabolism. A large number of metabolites have been isolated and some of the metabolites are active, particularly 7-hydroxychlorpromazine, although less so than the parent drug; several metabolites may be detected in plasma at concentrations similar to those of chlorpromazine during chronic treatment. About 20 to 70% of an oral dose is excreted in the urine as metabolites, mostly conjugated, with 5% of the dose as the sulfoxide, and less than 1% as unchanged drug; about 5% of a dose is eliminated in the faeces as metabolites. Chlorpromazine metabolites have been detected in urine up to 18 months after discontinuation of long-term treatment. The monodesmethyl, 7-hydroxy, and sulfoxide metabolites are taken up by erythrocytes along with traces of the parent drug and its *N*-oxide. Chlorpromazine is widely distributed in the body. It crosses the blood–brain barrier with levels in the brain higher than those in plasma. Chlorpromazine and its metabolites cross the placenta and are found in breast milk.

Therapeutic concentration. Plasma concentrations vary considerably between individual subjects.

Peak plasma concentrations of 0.010 to 0.026 mg/L (mean 0.018) were reported 3 h after administration of a single oral dose of 150 mg to 6 subjects [L. E. Hollister *et al.*, *Clin. Pharmacol. Ther.*, 1970, *11*, 49–59].

Following daily oral doses of 200 to 600 mg to 10 subjects, minimum steady-state plasma concentrations of 0.002 to 0.122 mg/L (mean 0.03) of chlorpromazine were reported; monodesmethylchlorpromazine and 7-hydroxychlorpromazine plasma concentrations averaged 16% and 30%, respectively, of the chlorpromazine plasma concentration, but there were considerable intersubject variations [G. Alfredsson *et al.*, *Psychopharmacology*, 1976, *48*, 123–131].

Toxicity. Severe toxic symptoms have occurred with doses of less than 0.1 g. Overdosage with chlorpromazine is a fairly common occurrence, but fatalities are relatively rare. Blood concentrations in the region of 0.5 to 2 mg/L are associated with toxic effects and concentrations of 2 mg/L or greater may be lethal.

In a review of 8 fatal cases, blood concentrations of 3 to 35 mg/L (mean 17), and liver concentrations of 54 to 2110 µg/g (mean 366) were reported [R. Bonnichsen *et al.*, *Z. Rechtsmed.*, 1970, *67*, 158–169].

The following tissue distribution was reported in 2 fatalities: blood 4.2 and 6.7 mg/L, brain 126 and 148 µg/g, kidney 134 and 162 µg/g, liver 240 and 280 µg/g, urine 62 and 78 mg/L [A. Coutselinis *et al.*, *Forensic Sci.*, 1974, *4*, 191–194].

A patient with renal failure died suddenly following the administration of chlorpromazine 780 mg daily for 5 days. Blood concentrations of 1.534 mg/L were reported [P. G. Dorson and M. L. Crismon, *Drug Intell. Clin. Pharm.*, 1988, *22*, 776–778].

Bioavailability. About 20 to 30% but reduced during chronic therapy.

Half-life. Plasma half-life, 7 to 120 h; mean values are usually in the range 15 to 30 h.

Volume of distribution. About 21 L/kg.

Clearance. Plasma, about 8.6 mL/min/kg.

Protein binding. In plasma, about 95 to 98%.

Note. For a review of the pharmacokinetics of antipsychotics see T. B. Cooper, *Clin. Pharmacokinet.*, 1978, *3*, 14–38.

Dose. 75 to 300 mg of chlorpromazine hydrochloride daily; up to 1 g or more daily has been given to psychotic patients.

Chlorpropamide

Antidiabetic

Synonyms. Chlorglypropamide; P-607.

Proprietary names. Chloromide; Chloronase; Diabetoral; Diabinese; Glymese; Insulase; Melitase; Mellinese; Novopropamide; Promide; Stabinol.

4-Chloro-*N*-[(propylamino)carbonyl]benzenesulfonamide
$C_{10}H_{13}ClN_2O_3S$=276.7
CAS—94-20-2

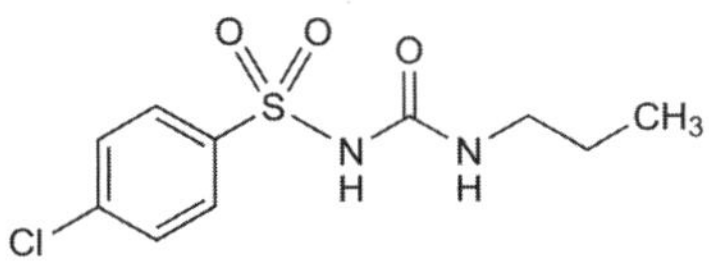

A white crystalline powder. M.p. 126° to 130°.
Practically insoluble in water; soluble 1 in 12 of ethanol, 1 in 5 of acetone, 1 in 9 of chloroform, and 1 in 200 of ether.

Dissociation Constant. pK_a 5.0 (20°).

Partition Coefficient. Log *P* (octanol/water), 2.3.

Colour Tests. Koppanyi–Zwikker Test—violet; Mercurous Nitrate—black.

Thin-layer Chromatography. System TA—Rf 72; system TB—Rf 00; system TD—Rf 38; system TE—Rf 10; system TF—Rf 43; system TT—Rf 84; system TU—Rf 43; system TV—Rf 03; system TAD—Rf 49; system TAE—Rf 87; system TAF—Rf 88; system TAJ—Rf 65; system TAK—Rf 78; system TAL—Rf 06.

Gas Chromatography. System GA—chlorpropamide RI 1791, chlorpropamide-Me RI 2165, chlorpropamide-Me_2 RI 2250.

High Performance Liquid Chromatography. System HX—RI 450; system HY—RI 411 and 413; system HZ—retention time 5.0 min; system HAA—retention time, 17.7 min.

Ultraviolet Spectrum. Methanolic acid—232 nm (A_1^1=598a).

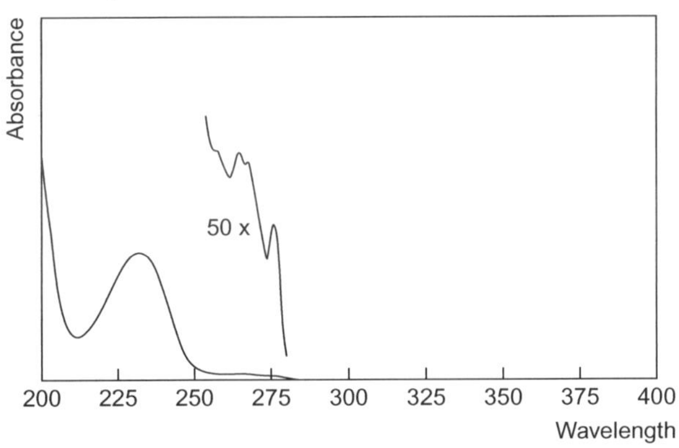

Infra-red Spectrum. Principal peaks at wavenumbers 1661, 1159, 1553, 757, 1086, 909 cm^{-1} (KBr disk).

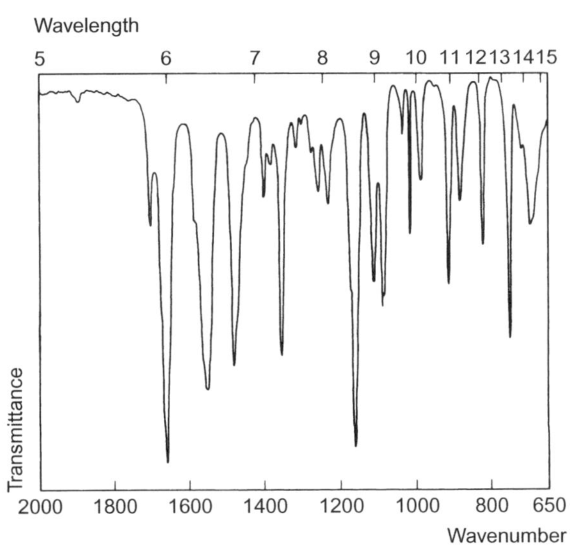

Mass Spectrum. Principal ions at *m/z* 111, 175, 75, 85, 30, 276, 127, 113.

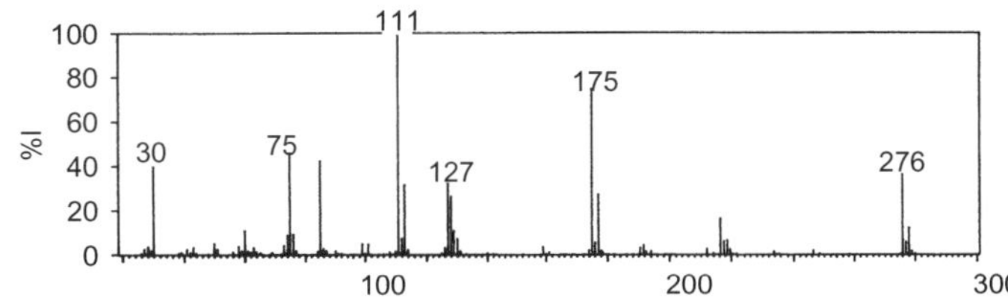

Quantification

Gas chromatography. In plasma: chlorpropamide or tolbutamide, limit of detection 50 µg/L, FID—K. K. Midha *et al.*, *J. Pharm. Sci.*, 1976, *65*, 576–579. In blood or plasma: chlorpropamide or tolbutamide, limit of detection 1 mg/L, ECD—S. B. Matin and M. Rowland, *J. Pharm. Pharmacol.*, 1973, *25*, 186–187.

High performance liquid chromatography. In serum: chlorpropamide or tolbutamide, limit of detection 7 mg/L for chlorpropamide, UV detection—R. E. Hill and J. Crechiolo, *J. Chromatogr.* 1978, *145 B*, *Biomed. Appl.*, *2*, 165–168. In urine: chlorpropamide and metabolites, using initial separation by thin-layer chromatography, UV detection—J. A. Taylor, *Clin. Pharmacol. Ther.*, 1972, *13*, 710–718.

Disposition in the Body. Rapidly and completely absorbed after oral administration. The main metabolic reactions are hydroxylation at the 2- and 3-positions of the propyl substituent in the side-chain, *N*-dealkylation and hydrolysis to form the sulfonamide metabolite. About 80% of a single oral dose is excreted in the urine in 7 days. During chronic therapy, up to 100% of a dose is excreted in the urine in 24 h, with about 18% of the dose as unchanged drug, 2% as 4-chlorobenzenesulfonamide, 20% as 4-chlorobenzenesulfonylurea, 55% as 2-hydroxychlorpropamide, and 2% as 3-hydroxychlorpropamide.

Therapeutic concentration. In plasma, usually in the range 30 to 250 mg/L.

Following single oral doses of 250 mg to 6 subjects, peak plasma concentrations of 23.9 to 39.4 mg/L (mean 28) were attained in 1 to 7 h. After daily oral doses of 250 to 500 mg to 4 subjects, steady-state plasma concentrations of 75.5 to 245.5 mg/L (mean 142) were reported; plasma concentrations of 4-chlorobenzenesulfonylurea and 2-hydroxychlorpropamide ranged from 3 to 6 mg/L and <1 to 9 mg/L, respectively. [J. A. Taylor, *Clin. Pharmacol. Ther.*, 1972, *13*, 710–718.]

Toxicity. Prolonged hypoglycaemic coma has been reported after overdosage but fatalities are comparatively rare, although some instances of fatal blood dyscrasias have been reported. Peak plasma concentrations of 200 to 750 mg/L have been observed in comatose subjects.

Half-life. Plasma half-life, 20 to 45 h (mean 35); increased in renal impairment.

Volume of distribution. About 0.1 to 0.3 L/kg.

Protein binding. In plasma, 60 to 95%.

Dose. 100 to 500 mg daily.

Chlorprothixene

Tranquilliser

Synonyms. N-714; Ro-4-0403.
Proprietary names. Taractan; Tarasan; Truxal; Truxaletten. It is also an ingredient of Silgastrin-T.
(*Z*)-3-(2-Chloro-9*H*-thioxanthen-9-ylidene)-*N*,*N*-dimethyl-1-propanamine
$C_{18}H_{18}ClNS$=315.9
CAS—113-59-7

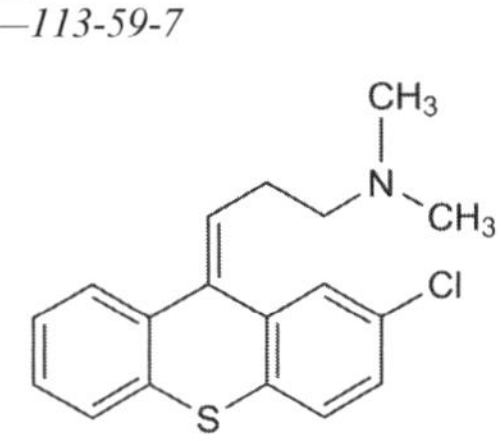

A pale yellow crystalline powder. M.p. 97° to 98°. Protect from light.

Soluble 1 in 1700 of water, 1 in 29 of ethanol, 1 in 18 of acetone, 1 in 2 of chloroform, and 1 in 14 of ether. Incompatible with acids and alkalis.

Chlorprothixene Hydrochloride

Proprietary names. Cloxan; Truquil.
$C_{18}H_{18}ClNS,HCl=352.4$
CAS—6469-93-8
White or almost white crystalline powder. M.p. 221°. Protect from light. Freely soluble in water at pH 6 to 6.5, slightly soluble in dichloromethane.

Chlorprothixene Mesilate

Synonym. Chlorprothixene Mesylate
$C_{18}H_{18}ClNS,CH_3SO_3H,H_2O=430.0$

Dissociation Constant. pK_a 8.8.

Partition Coefficient. Log *P* (octanol/water), 5.18.

Colour Tests. Formaldehyde–Sulfuric Acid—red (orange fluorescence under ultraviolet light); Liebermann's Test—red; Mandelin's Test—red; Marquis Test—red-orange; Sulfuric Acid—orange (fluoresces under ultraviolet light).

Thin-layer Chromatography. System TA—Rf 56; system TB—Rf 51; system TC—Rf 51; system TE—Rf 74; system TL—Rf 25; system TAE—Rf 34; system TAF—Rf 51; system TAJ—Rf 20; system TAK—Rf 08; system TAL—Rf 65. (Acidified iodoplatinate solution, positive.)

Gas Chromatography. System GA—chlorprothixene RI 2492, M (OH-dihydro-) isomer 1 RI 2750, M (OH-dihydro-) isomer 2 RI 2790, M (OH-methoxy-dihydro-) RI 2810, M (*N*-oxide)-$(CH_3)_2NOH$ RI 2410, M (*N*-oxide sulfoxide)-$(CH_3)_2NOH$ RI 2560, M (sulfoxide) RI 2720, Art (dihydro-) RI 2490, Art (Cl-thioxanthenone) RI 2260; system GB—chlorprothixene RI 2608; system GF—RI 2910.

High Performance Liquid Chromatography. System HA—*k* 3.0; system HX—RI 459; system HY—RI 353; system HZ—retention time 10.1 min; system HAX—retention time 17.6 min; system HAY—retention time 8.3 min.

Column: RP-100 CN (Nucleosil, 250 × 4.6 mm i.d., 5 μm). Mobile phase: acetonitrile:pyridine:sodium acetate (0.14 M, pH 3.1) (698:2:300), flow rate 0.9 mL/min. Electrochemical detection. Retention time: 10.2 min. [M. Bagli *et al.*, *J. Chromatogr.* 1994, *657 B Biomed. Appl.*, 141–148.]

Ultraviolet Spectrum. Aqueous acid—230 nm (A_1^1=1096b), 268, 324 nm.

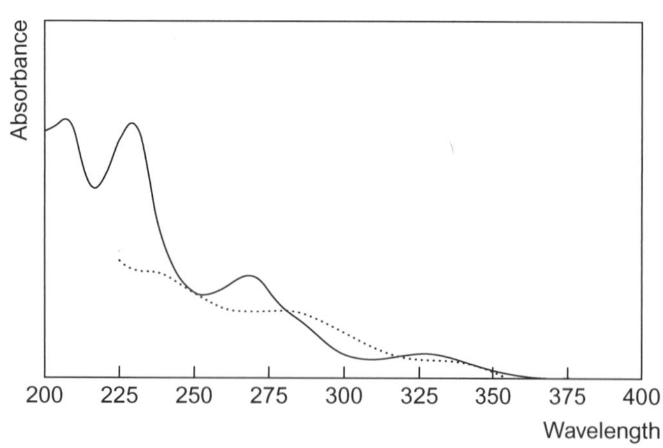

Infra-red Spectrum. Principal peaks at wavenumbers 776, 1104, 832, 746, 1030, 1170 cm^{-1} (KBr disk).

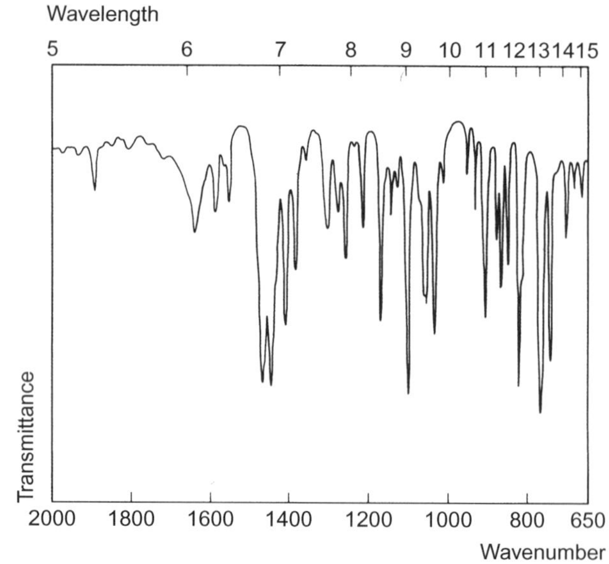

Mass Spectrum. Principal ions at *m/z* 58, 59, 221, 30, 42, 222, 255, 43.

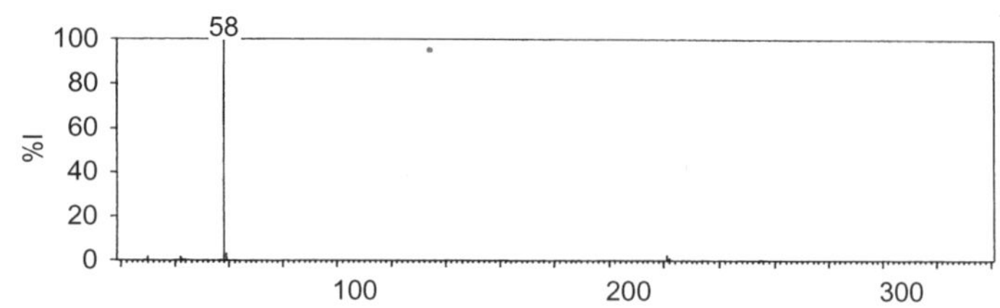

Quantification

High performance liquid chromatography. In plasma: limit of quantification 5 μg/L, UV detection (λ=229 nm)—M. A. Brooks *et al.*, *J. Chromatogr.*, 1985, *337*, 351–362. In serum: limit of detection 0.5 μg/L, electrochemical detection—M. Bagli *et al.*, *J. Chromatogr.* 1994, *657 B Biomed. Appl.*, 141–148.

Spectrofluorimetry. In plasma—T. Mjörndal and L. Oreland, *Acta Pharmacol. Toxicol.*, 1971, *29*, 295–302. In blood: limit of detection 1 μg/L—J. Raaflaub, *Experientia*, 1975, *31*, 557–558.

Ultraviolet spectrophotometry. In blood, liver, or urine: chlorprothixene and metabolites, limit of detection 500 ng/g, separation by thin-layer chromatography—H. Christensen, *Acta Pharmacol. Toxicol.*, 1974, *34*, 16–26.

Disposition in the Body. Readily absorbed after oral administration, but undergoes extensive first-pass metabolism. The major metabolite is the sulfoxide, but *N*-demethylation and *N*-oxidation also occur. Chlorprothixene and its sulfoxide metabolites are distributed into breast milk. After daily oral doses, up to about 30% is excreted in the urine in 24 h as chlorprothixene sulfoxide, and up to about 40% is eliminated in the faeces also as the sulfoxide.

Therapeutic concentration

Following a single oral dose of 30 mg to one subject, a peak blood concentration of about 0.01 mg/L was attained in 4 h. [J. Raaflaub, *Experientia*, 1975, *31*, 557–558.]

Oral administration of a single 100 mg dose of chlorprothixene, in the form of a solution (base), suspension (base), or tablets (hydrochloride), to 8 subjects, produced respective peak plasma chlorprothixene concentrations of 22.4 to 65.7 μg/L (mean 31.6) at 3.0 h, 13.3 to 70.6 μg/L (mean 24.2) at 2.88 h and 13.4 to 52.6 μg/L (mean 25.8) at 2.5 h. [M. Bagli *et al.*, *Arzneimittelforschung*, 1996, *46*, 247–250.]

Toxicity. The estimated minimum lethal dose is 2.5 g, although recovery has occurred after the ingestion of 12 g.

2 to 12 h after a suicidal ingestion of about 10 g of chlorprothixene, a 31-year-old female had the following plasma concentrations: chlorprothixene 10 mg/L, desmethylchlorprothixene 8 mg/L, and chlorprothixene sulfoxide 1 mg/L. After 4 h haemoperfusion, the levels were: chlorprothixene 0.1 mg/

L, desmethylchlorprothixene 0.1 mg/L, and chlorprothixene sulfoxide was not detected. [C. Koppel *et al.*, *Intensive Care Med.*, 1987, *13*, 358–360.]

In 6 fatalities attributed to the ingestion of about 2.5 to 4 g of chlorprothixene, the following postmortem concentrations were reported: blood, chlorprothixene <0.1 to 0.4 mg/L, total metabolites <0.1 to 0.6 mg/L; liver, chlorprothixene 5 to 42 µg/g (mean 18), total metabolites 14 to 67 µg/g (mean 25); in 1 case a urine concentration of total thioxanthenes of 15 mg/L was also reported; desmethylchlorprothixene was the major metabolite in the liver. Alcohol was also detected in 3 cases. [H. Christensen, *Acta Pharmacol. Toxicol.*, 1974, *34*, 16–26.]

In a fatality involving the ingestion of up to 4 g of chlorprothixene, the following postmortem tissue concentrations were reported (mg/L):

	Chlorprothixene	Chlorprothixene sulfoxide
Blood	0.1	0.6
Bile	3.9	7.0
Urine	0.4	3.4

[A. Poklis *et al.*, *J. Anal. Toxicol.*, 1983, *7*, 29–32.]

Bioavailability. About 40%.

Half-life. Plasma half-life, about 8 to 12 h.

Volume of distribution. About 10 to 20 L/kg.

Clearance. Plasma clearance, about 14 to 20 mL/min/kg.

Dose. 45 to 200 mg daily in divided doses; up to 600 mg daily has been given.

Chlorpyrifos

Acaricide, Insecticide

Synonyms. Chlorpyrifos-ethyl; Dowco 179; ENT-27311.
Proprietary names. Affront; Brodan; Bullet; Detmol UA; Dursban; Empire; Eradex; Ethion; Lorsban; Paqeant; Piridane; Pyrinex; Scout; Stipend.
Phosphorothioic acid *O*,*O*-diethyl *O*-(3,5,6-trichloro-2-pyridinyl) ester
$C_9H_{11}Cl_3NO_3PS$=350.6
CAS—2921-88-2

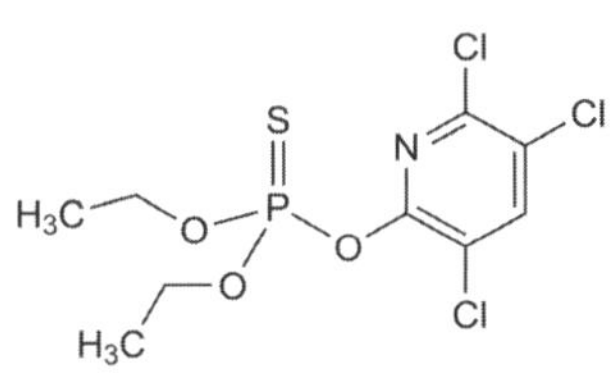

Off-white to pale yellow granular crystals. M.p. 41° to 42°.
It is practically insoluble in water (2 mg/L at 24°); readily soluble in organic solvents: acetone (6500 g/kg at 25°), benzene (7900 g/kg at 25°), chloroform (6300 g/kg at 25°), carbon disulfide (5900 g/kg at 25°), diethyl ether (5100 g/kg at 25°), xylene (5000 g/kg at 25°), methanol (450 g/kg at 25°), methylene chloride, and ethylene dichloride.

Chlorpyrifos-methyl

Synonyms. Dowco 214; ENT-27520; NSC-60380; OMS-1155.
Proprietary names. Douco 214; Dusban-methyl; Graincote; Noltron; Reldan; Smite; Turmar; Zertell.
$C_7H_7Cl_3NO_3PS$=322.5
CAS—5598-13-0
A colourless, crystalline solid. M.p. 45.5° to 46.5°. It is soluble in water (5 mg/L at 25°); very soluble in organic solvents: acetone (6400 g/kg at 24°), benzene (5200 g/kg at 24°), diethyl ether (4800 g/kg at 24°), chloroform (3500 g/kg at 24°), methanol (390 g/kg at 24°), and hexane (230 g/kg at 24°).

Partition Coefficient. Log *P* (octanol/water), 4.96.

Thin-layer Chromatography. System TE—chlorpyrifos Rf 99; system TX—chlorpyrifos Rf 64, chlorpyrifos-methyl Rf 56; system TY—chlorpyrifos Rf 95, chlorpyrifos-methyl Rf 89; system TAB—chlorpyrifos-methyl Rf 60; system TAC—chlorpyrifos-methyl Rf 35; system TAE—chlorpyrifos RF 85.

Gas Chromatography. System GA—chlorpyrifos RI 1955, chlorpyrifos-methyl RI 1847; system GKA—chlorpyrifos-methyl RI 1866; system GKB—chlorpyrifos-methyl RI 2060; system GKC—chlorpyrifos-methyl RI 2234.

Column: DB-17 (30 × 0.25 mm i.d., 0.5 µm film thickness). Column temperature: 80° for 1 min, to 180° at 25°/min, to 250° at 20°/min, held for 5 min, to 320° held for 2 min. Carrier gas: helium. MS detection (SIM *m/z* at 297, 302, 313, 318). IS : Chlorpyrifos-$^{13}C_2$-^{15}N. Retention time: 9.26 min. [K. A. Brzak *et al.*, *J. Anal. Toxicol.*, 1998, *22*, 203–210.]

High Performance Liquid Chromatography. System HAO—chlorpyrifos-methyl *k* 6.18.

Ultraviolet Spectrum. Aqueous acid—230, 289 nm.

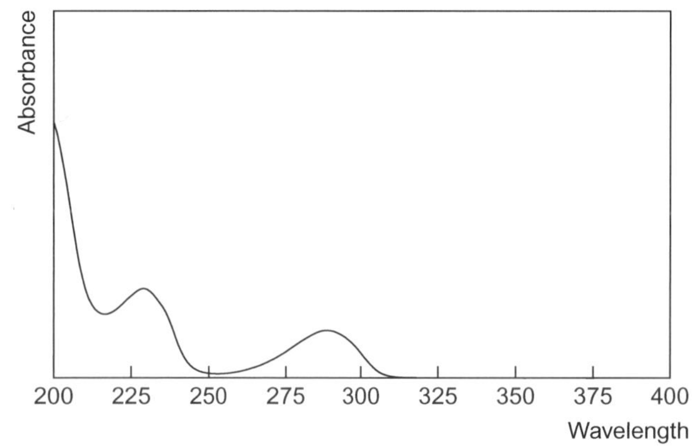

Infra-red Spectrum. Principal peaks at wavenumber 1406, 1038, 850, 967, 1166, 1271 cm^{-1}.

Quantification

Gas chromatography. In blood and urine: limit of quantification 10 µg/L, FPD or ECD—R. J. Nolan *et al.*, *Toxicol. Appl. Pharmacol.*, 1984, *73*, 8–15.

Gas chromatography–mass spectrometry. In blood: limit of quantification 1 µg/L—K. A. Brzak *et al.*, *J. Anal. Toxicol.*, 1998, *22*, 203–210. In urine: limit of detection of TCP metabolite is 0.5 µg/L—M. J. Bartels and P. E. Kastl, *J. Chromatogr.*, 1992, *575(1)*, 69–74.

High performance liquid chromatography. In serum and urine: limit of detection of chlorpyrifos and metabolites is 1.5 µg/L serum and 0.5 µg/L urine. MS/MS detection—J. V. Sancho *et al.*, *Rapid Commun. Mass Spectrom.*, 2000, *14(16)*, 1485–1490.

Disposition in the Body. Chlorpyrifos is readily absorbed into the bloodstream from the gastrointestinal tract, through the lungs and through the skin. The major metabolites observed are 3,5,6-trichloro-2-pyridinol (TCP), diethylphosphate, and diethylthio-phosphate. Chlorpyrifos and its metabolites are eliminated rapidly from the body via urine and faeces. The majority of an ingested dose is recovered in urine as the metabolites whereas only 1% of the compound absorbed through dermal exposure is detected as metabolites in urine. No significant bioaccumulation has been observed.

Blood concentration
6 male, healthy Caucasian volunteers were administered a single oral dose of 0.5 mg/kg bodyweight followed by topical exposure of 0.5 mg/kg 4 weeks later. Following both doses, blood chloripyrifos concentrations of <30 µg/L were observed. The maximum TCP blood concentration was on average 930 µg/L (range, 510 to 1350 µg/L) 6 h after oral administration, and 63 µg/L (range, 29 to 122 µg/L) 24 h after topical administration. [R. J. Nolan *et al.*, *Toxicol. Appl. Pharmacol.*, 1984, *73*, 8–15.]

Toxicity. Chlorpyrifos is very toxic and affects the central nervous, cardiovascular, and respiratory systems. It is irritating to skin and eyes. Doses up to 28 g may be fatal. No toxic effects have been observed with doses of 0.1 mg/kg body weight daily taken over 4 weeks. This dose is deemed the acceptable daily intake. A toxic dose of 300 mg/kg body weight has effects on the peripheral nervous system.

Half-life. Chlorpyrifos, 1 day; TCP, 26.9 h (oral dose) and 30 h (dermal exposure).

Volume of distribution. TCP, 181 mL/kg.

Chlorquinaldol

Antibacterial/Antifungal

Synonyms. Chlorchinaldol; Hydroxydichloroquinaldine.
Proprietary names. Afungil; Gyno-Sterosan; Gynothérax; Quesil; Siogen(o); Siosteran; Soprosan; Sterosan; Steroxin.
5,7-Dichloro-2-methyl-8-quinolinol
$C_{10}H_7Cl_2NO$=228.1
CAS—72-80-0

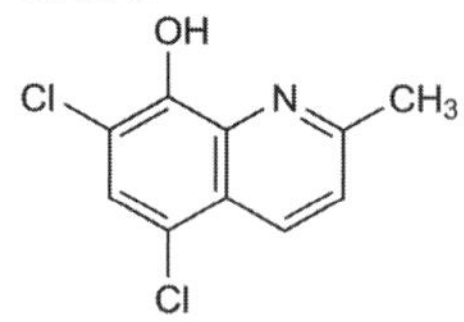

A green or yellowish-brown crystalline powder. M.p. about 113°.
Practically insoluble in water; soluble 1 in 100 of ethanol, 1 in 20 of chloroform, and 1 in 33 of ether; soluble in acetone, benzene, and glacial acetic acid.

Partition Coefficient. Log *P* (octanol/water), 3.5.

Colour Test. Ferric Chloride—blue-green.

Thin-layer Chromatography. System TA—Rf 71. (Acidified iodoplatinate solution, positive.)

Gas Chromatography. System GA—RI 1802.

Ultraviolet Spectrum. Aqueous acid—263 nm (A^1_1=2100b), 330 nm (A^1_1=132b); aqueous alkali—263 nm (A^1_1=1410b), 345 nm (A^1_1=186b); methanol—251 nm (A^1_1=1900b), 315 nm (A^1_1=146b).

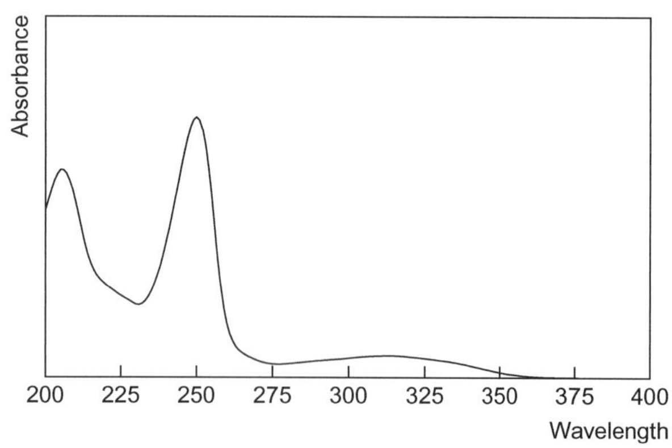

Infra-red Spectrum. Principal peaks at wavenumbers 1656, 1739, 1605, 758, 1111, 1153 cm^{-1} (KBr disk).

Uses. Chlorquinaldol is used topically in a concentration of 3%; it has been used as 200 mg vaginal tablets.

Chlortalidone

Diuretic

Synonyms. Chlorthalidone; G-33182; Phthalamudine.
Proprietary names. Hydro-long; Hygroton; Igrolina; Novothalidone; Renon; Uridon; Urolin; Zambesil. It is an ingredient of Kalspare, Lopresoretic, Regroton, and Tenoret(ic).
2-Chloro-5-(2,3-dihydro-1-hydroxy-3-oxo-1*H*-isoindol-1-yl)-benzenesulfonamide
$C_{14}H_{11}ClN_2O_4S$=338.8
CAS—77-36-1

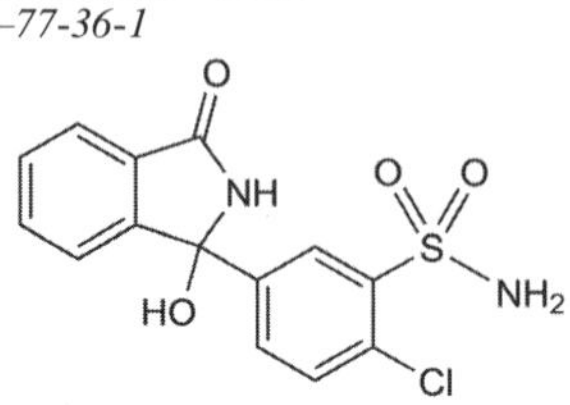

A white or yellowish-white crystalline powder. M.p. about 220°, with decomposition.
Practically insoluble in water; soluble 1 in 150 of ethanol, 1 in 650 of chloroform, and 1 in 25 of methanol; slightly soluble in ether; soluble in solutions of alkali hydroxides.

Dissociation Constant. pK_a 9.4.

Partition Coefficient. Log *P* (octanol/water), 0.8.

Colour Tests. Koppanyi–Zwikker Test—violet; Marquis Test—yellow.

Thin-layer Chromatography. System TD—Rf 04; system TE—Rf 42; system TF—Rf 40; system TAD—Rf 23; system TAE—Rf 88; system TAF—Rf 83; system TAJ—Rf 17; system TAK—Rf 10; system TAL—Rf 63.

Gas Chromatography. System GA—chlortalidone RI 2145, chlortalidone-Me_4 RI 2630; system GX—chlortalidone-Me_4 retention time 7.7 min; system GY—chlortalidone-Me_4 retention time 4.8 min.

High Performance Liquid Chromatography. System HN—*k* 1.28; system HX—RI 367; system HY—RI 308; system HZ—retention time, 2.3 min.

Ultraviolet Spectrum. Ethanol—275 nm (A^1_1=57a), 284 nm (A^1_1=45a).

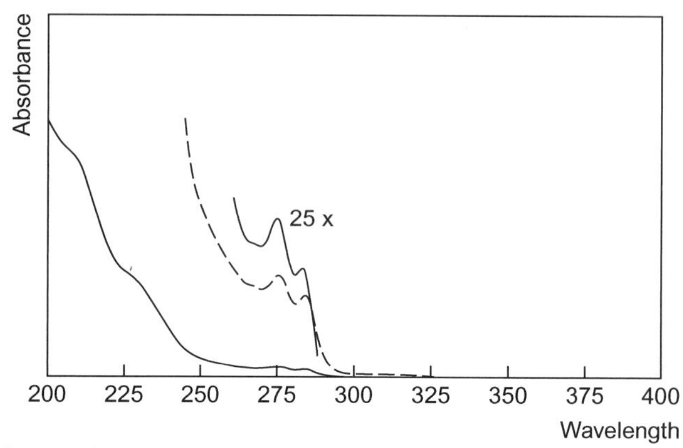

Infra-red Spectrum. Principal peaks at wavenumbers 1685, 1033, 1160, 845, 1190, 1310 cm^{-1} (KBr disk).

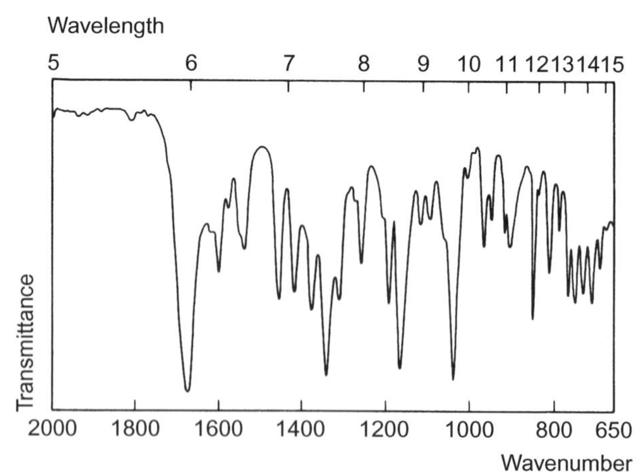

Mass Spectrum. Principal ions at *m/z* 76, 239, 104, 240, 285, 241, 50, 75.

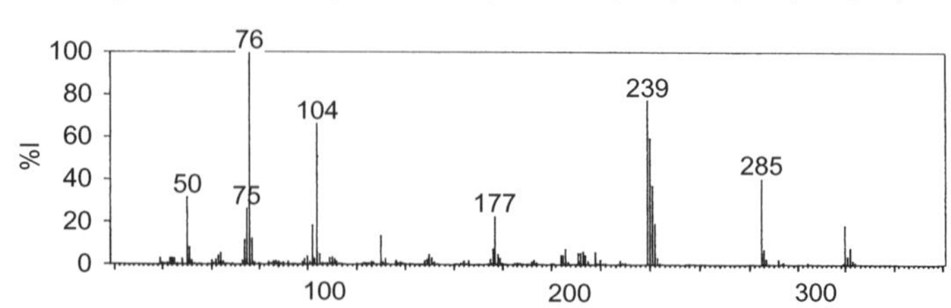

Quantification

Gas chromatography. In plasma, erythrocytes or urine: limit of detection 10 μg/L in plasma, AFID—H. L. J. Fleuren and J. M. van Rossum, *J. Chromatogr.*, 1978, *152*, 41–54.

High performance liquid chromatography. In blood, plasma or urine: limit of detection 30 µg/L , UV detection—P. J. M. Guelen *et al.*, *J. Chromatogr.* 1980, *181 B Biomed. Appl.*, *7*, 497–503. In blood or urine: limit of detection 100 µg/L , UV detection—T. R. MacGregor *et al.*, *Ther. Drug Monit.*, 1984, *6*, 83–90. In plasma: limit of quantification 10 µg/L, UV detection—C. Giachetti *et al.*, *J. Chromatogr. B Biomed. Sci. Appl.*, 1997, *698(1–2)*, 187–194. In urine: limit of quantification 0.1 mg/L and limit of detection 0.02 mg/L, UV detection (λ=214 nm)—S. Salado *et al.*, *J. Chromatogr. B Biomed. Sci. Appl.*, 1997, *690(1–2)*, 195–202.

Disposition in the Body. Readily but incompletely absorbed after oral administration. It does not appear to be significantly metabolised. After a single dose, about 25 to 40% is excreted in the urine as unchanged drug and about 1% is eliminated in the bile; the quantity excreted in the urine appears to be dose-dependent. During daily therapy, about 50% of the daily dose is excreted unchanged in the urine in 24 h and about 25% is eliminated in the faeces.

Therapeutic concentration

After single oral doses of 50 to 75 mg given to 7 subjects, peak plasma concentrations of 0.14 to 0.26 mg/L were attained in 1 to 3 h. [H. L. J. Fleuren *et al.*, *Eur. J. Clin. Pharmacol.*, 1979, *15*, 35–50.]

Following daily oral doses of 50 mg to 10 subjects, steady-state plasma concentrations of 0.2 to 1.4 mg/L (mean 0.5) were reported. [P. Collste *et al.*, *Eur. J. Clin. Pharmacol.*, 1976, *9*, 319–325.]

Bioavailability. About 65%.

Half-life. Plasma half-life, 35 to 70 h (mean 48), increased in elderly subjects.

Volume of distribution. About 4 L/kg.

Clearance. Plasma clearance, about 1 to 2 mL/min/kg.

Distribution in blood. Plasma : whole blood ratio, about 0.04 at therapeutic concentrations.

Protein binding. In plasma, about 75%.

Note. For a review of the pharmacokinetics of diuretics, see B. Beerman and M. Groschinsky-Grind, *Clin. Pharmacokinet.*, 1980, *5*, 221–245.

Dose. Usually 50 mg daily or 100 to 200 mg on alternate days.

Chlortetracycline

Antibacterial

Proprietary names. Acronize; Biomitsin; Orospray.
[4*S*-(4α,4aα,5aα,6β,12aα)]-7-Chloro-4-dimethylamino-1,4,4a,5,5a,6,11,-12a-octahydro-3,6,10,12,12a-pentahydroxy-6-methyl-1,11-dioxo-2-naphthacenecarboxamide
$C_{22}H_{23}ClN_2O_8$=478.9
CAS—57-62-5

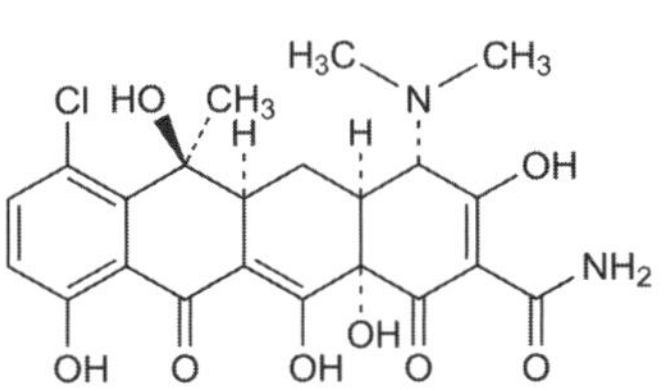

A yellow crystalline powder. M.p. 168° to 169°.
Very slightly soluble in water; very soluble in aqueous solutions above pH 8.5; slightly soluble in ethanol, acetone, ethyl acetate, and benzene; practically insoluble in ether.

Chlortetracycline Calcium

CAS—5892-31-9
A white powder.
Practically insoluble in water.

Chlortetracycline Hydrochloride

Synonym. Biomycin
Proprietary names. Aureomycin(e); Chlortet. It is an ingredient of Aureocort and Deteclo.
$C_{22}H_{23}ClN_2O_8$,HCl=515.3
CAS—64-72-2
Yellow crystals. M.p. about 210°, with decomposition.
Soluble 1 in 75 to 1 in 110 of water and 1 in 250 to 1 in 560 of ethanol; practically insoluble in acetone, chloroform, and ether; soluble in solutions of alkali hydroxides and carbonates.

Dissociation Constant. pK_a 3.3, 7.4, 9.3 (25°).

Partition Coefficient. Log *P* (octanol/pH 7.5), −0.9.

Colour Tests. Benedict's Reagent—red; Formaldehyde–Sulfuric Acid—orange-brown; Mandelin's Test—violet-brown→yellow; Marquis Test—yellow→green; Sulfuric Acid—brown-blue.

Thin-layer Chromatography. System TA—Rf 05, streaking. (Location under ultraviolet light, orange fluorescence; acidified potassium permanganate solution, positive.)

High Performance Liquid Chromatography. System HY—RI 280 and 282.

Ultraviolet Spectrum. Aqueous acid—266 nm (A_1^1=386a), 359 nm; aqueous alkali—253, 284, 346 nm. (See below)

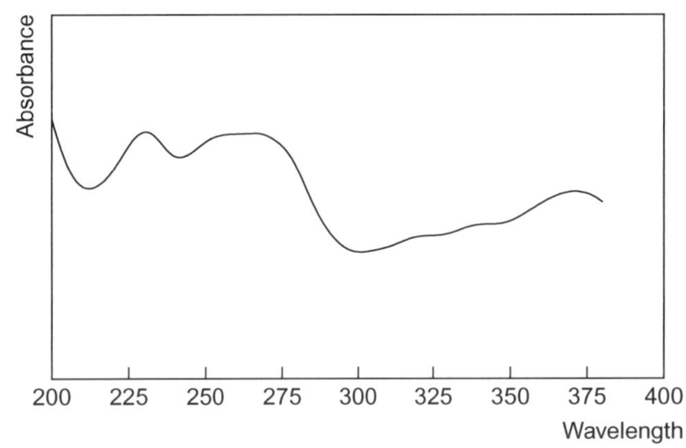

Infra-red Spectrum. Principal peaks at wavenumbers 1622, 1580, 1666, 1311, 1041, 1227 cm^{-1} (chlortetracycline hydrochloride, KBr disk). Polymorphism may occur.

Disposition in the Body. Readily absorbed after oral administration but rapidly inactivated in the body. It is eliminated mainly by biliary excretion with only about 15% of a dose being excreted in the urine as unchanged drug.

Half-life. Plasma half-life, about 6 h.

Protein binding. In plasma, about 47%.

Dose. 1 to 2 g of chlortetracycline hydrochloride daily.

Chlorzoxazone

Muscle Relaxant

Synonym. Chlorobenzoxazolinone
Proprietary names. Biomioran; Paraflex. It is an ingredient of Parafon.
5-Chloro-2(3*H*)-benzoxazolone
$C_7H_4ClNO_2$=169.6
CAS—95-25-0

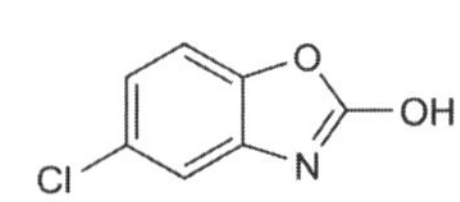

Colourless crystals or white crystalline powder. M.p. 190° to 194°.
Sparingly soluble in water; soluble 1 in 20 of ethanol, 1 in 250 of chloroform, and 1 in 60 of ether; soluble in acetone, methanol, and isopropanol; freely soluble in aqueous solutions of alkali hydroxides and ammonia.

Dissociation Constant. pK_a 8.0 (20°).

Partition Coefficient. Log *P* (octanol/water), 1.6.

Colour Test. Koppanyi–Zwikker Test—violet.

Thin-layer Chromatography. System TA—Rf 85; system TB—Rf 00; system TC—Rf 51; system TD—Rf 54; system TE—Rf 33; system TF—Rf

61; system TL—Rf 47; system TAD—Rf 56; system TAE—Rf 88; system TAF—Rf 90; system TAJ—Rf 51; system TAK—Rf 61; system TAL—Rf 92.

Gas Chromatography. System GA—chlorzoxazone RI 1728, chlorzoxazone-Me RI 1750.

High Performance Liquid Chromatography. System HX—RI 397.

Ultraviolet Spectrum. Aqueous acid—280 nm (A_1^1=306a); aqueous alkali—243 nm (A_1^1=580a), 287 nm (A_1^1=409a).

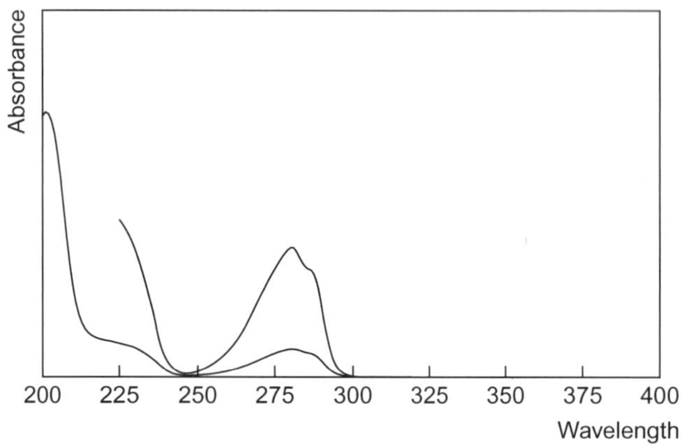

Infra-red Spectrum. Principal peaks at wavenumbers 1762, 801, 962, 1149, 840, 1300 cm^{-1} (KBr disk).

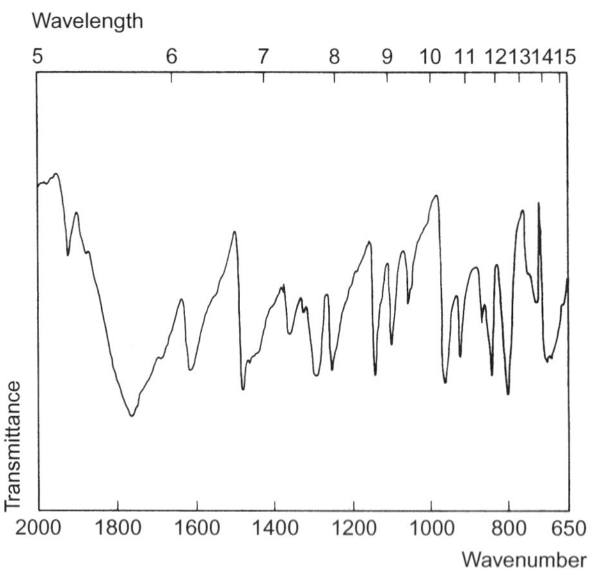

Mass Spectrum. Principal ions at *m/z* 169, 78, 171, 113, 115, 63, 51, 170.

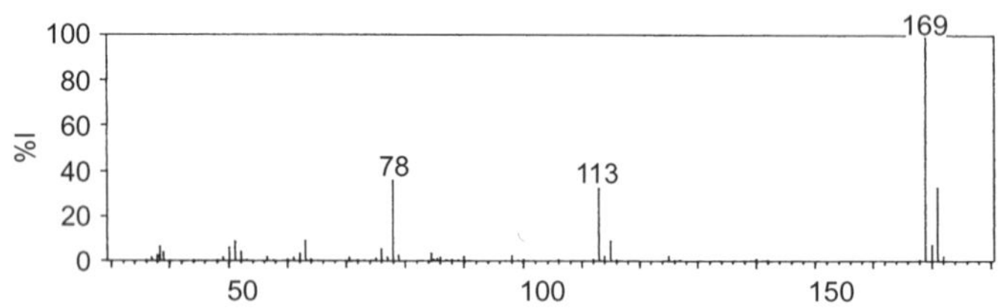

Quantification

Spectrofluorimetry. In plasma or urine: limits of detection 60 μg/L and 130 μg/L respectively—J. T. Stewart and C. Chan, *J. Pharm. Sci.*, 1979, *68*, 910–912.

Gas chromatography–mass spectrometry. In plasma: limit of quantification 5 μg/L—C. B. Eap *et al.*, *J. Chromatogr. B Biomed. Sci. Appl.*, 1998, *705(1)*, 139–144.

High performance liquid chromatography. In plasma: chlorzoxazone and 6-hydroxychlorzoxazone, limit of detection 80 ng, UV detection—I. L. Honigberg *et al.*, *J. Pharm. Sci.*, 1979, *68*, 253–255. In plasma and urine: limit of quantification 100 μg/L, UV detection (λ=283 nm)—R. F. Frye and D. D. Stiff, *J. Chromatogr. B Biomed. Sci. Appl.*, 1996, *686(2)*, 291–296. In serum: limit of quantification 0.5 mg/L and limit of detection 0.1 mg/L, UV detection (λ=230 nm)—A. Haque and J. T. Stewart, *Biomed. Chromatogr.*, 1997, *11(4)*, 236–239. In serum: limit of quantification 0.01 mg/L, UV detection (λ=287 nm)—E. Tanaka, *J. Pharm. Biomed. Anal.*, 1998, *16(5)*, 899–904.

Disposition in the Body. Absorbed after oral administration and rapidly metabolised to 6-hydroxychlorzoxazone. Up to 90% of a dose is excreted in the urine in 48 h as conjugates of the 6-hydroxy metabolite; less than 1% is excreted as unchanged drug; 5-chloroacetanilide and 6-hydroxybenzoxazol-2(3*H*)-one have also been detected in urine.

Therapeutic concentration

Following a single oral dose of 750 mg of chlorzoxazone and 900 mg of paracetamol, a mean peak plasma concentration of 36.3 mg/L of chlorzoxazone was attained in 0.7 h. [R. K. Desiraju *et al.*, *J. Pharm. Sci.*, 1983, *72*, 991–994.]

Half-life. Plasma half-life, about 1 h.

Dose. 0.75 to 3 g daily.

Cholesterol

Synonym. Cholesterin
(3*β*)-Cholest-5-en-3-ol
$C_{27}H_{46}O$=386.7
CAS-57-88-5

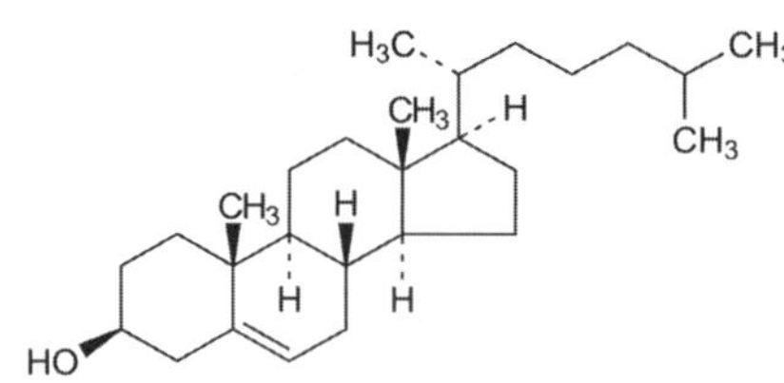

White or faintly yellow, pearly leaflets, needles, powder, or granules. It acquires a yellow to pale tan colour on prolonged exposure to light. M.p. 147° to 150°.
Practically insoluble in water; slowly soluble 1 in 100 of ethanol and 1 in 50 of dehydrated alcohol; soluble 1 in 2.8 of ether and 1 in 4.5 of chloroform; soluble in acetone, benzene and dioxan.

Partition Coefficient. Log *P* (octanol/water), 8.7.

Colour Tests. Antimony Pentachloride—orange→brown; Naphthol–Sulfuric Acid—yellow-brown/violet; Sulfuric Acid—orange.
To a solution of 10 mg in 1 mL of chloroform add 1 mL of sulfuric acid; chloroform layer—red, sulfuric acid layer—green fluorescence.
Dissolve about 5 mg in 2 mL of chloroform, add 1 mL of acetic anhydride and 1 drop of sulfuric acid—pink→red→blue→green.

Thin-layer Chromatography. System TB—Rf 22; system TC—Rf 64; system TD—Rf 61; system TE—Rf 76; system TF—Rf 60; system TL—Rf 69; system TAD—Rf 64; system TAE—Rf 84; system TAF—Rf 96; system TAJ—Rf 65; system TAK—Rf 78; system TAL—Rf 96; system TAM—Rf 96.

Gas Chromatography. System GA—cholesterol RI 3088, cholesterol-H_2O RI 3030; system GE—RRT 1.35 (relative to phenytoin).

Infra-red Spectrum. Principal peaks at wavenumbers 1059, 1022, 800, 959, 952, 839 cm^{-1} (Nujol mull).

Mass Spectrum. Principal ions at *m/z* 386, 368, 43, 55, 275, 81, 57, 95.

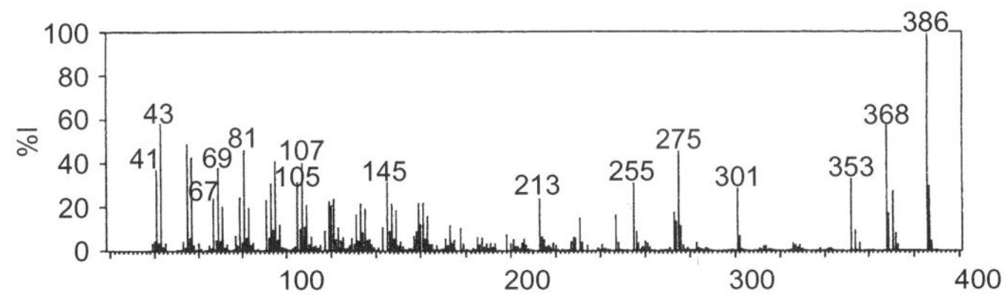

Quantification.
High performance liquid chromatography. In semen: light scattering detection—G. Grizard *et al., J. Chromatogr. Biomed. B Sci. Appl.*, 2000, *740(1)*, 101–107.

Choline

Proprietary names. Choline and its salts are ingredients of many preparations, see *Martindale, The Complete Drug Reference*, 3rd Edn, London, Pharmaceutical Press, 2002.
2-Hydroxy-*N*,*N*,*N*-trimethylethanaminium
$[C_5H_{14}NO]^+ = 104.2$
CAS—62-49-7 (cation)

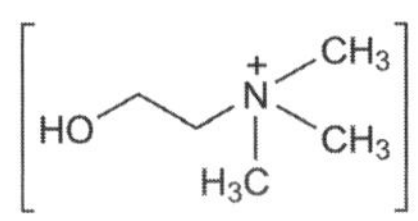

A colourless, viscid, hygroscopic, strongly alkaline liquid.
Very soluble in water and ethanol; practically insoluble in ether.

Choline Bitartrate
Synonym. Choline Acid Tartrate
$C_9H_{19}NO_7 = 253.3$
CAS—87-67-2
A white, hygroscopic, crystalline powder.
Very soluble in water; slightly soluble in ethanol; practically insoluble in chloroform and ether.

Choline Chloride
Proprietary name. Becholine
$C_5H_{14}ClNO = 139.6$
CAS—67-48-1
White, very hygroscopic crystals.
Very soluble in water and ethanol; practically insoluble in chloroform and ether.

Choline Dihydrogen Citrate
Synonym. Choline Citrate
Proprietary name. Neurotropan
$C_{11}H_{21}NO_8 = 295.3$
CAS—77-91-8
Colourless, translucent, hygroscopic crystals or white crystalline powder. M.p. 105.0° to 107.5°.
Soluble 1 in 1 of water and 1 in 45 of ethanol; practically insoluble in benzene, chloroform, and ether.

Choline Hydroxide
Synonyms. Bursine; Fagine; Gossypine; Sincaline; Vidine.
$C_5H_{15}NO_2 = 121.2$
Strongly alkaline liquid.
Very soluble in water, alcohol. Insoluble in ether.

Dissociation Constant. pK_a 8.9.

Thin-layer Chromatography. System TA—Rf 02; system TN—Rf 60; system TO—Rf 60. (Acidified iodoplatinate solution, positive; acidified potassium permanganate solution, positive.)

Ultraviolet Spectrum. No significant absorption, 230 to 360 nm.

Infra-red Spectrum. Principal peaks at wavenumbers 1636, 1620, 953, 1075, 1040, 860 cm^{-1} (choline chloride, thin film).

Quantification
Colorimetry. In urine—S. Eksborg and B. A. Persson, *Acta Pharm. Suec.*, 1971, *8*, 605–608.

High performance liquid chromatography. In plasma: electrochemical detection—T. Fossati *et al., J. Chromatogr. B Biomed. Appl.*, 1994, *656*, 59–64.In plasma and peritoneal dialysis effluent: electrochemical detection—L. E. Webb *et al., Clin. Biochem.*, 1993, *26*, 173–177.

High performance liquid chromatography and gas chromatography. In plasma: choline and metabolites—E. A. Pomfret *et al., Anal. Biochem.*, 1989, *180*, 85–90.

High performance liquid chromatography–mass spectrometry. In tissues: choline and metabolites—H. Koc *et al., Anal. Chem.*, 2002, *74*, 4734–4740.

Disposition in the Body. Choline is a metabolite of suxamethonium chloride and suxethonium bromide.

Dose. Choline has been given in doses of 2 to 4 g daily.

Choline Alfoscerate

Nootropic

Synonym. L-α-Glycerylphosphorylcholine
Proprietary names. Brezal; Delecit; Gliatilin.
(*R*)-2-[[(2,3-Dihydroxypropoxy)hydroxyphosphinyl]oxy]-*N*,*N*,*N*-trimethylethanaminium hydroxide inner salt
$C_8H_{20}NO_6P = 257.2$
CAS—28319-77-9

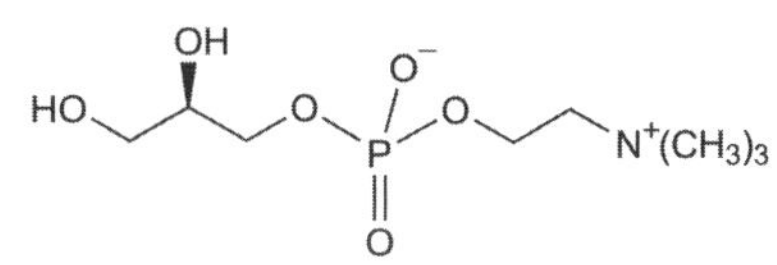

White crystals. M.p. 142.5°.

Partition Coefficient. Log *P* (octanol/water), −5.15.

High Performance Liquid Chromatography. Column: (analytical) RP cyano (Spheri-5, 5 μm, 100 × 4.6 mm i.d.), (bioreactor) anion-exchange cartridge (Aquapore AX-300, 7 μm, 30 × 2.1 mm i.d.). Mobile phase: sodium hydrogen phosphate (20 mM) and tetramethylammonium chloride (10 mM) solution, pH adjusted to 7.1 with phosphoric acid (65%). Flow rate, 0.7 mL/min. Electrochemical detection: platinum electrode at +300 mV. Retention time: choline, 5 min. [T. Fossati *et al., J. Chromatogr.*, 1994, *656, Biomed. Appl.*, 59–64].

Column: RP cyano (Spheri-10, 10 μm, 30 × 4.6 mm), (bioreactor) anion-exchange cartridge (Aquapore AX-300, 7 μm, 30 × 2.1 mm i.d.). Mobile phase: sodium hydrogen phosphate (15 mM) and tetramethylammonium chloride (0.5 mM) solution, pH 7. Electrochemical detection: platinum electrode against Ag/AgCl electrode at +0.5 V. Retention time: choline, 3.1 min. [G. Abbiati *et al., J. Chromatogr.* 1991, *566, Biomed. Appl.*, 445–451].

Quantification
Gas chromatography–mass spectrometry. In blood: limit of quantification 0.3 pg/L—Y. Hasegawa *et al., J. Chromatogr.*, 1982, *239*; 335–342.

High performance liquid chromatography. In plasma: limit of quantification 3.58 μg/L. Electrochemical detection—T. Fossati *et al., J. Chromatogr.* 1994, *656*; *Biomed. Appl.*, 59–64.

Disposition in the Body. Choline alfoscerate is completely absorbed after oral administration and is widely metabolised after intramuscular or oral administration. It is rapidly cleaved by glycerylphosphorylcholine diesterase to glycerophosphate and choline, the main plasma metabolite, which is detectable until 6 to 8 h after administration.

Therapeutic concentration
Twelve healthy males aged between 20 and 29 years were administered, intramuscularly, with a 1 g dose of L-α-glycerylphosphorylcholine. Choline levels in plasma reached 35.5 ± 3.5 μmol/L at 0.25 h and 35.8 ± 3.5 μmol/L at 0.5 h and mean endogenous plasma levels ranged from 10.6 to 12.0 μg/L. [G. Gatti *et al., Int. J. Clin. Pharm. Ther. Toxicol.*, 1992, *30(9)*, 331–335].

Half-life. Terminal half-life of free choline derived from L-α-glycerylphosphorylcholine is 1.37 h.

Clearance. 42.7 ± 2.7 μmol/l/h.

Chorionic Gonadotropin

Gonad Stimulating Hormone

Synonyms. CG; Choriogonadotropin; Chorionic Gonadotropin; Gonadotrophinum Chorionicum.
Proprietary names. APL; Choragon; Chorex; Choron; Gonadotraphon LH; Gonasi HP; Gonic; Physex; Predalon; Pregnesin; Pregnyl; Primogonyl; Profasi.
Sialoglycoprotein = approx. 37 000
CAS—9002-61-3

Molecular structure. α-Subunit consists of 96 amino acids and 2 carbohydrate moieties, and the β-subunit consists of 149 amino acid residues at the C-terminal region.
It is a white or almost white amorphous powder, which needs to be protected from light. It is soluble in water, aqueous glycerol and glycols; insoluble in anhydrous organic solvents.

Quantification

Fluoroimmunoassay. In serum or urine: limit of detection 2.7 International Units (IU)/L and 4.9 IU/L, respectively—D. A. Cowan *et al.*, *J. Endocrinol.*, 1991, 131, 147–154.

Disposition in the Body. Distributed primarily to the gonads. 20 to 30% of intramuscular dose is excreted in urine within 5 to 6 days. The β-subunit of chorionic gonadotrophin is metabolised in the liver to a smaller component of molecular weight 12 000 to 17 500. Normally present in males and non-pregnant females < 10 IU/L.

Therapeutic concentration

18 pituitary-suppressed healthy females, aged between 18 and 26 years, were administered with single dose human chorionic gonadotrophin injections of 5000 and 10 000 IU (intramuscularly) and 10 000 IU (subcutaneously). Mean serum peak concentrations reached 156 IU/L, 307 IU/L and 339 IU/L, respectively, 20 h after injection. [B. M. Mannaerts *et al.*, *Hum. Reprod.*, 1998, *13(6)*, 1461–1464].

Toxicity. Dose of 36 mg/kg (female) can cause reproductive side effects and changes in female fertility.

Half-life. Blood concentrations decline in a biphasic manner. Half-lives between 6 and 11, and 23 and 38 h, respectively.

Clearance. Metabolic clearance is 3.4 mL/min for men and 3.9 mL/min for women.

Dose. Infertility treatment (female): single dose between 5000 and 10 000 IU, intramuscular injection, followed by up to 3 repeat injections of 5000 IU each, within 9 days. Infertility treatment (male): single dose between 500 and 4000 units twice/three times a week. Prepubertal cryptorchidism treatment: single dose between 500 and 4000 IU three times a week, for 6 to 10 weeks. Delayed puberty treatment (male): initial dose of 500 to 1500 IU administered twice weekly, 4 to 6 weeks.

Ciclosporin

Immunosuppressant

Synonyms. Cyclosporin; Cyclosporin A; Cyclosporine.
Proprietary names. Neoral; Sandimmun; Sandimmune, SangCya.
[*R*-[*RR**(E)]]-Cyclic(L-alanyl-D-alanyl-*N*-methyl-L-leucyl-*N*-methyl-L-leucyl-*N*-methyl-L-valyl-3-hydroxy-*N*,4-dimethyl-L-2-amino-6-octenoyl-L-α-amino-butyryl-*N*-methylglycyl-*N*-methyl-L-leucyl-L-valyl-*N*-methyl-L-leucyl)
$C_{62}H_{111}N_{11}O_{12}$ = 1202.6
CAS—59865-13-3

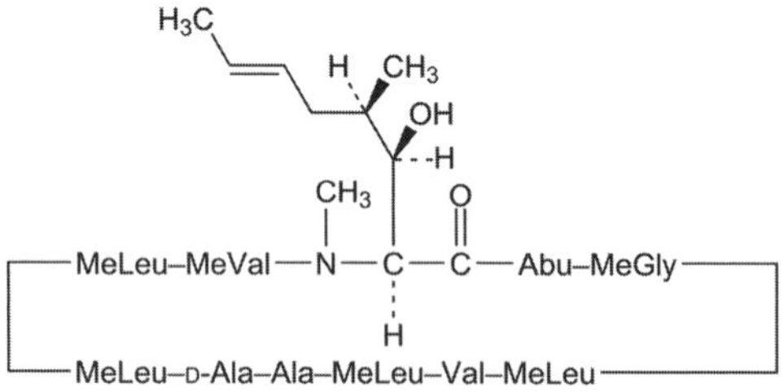

Cyclosporin A

A white or almost white powder. Soluble in methanol, ethanol, ether, chloroform and methylene chloride. It is practically insoluble in water and saturated hydrocarbons.

High Performance Liquid Chromatography. Column: C_8 (Alltima, 100 × 2.1 mm i.d., 5 μm) at 70°. Mobile phase: 72% methanol:28% 50 mM ammonium acetate buffer (pH 5.1), 0.3 mL/min flow rate. Electron spray tandem mass spectrometry detection. Retention time: 11.8 min. [P. J. Taylor *et al.*, *J. Chromatogr. B.*, 1998, *705*, 289–294].

Column: Spherisorb S5 CN (250-4 phasesep, 250 × 4.6 mm, 5 μm) at 50°. Mobile phase: hexane:isopropanol (90:10), 1.45 mL/min flow rate. UV detection (λ = 212 nm). Retention times: ciclosporin, 8.9 min; metabolites, 11.0, 12.9 and 16.3 min. [G. Khoschsorur *et al.*, *J. Chromatogr. B*, 1997, *690*, 367–372].

Column: RP-18 (RP Velosep, (400 × 3.2 mm, 3 μm). Mobile phase: 50% acetonitrile:11% methanol:39% 0.01 M dipotassium hydrogen orthophosphate buffer (pH 6.5), 1.5 mL/min flow rate. UV detection (dual wavelength, 220 and 230 nm). Retention time: 2.5 min. [P. Salm *et al.*, *Ther. Drug Monit.*, 1993, *15*, 65–69].

Column: (analytical) Si 60 silica (250 × 4 mm, 5 μm) at 60°; (pre-column) Si 60 silica (10 mm). Mobile phase: hexane:ethanol (85:15), 1.5 mL/min flow rate. UV detection (λ = 210 nm). Retention time: 3.4 min. [J.-M. Poirier *et al.*, *Ther. Drug Monit.*, 1994, *16*, 388–389].

Quantification

High performance liquid chromatography. In whole blood: limit of detection 5 μg/L, MS detection—P. J. Taylor *et al.*, *J. Chromatogr. B*, 1998, *705*, 289–294. In whole blood: limit of detection 0.01 mg/L, UV detection (λ = 212 nm)—G. Khoschsorur *et al.*, *J. Chromatogr. B*, 1997, *690*, 367–372. In whole blood: limit of detection 45 μg/L, UV detection (λ = 220, 230 nm)—P. Salm *et al.*, *Ther. Drug Monit.*, 1993, *15*, 65–69. In whole blood: limit of quantification 25 μg/L, UV detection (λ = 210 nm)—J.-M. Poirier *et al.*, *Ther. Drug Monit.*, 1994, *16*, 388–389.

Disposition in the Body. After oral administration of conventional formulations absorption is very variable; absolute bioavailability can vary from less than 10% in liver transplant patients to up to 89% in some renal transplant patients. Peak blood and plasma concentrations are achieved about 3.5 h after an oral dose. Following administration of a microemulsion formulation, peak concentrations are achieved after about 1.5 to 2 h and bioavailability is greater than with conventional formulations although is still very variable. Ciclosporin is widely distributed throughout the body. In blood, the distribution is concentration dependent (see below). It is extensively metabolised by CYP4503A mainly in the liver (some also in the gastro-intestinal tract and kidney) and excreted primarily in faeces via the bile; only about 6% is excreted in the urine. The low oral bioavailability of ciclosporin is due to first-pass metabolism in the gastro-intestinal wall rather than the liver. It crosses the placenta and is distributed into breast milk. Dialysis does not affect clearance significantly.

Therapeutic concentration

9 paediatric patients undergoing liver transplants, aged between 0.5 and 11 years, were administered with a 10.1 mg/kg intravenous dose over 24 h. The peak concentration was 0.834 mg/L after 4.4 h. The same children administered with an oral dose of 30 mg/kg reached peak plasma concentrations of 1.356 mg/L 2.6 h after ingestion. [S. P. Dunn *et al.*, *Transplantation*, 1995, *60(12)*, 1438–1442.]

54 paediatric patients, with a mean age of 13.2 years, were administered with an oral 7.8 mg/kg dose under steady state conditions. Peak concentrations of 0.588 mg/L were reached 2.4 h after ingestion. [H. Humbert *et al.*, *Transplant Proc.*, 1994, *26*, 2791–2797].

Toxicity. Nephrotoxicity is the major toxic effect; doses must be adjusted individually and kidney function must be monitored during therapy.

A 31-year-old woman accidentally received 5000 mg (92.6 mg/kg) of ciclosporin orally as a single dose on day 80 post kidney transplant. She developed a severe headache, intractable vomiting and felt drunk. By 72 h post ingestion all symptoms had subsided. At 18 h post dose serum-ciclosporin concentration was 2.6 mg/L. At 30 h post dose, whole blood-ciclosporin concentration was 1.775 mg/L. There was little evidence of nephrotoxicity and no evidence of hepatotoxicity. There were no long-term sequelae. [T. J. Schroeder *et al.*, *Transplantation*, 1986, *41*, 406–409].

A 43-year-old man with multiple sclerosis took 25 g of ciclosporin over an 8-day period when he misunderstood instructions. Symptoms included burning sensation in mouth and feet, altered taste, hyperaesthesia of the hands, sore gums, facial flushing, sensation of abdominal swelling, foot swelling, and mild stomach upset. Whole blood-ciclosporin concentration measured the day after discontinuation of ciclosporin was 1.778 mg/L. There was no evidence of hepatotoxicity or nephrotoxicity. [R. W. Baumhefner *et al.*, *Lancet*, 1987, *2*, 332].

A 31-year-old man was given an overdose of 1.1 mg/kg/h for 33 h on day 19 post kidney transplant. He developed severe abdominal pain that was considered to be due to the toxic levels of ciclosporin. There was also hepatotoxicity. Blood-ciclosporin concentration measured 10 h after stopping ciclosporin was 2 mg/L. It was estimated that concentrations were higher than 4 mg/L for the duration of the infusion. There was little evidence of nephrotoxicity. [Y. Kokado *et al.*, *Transplantation*, 1989, *47*, 1096–1097].

Half-life. Terminal, ranged from 6.3 h (healthy adults); 20.4 h (patients with severe liver disease).

Volume of distribution. 2 to 5 L/kg; apparent, 13 L/kg.

Clearance. Blood clearance, 0.71 L/h/kg (paediatrics); 0.34 L/h/kg (adults).

Distribution in blood. This is concentration and temperature dependent. Approx. 40% is taken up in erythrocytes and the remainder extensively binds plasma proteins. At high concentrations the binding to blood cells becomes saturated.

Protein binding. In plasma, 90% (mostly to lipoprotein).

Note. For reviews, see G. F. Cooney *et al.*, *Clin. Pharmacokinet.*, 1997, *32*, 481–495 and D. W. Holt and A. Johnston, *Ther. Drug Monit.*, 1995, *17*, 625–630.

Dose. Organ transplantation: initially 10 to 15 mg/kg orally daily in two divided doses; the intravenous dose is one-third of the oral dose; maintenance dose, 2 to 6 mg/kg daily. Bone marrow transplant: maintenance dose, 12.5 mg/kg orally daily (3 to 6 months). Psoriasis and atopic dermatitis: 2.5 to 5.0 mg/kg orally daily. Rheumatoid arthritis: 2.5 to 4.0 mg/kg orally daily. Nephrotic syndrome: 5 mg/kg orally daily (adults); 6 mg/kg (children).

Cidofovir

Antiviral

Synonym. (*S*)-HPMPC, GS-504
Proprietary name. Vistide
(*S*)-[[2-(4-Amino-2-oxo-1(2*H*)-pyrimidinyl)-1-(hydroxymethyl)ethoxy] methyl]-phosphonic acid
$C_8H_{14}N_3O_6P$=279.2
CAS—113852-37-2

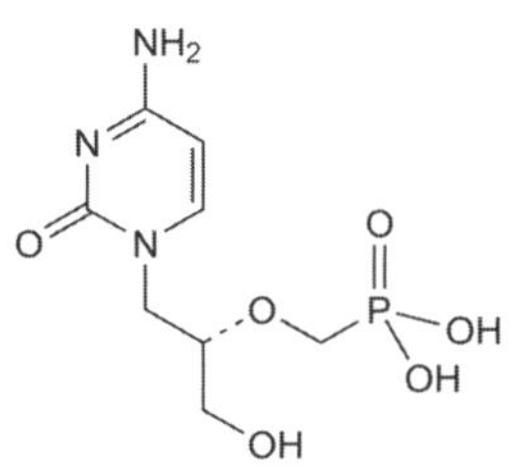

A fluffy white powder. M.p. 260° with decomposition. It is soluble in water at 170 g/l.

High Performance Liquid Chromatography. Column: (analytical) C_8 (Zorbax, 250 × 4.6 mm i.d., 5 µm); (guard) C_8 (Zorbax, 40 × 6.0 mm). Mobile phase: (A) acetonitrile:phosphate buffer (100 mM, pH 7.2) with 5 mM tetrabutylammonium dihydrogen phosphate (TBAHP) (5:95); (B) acetonitrile:phosphate buffer (100 mM, pH 7.2) with 5 mM TBAHP (15:85). Linear gradient—100% (A) to 100% (B) over 9 min, flow rate 1.4 mL/min. UV detection (λ=274 nm). Retention time: 6.0 min.

Column: (analytical) ODS-IP (Beckman Ultrasphere, 150 × 4.6 mm); (guard) RP-18 (Newguard, 15 × 3.2 mm). Mobile phase: acetonitrile:methanol:water containing 5 mM octyltriethylammonium phosphate (5:5:90), flow rate 2.0 mL/min. UV detection (λ= 274 nm). Retention time: 6.6 min. [K. C. Cundy *et al.*, *Antimicrob. Agents Chemother.*, 1995, *39(6)*, 1247–1252].

Column: ODS-2 (Prodigy, 100 × 4.6 mm, 5 µm). Mobile phase: Q12 (6 mmol/L) and phosphoric acid (12 mmol/L) in acetonitrile:water (30:70), final pH 3.0 to 3.1, 3 mL/min flow rate. Fluorescence detection (λ_{ex} = 305 nm, λ_{em} = 370 nm). Retention time: 3.1 min. [E. J. Eisenberg and K. C. Cundy, *J. Chromatogr.* 1996, *679*; *Biomed. Appl.*, 119–127].

Quantification
High performance liquid chromatography. In plasma: limit of detection 5 µg/L, fluorescence detection—E. J. Eisenberg and K. C. Cundy, *J. Chromatogr.* 1996, *679*; *Biomed. Appl.*, 119–127. In serum and urine: limit of quantification 0.22 mg/L and 1.0 mg/L, respectively—K. C. Cundy *et al.*, *Antimicrob. Agents Chemother.*, 1995, *39(6)*, 1247–1252.

Disposition in the Body. Cidofovir is administered intravenously. It is excreted largely unchanged in urine by glomerular filtration and tubular secretion. About 80 to 100% of a dose is recovered unchanged in urine over 24 h. No active metabolites are detected in serum. It is given concurrently with prehydration and oral probenecid to block the tubular secretion and thus reduce high concentrations in the kidney, since cidofovir is nephrotoxic.

Therapeutic concentration

39 HIV-infected males and 3 females, aged between 28 and 55 years, mean 39 years, were intravenously administered with 1 (no of subjects, n=5), 3 (n=10), 5 (n=2) or 10 (n=8) mg/kg cidofovir. Peak serum concentrations of the drug were 3.12, 7.34, 11.5 and 23.56 mg/L, respectively, for the 4 doses observed at the end of infusion. In the same study, cidofovir was also administered to the patients along with a high dose of probenecid. A 3 mg/kg dose of cidofovir produced a peak concentration of 8.08 mg/L; 5 mg/kg, 26.07 mg/L and 7.5 mg/kg dose, 42.95 mg/L, respectively. [K. C. Cundy *et al.*, *Antimicrob. Agents Chemother.*, 1995, *39(6)*, 1247–1252].

Toxicity. Dose-dependent nephrotoxicity is the major adverse effect. A 5 mg/kg dose twice weekly is not well tolerated with resulting renal toxicity. (5 mg/kg weekly or 7.5 mg/kg every 3 weeks is feasible).

Half-life. Plasma half-life of cidofovir, 2.2 h; active metabolite, cidofovir diphosphate, 17 to 65 h.

Volume of distribution. Steady state, mean, 490 mL/kg; 356 mL/kg (with probenecid).

Clearance. Serum, mean, 148 mL/h/kg; 125 mL/h/kg (with probenecid).

Protein binding. Less than 10% (*in vitro*) bound to plasma or serum proteins.

Note. For a review of cidofovir, see M. A. Poklis *et al.*, *Antimicrob. Agents Chemother.*, 1995, *39*, 882–886.

Dose. 5 mg/kg intravenously once every 2 weeks (maintenance dose) together with probenecid and prehydration.

Cilazapril

ACE Inhibitor

Synonyms. Cilazapril monohydrate, Ro-31-2848/006
Proprietary names. Dynorm; Inhibace; Initiss; Justor; Vascace
[1*S*-[1α,9α(*R**)]]-9-[[1-(Ethoxycarbonyl)-3-phenylpropyl]amino] octahydro-10-oxo-6*H*-pyridazino[1,2-a][1,2]diazepine-1-carboxylic acid monohydrate
$C_{22}H_{31}N_3O_5.H_2O$=435.5
CAS—92077-78-6

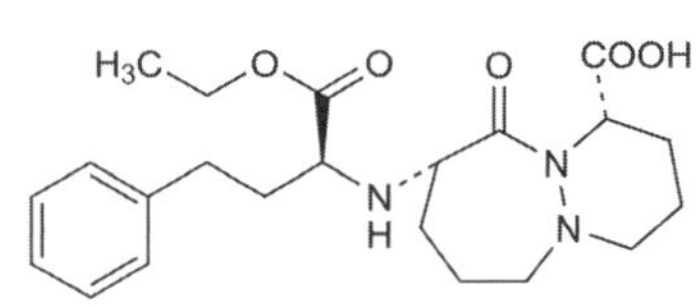

Crystals (from aqueous ethanol).M.p. 95° to 97°.

Thin-Layer Chromatography. System TE—Rf 3; system TF—Rf 0.

Gas Chromatography. System GP—RI 3010 (cilazapril-ME); RI 2960 (M (cilazaprilate)-ME3).

High Performance Liquid Chromatography. System HX—RI 420; system HZ—cilazapril, retention time 4.5 min; cilazaprilate, retention time 1.7 min; system HAA—retention time 14.4 min.

Column: (analytical) C_{18} (µBondapak, 300 × 3.9 mm i.d., 10 µm), (precolumn insert) µBondapak Guard-pak, at 40°. Mobile phase: methanol:phosphoric acid (5 mM) (50:50), 1.0 mL/min flow rate. Electrochemical detection. Retention time: cilazapril, 5.1 min; cilazaprilate, 8.4 min. [J. A. Prieto *et al.*, *J. Chromatogr. B Biomed. Sci. Appl.*, 1998, *714*, 285–292].

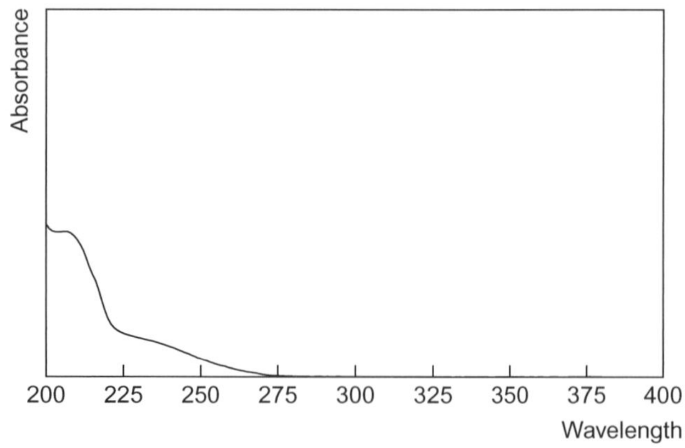

Mass Spectrum. Principal ions at *m/z* 211, 143, 91, 283, 197, 70, 344, 97.

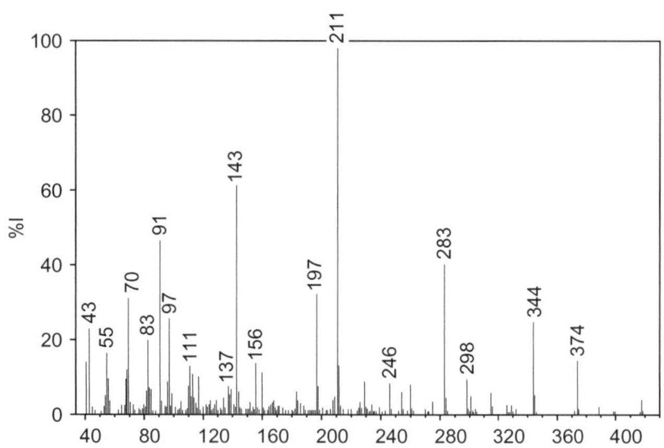

Quantification

High performance liquid chromatography. In urine and pharmaceutical products: limit of detection 50 µg/L for cilazapril and 40 µg/L for cilazaprilate; limit of quantification 0.17 mg/L and 0.14 mg/L, respectively. Electrochemical detection— J. A. Prieto *et al.*, *J. Chromatogr. B Biomed. Appl.*, 1998, *714*, 285–292.

Enzymic immunoassay. In plasma or serum: limit of detection 30 ng/L for cilazapril and 30 µg/L for cilazaprilate—H. Tanaka *et al.*, *J. Pharm. Sci.*, 1987, *76(3)*, 224–227.

Disposition in the Body. After oral administration and rapid absorption, cilazapril is hydrolysed in the liver to its diacid, cilazaprilate (active ACE inhibitor), and no further metabolism occurs. Excretion is biphasic and occurs almost exclusively in the kidneys with approx. 53% cilazaprilate being recovered in urine after oral administration of cilazapril. Rapid elimination of cilazaprilate occurs with unbound drug eliminated within 8 h. Both cilazapril and cilazaprilate are removed to a limited extent by haemodialysis.

Therapeutic concentration

12 healthy males, between 19 and 38 years old, were administered a single 2.5 mg oral dose of cilazapril at weekly intervals. A mean maximum plasma concentration of 0.082 mg/L at 0.83 h was observed for cilazapril and 0.036 mg/L at 1.7 h for cilazaprilate. [P.E.O. Williams *et al.*, *Br. J. Clin. Pharmacol.*, 1989, *27 (suppl. 1)*, 181–188]; [P.E.O. Williams *et al.*, *Br. J. Clin. Pharmacol.*, 1989, *27 (suppl. 1)*, 211–215].

Toxicity. Skin rashes and allergies have been noted in women administered the low toxic dose of 15 mg/kg at 22 week intervals. It is a poison by intravenous routes and moderately toxic by subcutaneous and intraperitoneal routes.

Bioavailability. About 60%.

Half-life. Initial half-life of 1.3 to 1.8 h and a terminal phase elimination half-life of 40 to 50 h for cilazaprilate. Effective half-life (steady state reached) is approx. 9 h.

Volume of distribution. Apparent mean volume of distribution for cilazaprilate is 29 to 46 L.

Clearance. Plasma clearance, of cilazaprilate is 14 to 24 L/h, after a single oral dose of 2.5 to 10 mg cilazapril, and in patients with moderate essential hypertension clearance is 14 to 16 L/h, after a single oral dose of 5 to 20 mg.

Protein binding. 24%.

Dose. An initial daily dose of 1.25 mg for 2 days; gradually increasing to 5 mg/day depending on blood pressure response. A single dose is usually between 2.5 and 5 mg/day.
Patients with creatinine clearance > 40 mL/min, receive an initial daily dose of 1 mg; patients with clearance between 10 and 40 mL/min have an initial daily dose of 0.5 mg and following doses with a maximum of 2.5 mg. Patients with clearance < 10 mL/min receive a 0.25 to 0.5 mg/day dose once or twice a week.

Cilostazol

Antithrombotic

Synonyms. OPC-21; OPC-13013.
Proprietary names. Pletaal; Pletal.
6-[4-(1-Cyclohexyl-1*H*-tetrazol-5-yl)butoxyl]-3,4-dihydro-2(1*H*)-quinolinone
$C_{20}H_{27}N_5O_5$=369.5
CAS—73963-72-1

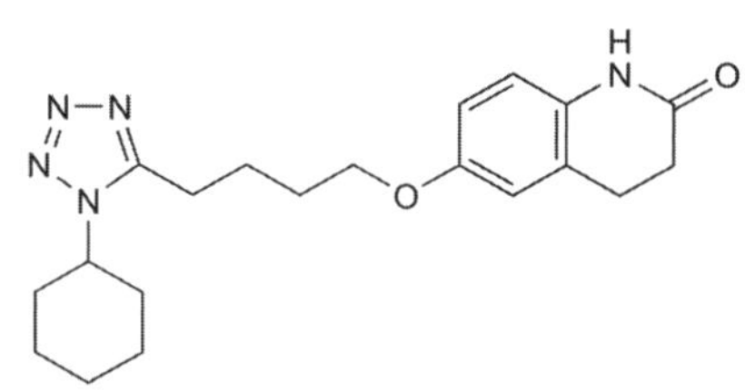

White to off-white crystals or crystalline powder. M.p. 160°. It is freely soluble in acetic acid, chloroform, *N*-methyl-2-pyrrolidone and DMSO; slightly soluble in methanol and ethanol; practically insoluble in ether, water, 0.1 M hydrochloric acid and 0.1 M sodium hydroxide.

Partition Coefficient. Log *P* (octanol/water), 4.04.

Ultraviolet Spectrum. methanol—257 nm.

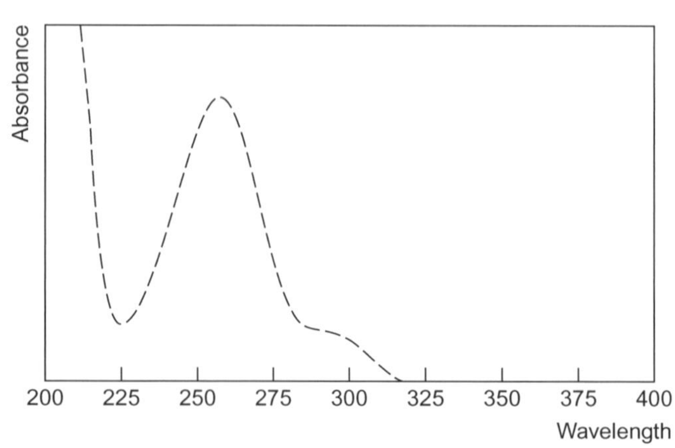

Infra-red Spectrum. Principal peaks at wavenumbers 1667, 1505, 1246, 1039, 2932, 2867 cm^{-1}.

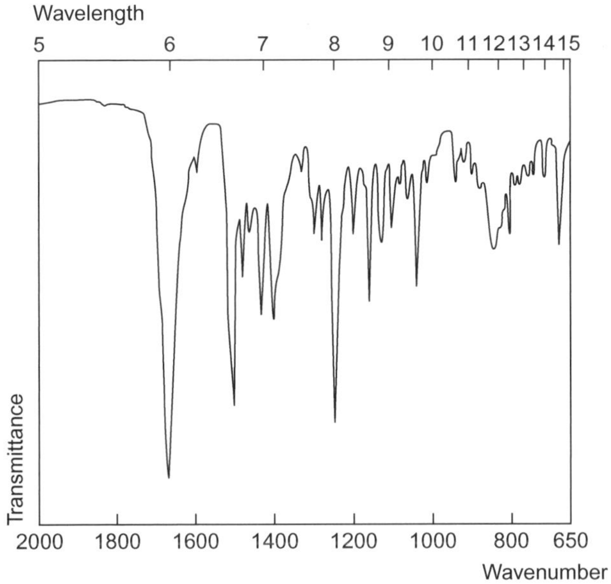

Mass Spectrum. Principal ions at m/z 125, 207, 55, 369, 41, 126, 134, 163.

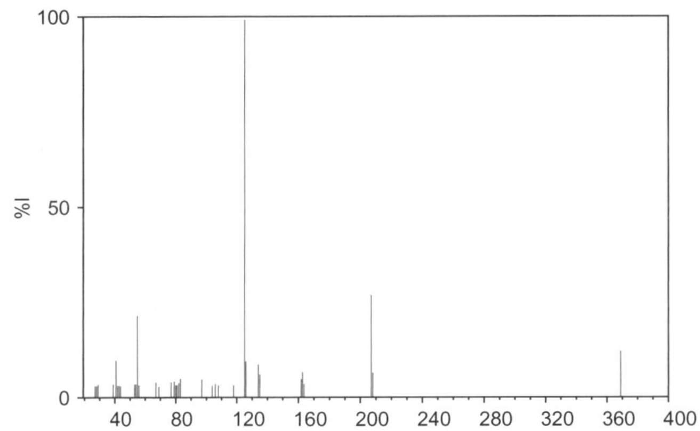

Disposition in the Body. Cilostazol is absorbed at a moderate rate after oral administration. Absorption is increased if the drug is administered with a high fat meal. Mean peak plasma concentrations are observed 2.4 h after administration and the drug is extensively metabolised by hepatic cytochrome P450 enzymes (mainly 3A4). A number of metabolites are produced, two of which are active; 3,4-dehydrocilostazol (the most active metabolite accounting for at least 50% of the pharmacological activity) and 4′-*trans*-hydroxycilostazol. In plasma, 56% of the dose is detected as the unchanged drug, 15% 3,4-dehydrocilostazol and 4% 4′-*trans*-hydroxy-cilostazol. The primary elimination route is urine with 74% of the dose excreted in this way; <2% as the 3,4-dehydrocilostazol metabolite and 30% 4′-*trans*-hydroxycilostazol. No unchanged drug is detected in urine. It is extensively distributed in tissues.

Therapeutic concentration

20 healthy non-smoking males, with a mean age of 24 years, were administered with single doses of 50, 100 and 200 mg. 26 patients (male and female) with intermittent claudication (a complex of symptoms) resulting from peripheral arterial disease (PAD), with a mean age of 68 years, were administered with a dose of 100 mg. The mean peak plasma concentration of cilostazol was 1.223 mg/L for the healthy individuals and 1.332 mg/L for the patients which were observed 2.5 h (range 1 to 5) and 2 h (range 1 to 6) after administration, respectively. Mean peak concentrations for the metabolite OPC-13015 were 0.406 mg/L and 0.426 mg/L, respectively, for the healthy individuals and the patients. These levels were reached at about 3 h (range 1 to 6). Mean peak concentrations for the metabolite OPC-13213 were 0.125 mg/L and 0.224 mg/L, respectively, for the healthy individuals and the patients. These levels were reached at about 3 h (range 1 to 8 and 1 to 5, respectively). [S. L. Bramer *et al.*, *Clin. Pharmacokinet.*, 1999, *37 (suppl. 2)*, 1–11].

Half-life. 11 to 13 h.

Volume of distribution. 2.76 L/kg.

Clearance. Oral, 0.18 L/h/kg. Relatively low plasma clearance.

Protein binding. Approx. 95 to 98%.

Dose. The recommended dose is 100 mg daily but reduced to 50 mg if co-administered.

Cimetidine

Histamine H_2-Receptor Antagonist

Synonym. SKF-92334
Proprietary names. Acibilin; Dyspanet; Edalene; Gimal; Gimetum; Peptol; Tagamet; Tratul; Ulcomet; Ulhys.
N-Cyano-*N*′-methyl-*N*″-[2-[[(5-methyl-1*H*-imidazol-4yl)methyl]thio]-ethyl]guanidine
$C_{10}H_{16}N_6S = 252.4$
CAS—51481-61-9

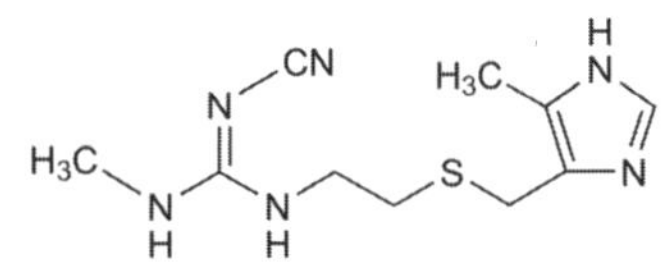

A crystalline powder. M.p. 141° to 143°.
Soluble 1 in about 88 of water.

Dissociation Constant. pK_a 6.8.

Partition Coefficient. Log *P* (octanol/water), 0.4.

Colour Tests. Nessler's Reagent (100°)—black; Sodium Picrate—red.

Thin-layer Chromatography. System TA—Rf 54; system TB—Rf 00; system TC—Rf 09; system TE—Rf 27; system TL—Rf 12; system TAE—Rf 53; system TAF—Rf 55; system TAJ—Rf 00; system TAK—Rf 00; system TAL—Rf 08.

Gas Chromatography. System GA—not eluted.

High Performance Liquid Chromatography. System HA—*k* 0.4; system HX—RI 251; system HY—RI 226; system HZ—retention time, 1.8 min; system HAA—retention time, 3.6 min.

Ultraviolet Spectrum. No significant absorption, 230 to 360 nm.

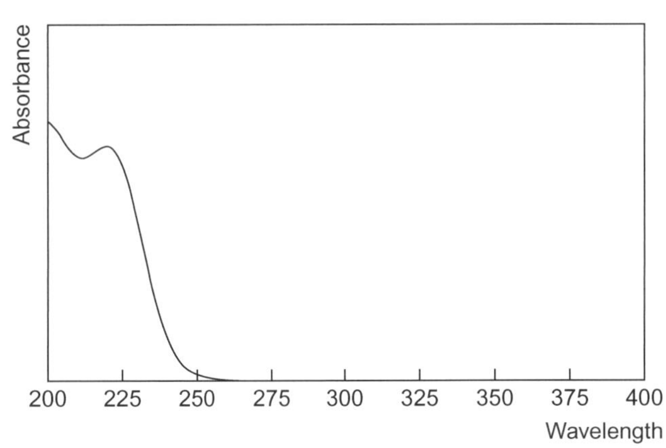

Infra-red Spectrum. Principal peaks at wavenumbers 1588, 1620, 1208, 1082, 1160, 1503 cm^{-1} (KBr disk). Polymorphism may occur. (See below)

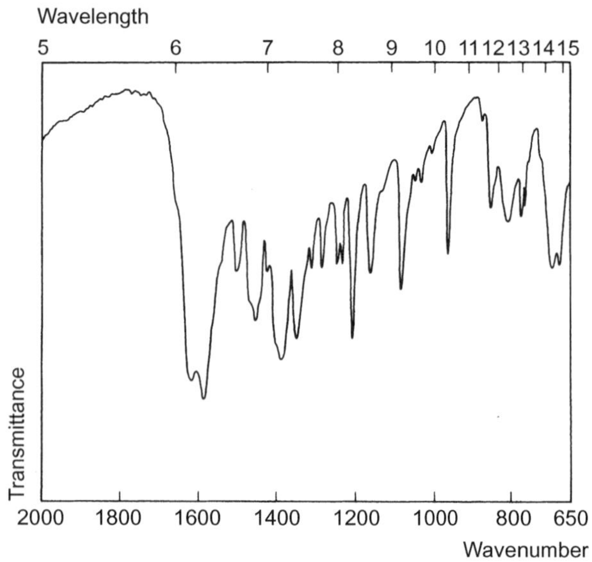

Mass Spectrum. Principal ions at *m/z* 30, 57, 82, 116, 99, 53, 55, 42.

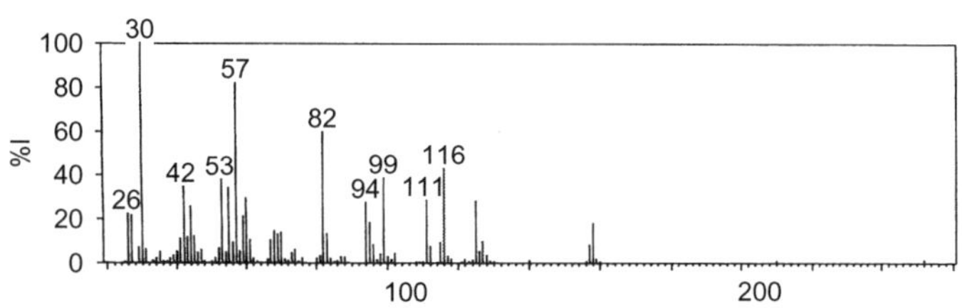

Quantification

High performance liquid chromatography. In serum or urine: cimetidine and metabolites, limit of detection 50 µg/L for cimetidine, UV detection—J. A. Ziemniak *et al.*, *Clin. Chem.*, 1981, *27*, 272–275. In plasma or urine: limit of detection 25 µg/L, UV detection—M. S. Ching *et al.*, *J. Pharm. Sci.*, 1984, *73*, 1015. In plasma: limit of quantification 50 µg/L and limit of detection 15 µg/L, UV detection (λ=228 nm)—M. T. Kelly *et al.*, *J. Chromatogr.* 1995, *668(1) B Biomed. Appl.*, 117–123. In plasma: lower limit of quantification 0.1 mg/L, UV detection (λ=234 nm)—J. Hempenius *et al.*, *J. Chromatogr. B Biomed. Sci. Appl.*, 1998, *714(2)*, 361–368. In plasma: limit of quantification 5 µg/L, MS detection—K. Xu *et al.*, *Biomed. Chromatogr.*, 1999, *13(7)*, 455–461.

Disposition in the Body. Rapidly absorbed after oral administration. About 50 to 80% of an intravenous dose is excreted in the urine as unchanged drug in 24 h, together with about 10% as the sulfoxide metabolite and about 5% as the 5-hydroxymethyl derivative. Up to about 10% of the dose is eliminated in the faeces.

Therapeutic concentration. In plasma, usually in the range 0.5 to 1.5 mg/L.

A single oral dose of 200 mg administered to 20 subjects resulted in peak blood concentrations of 0.6 to 1.9 mg/L (mean 1.1) in 1 to 2 h. [A. Redolfi *et al.*, *Eur. J. Clin. Pharmacol.*, 1979, *15*, 257–261.]

Following oral administration of 200 mg five times a day to 10 subjects, minimum steady-state plasma concentrations of 0.26 to 0.80 mg/L (mean 0.4) were reported; steady-state plasma concentrations of the sulfoxide metabolite ranged from 0.07 to 0.21 mg/L (mean 0.12). [R. Larsson, *Br. J. Clin. Pharmacol.*, 1982, *13*, 163–170.]

Toxicity. Cimetidine appears to be relatively non-toxic; recovery has occurred after ingestion of 24 g in one dose, and ingestion of 60 g during 5 days caused no untoward effects. During chronic therapy, toxic effects are reportedly associated with trough plasma concentrations greater than 1.3 mg/L.

In 3 cases of overdose caused by the ingestion of 5.2, 16, and 19.6 g of cimetidine, plasma concentrations of 37, 57, and 36 mg/L, respectively, were reported 2 to 3 h after ingestion; the subjects all recovered. [R. N. Illingworth and D. R. Jarvie, *BMJ*, 1979, *1*, 453–454.]

In a fatality caused by the ingestion of cimetidine and diazepam, postmortem blood concentrations of 110 mg/L of cimetidine and 5.8 mg/L of diazepam were reported. [J. Hiss *et al.*, *Lancet*, 1982, *2*, 982.]

Bioavailability. About 70% but there is considerable intersubject variation.

Half-life. Plasma half-life, 1 to 3 h.

Volume of distribution. About 1 to 2 L/kg.

Clearance. Plasma clearance, about 9 mL/min/kg; considerably reduced in elderly patients.

Distribution in blood. Plasma : whole blood ratio, about 1.0.

Protein binding. In plasma, 13 to 26%.

Note. For a review of the pharmacokinetics of cimetidine see A. Somogyi and R. Gugler, *Clin. Pharmacokinet.*, 1983, *8*, 463–495.

Dose. 0.8 to 1.6 g daily; maximum of 2.4 g daily.

Cinchocaine

Local Anaesthetic

Synonyms. Cincainum; Dibucaine.
Proprietary name. Nupercainal. It is an ingredient of many proprietary preparations—see *Martindale, The complete drug reference*, 33rd Edn., Pharmaceutical Press, London, 2002.
2-Butoxy-*N*-[2-(diethylamino)ethyl]-4-quinolinecarboxamide
$C_{20}H_{29}N_3O_2$=343.5
CAS—85-79-0

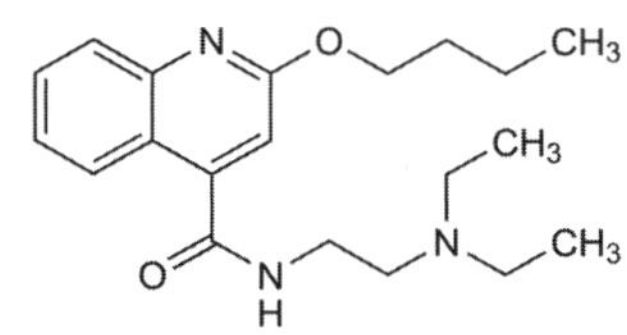

A white, somewhat hygroscopic powder. M.p. 64°.
Soluble 1 in 4600 of water, 1 in less than 1 of ethanol and of chloroform, and 1 in 1.5 of ether.

Cinchocaine Hydrochloride

Synonyms. Cincaini Chloridum; Percainum; Sovcainum.
Proprietary names. Cincain; Doloposterine N; Nupercainal; Nupercaine.
$C_{20}H_{29}N_3O_2$,HCl=379.9
CAS—61-12-1
Fine, white, hygroscopic, crystals or white crystalline powder. M.p. 90° to 98°, with decomposition.
Soluble 1 in 0.5 of water; freely soluble in ethanol, acetone and chloroform; insoluble in ether and oils.

Dissociation Constant. pK_a 7.5 (20°).

Partition Coefficient. Log *P* (octanol/water), 4.4.

Colour Test. Mercurous Nitrate—black

Thin-layer Chromatography. System TA—Rf 63; system TB—Rf 25; system TC—Rf 34; system TE—Rf 67; system TL—Rf 35; system TAE—Rf 42. (Acidified iodoplatinate solution, positive.)

Gas Chromatography. System GA—RI 2890; system GQ—retention time 10.4 min.

High Performance Liquid Chromatography. System HA—*k* 1.9; system HR—*k* 5.51; system HY—RI 371.

Ultraviolet Spectrum. Aqueous acid—247 nm (A_1^1=720a), 319 nm (A_1^1=260a); aqueous alkali—238, 325 nm.

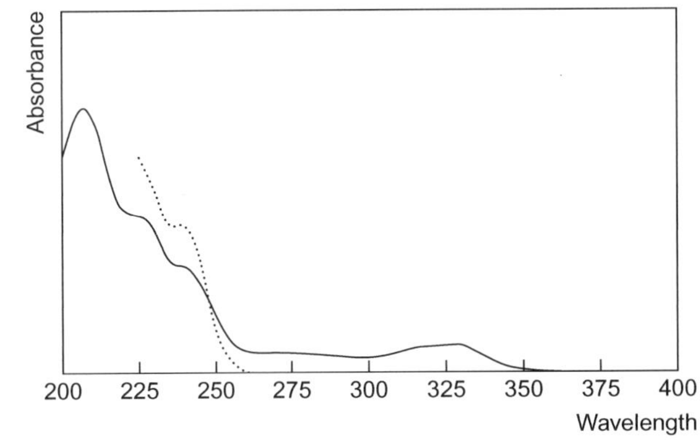

Infra-red Spectrum. Principal peaks at wavenumbers 1598, 1643, 1540, 766, 1236, 1574 cm^{-1} (KBr disk).

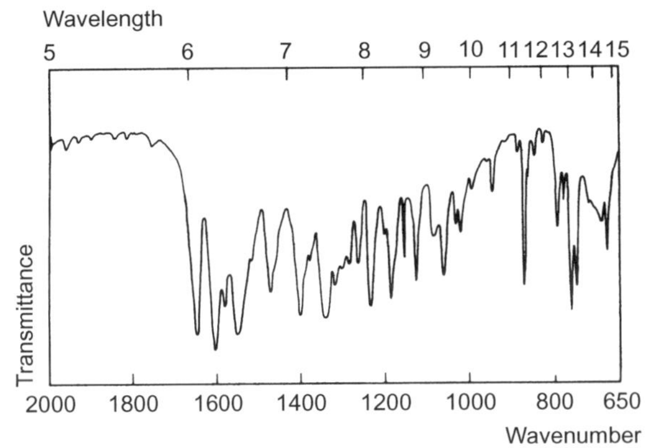

Mass Spectrum. Principal ions at *m/z* 86, 87, 58, 149, 111, 99, 57, 41 (no peaks above 210).

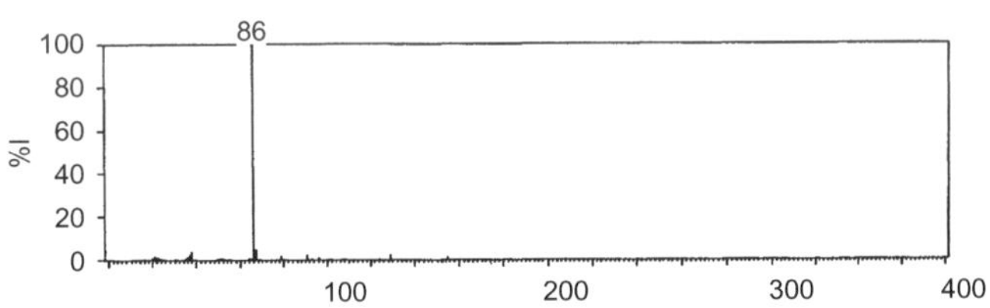

Quantification

Gas chromatography–mass spectrometry. In plasma and urine: limit of quantification 100 μg/L and limit of detection 80 μg/L (SIM, *m/z* 86)—T. Ohhima and T. Takayasu, *J. Chromatogr. B Biomed. Sci. Appl.*, 1999, *726(1–2)*, 185–194. In serum: limit of detection 1 μg/L—D. Alkalay *et al.*, *Analyt. Lett.* (Part B), 1981, *14*, 1745–1756.

Disposition in the Body

Toxicity. Cinchocaine is more toxic than procaine by injection, and more toxic than cocaine by local application.

An 18-month-old girl died 7 h after ingesting an estimated 150 mg (15 mg/kg) cinchocaine contained in a tube of ointment; cinchocaine levels were not obtained at autopsy. In a second fatality, involving a 2-year-old boy who ingested an unknown quantity of cinchocaine cream, the postmortem blood cinchocaine level was 1.3 mg/L. A third fatality was reported—a 21-month-old girl who ingested three-quarters of a 1 oz tube of cinchocaine ointment (approx. 225 mg; 19 mg/kg)—in which death occurred 3 h after the ingestion; no autopsy was performed. [P. S. Dayan *et al.*, *Ann. Emerg. Med.*, 1996, *28*, 442–445.]

In a fatality involving the ingestion of cinchocaine, the following postmortem tissue concentrations were reported: blood 0.6 mg/L, kidney 5.7 μg/g, liver 25 μg/g; ethanol was also detected in blood at a concentration of 1500 mg/L. [T. Borkowski and W. Gubala, *Bull. Int. Assoc. Forensic Toxicol.*, 1976, *12(3)*, 18.]

Half-life. Plasma half-life, about 11 h.

Use. Cinchocaine is used in concentrations of 0.1 to 1%, for surface anaesthesia.

Cinchonidine

Antimalarial

Synonyms. Cinchonatine; α-Quinidine.
(8α,9*R*)-Cinchonan-9-ol
$C_{19}H_{22}N_2O=294.4$
CAS—485-71-2

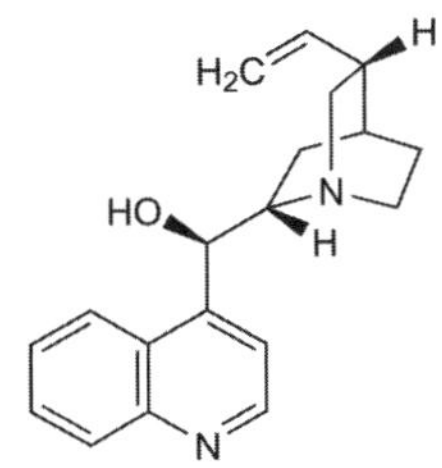

An alkaloid present in the bark of various species of *Cinchona* (Rubiaceae). Cinchonidine is the (−)-stereoisomer of cinchonine; quinine is its (−)-6′-methoxy derivative.

White crystals or powder. M.p. about 210°, with decomposition.

Practically insoluble in water; soluble 1 in 10 of ethanol; soluble in chloroform; moderately soluble in ether.

Cinchonidine Sulfate

$(C_{19}H_{22}N_2O)_2,H_2SO_4,7H_2O=813.0$
CAS—524-61-8 (anhydrous)

Colourless, shining, silky crystals. M.p. about 207° (anhydrous salt).

Soluble 1 in 100 of water and 1 in 60 of ethanol; practically insoluble in chloroform and ether.

Dissociation Constant. pK_a 4.0, 8.2 (25°).

Partition Coefficient. Log *P* (octanol/water), 2.8.

Thin-layer Chromatography. System TA—Rf 49; system TB—Rf 06; system TC—Rf 8; system TE—Rf 44; system TL—Rf 06; system TAE—Rf 24; system TAF—Rf 55; system TAJ—Rf 00; system TAK—Rf 00; system TAL—Rf 70. (Dragendorff spray, positive; acidified iodoplatinate solution, positive.)

Gas Chromatography. System GA—RI 2590.

High Performance Liquid Chromatography. System HA—*k* 3.1; system HX—RI 306; system HY—RI 214.

Ultraviolet Spectrum. Aqueous acid—236 nm ($A_1^1=1208a$), 316 nm.

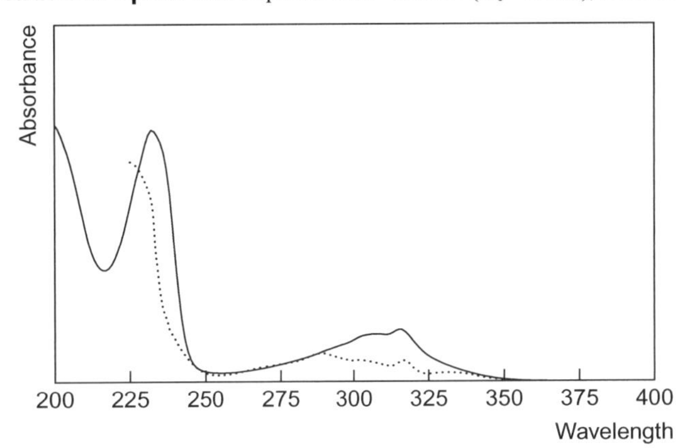

Infra-red Spectrum. Principal peaks at wavenumbers 754, 899, 1090, 800, 877, 1587 cm^{-1} (KBr disk).

Mass Spectrum. Principal ions at *m/z* 136, 81, 137, 42, 41, 55, 130, 128.

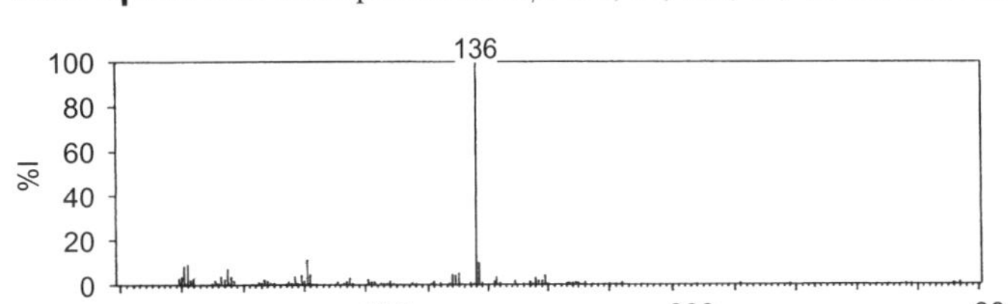

Disposition in the Body. Metabolised by 2′-hydroxylation of the quinoline nucleus followed by 2-hydroxylation of the quinuclidine ring; both 2′-hydroxycinchonidine and 2,2′-dihydroxycinchonidine have been detected in urine.

Dose. Cinchonidine sulfate was formerly given in doses of 60 to 600 mg.

Cinchonine

Antimalarial

(9*S*)-Cinchonan-9-ol
$C_{19}H_{22}N_2O$=294.4
CAS—118-10-5

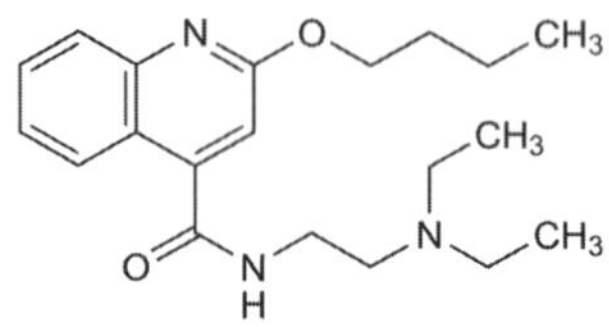

An alkaloid present in the bark of various species of *Cinchona* (Rubiaceae). Cinchonine is the (+)-stereoisomer of cinchonidine; quinidine is its (+)-6′-methoxy derivative.
White shining prisms or needles. M.p. 264°, subliming at 220°.
Practically insoluble in water; soluble 1 in 60 in ethanol, 1 in 110 of chloroform, and 1 in 500 of ether.

Cinchonine Hydrochloride

$C_{19}H_{22}N_2O,HCl,2H_2O$=366.9
CAS—5949-11-1 (anhydrous)
White microcrystalline flakes or needles. M.p. about 215°, with decomposition (anhydrous salt).
Soluble 1 in 20 of water, 1 in 1.5 of ethanol, 1 in 20 of chloroform, and 1 in 300 of ether.

Dissociation Constant. pK_a 4.1, 8.2 (25°).

Partition Coefficient. Log *P* (octanol/water), 2.7.

Thin-layer Chromatography. System TA—Rf 49; system TB—Rf 06; system TC—Rf 12; system TE—Rf 44; system TL—Rf 05; system TAE—Rf 19; system TAF—Rf 61. (Dragendorff spray, positive; acidified iodoplatinate solution, positive.)

Gas Chromatography. System GA—RI 2590.

High Performance Liquid Chromatography. System HX—RI 304; system HY—RI 209; system HAA—retention time, 10.2 min.

Ultraviolet Spectrum. Aqueous acid—235 nm (A_1^1=1208a), 315 nm; aqueous alkali—288, 302, 315 nm.

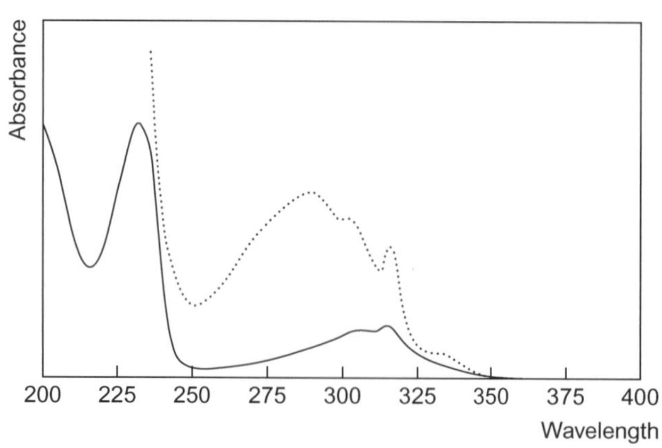

Infra-red Spectrum. Principal peaks at wavenumbers 760, 1110, 1505, 1590, 990, 909 cm^{-1} (KBr disk).

Mass Spectrum. Principal ions at *m/z* 136, 294, 81, 159, 55, 42, 41, 143.

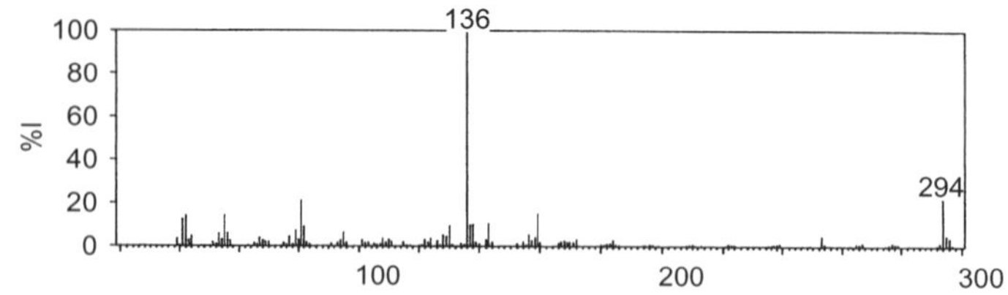

Disposition in the Body. Rapidly and almost completely absorbed from the gastro-intestinal tract, peak plasma concentrations being attained in 1 to 2 h. Metabolised by 2′-hydroxylation of the quinoline nucleus followed by 2-hydroxylation of the quinuclidine ring. About 55% of a dose is excreted as 2′-hydroxycinchonine, 22% as 2,2′-dihydroxycinchonine, and 5% as unchanged cinchonine.

Dose. Cinchonine hydrochloride was formerly given in doses of 60 to 600 mg.

Cinchophen

Analgesic

Synonyms. Acifenokinolin; Phenylcinchoninic Acid; Quinophan.
Proprietary names. Atophan; Quinophan; Phenoquin; Agotan; Rhematan; Tophol; Tophosan.
2-Phenyl-4-quinolinecarboxylic acid
$C_{16}H_{11}NO_2$=249.3
CAS—132-60-5

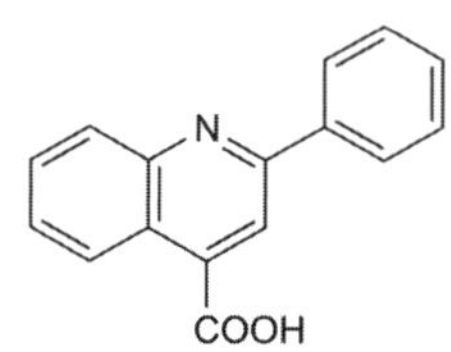

White or yellowish crystals or powder. M.p. 213° to 216°.
Practically insoluble in water; soluble 1 in 120 of ethanol, 1 in 40 of acetone, 1 in 400 of chloroform, and 1 in 100 of ether.

Partition Coefficient. Log *P* (octanol/water), 3.8.

Colour Tests. Liebermann's Test—red-orange; Marquis Test—yellow; Sulfuric Acid—yellow.

Thin-layer Chromatography. System TA—Rf 75; system TB—Rf 00; system TC—Rf 02; system TD—Rf 00; system TE—Rf 08; system TF—Rf 00; system TL—Rf 00; system TAD—Rf 07; system TAE—Rf 82; system TAF—Rf 72. (Acidified iodoplatinate solution, positive.)

Gas Chromatography. System GA—not eluted.

Ultraviolet Spectrum. Aqueous acid—243 nm (A_1^1=610b), 268, 344 nm; aqueous alkali—259, 330 nm.

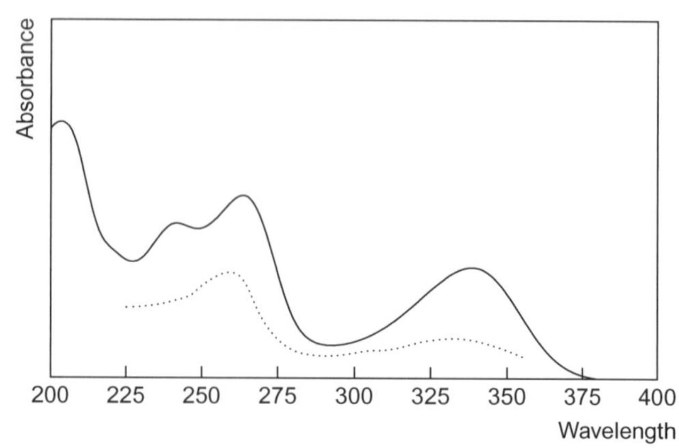

Infra-red Spectrum. Principal peaks at wavenumbers 759, 1250, 1698, 699, 731, 1199 cm^{-1} (KBr disk).

Disposition in the Body. Readily absorbed after oral administration and extensively metabolised; less than 5% of a dose is excreted in the urine unchanged.

Half-life. Plasma half-life, about 4 h.

Dose. Cinchophen was formerly given in doses of 300 to 600 mg.

Cineole

Essential Oil

Synonyms. Cajuputol; Eucalyptol.
1,3,3-Trimethyl-2-oxabicyclo[2.2.2]octane
$C_{10}H_{18}O$ = 154.3
CAS—470-82-6

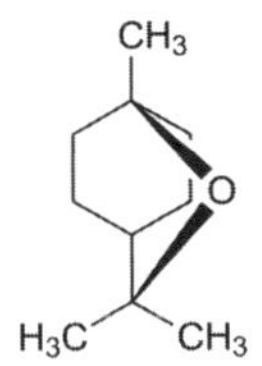

Cineole is obtained from eucalyptus oil, cajuput oil, and other oils.
A colourless liquid with an aromatic camphoraceous odour. Mass per mL 0.922 to 0.924 g. F.p. not lower than 0°. B.p. 176° to 177°. Refractive index (at 20°) 1.456 to 1.460.
Practically insoluble in water; miscible with ethanol, chloroform, ether, and glacial acetic acid.

Partition Coefficient. Log *P* (octanol), 2.7.

Gas Chromatography. System GB—RI 1063; system GO—retention time 11.2 min.

Infra-red Spectrum. Principal peaks at wavenumbers 980, 1075, 1219, 847, 1162, 1052 cm^{-1}.

Cinnarizine

Antihistamine

Synonyms. Ginnipirine; S16-MD.
Proprietary names. Aplactan; Aplexal; Carecin; Cerepar; Cinnacet; Gigantēn; Hilactan; Ixertol; Katoseran; Midronal; Olamin; Sepan; Stugeron.
1-(Diphenylmethyl)-4-(3-phenyl-2-propenyl)piperazine
$C_{26}H_{28}N_2$ = 368.5
CAS—298-57-7

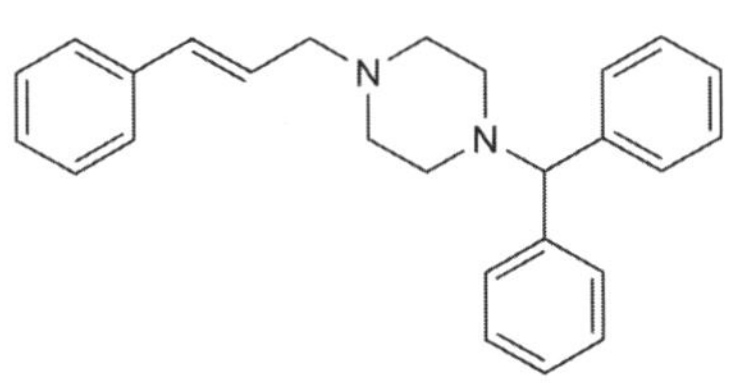

Practically insoluble in water; soluble in dilute hydrochloric acid.

Partition Coefficient. Log *P* (octanol/water), 5.8.

Thin-layer Chromatography. System TA—Rf 76; system TB—Rf 54; system TC—Rf 78; system TE—Rf 86; system TL—Rf 65; system TAE—Rf 79; system TAF—Rf 87. (Acidified iodoplatinate solution, positive.)

Gas Chromatography. System GA—cinnarizine RI 3050, M (desalkyl-) (norcyclizine) RI 2120, M (benzophenone) (BPH) RI 1610, M (OH-BPH) isomer 1 RI 2065, M (OH-BPH) isomer 2 RI 2080, M (OH-methoxy-BPH) isomer 1 RI 2050, M (OH-methoxy-BPH) isomer 2 RI 2070, M (carbinol) RI 1750; system GB—cinnarizine RI 3233, M (desalkyl-) RI 2128, M (BPH) RI 1673.

High Performance Liquid Chromatography. System HA—*k* 0.8; system HX—RI 560; system HZ—retention time 22.0 min; system HAA—retention time 19.3 min.

Ultraviolet Spectrum. Aqueous acid—254 nm (A^1_1 = 584a).

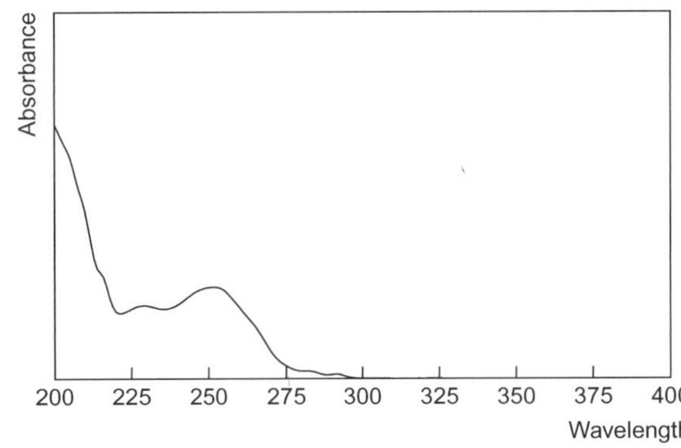

Infra-red Spectrum. Principal peaks at wavenumbers 702, 691, 1138, 964, 740, 1000 cm^{-1} (KBr disk).

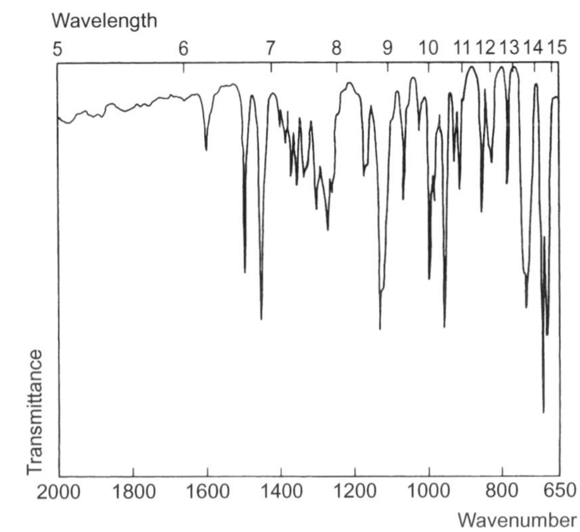

Mass Spectrum. Principal ions at *m/z* 201, 117, 167, 202, 251, 165, 118, 115.

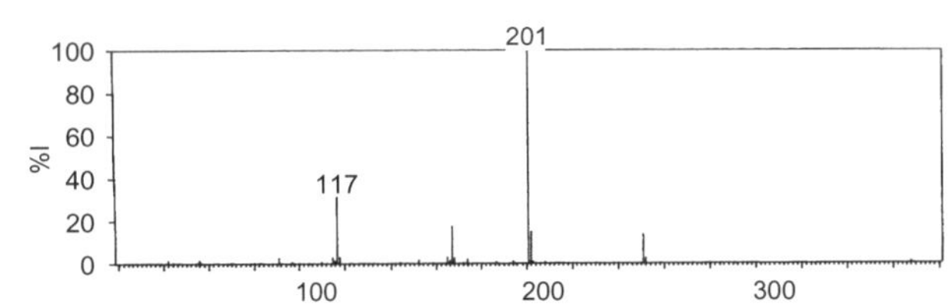

Quantification

Gas chromatography. In plasma or urine: limit of detection 0.5 µg/L, AFID—R. Woestenborgh *et al.*, *J. Chromatogr.* 1982, *232 B Biomed. Appl.*, *21*, 85–91.

High performance liquid chromatography. In plasma: limit of detection 20 µg/L, UV detection—V. Nitsche and H. Mascher, *J. Chromatogr.* 1982, *227(16) B Biomed. Appl.*, 521–524. In serum: limit of detection 16 µg/L, UV detection (λ = 250 nm)—S. S. Hassan *et al.*, *J. Pharm. Biomed. Anal.*, 2002, *28(3–4)*, 711–719.

Thin layer chromatography. In serum: limit of detection 10 µg/L—S. S. Hassan *et al.*, *J. Pharm. Biomed. Anal.*, 2002, *28(3–4)*, 711–719.

Disposition in the Body

Therapeutic concentration

Following a single oral dose of 50 mg to 6 subjects, a mean peak plasma concentration of 0.08 mg/L was attained in 2.3 h. [H. K. L. Hundt *et al.*, *J. Chromatogr.* 1980, *183(9) B Biomed. Appl.*, 378–382.]

6 young, healthy males were administered 75 mg cinnarizine as a tablet. Peak plasma drug concentrations reached a mean of 275 µg/L 3 h after dosing. [G. Castaneda-Hernandez *et al.*, *Arzneimittelforschung*, 1993, *43(5)*, 539–542.]

Half-life. Plasma half-life, about 5 h.

Dose. Usually 45 to 90 mg daily; doses of 150 to 225 mg daily are given in peripheral arterial disease.

Ciprofibrate

Lipid Regulator

Synonym. Win-35833
Proprietary names. Bi-Lipanor; Ciprol; Hyperlipen; Lipanor; Modalim.
2-[4-(2,2-Dichlorocyclopropyl)phenoxy]-2-methylpropanoic acid
$C_{13}H_{14}Cl_2O_3$=289.2
CAS—52214-84-3

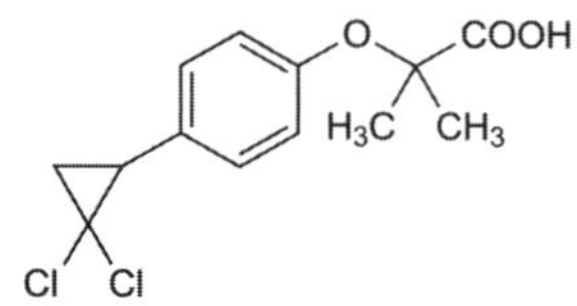

A pale cream solid. M.p. 114° to 116°.

Partition Coefficient. Log *P* (octanol/water), 3.94.

High Performance Liquid Chromatography. System HAA—retention time 21.2 min.

Column: (analytical) RP Shimpack CLC-ODS RP-C_{18} (250 × 4.6 mm i.d., 5 μm); (guard) Shimpack G-ODS (10 × 4 mm, 5 μm). Mobile phase: acetonitrile:0.02 M H_3PO_4 (55:45), 2.0 mL/min flow rate for the first 8 min then 2.5 mL/min until the end. UV detection (λ=232 nm). Retention time: 4.9 min. [L. D. Masnatta *et al.*, *J. Chromatogr.* 1996, *687; Biomed. Appl.*, 437–442].

Ultraviolet Spectrum. ethanol—232 nm.

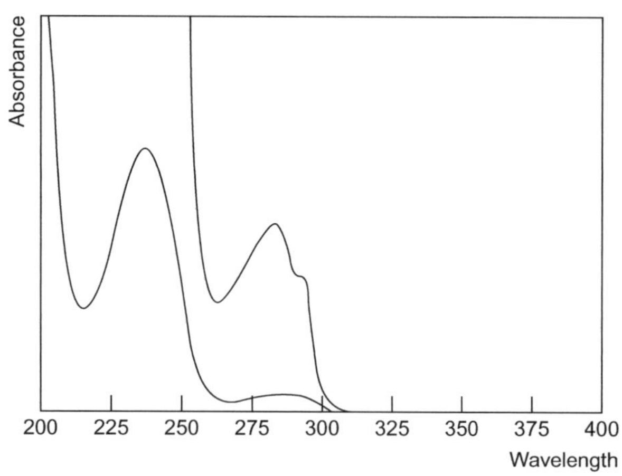

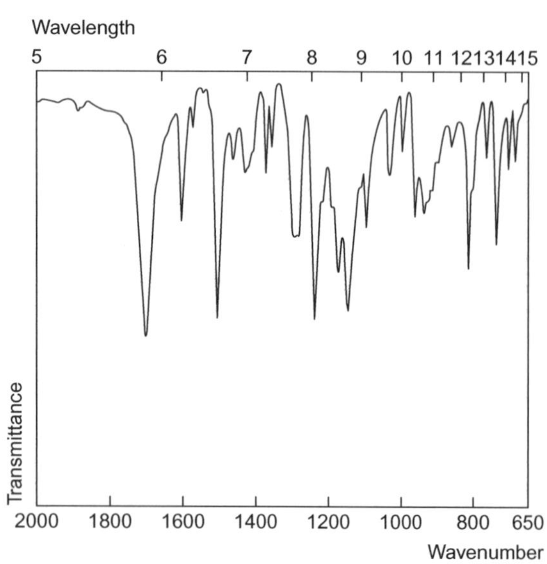

Mass Spectrum. Principal ions at *m/z* 131, 167, 41, 103, 43, 132, 77, 289.

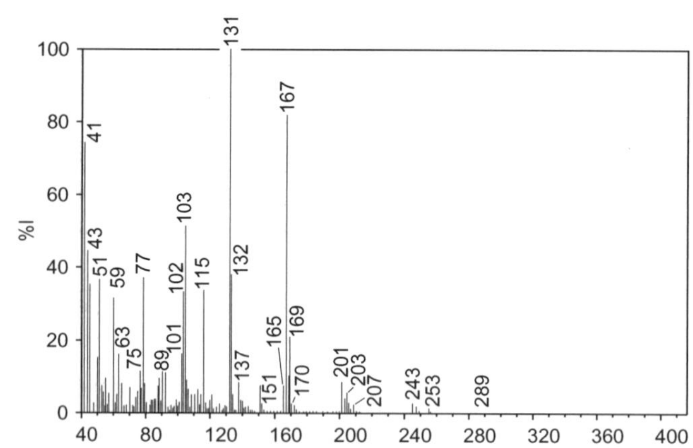

Quantification

High performance liquid chromatography. In plasma: limit of detection 0.69 mg/L, UV detection—G. B. Park *et al.*, *J. Chromatogr.*, 1982, *227; Biomed. Appl.*, *16*, 534–539. In plasma: limit of detection 0.25 mg/L, UV detection (λ=232 nm)—L. D. Masnatta *et al.*, *J. Chromatogr.* 1996, *687; Biomed. Appl.*, 437–442.

Disposition in the Body. Ciprofibrate is readily absorbed after oral administration; peak plasma concentrations occur within 1 to 4 h. About 30 to 75% of a single dose is excreted in urine as the unchanged drug (20 to 25% of total excreted) and as glucuronide conjugates, in 72 h. It is not removed by dialysis.

Therapeutic concentration

Group 1: 6 patients with normal renal function, creatinine clearance 89 to 133 mL/min/1.73 m^2, aged 24 to 37 years; group 2: mild renal insufficiency, creatinine clearance 39 to 60 mL/min 1.73 m^2, aged 25 to 66 years; group 3: severe insufficiency, creatinine clearance 11 to 30 mL/min/1.73 m^2, aged 37 to 60 years; group 4: haemodialysis patients, 44 to 70 years old. Each group was administered with 100 mg ciprofibrate in a fasting state. The peak concentrations were 24, 22 and 17 mg/L for the first three groups observed at 1.3, 2.3 and 2.8 h. [N. Ferry *et al.*, *Br. J. Clin. Pharmacol.*, 1989, *28(6)*, 675–681].

Half-life. Plasma, 81 h in healthy individuals; 117 h (patients with mild renal failure; 154 h (patients undergoing haemodialysis); 172 h (severe renal failure).

Protein binding. In plasma, 95% bound to albumin.

Note. For reviews of ciprofibrate see D. J. Betteridge, *Postgrad. Med. J.*, 1993, *69*, *Suppl.*, *1*, S42–S49, and G. Turpin and E. Bruckert, *Atherosclerosis*, 1996, *124*, *Suppl.*, S83–S87.

Dose. 100 mg daily.

Ciprofloxacin

Antibacterial

Synonym. Bay-q-3939
Proprietary names. Ciflox; Cipro; Ciprobay; Ciproxin; Ciproxine; Plenolyt; Septocipro.
1-Cyclopropyl-6-fluoro-1,4-dihydro-4-oxo-7-(1-piperazinyl)-3-quinolinecarboxylic acid
$C_{17}H_{18}FN_3O_3$=331.4
CAS—85721-33-1

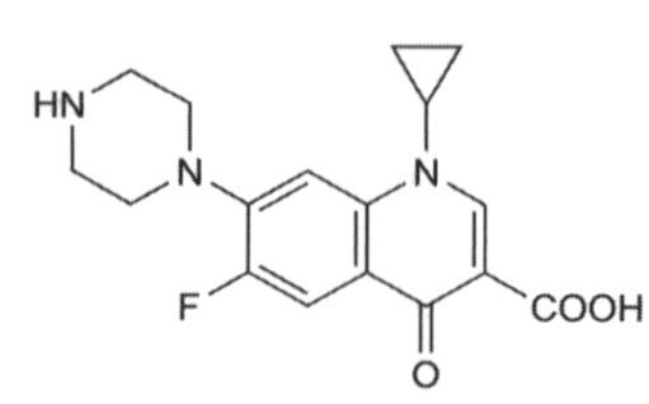

M.p. 255° to 257°, with decomposition. It is practically insoluble in water; very slightly soluble in ethanol and in methylene chloride; soluble in dilute acetic acid.

Ciprofloxacin Hydrochloride

Synonym. Bay-o-9867

Proprietary names. Baycip; Belmacina; Catex; Ceprimax; Cetraxal; Ciflox; Ciloxan; Cipro; Ciprobay; Ciproxin; Ciproxine; Cunesin; Estecina; Flociprin; Globuce; Huberdoxina; Inkamil; Quipro; Rigoran; Sepcen; Septocipro; Tam; Velmonit.

$C_{17}H_{18}FN_3O_3.HCl,H_2O$=385.8

CAS—86483-48-9 (anhydrous); 86393-32-0 (monohydrate)

Faintly yellowish to light yellow crystals. M.p. 318° to 320°. It is sparingly soluble to soluble in water; slightly soluble in acetic acid and in methanol; very slightly soluble in ethanol; practically insoluble in acetone, in acetonitrile, in ethyl acetate, in hexane and in methylene chloride.

Ciprofloxacin Lactate

Proprietary Names. Baycip; Ciprobay; Ciproxin; Ciproxine; Flociprin; Rigoran; Septocipro; Velmonit.

$C_{17}H_{18}FN_3O_3,C_3H_6O_3$=421.4

CAS—97867-33-9

Partition Coefficient. Log *P* (octanol/water), 0.28.

Thin-Layer Chromatography. System TE—Rf 00; system TF—Rf 00.

High Performance Liquid Chromatography. System HX—RI 318; system HY—RI 260; system HZ—retention time 1.8 min; system HAA—retention time 9.1 min.

Column: ODS Hypersil (100 × 4.6 mm i.d., 5 µm). Mobile phase: methanol:aqueous 0.01 M dihydrogen potassium phosphate buffer, adjusted to pH 3.5 with 30 drops/L triethylamine (90:10), 1 mL/min flow rate. UV diode array detection. Retention time: 1.1 min. [T. Mills and J. C. Roberson, *Instrumental Data for Drug Analysis*, 1993, CRC Press, Boca Raton, US. 2nd Edn, Vol. 5, pp. 104–105].

Ultraviolet Spectrum. Aqueous acid (0.2 M NH_2SO_4)—277, 315 nm; basic—272, 322, 334 nm.

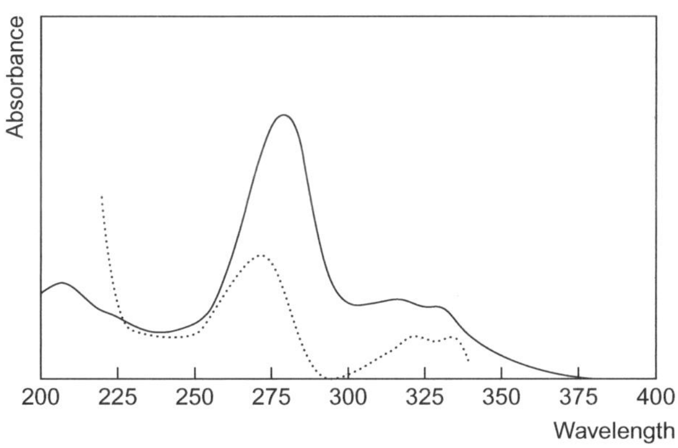

Infra-red Spectrum. Principal peaks at wavenumbers 1703, 1619, 1267 cm^{-1} (KBr pellets).

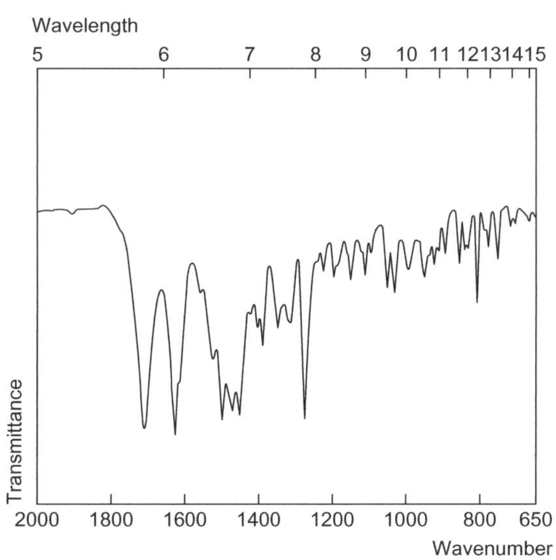

Mass Spectrum. Principal ions at *m/z* 287, 245, 289, 331, 56, 29, 41, 57.

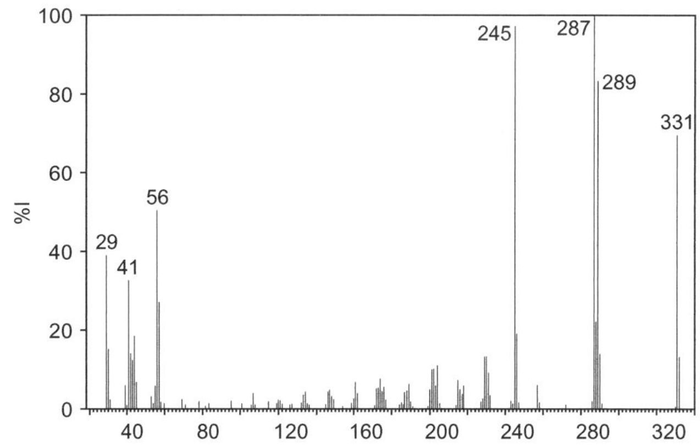

Quantification

High performance liquid chromatography. In plasma, serum and urine: limit of quantification is 0.05 mg/L for ciprofloxacin and 0.01, 0.05 and 0.5 mg/L for its metabolites, M1, M2 and M3, respectively—G. J. Krol *et al.*, *J. Pharm. Biomed. Anal.*, 1995, *14(1–2)*, 181–190. In serum, urine, saliva or sputum: limit of detection 0.05 mg/L, UV detection—G. Mack, *J. Chromatogr.*, 1992, *582*; *Biomed. Appl.*, *120*, 263–267. In serum: limit of detection 0.1 mg/L, UV detection—L. Pou-Clave *et al.*, *J. Chromatogr.*, 1991, *563*; *Biomed. Appl.*, *101*, 211–215. In plasma, whole blood or erythrocytes: limit of detection 0.025 mg/L, fluorescence detection—P. Teja-Isavadharm *et al.*, *Ther. Drug Monit.*, 1991, *13*, 263–267. In serum, urine or sputum: limit of detection 0.02 mg/L, fluorescence detection—C. M. Myers and J. L. Blumer, *J. Chromatogr.*, 1987, *422*; *Biomed. Appl.*, *66*, 153–164. In serum or urine: limit of detection 0.01 mg/L, fluorescence detection—I. Nilsson-Ehle, *J. Chromatogr.*, 1987, *416*; *Biomed. Appl.*, *60*, 207–211. In serum, urine, blister fluid, sputum or saliva: limit of detection 0.06 mg/L, UV detection—F. Vallée *et al.*, *Ther. Drug Monit.*, 1986, *8*, 340–345. In serum, urine or bile: limit of detection 0.01 mg/L, 0.5 mg/L and 0.2 mg/L, respectively, UV detection—F. Jehl *et al.*, *J. Chromatogr.*, 1985, *339*; *Biomed. Appl.*, *40*, 347–357. In serum or urine: limit of detection 0.08 mg/L, fluorescence detection—D. E. Nix *et al.*, *Clin. Chem.*, 1985, *31*, 684–686.

Capillary electrophoresis. In plasma: limit of detection 0.02 mg/L, fluorescence detection—K. H. Bannefeld *et al.*, *J. Chromatogr. Biomed. Sci. Appl.*, 1997, *692*, 453–459.

Disposition in the Body. Ciprofloxacin is rapidly and well absorbed after oral administration. It is widely distributed and it diffuses into CSF (cerebrospinal fluid); concentrations are usually less than 10% of peak plasma concentrations although higher concentrations are found if the meninges are inflamed. It crosses the placenta and is distributed into breast milk. The drug is eliminated principally by urinary excretion (active tubular secretion as well as glomerular filtration). Non-renal clearance may account for about a third of elimination (hepatic metabolism, biliary excretion, and possibly transluminal secretion across intestinal mucosa). Active metabolites have been identified. About 40 to 50% of an oral dose is excreted unchanged in urine with about 15% excreted as metabolites. Up to 70% of a parenteral dose may be excreted unchanged within 24 h and 10% as metabolites. Faecal excretion over 5 days has accounted for 20 to 35% of an oral dose and 15% of an intravenous dose. Only small amounts are removed by haemodialysis or peritoneal dialysis.

Therapeutic concentration. The trough serum therapeutic concentration range is 0.05 to 0.5 mg/L and peak, 1 to 5 mg/L.

Single oral doses of 500 mg administered to 7 people undergoing orthopaedic surgery produced mean concentrations of 1.4 mg/L (serum), 0.4 µg/g (bone) and 1.1 µg/g (muscle). [I. W. Fong *et al.*, *Antimicrob. Agents Chemother.*, 1986, *29*, 405–408].

Toxicity

A 29-year-old woman was presented to hospital the day after ingesting 21 g of ciprofloxacin. She had vomited about 3 h after swallowing the tablets. The serum-ciprofloxacin concentration at presentation was 12 mg/L. 12 h later she developed oliguric acute renal failure. She made a full recovery following treatment with steroids, and hydration and acidification of urine. [M. J. George *et al.*, *Arch. Intern. Med.*, 1991, *151*, 620].

Bioavailability. 70%.

Half-life. Plasma, 3.5 to 4.5 h.

Volume of distribution. 1.8 to 5.0 L/kg.

Clearance. Plasma, 35 L/h.

Protein binding. In plasma, 20 to 40%.

Note. For reviews of ciprofloxacin, see D. M. Campoli-Richards *et al.*, *Drugs*, 1988, *35*, 373–447 and K. Vance-Bryan *et al.*, *Clin. Pharmacokinet.*, 1990, *19*, 434–461.

Dose. The equivalent of up to 1500 mg of ciprofloxacin daily by mouth; up to 800 mg daily may be given intravenously.

Cisapride

Peristaltic Stimulant

Proprietary names. Alimix; Arcasin; Cyprid; Fisiogastrol; Kelosal; Kinet; Prepulsid; Propulsid; Propulsin; Pulsitil; Trautil.
cis-4-Amino-5-chloro-*N*-[1-[3-(4-fluorophenoxy)propyl]-3-methoxy-4-piperidinyl]-2-methoxybenzamide
$C_{23}H_{29}ClFN_3O_4$=466.0
CAS—81098-60-4

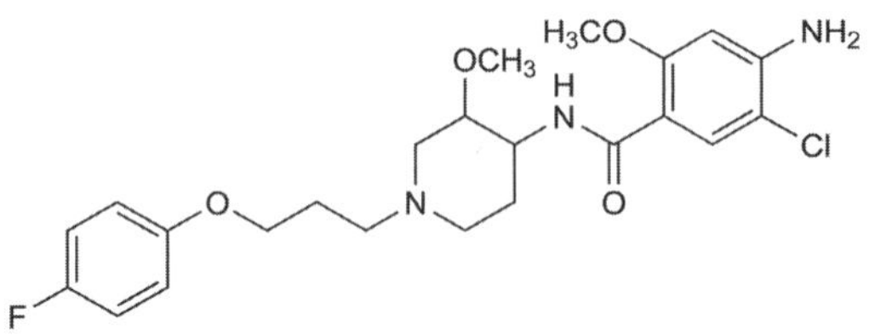

A white or almost white powder; it exhibits polymorphism. It is practically insoluble in water; freely soluble in dimethylformamide; soluble in dichloromethane; sparingly soluble in methanol.

Cisapride Monohydrate

Synonym. R-51619
Proprietary names. Acenalin; Alimix; Cipril; Prepulsid; Propulsin; Risamal.
$C_{23}H_{29}ClFN_3O_4.H_2O$=484.0
Crystals from 2-propanol. M.p. 109.8°.

Partition Coefficient. Log *P* (octanol/water), 3.09.

Thin-layer Chromatography. System TB—Rf 00; system TE—Rf 62; system TAE—Rf 66.

High Performance Liquid Chromatography. System HX—RI 431; system HY—RI 317; system HZ—retention time 5.2 min; system HAA—retention time 14.6 min; system HAX—retention time 10.9 min; system HAY—retention time 5.8 min.

Column: C_{18} RP (NovaPak, 150 × 3.9 mm i.d., 4 µm). Mobile phase: acetonitrile:methanol:sodium phosphate buffer (0.015 M, adjusted to pH 2.2 with 85% orthophosphoric acid) (68:19.4:12.6), 0.8 mL/min flow rate. UV detection (λ 276 nm). *k* values: cisapride, 2.7 (retention time, 4.3 min); norcisapride, 3.7 (5.3 min). [S. Cisternino *et al.*, *J. Chromatogr. Biomed. Sci. Appl.*, 1998, *714*, 395–398].

Ultraviolet Spectrum. Aqueous acid (0.2 M H_2SO_4)—273, 307 nm; basic—275, 308 nm.

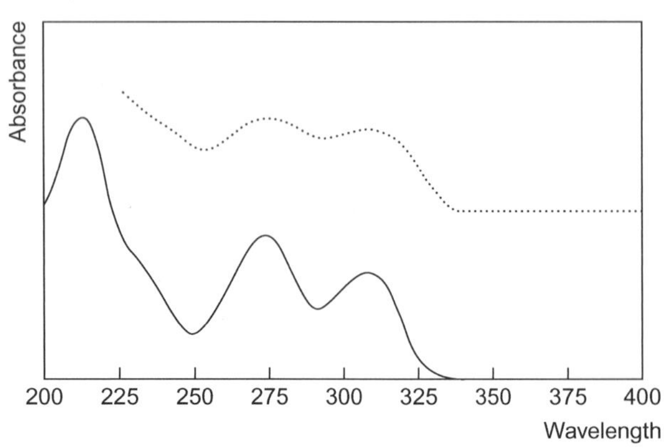

Infra-red Spectrum. Principal peaks at wavenumbers 1499, 1203, 823 cm^{-1} (KBr pellets).

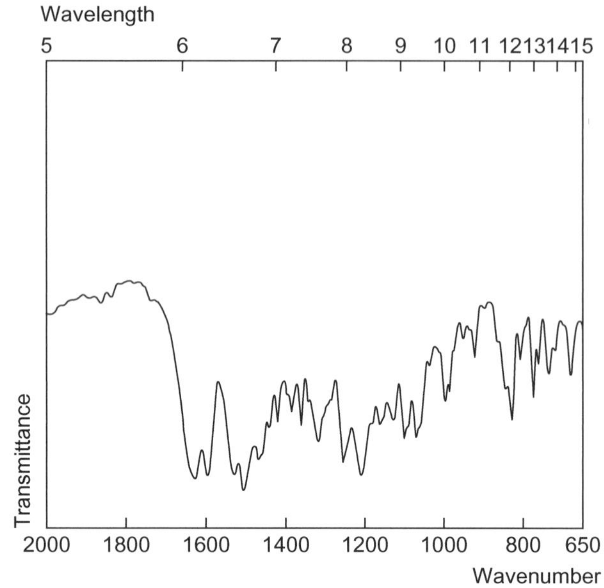

Mass Spectrum. Principal ions at *m/z* 232, 184, 233, 201, 186, 433, 95, 120.

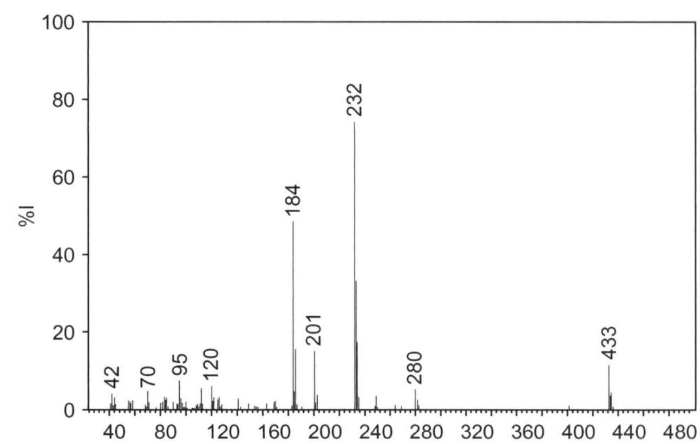

Quantification

High performance liquid chromatography. In plasma: limit of detection 1 µg/L, UV detection—R. Woestenborghs *et al.*, *J. Chromatogr.*, 1988, *424*; *Biomed. Appl.*, *68*, 195–200. In neonate plasma: limit of detection 8 µg/L, fluorescence detection—Y. Preechagoon and B. G. Charles, *J. Chromatogr.*, 1995, *670*; *Biomed. Appl.*, 139–143. In plasma: cisapride and norcisapride, limit of detection 10 µg/L, UV detection—S. Cisternino *et al.*, *J. Chromatogr. Biomed. Sci. Appl.*, 1998, *714*, 395–398. In urine: norcisapride, limit of detection 50 µg/L, fluorescence detection—R. S. Addison *et al.*, *J. Chromatogr. Sci.*, 1999, *37*, 61–64.

Disposition in the Body. Cisapride is readily absorbed after oral administration, and the presence of food enhances absorption. It undergoes extensive metabolism in the liver and gut wall mainly via the cytochrome P450 isoenzyme CYP3A4. The main metabolic pathways are oxidative *N*-dealkylation, producing the major metabolite norcisapride, and aromatic hydroxylation to 3-fluoro-4-hydroxycisapride and 4-fluoro-2-hydroxycisapride. More than 90% of a dose is excreted as metabolites in urine and faeces in approximately equal amounts. 4 to 6% of a dose is recovered as the unchanged drug in faeces and 0.2% in urine. A small amount is distributed into breast milk with approx. 0.1% of a dose being detected (milk:serum ratio, 0.045). It is not removed by haemodialysis.

Bioavailability. 35 to 40%.

Therapeutic concentration. Mean peak plasma concentrations of 45 to 65 µg/L were reached about 1 to 2 h after administration of 10 mg given orally to healthy volunteers 15 min prior to food intake. Peak plasma concentrations of 49 µg/L were observed in the fasting state and 60 µg/L after the meal. [Janssen Pharmaceutica data files].

Toxicity. Rare cases of cardiac arrhythmia, including ventricular tachycardia, ventricular fibrillation, and torsade de pointes, and QT interval prolongation have been reported.

A prolonged QT interval developed in 6 infants aged 11 to 70 days (weighing 1.2 to 4.0 kg) who were given cisapride 1.0 to 1.6 mg/kg daily. Correction of the QT interval occurred following cessation of cisapride in 5 of the infants and dose reduction to 0.8 mg/kg in another. (No plasma-cisapride concentrations were reported.) [A. Bedu *et al.*, *J. Pediatr.*, 1997, *130*, 164].

Half-life. Plasma, 7 to 10 h.

Volume of distribution. Approx. 2.4 L/kg.

Clearance. Plasma clearance, approx. 100 mL/min.

Protein binding. In plasma, 98% mainly to albumin.

Note. For a review of cisapride see R. W. McCallum *et al.*, *Drugs*, 1988, *36*, 652–681.

Dose. Usually 5 to 10 mg three or four times daily.

Cisatracurium

Skeletal Muscle Relaxant

(1*R*,1′*R*,2*R*,2′*R*)-2,2′-[1,5-Pentanediylbis[oxy(3-oxo-3,1-propanediyl)]] bis[1-[(3,4-dimethoxyphenyl)methyl]-1,2,3,4-tetrahydro-6,7-dimethoxy-2-methylisoquinolinium]
$C_{53}H_{72}N_2O_{12}$=929.2

Cisatracurium Besilate

Synonyms. Cisatracurium besylate; 51W89.
Proprietary name. Nimbex, dibenzenesulfonate.
$C_{65}H_{82}N_2O_{18}S_2$=1243.5
CAS—96946-42-8

Partition Coefficient. Log *P* (octanol/water), −2.12.

Quantification

High performance liquid chromatography. In plasma: limit of quantification 0.01 mg/L, fluorescence detection—A. H. Boyd *et al.*, *Br. J. Anaesth.*, 1996, *76*, 382–388.

Disposition in the Body. After intravenous administration it is inactivated in plasma by Hofmann elimination, a non-enzymatic breakdown process (pH and temperature dependent) to form a monoquaternary acrylate metabolite and laudanosine, neither of which has neuromuscular blocking activity. This elimination process contributes to 77% of the clearance of the drug. The acrylate metabolite may also undergo further metabolism to its corresponding alcohol and then more laudanosine. Laudanosine (which may have some stimulatory action on the CNS (central nervous system)) is further metabolised to desmethyl metabolites that are conjugated with glucuronic acid. Cisatracurium is excreted mainly as metabolites in urine and faeces; less than 10% is excreted as the unchanged drug. About 40% of a dose is eliminated in faeces.

Therapeutic concentration.

The mean peak plasma-laudanosine concentration was 0.71 mg/L (range 0.21 to 1.26) following an infusion of cisatracurium at 0.19 (0.16 to 0.21) mg/kg/h in 6 intensive care patients, critically ill, sedated and requiring neuromuscular blocking drug to assist mechanical ventilation (> 18 years old). Following a mean atracurium infusion of 0.47 (range 0.3 to 0.74) mg/kg/h, the mean concentration was 2.31 mg/L (range 0.78 to 4.40). [A. H. Boyd *et al.*, *Br. J. Anaesth.*, 1996, *76*, 382–388].

The mean peak plasma concentration of laudanosine was 23.1 µg/L 4 min after a 0.1 mg/kg cisatracurium dose administered intravenously to 15 healthy subjects, with a mean age of 42.9 years (range 21.8 to 64.0) undergoing elective surgery. 17 Patients with end-stage chronic renal failure, most of them scheduled for dialysis-access procedures with a mean age of 43.9 years (range 25.7 to 62.4) were administered with the same dose and mean concentrations were 0.031 mg/L at 150 min. [N. B. Eastwood *et al.*, *Br. J. Anaesth.*, 1995, *75*, 431–435].

Peak plasma concentrations of laudanosine following administration of 0.1 mg/kg intravenous bolus of cisatracurium to 10 subjects ranged from 0.013 to 0.086 mg/L (mean 0.038 mg/L). Following administration of 0.2 mg/kg intravenous bolus to 10 subjects peak plasma-laudanosine concentrations ranged from 0.066 to 0.174 mg/L (mean 0.103 mg/L). [C. A. Lien *et al.*, *Anesthesiology*, 1996, *84*, 300–308].

Half-life. Plasma, 22 to 35 min.

Volume of distribution. Steady state, 0.11 to 0.16 L/kg; increased in the elderly 17 to 37% and in patients with end-stage liver failure (21%).

Clearance. Plasma, 4.6 to 5.7 mL/min/kg; decreases in those with renal failure and increases in patients with end-stage liver disease.

Note. For a review of cisatracurium see H. M. Bryson and D. Faulds, *Drugs*, 1997, *53*, 848–866.

Dose. The equivalent of 0.15 or 0.2 mg/kg of cisatracurium intravenously for intubation followed by 0.03 mg/kg every 20 min for maintenance.

Cisplatin

Antineoplastic

Synonyms. CACP; CDDP; *cis*-DPP; Cisplatinum; CPDC; DDP; NSC-119875; Peyrone's salt; Platinum diamminodichloride.
Proprietary names. Abiplatin; Cisplatyl; Citoplatino; Lederplatin; Neoplatin; Norplatin; Placis; Platamine; Platiblastin; Platiblastine; Platinex; Platinol; Platistil; Platistin; Platosin; Randa.
cis-Diamminedichloroplatinum
$(NH_3)_2.PtCl_2$=300.1
CAS—15663-27-1

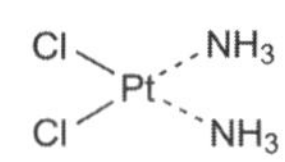

A yellow powder or yellow or orange-yellow crystals. M.p. 270°, with decomposition.
It is slightly soluble in water (0.253 g/100 g at 25°); sparingly soluble in dimethylformamide; practically insoluble in ethanol and most common organic solvents, except *N*,*N*-dimethylformamide, *N*,*N*-dimethylacetamide and dimethylsulfoxide.

Partition Coefficient. Log *P* (octanol/water), −2.19.

High Performance Liquid Chromatography. Column: anionic exchange resin (150 × 4.6 mm i.d., 5 µm). Mobile phase: acetonitrile:sodium chloride (10 mM) (85:15), 0.7 mL/min flow rate. UV detection (λ=290 nm). Retention time: 11 min (derivative). [M. Kinoshita *et al.*, *J. Chromatogr.*, 1990, *529*; *Biomed. Appl.*, *94*, 462–467].

Ultraviolet Spectrum. Aqueous acid (0.1 M hydrochloric acid)—203 (A^1_1=173b), 285 (A^1_1=3.63b), 301 (A^1_1=4.33b), 362 (A^1_1=0.806b).

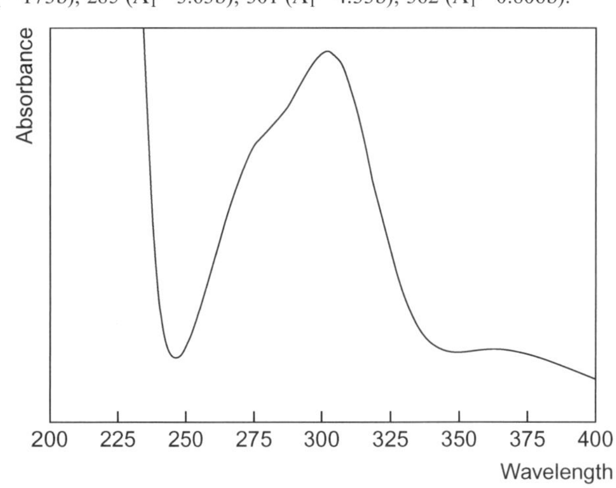

Mass Spectrum. Principal ions at *m/z* 300, 302, 298, 299, 301, 193, 207, 264.

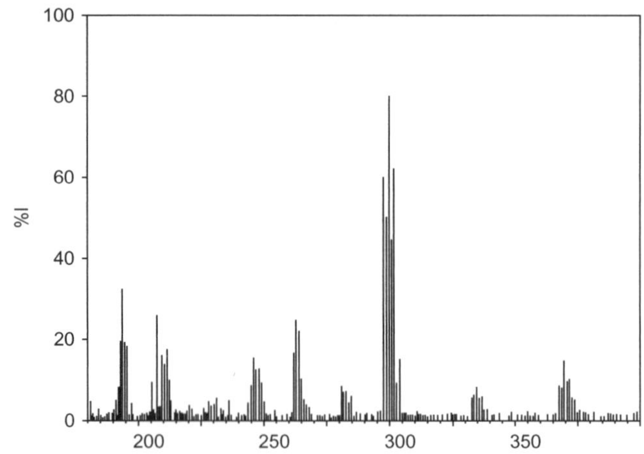

Quantification

High performance liquid chromatography. In plasma: limit of detection 0.062 mg/L, electrochemical detection—P. J. Parsons and A. F. LeRoy, *J. Chromatogr.*, 1986, *378*; *Biomed. Appl.*, *51*, 395–408. In plasma or urine: limit of detection 0.08 mg/L, UV detection (λ=290 nm)—M. Kinoshita *et al.*, *J. Chromatogr.*, 1990, *529*; *Biomed. Appl.*, *94*, 462–467. In plasma: limit of detection 2.5 μg/L, UV detection—P. A. Reece *et al.*, *J. Chromatogr.*, 1984, *306*; *Biomed. Appl.*, *31*, 417–423. In plasma: limit of detection 0.1 mg/L, UV detection (λ=254 nm)—P. A. Andrews *et al.*, *Anal. Biochem.*, 1984, *143*, 46–56.

High performance liquid chromatography–Mass spectrometry. In plasma: cisplatin and metabolites, limit of detection 0.035 mg/L, atomic emission spectroscopy—W. A. De Waal *et al.*, *J. Chromatogr.*, 1987, *407*, 253–272.

Disposition in the Body. Following intravenous administration, cisplatin concentrates in the liver, kidneys, and the large and small intestines. Penetration into CNS (central nervous system) is poor. It is distributed into breast milk. The chlorine atoms in cisplatin undergo chemical displacement reactions with water and sulfhydryl groups (for example, on proteins) rather than undergoing enzyme-catalysed metabolism. Excretion is mainly in urine but is incomplete and prolonged; up to 50% of a dose has been reported to be excreted in urine over 5 days and platinum may be detected in tissue for several months afterwards. There is some excretion in faeces via bile. Cisplatin is well absorbed following intraperitoneal administration.

Therapeutic concentration. The peak plasma therapeutic concentration is 1 to 5 mg/L (free fraction).

Toxicity. The trough toxic concentration is 0.1 mg/L (free fraction).

A 59-year-old male received an accidental overdose of 300 mg/m^2 over 3 days. He developed severe emesis, myelosuppression, renal failure, mental deterioration, dim vision and hepatic toxicity. Three days later the plasma-platinum concentration was 2.679 mg/L. Plasmapheresis was employed to reduce plasma-platinum concentrations and all symptoms resolved. (H. K. Jung *et al.*, *Korean J. Intern. Med.*, 1995, *10*, 150–154).

A 68-year-old woman received 280 mg/m^2 cisplatin without hydration when it was accidentally substituted for carboplatin. She developed severe emesis, myelosuppression, nephrotoxicity, ototoxicity, central neurotoxicity, visual loss and hepatic toxicity. On day 13 after the overdose, the plasma-platinum concentration was 2.6 mg/L. Plasmapheresis was performed to reduce plasma-platinum concentrations, but the patient required a kidney and bone-marrow transplant and remained deaf. (G. Chu *et al.*, *Cancer*, 1993, *72*, 3707–3714).

Half-life. Plasma, unbound cisplatin 25 to 48 min; protein-bound platinum, 58 to 73 h.

Volume of distribution. 11 to 12 L/m^2, also reported as 20 to 80 L.

Clearance. Plasma, 15 to 16 L/h/m^2.

Protein binding. In plasma, majority is bound.

Dose. Up to 120 mg/m^2 body-surface area by intravenous infusion as a single dose, or 15 to 20 mg/m^2 by infusion daily for 5 consecutive days, every 3 to 4 weeks.

Citalopram

Antidepressant

Synonyms. Lu 10-171; nitalapram.
1-[3-(Dimethylamino)propyl]-1-(4-fluorophenyl)-1,3-dihydro-5-isobenzofurancarbonitrile
$C_{20}H_{21}FN_2O$=324.4
CAS—*59729-33-8*

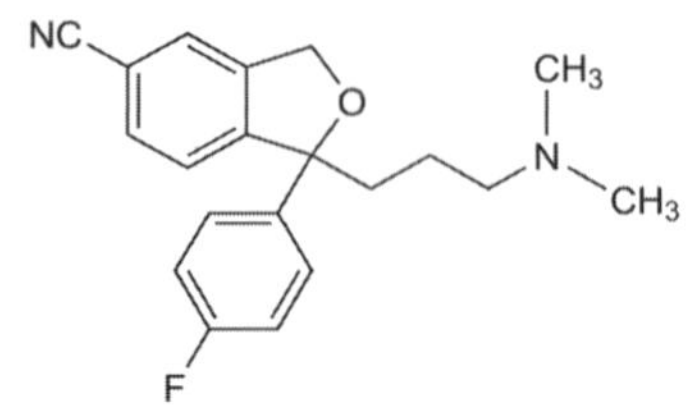

Citalopram Hydrobromide

Synonym. Lu 10-171-B
Proprietary names. Cipramil; Seropram.
$C_{20}H_{21}FN_2O$,HBr=405.3
CAS—*59729-32-7*

A white to off-white, crystalline solid with M.p. 186°. It is sparingly soluble in water; soluble in ethanol (96%); freely soluble in chloroform; practically insoluble in diethylether.

Dissociation Constant. pK_a 9.5 (hydrobromide).

Partition Coefficient. Log *P* (octanol/phosphate buffer pH 7.4), 1.57 (hydrobromide); log *P* (octanol/water), 3.74.

Thin-layer Chromatography. System TB—Rf 22; system TE—Rf 60; system TAE—Rf 19.

Gas Chromatography. System GB—RI 2499 (citalopram); RI 2526 (norcitalopram); system GM—RRT 1.121 (citalopram); RRT 1.231 (norcitalopram), relative to iprindole.

Column: fused-silica capillary (Permabond SE-54-DF-0.25, 25 m × 0.25 mm i.d., 0.27 μm film thickness). Column temperature: 160° increased to 260° at 30°/min. Carrier gas: helium, 60 mL/min flow rate. Detection: nitrogen–phosphorous. Retention times (relative to amitriptyline, internal standard): citalopram, 1.27; didesmethylcitalopram, 1.27; desmethylcitalopram, 1.32. [P. Reymond *et al.*, *J. Chromatogr.*, 1993, *616*, 221–228].

Column: fused-silica capillary (Permabond SE-54-DF-0.25, 25 m × 0.25 mm, 0.27 μm). Column temperature: 160° increased to 260° at 30°/min. Carrier gas: helium, 60 mL/min flow rate. MS detection. Retention times: citalopram, 8.35 min; desmethylcitalopram, 8.72 min; didesmethylcitalopram, 8.52 min. [P. Reymond *et al.*, *J. Chromatogr.*, 1993, *616*, 221–228].

High Performance Liquid Chromatography. System HX—RI 403; system HZ—retention time: citalopram, 4.5 min; desmethylcitalopram, 3.7 min.

Column: C_{18} (Supelco, 250 × 4.6 mm i.d.). Mobile phase: 44 mM potassium dihydrogen phosphate buffer containing 1.5 mL triethylamine/1000 mL, adjusted to pH 2.5 with phosphoric acid:acetonitrile (55:45), 1.5 mL/min flow rate. UV detection (λ 240 nm). Retention time: citalopram, 5.56 min; desmethylcitalopram, 5.06 min; didesmethylcitalopram, 4.51 min. [O. V. Olesen and K. Linnet, *J. Chromatogr.* 1996, *675*; *Biomed. Appl.*, 83–88].

Column: acetylated β-Cyclobond (250 × 4.6 mm, 5 μm). Mobile phase: 20% acetonitrile or 65% methanol with 1% DEA buffer, adjusted to pH 6.1 with acetic acid, 0.8 mL/min flow rate. Fluorimetric detection (λ_{ex}=240 nm, λ_{em}=296 nm). Retention times: citalopram (*S*-(+)-), 15.5 min; (*R*-(−)-), 16.6 min; desmethylcitalopram (*S*-(+)-), 12.2 min; (*R*-(−)-), 12.9 min; didesmethylcitalopram (*S*-(+)-), 10.6 min; (*R*-(−)-), 11.1 min. [B. Rochat *et al.*, *Ther. Drug Monit.*, 1995, *17(3)*, 273–279].

Ultraviolet Spectrum. Aqueous acid (0.1 M hydrochloric acid)—205, 238 nm (hydrobromide); (methanol)—209, 237, 270 nm.

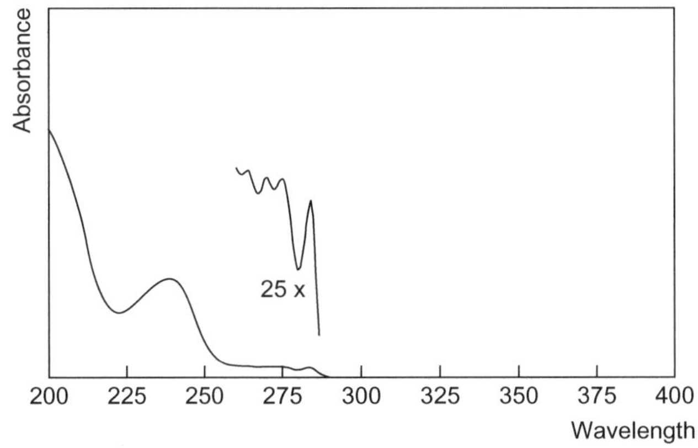

Infrared Spectrum. Principal peaks at wavenumbers 834, 1507, 1034, 1226, 1160, 1601 cm^{-1}.

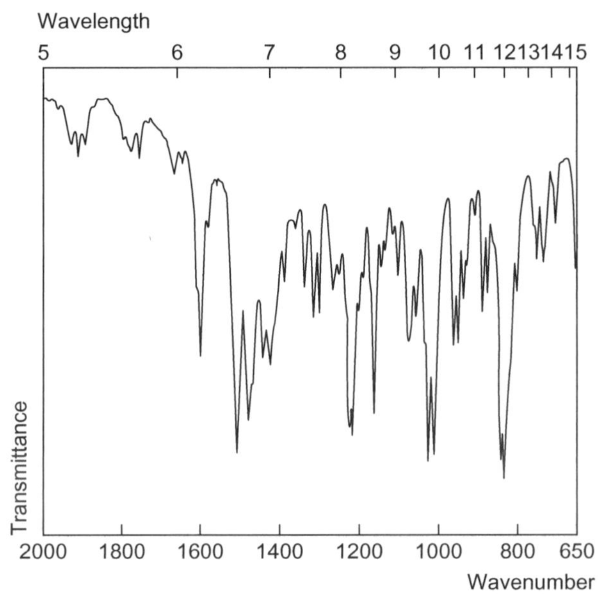

Mass Spectrum. Principal ions at *m/z* 58, 238, 208, 42, 324, 190; *m/z* 44, 238, 310, 138, 208, 57 (desmethylcitalopram).

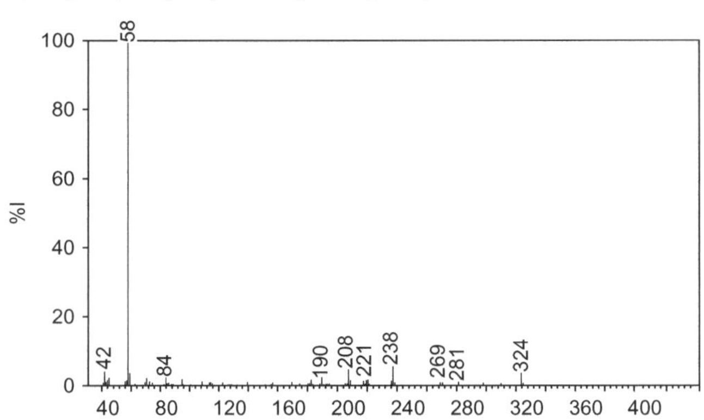

Quantification

Gas chromatography–mass spectrometry. In plasma: limit of quantification 1 µg/L—P. Reymond *et al.*, *J. Chromatogr.*, 1993, *616*, 221–228.

High performance liquid chromatography. In plasma: limit of detection 0.8 µg/L. UV detection (λ=239 nm)—P. P. Rop *et al.*, *J. Chromatogr.*, 1990, *527*, 226–232. In plasma: limit of detection 4 to 5 µg/L, UV detection—P. P. Rop *et al.*, *J. Chromatogr.*, 1985, *338*, 171–178. In plasma: limit of detection about 1 µg/L (for each enantiomer), UV detection—D. Haupt, *J. Chromatogr. B*, 1996, *685*, 299–305. In serum: limit of quantification about 2 µg/L, UV detection (λ=240 nm)—O. V. Olesen and K. Linnet, *J. Chromatogr. B*, 1996, *675*, 83–88. In plasma: limit of quantification 3 µg/L, fluorescence detection (λ_{ex}=240 nm, λ_{em}=296 nm)—B. Rochat *et al.*, *Ther. Drug Monit.*, 1995, *17*, 273–279.

Disposition in the Body. Citalopram is readily absorbed after oral administration with a bioavailability of about 80%; peak plasma concentrations occur after about 2 to 4 h. Metabolised by *N*-demethylation, deamination and oxidation to desmethylcitalopram, didesmethylcitalopram, citalopram-*N*-oxide and a propionic acid derivative. The metabolites have some pharmacological activity although they do not contribute to the overall antidepressant effect of citalopram. Unlike some other selective serotonin reuptake inhibitors, it has only a mild inhibitory effect on CYP2D6. About 12% of the daily dose is excreted unchanged in urine and an equal amount as the main active metabolite, desmethylcitalopram. Also present are an amino metabolite and a conjugated propionic acid derivative. Approximately 65% of a dose is unaccounted for and could possibly be present in faeces or undergo a number of different metabolic pathways. It is distributed into breast milk in very small amounts. Extensive tissue binding has been observed and accumulation can occur with repeated dosing.

Therapeutic concentration. The therapeutic concentration range is 20 to 200 µg/L.

12 healthy male volunteers, aged between 18 and 40 years, were administered with 20 or 40 mg daily for 9 days. The mean plasma concentration was 91 µg/L with a range of 45 to 126 µg/L. The mean didesmethylcitalopram concentration was 19 to 50 µg/L. [M. Lader *et al.*, *Eur. J. Clin. Pharmacol.*, 1986, *31*, 183–190].

Patients suffering from severe depression were administered with 20 mg daily for 12 weeks and the steady state concentrations for citalopram was 40 µg/L; desmethylcitalopram, 12 µg/L and didesmethylcitalopram, 2 µg/L. For those given 40 mg daily, steady state concentrations were 67, 22 and 4 µg/L for the drug and its two metabolites, respectively. [S. A. Montgomery *et al.*, *Int. Clin. Psychopharmacol.*, 1993, *8*, 181–188].

Toxicity. The lethal concentration is 500 µg/L.

Citalopram plasma concentrations were six times greater than the therapeutic concentrations in a patient who attempted suicide. There were no significant changes in unconsciousness, electrocardiogram or blood pressure. [O. L. Pedersen *et al.*, *Psychopharmacology (Berl.)*, 1982, *77*, 199–204].

A 41-year old Caucasian man was found dead at his home; he had a history of depression and suicide attempts. Surrounding the man was a number of medication bottles and a bottle of whiskey. Toxicological analysis showed that the man had ethanol, lormetazepam, cotinine, caffeine, moclobemide and citalopram in his urine and blood. Citalopram was detected in blood at a concentration of 4.47 mg/L and in urine, 19.7 mg/L. Its metabolite, desmethylcitalopam, was found at concentrations of 0.42 mg/L and 1.22 mg/L in the two fluids, respectively. The cause of death was determined as the synergistic toxicity of moclobemide and citalopram; and death was ruled as multiple drug intoxication. [R. Dams *et al.*, *J. Anal. Toxicol.*, 2001, *25(2)*, 147–151].

Bioavailability. About 80%.

Half-life. Plasma, 33 h (parent drug); desmethylcitalopram, 48 h; didesmethylcitalopram, 96 h; in the elderly, 3.75 days.

Volume of distribution. 12 to 16 L/kg.

Clearance. Plasma, 0.33 L/min in the young and 0.08 L/min in the elderly.

Protein binding. In plasma, 50%.

Note. For reviews of citalopram see P. Baumann, *Clin. Pharmacokinet.*, 1996, *31*, 444–469, S. H. Preskorn, *Clin. Pharmacokinet.*, 1997, *32*, *Suppl. 1*, 1–21, and R. J. Milne and K. L. Goa, *Drugs*, 1991, *41*, 450–477.

Dose. The usual starting dose is 20 mg or, more frequently, 40 mg, which may be increased up to 60 mg daily of citalopram, given as the hydrobromide.

Cladribine

Antineoplastic

Synonyms. 2-CdA; CldAdo; NSC-105014-F.
Proprietary names. Leustat; Leustatin; Leustatine.
2-Chloro-2′-deoxyadenosine
$C_{10}H_{12}ClN_5O_3$=285.7

CAS—4291-63-8

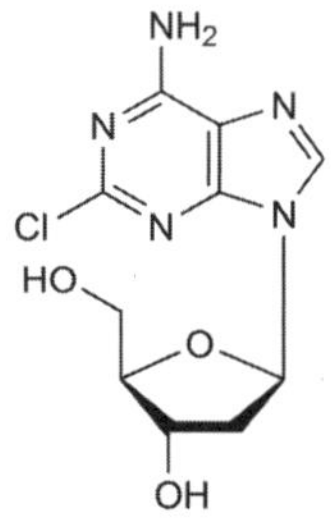

Crystals from water which soften at 210° to 215° and when solidified, turn brown. Also reported as crystals from ethanol with m.p. 220° (soften), that re-solidify, turn brown and do not melt <300°.

High Performance Liquid Chromatography. Column: (analytical) Supelcosil LC-8-DB (330 × 4.6 mm i.d., 3 μm); (guard) LC-8-DB 2. Mobile phase: methanol:5 mM ammonium acetate (25:75), 1.0 mL/min flow rate. Tandem MS detection (positive ion mode). Retention time: 1.5 min. [M. D. Moyer *et al.*, *J. Pharm. Biomed. Analysis*, 1998, *17*, 45–51].

Column: C_{18} (80 × 4.6 mm, 3 μm). Mobile phase: 10 mM phosphate buffer, pH 3 with 11% methanol and 7% acetonitrile, 1 mL/min flow rate. UV detection (λ 265 nm). *k* value: cladribine, 4.8; 2-chloro-2′-deoxyadenosine (metabolite), 2.2. [F. Albertioni *et al.*, *Ther. Drug Monit.*, 1994, *16*, 413–418].

Ultraviolet Spectrum. Aqueous acid (0.1 M hydrochloric acid)—265 nm; aqueous alkali (0.1 M sodium hydroxide)—265 nm.

Quantification

High performance liquid chromatography. In plasma or urine: cladribine, limit of detection 1 nmol/L in plasma and 100 nmol/L in urine, UV detection (λ=265 nm)—F. Albertioni *et al.*, *Ther. Drug Monit.*, 1994, *16*, 413–418. In plasma: limit of detection 1 μg/L—J. Liliemark *et al.*, *Biomed. Chromatogr.*, 1991, *5*, 262–264.

High performance liquid chromatography–mass spectrometry. In plasma: limit of detection 0.1 μg/L—M. D. Moyer *et al.*, *J. Pharm. Biomed. Anal.*, 1998, *17*, 45–51.

Disposition in the Body. Cladribine is extensively distributed after intravenous administration and undergoes metabolism in cells containing deoxycytidine kinase activity to form 2-chloro-2′-deoxyadenosine-5′-triphosphate. Other metabolites include, 5′-monophosphate and 2-chloroadenine (CAde), the major metabolite identified in plasma. It penetrates into CSF (cerebrospinal fluid); concentrations are about 25% of those in plasma. About 21 to 32% of an intravenous dose is excreted unchanged in urine within 24 h with 1.5% as CAde. After oral administration, 25% of the dose is excreted in urine with 3.8% the metabolite, CAde.

Therapeutic concentration

A mean steady-state plasma concentration of 22.5 ng/L was reported during intravenous infusion of 0.14 mg/kg/day over 24 h for 5 days in 12 subjects. The mean peak concentration was 198 ng/L (range 70 to 381 ng/L) observed during the 2 h infusion, which decreased to the steady state levels with a mean of 6.3 h after the end of infusion. The volunteers were either diagnosed with chronic lymphocytic leukaemia, non-Hodgkins lymphoma or hairy cell leukaemia. [J. Liliemark and G. Juliusson, *Cancer Res.*, 1991, *51*, 5570–5572].

Intravenous infusion of 8.9 mg/m^2/24 h for 5 days in 25 patients, aged between 8 months and 23 years, produced steady-state plasma concentrations ranging from 23.2 to 84.5 ng/L (mean 37.7 ng/L) at 12 h. Mean CSF concentration was 6.1 ng/L. These patients suffered from relapsed haematological malignancies, acute myeloid leukaemia or acute lymphoid leukaemia. [C. M. Kearns *et al.*, *Cancer Res.*, 1994, *54*, 1235–1239].

Toxicity. Cladribine has considerable bone marrow toxicity (haemopoietic stem cell toxicity). In a phase I study, patients were administered with doses >0.26 mg/kg daily for 10 to 14 days. Both renal and central nervous system toxicity was observed, with some patients requiring haemodialysis due to severity of toxicity. Toxicity was not observed with doses of 0.9 mg/kg daily for 7 days. [E. Beutler, *Lancet*, 1992, *340*, 952–956].

Half-life. Plasma, from 3 to 22 h

Volume of distribution. Approx. 9.2 to 12.7 L/kg; 356.6 L/m^2.

Clearance. Plasma clearance, approx. 26 to 45 L/h/m^2; mean, 1.44 L/h/kg.

Protein binding. In plasma, 20%.

Note. For reviews of cladribine see E. Beutler, *Lancet*, 1992, *340*, 952–956, H. M. Bryson and E. M. Sorkin, *Drugs*, 1993, *46*, 872–894, and A. Saven and L. D. Piro, *Ann. Intern. Med.*, 1994, *120*, 784–791.
For a review of the pharmacokinetics of cladribine see J. Liliemark, *Clin. Pharmacokinet.*, 1997, *32*, 120–131.

Dose. In chronic lymphocytic leukaemia 120 μg/kg daily for 5 consecutive days of a 28-day cycle, in hairy-cell leukaemia 90 μg/kg daily for 7 days.

Clarithromycin

Antibacterial

Synonyms. 6-*O*-Methylerythromycin, A-56268.
Proprietary names. Biaxin; Biaxin HP; Biclar; Bremon; Cyllind; Klacid; Klaciped; Klaricid; Kofron; Macladin; Maclar; Mavid; Naxy; Veclam; Zeclar.
(2*R*,3*S*,4*S*,5*R*,6*R*,8*R*,10*R*,11*R*,12*S*,13*R*)-3-(2,6-Dideoxy-3-*C*,3-*O*-dimethyl-α-L-*ribo*hexopyranosyloxy)-11,12-dihydroxy-6-methoxy-2,4,6,8,10,12-hexamethyl-9-oxo-5-(3,4,6-trideoxy-3-dimethylamino-β-D-*xylo*hexopyranosyloxy)pentadecan-13-olide
$C_{38}H_{69}NO_{13}$=748.0
CAS—81103-11-9

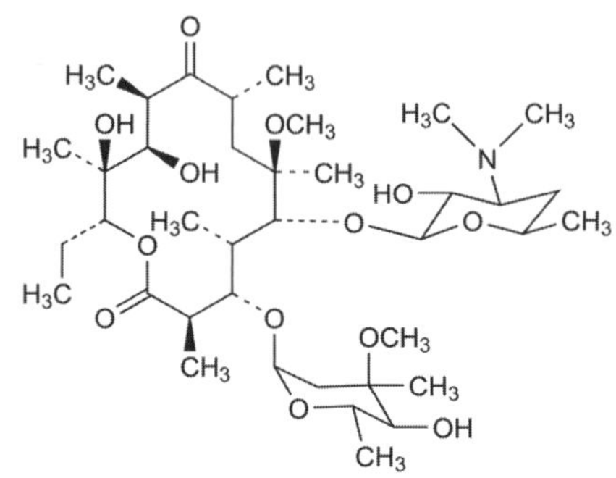

A white to off-white crystalline powder. Crystals, m.p. 217° to 220° from chloroform and diisopropyl ether; m.p. 222° to 225° from ethanol. It is practically insoluble in water; soluble in acetone; slightly soluble in acetonitrile, ethanol, and methanol.

High Performance Liquid Chromatography. System HBA—retention time 15.7 min; system HBB—retention time 6.8 min.

Column: (analytical) C_{18} (Nucleosil 100-3, 150 × 4.6 mm i.d., 3 μm); (pre-column) C_{18} (Nucleosil 120-5, 10 × 4 mm, 5 μm) at 60°. Mobile phase: methanol:15 mM potassium dihydrogen phosphate buffer, adjusted to pH 6.0 with potassium hydroxide (70:30), 1.2 mL/min flow rate. UV detection (λ=220 nm). Retention time: 10.2 min. [J. Macek *et al.*, *J. Chromatogr. B, Biomed. Sci. Appl.*, 1999, *723*, 233–238].

Ultraviolet Spectrum. Aqueous acid (0.2 M H_2SO_4)—283 nm; basic—282 nm.

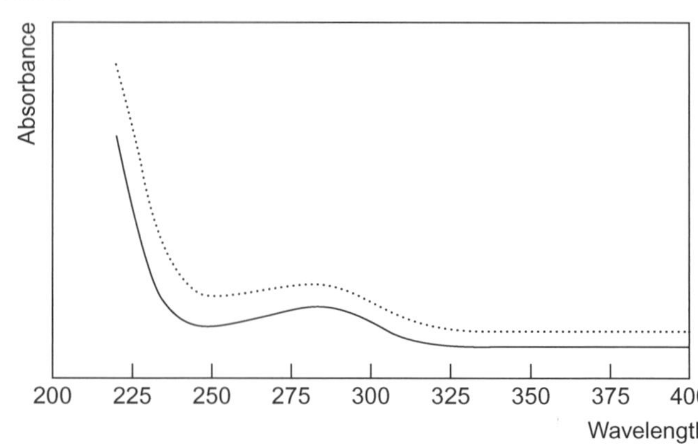

Infra-red Spectrum. Principal peaks at wavenumbers 1052, 1170, 1108, 1734 cm^{-1} (KBr pellet).

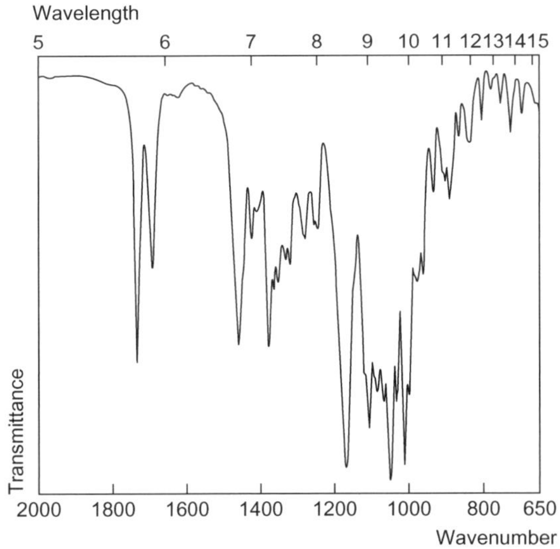

Quantification

High performance liquid chromatography. In plasma or urine: clarithromycin and 14-hydroxyclarithromycin, limit of detection 0.03 mg/L, electrochemical detection—S.-Y. Chu *et al.*, *J. Chromatogr.*, 1991, *571*; *Biomed. Appl.*, *109*, 199–208. In serum: limit of detection 0.2 mg/L, fluorescence detection (λ_{ex}=255 nm, λ_{em} = 315 nm)—J. Sastre Toraño and H.-J. Guchelaar, *J. Chromatogr. B, Biomed. Sci. Appl.*, 1998, *720*, 89–97. In plasma: limit of detection 0.03 mg/L, electrochemical detection—F. Kees *et al.*, *J. Chromatogr. A*, 1998, *812*, 287–293. In plasma: limit of quantification is 0.1 mg/L, electrochemical detection—C. Taninaka *et al.*, *J. Chromatogr. B, Biomed. Sci. Appl.*, 2000, *738*, 405–411. In plasma: limit of quantification 0.5 mg/L, UV detection (λ=220 nm)—J. Macek *et al.*, *J. Chromatogr. B, Biomed. Sci. Appl.*, 1999, *723*, 233–238.

Note. For a review of methods for the determination of macrolides in biological fluids see I. Kanfer *et al.*, *J. Chromatogr. A*, 1998, *812*, 255–286.

Disposition in the Body. Clarithromycin is rapidly absorbed from the gastro-intestinal tract after oral administration with a bioavailability of about 55%. It undergoes first-pass metabolism. Pharmacokinetics are nonlinear and dose dependent with high doses producing disproportionate increases in plasma concentrations owing to saturation of metabolic pathways. Widely distributed and tissue concentrations exceed plasma concentrations. Readily enters leukocytes and macrophages. It is distributed into breast milk. Undergoes extensive metabolism in the liver by demethylation, hydroxylation and hydrolysis. The principal metabolite is 14-hydroxyclarithromycin and this also has antibacterial activity. At steady state, about 20% and 30%, respectively of a 250 mg or 500 mg dose is excreted in the urine as unchanged drug. Excretion in urine and faeces occurs in a dose-dependent manner: at low doses the two fractions are similar; at high doses urinary excretion is predominant. Not significantly removed by haemodialysis or peritoneal dialysis.

Therapeutic concentration

16 patients, aged between 31 and 67 years (mean 50.1 years) were administered with a single nasogastric dose of 500 mg clarithromycin suspension on days 1 and 4 with at least 72 h 'wash-out' between doses. The mean peak plasma concentration of clarithromycin was 2.1 mg/L on day 1 and 2.3 mg/L on day 4, observed at 3.5 and 3.3 h, respectively. The mean concentrations for the metabolite, 14-hydroxyclarithromycin, were 0.9 mg/L at 4.4 h and 1.0 mg/L at 4.3 h, on days 1 and 4, respectively. [D. N. Fish and E. Abraham, *Antimicrob. Agents Chemother.*, 1999, *43(5)*, 1277–1280].

17 healthy males aged 18 to 40 years (mean 29 years) and 17 healthy males aged 20 to 39 years (mean 31 years) were administered with 250 and 500 mg doses, respectively, every 12 h for 7 doses after an overnight fast. The peak plasma concentrations for the 250 mg dose were 0.78 (0.4 to 1.22), 1.01 (0.67 to 1.67) and 1.14 (0.51 to 1.72) mg/L for a single dose and multiple dosing (dose 5 and 7), respectively. These were observed at 1.8, 2.1 and 2.0 (range of 0.5 to 4) h. For the 500 mg single dose, a concentration of 2.12 (0.78 to 3.54) mg/L was observed at 2 (1 to 3) h and for the multiple dosing 2.67 (095 to 4.71) mg/L at 2.6 (1 to 6) h for dose 5; and 2.85 (0.98 to 4.85) mg/L at 2.6 h (range, 1 to 4 h) for dose 7. [S.-y. Chu *et al.*, *J. Clin. Pharmacol.*, 1993, *33*, 719–726].

12 healthy, young volunteers with mean age 23.2 (21 to 29) years and 12 healthy, elderly individuals (mean 73.6 years; range, 65 to 81 years) were administered with 500 mg clarithromycin every 12 h for 5 doses. The subjects were in fasting state and fasted for an additional 2 h after dosing. The mean drug peak plasma concentrations were 2.41 (range 1.58 to 4.09) mg/L and 3.28 (1.75 to 4.55) mg/L for the young and elderly, respectively, observed at approximately 2 h (slightly later in the elderly). Peak concentrations for the metabolite, 14-hydroxyclarithromycin, were 0.66 (0.29 to 1.06) mg/L for the young and 1.33 (0.72 to 2.05) mg/L for the elderly. [S.-y. Chu *et al.*, *J. Clin. Pharmacol.*, 1992, *32*, 1045–1049].

Bioavailability. About 55%.

Half-life. Plasma half-life is dose dependent: clarithromycin about 3 to 4 h in subjects taking 250 mg twice daily and about 5 to 7 h in subjects taking 500 mg twice daily; 14-hydroxyclarithromycin 5 to 6 h in subjects taking 250 mg twice daily and about 7 h in subjects taking 500 mg twice daily. Plasma half-life is increased in subjects with impaired renal function: clarithromycin half-life is about 22 h and 14-hydroxyclarithromycin half-life is about 47 h when creatinine clearance is less than 30 mL/min.

Volume of distribution. Apparent, 175 L.

Clearance. Total body, 29.2 to 58.1 L/h.

Protein binding. In plasma, about 80% at therapeutic concentrations (free clarithromycin fraction increases at serum concentrations >1 mg/L suggesting saturation of binding process).

Note. For a review of the pharmacokinetics of clarithromycin see F. Fraschini *et al.*, *Clin. Pharmacokinet.*, 1993, *25*, 189–204. For reviews of clarithromycin see D. H. Peters and S. P. Clissold, *Drugs*, 1992, *44*, 117–164 and L. B. Barradell *et al.*, *Drugs*, 1993, *46*, 289–312.

Dose. Usually 250 or 500 mg twice daily.

Clefamide

Anti-amoebic

Synonym. Chlorophenoxamide
Proprietary name. Mebinol
2,2-Dichloro-*N*-(2-hydroxyethyl)-*N*-[[4-(4-nitrophenoxy)phenyl]methyl]-acetamide
$C_{17}H_{16}Cl_2N_2O_5$=399.2
CAS—3576-64-5

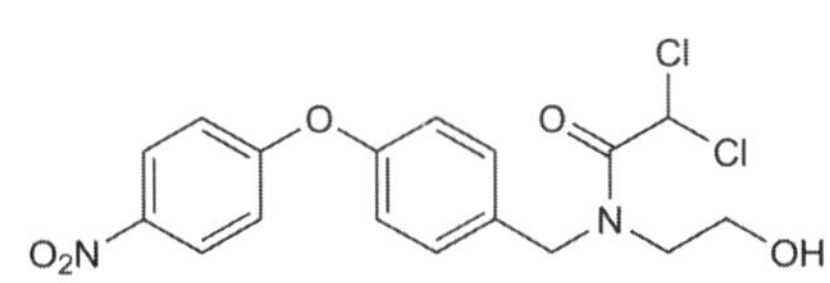

A lemon-yellow crystalline powder. M.p. 134° to 137°.
Practically insoluble in water; soluble 1 in 100 of ethanol, 1 in 40 of acetone, and 1 in 80 of chloroform.

Partition Coefficient. Log *P* (octanol/water), 3.2.

Colour Tests. Mandelin's Test—green→brown; Marquis Test—yellow; Sulfuric Acid—yellow.

Thin-layer Chromatography. System TA—Rf 69; system TB—Rf 00; system TC—Rf 56; system TL—Rf 68. (Acidified iodoplatinate solution, positive.)

Ultraviolet Spectrum. Ethanol—303 nm (A_1^1=310b). (See below)

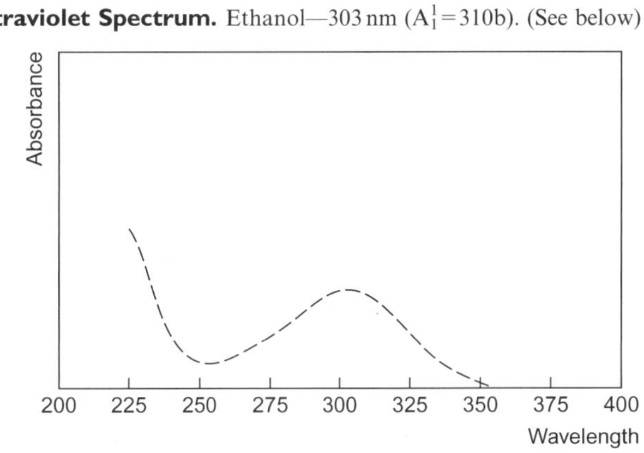

Infra-red Spectrum. Principal peaks at wavenumbers 1244, 1666, 1510, 1595, 1078, 880 cm^{-1} (KBr disk).

Mass Spectrum. Principal ions at *m/z* 228, 182, 363, 88, 229, 76, 276, 257.

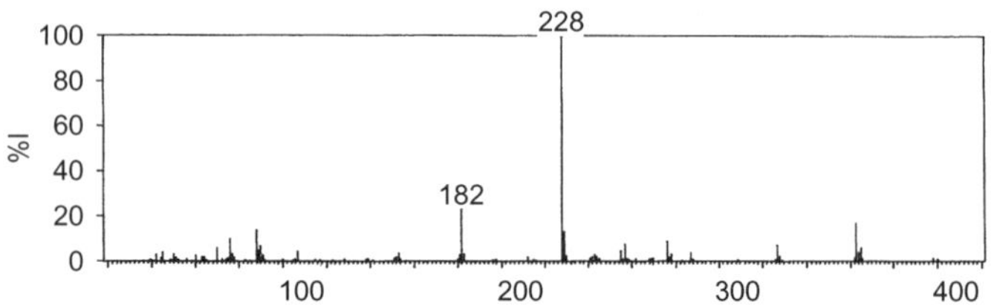

Disposition in the Body. Poorly absorbed after oral administration.

Dose. Clefamide has been given in doses of 1.5 to 2.25 g daily.

Clemastine

Antihistamine

Synonyms. Meclastine; Mecloprodin.
(2*R*)-2-[2-[(1*R*)-1-(4-Chlorophenyl)-1-phenylethoxy]ethyl]-1-methylpyrrolidine
$C_{21}H_{26}ClNO$=343.9
CAS—15686-51-8

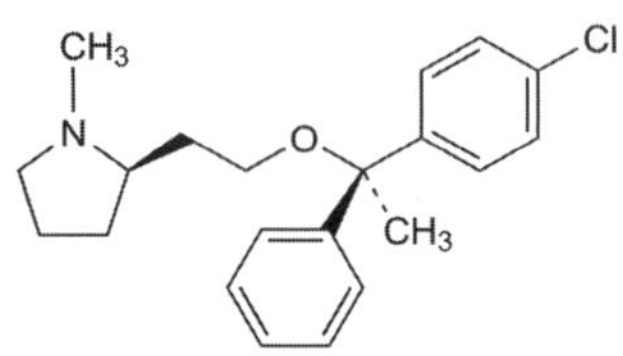

Soluble in chloroform.

Clemastine Fumarate

Proprietary names. Aller-eze; Alginan; Tavegil; Tavegyl; Tavist; Xolamin.
$C_{21}H_{26}ClNO,C_4H_4O_4$=460.0
CAS—14976-57-9
A white crystalline powder. M.p. 177° to 178°.
Slightly soluble in dilute acetic acid; soluble in methanol.

Colour Tests. Liebermann's Test—brown; Mandelin's Test—yellow-brown; Marquis Test—yellow (green rim); Sulfuric Acid—yellow (green rim).

Thin-layer Chromatography. System TA—Rf 46; system TB—Rf 49; system TC—Rf 25; system TE—Rf 58; system TL—Rf 09; system TAE—Rf 88; system TAF—Rf 49. (Acidified iodoplatinate solution, positive.)

Gas Chromatography. System GA—clemastine RI 2425, M (OH-methoxy-carbinol)-H_2O RI 2220; system GF—RI 2710.

High Performance Liquid Chromatography. System HA—*k* 3.7; system HX—RI 501; system HZ—retention time, 14.0 min.

Ultraviolet Spectrum. Aqueous acid—257 nm (A^1_1=27b).

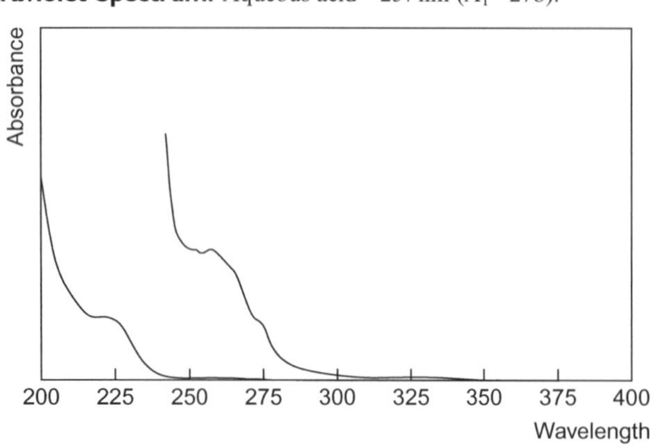

Infra-red Spectrum. Principal peaks at wavenumbers 1090, 1011, 700, 763, 1121, 1210 cm^{-1} (KBr disk).

Mass Spectrum. Principal ions at *m/z* 84, 128, 179, 42, 85, 178, 214, 98.

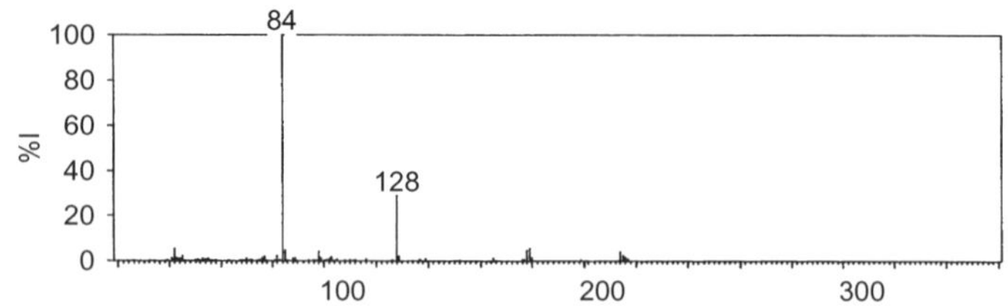

Quantification

Gas chromatography. In plasma: limit of detection 1 µg/L, ECD—R. Tham *et al.*, *Arzneimittelforschung*, 1978, *28*, 1017–1020. In plasma: limit of detection 0.06 µg/L, NPD—N. N. Davydova *et al.*, *J. Chromatogr. B Biomed. Sci. Appl.*, 2000, *744(1)*, 177–181.

Disposition in the Body

Therapeutic concentration

Following a single oral dose equivalent to 2 mg of clemastine to 12 subjects, peak plasma concentrations of about 0.002 mg/L were attained in 3 to 5 h. [R. Tham *et al.*, *Arzneimittelforschung*, 1978, *28*, 1017–1020.]

19 healthy men and women, aged 19 to 56 years, were orally administered a single 2.68 mg clemastine fumarate dose and in addition received the same dose three times daily for 3 days in a multidose study. The mean peak plasma concentrations reached were 0.75 µg/L for the single dose and 1.75 µg/L for the multiple dose. Each observed approximately 3.4 h after dosing. [N. N. Davydova *et al.*, *J. Chromatogr. B Biomed. Sci. Appl.*, 2000, *744(1)*, 177–181.]

Dose. The equivalent of 2 to 6 mg of clemastine daily.

Clemizole

Antihistamine

1-[(4-Chlorophenyl)methyl]-2-(1-pyrrolidinylmethyl)-1*H*-benzimidazole
$C_{19}H_{20}ClN_3$=325.8
CAS—442-52-4

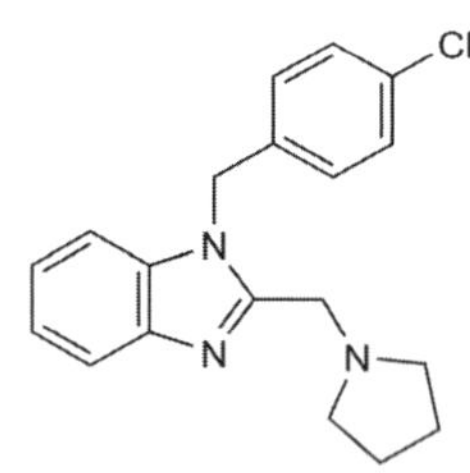

Crystals. M.p. 167°.

Clemizole Hydrochloride

Proprietary name. Allercur
$C_{19}H_{20}ClN_3,HCl$=362.3
CAS—1163-36-6
A white crystalline powder. M.p. about 246°.
Sparingly soluble in water; soluble in ethanol and chloroform; practically insoluble in ether.

Partition Coefficient. Log *P* (octanol/water), 4.4.

Thin-layer Chromatography. System TA—Rf 78; system TB—Rf 33; system TC—Rf 69; system TE—Rf 78; system TL—Rf 52; system TAE—Rf 76; system TAF—Rf 73. (Dragendorff spray, positive; acidified iodoplatinate solution, positive.)

Gas Chromatography. System GA—clemizole RI 2620, M (oxo-) RI 2965.

High Performance Liquid Chromatography. System HA—*k* 4.8 (tailing peak); system HX—RI 420.

Ultraviolet Spectrum. Aqueous acid—275 nm (A^1_1=330a); aqueous alkali—254 nm (A^1_1=253b), 269, 275, 283 nm.

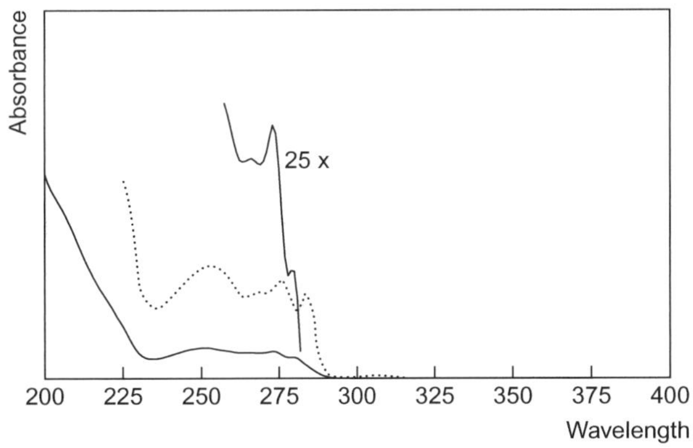

Infra-red Spectrum. Principal peaks at wavenumbers 748, 765, 740, 833, 1111, 1010 cm^{-1} (KBr disk).

Mass Spectrum. Principal ions at *m/z* 131, 256, 125, 42, 255, 89, 258, 257.

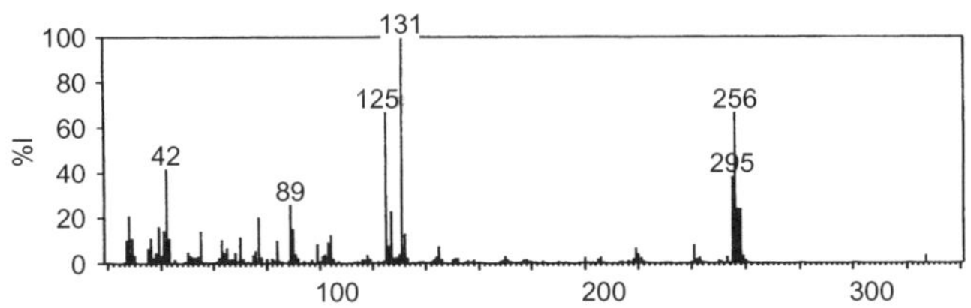

Dose. 40 to 160 mg of clemizole hydrochloride daily.

Clenbuterol

Beta-adrenergic Agonist

Synonym. NAB-365
4-Amino-3,5-dichloro-α-[[(1,1-dimethylethyl)amino]methyl] benzenemethanol
$C_{12}H_{18}Cl_2N_2O=277.2$
CAS—*37148-27-9*

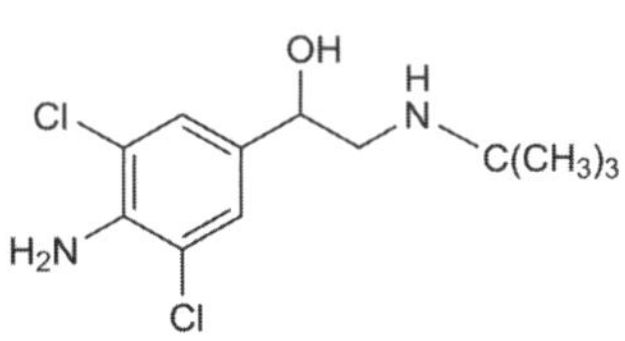

Clenbuterol Hydrochloride
Synonym. NAB-365Cl
Proprietary names. Broncodil; Clenasma; Contrasmina; Contraspasmin; Monores; Prontovent; Spiropent; Ventolase; Ventipulmin.
CAS—*21898-19-1*
A colourless, microcrystalline powder. M.p. 174° to 175.5°. It is very soluble in water, methanol and ethanol; slightly soluble in chloroform; insoluble in benzene.

Partition Coefficient. Log *P* (octanol/water), 2.00.

Thin-layer Chromatography. System TAE—Rf 22 (clenbuterol); Rf 30 (M-hydroxy); Rf 87 (M#2); Rf 87 (M#3); system TB—Rf 13 (clenbuterol); Rf 01 (M-hydroxy); Rf 00 (M#2); Rf 00 (M#3); system TE—Rf 58 (clenbuterol); Rf 43 (M-hydroxy); Rf 02 (M#2); Rf 06 (M#3); system TF—Rf 00 (M#2); Rf 19 (M#3).

Plate: silica gel 60 (Merck, 10 × 10 cm). Mobile phase: ethyl acetate:methanol:propionic acid (8:1:1) (solvent system 1) and ethyl acetate:methanol:ammonia (8.5:1:0.5) (solvent system 2). Developed with Ehrlich's reagent. Rf 0.40 (solvent system 1) and Rf 0.51 (solvent system 2). [D. Courtheyn *et al.*, *J. Chromatogr.* 1991, *564*; *Biomed. Appl.*, 537–549].

Gas Chromatography. System GA—RI 2100 (clenbuterol); RI 1895 (Art (-H_2O)); RI 2160 (Art); system GAI—retention time relative to 17α-methyl-5α-androstan-3β, 0.57.

Column: HP Ultra 1 (25 m × 0.2 mm i.d., 0.11 μm film thickness). Column temperature: 80° for 2 min, 20°/min up to 160°, then 2°/min to 190° and 30°/min to 300°, held for 10 min. Injector temperature: 290°. Carrier gas: helium, flow rate 1.0 mL/min. Detection: mass spectrometer (EI, SIM at *m/z* 86, 243, 262, 264, 266, 277). Retention time: clenbuterol–mono-TMS (trimethylsilyl) derivative 15.42 min. [D. Courtheyn *et al.*, *J. Chromatogr.* 1991, *564*; *Biomed. Appl.*, 537–549].

Column: 1% phenylmethylsilicone (HP 1-MS, 15 m × 0.25 mm i.d., 0.25 μm). Column temperature: 150° for 1 min, 15°/min to 215°, 35°/min to 300°, held for 2 min. Carrier gas: helium, 1.1 mL/min flow rate. MS detection (FS mode). Internal standard: brombuterol. Retention time: 5.09 min. [I. K. Abukhalaf *et al.*, *Biomed. Chromatogr.*, 2000, *14*, 99–105].

High Performance Liquid Chromatography. System HAW—*k* 6.1 (column (a)); *k* 5.0 (column (b)); system HAA—retention time 10.8 min; system HX—RI 326 (clenbuterol); RI 297 (M-hydroxy); RI 346 (M#2); RI 419 (M#3); system HY—RI 282.

Ultraviolet Spectrum. Aqueous acid (0.2 M H_2SO_4)—242, 295 nm; basic—240, 295 nm.

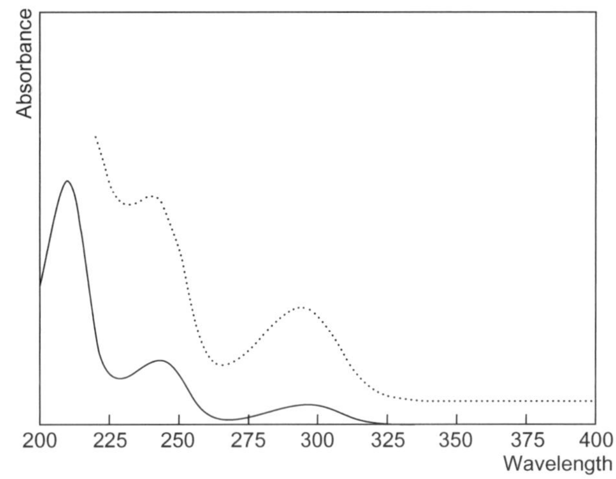

Infra-red Spectrum. Principal peaks at wavenumbers 1414, 774, 640 cm^{-1} (KBr pellets).

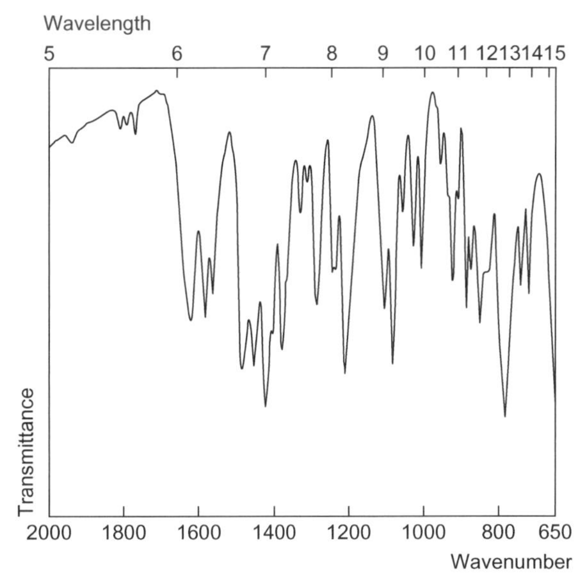

Mass Spectrum. Principal ions at *m/z* 86, 57, 41, 127, 190, 243, 90, 174.

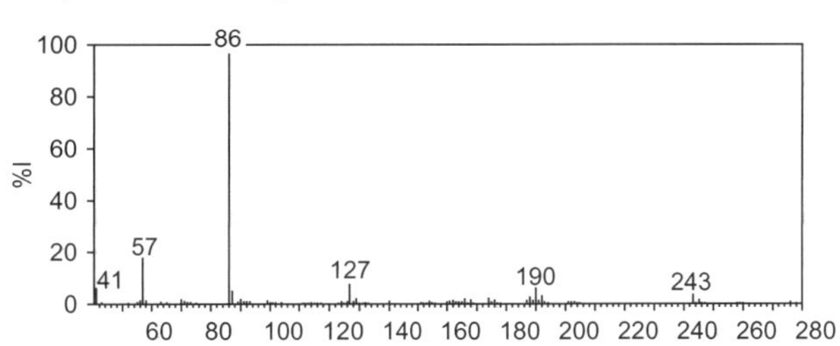

Quantification

Gas chromatography–mass spectrometry. In plasma: limit of detection is 0.5 µg/L and limit of quantification is 1.5 µg/L. In urine: 0.2 and 0.7 µg/L, respectively—I. K. Abukhalaf *et al.*, *Biomed. Chromatogr.*, 2000, *14*, 99–105.

Enzyme immunoassay (EIA). In hair: limit of detection 0.05 µg/L—A. Gleixner *et al.*, *Clin Chem.*, 1996, *42(11)*, 1869–1870. In urine: limit of detection < 5 µg/L—M. E. Ploum *et al.*, *J. Chromatogr.* 1991, *564*; *Biomed. Appl.*, 413–427.

Disposition in the Body. Clenbuterol is rapidly and almost completely absorbed after oral administration, and extensively metabolised by first-pass sulfation. Excretion is mainly via the kidneys for intravenous administration and biotransformation for oral administration. No accumulation observed.

Therapeutic concentration.

Healthy males were orally administered 20, 40 and 80 µg doses of clenbuterol. Plasma levels reached maximum values of 0.1, 0.2 and 0.35 µg/L, respectively, within 2.5 h and lasted over 6 h. After repeated oral administration (twice a day), plasma levels reached 0.2 to 0.3 µg/L and 0.5 to 0.6 µg/L for doses of 20 and 40 µg, respectively. [I. Yamamoto *et al.*, *J. Pharmacobiodyn.*, 1985, *8(5)*, 385–391].

Toxicity

A 21-year-old body builder drank orange juice 'spiked' with 48 tablets (4.8 g) of clenbuterol and admitted with tachycardia, headache, dizziness, tremor, sweats, muscle weakness and agitation. [Z. Chodorowski and J. Sein Anand, *Przegl. Lek.*, 1997, *54*, 763–764].

Half-life. In plasma, estimated to be approx. 35 h.

Protein binding. Clenbuterol binds plasma protein approx. 89 to 98%, after a single dose of 80 µg.

Dose. A dose of 20 µg is administered by mouth twice daily and up to 40 µg has been reported. Clenbuterol hydrochloride can be used as an inhaler with a dosage of 20 µg three times a day.

Clidinium Bromide

Anticholinergic

Synonym. Ro-2-3773

Proprietary names. Quarzan. It is an ingredient of Librax(in).

3-[(Hydroxydiphenylacetyl)oxy]-1-methyl-1-azoniabicyclo[2.2.2]octane bromide

$C_{22}H_{26}BrNO_3$=432.4

CAS—7020-55-5 (clidinium); 3485-62-9 (bromide)

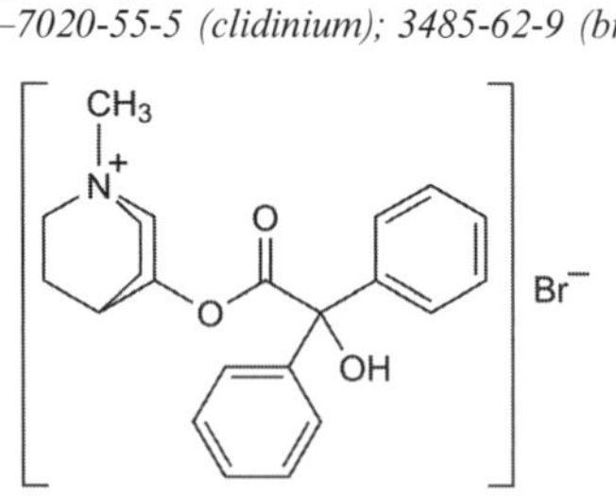

A white crystalline powder. M.p. about 242°.

Soluble in water and ethanol; slightly soluble in ether.

Partition Coefficient. Log *P* (octanol/water), −0.5.

Colour Tests. The following tests are performed on the nitrate (see p. 128): Liebermann's Test—orange→brown; Mandelin's Test—brown; Marquis Test—orange→blue; Sulfuric Acid—orange.

Thin-layer Chromatography. System TA—Rf 02; system TB—Rf 00; system TE—Rf 01; system TF—Rf 70; system TAE—Rf 03. (Acidified iodoplatinate solution, positive.)

High Performance Liquid Chromatography. System HX—RI 379; system HAA—retention time, 13.3 min (clidinium).

Ultraviolet Spectrum. Aqueous acid—253 nm (A^1_1=10b), 259 nm (A^1_1=11b); methanol—252 nm, 258 nm (A^1_1=10.4a), 264 nm.

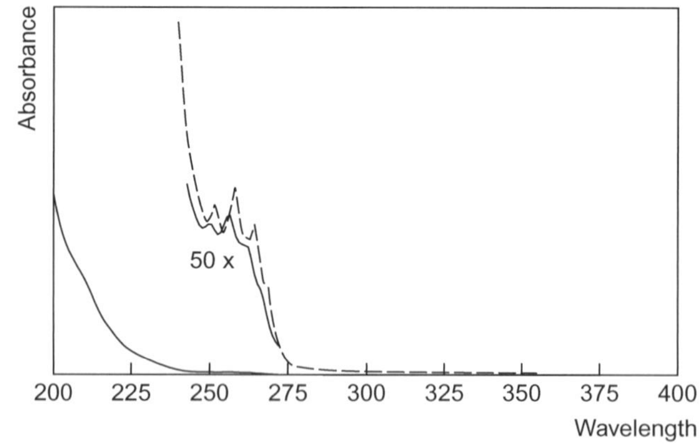

Infra-red Spectrum. Principal peaks at wavenumbers 1730, 1240, 769, 1190, 712, 1011 cm^{-1}.

Mass Spectrum. Principal ions at *m/z* 105, 77, 96, 183, 51, 42, 182, 94.

Disposition in the Body. The major metabolite is 3-hydroxy-1-methylquinuclidinium bromide.

Dose. 7.5 to 20 mg daily.

Clindamycin

Antibiotic

Synonyms. Chlorodeoxylincomycin; (7*S*)-Chloro-7-deoxylincomycin; U-21251.

Note. The name Clinimycin was formerly used for clindamycin and has also been used for a preparation of oxytetracycline.

(2*S*-*trans*)-Methyl-7-chloro-6,7,8-trideoxy-6-[[(1-methyl-4-propyl-2-pyrrolidinyl)carbonyl]amino]-1-thio-L-*threo*-α-D-*galacto*-octopyranoside

$C_{18}H_{33}ClN_2O_5S$=425.0

CAS—18323-44-9

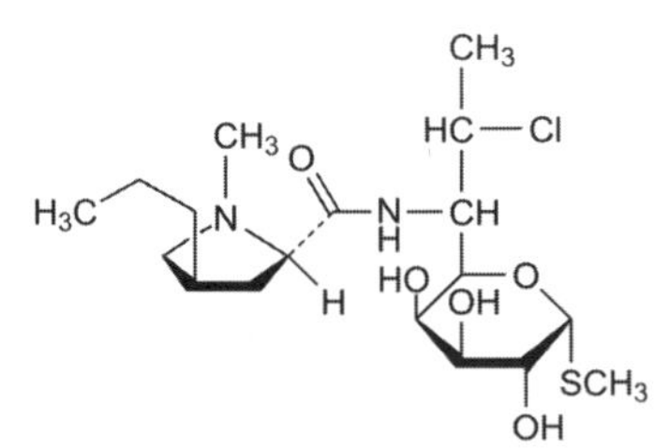

A yellow, amorphous solid.

Clindamycin Hydrochloride

Proprietary names. Cleocin; Dalacin C; Dalacin(e); Sobelin (all as capsules).

$C_{18}H_{33}ClN_2O_5S,HCl,H_2O$=479.5

CAS—21462-39-5 (anhydrous); 58207-19-5 (monohydrate)

A white crystalline powder. M.p. 141° to 143°.

Soluble 1 in 2 of water and 1 in 200 of ethanol; freely soluble in methanol; very slightly soluble in chloroform.

Clindamycin Palmitate Hydrochloride

Proprietary names. Cleocin; Dalacin; Dalacin C; Sobelin (all as granules for oral suspension).

$C_{34}H_{63}ClN_2O_6S,HCl$=699.9

CAS—36688-78-5 (palmitate); 25507-04-4 (palmitate hydrochloride)

A white amorphous powder. It hydrolyses in solutions above pH 6.0.

Freely soluble in water, ethanol, chloroform, and ether.

Clindamycin Phosphate

Proprietary names. Cleocin; Dalacin; Dalacin C; Sobelin (all as injection).

$C_{18}H_{34}ClN_2O_8PS$=505.0

CAS—24729-96-2

A white, hygroscopic, crystalline powder.

Soluble 1 in 2.5 of water; slightly soluble in dehydrated alcohol; practically insoluble in chloroform and ether.

Dissociation Constant. pK_a 7.7 (25°).

Partition Coefficient. Log *P* (octanol/water), 2.2.

Colour Tests. Palladium Chloride—yellow; Sodium Nitroprusside (Method 2)—violet.

Thin-layer Chromatography. System TA—Rf 72; system TB—Rf 00; system TE—Rf 28; system TAE—Rf 81. (Acidified iodoplatinate solution, positive.)

High Performance Liquid Chromatography. System HX—RI 354; system HY—RI 291; system HAA—retention time, 12.0 min.

Ultraviolet Spectrum. No significant absorption, 230 to 360 nm.

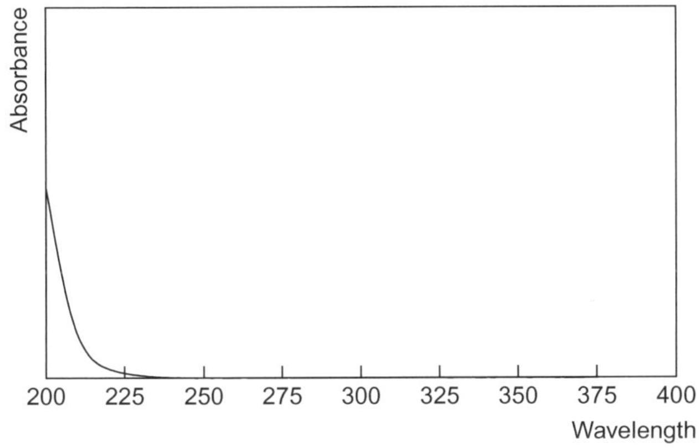

Infra-red Spectrum. Principal peaks at wavenumbers 1513, 1664, 1080, 1050, 1302, 1250 cm^{-1} (KBr disk).

Quantification

High performance liquid chromatography. In plasma, MS–MS detection—G. N. Rechberger *et al.*, *Rapid Commun. Mass Spectrom.*, 2003, *17(2)*, 135–139. In serum and bone tissue: limit of quantification 0.1 mg/L and 0.1 µg/g, respectively, MS detection (*m/z* 405 to 425)—J. Martens-Lobenhoffer and P. Banditt, *J. Chromatogr. B Biomed. Sci. Appl.*, 2001, *755(1–2)*, 143–149. In plasma: limit of quantification 0.05 mg/L, MS–MS detection—L. L. Yu *et al.*, *J. Chromatogr. B Biomed Sci. Appl.*, 1999, *724(2)*, 287–294.

Dose. The equivalent of 0.6 to 1.8 g of clindamycin daily.

Clioquinol

Anti-amoebic

Synonyms. Chinoform; Chloroiodoquine; Cliochinolum; Iodochlorhydroxyquin; Iodochlorhydroxyquinoline; Quiniodochlor; Vioformo.
Proprietary names. Amebil; Budoform; Eczecidin; Enteroquinol; Entero-Valodon; Entero-Vioform; Nioform; Rometin; Vioform. It is an ingredient of Oralcer and Unidiarea.
5-Chloro-7-iodo-8-quinolinol
C_9H_5ClINO=305.5
CAS—130-26-7

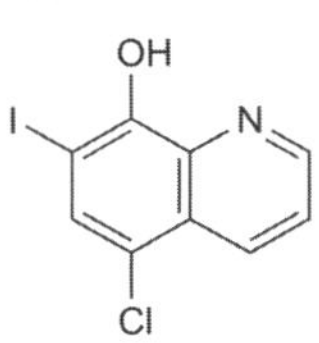

A yellowish-white to brownish-yellow, voluminous powder. It darkens on exposure to light. M.p. 178° to 179°, with decomposition.
Almost insoluble in water, ethanol, and ether; soluble 1 in 43 of boiling ethanol, 1 in 128 of chloroform, 1 in 17 of boiling ethyl acetate, 1 in 170 of cold acetic acid, and 1 in 13 of boiling acetic acid; soluble in dimethylformamide.

Partition Coefficient. Log *P* (octanol/water), 3.5.

Thin-layer Chromatography. System TA—Rf 56; system TB—Rf 00; system TC—Rf 05; system TE—Rf 30; system TL—Rf 09; system TAD—Rf 70; system TAE—Rf 40; system TAF—Rf 88.

Gas Chromatography. System GA—RI 1975.

Ultraviolet Spectrum. Methanol—255 nm (A_1^1=1196a), 325 nm.

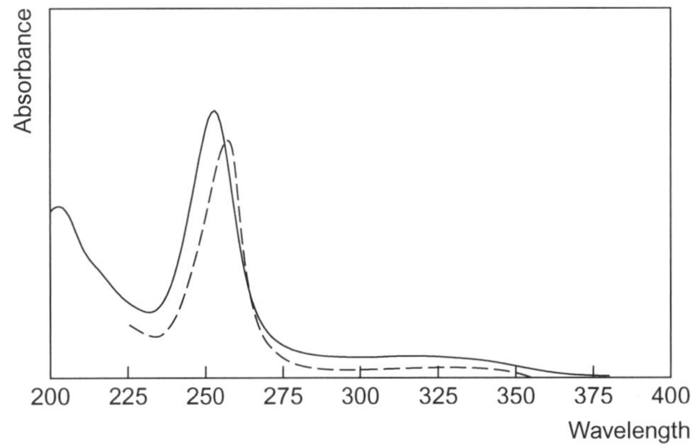

Infra-red Spectrum. Principal peaks at wavenumbers 953, 1198, 808, 784, 1266, 728 cm^{-1} (KBr disk).

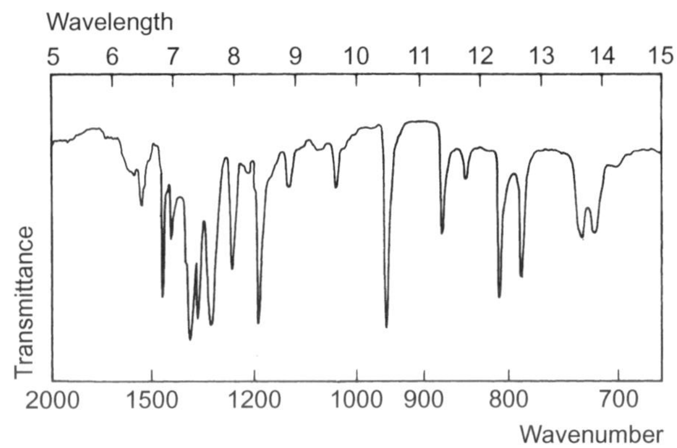

Mass Spectrum. Principal ions at *m/z* 305, 150, 307, 115, 152, 114, 306, 123.

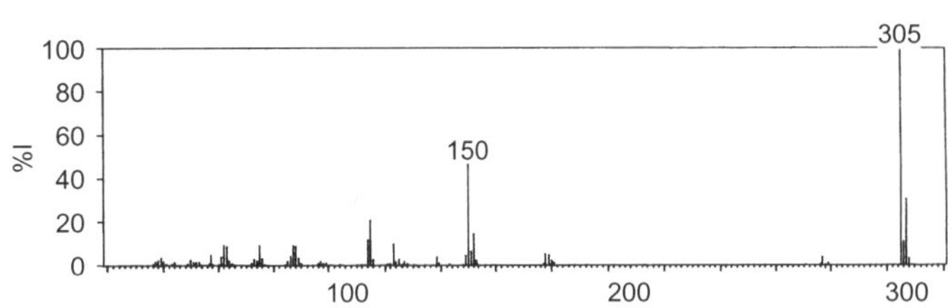

Quantification

Gas chromatography. In plasma: limit of detection 50 µg/L, ECD—A. Sioufi and F. Pommier, *J. Chromatogr.* 1981, *226(15) B Biomed. Appl.*, 219–223.

High performance liquid chromatography. In plasma or urine: limit of detection 600 µg/L, UV detection—K. Hayakawa *et al.*, *J. Chromatogr.* 1982, *229(18) B Biomed. Appl.*, 159–165.

Disposition in the Body. Poorly absorbed after oral administration. About 25% of a dose is excreted in the urine in 24 h as glucuronide and sulfate conjugates.

Therapeutic concentration

Following single oral doses of 250 and 1500 mg to 6 subjects, peak plasma concentrations of 1.7 to 8.3 mg/L (mean 5.2) and 14.6 to 34.8 mg/L (mean 23), respectively, were attained in 2 to 4 h. [D. B. Jack and W. Riess, *J. Pharm. Sci.*, 1973, *62*, 1929–1932.]

Half-life. Plasma half-life, 11 to 14 h.

Dose. Usually 0.75 to 1.5 g daily.

Clioxanide

Anthelmintic (Veterinary)

Synonyms. CI-633; SYD-230.
2-(Acetyloxy)-*N*-(4-chlorophenyl)-3,5-diiodobenzamide
$C_{15}H_{10}ClI_2NO_3=541.5$
CAS—14437-41-3

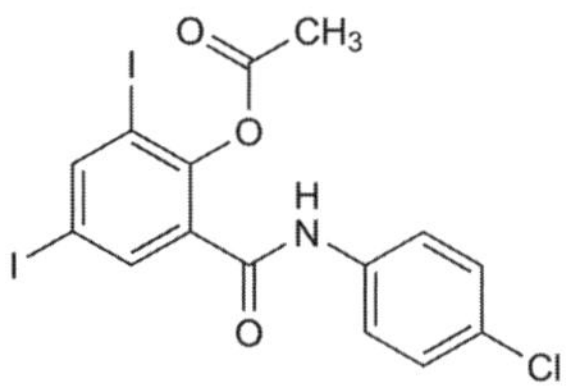

A white crystalline powder. M.p. 215° to 216°.
Sparingly soluble in water; moderately soluble in ethanol and acetone; soluble in chloroform.

Partition Coefficient. Log *P* (octanol/water), 5.3.

Colour Tests. Iodine Test—positive; Mandelin's Test—red-brown.

Thin-layer Chromatography. System TA—Rf 79. (Acidified potassium permanganate solution, positive.)

Gas Chromatography. System GA—not eluted.

Ultraviolet Spectrum. Ethanol—233 nm (A^1_1=625b); aqueous alkali—240 nm (A^1_1=561b), 282 nm (A^1_1=270b), 362 nm(A^1_1=172b).

Infra-red Spectrum. Principal peaks at wavenumbers 1190, 1647, 1520, 1309, 1764, 816 cm^{-1} (Nujol mull).

Clobazam

Tranquilliser

Synonyms. H-4723; HR-376; LM-2717.
Proprietary names. Castilium; Clarmyl; Clopax; Frisium; Noiafren; Urbadan; Urbanil; Urbanol; Urbanyl.
7-Chloro-1-methyl-5-phenyl-1*H*-1,5-benzodiazepine-2,4(3*H*,5*H*)-dione
$C_{16}H_{13}ClN_2O_2=300.8$
CAS—22316-47-8

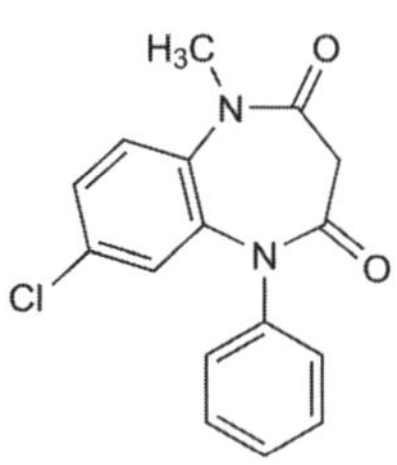

White crystalline powder. M.p. 180° to 182°.
Practically insoluble in water; sparingly soluble in ethanol; freely soluble in acetone and chloroform.

Partition Coefficient. Log *P* (octanol/water), 2.12.

Colour Test. Aromaticity (Method 2)—colourless (heat for 3 min)/red.

Thin-layer Chromatography. System TA—Rf 62; system TB—Rf 08; system TC—Rf 70; system TD—Rf 53; system TE—Rf 75; system TF—Rf 47; system TL—Rf 62; system TAD—Rf 70; system TAE—Rf 84; system TAF—Rf 85.

Gas Chromatography. System GA—clobazam RI 2558, M (nor-) RI 2747, M (OH-) RI 3000, M (OH-MeO-) RI 3255; system GB—clobazam RI 2683, M (nor-) RI 2759; system GG—RI 3147.

Column: HP-5 cross-linked 5% phenylmethylsilicone (5.0 m × 0.53 mm i.d., 2.65 µm film thickness). Carrier gas: helium, flow rate 10 mL/min. Column, injector, and detector temperatures: 250°, 300°, and 350°, respectively. IS: nitrazepam. Detection: ^{63}Ni electron capture. Retention time: clobazam, 1.86 min; norclobazam, 2.2 min; IS, 3.2 min. [D. F. LeGatt and D. P. McIntosh, *Clin. Biochem.*, 1993, *26*, 159–163.]

High Performance Liquid Chromatography. System HI—clobazam *k* 3.91, M (nor-) *k* 3.06; system HK—clobazam *k* 0.03, M (nor-) *k* 0.01; system HX—RI 488; system HY—RI 455; system HZ—clobazam retention time 6.2 min; system HAA—retention time 19.2 min; system HAK—retention time 9.3 min; system HAL—retention time 7.8 min; system HAM—not detected; system HAX—retention time 7.2 min; system HAY—retention time 7.1 min; system HBH—*k* 4.14; system HBI—*k* 1.09.

Column: RP C_8 (Ultrasphere, 250 × 4.6 mm i.d., 5 µm). Mobile phase: acetate buffer (20 mM, pH 5.5):acetonitrile:triethylamine (70:30:0.01), flow rate 1.8 mL/min. IS: methoxycarbamazepine. Retention time(s): clobazam, 13.5 min; IS, 6.5 min. [A. Bolner *et al.*, *J. Chromatogr. B Biomed. Sci. Appl.*, 2001, *750*, 177–180.]

Column: (analytical) RP C_{18} (Lichrosorb, 250 × 4.0 mm i.d., 10 µm), (guard) RP C_{18} (Lichrosorb, 4.0 × 4.0 mm i.d., 5 µm). Mobile phase: methanol:acetonitrile:potassium dihydrogen phosphate (0.1 M, pH 3.6) (23:20:57), flow rate 2 mL/min. IS: nordazepam. Retention time(s): clobazam, 12 min; IS, 15 min; clonazepam, 7.5 min. [J. Knapp *et al.*, *J. Chromatogr. Sci.*, 1999, *37*, 145–149.]

Ultraviolet Spectrum. Aqueous acid—230 nm (A^1_1=1373b), 289 nm (A^1_1=76b); aqueous alkali—286 nm (A^1_1=193b).

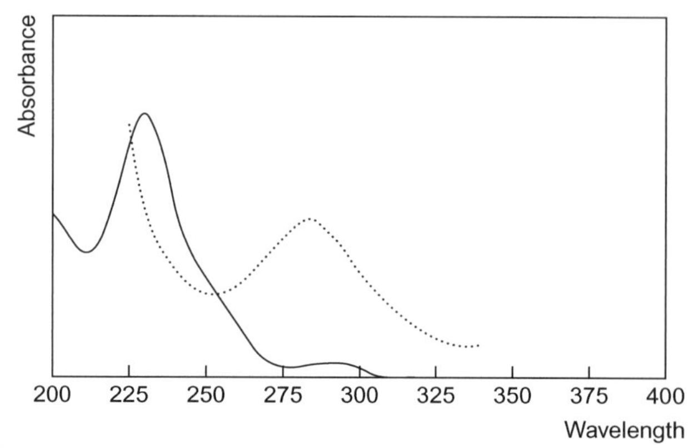

Infra-red Spectrum. Principal peaks at wavenumbers 1684, 1664, 704, 1490, 764, 845 cm^{-1} (KBr disk).

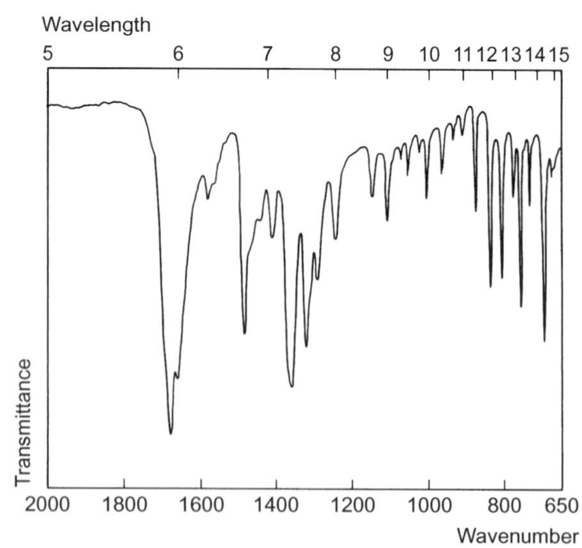

Mass Spectrum. Principal ions at *m*/*z* 300, 258, 77, 259, 283, 302, 231, 256; desmethylclobazam 286, 244, 77, 218, 51, 217, 288, 215.

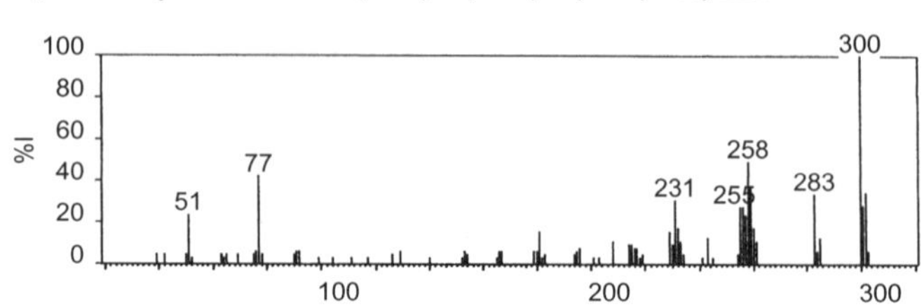

Quantification

Gas chromatography. In plasma: limits of detection 3 µg/L for clobazam and 5 µg/L for desmethylclobazam, ECD—D. J. Greenblatt, *J. Pharm. Sci.*, 1980, *69*, 1351–1352. In plasma or whole blood: clobazam and other benzodiazepines, NPD and ECD—P. Lillsunde and T. Seppala, *J. Chromatogr.*, 1990, *533*, 97–110. In serum: clobazam and norclobazam, ECD—D. F. LeGatt and D. P. McIntosh, *Clin. Biochem.*, 1993, *26*, 159–163.

Gas chromatography–mass spectrometry. In plasma: clobazam and other benzodiazepines, limits of detection 1 to 5 µg/L—C. Drouet-Coassolo *et al.*, *J. Chromatogr.*, 1989, *487*, 295–311.

High performance liquid chromatography. In plasma: limit of detection 50 µg/L for clobazam and 100 µg/L for desmethylclobazam, UV detection—A. Brachet-Liermain *et al.*, *Ther. Drug Monit.*, 1982, *4*, 301–305. In plasma: limits of detection 15 µg/L and 30 µg/L for clobazam and desmethylclobazam, respectively, UV detection (λ=235 nm)—J. M. Streete *et al.*, *Ther. Drug Monit.*, 1991, *13*, 339–344. In plasma: clobazam, diazepam, and their metabolites—C. Lacroix *et al.*, *J. Chromatogr.*, 1993, *617*, 285–290. In plasma and serum: limit of detection 4.6 µg/L, UV detection (DAD)—K. K. Akerman, *Scand. J. Clin. Lab. Invest.*, 1996, *56*, 609–614. In plasma: UV detection—J. Knapp *et al.*, *J. Chromatogr. Sci.*, 1999, *37*, 145–149. In serum or urine: clobazam and *N*-desmethylclobazam, limits of quantification 2 µg/L and 1 µg/L, respectively, UV detection—P. K. Kunicki, *J. Chromatogr. B Biomed. Sci. Appl.*, 2001, *750*, 41–49. In plasma: limit of quantification 5 µg/L, UV detection—A. Bolner *et al.*, *J. Chromatogr. B Biomed. Sci. Appl.*, 2001, *750*, 177–180.

Disposition in the Body. Readily absorbed after oral administration; peak plasma concentrations reached after 1 to 4 h. Clobazam is highly lipophilic and rapidly crosses the blood–brain barrier. It is metabolised in the liver by demethylation and hydroxylation. Metabolites found in the serum include *N*-desmethylclobazam (norclobazam), which is thought to be active, 4′-hydroxyclobazam, and 4′-hydroxydesmethylclobazam. About 90% of a dose is excreted in the urine in 17 days and about 2% is eliminated in the faeces.

Therapeutic concentration

After a single oral dose of 20 mg, administered to 16 subjects, peak serum concentrations of 0.30 to 0.95 mg/L (mean 0.57) were attained in about 1.3 h. [H. R. Och *et al.*, *Eur. J. Clin. Pharmacol.*, 1984, *26*, 499–503.]

Following daily oral doses of 10 mg to 7 young male and 6 elderly male subjects, the mean steady-state plasma concentrations for the 2 groups were: clobazam 0.12 to 0.25 mg/L (mean 0.17) and 0.17 to 0.41 mg/L (mean 0.3); desmethylclobazam 0.12 to 0.25 mg/L (mean 0.16) and 0.21 to 12.8 mg/L (mean 3.9), respectively. The corresponding steady-state plasma concentrations in 5 young female and 6 elderly female subjects, receiving the same dosage schedule, were: clobazam 0.19 to 0.27 mg/L (mean 0.23) and 0.16 to 0.32 mg/L (mean 0.23); desmethylclobazam 0.22 to 1.37 mg/L (mean 0.7) and 0.17 to 4.13 mg/L (mean 1.0), respectively. [D. J. Greenblatt *et al.*, *Clin. Pharmacokinet.*, 1983, *8*, 83–94.]

Toxicity. Up to 300 mg has been ingested without serious toxic effects.

Postmortem concentrations for clobazam in serum and liver in a 6-year-old male were 0.1 mg/L and 0.4 µg/g. Desmethylclobazam concentrations were also reported as 1.5 mg/L in serum, 8.6 µg/g in liver, and 3.6 µg/g in the brain. [A. D. Fraser *et al.*, *J. Forensic Sci.*, 1988, *33*, 1058–1063.]

Half-life. Plasma half-life, clobazam 10 to 58 h (mean 25), desmethylclobazam, about 40 h. The half-life may be prolonged considerably in elderly subjects.

Volume of distribution. About 1 L/kg.

Clearance. Plasma clearance, about 0.5 mL/min/kg.

Protein binding. In plasma, about 85%.

Note. For a review of the pharmacokinetics of clobazam, see R. N. Brogden *et al.*, *Drugs*, 1980, *20*, 161–178. For a review of the pharmacokinetics of benzodiazepines, see D. J. Greenblatt *et al.*, *Clin. Pharmacokinet.*, 1983, *8*, 233–252.

Dose. Adults, usually 20 to 30 mg; in severe conditions up to 60 mg daily; children (3 years and over), no more than 30 mg daily.

Clobetasol Propionate

Corticosteroid

Proprietary names. Dermoval; Dermovat(e); Dermoxin.

(11*β*,16*β*)-21-Chloro-9-fluoro-11,17-dihydroxy-16-methylpregna-1,4-diene-3,20-dione-17-propionate

$C_{25}H_{32}ClFO_5$=467.0

CAS—25122-41-2 (clobetasol); 25122-46-7 (propionate)

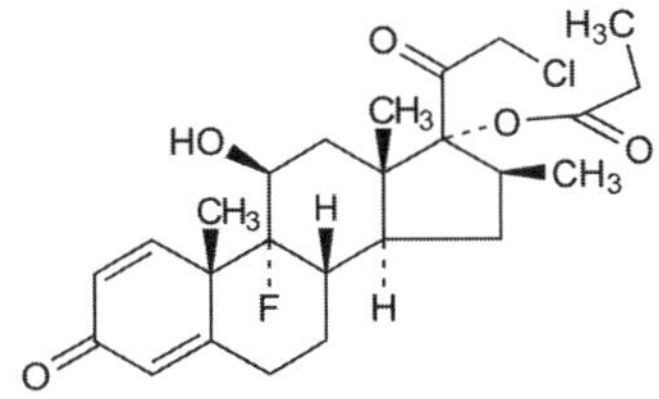

A white to creamy-white, crystalline powder. M.p. 195.5° to 197°.

Practically insoluble in water; soluble 1 in 100 of ethanol and 1 in 1000 of ether; soluble in acetone and chloroform.

Partition Coefficient. Log *P* (octanol/water), 3.5.

High Performance Liquid Chromatography. System HY—RI 636.

Ultraviolet Spectrum. Methanol—239 nm (A^1_1=390b).

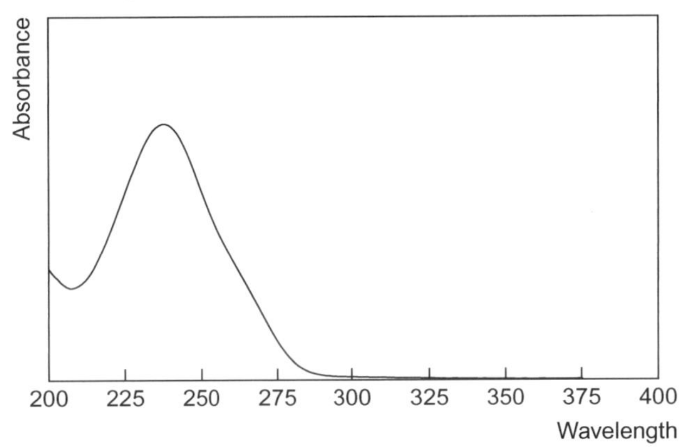

Infra-red Spectrum. Principal peaks at wavenumbers 1666, 1612, 1724, 884, 1063, 1010 cm^{-1}.

Use. Topically in a concentration of 0.05%.

Clobetasone Butyrate

Corticosteroid

Proprietary names. Emovat(e); Eumovate. It is an ingredient of Trimovate.

(16*β*)-21-Chloro-9-fluoro-17-hydroxy-16-methylpregna-1,4-diene-3,11,20-trione-17-butyrate

$C_{26}H_{32}ClFO_5$=479.0

CAS—54063-32-0 (clobetasone); 25122-57-0 (butyrate)

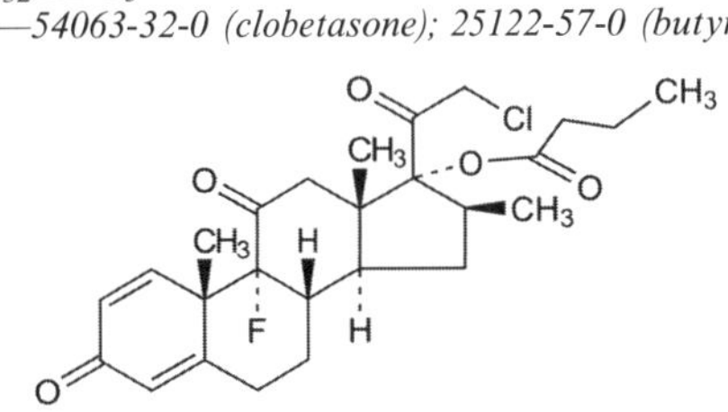

A white crystalline powder. M.p. 90° to 100°.

Practically insoluble in water; soluble in many organic solvents.

Partition Coefficient. Log *P* (octanol/water), 3.8.

Ultraviolet Spectrum. Methanol—236 nm (A^1_1=330b).

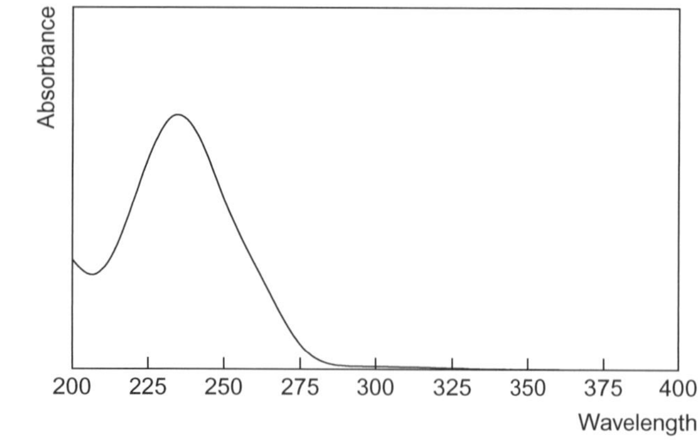

Mass Spectrum. Principal ions at *m/z* 331, 43, 71, 332, 121, 147, 131, 41 (clobetasone).

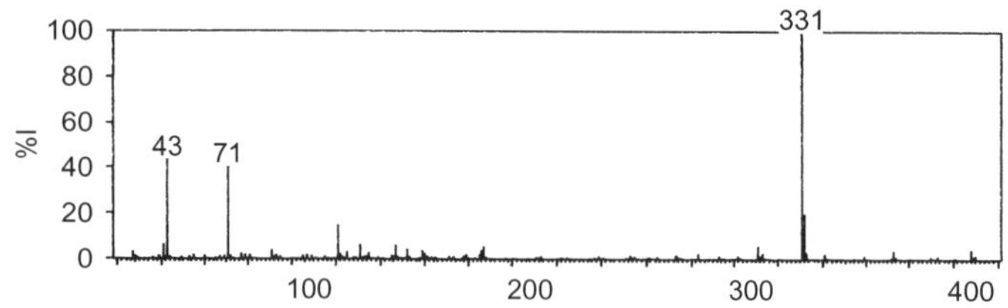

Use. Topically in a concentration of 0.05%.

Clodantoin

Antifungal

Synonym. Chlordantoin
Proprietary name. Sporostacin
5-(1-Ethylpentyl)-3-[(trichloromethyl)thio]-2,4-imidazolidinedione
$C_{11}H_{17}Cl_3N_2O_2S = 347.7$
CAS—5588-20-5

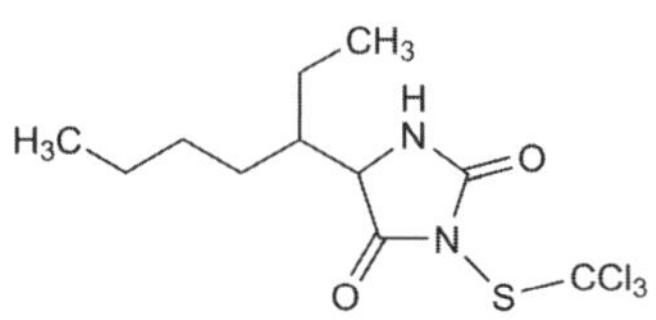

Partition Coefficient. Log *P* (octanol/water), 3.7.

Ultraviolet Spectrum. No significant absorption, 230 to 360 nm.

Infra-red Spectrum. Principal peaks at wavenumbers 1730, 1786, 730, 1059, 766, 1309 cm^{-1}.

Use. Topically in a concentration of 1%.

Clodronic Acid

Calcium Regulator

Synonyms. Clondronate; DMDP.
(Dichloromethylene)bisphosphonic acid
$CH_4Cl_2O_6P_2 = 244.9$
CAS—10596-23-3

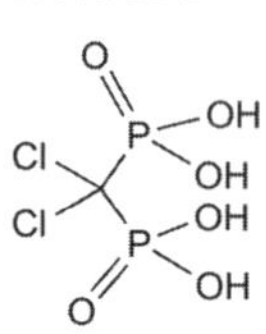

M.p. 249° to 251°.

Disodium Clodronate

Synonyms. Clodronate disodium; clodronate sodium; sodium clodronate; BM-06.011; Cl_2MDP.
Proprietary names. Ascredar; Bonefos; Clasteon; Clastoban; Difosfonal; Lodronat; Loron; Lytos; Mebonat; Ostac; Ossiten.
$CH_2Cl_2Na_2O_6P_2 = 288.9$
CAS—22560-50-5

Partition Coefficient. Log *P* (octanol/water), 0.67.

Gas Chromatography. Column: OV-1 (25 m × 0.31 mm i.d., 0.1 μm film thickness). Column temperature: 120° to 230° at 10°/min. Injector temperature: 250°. Carrier gas: methane. MS detection (EI). Retention time: clodronate (TMS (trimethylsilyl) derivative), 7.2 min. [S. Auriola *et al.*, *J. Pharm. Biomed. Anal.*, 1989, *7*, 1623–1629].

High Performance Liquid Chromatography. Column: (analytical) anion exchange HPIC AS7 (250 × 4.0 mm i.d., 10 μm); (guard) anion exchange AG7, (50 × 4.0 mm, 10 μm). Mobile phase: 30 mM nitric acid solution, pH adjusted with sodium hydroxide, 1.0 mL/min flow rate. UV detection (λ = 550 nm). *k* values: 7.16 (pH 2.7); 7.36 (pH 2.4); 5.82 (pH 2.1); 5.18 (pH 1.8). [V. Virtanen and L. H. J. Lajunen, *J. Chromatogr.*, 1993, *617*; *Biomed. Appl.*, *128*, 291–298].

Quantification

Gas chromatography–mass spectrometry. In urine: limit of detection 0.025 mg/L—S. Auriola *et al.*, *J. Pharm. Biomed. Anal.*, 1989, *7*, 1623–1629.

High performance liquid chromatography. In urine: limit of detection 0.3 mg/L, UV detection (λ = 550 nm)—V. Virtanen and L. H. J. Lajunen, *J. Chromatogr.*, 1993, *617*; *Biomed. Appl.*, *128*, 291–298.

Disposition in the Body. Clodronate is poorly absorbed after oral administration and absorption is reduced by food, especially products containing calcium or other polyvalent cations; bioavailability is only 1 to 4% and varies between different formulations. It is not metabolised. Over 70% of an intravenous dose is excreted unchanged in the urine within 24 h, 5% in faeces, and the remainder is sequestered in bone tissue from where it is eliminated very slowly.

Therapeutic concentration

20 patients with tumour-related bone disease of varying stages, 15 of which were women and 5 men with a mean age of 61 years (range 36 to 78), were administered with 300 mg clodronate over 2 to 3 h. The peak serum concentration was 11.8 mg/L after 2 h which decreased to 0.4 mg/L over 24 h. [N. O'Rourke *et al.*, *Drug Invest.*, 1994, *7*, 26–33].

6 patients, 3 females and 2 males with Paget's disease and 1 male with prostatic cancer, were administered with 300 mg as a 3 h infusion daily for 5 consecutive days. A peak serum disodium clodronate concentration of 5.7 mg/L was observed in the males and 10.1 mg/L for the females. [H. Hanhijarvi *et al.*, *Int. J. Clin. Pharmacol. Ther. Toxicol.*, 1989, *27(12)*, 602–606].

Bioavailability. About 1 to 2%.

Half-life. Plasma, 2 h; also reported as 5.6 h.

Volume of distribution. 0.2 to 0.7 L/kg.

Clearance. Plasma, 5 to 15 L/h.

Protein binding. In plasma, 36%.

Note. For a review of clodronic acid see G. L. Plosker and K. L. Goa, *Drugs*, 1994, *47*, 945–982.

Dose. Up to 3.20 g of disodium clodronate (in capsule form) daily by mouth or up to 2.08 g of disodium clodronate (in tablet form) daily. By intravenous infusion, 300 mg of disodium clodronate daily for not more than 10 days, or a single dose of 1.5 g infused over 4 h.

Clofazimine

Antileprotic

Synonyms. B-663; G-30320; Riminophenazine.
Proprietary name. Lampren(e)
N,5-Bis(4-chlorophenyl)-3,5-dihydro-3-[(1-methylethyl)imino]-2-phenazinamine
$C_{27}H_{22}Cl_2N_4 = 473.4$
CAS—2030-63-9

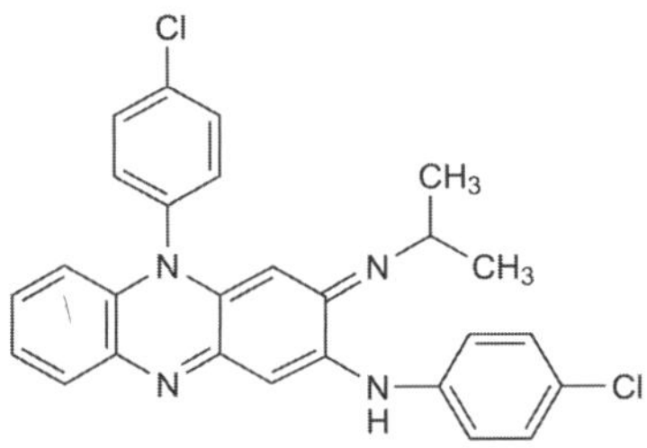

Dark red crystals or orange-red microcrystalline powder. M.p. 210° to 212°.
Practically insoluble in water; soluble 1 in 700 of ethanol, 1 in 15 of chloroform, and 1 in 1000 of ether; soluble in dilute acetic acid and dimethylformamide.

Dissociation Constant. pK_a 8.5.

Partition Coefficient. Log *P* (octanol/water), 7.7.

Colour Tests. Mandelin's Test—yellow-brown; Marquis Test—violet; Sulfuric Acid—violet.

Thin-layer Chromatography. System TA—Rf 70; system TB—Rf 57; system TC—Rf 59; system TE—Rf 86; system TL—Rf 68; system TAE—Rf 33; system TAF—Rf 86. (Acidified iodoplatinate solution, positive.)

Gas Chromatography. System GA—not eluted.

Ultraviolet Spectrum. Methanolic acid—283 nm (A^1_1 = 1300b).

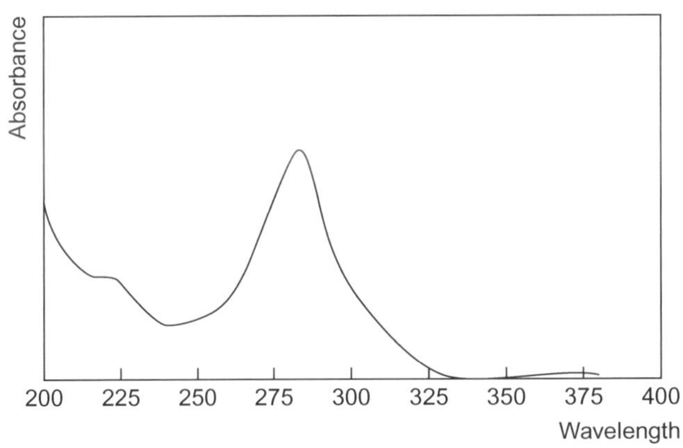

Infra-red Spectrum. Principal peaks at wavenumbers 1508, 1560, 1295, 1587, 747, 1083 cm^{-1} (KBr disk).

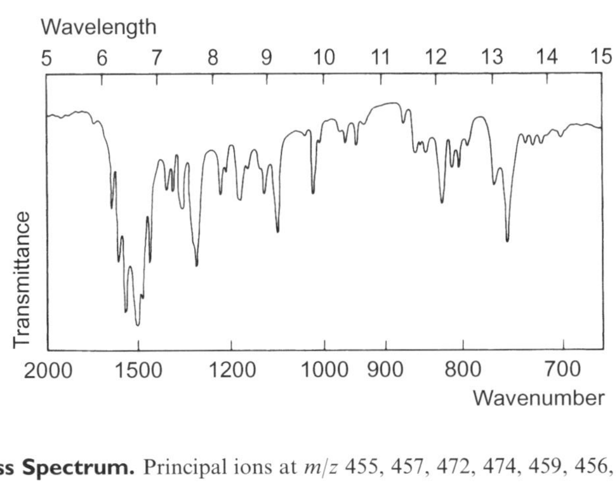

Mass Spectrum. Principal ions at *m/z* 455, 457, 472, 474, 459, 456, 458, 473.

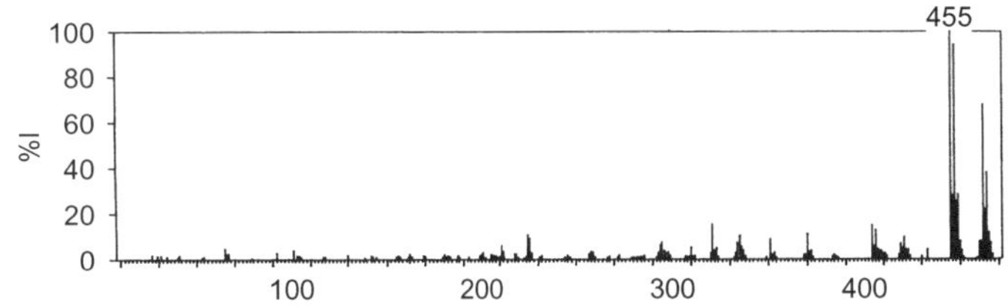

Quantification

High performance liquid chromatography. In plasma: limit of detection 10 µg/L, UV detection—J. H. Peters *et al.*, *J. Chromatogr.* 1982, *229(18) B Biomed. Appl.*, 503–508. In urine, MS detection—D. R. Krishna *et al.*, *Arzneimittelforschung*, 1997, *47(3)*, 303–306. In tissue and serum—K. Borner *et al.*, *Int. J. Antimicrob. Agents*, 1999, *11(1)*, 75–79.

Thin-layer chromatography. In plasma: limit of detection 5 µg/L—Z. Lanyi and J. P. Dubois, *J. Chromatogr.* 1982, *232(21) B Biomed. Appl.*, 219–223. In urine—D. R. Krishna *et al.*, *Arzneimittelforschung*, 1997, *47(3)*, 303–306.

Disposition in the Body. Incompletely absorbed after oral administration. It is stored in body tissues and only very slowly excreted in the urine. 3-(*p*-Hydroxy)clofazimine and a 3-glucuronide conjugate have been detected in the urine, each accounting for less than 0.5% of a daily dose.

Therapeutic concentration

Following single oral doses of 200 mg and 400 mg to 1 subject, peak plasma concentrations of 0.07 mg/L and 0.16 mg/L were attained in 8 and 4 h, respectively; plasma concentrations of clofazimine were still detectable at 264 h. [Z. Lanyi and J. P. Dubois, *J. Chromatogr.* 1982, *232(21) B Biomed. Appl.*, 219–223.]

Dose. 50 to 100 mg daily; 300 mg daily for lepra reactions.

Clofedanol

Cough Suppressant

Synonym. Clophedianol
2-Chloro-α-[2-(dimethylamino)ethyl]-α-phenylbenzenemethanol
$C_{17}H_{20}ClNO$ = 289.8
CAS—791-35-5

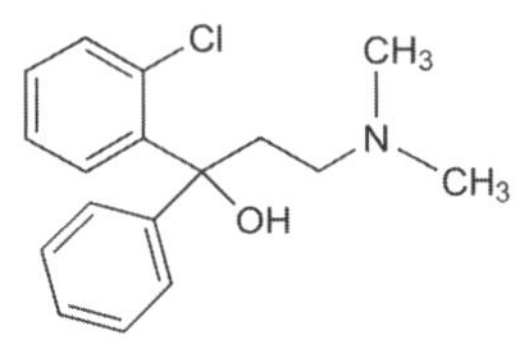

M.p. 120°.

Clofedanol Hydrochloride

Proprietary names. Detigon; Pectolitan.
$C_{17}H_{20}ClNO,HCl$ = 326.3
CAS—511-13-7
Crystals. M.p. 190° to 191°.
Freely soluble in water and ethanol; sparingly soluble in ether, benzene, and ethyl acetate.

Partition Coefficient. Log *P* (octanol/water), 3.5.

Colour Tests. Mandelin's Test—green-blue; Marquis Test—red-violet→brown.

Thin-layer Chromatography. System TA—Rf 52; system TB—Rf 41; system TC—Rf 37; system TL—Rf 29; system TAE—Rf 32. (Acidified iodoplatinate solution, positive.)

Gas Chromatography. System GA—clofedanol RI 2090, clofedanol-H_2O RI 2085, M (2-Cl-benzophenone) RI 1720, M (OH-)-H_2O RI 2130, M (aldehyde) RI 1900, M (nor)-H_2O RI 2090.

Ultraviolet Spectrum. Aqueous acid—259 (A^1_1 = 14.6a), 265 nm. No alkaline shift.

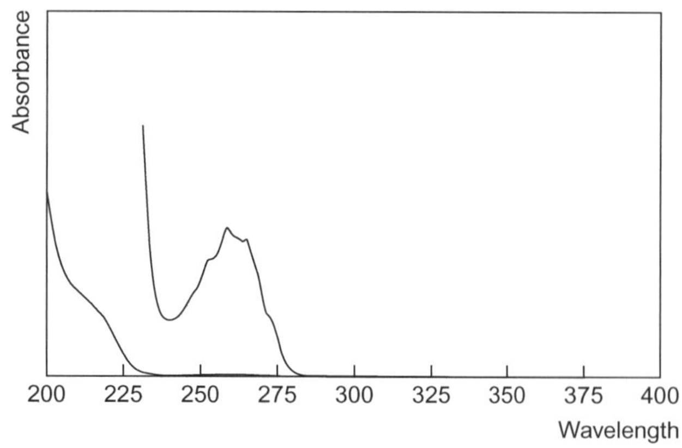

Infra-red Spectrum. Principal peaks at wavenumbers 756, 700, 1035, 770, 1190, 735 cm^{-1}(KBr disk).

Mass Spectrum. Principal ions at *m/z* 58, 254, 45, 44, 77, 42, 59, 72.

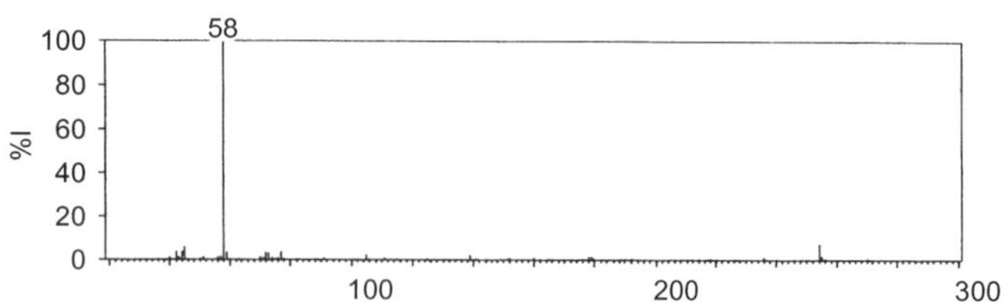

Dose. 75 to 100 mg of clofedanol hydrochloride daily.

Clofenotane

Pesticide

Synonyms. Chlorophenothane; Chlorphenothanum; Dicophane; DDT; Dichlorodiphenyltrichloroethane; Dichophanum; Parachlorocidum; Penticidum.

Clofenotane contains about 70% of 1,1,1-trichloro-2,2-bis(4-chlorophenyl)ethane (*pp'*-DDT) together with varying quantities of an isomer, 1,1,1-trichloro-2-(2-chlorophenyl)-2-(4-chlorophenyl)ethane (*op'*-DDT) and other related compounds.

$C_{14}H_9Cl_5$=354.5

CAS—50-29-3

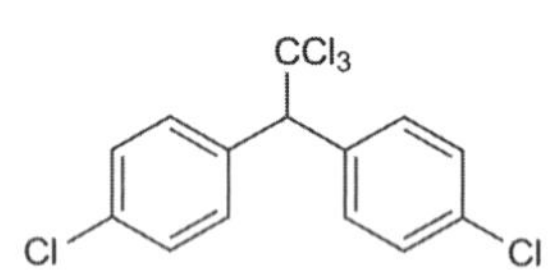

White or nearly white crystals, small granules, flakes, or powder. M.p. about 109°. The technical product is a waxy solid of indefinite melting point.

Practically insoluble in water; soluble 1 in 50 of ethanol, 1 in 6 of boiling ethanol, 1 in 2.5 of acetone, 1 in 3.5 of chloroform, and 1 in 4 of ether.

Partition Coefficient. Log *P* (octanol/water), 6.9.

Colour Tests. Liebermann's Test—brown; Nitric–Sulfuric Acid—red→orange→green.

Heat a small quantity with a 0.5% solution of hydroquinone in sulfuric acid—red.

Note. Clofenotane does not react to the Fujiwara Test.

Thin-layer Chromatography. System TD—Rf 82; system TE—Rf 87; system TF—Rf 74; system TAD—Rf 80; system TAJ—Rf 95; system TAK—Rf 93; system TAL—Rf 97.

Gas Chromatography. System GA—*pp'*-DDT RI 2314, *op'*-DDT RI 2218 and 2275, *pp'*-DDE RI 2140, *op'*-DDE RI 2090; system GK—*pp'*-DDT RRT 1.32, *op'*-DDT RRT 1.24 (both relative to caffeine).

Ultraviolet Spectrum. Methanol—236 (A^1_1=510b), 267 nm (A^1_1=19b).

Infra-red Spectrum. Principal peaks at wavenumbers 775, 790, 1500, 1100, 1022, 850 cm^{-1} (KBr disk).

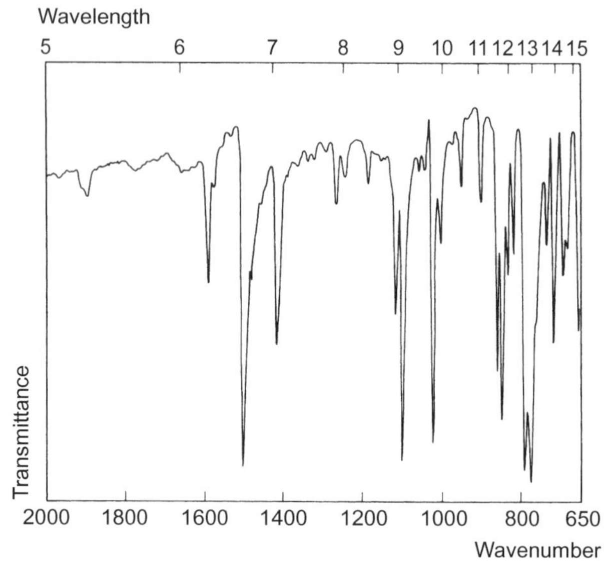

Mass Spectrum. Principal ions at *m/z* 235, 237, 165, 236, 75, 239, 82, 199 (pp'-DDT).

Quantification

Gas chromatography. In serum: clofenotane and metabolites, ECD—W. E. Dale *et al.*, *J. Assoc. Off. Anal. Chem.*, 1970, *53*, 1287–1292. In blood or tissues: clofenotane and metabolites, limit of detection, blood <1 mg/L, tissues <5 ng/g, ECD—J. L. Radomski and A. Rey, *J. Chromatogr. Sci.*, 1970, *8*, 108–114. In urine: dichlorodiphenylacetic acid (DDA), limit of detection 50 pg, ECD—H. Della Fiorentina *et al.*, *J. Chromatogr.*, 1978, *157*, 421–426.

Disposition in the Body. Clofenotane dry powder is poorly absorbed from the gastro-intestinal tract and is not absorbed through the skin. Solutions of clofenotane in oils are rapidly absorbed through intact skin and are also readily absorbed from the gastro-intestinal tract. Clofenotane is metabolised to a small extent by dehydrochlorination to dichlorodiphenyldichloroethylene (DDE) which is less toxic; DDE does not appear to be metabolised further and is stored indefinitely in adipose tissues. Most of the DDE present in human fat is thought to result from preformed DDE taken in the diet rather than being due to ingestion of clofenotane. The major metabolic route for clofenotane is dechlorination to dichlorodiphenyldichloroethane (DDD) followed by degradation to dichlorodiphenylacetic acid (DDA) which is the major urinary excretion product. Urinary concentrations of DDA are indicative of storage of DDT in adipose tissue.

Blood concentration

The following tissue concentrations of total DDT plus metabolites were reported in 35 industrially exposed subjects: blood 0.11 to 2.2 µg/mL (mean 0.6), fat 38 to 647 µg/g (mean 204), urine 0.05 to 3.4 µg/mL (mean 1.3); DDE accounted for about 40% of the material stored in fat and 6% of the urinary material compared to about 80% and 60%, respectively, reported for members of the general population. [E. R. Laws *et al.*, *Arch. Environ. Health*, 1967, *15*, 766–775.]

Fat residues ranging from 0.04 to 17 µg/g (mean 2.6) of total DDT were reported in 236 subjects, without occupational exposure, in the United Kingdom in 1976–77. [D. C. Abbott *et al.*, *BMJ*, 1981, *283*, 1425–1428.]

Toxicity. The estimated minimum lethal dose is 30 g but a single oral dose of 10 mg/kg may produce toxic symptoms; the maximum permissible atmospheric concentration is 1 mg/m^3 and the maximum acceptable daily intake is 5 µg/kg. The toxicity of some of the organic solvents, such as kerosene, used in the application of clofenotane has probably contributed to clofenotane fatalities.

Clofibrate

Lipid-regulating Agent

Synonyms. Ethyl Chlorophenoxyisobutyrate; Ethyl Clofibrate.
Proprietary names. Amotril; Atheropront; Atromidin; Atromid-S; Azionyl; Claripex; Clofibral; Clofirem; Lipavlon; Liprin(al); Normolipol; Novofibrate; Regelan; Skleromexe.
2-(4-Chlorophenoxy)-2-methylpropionic acid ethyl ester
$C_{12}H_{15}ClO_3$=242.7
CAS—637-07-0

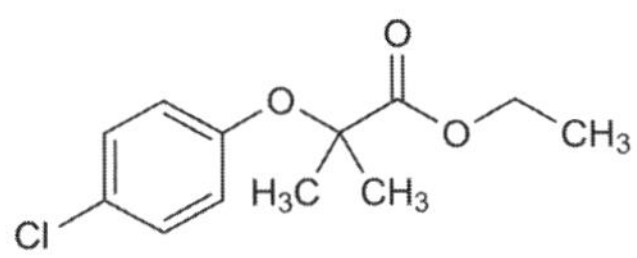

A clear, colourless to pale yellow liquid. Mass per mL 1.138 to 1.144 g. Practically insoluble in water; miscible with ethanol, acetone, chloroform, and ether.

Dissociation Constant. pK_a 3.0 (clofibric acid).

Partition Coefficient. Log *P* (octanol/water), 3.6.

Colour Tests. Liebermann's Test—violet-brown; Marquis Test—blue (deepening).

Thin-layer Chromatography. System TD—Rf 75; system TE—Rf 84; system TF—Rf 66; system TAD—Rf 71; system TAE—Rf 81; system TAJ—Rf 90; system TAK—Rf 80; system TAL—Rf 97.

Gas Chromatography. System GA—clofibrate RI 1542, M (clofibric acid) RI 1640.

High Performance Liquid Chromatography. System HAA—retention time, 18.3 min.

Ultraviolet Spectrum. Dehydrated alcohol—280 nm (A^1_1=43b), 288 nm (A^1_1=31b).

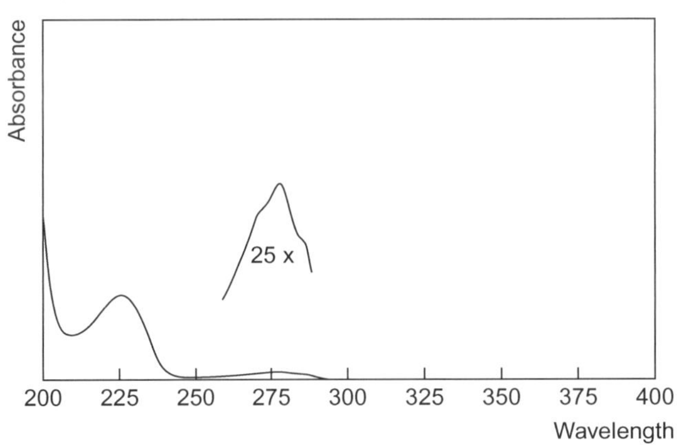

Infra-red Spectrum. Principal peaks at wavenumbers 1140, 1238, 1735, 1175, 1282, 1090 cm^{-1} (KBr disk).

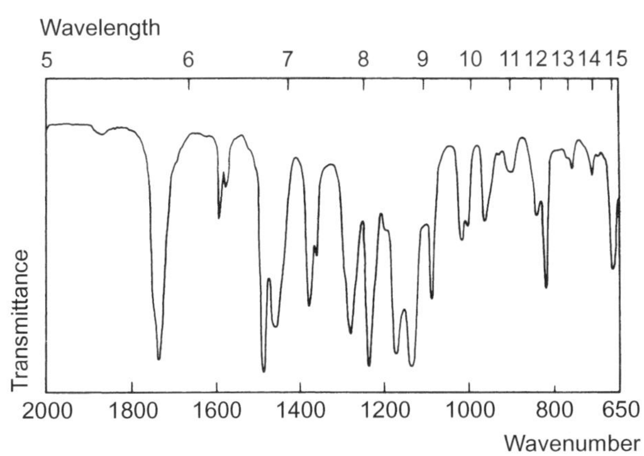

Mass Spectrum. Principal ions at *m/z* 128, 130, 169, 87, 41, 129, 242, 171.

Quantification

Gas chromatography. In plasma: limit of detection 1 mg/L for clofibrate and clofibric acid, FID—M. S. Wolf and J. J. Zimmerman, *J. Pharm. Sci.*, 1980, *69*, 92–93.

High performance liquid chromatography. In plasma, saliva or urine: limit of detection 500 µg/L for clofibric acid, UV detection—T. D. Bjornsson *et al.*, *J. Chromatogr.*, 1977, *137*, 145–152. In plasma or urine: limit of detection 10 mg/L for clofibric acid and 1.5 mg/L for the glucuronide, UV detection—J. R. Veenendaal and P. J. Meffin, *J. Chromatogr.* 1981, *223(12) B Biomed. Appl.*, 147–154. In plasma: limit of detection clofibrate 1.1 mg/L and clofibric acid 1.5 mg/L, respectively, and limit of quantification 3.6 and 4.9 mg/L, respectively, UV detection (λ=223 nm)—J. Barra *et al.*, *J. Chromatogr.* 1994, *661(1) B Biomed. Appl.*, 178–182.

Disposition in the Body. Readily and almost completely absorbed after oral administration. Rapidly hydrolysed by serum enzymes to clofibric acid, 2-(4-chlorophenoxy)-2-methylpropionic acid (active), which is conjugated with glucuronic acid. About 50 to 85% of a dose is excreted in the urine in 48 h, mostly as conjugated clofibric acid.

Therapeutic concentration

After a single oral dose of 1 g, given to 8 subjects, peak plasma concentrations of 43 to 79 mg/L (mean 55) of clofibric acid were attained in 2 to 8 h. [L. F. Chasseaud *et al.*, *J. Clin. Pharmacol.*, 1974, *14*, 382–386.]

After a single oral dose of 2 g, given to 5 subjects, a mean plasma concentration of 151 mg/L of clofibric acid was attained in 4 to 6 h; a mean steady-state plasma concentration of 122 mg/L of clofibric acid was achieved after administering 1 g twice daily to 5 subjects. [R. Gugler, *Clin. Pharmacol. Ther.*, 1978, *24*, 432–438.]

Toxicity.

A 15-year-old boy who took 24.5 g of clofibrate in a suicide attempt complained of headache, pain in the arms, and inability to walk, but no evidence of toxicity was found in the following 5 days. [A. H. Greenhouse, *JAMA*, 1968, *204*, 402–403.]

Half-life. Plasma half-life, clofibric acid 12 to 25 h but may be decreased when free fatty acid concentrations are high; longer half-lives have been reported after repeated doses, and in subjects with renal impairment.

Volume of distribution. Clofibric acid, about 0.1 to 0.2 L/kg.

Protein binding. In plasma, clofibric acid, about 95 to 98%. This may be reduced in the presence of high free fatty acid concentrations and is progressively reduced at plasma concentrations greater than 50 mg/L.

Note. For a summary of the clinical pharmacokinetics of clofibrate see L. B. Sheiner *et al.*, *J. Pharmacokinet. Biopharm.*, 1981, *9*, 84–87.

Dose. 20 to 30 mg/kg daily, by mouth.

Clomethiazole

Hypnotic/Sedative

Synonym. Chlormethiazole
Proprietary names Distraneurin(e); Hemineurin(e); Heminevrin (includes proprietary names of Clomethiazole Edisilate).
5-(2-Chloroethyl)-4-methylthiazole
C_6H_8ClNS=161.7
CAS—533-45-9

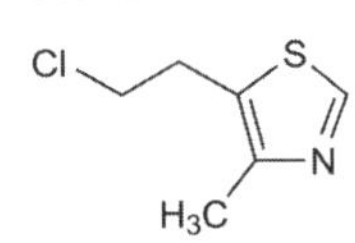

A colourless to slightly yellow-brown, oily, viscous liquid.
Soluble 1 in 100 of water; miscible with ethanol, chloroform, and ether.

Clomethiazole Edisilate

Synonyms. Chlormethiazole Edisylate; Chlormethiazole Ethanedisulphonate.
$C_{14}H_{22}Cl_2N_2O_6S_4$=513.5
CAS—1867-58-9
A white crystalline powder. M.p. 126° to 129°.
Freely soluble in water and warm ethanol; practically insoluble in ether.

Dissociation Constant. pK_a 3.2.

Partition Coefficient. Log *P* (octanol/water), 2.1.

Colour Test. Sodium Nitroprusside (Method 3) —violet.

Thin-layer Chromatography. System TA—Rf 64; system TB—Rf 44; system TC—Rf 69; system TE—Rf 76; system TL—Rf 58; system TAE—Rf 80; system TAF—Rf 85. (Acidified iodoplatinate solution, positive.)

Gas Chromatography. System GA—clomethiazole RI 1227, M (1-OH-ethyl-) RI 1560, M (2-OH-) RI 1365, M (deschloro-) RI 1185, M (deschloro-2-OH-) RI 1160, M (deschloro-2-OH-ethyl-) RI 1380, M (deschloro-COOH-) RI 1235, M (deschloro-di-OH-) RI 1685; system GB—clomethiazole RI 1269.

High Performance Liquid Chromatography. System HA—*k* 0.1; system HX—RI 395; system HY—RI 292; system HAA—retention time 16.0 min.

Ultraviolet Spectrum. Aqueous acid—258 (A^{1}_{1}=288a); aqueous alkali—250 nm (A^{1}_{1}=270b).

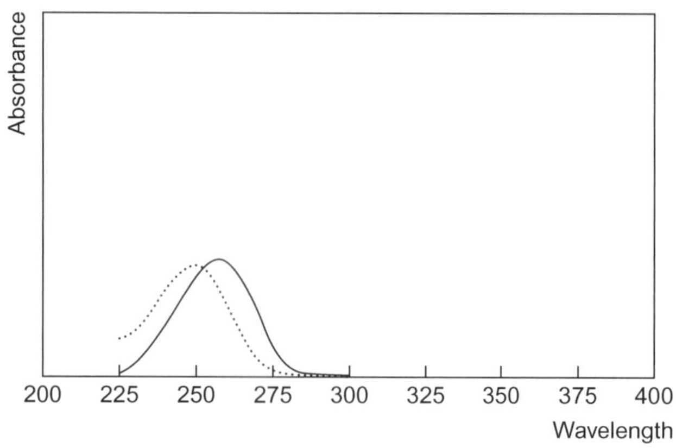

Infra-red Spectrum. Principal peaks at wavenumbers 1190, 1227, 1041, 1031, 779, 823 cm^{-1} (clomethiazole edisilate, KBr disk).

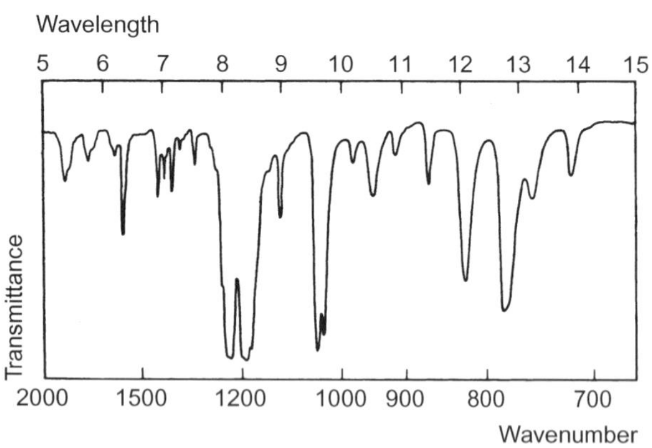

Mass Spectrum. Principal ions at *m/z* 112, 161, 85, 45, 163, 113, 114, 59.

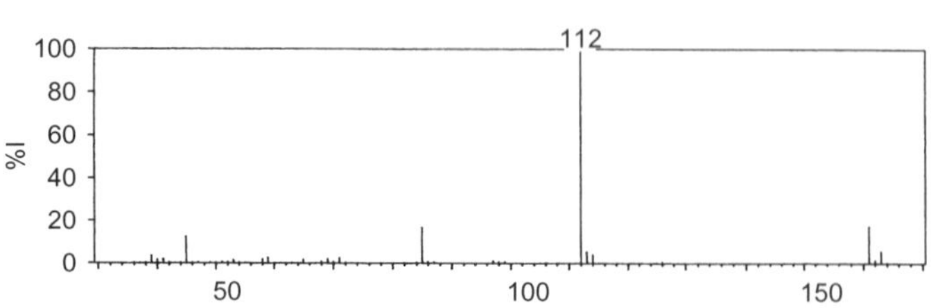

Quantification

Gas chromatography. In blood or plasma: clomethiazole and two metabolites, limit of detection 32 ng for clomethiazole in plasma, AFID—S. E. Tsuei *et al.*, *J. Chromatogr.* 1980, *182*(8) *B Biomed. Appl.*, 55–62. In plasma or urine: limit of detection 50 µg/L for clomethiazole edisilate, FID—R. G. Moore *et al.*, *Eur. J. Clin. Pharmacol.*, 1975, *8*, 353–357.

Gas chromatography–mass spectrometry. In blood or plasma: limit of detection 1 µg/L—K. G. Jostell *et al.*, *Acta Pharmacol. Toxicol.*, 1978, *43*, 180–189. In plasma: clomethiazole and two metabolites, limit of detection 1 µg/L for clomethiazole—R. L. Nation *et al.*, *Eur. J. Clin. Pharmacol.*, 1977, *12*, 137–145.

High performance liquid chromatography. In plasma: limit of detection 200 µg/L, UV detection—R. Hartley *et al.*, *J. Chromatogr.* 1983, *276*(27) *B Biomed. Appl.*, 471–477. In plasma: limit of detection 50 µg/L, UV detection—R. Hartley *et al.*, *J. Chromatogr.*, 1987, *415*, 357–364.

Disposition in the Body. Rapidly absorbed after oral administration but extensively metabolised. A considerable number of metabolites have been identified in small quantities in urine. Less than 5% of a dose is excreted unchanged in the urine, and up to about 14% is excreted as 4-methylthiazole-5-acetic acid. Other metabolites identified in the urine include 5-(1-hydroxy-2-chloroethyl)-4-methylthiazole and 5-(2-hydroxyethyl)thiazole-4-carbolactone (which appear to be more abundant than 4-methylthiazole-5-acetic acid), together with 5-acetyl-4-methylthiazole, 5-(1-hydroxyethyl)-4-methylthiazole, and 5-(2-hydroxyethyl)-4-methylthiazole in both free and conjugated forms. 5-Ethyl-2-hydroxy-4-methylthiazole has been found in the tissues following overdoses of clomethiazole. 5-(1-Hydroxyethyl)-4-methylthiazole and 5-acetyl-4-methylthiazole may be present in the plasma at concentrations similar to, or greater than, those of unchanged drug. Clomethiazole crosses the placenta and is found in breast milk.

Therapeutic concentration. In plasma, usually in the range 0.1 to 2.8 mg/L.

Following single oral doses of 192 mg to 6 subjects, peak plasma concentrations of 0.10 to 0.55 mg/L (mean 0.27) were attained in about 0.6 h. [P. J. Pentikainen *et al.*, *Eur. J. Clin. Pharmacol.*, 1980, *17*, 275–284.]

Toxicity. Toxic effects are associated with plasma concentrations of 1.6 to 13 to 26 mg/L, and fatalities with concentrations of 8 to 50 to 170 mg/L.

In a report of 9 cases of fatal overdose, in which doses of about 10 to 50 g had been ingested, postmortem blood concentrations of 25 to 80 mg/L (mean 56) were found; in a further 6 fatalities due to clomethiazole and alcohol ingestion, postmortem blood concentrations ranged from 5 to 47 mg/L (mean 21). [S. Jakobsson and M. Möller, *Forensic Sci.*, 1972, *1*, 114.]

In a report of 2 cases of fatal overdose, postmortem concentrations were: blood 21 and 214 mg/L, liver blood 21 and 100 mg/L, bile 38 and 143 mg/L, urine 5 and 114 mg/L; in 3 further cases blood concentrations were reported to be 3.4, 50, and 75 mg/L. [A. E. Robinson and R. D. McDowall, *Forensic Sci. Int.*, 1979, *14*, 49–55.]

Note. For a review of clomethiazole fatalities, see E. Klug and V. Schneider, *Z Rechtsmed.*, 1984, *93*, 89–94.

Half-life. Plasma half-life, about 3 to 7 h, increased in elderly subjects and in patients with liver disease.

Volume of distribution. About 3 to 12 L/kg (mean 8).

Clearance. Plasma clearance, 10 to 25 mL/min/kg.

Distribution in blood. Plasma:whole blood ratio, about 1.2.

Protein binding. In plasma, about 60 to 70%.

Note. For a review of clomethiazole toxicity see A. Houston *et al.*, *Human Toxicol.*, 1983, *2*, 361–369.

Dose. Clomethiazole as Heminevrin (Astra) is given in doses of 2 to 3 capsules daily. In alcohol withdrawal, an initial dose of 9 to12 capsules is given on the first day in a hospital or specialist centre, with dosage gradually reduced over the following 5 days.

Note. Due to variations in bioavailability: for an equivalent therapeutic effect, one capsule (192 mg clomethiazole base) ≡ 5 mL syrup (250 mg/5 mL clomethiazole edisilate) ≡ one tablet (500 mg edisilate).

Clomifene

Induction of Ovulation

Synonyms. Chloramiphene; Clomiphene.

A mixture of the *E* and *Z* isomers of 2-[4-(2-Chloro-1,2-diphenylethenyl)phenoxy]-*N*,*N*-diethylethanamine.

Clomifene may be separated into its *E* and *Z* isomers, enclomifene and zuclomiphene.
$C_{26}H_{28}ClNO = 406.0$
CAS—911-45-5; 15690-57-0 (E); 15690-55-8 (Z)

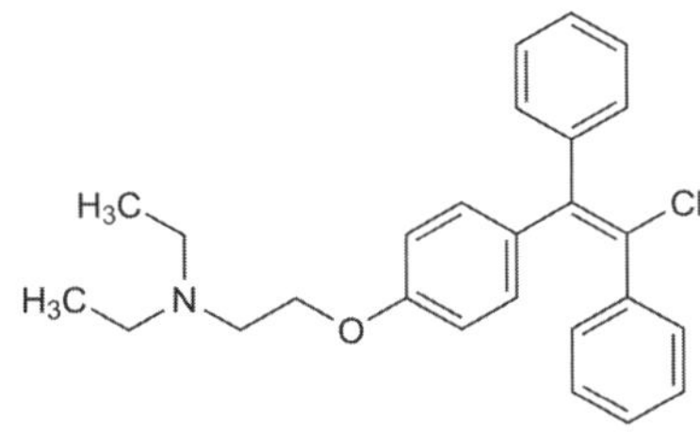

A white to pale yellow solid. M.p. 111° to 115°.
Sparingly soluble in water and ethanol; slightly soluble in chloroform.

Clomifene Citrate
Proprietary names. Clomid; Clomivid; Dyneric; Serophene.
$C_{26}H_{28}ClNO,C_6H_8O_7 = 598.1$
CAS—50-41-9; 7599-79-3 (E); 7619-53-6 (Z)
A white to pale yellow powder. M.p. 116.5° to 118°.
Soluble 1 in 900 of water, 1 in 40 of ethanol, and 1 in 800 of chloroform; freely soluble in glacial acetic acid and methanol; insoluble in ether.

Partition Coefficient. Log *P* (octanol/water), 6.7.

Colour Tests. Liebermann's Test—brown; Mandelin's Test—violet →orange-brown; Marquis Test—violet-brown.

Thin-layer Chromatography. System TA—Rf 60; system TB—Rf 56; system TC—Rf 52; system TE—Rf 82; system TL—Rf 35; system TAE—Rf 30. (Acidified iodoplatinate solution, positive.)

Gas Chromatography. System GA—RI 2930.

Ultraviolet Spectrum. Aqueous acid—235 nm ($A_1^1 = 464b$), 292 nm ($A_1^1 = 259b$).

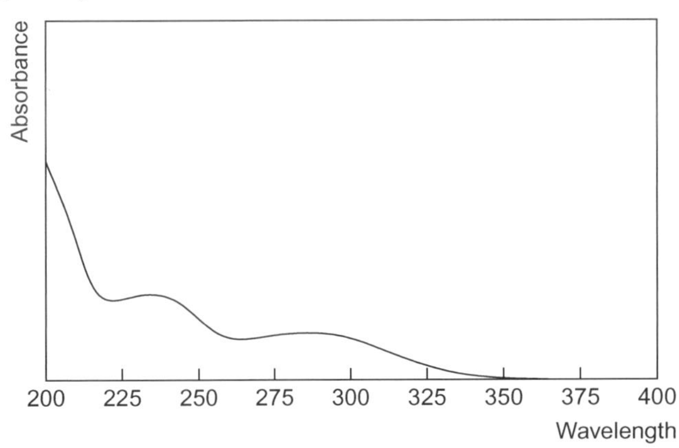

Infra-red Spectrum. Principal peaks at wavenumbers 1590, 1111, 1245, 1505, 700, 1170 cm^{-1}.

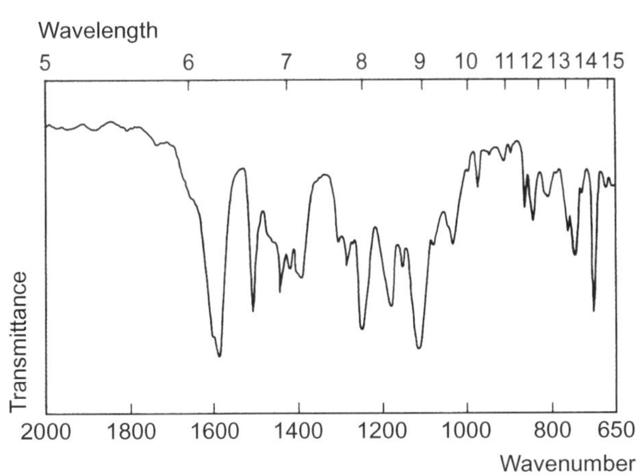

Mass Spectrum. Principal ions at *m/z* 86, 87, 100, 30, 58, 44, 42, 29.

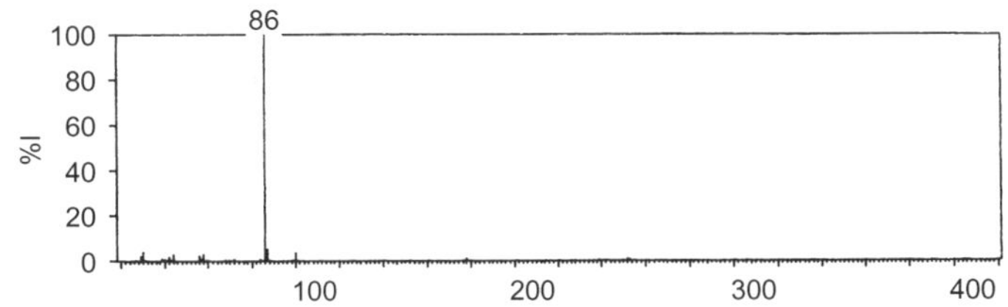

Quantification
High performance liquid chromatography. In plasma: limit of detection 350 ng/L, photolysis and fluorescence detection—P. J. Harman *et al., J. Chromatogr.* 1981, *225(14) B Biomed. Appl.*, 131–138. In plasma: limit of quantification 0.75 µg/L for *cis*-clomiphene and 1.25 µg/L for *trans*-clomiphene, fluorescence detection ($\lambda_{ex} = 247$ nm; $\lambda_{em} = 378$ nm)—I. Urmos *et al., J. Chromatogr.*, 1993, *617(1)*, 168–172.

Disposition in the Body. Absorbed after oral administration and slowly excreted in the bile; enterohepatic circulation occurs.

Half-life. Biological half-life, about 5 days.

Dose. 50 mg of clomifene citrate daily, for 5 days; up to 250 mg daily has been given.

Clomipramine

Antidepressant

Synonyms. Chlorimipramine; Monochlorimipramine.
3-Chloro-10,11-dihydro-*N*,*N*-dimethyl-5*H*-dibenz[*b*,*f*]azepine-5-propanamine
$C_{19}H_{23}ClN_2 = 314.9$
CAS—303-49-1

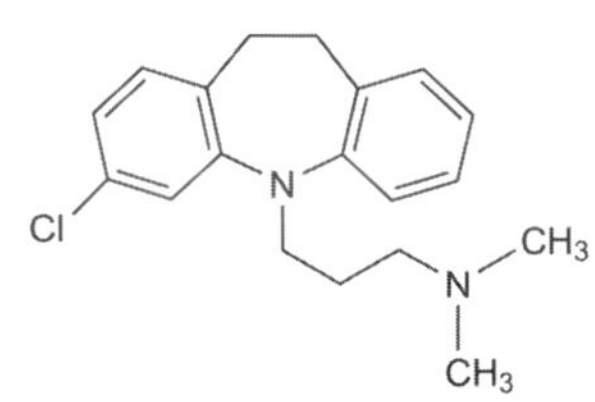

Clomipramine Hydrochloride
Proprietary name. Anafranil
$C_{19}H_{23}ClN_2,HCl = 351.3$
CAS—17321-77-6
A white or slightly yellow crystalline powder. M.p. about 192°.
Soluble 1 in 8 of water, 1 in 5 of ethanol, 1 in 3 of chloroform, and 1 in 100 of ether.

Partition Coefficient. Log *P* (octanol/water), 5.2.

Colour Tests. Forrest Reagent—blue; FPN Reagent—blue; Liebermann's Test—blue; Mandelin's Test—blue.

Thin-layer Chromatography. System TA—Rf 51; system TB—Rf 53; system TC—Rf 34; system TE—Rf 72; system TL—Rf 18; system TAE—Rf 26; system TAF—Rf 54; system TAJ—Rf 18; system TAK—Rf 16; system TAL—Rf 75. (Acidified iodoplatinate solution, strong reaction.)

Gas Chromatography. System GA—clomipramine RI 2415, M (nor-) RI 2432, M (*N*-oxide) RI 2146, M (ring) RI 2230, M (8-OH) RI 2727, M (8-OH-nor) RI 2762, M (2-OH-) RI 2569, M (10-OH-) RI 2574; system GB—clomipramine RI 2511, M (nor-) RI 2540, M (*N*-oxide) RI 2150, M (ring) RI 2335, M (8-OH-) RI 2843, M (8-OH-nor-) RI 2880, M (2-OH-) RI 2735, M (10-OH-) RI 2698; system GF—RI 2795; system GM—clomipramine RRT 1.172, M (nor-) RRT 1.374 (relative to iprindole).

High Performance Liquid Chromatography. System HA—clomipramine *k* 3.4, monodesmethylclomipramine *k* 2.0; system HF—*k* 9.92; system HX—RI 462; system HY—RI 405; system HZ—retention time, 10.2 min; system HAA—retention time, 16.4 min.

Ultraviolet Spectrum. Aqueous acid—251 nm ($A_1^1 = 253a$).

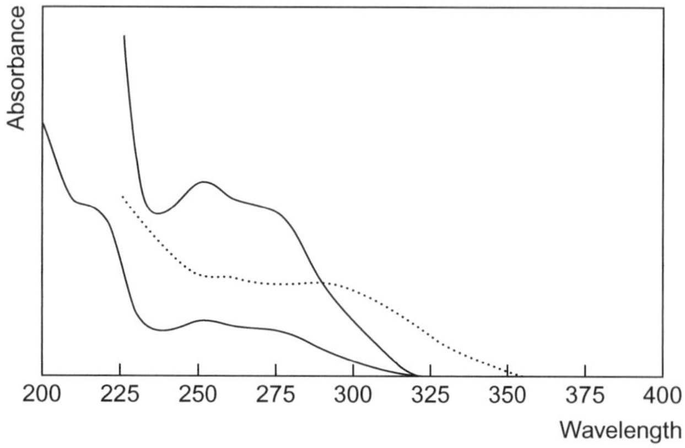

Infra-red Spectrum. Principal peaks at wavenumbers 752, 1225, 805, 842, 1212, 1237 cm^{-1} (clomipramine hydrochloride, KBr disk).

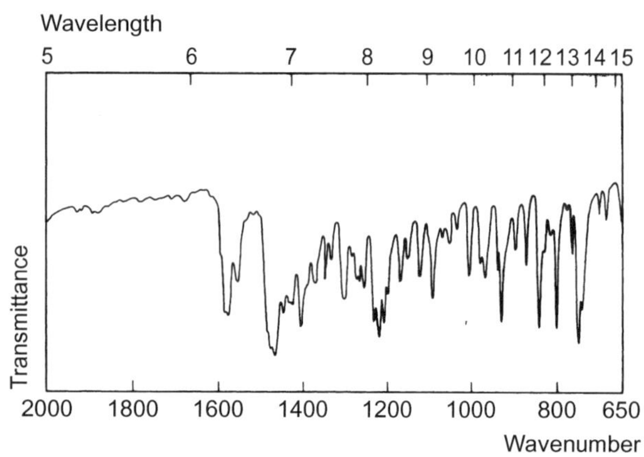

Mass Spectrum. Principal ions at *m/z* 58, 85, 269, 268, 270, 271, 314, 242; monodesmethylclomipramine 44, 71, 268, 227, 193, 42, 269, 229; 8-hydroxyclomipramine 58, 85, 86, 57, 84, 70, 43, 268.

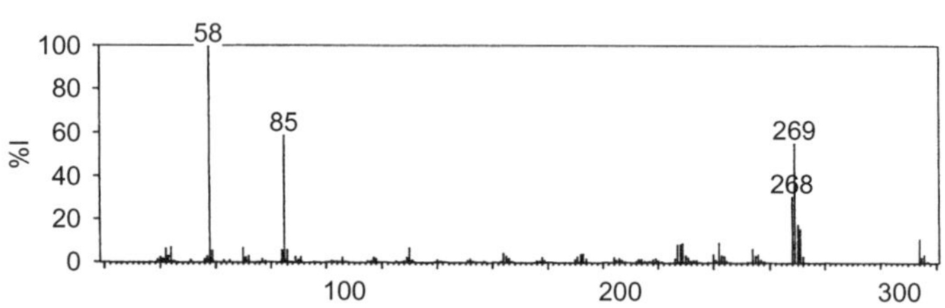

Quantification

Gas chromatography. In plasma: limit of detection 5 ng, AFID—L. Gifford *et al.*, *J. Chromatogr.*, 1975, *105*, 107–113. In serum: limit of detection 5 µg/L—M. L. Rao *et al.*, *Clin. Chem.*, 1994, *40(6)*, 929–933.

High performance liquid chromatography. In plasma or blood: limit of detection 5 µg/L for clomipramine and 10 µg/L for monodesmethylclomipramine, UV detection—J. Godbillon and S. Gauron, *J. Chromatogr.*, 1981, *204*, 303–311. In serum: limit of quantification 15 µg/L, UV (λ=260 nm)—H. Weigmann *et al.*, *J. Chromatogr. B Biomed. Sci. Appl.*, 1998, *710*, 227–233. In plasma: limit of detection 10 µg/L, UV (λ=254 nm)—L. Palego *et al.*, *Prog. Neuropsychopharmacol. Biol. Psychiatry*, 2001, *25*, 519–533. In plasma: lower limit of detection 1 to 2 µg/L and limit of quantification 5 µg/L, UV detection (λ=214 nm)—R. Pirola *et al.*, *J. Chromatogr. B Biomed. Sci. Appl.*, 2002, *772*, 205–210.

Fluorescence polarization immunoassay. In serum: limit of detection 20 µg/L—M. L. Rao *et al.*, *Clin. Chem.*, 1994, *40*, 929–933.

Disposition in the Body. Rapidly and completely absorbed after oral administration, but undergoes extensive first-pass *N*-demethylation to the major active metabolite, monodesmethylclomipramine. Clomipramine and monodesmethylclomipramine are further metabolised by 8-hydroxylation, *N*-oxidation, and conjugation. About 10 to 15% of a dose is excreted in the urine in 24 h, of which less than 0.2% is unchanged clomipramine or monodesmethylclomipramine. A total of 45 to 60% of a dose is excreted in the urine over a period of 14 days and about 20 to 30% is slowly eliminated in the faeces.

Therapeutic concentration. Plasma concentrations of clomipramine and the desmethyl metabolite vary considerably between individual patients. Steady-state concentrations of clomipramine are usually achieved in about 1 to 2 weeks, but monodesmethylclomipramine may continue to accumulate for 6 weeks or longer. 8-Hydroxyclomipramine and 8-hydroxydesmethylclomipramine have been detected in plasma at significant concentrations during high-dose chronic treatment.

After a single oral dose of 50 mg, given to 5 subjects, peak plasma concentrations of clomipramine of 0.02 to 0.07 mg/L (mean 0.05) were attained in 2 to 4 h; peak plasma concentrations of monodesmethylclomipramine of 0.05 to 12 µg/L (mean 5) were attained in 4 to 24 h. [R. Jones and D. Luscombe, *Postgrad. Med. J.*, 1976, *52*, *Suppl. 3*, 62–67.]

Steady-state plasma concentrations of 0.10 to 0.48 mg/L (mean 0.23) were reported after daily oral doses of 150 mg given to 17 subjects; the steady-state concentration of monodesmethylclomipramine was 0.24 to 0.96 mg/L (mean 0.45). [S. Montgomery *et al.*, *Postgrad. Med. J.*, 1980, *56*, *Suppl. 1*, 130–133.]

Toxicity. Toxic effects have been associated with blood concentrations greater than 0.4 mg/L of clomipramine plus monodesmethylclomipramine.

In 2 fatalities caused by clomipramine, postmortem concentrations were: blood 1 mg/L, trace; brain 4.5 µg/g; liver 30, 22 µg/g; urine 25 mg/L. [M. T. Haqqani and D. R. Gutteridge, *Forensic Sci.*, 1974, *3*, 83–87.]

In a fatality caused by clomipramine overdose, the following postmortem concentrations were reported: blood, clomipramine 0.54 mg/L and monodesmethylclomipramine 0.58 mg/L; urine, clomipramine 0.35 mg/L and monodesmethylclomipramine 0.70 mg/L. [R. C. Meatherall *et al.*, *J. Anal. Toxicol.*, 1983, *7*, 168–171.]

A 31-year-old man suffering from mental illness died in hospital after a suicide attempt. Postmortem clomipramine and *N*-desmethylclomipramine concentrations ranged from 0.48 to 1.61 mg/L in the brain and 0.26 to 1.32 mg/L in the heart. Blood clomipramine concentration was 1.61 mg/L in heart and 0.48 mg/L in brain. Liver concentration was 3.95 mg/kg and 2.36 mg/kg in kidney. These results may reflect a postmortem drug redistribution. [G. Romano and G. Di Bono, *J. Forensic Sci.*, 1994, *39(3)*, 877-882.]

In 10 overdose cases, postmortem blood concentrations of 0.21 to 4.9 mg/L were observed and liver concentrations were 7.0 to 320.0 mg/kg. A 41-year-old female suffering from depression was found dead and clomipramine concentrations were detected in blood at 3.3 mg/L and 280 mg/kg in liver. A 29-year-old man also suffering from depression showed concentrations of 1.8 mg/L and 320 mg/kg, respectively. [I. M. McIntyre *et al.*, *J. Forensic Sci.*, 1994, *39(2)*, 486-496.]

For details of a fatality involving the ingestion of clomipramine and trimipramine, see under Trimipramine.

Half-life. Plasma half-life, 20 to 84 h (mean 36); decreased in children.

Distribution in blood. Plasma : whole blood ratio, 1.2.

Protein binding. In plasma, clomipramine 90 to 95%, monodesmethylclomipramine 97 to 99%.

Note. For a review of the pharmacokinetics of tricyclic antidepressants see G. Molnar and R. N. Gupta, *Biopharm. Drug Dispos.*, 1980, *1*, 283–305.

Dose. 10 to 150 mg of clomipramine hydrochloride daily.

Clomocycline

Antibacterial

Synonyms. Chlormethylencycline; N^2-(Hydroxymethyl)chlortetracycline; Methylolchlortetracycline.

7-Chloro-4-(dimethylamino)-1,4,4a,5,5a,6,11,12a-octahydro-3,6,10,12,12a-pentahydroxy-*N*-(hydroxymethyl)-6-methyl-1,11-dioxo-2-naphthacenecarboxamide

$C_{23}H_{25}ClN_2O_9$=508.9

CAS—1181-54-0

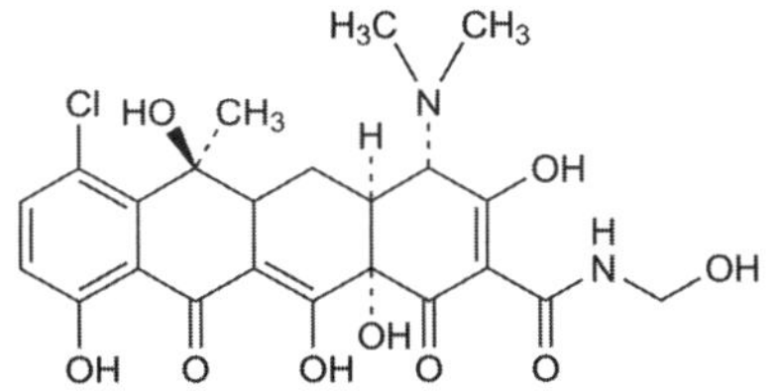

A yellow powder. It is sensitive to light and air, and undergoes decomposition between 145° and 170° without a definite melting point.

Clomocycline Sodium
Proprietary name. Megaclor
$C_{23}H_{24}ClN_2NaO_9$=530.9
A yellow powder. It is sensitive to light and air, and undergoes decomposition without melting.
Very soluble in water; soluble 1 in 250 of ethanol; practically insoluble in chloroform and ether.

Partition Coefficient. Log *P* (octanol/water), −1.5.

Colour Tests. Benedict's Reagent—red; Formaldehyde–Sulfuric Acid—orange-brown; Liebermann's Test—black; Mandelin's Test—violet→brown; Marquis Test—orange-brown; Sulfuric Acid—blue-black.

Thin-layer Chromatography. System TA—Rf 05, streaking. (Acidified potassium permanganate solution, strong reaction.)

Ultraviolet Spectrum. Aqueous acid—229, 268 nm (A^1_1=350b); aqueous alkali—251, 283 nm.

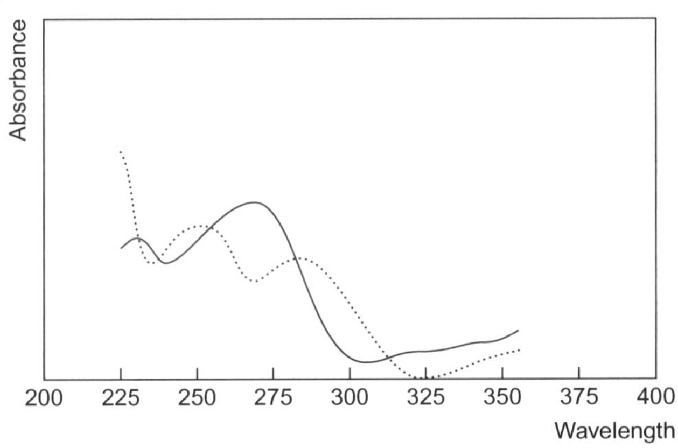

Infra-red Spectrum. Principal peaks at wavenumbers 1600, 1634, 1501, 1307, 1205, 1235 cm^{-1} (clomocycline sodium, KBr disk).

Dose. 0.68 to 1.36 g of clomocycline sodium daily.

Clonazepam

Anticonvulsant

Synonyms. Clonazepamum; Ro-5-4023.
Proprietary names. Antelepsin; Clonapam; Clonex; Clonopin; Iktorivil; Kenoket; Klonopin; Paxam; Rivotril.
5-(2-Chlorophenyl)-1,3-dihydro-7-nitro-2*H*-1,4-benzodiazepin-2-one
$C_{15}H_{10}ClN_3O_3$=315.7
CAS—1622-61-3

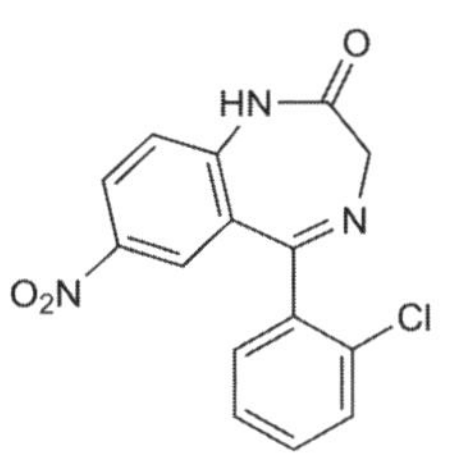

A white to light yellow crystalline powder. M.p. 236.5° to 238.5°. Protect from light.

Solubility in mg/mL at 25°: acetone 31, chloroform 15, methanol 8.6, ether 0.7, benzene 0.5, water <0.1.

Dissociation Constant. pK_a 1.5, 10.5.

Partition Coefficient. Log *P* (octanol/water), 2.41.

Colour Test. Formaldehyde–Sulfuric Acid—orange.

Thin-layer Chromatography. System TA—Rf 72; system TB—Rf 00; system TC—Rf 53; system TD—Rf 35; system TE—Rf 67; system TF—Rf 45; system TL—Rf 61; system TAD—Rf 56; system TAE—Rf 85; system TAF—Rf 87; system TAJ—Rf 50; system TAK—Rf 53; system TAL—Rf 91. (Acidified iodoplatinate solution, positive; acidified potassium permanganate solution, positive.)

Gas Chromatography. System GA—clonazepam RI 2823, M (7-amino-) RI 2890, M (amino-OH-) RI 2935; system GB—clonazepam RI 3000, clonazepam-TMS RI 2781, M (7-amino-) RI 2996, M (7-amino-)-TMS_2 RI 2742; system GG—RI 3600.

High Performance Liquid Chromatography. System HI—*k* 2.85; system HK—*k* 0.35; system HX—RI 465; system HY—RI 403; system HZ—retention time 4.6 min; system HAA—retention time 17.4 min; system HAF—retention time 5.3 min; system HAK—retention time 6.2 min; system HAL—retention time(s): clonazepam 4.33 min, 7-acetamidoclonazepam 1.45 min, 7-aminoclonazepam 1.55 min; system HAM—retention time 4.3 min; system HAX—retention time 6.5 min; system HAY—retention time 6.0 min; system HAZ—*k* 0.79; system HBH—*k* 2.92; system HBI—*k* 0.79.

Ultraviolet Spectrum. Aqueous acid—273 nm (A^1_1=645b); methanol—245 nm (A^1_1=460b), 309 nm (A^1_1=360b).

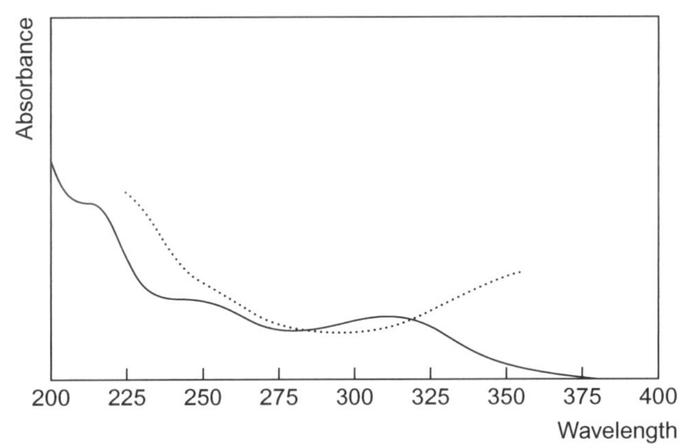

Infra-red Spectrum. Principal peaks at wavenumbers 1685, 1610, 748, 1255, 1578, 1532 cm^{-1} (KBr disk).

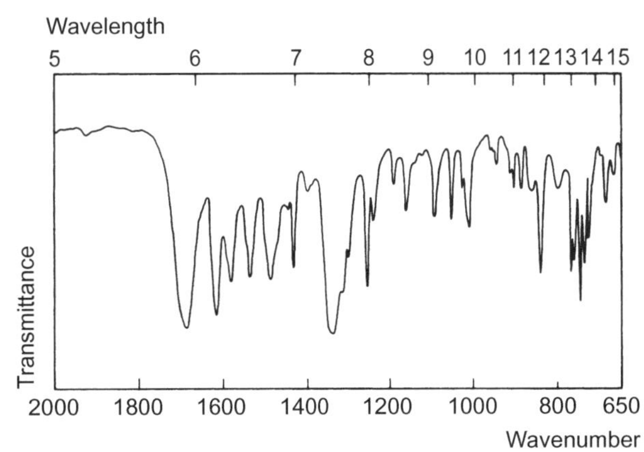

Mass Spectrum. Principal ions at *m/z* 280, 314, 315, 286, 234, 288, 316, 240; 7-acetamidoclonazepam 43, 327, 299, 298, 292, 329, 328, 256; 7-aminoclonazepam 285, 256, 257, 258, 44, 287, 110, 220.

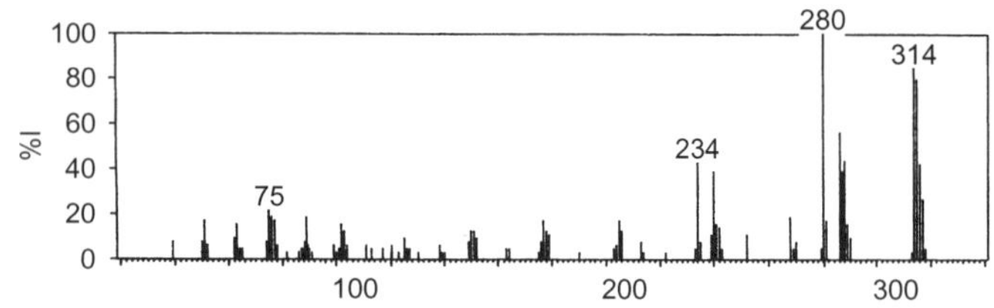

Quantification

Gas chromatography. In plasma: limit of detection 1 µg/L, ECD—A. G. de Boer *et al.*, *J. Chromatogr.* 1978, *145*(2) *B Biomed. Appl.*, 105–114. In plasma: limit of detection 5 µg/L, AFID—A. K. Dhar and H. Kutt, *J. Chromatogr.* 1981, *222*(11) *B Biomed. Appl.*, 203–211. In plasma or whole blood: clonazepam and other benzodiazepines, ECD and NPD—P. Lillsunde and T. Seppala, *J. Chromatogr.*, 1990, *533*, 97–110. In plasma: ECD, comparison with HPLC—D. de Carvalho and V. L. Lanchote, *Ther. Drug Monit.*, 1991, *13*, 55–63. In urine: clonazepam and other benzodiazepines, limits of detection 2 to 20 µg/L, ECD—F. Guan *et al.*, *J. Anal. Toxicol.*, 1999, *23*, 54–61.

Gas chromatography–mass spectrometry. In urine: clonazepam and other benzodiazepines—D. A. Black *et al.*, *J. Anal. Toxicol.*, 1994, *18*, 185–188 and D. A. Black *et al.*, *J. Anal. Toxicol.*, 1995, *19*, 58–59. In plasma: limit of detection 0.1 µg/L—D. Song *et al.*, *J. Chromatogr.* 1996, *686 B Biomed. Appl.*, 199–204. In hair: clonazepam and 7-aminoclonazepam—A. Negrusz *et al.*, *J. Anal. Toxicol.*, 2000, 24, 614–620.

High performance liquid chromatography. In plasma: clonazepam, 7-acetamidoclonazepam and 7-aminoclonazepam, limit of detection 10 µg/L, UV detection—I. Petters *et al.*, *J. Chromatogr.* 1984, *306*(31) *B Biomed. Appl.*, 241–248. In serum: limit of detection about 2 µg/L—K. Furuno *et al.*, *Acta Med. Okayama*, 1991, *45*, 123–127. In plasma: limit of detection 2 µg/L, UV detection—B. C. Sallustio *et al.*, *Ther. Drug Monit.*, 1994, *16*, 174–178. In postmortem blood: clonazepam and other benzodiazepines and their 7-amino- metabolites, limits of detection 1 to 8 µg/L, UV detection—M. D. Robertson and O. H. Drummer, *J. Chromatogr.* 1995, *667 B Biomed. Appl.*, 179–184. In serum: clonazepam and other benzodiazepines, UV detection—E. Tanaka *et al.*, *J. Chromatogr.* 1996, *682 B Biomed. Appl.*, 173–178; E. Tanaka *et al.*, *J. Chromatogr. B. Biomed. Appl.*, 1998, *709*, 324. In serum or plasma: clonazepam and other benzodiazepines, limit of detection 1.6 µg/L, UV detection—K. K. Akerman *et al.*, *Clin. Chem.*, 1996, *42*, 1412–1416. In plasma: UV detection—C. Le Guellec *et al.*, *J. Chromatogr. B Biomed. Sci. Appl.*, 1998, *719*, 227–233. In whole blood: clonazepam and other benzodiazepines, limit of quantification for clonazepam 25 µg/L, diode-array detection—A. El Mahjoub and C. Staub, *J. Anal. Toxicol.*, 2001, *25*, 209–314. In hair: clonazepam and other benzodiazepines, limit of quantification for clonazepam 0.5 µg/g, photodiode-array detection—A. El Mahjoub and C. Staub, *Forensic Sci. Int.*, 2001, *123*, 17–25. In urine: clonazepam and other benzodiazepines, limit of detection for clonazepam 600 µg/L, UV detection—W. M. Mullett and J. Pawliszyn, *Anal. Chem.*, 2002, *74*, 1081–1087.

Radioimmunoassay. In plasma: limit of detection 5 µg/L—W. Dixon *et al.*, *J. Pharm. Sci.*, 1977, *66*, 235–237.

Disposition in the Body. Rapidly absorbed after oral administration with peak plasma levels found after about 4 h. The major metabolic reaction catalysed by cytochrome P450 isoenzyme CYP3A4, is reduction of the nitro group to 7-aminoclonazepam, followed by acetylation to 7-acetamidoclonazepam; 7-aminoclonazepam is slightly active and is found in plasma at concentrations similar to those of clonazepam. 3-Hydroxylation of clonazepam and its two metabolites may also occur, followed by conjugation with glucuronic acid or sulfate. Clonazepam crosses the placental barrier and is excreted in breast milk. Less than 1% of a dose is excreted unchanged in the urine in 24 h. Urinary excretion accounts for up to 70% of a dose, as both free and conjugated metabolites, over a period of 7 days, of which about 50% consists of 7-aminoclonazepam and 7-acetamidoclonazepam.

Therapeutic concentration. In plasma, usually in the range 0.02 to 0.07 mg/L.

A single oral dose of 2 mg given to 8 subjects produced peak plasma concentrations of 0.007 to 0.024 mg/L (mean 0.017) in 1 to 4 h. [A. Berlin and H. Dahlström, *Eur. J. Clin. Pharmacol.*, 1975, *9*, 155–159.]

After daily oral dosing of 25 subjects with 6 mg per day, steady-state plasma concentrations of 0.029 to 0.075 mg/L of clonazepam, 0.023 to 0.137 mg/L of 7-aminoclonazepam, and < 0.003 to 0.013 mg/L of 7-acetamidoclonazepam were reported. [J. Naestoft and N.-E. Larsen, *J. Chromatogr.*, 1974, *93*, 113–122.]

In 4 children whose epilepsy was unsatisfactorily controlled with valproate therapy, a single oral dose of clonazepam 0.05 mg/kg produced peak plasma concentrations of 0.025 to 0.114 mg/L at 1 to 1.5 h; valproate concentrations remained within the therapeutic range and were unaffected by clonazepam. [L. Wang and X. D. Wang, *Ther. Drug Monit.*, 2002, *24*, 532–536.]

Toxicity. Toxicity is associated with plasma concentrations greater than 0.1 mg/L.

Bioavailability. About 98%.

Half-life. Plasma half-life, 20 to 40 h.

Volume of distribution. About 3 L/kg.

Clearance. Plasma clearance, about 1.5 mL/min/kg.

Protein binding. In plasma, about 86%.

Note. For reviews of the pharmacokinetics of clonazepam, see A. Berlin and H. Dahlstrom, *Eur. J. Clin. Pharmacol.*, 1975, *9*, 155–159 and R. M. Pinder *et al.*, *Drugs*, 1976, *12*, 321–361.

Dose. 4 to 8 mg daily.

Clonidine

Antihypertensive

Synonyms. Chlophazoline; ST-155-BS.
N-(2,6-Dichlorophenyl)-4,5-dihydro-1*H*-imidazol-2-amine
$C_9H_9Cl_2N_3$=230.1
CAS—4205-90-7

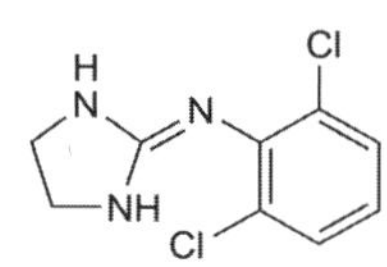

A white powder. M.p. 130°.
Soluble 1 in 8 of chloroform and 1 in 50 of ether.

Clonidine Hydrochloride

Synonym. ST-155
Proprietary names. Aruclonin; Atensina; Barclyd; Caprysin; Catanidin; Catapres(an); Clonistada; Clonnirit; Dispaclonidin; Dixarit; Duraclon; Edolglau; Haemiton; Isoglaucon; Mirfat; Normopresan; Paracefan; Tenso-Timelets. It is an ingredient of Clorpres, Combipres, Combipresan, and Dilapres.
$C_9H_9Cl_2N_3$,HCl=266.6
CAS—4205-91-8
A white crystalline powder. M.p. 305°.
Soluble 1 in 13 of water, 1 in 25 of ethanol, 1 in 38 of dehydrated alcohol, and 1 in 5000 of chloroform; practically insoluble in ether.

Dissociation Constant. pK_a 8.05.

Partition Coefficient. Log *P* (octanol/water), 1.59.

Colour Test. Liebermann's Test—yellow (→orange at 100°).

Thin-layer Chromatography. System TA—Rf 62; system TB—Rf 08; system TC—Rf 31; system TE—Rf 70; system TL—Rf 53; system TAE—Rf 44; system TAF—Rf 76; system TAJ—Rf 09; system TAK—Rf 02; system TAL—Rf 51. (Acidified iodoplatinate solution, positive.)

Gas Chromatography. System GA—clonidine RI 2090, art (dichlorophenylisocyanate) RI 1350, art (dichlorophenylmethylcarbamate) RI 1500; system GB—clonidine RI 2165.

High Performance Liquid Chromatography. System HA—*k* 1.2; system HX—RI 258; system HY—RI 194; system HZ—retention time 2.5 min; system HAA—retention time 6.1 min; system HAX—retention time 7.8 min; system HAY—retention time 4.3 min.

Ultraviolet Spectrum. Aqueous acid—271 nm (A^1_1=21a), 278 nm.

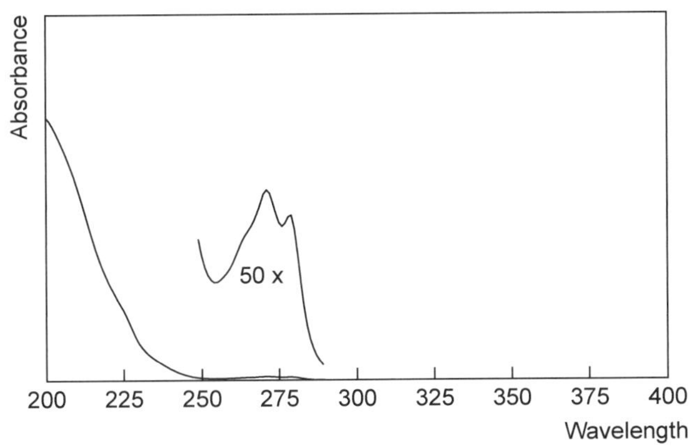

Infra-red Spectrum. Principal peaks at wavenumbers 1653, 1610, 778, 795, 1295, 1568 cm^{-1} (clonidine hydrochloride, KBr disk).

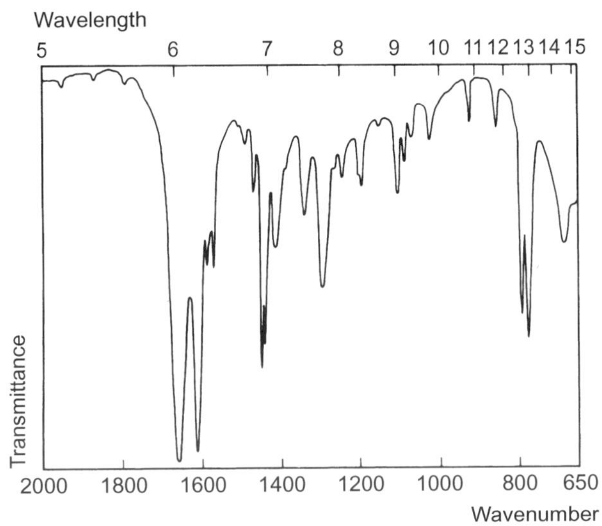

Mass Spectrum. Principal ions at *m/z* 229, 30, 231, 172, 194, 174, 200, 230.

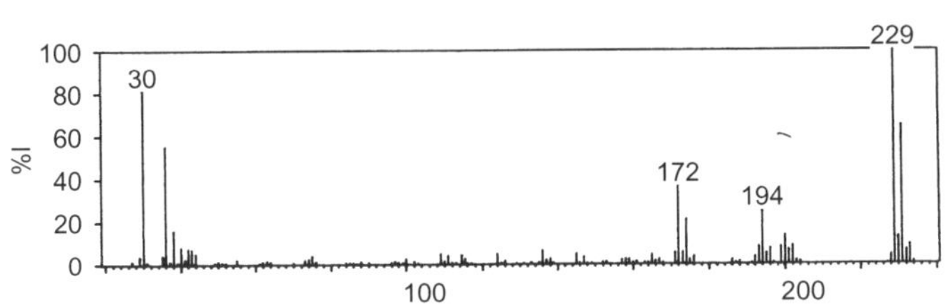

Quantification

Gas chromatography. In plasma or urine: limit of detection 25 ng/L in plasma, ECD—L.-C. Chu *et al.*, *J. Pharm. Sci.*, 1979, *68*, 72–74. In plasma: limit of detection 100 ng/L, ECD—P. O. Edlund, *J. Chromatogr.*, 1980, 187, 161–169.

Gas chromatography–mass spectrometry. In plasma or urine: limit of detection 100 ng/L in plasma—S. Murray *et al.*, *Biomed. Mass Spectrom.*, 1981, *8*, 500–502. In plasma: limit of detection 5 ng/L—J. Girault and J. B. Fourtillan, *Biomed. Environ. Mass Spectrom.*, 1988, *17*, 443–448. In plasma: limit of detection 0.025 µg/L—T. Yamahata *et al.*, *J. Chromatogr.* 1994, *653 B Biomed. Appl.*, 92–97.

Radioimmunoassay. In plasma: limit of detection 100 ng/L—D. Arndts *et al.*, *Arzneimittelforschung*, 1979, *29*, 532–538.

Disposition in the Body. Well absorbed after oral administration; peak plasma concentrations reached within 3 to 5 h. About 40 to 60% of a single dose is excreted in the urine as unchanged drug in 24 h, and about 20% of a dose is eliminated in the faeces in 4 days, probably via enterohepatic circulation. Several inactive metabolites have been detected in urine in small quantities. Clonidine is absorbed through the skin, therapeutic concentration being achieved 2 or 3 days after application of a transdermal delivery system, and are maintained for about 8 h after removal. Clonidine crosses the placental barrier.

Therapeutic concentration

In 31 cancer patients given clonidine 0.030 mg/h by continuous epidural infusion, for 14 days, steady-state plasma concentrations of 0.22 to 6.23 µg/L (mean 0.00219) on day 8 and 0.61 to 6.51 µg/L (mean 0.0025) on day 15 were reported; no accumulation in the plasma appeared to occur. [G. Boswell *et al.*, *Clin. Ther.*, 1997, *19*, 1024–1030.]

Following oral administration of clonidine 0.075 mg every 12 h for 3 days to 8 subjects, a peak plasma concentration of 0.39 µg/L was attained at 75 h after the seventh dose. In the same subjects, when clonidine was applied transdermally to the chest wall for 3 days (as a patch containing 6 mg), the peak plasma concentration was not significantly different (0.30 at 68 h). [A. Fujimura *et al.*, *J. Clin. Pharmacol.*, 1994, *34*, 260–265.]

Following rectal administration of 2.5 µg/kg clonidine to 10 infants (aged 14 to 48 month), peak plasma concentrations of 0.62 to 0.88 µg/L (mean 0.77) were obtained at 29 to 70 min (mean 52). [P. A. Lonnqvist *et al.*, *Anesthesiology*, 1994, *81*, 1097–1101.]

Toxicity. Serious toxic effects have been reported after ingestion of doses of 0.4 to 4 mg by children and 4 to 11 mg by adults. However, recovery is usually rapid.

17 h after a 5-year-old child, weighing 17.5 kg, ingested an overdose of 50 mg clonidine hydrochloride, the serum concentration was 0.064 mg/L, the highest reported in a paediatric patient. Following supportive treatment and administration of atropine and naloxone, the child recovered and was discharged without sequelae 42 h after admission. The overdose resulted from a pharmacy compounding error so that the child ingested 5 mL of a medication containing approx. 50 mg of clonidine instead of 0.05 mg/5 mL. [M. J. Romano and A. Dinh, *Pediatrics*, 2001, *108*, 471–472.]

A 9-month-old child was admitted to hospital with a decreased level of consciousness and within a few hours developed apnoea and pinpoint pupils. The child was discharged 36 h after admission, following treatment with naloxone. Further investigation led to the theory that, the evening before admission, the elderly babysitter's clonidine patch had accidentally fallen into the baby's playpen where the baby subsequently sucked on it (despite the babysitter's denial of any involvement); the baby's clonidine level was determined to be 0.011 mg/L but the results were not available until nearly 2 weeks after discharge. [M. E. Kraft, *J. Emerg. Nurs.*, 1998, *24*, 457–459.]

2 women were accidentally given doses of 25 mg instead of 0.025 mg; plasma concentrations of 0.025 and 0.027 mg/L were reported on admission and at 24 h, respectively, and decreased with a half-life of 22 h; the subjects recovered with treatment. [J. A. Rotellar *et al.*, *Lancet*, 1981, *1*, 1312.]

In a fatality due to clonidine overdose, the following postmortem concentrations were reported: blood 0.023 mg/L, brain 0.024 µg/g, kidney 0.086 µg/g. [I. Lukkari *et al.*, *Bull. Int. Assoc. Forensic Toxicol.*, 1983, *17(2)*, 13–14.]

Bioavailability. Reported as 75% to 95 %.

Half-life. Plasma half-life, 10 to 25 h.

Volume of distribution. 2.1 to 5.6 L/kg.

Protein binding. In plasma, about 20 to 40%.

Note. For a review of the pharmacokinetics of clonidine, see D.T. Lowenthal *et al.*, *Clin. Pharmacokinet.*, 1988, *14*, 287–310.

Dose. Usually 0.2 to 1.2 mg of clonidine hydrochloride daily; doses of 1.8 mg or more daily may be given.

Clonixin

Analgesic

2-[(3-Chloro-2-methylphenyl)amino]-3-pyridinecarboxylic acid

$C_{13}H_{11}ClN_2O_2$ = 262.7

CAS—17737-65-4

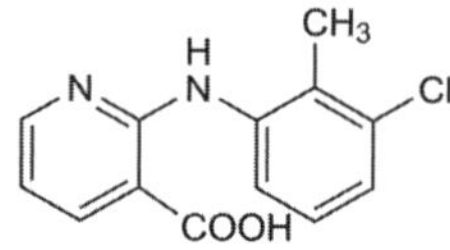

A colourless or cream-coloured solid. M.p. about 234°.

Partition Coefficient. Log *P* (octanol/water), 4.6.

Thin-layer Chromatography. System TG—Rf 30; system TAJ—Rf 40; system TAK—Rf 14; system TAL—Rf 80. (Ludy Tenger reagent, orange.)

Gas Chromatography. System GD—RRT of methyl derivative 1.61 (relative to n-$C_{16}H_{34}$).

High Performance Liquid Chromatography. System HV—RRT 0.87 (relative to meclofenamic acid); system HY—RI 345.

Ultraviolet Spectrum. Methanol—289 nm (A_1^1=950b), 335 nm.

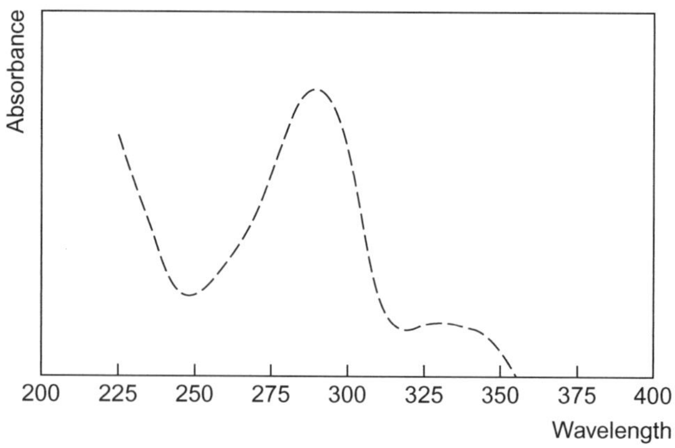

Quantification

High performance liquid chromatography. In plasma and urine: limit of quantification 10 µg/L and 20 µg/L—A. Bica *et al.*, *J. Chromatogr. A*, 2000, *889(1–2)*, 135–141.

Disposition in the Body. Rapidly absorbed after oral administration. Metabolised by hydroxylation to 4′-hydroxy-, 5′-hydroxy-, and 2′-hydroxymethyl derivatives. About 60% of a dose is excreted in the urine in 24 h.

Therapeutic concentration

Following a single oral dose of 750 mg to 12 subjects, peak serum concentrations of 29 to 66 mg/L (mean 46) were attained in about 1.7 h. [D. E. Furst and H. E. Paulus, *Clin. Pharmacol. Ther.*, 1975, *17*, 622–626.]

Half-life. Plasma half-life, about 1.5 h.

Dose. Clonixin has been given in doses of 600 mg.

Clopamide

Antihypertensive/Diuretic

Synonyms. Chlosudimeprimyl; DT-327.
Proprietary names. Brinaldix. It is an ingredient of Viskaldix.
rel-3-(Aminosulfonyl)-4-chloro-*N*-[(2*R*,6*S*)-2,6-dimethyl-1-piperidinyl]benzamide
$C_{14}H_{20}ClN_3O_3S$=345.9
CAS—636-54-4

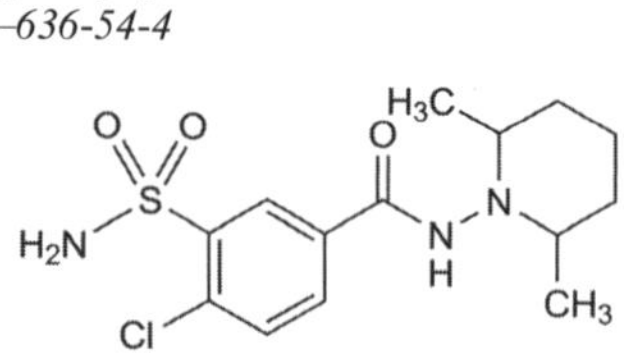

A white crystalline powder. M.p. about 246°.
Soluble 1 in about 250 of water, 1 in about 100 of dehydrated alcohol, 1 in about 250 of chloroform, and 1 in 35 of methanol.

Partition Coefficient. Log *P* (octanol/water), 1.9.

Colour Tests. Koppanyi–Zwikker Test—violet; Mercurous Nitrate—black.

Thin-layer Chromatography. System TA—Rf 79; system TD—Rf 19; system TE—Rf 55; system TF—Rf 38; system TAD—Rf 39. (Acidified iodoplatinate solution, strong reaction.)

Gas chromatography. System GA—clopamide not eluted, clopamide-Me_2 RI 2805, clopamide-ME_3 RI 2600, Art (-SO_2NH) RI 2195; system GX—clopamide-Me_2 retention time 7.0 min.

High Performance Liquid Chromatography. System HN—*k* 4.01; system HX—RI 377; system HY—RI 310.

Ultraviolet Spectrum. Aqueous acid—242 (A_1^1=346b); methanol—232, 277 (A_1^1=48b), 286 nm (A_1^1=36b).

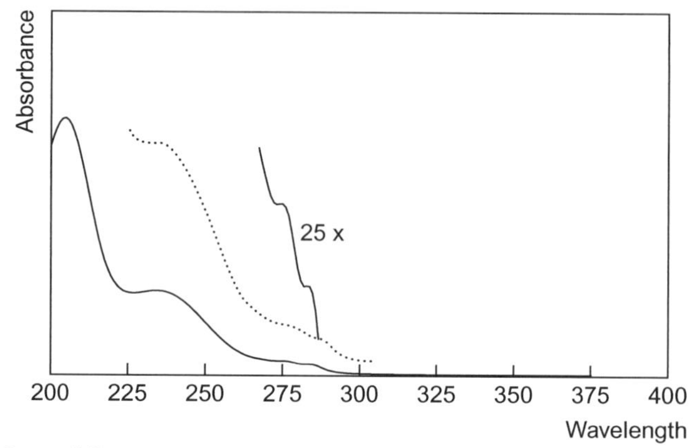

Infra-red Spectrum. Principal peaks at wavenumbers 1663, 1172, 1038, 1532, 1285, 928 cm^{-1}.

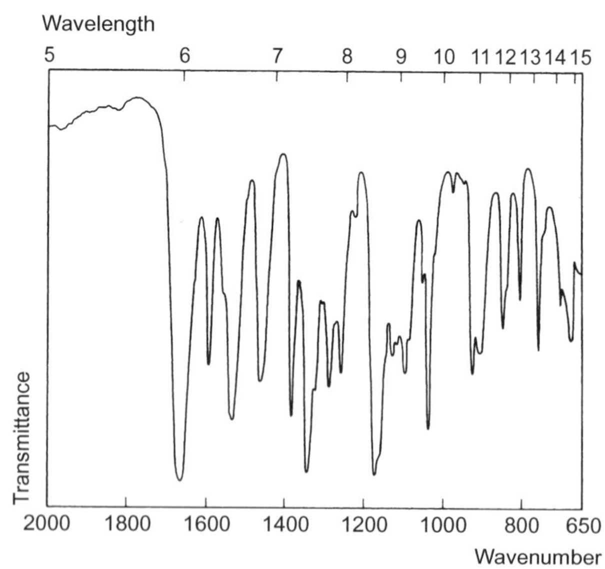

Mass Spectrum. Principal ions at *m/z* 111, 127, 55, 83, 59, 41, 112, 42; clopamide-Me_2 *m/z* 111, 112, 127, 55, 139, 358; clopamide-Me_3 *m/z* 372, 374, 387, 373, 264, 245; Art (-SO_2NH) *m/z* 111, 127, 139, 83, 96, 251.

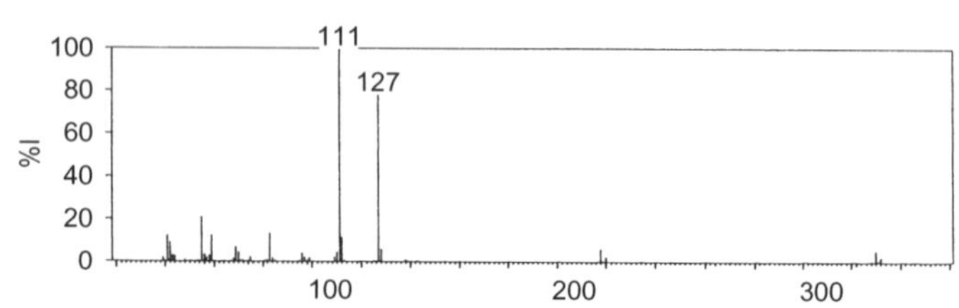

Quantification

Gas-liquid chromatography–mass spectrometry. In plasma: limit of detection 10 mg/L—W. Stuber *et al.*, *J. Pharm. Sci.*, 1989, *78(8)*, 679–682.

Disposition in the Body

Therapeutic concentration

Eight healthy volunteers were administered 5 mg clopamide and a mean peak plasma concentration of 197 mg/L was reached after 1.1 h. [W. Stuber *et al.*, *J. Pharm. Sci.*, 1989, *78(8)*, 679–682.]

Dose. 20 to 60 mg daily.

Clopenthixol

Tranquilliser

Synonym. Cloperphenthixan

4-[3-(2-Chloro-9*H*-thioxanthen-9-ylidene)propyl]-1-piperazine-ethanol

$C_{22}H_{25}ClN_2OS$=401.0

CAS—982-24-1

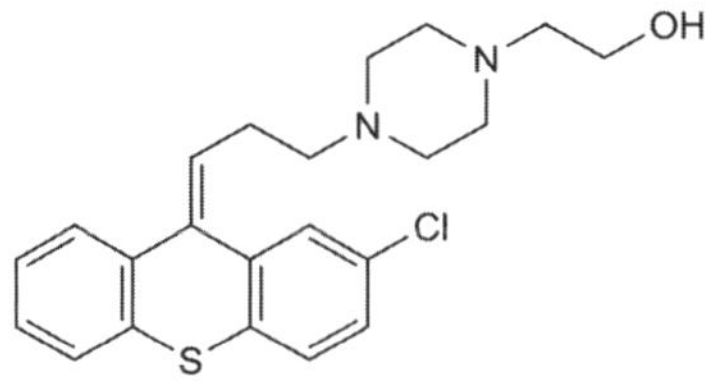

cis-isomer

Colourless syrup. Sparingly soluble in ether. Readily soluble in methanol.

Clopenthixol Decanoate

Proprietary name. Clopixol (injection)

$C_{32}H_{43}ClN_2O_2S$=555.2

A yellowish oily liquid.

Practically insoluble in water; soluble in ethanol, chloroform, and ether.

Clopenthixol Hydrochloride

Proprietary names. Ciatyl; Clopixol (tablets); Sordinol.

$C_{22}H_{25}ClN_2OS,2HCl$=473.9

CAS—633-59-0

Crystals. M.p. about 257°, with decomposition.

Freely soluble in water; sparingly soluble in ethanol.

Partition Coefficient. Log *P* (octanol/water), 4.2.

Colour Tests. Formaldehyde–Sulfuric Acid—red (orange fluorescence under UV light); Liebermann's Test—red; Sulfuric Acid—orange (fluoresces under UV light).

Thin-layer Chromatography. System TA—Rf 56; system TB—Rf 07; system TC—Rf 32; system TE—Rf 44; system TL—Rf 11; system TAE—Rf 45. (Acidified iodoplatinate solution, positive.)

Gas Chromatography. System GA—clopenthixol *cis*-isomer (zuclopenthixol) RI 3400; clopenthixol-AC RI 3460, M (*N*-oxide)-$C_6H_{14}N_2O_2$ RI 2410, M (desalkyl-)-AC RI 3490, M (desalkyl-dihydro-)-AC RI 3450, Art-(Cl-thioxanthenone) RI 2260.

High Performance Liquid Chromatography. System HX—RI 448; system HY—RI 411.

Ultraviolet Spectrum. Aqueous acid—231 (A_1^1=891a), 269, 325 nm.

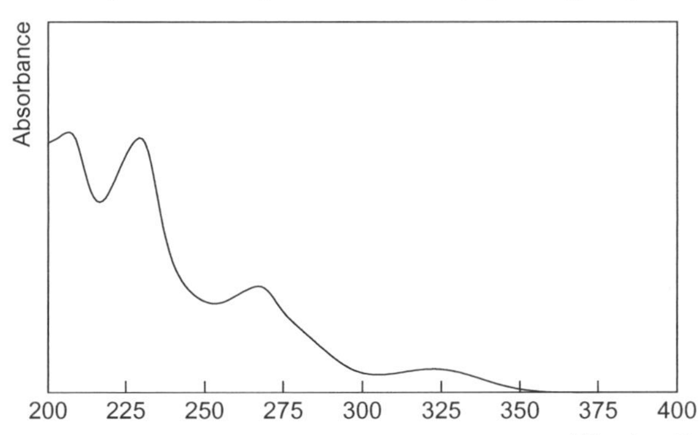

Infra-red Spectrum. Principal peaks at wavenumbers 1150, 1090, 757, 740, 1052, 1123 cm^{-1} (KBr disk).

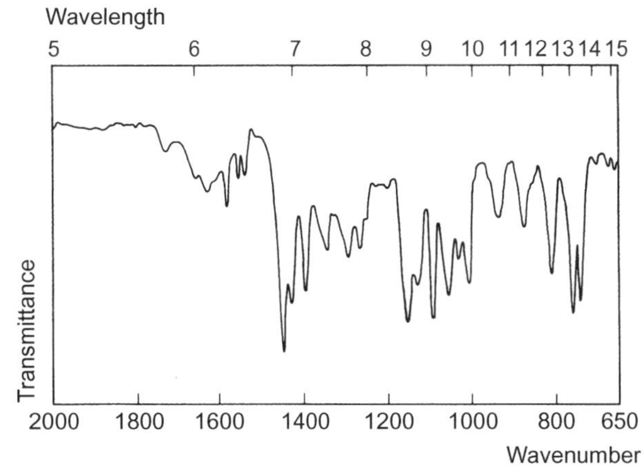

Mass Spectrum. Principal ions at *m/z* 143, 70, 100, 144, 42, 56, 98, 221.

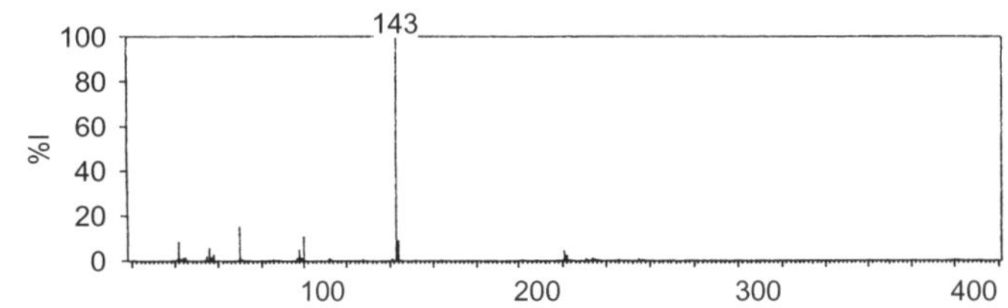

Quantification

Spectrofluorimetry. In serum: clopenthixol decanoate, clopenthixol, and des-(2-hydroxyethyl)clopenthixol, limit of detection about 3 μg/L for clopenthixol decanoate and about 2 μg/L for clopenthixol and the metabolite—K. Overø, *Acta Psychiat. Scand.*, 1980, *61*, Suppl. 279, 92–103.

High performance liquid chromatography. In serum: *cis*- and *trans*-clopenthixol and des-(2-hydroxyethyl)clopenthixol, limit of detection 500 ng/L for clopenthixol and 2.5 μg/L for the metabolite, UV detection—T. Aaes-Jørgensen, *J. Chromatogr.* 1980, *183(9) Biomed. Appl.*, *9*, 239–245. In urine and plasma: limit of detection 0.05 μg/L drug and 0.2 μg/L metabolite, fluorescence detection (λ_{ex}=260 nm; λ_{em}=435 nm)—B. B. Hansen and S. H. Hansen, *J. Chromatogr. B Biomed. Sci. Appl.*, 1994, *658(2)*, 319–325.

Disposition in the Body. Clopenthixol decanoate is slowly absorbed after injection to give peak serum concentrations of clopenthixol and the des-(2-hydroxyethyl) metabolite after about 3 to 7 days. Clopenthixol, the des-(2-hydroxyethyl) metabolite, and their sulfoxide metabolites have been detected in urine together with small amounts of clopenthixol glucuronide.

Therapeutic concentration

A mean minimum steady-state serum concentration of 0.004 mg/L of clopenthixol was reported in 24 subjects, who had been receiving average doses of 200 mg intramuscularly every 4 weeks, for 5 to 6 months. [S. J. Dencker *et al.*, *Acta Psychiat. Scand.*, 1980, *61*, Suppl. 279, 55–63.]

Following an oral dose of 30 mg of clopenthixol to 1 subject, a peak serum concentration of about 0.005 mg/L of *cis*-clopenthixol was attained in about 3 h; the peak concentration of the inactive *trans*-isomer was slightly higher and was attained after 4 h; the serum concentrations declined slowly and were still measurable after 48 h; only traces of the des-(2-hydroxyethyl) metabolite were detected. [T. Aaes-Jørgensen, *J. Chromatogr.* 1980, *183 B Biomed. Appl.*, *9*, 239–245.]

Toxicity

A 26-year-old man with mental illness and drug addiction was found dead. The total clopenthixol in peripheral blood was 0.455 mg/L, 0.7 mg/L in cardiac blood, 31.56 mg/L in gastric contents, and 0.735 mg/L in urine. The *cis*(*Z*)-isomer of the drug was found at a concentration of 0.455, 29.88, and 0.505 mg/L in cardiac blood, gastric contents, and urine, respectively. The *trans*(*E*)-isomer was found at concentrations of 0.245, 1.68 and 0.23 mg/L, respectively. [P. P. Rop, *J. Anal. Toxicol.*, 2001, *25(5)*, 348–352.]

A 16-year-old female was found dead. The *cis*(*Z*)-clopenthixol concentrations were 0.391, 0.957, and 105.4 mg/L, 0.75, 1.413, 5.21, and 0.12 ng/g in blood, urine, gastric contents, liver, kidney, lung, and brain, respectively. The *trans*(*E*)-clopenthixol concentrations were 0.275, 0.832, and 7.430 mg/L, 0.837, 2.380, 9.758, and 0.058 ng/g, respectively. [A. Tracqui *et al.*, *J. Anal. Toxicol.*, 1997, *21(4)*, 314–318.]

Dose. The equivalent of 20 to 150 mg of clopenthixol daily; up to 250 mg daily has been given.

Clopidogrel

Anti-platelet

Synonym. SR-25990

(αS)-α-(2-Chlorophenyl)-6,7-dihydrothieno[3,2-*c*]pyridine-5-(4*H*)-acetic acid methyl ester

$C_{16}H_{16}ClNO_2S = 321.8$

CAS—113665-84-2; 94188-84-8

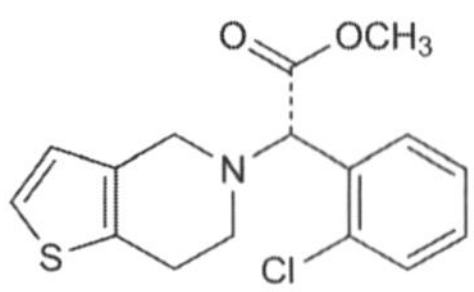

Clopidogrel Bisulfate

Synonyms. Clopidogrel Bisulphate; Clopidogrel Hydrogen Sulphate; SR-25990C

Proprietary name. Plavix

$C_{16}H_{16}ClNO_2S, H_2SO_4 = 419.9$

CAS—120202-66-6

A white to off-white powder. M.p. 184°. It is practically insoluble in water at neutral pH; freely soluble in water at pH 1, and in methanol; sparingly soluble in methylene chloride; practically insoluble in ethyl ether.

Gas Chromatography. Column: DB1 (30 m × 0.25 mm i.d., 0.1 μm film thickness). Column temperature: 120° then up to 290° at 30°/min, held for 3 min. Injector temperature: 290°. Carrier gas: helium, flow rate 40 cm/s. MS detection (CI (chemical ionisation), FS (full scan) mode). Retention time: clopidogrel (carboxylic acid derivative), 6.5 min. [P. Lagorce *et al.*, *J. Chromatogr. B, Biomed. Sci. Appl.*, 1998, *720*, 107–117].

Ultraviolet Spectrum. Aqueous acid—270, 278, 308 nm.

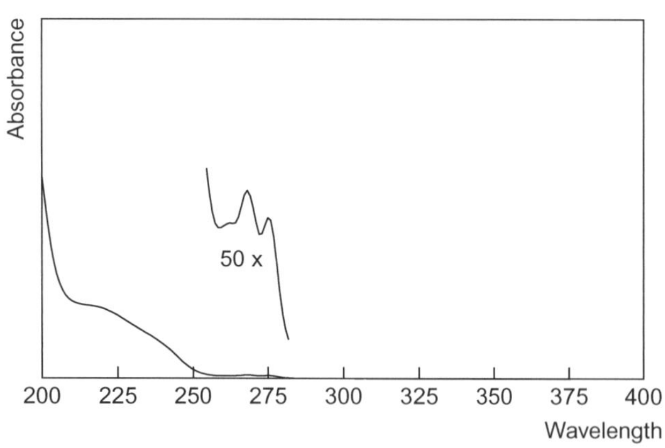

Mass Spectrum. Principal ions at *m/z* 262, 264, 110, 138, 125, 152, 89, 77 (clopidogrel bisulfate).

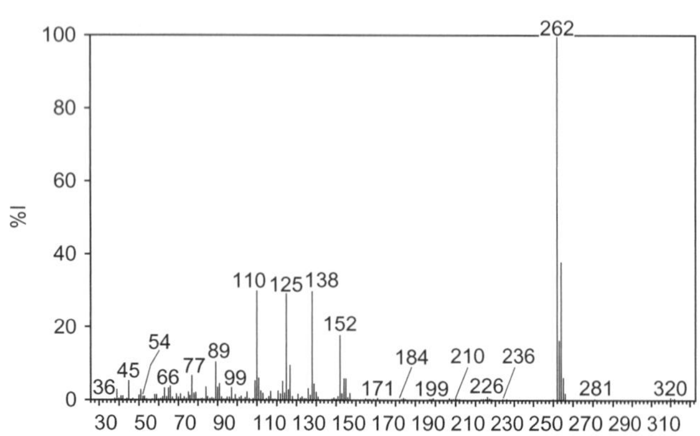

Quantification

Gas chromatography–mass spectrometry. In plasma and serum: limit of quantification 5 μg/L—P. Lagorce *et al.*, *J. Chromatogr. B, Biomed. Sci. Appl.*, 1998, *720*, 107–117.

Disposition in the Body. After oral administration, clopidogrel is rapidly, but incompletely (approx. 50%), absorbed. It is extensively metabolised in the liver to produce two metabolites, the main circulating metabolite (85%) being the inactive carboxylic acid derivative. Clopidogrel is oxidised to 2-oxo-clopidogrel with further hydrolysis to produce the active thiol derivative, which has not yet been identified in plasma. Clopidogrel and its metabolites are equally excreted in urine and faeces.

Therapeutic concentration

12 healthy males were administered with single oral doses of 50, 75, 100 and 150 mg. Plasma concentrations of the parent drug were very low, less than the quantification limit (0.00025 mg/L) and peak concentrations of the inactive metabolite reached approx. 1.6, 2.9, 3.1 mg/L, respectively, within 0.8 to 1 h. Steady state values (between 0.8 and 0.11 mg/L) were reached by the eighth day (75 mg/day). [H. Caplain *et al.*, *Semin. Thromb. Hemost.*, 1999, *25*, 25–28].

Toxicity. A single case of deliberate overdose, during clinical trials, has been reported. A 34-year-old woman swallowed a single dose of 1050 mg (equivalent to 14 standard 75 mg tablets) clopidogrel with no associated undesirable effects. No special therapy was needed.

Half-life. The elimination half-life of the inactive metabolite is approx. 8 h.

Clearance. 10 mg/L/h.

Protein binding. Clopidogrel and its inactive metabolite bind plasma proteins 98% and 94%, respectively.

Dose. A single oral daily dose of 75 mg.

Clopidol

Coccidiostat (Veterinary)

Synonyms. Clopindol; Meticlorpindol.

Proprietary name. Coyden

3,5-Dichloro-2,6-dimethyl-4-pyridinol

$C_7H_7Cl_2NO = 192.0$

CAS—2971-90-6

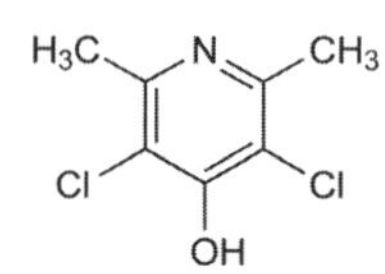

A white crystalline powder. M.p. greater than 320°.

Practically insoluble in water; slightly soluble in ethanol; soluble in methanol.

Partition Coefficient. Log *P* (octanol/water), 2.7.

Ultraviolet Spectrum. Ethanol—269 nm ($A_1^1 = 460b$).

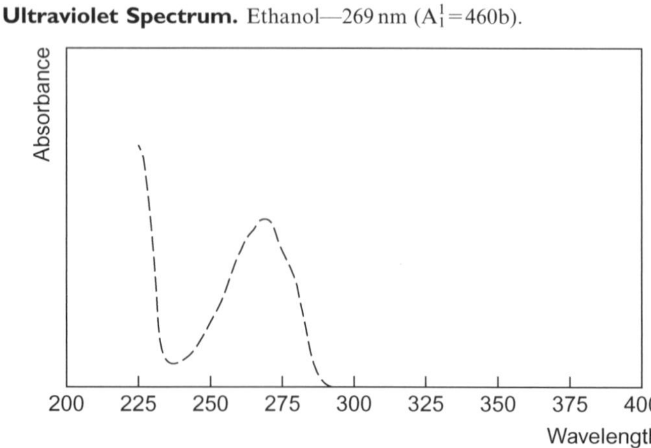

Infra-red Spectrum. Principal peaks at wavenumbers 1538, 1504, 753, 1618, 762, 1095 cm^{-1} (KBr disk).

Cloral Betaine *Hypnotic/Sedative*

1-Carboxy-*N*,*N*,*N*-trimethanaminium inner salt compound with 2,2,2-trichloro-1,1-ethanediol (1 : 1)
The adduct formed by cloral hydrate, $CCl_3{\cdot}CH(OH)_2$, and betaine, $C_5H_{11}NO_2$, containing about 58% of cloral hydrate.
$C_7H_{12}Cl_3NO_3,H_2O=282.6$
CAS—2218-68-0
A white crystalline powder. M.p. about 124°, with decomposition.
Soluble 1 in 1 of water and 1 in 4 of ethanol; practically insoluble in chloroform and ether.

Ultraviolet Spectrum. No significant absorption, 230 to 360 nm.

Infra-red Spectrum. Principal peaks at wavenumbers 840, 1630, 1085, 1130, 730, 1500 cm^{-1} (KBr disk).

Mass Spectrum. Principal ions at *m/z* 81, 83, 46, 110, 82, 112, 84, 117.

Dose. Usually 0.87 to 2.61 g daily, but doses of up to 3.5 g may be necessary.

Cloral Hydrate *Hypnotic/Sedative*

Synonym. Cloral; Chloral Hydrate
Proprietary names. Aquachloral; Chloradorm; Chloraldurat; Chloralex; Chloralvan; Dormel; Elix-Nocte; Escre; Medianox; Noctec; Novo-chlorhydrate; Nycton; Rectules; Somnos; Welldorm. Also an ingredient of Babygencal; Dermophil Indien; Synthol.
2,2,2-Trichloro-1,1-ethanediol
$C_2H_3Cl_3O_2=165.4$
CAS—302-17-0

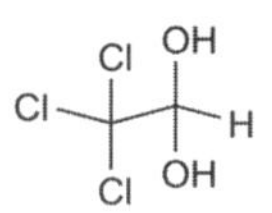

Colourless or white crystals which volatilise slowly on exposure to air and are decomposed by caustic alkalis, liberating chloroform. It liquefies between 50° and 58°. It boils at 98° with dissociation into water and trichloroacetaldehyde.
1 mL of water dissolves the following amounts of cloral hydrate: 2.4 g at 0°, 8.3 g at 25°, 14.3 g at 140°. Soluble: 1 in 0.2 of ethanol, 1 in 1.3 of alcohol, 1 in 2 of chloroform, 1 in 1.4 olive oil, 1 in 0.5 glycerol, 1 in 68 g carbon disulfide and 1 in 1.5 of ether. Freely soluble in acetone and methylethyl ketone. Moderately or sparingly soluble in turpentine, petroleum ether, carbon tetrachloride, benzene, and toluene. Ethanolic solutions may deposit crystals of cloral ethanolate.

Dissociation Constant. pK_a 10.0.

Partition Coefficient. Log *P* (octanol/water), 0.99.

Colour Tests. Fujiwara Test—red; Palladium Chloride—black.

Gas Chromatography. System GA—RI 695 (tailing peak); system GI—retention time 12.5 min (tailing peak).

Ultraviolet Spectrum. No significant absorption, 230 to 360 nm.

Infra-red Spectrum. Principal peaks at wavenumbers 835, 1083, 1300, 970, 1620 cm^{-1}.

Mass Spectrum. Principal peaks at *m/z* 82, 47, 84, 29, 111, 83, 113, 85; trichloroacetic acid 44, 83, 85, 36, 28, -, -, -; trichloroethanol 31, 49, 77, 113, 115, 82, 51, 117.

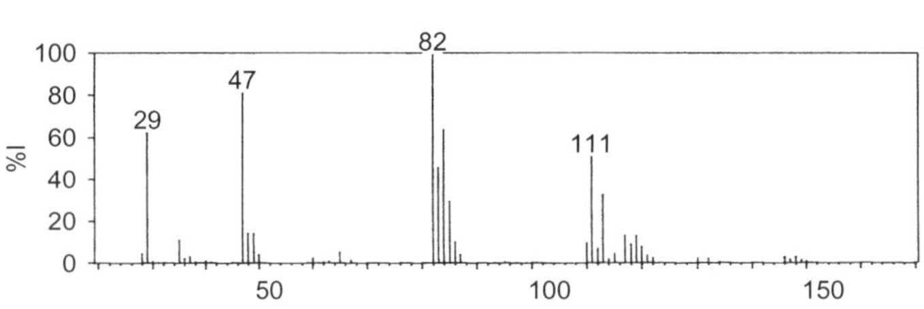

Quantification

Ultraviolet spectrophotometry. In blood or urine: trichloroethanol (modified Fujiwara reaction)—A. J. McBay *et al.*, *J. Anal. Toxicol.*, 1980, *4*, 99–101.

Gas chromatography. In blood: ECD—E. Meyer *et al.*, *J. Anal. Toxicol.*, 1995, *19*, 124–126. In plasma or urine: trichloroethanol, ECD—D. J. Berry, *J. Chromatogr.*, 1975, *107*, 107–114. In blood or urine: cloral hydrate, trichloroethanol, and trichloroacetic acid, head-space analysis, limit of detection 500 μg/L for cloral hydrate and trichloroethanol, ECD—D. D. Breimer *et al.*, *J. Chromatogr.*, 1974, *88*, 55–63.

Gas chromatography–mass spectrometry. In plasma: cloral hydrate and metabolites. MS detection—Z. Yan *et al.*, *J. Pharm. Biomed. Anal.*, 1999, *19*, 309–318.

Disposition in the Body. Readily absorbed following oral administration. It is rapidly metabolised by reduction to trichloroethanol, the major active metabolite, which is further metabolised by conjugation with glucuronic acid to give urochloralic acid and by oxidation to trichloroacetic acid, the major urinary metabolite. Trichloroethanol passes into the CSF, into breast milk, and across the placenta. About 10 to 30% of a dose is excreted in the urine as urochloralic acid and up to 5% as trichloroethanol in 24 h. Trichloroacetic acid is slowly excreted in urine over several days; a small amount of urochloralic acid may be excreted in the bile.

Therapeutic concentration. Cloral hydrate is difficult to detect in body fluids after normal doses. The plasma concentration of trichloroethanol is usually in the range 1.5 to 15 mg/L. Trichloroacetic acid and urochloralic acid are present in plasma at concentrations similar to, or greater than, those of trichloroethanol. When alcohol has been taken, peak plasma concentrations of trichloroethanol are increased and remain elevated for about 6 h after ingestion, and those of trichloroacetic acid are decreased. Trichloroacetic acid accumulates in the plasma during chronic administration of cloral hydrate.

Following a single oral dose of 825 mg to 5 subjects, peak plasma trichloroethanol concentrations of 7.6 to 12.2 mg/L (mean 9.7) were attained in 0.5 to 1 h. [D. J. Berry, *J. Chromatogr.*, 1975, *107*, 107–114.]

Toxicity. Fatalities have occurred following the ingestion of 1.25 and 3 g but recovery has occurred after ingestion of 30 g. Plasma concentrations greater than 40 mg/L of trichloroethanol are likely to produce toxic effects; fatalities have been reported at blood concentrations of 20 to 495 mg/L (mean 155) of trichloroethanol.

In a fatality caused by the admistration of cloral hydrate, lidocaine, and nitrous oxide, postmortem trichloroethanol concentrations were: plasma, 79.0 mg/L; urine, 31.0 mg/L; gastric contents, 454.0 mg/L; bile, 111.0 mg/L; vitreous humour, 40.2 mg/L; CSF, 68.3 mg/L; and liver, 164 mg/kg. Lidocaine concentrations ranged from 3.7 mg/L in urine to 19.0 mg /L in bile. Nitrous oxide was measured at 4.4 mL/L in blood. [D. A. Engelhart *et al*, *J. Anal. Toxicol.*, 1998, *22*, 246–247.]

In 4 fatalities known to involve the acute ingestion of 15 to 30 g of cloral hydrate, postmortem blood trichloroethanol concentrations ranged from 100 to 640 mg/L (mean 265). [R. C. Baselt and R. H. Cravey, *J. Anal. Toxicol.*, 1977, *1*, 81–103.]

In a fatality due to the ingestion of cloral hydrate, the following postmortem tissue concentrations of trichloroethanol were reported: blood 55 mg/L, brain 91 mg/kg, liver 200 mg/kg, urine 30 mg/L. [A. Poklis *et al.*, *Bull. Int. Assoc. Forensic Toxicol.*, 1973, *9(3 and 4)*, 8–9.]

Half-life. Plasma half-life, cloral hydrate about 4 min, trichloroethanol about 7 to 11 h, urochloralic acid about 7 h, trichloroacetic acid about 4 days.

Volume of distribution. Trichloroethanol, about 0.6 L/kg.

Distribution in blood. Plasma:whole blood ratio, trichloroethanol, about 0.9.

Protein binding. In plasma, trichloroethanol 35% and trichloroacetic acid 94%.

Note. For a review of the pharmacokinetics of sedatives in neonates see E. Jacqz-Aigrain and P. Burtin, *Clin. Pharmacokinet.*, 1996, *31*, 423–443; for a review of the pharmacokinetics of hypnotic drugs see D. D. Breimer, *Clin. Pharmacokinet.*, 1977, *2*, 93–109.

Dose. 0.5 to 2 g daily. Children may be given 30 to 50 mg/kg body-weight with a maximum single dose of 1 g.

Clorazepic Acid

Tranquilliser

7-Chloro-2,3-dihydro-2-oxo-5-phenyl-1*H*-1,4-benzodiazepine-3-carboxylic acid
$C_{16}H_{11}ClN_2O_3$=314.7
CAS—23887-31-2

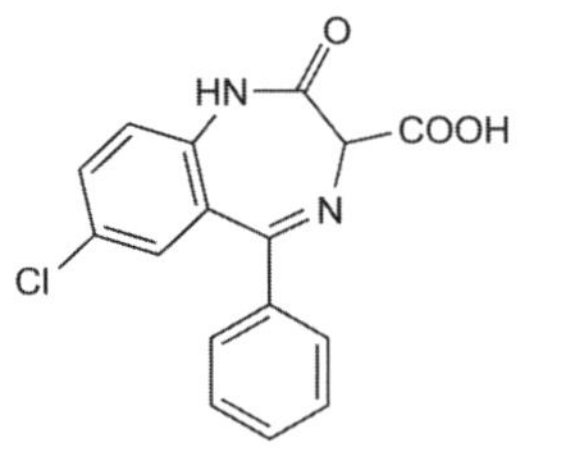

Clorazepate Dipotassium

Synonyms. Abbott 35616; AH-3232; CB-4306; Clorazepate Dipotassium; Potassium Clorazepate.
Proprietary names. Belseren; Clorazecaps; Clorazetabs; Dorken; Gen-Xene; Medipax; Mendon; Nansius; Novo-Clopate; Transene; Tranxen(e); Tranxilen(e); Tranxilium. It is an ingredient of Dorken and Noctran.
$C_{16}H_{10}ClKN_2O_3$,KOH=408.9
CAS—57109-90-7
A fine off-white powder.
Freely soluble in water, very poorly soluble in ethanol. Practically insoluble in ether and chloroform. In aqueous solution, it converts to the monopotassium salt.

Clorazepate Monopotassium

Synonym. CB-4311
Proprietary name. Azene
$C_{16}H_{10}ClKN_2O_3$=352.8
CAS—5991-71-9
A fine, off-white powder.
Very soluble in water; practically insoluble in organic solvents.

Dissociation Constant. pK_a 3.5, 12.5.

Partition Coefficient. Log *P* (octanol/water), 2.05.

Colour Test. Formaldehyde–Sulfuric Acid—orange.

Thin-layer Chromatography. System TA—Rf 84; system TB—Rf 03; system TC—Rf 56; system TD—Rf 34; system TE—Rf 68; system TF—Rf 46; system TL—Rf 60; system TAD—Rf 57; system TAE—Rf 83; system TAF—Rf 87.

Gas Chromatography. System GA—clorazepic acid RI 2457, nordazepam RI 2490, oxazepam RI 2325; system GB—clorazepic acid RI 2618, nordazepam RI 2625, oxazepam RI 2438; system GG—clorazepic acid RI 3125, nordazepam RI 3041, oxazepam RI 2803.

High Performance Liquid Chromatography. System HI—*k* 1.17; system HK—*k* 2.00; system HX—RI 475; system HY—RI 388; system HZ—retention time 5.6 min; system HAA—clorazepate retention time 18.4 min; system HBH—*k* 8.22; system HBI—*k* 1.84.

Ultraviolet Spectrum. Dipotassium clorazepate: aqueous acid—237 nm (A_1^1=747b), 287 nm.

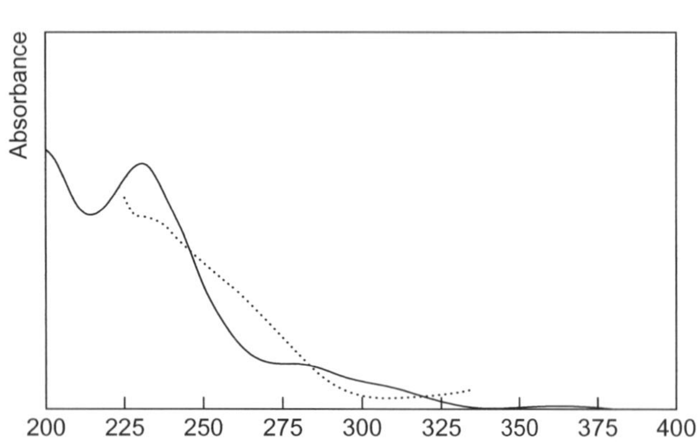

Infra-red Spectrum. Principal peaks at wavenumbers 1597, 1548, 1300, 702, 1230, 830 cm^{-1} (dipotassium clorazepate, KBr disk).

Mass Spectrum. Principal ions at *m/z* 242, 43, 270, 269, 241, 103, 243, 76.

Quantification
Gas chromatography. In blood or urine: clorazepic acid and desmethyldiazepam, limits of detection 4 μg/L in blood and 5 μg/L in urine, ECD; also oxazepam in urine 25 μg/L, ECD—M. A. Brooks *et al., J. Chromatogr.*, 1977, *135*, 123–131.

High performance liquid chromatography. In plasma: clorazepate dipotassium and desmethyldiazepam, UV detection—P. Colin et al., *J. Chromatogr.* 1983, 273(24) *B Biomed. Appl.*, 367–377.

Disposition in the Body. Rapidly decarboxylated below pH 4 to the active metabolite desmethyldiazepam (nordazepam), and thus is absorbed mainly as desmethyldiazepam after oral administration; this is then hydroxylated to form oxazepam which is conjugated with glucuronic acid. Up to about 10% of a dose is excreted in urine in 24 h, mainly as oxazepam glucuronide, together with small amounts of unchanged clorazepate and conjugated desmethyldiazepam. Oxazepam glucuronide is still detectable in urine 12 days after a single dose. Small amounts of clorazepic acid and its metabolites are excreted in breast milk.

Therapeutic concentration

Following a single oral dose of 15 mg to 4 subjects, peak blood concentrations of desmethyldiazepam of 0.14 to 0.18 mg/L (mean 0.16) were attained in 0.5 to 1 h; peak blood-clorazepate concentrations of 0.03 to 0.11 mg/L (mean 0.06) were reported at about 1 h. [C. W. Abruzzo *et al., J. Pharmacokinet. Biopharm.*, 1977, *5*, 377–390.]

Average steady-state serum concentrations of 0.40 to 0.61 mg/L (mean 0.48) of desmethyldiazepam were reported in 7 patients receiving daily oral doses of 0.6 mg/kg. [A. J. Wilensky *et al., Clin. Pharmacol. Ther.*, 1978, *24*, 22–30.]

Toxicity. Fatalities from overdosage are rare and recovery from an overdose of 600 mg has been reported.

Half-life. Plasma half-life, clorazepate about 2 h, desmethyldiazepam about 40 to 100 h but there is considerable intersubject variation—see under Nordazepam.

Volume of distribution. Desmethyldiazepam 0.5 to 2.5 L/ kg, increased in elderly subjects.

Clearance. Plasma clearance, desmethyldiazepam about 0.1 to 0.3 mL/min/kg.

Distribution in blood. Plasma:whole blood ratio, desmethyldiazepam 1.7.

Protein binding. In plasma, desmethyldiazepam about 91%.

Dose. 7.5 to 22.5 mg of dipotassium clorazepate daily; up to 60 mg daily has been given.

Clorexolone

Diuretic

Proprietary name. Flonatril; Nefrolan
6-Chloro-2-cyclohexyl-2,3-dihydro-3-oxo-1*H*-isoindole-5-sulfonamide
$C_{14}H_{17}ClN_2O_3S$=328.8
CAS—2127-01-7

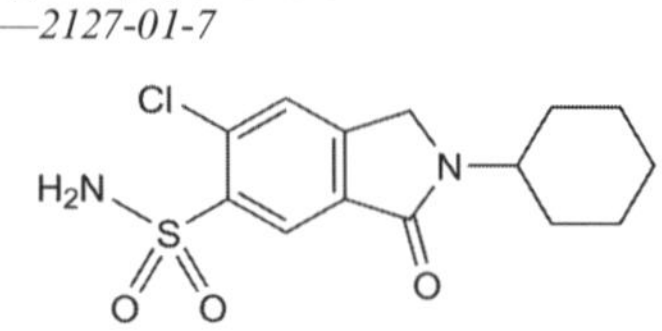

A white crystalline powder. M.p. 266° to 268°.
Very slightly soluble in water; soluble in dimethylformamide, methanol, and solutions of alkali hydroxides.

Partition Coefficient. Log *P* (octanol/water), 2.0.

Colour Test. Koppanyi–Zwikker Test—violet.

Thin-layer Chromatography. System TA—Rf 76; system TD—Rf 31; system TE—Rf 60; system TF—Rf 51; system TAD—Rf 47; system TAE—Rf 79. (Acidified iodoplatinate solution, positive.)

Gas Chromatography. System GA—RI 3194.

High Performance Liquid Chromatography. System HN—*k* 7.26; system HY—RI 391.

Ultraviolet Spectrum. Ethanol—252 nm (A_1^1=246a).

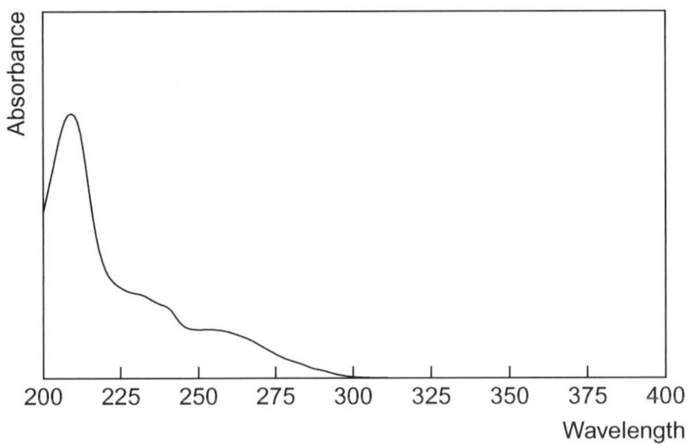

Infra-red Spectrum. Principal peaks at wavenumbers 1661, 1172, 1234, 1149, 978, 1613 cm^{-1} (KBr disk).

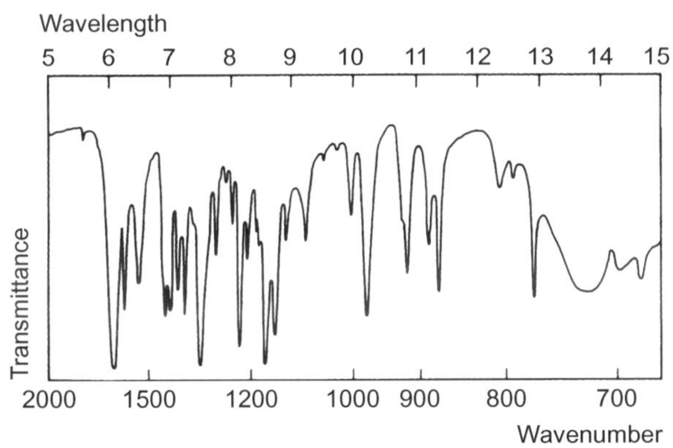

Mass Spectrum. Principal ions at *m/z* 247, 285, 328, 249, 41, 287, 330, 55.

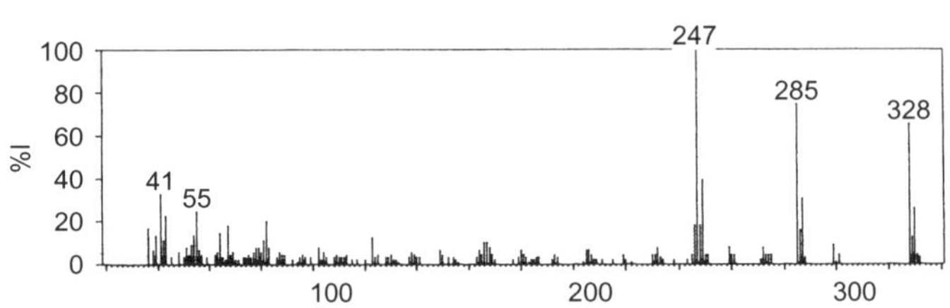

Disposition in the Body. Absorbed after oral administration. It is almost completely excreted in the urine in 48 h as three cyclohexane ring-hydroxylated metabolites.

Dose. 10 to 100 mg daily.

Clorgiline

Antidepressant

Synonym. Clorgyline
N-[3-(2,4-Dichlorophenoxy)propyl]-*N*-methylprop-2-ynylamine
$C_{13}H_{15}Cl_2NO$=272.2
CAS—17780-72-2

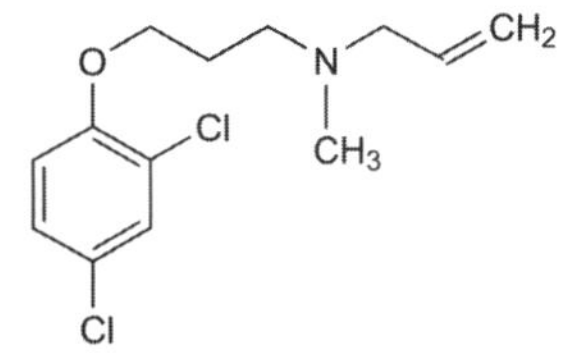

Clorgiline Hydrochloride

$C_{13}H_{15}Cl_2NO,HCl$=308.6
CAS—17780-75-5
A white crystalline powder. M.p. 102° to 103°.
Very soluble in water; soluble in chloroform.

Colour Test. Liebermann's Test—black.

Thin-layer Chromatography. System TA—Rf 67; system TB—Rf 42; system TC—Rf 70; system TL—Rf 59. (Acidified iodoplatinate solution, positive.)

Gas Chromatography. System GA—RI 1883.

Ultraviolet Spectrum. Aqueous acid—228 (A_1^1=310b), 282 nm.

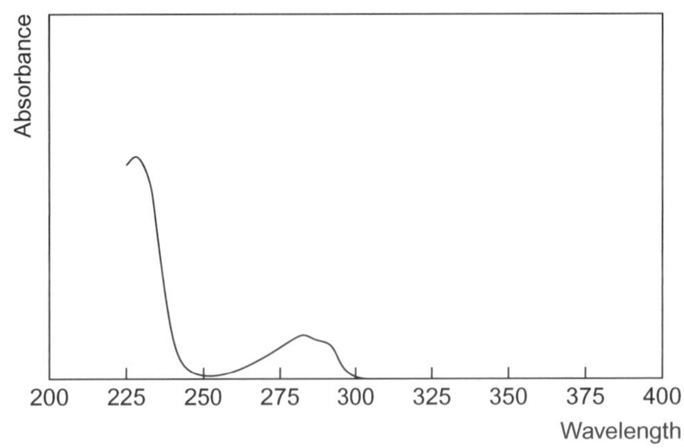

Infra-red Spectrum. Principal peaks at wavenumbers 1280, 1250, 1055, 1099, 801, 1124 cm^{-1}.

Dose. Clorgiline hydrochloride has been tried in doses of 10 to 30 mg daily.

Cloricromen

Antithrombotic/Vasodilator (Coronary)

Synonym. 8-Chlorocarbocromen; AD_6.
[[8-Chloro-3-[2-(diethylamino)ethyl]-4-methyl-2-oxo-2*H*-1-benzopyran-7-yl]oxy]acetic acid ethyl ester
$C_{20}H_{26}ClNO_5$=395.9
CAS—68206-94-0

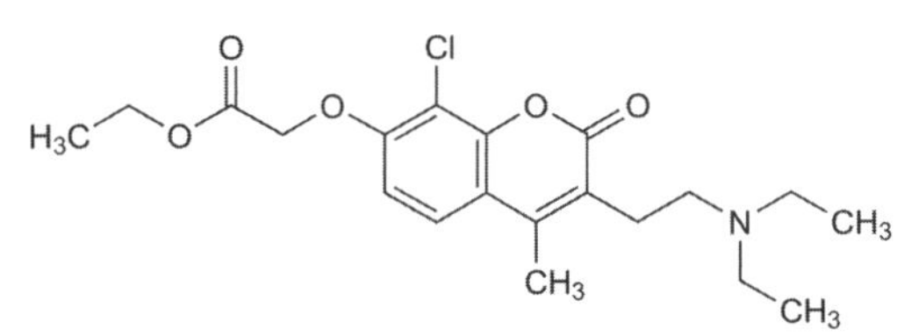

Crystals. M.p. 147° to 148° (from ethyl acetate).

Cloricromen Hydrochloride

Proprietary names. Cromocap; Proendotel.
$C_{20}H_{25}ClNO_5,HCl$=432.3
CAS—74697-28-2
M.p. 219° to 220°.

Quantification

High Performance Liquid Chromatography. In biological samples: fluorescence detection (λ_{ex}=310 nm; λ_{em}=390 nm)—R. Mariot *et al.*, *J. Chromatogr.*, 1992, *576*, 143–148.

Note. For studies on the molecular aspects of cloricromen distribution in human platelets and its pharmacological effects, see R. A. Travagli *et al.*, *Thromb. Res.*, 1989, *54*, 327–338.

Dose. Orally, 100 mg two or three time daily or IV in a dose of 30 mg daily.

Clorprenaline

Sympathomimetic

Synonyms. Chlorprenaline; Isoprofenamine; Isoprophenamine.
2-Chloro-α-[[(1-methylethyl)amino]methyl]benzenemethanol
$C_{11}H_{16}ClNO=213.7$
CAS—3811-25-4

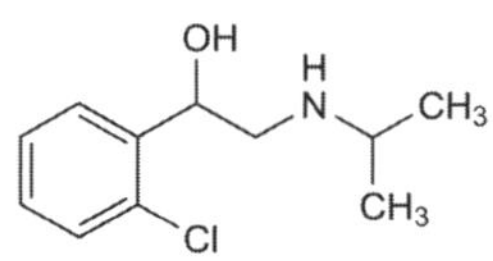

Soluble in chloroform.

Clorprenaline Hydrochloride

Proprietary names. Broncon; Clopinerin; Conselt; Fusca; Katulein; Pentadoll; Restanolon.
$C_{11}H_{16}ClNO,HCl,H_2O=268.2$
CAS—6933-90-0 (anhydrous); 5588-22-7 (monohydrate)
White crystals. M.p. 163° to 164° (monohydrate).
Soluble in water.

Partition Coefficient. Log *P* (octanol/water), 1.82.

Thin-layer Chromatography. System TA—Rf 57; system TB—Rf 18; system TC—Rf 15; system TL—Rf 20. (Acidified potassium permanganate solution, positive.)

Gas Chromatography. System GA—RI 1604; system GB—RI 1614; system GC—RI 1880.

High Performance Liquid Chromatography. System HA—*k* 1.1.

Ultraviolet Spectrum. Aqueous acid—262, 266 nm ($A_1^1=10.1$b).

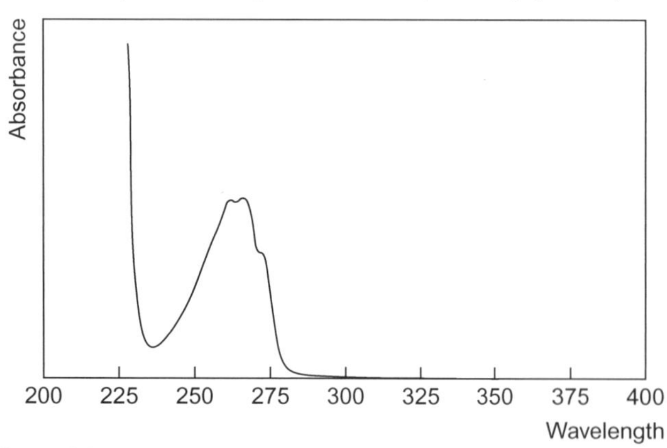

Infra-red Spectrum. Principal peaks at wavenumbers 1075, 775, 1587, 1041, 1030, 1123 cm^{-1}.

Mass Spectrum. Principal ions at *m/z* 72, 30, 43, 77, 73, 51, 41, 27.

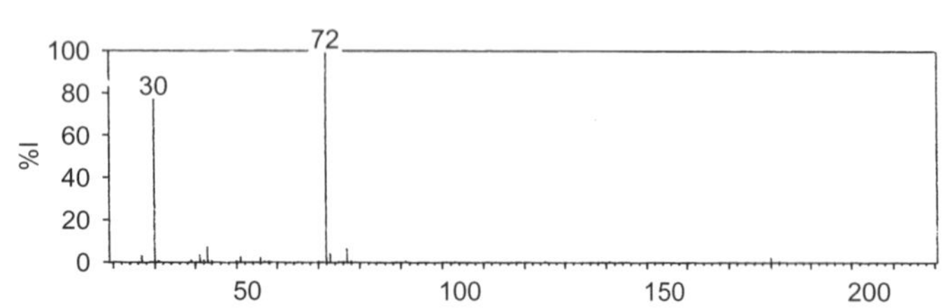

Quantification

High performance liquid chromatography. In plasma: clorprenaline enantiomers, limit of quantification 1 ng—T. Miwa *et al.*, *J. Chromatogr.*, 1991, *566*, 163–171.

Dose. Clorprenaline hydrochloride has been given in doses of 30 to 80 mg daily.

Clospipramine

Anti-psychotic

Synonym. Mosapramine.
1′-[3-(3-Chloro-10,11-dihydro-5*H*-dibenz[*b,f*]azepin-5-yl)propyl]-hexahydrospiro[imidazo[1,2-*a*]pyridine-3(2*H*),4′-piperidin]-2-one
$C_{28}H_{35}ClN_4O=479.1$
CAS—89419-40-9

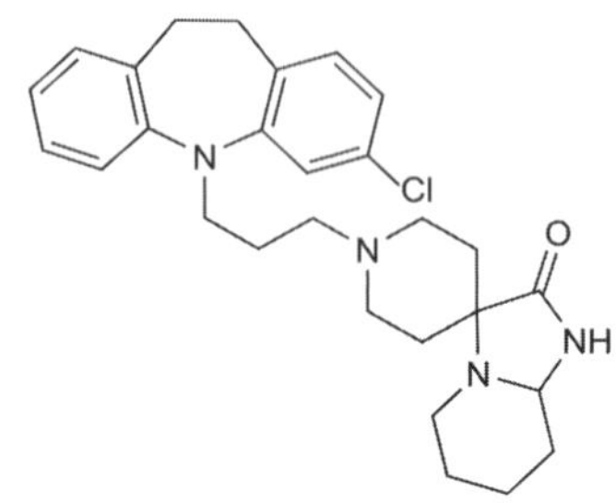

Clospipramine Dihydrochloride

Synonym. Mosapramine dihydrochloride.
Proprietary names. Cremin; Y-516.
$C_{28}H_{35}ClN_4O.2HCl=552.0$
CAS—98043-60-8
A white to slightly creamy white, odourless crystalline powder. M.p. 271°. It is freely soluble in formic acid; slightly soluble in water, methanol, ethanol and dimethylformamide; practically insoluble in acetonitrile, acetic anhydride and ether.

Quantification

High performance liquid chromatography. In plasma and urine: limit of detection of clospipramine is 1 μg/L and 20 μg/L, respectively. UV detection (λ=257 nm)—J. Ishigooka *et al.*, *Psychopharmacology*, 1989, *97*, 303–308.

Disposition in the Body. Clospipramine dihydrochloride is metabolised, mainly in the liver, by hydrogenation at the spiroamine site and hydroxylation at the iminodibenzyl ring to produce two metabolites. Excretion is mainly via bile but drug has also been recovered in faeces and urine (rate urinary excretion <0.5%).

Therapeutic concentration

5 healthy males, aged between 22 and 44 years, were administered orally with single doses of 6.25, 12.5 and 25 mg. Plasma concentrations reached a maximum of 7.9 ± 1.7 μg/L within 6.0 ± 1.4 h. Plasma concentrations are dose dependent and decrease in a monophasic manner. [J. Ishigooka *et al.*, *Psychopharmacology*, 1989, *97*, 303–308].

Half-life. 15 h.

Clearance. 130 to 170 L/h.

Dose. Usual dose of 30 to150 mg/day is administered as three separate doses. Dose may be increased to 300 mg/day.

Clostebol

Anabolic Steroid

Synonym. 4-Chlorotestosterone
(17*β*)-4-Chloro-17-hydroxyandrost-4-en-3-one
$C_{19}H_{27}ClO_2=322.9$
CAS—1093-58-9

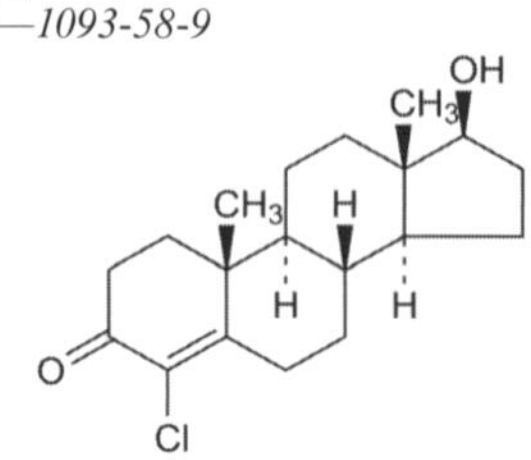

Crystals. M.p. 188° to 190° (from acetone and hexane).

Clostebol Acetate

Synonyms. Chlortestosterone Acetate; 4-Chlorotestosterone Acetate.
Proprietary names. Alfa-Trofodermine; Macrobin; Megagrisent Mono; Steranabol; Trofodermin; Trofoseptine.
$C_{21}H_{29}ClO_3$=364.9
CAS—855-19-6
M.p. 228° to 230°.
Soluble in ethanol.

Partition Coefficient. Log *P* (octanol/water), 3.76.

Colour Test. Zimmerman Test—blue

Gas Chromatography. System GA—clostebol acetate RI 2965, clostebol acetate-TMS RI 2870, clostebol enol-TMS_2 RI 2830, clostebol-HCl-AC RI 2700, clostebol-HCl-TMS RI 2675, clostebol-HCl enol-TMS_2 RI 2640.

Column: silica cross linked with 5% phenylmethylsilicone (DB5 or Ultra 2). Column temperature: 100°, held 1 min, 100° to 230° at 40°/min, 230° to 280° at 5°/min, held 15 min. Carrier gas: helium. MS detection. Internal standard: 4-chloroandrost-4-en-3α-ol-17-one. Retention time: 15.6 min. [D. Debruyckere *et al.*, *Anal. Chim. Acta*, 1994, *291*, 155–160.]

Column: methyl silicone (HP1, 0.2 mm i.d., 0.33 µm film thickness). Column temperature: 280°. Carrier gas: helium, flow rate 0.9 mL/min. MS detection. RI: 3023. [T. Mills and J. C. Roberson, *Instrumental Data for Drug Analysis*, 2nd Edn., CRC Press, Boca Raton, FL, Vol. 5, 1993, pp. 126–127.]

High Performance Liquid Chromatography. System HAR—clostebol acetate RRT 1.90 (relative to testosterone).

Column: ODS Hypersil (100 × 4.6 mm i.d., 5 µm). Mobile phase: methanol:aqueous 0.01 M dihydrogen potassium phosphate buffer, adjusted to pH 3.5 with 85% phosphoric acid (90:10), flow rate 1 mL/min. UV diode array detection. Retention time: 4.6 min. [T. Mills and J. C. Roberson, *Instrumental data for drug analysis*, 2nd Edn., CRC Press, Vol. 5, pp. 126–127.]

Ultraviolet Spectrum. (Clostebol acetate) ethanol—254 nm.

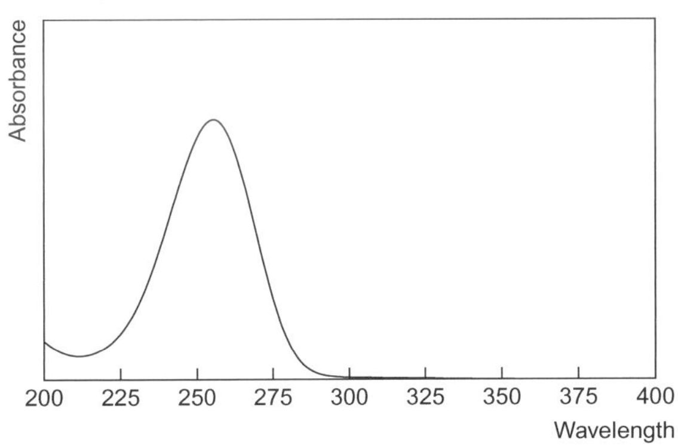

Infra-red Spectrum. Clostebol acetate: principal peaks at wavenumbers 1727, 1683, 1251 cm^{-1} (KBr disks).

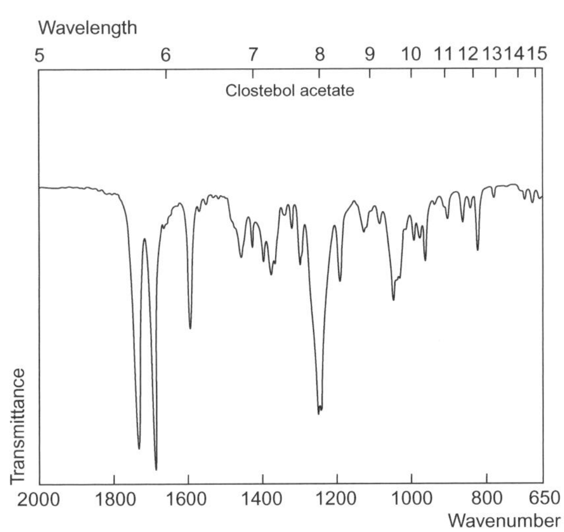

Mass Spectrum. Clostebol acetate: principal ions at *m/z* 43, 147, 158, 91, 328, 55, 93, 79.

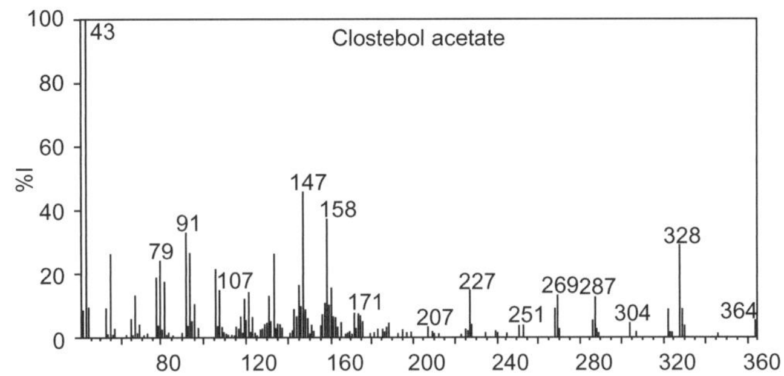

Quantification

Gas chromatography–mass spectrometry. In urine: limit of quantification 0.8 µg/L—M. Walshe *et al.*, *Analyst*, 1998, *123*, 2687–2691.

Enzyme immunoassay. In urine: limit of quantification 25 µg/L—M. Walshe *et al.*, *Analyst*, 1998, *123*, 2687–2691.

Disposition in the Body. A high percentage of clostebol acetate is absorbed after oral administration and possibly inactivated. Clostebol is metabolised to 4-chloro-Δ-4-androstene-3α-ol-17-one, which can be detected in urine along with additional 17-ketosteroid metabolites and 4-chlorotestosterone alcohol. Free 4-chlorotestosterone acetate can be detected in faeces but never in urine. Distributed in breast milk.

Dose. 30 mg dose administered weekly (intramuscular injection) or 15 mg 2 or 3 times daily (orally).

Clotiapine

Tranquilliser

Synonym. Clothiapine
Proprietary names. Entumin(e); Entumin.
2-Chloro-11-(4-methyl-1-piperazinyl)dibenzo[*b,f*][1,4]thiazepine
$C_{18}H_{18}ClN_3S$=343.9
CAS—2058-52-8

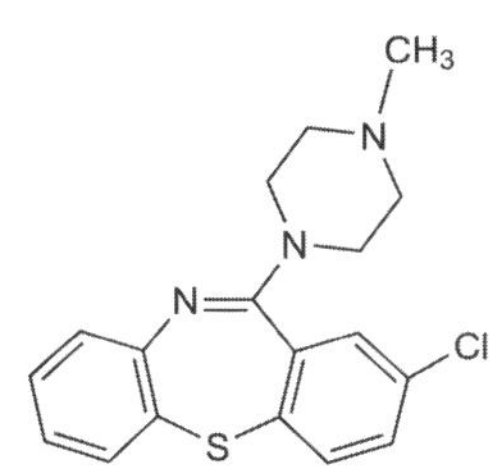

Crystals. M.p. 116° to 122°.
Soluble 1 in 10 of hydrochloric acid.

Partition Coefficient. Log *P* (octanol/water), 3.8.

Thin-layer Chromatography. System TA—Rf 59; system TB—Rf 41; system TC—Rf 59; system TL—Rf 23. (Acidified iodoplatinate solution, positive.)

Gas chromatography. System GA—clotiapine RI 2712, M (OH-)-AC RI 3000, M (nor-)-AC RI 3030, M (nor-OH-)-AC_2 RI 3400, M (oxo-) RI 3030; system GB—clotiapine RI 2833, M (nor-) RI 2882.

High Performance Liquid Chromatography. System HY—RI 348.

Ultraviolet Spectrum. Aqueous acid—213, 297 nm.

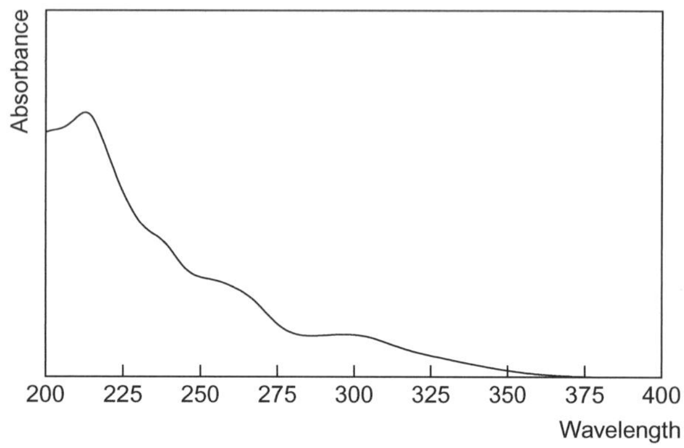

Infra-red Spectrum. Principal peaks at wavenumbers 1596, 1570, 1548, 1295, 757, 1234 cm^{-1} (KBr disk).

Mass Spectrum. Principal ions at *m/z* 83, 70, 273, 244, 209, 42, 71, 43.

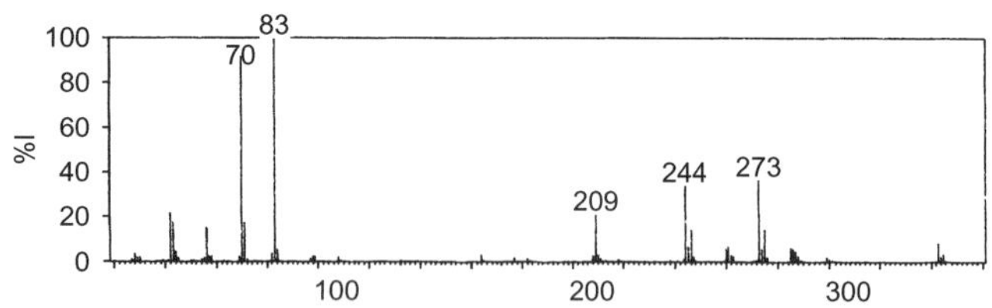

Dose. Clotiapine has been given in doses of 40 to 120 mg daily.

Clotrimazole

Antifungal

Synonym. Chlortritylimidazol
Proprietary names. Canesten; Eparol; Gyne-Lotrimin; Lotrimin; Mycelex; Trimysten.
1-[(2-Chlorophenyl)diphenylmethyl]-1*H*-imidazole
$C_{22}H_{17}ClN_2$=344.8
CAS—23593-75-1

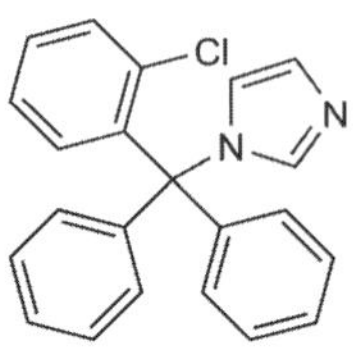

A white to pale yellow crystalline powder. M.p. 147° to 149°.
Slightly soluble in water, benzene, and toluene; freely soluble in ethanol; soluble in acetone, chloroform, and ethyl acetate; slightly soluble in ether.

Partition Coefficient. Log *P* (octanol/water), 6.3.

Thin-layer Chromatography. System TE—Rf 76; system TAD—Rf 68; system TAE—Rf 80.

Gas Chromatography. System GA—RI 2800.

Ultraviolet Spectrum. Methanol—254, 260 nm (A^1_1=20b).

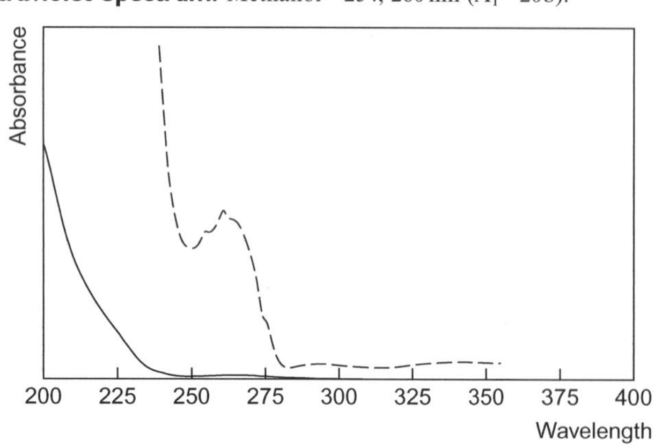

Infra-red Spectrum. Principal peaks at wavenumbers 765, 752, 708, 1075, 741, 1205 cm^{-1} (KBr disk). (See below)

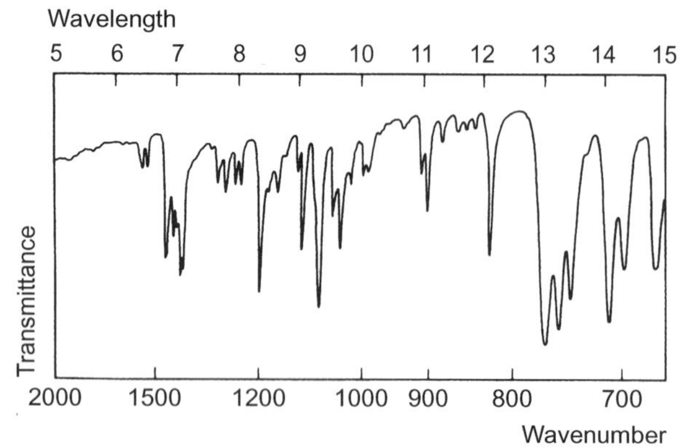

Mass Spectrum. Principal ions at *m/z* 277, 279, 165, 278, 241, 239, 242, 240.

Uses. Topically in a concentration of 1 or 2% or as vaginal tablets.

Cloxacillin

Antibiotic

(2*S*,5*R*,6*R*)-6-[[[3-(2-Chlorophenyl)-5-methyl-4-isoxazolyl]carbonyl]-amino]-3,3-dimethyl-7-oxo-4-thia-1-azabicyclo[3.2.0]heptane-2-carboxylic acid
$C_{19}H_{18}ClN_3O_5S$=435.9
CAS—61-72-3

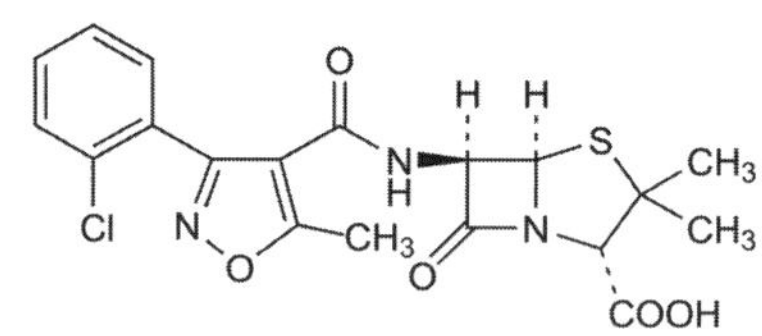

Cloxacillin Sodium

Proprietary names. Austrastaph; Bactopen; Cloxapen; Cloxilean; Cloxypen; Ekvacillin; Novocloxin; Orbenin(e); Staphybiotic; Tegopen. It is an ingredient of Ampiclox.
$C_{19}H_{17}ClN_3NaO_5S,H_2O$=475.9
CAS—642-78-4 (anhydrous); 7081-44-9 (monohydrate)
A white, hygroscopic, crystalline powder. M.p. 170° with decomposition.
Soluble 1 in 2.5 of water, 1 in 30 of ethanol, and 1 in 500 of chloroform. Soluble in pyridine and ethylene glycol.

Dissociation Constant. pK_a 2.7 (25°).

Partition Coefficient. Log *P* (octanol/water), 2.5.

Ultraviolet Spectrum. No significant absorption between 200 and 400 nm.

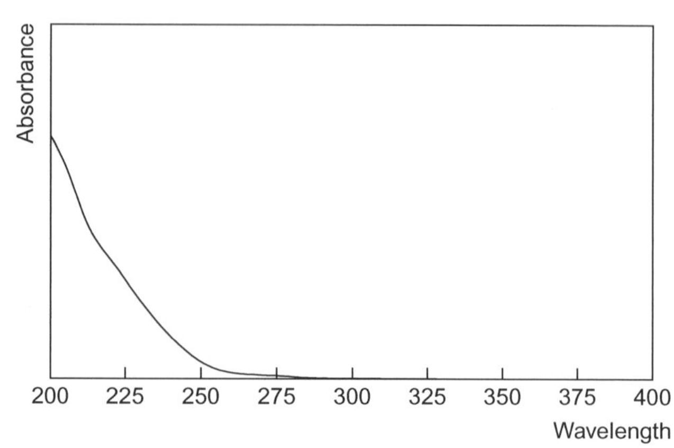

Infra-red Spectrum. Principal peaks at wavenumbers 1598, 1620, 1765, 1495, 1659, 771 cm^{-1} (cloxacillin sodium, KBr disk).

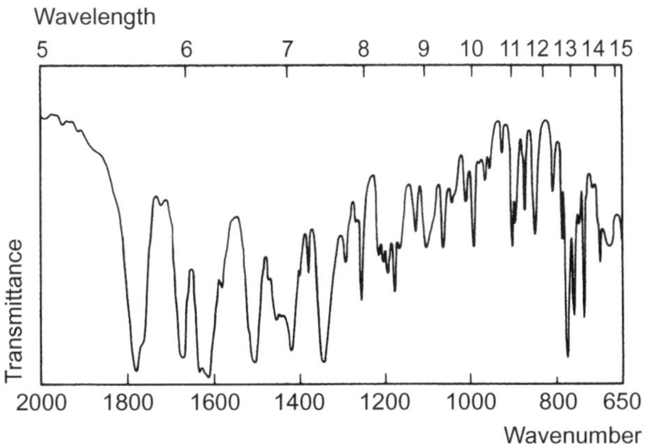

Quantification

High performance liquid chromatography. In serum or urine: limit of detection 50 mg/L, UV detection—F. W. Teare *et al.*, *J. Pharm. Sci.*, 1982, *71*, 938–941. In serum: limit of detection 500 mg/L, UV detection—S. J. Soldin *et al.*, *Ther. Drug Monit.*, 1980, *2*, 417–422.

Disposition in the Body. Incompletely absorbed after oral administration. About 35% of an oral dose is excreted in the urine unchanged in 12 h, together with about 11% as penicilloic acid; about 10% of a dose is excreted in the bile.

Half-life. Plasma half-life, about 0.5 to 1.5 h.

Volume of distribution. About 0.1 L/kg.

Protein binding. In plasma, about 94%.

Dose. Usually the equivalent of 2 g of cloxacillin daily.

Clozapine

Antipsychotic

Synonyms. Clozapinum; HF-1854.
Proprietary names. Clopine; Clopsine; Clozaril; Elcrit; Froidir; Leponex.
8-Chloro-11-(4-methyl-1-piperazinyl)-5*H*-dibenzo[*b*,*e*][1,4]diazepine
$C_{18}H_{19}ClN_4$=326.8
CAS—5786-21-0

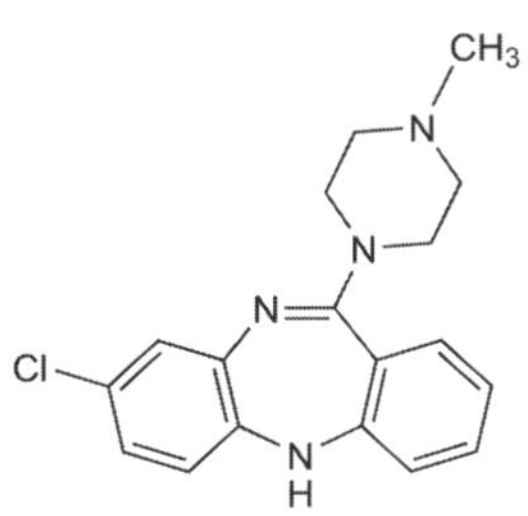

Yellow crystals. M.p. about 183°.
Soluble in chloroform; slightly soluble in acetone, acetonitrile, ethyl acetate, and ethanol; practically insoluble in water.

Dissociation Constant. pK$_a$ 3.70, 7.60.

Partition Coefficient. Log *P* (octanol/water), 3.23.

Colour Tests. Formaldehyde–Sulfuric Acid—yellow.
Cold nitric acid gives a red colour.

Thin-layer Chromatography. System TA—Rf 57; system TB—Rf 04; system TC—Rf 38; system TD—Rf 04; system TE—Rf 55; system TF—Rf 05; system TL—Rf 17; system TAD—Rf 29; system TAE—Rf 42.

Gas Chromatography. System GA—clozapine RI 2895, M (nor-) RI 3105, M (nor-acetyl-) RI 3490; system GB—clozapine RI 3024, M (nor-) RI 3092, M (nor-acetyl-) RI 3609; system GG—RI 3455.

High Performance Liquid Chromatography. System HX—RI 368; system HY—RI 284; system HZ—retention time 3.9 min; system HAX—retention time 10.9 min; system HAY—retention time 5.2 min.

Ultraviolet Spectrum. Aqueous acid—245, 297 nm; aqueous alkali—238, 261, 297 nm.

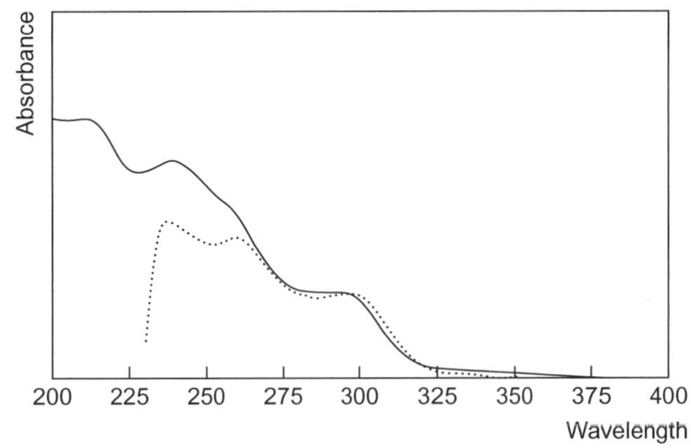

Infra-red Spectrum. Principal peaks at wavenumbers 1600, 1560, 758, 1136, 1101, 1117 cm^{-1}.

Mass Spectrum. Principal ions at *m/z* 243, 256, 70, 245, 192, 227, 258, 326.

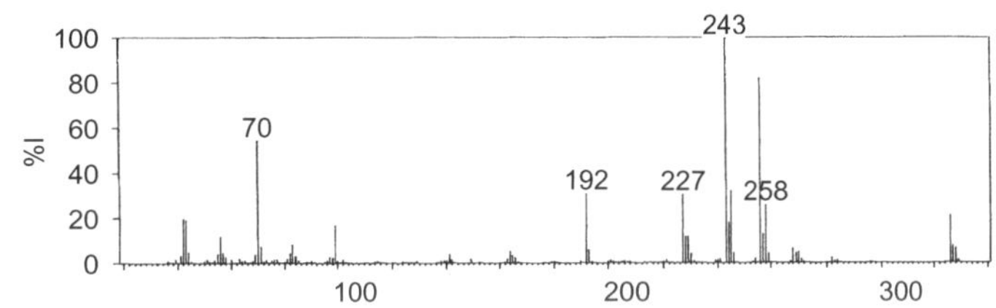

Quantification

Gas chromatography. In serum:, limits of quantification 1 to 2 µg/L, nitrogen-specific detection—K. Richter, *J. Chromatogr.*, 1988, *434*, 465–468. In plasma or serum: limit of quantification 35 µg/L, nitrogen-specific detection—T. A. Jennison *et al.*, *J. Anal. Toxicol.*, 1995, *19*, 537–541 and T. A. Jennison *et al.*, *J. Anal. Toxicol.*, 1997, *21*, 73–75. In serum: clozapine and *N*-desmethylclozapine, UV detection—R. N. Gupta, *J. Chromatogr.* 1995, *673 B Biomed. Appl.*, 311–315.

Gas chromatography–mass spectrometry. In plasma: clozapine and norclozapine, limits of quantification 1 µg/L and 5 µg/L, respectively—U. Bondesson and L. H. Lindstrom, *Psychopharmacology (Berl.)*, 1988, *95*, 472–475. In blood or urine: limits of detection 25 µg/L and 30 µg/L, respectively—A. B. Melent'ev and I. V. Kurochkina, *Sud. Med. Ekspert*, 1999, *42*, 27–29.

High performance liquid chromatography. In plasma: clozapine and norclozapine, limits of detection 15 µg/L and 30 µg/L, respectively—M. J. Lovdahl *et al.*, *Ther. Drug Monit.*, 1991, *13*, 69–72. In serum: clozapine and its metabolites, limits of detection 5 µg/L and 10 to 20 µg/L, respectively, UV detection—H. Weigmann and C. Hiemke, *J. Chromatogr.*, 1992, *583*, 209–216. In plasma: clozapine and norclozapine, limits of detection 2 µg/L and 1 µg/L, respectively, UV detection—M. C. Chung *et al.*, *J. Chromatogr.*, 1993, *613*, 168–173. In plasma or serum: clozapine and norclozapine, limit of detection <0.5 µg/L, UV detection—P. T. McCarthy *et al.*, *Biomed. Chromatogr.*, 1995, *9*, 36–41. In serum: clozapine and its metabolites, limits of quantification 0.5 µg/L for clozapine and norclozapine and 5 µg/L for clozapine-*N*-oxide, electrochemical detection—E. Schulz *et al.*, *Pharmacopsychiatry*, 1995, *28*, 20–25. In serum: clozapine and norclozapine, limit of quantification 25 µg/L—D. J. Freeman *et al.*, *Ther. Drug Monit.*, 1996, *18*, 688–692. In plasma or red blood cells: clozapine and its major metabolites, limits of quantification 20 µg/L for clozapine and norclozapine and 30 µg/L for clozapine-*N*-oxide, UV detection—C. Guitton *et al.*, *J. Chromatogr. B Biomed. Sci. Appl.*, 1997, *690*, 211–222. In plasma: clozapine and norclozapine, limits of detection 16.3 µg/L and 18 µg/L, respectively—K. Johansen *et al.*, *J. Chromatogr. B Biomed. Sci. Appl.*, 1997, *690*, 223–231. In serum or urine: clozapine and its metabolites, limits of quantification 10 µg/L and 20 to 30 µg/L, respectively, UV detection—H. Weigmann *et al.*, *Ther. Drug Monit.*, 1997, *19*, 480–488. In plasma or serum: clozapine and norclozapine, limit of detection 4.9 µg/L, diode-array detection—K. K. Akerman, *J. Chromatogr. B Biomed. Sci. Appl.*, 1997, *696*, 253–259. In plasma: clozapine and norclozapine, limit of detection 5 µg/L, UV detection—L. Edno *et al.*, *J. Pharm. Biomed. Anal.*, 1997, *16*, 311–318. In plasma: clozapine and its metabolites, limits of quantification 2 µg/L for clozapine and norclozapine and 5 µg/L for clozapine-*N*-oxide, UV detection—A. Avenoso *et al.*, *J. Chromatogr. B Biomed. Sci. Appl.*, 1998, *714*, 299–308. In plasma: clozapine and norclozapine, limit of quantification 20 µg/L, UV detection—F. Coudore *et al.*, *J. Anal. Toxicol.*, 1999, *23*, 195–199. In plasma: limit of detection 30 µg/L, NPD—S. Ulrich *et al.*, *J. Chromatogr. B Biomed. Sci. Appl.*, 1999, *731*, 231–240. In plasma: clozapine and norclozapine, limit of quantification 25 µg/L, UV detection—A. Llerena *et al.*, *J. Chromatogr. B. Biomed. Sci. Appl.*, 2001, *755*, 349–354. In serum: clozapine and its metabolites, limits of quantification 10 to 20 µg/L, UV detection—H. Weigmann *et al.*, *J. Chromatogr. B. Biomed. Sci. Appl.*, 2001, *759*, 63–71. In plasma: clozapine and its metabolites, limits of quantification 12.5 µg/L for clozapine and its *N*-oxide and 10 µg/L for norclozapine, UV detection—Y. Y. Liu *et al.*, *Biomed. Chromatogr.*, 2001, *15*, 280–286. In serum: clozapine and some antidepressants, UV and fluorescence detection—R. Waschgler *et al.*, *Int. J. Clin. Pharmacol. Ther.*, 2002, *40*, 554–559.

High performance liquid chromatography–mass spectrometry. In plasma: clozapine and its metabolites—M. Kollroser and C. Schober, *Rapid Commun. Mass Spectrom.*, 2002, *16*, 1266–1272.

Disposition in the Body. Clozapine undergoes a moderate first-pass metabolism and is almost completely metabolised before excretion via *N*-demethylation, *N*-oxidation, oxidation of the chlorine-containing ring, and thiomethyl conjugation. Metabolism is catalysed by cytochrome P450 isoenzyme CYP1A2. Only the desmethyl metabolite (norclozapine) shows any pharmacological actions but these are considerably weaker and of shorter duration than the parent drug. Only trace amounts of unchanged drug are detected in the urine and faeces. Approx. 50% of the administered dose are excreted as metabolites in the urine and 30% in the faeces.

Therapeutic concentration

After administration of clozapine at a dosage of up to 500 mg daily for 12 weeks to 45 schizophrenic patients, mean steady-state plasma concentrations of clozapine and norclozapine were reported to be 0.472 and 0.201 mg/L, respectively, in those who responded to treatment and 0.328 and 0.156 mg/L in those unresponsive to treatment. A cut-off value of 0.350 to 0.400 mg/L distinguished responders from non-responders although the incidence of adverse effects was twice as high at concentrations above 0.350 mg/L compared with those below. [E. Spina *et al.*, *Psychopharmacology (Berl.)*, 2000, *148*, 83–89.]

26 subjects treated with clozapine 200 to 700 mg daily for psychosis had concentrations of 0.030 to 1.016 mg/L in plasma (22 subjects), 0.17 to 34.24 µg/g in hair (23 subjects), and 0.049 to 5.609 µg/patch in sweat (20 subjects); a better dose–concentration relationship was observed between daily dose and hair or sweat concentrations than plasma concentration. [V. Crimele *et al.*, *Forensic Sci. Int.*, 2000, *107*, 289–300.]

In 12 subjects titrated over 10 to 14 days to a target dose of 6 mg/kg daily, the mean clozapine plasma concentration achieved after 5 days at the target dose was 0.584 mg/L; a wide variation was apparent (±0.417 mg/L). [J. A. Bennett and P. E. Keck, *Ann. Clin. Psychiatry*, 1996, *8*, 19–21.]

After administration of an oral dose of clozapine 200 mg to 10 schizophrenic patients, average peak plasma concentrations of 0.386 mg/L were attained in 1.0 to 6.3 h (mean 3). [Y. F. Cheng *et al.*, *Eur. J. Clin. Pharmacol.*, 1988, *34*, 445–449.]

Toxicity

In 3 fatalities involving clozapine, tissue concentrations were reported as follows: 3.6, 2.6, and 13 µg/g in the blood and 28, 19, and 85 µg/g in the liver. The concentrations of desmethylclozapine were: –, 1.1, and 3.1 µg/g in the blood and –, 18, and 50 µg/g in the liver. [K. Worm *et al.*, *Int. J. Legal Med.*, 1993, *106*, 115–118.]

A 25-year-old male who died several hours after the ingestion of an estimated 2 g clozapine had the following postmortem tissue concentrations: blood 5.81 µg/L, liver 42.9 mg/kg, urine 1.13 µg/L, gastric contents 6.5 mg (total); the antemortem blood concentration was 1.94 µg/L at approx. 4 h after the ingestion. [J. E. Meeker *et al.*, *J. Anal. Toxicol.*, 1992, *16*, 54–56.]

The following body-fluid concentrations were reported in a 15-year-old girl who died following ingestion of an unknown quantity of 100 mg clozapine tablets in a suicide attempt:

	Clozapine (mg/L)	*N*-Desmethyl-clozapine (mg/L)
Antemortem peripheral blood	9.4	0.6
Postmortem peripheral blood	8.8	0.5
Heart blood	12.0	1.5
Cerebrospinal fluid	0.2	not detected
Vitreous humour	1.3	not detected
Stomach content	2410	172
Bile	1844	75

[T. Keller *et al.*, *Forensic Sci. Int.*, 1997, *86*, 119–125.]

A 19-year-old female who survived despite ingesting 5 g clozapine, had a plasma concentration of 3.8 mg/L 2.5 h after the ingestion. The only symptoms were somnolence with intermittent periods of agitation and a mild anticholinergic syndrome. [K. Broich *et al.*, *Pharmacopsychiatry*, 1998, *31*, 149–151.]

Bioavailability. Approx. 50 to 60%.

Half-life. 6 to 17 h.

Volume of distribution. 2 to 7 L/kg. Also reported as 1.6 L/kg.

Protein binding. About 95%.

Note. For a review of the pharmacokinetics and pharmacodynamics of clozapine, see M. W. Jann *et al.*, *Clin. Pharmacokinet*, 1993, *24*, 161–176 and for discussions on therapeutic drug monitoring in clozapine therapy, see O. V. Olesen, *Clin. Pharmacokinet.*, 1998, *34*, 497–502 and D. J. Freeman and L. K. Oyewumi, *Clin. Pharmacokinet.*, 1997, *32*, 93–100.

Dose. In schizophrenia, initially 12.5 mg once or twice daily, increased gradually to 200 to 400 mg daily; maximum daily dose 900 mg; usual maintenance dose 150 to 300 mg daily.

Cocaine

Local Anaesthetic

Synonyms. Cocaina; Methyl Benzoylecgonine.
Note. For names used to describe various forms of cocaine—see *Martindale, The complete drug reference*, 33rd Edn., Pharmaceutical Press, London, 2002.
Methyl-[1*R*-(*exo*,*exo*)]-3-(benzoyloxy)-8-methyl-8-azabicyclo[3.2.1]-octane-2-carboxylate
$C_{17}H_{21}NO_4$=303.4
CAS—50-36-2

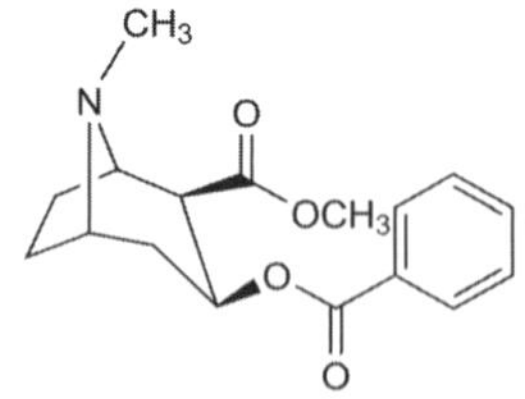

An alkaloid obtained from coca, the dried leaves of *Erythroxylum coca* and other species of *Erythroxylum* (Erythroxylaceae) or by synthesis from ecgonine.
A white crystalline, slightly volatile, powder. M.p. 98°.
Soluble 1 in 600 of water (1 in 270 of water at 80°), 1 in 6.5 of ethanol, 1 in 0.7 of chloroform, and 1 in 3.5 of ether; also soluble in acetone, ethyl acetate, and carbon disulfide.

Cocaine Hydrochloride

Synonyms. Cocainium Chloratum; Cocaini Hydrochloridum.
$C_{17}H_{21}NO_4,HCl$=339.8
CAS—53-21-4
Hygroscopic colourless crystals or white crystalline powder. M.p. about 195°, with decomposition.

Soluble 1 in 0.4 of water, 1 in 3.2 of cold alcohol and 1 in 2 of hot alcohol, and 1 in 12.5 of chloroform; also soluble in glycerol and acetone; practically insoluble in ether.

Dissociation Constant. pK_a 8.6 (20°).

Partition Coefficient. Log *P* (octanol/water), 2.3.

Colour Test. *p*-Dimethylaminobenzaldehyde (100° for 3 min)—red; cobalt thiocyanate—blue

Thin-layer Chromatography. System TA—Rf 65; system TB—Rf 45; system TC—Rf 47; system TE—Rf 77; system TL—Rf 54; system TAE—Rf 35; system TAF—Rf 30; system TAJ—Rf 13; system TAK—Rf 00; system TAL—Rf 02. (Dragendorff spray, positive; acidified iodoplatinate solution, positive.)

Plate: silica 60 F_{254} (10 × 10 cm). Mobile phase: hexane:toluene: diethylamine (65:20:5). UV detection. Rf 0.36. [L. Antonilli *et al.*, *J. Chromatogr. B Biomed. Sci. Appl.*, 2001, *751*, 19–27].

Gas Chromatography. System GA—cocaine RI 2187, M (benzoylecgonine) RI 2570, M (ecgonine) not eluted, M (anhydroecgonine methylester) RI 1280, M (methylecgonine) RI 1472, M (nor-) RI 2162, M (*m*-OH-) RI 2460, M (OH-methoxy-) RI 2670, M (cocaethylene) RI 2250, M (norcocaethylene) RI 2115; system GB—cocaine RI 2289, M (ecgonine) not eluted, M (anhydroecgonine methylester) RI 1430, M (norecgonine) RI 1472, M (methylecgonine) RI 1530, M (ethylecgonine) RI 1602, M (nor-) RI 2259, M (benzoylecgonine) RI 2663, M (*m*-OH-) RI 2608, M (*p*-OH-) RI 2650, M (OH-methoxy-) RI 2729, M (cocaethylene) RI 2345, M (norcocaethylene) RI 2317, M (OH-cocaethylene) RI 2709, M (OH-methoxycocaethylene) RI 2779, M (methoxycocaethylene) RI 2663; system GF—RI 2550; system GQ—retention time, 7.85 min; system GAK—retention time 12.7 min.

High Performance Liquid Chromatography. System HA—cocaine *k* 2.8, benzoylecgonine *k* 0.9 (tailing peak), ecgonine *k* 1.1; system HQ—cocaine *k* 2.68, benzoylecgonine *k* 5.68; system HX—RI 348; system HY—RI 289; system HZ—retention time, 3.3 min; system HAA—retention time, 11.9 min; system HAX—retention time 10.0 min; system HAY—retention time 5.0 min; system HBC—retention time 5.2 min.

Column: LiChrocart-LiCrospher 100 RP-18 (250 × 4 mm i.d., 5 μm)l precolumn, 100 RP-18 (4 × 4 mm i.d., 5 μm). Mobile phase: (A)—0.045 M ammonium acetate solution in HPLC-grade water:methanol: acetonitrile (80:10:10); (B)—0.045 M ammonium acetate solution in water:methanol:acetonitrile (20:40:40). Elution programme: 100 to 47.2% (A) in 20 min, flow rate 1 mL/min. UV detection, (λ = 235 nm). Retention time: 14.8 min. [L. Antonilli *et al.*, *J. Chromatogr. Biomed. Sci. Appl.*, 2001, *751*, 19–27.]

Ultraviolet Spectrum. Aqueous acid—233 nm (A^{1}_{1} = 430a), 275 nm.

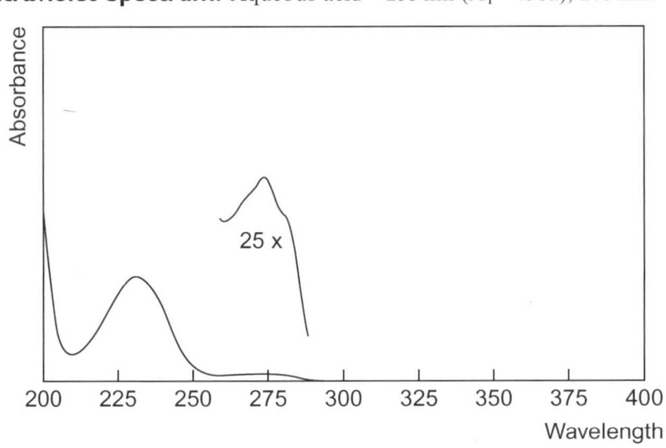

Infra-red Spectrum. Principal peaks at wavenumbers 1710, 1738, 1275, 1110, 712, 1037 cm^{-1} (KBr disk).

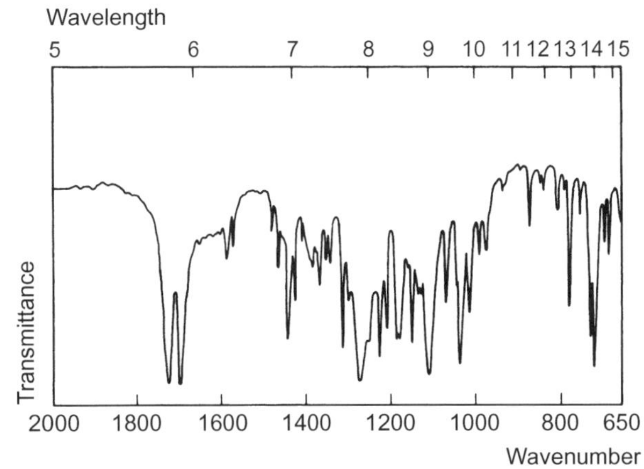

Mass Spectrum. Principal ions at *m/z* 82, 182, 83, 105, 303, 77, 94, 96; benzoylecgonine 124, 82, 168, 77, 105, 42, 94, 83.

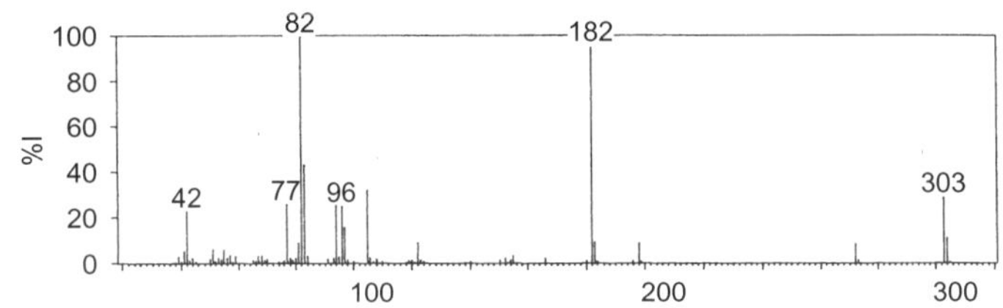

Quantification

Gas chromatography. In whole blood or plasma: limit of detection 20 μg/L, AFID—B. H. Dvorchik *et al.*, *J. Chromatogr.*, 1977, *135*, 141–148. In plasma, urine, or erythrocytes: ECD—J. I. Javaid *et al.*, *J. Chromatogr.*, 1978, *152*, 105–113. In plasma: cocaine and benzoylecgonine, limit of quantification 4 μg/L, NPD—L. Virag *et al.*, *J. Chromatogr. 1994, 658 B Biomed. Appl.*, 135–141. In urine: limit of detection 5 μg/L—M. Farina *et al.*, *Forensic Sci. Int.*, 2002, *127*, 204–207.

Gas chromatography–mass spectrometry. In meconium: cocaine and benzoylecgonine, limits of quantification < 0.25 mg/kg and 0.56 mg/kg respectively—G. D. Clark *et al.*, *J. Anal. Toxicol.*, 1992, *16*, 261–263. In biological samples: cocaine, opioids, and metabolites—E. J. Cone and W. D. Darwin, *J. Chromatogr.*, 1992, *580*, 43–61. In blood or urine: cocaine and benzoylecgonine, limits of detection 20 to 40 μg/L—R. E. Aderjan *et al.*, *J. Anal. Toxicol.*, 1993, *17*, 51–55. In urine: benzoylecgonine, limit of quantification 150 μg/L—J. Gerlits, *J. Forensic Sci.*, 1993, *38*, 1210–1214. In urine or meconium: cocaine and metabolites, limit of detection 11 μg/L—N. Lombardero *et al.*, *Ann. Clin. Lab. Sci.*, 1993, *23*, 385–394. In whole blood, plasma, or meconium: cocaine and metabolites—G. M. Abusada *et al.*, *J. Anal. Toxicol.*, 1993, *17*, 353–358. In hair: cocaine, benzoylecgonine and other drugs of abuse, limit of detection < 0.1 μg/g—M. R. Moeller *et al.*, *Forensic Sci. Int.*, 1993, *63*, 185–206. In postmortem blood: cocaine and benzoylecgonine, limit of detection 2.5 μg/L—M. R. Corburt and E. M. Koves, *J. Forensic Sci.*, 1994, *39*, 136–149. In brain tissue: cocaine and its metabolites, limit of quantification 50 μg/kg—A. Hernandez *et al.*, *Forensic Sci. Int.*, 1994, *65*, 149–156. In plasma, saliva, or urine: cocaine and its metabolites, limit of detection for cocaine about 1 μg/L—E. J. Cone *et al.*, *Clin. Chem.*, 1994, *40*, 1299–1305. In urine: cocaine and diamorphine and its metabolites, limit of detection 50 μg/L—N. De Giovanni *et al.*, *J. Chromatogr.* 1994, *658 Biomed Appl.*, 69–73. In hair, plasma, saliva, and urine: limit of detection 0.1 μg/g in hair and 1 μg/L in plasma, saliva, and urine—W. L. Wang *et al.*, *J. Chromatogr.*, 1994, *660*; *Biomed. Appl.*, 279–290. In urine: limit of detection 1 to 2 μg/L for cocaine and its metabolites—R. de la Torre *et al.*, *J. Pharm. Biomed. Anal.*, 1995, *13*, 305–312. In hair: limit of detection 0.05 μg/g cocaine, 0.2 μg/g benzoylecgonine, and 0.8 μg/g ecgonine methylester using a 30 mg sample—P. Kintz and P. Mangin, *Forensic Sci. Int.*, 1995, *73*, 93–100. In urine: cocaine and its metabolites, limit of detection for cocaine 1 μg/L—S. Cardenas *et al.*, *Rapid Commun. Mass Spectrom.*, 1996, *10*, 631–636. In postmortem blood: ecgonine and other cocaine metabolites—D. Smirnow and B. K. Logan, *J. Anal. Toxicol.*, 1996, *20*, 463–467 and 2001, *25*, 219–230. In hair: cocaine, its metabolites, and opioids, limit of detection 0.12 to 0.28 μg/g—Y. Gaillard and G. Pepin, *Forensic Sci. Int.*, 1997, *86*, 49–59. In urine: limit of detection 5 µg/L—D. Garside *et al.*, *J. Chromatogr. B. Biomed. Sci. Appl.*, 1997, *692*, 61–65. In hair: cocaine, opioids, and their metabolites, limit of quantification 500 µg/g—K. M. Hold *et al.*, *J. Chromatogr. Sci.*, 1998, *36*, 125–130. In hair—K. M. Hold *et al.*, *J. Anal. Toxicol.*, 1998, *22*, 414–417. In urine: *m*-hydroxybenzoylecgonine, limit of quantification 5 µg/L—M. A. elSohly *et al.*, *Clin. Lab. Med.*, 1998, *18*, 699–704. In urine: limit of detection 5 µg/L—K. L. Preston *et al.*, *J. Anal. Toxicol.*, 1999, *23*, 131–322. In plasma and urine: limit of quantification 100 µg/L and limit of detection 80 µg/L (SIM, *m/z* 82)—T. Ohhima and T. Takayasu, *J. Chromatogr. B. Biomed. Sci. Appl.*, 1999, *726*, 185–194. In biological samples: cocaine *N*-oxide—P. P. Wang and M. G. Bartlett, *J. Anal. Toxicol.*, 1999, *23*, 62–66. In urine: benzoylecgonine, limit of detection 30 µg/L—B. J. Hall *et al.*, *J. Forensic Sci.*, 1999, *44*, 527–534. In hair: cocaine and opioids, and other drugs of abuse—S. Pichini *et al.*, *J. Anal. Toxicol.*, 1999, *23*, 343–348; C. Girod and C. Staub, *Forensic Sci. Int.*, 2000, *107*, 261–271; W. E. Brewer *et al.*, *Anal. Chem.*, 2001, *73*, 2371–2376; L. Skender *et al.*, *Forensic Sci. Int.*, 2002, *125*, 120–126. In sweat: cocaine, codeine, and their metabolites—M. A. Huestis *et al.*, *J. Chromatogr. B. Biomed. Sci. Appl.*, 1999, *733*, 247–264. In postmortem blood: cocaine and its metabolites and cocaethylene, limit of detection for cocaine 25 µg/L—A. A. Chasin and A. F. Midio, *Forensic Sci. Int.*, 2000, *109*, 1–13. In serum: cocaine, its metabolites, and other drugs of abuse—W. Weinmann *et al.*, *Int. J. Legal Med.*, 2000, *113*, 229–235. In urine: cocaine and other drugs of abuse, limits of detection 3 to 12 µg/L—V. Karacic and L. Skender, *Arh. Hig. Rada. Toksikol.*, 2000, *51*, 389–400. In hair: cocaine and its metabolites, limit of detection 0.01 µg/g—J. A. Bourland *et al.*, *J. Anal. Toxicol.*, 2000, *24*, 489–495. In breast milk: cocaine and its metabolites, limits of detection 2.5 to 10 µg/L—R. E. Winecker *et al.*, *J. Forensic Sci.*, 2001, *46*, 1221–1223.

High performance liquid chromatography. In plasma or tissues: cocaine and metabolites, limit of detection < 1000 µg/L, UV detection—M. A. Evans and T. Morarity, *J. Anal. Toxicol.*, 1980, *4*, 19–22. In brain tissue: cocaine and benzoylecgonine—S. P. Browne *et al.*, *J. Forensic Sci.*, 1991, *36*, 1662–1665. In urine: cocaine and its metabolites, limit of quantification 200 µg/L, UV detection—I. M. Roy *et al.*, *J. Pharm. Biomed. Anal.*, 1992, *10*, 943–948. In amniotic fluid: cocaine and benzoylecgonine—C. Moore *et al.*, *Forensic Sci. Int.*, 1992, *56*, 177–181. In urine: benzoylecgonine and ecgonine, limits of detection 0.11 µg/L and 46.3 µg/L, respectively, fluorescence detection—K. Nakashima *et al.*, *J. Chromatogr.*, 1992, *584*, 275–279. In meconium: cocaine metabolites, limit of quantification 50 ng/g—L. J. Murphy *et al.*, *J. Chromatogr.*, 1993, *613*, 330–335. In hair: limit of detection 15 ng/g, UV detection—F. Tagliaro *et al.*, *Forensic Sci. Int.*, 1993, *63*, 227–238. In biological samples: cocaine and benzoylecgonine, photodiode-array detection—M. Balikova and J. Vecerkova, *J. Chromatogr.*, 1994, *656 B Biomed. Appl.*, 267–273. In plasma or hair: limit of detection 1 µg/L, fluorescence detection—F. Tagliaro *et al.*, *J. Chromatogr. A.* 1994, *674*, 207–215. In hair: cocaine and other drugs of abuse, electrochemical detection—G. Achilli *et al.*, *J. Chromatogr. A.* 1996, *729*, 273–277. In plasma or urine: cocaine and benzoylecgonine, UV detection—P. Fernandez *et al.*, *J. Anal. Toxicol.*, 1996, *20*, 224–228. In urine: cocaine and metabolites, diode-array detection—K. M. Klauwaert *et al.*, *Anal. Chem.*, 1996, *68*, 3021–3028. In hair: cocaine and its metabolites, fluorescence detection—K. M. Klauwaert *et al.*, *Forensic Sci. Int.*, 2000, *110*, 157–166. In hair: cocaine and its metabolites, fluorescence detection and MS—K. M. Clauwaert *et al.*, *Anal. Chem.*, 1998, *70*, 2336–2344. In urine: limit of detection 25 µg/L and limit of quantification 100 µg/L, UV detection ($\lambda = 235$ nm)—L. Antonilli *et al.*, *J. Chromatogr. B Biomed. Sci. Appl.*, 2001, *751*, 19–27.

High performance liquid chromatography–mass spectrometry. In urine: cocaine and its metabolites—M. Nishikawa *et al.*, *Forensic Sci. Int.*, 1994, *66*, 149–158. In dried blood spots on filter paper: benzoylecgonine, limit of detection 2 µg/L—C. S. Sosnoff *et al.*, *J. Anal. Toxicol.*, 1996, *20*, 179–184. In plasma, blood or urine: limit of quantification 5 µg/L—A. Cailleux *et al.*, *J. Anal. Toxicol.*, 1999, *23*, 620–624. In urine: cocaine and ecgonine methyl ester—S. R. Needham *et al.*, *J. Chromatogr. B Biomed. Sci. Appl.*, 2000. *748*, 77–87. In plasma: cocaine and its metabolites—A. Klingmann *et al.*, *J. Anal. Toxicol.*, 2001, *25*, 425–430. In urine: limit of detection 0.5 µg/L, tandem MS—P. M. Jeanville *et al.*, *J. Anal. Toxicol.*, 2001, *25*, 69–75 and *J. Am. Soc. Mass Spectrom.*, 2000, *11*, 257–263.

Disposition in the Body. Cocaine is normally only used as a surface anaesthetic in the eye, ear, nose, and throat because of the possibility of systemic toxic effects when given by other routes. Addicts may inject it or use it as a snuff; it is, however, increasingly misused in its smokeable form, i.e., the freebase form known as 'crack cocaine' owing to the rapid absorption of the substance from the lungs. It is less toxic when taken orally owing to hydrolysis in the gastro-intestinal tract. The main metabolites are benzoylecgonine, ecgonine, and ecgonine methyl ester, all of which are inactive; some norcocaine, an active metabolite, may also be produced; other metabolites that have been reported are ethylecgonine, hydroxycocaine, and methylecgonidine. When taken in combination with alcohol, a cocaethylene metabolite is also produced. About 1 to 9% of a daily intravenous dose of 120 mg of cocaine is excreted unchanged in the urine, together with 35 to 55% as benzoylecgonine; the excretion of unchanged drug is increased when the urine is acid; some ecgonine may also be present. After an intranasal dose of 1.5 mg/kg, up to 4% of the dose is excreted in the urine unchanged in 24 h, and 16 to 36% of the dose is excreted as benzoylecgonine. About 30 to 60% of an oral, intranasal, or intravenous dose is excreted in the urine as ecgonine methyl ester. Elimination of cocaine and metabolites in urine is typically complete within 48 h of dosing; in plasma, it is usually in the range of 18 to 24 h. No unchanged drug is eliminated in the faeces. Cocaine crosses the placenta and is found in breast milk.

Therapeutic concentration

6 males with a history of cocaine abuse were administered with a single cocaine dose by the following routes: 25 mg cocaine hydrochloride (intravenous), 32 mg cocaine hydrochloride (intranasal), and 42 mg cocaine base (smoked). Plasma concentrations of benzoylecgonine (BZE), ecgonine methyl ester (EME), norcocaine (NCOC), benzoylnorecgonine (BNE), *meta*- and *para*-hydroxycocaine (*m*-HOCOC, *p*-HOCOC), *meta*- and *para*-hydroxybenzoylecgonine (*m*-HOBZE, *p*-HOBZE), and anhydroecgonine methyl ester (AEME) were determined by GC–MS and were as follows:

	Intravenous (n=6)		**Intranasal (n=6)**		**Smoked (n=5)**	
	Plasma conc. (µg/L)	**Time (h)**	**Plasma conc. (µg/L)**	**Time (h)**	**Plasma conc. (µg/L)**	**Time (h)**
Cocaine	775	3.9	412	5.1	707	2.6
BZE	15 611	5.6	13 681	7.8	9 395	4.1
EME	4 968	5	5 831	5	3 193	4.1
NCOC	19	5.1	11	4.3	4	3.3
BNE	255	0.6	409	8.5	160	5.1
m-HOCOC	43	0.08	47	5.3	48	3.7
p-HOCOC	6	0.01	7	4.6	1	4.8
m-HOBZE	131	0.45	208	10.2	131	6.9
p-HOBZE	247	0.43	353	7.5	258	4.1
AEME	0	n/a	0	n/a	23	2.3

Total percentage dose excreted in urine for the intravenous, intranasal and smoked routed were 57.1, 45.4, and 24.9%, respectively.

[E.J. Cone *et al.*, *Ther. Drug Monit.*, 1998, *20*, 556–560.]

10 volunteers were administered single and multiple doses of cocaine; intravenously and by inhalation. On 4 separate study days, the volunteers smoked 2 doses of 25 mg cocaine with a 14 min interval (day 1); smoked 2 doses 50 mg cocaine (day 2); were intravenously administered 2 doses of 16 mg cocaine with a 14 min period in between (day 3); and 2 doses of 32 mg, again intravenously (day 4). Plasma concentrations of cocaine and benzoylecgonine were determined and were as follows (n = 10):

			Cocaine	**Benzoylecgonine**
Intravenous	2 × 16 mg	conc. (mg/L)	0.23	0.24
		time (min)	18	90
	2 × 32 mg	conc. (mg/L)	0.47	0.4
		time (min)	18	90
Smoked	2 × 25 mg	conc. (mg/L)	0.21	0.2
		time (min)	18	60
	2 × 50 mg	conc. (mg/L)	0.38	0.35
		time (min)	18	90

After multiple dosing in 3 volunteers (316 mg dose administered over 90 min), the peak plasma cocaine concentration was 1.2 mg/L

[D. S. Isenschmid *et al.*, *J. Anal. Toxicol.*, 1992, *16(5)*, 311–314.]

Toxicity. The estimated minimum lethal dose is 1.2 g but susceptible persons have died from doses as small as 30 mg when applied to mucous membranes; addicts may be able to tolerate up to 5 g a day. Toxic effects have been noted with blood concentrations in the range 0.25 to 5 mg/L and fatalities have occurred with concentrations of 1 mg/L or more.

Postmortem concentrations of cocaine and benzoylecgonine in a 27-year-old man who died following the rupture, in his gastro-intestinal tract, of 4 cocaine-containing packages were reported as: blood 4.0 and 17.0 mg/L, urine 152.0 and 512 mg/L, bile 99.8 and 54.0 mg/L, vitreous humour 7.1 and 5.8 mg/L, brain 7.5 and 3.5 mg/g, hair 55.5 and 27.7 µg/g. [C. Furnari *et al.*, *J. Forensic Sci.*, 2002, *47*, 208–210.]

A 17-year-old male drug dealer died about 90 min after swallowing a package containing cocaine; the following postmortem tissue concentrations were reported for cocaine, benzoylecgonine, and ecgonine methyl ester, respectively: blood 98.1, 86.1, and 51.4 mg/L, liver 128.1, 134.3, and 20.3 µg/g, kidney 92.5, 8.6, and 6.2 µg/g, brain 99.1, 32.1, and 17.6 µg/g, spleen 72.6, 4.7 and 6.9 µg/g, lung 121.3, 89.4, and 36.4 µg/g, urine 10, 3.3, and 4.2 mg/L. [V. Fineschi *et al.*, *Forensic Sci. Int.*, 2002, *126*, 7–10.]

A teenage drug courier who died after a 12 h flight was found to have 24 packages of cocaine in her intestinal tract, several of which had burst or become damaged. Her postmortem blood concentration of cocaine was 104 mg/L. [F. Patel, *Forensic Sci. Int.*, 1996, *79*, 167–174.]

A blood cocaine concentration of 330 mg/L was found in a 26-year-old female who died as a result of cocaine intoxication; the concentrations of benzoylecgonine and ecgonine methyl ester were 50 and 18 mg/L, respectively. Such high concentrations suggested a massive administration but the manner of death was undetermined. [F. J. Peretti *et al.*, *Forensic Sci. Int.*, 1990, *48*, 135–138.]

Half-life. Plasma half-life, 0.7 to 1.5 h (dose-dependent).

Volume of distribution. About 1 to 3 L/kg.

Clearance. Plasma clearance, 10 to 32 mL/min/kg (dose-dependent).

Note. For a review of cocaine pathophysiology and clinical toxicology, see M. S. Boghdadi and R. J. Henning, *Heart Lung*, 1997, *26*, 466–483; for a review of the effects of concurrent use of alcohol and cocaine, see E. J. Pennings *et al.*, *Addiction*, 2002, *97*, 773–783; for a review of prenatal cocaine exposure, see R. W. Keller Jr and A. Snyder-Keller, *Ann. N. Y. Acad. Sci.*, 2000, *909*, 217–232; for a review of cocaine metabolism in humans after use of alcohol, see J. Carni *et al.*, *Recent Dev. Alcohol*, 1998, *14*, 437–455.

Use. Cocaine hydrochloride is used in concentrations of 1 to 25%, for local anaesthesia.

Codeine

Narcotic Analgesic

Synonyms. Codeinum; Methylmorphine; Metilmorfina; Morphine Methyl Ether.
Proprietary names. Codicaps; Eulyptan; Pneumogenol.
(5α,6α)-7,8-Didehydro-4,5-epoxy-3-methoxy-17-methylmorphinan-6-ol monohydrate
$C_{18}H_{21}NO_3,H_2O$=317.4
CAS—76-57-3 (anhydrous); 6059-47-8 (monohydrate)

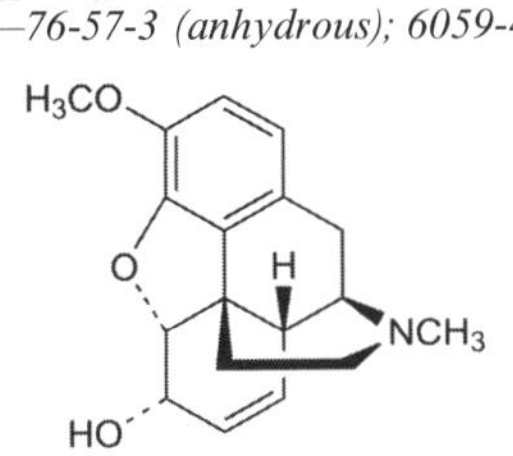

An alkaloid obtained from opium or prepared by methylation of morphine. Colourless crystals or white crystalline powder which effloresces slowly in dry air and is affected by light. M.p. 154° to 156°.
Soluble 1 in 120 of water, 1 in 15 of boiling water, 1 in 2 of ethanol, 1 in 0.5 of chloroform, 1 in 13 of benzene, and 1 in 18 of ether; freely soluble in amyl alcohol, methanol, and dilute acids; almost insoluble in petroleum ether or in solutions of alkali hydroxides.

Codeine Hydrochloride

$C_{18}H_{21}NO_3,HCl$=335.8
CAS—1422-07-7 (anhydrous)
A white crystalline powder. M.p. about 280°, with some decomposition.
Soluble 1 in 20 of water, 1 in 180 of ethanol, and 1 in 800 of chloroform.

Codeine Phosphate

Synonyms. Codeine Phosphate Hemihydrate; Codeini Phosphas; Methylmorphine Phosphate
Proprietary names. Actacode; Bromophar; Bronchodine; Bronchosedal; Codant; Codedrill; Codenfan; Codicompren; Evacode; Galcodine; Glottyl; Paderyl; Toularynx; Tricodein; Tryasol; Tussoret.
Codeine phosphate is an ingredient of many proprietary preparations—see *Martindale, The complete drug reference*, 33rd Edn., Pharmaceutical Press, London, 2002
$C_{18}H_{21}NO_3,H_3PO_4,\frac{1}{2}H_2O$=406.4
CAS—52-28-8 (anhydrous); 41444-62-6 (hemihydrate); 5913-76-8 (sesquihydrate)
Small colourless crystals or white crystalline powder.
Soluble 1 in 4 of water, 1 in 450 of ethanol, and 1 in 125 of boiling ethanol; practically insoluble in chloroform and ether.

Codeine Sulfate

Synonym. Codeine Sulphate
Proprietary name. It is an ingredient of Bepro
$(C_{18}H_{21}NO_3)_2,H_2SO_4,3H_2O$=750.9
CAS—1420-53-7 (anhydrous); 6854-40-6 (trihydrate)
White crystals or crystalline powder.
Soluble 1 in 30 of water and 1 in 1300 of ethanol; practically insoluble in chloroform and ether.

Dissociation Constant. pK_a 8.2 (20°).

Partition Coefficient. Log *P* (octanol/pH 7.4), 0.6.

Colour Tests. Liebermann's Test—black; Mandelin's Test—green; Marquis Test—violet

Thin-layer Chromatography. System TA—Rf 33; system TB—Rf 06; system TC—Rf 18; system TE—Rf 35; system TL—Rf 03; system TAE—Rf 21; system TAF—Rf 22; system TAJ—Rf 10; system TAK—Rf 00; system TAL—Rf 26. (Dragendorff spray, positive; acidified iodoplatinate solution, positive; Marquis reagent, violet.)

Gas Chromatography. System GA—codeine RI 2375, codeine-AC RI 2503, codeine-PFP RI 2430, codeine-TFA RI 2280, codeine-TMS RI 2520, M (nor-) RI 2388, M (nor-)-AC_2 RI 2945, morphine RI 2445; system GB—codeine RI 1511, codeine-AC RI 2645, codeine-TMS RI 2592, M (nor-) RI 2535, M (nor-)-TMS_2 RI 2631; system GC—codeine RI 2681, morphine RI 2542; system GF—RI 2860; system GM—codeine RRT 1.519, codeine-AC RRT 1.449 (both relative to iprindole).

Column: HP-5 capillary 95% dimethylsiloxane, 5% diphenylsiloxane (25 m × 0.25 mm i.d., 0.25 µm film thickness). Column temperature: 120°; held, 2 min; increased to 280° at 20°/min; held, 10 min. Carrier gas: helium, flow rate 1 mL/min. MS detection, SIM (*m/z* 282, 395). Retention time: 13.2 min. [F. Pragst *et al.*, *J. Anal. Toxicol.*, 1999, *23*, 168–171.]

Column: DB-17 fused-silica capillary (30 m × 0.25 mm i.d., 0.25 µm film thickness). Column temperature: 130°, held 2 min; increased to 300° at 8°/min. Carrier gas: helium. NPD. RT: 23.9 min. [H. Seno *et al.*, *J. Chromatogr.*, 1995, *673(2)*, *Biomed. Appl.* 189–195].

High Performance Liquid Chromatography. System HA—codeine *k* 4.8 (tailing peak), morphine *k* 3.8 (tailing peak), M (nor-) *k* 3.1 (tailing peak); system HC—codeine *k* 1.21, morphine *k* 1.30, M (nor-) *k* 3.51; system HS—codeine *k* 1.90, morphine *k* 5.16; system HX—RI 266; system HY—RI 237; system HZ—retention time 1.9 min; system HAA—retention time 5.0 min; system HAM—not detected; system HAX—retention time 6.1 min; system HAY—retention time 3.4 min.

Column: Basic C_8 (150 × 4.6 mm i.d., 3 µm). Mobile phase: acetonitrile:ammonium phosphate dibasic (5 mM), adjusted to pH 5.8 with phosphoric acid (8:92), flow rate 1.0 mL/min. Fluorescence detection (λ_{ex} = 214 nm, λ_{em} = 345 nm). Retention time: 15 min. [B. Weingarten *et al.*, *J. Chromatogr. A*, 1995, *696(1)*, 83–92.]

Column: µPorasil (300 × 3.9 mm i.d., 10 µm): pre-column, silica (15 × 3.2 mm i.d., 7 µm). Mobile phase: sodium acetate buffer (5 mM, pH 3.75):acetonitrile (25:75), flow rate 1.2 mL/min. ECD. Retention time: 8.2 min (k, 3.76). [W. J. Liaw *et al.*, *J. Chromatogr. B Biomed. Sci. Appl.*, 1998, *714(2)*, 237–245.]

Column: Hypersil BDS C_{18} (100 × 4.6 mm i.d., 3 µm). Mobile phase: potassium dihydrogen phosphate (10 mM, pH 3):acetonitrile (93:7), flow rate 1.0 mL/min. UV detection (λ = 212 nm). Retention time: codeine, 6.4 min; norcodeine, 5.5 min. [J. A. Pascual and J. Sanagustin, *J. Chromatogr. B Biomed. Sci. Appl.*, 1999, *724(2)*, 295–302.]

Ultraviolet Spectrum. Aqueous acid—285 nm (A_1^1=55a). No alkaline shift.

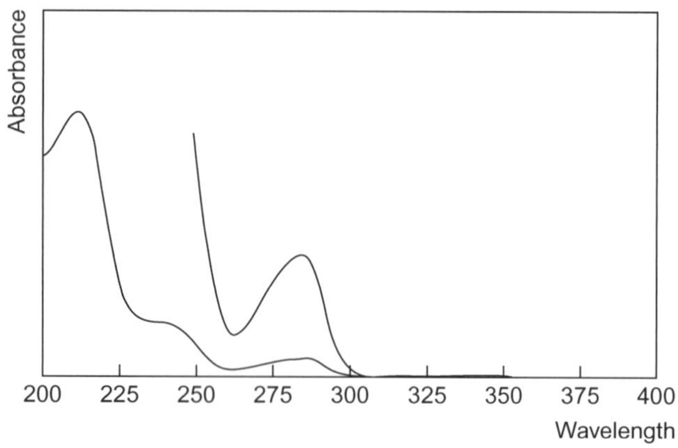

Infra-red Spectrum. Principal peaks at wavenumbers 1052, 1268, 1500, 1111, 793, 934 cm^{-1} (KBr disk).

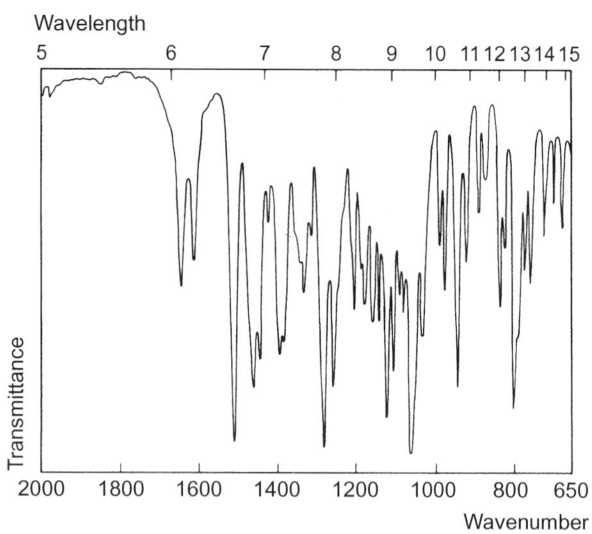

Mass Spectrum. Principal ions at *m/z* 299, 42, 162, 124, 229, 59, 300, 69; morphine 285, 162, 42, 215, 286, 124, 44, 284; norcodeine 285, 81, 215, 148, 286, 164, 110, 115.

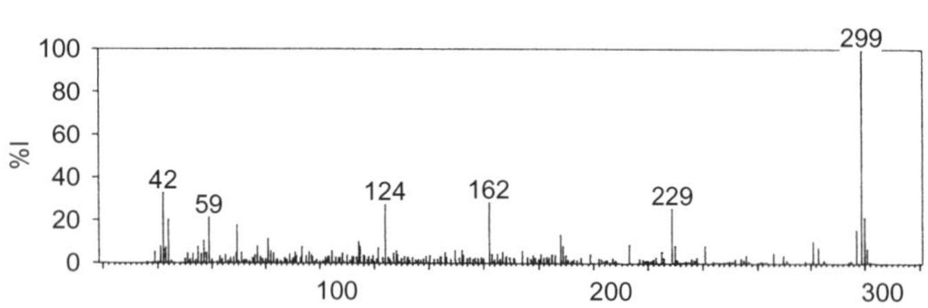

Quantification

Gas chromatography. In urine: codeine, morphine and 6-monoacetylmorphine, NPD, FID—T. Vu-Duc and A. Vernay, *Biomed. Chromatogr.*, 1990, *4*, 65–69. In blood or bile: codeine and morphine, limit of detection for codeine 0.1 mg/L, NPD—H. M. Lee and C. W. Lee, *J. Anal. Toxicol.*, 1991, *15*, 182–187. In biological fluids: limit of detection 5 µg/L for codeine and 1 µg/L for morphine, ECD—P. O. Edlund, *J. Chromatogr.*, 1981, *206*, 109–116. In plasma or urine: codeine and dihydrocodeine, limit of detection 2.5 µg/L, SID—H. Seno *et al.*, *J. Chromatogr.* 1995, *673 B Biomed. Appl.*, 189–195.

Gas chromatography–mass spectrometry. In blood: codeine and other opioids, limit of detection for codeine 8.3 µg/L—H. Gjerde *et al.*, *Forensic Sci. Int.*, 1991, *51*, 105–110. In plasma or whole blood: codeine and other opioids—M. Krogh *et al.*, *J. Chromatogr.*, 1993, *621*, 41–48. In serum, blood, and postmortem blood: codeine and other opioids, limit of detection <1 µg/L—F. Musshoff and T. Daldrup, *Int. J. Legal Med.*, 1993, *106*, 107–109. In hair, plasma, saliva, or urine: limit of detection 0.3 µg/g in hair and 5 µg/L in plasma, saliva, and urine, SIM (norcodeine, 429, 250, and 292)—W. L. Wang *et al.*, *J. Chromatogr.* 1994, *660 B Biomed. Appl.*, 279–290. In plasma: codeine and other opioids, limit of detection <1 pg—D. G. Watson *et al.*, *J. Pharm. Biomed. Anal.*, 1995, *13*, 27–32. In hair: codeine and other opioids and cocaine, limit of detection for codeine 0.1 µg/g, using a 30 mg hair sample, SIM—P. Kintz and P. Mangin, *Forensic Sci. Int.*, 1995, *73*, 93–100. In hair: codeine and its major metabolites, limit of detection 10 pg—D. Wilkins *et al.*, *J. Anal. Toxicol.*, 1995, *19*, 269–274. In plasma or whole blood: codeine and other opioids, limit of detection <5 µg/L—A. Geier *et al.*, *Int. J. Legal Med.*, 1996, *109*, 80–83. In urine: limit of detection 2.0 µg/L and limit of quantification 10.0 µg/L, SIM—C. L. O'Neal and A. Poklis, *J. Anal. Toxicol.*, 1997, *21*, 427–432. In urine: codeine and other opioids—L. A. Broussard *et al.*, *Clin. Chem.*, 1997, *43*, 1029–1032. In hair: limit of quantification 0.5 mg/g, SIM—K. M. Hold *et al.*, *J. Chromatogr. Sci.*, 1998, *36*, 125–130. In urine: codeine and other opioids—M. Cremese *et al.*, *J. Forensic Sci.*, 1998, *43*, 1220–1224. In urine: codeine and morphine, limit of detection for codeine 6 µg/L—B. D. Paul *et al.*, *Clin. Chem.*, 1999, *45*, 510–519. In cerebrospinal fluid, urine, or vitreous humour: limit of quantification 1 µg/L, SIM—F. Pragst *et al.*, *J. Anal. Toxicol.*, 1999, *23*, 168–172. In urine: codeine and other opioids, limit of quantification 25 µg/L and limit of detection 10 µg/L for codeine and hydrocodone—R. Meatherall, *J. Anal. Toxicol.*, 1999, *23*, 177–186. In serum: codeine and morphine, limit of quantification for codeine 0.15 µg/L—U. Hofmann *et al.*, *J. Chromatogr. B Biomed. Sci. Appl.*, 1999, *727*, 81–88. In hair: codeine and other opioids—S. Pichini *et al.*, *J. Anal. Toxicol.*, 1999, *23*, 343–348; L. Skender *et al.*, *Forensic Sci. Int.*, 2002, *125*, 120–126. In serum: codeine and other drugs of abuse—W. Weinmann *et al.*, *Int. J. Legal Med.*, 2000, *113*, 229–235. In hair: codeine, other opioids, and cocaine—W. E. Brewer *et al.*, *Anal. Chem.*, 2001, *73*, 2371–2376. In hair or oral fluids: codeine and other opioids—J. Jones *et al.*, *J. Anal. Toxicol.*, 2002, *26*, 171–175. In urine: codeine and other opioids—C. Meadway *et al.*, *Forensic Sci. Soc.*, 2002, *127*, 136–141.

High performance liquid chromatography. In biological samples: codeine and its metabolites, electrochemical detection—C. P. Verwey-van Wissen *et al.*, *J. Chromatogr.*, 1991, *570*, 309–320. In plasma, urine, or cerebrospinal fluid: limit of detection 500 ng/L, optical scanning detection—G. Chari *et al.*, *J. Chromatogr.*, 1991, *571*, 263–270 and G. Chari *et al.*, *J. Chromatogr.*, 1992, *579*, 189–190 and G. Chari *et al.*, *J. Chromatogr.*, 1992, *579*, 191–192. In plasma or urine: limit of quantification 5 µg/L and 20 µg/L, respectively, for codeine and its metabolites, ECD—T. B. Vree *et al.*, *Biopharm. Drug Dispos.*, 1992, *13*, 445–460. In urine: limit of detection 50 µg/L, UV and ECD—J. Gerostamoulos *et al.*, *J. Chromatogr.*, 1993, *617*, 152–156. In blood or bile: codeine and morphine, limits of quantification in blood 5 mg/L and in urine 0.1 mg/L, UV and fluorescence detection—K. L. Crump *et al.*, *J. Anal. Toxicol.*, 1994, *18*, 208–212. In plasma: limit of detection 5 µg/L, fluorescence detection (λ_{ex} = 214 nm, λ_{em} = 345 nm)—B. Weingarten *et al.*, *J. Chromatogr. A.*, 1995, *696*, 83–92. In plasma or urine: codeine and its metabolites, limit of detection for codeine 6.4 µg/L, UV detection and electrochemical detection—J. O. Svensson *et al.*, *J. Chromatogr.* 1995, *674 B Biomed. Appl.*, 49–55. In hair: codeine and drugs of abuse, electrochemical detection—G. Achilli *et al.*, *J. Chromatogr. A*, 1996, *729*, 273–277. In plasma: codeine and morphine, limit of quantifiaction 50 µg/L, UV detection—M. Friermuth and J. C. Plasse, *J. Pharm. Biomed. Anal.*, 1997, *15*, 759–764. In plasma or urine: codeine and its metabolites, limit of detection for codeine 6.4 µg/L, UV and electrochemical detection—H. He *et al.*, *J. Chromatogr. B Biomed. Sci. Appl.*, 1998, *708*, 185–193. In plasma: limit of detection 0.5 µg/L, UV detection, (λ = 212 nm)—J. A. Pascual and J. Sanagustin, *J. Chromatogr. B Biomed. Sci. Appl.*, 1999, *724*, 295–302. In plasma: limit of detection 0.14 µg/L, ECD—W. J. Liaw *et al.*, *J. Chromatogr. B Biomed. Sci. Appl.*, 1998, *714*, 237–245.

High performance liquid chromatography—Mass spectrometry. In blood, cerebrospinal fluid, serum, urine, or vitreous humour: limits of detection 5 µg/L codeine and 200 µg/L 6-glucuronide—M. J. Bogusz *et al.*, *J. Chromatogr. B Biomed. Sci. Appl.*, 1997, *703*, 115–127. In serum: 4 µg/L—P. Zuccaro *et al.*, *J. Anal. Toxicol.*, 1997, *21*, 268–277. In blood: limit of quantification 1 µg/L for codeine and the 6-glucuronide metabolite—A. Dienes-Nagy *et al.*, *J. Chromatogr. A*, 1999, *854*, 109–118.

Review. Analysis of opioids by GC–MS—R. Wasels and F. Belleville, *J. Chromatogr. A*, 1994, *674*, 225–234.

Disposition in the Body. Well absorbed after oral administration, with peak plasma levels occurring after about 1 h; metabolised in the liver by *O*-demethylation involving P450 isoenzyme CYP2D6 to form morphine, *N*-demethylation to form norcodeine, and conjugation to form glucuronides and sulfates of both unchanged drug and its metabolites. After an oral dose, about 86% is excreted in the urine in 24 h; of the excreted material, 40 to 70% is free or conjugated codeine, 5 to 15% is free or conjugated morphine, 10 to 20% is free or conjugated norcodeine, and trace amounts may be free or conjugated normorphine; some of the dose is excreted in the bile and trace amounts are found in the faeces; unchanged drug accounts for 6 to 8% of the dose in urine in 24 h but this may increase to about 10% when the urinary pH is decreased. After an intramuscular dose, 15 to 20% is excreted unchanged in acid urine in 24 h. Small amounts of hydrocodone, norhydrocodone, 6α-hydrocodol, and 6β-hydrocodol have also been detected in urine.

Therapeutic concentration

13 healthy adult volunteers with a mean age of 36.5 years (33 to 44 years old) were administered 150 mg of a sustained-release formulation of codeine every 12 h for 5 doses and an immediate-release codeine phosphate dose of 60 mg every 4 h for the first 3 doses followed by 30 mg every 4 h for 12 doses. After a single dose, the peak plasma concentration was 217.8 (range, 112.1 to 375.7) μg/L for the sustained-release formulation and 138.8 (49.7 to 221.3) μg/L for the immediate release. These concentrations were observed at 2.3 (1.0 to 4.5) and 1.1 (0.5 to 2.0) h, respectively. The mean steady-state concentrations were 263.8 (172.9 to 453.0) and 222.9 (129.8 to 274.6) μg/L, respectively, for the sustained-release and immediate-release formulations of codeine at 3.2 (1.5 to 5.0) and 1.1 (0.5 to 1.5) h. [C. J. Band *et al.*, *J. Clin. Pharmacol.*, 1994, *34(9)*, 938–943.]

8 healthy male and female volunteers, aged 20 to 50 years, were administered an oral dose of 30 mg codeine phosphate (equivalent to 22 mg codeine). The mean peak codeine plasma concentration was 66.9 (range, 34.0 to 118.8) μg/L; codeine-6-phosphate, 968.0 (693.0 to 1518.0) μg/L; morphine-3-glucuronide, 53.5 (32.2 to 71.3) μg/L. These concentrations were observed after 2 h. [T. B. Vree *et al.*, *Biopharm. Drug Dispos.*, 1992, *13*, 445–460.]

In 11 women undergoing hysterectomy, using patient-controlled analgesia as a means of administering codeine, there was a 9-fold variation in the minimum plasma concentrations consistent with pain relief (40 to 350 μg/L). 2 patients did not experience pain relief, 1 of whom had been classified as a poor metaboliser of dextromethorphan. In the 9 responding patients, the effective dose varied from 4.8 to 25.3 mg/h. [K. Persson *et al.*, *Br. J. Clin. Pharmacol.*, 1995, *39*, 182–186.]

Toxicity. The estimated minimum lethal dose is 800 mg, but codeine is much less toxic than morphine and death directly attributable to codeine is rare; in most fatalities involving codeine, other drugs and/or alcohol is also present. Drug addicts may use doses up to 10 times normal before showing toxic effects, whilst children may show toxicity with only 1/20th of the dose.

Of 107 drug-related deaths involving codeine, it was considered to be the major poison in 6 deaths. The mean total concentration of codeine in femoral blood was 4.0 mg/L (range 2.1 to 8.0), with the mean concentration of free codeine being 1.3 mg/L (range 0.4 to 2.8). In the remaining 101 cases involving a combination of codeine and other drugs (most often paracetamol, diazepam, salicylates, or ethanol), the mean total and free codeine blood concentration was 1.8 mg/L (range 0.04 to 26.00) and 0.82 mg/L (range 0.02 to 9.00), respectively. In the absence of other contributing factors total and free codeine concentrations of >2.0 and >0.4 mg/L, respectively, may be sufficient to cause death. [J. Gerostamoulos *et al.*, *Am. J. Forensic Med. Pathol.*, 1996, *17*, 327–335.]

In 39 fatal cases in which codeine was implicated, the postmortem blood concentrations for codeine ranged from <0.1 mg/L to 8.8 mg/L (mean, 1.2) and for morphine from <0.1 mg/L to 0.7 mg/L (mean, 0.16); in 22 of these cases, the following concentrations, mg/L or μg/g (mean), in other tissues and fluids were reported:

	Codeine	Morphine
Bile	0.5–43 (11)	<0.1–119 (33)
Kidney	<0.1–36.3 (7)	<0.1–12.4 (2)
Liver	<0.1–45 (5)	<0.1–6.4 (2)
Urine	3.2–229 (60)	<0.1–69.8 (20)

In all cases, other drugs were also present. [G. R. Nakamura *et al.*, *J. Forensic Sci.*, 1976, *21*, 518–524.]

In 2 fatalities involving the ingestion of large numbers of codeine tablets, postmortem blood concentrations of codeine of 15 and 48 mg/L were reported; urine concentrations were 155 and 370 mg/L; in both cases alcohol had also been ingested and in one case a low concentration of salicylate was also found in the blood. [M. A. Peat and A. Sengupta, *Forensic Sci.*, 1977, 9, 21–32.]

Bioavailability. About 50%.

Half-life. Plasma half-life, 2 to 4 h.

Volume of distribution. About 2.5 to 3.5 L/kg.

Clearance. Plasma clearance, 10 to 15 mL/min/kg.

Protein binding. In plasma, about 7 to 25%.

Dose. For pain relief, 30 to 60 mg every 4 h to a usual maximum of 240 mg daily.

Co-dergocrine Mesilate

Vasodilator

Synonyms. Co-dergocrine Methanesulfonate; DEA; DHAE; Dihydroergotoxine Mesilate; Dihydrogenated Ergot Alkaloids; Hydrogenated Ergot Alkaloids.

Proprietary names. Circanol; Deapril-ST; Hydergin(e); Progeril.

A mixture in equal proportions of dihydroergocornine mesilate ($C_{31}H_{41}N_5O_5,CH_4O_3S$=659.8), dihydroergocristine mesilate ($C_{35}H_{41}N_5O_5,CH_4O_3S$=707.8), and α- and β-dihydroergocryptine mesilates ($C_{32}H_{43}N_5O_5,CH_4O_3S$=673.8) in the ratio 2:1.

CAS—11032-41-0 (co-dergocrine); 8067-24-1 (mesilate)

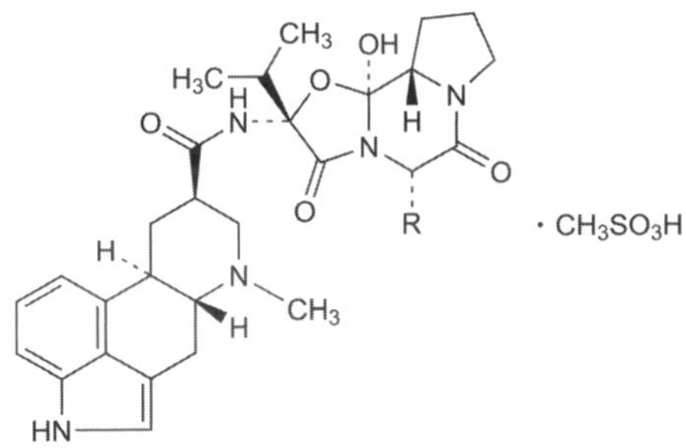

A white to yellowish-white powder. M.p. 196° to 206°, with decomposition. Soluble 1 in 50 of water, 1 in 30 of ethanol, 1 in 10 of acetone, and 1 in 100 of chloroform; practically insoluble in ether.

Dissociation Constant. pK_a 6.9 (24°).

Thin-layer Chromatography. Co-dergocrine: system TA—Rf 66; system TB—Rf 01; system TC—Rf 48; system TL—Rf 29; system TM—Rf 64.

High Performance Liquid Chromatography. System HP—dihydroergocristine *k* 18.3, dihydroergocryptine *k* 15.9.

Infra-red Spectrum. Principal peaks at the following wavenumbers (all KBr disk):
Dihydroergocornine 1633, 1662, 1720, 1705, 1558, 768 cm^{-1}.
Dihydroergocristine 1635, 1728, 1510, 1215, 760, 1540 cm^{-1}.
Dihydroergocryptine mesilate 1633, 1210, 1172, 1048, 1675, 1732 cm^{-1}.

Mass Spectrum. Principal ions at the following *m/z*:
Co-dergocrine 70, 154, 125, 41, 43, 155, 42, 225.
Dihydroergocornine 70, 71, 269, 154, 195, 55, 59, 57.
Dihydroergocristine 125, 70, 91, 153, 41, 244, 43, 71.
Dihydroergocryptine 154, 70, 155, 167, 223, 225, 349, 153.

Quantification

High performance liquid chromatography. In plasma: limit of detection 700 ng/L, fluorescence detection—L. Zecca *et al.*, *J. Chromatogr.*, 1983, *272(23) B Biomed. Appl.*, 401–405.

Radioimmunoassay. In plasma: limit of detection 10 ng/L—W. Loh and B. G. Woodcock, *Arzneimittelforschung*, 1983, *33*, 568–570.

Disposition in the Body. Poorly absorbed after oral administration.

Therapeutic concentration

Following a single oral dose of 4.5 mg to 8 subjects, peak plasma concentrations of 0.3 to 1.1 μg/L (mean 0.0006) were attained in 0.2 to 1.2 h. [B. G. Woodcock *et al.*, *Clin. Pharmacol. Ther.*, 1982, *32*, 622–627.]

Bioavailability. 5 to 12%.

Half-life. Plasma half-life, 8 to 25 h (mean 13).

Volume of distribution. 10 to 20 L/kg.

Clearance. Plasma clearance, 20 to 30 mL/min/kg.

Dose. Up to 4.5 mg daily, by mouth; 0.75 to 3 mg daily, sublingually.

Colchicine

Gout Suppressant

Synonym. Colchicinum

Proprietary names. Colchineos; Colchiquim; Colcin; Colgout; Coluric; Ticolcin. It is also an ingredient of ColBenemid, Colchimax, Gripponyl, and Proben-C.

N-[(7*S*)-5,6,7,9-Tetrahydro-1,2,3,10-tetramethoxy-9-oxobenzo[*a*]-heptalen-7-yl]acetamide

$C_{22}H_{25}NO_6$=399.4

CAS—64-86-8

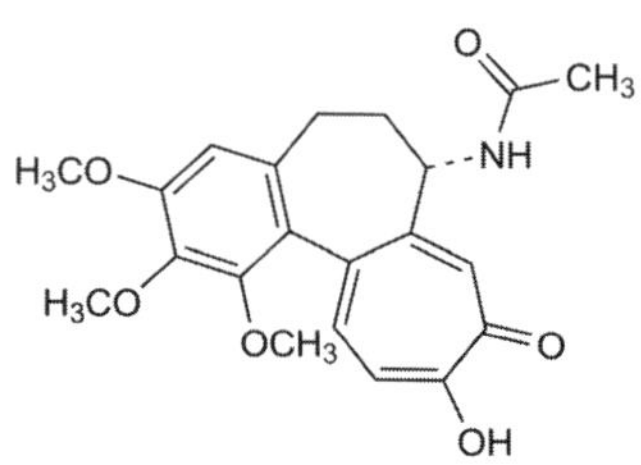

An alkaloid obtained from the corm and seeds of the meadow saffron, *Colchicum autumnale* (Liliaceae) and other *Colchicum* species.

Pale yellow to greenish-yellow crystals or amorphous scales or powder, darkening on exposure to light. M.p. 142° to 150°.

Soluble 1 in about 20 of water, but moderately concentrated aqueous solutions may deposit crystals of a sesquihydrate, which is less soluble in cold water than the anhydrous alkaloid. Freely soluble in ethanol and chloroform; soluble 1 in 220 of ether and 1 in 100 benzene; practically insoluble in petroleum ether.

Dissociation Constant. pK_a 12.35 (20°).

Partition Coefficient. Log *P* (octanol/water), 1.3.

Colour Tests. Liebermann's Test—green; Mandelin's Test—green; Marquis Test—yellow

Thin-layer Chromatography. System TA—Rf 55; system TB—Rf 00; system TC—Rf 37; system TE—Rf 33; system TL—Rf 12; system TAE—Rf 69; system TAF—Rf 63; system TAJ—Rf 39; system TAK—Rf 08; system TAL—Rf 73. (Van Urk reagent, yellow.)

Gas Chromatography. System GA—RI 3200.

High Performance Liquid Chromatography. System HA—*k* 0.2; system HX—RI 382; system HY—RI 327; system HZ—retention time 2.1 min; system HAX—retention time 5.1 min; system HAY—retention time 4.1 min.

Column: (analytical) C_{18} ODS (Hypersil, 125 × 4.6 mm i.d., 5 μm), (guard) C_{18} ODS (10 × 4.6 mm i.d.). Mobile phase: acetonitrile:ammonium sulfate (0.03 M, with 1% TEA, adjusted to pH 3.0 with phosphoric acid); (25:75) for 5 min, gradient to (40:60) in 5 min, held for 10 min; flow rate 1 mL/min. IS: methylclonazepam. UV detection (λ=340 nm). Retention time(s): colchicine, 8.1 min; IS, 18.0 min. [B. Dehon *et al.*, *Biomed. Chromatogr.*, 1999, *13*, 235–238.]

Column: (analytical) RP C_{18} (Novapak, 150 × 4.6 mm i.d., 5 μm), (guard) RP C_{18} (Novapak). Mobile phase: potassium dihydrogen phosphate (0.1 M, with 5 μM pentane sulfonic acid, pH 6.0):methanol:acetonitrile (60:26.6:13.4), flow rate 0.8 mL/min. UV detection (λ=245 nm). Retention time: 6.6 min. [I. M. McIntyre *et al.*, *J. Forensic Sci.*, 1994, *39*, 280–286.]

Ultraviolet Spectrum. Ethanol—243 nm (A^1_1=730a), 350 nm (A^1_1=425a).

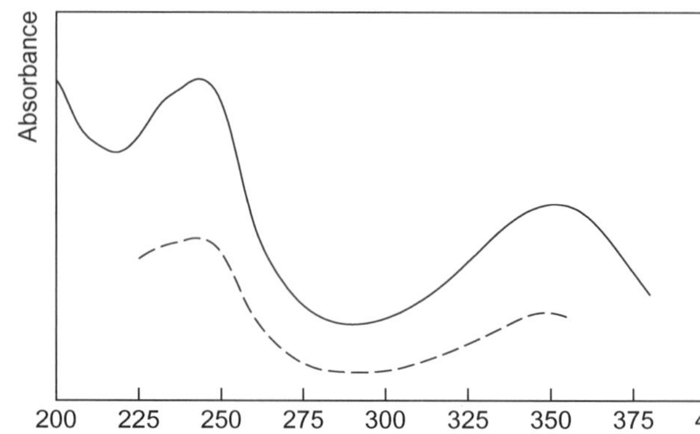

Infra-red Spectrum. Principal peaks at wavenumbers 1250, 1550, 1588, 1610, 1090, 1655 cm^{-1} (KBr disk).

Mass Spectrum. Principal ions at *m/z* 312, 43, 399, 297, 356, 281, 371, 311.

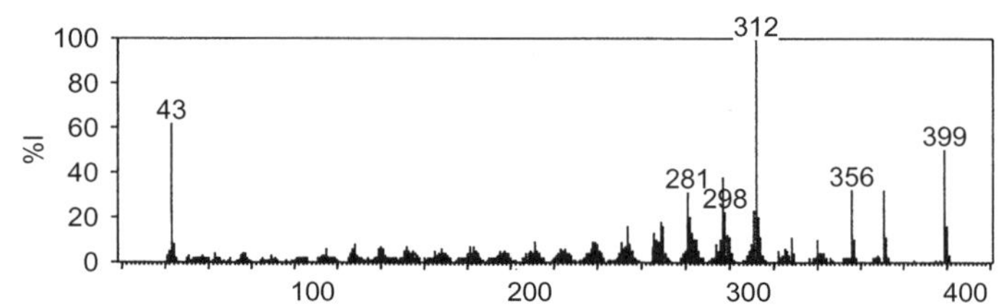

Quantification

Spectrofluorimetry. In plasma or urine—R. Bourdon and M. Galliot, *Ann. Biol. Clin. (Paris)*, 1976, *34*, 393–401.

High performance liquid chromatography. In plasma: limit of detection 5 μg/L, UV detection—D. Jarvie *et al.*, *Clin. Toxicol.*, 1979, *14*, 375–381. In whole blood: limit of detection 10 μg/L, UV detection—Y. H. Caplan *et al.*, *J. Anal. Toxicol.*, 1980, *4*, 153–155. In serum or urine: limits of detection 0.4 μg/L and 4.0 μg/L for desacetylcolchicine and colchicine, respectively (λ=254 nm)—R. J. Ko *et al.*, *J. Chromatogr.*, 1990, *525*, 411–418. In blood: limit of detection 1.0 μg/L, UV detection (λ=350 nm)—P. Kintz *et al.*, *J. Anal. Toxicol.*, 1997, *21*, 70–72. In tissue: limit of detection 5 ng/g, UV detection (λ=340 nm)—B. Dehon *et al.*, *Biomed. Chromatogr.*, 1999, *13*, 235–238.

High performance liquid chromatography–mass spectrometry. In blood, plasma, or urine: limit of detection 0.6 μg/L—A. Tracqui *et al.*, *J. Chromatogr.* 1996, *675 B Biomed. Anal.*, 235–242.

Radioimmunoassay. In serum: limit of detection 350 ng/L—J. M. Scherrmann *et al.*, *J. Pharm. Pharmacol.*, 1980, *32*, 800–802. In plasma: limit of detection 0.2 μg/L, comparison of three RIAs—A. Sabouraud *et al.*, *Ther. Drug Monit.*, 1994, *16*, 179–185.

Disposition in the Body. Readily absorbed after oral administration with peak plasma concentrations reached within 2 h. It is partially deacetylated in the liver to desmethylcolchicine. Most of the drug is excreted in the faeces but 10 to 20% is excreted in the urine. Colchicine is excreted in the bile and undergoes enterohepatic circulation. Colchicine is distributed in the kidney, liver, and spleen, but little is found in the heart, skeletal muscle, and brain.

Therapeutic concentration

In 30 patients treated for familial Mediterranean fever with colchicine 0.5 to 2 mg daily, there was a large inter-subject variability in plasma colchicine concentration (0.13 to 1.75 μg/L 24 h after a dose of 1 mg daily). [O. Chappey *et al.*, *Br. J. Clin. Pharmacol.*, 1994, *38*, 87–89.]

After administration of a single oral dose of 1 mg colchicine to 8 patients with chronic liver disease, a mean peak plasma concentration of 3.6 μg/L (range 0.4 to 10.0) was attained at 2.16 h. Repeated administration resulted in comparable values. Concentrations in bile were higher (2.025 mg/L). [J. Rudi *et al.*, *Scand. J. Gastroenterol.*, 1994, *29*, 346–351.]

Steady-state serum concentrations of 0.3 to 2.4 µg/L were reported after daily oral doses of 1 mg given to 8 subjects. [H. Halkin *et al.*, *Clin. Pharmacol. Ther.*, 1980, *28*, 82–87.]

Toxicity. The minimum lethal dose in man is about 6 mg although recovery has occurred after much larger doses.

A 73-year-old man was hospitalised 8 h after receiving a 1 mg intravenous dose of colchicine for gouty arthritis and died 10 h later; he had consumed 8 × 0.6 mg colchicine tablets over the previous 8 days. The following postmortem colchicine tissue concentrations were reported: cardiac blood 50 µg/L, vitreous humour 10 µg/L, liver 0.575 µg/g, bile 12 000 µg/L, gastric contents 4.4 µg in 60 g. [G. R. Jones *et al., J. Anal. Toxicol.*, 2002, *26*, 365–369.]

After ingestion of about 40 flowers of *Colchicum autumnale* L., a 44-year-old man was admitted 2 h later with nausea, vomiting, and abdominal pains followed by diarrhoea after 14 h. Maximal colchicine levels were 4.34 µg/L at 13 h in plasma and 5.43 µg/L at 16 h in erythrocytes. [V. C. Danel *et al., J. Toxicol. Clin. Toxicol.*, 2001, *39*,409–411.]

In a reported fatality following the ingestion of colchicine tablets, a 42-year-old man had the following levels in blood and postmortem tissues: plasma, 4.5 µg/L (after 24 h); kidney, 396 µg/g; liver, 347 µg/g; heart, 334 µg/g; lung, 58 µg/g; muscle, 10 µg/g; and brain, 5 µg/g. [B. Dehon *et al., Biomed. Chromatogr.*, 1999, *13*, 235–238.]

In a suicidal overdose resulting from the ingestion of colchicine tablets, the femoral blood level was 62 µg/L and the maximum concentration found in bile was 2921 µg/L. [P. Kintz *et al., J. Anal. Toxicol.*, 1997, *21*, 70–72.]

Half-life. Plasma half-life, about 1 h.

Volume of distribution. About 0.7 to 2 L/kg.

Protein binding. In plasma, about 30 to 50%.

Dose. For an acute attack of gout, 1 mg initially, followed by 500 µg every 2 or 3 h; maximum total dose of 6 mg; a second course may be taken after an interval of at least 3 days.

Colecalciferol

Vitamin

Synonyms. Activated 7-Dehydrocholesterol; Cholecalciferol; Vitamin D_3.
Proprietary names. D-Mulsin; D_3-Vicotrat forte; Neo-Dohyfral D_3.
(3*β*,5*Z*,7*E*)-9,10-Secocholesta-5,7,10(19)-trien-3-ol
$C_{27}H_{44}O$=384.6
CAS—67-97-0

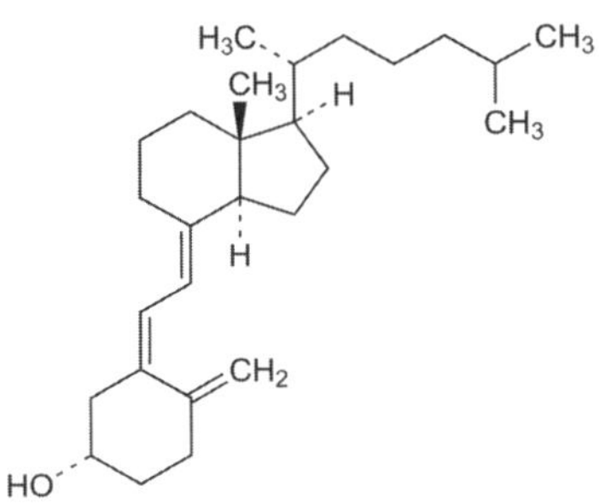

White crystals. It is affected by air and light and should be stored in a cool place in hermetically sealed containers in which the air has been replaced by an inert gas. Solutions in volatile solvents are unstable. M.p. about 84°. Practically insoluble in water; freely soluble in ethanol, chloroform, and ether.

Partition Coefficient. Log *P* (octanol/water), 10.2.

Colour Test. To a 10% solution in chloroform, add 0.3 mL of acetic anhydride and 0.1 mL of sulfuric acid—red→violet→blue-green.

Gas Chromatography. System GA—colecalciferol RI 3150, colecalciferol-H_2O RI 3130.

Ultraviolet Spectrum. Ethanol—265 nm (A^1_1=480a).

Infra-red Spectrum. Principal peaks at wavenumbers 1052, 894, 901, 967, 862, 1075 cm^{-1} (KBr disk).

Quantification

High performance liquid chromatography. In plasma: colecalciferol, ergocalciferol and the 25-hydroxy metabolites, limit of detection 500 ng/L, UV detection—G. Jones, *Clin. Chem.*, 1978, *24*, 287–298.

Disposition in the Body. Well absorbed after oral administration and subject to enterohepatic circulation; decreased absorption may occur in subjects with impaired liver and biliary function. Metabolised by hydroxylation to active metabolites. The major metabolite is 25-hydroxycolecalciferol which is formed in the liver. This is further metabolised by 1α- or 24-hydroxylation in the kidneys. Most of a dose is excreted in the bile and eliminated in the faeces; about 25% of a dose is excreted as conjugates. Unchanged colecalciferol does not appear to be excreted in the urine.

Blood concentration. Normal serum concentrations of 25-hydroxycolecalciferol are about 15 to 40 µg/L, but there are considerable intersubject and seasonal variations.

Half-life. Plasma half-life, about 1 to 2 days; after intravenous administration a terminal elimination half-life of about 18 days has been reported.

Protein binding. Bound to some extent to globulins and to lipoproteins.

Dose. 0.025 to 5 mg daily.

Colfosceril Palmitate

Lung Surfactant

Synonyms. Dipalmitoyl phosphatidylcholine, DPCC.
Proprietary names. Exosurf Neonatal; Exosurf Neonate.
(7*R*)-4-Hydroxy-*N*,*N*,*N*-trimethyl-10-oxo-7-[(1-oxohexadecyl)oxy]-3,5,9-trioxa-4-phosphapentacosan-1-aminium inner salt 4-oxide
$C_{40}H_{80}NO_8P$=734.0
CAS—63-89-8

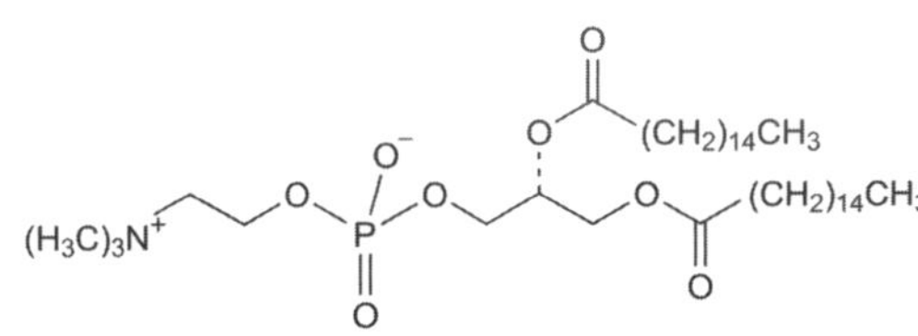

A sterilised lyophilised powder. M.p. 234° to 235°. Readily soluble in chloroform, hot di-isobutyl ketone, hot dioxane. Solubility at 22° to 23° (g/100 mL): ethanol 1.5, ether 0.02, acetone 0.02, pyridine 1.1, acetic acid 4.0, methanol 1.4.

Partition Coefficient. Log *P* (octanol/water), 9.81.

Thin-layer Chromatography. Plate: silica gel (LK5, 20 × 20 cm). Mobile phase: chloroform:methanol:1-propanol:potassium chloride (0.25%):ethyl acetate (25:13:25:9:25 mL). Reference compounds: phosphatidylcholine, sphingomyelin, phosphatidylinositol, phosphatidylethanolamine, phosphatidylserine and phosphatidyl-glycerol. Detection by spraying with cupric acetate (3%):phosphoric acid (8%). Rf 0.35.

Plate: silica gel (LK5, 20 × 20 cm). Mobile phase: chloroform:methanol:2-propanol:potassium chloride (0.25%):triethylamine (30:9:25:6:18 mL). Rf 0.26.

Plate: LHPK (HPTLC) (10 × 10 cm). Mobile phase: chloroform:methanol:2-propanol:water:triethylamine (30:9:27:8:25 mL). Rf 0.23.

Plate: LHPK (HPTLC) (10 × 10 cm). Mobile phase: chloroform:ethanol:water:triethylamine (30:34:7:35 mL). Rf 0.21. [J. C. Touchstone *et al.*, *Lipids*, 1980, *15(1)*, 61–62].

High Performance Liquid Chromatography. Column: ODS silica (Apex II, 25 cm). Mobile phase: choline chloride (40 mM) in methanol:water (92.5:7.5), 1.0 mL/min flow rate. Fluorescence detection (λ_{ex}=340 nm, λ_{em}=460 nm). Retention time: colfosceril palmitate, 39.7 min. [M. R. Ashton *et al.*, *Arch. Dis. Child.*, 1992, *67*, 383–387].

Quantification
High performance liquid chromatography. In endotracheal tube aspirate: limit of detection 0.2 ng/L, fluorescence detection—M. R. Ashton *et al.*, *Arch. Dis. Child.*, 1992, *67*, 383–387.

Disposition in the Body. Colfoscerol palmitate is absorbed from the alveolus into the lung tissue where it is reused for further phospholipid synthesis and secreted into the alveolus as new surfactant. Metabolism occurs and the products are incorporated into the body pools. Elimination is mainly through expired air with a small amount in faeces and urine.

Therapeutic concentration
22 infants of less than 34 weeks' gestation and ventilated from day 1 for respiratory distress syndrome, were administered two doses of 67.5 mg colfosceril palmitate (DPPC) in the first 24 h. Percentage DPPC (of total phosphatidylcholine) reached 100% within 2 days. [M. R. Ashton *et al.*, *Arch. Dis. Child.*, 1992, *67*, 383–387].

Toxicity. Associated with cytotoxicity.

Half-life. Mean half-life of the phosphatidylcholine component, 30 h.

Dose. A single dose of 67.5 mg/kg birth weight of colfoscerol palmitate is administered. Doses may be repeated 12 and 24 h later.

Conessine

Anti-amoebic

(3*β*)-*N*,*N*-Dimethylcon-5-enin-3-amine
$C_{24}H_{40}N_2$=356.6
CAS—546-06-5

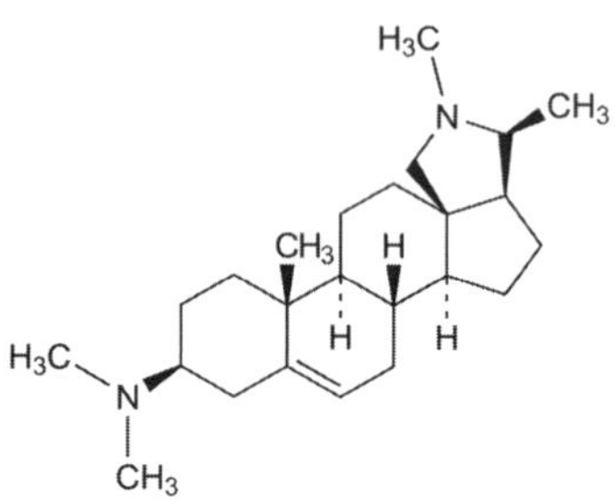

An alkaloid obtained from the seeds of *Holarrhena antidysenterica* (Apocynaceae).
A white crystalline powder. M.p. 127° to 129°.
Sparingly soluble in water.

Conessine Hydrobromide
Synonym. Conessine Bromide
$C_{24}H_{40}N_2$,2HBr=518.4
CAS—5913-82-6
White acicular crystals or microcrystalline powder. M.p. 340°, with decomposition.
Soluble 1 in 5 of water and 1 in 11 of ethanol (90%); very slightly soluble in ether; practically insoluble in petroleum ether.

Partition Coefficient. Log *P* (octanol/water), 5.1.

Colour Tests. Mandelin's Test—yellow; Marquis Test—yellow→orange.

Thin-layer Chromatography. System TA—Rf 28; system TB—Rf 49; system TC—Rf 03; system TL—Rf 03. (Acidified iodoplatinate solution, positive.)

Ultraviolet Spectrum. No significant absorption, 230 to 360 nm.

Mass Spectrum. Principal ions at *m*/*z* 84, 71, 85, 82, 80, 341, 70, 356.

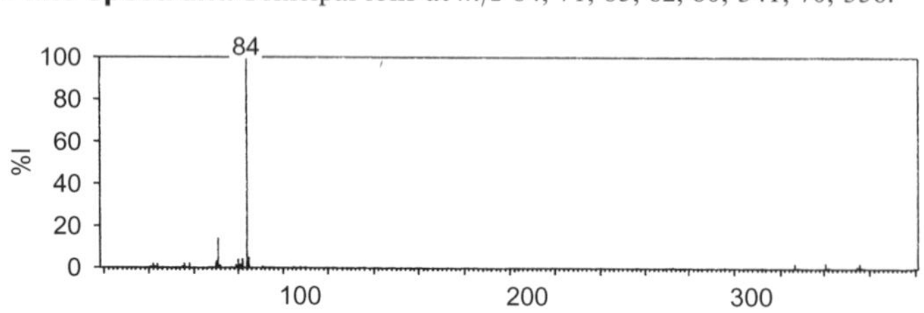

Dose. Conessine hydrobromide was formerly given in doses of 300 to 500 mg daily.

Coniine

Alkaloid

Synonyms. Cicutine; Conicine; Conine.
(2*S*)-2-Propylpiperidine
$C_8H_{17}N$=127.2
CAS—458-88-8

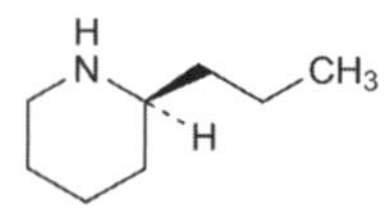

An alkaloid obtained mainly from the fruits and leaves of hemlock, *Conium maculatum* (Umbelliferae).
An almost colourless volatile liquid. F.p. −2°. B.p. 166°.
Soluble 1 in 100 of water; miscible with ethanol and ether; slightly soluble in chloroform.

Coniine Hydrobromide
$C_8H_{17}N$,HBr=208.1
CAS—637-49-0
Colourless crystals. M.p. about 211°.
Soluble 1 in 2 of water and 1 in 3 of ethanol; soluble in chloroform and ether.

Dissociation Constant. pK_a 11.0 (25°).

Partition Coefficient. Log *P* (octanol/water), 2.6.

Thin-layer Chromatography. System TA—Rf 26; system TB—Rf 39; system TC—Rf 13; system TE—Rf 37; system TL—Rf 05; system TAE—Rf 05; system TAF—Rf 70. (Acidified iodoplatinate solution, positive.)

Gas Chromatography. System GA—not eluted.

High Performance Liquid Chromatography. System HX—RI 214.

Ultraviolet Spectrum. Aqueous acid—266 (A_1^1=6b); aqueous alkali—262, 268 nm.

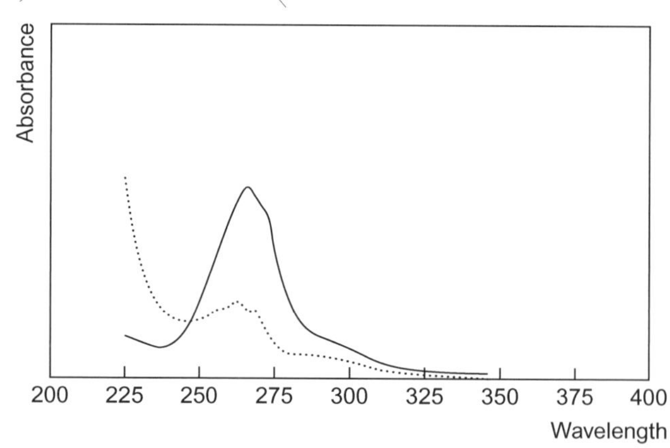

Infra-red Spectrum. Principal peaks at wavenumbers 1033, 1007, 1575, 1300, 1078, 1139 cm^{-1} (coniine hydrobromide, Nujol mull).

Mass Spectrum. Principal ions at *m*/*z* 84, 82, 80, 56, 43, 28, 30, 41.

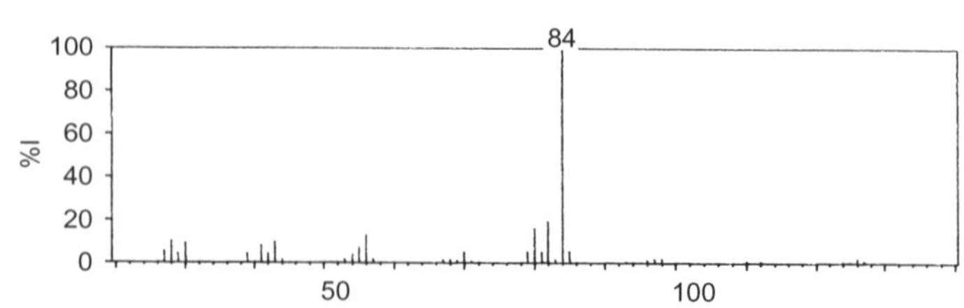

Disposition in the Body
Toxicity. Coniine is well absorbed from the gastro-intestinal tract and is very poisonous; the estimated minimum lethal dose is 150 mg and toxic symptoms may occur after ingestion of 60 mg. Death may occur within 30 min or be delayed 3 to 12 h. Coniine resembles nicotine in its peripheral action but produces more pronounced paralysis of the CNS and of the skeletal muscle nerve endings.

Cortisone

Corticosteroid

Synonyms. Compound E; 11-Dehydro-17-hydroxycorticosterone.
17,21-Dihydroxypregn-4-ene-3,11,20-trione
$C_{21}H_{28}O_5$=360.4
CAS—53-06-5

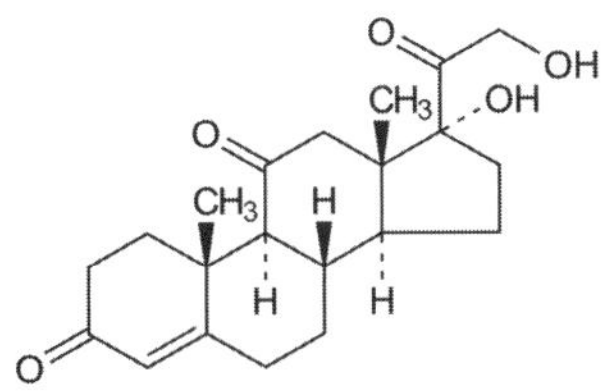

Crystals. M.p. 217° to 224°, with some decomposition.
Very slightly soluble in water; fairly soluble in ethanol and acetone; sparingly soluble in chloroform and ether.

Cortisone Acetate

Synonym. Cortisone 21-Acetate
Proprietary names. Adreson; Cortate; Cortelan; Cortisol; Cortison; Cortistab; Cortisyl; Cortone; Cortone Acetate; Sterop.
Note. The name Cortisol is also applied to hydrocortisone.
$C_{23}H_{30}O_6$=402.5
CAS—50-04-4
A white crystalline powder. M.p. 235° to 238°, with decomposition.
Soluble 1 in 5000 of water, 1 in 300 to 1 in 350 of ethanol, and 1 in 4 of chloroform; slightly soluble in ether.

Partition Coefficient. Log *P* (octanol/water), 1.5.

Colour Tests. Naphthol–Sulfuric Acid—orange-brown/orange; Sulfuric Acid—yellow (green fluorescence under UV light).

Thin-layer Chromatography. Cortisone acetate: system TA—Rf 90; system TB—Rf 03; system TE—Rf 68; system TP—Rf 72; system TQ—Rf 28; system TR—Rf 55; system TS—Rf 00; system TAE—Rf 87; system TAJ—Rf 51; system TAK—Rf 09; system TAL—Rf 83; system TAM—Rf 91. (DPST solution.)

High Performance Liquid Chromatography. System HT—*k* 2.4; system HY—RI 372.

Ultraviolet Spectrum. Cortisone acetate: ethanol—240 nm (A^1_1=390a).

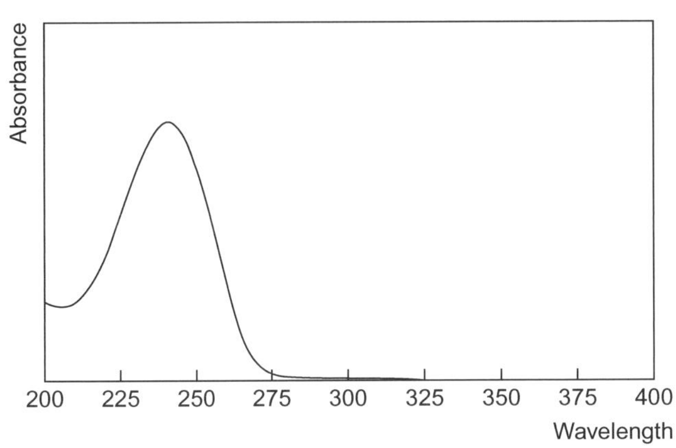

Infra-red Spectrum. Principal peaks at wavenumbers 1700, 1660, 1235, 1720, 1275, 1750 cm^{-1} (cortisone acetate, KBr disk).

Quantification

High performance liquid chromatography. In plasma and urine: limit of detection 0.1 mg/L, fluorescence detection—N. Shibata *et al.*, *J. Chromatogr. B Biomed. Sci. Appl.*, 1998, *706*, 191–199. In hair: limit of detection 0.03 to 0.17 mg/g, MS—V. Cirimele *et al.*, *Forensic Sci. Int.*, 2000, *107*, 381–388. In urine: limit of detection 2 mg/L, MS/MS—R. L. Taylor *et al.*, *Clin. Chem.*, 2002, *48*, 1511–1519.

Dose. 25 to 50 mg of cortisone acetate daily.

Cotarnine

Haemostatic

5,6,7,8-Tetrahydro-4-methoxy-6-methyl-1,3-dioxolo[4,5-*g*]isoquinolin-5-ol
$C_{12}H_{15}NO_4$=237.3
CAS—82-54-2

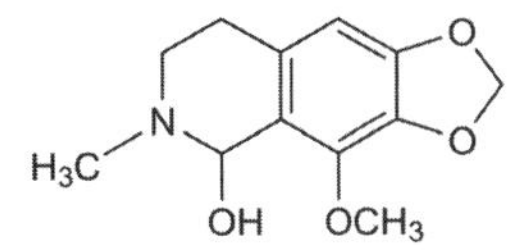

An alkaloid obtained by oxidising noscapine with nitric acid. Crystals. M.p. 132° to 137°, with decomposition.
Slightly soluble in water; soluble in dilute acids, ethanol, chloroform, benzene, and ether.

Cotarnine Chloride

Synonyms. Cotarnine Hydrochloride; Stypticine.
$C_{12}H_{14}ClNO_3,2H_2O$=291.7
CAS—10018-19-6 (anhydrous); 16210-52-9 (dihydrate)
A pale yellow deliquescent powder. M.p. 197°. When heated to decomposition, highly toxic fumes are evolved.
Soluble in water, ethanol, and chloroform; practically insoluble in ether.

Partition Coefficient. Log *P* (octanol/water), 0.6.

Colour Tests. Liebermann's Test—black; Mandelin's Test—red-orange→brown.

Thin-layer Chromatography. System TA—Rf 02; system TB—Rf 38; system TC—Rf 01; system TE—Rf 26; system TL—Rf 00; system TAE—Rf 01; system TAF—Rf 22. (Acidified iodoplatinate solution, positive.)

Gas Chromatography. System GA—RI 1808.

High Performance Liquid Chromatography. System HA—*k* 8.2 (tailing peak).

Ultraviolet Spectrum. Aqueous acid—253 (A^1_1=582b), 332 (A^1_1=666b); aqueous alkali—286, 330 nm.

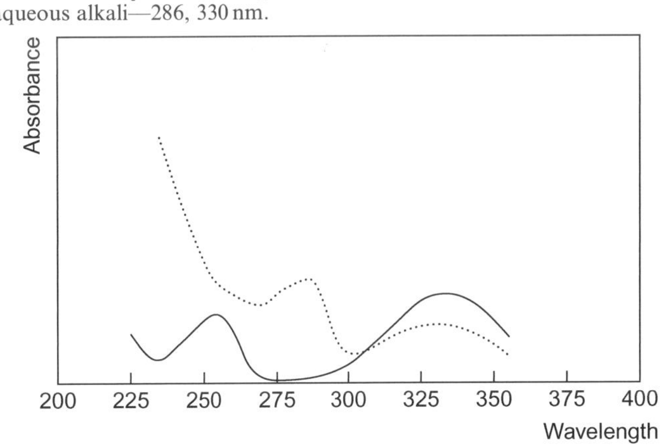

Infra-red Spectrum. Principal peaks at wavenumbers 1605, 1086, 1490, 1655, 1505, 1300 cm^{-1} (cotarnine chloride, KCl disk).

Dose. Cotarnine chloride was formerly given in doses of 20 to 100 mg.

Coumaphos

Ectoparasiticide, Insecticide, Nematicide

Synonyms. Bayer 21/199; Coumafos; ENT 17957; OMS 485.
Proprietary names. Agridip; Asunthol; Baymix; Checkmite; Co-Ral; Diolice; Meldane; Muscatox; Negasunt; Perizin; Resitox; Suntol; Umbethion.
Phosphorothioic acid *O*-(3-chloro-4-methyl-2-oxo-2*H*-1-benzopyran-7-yl) *O,O*-diethyl ester
$C_{14}H_{16}ClO_5PS$=362.8
CAS—56-72-4

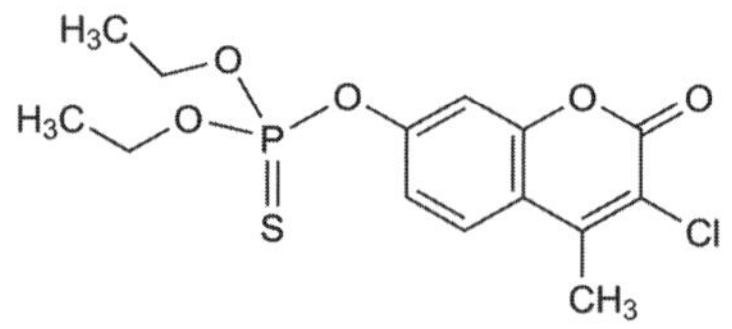

A white to tan to grey coloured crystalline solid. M.p. 95° (90° to 92° in the technical state).
It is practically insoluble in water; limited solubility in most organic solvents; soluble in chloroform.

Partition Coefficient. Log *P* (octanol/water), 4.13.

Thin-layer Chromatography. System TX—Rf 27; system TY—Rf 61.

Gas Chromatography. System GA—RI 2573.

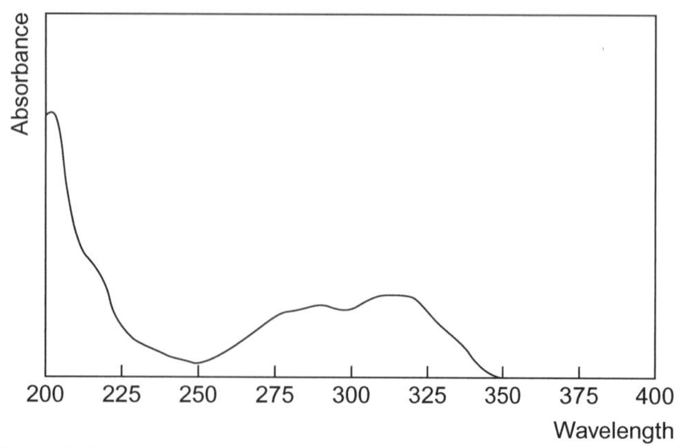

Infra-red Spectrum. Principal peaks at wavenumber 1774, 1046, 1004, 888, 1609, 1151 cm^{-1}.

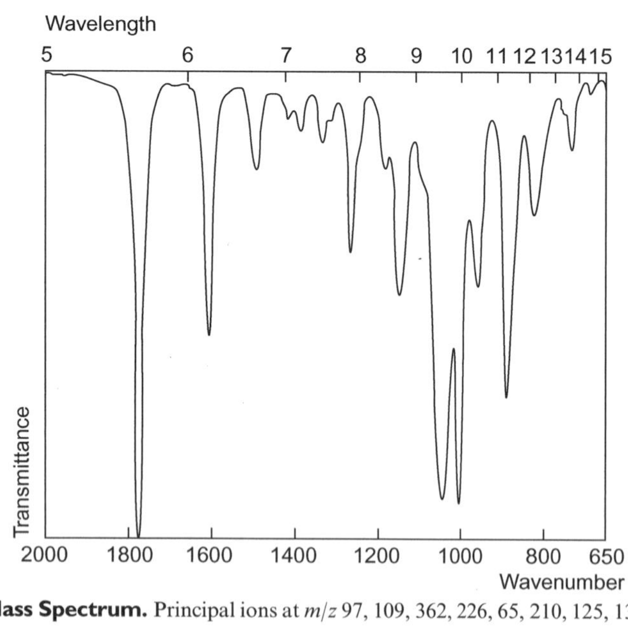

Mass Spectrum. Principal ions at *m*/*z* 97, 109, 362, 226, 65, 210, 125, 137.

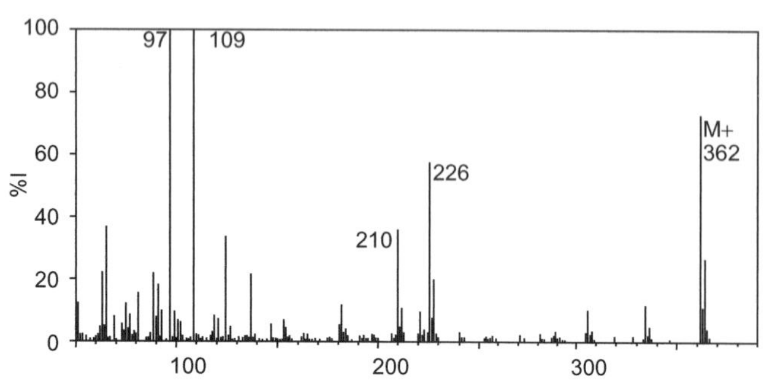

Disposition in the Body. Coumaphos is readily absorbed through the skin. It is rapidly broken down in the body into non-toxic products which are eliminated via urine (the majority) and faeces. There is no evidence of bioaccumulation.

Toxicity. Coumaphos is highly toxic if ingested or inhaled, and is moderately toxic via skin contact and if administered via intraperitoneal routes.

Coumatetralyl

Rodenticide

Proprietary name. Racumin
4-Hydroxy-3-(1,2,3,4-tetrahydro-1-naphthyl)coumarin
$C_{19}H_{16}O_3$=292.3
CAS—5836-29-3

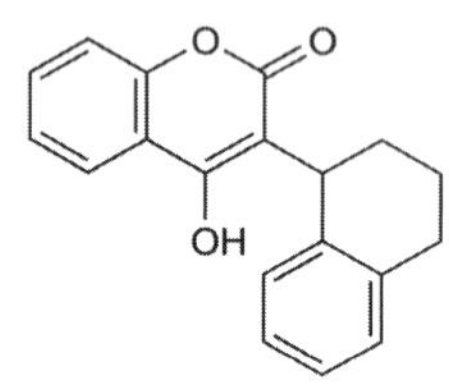

A yellowish-white crystalline powder. M.p. 172° to 176°.
Practically insoluble in water; soluble in ethanol and acetone; slightly soluble in ether.

Dissociation Constant. pK_a 4.8.

Partition Coefficient. Log *P* (octanol/water), 3.5.

Thin-layer Chromatography. System TD—Rf 73; system TE—Rf 13; system TF—Rf 74; system TX—Rf 14; system TY—Rf 30. (Location under UV light, pink fluorescence; acidified potassium permanganate solution, positive.)

Gas Chromatography. System GA—coumatetralyl RI 2635, coumatetralyl-HY RI 2250, coumatetralyl-Me-HY RI 2300, coumatetralyl isomer-1-Me RI 2655, coumatetralyl isomer-2-Me RI 2690, M (OH-) isomer-1-ME RI 2910, M (OH-) isomer-2-Me_2 RI 2925, M (OH-) isomer-3-Me_2 RI 2935, M (OH-) isomer-4-Me_2 RI 2990, M (di-OH-) isomer-1-Me_2 RI 3005, M (OH-methoxy-)-Me_2 RI 3070, M (di-OH-) isomer-2-Me_2 RI 3085, M (di-OH-) isomer-3-Me_3 RI 3105, M (tri-OH-)-H_2O-Me_2 RI 3175.

High Performance Liquid Chromatography. System HY—RI 598; system HAA—retention time 5.0 min.

Ultraviolet Spectrum. Aqueous acid—273, 283, 309; aqueous alkali—311 nm.

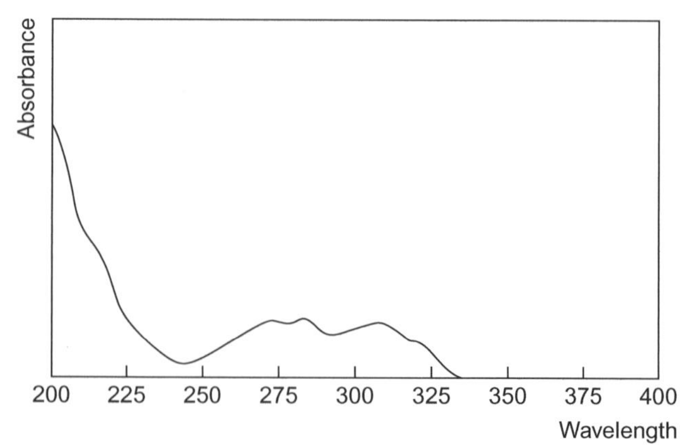

Infra-red Spectrum. Principal peaks at wavenumbers 1615, 762, 740, 1685, 1250, 1570 cm^{-1}.

Mass Spectrum. Principal ions at *m*/*z* 292, 121, 188, 130, 115, 91, 128, 129.

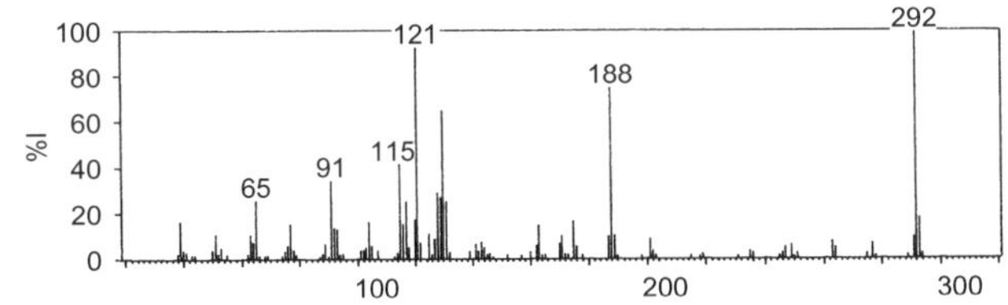

Quantification

High performance liquid chromatography. In serum and liver: 1 mg/L and 1 ng/g, respectively, fluorescence detection (λ_{ex}=318 nm; λ_{em}=390 nm) — T. Chalermchaikit *et al.*, *J. Anal. Toxicol.*, 1993, *17(1)*, 56–61.

Thin layer chromatography. In blood and liver samples: limit of detection 0.2 mg/L and 0.2 mg/g, respectively, and limit of quantification 0.5 mg/L—P. J. Berny *et al.*, *J. Anal. Toxicol.*, 1995, *19(7)*, 576–580.

Cresol

Disinfectant

Synonyms. Cresylic Acid; Tricresol. It is an ingredient of Lysol (Cresol and Soap Solution containing 50% v/v of cresol).
Note. The use of the name Lysol is limited. In some countries it is a trademark applied to a product of different composition.
Proprietary name. It is an ingredient of Lyseptol.
Cresol is a mixture of *o*-, *m*-, and *p*-cresols ($CH_3C_6H_4OH$=108·1), in which the *m*-isomer predominates, and of other phenols obtained from coal tar.
CAS—1319-77-3; 95-48-7 (o-cresol); 108-39-4 (m-cresol);106-44-5 (p-cresol)

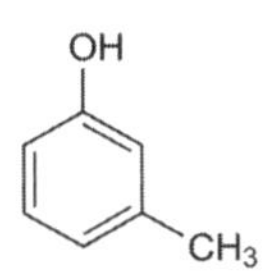

m-cresol

An almost colourless to pale brownish-yellow liquid, becoming darker with age or on exposure to light. Mass per mL 1.029 to1.044 g. B.p. 195° to 205°. Almost completely soluble 1 in 50 of water; miscible with ethanol, benzene, chloroform, glycerol, petroleum ether, and ether. Soluble in solutions of fixed alkali hydroxides.

Dissociation Constant. pK_a *m*-cresol 10.1, *o*-cresol 10.3, *p*-cresol 10.3 (25°).

Partition Coefficient. Log *P* (octanol/water), 2.0.

Colour Tests. Folin–Ciocalteau Reagent—blue; Liebermann's Test—black; Potassium Dichromate—brown (*o*-cresol 30 s, *m*-cresol 2 min).
Heat with about an equal quantity of phthalic anhydride and a few drops of sulfuric acid until the mixture is orange-brown; cool the mixture with a few drops of water and make alkaline with sodium hydroxide solution—red with *o*-cresol and blue-violet with *m*-cresol.

Thin-layer Chromatography. System TAJ—*m*-cresol RF 69, *o*-cresol RF 73, *p*-cresol RF 66; system TAK—*m*-cresol RF 78, *o*-cresol RF 82, *p*-cresol RF 78; system TAL—*m*-, *o*-, *p*-cresol RF 96.

Gas Chromatography. System GA—*m*-cresol RI 1065, *o*-cresol RI 1040, *p*-cresol RI 1060, *p*-cresol-AC RI 1110.

Ultraviolet Spectrum. Aqueous alkali—239 (A^1_1=949b), 290 (A^1_1=251b); ethanol—275 (A^1_1=163b), 279 nm(A^1_1=145b).

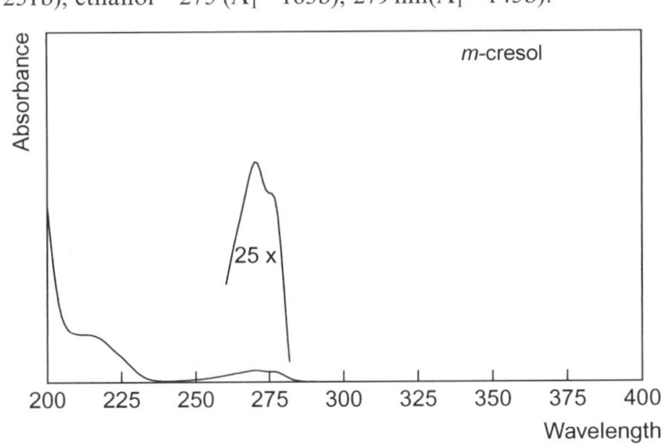

Infra-red Spectrum. Principal peaks at wavenumbers 1209, 816, 1515, 741, 1176, 1105 cm^{-1} (*p*-cresol, Nujol mull).

Mass Spectrum. Principal ions at *m/z* 107, 108, 77, 79, 51, 39, 53, 50 (*p*-cresol).

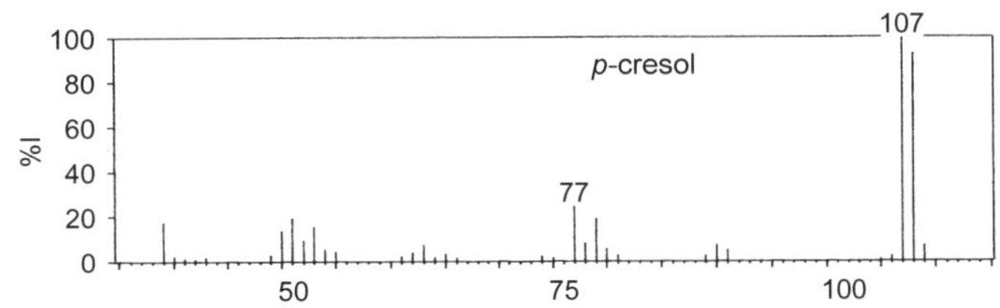

Quantification

Gas chromatography. In blood, urine or tissues: limit of detection 20 mg/L, FID—A. M. Bruce *et al.*, *Med. Sci. Law*, 1976, *16*, 171–176. In urine: ECD—R. L. Dills *et al.*, *J. Chromatogr. B Biomed. Sci. Appl.*, 1997, *703(1–2)*, 105–113. In urine: FID—L. C. Amorim *et al.*, *J. Toxicol. Environ. Health*, 1997, *50(4)*, 401–407. In biological fluids—M. Yashiki *et al.*, *Forensic Sci. Int.*, 1990, *47(1)*, 21–29.

High performance liquid chromatography. In serum: limit of detection *p*-cresol 0.14 mg/L, fluorescence detection (λ_{ex}=284 nm; λ_{em}=310 nm)—R. De Smet *et al.*, *Clin. Chim. Acta*, 1998, *278(1)*, 1–21. In urine and faeces: limit of detection 0.8 mg, UV detection (λ = 270 nm) —A. M. Birkett *et al.*, *J. Chromatogr. Biomed. Sci. Appl.*, 1995, *674(2)*, 187–191. In urine: limit of detection 0.2 mg/L, UV detection (λ = 271 nm) —J. Schlatter and A. Astier, *Biomed. Chromatogr.*, 1995, *9(6)*, 302–304.

Disposition in the Body. Absorbed after ingestion, and through the skin and mucous membranes. It is metabolised by conjugation and oxidation; *p*-cresol is endogenously produced in normal subjects, and may be present in urine at concentrations of 20 to 200 mg/L (mainly in conjugated form).

Toxicity. The estimated minimum lethal dose is 2 g, and the maximum permissible atmospheric concentration is 5 ppm.

In 2 fatalities due to the ingestion of cresol, the following postmortem tissue concentrations were reported: blood 71, 190 mg/L; brain 2.8, – μg/g; kidney 396, – μg/g; liver 900, 480 μg/g; urine –, 304 mg/L. [A. M. Bruce *et al.*, *Med. Sci. Law*, 1976, *16*, 171–176.]

A 65-year-old man with schizophrenia died 15 min after he ingested a large volume of saponated cresol solution. Free *p*-cresol was detected in heart blood at a concentration of 458.8 mg/L and *m*-cresol at 957.3 mg/L; and the glucuronic acid conjugated forms at 38.2 and 85.6 mg/L, respectively. 250 mL of a cresol-odour-emitting fluid was also present in the stomach. [J. Monma-Ohtaki *et al.*, *Forensic Sci. Int.*, 2002, *126(1)*, 77–81.]

A 46-year-old man ingested 100 mL of saponated cresol solution and was admitted to hospital. The serum concentrations of *p*-cresol and *m*-cresol were 43.3 mg/g and 73.8 mg/g, respectively, and the total concentration of cresol was 117 mg/g. Although levels were in the fatal ranges the individual recovered after hospital treatment. [M. Yashiki *et al.*, *Forens. Sci. Int.*, 1990, *47(1)*, 21–29.]

Cropropamide

Respiratory Stimulant

Synonym. It is an ingredient of Prethcamide which is a mixture of equal parts by weight of cropropamide and crotetamide.
Proprietary names. It is an ingredient of Micoren and of Respirot.
N-[1-[(Dimethylamino)carbonyl]propyl]-*N*-propyl-2-butenamide
$C_{13}H_{24}N_2O_2$=240.3
CAS—633-47-6 (cropropamide); 8015-51-8 (prethcamide)

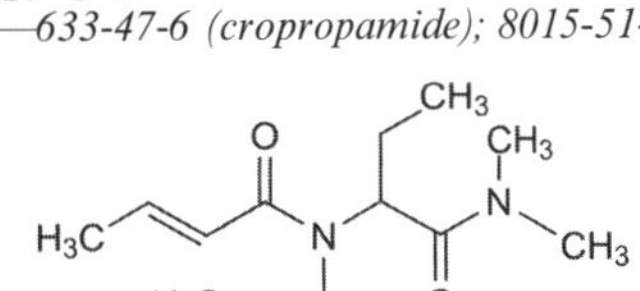

A liquid.
Easily soluble in water and ether; miscible with ethanol.

Partition Coefficient. Log *P* (octanol/water), 1.6.

Thin-layer Chromatography. System TA—Rf 70; system TB—Rf 29; system TC—Rf 69; system TE—Rf 74; system TL—Rf 57; system TAE—Rf 25; system TAF—Rf 83. (Acidified potassium permanganate solution, positive.)

Gas Chromatography. System GA—RI 1738.

High Performance Liquid Chromatography. System HZ—Retention time(s), 3.3 min.

Ultraviolet Spectrum. No significant absorption, 230 to 360 nm.

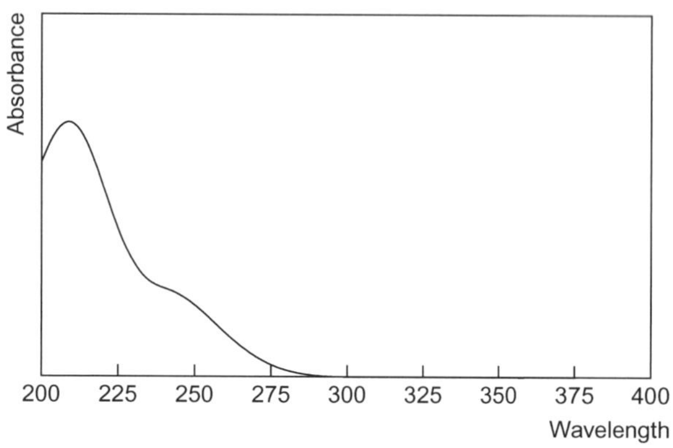

Infra-red Spectrum. Principal peaks at wavenumbers 1654, 1617, 1219, 1282, 1098, 1123 cm^{-1} (KBr disk).

Dose. Prethcamide (cropropamide and crotetamide) is usually given in doses of 1.2 to 1.6 g daily.

Crotamiton

Acaricide/Antipruritic

Proprietary names. Crotamitex; Eurax; Euraxil.
N-Ethyl-*N*-(2-methylphenyl)-2-butenamide
$C_{13}H_{17}NO = 203.3$
CAS—483-63-6

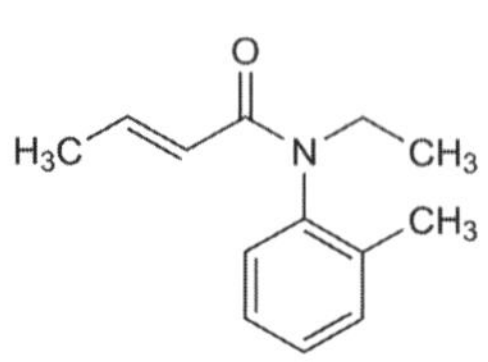

A colourless or pale yellow, oily liquid.
Soluble 1 in 400 of water; miscible with ethanol, ether, and methanol.

Partition Coefficient. Log *P* (octanol/water), 2.7.

Thin-layer Chromatography. System TA—Rf 83; system TE—Rf 83; system TAE—Rf 84. (Acidified iodoplatinate solution, positive.)

Gas Chromatography. System GA—RI 1600.

Ultraviolet Spectrum. No significant absorption, 230 to 360 nm.

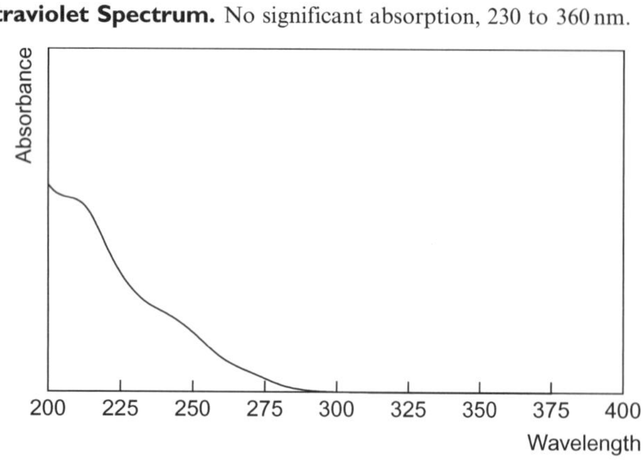

Infra-red Spectrum. Principal peaks at wavenumbers 1656, 1623, 1235, 1280, 1316, 1590 cm^{-1} (thin film).

Use. Topically in a concentration of 10%.

Crotetamide

Respiratory Stimulant

Synonyms. Crotethamide. It is an ingredient of Prethcamide which is a mixture of equal parts by weight of cropropamide and crotetamide.
Proprietary names. It is an ingredient of Micoren and of Respirot.
N-[1-[(Dimethylamino)carbonyl]propyl]-*N*-ethyl-2-butenamide
$C_{12}H_{22}N_2O_2 = 226.3$
CAS—6168-76-9 (crotetamide); 8015-51-8 (prethcamide)

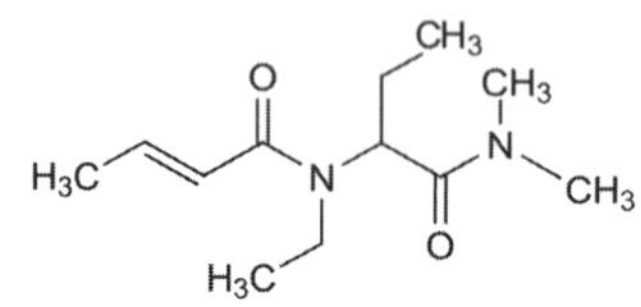

A liquid.
Easily soluble in water and ether; miscible with ethanol.

Partition Coefficient. Log *P* (octanol/water), 1.1.

Thin-layer Chromatography. System TA—Rf 68; system TB—Rf 28; system TC—Rf 67; system TE—Rf 69; system TL—Rf 55; system TAE—Rf 83; system TAF—Rf 79. (Acidified potassium permanganate solution, positive.)

Gas Chromatography. System GA—RI 1688.

High Performance Liquid Chromatography. System HX—RI 366; system HZ—Retention time(s), 2.6 min.

Ultraviolet Spectrum. No significant absorption, 230 to 360 nm.

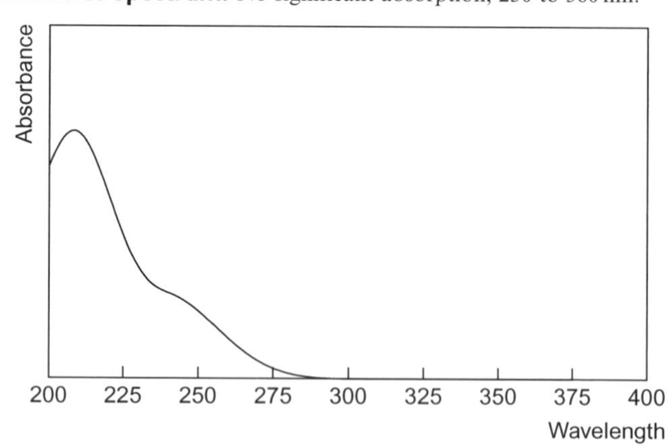

Infra-red Spectrum. Principal peaks at wavenumbers 1655, 1617, 1234, 1098, 1282, 1123 cm^{-1} (KBr disk).

Dose. See under Cropropamide.

Cryofluorane

Aerosol Propellent/Refrigerant

Synonyms. Dichlorotetrafluoroethane; Propellent 114; Refrigerant 114; Tetrafluorodichloroethane.
Proprietary names. Arcton 33; Arcton 114.
1,2-Dichloro-1,1,2,2-tetrafluoroethane
$CClF_2{\cdot}CClF_2 = 170.9$
CAS—76-14-2

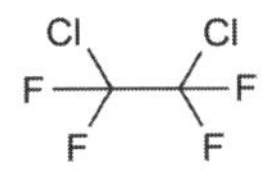

A colourless non-flammable gas which, when liquefied by compression, forms a clear colourless liquid. B.p. about 3.5°.
In the liquid state it is practically immiscible with water, but miscible with dehydrated alcohol.

Partition Coefficient. Log *P* (octanol/water), 2.8.

Gas Chromatography. System GA—RI 361; system GI—Retention time 2.0 min.

Mass Spectrum. Principal ions at *m/z* 85, 135, 87, 137, 31, 101, 100, 50.

Cyanide

Synonyms. Cyanide (1 −); cyanide anion; cyanide ion; cyanides; isocyanide.
CN = 26.0177
CAS—57-12-5
A white solid with a faint almond odour. Water solubility 9.54 mg/L (25°).

Partition Coefficient. Log *P* (octanol/water), −0.69.

Colour Test. Sodium picrate—orange-red/red; limit of detection 25 to 135 µg/L.

Gas Chromatography. Column: PLOT fused-silica (Supel-Q, 30 m × 0.32 mm i.d.). Column temperature: 1 min hold at −30°, 10°/min from −30° to 160°. Injector temperature: 150°. Carrier gas: helium, 3.0 mL/min flow rate. Detection: nitrogen–phosphorous and mass spectrometry (EI, SIM). Retention time: cyanide 9.0 min. [I. Akira *et al.*, *Anal. Chem.*, 1998, 70, 4873–4876].

Column: silica (CP Sil 8B methyl silicone, 50 m × 0.23 mm, film thickness 1.2 µm). Column temperature: 60°. Carrier gas: helium, flow rate 2 mL/min. Split ratio 1:20. ECD. Retention time: cyanogen chloride, 2.7 min. [M. Odoul *et al.*, *J. Anal. Toxicol.*, 1994, 18, 205–207].

High Performance Liquid Chromatography. Column: RP18 (Hypersil ODS, 5 µm, 100 × 2.1 mm i.d.). Mobile phase: deionised water:acetonitrile (92:8), 0.4 mL/min flow rate. Fluorescence detection (λ_{ex} = 418 nm, λ_{em} = 460 nm). Retention time: 1-cyano-2-substituted benzoisoindole derivative, 1.7 min. [D. Felscher and M. Wulfmeyer, *J. Anal. Toxicol.*, 1998, *22*, 363–366].

Column: C_{18} (Kromasil KR 100-5, 250 × 4.6 mm, 5 µm) with C_{18} precolumn (Kromasil, 10 × 3.2 mm, 5 µm). Mobile phase: methanol:orthophosphoric acid (50 mM, pH 2.3) (1:1.3), 0.5 mL/min flow rate. Fluorimetric detection (λ_{ex} = 385 nm, λ_{em} = 476 nm). Retention times: *N*-carbamylcysteine–DACM derivative, 12 min; cysteine–DACM derivative, 22 and 24 min. [P. Lundquist *et al.*, *Anal. Biochem.*, 1995, *228*, 27–34].

Mass Spectrum. Principal ions at *m/z* 27, 26, 12, 28, 13, 14 (HCN).

Quantification
Gas chromatography. In whole blood: limit of detection 5 µg/L, ECD—M. Odoul *et al.*, *J. Anal. Toxicol.*, 1994, *18*, 205–207.

Gas chromatography–mass spectrometry. In whole blood: limit of detection 2 µg/L—I. Akira *et al.*, *Anal. Chem.*, 1998, *70*, 4873–4876.

High performance liquid chromatography. In whole blood: limit of detection 2 µg/L, fluorescence detection (λ_{ex} = 418 nm, λ_{em} = 460 nm)—D. Felscher and M. Wulfmeyer, *J. Anal. Toxicol.*, 1998, *22*, 363–366. In urine: limit of detection 0.3 µg/L, fluorescence detection (λ_{ex} = 385 nm, λ_{em} = 476 nm)—P. Lundquist *et al.*, *Anal. Biochem.*, 1995, *228*, 27–34.

Bioassay. In serum: limit of detection is 100 µg/L—T. Fonong, *Analyst*, 1987, *112*, 1033–1035.

Disposition in the Body. Cyanide is metabolised to thiocyanate after reacting with a sulfur donor, for example, thiosulfate. Up to 80% of a cyanide dose is converted this way. An alternative metabolic pathway is the formation of 2-aminothiazoline-4-carboxylic acid (ATC) when cyanide reacts with cystine (when exposure rate exceeds cyanide-to-thiocyanate conversion rate). Cyanide is excreted through the lungs and kidneys.

Therapeutic concentration A smoker can have cyanide levels of ⩾500 µg/L in whole blood. For normal red blood cell cyanide, levels can be <26 µg/L.

In healthy volunteers, endogenous cyanide concentration were found to be approx. 8.41 ± 3.09 µg/L. [I. Akira *et al.*, *Anal. Chem.*, 1998, *70*, 4873–4876].

Toxicity. Cyanide can be fatal at plasma concentrations of 260 µg/L and above. The toxic concentration is 500 µg/L; lethal concentration, 4 to 5 mg/L; also reported to be as low as 1 mg/L.

Half-life. Cyanide has a half-life of 0.7 to 2.1 h.

Volume of distribution. Volume of distribution for cyanide is 0.4 L/kg.

Distribution in blood. Cyanide is concentrated in the erythrocytes. 98% of cyanide is found in red blood cells and 2% in plasma.

Protein binding. Binds to methaemoglobin, present in haemoglobin.

Cyanocobalamin

Haemopoietic Vitamin

Synonyms. Cobamin; Cycobemin; Vitamin B_{12}.
Proprietary names. Anacobin; Bedoz; Berubigen; Betalin 12; Bio-12; Cyanabin; Cytacon; Cytamen; Hepacon-B12; Neo-Rubex; Redisol; Rubesol; Rubion; Rubramin; Ruvite; Sytobex. It is an ingredient of Ce-Cobalin, Hepanorm and Reactivan.
5,6-Dimethylbenzimidazolyl cyanocobamide
$C_{63}H_{88}CoN_{14}O_{14}P$ = 1355.4
CAS—68-19-9

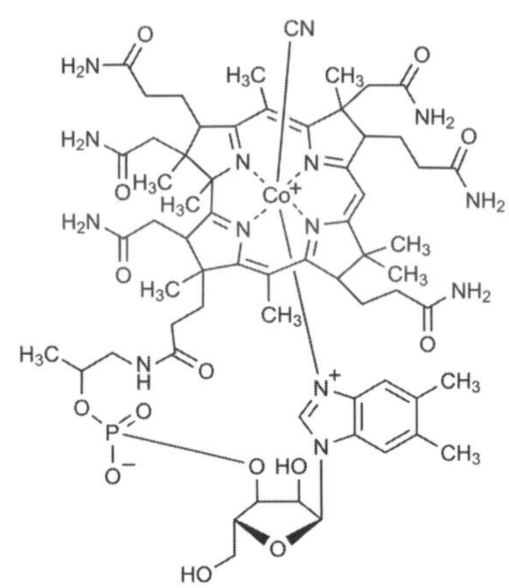

Dark red hygroscopic crystals or powder.
Soluble 1 in 80 of water and 1 in 180 of ethanol (90%); practically insoluble in chloroform and ether.

Partition Coefficient. Log *P* (octanol/water), 3.6.

High Performance Liquid Chromatography. System HAA—Retention time(s), 3.8 min.

Ultraviolet Spectrum. Water—278 (A^1_1 = 119a), 361 (A^1_1 = 207a), 550 nm (A^1_1 = 63a).

Infra-red Spectrum. Principal peaks at wavenumbers 1660, 1497, 1575, 1070, 1150, 1220 cm^{-1} (KBr disk).

Dose. Initially 0.25 to 1 mg intramuscularly, on alternate days.

Cyclandelate

Vasodilator

Proprietary names. Cyclobral; Cyclospasmol; Spasmocyclon.
α-Hydroxybenzeneacetic acid 3,3,5-trimethylcyclohexyl ester
$C_{17}H_{24}O_3$ = 276.4
CAS—456-59-7

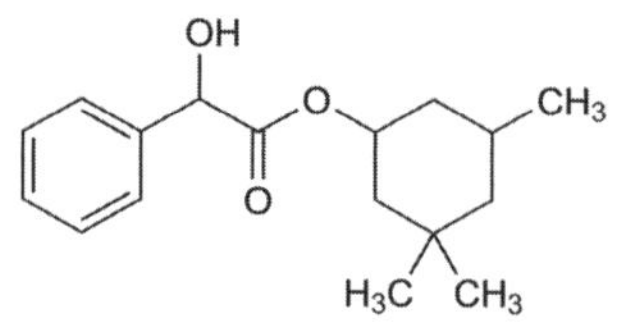

A white amorphous powder, which may sublime on storage into a crystalline form resembling cotton wool. M.p. 55.0° to 56.5°.
Practically insoluble in water; soluble 1 in about 1 of ethanol; very soluble in chloroform and ether; freely soluble in acetonitrile, ethyl acetate, dimethylformamide and toluene.

Partition Coefficient. Log *P* (octanol/water), 4.1.

Colour Tests. Liebermann's Test—orange; Marquis Test—orange (slow).

Thin-layer Chromatography. System TB—Rf 37; system TD—Rf 74; system TE—Rf 80; system TF—Rf 77; system TAD—Rf 73; system TAE—Rf 87; system TAF—Rf 95; system TAJ—Rf 81; system TAK—Rf 71; system TAL—Rf 95.

Gas Chromatography. System GA—RI 1903.

High Performance Liquid Chromatography. System HAA—Retention time(s), 26.4 min.

Ultraviolet Spectrum. Methanol—252, 258 (A^1_1=7.6b), 264 nm.

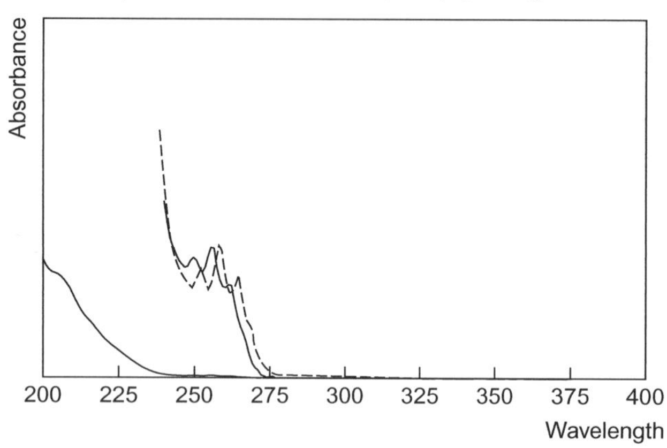

Infra-red Spectrum. Principal peaks at wavenumbers 1734, 1192, 1212, 1274, 1104, 1074 cm^{-1} (KBr disk).

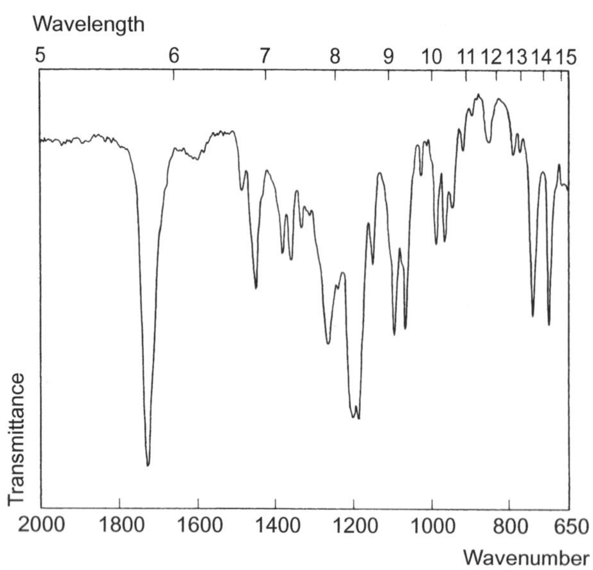

Mass Spectrum. Principal ions at *m/z* 107, 69, 125, 83, 79, 55, 41, 77.

Dose. 1.6 g daily.

Cyclazocine

Narcotic Antagonist

3-(Cyclopropylmethyl)-1,2,3,4,5,6-hexahydro-6,11-dimethyl-2,6-methano-3-benzazocin-8-ol
$C_{18}H_{25}NO$=271.4
CAS—3572-80-3

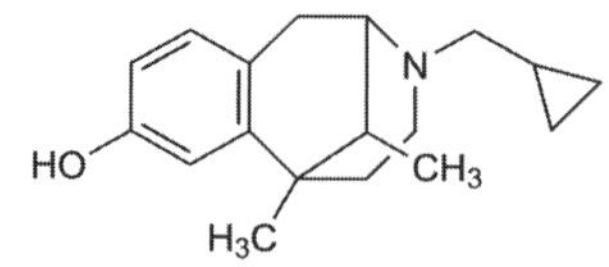

Crystals. M.p. 201° to 204°.
Soluble in chloroform and dilute acetic acid.

Partition Coefficient. Log *P* (octanol/pH 7.4), 1.3.

Colour Tests. Liebermann's Test—black; Mandelin's Test—green; Marquis Test—brown→green.

Thin-layer Chromatography. System TA—Rf 53; system TB—Rf 15; system TC—Rf 13; system TE—Rf 65; system TL—Rf 25; system TAE—Rf 24; system TAF—Rf 74; system TAJ—Rf 06; system TAK—Rf 05; system TAL—Rf 60. (Acidified iodoplatinate solution, strong reaction.)

High Performance Liquid Chromatography. System HA—*k* 2.1; system HY—RI 289.

Ultraviolet Spectrum. Aqueous acid—277 nm; aqueous alkali—237, 298 nm.

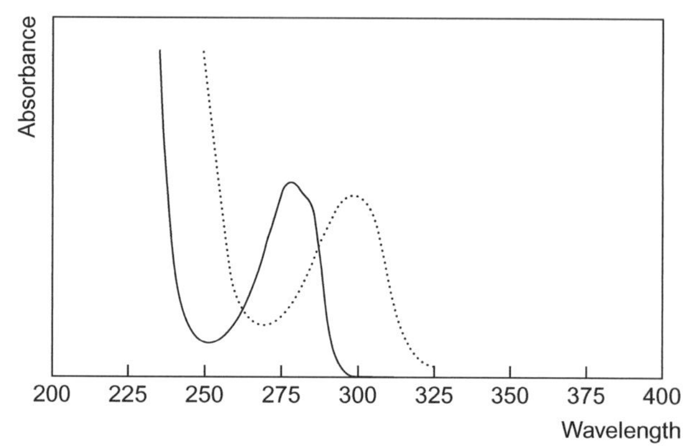

Infra-red Spectrum. Principal peaks at wavenumbers 1570, 1255, 1304, 754, 1227, 1241 cm^{-1} (KBr disk).

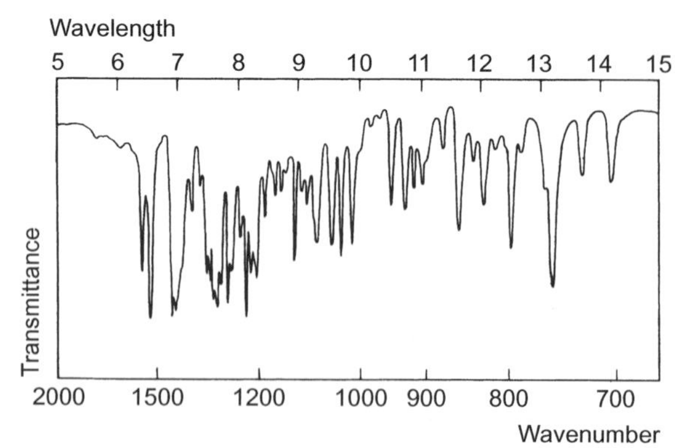

Mass Spectrum. Principal ions at *m/z* 230, 271, 55, 256, 164, 270, 71, 124.

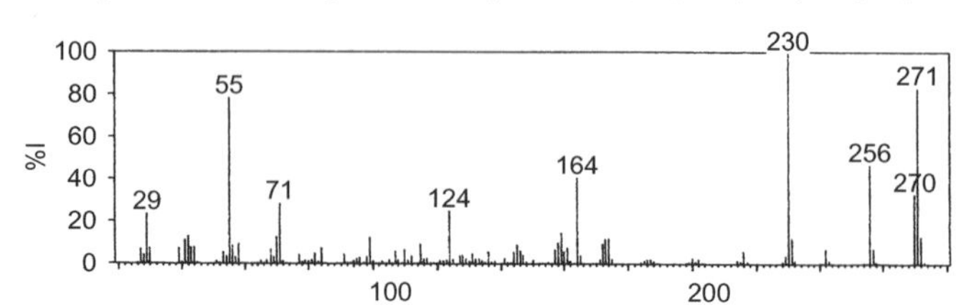

Quantification

Gas chromatography. In urine: cyclazocine and norcyclazocine, limit of detection 40 ng, FID—R. F. Kaiko and C. E. Inturrisi, *J. Chromatogr.*, 1974, *100*, 63–72.

Gas chromatography–mass spectrometry. In plasma: comparison with radioimmunoassay, limits of detection 110 ng/L and 20 ng/L, respectively—J. E. Peterson *et al.*, *J. Pharm. Sci.*, 1979, *68*, 1447–1450.

Disposition in the Body. Cyclazocine is absorbed after oral administration. About 20% of a dose is excreted in the urine unchanged together with 24% as conjugated cyclazocine, 4% as norcyclazocine, and 11% as conjugated norcyclazocine.

Dose. Cyclazocine has been given in maintenance doses of about 4 mg daily; doses of 10 mg have been given to extend the effect to 48 h.

Cyclizine

Antihistamine/Anti-emetic

Synonyms. Compd 47-83; Wellcome prepn 47-83.
1-Diphenylmethyl-4-methylpiperazine
$C_{18}H_{22}N_2$=266.4
CAS—82-92-8

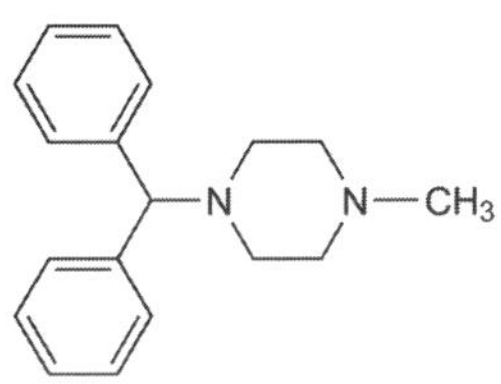

A white or creamy-white light-sensitive crystalline powder. M.p. 105.5° to 107.5° (from petroleum ether).
Practically insoluble in water; soluble 1 in 6 of ethanol, 1 in 1 of chloroform, and 1 in 6 of ether. Dissolves in most organic solvents and in dilute acids.

Cyclizine Hydrochloride
Synonym. Cyclizinium Chloride
Proprietary names. Covamet; Echnatol; Emitex; Fortravel; Marezine (tablets); Marzine; Medazine; Nauzine; Norizine; Ryccard; Triazine; Valoid (tablets). It is an ingredient of Cyclimorph, Diconal, Igril, Megral, Migral, Migril, Vertipam, and Wellconal.
$C_{18}H_{22}N_2$,HCl=302.8
CAS—303-25-3
A white crystalline powder, or small colourless crystals. M.p. about 285°, with decomposition.
Soluble 1 in about 125 of water, 1 in about 120 of ethanol, and 1 in 75 of chloroform; practically insoluble in ether.

Cyclizine Lactate
Proprietary names. Marezine (injection); Valoid (injection).
$C_{18}H_{22}N_2$,$C_3H_6O_3$=356.5
CAS—5897-19-8
Freely soluble in water.

Cyclizine Tartrate
$C_{18}H_{22}N_2$, $C_4H_6O_6$=416.5

Dissociation Constant. pK_a 2.4, 7.8.

Partition Coefficient. Log *P* (octanol/water), 2.97.

Colour Tests. Liebermann's Test—orange; Marquis Test—yellow

Thin-layer Chromatography. System TA—Rf 57; system TB—Rf 48; system TC—Rf 41; system TE—Rf 68; system TL—Rf 16; system TAE—Rf 39; system TAF—Rf 52; system TAJ—Rf 23; system TAK—Rf 11; system TAL—Rf 72. (Dragendorff spray, positive; acidified iodoplatinate solution, positive; Marquis reagent, yellow.)

Gas Chromatography. System GA—cyclizine RI 2025, M (nor-) RI 2120, M (benzophenone) RI 1610; system GB—cyclizine RI 2104, M (nor-) RI 2128, M (benzophenone) RI 1673; system GC—RI 2348; system GF—RI 2320.

Column: OV-17 fused silica (15 m × 0.25 mm i.d., 0.2 µm film thickness). Column temperature: 100° to 260° at 10°/min, held at 260° for 11 min. Injector temperature: 230°. IS: diphenhydramine. Detection: MS (TIC), *m/z* 56 and 58 for cyclizine and diphenhydramine, respectively. Retention time: cyclizine, 12.2 min; diphenhydramine, 10.5 min. [R. C. Backer *et al.*, *J. Anal. Toxicol.*, 1989, *13*, 308–309.]

High Performance Liquid Chromatography. System HA—cyclizine *k* 2.9, norcyclizine *k* 2.2; system HX—RI 405; system HZ—retention time 4.8 min; system HAX—retention time 12.4 min; system HAY—retention time 5.8 min.

Column: (analytical) ODS C_{18} (Techil, 150 × 4.1 mm i.d., 5 µm), (guard) glass bead packed pre-column kit (Uptight), at 30°. Mobile phase: phosphate buffer (0.05 M, pH 3.0):acetonitrile (70:30), flow rate 1 mL/min. IS: chlorcyclizine hydrochloride. Electrochemical detection. Retention time(s): norcyclizine, 5 min; cyclizine, 6 min; IS, 12 min. [R. B. Walker and I. Kanfer, *J. Chromatogr.* 1995, *672 B Biomed. Appl.*, 172–177].

Ultraviolet Spectrum. Aqueous acid—257, 262 nm (A_1^1=28a), 268 nm; aqueous alkali—260 nm (A_1^1=16b). (See below.)

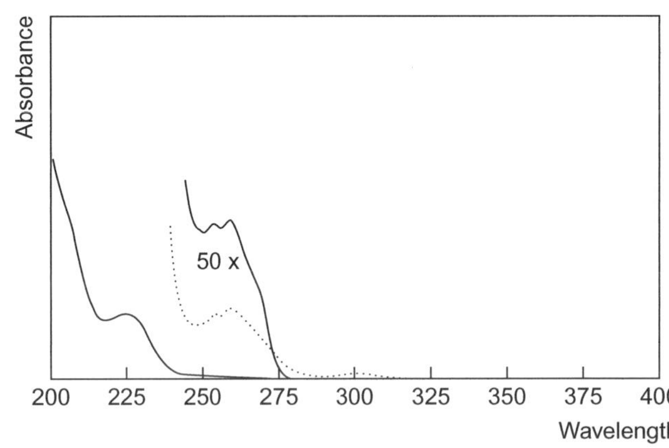

Infra-red Spectrum. Principal peaks at wavenumbers 716, 756, 701, 984, 1125, 1496 cm^{-1} (cyclizine hydrochloride, KBr disk). (See below.)

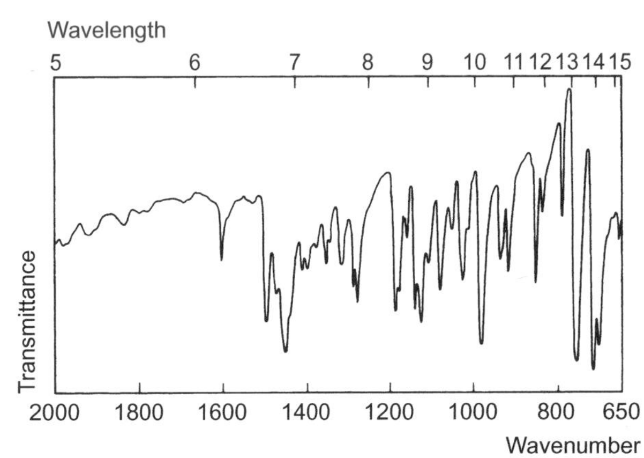

Mass Spectrum. Principal ions at *m/z* 99, 56, 167, 207, 194, 266, 195, 165.

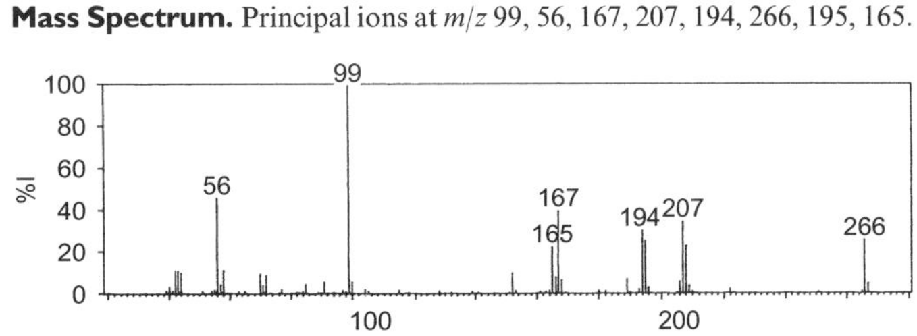

Quantification

Gas chromatography. In plasma or urine: cyclizine and norcyclizine, limit of detection 10 µg/L for cyclizine, AFID—G. Land *et al.*, *J. Chromatogr.*, 1981, *222*(11) *B Biomed. Appl.*, 135–140. In blood or urine: limit of detection 10 µg/L and 5 µg/L, respectively, AFID—D. S. Griffin and R. C. Baselt, *J. Anal. Toxicol.*, 1984, 8, 97–99.

High performance liquid chromatography. In serum or urine: cyclizine and norcyclizine, limit of detection 1 μg/L, coulometric detection—R. B. Walker and I. Kanfer, *J. Chromatogr.* 1995, *672 B Biomed. Appl.*, 172–177.

Disposition in the Body. Cyclizine is absorbed from the gastro-intestinal tract with an onset of action within 2 h. It is extensively metabolised by *N*-demethylation to form the relatively inactive norcyclizine, a metabolite that is widely distributed throughout the tissues and especially in lungs, kidneys, liver, and spleen. Less than 1% of the total oral dose is eliminated in the urine.

Therapeutic concentration

Following a single oral dose of 50 mg of cyclizine hydrochloride to 1 subject, a peak blood concentration of 0.069 mg/L was attained in 2 h. [D. S. Griffin and R. C. Baselt, *J. Anal. Toxicol.*, 1984, 8, 97–99.]

On the first day after termination of therapy with oral doses of 50 mg thrice daily to 4 subjects, plasma concentrations of norcyclizine were in the range of 0.004 to 0.022 mg/L (mean 0.014). [R. Kuntzman *et al.*, *J. Pharmacol. Exp. Ther.*, 1967, *158*, 332–339.]

Toxicity

In a fatality resulting from a cyclizine overdose, 80 mg/L cyclizine in blood was detected in a 17-year-old female. Norcyclizine was not detected. [R. C. Backer *et al.*, *J. Anal. Toxicol.*, 1989, *13*, 308–309.]

In a fatality attributed principally to cyclizine, postmortem concentrations were: blood 15 mg/L, liver 108 μg/g; doxepin was also detected at concentrations of 0.7 mg/L and 6 μg/g in the blood and liver, respectively. [J. F. Lewin *et al.*, *Bull. Int. Assoc. Forensic Toxicol.*, 1981, *16(2)*, 23–24.]

For case histories involving the injection of cyclizine with dipipanone, see under Dipipanone.

Half-life. Plasma half-life, cyclizine about 24 h.

Protein binding. In plasma, norcyclizine about 60%.

Dose. Adults, up to 150 mg of cyclizine hydrochloride daily; children (6 to 12 years), up to 75 mg daily, in divided doses.

Cyclobarbital

Hypnotic/Barbiturate

Synonyms. Ciclobarbital; Cyclobarbitalum; Cyclobarbitone; Ethylhexabital; Hexemalum; Tetrahydrophenobarbital.
Proprietary names. Cavonyl; Cyclodorm; Cyklodorm; Fanodormo; Irifan; Namuron; Palinum; Phanodorm; Phanodorn; Philodorm; Prälumin; Pro-Sonil; Sonaform.
Note. The name ciclobarbital has been applied to hexobarbital.
5-(1-Cyclohexen-1-yl)-5-ethyl-2,4,6(1*H*,3*H*,5*H*)-pyrimidinetrione
$C_{12}H_{16}N_2O_3$=236.3
CAS—52-31-3

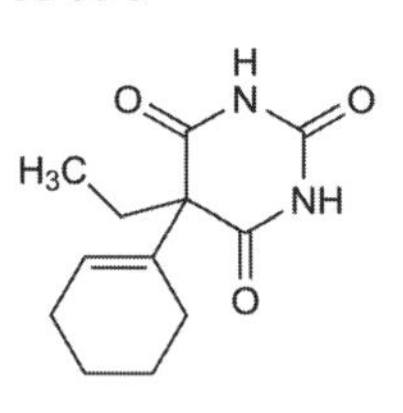

A white crystalline powder, which gradually decomposes on storage. M.p. 171° to 174°.
Soluble 1 in 800 of water, 1 in 5 of ethanol, 1 in 20 of chloroform, and 1 in 20 of ether.

Cyclobarbital Calcium

Synonyms. Ciclobarbital Calcium; Cyclobarbitone Calcium; Hexemalcalcium.
Proprietary name. It is an ingredient of Domidorm.
$(C_{12}H_{15}N_2O_3)_2Ca$=510.6
CAS-143-76-0
A white or slightly yellowish, crystalline powder.
Soluble 1 in 70 of water, 1 in 500 of 95% alcohol. Practically insoluble in ether and chloroform.

Dissociation Constant. pK_a 7.6 (20°).

Partition Coefficient. Log *P* (octanol/water), 1.77.

Colour Tests. Koppanyi–Zwikker Test—violet; Mercurous Nitrate—black; Vanillin Reagent—brown-red/green.

Thin-layer Chromatography. System TD—Rf 50; system TE—Rf 40; system TF—Rf 64; system TH—Rf 59; system TAD—Rf 58; system TAE—Rf 88. (Mercuric chloride–diphenylcarbazone reagent, positive; mercurous nitrate spray, black; acidified potassium permanganate solution, yellow-brown; Zwikker's reagent, pink.)

Gas Chromatography. System GA—cyclobarbital RI 1955, cyclobarbital-Me_2 RI 1845, M (oxo-) RI 2190, M (oxo-)-Me_2 RI 2050; system GF—RI 2825; system GAJ—cyclobarbital RRT 1.142 (relative to methylphenobarbital).

High Performance Liquid Chromatography. System HG—*k* 5.25; system HH—*k* 2.61; system HX—RI 384; system HY—RI 352; system HZ—retention time 3.2 min.

Ultraviolet Spectrum. Borax buffer 0.05 M (pH 9.2)—239 nm (A^1_1=410a); 1 M sodium hydroxide (pH 13)—256 nm (A^1_1=320b).

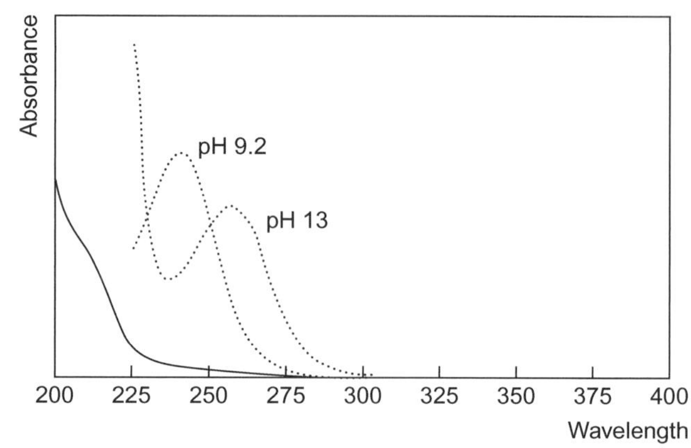

Infra-red Spectrum. Principal peaks at wavenumbers 1693, 1725, 1745, 1300, 1210, 830 cm^{-1} (KBr disk).

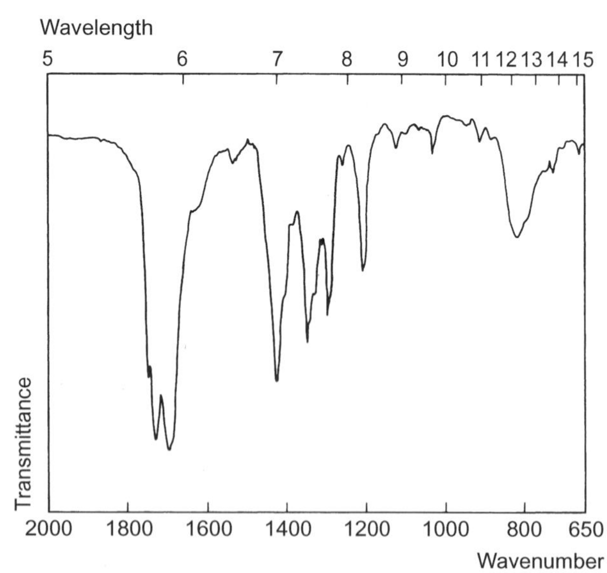

Mass Spectrum. Principal ions at *m/z* 207, 141, 81, 79, 67, 80, 41, 77.

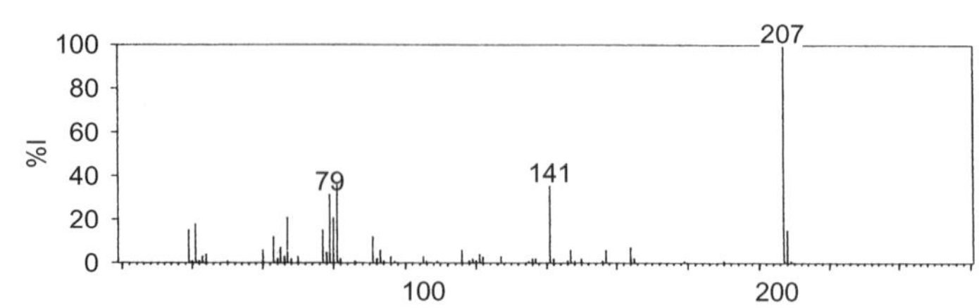

Quantification. See under Amylobarbital.

Disposition in the Body. Rapidly absorbed after oral administration. The main metabolic reaction appears to be oxidation to ketocyclobarbital [5-(3-oxocyclohex-1-enyl)-5-ethylbarbituric acid]. Less than 10% of a dose is excreted in the urine unchanged.

Therapeutic concentration. In plasma, usually in the range 2 to 10 mg/L.

After a single oral dose of 300 mg of the calcium salt, given to 6 subjects, peak plasma concentrations of 7.4 to 10.3 mg/L (mean 8.7) were attained in 0.7 to 2.5 h. [D. D. Breimer and A. C. M. Winten, *Eur. J. Clin. Pharmacol.*, 1976, *9*, 443–450.]

Toxicity. The estimated minimum lethal dose is 2 g. Severe toxic effects are associated with blood concentrations greater than 10 mg/L.

Half-life. Plasma half-life, 8 to 17 h (mean 12), increased in subjects with liver disease.

Volume of distribution. About 0.5 L/kg.

Clearance. Plasma clearance, about 0.5 mL/min/kg.

Protein binding. In plasma, about 70%.

Dose. 100 to 400 mg of cyclobarbital calcium, as a hypnotic.

Cyclobenzaprine

Muscle Relaxant

Synonyms. CBZ; Mk-130; Proheptatriene; Ro-4-1577; RP-9715.
3-(5*H*-Dibenzo[*a,d*]cyclohepten-5-ylidene)-*N,N*-dimethyl-1-propanamine
$C_{20}H_{21}N$=275.4
CAS—303-53-7

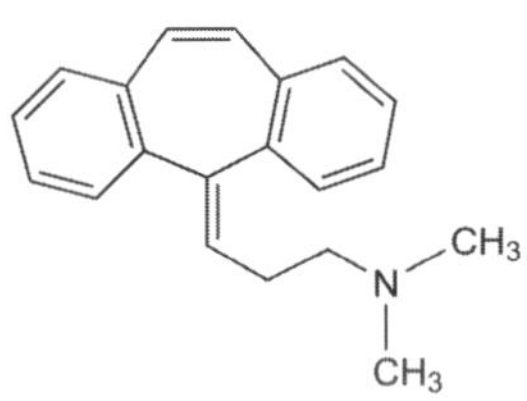

Cyclobenzaprine Hydrochloride

Proprietary name. Flexeril
$C_{20}H_{21}N,HCl$=311.9
CAS—6202-23-9
A white crystalline powder. M.p. 215° to 219°.
Freely soluble in water and ethanol; sparingly soluble in isopropanol; slightly soluble in chloroform and methylene chloride; practically insoluble in hydrocarbons.

Partition Coefficient. Log *P* (octanol/water), 4.8.

Thin-layer Chromatography. System TE—Rf 69.

Gas Chromatography. System GA—RI 2195.

High Performance Liquid Chromatography. System HY—RI 378; system HAX—retention time 15.5 min; system HAY—retention time 7.1 min.

Ultraviolet Spectrum. Aqueous acid—290 nm (A^1_1=407b). No alkaline shift.

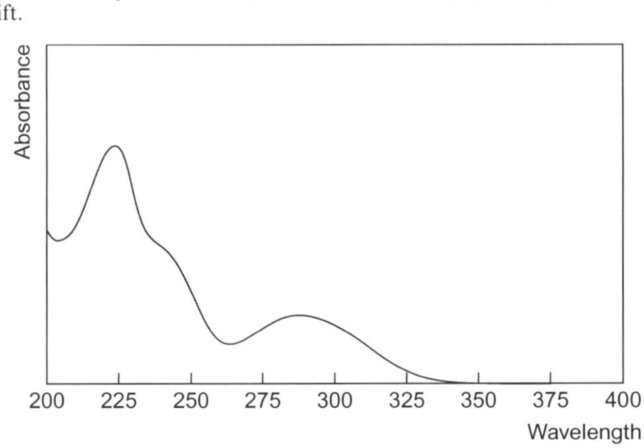

Infra-red Spectrum. Principal peaks at wavenumbers 764, 778, 800, 968, 988, 880 cm^{-1} (KBr disk). (See below)

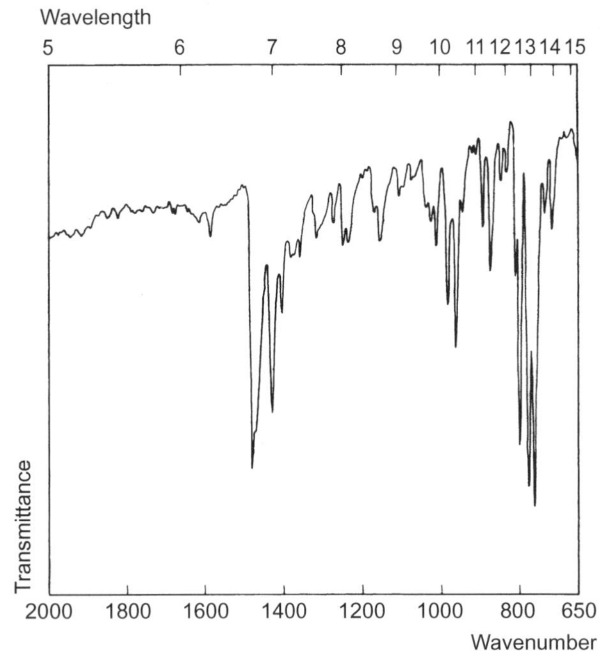

Mass Spectrum. Principal ions at *m/z* 58, 59, 42, 215, 202, 57, 189, 43.

Quantification

Gas chromatography. In plasma or urine: limit of detection 10 mg/L, FID—H. B. Hucker and S. C. Stauffer, *J. Pharm. Sci.*, 1976, *65*, 1253–1255. In plasma: limit of detection 2 mg/L, AFID—H. B. Hucker and S. C. Stauffer, *J. Chromatogr.*, 1976, *124*, 164–168.

High performance liquid chromatography. In plasma and urine: limit of quantification 0.5 mg/L, UV detection (λ = 226 nm); 0.1 mg/L, MS/MS (*m/z* 276/215) —M. Constanzer *et al.*, *J. Chromatogr. B Biomed. Sci. Appl.*, 1995, *666(1)*, 117–126.

Disposition in the Body. Irregularly absorbed after oral administration, and extensively metabolised. The major metabolites are a glucuronide conjugate and 10,11-dihydroxynortriptyline; monodesmethylcyclobenzaprine is a minor metabolite. About 50% of an oral dose is excreted in the urine in 5 days, with less than 1% as unchanged drug. About 14% of a dose is eliminated in the faeces.

Therapeutic concentration

After a single oral dose of 40 mg to 4 subjects, peak plasma concentrations of about 0.027 mg/L were attained in 4 h; following oral doses of 20 mg three times a day to 9 subjects, a mean peak plasma concentration of 0.034 mg/L was reported 6 h after the first dose on the fourth day. [H. B. Hucker *et al.*, *J. Clin. Pharmacol.*, 1977, *17*, 719–727.]

Toxicity

In a fatality where cyclobenzaprine was the suspected cause of death, the following postmortem tissue concentrations were reported: blood 0.46 mg/L, bile 12.0 mg/L, liver 12.4 μg/g, urine 3.2 mg/L; low concentrations of morphine and diazepam were also detected. [B. K. Beck and T. Lamoreaux, *Bull. Int. Assoc. Forensic Toxicol.*, 1979, *14(3)*, 27.]

A 35-year-old woman was found dead in her bath. Cyclobenzaprine was found at a concentration of 1.8 mg/L in the blood along with ethanol at 21.5 mg/L. [C. L. Winek *et al.*, *Forensic Sci. Int.*, 1999, *100(1–2)*, 105–108.]

A 19-year-old man died 7 h after admission to hospital, after being found with a number of medicine bottles. Cyclobenzaprine was found in his blood at a concentration of 0.3 mg/L as well as phenylpropanolamine (2.5 mg/L), chlorpheniramine (0.2 mg/L), lidocaine (6.6 mg/L), phenytoin (19 mg/L), and ibuprofen (130 mg/L). Cause of death was cyclobenzaprine and ibuprofen intoxication. [B. Levine *et al.*, *Am. J. Forensic Med. Pathol.*, 1993, *14(3)*, 246–248.]

Half-life. Plasma half-life, about 1 to 3 days.

Protein binding. In plasma, about 93%.

Dose. Usually 30 mg of cyclobenzaprine hydrochloride daily; maximum of 60 mg daily.

Cyclofenil

Induction of Ovulation

Synonyms. F-6066; H-3452; ICI-48213.
Proprietary names. Fertodur; Ondogyne; Ondonid; Rehibin; Sexovid.
4-[[4-(Acetyloxy)phenyl]cyclohexylidenemethyl]phenol acetate
$C_{23}H_{24}O_4$=364.4
CAS—2624-43-3

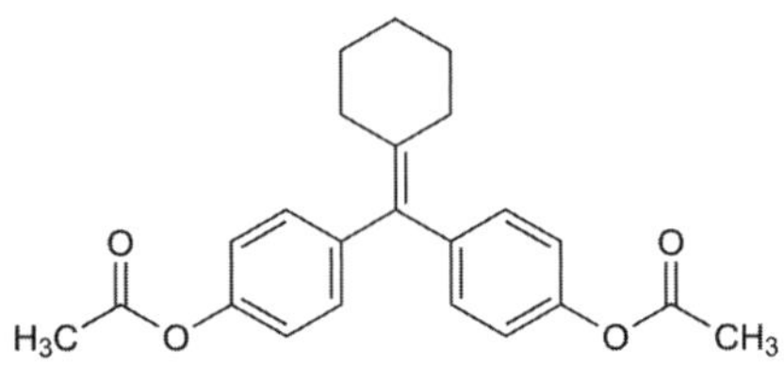

A white crystalline powder. M.p. 137° to 140°.
Practically insoluble in water; soluble 1 in 250 of ethanol, 1 in 2 of chloroform and 1 in 30 of ether.

Partition Coefficient. Log *P* (octanol/water), 5.4.

Ultraviolet Spectrum. Acid ethanol—247 nm; alkaline ethanol—262 nm.

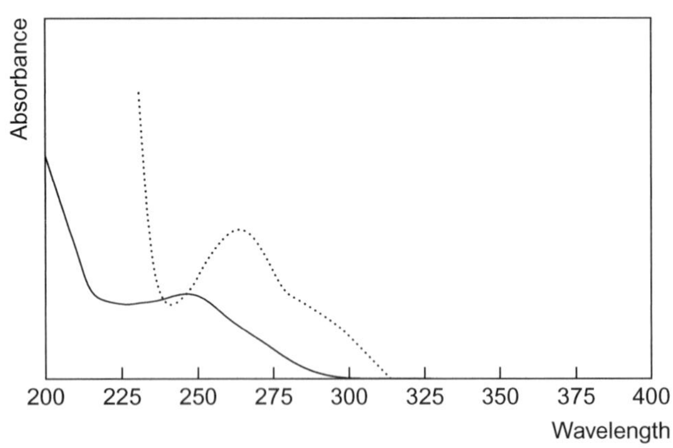

Infra-red Spectrum. Principal peaks at wavenumbers 1204, 1219, 1754, 917, 1162, 1492 cm^{-1}.

Dose. 200 to 400 mg daily; doses of 800 mg daily have been given in 5-day courses.

Cycloguanil

Antimalarial

Synonyms. Chlorguanide triazine; TCl; M-10580; D-20.
1-(4-Chlorophenyl)-1,6-dihydro-6,6-dimethyl-1,3,5-triazine-2,4-diamine
$C_{11}H_{14}ClN_5$=251.7
CAS—516-21-2

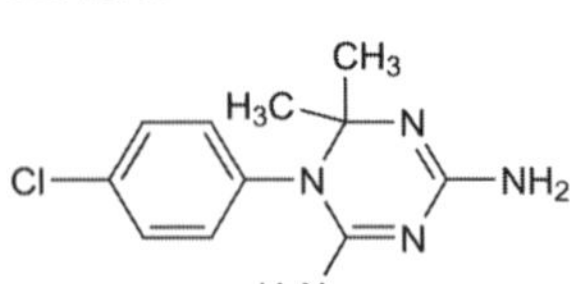

Crystals. M.p. 146°.

Cycloguanil Embonate
Synonym. Cycloguanil Pamoate
$(C_{11}H_{14}ClN_5)_2,(C_{23}H_{16}O_6)$=891.8
CAS—609-78-9
A pale greenish-yellow, crystalline powder. M.p. 231° to 234°.
Practically insoluble in water; sparingly soluble in dimethylformamide.

Partition Coefficient. Log *P* (octanol/water), 1.0.

High Performance Liquid Chromatography. System HAA—retention time 10.8 min.

Ultraviolet Spectrum. Methanol—237m (A_1^1=2250b), 278, 289 (A_1^1=180b), 301 nm.

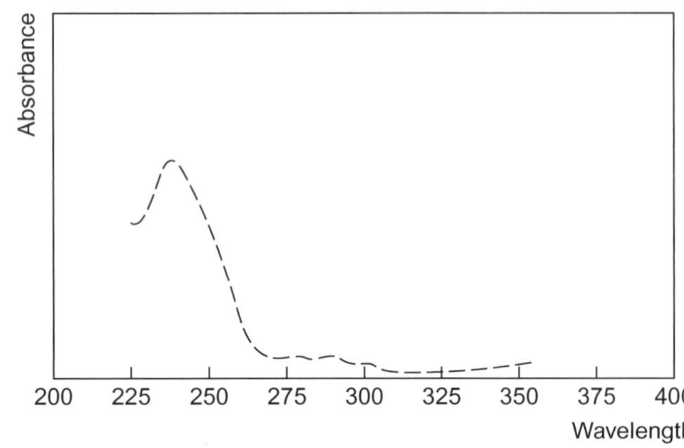

Infra-red Spectrum. Principal peaks at wavenumbers 1673, 1515, 1628, 1570, 760, 1224 cm^{-1} (KBr disk).

Quantification. See also under Proguanil.

High performance liquid chromatography. In plasma and urine: limit of detection 1 and 5 mg/L, respectively—M. Kusaka *et al.*, *Am. J. Trop. Med. Hyg.*, 1996, *54(2)*, 189–196. In whole blood: limit of quantification 15 mg/L, UV detection—J. A. Kolawole *et al.*, *J. Chromatogr. B Biomed. Sci. Appl.*, 1995, *674(1)*, 149–154.

Disposition in the Body. Slowly absorbed after IM administration and excreted mainly in the urine.
Cycloguanil is the active metabolite of proguanil.

Dose. The equivalent of 5 to 6 mg/kg of cycloguanil, IM, every 4 months.

Cyclomethycaine

Local Anaesthetic

4-(Cyclohexyloxy)benzoic acid 3-(2-methyl-1-piperidinyl)propyl ester
$C_{22}H_{33}NO_3$=359.5
CAS—139-62-8 (cyclomethycaine); 537-61-1 *(hydrochloride)*

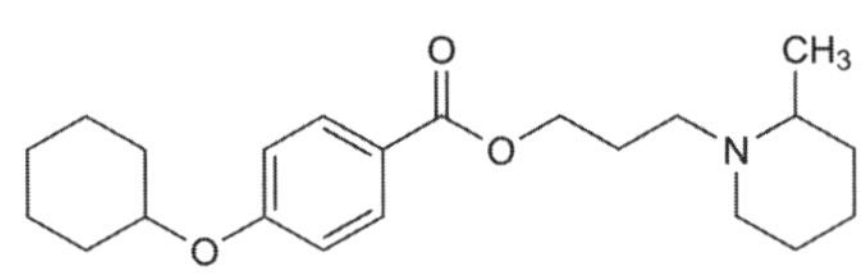

A white crystalline powder.
Sparingly soluble in water, ethanol and ether; very slightly soluble in chloroform.

Cyclomethycaine Sulfate
Proprietary name. Surfacaine
$C_{22}H_{33}NO_3,H_2SO_4$=457.6
CAS—50978-10-4
A white crystalline powder. M.p. 162° to 166°.
Soluble 1 in 50 of water, 1 in 50 of ethanol and 1 in about 227 of chloroform.

Partition Coefficient. Log *P* (octanol/water), 6.2.

Colour Test. Mandelin's test—green→brown.

Thin-layer Chromatography. System TA—Rf 58; system TB—Rf 55; system TC—Rf 36; system TL—Rf 25. (Acidified iodoplatinate solution, positive.)

High Performance Liquid Chromatography. System HR—*k* 10.31; system HY—RI 413.

Ultraviolet Spectrum. Aqueous acid—261 nm (A_1^1=508a).

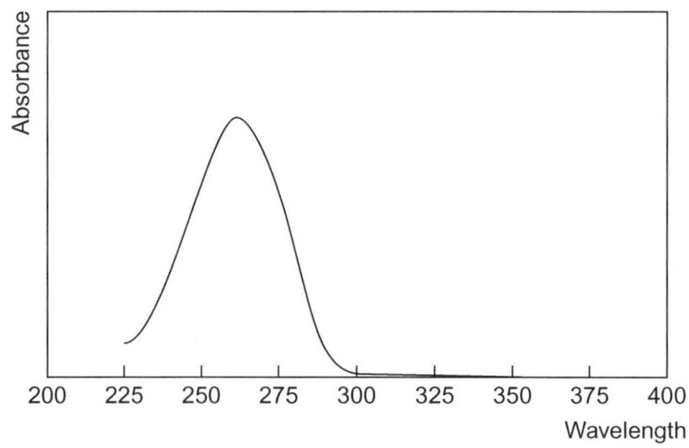

Infra-red Spectrum. Principal peaks at wavenumbers 1704, 1605, 1253, 775, 1170, 1235 cm^{-1} (cyclomethycaine sulfate, Nujol mull).

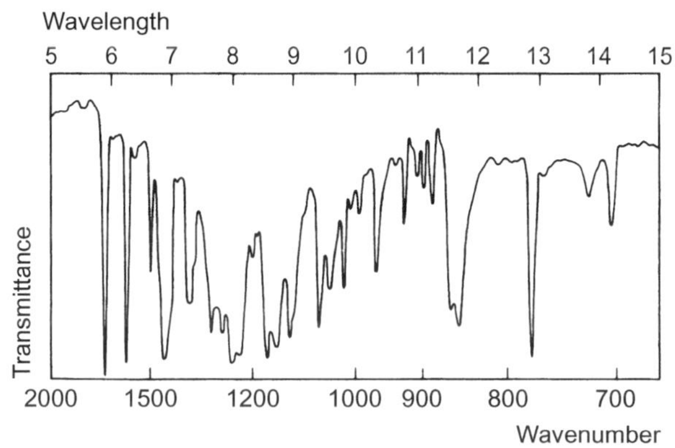

Mass Spectrum. Principal ions at *m/z* 112, 344, 121, 41, 67, 55, 54, 345.

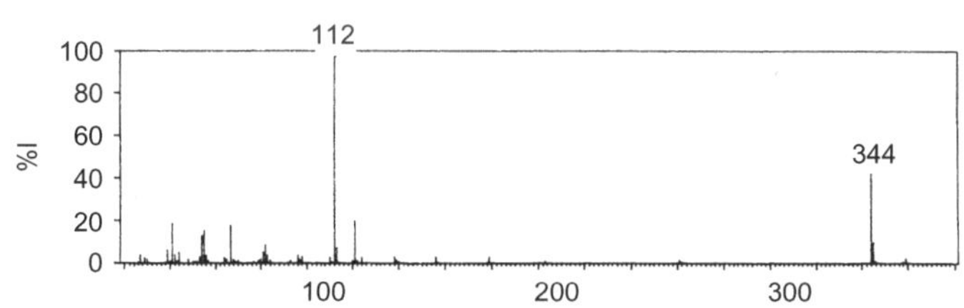

Use. Cyclomethycaine sulfate has been used in concentrations of 0.5 to 1%.

Cyclopentamine

Sympathomimetic

Synonym. Cyclopentadrin
N,α-Dimethylcyclopentaneethanamine
$C_9H_{19}N = 141.3$
CAS—102-45-4

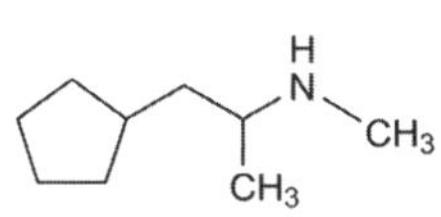

Cyclopentamine Hydrochloride

Synonym. Cyclopentaminium Chloride
Proprietary name. It is an ingredient of Co-Pyronil.
$C_9H_{19}N,HCl = 177.7$
CAS—3459-06-1
A white crystalline powder. M.p. 113° to 115°.
Soluble 1 in 1 of water, 1 in 2 of ethanol, and 1 in 1 of chloroform; slightly soluble in ether.

Partition Coefficient. Log *P* (octanol/water), 3.0.

Thin-layer Chromatography. System TA—Rf 20; system TB—Rf 32; system TC—Rf 10; system TE—Rf 66; system TL—Rf 02; system TAE—Rf 06; system TAF—Rf 68. (Dragendorff spray, positive; acidified iodoplatinate solution, positive; Ninhydrin spray, positive; Acidified potassium permanganate solution, positive.)

Gas Chromatography. System GA—cyclopentamine RI 1230; cyclopentamine-AC RI 1680.

High Performance Liquid Chromatography. System HA—*k* 1.7.

Ultraviolet Spectrum. No significant absorption, 230 to 360 nm.

Infra-red Spectrum. Principal peaks at wavenumbers 1585, 1020, 1050, 1100, 1082, 115 cm^{-1}.

Mass Spectrum. Principal ions at *m/z* 58, 41, 30, 126, 59, 69, 56, 44.

Disposition in the Body
Toxicity. The estimated minimum lethal dose for children up to 2 years is 200 mg when applied to the mucous membranes; the minimum lethal dose for adults may be at least 10 times greater.

Dose. Cyclopentamine hydrochloride has been used as a 0.5 or 1% nasal solution. It has been given in doses of 25 mg intramuscularly, or 5 to 10 mg intravenously.

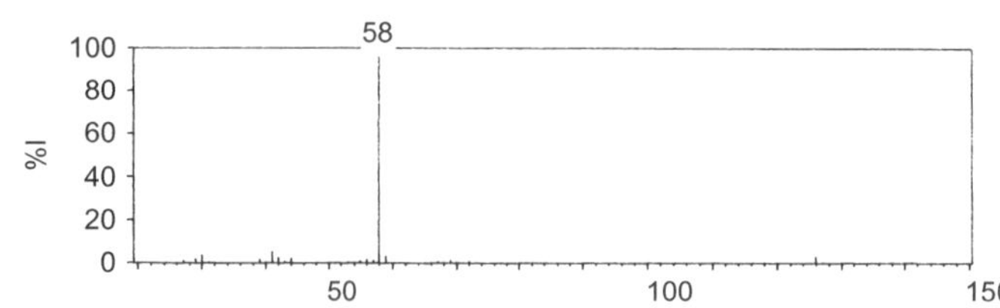

Cyclopenthiazide

Diuretic

Proprietary names. Navidrex. It is an ingredient of Trasidrex.
6-Chloro-3-(cyclopentylmethyl)-3,4-dihydro-2*H*-1,2,4-benzothiadiazine-7-sulfonamide 1,1-dioxide
$C_{13}H_{18}ClN_3O_4S_2 = 379.9$
CAS—742-20-1

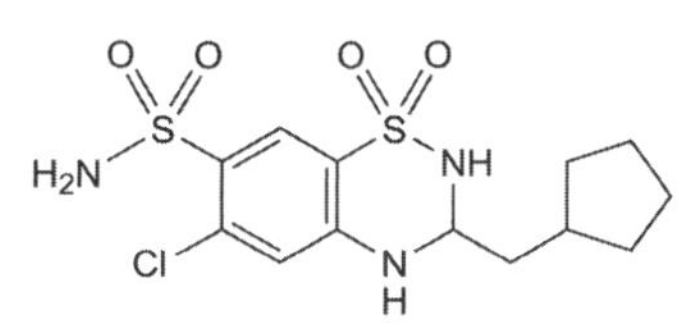

A white powder. M.p. 235°, with decomposition.
Practically insoluble in water; soluble 1 in 12 of ethanol and 1 in 600 of chloroform; soluble in ether.

Partition Coefficient. Log *P* (octanol/water), 1.3.

Colour Tests. Koppanyi–Zwikker Test—violet; Liebermann's Test—brown-green; Sulfuric Acid—yellow.

Thin-layer Chromatography. System TD—Rf 21; system TE—Rf 66; system TF—Rf 62; system TAD—Rf 27.

Gas Chromatography. System GY—cyclopenthiazide-Me_4 Retention time(s) 6.3 min.

High Performance Liquid Chromatography. System HN—*k* 16.45; system HY—RI 453.

Ultraviolet Spectrum. Aqueous acid—274 ($A^1_1 = 556a$), 319 nm. No alkaline shift.

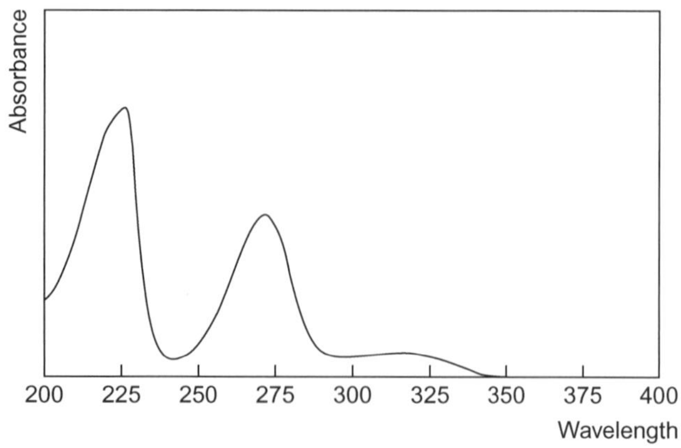

Infra-red Spectrum. Principal peaks at wavenumbers 1168, 1138, 1605, 1309, 1511, 1060 cm^{-1} (KBr disk).

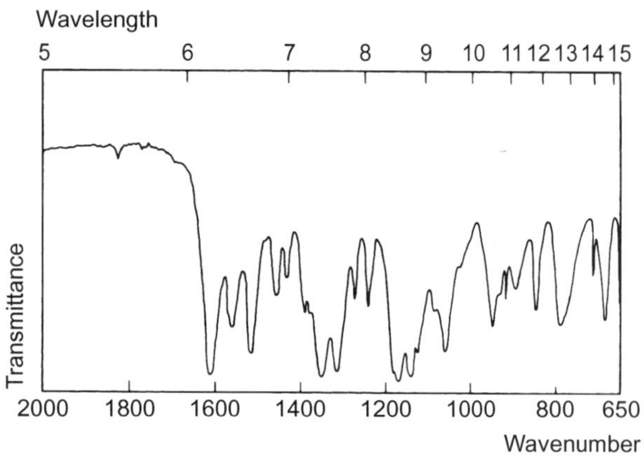

Mass Spectrum. Principal ions at *m/z* 296, 41, 44, 110, 298, 285, 55, 268.

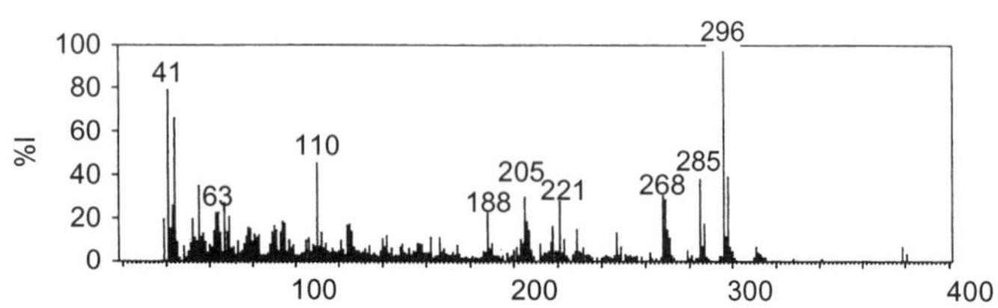

Dose. 250 to 500 μg daily; maximum of 1.5 mg daily.

Cyclopentobarbital

Sedative/Barbiturate

Synonyms. Cyclopentenylallyl Barbituric Acid; Cyclopentobarbitone.
Proprietary name. Cyclopal
5-(2-Cyclopenten-1-yl)-5-(2-propenyl)-2,4,6(1*H*,3*H*,5*H*)-pyrimidinetrione
$C_{12}H_{14}N_2O_3$=234.3
CAS—76-68-6

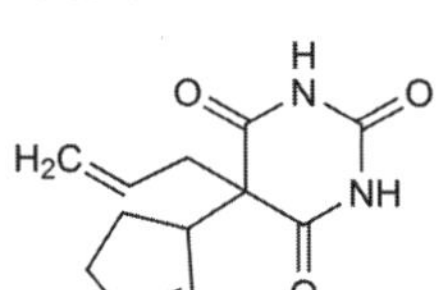

Crystals. M.p. 139° to 140°.
Slightly soluble in cold water; moderately soluble in hot water; freely soluble in ethanol and organic solvents.

Dissociation Constant. pK_a 7.8.

Partition Coefficient. Log *P* (octanol/water), 1.5.

Colour Test. Vanillin Reagent—brown-red/green.

Thin-layer Chromatography. System TD—Rf 50; system TE—Rf 39; system TF—Rf 65; system TH—Rf 62; system TAD—Rf 59; system TAE—Rf 90; system TAJ—Rf 66; system TAK—Rf 63; system TAL—Rf 90.

Gas Chromatography. System GA—cyclopentobarbital RI 1865; cyclopentobarbital-Me_2 RI 1775.

High Performance Liquid Chromatography. System HG—*k* 6.00; system HH—*k* 3.84; system HX—RI 391; system HY—RI 352.

Ultraviolet Spectrum. Borax buffer 0.05 M (pH 9.2)—241 nm (A^1_1=411a); 1 M sodium hydroxide (pH 13)—254 nm (A^1_1=306b).

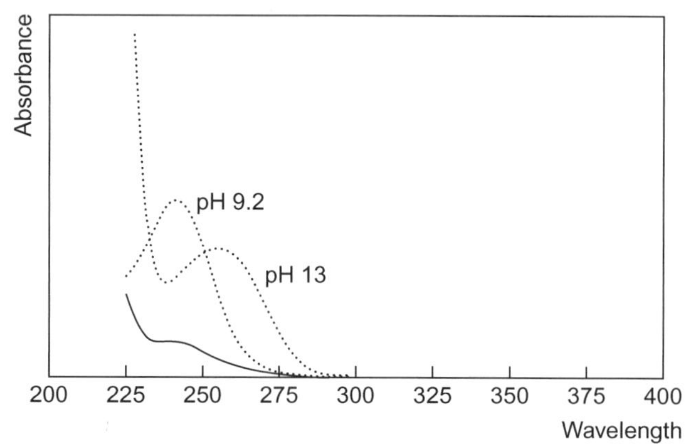

Infra-red Spectrum. Principal peaks at wavenumbers 1700, 1755, 1212, 815, 1319, 848 cm^{-1} (KBr disk).

Mass Spectrum. Principal ions at *m/z* 67, 193, 66, 41, 169, 39, 65, 77.

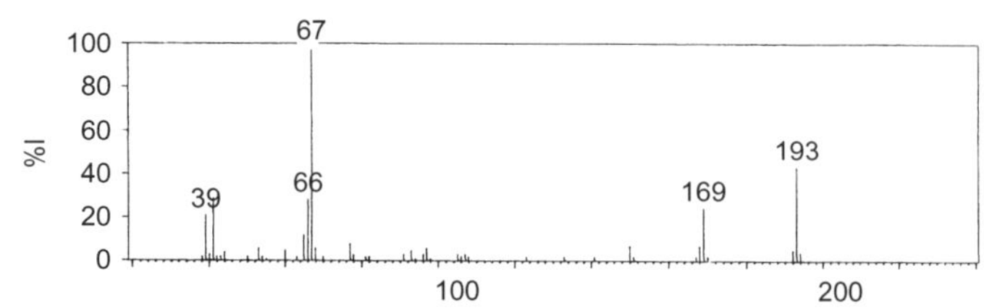

Dose. Cyclopentobarbital has been given in a dose of 100 to 200 mg.

Cyclopentolate

Anticholinergic

α-(1-Hydroxycyclopentyl)benzeneacetic acid 2-(dimethylamino)ethyl ester
$C_{17}H_{25}NO_3$=291.4
CAS—512-15-2

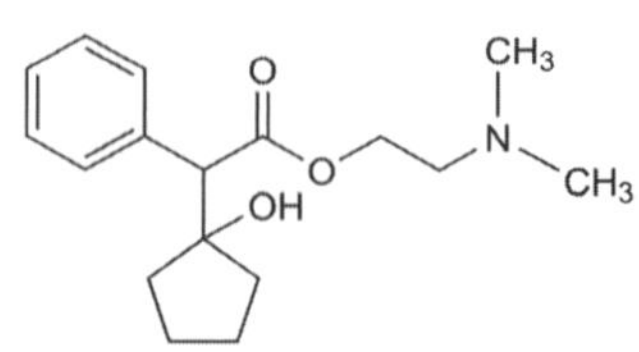

Cyclopentolate Hydrochloride

Proprietary names. Cyclogyl; Cyclopen; Mydplegic; Mydrilate; Skiacol P.O.S.; Zyklolat.
$C_{17}H_{25}NO_3,HCl$=327.9
CAS—5870-29-1
A white crystalline powder. M.p. 135° to 138°.
Soluble 1 in less than 1 of water and 1 in 5 of ethanol; practically insoluble in ether.

Dissociation Constant. pK_a 7.9.

Partition Coefficient. Log *P* (octanol/water), 2.5.

Colour Test. Mandelin's Test—brown.

Thin-layer Chromatography. System TA—Rf 57; system TB—Rf 32; system TC—Rf 39; system TE—Rf 64; system TL—Rf 26; system TAE—Rf 46; system TAJ—Rf 23; system TAK—Rf 02; system TAL—Rf 42.

Gas Chromatography. System GA—cyclopentolate RI 2022, cyclopentolate-H_2O RI 2000; system GB—cyclopentolate RI 2092, cyclopentolate-H_2O RI 1551.

High Performance Liquid Chromatography. System HA—*k* 1.6 (tailing peak); system HX—RI 353; system HY—RI 287; system HZ—retention time 3.2 min.

Ultraviolet Spectrum. Aqueous acid—252 (A^1_1=5a), 258 (A^1_1=6a), 264 nm (A^1_1=5a). No alkaline shift.

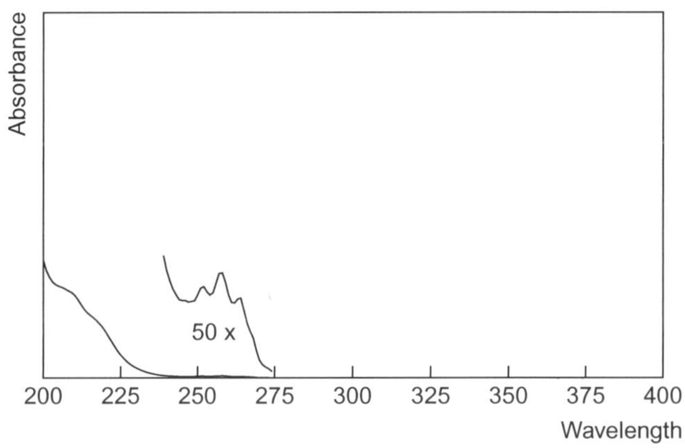

Infra-red Spectrum. Principal peaks at wavenumbers 1148, 1733, 704, 1199, 735, 990 cm^{-1} (cyclopentolate hydrochloride, KBr disk).

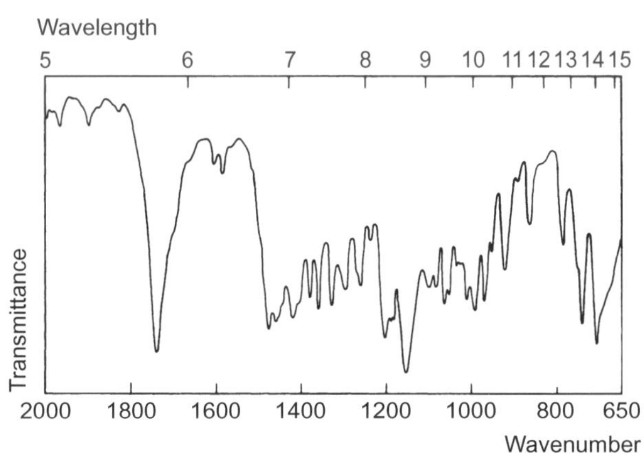

Mass Spectrum. Principal ions at *m/z* 58, 71, 72, 207, 42, 91, 59, 118; cyclopentolate-H_2O *m/z* 58, 71, 91, 115, 129, 273.

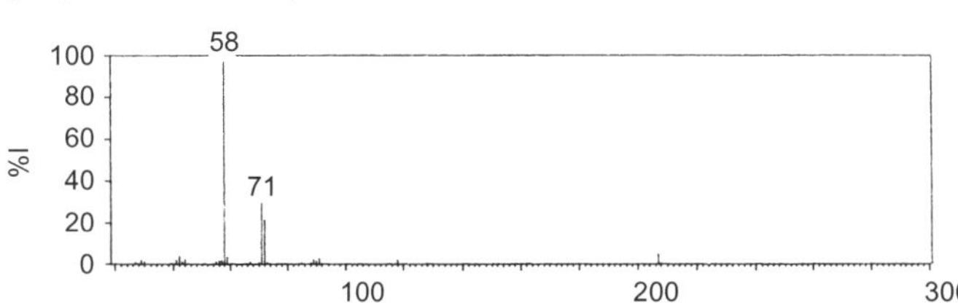

Disposition in the Body

Therapeutic concentration

Eight healthy volunteers were administered 30 mL 1% cyclopentolate hydrochloride or cyclopentolate polygalacturonate in saline or acetate buffer in one eye. Peak plasma concentrations of 3 mg/L were reached within 30 min with both formulations. [K. Lahdes *et al.*, *Br. J. Clin. Pharmacol.*, 1993, *35(5)*, 479–483.]

Half-life. Elimination, 111 min.

Use. Cyclopentolate hydrochloride is used as a 0.5 to 1% ophthalmic solution.

Cyclophosphamide

Antineoplastic

Proprietary names. Cytoxan; Endoxan(a); Procytox; Sendoxan.
N,N-Bis(2-chloroethyl)tetrahydro-2*H*-1,3,2-oxazaphosphorin-2-amine-2-oxide monohydrate
$C_7H_{15}Cl_2N_2O_2P,H_2O$=279.1
CAS—50-18-0 (anhydrous); 6055-19-2 (monohydrate)

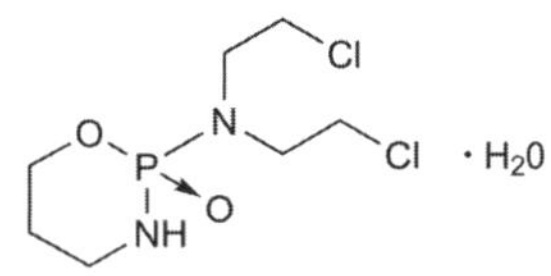

A fine, white, crystalline powder which discolours on exposure to light. M.p. 41° to 45°. It liquefies upon loss of its water of crystallisation. In aqueous solutions, at temperatures above 30°, hydrolysis occurs with removal of chlorine.
Soluble 1 in 25 of water and 1 in 1 of ethanol; slightly soluble in benzene, ethylene glycol, carbon tetrachloride, and dioxane; sparingly soluble in ether and acetone.

Partition Coefficient. Log *P* (octanol/water), 0.6.

Colour Test. Phosphorus Test—yellow precipitate.

Thin-layer Chromatography. System TAE—Rf 74.

Gas Chromatography. System GA—cyclophosphamide RI 2065, cyclophosphamide-HCl RI 1975.

Ultraviolet Spectrum. No significant absorption, 230 to 360 nm.

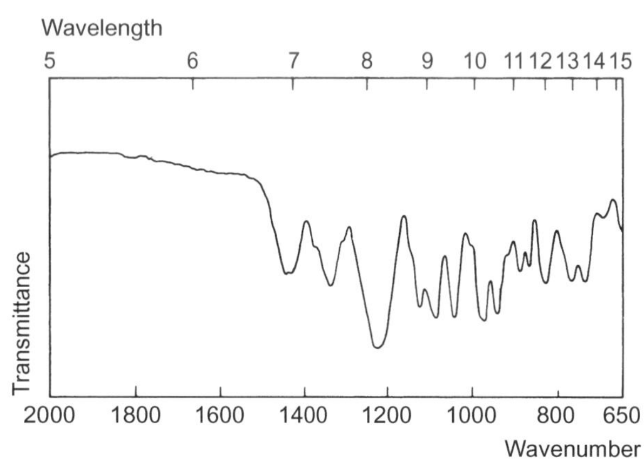

Infra-red Spectrum. Principal peaks at wavenumbers 1225, 1044, 975, 1088, 945, 1128 cm^{-1} (KBr disk). (See below)

Quantification

Gas chromatography. In plasma: limit of detection 10 µg/L, AFID—N. Van den Bosch and D. De Vos, *J. Chromatogr.* 1980, *183(9) B Biomed. Appl.*, 49–56. In plasma or urine: limit of detection 10 µg/L, AFID—T. Facchinetti *et al.*, *J. Chromatogr.* 1978, *145 B Biomed. Appl.*, *2*, 315–318. In plasma: cyclophosphamide metabolites (phosphoramide mustard and nornitrogen mustard), AFID—F. D. Juma *et al.*, *Br. J. Clin. Pharmacol.*, 1980, *10*, 327–335. In plasma: limit of detection 1 mg/L and limit of quantification 5 mg/L, NPD—A. D. Huitema *et al.*, *J. Chromatogr. B Biomed. Sci. Appl.*, 2001, *757(2)*, 349–357. In plasma: NPD—T. F. Kalhorn *et al.*, *J. Chromatogr. B Biomed. Sci. Appl.*, 1999, *732(2)*, 287–298.

Gas chromatography–mass spectrometry. In urine: limit of detection >0.25 mg/L—P. J. Sessink *et al.*, *J. Chromatogr.*, 1993, *616(2)*, 333–337.

High performance liquid chromatography–mass spectrometry. In urine: cyclophosphamide, 4-ketocyclophosphamide and carboxyphosphamide, limit of detection 10 pg—U. Bahrand H.-R. Schulten, *Biomed. Mass*

Spectrom., 1981, *8*, 553–557. In plasma: limit of quantification 60 µg/L, fluorescence detection (λ_{ex}=350 nm; λ_{em}=550 nm)—L. Griskevicius *et al.*, *Ther. Drug Monit.*, 2002, *24(3)*, 405–409. In plasma: limit of detection 40 µg/L and limit of quantification 50 µg/L, UV detection (λ = 276 nm) — A. D. Huitema *et al.*, *J. Chromatogr. B Biomed. Sci. Appl.*, 2000, *745(2)*, 345–355. In plasma: limit of detection 15 µg/L and 30 µg/L metabolites—F. Baumann *et al.*, *J. Chromatogr. B Biomed. Sci. Appl.*, 1999, *729(1–2)*, 297–305.

Disposition in the Body. Well absorbed after oral administration. The parent drug is inactive, but is converted into active metabolites by the liver. The drug and metabolites are widely distributed in the body. It is oxidised to 4-hydroxycyclophosphamide, which is in equilibrium with aldophosphamide, both of which are cytotoxic. 4-Hydroxycyclophosphamide can be oxidised further to 4-ketocyclophosphamide (inactive). Aldophosphamide may be converted to the cytotoxic metabolites phosphoramide mustard and acrolein, or oxidised to inactive carboxyphosphamide. Carboxyphosphamide may be converted to nornitrogen mustard, an active alkylating agent at acid pH. Up to 95% of a dose is excreted in the urine, mostly during the first 48 h, with up to 25% as unchanged drug and the rest as metabolites. Small amounts are excreted in the bile and faeces.

Therapeutic concentration

After a single IV dose of 9.4 mg/kg to a patient, a plasma concentration of about 26 mg/L of cyclophosphamide was attained immediately after injection, and this fell to about 13 mg/L after 2 h. After single IV doses of 9 to 12 mg/kg and 40 mg/kg, peak plasma concentrations of unbound alkylating metabolites of about 0.3 to 2 mg/L (8 studies) and about 2 to 6 mg/L (7 studies), respectively, were achieved, usually after 2 to 3 h. [C. M. Bagley, jun., *et al.*, Cancer Res., 1973, *33*, 226–233.]

Six male and female patients, mean age 52.8 years, were administered an IV bolus of 0.3 to 0.75 (mean, 0.55) g/m^2 cyclophosphamide. 1 h after dose, the mean serum concentration of *R*-cyclophosphamide was 13.49 mg/L and *S*-cyclophosphamide 12.89 mg/L; and 2.08 and 2.25 mg/L 20 h after dosing. [S. A. Corlett and H. Chrystyn, *J. Chromatogr. B Biomed. Sci. Appl.*, 1996, *682(2)*, 337–342.]

Bioavailability. Greater than 75%.

Half-life. Plasma half-life, about 3 to 12 h (mean 7).

Volume of distribution. About 0.7 L/kg.

Clearance. Plasma clearance, about 1 mL/min/kg.

Saliva. Plasma:saliva ratio, about 1.6.

Protein binding. In plasma, cyclophosphamide about 12 to 24%, alkylating metabolites about 50 to 60%.

Note. For a review of the pharmacokinetics of cyclophosphamide, see L. B. Grochow and M. Colvin, *Clin. Pharmacokinet.*, 1979, *4*, 380–394.

Dose. Regimens usually range from 2 to 6 mg/kg daily, by mouth or intravenously, to 60 to 80 mg/kg as a single IV dose every 3 to 4 weeks.

Cycloserine

Antibiotic/Tuberculostatic

Synonym. D-Cycloserine
Proprietary names. Closina; Seromycin.
D-4-Amino-3-isoxazolidinone
$C_3H_6N_2O_2$=102.1
CAS—68-41-7

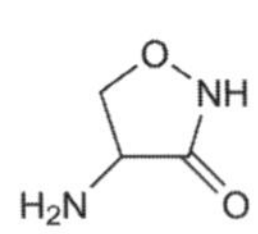

An antimicrobial substance produced by the growth of certain strains of *Streptomyces orchidaceus* or *S. garyphalus*, or obtained by synthesis.
A white or pale yellow, hygroscopic, crystalline powder. It is unstable in neutral or acid solutions. M.p. 155° to 156°, with decomposition.
Soluble 1 in 10 of water and 1 in 50 of ethanol; slightly soluble in chloroform, ether, and propylene glycol.

Dissociation Constant. pK_a 4.5, 7.4 (25°).

Partition Coefficient. Log *P* (octanol/water), −1.7.

Colour Test. Mercurous Nitrate—black.

Thin-layer Chromatography. System TA—Rf 44; system TB—Rf 01; system TC—Rf 01; system TL—Rf 02. (Acidified iodoplatinate solution, positive.)

Ultraviolet Spectrum. No significant absorption, 230 to 360 nm.

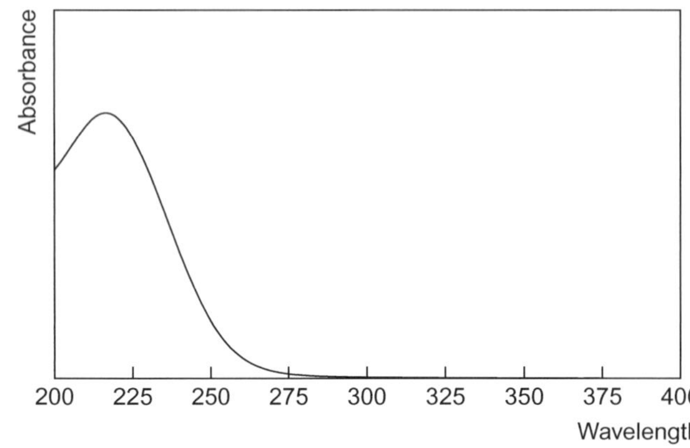

Infra-red Spectrum. Principal peaks at wavenumbers 1577, 1550, 1526, 1620, 934, 877 cm^{-1} (KBr disk).

Mass Spectrum. Principal ions at *m/z* 43, 29, 28, 59, 30, 42, 74, 102.

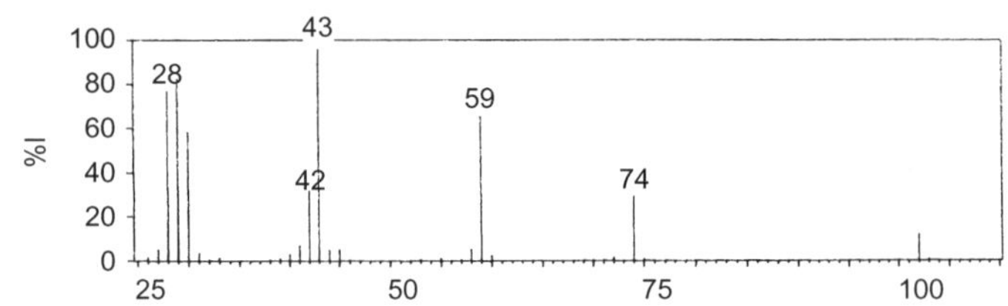

Quantification

High performance liquid chromatography. In plasma: limit of detection 10 mg/L, fluorescence detection (λ_{ex}=381 nm; λ_{em}=450 nm) —V. David *et al.*, *J. Chromatogr. B Biomed. Sci. Appl.*, 2001, *761(1)*, 27–33.

Disposition in the Body. Readily absorbed after oral administration and widely distributed throughout body fluids and tissues. About 65% of a dose is excreted in the urine unchanged in 72 h, mostly in the first 24 h.

Therapeutic concentration

After oral administration of 750 mg, divided into three 6-hourly doses to 11 subjects, followed by a single dose of 500 mg the next morning, peak serum concentrations of 22 to 34 mg/L (mean 28) were reported 2 to 4 h after the last dose. [M. J. Mattila *et al.*, *Scand. J. Resp. Dis.*, 1969, *50*, 291–300.]

Toxicity

A female subject who ingested a non-fatal overdose of 3 g, had a peak plasma concentration of 91 mg/L on admission to hospital; following peritoneal dialysis for 20 h, the plasma concentration declined to 25 mg/L. [R. Atkins *et al.*, *BMJ*, 1965, *1*, 907–908.]

Half-life. Plasma half-life, 4 to 30 h (mean 10).

Protein binding. In plasma, less than 20%.

Dose. 0.25 to 1 g daily.

Cyclothiazide

Diuretic

Proprietary names. Anhydron; Doburil.
3-Bicyclo[2.2.1]hept-5-en-2-yl-6-chloro-3,4-dihydro-2*H*-1,2,4-benzothiadiazine-7-sulfonamide 1,1-dioxide
$C_{14}H_{16}ClN_3O_4S_2$=389.9
CAS—2259-96-3

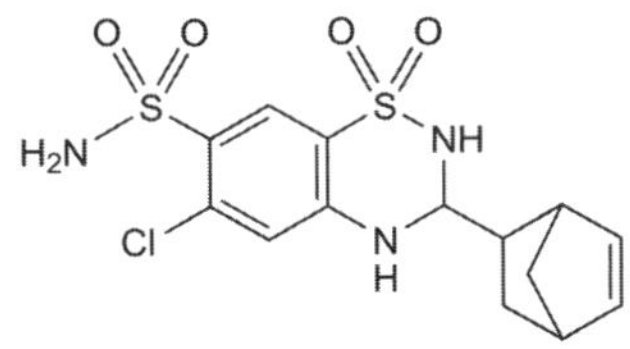

A white powder. M.p. 217° to 225°.
Practically insoluble in water; soluble 1 in 70 of ethanol and 1 in 30 of methanol; freely soluble in acetone; practically insoluble in chloroform and ether.

Partition Coefficient. Log *P* (octanol/water), 2.0.

Colour Tests. Koppanyi–Zwikker Test—violet; Liebermann's Test—brown; Sulfuric Acid—orange→red-brown.

Thin-layer Chromatography. System TA—Rf 77; system TD—Rf 18; system TE—Rf 59; system TF—Rf 60; system TAD—Rf 26. (Acidified potassium permanganate solution, positive.)

High Performance Liquid Chromatography. System HN—*k* 10.78, 11.91, and 12.81; system HY—RI 433.

Ultraviolet Spectrum. Aqueous acid—272 (A_1^1=549b), 314 nm.

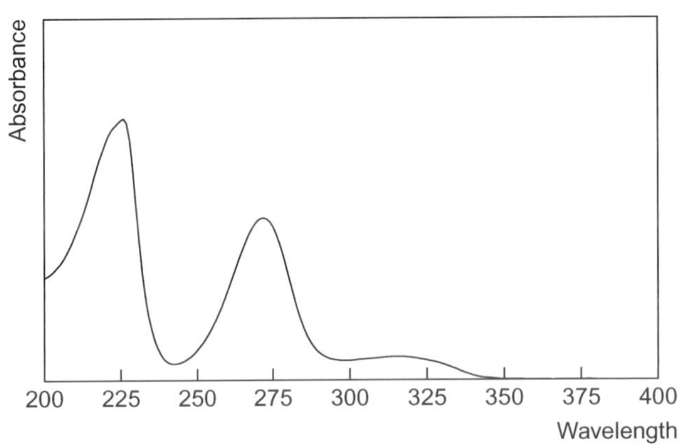

Infra-red Spectrum. Principal peaks at wavenumbers 1596, 1153, 1168, 1307, 1500, 1075 cm^{-1} (KBr disk).

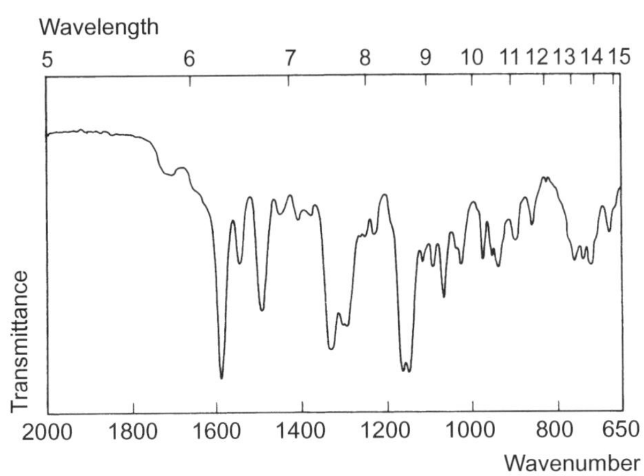

Mass Spectrum. Principal ions at *m*/*z* 66, 120, 39, 65, 269, 205, 118, 77.

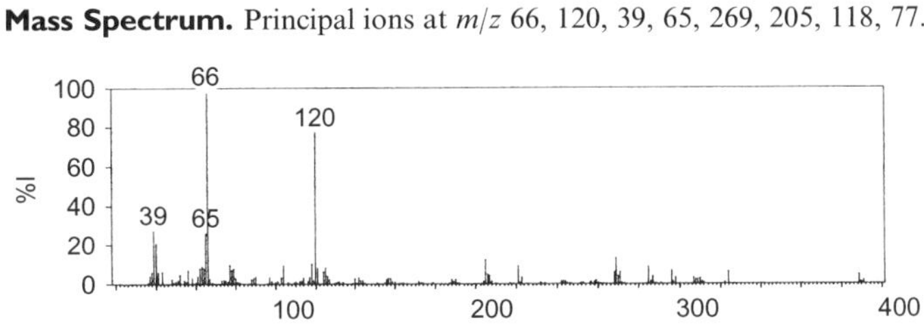

Dose. 1 to 2 mg daily; up to 6 mg daily may be given.

Cycrimine

Anticholinergic

1-Cyclopentyl-1-phenyl-3-piperidinopropan-1-ol
$C_{19}H_{29}NO$=287.4
CAS—77-39-4

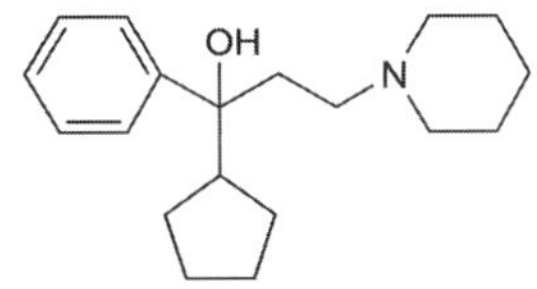

M.p. 90° to 96°.

Cycrimine Hydrochloride

Synonym. Cycriminium Chloride
Proprietary name. Pagitane Hydrochloride
$C_{19}H_{29}NO,HCl$=323.9
CAS—126-02-3
A white solid. M.p. about 242°, with decomposition.
Soluble 1 in 175 of water, 1 in 50 of ethanol, and 1 in 35 of chloroform; practically insoluble in ether.

Partition Coefficient. Log *P* (octanol/water), 2.0 (hydrochloride).

Colour Tests. Liebermann's Test—red-orange; Mandelin's Test—red-brown; Marquis Test—orange→red.

Thin-layer Chromatography. System TA—Rf 66; system TB—Rf 67; system TC—Rf 61; system TL—Rf 60. (Acidified iodoplatinate solution, positive.)

Gas Chromatography. System GA—RI 2114.

Ultraviolet Spectrum. Aqueous acid—251, 256 nm (A_1^1=6b), 263 nm.

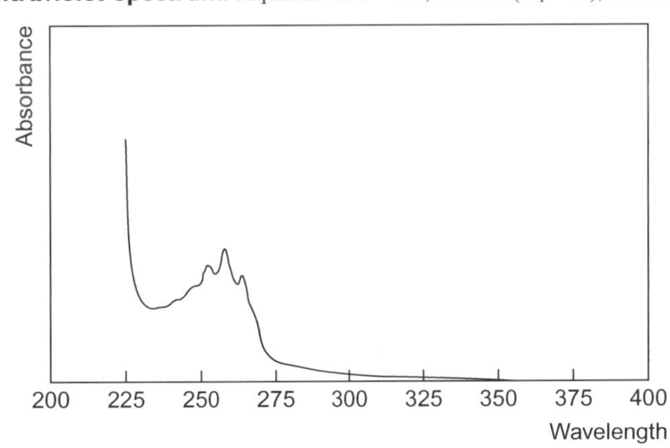

Infra-red Spectrum. Principal peaks at wavenumbers 696, 1117, 755, 751, 1030, 1298 cm^{-1} (KBr disk).

Mass Spectrum. Principal ions at *m*/*z* 98, 41, 42, 55, 99, 77, 69, 44.

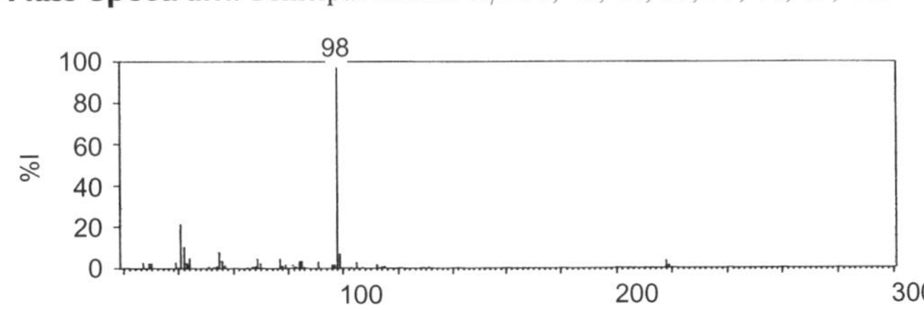

Quantification

Gas chromatography–mass spectrometry. In biological fluids: limit of detection 50 to 100 ng/L, flame thermionic detection—J. A. Owen *et al.*, *J. Chromatogr.*, 1989, *494*, 135–142.

Dose. Usually 3.75 to 20 mg of cycrimine hydrochloride daily.

Cyfluthrin

Insecticide

Synonyms. β-Cyfluthrin; Cyfoxylate; BAY FCR 1272; BAY-VI-1704; FCR 1272; FCR 4545.
Proprietary names. Attatox; Baythroid; Baythroid H; Bulldock; Contur; Eulan SP; Laser; Responsar; Solfac; Tempo; Tempo H.
Cyano-(4-fluoro-3-phenoxy-phenyl)methyl-3-(2,2-dichloroethenyl)-2,2-dimethylcyclopropanecarboxylate
$C_{22}H_{18}Cl_2FNO_3$=434.3
CAS—68359-37-5

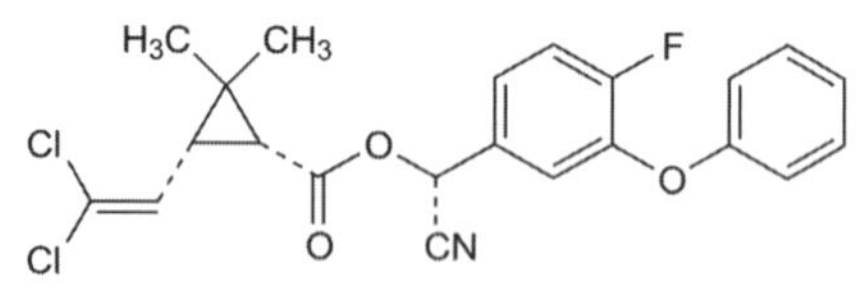

(1*R*,3*R*,α*R*)-form

A yellowish brown oil. M.p. 60°.
It is soluble in water (0.002 g/L at 20°), 2-propanol (20 to 50 g/L), methylene chloride (>200 g/L), hexane (10 to 20 g/L), and toluene.

Partition Coefficient. Log *P* (octanol/water), 5.95.

Thin-layer Chromatography. System TX—Rf 37; system TY—Rf 89.

Gas Chromatography. System GA—RI 2749.

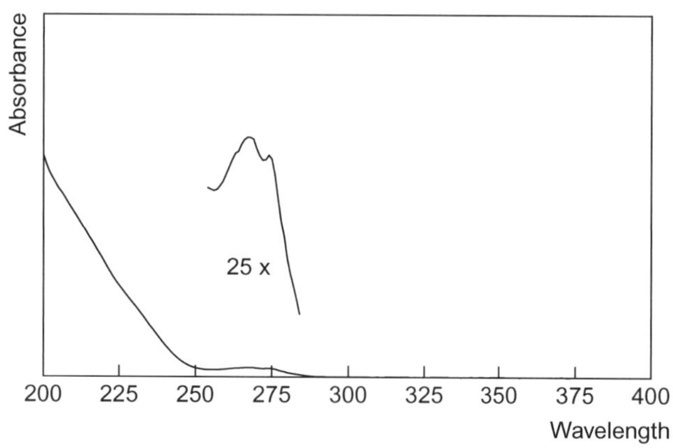

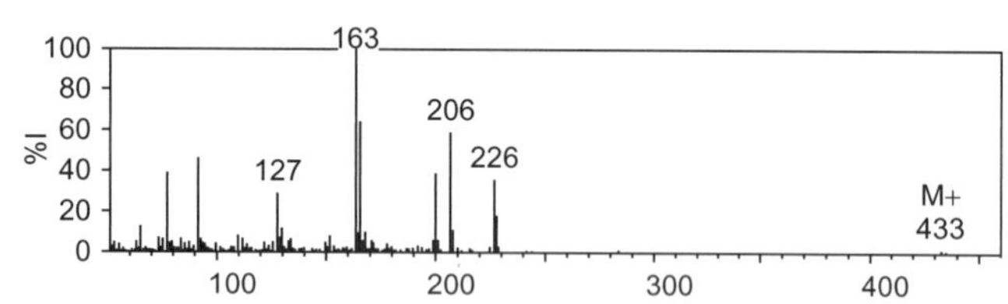

Quantification
Gas chromatography–mass spectrometry. In urine and plasma: limit of detection of the metabolites, DCCA and FPBA, 0.5 μg/L in urine and 5.0 μg/L in plasma—G. Leng *et al.*, *Sci. Total Environ.*, 1997, *199(1–2)*, 173–181.

Disposition in the Body. Cyfluthrin is rapidly metabolised in the liver and metabolites include *cis*-(3(2,2-dichlorovinyl)-2,2-dimethylcyclopropane-carboxylic acid (*cis*-DCCA), *trans*-DCCA, and 4-fluoro-3-phenoxybenzoic acid (FPBA). It is eliminated fairly quickly in urine (approx. 60%) and faeces (approx. 20%) within 24 h. 98% of the dose is eliminated within 48 h.

Toxicity. Moderately toxic and is an irritant to human skin especially facial skin. Toxic effects have a delay of 1 to 2 h after exposure.

A 64-year-old man was found unconscious at home with one empty bottle and one half-filled bottle containing emulsion (with 35 mL cyfluthrin). Toxicological analysis showed that there was a concentration of 10 mg/L cyfluthrin in the man's blood, a total of 14 mg cyfluthrin in his stomach, 4 μg cyfluthrin/g in liver, and 7 mg/L in his urine. [K. Hon *et al.*, *TIAFT Bulletin Case Notes*, 1988, *20(1)*.]

Half-life. *cis*-DCCA, 6.9 h; *trans*-DCCA, 6.2 h; FPBA, 5.3 h.

Cyproheptadine

Antihistamine

4-(5*H*-Dibenzo[*a*,*d*]cyclohepten-5-ylidene)-1-methylpiperidine
$C_{21}H_{21}N$=287.4
CAS—129-03-3

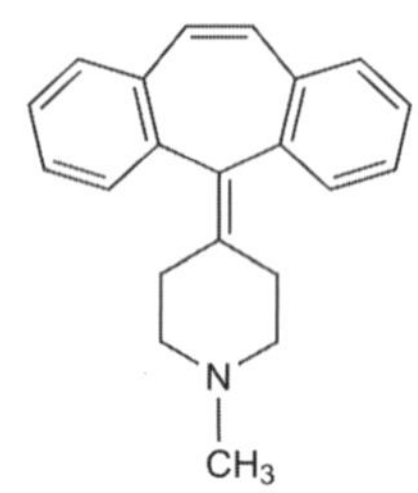

Crystals. M.p. about 113°.

Cyproheptadine Hydrochloride

Proprietary names. Antegan; Nuran; Periactin(e); Periactinol; Vimicon.
$C_{21}H_{21}N,HCl,1\frac{1}{2}H_2O$=350.9
CAS—969-33-5 (anhydrous); 41354-29-4 (sesquihydrate)
A white to slightly yellow, crystalline powder. M.p. 214° to 216°, with decomposition.
Soluble 1 in 275 of water, 1 in 35 of ethanol, 1 in about 16 of chloroform, and 1 in 1.5 of methanol; practically insoluble in ether.

Partition Coefficient. Log *P* (octanol/pH 7.4), 3.2.

Colour Tests. Mandelin's Test—violet-brown; Marquis Test—grey-green; Sulfuric Acid—violet.

Thin-layer Chromatography. System TA—Rf 51; system TB—Rf 45; system TC—Rf 44; system TE—Rf 64; system TL—Rf 13; system TAE—Rf 30; system TAF—Rf 50; system TAJ—Rf 18; system TAK—Rf 16; system TAL—Rf 76. (Acidified iodoplatinate solution, positive.)

Gas Chromatography. System GA—cyproheptadine RI 2355, M (OH-) RI 3060, M (nor-) RI 2400, M (oxo-) RI 2960, M (nor-OH-)-H_2O RI 2450; system GB—cyproheptadine RI 2460, M (nor-OH-)-H_2O RI 2608; system GC—RI 2307; system GF—RI 2710.

High Performance Liquid Chromatography. System HA—*k* 3.2; system HY—RI 354; system HZ—retention time 6.5 min; system HAA—retention time 15.0 min.

Ultraviolet Spectrum. Aqueous acid—286 (A_1^1=433a); aqueous alkali—284 nm (A_1^1=377b).

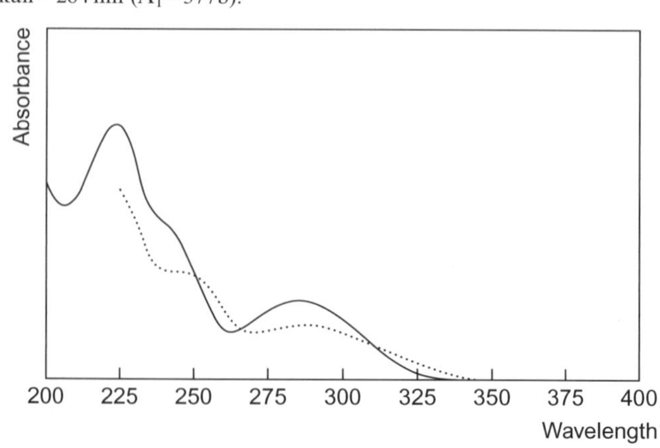

Infra-red Spectrum. Principal peaks at wavenumbers 777, 756, 815, 786, 1640, 960 cm^{-1} (cyproheptadine hydrochloride, KBr disk).

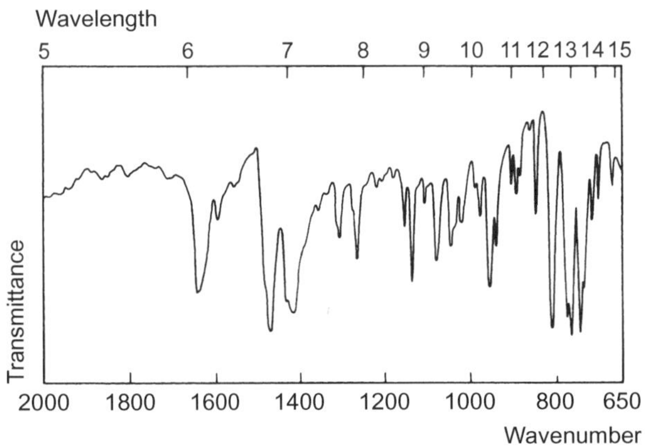

Mass Spectrum. Principal ions at *m/z* 287, 96, 286, 215, 70, 44, 58, 42; M (OH-) *m/z* 303, 203, 202, 217, 304, 205; M (nor-) *m/z* 273, 215, 216, 231, 229, 272; M (oxo-) *m/z* 229, 215, 202, 242, 301, 258; M (nor-OH-)-H_2O *m/z* 271, 272, 270, 165, 193, 241.

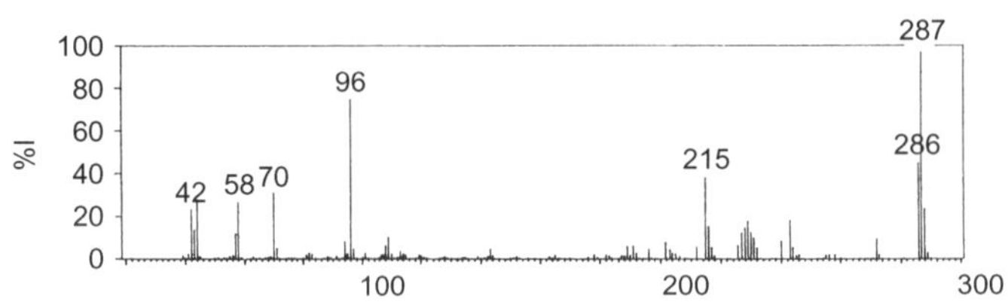

Quantification

Gas chromatography. In plasma or urine: limit of detection 3 µg/L, AFID—H. B. Hucker and J. E. Hutt, *J. Pharm. Sci.*, 1983, *72*, 1069–1070.

High performance liquid chromatography. In urine: limit of quantification 50 µg/L and limit of detection 15 µg/L, UV (λ = 254 nm) —J. E. Kountourellis and K. O. Ebete, *J. Chromatogr. B Biomed. Sci. Appl.*, 1995, *664(2)*, 468–471.

Disposition in the Body. Absorbed after oral administration and extensively distributed throughout the tissues. Metabolised by aromatic ring hydroxylation, *N*-demethylation, heterocyclic ring oxidation, and glucuronic acid conjugation; the major metabolite in urine is a quaternary ammonium glucuronide conjugate. About 67 to 77% of a dose is excreted in the urine in 6 days, the remainder being eliminated in the faeces. Of the excreted material, 58 to 65% is conjugated with glucuronic acid, 9 to 11% is conjugated with sulfate, 20 to 26% is excreted as polar material not hydrolysable by glucuronidase or sulfatase, and about 5% is unconjugated.

Therapeutic concentration

After a single oral dose of 5 mg to 2 subjects, peak plasma concentrations of cyproheptadine metabolites of 0.036 and 0.05 mg/L were attained in 6 to 9 h; unchanged drug was not detected. [K. L. Hintze *et al.*, *Drug Met. Disp.*, 1975, *3*, 1–9.]

Toxicity

A 28-year-old man was found dead. The heart blood concentration of cyproheptadine was 0.46 mg/L and ethanol was detected at 0.9 g/L. Cyproheptadine was also detected at concentrations of 8.1 mg/L, 1.8 mg/kg, 7.6 mg/kg, 0.75 mg/L, and 2.3 mg in bile, kidney, liver, urine, and stomach contents, respectively. [B. Levine *et al.*, *J. Anal. Toxicol.*, 1998, *22(1)*, 72–74.]

Dose. 12 to 16 mg of anhydrous cyproheptadine hydrochloride daily; maximum of 32 mg daily.

Cytarabine

Antineoplastic

Synonyms. Arabinosylcytosine; Ara-C; Cytosine Arabinoside.
Proprietary names. Alexan; Aracytin(e); Cytosar; Cytosar-U; Udicil.
4-Amino-1-*β*-D-arabinofuranosyl-2(1*H*)-pyrimidinone
$C_9H_{13}N_3O_5$=243.2
CAS—147-94-4

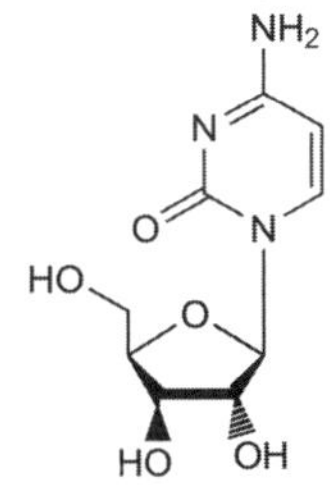

A white crystalline powder. M.p. 212° to 213°.
Soluble 1 in 10 of water, 1 in 1000 of ethanol, and 1 in 1000 of chloroform.

Cytarabine Hydrochloride
$C_9H_{13}N_3O_5$,HCl=279.7
CAS—69-74-9
A white crystalline powder.
Soluble 1 in 1 of water; less soluble in organic solvents.

Dissociation Constant. pK_a 4.3.

Partition Coefficient. Log *P* (octanol/water), −2.5.

Thin-layer Chromatography. System TA—Rf 05; system TB—Rf 00; system TC—Rf 01; system TL—Rf 01; system TAD—Rf 00; system TAE—Rf 69. (Acidified potassium permanganate solution, positive.)

Ultraviolet Spectrum. Aqueous acid—280 (A^1_1=555a); aqueous alkali—274 nm.

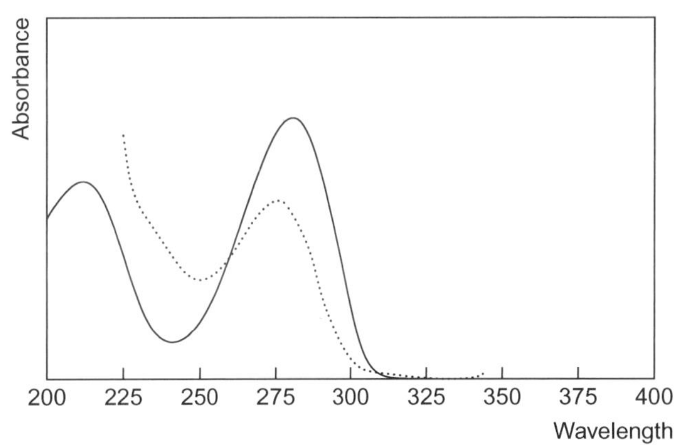

Infra-red Spectrum. Principal peaks at wavenumbers 1075, 1027, 1145, 1109, 1178, 1002 cm^{-1} (KBr disk).

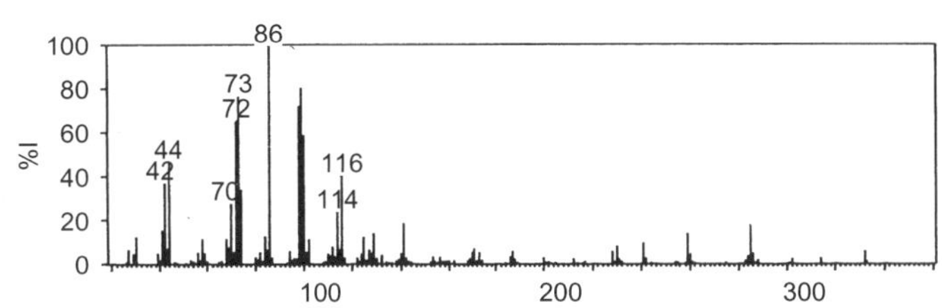

Quantification

Gas chromatography. In plasma: limit of detection 40 µg/L, AFID—J. Boutagy and D. J. Harvey, *J. Chromatogr.* 1978, *146(3) B Biomed. Appl.*, 283–296.

High performance liquid chromatography. In plasma: limit of detection 20 µg/L, UV detection—R. W. Bury and P. J. Keary, *J. Chromatogr.* 1978, *146 B Biomed. Appl.*, 350–353. In plasma, urine, or cerebrospinal fluid: limit of detection 20 µg/L, UV detection—J. A. Sinkule and W. E. Evans, *J. Chromatogr.* 1983, *274(25) B Biomed. Appl.*, 87–93.

Dose. 2 to 4 mg/kg daily, intravenously.

Cytisine

Alkaloid

Synonyms. Baptitoxine; Cytiton; Laburnine; Sophorine; Ulexine.
(1*R*)-1,2,3,4,5,6-Hexahydro-1,5-methano-8*H*-pyrido[1,2-*a*][1,5]diazocin-8-one
$C_{11}H_{14}N_2O = 190.2$
CAS—485-35-8

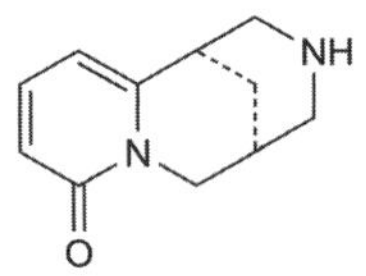

An alkaloid found in all parts of the laburnum, *Laburnum anagyroides* (Leguminosae), particularly in the pods and seeds, and in some other leguminous plants.
A white or slightly yellowish crystalline powder. M.p. 154° to 157°.
Soluble 1 in 1.3 of water, 1 in 13 of acetone, 1 in 30 of benzene, 1 in 10 of ethyl acetate, 1 in 3.5 of ethanol, and 1 in 2 of chloroform; practically insoluble in petroleum ether.

Partition Coefficient. Log *P* (octanol/water), 0.6.

Thin-layer Chromatography. System TA—Rf 40; system TB—Rf 01; system TC—Rf 10; system TL—Rf 02. (Acidified iodoplatinate solution, positive.)

Ultraviolet Spectrum. Aqueous acid—232, 302 nm (A^1_1=344b).

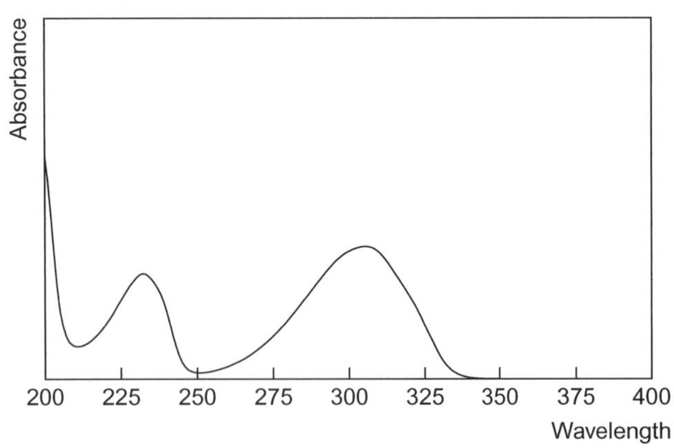

Infra-red Spectrum. Principal peaks at wavenumbers 1650, 1540, 1565, 1140, 790, 1311 cm^{-1} (KBr disk).

Mass Spectrum. Principal ions at *m/z* 44, 146, 147, 39, 41, 190, 42, 148.

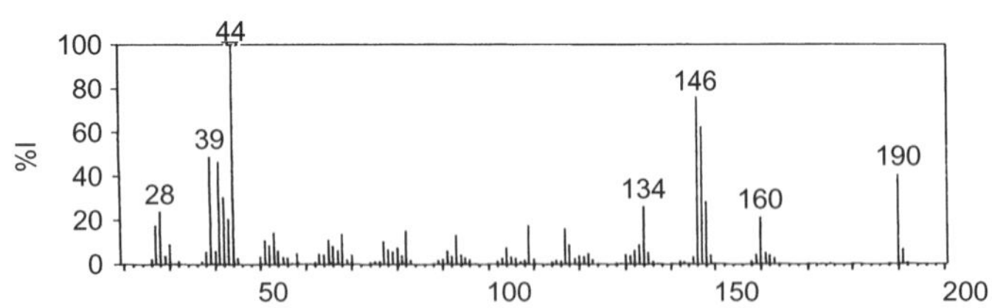

Quantification

Ultraviolet spectrophotometry. In blood—H. G. H. Richards and A. Stephens, *Med. Sci. Law*, 1970, *10*, 260–266.

Disposition in the Body

Toxicity. Cytisine is a highly toxic alkaloid which resembles nicotine in its actions. Fatalities have occurred after the ingestion of laburnum seeds, but recovery is more usual.

> In a fatality due to the ingestion of laburnum seeds (estimated amount ingested 50 mg), a blood concentration of 6.8 mg/L of cytisine was reported; the stomach contained 23 laburnum pods [H. G. H. Richards and A. Stephens, *Med. Sci. Law*, 1970, *10*, 260–266].

Note. For reviews of laburnum poisoning in children see R. G. Mitchell, *Lancet*, 1951, *2*, 57–58, and A. Bramley and R. Goulding, *BMJ*, 1981, *283*, 1220–1221.

Dactinomycin

Antineoplastic

Synonyms. Actinomycin C_1; Actinomycin D; Meractinomycin; NSC-3053.
Proprietary names. Cosmegen
[2-Amino-*N*,*N*′-bis[hexadecahydro-2,5,9-trimethyl-6,13-bis(1-methylethyl)-1,4,7,11,14-pentaoxo-1*H*-pyrrolo-[2,1-i][1,4,7,10,13]oxatetra-azacyclohexadecin-10-yl]-4,6-dimethyl-3-oxo]-3*H*-phenoxazine-1,9-dicarboxamide
$C_{62}H_{86}N_{12}O_{16} = 1255.5$
CAS—50-76-0

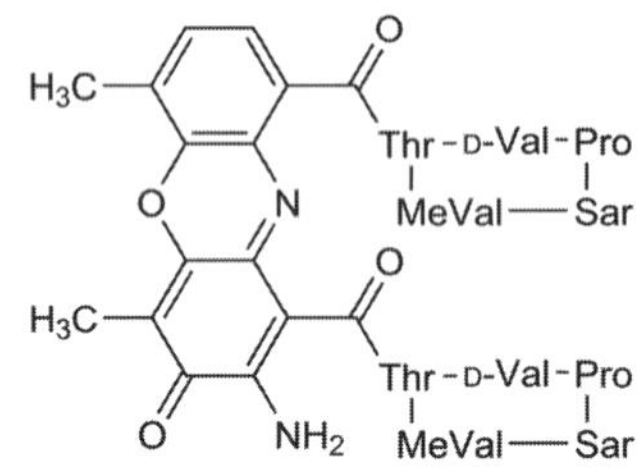

A bright red, somewhat hygroscopic, crystalline powder. Crystals from absolute alcohol. M.p. 241.5° to 243°, with decomposition. Dilute solutions are very sensitive to light. It is soluble in water at 10°, slightly soluble in water at 37°; freely soluble in ethanol; very slightly soluble in ether.

Partition Coefficient. Log *P* (octanol/water), −0.91.

High Performance Liquid Chromatography. Column: (analytical) ODS Hypersil Si-10 (300 × 4.0 mm i.d., 10 μm) with 5 cm guard filled with Porasil A. Mobile phase: methanol with 1% NHOH:methylene chloride (2:98), flow rate 2 mL/min. UV detection. Retention time: 5.0 min. [T. Mills and J. C. Roberson, *Instrumental Data for Drug Analysis*, 1993, CRC Press, Boca Raton, US. 2nd Edn, Vol. 1, pp. 580–581].

Ultraviolet Spectrum. Ethanol—240 nm.

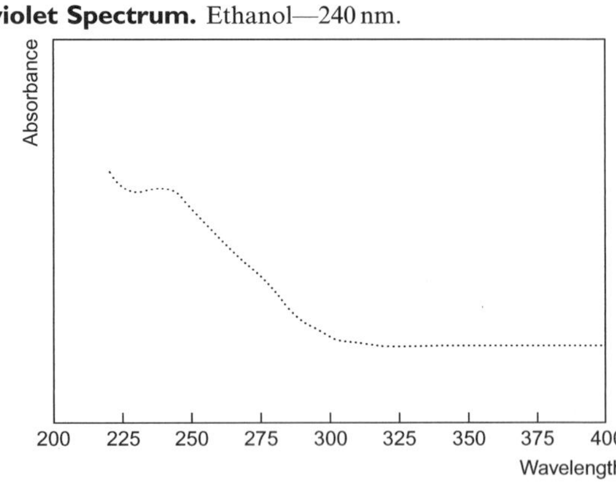

Infra-red Spectrum. Principal peaks at wavenumbers 1745, 1668, 1590, 1195 cm^{-1} (KBr pellets).

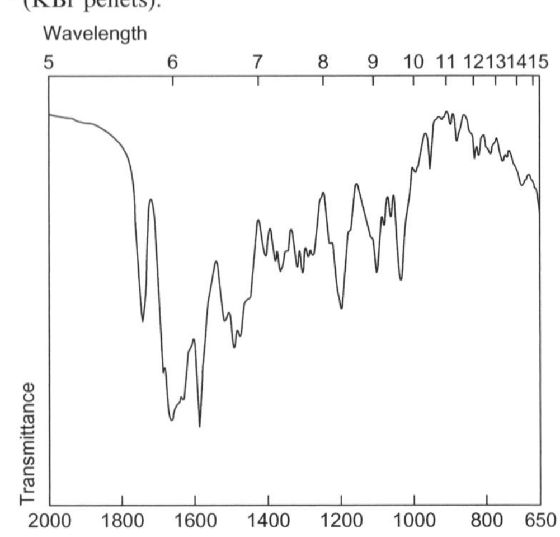

Disposition in the Body. Dactinomycin is rapidly distributed following intravenous administration and concentrates in bone marrow and nucleated cells. It does not cross the blood–brain barrier. The drug undergoes minimal metabolism and is slowly excreted in urine (about 10% as unchanged drug) and via bile in faeces (about 50% as the unchanged drug).

Half-life. Plasma, 36 h.

Dose. Usually 500 µg intravenously daily for a maximum of 5 days.

Danazol

Androgen

Synonym. Win-17757
Proprietary names. Azol; Cyclomen; Danatrol; Danazant; Danocrine; Danokrin; Danol; Ladazol; Mastodanatrol; Winobanin.
17α-Pregna-2,4-dien-20-yno[2,3-*d*]isoxazol-17β-ol
$C_{22}H_{27}NO_2 = 337.5$
CAS—17230-88-5

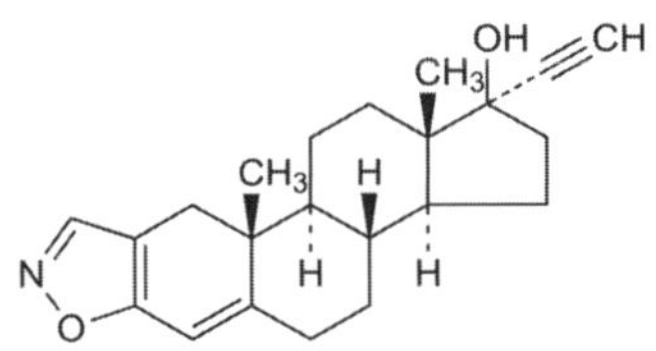

A white or pale yellow crystalline powder. M.p. 224.4° to 226.8°, with decomposition. It is practically insoluble in water and in light petroleum; sparingly soluble in ethanol and in benzene; freely soluble in chloroform; slightly soluble in ether; soluble in acetone.

Partition Coefficient. Log *P* (octanol/water), 4.21.

Gas Chromatography. Column: 3% OV-1 Chromosorb WHP 80/100 mesh (4 feet × 1/4 inch). Column temperature: 280°. Carrier gas: nitrogen, 32 mL/min flow rate. Detection: flame ionisation. Retention index: 3126. [T. Mills and J. C. Roberson, *Instrumental Data for Drug Analysis*, 1993, CRC Press, Boca Raton, US. 2nd Edn, Vol. 1, pp. 582–583].

High Performance Liquid Chromatography. System HY—RI 711.

Column: (1)-C_8 (Spherisorb, 150 × 3.9 mm i.d., 5 µm); (2)-ODS-2 (Spherisorb, 150 × 4.6 mm, 5 µm). Mobile phase: acetonitrile:water (55:45), 1.6 mL/min flow rate. UV detection (λ = 285 nm). Retention time: 9.5 min. [K. Selinger *et al.*, *J. Pharm. Biomed. Anal.*, 1990, *8(1)*, 79–84].

Column: ODS Hypersil Si-10 (300 × 4.0 mm i.d., 10 µm film thickness). Mobile phase: methanol with 1% NHOH:methylene chloride (10:90), flow rate 2 mL/min. UV detection (λ = 254 nm). Retention time: 5.5 min. [T. Mills and J. C. Roberson, *Instrumental Data for Drug Analysis*, 1993, CRC Press, Boca Raton, US. 2nd Edn, Vol. 1, pp. 582–583].

Ultraviolet Spectrum. Ethanol—228 , 254 nm.

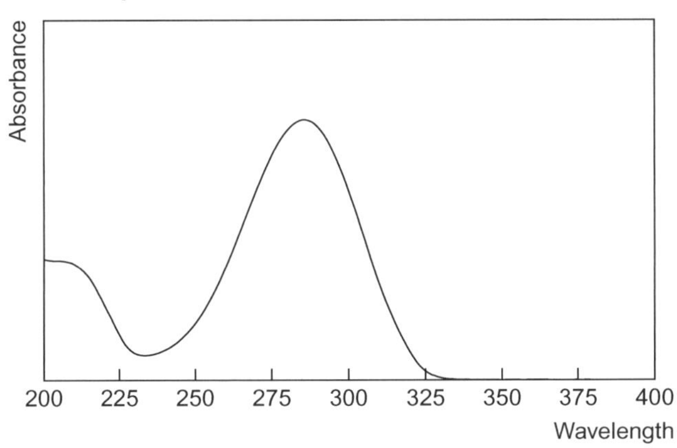

Infra-red Spectrum. Principal peaks at wavenumbers 1597, 1470, 1062, 843 cm^{-1}.

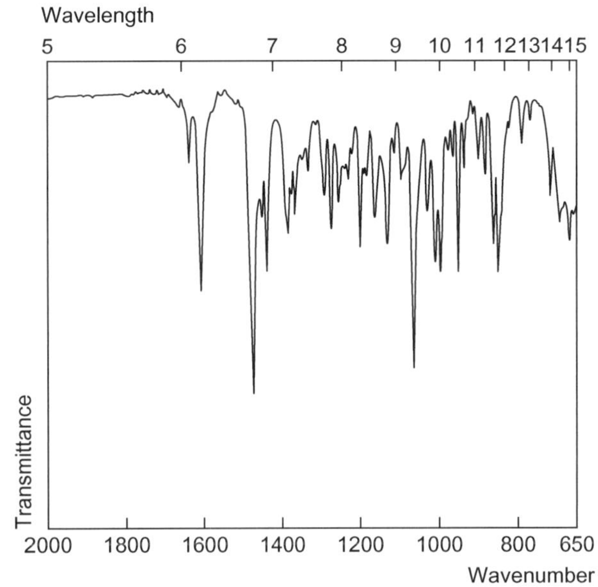

Mass Spectrum. Principal ions at *m/z* 91, 79, 77, 55, 67, 93, 270, 105, 147, 131, 337.

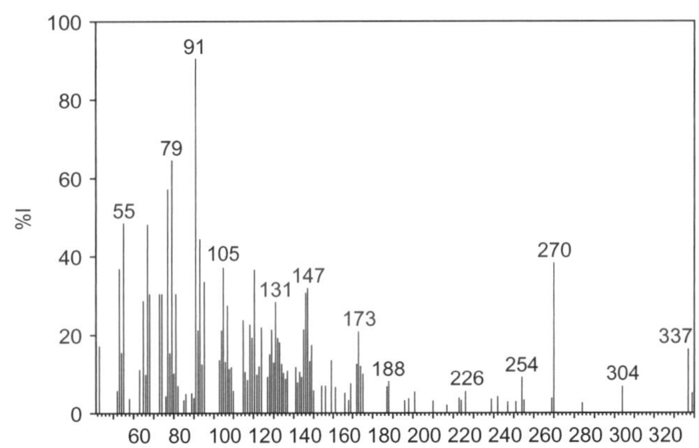

Quantification

High performance liquid chromatography. In plasma: limit of detection 2 µg/L, UV detection—W. D. Hooper *et al.*, *J. Chromatogr.*, 1987, *416*; *Biomed. Appl.*, *60*, 347–352. In serum: limit of detection 1.5 µg/L, UV detection—G. A. Nygard *et al.*, *J. Chromatogr.*, 1987, *415*; *Biomed. Appl.*, *59*, 438–444. In serum: limit of detection is 1 µg/L. UV detection (λ = 285 nm)—K. Selinger *et al.*, *J. Pharm. Biomed. Anal.*, 1990, *8(1)*, 79–84.

Disposition in the Body. Danazol is absorbed following oral administration; absorption is increased markedly if taken with food. It is metabolised in the liver to inactive metabolites, including 2-hydroxymethylethisterone, that are then excreted in urine.

Therapeutic concentration

24 healthy females, aged between 18 and 41 years (mean 26 years), were administered with 50, 100, 200 or 400 mg doses after an overnight fast, for 3 weeks. Steady state plasma concentrations were 83, 115, 183 and 193 µg/L, respectively, observed after 1 to 2 h. [G. O. Potts *et al.*, *Drugs*, 1980, *19*, 321–330].

15 healthy, sterile, premenopausal females, aged 18 to 45 years, were orally administered with a single dose of 200 mg danazol on two separate occasions, 14 days apart. Mean peak serum concentrations reached 51.5 µg/L on the first treatment at 2.3 h and 54.3 µg/L at 2.7 h on the second occasion. [K. Selinger *et al.*, *J. Pharm. Biomed. Anal.*, 1990, *8(1)*, 79–84].

15 healthy young males, aged 18 to 26 years (mean 22.3 years), were administered with 400 mg danazol following an overnight fast; two different formulations were used. The peak plasma concentrations ranged from 34.1 to 170 (mean 73.6) µg/L for formulation produced by Alphapharm and 30.8 to 143 (mean 69.6) µg/L for the Winthrop

formulation. These were observed at 2 h and 2.47 h, respectively, for the two formulations. [W. D. Hooper *et al.*, *Biopharm. Drug Dispos.*, 1991, *12*, 577–582].

Half-life. Plasma half-life, 4.5 h (healthy women); 9.4 h (healthy males).

Clearance. Total body, mean, 710 L/h (healthy males).

Note. For a review of danazol, see G. O. Potts *et al.*, *Drugs*, 1980, *19*, 321–330.

Dose. Up to 800 mg daily.

Dantrolene *Muscle Relaxant*

1-[[[5-(4-Nitrophenyl)-2-furanyl]methylene]amino]-2,4-imidazolidinedione
$C_{14}H_{10}N_4O_5$=314.3
CAS—7261-97-4

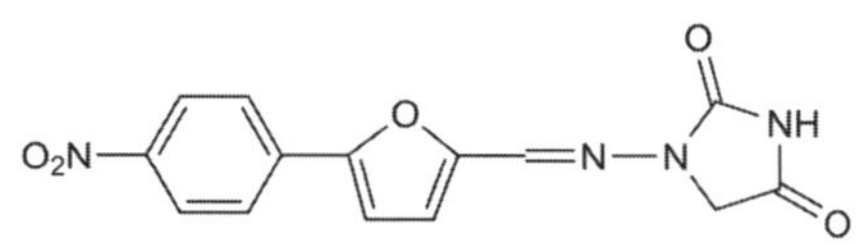

Crystals. M.p. 279° to 280°.
Practically insoluble in water.

Dantrolene Sodium
Proprietary names. Dantamacrin; Dantrium.
$C_{14}H_9N_4NaO_5,3\frac{1}{2}H_2O$=399.3
CAS—14663-23-1 (anhydrous); 24868-20-0 (hemiheptahydrate)
An orange powder.
Slightly soluble in water; its solubility increases in alkaline solution. Soluble 1 in 40 to 1 in 50 of acetone, and 1 in 25 of propylene glycol.

Dissociation Constant. pK_a 7.5.

Partition Coefficient. Log *P* (octanol/water), 1.7.

Thin-layer Chromatography. System TD—Rf 19; system TE—Rf 09; system TF—Rf 36; system TAD—Rf 50; system TAJ—Rf 46; system TAK—Rf 24; system TAL—Rf 90.

High Performance Liquid Chromatography. System HZ—Retention time, 4.0 min; system HAX—Retention time, 6.0 min; system HAY—Retention time, 5.2 min.

Ultraviolet Spectrum. Dantrolene sodium: aqueous alkali—314 nm (A^1_1=487b).

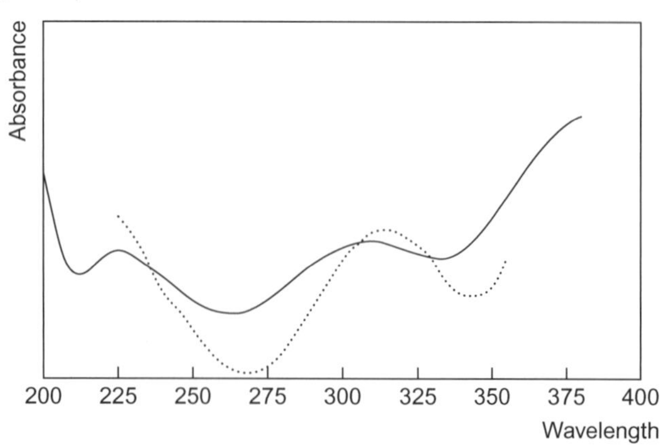

Infra-red Spectrum. Principal peaks at wavenumbers 1600, 1225, 1510, 850, 1713, 1108 cm^{-1} (dantrolene sodium, KBr disk).

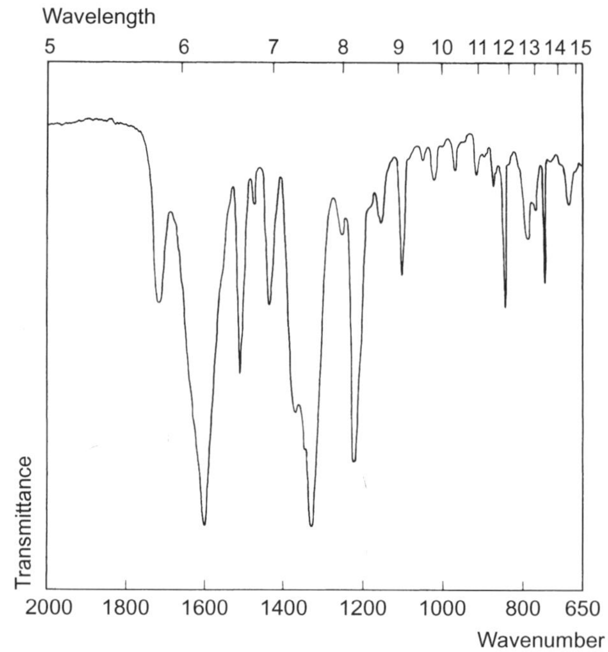

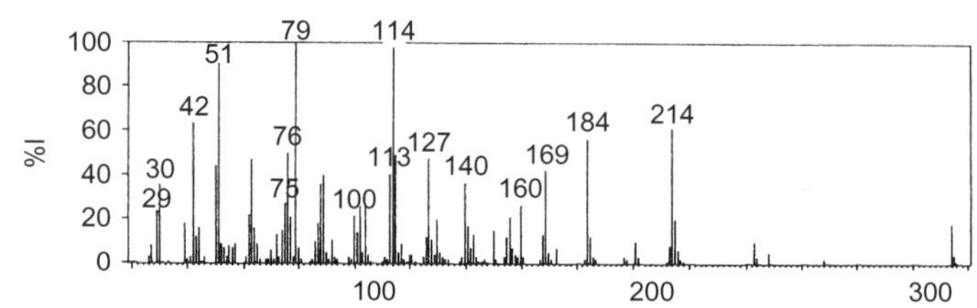

Quantification

Spectrofluorimetry. In plasma, blood, urine or tissues: limit of detection 100 μg/L in plasma, blood and urine, 400 mg/L in bile and tissues—R. D. Hollifield and J. D. Conklin, *J. Pharm. Sci.*, 1973, *62*, 271–274.

High performance liquid chromatography In plasma and urine: metabolite—E. W. Wuis *et al.*, *J. Chromatogr.*, 1990, *526*, 575–580. In plasma or urine: dantrolene, 5-hydroxydantrolene and *p*-acetamidodantrolene, limit of detection 20 mg/L, UV detection—E. W. Wuis *et al.*, *J. Chromatogr.*, 1982, 231; *B Biomed. Appl.*, *20*, 401–409.

Disposition in the Body. Slowly and incompletely absorbed after oral administration. Metabolised by oxidation to 5-hydroxydantrolene, which is active, and by reduction followed by acetylation to form the *p*-acetamido derivative. About 20% of an oral dose is excreted in the urine as metabolites, mainly the 5-hydroxy derivative; less than 5% of a dose is excreted in the urine as unchanged drug; up to about 50% of a dose may be excreted in the bile.

Therapeutic concentration

Following a single oral dose of 100 mg to 8 subjects, peak plasma concentrations of 0.7 to 1.7 mg/L (mean 1.2) of dantrolene and 0.2 to 0.5 mg/L (mean 0.4) of 5-hydroxydantrolene were attained in about 1 to 8 h and 1 to 22 h respectively [W. J. Meyler *et al.*, *Eur. J. Clin. Pharmacol.*, 1979, *16*, 203–209].

In 4 subjects receiving daily oral doses of 25 to 50 mg 2 to 4 times a day, plasma-dantrolene concentrations were fairly stable and remained between about 0.03 and 0.1 mg/L; concentrations in an additional 2 subjects fluctuated between about 0.03 and 0.2 mg/L; plasma concentrations of 5-hydroxydantrolene and *p*-acetamidodantrolene ranged from about 0.1 to 0.3 mg/L [J. J. Vallner *et al.*, *Curr. Ther. Res.*, 1979, *25*, 79–91].

Toxicity. Fatalities due to liver damage have been reported.

Half-life. Plasma half-life, dantrolene 4 to 22 h (mean 9), 5-hydroxydantrolene 8 to 29 h (mean 16).

Note. For a review of the pharmacokinetics of dantrolene see R. M. Pinder *et al.*, *Drugs*, 1977, *13*, 3–23.

Dose. Initially 25 mg of dantrolene sodium daily, increased to a maximum of 400 mg daily.

Dantron

Purgative

Synonyms. Antrapurol; Chrysazin; Chryzacin; Danthron; Dianthon; Dioxyanthrachinonum.
Proprietary names. Dorbane; Duolax; Modane; Roydan. It is an ingredient of Dorbanex, Dorbantyl, Doxidan, Normacol X, and Normax.
1,8-Dihydroxy-9,10-anthracenedione
$C_{14}H_8O_4$=240.2
CAS—117-10-2

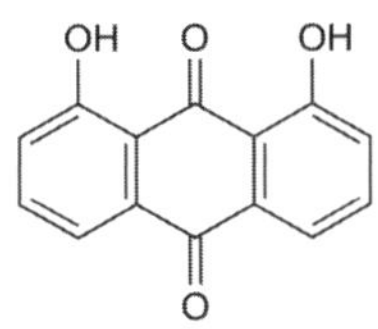

An orange crystalline powder. M.p. 193° to 197°.
Almost insoluble in water; soluble 1 in 2500 of ethanol, 1 in 30 of chloroform, and 1 in 500 of ether; very slightly soluble in aqueous solutions of alkali hydroxides.

Partition Coefficient. Log *P* (octanol/water), 3.9.

Colour Tests. When dissolved in sulfuric acid—red; dilution with water gives a yellow precipitate.

Thin-layer Chromatography. System TD—Rf 80; system TE—Rf 43; system TF—Rf 69; system TAD—Rf 78.

Gas Chromatography. System GA—dantron-Me RI 2435, dantron-Me_2 RI 2475, dantron-AC RI 2460, dantron-AC_2 RI 2595, dantron-TMS RI 2465, dantron-TMS_2 RI 2530; system GB—dantron-TMS RI 2574, dantron-TMS_2 RI 2611.

High Performance Liquid Chromatography. System HY—RI 603.

Ultraviolet Spectrum. Methanol—252 (A^1_1=915a), 283; alkaline methanol—280 nm (A^1_1=510a).

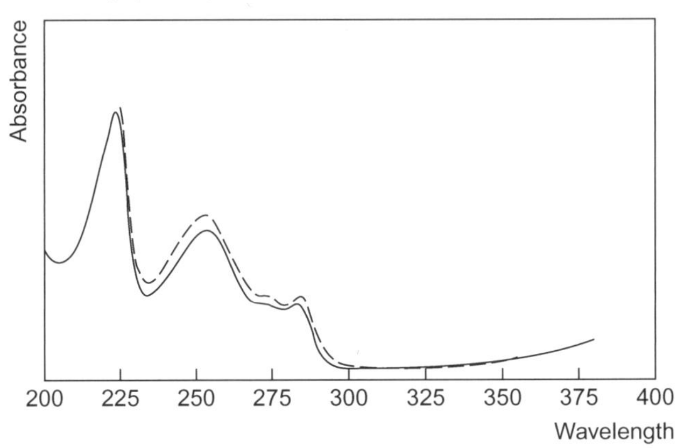

Infra-red Spectrum. Principal peaks at wavenumbers 1264, 740, 1620, 1597, 1152, 1197 cm^{-1} (KBr disk).

Mass Spectrum. Principal ions at *m/z* 240, 212, 241, 184, 138, 92, 128, 63.

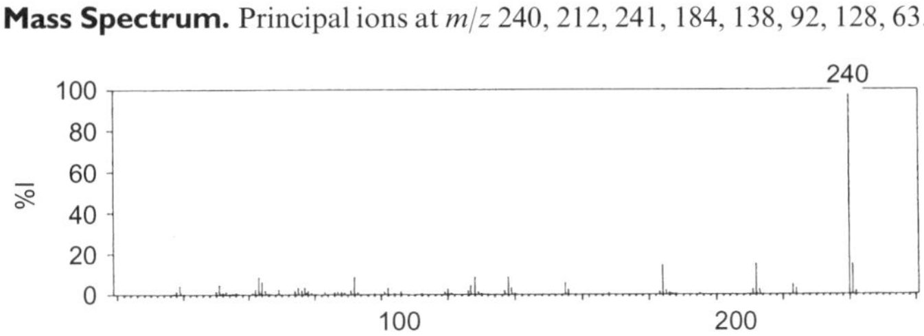

Dose. 50 to 150 mg daily.

Dapsone

Antileprotic

Synonyms. DADPS; DDS; Diaphenylsulfone; Disulone; Sulphonyldianiline.
Proprietary names. Avlosulfon; Cryosulfone; Diphenasone; Disulone; Eporal; Navophone. It is an ingredient of Maloprim.
4,4′-Sulfonylbisbenzeneamine
$C_{12}H_{12}N_2O_2S$=248.3
CAS—80-08-0

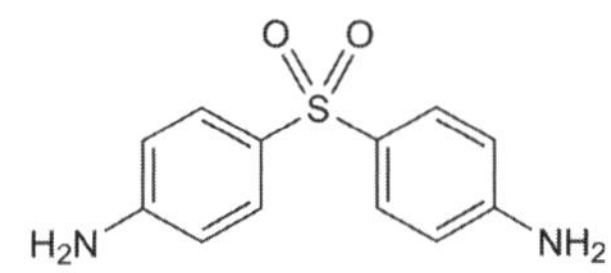

A white or slightly yellowish-white crystalline powder. It discolours on exposure to light but this is not accompanied by significant decomposition. M.p. 175° to 181°.
Soluble 1 in 7000 of water and 1 in about 36 of ethanol; soluble in acetone and dilute mineral acids.

Dissociation Constant. pK_a 1.3, 2.5.

Partition Coefficient. Log *P* (octanol/water), 2.0.

Gas Chromatography. System GA—RI 2880.

High Performance Liquid Chromatography. System HY—RI 298; system HZ—retention time 2.6 min; system HAA—retention time 12.6 min.

Ultraviolet Spectrum. Aqueous acid—288 (A^1_1=350b); aqueous alkali—256, 292 nm.

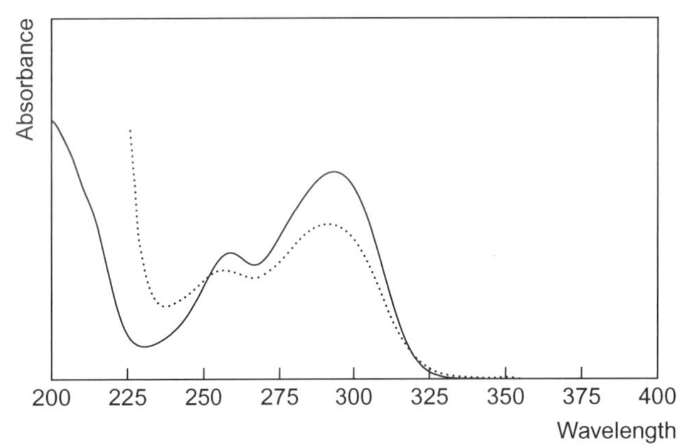

Infra-red Spectrum. Principal peaks at wavenumbers 1150, 1276, 1592, 1107, 685, 1633 cm^{-1} (KBr disk).

Mass Spectrum. Principal ions at *m/z* 108, 248, 140, 65, 92, 141, 109, 80.

Quantification

Gas chromatography. In plasma: dapsone and monoacetyldapsone, ECD—H. P. Burchfield *et al.*, *Anal. Chem.*, 1973, *45*, 916–920.

High performance liquid chromatography. In raw material, dosage forms or biological fluids: detection limit 10 pg using fluorescence detection and 250 pg using UV detection—C. A. Mannan *et al.*, *J. Pharm. Sci.*, 1977, *66*, 1618–1623. In plasma: dapsone and monoacetyldapsone, limit of detection 5 mg/L, UV detection—C. R. Jones and S. M. Ovenell, *J. Chromatogr.* 1979, *163 B Biomed. Appl.*, *5*, 179–185. In serum: dapsone and monoacetyldapsone, limit of detection 200 mg/L, UV detection—J. Zuidema *et al.*, *J. Chromatogr.* 1980, *182 B Biomed. Appl.*, *8*, 130–135. In blood: limit of quantification 20 mg/L for dapsone and 15 mg/L for monoacetyldapsone—A. M. Ronn *et al.*, *Ther. Drug. Monit.*, 1995, *17(1)*, 79–83. In plasma: limit of detection 0.002 mg/L for dapsone and 0.047 mg/L for hydroxylamino-dapsone, UV detection (λ = 295 nm)—S. Kwadijk and J. S. Torano, *Biomed. Chromatogr.*, 2002, *16(3)*, 203–208. In serum and saliva: limit of detection 25 mg/L, UV detection (λ = 295 nm) and 0.2 mg/L, ECD—J. Moncrieff, *J. Chromatogr. B Biomed. Sci. Appl.*, 1994, *654(1)*, 103–110.

Thin-layer chromatography. In plasma or saliva: limit of detection 20 mg/L—R. A. Ahmad and H. J. Rogers, *Eur. J. Clin. Pharmacol.*, 1980, *17*, 129–133.

Disposition in the Body. Slowly and almost completely absorbed after oral administration and widely distributed throughout the body. It is acetylated to monoacetyldapsone, the extent of which is genetically determined. It is also metabolised by *N*-oxidation to mono-*N*-hydroxy-dapsone, together with glucuronic acid and sulfate conjugation of dapsone and the metabolites. Enterohepatic recycling occurs. About 70 to 90% of a dose is excreted in the urine, about 10 to 20% as unchanged drug, about 50% as dapsone conjugates, and about 30% as *N*-oxidation products (mostly conjugated). Small amounts are eliminated in the faeces. About 30 to 50% of a single dose is excreted in the urine within 24 h and more than 70% in 3 days, but there is wide individual variation.

Therapeutic concentration

After a single oral dose of 50 mg to 6 subjects, plasma concentrations of dapsone were 1.02 to 1.44 mg/L (mean 1.24) in 3 slow acetylators, and 1.03 to 1.48 mg/L (mean 1.23) in 3 rapid acetylators, after 4 h. The concentrations of monoacetyldapsone were 0.15 to 0.38 mg/L (mean 0.25) in the slow acetylators and 0.63 to 1.66 mg/L (mean 0.98) in the rapid acetylators, after 4 h. [J. T. Biggs and L. Levy, *Proc. Soc. Exp. Biol. Med.*, 1971, *137*, 692–695.]

Toxicity. Toxic effects are likely to occur at serum concentrations above 10 mg/L.

In 1 case of fatal overdosage, a 22-month-old child died 55 h after ingesting about 5 g of dapsone. The concentrations in the plasma and cerebrospinal fluid were 150 mg/L and 33 mg/L, respectively, 42 h after ingestion. Post-mortem concentrations were: blood 135 mg/L, brain 90 μg/g, liver 165 μg/g, and urine 400 mg/L. [R. Davies, *Lancet*, 1950, *1*, 905–906.]

Half-life. Plasma half-life, 10 to 50 h (mean 24).

Protein binding. In plasma, dapsone 50 to 80%, monoacetyldapsone 98 to 100%.

Dose. 50 to 100 mg daily.

Daunorubicin

Antineoplastic

Synonyms. Daunomycin; Leukaemomycin C; RP-13057; Rubidomycin.
Proprietary name. Cerubidin
(8*S*-*cis*)-8-Acetyl-10-[(3-amino-2,3,6-trideoxy-α-L-*lyxo*-hexopyranosyl)oxy]-7,8,9,10-tetrahydro-6,8,11-trihydroxy-1-methoxy-5,12-naphthacenedione
$C_{27}H_{29}NO_{10} = 527.5$
CAS—20830-81-3

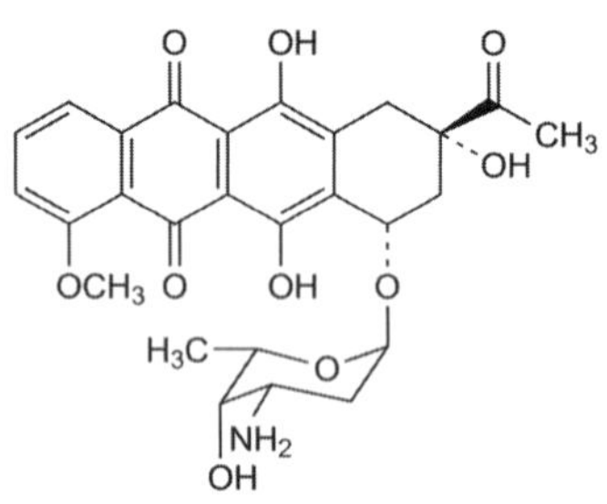

M.p. 208° to 209°.

Daunorubicin Hydrochloride

Proprietary names. Cerubidine; Daunoblastin; Ondena.
$C_{27}H_{29}NO_{10},HCl = 564.0$
CAS—23541-50-6
An orange-red, hygroscopic crystalline powder. Decomposes at 188° to 190°. It is freely soluble in water, methanol and aqueous alcohol; slightly soluble in ethanol; very slightly soluble in chloroform; practically insoluble in acetone, chloroform, ether and benzene.

Daunorubicin Lactate

Proprietary name. Daunoxome
$C_{27}H_{29}NO_{10},C_6H_8O_7 = 719.6$

Dissociation Constant. pK_a 10.3.

Partition Coefficient. Log *P* (octanol/water), 1.83.

High Performance Liquid Chromatography. Column: ODS Hypersil Si-10 (300 × 4 mm i.d., 10 μm film thickness). Mobile phase: methanol with 1% NHOH:methylene chloride (10:90), flow rate 2 mL/min. UV detection (λ = 254 nm). Retention time: 4.0 min. [T. Mills and J. C. Roberson, *Instrumental Data for Drug Analysis*, 1993, CRC Press, Boca Raton, US. 2nd Edn, Vol. 1, pp. 588–589].

Ultraviolet Spectrum. Ethanol—234, 251, 288 nm

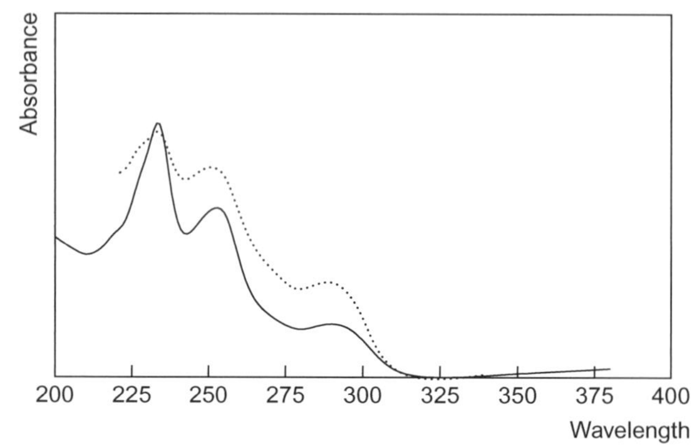

Infra-red Spectrum. Principal peaks at wavenumbers 1703, 1618, 1576, 1407 cm^{-1} (KBr pellets).

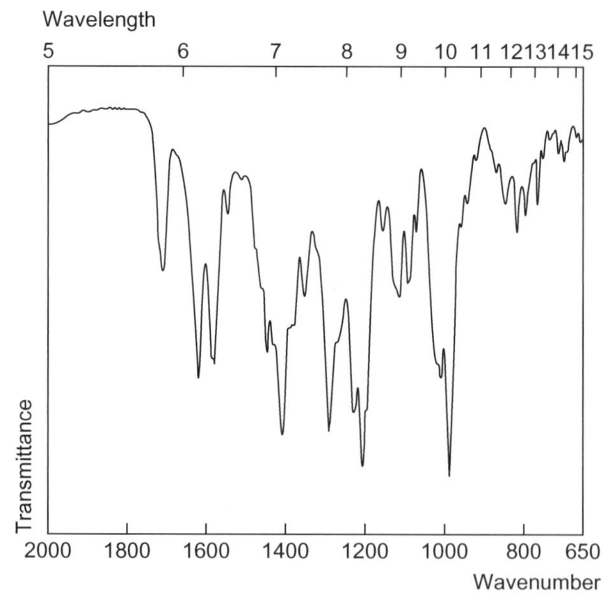

Mass Spectrum. Principal ions at *m*/*z* 43, 398, 337, 72, 309, 95, 362, 217.

Quantification

High performance liquid chromatography. In plasma or tissue: daunorubicin and metabolites, detection range 200 to 900 μg/L in plasma, fluorescence detection—J. de Jong *et al.*, *J. Chromatogr.*, 1990, *529*; *Biomed. Appl.*, *94*, 359–368. In plasma (and other biological fluids): daunorubicin and metabolites, limit of detection < 10 μg/L in plasma, electrochemical detection—C. Akpofure *et al.*, *J. Chromatogr.*, 1982, *232*, 377–383. In plasma: daunorubicin and metabolites, limit of detection 5 μg/L, fluorescence detection—P. Galettis *et al.*, *Br. J. Cancer*, 1994, *70*, 324–329.

Disposition in the Body. Conventional formulations of daunorubicin are rapidly distributed into body tissues following intravenous administration, particularly liver, lungs, kidneys, spleen and heart. It does not cross the blood–brain barrier. It is rapidly metabolised in the liver and excreted in bile (about 40%) and urine as the unchanged drug and metabolites. The major metabolite, daunorubicinol, has antineoplastic activity. A liposomal formulation of daunorubicin is also available that differs in its pharmacokinetic characteristics. Following intravenous administration it remains largely confined within the vascular fluid volume and therefore plasma clearance is higher. The values below apply to the conventional formulation.

Therapeutic concentration

Patients diagnosed with a variety of disseminated solid malignancies with normal renal function, were administered either with an 80 mg/m^2 intravenous dose or with 120 mg/m^2. Plasma concentrations after 15, 30 and 60 min were 400, 290 and 250 µg/L, respectively, for the 80 mg/m^2 dose and 650, 400 and 320 µg/L for the 120 mg/m^2 dose. [D. S. Alberts *et al.*, *Clin. Pharmacol. Ther.*, 1971, *12*, 96–104].

Toxicity. Cardiotoxicity, both acute and chronic, is the main major dose-limiting adverse effect. It is more likely to occur if the total cumulative dose exceeds 550 mg/m^2 in adults or 300 mg/m^2 in children.

Daunorubicin concentrations were measured at autopsy in 2 subjects who died 16 and 19 h after receiving doses of 120 mg/m^2 and 140 mg/m^2, respectively. The following concentrations of the two doses in different organs were: 18.4 and 38 µg/g (kidney), 10.0 and 13.0 µg/g (spleen), 8.3 and 12.0 µg/g (liver), 6.5 and 10.0 µg/g (lung), 4.4 and 6.5 µg/g (heart), 4.0 and 7.3 µg/g (ileum). [D. S. Alberts *et al.*, *Clin. Pharmacol. Ther.*, 1971, *12*, 96–104].

Half-life. Plasma, daunorubicin, 18.5 h; daunorubicinol, 26.7 h.

Volume of distribution. Approx. 1000 L; 1055 L or 619 L/m^2 (80 mg/m^2); 897 L or 511 L/m^2 (120 mg/m^2).

Clearance. Plasma clearance, 230 mL/min.

Dose. Usually up to 45 mg/m^2 body surface intravenously daily to a maximum cumulative dose of 550 mg/m^2.

Debrisoquine

Antihypertensive

Synonym. Isocaramidine

3,4-Dihydro-2(1*H*)-isoquinolinecarboximidamide

$C_{10}H_{13}N = 175.2$

CAS—1131-64-2

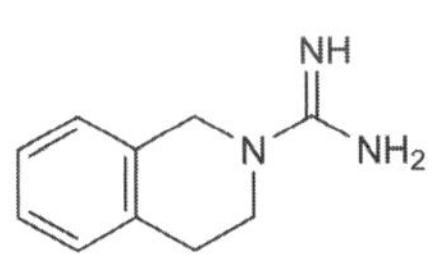

Debrisoquine Sulfate

Proprietary name. Declinax

$(C_{10}H_{13}N_3)_2, H_2SO_4 = 448.5$

CAS—581-88-4

A white crystalline powder. M.p. about 274°, with decomposition.

Soluble 1 in 40 of water; very slightly soluble in ethanol; practically insoluble in chloroform and ether.

Dissociation Constant. pK_a 11.9.

Partition Coefficient. Log *P* (octanol/water), 0.8.

Colour Tests. Mandelin's Test—green; Marquis Test—red-brown.

Thin-layer Chromatography. System TA—Rf 01; system TB—Rf 00; system TC—Rf 00; system TL—Rf 00; system TAJ—Rf 00; system TAK—Rf 03; system TAL—Rf 36. (Acidified iodoplatinate solution, positive.)

Gas Chromatography. System GA—not eluted; system GB—not eluted.

High Performance Liquid Chromatography. System HA—*k* 1.2; system HY—RI 245.

Ultraviolet Spectrum. Aqueous acid—262 (A^1_1=17.7a), 270 nm. No alkaline shift.

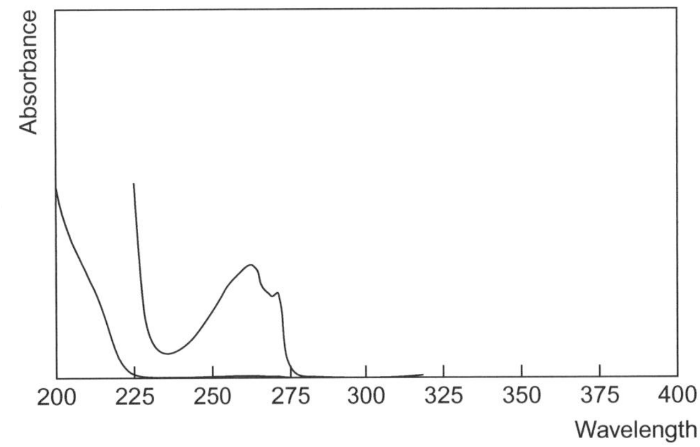

Infra-red Spectrum. Principal peaks at wavenumbers 1614, 1090, 1650, 1583, 750, 715 cm^{-1} (debrisoquine sulfate, KBr disk).

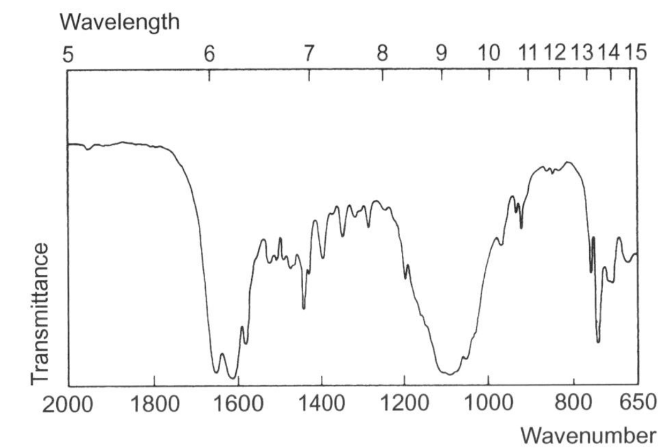

Mass Spectrum. Principal ions at *m/z* 132, 104, 44, 175, 103, 117, 43, 130.

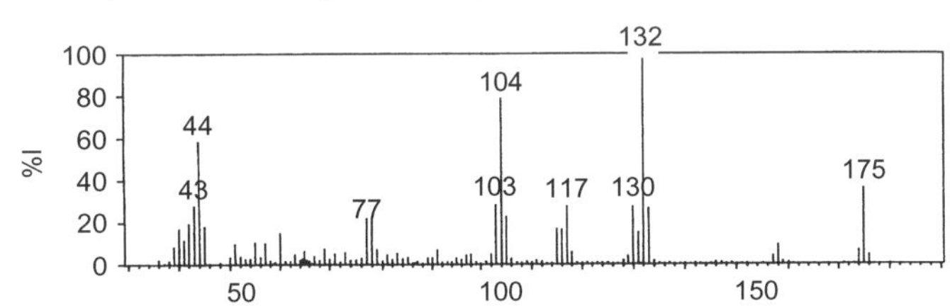

Quantification

Gas chromatography. In blood, plasma, saliva, or urine: debrisoquine and 4-hydroxydebrisoquine, limit of detection 3 µg/L, AFID—M. S. Lennard *et al.*, *J. Chromatogr.*, 1977, *133*, 161–166. In urine: ECD—J. R. Idle *et al.*, *Br. J. Clin. Pharmacol.*, 1979, *7*, 257–266.

Gas chromatography–mass spectrometry. In plasma: limit of detection 1 µg/L for debrisoquine and 5 µg/L for 4-hydroxydebrisoquine—S. L. Malcolm and T. R. Marten, *Anal.Chem.*, 1976, *48*, 807–809.

High performance liquid chromatography. In urine—V. A. Pereira *et al.*, *Braz. J. Med. Biol. Research*, 2000, *33(5)*, 509–514. In urine: limit of detection 30 µg/L for drug and 20 µg/L for metabolite, limit of quantification 50 µg/L, fluorescence detection (λ_{ex}=208 nm; λ_{em}=562 nm)—R. F Frye and R. A. Branch, *J. Chromatogr. B Biomed. Sci. Appl.*, 1996, *677(1)*, 178–182. In urine—A. Bozkurt *et al.*, *J. Pharm. Biomed. Anal.*, 1993, *11(8)*, 745–749.

Disposition in the Body. Rapidly absorbed after oral administration. The main metabolic reaction is 4-hydroxylation; aromatic hydroxylation at positions 5, 6, 7, and 8 also occurs and acidic ring-opened metabolites are also formed. There is no evidence of glucuronic acid conjugation in man. The extent of 4-hydroxylation of debrisoquine is genetically determined. About 75% of a dose is excreted in the urine in 24 h. Excretion of unchanged drug ranges from 8 to 80% of a dose. About 90% of the population are extensive metabolisers of debrisoquine and, in these subjects, about 10 to 40% of a dose is excreted as 4-hydroxydebrisoquine; the remaining 10% are poor metabolisers and excrete less than 2% as the 4-hydroxy metabolite. Acidic ring-opened metabolites account for up to 15% of a dose and the 5-, 6-, 7-, and 8-hydroxy metabolites for about 7%. About 12% of a dose is eliminated in the faeces.

Therapeutic concentration

Following a single oral dose of 20 mg to 3 subjects, peak plasma concentrations of 0.010, 0.013, and 0.024 mg/L of debrisoquine were reported at 1.5 to 3.5 h; peak concentrations of the 4-hydroxy metabolite averaging 0.035 mg/L were attained in 1.5 to 2.5 h. The 4-hydroxy metabolite was eliminated more rapidly than debrisoquine and was not detectable after 24 h. [J. H. Silas *et al.*, *Br. J. Clin. Pharmacol.*, 1978, *5*, 27–34.]

Maximum steady-state plasma concentrations of 0.015 to 0.18 mg/L (mean 0.08), and 0 to 0.05 mg/L (mean 0.02) for debrisoquine and 4-hydroxydebrisoquine respectively, were reported in 13 patients receiving daily oral doses of 40 mg. [J. H. Silas *et al.*, *BMJ*, 1977, *1*, 422–425.]

Half-life. Plasma half-life, debrisoquine about 16 to 30 h, 4-hydroxydebrisoquine about 10 h.

Distribution in blood. Plasma:whole blood ratio, 0.45.

Protein binding. In plasma, about 25%.

Dose. The equivalent of 10 to 120 mg of debrisoquine daily; up to 300 mg or more daily may be given.

Decamethonium Bromide

Muscle Relaxant

Synonym. C-10
Proprietary name. Syncurine
N,N,N,N′,N′,N′-Hexamethyl-1,10-decanediaminium dibromide
$C_{16}H_{38}Br_2N_2$ = 418.3
CAS—156-74-1 (decamethonium); 541-22-0 (bromide)

A white, hygroscopic, crystalline powder. M.p. about 265°, with decomposition.
Freely soluble in water and ethanol; very slightly soluble in chloroform; practically insoluble in ether.

Partition Coefficient. Log *P* (octanol/water), −4.8.

Thin-layer Chromatography. System TA—Rf 00; system TN—Rf 56; system TO—Rf 16. Decamethonium: system TA—Rf 00; system TB—Rf 00; system TC—Rf 00; system TE—Rf 00; system TL—Rf 00; system TAE—Rf 00; system TAF—Rf 02. (Acidified iodoplatinate solution, positive.)

High Performance Liquid Chromatography. System HX—RI 56 (decamethonium).

Ultraviolet Spectrum. Aqueous acid—227 nm (A^1_1 = 584b).

Infra-red Spectrum. Principal peaks at wavenumbers 1627, 910, 965, 1030, 1136, 1063 cm^{-1} (KBr disk).

Dose. Initially 2 to 2.5 mg by IV injection.

Decoquinate

Coccidiostat (Veterinary)

Synonym. M&B 15497
Proprietary name. Deccox
6-Decyloxy-7-ethoxy-4-hydroxy-3-quinolinecarboxylic acid ethyl ester
$C_{24}H_{35}NO_5$ = 417.5
CAS—18507-89-6

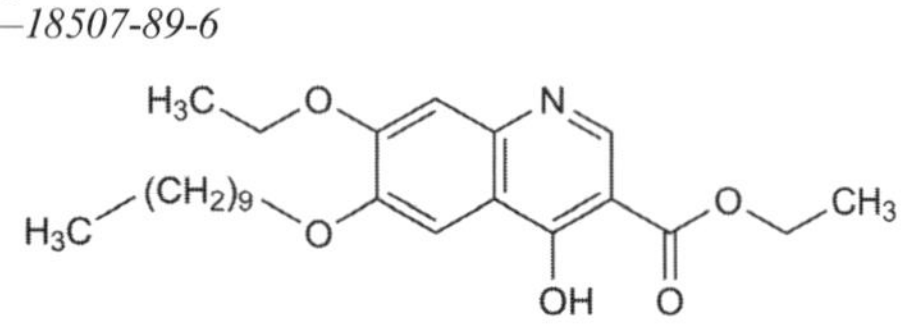

A cream to buff-coloured microcrystalline powder. M.p. about 242°.

Practically insoluble in water and ethanol; slightly soluble in chloroform and ether; soluble in acetone.

Partition Coefficient. Log *P* (octanol/water), 7.8.

Colour Tests. Liebermann's Test—orange (slow); Mandelin's Test—red-brown.

Gas Chromatography. System GA—not eluted.

Ultraviolet Spectrum. Methanolic acid—265 nm (A^1_1 = 1000b).

Infra-red Spectrum. Principal peaks at wavenumbers 1695, 1613, 1497, 1263, 1205, 1558 cm^{-1} (KBr disk).

Deferiprone

Iron Chelator

Synonyms. BRN-1447108; CP20; L1.
Proprietary name. Kelfer
1,2-Dimethyl-3-hydroxypyrid-4-one
$C_7H_9NO_2$ = 139.2
CAS—30652-11-0

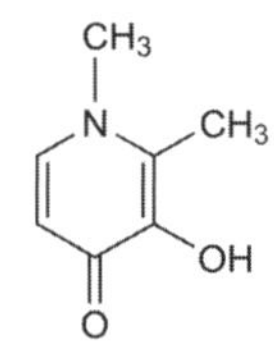

M.p. 271° to 273°. Maximum water solubility of 16 to 18 g/L at 24°.

Dissociation Constant. pK_a 3.5.

Partition Coefficient. Log *P* (octanol/water), −0.77; log *P* (*n*-octanol/Tris HCl, pH 7.4), 0.0009.

High Performance Liquid Chromatography. Column: Hypercarb (Shandon, 100 × 4.7 mm i.d., 7 µm). Mobile phase: disodium phosphate (10 mM) and ethylenediaminetetra-acetate (EDTA) (2 mM), adjusted to pH 3 with 20% phosphoric acid:acetonitrile (88:12), 1.0 mL/min flow rate. UV detection (λ = 280 nm). Retention time: 5.38 min. [J. Klein *et al.*, *Ther. Drug Monit.*, 1991, *13*, 51–54].

Column: Hypercarb-PGC (100 × 4.6 mm i d., 7 µm). Mobile phase: phosphate buffer (10 mM, pH 2.9) containing EDTA (2 mM) and acetonitrile (88:12). UV detection (λ = 275 nm). Retention time: 4 min. [S. Singh *et al.*, *Drug Metab. Dispos.*, 1991, *20*, 256–261].

Ultraviolet Spectrum. Aqueous acid—279 nm.

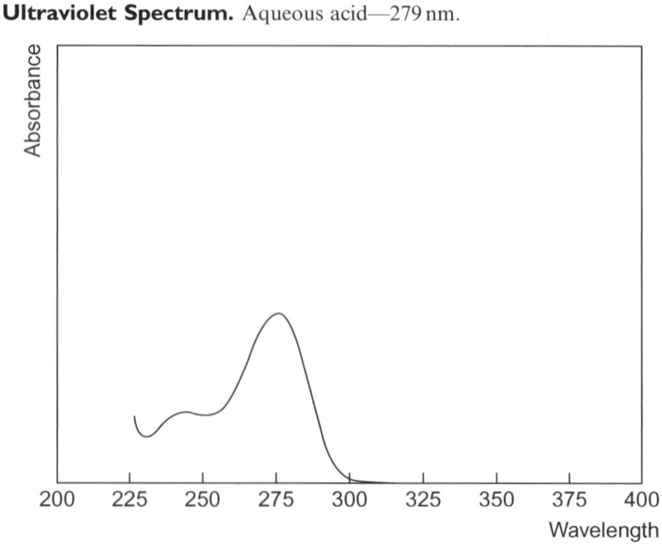

Mass Spectrum. (Deferiprone-*O*-methylated metabolite) Principal ions at *m*/*z* 154, 31, 29, 139, 133, 43, 27.

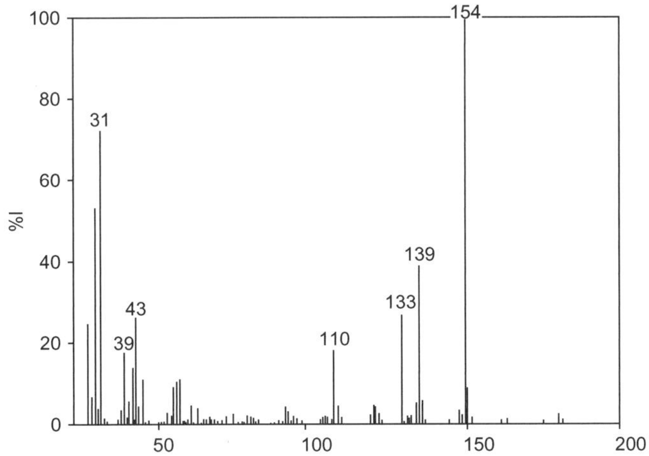

Quantification

High performance liquid chromatography. In urine: limit of detection is 120 mg/L. UV detection (λ=280 nm)—G. J. Kontoghiorghes *et al.*, *Clin. Pharmacol. Ther.*, 1990, *48*, 255–261. In plasma: limit of detection 0.5 mg/L. UV detection (λ=280 nm)—J. Klein *et al.*, *Ther. Drug Monit.*, 1991, *13*, 51–54.

Bioassay. In serum and saliva: limit of detection is 0.5 mg/L—E. Pope *et al.*, *Ther. Drug Monit.*, 1997, *19*, 95–97.

Disposition in the Body. Deferiprone is rapidly absorbed and more than 85% of an administered dose is metabolised in the liver by glucuronidation to a conjugate lacking chelating properties. Deferiprone is excreted mainly in urine (approx. 80% recovered) as the parent drug, its conjugate and bound to iron. Only a small proportion of the drug is found unchanged in urine within 24 h. Excretion of the glucuronide is slower than that of the parent drug. Other metabolites include an *O*-methyl metabolite, 2-hydroxylmethyl metabolite and its glucuronide.

Therapeutic concentration

4 males and 5 females with homozygous β-thalassemia, aged between 11 and 18.5 years, were administered with a mean dose of 75.7 ± 1.73 mg/kg deferiprone daily for 3 to 13 months. A mean peak plasma concentration of 11.3 mg/L was reached within 1 h. [E. Pope *et al.*, *Ther. Drug Monit.*, 1997, *19*, 95–97].

Half-life. 1 to 2.5 h.

Volume of distribution. Steady state, 1.55 to 1.73 L/kg; healthy volunteers, 72.8 L/kg; patients with β-thalassemia, 115.1 L/kg.

Clearance. Healthy volunteers, 34.8 L/h; patients with β-thalassemia, 39.6 L/h.

Protein binding. 24.8 to 42.6% depending on dose administered.

Dose. A usual dose of 25 mg/kg is administered three times a day, with a maximum of 100 mg/kg daily.

Deflazacort

Anti-inflammatory

Synonyms. L5458; DL-458-IT; MDL-458.
Proprietary names. Azacort; Calcort; Deflan; Dezacor; Flantadin; Lantadin: Oxazacort; Zamane.
(11*β*,16*β*)-21-(Acetyloxy)-11-hydroxy-2′-methyl-5′*H*-pregna-1,4-dieno [17,16-*d*]oxazole-3,20-dione
$C_{25}H_{31}NO_6$ = 441.5
CAS—14484-47-0

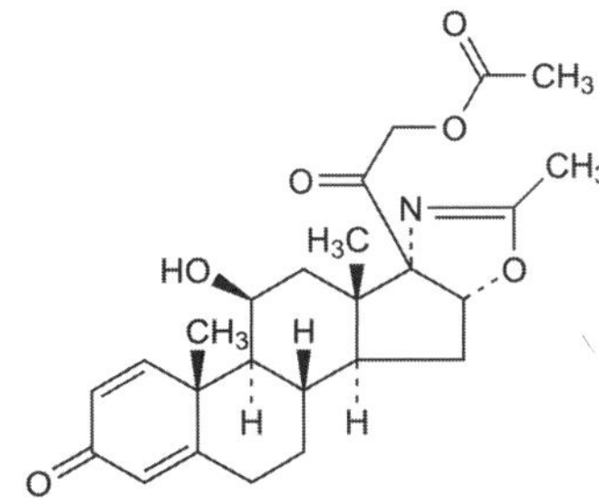

White crystals (acetone:hexane). M.p. 255° to 256.5°.

Partition Coefficient. Log *P* (octanol/water), 1.31.

High Performance Liquid Chromatography. Column: 5-ODS (Hypersil, 200 × 4.6 mm i.d., 5 μm at 30°, or Spherisorb, 150 × 4.6 mm i.d., 5 μm at 20°). Mobile phase: water:tetrahydrofuran (77:23) 1.0 mL/min flow rate (Hypersil) or (80:20) 1.2 mL/min flow rate (Spherisorb). UV detection (λ=245 nm). *k* values: deflazacort, 15.5 (Hypersil), 13.8 (Spherisorb); 21-hydroxydeflazacort, 4.6, 3.8. [A. Santos-Montes *et al.*, *J. Chromatogr.* 1994, *657*, *Biomed. Appl.*, 248–253].

Column: ODS (Hypersil, 250 × 4.6 mm i. d., 5 μm) with μBondapak C_{18} guard at 40°. Mobile phase: isopropanol:acetate buffer (solvent A, 0.05 M, pH 4.5) (10:90). Solvent A composition decreased from 90% to 30% for 25 min and held for 5 min, increased to 90% for 5 min and held for 15 min. Retention time: 21-hydroxydeflazacort, 6.1 min; deflazacort-6-β-hydroxide, 28.3 min. [H. Hitara *et al.*, *J. Chromatogr.* 1994, *658*; *Biomed. Appl.*, 55–61].

Ultraviolet Spectrum. Methanol—242 nm.

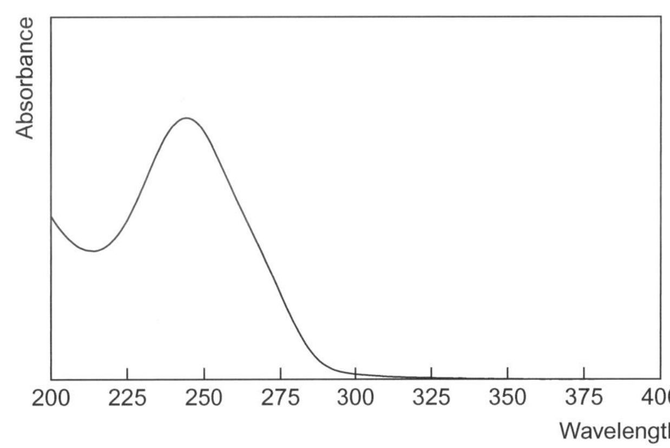

Quantification

High performance liquid chromatography. In plasma: detection range 1.0 to 500 μg/L for metabolite, 21-desacetyldeflazacort, UV detection—N. Rao *et al.*, *Biopharm. Drug Dispos.*, 1996, *17*, 753–760. In urine: limit of detection 0.4 μg/L, UV detection (λ=245 nm)—A. Santos-Montes *et al.*, *J. Chromatogr.* 1994, *657*, *Biomed. Appl.*, 248–253.

Disposition in the Body. Deflazacort is well absorbed from the gastrointestinal tract and is immediately converted by plasma esterases to its active metabolite, 21-desacetyldeflazacort with further metabolism to deflazacort-6-β-hydroxide. Elimination is mainly via the kidneys, with 70% of the administrated dose recovered in the urine and the remaining 30% in faeces.

Therapeutic concentration

23 healthy males, approx. 25 years old, were orally administered with 3, 6 and 36 mg doses of deflazacort (tablets and aqueous suspensions). Peak plasma concentrations of active metabolite, 21-desacetyldeflazacort, were 10.4 ± 5.0, 19.8 ± 7.5, 132.6 ± 52.5 μg/L, respectively, and were reached within 1.5 to 2 h. [N. Rao *et al.*, *Biopharm. Drug Dispos.*, 1996, *17*, 753–760].

Bioavailability. Approx. 68%.

Half-life. 1.9 to 2.3 h.

Volume of distribution. Deflazacort-6-β-hydroxide, 83 L.

Clearance. 83.9 ± 24.5 (36 mg dose) to 97.1 ± 47.7 L/h (3 mg dose).

Protein binding. 40% plasma protein binding.

Note. For a review of pharmacokinetics data see N. Rao *et al.*, *Biopharm. Drug Dispos.*, 1996, *17*, 753–760.

Dose. By oral administration, initial dose up to 120 mg/kg body weight and a usual maintenance dose of 3 to 18 mg/kg. Between 0.25 and 1.5 mg/kg body weight for children.

Dehydroemetine

Antiprotozoal

2,3-Didehydro-6′,7′,10,11-tetramethoxyemetan
$C_{29}H_{38}N_2O_4$=478.6
CAS—4914-30-1

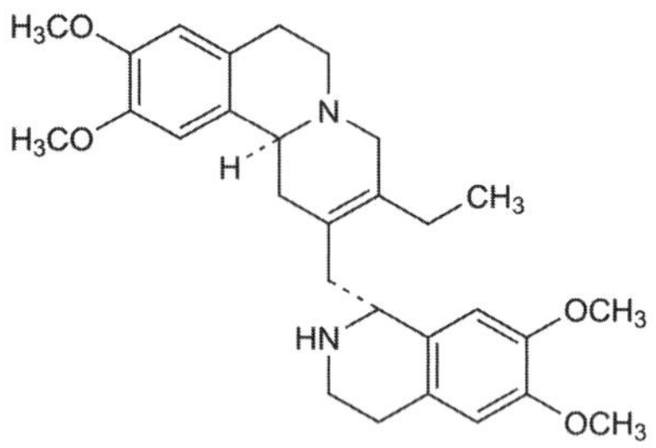

Dehydroemetine Hydrochloride
Proprietary name. Dametine
$C_{29}H_{38}N_2O_4$,2HCl=551.6
CAS—2228-39-9
A white crystalline powder.
Soluble 1 in 30 of water.

Partition Coefficient. Log *P* (octanol/water), 5.2.

Colour Test. Marquis Test—orange.

Thin-layer Chromatography. System TA—Rf 43; system TB—Rf 06; system TC—Rf 21; system TL—Rf 02. (Acidified iodoplatinate solution, positive.)

Ultraviolet Spectrum. Aqueous acid—230 nm (A_1^1=290a), 283 nm.

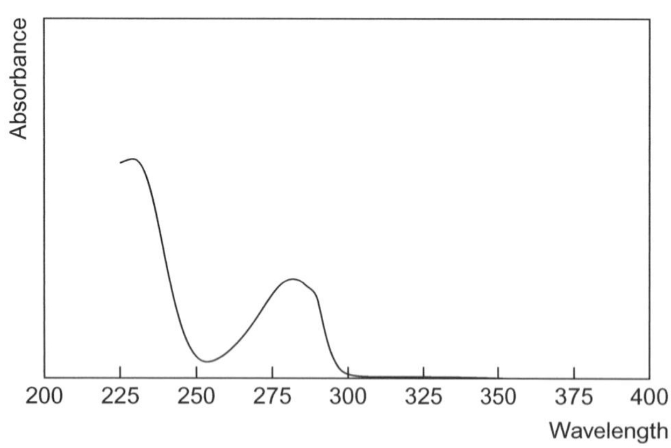

Infra-red Spectrum. Principal peaks at wavenumbers 1121, 1222, 1508, 1252, 1205, 1022 cm^{-1} (dehydroemetine hydrochloride, KBr disk).

Mass Spectrum. Principal ions at *m/z* 192, 193, 287, 176, 191, 286, 270, 285.

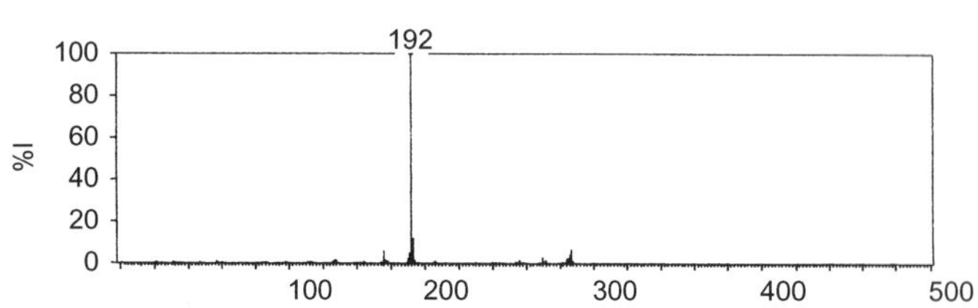

Dose. 60 to 180 mg of dehydroemetine hydrochloride daily, intramuscularly.

Dehydroepiandrosterone

Endogenous Steroid

Synonyms. Dehydroisoandrosterone; DHEA; Prasterone.
Proprietary names. Astenile; Deandros; Diandrone; Psicosterone.
3(*β*)-3-Hydroxyandrost-5-en-17-one
$C_{19}H_{28}O_2$=288.4
CAS—53-43-0

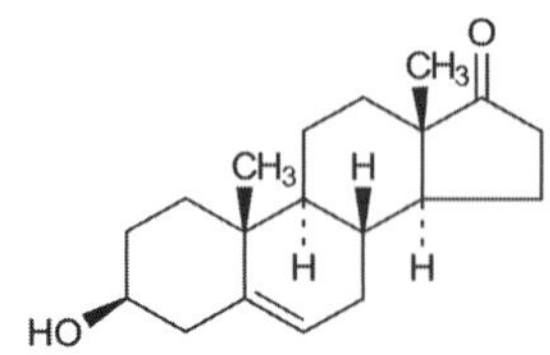

Dimorphous needles with M.p. 140° to 141° or leaflets with M.p. 152° to 153°.
Soluble in water (solubility is 63.45 mg/L at 25°), benzene, alcohol, and ether; sparingly soluble in chloroform and petroleum ether.

Dehydroepiandrosterone sodium sulfate
Synonyms. DHA-S Sodium; DHEAS; Sodium Dehydroepiandrosterone Sulfate; Prasterone Sodium Sulfate.
Proprietary name. Mylis
$C_{19}H_{27}NaO_5S$=390.5
CAS—1099-87-2
A white crystalline powder with M. p. 154°.
Soluble in methanol; slightly soluble in water and absolute ethanol; practically insoluble in acetone, chloroform, and benzene.

Dehydroepiandrosterone Sodium Sulfate Dihydrate
$C_{19}H_{27}NaO_5S,2H_2O$=426.6

Dehydroepiandrosterone Sulfate
Synonyms. DHA-S; Dehydroepiandrosterone Sulfate; Prasterone Sulfate.
$C_{19}H_{28}O_5S$=368.5
CAS—651-48-9

Dehydroepiandrosterone Enantate
Synonyms. Dehydroepiandrosterone Heptanoate; Prasterone Enanthate; Prasterone Heptanoate.
$C_{26}H_{40}O_3$=400.6
CAS—23983-43-9

Partition Coefficient. Log *P* (octanol/water), 3.23.

Thin-layer Chromatography. Plate: silica gel G-Merck (20 × 20 cm). Mobile phase: hexane:ether:acetic acid (1:9:0.1). Developed with colour developing reagents. Rf 0.60. [R. F. Frye *et al.*, *J. Clin. Pharmacol.*, 2000, *40*, 596–605.]

Gas Chromatography. System GA—DHEA RI 2530, DHEA-H_2O RI 2595, DHEA enol-TMS_2 RI 2580; system GAR—DHEA retention time 11.8 min.

Column: 5% phenyl–95% methylsiloxane (30 m × 0.25 mm i.d., 0.25 μm film thickness). Column temperature: 150°, held for 1 min, 30°/min to 295°, held for 8 min. Injector temperature: 270°. Splitless injection. Carrier gas: helium, flow rate 1.0 mL/min. MS detection (EI). Internal standard: testosterone-d_3. Retention time: dehydroepiandrosterone, 7.0 min; testosterone, 7.4 min. [P. Kintz *et al.*, *J. Anal. Toxicol.*, 1999, *23*, 424–428.]

Column: methyl silicone (HP1, 0.2 mm i.d., 0.33 μm film thickness). Column temperature: 280°. Carrier gas: helium, flow rate 0.9 mL/min. MS detection. RI: 2588. [T. Mills and J. C. Roberson, *Instrumental data for drug analysis*, 2nd Edn., CRC Press, Boca Raton, FL, Vol. 5, 1993, pp. 340–341.]

High Performance Liquid Chromatography. System HATb—RRT 1.13 (relative to testosterone).

Column: 5C_4 (Wakosil, 300 × 4.0 mm i.d.). Mobile phase: acetonitrile:water (7:3), flow rate 0.8 mL/min. Fluorescence detection (λ_{ex}=495 nm, λ_{em}=516 nm). Retention time: 7.7 min. [M. Katayama *et al.*, *Analyst*, 1998, *123*, 2339–2342.]

Column: ODS Hypersil (100 × 4.6 mm i.d., 5 μm). Mobile phase: methanol:aqueous 0.01 M dihydrogen potassium phosphate buffer, adjusted to pH 3.5 with 85% phosphoric acid (90:10), flow rate 1 mL/min. UV diode array detection. Retention time: 2.4 min. [T. Mills and J. C. Roberson, *Instrumental data for drug analysis*, 2nd Edn., CRC Press, Boca Raton, FL, Vol. 5, 1993, pp. 340–341.]

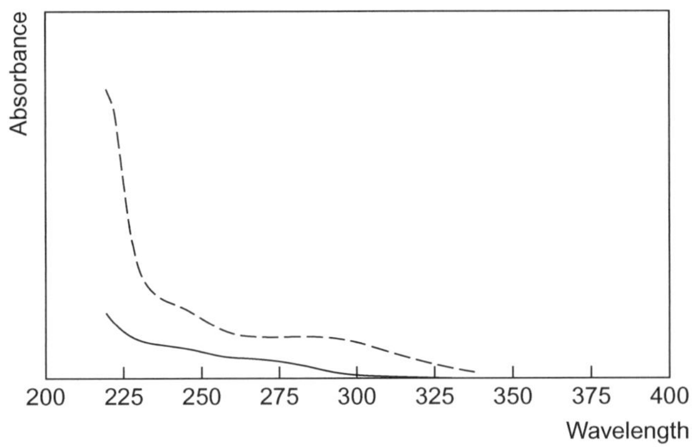

Infra-red Spectrum. Principal peak at wavenumbers 1725, 1372, 1062 cm^{-1} (KBr disks).

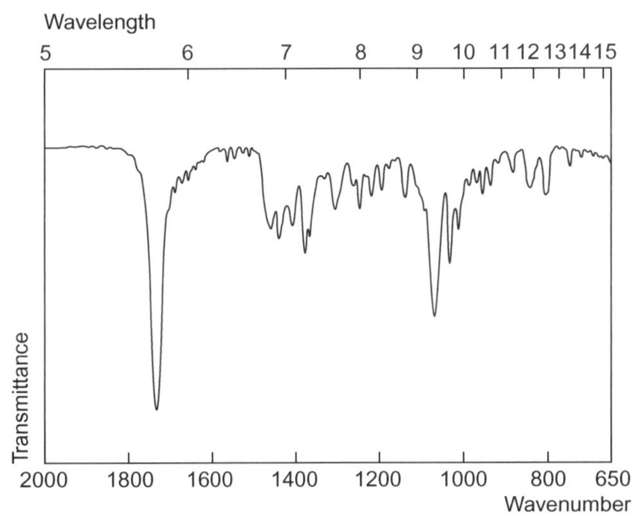

Mass Spectrum. Principal ions at *m/z* 288, 91, 107, 105, 255, 79, 203, 93.

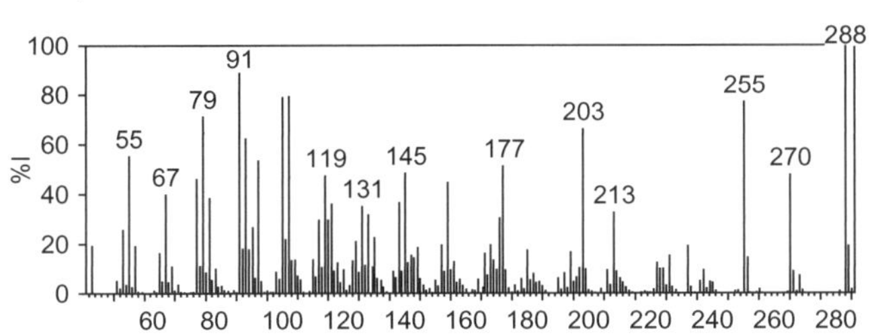

Quantification

Gas chromatography–mass spectrometry. In hair: limit of detection 0.5 ng/g—P. Kintz *et al., J. Anal. Toxicol.*, 1999, *23*, 424–428. In hair: limit of detection 0.02 ng/g—M. H. Choi and B. C. Chung, *Analyst*, 1999, *124*, 1297–1301.

High performance liquid chromatography. In serum: limit of detection 1.2 pg/L—M. Katayama *et al., Analyst*, 1998, *123*, 2339–2342. In plasma: limit of detection 3 μg/L and limit of quantification 10 μg/L—A. Marwah *et al., J. Chromatogr. B Biomed. Sci. Appl.*, 1999, *721*, 197–205.

Disposition in the Body. Both DHEA and DHEA-S are widely distributed throughout the body. DHEA is metabolised to androsterone and etiocholanolone, the most abundant metabolites found in urine after a single oral dose. Other metabolites include androstenedione, product from 3β-hydrosteroid dehydrogenase (HD), and testosterone (17β-HD). Men and women metabolise DHEA and DHEA-S differently, which may result in varying concentrations of other androgenic and estrogenic steroids being detected in the body.

Therapeutic concentration

6 healthy men and 7 women were administered with a 200 mg single dose of dehydroepiandrosterone and multiple doses. Men: peak plasma concentrations of 22.4 ± 1.6 μg/L DHEA, 7015 ± 625 μg/L DHEA-S were reached within 1.3 ± 0.6 h and 3.3 ± 1.8 h, respectively. Women: peak plasma concentrations of 27.2 ± 2.9 μg/L DHEA and 7467 ± 645 μg/L DHEA-S were seen 1.4 ± 0.7 and 2.1 ± 0.7 h after administration. After multiple dosing, peak plasma concentrations and time to peak remained relatively constant. [R. F. Frye *et al., J. Clin. Pharmacol.*, 2000, *40*, 596–605.]

Toxicity. Dehydroepiandrosterone sodium sulfate and its dihydrate both have low toxicity at 4 mg/kg with gastro-intestinal and skin effects, for example, rashes and haemorrhages. It is moderately toxic by intraperitoneal and subcutaneous routes, and can be a poison by the intravenous route.

Half-life. DHEA: (men) 6 to 7.5 h, (women) 7 to 11.5 h; DHEA-S: (men and women) 20 to 27 h.

Dose. 25 to 50 mg daily is generally recommended as a supplementation dose for a normal population, but body builders are recommended up to 1000 mg daily by some suppliers.

Delavirdine

Antiviral

Synonym. U-90152

1-[3-[(1-Methylethyl)amino]-2-pyridinyl]-4-[[5-[(methylsulfonyl)amino]-1*H*-indol-2-yl]carbonyl]piperazine

$C_{22}H_{28}N_6O_3S = 456.6$

CAS—136817-59-9

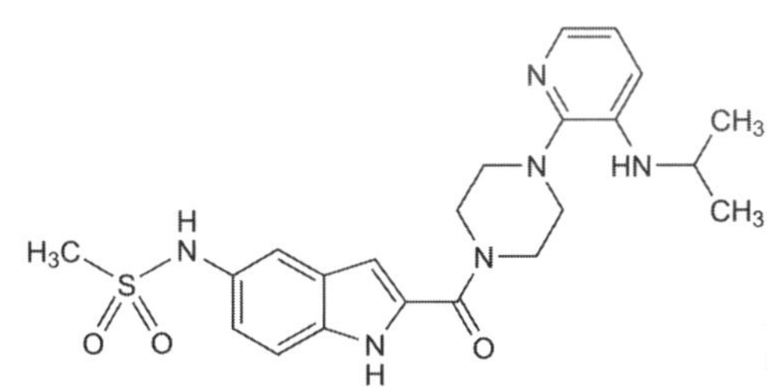

Crystals from ethyl acetate and hexane. M.p. 226° to 228°.

Delavirdine monomethanesulfonate

Synonyms. Delavirdine mesylate; U-90152S.

Proprietary name. Rescriptor

$C_{22}H_{28}N_6O_3S.CH_4O_3S = 552.7$

CAS—147221-93-0

Dissociation Constant. pK_a 4.5.

High Performance Liquid Chromatography. System HAE—retention time 6.3 min.

Column: (analytical) cyano (DuPont Zorbax SB CN); (guard) cyano (Brownlee CN). Mobile phase: potassium dihydrogen phosphate (10 mM, pH 6):acetonitrile (67:33). Fluorescence detection (λ_{ex} = 295 nm, λ_{em} = 418 nm). Retention time: delavirdine, 7.9 min; desalkyl delavirdine, 2.7 min. [M. T. Borin *et al., Antimicrob. Agents Chemother.*, 1997, *41(9)*, 1892–1897].

Column: (analytical) Zorbax SB C_{18} (75 × 4.6 mm, 3.5 μm); (guard) Chromguard C_{18} (10 × 3 mm). Mobile phase: citrate buffer (25 mM):acetonitrile (82:18), adjusted to pH 2.7 with 2 M hydrochloric acid. 1.5 mL/min flow rate. Fluorescence detection (λ_{ex} = 300 nm, λ_{em} = 425 nm). Retention time: 19.2 min. [A. L. Veldkamp *et al., J. Chromatogr. Biomed. Sci. Appl.*, 1999, *727(1-2)*, 151–157].

Quantification

High performance liquid chromatography. In plasma: limit of quantification is 75 μg/L. UV detection (λ = 260 nm)—V. Proust *et al., J. Chromatogr.*

Biomed. Sci. Appl., 2000, *742*, 453–458. In plasma: limit of quantification 50 µg/L and limit of detection 10 µg/L, fluorescence detection (λ_{ex}=300 nm, λ_{em}=425 nm)—A. L. Veldkamp *et al.*, *J. Chromatogr. Biomed. Sci. Appl.*, 1999, *727(1-2)*, 151–157. In serum: limit of detection is 110 µg/L. UV detection—V. A. Simon *et al.*, *J. Chromatogr. A*, 2001, *913(1-2)*, 447–453.

Disposition in the Body. Delavirdine is rapidly absorbed after oral administration and is extensively metabolised in the liver by the cytochrome P450 3A isoenzymes. Absorption is at least 45%. It is excreted as the metabolites in urine and faeces with <5% as the unchanged drug in urine.

Therapeutic concentration

13 HIV (human immunodeficiency virus)-positive volunteers, with a mean CD4 count of 260 cells/mm^3 (range 192 to 402 cells/mm^3) and mean age of 39 years (range 24 to 50 years) were administered 300 mg delavirdine mesylate orally every 8 h for 30 days, 2 h after or 1 h before meals. Steady state concentrations were observed by day 11 and averaged 19 µg/L for delavirdine and 2.6 µg/L for desalkyl delavirdine. For the parent drug, peak plasma concentrations reached 31 (22 to 44) µg/L on day 15, 26 (20 to 36) µg/L on day 16 and 28 (18 to 40) µg/L on day 30. These concentrations were observed at 1.0 (1.0 to 1.5), 2.0 (0.75 to 2.5) and 0.75 to 1.0 h, respectively. For desalkyl delavirdine, peak concentrations were 3.2 (2.9 to 4.2), 2.8 (2.3 to 4.0) and 2.8 (2.5 to 4.5) µg/L for days 15, 16 and 30 observed at approx. 2.5 h (0.75 to 6.0 h). [M. T. Borin *et al.*, *Antimicrob. Agents Chemother.*, 1997, *41(9)*, 1892–1897].

Half-life. 2 to 11 h.

Protein binding. 98%.

Dose. The usual dose is 400 mg three times daily.

Deltamethrin

Ectoparasiticide, Insecticide

Synonyms. Decamethrin; Deltamethrine; Esbecythrin; FMC-45498; NRDC-161; OMS 1998; RU-22974.
Proprietary names. Butofin; Butoss; Butox; Cislin; Crackdown; Cresus; Decis; Decis-Prime; Delsekte; Hunter; K-Othrin; K-Otek.
(*S*)-α-Cyano-3-phenoxybenzyl-(1*R*)-*cis*-3-(2,2-dibromovinyl)-2,2-dimethylcyclopropanecarboxylate
$C_{22}H_{19}Br_2NO_3$=505.2
CAS—52918-63-5

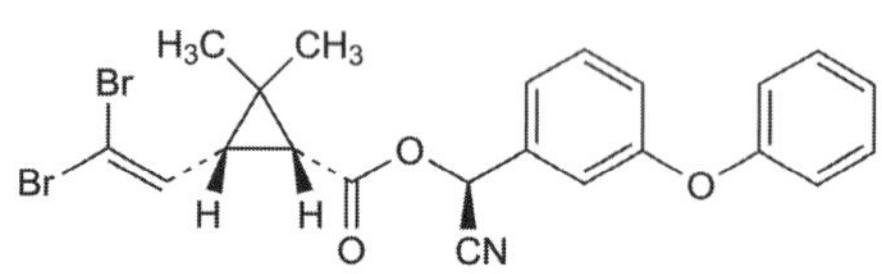

A colourless, crystalline powder or white/slightly beige powder. M.p. 98° to 101°.
It is soluble in kerosene and isoalkanes (<0.5 g/100 g at 20°), isopropanol (<0.6 g/100 g at 20°), ethanol (1.5 g/100 g at 20°), xylene (25 g/100 g at 20°), methylene chloride (70 g/100 g at 20°), toluene (250 g/L at room temperature), acetone (500 g/L at room temperature), benzene and dimethyl sulfoxide (450 g/L at room temperature), cyclohexane (750 g/L at room temperature), and dioxane (900 g/L at room temperature); practically insoluble in water (2 µg/L at 20°).

Partition Coefficient. Log *P* (octanol/water), 4.6 (25°).

Thin-layer Chromatography. System TX—Rf 40; system TY—Rf 90; system TZ—Rf 95; system TAA—Rf 72.

Plate: silica gel G (0.25 mm thickness). Mobile phase: cyclohexane:toluene (6:4). Developed by spraying with 20% sodium hydroxide solution, 1% copper (II) acetate solution, and 1% phosphomolybdic acid solution, and 0.1% *o*-toluidine reagent 5 min later. Rf 0.31. [V. B. Patil *et al.*, *Analyst*, 1992, *17*, 75–76.]

Gas Chromatography. System GA—deltamethrin RI 2900, M (COOH-)-Me RI 1540, M (desacyl-)-HCN RI 1700, M (desacyl-)-Me RI 2590; system GKD—retention time 5.8 min.

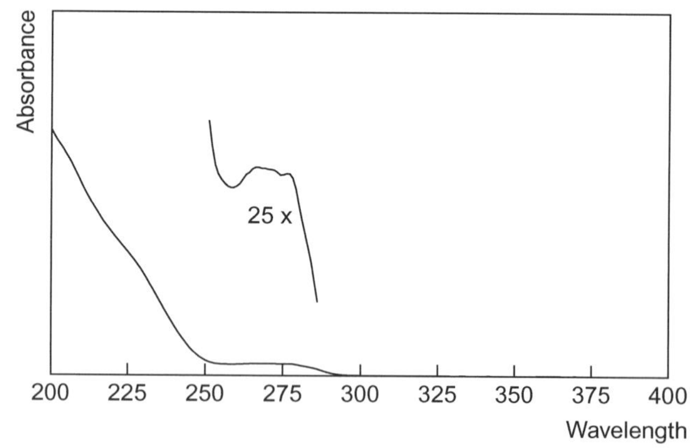

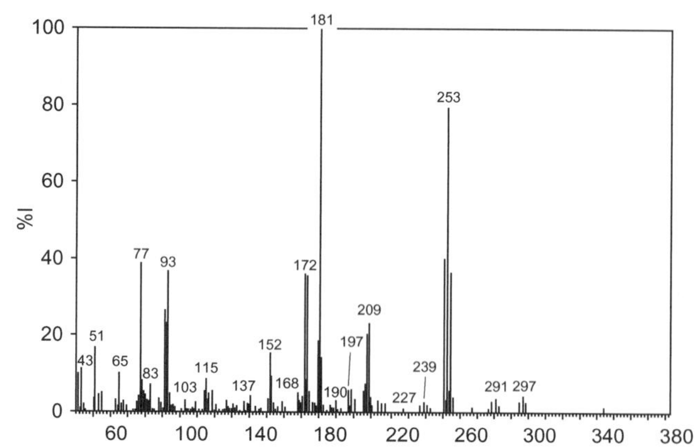

Quantification

Gas chromatography. In urine: limit of detection of deltamethrin 200 mg/L—Y-Q. Wu *et al.*, *Biomed. Env. Sci.*, 1994, *7(3)*, 216–221. In plasma and urine: limit of detection 2 mg/L—L. Junting and F. Chuichang, *Forensic Sci. Int.*, 1991, *51*, 89–93.

Gas chromatography–mass spectrometry. In urine: limit of detection 0.2 µg/L—K-H. Kuhn *et al.*, *Chromatographia*, 1996, *43(5/6)*, 285. In urine: limit of detection for the metabolites 0.3 to 0.5 µg/L—J. Angerer and A. Ritter, *J. Chromatogr. B Biomed. Sci. Appl.*, 1997, *695*, 217–226.

Disposition in the Body. Deltamethrin is hydrolysed by liver microsomal enzymes to three metabolites: 3-(2,2-dibromovinyl)-2,2-cyclopropane carboxylic acid, 3-phenoxy-benzylhydroxy-ethyl acetate, and 3-phenoxylbenzoic acid. All three metabolites have been detected in urine.

Toxicity. There have been many cases of dermal deltamethrin poisoning due to inadequate handling of the chemical during agricultural use. Cases of accidental and suicidal poisoning have also been observed with oral doses between 2 and 250 mg/kg. A dose of 100 to 250 mg/kg can result in coma, even though short-lived (15 to 20 min). The allowed daily intake is 0.01 mg/kg.

Demecarium Bromide

Anticholinesterase

Synonym. BC-4
Proprietary names. Humorsol; Tosmilen(e).
3,3′-[1,10-Decanediylbis[(methylimino)carbonyloxy]]bis[*N*,*N*,*N*-trimethylbenzeneaminium]dibromide
$C_{32}H_{52}Br_2N_4O_4$=716.6
CAS—56-94-0

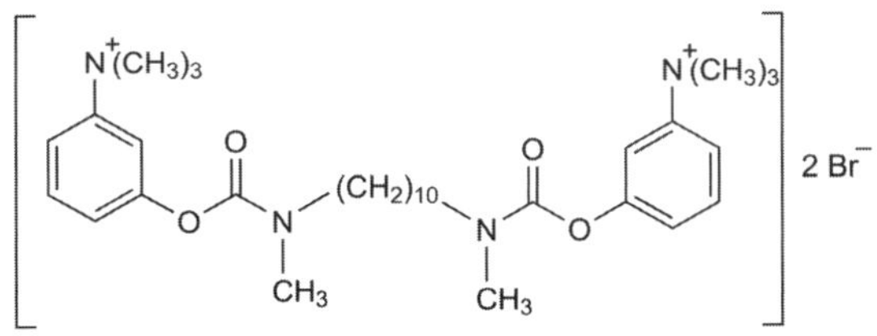

A white or slightly yellow, slightly hygroscopic, crystalline powder. M.p. 162° to 167°, with decomposition.
Freely soluble in water and ethanol; sparingly soluble in acetone; insoluble in ether.

Partition Coefficient. Log *P* (octanol/water), −1.8.

Thin-layer Chromatography. System TA—Rf 00. (Acidified iodoplatinate solution, positive.)

Ultraviolet Spectrum. Aqueous acid—259 nm (A^1_1=14b), 265 nm. No alkaline shift.

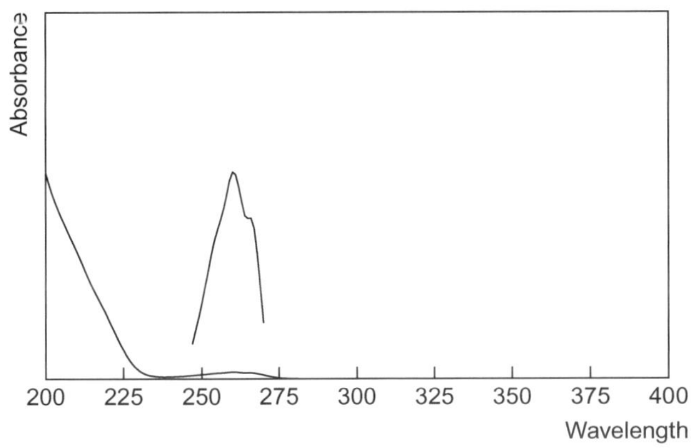

Infra-red Spectrum. Principal peaks at wavenumbers 1724, 1216, 1149, 1178, 1124, 943 cm^{-1} (KBr disk).

Use. As a 0.25 to 0.5% ophthalmic solution.

Demeclocycline

Antibacterial

Synonyms. Demethylchlortetracycline; DMCT; RP-10192.
Proprietary name. Ledermycin (drops and syrup)
[4*S*-(4α,4aα,5aα,6β,12aα)]-7-Chloro-4-(dimethylamino)-1,4,4a,5,5a,6,11,12a-octahydro-3,6,10,12,12a-pentahydroxy-1,11-dioxo-2-naphthacenecarboxamide
$C_{21}H_{21}ClN_2O_8$=464.9
CAS—127-33-3

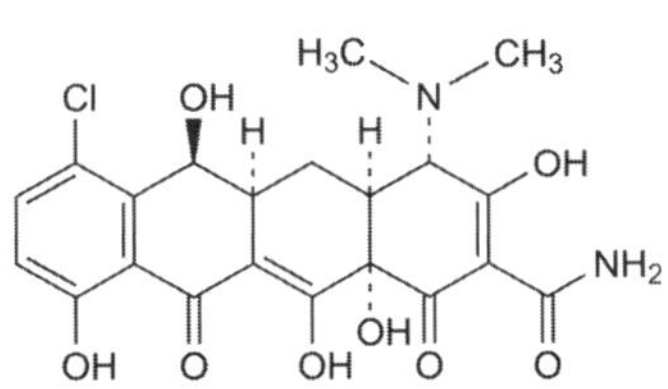

A yellow crystalline powder.
Sparingly soluble in water; soluble 1 in 200 of ethanol and 1 in 40 of methanol; soluble in dilute hydrochloric acid and in solutions of alkali hydroxides and carbonates.

Demeclocycline Hydrochloride

Proprietary names. Declomycin; Ledermycin(e) (capsules and tablets). It is an ingredient of Declostatin and Deteclo.
$C_{21}H_{21}ClN_2O_8,HCl$=501.3
CAS—64-73-3
A yellow, amphoteric, crystalline powder.
Soluble 1 in 30 to 1 in 60 of water, 1 in 45 to 1 in 200 of ethanol and 1 in 50 of methanol; practically insoluble in chloroform and ether; soluble in aqueous solutions of alkali hydroxides and carbonates.

Dissociation Constant. pK_a 3.3, 7.2, 9.3 (25°).

Partition Coefficient. Log *P* (octanol/pH 7.5), −1.3.

Colour Tests. Benedict's Reagent—red; Formaldehyde–Sulfuric Acid—orange→brown-red; Mandelin's Test—violet-brown; Marquis Test—yellow→green; Nessler's Reagent—brown; Sulfuric Acid—brown-blue.

Thin-layer Chromatography. System TA—Rf 05, streaking; system TAJ—Rf 00; system TAK—Rf 00; system TAL—Rf 04. (Location under ultraviolet light, orange fluorescence; acidified potassium permanganate solution, positive.)

High Performance Liquid Chromatography. System HY—RI 273.

Ultraviolet Spectrum. Aqueous acid—268 nm (A^1_1=398a); aqueous alkali—241 nm (A^1_1=364b), 276 nm (A^1_1=304b), 388 nm (A^1_1=385b).

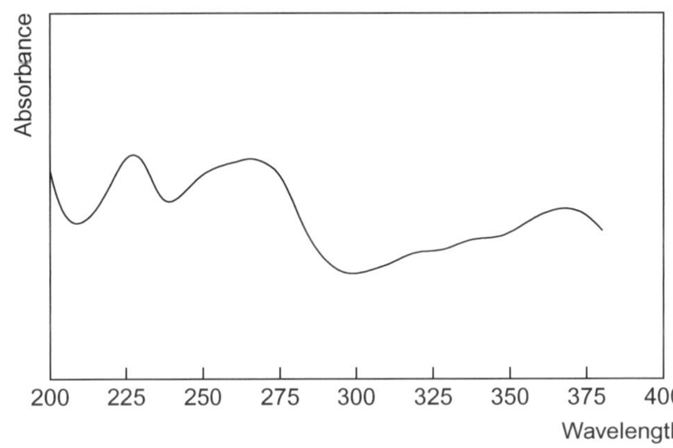

Infra-red Spectrum. Principal peaks at wavenumbers 1616, 1573, 1660, 1190, 1298, 1315 cm^{-1} (KBr disk).

Disposition in the Body. Readily absorbed after oral administration and slowly excreted in the urine.

Half-life. Plasma half-life, about 10 to 15 h.

Protein binding. In plasma, 40 to 90%.

Dose. Usually 600 mg of demeclocycline hydrochloride daily; up to 1.2 g daily has been given.

Demeton-*S*

Pesticide

Synonyms. Isosystox; Mercaptofos Teolovy.
O,O-Diethyl-*S*-[2-(ethylthio)ethyl] phosphorothioate
$C_8H_{19}O_3PS_2$=258.3
CAS—126-75-0

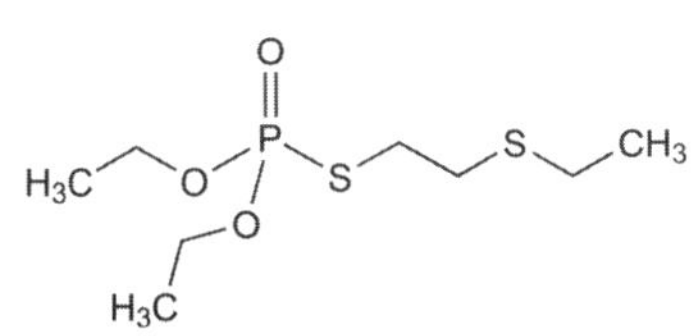

A colourless oil.
Soluble 1 in 500 of water; soluble in most organic solvents.

Demeton-*S*-methyl

Synonyms. Methyl-mercaptofos Teolovy; Metaisosystox.
Note. The name Demeton-methyl used to be applied to a mixture of demeton-*S*-methyl and demeton-*O*-methyl but this mixture has been replaced by demeton-*S*-methyl.
Proprietary names. Azotox; Demetox; DSM; Duratox; Metasystox 55.
$C_6H_{15}O_3PS_2$=230.3

CAS—919-86-8
A pale yellow oil of low viscosity. In solution or upon storage, demeton-*S*-methyl is oxidised to the sulfoxide and the sulfone. Refractive index 1.5065. Soluble 1 in 300 of water; soluble in most organic solvents.

Partition Coefficient. Log *P* (octanol/water), 2.1.

Colour Tests. Palladium Chloride—brown-orange; Phosphorus Test—yellow.

Thin-layer Chromatography. Demeton-*S*-methyl: system TE—Rf 81; system TX—Rf 18; system TY—Rf 13; system TAE—Rf 86.

Gas Chromatography. System GA—Demeton RI 1684, demeton-*S*-methyl RI 1628, demeton-*S*-methylsulfone RI 1866, demeton-*S*-methylsulfoxide RI 1860; system GK—RRT 0.70 (relative to caffeine).

High Performance Liquid Chromatography. Demeton-*S*-methyl: system HY—RI 353.

Infra-red Spectrum. Principal peaks at wavenumbers 1020, 1250, 775, 793, 826, 1190 cm^{-1} (demeton-*S*-methyl).

Mass Spectrum. Principal ions at *m/z* 88, 60, 109, 142, 79, 47, 111, 61 (demeton-*S*-methyl).

Disposition in the Body. Demeton-*S* and demeton-*S*-methyl are very readily absorbed by all routes and have a particularly high toxicity following percutaneous absorption. They are rapidly hydrolysed in the tissues to the corresponding sulfoxide and sulfone.

Toxicity. Demeton-*S* and demeton-*S*-methyl exert a direct inhibitory action on cholinesterase. The estimated minimum lethal dose is 5 g but exposure to 300 mg daily may be dangerous.

In a fatality due to the ingestion of demeton-*S*-methyl, the following postmortem tissue concentrations were reported: blood 10 mg/L, bile 58 mg/L, kidney 5 µg/g, liver 17 µg/g, urine 121 mg/L. [R. A. Hall and E. D. Carson, *Bull. Int. Assoc. Forensic Toxicol.*, 1970, *7*(3), 6.]

Demoxepam

Tranquilliser

Synonym. Chlordiazepoxide Lactam
7-Chloro-1,3-dihydro-5-phenyl-2*H*-1,4-benzodiazepin-2-one 4-oxide
$C_{15}H_{11}ClN_2O_2$=286.7
CAS—963-39-3

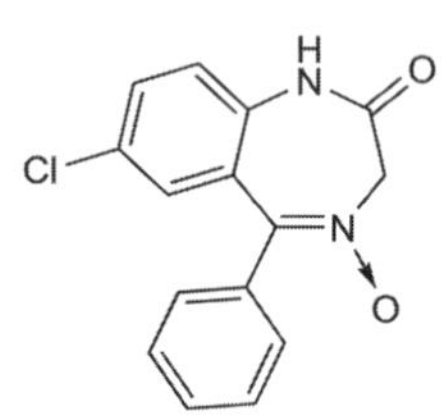

A white crystalline powder.
Soluble in chloroform.

Dissociation Constant. pK_a 4.5, 10.6.

Partition Coefficient. Log *P* (octanol/pH 7.4), 1.5.

Colour Test. Formaldehyde–Sulfuric Acid—orange.

Thin-layer Chromatography. System TA—Rf 63; system TB—Rf 00; system TC—Rf 35; system TD—Rf 15; system TE—Rf 41; system TF—Rf 24; system TL—Rf 51; system TAD—Rf 42; system TAE—Rf 81; system TAF—Rf 83; system TAJ—Rf 42; system TAK—Rf 38; system TAL—Rf 89. (Acidified iodoplatinate solution, positive; acidified potassium permanganate solution, positive.)

Gas Chromatography. System GA—demoxepam RI 2529, oxazepam RI 2325; system GB—demoxepam RI 2806, oxazepam RI 2438; system GG—demoxepam RI 3043, oxazepam RI 2803.

High Performance Liquid Chromatography. System HI—demoxepam *k* 2.42, oxazepam *k* 4.62; system HK—demoxepam *k* 0.03, oxazepam *k* 0.73; system HX—RI 416; system HY—RI 341; system HZ—retention time 3.1 min; system HAX—retention time 5.8 min; system HAY—retention time 5.1 min.

Ultraviolet Spectrum. Aqueous acid—237, 305; aqueous alkali—243, 255, 310; methanol—236 (A_1^1=1340b), 310 nm.

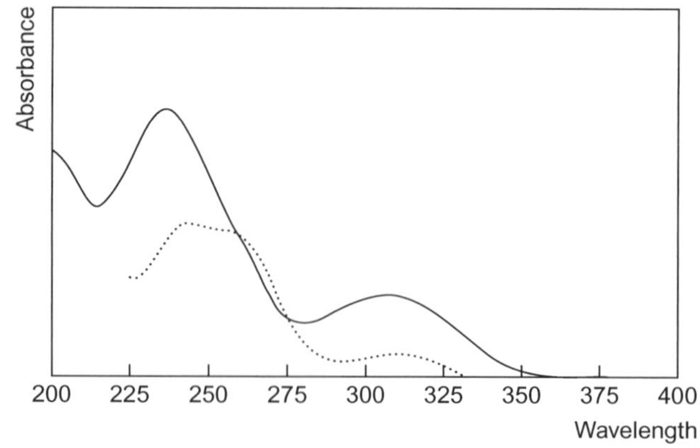

Infra-red Spectrum. Principal peaks at wavenumbers 1678, 690, 1240, 1265, 755, 717 cm^{-1}.

Mass Spectrum. Principal ions at m/z 285, 286, 269, 287, 241, 242, 77, 270.

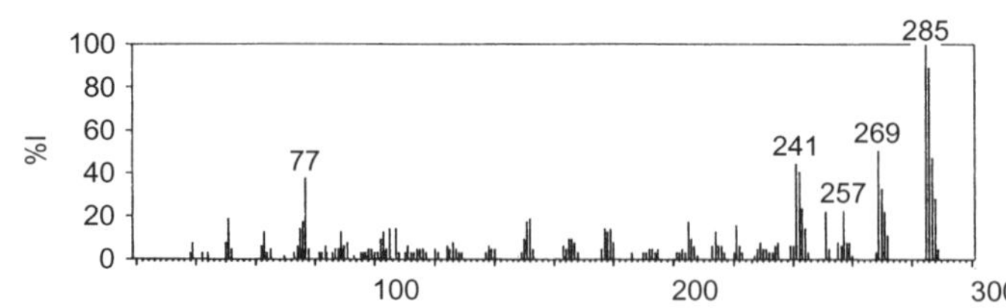

Quantification

Gas chromatography. In serum: demoxepam and chlordiazepoxide, ECD—S. R. Sun and D. J. Hoffman, *J. Pharm. Sci.*, 1978, *67*, 1647–1648.

High performance liquid chromatography. In plasma: limit of detection 0.075 to 0.125 mg/L—D. J. Garretty *et al.*, *Ann. Clin. Biochem.*, 1998, *35*, 528–533. In urine: limit of detection 250 ng on column—H. Essien *et al.*, *J. Chromatogr. B Biomed. Appl.*, 1996, *683*, 199–208.

Disposition in the Body. Well absorbed after oral administration. About 10% of a dose is excreted in the urine in 24 h and about 60% in 7 days, including about 27% as unchanged demoxepam and about 5% as conjugated oxazepam. Other urinary metabolites include the 5-(4-hydroxyphenyl) and 9-hydroxy derivatives. Approximately 15% of the dose is eliminated in the faeces in 7 days with about 2% as desmethyldiazepam. Demoxepam is a metabolite of chlordiazepoxide.

Therapeutic concentration

Following a single oral dose of 20 mg of demoxepam given to 6 subjects, peak plasma concentrations of 0.50 to 0.74 µg/mL (mean 0.6) were attained in 2 to 8 h. [M. A. Schwartz *et al.*, *J. Pharm. Sci.*, 1971, *60*, 1500–1503.]

Half-life. Plasma half-life, 14 to 95 h (mean 40).

Denatonium Benzoate

Alcohol Denaturant

Proprietary name. Bitrex
N-[2-[(2,6-Dimethylphenyl)amino]-2-oxoethyl]-*N*,*N*-diethylbenzenemethanaminium benzoate
$C_{28}H_{34}N_2O_3$=446.6
CAS—3734-33-6

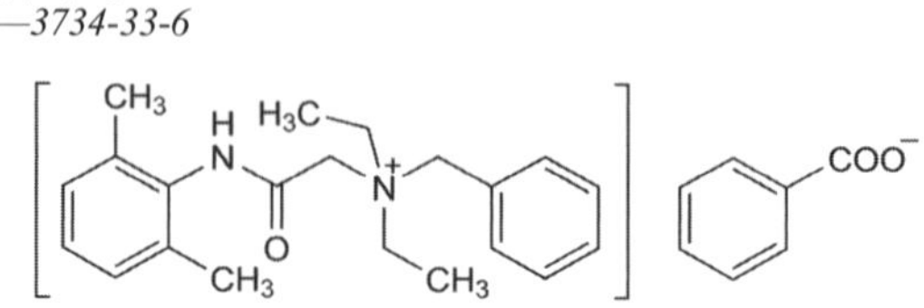

A white crystalline powder. M.p. 166° to 170°.

Soluble in water; soluble 1 in about 2 of ethanol and 1 in about 3 of chloroform; sparingly soluble in acetone; practically insoluble in ether.

Partition Coefficient. Log *P* (octanol/water), 1.8.

Colour Test. Mandelin's Test—violet

Thin-layer Chromatography. System TA—Rf 10; system TB—Rf 00; system TE—Rf 03; system TF—Rf 25; system TAE—Rf 01. (Acidified iodoplatinate solution, positive.)

High Performance Liquid Chromatography. System HX—RI 422.

Ultraviolet Spectrum. Aqueous acid—263 nm (A^1_1=36b), 269 nm.

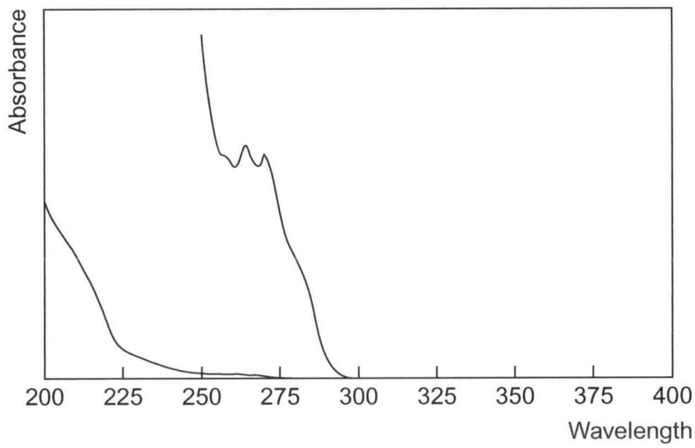

Infra-red Spectrum. Principal peaks at wavenumbers 1550, 1596, 1680, 719, 704, 757 cm^{-1}.

Deptropine

Antihistamine

Synonym. Dibenzheptropine

endo-3-[(10,11-Dihydro-5*H*-dibenzo[*a*,*d*]cyclohepten-5-yl)oxy]-8-methyl-8-azabicyclo[3.2.1]octane

$C_{23}H_{27}NO$=333.5

CAS—604-51-3

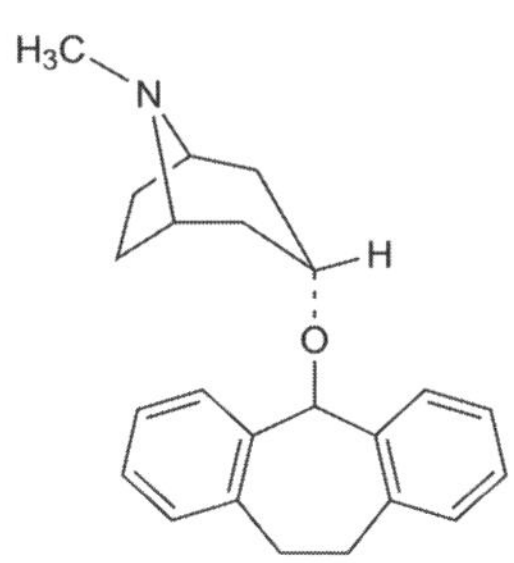

Deptropine Citrate

Proprietary names. Brontine. It is an ingredient of Brontisol.

$C_{23}H_{27}NO,C_6H_8O_7$=525.6

CAS—2169-75-7

A white to off-white microcrystalline powder.

Very slightly soluble in water and ethanol; soluble 1 in 100 of methanol; practically insoluble in chloroform and ether.

Partition Coefficient. Log *P* (octanol/water), 5.3.

Colour Tests. Mandelin's Test—yellow; Marquis Test—yellow.

Thin-layer Chromatography. System TA—Rf 13; system TB—Rf 26; system TC—Rf 04; system TE—Rf 36; system TL—Rf 01; system TAE—Rf 01. (Acidified potassium permanganate solution, positive.)

Gas Chromatography. System GA—RI 2615.

High Performance Liquid Chromatography. System HA—*k* 5.0 (tailing peak); system HX—RI 471; system HZ—Retention time, 10.3 min.

Ultraviolet Spectrum. Methanol—266 nm (A^1_1=18.6b), 272 nm.

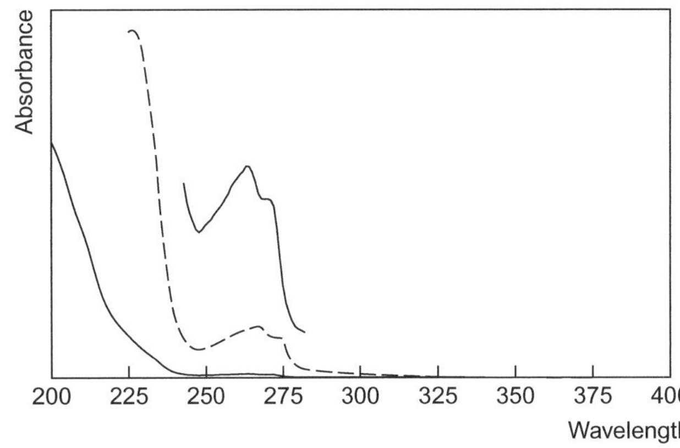

Infra-red Spectrum. Principal peaks at wavenumbers 1059, 1040, 751, 760, 738, 1114 cm^{-1} (KBr disk).

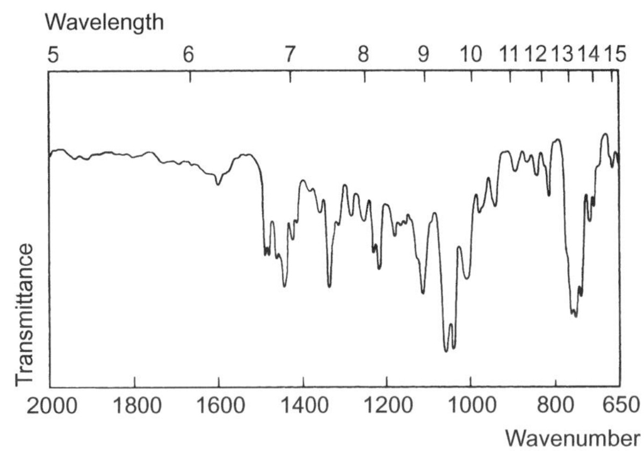

Mass Spectrum. Principal ions at *m/z* 83, 140, 82, 124, 43, 96, 97, 42.

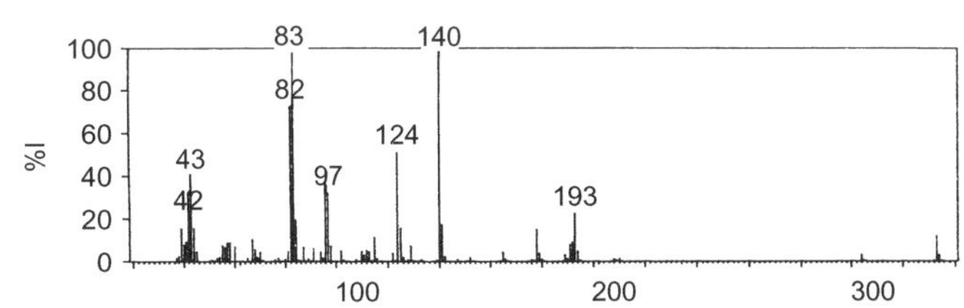

Dose. 2 mg of deptropine citrate daily.

Dequalinium Chloride

Antibacterial/Antifungal

Synonyms. Decalinium Chloride; Decaminum.

Proprietary names. Dequadin; Dequavagyn; Labosept; Optipect Halstabletten; Phylletten; Sorot.

1,1′-(1,10-Decanediyl)bis-[4-amino-2-methylquinolinium chloride]

$C_{30}H_{40}Cl_2N_4$=527.6

CAS—6707-58-0 (dequalinium); 522-51-0 (chloride)

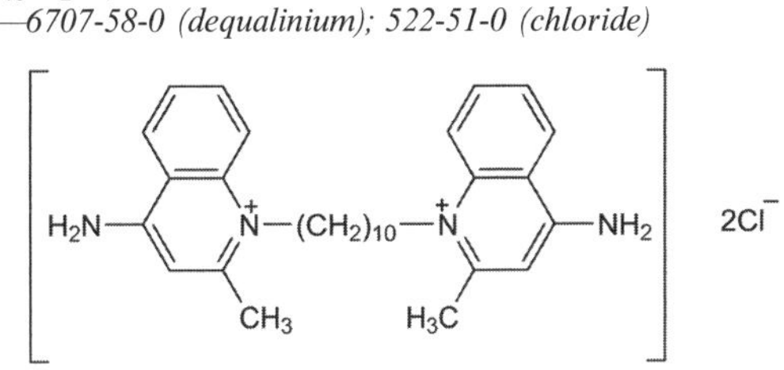

A creamy-white powder. M.p. about 315°, with decomposition.

Slightly soluble in water; soluble 1 in 30 of boiling water, 1 in 60 of methanol and 1 in 200 of propylene glycol.

Dequalinium Acetate
$C_{34}H_{46}N_4O_4$=574.8
CAS—4028-98-2
A white or pinkish-buff, slightly hygroscopic powder. M.p. about 280°, with decomposition.
Soluble 1 in 2 of water and 1 in 12 of ethanol.

Partition Coefficient. Log *P* (octanol/water), 4.3.

Colour Tests. Aromaticity (Method 2)—red/brown-violet; Liebermann's Test—yellow (→orange at 100°).

Thin-layer Chromatography. System TA—Rf 03. (Acidified iodoplatinate solution, positive.)

Ultraviolet Spectrum. Water—240 nm (A^1_1=812b), 326 nm (A^1_1=469b), 335 nm (A^1_1=406b); aqueous acid—241, 330 nm.

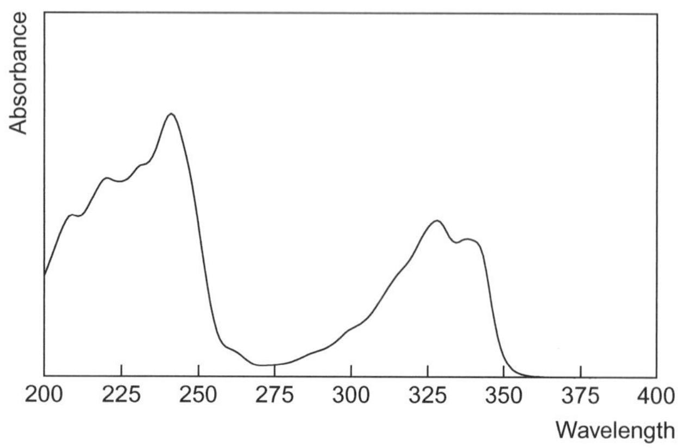

Infra-red Spectrum. Principal peaks at wavenumbers 1605, 1660, 765, 1560, 1540, 1307 cm^{-1} (KCl disk).

Dose. Lozenges containing 250 µg of dequalinium chloride are available.

Deserpidine

Antihypertensive

Synonyms. Canescine; 11-Demethoxyreserpine.
Proprietary names. Harmonyl. It is an ingredient of Enduronyl.
Methyl-(3*β*,16*β*,17*α*,18*β*,20*α*)-17-methoxy-18-[(3,4,5-trimethoxybenzoyl)oxy]-3,20-yohimban-16-carboxylate
$C_{32}H_{38}N_2O_8$=578.7
CAS—131-01-1

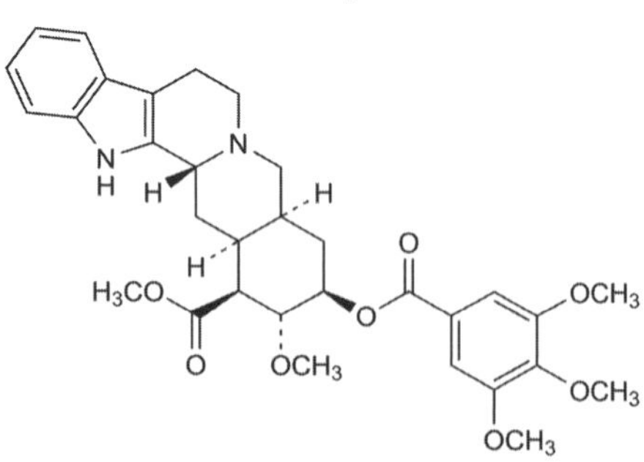

An alkaloid isolated from the root of *Rauwolfia canescens* (Apocynaceae).
Crystals. M.p. 230° to 234°, with decomposition.
Practically insoluble in water; soluble in hot ethanol and chloroform.

Partition Coefficient. Log *P* (octanol/water), 3.2.

Colour Tests. Mandelin's Test—blue→green; Marquis Test—grey-green.

Thin-layer Chromatography. System TA—Rf 72; system TB—Rf 03; system TC—Rf 77; system TE—Rf 81; system TL—Rf 66; system TAE—Rf 73. (Acidified iodoplatinate solution, positive.)

High Performance Liquid Chromatography. System HA—*k* 0.4.

Ultraviolet Spectrum. Aqueous acid—269 nm; aqueous alkali—275 nm.

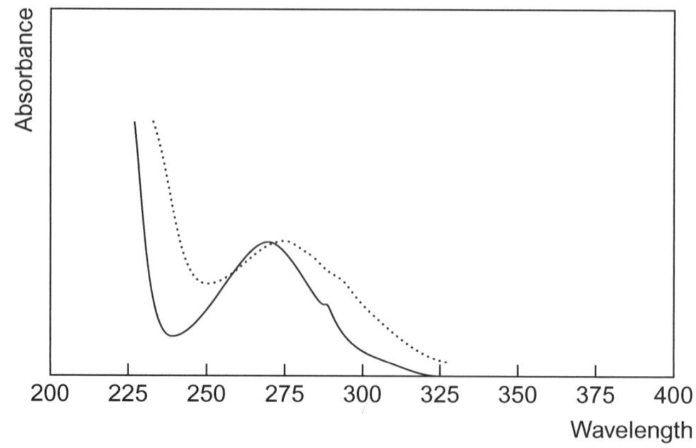

Infra-red Spectrum. Principal peaks at wavenumbers 1225, 1127, 1715, 1100, 1184, 1590 cm^{-1} (KBr disk).

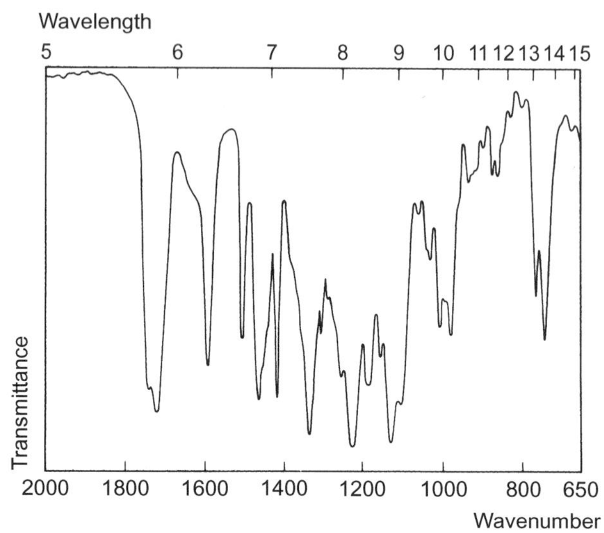

Mass Spectrum. Principal ions at *m*/*z* 578, 195, 577, 367, 351, 579, 366, 365.

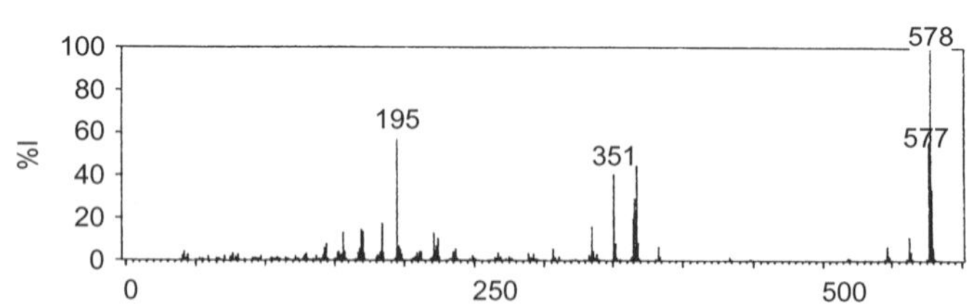

Dose. 0.25 to 1 mg daily.

Desferrioxamine

Chelating Agent

Synonyms. Deferoxamine; DFM; DFOM.
N′-[5-[[4-[[5-(Acetylhydroxyamino)pentyl]amino]-1,4-dioxobutyl]-hydroxyamino]pentyl]-*N*-(5-aminopentyl)-*N*-hydroxybutanediamide
$C_{25}H_{48}N_6O_8$=560.7
CAS—70-51-9

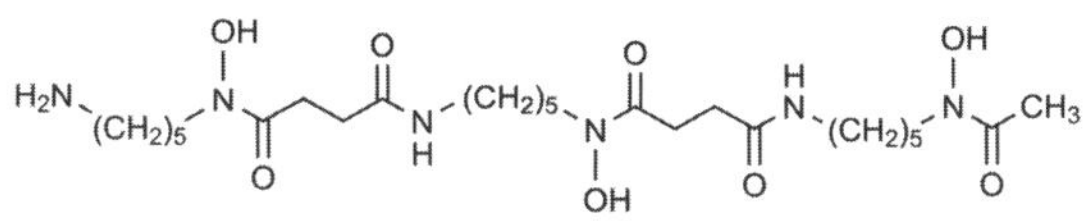

Desferrioxamine Mesilate
Synonyms. Deferoxamine Mesilate; Desferrioxamine B Mesilate; Desferrioxamine Methanesulfonate.
Proprietary name. Desferal
$C_{25}H_{48}N_6O_8,CH_3SO_3H = 656.8$
CAS—138-14-7
A white to cream-coloured powder.
Soluble 1 in 5 of water and 1 in 20 of ethanol; practically insoluble in dehydrated alcohol, chloroform, and ether.

Partition Coefficient. Log *P* (octanol/water), −2.5.

Colour Test. Mandelin's Test—blue→violet.

Thin-layer Chromatography. System TA—Rf 08, streaking. (Acidified potassium permanganate solution, positive.)

Ultraviolet Spectrum. No significant absorption, 230 to 360 nm.

Infra-red Spectrum. Principal peaks at wavenumbers 1628, 1195, 1562, 1265, 1149, 1041 cm^{-1} (KBr disk).

Quantification
High performance liquid chromatography. In plasma: limit of detection desferrioxamine 0.313 mg/L and ferrioxamine 0.039 mg/L, limit of quantification 1.0 mg/L and 5.0 mg/L, respectively, UV detection (λ = 430 nm)—H. J. Kraemer and H. Breithaupt, *J. Chromatogr. B Biomed. Sci. Appl.*, 1998, *710*, 191–204.

Disposition in the Body. Poorly absorbed after oral administration. It specifically chelates ferric iron to an octahedral complex, ferrioxamine, which is readily excreted in the urine. Theoretically, 100 mg of desferrioxamine can chelate approximately 8.5 mg of iron. About 13 to 65% of a ^{59}Fe-labelled dose is excreted in the urine in 24 h.

Dose. In acute iron poisoning: 5 g of desferrioxamine mesilate by mouth, with 2 g IM, and up to 15 mg/kg/h by IV infusion.

Desflurane

General Anaesthetic

Synonym. I-653
Proprietary name. Suprane
2-(Difluoromethyl)-1,2,2,2-tetrafluoroethyl ether
$C_3H_2F_6O = 168.0$
CAS—57041-67-5

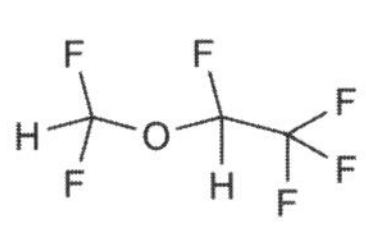

A non-flammable colourless volatile liquid with a slight non-pungent odour. B.p. 23.5°. Density 1.44.

Partition Coefficient. Log *P* (oil/gas), 18.7 (37°); log *P* (blood/gas), 0.424 (37°); log *P* (octanol/water), 1.20.

Gas Chromatography. Column: PoraPLOT Q (25 m × 0.32 mm, 10 μm film thickness). Column temperature: 30° for 2 min, to 250° at 15°/min and held for 5 min. Injector and detector temperatures: 250° and 270°, respectively. Carrier gas: helium, flow rate 3.8 mL/min. Detection: flame ionisation/FTIR (Fourier transform infra-red). Reference compound: diethyl ketone. Retention time: (relative to diethyl ketone) 0.65. [I. Ojanpera *et al.*, *J. Anal. Toxicol.*, 1998, *22*, 290–295].

Infra-red Spectrum. Principal peaks at wavenumbers 1219, 1180, 1112, 1135, 1304, 696 cm^{-1}.

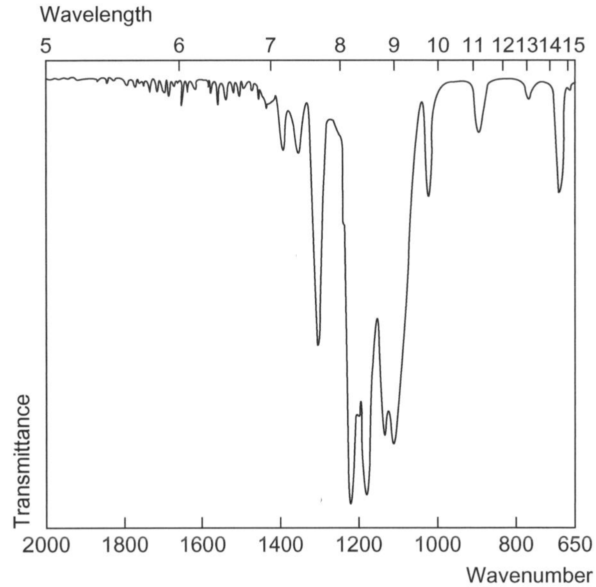

Mass Spectrum. Principal ions at *m/z* 51, 29, 101, 149, 31, 69, 99, 32.

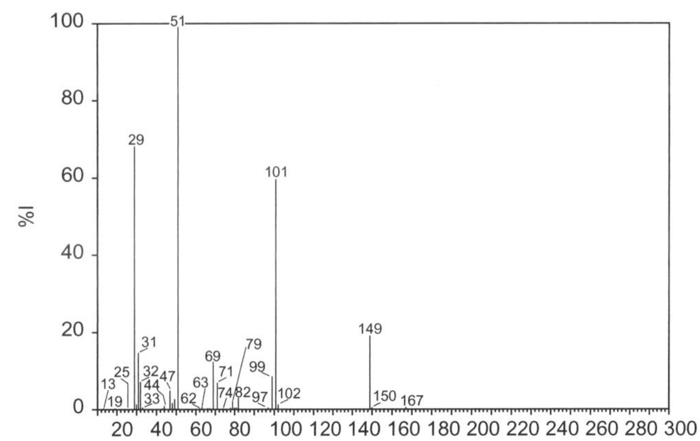

Quantification
Gas chromatography. In blood: limit of quantification 0.13 mg/L, FTIR detection—I. Ojanpera *et al.*, *J. Anal. Toxicol.*, 1998, *22*, 290–295.

Disposition in the Body. Absorption, distribution and elimination following inhalation are more rapid than for other halogenated anaesthetics such as isoflurane or halothane. This is due to the low blood/gas coefficient of desflurane. About 0.02% of administered desflurane is metabolised in the liver; trifluoroacetic acid has been detected in the serum and urine of patients given desflurane. The majority of desflurane is excreted mainly unchanged through the lungs. A very small amount diffuses through the skin.

Therapeutic concentration
The mean maximum serum concentration of trifluoroacetic acid in 13 subjects was 0.38 μmol/L at 24 h after exposure to desflurane for a mean of 6.81 h. Concentrations remained elevated for 6 days after exposure. [T. S. Sutton *et al.*, *Anesth. Analg.*, 1991, *73*, 180–185].

Clearance. Plasma clearance, 4.6 L/min; pulmonary, 4.11 L/min.

Note. For a review of desflurane, see D. D. Koblin, *Anesth. Analg.*, 1992, *74*, *Suppl. 4S*, S10–S16 and J. E. Caldwell, *Clin. Pharmacokinet.*, 1994, *27*, 6–18.

Dose. Using a calibrated vaporiser, concentrations of 4 to 11% are required for induction of anaesthesia. For maintenance, concentrations between 2 and 6% (in nitrous oxide); 2.5 to 8.5% (in oxygen or oxygen-enriched air); maximum, 17%.

Desipramine

Antidepressant

Synonyms. Desmethylimipramine; DMI; Norimipramine.
10,11-Dihydro-*N*-methyl-5*H*-dibenz[*b,f*]azepine-5-propanamine
$C_{18}H_{22}N_2$=266.4
CAS—50-47-5

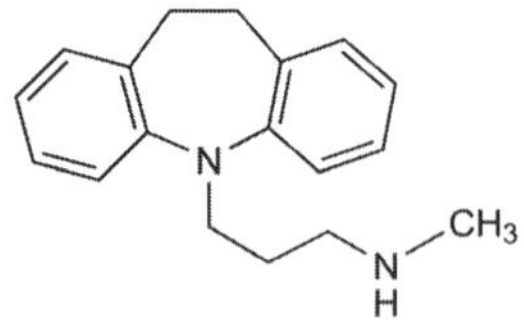

Desipramine Hydrochloride

Synonyms. Desipramini Hydrochloridum; EX-4355; G-35020; JB-8181; NSC-114901; RMI-9384A.
Proprietary names. Deprexan; Norpramin; Nortimil; Pertofran(e); Petylyl.
$C_{18}H_{22}N_2$,HCl=302.8
CAS—58-28-6
A white crystalline powder. M.p. 215° to 216°.
Soluble 1 in 20 of water, 1 in 20 of ethanol, and 1 in about 4 of chloroform; practically insoluble in ether; freely soluble in methanol.

Dissociation Constant. pK_a 10.2 (24°).

Partition Coefficient. Log *P* (octanol/pH 7.4), 1.4.

Colour Tests. Forrest Reagent—blue; Mandelin's Test—yellow→blue.

Thin-layer Chromatography. System TA—Rf 26; system TB—Rf 19; system TC—Rf 11; system TE—Rf 40; system TL—Rf 03; system TAE—Rf 07; system TAF—Rf 71; system TAJ—Rf 07; system TAK—Rf 23; system TAL—Rf 72. (Dragendorff spray, positive; FPN reagent, blue; acidified iodoplatinate solution, positive; Marquis reagent, blue.)

Gas Chromatography. System GA—desipramine RI 2235, M (2-OH-) RI 2553, M (ring) RI 1930, M (ring-OH-) RI 2240, M (ring-di-OH-) RI 2600, M (acetyl-) RI 2670, M (ring-OH-methoxy-) RI 2390; system GB—desipramine RI 2338, M (2-OH-) RI 2669, M (10-OH-) RI 2521, M (ring) RI 2014, M (ring-OH-) RI 2335, M (di-OH-) RI 2995, M (acetyl-) RI 2811, M (OH-methoxy-) RI 2749; system GM—desipramine RRT 0.896 (relative to iprindole); system GS—retention time 18.7 min.

High Performance Liquid Chromatography. System HA—desipramine *k* 2.1, didesmethylimipramine *k* 1.3, 2-hydroxydesipramine *k* 1.2; system HF—*k* 3.60; system HX—RI 424; system HY—RI 361; system HZ—retention time 5.9 min; system HAA—retention time 14.9 min; system HAM—retention time 9.1 min; system HAX—retention time 13.0 min; system HAY—retention time 6.3 min; system HAZ—desipramine *k* 1.52, M (2-OH-) *k* 0.39.

Ultraviolet Spectrum. Aqueous acid—250 nm (A^1_1=308a). No alkaline shift.

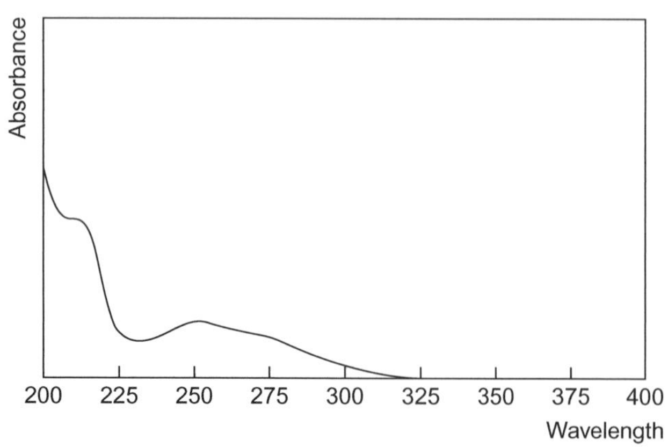

Infra-red Spectrum. Principal peaks at wavenumbers 746, 741, 763, 1230, 1590, 1104 cm^{-1} (desipramine hydrochloride, KBr disk).

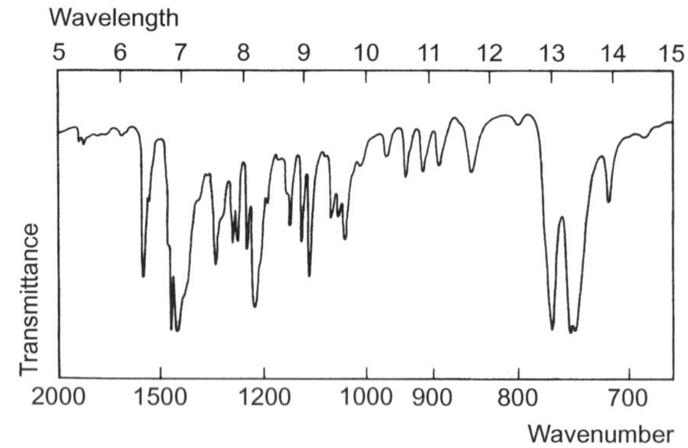

Mass Spectrum. Principal ions at *m/z* 235, 195, 208, 44, 234, 193, 194, 71; 2-hydroxydesipramine 44, 209, 211, 250, 210, 224, 42, 251.

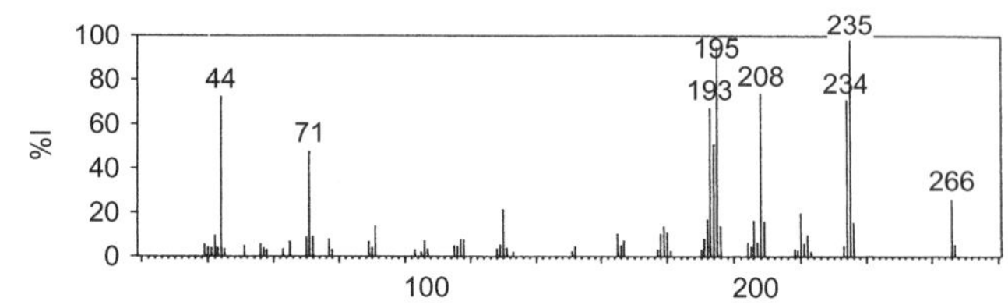

Quantification. See also under Imipramine.

Gas chromatography. In plasma or serum: limit of detection 1 µg/L, AFID—E. Antal *et al.*, *J. Chromatogr.* 1980, *183*(9) *B Biomed. Appl.*, 149–157. In plasma: desipramine and other antidepressants and metabolites, limit of quantification for desipramine 90 µg/L, NPD—S. Ulrich and J. Martens, *J. Chromatogr. B Biomed. Sci. Appl.*, 1997, *696*, 217–234. In plasma: desipramine and other tricyclic antidepressants, limits of detection 1.2 to 5.8 µg/L, NPD—R. de la Torre *et al.*, *Ther. Drug Monit.*, 1998, *20*, 340–346. In whole blood: desipramine and other antidepressants, limits of detection 39 to 153 µg/L, NPD —M. A. Martinez *et al.*, *J. Anal. Toxicol.*, 2002, *26*, 296–302.

Gas chromatography–mass spectrometry. In plasma: desipramine and other tricyclic antidepressants, limit of quantification 25 µg/L—B. A. Way *et al.*, *J. Anal. Toxicol.*, 1998, *22*, 374–382.

High performance liquid chromatography. In plasma: desipramine, imipramine, and metabolites, UV and coulometric detection—J. P. Foglia *et al.*, *J. Chromatogr.*, 1991, *572*, 247–258. In serum or plasma: desipramine and other tricyclic antidepressants, UV detection—M. P. Segatti *et al.*, *J. Chromatogr.*, 1991, *536*, 319–325; R. H. Queiroz *et al.*, *Pharm. Acta Helv.*, 1995, *70*, 181–186; R. Theurillat and W. Thormann, *J. Pharm. Biomed. Anal.*, 1998, *18*, 751–760. In plasma or urine: desipramine, imipramine and their metabolites, limit of detection for desipramine 0.3 µg/L, UV detection—E. Koyama *et al.*, *Ther. Drug Monit.*, 1993, *15*, 224–235. In plasma: desipramine and lofepramine, limit of quantification for desipramine 6.7 µg/L, UV detection—T. Elm and E. L. Hansen, *J. Chromatogr.* 1995, *665 B Biomed. Appl.*, 355–361. In biological samples: desipramine and other antidepressants, UV detection—E. Tanaka *et al.*, *J. Chromatogr. B Biomed. Sci. Appl.*, 1997, *692*, 405–412. In plasma or urine: desipramine, imipramine and their metabolites, limit of quantification for desipramine 3 µg/L, electrochemical detection—A. G. Chen *et al.*, *J. Chromatogr. B Biomed. Sci. Appl.*, 1997, *693*, 153–158.

High performance liquid chromatography–mass spectrometry. In plasma: desipramine and other tricyclic antdepressants, limit of quantification 5 µg/L, TOF–MS—H. Zhang *et al.*, *J. Mass Spectrom.*, 2000, *35*, 423–431.

Disposition in the Body. Well absorbed after oral administration. Metabolised by aromatic hydroxylation and possibly hydroxylamine formation; *N*-demethylation to form didesmethylimipramine may occur to a minor extent. 2-Hydroxydesipramine, the major metabolite, is active. Less than 5% of a dose is excreted in urine in 24 h as unchanged drug; the urinary excretion of unchanged drug is pH-dependent and is increased in acidic urine; the hydroxylated metabolites are excreted mainly as glucuronide conjugates. The extent of 2-hydroxylation is genetically determined. Desipramine is the major active metabolite of imipramine and lofepramine.

Therapeutic concentration. Plasma concentrations vary considerably between individual subjects.

After administration of a single oral dose of 50 mg to 4 subjects, peak plasma-desipramine concentrations of 0.008 to 0.015 mg/L (mean 0.012) were attained in 3 to 6 h; peak plasma concentrations of 2-hydroxydesipramine of 0.011 to 0.013 mg/L were attained in about 2 to 4 h. [C. L. De Vane *et al.*, *Eur. J. Clin. Pharmacol.*, 1981, *19*, 61–64.]

Following daily oral doses of about 2.5 mg/kg to 47 subjects, minimum steady-state plasma concentrations of 0.02 to 0.88 mg/L (mean 0.17) of desipramine and 0.007 to 0.13 mg/L (mean 0.04) of 2-hydroxydesipramine were reported. [J. L. Bock *et al.*, *Clin. Pharmacol. Ther.*, 1983, *33*, 322–328.]

Of 34 elderly patients treated for depression with desipramine for 4 weeks at a fixed dosage regimen, 12 non-responders received a second period of treatment at an increased dose. In patients aged over 74 years ($n = 16$), a daily dose of 2.45 mg/kg resulted in a mean plasma level of 0.118 mg/L for desipramine and 0.072 mg/L for hydroxydesipramine; in patients aged less than 60 years ($n=45$, including some patients from previously published work), a daily dose of 2.6 mg/kg resulted in a mean plasma level of 0.142 mg/L for desipramine and 0.041 mg/L for hydroxydesipramine. A plasma concentration of 0.105 mg/L significantly separated responders from non-responders, although the response rate was still low relative to rates in prior studies of younger patients. [J. C. Nelson *et al.*, *J. Clin. Psychopharmacol.*, 1995, *15*, 99–105.]

Toxicity. Plasma concentrations greater than 0.4 mg/L may produce toxic effects. Fatalities are comparatively rare, but may occur with plasma concentrations greater than 10 mg/L.

Recovery has occurred in 2 subjects after the ingestion of up to 2 g; peak plasma concentrations of 1.56 mg/L and 1.58 mg/L were reported. [J. T. Biggs, *JAMA*, 1977, *238*, 135–138.]

In 1 fatal case, a blood concentration of 3 mg/L and a liver concentration of 140 mg/kg were reported. [R. C. Baselt and R. H. Cravey, *J. Anal. Toxicol.*, 1977, *1*, 81–103.]

The following postmortem concentrations were found after the death of a 2-year-old child: blood 8 mg/L, liver blood 22 mg/L, bile 67 mg/L, urine 2 mg/L. [A. E. Robinson *et al.*, *J. Anal. Toxicol.*, 1979, *3*, 3–13.]

Half-life. Plasma half-life, 10 to 35 h.

Protein binding. In plasma, about 70 to 90%.

Note. For a review of tricyclic antidepressant overdose, see G. W. Kerr *et al.*, *Emerg. Med. J.*, 2001, *18*, 236–241. For a review of the clinical pharmacokinetics of imipramine and desipramine, see F. R. Sallee and B. G. Pollock, *Clin. Pharmacokinet.*, 1990, *18*, 346–364. For a review of the pharmacokinetics of tricyclic antidepressants, see G. Molnar and R. N. Gupta, *Biopharm. Drug Dispos.*, 1980, *1*, 283–305.

Dose. 25 to 200 mg of desipramine hydrochloride daily; up to 300 mg daily has been given.

Deslanoside

Cardiac Glycoside

Synonyms. Deacetyl-lanatoside C; Desacetyl-lanatoside C.
Proprietary names. Cedilanid-D; Cedilanid(e); Desace.
Note. The name Cedilanid(e) is also applied to preparations of lanatoside C.
(3β,5β,12β)-3-[(*O*-β-D-Glucopyranosyl-(1→4)-*O*-2,6-dideoxy-β-D-*ribo*-hexopyranosyl-(1→4)-*O*-2,6-dideoxy-β-D-*ribo*-hexopyranosyl-(1→4)-2,6-dideoxy-β-D-*ribo*-hexopyranosyl)oxy]-12,14-dihydroxycard-20(22)-enolide
$C_{47}H_{74}O_{19}=943.1$
CAS—17598-65-1

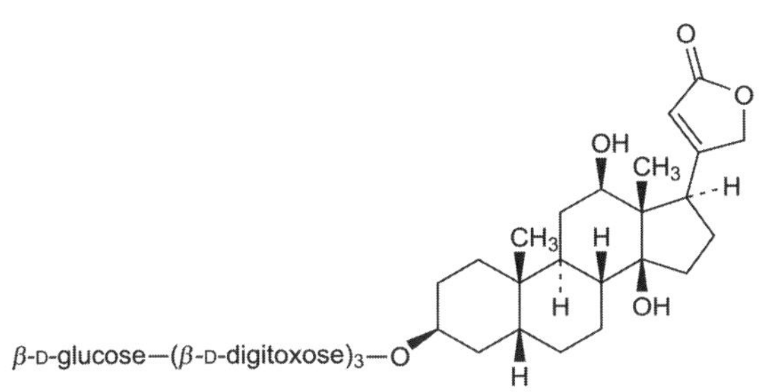

White hygroscopic crystals or crystalline powder. M.p. about 220°.

Practically insoluble in water; soluble 1 in 2500 of ethanol and 1 in 200 of methanol; very slightly soluble in chloroform; practically insoluble in ether.

Colour Test. Dissolve 2 to 3 mg in 5 mL of a solution containing 0.5 mL of a 9% ferric chloride solution and 100 mL of acetic acid; underlay with 5 mL of sulfuric acid—intense blue in the acetic acid layer and a brown ring free from red at the junction of the two liquids (see also Lanatoside C). (Perchloric acid solution, followed by examination under UV light, blue fluorescence; *p*-anisaldehyde reagent, blue.)

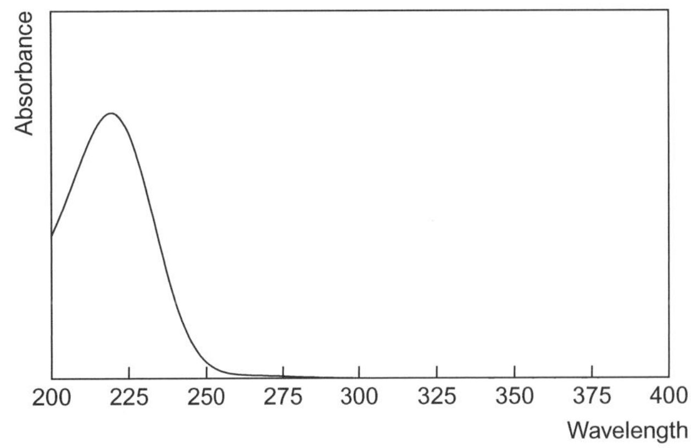

Disposition in the Body. Incompletely absorbed after oral administration and metabolised to digoxin. After IV administration, about 80% of a single dose is excreted in the urine in 72 h, mostly as unchanged drug, and about 10% of a dose is eliminated in the faeces. During maintenance treatment, about 30% of a daily dose is excreted in the 24-h urine. After oral administration digoxin accounts for about 50% of the total urinary excretion material.
Deslanoside is a metabolite of lanatoside C.

Therapeutic concentration

After an IV dose of 400 µg given to 5 subjects, a mean plasma concentration of 0.03 mg/L was reported at 15 min, declining to 0.001 mg/L at 48 h; after an oral dose of 800 µg given to 5 subjects, a mean peak plasma concentration of 0.003 mg/L was attained in 2 h. [A. Marzo *et al.*, *Farmaco, Edn Prat.*, 1982, *37*, 28–37.]

Half-life. Plasma half-life, about 33 h.

Distribution in blood. Plasma:whole blood ratio, 1.4.

Protein binding. In plasma, weakly bound.

Dose. For rapid digitalisation, 0.8 to 1.6 mg intravenously.

Desmetryne

Herbicide

Proprietary name. Semeron 25 WP
2-Isopropylamino-4-methylamino-6-methylthio-1,3,5-triazine
$C_8H_{15}N_5S=213.3$
CAS—1014-69-3

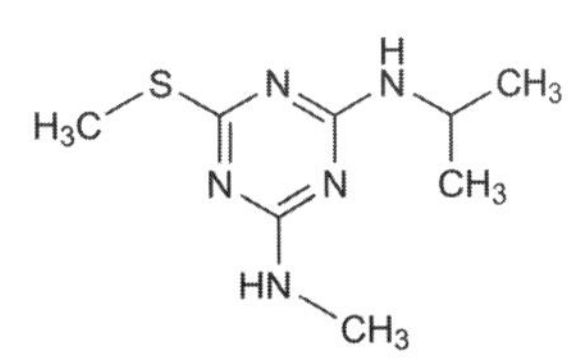

A white crystalline solid. M.p. 84° to 86°.
Very slightly soluble in water; readily soluble in organic solvents.

Dissociation Constant. pK_a 4.0.

Partition Coefficient. Log P (octanol/water), 2.4.

Thin-layer Chromatography. System TA—Rf 73; system TX—Rf 21; system TY—Rf 16. (Dragendorff spray, positive.)

Gas Chromatography. System GA—RI 1800; system GK—RRT 0.95 (relative to caffeine).

Ultraviolet Spectrum. Aqueous acid—258 nm (A_1^1=450b).

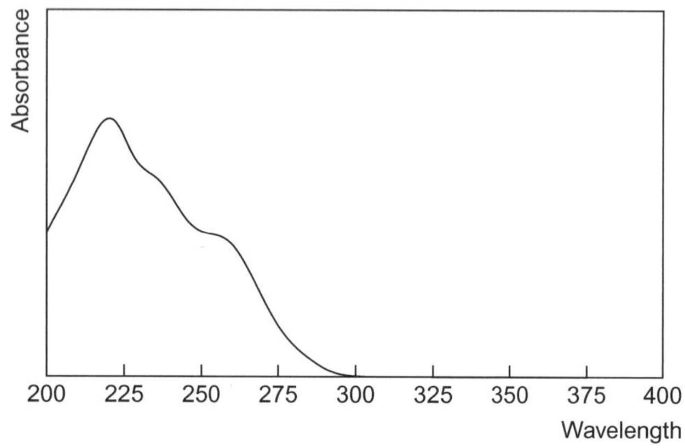

Infra-red Spectrum. Principal peaks at wavenumbers 1531, 1587, 1258, 806, 1292, 1163 cm^{-1} (KBr disk).

Mass Spectrum. Principal ions at *m/z* 213, 57, 58, 198, 82, 171, 43, 99.

Desonide

Anti-inflammatory Corticosteroid

Synonyms. Desfluorotriamcinolone Acetonide; 16-Hydroxyprednisolone-16,17-Acetonide.
Proprietary names. Apolar; Locapred; Tridesilon; Tridésonit.
(11β,16α)-11,21-Dihydroxy-16,17-[(1-methylethylidene)bis(oxy)]pregna-1,4-diene-3,20-dione
$C_{24}H_{32}O_6$=416.5
CAS—638-94-8

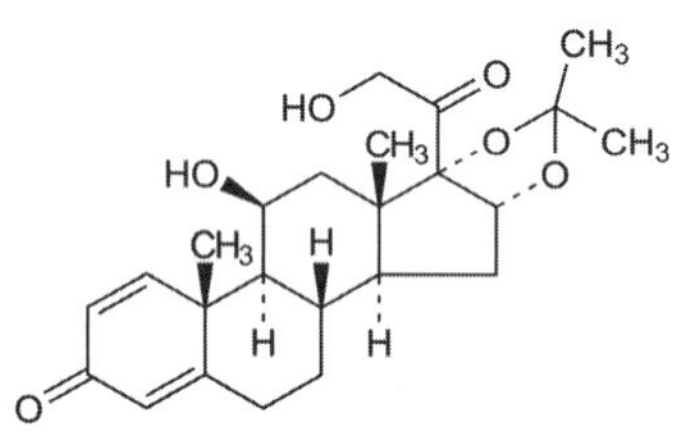

White powder or crystals.

Partition Coefficient. Log *P* (octanol/water), 2.8.

Ultraviolet Spectrum. Methanol—243 nm (A_1^1=450b).

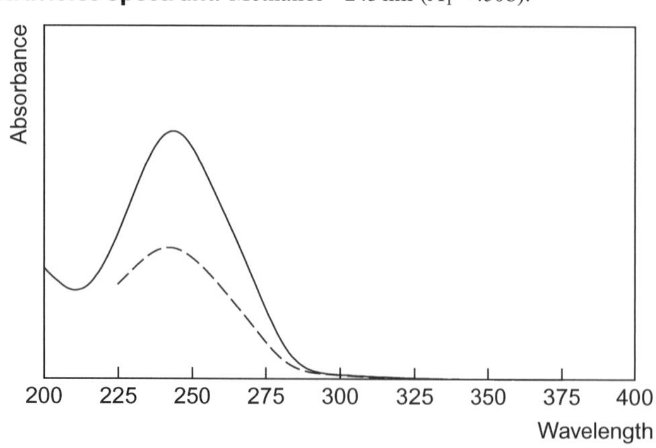

Infra-red Spectrum. Principal peaks at wavenumbers 1639, 1052, 1612, 1086, 1265, 1694 cm^{-1}.

Use. Topically as a 0.05% cream or ointment.

Desoxycortone

Corticosteroid

Synonyms. Decortone; Deoxycorticosterone; Deoxycortone; Desoxycorticosterone; 21-Hydroxyprogesterone.
21-Hydroxypregn-4-ene-3,20-dione
$C_{21}H_{30}O_3$=330.5
CAS—64-85-7

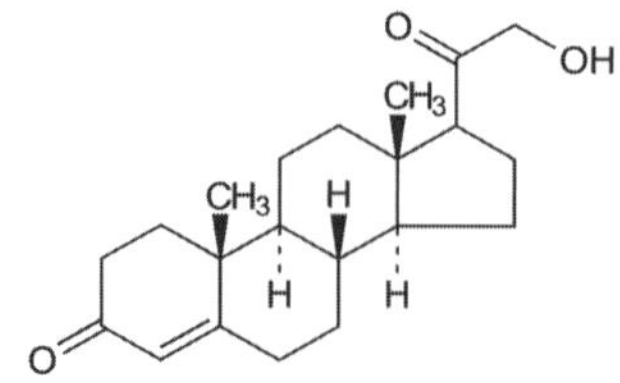

Crystals. M.p. 141° to 142°.
Freely soluble in ethanol and acetone.

Desoxycortone Acetate

Proprietary names. Cortiron; Doca; Percorten; Syncortyl. It is an ingredient of Plex-Hormone.
$C_{23}H_{32}O_4$=372.5
CAS—56-47-3
Colourless crystals or white or creamy-white crystalline powder. M.p. 155° to 161°.
Practically insoluble in water; soluble 1 in 50 of ethanol, 1 in 30 of acetone, 1 in 1.5 of chloroform and 1 in 170 of ether; slightly soluble in dioxane and propylene glycol.

Desoxycortone Pivalate

Synonyms. Desoxycortone Trimethylacetate; Desoxycorticosterone Pivalate.
Proprietary name. Percorten M
$C_{26}H_{38}O_4$=414.6
CAS—808-48-0
A white or creamy-white crystalline powder. M.p. 198° to 206°. A solution in dioxan is dextrorotatory.
Practically insoluble in water; soluble 1 in 350 to 1 in 500 of ethanol, 1 in 3 of chloroform and 1 in 60 of dioxan; slightly soluble in ether.

Partition Coefficient. Log *P* (octanol/water), 2.9.

Colour Tests. Antimony Pentachloride—orange; Naphthol–Sulfuric Acid—orange-red/blue-black; Sulfuric Acid—yellow (green-yellow fluorescence under ultraviolet light).

Thin-layer Chromatography. Desoxycortone acetate: system TP—Rf 86; system TQ—Rf 52; system TR—Rf 98; system TS—Rf 95; system TAJ—Rf 78; system TAK—Rf 71; system TAL—Rf 96; system TAM—Rf 91. (DPST solution.)

Ultraviolet Spectrum. Desoxycortone acetate: ethanol—240 nm (A_1^1=445a).

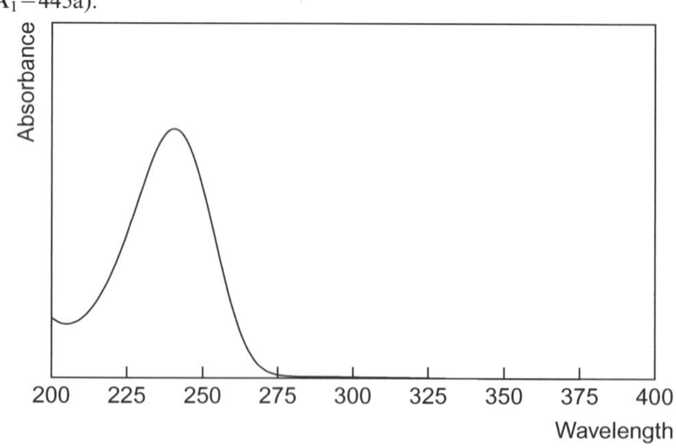

Infra-red Spectrum. Principal peaks at wavenumbers 1242, 1667, 1744, 1718, 1203, 1610 cm^{-1} (desoxycortone acetate, KBr disk).

Mass Spectrum. Principal ions at *m/z* 43, 55, 299, 91, 147, 79, 253, 271 (desoxycortone acetate).

Dose. Usually 1 to 5 mg of desoxycortone acetate daily, intramuscularly; sublingual doses of 2 to 10 mg daily have also been given.

Dexamethasone

Corticosteroid

Synonyms. Desamethasone; 9α-Fluoro-16α-methylprednisolone.
Proprietary names. Aeroseb-Dex; Decaderm; Decadron (elixir and tablets); Decalix; Decaspray; Dexacortisyl; Dexalocal; Dexasone (tablets); Dexone; Dezone (tablets); Fortecortin (tablets); Hexadrol (tablets); Maxidex; Millicorten; Miral; Oradexon (tablets). It is an ingredient of Maxitrol.
(11β,16α)-9-Fluoro-11,17,21-trihydroxy-16-methylpregna-1,4-diene-3,20-dione
$C_{22}H_{29}FO_5$=392.5
CAS—50-02-2

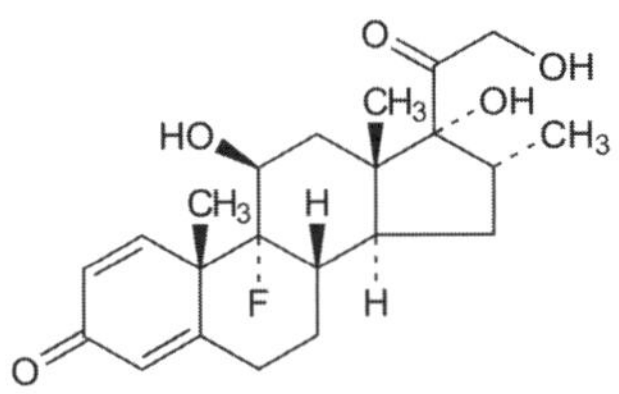

Dexamethasone is a synthetic glucocorticoid and is an isomer of betamethasone.
A white crystalline powder. M.p. 268° to 271°, with decomposition. A solution in dioxan is dextrorotatory.
Practically insoluble in water; soluble 1 in 42 of ethanol and 1 in 165 of chloroform; soluble in acetone; sparingly soluble in methanol; very slightly soluble in ether.

Dexamethasone Acetate

Synonym. Dexamethasone 21-acetate
Proprietary names. Decadron-LA; Dexacen-La-8; Dexasone L.A.; Fortecortin (suspension for injection).
$C_{24}H_{31}FO_6$=434.5
CAS—1177-87-3 (anhydrous); 55812-90-3 (monohydrate)
A white powder. M.p. about 225°, with decomposition.
Practically insoluble in water; soluble 1 in 40 of ethanol, 1 in 25 of dehydrated alcohol, 1 in 33 of chloroform, and 1 in 1000 of ether; freely soluble in acetone and methanol.

Dexamethasone Isonicotinate

Synonym. Dexamethasone 21-isonicotinate
Proprietary names. Auxison(e). It is an ingredient of Dexa-Rhinaspray.
$C_{28}H_{32}FNO_6$=497.6
CAS—2265-64-7
Crystals. M.p. 250° to 252°.

Dexamethasone Sodium Phosphate

Synonym. Sodium 9α-fluoro-16α-methylprednisolone 21-phosphate
Proprietary names. Dalaron; Decadron (injection); Decasone; Dexacen-4; Dexasone (injection); Dezone (injection); Fortecortin (injection); Hexadrol (injection); Novadex; Oradexon (injection); Savacort-D; Turbinaire Decadron.
$C_{22}H_{28}FNa_2O_8P$=516.4
CAS—2392-39-4
A white or slightly yellow, very hygroscopic, crystalline powder. M.p. 233° to 235°.
Soluble 1 in 2 of water; sparingly soluble in dehydrated alcohol; practically insoluble in chloroform and ether.

Dexamethasone Tebutate

Synonyms. Dexamethasone butylacetate; Dexamethasone TBA; Dexamethasone tertiary butylacetate.
Proprietary name. Decadron-TBA
$C_{28}H_{39}FO_6$=490.6
CAS—24668-75-5
Practically insoluble in water; soluble in ethanol and acetone.

Partition Coefficient. Log *P* (octanol/water), 1.8.

Colour Tests. Antimony Pentachloride—green; Naphthol–Sulfuric Acid—yellow-green/yellow; Sulfuric Acid—orange-pink.

Thin-layer Chromatography. System TP—Rf 32; system TQ—Rf 08; system TR—Rf 00; system TS—Rf 00; system TAJ—Rf 38; system TAK—Rf 07; system TAL—Rf 75; system TAM—Rf 66. (DPST solution.)

Gas Chromatography. System GA—RI 2970.

High Performance Liquid Chromatography. System HT—*k* 4.8; system HY—RI 381; system HZ—retention time 3.4 min; system HAA—retention time 13.1 min.

Ultraviolet Spectrum. Methanol—240 nm (A_1^1=385a).

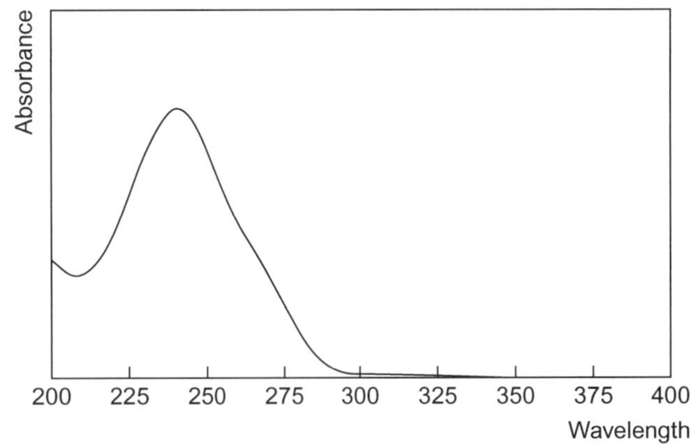

Infra-red Spectrum. Principal peaks at wavenumbers 1663, 896, 1622, 1695, 1052, 1603 cm^{-1}.

Mass Spectrum. Principal ions at *m/z* 121, 122, 315, 43, 147, 223, 135, 41.

Quantification
Gas chromatography–mass spectrometry. In plasma, synovial fluid and tissues: limit of detection 0.1 μg/L—J. Girault *et al.*, *Biomed. Env. Mass Spectrom.*, 1990, *19(5)*, 295–302.

High performance liquid chromatography. In serum and urine—B. C. McWhinney *et al.*, *Clin. Chem.*, 1996, *42*, 979–981. In plasma: limit of quantification 15 μg/L, UV detection (λ = 240 nm)—P. N. Schild and B. G. Charles, *J. Chromatogr. B Biomed. Sci. Appl.*, 1994, *658(1)*, 189–192. In plasma or tissues: limit of detection 10 ng in plasma, UV detection—B. Cham *et al.*, *Ther. Drug Monit.*, 1980, *2*, 373–377.

Disposition in the Body. Rapidly absorbed after oral administration. Up to 65% of a dose is excreted in the urine in 24 h, mainly as metabolites.

Therapeutic concentration
Seven extremely low birth weight infants, mean gestational age 25.6 weeks, suffering from bronchoplumonary dysplasia, were administered an IV bolus dose of 0.369 mg/kg dexamethasone sodium phosphate. A mean peak concentration of 250.5 μg/L was reached. [B. Charles *et al.*, *Dev. Pharmacol. Ther.*, 1993, *20(3–4)*, 205–210.]

Half-life. Plasma half-life, about 2 to 5 h.

Volume of distribution. About 1 L/kg.

Distribution in blood. Plasma:whole blood ratio, 1.2.

Protein binding. In plasma, about 67%.

Dose. 0.5 to 9 mg daily.

Dexamfetamine

Central Stimulant

Synonyms. Dexamphetamine; Dextroamphetamine.
Proprietary names. It is an ingredient of Biphetamine and Durophet.
(αS)-α-Methylbenzeneethanamine
$C_9H_{13}N$=135.2
CAS—51-64-9

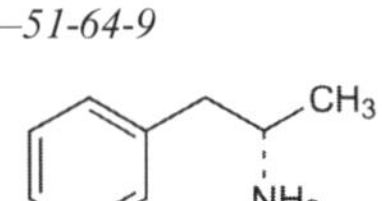

Dexamfetamine Phosphate

Synonyms. Dextroamphetamine Phosphate; Monobasic Dextroamphetamine Phosphate.
$C_9H_{13}N,H_3PO_4$=233.2
CAS—7528-00-9
A white crystalline powder.

Soluble 1 in 20 of water; slightly soluble in ethanol; practically insoluble in chloroform and ether.

Dexamfetamine Sulfate
Synonym. Dextro Amfetamine Sulfate
Proprietary names. Dexampex; Dexedrine; Diphylets; Ferndex. It is an ingredient of Dexamyl and Eskatrol.
$(C_9H_{13}N)_2,H_2SO_4$=368.5
CAS—51-63-8
A white or almost white crystalline powder. M.p. >300°.
Soluble 1 in 9 to 1 in 10 of water and 1 in 800 of ethanol; practically insoluble in ether.

Dissociation Constant. pK_a 9.9.

Partition Coefficient. Log *P* (octanol/water), 1.8.
For analytical data and quantification see under Amfetamine.

Disposition in the Body. Well absorbed after oral administration. It is approximately twice as potent as amfetamine. For information on metabolism, excretion and pharmacokinetics, see under Amfetamine.

Dose. 5 to 60 mg of dexamphetamine sulfate daily.

Dexbrompheniramine

Antihistamine

(+)-γ-(4-Bromophenyl)-*N*,*N*-dimethyl-2-pyridinepropanamine
$C_{16}H_{19}BrN_2$=319.2
CAS—132-21-8

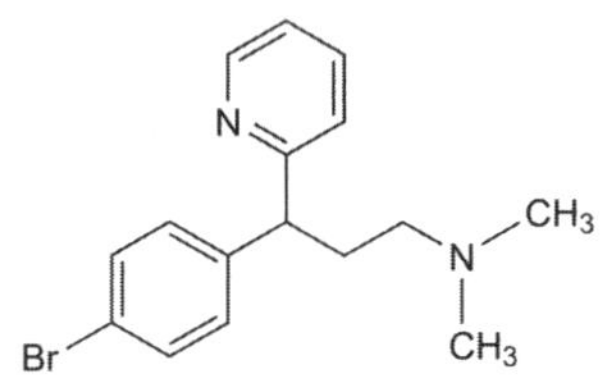

An oily liquid.

Dexbrompheniramine Maleate
Proprietary names. It is an ingredient of Disophrol, Drixoral and Halin.
$C_{16}H_{19}BrN_2,C_4H_4O_4$=435.3
CAS—2391-03-9
A white crystalline powder. M.p. 103° to 113°.
Soluble 1 in 1.2 of water, 1 in 2.5 of ethanol and 1 in 2 of chloroform; very slightly soluble in ether.
For analytical data see under Brompheniramine.

Disposition in the Body. See under Brompheniramine. Dexbrompheniramine is approximately twice as potent as brompheniramine.

Toxicity
The following post-mortem concentrations of dexbrompheniramine were reported in a fatality involving the ingestion of dexbrompheniramine and 3 other drugs: blood 0.2 mg/L, liver 4.5 μg/g [R. C. Baselt and E. M. Gross, *J. Anal. Toxicol.*, 1977, *1*, 168–170].

Dose. Usually 8 mg of dexbrompheniramine maleate daily; up to 18 mg daily has been given in sustained-release preparations.

Dexchlorphenamine

Antihistamine

Synonym Dexchlorpheniramine
(+)-γ-(4-Chlorophenyl)-*N*,*N*-dimethyl-2-pyridinepropanamine
$C_{16}H_{19}ClN_2$=274.8
CAS—25523-97-1

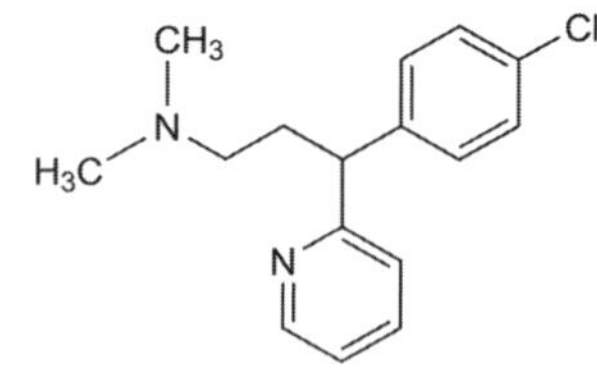

An oily liquid.
Soluble in chloroform.

Dexchlorphenamine Maleate
Proprietary names. Destral; Polaramin(e).
$C_{16}H_{19}ClN_2,C_4H_4O_4$=390.9
CAS—2438-32-6
A white crystalline powder. M.p. 113° to 115°.
Soluble 1 in 1.1 of water, 1 in 2 of ethanol and 1 in 1.7 of chloroform; very slightly soluble in ether.
For analytical data see under Chlorphenamine.

Disposition in the Body. See under Chlorphenamine. Dexchlorphenamine is more potent than chlorphenamine.

Dose. 6 to 8 mg of dexchlorphenamine maleate daily; up to 18 mg daily has been given in sustained-release preparations.

Dexketoprofen

NSAID

(*S*)-(+)-2-(3-Benzoylphenyl)propionic acid
$C_{16}H_{14}O_3$=254.3
CAS—22161-81-5

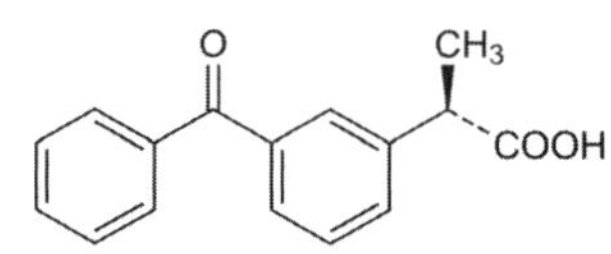

A white to off-white crystalline powder. M.p. 92° to 97°. Practically insoluble in water; freely soluble in alcohol, acetone and dichloromethane.

Dexketoprofen trometamol
Proprietary names. Enantyrum; Ketesse: Nosatal; Quiralem; Sympal; Viaxel.
$C_{16}H_{14}O_3.C_4H_{11}NO_3$=375.4
CAS—156604-79-4
A white crystalline powder with m.p. 103° to 107°. It is very soluble in water, methanol and dimethyl sulfoxide; fairly soluble in ethanol; slightly soluble in isopropyl alcohol; virtually insoluble in chloroform, ethyl ether and hexane.

For analytical data see under Ketoprofen.

Quantification
High performance liquid chromatography. In plasma: limit of quantification is 0.01 mg/L (reverse-phase column) and 0.08 mg/L (chiral column)—M. J. Barbanoj *et al.*, *J. Clin. Pharmacol.*, 1998, *38*, 33S–40S.

Disposition in the Body. Dexketoprofen is rapidly absorbed and metabolised to produce an acyl-glucuronide conjugate metabolite, which is easily hydrolysed in plasma and alkali conditions. The drug is excreted in urine as the conjugate and also as the unaltered form when the glucuronide undergoes hydrolysis, so the metabolic transfer is reversed. Between 73 and 82% of a dose is recovered in urine within the first 12 h.

Therapeutic concentration
9 healthy males and 9 females, aged between 19 and 34 years, were administered a single dose of dexketoprofen (25 mg) and a single dose of dexketoprofen trometamol (25 mg), equivalent to 25 mg dexketoprofen. For dexketoprofen, peak plasma concentrations of 2.02 ± 0.69 mg/L were reached within 0.5 to 3 h. For dexketoprofen trometamol, peak concentrations were 3.70 ± 0.72 mg/L 0.25 to 0.75 h after administration. [M. J. Barbanoj *et al.*, *J. Clin. Pharmacol.*, 1998, *38*, 33S–40S].

Toxicity. Gastro-intestinal toxicity can occur with potentially life threatening bleeding and perforations.

Half-life. 1.2 to 2.5 h.

Volume of distribution. Approx. 0.25 L/kg.

Clearance. Approx. 0.10 L/kg/h.

Protein binding. Dexketoprofen is bound 99.2%.

Dose. The usual dose is 12.5 mg every 4 to 6 h or 25 mg every 8 h. A maximum dose of 75 mg daily may be administered. In the elderly, a maximum dose of 50 mg daily may be given.

Dexmedetomidine

Analgesic/Anxiolytic/Sedative

Synonyms. D-form of Medetomidine; MPV-1440; (*S*)-Medetomidine.
Proprietary name. Precedex
4-[(1*S*)-1-(2,3-Dimethylphenyl)ethyl]-*1H*-imidazole
$C_{13}H_{16}N_2 = 200.3$
CAS—113775-47-6

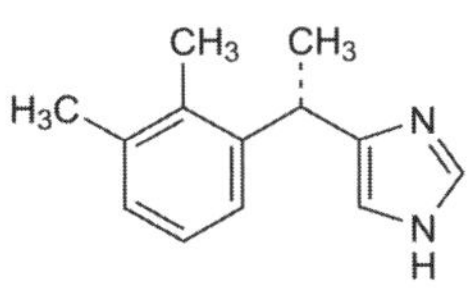

Quantification

Gas chromatography–mass spectrometry. In serum: limit of quantification 0.01 μg/L—L. Vuorilehto *et al.*, *J. Chromatogr.*, 1989, *497*, 282–287.

Therapeutic concentration

9 healthy male volunteers, mean age 23 years, were fasted overnight and supplied with a standard light breakfast prior to treatment with a transdermal patch (625 μg dexmedetomide base) which was placed on the forehead for 12 h or an intravenous dose of dexmedetomide hydrochloride. The intravenous dose was administered at a constant-rate infusion of 2 μg/kg for over 5 min. The mean peak plasma concentration for the transdermal patch was 0.51 μg/L (range 0.21 to 0.79 μg/L) observed at 6 (3 to 8) h. For the intravenous dose, a peak concentration of approx. 3.5 μg/L was reached by the end of the infusion. [K. T. Kivisho *et al.*, *Eur. J. Clin. Pharmacol.*, 1994, *46*, 345–349].

6 healthy males, 21 to 23 years old, were administered 0.5, 1.0 and 1.5 μg/kg doses of dexmedetomide after an overnight fast and standard light breakfast. At least 48 h was allowed between each dose. The peak plasma concentrations were 0.137, 0.257 and 0.335 μg/L for the three doses observed at 1.66, 1.57 and 1.63 h. [H. Scheinin *et al.*, *Clin. Pharmacol. Ther.*, 1992, *52*, 537–546].

Half-life. Mean, 2.1 h.

Volume of distribution. Apparent, mean, 2.30 L/kg.

Clearance. Total plasma, mean, 0.80 L/min.

Dexpanthenol

Vitamin B Activity

Synonyms. Dextro-Pantothenyl Alcohol; Pantothenol.
Proprietary names. Bepanthen(e); Ilopan; Motilyn; Panthoderm.
2,4-Dihydroxy-*N*-(3-hydroxypropyl)-3,3-dimethylbutanamide
$C_9H_{19}NO_4 = 205.3$
CAS—81-13-0

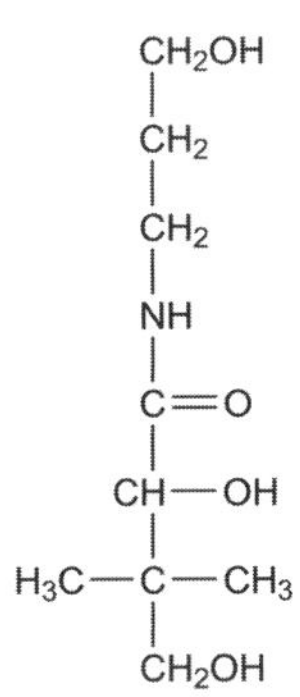

A clear, colourless or slightly yellow, hygroscopic, viscous liquid.
Freely soluble in water, ethanol and methanol; soluble 1 in 70 of chloroform and 1 in 200 of ether.

Partition Coefficient. Log *P* (octanol/water), −1.9.

Thin-layer Chromatography. System TA—Rf 70. (Acidified potassium permanganate solution, positive, developing slowly.)

Gas Chromatography. System GA—RI 1807.

Ultraviolet Spectrum. No significant absorption, 230 to 360 nm.

Infra-red Spectrum. Principal peaks at wavenumbers 1629, 1035, 1064, 1520, 1282, 1250 cm^{-1} (thin film).

Dose. Dexpanthenol has been given in doses of 250 to 500 mg intramuscularly.

Dexrazoxane

Cardioprotective

Synonyms. ADR-529; ICRF-187; NSC-169780; 2,6-Piperazinedione.
Proprietary names. Cardioxane; Eucardian; Zinecard.
(+)-(*S*)-4,4′-(1-Methyl-1,2-ethanediyl)bis-2,6-piperazinedione
$C_{11}H_{16}N_4O_4 = 268.3$
CAS—24584-09-6

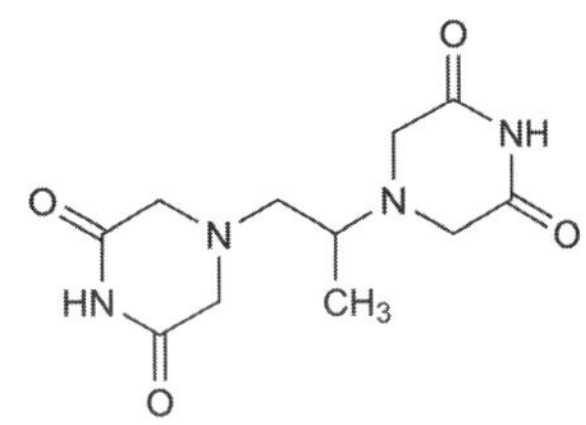

A whitish crystalline powder with m.p. 191° to 197°. It is sparingly soluble in water (approx. 14 g/L) and 0.1 M hydrochloric acid; slightly soluble in ethanol, methanol; practically insoluble in non-polar organic solvents.

Dissociation Constant. pK_a 2.1.

Partition Coefficient. Log *P* (octanol/water), 0.025.

High Performance Liquid Chromatography. Column: ODS2 (LKB Spherisorb, 3 μm). Mobile phase: ammonium formate (0.15 M, pH 7.4):methanol, composition increased linearly from 0 to 8% in 10 min, then to 80% in 20 min. 1 mL/min flow rate. Retention times: dexrazoxane, 17.1 min; diacid–diamide derivative, 3.7 min; monoacid–monoamide derivatives, 4.8 min; 4.1 min. [T. G. Burke *et al.*, *J. Pharm. Sci.*, 1991, *80*, 338–340].

Disposition in the Body. Dexrazoxane is distributed rapidly throughout the body and is hydrolysed, by dihydropyrimidine amidohydrolase (DHPase) to 1-ring and 2-ring open EDTA (ethylenediamminetetraacetate)-like products. Metabolites (active) include a diacid–diamide cleavage product and the two monoacid–monoamide ring products. Dexrazoxane is excreted in urine as the unchanged drug and the metabolites. Approximately 42% of a dose is recovered in urine.

Therapeutic concentration

Mean peak plasma concentrations can be detected at the end of a 15-min infusion and reach 0.0365 mg/L with a 500 mg/m^2 dose. [Pharmacie and UpJohn Company, Zinecard® (dexrazoxane for injection) prescribing information].

Toxicity. Haematological toxicity can occur, caused by chemotherapy, but is more common in dexrazoxane-treated patients. Dose-limiting leucopenia has been observed with doses > 4000 mg/m^2 dexrazoxane (on its own) but there is no evidence of cumulative toxicity.

Half-life. 2.1 to 2.5 h.

Volume of distribution. 22.0 to 22.4 L/m^2 (or 0.5 to 1.3 L/kg), tends to be higher in children compared with adults.

Clearance. Between 6.25 and 7.88 L/h/m^2, tends to be higher in children than adults.

Protein binding. < 2%.

Dose. In the USA: dexrazoxane is administered with doxorubicin or epirubicin in a 10:1 ratio; 500 mg/m^2 dose of dexrazoxane with 50 mg/m^2 doxorubicin or 1000 mg/m^2 with 100 mg/m^2 epirubicin. In Europe: the ratio is 20:1 with a maximum dose of 1000 mg/m^2 each cycle.

Dextromethorphan

Cough Suppressant

Synonyms. Deoxydihydrothebacodine; Methorphan.
(+)-3-Methoxy-17-methylmorphinan
$C_{18}H_{25}NO = 271.4$
CAS—125-71-3

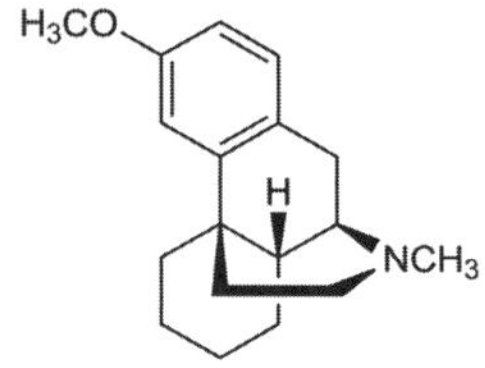

An almost white or slightly yellow crystalline powder. M.p. 109° to 113°. Practically insoluble in water; freely soluble in chloroform.

Dextromethorphan Hydrobromide

Synonyms. Ro-1-5470/5; Demorphan hydrobromide.
Proprietary names. Benylin Adult; Benylin DM; Benylin Pediatric; Benylin Dry Coughs Non-Drowsy; Creo-Terpin; Delsym; DexAlone; Diabe-Tuss DM; Franolyn Sedative; Hold DM; Nirolex for Dry Coughs; Pertussin; Robitussin for Dry Coughs; Robitussin Junior; Silphen DM; Strepsils Cough; Suppress; Trocal; Vicks Vaposray for Dry Coughs. It is an ingredient of many proprietary preparation—see *Martindale, The complete drug reference*, 33rd Edn., Pharmaceutical Press, London, 2002.
$C_{18}H_{25}NO,HBr,H_2O = 370.3$
CAS—125-69-9 (anhydrous); 6700-34-1 (monohydrate)
A white crystalline powder. M.p. 122° to 124°, with decomposition.
Soluble in water: 1 in 60 to 1 in 65 at 25°, 1 in 20 at 50°, 1 in 4 at 85°. Also soluble 1 in 10 of glycerol and 1 in 10 of ethanol; freely soluble in chloroform with the separation of water; practically insoluble in ether.

Dissociation Constant. pK_a 8.3.

Colour Tests. Aromaticity (Method 2) —yellow/orange-red; Liebermann's Test—black.

Thin-layer Chromatography. System TA—Rf 33; system TB—Rf 42; system TC—Rf 18; system TE—Rf 47; system TL—Rf 06; system TAE—Rf 10; system TAF—Rf 42. (Acidified iodoplatinate solution, positive.)

Gas Chromatography. System GA—dextromethorphan RI 2138, dextrorphan RI 2240.

High Performance Liquid Chromatography. System HA—dextromethorphan *k* 5.6 (tailing peak), dextrorphan *k* 4.7 (tailing peak); system HX—RI 377; system HY—RI 298; system HAA—rertention time 13.3 min.

Ultraviolet Spectrum. Aqueous acid—278 nm ($A^1_1 = 70a$). No alkaline shift.

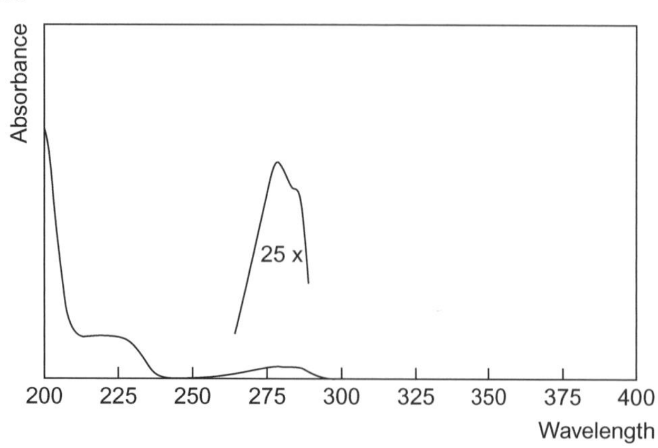

Infra-red Spectrum. Principal peaks at wavenumbers 1496, 1242, 1040, 1300, 1280, 1070 cm^{-1} (dextromethorphan hydrobromide, KBr disk).

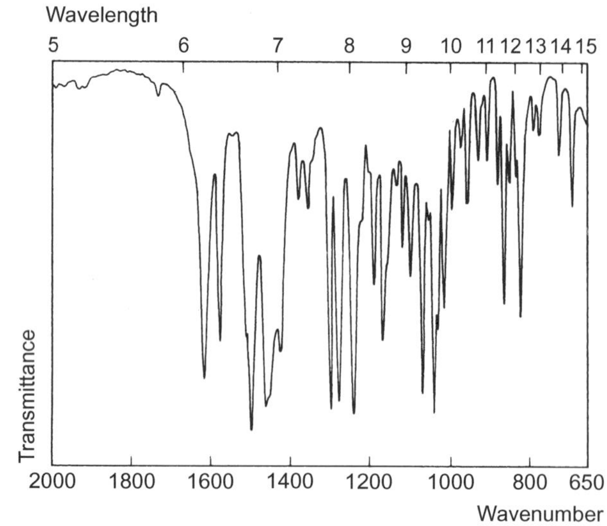

Mass Spectrum. Principal ions at *m/z* 59, 271, 150, 270, 31, 214, 42, 171; dextrorphan 59, 257, 150, 256, 31, 76, 42, 157.

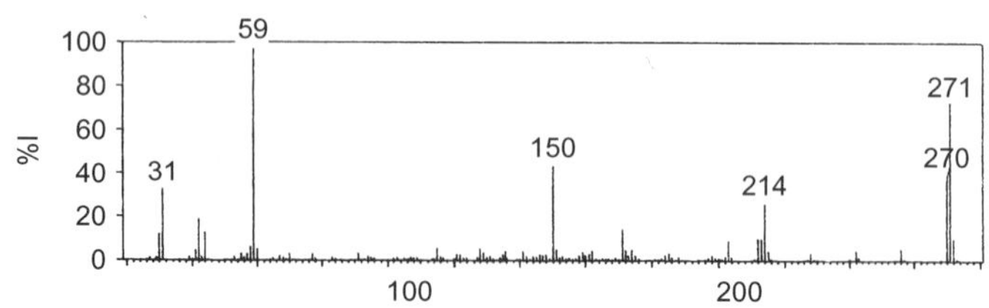

Quantification

Spectrofluorimetry. In plasma: dextrorphan—G. Ramachander *et al., J. Pharm. Sci.*, 1977, *66*, 1047–1048.

Gas chromatography. In serum: dextromethorphan, limit of detection 1 µg/L, ECD—J. W. Barnhart and E. N. Massad, *J. Chromatogr.* 1979, *163*(5) *B Biomed. Appl.*, 390–395. In liver microsomes: dextrorphan, ECD—M. Salsali *et al., J. Pharmacol. Toxicol. Methods*, 1999, *41*, 143–146. In urine: dextromethorphan and dextrorphan, limits of detection 81 µg/L and 40 µg/L, FID—Y. J. Wu *et al., J. Chromatogr. B Anal. Technol. Biomed. Life Sci.*, 2003, *784*, 219–224.

Gas chromatography–mass spectrometry. In urine: dextromethorphan and its metabolites, limit of detection for dextromethorphan 10 ng—Y. X. Xu *et al., Yao Xue Xue Bao*, 1993, *28*, 156–159.

High performance liquid chromatography. In plasma: dextrorphan, limit of detection 20 µg/L, fluorescence detection—R. Gillilan *et al., Anal. Lett.* (Part B), 1980, *13*, 381–387. In urine: dextromethorphan and metabolites, limit of detection 17 to 90 µg/L in non-hydrolysed urine and 110 to 210 µg/L in hydrolysed urine, UV detection—Y. H. Park *et al., J. Pharm. Sci.*, 1984, *73*, 24–29. In urine: dextromethorphan and dextrorphan, limits of quantification 50 µg/L—P. S. Marshall *et al., Ther. Drug Monit.*, 1992, *14*, 402–407. In urine: dextromethorphan and dextrorphan, limit of detection for dextromethorphan 20 µg/L, fluorescence detection, also UV detection—Y. W. Lam and S. Y. Rodriguez, *Ther. Drug Monit.*, 1993, *15*, 300–304. In urine: dextromethorphan and its metabolites, limit of quantification for dextromethorphan 2 µg/L, fluorescence detection—D. R. Jones *et al., J. Chromatogr.* 1996, *678 B Biomed. Appl.*, 105–111. In plasma: dextromethorphan and its metabolites, limit of quantification about 5 µg/L, fluorescence detection—S. Hartter *et al., Ther. Drug Monit.*, 1996, *18*, 297–303. In urine: dextromethorphan and its metabolites, limit of quantification 25 µg/L, fluorescence detection—R. A. Bartoletti *et al., J. Pharm. Biomed. Anal.*, 1996, *14*, 1281–1286. In urine: dextromethorphan and dextrorphan, limit of detection for dextromethorphan 23 µg/L, fluorescence detection—W. M. Cai *et al., Yao Xue Xue Bao*, 1997, *32*, 861–864. In urine: dextromethorphan and dextrorphan, limit of quantification about 50 µg/L, fluorescence detection—B. Mistry *et al., J. Pharm. Biomed. Anal.*, 1998, *16*, 1041–1049. In urine or microsomal preparations: dextromethorphan and its metabolites, limit of detection 2.7 µg/L, fluorescence detection—E. K. Bendriss *et al.*, *J. Chromatogr. B Biomed. Sci. Appl.*, 2001, *754*, 209–215.

High performance liquid chromatography–mass spectrometry. In plasma: dextromethorphan and dextrorphan, limit of quantification 5 ng/L—T. H. Eichhold *et al.*, *J. Mass Spectrom.*, 1997, *32*, 1205–1211. In plasma: limit of quantification 50 ng/L—T. H. Eichhold *et al.*, *J. Chromatogr. B Biomed. Sci. Appl.*, 1997, *698*, 147–154. In urine: dextromethorphan and its metabolites, limit of quantification for dextromethorphan 1 µg/L—S. S. Vengurlekar *et al.*, *J. Pharm. Biomed. Anal.*, 2002, *30*, 113–124.

Disposition in the Body. Well absorbed after oral administration. Metabolised by *N*- and *O*-demethylation followed by sulfate or glucuronic acid conjugation; *O*-demethylation involves the cytochrome P450 isoenzyme CYP2D6. The major metabolite is dextrorphan, (+)-3-hydroxy-*N*-methylmorphinan which has some activity; (+)-3-hydroxymorphinan has also been identified. About 50% of a dose is excreted in the urine in 24 h, mostly as the glucuronide and sulfate conjugates of the metabolites; about 8% of a dose is excreted as unchanged drug in 6 h.

Therapeutic concentration

Following a single oral dose of 30 mg to 6 subjects, a mean peak plasma concentration of 0.38 mg/L of conjugated dextrorphan was attained in 2 h. [G. Ramachander *et al.*, *J. Pharm. Sci.*, 1977, *66*, 1047–1048.]

After an oral dose of 20 mg of dextromethorphan hydrobromide given to 12 subjects, peak serum concentrations of less than 0.001 to 0.008 mg/L (mean 0.0018) of dextromethorphan were attained in about 2.5 h. [J. W. Barnhart and E. N. Massad, *J. Chromatogr.* 1979, *163*(5) *B Biomed. Appl.*, 390–395.]

Toxicity. The estimated minimum lethal dose is 0.5 g.

Of 2 cases of death following dextromethorphan intake in young people, the first was by suicide. In this case, an 18-year-old girl was found dead, with two empty bottles of tablets containing 30 mg dextromethorphan in her handbag (the quantity of tablets contained therein was not stated). The following blood and liver concentrations were reported, respectively: dextromethorphan 9.2 and 31.2 µg/g, dextrorphan 2.9 and 11.5 µg/g. In the second case, a 27-year-old man, in whom it was not known whether the overdose was intentional, the following blood and liver concentrations were reported: dextromethorphan 3.3 and 230 µg/g, dextrorphan 1.5 and 29.2 µg/g. [L. Rammer *et al.*, *Forensic Sci. Int.*, 1988, *37*, 233–236.]

Half-life. Reported as 3.2 to 3.6 h in rapid metabolisers.

Volume of distribution. Reported as 255 to 316 L/kg.

Dose. Up to 120 mg of dextromethorphan hydrobromide daily in divided doses.

Dextromoramide

Narcotic Analgesic

Synonyms. R-875; SKF-5137; Dextrodiphenopyrine; *d*-Moramid; Pyrrolamidol.

1-[(3*S*)-3-Methyl-4-(4-morpholinyl)-1-oxo-2,2-diphenylbutyl]pyrrolidine

$C_{25}H_{32}N_2O_2 = 392.5$

CAS—357-56-2

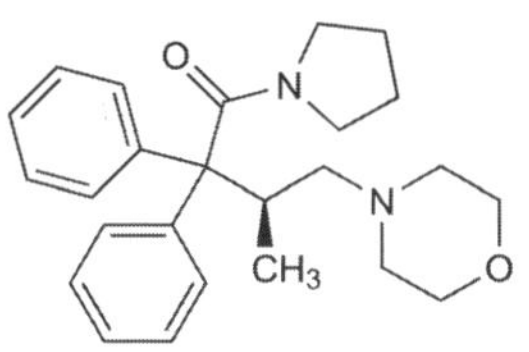

A white amorphous or microcrystalline powder. M.p. 180° to 184°.
Practically insoluble in water; solubility (g/100 mL): in ethanol 50, in methanol 40, in acetone 50, in ethyl acetate 40, in benzene 5, in chloroform 5; slightly soluble in ether.

Dextromoramide Tartrate

Synonyms. Dextromoramide Acid Tartrate; Dextromoramide Hydrogen Tartrate; Dextromoramidi Tartras.

Proprietary names. Dimorlin; Jetrium; Palfium; Palphium.

$C_{25}H_{32}N_2O_2,C_4H_6O_6 = 542.6$

CAS—2922-44-3

A white amorphous or crystalline powder. M.p. 189° to 192°, with slight decomposition.

Soluble 1 in 1 of ethanol, 1 in 1 acetone, 1 in 25 of water, and 1 in 40 of methanol; slightly soluble in chloroform and isopropyl alcohol; very slightly soluble in ether.

Partition Coefficient. Log *P* (octanol/water), 3.61.

Colour Test. Liebermann's Test (100°)—green.

Thin-layer Chromatography. System TA—Rf 73; system TB—Rf 42; system TC—Rf 71; system TE—Rf 79; system TL—Rf 60; system TAE—Rf 72; system TAF—Rf 78. (Dragendorff spray, positive; acidified iodoplatinate solution, positive.)

Gas Chromatography. System GA—dextromoramide RI 2940, M (OH-) RI 3095, M (OH-)-AC RI 3210, M (methoxy-) RI 3269; system GB—dextromoramide RI 3094, M (OH-) RI 3310; system GC—RI 3625.

High Performance Liquid Chromatography. System HA—*k* 0.7; system HC—*k* 0.09; system HX—RI 440; system HY—RI 390; system HAA—retention time 15.8 min.

Ultraviolet Spectrum. Aqueous acid—254, 259 (A^{1}_{1}=10.6a), 264 nm. No alkaline shift.

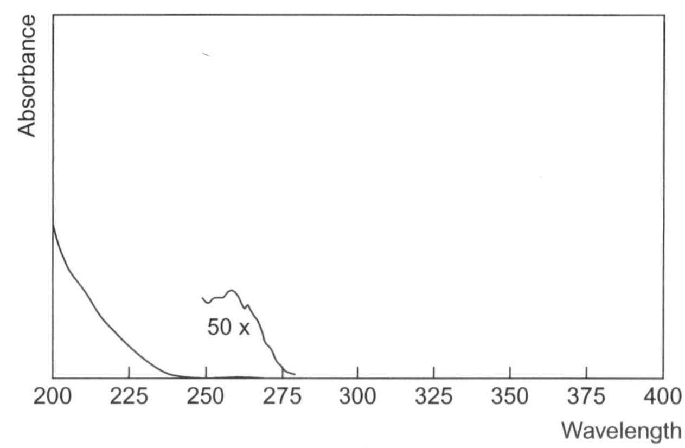

Infra-red Spectrum. Principal peaks at wavenumbers 1623, 703, 1107, 717, 858, 1002 cm^{-1} (Nujol mull).

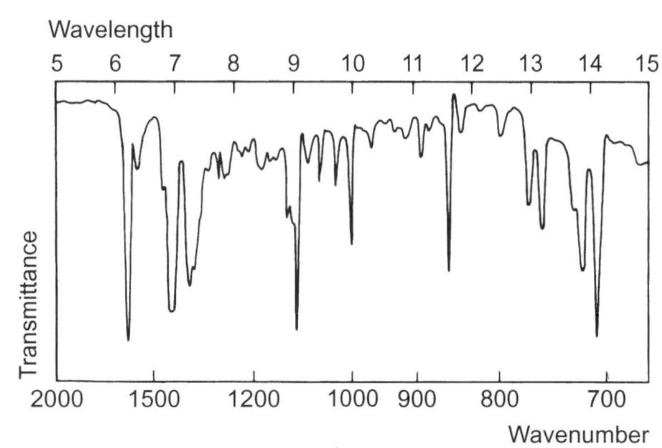

Mass Spectrum. Principal ions at *m/z* 100, 265, 128, 266, 44, 98, 56, 101.

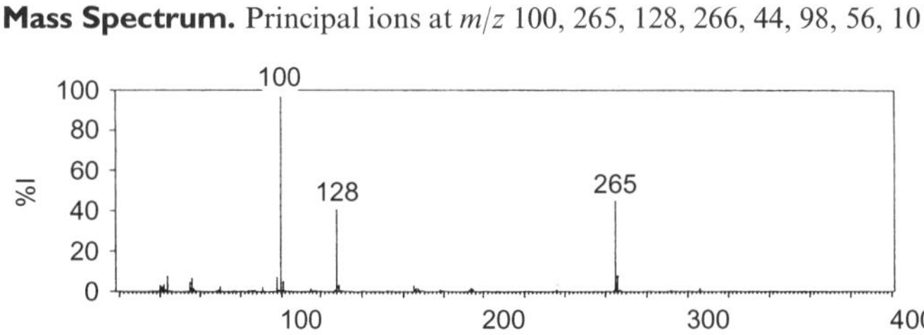

Quantification

Gas chromatography. In plasma: dextromoramide and other narcotic analgesics, limit of quantification 10 µg/L, nitrogen selective detection—P. Kintz *et al.*, *Methods Find. Exp. Clin. Pharmacol.*, 1990, *12*, 193–196.

Gas chromatography–mass spectrometry. In plasma or urine, limits of detection 0.5 μg/L and 0.3 μg/L respectively—P. Kintz *et al.*, *J. Anal. Toxicol.*, 1990, *14*, 252–253.

High performance liquid chromatography. In plasma or whole blood: UV detection—P. P. Rop *et al.*, *J. Chromatogr.*, 1992, *573*, 87–92. In postmortem blood: dextromoramide and dextropropoxyphene and its metabolite, photodiode-array detection—P. P. Rop *et al.*, *J. Chromatogr.*, 1993, *615*, 357–364. In plasma: dextromoramide in presence of methadone, UV detection—J. G. Ufkes *et al.*, *Pharm. World Sci.*, 1998, *20*, 83–87.

Disposition in the Body. Absorbed after oral administration. Metabolic reactions may include *N*-oxidation, hydroxylation, and amide hydrolysis; it is possible that 2-hydroxydextromoramide is a major metabolite. Excreted in the urine, partly as unchanged drug.

Therapeutic concentration

In 3 cancer patients receiving treatment with IV dextromoramide, 5 mg one to three times daily, the plasma level on the 4th day of treatment was 13.85 μg/L just before the first daily dose and 84.28 μg/L just after dosing. In one patient, the whole blood concentration was undetectable just before the dose and was 76 μg/L 30 min after dosing. [P. P. Rop *et al.*, *J. Chromatogr.*, 1992, *573*, 87–92.]

Toxicity. The estimated minimum lethal dose is 500 mg. Fatalities have occurred at blood concentrations greater than 0.04 mg/L.

In a fatality resulting from the abuse of dextromoramide and propoxyphene, the postmortem whole blood concentrations were 0.194 mg/L dextromoramide, 0.614 mg/L propoxyphene, and 1.1 mg/L norpropoxyphene. [P. P. Rop *et al.*, *J. Chromatogr.*, 1993, *61*, 357–364.]

A 38-year-old man was found in his car suffering from a heart attack. Serum analysis confirmed the presence of dextromoramide (Palfium), methadone, and lidocaine (lignocaine). The serum concentrations at admission to the hospital were: 1.9 mg/L of dextromoramide, 0.4 mg/L of methadone, and 0.4 mg/L of lidocaine. [E. Brewer, *J. Forensic Sci.*, 1990, *35*, 483–489.]

In 2 fatalities involving overdose resulting from the abuse of dextromoramide, the whole blood concentrations were 0.984 mg/L and 0.871 mg/L. [P. Kintz *et al.*, *J. Anal. Toxicol.*, 1989, *13*, 238–239.]

The following postmortem tissue concentrations were reported in a 31-year-old female who died after IV injection of dextromoramide: blood 1.526 mg/L, bile 0.494 mg/L, gastric contents (30 mL) 0.018 mg, kidney 0.131 μg/g, brain 0.065 μg/g, liver 0.391 μg/g; no other drugs were detected. [P. Kintz *et al.*, *J. Toxicol. Clin. Toxicol.*, 1989, *27*, 385–388.]

Dose. The equivalent of 5 to 20 mg of dextromoramide, repeated as necessary.

Dextropropoxyphene

Narcotic Analgesic

Synonym. Propoxyphene

(αS)-α-[(1R)-2-(Dimethylamino)-1-methylethyl]-α-phenylbenzene-ethanol propanoate

$C_{22}H_{29}NO_2=339.5$

CAS—469-62-5

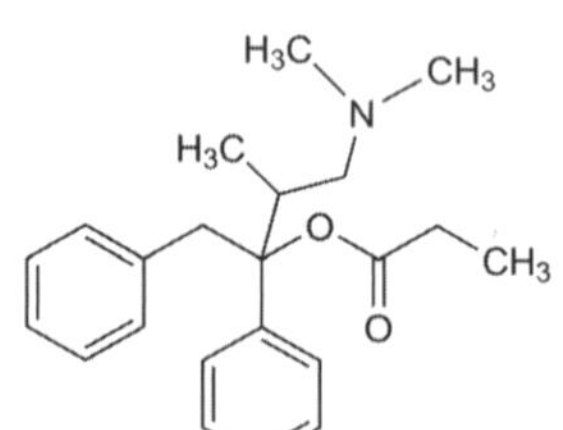

Crystals. M.p. 75° to 76°.
Very slightly soluble in water.

Dextropropoxyphene Hydrochloride

Synonym. Propoxyphene Hydrochloride

Proprietary names. Algaphan; Algodex; Antalvic; Daraphen; Darvon; Depronal; Depronal SA; Develin; Dolene; Dolocap; Erantin; Mardon; Novopropoxyn; Pro-65; Proxagesic; SK-65; 642 Tablets. It is an ingredient of Cosalgesic, Dextrogesic, and Distalgesic.

$C_{22}H_{29}NO_2,HCl=375.9$

CAS—1639-60-7

A white or slightly yellow powder. M.p. 163° to 169°.

Soluble 1 in 0.3 of water, 1 in 1.5 of ethanol, and 1 in 0.6 of chloroform; soluble in acetone; practically insoluble in benzene and ether.

Dextropropoxyphene Napsilate

Synonym. Propoxyphene Napsilate

Proprietary names. Darvon-N; Doloxene. It is an ingredient of Darvocet-N, Distalgesic Soluble, Dolasan, and Napsalgesic.

$C_{22}H_{29}NO_2,C_{10}H_8O_3S,H_2O=565.7$

CAS—17140-78-2 (anhydrous); 26570-10-5 (monohydrate)

A white powder. M.p. 158° to 165°.

Practically insoluble in water; soluble 1 in 13 to 1 in 15 of ethanol, and 1 in 3 of chloroform; soluble in acetone and methanol.

Dissociation Constant. pK_a 6.3.

Partition Coefficient. Log *P* (octanol/water), 4.2.

Colour Tests. Liebermann's Test—brown; Mandelin's Test—grey-brown; Marquis Test—black-violet→green.

Thin-layer Chromatography. System TA—Rf 68; system TB—Rf 59; system TC—Rf 55; system TAJ—Rf 33; system TAK—Rf 04; system TAL—Rf 51. (Dragendorff spray, positive; acidified iodoplatinate solution, positive; Marquis reagent, violet.)

Gas Chromatography. System GA—dextropropoxyphene RI 2188, norpropoxyphene RI 2214, M (nor-amide) RI 2526, M (nor-*N*-proponyl-) RI 2400, M (nor-)-AC RI 2365; system GB—dextropropoxyphene RI 2268, norpropoxyphene RI 2487, M (nor-amide) RI 2673, M (nor-*N*-proponyl-) RI 2514; system GC—dextropropoxyphene RI 2173; system GF—dextropropoxyphene RI 2370, norpropoxyphene RI 3025; system GM—RRT (relative to iprindole): dextropropoxyphene 1.220, norpropoxyphene 1.248, M (nor-amide) 1.969, M (nor-*N*-proponyl-) 1.300.

High Performance Liquid Chromatography. System HA—dextropropoxyphene *k* 1.9, norpropoxyphene *k* 1.3; system HC—*k* 0.19; system HY—RI 374; system HZ—retention time 7.6 min; system HAA—retention time 15.8 min.

Ultraviolet Spectrum. Aqueous acid—252, 257 ($A_1^1=12a$), 263 nm. No alkaline shift.

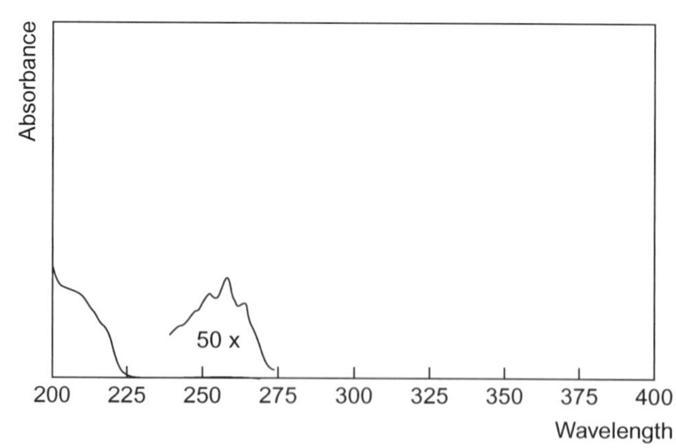

Infra-red Spectrum. Principal peaks at wavenumbers 1730, 1175, 725, 704, 776, 1026 cm^{-1} (Nujol mull).

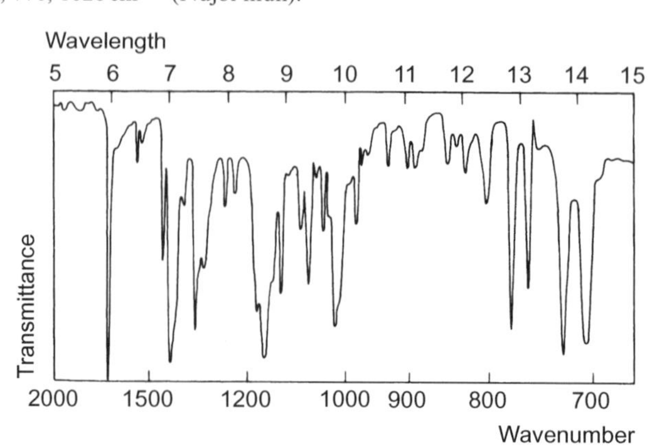

Mass Spectrum. Principal ions at *m/z* 58, 117, 208, 115, 193, 91, 179, 130 (no peaks above 210); norpropoxyphene 44, 208, 117, 58, 193, 130, 57, 29.

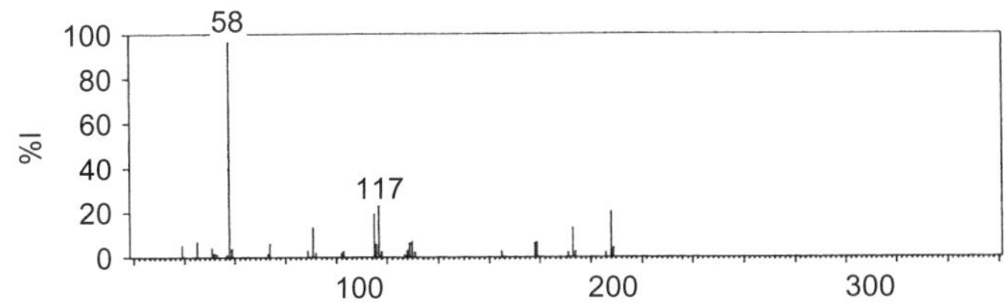

Quantification

Gas chromatography. In plasma: dextropropoxyphene and norpropoxyphene, FID—M. Cleeman, *J. Chromatogr.*, 1977, *132*, 287–294. In plasma: review of thermal decomposition of dextropropoxyphene during gas chromatography—B. J. Millard *et al.*, *J. Pharm. Sci.*, 1980, *69*, 1177–1179. In plasma or urine: limit of detection 50 µg/L for dextropropoxyphene and 100 µg/L for norpropoxyphene, AFID—P. A. Margot *et al.*, *J. Chromatogr. Sci.*, 1983, *21*, 201–204. In plasma: limit of detection dextropropoxyphene 6 µg/L and norpropoxyphene 12 µg/L—P. Kintz *et al.*, *J. Toxicol. Clin. Exp.*, 1990, *10(2)*, 89–94. In urine: limit of detection 27 µg/L for dextropropoxythene and for norpropoxythene 48 µg/L; limit of quantification 90 and 160 µg/L, respectively, FID—G. Amalfitano *et al.*, *J. Anal. Toxicol.*, 1996, *20(7)*, 547–554.

Gas chromatography–mass spectrometry. In hair and whole blood: limit of detection 0.05 µg/g and 0.07 mg/L, respectively, SIM—Y. Gaillard and G. Pepin, *J. Chromatogr. B Biomed. Sci. Appl.*, 1998, *709(1)*, 69–77. In hair: limit of detection dextropropoxyphene 26.4 µg/g and norpropoxyphene 71.0 µg/g—F. Mersch *et al.*, *Forensic Sci. Int.*, 1997, *84(1–3)*, 237–242.

High performance liquid chromatography. In hair: limit of detection dextropropoxyphene <1.0 µg/g and norpropoxyphene 1.5 µg/g—F. Mersch *et al.*, *Forensic Sci. Int.*, 1997, *84(1–3)*, 237–242. In plasma or breast milk: dextropropoxyphene and norpropoxyphene, limit of detection 20 µg/L, UV detection—R. L. Kunka *et al.*, *J. Pharm. Sci.*, 1985, *74*, 103–104.

Disposition in the Body. Readily and completely absorbed but undergoes considerable first-pass metabolism. Rapidly distributed and concentrated in the brain, lungs, liver, and kidneys. The main metabolic reaction is *N*-demethylation which produces norpropoxyphene, the major metabolite, and also dinorpropoxyphene which is dehydrated to cyclic dinorpropoxyphene. Norpropoxyphene has less than half the activity of dextropropoxyphene. In 24 h, about 35% of a dose is excreted in urine with about 13% of the dose as norpropoxyphene and up to 5% as unchanged drug. A total of 60 to 70% of a dose is excreted in urine in about 5 days; about 18% of the dose may be eliminated in the faeces over the same period.

Therapeutic concentration. In plasma, usually in the range 0.05 to 0.75 mg/L.

Peak plasma concentrations of dextropropoxyphene of 0.17 to 0.37 mg/L (mean 0.23) were attained 2 h after administration of a single oral dose of 130 mg to 6 subjects; peak norpropoxyphene concentrations of 0.19 to 0.42 mg/L (mean 0.27) were attained in 4 h. [K. Verebely and C. E. Inturrisi, *Clin. Pharmacol. Ther.*, 1974, *15*, 302–309.]

Following daily oral dosing of 195 mg to 3 subjects, steady-state plasma concentrations were: dextropropoxyphene 0.24 to 0.75 mg/L (mean 0.4); norpropoxyphene 0.6 to 3.0 mg/L (mean 1.5). [K. Verebely and C. E. Inturrisi, *J. Chromatogr.*, 1973, *75*, 195–205.]

Toxicity. The estimated minimum lethal dose is 0.5 g. Addicts can ingest 10 times the normal dosage before showing toxicity whereas children show toxic symptoms after only one-twentieth of the normal dose. Blood concentrations in the region of 1 mg/L are likely to cause toxic reactions; concentrations of 2 mg/L or more may be lethal.

In a review of a number of fatalities, blood concentrations in 23 cases ranged from 1 to 60 mg/L (mean 13) and liver concentrations in 73 cases ranged from 5 to 550 mg/kg (mean 97). [R. H. Cravey *et al.*, *J. Forensic Sci.*, 1974, *19*, 72–80.]

In 6 fatalities attributed to dextropropoxyphene overdose, the following postmortem tissue concentrations, mg/L or mg/kg (mean, *n*), were reported:

	Dextropropoxyphene	Norpropoxyphene
Blood	1.1–4.9 (3.5, *6*)	1.4–5.9 (3.5, *6*)
Brain	2.8–25.2 (14, *4*)	4.0–9.1 (6, *4*)
Liver	5.7–229 (117, *6*)	24.2–73.2 (50, *6*)
Urine	1.5–60.2 (17, *5*)	1.6–287 (68, *5*)

[A. J. McBay, *Clin. Chem.*, 1976, *22*, 1319–1321.]

30 hair samples from deceased drug addicts were analysed and the mean dextropropoxyphene concentration was 8.7 µg/g (range 0.24 to 27.41) and mean norpropoxyphene 24.1 (range 0.36 to 68.94) µg/g. [Y. Gaillard and G. Pepin, *J. Chromatogr. B Biomed. Sci. Appl.*, 1998, *709(1)*, 69–77.]

Bioavailability. About 40%.

Half-life. Plasma half-life, dextropropoxyphene 8 to 24 h (mean 15), norpropoxyphene 20 to 50 h (mean 29).

Volume of distribution. About 16 L/kg.

Clearance. Plasma clearance, about 15 mL/min/kg.

Protein binding. In plasma, about 70 to 80%.

Note. For a review of dextropropoxyphene pharmacokinetics and overdose, see R. J. Young, *Drugs*, 1983, *26*, 70–79.

Dose. Usually 195 to 260 mg of dextropropoxyphene hydrochloride, or 300 to 400 mg of the napsilate, daily.

Dextrorphan

Cough Suppressant

Synonym. Ro-1-6794

(+)-17-Methylmorphinan-3-ol

$C_{17}H_{23}NO$=257.4

CAS—125-73-5

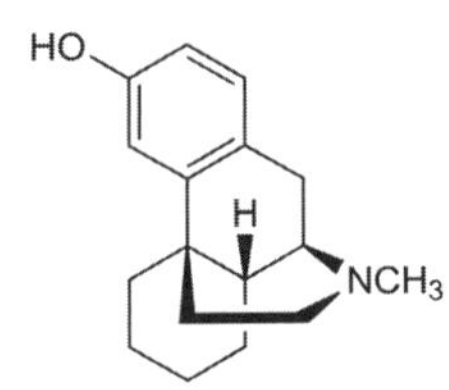

Crystals. M.p. 198° to 199°.

Partition Coefficient. Log *P* (octanol/water), 3.1.

Thin-layer Chromatography. System TA—Rf 35; system TB—Rf 14; system TC—Rf 04; system TE—Rf 42; system TL—Rf 03; system TAE—Rf 10; system TAF—Rf 49. (Dragendorff spray, positive; acidified iodoplatinate solution, positive.)

Gas Chromatography. System GA—dextrorphan RI 2230, dextrorphan-AC RI 2280, dextrorphan-PFP RI 2060, dextrorphan-TFA RI 2015, dextrorphan-TMS RI 2230, M (nor-) RI 2241, M (nor-)-AC_2 RI 2710, M (OH-)-AC_2 RI 2555; system GB—dextrorphan RI 2323, M (nor-) RI 2328.

High Performance Liquid Chromatography. System HA—*k* 4.7 (tailing peak); system HX—RI 325.

Ultraviolet Spectrum. Aqueous acid—279 (A_1^1=79a); aqueous alkali—240 (A_1^1=339a), 299 nm (A_1^1=119a).

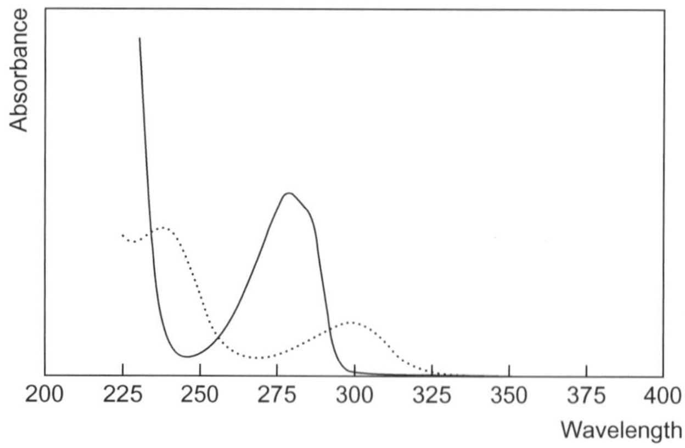

Infra-red Spectrum. Principal peaks at wavenumbers 1240, 1495, 1280, 1580, 756, 1610 cm^{-1} (KBr disk).

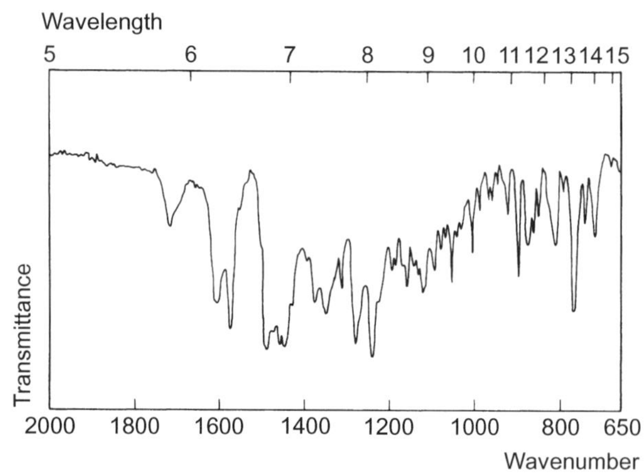

Mass Spectrum. Principal ions at *m/z* 59, 257, 150, 256, 31, 76, 42, 157; M (nor-) *m/z* 243, 157, 136, 198, 200, 242; M (OH-)-AC_2 *m/z* 357, 231, 356, 355, 298, 315.

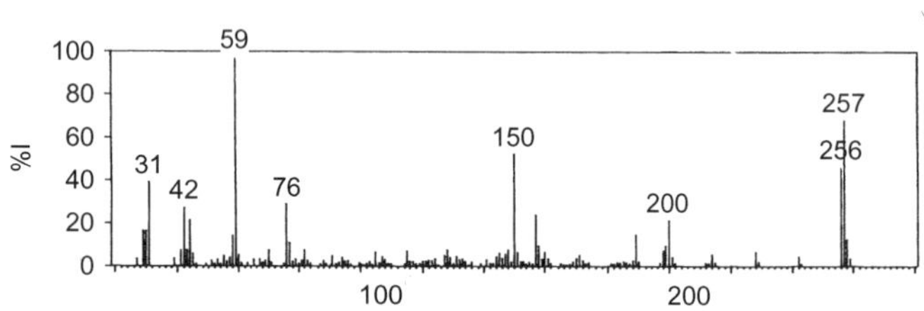

Quantification See under Dextromethorphan.

High Performance Liquid Chromatography. In plasma: limit of quantification 5 ng/L, MS/MS detection—T. H. Eichhold *et al.*, *J. Mass Spectrom.*, 1997, *32(11)*, 1205–1211. In plasma: limit of detection 20 µg/L, fluorescence detection (λ_{ex}=280 nm; λ_{em}=315 nm)—S. Stavchansky *et al.*, *J. Pharm. Biomed. Anal.*, 1995, *13(7)*, 919–925. In urine: limit of detection dextromethorphan 0.02 mg/L, fluorescence detection (λ_{ex}=280 nm; λ_{em}=310 nm)—Y. W. Lam and S. Y. Rodriguez, *Ther. Drug Monit.*, 1993, *15(4)*, 300–304.

Disposition in the Body. Dextrorphan is the major metabolite of dextromethorphan but has less antitussive activity.

Diamfenetide

Anthelmintic (Veterinary)

Synonym. Diamphenethide
Proprietary name. Coriban
N,N'-[Oxybis(2,1-ethanediyloxy-4,1-phenylene)]bisacetamide
$C_{20}H_{24}N_2O_5$=372.4
CAS—36141-82-9

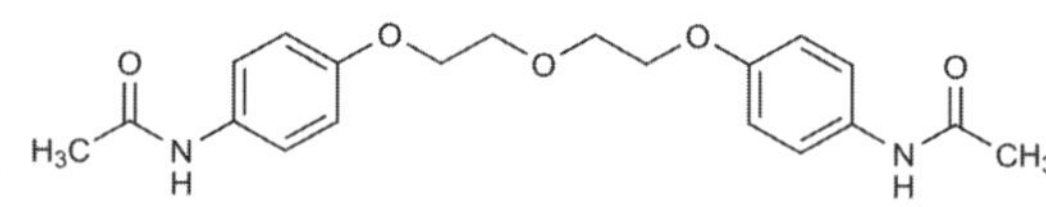

A white to pale buff-coloured powder.
Practically insoluble in water; soluble 1 in 160 of ethanol, 1 in 500 of chloroform and 1 in 150 of methanol; practically insoluble in ether.

Partition Coefficient. Log *P* (octanol/water), 1.8.

Colour Test. Mandelin's Test—grey-green.

Thin-layer Chromatography. System TA—Rf 81. (Acidified iodoplatinate solution, positive.)

Ultraviolet Spectrum. Aqueous acid—244 nm.

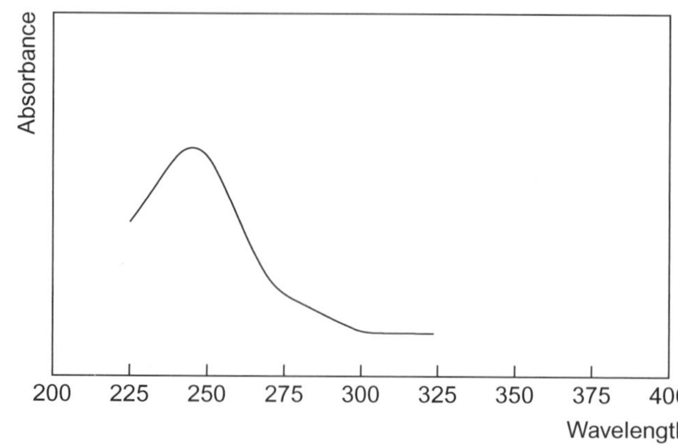

Infra-red Spectrum. Principal peaks at wavenumbers 1653, 1508, 1529, 1238, 1136, 1597 cm^{-1} (KBr disk).

Diamorphine

Narcotic Analgesic

Synonyms. Acetomorphine; Diacetylmorphine; Heroin.
(5α,6α)-7,8-Didehydro-4,5-epoxy-17-methylmorphinan-3,6-diol diacetate (ester)
$C_{21}H_{23}NO_5$=369.4
CAS—561-27-3

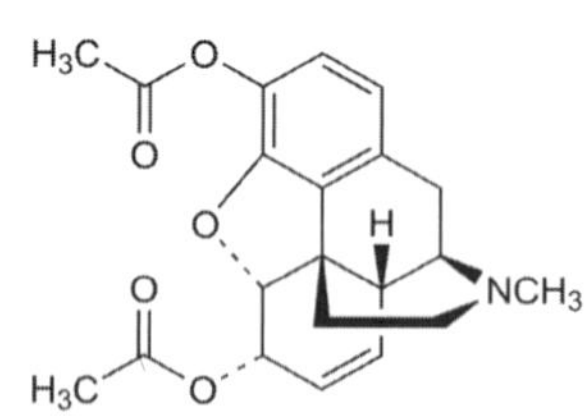

White crystals. M.p. 173°. It is rapidly hydrolysed by alkalis.
Soluble 1 in 1700 of water, 1 in 31 of ethanol, 1 in 1.5 of chloroform, and 1 in 100 of ether.

Diamorphine Hydrochloride

Proprietary names. Diagesil; Diamorf.
$C_{21}H_{23}NO_5,HCl,H_2O$=423.9
CAS—1502-95-0 (hydrate)
An almost white crystalline powder. M.p. 229° to 233°.
Soluble 1 in 2 of water, 1 in 11 of ethanol, and 1 in 1.6 of chloroform; insoluble in ether.
Diamorphine hydrolyses in aqueous solution to 3-*O*- and 6-*O*-monoacetylmorphine and morphine to a significant extent at room temperature.

Dissociation Constant. pK_a 7.6 (23°).

Partition Coefficient. Log *P* (octanol/water), 1.58.

Colour Tests. Liebermann's Test—black; Mandelin's Test—blue-grey; Marquis Test—violet

Thin-layer Chromatography. System TA—Rf 47; system TB—Rf 15; system TC—Rf 38; system TE—Rf 49; system TL—Rf 04; system TAE—Rf 26; system TAF—Rf 33; system TAJ—Rf 25; system TAK—Rf 05; system TAL—Rf 64. (Dragendorff spray, positive; acidified iodoplatinate solution, positive; Marquis reagent, violet.)

Gas Chromatography. System GA—diamorphine RI 2615, 6-monoacetylmorphine RI 2525, 3-monoacetylmorphine RI 2495, morphine RI 2445; system GB—diamorphine RI 2769, 6-monoacetylmorphine RI 2646, 3-monoacetylmorphine RI 2625, morphine RI 2564; system GAK—retention time 14.2 min.

High Performance Liquid Chromatography. System HA—diamorphine *k* 3.0 (tailing peak), 6-monoacetylmorphine *k* 3.6 (tailing peak), morphine *k* 3.8 (tailing peak); system HC—diamorphine *k* 0.66, 6-monoacetylmorphine *k* 0.80, morphine *k* 1.30; system HS—diamorphine *k* 0.35, 6-monoacetylmorphine *k* 1.00, morphine *k* 5.16; system HX—RI 340; system HY—RI 282; system HAX—retention time 7.9 min; system HAY—retention time 4.1 min; system HBC—retention time 2.9 min.

Ultraviolet Spectrum. Aqueous acid—279 nm (A_1^1=46a); aqueous alkali—299 nm (A_1^1=69a).

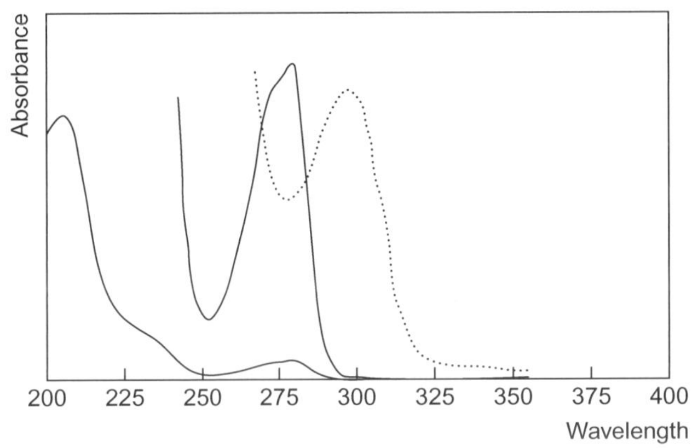

Infra-red Spectrum. Principal peaks at wavenumbers 1245, 1764, 1178, 1215, 911, 1736 cm^{-1} (diamorphine hydrochloride, Nujol mull). Two polymorphic forms may occur.

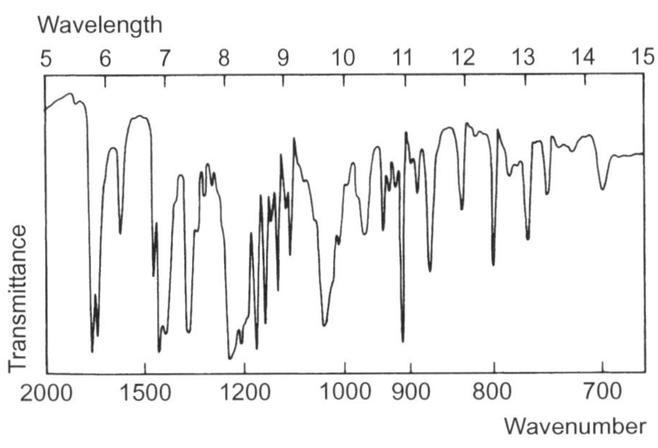

Mass Spectrum. Principal ions at *m/z* 327, 43, 369, 268, 310, 42, 215, 204; 6-monoacetylmorphine 327, 268, 42, 43, 215, 44, 328, 269; morphine 285, 162, 42, 215, 286, 124, 44, 284.

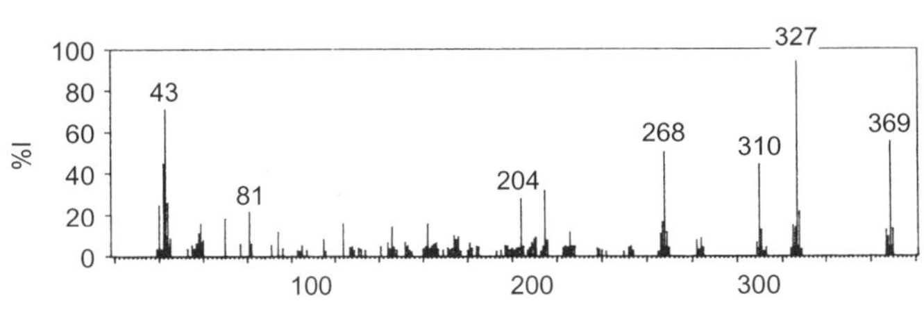

Quantification. (See also 6-monoacetylmorphine for additional systems.)

Gas chromatography. In blood: diamorphine and 6-monoacetylmorphine, limit of detection 100 µg/L, AFID—D. A. Smith and W. J. Cole, *J. Chromatogr.*, 1975, *105*, 377–381. In illicit heroin samples—G. Machata and W. Vycudlik, *J. Anal. Toxicol.*, 1980, *4*, 318–321.

Gas chromatography–mass spectrometry. In blood, plasma, saliva, or urine: diamorphine and its metabolites, limit of quantification 1 µg/L—B. A. Goldberger *et al.*, *Clin. Chem.*, 1993, *39*, 670–675. In hair: diamorphine and its metabolites—A. Polettini *et al.*, *Forensic Sci. Int.*, 1993, *63*, 217–225. In urine: metabolites, limit of detection 50 µg/L—N. De Giovanni *et al.*, *J. Chromatogr.*, 1994, *658 B Biomed. Appl.*, 69–73. In hair, plasma, saliva, or urine: limit of detection 0.1 µg/g in hair (diamorphine); 0.5 µg/g (normorphine) and 1 µg/L in plasma, saliva, and urine (diamorphine); 5 µg/L (normorphine)—W. L. Wang *et al.*, *J. Chromatogr.*, 1994, *660*; *Biomed. Appl.*, 279–290. In hair: diamorphine, other opioids, and cocaine—S. Pichini *et al.*, *J. Anal. Toxicol.*, 1999, *23*, 343–348. In meconium: diamorphine metabolites, limits of detection 2.5 to 20 ng/g—M. Y. Salem *et al.*, *J. Anal. Toxicol.*, 2001, *25*, 93–98.

High performance liquid chromatography. In illicit samples, using reversed phase ion-pair chromatography—I. S. Lurie *et al.*, *J. Forensic Sci.*, 1982, *27*, 519–526. In blood: diamorphine, 6-monoacetylmorphine, and morphine, limit of detection 12.5 µg/L, UV detection—J. G. Umans *et al.*, *J. Chromatogr.* 1982, *233 B Biomed. Appl.*, *22*, 213–225. In postmortem tissues and fluids: diamorphine, morphine, and hydromorphone, electrochemical detection—W. R. Sawyer *et al.*, *J. Forensic Sci.*, 1988, *33*, 1146–1155 and 1990, *35*, 520-523. In urine: heroin metabolites, limits of detection 4 to 20 µg/L—A. S. Low and R. B. Taylor, *J. Chromatogr.* 1995, *663 B Biomed. Appl.*, 225–233. In plasma: diamorphine and morphine and their metabolites, limit of quantification 25 µg/L, diode-array detection—D. Bourquin *et al.*, *J. Chromatogr. B. Biomed. Sci. Appl.*, 1997, *694*, 233–238.

High performance liquid chromatography–mass spectrometry. In serum: limit of quantification is 0.5 µg/L—P. Zuccaro *et al.*, *J. Anal. Toxicol.*, 1997, *21*, 268–277.

Disposition in the Body. Readily absorbed after oral administration or by injection. Following injection, it is rapidly hydrolysed to 6-monoacetylmorphine in blood and then more slowly metabolised to morphine which is the major active metabolite; normorphine is also formed to a minor extent; small quantities of codeine are occasionally seen in the urine of addicts, but this is thought to arise from the presence of acetylcodeine as an impurity in illicit heroin samples. The blood concentration of morphine depends on the route of administration of the drug, dose, time since last dose, and individual's metabolism. Orally administered diamorphine undergoes extensive first-pass metabolism to morphine. All metabolites may be conjugated with glucuronic acid. Up to 80% of a dose is excreted in the urine in 24 h, mainly as morphine-3-glucuronide with about 5 to 7% of the dose as free morphine, 1% as 6-monoacetylmorphine, 0.1% as unchanged drug, and trace amounts of other metabolites; after inhalation, 14 to 20% of the dose appears in the urine; morphine metabolites are excreted in the bile. Diamorphine crosses the blood–brain barrier within 15 to 20 s and achieves relatively high brain levels; 68% of an intravenous dose is absorbed into the brain.

Therapeutic concentration. Because of its rapid hydrolysis, diamorphine is difficult to detect in plasma. Morphine plasma concentrations are usually in the range 0.01 to 0.07 mg/L.

26 newborn premature neonates, with a gestational age of 26 to 40 weeks (mean 30.7 weeks), were administered with a loading dose of 50 µg/kg diamorphine over a 30 min period followed by a 15 µg/kg/h intravenous infusion for 14 to 149 h (mean 60.2 h). The mean steady-state plasma morphine concentration, after the 15 µg/kg/h dose, was 62.5 µg/L (20 to 98 µg/L). [D. A. Barrett *et al.*, *Br. J. Clin. Pharmacol.*, 1991, *32(1)*, 31–37.]

19 new-born infants of 24 to 41 weeks' gestation (mean 29.7 weeks), who were on ventilation, were administered with a loading dose of 50 µg/kg or 200 µg/kg diamorphine followed by 15 µg/kg/h as an intravenous infusion. The mean steady-state plasma morphine concentration was 86 µg/L after the 50 µg/kg and 200 µg/kg dose (20 to 215 µg/L for the 50 µg/kg loading dose and 14 to 146 µg/L for the 200 µg/kg dose). For morphine-3-glucuronide, steady-state was 703 µg/L (135 to 1237 µg/L and 45 to 1401 µg/L for the two loading doses, respectively) and morphine-6-glucuronide, 48 µg/L (35 to 91 µg/L for 50 µg/kg and 11 to 120 µg/L for 200 µg/kg). [D. A. Barrett *et al.*, *Br. J. Clin. Pharmacol.*, 1996, *41(6)*, 531–537.]

Diamorphine was detected in blood 2 minutes after an intravenous dose of 4 to 5 mg given to 4 subjects, but declined to a blood concentration of less than 0.01 mg/L within 10 to 15 minutes (C. E. Inturrisi *et al.*, *New. Engl. J. Med.*, 1984, *310*, 1213–1217).

Toxicity. Diamorphine is 2 to 3 times more potent than morphine. The estimated minimum lethal dose is 200 mg, but addicts may be able to tolerate up to 10 times as much; fatalities have occurred after doses of 10 mg.

A 17-year-old pregnant girl, a known drug abuser, was found dead in a public toilet with needle puncture marks. Postmortem examination carried out 48 h after death showed massive brain and lung oedema associated with an acute intoxication. In her femoral vein blood a 6-Monoacetylmorphine concentration of 4 µg/L was detected as well as 280 µg/L morphine and 20 µg/L codeine. In her urine 1170 µg/L was found. These were all consistent with a recent heroin intake. 6-monoacetylmorphine, morphine, morphine-3-glucuronide, and codeine were all detected in the fetus' amniotic fluid, brain and lung at high concentrations. [L. Potsch *et al.*, *Ther. Drug Monit.*, 1999, *21*, 593–597.]

A 40-year-old man with a long history of drug abuse was found dead after an overdose of heroin. Heroin was detected at a concentration of 0.109 mg/L in blood and 17 ng/g in gastro-intestinal content. Its metabolite, 6-monoacetylmorphine, was found at concentrations of 0.168 mg/L and 12 ng/g, respectively and morphine at 1.14 mg/L in blood and 425 ng/g in the gastro-intestinal contents. Morphine was also found in urine at a concentration of 3.65 mg/L. [P.P. Rop *et al.*, *J. Anal. Toxicol.*, 1997, *21(3)*, 232–235.]

Of 10 fatalities resulting from heroin overdoses via non-injection routes, 4 cases involved inhalation ('chasing'), 4 involved nasal administration ('snorting'), and 2 involved oral ingestion; in one case the deceased was observed to smoke a heroin cigarette and then snort heroin immediately before losing conciousness. In 9 of the cases, venepuncture marks were detected postmortem. The median blood morphine concentration was 0.31 mg/L (range 0.06 to 0.99). Drugs other than morphine were also detected in 7 cases (alcohol (4), cocaine (2), dosulepin, methadone and paracetamol (1 each)). [S. Darke and J. Ross, *Addiction*, 2000, *95*, 569–573.]

A 46-year-old man died after injecting heroin into his penis. The concentration of morphine in body fluids at postmortem were: blood 0.68 mg/L, urine 0.49 mg/L, bile 0.32 mg/L, and vitreous humour 0.062 mg/L; ethanol was also detected in these fluids. [C. L. Winek *et al.*, *Am. J. Forensic Med. Pathol.*, 1999, *20*, 90–92.]

Of 10 deaths involving heroin body-packers, 4 had morphine blood concentrations <1 mg/L. In the others, morphine concentrations were 4.4, 6.7, 35.8, 39.4, and 52.6 mg/L, respectively. One victim, who died of peritonitis, had no detectable morphine in the blood. [C. V. Wetli *et al.*, *Am. J. Forensic Med. Pathol.*, 1997, *18*, 312–318.]

Half-life. Plasma half-life, diamorphine about 3 min, 6-monoacetylmorphine about 6 to 25 min, morphine about 2 to 3 h.

Volume of distribution. Diamorphine, 25 L/kg. Morphine about 3 to 5 L/kg.

Clearance. Plasma clearance, morphine about 15 to 20 mL/min/kg; new-born infants (24 to 41 weeks' gestation), 4.6 mL/min/kg.

Protein binding. In plasma, morphine about 20 to 35%.

Note. For a review of the pharmacokinetics and pharmacodynamics of smoked heroin, see A. J. Jenkins *et al.*, *J. Anal. Toxicol.*, 1994, *18*, 317–330. For reports of heroin use when driving, see G. Ceder and A. W. Jones, *J. Forensic Sci.*, 2002, *47*, 366–368. For a review of the metabolism and excretion of diamorphine, see U. Boerner *et al.*, *Drug Metab. Rev.*, 1975, *4*, 39–73. For a review of fatal heroin overdose, see S. Darke and D. Zador, *Addiction*, 1996, *91*, 1765–1772; for a review of the formation and clearance of active and inactive metabolites of opiates in humans, see R. E. Aderjan and G. Skopp, *Ther. Drug Monit.*, 1998, *20*, 561–569.

Dose. For acute pain, 5 to 10 mg of diamorphine hydrochloride every 4 h by subcutaneous or intramuscular injection.

Diamthazole

Antifungal

Synonyms. Amycazol; Dimazole.

6-[2-(Diethylamino)ethoxy]-*N*,*N*-dimethyl-2-benzothiazolamine

$C_{15}H_{23}N_3OS = 293.4$

CAS—95-27-2

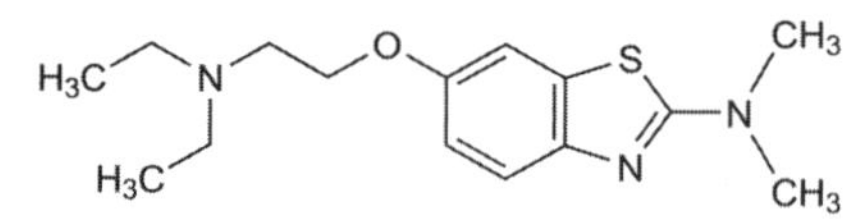

Diamthazole Hydrochloride

Proprietary name. Asterol

$C_{15}H_{23}N_3OS,2HCl = 366.4$

CAS—136-96-9

A white, hygroscopic, crystalline powder. M.p. 240° to 243°.

Soluble in water, ethanol and methanol; very slightly soluble in chloroform and ether.

Partition Coefficient. Log *P* (octanol/water), 2.5 (hydrochloride).

Colour Test. Liebermann's Test—green.

Thin-layer Chromatography. System TA—Rf 52; system TB—Rf 30; system TC—Rf 30. (Acidified iodoplatinate solution, positive.)

Ultraviolet Spectrum. Aqueous acid—270 nm ($A_1^1 = 370b$), 293 nm.

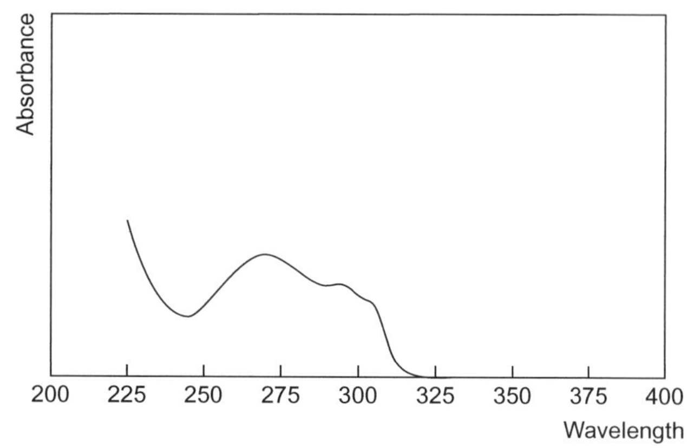

Infra-red Spectrum. Principal peaks at wavenumbers 1015, 1041, 667, 1548, 1602, 1190 cm^{-1} (KBr disk).

Mass Spectrum. Principal ions at *m/z* 86, 100, 44, 30, 29, 42, 58, 56.

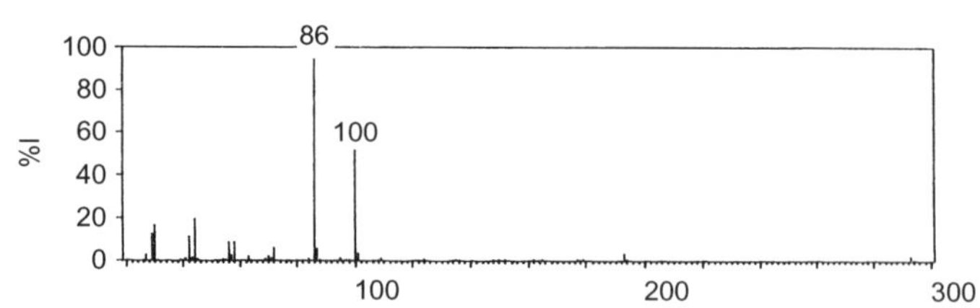

Use. Diamthazole hydrochloride has been used in a concentration of 5%.

Diaveridine

Coccidiostat (Veterinary)

Proprietary name. It is an ingredient of Saquadil.

5-[(3,4-Dimethoxyphenyl)methyl]-2,4-pyrimidinediamine

$C_{13}H_{16}N_4O_2 = 260.3$

CAS—5355-16-8

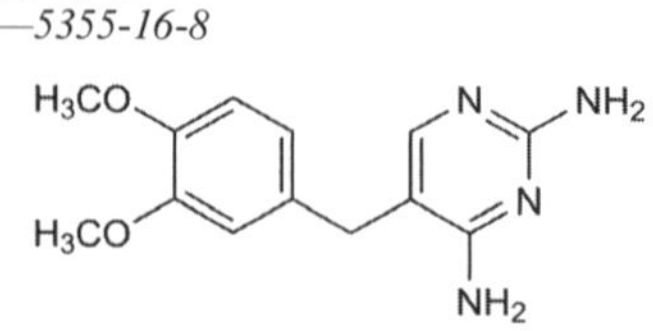

A white or creamy-white crystalline powder. M.p. 233°.

Very slightly soluble in water and ethanol; soluble 1 in 600 of chloroform.

Partition Coefficient. Log *P* (octanol/water), 1.0.

Colour Tests. Mandelin's Test—green; Marquis Test—grey→violet-brown.

Thin-layer Chromatography. System TA—Rf 58. (Acidified iodoplatinate solution, positive.)

High Performance Liquid Chromatography. System HAA—Retention time, 7.0 min.

Ultraviolet Spectrum. Aqueous acid—276 nm (A_1^1=300a).

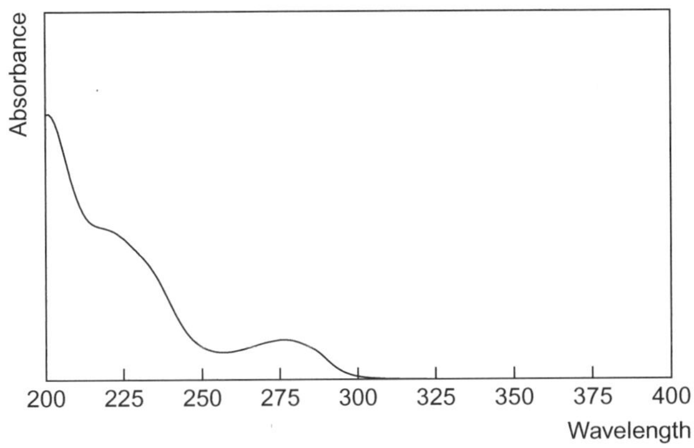

Infra-red Spectrum. Principal peaks at wavenumbers 1630, 1645, 1598, 1250, 1510, 1570 cm^{-1} (KBr disk).

Diazepam

Tranquilliser

Synonyms. Diazepamum; LA-III; NSC-77518; Ro-5-2807; Wy-3467.
Proprietary names. Antenex; Anxicalm; Apozepam; Dialar; Diapam; Diazemuls; Diazep; Ducene; Faustan; Gewacalm; Hexalid; Lamra; Med-ipam; Novazam; Novodipam; Pro-Pam; Psychopax; Rimapam; Serenack; Stesolid; Tensium; Tranquase; Umbrium; Valaxona; Valclair; Valiquid; Valium; Vivol.
7-Chloro-1,3-dihydro-1-methyl-5-phenyl-2*H*-1,4-benzodiazepin-2-one
$C_{16}H_{13}ClN_2O$=284.7
CAS—439-14-5

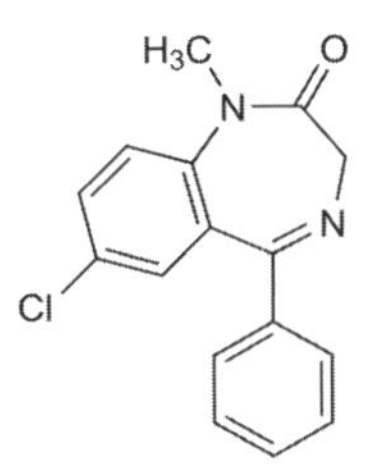

A white or yellow crystalline powder. M.p. 131° to 135°.
Slightly soluble in water; soluble 1 in 25 of ethanol, 1 in 2 of chloroform, and 1 in 39 of ether.

Dissociation Constant. pK_a 3.3 (20°).

Partition Coefficient. Log *P* (octanol/pH 7.4), 2.7.

Colour Test. Formaldehyde–Sulfuric Acid—orange.

Thin-layer Chromatography. System TA—Rf 75; system TB—Rf 27; system TC—Rf 73; system TD—Rf 58; system TE—Rf 76; system TF—Rf 49; system TL—Rf 59; system TAD—Rf 72; system TAE—Rf 82; system TAF—Rf 85; system TAJ—Rf 67; system TAK—Rf 48; system TAL—Rf 96. (Dragendorff spray, positive; FPN reagent, yellow; acidified iodoplatinate solution, positive; Marquis reagent, yellow.)

Gas Chromatography. System GA—diazepam RI 2428, nordazepam RI 2490, oxazepam RI 2325, temazepam RI 2595; system GB—diazepam RI 2556, nordazepam RI 2625, oxazepam RI 2438, temazepam RI 2727; system GF—diazepam RI 3045; system GG—diazepam RI 2940, nordazepam RI 3041, oxazepam RI 2803, temazepam RI 3125.

High Performance Liquid Chromatography. System HA—diazepam *k* 0.1, nordazepam *k* 0.2; system HI—diazepam *k* 9.47, nordazepam *k* 8.00, oxazepam *k* 4.62, temazepam *k* 5.68; system HJ—diazepam *k* 2.29; system HK—diazepam *k* 2.49, nordazepam *k* 1.99, oxazepam *k* 0.73, temazepam *k* 0.60; system HX—RI 528; system HY—RI 429; system HZ—retention time 8.4 min; system HAA—retention time 20.3 min; system HAL—retention time 13.2 min; system HAF—retention time 29.8 min; system HAX—diazepam retention time 7.7 min, nordazepam 6.7 min, oxazepam 6.0 min, temazepam 8.9 min; system HAY—diazepam retention time 8.8 min, nordazepam 6.8 min, oxazepam 4.5 min, temazepam 6.7 min; system HAM—diazepam retention time 10.3 min, oxazepam 3.4 min and 4.4 min; system HAZ—*k* 2.25; system HBH—diazepam *k* 10.4, nordazepam *k* 8.97, oxazepam *k* 5.42, temazepam *k* 6.80; system HBI—diazepam *k* 2.29, nordazepam *k* 1.89, oxazepam *k* 1.25, temazepam *k* 1.49.

Ultraviolet Spectrum. Aqueous acid—242 (A_1^1=1020a), 284, 366 nm.

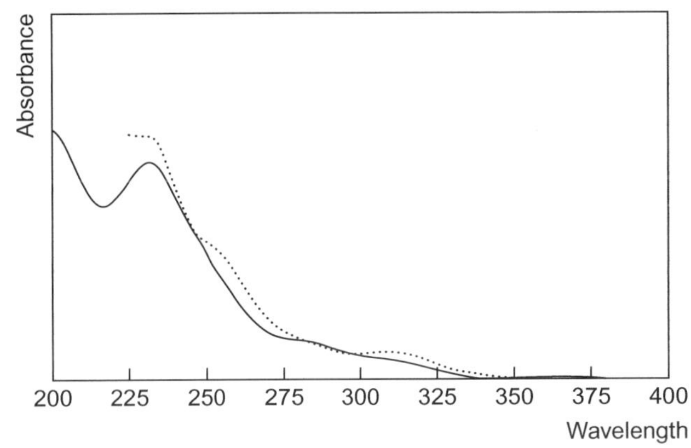

Infra-red Spectrum. Principal peaks at wavenumbers 1681, 1313, 705, 840, 1125, 740 cm^{-1} (KBr disk).

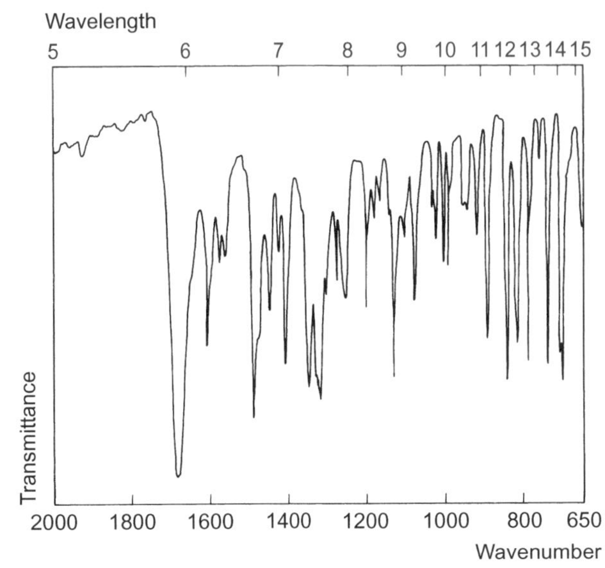

Mass Spectrum. Principal ions at *m*/*z* 256, 283, 284, 285, 257, 255, 258, 286; desmethyldiazepam (nordazepam) 242, 269, 270, 241, 243, 271, 244, 272; oxazepam 257, 77, 268, 239, 205, 267, 233, 259; temazepam 271, 273, 300, 272, 256, 77, 255, 257.

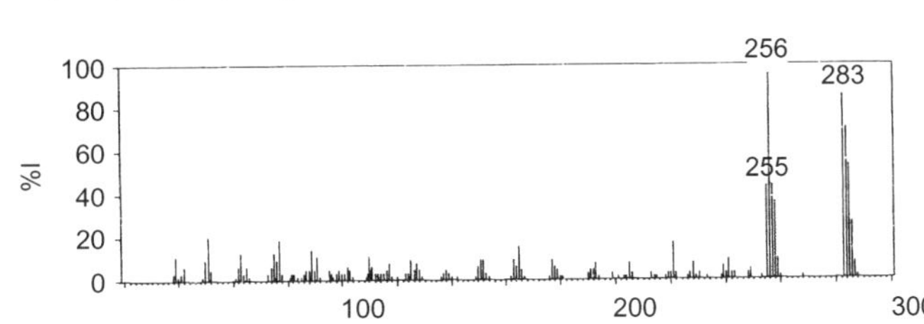

Quantification

Gas chromatography. In plasma or blood: diazepam and other benzodiazepines, ECD and NPD—P. Lillsunde and T. Seppala, *J. Chromatogr.*, 1990, *30*, 97–110. In blood: diazepam and other benzodiazepines, limits of detection >5.6 µg/L, ECD—H. Gjerde *et al.*, *J. Pharm. Biomed. Anal.*, 1992, *10*, 317–322. In plasma: diazepam and other benzodiazepines, ECD and NPD—Y. Gaillard *et al.*, *J. Chromatogr.*, 1993, *622*, 197–208. In plasma: limit of detection 2.9 µg/L, NPD—M. Krogh *et al.*, *J. Chromatogr. B Biomed. Sci. Appl.*, 1997, *689*, 357–364. In plasma or urine: diazepam and other benzodiazepines, limits of detection >2.9 µg/L—K. J. Reubsaet *et al.*, *J. Pharm. Biomed. Anal.*, 1998, *18*, 667–680. In plasma or urine: diazepam and *N*-desmethyldiazepam, limits of detection 5.8 to 31.0 µg/L, NPD—H. G. Ugland *et al.*, *J. Chromatogr. B Biomed. Sci. Appl.*, 2000, *749*, 85–92.

Gas chromatography–mass spectrometry. In blood: diazepam and other benzodiazepines, limits of detection 0.2 to 20 µg/L—H. Inoue *et al.*, *Forensic Sci. Int.*, 2000, *113*, 367–373.

High performance liquid chromatography. In serum: diazepam and oxazepam—A. Goldnik *et al.*, *Acta Pol. Pharm.*, 1993, *50*, 421–422. In plasma: diazepam and desmethyldiazepam—F. Kamali, *J. Pharm. Biomed. Anal.*, 1993, *11*, 625–627. In plasma: diazepam, clobazam, and their metabolites—C. Lacroix *et al.*, *J. Chromatogr.*, 1993, *617*, 285–290. In plasma: diazepam, and theophylline, limit of quantification for diazepam 0.1 ng, UV detection—H. Iwase *et al.*, *J. Chromatogr.* 1994, *655 B Biomed. Appl.*, 73–81 and H. Iwase *et al.*, *J. Chromatogr.* 1994, *660 B Biomed. Appl.*, 422. In urine: diazepam metabolites, limit of detection 2 µg/L—K. Chiba *et al.*, *J. Chromatogr. B Biomed. Appl.*, 1995, *668*, 77–84. In serum: diazepam and nitrazepam, limit of quantification 1 µg/L—B. Welk, *Acta Pol. Pharm.*, 1996, *53*, 3–6. In serum: diazepam and other benzodiazepines, UV detection—E. Tanaka *et al.*, *J. Chromatogr. B Biomed. Appl.*, 1996, *682*, 173–178 and E. Tanaka *et al.*, *J. Chromatogr. B Biomed. Appl.*, 1998, *709*, 324. In plasma or urine: limit of quantification and detection is 10 µg/L for diazepam and *N*-desmethyldiazepam, UV detection (λ = 232 nm)—R. M. Azzam *et al.*, *J. Chromatogr. B Biomed. Sci. Appl.*, 1998, *708*, 304–309. In plasma: diazepam and nordazepam—J. Atta-Politou *et al.*, *J. Pharm. Biomed. Anal.*, 1999, *20*, 389–396. In urine: diazepam and other benzodiazepines—M. Segura *et al.*, *J. Anal. Toxicol.*, 2001, *25*, 130–136. In whole blood: diazepam and other benzodiazepines, limit of quantification for diazepam 25 µg/L, diode-array detection—A. El Mahjoub and C. Staub, *J. Anal. Toxicol.*, 2001, *25*, 209–214. In plasma: limit of detection 5 µg/L, UV detection—S. N. Muchoh *et al.*, *J. Chromatogr. B Biomed. Sci. Appl.*, 2001, *761*, 255–259. In hair: diazepam and other benzodiazepines, limit of quantification for diazepam 0.5 ng/mg, photodiode-array detection—A. El Mahjoub and C. Staub, *Forensic Sci. Int.*, 2001, *123*, 17–25. In urine: diazepam and other benzodiazepines, limit of detection for diazepam 46 µg/L, UV detection—W. M. Mullett and J. Pawliszyn, *Anal. Chem.*, 2002, *74*, 1081–1087.

High performance liquid chromatography–mass spectrometry. In serum or urine: diazepam and other benzodiazepines, limit of quantification 2 µg/L—M. Kleinschnitz *et al.*, *J. Chromatogr.* 1996, *676 B Biomed. Appl.*, 61–67.

Disposition in the Body. Rapidly and completely absorbed after oral administration, with peak plasma levels occurring within about 30 to 90 min. The main metabolic reactions are *N*-demethylation, 3-hydroxylation, and glucuronic acid conjugation. The major active metabolite is desmethyldiazepam [nordazepam] which accumulates during chronic dosing; other metabolites include oxazepam and temazepam, both of which are active. The formation of nordazepam and oxazepam is catalysed by the P450 isoenzymes CYP2C19 and CYP3A. Only small traces of unchanged diazepam are excreted in the urine and the relative amounts of metabolites are variable and appear to be dose-dependent. About 70% of a dose is excreted in the urine, mainly as oxazepam glucuronide and conjugated desmethyldiazepam, together with smaller amounts of conjugated temazepam. About 10% of the dose may be eliminated in the faeces. Diazepam and its metabolites cross the blood–brain barrier and the placeta; they are also found in breast milk.
Diazepam is a metabolite of ketazolam and medazepam.

Therapeutic concentration. In plasma, usually in the range 0.1 to 1.0 mg/L. After discontinuation of chronic therapy, concentrations of desmethyldiazepam may be substantially higher than diazepam and both unchanged drug and metabolite are still detectable 7 days after cessation of dosing.

Following a single oral dose of 10 mg to 4 subjects, peak blood concentrations of 0.14 to 0.19 mg/L (mean 0.15) were attained in 1 to 1.5 h; average peak concentrations of 0.03 mg/L of desmethyldiazepam were attained after 24 h. [S. A. Kaplan *et al.*, *J. Pharm. Sci.*, 1973, *62*, 1789–1796.]

After chronic daily oral dosing of 5 mg twice daily to 15 subjects, steady-state plasma concentrations were: diazepam 0.09 to 0.37 mg/L (mean 0.23), desmethyldiazepam 0.13 to 0.46 mg/L (mean 0.29), oxazepam 0.01 to 0.03 mg/L (mean 0.02), temazepam 0.01 to 0.05 mg/L (mean 0.03). [I. A. Zingales, *J. Chromatogr.*, 1973, *75*, 55–78.]

After intranasal administration of diazepam to 9 healthy subjects (20 mg/mL solution; 100 µL into 1 nostril ≡ 2 mg dose), a mean serum plasma concentration of 0.039 mg/L was attained in 18 min; this equated to 32.9% of the concentration that was attained 10 min after the same dose given IV to the same subjects. [S. Gizurarson *et al.*, *Biol. Pharm. Bull.*, 1999, *22*, 425–427.]

Toxicity. Toxic effects may be produced by blood concentrations greater than 1.5 mg/L; fatalities caused by diazepam alone are rare, but may occur at blood concentrations greater than 5 mg/L.

In a review of 914 drug-related deaths in which diazepam was involved it was found to be the sole cause of death in only 2 cases; postmortem concentrations of diazepam in the 2 cases were: blood 5 and 19 mg/L, liver 13 mg/kg in the first case. [B. S. Finkle *et al. JAMA.*, 1979, *242*, 429–434.]

In a fatality due to diazepam and alcohol ingestion, postmortem tissue-diazepam concentrations were: blood 1.3 mg/L, bile 4.5 mg/L, brain 2.4 µg/g, kidney 11.7 mg/kg, liver 11.4 mg/kg, urine 6.6 mg/L. [R. K. Simon, *Bull. Int. Assoc. Forensic Toxicol.*, 1976, *12(1)*, 19–20.]

Half-life. Plasma half-life, diazepam 20 to 40 h, desmethyldiazepam about 40 to 100 h but there is considerable intersubject variation— see under Nordazepam. The plasma half-life appears to be increased in elderly subjects and neonates, and in subjects with liver disease; sex differences have also been suggested.

Volume of distribution. Diazepam and desmethyldiazepam 0.5 to 2.5 L/kg, increased in elderly subjects.

Clearance. Plasma clearance, diazepam about 0.3 to 0.5 mL/min/kg, desmethyldiazepam about 0.1 to 0.3 mL/min/kg.

Distribution in blood. Plasma:whole blood ratio, diazepam 1.8, desmethyldiazepam 1.7.

Protein binding. In plasma, diazepam 98 to 99%, desmethyldiazepam about 97%.

Note. For reviews of the clinical pharmacokinetics of diazepam, see M. Mandelli *et al.*, *Clin. Pharmacokinet.*, 1978, *3*, 72–91 and H. Friedman *et al.*, *Clin. Pharmacol. Ther.*, 1992, *52*, 139–150.

Dose. Usually 5 to 30 mg daily.

Diazoxide

Antihypertensive/Hyperglycaemic

Synonym. SRG-95213
Proprietary names. Eudemine; Hyperstat; Hypertonalum; Proglicem; Proglycem.
7-Chloro-3-methyl-2*H*-1,2,4-benzothiadiazine 1,1-dioxide
$C_8H_7ClN_2O_2S$ = 230.7
CAS—364-98-7

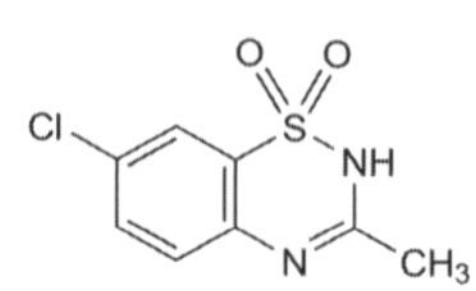

A white or creamy-white crystalline powder. M.p. 330° to 331°.
Practically insoluble in water, chloroform and ether; soluble 1 in 250 of ethanol; very soluble in solutions of alkali hydroxides; freely soluble in dimethylformamide.

Dissociation Constant. pK_a 8.7.

Partition Coefficient. Log *P* (octanol/water), 1.2.

Thin-layer Chromatography. System TA—Rf 82; system TB—Rf 01; system TC—Rf 28; system TE—Rf 20; system TL—Rf 41; system TAE—Rf 84; system TAJ—Rf 37; system TAK—Rf 13; system TAL—Rf 75.

Gas Chromatography. System GA—not eluted; system GB—not eluted.

High Performance Liquid Chromatography. System HA—*k* 0.1; system HX—RI 368; system HY—RI 299.

Ultraviolet Spectrum. Aqueous alkali—280 nm (A^1_1 = 585a).

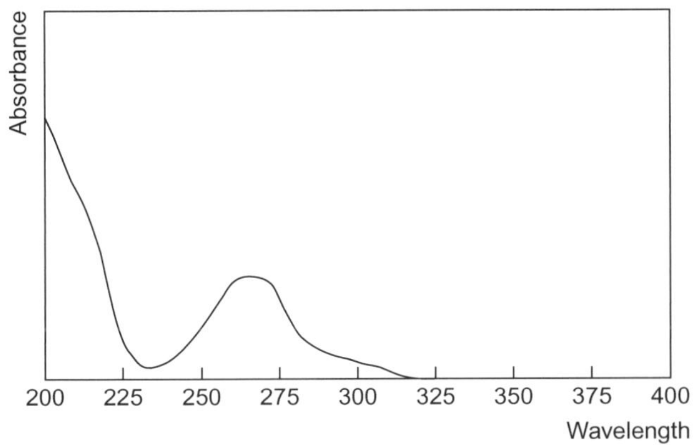

Infra-red Spectrum. Principal peaks at wavenumbers 1139, 1294, 1166, 1495, 1112, 812 cm^{-1} (KBr disk).

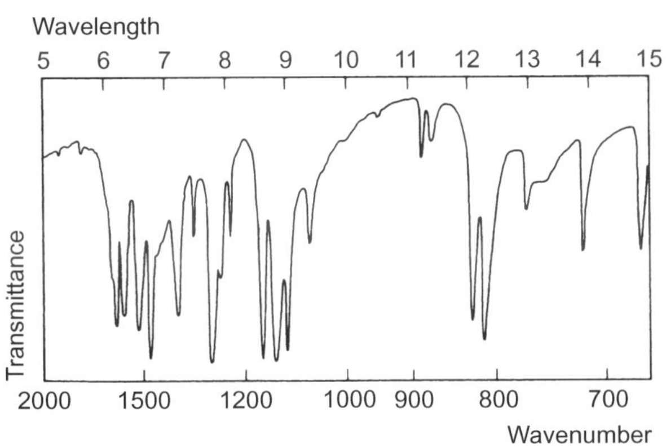

Mass Spectrum. Principal ions at *m/z* 125, 189, 230, 127, 191, 63, 232, 90.

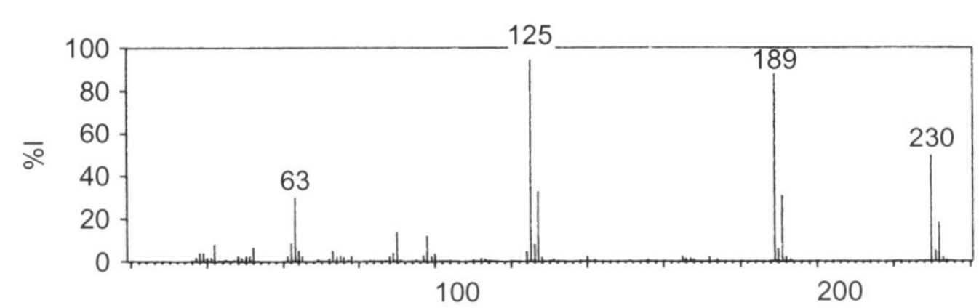

Quantification

Gas chromatography–mass spectrometry. In plasma or urine: limit of detection 10 μg/L—W. Sadee *et al.*, *J. Pharmacokinet. Biopharm.*, 1973, *1*, 295–305.

High performance liquid chromatography. In plasma or urine: limit of detection 100 μg/L, UV detection—T. B. Vree *et al.*, *J. Chromatogr.*, 1979, *164*; *Biomed. Appl.*, *6*, 228–234.

Thin-layer chromatography–ultraviolet spectrophotometry. In plasma, urine or faeces: diazoxide and metabolites—A. W. Pruitt *et al.*, *J. Pharmacol. Exp. Ther.*, 1974, *188*, 248–256.

Disposition in the Body. Readily absorbed after oral administration. Metabolised by oxidation to the 3-hydroxymethyl derivative which is conjugated with sulfate or further metabolised to the 3-carboxy derivative. About 90% of a dose is excreted in the urine in 5 to 6 days, of which 6 to 50% is unchanged drug; the 3-hydroxymethyl and 3-carboxy metabolites each account for about 20 to 30% of the excreted material; the amount of unchanged drug excreted in the urine appears to be reduced in hypertensive patients; about 2% of a dose is eliminated in the faeces.

Therapeutic concentration. In plasma, usually in the range 15 to 50 mg/L.

Following a single oral dose of 300 mg to 2 subjects, peak plasma concentrations of about 15 to 20 mg/L were attained in 3 to 6 h [A. W. Pruitt *et al.*, *Clin. Pharmacol. Ther.*, 1973, *14*, 73–82].

Toxicity. Toxic effects may be associated with plasma concentrations greater than 100 mg/L.

Half-life. Plasma half-life, adults, about 20 to 70 h; appears to be lower in children.

Volume of distribution. About 0.2 to 0.3 L/kg.

Clearance. Plasma clearance, about 0.1 mL/min/kg.

Distribution in blood. Plasma : whole blood ratio, about 1.7.

Protein binding. In plasma, about 90%; decreased in subjects with renal impairment.

Note. For a review of the pharmacokinetics of diazoxide see R. M. Pearson, *Clin. Pharmacokinet.*, 1977, *2*, 198–204.

Dose. In the treatment of intractable hypoglycaemia: initially 5 mg/kg daily, by mouth. In hypertensive crises: 300 mg intravenously.

Dibenzepin

Antidepressant

10-[2-(Dimethylamino)ethyl]-5,10-dihydro-5-methyl-11*H*-dibenzo[*b*,*e*]-[1,4]diazepin-11-one
$C_{18}H_{21}N_3O = 295.4$
CAS—4498-32-2

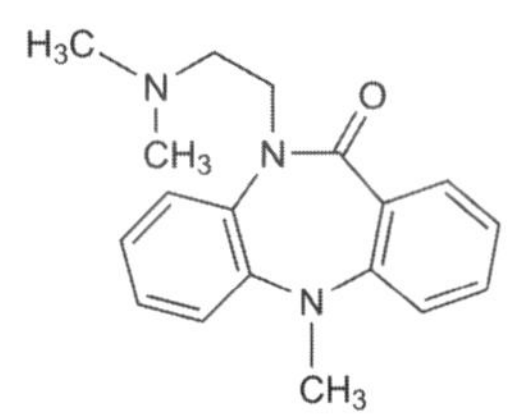

M.p. 116° to 117°.

Dibenzepin Hydrochloride

Proprietary names. Deprex; Écatril; Noveril.
Note. Deprex is also used as a proprietary name for amitriptyline hydrochloride.
$C_{18}H_{21}N_3O,HCl = 331.8$
CAS—315-80-0
A colourless, fine crystalline powder. M.p. 238°.
Soluble 1 in 16 of water; soluble in ethanol and chloroform.

Partition Coefficient. Log *P* (octanol/pH 7.4), 1.7.

Colour Test. Mandelin's Test—green.

Thin-layer Chromatography. System TA—Rf 54; system TB—Rf 22; system TC—Rf 35; system TE—Rf 55; system TL—Rf 14; system TAE—Rf 38; system TAF—Rf 22. (Acidified iodoplatinate solution, positive.)

Gas Chromatography. System GA—dibenzepin RI 2450, M (nor-) RI 2449, M (di-nor) RI 2406, M (ter-nor-) RI 2680, M (N_5-desmethyl-) RI 2455, M (OH-) isomer-1-AC RI 2600, M (OH-) isomer-2-AC RI 2770; system GB—dibenzepin RI 2566; system GF—RI 2885; system GM—dibenzepin RRT 1.735 (relative to iprindole).

High Performance Liquid Chromatography. System HA—*k* 2.8; system HF—*k* 0.50; system HX—RI 361; system HY—RI 300.

Ultraviolet Spectrum. Aqueous acid—203, 223 nm.

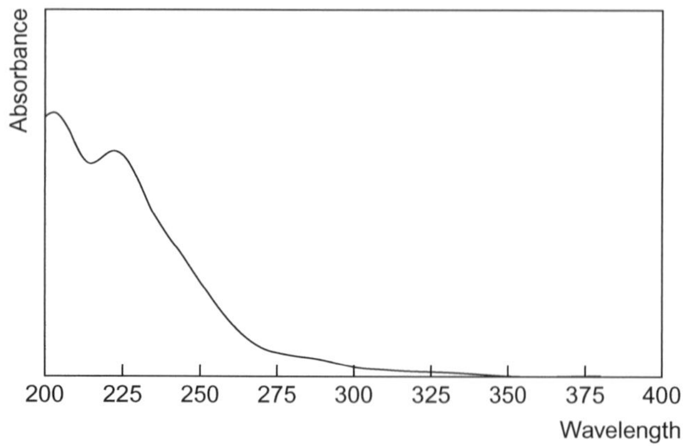

Infra-red Spectrum. Principal peaks at wavenumbers 1639, 775, 761, 1603, 1250, 1316 cm^{-1} (dibenzepin hydrochloride, KBr disk).

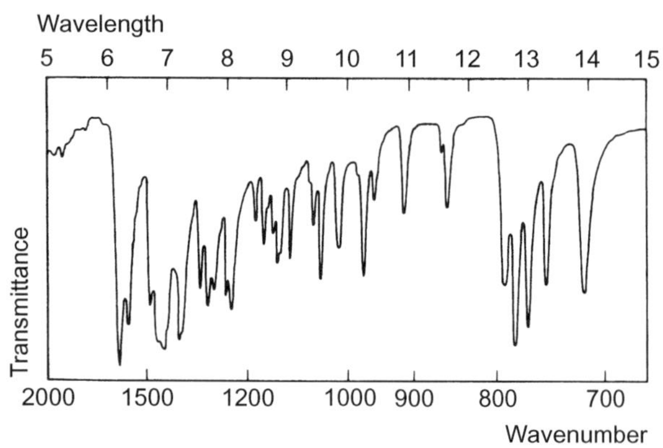

Mass Spectrum. Principal ions at *m/z* 58, 224, 209, 71, 225, 72, 210, 180.

Quantification

Ultraviolet spectrophotometry. In blood, urine, or tissues: limit of detection 500 ng/g for dibenzepin and desmethyl metabolites—H. Christensen and S. Felby, *Acta Pharmacol. Toxicol.*, 1975, *37*, 393–401.

Gas chromatography. In blood, urine, or tissues: dibenzepin and desmethyl metabolites, limit of detection 300 ng/g, AFID—H-J. Schlicht and H-P. Gelbke, *J. Chromatogr.*, 1978, *166*, 599–603.

High performance liquid chromatography. In plasma, MS/MS detection—M. Kollroser and C. Schober, *Ther. Drug Monit.*, 2002, *24(4)*, 537–544.

Disposition in the Body. Readily absorbed after oral administration; rapidly and extensively metabolised, mainly by *N*-demethylation. About 20 to 30% of a dose is excreted in the urine as free and conjugated desmethyl metabolites in 24 h, together with about 1% of the dose as unchanged drug.

Therapeutic concentration

During daily oral treatment with doses of 8 mg/kg of dibenzepin hydrochloride given to 12 patients for 22 days, mean plasma concentrations of 0.18 mg/L of dibenzepin and 0.28 mg/L of *N*-monodesmethyldibenzepin (demethylated in the side-chain) were reported, determined 4 h after a dose. Plasma concentrations declined slightly during therapy. [R. Gauch and J. Modestin, *Arzneimittelforschung*, 1973, *23*, 687–690.]

Toxicity. The estimated minimum lethal dose is about 3 g; doses greater than 1.5 g may result in serious poisoning. Patients liable to arrhythmias are particularly susceptible to toxic effects.

The following tissue disposition of total dibenzepin and metabolites was reported in 6 suicides due to the ingestion of dibenzepin: blood 23 to 147 µg/g (mean 73), liver 255 to 566 µg/g (mean 386), urine 63 to 695 µg/g (mean 230, 4 cases). [H. Christensen and S. Felby, *Acta Pharmacol. Toxicol.*, 1975, *37*, 393–401.]

In a fatality due to the ingestion of 3.6 g of dibenzepin, the following postmortem tissue concentrations were reported for dibenzepin and total desmethyl metabolites, respectively: blood 23, - mg/L; bile 113, 137 mg/L; brain 42, 12 µg/g; kidney 63, 38 µg/g; liver 130, 134 µg/g; urine 350, 258 mg/L. [H.-J. Schlicht and H.-P. Gelbke, *J. Chromatogr.*, 1978, *166*, 599–603.]

Half-life. Plasma half-life, about 4 h (dibenzepin plus desmethyl metabolites).

Dose. 240 to 560 mg of dibenzepin hydrochloride daily.

Dibrompropamidine

Antibacterial/Antifungal

4,4′-[1,3-Propanediylbis(oxy)]bis(3-bromobenzenecarboximidamide)
$C_{17}H_{18}Br_2N_4O_2$=470.2
CAS—496-00-4

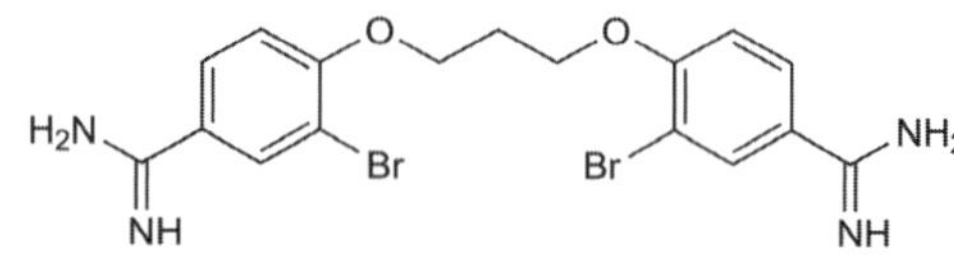

Dibrompropamidine Isetionate

Proprietary names. Brolene (eye ointment); Brulidine.
$C_{17}H_{18}Br_2N_4O_2,2C_2H_6O_4S$=722.4
CAS—614-87-9
A white crystalline powder. M.p. 226°.
Soluble 1 in 2 of water and 1 in 60 of ethanol; soluble in glycerol; practically insoluble in chloroform and ether.

Colour Tests. Aromaticity (Method 2)—yellow/brown; Liebermann's Test—black.

Thin-layer Chromatography. System TA—Rf 01. (Acidified iodoplatinate solution, positive.)

Ultraviolet Spectrum. Aqueous acid—261 nm (A^1_1=512a).

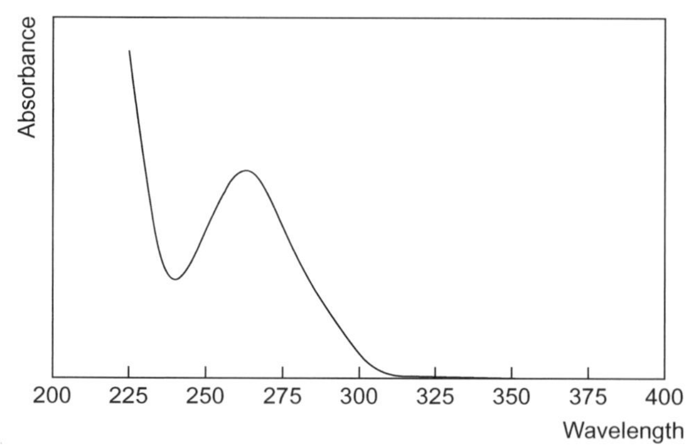

Infra-red Spectrum. Principal peaks at wavenumbers 1190, 1654, 1266, 1047, 1600, 1306 cm^{-1} (dibrompropamidine isetionate, KBr disk).

Use. Dibrompropamidine isetionate is used in a concentration of 0.15%.

Dibutyl Phthalate

Insect Repellent

Synonyms. Butyl Phthalate; DBP.
1,2-Benzenedicarboxylic acid dibutyl ester
$C_{16}H_{22}O_4$=278.3
CAS—84-74-2

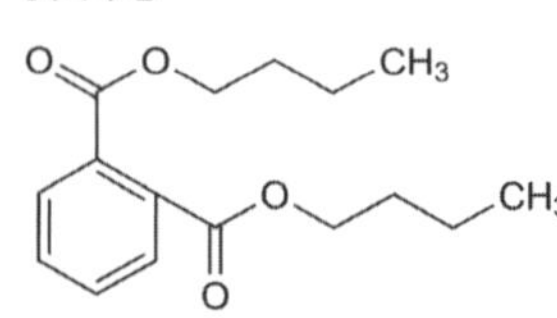

A clear, colourless or faintly yellow, somewhat viscous liquid. Mass per mL about 1.045 g. B.p. 340°. Refractive index 1.492 to 1.495.
Soluble 1 in 2500 of water; very soluble in ethanol, ether, acetone, and benzene.

Partition Coefficient. Log *P* (octanol/water), 4.5.

Gas Chromatography. System GA—RI 1913.

Ultraviolet Spectrum. Methanol—274 nm (A_1^1=45b).

Mass Spectrum. Principal ions at *m/z* 149, 41, 29, 57, 56, 104, 32, 65.

Dicamba

Herbicide

Synonym. Dianat
Proprietary names. Banfel; Banvel; Banvel-CST; Banvel-D; Banvel XG; Dianat; Dicazin; Fallowmaster; Killes; Mediben; Metambane; Tracker; Trooper; Velsicol. It is also an ingredient in Banlene and Cambilene.
3,6-Dichloro-2-methoxybenzoic acid.
$C_8H_6Cl_2O_3$=221.0
CAS—1918-00-9

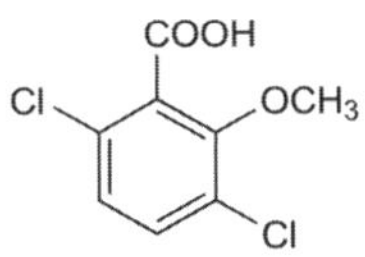

Pure dicamba is a white crystalline solid and the technical acid is a pale buff crystalline solid. M.p. 114° to 116°.
It is soluble in ethanol (922 g/L at 25°), cyclohexane (916 g/L at 25°), acetone (810 g/L at 25°), dichloromethane (260 g/L at 25°), toluene (130 g/L at 25°), and xylene (78 g/L at 25°); very slightly soluble in dioxane and water (8.3 g/L at 25°).

Dissociation Constant. pK_a 1.97 (also reported as 1.90 and 1.87 at 25°).

Partition Coefficient. Log *P* (octanol/water), 2.21.

Thin-layer Chromatography. System TX—Rf 41; system TY—Rf 70; system TAB—Rf 04; system TAC—Rf 05.

Gas Chromatography. System GA—dicamba RI 1795, 2,5-dichloromethoxybenzene RI 1200, dicamba-Me RI 1525; system GK—dicamba RRT 0.49 (relative to caffeine).

Column: DB-1 (2.0 m × 0.25 mm i.d., 0.25 μm film thickness). Column temperature: 120°, held for 0.3 min, to 180° at 15°/min. Carrier gas: hydrogen, 1.9 mL/min. FID. Retention time: 1.3 min. [Z. Liu *et al.*, *Anal. Chem.*, 1994, *66*, 3086–3092.]

High Performance Liquid Chromatography. Column: (analytical) RP C_{18} (Econosphere, 150 × 4.6 mm i.d., 5 μm), (guard) C-18 (10 × 4.6 mm i.d.). Mobile phase: (A:B) acetonitrile:acetic acid solution (2% v/v). Elution programme: (A:B) (25:75) for 5 min, to (40:60) over 10 min, held 5 min, flow rate 1.5 mL/min. Retention time: 6.1 min. [R. D. Larson and J. E. Houglum, *J. Assoc. Off. Anal. Chem.*, 1991, *74(4)*, 679–681.]

Ultraviolet Spectrum. Aqueous solution (neutral)—274; acetonitrile—205, 230, 278 nm.

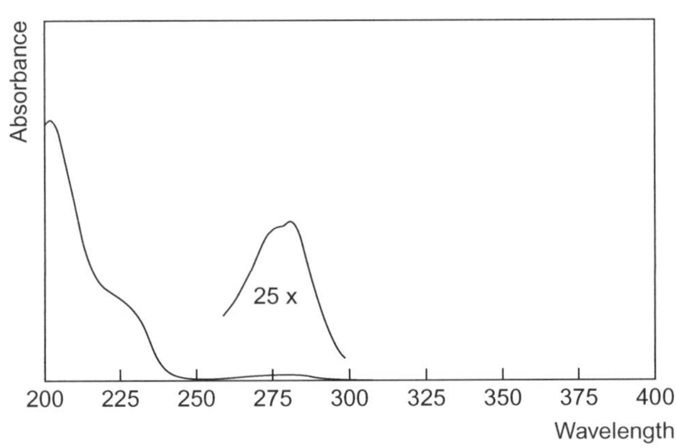

Infra-red Spectrum. Principal peaks at wavenumber 1778, 1169, 1019, 1094, 1402 cm^{-1}.

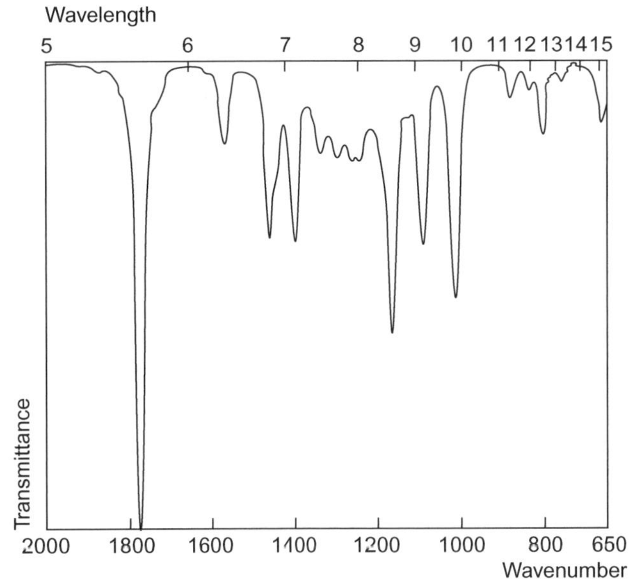

Mass Spectrum. Principal ions at *m/z* 173, 175, 220, 73, 222, 174, 191, 62.

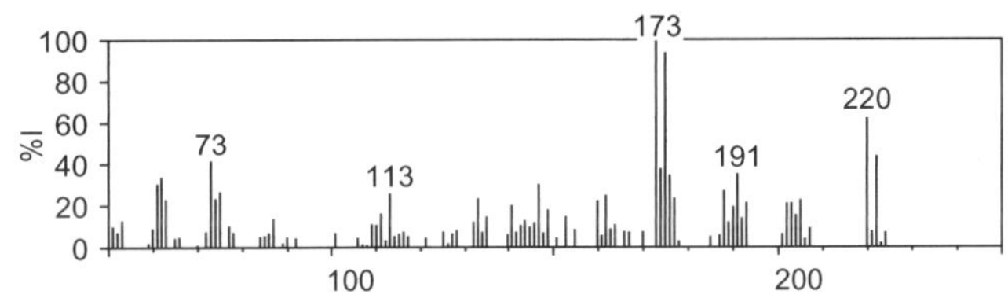

Quantification

Gas chromatography. In urine: limit of detection of dicamba 0.017 mg/L, ECD—R. Grover *et al.*, *J. Env. Sci. Health*, 1985, *20(1)*, 113–128.

High performance liquid chromatography. In solution: limit of detection <1 mg/L, UV detection (λ=274 nm)—A. M. Fogarty *et al.*, *J. Liq. Chromatogr.*, 1994, *17(12)*, 2667–2674.

Disposition in the Body. Dicamba is rapidly and almost completely absorbed into the bloodstream from the gastro-intestinal tract. It is distributed to tissues around the body and does not bioaccumulate. There is no evidence that it is absorbed through the skin. Dicamba is excreted mainly in urine as the unmetabolised state but can also be detected in faeces.

Toxicity. Dicamba is moderately toxic by ingestion and slightly toxic by inhalation and dermal exposure. It can be irritating, corrosive, and cause severe and permanent damage to the eyes. The Environmental Protection Agency (EPA) has established a Lifetime Health Advisory (LHA) level of 200 μg/L of dicamba in drinking water.

A 61-year-old woman committed suicide by ingesting an unknown quantity of Killes, containing 9 g/L dicamba. Postmortem toxicological analysis showed that the woman's blood dicamba concentration was 170 mg/L, 140 mg/L in her bile, and in her liver a concentration of <100 mg/kg was found. (2,4-Dichlorophenoxy) acetic acid and mecoprop were also detected. [A. D. Fraser *et al.*, *J. Forensic Sci.*, 1984, *29(4)*, 1237–1241.]

Protein binding. Dicamba is highly protein bound in plasma.

Dichloralphenazone

Hypnotic/Sedative

Synonym. Dichloralantipyrine
Proprietary names. Bonadorm; Chloralol; Welldorm. It is an ingredient of Midrid and Paedo-Sed.
A complex of cloral hydrate and phenazone.
$C_{15}H_{18}Cl_6N_2O_5$=519.0
CAS—480-30-8

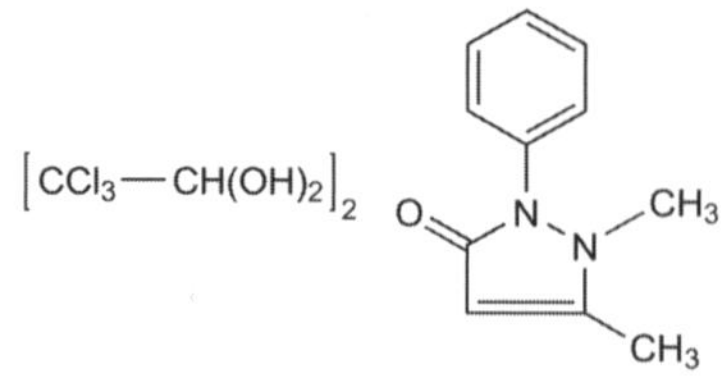

A white microcrystalline powder. M.p. 64° to 67°.
Soluble 1 in 10 of water, 1 in 1 of ethanol and 1 in 2 of chloroform; soluble in dilute acids.

Note. It is decomposed by dilute alkalis with the liberation of chloroform. In aqueous and ethanolic solutions it dissociates into cloral hydrate and phenazone.

Partition Coefficient. Log *P* (octanol/water), 0.6.

Gas Chromatography. System GA—dichloralphenazone RI 1855, M (4-OH-phenazone) RI 1855.

Ultraviolet Spectrum. Phenazone: aqueous acid—230 nm (A^1_1=590b); aqueous alkali—242 nm (A^1_1=494a), 256 nm.

Infra-red Spectrum. Principal peaks at wavenumbers 1656, 767, 1587, 1562, 1315, 1298 cm^{-1} (KBr disk).

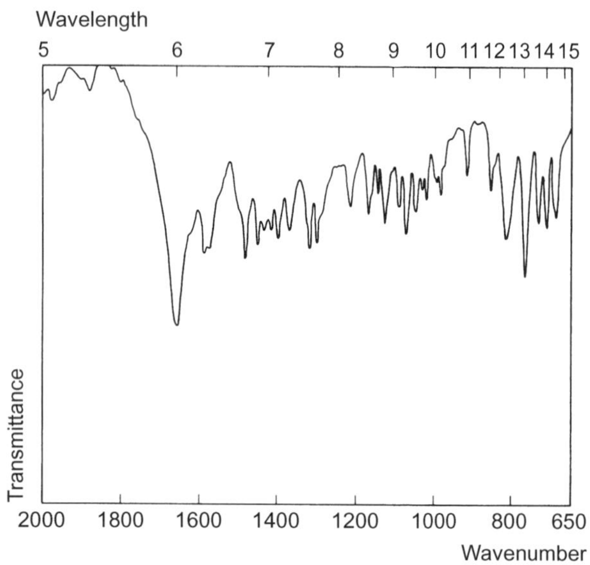

Mass Spectrum. Principal ions at *m*/*z* 188, 47, 82, 96, 29, 77, 84, 56.

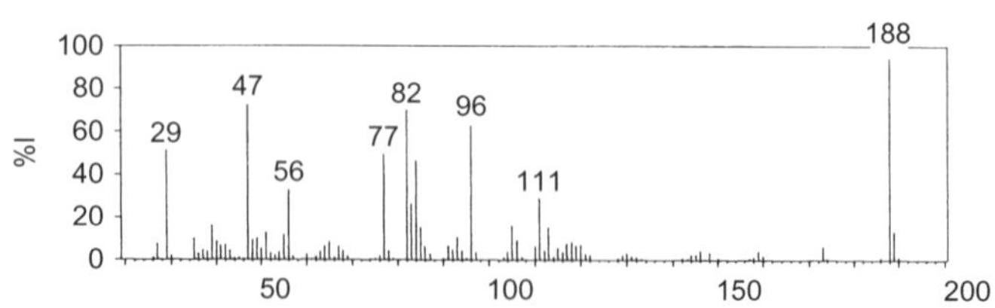

Quantification. See under Cloral Hydrate and Phenazone.

Disposition in the Body. After administration, dichloralphenazone acts as a mixture of cloral hydrate and phenazone and reference should be made to the entries under these substances.

Toxicity
Blood concentrations of 20 mg/L of trichloroethanol and 40 mg/L of phenazone were reported in a comatose subject following an overdose of dichloralphenazone; the subject eventually recovered [R. J. Armstrong and H. M. Stone, *Bull. Int. Assoc. Forensic Toxicol.*, 1972, *8*(4), 8–9].

Dose. 0.65 to 1.95 g daily.

Dichlorodifluoromethane *Aerosol Propellent/Refrigerant*

Synonyms. Difluorodichloromethane; Propellent 12; Refrigerant 12.
Proprietary names. Arcton 12. It is an ingredient of PR Spray and Skefron.
CCl_2F_2=120.9
CAS—75-71-8

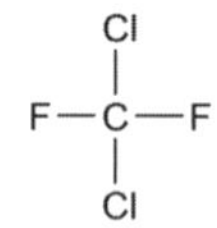

A colourless non-flammable gas which, when liquefied by compression, forms a clear colourless liquid. F.p. −155°. B.p. about −29.8°.

Partition Coefficient. Log *P* (octanol/water), 2.2.

Gas Chromatography. System GA—RI 305; system GI—Retention time 0.9 min.

Mass Spectrum. Principal ions at *m*/*z* 85, 87, 101, 50, 103, 31, 66, 35.

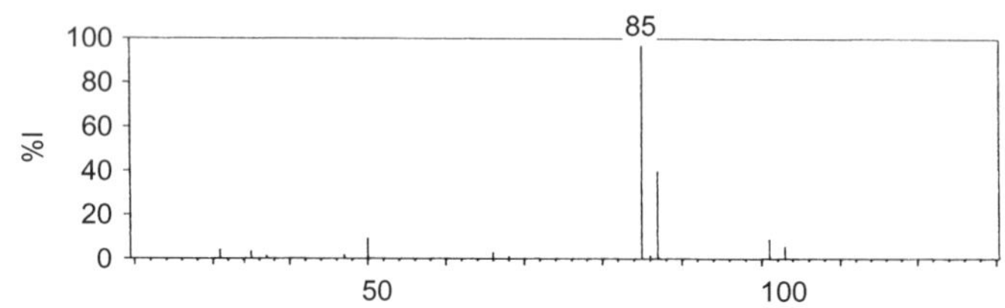

Dichlorophen *Anthelmintic*

Synonym. Di-phenthane-70
Proprietary names. Anthiphen; Dicestal (vet.); Ovis; Plath-Lyse; Wespuril.
2,2′-Methylenebis[4-chlorophenol]
$C_{13}H_{10}Cl_2O_2$=269.1
CAS—97-23-4

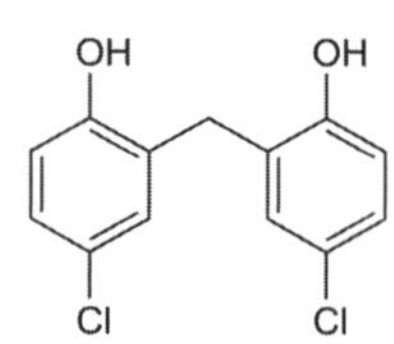

A white or slightly cream-coloured powder. M.p. about 175°.
Practically insoluble in water; soluble 1 in 1 of ethanol and 1 in less than 1 of ether; soluble in methanol, isopropyl ether, and petroleum ether; sparingly soluble in toluene.

Dissociation Constant. pK_a 7.6.

Partition Coefficient. Log *P* (octanol/water), 4.3.

Colour Tests. Aromaticity (Method 2) —yellow/brown; Folin–Ciocalteu Reagent—blue; Liebermann's Test—violet-brown; Millon's Reagent—red.

Thin-layer Chromatography. System TD—Rf 59; system TE—Rf 34; system TF—Rf 67; system TX—Rf 12; system TY—Rf 16; system TAD—Rf 57; system TAE—Rf 91.

Gas Chromatography. System GA—dichlorophen RI 2140, dichlorophen-AC_2 RI 2250, dichlorophen-Et_2 RI 2225, dichlorophen-Me_2 RI 2245.

High Performance Liquid Chromatography. System HY—RI 591.

Ultraviolet Spectrum. Aqueous acid—282; aqueous alkali—245 (A^1_1=650a), 304 nm.

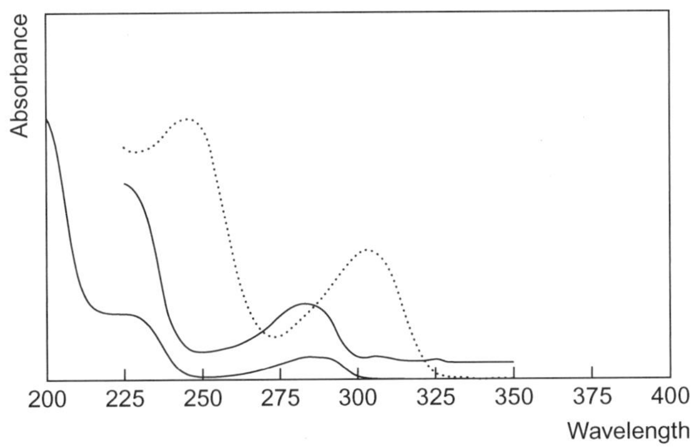

Infra-red Spectrum. Principal peaks at wavenumbers 1226, 817, 1111, 1162, 1245, 1170 cm^{-1} (KBr disk).

Mass Spectrum. Principal ions at *m/z* 128, 141, 268, 130, 270, 77, 143, 233.

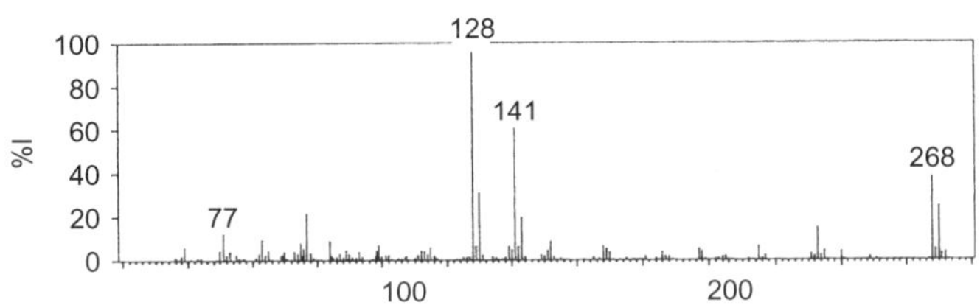

Disposition in the Body

Toxicity

An acute fatality was reported with a blood concentration of 9.77 mg/L dichlorophen. No other drugs or alcohol were detected. [P. Kintz *et al.*, *Int. J. Legal Med.*, 1997, *110(2)*, 95–96.]

Dose. Usually 6 g daily for 2 or 3 days; a single dose of 9 g has also been given.

Dichlorophenoxyacetic Acid

Herbicide

Synonym. 2,4-D

Proprietary names. Cornox D; Destox; Dicotox; Dioweed; Dormone; Fernimine; For-ester; Iso-planatox; Palormone D; Silvapron D; Syford; Vigon-DC. It is an ingredient of Econal, Nettle Ban, Spontox, and Stancide BWK 75.

(2,4-Dichlorophenoxy)acetic acid

$C_8H_6Cl_2O_3$=221.0

CAS—94-75-7

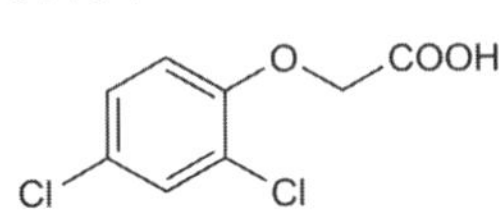

A white powder which is corrosive. M.p. about 140°.

Almost insoluble in water; soluble in aqueous solutions of alkalis and in alcohols.

Dissociation Constant. pK_a 2.7.

Partition Coefficient. Log *P* (octanol/water), 2.8.

Thin-layer Chromatography. System TD—Rf 04; system TE—Rf 04; system TF—Rf 06; system TX—Rf 00; system TY—Rf 02; system TAB—Rf 02; system TAC—Rf 03.

Gas Chromatography. System GA—2,4-D RI 1800, M (2,4-dichlorophenol) RI 1320; 2,4-D-Me RI 1593, 2,4-D-butyl ester RI 1840, 2,4-D-isobutyl ester RI 1805, 2,4-D-isopropyl ester RI 1700, 2,4-Dichlorophenoxybutyric acid-Me RI 1835; system GK—RRT 0.65 (relative to caffeine). Dichlorophenoxyacetic acid iso-octil ester: system GK—RRT 1.12, 1.18 (relative to caffeine).

Ultraviolet Spectrum. Ethanol—284 (A_1^1=95b), 292 nm.

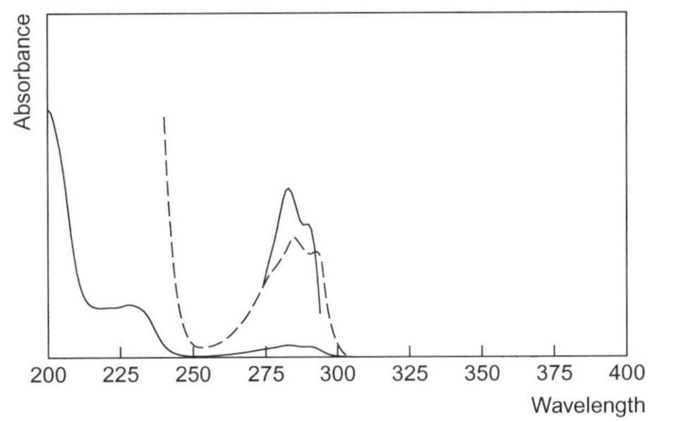

Infra-red Spectrum. Principal peaks at wavenumbers 1090, 1230, 795, 1264, 1247, 1724 cm^{-1} (Nujol mull). (See below)

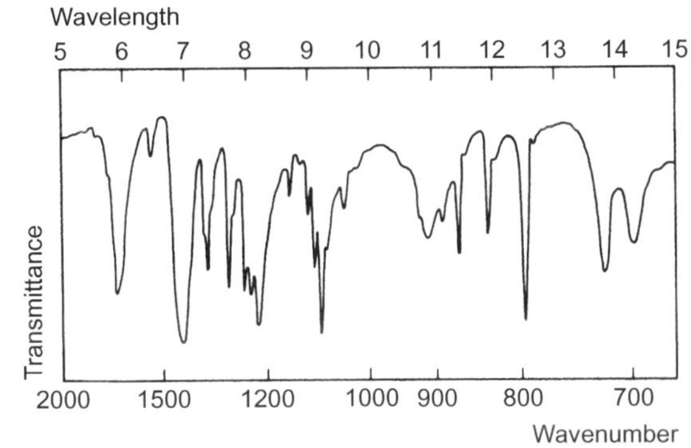

Mass Spectrum. Principal ions at *m/z* 199, 45, 175, 145, 111, 109, 234, 133 (dichlorophenoxyacetic acid methyl ester).

Quantification

Gas chromatography. In plasma or urine: FID—J. D. Kohli *et al.*, *Xenobiotica*, 1974, *4*, 97–100. In urine: limit of detection 100 μg/L, ECD—A. E. Smith and B. J. Hayden, *J. Chromatogr.*, 1979, *171*, 482–485.

High performance liquid chromatography. In plasma: limit of detection 0.5 mg/L, UV detection (λ = 284 nm) —T. Keller *et al.*, *Forensic Sci. Int.*, 1994, *65(1)*, 13–18.

Disposition in the Body. Readily absorbed after ingestion but poorly absorbed through the skin. After ingestion, about 80% is excreted in the urine unchanged in 4 days, and about 13% is excreted as conjugates.

Blood concentration

After ingestion of 5 mg/kg by 6 subjects, average peak plasma concentrations of about 35 mg/L were attained in 7 to 24 h. [J. D. Kohli *et al.*, *Xenobiotica*, 1974, *4*, 97–100.]

Toxicity. The estimated minimum lethal dose is 7 g. The maximum permissible atmospheric concentration is 10 mg/m^3 and the maximum acceptable daily intake is 300 μg/kg. Dichlorophenoxyacetic acid is very irritating to the eyes, nose, and throat.

The following postmortem tissue concentrations have been reported in 4 fatalities involving ingestion of dichlorophenoxyacetic acid: blood 126 to 826 mg/L (mean 447, 4 cases), bile 573 mg/L (1 case), brain 13 and 66 μg/g (2 cases), kidney 62 to 82 μg/g (mean 69, 3 cases), liver 21 to 183 μg/g (mean 134, 4 cases), urine 111 and 264 mg/L (2 cases). [K. Nielsen *et al.*, *Acta Pharmacol. Toxicol.*, 1965, *22*, 224–234; A. Coutselenis *et al.*, *Forensic Sci.*, 1977, *10*, 203–204; J. E. Ryall, *Bull. Int. Assoc. Forensic Toxicol.*, 1978, *14(2)*, 17–18; M. Watson, *Bull. Int. Assoc. Forensic Toxicol.*, 1978, *14(2)*, 18.]

A 49-year-old man ingested an unknown amount of dichlorophenoxyacetic acid solution (500 g/L) and later died after hospital treatment. The concentrations of the herbicide in lung, liver, kidney, heart, pancreas, muscle, brain, and stomach contents were 535, 386, 370, 361, 298, 273, and 185 mg/kg and 125 mg/L, respectively. The herbicide was detected in blood before treatment at a concentration of 389 mg/L and in plasma 750 mg/L. [T. Keller *et al.*, *Forensic Sci. Int.*, 1994, *65(1)*, 13–18.]

Half-life. Plasma half-life, about 12 to 33 h.

Volume of Distribution. About 0.1 L/kg.

Dichlorvos

Insecticide

Synonyms. DDVP; Dichlorfos; Dichlorovos; Dichlorphos; ENT-20738; NSC-6738; OMS-14; SD-1750.

Proprietary names. Astrobat; Atgard; Canogard; Dedevap; Dichlorman; Divipan; Equigard; Equigal; Estrosol; Herkol; Nogos; Nuvan; Prosvit; Task; Vapona; Verdisol.

Phosphoric acid 2,2-dichloroethenyl dimethyl ester

$C_4H_7Cl_2O_4P$=221.0

CAS—62-73-7

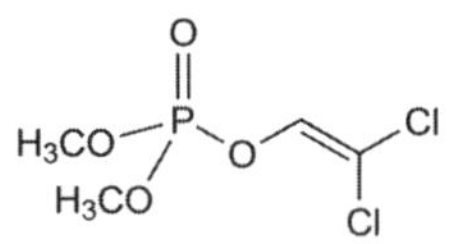

A colourless to amber, oily liquid. M.p. <25°. B.p. 140° at 20 mmHg.
It is soluble in water (8000 mg/L at 20°) and glycerol (0.5 g/100 mL); very soluble in dichloromethane, 2-propanol, and toluene; soluble in ethanol, chloroform, acetone, and kerosene; miscible with many organic solvents and aerosol propellents; moderately soluble in diesel oil, kerosene, isoparaffinic hydrocarbons, and mineral oils.

Partition Coefficient. Log *P* (octanol/water), 1.47.

Thin-layer Chromatography. System TE—Rf 83; system TX—Rf 20; system TY—Rf 20; system TZ—Rf 75; system TAA—Rf 36; system TAB—Rf 00; system TAC—Rf 00.

Gas Chromatography. System GA—RI 1275; system GK—RRT 0.23 (relative to caffeine).

High Performance Liquid Chromatography. System HAO—*k* 5.22; system HAP—*k* 0.86.

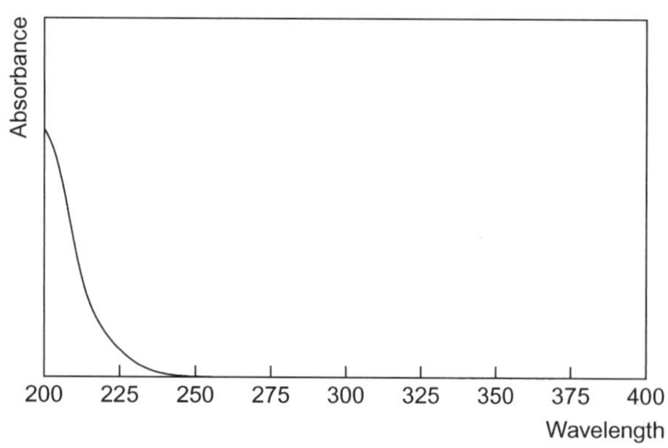

Infra-red Spectrum. Principal peaks at wavenumber 1061, 1158, 850, 978, 1320 cm^{-1}.

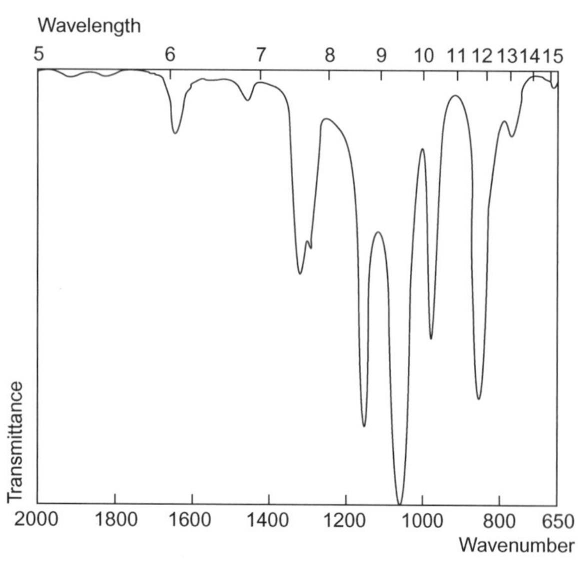

Mass Spectrum. Principal ions at *m/z* 109, 79, 185, 47, 145, 187, 83, 93.

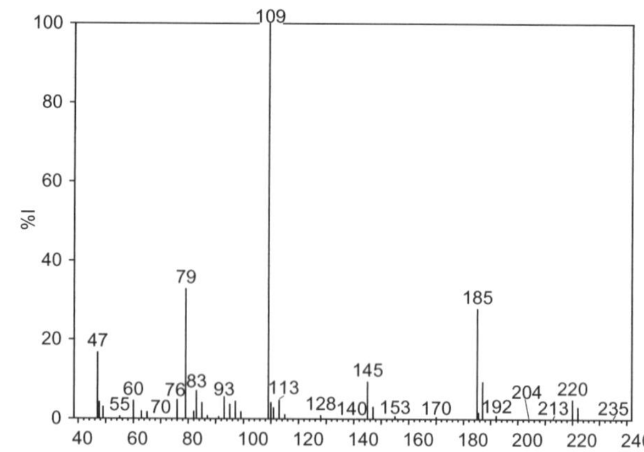

Quantification

Gas chromatography. In blood and urine: limit of quantification 1 µg/L, ECD—R. Heinig *et al.*, *J. Chromatogr. B Biomed. Sci. Appl.*, 2000, *741(2)*, 257–269. In blood: limit of detection 14 µg/L—R. Garcia-Repetto *et al.*, *Vet. Hum. Toxicol.*, 1995, *37(4)*, 306–309.

Gas chromatography–mass spectrometry. In serum: limit of detection of the metabolite, dimethylphosphate (DMP), 60 µg/L—F. A. Tarbah *et al.*, *TIAFT Poster Session, 4*, 1998. In blood: limit of quantification 50 µg/L—T. Villen *et al.*, *J. Chromatogr.*, 1990, *529*, 309–317. In blood and urine: limit of quantification 2.5 µg/L—R. Heinig *et al.*, *J. Chromatogr. B Biomed. Sci. Appl.*, 2000, *741(2)*, 257–269.

High performance liquid chromatography. In plasma: limit of quantification 40 µg/L for dichlorvos—L. K. Unni *et al.*, *J. Chromatogr. B Biomed. Sci. Appl.*, 1992, *573*, 99–103.

Disposition in the Body. Dichlorvos is easily absorbed through the skin. It is absorbed after ingestion and rapidly moved to the liver where it is quickly detoxified by degrading enzymes, found in tissues and blood plasma. It is distributed in tissues especially kidneys, liver, stomach, and intestines. It is rapidly metabolised and eliminated from the body via expired air and urine. One metabolite is dimethylphosphate (DMP) which is common for some of the organophosphate compounds and another is dichloroacetaldehyde. It does not accumulate in tissues.

Toxicity. Dichlorvos is highly toxic by inhalation, dermal absorption, and ingestion. Severe poisoning will affect the CNS. A lethal oral dose of 400 mg/kg body weight has been reported and a toxic dose of 300 mg/kg. The allowed daily intake is 0.04 mg/kg.

A 72-year-old woman was found dead after ingesting dichlorvos. A 500 mL bottle of dichlorvos was found beside the body (concentration 75%). 250 mL of a volatile fluid was found in the stomach which was equivalent to 300 g dichlorvos. Dichlorvos was detected in the spleen (3.34 mg/g), heart (815 µg/g), urine (4.5 mg/L), blood (29 mg/L), brain (9.7 µg/g), lung (81 µg/g), kidney (80 µg/g), and liver (20 µg/g). [K. Shimizu *et al.*, *Forensic Sci. Int.*, 1996, *83(1)*, 61–66.]

Half-life. Approx. 25 min.

Clearance. Oral clearance, in healthy volunteers, is approximately 1558 L/h.

Diclofenac

Analgesic

Synonym. Diclophenac

2-[(2,6-Dichlorophenyl)amino]benzeneacetic acid

$C_{14}H_{11}Cl_2NO_2$=296.2

CAS—15307-86-5

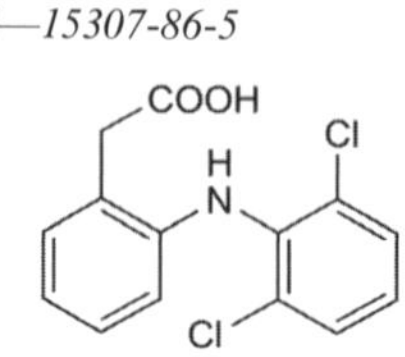

Crystals. M.p. 156° to 158°.

Diclofenac Sodium

Synonyms. Diclofenacum Natricum; GP-45840.

Proprietary names. Acoflam; Arthrotec; Cataflam; Dicloflex; Diclomax; Diclotard; Diclovol; Diclozip; Econac; Flamatak; Flamrase; Flexotard; Isclofen; Lofensaid; Motifene; Pennsaid; Rheumatac; Rhumalgan; Slofenac; Solaraze; Volraman; Volsaid; Voltaren(e); Voltarol.

$C_{14}H_{10}Cl_2NNaO_2$=318.1

CAS—15307-79-6

Crystals. M.p. 283° to 285°.

Solubility at 25° (mg/mL): deionised water (pH 5.2) >9; methanol >24; acetone 6; acetonitrile <1; cyclohexane <1.

Dissociation Constant. pK_a 4.2.

Partition Coefficient. Log *P* (octanol/water), 4.5.

Colour Tests. Liebermann's Test—red-brown; Mandelin's Test—red-brown; Marquis Test—brown (slow).

Thin-layer Chromatography. System TA—Rf 90; system TD—Rf 25; system TE—Rf 12; system TF—Rf 27; system TG—Rf 29; system TAD—Rf 47; system TAE—Rf 90; system TAJ—Rf 40; system TAK—Rf 64; system TAL—Rf 84. (Chromic acid solution, red.)

Gas Chromatography. System GA—diclofenac RI 2271, diclofenac-Me RI 2195, diclofenac-Me_2 RI 2220, M (OH-)-Me_2 RI 2460; system GB—RI 2231; system GD—diclofenac-Me RRT 1.42 (relative to n-$C_{16}H_{34}$); system GL—diclofenac-Me RI 2200, M (OH-)-Me_2 RI 2460.

High Performance Liquid Chromatography. System HD—*k* 11.5; system HV—RRT 0.85 (relative to meclofenamic acid); system HX—RI 616; system HY—RI 592; system HZ—retention time 14.8 min; system HAA—retention time 22.1 min; system HAX—retention time 8.7 min; system HAY—retention time 10.0 min.

Ultraviolet Spectrum. Aqueous acid—273 nm (A^1_1=309b); aqueous alkali—275 nm (A^1_1=351b).

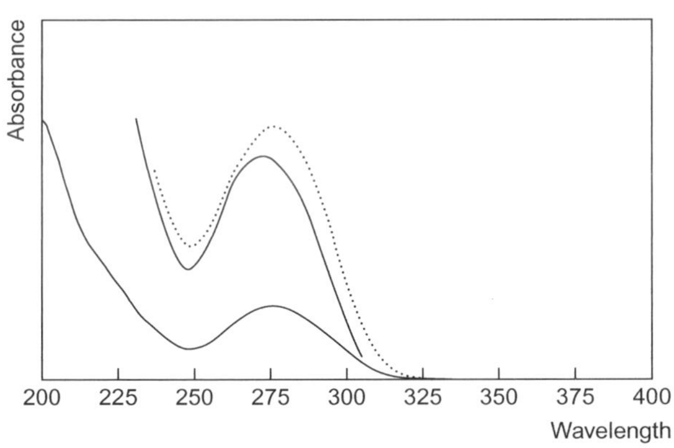

Infra-red Spectrum. Principal peaks at wavenumbers 1572, 756, 1504, 775, 1286, 1308 cm^{-1} (diclofenac sodium, KBr disk).

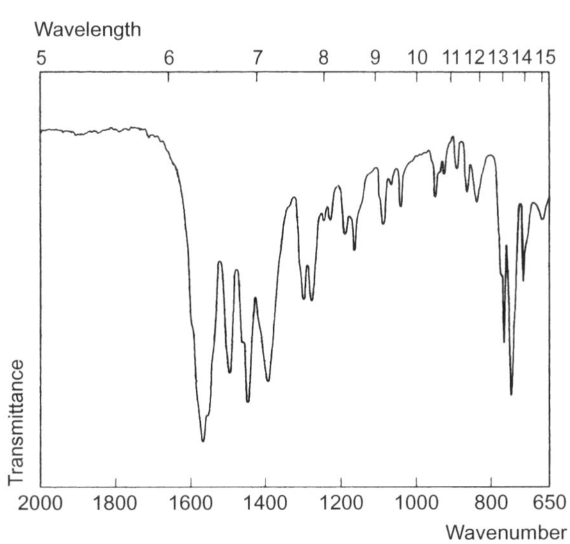

Mass Spectrum. Principal ions at *m/z* 214, 216, 242, 295, 215, 297, 179, 178.

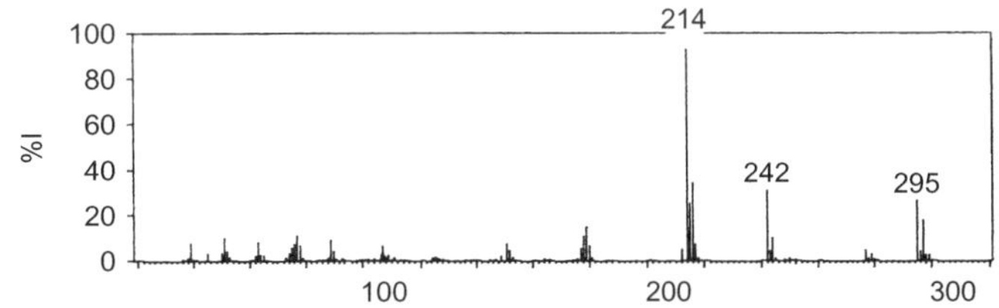

Quantification

Gas chromatography. In plasma: limit of detection 100 µg/L, ECD—M. Ikeda *et al.*, *J. Chromatogr.* 1980, *183*(9) *B Biomed. Appl.*, 41–47. In urine: diclofenac and hydroxy metabolites, ECD—W. Schneider and P. H. Degen, *J. Chromatogr.*, 1981, *217*, 263–271.

Gas chromatography–mass spectrometry. In plasma: limit of detection 2 µg/L, SIM—M. Del Puppo *et al.*, *Biol. Mass Spectrom.*, 1991, *20*, 426–430. In plasma or urine: limit of detection 100 ng/L—A. Sioufi *et al.*, *J. Chromatogr.*, 1991, *571*, 87–100. In plasma: limit of detection 0.2 µg/L—M. R. Borenstein *et al.*, *J. Chromatogr.* 1996, *685 B Biomed. Appl.*, 59–66. In urine: diclofenac and other NSAIDs—B. M. el Haj *et al.*, *Forensic Sci. Int.*, 1999, *105*, 141–153. In urine: diclofenac and other NSAIDs, limits of detection 10 to 50 µg/L—H. H. Maurer *et al.*, *J. Anal. Toxicol.*, 2001, *25*, 237–244.

High performance liquid chromatography. In plasma: limit of detection 5 µg/L, UV detection—K. K. H. Chan *et al.*, *Anal. Lett. (Part B)*, 1982, *15*, 1649–1663. In plasma: limit of detection 6 µg/L, fluorescence detection—B. Wiese and J. Hermansson, *J. Chromatogr.*, 1991, *567*, 175–183. In plasma: limit of quantification 5 µg/L, UV detection—L. A. Brunner and R. C. Luders, *J. Chromatogr. Sci.*, 1991, *29*, 287–291. In plasma or cerebrospinal fluid: limit of detection <1 µg/L, electrochemical detection—L. Zecca *et al.*, *J. Chromatogr.*, 1991, *567*, 425–432. In plasma: limit of detection 1 µg/L, UV detection—S. R. Santos *et al.*, *Braz. J. Med. Biol. Res.*, 1992, *25*, 125–128. In serum: limit of quantification 20 µg/L, fluorescence detection—J. Moncrieff, *J. Chromatogr.*, 1992, *577*, 185–189. In plasma or synovial fluid: diclofenac and other NSAIDs—I. S. Blagbrough *et al.*, *J. Chromatogr.*, 1992, *578*, 251–257. In plasma: limit of detection <2.5 µg/L, UV detection—R. B. Miller, *J. Chromatogr.*, 1993, *616*, 283–290. In plasma or urine: limit of detection 0.2 mg/L, UV detection—A. Avgerinos *et al.*, *J. Chromatogr.*, 1993, *619*, 324–329. In serum: limit of detection 10 µg/L—S. Y. Zhang *et al.*, *Yao Xue Xue Bao*, 1994, *29*, 228–231. In aqueous humour: diclofenac and flurbiprofen, limit of detection for diclofenac 0.3 ng, UV detection—M. Riegel and P. P. Ellis, *J. Chromatogr.* 1994, *654 B Biomed. Appl.*, 140–145. In plasma: limit of detection 3 µg/L, UV detection—A. Hanses *et al.*, *Arch. Pharm. (Weinheim)*, 1995, *328*, 257–260. In urine: diclofenac and its metabolites, limit of quantification 0.4 mg/L—R. J. Sawchuk *et al.*, *Pharm. Res.*, 1995, *12*, 756–762. In urine: diclofenac and other NSAIDs, limit of detection for diclofenac 0.05 mg/L, UV detection—T. Hirai *et al.*, *J. Chromatogr. B Biomed. Sci. Appl.*, 1997, *692*, 375–388. In serum or aqueous humour: limit of detection 1 µg/L, UV detection—O. Kuhlmann and G. J. Krauss, *J. Pharm. Biomed. Anal.*, 1997, *16*, 553–559. In plasma: diclofenac and flurbiprofen—G. Giagoudakis and S. L. Markantonis, *J. Pharm. Biomed. Anal.*, 1998, *17*, 897–901. In aqueous humour: diclofenac and oxybuprocaine, limit of detection for diclofenac 500 ng/L, electrochemical detection—O. Kuhlmann *et al.*, *J. Pharm. Biomed. Anal.*, 1998, *17*, 1351–1356. In urine: diclofenac and other NSAIDs, limit of quantification for diclofenac 0.02 mg/L, UV detection—A. Bakkali *et al.*, *J. Chromatogr. B Biomed. Sci. Appl.*, 1999, *729*, 139–145. In plasma: diclofenac and aceclofenac, limit of detection 10 µg/L—H. S. Lee *et al.*, *J. Pharm. Biomed. Anal.*, 2000, *23*, 775–781. In plasma: limit of detection 5 µg/L—C. Arcelloni *et al.*, *J. Chromatogr. B Biomed. Sci. Appl.*, 2001, *763*, 195–200.

Disposition in the Body. Well absorbed after oral administration but undergoes significant first-pass metabolism. Up to about 70% of a dose is excreted in the urine in 3 days, including 20 to 40% as glucuronide and sulfate conjugates of the major metabolite 4′-hydroxydiclofenac (active) and up to about 15% as conjugates of unchanged diclofenac. Other metabolites identified in the urine include 5-hydroxydiclofenac (about 12% of the dose), 3′-hydroxydiclofenac, and 4′,5-dihydroxydiclofenac. About 10 to 20% of a dose is excreted in the bile as 4′-hydroxydiclofenac and less than 5% as unchanged drug. Diclofenac enters the synovial fluid and maximum concentrations are measured 2 to 4 h after the peak plasma levels have been reached. Diclofenac is excreted in breast milk but in quantities so small that no adverse effects on breast-fed infants would be expected.

Therapeutic concentration

Following oral administration of 50 mg of diclofenac sodium three times a day to 4 subjects, peak plasma concentrations of 0.1 to 2.2 mg/L (mean 0.8) of diclofenac and 0.3 to 2.0 mg/L (mean 1.2) of 4′-hydroxydiclofenac were reported 3 h after a dose; peak concentrations in synovial fluid of 0.1 to 0.6 mg/L (mean 0.3) of diclofenac and 0.2 to 1.0 mg/L (mean 0.6) of 4′-hydroxydiclofenac were attained in 3 h; concentrations in synovial fluid exceeded those in plasma after 4 h. [P. D. Fowler *et al., Eur. J. Clin. Pharmacol.*, 1983, *25*, 389–394.]

Diclofenac was administered as a single oral 150 mg dose to healthy subjects ($n = 6$) and to patients with either chronic active hepatitis ($n = 6$) or alcoholic cirrhosis (n=6). Peak plasma concentrations of diclofenac, 3′-hydroxydiclofenac, 4′-hydroxydiclofenac, and 3′-hydroxy-4′,5-methoxydiclofenac of 5.699, 0.412, 2.613, and 0.385 mg/L were attained at 0.63, 0.79, 0.88, and 5.8 h, respectively, in healthy subjects. The equivalent respective values in patients with hepatitis were: 6.574, 0.392, 2.786, and 0.306 mg/L at 0.42, 0.58, 0.50, and 4.0 h and in patients with cirrhosis were: 11.59, 0.264, 2.481, and 0.191 mg/L at 0.33, 1.04, 0.75, and 7.0 h. [J. S. Lill *et al., J. Clin. Pharmacol.*, 2000, *40*, 250–257.]

In 20 healthy subjects given a single oral dose of diclofenac 100 mg as 2 different sustained-release tablets, respective peak plasma concentrations of 1.161 and 0.799 mg/L were attained in 4.2 and 4.5 h. [S. Zmeili *et al., Int. J. Clin. Pharmacol. Ther.*, 1996, *34*, 564–570.]

Toxicity

A 19-year-old man was admitted to hospital following the ingestion of 1.5 g of diclofenac sodium and 4 g of chlormezanone. Plasma diclofenac concentrations of 60.1 mg/L and 0.19 mg/L were reported at 7 and 15 h, respectively; chlormezanone could not be determined. The subject recovered after about 2 days. [P. Netter *et al., Eur. J. Clin. Pharmacol.*, 1984, *26*, 535–536.]

Bioavailability. About 50 to 60%

Half-life. Plasma half-life, about 1 to 2 h; synovial fluid half-life 3 to 6 h.

Volume of distribution. 0.17 L/kg.

Clearance. Plasma clearance, about 4 mL/min/kg.

Protein binding. In plasma, more than 99%.

Note. For reviews of diclofenac see R. W. Brogden *et al., Drugs*, 1980, *20*, 24–48 and N. M. Davies and K. E. Anderson, *Clin. Pharmacokinet.*, 1997, *33*, 184–213.

Dose. 75 to 150 mg of diclofenac sodium daily in divided doses.

Thin-layer Chromatography. System TA—Rf 82; system TD—Rf 14; system TE—Rf 33; system TF—Rf 64; system TAD—Rf 23. (Acidified iodoplatinate solution, positive.)

Ultraviolet Spectrum. Aqueous acid—286 nm (A^1_1=60a), 296 nm.

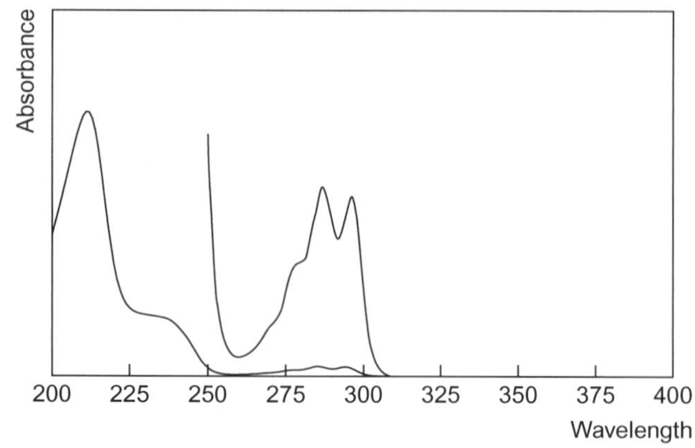

Infra-red Spectrum. Principal peaks at wavenumbers 1162, 1176, 882, 702, 907, 1123 cm^{-1} (KBr disk).

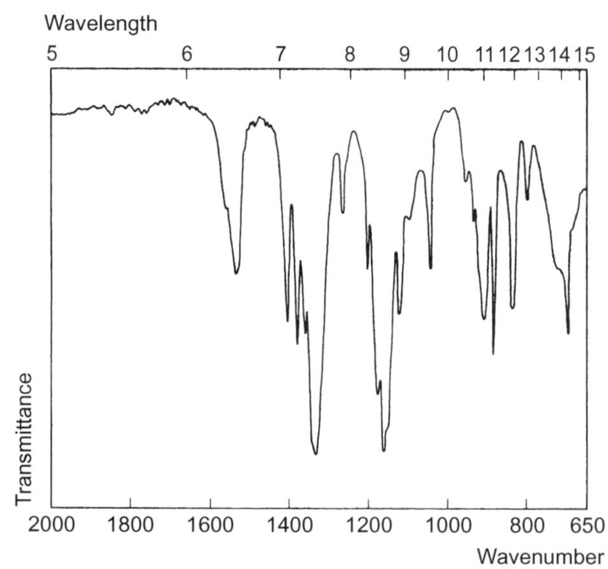

Mass Spectrum. Principal ions at m/z 304, 306, 64, 74, 109, 177, 176, 48.

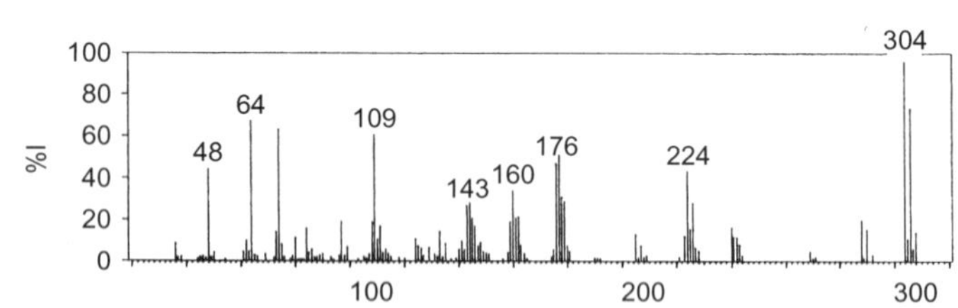

Quantification

Gas chromatography. In rabbit serum: limit of detection 20 μg/L, ECD—C. Schmitt *et al., J. Pharm. Sci.*, 1979, *68*, 381–383.

Dose. 100 to 200 mg daily in the treatment of glaucoma.

Diclofenamide

Carbonic Anhydrase Inhibitor

Synonyms. DCPA; Dichlorophenamide; Dichlorphenamide.
Proprietary names. Daranide; Oralcon; Oratrol.
4,5-Dichloro-1,3-benzenedisulfonamide
$C_6H_6Cl_2N_2O_4S_2$=305.2
CAS—120-97-8

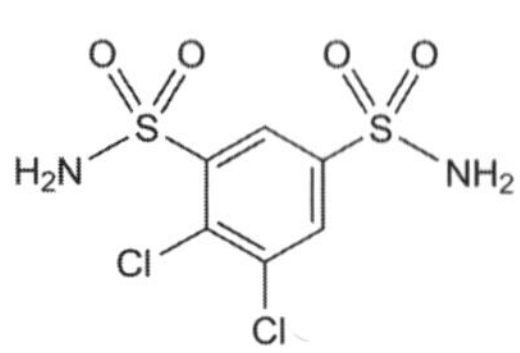

A white crystalline powder. M.p. about 240°.
Practically insoluble in water and chloroform; soluble 1 in 30 of ethanol; slightly soluble in ether; freely soluble in pyridine; soluble in solutions of alkali hydroxides and carbonates.

Dissociation Constant. pK_a 7.4, 8.6.

Partition Coefficient. Log *P* (ether/pH 7.4), 1.0.

Colour Test. Koppanyi–Zwikker Test—violet.

Dicoumarol

Anticoagulant

Synonyms. Bishydroxycoumarin; Dicoumarin; Dicumarol; Melitoxin.
Proprietary name. Dufalone
3,3′-Methylenebis[4-hydroxy-2*H*-1-benzopyran-2-one]

$C_{19}H_{12}O_6$=336.3
CAS—66-76-2

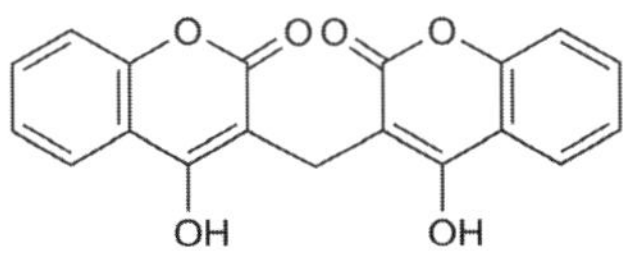

A white or creamy-white crystalline powder. M.p. 287° to 293°.
Practically insoluble in water, ethanol and ether; slightly soluble in benzene and chloroform; freely soluble in solutions of alkali hydroxides.

Dissociation Constant. pK_a 4.4, 8.0.

Partition Coefficient. Log *P* (octanol/water), 2.1.

Thin-layer Chromatography. System TB—Rf 00; system TD—Rf 18; system TE—Rf 30; system TF—Rf 32; System TAD—Rf 33; system TAE—Rf 88; system TAJ—Rf 60; system TAK—Rf 80; system TAL—Rf 96. (Acidified potassium permanganate solution, positive.)

Gas Chromatography. System GA—not eluted.

High Performance Liquid Chromatography. System HX—RI 599.

Ultraviolet Spectrum. Aqueous alkali—314 nm (A_1^1=756a).

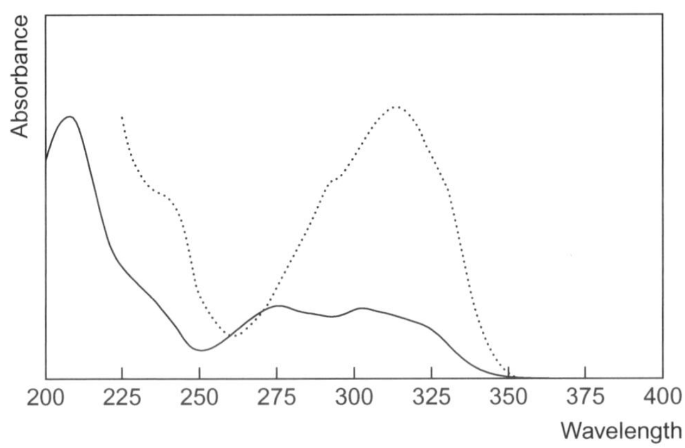

Mass Spectrum. Principal ions at *m/z* 336, 121, 120, 215, 162, 92, 337, 187.

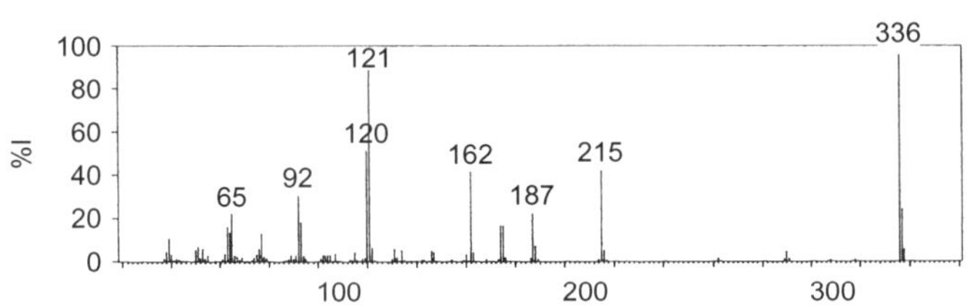

Quantification

Ultraviolet spectrophotometry. In plasma: limit of detection 2 mg/L—R. Nagashima *et al.*, *J. Pharm. Sci.*, 1968, *57*, 58–67.

Disposition in the Body. Slowly and irregularly absorbed after oral administration. It is extensively metabolised with less than 1% of a dose being excreted in the urine as unchanged drug.

Therapeutic concentration

After a single oral dose of 150 mg to 8 subjects, a mean peak plasma concentration of 16.7 mg/L was attained in 12 h [H. M. Solomon and J. J. Schrogie, *Clin. Pharmacol. Ther.*, 1967, *8*, 65–69].

Following daily oral administration of 2 mg/kg to 3 subjects, plasma concentrations of 44 to 59 mg/L (mean 53) were reported on the 6th day [E. S. Vesell and J. G. Page, *J. Clin. Invest.*, 1968, *47*, 2657–2663].

Toxicity. Fatalities, usually due to severe haemorrhage, have been reported following daily oral doses of 100 mg or more.

Half-life. Plasma half-life, dose-dependent and may range from 7 to 100 h.

Protein binding. In plasma, more than 99%.

Dose. Maintenance, 25 to 150 mg daily.

Dicycloverine

Anticholinergic

Synonym. Dicyclomine
[1,1′-Bicyclohexyl]-1-carboxylic acid 2-(diethylamino)ethyl ester
$C_{19}H_{35}NO_2$=309.5
CAS—77-19-0

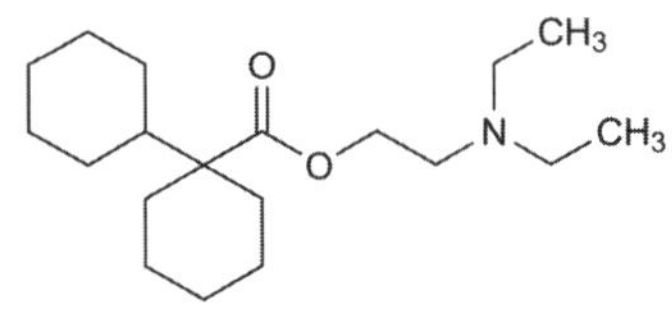

Dicycloverine Hydrochloride

Proprietary names. Antispas; Bentyl; Bentylol; Byclomine; Clomin; Dibent; Diclomin; Dicomin; Dilomine; Formulex; Lomine; Medicyclomine; Merbentyl; Notensyl; Optimal; Or-Tyl; Wyovin. It is an ingredient of Anacidron, Diarrest, Kolanticon, Kolantyl, and Ovol.
$C_{19}H_{35}NO_2$,HCl=346.0
CAS—67-92-5
A white crystalline powder. M.p. 164° to 166° (from butanone).
Soluble 1 in 20 of water, 1 in 5 of ethanol, and 1 in 2 of chloroform; very slightly soluble in ether.

Partition Coefficient. Log *P* (octanol/water), 3.98 (hydrochloride).

Thin-layer Chromatography. System TA—Rf 68; system TB—Rf 67; system TC—Rf 64; system TE—Rf 84; system TL—Rf 54; system TAE—Rf 55; system TAJ—Rf 42; system TAK—Rf 25; system TAL—Rf 84. (Acidified iodoplatinate solution, positive.)

Gas Chromatography. System GA—RI 2111; system GB—RI 2175; system GF—RI 2265.

High Performance Liquid Chromatography. System HA—*k* 1.1; system HY—RI 575.

Ultraviolet Spectrum. Aqueous acid—218, 252, 280 nm.

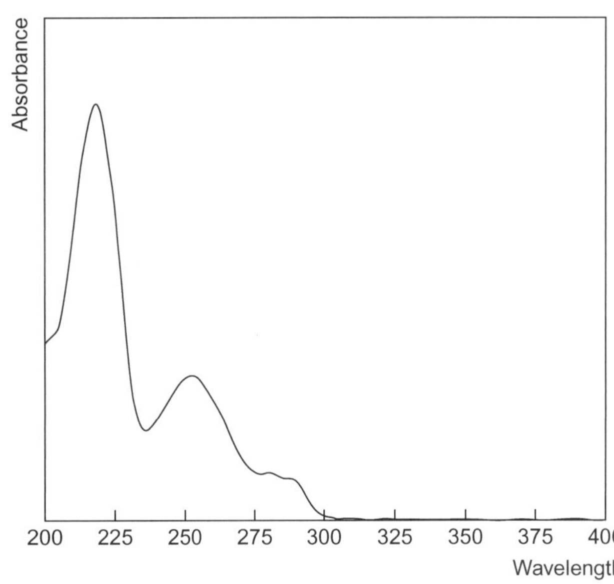

Infra-red Spectrum. Principal peaks at wavenumbers 1714, 1214, 1136, 1197, 1184, 1155 cm^{-1} (dicycloverine hydrochloride, KBr disk).

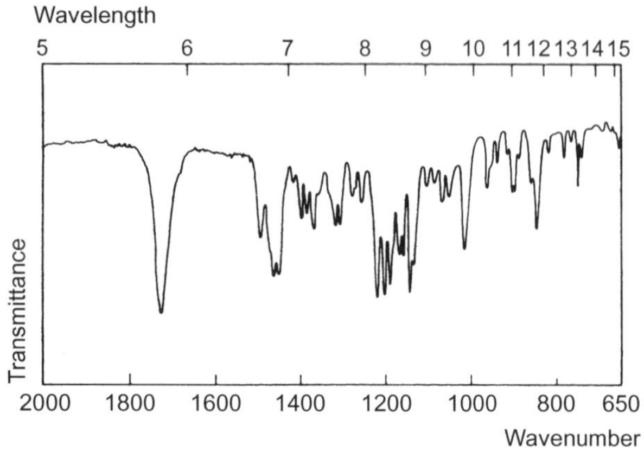

Mass Spectrum. Principal ions at *m/z* 86, 71, 99, 58, 55, 56, 100, 87.

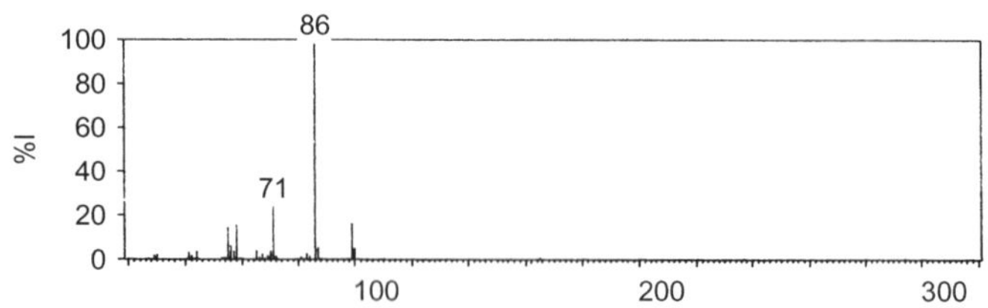

Quantification

Gas chromatography. In plasma: limit of detection 1 μg/L, AFID—P. J. Meffin *et al.*, *Anal. Chem.*, 1973, *45*, 1964–1966. In plasma: nitrogen-selective detection—B. J. Walker *et al.*, *J. Chromatogr.*, 1987, *416*, 150–153.

Disposition in the Body. Rapidly absorbed after oral administration. About 80% of a dose is excreted in the urine and 10% is eliminated in the faeces.

Therapeutic concentration

After a single oral dose of 20 mg to 1 subject, a peak plasma concentration of about 0.02 mg/L was attained in about 1.5 h; following administration of 40 mg to the same subject as a sustained-release preparation, a maximum plasma concentration of about 0.08 mg/L was reported after about 2.5 h. [P. J. Meffin *et al.*, *Anal. Chem.*, 1973, *45*, 1964–1966.]

Toxicity. Fatalities have been reported in children after the ingestion of about 0.2 g of a sustained-release preparation.

A blood concentration of 0.505 mg/L (nearly 10 times the reported adult therapeutic level) was reported in a fatality involving an infant. [J. C. Garriott *et al.*, *J. Toxicol. Clin. Toxicol.*, 1984, *22*, 455–462.]

Half-life. Plasma half-life, about 5 h.

Dose. 30 to 80 mg of dicycloverine hydrochloride daily; in the USA doses of up to 160 mg daily in divided doses have been recommended.

Didanosine

Antiviral

Synonyms. DDI; ddI; ddIno; Dideoxyinosine; NSC-612049, BMY-40900.
Proprietary name. Videx
2′,3′-Dideoxyinosine $C_{10}H_{12}N_4O_3$ = 236.2
CAS—69655-05-6

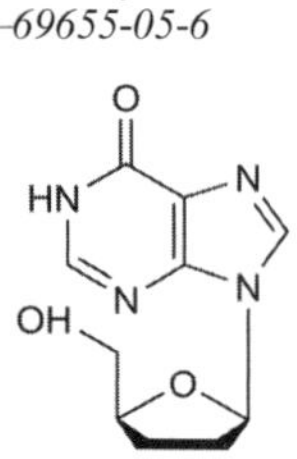

A white crystalline powder with m.p. 160° to 163°. It is unstable in acidic solutions.

Dissociation Constant. pK_a 9.12.

Partition Coefficient. Log *P* (octanol/water), −1.24.

High Performance Liquid Chromatography. System HAD—*k* 3.2.

Column: NovaPak (100 × 8 mm i.d., 4 μm). Mobile phase: 5% acetonitrile in 0.1% heptafluorobutyric acid in deionised, distilled water, 2.0 mL/min flow rate. UV detection (λ = 252 and 260 nm). Retention time: 8.4 min. [M. E. Carpen *et al.*, *J. Chromatogr.*, 1990, *526*; *Biomed. Appl.*, *91*, 69–75].

Column: (analytical-plasma) ODS (Ultrasphere, 250 × 4.6 mm, 5 μm); (urine) C_8 (Zorbax, 250 × 4.6 mm, 5 μm); (guard) ODS (Whatman Pellicular, 2.3 × 0.4 cm). Mobile phase (plasma): 15% methanol in 50 mM potassium phosphate buffer containing 0.05% TEA (pH 4.0), 0.7 mL/min flow rate; (urine) 3.9% methoxyethanol in 18.3 mM potassium phosphate buffer (pH 7.2), 1.0 mL/min. UV detection (λ = 254 nm). Retention time: (plasma) 11.2 min; (urine) 15.3 min. [C. A. Knupp *et al.*, *J. Chromatogr. B*, 1990, *533*, 282–290].

Ultraviolet Spectrum. Aqueous acid (pH 2)—248 nm; (ethanol)—246, 250 nm; aqueous alkali (pH 12)—254 nm.

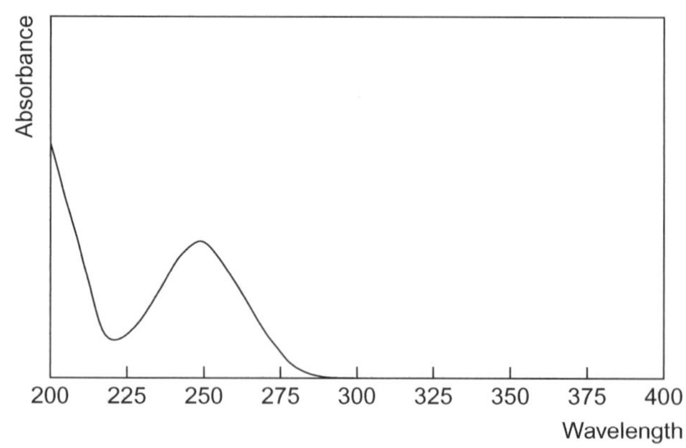

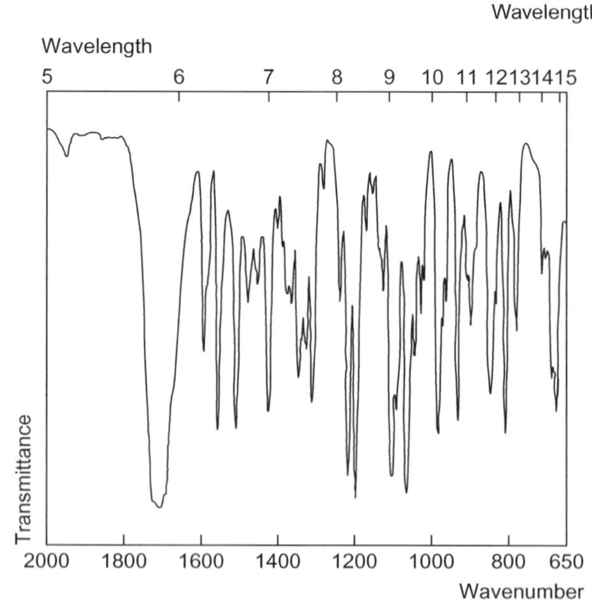

Quantification

High performance liquid chromatography. In CSF (cerebrospinal fluid), plasma, or urine: limit of detection 0.1 μg/L, UV detection—M. E. Carpen *et al.*, *J. Chromatogr.*, 1990, *526*; *Biomed. Appl.*, *91*, 69–75. In plasma: limit of detection 50 μg/L, UV detection—N. Frijus-Plessen *et al.*, *J. Chromatogr.*, 1990, *534*; *Biomed. Appl.*, 99, 101–107. In plasma or urine: limit of detection 25 μg/L and 1000 μg/L, respectively, UV detection—C. A. Knupp *et al.*, *J. Chromatogr.*, 1990, *533*; *Biomed. Appl.*, *98*, 282–290. In serum: free didanosine, limit of detection 25 μg/L, UV detection—M. L. Rosell-Rovira *et al.*, *J. Chromatogr.* 1996, *675*, *Biomed. Appl.*, 89–92. In plasma: limit of quantification is 10 μg/L—G. Aymard *et al.*, *J. Chromatogr. Biomed. Sci. Appl.*, 2000, *744*, 227–240. In serum: limit of detection is 120 μg/L, UV detection—V. A. Simon *et al.*, *J. Chromatogr. A*, 2001, *913(1-2)*, 447–453.

Disposition in the Body. Didanosine is rapidly absorbed and reduced by 50% in the presence of food. It is hydrolysed in the acid medium of the stomach and is therefore given by mouth with pH buffers or antacids. Concentrations in CSF are about 20% of those in plasma 1 h after intravenous infusion. It crosses the placenta; is detected in amniotic fluid and fetal blood and crosses the blood–brain barrier; detected in CSF. The drug is extensively metabolised to the active antiviral metabolite dideoxyadenosine triphosphate, as well as uric acid. Acid hydrolysis may also occur to produce hypoxanthine. About 35 to 60% of a dose is excreted unchanged in urine by glomerular filtration and active tubular secretion. It is partially cleared by haemodialysis but not by peritoneal dialysis.

Therapeutic concentration. Mean peak plasma concentrations of 1.6 mg/L (range 0.6 to 2.9 mg/L) are produced after a single dose of 375 mg of a buffered powder for oral solution. Mean peak plasma concentrations of 1.6 mg/L (range 0.5 to 2.6 mg/L) are produced after administration of a single dose of 300 mg of a buffered chewable/dispersible tablet.

Groups of three to four patients diagnosed having AIDS (acquired immunodeficiency syndrome) or poor-prognosis AIDS-related complex were administered 0.2, 0.4, 0.8, 1.6, 3.2 or 6.4 mg/kg intravenous doses over 90 min or the equivalent oral doses. Peak concentrations were 0.6, 1.5, 1.8, 4.6, 10.5 and 18.5 μmol/L for the intravenous doses and 0.3, 0.8, 1.2, 2.8, 6.2 and 9.2 μmol/L for the oral doses, respectively. [N. R. Harman *et al.*, *Clin. Pharmacol. Ther.*, 1990, *47*, 647–654].

Toxicity

In phase I clinical studies, 12 out of 92 patients suffered from peripheral neuropathy (the most frequent serious toxic effect), which is dose related, when administered doses of 12 mg/kg daily for 6 weeks. This is believed to be due to accumulation of the drug above concentrations of 1250 mg/kg. Pancreatitis, in some cases fatal, has developed during therapy with didanosine; 8 out of 92 patients being treated with > 12.5 mg/kg daily for 5 to 8.5 months suffered from pancreatitis. [D. Faulds and R. N. Brogden, *Drugs*, 1992, *44*, 94–116].

A 36-year-old man with Gilbert Syndrome, AIDS and a history of severe myelosuppression when administered with zidovudine was treated with 12 mg/kg once daily didanosine instead. Treatment was stopped after 15 weeks owing to side effects but was resumed after 6 weeks. 3 months after treatment was restarted, the man was admitted to hospital with nausea, anorexia and abdominal pain. A CT scan showed he had a fatty liver with an enlarged globular pancreas. Renal dysfunction was observed the day before he died, caused by fulminent hepatic failure (a complication of treatment). [K. Kew Lai *et al.*, *Ann. Intern Med.*, 1991, *115(4)*, 283–284].

Bioavailability. Bioavailability is substantially reduced by administration with or after food and varies considerably between patients; it is reported to range from 20 to 40% depending on the formulation used.

Half-life. Plasma, didanosine, 30 min to 4 h; dideoxyadenosine triphosphate, more than 12 h; increased in patients with renal impairment.

Volume of distribution. Mean, 1.01 L/kg in adults (range 0.76 to 1.29 L/kg); 24 L/m^2 in children.

Clearance. Plasma clearance, 600 to 800 mL/min in adults; 510 mL/min/m^2 in children. Total body, 0.08 L/kg/h.

Protein binding. In plasma, less than 5%.

Note. For reviews of didanosine see M. J. Shelton *et al.*, *Ann. Pharmacother.*, 1992, *26*, 660–670, D. Faulds and R. N. Brogden, *Drugs*, 1992, *44*, 94–116, J. J. Lipsky, *Lancet*, 1993, *341*, 30–32, and C. M. Perry and J. A. Balfour, *Drugs*, 1996, *52*, 928–962.
For a review of the pharmacokinetics of antiviral nucleoside analogues see G. D. Morse *et al.*, *Clin. Pharmacokinet.*, 1993, *24*, 101–123.

Dose. Adults with body weight ⩾ 60 kg: 200 mg (tablets) or 250 mg (solution) every 12 h; ⩽ 60 kg: 125 mg (tablets) or 167 mg (solution). Children: 25 to 100 mg (tablet) or 31 to 125 mg (powder formulation) twice daily, depending on body surface area.

Dieldrin

Insecticide

Proprietary name. Dilstan EC-15
Dieldrin contains about 85% of HEOD, (1aα,2β,2aα,3β,6β,6aα,7β,7aα)-3,4,5,6,9,9-hexachloro-1a,2,2a,3,6,6a,7,7a-octahydro-2,7:3,6-dimethanonaphth[2,3-*b*]oxirene, the remaining 15% being mainly chlorinated organic compounds related to HEOD.
$C_{12}H_8Cl_6O=380.9$
CAS—60-57-1 (HEOD)

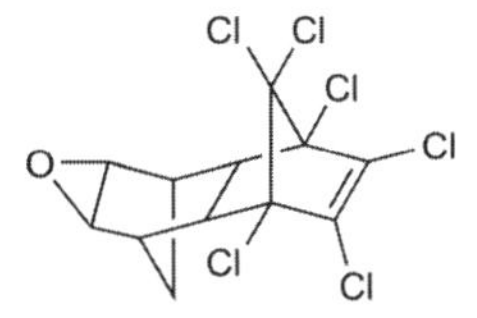

A light-tan, flaky, crystalline solid. M.p. 176° to 177°.
Practically insoluble in water; soluble 1 in 4 of ethanol, 1 in 40 of carbon tetrachloride, and 1 in 1 of methanol; moderately soluble in chloroform.

Partition Coefficient. Log *P* (octanol/water), 5.4.

Colour Tests. Nitric–Sulfuric Acid—pink; Sulfuric Acid–Fuming Sulfuric Acid—red.

Thin-layer Chromatography. System TB—Rf 60; system TE—Rf 89; system TF—Rf 74; system TX—Rf 65; system TY—Rf 87; system TAB—Rf 51; system TAC—Rf 27; system TAE—Rf 89.

Gas Chromatography. System GA—RI 2110; system GK—RRT 1.13 (relative to caffeine).

Ultraviolet Spectrum. No significant absorption, 230 to 360 nm.

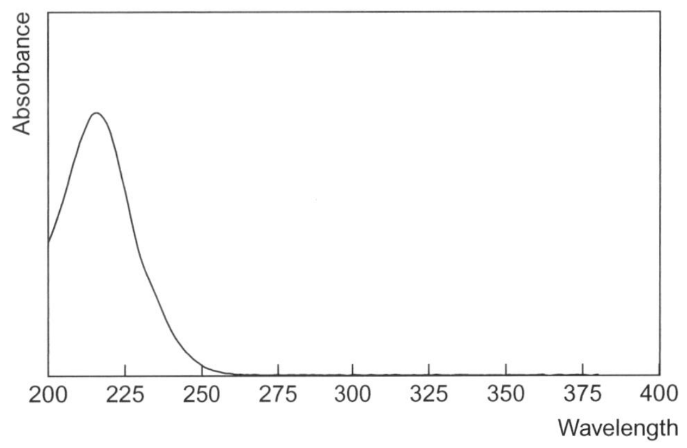

Infra-red Spectrum. Principal peaks at wavenumbers 848, 811, 1038, 700, 1005, 912 cm^{-1} (KCl disk).

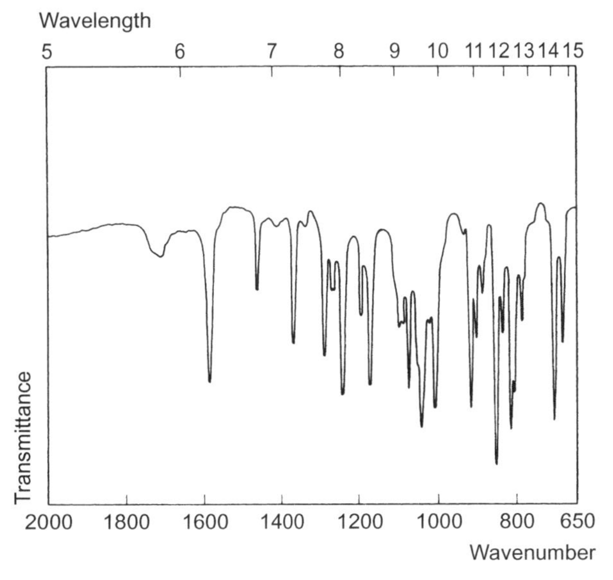

Mass Spectrum. Principal ions at *m*/*z* 79, 82, 81, 263, 77, 108, 265, 80.

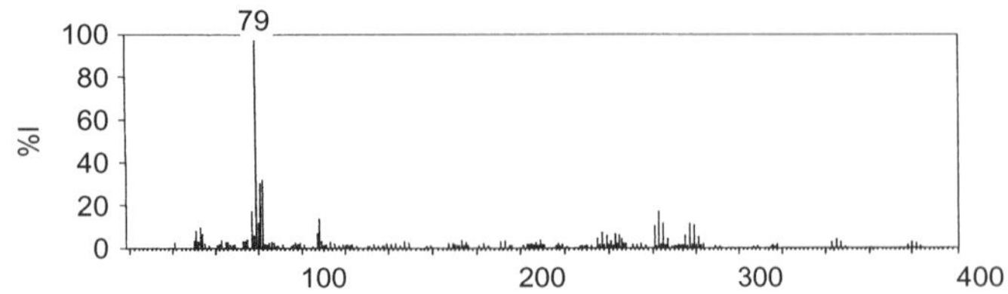

Quantification

Gas chromatography. In blood or tissues: ECD—A. Steentoft, *Med., Sci. Law*, 1979, *19*, 268–269. In serum and plasma: limit of detection 0.1 to 0.7 µg/L, ECD—J. J. Saady and A. Poklis, *J. Anal. Toxicol.*, 1990, *14(5)*, 301–304.

Gas chromatography–mass spectrometry. In serum—J. Dmitrovic *et al.*, *Toxicol. Letters*, 2002, *134(1–3)*, 253–258.

Disposition in the Body. Both dieldrin powder and solutions are readily absorbed after oral administration, through the lungs, and through intact skin. Dieldrin is selectively stored in body fat and persists for several weeks after cessation of exposure. It is eliminated in the faeces mainly as unknown hydrophilic metabolites; a small amount is excreted in the urine as metabolites but very little as unchanged dieldrin.
Dieldrin is a metabolite of aldrin.

Blood concentration. Blood concentrations averaging 0.001 mg/L have been reported in subjects with no occupational exposure to dieldrin.

Serum concentrations ranging from 0.001 to 0.137 mg/L (mean 0.02) were reported in 71 industrially exposed workers, and fat concentrations of 0.6 to 32 µg/g (mean 6) were reported in 28 of these subjects. [W. T. Hayes and A. Curley, *Arch. Environ. Health*, 1968, *16*, 155–162.]

Steady-state blood concentrations of about 0.007 and 0.02 mg/L were reported in 2 groups of 3 subjects who received doses of 0.05 mg and 0.21 mg daily for 2 years; maximum fat concentrations of 1.3 to 1.6 µg/g and 2.2 to 4.9 µg/g were reported in the same subjects. [C. G. Hunter *et al.*, *Arch. Environ. Health*, 1969, *18*, 12–21.]

Fat residues in 236 non-exposed subjects were reported to be in the range <0.01 to 0.5 µg/g (mean 0.1). [D. C. Abbott *et al.*, *BMJ*, 1981, *283*, 1425–1428.]

Toxicity. The estimated minimum lethal dose is 5 g; ingestion of 10 mg/kg may produce toxic effects. The maximum permissible atmospheric concentration is 0.25 mg/m^3 and the maximum acceptable daily intake is 0.1 µg/kg. Blood concentrations greater than 0.15 µg/mL are usually toxic. Several fatalities due to accidental or deliberate ingestion of dieldrin have been reported.

A serum concentration of 0.27 mg/L and a fat concentration of 47 µg/g were reported 3 days after ingestion of dieldrin by a 4-year-old boy who survived. [L. K. Garrettson and A. Curley, *Arch. Environ. Health*, 1969, *19*, 814–822.]

In a fatality due to the ingestion of dieldrin, postmortem blood and liver concentrations of 0.5 mg/L and 29 µg/g, respectively, were reported. [A. Steentoft, *Med., Sci. Law*, 1979, *19*, 268–269.]

Half-life. Blood half-life, 50 to 170 days (mean 97).

Distribution in blood. Plasma:whole blood ratio, about 1.5.

Protein binding. In plasma, more than 99%.

Dienestrol

Oestrogen

Synonyms. Dehydrostilbestrol; Dienoestrol; Oestrodienolum.
Proprietary names. Cycladiene; DV; Estraguard; Hormofemin.
4,4′-(1,2-Diethylidene-1,2-ethanediyl)bisphenol
$C_{18}H_{18}O_2$=266.3
CAS—84-17-3; 13029-44-2 (E,E)

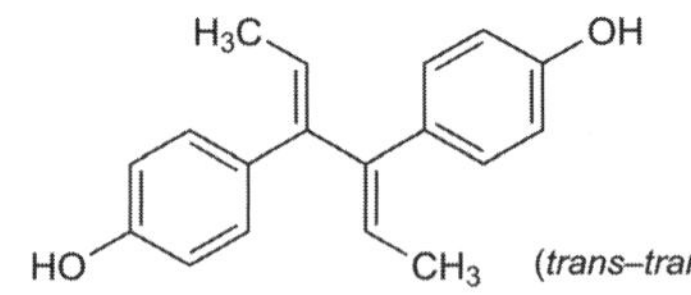

(trans–trans)-form

White crystals or crystalline powder. M.p. 227° to 234°.
Practically insoluble in water; soluble 1 in 8 of ethanol, 1 in 5 of acetone and 1 in 15 of ether; freely soluble in propylene glycol; soluble in chloroform and aqueous solutions of alkali hydroxides.
Caution. Dienestrol is a powerful oestrogen. Contact with the skin or inhalation should be avoided.

Partition Coefficient. Log *P* (octanol/water), 5.3.

Colour Tests. Antimony Pentachloride—red; Naphthol–Sulfuric Acid—orange-brown/yellow; Sulfuric Acid—orange-red.
Dissolve about 0.5 mg in 0.2 mL of acetic acid, add 1 mL of phosphoric acid, and heat on a water-bath for 3 min—violet, becoming slightly more blue on dilution with 3 mL of acetic acid. (This test distinguishes dienestrol from diethylstilbestrol, which produces a yellow colour.)

Thin-layer Chromatography. System TP—Rf 72; system TQ—Rf 25; system TR—Rf 34; system TS—Rf 05, streaking may occur.

High Performance Liquid Chromatography. System HY—RI 535.

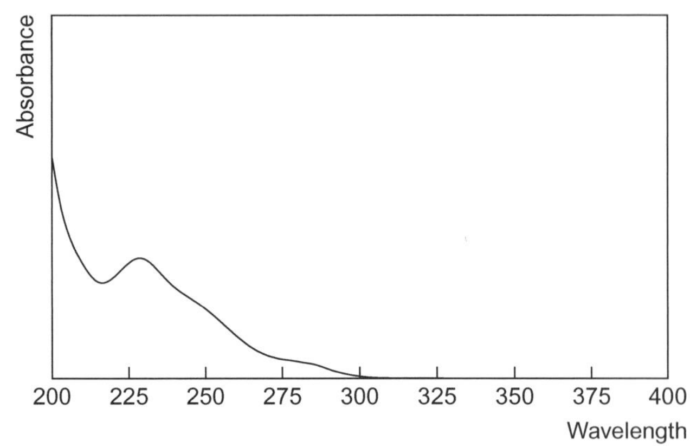

Infra-red Spectrum. Principal peaks at wavenumbers 1206, 827, 1173, 1510, 1248, 775 cm^{-1} (KBr disk).

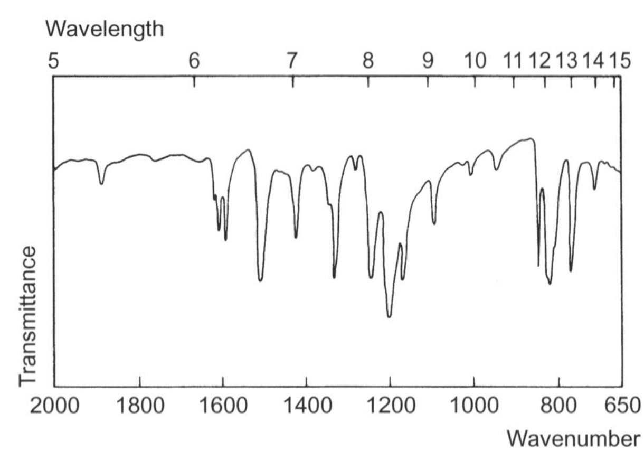

Disposition in the Body. Readily absorbed after oral administration. It is excreted in the urine mainly as a glucuronide conjugate.

Dose. Dienestrol has been given by mouth in doses of 0.5 to 30 mg daily. It is used as a 0.01 to 0.025% vaginal cream.

Diethazine

Anticholinergic

Synonyms. Eazamine; RP-2987.
N,N-Diethyl-10*H*-phenothiazine-10-ethanamine
$C_{18}H_{22}N_2S$=298.4

CAS—60-91-3

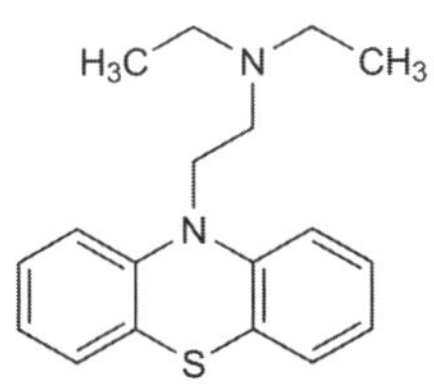

An oily liquid.

Diethazine Hydrochloride
$C_{18}H_{22}N_2S,HCl=334.9$
CAS—341-70-8
A white or slightly cream-coloured crystalline powder. M.p. 184° to 186°.
Soluble 1 in 5 of water, 1 in 6 of ethanol and 1 in 5 of chloroform; practically insoluble in ether.

Dissociation Constant. pK_a 9.1 (20°).

Partition Coefficient. Log *P* (octanol/water), 5.9.

Colour Tests. Formaldehyde–Sulfuric Acid—red-violet; Forrest Reagent—red; FPN Reagent—orange; Mandelin's Test—green→violet (excess reagent); Marquis Test—violet-brown.

Thin-layer Chromatography. System TA—Rf 58; system TB—Rf 57; system TC—Rf 51; system TE—Rf 77; system TL—Rf 39; system TAE—Rf 33; system TAF—Rf 54. (Acidified iodoplatinate solution, positive.)

Gas Chromatography. System GA—RI 2377.

High Performance Liquid Chromatography. System HA—*k* 3.4; system HAX—Retention time 15.1 min; system HAY—Retention time 7.4 min.

Ultraviolet Spectrum. Aqueous acid—250 nm ($A_1^1=1200b$), 298 nm; aqueous alkali—265 nm.

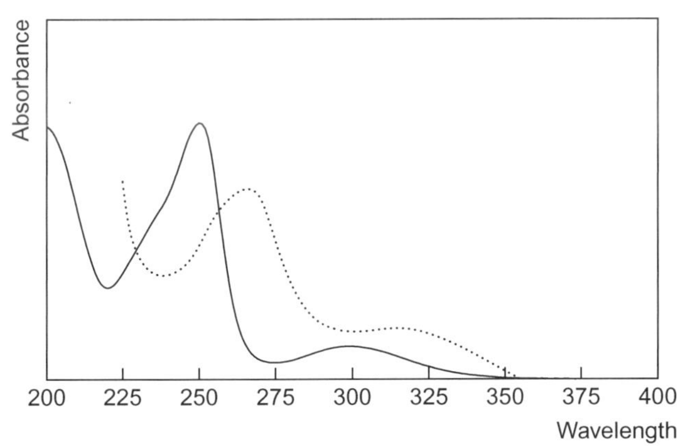

Infra-red Spectrum. Principal peaks at wavenumbers 748, 1245, 1587, 1282, 1562, 1219 cm^{-1} (KBr disk).

Mass Spectrum. Principal ions at *m/z* 86, 298, 87, 30, 58, 299, 212, 180.

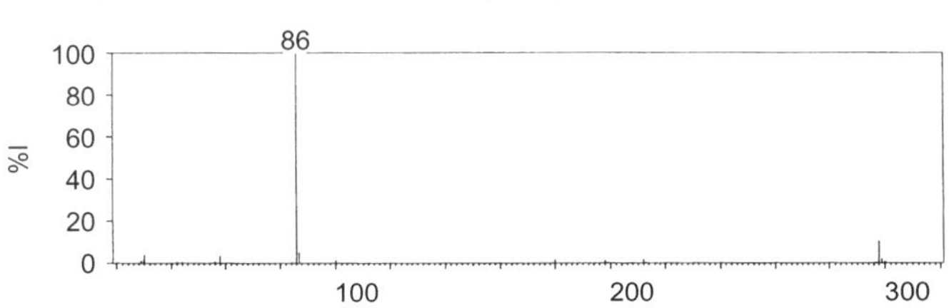

Dose. Diethazine hydrochloride has been given in doses of 0.15 to 1.5 g daily.

Diethyl Phthalate

Plasticiser/Solvent

Synonym. Ethyl Phthalate
Diethyl-1,2-benzenedicarboxylate
$C_{12}H_{14}O_4=222.2$
CAS—84-66-2

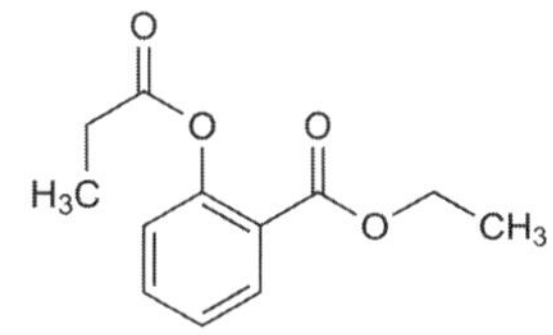

A clear, colourless, somewhat viscous liquid. Mass per mL about 1.117 g. B.p. about 295°. Refractive index 1.500 to 1.505.
Practically insoluble in water; miscible with ethanol and ether.

Partition Coefficient. Log *P* (octanol/water), 2.4.

Gas Chromatography. System GA—RI 1564.

Infra-red Spectrum. Principal peaks at wavenumbers 1733, 1287, 1086, 1132, 744, 1044 cm^{-1} (thin film).

Mass Spectrum. Principal ions at *m/z* 149, 177, 150, 65, 76, 105, 176, 104.

Diethylcarbamazine

Antifilarial

N,N-Diethyl-4-methyl-1-piperazinecarboxamide
$C_{10}H_{21}N_3O=199.3$
CAS—90-89-1

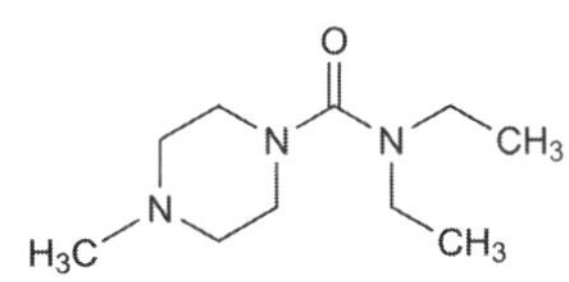

A crystalline powder. M.p. 47° to 49°.
Soluble in water, ethanol, chloroform, and ether.

Diethylcarbamazine Citrate
Synonyms. Diethylcarbamazine Acid Citrate; Ditrazini Citras.
Proprietary names. Banocide; Hetrazan; Notézine.
$C_{10}H_{21}N_3O,C_6H_8O_7=391.4$
CAS—1642-54-2
A white, crystalline, slightly hygroscopic powder. M.p. 141° to 143°.
Freely soluble in water; soluble 1 in 35 of ethanol; practically insoluble in acetone, benzene, chloroform, and ether.

Dissociation Constant. pK_a 7.7 (20°).

Partition Coefficient. Log *P* (octanol/water), 0.4.

Thin-layer Chromatography. System TA—Rf 52; system TB—Rf 17; system TC—Rf 26; system TL—Rf 05. (Dragendorff spray, positive.)

Gas Chromatography. System GA—RI 1497.

High Performance Liquid Chromatography. System HA—*k* 1.4; system HX—RI 219; system HY—RI 192.

Ultraviolet Spectrum. No significant absorption, 230 to 360 nm.

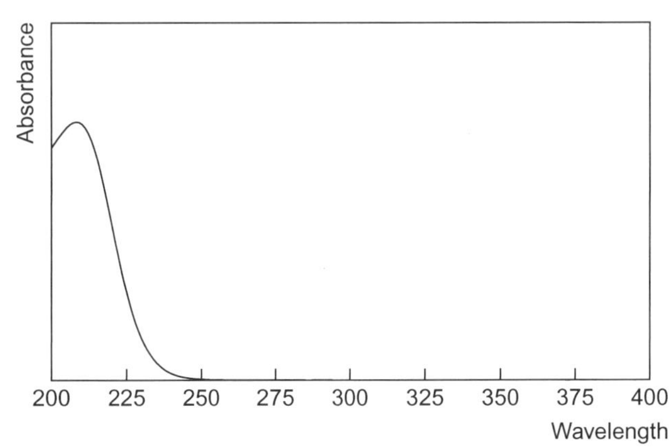

Infra-red Spectrum. Principal peaks at wavenumbers 1618, 1258, 1217, 1712, 1105, 1149 cm^{-1} (KBr disk).

Mass Spectrum. Principal ions at *m/z* 71, 72, 58, 100, 83, 56, 70, 44.

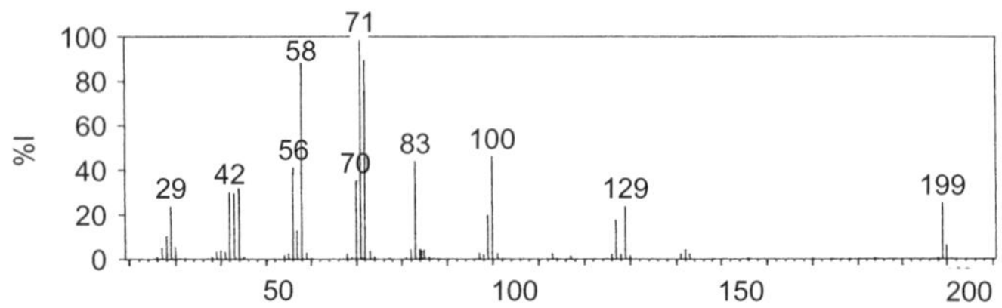

Quantification

Gas chromatography. In plasma: limit of detection 60 µg/L and limit of quantification 70 µg/L, FID—J. R. Miller Jnr and L. Fleckenstein, *J. Pharm. Biomed. Anal.*, 2001, *26(4)*, 665–674. In plasma: limit of detection 4 µg/L, nitrogen specific detector—S. Lee *et al., J. Chromatogr. B Biomed. Sci. Appl.*, 1997, *704(1–2)*, 181–185. In plasma or urine: limit of detection 10 µg/L, AFID—G. D. Allen *et al., J. Chromatogr.* 1979, *164 B Biomed. Appl., 6*, 521–526.

Immunoassay. In biological fluids—Y. Mitsui *et al., Trop. Med. Int. Health*, 1996, *1(4)*, 528–534.

Disposition in the Body. Readily absorbed after oral administration. About 50% of a dose is excreted in the urine as unchanged drug and 10% as the *N*-oxide metabolite in 48 h; the excretion of unchanged drug is pH-dependent being increased in acidic urine (pH 5) but decreasing to less than 10% in alkaline urine (pH 8).

Therapeutic concentration

Following a single oral dose of 50 mg to 5 subjects, peak plasma concentrations of 0.08 to 0.20 mg/L were attained in about 1 to 2 h; a secondary rise in plasma concentrations was observed at 3 to 9 h. [G. Edwards *et al., Clin. Pharmacol. Ther.*, 1981, *30*, 551–557.]

Half-life. Plasma half-life, about 10 h under alkaline urinary pH conditions or 3 h if an acidic urinary pH is maintained.

Protein binding. In plasma, not significantly bound.

Dose. 1 to 6 mg/kg of diethylcarbamazine citrate daily, by mouth.

Diethylpropion

Anorectic

Synonym. Amfepramone

2-(Diethylamino)-1-phenyl-1-propanone

$C_{13}H_{19}NO=205.3$

CAS—90-84-6

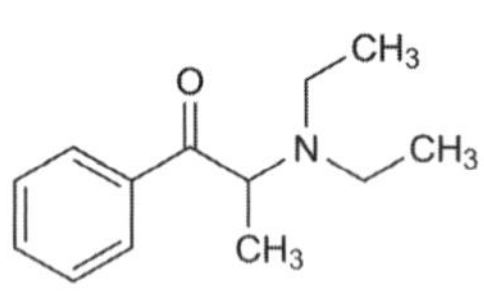

Diethylpropion Hydrochloride

Proprietary names. Anorex; Atractil; Dobesin; Dietec; D.I.P.; Dualid S; Hipofagin S; Ifa Norex; Inibex S; Moderatan Diffucap; Neobes; Prefamone; Regenon; Tenuate Dospan.

Note. The name Tepanil is also applied to phenylpropanolamine hydrochloride.

$C_{13}H_{19}NO,HCl=241.8$

CAS—134-80-5

A white to off-white, fine, crystalline powder. M.p. 168°, with decomposition. Soluble 1 in 0.5 of water, 1 in 3 of ethanol, and 1 in 3 of chloroform; practically insoluble in ether.

Partition Coefficient. Log *P* (octanol/water), 3.04.

Colour Test. Liebermann's Test—yellow

Thin-layer Chromatography. System TA—Rf 76; system TB—Rf 62; system TC—Rf 63; system TE—Rf 85; system TL—Rf 64; system TAE—Rf 55; system TAF—Rf 56; system TAJ—Rf 44; system TAK—Rf 02; system TAL—Rf 35. (Dragendorff spray, positive; FPN reagent, pink; acidified iodoplatinate solution, positive; Marquis reagent, violet-brown.)

Gas Chromatography. System GA—diethylpropion RI 1486, M (phenylpropanolamine) RI 1360; system GB—diethylpropion RI 1532, M (phenylpropanolamine) RI 1352, M (diethylnorephedrine) RI 1599, M (ethylnorephedrine) RI 1457, M (*N*-desethyl-) RI 1423, M (*N*-didesethyl-) RI 1338; system GC—diethylpropion RI 1715, M (norephedrine) RI 1383; system GF—diethylpropion RI 1655.

High Performance Liquid Chromatography. System HA—diethylpropion *k* 1.7, M (norephedrine) *k* 0.9; system HC—diethylpropion *k* 0.16, M (norephedrine) *k* 0.70; system HY—RI 230; system HZ—retention time 2.8 min.

Ultraviolet Spectrum. Aqueous acid—253 nm (A_1^1=673a); aqueous alkali—246 nm.

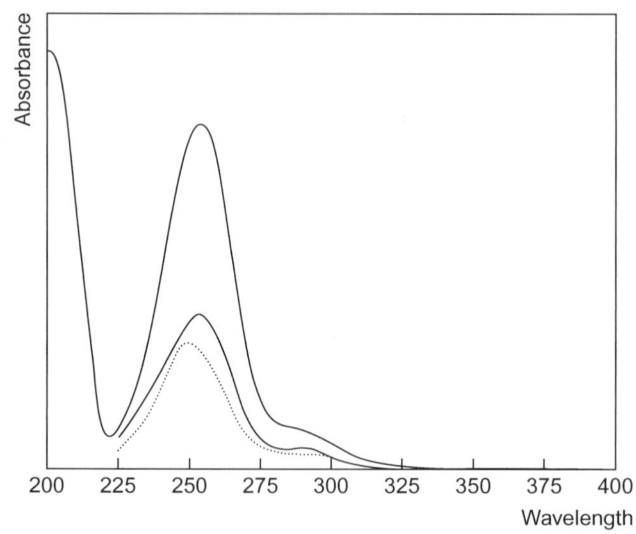

Infra-red Spectrum. Principal peaks at wavenumbers 701, 1230, 1682, 1287, 973, 1594 cm^{-1} (diethylpropion hydrochloride, KBr disk).

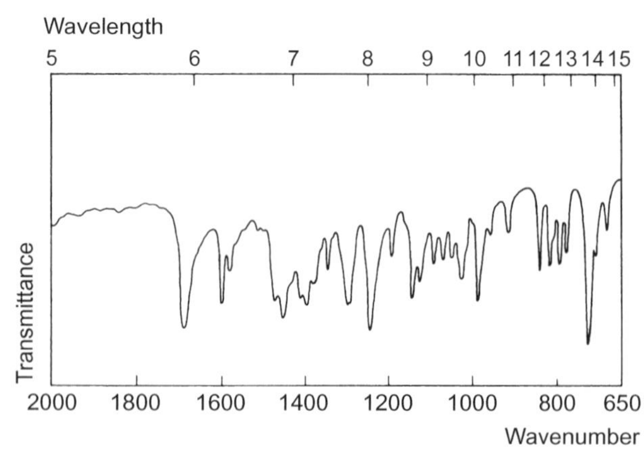

Mass Spectrum. Principal ions at *m/z* 100, 44, 72, 101, 77, 56, 42, 105 (no peaks above 110); norephedrine 44, 77, 79, 51, 45, 42, 107, 105.

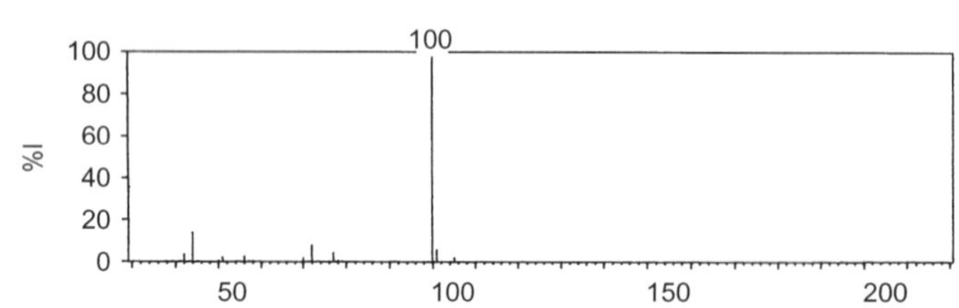

Quantification

Gas chromatography. In urine: diethylpropion and metabolites, limit of detection 300 µg/L, FID—B. Testa and A. H. Beckett, *J. Chromatogr.*, 1972, *71*, 39–54.

Gas chromatography–mass spectrometry. In plasma: limit of detection 600 ng/L—G. J. Wright *et al.*, *Drug Metab. Rev.*, 1975, *4*, 267–276.

High performance liquid chromatography. In plasma: diethylpropion enantiomers—B. Mey *et al.*, *Chirality*, 1998, *10*, 307–315.

Disposition in the Body. Readily absorbed after oral administration. Metabolised by *N*-dealkylation, reduction, deamination, and *N*-hydroxylation primarily to active metabolites; keto reduction is stereoselective resulting in the formation of *threo*-hydroxylated metabolites; glucuronide formation also occurs along with the formation of hippuric and mandelic acids. About 80 to 90% of a dose is excreted in the urine; the amount excreted in the urine is reduced when the urine is alkaline; of the urinary excreted material, *N*-ethylaminopropiophenone, norephedrine (phenylpropanolamine), and hippuric acid are the main metabolites together with small amounts of unchanged drug, aminopropiophenone, *N*-diethylnorephedrine, and *N*-ethylnorephedrine. Diethylpropion crosses the blood–brain barrier and the placenta. The drug and its metabolites are distributed into breast milk.

Therapeutic concentration

Following a single oral dose of 75 mg to 5 subjects, a mean peak plasma concentration of 0.007 mg/L was attained in 0.5 h; total concentrations of the monodesethyl and didesethyl metabolites reached an average peak of 0.19 mg/L at 2 h. [G. J. Wright *et al.*, *Drug Metab. Rev.*, 1975, *4*, 267–276.]

Toxicity. The estimated minimum lethal doses are 200 mg for a child and 2 g for an adult.

The following disposition was reported in a case of fatal overdose resulting from the injection of illicit diethylpropion tablets: blood 5.4 mg/L, bile 14.4 mg/L, kidney 0.9 μg/g, liver 0.9 μg/g, injection site 43.2 μg/g. [R. R. Fysh and J. F. Taylor, *Bull. Int. Assoc. Forensic Toxicol.*, 1978, *14(2)*, 16–17.]

Half-life. Derived from urinary excretion data, 1.5 to 3 h in subjects whose urines are acidic.

Dose. Usually 75 mg of diethylpropion hydrochloride daily.

Diethylstilbestrol

Antineoplastic (hormonal)

Synonyms. DES; Diethylstilboestrol; Stilbol.
Proprietary names. Apstil; Distilbene.
4,4′[(*1E*)-1,2-Diethyl-1,2-ethenediyl]bisphenol
$C_{18}H_{20}O_2$=268.4
CAS—56-53-1

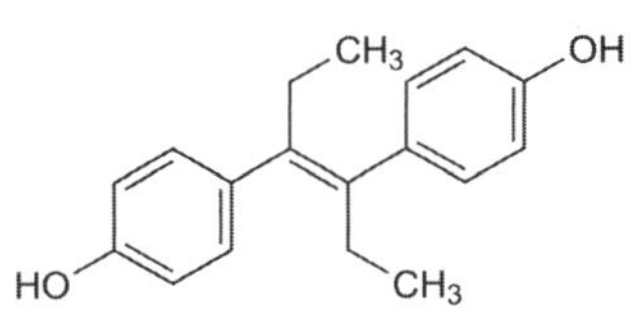

A white crystalline powder. M.p. 169° to 172°.
Practically insoluble in water; soluble 1 in 5 of ethanol, 1 in 200 of chloroform and 1 in 3 of ether; soluble in acetone and methanol; soluble in fatty oils and alkali hydroxides.

Caution. Diethylstilbestrol is a powerful oestrogen. Contact with the skin or inhalation should be avoided.

Diethylstilbestrol Diphosphate

Synonyms. Fosfestrol; Phosphoestrolum.
Proprietary names. Honvan; Stilphostrol (tablets)

Note. Fosfestrol Sodium (the tetra-sodium salt of diethylstilbestrol diphosphate) is available under the proprietary names Honvan, Honvol, Ronvan, ST-52, and Stilphostrol (injection).
$C_{18}H_{22}O_8P_2$=428.3
CAS—522-40-7
An off-white crystalline powder which decomposes at about 204° to 206°.
Sparingly soluble in water; soluble in ethanol and dilute alkalis.

Diethylstilbestrol Dipropionate

Proprietary names. Cyren B; Dibestil
$C_{24}H_{28}O_4$=380.5
CAS—130-80-3
Colourless crystals or white crystalline powder. M.p. 104°.
Slightly soluble in water and dilute mineral acids; soluble 1 in 100 of ethanol (90%) and 1 in 6 of ether; freely soluble in acetone and chloroform.

Partition Coefficient. Log *P* (octanol/water), 5.1.

Colour Tests. Antimony pentachloride—red; Naphthol–Sulfuric acid—yellow/orange; Sulfuric acid—orange.
Dissolve about 0.5 mg in 0.2 mL of acetic acid, add 1 mL of phosphoric acid acid, and heat on a water-bath for 3 min—yellow, disappearing on dilution with 3 mL of acetic acid. (This test distinguishes diethylstilbestrol from dienestrol, which produces a violet colour.)

Thin-layer Chromatography. System TB—Rf 3; system TE—Rf 73; system TF—Rf 68; system TP—Rf 65, streaking may occur; system TQ—Rf 10, streaking may occur; system TR—Rf 18, streaking may occur; system TS—Rf 03; system TAE—Rf 92; system TAF—Rf 92.

Gas Chromatography. System GA—RI 2298.

High Performance Liquid Chromatography. System HX—592; system HY—RI 559; system HAA—Retention time(s) 20.9 min.

Ultraviolet Spectrum. Ethanol—241 nm (A_1^1=600a).

Infra-red Spectrum. Principal peaks at wavenumbers 1205, 1176, 833, 1250, 1512, 1610 cm^{-1} (KBr disk).

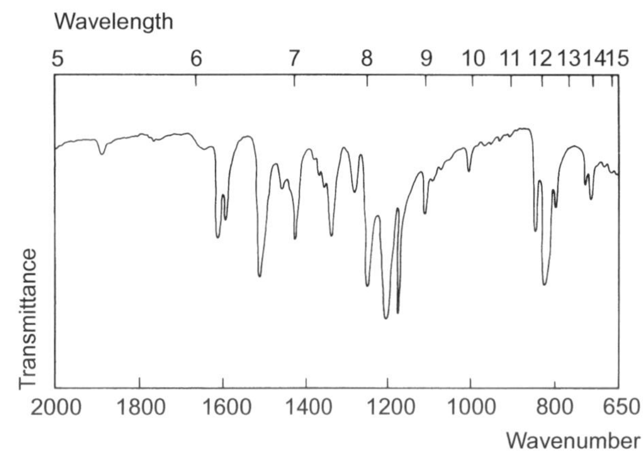

Mass Spectrum. Principal ions at *m/z* 107, 145, 268, 238, 121, 133, 159, 224.

Quantification

Gas chromatography. In blood, plasma, serum, bile or tissues: FID—K. A. Kohrman and J. MacGee, *J. Assoc. Off. Anal. Chem.*, 1977, *60*, 5–8.

High performance liquid chromatography. In plasma, urine or tissues: UV detection—G. D. Newport *et al.*, *J. Liq. Chromatogr.*, 1980, *3*, 1053–1070.

Dose. 0.1 to 2 mg daily; doses of 15 mg daily may be given.

Diethylthiambutene

Narcotic Analgesic (Veterinary)

Synonyms. Thiambutene; 191C49.
N,*N*-Diethyl-1-methyl-3,3-di-2-thienylallylamine
$C_{16}H_{21}NS_2$=291.5
CAS—86-14-6

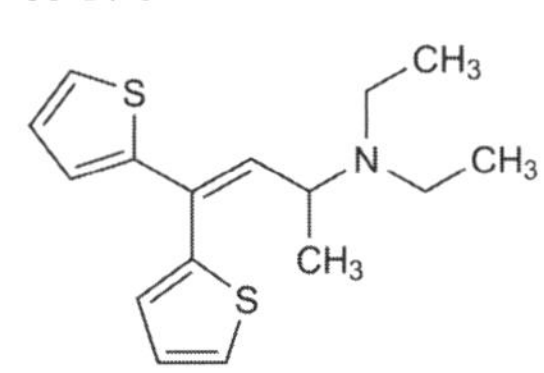

Diethylthiambutene Hydrochloride

$C_{16}H_{21}NS_2$,HCl=327.9
CAS—132-19-4
A white crystalline powder. M.p. 152° to 153°.
Soluble 1 in 2 of water and 1 in 1 of ethanol; practically insoluble in ether.

Partition Coefficient. Log *P* (octanol/water), 4.5.

Colour Tests. Liebermann's Test (100°)—orange; Mandelin's Test—green→green-blue; Marquis Test—violet; Sulfuric Acid—orange.
Cold nitric acid gives a pink-brown colour changing to green.

Thin-layer Chromatography. System TA—Rf 70; system TB—Rf 60; system TC—Rf 43; system TE—Rf 81; system TL—Rf 43; system TAE—Rf 40. (Dragendorff spray, positive; acidified iodoplatinate solution, positive; Marquis reagent, red-violet.)

Gas Chromatography. System GA—RI 2008.

High Performance Liquid Chromatography. System HA—*k* 2.0.

Ultraviolet Spectrum. Aqueous acid—268, 288 nm (A^1_1=362a); aqueous alkali—295 nm.

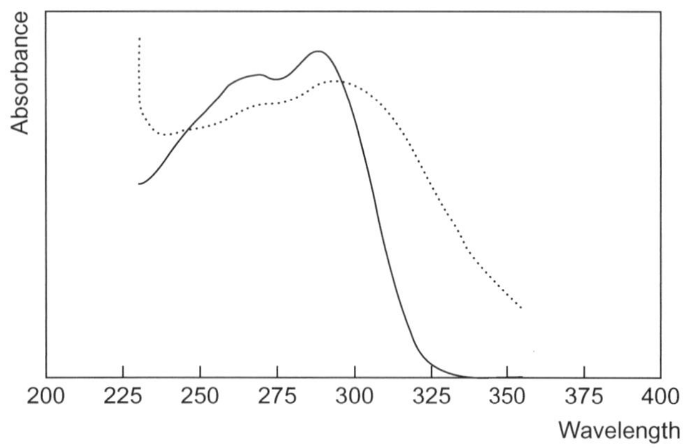

Infra-red Spectrum. Principal peaks at wavenumbers 716, 743, 851, 833, 1244, 1618 cm^{-1} (diethylthiambutene hydrochloride, KBr disk).

Mass Spectrum. Principal ions at *m/z* 276, 111, 219, 42, 277, 97, 29, 100.

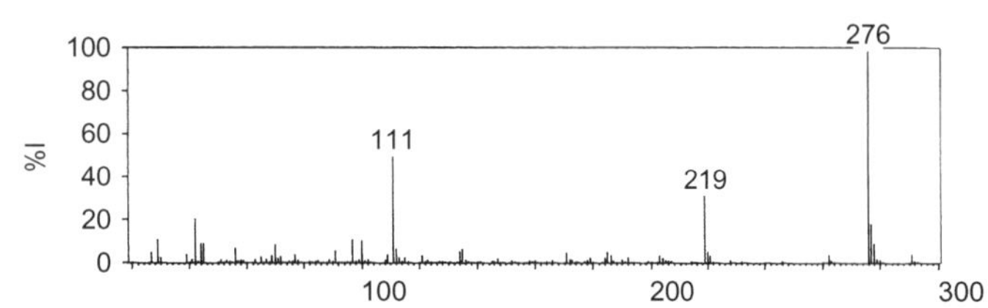

Diethyltoluamide

Insect Repellent

Synonym. DEET
Proprietary names. Autan; Detamide; Dieltamid; Flypel; Metadelphene; Off; Repel.
N,N-Diethyl-3-methylbenzamide
$C_{12}H_{17}NO$=191.3
CAS—134-62-3

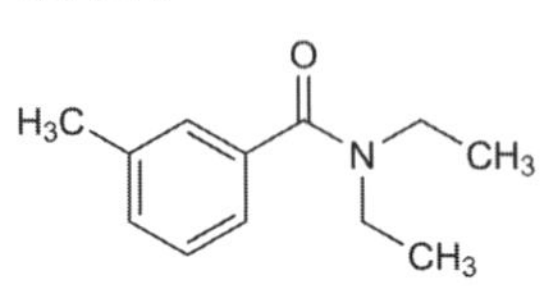

A colourless or faintly yellow liquid. Wt per mL 0.997 to 1.000 g.
Practically insoluble in water; freely soluble in ethanol, benzene, chloroform, and ether; sparingly soluble in petroleum ether.

Partition Coefficient. Log *P* (octanol/water), 2.2.

Thin-layer Chromatography. System TA—Rf 73. (Acidified iodoplatinate solution, positive.)

Gas Chromatography. System GA—RI 1583.

Ultraviolet Spectrum. No significant absorption, 230 to 360 nm.

Infra-red Spectrum. Principal peaks at wavenumbers 1629, 1284, 794, 1305, 1581, 1095 cm^{-1} (KBr disk).

Quantification
Gas chromatography–mass spectrometry. In urine: diethyltoluamide and metabolites—A. Wu *et al.*, *J. High Resolut. Chromatogr. Chromatogr. Commun.*, 1979, *2*, 558–562.

Disposition in the Body
Toxicity
Two patients ingested large amounts of a concentrated (between 47.5 and 95%) insect repellent containing DEET. Serum concentrations were 168 mg/L and 240 mg/L. [M. Tenenbein, *JAMA*, 1987, *258(11)*, 1509–1511.]

Use. As a 50 to 75% solution.

Diethyltryptamine

Hallucinogen

Synonyms. D.E.T.; *N,N*-Diethyltryptamine.
N,N-Diethyl-1*H*-indole-3-ethanamine
$C_{14}H_{20}N_2$=216.3
CAS—61-51-8

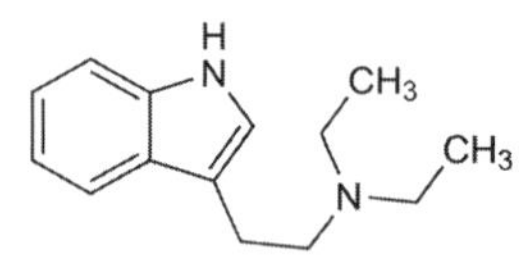

An orange oily liquid.
Soluble in ethanol and chloroform.

Diethyltryptamine Hydrochloride
A white crystalline powder. M.p. 87° to 89°.
Soluble in water.

Colour Tests. Mandelin's Test—grey-green→yellow; Marquis Test—yellow→brown.

Thin-layer Chromatography. System TA—Rf 46; system TB—Rf 15; system TC—Rf 10; system TE—Rf 63; system TL—Rf 11; system TAE—Rf 14; system TAF—Rf 56; system TAJ—Rf 02; system TAK—Rf 03; system TAL—Rf 41. (Dragendorff spray, positive; acidified iodoplatinate solution, positive; Marquis reagent, brown.)

Gas Chromatography. System GA—RI 1910.

High Performance Liquid Chromatography. System HY—RI 276.

Ultraviolet Spectrum. Aqueous acid—278 nm (A^1_1=270a), 287 nm.

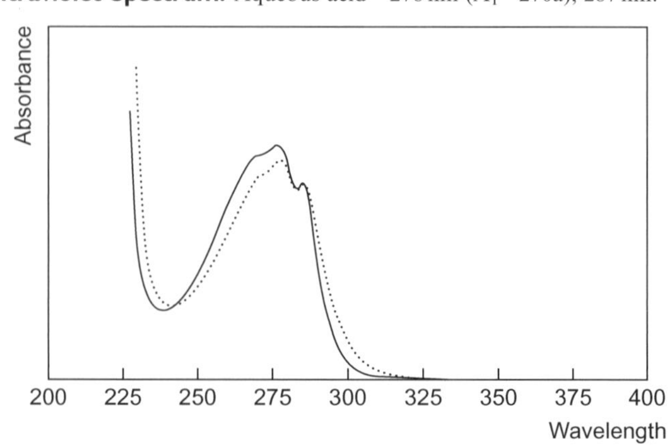

Infra-red Spectrum. Principal peaks at wavenumbers 740, 1111, 1063, 1086, 1234, 724 cm^{-1}.

Mass Spectrum. Principal ions at *m/z* 86, 30, 58, 29, 130, 87, 77, 42.

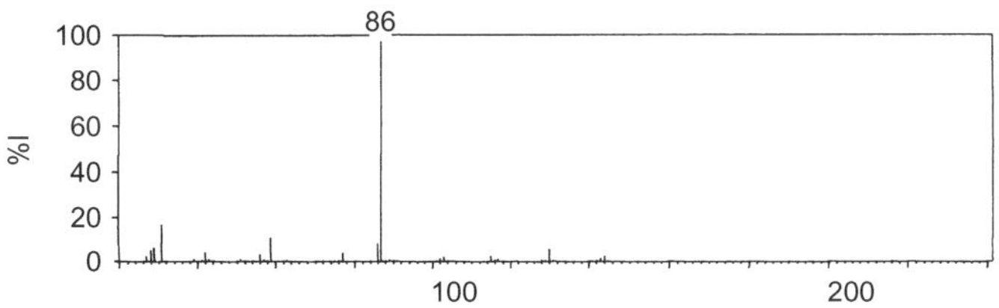

Difenidol

Anti-emetic

Synonym. Diphenidol
Proprietary names. Dicavin; Hemitiken; Laudifen; Nautrol; Normitrol; Serratol; Vernausin.
α,α-Diphenyl-1-piperidinebutanol
$C_{21}H_{27}NO=309.4$
CAS—972-02-1

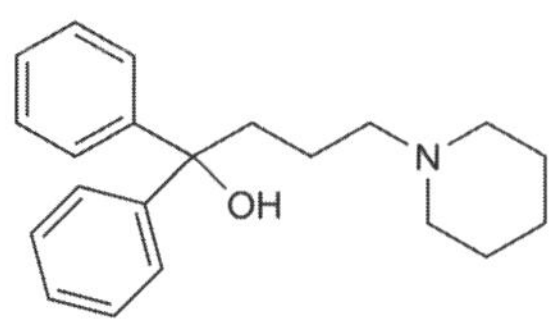

M.p. 103° to 104°.

Difenidol Hydrochloride

Proprietary names. Cephadol; Normavom; Vontril; Vontrol.
$C_{21}H_{27}NO,HCl=345.9$
CAS—3254-89-5
A white crystalline powder. M.p. 214° to 221°, with decomposition.
Soluble in water, ethanol, and chloroform; freely soluble in methanol; practically insoluble in ether, benzene, and petroleum ether.

Partition Coefficient. Log *P* (octanol/water), 4.7.

Colour Tests. Liebermann's Test—brown; Mandelin's Test—yellow; Marquis Test—yellow; Sulfuric Acid—orange.

Thin-layer Chromatography. System TA—Rf 61; system TB—Rf 56; system TC—Rf 45; system TE—Rf 91; system TL—Rf 51; system TAJ—Rf 24; system TAK—Rf 13; system TAL—Rf 67. (Acidified iodoplatinate solution, positive.)

Gas Chromatography. System GA—RI 2384.

High Performance Liquid Chromatography. System HAX—retention time 12.1 min; system HAY—retention time 6.1 min.

Ultraviolet Spectrum. Aqueous acid—252, 258 nm.

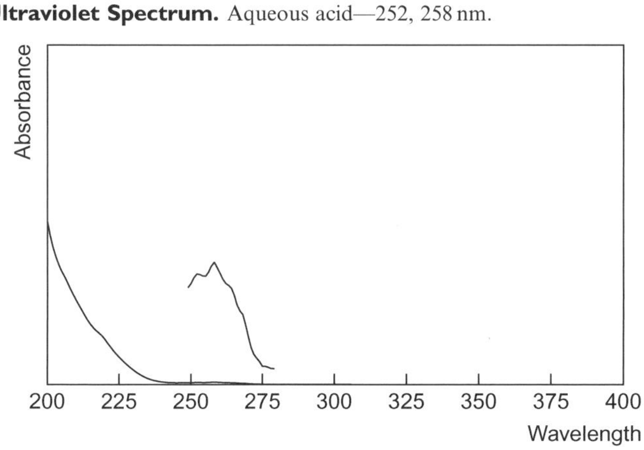

Infra-red Spectrum. Principal peaks at wavenumbers 697, 701, 749, 773, 1123, 1219 cm^{-1} (KBr disk).

Mass Spectrum. Principal ions at *m/z* 98, 99, 105, 77, 55, 41, 127, 111.

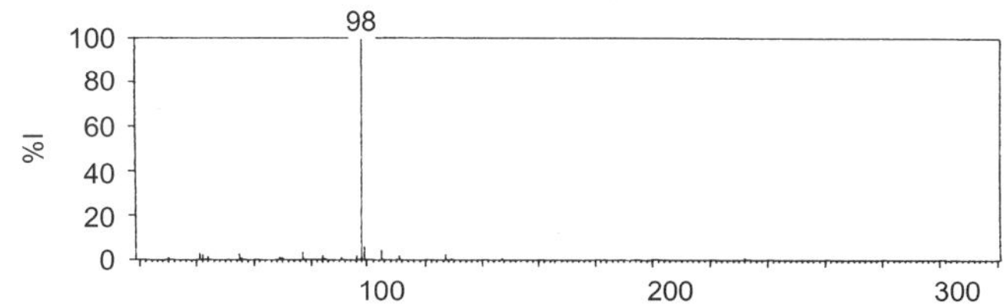

Disposition in the Body. Absorbed from the gastro-intestinal tract; peak blood concentrations are attained in 1.5 to 3 h. It is excreted in the urine and faeces.

Toxicity

Analysis of 21 cases of difenidol overdose showed that the average amount ingested was 222.5 mg (range 25 to 800); adults ingested 150 to 700 mg, children ingested 25 to 800 mg. Toxicity was severe in 4 children, one of whom died (a 2½-year-old boy who ingested 225 mg (15 mg/kg)). [C. C. Yang and J. F. Deng, *J. Toxicol. Clin. Toxicol.*, 1998, *36*, 33–39.]

Dose. The equivalent of 25 to 50 mg of difenidol every 4 h; maximum of 300 mg daily.

Diflunisal

Analgesic

Proprietary names. Aflogos; Artrodol; Biartac; Difludol; Diflusal; Dolobid; Dolobis; Donobid; Fluniget.
2′,4′-Difluoro-4-hydroxy-[1,1′-biphenyl]-3-carboxylic acid
$C_{13}H_8F_2O_3=250.2$
CAS—22494-42-4

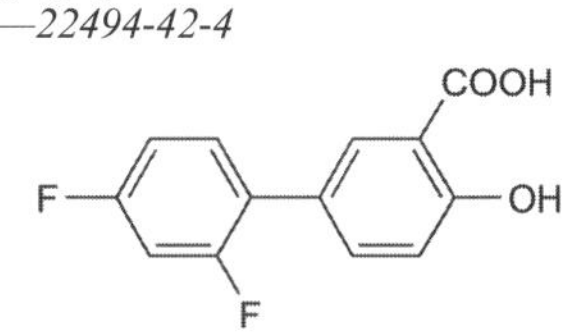

White crystals or crystalline powder. M.p. about 212°.
Sparingly soluble in water; soluble in ethanol, ether, and dilute alkalis.

Partition Coefficient. Log *P* (octanol/water), 4.4.

Colour Tests. Ferric Chloride—violet; Folin–Ciocalteu Reagent—blue; McNally's Test—violet

Thin-layer Chromatography. System TD—Rf 08; system TE—Rf 16; system TF—Rf 05; system TG—Rf 37; system TAD—Rf 18; system TAE—Rf 89; system TAJ—Rf 06; system TAK—Rf 69; system TAL—Rf 69. (Chromic acid solution, blue-grey.)

Gas Chromatography. System GA—diflunisal RI 2095, diflunisal-Me RI 2050, diflunisal-Me_2 RI 1990; system GD—RRT of methyl derivative 1.20 (relative to n-$C_{16}H_{34}$).

High Performance Liquid Chromatography. System HD—*k* 4.1; system HV—RRT 0.77 (relative to meclofenamic acid); system HX—RI 508; system HY—RI 583; system HZ—retention time 5.4 min; system HAX—retention time 5.9 min; system HAY—retention time 6.0 min.

Ultraviolet Spectrum. Acid methanol—251 nm ($A_1^1=560a$), 315 nm ($A_1^1=130a$); aqueous alkali—277 nm.

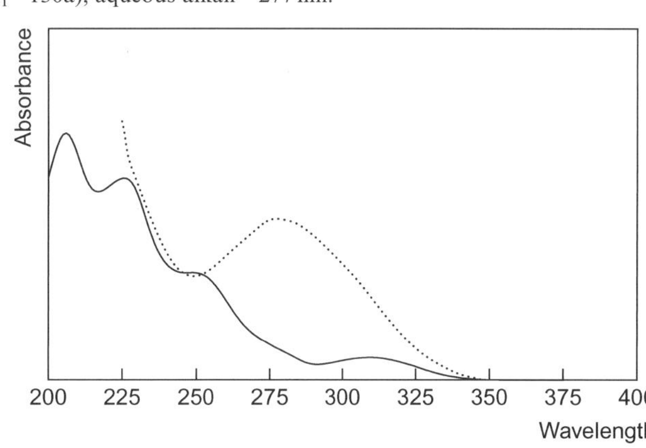

Infra-red Spectrum. Principal peaks at wavenumbers 1683, 1492, 1248, 1220, 1150, 978 cm^{-1} (KBr disk). Two polymorphic forms may occur.

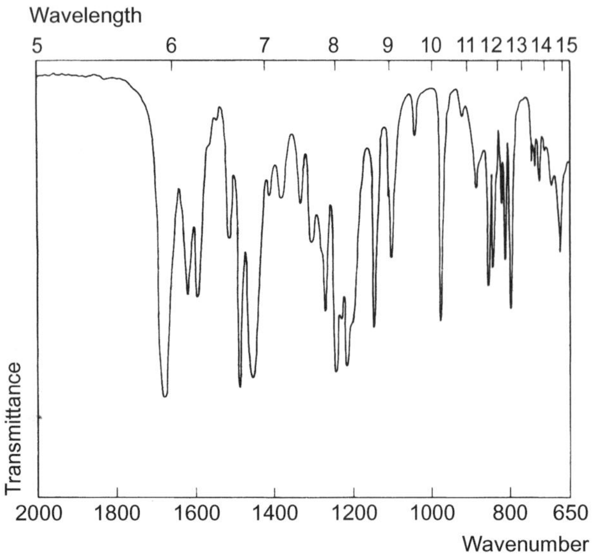

Mass Spectrum. Principal ions at *m/z* 232, 250, 175, 204, 176, 233, 102, 78.

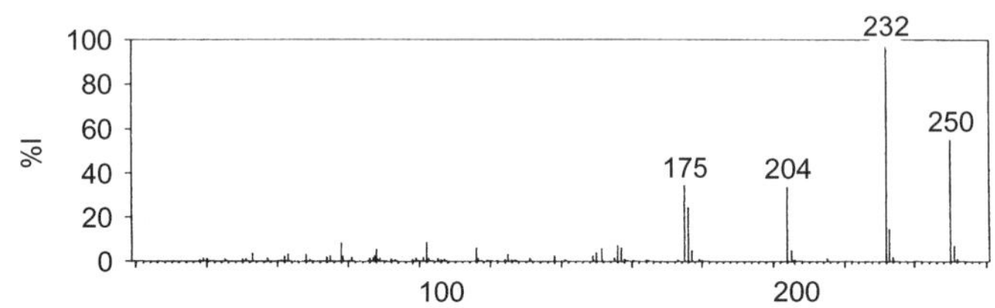

Quantification

Spectrofluorimetry. In plasma: limit of detection 500 ng—D. J. Tocco *et al.*, *Drug Metab. Dispos.*, 1975, *3*, 453–466.

Gas chromatography. In plasma or urine: limit of detection 1 mg/L, FID—D. J. Tocco *et al.*, *Drug Metab. Dispos.*, 1975, *3*, 453–466.

Gas chromatography–mass spectrometry. In urine: diflunisal and some NSAIDs—B. M. el Haj *et al.*, *Forensic Sci. Int.*, 1999, *105*, 141–153.

High performance liquid chromatography. In plasma or urine: limit of detection 50 µg/L, fluorescence detection—J. E. Ray and R. O. Day, *J. Pharm. Sci.*, 1983, *72*, 1403–1405. In urine: diflunisal glucuronides—D. G. Musson *et al.*, *J. Chromatogr.*, 1985, *337*, 363–378. In serum or urine: diflunisal and its glucuronides—J. Hansen-Moller *et al.*, *J. Chromatogr.*, 1987, *420*, 99–109. In plasma or serum: in overdose, diflunisal and other NSAIDs, UV detection—P. J. Streete, *J. Chromatogr.*, 1989, *495*, 179–193. In urine: diflunisal and its glucuronide and sulfate conjugates, limit of detection for diflunisal 0.1 mg/L, fluorescence detection—G. R. Loewen *et al.*, *J. Pharm. Sci.*, 1989, *78*, 250–255.

Disposition in the Body. Well absorbed after oral administration. Up to about 80% of a dose is excreted in the urine in 24 h, mostly as the ester and ether glucuronides. Less than 3% of a dose is eliminated in the faeces.

Therapeutic concentration

After a single oral dose of 500 mg given to 5 subjects, peak plasma concentrations of 58 to 92 mg/L (mean 77) were attained in 2 h. [R. Verbeeck *et al.*, *Br. J. Clin. Pharmacol.*, 1979, *7*, 273–282.]

Following oral administration of 500 mg twice daily to 6 subjects, steady-state plasma concentrations of 66 to 183 mg/L were reported. [E. Wählin-Boll *et al.*, *Eur. J. Clin. Pharmacol.*, 1981, *20*, 375–378.]

After administration of diflunisal as either a single oral dose of 1000 mg daily or two doses of 500 mg daily to 13 subjects, mean peak plasma concentrations of 186 and 150 mg/L, respectively, were achieved in 2.5 and 1.9 h. Steady-state plasma concentrations were 118 and 116 mg/L in the respective groups. [P. Mohaverian *et al.*, *Pharmacotherapy*, 1985, *5*, 336–339.]

Toxicity. Diflunisal appears to be relatively non-toxic.

A 47-year-old woman went into a coma after ingesting 29 g of diflunisal but subsequently recovered uneventfully. [H. P. Upadhyay and S. K. Gupta, *BMJ*, 1978, *2*, 640.]

In a fatality involving the ingestion of diflunisal, the following postmortem tissue concentrations were reported: blood 260 mg/L, bile 71 mg/L, kidney 350 µg/g, liver 400 µg/g, stomach contents 34 g, urine 78 mg/L. [B. Levine *et al.*, *Forensic Sci. Int.*, 1987, *35*, 45–50.]

Half-life. Plasma half-life, about 5 to 12 h (dose-dependent).

Volume of distribution. About 0.1 L/kg.

Clearance. Plasma clearance, about 0.1 mL/min/kg.

Protein binding. In plasma, about 99%.

Note. For a review of the pharmacokinetics of diflunisal, see R. N. Brogden *et al.*, *Drugs*, 1980, *19*, 84–106.

Dose. 0.5 to 1 g daily.

Digitoxin

Cardiac Glycoside

Synonyms. Digitaline Cristallisée; Digitoxoside.
Proprietary names. Asthenthilo; Coramedan; Crystodigin; Digimerck; Digitaline Nativelle; Digitox; Digitrin; Ditaven; Purodigin; Tardigal; Variplastic.
(3β,5β)-3-[(*O*-2,6-Dideoxy-β-D-*ribo*-hexopyranosyl-(1→4)-*O*-2,6-dideoxy-β-D-*ribo*-hexopyranosyl-(1→4)-2,6-dideoxy-β-D-*ribo*-hexopyranosyl)oxy]-14-hydroxycard-20(22)-enolide
$C_{41}H_{64}O_{13}$=764.9
CAS—71-63-6

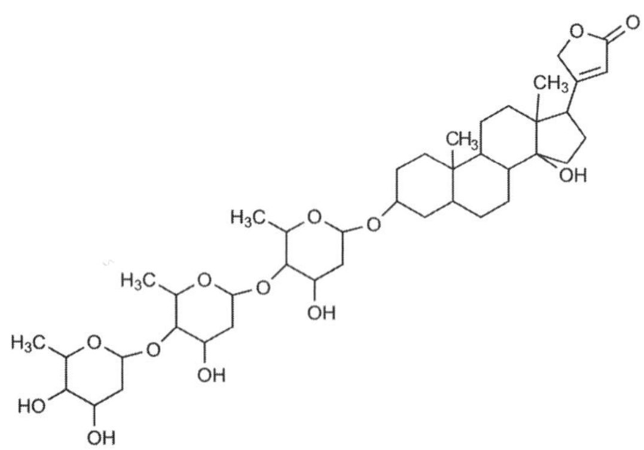

A glycoside obtained from suitable species of *Digitalis* (Scrophulariaceae). A white or pale buff-coloured, microcrystalline powder. M.p. about 256°. Practically insoluble in water; soluble 1 in 60 of ethanol, 1 in 40 of chloroform, and 1 in 400 of ethyl acetate; sparingly soluble in ether, petroleum ether, and methanol; freely soluble in a mixture of equal volumes of chloroform and methanol.

Partition Coefficient. Log *P* (octanol/water), 1.8.

Colour Test. Antimony Pentachloride—yellow→brown→black-violet.

Thin-layer Chromatography. System TD—Rf 03; system TE—Rf 36; system TF—Rf 10; system TAD—Rf 42; system TAE—Rf 88; system TAJ—Rf 35; system TAK—Rf 01; system TAL—Rf 78. (Perchloric acid solution, followed by examination under ultraviolet light, red fluorescence; *p*-anisaldehyde reagent, blue.)

Gas Chromatography. System GA—RI 1902.

High Performance Liquid Chromatography. System HM—*k* 5.4; system HY—RI 468; system HAA—retention time 18.7 min. For further information on allied compounds and metabolites, see Chapter 29.

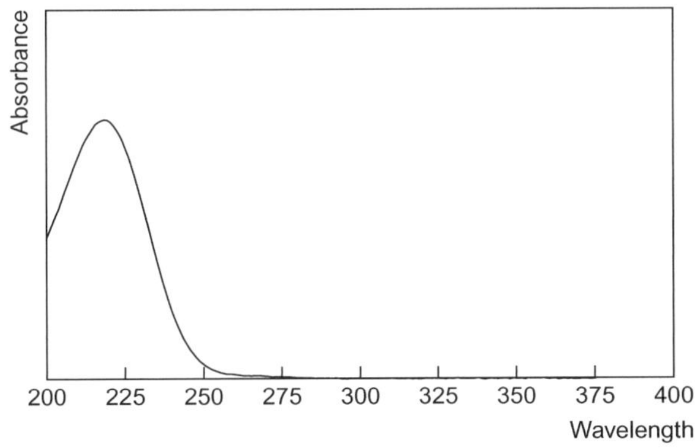

Infra-red Spectrum. Principal peaks at wavenumbers 1072, 1058, 1010, 1740, 1168, 990 cm^{-1} (KBr disk).

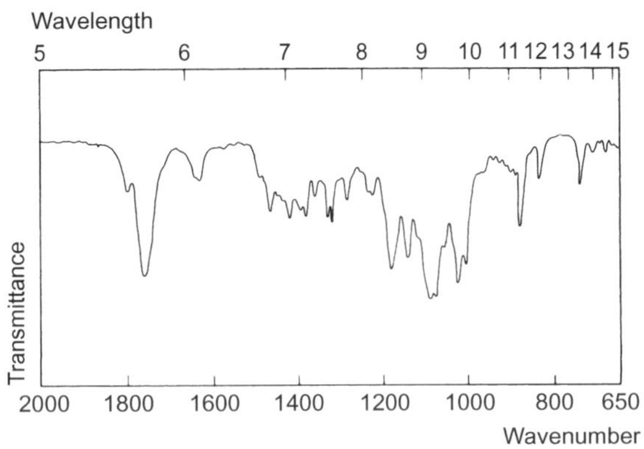

Mass Spectrum. Principal ions at *m/z* 43, 29, 39, 41, 45, 57, 68, 58.

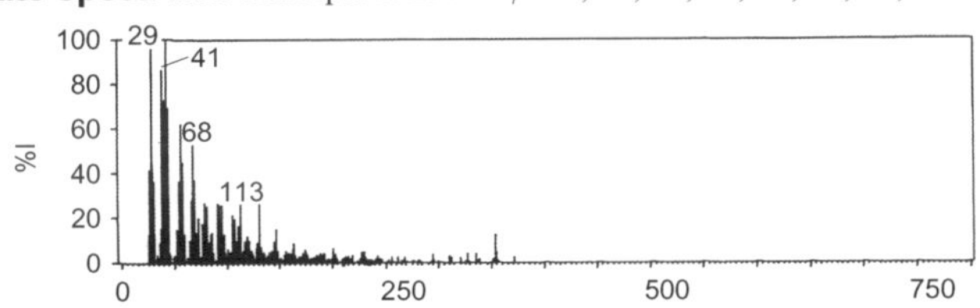

Quantification

High performance liquid chromatography–mass spectrometry. In plasma: digitoxin and other cardiac glycosides, limits of detection 0.15 to 0.6 µg/L—A. Tracqui *et al.*, *J. Chromatogr. B. Biomed. Sci. Appl.*, 1997, *692*, 101–109. In blood or urine: digoxin and other cardiac glycosides—F. Guan *et al.*, *Anal. Chem.*, 1999, *71*, 4034–4043.

High performance liquid chromatography–radioimmunoassay. In tissues: digitoxin, digoxin, and their active metabolites—J. Plum and T. Daldrup, *J. Chromatogr.*, 1986, *377*, 221–231. In urine: digitoxin and its metabolites—S. R. Santos *et al.*, *J. Chromatogr.* 1987, *419*, 155–164.

Thin-layer chromatography. In serum: limit of detection 1 to 2 ng—D. B. Faber *et al.*, *J. Chromatogr.* 1977, *143(1) B Biomed. Appl.*, 95–103.

Radioimmunoassay. In serum, urine, or cerebrospinal fluid: limit of detection 5 µg/L—A. K. Nore *et al.*, *Clin. Chem.*, 1980, *26*, 321–323.

Fluoroimmunoassay. In serum: limit of detection 1 µg/L—M. H. H. Al-Hakiem *et al.*, *Clin. Chem.*, 1982, *28*, 1364–1366.

Disposition in the Body. Readily absorbed after oral administration. High concentrations are found in the kidney, ventricular myocardium, liver, and skeletal muscle. Extensively metabolised by hydrolysis to digitoxigenin bisdigitoxoside, digitoxigenin monodigitoxoside, and digitoxigenin, and by hydroxylation to digoxin and the corresponding digoxigenin derivatives, all of which are active. Epimerisation to the inactive metabolites, epidigitoxigenin and epidigoxigenin, followed by glucuronide conjugation also occurs; dihydrodigitoxin has also been detected in plasma. About 60 to 80% of a single dose is excreted in the urine over a period of 3 weeks, mainly as metabolites, and up to 20% is eliminated in the faeces. The excretion of digitoxin and its active and inactive metabolites is very variable and is independent of dose and route of administration. About 20 to 50% of a dose appears to be excreted as unchanged drug in urine and faeces in variable proportions, and the amount of unchanged drug in the urine has been reported to be greater during maintenance treatment than in single dose studies.

Digitoxin is a metabolite of acetyldigitoxin.

Therapeutic concentration. In serum, usually in the range 0.01 to 0.03 mg/L.

After a single oral dose of 20 µg/kg, given to 6 children, peak serum concentrations of 0.02 to 0.05 mg/L were attained in 1.5 to 2.5 h. [A. Larsen and L. Storstein, *Clin. Pharmacol. Ther.*, 1983, *33*, 717–726.]

Following daily oral doses of 0.1 mg to 7 subjects, steady-state serum concentrations of 9 to 26 µg/L (mean 17) were reported. [K. Haustein, *Eur. J. Clin. Pharmacol.*, 1981, *19*, 45–51.]

Toxicity. The estimated minimum lethal dose is 3 mg. Toxic effects are usually associated with serum concentrations of about 0.03 mg/L or more.

A subject who ingested 10 mg of digitoxin recovered following treatment with activated charcoal; a plasma concentration of 0.26 mg/L was reported 4 h after the dose, decreasing to 0.027 mg/L at 80 h. [S. Pond *et al.*, *Lancet*, 1981, *2*, 1177–1178.]

Following a massive digitoxin overdose in a 20-month-old girl, an initial serum level of 0.629 mg/L was reported. After 6 doses of digoxin-specific antibody fragments, digitoxin was undetectable in the serum but reappeared on days 6 and 7. [K. Schmitt *et al.*, *Pediatr. Cardiol.*, 1994, *15*, 48–49.]

In a 65-year-old female who died almost 15 h after ingesting 7 mg of digitoxin, the plasma concentration just before death was 0.212 mg/L. [J. Krappweis *et al.*, *Eur. J. Med. Res.*, 1996, *25*, 551–553.]

Half-life. Plasma half-life, 3 to 16 days (mean 7).

Bioavailability. Greater than 90%.

Volume of distribution. 0.4 to 0.8 L/kg (mean 0.6); increased in children.

Clearance. Plasma clearance, about 0.04 mL/min/kg; increased in children.

Distribution in blood. Plasma:whole blood ratio, about 1.7.

Protein binding. In plasma, about 95%.

Note. For a review of the clinical pharmacokinetics of digitoxin, see D. Perrier *et al.*, *Clin. Pharmacokinet.*, 1977, *2*, 292–311.

Dose. Maximum initial total dose of 1.6 mg over 1 to 2 days; maintenance, 50 to 200 µg daily.

Digoxin

Cardiac Glycoside

Synonyms. Digoxinum; Digoxosidum.

Proprietary names. Digacin; Digomal; Digosin; Digoxin(e) Nativelle; Dilanacin; Dogoxine; Eudigox; Grexin; Hemigoxine Nativelle; Lanacordin; Lanacrist; Lanicor; Lanoxin(e); Lanoxicaps; Lenoxin; Malpluxin; Neo-Dioxanin; Novodigal; Prodigox; Purgoxin; Rougoxin; Toloxin.

(3β,5β,12β)-3-[(*O*-2,6-Dideoxy-β-D-*ribo*-hexopyranosyl-(1→4)-*O*-2,6-dideoxy-β-D-*ribo*-hexopyranosyl-(1→4)-2,6-dideoxy-β-D-*ribo*-hexopyranosyl)oxy]-12,14-dihydroxycard-20(22)-enolide

$C_{41}H_{64}O_{14}$=780.9

CAS—20830-75-5

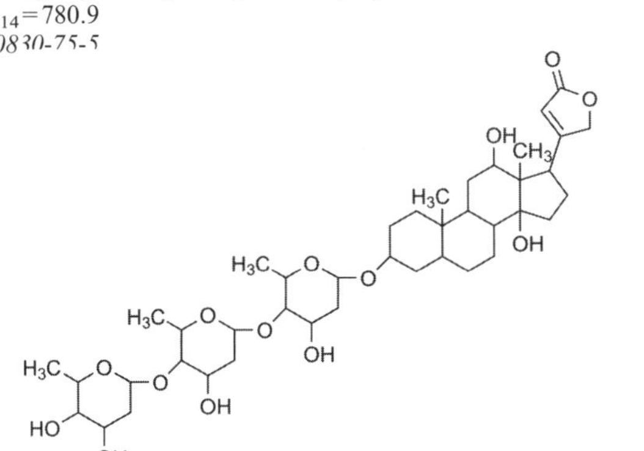

A glycoside obtained from the leaves of *Digitalis lanata* (Scrophulariaceae). Colourless crystals or a white powder. M.p. about 240°, with decomposition.

Practically insoluble in water, dehydrated alcohol, ether, acetone, and ethyl acetate; soluble 1 in 122 of ethanol (80%) and 1 in 4 of pyridine; slightly soluble in chloroform; freely soluble in a mixture of equal volumes of chloroform and methanol.

Metildigoxin
Synonyms. Medigoxin; β-Methyldigoxin.
Proprietary names. Cardiolan; Lanirapid; Lanitop; Miopat.
4‴-*O*-Methyldigoxin
$C_{42}H_{66}O_{14}$=795.0
CAS—30685-43-9
Crystals. M. p. 227° to 231°.

α-Acetyldigoxin
Proprietary names. Lanatilin; Sandolanid.
$C_{43}H_{66}O_{15}$=823.0
CAS—5511-98-8
Prisms. M.p. 225° with decomposition. Very sparingly soluble in ethyl acetate.

β-Acetyldigoxin
Proprietary names. Corotal; Digostad; Digotab; Digox; Gladixol N; Kardiamed; Longdigox; Novodigal (β-acetyldigoxin or digoxin); Stillacor.
CAS—5355-48-6
Needles. Sparingly soluble in ethyl acetate.

Partition Coefficient. Log *P* (octanol/water), 1.26.

Colour Test. Antimony Pentachloride—yellow→brown→black-violet.

Thin-layer Chromatography. System TD—Rf 01; system TE—Rf 33; system TF—Rf 05; system TAD—Rf 28; system TAE—Rf 85. (Perchloric acid solution, followed by examination under UV light, blue fluorescence; *p*-anisaldehyde reagent, blue.)

High Performance Liquid Chromatography. System HM—*k* 11.3; system HY—RI 347; system HAA—retention time 13.9 min. For further information on allied compounds and metabolites, see Chapter 29.

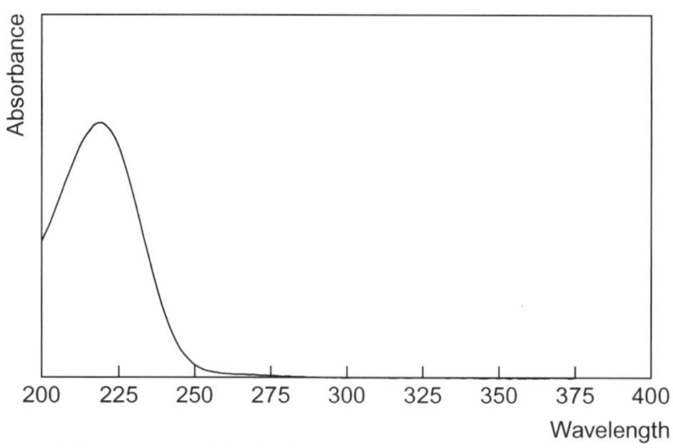

Infra-red Spectrum. Principal peaks at wavenumbers 1075, 1709, 1055, 1020, 1160, 1110 cm^{-1} (KBr disk).

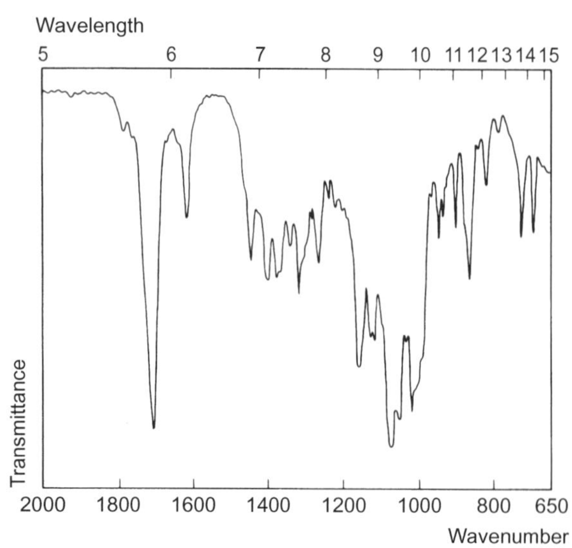

Mass Spectrum. Principal ions at *m/z* 73, 58, 57, 43, 41, 39, 29, 45 (no peaks above 360).

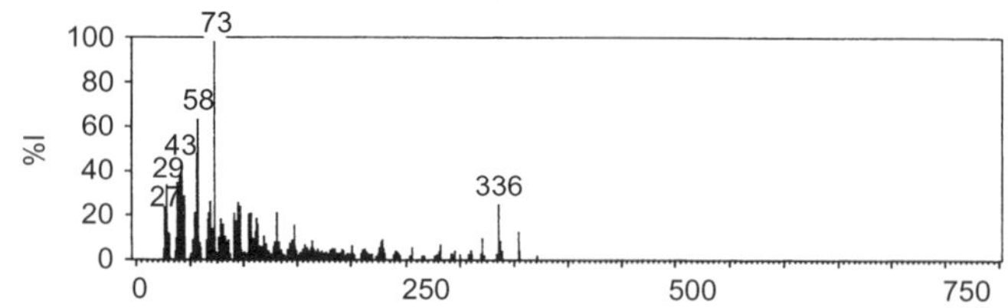

Quantification

High performance liquid chromatography. In urine: tritiated digoxin and metabolites, limit of detection 8 ng/L for digoxin—M. H. Gault *et al.*, *J. Chromatogr.* 1980, *182(8) B Biomed. Appl.*, 465–472. In serum: digoxin and its metabolites, limit of detection 160 ng/L, immunochemical detection—A. J. Oosterkamp *et al.*, *J. Chromatogr.* 1994, *653 B Biomed. Appl.*, 55–61. In serum: digoxin and its metabolites, fluorescence detection—M. C. Tzou *et al.*, *J. Pharm. Biomed. Anal.*, 1995, *13*, 1531–1540.

High performance liquid chromatography–mass spectrometry. In plasma: digoxin and related cardiac glycosides, limits of detection 0.15 to 0.6 μg/mL—A. Tracqui *et al.*, *J. Chromatogr. B Biomed. Sci. Appl.*, 1997, *692*, 101–109. In blood or urine: digoxin and other cardiac glycosides—F. Guan *et al.*, *Anal. Chem.*, 1999, *71*, 4034–4043.

High pressure liquid chromatography–radioimmunoassay. In plasma: digoxin and metabolites—H. A. Nelson *et al.*, *J. Chromatogr.* 1979, *163(5) B Biomed. Appl.*, 169–177.

Radioimmunoassay. In haemolysed blood—S. M. Fletcher *et al.*, *J. Forensic Sci. Soc.*, 1979, *19*, 183–188. In serum or urine: dihydrodigoxin, limit of detection 250 ng/L—V. P. Butler *et al.*, *J. Pharmacol. Exp. Ther.*, 1982, *221*, 123–131.

Disposition in the Body. The absorption of digoxin after oral administration is variable and subject to bioavailability differences. Absorption occurs mainly in the small intestine and is delayed in the presence of food. Digoxin is rapidly distributed throughout the body and less than 20% of the total digoxin in the body is located in the blood. High concentrations are found in the heart, brain, and kidneys, but the skeletal muscles form the largest digoxin store. Concentrations in the myocardium are higher than in plasma. Digoxin is also found in the CSF and it also crosses the placenta. Small amounts of digoxin are excreted in breast milk. Digoxin is metabolised by stepwise removal of the sugar moieties to form digoxigenin, which is further metabolised to inactive metabolites which may be excreted in the free or conjugated form. Reduction to dihydrodigoxin, which is relatively inactive, also occurs. Up to 80% of a dose is excreted in the urine in 7 days with 27% of the dose in the first 24 h; the remainder is eliminated in the faeces via the bile. In most patients, 80 to 90% of the material excreted in the urine is unchanged, up to 10% is in the dihydro form, and a small amount includes digoxigenin and the mono- and bisdigitoxosides. In about 10% of patients, however, between 20 and 55% is excreted as metabolites, mainly dihydrodigoxin. Of the material excreted in the bile, about 50% is unchanged, about 25% is digoxin bisdigitoxoside, about 25% is digoxin monodigitoxoside, and about 1% is digoxigenin.
Digoxin is a metabolite of deslanoside, digitoxin, lanatoside C, and metildigoxin.

Therapeutic concentration. In serum, usually in the range 1 to 2.5 μg/L. Blood concentrations are significantly lower in hyperthyroidism, but increased in hypothyroidism and in patients with renal failure; children tolerate higher serum concentrations than adults.

In a *post-hoc* analysis of a trial involving 3782 subjects, a serum digoxin concentration in the range 0.5 to 0.8 μg/L was found to be optimal for treating heart failure in men with a left ventricular ejection fraction of 45% or less; the daily dose of digoxin was in the range 0.125 to 0.500 mg, with 75% of subjects receiving 0.250 mg daily. [S. S. Rathore *et al.*, *JAMA*, 2003, *289*, 871–878.]

Following a single oral dose of 0.25 mg to 6 subjects, a mean peak serum concentration of 1 μg/L was attained in 1 h. [J. C. Panisset *et al.*, *Can. Med. Assoc. J.*, 1973, *109*, 700–702.]

Steady-state plasma concentrations of 0.4 to 2.1 μg/L (mean 1.1) were reported in 14 patients on an oral daily dosage of 0.125 to 0.250 mg. [J. Gayes and D. Greenblatt, *J. Clin. Pharmacol.*, 1978, *5*, 92–93.]

Toxicity. Toxic effects are usually associated with serum concentrations of 1.4 to 2.8 to 7 μg/L and fatalities with concentrations of 1.5 to 10 to 30 μg/L.

In an overdose fatality involving digoxin in a suicidal 82-year-old man, blood concentrations of 12.2 to 13.2 μg/L were reported approximately 2.5 h after ingestion of the drug [M. S. Rodriguez-Calvo *et al.*, *Med. Sci. Law*, 2002, *42*, 265–268.]

Total and free serum digoxin concentrations of 17.1 and 12.4 μg/L, respectively, were reported in a 2-year-old child 4 h after ingestion of 22.5 to 23 mg digoxin. Following gastro-intestinal decontamination and treatment with digoxin-specific Fab fragments, serum levels reduced to 0.11 mg/L within 40 min. [G. L. Kearns *et al.*, *J. Clin. Pharmacol.*, 1989, *29*, 901–908.]

The following distribution was observed in a 3-day-old child who received a total of 4 mg of digoxin and died several hours later: blood 0.03 mg/L, brain 0.9 ng/g, kidney 0.13 μg/g, liver 0.034 μg/g. [M. Selesky *et al.*, *J. Forensic Sci.*, 1977, *22*, 409–417.]

In 7 fatalities involving ingestion of digoxin, postmortem 'serum' concentrations of 0.007 to 0.024 mg/L (mean 0.013) were reported; in a fatality involving IM injection of 1 mg of digoxin in an infant, a postmortem 'serum' concentration of 0.071 mg/L was reported. [A. C. Moffat, *Acta Pharmacol. Toxicol.*, 1974, *35*, 386–394.]

Bioavailability. About 70% from tablets (BP or USP specifications), 80% from elixirs, and over 90% from liquid-filled soft gelatin capsules.

Half-life. Plasma half-life, about 20 to 50 h, prolonged in subjects with renal impairment.

Volume of distribution. About 5 to 10 L/kg.

Clearance. Plasma clearance, about 1 to 4 mL/min/kg.

Distribution in blood. Plasma:whole blood ratio, 0.93.

Protein binding. In plasma, about 22 to 30%.

Note. For reviews of the pharmacokinetics of digoxin, see E. Iisalo, *Clin. Pharmacokinet.*, 1977, *2*, 1–16, J. K. Aronson, *Clin. Pharmacokinet.*, 1980, *5*, 137–149, and A. D. Mooradian, *Clin. Pharmacokinet.*, 1988, *15*, 165–179.

Dose. 125 to 500 μg daily. For rapid digitalisation, an initial dose of 0.75 to 1.5 mg may be given.

Dihydralazine

Antihypertensive

Synonym. Dihydrallazine
2,3-Dihydro-1,4-phthalazinedione dihydrazone
$C_8H_{10}N_6$=190.2
CAS—484-23-1

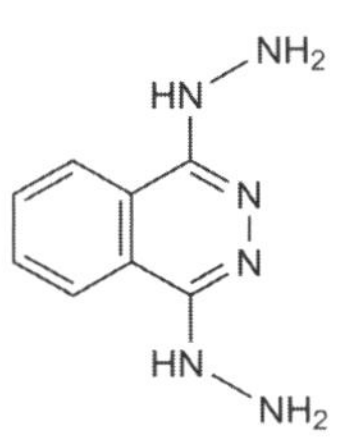

Orange crystalline needles. M.p. about 180° with decomposition.

Dihydralazine Sulfate

Proprietary names. Depressan; Dihyzin; Nepresol; Nepressol.
$C_8H_{10}N_6,H_2SO_4$=288.3
CAS—7327-87-9
A white to slightly yellow crystalline powder. M.p. 233° with decomposition.
Slightly soluble in water; practically insoluble in ethanol, chloroform, and methanol.

Partition Coefficient. Log *P* (octanol/water), −1.8.

Colour Tests. Mandelin's Test—yellow; Nessler's Reagent—black

Thin-layer Chromatography. System TA—Rf 55; system TB—Rf 34; system TC—Rf 02; system TE—Rf 18; system TL—Rf 01; system TAE—Rf 00.

High Performance Liquid Chromatography. System HX—RI 39.

Ultraviolet Spectrum. Aqueous acid—240, 274, 306 nm (A^1_1=323a).

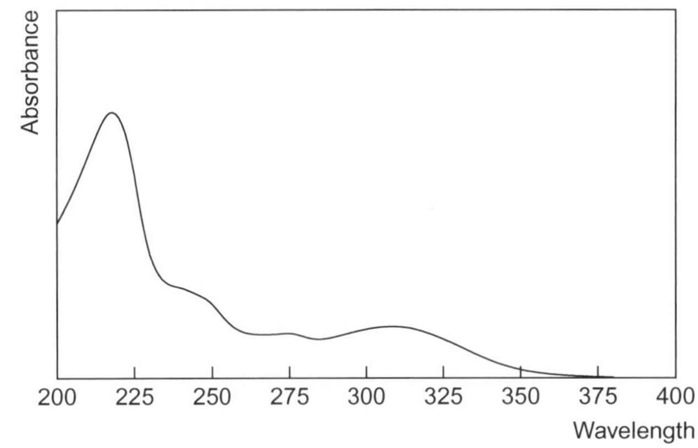

Infra-red Spectrum. Principal peaks at wavenumbers 1608, 1575, 1537, 1136, 769, 1100 cm^{-1} (KBr disk).

Quantification

Gas chromatography. In plasma: dihydralazine plus acid-labile hydrazones, limit of detection 5 μg/L, ECD—P. H. Degen *et al.*, *J. Chromatogr.* 1982, *233(22) B Biomed. Appl.*, 375–380.

Dose. Dihydralazine sulfate has been given in doses of 12.5 to 150 mg daily.

Dihydrocodeine

Narcotic Analgesic

Synonyms. Dihydroneopine; Drocode; Hydrocodeine.
Proprietary name. Remedacen (Dihydrocodeine Polistirex)
(5α,6α)-4,5-Epoxy-3-methoxy-17-methylmorphinan-6-ol
$C_{18}H_{23}NO_3$=301.4
CAS—125-28-0

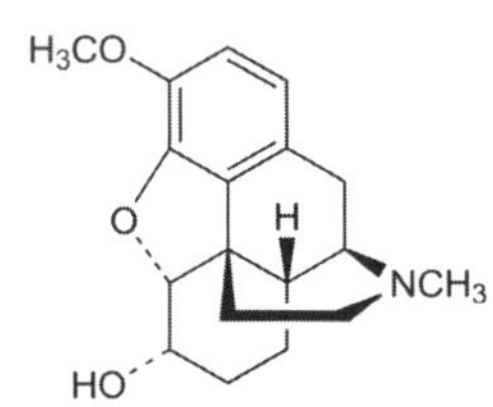

Crystals. M.p. 112° to 113°.

Dihydrocodeine Phosphate

$C_{18}H_{23}NO_3,H_3PO_4$=399.4
CAS—24204-13-5
A white to yellowish-white crystalline powder.
Soluble 1 in 3 of water; slightly soluble in ethanol.

Dihydrocodeine Tartrate

Synonyms. Dihydrocodeine Acid Tartrate; Dihydrocodeine Bitartrate; Drocode Bitartrate; Hydrocodeine Bitartrate.
Proprietary names. Codicontin; Codilol; Contugesic; DF 118; DHC; Dicodin; Didor; Fortuss; Hydol; Hydrocodeinon; Paracodin(a); Paracodine; Rikodeine; Tiamon Mono; Tosidrin. It is an ingredient of DHC Plus, Galake, Panlor DC, Paramol, Remedeine, and Synalgos-DC.
$C_{18}H_{23}NO_3,C_4H_6O_6$=451.5
CAS—5965-13-9
Colourless crystals or white crystalline powder. M.p. 192° to 193° (anhydrous), 186° to 190° (commercial medicinal grade).
Soluble 1 in 4.5 of water; sparingly soluble in ethanol; practically insoluble in ether.

Dissociation Constant. pK_a 8.8 (25°).

Partition Coefficient. Log *P* (ether/pH 7.0), −1.5.

Colour Tests. Mandelin's Test—grey-green; Marquis Test—violet

Thin-layer Chromatography. System TA—Rf 26; system TB—Rf 08; system TC—Rf 13; system TE—Rf 29; system TL—Rf 02; system TAE—Rf 11; system TAF—Rf 19; system TAJ—Rf 06; system TAK—Rf 00; system TAL—Rf 38. (Dragendorff spray, positive; acidified iodoplatinate solution, positive; Marquis reagent, blue-violet.)

Gas Chromatography. System GA—dihydrocodeine RI 2390, dihydrocodeine-AC RI 2445, dihydrocodeine-PFP RI 2360, dihydrocodeine-TFA RI 2265, dihydrocodeine-TMS RI 2480, M (nor-)-AC_2 RI 2750; system GB—dihydrocodeine RI 2511, dihydrocodeine-TMS RI 2496, M (nor-) RI 2599, M (nor-)-TMS_2 RI 2559; system GC—RI 2702; system GF—RI 2840; system GM—dihydrocodeine RRT 1.493 (relative to iprindole).

High Performance Liquid Chromatography. System HA—*k* 7.2 (tailing peak); system HC—*k* 2.50; system HX—RI 261; system HY—RI 208; system HZ—retention time 2.0 min; system HAA—retention time 4.7 min.

Ultraviolet Spectrum. Aqueous acid—283 nm (A_1^1=47a). No alkaline shift.

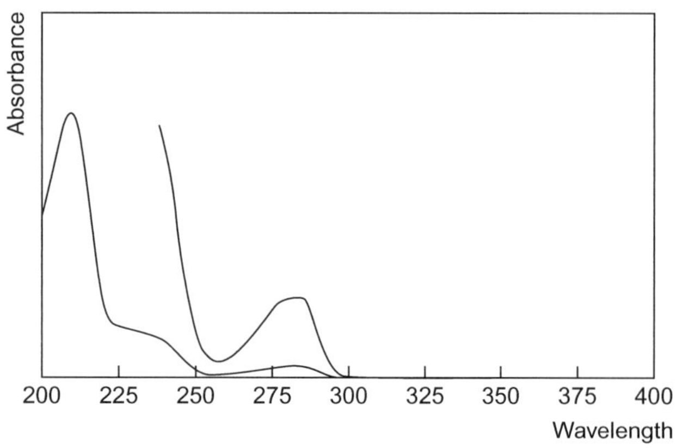

Infra-red Spectrum. Principal ions at wavenumbers 1495, 1271, 1040, 1250, 1055, 1149 cm^{-1} (Nujol mull).

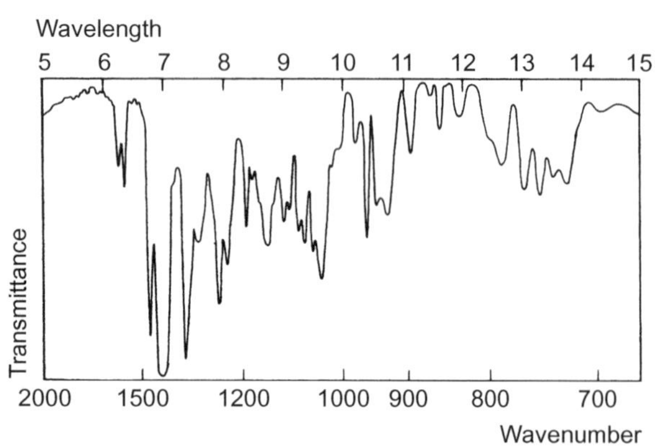

Mass Spectrum. Principal ions at *m/z* 301, 44, 42, 59, 164, 70, 302, 242.

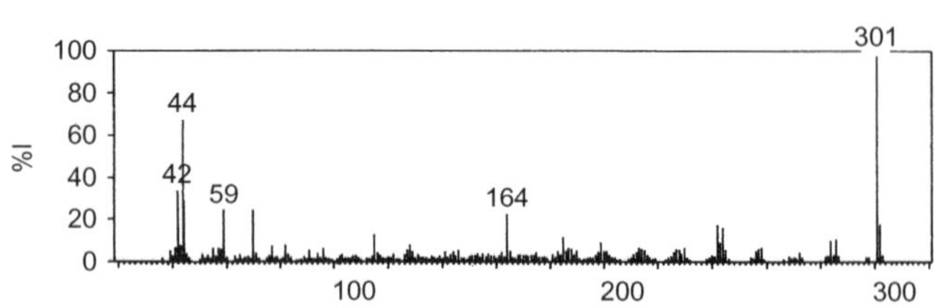

Quantification

Gas chromatography. In blood, bile, liver blood, or urine: FID—M. A. Peat and A. Sengupta, *Forensic Sci.*, 1977, *9*, 21–32. In plasma: limit of quantification 20 μg/L—D. A. Cowan *et al.*, *J. Pharm. Sci.*, 1988, *77*, 606–609. In plasma or urine: dihydrocodeine and codeine, limit of detection 2.5 μg/L, SID (comparison with nitrogen-phosphorus detection)—H. Seno *et al.*, *J. Chromatogr.* 1995, *673 B Biomed. Appl.*, 189–195 In blood: dihydrocodeine and other opioids, limit of quantification 10 μg/L, electron ionisation detection—S. Mykkanen *et al.*, *J. Anal. Toxicol.*, 2000, *24*, 122–126.

Gas chromatography–mass spectrometry. In hair: dihydrocodeine and other opioids—H. Sach *et al.*, *Int. J. Legal Med.*, 1993, *105*, 247–250. In serum, blood, or postmortem blood: dihydrocodeine morphine and codeine, limit of detection <1 μg/L—F. Musshoff and T. Daldrup, *Int. J. Legal Med.*, 1993, *106*, 107–109. In serum: dihydrocodeine and dihydromorphine, limits of quantification 2 μg/L and 40 ng/L, respectively—U. Hofmann *et al.*, *J. Chromatogr.* 1995, *663 B Biomed. Appl.*, 59–65. In plasma or whole blood: dihydrocodeine and other opioids, limit of detection <5 μg/L—A. Geier *et al.*, *Int. J. Legal Med.*, 1996, *109*, 80–83. In urine: dihydrocodeine and other opioids—C. Meadway *et al.*, *Forensic Sci. Int.*, 2002, *127*, 136–141.

High performance liquid chromatography. In urine: limit of quantification 2 μg/L—D. A. Cowan *et al.*, *J. Pharm. Sci.*, 1988, *77*, 606–609. In urine: dihydrocodeine and other opioids, limits of detection 4 to 20 μg/L (comparison with enzyme immunoassay)—A. S. Low and R. B. Taylor, *J. Chromatogr.* 1995, *663 B Biomed. Appl.*, 225–233. In hair: dihydrocodeine and other opioids and drugs of abuse, electrochemical detection—G. Achilli *et al.*, *J. Chromatogr. A*, 1996, *729*, 273–277. In postmortem blood: dihydrocodeine and its main metabolites, fluorescence detection—K. Klinder *et al.*, *Int. J. Legal Med.*, 1999, *112*, 155–158.

Review. In biological samples: dihydrocodeine and drugs of abuse and their metabolites, methods of quantification—M. R. Moeller *et al.*, *J. Chromatogr. B Biomed. Sci. Appl.*, 1998, *713*, 91–109.

Disposition in the Body. It undergoes extensive first-pass metabolism in the gut wall or liver. Metabolism includes *N*-demethylation to form nordihydrocodeine, *O*-demethylation producing dihydromorphine, 6-keto reduction, and conjugation. After an oral dose of 52 mg, 20 to 30% is excreted in the urine in 24 h; this is increased to about 35% when the urine is acid. After an intramuscular dose of about 43 mg under conditions of controlled acidic urinary pH, 40 to 60% is excreted in the urine in 24 h. About 30 to 45% of the urinary excreted material is conjugated.

Therapeutic concentration

Following single oral doses of 30 mg and 60 mg to 7 subjects, mean peak plasma concentrations of 0.072 and 0.146 mg/L were attained in 1.7 h; the corresponding peak plasma concentrations of acidic metabolites were 0.56 and 1.48 mg/L. [F. J. Rowell *et al.*, *Eur. J. Clin. Pharmacol.*, 1983, *25*, 419–424.]

Following a single oral dose of dihydrocodeine 60 mg to 12 subjects, peak plasma dihydrocodeine concentrations of 0.094 to 0.112 mg/L (mean 0.103) and dihydromorphine concentrations of 0.001 to 0.002 mg/L (mean 0.0014) were attained in about 5 h; multiple dosing at 60 mg twice daily for 2 days, then 90 mg twice daily for 2 days, and then 120 mg twice daily for 2 days produced minimum steady-state dihydrocodeine concentrations of 0.047 to 0.065 mg/L (mean 0.056), 0.073 to 0.104 mg/L (mean 0.085), and 0.11 to 0.156 mg/L (mean 0.133), respectively. [S. Ammon *et al.*, *Br. J. Clin. Pharmacol.*, 1999, *48*, 317–322.]

Toxicity. The estimated minimum lethal dose is 0.5 g, but addicts may be able to tolerate up to ten times as much, whereas 25 mg may be fatal in children.

In a fatality attributed to an oral overdose of dihydrocodeine, the following postmortem tissue concentrations were reported: blood 12 mg/L, bile 5340 mg/L, liver 620 mg/kg, urine 570 mg/L; chlordiazepoxide was also detected. In a second case in which the death of an addict occurred rapidly after an intravenous overdose of dihydrocodeine, the postmortem concentrations were: blood 720 mg/L, bile 3 mg/L, liver blood 364 mg/L, urine 7 mg/L; pentobarbital and paracetamol were also detected. [M. A. Peat and A. Sengupta, *Forensic Sci.*, 1977, *9*, 21–32.]

In 4 fatalities caused by ingestion of dihydrocodeine, postmortem blood concentrations of 7.2 to 12.0 mg/L (mean 9.0) were reported. [S. C. Patterson, *Forensic Sci. Int.*, 1985, *27*, 129–133.]

A 30-year-old man who had been undergoing long-term substitution therapy with dihydrocodeine, died of unkown causes. Autopsy 3.5 h after death revealed, in addition to diazepam and nordazepam, the following tissue concentrations (in mg/L or mg/kg):

	Left femoral vein (WB⁺)	Left ventricle (WB⁺)	Liver	Kidney	Cerebrum
Dihydrocodeine	1.910	2.695	1.282	10.557	0.802
Dihydrocodeine-6-glucuronide	1.689	1.759	1.955	27.609	–
N-Nordihydrocodeine	0.199	0.226	0.364	4.938	1.369
Dihydromorphine	0.152	0.182	–	2.080	–
Dihydromorphine-3-glucuronide	0.658	0.580	–	–	–
Dihydromorphine-6-glucuronide	0.093*	0.132*	–	1.330	–

*serum; ⁺ WB, whole blood.

[G. Skopp *et al.*, *Forensic Sci. Int.*, 1998, *95*, 99–107.]

In 3 fatalities involving dihydrocodeine, the femoral blood concentrations of dihydrocodeine and its metabolites *post mortem* were: dihydrocodeine 18.45, 1.92, and 2.36 mg/L; dihydrocodeine-6-glucuronide 7.18, 2.68, and 1.61 mg/L; nordihydrocodeine 2.21, 0.27, and 0.12 mg/L; dihydromorphine 0.21, 0.18, and 0.16 mg/L; dihydromorphine-3-glucuronide 1.08, 1.04, and 0.31 mg/L; dihydromorphine-6-glucuronide 0.08, 0.08, and 0.07 mg/L. In the first 2 cases diazepam and nordazepam were also detected and in the 3rd case cloral hydrate and trichlorethanol had also been ingested. [K. Klinder *et al.*, *Int. J. Legal Med.*, 1999, *112*, 155–158.]

In a 16-year-old male who died owing to drowning and cold exposure following a drug overdose, the following concentrations of diphenhydramine, free dihydrocodeine, and total dihydrocodeine were found, respectively, approx. 9 days after death: femoral venous blood 1.89, 3.27, and 3.30 mg/ L; right cardiac chamber blood 0.294, 0.237, and 0.240 mg/L; urine 22.6, 37.3, and 43.1 mg/L; stomach 0.029, 0.018, and 0.024 mg; femoral muscle 0.270, 0.246, and 0.314 µg/g. [F. Moriya and Y. Hashimoto, *Forensic Sci. Int.*, 2001, *123*, 248–253.]

Bioavailability. About 20%

Half-life. Plasma half-life, about 4 h.

Volume of distribution. About 1 L/kg.

Clearance. Plasma clearance, about 4 mL/min/kg.

Dose. 30 to 60 mg of dihydrocodeine tartrate every 4 to 6 h up to maximum of 240 mg daily.

Dihydroergotamine

Treatment of Migraine

9,10-Dihydro-12′-hydroxy-2′-methyl-5′-(phenylmethyl)ergotaman-3′,6′,18-trione
$C_{33}H_{37}N_5O_5$=583.7
CAS—5111-12-6

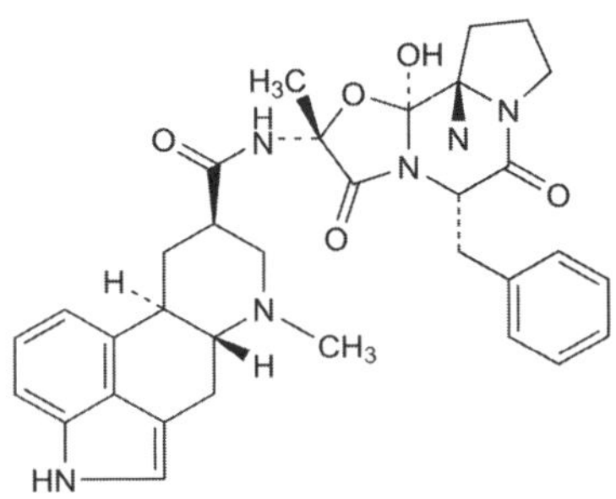

White crystals. M.p. 239°.
Practically insoluble in water; sparingly soluble in ethanol, methanol, benzene and chloroform.

Dihydroergotamine Mesilate

Synonym. Dihydroergotamine Methanesulphonate
Proprietary names. DET MS; D.H.E. 45; Dihydergot; Ikaran; Séglor; Tonopres.
$C_{33}H_{37}N_5O_5,CH_3SO_3H$=679.8
CAS—6190-39-2
A white to slightly yellowish, or an off-white to slightly red, microcrystalline powder.
Soluble 1 in 125 of water, 1 in 90 of ethanol, 1 in 175 of chloroform and 1 in 2600 of ether; soluble in acetone.

Dihydroergotamine Tartrate

$(C_{33}H_{37}N_5O_5)_2,C_4H_6O_6$=1317.4
CAS—5989-77-5
Colourless crystals or a white crystalline powder. M.p. about 203°, with decomposition.
Very slightly soluble in water; sparingly soluble in ethanol; soluble in pyridine.

Dissociation Constant. pK_a 6.9 (24°).

Colour Tests. *p*-Dimethylaminobenzaldehyde—violet; Mandelin's Test—violet-brown; Marquis Test—grey-brown.

Thin-layer Chromatography. System TA—Rf 60; system TB—Rf 01; system TC—Rf 28; system TE—Rf 42; system TL—Rf 14; system TM—Rf 40; system TAE—Rf 58; system TAJ—Rf 33; system TAK—Rf 03; system TAL—Rf 84. (Van Urk reagent, blue.)

Gas Chromatography. System GA—RI 2315.

High Performance Liquid Chromatography. System HA—*k* 0.6; system HP—*k* 11.4; system HX—RI 411; system HZ—Retention time, 3.4 min.

Ultraviolet Spectrum. Aqueous acid—280 nm (A^1_1 = 108a). No alkaline shift. (See below.)

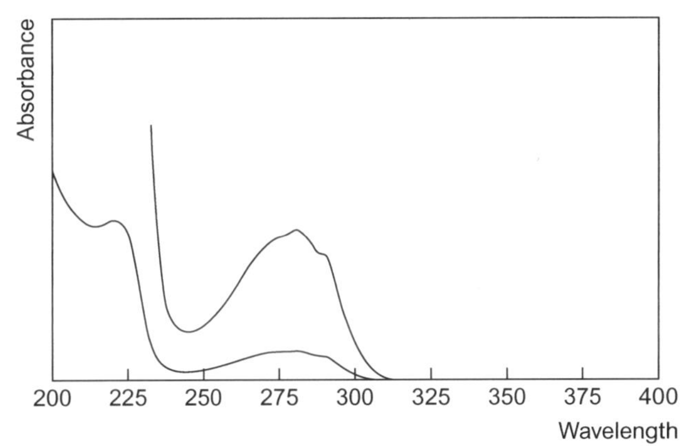

Infra-red Spectrum. Principal peaks at wavenumbers 1660, 1210, 1712, 1053, 1140, 768 cm^{-1} (KBr disk). (See below.)

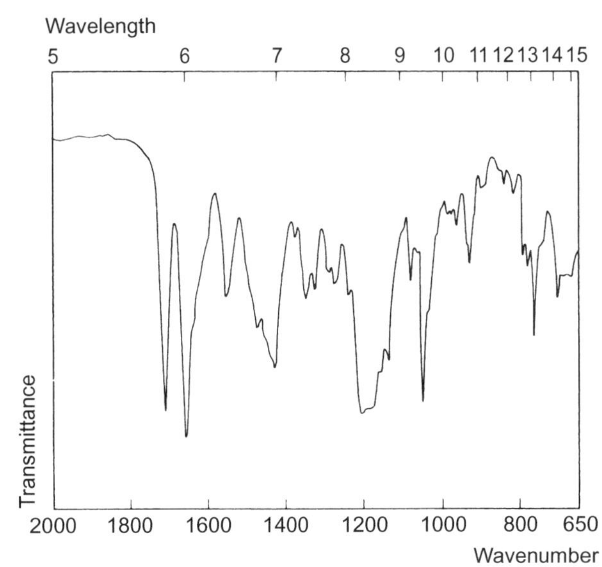

Mass Spectrum. Principal ions at *m/z* 70, 125, 91, 153, 43, 41, 44, 244 (no peaks above 340).

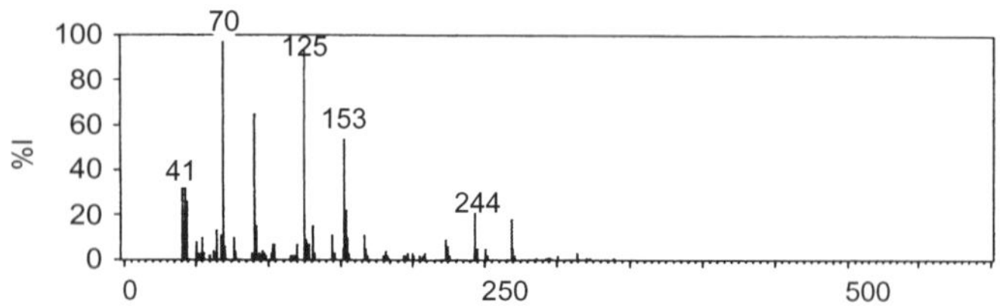

Quantification

High performance liquid chromatography. In plasma: limit of quantification 0.1 μg/L, fluorescence detection—M. Murday *et al.*, *J. Chromatogr. B Biomed. Sci. Appl.*, 1999, *735*, 151–157. In plasma: limit of detection 0.08 μg/L, fluorescence detection (λ_{ex}=277 nm, λ_{em}=348 nm)—S. G. Romeijn *et al.*, *J. Chromatogr. B Biomed. Sci. Appl.*, 1997, *692*, 227–232. In plasma and urine: dihydroergotamine and metabolites, limit of detection 0.1 mg/L, fluorescence detection—H. Humbert *et al.*, *J. Chromatogr.*, 1987, *417*, 319–329.

Radioimmunoassay. In plasma—J. Rosenthaler and H. Munzer, *Experientia*, 1979, *32*, 234–240.

Disposition in the Body. Poorly absorbed after oral administration and undergoes extensive first-pass metabolism with considerable intersubject variation. After oral administration less than 5% of a dose is excreted in the urine unchanged in 24 h, compared to about 11% after intravenous administration. The major metabolite is the 8′-hydroxy derivative, which is active.

Therapeutic concentration

Following single oral doses of 10, 20 and 30 mg to 6 subjects, mean plasma concentrations of about 0.0002, 0.0006 and 0.001 mg/L, respectively, were attained in about 0.5 to 1 h [P. J. Little *et al.*, *Br. J. Clin. Pharmacol.*, 1982, *13*, 785–790].

Note. For a study of the pharmacokinetics of dihydroergotamine administered by nasal spray, see H. Humbert *et al.*, *Clin. Pharmacol. Ther.*, 1996, *60*, 265–275.

Bioavailability. Less than 5%.

Half-life. Plasma half-life, about 2 to 4 h; a longer terminal elimination half-life of about 20 to 30 h has also been reported.

Volume of distribution. 6 to 23 L/kg (mean 14).

Clearance. Plasma clearance, 7 to 22 mL/min/kg (mean 15).

Note. For a review of the current uses of ergotamine and dihydroergotamine see P. Tfelt-Hansen, *Curr. Med. Red. Opin.*, 2001, *17 Suppl. 1*, S30–S34.

Dose. 1 to 3 mg of dihydroergotamine mesilate, repeated if necessary to a maximum of 10 mg daily.

Dihydromorphine

Narcotic Analgesic

(5α,6α)-4,5-Epoxy-17-methylmorphinan-3,6-diol
$C_{17}H_{21}NO_3$=287.4
CAS—509-60-4

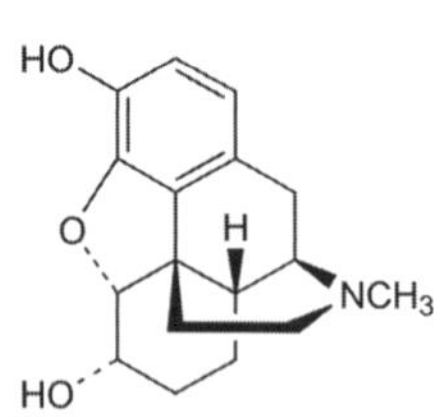

White crystals. M.p. of the hydrated compound, 157°, with decomposition. Practically insoluble in water; soluble in acetone, ethanol, and chloroform.

Dihydromorphine Hydrochloride
$C_{17}H_{21}NO_3$,HCl=323.8
CAS—1421-28-9
Crystals.
Very soluble in water; sparingly soluble in ethanol.

Dissociation Constant. pK_a 8.6.

Partition Coefficient. Log *P* (octanol/pH 7.4), −1.0.

Colour Tests. Mandelin's Test—grey; Marquis Test—red-violet.

Thin-layer Chromatography. System TA—Rf 25; system TB—Rf 02; system TC—Rf 03; system TE—Rf 18; system TL—Rf 01; system TAE—Rf 12; system TAJ—Rf 00; system TAK—Rf 00; system TAL—Rf 25. (Dragendorff spray, positive; acidified iodoplatinate solution, positive; Marquis reagent, violet.)

Gas Chromatography. System GA—dihydromorphine RI 2400, dihydromorphine-AC_2 RI 2545, dihydromorphine-PFP_2 RI 2330, dihydromorphine-TMS_2 RI 2520, M (nor-)-AC_3 RI 2790; system GB—dihydromorphine RI 2527, dihydromorphine-TMS_2 RI 2518; system GC—RI 2504.

High Performance Liquid Chromatography. System HA—*k* 5.7 (tailing peak); system HC—*k* 2.75; system HX—RI 237; system HY—RI 156.

Ultraviolet Spectrum. Aqueous acid—283 nm (A_1^1=45a); aqueous alkali—297 nm (A_1^1=82b).

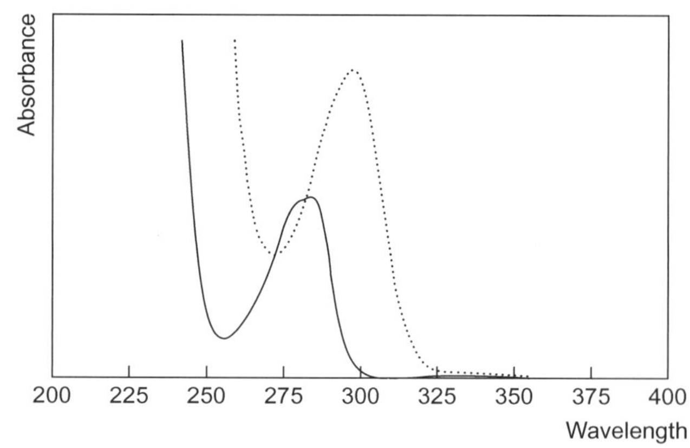

Infra-red Spectrum. Principal peaks at wavenumbers 1245, 760, 940, 747, 1085, 1145 cm^{-1} (KBr disk).

Mass Spectrum. Principal ions at *m/z* 287, 70, 44, 164, 42, 288, 59, 230.

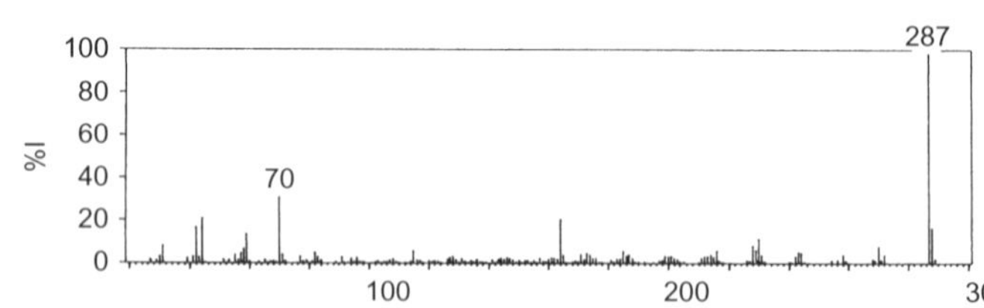

Quantification.

Gas chromatography–mass spectrometry. In serum: dihydromorphine and dihydrocodeine, limits of detection <40 ng/L—U. Hofmann *et al.*, *J. Chromatogr.* 1995, *663 B Biomed. Appl.*, 59–65.

Dihydrostreptomycin

Antibiotic

O-2-Deoxy-2-(methylamino)-α-L-glucopyranosyl-(1→2)-*O*-5-deoxy-3-*C*-(hydroxymethyl)-α-L-lyxofuranosyl-(1→4)-*N*,*N*′-bis-(aminoiminomethyl)-D-streptamine
$C_{21}H_{41}N_7O_{12}$=583.6
CAS—128-46-1

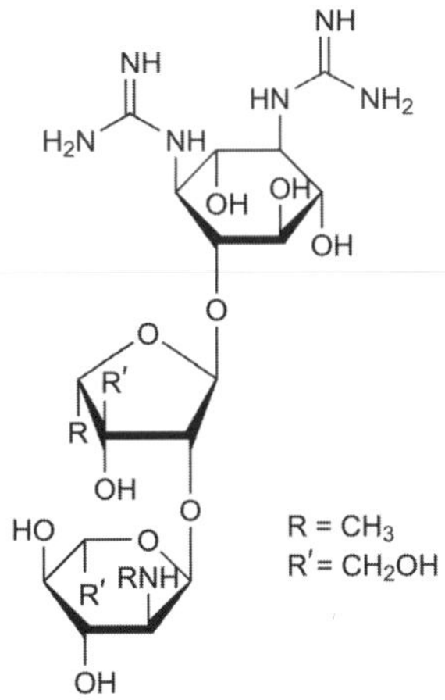

Dihydrostreptomycin Sulfate

Proprietary names. It is an ingredient of Citrocil, Cilinafosal DHD Estrep, Estrefen, Estreptoenterol, Fluocal com Pectina, Salitanol Estreptomicina, and Sulfintestin Neomicina.
$(C_{21}H_{41}N_7O_{12})_2,3H_2SO_4$=1461.4
CAS—5490-27-7
A white hygroscopic solid. M.p. 255° to 265° with decomposition.
Very soluble in water; practically insoluble in ethanol, chloroform, and ether.

Dissociation Constant. pK_a 7.8.

Partition Coefficient. Log *P* (octanol/water), −7.5.

Colour Tests. Nessler's Reagent—yellow→brown; Palladium Chloride—brown (slow).

Thin-layer Chromatography. System TA—Rf 01; system TAE—Rf 00. (Acidified potassium permanganate solution, positive.)

Ultraviolet Spectrum. No significant absorption, 230 to 360 nm.

Infra-red Spectrum. Principal peaks at wavenumbers 1111, 1666, 1052, 1724, 1250, 1515 cm^{-1}.

Dose. The equivalent of 0.5 to 1 g of dihydrostreptomycin has been given daily, intramuscularly.

Dihydrotachysterol

Vitamin D Activity

Synonym. Dichysterol
Proprietary names. AT 10; Calcamine; Dihydral; Dygratyl; Hytakerol; Parterol; Tachyrol.
(3*β*,5*E*,7*E*,10*α*,22*E*)-9,10-Secoergosta-5,7,22-trien-3-ol
$C_{28}H_{46}O$=398.7
CAS—67-96-9

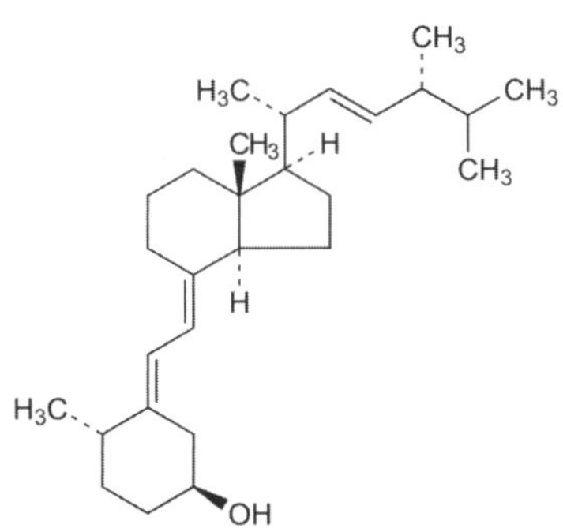

Colourless crystals or white crystalline powder. M.p. 123° to 129°. May also occur in a form melting at about 113°.
Practically insoluble in water; soluble 1 in 20 of ethanol, 1 in 0.7 of chloroform, and 1 in 3 of ether.

Partition Coefficient. Log *P* (octanol/water), 10.4.

Ultraviolet Spectrum. Methanol—242, 251 nm (A_1^1=990a), 261 nm.

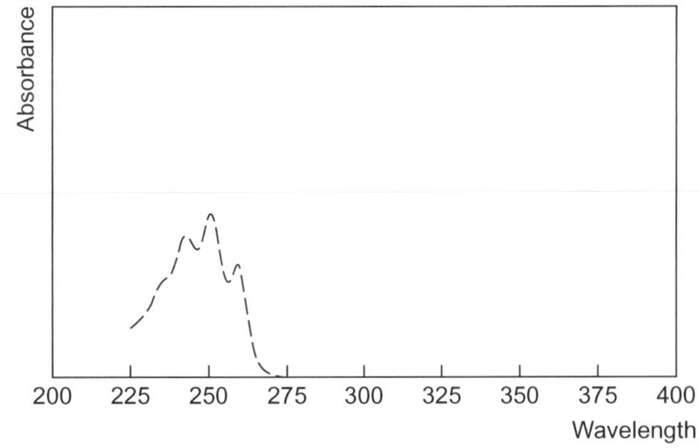

Infra-red Spectrum. Principal peaks at wavenumbers 1056, 967, 1018, 1009, 870, 980 cm^{-1} (KBr disk).

Dose. Initially 0.25 to 2.5 mg daily.

Diiodohydroxyquinoline

Anti-amoebic

Synonyms. Diiodohydroxyquin; Diodoxyquinoléine; Iodoquinol.
Proprietary names. Amabagyl; Antidifar; Carsuquin; Diameb; Diodolina; Diodoquin; Direxiode; Diyomex; Diyosul; Diyowil; Drioquilen; Dysetrin; Embequin; Entero-Diyod; Entodiba; Flanoquin; Floraquin; Moebiquin; Sebaquin; Versamiv; Yodoxin; Yopin.
5,7-Diiodo-8-quinolinol
$C_9H_5I_2NO$=397.0
CAS—83-73-8

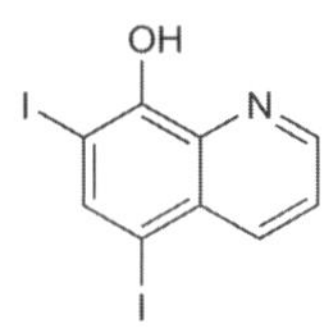

A light yellowish to tan-coloured microcrystalline powder, not readily wetted in water. M.p. 200° to 215°, with decomposition.
Almost insoluble in water; sparingly soluble in ethanol, acetone, and ether; soluble in hot pyridine and hot dioxane.

Partition Coefficient. Log *P* (octanol/water), 4.0.

Colour Test. Heat a few crystals with 1 mL of sulfuric acid—violet iodine vapour.

Thin-layer Chromatography. System TD—Rf 17; system TE—Rf 28; system TF—Rf 19; system TAD—Rf 72.

Ultraviolet Spectrum. Dilute 5 mL of a 0.01% solution in dioxan to 100 mL with dehydrated alcohol—258 nm (A_1^1=1060b).

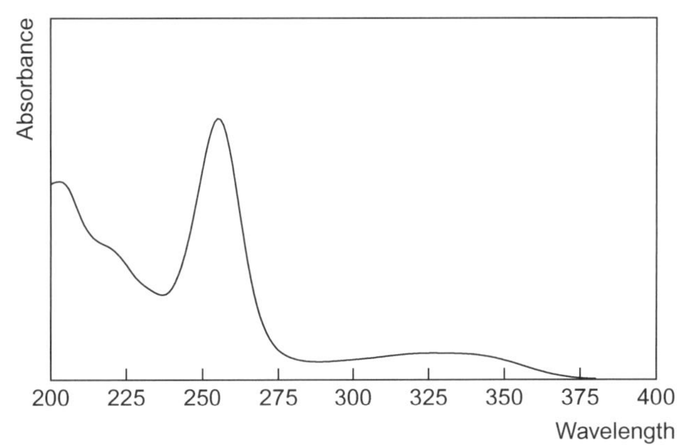

Infra-red Spectrum. Principal peaks at wavenumbers 1204, 781, 806, 920, 1265, 869 cm^{-1} (KBr disk).

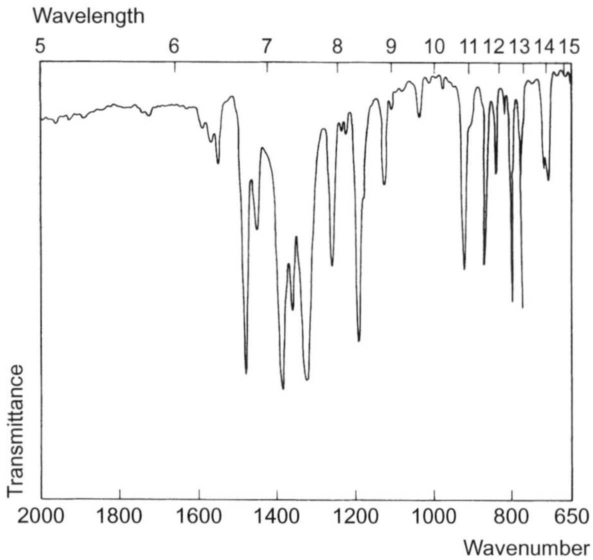

Mass Spectrum. Principal ions at *m/z* 397, 115, 242, 398, 88, 143, 271, 62.

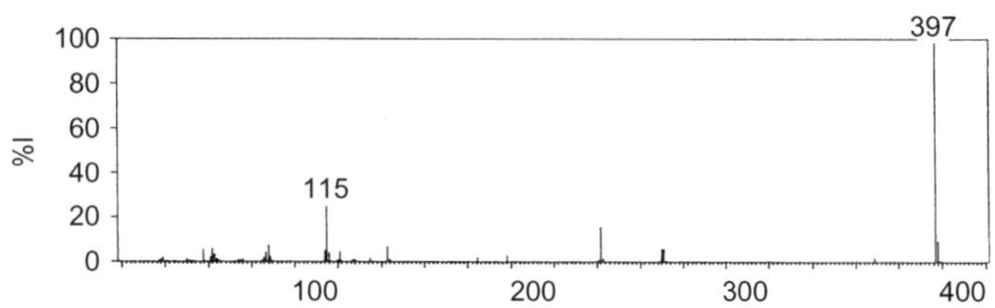

Quantification

Colorimetry. In urine: limit of detection 10 mg/L—L. Berggren and O. Hansson, *Clin. Pharmacol. Ther.*, 1968, *9*, 67–70.

Disposition in the Body. Incompletely and irregularly absorbed from the small intestine. About 5% of a dose is excreted in the urine as the glucuronide conjugate in 10 h.

Dose. Usually 1.8 g daily.

Diloxanide

Anti-amoebic

Synonym. Diloxan

2,2-Dichloro-*N*-(4-hydroxyphenyl)-*N*-methylacetamide

$C_9H_9Cl_2NO_2$=234.1

CAS—579-38-4

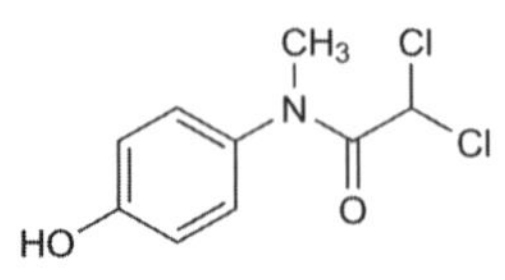

A white crystalline powder. M.p. 175°.

Slightly soluble in water; soluble 1 in 8 of ethanol, 1 in 35 of chloroform, and 1 in 66 of ether.

Diloxanide Furoate

Proprietary names. Furamid(e). It is an ingredient of Entamizole.

$C_{14}H_{11}Cl_2NO_4$=328.2

CAS—3736-81-0

A white crystalline powder. M.p. 114° to 116°.

Very slightly soluble in water; soluble 1 in 100 of ethanol, 1 in 2.5 of chloroform, and 1 in 130 of ether.

Partition Coefficient. Log *P* (octanol/water), 1.8.

Colour Tests. Folin–Ciocalteau Reagent—blue; Liebermann's Test—yellow

Thin-layer Chromatography. System TA—Rf 66; system TB—Rf 16; system TC—Rf 74; system TL—Rf 67. (Acidified iodoplatinate solution, positive.)

Gas Chromatography. System GA—RI 2420.

High Performance Liquid Chromatography. System HY—RI 500.

Ultraviolet Spectrum. Diloxanide furoate: aqueous acid—262 nm (A^{1}_{1}=224b); ethanol—258 nm (A^{1}_{1}=705a). Diloxanide: ethanol—278 nm (A^{1}_{1}=104a).

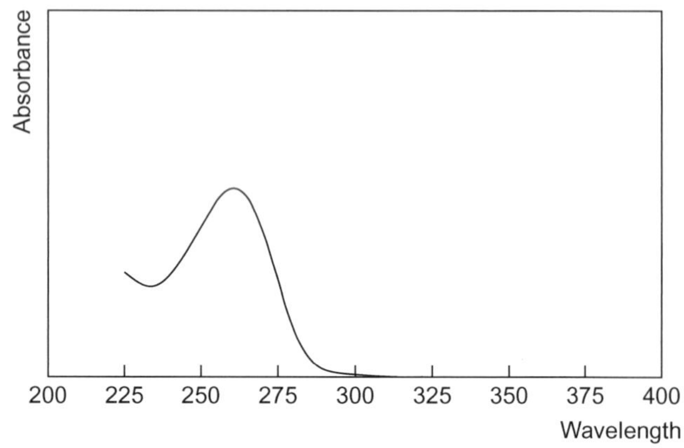

Infra-red Spectrum. Principal peaks at wavenumbers 1678, 1197, 1093, 1290, 1727, 1167 cm^{-1} (KBr disk).

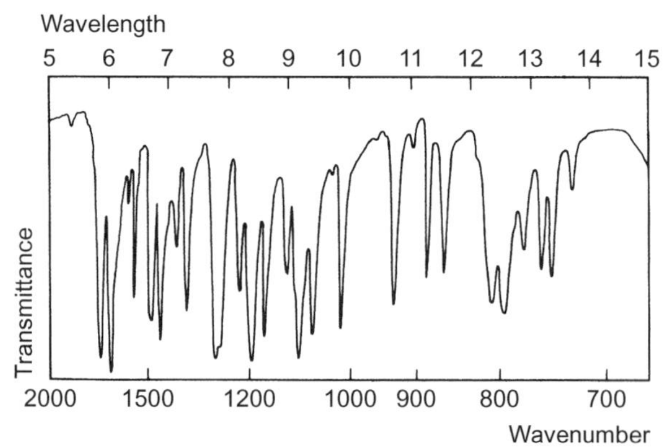

Mass Spectrum. Principal ions at *m/z* 95, 327, 39, 329, 96, 122, 244, 67 (diloxanide furoate).

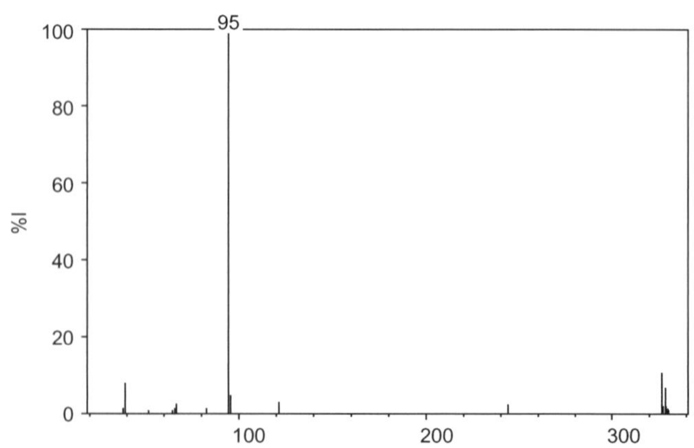

Disposition in the Body. After oral administration diloxanide furoate is hydrolysed to diloxanide and then readily absorbed; it is excreted in the urine and faeces.

Dose. 1.5 g of diloxanide furoate daily.

Diltiazem

Antihypertensive

Proprietary name. Dilzem

(2*S-cis*)-3-(Acetyloxy)-5-[2-(dimethylamino)ethyl]-2,3-dihydro-2-(4-methoxyphenyl)-1,5-benzothiazepin-4-(5*H*)-one

$C_{22}H_{26}N_2O_4S = 414.5$

CAS—42399-41-7

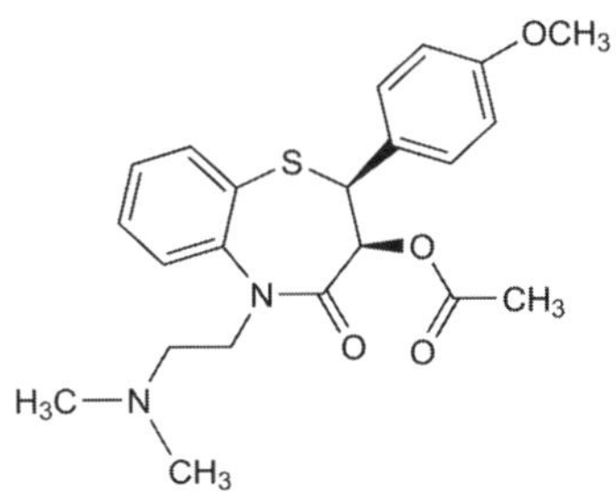

Diltiazem Hydrochloride

Synonyms. Diltiazem hydrochloridum; Latiazem hydrochloride; CRD-401; MK-793 (diltiazem maleate).

Proprietary names. Adizem; Altiazem; Angiozem; Angitil; Calazem; Calcicard; Cardizem; Dilacar; Dilcardia; Slozem; Tiazac; Tildiem; Viazam; Zemtard.

$C_{22}H_{26}N_2O_4S,HCl = 451.0$

CAS—33286-22-5

A white, odourless, crystalline powder or small crystals. It is freely soluble in water, chloroform, dichloromethane, formic acid and methyl alcohol; sparingly soluble in dehydrated alcohol; practically insoluble in ether. M.p. 207.5° to 212.0°.

Partition Coefficient. Log *P* (octanol/water), 2.79.

Thin-Layer Chromatography. System TE—Rf 56; system TAE—Rf 47.

Plates: Silica (Merck 60). Mobile phase: Ethyl acetate:methanol:ammonia (80:10:10). Reference compounds: diltiazem hydrochloride Rf 0.54. [P. V. Devarajan *et al.*, *J. Chromatogr. Biomed. Sci. Appl.*, 1998, *706*, 362–366].

Gas Chromatography. System GA—RI 2949 diltiazem; RI 2990 M (desacetyl-); RI 3050 M (O-desmethyl-); system GB—RI 3076 diltiazem; RI 3092 M (desacetyl-); RI 3147 M (*O*-desmethyl-); RI 3114 M (*N*-desmethyl-).

Column: 1% OV-17 on 100-120 mesh Chromosorb W (glass, 2 m × 3 mm, i.d.). Column temperature: 280°. Injector and detector temperature: 300°. Carrier gas: nitrogen at 50 mL/min. Reference compound: flurazepam. ECD. Retention time: 4.2 min. [T. Alebic-Kolbah and F. Plavsic, *J. Pharm. Biomed. Anal.*, 1990, *8*, 915–918].

Column: HP-1 (Hewlett-Packard, 12.5 m × 0.2 mm, 0.33 µm film thickness). Column temperature: held at 50° for 1 min, increased to 190° at 25°/min and held for 3 min, increased to 280° at 10°/min, held 12 min. Carrier gas: helium, 1.0 mL/min. MS detection. Retention time: 18.9 min. [J. R. Kalin *et al.*, *J. Anal. Toxicol.*, 1994, *18*, 180].

High Performance Liquid Chromatography. System HAV—diltiazem, *k* 6.1; deacetyldiltiazem, 3.6; desmethyldiltiazem, 5.1; system HAA—retention time 14.0 min; system HAX—diltiazem, 11.1 min, desacetyldiltiazem, 9.3 min; system HAY—diltiazem, 5.4 min, desacetyldiltiazem, 4.6 min; system HY—RI 361; system HZ—retention time 4.5 min.

Column: C_{18} R-P (Supelcosil, 250 × 4.6 mm, i.d., 5 µm), C_{18} cartridge guard column. Mobile phase: methanol:ammonium acetate buffer (0.04 M):acetonitrile (38:36:26), containing 0.08% triethylamine, pH 7.5 at flow rate 1.2 mL/min. UV detection (λ = 237 nm). Retention times for metabolites M_6, M_B, M_4, M_X, M_2, M_A and M_1: 3.6, 4.1, 4.7, 5.6, 7.8, 9.4 and 10.6 min, respectively. Diltiazem, 13.1 min. [P. K. F. Yeung *et al.*, *Ther. Drug Monit.*, 1996, *18*, 40–45].

Column: (analytical) RP-8 (LiChrosorb, 300 × 4.1 mm i.d., 10 µm), (guard) C_8 (23 × 3.6 mm i.d., 10 µm). Mobile phase: 40% acetonitrile in 0.01 M dibasic sodium phosphate and 0.1% triethanolamine dissolved in ultra-pure deionised water, adjusted to pH 3 with orthophosphoric acid. Flow rate, 1.2 mL/min. UV detection (λ = 237 nm). Retention time: 5.6 min. [R. S. Chaudhary *et al.*, *J. Chromatogr.* 1993, *614*; *Biomed. Appl.*, 261–266].

Ultraviolet Spectrum. Aqueous acid (0.2 M H_2SO_4)—236 nm; basic—237 nm.

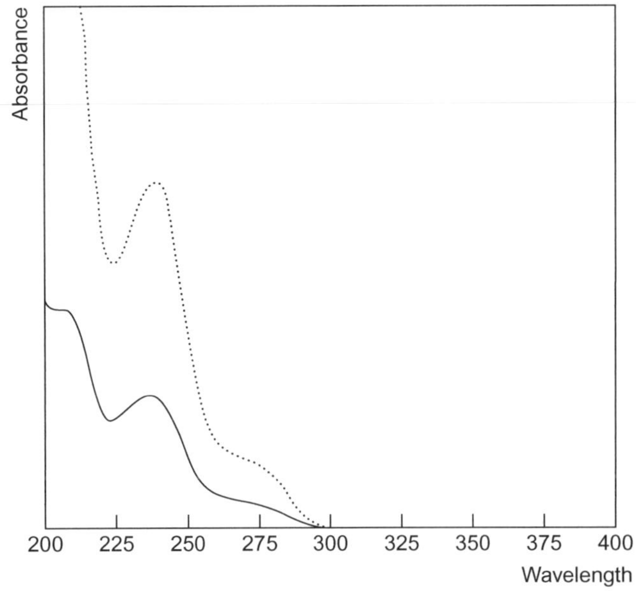

Infra-red Spectrum. Principal peaks at 1682, 1512, 1252, 1033 cm^{-1}.

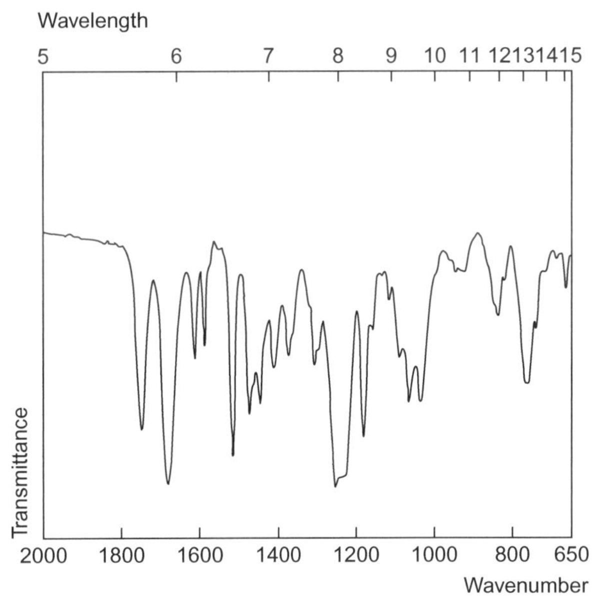

Mass Spectrum. Principal ions at *m*/*z* 58, 71, 73, 121, 150, 136, 43, 161.

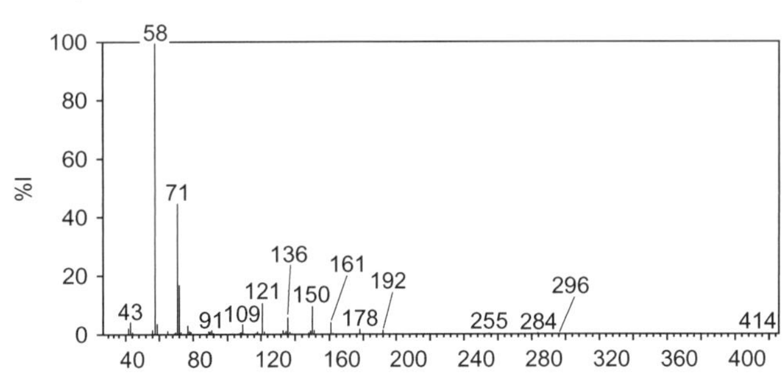

Quantification

Gas chromatography. In serum: limit of detection 2 mg/L, ECD—T. Alebic-Kolbah and F. Plavsic, *J. Pharm. Biomed. Anal.*, 1990, *8*, 915–918.

Gas chromatography–mass spectrometry. In urine: lower limit of quantification 0.1 mg/L—J. R. Kalin *et al.*, *J. Anal. Toxicol.*, 1994, *18*, 180–182.

High performance liquid chromatography. In plasma: limit of detection for diltiazem and metabolites < 10 mg/L, UV detection (λ=237 nm)—P. K. F. Yeung *et al.*, *Ther. Drug Monit.*, 1996, *18*, 40–45. In serum: limit of detection 2.5 mg/L. UV detection (λ=237 nm)—R. S. Chaudhary *et al.*, *J. Chromatogr.* 1993, *614*; *Biomed. Appl.*, 261–266.

Disposition in the Body. After oral administration, diltiazem is rapidly absorbed (approx. 90%) from the gastro-intestinal tract and undergoes extensive first-pass hepatic metabolism via deacetylation, *N*-demethylation, *O*-demethylation and oxidative deamination. Metabolites are A_1, M_A, M_B, M_X, M_1, M_2, M_4 and M_6. 2 to 4% of administered dose appears unchanged in the urine. Metabolites are excreted via bile, urine and faeces, and it can be found in breast milk.

Therapeutic concentration. Average optimum dose 180 to 360 mg daily with a blood therapeutic level 0.05 to 0.20 mg/L. The serum therapeutic concentration range is 0.05 to 0.4 mg/L.

6 healthy males and 6 females were administered orally with a single 120 mg dose of diltiazem. Peak serum levels reached 0.194 ± 0.094 and 0.181 ± 0.048 mg/L for male and females, respectively within 2.2 ± 0.8 h. [D. Saenz-Campos *et al.*, *Int. J. Clin. Phamacol. Ther. Toxicol.*, 1995, *33*, 397–400].

Toxicity. Toxic dose for adults is 2 g and 6 mg/kg for children, and it affects the skin causing, for example, rashes. It is a poison by subcutaneous, intravenous and intraperitoneal routes and moderately toxic by ingestion. Overdose is associated with bradycardia with or without atrioventricular conduction defects and hypotension. A serum toxic concentration is 0.8 mg/L and a concentration of 2 to 6 mg/L has been associated with fatalities.

A 58-year-old took 10.8 g diltiazem and was admitted with hypotension and complete heart block. Dopamine, isoprendine and calcium chloride were required to maintain blood pressure. ECG (electrocardiogram) converted to sinus rhythm after 31 h. Plasma concentrations were 1.67 mg/L 43 h after oral administration and decreased to 0.012 mg/L over the following 55 h. [N. Malcolm *et al.*, *Drug Intell. Clin. Pharm.*, 1986, *20*, 888].

A suicidal 39-year-old man was found dead and the coroner decided it was due to cardiac failure. Toxicological analysis of blood from around his heart and urine was requested because the previous night he had been threatening to commit suicide and the police had been called in. Analysis showed that he had more than 30 times the recommended therapeutic dose of diltiazem. [J. R. Kalin *et al.*, *J. Anal. Toxicol.*, 1994, *18*, 180].

Bioavailability. About 30 to 40%.

Half-life. 3 to 7 h.

Volume of distribution. 3.1 L/kg for oral administration and 11.1 L/kg intravenously. Mean apparent volume of distribution at steady state also reported as 360 to 391 L.

Clearance. Total clearance, 12 to 21 mL/min/kg after oral administration and 16 mL/min/kg after intravenous injection; also reported as 65 L/h.

Distribution in blood. 14 to 23% unbound drug in serum.

Protein binding. 80 to 85% bound to plasma proteins but only 30 to 40% bound to albumin.

Dose. For angina pectoris: initial dose of 60 mg diltiazem hydrochloride three times a day, which can be increased to 360 mg a day if necessary. (Reduced to 60 mg twice daily for the elderly). For hypertension: initial dose of 60 to 120 mg twice daily, which can be increased, if necessary, to 360 mg/kg daily. For cardiac arrhythmia: 0.25 mg/kg body weight followed by 0.35 mg/kg after 15 min, if required.

Dimefline

Respiratory Stimulant

8-[(Dimethylamino)methyl]-7-methoxy-3-methyl-2-phenyl-4*H*-1-benzopyran-4-one
$C_{20}H_{21}NO_3$=323.4
CAS—1165-48-6

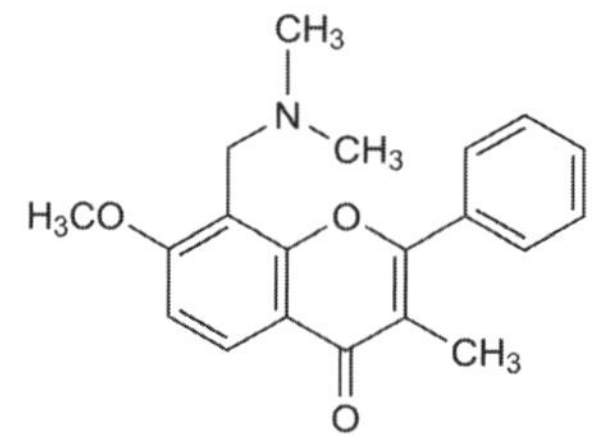

Dimefline Hydrochloride
Proprietary name. Remeflin
$C_{20}H_{21}NO_3,HCl$=359.9
CAS—2740-04-7
A white crystalline powder. M.p. 213° with decomposition.
Soluble in water and ethanol; practically insoluble in chloroform and ether.

Partition Coefficient. Log *P* (octanol/water), 3.6.

Colour Test. Liebermann's Test—orange

Thin-layer Chromatography. System TA—Rf 59; system TB—Rf 15; system TC—Rf 48; system TL—Rf 24. (Acidified iodoplatinate solution, positive.)

Gas Chromatography. System GA—RI 2555.

Ultraviolet Spectrum. Aqueous acid—309 nm (A_1^1=950b).

Infra-red Spectrum. Principal peaks at wavenumbers 1637, 1278, 1602, 1081, 699, 1136 cm^{-1} (KBr disk).

Mass Spectrum. Principal ions at *m/z* 279, 163, 323, 58, 277, 308, 280, 322.

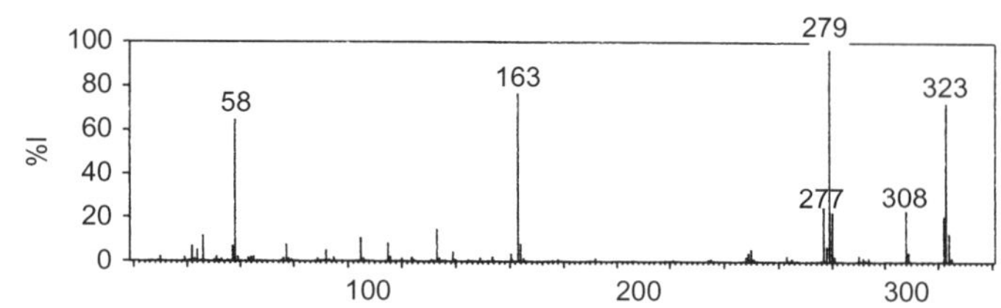

Quantification

Gas chromatography. In urine: limit of detection 10 µg/L, nitrogen specific detection—F. T. Delbeke and M. Debackere, *J. Pharm. Biomed. Anal.*, 1991, *9*, 23–28.

Dose. Dimefline hydrochloride has been given in doses of 16 to 48 mg daily.

Dimenhydrinate

Antihistamine

Synonyms. Chloranautine; Diphenhydramine Teoclate; Diphenhydramine Theoclate; Dimenhydrinatum.
Proprietary names. Amosyt; Antemin; Calm-X; Dimen; Dimetabs; Dinate; Dramamine; Dramanate; Dramilin; Dymenate; Emedyl; Gravol; Hydrate; Lomarin; Marmine; Motozina; Nauseatol; Nausex; Nausicalm; Reisegold; Reisetabletten-ratiopharm; RubieMen; Superpep; Tega-Vert; Travamine; Travel-Gum; Trawell; Triptone; Vagomine; Valontan; Vertab; Vertigo-Vomex; Vertirosan; Vomacur; Xamamina.
8-Chloro-3,7-dihydro-1,3-dimethyl-1*H*-purine-2,6-dione compound with 2-(diphenylmethoxy)-*N*,*N*-dimethylethanamine (1:1)
$C_{17}H_{21}NO,C_7H_7ClN_4O_2$=470.0
CAS—523-87-5

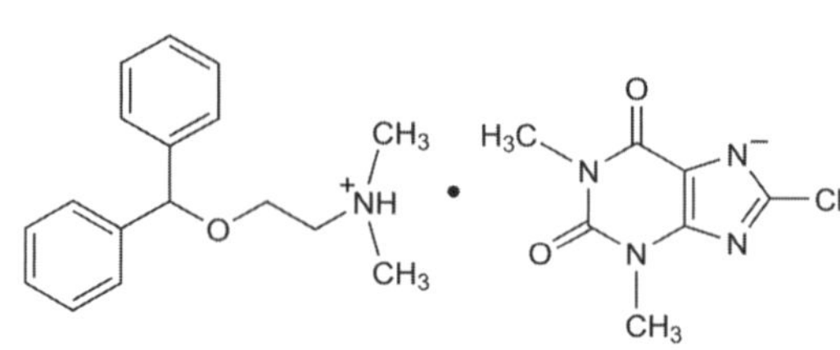

A white crystalline powder. M.p. 102° to 107°.

Solubility in water about 3 mg/mL; soluble 1 in 2 of ethanol and 1 in 2 of chloroform; soluble in benzene; almost insoluble in ether.

Partition Coefficient. Log *P* (octanol/water), −0.4.

Thin-layer Chromatography. System TA—Rf 55 and 88; system TB—Rf 45 and 00; system TC—Rf 33 and 10; system TE—Rf 68 and 02; system TL—Rf 15 and 10; system TAE—Rf 28 and 87; system TAF—Rf 48 and 46.

Gas Chromatography. System GA—RI 1844.

High Performance Liquid Chromatography. System HY—RI 182.

Ultraviolet Spectrum. Aqueous acid—208, 276 (A_1^1=268a); aqueous alkali—278 nm.

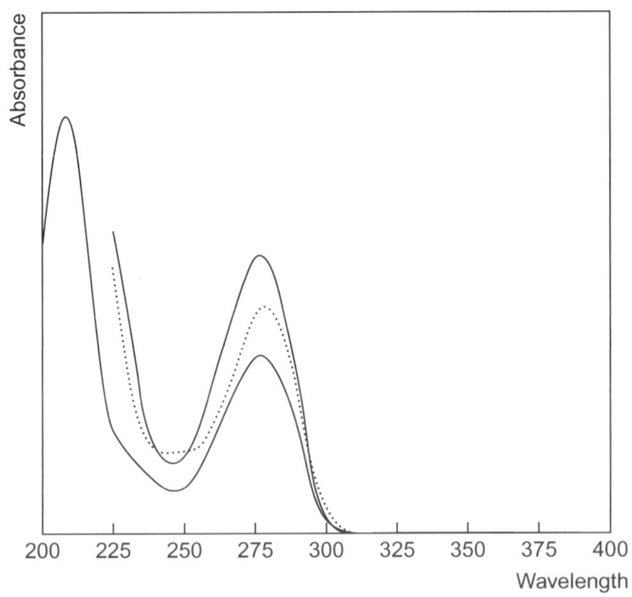

Infra-red Spectrum. Principal peaks at wavenumbers 1640, 1685, 1118, 755, 712, 1255 cm^{-1} (KBr disk).

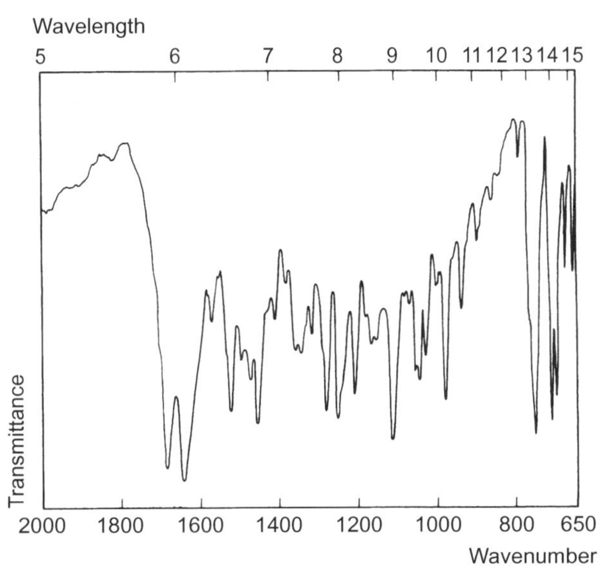

Mass Spectrum. Principal ions at *m/z* 58, 73, 45, 43, 57, 167, 44, 165.

Quantification

High performance liquid chromatography. In serum: limit of detection 50 µg/mL, UV detection—G. Skofitsch and F. Lembeck, *Arzneimittel-forschung*, 1983, *33*, 1674–1676.

Toxicity

In a 4-month-old infant to whom a dimenhydrinate overdose was intentionally administered, repeated analysis of the serum at 6 h post-ingestion revealed diphenhydramine levels of 4.8 mg/L. The infant presented with status epilepticus, coma, and ventricular dysrhythmias but recovered after IV administration of sodium bicarbonate. [M. Farrell *et al.*, *J. Toxicol. Clin. Toxicol.*, 1991, *29*, 527–535.]

A 19-year-old female died after ingesting 5 g of dimenhydrinate in a suicidal gesture; within an hour of the ingestion, status epilepticus and ventricular dysrhythmias presented. Diphenhydramine concentrations in the urine were 10.8 mg/L. [R. E. Winn and K. P. McDonnell, *Ann. Emerg. Med.*, 1993, *22*, 1481–1484.]

Dose. 50 to 100 mg three or four times daily.

Dimercaprol

Chelating Agent

Synonyms. BAL; British Anti-Lewisite; Dimercaptopropanol.
Proprietary name. Sulfactin
2,3-Dimercapto-1-propanol
$C_3H_8OS_2$=124.2
CAS—59-52-9

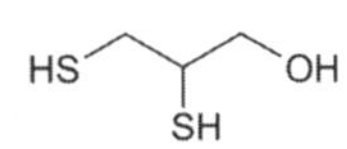

A clear, colourless, or slightly yellow liquid. Relative density 1.239 to 1.259. Refractive index 1.568 to 1.574.
Soluble 1 in 20 of water; miscible with ethanol, ether, and methanol; soluble in vegetable oils.

Dissociation Constant. pK_a 8.6 (25°).

Partition Coefficient. Log *P* (octanol/water), 0.2.

Colour Test. Palladium Chloride—yellow

Ultraviolet Spectrum. No significant absorption, 230 to 360 nm.

Infra-red Spectrum. Principal peaks at wavenumbers 1022, 1050, 990, 1270, 1235, 1170 cm^{-1} (thin film).

Dose. 2.5 to 4 mg/kg, intramuscularly, up to 6 times daily as an antidote to arsenic, gold, and mercury poisoning.

Dimethadione

Anticonvulsant

5,5-Dimethyl-2,4-oxazolidinedione
$C_5H_7NO_3$=129.1
CAS—695-53-4

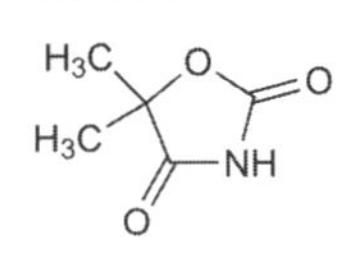

Crystals. M.p. 76° to 77°.

Dissociation Constant. pK_a 6.1 (37°).

Partition Coefficient. Log *P* (octanol/water), 0.2.

Colour Tests. Koppanyi–Zwikker Test—violet; Mercurous Nitrate—black

Gas Chromatography. System GA—RI 1060.

Ultraviolet Spectrum. No significant absorption, 230 to 360 nm.

Infra-red Spectrum. Principal peaks at wavenumbers 1740, 1760, 1815, 1188, 1280, 1007 cm^{-1}.

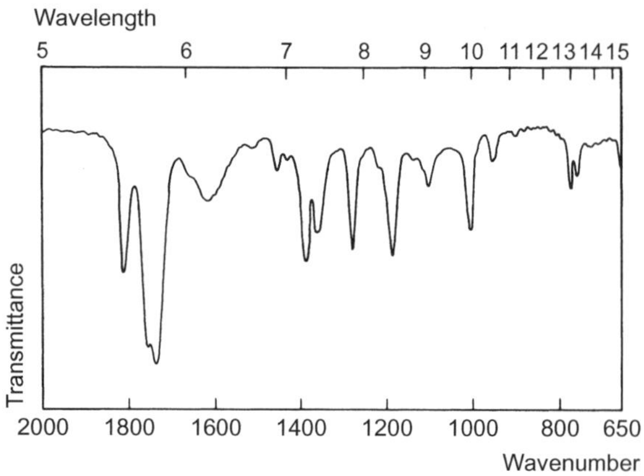

Quantification. See under Trimethadione.

Disposition in the Body. Dimethadione is the active metabolite of trimethadione. It is very slowly excreted in the urine over a period of several days, the rate of excretion being increased in alkaline urine.

Toxicity. Toxic effects may be associated with plasma concentrations greater than 1 g/L.

Half-life. Derived from urinary excretion data, 6 to 13 days.

Dimethisterone

Progestational Steroid

Synonym. 6α,21-Dimethylethisterone
(6α,17β)-17-Hydroxy-6-methyl-17-(1-propynyl)androst-4-en-3-one monohydrate
$C_{23}H_{32}O_2,H_2O = 358.5$
CAS—79-64-1 (anhydrous); 41354-30-7 (monohydrate)

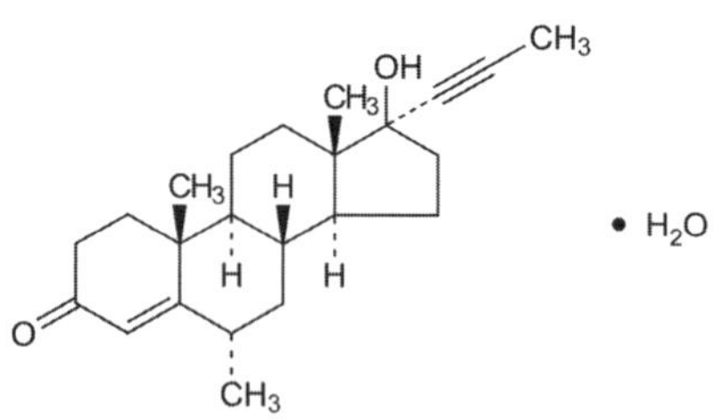

A white crystalline powder. M.p. 102° (anhydrous).
Practically insoluble in water; soluble 1 in 3 of ethanol, 1 in 0.7 of chloroform, and 1 in 1 of pyridine; slightly soluble in acetone.

Partition Coefficient. Log *P* (octanol/water), 4.4.

Colour Tests. Antimony Pentachloride—brown; Naphthol–Sulfuric Acid—red-brown/brown-green; Sulfuric Acid—orange-red.

Thin-layer Chromatography. System TP—Rf 80; system TQ—Rf 42; system TR—Rf 91; system TS—Rf 95.

Ultraviolet Spectrum. Dimethisterone anhydrous: dehydrated alcohol—240 nm (A^1_1=467a).

Infra-red Spectrum. Principal peaks at wavenumbers 1658, 1605, 1275, 876, 1281, 1241 cm^{-1} (KBr disk).

Mass Spectrum. Principal ions at *m/z* 67, 137, 91, 138, 55, 79, 41, 95.

Dose. Dimethisterone has been given in doses of 15 mg daily.

Dimethoate

Pesticide

Synonym. Fosfamid
Proprietary names. Cygon; Fostion MM; Rogor E; Roxion.
Phosphorodithioic acid *O*,*O*-dimethyl-*S*-[2-(methylamino)-2-oxoethyl] ester
$C_5H_{12}NO_3PS_2 = 229.3$
CAS—60-51-5

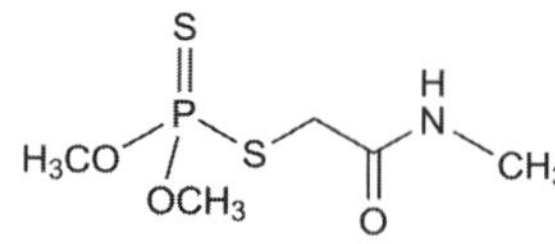

A white solid. M.p. 52° to 52.5°.
Soluble 1 in 40 of water; freely soluble in most organic solvents except saturated hydrocarbons.

Partition Coefficient. Log *P* (octanol/water), 0.8.

Colour Tests. Palladium Chloride—yellow; Phosphorus Test—yellow

Thin-layer Chromatography. System TE—Rf 99; system TL—Rf 01; system TW—Rf 19; system TX—Rf 04; system TY—Rf 04; system TZ—Rf 37; system TAA—Rf 08; system TAB—Rf 03; system TAE—Rf 80.

Gas Chromatography. System GA—dimethoate RI 1725, M (OH-) RI 1430, M (COOH-)-Me RI 1400; system GK—dimethoate, RRT 0.86 (relative to caffeine).

High Performance Liquid Chromatography. System HY—RI 289; system HZ—retention time 2.8 min.

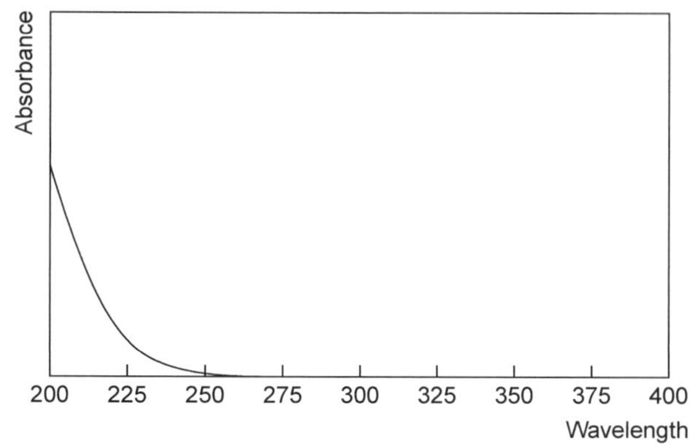

Infra-red Spectrum. Principal peaks at wavenumbers 1010, 1666, 819, 666, 1538, 1176 cm^{-1}.

Mass Spectrum. Principal ions at *m/z* 87, 93, 125, 58, 47, 63, 79, 42.

Quantification
Gas chromatography. In blood: FPD—T. Kojima *et al.*, *Forensic Sci. Int.*, 1990, *48*, 79–88.

Disposition in the Body
Toxicity
In a 57-year-old male who became semi-comatose after ingesting not more than 22 g of formothion, blood levels of dimethoate at approximately 1.5 and 6 h after ingestion were 21.4 and 12.7 μg/g, respectively. [T. Kojima *et al.*, *Forensic Sci. Int.*, 1990, *48*, 79–88.]

Dimethoxanate

Cough Suppressant

10*H*-Phenothiazine-10-carboxylic acid 2-[2-(dimethylamino)ethoxy]ethyl ester
$C_{19}H_{22}N_2O_3S = 358.5$
CAS—477-93-0

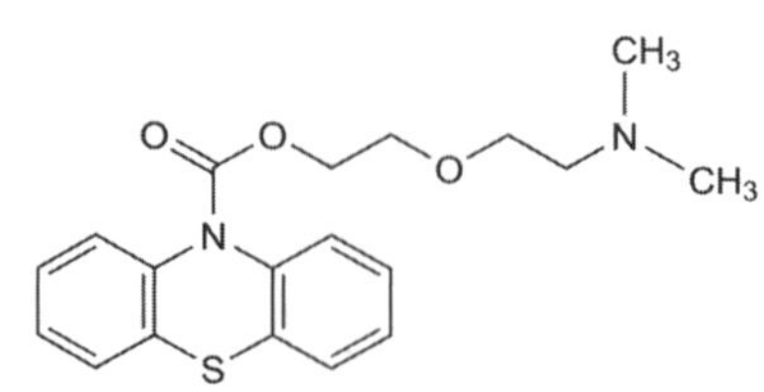

Dimethoxanate Hydrochloride
Proprietary name. Cotrane
$C_{19}H_{22}N_2O_3S,HCl = 394.9$

CAS—518-63-8
Crystals. M.p. 161° to 163°, with decomposition.

Partition Coefficient. Log *P* (octanol/water), 4.1.

Colour Tests. Mandelin's Test—green→brown; Marquis Test—violet.

Thin-layer Chromatography. System TA—Rf 39; system TB—Rf 18; system TC—Rf 24; system TE—Rf 49; system TL—Rf 06; system TAE—Rf 21; system TAF—Rf 38; system TAJ—Rf 10; system TAK—Rf 84; system TAL—Rf 49. (Dragendorff spray, positive; FPN reagent, violet; acidified iodoplatinate solution, positive; Marquis reagent, brown; ninhydrin spray, positive.)

Gas Chromatography. System GA—RI 2029.

High Performance Liquid Chromatography. System HA—*k* 5.8 (tailing peak).

Ultraviolet Spectrum. Aqueous acid—254 nm (A_1^1=24b). No alkaline shift.

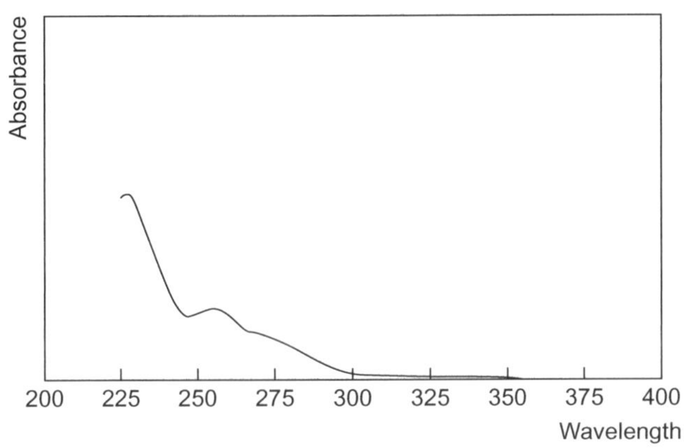

Infra-red Spectrum. Principal peaks at wavenumbers 1718, 1317, 1217, 1250, 763, 1298 cm^{-1} (KBr disk).

Mass Spectrum. Principal ions at *m/z* 58, 116, 198, 199, 72, 59, 42, 44.

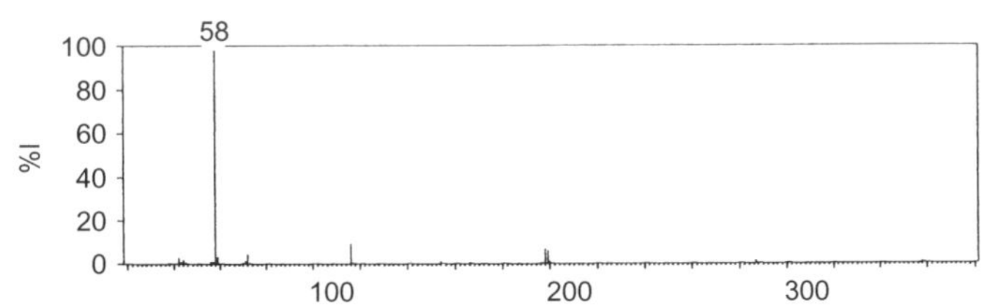

Dose. Dimethoxanate hydrochloride has been given in doses of 75 to 200 mg daily.

Dimethyl Phthalate

Insect Repellent

Synonyms. DMP; Methyl Phthalate.
Proprietary names. Avolin; Fermine; Mipax; Palitinol M.
1,2-Benzenedicarboxylic acid dimethyl ester
$C_{10}H_{10}O_4$=194.2
CAS—131-11-3

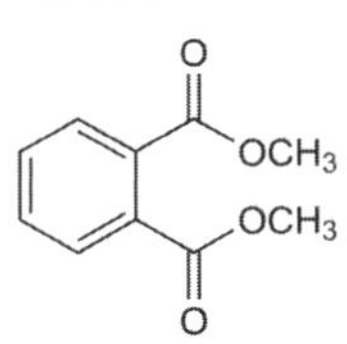

A colourless liquid. Mass per mL 1.186 to 1.192 g. B.p. about 280°, with decomposition. Refractive index 1.515 to 1.517.
Soluble 1 in 250 of water; miscible with ethanol, ether, chloroform, and most organic solvents; practically insoluble in petroleum ether and other paraffin hydrocarbons.

Partition Coefficient. Log *P* (octanol/water), 1.6.

Gas Chromatography. System GA—RI 1406.

High Performance Liquid Chromatography. System HAA—retention time 17.0 min.

Ultraviolet Spectrum. Ethanol—275 nm (A_1^1=75b).

Mass Spectrum. Principal ions at *m/z* 163, 77, 164, 135, 194, 76, 92, 50.

Use. Topically in concentrations of at least 40%.

Dimethyl Sulfoxide

Solvent

Synonyms. Dimethyl Sulphoxide; Dimexide; DMSO; Methyl Sulfoxide.
Proprietary names. Deltan; Dolicur; Dolmoso; Kemsol; Rheumabene; Rimso-50. It is an ingredient of Herpid and Iduridin.
C_2H_6OS=78.1
CAS—67-68-5

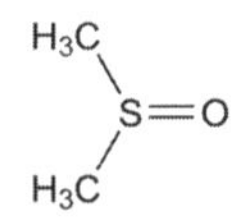

A colourless, hygroscopic, viscous liquid. Mass per mL 1.099 to 1.101 g. F.p. not lower than 18.3°. B.p. 189° to 192°. Refractive index 1.478 to 1.479.
Soluble in water, ethanol, acetone, benzene, chloroform, ether, and most organic solvents.

Partition Coefficient. Log *P* (octanol/water), −1.4.

Colour Tests. 1% potassium permanganate solution—decolorises; cautiously add 1.5 mL dropwise to 2.5 mL of hydriodic acid cooled in ice and filter rapidly—unstable violet residue which is soluble in chloroform giving a red solution.

Gas Chromatography. System GA—RI 784.

Ultraviolet Spectrum. No significant absorption, 230 to 360 nm.

Mass Spectrum. Principal ions at *m/z* 63, 78, 45, 61, 46, 62, 48, 47.

Quantification

Gas chromatography. In serum or urine: dimethyl sulfoxide and sulfone metabolite, FID—H. B. Hucker *et al.*, *J. Pharmacol. Exp. Ther.*, 1967, *155*, 309–317. In plasma, serum, urine, or cerebrospinal fluid: limit of detection 10 μg/mL, FID—S. E. Garretson and J. P. Aitchison, *J. Anal. Toxicol.*, 1982, *6*, 76–81.

Disposition in the Body. Readily absorbed after injection or after oral or percutaneous administration. Widely distributed throughout the body. It is oxidised to dimethyl sulfone. After an oral dose, about 30 to 70% is excreted in the urine unchanged and about 20% as the sulfone; after percutaneous administration, about 13% is excreted unchanged and about 18% as the sulfone; about 3% of a dose is eliminated through the lungs as dimethyl sulfide.

Blood concentration

After an oral dose of 1 g/kg to 6 subjects, peak serum concentrations of dimethyl sulfoxide of 1029 to 3380 mg/L (mean 2200) were attained in 1 to 4 h, and peak concentrations of the sulfone metabolite of 260 to 600 mg/L were reported after about 72 h. After percutaneous administration of 1 g/kg to 2 subjects, peak serum concentrations of about 500 mg/L of dimethyl sulfoxide and 350 mg/L of the sulfone metabolite were reported after 4 to 8 h and 36 to 72 h, respectively. [H. B. Hucker *et al.*, *J. Pharmacol. Exp. Ther.*, 1967, *155*, 309–317.]

The mean peak plasma dimethyl sulfoxide concentration in 10 subjects undergoing peripheral blood stem-cell transplants (cryopreserved with 10% v/v dimethyl sulfoxide; patients received infusions containing 254 to 824 mmol over 20 to 120 min) was 19.1 mmol/L (0.5 mg/L) 5 min after the end of the infusion. Plasma dimethyl sulfone concentrations increased during the first 24 h, plateaued at 4.4 mmol/L and remained at this level until 48 h. Dimethyl sulfide concentrations were at steady state by 5 min and remained between 3 and 5 mmol/L for 48 h. [M. J. Egorin *et al.*, *J. Clin. Oncol.*, 1998, *16*, 610–615.]

Toxicity. Dimethyl sulfoxide has low systemic toxicity, but gives local toxic effects.

Half-life. Plasma half-life, dimethyl sulfoxide about 10 to 20 h, sulfone metabolite about 70 h.

Dimethylamfetamine

Central Stimulant

Synonym. Dimethylamphetamine
N,N,α-Trimethylbenzeneethanamine
$C_{11}H_{17}N$=163.3
CAS—4075-96-1

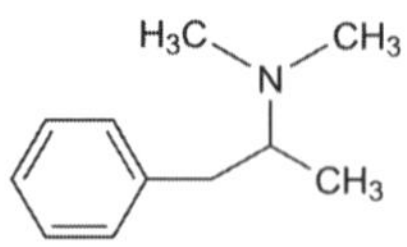

Dissociation Constant. pK_a 9.8.

Gas Chromatography. System GA—RI 1235; system GC—RI 1429.

High Performance Liquid Chromatography. System HB—*k* 11.08; system HC—*k* 1.89.

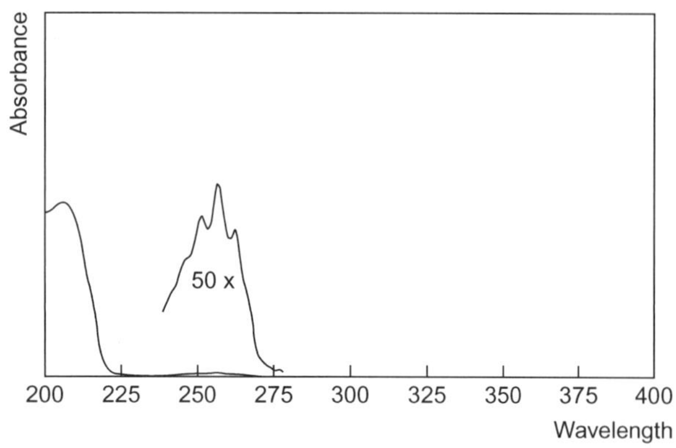

Mass Spectrum. Principal ions at *m/z* 72, 91, 73, 44, 42, 56, 70, 65.

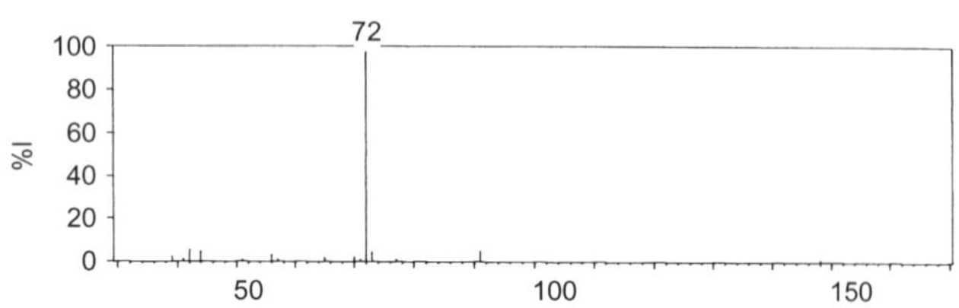

Disposition in the Body. Dimethylamfetamine is metabolised to metamfetamine.

Quantification

High performance liquid chromatography–mass spectrometry. In urine: dimethylamfetamine and its metabolites, limit of detection for dimethylamfetamine 5 μg/L—M. Katagi *et al.*, *J. Anal. Toxicol.*, 2000, *24*, 354–358.

Dimethyltryptamine

Hallucinogen

Synonyms. Businessman's Trip; *N,N*-Dimethyltryptamine; DMT.
N,N-Dimethyl-1*H*-indole-3-ethanamine
$C_{12}H_{16}N_2$=188.3
CAS—61-50-7

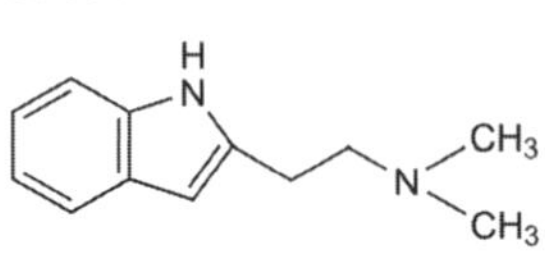

An active principle obtained from the seeds and leaves of *Piptadenia peregrina* (Mimosaceae). Crystals. M.p. 44.6° to 46.8°.

Freely soluble in dilute acetic acid and dilute mineral acids.

Dimethyltryptamine Hydrochloride

A white crystalline powder. M.p. 165° to 168°.
Soluble in water.

Dissociation Constant. pK_a 8.7 (ethanol–water).

Partition Coefficient. Log *P* (octanol/water), 1.9.

Colour Test. Marquis Test—orange

Thin-layer Chromatography. System TA—Rf 40; system TB—Rf 09; system TC—Rf 09; system TE—Rf 50; system TL—Rf 06; system TAE—Rf 14; system TAF—Rf 39. (Dragendorff spray, positive; acidified iodoplatinate solution, positive; Marquis reagent, grey-brown; Van Urk reagent, blue.)

Gas Chromatography. System GA—RI 1753.

High Performance Liquid Chromatography. System HY—RI 228.

Ultraviolet Spectrum. Aqueous acid—279 nm (A_1^1=327a), 288 nm.

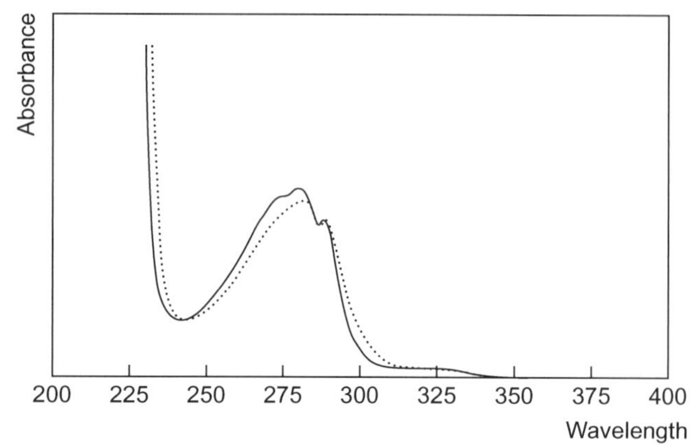

Infra-red Spectrum. Principal peaks at wavenumbers 743, 1113, 1235, 1050, 812, 1010 cm^{-1} (KBr disk).

Mass Spectrum. Principal ions at *m/z* 58, 188, 130, 59, 42, 143, 129, 115.

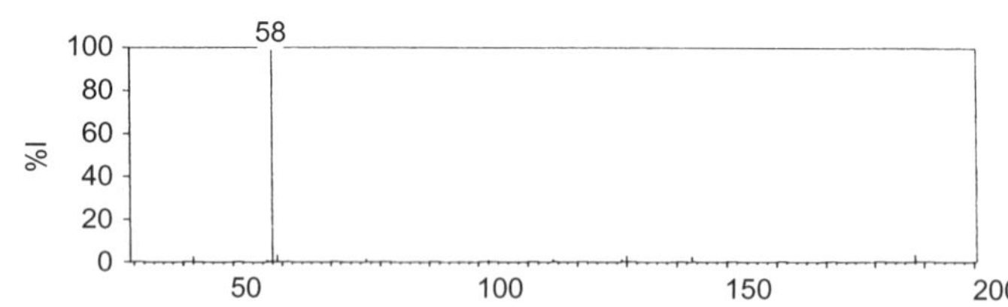

Quantification

Gas chromatography. In blood and urine: limit of detection 0.5 μg/L, SID—A. Ishii *et al.*, *J. Anal. Toxicol.*, 1997, *21*, 36–40. In plasma: *N,N*-dimethyltryptamine and *β*-carboline alkaloids, limit of quantification for *N,N*-dimethyltryptamine 1.6 μg/L—M. Yritia *et al.*, *J. Chromatogr. B Anal. Technol. Biomed. Life Sci.*, 2002, *779*, 271–281.

Gas chromatography–mass spectrometry. In blood: limit of detection 10 ng/L—R. W. Walker *et al.*, *J. Chromatogr.* 1979, *162*(4) *B Biomed. Appl.*, 539–546. In urine: limit of detection 100 ng/L—M. Räisänen and J. Kärrkkäinen, *J. Chromatogr.* 1979, *162*(4) *B Biomed. Appl.*, 579–584.

High performance liquid chromatography. In plasma: limit of quantification 2 μg/L, fluorescence detection (λ_{ex}=232 nm, λ_{em}=351 nm, or λ_{ex}=340, λ_{em}=495 nm)—J. C. Callaway *et al.*, *J. Anal. Toxicol.*, 1996, *20*, 492–497. In urine: limit of detection 0.1 μg/L. MS–MS detection—T. Forsstrom *et al.*, *Scand. J. Clin. Lab. Invest.*, 2001, *61*, 547–556.

Disposition in the Body. It is inactive when taken orally. After intramuscular injection it is rapidly and extensively metabolised, primarily to indol-3-ylacetic acid. About 33% of a dose is excreted in the urine in 6 h as free and conjugated (glucuronide) indol-3-ylacetic acid; less than 0.1% of a dose is excreted unchanged in the urine in 24 h.

Blood concentration. Plasma concentrations of endogenous dimethyltryptamine are generally less than 0.001 mg/L.

15 male volunteers, between the age of 26 to 48 years were administered 2 mL/kg of hoasca tea, an Amazonian sacramental beverage. The tea alkaloid content was determined to be as follows: DMT, 0.24 mg/mL; harmine, 1.70 mg/mL; harmaline, 0.20 mg/mL; tetrahydroharmine, 1.07 mg/mL. DMT peak plasma concentration was 15.8 μg/L (mean) after 107.5 min which coincided with peak times of psychoactivity. [J. C. Callaway *et al.*, *J. Ethnopharmacol.*, 1999, *65*, 243–256.]

After intramuscular injection of 0.7 mg/kg to 11 subjects, peak blood concentrations averaged 0.1 mg/L at 0.17 h, coinciding with the maximum psychoactive effects. [J. Kaplan *et al.*, *Psychopharmacologia*, 1974, *28*, 239–245.]

Toxicity. Dimethyltryptamine produces hallucinations and perceptual distortion similar to the effects of lysergide.

Dimetindene

Antihistamine

Synonyms. Dimethindene; Dimethpyrindene; Dimethylpyrindene.
N,*N*-Dimethyl-3-[1-(2-pyridinyl)ethyl]-1*H*-indene-2-ethanamine
$C_{20}H_{24}N_2$=292.4
CAS—5636-83-9

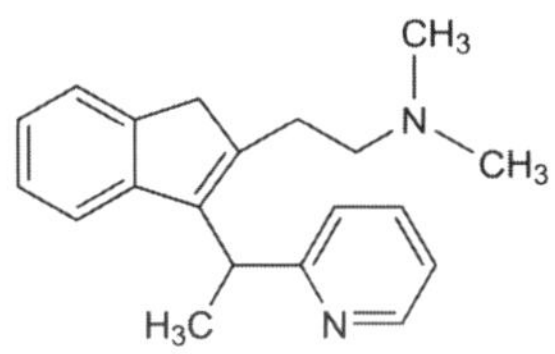

Dimetindene Maleate

Proprietary names. Fenistil; Neostil. It is an ingredient of Vibrocil.
$C_{20}H_{24}N_2,C_4H_4O_4$=408.5
CAS—3614-69-5
A white to off-white crystalline powder. M.p. 159° to 161°.
Soluble 1 in 63 of water, 1 in 185 of ethanol, and 1 in 10 of chloroform; practically insoluble in ether.

Partition Coefficient. Log *P* (octanol/water), 5.0.

Colour Tests. Cyanogen Bromide—orange-pink; Mandelin's Test—green; Marquis Test—violet→blue.

Thin-layer Chromatography. System TA—Rf 42; system TB—Rf 36; system TC—Rf 13; system TE—Rf 47; system TL—Rf 06; system TAE—Rf 10; system TAJ—Rf 04; system TAK—Rf 00; system TAL—Rf 40. (Acidified iodoplatinate solution, positive.)

Gas Chromatography. System GA—RI 2275; system GB—RI 2376; system GC—RI 2669.

High Performance Liquid Chromatography. System HA—*k* 5.1; system HX—RI 338; system HY—RI 288.

Ultraviolet Spectrum. Aqueous acid—260 nm (A_1^1=613b).

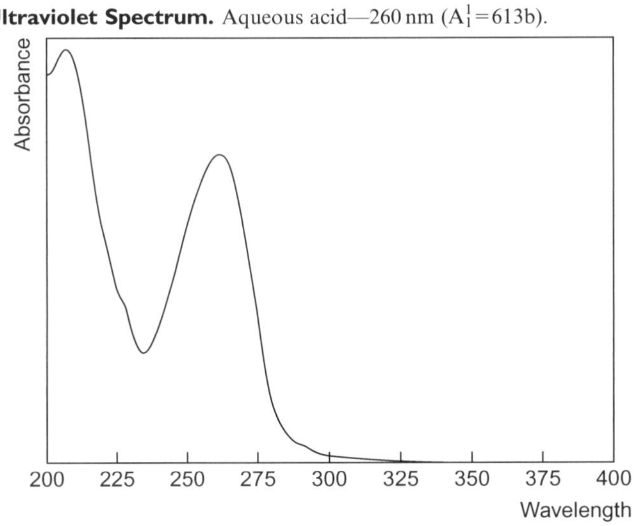

Infra-red Spectrum. Principal peaks at wavenumbers 763, 1590, 724, 747, 1570, 1050 cm^{-1}.

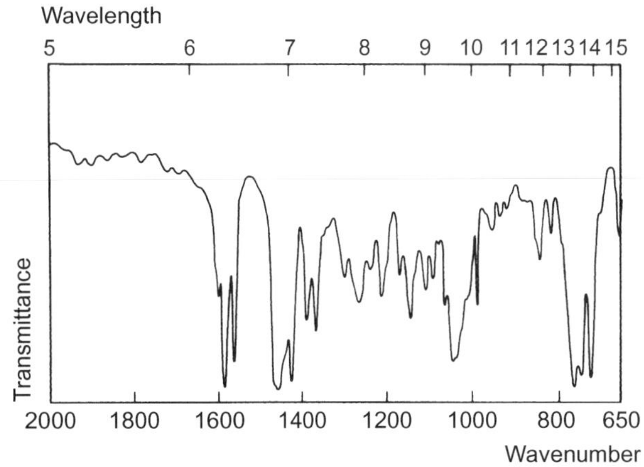

Mass Spectrum. Principal ions at *m/z* 58, 59, 72, 45, 292, 218, 42, -.

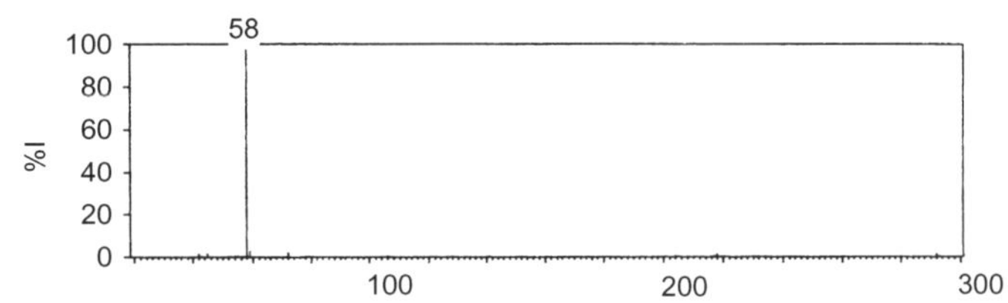

Quantification.
Gas chromatography. In serum or urine: limit of detection 10 μg/L, FID—M. M. Wermeille and G. A. Huber, *J. Chromatogr.* 1982, *228(17) B Biomed. Appl.*, 187–194.

Gas chromatography–mass spectrometry. In plasma—G. Kauert *et al.*, *J. Chromatogr.*, 1993, *617*, 318–323.

High performance liquid chromatography. In urine: dimetindene and *N*-desmethyldimetindene—S. Radler and G. Blaschke, *J. Chromatogr.*, 1991, *567*, 229–239. In urine: limit of detection <5 nmol/L—D. Chollet *et al.*, *J. Chromatogr.*, 1993, *629*, 89–93. In urine: dimetindene and its major metabolites—D. Prien and G. Blaschke, *J. Chromatogr. B Biomed. Sci. Appl.*, 1997, *688*, 309–318. In tears: limit of detection <12 μg/L—D. F. Chollet *et al.*, *J. Chromatogr. B Biomed. Sci. Appl.*, 1998, *707*, 334–347.

Dose. Up to 6 mg of dimetindene maleate daily.

Dimetotiazine

Antihistamine

Synonyms. Dimethiotazine; Dimethothiazine; Fonazine.
10-[2-(Dimethylamino)propyl]-*N*,*N*-dimethyl-10*H*-phenothiazine-2-sulfonamide
$C_{19}H_{25}N_3O_2S_2$=391.6
CAS—7456-24-8

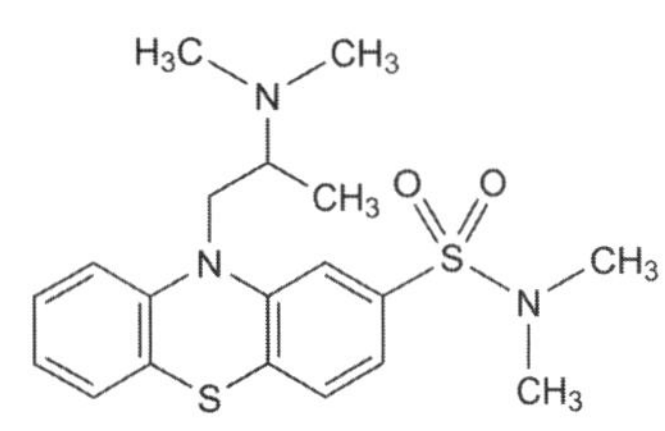

Dimetotiazine Mesilate

Proprietary names. Banistyl; Bonpac; Calsekin; Migristene; Neomestine; Promaquid; Yoristen.
$C_{19}H_{25}N_3O_2S_2,CH_3SO_3H$=487.7
CAS—7455-39-2; 13115-40-7
A white crystalline powder. M.p. about 175°.
Very soluble in water; practically insoluble in ether.

Partition Coefficient. Log *P* (octanol/water), 3.5.

Colour Tests. Formaldehyde–Sulfuric Acid—yellow; Forrest Reagent—red; FPN Reagent—red; Mandelin's Test—red-violet; Marquis Test—red.

Thin-layer Chromatography. System TA—Rf 56; system TB—Rf 13; system TC—Rf 48; system TL—Rf 28; system TAE—Rf 43. (Acidified iodoplatinate solution, positive.)

Gas Chromatography. System GA—dimetotiazine RI 3060, M (nor-) RI 3150, M (OH-)-AC RI 3200, M (bis-nor-)-AC RI 3380, M (nor-)-AC RI 3360; system GB—RI 3096.

High Performance Liquid Chromatography. System HA—*k* 2.1.

Ultraviolet Spectrum. Aqueous acid—235, 262 (A^1_1=675a); aqueous alkali—268 nm (A^1_1=808b).

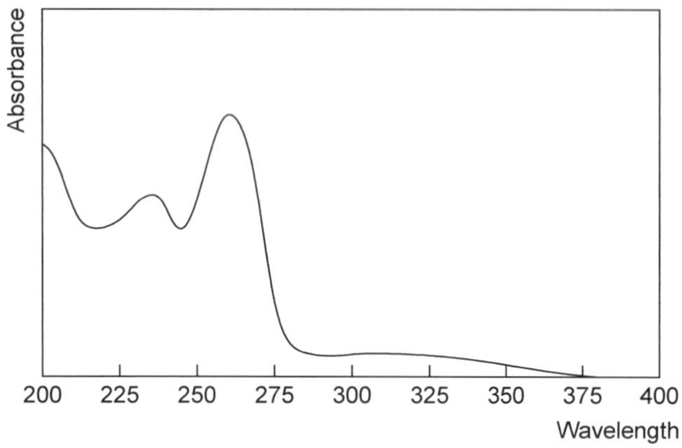

Infra-red Spectrum. Principal peaks at wavenumbers 1205, 1190, 1057, 1160, 1220, 717 cm^{-1} (dimetotiazine mesilate, KBr disk).

Mass Spectrum. Principal ions at *m/z* 72, 73, 320, 71, 70, 56, 210, 198.

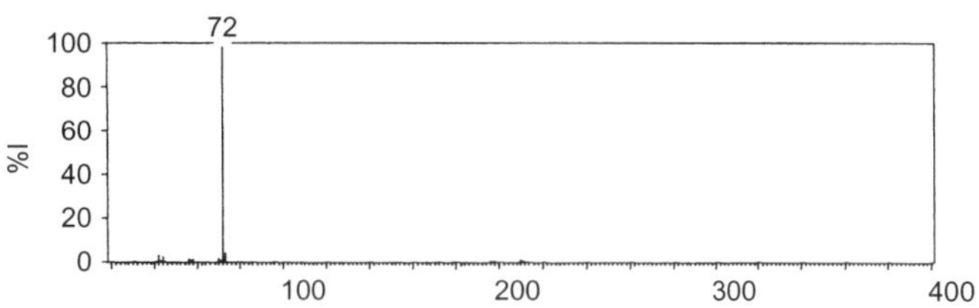

Dose. Usually the equivalent of 60 to 120 mg of dimetotiazine daily.

Dimetridazole

Antiprotozoal (Veterinary)

Proprietary names. Dimetrasol; Emtryl; Unizole.
1,2-Dimethyl-5-nitro-1*H*-imidazole
$C_5H_7N_3O_2$=141.1
CAS—551-92-8

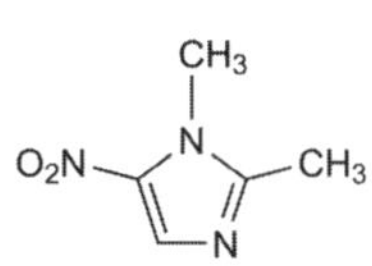

An almost white to brownish-yellow powder, which darkens on exposure to light. M.p. 138° to 141°.
Sparingly soluble in cold water; soluble 1 in 30 of ethanol, 1 in 5 of chloroform, and 1 in 170 of ether.

Dimetridazole Hydrochloride
$C_5H_7N_3O_2$,HCl=177.6
CAS—25332-20-1
Crystals. M.p. 195°.
Freely soluble in water and ethanol; sparingly soluble in acetone.

Partition Coefficient. Log *P* (octanol/water), 0.3.

Colour Test. Methanolic Potassium Hydroxide—violet (when boiled).

Thin-layer Chromatography. System TA—Rf 63. (Acidified potassium permanganate solution, strong reaction.)

Gas Chromatography. System GA—RI 1353.

High Performance Liquid Chromatography. System HAA—retention time 10.0 and 10.1 min.

Ultraviolet Spectrum. Aqueous acid—317, 226 nm; aqueous alkali—322 nm (A^1_1=500b).

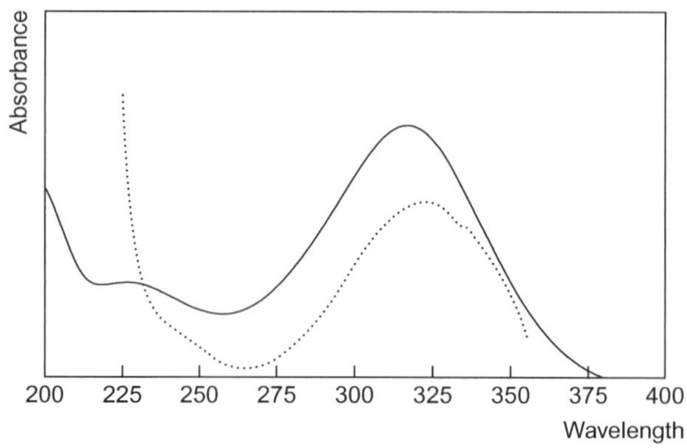

Infra-red Spectrum. Principal peaks at wavenumbers 1181, 1258, 1515, 825, 746, 1119 cm^{-1} (KBr disk).

Diminazene

Antiprotozoal/Antibacterial

4,4′-(1-Triazene-1,3-diyl)bis(benzenecarboximidamide)
$C_{14}H_{15}N_7$=281.3
CAS—536-71-0

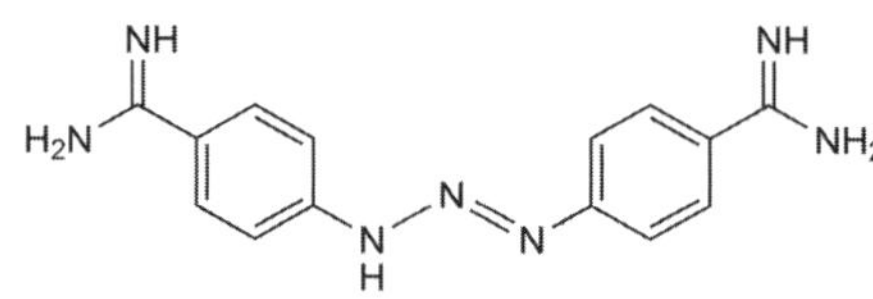

Diminazene Aceturate
Proprietary names. Azidin; Berenil; Ganasag; Pirocide.
$C_{22}H_{29}N_9O_6$,$4H_2O$=587.6
CAS—908-54-3 (anhydrous)
A yellow powder. M.p. 217°, with decomposition.
Soluble 1 in 14 of water; slightly soluble in ethanol; very slightly soluble in chloroform and ether.

Partition Coefficient. Log *P* (octanol/water), 1.5 (aceturate).

Thin-layer Chromatography. System TA—Rf 00; system TB—Rf 00; system TC—Rf 00; system TL—Rf 00 (aceturate). (Acidified iodoplatinate solution, positive.)

Ultraviolet Spectrum. Diminazene aceturate: aqueous acid—257 (A^1_1=305a); aqueous alkali—247 nm (broad) (A^1_1=239 b).

Infra-red Spectrum. Principal peaks at wavenumbers 1610, 1635, 1588, 1171, 1267, 1198 cm^{-1} (KBr disk).

Mass Spectrum. Principal ions at *m/z* 30, 43, 72, 102, 73, 42, 118, 99.

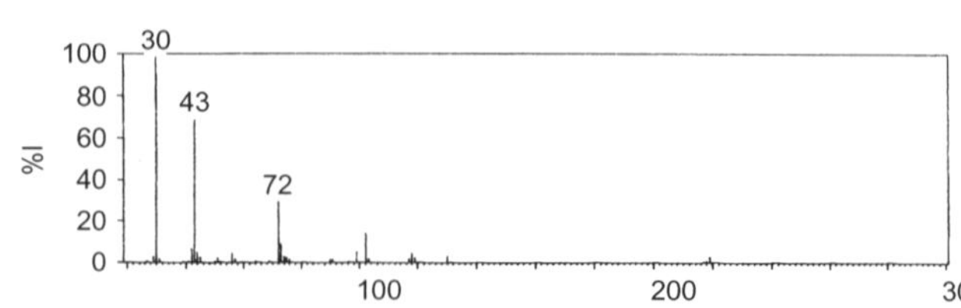

Dimoxyline

Antispasmodic

Synonym. Dioxyline
1-(4-Ethoxy-3-methoxybenzyl)-6,7-dimethoxy-3-methylisoquinoline

$C_{22}H_{25}NO_4$=367.4
CAS—147-27-3

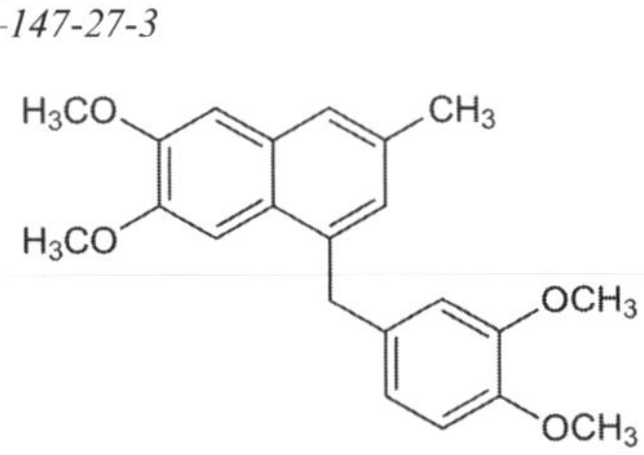

Crystals. M.p. 124° to 125°.

Dimoxyline Phosphate
Proprietary names. Paveril Phosphate; Paverona.
$C_{22}H_{25}NO_4,H_3PO_4$=465.4
CAS—5667-46-9
A white crystalline powder. M.p. about 198°, with decomposition.
Soluble 1 in 25 of water and 1 in 320 of ethanol.

Partition Coefficient. Log *P* (octanol/water), 4.7.

Colour Tests. Mandelin's Test—green; Marquis Test—brown.

Thin-layer Chromatography. System TA—Rf 68; system TB—Rf 16; system TC—Rf 75; system TE—Rf 87; system TL—Rf 58; system TAJ—Rf 64; system TAK—Rf 10; system TAL—Rf 93. (Acidified iodoplatinate solution, positive.)

Gas Chromatography. System GA—RI 2895.

Ultraviolet Spectrum. Aqueous acid—285, 309 (A^1_1=179b), 335 nm.

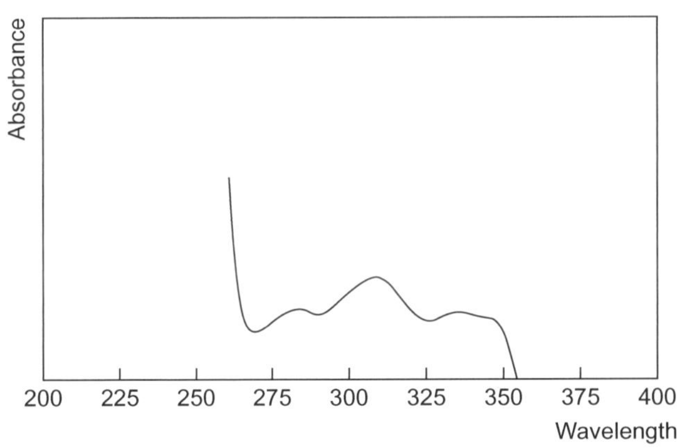

Infra-red Spectrum. Principal peaks at wavenumbers 1504, 1247, 1208, 1145, 1225, 865 cm^{-1} (KCl disk).

Mass Spectrum. Principal ions at *m/z* 352, 367, 338, 366, 29, 368, 353, 339.

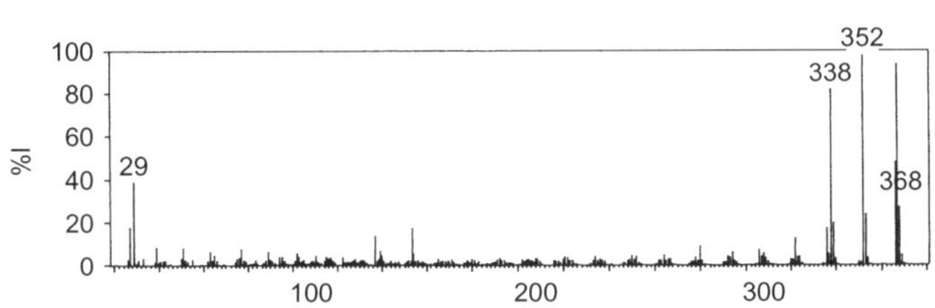

Disposition in the Body. Absorbed from the gastro-intestinal tract. Metabolised in the liver and excreted in the urine.

Dose. 0.3 to 1.6 g of dimoxyline phosphate daily.

Dimpylate

Pesticide

Synonym. Diazinon
Proprietary names. Basudin; Diazitol.
Phosphorothioic acid *O*,*O*-diethyl *O*-[6-methyl-2-(1-methylethyl)-4-pyrimidinyl]ester
$C_{12}H_{21}N_2O_3PS$=304.4
CAS—333-41-5

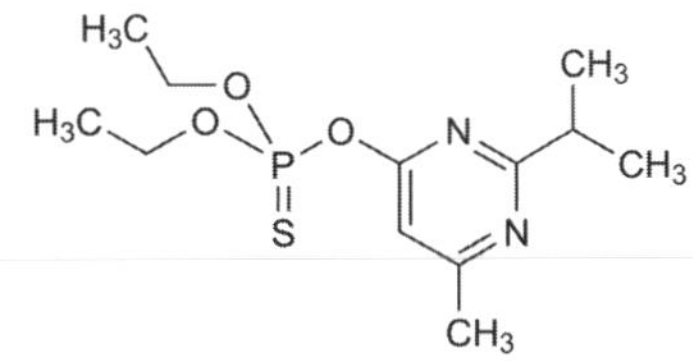

The pure compound is a colourless liquid; the technical grade is a pale to dark brown liquid. It is stable in alkaline solutions but is slowly hydrolysed in water and dilute acids.
Slightly soluble in water; miscible with ethanol, ether, and petroleum oils.

Partition Coefficient. Log *P* (octanol/water), 3.8.

Colour Tests. Palladium Chloride—orange-brown; Phosphorus Test—yellow.

Thin-layer Chromatography. System TE—Rf 39; system TF—Rf 64; system TW—Rf 82; system TX—Rf 47; system TY—Rf 50; system TZ—Rf 76; system TAA—Rf 21; system TAB—Rf 30; system TAC—Rf 20; system TAE—Rf 81.

Gas Chromatography. System GA—RI 1760; system GK—RRT 0.79 (relative to caffeine).

High Performance Liquid Chromatography. System HAA—Retention time 25.8 min; system HX—RI 618; system HY—RI 628; system HZ—Retention time 33.2 min.

Ultraviolet Spectrum. Hexane—248 nm (A^1_1=170b).

Infra-red Spectrum. Principal peaks at wavenumbers 1020, 1587, 971, 1562, 823, 1159 cm^{-1}.

Mass Spectrum. Principal ions at *m/z* 137, 179, 152, 93, 153, 199, 97, 43.

Quantification
Gas chromatography. In postmortem tissues: FID or ECD—A. Poklis *et al.*, *Forensic Sci. Int.*, 1980, *15*, 135–140.

Disposition in the Body. Rapidly absorbed from the lungs and through the skin.

Toxicity. The estimated minimum lethal dose is 25 g.

In 2 fatalities due to dimpylate ingestion, postmortem tissue concentrations were: blood 0.7, 33 mg/L, brain 12, 62 µg/g, kidney 3, - µg/g, liver 30, 345 µg/g, adipose tissue 37, - µg/g. [W. H. Wall, *Bull. Int. Assoc. Forensic Toxicol.*, 1981, *16(2)*, 27–28.]

In a fatality attributed to dimpylate, the following postmortem tissue concentrations were reported: blood 277 mg/L, bile 200 mg/L, brain 2 µg/g, kidney 0.1 µg/g, liver 4 µg/g. [A. Poklis *et al.*, *Forensic Sci. Int.*, 1980, *15*, 135–140.]

Dinitolmide

Coccidiostat (Veterinary)

Synonyms. Dinitrotoluamide; Methyldinitrobenzamide; Zoalene.
Proprietary name. Zoamix
2-Methyl-3,5-dinitrobenzamide
$C_8H_7N_3O_5$=225.2
CAS—148-01-6

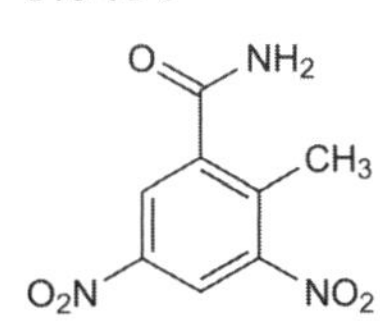

A cream-coloured to light tan-coloured powder. M.p. 177° to 181°.
Practically insoluble in water; soluble 1 in 100 of ethanol, 1 in 15 of acetone, 1 in 650 of chloroform, and 1 in 850 of ether.

Partition Coefficient. Log *P* (octanol/water), 0.2.

Colour Tests. Methanolic Potassium Hydroxide—green; Nessler's Reagent—brown-orange.

Thin-layer Chromatography. System TA—Rf 75. (Acidified iodoplatinate solution, positive, developing slowly.)

Infra-red Spectrum. Principal peaks at wavenumbers 1527, 1672, 1612, 738, 1595, 1289 cm^{-1} (KBr disk).

Dinitro-orthocresol

Insecticide/Herbicide

Synonyms. Dinitrocresol; Dinitrol; Ditrosol; DN; DNC; DNOC; KIII; KIV.
Proprietary names. Effusan; Lipan; Selinon; Sinox.
2-Methyl-4,6-dinitrophenol
$C_7H_6N_2O_5$=198.1
CAS—534-52-1

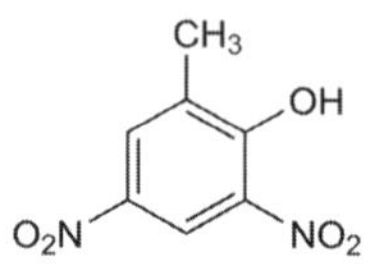

Yellowish crystals. M.p. 86°.
Soluble 1 in 7500 of water; readily soluble in alkaline aqueous solutions, ether, acetone, ethanol, and most organic solvents; sparingly soluble in petroleum ether.
Caution. It is explosive and is usually moistened with up to 10% of water to reduce the hazard.

Dissociation Constant. pK_a 4.3 (21°).

Partition Coefficient. Log *P* (octanol/water), 2.1.

Colour Test. Methanolic Potassium Hydroxide—orange (100°).

Thin-layer Chromatography. System TF—Rf 25; system TX—Rf 6; system TY—Rf 38.

Gas Chromatography. System GA—RI 1660. Dinitro-orthocresol methyl ether: system GK—RRT 0.74 (relative to caffeine).

Ultraviolet Spectrum. Aqueous acid—271 (A_1^1=631b); aqueous alkali—265 nm (A_1^1=251b).

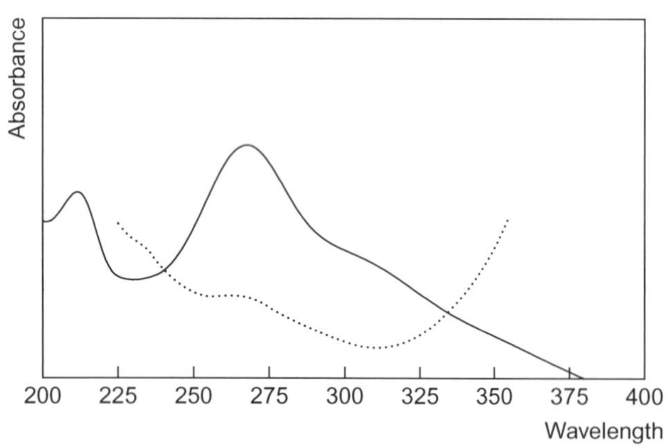

Infra-red Spectrum. Principal peaks at wavenumbers 1605, 1232, 1090, 1218, 1546, 1156 cm^{-1} (Nujol mull).

Mass Spectrum. Principal ions at *m/z* 182, 165, 89, 90, 212, 51, 65, 91 (dinitro-orthocresol methyl ether).

Quantification
Colorimetry. In blood or tissues—M. L. Fenwick and V. H. Parker, *Analyst*, 1955, *80*, 774–776.

Disposition in the Body. Absorbed through the skin, by inhalation, or by accidental ingestion. It acts as a cumulative poison causing an increase in the metabolic rate, and it is eliminated slowly over a period of weeks. After ingestion, less than 5% is excreted unchanged in the urine.

Toxicity. The acute toxic dose is about 200 mg and the maximum permissible atmospheric concentration is 0.2 mg/m^3. Blood concentrations greater than about 50 mg/L are associated with severe toxicity.

Note. For a review of poisoning by dinitro-orthocresol see P. L. Bidstrup *et al.*, *Lancet*, 1952, *1*, 794–795.

Diperodon

Local Anaesthetic

Synonym. Diperocaine
Proprietary name. Diothane
3-Piperidinopropylene bis(phenylcarbamate) monohydrate
$C_{22}H_{27}N_3O_4,H_2O$=415.5
CAS—101-08-6 (anhydrous); 51552-99-9 (monohydrate)

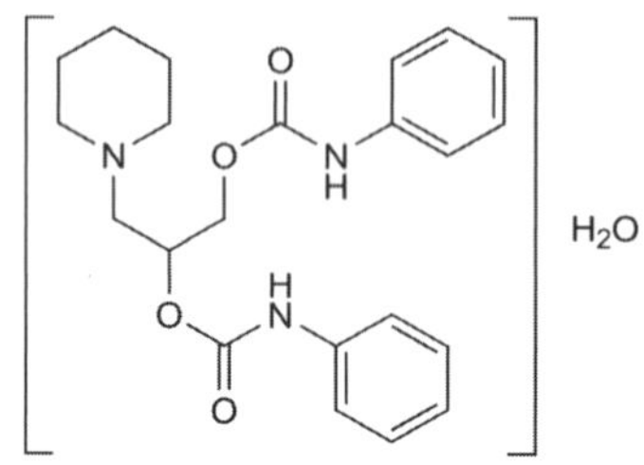

A white to cream-coloured powder.
Practically insoluble in water; soluble 1 in 3 of ethanol, 1 in 10 of chloroform, 1 in 4 of ether, and 1 in 1 of methanol.

Diperodon Hydrochloride
$C_{22}H_{27}N_3O_4,HCl$=433.9
CAS—537-12-2
A white crystalline powder. M.p. about 198°.
Soluble 1 in 100 of water; soluble in ethanol; slightly soluble in acetone; practically insoluble in ether.

Partition Coefficient. Log *P* (octanol/water), 2.6 (hydrochloride).

Colour Tests. Liebermann's Test—brown; Mandelin's Test—red→green.

Thin-layer Chromatography. System TA—Rf 70; system TB—Rf 15; system TC—Rf 58; system TL—Rf 66. (Acidified iodoplatinate solution, positive.)

Gas Chromatography. System GA—RI 2370.

High Performance Liquid Chromatography. System HR—*k* 2.48.

Ultraviolet Spectrum. Aqueous acid—232 nm (A_1^1=1320b).

Infra-red Spectrum. Principal peaks at wavenumbers 1210, 1705, 1530, 1600, 1305, 1050 cm^{-1} (KBr disk).

Mass Spectrum. Principal ions at *m/z* 98, 119, 91, 99, 124, 64, 41, 55.

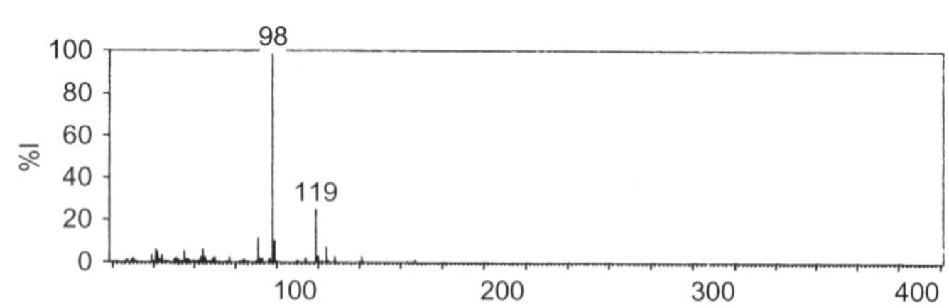

Quantification
High performance liquid chromatography. In blood: limit of detection 5 µg/mL—J. Cizmarik *et al.*, *Acta Pol. Pharm.*, 1996, *53*, 167–169.

Use. Diperodon has been applied topically in a concentration of 1%.

Diphemanil Metilsulfate

Anticholinergic

Synonyms. Diphemanil Methylsulfate; Diphenmethanil Methylsulfate; Vagophemanil Methylsulfate.
Proprietary name. Prantal
4-(Diphenylmethylene)-1,1-dimethylpiperidinium methyl sulfate
$C_{20}H_{24}N,CH_3SO_4$=389.5
CAS—62-97-5

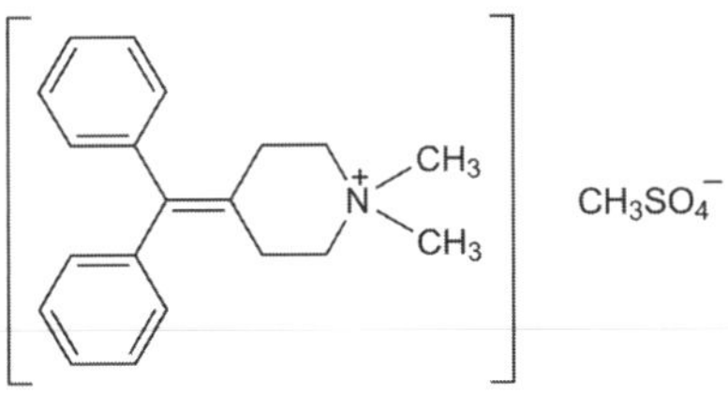

A white, hygroscopic, crystalline powder. M.p. 194° to 195°.
Soluble 1 in 33 of water, 1 in 33 of ethanol, and 1 in 33 of chloroform; very slightly soluble in ether.

Partition Coefficient. Log *P* (octanol/water), 2.6.

Colour Tests. Liebermann's Test—brown; Mandelin's Test—brown; Marquis Test—orange-red; Sulfuric Acid—orange.

Thin-layer Chromatography. System TA—Rf 02. (Acidified iodoplatinate solution, positive.)

Infra-red Spectrum. Principal peaks at wavenumbers 708, 1250, 1230, 1010, 765, 699 cm^{-1} (KBr disk).

Dose. 400 to 800 mg daily.

Diphenadione

Anticoagulant/Rodenticide

Synonym. Diphacinone
Proprietary name. Diphacin (rodenticide)
2-(Diphenylacetyl)-1*H*-indene-1,3(2*H*)-dione
$C_{23}H_{16}O_3$=340.4
CAS—82-66-6

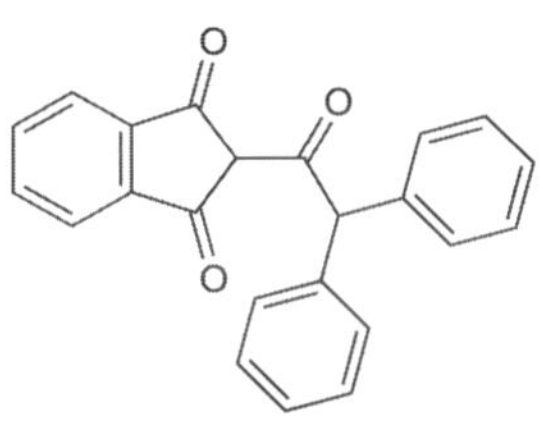

Yellow crystals or crystalline powder. M.p. 144° to 150°.
Practically insoluble in water; soluble 1 in less than 100 of ethanol and chloroform; soluble in ether, acetone, and glacial acetic acid; slightly soluble in benzene.

Partition Coefficient. Log *P* (octanol/water), 4.8.

Colour Tests. Liebermann's Test—orange-brown; Methanolic Potassium Hydroxide—yellow; Sulfuric Acid—yellow.

Thin-layer Chromatography. System TD—Rf 11; system TE—Rf 46; system TF—Rf 33; system TAD—Rf 53; system TAJ—Rf 51; system TAK—Rf 74; system TAL—Rf 91. (Acidified potassium permanganate solution, positive.)

Gas Chromatography. System GA—RI 2934.

Ultraviolet Spectrum. Aqueous acid—336 nm (A^1_1=675b). No alkaline shift.

Mass Spectrum. Principal ions at *m/z* 173, 340, 168, 167, 165, 341, 174, 322.

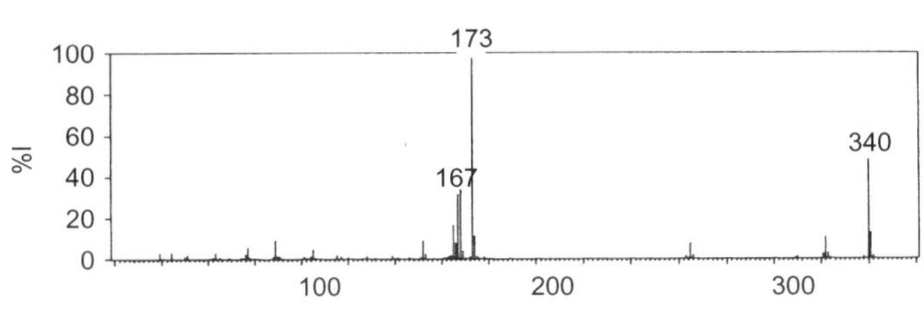

Dose. Maintenance, 2.5 to 5 mg daily.

Diphenhydramine

Antihistamine

Synonym. Benzhydramine
2-Diphenylmethoxy-*N*,*N*-dimethylethanamine
$C_{17}H_{21}NO$=255.4
CAS—58-73-1

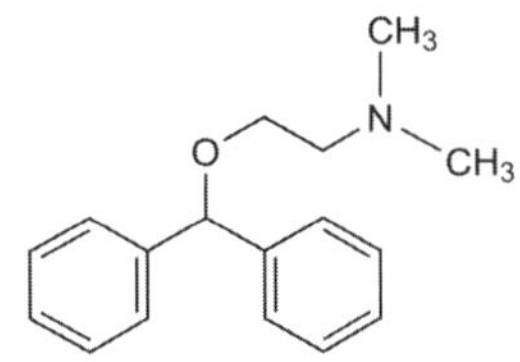

Note. Diphenhydramine is an isomer of phenyltoloxamine.

Diphenhydramine Di(acefyllinate)

Synonyms. Benzhydramine Di(acefyllinate); Bietanautine.
Proprietary name. Nautamine
$C_{17}H_{21}NO,2C_9H_{10}N_4O_4$=731.8
CAS—6888-11-5

Diphenhydramine Hydrochloride

Synonyms. Benzhydramine Hydrochloride; Dimedrolum.
Proprietary names. Aller-Dryl; Aller-eze; Allermax; Banophen Allergy; Benadryl; Bidramine; Dermamycin; Diphen; Diphenhist; Dormin; Dreemon; Dytuss; Genahist; Histergan; Hyrexin; Medinex; Nightcalm; Nytol; Paxidorm; Siladryl; Silphen; Sleep Aid; Sleepeaze; Sleepia; Pheramin; Sominex; Somnium; Tusstat; Twilite. It is an ingredient of many proprietary preparations—see *Martindale, The complete drug reference*, 33rd Edn, London, Pharmaceutical Press, 2002.
$C_{17}H_{21}NO,HCl$=291.8
CAS—147-24-0
A white crystalline powder which slowly darkens on exposure to light. M.p. 166° to 170°.
Soluble 1 in 1 of water, 1 in 2 of ethanol, 1 in 50 of acetone, and 1 in 2 of chloroform; very slightly soluble in benzene and in ether.

Dissociation Constant. pK_a 9.0 (25°).

Partition Coefficient. Log *P* (octanol/water), 3.3.

Colour Tests. Liebermann's Test—brown-orange; Mandelin's Test—yellow; Marquis Test—yellow; Sulfuric Acid—orange.

Thin-layer Chromatography. System TA—Rf 55; system TB—Rf 44; system TC—Rf 33; system TE—Rf 65; system TL—Rf 15; system TAE—Rf 27; system TAF—Rf 48. (Dragendorff spray, positive; FPN reagent, pink; acidified iodoplatinate solution, positive; Marquis reagent, yellow; ninhydrin spray, positive.)

Gas Chromatography. System GA—diphenhydramine RI 1870, M (nor-) RI 1520, M (nor-acetyl-) RI 2265, M (di-nor-acetyl) RI 2240, M (methoxy) RI 2010, M (diphenylmethanol) RI 1645, M (OH-) RI 1890, M (di-OH-) RI 1895, M (desamino-OH-) RI 1760, M (benzophenone) (BPH) RI 1610, M (OH-BPH) isomer 1 RI 2065, M (OH-BPH) isomer 2 RI 2080, M (OH-methoxy-BPH) isomer 1 RI 2050, M (OH-methoxy-BPH) isomer 2 RI 2070, system GB—diphenhydramine RI 1928, M (nor-) RI 1922, M (nor-acetyl-) RI 2360, M (di-nor-acetyl-) RI 2240; M (desamino-) RI 1883, M (methoxy-) RI 2239, M (diphenylmethane) RI 1465, M (diphenylmethanol) RI 1645, M (4-phenylmethylphenol) RI 1780, system GC—RI 2378; system GF—RI 2105.

High Performance Liquid Chromatography. System HA—*k* 3.3; system HX—RI 393; system HY—RI 336; system HAX—retention time 12.2 min; system HAY—retention time 6.0 min.

Ultraviolet Spectrum. Aqueous acid—252, 257 nm (A^1_1= 17 a).

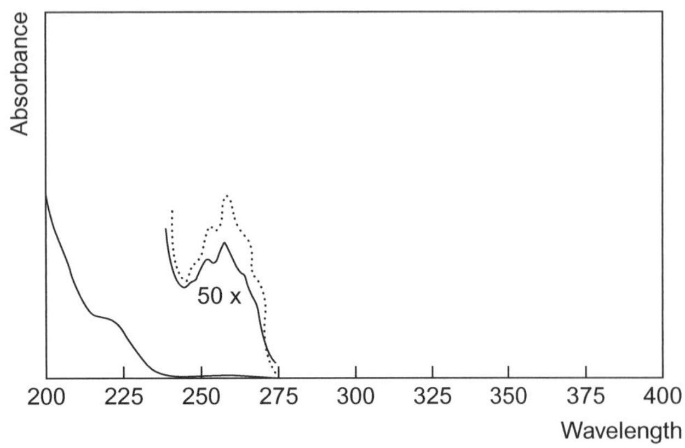

Infra-red Spectrum. Principal peaks at wavenumbers 713, 754, 1103, 1017, 1180, 991 cm^{-1} (diphenhydramine hydrochloride, KBr disk).

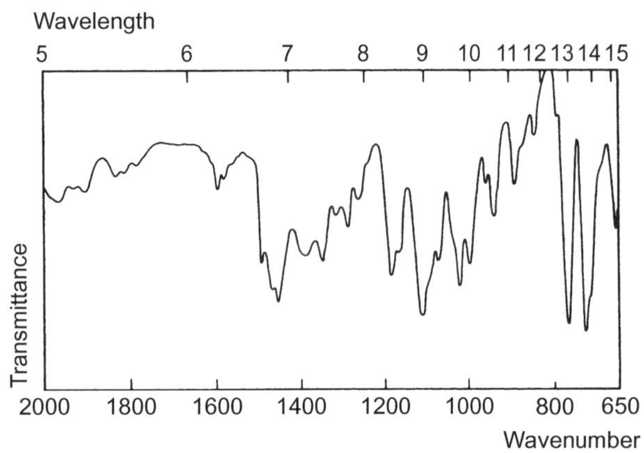

Mass Spectrum. Principal ions at *m/z* 58, 73, 45, 167, 165, 166, 44, 152 (no peaks above 200); didesmethyldiphenhydramine 30, 167, 45, 168, 165, 183, 166, 152; monodesmethyldiphenhydramine 44, 167, 168, 165, 183, 105, 152, 77.

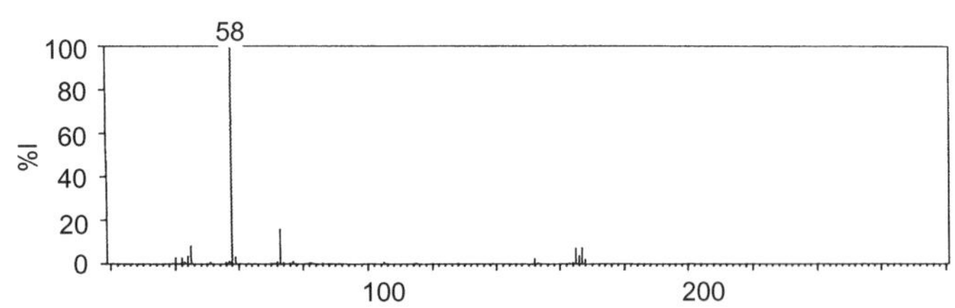

Quantification

Gas chromatography. In blood, urine, or tissues: FID—R. C. Backer *et al., J. Anal. Toxicol.*, 1977, *1*, 227–228.
In serum: limit of detection 2.5 µg/L, AFID—D. Lutz *et al., J. Clin. Chem. Clin. Biochem.*, 1983, *21*, 595–597. In blood or urine: diphenhydramine and other antihistamines, limits of detection 100 to 250 ng/L, SID—H. Hattori *et al., J. Chromatogr.*, 1992, *581*, 213–218. In blood or urine: diphenhydramine and other antihistamines, limits of detection 76 to 473 µg/L in blood and 13 to 186 µg/L in urine, FID—M. Nishikawa *et al., J. Chromatogr. Sci.*, 1997, *35*, 275–279.

High performance liquid chromatography. In urine: *N*-glucuronides of diphenhydramine and amitriptyline—D. Fischer and U. Breyer-Pfaff, *J. Pharm. Pharmacol.*, 1995, *47*, 534–538.

Disposition in the Body. Readily absorbed after oral administration, but undergoes extensive first-pass metabolism by *N*-dealkylation and oxidative deamination to form monodesmethyl and didesmethyl metabolites, and diphenylmethoxyacetic acid which may be conjugated with glutamine or glycine. Up to 65% of a dose is excreted in the urine in 96 h. The major urinary metabolite appears to be diphenylmethoxyacetic acid in free or conjugated form; very little is excreted as unchanged drug. Diphenhydramine crosses the placenta and is excreted in breast milk.

Therapeutic concentration. In plasma, usually in the range 0.1 to 1.0 mg/L.

Following a single oral dose of 100 mg of diphenhydramine hydrochloride to 4 subjects, peak plasma concentrations of 0.08 to 0.16 mg/L (mean 0.11) were obtained 2 to 4 h after administration; total amine concentrations were approximately 50% higher due to the presence of *N*-dealkylated metabolites. After single oral doses of 100 mg to a further 4 subjects, the concentration of acidic metabolites increased over a period of 24 h to about 2 mg/L. After multiple oral doses of 50 mg of diphenhydramine hydrochloride four times daily to 4 subjects, maximum steady-state plasma diphenhydramine concentrations of 0.10 to 0.27 mg/L were reported; the maximum steady-state amine concentrations were between 0.17 and 0.37 mg/L. [A. J. Glazko *et al., Clin. Pharmacol. Ther.*, 1974, *16*, 1066–1076.]

Toxicity. The estimated minimum lethal dose is 3 g. Toxic effects may be produced by plasma concentrations greater than 1 mg/L.

In 4 fatalities due to overdosage of diphenhydramine, the following postmortem concentrations were obtained: blood 8 to 31 mg/L (mean 20), brain 8 and 32 µg/g (2 cases), kidney 13 µg/g (1 case), liver 23 to 47 µg/g (mean 34), urine 40 and 6.4 mg/L (2 cases). [R. C. Backer *et al., J. Anal. Toxicol.*, 1977, *1*, 227–228; R. C. Baselt and R. H. Cravey, *J. Anal. Toxicol.*, 1977, *1*, 81–103; C. Peclet *et al., Bull. Int. Assoc. Forensic Toxicol.*, 1981, *16*(1), 26–27.]

In 2 fatalities attributed to diphenhydramine, the following postmortem tissue concentrations were reported (mg/L or µg/g):

	Diphenhydramine	Diphenylmethoxyacetic acid
Blood	19.7, 6.9	3.0, 15.3
Heart blood	50, 14.7	3.6, 19
Kidney	114, –	–, –
Liver	260, –	–, –
Lung	460, –	–, –
Urine	34.9, 376	0.3, 20.4

In the first case death occurred within 3 h whereas the second subject survived for 12 h after ingestion. [R. Aderjan *et al., Z. Rechtsmed.*, 1982, *88*, 263–270.]

In 4 cases of suicidal diphenhydramine overdose, blood levels ranged from 5 to 35 mg/L. [S. B. Karch, *Am. J. Forensic. Med. Pathol.*, 1998, *19*, 143–147.]

In a 16-year-old male who died due to drowning and cold exposure following a drug overdose, the following concentrations of diphenhydramine, free dihydrocodeine, and total dihydrocodeine were found, respectively, approximately 9 days after death: femoral venous blood 1.89, 3.27, and 3.30 mg/ L, right cardiac chamber blood 0.294, 0.237, and 0.240 mg/L, urine 22.6, 37.3, and 43.1 mg/L, stomach 0.029, 0.018, and 0.024 mg, femoral muscle 0.270, 0.246, and 0.314 µg/g. [F. Moriya and Y. Hashimoto., *Forensic Sci. Int.*, 2001, *123*, 248–253.]

A 35-year-old female who underwent emergency charcoal haemoperfusion and haemodialysis 4.5 h after ingesting 16 g (approx. 20 mg/kg) diphenhydramine, had blood concentrations of 3.3 mg/L immediately before haemoperfusion and 2.56 mg/L immediately after. [M. E. Mullins *et al., Ann. Emerg. Med.*, 1999, *33*, 104–107.]

Bioavailability. About 50 to 70%.

Half-life. Plasma half-life, 2.4 to 9.3 h.

Volume of distribution. 4.5 to 8 L/kg.

Clearance. Plasma clearance, about 6 to 10 mL/min/kg.

Distribution in blood. Plasma:whole blood ratio, about 1.3.

Saliva. Plasma:saliva ratio, about 3.

Protein binding. In plasma, about 80%.

Dose. 75 to 200 mg of diphenhydramine hydrochloride daily in divided doses.

Diphenoxylate

Narcotic Antidiarrhoeal

1-(3-Cyano-3,3-diphenylpropyl)-4-phenyl-4-piperidinecarboxylic acid ethyl ester
$C_{30}H_{32}N_2O_2$=452.6
CAS—915-30-0

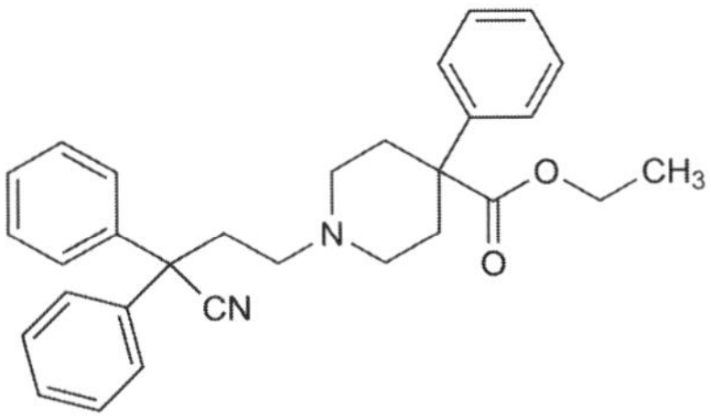

Diphenoxylate Hydrochloride

Proprietary names. Dhamotil; Diarphen; Diarsed; Diastop; Dilomil; Eldox; Erlotyl; Intard; Lofenoxal; Logen, Lomotil; Lonox; Lotharin; Reasec; Remodil; Retardin; Tropergen.
Note. Preparations of diphenoxylate hydrochloride usually contain subclinical amounts of atropine sulfatein an attempt to prevent abuse by deliberate overdosage.
$C_{30}H_{32}N_2O_2$,HCl=489.1
CAS—3810-80-8
A white crystalline powder. M.p. 220.5° to 222°.
Sparingly soluble in water; soluble 1 in 50 of ethanol and 1 in 2.5 of chloroform; soluble in methanol; practically insoluble in ether.

Dissociation Constant. pK_a 7.1.

Partition Coefficient. Log *P* (octanol/water), 6.3.

Colour Test. Sodium Picrate—orange.

Thin-layer Chromatography. System TA—Rf 74; system TB—Rf 42; system TC—Rf 84; system TE—Rf 87; system TL—Rf 70; system TAE—Rf 90; system TAF—Rf 92. (Dragendorff spray, positive; acidified iodoplatinate solution, positive; Marquis reagent, orange.)

Gas Chromatography. System GA—RI 3514; system GB—RI 3670; system GM—not eluted.

High Performance Liquid Chromatography. System HA—diphenoxylate *k* 0.2, diphenoxylic acid *k* 0.6 (tailing peak); system HY—RI 385; system HZ—retention time 27.4 min; system HAY—retention time 14.1 min.

Ultraviolet Spectrum. Methanol—252, 258 (A^1_1=14a), 264 nm.

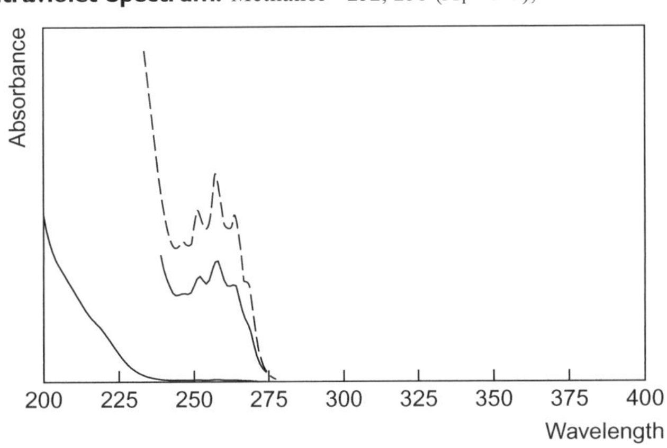

Infra-red Spectrum. Principal peaks at wavenumbers 1728, 697, 1183, 1120, 1215, 1495 cm^{-1} (KBr disk).

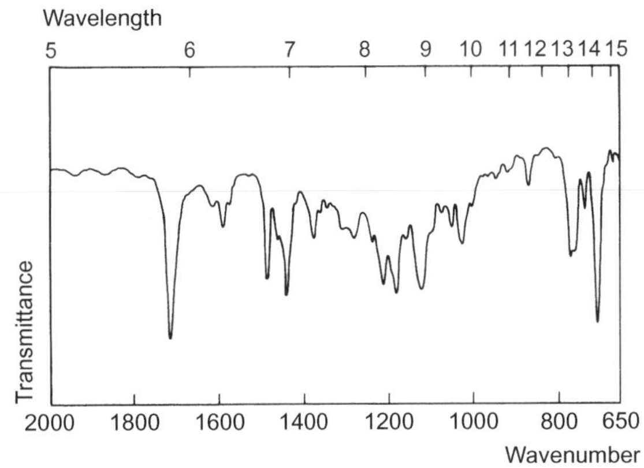

Mass Spectrum. Principal ions at *m/z* 246, 42, 247, 91, 103, 165, 115, 56; diphenoxylic acid 218, 42, 219, 91, 165, 155, 193, 115.

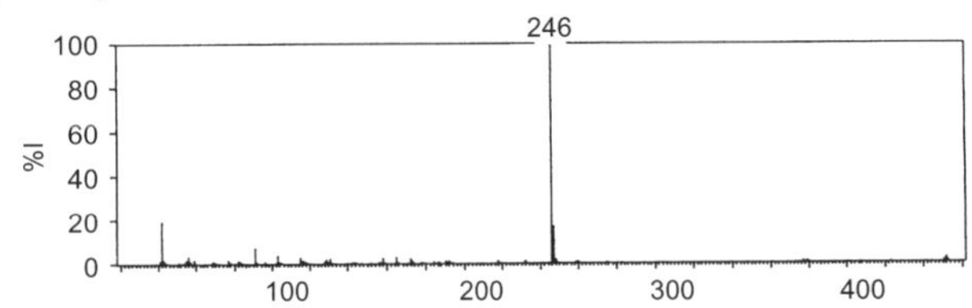

Quantification

Gas chromatography. In plasma or urine: TCD—S. Abu al Ragheb *et al.*, *Med. Sci. Law*, 1982, *22*, 210–214.

Gas chromatography–mass spectrometry. In plasma: diphenoxylic acid, limit of detection 20 mg/L—G. C. Ford *et al.*, *Biomed. Mass Spectrom.*, 1976, *3*, 45–47.

Disposition in the Body. Rapidly absorbed after oral administration but it is usually administered together with a small quantity of atropine and this may delay absorption, especially with high doses. It is extensively metabolised by hydrolysis, hydroxylation, and conjugation with glucuronic acid. The major metabolites are diphenoxylic acid (difenoxin), which is active, and hydroxydiphenoxylic acid in both free and conjugated forms. About 14% and 50% of a dose, respectively, is excreted in the urine and faeces in 96 h; less than 0.1% of a dose is excreted in the urine as unchanged drug in 24 h.

Therapeutic concentration

After an oral dose of 5 mg, peak plasma concentrations of diphenoxylate of about 0.01 mg/L were attained in 2 h and peak concentrations of diphenoxylic acid of about 0.04 mg/L were attained in the same period. [A. Karim *et al.*, *Clin. Pharmacol. Ther.*, 1972, *13*, 407–419.]

Toxicity. Diphenoxylate has addiction-producing properties. The estimated minimum lethal dose is 0.2 g although recovery has occurred after the ingestion of 0.75 g.

A postmortem blood concentration of 0.34 µg/mL was reported in a 3½-year-old child who died after ingesting diphenoxylate. [S. Abu al Ragheb *et al.*, *Med. Sci. Law*, 1982, *22*, 210–214.]

Half-life. Plasma half-life, diphenoxylate about 2.5 h, diphenoxylic acid about 4 h.

Volume of distribution. About 4 L/kg.

Dose. Initially 10 mg of diphenoxylate hydrochloride, followed by 5 mg every 6 h.

Diphenyl

Fungistatic

Synonym. Phenylbenzene
1,1′-Biphenyl
$C_{12}H_{10}$=154.2
CAS—92-52-4

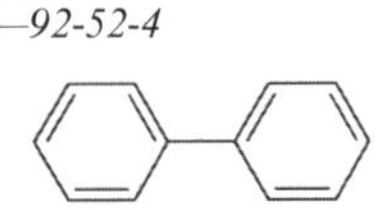

A white crystalline powder. M.p. 69° to 71°. B.p. 254° to 255°.

Practically insoluble in water; soluble in ethanol and ether.

Partition Coefficient. Log *P* (octanol/water), 4.0.

Gas Chromatography. System GA—RI 1389.

Infra-red Spectrum. Principal peaks at wavenumbers 740, 710, 1573, 1175, 1018, 918 cm^{-1} (KBr disk).

Diphenylpyraline

Antihistamine

Synonym. Diphenylpyrilene
4-(Diphenylmethoxy)-1-methylpiperidine
$C_{19}H_{23}NO$=281.4
CAS—147-20-6

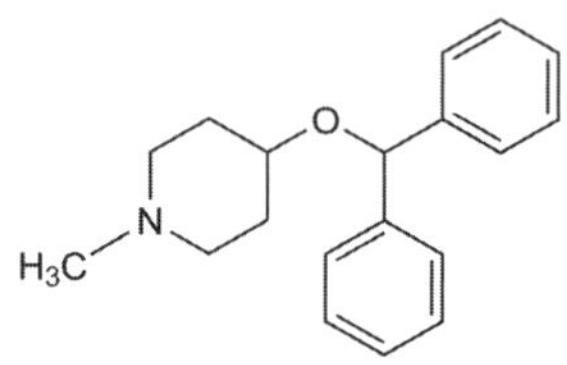

Diphenylpyraline Hydrochloride
Proprietary names. Arbid-N; Dayfen; Diafen; Hispril; Histryl; Histyn; Kolton (gel); Lergoban; Lergobine. It is an ingredient of Eskornade.
$C_{19}H_{23}NO,HCl$=317.9
CAS—132-18-3
A white crystalline powder. M.p. 204° to 209°.
Soluble 1 in 1 of water, 1 in 3 of ethanol, and 1 in 2 of chloroform; soluble in isopropanol; practically insoluble in ether and benzene.

Diphenylpyraline Hydrobromide
$C_{19}H_{23}NO,HBr$=362.3
CAS—132-18-3
Crystals M.p. 201° to 202°.
Soluble in water and ethanol

Partition Coefficient. Log *P* (octanol/water), 3.9.

Colour Tests. Liebermann's Test—red-orange; Mandelin's Test—yellow; Marquis Test—yellow.

Thin-layer Chromatography. System TA—Rf 46; system TB—Rf 42; system TC—Rf 28; system TE—Rf 68; system TL—Rf 8; system TAE—Rf 23; system TAF—Rf 49; system TAJ—Rf 61; system TAK—Rf 50; system TAL—Rf 92. (Dragendorff spray, positive; FPN reagent, pink; acidified iodoplatinate solution, positive; Marquis reagent, brown; ninhydrin spray, positive.)

Gas Chromatography. System GA—Diphenylpyraline RI 2100, M (benzophenone) (BPH) RI 1610, M (OH-BPH) isomer-1 RI 2065, M (OH-BPH) isomer 2 RI 2080, M (OH-methoxy-BPH) isomer-1 RI 2050, M (OH-methoxy-BPH) isomer-2 RI 2070; system GB—RI 2128; system GC—RI 2447; system GF—RI 2405.

High Performance Liquid Chromatography. System HA—*k* 3.3 (tailing peak); system HX—RI 401.

Ultraviolet Spectrum. Aqueous acid—253, 258 nm (A_1^1=17a).

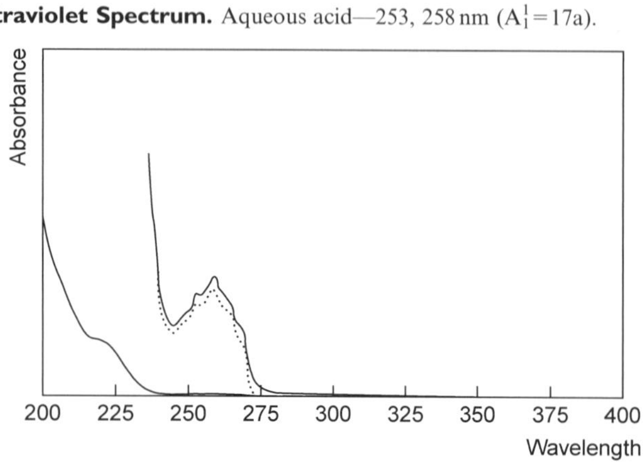

Infra-red Spectrum. Principal peaks at wavenumbers 1070, 709, 1050, 696, 765, 1101 cm^{-1} (diphenylpyraline hydrochloride, KCl disk).

Mass Spectrum. Principal ions at *m/z* 99, 114, 98, 167, 70, 165, 57, 43.

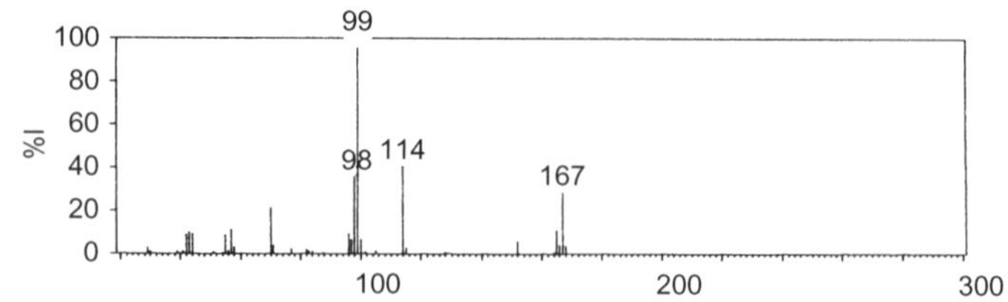

Quantification
Gas chromatography. In urine: FID—G. Graham and A. G. Bolt, *J. Pharmacokinet. Biopharm.*, 1974, *2*, 191–195. In blood or urine: diphenylpyraline and other antihistamines, limits of detection 76–473 mg/L in blood and 13–186 mg/L in urine, FID—M. Nishikawa *et al.*, *J. Chromatogr. Sci.*, 1997, *35*, 275–279.

High performance liquid chromatography. In plasma or urine: limit of detection 15 mg/L, UV detection—K. O. Ebete and J. E. Koundourellis, *J. Chromatogr. B Biomed. Appl.*, 1996, *677*, 319–323.

Disposition in the Body. Absorbed after oral administration. Less than 10% of a dose is excreted in the urine as unchanged drug. Possible metabolites include the *N*-oxide and *N*-desmethyldiphenylpyraline.

Half-life. Derived from urinary excretion data, 24 to 40 h.

Dose. 10 to 20 mg of diphenylpyraline hydrochloride daily.

Dipipanone

Narcotic Analgesic

Synonyms. Phenylpiperone; Piperidyl Methadone; Piperidylamidone.
4,4-Diphenyl-6-(1-piperidinyl)-3-heptanone
$C_{24}H_{31}NO$=349.5
CAS—467-83-4

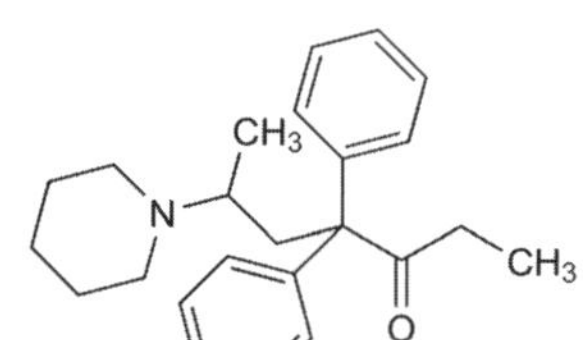

Dipipanone Hydrochloride
Proprietary names. It is an ingredient of Diconal and Wellconal.
$C_{24}H_{31}NO,HCl,H_2O$=404.0
CAS—856-87-1
A white crystalline powder. M.p. 123° to 126° (also reported as 126° to 127°).
Soluble 1 in 40 of water, 1 in 1.5 of ethanol, and 1 in 6 of acetone; practically insoluble in ether.

Dissociation Constant. pK_a 8.5 (25°).

Partition Coefficient. Log *P* (octanol/water), 5.5.

Colour Test. Mandelin's Test—green→blue.

Thin-layer Chromatography. System TA—Rf 66; system TB—Rf 67; system TC—Rf 33; system TE—Rf 87; system TL—Rf 70; system TAE—Rf 27; system TAF—Rf 72. (Dragendorff spray, positive; acidified iodoplatinate solution, positive.)

Gas Chromatography. System GA—RI 2474; system GB—RI 2586; system GC—RI 2894; system GF—RI 2710; system GM—RRT 1.309 (relative to iprindole).

High Performance Liquid Chromatography. System HA—*k* 2.2; system HC—*k* 1.61; system HX—RI 500; system HY—RI 363.

Ultraviolet Spectrum. Aqueous acid—259, 265, 293 nm (A_1^1=15.6a).

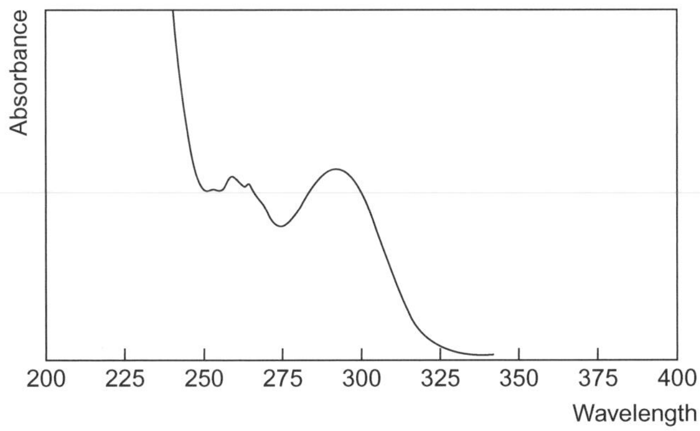

Infra-red Spectrum. Principal peaks at wavenumbers 1708, 698, 1491, 1110, 1092, 1030 cm^{-1} (KBr disk).

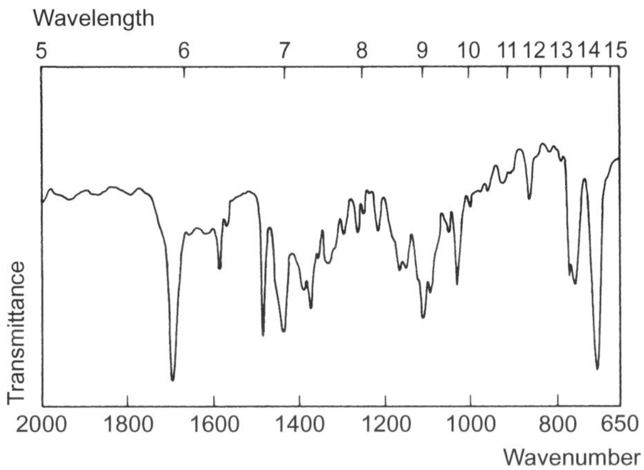

Mass Spectrum. Principal ions at *m/z* 112, 264, 113, 91, 179, 110, 178, 115.

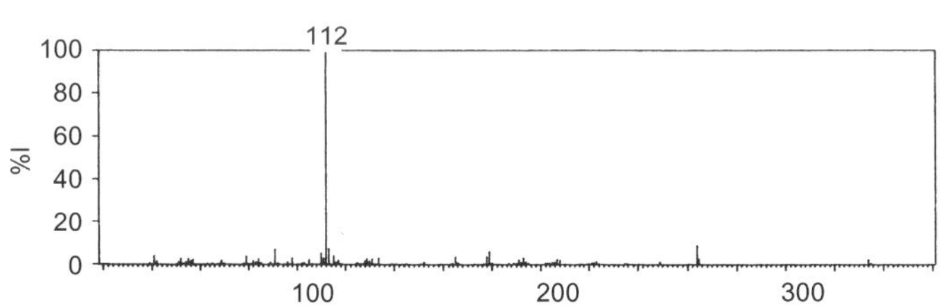

Disposition in the Body. Absorbed after oral administration with rapid onset of action. It is metabolised in the liver and excreted in the urine and faeces. Prolonged use of dipipanone may produce dependence of the morphine type.

Toxicity. The estimated minimum lethal dose is 0.1 g.

In two fatalities following IV injection of Diconal (dipipanone with cyclizine), the following postmortem tissue concentrations (mg/L or µg/g) were reported:

	Cyclizine	Dipipanone
Blood	2.0, 0.5	6.2, 0.5
Bile	20, –	–, –
Liver	3.0, –	5.2, –
Urine	0.5, 9.5	–, 18.5

In 34 addicts, urinary concentrations of free dipipanone ranged from 0 to 5.2 mg/L (mean 1.6). [T. M. T. Sheehan *et al.*, *The Abuse of Preparations Containing Dipipanone and Cyclizine, in Forensic Toxicology (Proceedings of the European Meeting of the International Association of Forensic Toxicologists)*, J. S. Oliver (Ed.), London, Croom Helm, 1979.]

Dose. 10 to 30 mg of dipipanone hydrochloride every 6 h.

Diprenorphine

Narcotic Antagonist (Veterinary)

(5α,7α-17-(Cyclopropylmethyl)-4,5-epoxy-18,19-dihydro-3-hydroxy-6-methoxy-α,α-dimethyl-6,14-ethenomorphinan-7-methanol
$C_{26}H_{35}NO_4$=425.6
CAS—14357-78-9

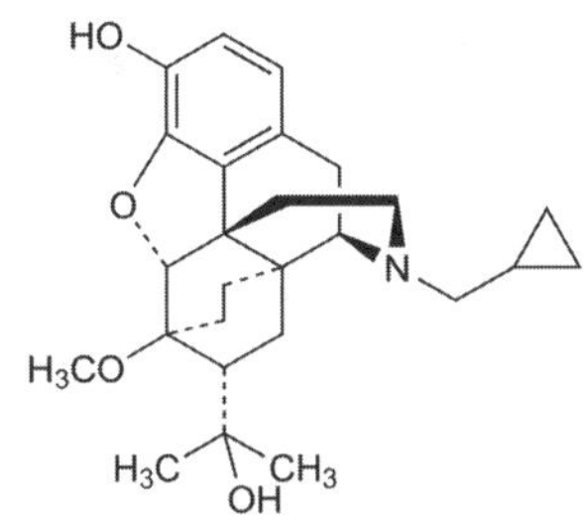

A white microcrystalline powder. M.p. 190° to 192°.

Diprenorphine Hydrochloride
Proprietary name. Revivon
$C_{26}H_{35}NO_4$,HCl=462.0
CAS—16808-86-9
A white crystalline powder.
Soluble 1 in 30 of water, 1 in 160 of ethanol, and 1 in 2500 of chloroform; practically insoluble in ether.

Colour Tests. Liebermann's Test—black; Mandelin's Test—grey; Marquis Test—grey-violet.

Thin-layer Chromatography. System TA—Rf 70. (Acidified iodoplatinate solution, positive.)

Gas Chromatography. System GB—RI 3385; system GM—not eluted.

High Performance Liquid Chromatography. System HA—*k* 0.6; system HY—RI 301.

Ultraviolet Spectrum. Aqueous acid—230 (A_1^1=158b), 286 (A_1^1=36a); aqueous alkali—246 (A_1^1=184b), 299 nm (A_1^1=58a).

Infra-red Spectrum. Principal peaks at wavenumbers 1160, 947, 1311, 1092, 1078, 934 cm^{-1} (KBr disk).

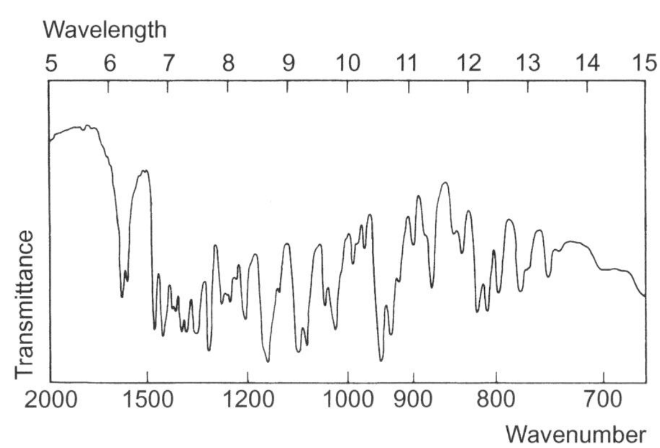

Diprophylline

Xanthine Bronchodilator

Synonyms. Dihydroxypropyltheophyllinum; Diprophyllinum; Dyphylline; Glyphyllinum; Hyphylline.
Proprietary names. Asthmolysin; Austrophyllin; Dilor; Droxine; Dyflex; Dylix; Isophyllen; Katasma; Lufyllin; Neothyllin(e); Neufil.
7-(2,3-Dihydroxypropyl)-3,7-dihydro-1,3-dimethyl-1*H*-purine-2,6-dione

$C_{10}H_{14}N_4O_4$=254.2
CAS—479-18-5

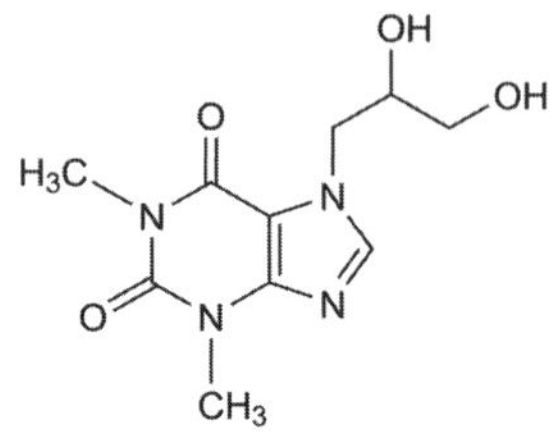

A white crystalline powder. M.p. 158°.
Soluble 1 in 3 of water and 1 in 50 of ethanol; slightly soluble in chloroform; practically insoluble in ether.

Partition Coefficient. Log *P* (octanol/water), −1.5.

Colour Test. Amalic Acid Test—yellow/violet.

Thin-layer Chromatography. System TA—Rf 48; system TB—Rf 00; system TC—Rf 12; system TE—Rf 25; system TL—Rf 12; system TAE—Rf 70; system TAF—Rf 59. (Acidified potassium permanganate solution, positive.)

Gas Chromatography. System GA—diprophylline RI 2280, diprophylline-AC_2 RI 2455.

High Performance Liquid Chromatography. System HX—RI 275; system HY—RI 227; system HAA—retention time 3.6 min.

Ultraviolet Spectrum. Aqueous acid—206, 273 nm (A_1^1=380a). No alkaline shift. (See below)

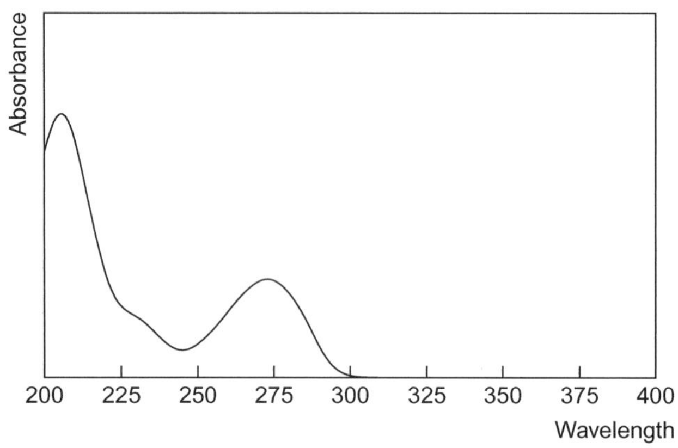

Infra-red Spectrum. Principal peaks at wavenumbers 1660, 1700, 1039, 747, 1562, 1234 cm^{-1} (KBr disk). (See below)

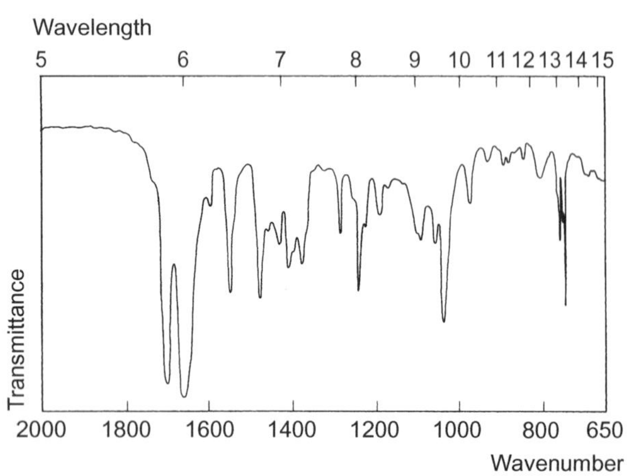

Mass Spectrum. Principal ions at *m/z* 180, 223, 194, 254, 109, 95, 193, 166.

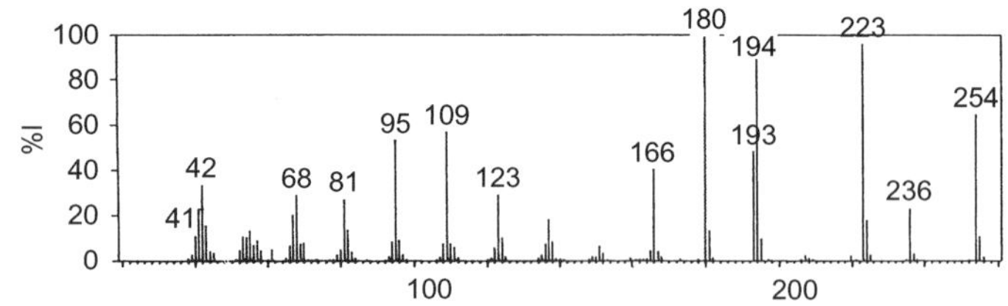

Quantification

Gas Chromatography. In serum or saliva: FID—Z. K. Shihabi and R. P. Dave, *Clin. Chem.*, 1977, *23*, 942–943.

High Performance Liquid Chromatography. In plasma, saliva, or urine: limit of detection 25 μg/L for plasma and 50 μg/L for saliva—L. Gisclon *et al.*, *Res. Commun. Chem. Path. Pharmacol.*, 1979, *23*, 523–531. In serum: limit of detection 1 mg/L, UV detection—N. Paterson, *J. Chromatogr.*, 1982, *232(21) B Biomed. Appl.*, 450–455. In serum: diprophylline and theophylline, limit of detection 0.25 mg/L, UV detection—M. B. Kester *et al.*, *J. Chromatogr.*, 1987, *416*, 91–97. In serum: diprophylline and doxophylline, UV detection—F. Tagliaro *et al.*, *Clin. Chem.*, 1990, *36*, 113–115.

Disposition in the Body. Rapidly and almost completely absorbed after oral administration. About 83% of a dose is excreted in the urine as unchanged drug in 24 h; less than 1% of a dose is eliminated in the faeces. It is also rapidly absorbed from IM injection sites. Diprophylline is excreted in breast milk.

Therapeutic concentration. In plasma, usually in the range 10 to 20 mg/L.

After a single oral dose of 1.2 g to 6 subjects, peak plasma concentrations of 18 to 29 mg/L (mean 22) were attained in about 0.5 h and peak saliva concentrations of 7 to 17 mg/L (mean 12) were reported at 0.7 h. [L. G. Gisclon *et al.*, *Am. J. Hosp. Pharm.*, 1979, *36*, 1179–1184.]

Toxicity. Plasma concentrations greater than 20 μg/mL may produce toxic effects.

Bioavailability. About 90%.

Half-life. Plasma half-life, about 2 h.

Volume of distribution. About 0.8 L/kg.

Clearance. Plasma clearance, about 5 mL/min/kg.

Dose. 15 mg/kg body weight every 6 h.

Dipyridamole

Antithrombotic/Anti-anginal Vasodilator

Proprietary names. Agremol; Atrombin; Cardoxin; Cerebrovase; Cleridium; Coronarine; Corosan; Curantyl N; Dipyridan; Dipyrin; Fluxocor; Miosen; Modaplate; Natyl; Novo-Dipiradol; Perkod; Persantin(e); Plato; Posanin; Procardin; Procor; Protangix; Pytazen.
2,2′,2″,2‴-[(4,8-Di-1-piperidinylpyrimido[5,4-*d*]pyrimidine-2,6-diyl)-dinitrilo]tetrakisethanol
$C_{24}H_{40}N_8O_4$=504.6
CAS—58-32-2

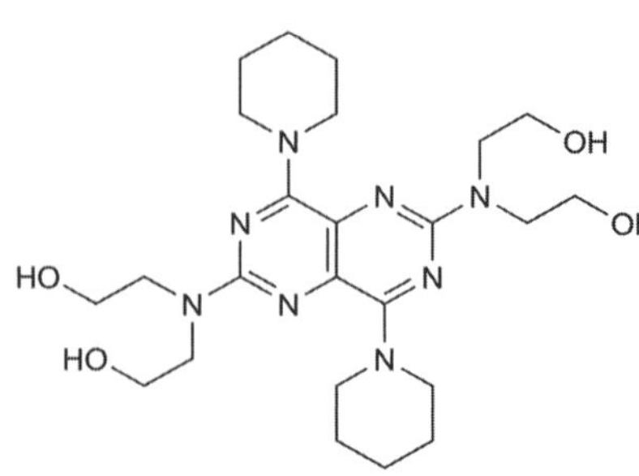

An intensely yellow crystalline powder. Solutions have a yellowish-blue fluorescence. M.p. 164° to 167°.
Slightly soluble in water; very soluble in methanol, ethanol, and chloroform; soluble in dilute acids; practically insoluble in ether.

Dissociation Constant. pK_a 6.4.

Partition Coefficient. Log *P* (octanol/water), 2.7.

Colour Tests. Mandelin's Test—violet; Marquis Test—orange.

Thin-layer Chromatography. System TA—Rf 68; system TB—Rf 00; system TC—Rf 37; system TE—Rf 44; system TL—Rf 42; system TAE—Rf 82; system TAF—Rf 87. (Acidified iodoplatinate solution, positive.)

Gas Chromatography. System GA—RI 1640.

High Performance Liquid Chromatography System HA—*k* 0.2; system HX—RI 393; system HY—RI 335; system HZ—retention time 3.0 min; system HAA—retention time 13.2 min; system HAX—retention time 8.6 min; system HAY—retention time 4.8 min.

Ultraviolet Spectrum. Acid methanol—230, 285 (A^1_1=650a); aqueous alkali—295 nm.

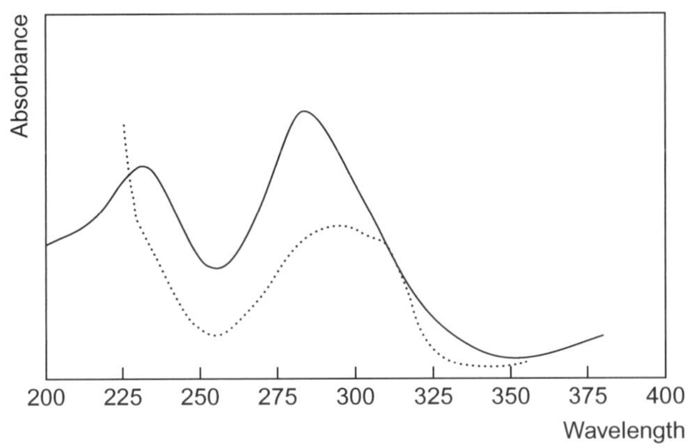

Infra-red Spectrum. Principal peaks at wavenumbers 1526, 1214, 1010, 1076, 1041, 1251 cm^{-1} (KBr disk).

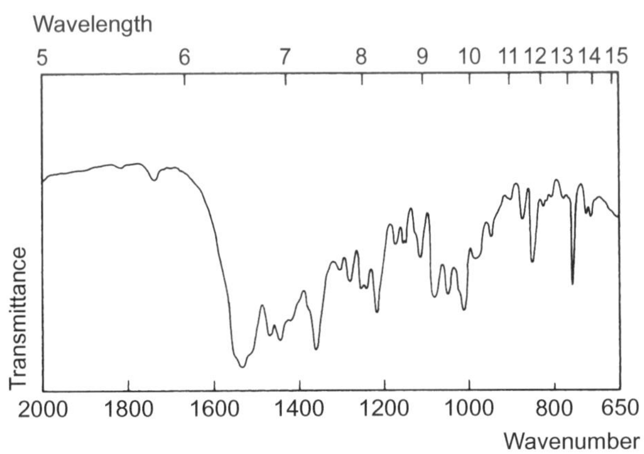

Mass Spectrum. Principal ions at *m/z* 504, 473, 429, 505, 221, 474, 84, 430.

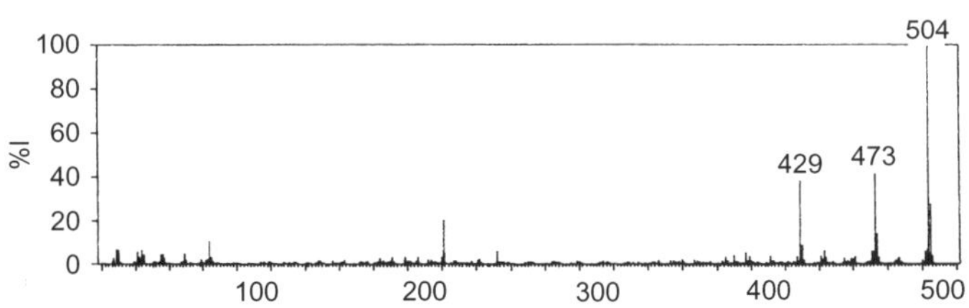

Quantification

Spectrofluorimetry. In serum—J. M. Steyn, *J. Chromatogr.* 1979, *164(6) B Biomed. Appl.*, 487–494.

High performance liquid chromatography In plasma or whole blood: fluorescence detection—K. M. Wolfram and T. D. Bjornsson, *J. Chromatogr.* 1980, *183(9) B Biomed. Appl.*, 57–64. In plasma: limit of detection 2 µg/mL, UV detection—J. Rosenfeld *et al.*, *J. Chromatogr.* 1982, *231(20) B Biomed. Appl.*, 216–221. In plasma: UV detection—M. Barberi *et al.*, *J. Chromatogr.*, 1991, *565*, 511–555.

Disposition in the Body. Readily absorbed after oral administration. Eliminated mainly in the faeces; excretion may be delayed due to entero-hepatic circulation. Small amounts are excreted in the urine as the glucuronide conjugate.

Therapeutic concentration

After a single oral dose of 100 mg given to 6 subjects, peak serum concentrations of about 2 mg/L were attained in 1 h. [F. Nielsen-Kudsk and A. K. Pederson, *Acta Pharmacol. Toxicol.*, 1979, *44*, 391–399.]

Following oral administration of 50 mg three times a day to 10 subjects, maximum steady-state plasma concentrations of 0.4 to 2.6 mg/L (mean 1.4) were reported; trough concentrations were 0.1 to 1.5 mg/L (mean 0.7). In 10 subjects given 75 mg twice daily, the corresponding maximum and minimum steady-state concentrations were 0.5 to 4 mg/L (mean 1.7) and 0.1 to 2.6 mg/L (mean 0.9). [C. Mahony *et al.*, *J. Clin. Pharmacol.*, 1983, *23*, 123–126.]

Toxicity

A 23-year-old female who suffered profound shock after deliberately ingesting 1750 mg of dipyridamole was successfully treated with amino-phylline and dopamine. [Z. C. Chen *et al.*, *Int. J. Cardiol.*, 1994, *46*, 75–78.]

Half-life. Plasma half-life, about 12 h.

Volume of distribution. About 2.5 L/kg.

Clearance. Plasma clearance, about 2 mL/min/kg.

Protein binding. In plasma, more than 90%.

Dose. 300 to 600 mg daily (antithrombotic); 150 mg daily (anti-anginal).

Dipyrone

Analgesic

Synonyms. NSC-73205; Aminopyrine-sulfonate Sodium; Analginum; Metamizole; Metamizole Sodium; Metamizolum Natricum; Methampyrone; Methylmelubrin; Natrium Novaminsulfonicum; Noramidazophenum; Noraminophenazonum; Novamidazofen; Sodium Noramidopyrine Methanesulphonate; Sulpyrine.

Proprietary names. Algi; Analgin; Baralgin; Berlosin; Conmel; Dolemicin; Dolocalma; Inalgon Neu; Lasain; Metilon; Minalgin; Neo Melubrina; Nevralgina; Nolotil; Novalgin(e); Novaminsulfon; Optalgin; Pyril; Trisalgina; Unagen. It is an ingredient of many proprietary preparations—see *Martindale, The complete drug reference*, 33rd Edn., London, Pharmaceutical Press, 2002.

Sodium-[(2,3-dihydro-1,–5-dimethyl-3-oxo-2-phenyl-1*H*-pyrazol-4-yl) methylamino]methanesulphonate monohydrate

$C_{13}H_{16}N_3NaO_4S,H_2O$=351.4

CAS—68-89-3 (anhydrous); 5907-38-0 (monohydrate)

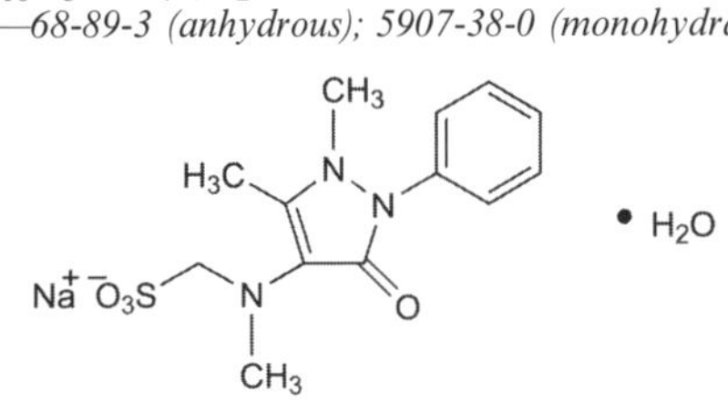

A white or yellowish-white crystalline powder. M.p. 172°.

Soluble 1 in 1.5 of water and 1 in 30 of ethanol; practically insoluble in ether, acetone, benzene, and chloroform.

Colour Tests. Ferric Chloride—violet; Folin–Ciocalteau Reagent—blue; Liebermann's Test (100°)—blue; Mandelin's Test—brown; Nitrous Acid—transient blue.

Thin-layer Chromatography. System TA—Rf 84; system TB—Rf 00; system TC—Rf 01; system TD—Rf 00; system TE—Rf 02; system TF—Rf 00; system TL—Rf 02; system TAD—Rf 02; system TAE—Rf 85; system TAF—Rf 59; system TAJ—Rf 00; system TAK—Rf 00; system TAL—Rf 24. (Acidified iodoplatinate solution, white.)

Gas Chromatography. System GA—M (bis-desalkyl-) RI 1955, M (desalkyl-)-AC RI 2395; system GB—dipyrone RI 2069.

High Performance Liquid Chromatography. System HD—*k* 0.1; system HW—*k* 0.45; system HX—RI 316; system HY—RI 194; system HZ—retention time 1.4 min.

Ultraviolet Spectrum. Aqueous acid—258 nm (A_1^1=266a).

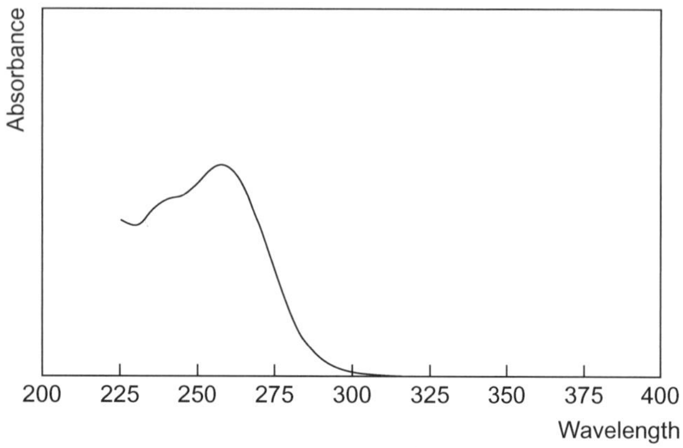

Infra-red Spectrum. Principal peaks at wavenumbers 1672, 1064, 1179, 1163, 1208, 1639 cm^{-1} (KBr disk).

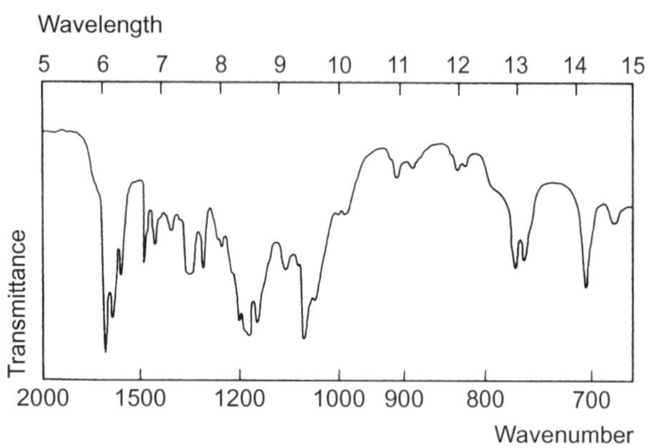

Mass Spectrum. Principal ions at *m/z* 56, 42, 83, 57, 77, 51, 97, 54.

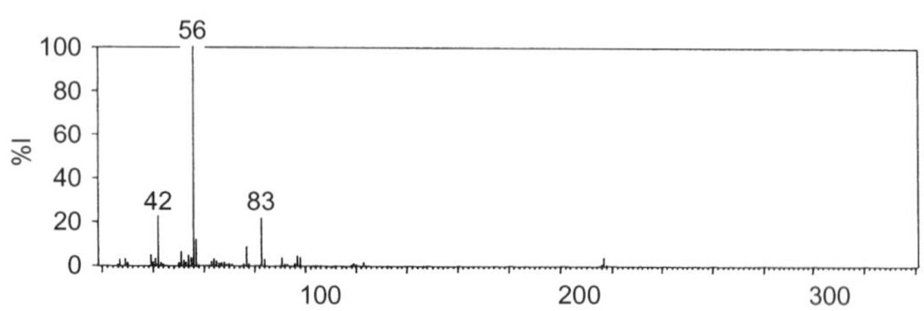

Quantification

High performance liquid chromatography. In plasma or urine: limits of detection 1 mg/L for dipyrone and 250 µg/L for 4-methylaminophenazone, UV detection—G. Asmardi and F. Jamali, *J. Chromatogr.*, 1983, *277* (28) *B Biomed. Appl.*, 183–189. In plasma or urine: dipyrone metabolites, limits of detection 0.1 mg/L in plasma and 2 mg/L in urine, UV detection—D. Damm, *Arzneimittelforschung*, 1989, *39*, 1415–1417. In urine: dipyrone and its metabolites and aminopyrine, UV detection—J. A. Agundez *et al.*, *Ther. Drug Monit.*, 1994, *16*, 316–322.

Disposition in the Body. Rapidly hydrolysed in gastric juice after oral administration to the active metabolite 4-methylamino-phenazone, which is metabolised after absorption to 4-formylamino-phenazone, 4-amino-phenazone, and 4-acetylamino-phenazone. About 70% of a dose is excreted in the urine in 24 h as metabolites. Dipyrone metabolites are excreted in breast milk.

Therapeutic concentration

Following a single oral dose of 1 g given to 12 slow acetylators and 11 rapid acetylators (determined with reference to dapsone), the following mean peak plasma concentrations (mg/L, time in h) were reported:

	Slow acetylators	Rapid acetylators
4-Acetylaminophenazone	1.6 (16.1)	4.4 (10.0)
4-Aminophenazone	2.7 (6.7)	1.6 (3.2)
4-Formylaminophenazone	1.8 (7.7)	2.5 (6.6)
4-Methylaminophenazone	10.0 (1.6)	11.0 (1.2)

[M. Levy *et al.*, *Eur. J. Clin. Pharmacol.*, 1984, *27*, 453–458.]

In 12 subjects given single oral doses of a test and reference preparation of dipyrone 1 g, the mean peak plasma concentrations of 4-methylamino-phenazone, 4-formylamino-phenazone, 4-amino-phenazone, and 4-acetylamino-phenazone were 17.19 and 16.92 mg/L (test and reference), 1.6 and 1.84 mg/L, 2.94 and 2.89 mg/L, and 1.93 and 1.86 mg/L at 1.42 and 1.46 h, 6.2 and 7.0 h, 4.4 and 4.4 h, and 11.3 and 11.6 h, respectively. 4 of the subjects were rapid and 8 were slow acetylators; the peak plasma concentration (or the test preparation) differed significantly between the two acetylator types only for 4 amino-phenazone (16.98 vs 18.52 for slow vs rapid acetylators) and 4-acetyl-amino-phenazone (1.38 vs 4.38 mg/L). [N. Bacracheva *et al.*, *Arzneimittelforschung*, 1995, *45*, 282–285.]

Toxicity. The estimated minimum lethal dose is 5 g, but fatalities from acute poisoning are rare.

A 56-year-old man died after ingesting up to 20 g dipyrone, 2 g baclofen, and 0.15 g oxybutynin; terazosin, aspirin, defibrotide, and laxatives also may have been ingested. Postmortem examination, performed a few hours after death, revealed dipyrone, baclofen, and oxybutynin concentrations, respectively, of 106, 669, and 0.1 mg/L in the blood and 774 mg/L, 215 mg/L, and trace amounts in the urine. [N. De Giovanni and E. d'Aloha, *Forensic Sci. Int.*, 2001, *123*, 26–32.]

Half-life. Plasma half-life, 4-acetylamino-phenazone about 10.6 h, 4-amino-phenazone about 5 h, 4-formylamino-phenazone about 10 h, and 4-methylamino-phenazone about 3.3 h.

Dose. 0.5 to 4 g daily in divided doses.

Diquat

Herbicide

Synonym. Deiquat

6,7-Dihydrodipyrido[1,2-*a*:2′,1′-*c*]pyrazinediium ion

$C_{12}H_{12}N_2$=184.2

CAS—2764-72-9

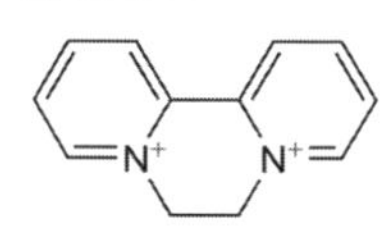

Diquat Dibromide

Proprietary names. Aquacide; Reglone. It is an ingredient of Pathclear and Weedol.

$C_{12}H_{12}Br_2N_2$=344.0

CAS—85-00-7

Yellow crystals. M.p. about 335°.

Soluble in water.

Note. Unless otherwise stated, the analytical information given below refers to diquat dibromide.

Partition Coefficient. Log *P* (octanol/water), 2.4.

Colour Test. Sodium Dithionite—green.

Thin-layer Chromatography. System TA—Rf 00; system TE—Rf 94; system TL—Rf 00; system TAB—Rf 00; system TAC—Rf 00; system TAE—Rf 00; system TAF—Rf 00; system TAJ—Rf 98; system TAK—Rf 04; system TAL—Rf 98. (Acidified iodoplatinate solution, positive.)

Gas Chromatography. System GA—Diquat dibromide, not eluted; system GK—monoene reduction product RRT 0.40, diene reduction product RRT 0.49 (both relative to caffeine).

High Performance Liquid Chromatography. System HX—RI 0; system HAO—diquat dibromide, *k* 99.9; system HAP—diquat dibromide, *k* 0.

Ultraviolet Spectrum. Aqueous acid—310 nm (A_1^1 = 518b).

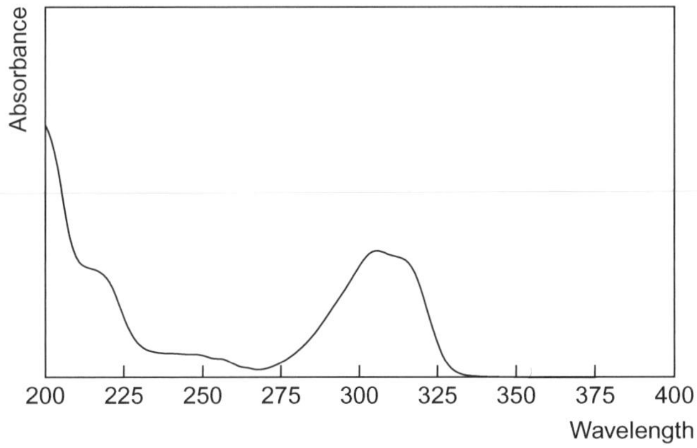

Infra-red Spectrum. Principal peaks at wavenumbers 1522, 1498, 1140, 1166, 1097, 1632 cm^{-1} (KBr disk).

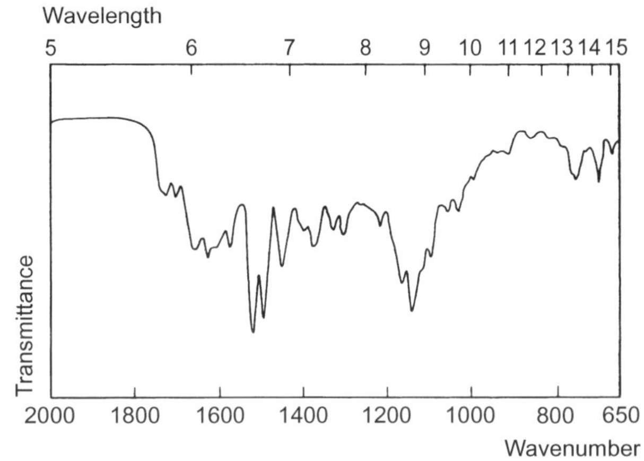

Mass Spectrum. Principal ions at *m/z* 83, 108, 96, 54, 111, 192, 84, 55 (monoene reduction product); 54, 108, 81, 190, 111, 135, 83, 80 (diene reduction product).

Quantification

Gas chromatography. In blood or urine: diquat and paraquat, FID—S. Kawase *et al.*, *J. Chromatogr.*, 1984, *282*, 231–240.

High performance liquid chromatography. In urine: diquat and paraquat, limit of detection <1 mg/L, UV detection—R. Gill *et al.*, *J. Chromatogr.*, 1983, *255*, 483–490. In biological materials: diquat dichloride and paraquat dichloride, limit of detection 0.05 μg/g, UV detection—S. Ito *et al.*, *J. Chromatogr.*, 1993, *617*, 119–123. In blood, bile, liver and kidney tissue, or urine: diquat and paraquat—C. Madhu *et al.*, *J. Chromatogr. B Biomed. Appl.*, 1995, *674*, 193–196.

Disposition in the Body. Absorbed from the gastro-intestinal tract; slightly absorbed through the skin.

Toxicity. Diquat produces similar adverse effects to those of paraquat except that it does not seem to cause the progressive fibrosis in the lungs. A fatality after ingestion of about 2 g has been reported and the ingestion of about 20 to 50 mL of a 20% concentrate has caused death within 2 to 7 days. The maximum permissible atmospheric concentration is 0.5 mg/m^3 (as the dibromide) and the maximum acceptable daily intake (as the dichloride) is 5 μg/kg.

A young man drank several mouthfuls of a 20% concentrate of diquat and died 7 days later. The following postmortem concentrations were reported: blood 0.6 mg/L, heart 0.11 μg/g, kidney 1.19 μg/g, liver 0.33 μg/g, lung 0.56 μg/g, and spleen 1.04 μg/g [H. Schönborn *et al.*, *Arch. Toxicol.*, 1971, *27*, 204–216.]

A 44-year-old woman ingested an unknown quantity of diquat and died about 16 h after being found. The following postmortem concentrations were reported: kidney 11.6 μg/g and liver 5.1 μg/g. [L. K. Pannell and B. M. Thomson, *Bull. Int. Assoc. Forensic Toxicol.*, 1981, *16*(2), 24–25.]

A 37-year-old man died 26 h after ingesting 300 mL of diquat solution (equivalent to 60 g diquat ion) in a suicide attempt. 4 h after ingestion, the concentration of diquat in the serum was 64 mg/L. Postmortem tissue concentrations were (μg/g): kidney 4.5, lung 3.4, liver 2.3, brain 1.6, heart 1.1. [P. Hantson *et al.*, *J. Toxicol. Clin. Toxicol.*, 2000, *38*, 149–152.]

Note. For a review of diquat poisoning see G. M. Jones and J. A. Vale, *J. Toxicol. Clin. Toxicol.*, 2000, *38*, 123–138.

Disopyramide

Anti-arrhythmic

Proprietary names. Dicorynan; Dimodan; Disofarin; Disonorm; Durbis (capsules); Isomide; Isorythm; Ritmodan; Rythmodan (capsules).

α-[2-[Bis(1-methylethyl)amino]ethyl]-α-phenyl-2-pyridineacetamide

$C_{21}H_{29}N_3O$=339.5

CAS—3737-09-5

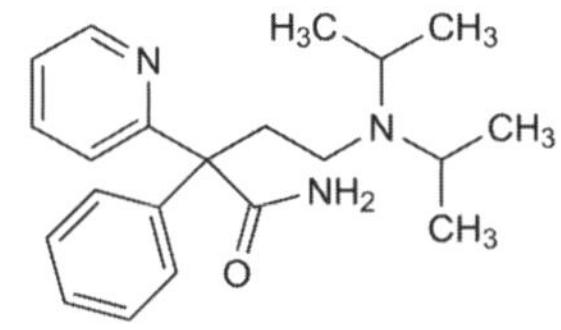

A white powder. M.p. about 95°.

Soluble 1 in 200 of water, 1 in 10 of ethanol, 1 in 5 of chloroform, and 1 in 5 of ether.

Disopyramide Phosphate

Proprietary names. Dicorantil; Dirythmin; Dirytmin; Diso-Duriles; Disomet; Disonorm; Durbis (injection); Isomide; Isorythm; Norpace; Ritmodan; Ritmoforine; Rythmical; Rythmodan (injection and tablets); Rythmodul.

$C_{21}H_{29}N_3O,H_3PO_4$=437.5

CAS—22059-60-5

A white powder. M.p. about 205°, with decomposition.

Soluble 1 in 20 of water and 1 in 50 of ethanol; practically insoluble in chloroform and ether.

Dissociation Constant. pK_a 8.4.

Partition Coefficient. Log *P* (octanol/water), 2.6.

Thin-layer Chromatography. System TA—Rf 45; system TB—Rf 07; system TC—Rf 08; system TE—Rf 60; TL—Rf 13; system TAE—Rf 09; system TAF—Rf 07.

Gas Chromatography. System GA—disopyramide RI 2505, disopyramide-CHNO RI 2030, M (*N*-desalkyl-)-CHNO-AC RI 2330, M (*N*-desalkyl-)-AC RI 2640, M (bis-desalkyl-)-NH_3 RI 2245; system GB—disopyramide RI 2608, M (*N*-desalkyl-) RI 2286; system GF—RI 2910.

High Performance Liquid Chromatography. System HA—disopyramide *k* 2.4, *N*-monodesisopropyldisopyramide *k* 1.8; system HX—RI 345; system HY—RI 281; system HZ—retention time 3.0 min; system HAA—retention time 11.4 min; system HAX—retention time 9.6 min; system HAY—retention time 4.9 min.

Ultraviolet Spectrum. Aqueous acid—263, 269 (A^1_1=199a); aqueous alkali—261 nm.

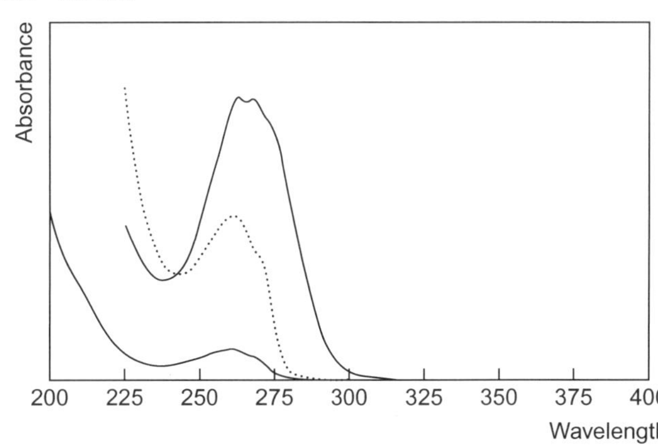

Infra-red Spectrum. Principal peaks at wavenumbers 1664, 1585, 697, 1163, 1562, 760 cm^{-1} (KBr disk).

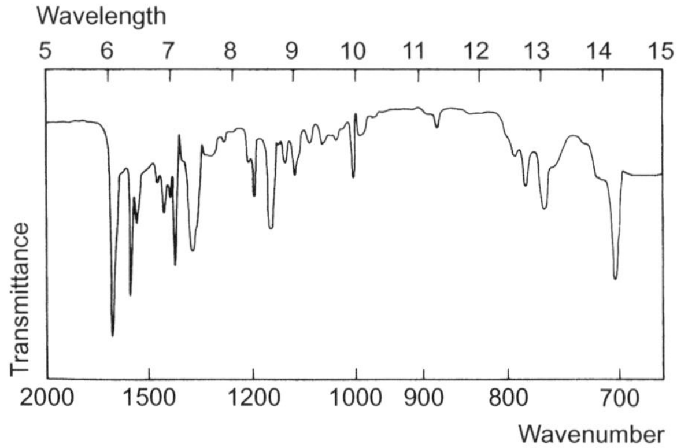

Mass Spectrum. Principal ions at *m/z* 195, 212, 114, 30, 194, 72, 44, 43 (no peaks above 240).

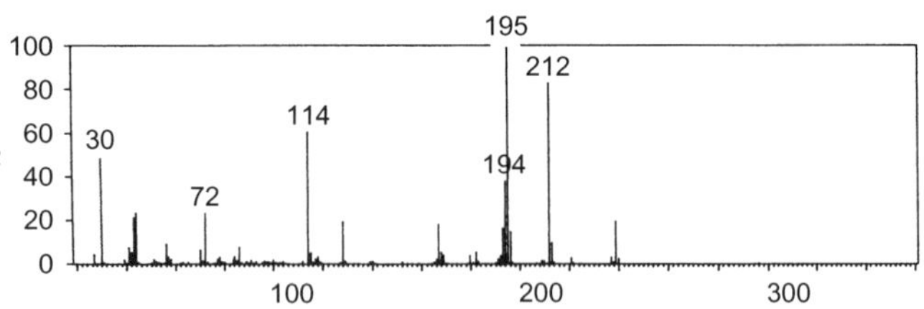

Quantification

Gas chromatography. In plasma: limit of detection 100 mg/L, FID—E. N. Foster and P. R. Reid, *J. Chromatogr.*, 1979, *178*, 571–574. In plasma, urine or postmortem tissues: FID—R. W. Michalek *et al.*, *J. Anal. Toxicol.*, 1982, *6*, 255–257. In serum: limit of detection 100 mg/L for disopyramide and the desalkyl metabolite, AFID—J. E. Bredesen, *Clin. Chem.*, 1980, *26*, 638–640.In plasma: nitrogen/phosphorus selective detection—R. P. Kapil *et al.*, *Res. Commun. Chem. Pathol. Pharmacol.*, 1985, *48*, 153–156. In plasma: FID—M. P. Quaglio *et al.*, *Boll. Chim. Farm.*, 1995, *134*, 34–38.

High performance liquid chromatography. In plasma or urine: disopyramide and the desalkyl metabolite, limit of detection 50 mg/L, UV detection—C. Charette *et al.*, *J. Chromatogr.* 1983, *274 B Biomed. Appl.*, *25*, 219–230. In serum: disopyramide and its active metabolite mono-*N*-dealkyldisopyramide, limit of detection 50 mg/L—L. H. Wang *et al.*, *Ther. Drug Monit.*, 1986, *8*, 85–89. In serum: UV detection—E. H. Taylor *et al.*, *Ther. Drug Monit.*, 1986, *8*, 219–222. In serum: disopyramide, other anti-arrhythmic drugs and their active metabolites, limit of detection 0.1 to 0.2 mg/L—H. F. Proelss and T. B. Townsend, *Clin. Chem.*, 1986, *32*, 1311–1317. In biological material: disopyramide and lidocaine and their active monodealkylated metabolites, limit of detection 0.3 µmol/L, UV detection—H. R. Angelo *et al.*, *Scand J. Clin. Lab. Invest.*, 1986, *46*, 623–627. In plasma or urine: disopyramide and its active metabolite mono-*N*-dealkyldisopyramide, limits of detection 0.01 to 0.025 mg/mL, UV detection—H. Echizen *et al.*, *Clin. Chem.*, 1990, *36*, 1300–1304. In plasma or urine: disopyramide and its mono-*N*-dealkylated metabolite enantiomers, limits of detection for disopyramide enantiomers 40 µg/L and 80 µg/L—H. Takahashi *et al.*, *J. Chromatogr.*, 1990, *529*, 347–358. In plasma: disopyramide and other anti-arrhythmic drugs, UV or fluorescence detection—R. Verbesselt *et al.*, *Ther. Drug Monit.*, 1991, *13*, 157–165. In serum: disopyramide and its active metabolite mono-*N*-dealkylated disopyramide, UV detection—F. Mayer *et al.*, *J. Chromatogr.*, 1991, *572*, 339–345. In plasma or urine: disopyramide and mono-*N*-dealkyldisopyramide enantiomers, limits of detection in plasma 12.5 µg/L, UV detection—R. Bortocan *et al.*, *J. Chromatogr. B Biomed. Sci. Appl.*, 2000, *744*, 299–306.

Disposition in the Body. Rapidly and almost completely absorbed after oral administration and widely distributed throughout the body.The major metabolite, *N*-monodesisopropyldisopyramide, is about one half as active as disopyramide. Up to about 50 to 60% of a dose is excreted in the urine in 5 days as unchanged drug, with about 20 to 30% as the desalkyl metabolite; about 10 to 15% of a dose is eliminated in the faeces.

Therapeutic concentration. In plasma, usually in the range 2 to 5 mg/L.

After a single oral dose of 100 mg of disopyramide phosphate to 6 subjects, peak plasma concentrations of 1.8 to 3.6 mg/L (mean 2.7) were attained in about 2 h. [R. E. Ranney *et al.*, *Arch. Int. Pharmacodyn. Thér.*, 1971, *191*, 162–188.]

Following oral daily doses averaging 6 mg/kg to 63 subjects, mean steady-state plasma concentrations of 3.3 mg/L for disopyramide and 0.99 mg/L for the desalkyl metabolite were reported; plasma concentrations were higher in 17 subjects with renal dysfunction (mean 4.3), but lower in subjects concurrently taking enzyme-inducing drugs. [M. Aitio, *Br. J. Clin. Pharmacol.*, 1981, *11*, 369–376.]

Toxicity. Toxic effects are usually associated with plasma concentrations greater than about 8 mg/L.

In a fatality due to the ingestion of about 15 g of disopyramide, the following postmortem tissue concentrations were reported: blood 57 mg/L, brain 29 µg/g, liver 115 µg/g, urine 1500 mg/L. [R. W. Michalek *et al.*, *J. Anal. Toxicol.*, 1982, *6*, 255–257.]

In 2 cases of suicide by means of disopyramide ingestion, the postmortem blood concentrations were 146 mg/L (amount ingested unknown) and 63 mg/L (3.6 g apparently ingested). [L. Sathyavagiswaran, *J. Forensic Sci.*, 1987, *32*, 1813–1318.]

In a 4-year-old child who died after accidental ingestion of disopyramide and sulindac, postmortem tissue concentrations were (for disopyramide and sulindac, respectively): blood 41.3 and 12.2 mg/L, bile 435 and 1251 mg/L, liver 98.2 and 12.4 µg/g, gastric content 15 and 70 mg, urine 430 and 29.8 mg/L. [P. Singer and A. Mozayani, *J. Anal. Toxicol.*, 1995, *19*, 529–530.]

Bioavailability. About 80%.

Half-life. Plasma half-life, disopyramide 3 to 11 h (dose-dependent), increased in subjects with renal impairment; desalkyl metabolite about 13 h.

Volume of distribution. About 0.7 L/kg (dose-dependent); unbound drug about 2 L/kg.

Clearance. Plasma clearance, about 0.5 to 2 mL/min/kg (dose-dependent); unbound drug about 6 mL/min/kg.

Protein binding. In plasma, disopyramide about 35 to 80% (concentration-dependent), desalkyl metabolite about 30 to 70% (concentration-dependent); considerable intersubject variation occurs.

Note. For reviews of disopyramide see R. C. Heel *et al.*, *Drugs*, 1978, *15*, 331–368 and A. Karim *et al.*, *J. Pharmacokinet. Biopharm.*, 1982, *10*, 465–494.

Dose. 300 to 800 mg daily.

Distigmine Bromide

Anticholinesterase

Synonyms. Bispyridostigmine Bromide; Hexamarium Bromide.
Proprietary names. Tonus; Ubretid.
3,3′-[1,6-Hexanediylbis[(methylimino)carbonyl]oxy]bis[1-methylpyridinium]dibromide
$C_{22}H_{32}Br_2N_4O_4$ = 576.3
CAS—15876-67-2

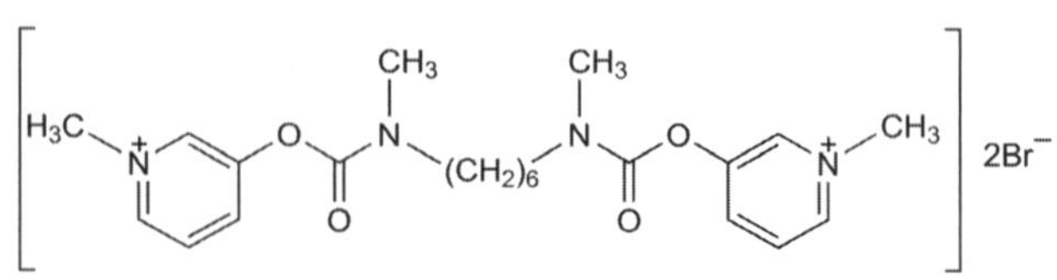

A crystalline powder. Decomposes at 149°.
Freely soluble in water.

Partition Coefficient. Log *P* (octanol/water), −0.4.

Thin-layer Chromatography. System TA—Rf 00; system TE—Rf 03; system TAE—Rf 02. (Acidified iodoplatinate solution, positive.)

Ultraviolet Spectrum. Aqueous acid—270 nm (A_1^1 = 160a).

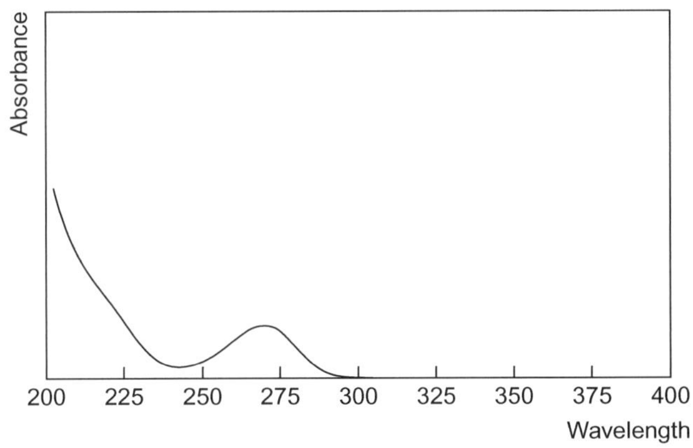

Infra-red Spectrum. Principal peaks at wavenumbers 1735, 1255, 1170, 1507, 1135, 1295 cm^{-1} (KBr disk).

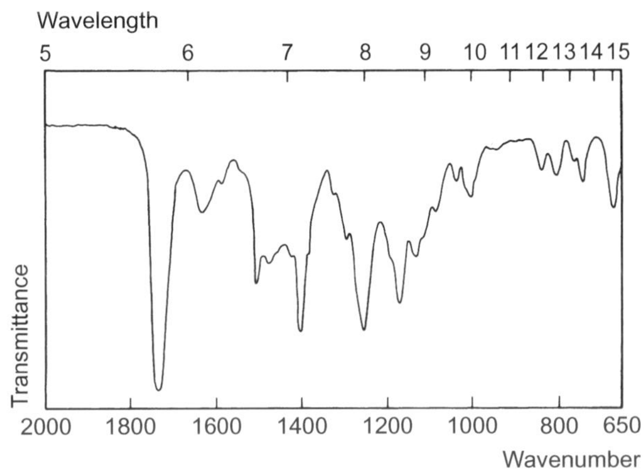

Disposition in the Body. Poorly absorbed after oral administration. Less than 5% of an oral dose is excreted in the urine in 24 h, compared to 50% of an IM dose.

Dose. 5 to 20 mg daily, by mouth.

Disulfamide

Diuretic

Synonym. Disulphamide
Proprietary names. Disamide; Natirene.
4-Chloro-6-methyl-1,3-benzenedisulfonamide
$C_7H_9ClN_2O_4S_2$=284.7
CAS—671-88-5

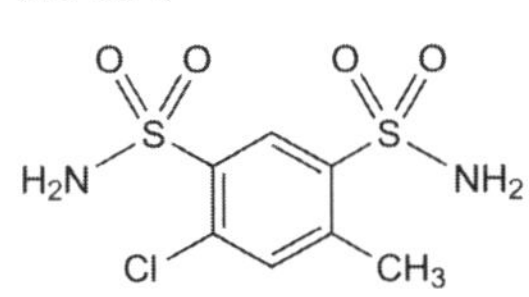

A white or creamy-white crystalline powder. M.p. 260°.
Soluble 1 in 500 of cold water, 1 in 50 of boiling water, 1 in 50 of ethanol, and 1 in 1000 of ether; slightly soluble in chloroform.

Partition Coefficient. Log *P* (octanol/water), 1.0.

Ultraviolet Spectrum. Aqueous acid—235 (A^{1}_{1}=336b), 276, 285 nm.

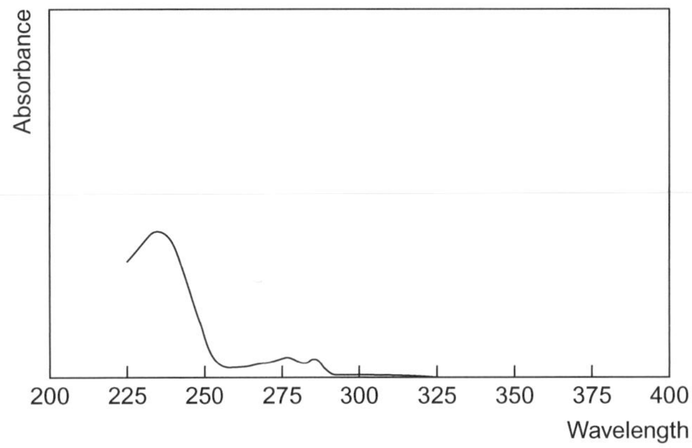

Infra-red Spectrum. Principal peaks at wavenumbers 1320, 1172, 1552, 965, 675, 1550 cm^{-1} (KBr disk).

Dose. Disulfamide has been given in doses of 100 to 200 mg daily.

Disulfiram

Alcohol Deterrent

Synonyms. Éthyldithiourame; TTD.
Proprietary names. Antabus(e); Difaram; Esperal; Etabus; Etiltox; Refusal; Tetradin.
Tetraethylthioperoxydicarbonic diamide
$C_{10}H_{20}N_2S_4$=296.5
CAS—97-77-8

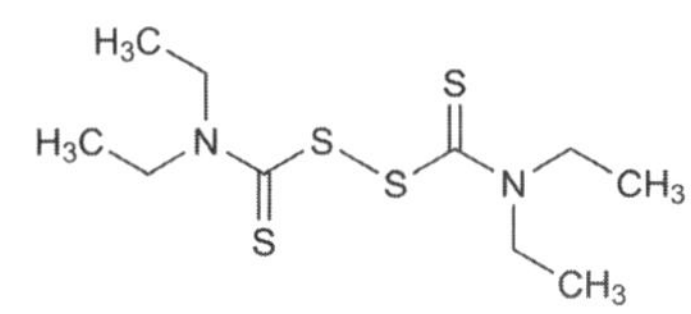

A white powder. M.p. 70°.
Practically insoluble in water; soluble 1 in 65 of ethanol, 1 in 2 of chloroform, and 1 in 20 of ether; soluble in acetone, benzene, and carbon disulfide.

Partition Coefficient. Log *P* (octanol/water), 3.9.

Colour Tests. Palladium Chloride—orange.
Dissolve 50 mg in 5 mL of ethanol and add 1 mL of potassium cyanide solution—yellow→green→blue-green.

Thin-layer Chromatography. System TA—Rf 71; system TB—Rf 21; system TC—Rf 78; system TE—Rf 78; system TL—Rf 69; system TAE—Rf 78; system TAF—Rf 81.

Gas Chromatography. System GA—RI 2141 (on packed column; not eluted on capillary column).

High Performance Liquid Chromatography. system HX—RI 741; system HY—RI 734; System HAA—retention time 25.1 min.

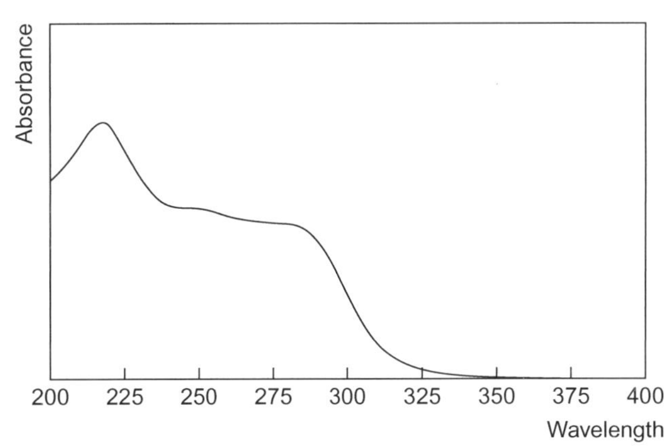

Infra-red Spectrum. Principal peaks at wavenumbers 1267, 1193, 1492, 1147, 966, 913 cm^{-1} (Nujol mull).

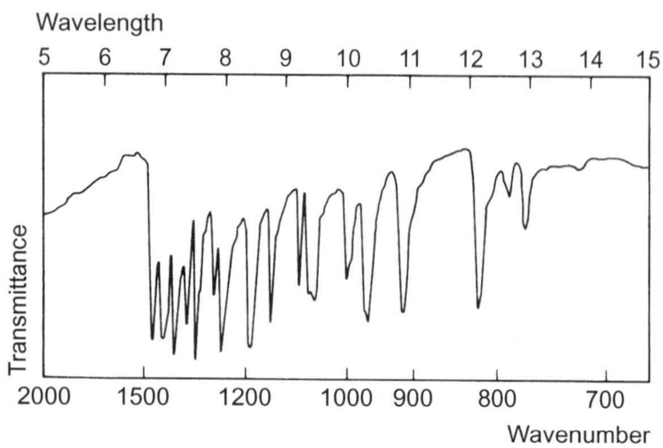

Mass Spectrum. Principal ions at *m/z* 116, 88, 29, 44, 60, 148, 56, 27.

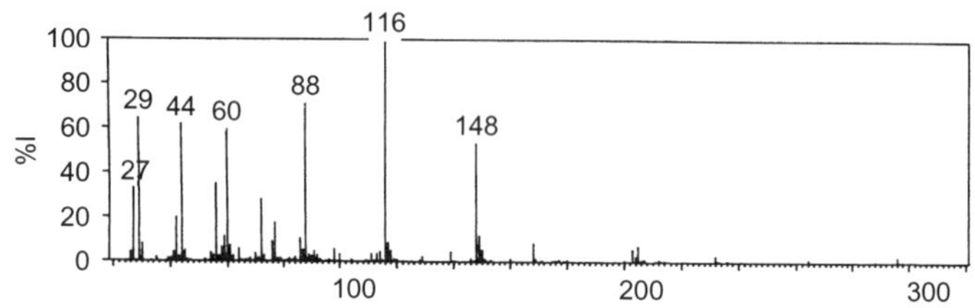

Quantification

Gas chromatography. In blood: disulfiram and metabolites, limit of detection 10 μg/L using head-space analysis and FPD—A. M. Sauter and J. P. von Wartburg, *J. Chromatogr.*, 1977, *133*, 167–172.

High performance liquid chromatography. In plasma or urine: disulfiram and metabolites, limit of detection 200 μg/L, UV detection—J. C. Jensen and M. D. Faiman, *J. Chromatogr.* 1980, *181(7) B Biomed. Appl.*, 407–416. In plasma: disulfiram and dithiocarbamate metabolites, limit of detection 50 μg/L, UV detection—P. D. Masso and P. A. Kramer, *J. Chromatogr.* 1981, *224 B Biomed. Appl.*, *13*, 457–464. In plasma: disulfiram and its metabolites—B. Johansson, *J. Chromatogr.*, 1986, *378*, 419–429.

Disposition in the Body. Disulfiram produces hypersensitivity to alcohol by inhibiting the oxidation of acetaldehyde, the primary metabolite of alcohol; the concentrations of acetaldehyde in the blood and expired air are increased by 5 to 10 times. Disulfiram is incompletely absorbed after oral administration; the maximum effect usually occurs about 12 h after ingestion, possibly because it is highly lipid soluble and is likely to be initially localised in fat. The metabolites include diethyldithiocarbamic acid, methyl diethyldithiocarbamate, diethylamine, carbon disulfide, and inorganic sulfate; glucuronide conjugation may occur. Up to about 20% of a dose is eliminated unchanged in the faeces, up to 50% of a dose may be excreted from the lungs as carbon disulfide, and the remainder is slowly excreted as metabolites in the urine; about 20% of a dose is still present in the body up to 7 days after ingestion.

Therapeutic concentration

Following a single oral dose of 250 mg to 15 subjects, mean peak plasma concentrations of 0.38 mg/L of disulfiram, 0.77 mg/L of diethyldithiocarbamic acid, 0.30 mg/L of methyl diethyldithiocarbamate, and 1.7 mg/L of diethylamine were attained in about 9 h; a mean peak plasma concentration of 22 mg/L of carbon disulfide was reported at 6 h; there was considerable intersubject variability in the plasma concentrations. [M. D. Faiman *et al.*, *Clin. Pharmacol. Ther.*, 1984, *36*, 520–526.]

Toxicity. Severe toxic reactions may occur after administration of disulfiram if the blood concentration of acetaldehyde is greater than 5 mg/L; with very high concentrations of alcohol in the blood the administration of as little as 0.5 to 1 g of disulfiram has proved fatal in some cases. Fatalities due to disulfiram-induced hepatitis have been reported and there have also been reports of severe phenytoin intoxication after simultaneous administration.

In a fatality due to ingestion of disulfiram and alcohol, postmortem blood concentrations of 8 mg/L of sodium diethyldithiocarbamate and 9600 mg/L of ethanol were reported. [F. Martens and A. Heyndrickx, *Bull. Int. Assoc. Forensic Toxicol.*, 1975, *11*(2), 18–19.]

Half-life. Plasma half-life, disulfiram about 7 h, diethyldithiocarbamic acid about 15 h, carbon disulfide about 9 h.

Note. For a review of disulfiram see J. F. Brien *et al.*, *Drug Met. Rev.*, 1983, *14*, 113–126 and B. Johansson, *Acta Psychiatr. Scand Suppl.*, 1992, *369*, 15–26.

Dose. 800 mg on the first day, reducing to a maintenance dose of 100 to 200 mg daily.

Disulfoton

Insecticide

Synonyms. Bay-19639; Bay-S276; Dithiodemeton; ENT-23347; Ethylthiodemeton; Thiodemeton; Thiometon-ethyl.

Proprietary names. Dimaz; Disipton; Dithiosystox; Di-syston; Disystox; Ekatin TD; Frumen AL; Frumin G; Frumin AL; Solvigram; Solvirex; Terraclor Super-X.

Phosphorodithioic acid *O*,*O*-diethyl-*S*-[2-(ethylthio)ethyl] ester

$C_8H_{19}O_2PS_3$ = 274.4

CAS—298-04-4

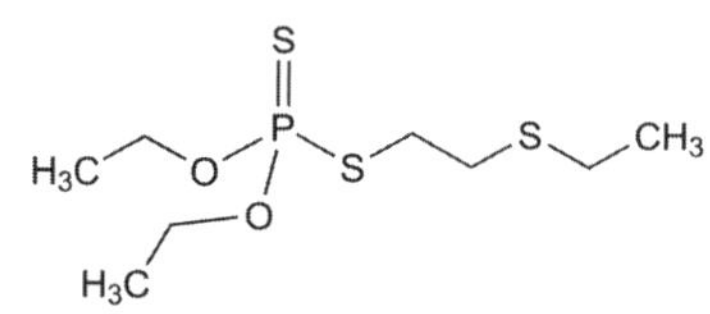

A pale yellow liquid or solid. M.p. 108°. B.p. 62° at 0.01 mmHg.
It is insoluble in water (25 mg/L at 23°, 16.3 mg/L at 20°); soluble in most organic solvents and fatty oils.

Partition Coefficient. Log *P* (octanol/water), 4.02.

Thin-layer Chromatography. System TX—Rf 58; system TY—Rf 89; system TAB—Rf 52; system TAC—Rf 35.

Gas Chromatography. System GA—disulfoton RI 2749, M (sulphone) RI 2077, M (sulphoxide) RI 1303; system GK—disulfoton RRT 0.86 (relative to caffeine); system GKA—RI 1776; system GKB—RI 1906; system GKC—RI 2080.

High Performance Liquid Chromatography. System HY—RI 691; system HAO—*k* 0.10; system HAP—*k* 6.48.

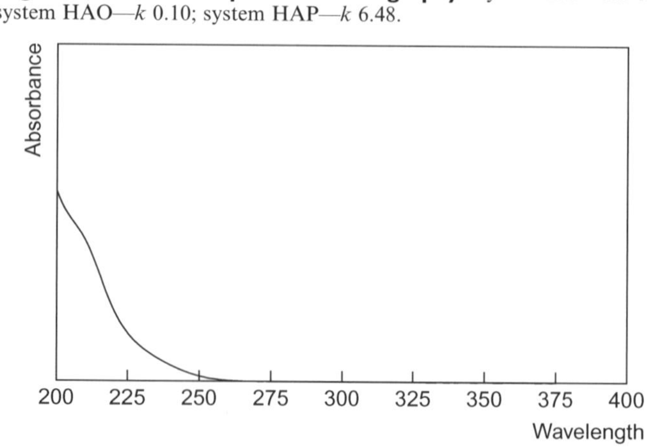

Infra-red Spectrum. Principal peaks at wavenumber 1031, 952, 666, 798, 2983, 2941 cm^{-1}.

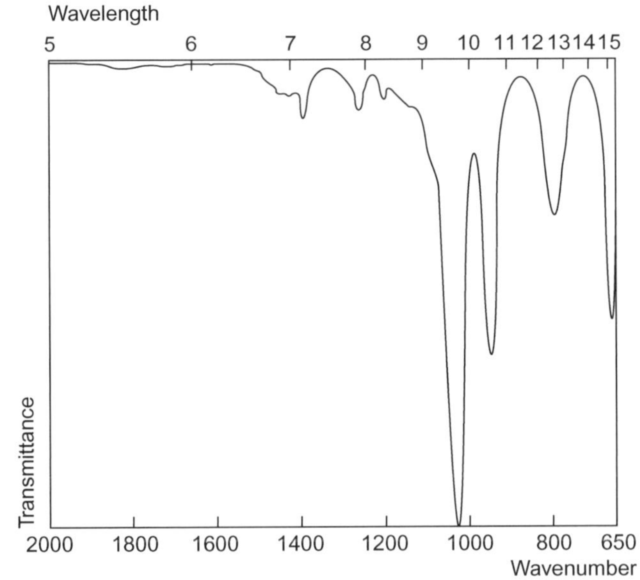

Mass Spectrum. Principal ions at *m/z* 88, 89, 97, 61, 60, 153, 186, 125.

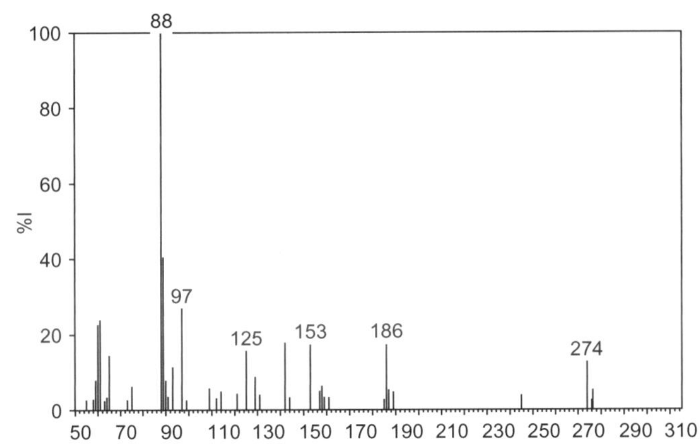

Disposition in the Body. Disulfoton is rapidly absorbed after oral ingestion, from the gastro-intestinal tract. It is metabolised to the sulfoxide and sulfone metabolites, and corresponding phosphorothioate metabolites and derivatives of *O,O*-diethylhydrophosphate and 2-ethylthioethylmercaptan. It is excreted mainly via urine (approx. 80%) and, also, faeces and expired air.

Toxicity. Disulfoton is very highly toxic by all routes of exposure. The allowed daily intake is 0.2 µg/kg body weight and a blood disulfoton level of 1.45 nmol/g is associated with fatality. A lethal adult dose is estimated to be between 500 mg and 4 g.

A 75-year-old woman was admitted into hospital after an attempted suicide. She had ingested a large amount of granular Di-Syston, containing 5% disulfoton. On admission, the total disulfoton and metabolites plasma concentration was 1.095 mg/L which decreased to 505 µg/L after gastric lavage. A peak concentration (1.322 mg/L) was not reached, however, until 56 h post-ingestion, because of the prolonged absorption of the organophosphate from the granules present in the stomach. These concentrations indicate a severe level of disulfoton intoxication. [K. Futagami *et al.*, *J. Toxicol. Clin. Toxicol.*, 1995, *33(2)*, 151–155.]

An 87-year-old man was admitted to hospital after ingesting 3 or 4 heaped tablespoonfuls of Di-Syston (disulfoton) dissolved in water. He was unconscious, had difficulty breathing and did not respond well to pain stimuli, but made a full recovery after treatment. The concentration of disulfoton in his blood was 25.4 ng/g and the total of metabolites was 4.92 nmol/g (corresponding to 1.35 µg/g disulfoton), indicating a severe level of disulfoton intoxication. The concentration of the pesticide in the stomach contents on admission to hospital was 32.9 µg/g. [M. Yashiki *et al.*, *Forensic Sci. Int.*, 1990, *48*, 145–154.]

Dithranol

Dermatological Agent

Synonyms. Anthralin; Dioxyanthranol.
Proprietary names. Anthra-Derm; Anthraforte; Anthrascalp; Anthranol; Antranol; Desmoline; Dithrocream; Drithocreme; Dritho-Scalp; Lasan; Micanol; Psoricreme; Psoriderm; Timicolid. It is an ingredient of Psoradrate and Psorin.
1,8-Dihydroxy-9(10*H*)-anthracenone
$C_{14}H_{10}O_3 = 226.2$
CAS—1143-38-0

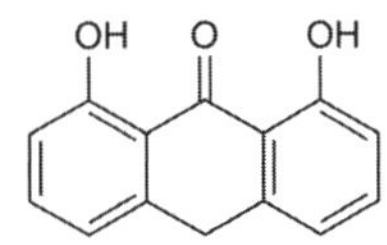

A yellow to yellowish-brown crystalline powder. M.p. 176° to 181°. Practically insoluble in water; slightly soluble in ethanol, glacial acetic acid, and ether; soluble in acetone, benzene, and chloroform.
Caution. Dithranol is a powerful irritant and should be kept away from the eyes and tender parts of the skin.

Dithranol Triacetate

Synonym. Dithranol Acetate
Proprietary name. Exolan (cream)
$C_{20}H_{16}O_6 = 352.3$
CAS—16203-97-7

Partition Coefficient. Log *P* (octanol/water), 4.4.

High Performance Liquid Chromatography. System HY—RI 703.

Ultraviolet Spectrum. Aqueous alkali—276 (A_1^1=490b); methanol—256 (A_1^1=467b), 288 (A_1^1=358b), 360 nm (A_1^1=418b).

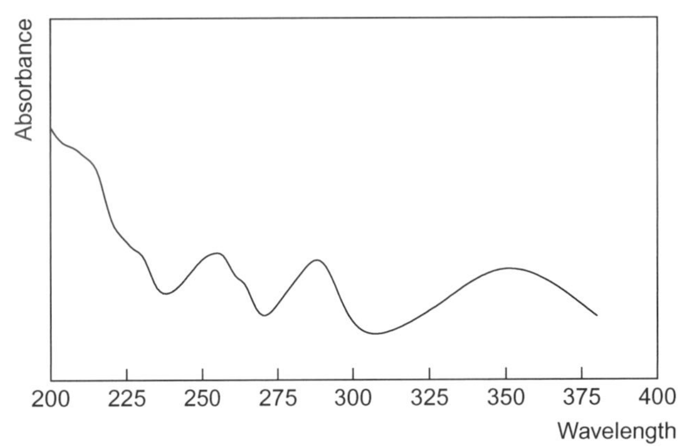

Infra-red Spectrum. Principal peaks at wavenumbers 1598, 1278, 1615, 1222, 1168, 1635 cm^{-1} (KCl disk).

Use. Topically in concentrations of 0.05 to 1%.

Ditiocarb

Immunomodulator/Chelator

Synonyms. Dithiocarb; Diethylcarbamodithioc acid.
Diethyldithiocarbamic acid.
$C_5H_{10}NS_2 = 148.3$

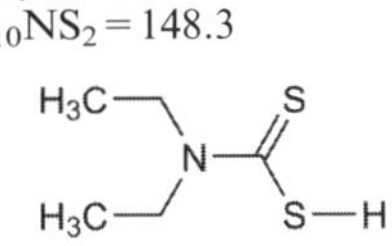

Ditiocarb Sodium

Synonyms. ACS; DEDC; DEDK; DeDTC; DDTC; DTC; Diethylcarbamodithioc acid sodium salt; Dithiocarb sodium; DRG-0066; SDDC; Sodium diethyldithiocarbamate; Dithiocarb
Proprietary name. Imuthiol
$C_5H_{10}NNaS_2 = 171.3$

CAS—148-18-5
A white, slightly brown or slightly pink crystalline powder. M.p. 95°. Soluble in water (⩾ 10 g/100 mL at 14°).

Ditiocarb Sodium Trihydrate
$C_5H_{10}NNaS_2,3H_2O = 225.3$
A powder comprising thin, irregular, plate-like crystals. M.p. 94° to 102°. It is freely soluble in water; soluble in ethanol, methanol and acetone; insoluble in ether and benzene.

Partition Coefficient. Log *P* (octanol/water), −1.43.

Infra-red Spectrum. (Ditiocarb sodium) Principal peaks at wavenumbers 1477, 1202, 984, 914 cm^{-1} (KBr pellets).

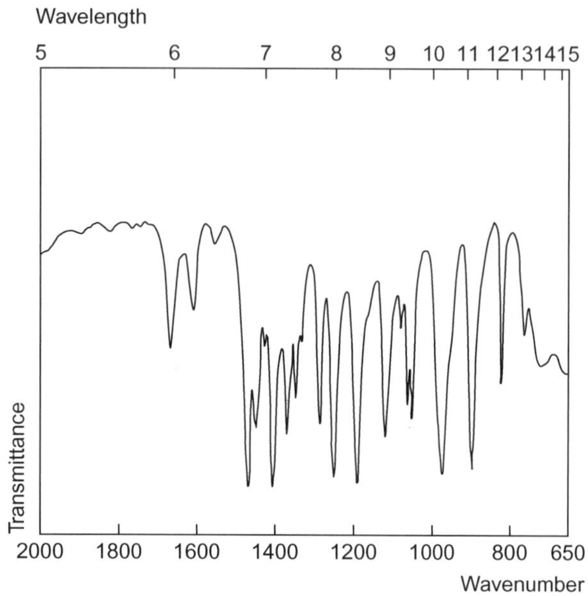

Quantification
High performance liquid chromatography. In plasma: limit of detection 0.5 mg/L—W. M. Awni *et al., J. Clin. Pharmacol.*, 1994, *34*, 1183–1190.

Disposition in the Body. Ditiocarb is well absorbed and metabolised in the liver to its glucuronide, methyl ester and diethylamine metabolites, carbon disulfide and sulfate ions. Excretion is via urine with carbon disulfide being excreted in exhaled breath. Approximately 80% of an oral dose is detected in plasma 20 min after administration. Ditiocarb is eliminated rapidly from the body with 60% of a dose being excreted within 3 h.

Therapeutic concentration
18 healthy male volunteers, aged between 18 and 35 years, of white, black and Native American origin were administered with either a 200 mg/m^2/h dose of DDTC or 400 mg/m^2/h, over 4 h. Mean steady state concentrations of diethyldithiocarbamate were 0.027 mg/L for the lower dose and 0.075 mg/L for the higher dose. [W. M. Awni *et al., J. Clin. Pharmacol.*, 1994, *34*, 1183–1190].

Half-life. Approx. 20 min.

Volume of distribution. Mean, 0.287 L/kg (200 mg/m^2/h dose); 0.211 L/kg (400 mg/m^2/h dose).

Clearance. Mean plasma clearance, 25.5 mL/min/kg (200 mg/m^2/h dose); 16.9 mL/min/kg (400 mg/m^2/h dose).

Diuron

Herbicide

Proprietary names. Karmex; Urox D. It is an ingredient of Dexuron and Krovar.
N'-(3,4-Dichlorophenyl)-*N*,*N*-dimethylurea
$C_9H_{10}Cl_2N_2O = 233.1$
CAS—330-54-1

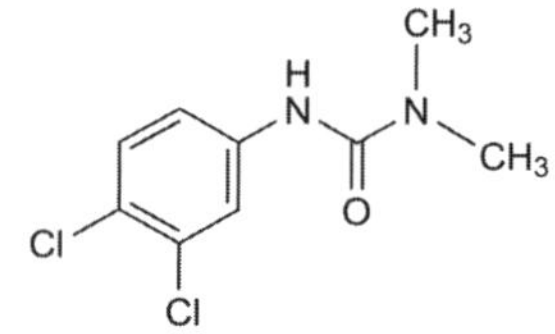

Crystals. M.p. 158° to 159°.
Practically insoluble in water; soluble in acetone; sparingly soluble in hydrocarbon solvents.

Partition Coefficient. Log *P* (octanol/water), 2.7.

Colour Tests. Liebermann's Test—orange; Marquis Test—pink-orange.

Gas Chromatography. System GA—diuron RI 1850, diuron-ME RI 1880, 3,4-dichloroaniline RI 1405; system GK—3,4-dichloroaniline RRT 0.36 and 3,4-dichlorophenyl isocyanate RRT 0.13 (both relative to caffeine).

High Performance Liquid Chromatography. System HY—RI 417; system HZ—retention time 5.8 min; system HAA—retention time 18.5 min.

Ultraviolet Spectrum. Ethanol—250 (A^1_1 = 1124b), 287 nm.

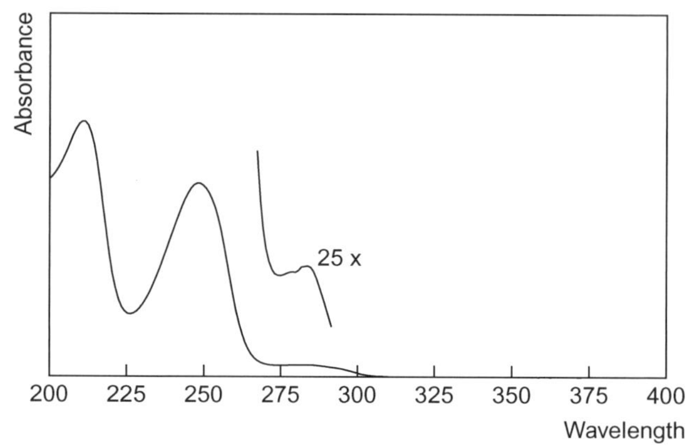

Mass Spectrum. Principal ions at *m/z* 72, 44, 73, 42, 232, 187, 124, 45.

Quantification
Gas chromatography. In urine: dichloroanilines as markers for diuron and other herbicides, some pesticides, and fungicides, limits of detection 0.03 µg/L and 0.05 µg/L with MS detection and ECD respectively—K. Wittke *et al., J. Chromatogr. B Biomed. Sci. Appl.*, 2001, *755*, 215–228.

High performance liquid chromatography. In blood or urine: diuron and its metabolites—M. Van Boven *et al., J. Anal. Toxicol.*, 1990, *14*, 231–234.

Dixyrazine

Tranquilliser

Synonym. UCB-3412
Proprietary name. Esucos
2-[2-[4-[2-Methyl-3-(10*H*-phenothiazin-10-yl)propyl]-1-piperazinyl]-ethoxy]ethanol
$C_{24}H_{33}N_3O_2S = 427.6$
CAS—2470-73-7

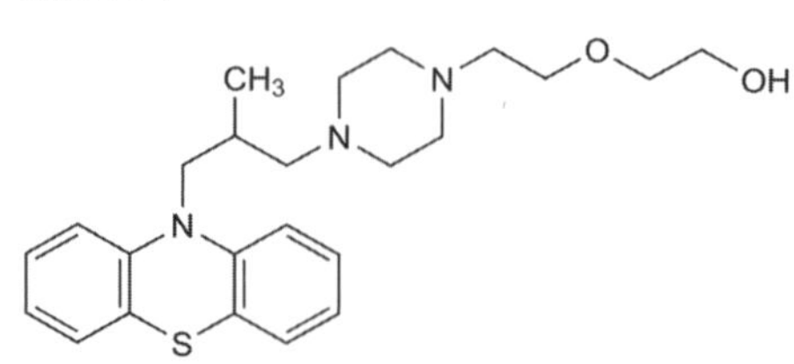

A white to slightly greyish or yellowish powder.
Very slightly soluble in water; soluble in ethanol, chloroform, and ether.

Dissociation Constant. pK_a 7.8 (25°).

Partition Coefficient. Log *P* (octanol/water), 3.3.

Thin-layer Chromatography. System TE—Rf 49; system TAE—Rf 47.

Gas Chromatography. System GA—dixyrazine RI 3220, M (phenothiazine) RI 2020, dixyrazine-AC RI 3530, M (*N*-desalkyl-)-AC RI 3355, M (*O*-desalkyl-)-AC RI 3350, M (amino-)-AC RI 2765.

Ultraviolet Spectrum. Methanol—255 nm (A_1^1=980b), 305 nm.

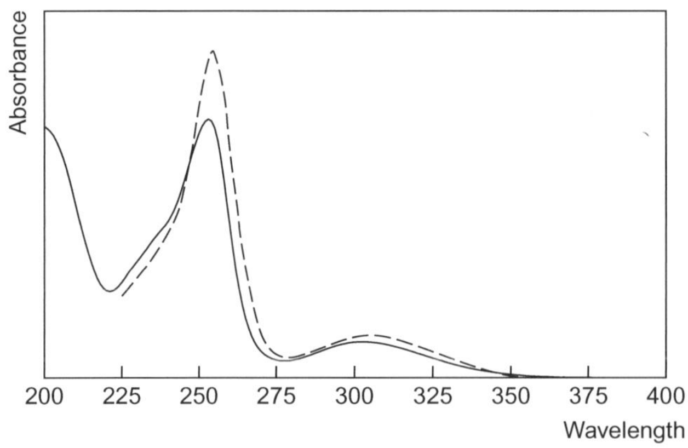

Mass Spectrum. Principal ions at *m*/*z* 212, 42, 187, 45, 70, 180, 56, 98.

Quantification
Gas chromatography–mass spectrometry. In plasma or serum: limit of detection 400 ng/L—G. Brante *et al.*, *Eur. J. Clin. Pharmacol.*, 1981, *20*, 307–310.

Dose. 20 to 75 mg daily.

Dobutamine

Sympathomimetic

4-[2-[[3-(4-Hydroxyphenyl)-1-methylpropyl]amino]ethyl]-1,2-benzenediol
$C_{18}H_{23}NO_3$=301.4
CAS—34368-04-2

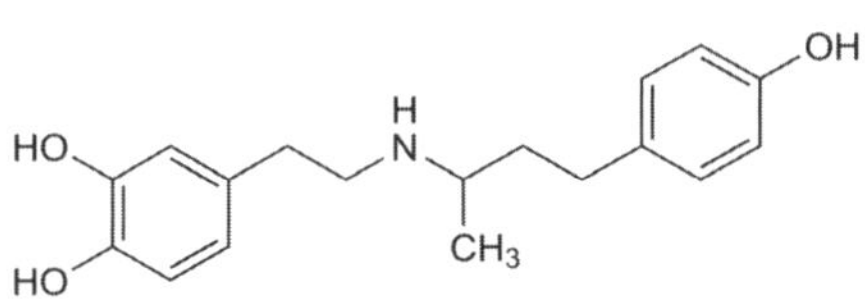

Dobutamine Hydrochloride

Proprietary names. Butamine; Cryobutol; Dobucard; Dobuject; Dobutam; Dobutina; Dobutrex; Inotrex; Kardion; Oxiken; Posiject.
$C_{18}H_{23}NO_3$,HCl=337.8
CAS—49745-95-1
A white powder. M.p. 184° to 186°.
Sparingly soluble in water and ethanol; soluble in methanol and pyridine.

Dissociation Constant. pK_a 9.5.

Colour Tests. Ammoniacal Silver Nitrate—black; *p*-Dimethylaminobenzaldehyde—orange/violet; Ferric Chloride—green; Folin–Ciocalteau Reagent—blue; Methanolic Potassium Hydroxide—brown-pink; Millon's Reagent—red; Nessler's Reagent—black; Palladium Chloride—orange→brown; Potassium Dichromate—green-brown.

Thin-layer Chromatography. System TA—Rf 52; system TB—Rf 00; system TC—Rf 01; system TE—Rf 49; system TL—Rf 03; system TAE—Rf 87.

Gas Chromatography. System GA—dobutamine-AC_4 RI 3495, M (*N*-desalkyl-*O*-methyl-)-AC_2 RI 2070, M (*N*-desalkyl-*O*-methyl-)-AC RI 2330, M (*O*-methyl-) RI 3200, M (*O*-methyl-)-AC_2 RI 3100, M (*O*-methyl-)-AC_3 RI 3350.

High Performance Liquid Chromatography. System HX—RI 308; system HAX—retention time 6.6 min; system HAY—retention time 3.8 min.

Ultraviolet Spectrum. Aqueous acid—279 (A_1^1=131b); aqueous alkali—236, 292 nm.

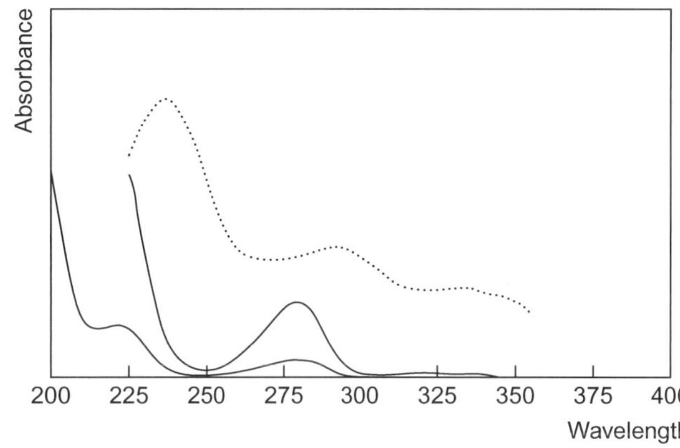

Infra-red Spectrum. Principal peaks at wavenumbers 1520, 1280, 1266, 1190, 1200, 1220 cm^{-1} (dobutamine hydrochloride, KBr disk).

Mass Spectrum. Principal ions at *m*/*z* 58, 107, 30, 178, 77, 56, 57, 137.

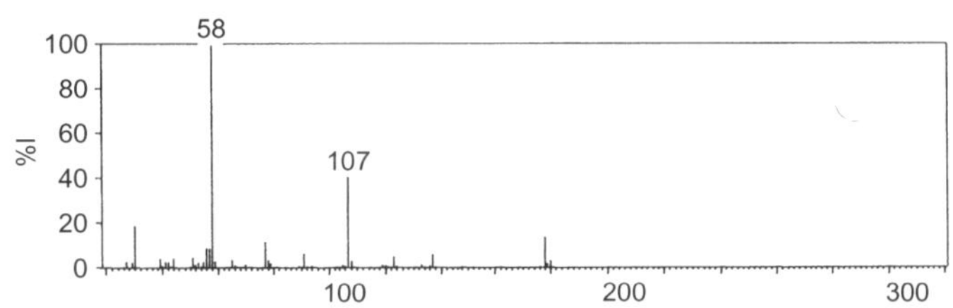

Quantification
High performance liquid chromatography. In equine plasma: limit of detection 100 µg/L, electrochemical detection—G. E. Hardee and J. W. Lai, *Anal. Lett. (Part B)*, 1983, *16*, 69–75. In plasma: limit of detection 1 µg/L, electrochemical detection—R. Dixon *et al.*, *Res. Commun. Chem. Pathol. Pharmacol.*, 1985, *48*, 313–316. In plasma: fluorescence detection—R. Knoll and M. Brandl, *Anasth. Intensivther. Notfallmed.*, 1986, *21*, 34–37. In plasma or urine: limits of detection 0.3 to 0.8 pg, fluorescence detection—G. Alberts *et al.*, *J. Chromatogr.*, 1992, *583*, 236–240. In plasma: limit of detection $<$0.1 µg/L, electrochemical detection—H. Husseini *et al.*, *J. Chromatogr.*, 1993, *620*, 164–168. In plasma: limit of detection 5 µg/L, fluorescence detection—C. Leflour *et al.*, *Biomed. Chromatogr.*, 1994, *8*, 309–312.

Disposition in the Body. Inactive after oral administration. After IV administration, it is rapidly metabolised by glucuronide conjugation and 3-*O*-methylation to inactive metabolites which are excreted in the urine, mostly in the first 2 hours.

Half-life. Plasma half-life, about 2 min.

Dose. Usually 2.5 to 10 µg/kg/min of dobutamine hydrochloride, by IV infusion.

Docetaxel

Antineoplastic

Synonyms. RP-56976; *N*-debenzoyl-*N*-*tert*-butoxycarbonyl-10-deacetyl taxol.
Proprietary name. Taxotere
(α*R*,β*S*)-β-[[(1,1-Dimethylethoxy)carbonyl]amino]-α-hydrobenzenepropanoic acid (2a*R*,4*S*,4a*S*,6*R*,9*S*,11*S*,12*S*,12a*R*,12b*S*)-12b-(acetyloxy)-12-(benzoyloxy)-2a,3,4,4a,5,6,9,10,11,12,12a,12b-dodecahydro-4,6,11-trihydroxy-4a,8,13,13-tetramethyl-5-oxo-7,11-methano-1*H*-cyclodeca[3,4]benz[1,2-*b*]oxet-9-yl ester
$C_{43}H_{53}NO_{14}$=807.9
CAS—114977-28-5

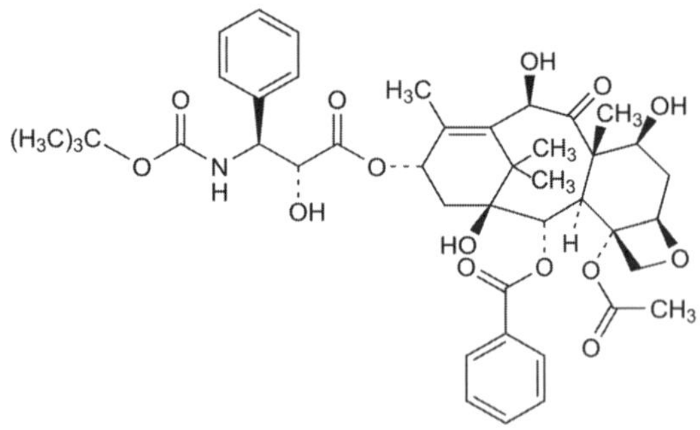

A white to almost white powder with m.p. 232°.

Docetaxel trihydrate
$C_{43}H_{59}NO_{17}$ = 861.9
CAS—148408-66-6

High Performance Liquid Chromatography. Column: RP-CSC-C_8 (Nucleosil, 150 × 4.6 mm i.d., 5 μm). Mobile phase: phosphate buffer (30 mM, pH 3.0):acetonitrile (47:53), 1.3 mL/min flow rate. UV detection (λ=227 nm). Retention time: 7.2 min. [M. R. Rouini *et al.*, *J. Pharm. Biomed. Anal.*, 1998, *17*, 1243–1247].

Column: (analytical) Inertsil ODS-80A (150 × 4.6 mm i.d., 5 μm), (guard) 100 RP-18 endcapped (Lichrospher, 4.0 × 4.0 mm, 5 μm) at 60°. Mobile phase: water:methanol:tetrahydrofuran:ammonium hydroxide (37.5:60:2.5:0.1), adjusted to pH 6.0 with formic acid, 1.0 mL/min flow rate. UV detection (λ=230 nm). Retention time: 8.5 min. [W. J. Loos *et al.*, *J. Chromatogr. Biomed. Sci. Appl.*, 1997, *693*, 437–441].

Ultraviolet Spectrum. Aqueous acid (ethanol)—230, 275, 283 nm.

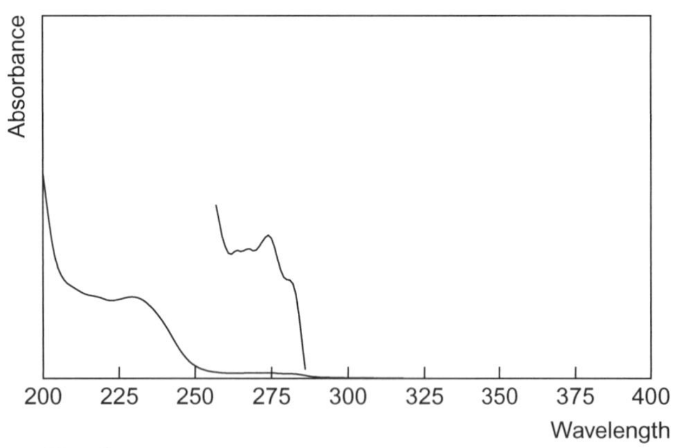

Quantification

High performance liquid chromatography. In plasma: limit of detection of docetaxel is 2.5 μg/L and limit of quantification 5 μg/L. UV detection (λ=227 nm)—M. R. Rouini *et al.*, *J. Pharm. Biomed. Anal.*, 1998, *17*, 1243–1247. In plasma: limit of quantification is 10 μg/L. UV detection (λ=227 nm)—W. J. Loos *et al.*, *J. Chromatogr. Biomed. Sci. Appl.*, 1997, *693*, 437–441.

Disposition in the Body. Docetaxel is rapidly distributed throughout the body into body tissue and is extensively metabolised by the hepatic cytochromes of the CYP3A group. Excretion is mainly in faeces (75%) as one major and three minor inactive metabolites and a very low amount of the unchanged drug.

Therapeutic concentration

4 patients with solid tumours, both male and female, were administered with an intravenous dose of 100 mg/m^2 docetaxel over 1 to 2 h. A peak plasma concentration of 2.41 mg/L was reached by the end of infusion. [J. M. Extra *et al.*, *Cancer Res.*, 1993, *53*, 1037–1042].

In another study, 7 patients administered with a 100 mg/m^2 dose reached peak plasma concentrations of 3.67 mg/L. [M. S. Aapro *et al.*, *Ann. Oncol.*, 1992, *3*, *Suppl. 5*, 53].

Toxicity. The maximum tolerated dose is 90 mg/m^2 as a 24-h infusion. Development of severe peripheral neurotoxicity has been observed in 4.1% of patients.

Half-life. Approx. 11 h.

Volume of distribution. 95 to 150 L/m^2 (from various studies), also reported as 113 L.

Clearance. 17 to 22 L/h/m^2 (as reported in various literature).

Distribution in blood. Little interaction with red blood cells.

Protein binding. > 95%.

Dose. Doses between 55 and 100 mg/m^2 body surface are administered for 1 h every 3 weeks; the greater dose is the usual dose. Lower doses are given if adverse reactions are observed during treatment. Patients with hepatic impairment: 75 mg/m^2.

Docusate Sodium *Anionic Surfactant*

Synonyms. Dioctyl Sodium Sulfosuccinate; DSS; Sodium Dioctyl Sulphosuccinate.
Proprietary names. Colace; Coloxyl; Dialose; Dioctyl; Disonate; Docusoft; Docusol; DOK; Modane Soft; Molcer; Norgalax; Regulex; Silace; Waxsol. It is an ingredient of Capsuvac, Klyx, Migraleve, and Normax.
Sodium 1,4-bis(2-ethylhexyl) sulfosuccinate
$C_{20}H_{37}NaO_7S$=444.6
CAS—10041-19-7 [1,4-bis(2-ethylhexyl) sulfosuccinate]; 577-11-7 (sodium salt)

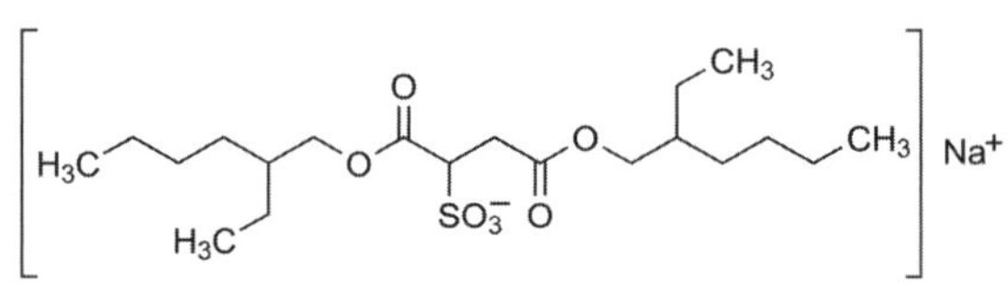

White, hygroscopic, waxy masses or flakes.
Slowly soluble 1 in 70 of water, higher concentrations forming a thick gel; soluble 1 in 3 of ethanol, 1 in 1 of chloroform, and 1 in 1 of ether; soluble in carbon tetrachloride, petroleum ether, naphtha, xylene, dibutyl phthalate, liquid petrolatum, acetone, and vegetable oils.

Docusate Calcium
Synonym. Dioctyl Calcium Sulfosuccinate
Proprietary names. Surfak. It is an ingredient of Doxidan.
$C_{40}H_{74}CaO_{14}S_2$=883.2
CAS—128-49-4
A white amorphous solid.
Soluble 1 in 3300 of water; freely soluble in ethanol, chloroform, and ether; soluble in mineral and vegetable oils and liquid polyethylene glycol; practically insoluble in glycerol.

Docusate Potassium
Synonym. Dioctyl Potassium Sulfosuccinate
Proprietary names. Dialose; Kasof.
$C_{20}H_{37}KO_7S$=460.7
CAS—7491-09-0
A white amorphous solid.
Sparingly soluble in water; soluble in ethanol; very soluble in light petroleum.

Partition Coefficient. Log *P* (octanol/water), 6.1.

Colour Tests. To 5 mL of a 0.1% solution add 1 mL of dilute sulfuric acid, 10 mL of chloroform, and 0.2 mL of dimethyl yellow solution, and shake—the chloroform layer is coloured red. Add 50 mg of cetrimide and shake—the colour of the chloroform layer changes to yellow.

Infra-red Spectrum. Principal peaks at wavenumbers 1724, 1250, 1052, 1020, 1612, 1086 cm^{-1}.

Disposition in the Body. Absorbed after oral administration and excreted in the bile. It is excreted in breast milk.

Dose. 50 to 500 mg daily as a laxative.

Dodecyl Gallate *Antoxidant*

Synonym. Lauril Gallate
Proprietary names. Progallin LA. It is an ingredient of Embanox 7.
Dodecyl 3,4,5-trihydroxybenzoate

$C_{19}H_{30}O_5$=338.4
CAS—1166-52-5

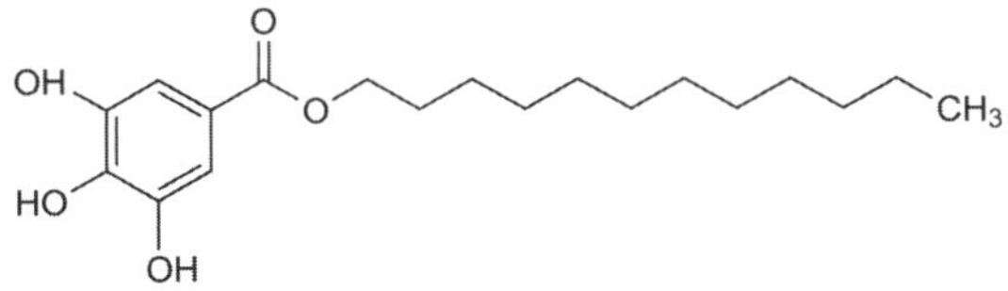

A white or creamy-white powder. M.p. 96° to 97.5°.
Practically insoluble in water; soluble 1 in 3.5 of ethanol, 1 in 60 of chloroform, and 1 in 4 of ether.

Colour Tests. Ammoniacal Silver Nitrate—black; Ferric Chloride—blue; Folin–Ciocalteau Reagent—blue; Methanolic Potassium Hydroxide—orange; Nessler's Reagent—black.

Ultraviolet Spectrum. Methanol—275 nm (A_1^1=300b).

Dofamium Chloride

Cationic Disinfectant

Synonym. Phenamylium Chloride
Dimethyl [2-(*N*-methyldodecanamido)ethyl][(phenylcarbamoyl)methyl]ammonium chloride
$C_{25}H_{44}ClN_3O_2$=454.1
CAS—54063-35-3

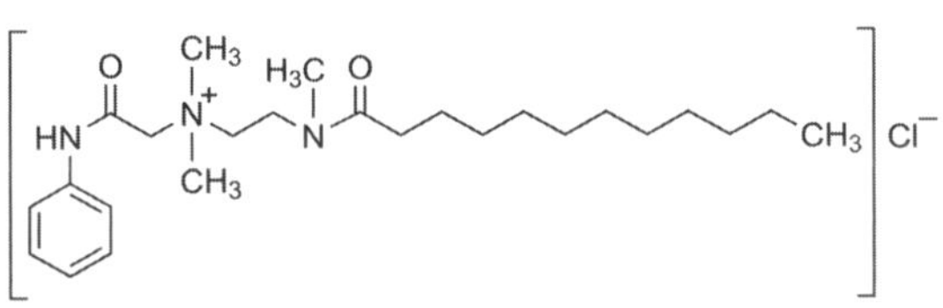

A white crystalline powder.
Soluble in water.

Colour Test. Mandelin's Test—red→brown.

Thin-layer Chromatography. System TA—Rf 03. (Acidified iodoplatinate solution, positive.)

Gas Chromatography. System GA—RI 1676, 1898, and 1974.

Ultraviolet Spectrum. Aqueous acid—244 nm (A_1^1=242b).

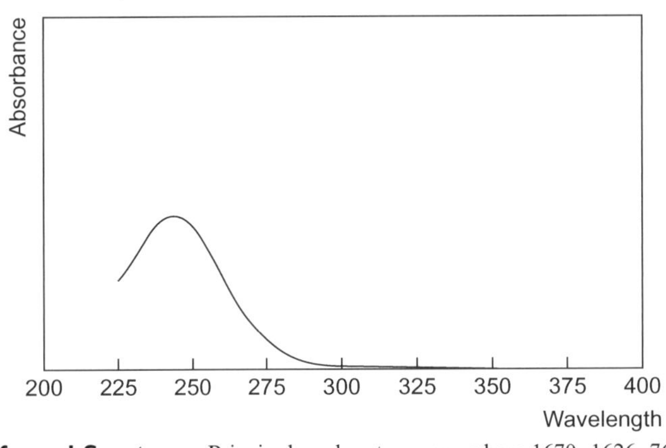

Infra-red Spectrum. Principal peaks at wavenumbers 1670, 1626, 760, 1538, 1592, 1298 cm^{-1}.

Dofetilide

Anti-arrhythmic

Synonym. UK-68798
Proprietary name. Tikosyn
N-[4-[2-[Methyl[2-[4-[(methylsulfonyl)amino]phenoxy]ethyl]amino]-ethyl]phenyl]methane sulfonamide
$C_{19}H_{27}N_3O_5S$=441.6
CAS—115256-11-6

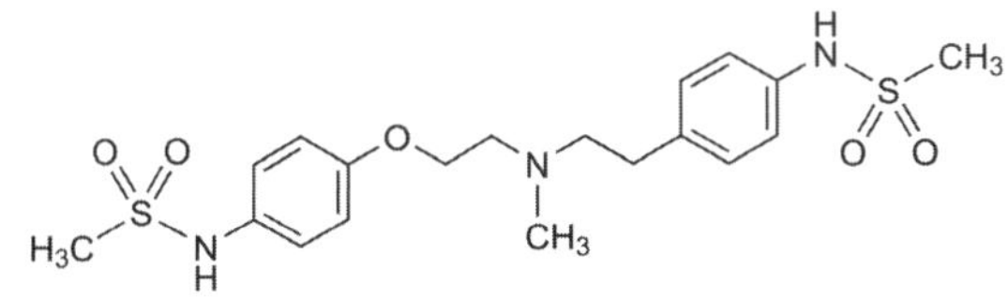

A white to off-white crystalline solid. M.p. 161°. It is very slightly soluble in water and propan-2-ol; soluble in 0.1 M sodium hydroxide, acetone and 0.1 M hydrochloric acid.

Dissociation Constant. pK_a 7.0; 9.0; 9.6.

Partition Coefficient. Log *P* (octanol/buffer pH 7.4), 0.96.

High Performance Liquid Chromatography. Column: silica (Spherisorb, 250 × 4.6 mm i.d., 5 µm). Mobile phase: acetonitrile:ammonium phosphate buffer, pH 7.0 (35:65), 1.0 mL/min flow rate. UV detection (λ=230 nm). Retention times: dofetilide, 8.5 min; *N*-desmethyl metabolite, 7.5 min. [D. K. Walker *et al.*, *J. Chromatogr.* 1991, *568(2)*; *Biomed. Appl.*, 475–480].

Quantification

High performance liquid chromatography. In urine: limit of detection is 2.5 µg/L, UV detection (λ=230 nm)—D. K. Walker *et al.*, *J. Chromatogr.* 1991, *568(2)*; *Biomed. Appl.*, 475–480.

Disposition in the Body. Dofetilide is almost completely absorbed after oral administration and peak plasma concentrations are observed after 3 h. The presence of food increases the time taken to reach these concentrations but does not alter the oral bioavailability. Steady state concentrations are reached within 2 to 3 days. It is metabolised, in the liver, by *N*-oxidation and *N*-dealkylation to essentially inactive metabolites. Approximately 80% of an administered dose is excreted in urine; mostly as the unchanged drug (80%) and the rest as inactive or minimal activity metabolites. No quantifiable amounts of metabolites have been detected in plasma but five have been detected in urine.

Therapeutic concentration

18 male and female patients with coronary artery disease, mean age 55 years (range 42 to 65 years), were administered with doses of 1.5, 3.0 and 4.5 µg/kg dofetilide at a constant infusion rate over 10 min. The mean peak plasma concentrations were 1.74 (0.70 to 2.51) µg/L, 3.35 (2.7 to 3.86) µg/L and 5.11 (3.25 to 6.47) µg/L for the three doses. These concentrations were observed at the end of the infusion period. [M. Sedgwick *et al.*, *Br. J. Clin. Pharmacol.*, 1991, *31*, 515–519].

10 healthy males (mean age 23.4 years; range 19 to 30 years) were administered 0.5 mg dofetilide orally and 0.5 mg intravenously as a continuous infusion over a 30-min period. A wash-out period of 1 week was allowed between treatments. The peak plasma concentrations were 1.9 (range, 1.3 to 2.4) µg/L for the oral dose, observed at 2.6 (1.5 to 4.0) h, and 6.0 (3.7 to 8.2) µg/L for the intravenous dose. [F. Le Coz *et al.*, *Clin. Pharmacol. Ther.*, 1995, *57(5)*, 533–542].

Healthy males aged 18 to 45 years (mean 25 years) were divided into three groups and treated with dofetilide. Group 1: 1.0 mg daily (0.33 mg three times a day) and 0.5 mg twice daily; group 2: 1.5 mg daily (0.5 mg three times daily) and 0.75 mg twice daily; group 3: 2.5 mg daily (1.25 mg twice daily) and 0.83 mg three times daily. Each volunteer participated in a 5-day dosing period with a 6-day washout in between. For group 1, the peak plasma concentrations were 1.7 µg/L for the 0.33 mg dose on day 1 and 2.64 µg/L for the 0.5 mg dose. These concentrations were observed at 2.29 and 2.00 h, respectively. On day 5, the concentrations were 3.04 and 3.80 µg/L for the two doses, observed at 2 h. For group 2, peak plasma concentrations were 2.26 µg/L for the 0.5 mg dose on day 1 and 3.54 µg/L for the 0.75 mg dose, observed at 2.13 h. On day 5, the concentrations were 4.78 and 5.23 µg/L for the two doses, observed at 2.0 and 1.88 h, respectively. For group 3, concentrations reached 3.55 µg/L for the 0.83 mg dose on day 1 and 5.47 µg/L for the 1.25 mg dose. These were observed at 2.29 and 1.57 h, respectively. On day 5, concentrations were 7.71 and 10.07 µg/L for the two doses, observed at 2.14 and 1.57 h, respectively. Steady state concentrations were reached by day 3. [M. J. Allen *et al.*, *Br. J. Clin. Pharmacol.*, 2000, *50(3)*, 247–253].

Toxicity

In some patients, dofetilide can cause an abnormal heartbeat which in rare instances can result in death. Symptoms are fast beating of the heart, dizziness and fainting which usually occur in the first few days of treatment. [As described in the Patient Information Leaflet, Pfizer Ltd.].

Above the recommended therapeutic dose, 500 μg twice daily, the degree of QT prolongation and the subsequent risk of cardiac arrhythmia is considered unacceptable. [M. J. Allen *et al.*, *Br. J. Clin. Pharmacol.*, 2000, *50(3)*, 247–253].

Bioavailability. 92 to 99%.

Half-life. Plasma elimination, 6.2 to 9.7 h; half-life increases with renal impairment.

Volume of distribution. 226 to 249 L; 3.8 L/kg.

Clearance. Systemic clearance, 0.35 L/h/kg; plasma, 4.7 mL/min/kg; 20.8 to 28.2 L/h; clearance decreases with renal impairment.

Protein binding. 60 to 70%.

Dose. The recommended oral dose is 500 μg twice daily (normal renal function); 250 μg twice daily (creatinine clearance, 40 to 60 mL/min); 125 μg twice daily (creatinine clearance, 20 to 40 mL/min).

Dolasetron

Anti-emetic

Synonym. MDL-73147
1*H*-Indole-3-carboxylic acid (2α,6α,8α,9a*β*)-octahydro-3-oxo-2,6-methano-2*H*-quinolizin-8-yl ester
$C_{19}H_{20}N_2O_3$ = 324.4
CAS—115956-12-2

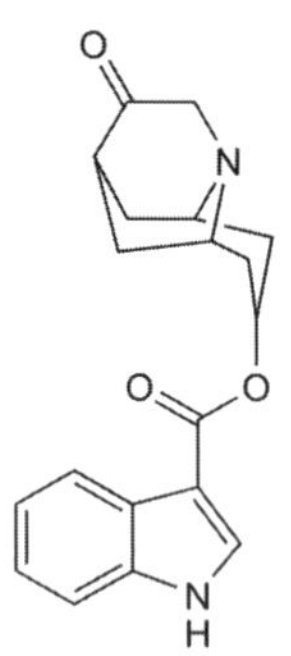

Dolasetron Methanesulfonate

Synonyms. Dolasetron mesylate; MDL-73147EF.
Proprietary names. Anzemet
$C_{19}H_{20}N_2O_3,CH_3SO_3H$ = 420.5
CAS—115956-13-3
A white to off-white powder. M.p. 278°. It is freely soluble in water and propylene glycol; slightly soluble in ethanol and normal saline.

Gas Chromatography. Column: DB-5 (7.5 m × 0.32 mm i.d., 0.25 μm film thickness). Column temperature: 170°, held 1 min, increased to 270° at 20°/min, held 2 min. Injector temperature: 275°. MS detection. Retention time: 6.45 min. [T. A. Gillespie *et al.*, *J. Pharm. Biomed. Anal.*, 1993, *11(10)*, 955–962].

High Performance Liquid Chromatography. Column: CN Spherisorb (150 × 4.6 mm i.d., 3 μm). Mobile phase: acetonitrile:ammonium acetate buffer (0.05 M, pH adjusted to 7.5 with ammonium hydroxide) (24:76), 0.8 mL/min flow rate. UV detection (λ = 280 nm). Internal standard (IS): methyl analogue of reduced dolasetron. Retention time: dolasetron, 7.2 min; IS 19.5 min. [T. A. Gillespie *et al.*, *J. Pharm. Biomed. Anal.*, 1993, *11(10)*, 955–962].

Column: (analytical) Nucleosil C_4 (250 × 4.6 mm, 5 μm), stainless steel; (guard) μBondapak C_{18} (40 × 6 mm, 10 μm). Mobile phase: (A)-acetonitrile:ammonium acetate (0.05 M) (10:90); (B)-acetonitrile:ammonium acetate (0.05 M) (60:40), pH adjusted to 4.7 with addition of glacial acetic acid (both mobile phases). Gradient elution—100% A to 100% B over 30 min, 1.0 mL/min flow rate. UV detection (λ = 280 mn). Retention time (*k*): hydrodolasetron, 18.9 min (8.95). [P. Sanwald *et al.*, *J. Chromatogr.* 1994, *661, Biomed. Appl.*, 101–107].

Column: (analytical) Ultrasphere IP(C_{18}) (150 × 4.6 mm i.d., 5 μm); (guard) μBondapak C_{18} (40 × 6 mm i.d., 10 μm). Mobile phase: sodium dihydrogenphosphate (0.05 M, adjusted to pH 2.5 with orthophosphoric acid):*n*-butanol:acetonitrile (89:6:5), 0.7 mL/min flow rate. Fluorescence detection (λ_{ex} = 285 nm, λ_{em} = 345 nm). Retention time: dolasetron mesylate, 7.6 min (retention factor, 3.2); hydrodolasetron, 8.7 min (3.9). [N. D. Huebert *et al.*, *J. Chromatogr.* 1996, *685(2)*; *Biomed. Appl.*, 291–297].

Ultraviolet Spectrum. Aqueous acid—229, 282 nm.

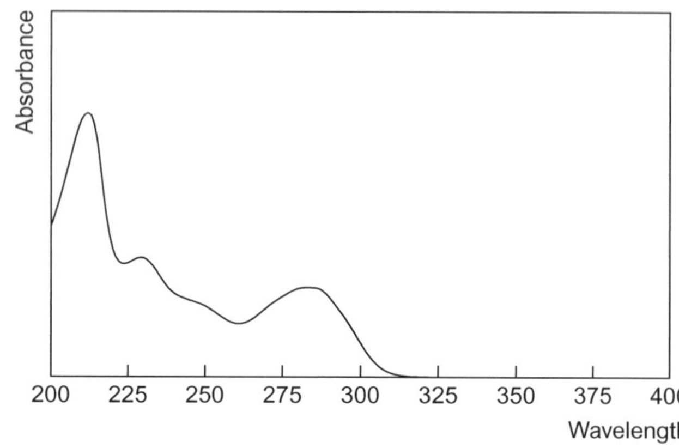

Mass Spectrum. Principal ions at *m/z* 134, 93, 135, 144, 94, 116, 296, 136.

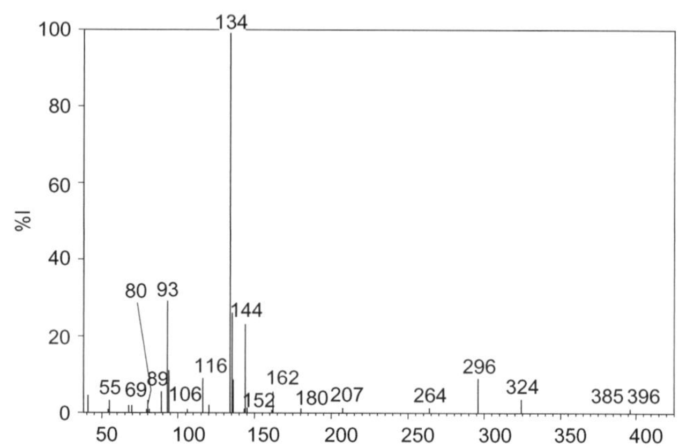

Quantification

Gas chromatography–mass spectrometry. In plasma: limit of quantification 2 μg/L—T. A. Gillespie *et al.*, *J. Pharm. Biomed. Anal.*, 1993, *11(10)*, 955–962.

High performance liquid chromatography. In plasma and urine: limit of quantification is 4 μg/L for dolasetron and 2 μg/L for hydrodolasetron in plasma and 20 μg/L for both in urine. Fluorescence detection (λ_{ex} = 285 nm, λ_{em} = 345 nm)—N. D. Huebert *et al.*, *J. Chromatogr.* 1996, *685(2)*; *Biomed. Appl.*, 291–297. In plasma: limit of quantification is 200 μg/L. UV detection (λ = 280 nm)—P. Sanwald *et al.*, *J. Chromatogr.* 1994, *661*; *Biomed. Appl.*, 101–107. In plasma: limit of quantification is 1.7 μg/L. Fluorescence detection (λ_{ex} = 274 nm, λ_{em} = 345 nm)—J. S. McElvain *et al.*, *J. Pharm. Biomed. Anal.*, 1997, *15(4)*, 485–492. In plasma: limit of quantification is 10 μg/L. UV detection (λ = 280 nm)—T. A. Gillespie *et al.*, *J. Pharm. Biomed. Anal.*, 1993, *11(10)*, 955–962.

Disposition in the Body. Dolasetron is rapidly absorbed and subsequently metabolised to hydrodolasetron (with the most clinically relevant activity) by carbonyl reductase. The metabolite appears rapidly in plasma with peak concentrations appearing within the hour; the parent drug is rarely detected. Food does not affect the abosorption of the drug. Hydrodolasetron undergoes additional hydroxylation (cytochrome P450 isoenzyme, CYP2D6) and *N*-oxidation (by flavin mono-oxygenase and isoenzyme, CYP3A). It is excreted in urine as hydrodolasetron (53% of administered intravenous dose) and other metabolites including hydroxylated glucuronides and *N*-oxide. Approximately two-thirds of an administered dose is detected in urine and the remainder in faeces.

Therapeutic concentration

Group 1: 6 healthy volunteers with a mean age 41.5 years (34 to 53 years); group 2: 7 patients with mild hepatic impairment (Child-Pugh class A), mean age 40.7 (34 to 46 years); group 3: 4 patients with moderate to severe impairment (class B or C1), mean age 48.5 (42 to 52) years. All participants had creatinine clearance >70 mL/min and were fasted overnight before treatment. Each subject was administered a single 150 mg oral and an intravenous dose of dolasetron mesylate over a 10-min infusion period. A 7-day washout period was allowed between the two doses. For the oral doses of the drug, mean peak plasma dolasetron concentrations were 6 (range 0 to 12) μg/L, 37 (0 to 138) μg/L and 214 (137 to 289) μg/L for groups 1, 2 and 3, respectively. These concentrations were observed between 0.25 and 1.0 h. The mean peak hydrodolasetron concentrations were 347 (range 170 to 526) μg/L, 387 (258 to 542) μg/L and 410 (374 to 466) μg/L for the three groups, observed between 0.5 and 2.0 h. After intravenous administration of dolasetron, peak plasma concentrations were 3055 (2358 to 5584) μg/L for group 1, 2098 (792 to 4025) μg/L for group 2 and 3299 (2371 to 4871) μg/L for group 3. These concentrations were observed at 0.18 h (0.1 to 0.28 h). Peak hydrodolasetron concentrations were 424 (339 to 492) μg/L, 473 (375 to 610) μg/L and 396 (278 to 602) μg/L for the three groups, respectively, observed at 0.25 to 1.0 h. [K. Stubbs *et al.*, *J. Clin. Pharmacol.*, 1997, *37(10)*, 926–936].

Group 1: 12 male and female patients with mild to moderate renal impairment (creatinine clearance, 41 to 80 mL/min), mean age 62.8 years; group 2: 12 patients with moderate to severe renal impairment (creatinine clearance, 11 to 40 mL/min), mean age 50.7 years; group 3: 12 patients, mean age 51.8 years, with end-stage renal impairment undergoing chronic haemodialysis (creatinine clearance ⩽10 mL/min); group 4: 24 healthy male volunteers (creatinine clearance, >80 mL/min), mean age 23.8 years. All subjects were fasted overnight and administered 200 mg dolasetron mesylate orally and intravenously as a 10-min infusion, with a 7-day washout period between doses. Peak plasma hydrodolasetron concentrations were 775.7, 812.8, 866.5 and 646.9 μg/L for groups 1, 2, 3 and 4, respectively, following the intravenous dose. these concentrations were observed at 0.72, 0.77, 0.69 and 0.67 h, respectively. After the oral dose, concentrations were 742.7, 680.9, 700.8 and 601.2 μg/L at 0.81, 0.79, 0.72 and 0.74 h, respectively, for the four groups. [D. C. Dimmitt *et al.*, *J. Clin. Pharmacol.*, 1998, *38*, 798–806].

Toxicity. Symptoms of acute toxicity include tremors, depression and convulsions. Dolasetron has been associated with electrocardiogram interval changes; magnitude and frequency are dependent on the concentration of the metabolite, hydrodolasetron, in the blood. This can lead to cardiovascular effects including heart block and cardiac arrhythmias.

Bioavailability. 75%.

Half-life. Hydrodolasetron, 8.1 h.

Volume of distribution. 1.4 L/kg (patients with mild to moderate renal impairment); 1.5 L/kg (moderate to severe renal impairment); 3.65 L/kg (end-stage renal impairment); 1.03 L/kg (healthy individuals). Hydrodolasetron, 5.8 L/kg.

Clearance. Systemic clearance, 55.7 mL/min/kg (patients with mild to moderate renal impairment); 117.5 mL/min/kg (moderate to severe renal impairment); 66.1 mL/min/kg (end-stage renal impairment); 114.9 mL/min/kg (healthy individuals). Apparent clearance, hydrodolasetron, 9.4 to 13.4 mL/min/kg.

Protein binding. 69 to 77%.

Dose. Orally: adults, 100 mg 1 h before chemotherapy or within 2 h before surgery. Children (2 to 16 years old), 1.8 mg/kg body weight within 1 h of chemotherapy; a maximum of 100 mg; alternatively, 1.2 mg/kg body weight within 2 h before surgery.
By injection: adults, 100 mg 30 min before chemotherapy; alternatively, 12.5 mg 15 min before anaesthesia has finished before surgery. Children (2 to 16 years old), 1.8 mg/kg 30 min before chemotherapy, maximum 100 mg; alternatively, 0.35 mg/kg 15 min before the end of anaesthesia, maximum 12.5 mg.

DOM

Hallucinogen

Synonyms. 2,5-Dimethoxy-4-methylamfetamine; 2,5-Dimethoxy-4-metamfetamine.
2,5-Dimethoxy-α,4-dimethylbenzeneethanamine
$C_{12}H_{19}NO_2$=209.3
CAS—15588-95-1

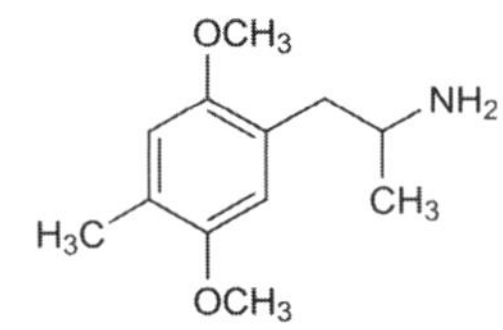

DOM is reported to be the active principle of the hallucinogenic preparation known as STP. (STP has also been used as a synonym for DOM.)
M.p. 60.5° to 61.0°.
Practically insoluble in water; soluble in chloroform.

DOM Hydrochloride
$C_{12}H_{19}NO_2$, HCl=245.7
CAS—15589-00-1
White crystals. M.p. 189° to 189.5° (from isopropanol/ether).

Partition Coefficient. Log *P* (octanol/water), 2.2.

Colour Test. Marquis Test—yellow

Thin-layer Chromatography. System TA—Rf 51; system TB—Rf 15; system TC—Rf 17; system TE—Rf 41; system TL—Rf 16; system TAE—Rf 09; system TAF—Rf 76. (Dragendorff spray, positive; FPN reagent, positive; acidified iodoplatinate solution, positive; Marquis reagent, yellow; ninhydrin spray, positive; acidified potassium permanganate solution, positive.)

Gas Chromatography. System GA—DOM RI 1616, DOM-PFP RI 1730, DOM-AC RI 2020, DOM-AC_2 RI 2090, art (formyl) RI 1565, M (*O*-desmethyl-)-PFP_2 RI 1780, M (OH-)-AC_2 RI 2260, M (desamino-oxo-OH-)-PFP_2 RI 2045, M (desamino-oxo-OH-)-AC_2 RI 2560; system GB—RI 1652.

High Performance Liquid Chromatography. System HC—*k* 1.13; system HX—RI 340.

Ultraviolet Spectrum. Aqueous acid—289 nm (A_1^1=221b).

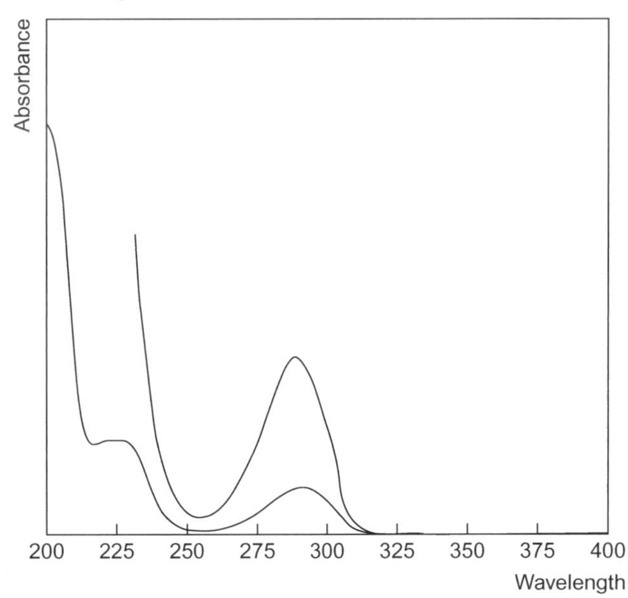

Infra-red Spectrum. Principal peaks at wavenumbers 1208, 1041, 1541, 1515, 1634, 1094 cm^{-1}.

Mass Spectrum. Principal ions at *m/z* 44, 166, 151, 57, 43, 91, 135, 209.

Disposition in the Body. About 20% of an ingested dose is excreted in the urine unchanged in 24 h; peak urinary excretion occurs 3 to 6 h after ingestion.

Domiphen Bromide

Cationic Disinfectant

Synonym. Phenododecinium Bromide
Proprietary names. Antiseptique Pastilles; Bradoral; Bronchodex Pastilles; Neobradoral; Oraseptic. It is an ingredient of Bradosol.

It consists chiefly of *N*,*N*-dimethyl-*N*-(2-phenoxyethyl)-1-dodecanaminium bromide
$C_{22}H_{40}BrNO=414.5$
CAS—13900-14-6 (domiphen); 538-71-6 (bromide)

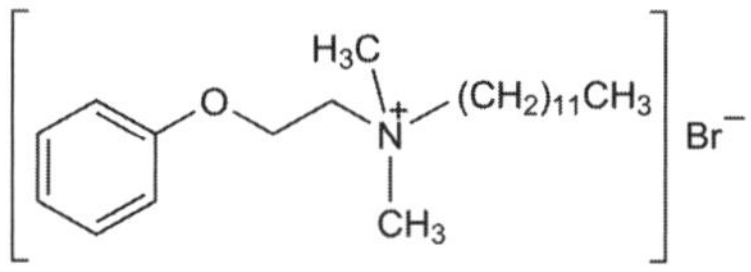

Colourless or faintly yellow crystalline flakes. M.p. 112° to 113°.
Soluble 1 in less than 2 of water and of ethanol, and 1 in 30 of acetone; soluble in ethyl acetate and chloroform; very slightly soluble in benzene.

Partition Coefficient. Log *P* (octanol/water), 4.2.

Colour Test. Dissolve 10 mg in 10 mL of water, add 0.1 mL of a 0.5% aqueous eosin solution and 100 mL of water—pink.

Thin-layer Chromatography. System TA—Rf 05. (Acidified iodoplatinate solution, positive.)

Gas Chromatography. System GA—RI 2310.

High Performance Liquid Chromatography. System HY—RI 506 (domiphen).

Ultraviolet Spectrum. Methanol—268 (A^{1}_{1}=30a), 277 nm.

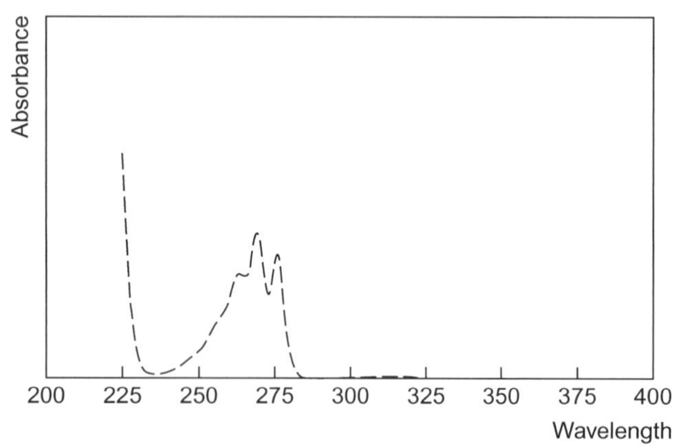

Infra-red Spectrum. Principal peaks at wavenumbers 1228, 752, 1500, 1600, 689, 1080 cm^{-1} (KBr disk).

Dose. Lozenges containing 500 µg of domiphen bromide are available.

Donepezil

Nootropic

Synonym. ER-4111
2,3-Dihydro-5,6-dimethoxy-2-[[1-(phenylmethyl)-4-piperidinyl]methyl]-1*H*-inden-1-one
$C_{24}H_{29}NO_3=379.5$
CAS—120014-06-4

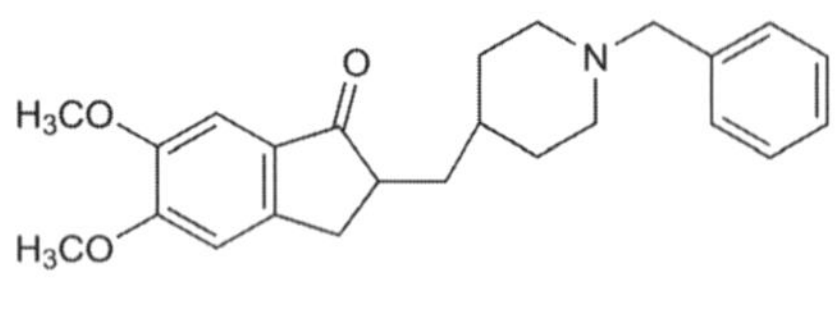

Donepezil Hydrochloride
Synonyms. BNAG; E2020.
Proprietary names. Aricept; Memac.
$C_{24}H_{29}NO_3,HCl=416.0$
CAS—120011-70-3
A white to off-white solid with m.p. 224°. It is soluble in water (55 g/L at 25°); freely soluble in chloroform and glacial acetic acid.

Dissociation Constant. pK_a 8.90.

High Performance Liquid Chromatography. Column: C_{18} (Nucleosil, 250 × 4.6 mm i.d., 5 mm). Mobile phase: acetonitrile (60%):sodium dodecyl sulfate (5 mmol/L, pH 3.5). UV detection. Retention time: donepezil hydrochloride, 7 min. [A. Ohnishi *et al*, *J. Clin. Pharmacol.*, 1993, *33*, 1086–1091].

Ultraviolet Spectrum. Aqueous acid—230, 271, 316 nm. No alkaline shift.

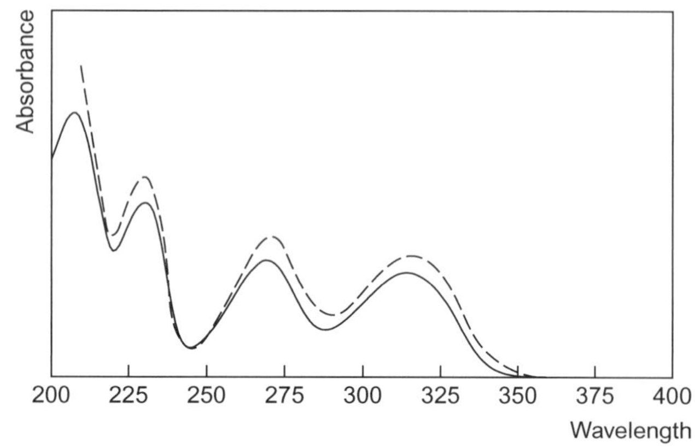

Infra-red Spectrum. Principal peaks at wavenumbers 1605, 1589, 1500, 749, 702 cm^{-1}.

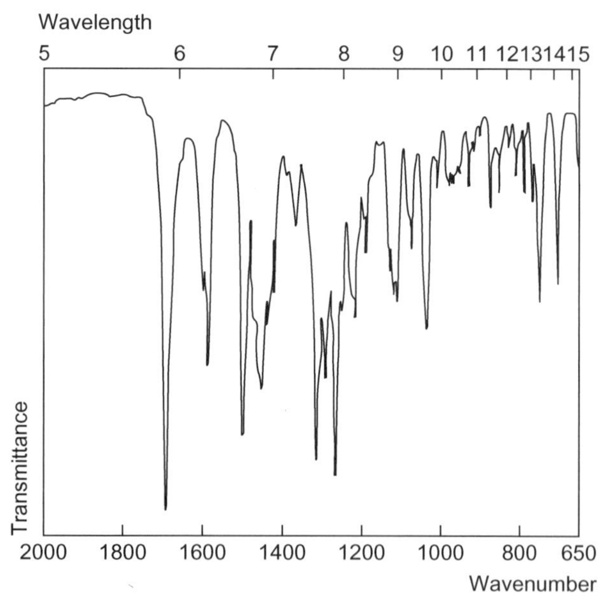

Mass Spectrum. Principal ions at *m*/*z* 288, 379, 91, 175, 172, 189, 378, 191.

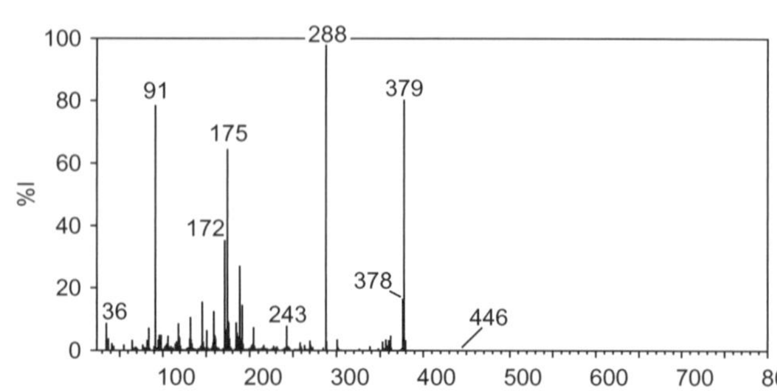

Quantification

High performance liquid chromatography. In plasma and urine: limit of detection, for donepezil hydrochloride, 0.5 µg/L and 2.0 µg/L, respectively and for its metabolites 5.0 µg/L, UV detection—A. Ohnishi *et al.*, *J. Clin.*

Pharmacol., 1993, *33*, 1086–1091. In serum: limit of quantification 0.02 µg/L. MS-MS detection—K. Matsui *et al.*, *J. Chromatogr. Biomed. Sci. Appl.*, 1999, *729*, 147–155.

Disposition in the Body. Donepezil is well absorbed from the gastro-intestinal tract after oral administration and is partially metabolised in the liver by cytochrome P450. *O*-Dealkylation followed by hydroxylation and partial subsequent glucuronidation or hydrolysis produces four major metabolites which are known to be active, and several minor metabolites. Over 10 days, 57% of a single dose is recovered as metabolites in urine and 15% in faeces; 17% of the drug remains unchanged and is excreted in urine; 28% is unrecovered, possibly owing to accumulation.

Therapeutic concentration

48 healthy males (non-smokers) were administered a single dose of donepezil, 2, 4 or 6 mg. Maximum plasma concentrations reached 3.2 ± 0.6, 6.9 ± 0.7, 11.6 ± 2.8 µg/L, respectively. Plasma concentration rises in proportion to the dose (the same for multiple dose studies). These concentrations were reached within 1.7 to 6.6 h. [S. L. Rogers and L. T. Friedhoff, *Br. J. Clin. Pharmacol.*, 1998, *46 Suppl. 1*, 1–6].

Half-life. Elimination, approx. 50 to 60 h (single dose); 75 h (steady state); 104 h (elderly).

Volume of distribution. 13.6 to14.8 L/kg.

Clearance. Body clearance, 0.12 L/h/kg.

Protein binding. Donepezil is bound approx. 95% to plasma proteins.

Dose. A 5 mg dose is administered once daily. After 4 to 6 weeks the dose can be increased to 10 mg daily, if necessary.

Dopamine

Sympathomimetic

Synonym. 3-Hydroxytyramine
4-(2-Aminoethyl)-1,2-benzenediol
$C_8H_{11}NO_2$ = 153.2
CAS—51-61-6

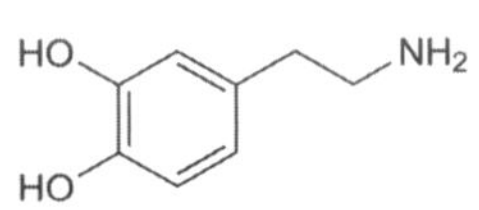

Crystals.

Dopamine Hydrochloride

Proprietary names. Abbodop; Cordodopa; Dopamex; Dopaminex; Docard; Dopmin; Drynalken; Drynalquin; Dynatra; Dynos; Giludop; Inopin; Inovan; Intropin; Inotropisa; Medopa; Revimine; Revivan; Zetarina.
$C_8H_{11}NO_2$,HCl = 189.6
CAS—62-31-7
A white crystalline powder. M.p. about 241°, with decomposition.
Freely soluble in water; soluble in methanol and ethanol; practically insoluble in ether, petroleum ether, chloroform, benzene, and toluene.

Dissociation Constant pK_a 8.8, 10.6 (20°).

Partition Coefficient. Log *P* (octanol/water), −1.0.

Colour Tests. Ammoniacal Silver Nitrate—orange-brown/black; *p*-Dimethylaminobenzaldehyde—orange/violet; Ferric Chloride—green; Folin–Ciocalteau Reagent—blue; Marquis Test—brown-violet; Methanolic Potassium Hydroxide—blue→orange→brown; Nessler's Reagent—black; Potassium Dichromate—green→brown (30 s).

Thin-layer Chromatography. System TA—Rf 18, streaking; system TB—Rf 00; system TC—Rf 00; system TE—Rf 43; system TL—Rf 00; system TAE—Rf 14; system TAF—Rf 59; system TAJ—Rf 00; system TAK—Rf 00; system TAL—Rf 07. (Acidified potassium permanganate solution, positive.)

Gas Chromatography. System GA—dopamine RI 2175, M (*O*-methyl-)-AC_2 RI 2070, M (*O*-methyl-)-AC.

High Performance Liquid Chromatography. System HA—*k* 2.7 (tailing peak); system HZ—retention time 1.7 min.

Ultraviolet Spectrum. Aqueous acid—280 nm (A_1^1 = 178a).

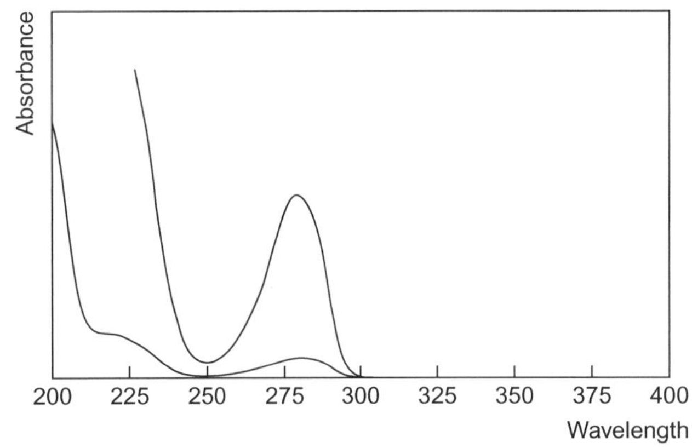

Infra-red Spectrum. Principal peaks at wavenumbers 1503, 1287, 1190, 1174, 813, 1115 cm^{-1} (KBr disk).

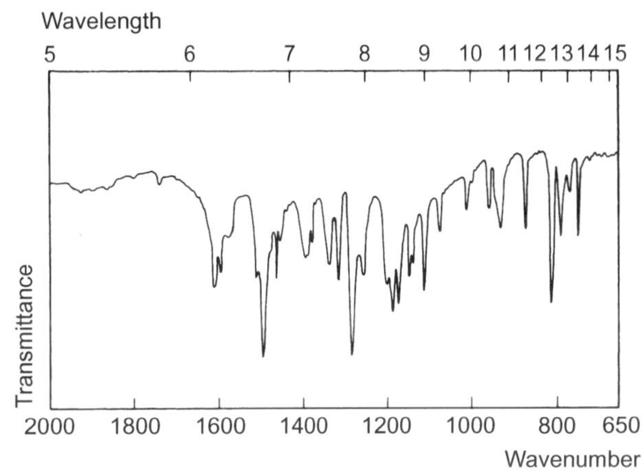

Quantification. See under Levodopa.

Disposition in the Body. Dopamine is a naturally occurring catecholamine and is considered to be the metabolic precursor of noradrenaline. It is inactivated after oral administration. It is excreted mainly as 3,4-dihydroxyphenylacetic acid (DOPAC) and 3-methoxy-4-hydroxyphenylacetic acid (homovanillic acid); noradrenaline (norepinephrine) and 3-methoxytyramine are also metabolites.
Dopamine is a metabolite of levodopa.

Dose. Initially 2 to 5 µg/kg/min of dopamine hydrochloride, by IV infusion.

Dopexamine

Beta-adrenergic Agonist

Synonym. FPL-60278
4-[2-[[6-(Phenylethylamino)hexyl]amino]ethyl]pyrocatechol
$C_{22}H_{32}N_2O_2$ = 356.5
CAS—86197-47-9

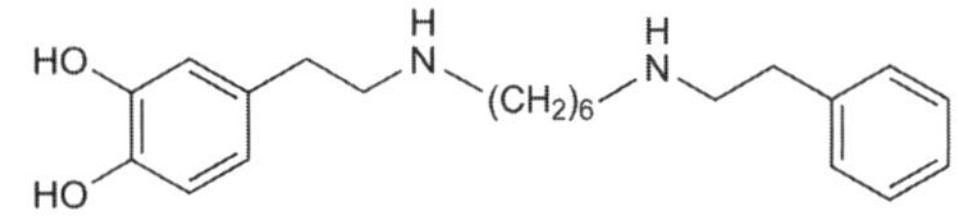

Dopexamine Dihydrochloride

Synonym. FPL-60278AR
Proprietary name. Dopacard
$C_{22}H_{32}N_2O_2$,2HCl = 429.4
CAS—86484-91-5

Partition Coefficient. Log *P* (octanol/water), 4.27.

Thin-Layer Chromatography. System TB—Rf 00; system TE—Rf 16; system TAE—Rf 00.

High Performance Liquid Chromatography. System HX—RI 289.

Columns: (pre-column) silica (250 × 4.6 mm i.d., 25 to 40 μm) connected before autosampler to condition mobile phase; (analytical) ODS silica (Hypersil, 250 × 4.9 mm i.d., 5 μm). Column temperature: 37° to 43°. Mobile phase: methanol:sodium heptane-1-sulfonate (4.04 g/L), disodium EDTA (1 mmol/L), orthophosphoric acid (10 ml/L) and di-isopropylamine (22.5 ml/L) (49:51). 1.2 mL/min flow rate. Electrochemical detection. Retention time: dopexamine hydrochloride, 7.0 to 7.3 min. [P. R. Baker *et al.*, *J. Chromatogr.* 1995, *667*; *Biomed. Appl.*, 283–290].

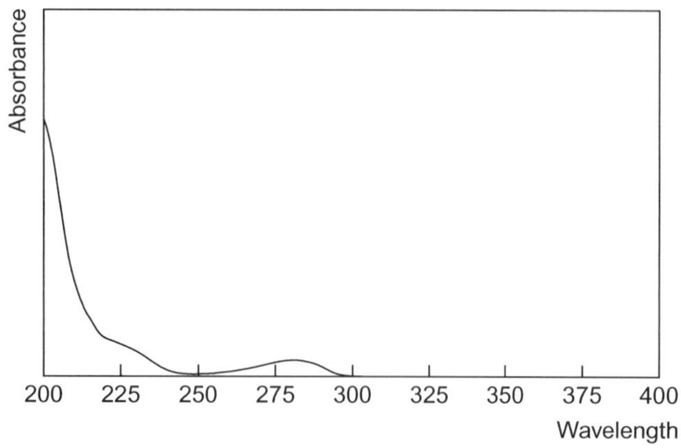

Quantification

High performance liquid chromatography. In whole blood: limit of quantification 5 μg/L, electrochemical detection—P. R. Baker *et al.*, *J. Chromatogr.* 1995, *667*; Biomed. Appl., 283–290.

Disposition in the Body. Dopexamine is extensively metabolised by *O*-methylation of the catechol-hydroxy moiety and subsequent sulfate conjugation. Elimination from blood occurs quickly. Two pharmacologically inactive metabolites are produced and both are excreted in urine and faeces, along with the unchanged drug. The major metabolite is the 2-methoxy, 1-sulfate metabolite and accounts for more than 90% of an administered dose. Over 12 days, 50% drug is excreted in urine and 20% in faeces.

Therapeutic concentration

10 healthy volunteers were administered dopexamine hydrochloride (total dose 180 μg/kg) over 60 min by intravenous infusion. There was a proportional increase in plasma concentration with a peak at 124 mg/L after 1 h. Plasma concentrations rapidly decreased when the infusion was stopped. [A. Filton and P Banfield, *Drugs*, 1990, *39(2)*, 308–330].

Toxicity. Overdose effects are short lived owing to short half-life with pharmacological actions including tachycardia, palpitations, tremors, nausea, vomiting and anginal pain.

Half-life. 7 min; 11 min in patients with cardiac failure.

Clearance. Plasma clearance, 36 mL/min/kg.

Dose. An initial dose of 0.5 μg/kg body weight/min is administered, which can be increased up to 1 μg/kg body weight/min, if necessary. Further increases occur in 0.5 to 1.0 μg/kg/min increments at intervals of not less than 15 min with a maximum dose of 6 μg/kg body weight/min.

Dosulepin

Antidepressant

Synonym. Dothiepin

3-Dibenzo[*b*,*e*]thiepin-11(6*H*)-ylidene-*N*,*N*-dimethyl-1-propanamine

$C_{19}H_{21}NS$=295.4

CAS—113-53-1

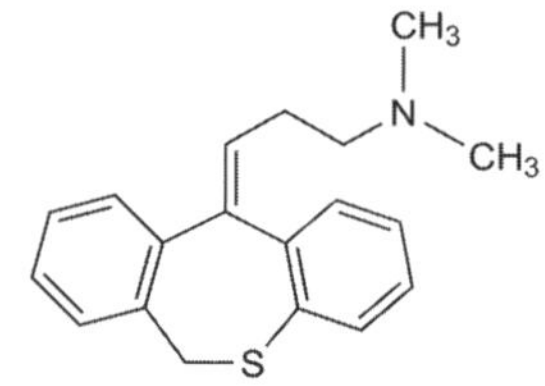

M.p. 55° to 57°.

Dosulepin Hydrochloride

Proprietary names. Dopin; Dopress; Dothapax; Dothep; Jardin; Prepadine; Prothiaden; Protiaden(e); Thaden; Xerenal.

$C_{19}H_{21}NS,HCl$=331.9

CAS—897-15-4

A white to faintly yellow crystalline powder. M.p. 218° to 221°.

Soluble 1 in 2 of water, 1 in 8 of ethanol, and 1 in 2 of chloroform; practically insoluble in ether.

Partition Coefficient. Log *P* (octanol/buffer pH 7.4), 2.8.

Colour Tests. Liebermann's Test—red-brown; Mandelin's Test—green; Marquis Test—brown; Sulfuric Acid—violet.

Thin-layer Chromatography. System TA—Rf 51; system TB—Rf 49; system TC—Rf 42; system TE—Rf 65; system TF—dothiepin *S*-oxide Rf 00; system TL—Rf 16; system TAE—Rf 27; system TAF—Rf 41. (Acidified iodoplatinate solution, positive.)

Gas Chromatography. System GA—dosulepin RI 2380, M (OH-) RI 2500; M (nor-) RI 2421; M (*N*-oxide) RI 2100; M (OH-*N*-oxide) RI 2130; M (sulfoxide) RI 2392; M (norsulfoxide) RI 2421; system GB—dosulepin RI 2486; M (nor-) RI 2507; M (sulfoxide) RI 2533; M (norsulfoxide) RI 2839; system GF—dosulepin RI 2770, dosulepin sulfoxide RI 2820; system GM—dosulepin RRT 1.259; M (nor-) RRT 1.450 (both relative to iprindole).

High Performance Liquid Chromatography. System HA—dosulepin *k* 3.2, M (sulfoxide) *k* 4.6 (tailing peak), M (nor-) *k* 2.2; system HF—*k* 3.60; system HX—RI 428; system HY—RI 367; system HZ—retention time 5.7 min.

Ultraviolet Spectrum. Aqueous acid—230 nm (A_1^1=770a), 303 nm.

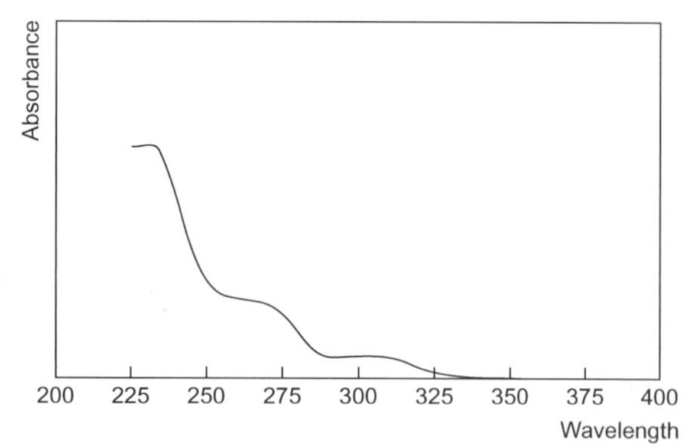

Infra-red Spectrum. Principal peaks at wavenumbers 763, 727, 747, 1252, 963, 717 cm^{-1} (dosulepin hydrochloride, KBr disk).

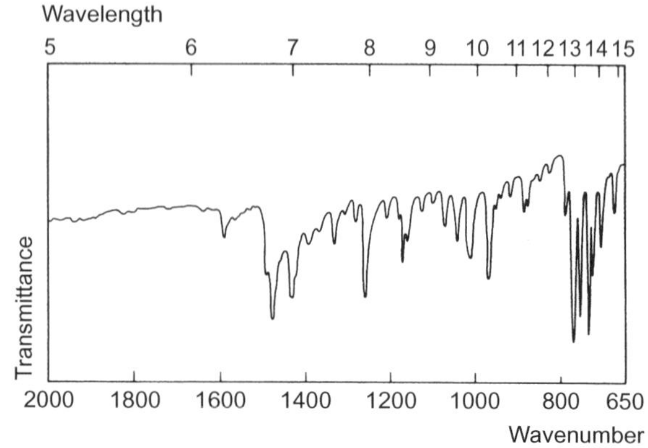

Mass Spectrum. Principal ions at *m/z* 58, 236, 40, 202, 235, 203, 42, 44; desmethyldosulepin 44, 204, 203, 202, 41, 221, 57, 55; dosulepin sulfoxide 58, 44, 31, 59, 57, 42, 45, 40.

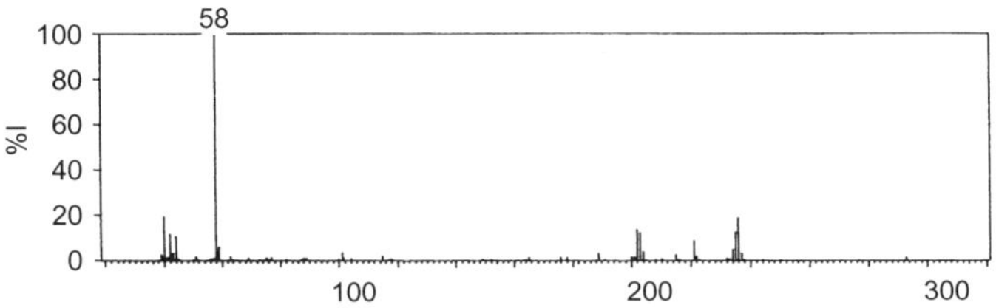

Quantification

Gas chromatography. In plasma: limit of detection 4 ng, AFID—L. A. Gifford *et al.*, *J. Chromatogr.*, 1975, *105*, 107–113.

Gas chromatography–mass spectrometry. In plasma or whole blood: dosulepin, monodesmethyldosulepin, and dosulepin sulfoxide, limit of detection 1 µg/L—K. P. Maguire *et al.*, *J. Chromatogr.* 1981, *222*(11) *B Biomed. Appl.*, 399–408. In biological fluids, tissues, or hair—V. Cirimele *et al.*, *Forensic Sci. Int.*, 1995, *76*, 205–209.

High performance liquid chromatography. In plasma or serum: dosulepin and monodesmethyldosulepin, limit of detection 10 µg/L, UV detection—R. R. Brodie *et al.*, *J. Int. Med. Res.*, 1977, *5*, 387–390. In plasma: dosulepin and its major metabolites—P. J. Taylor *et al.*, *J. Chromatogr.*, 1992, *581*, 152–155. In postmortem or clinical specimens: dosulepin and other antidepressants and metabolites, limit of detection in blood 50 µg/L, UV detection—I. M. McIntyre *et al.*, *J. Chromatogr.*, 1993, *621*, 215–223. In biological fluids, tissues, or hair, diode-array detection—V. Cirimele *et al.*, *Forensic Sci. Int.*, 1995, *76*, 205–209. In biological samples: dosulepin and other antidepressants, UV detection—E. Tanaka *et al.*, *J. Chromatogr. B Biomed. Sci. Appl.*, 1997, *692*, 405–412.

Disposition in the Body. Well absorbed after oral administration. The main metabolic reactions are demethylation to desmethyldosulepin (northiaden) and oxidation to dosulepin sulfoxide. About 50 to 60% of a dose is excreted in the urine in 24 h, mainly as metabolites, and 15 to 40% of a dose is eliminated in the faeces in the same period. Enterohepatic circulation has been reported. Small amounts may be excreted in breast milk

Therapeutic concentration. Plasma concentrations vary considerably between individual subjects.

Following a single oral dose of 75 mg to 7 subjects, peak plasma concentrations of 0.03 to 0.07 mg/L (mean 0.05) of dosulepin and 0.003 to 0.02 mg/L (mean 0.01) of monodesmethyldosulepin were attained in about 3 h and 6 h respectively. Peak blood concentrations of dosulepin sulfoxide of 0.03 to 0.15 mg/L (mean 0.08) were reported in 4 subjects at 5 h. [K. P. Maguire *et al.*, *Br. J. Clin. Pharmacol.*, 1981, *12*, 405–409.]

Following oral administration of 25 mg given 3 times a day to 5 subjects for 12 days, minimum steady-state serum concentrations of 0.02 to 0.06 mg/L (mean 0.04) of dosulepin, and <0.01 to 0.05 mg/L (mean 0.02) of monodesmethyldosulepin, were reported. [B. R. S. Nakra *et al.*, *J. Int. Med. Res.*, 1977, *5*, 391–397.]

Toxicity. Fatalities have been associated with blood concentrations of 1 to 5 to 19 mg/L.

A 36-year-old female was admitted to hospital 3 h after the ingestion of 2 to 3 g of dosulepin with alcohol. After 24 h, following treatment by haemoperfusion, she appeared to be recovering but toxic symptoms reappeared after 48 h followed by death 56 h after ingestion. The following plasma concentrations were reported (mg/L):

Hours after ingestion	Dosulepin	Monodesmethyldosulepin
4.5	2.51	0
6.0	1.88	0.13
17.5	1.07	0.32
57.5*	4.54	1.28

* postmortem

[L. Bloodworth *et al.*, *Postgrad. Med. J.*, 1984, *60*, 442–444.]

In 8 cases of overdose with dosulepin, all had high initial levels of dosulepin (0.819 to 3.851 mg/L), dosulepin-*S*-oxide (0.655 to 2.162 mg/L), nordosulepin (0.088 to 0.422 mg/L), and nordosulepin-*S*-oxide (0.176 to 0.530 mg/L); all patients survived following treatment with repeated-dose activated charcoal. [K. F. Bett *et al.*, *Ther. Drug Monit.*, 1991, *13*, 485–489.]

In 2 cases of suicide involving dosulepin ingestion (765 and 1875 mg, respectively), initial blood concentrations were 0.26 to 1.85 and 4.08 to 23.98 mg/L. Pulmonary artery concentrations rose over 18 h (0.32 rising to 0.9, and 6.54 rising to 19.53 mg/L) with peripheral blood concentrations remaining stable. Postmortem tissue concentrations in the respective cases were: liver 4.3 and 52 µg/g, heart 2.92 and 16.8 µg/g, lung 18.6 and 73.9, and skeletal muscle 1.1 and 8.98 µg/g. Mean dosulepin levels in thoracic blood rose from 0.43 mg/L at 0 h *postmortem* to 1.73 at 8 h and then fell to 0.61 mg/L at 12 h, probably reflecting redistribution from the lungs. [D. J. Pounder *et al.*, *Am. J. Forensic. Med. Pathol.*, 1994, *15*, 231–235.]

The following postmortem tissue concentrations were reported in a 22-year-old man suspected of ingesting up to 4.5 g of dosulepin (mg/L or µg/g): blood 5.75, urine 7.42, bile 110, gastric contents 373, liver 45.2, kidney 10.4, heart 16.0, brain 2.77, hair of head 1.89, axillary hair 1.17. [V. Cirimele *et al.*, *Forensic Sci. Int.*, 1995, *76*, 205–209.]

In a 32-year-old man who committed suicide by ingesting an unknown quantity of dosulepin, the following postmortem tissue concentrations of dosulepin and desmethyldosulepin, respectively, were reported: peripheral blood 7.28 and 2.03 mg/L, heart blood 6.98 and 1.63 mg/L, urine 12.58 and 3.71 mg/L, vitreous humour 0.28 and 0.02 mg/L, stomach contents 65.41 and 1.01 mg/L, bile 12.24 and 1.06 mg/L; diazepam and desmethyldiazepam were also detected in tissues. [T. Keller *et al.*, *Forensic Sci. Int.*, 2000, *109*, 159–166.]

Half-life. Plasma half-life, dosulepin 11 to 40 h (mean 22), monodesmethyldosulepin 22 to 60 h (mean 33), dosulepin sulfoxide 13 to 35 h (mean 20).

Distribution in blood. Plasma:whole blood ratio, about 1.4.

Note. For a review of the pharmacokinetics of tricyclic antidepressants, see G. Molnar and R. N. Gupta, *Biopharm. Drug Disp.*, 1980, *1*, 283–305.

Dose. 75 to 150 mg of dosulepin hydrochloride daily; up to 225 mg daily has been given.

Doxacurium Chloride

Muscle Relaxant

Synonym. BW-A938U
Proprietary name. Nuromax
[1α,2β(1′*S**,2′*R**)]-2,2′-[(1,4-Dioxo-1,4-butanediyl)bis(oxy-3,1-propanediyl)]bis[1,2,3,4-tetrahydro-6,7,8-trimethoxy-2-methyl-1-[(3,4,5-trimethoxyphenyl)methyl]isoquinolinium] dichloride
$C_{56}H_{78}Cl_2N_2O_{16}$ = 1106.1
CAS—106819-53-8 (*meso* isomer)*; 83348-52-1* (*total racemate*)

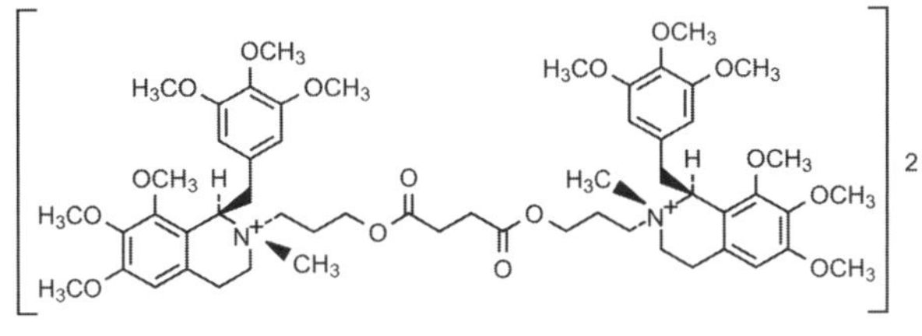

An amorphous solid which is soluble in water.

High Performance Liquid Chromatography. Column: S5C1 (Spherisorb, 150 × 4.6 mm i.d., 5 µm). Mobile phase: monobasic potassium phosphate (0.05 M, pH 3):acetonitrile containing 0.5% methanol (30:70), 1.0 mL/min flow rate. UV detection (λ=210 nm). Retention time: 6.7 min. [R. DeAngelis *et al.*, *J. Chromatogr.* 1990, *525*; *Biomed. Appl.*, 389–400].

Quantification

High performance liquid chromatography. In plasma and urine: limit of quantification is 10 µg/L. UV detection (λ=210 nm)—R. DeAngelis *et al.*, *J. Chromatogr.*, 1990, *525(2)*, 389–400. In plasma and urine: limit of quantification 4 µg/L. UV detection—L. P. Gariepy *et al.*, *Clin. Pharmacol. Ther.*, 1993, *53(3)*, 340–347.

Disposition in the Body. Doxacurium is excreted in urine and bile, mostly as the unchanged parent drug. It is distributed primarily in extracellular fluids as it is a large polar compound. It is not metabolised by plasma cholinesterase or hepatic enzymes. The drug is rapidly cleared from the body and is eliminated mainly in urine (70%) and also via bile. In healthy individuals, 24 to 38% of a dose is recovered unchanged in urine within 6 to 12 h after administration.

Therapeutic concentration

9 healthy, young subjects (aged 19 to 39 years) and 9 healthy, elderly subjects (70 to 83 years) were administered 30 µg/kg doxacurium chloride (equivalent to 25 µg/kg doxacurium base) after induction of anaesthesia. In the younger subjects the mean plasma concentration reached 337 µg/L at 2 min and then declined to 5 µg/L over 360 min after injection. In the elderly subjects, however, their peak concentration of 336 µg/L declined to 8 µg/L after 480 min. [L. P. Gariepy *et al.*, *Clin. Pharmacol. Ther.*, 1993, *53(3)*, 340–347].

Half-life. Approx. 1.7 to 2 h (healthy individuals); 3.7 h (patients with renal insufficiency).

Volume of distribution. Steady state, 0.23 (0.12 to 0.29) L/kg.

Clearance. Plasma, 2.5 mL/kg/min.

Protein binding. Approx. 28 to 34% (plasma proteins).

Dose. The initial dose is 50 µg/kg body weight intravenously, followed by a maintenance dose of 5 to 10 µg/kg. A dose of 80 µg/kg may also be used.

Doxapram

Respiratory Stimulant

1-Ethyl-4-[2-(4-morpholinyl)ethyl]-3,3-diphenyl-2-pyrrolidinone
$C_{24}H_{30}N_2O_2$=378.5
CAS—309-29-5

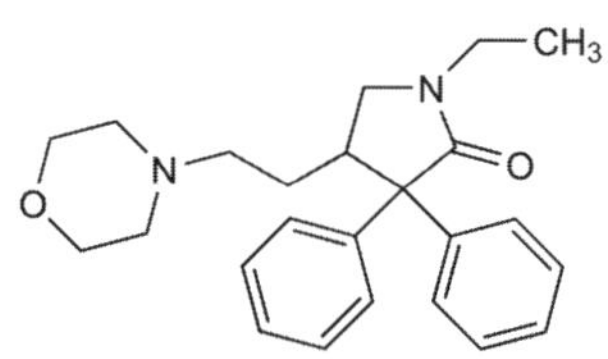

Doxapram Hydrochloride
Proprietary names. Dopram; Doxapril; Stimulexin.
$C_{24}H_{30}N_2O_2$,HCl,H_2O=433.0
CAS—113-07-5 (anhydrous); 7081-53-0 (monohydrate)
A white crystalline powder. M.p. about 220°.
Soluble 1 in 50 of water; sparingly soluble in ethanol; slightly soluble in chloroform; practically insoluble in ether.

Partition Coefficient. Log *P* (octanol/water), 3.4.

Colour Tests. Liebermann's Test—orange; Mandelin's Test—blue.

Thin-layer Chromatography. System TA—Rf 64; system TB—Rf 20; system TC—Rf 70; system TE—Rf 72; system TL—Rf 54; system TAE—Rf 69; system TAJ—Rf 60; system TAK—Rf 03; system TAL—Rf 73. (Acidified iodoplatinate solution, positive.)

Gas Chromatography. System GA—RI 2906; system GB—doxapram RI 3046, M (keto-) RI 3018; system GC—RI 2230.

High Performance Liquid Chromatography. System HA—*k* 0.4; system HY—RI 312; system HZ—retention time 3.2 min; system HAX—retention time 8.7 min; system HAY—retention time 4.6 min.

Ultraviolet Spectrum. Aqueous acid—253, 259 (A_1^1=12c), 265 nm.

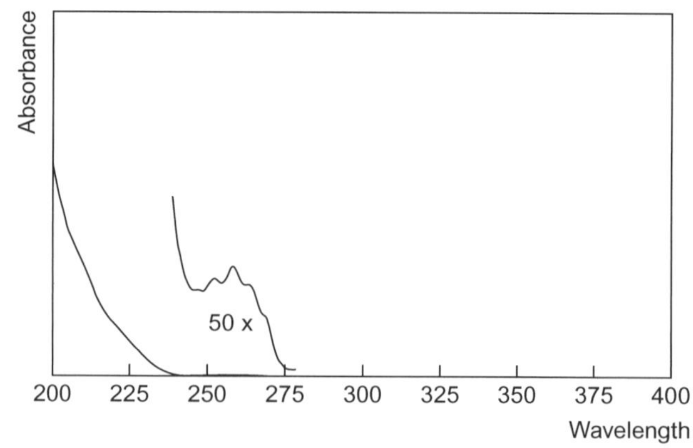

Infra-red Spectrum. Principal peaks at wavenumbers 1683, 753, 710, 1253, 696, 764 cm^{-1} (doxapram hydrochloride, KBr disk).

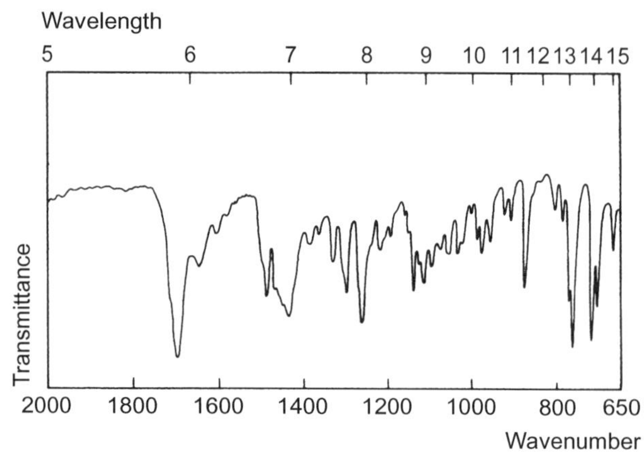

Mass Spectrum. Principal ions at *m/z* 100, 113, 56, 101, 87, 378, 194, 91.

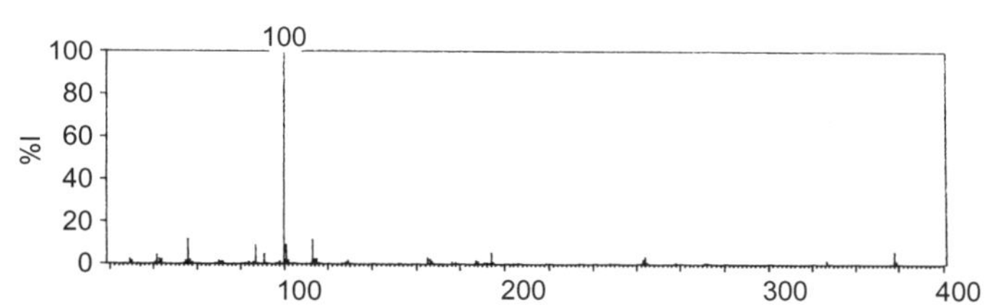

Quantification

Gas chromatography. In plasma: limit of detection 10 µg/L, AFID—R. H. Robson and L. F. Prescott, *J. Chromatogr.* 1977, *143(1) B Biomed. Appl.*, 527–529. In blood, plasma or urine: mass spectrometric detection (blood or plasma), FID (urine)—H. Nichol *et al.*, *J. Chromatogr.*, 1980, *182*, 191–200.

Disposition in the Body. Readily absorbed after oral administration. The major metabolite is the 2-ketomorpholino derivative.

Therapeutic concentration

Following an IV injection of 1.5 mg/kg to 6 subjects, plasma concentrations of 1.6 to 4.3 mg/L (mean 2.6) were reported after 2 min declining to 0.6 to 1.5 mg/L (mean 0.9) at 2 h. Following IV infusion of 6.5 mg/kg to 6 subjects, peak plasma concentrations of 3.3 to 5.2 mg/L (mean 4.1) were reported at the end of the infusion; peak concentrations of the 2-ketomorpholino metabolite of 1.1 to 2.0 mg/L (mean 1.6) were attained 0.2 to 2 h after the end of the infusion. [J. A. Clements *et al.*, *Eur. J. Clin. Pharmacol.*, 1979, *16*, 411–416.]

In 18 premature infants, a steady-state plasma concentration of approx. 1.5 mg/L was achieved by IV administration of a loading dose of 5.5 mg/kg and a maintenance infusion of 1/mg/h. [F. Jamali *et al.*, *Dev. Pharmacol. Ther.*, 1988, *11*, 253–257.]

Bioavailability. About 60%.

Half-life. Plasma half-life, about 7 h.

Volume of distribution. About 3 L/kg.

Clearance. Plasma clearance, about 5 mL/min/kg.

Dose. 1 to 1.5 mg/kg of doxapram hydrochloride by IV injection.

Doxazosin

Antihypertensive

Synonym. UK-33274
1-(4-Amino-6,7-dimethoxy-2-quinazolinyl)-4-[(2,3-dihydro-1,4-benzodioxin-2-yl)carbonyl]piperazine
$C_{23}H_{25}N_5O_5$=451.5
CAS—74197-85-8

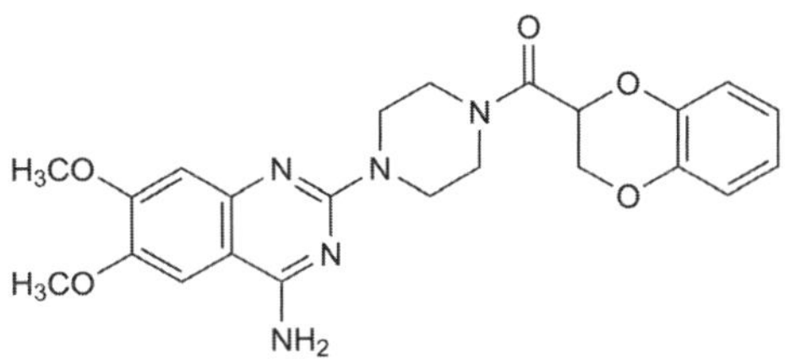

Doxazosin Hydrochloride

$C_{23}H_{25}N_5O_5,HCl$=488.0
CAS—70918-01-3
A crystalline powder. M.p. 289° to 290°.

Doxazosin Mesilate

Synonyms. Doxazosin Mesylate; UK-33274-27.
Proprietary names. Aldafil; Benur; Cardenalin; Cardular; Cardura; Carduran; Dedralen; Diblocin; Normothen; Progandol; Prostadilate; Supressin.
$C_{23}H_{25}N_5O_5,CH_3SO_3H$=547.6
CAS—77883-43-3
It is freely soluble in dimethylsulfoxide; soluble in dimethylformamide; slightly soluble in methanol, ethanol, and water (0.8% solubility at 25°); very slightly soluble in acetone and methylene chloride.

Partition Coefficient. Log *P* (octanol/water), 2.09.

Thin-layer Chromatography. System TB—Rf 00; system TE—Rf 73; system TAE—Rf 71.

Gas Chromatography. System GB—RI 3054.

High Performance Liquid Chromatography. System HX—RI 403.

Column: ODS (Spherisorb, 125 × 5 mm i.d., 5 μm). Mobile phase: methanol:tetramethyl ammonium chloride (0.02 M)/sodium heptane sulfonate (0.01 M) buffer (70:30), flow rate 1.0 mL/min. Retention time: 5.2 min. [B. Kaye *et al.*, *Br. J. Clin. Pharmacol.*, 1986, *21*, 19S–25S.]

Ultraviolet Spectrum. Aqueous acid—246, 331 nm (doxazosin); Ethanol—250, 275, 282 nm (Doxazosin mesilate).

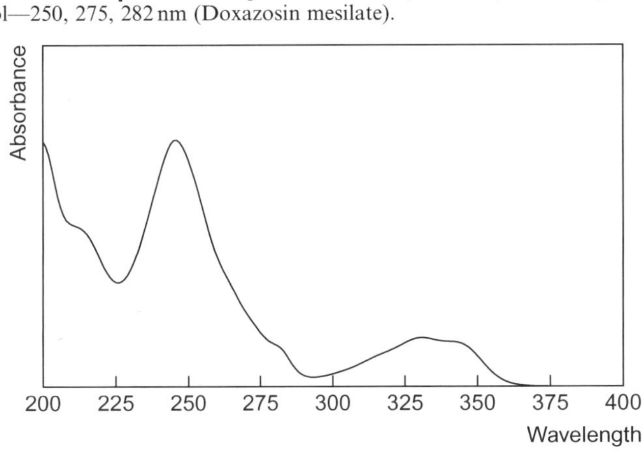

Mass Spectrum. Principal ions at *m/z*: 233, 45, 245, 316, 451, 259, 42, 96.

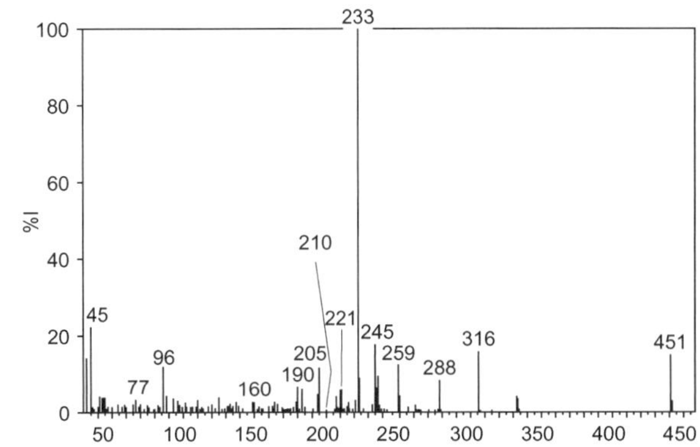

Quantification

High performance liquid chromatography. In plasma: limit of quantification 0.2 μg/L—V. Vashi *et al., J. Clin. Pharmacol.*, 1996, *36*, 325–331. In plasma: limit of determination 1 μg/L—G. P. Jackman *et al., J. Chromatogr.* 1991, *566 B Biomed. Appl.*, 234–238.

Disposition in the Body. Doxazosin is well absorbed and extensively metabolised in the liver by *O*-demethylation or hydroxylation. Enterohepatic recycling occurs as a large amount of the drug is excreted in faeces as its metabolites and a small amount of the unchanged drug. The remainder of the drug can be found in urine, approx. 9%. 16% of an oral dose is found as the 6-*O*-demethylation metabolite, 7% as the 7-*O*-demethylation metabolite, 5% as the 6′-hydroxy metabolite, and 7% as the 7′-hydroxymetabolite. Other metabolites include 2-piperazinyl and 2-amino compounds.

Therapeutic concentration

5 men and 5 women patients with essential hypertension were administered with a 1 mg dose of doxazosin. Peak plasma concentrations of 15.7 ± 2.7 μg/L were reached within 2.1 ± 0.4 h. After multiple dosing of the same dosage, over 2 weeks, peak concentrations reached 19.3 ± 2.3 μg/L still within 1.9 ± 0.2 h. [B. Kaye *et al., Br. J. Clin. Pharmacol.*, 1986, *21*, 19S–25S.]

Toxicity

A 32-year-old woman with chronic renal failure and depression took a 60 mg dose of doxazosin and died owing to a grand mal seizure resulting from hypotension. Blood analysis showed a doxazosin level of 0.9 g/L. [www.Rxlist.com]

Bioavailability. 65%.

Half-life. 16 to 22 h.

Volume of distribution. 1.01 L/kg (in young adults, aged approx. 29 years); 1.71 L/kg (elderly, aged 71 years).

Clearance. 1.2 mL/min/kg.

Protein binding. Approx. 98%.

Dose. Initially a dose of 1 mg daily is administered, which can be increased over time to a maximum of 16 mg daily.

Doxepin

Antidepressant

A mixture of the *cis*- and *trans*-isomers of 3-dibenz[*b*,*e*]oxepin-11(6*H*)-ylidene-*N*,*N*-dimethyl-1-propanamine.
$C_{19}H_{21}NO$=279.4
CAS—1668-19-5

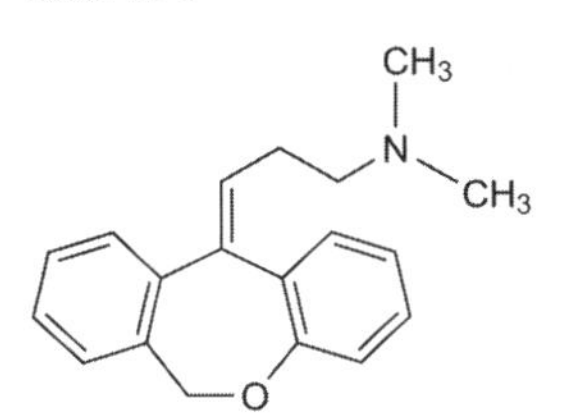

An oily liquid.

Doxepin Hydrochloride
Synonyms. NSC-108160; P-3693A.
Proprietary names. Anten; Aponal; Deptran; Desidoxepin; Doneurin; Doxal; Gilex; Mareen; Quitaxon; Sinequan; Sinquan(e); Xepin; Zonalon.
$C_{19}H_{21}NO,HCl = 315.8$
CAS—1229-29-4
A white crystalline powder. M.p. 184° to 186°, also reported as 188° to 189°. Soluble 1 in 1.5 of water, 1 in 1 of ethanol, and 1 in 2 of chloroform; very slightly soluble in ether.

Dissociation Constant. pK_a 9.0 (25°).

Partition Coefficient. Log *P* (octanol/buffer pH 7.4), 2.4.

Colour Tests. Liebermann's Test—black; Mandelin's Test—brown; Marquis Test—brown; Sulfuric Acid—orange.

Thin-layer Chromatography. System TA—Rf 51; system TB—Rf 48; system TC—Rf 37; system TE—Rf 63; system TL—Rf 13; system TAE—Rf 24; system TAF—Rf 45; system TAJ—Rf 23; system TAK—Rf 14; system TAL—Rf 71. (Acidified iodoplatinate solution, positive.)

Gas Chromatography. System GA—doxepin (*cis* and *trans*) RI 2220, M (*cis-N*-oxide) RI 1970, M (*cis*-nor-) RI 2245, M (*trans*-nor-) RI 2245, M (*cis*-OH-) RI 2535, M (*trans*-OH-) RI 2560, M (*cis*-nor-OH-) RI 2540, M (OH-dihydro-) RI 2530; system GB—doxepin-*cis* isomer RI 2301; doxepin-*trans* isomer RI 2321, M (*cis-N*-oxide) RI 2077, M (*trans-N*-oxide) RI 2081, M (*cis*-nor) RI 2333, M (*trans*-nor) RI 2339, M (*cis*-OH-) RI 2528, M (*trans*-OH-) RI 2544, M (*cis*-nor-OH-) RI 2644, M (*trans*-nor-OH-) RI 2671; system GF—RI 2570; system GM—doxepin-*cis* isomer RRT 0.788; doxepin-*trans* isomer RRT 0.823, M (*cis*-nor-) RRT 0.830, M (*trans*-nor-) RRT 0.933 (all relative to iprindole); system GS—doxepin-*cis* isomer retention time 17.2 min; doxepin-*trans* isomer retention time 17.6 min; chloramitriptyline (IS) retention time 21.2 min.

High Performance Liquid Chromatography. System HA—doxepin *k* 3.7, M (nor-) *k* 2.2; system HF—*k* 2.27; system HX—RI 404; system HY—RI 316; system HZ—doxepin retention time 5.0 min, M (nor-) retention time 4.6 min; system HAA—retention time 14.1 min; system HAX—retention time 12.9 min; system HAY—retention time 6.1 min.

Ultraviolet Spectrum. Aqueous acid—292 nm ($A^1_1 = 231a$).

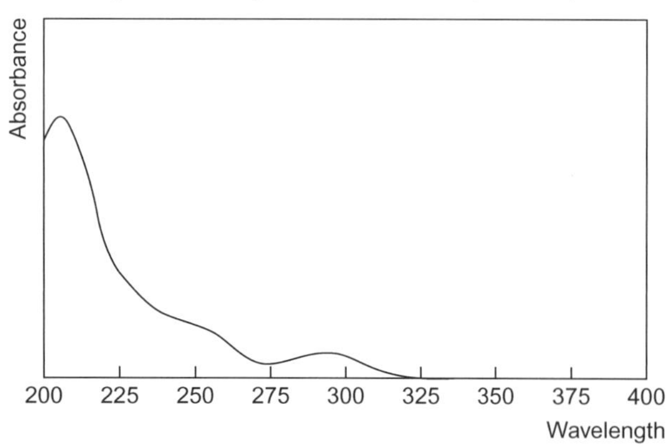

Infra-red Spectrum. Principal peaks at wavenumbers 750, 1006, 768, 1198, 1290, 1219 cm^{-1} (doxepin hydrochloride, KBr disk).

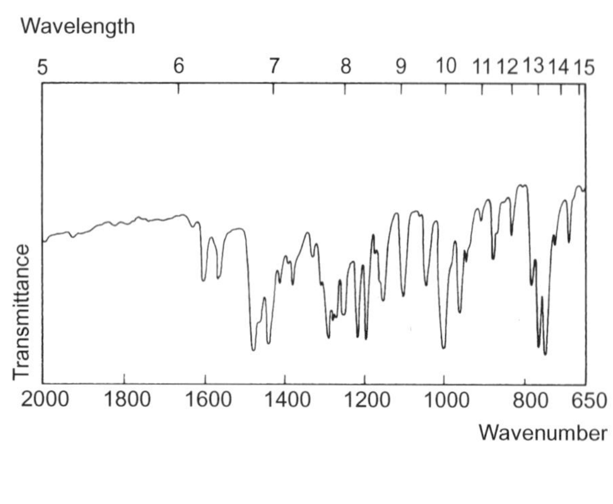

Mass Spectrum. Principal ions at *m/z* 58, 220, 219, 59, 191, 189, 42, 205.

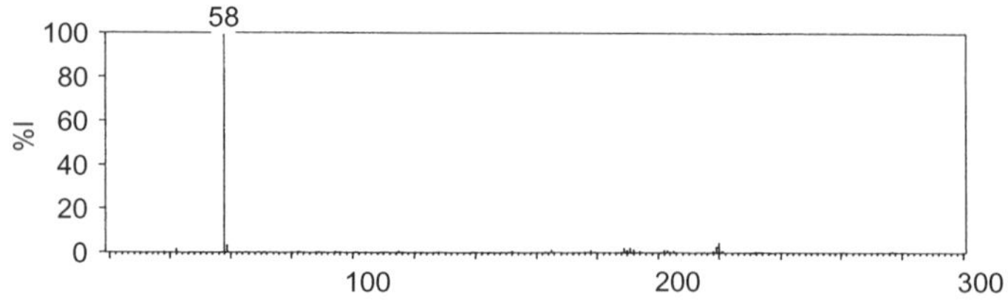

Quantification
Gas chromatography. In plasma: limit of detection 10 µg/L, FID—J. E. O'Brien and O. N. Hinsvark, *J. Pharm. Sci.*, 1976, *65*, 1068–1069. In plasma: limit of detection 2 µg/L for doxepin and 1 µg/L for monodesmethyldoxepin, AFID—M. T. Rosseel *et al.*, *J. Pharm. Sci.*, 1978, *67*, 802–805. In plasma: limit of detection 2.5 µg/L, ECD—J. E. Wallace *et al.*, *J. Anal. Toxicol.*, 1978, *2*, 44–49.

Gas chromatography–mass spectrometry. In blood, urine, or tissues: doxepin and monodesmethyldoxepin—G. de Groot *et al.*, *J. Anal. Toxicol.*, 1978, *2*, 13–17. In hair: doxepine and desmethyldoxepin, limit of detection <0.25 µg/g—A. Negrusz *et al.*, *J. Anal. Toxicol.*, 1998, *22*, 531–536. In hair: doxepin and other antidepressant and antipsychotic drugs—M. Shen *et al.*, *Forensic Sci. Int.*, 2002, *126*, 153–161.

High performance liquid chromatography. In plasma: limit of detection 5 µg/L for doxepin and monodesmethyldoxepin, UV detection—R. D. Faulkner and C. Lee, *J. Pharm. Sci.*, 1983, *72*, 1165–1167. In serum: doxepin and desmethyldoxepin enantiomers—M. Adamczyk *et al.*, *Ther. Drug Monit.*, 1995, 17, 371–376. In plasma or urine: doxepin and desmethyldoxepin enantiomers, limit of detection <1 µg/L, UV detection—J. Yan *et al.*, *J. Chromatogr. B Biomed. Sci. Appl.*, 1997, *691*, 131–138. In biological samples: doxepin and other antidepressants, UV detection—E. Tanaka *et al.*, *J. Chromatogr. B Biomed. Sci. Appl.*, 1997, *692*, 405–412.

High performance liquid chromatography–mass spectrometry. In plasma: doxepin and desmethyldoxepin—D. Badenhorst *et al.*, *J. Chromatogr. B Biomed. Sci. Appl.*, 2000, *742*, 91–98. In plasma: doxepin and other antidepressants—M. Kollroser and C. Schober, *Ther. Drug Monit.*, 2002, *24*, 537–544.

Radioimmunoassay. In serum or plasma: doxepin and monodesmethyldoxepin, limit of detection 2.5 µg/L—R. Virtanen *et al.*, *Acta Pharmacol. Toxicol.*, 1980, *47*, 274–278.

Disposition in the Body. Well absorbed after oral administration, but undergoes extensive first-pass demethylation. Other metabolic reactions include *N*-oxidation, aromatic hydroxylation, and glucuronic acid conjugation. Monodesmethyldoxepin is an active metabolite. Doxepin is excreted in the urine, chiefly as metabolites and conjugated metabolites; less than 1% of a dose is excreted in the urine as unchanged drug in 24 h. It is also absorbed through the skin if applied topically. It crosses the blood–brain barrier and the placenta. Both doxepin and its active metabolite, desmethyldoxepin, are excreted in breast milk.

Therapeutic concentration. In plasma, usually in the range 0.02 to 0.15 mg/L.

After a single oral dose of 75 mg given to 7 subjects, peak plasma concentrations of 0.01 to 0.05 mg/L (mean 0.03) of doxepin were attained in 2 to 4 h and peak plasma concentrations of 0.005 to 0.014 mg/L (mean 0.01) of monodesmethyldoxepin were reported at 2 to 10 h. [V. E. Ziegler *et al.*, *Clin. Pharmacol. Ther.*, 1978, *23*, 573–579.]

Analysis of data from a serum-level databank from German and US sources showed the mean steady-state serum concentration of doxepin plus desmethyldoxepin to be 0.089 (±0.075) mg/L following a daily dose of 143 (±30) mg doxepin. [S. Leucht *et al.*, *J. Clin. Psychopharmacol.*, 2001, *21*, 432–439.]

A retrospective analysis of data from 114 psychiatric patients treated with doxepin 25 to 400 mg daily for 22 to 306 days (92% by the oral route; 8% by the IV route) revealed doxepin plasma concentration to be 0.011 to 0.295 mg/L (mean 0.077) and desmethyldoxepin to be 0.037 to 0.43 mg/L (mean 0.066). [M. Meyer-Barner *et al.*, *Eur. J. Clin. Pharmacol.*, 2002, *58*, 253–257.]

Toxicity. Doses in excess of 500 mg are likely to produce severe toxic effects and the estimated minimum lethal dose is 1 g. Blood concentrations

>0.1 mg/L may be associated with toxic reactions and fatalities have been associated with blood concentrations of 1 to 18 mg/L (mean 8).

In 5 deaths due to overdosage of doxepin, the postmortem blood concentrations ranged from 9 to 19 mg/L (mean 13) and, in 3 of these cases, liver concentrations of 71, 75, and 500 µg/g were reported. [J. S. Oliver and A. A. Watson, *Med. Sci. Law*, 1974, *14*, 280–283.]

In a report of 4 fatalities attributed to overdose of doxepin, the following postmortem blood and tissue concentrations, mg/L or mg/kg (mean), were found:

	Doxepin	Monodesmethyldoxepin
Blood	0.7–29 (9.3)	0.1–6.2 (1.7)
Bile	38–195 (95)	1.0–19 (7.1)
Brain	9–21 (14)	1.5–22 (7.2)
Kidney	3.3–19 (12)	0.5–9.0 (3.0)
Liver	22–38 (32)	1.2–20 (7.5)
Urine	2.1–12 (7.5)	0.7–6.4 (2.8)

[G. de Groot *et al.*, *J. Anal. Toxicol.*, 1978, *2*, 18–20.]

In a young female fatality, femoral blood drug concentrations were: paroxetine 0.176 mg/L, doxepin 82.12 mg/L, and desmethyldoxepin 0.34 mg/L. [F. Musshoff *et al.*, *Arch. Kriminol.*, 1999, *204*, 28–32.]

Bioavailability. 15 to 45%.

Half-life. Plasma half-life, doxepin 8 to 24 h (mean 17), desmethyldoxepin 33 to 80 h (mean 51).

Volume of distribution. About 20 to 24 L/kg.

Clearance. Plasma clearance, about 15 mL/min/kg.

Distribution in blood. Plasma:whole blood ratio, doxepin about 0.8 but there is considerable intersubject variation; monodesmethyldoxepin about 0.6.

Protein binding. In plasma, about 80%.

Note. For a review of the pharmacokinetics of tricyclic antidepressants, see G. Molnar and R. N. Gupta, *Biopharm. Drug Dispos.*, 1980, *1*, 283–305.

Dose. The equivalent of 30 to 300 mg of doxepin daily by mouth.

Doxorubicin

Antineoplastic

Synonyms. Adriamycin; 14-Hydroxydaunorubicin.
(8*S*-*cis*)-10-[(3-Amino-2,3,6-trideoxy-α-L-lyxo-hexopyranosyl)oxy]-7,8,9,10-tetrahydro-6,8,11-trihydroxy-8-(hydroxyacetyl)-1-methoxy-5,12-naphthacenedione
$C_{27}H_{29}NO_{11}$ = 543.5
CAS—23214-92-8

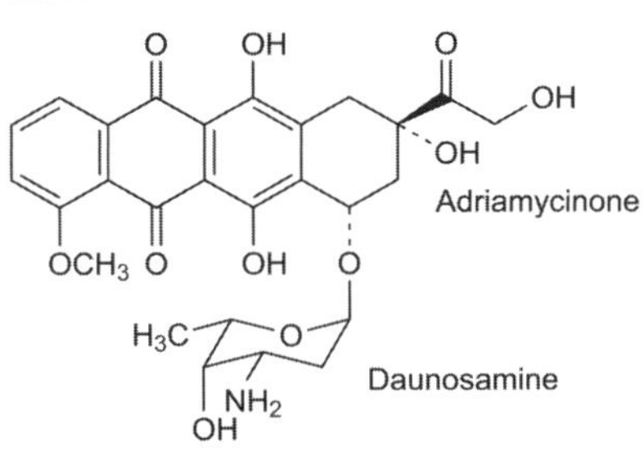

An antibiotic isolated from *Streptomyces peucetius var. caesius*. M.p. 229° to 231°.

Doxorubicin Hydrochloride

Proprietary names. Adriamycin; Adriblastin(a); Adriblastine; Adrim; Adrimedac; Caelyx; Doxil; DOXO-cell; Doxolem; Doxorubin; Doxotec; Farmiblastina; Fauldoxo; Ribodoxo-L; Rubex.
$C_{27}H_{29}NO_{11}$,HCl = 580.0
CAS—25316-40-9
An orange-red, hygroscopic, crystalline powder. M.p. 204° to 205°, with decomposition. Soluble in water, methanol, and aqueous alcohols; soluble 1 in 75 of ethanol; practically insoluble in acetone, benzene, chloroform, ethyl ether, petroleum ether, ether, and other organic solvents.
Caution. Doxorubicin hydrochloride is irritant; avoid contact with skin and mucous membranes.

Dissociation Constant. pK_a 8.2, 10.2.

Partition Coefficient. Log *P* (octanol/water), 1.3.

Colour Tests. Mandelin's Test—green; Marquis Test—violet.

Thin-layer Chromatography. System TA—Rf 12; system TE—Rf 00; system TF—Rf 00. (Visible red streak.)

High Performance Liquid Chromatography. System HX—RI 370; system HAA—retention time 12.1 min.

Ultraviolet Spectrum. Aqueous acid—233, 253, 290; aqueous alkali—253; methanol—233 (A_1^1 = 702b), 253, 290 nm.

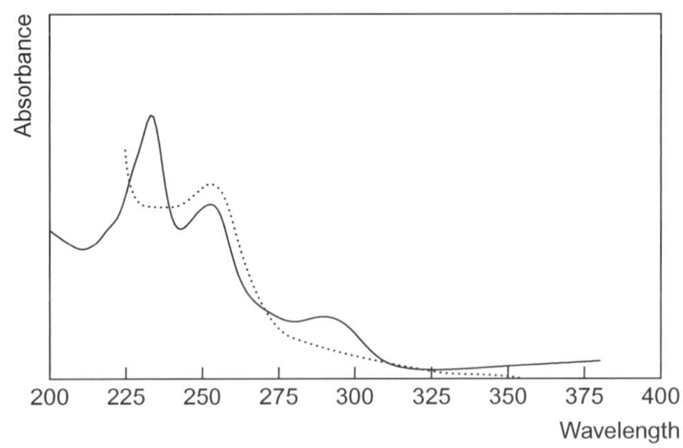

Infra-red Spectrum. Principal peaks at wavenumbers 1282, 990, 1010, 1587, 1612, 1204 cm^{-1} (doxorubicin hydrochloride).

Quantification

High performance liquid chromatography. In plasma: doxorubicin and daunorubicin, limit of detection 10 µg/L, UV detection—A. Mikan *et al.*, *Biomed. Chromatogr.*, 1990, *4*, 154–156. In plasma: doxorubicin and metabolites, fluorescence detection—J. H. Beijnen *et al.*, *J. Pharm. Biomed. Anal.*, 1991, *9*, 995–1002. In plasma or tissues: limit of detection <25 µg/L, fluorescence detection—S. K. Cox *et al.*, *J. Chromatogr.*, 1991, *564*, 322–329. In plasma: doxorubicin and its metabolites, limits of detection 1 to 2 nM, fluorescence detection—A. Andersen *et al.*, *Ther. Drug Monit.*, 1993, *15*, 455–461. In plasma: doxorubicin, epirubicin, and principal metabolites, limit of detection <1 µg/L, electrochemical detection—R. Ricciarello *et al.*, *J. Chromatogr. B Biomed. Sci. Appl.*, 1998, *707*, 219–225. In plasma: doxorubicin and doxorubicinol, limit of detection <1 µg/L, fluorescence detection—P. de Bruijn *et al.*, *Anal. Biochem.*, 1999, *266*, 216–221.

Dose. 1.2 to 2.4 mg/kg, IV, as a single dose every 3 weeks.

Doxycycline

Antibiotic

Synonym. Doxycycline Monohydrate
Proprietary names. Cyclodox; Doximed; Doxy; Doxybene; Doxycline; Doxyderma; Doxydoc; Doxy-HP; Doxymerck; Doxymono; Doxysol; Doxystad; Idocyklin; Vibradox; Vibramycin-D; Vibramycine N; Vibra-S; Vibravenös.
[4*S*-(4α,4aα,5α,5aα,6α,12aα)]-4-(Dimethylamino)-1,4,4a,5,5a,6,11,12a-octahydro-3,5,10,12,12a-pentahydroxy-6-methyl-1,11-dioxo-2-naphthacenecarboxamide monohydrate
$C_{22}H_{24}N_2O_8$,H_2O = 462.5
CAS—564-25-0 (anhydrous); 17086-28-1 (monohydrate)

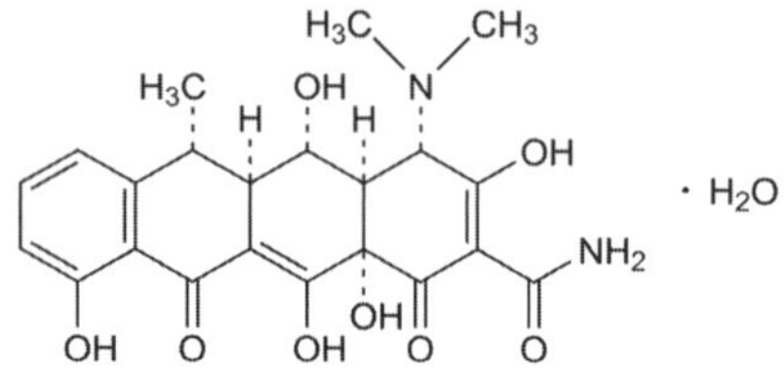

A yellow crystalline powder.
Very slightly soluble in water; sparingly soluble in ethanol; practically insoluble in chloroform and ether; freely soluble in dilute acids and alkali hydroxides.

Doxycycline Hydrochloride

Synonyms. Doxycycline Hyclate; Doxycyclini Chloridum.
Proprietary names. Atridox; Demix; Doxi Crisol; Doxi Sergo; Doxibiotic; Doxiclat; Doxylar; Doximycin; Doxin(a); Doxine; Doxitab; Doxiten; Doxitin; Doxy; Doxybene; Doxybiocin; Doxycap; Doxychel; Doxyclin(e); Doxycyl; Doxylar; Dumoxin; Idocyklin; Periostat; Ramysis; Vibramycin(e); Vibra-Tabs; Vibraveineuse; Vibravenos.
$C_{22}H_{24}N_2O_8$,HCl,½C_2H_5OH,½H_2O=512.9
CAS—10592-13-9 ($C_{22}H_{24}N_2O_8$,HCl); 24390-14-5 ($C_{22}H_{24}N_2O_8$,HCl, ½C_2H_5OH,½H_2O)
A yellow crystalline powder. M.p. about 200°, with decomposition.
Soluble 1 in 3 of water, 1 in 60 of ethanol, and 1 in 4 of methanol; practically insoluble in chloroform and ether.

Dissociation Constant. pK_a 3.5, 7.7, 9.5 (20°).

Partition Coefficient. Log *P* (octanol/water), −0.02.

Colour Tests. Benedict's Reagent—red; Formaldehyde–Sulfuric Acid—yellow; Mandelin's Test—green→yellow; Marquis Test—yellow; Sulfuric Acid—yellow.

Thin-layer Chromatography. System TA—Rf 12, streaking; system TAE—Rf 88. (Acidified iodoplatinate solution, positive.)

High Performance Liquid Chromatography. System HY—RI 291.

Ultraviolet Spectrum. Aqueous acid—269 (A^1_1=412b), 346 nm.

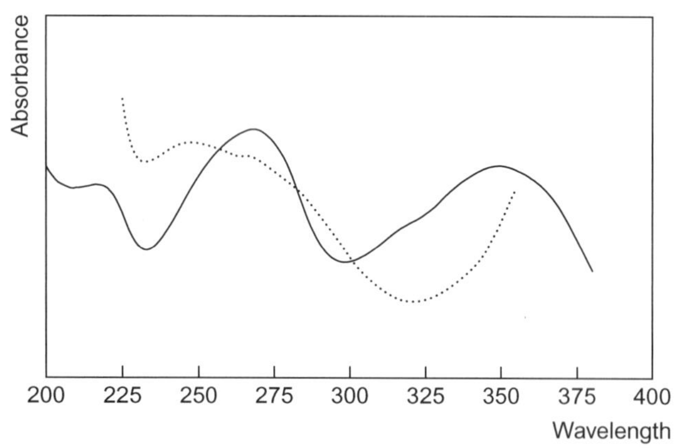

Infra-red Spectrum. Principal peaks at wavenumbers 1580, 1613, 1660, 1244, 1220, 1040 cm^{-1} (doxycycline hydrochloride, KBr disk).

Quantification

High performance liquid chromatography. In serum or urine: limit of detection 50 μg/L in serum, UV detection—A. P. De Leenheer and H. J. C. Nelis, *J. Pharm. Sci.*, 1979, *68*, 999–1002. In plasma or urine, limit of detection <25 μg/L, UV detection—J. M. Prevosto *et al.*, *Ann. Biol. Clin. (Paris)*, 1995, *53*, 29–32. In plasma or tissue: limit of detection in plasma 0.125 mg/L—B. Axisa *et al.*, *J. Chromatogr. B Biomed. Sci. Appl.*, 2000, *744*, 359–365. In plasma: limit of detection 3 μg/L, UV detection—A. Zarghi *et al.*, *Boll. Chim. Farm.*, 2001, *140*, 112–114.

Disposition in the Body. Readily and almost completely absorbed after oral administration; peak plasma concentrations are attained in about 2 h. It does not appear to be significantly metabolised. About 40% of a dose is excreted in the urine unchanged in 72 h (about 24% in the first 24 h).

Half-life. Plasma half-life, about 22 h.

Protein binding. In plasma, about 82 to 90%.

Note. For a review of doxycycline see B. A. Cunha *et al.*, *Ther. Drug Monit.*, 1982, *4*, 115–135.

Dose. The equivalent of 100 to 200 mg of doxycycline daily; a 1-day course of 300 to 600 mg has also been given.

Doxylamine

Antihistamine

Synonym. Histadoxylamine
N,N-Dimethyl-2-[1-phenyl-1-(2-pyridinyl)ethoxy]ethanamine
$C_{17}H_{22}N_2O$=270.4
CAS—469-21-6

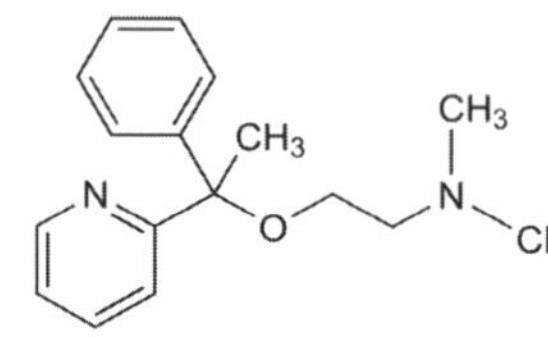

A liquid. B.p. about 140°.
Soluble in acids.

Doxylamine Succinate

Synonym. Doxylamine Hydrogen Succinate
Proprietary names. Decapryn; Donormyl; Dormidina; Dozile; Duebien; Gittalun; Hewedormir forte; Hoggar N; Lidene; Mereprine; Munleit; Noctyl; Restavit; Restwel; Sanalepsi N; Sedaplus; Somnil; Unisom.
It is an ingredient of many proprietary preparations—see *Martindale, The complete drug reference*, 33rd Edn., London, Pharmaceutical Press, 2002.
$C_{17}H_{22}N_2O$,$C_4H_6O_4$=388.5
CAS—562-10-7
A white or creamy-white powder. M.p. 100° to 104°.
Soluble 1 in 1 of water, 1 in 2 of ethanol, 1 in 2 of chloroform, and 1 in 370 of ether; slightly soluble in benzene.

Dissociation Constant. pK_a 4.4, 9.2.

Partition Coefficient. Log *P* (octanol/water), 2.4.

Colour Tests. Cyanogen Bromide—orange-pink; Liebermann's Test—red-orange; Marquis Test—violet; Sulfuric Acid—pink.

Thin-layer Chromatography. System TA—Rf 48; system TB—Rf 41; system TC—Rf 10; system TE—Rf 60; system TL—Rf 09; system TAE—Rf 12; system TAJ—Rf 00; system TAK—Rf 00; system TAL—Rf 08. (Acidified iodoplatinate solution, positive.)

Gas Chromatography. System GA—doxylamine RI 1910, M (carbinol)-H_2O RI 1560, M (OH-)-AC RI 2300, M (OH-carbinol-)-AC RI 2980, M (OH-methoxy-)-AC RI 2320, M (bis-nor-)-AC RI 2280, M (desamino-OH-)-AC RI 1960, M (nor-)-AC RI 2340; system GB—doxylamine RI 1970, M (nor-) RI 1974, M (carbinol)-H_2O RI 1670; system GF—RI 2170.

High Performance Liquid Chromatography. System HA—*k* 4.4; system HY—RI 259; system HAA—retention time 11.1 min.

Ultraviolet Spectrum. Aqueous acid—261 nm (A^1_1=335a). No alkaline shift.

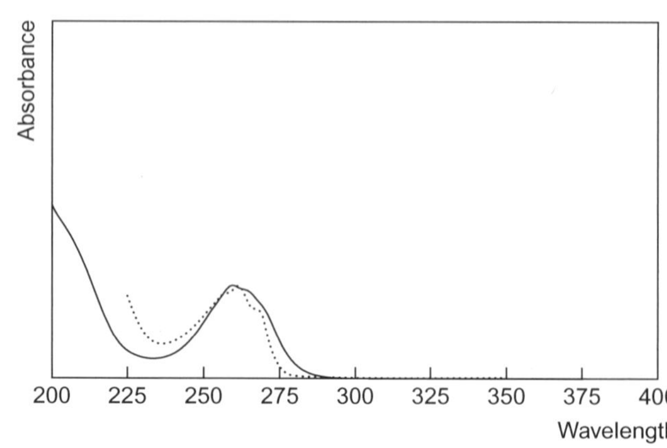

Infra-red Spectrum. Principal peaks at wavenumbers 700, 1590, 1123, 1086, 1041, 751 cm^{-1} (KBr disk).

Mass Spectrum. Principal ions at *m/z* 58, 71, 72, 167, 182, 42, 180, 59.

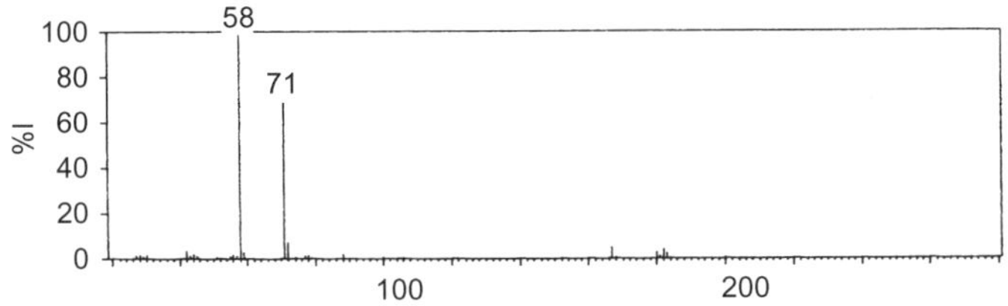

Quantification

Gas chromatography. In plasma: nitrogen-phosphorus detection—H. Friedman and D. J. Greenblatt, *J. Clin. Pharmacol.*, 1985, *25*, 448–451.

Gas chromatography–mass spectrometry. In plasma: limit of detection 100 µg/L—A. Cailleux *et al.*, *J. Chromatogr. Sci.*, 1981, *19*, 163–176.

High performance liquid chromatography. In plasma: limit of detection 5 µg/L, UV detection—K. J. Kohlhof *et al.*, *J. Pharm. Sci.*, 1983, *72*, 961–962.

Disposition in the Body. Absorbed after oral administration with 60 to 80% of a dose recovered in urine within 24 h.

Therapeutic concentration

Following a single oral dose of 25 mg in 16 subjects, a peak plasma level of 99 µg/L was obtained after 2.4 h. [H. Friedman and D. J. Greenblatt, *J. Clin. Pharmacol.*, 1985, *25*, 448–451.]

Toxicity

In 109 cases of doxylamine monointoxication, about 60% of the cases involved ingestion of 250 to 1000 mg (10 to 40 times the single therapeutic dose). For 23 of the cases, about 80% of doxylamine plasma levels were in the range 0.5 to 5.0 mg/L. [C. Koppel *et al.*, *Hum. Toxicol.*, 1987, *6*, 355–339.]

In a fatality involving doxylamine overdose, the blood concentration was 1.2 mg/L, with a nordoxylamine concentration of 0.52 mg/L; the concentration of doxylamine plus metabolites in urine was 25 mg/L. [T. J. Siek and W. A. Dunn, *J. Forensic Sci.*, 1993, *38*, 713–720.]

In 2 cases of suicide by means of doxylamine ingestion, the following tissue distribution was reported at postmortem examination: blood 140 and 100 mg/L (in case 1 and case 2, respectively), urine 180 mg/L and not reported, stomach contents 500 and 900 mg, liver 80, and 300 µg/g. [B. Bockholdt *et al.*, *Forensic Sci. Int.*, 2001, *119*, 138–140.]

Half-life. Elimination half-life, about 10 h.

Dose. Usually up to 150 mg of doxylamine succinate daily; usual hypnotic dose, 25 mg at night.

Droperidol

Antipsychotic/Tranquilliser

Proprietary names. Dehydrobenzperidol; Dridol; Droleptan; Inapsine; Paxical; Sintodian. It is an ingredient of Innovar and Thalamonal.

1-[1-[4-(4-Fluorophenyl)-4-oxobutyl]-1,2,3,6-tetrahydro-4-pyridinyl]-1,3-dihydro-2*H*-benzimidazol-2-one

$C_{22}H_{22}FN_3O_2 = 379.4$

CAS—548-73-2

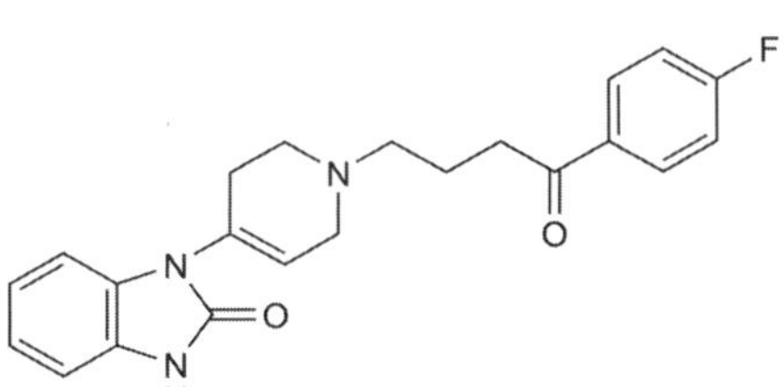

A white to light tan-coloured, amorphous or microcrystalline powder, which gradually darkens on exposure to light. M.p. 145° to 146.5°.

Practically insoluble in water; soluble 1 in 140 of ethanol, 1 in 4 of chloroform, and 1 in 500 of ether.

Dissociation Constant. pK_a 7.5.

Partition Coefficient. Log *P* (octanol/water), 3.5.

Colour Test. Mandelin's Test—blue→green.

Thin-layer Chromatography. System TA—Rf 67; system TB—Rf 02; system TC—Rf 48; system TE—Rf 58; system TL—Rf 36; system TAE—Rf 71; system TAF—Rf 73; system TAJ—Rf 37; system TAK—Rf 02; system TAL—Rf 46. (Acidified iodoplatinate solution, positive.)

Gas Chromatography. System GA—droperidol RI 3430, droperidol-Me RI 3370, M (benzimidazolone) RI 1950, M (benzimidazolone)-AC_2 RI 1730; system GB—droperidol, not eluted.

High Performance Liquid Chromatography. System HA—*k* 0.6; system HX—RI 385; system HY—RI 323; system HZ—retention time 3.5 min; system HAA—retention time 21.2 min; system HAX—retention time 8.6 min; system HAY—retention time 4.7 min.

Ultraviolet Spectrum. Aqueous acid—248 (A^1_1 = 443a), 276; aqueous alkali—246, 288 nm.

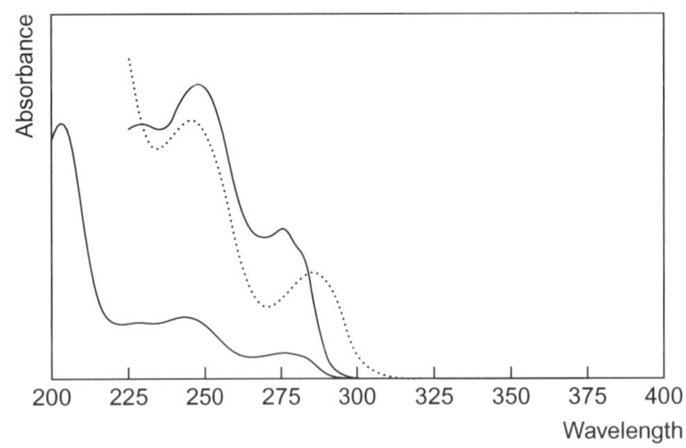

Infra-red Spectrum. Principal peaks at wavenumbers 1685, 1705, 1595, 1230, 752, 1156 cm^{-1} (KBr disk).

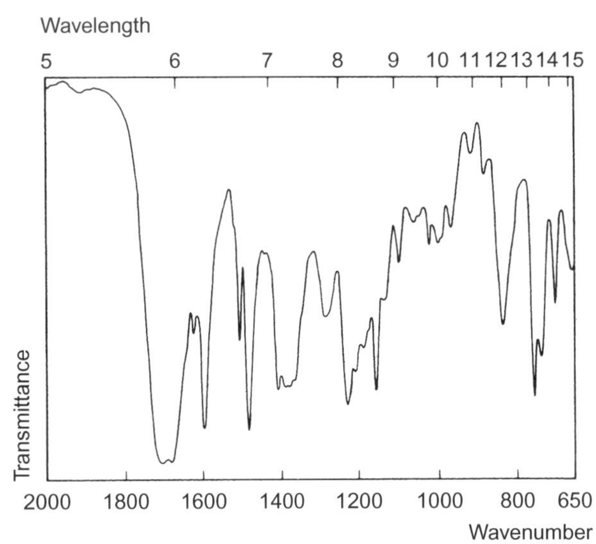

Mass Spectrum. Principal ions at *m/z* 246, 165, 42, 123, 199, 247, 214, 108.

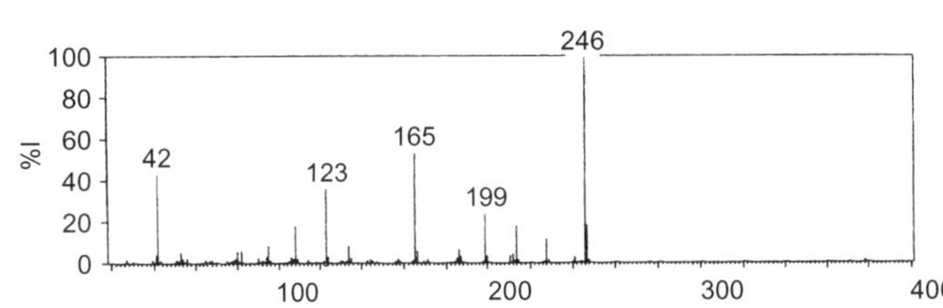

Quantification

Gas chromatography. In plasma: limit of detection 30 µg/L, FID—M. P. Quaglio *et al.*, *Boll. Chim. Farm.*, 1982, *121*, 276–284.

High performance liquid chromatography. In plasma: droperidol and flunitrazepam, limit of detection for droperidol 20 µg/L—J. Guichard *et al.*, *J. Chromatogr.*, 1993, *612*, 269–275. In plasma: limit of detection <2 µg/L—K. Kumar *et al.*, *J. Pharm. Biomed. Anal.*, 1996, *14*, 1529–1533.

Disposition in the Body. Absorbed after oral administration. About 75% of a dose is excreted in the urine with less than 10% as unchanged drug; about 22% of a dose is eliminated in the faeces.

Half-life. Plasma half-life, about 2 to 3 h.

Protein Binding. In plasma, about 85 to 90%.

Dose. 5 to 20 mg every 4 to 8 h.

Dropropizine

Cough Suppressant

Proprietary names. Atossion; Catabex; Domutussina; Eritos; Ribex; Tosofren; Tussiflex D; Vibral.
3-(4-Phenyl-1-piperazinyl)-1,2-propanediol
$C_{13}H_{20}N_2O_2$=236.3
CAS—17692-31-8

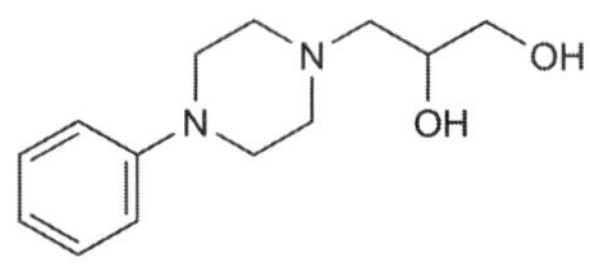

A white crystalline powder. M.p. 108° to 109°.
Soluble in chloroform and in dilute acetic acid.

Partition Coefficient. Log *P* (octanol/water), 0.1.

Colour Tests. Liebermann's Test—red-orange; Mandelin's Test—orange (slow).
Cold nitric acid gives a red colour.

Thin-layer Chromatography. System TA—Rf 65; system TB—Rf 01; system TE—Rf 34; system TAE—Rf 59. (Acidified iodoplatinate solution, strong reaction.)

Gas Chromatography. System GA—dropropizine RI 2205, dropropizine-AC_2 RI 2430, dropropizine-AC RI 2390.

High Performance Liquid Chromatography. System HX—RI 240; system HAA—retention time 7.2 min.

Ultraviolet Spectrum. Aqueous acid—238 nm (A^1_1=330a).

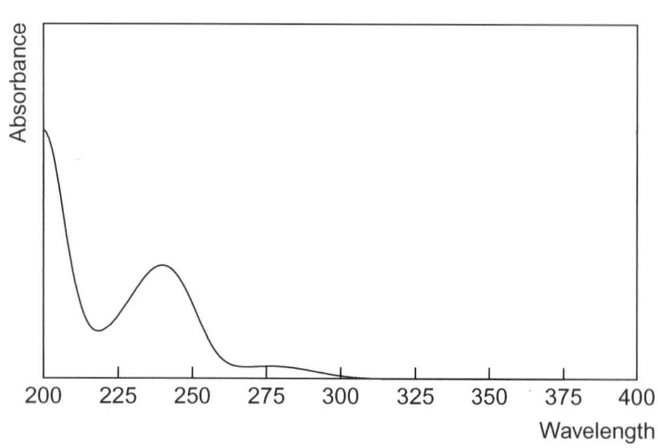

Infra-red Spectrum. Principal peaks at wavenumbers 1595, 1238, 1500, 760, 1060, 925 cm^{-1} (KBr disk).

Dose. Dropropizine has been given in doses of 90 to 120 mg daily.

Drostanolone Propionate

Anabolic Steroid

Synonym. Dromostanolone Propionate
Proprietary names. Drolban; Masterid; Masteril; Masteron; Permastril.
(2α,5α,17β)-17-Hydroxy-2-methyl-androstan-3-one propionate
$C_{23}H_{36}O_3$=360.5
CAS—58-19-5 (drostanolone); 521-12-0 (propionate)

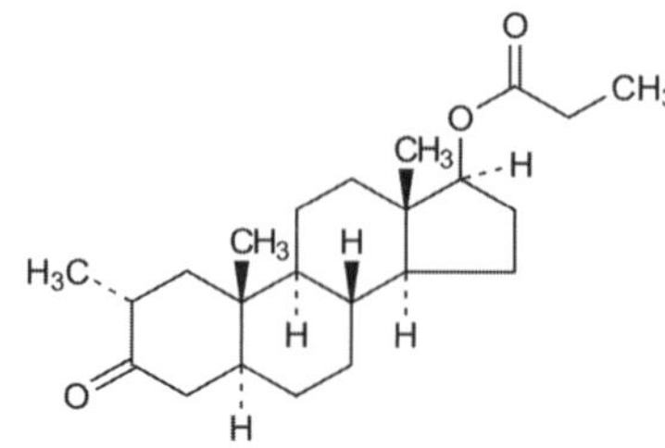

A white to creamy-white crystalline powder. M.p. 127° to 133°.
Practically insoluble in water; soluble 1 in 30 of ethanol, 1 in 2 of chloroform, and 1 in 20 of ether.

Partition Coefficient. Log *P* (octanol/water), 5.0.

Gas Chromatography. System GA—drostanolone RI 2555, drostanolone-AC RI 2700, drostanolone-TMS RI 2575, drostanolone-enol-TMS_2 RI 2625, drostanolone propionate RI 2985; system GAI—RRT 0.974 (relative to 17α-methyl-5α-androstan-3β,17β-diol)

Infra-red Spectrum. Principal peaks at wavenumbers 1715, 1200, 1735, 1035, 1087, 1265 cm^{-1} (KBr disk).

Dose. Usually 100 mg thrice weekly, by intramuscular injection.

Droxidopa

Dopaminergic

Synonyms. Threo-dopaserine; L-*threo*-DOPS; L-DOPS; L-*threo*-3-(3,4-dihydroxyphenyl)serine.
Proprietary name. Dops
threo-β,3-dihydroxy-L-tyrosine
$C_9H_{11}NO_5$=213.2
CAS—23651-95-8

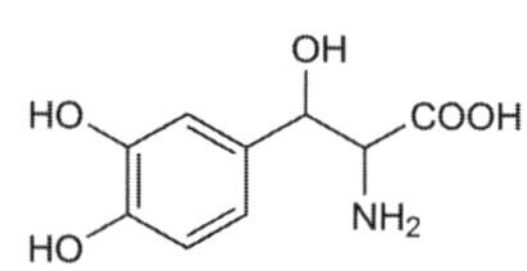

Crystals from ethanol and ether. M.p. 232° to 235°, with decomposition.

High Performance Liquid Chromatography. Column: ODS-T (Yanapak, 250 × 4 mm i.d.), $7C_{18}$ (Nucleosil) or 7ODS-H (Chemcosorb). Mobile phase: potassium phosphate (0.1 M, pH 3.10), 0.8 mL/min flow rate. Electrochemical detection. Retention time: 3.5 min. [T. Suzuki *et al.*, *Eur. J. Clin. Pharmacol.*, 1982, *23*, 463–468].

Column: C_{18} (Cp™ MicroSpher, 3 µm, 100 × 4.6 mm), at 35°. Mobile phase: disodium hydrogen phosphate (0.025 M), sodium dodecyl sulfate (0.347 mM), EDTA (0.269 mM):methanol (90:10), adjusted to pH 2.1 with phosphoric acid. Electrochemical detection. Retention time: D,L-*threo*-DOPS, 4.1 min.

Column: C_{18} (Cp™ MicroSpher, 3 µm, 100 × 4.6 mm). Mobile phase: (A) sodium phosphate (0.05 M, pH 6.5); (B) tetrahydrofuran (20 mL):methanol (10 mL):sodium phosphate (1 L). Elution programme: 0 to 100% B in 0 to 1 min, followed by isocratic elution with B, 1 mL/min flow rate. Fluorescence detection (λ_{ex}=344 nm, λ_{em}=442 nm). Retention time: D-*threo*-DOPS derivative (*o*-phthaldialdehyde and *N*-acetyl-L-cysteine), 7.14 min; L-*threo*-DOPS derivative, 7.90 min. [F. Boomsma *et al.*, *J. Chromatogr.* 1988, *427*; *Biomed. Appl.*, 219–227].

Quantification

High performance liquid chromatography. In plasma and urine: limit of detection 0.15 mg/L. Electrochemical detection—T. Suzuki *et al.*, *Eur. J.*

Clin. Pharmacol., 1982, *23*, 463–468. In plasma: limit of detection 0.01 mg/L (liquid–liquid extraction method) and 0.02 mg/L (deproteinisation method). Electrochemical detection/fluorescence detection—F. Boomsma *et al.*, *J. Chromatogr.* 1988, *427*; *Biomed. Appl.*, 219–227.

Disposition in the Body. Absorption of droxidopa is relatively slow after oral administration and it is converted to (–)-noradrenaline [(–)-norepinephrine] by aromatic L-amino acid decarboxylase, which is distributed in various tissues including the peripheral sympathetic nerves. Maximum plasma concentration is reached after 3 h. It is excreted in urine unchanged (20% of an oral dose is recovered within 12 h of administration) and as noradrenaline (norepinephrine), with approx. 1.5% of a dose being recovered over 24 h.

Therapeutic concentration

5 healthy males and 2 women, aged between 25 and 41 years, were administered a single 300 mg dose of droxidopa after overnight fasting. Peak plasma concentrations of droxidopa were reached within 3 h after administration at 1.50 ± 0.31 mg/L. A considerable amount remained in the blood 12 h after administration. [T. Suzuki *et al.*, *Eur. J. Clin. Pharmacol.*, 1982, *23*, 463–468].

Duteplase

Thrombolytic

Synonyms. SM-9527; t-PA; TPA; Fibrinokinase; Extrinsic Plasminogen Activator
Proprietary names. Actilyse; Actiplas; Prolysis; Solcot; Tiplagen
245-L-Methionine plasminogen activator (human tissue type2-chain form protein moiety)
$C_{2736}H_{4174}N_{914}O_{824}S_{46}$=64529.1
CAS—120608-46-0
Practically insoluble in solutions of low ionic strength at neutral pH.

Therapeutic concentration

24 patients with suspected acute myocardial infarction were divided into two dosing groups. Group 1: 9 patients, mean age 61 years, were administered a mean dose of 115.7 mg duteplase as an intravenous infusion at a rate of 33.3 mL/min for a mean of 81.3 min. Heparin was also administered intravenously as a bolus within 30 min of the start of the duteplase dose and continued for 48 h after the end of duteplase treatment. Group 2: 15 patients, mean age 53 years, were administered a lytic dose of 1.2 mg/kg (dose adjusted to nearest 5 kg body weight) duteplase over 60 min at an infusion rate of 30 mL/h, followed by a 0.12 mg/kg bolus over 1 min and a maintenance infusion of 0.69 mg/kg over 3 h at 5.6 mL/h. Heparin was also administered before duteplase treatment and for 3 h after. The mean total duteplase dose was 153.4 mg. The steady state plasma antigen concentration was 2335 µg/L for group 1 and 2319 µg/L after the lytic dose for group 2 and 434 µg/L after the maintenance dose. For the individuals in group 1, the mean time to reach 75% of the steady state concentration was 18 min and 27 min to reach 90%. For group 2, 75% of the steady state concentration was reached in 14 min and 90% in 22 min [R. W. Koster *et al.*, *Clin. Pharmacol. Ther.*, 1991, *50(3)*, 267–277].

Toxicity. High doses of duteplase are associated with an increased risk of serious bleeding.

A 47-year-old woman with acute myocardial infarction was treated with 162.5 mg oral aspirin, 0.4 million units/kg bolus duteplase, then 0.36 million units/kg over the first hour, followed by 0.7 million units/kg/h for 3 h and 12 500 units of subcutaneous heparin. This was the thrombolytic protocol. 9 h after duteplase was administered, the woman became hypotensive and tachycardic. She also developed a splenic haemorrhage and rupture resulting in removal of the spleen [J. Blankenship and M. Indeck, *N. Engl. J. Med.*, 1991, *325*, 969].

Half-life. Mean, 8 min.

Volume of distribution. Mean, 8.5 L.

Clearance. Mean, 685 mL/min.

Dyclonine

Local Anaesthetic

1-(4-Butoxyphenyl)-3-(1-piperidinyl)-1-propanone
$C_{18}H_{27}NO_2$=289.4
CAS—586-60-7

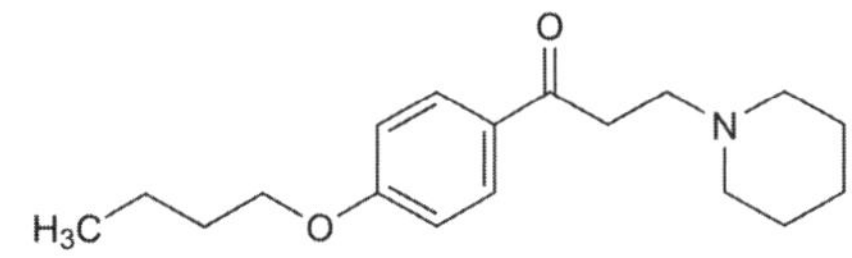

Dyclonine Hydrochloride
Synonym. Dyclonine Chloride
Proprietary names. Dyclone; Sucrets.
$C_{18}H_{27}NO_2$,HCl=325.9
CAS—536-43-6
White crystals or white crystalline powder. M.p. 175° to 176°.
Soluble 1 in 60 of water, 1 in 24 of ethanol, and 1 in 2.3 of chloroform; soluble in acetone; practically insoluble in ether.

Colour Tests. Aromaticity (Method 2)—yellow-orange; Liebermann's Test (100°)—orange.

Thin-layer Chromatography. System TA—Rf 60; system TB—Rf 49; system TC—Rf 40; system TL—Rf 25. (Acidified iodoplatinate solution, positive.)

Gas Chromatography. System GA—RI 1678.

High Performance Liquid Chromatography. System HR—*k* 2.78; system HY—RI 347.

Ultraviolet Spectrum. Aqueous acid—282 nm (A^1_1=580b).

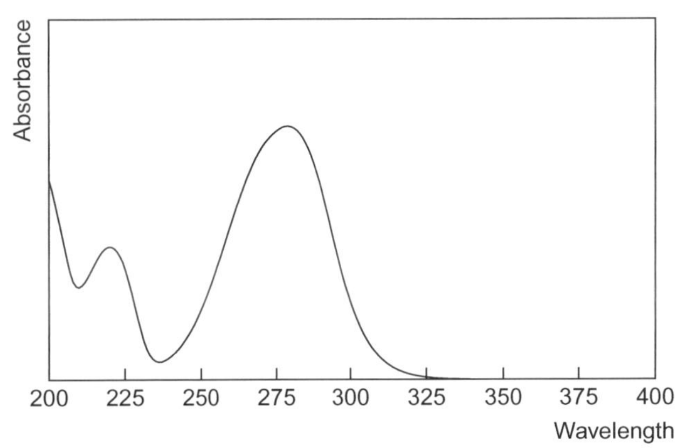

Infra-red Spectrum. Principal peaks at wavenumbers 1178, 1605, 1229, 1672, 1575, 965 cm^{-1} (dyclonine hydrochloride, KBr disk).

Use. Dyclonine hydrochloride is applied as a 0.5 or 1% solution.

Dydrogesterone

Progestational Steroid

Synonyms. Dehydroprogesterone; Didrogesteron; Isopregnenone.
Proprietary names. Biphaston; Dufaston; Duphaston; Gynorest. It is an ingredient of Femapak and Femoston.
(9β,10α)-Pregna-4,6-diene-3,20-dione
$C_{21}H_{28}O_2$=312.5
CAS—152-62-5

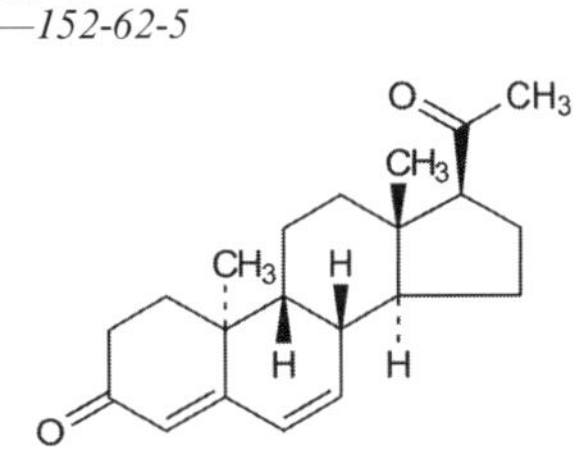

A white to pale yellow crystalline powder. M.p. 167° to 171°.
Practically insoluble in water; soluble 1 in 40 to 1 in 52 of ethanol, 1 in 17 of acetone, 1 in 2 of chloroform, and 1 in 140 of ether.

Partition Coefficient. Log *P* (octanol/water), 3.4.

Colour Tests. Antimony Pentachloride—orange; Naphthol–Sulfuric Acid—orange-red; Sulfuric Acid—orange (green-yellow fluorescence under ultraviolet light).

Thin-layer Chromatography. System TP—Rf 86; system TQ—Rf 53; system TR—Rf 96; system TS—Rf 98. (*p*-Toluenesulfonic acid solution, positive.)

Ultraviolet Spectrum. Dehydrated alcohol—286 nm (A^1_1=838a).

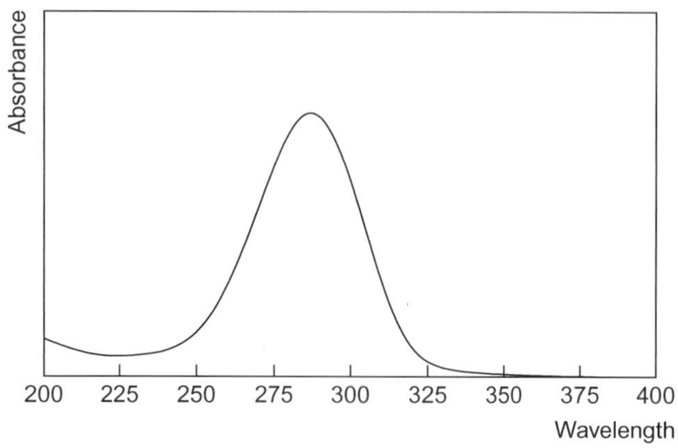

Infra-red Spectrum. Principal peaks at wavenumbers 1660, 1622, 1697, 1581, 1232, 1197 cm^{-1} (KBr disk).

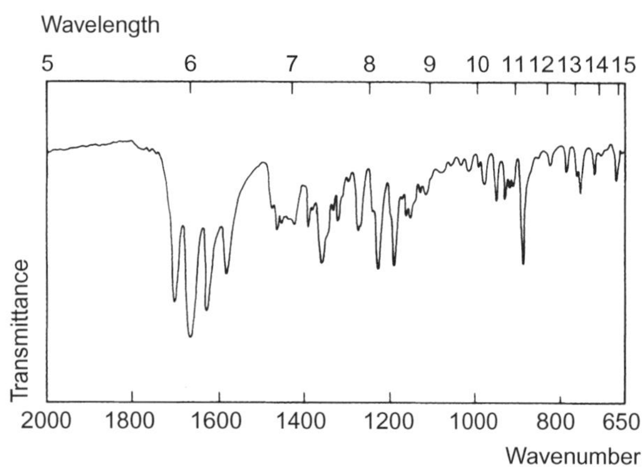

Mass Spectrum. Principal ions at *m/z* 43, 91, 227, 268, 312, 79, 55, 77.

Disposition in the Body. Rapidly absorbed after oral administration. The major metabolites are 20α-hydroxydydrogesterone and 21-hydroxydydrogesterone. About 50% of a dose is excreted in the urine in 24 h, as metabolites.

Dose. Usually 20 to 30 mg daily.

Ebastine

Antihistamine

Synonym. LAS-W-090
Proprietary names. Bastel; Bromselon; Ebastel; Evastel; Kestine.
1-[4-(1,1-Dimethylethyl)phenyl]-4-[4-(diphenylmethoxy)-1-piperidinyl]-1-butanone
$C_{32}H_{39}NO_2$=469.7
CAS—90729-43-4

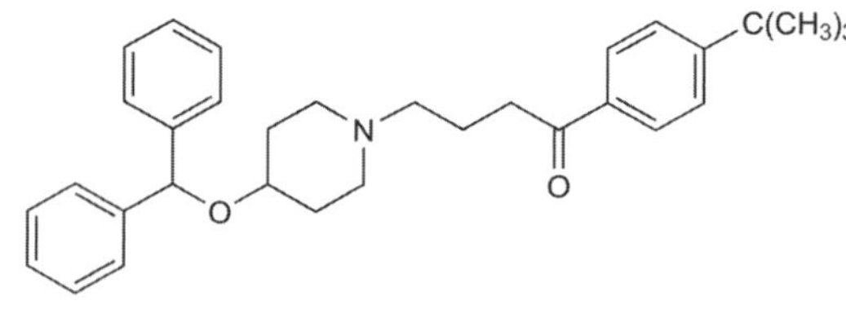

Ebastine Fumarate
$C_{32}H_{39}NO_6$, $C_4H_4O_4$=585.7
Crystals from ethanol with M.p. 197° to 198°.

Dissociation Constant. pK_a 10.32.

High Performance Liquid Chromatography. Column: ODS (250 × 4.0 mm i.d., 10 μm). Mobile phase: methanol:sodium acetate (0.02 M):glacial acetic acid: water (380:20:5.5:100), 2 mL/min flow rate. UV detection. Retention time: carebastine metabolite, 7.3 min [J. Vincent *et al.*, *Br. J. Clin. Pharmacol.*, 1988, *26*, 497–502]

Quantification
High performance liquid chromatography. In plasma: limit of detection for carebastine is 0.02 mg/L—J. Vincent *et al.*, *Br. J. Clin. Pharmacol.*, 1988, *26*, 497–502.

Disposition in the Body. Ebastine is extensively metabolised in the liver into the active metabolite, carebastine, a carboxylic acid metabolite. As metabolism is extensive, there is little parent drug present in plasma. Ebastine is excreted mainly in urine with 40% of a dose being recovered over a 24-h period. Approx. 6% can be detected in faeces.

Therapeutic concentration
9 healthy normotensive male volunteers, aged between 19 and 33 years, were administered with a 10 mg and a 50 mg dose of ebastine. Peak plasma concentrations of 0.099 ± 0.029 mg/L and 0.417 ± 0.0546 mg/L were reached within 3.61 ± 1.06 and 3.70 ± 0.76 h, respectively [J. Vincent *et al.*, *Br. J. Clin. Pharmacol.*, 1988, *26*, 497–502].

Bioavailability. Increases with consumption of food.

Half-life. 13 to 16 h.

Protein binding. Approx. 98%.

Dose. A usual dose of 10 mg daily is administered to adults, with a maximum of 20 mg. For children over 6 years, 5 mg daily is given.

Ecgonine

Alkaloid

Synonym. Laevo-ecgonine
[1*R*-(*exo*,*exo*)]-3-Hydroxy-8-methyl-8-azabicyclo[3.2.1]octane-2-carboxylic acid
$C_9H_{15}NO_3$=185.2
CAS—481-37-8

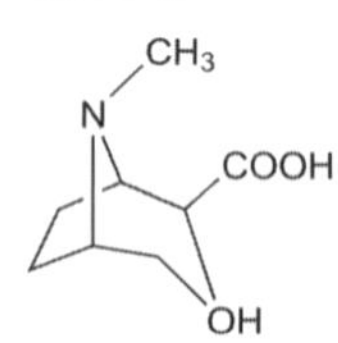

M.p. 198°, with decomposition; the dry substance melts at 205°.
Soluble in water; slightly soluble in ethanol; sparingly soluble in acetone, ether, benzene, chloroform, and petroleum ether.

Ecgonine Hydrochloride
$C_9H_{15}NO_3$,HCl=221.7
CAS—5796-31-6
Triclinic plates from water. M.p. 246°

Dissociation Constant. pK_a 2.8, 11.1.

Partition Coefficient. Log *P* (octanol/water), −3.8.

Thin-layer Chromatography. System TA—Rf 17; system TAL—Rf 05. (Acidified iodoplatinate solution, positive.)

Gas Chromatography. System GA—not eluted.

High Performance Liquid Chromatography. System HA—*k* 1.1.

Ultraviolet Spectrum. Ethanol—275 nm.

Infra-red Spectrum. Principal peaks at wavenumbers 1688, 1210, 1200, 1223, 1134, 1179 cm^{-1} (ecgonine hydrochloride, KBr disk).

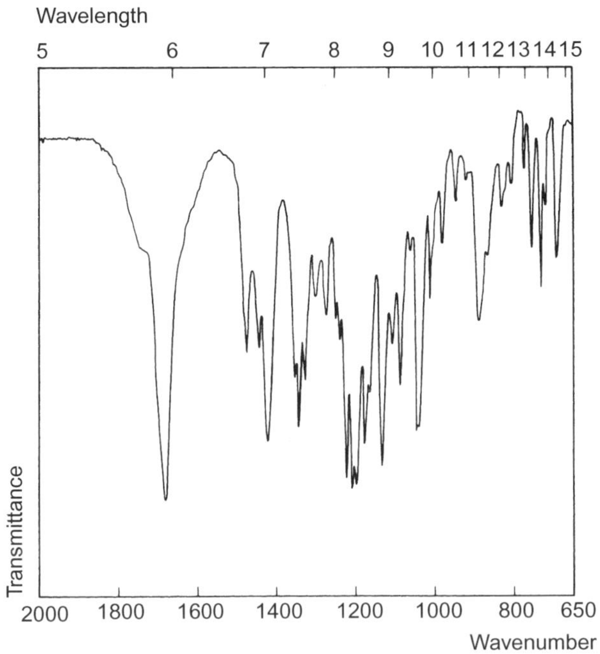

Mass Spectrum. Principal ions at *m/z* 82, 97, 42, 83, 96, 57, 94, 55.

Quantification. See also under Cocaine.

High performance liquid chromatography. In urine: ecgonine methyl ester and other cocaine metabolites, fluorescence detection—I. M. Roy *et al.*, *J. Pharm. Biomed. Anal.*, 1992, *10*, 943–948.

High performance liquid chromatography–mass spectrometry. In urine: ecgonine, ecgonine methyl ester, and other cocaine metabolites—M. Nishikawa *et al.*, *Forensic Sci. Int.*, 1994, *66*, 149–158. In urine: ecgonine methyl ester and cocaine, limit of detection for ecgonine methyl ester 2.8 pg—S. R. Needham *et al.*, *J. Chromatogr. B. Biomed. Sci. Appl.*, 2000, *748*, 77–87. In urine: ecgonine methyl ester, benzoylecgonine, and cocaine, limit of detection for ecgonine methyl ester 0.5 µg/L—P. M. Jeanville *et al.*, *J. Anal. Toxicol.*, 2001, *25*, 69–75. In plasma: ecgonine and cocaine and some other metabolites—A. Klingmann *et al.*, *J. Anal. Toxicol.*, 2001, *25*, 425–430.

Review. In blood, plasma, or serum: methods for monitoring drugs of abuse in cases of suspected driving under the influence of drugs—M. R. Moeller and T. Kraemer, *Ther. Drug Monit.*, 2002, *24*, 210–221.

Disposition in the Body. Ecgonine and its methyl ester are metabolites of cocaine.

Econazole

Antifungal

1-[2-[(4-Chlorophenyl)methoxy]-2-(2,4-dichlorophenyl)ethyl]-1*H*-imidazole
$C_{18}H_{15}Cl_3N_2O$ = 381.7
CAS—27220-47-9

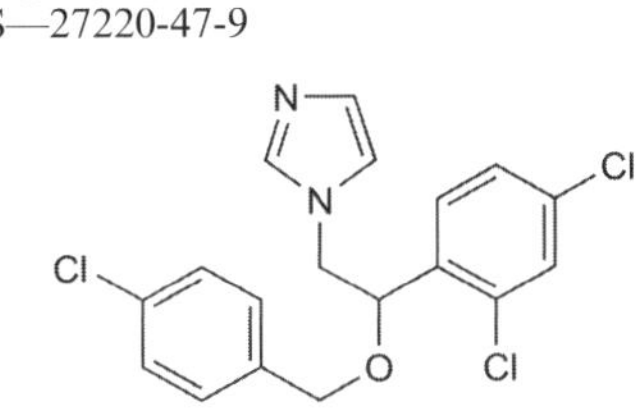

M.p. 86.8°.

Econazole Nitrate

Proprietary names. Dermazol(e); Eccelium; Eco Mi; Ecodergin; Ecoderm; Ecorex; Ecostatin; Ecosteril; Ecotam; Ecreme; Epi-Pevaryl; Gyno-Pevaryl; Ifenac; Micoespec; Micoseptil; Micostyl; Pevalip; Pevaryl; Sebolith; Spectazole. It is an ingredient of Econacort.
$C_{18}H_{15}Cl_3N_2O,HNO_3$ = 444.7
CAS—24169-02-6; 68797-31-9
A white crystalline powder. M.p. about 164°, with decomposition.
Very slightly soluble in water and ether; soluble 1 in 125 of ethanol, 1 in 60 of chloroform and 1 in 25 of methanol.

Thin-layer Chromatography. System TA—Rf 80; system TB—Rf 09; system TC—Rf 61; system TE—Rf 75; system TAE—Rf 78; system TAF—Rf 80.

Gas Chromatography. System GA—RI 3550.

High Performance Liquid Chromatography. System HX—RI 526; system HY—RI 385; system HAA—Retention time, 20.1 min.

Ultraviolet Spectrum. Methanolic acid—265 nm (A_1^1 = 12b), 271 nm (A_1^1 = 12.5a), 280 nm (A_1^1 = 7.6a).

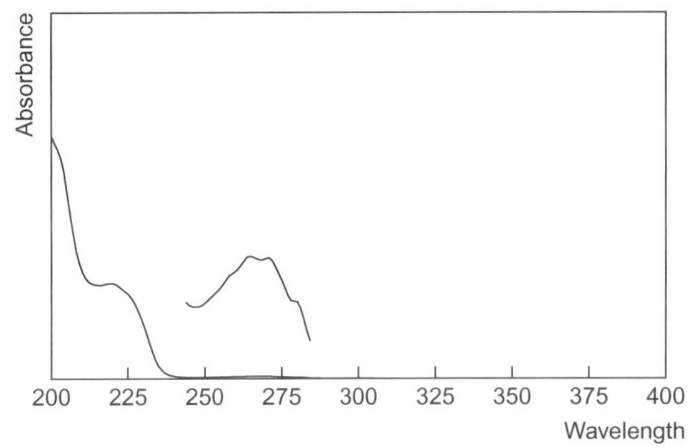

Infra-red Spectrum. Principal peaks at wavenumbers 1090, 1310, 805, 825, 1010, 1040 cm^{-1} (econazole nitrate, KBr disk).

Quantification
High performance liquid chromatography. In plasma: limit of detection 200 µg/L, UV detection—R. R. Brodie *et al.*, *J. Chromatogr.*, 1978, *155*, 209–213. In serum: econazole and other antifungal drugs—T. K. Ng *et al.*, *J. Antimicrob. Chemother.*, 1996, *37*, 465–472.

Disposition in the Body. About 10% of a topical dose is absorbed and after vaginal application about 5% of the dose is absorbed. Following oral administration, about 40% of the dose is excreted in the urine and 30% is eliminated in the faeces, in 5 days.

Blood concentration
A mean peak plasma concentration of 2.6 mg/L has been reported 2.5 h after oral administration of 250 mg of econazole to 8 subjects [R. C. Heel *et al.*, *Drugs*, 1978, *16*, 177–201].

Uses. Econazole nitrate is applied topically in a concentration of 1%, or as pessaries.

Ecothiopate Iodide

Anticholinesterase

Synonyms. Diethoxyphosphinylthiocholine Iodide; Echothiopate Iodide; Echothiophate Iodide; Ecostigmine Iodide.
Proprietary name. Phospholine Iodide
2-[(Diethoxyphosphinyl)thio]-*N*,*N*,*N*-trimethylethanaminium iodide
$C_9H_{23}INO_3PS$ = 383.2
CAS—6736-03-4 (ecothiopate); 513-10-0 (iodide)

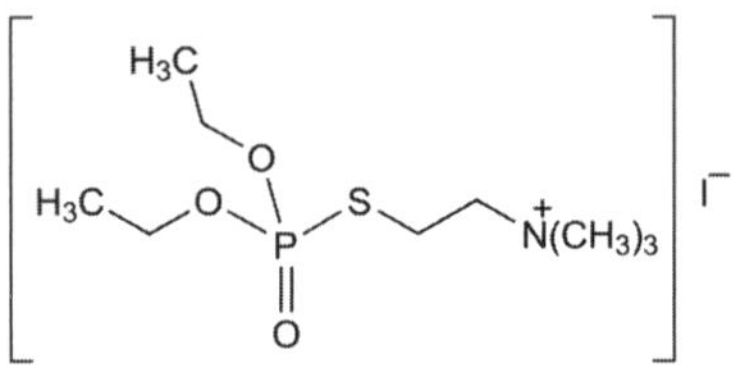

A white, hygroscopic, crystalline powder. M.p. 138° or 124° to 124.5°. Soluble in water, alcohol and chloroform.

Partition Coefficient. Log *P* (octanol/water), −2.2.

Colour Test. Palladium Chloride—orange

Thin-layer Chromatography. System TA—Rf 02. (Acidified iodoplatinate solution, positive.)

Use. As a 0.03 to 0.25% ophthalmic solution.

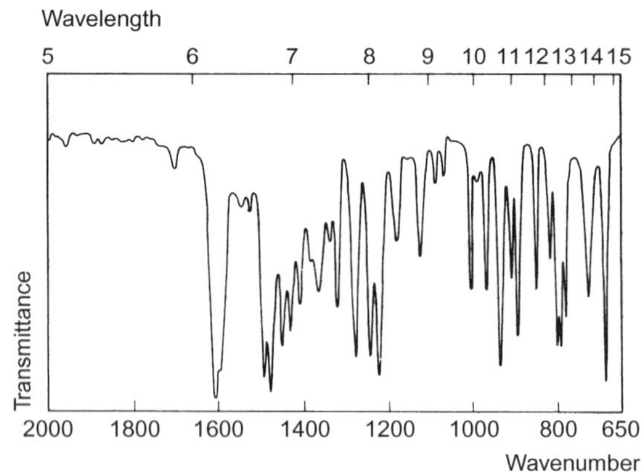

Disposition in the Body

Therapeutic concentration

Following intravenous injections of 100 µg/kg to 5 subjects, plasma concentrations of 0.8 to 3.9 mg/L (mean 1.6) were reported at 2 min, declining to 0.038 to 0.056 mg/L (mean 0.048) at 1 h [T. N. Calvey *et al.*, *Clin. Pharmacol. Ther.*, 1976, *19*, 813–820].

Toxicity. The estimated minimum lethal dose is 100 mg.

Half-life. Plasma half-life, about 0.5 h.

Dose. 2 to 10 mg intravenously, in the diagnosis of myasthenia gravis.

Edrophonium Chloride

Anticholinesterase

Proprietary names. Anticude; Camsilon; Enlon; Reversol; Tensilon.
N-Ethyl-3-hydroxy-*N*,*N*-dimethylbenzenaminium chloride
$C_{10}H_{16}ClNO$=201.7
CAS—312-48-1 (edrophonium); 116-38-1 (chloride)

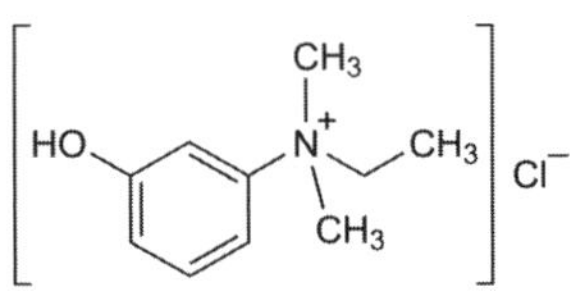

A white crystalline powder. M.p. 165° to 170°, with decomposition. Soluble 1 in 0.5 of water and 1 in 5 of ethanol; practically insoluble in chloroform and ether.

Partition Coefficient. Log *P* (octanol/water), −3.0.

Colour Test. Mandelin's Test—blue-green.

Thin-layer Chromatography. System TA—Rf 07. (Acidified iodoplatinate solution, positive.)

Ultraviolet Spectrum. Aqueous acid—273 nm (A_1^1=110a); aqueous alkali—240 nm (A_1^1=550b), 294 nm (A_1^1=170b).

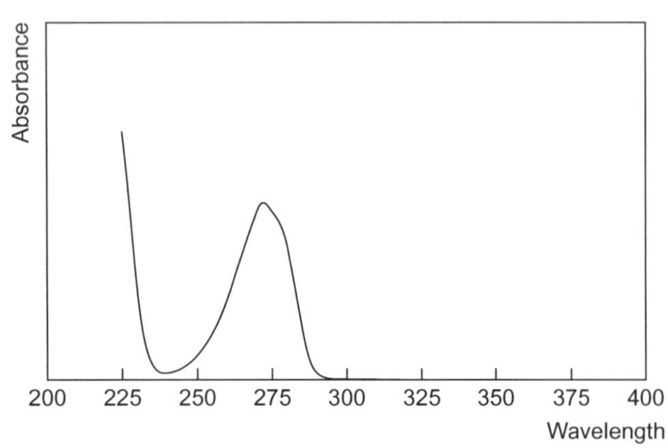

Infra-red Spectrum. Principal peaks at wavenumbers 1609, 690, 1217, 1495, 934, 1280 cm^{-1} (KBr disk).

Efavirenz

Antiviral

Synonyms. DMP-266; L-743726.
Proprietary name. Sustiva
(*S*)-6-Chloro-4-(cyclopropylethynyl)-1,4-dihydro-4-(trifluoromethyl)-2*H*-3,1-benzoxazin-2-one
$C_{14}H_9ClF_3NO_2$=315.7
CAS—154598-52-4

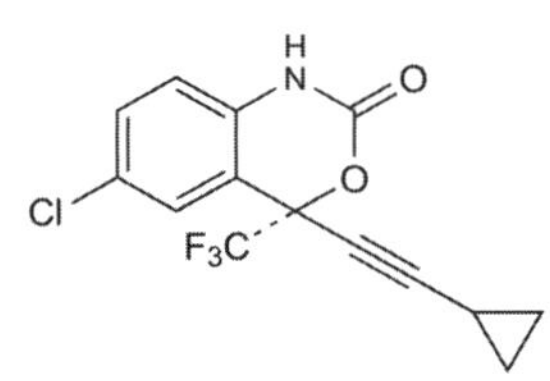

A white to slightly pink crystalline powder, which is practically insoluble in water (<10 g/L).

Dissociation Constant. pK_a 10.2.

High Performance Liquid Chromatography. System HAC—*k* 8.5; system HAE—retention time, 28.6 min.

Column: (analytical) C_{18} (Zorbak SB, 3.5 µm, 150 × 4.6 mm i.d.), (guard) (10 × 3 mm i.d.). Mobile phase: phosphate buffer (25 mM): acetonitrile (53:47), pH adjusted to 7.5 with diluted 2 M potassium hydroxide solution, 1.5 mL/min flow rate. UV detection (λ=246 nm). Retention time: 10.2 min [A. I. Veldkamp *et al.*, *J. Chromatogr. B Biomed. Sci. Appl.*, 1999, *734*, 55–61].

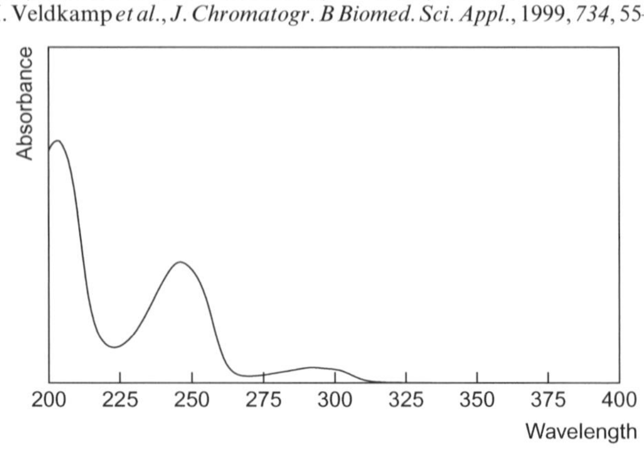

Mass Spectrum. Principal ions at *m/z* 246, 243, 180, 315, 248, 245, 182, 167.

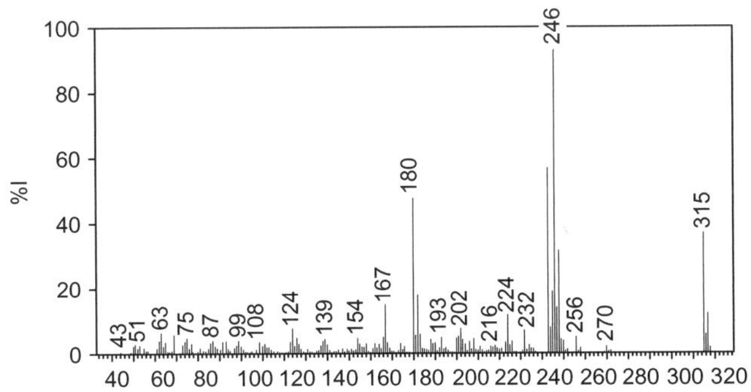

Quantification

High performance liquid chromatography. In serum: limit of detection 0.062 mg/L, UV detection—V. A. Simon *et al.*, *J. Chromatogr. A*, 2001, *913(1-2)*, 447–453. In plasma: limit of detection 0.1 mg/L. UV detection (λ=247 nm)—P. Villani *et al.*, *Ther. Drug Monit.*, 1999, *21(3)*, 346–350. In plasma: limit of detection 0.01 mg/L. UV detection (λ=246 nm)—A. I. Veldkamp *et al.*, *J. Chromatogr. B Biomed. Sci. Appl.*, 1999, *734(1)*, 55–61. In plasma: limit of quantification is 0.05 mg/L. UV detection (λ=241 nm)—G. Aymard *et al.*, *J. Chromatogr. B Biomed. Sci. Appl.*, 2000, *744*, 227–240.

Disposition in the Body. Efavirenz is metabolised by the cytochrome P450 system to hydroxylated metabolites, which can undergo subsequent glucuronidation to inactive metabolites. 14 to 34% of an administered dose can be recovered in urine as the metabolites and 16 to 61% in faeces as the parent drug. Efavirenz is known to cross the blood–brain barrier.

Therapeutic concentration

A single oral dose between 100 and 1600 mg was administered to uninfected volunteers and peak plasma concentrations between 0.51 and 2.9 mg/L were observed. These levels were reached after 5 h. A 600 mg dose administered to HIV-infected patients, however, produced a peak plasma concentration of 4.1 mg/L, which was reached within 3 to 5 h [DuPont Pharmaceutical Company, Sustiva (Efavirenz capsules) Prescribing Information, 1998, Sept. 17].

Toxicity. A mild to moderate rash with blistering and shedding is the main toxicology effect. Two incidents have been noted, where two patients accidentally took a total dose of 1200 mg and showed an increase in nervous system symptoms and involuntary muscle contractions.

Half-life. Elimination half-life for a single dose is 52 to 76 h, and 40 to 55 h for multiple doses.

Clearance. Mean plasma clearance, 0.18 L/h/kg.

Protein binding. >99% bound to plasma proteins, mainly albumin.

Dose. Adult: 600 mg daily. Child: between 200 and 400 mg daily depending on body weight (13 to 39 kg), >40 kg: adult dose.

Eflornithine

Antineoplastic/Antiprotozoal

Synonyms. DFMO; MDL-71782; RMI-71782.
2-(Difluoromethyl)-D,L-ornithine
$C_6H_{12}F_2N_2O_2$=182.2
CAS—67037-37-0

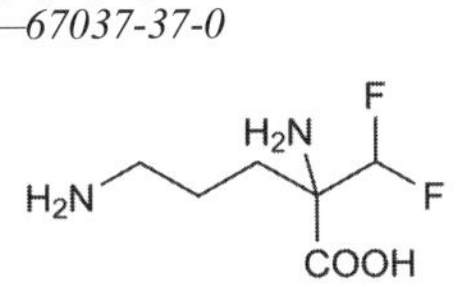

Eflornithine Hydrochloride
$C_6H_{13}ClF_2N_2O_2$=218.7
CAS—68278-23-9
Crystalline powder. M.p. 183°.

Eflornithine Hydrochloride Monohydrate
Synonym. MDL-71782A
Proprietary name. Ornidyl
$C_6H_{15}ClF_2N_2O_3$=236.6
CAS—96020-91-6
Crystalline powder. M.p. 183°.

High Performance Liquid Chromatography. Column: (analytical) RP C_8 (150 × 4.6 mm i.d., 5 μm), (guard) C_8 (15 × 4.6 mm i.d., 5 μm). Mobile phases: (A) sodium acetate (10 mM, adjusted to pH 4.18 with acetic acid (1.0 M)): tetrahydrofuran (95:5); (B) acetonitrile: tetrahydrofuran (90:10). Elution program: (A:B) (100:0) for 2 min, to (63.3:36.7) in 19 min, to (0:100) for 2 min at 1.5 mL/min, back to initial conditions in 2 min, held for 3 min. UV detection (λ=330 nm). Retention time: 14.7 min [J. L. Cohen *et al.*, *J. Pharm. Sci.*, 1989, *78(2)*, 114–116].

Quantification

High performance liquid chromatography. In serum: limit of detection 10 mg/L. UV detection (λ=330 nm)—J. L. Cohen *et al.*, *J. Pharm. Sci.*, 1989, *78(2)*, 114–116.

Enzyme-linked immunosorbant assay. In plasma: limit of detection 0.5 nmol/L—P. C. Gunaretna *et al.*, *J. Pharm. Biomed. Anal.*, 1994, *12(10)*, 1249–1257.

Disposition in the Body. Eflornithine is absorbed (approx. 60%) after oral administration and undergoes decarboxylation. >80% of the dose is excreted in urine, 40 to 45% of which remains unchanged. The drug is distributed into central spinal fluid.

Therapeutic concentration

6 healthy men, aged between 21 and 31 years, were administered an oral dose of 10 and 20 mg/kg body weight eflornithine, and a 10 mg/kg dose intravenously. Peak plasma concentrations of 31.4 to 51.0 nmol/L were reached, within 2 to 6 h, for the 10 mg/kg oral dose and 27.4 to 137.5 nmol/L for the 20 mg/kg dose (1.5 to 4 h) [K. D. Haegele *et al.*, *Clin. Pharmacol. Ther.*, 1981, *30*, 210–215].

Toxicity. Ototoxicity can occur and loss of hearing has been observed with a cumulative dose. Low toxicity via ingestion and intraperitoneal routes.

Bioavailability. Oral bioavailability, 55%.

Half-life. 3 to 4 h.

Volume of distribution. 0.33 to 0.37 L/kg.

Clearance. Total body clearance, 1.17 mL/min/kg.

Dose. A dose of 100 mg/kg body weight is administered every 6 h, intravenously, for at least 14 days, which may be followed by a 300 mg/kg body weight daily dose (orally) for 3 to 4 weeks. Dose is decreased for patients with impaired renal function.

Embutramide

Narcotic Analgesic

Proprietary names. It is an ingredient of Tanax (vet.) and T 61 (vet.).
N-(*β*,*β*-Diethyl-*m*-methoxyphenethyl)-4-hydroxybutyramide
$C_{17}H_{27}NO_3$=293.4
CAS—15687-14-6

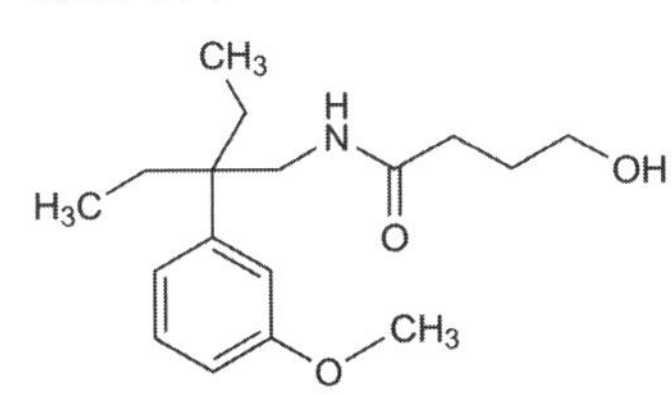

Crystals. M.p. 70°.

Colour Tests. Mandelin's Test—brown; Marquis Test—blue

Thin-layer Chromatography. System TA—Rf 72; system TE—Rf 59; system TAJ—Rf 53; system TAK—Rf 46. (Acidified potassium permanganate solution, positive.)

High Performance Liquid Chromatography. System HAA—Retention time, 17.4 min.

Ultraviolet Spectrum. Aqueous acid—271 nm (A^1_1=50b), 276 nm.

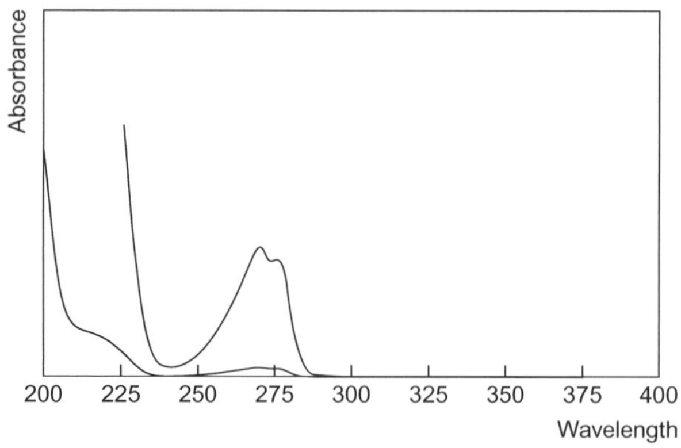

Infra-red Spectrum. Principal peaks at wavenumbers 1652, 1248, 1037, 1595, 1562, 1063 cm^{-1} (KBr disk).

Quantification

Gas chromatography–mass spectrometry. In body tissues or fluids—W. E. Braselton *et al.*, *Vet. Hum. Toxicol.*, 1988, *30*, 536–539. In blood, liver or kidney—M. Giorgi *et al.*, *J. Anal. Toxicol.*, 2001, *25*, 323–327.

High performance liquid chromatography. In blood, liver or kidney—M. Giorgi *et al.*, *J. Anal. Toxicol.*, 2001, *25*, 323–327.

Ultraviolet spectrophotometry. In blood or urine—E. Bertol *et al.*, *J. Pharm. Biomed. Anal.*, 1983, *1*, 373–377.

Disposition in the Body

Toxicity

In 3 fatalities caused by the injection of a preparation containing embutramide and mebezonium iodide, the following postmortem concentrations (mg/L) were reported:

	Embutramide	Mebezonium iodide
Blood	3.0, 15.5, 12.1	4.5, 6.0, 7.5
Urine	2.0, 6.3, 4.5	0.8, 2.0, 1.8

[E. Bertol *et al.*, *J. Pharm. Biomed. Anal.*, 1983, *1*, 373–377.]

A 58-year-old veterinarian died after ingesting about 30 mL of T-61 solution (a mixture of embutramide, mebezonium and tetracaine, used for animal euthanasia). The embutramide concentration in postmortem femoral blood was 43.0 mg/L [P. Kintz *et al.*, *J. Anal. Toxicol.*, 2002, *26*, 529–531.]

Emepronium Bromide

Anticholinergic

Proprietary names. Cetiprin; Uro-Ripirin.

N-Ethyl-*N*,*N*-α-trimethyl-γ-phenylbenzenepropanaminium bromide

$C_{20}H_{28}BrN = 362.4$

CAS—27892-33-7 (emepronium); 3614-30-0 (bromide)

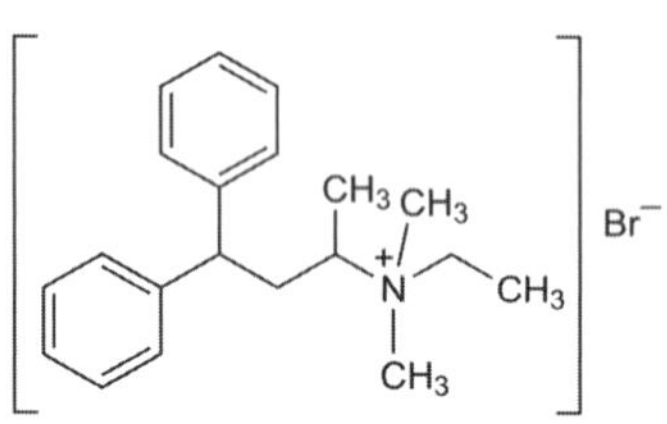

A white crystalline powder. M.p. 204°.

Soluble in water, ethanol and chloroform.

Partition Coefficient. Log *P* (octanol/water), 0.5.

Colour Test. Liebermann's Test—brown

Thin-layer Chromatography. System TA—Rf 05; system TB—Rf 00; system TE—Rf 02; system TAE—Rf 03. (Acidified iodoplatinate solution, strong reaction.)

Gas Chromatography. System GA—RI 1973.

High Performance Liquid Chromatography. System HA—*k* 5.2; system HX—RI 420.

Ultraviolet Spectrum. Aqueous acid—253, 258 nm ($A_1^1 = 13a$), 268 nm.

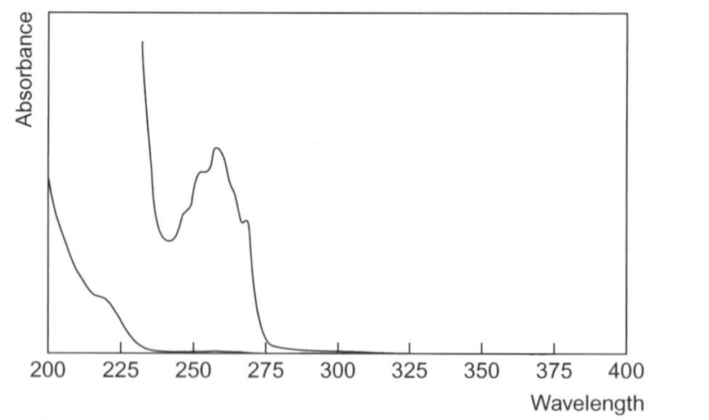

Infra-red Spectrum. Principal peaks at wavenumbers 708, 699, 752, 1102, 742, 1134 cm^{-1} (KBr disk).

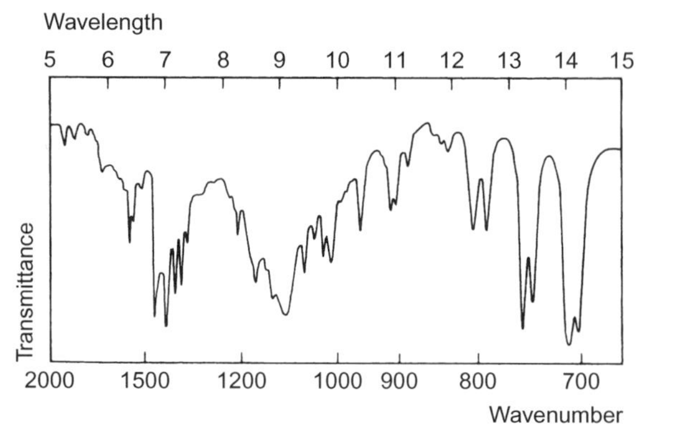

Quantification

Gas chromatography. In serum: limit of detection 200 ng/L, ECD—P. Hartvig *et al.*, *J. Pharm. Sci.*, 1976, *65*, 1707–1709.

Disposition in the Body. Poorly absorbed after oral administration; less than 5% of a dose is excreted in the urine in 24 h, partly as metabolites. After intramuscular administration, about 30% of a dose is excreted in the urine in 3 days and 45% is eliminated in the faeces in the same period.

Therapeutic concentration

Following a single oral dose of 150 mg to 5 subjects, peak serum concentrations of 0.017 to 0.10 mg/L were attained in about 2 h [J. Vessman *et al.*, *Acta Pharm. Suec.*, 1970, *7*, 363–372.]

Half-life. Plasma half-life, about 7 to 11 h.

Dose. 200 to 600 mg daily.

Emetine

Anti-amoebic

Synonyms. Ipecine; Methylcephaëline.

6′,7′,10,11-Tetramethoxyemetan

$C_{29}H_{40}N_2O_4 = 480.6$

CAS—483-18-1

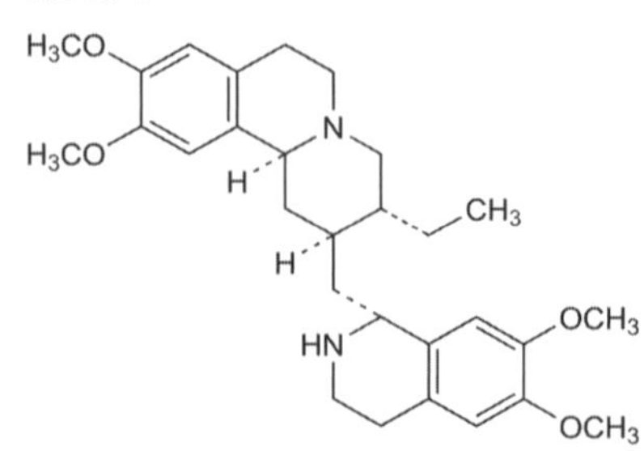

An alkaloid present in ipecacuanha, the dried root, or rhizome and roots, of *Cephaëlis ipecacuanha* (= *Uragoga ipecacuanha*) (Rubiaceae) or *C. acuminata*.

A white amorphous powder. M.p. 74°.

Slightly soluble in water; soluble in ethanol, chloroform and ether.

Emetine Hydrochloride
Synonym. Emetine Dihydrochloride
Proprietary names. It is an ingredient of Cophylac, Ipeca, Sano Tuss and Spirbon.
$C_{29}H_{40}N_2O_4,2HCl,7H_2O=679.7$
CAS—316-42-7 (anhydrous); 7083-71-8 (hydrate)
A white or very slightly yellow, crystalline powder. M.p. 235° to 255° with decomposition, after drying.
Soluble 1 in 8 of water, 1 in 12 of ethanol (90%) and 1 in 4 of chloroform; practically insoluble in ether.

Dissociation Constant. pK_a 7.4, 8.3 (25°).

Partition Coefficient. Log *P* (octanol/water), 5.2.

Colour Test. Liebermann's Test—black

Thin-layer Chromatography. System TA—Rf 54; system TB—Rf 13; system TC—Rf 34; system TE—Rf 53; system TL—Rf 12; system TAE—Rf 19; system TAJ—Rf 09; system TAK—Rf 02; system TAL—Rf 58. (Acidified iodoplatinate solution, positive.)

Gas Chromatography. System GA—RI 2505.

High Performance Liquid Chromatography. System HA—*k* 7.1 (tailing peak); system HX—RI 310; system HAA—Retention time, 9.4 min.

Ultraviolet Spectrum. Aqueous acid—230 nm (A_1^1=341a), 282 nm (A_1^1=158a).

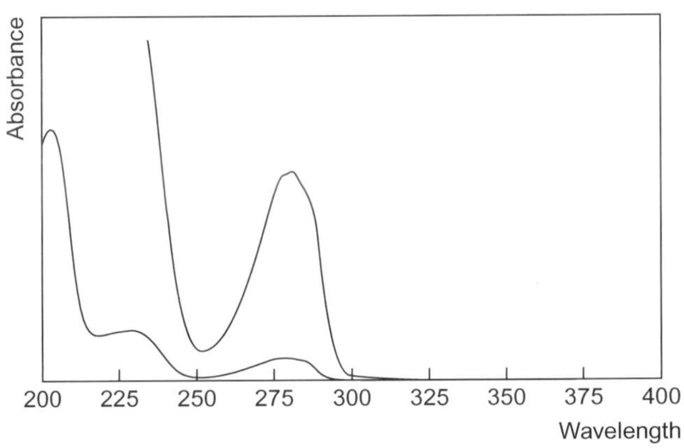

Infra-red Spectrum. Principal peaks at wavenumbers 1514, 1256, 1228, 1110, 1200, 1150 cm^{-1} (KBr disk).

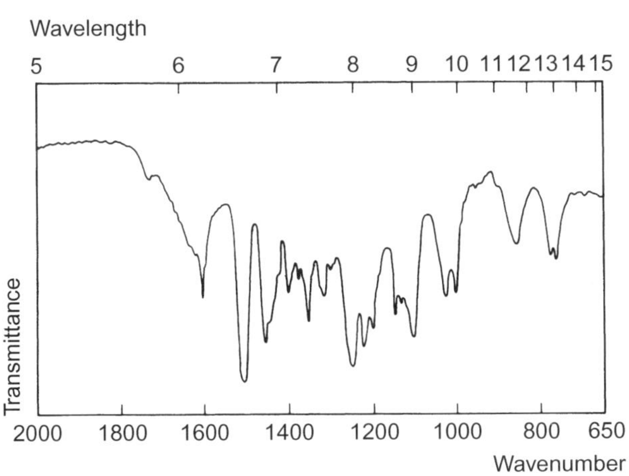

Mass Spectrum. Principal ions at *m/z* 192, 206, 272, 480, 288, 246, 205, 191.

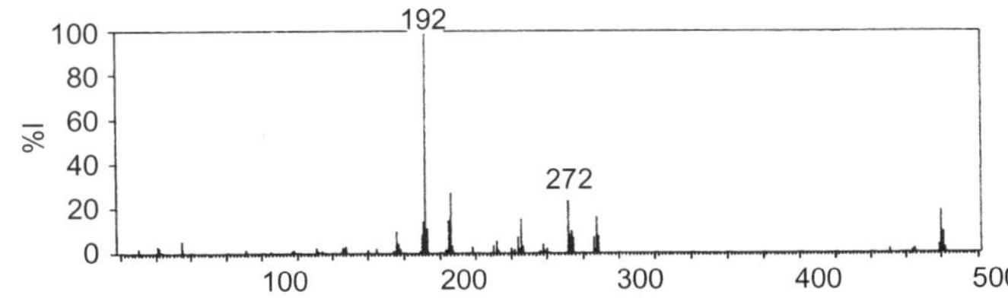

Quantification
High performance liquid chromatography. In plasma: limit of detection 10 µg/L, fluorescence detection—S. J. Bannister *et al.*, *J. Chromatogr.*, 1979, *176*, 381–390. In blood or urine: limit of detection 5 µg/L, fluorescence detection—D. J. Crouch *et al.*, *J. Anal. Toxicol.*, 1984, *8*, 63–65. In plasma or urine: emetine and cephaëline, limits of detection for emetine <2.5 µg/L in plasma and <5 µg/L in urine, fluorescence detection—T. Asano *et al.*, *J. Chromatogr. B. Biomed. Sci. Appl.*, 2001, *757*, 197–206.

Disposition in the Body. Rapidly absorbed after oral administration and after injection; concentrated in the liver, kidneys, lungs and spleen. It is excreted only very slowly in the urine and detectable concentrations are found up to 60 days after treatment.

Toxicity. The minimum lethal dose is 150 mg.

In a fatality which occurred after chronic ingestion of about 70 mg of emetine daily for 3 months, the following postmortem tissue concentrations were reported: blood 2.4 µg/g, bile 1.9 µg/g, kidney 7.4 µg/g, liver 14 µg/g [A. G. Adler *et al.*, *JAMA*, 1980, *243*, 1927–1928].

Dose. Up to 60 mg of emetine hydrochloride daily, subcutaneously or intramuscularly, for no longer than 10 days.

Emylcamate

Tranquilliser/Muscle Relaxant

3-Methyl-3-pentanol carbamate
$C_7H_{15}NO_2=145.2$
CAS—78-28-4

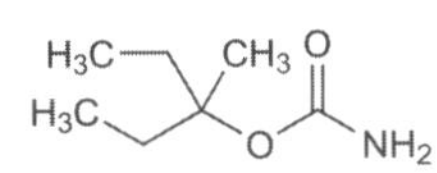

A white crystalline powder. M.p. 56° to 58°.
Soluble 1 in 250 of water; freely soluble in benzene, ethanol, ether and glycol ethers.

Partition Coefficient. Log *P* (octanol/water), 1.8.

Gas Chromatography. System GA—RI 1105.

Ultraviolet Spectrum. No significant absorption, 230 to 360 nm.

Infra-red Spectrum. Principal peaks at wavenumbers 1690, 1610, 1041, 1170, 1150, 1010 cm^{-1} (KCl disk).

Mass Spectrum. Principal ions at *m/z* 73, 43, 84, 55, 69, 41, 44, 85.

Dose. Emylcamate was formerly given in doses of 600 to 800 mg daily.

Enalapril

Antihypertensive

(*S*)-1-[*N*-[1-(Ethoxycarbonyl)-3-phenylpropyl]-L-alanyl]-L-proline
$C_{20}H_{28}N_2O_5=376.5$
CAS—75847-73-3

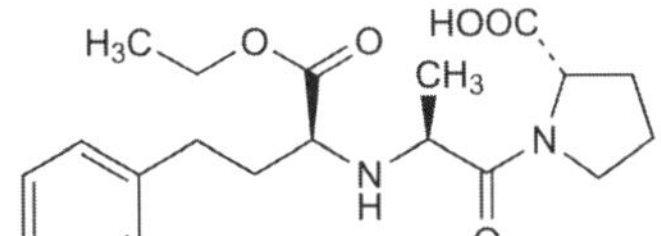

Enalapril Maleate
Synonyms. L-154; MK-421; 739-001D.
Proprietary names. Amprace; Bitensil; Cardiovet; Enacard; Enaloc; Enapren; Glioten; Hipoartel; Innovace; Lotrial; Olivin; Pres; Renitec; Reniten; Renivace; Vasotec; Xanef.
$C_{20}H_{28}N_2O_5, C_4H_4O_4=492.5$

CAS—76095-16-4
A white to off-white crystalline, odourless powder. M.p. 143° to 144.5°. Solubility in water is 0.025 g/mL, alcohol 0.08 g/mL, methanol 0.2 g/mL and dimethyl formamide >400 g/L. It is, also, slightly soluble in semi-polar organic solvents; practically insoluble in non-polar organic solvents.

Enalaprilat

Synonyms. Enalaprilic Acid; MK-422.
$C_{18}H_{24}N_2O_5$, $2H_2O$=384.4
CAS—76420-72-9 (anhydrous); 84680-54-6 (dihydrate)
A white to nearly white, hygroscopic crystalline powder, needles from water, M.p. 148° to 151°. It is soluble in water (1 in 200), methyl alcohol (1 in 68), dimethyl formamide (1 in 40); slightly soluble in isopropyl alcohol; very slightly soluble in acetone, alcohol and hexane; practically insoluble in chloroform.

Dissociation Constant. pK_a 2.97 and 5.35 (25°) (maleate).

Partition Coefficient. Log *P* (octanol/water), 2.45.

Colour Test. Bromothymol blue (acidic aqueous, pH 2: $CHCl_3$)—yellow.

Thin-layer Chromatography. System TB—Rf 00; system TD—Rf 00; system TE—Rf 00 (enalapril); Rf 00 (enalaprilat); system TF—Rf 00 (enalapril); Rf 00 (enalaprilat); system TAD—Rf 00; system TAE—Rf 85.

Plate: silica gel (Analtech GF, Whatman KLF or E Merck G60). Mobile phase: chloroform: methanol: acetic acid (90:10:1). Enalapril, Rf 0.6; enalaprilat, Rf 0.

Plate: silica gel (Analtech GF, Whatman KLF or E Merck G60). Mobile phase: *n*-butanol: water: acetic acid (3:1:1). Enalapril, Rf 0.7; enalaprilat, Rf 0.35.

Plate: silica gel (Analtech GF, Whatman KLF or E Merck G60). Mobile phase: *n*-butanol: toluene: water: acetone: acetic acid (1:1:1:1). Enalapril, Rf 0.55; enalaprilat, Rf 0.45. [D. P. Ip and G. S. Brenner. In: H. G. Brittain (ed.), *Analytical Profiles of Drug Substances and Excipients*, 1987, Vol. 16, Academic Press, New York, pp. 207–243].

Gas Chromatography. System GA—RI 2620 enalapril, RI 2650 enalapril-ME; RI 2730 M (enalaprilate-H_2O)-ME; system GP—RI 2675 enalapril-ME; RI 2680 M (enalaprilat)-ME3; RI 2735 M (enalaprilat-H_2O)-ME.

Column: silica (DB-1, 10 m × 0.25 mm i.d., 0.25 µm). Column temperature: 150°, held 1 min, and increased to 280° at 30°/min. Injector temperature: 280°. Carrier gas: helium. MS detection (NICI, SIM (selected-ion monitoring) at *m/z* 302, enalapril; 288 enalaprilat). Reference compound: RS-5139. Retention time: enalapril 4.58 min; enalaprilat 4.49 min [H. Shioya *et al.*, *Biomed. Chromatogr.*, 1992, *6*, 59–62].

High Performance Liquid Chromatography. System HX—RI 201; system HZ— retention time 1.5 min (enalaprilat); system HAA—retention time 3.4 min.

Column: Hypersil ODS (250 × 4.5 mm i.d., 5 µm). Mobile phase: sodium heptanesulfonate (20 mM, pH 2.5): acetonitrile (5% THF) (63:37), 1.0 mL/min flow rate. UV detection (λ=215 nm). Retention time: 10 min [D. Bonazzi *et al.*, *J. Pharm. Biomed. Anal.*, 1998, *16*, 431–438].

Ultraviolet Spectrum. Aqueous acid (0.2 M H_2SO_4)—257, 268 nm; (0.1 M phosphate buffer, pH 4.5: methanol (80:20)—229 nm (enalapril maleate).

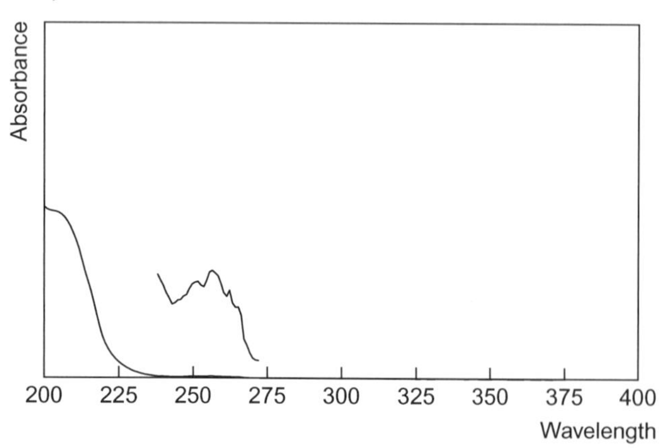

Infra-red Spectrum. Principal peaks at wavenumbers 1750, 1645, 1425, 1390, 1187 cm^{-1} (maleate).

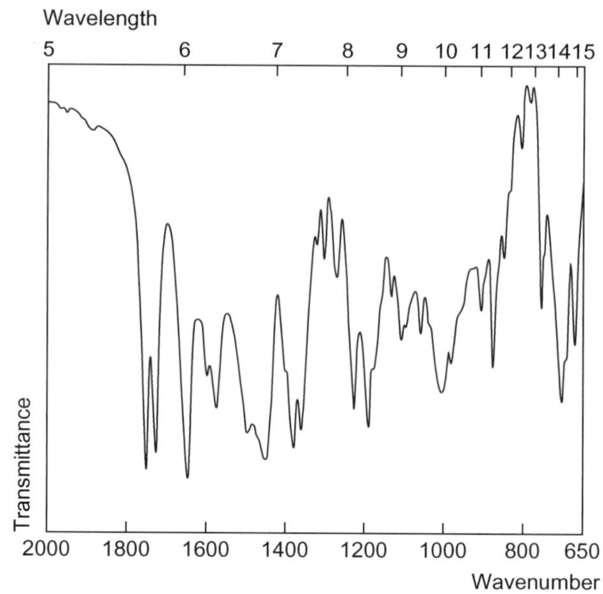

Mass Spectrum. Principal ions at *m/z* 91, 70, 208, 254, 117, 56, 160, 54 (maleate).

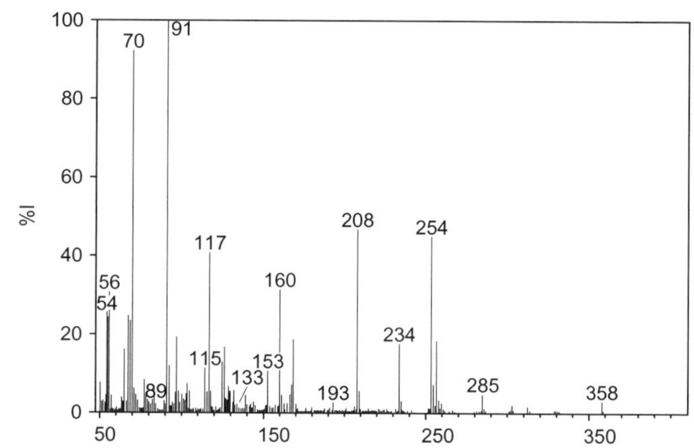

Quantification

Gas chromatography–mass spectrometry. In plasma and urine: limit of detection for both enalapril and enalaprilat is 0.2 µg/L and 2 µg/L, respectively—H. Shioya *et al.*, *Biomed. Chromatogr.*, 1992, *6(2)*, 59–62.

Fluoroimmunoassay. In serum: limit of detection 0.5 µg/L—A. S. Yuan and J. D. Gilbert, *J. Pharm. Biomed. Anal.*, 1996, *14(7)*, 773–781.

Disposition in the Body. After oral administration, 60% of a dose is absorbed, and rapidly and extensively hydrolysed in the liver to enalaprilat. Peak plasma concentrations of enalaprilat are achieved 3 to 4 h after oral dose. Enalapril is excreted in urine as the metabolite, enalaprilat, and the rest in faeces as the unchanged drug. After a single oral dose of 20 mg enalapril, enalapril and enalaprilat can be detected in breast milk with a concentration of 1 to 2.3 µg/L for the latter. Enalaprilat is removed by haemodialysis and peritoneal dialysis.

Therapeutic concentration. The serum therapeutic concentration range is 0.01 to 0.05 mg/L for the metabolite, desethylenalapril.

18 healthy, normotensive subjects: 9 males, aged between 21 and 39 years, 6 males and 3 females, 66 to 76 years old, were administered 10 mg enalapril maleate after an overnight fast. Peak plasma concentrations of 128 ± 63 nmol/L enalaprilat were reached, within 4 h, for the younger group and 199 ± 105 nmol/L, within 5 h, for the more elderly group [N. J. MacDonald *et al.*, *Br. J. Clin. Pharmacol.*, 1993, *36*, 205–209].

Toxicity. Treatment with enalapril can result in renal failure, with the possibility of death. Severe hypotension is the main toxic effect and loss of hearing has also been reported by some.

Bioavailability. Oral bioavailability, 53 to 74% (enalapril) and 36 to 44% (enalaprilat).

Half-life. Elimination half-life is approx. 2 h for enalapril and ⩾ 38 h for enalaprilat (also reported as 11 h).

Volume of distribution. 1.7 L/kg.

Protein binding. 50 to 60% bound.

Dose. An initial dose of 5 mg daily is administered, followed by a maintenance dose of 10 to 20 mg daily. The maximum dose is 40 mg daily. In patients with renal impairment, or those also taking a diuretic and the elderly: an initial dose of 2.5 mg daily is administered.

Enallylpropymal

Barbiturate

1-Methyl-5-(1-methylethyl)-5-(2-propenyl)-2,4,6(1*H*,3*H*,5*H*)-pyrimidinetrione
$C_{11}H_{16}N_2O_3$=224.3
CAS—1861-21-8

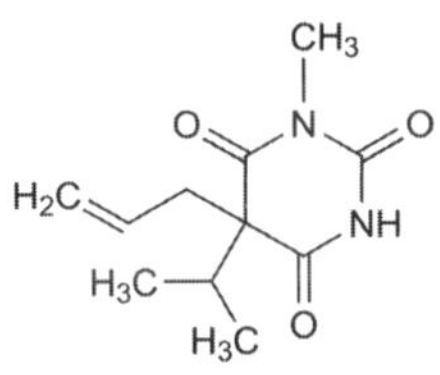

Crystals. M.p. 56° to 57°.
Soluble in organic solvents.

Partition Coefficient. Log *P* (octanol/water), 1.6.

Thin-layer Chromatography. System TD—Rf 71; system TE—Rf 58; system TF—Rf 71; system TH—Rf 87; system TAD—Rf 70.

Gas Chromatography. System GA—enallylpropymal RI 1560; enallylpropymal-Me$_2$ RI 1520.

High Performance Liquid Chromatography. System HG—*k* 8.65; system HH—*k* 6.96; system HY—RI 394.

Ultraviolet Spectrum. Borax buffer 0.05 M (pH 9.2)—245 nm (A^1_1=329b); 1 M sodium hydroxide (pH 13)—244 nm (A^1_1=362b).

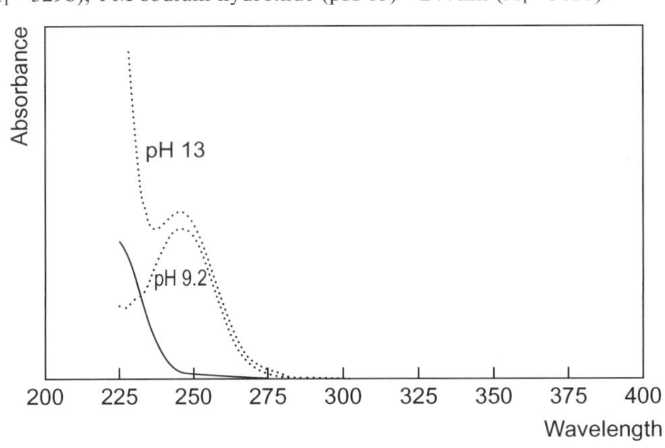

Infra-red Spectrum. Principal peaks at wavenumbers 1689, 1718, 1550, 1640, 1285, 672 cm^{-1}.

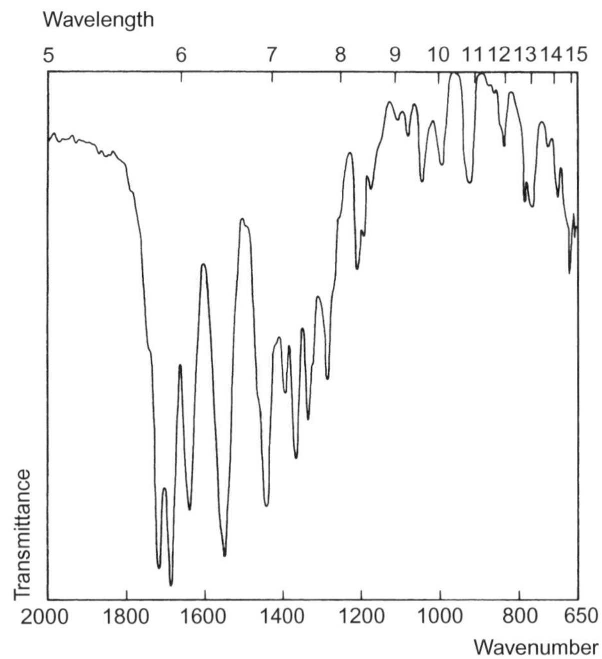

Mass Spectrum. Principal ions at *m/z* 181, 41, 182, 39, 124, 53, 138, 97.

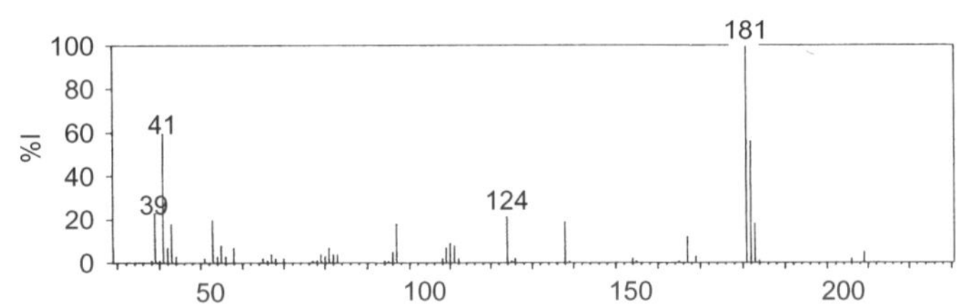

Encainide

Anti-arrhythmic

Synonym. MJ-9067-1
4-Methoxy-*N*-[2-[2-(1-methyl-2-piperidinyl)ethyl]phenyl]benzamide
$C_{22}H_{28}N_2O_2$=352.5
CAS—66778-36-7; 37612-13-8

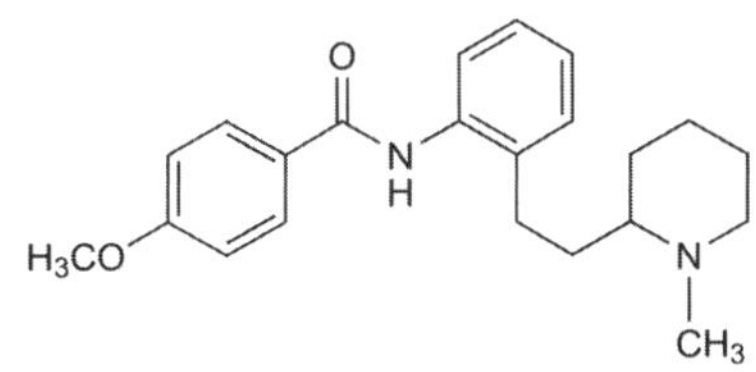

Encainide Hydrochloride
Synonym. MJ-9067
Proprietary names. Enkade; Enkaid.
$C_{22}H_{28}N_2O_2$, HCl=388.9
CAS—66794-74-9
Crystalline powder. M.p. 131.5° to 132.5°. It is freely soluble in water; slightly soluble in ethanol; insoluble in heptane.

Dissociation Constant. pK_a 10.2.

Partition Coefficient. Log *P* (octanol/water), 4.24.

Thin-layer Chromatography. System TB—Rf 28; system TE—Rf 54; system TAE—Rf 16.

Gas Chromatography. System GA—RI 3016.

High Performance Liquid Chromatography. System HX—RI 363; system HAX—retention time 9.4 min; system HAY—4.9 min.

Column: silica (Zorbax, 250 × 4 mm i. d., 5 to 6 µm). Mobile phase: absolute ethanol:water:methanesulfonic acid (500:60:0.2), 1.0 mL/min flow rate. UV detection (λ=254 nm). Retention times: encainide, 9.29 min; 3-methoxy-*o*-desmethyl encainide (MODE), 8.15 min; *o*-desmethyl encainide (ODE), 7.11 min; *N*-desmethyl encainide (NDE), 6.00 min. [M. J. Bartek *et al.*, *Ther. Drug Monit.*, 1988, *10(4)*, 446–452].

Column: phenyl (µBondapak, 300 × 3.9 mm i.d., 10 µm). Mobile phase: ethanol:water:methanesulfonic acid (500:30:0.1), 1.5 mL/min flow rate. UV detection (λ=254 nm). Retention times: encainide, 13.2 min; *N*-desmethyl encainide, 9.1 min; 3-methoxy-*o*-desmethyl encainide, 6.0 min; *o*-desmethyl encainide, 5.3 min. [K. Selinger and J. C. Crawhall, *J. Pharm. Biomed. Anal.*, 1989, *7(3)*, 355–359].

Column: (analytical) silica (Resolve, 150 mm × 4.6 mm i.d., 5 µm), (guard) 10 mm pre-column packed with same material. Mobile phase: methanol:water:methanesulfonic acid:triethylamine (400:4:0.02:0.02). Internal standard (IS): 4-methyl-propanolol. UV detection (λ=270 nm). Retention times: IS, 3.6 min; NDE, 4.5 min; ODE, 5.6 min; MODE, 6.3 min; encainide, 7.0 min [J-M Poirier *et al.*, *J. Chromatogr.*, 1990, *534*, *Biomed. Appl.*, 223–227].

Mass Spectrum. Principal ions at *m/z* 98, 135, 99, 70, 77, 97, 42, 112.

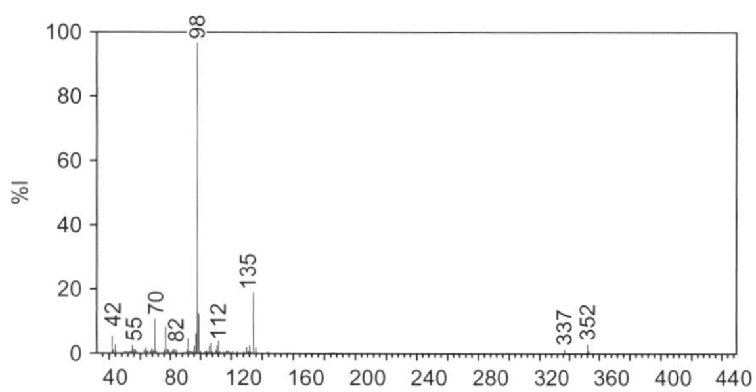

Quantification

High performance liquid chromatography. In plasma and urine: limit of detection 5 µg/L and 25 µg/L, respectively. UV detection (λ=254 nm)—M. J. Bartek *et al.*, *Ther. Drug Monit.*, 1988, *10(4)*, 446–452. In plasma: limit of detection 10 µg/L. UV detection (λ=254 nm)—K. Selinger and J. C. Crawhall, *J. Pharm. Biomed. Anal.*, 1989, *7(3)*, 355–359.

Disposition in the Body. Encainide is well absorbed and extensively metabolised in the liver to two active metabolites, (ODE) and (MODE). Inactive metabolites include (NDE) and sulfate and glucuronide conjugates. The extent of metabolism varies between individuals as there are extensive metabolisers and poor metabolisers. Approx. 7% of the Caucasian and Black population are poor metabolisers. Excretion varies between these individuals but is mainly via urine with approx. 30% of a dose present in faeces. 39% of an administered dose is found in the urine of poor metabolisers but only 4.9% for extensive metabolisers with 10.6% ODE and 3.6% MODE.

Therapeutic concentration. The serum therapeutic concentration range is 60 to 280 µg/L for the metabolite, MODE and 100 to 300 µg/L for ODE.

8 healthy individuals, extensive and poor metabolisers, were administered a 50 mg dose encainide every 8 h. The extensive metabolisers reached plasma concentrations of 18 ± 6 µg/L encainide, 115 ± 11 µg/L ODE, 94 ± 10 µg/L MODE and < 10 µg/L NDE. The poor metabolisers, however, had plasma concentrations of 450 µg/L encainide, 12 µg/L ODE and 80 µg/L NDE. No MODE was detected.

6 patients with hepatic disease were also studied with a dose of 50 mg encainide. Plasma concentrations of 63 ± 9 µg/L encainide, 87 ± 8 µg/L ODE and 113 ± 81 µg/L MODE were reached. No NDE was detected [D. M. Roden *et al.*, *Clin Pharmacokinet.*, 1988, *14*, 141–147].

Toxicity. Severe and potentially fatal ventricular tachycardia and cardiac arrest, congestive heart failure and seizures. Toxicity observed with ODE concentrations > 300 µg/L.

Bioavailability. 30% (extensive metabolisers) and 88% (poor metabolisers).

Half-life. For encainide, 2.5 h (extensive metabolisers) and 8 to 11 h (poor metabolisers). For ODE, 4 to 8 h and MODE, 12 to 20 h.

Volume of distribution. Approx. 265 L.

Protein binding. Encainide is bound 70 to 78%, ODE 75 to 85% and MODE 92%.

Dose. A usual dose of 100 to 200 mg daily is administered. In patients with renal clearance 10 to 50 mL/min: dose reduced by 50%, clearance < 10 mL/min: initially 25 mg daily, which can be increased to a maximum of 150 mg daily.

Endosulfan

Pesticide

Synonym. Benzoepin
Proprietary names. Malix; Thiodan; Thionex.
6,7,8,9,10,10-Hexachloro-1,5,5a,6,9,9a-hexahydro-6,9-methano-2,4,3-benzodioxathiepin-3-oxide
$C_9H_6Cl_6O_3S$=406.9
CAS—115-29-7; 959-98-8 (α); 33213-65-9 (β)

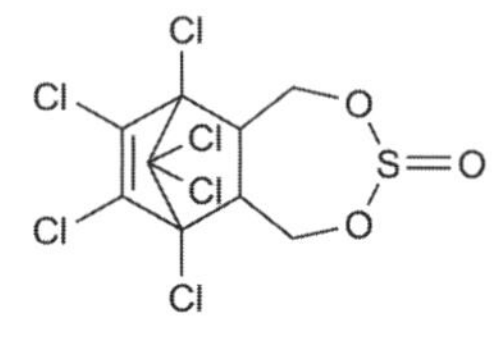

Endosulfan is a mixture of 2 stereoisomers: the α-isomer, M.p. 108° to 110°, accounts for about 70% of the technical grade and the *β*-isomer, M.p. 208° to 210°, for about 30%.
The technical grade is a brownish crystalline solid. M.p. 70° to 100°. Practically insoluble in water; soluble in most organic solvents.

Partition Coefficient. Log *P* (octanol/water), 3.8.

Thin-layer Chromatography. System TX—Rf 40; system TY—Rf 77; system TZ—Rf 77; system TAA—Rf 95.

Gas Chromatography. System GA—endosulfan RI 2090, endosulfan sulfate RI 2260, endosulfan II RI 2175; system GK—RRT 1.10 (relative to caffeine).

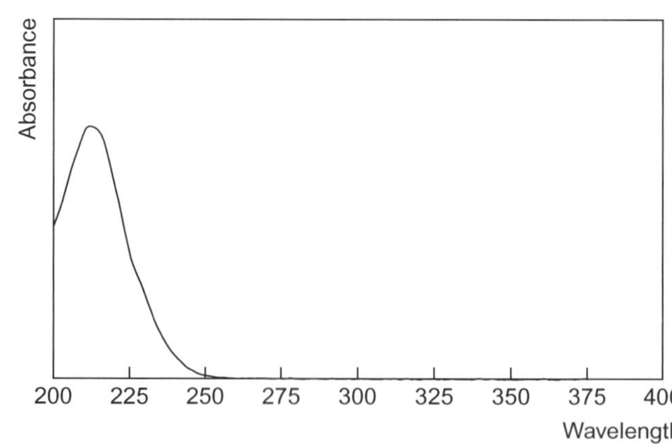

Mass Spectrum. Principal ions at *m/z* 195, 36, 237, 41, 241, 75, 239, 170.

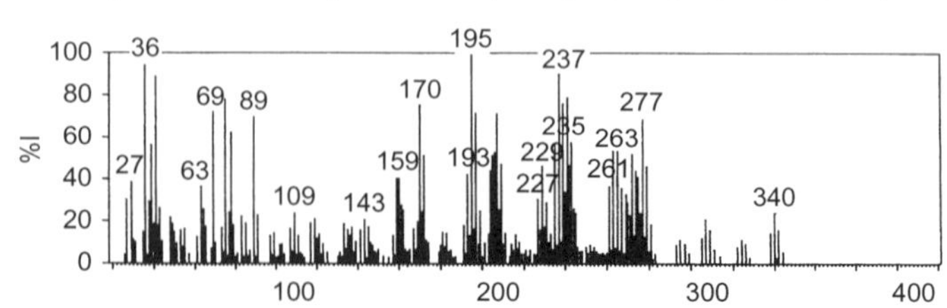

Quantification

Gas chromatography. In blood or tissues: ECD or FID—A. Coutselinis *et al.*, *Forensic Sci.*, 1976, *8*, 251–254. In blood: endosulfan and other pesticides, nitrogen–phosphorus detection or electrochemical detection—R. Garcia-Repetto *et al.*, *J. AOAC Int.*, 2001, *84*, 342–349 In blood: ECD—A. Ramesh and P. E. Ravi, *J. Environ. Monit.*, 2002, *4*, 190–193. In serum: α- and *β*-endosulfan and metabolites, ECD—J. L.Martinez Vidal *et al.*, *Anal. Bioanal. Chem.*, 2002, *372*, 766–775.

Gas chromatography–mass spectrometry. In serum, urine or tissues: limit of detection 2 ng for α-endosulfan—J. Demeter *et al.*, *Quant. Mass Spectrom.*

Life Sci., 1978, *2*, 471–481. In serum: α- and β-endosulfan and metabolites, limit of detection 0.05 μg—J. L.Martinez Vidal *et al.*, *Rapid Commun. Mass Spectrom.*, 2000, *14*, 939–946. In serum: endosulfan and its metabolites, limits of detection 6 to 19 ng/L—F. J. Arrebola *et al.*, *J. Chromatogr. Sci.*, 2001, *39*, 177–182. In serum: endosulfan and other pesticides—J. Dmitrovic *et al.*, *Toxicol. Lett.*, 2002, *134*, 253–258. In serum: α- and β-endosulfan and metabolites—J. L. Martinez Vidal *et al.*, *Anal. Bioanal. Chem.*, 2002, *372*, 766–775.

Disposition in the Body

Toxicity

In a death involving the ingestion of endosulfan dispersed in 55% xylene, the following concentrations of endosulfan were reported: blood 30 mg/L, liver 20 μg/g, kidney 2.0 μg/g, brain 0.3 μg/g; 0.5 g endosulfan and 0.4 g xylene were found in 50 mL stomach contents [B. C. Bernardelli and M. C. Gennari, *J. Forensic Sci.*, 1987, *32*, 1109–1112].

In 6 reported cases of acute endosulfan intoxication, the one fatality had a blood endosulfan level of 2.85 mg/L compared with a mean of 0.48 mg/L in the survivors [J. L. Blanco-Coronado *et al.*, *J. Toxicol. Clin. Toxicol.*, 1992, *30*, 575–583].

In a 43-year-old man who died 4 days after non-accidental ingestion of 100 mL of endosulfan (18 g, 260 mg/kg), the postmortem tissue concentrations of α-endosulfan, β-endosulfan, and endosulfan sulfate were, respectively (μg/g): adipose tissue 4.105, not found, not found; liver <0.050, <0.055, 3.034; brain 0.080, 0.069, 1.348; kidney 0.059, <0.050, 0.393; stomach content 3.541, 1.391, <0.080. Blood concentrations 2.5 h after ingestion were 644, 101 and 874 μg/L, respectively, and declined to 106, 27 and 347 μg/L at 7.5 h [F. T. Boereboom *et al.*, *J. Toxicol. Clin. Toxicol.*, 1998, *36*, 345–352].

Endrin

Insecticide

(1aα,2β,2aβ,3α,6α,6aβ,7β,7aα)-3,4,5,6,9,9-Hexachloro-1a,2,2a,3,6,6a,7,7a-octahydro-2,7:3,6-dimethanonaphth[2,3-b]oxirene

$C_{12}H_8Cl_6O = 380.9$

CAS—72-20-8

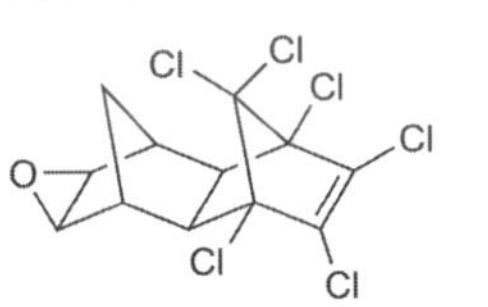

A white crystalline solid. M.p. 245°, with decomposition.
Practically insoluble in water; sparingly soluble in ethanol.

Partition Coefficient. Log *P* (octanol/water), 5.2.

Colour Tests. Nitric–Sulfuric Acid—pink; Sulfuric Acid–Fuming Sulfuric Acid—pink-orange.

Thin-layer Chromatography. System TX—Rf 71; system TY—Rf 90; system TAB—Rf 55; system TAC—Rf 35.

Gas Chromatography. System GA—RI 2183; system GK—RRT 1.19 (relative to caffeine).

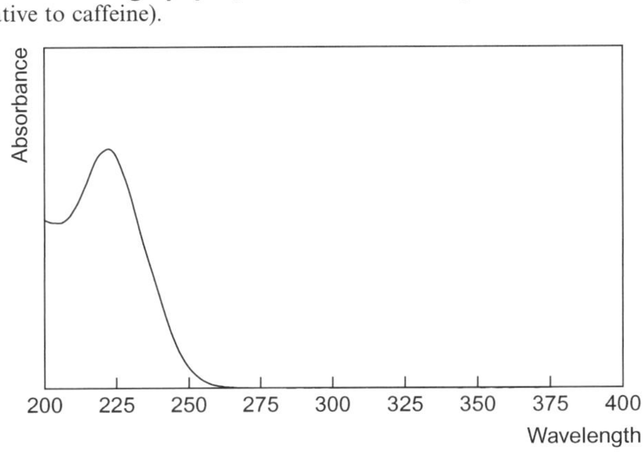

Infra-red Spectrum. Principal peaks at wavenumbers 851, 750, 724, 1049, 889, 1010 cm⁻¹ (Nujol mull).

Mass Spectrum. Principal ions at *m/z* 67, 81, 263, 36, 79, 82, 261, 265.

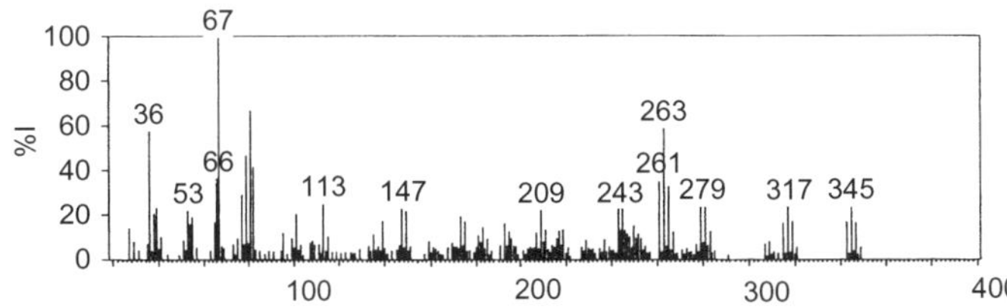

Quantification

Colorimetry. In blood, urine or tissues: limit of detection 4 mg/L—R. T. Sane and S. S. Kamat, *Forensic Sci. Int.*, 1981, *18*, 63–66.

Disposition in the Body

Toxicity

Endrin concentrations in blood 4 h, 6 days, and 11 days after ingestion of 12 g by a 49-year-old man were 450, 86 and 71 μg/L, respectively; corresponding dieldrin concentrations were 60, 19 and 19 μg/L. The man died on the 11th day following ingestion and postmortem tissue concentrations of endrin were: blood 0.071 mg/L, adipose tissue 89.5 μg/g, heart 0.87 μg/g, brain 0.89 μg/g, kidneys 0.55 μg/g, liver 1.32 μg/g [E. A. Runhaar *et al.*, *Hum. Toxicol.*, 1985, *4*, 241–247.]

In a fatality attributed to the ingestion of endrin by an 86-year-old female, postmortem tissue concentrations, approximately 20 h after death, were (mg/L or μg/g): femoral vein blood 0.353, left cardiac chamber blood 0.615, thoracic aorta blood 0.542, bile 2.06, myocardium 0.467, cerebrum 1.93, cerebrospinal fluid 0.515, vitreous humour 1.67, left hilus of lung 6.20, right hilus of lung 1.19, liver 13.8, kidney none detected, right femoral muscle 2.08, stomach content total of 66 mg [F. Moriya and Y. Hashimoto, *J. Forensic Sci.*, 1999, *44*, 1131–1135.]

Enflurane

General Anaesthetic

Synonyms. Anaesthetic Compound No. 347; Methylflurether.
Proprietary names. Alyrane; Efrane; Enfran; Enlirane; Ethrane; Etrane.
2-Chloro-1-(difluoromethoxy)-1,1,2-trifluoroethane

$C_3H_2ClF_5O = 184.5$

CAS—13838-16-9

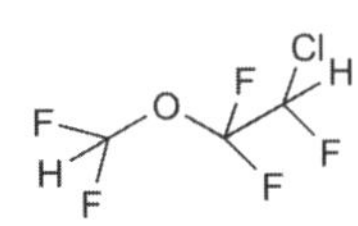

A colourless volatile liquid. B.p. 56.5°. Relative density 1.516 to 1.519.
Miscible with other organic liquids including fats and oils.

Partition Coefficient. Log *P* (octanol/water), 2.1.

Gas Chromatography. System GA—RI 462; system GI—Retention time 8.3 min; system GR—Retention time 3.7 min.

Quantification

Gas chromatography. In blood: limit of detection 1.5 mg/L, TCD—M. S. Miller and A. J. Gandolfi, *Anesthesiology*, 1979, *51*, 542–544. In tissues: limits of detection 200 to 300 ng/0.25 g, FID—H. Ise *et al.*, *J. Chromatogr. B. Biomed. Sci. Appl.*, 1997, *698*, 97–102. In blood: enflurane, isoflurane, halothane and sevoflurane, limits of detection 10 to 100 μg/L, FID—T. Kojima *et al.*, *J. Chromatogr. B. Biomed. Sci. Appl.*, 2001, *762*, 103–108.

Gas chromatography–mass spectrometry. In blood: enflurane, halothane, isoflurane and sevoflurane—K. Saito *et al.*, *J. Anal. Toxicol.*, 1995, *19*, 115–119. In tissues: limits of detection 200 to 300 ng/0.25 g—H. Ise *et al.*, *J. Chromatogr. B. Biomed. Sci. Appl.*, 1997, *698*, 97–102. In blood: enflurane, desflurane, isoflurane, halothane and sevoflurane—N. C. Yang *et al.*, *J. Chromatogr. B. Biomed Sci. Appl.*, 2001, *759*, 307–318.

Review. In vaporisers, exhaled and inhaled gas mixtures, body fluids and tissues: enflurane, halothane, isoflurane and nitrous oxide, a review of GC methods—A. Uyanik, *J. Chromatogr. B. Biomed. Sci. Appl.*, 1997, *693*, 1–9.

Disposition in the Body. Readily absorbed on inhalation. About 50% of a dose is exhaled unchanged in 18 h and more than 80% is exhaled in 5 days. Less than 5% of a dose is excreted in the urine as non-volatile metabolites. Difluoromethoxydifluoroacetic acid has been identified as a urinary metabolite.

Therapeutic concentration

In 10 subjects receiving anaesthesia with 0.5 to 2.5% of enflurane, a mean peak venous blood concentration of 95 mg/L was attained in 30 min, declining to 0.5 mg/L at 90 min after discontinuation of anaesthesia [I. M. Corall *et al.*, *Br. J. Anaesth.*, 1977, *49*, 881–885].

A mean peak serum-fluoride concentration of 0.2 mg/L was attained 3 h after induction in 18 subjects receiving 0.6 to 2% of enflurane [P. Duvaldestin *et al.*, *Clin. Pharmacol. Ther.*, 1981, *29*, 61–64].

Toxicity

A 21-year-old man found dead after apparent accidental intoxication with enflurane following its abuse had the following tissue concentrations 3½ days later: blood 130 mg/L, brain 350 mg/L, subcutaneous fat 100 mg/L [B. Jacob *et al.*, *J. Forensic Sci.*, 1989, *34*, 1408–1412].

Half-life. About 36 h.

Dose. For induction of anaesthesia, up to 4% of the vapour by inhalation; maintenance, 0.5 to 3%.

Enoxaparin

Anticoagulant

Synonyms. Enoxaparine; low molecular weight Heparin; PK10169; RP-54563
Proprietary name. Lovenox
Low molecular weight fragment of depolymerised heparin = approx. 4000 to 6000 Da
CAS—74011-58-8
Obtained by peroxide fragmentation of heparin sodium.

Enoxaparin Sodium

Synonyms. Enoxaparinum Natricum; Heparin Sodium.
Proprietary names. Clexane: Decipar; Klexane; Lovenox; Plancina; Trombenox; Ultraparin.
CAS—9041-08-1

Quantification

Bioassay. Antifactor II_a activity: in plasma—M. L. Larsen *et al.*, *Thromb. Res.*, 1987, *13*, 285.

Disposition in the Body. Enoxaparin is rapidly and completely absorbed after subcutaneous injection with a peak plasma activity reached in 1 to 5 h. It is metabolised in the liver by desulfation and depolymerisation. It is excreted via the kidneys and is found unchanged and as its metabolites in urine. Enoxaparin is poorly absorbed after oral administration.

Therapeutic concentration

12 healthy volunteers were administered with single doses of 20, 40, 60 and 80 mg enoxaparin. Peak plasma concentrations were between 1.6 and 7.5 mg/L and were reached between 2.3 and 4.0 h [A. M. Frydman *et al.*, *J. Clin. Pharmacol.*, 1988, *28*, 609–618].

Toxicity. Large oral doses should not lead to any serious effects. Accidental overdosing, by parenteral administration, may lead to haemorrhagic problems with severe bleeding. Risk of bleeding increases with plasma concentrations of antifactor $X_A > 0.4$ units/mL.

Bioavailability. About 92%.

Half-life. 4 to 5 h, 6 to 7 h in the elderly.

Volume of distribution. Between 5.2 and 9.3 L.

Clearance. Total body clearance varies from 0.8 to 1.9 L/h.

Protein binding. Enoxaparin binds endogenous plasma proteins, for example, histidine-rich glycoprotein and fibronectin.

Note. For a review of the pharmacokinetics of enoxaparin, see S. Noble *et al.*, *Drugs*, 1995, *49*, 388–410. For a review of low-molecular-weight heparins, see M. J. Cziraky and S. A. Spinler, *Clin Pharm.*, 1993, *12*, 892–899.

Dose. Dose ranges from 1 mg (100 International Units, IU)/kg body weight every 12 h with increases in 0.5 to 1 mg/kg body weight increments to a single dose of 40 mg (2000 IU) once daily.

Enoximone

Vasodilator/Inotrope

Synonyms. Fenoximone; MDL-17043; MDL-19438; RMI-17043; YMDL-17043.
Proprietary names. Perfan; Perfane.
1,3-Dihydro-4-methyl-5-[4-(methylthio)benzoyl]-2*H*-imidazol-2-one
$C_{12}H_{12}N_2O_2S = 248.3$
CAS—77671-31-9

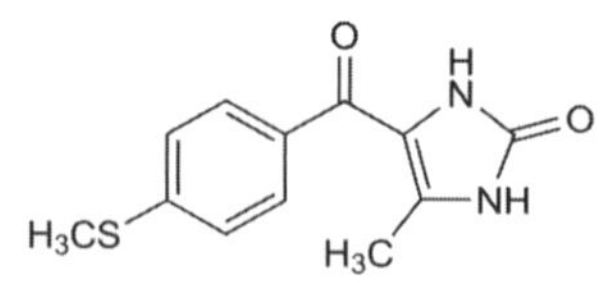

Crystalline powder, M.p. 255° to 258° with decomposition.

Partition Coefficient. Log *P* (octanol/water), 1.86.

High Performance Liquid Chromatography. Column: C_{18} ODS (Ultraspher, 150 × 4.6 mm i.d., 5 µm). Mobile phase: water:acetonitrile (86:14) for 3 min, to (10:90) in 6 min, back to original conditions in 1 min, 1 mL/min flow rate. UV detection (λ = 365 nm). Internal standard (IS): MDL 82249. Retention times: enoximone, 8.25 min; enoximone sulfoxide, 2.47 min; IS, 7.75 min [E. Tarral *et al.*, *Therapie*, 1990, *45*, 1–6].

Ultraviolet Spectrum. Aqueous acid—327 nm.

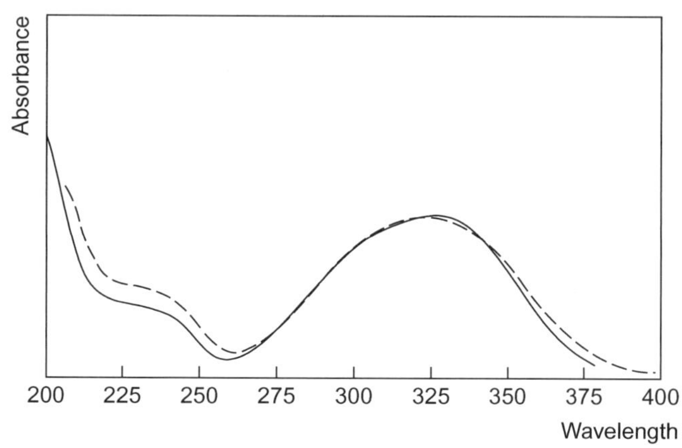

Infra-red Spectrum. Principal peaks at wavenumbers 1700, 1610, 1435, 1325, 830, 1090 cm^{-1}.

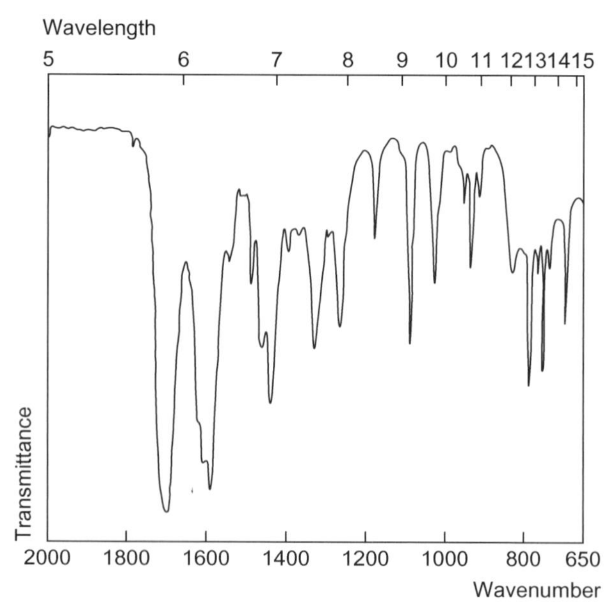

Mass Spectrum. Principal ions at *m/z* 42, 248, 247, 32, 151, 45, 201, 69.

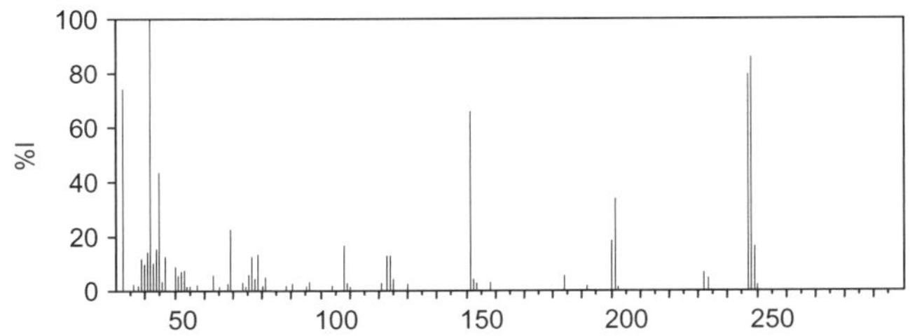

Quantification

High performance liquid chromatography. In serum: limit of quantification is 0.05 mg/L for enoximone and sulfoxide metabolite—K. Y. Chan *et al.*, *J. Chromatogr.*, 1984, *306*, 249–256. In serum: enoximone and metabolite, limit of detection 0.01 mg/L, UV detection (λ=335 nm)—J. D. Cooper and D. C. Turnell, *J. Chromatogr.*, 1986, *380*, *Biomed. Appl.*, *53*, 109–116. In plasma and urine: limit of quantification 0.005 and 0.01 mg/L for enoximone and the metabolites, respectively, in plasma and 0.5 and 1.0 mg/L in urine, UV detection (λ=340 nm)—S. Morita *et al.*, *J. Pharm. Sci.*, 1995, *84(2)*, 152–157.

Disposition in the Body. Following intravenous injection or infusion it undergoes metabolism in the liver to an active sulfoxide metabolite (piroximone). It is excreted primarily via the kidney, as metabolites in urine. After an intravenous dose, approx. 70% is excreted in urine as metabolites and 1% as the unchanged drug.

Therapeutic concentration

20 infants, aged between 0.6 and 49.7 weeks (median 6.0 weeks), were administered a loading dose of 1 mg/kg enoximone over 2 min, followed by an infusion of 10 μg/kg/min for a median time of 97 h (24 to 572 h). The infants were already anaesthetised for weaning from cardiopulmonary bypass. The maximum plasma concentration ranged between 0.708 and 6.893 mg/L (median 1.536 mg/L) [P. D. Booker *et al.*, *Br. J. Anaesth.*, 2000, *85(2)*, 205–210].

23 healthy male Japanese volunteers with a mean age of 22.0 years (range 20 to 27 years) were administered either a 0.25, 0.5 or 1.0 mg/kg single intravenous bolus dose at 2-weekly intervals; or a single 2.0 mg/kg dose; or a single 1.0 mg/kg bolus dose on day 1 followed by 3-hourly interval doses on day 2; or a single 10 μg/kg/min continuous infusion over a 4-h period. In the first part of the study, the peak concentrations for the 0.25, 0.5, 1.0 and 2.0 mg/kg dose were 0.31, 1.82, 3.40 and 5.38 mg/L, respectively observed at 0.06, 0.01 and 0.0 h. The sulfoxide metabolite concentrations were 0.23, 0.53, 1.08 and 1.82 mg/L at 0.25, 0.25, 0.17 and 0.19 h for the four doses, respectively. The multiple dosing with a 1 mg/kg dose produced peak concentrations of 2.35 mg/L at 3.21 h. The single 10 μg/kg/min dose produced concentrations of 0.51 mg/L at 4.0 h. [S. Morita *et al.*, *J. Pharm. Sci.*, 1995, *84(2)*, 152–157].

Toxicity. Severe supraventricular and ventricular arrhythmias can occur.

Half-life. In healthy volunteers, 1 to 4 h, in patients with heart failure, 6 h (bolus injections), 8 h (continuous infusion); infants (0.6 to 49.7 weeks) 1.4 to 10.9 h (median 6.4); sulfoxide, 2.9 to 17.7 h (median 7.4).

Volume of distribution. 1.1 to 3.6 L/kg; 1.4 to 15.5 L/kg (median 3.8) (infants aged 0.6 to 49.7 weeks).

Clearance. Plasma clearance, 3.7 to 13.0 mL/min/kg; 2.4 to 18.9 mL/min/kg (median 9.2) (infants aged 0.6 to 49.7 weeks).

Protein binding. In plasma, 85%.

Dose. Maximum of 24 mg/kg intravenously in 24 h.

Enoxolone

Dermatological Agent

Synonyms. Glycyrrhetic Acid; Glycyrrhetinic Acid.
Proprietary names. Arthrodont; PO 12. It is an ingredient of Gelclair.
(3*β*,20*β*)-3-Hydroxy-11-oxoolean-12-en-29-oic acid
$C_{30}H_{46}O_4$=470.7
CAS—471-53-4

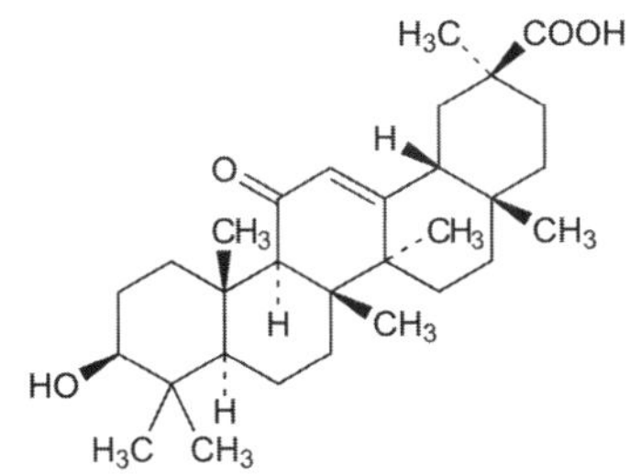

A white or faintly cream-coloured powder. M.p. 296°.
Very sparingly soluble in water; soluble in ethanol, ether, pyridine and acetic acid; freely soluble in chloroform and dioxane; practically insoluble in petroleum ether.

Partition Coefficient. Log *P* (octanol/water), 6.9.

Colour Tests. Antimony Pentachloride—orange-brown→violet; Naphthol–Sulfuric Acid—red-brown/orange; Sulfuric Acid—yellow

Thin-layer Chromatography. System TD—Rf 21; system TE—Rf 07; system TF—Rf 46; system TAD—Rf 47.

Ultraviolet Spectrum. Aqueous acid—254 nm; aqueous alkali—260 nm (A_1^1=338b).

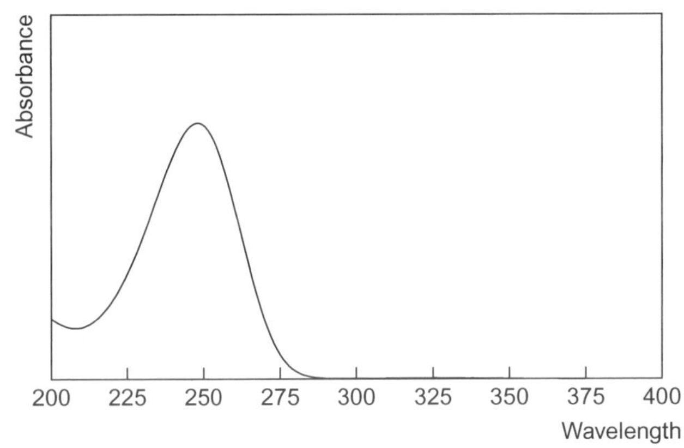

Mass Spectrum. Principal ions at *m/z* 303, 262, 135, 175, 41, 55, 43, 95.

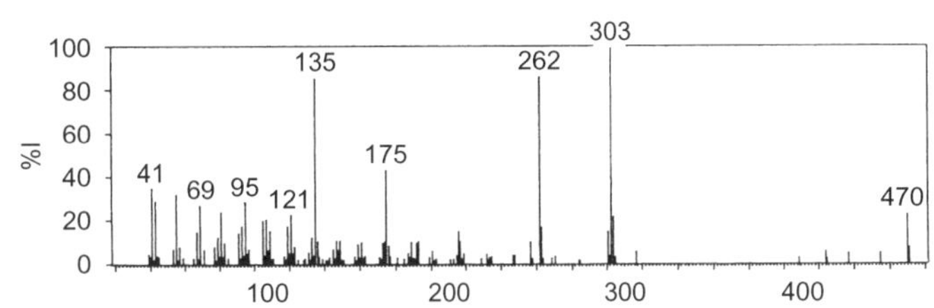

Disposition in the Body. Enoxolone is a metabolite of carbenoxolone.

Use. Has been used topically in a concentration of 2%.

Entacapone

Dopaminergic/Antiparkinsonian

Proprietary names. Comtan; Comtess.
(E)-2-Cyano-*N*,*N*-diethyl-3-(3,4-dihydroxy-5-nitrophenyl)acrylamide
$C_{14}H_{15}N_3O_5$=305.3
CAS—130929-57-6

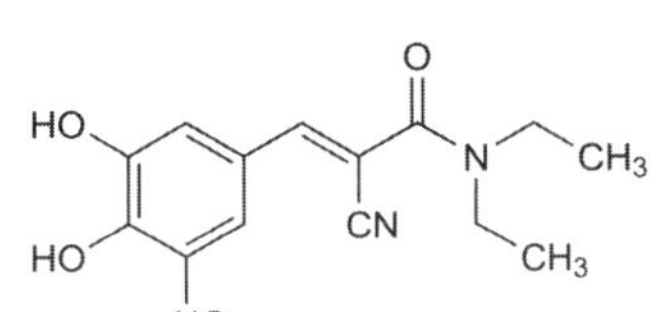

Powder. M.p. 153° to 156°.

Dissociation Constant. pK_a 4.5.

High Performance Liquid Chromatography. Column: ODS-2 silica (Spherisorb, 150 × 4.6 mm i.d., 5 μm). Mobile phase: sodium dihydrogen phosphate buffer (25 mM) and citric acid (10 mM) buffer (pH 2.2 with phosphoric acid):methanol (55:45), 1.0 mL/min flow rate. UV detection (λ=310 nm). Retention time: entacapone, 9.5 min; (Z)-entacapone, 5.8 min [T. Wikberg *et al.*, *Drug Metab. Dispos.*, 1993, *21*, 81–92].

Ultraviolet Spectrum. Neutral—306 nm.

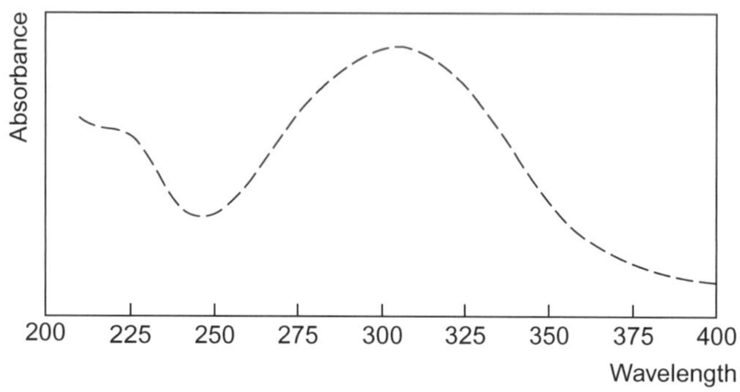

Infra-red Spectrum. Principal peaks at wavenumbers 2209, 1630, 1610, 1537 cm^{-1}.

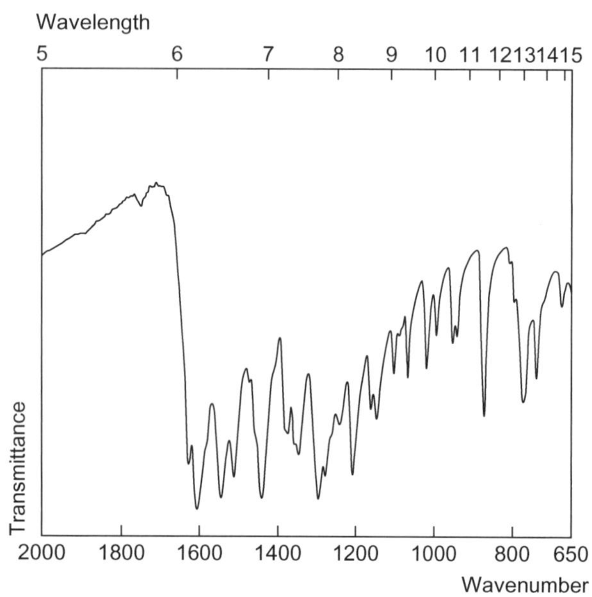

Mass Spectrum. Principal ions at *m*/*z* 58, 233, 29, 304, 72, 305, 159, 288.

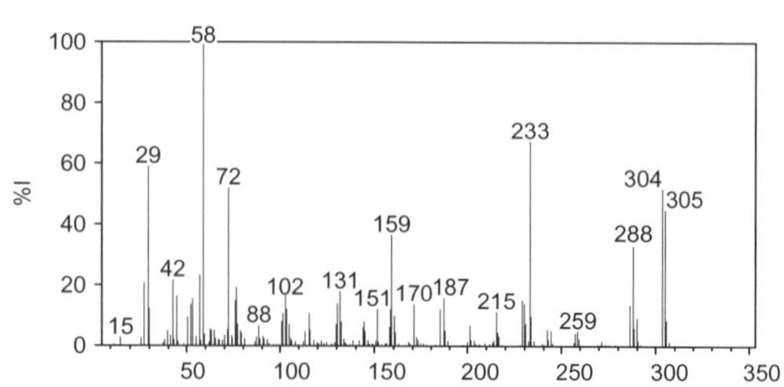

Quantification

High performance liquid chromatography. In urine: limit of detection is 0.5 mg/L, UV detection (λ=310 nm)—T. Wikberg *et al.*, *Drug Metab. Dispos.*,1993, *21*, 81–92. In plasma: limit of quantification 0.01 mg/L, amperometric detection—M. Karlson and T. Wikberg, *J. Pharm. Biomed. Anal.*, 1992, *10*, 593–600.

Disposition in the Body. Entacapone is rapidly absorbed from the gastro-intestinal tract and undergoes extensive first pass metabolism. Entacapone is converted to its (*cis*)-isomer, (*Z*)-entacapone, the main metabolite in plasma, followed by direct glucuronidation to inactive glucuronide conjugates. Four metabolites have been observed—M3, M6, M8 and M10. Elimination is mainly via faeces (80 to 90%) and the remainder in urine as glucuronide conjugates and (*Z*)-isomer.

Therapeutic concentration

12 healthy males were administered single oral doses of entacapone: 5, 25, 50, 100, 200, 400 and 800 mg. Peak plasma concentrations ranged from 62 to 7280 μg/L, with increasing dose, and were reached between 0.46 and 0.88 h [T. Keranen *et al.*, *Eur. J. Clin. Pharmacol.*, 1994, *46(2)*, 151–157].

Toxicity. No special hazard to humans, anaemia observed in repeated dose toxicity studies.

Bioavailability. Approx. 35% (oral).

Half-life. Elimination half-life, $t_{1/2}$ (α-phase) 0.27 to 0.37 h and (β-phase) 1.59 to 3.10 h.

Volume of distribution. 181 L.

Clearance. Total clearance, 800 mL/min.

Protein binding. Extensively binds plasma proteins and serum albumin approx. 98%.

Dose. A usual dose of 200 mg entacapone, up to ten times a day, with a maximum of 2000 mg.

Ephedrine

Sympathomimetic

Synonym. Hydrated Ephedrine
Proprietary name. It is an ingredient of Franolyn Expectorant
(α*R*)-α-[(1*S*)-1-(Methylamino)ethyl]benzenemethanol hemihydrate
$C_{10}H_{15}NO,½H_2O=174.2$
CAS—50906-05-3

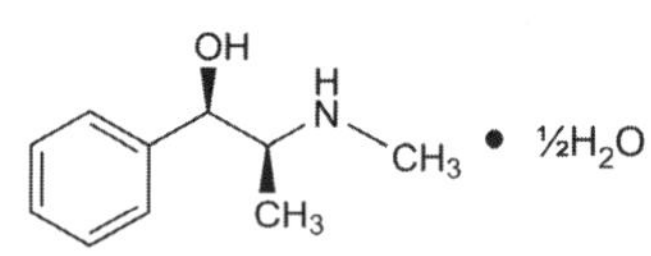

An alkaloid obtained from species of *Ephedra*, or prepared synthetically. Colourless crystals or white crystalline powder or granules which decompose on exposure to light. M.p. 40°; in warm weather it slowly volatilises. Soluble 1 in 20 of water and 1 in less than 1 of ethanol; soluble in chloroform with turbidity owing to separation of water; soluble in ether.

Anhydrous Ephedrine

Synonym. Ephedrine
Proprietary names. Ephed 20th; Kondon's Nasal; Tendrin.
$C_{10}H_{15}NO=165.2$
CAS—299-42-3
Unctuous deliquescent colourless crystals, or white crystalline powder. It rapidly absorbs carbon dioxide and decomposes on exposure to light. M.p. 38.1°.
Soluble 1 in 20 of water; very soluble in ethanol; soluble in chloroform; freely soluble in ether.

Ephedrine Hydrochloride

Synonyms. Ephedrine Chloride; Ephedrinium Chloratum; L-Ephedrinum Hydrochloricum.
Proprietary names. CAM. It is an ingredient of many proprietary preparations—see *Martindale, The complete drug reference*, 33rd Edn., Pharmaceutical Press, London, 2002.
$C_{10}H_{15}NO,HCl=201.7$
CAS—50-98-6
Colourless crystals or white crystalline powder. M.p. 217° to 220°.
Soluble 1 in 3 to 1 in 4 of water and 1 in 14 to 1 in 17 of ethanol; very slightly soluble in chloroform; practically insoluble in ether.

Ephedrine Sulfate

Proprietary names. Pretz-D. It is an ingredient of Franol Plus.
$(C_{10}H_{15}NO)_2,H_2SO_4=428.6$

CAS—134-72-5
Fine white crystals or powder which darken on exposure to light. M.p. 245°, with decomposition.
Soluble 1 in 1.3 of water and 1 in 90 of ethanol.

Dissociation Constant. pK_a 9.6 (25°).

Partition Coefficient. Log *P* (octanol/water), 1.1.

Colour Test. Liebermann's Test—red-orange.

Thin-layer Chromatography. System TA—Rf 30; system TB—Rf 05; system TC—Rf 05; system TE—Rf 25; system TL—Rf 01; system TAE—Rf 10; system TAF—Rf 64; system TAJ—Rf 00; system TAK—Rf 01; system TAL—Rf 29. (Dragendorff spray, positive; acidified iodoplatinate solution, positive; Marquis reagent, brown; ninhydrin spray, positive; acidified potassium permanganate solution, positive.)

Gas Chromatography. System GA—ephedrine RI 1365, ephedrine-TFA_2 RI 1345, ephedrine-PFP_2 RI 1370, ephedrine-TMS_2 RI 1620, ephedrine-AC_2 RI 1795, M (nor-) RI 1360, M (nor-)-TFA_2 RI 1355, M (nor-)-PFP_2 RI 1380, M (nor-) -TMS_2 RI 1555, M (nor-)-AC_2 RI 1805, M (OH-) RI 1875, M (OH-)-AC_3 RI 2145; system GB—ephedrine RI 1410, M (nor-) RI 1356; system GC—ephedrine RI 1467, M (nor-) RI 1383.

High Performance Liquid Chromatography. System HA—ephedrine *k* 1.0, M (nor-) *k* 0.9; system HB—ephedrine *k* 5.68, M (nor-) *k* 3.87; system HC—ephedrine *k* 1.79, M (nor-) *k* 0.70; system HX—RI 221; system HY—RI 227; system HZ—retention time 2.1 min; system HAA—retention time 5.7 min; system HAM—ephedrine not detected.

Ultraviolet Spectrum. Aqueous acid—251, 257 nm (A_1^1 = 12a), 263 nm. No alkaline shift.

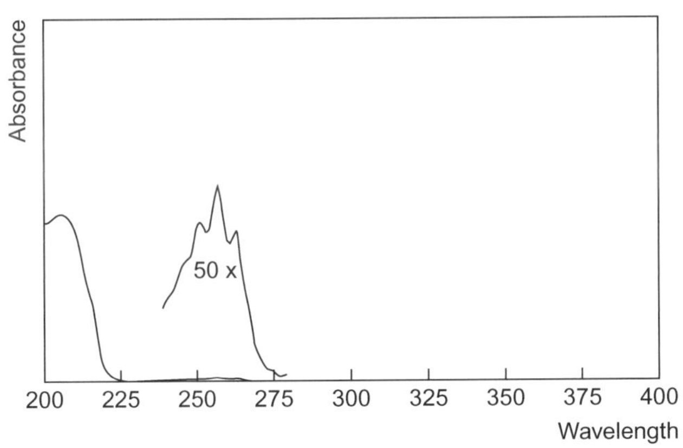

Infra-red Spectrum. Principal peaks at wavenumbers 994, 699, 754, 1049, 1242, 670 cm^{-1} (ephedrine hydrochloride, KBr disk).

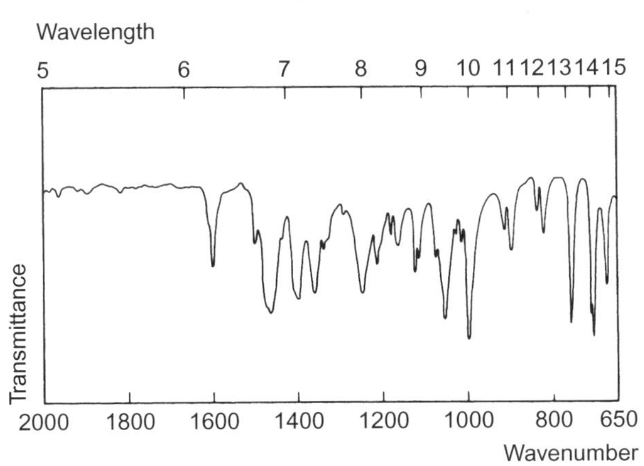

Mass Spectrum. Principal ions at *m/z* 58, 146, 56, 105, 77, 42, 106, 40; norephedrine 44, 77, 79, 51, 45, 42, 107, 105.

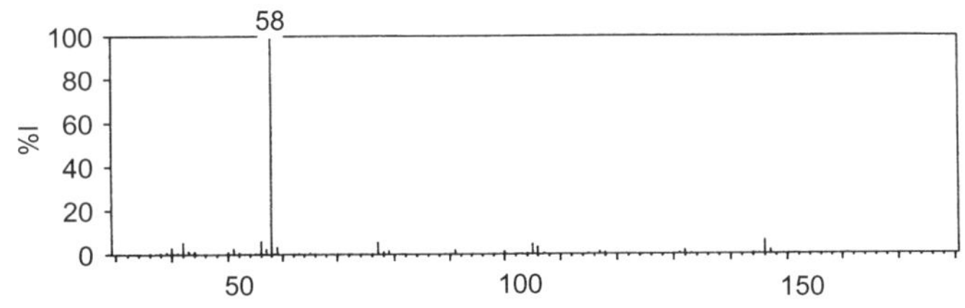

Quantification

Gas chromatography. In plasma or urine: limit of detection 2 µg/L in plasma, ECD—K. K. Midha *et al.*, *J. Pharm. Sci.*, 1979, *68*, 557–560.

Gas chromatography–mass spectrometry. In postmortem body fluids and tissues—R. Backer *et al.*, *J. Forensic Sci.*, 1997, *42*, 157–159.

High performance liquid chromatography. In urine: ephedrine and related drugs, UV detection—C. Imaz *et al.*, *J. Chromatogr.*, 1993, *631*, 201–205; P. J. van der Merwe *et al.*, *J. Chromatogr.* 1994, *661 B Biomed. Appl.*, 357–361. In plasma: ephedrine and pseudoephedrine, limit of detection 0.5 ng, fluorescence detection—G. Shao *et al.*, *Yao Xue Xue Bao*, 1995, *30*, 384–389. In plasma: ephedrine and norephedrine, limits of detection 2 µg/L and 5 µg/L, respectively, fluorescence detection—G. Aymard *et al.*, *J. Chromatogr. B Biomed. Sci. Appl.*, 2000, *744*, 25–31. In urine: ephedrine congeners—G. Gmeiner *et al.*, *J. Chromatogr. B Anal. Toxicol. Biomed. Life Sci.*, 2002, *768*, 214–221.

Disposition in the Body. Readily absorbed after oral or percutaneous administration. Metabolised by *N*-demethylation to norephedrine (phenylpropanolamine) and by oxidative deamination followed by conjugation. Accumulates in the liver, lungs, kidneys, spleen, and brain. About 90% of a dose is excreted in the urine in 24 h, with about 55 to 75% of the dose as unchanged drug, 8 to 20% as norephedrine, and 4 to 13% as deaminated metabolites such as benzoic acid, hippuric acid, and 1-phenylpropane-1,2-diol. In acidic urine, excretion of unchanged drug is increased slightly, whereas, in alkaline urine, about 20 to 35% of the dose is excreted unchanged and the proportion of norephedrine is increased.
Ephedrine is a metabolite of methylephedrine.

Therapeutic concentration. In plasma, usually in the range 0.035 to 0.08 mg/L.

After a single oral dose of 22 mg of the hydrochloride to 10 subjects, peak plasma concentrations of 0.04 to 0.14 mg/L (mean 0.08) were attained; after daily oral doses of 33 mg of the hydrochloride to 10 subjects, peak plasma concentrations of 0.07 to 0.12 mg/L (mean 0.08) were obtained. [J. F. Costello *et al.*, *Br. J. Clin. Pharmacol.*, 1975, *2*, 180P–181P.]

Ephedrine toxicity has been linked to nutritional supplements containing *Ephedra sinica* (ma huang) and a number of deaths have occurred. The pharmacokinetics of 3 commercially available ma huang products (mean ephedrine content per dose: 27, 25.6, and 23.6 mg, respectively) were compared with those of ephedrine hydrochloride capsules (25 mg dose) in 10 subjects. The mean peak plasma concentrations of ephedrine (and time at which the peak occurred) were: ephedrine hydrochloride 86 µg/L (at 2.81 h); ma huang products 100.1 µg/L (at 2.68 h), 86.2 µg/L (at 2.61 h), and 73.4 µg/L (at 3.05 h), respectively. [B. J. Gurley *et al.*, *Ther. Drug. Monit.*, 1998, *20*, 439–445.]

Toxicity. The estimated minimum lethal dose in children up to 2 years of age is 200 mg and for adults 2 g but fatalities are rare. Single doses of up to 400 mg have been given without causing serious toxic effects.

In a 28-year-old woman whose death was attributed to the ingestion of ephedrine with suicidal intent, the following postmortem tissue concentrations were reported: blood 11 mg/L, liver 24 µg/g, kidney 14 µg/g, brain 8.9 µg/g. Amitriptyline was also detected. [R. Backer *et al.*, *J. Forensic Sci.*, 1997, *42*, 157–159.]

Note. See Therapeutic concentration, above, for a comment on the toxicity of ephedrine-containing ma huang products.

Half-life. Plasma half-life, 3 to 6 h but may be increased when the urine is alkaline and decreased when it is acid.

Dose. 90 to 180 mg of ephedrine hydrochloride or sulfate daily by mouth in divided doses; in concentrations of 0.25 to 0.5% in nasal drops.

Epinastine

Antihistamine

Synonym. WAL-801
9,13b-Dihydro-1*H*-dibenz[*c*,*f*]imidazo[1,5-*a*]azepin-3-amine
$C_{16}H_{15}N_3$=249.3
CAS—80012-43-7

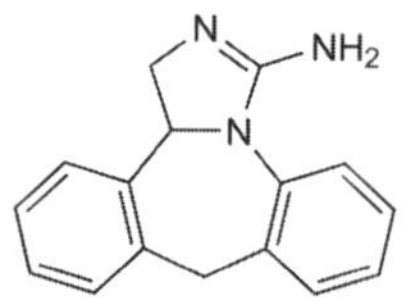

A crystalline powder. M.p. 205° to 208°.

Epinastine Hydrobromide
$C_{16}H_{15}N_3$, HBr=330.2
A crystalline powder. M.p. 284° to 286°.

Epinastine Hydrochloride
Synonym. WAL-801-Cl
Proprietary names. Alesion, Flurinol
$C_{16}H_{16}ClN_3$=285.8
CAS—108929-04-0
A crystalline powder. M.p. 273° to 275°. It is freely soluble in water.

Dissociation Constant. pK_a 11.2.

Partition Coefficient. Log *P* (octanol/water), 3.51; log *P* (octanol/aqueous buffer, pH 7.4 (20°)), −0.70.

High Performance Liquid Chromatography. Column: 5C18-MS (Cosmosil, 150 × 4.6 mm i.d.). Mobile phase: triethylamine (0.3%, adjusted to pH 4.5 with phosphoric acid):methanol (64:36), 1.3 mL/min flow rate. UV detection (λ=220 nm). Internal standard (IS): diphenidol. Retention time: epinastine, 8.1 min; IS, 14.8 min [H. Ohtani *et al.*, *J. Chromatogr.* 1996, *683, Biomed. Appl.*, 281–284].

Quantification
High performance liquid chromatography. In plasma: limit of detection for epinastine hydrochloride is 4 µg/L. UV detection (λ 220 nm)—H. Ohtani *et al.*, *J. Chromatogr.* 1996, *683*, *Biomed. Appl.*, 281–284.

Disposition in the Body. Epinastine is excreted mainly via urine and faeces unchanged.

Dose. A usual dose of 20 mg daily is administered.

Epirubicin

Antineoplastic

Synonyms. 4′-Epiadriamycin; 4′-epi-DX; 4′-Epidoxorubicin; IMI-28; Pidorubicin.
(8*S*,10*S*)-10-[(3-Amino-2,3,6-trideoxy-α-L-*arabino*-hexopyranosyl)oxy]-7,8,9,10-tetrahydro-6,8,11-trihydroxy-8-(hydroxyacetyl)-1-methoxy-5,12-naphthacenedione
$C_{27}H_{29}NO_{11}$=543.5
CAS—56420-45-2

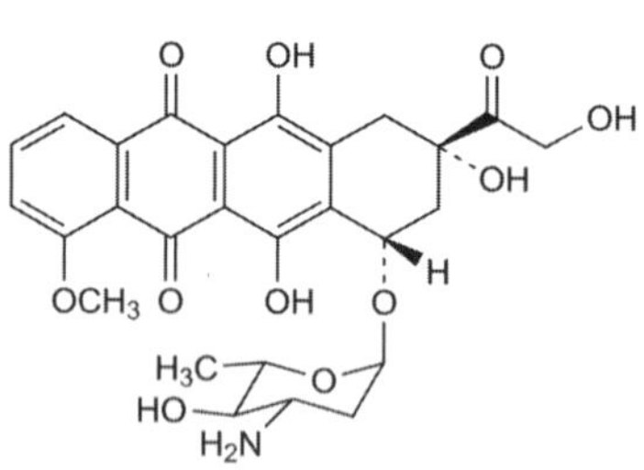

Epirubicin Hydrochloride
Proprietary names. Farmorubicin; Farmorubicina; Farmorubicine; Pharmorubicin.
$C_{27}H_{29}NO_{11}$,HCl=580.0
CAS—56390-09-1
Red–orange crystals. M.p. 185°, with decomposition.

Thin-layer Chromatography. System TE—Rf 00; system TF—Rf 00.

High Performance Liquid Chromatography. System HX—RI 379.

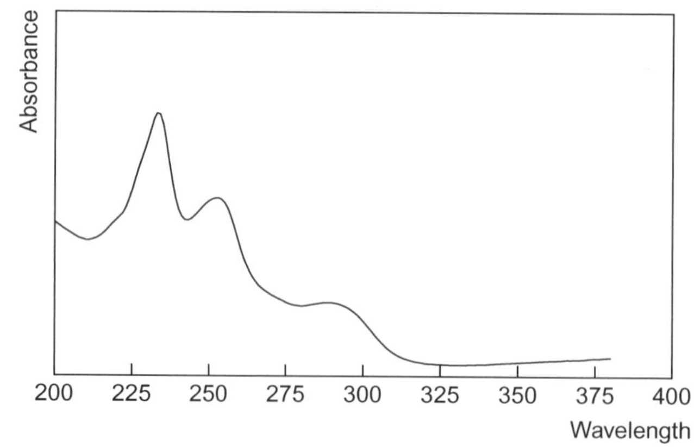

Quantification
High performance liquid chromatography. In plasma: limit of detection 1 µg>L. Fluorescence detection (λ_{ex}=480 nm, λ_{em}=580 nm)—N. A. Dobbs and C. J. Twelves, *J. Chromatogr.*, 1991, *572*; *Biomed. Appl.*, *110*, 211–217. In plasma: epirubicin and metabolites, limit of detection 5 µg>L for epirubicin, fluorescence detection—I. K. Barker *et al.*, *J. Chromatogr.* 1996, *681*, *Biomed. Appl.*, 323–329.

Disposition in the Body. Pharmacokinetics vary widely between patients. Epirubicin is rapidly and extensively distributed into body tissues after intravenous administration. High concentrations occur in tumour tissues. It also concentrates in red blood cells and therefore concentrations in blood are substantially higher than those in plasma. It does not cross the blood–brain barrier. Epirubicin undergoes extensive metabolism, primarily in the liver (but also in other organs and cells including red blood cells), to form epirubicinol (13-hydroxyepirubicin) which has a very low degree of cytotoxic activity and appreciable amounts of glucuronide derivatives. 7-Deoxyaglycones have also been detected in plasma of patients treated with epirubicin. Epirubicinol is eliminated mainly in bile. About 10 to 20% of a dose is recovered in urine within 48 h as the unchanged drug, epirubicinol, or as the glucuronide metabolite. 40% is recovered in bile in 72 h.

Therapeutic concentration. The serum therapeutic concentration range is 10 to 50 µg/L.

> 27 patients with nesopharyngeal carcinomas, were administered an intravenous dose of 75 mg/m^2 epirubicin rapidly. Peak plasma concentrations of 1860 µg>L were observed by the end of infusion [OY-P. Hu *et al.*, *Cancer Chemother. Pharmacol.*, 1989, *24*, 332–337].

Toxicity. Myelosuppression is the major acute dose-limiting toxicity and cardiotoxicity is the most important cumulative dose-limiting toxicity.

Half-life. Plasma half-life, 30 to 40 h.

Volume of distribution. Between 13 and 52 L/kg. Steady state, 1000 L/m^2.

Clearance. Plasma clearance, 50 L/h/m^2; 0.9 L/min.

Note. For reviews of epirubicin see G. L. Plosker and D. Faulds, *Drugs*, 1993, *45*, 788–856 and A. J. Coukell and D. Faulds, *Drugs.*, 1997, *53*, 453–482.
For a review of the pharmacokinetics of epirubicin see J. Robert, *Clin. Pharmacokinet.*, 1994, *26*, 428–438.

Dose. Usually 60 to 90 mg/m^2 as a single dose intravenously every 3 weeks. A total cumulative dose of 0.9 to 1 g/m^2 should not generally be exceeded because of the risk of cardiotoxicity.

Epithiazide

Diuretic

Synonym. Epitizide
Proprietary name. It is an ingredient of Dyta-Urese.
6-Chloro-3,4-dihydro-3-(2,2,2-trifluoroethylthiomethyl)-2*H*-1,2,4-benzothiadiazine-7-sulfonamide-1,1-dioxide
$C_{10}H_{11}ClF_3N_3O_4S_3$=425.8

CAS—1764-85-8

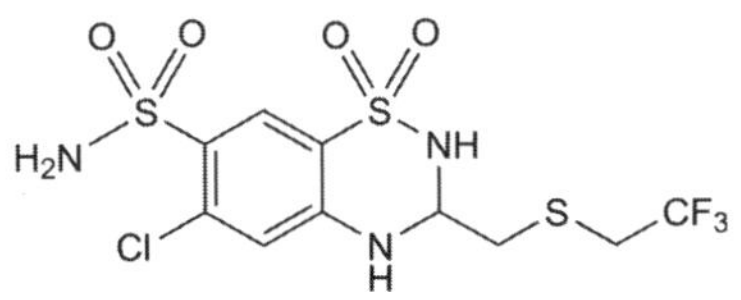

A white crystalline powder. M.p. 206° to 207°.
Practically insoluble in water; soluble in alkaline solutions.

Partition Coefficient. Log *P* (octanol/water), 0.8.

Thin-layer Chromatography. System TB—Rf 00; system TD—Rf 13; system TE—Rf 44; system TF—Rf 62; system TAD—Rf 25; system TAE—Rf 88; system TAJ—Rf 22; system TAK—Rf 05; system TAL—Rf 63.

Gas Chromatography. System GA—not eluted.

High Performance Liquid Chromatography. System HX—RI 457.

Ultraviolet Spectrum. Aqueous acid—272, 315 nm. (See below.)

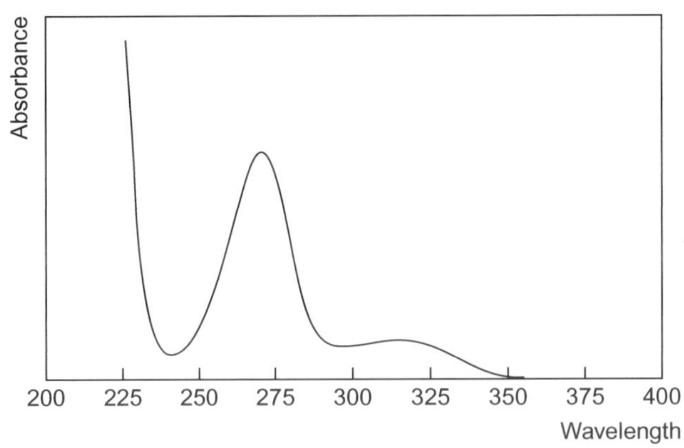

Infra-red Spectrum. Principal peaks at wavenumbers 1176, 1314, 1167, 1126, 1603, 1269 cm^{-1} (Nujol mull).

Dose. 8 to 12 mg daily.

Eptazocine

Analgesic

(*1S*)-2,3,4,5,6,7-Hexahydro-1,4-dimethyl-1,6-methano-1*H*-4-benzazonin-10-ol
$C_{15}H_{21}NO$=231.3
CAS—72522-13-5

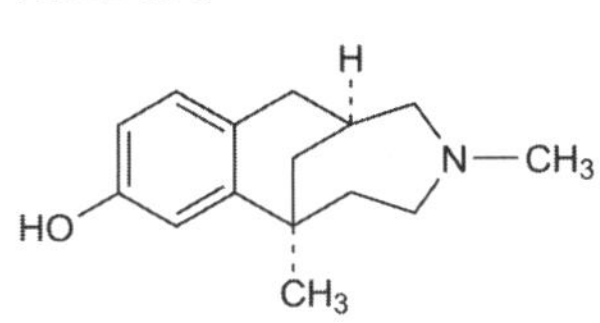

Eptazocine Hydrobromide

Synonym. ST-2121
Proprietary name. Sedapain
$C_{15}H_{22}BrNO$=312.2
CAS—72150-17-5
A crystalline powder. M.p. 207° to 210°.

High Performance Liquid Chromatography. Column: C_{18}-MS (Cosmosil, 150 × 4.6 mm i.d., 5 μm), at 25°. Mobile phase: sodium phosphate buffer (0.07 M, pH 3) containing sodium heptylsulfonate (5 mM):methanol (55:45), 0.8 mL/min flow rate. Fluorescence detection (λ_{ex}=278 nm, λ_{em}=324 nm). Internal standard (IS): methyleptazocine. Retention times: eptazocine, 4.9 min; IS, 7.2 min [T. Suzuki *et al.*, *Biol. Pharm. Bull.*, 2000, *23*, 1504–1510].

Ergocalciferol

Vitamin

Synonyms. Calciferol; Irradiated Ergosterol; Viosterol; Vitamin D_2.
Proprietary names. Drisdol; Endo D; Ostelin; Radiostol; Sterogyl; Vita-D-Grin.

Note. Ergocalciferol is also used as a rodenticide. It is an ingredient of Sorexa C.R.
(3*β*,5*Z*,7*E*,22*E*)-9,10-Secoergosta-5,7,10(19),22-tetraen-3-ol
$C_{28}H_{44}O$=396.7
CAS—50-14-6

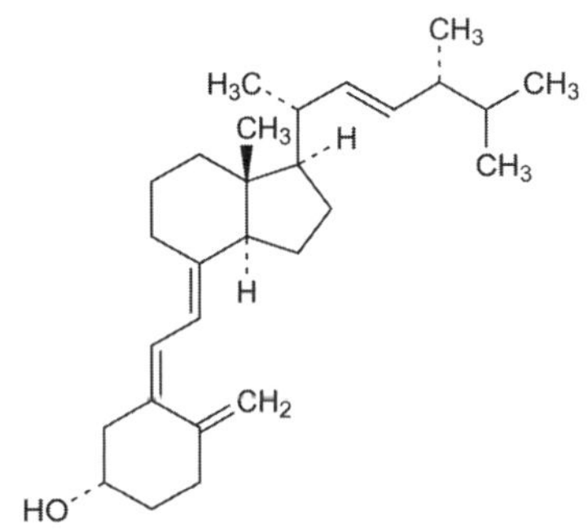

Colourless or slightly yellow crystals, or white or slightly yellow crystalline powder. M.p. 113° to 119°.
Practically insoluble in water; soluble 1 in 2 of ethanol, 1 in 10 of acetone, 1 in 0.7 of chloroform and 1 in 2 of ether.

Partition Coefficient. Log *P* (octanol/water), 10.4.

High Performance Liquid Chromatography. System HY—RI 276.

Ultraviolet Spectrum. Ethanol—265 nm (A^1_1=475b).

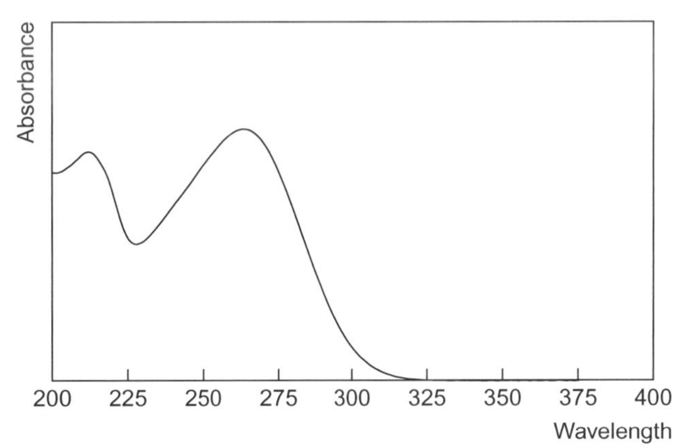

Infra-red Spectrum. Principal peaks at wavenumbers 973, 1059, 1079, 1712, 893, 1000 cm^{-1} (KBr disk).

Quantification. See under Colecalciferol.

Disposition in the Body. Well absorbed after oral administration; absorption may be decreased with impaired liver and biliary function, and extensive enterohepatic circulation occurs. Metabolised by 25-hydroxylation in the liver followed by 1α- or 24-hydroxylation in the kidney; possibly conjugated with glucuronic acid or sulfate. Excreted mainly in the bile together with small amounts of metabolites in the urine; unchanged ergocalciferol does not appear to be excreted in the urine.

Blood concentration. Normal serum concentrations of 25-hydroxyergocalciferol are about 0.01 to 0.04 mg/L but there are considerable intersubject and seasonal variations.

Half-life. About 40 days.

Protein binding. In blood, bound to α- and *β*-lipoproteins.

Dose. 0.025 to 5 mg daily.

Ergometrine

Ergot Alkaloid

Synonyms. Ergobasine; Ergonovine.
[8β (*S*)]-9,10-Didehydro-*N*-(2-hydroxy-1-methylethyl)-6-methylergoline-8-carboxamide
$C_{19}H_{23}N_3O_2$=325.4
CAS—60-79-7

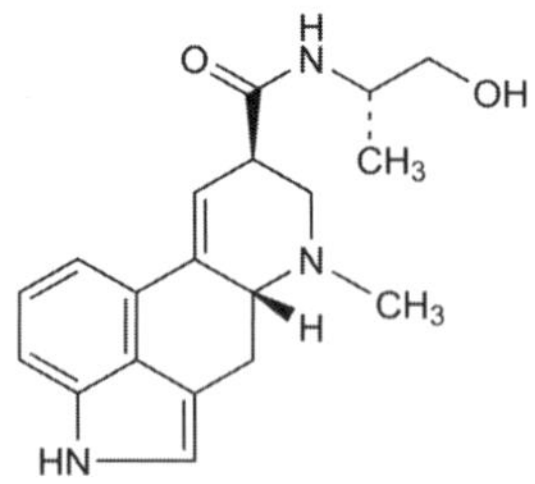

Colourless crystals. Solutions in water give a blue fluorescence. M.p. 162°. Slightly soluble in water; more soluble in ethanol; freely soluble in ethyl acetate and acetone; sparingly soluble in chloroform.

Ergometrine Maleate

Synonyms. Ergobasine Maleate; Ergometrinhydrogenmaleat; Ergonovine Bimaleate; Ergonovine Maleate; Ergostetrine Maleate; Ergotocine Maleate.
Proprietary names. Ergotrate. It is an ingredient of Syntometrine.
$C_{19}H_{23}N_3O_2,C_4H_4O_4$=441.5
CAS—129-51-1
A white or yellowish, slightly hygroscopic, microcrystalline powder. It darkens with age and on exposure to light. Solutions in water and ethanol give a blue fluorescence. M.p. 167°, with decomposition.
Soluble 1 in 36 of water and 1 in 100 of ethanol; practically insoluble in chloroform and ether.

Ergometrine Tartrate

Synonym. Ergonovinum Tartaricum
$(C_{19}H_{23}N_3O_2)_2,C_4H_6O_6$=800.9
CAS—129-50-0
White or slightly reddish-yellow, very light, matted masses of acicular crystals. Slightly soluble in water; soluble in ethanol; slightly soluble in chloroform and ether.

Dissociation Constant. pK_a 6.8 (20°).

Partition Coefficient. Log *P* (ether), −0.9.

Colour Tests. *p*-Dimethylaminobenzaldehyde—violet; Marquis Test—brown.

Thin-layer Chromatography. System TA—Rf 57; system TB—Rf 00; system TC—Rf 12; system TE—Rf 33; system TL—Rf 08; system TM—Rf 26; system TAE—RF 62; system TAF—Rf 60; system TAJ—Rf 17; system TAK—Rf 00; system TAL—Rf 37. (Van Urk reagent, blue.)

High Performance Liquid Chromatography. System HA—*k* 0.4; system HP—*k* 0.50; system HX—RI 292.

Ultraviolet Spectrum. Aqueous acid—313 nm (A^1_1=240a); aqueous alkali—310 nm.

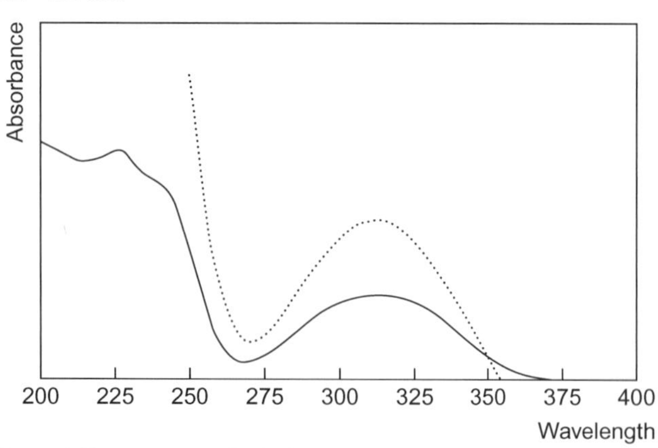

Infra-red Spectrum. Principal peaks at wavenumbers 1634, 754, 748, 1044, 1212, 1541 cm^{-1}.

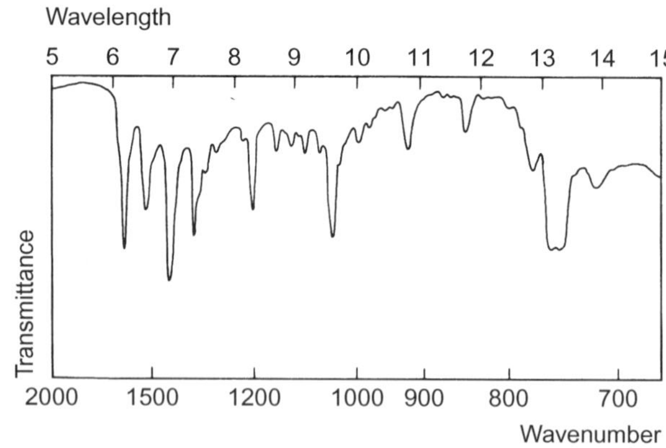

Mass Spectrum. Principal ions at *m*/*z* 221, 72, 325, 54, 196, 55, 207, 181.

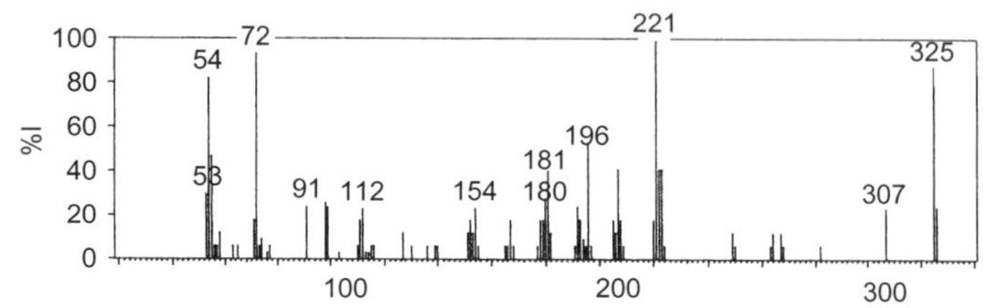

Quantification

High performance liquid chromatography. In plasma: limit of detection <75 ng/L, fluorescence detection—A. N. de Groot *et al.*, *J. Chromatogr.*, 1993, *613*, 158–161.

Disposition in the Body. More rapidly absorbed from the gastro-intestinal tract than ergotamine. Metabolised by hydroxylation and glucuronic acid conjugation and possibly *N*-demethylation. Peak plasma concentrations are attained within 60 to 90 min and are more than tenfold those achieved with an equivalent dose of ergotamine. It is less toxic than ergotamine. Ergometrine has been reported to be detected unchanged in urine up to 8 h after injection, the maximum concentration usually occurring 2 to 3 h after an injection. It is mainly excreted in the bile as 12-hydroxyergometrine glucuronide.

Dose. 0.4 to 1.5 mg of ergometrine maleate daily, by mouth; doses of 200 to 500 µg are given intramuscularly.

Ergotamine

Ergot Alkaloid

(5′α)-12′-Hydroxy-2′-methyl-(phenylmethyl)ergotaman-3′,6′,18-trione
$C_{33}H_{35}N_5O_5$=581.7
CAS—113-15-5

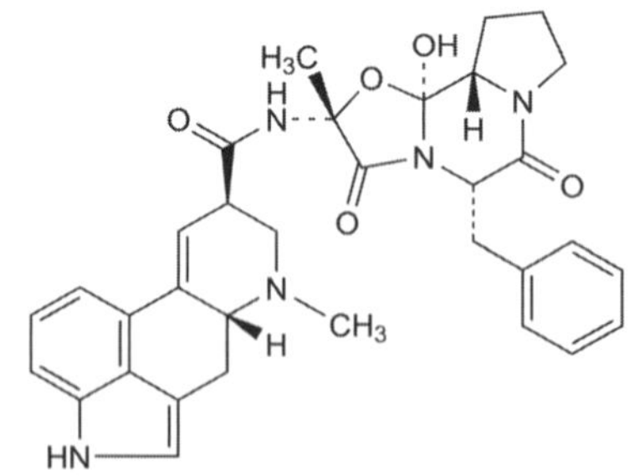

Hygroscopic crystals which darken and decompose on exposure to air, heat and light. M.p. 212° to 214°, with decomposition.
Almost insoluble in water; slightly soluble in ethanol; freely soluble in chloroform, pyridine and glacial acetic acid; moderately soluble in ethyl acetate; slightly soluble in benzene.

Ergotamine Tartrate

Proprietary names. Enxak; Ergodryl Mono; Ergokapton; Ergomar; Ergostat; Ergotan; Gynergen(e); Lingraine; Migrexa. It is an ingredient of Cafergot and Migril.
$(C_{33}H_{35}N_5O_5)_2,C_4H_6O_6$=1313.4

CAS—*379-79-3*
Colourless crystals or white or yellowish-white crystalline powder. M.p. about 180°, with decomposition.
Soluble 1 in about 500 of water and 1 in 500 of ethanol; practically insoluble in chloroform and ether.

Dissociation Constant. pK_a 6.4 (24°).

Partition Coefficient. Log *P* (octanol/water), 2.5.

Colour Tests. *p*-Dimethylaminobenzaldehyde—violet; Mandelin's Test—violet-brown; Marquis Test—brown.

Thin-layer Chromatography. System TA—Rf 63; system TB—Rf 01; system TC—Rf 34; system TE—Rf 44; system TL—Rf 23; system TM—Rf 48; system TAE—Rf 68; system TAF—Rf 64. (Van Urk reagent, blue.)

Gas Chromatography. System GA—RI 2366.

High Performance Liquid Chromatography. System HA—*k* 0.4; system HP—*k* 9.58; system HX—RI 416; system HZ—Retention time, 3.4 min.

Ultraviolet Spectrum. Aqueous acid—316 nm (A^1_1 = 133a); aqueous alkali—310 nm (A^1_1 = 148b).

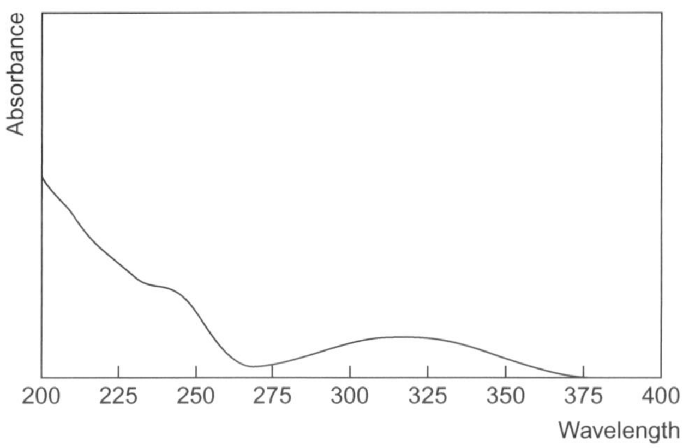

Infra-red Spectrum. Principal peaks at wavenumbers 1631, 1712, 750, 1208, 1136, 1160 cm^{-1} (KBr disk). (See below.)

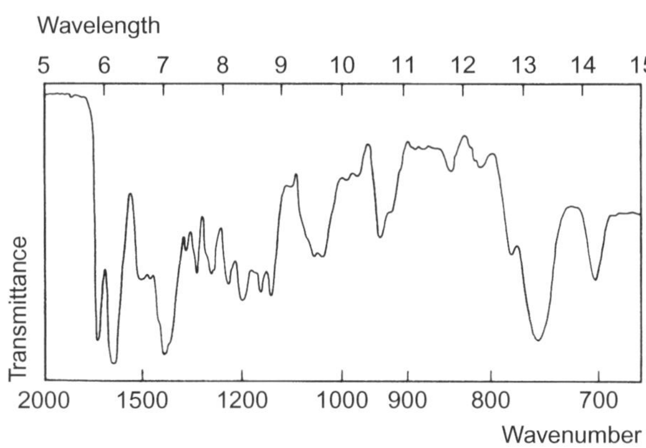

Mass Spectrum. Principal ions at *m/z* 125, 44, 70, 91, 41, 40, 244, 153 (no peaks above 250).

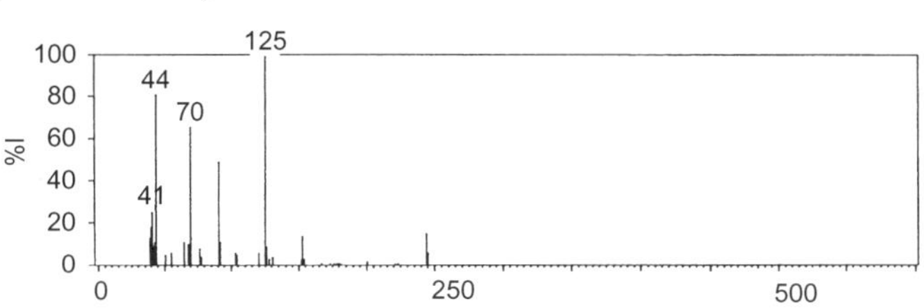

Quantification

Gas chromatography–mass spectrometry. In plasma or serum: limit of detection <50 ng/L—N. Feng *et al.*, *J. Chromatogr.*, 1992, *575*, 289–294.

High performance liquid chromatography. In plasma or serum: ergotamine and methylergometrine, limit of detection 100 ng/L, fluorescence detection—P. O. Edlund, *J. Chromatogr.*, 1981, *226*; *Biomed. Appl.*, *15*, 107–115.

Radioimmunoassay. In plasma—H. F. Schran *et al.*, *Clin. Chem.*, 1979, *25*, 1928–1933.

Disposition in the Body. Poorly absorbed after oral administration; the extent and rate of absorption is increased if caffeine is administered concurrently. Ergotamine is rapidly metabolised in the liver and is excreted mainly in the bile as metabolites; only traces of unchanged drug are excreted in the urine or faeces.

Therapeutic concentration

After a single oral dose of 2 mg of ergotamine tartrate administered to 11 subjects, peak plasma concentrations of 0.0001 to 0.0009 mg/L (mean 0.0006) were attained in 0.5 to 3 h; following an intramuscular dose of 0.5 mg given to 10 subjects, peak plasma concentrations of 0.0009 to 0.004 mg/L (mean 0.002) were attained in about 0.5 h [V. Ala-Hurula *et al.*, *Eur. J. Clin. Pharmacol.*, 1979, *15*, 51–55].

After intramuscular injection of ergotamine tartrate 0.5 mg (3.6 to 3.9 μg/kg) into 10 subjects with migraine, the steady-state plasma concentration resulting in 50% of maximal effect was calculated to be 0.24 μg/L [P. Tfelt-Hansen and L. Paalzow, *Clin. Pharmacol. Ther.*, 1985, *37*, 29–35].

Toxicity. Ergotamine is highly toxic; in large repeated doses it can produce all the symptoms of ergot poisoning. Fatal poisoning has occurred after the oral administration of 26 mg of ergotamine over a period of several days, and also following single injections of only 0.5 to 1.5 mg.

In 12 cases of non-fatal ergotamine overdose, plasma concentrations of 0 to 0.003 mg/L (mean 0.0008) were reported 1.7 to 5 h after ingestion [D. Lamb *et al.*, *Hum. Toxicol.*, 1983, *2*, 424].

Half-life. Plasma half-life, about 2 h.

Volume of distribution. About 2 L/kg.

Clearance. Plasma clearance, about 5 to 18 mL/min/kg (mean 11).

Dose. Not more than 8 mg of ergotamine tartrate in a day or 12 mg in any one week.

Ergotoxine

Ergot Derivative

Synonym. Ecboline
Ergotoxine is a mixture of the 3 isomorphous alkaloids ergocornine, ergocristine and ergocryptine.
$C_{31}H_{39}N_5O_5$ = 561.7
CAS—*006-25-5*
Crystals. M.p. 190° with decomposition.
Almost insoluble in water; very soluble in alcohol, acetone, chloroform and ethyl acetate; slightly soluble in ether.

Ergotoxine Esilate

Synonym. Ergotoxine Ethanesulfonate
$C_{31}H_{39}N_5O_5,C_2H_5SO_3H$ = 671.8
CAS—*8047-28-7*
Colourless crystals which decompose at 209°.
Almost insoluble in water; slightly soluble in ethanol; soluble in methanol.

Colour Test. *p*-Dimethylaminobenzaldehyde—violet.

Thin-layer Chromatography. System TA—Rf 66; system TB—Rf 01; system TC—Rf 62; system TL—Rf 48; system TM—Rf 67. (Acidified potassium permanganate solution, strong reaction; Van Urk reagent, blue.)

Gas Chromatography. System GA—ergocristine RI 2495, ergocryptine RI 2184.

High Performance Liquid Chromatography. System HA—ergocornine *k* 0.4, ergocristine *k* 0.3, ergocryptine *k* 0.4; system HP—ergocornine *k* 10.2, ergocristine *k* 17.3, ergocryptine *k* 15.2.

Infra-red Spectrum. Principal peaks at wavenumbers 1639, 1721, 758, 1534, 1212, 1294 cm^{-1} (KBr disk).

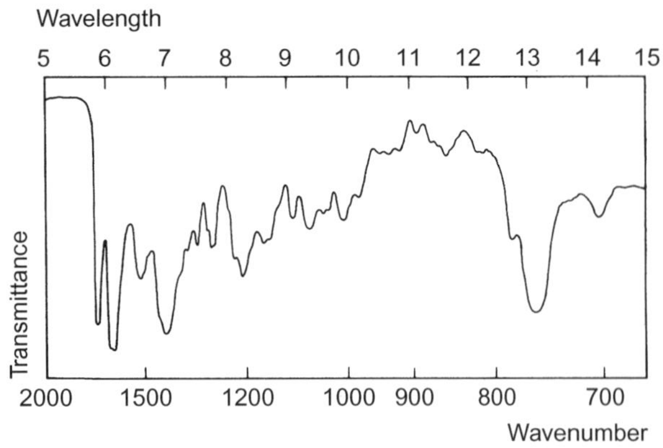

Mass Spectrum. Principal ions at *m/z* 43, 70, 29, 71, 27, 154, 41, 267; ergocornine 43, 70, 71, 54, 44, 154, 267, 55; ergocristine 70, 125, 71, 91, 153, 267, 154, 221; ergocryptine 43, 70, 71, 154, 41, 209, 69, 267.

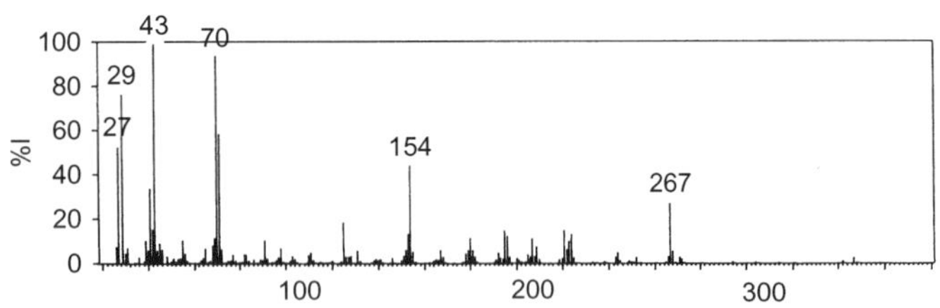

Dose. Ergotoxine esilate was formerly given parenterally in doses of 0.5 to 1 mg.

Erythromycin

Antibiotic

Proprietary names. Abboticine; Ak-Mycin; Akne-Mycin; ATS; Del-Mycin; E-Base; E/Gel; Emgel; Emu-V; E-Mycin; Eratrex; Eromycin; Eryacne; Eryc; Erycen; Erycette; Erycinum;Eryderm; Erygel; Erymax; Ery-Tab; Erythrocin; Erythromid; Ilosone; Ilotycin; Novo-Rythro; PCE; Retcin; Robimycin; Rommix; Ronmix; Staticin; Stiemycin; Theramycin Z; Toloryth; T-Stat.
Erythromycin and its salts are ingredients of many preparations—see *Martindale, The Complete Drug Reference*, 33rd Edn., Pharmaceutical Press, London, 2002.
$C_{37}H_{67}NO_{13}$=733.9
CAS—114-07-8 (erythromycin A)

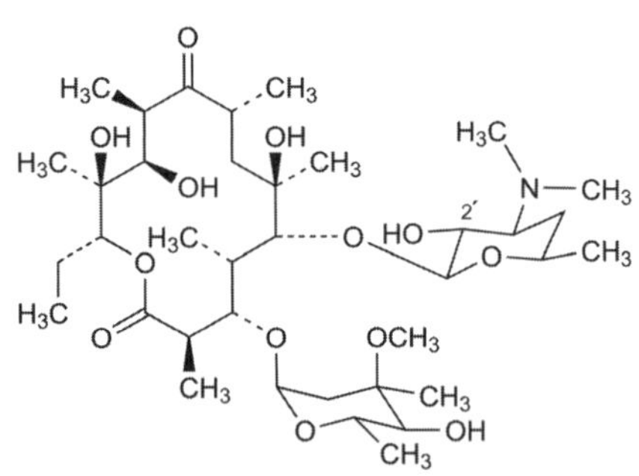

An antimicrobial substance produced by the growth of certain strains of *Streptomyces erythreus*. It is a mixture consisting largely of erythromycin A with lesser amounts of erythromycins B and C.
White or slightly yellow, slightly hygroscopic, crystals or powder. M.p. 135° to 140°.
Soluble 1 in 1000 of water, less soluble at higher temperatures; soluble 1 in 5 of ethanol; freely soluble in acetone, chloroform, acetonitrile and ethyl acetate; moderately soluble in ether, ethylene dichloride and amyl acetate.

Erythromycin Estolate

Synonyms. Erythromycin Propionate Laurilsulfate; Propionyl Erythromycin Laurilsulfate.
Proprietary names. E-Mycin; Erymin; Eromycin; Ilosone.
$C_{40}H_{71}NO_{14},C_{12}H_{26}O_4S$=1056.4
CAS—3521-62-8
A white crystalline powder. M.p. 135° to 140°, with decomposition.
Practically insoluble in water; soluble 1 in 2 of ethanol, 1 in 15 of acetone and 1 in 10 of chloroform.

Erythromycin Ethylsuccinate

Proprietary names. Abboticin(e); Arpimycin; EES; E-Mycin; Eromycin; Ery; Erymax; Erymin; Ery-Ped; Erythrocin(e) Erythroped.
$C_{43}H_{75}NO_{16}$=862.1
CAS—41342-53-4; 1264-62-6
A white or slightly yellow crystalline powder.
Very slightly soluble in water; freely soluble in ethanol and chloroform.

Erythromycin Gluceptate

Synonym. Erythromycin Glucoheptonate
Proprietary name. Ilotycin
$C_{37}H_{67}NO_{13},C_7H_{14}O_8$=960.1
CAS—23067-13-2
A white, slightly hygroscopic powder. M.p. 95° to 140°.
Freely soluble in water, ethanol, methanol, acetone, propylene glycol and dioxane; slightly soluble in chloroform; practically insoluble in ether, carbon tetrachloride, toluene and benzene.

Erythromycin Lactobionate

Proprietary names. Abboticin; Eryc; Erycinum; Erymax; Erythrocin(e).
$C_{37}H_{67}NO_{13},C_{12}H_{22}O_{12}$=1092
CAS—3847-29-8
White or slightly yellow crystals or powder. M.p. 145° to 150°.
Freely soluble in water, ethanol and methanol; slightly soluble in chloroform and ether.

Erythromycin Propionate

Proprietary names. Ery; Propiocine.
$C_{40}H_{71}NO_{14}$=790.0
CAS—134-36-1
A white powder.
Very slightly soluble in water; readily soluble in acetone, ethyl acetate, ethanol and chloroform.

Erythromycin Stearate

Proprietary names. Abboticin(e); Eramycin; Eromycin; Erotab; Erycin; Erycinum; Erythrocin(e).
$C_{37}H_{67}NO_{13},C_{18}H_{36}O_2$=1018.4
CAS—643-22-1
White or slightly yellow crystals or powder.
Practically insoluble in water; slightly soluble in ethanol, chloroform and ether.

Dissociation Constant. pK_a 8.9.

Partition Coefficient. Log *P* (octanol/water), 3.1.

Colour Test. Marquis Test—brown.

Thin-layer Chromatography. System TA—Rf 55; system TB—Rf 11; system TE—Rf 46; system TAE—Rf 24; system TAJ—Rf 04; system TAK—Rf 02; system TAL—Rf 42.

Infra-red Spectrum. Principal peaks at wavenumbers 1050, 1168, 1074, 1010, 1108, 1734 cm^{-1} (KBr disk).

Quantification

High performance liquid chromatography. In serum: erythromycin and erythromycin ethylsuccinate, limits of detection <10 μg/L, derivatisation and fluorescence detection—K. Tsuji, *J. Chromatogr.*, 1978, *158*, 337–348. In plasma or gastric juice: electrochemical detection—H. Toreson and B. M. Eriksson, *J. Chromatogr.*, 1995, *673*, *Biomed. Appl.*, 81–89. In serum: erythromycin and other macrolide antibiotics, fluorescence detection—J. Satre Torano and H. J. Guchelaar, *J. Chromatogr. B. Biomed. Sci. Appl.*, 1998, *720*, 89–97.

High performance liquid chromatography–mass spectrometry. In plasma: limit of detection <0.5 μg/L—X. Li *et al.*, *J. Pharm. Biomed. Anal.*, 1998, *16*, 961–970.

Review. Analysis of macrolide antibiotics—I. Kanfer *et al.*, *J. Chromatogr.*, 1998, *812*, 255–286.

Disposition in the Body. Erythromycin base is destroyed by gastric acid; erythromycin stearate is hydrolysed in the intestine and absorbed as free erythromycin; the estolate is absorbed as the ester and then hydrolysed.

About 5 to 10% of a dose is excreted in the urine unchanged and large amounts of unchanged drug are excreted in the bile.

Therapeutic concentration

Following single oral doses of 250 mg, 500 mg and 1 g of a preparation containing enteric-coated pellets of erythromycin base to 23 subjects, mean peak serum concentrations of 1.9, 3.8 and 6.5 mg/L, respectively, were attained in about 2 h. After a single oral dose of 500 mg of erythromycin stearate to the same subjects, a mean peak serum concentration of 2.9 mg/L was attained in about 2 h [K. Josefsson *et al.*, *Br. J. Clin. Pharmacol.*, 1982, *13*, 685–691].

Following oral administration of 250 mg of erythromycin four times a day to 16 subjects, maximum and minimum steady-state plasma concentrations of 1.7 and 0.45 mg/L were reported on the third day, compared to 1.34 and 0.58 mg/L respectively, following repeated oral administration of erythromycin estolate [A. R. DiSanto *et al.*, *J. Clin. Pharmacol.*, 1980, *20*, 437–443].

Half-life. Plasma half-life, about 1 to 3 h (dose-dependent).

Volume of distribution. About 0.7 L/kg.

Clearance. Plasma clearance, about 7 mL/min/kg.

Distribution in blood. Plasma:whole blood ratio, 0.43.

Protein binding. In plasma, erythromycin about 70 to 80%, erythromycin propionate about 90 to 99%, erythromycin stearate about 90%.

Dose. 1 to 4 g daily.

Esmolol

Beta-blocker

4-[2-Hydroxy-3-[(1-methylethyl)amino]propoxy]benzenepropanoic acid methyl ester

$C_{16}H_{25}NO_4$=295.4

CAS—84057-94-3

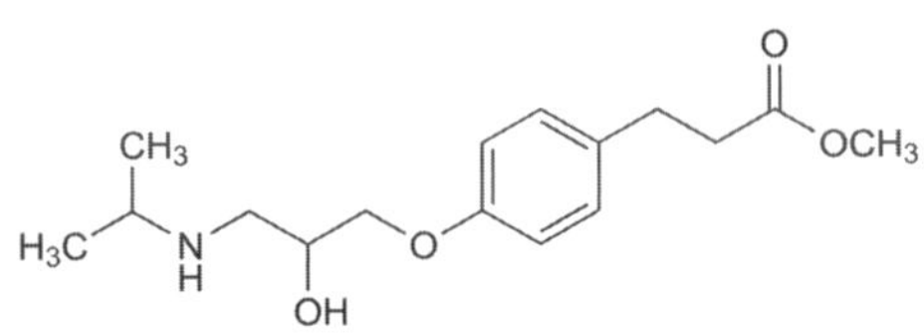

Esmolol is an oil, which gradually becomes crystalline at room temperature. M.p. 48° to 50°.

Esmolol Hydrochloride

Synonym. ASL-8052

Proprietary name. Brevibloc

$C_{16}H_{25}NO_4$, HCl=331.8

CAS—81161-17-3

A white to off-white crystalline powder, which is relatively hydrophilic. M.p. 85° to 86°. It is very soluble in water; freely soluble in alcohol.

Dissociation Constant. pK_a 9.5.

Partition Coefficient. Log *P* (octanol/water, pH 7), 0.42.

Gas Chromatography. System GB—RI 2311 (esmolol); RI 2395 (Art).

High Performance Liquid Chromatography. Columns: (A)-C_{18} (μBondapak, 300 × 3.9 mm i.d.); (B)-Spherisorb phenyl (250 × 4 mm, 10 μm). Mobile phases: (A)-phosphate buffer:acetonitrile (65:35), pH 6.9; (B)-10 mmol/L sodium acetate:acetonitrile:glacial acetic acid, pH 3.4 (91:8:1), 2.0 mL/min flow rate. UV detection (system A: λ=229 nm; system B: λ=280 nm). Retention times: esmolol (eluted with column and mobile phase (A)), 6.1 min; de-esterified metabolite (eluted with column and mobile phase (B)), 10.8 min [R. Archari *et al.*, *Clin. Chem.*, 1986, *32(2)*, 374–376].

Column: cyano-bonded silica (300 × 3.9 mm i.d., 10 μm). Mobile phase: acetonitrile:glacial acetic acid:sodium acetate trihydrate (0.068%) (150:10:840), 2 mL/min flow rate. UV detection (λ=280 nm). Retention time: esmolol hydrochloride, 7.71 min; esmolol, 5.14 min [Y-C. Lee *et al.*, *J. Pharm. Sci.*, 1984, *73(11)*, 1660–1661].

Column: CN (Radial-Pak, 100 × 5 mm i.d., 10 μm), C_{18} guard column (Whatman, 37 to 53 μm, 30 × 3.2 mm). Mobile phase: methanol:potassium dihydrogen phosphate buffer (0.06 M):triethylamine, adjusted to pH 3.15 with phosphoric acid (85%) (25:75:0.1), 1.8 mL/min flow rate. UV detection (λ=221 nm). Retention time: 2.6 min [C-D. Fan *et al.*, *J. Chromatogr.*, 1991, *570*, *Biomed. Appl.*, 217–223].

Ultraviolet Spectrum. Aqueous acid—223, 275, 281 nm.

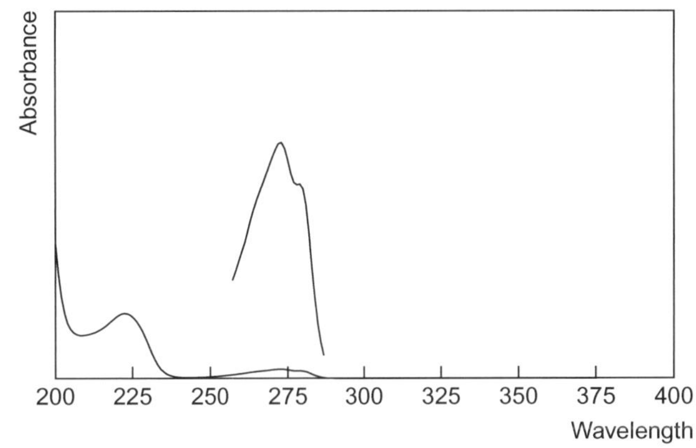

Mass Spectrum. Principal ions at *m/z* 72, 107, 56, 116, 43, 73, 41, 251.

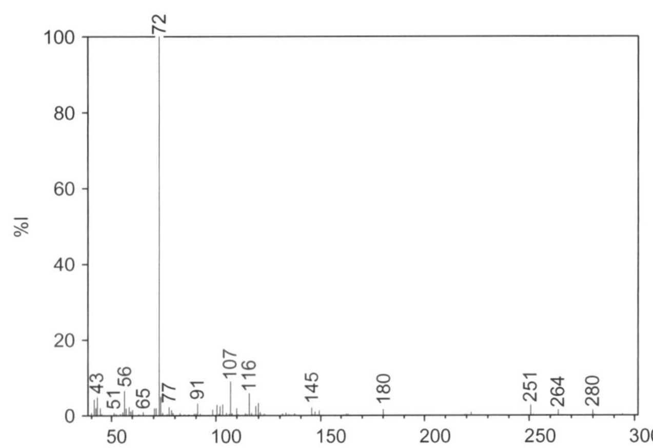

Quantification

Gas chromatography–mass spectrometry. In blood: limit of detection 2.5 μg/L—C. Y. Sum and A. Yacobi, *J. Pharm. Sci.*, 1984, *73*, 1177–1179.

High performance liquid chromatography. In solution: limit of quantification is 10 mg/L. UV detection (λ=280 nm)—Y-C. Lee *et al.*, *J. Pharm. Sci.*, 1984, *73(11)*, 1660–1661. In urine: esmolol and metabolite, limit of detection 0.025 mg/L for esmolol and 1.0 mg/L for metabolite, UV detection (λ=229, 280 nm)—R. Achari *et al.*, *Clin. Chem.*, 1986, *32*, 374–376. In blood: esmolol and metabolites, limit of detection 0.05 mg/L, UV detection—A. L. Sintetos *et al.*, *Clin. Pharmacol. Ther.*, 1987, *41*, 112–117. In blood: limit of detection 0.025 mg/L, UV detection—R. Achari *et al.*, *J. Chromatogr.*, 1988, *424*, *Biomed. Appl.*, *68*, 430–434. In blood: limit of detection 5 μg/L and limit of quantification 10 μg/L, UV detection (λ=221 nm)—C.-D. Fan *et al.*, *J. Chromatogr.*, 1991, *570*, *Biomed. Appl.*, *108*, 217–223.

Disposition in the Body. Esmolol is rapidly hydrolysed, in red blood cells, by esterases. An acidic de-esterified metabolite (ASL-8123, with very little beta-blocking activity), methanol and a number of inactive metabolites are produced. Excretion is primarily via urine primarily as the de-esterified metabolite (71 to 83%) and less than 2% of the drug appearing unchanged and the rest as the inactive metabolites. The remainder of the dose can be recovered in faeces. Only small amounts of the metabolite are removed by dialysis. The metabolite accumulates in patients with renal failure.

Therapeutic concentration

8 healthy male volunteers, aged between 21 and 27 years, were administered continuous intravenous doses of 50, 150 and 400 μg/kg/min for 2 h. Peak plasma concentrations of 77.9 mg/L ASL-8123 (mean) were reached within 26 min after infusion was stopped. Steady state concentrations of the parent

drug esmolol reached 1.59 mg/L (mean). [A. Yacobi *et al.*, *J. Pharm. Sci.*, 1983, *72*, 710–711].

9 male volunteers with cirrhosis and 3 healthy males, aged between 23 and 65 years, were administered 200 µg/kg/min esmolol over 4 h. Mean steady state esmolol concentrations were 1.68 mg/L for the healthy individuals and 1.41 mg/L for those with cirrhosis. These concentrations were observed during infusion and rapidly decreased once the infusion had completed. Mean concentrations of the metabolite were 39.2 and 56.0 mg/L for the healthy individuals and cirrhosis patients, respectively. These were seen after approx. 4 h. [K. N. Buchi *et al.*, *J. Clin. Pharmacol.*, 1987, *27*, 880–884].

Toxicity. Massive accidental overdosing has occurred due to dilution errors, which has resulted in cardiac arrest, death and permanent disability. A concentration between 12.5 and 50 mg/kg is associated with fatalities.

Half-life. Approx. 9 min for esmolol; increases in patients with liver failure, up to 16 min; 3.7 h for the metabolite.

Volume of distribution. 1.0 to 2.4 L/kg; increases in patients with renal failure, up to 3.4 L/kg; 0.41 L/kg (metabolite).

Clearance. Plasma clearance, 20 L/kg/h; 0.08 L/h/kg or 1.28 mL/min/kg (metabolite).

Protein binding. Esmolol is 55% bound and the metabolite (ASL-8123) 10%.

Note. For a general review of esmolol, see P. Benfield and E.M. Sorkin, *Drugs*, 1987, *33*, 392–412.

Dose. An initial loading dose of 500 µg/kg body weight is administered. A maintenance dose of 50 µg/kg/min is used, which can be increased if necessary to a maximum of 200 µg/kg/min.

Estradiol

Estrogen

Synonyms. Beta-estradiol; Dihydrofolliculine; Dihydrotheelin; Dihydroxyoestrin; Oestradiol.
Proprietary names. Estrace; Farmacyrol; Gynoestryl; Oestrogel; Progynon. It is an ingredient of Hormonin and Trisequens.
(17*β*)-Estra-1,3,5(10)-triene-3,17-diol
$C_{18}H_{24}O_2$=272.4
CAS—50-28-2

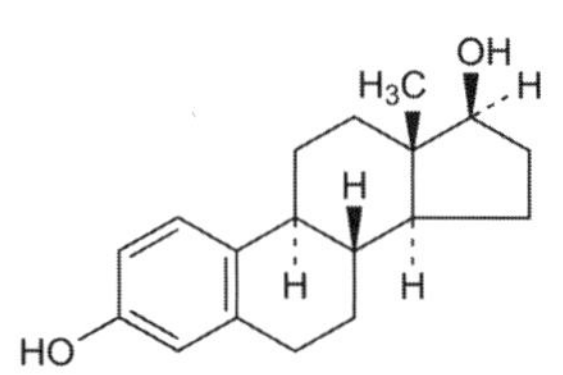

White or creamy-white, hygroscopic crystals or crystalline powder. M.p. 173° to 179°.
Almost insoluble in water; soluble 1 in 28 of ethanol, 1 in 17 of acetone, 1 in 435 of chloroform and 1 in 150 of ether; soluble in dioxan and solutions of alkali hydroxides.

Estradiol Benzoate

Synonyms. Oestradiol Benzoate; Estradiol Monobenzoate.
Proprietary names. Benzo-Gynoestryl 5; Benztrone; Gynécormone; Oestramine; Ovocyclin M; Progynon B. It is an ingredient of Mixogen (injection) and Plex-Hormone (injection).
$C_{25}H_{28}O_3$=376.5
CAS—50-50-0
Colourless crystals or white or creamy-white crystalline powder. M.p. 190° to 198°.
Practically insoluble in water; slightly soluble in ethanol; soluble 1 in 5 of chloroform and 1 in 150 of ether; soluble in acetone and dioxan.

Estradiol Cipionate

Synonyms. Oestradiol Cipionate; Estradiol Cyclopentylpropionate.
Proprietary names. Depo-Estradiol Cipionate; Neoginon Depositum.
$C_{26}H_{36}O_3$=396.6
CAS—313-06-4
A white crystalline powder. M.p. 149° to 153°.
Practically insoluble in water; soluble 1 in 40 of ethanol and 1 in 7 of chloroform; soluble in acetone, ether and dioxan.

Estradiol Undecylate

Synonyms. Oestradiol Undecylate; Estradiol Undecanoate.
Proprietary names. Progynon Depot; Progynon-Retard.
$C_{29}H_{44}O_3$=440.7
CAS—3571-53-7

Estradiol Valerate

Synonym. Oestradiol Valerate
Proprietary names. Delestrogen; Femogex; Östrogynol sine; Primogyn Depot; Progynon Depot; Progynova. It is an ingredient of Cyclacur and Cyclo-Progynova.
$C_{23}H_{32}O_3$=356.5
CAS—979-32-8
A white crystalline powder. M.p. 144° to 145°.
Practically insoluble in water; soluble in dioxan and methanol.

Partition Coefficient. Log *P* (octanol/water), 4.0.

Colour Tests. Antimony pentachloride—brown; Liebermann's test—black; Naphthol–sulfuric acid—blue-green, yellow dichroism/orange; Sulfuric acid—yellow (green fluorescence under ultraviolet light).

Thin-layer Chromatography. Estradiol benzoate: system TP—Rf 79; system TQ—Rf 32; system TR—Rf 96; system TS—Rf 79. Estradiol: system TD—Rf 61; system TE—Rf 78; system TF—Rf 58; system TAD—Rf 64; system TAJ—Rf 55; system TAK—Rf 58; system TAL—Rf 91; system TAM—Rf 09.

Gas Chromatography. System GA—RI 2659.

High Performance Liquid Chromatography. System HX—RI 896; system HY—RI 456; system HAA—retention time 18.2 min.

Ultraviolet Spectrum. Estradiol benzoate: ethanol—231 nm (A^1_1=490b).

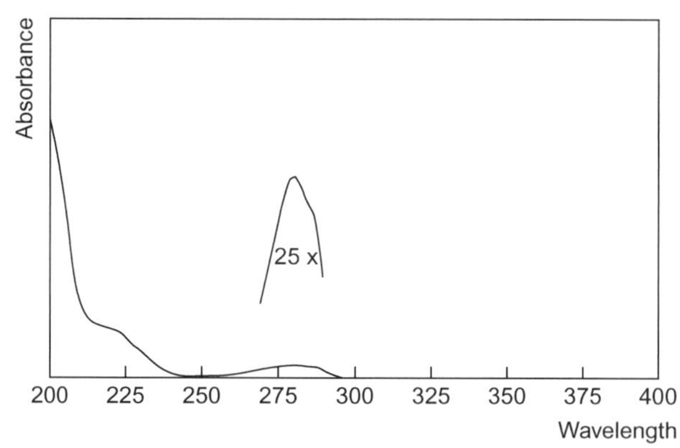

Infra-red Spectrum. Principal peaks at wavenumbers 1245, 1054, 1227, 1493, 1276, 821 cm^{-1} (KBr disk).

Quantification

Gas chromatography–mass spectrometry. In urine: estradiol, estriol and estrone—X. Xiao and D. McCalley, *Rapid Commun. Mass Spectrom.*, 2000, *14*, 1991–2001.

High performance liquid chromatography. In serum: estradiol and estriol, fluorescence detection (comparison with radioimmunoassay)—Z. Kondo *et al.*, *J. Lab. Clin. Med.*, 1990, *4*, 410–413. In serum: limit of detection 0.14 µg/L, fluorescence detection—K. H. DeSilva *et al.*, *Biomed. Chromatogr.*, 1996, *10*, 318–324.

High performance liquid chromatography–radioimmunoasssay. In serum: estradiol and estrone, limits of detection 0.64 µg/L and 1.04 µg/L, respectively—T. Yasui *et al.*, *J. Clin. Lab. Anal.*, 1999, *13*, 266–272.

Mass spectrometry. In serum: estradiol, estrone and other sex hormones (comparison with radioimmunoassay)—J. F. Dorgan *et al.*, *Steroids*, 2002, *67*, 151–158.

Therapeutic concentration

Mean serum estradiol concentrations in 25 subjects given 2 mg estradiol, 1 mg estriol and 1 mg norethisterone acetate for 4 months to 6 years were 138 (range 53 to 279) ng/L; concentrations remained relatively even, reaching a broad maximum between 2 and 14 h after intake. [I. Klehr-Bathmann and H. Kuhl, *Maturitas*, 1995, *21*, 245–250].

Following application of estradiol from a transdermal gel to 23 subjects at a dose of 0.5, 1.0 and 1.5 mg daily, mean peak serum levels of 39.0, 67.3 and

158.5 ng/L, respectively, were attained at 7, 6, and 3 h. [A. Järvinen *et al.*, *Maturitas*, 2000, *35*, 51–56].

Dose. Up to 2 mg daily, by mouth.

Estriol

Oestrogen

Synonyms. Oestriol; Theelol.
Proprietary names. Hormomed; Ovestin. It is an ingredient of Hormonin and Trisequens.
(16α,17β)-Estra-1,3,5(10)-triene-3,16,17-triol
$C_{18}H_{24}O_3$=288.4
CAS—50-27-1

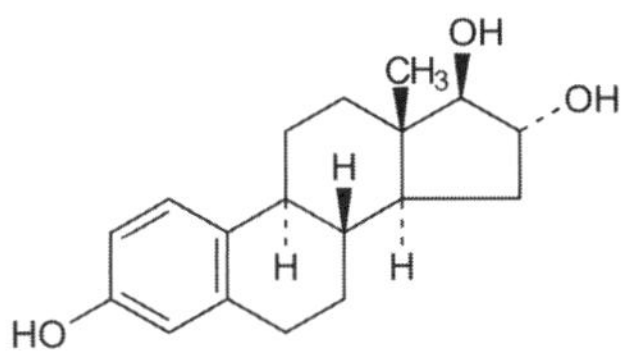

A white crystalline powder. M.p. about 280°.
Practically insoluble in water; soluble 1 in about 500 of ethanol; soluble in acetone, chloroform, dioxan and ether; freely soluble in pyridine and in solutions of fixed alkali hydroxides.

Dissociation Constant. pK_a 10.4.

Partition Coefficient. Log *P* (octanol/water), 2.4.

Colour Tests. Antimony pentachloride—brown; Liebermann's test—black; Naphthol–sulfuric acid—green, yellow dichroism/orange; Sulfuric acid—no initial colour (yellow-green fluorescence under ultraviolet light).

Gas Chromatography. System GA—RI 2955.

High Performance Liquid Chromatography. System HAA—retention time 13.1 min.

Ultraviolet Spectrum. Ethanol—280 nm.

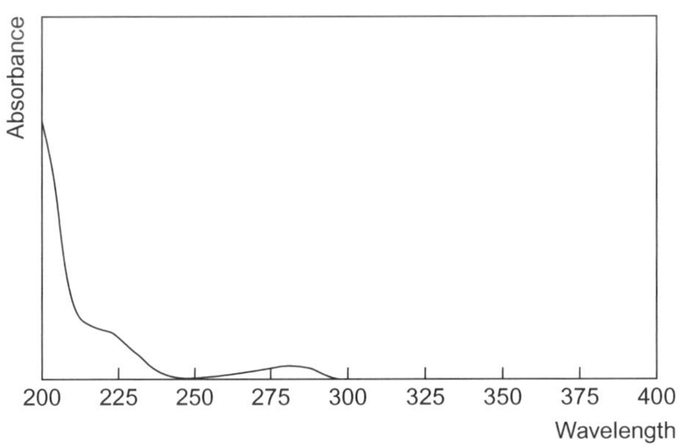

Infra-red Spectrum. Principal peaks at wavenumbers 1228, 1067, 917, 1147, 1250, 1605 cm^{-1} (Nujol mull).

Quantification. See also Estradiol.

High performance liquid chromatography. In urine: UV detection—L. Ke and Y.S. Yuan, *Biomed. Chromatogr.*, 1989, *3*, 196–198. In serum: estriol and estriol 3-sulfate, limits of detection 2.5 μg/L and 295 μg/L, respectively, UV and electrochemical detection—N. Tagawa *et al.*, *J. Chromatogr. B, Biomed. Sci. Appl.*, 1999, *723*, 39–45.

Dose. 0.25 to 1 mg daily.

Estrone

Oestrogen

Synonyms. Oestrone; Folliculin; Ketohydroxyoestrin.
Proprietary names. Cristallovar; Femogen; Kolpon; Oestrilin (vaginal preparations). It is an ingredient of Hormonin.
3-Hydroxyestra-1,3,5(10)-trien-17-one
$C_{18}H_{22}O_2$=270.4
CAS—53-16-7

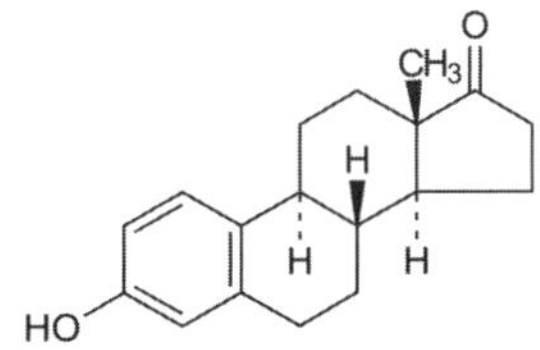

Colourless crystals or white to creamy-white crystalline powder. M.p. about 260°, with decomposition.
Practically insoluble in water; soluble 1 in 250 of ethanol, 1 in 50 of acetone and 1 in 110 of chloroform; soluble in dioxan, pyridine, fixed alkali hydroxide solutions; slightly soluble in ether.

Partition Coefficient. Log *P* (octanol/water), 3.1.

Colour Tests. Antimony pentachloride—brown; Liebermann's test—black; Naphthol–sulfuric acid—green, yellow dichroism/orange; Sulfuric acid—green-yellow (green fluorescence under ultraviolet light).

Thin-layer Chromatography. System TB—Rf 09; system TE—Rf 76; system TF—Rf 68; system TAE—Rf 87; system TAJ—Rf 63; system TAK—Rf 66; system TAL—Rf 91; system TAM—Rf 95.

Gas Chromatography. System GA—RI 2612.

High Performance Liquid Chromatography. System HX—RI 544; system HY—RI 521.

Ultraviolet Spectrum. Methanol—280 nm (A_1^1=78a).

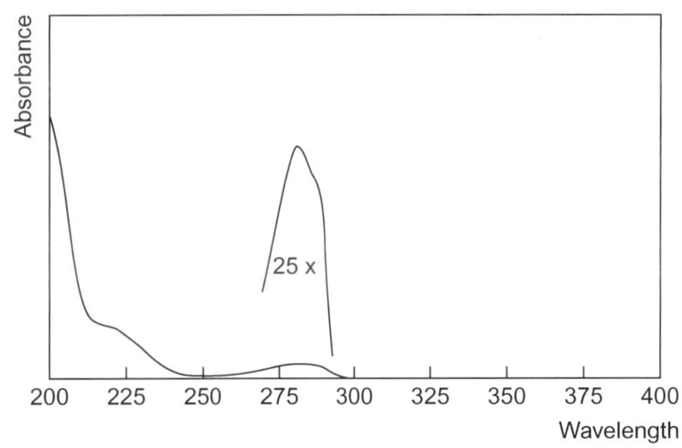

Infra-red Spectrum. Principal peaks at wavenumbers 1282, 820, 1709, 1244, 921, 1493 cm^{-1}.

Quantification. See under Estradiol.

Dose. Estrone has been given in doses of 0.1 to 5 mg daily by intramuscular injection.

Etafedrine

Sympathomimetic

Synonym. Ethylephedrine
α-[1-(Ethylmethylamino)ethyl]benzenemethanol
$C_{12}H_{19}NO$=193.3
CAS—7681-79-0; 48141-64-6

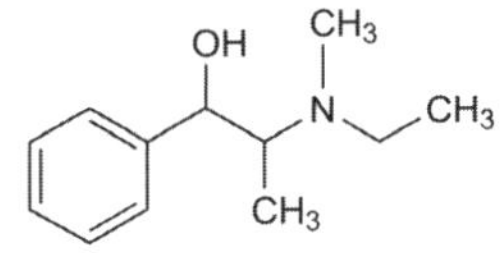

Etafedrine Hydrochloride

Proprietary names. It is an ingredient of Calmydone, Dalmacol, and some Nethaprin and Revenil preparations.
$C_{12}H_{19}NO,HCl$=229.8
CAS—5591-29-7
Crystals. M.p. 183° to 184°.

Soluble 1 in 1.5 of water and 1 in 8 of ethanol.

Partition Coefficient. Log *P* (octanol/water), 1.4.

Thin-layer Chromatography. System TA—Rf 44; system TB—Rf 35; system TC—Rf 09; system TE—Rf 56; system TL—Rf 15; system TAE—Rf 14; system TAJ—Rf 04; system TAK—Rf 06; system TAL—Rf 49. (Acidified potassium permanganate solution, positive.)

Gas Chromatography. System GA—RI 1519; system GB—RI 1510; system GC—RI 1737.

High Performance Liquid Chromatography. System HA—*k* 1.9.

Ultraviolet Spectrum. Aqueous acid—251, 257 nm (A^1_1=10a), 263 nm. (See below.)

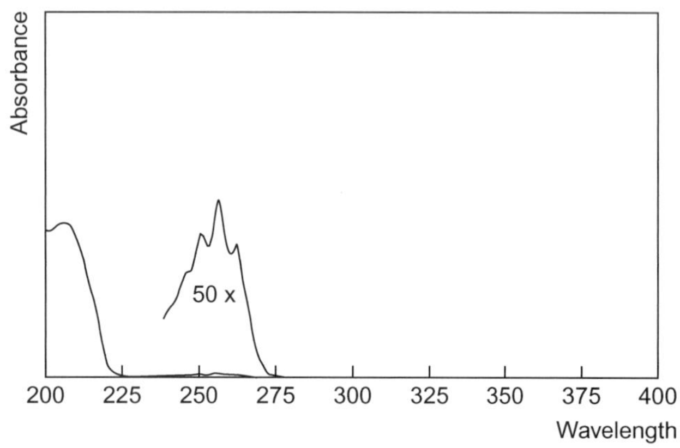

Infra-red Spectrum. Principal peaks at wavenumbers 697, 1051, 1020, 1000, 740, 1115 cm^{-1} (KBr disk).

Mass Spectrum. Principal ions at *m/z* 86, 58, 87, 42, 56, 77, 44, 43.

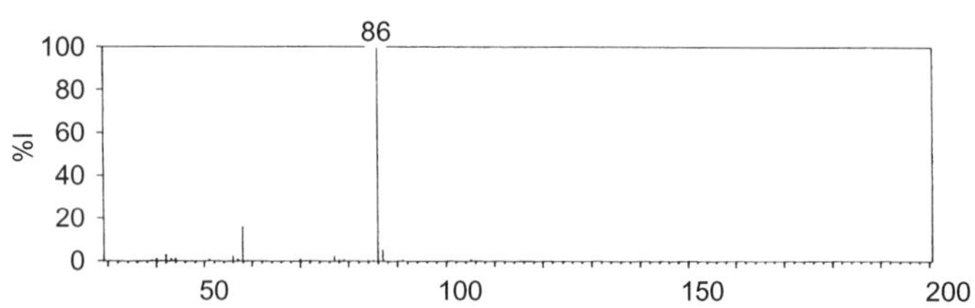

Dose. 80 to 200 mg of etafedrine hydrochloride daily.

Etamiphylline

Xanthine Bronchodilator

Synonym. Etamphyllin

7-[2-(Diethylamino)ethyl]-3,7-dihydro-1,3-dimethyl-1*H*-purine-2,6-dione

$C_{13}H_{21}N_5O_2$=279.3

CAS—314-35-2

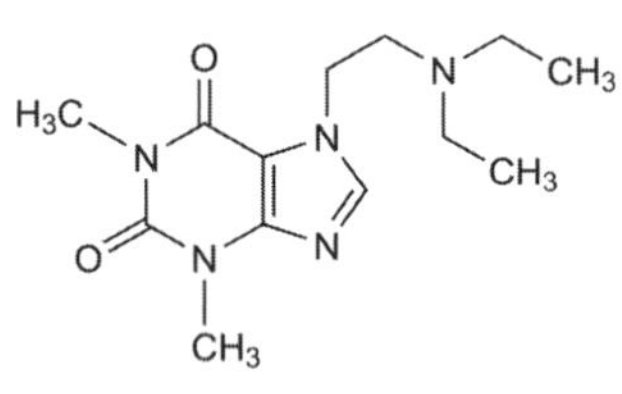

A waxy solid. M.p. 75°.

Very soluble in water and acetone; slightly soluble in ethanol and ether.

Etamiphylline Camsilate

Synonym. Diétamiphylline Camphosulfonate

Proprietary names. Camphophyline. It is an ingredient of Longtussin and Solufilina Sedante.

$C_{23}H_{37}N_5O_6S$=511.6

CAS—19326-29-5

A white crystalline powder. M.p. 174°.

Very soluble in water; soluble in ethanol and chloroform; very slightly soluble in ether.

Partition Coefficient. Log *P* (octanol/water), 0.8.

Colour Test. Amalic Acid Test—yellow/pink.

Thin-layer Chromatography. System TA—Rf 54; system TB—Rf 12; system TC—Rf 39; system TE—Rf 74; system TL—Rf 17; system TAJ—Rf 28; system TAK—Rf 02; system TAL—Rf 44. (Acidified iodoplatinate solution, positive.)

Gas Chromatography. System GA—etamiphylline RI 2210, M (desethyl-)-AC RI 2560.

High Performance Liquid Chromatography. System HA—*k* 1.2.

Ultraviolet Spectrum. Water—274 nm (A^1_1=320b).

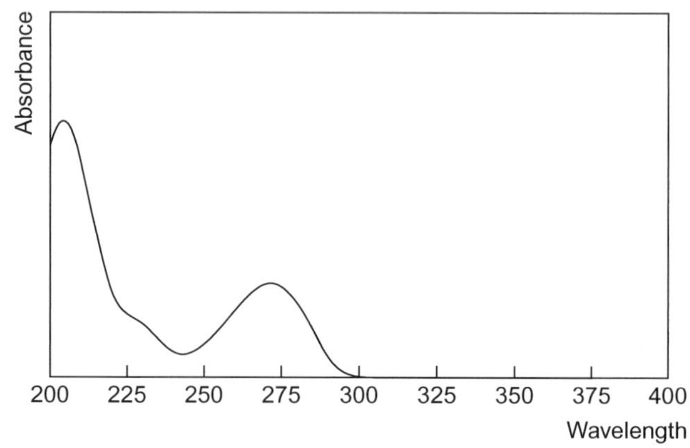

Infra-red Spectrum. Principal peaks at wavenumbers 1656, 1706, 748, 1543, 1220, 1600 cm^{-1}.

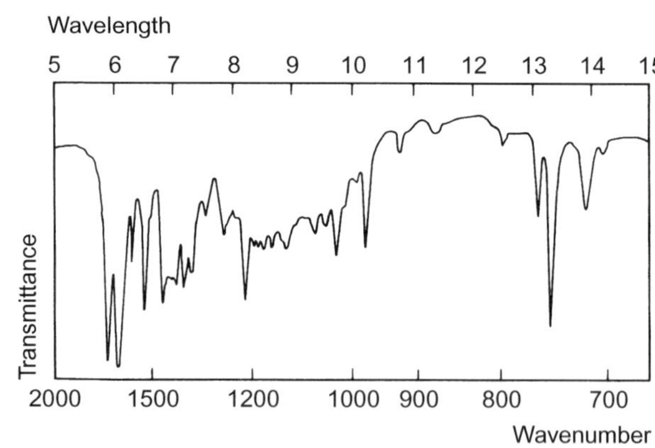

Mass Spectrum. Principal ions at *m/z* 86, 109, 30, 151, 87, 81, 99, 58.

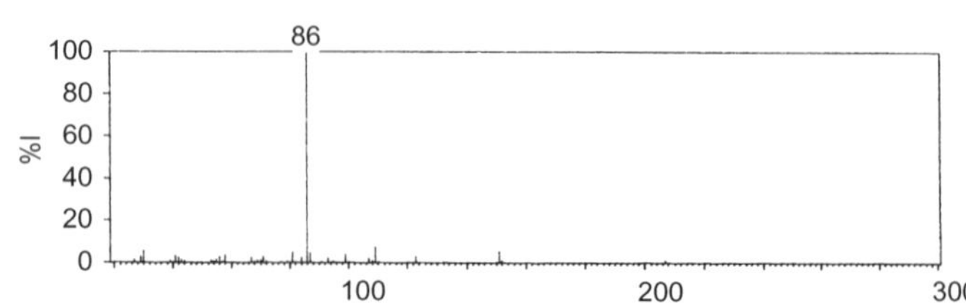

Dose. 0.3 to 1.2 g of etamiphylline camsilate daily.

Etamivan

Respiratory Stimulant

Synonyms. Ethamivan; Vanillic Acid Diethylamide; Vanillic Diethylamide.

Proprietary names. Cardiovanil; Emivan; Vandid.

N,N-Diethyl-4-hydroxy-3-methoxybenzamide

$C_{12}H_{17}NO_3$=223.3

CAS—304-84-7

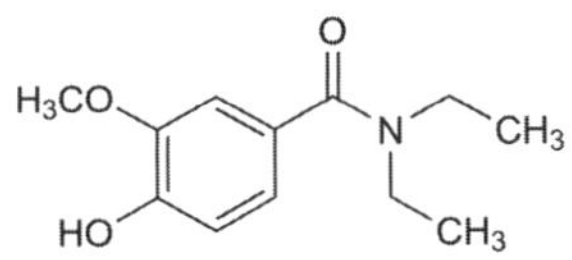

A white crystalline powder. M.p. 94° to 99°.
Soluble 1 in 100 of water, 1 in 2 of ethanol, 1 in 1.5 of chloroform and 1 in 50 of ether.

Partition Coefficient. Log *P* (octanol/water), 1.1.

Colour Tests. Ferric Chloride—green; Folin–Ciocalteu Reagent—blue; Liebermann's Test—black

Thin-layer Chromatography. System TA—Rf 94; system TD—Rf 38; system TE—Rf 41; system TF—Rf 35; system TAD—Rf 59; system TAE—Rf 85; system TAJ—Rf 60; system TAK—Rf 48; system TAL—Rf 96.

Gas Chromatography. System GA—etamivan RI 1900, etamivan-AC RI 1970; system GC—RI 2409.

Ultraviolet Spectrum. Aqueous acid—280 nm (A_1^1=153a).

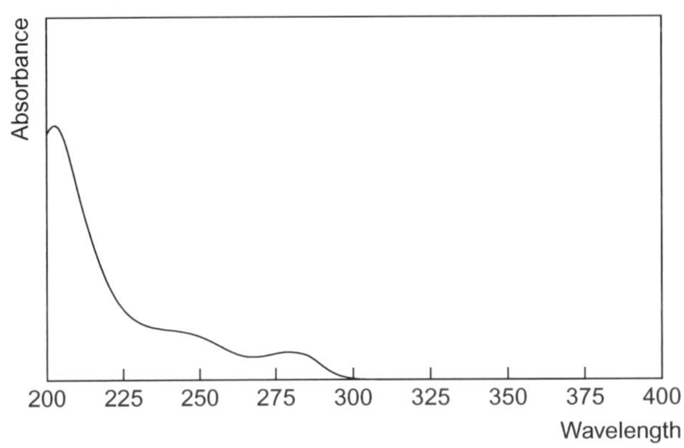

Infra-red Spectrum. Principal peaks at wavenumbers 1608, 1270, 1585, 1240, 1300, 1543 cm^{-1} (KBr disk).

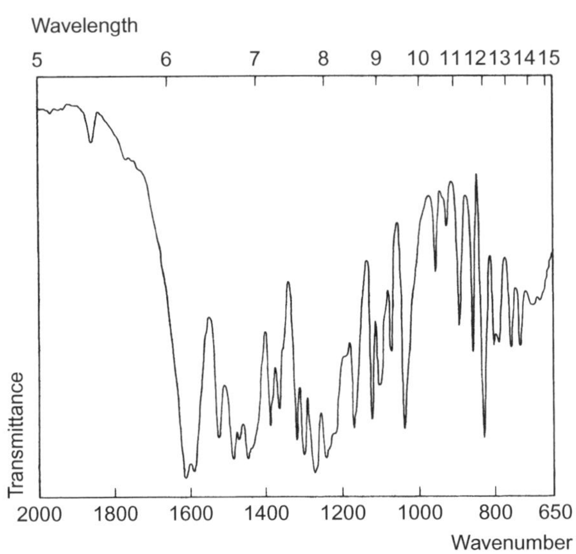

Mass Spectrum. Principal ions at *m/z* 151, 72, 223, 123, 222, 152, 52, 29.

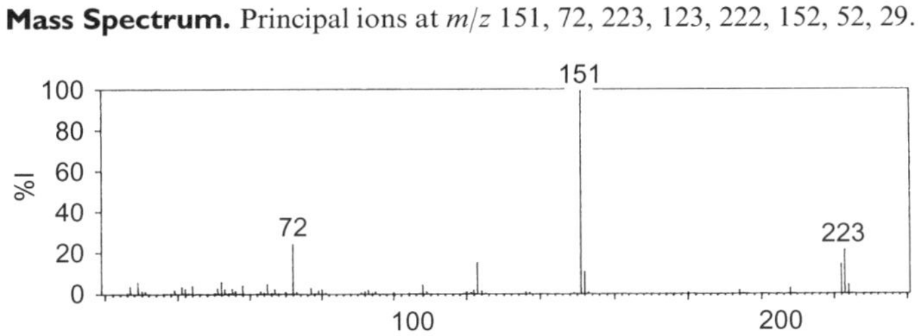

Quantification
High performance liquid chromatography. In urine: etamivan and other drugs of abuse—C. Ma *et al.*, *Yao Xue Xue Bao*, 1998, *33*, 764–767.

Dose. Etamivan has been given intravenously in doses of up to 10 mL of a 5% solution; doses of 40 to 240 mg daily have been given by mouth.

Etebenecid

Uricosuric

Synonym. Ethebenecid
4-Diethylsulfamoylbenzoic acid
$C_{11}H_{15}NO_4S$=257.3
CAS—1213-06-5

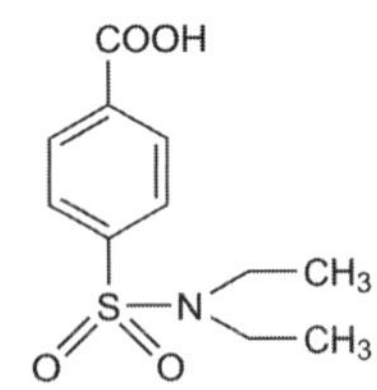

Crystals. M.p. 192° to 194°.

Dissociation Constant. pK_a 3.3 (25°).

Partition Coefficient. Log *P* (octanol/water), 1.9.

Ultraviolet Spectrum. Methanol—246 nm (A_1^1=460b).

Infra-red Spectrum. Principal peaks at wavenumbers 1694, 729, 1162, 1282, 1298, 934 cm^{-1}.

Dose. Etebenecid has been given in doses of 1 to 3 g daily.

Etenzamide

Analgesic

Synonyms. Aethoxybenzamidum; Ethenzamide; Ethoxybenzamide; Ethylsalicylamide; HP-209; Salicylamide *O*-Ethyl Ether.
Proprietary names. Simil NF; Trancalgyl. It is an ingredient of Algopriv; Antifohnon-N; Cephyl; Coldadolin; Dolmix; Glutisal; Helopyrin; Kata-grip; Kolton grippale N; Nicaphlogyl; Nisicur; Seltoc; Seranex sans codeine.
2-Ethoxybenzamide
$C_9H_{11}NO_2$=165.2
CAS—938-73-8

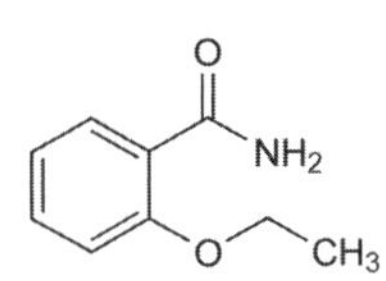

A white crystalline powder. M.p. 132° to 134°.
Practically insoluble in cold water; slightly soluble in boiling water and in ether; soluble in ethanol and acetone; freely soluble in chloroform.

Partition Coefficient. Log *P* (octanol/water), 0.8.

Colour Tests. Liebermann's Test—brown; Mandelin's Test—green-brown; Marquis Test—red; Nessler's Reagent—brown-orange (weak).

Thin-layer Chromatography. System TA—Rf 64; system TB—Rf 03; system TC—Rf 59; system TE—Rf 76; system TL—Rf 55; system TAE—Rf 87. (Acidified iodoplatinate solution, positive.)

Gas Chromatography. System GA—etenzamide RI 1560, M (desethyl)/ salicylamide RI 1414, M (desethyl-)-AC RI 1660.

High Performance Liquid Chromatography. System HD—*k* 0.55; system HW—*k* 4.6; system HY—RI 303.

Ultraviolet Spectrum. Aqueous acid—234 nm (A_1^1=540c), 293 nm.

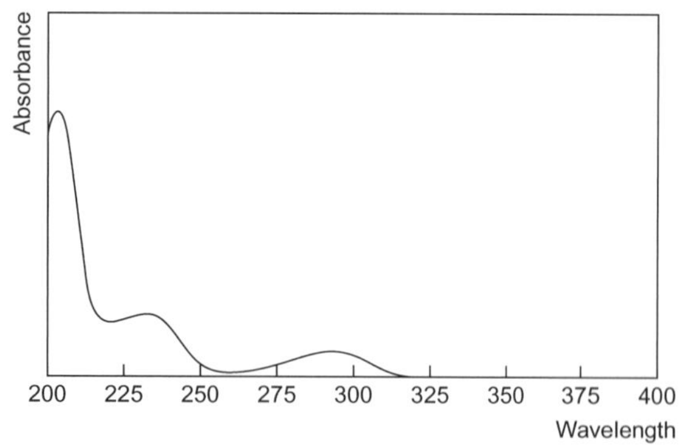

Infra-red Spectrum. Principal peaks at wavenumbers 1634, 1233, 753, 1276, 1114, 1587 cm^{-1} (KBr disk).

Mass Spectrum. Principal ions at *m/z* 120, 92, 105, 148, 150, 121, 133, 65.

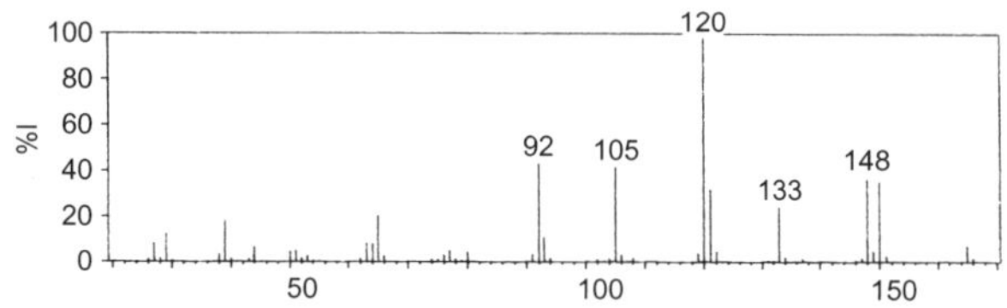

Dose. Etenzamide has been given in doses of up to 4 g daily in divided doses.

Ethacridine

Disinfectant

7-Ethoxy-3,9-acridinediamine
$C_{15}H_{15}N_3O=253.3$
CAS—442-16-0

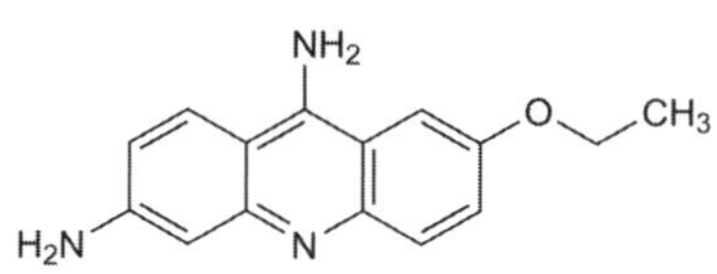

Orange crystals. M.p. 226°.

Ethacridine Lactate

Synonyms. Acrinol; Acrinol Lactate; Aethacridinium Lacticum; Ethacrindini Lactas; Lactoacridine.
Proprietary names. Metifex; Rivanol; Urocridin; Uroseptol; Vucine.
$C_{15}H_{15}N_3O,C_3H_6O_3=343.4$
CAS—1837-57-6
A yellow crystalline powder. It forms yellow fluorescent solutions. M.p. about 245°, with decomposition.
Slowly soluble 1 in 15 of water, 1 in 9 of boiling water and 1 in about 150 of ethanol.

Partition Coefficient. Log *P* (octanol/water), 2.1.

Colour Test. Marquis Test—orange→red.

Thin-layer Chromatography. System TA—Rf 60; system TAE—Rf 07. (Van Urk reagent, yellow.)

Ultraviolet Spectrum. Aqueous acid—268 nm ($A^1_1=2062a$).

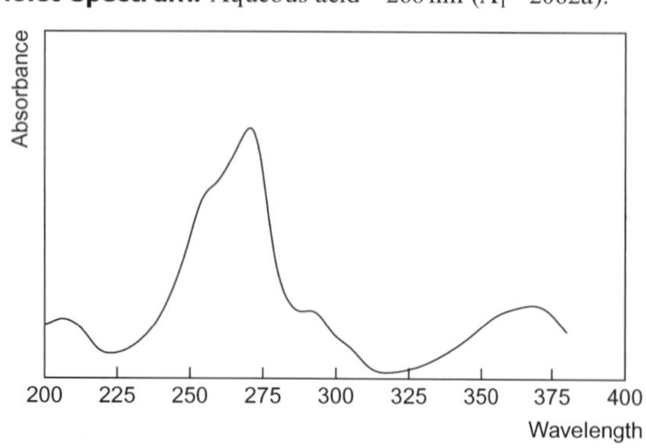

Infra-red Spectrum. Principal peaks at wavenumbers 1113, 1630, 1495, 1226, 1591, 1034 cm^{-1} (KBr disk).

Dose. Ethacridine lactate has been given, by mouth, in doses of 200 to 600 mg daily.

Ethambutol

Antituberculous Agent

Synonym. EMB
2,2′-(1,2-Ethanediyldiimino)bis-1-butanol
$C_{10}H_{24}N_2O_2=204.3$
CAS—74-55-5

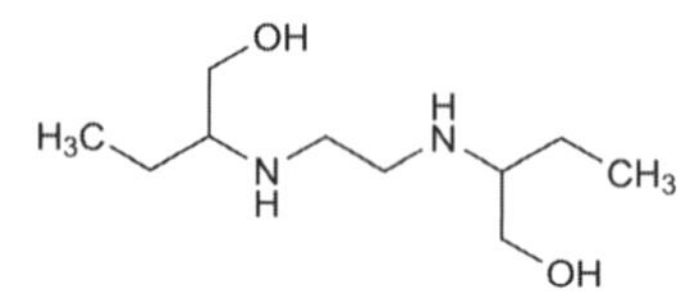

M.p. 87.5° to 88.8°.
Sparingly soluble in water; soluble in chloroform and methylene chloride.

Ethambutol Hydrochloride

Proprietary names. Dexambutol; EMB; Etapiam; Etibi; Lambutol; Miambutol; Myambutol; Mycrol; Myrin; Oributol; Servabutol; Tambutec; Tobutol; Tubetam; Turresis. It is an ingredient of Mynah.
$C_{10}H_{24}N_2O_2,2HCl=277.2$
CAS—1070-11-7
A white, crystalline, hygroscopic powder. M.p. 198.5° to 200.3° also reported as 201.8° to 202.6°.
Soluble 1 in 1 of water, 1 in 4 of ethanol, 1 in 850 of chloroform and 1 in 9 of methanol; very slightly soluble in ether.

Dissociation Constant. pK_a 6.3, 9.5 (20°).

Partition Coefficient. Log *P* (octanol/water), −0.4.

Thin-layer Chromatography. System TA—Rf 30; system TB—Rf 03; system TC—Rf 02; system TE—Rf 76; system TL—Rf 02; system TAD—Rf 00; system TAE—Rf 12; system TAJ—Rf 00; system TAK—Rf 00; system TAL—Rf 20. (Acidified potassium permanganate solution, positive.)

Ultraviolet Spectrum. No significant absorption, 230 to 360 nm.

Infra-red Spectrum. Principal peaks at wavenumbers 1090, 1061, 1142, 987, 1050, 1009 cm^{-1} (KBr disk).

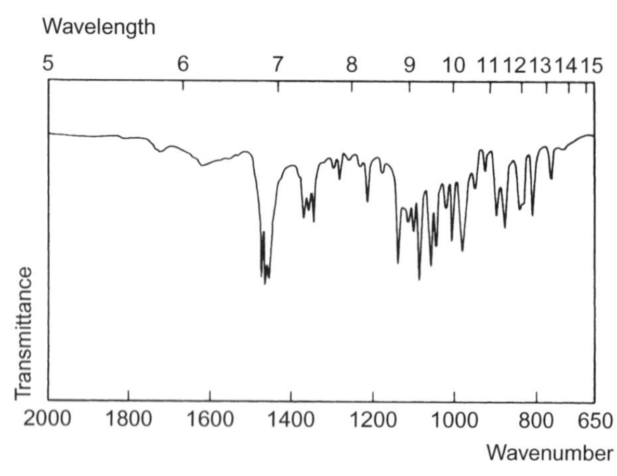

Mass Spectrum. Principal ions at *m/z* 102, 30, 72, 44, 116, 55, 173, 71.

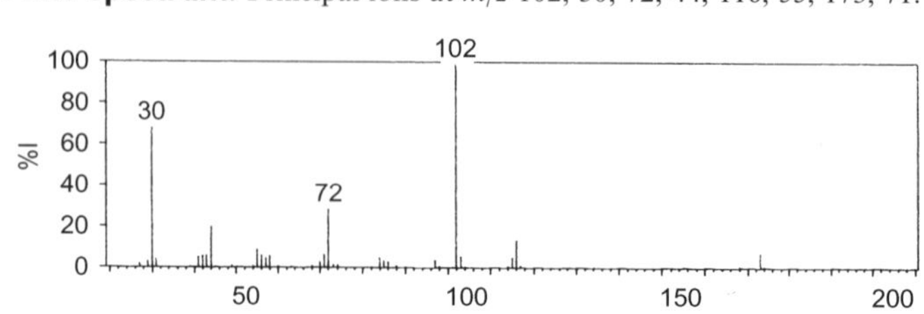

Quantification

Gas chromatography. In plasma: limit of detection 10 µg/L, ECD—C. S. Lee and L. H. Wang, *J. Pharm. Sci.*, 1980, *69*, 362–363.

Gas chromatography–mass spectrometry. In plasma: limit of detection 36 µg/L—M. R. Holdiness *et al.*, *J. Chromatogr.*, 1981, *224*, 415–422.

High performance liquid chromatography. In plasma or urine: limits of detection <10 µg/L and <10 mg/L respectively, fluorescence detection—M. Breda *et al.*, *J. Chromatogr. A.*, 1996, *729*, 301–307. In plasma: limit of detection <0.2 mg/L, UV detection—P. Chenevier *et al.*, *J. Chromatogr. B. Biomed. Sci. Appl.*, 1998, *708*, 310–315.

High performance liquid chromatography–mass spectrometry. In plasma, bronchoalveolar lavage fluid, or alveolar cells: limits of detection 0.05 mg/L in plasma and 0.005 mg/L in bronchoalveolar lavage and alveolar cells—J. E. Conte *et al.*, *J. Chromatogr. Sci.*, 2002, *40*, 113–118.

Disposition in the Body. Readily absorbed after oral administration. About 50 to 70% of a dose is excreted in the urine as unchanged drug in 24 h, and up to 15% may be excreted as inactive aldehyde and carboxylic acid metabolites; up to 20% of an oral dose may be eliminated in the faeces.

Therapeutic concentration. In plasma, usually in the range 2.5 to 6.5 mg/L.

After a single oral dose of 15 mg/kg to 6 subjects, peak plasma concentrations of 3.2 to 5.6 mg/L (mean 4) were attained in 2 to 4 h [C. S. Lee *et al.*, *Clin. Pharmacol. Ther.*, 1977, *22*, 615–621].

Toxicity. Toxic effects are usually associated with plasma concentrations greater than 6 mg/L.

In a fatality caused by the ingestion of ethambutol and rifampicin, the following postmortem concentrations were reported for ethambutol and rifampicin, respectively: blood 84 and 182 mg/L, urine 6800 and 3300 mg/L; low concentrations of ethanol were also detected [D. B. Jack *et al.*, *Lancet*, 1978, *2*, 1107–1108].

Half-life. Plasma half-life, about 10 to 15 h.

Clearance. Plasma clearance, about 9 mL/min/kg.

Distribution in blood. Plasma:whole blood ratio, 0.6 to 0.9.

Protein binding. In plasma, about 10 to 40% (concentration-dependent).

Dose. 15 to 25 mg/kg of ethambutol hydrochloride daily; 50 mg/kg has been given twice weekly.

Ethanol

Central Depressant

Synonyms. Alcohol; Ethyl Alcohol.
$CH_3{\cdot}CH_2OH = 46.07$
CAS—64-17-5

Ethanol of the *British Pharmacopoeia* is Dehydrated Alcohol (Absolute Alcohol) which contains 99.4 to 100% of C_2H_6O, sp.gr. 0.7904 to 0.7935 (20°/20°). Ethanol (96%) of the *B.P.* contains 96.0 to 96.6% of C_2H_6O, sp.gr. 0.8062 to 0.8087 (20°/20°). Rectified Spirit is ethanol (90%). In the *United States Pharmacopeia*, Alcohol contains 94.9 to 96.0% of C_2H_6O, sp.gr. 0.812 to 0.816 (15.56°).

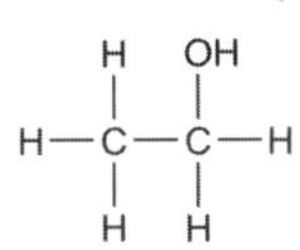

A clear, colourless, mobile, volatile, readily flammable, hygroscopic liquid. Ethanol (96%) boils at about 78°.
Miscible with water, chloroform and ether.

Industrial Methylated Spirit

Synonym. IMS
A mixture of ethanol, of an appropriate strength, 95 parts by volume with wood naphtha 5 parts by volume.
Note. Two other classes of methylated spirits are recognised in the United Kingdom: mineralised methylated spirits and denatured ethanol. Mineralised methylated spirits is ethanol of an appropriate strength, 90 parts by volume mixed with wood naphtha 9.5 parts by volume and crude pyridine 0.5 parts by volume, and to every 2000 L of this mixture is added 7.5 L of mineral naphtha (petroleum oil) and 3.0 g of methyl violet. Denatured ethanol is ethanol, of a strength not less than 85%, 98 parts by volume mixed with propanol 2 parts by volume, and to the resulting mixture is added denatonium benzoate 10 mg/L, or solid quassin 120 mg/L, or sucrose octa-acetate 4000 mg/L.
Surgical Spirit (*B.P.*) is a mixture of castor oil 2.5 mL, diethyl phthalate 2 mL and methyl salicylate 0.5 mL, diluted to 100 mL with industrial methylated spirit.
Rubbing Alcohol (*U.S.P.*) is a mixture of acetone 8 volumes, methyl isobutyl ketone 1.5 volumes and Alcohol 100 volumes; the mixture contains not less than 3550 µg/L of sucrose octa-acetate or 14 mg/L of denatonium benzoate.

Dissociation Constant. pK_a, 15.9 (25°).

Partition Coefficient. Log *P* (octanol/water), −0.3.

Colour Test. Potassium Dichromate (Method 2)—green.

Gas Chromatography. System GA—RI 421; system GI—Retention time 1.9 min.

Mass Spectrum. Principal ions at *m/z* 31, 45, 29, 27, 46, 43, 30, 42.

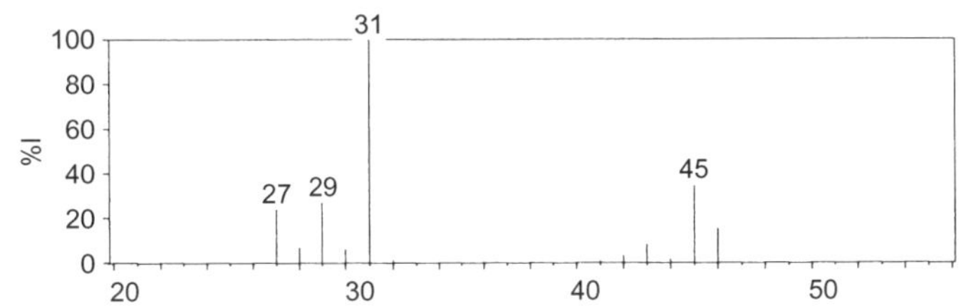

Quantification

Alcohol dehydrogenase method. In blood: limit of detection 500 mg/L—A. Poklis and M. A. Mackell, *Clin. Chem.*, 1982, *28*, 2125–2127.

Gas chromatography. In blood or urine: direct injection, FID—B. R. Manno and J. E. Manno, *J. Anal. Toxicol.*, 1978, *2*, 257–261. In biological materials: head-space analysis, limit of detection ethanol 125 µg, acetaldehyde 1 µg, FID—C. L. Mendenhall *et al.*, *J. Chromatogr.*, 1980, *190*, 197–200. In breath: ethanol and other volatile substances, ion-trap detection—Y. Ghoos *et al.*, *Biomed. Environ. Mass Spectrom.*, 1989, *18*, 613–616. In blood: blood gas sampler—K. Goto and S. Ikemoto, *Nippon Hoigaku Zasshi*, 1991, *45*, 393–399. In blood: ethanol and acetaldehyde, head-space analysis, FID—D. G. McCarver-May and L Durisin, *J. Anal. Toxicol.*, 1997, *21*, 134–141. In blood, serum, urine or faecal supernatants: limit of detection 0.1 mg/L—A. Tangerman, *Clin. Chem.*, 1997, *43*, 1003–1009. In blood or urine: ethanol, acetaldehyde and acetate, head-space analysis—S. Tsukamoto *et al.*, *Nihon Arukoru Yakubutsu Igakkai Zasshi*, 1998, *33*, 200–209. In blood: ethanol and other volatile compounds, head-space analysis, FID—D. Zuba *et al.*, *J. Chromatogr. B. Anal. Technol. Biomed. Life Sci.*, 2002, *773*, 75–82.

Gas chromatography–mass spectrometry. In plasma: limit of detection 5 ng—W. E. Pereira *et al.*, *Clin. Chim. Acta*, 1974, *51*, 109–112.

High performance liquid chromatography. In blood or serum: UV detection—S. Pellegrino *et al.*, *J. Chromatogr. B. Biomed. Sci. Appl.*, 1999, *729*, 103–110.

Reviews. In breath—M. F. Mason and K. M. Dubowski, *J. Forensic Sci.*, 1976, *21*, 9–41. In blood—R. H. Cravey and N. C. Jain, *J. Chromatogr. Sci.*, 1974, *12*, 209–213 and P. Fabiani, *Pharm. Biol.*, 1979, *13*, 39–40.

Disposition in the Body. Readily absorbed from the stomach and small intestine after oral administration but absorption may be delayed by the presence of food; rapidly distributed throughout the body fluids. Metabolised in the liver by alcohol dehydrogenase to acetaldehyde and then further oxidised to acetate and carbon dioxide. More than 90% is metabolised and is excreted by the lungs and in the urine, saliva, sweat and other secretions together with unchanged alcohol. The body can metabolise about 10 to 15 mL per hour. The rate of metabolism may be accelerated following repeated excessive use.

Blood concentration

After administration of 15, 30, 45 and 60 mL of 95% ethanol to 8 fasting subjects, peak blood concentrations of 25 to 290 mg/L (mean 199), 180 to 620 mg/L (mean 440), 410 to 860 mg/L (mean 680) and 630 to 1120 mg/L (mean 860), respectively, were attained in 0.3, 0.5, 0.8 and 1 h [P. K. Wilkinson *et al.*, *J. Pharmacokinet. Biopharm.*, 1977, *5*, 207–224].

After administration of 0.5 g/kg of ethanol to 4 subjects, blood-acetaldehyde concentrations of 20 to 60 mg/L were reported after 40 to 80 min [J. M. Christensen *et al.*, *Clin. Chim. Acta*, 1981, *116*, 389–395].

Toxicity. The minimum lethal dose is about 500 mL of 50% spirit ingested in about 1 h. In the UK it is illegal to be in charge of a motor vehicle with a concentration greater than 800 mg/L in the blood or 1070 mg/L in the urine or 0.35 mg/L in the breath. Toxic effects are associated with blood concentrations of 840 to **2400** to 4500 mg/L, and subjects with concentrations of 3000 mg/L or more are considered to be clinically drunk. Blood concentrations of 2250 to **4000** to 6030 mg/L have been associated with fatalities. The maximum permissible atmospheric concentration is 1000 ppm.

In 10 fatalities caused by the ingestion of ethanol, the following postmortem tissue concentrations were reported: blood 4230 to 17 660 mg/L (mean 7410), bile 1250 to 27 950 mg/L (mean 7860), brain 3100 to 9120 µg/g (mean 4430), kidney 2850 to 10 430 µg/g (mean 4830), liver 2450 to 11 610 µg/g (mean 4470), urine 4850 to 9400 mg/L (mean 6190) [G. Christopoulos *et al.*, *J. Chromatogr.*, 1973, *87*, 455–472].

An unusual distribution of ethanol in a dead 48-year-old man with a history of alcoholism was: femoral blood (2 samples) 2.57 and 2.73 g/L, heart blood 6.43 g/L, vitreous humour 7.63 g/L, urine 840 µg/g, bile 6.16 g/L, liver 2.50 mg/g, gastric contents 2.47 g/53 g. It was proposed that agonal or postmortem aspiration of ethanol-rich vomitus and postmortem fermentation could account for the elevated concentrations in heart blood and bile; high vitreous ethanol could have resulted from diffusion in the agonal phase or postmortem. [P. P. Singer and G. R. Jones, *J. Anal. Toxicol.*, 1997, *21*, 506–508].

Analysis of the blood of 169 acutely poisoned alcoholics on hospital admission showed the mean blood ethanol concentrations to be 3.14 g/L (range 0.76 to 6.6) [D. Zuba *et al.*, *Alcohol*, 2002, *26*, 17–22].

Half-life. Plasma half-life, dose-dependent.

Volume of distribution. About 0.6 L/kg.

Distribution in blood. Plasma:whole blood ratio, 1.2.

Saliva. Plasma:saliva ratio, about 0.93.

Protein binding. In plasma, not significantly bound.

Note. For a review of the clinical pharmacokinetics of ethanol see N. H. Holford, *Clin. Pharmacokinet.*, 1987, *13*, 273–292.

Ethchlorvynol

Hypnotic

Synonyms. *β*-Chlorovinyl Ethyl Ethynyl Carbinol; *E*-Ethchlorvynol.
Proprietary name. Placidyl
1-Chloro-3-ethyl-1-penten-4-yl-3-ol
$C_7H_9ClO = 144.6$
CAS—113-18-8

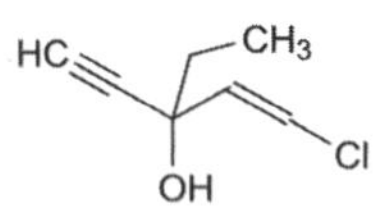

A colourless to yellow, slightly viscous liquid which darkens on exposure to air and light. Mass per mL about 1.072 g. Refractive index, at 20°, 1.4770 to 1.4805.
Practically immiscible with water; miscible with ethanol, chloroform, ether, and most other organic solvents.

Partition Coefficient. Log *P* (octanol/water), 1.6.

Colour Test. Ammoniacal Silver Nitrate—white precipitate/yellow.

Thin-layer Chromatography. System TB—Rf 00; system TD—Rf 81; system TF—Rf 74; system TAD—Rf 82; system TAE—Rf 87; system TAJ—Rf 73; system TAK—Rf 77; system TAL—Rf 96.

Gas Chromatography. System GA—RI 1015; system GB—RI 1060; system GI—retention time 35.2 min.

Infra-red Spectrum. Principal peaks at wavenumbers 935, 950, 830, 1010, 1063, 980 cm^{-1}.

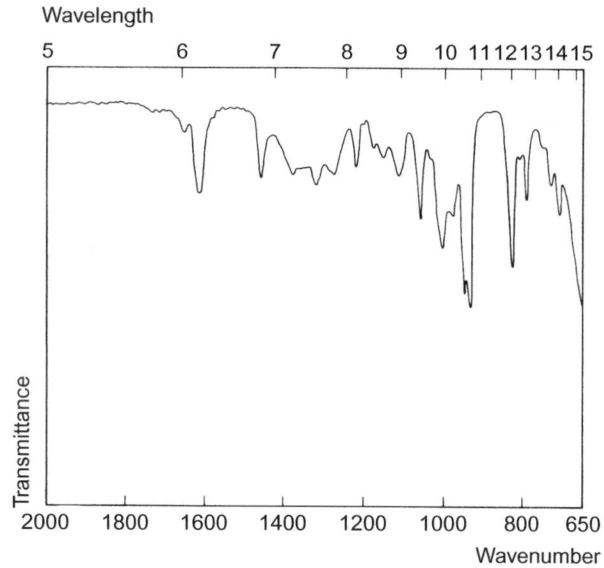

Mass Spectrum. Principal ions at *m/z* 115, 117, 89, 53, 109, 51, 91, 39.

Quantification

Ultraviolet spectrophotometry. In blood, serum, or urine—J. E. Wallace *et al.*, *Clin. Chem.*, 1974, *20*, 159–162.

Gas chromatography. In blood or urine: limit of detection 1 mg/L, FID—H. H. McCurdy, *J. Anal. Toxicol.*, 1977, *1*, 164–165. In plasma or urine: limit of detection 2 mg/L, FID—R. J. Flanagan and T. D. Lee, *J. Chromatogr.*, 1977, *137*, 119–126.

Review. For an evaluation of gas chromatographic and colorimetric methods, see R. R. Bridges and T. A. Jennison, *J. Anal. Toxicol.*, 1984, *8*, 263–268.

Disposition in the Body. Rapidly absorbed after oral administration. It is extensively metabolised; the major metabolite found in the blood and urine of poisoned patients is 1-chloro-3-ethynylpent-1-ene-3,4-diol; other metabolites include 1-chloro-3-ethynylpent-1-ene-3,5-diol and 1-chloro-3-ethylpent-1-ene-3,4-diol. Ethchlorvynol is highly localised in the tissues, particularly in adipose tissue, and is released very slowly. Less than 0.1% of a dose is excreted in the urine in 24 h as unchanged drug or its glucuronide conjugate. Ethchlorvynol crosses the placenta.

Therapeutic concentration. In plasma, usually in the range 5 to 20 mg/L.

Following a single oral dose of 500 mg to 8 subjects, a mean peak plasma concentration of 6.5 mg/L was attained in 1 h. [L. M. Cummins *et al.*, *J. Pharm. Sci.*, 1971, *60*, 261–263.]

Toxicity. The estimated minimum lethal dose is 15 g, although death has occurred after the acute ingestion of 2.5 g. Plasma concentrations greater than about 20 mg/L are associated with toxic effects. Prolonged use of ethchlorvynol may lead to dependence of the barbiturate–alcohol type.

In a review of 13 fatalities due to overdosage with ethchlorvynol, postmortem blood concentrations were in the range 14 to 400 mg/L (mean 119) [C. J. Rehling, Poison residues in human tissues, in *Progress in chemical toxicology*, Vol. 3, A. Stolman (Ed.), New York, Academic Press, 1967, pp. 363–386.]

In 3 fatalities due to ethchlorvynol, the following postmortem tissue concentrations were reported: blood 85, 22 and 66 mg/L; brain 57, –, 285 µg/g; kidney 54, 63, and 860 µg/g; liver 70, 60, and 507 µg/g; adipose tissue 1040 and 142 µg/g (2 cases). [R. H. Cravey and R. C. Baselt, *J. Forensic Sci.*, 1968, *13*, 532–536 and C. L. Winek, *Forensic Sci. Int.*, 1981, *17*, 219–224.]

Toxicological analysis of body fluids and tissues of a 54-year-old female fatality who had already been embalmed revealed an ethchlorvynol concentration of 112 mg/L in the bile; phenobarbital (32.8 mg/L) was also found in the bloody fluid from the heart. [C. L. Winek *et al.*, *Forensic Sci. Int.*, 1988, *37*, 161–166.]

In 2 fatalities involving ethchlorvynol overdose, the following postmortem tissue concentrations were reported: blood 198.2 and 29.0 mg/L, urine 261.8 and 10.6 mg/L, bile 361.8 and 22.7 mg/L, eye fluid 10.0 and not reported, liver 620.0 and 21.3 µg/g, kidney not reported and 17.3 µg/g, stomach contents (total) 130 g and 533 mg. In case 1 ethanol, diazepam, and nordazepam were also detected; in case 2 diazepam, nordazepam, and hydrocodone were also present. [C. L. Winek *et al.*, *J. Forensic Sci.*, 1989, *34*, 687–690.]

Half-life. Distribution half-life, about 1 to 3 h and elimination half-life of 10 to 20 h, increased in overdose cases.

Volume of distribution. About 2 to 3 L/kg.

Distribution in blood. Plasma:whole blood ratio, about 1.1.

Protein binding. In plasma, about 60%.

Dose. 0.2 to 1 g, as a hypnotic.

Ether

General Anaesthetic

Synonyms. Diethyl Oxide; Ethyl Ether; Ethyl Oxide.
1,1′-Oxybisethane
$(C_2H_5)_2O$ = 74.12
CAS—60-29-7

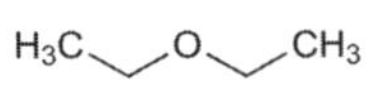

A clear, colourless, volatile, flammable, very mobile liquid. B.p. 34° to 36°. Soluble 1 in 10 to 1 in 12 of water; miscible with ethanol, chloroform, benzene and petroleum ether.
Anaesthetic Ether (*B.P.*) is highly purified ether containing not more than 0.002% of a stabiliser such as propyl gallate or hydroquinone.
Solvent Ether (*B.P.*) is not so highly purified and is without a stabiliser.
Caution. Ether is very volatile and flammable, and mixtures of its vapour with oxygen, nitrous oxide or air at certain concentrations are explosive. It should not be used in the presence of an open flame or any electrical apparatus liable to produce a spark; precautions should be taken against the production of static electrical discharge. Explosive peroxides are generated by the atmospheric oxidation of solvent ether and it is dangerous to distil a sample which contains peroxides.

Dissociation Constant. pK_a, −3.6.

Partition Coefficient. Log *P* (octanol/water), 0.9.

Gas Chromatography. System GA—RI 515; system GI—Retention time 5.9 min.

Mass Spectrum. Principal ions at *m/z* 31, 59, 29, 45, 74, 27, 41, 43.

Disposition in the Body. Absorbed into the circulation after inhalation; the blood:gas partition coefficient is high (about 12). About 90% of a dose is slowly exhaled unchanged and very little is metabolised; a small amount may be excreted unchanged in the urine. Acetaldehyde is believed to be a minor metabolite.

Therapeutic concentration. In plasma, during anaesthesia, usually in the range 500 to 1500 mg/L.

Toxicity. The estimated minimum lethal oral dose is 30 mL; the maximum permissible atmospheric concentration is 400 ppm. Atmospheric concentrations of 2000 ppm may cause dizziness and 100 000 ppm may be rapidly fatal.

In 4 elderly persons who died after being given ether with other medication, ether concentrations (mg/L or µg/g) immediately after operation were: blood 600, 3750, 2880, 190; brain 700, 610, 2720, 310; liver 400, 1280, 260, 230; lung 200, 1580, 210, –; in the second case the urine contained 340 mg/L [J. E. Campbell, *J. Forensic Sci.*, 1960, *5*, 501–549].

A 24-year-old man became severely comatose after attempting suicide by injecting 5 mL ether into his left cubital vein. Ether was identified by gas chromatography [N. Serrano *et al.*, *Intensive Care Med.*, 1999, *25*, 337–338].

Dose. For induction of anaesthesia, 10 to 20% of the vapour by inhalation; maintenance, 3 to 10%.

Ethiazide

Diuretic

6-Chloro-3-ethyl-3,4-dihydro-2*H*-1,2,4-benzothiadiazine-7-sulfonamide-1,1-dioxide
$C_9H_{12}ClN_3O_4S_2$ = 325.8
CAS—1824-58-4

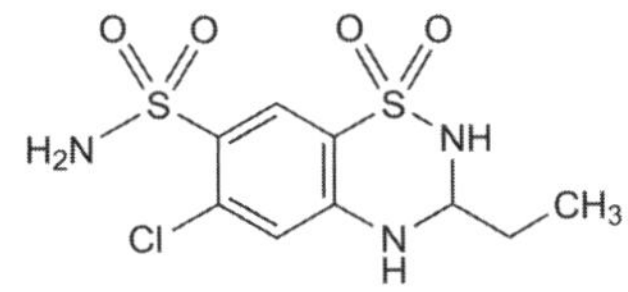

Crystals. M.p. 269° to 270°.

Partition Coefficient. Log *P* (octanol/water), 0.3.

Thin-layer Chromatography. System TD—Rf 11; system TE—Rf 50; system TF—Rf 50; system TL—Rf 22.

Ultraviolet Spectrum. Aqueous acid—272 nm (A^1_1 = 345b).

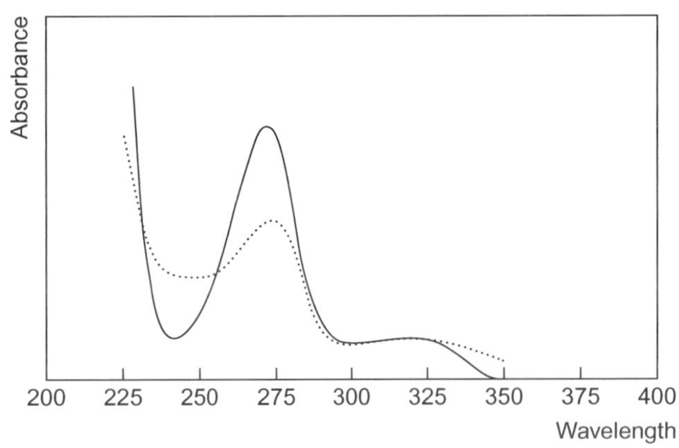

Infra-red Spectrum. Principal peaks at wavenumbers 1163, 1172, 1603, 1312, 781, 1510 cm^{-1} (Nujol mull).

Mass Spectrum. Principal ions at *m/z* 296, 298, 205, 221, 64, 63, 41, 125.

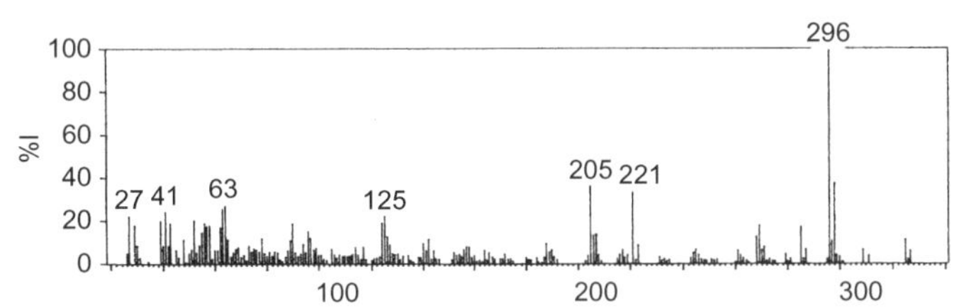

Dose. Usually 5 to 10 mg daily.

Ethinamate

Hypnotic

Proprietary names. Valamin; Valmid; Valmidate.
1-Ethynylcyclohexanol carbamate
$C_9H_{13}NO_2$ = 167.2
CAS—126-52-3

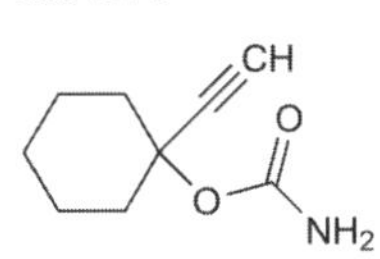

A white powder. M.p. 96° to 98°.
Soluble 1 in 400 of water and 1 in about 3 of ethanol; freely soluble in chloroform and ether.

Partition Coefficient. Log *P* (octanol/water), 1.9.

Colour Test. Ammoniacal Silver Nitrate—yellow/brown.

Thin-layer Chromatography System TA—Rf 76; system TB—Rf 05; system TD—Rf 49; system TE—Rf 76; system TF—Rf 59; system TAD—Rf 58; system TAE—Rf 86; system TAF—Rf 87; system TAJ—Rf 58; system TAK—Rf 69; system TAL—Rf 91. (Furfuraldehyde reagent, positive; acidified potassium permanganate solution, positive.)

Gas Chromatography. System GA—RI 1365.

Ultraviolet Spectrum. No significant absorption, 230 to 360 nm.

Infra-red Spectrum. Principal peaks at wavenumbers 1713, 1041, 1694, 1030, 1052, 1250 cm^{-1} (KBr disk).

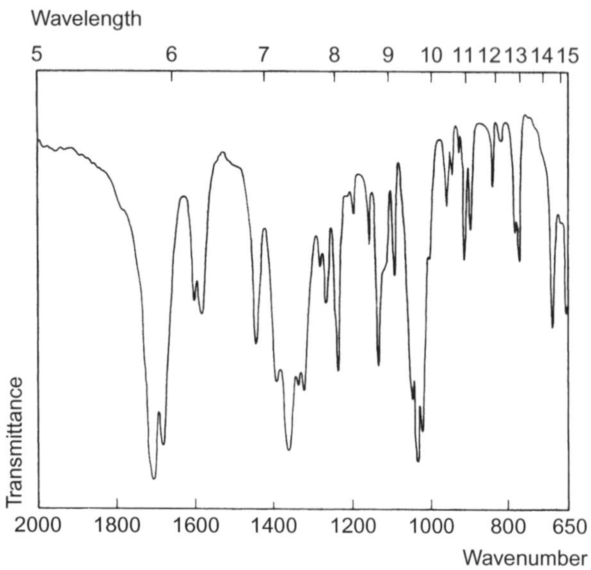

Mass Spectrum. Principal ions at *m/z* 91, 81, 106, 78, 39, 95, 68, 43.

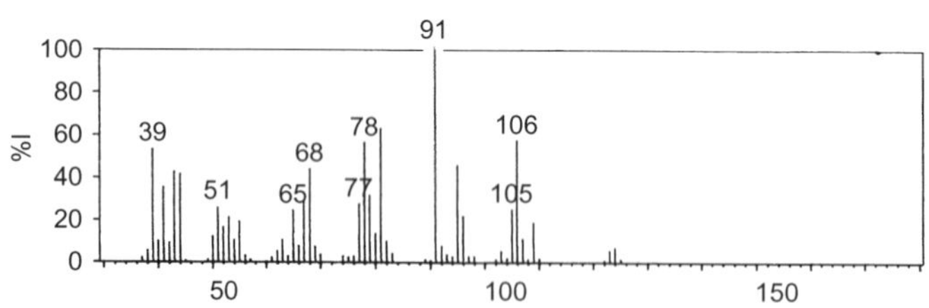

Quantification

Gas chromatography. In plasma or urine: ethinamate and *trans*-4-hydroxyethinamate, limit of detection 500 μg/L for ethinamate in plasma, FID—J. W. Kleber *et al.*, *J. Pharm. Sci.*, 1977, *66*, 992–994.

Disposition in the Body. Rapidly absorbed after oral administration. Metabolised by hydroxylation to 4-hydroxyethinamate, which exists as stereoisomers, and conjugated with glucuronic acid. About 40% of a dose is excreted in the urine in 24 h as *trans*-4-hydroxyethinamate or its glucuronide conjugate; only a small amount is excreted unchanged in the urine; 3- and 2-hydroxyethinamate have also been detected in urine.

Therapeutic concentration. In plasma, usually in the range 5 to 10 mg/L.

After a single oral dose of 1 g to 8 subjects, peak blood concentrations of 3.8 to 11.7 mg/L (mean 6.5) were attained in 1 to 2 h. [J. M. Clifford *et al.*, *Clin. Pharmacol. Ther.*, 1974, *16*, 376–389.]

Toxicity. The estimated minimum lethal dose is 15 g but recovery has occurred after ingestion of as much as 28 g. Prolonged use of ethinamate may lead to dependence of the barbiturate–alcohol type. Blood concentrations greater than 100 mg/L have been associated with fatalities.

Half-life. Plasma half-life, about 2 h.

Dose. 0.5 to 1 g, as a hypnotic.

Ethinylestradiol

Estrogen

Synonyms. Ethinyl Estradiol; Ethinyloestradiol; Etinilestradiol.
Proprietary names. Estigyn; Estinyl; Etifollin; Farmacyrol; Feminone; Gynolett; Lynoral; Primogyn C; Progynon C; Turisteron.
Ethinylestradiol is an ingredient of many oral contraceptives—see *Martindale, The Complete Drug Reference*, 33rd Edn., Pharmaceutical Press, London, 2002.
(17α)-19-Norpregna-1,3,5(10)-trien-20-yne-3,17-diol
$C_{20}H_{24}O_2$=296.4
CAS—57-63-6

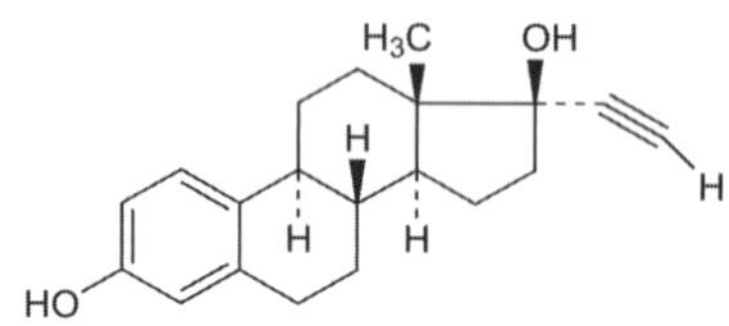

A fine, white to slightly yellowish-white, crystalline powder. There are two forms, one melts at 141° to 146° and the other at 182° to 184°.
Practically insoluble in water; soluble 1 in 5 of acetone, 1 in 4 of dioxane, 1 in 6 of ethanol, 1 in 20 of chloroform and 1 in 4 of ether.
Caution. Ethinylestradiol is a powerful estrogen. Contact with the skin or inhalation should be avoided.

Partition Coefficient. Log *P* (octanol/water), 3.7.

Colour Tests. Ammoniacal Silver Nitrate—white precipitate/yellow; Antimony Pentachloride—brown→black; Liebermann's Test—black; Naphthol–Sulfuric Acid—brown-red/pink; Sulfuric Acid—red-orange.

Thin-layer Chromatography. System TA—Rf 90; system TB—Rf 04; system TE—Rf 71; system TP—Rf 72; system TQ—Rf 30; system TR—Rf 40; system TS—Rf 40, streaking may occur; system TAE—Rf 86; system TAJ—Rf 55; system TAK—Rf 58; system TAL—Rf 91; system TAM—Rf 94.

Gas Chromatography. System GA—RI 2719.

High Performance Liquid Chromatography. System HX—RI 539.

Ultraviolet Spectrum. Ethanol—281 nm (A^1_1=70a).

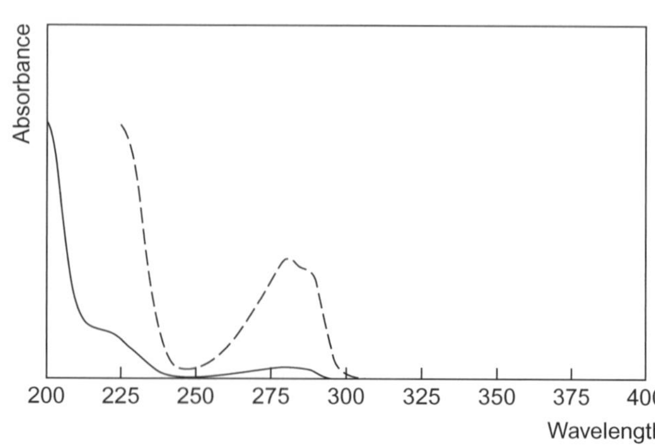

Infra-red Spectrum. Principal peaks at wavenumbers 1252, 1505, 1298, 1285, 1020, 1060 cm^{-1} (KBr disk).

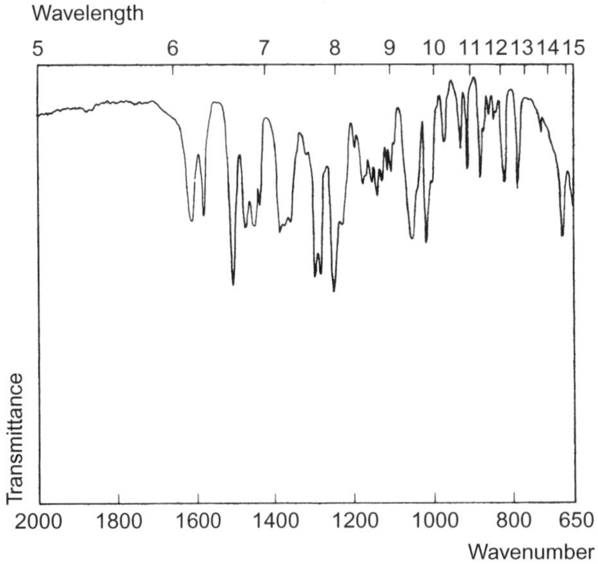

Mass Spectrum. Principal ions at *m/z* 213, 160, 159, 296, 133, 145, 212, 157.

Quantification

Radioimmunoassay. In serum: comparison with GC–MS—W. Kuhnz *et al.*, *Arzneimittelforschung*, 1993, *43*, 16–21. In plasma—A. L. Agasan *et al.*, *J. Immunol. Methods*, 1994, *177*, 251–260.

High performance liquid chromatography–radioimmunoassay. In plasma: limit of detection <2 ng/L—R. L. Tracey *et al.*, *J. Pharm. Biomed. Anal.*, 1994, *12*, 1303–1310.

Disposition in the Body

Therapeutic concentration. Application of a 20 cm^2 contraceptive patch, releasing ethinylestradiol 20 μg and norelgestromin 150 μg daily, to the abdomen, arm, buttock or torso of 37 subjects produced respective mean peak plasma ethinylestradiol concentrations of 58.7, 69.5, 66.3 and 71.2 ng/L at 48 h; corresponding peak plasma concentrations of norelgestromin (at 72 h) were 0.88, 1.18, 1.17 and 1.07 μg/L) [L. S. Abrams *et al.*, *Br. J. Clin. Pharmacol.*, 2002, *53*, 141–146].

Dose. 10 to 150 μg daily; up to 2 mg daily may be given.

Ethionamide

Antituberculous Agent

Synonym. Etionamida
Proprietary names. Ethatyl; Trescatyl.
2-Ethyl-4-pyridinecarbothioamide
$C_8H_{10}N_2S$ = 166.2
CAS—536-33-4

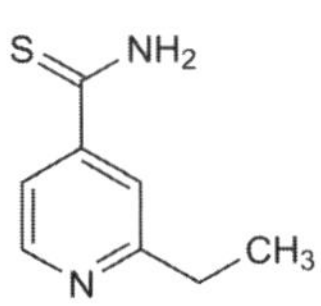

A bright yellow crystalline powder, darkening on exposure to light. M.p. 158° to 165°.

Very sparingly soluble in water; freely soluble in pyridine; soluble 1 in 30 of ethanol, 1 in 45 of acetone, 1 in 350 of chloroform and 1 in 600 of ether; sparingly soluble in methanol.

Partition Coefficient. Log *P* (octanol/water), 1.5.

Colour Tests. Nessler's Reagent—brown-orange; Palladium Chloride—brown

Thin-layer Chromatography. System TA—Rf 65; system TB—Rf 00; system TC—Rf 36; system TL—Rf 55. (Acidified iodoplatinate solution, positive.)

Gas Chromatography. System GA—RI 1756.

Ultraviolet Spectrum. Aqueous acid—230 nm (A^1_1 = 635a), 275 nm; aqueous alkali—277 nm.

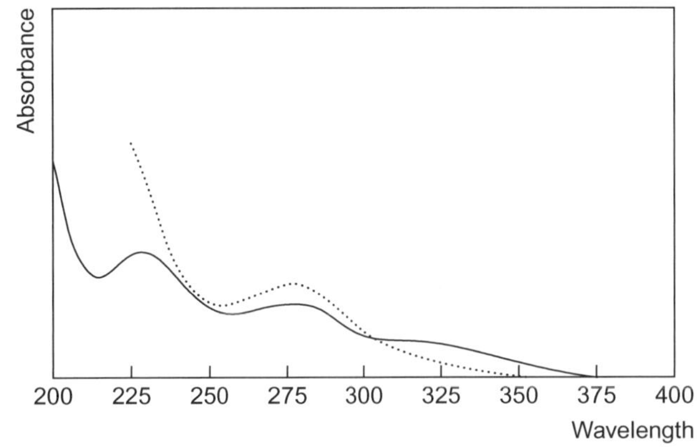

Infra-red Spectrum. Principal peaks at wavenumbers 1588, 808, 865, 1275, 1140, 880 cm^{-1} (KBr disk).

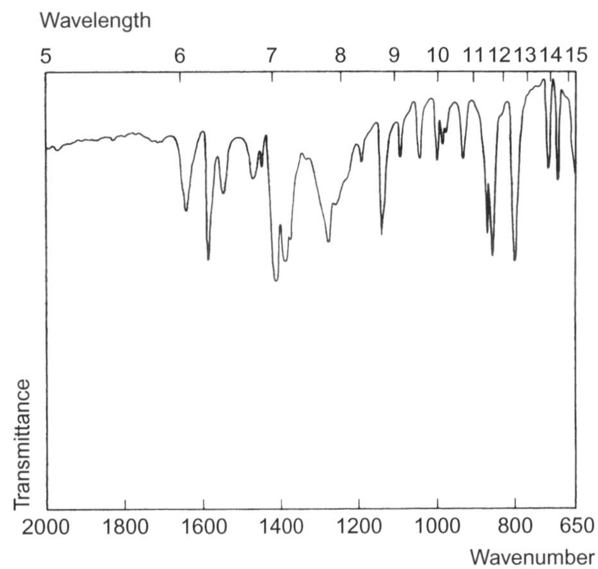

Mass Spectrum. Principal ions at *m/z* 166, 165, 167, 138, 133, 105, 60, 106.

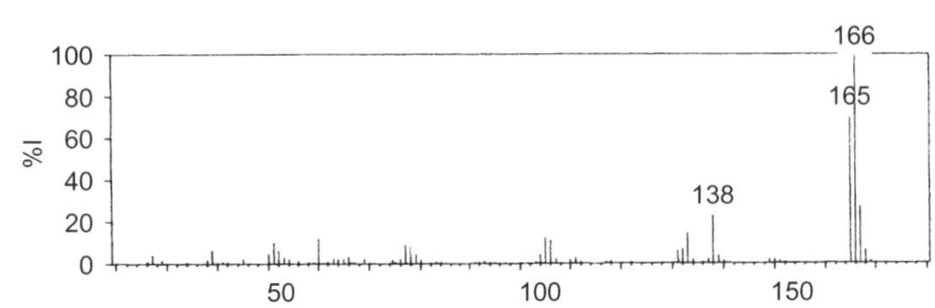

Quantification

High performance liquid chromatography. In plasma, serum or urine: limit of detection 10 μg/L, UV detection—P. J. Jenner and G. A. Ellard, *J. Chromatogr.*, 1981, *225*; *Biomed. Appl.*, *14*, 245–251. In serum—C. A. Peloquin *et al.*, *J. Chromatogr.*, 1991, *563*, 472–475. In serum: ethionamide and other antitubercular drugs, limit of detection <94 μg/L—M. C. Gennaro *et al.*, *J. Chromatogr. B. Biomed. Sci. Appl.*, 2001, *754*, 477–486.

High performance liquid chromatography–mass spectrometry. In plasma, bronchoalveolar lavage, or alveolar cells: limits of detection in plasma

0.05 mg/L and 0.005 mg/L in bronchoalveolar lavage and alveolar cells—J. E. Conte *et al.*, *J. Chromatogr. B. Biomed. Sci. Appl.*, 2001, *753*, 343–353.

Disposition in the Body. Readily absorbed after oral administration and widely distributed throughout the body. Peak plasma concentrations are attained 2 to 3 h after a dose. It is extensively metabolised and is excreted in the urine mainly as metabolites with little unchanged drug. The metabolites include ethionamide sulfoxide, 2-ethylisonicotinic acid and 2-ethylisonicotinamide.

Therapeutic concentration

Administration of a single oral 500 mg dose of ethionamide to 16 subjects resulted in a mean maximum plasma concentration of 2.3 mg/L (range 0.99 to 6.10) at 1.7 h (0.75 to 3.00) in the fasting state; this was not statistically changed when ethionamide was given with food, orange juice or antacids [B. Auclair *et al.*, *Antimicrob. Agents Chemother.*, 2001, *45*, 810–814].

Dose. 0.5 to 1 g daily.

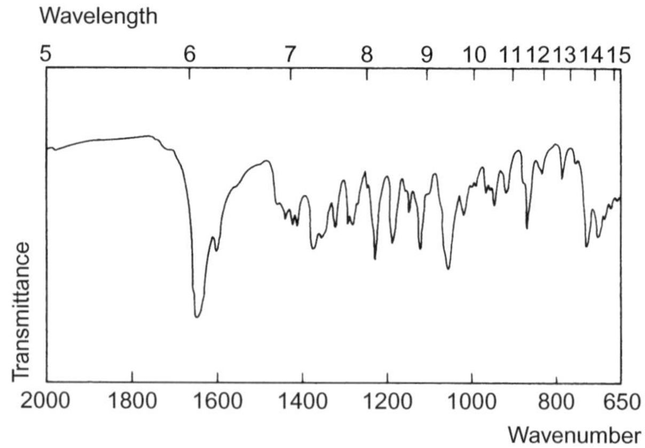

Mass Spectrum. Principal ions at *m/z* 122, 121, 91, 147, 161, 43, 107, 120.

Dose. 25 to 100 mg daily.

Ethisterone

Progestational Steroid

Synonyms. Aethisteron; Anhydrohydroxyprogesterone; Ethinyltestosterone; Praegnin; Pregneninolone; Pregnin.

Proprietary names. Etherone; Gestone-Oral; Lutocyclin; Lutocyclol; Ora-Lutin; Progesterol; Pranone; Syngestrotabs; Trosinone.

17α-Hydroxypregn-4-en-20-yn-3-one

$C_{21}H_{28}O_2$=312.4

CAS—434-03-7

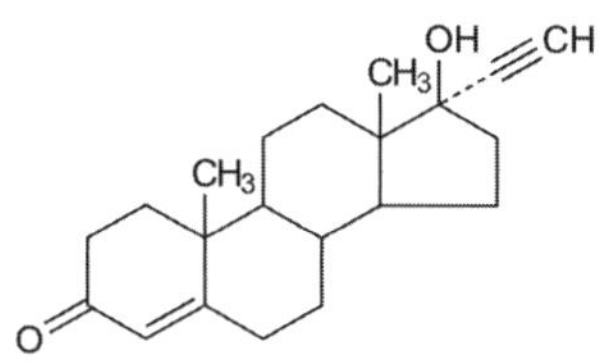

A white, slightly hygroscopic, crystalline powder. M.p. 272° to 276°.

Practically insoluble in water; soluble 1 in 1000 of ethanol, 1 in 750 of acetone, 1 in 110 of chloroform, 1 in 3000 of ether and 1 in 35 of pyridine.

Partition Coefficient. Log *P* (octanol/water), 3.1.

Thin-layer Chromatography. System TP—Rf 78; system TQ—Rf 39; system TR—Rf 80; system TS—Rf 00.

High Performance Liquid Chromatography. System HATb—RRT 0.84 (relative to testosterone).

Ultraviolet Spectrum. Dehydrated alcohol—240 nm (A^1_1=520a).

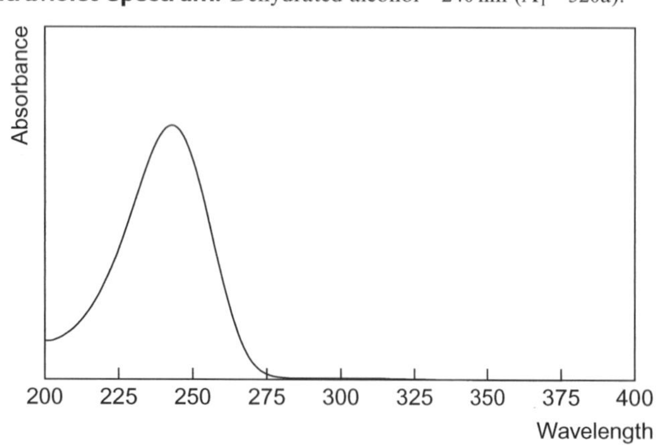

Infra-red Spectrum. Principal peaks at wavenumbers 1660, 1060, 1235, 1612, 1127, 723 cm^{-1} (KBr disk).

Ethoheptazine

Narcotic Analgesic

Synonym. Heptacyclazine

Ethylhexahydro-1-methyl-4-phenyl-1*H*-azepine-4-carboxylate

$C_{16}H_{23}NO_2$=261.4

CAS—77-15-6

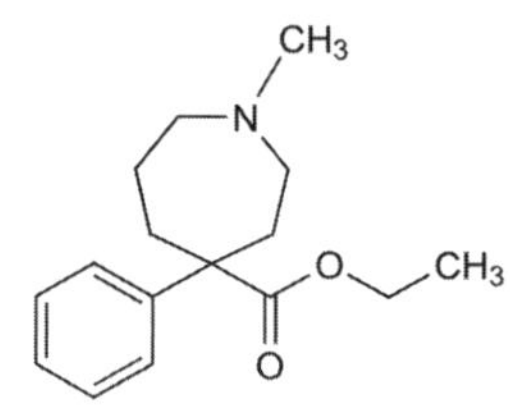

A liquid.

Ethoheptazine Citrate

Proprietary names. Zactane. It is an ingredient of Equagesic.

$C_{16}H_{23}NO_2,C_6H_8O_7$=453.5

CAS—6700-56-7

A white powder. M.p. about 140°.

Soluble in water and ethanol; practically insoluble in ether.

Dissociation Constant. pK_a 8.5.

Partition Coefficient. Log *P* (octanol/water), 3.5.

Colour Test. Marquis Test—orange

Thin-layer Chromatography. System TA—Rf 40; system TB—Rf 45; system TC—Rf 19; system TE—Rf 55; system TL—Rf 04; system TAE—Rf 12; system TAF—Rf 41; system TAJ—Rf 08; system TAK—Rf 12; system TAL—Rf 65. (Dragendorff spray, positive; acidified iodoplatinate solution, positive; Marquis reagent, orange; acidified potassium permanganate solution, positive.)

Gas Chromatography. System GA—RI 1857; system GB—RI 1923; system GC—RI 1630; system GF—RI 2110.

High Performance Liquid Chromatography. System HA—*k* 3.3; system HC—*k* 1.55; system HX—RI 359.

Ultraviolet Spectrum. Aqueous acid—251, 257 nm (A^1_1=8c), 263 nm. No alkaline shift.

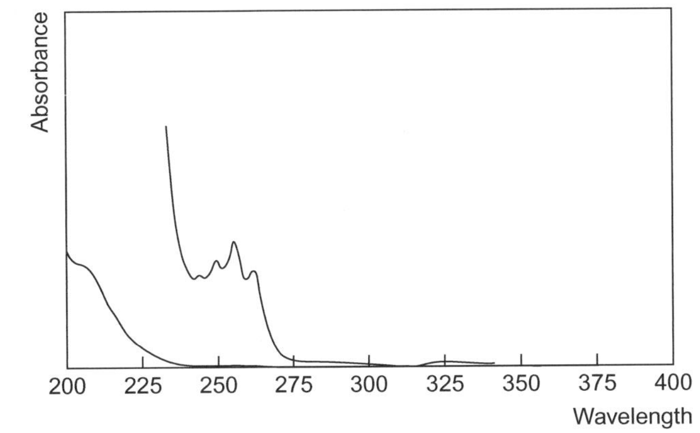

Infra-red Spectrum. Principal peaks at wavenumbers 1727, 1193, 1094, 695, 1248, 1030 cm^{-1} (KBr disk).

Mass Spectrum. Principal ions at *m/z* 57, 58, 70, 42, 44, 188, 84, 43.

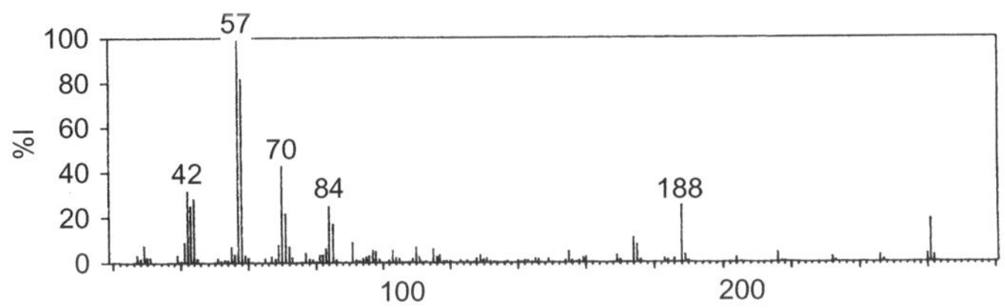

Quantification

Gas chromatography. In plasma or postmortem tissues: limit of detection 1 mg/L, AFID—R. H. Drost *et al.*, *J. Chromatogr.*, 1983, *277*; *Biomed. Appl.*, *28*, 352–355.

Disposition in the Body. Readily absorbed after oral administration; peak blood concentrations are attained within 1 h of a dose. It is extensively metabolised and is excreted in the urine.

Toxicity. The estimated minimum lethal dose is 1 g.

In a fatality caused by the ingestion of an unknown amount of ethoheptazine, the following postmortem concentrations were reported: blood 15 µg/g, brain 4.5 µg/g, kidney 2.4 µg/g, liver 10.0 µg/g, spleen 3.1 µg/g [R. H. Drost *et al.*, *J. Chromatogr.*, 1983, *277*; *Biomed. Appl.*, *28*, 352–355].

Dose. 225 to 600 mg of ethoheptazine citrate daily.

Ethomoxane

Tranquilliser

N-Butyl-8-ethoxy-1,4-benzodioxan-2-ylmethylamine
$C_{15}H_{23}NO_3$=265.4
CAS—3570-46-5

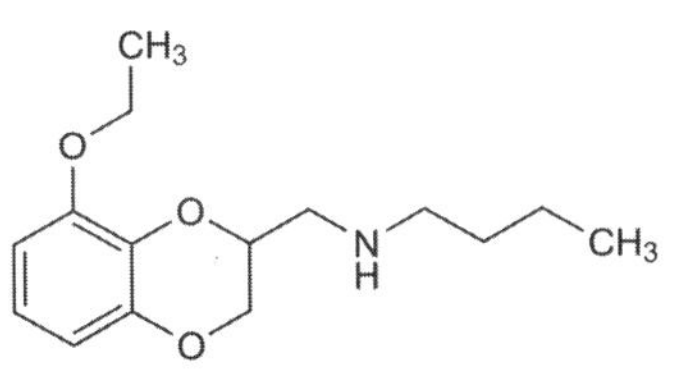

A liquid.

Ethomoxane Hydrochloride

$C_{15}H_{23}NO_3$,HCl=301.8
CAS—6038-78-4
Crystals. M.p. 196° to 197°.

Colour Tests. Mandelin's Test—red-brown; Marquis Test—red-violet.

Thin-layer Chromatography. System TA—Rf 60; system TB—Rf 34; system TC—Rf 47; system TL—Rf 36. (Acidified iodoplatinate solution, positive.)

Gas Chromatography. System GA—RI 1975.

Ultraviolet Spectrum. Aqueous acid—267 nm (A_1^1=23.5a).

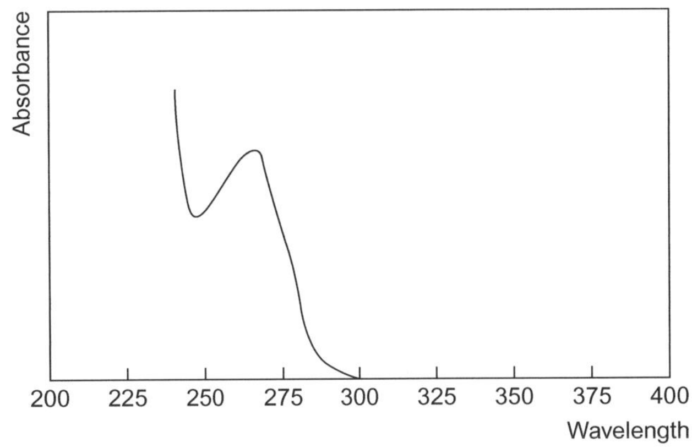

Infra-red Spectrum. Principal peaks at wavenumbers 1120, 1279, 1594, 1493, 1097, 1252 cm^{-1} (KBr disk).

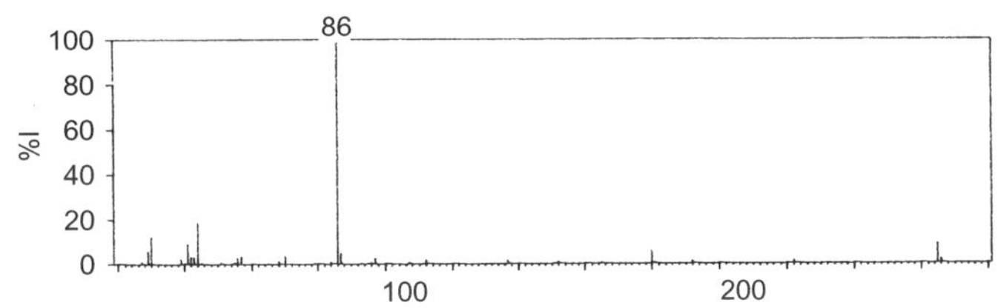

Mass Spectrum. Principal ions at *m/z* 86, 44, 30, 265, 41, 180, 29, 87.

Ethosuximide

Anticonvulsant

Synonym. Ethosuccimide
Proprietary names. Emeside; Ethymal; Petinimid; Petnidan; Pyknolepsinum; Simatin; Suxilep; Suxinutin; Zarondan; Zarontin.
3-Ethyl-3-methyl-2,5-pyrrolidinedione
$C_7H_{11}NO_2$=141.2
CAS—77-67-8

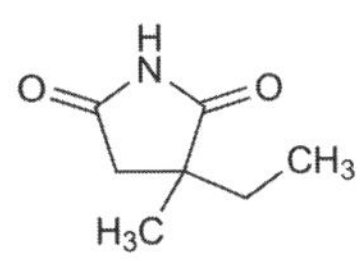

A white powder or waxy solid. M.p. 46° to 52°.
Soluble 1 in 4.5 of water and 1 in less than 1 of ethanol, chloroform and ether.

Dissociation Constant. pK_a 9.5 (20°).

Partition Coefficient. Log *P* (octanol/water), 0.4.

Colour Test. Koppanyi–Zwikker Test—violet.

Thin-layer Chromatography. System TA—Rf 70; system TB—Rf 05; system TD—Rf 50; system TE—Rf 66; system TF—Rf 53; system TAD—Rf 59; system TAE—Rf 84.

Gas Chromatography. System GA—ethosuximide RI 1205, M (3-OH) RI 1322, M (OH-ethyl) RI 1370, M (oxo-) RI 1270; system GB—ethosuximide RI 1258, M (OH-ethyl) RI 1436, M (3-OH) RI 1395; system GE—ethosuximide RRT 0.18 (relative to phenytoin); system GAJ—ethosuximide RRT 0.453 (relative to methylphenobarbital).

High Performance Liquid Chromatography. System HE—*k* 0.91; system HX—RI 301; system HY—RI 276; system HZ—Retention time, 2.3 min; System HAA—Retention time, 10.5 min.

Ultraviolet Spectrum. Aqueous acid—244 nm (A_1^1=9.9b).

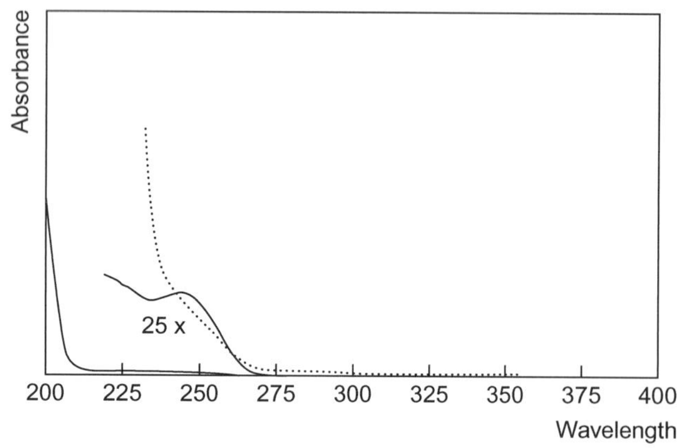

Infra-red Spectrum. Principal peaks at wavenumbers 1700, 1777, 1208, 1130, 1303, 730 cm^{-1} (KBr disk).

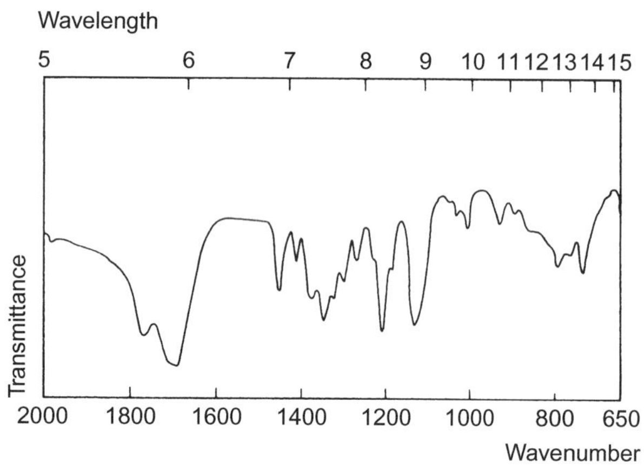

Mass Spectrum. Principal ions at *m/z* 113, 70, 55, 42, 41, 39, 85, 69; M (OH-ethyl) *m/z* 113, 85, 98, 69, 71, 142; M (3-OH-) *m/z* 71, 86, 129, 139, 142, 157; M (oxo-) *m/z* 70, 155, 55, 113, 69, 98.

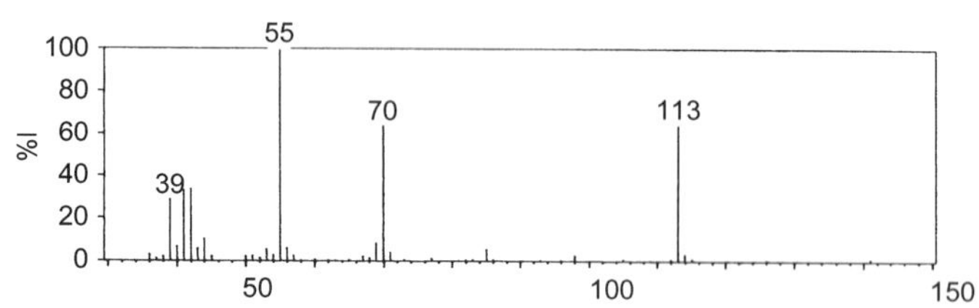

Quantification

Gas chromatography. In plasma or serum: limit of detection 500 μg/L, ECD—J. E. Wallace *et al.*, *Clin. Chem.*, 1979, *25*, 252–255. In plasma or urine: ethosuximide and phensuximide, limit of detection 2.5 mg/L, FID—E. van der Kleijn *et al.*, *J. Pharm. Pharmacol.*, 1973, *25*, 324–327.

Gas chromatography–mass spectrometry. In blood or liver: ethosuximide and other antiepileptic drugs—D. J. Speed *et al.*, *J. Anal. Toxicol.*, 2000, *24*, 685–690. In plasma or urine: ethosuximide enantiomers, limit of detection <2.5 mg/L—L. Sghendo *et al.*, *J. Chromatogr. B. Anal. Technol. Biomed. Life Sci.*, 2002, *772*, 307–315.

High performance liquid chromatography. In plasma or serum: ethosuximide and other anticonvulsants, limit of detection about 2 mg/L, UV detection—J. A. Christofides and D. E. Fry, *Clin. Chem.*, 1980, *26*, 499–501. In serum: ethosuximide and other anticonvulsants, limit of detection 1 mg/L, UV detection—P. M. Kabra *et al.*, *J. Anal. Toxicol.*, 1978, *2*, 127–133. In plasma: ethosuximide and other antiepileptic drugs, UV detection—K. M. Matar *et al.*, *Ther. Drug Monit.*, 1999, *21*, 559–566. In plasma: limit of detection about 0.9 μM—S. H. Chen *et al.*, *J. Chromatogr. B. Biomed. Sci. Appl.*, 1999, *729*, 111–117.

Disposition in the Body. Readily absorbed after oral administration. Metabolised by hydroxylation to 3-hydroxyethosuximide and 1-hydroxyethylethosuximide; the latter is further oxidised to produce 2-acetyl-2-methylsuccinimide; an additional metabolite, 2-carboxymethyl-2-methylsuccinimide has also been reported. None of the metabolites is pharmacologically active. About 25% of a dose is excreted in the urine in 24 h as 1-hydroxyethylethosuximide glucuronide and about 14% as the unconjugated metabolite. Up to about 20% of a dose is excreted as unchanged drug in the urine over a 9 day period.

Therapeutic concentration. In plasma, usually in the range 40 to 100 mg/L.

After a single oral dose of 500 mg to 5 children, peak plasma concentrations of 28 to 51 mg/L (mean 39) were attained in 3 to 7 h [R. A. Buchanan *et al.*, *J. Clin. Pharmacol.*, 1969, *9*, 393–398].

Steady-state serum concentrations of 31 to 68 mg/L (mean 49) were reported in 5 young adults receiving daily oral doses of 1 g [E. B. Solow and J. B. Green, *Clin. Chim. Acta*, 1971, *33*, 8–90].

Toxicity. The estimated minimum lethal dose is 5 g. Toxic effects may be observed at plasma concentrations greater than about 100 mg/L.

In a fatality involving ethosuximide, the following postmortem tissue concentrations were reported: blood 250 mg/L, liver 280 μg/g, urine 120 mg/L; phenobarbital was also detected [M. Rousseau *et al.*, *Bull. Int. Assoc. Forensic Toxicol.*, 1980, 15(2), 5–6].

Half-life. Plasma half-life, 40 to 60 h in adults and about 30 h in children.

Volume of distribution. About 0.7 L/kg.

Saliva. Plasma:saliva ratio, about 1.1.

Protein binding. In plasma, not significantly bound.

Dose. 0.5 to 2 g daily.

Ethotoin

Anticonvulsant

Proprietary name. Peganone
3-Ethyl-5-phenyl-2,4-imidazolidinedione
$C_{11}H_{12}N_2O_2$=204.2
CAS—86-35-1

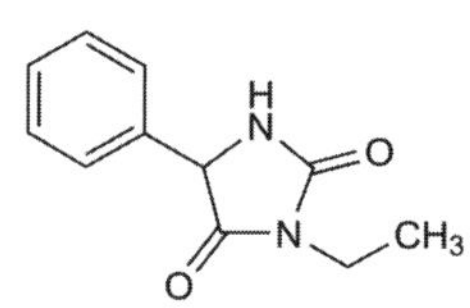

A white crystalline powder. M.p. about 90°.
Sparingly soluble in cold water, more soluble in hot water; soluble 1 in 4 of dehydrated alcohol, 1 in 1.5 of chloroform and 1 in 25 of ether; freely soluble in benzene and dilute aqueous solutions of alkali hydroxides.

Dissociation Constant. pK_a 8.5.

Partition Coefficient. Log *P* (octanol/water), 1.0.

Thin-layer Chromatography. System TA—Rf 88; system TD—Rf 53; system TE—Rf 71; system TF—Rf 54; system TAD—Rf 60; system TAJ—Rf 61; system TAK—Rf 66; system TAL—Rf 91.

Gas Chromatography. System GA—RI 1800; system GB—RI 1751; system GE—RRT 0.57 (relative to phenytoin); system GAJ—RRT 0.940 (relative to methylphenobarbital).

High Performance Liquid Chromatography. System HE—*k* 2.81.

Ultraviolet Spectrum. Dehydrated alcohol—259 nm (A_1^1=11b), 265 nm (A_1^1=8b).

Infra-red Spectrum. Principal peaks at wavenumbers 1716, 700, 760, 820, 1780, 1100 cm^{-1} (KBr disk).

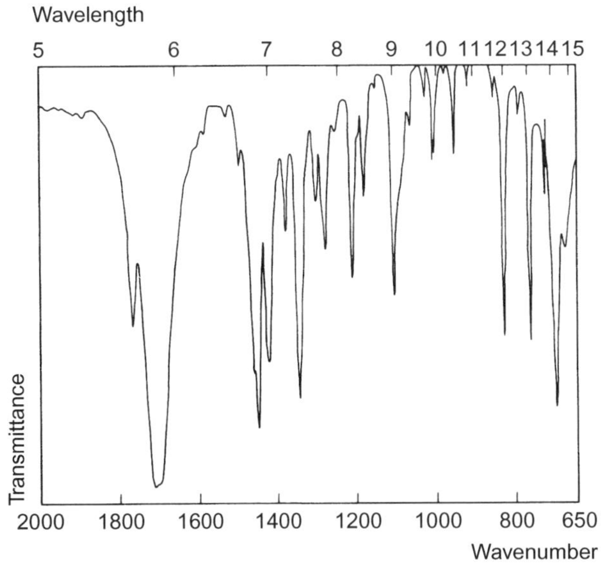

Mass Spectrum. Principal ions at *m/z* 104, 105, 204, 77, 78, 133, 51, 132.

Quantification
Gas chromatography. In serum: limit of detection 1 mg/L, FID—N.-E. Larsen and J. Naestoft, *J. Chromatogr.*, 1974, *92*, 157–161.

Gas chromatography–mass spectrometry. In urine: ethotoin and some metabolites, limit of detection 5 mg/L—J. Naestoft and N.-E. Larsen, *J. Chromatogr.*, 1977, *143*; *Biomed. Appl.*, *1*, 161–169.

Disposition in the Body. Readily absorbed after oral administration. Extensively metabolised by *N*-desethylation and ring cleavage, 5-hydroxylation and *p*-hydroxylation of the phenyl ring. During chronic therapy, less than 5% of the dose is excreted in the urine in 24 h as unchanged drug, together with 5 to 14% of the dose as desethylethotoin, 17 to 35% as 5-hydroxyethotoin, 14 to 32% as conjugated *p*-hydroxyethotoin and small amounts of other phenyl-substituted oxidation products. 2-Phenylhydantoic acid may account for about 10% of the dose.

Therapeutic concentration. In plasma, usually in the range 6 to 20 mg/L.

Following single oral doses of 500, 1500 and 2500 mg to 5 subjects, peak plasma concentrations of 9 to 15 mg/L (mean 12), 30 to 59 mg/L (mean 42) and 37 to 75 mg/L (mean 54), respectively, were attained in about 1.5, 3.5 and 3.5 h [M. C. Meyer *et al.*, *Clin. Pharmacol. Ther.*, 1983, *33*, 329–334].

During daily oral dosing with 30 mg/kg to 7 subjects, minimum steady-state plasma concentrations of 4.5 to 14 mg/L (mean 10) were reported; following daily oral treatment with 60 mg/kg to 6 subjects, minimum steady-state plasma concentrations of 14 to 50 mg/L (mean 30) were reported [O. Sjö *et al.*, *Clin. Exp. Pharmacol. Physiol*, 1975, *2*, 185–192].

Toxicity. The estimated minimum lethal dose is 5 g.

Half-life. Plasma half-life, 3 to 11 h (dose-dependent).

Dose. Initially 1 g daily, increasing to 2 to 3 g daily.

Ethoxzolamide

Carbonic Anhydrase Inhibitor/Diuretic

Synonym. Ethoxyzolamide
Proprietary names. Cardrase; Ethamide; Glaucotensil; Redupresin.
6-Ethoxy-2-benzothiazolesulfonamide
$C_9H_{10}N_2O_3S_2$=258.3
CAS—452-35-7

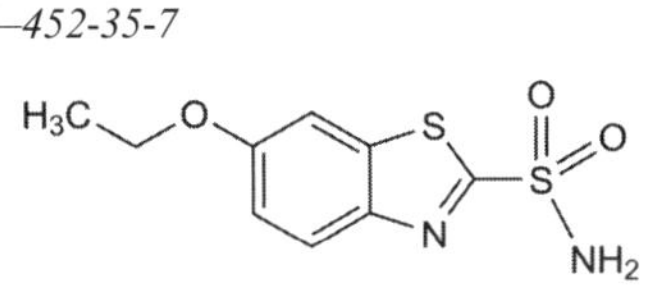

A white or slightly yellow crystalline powder. M.p. 189° to 195°.
Practically insoluble in water; slightly soluble in ethanol, chloroform and ether.

Dissociation Constant. pK_a 8.1.

Partition Coefficient. Log *P* (octanol/pH 7.4), 2.2.

Colour Tests. Koppanyi–Zwikker Test—violet; Liebermann's Test—yellow; Marquis Test—yellow

Thin-layer Chromatography. System TA—Rf 76; system TD—Rf 43; system TE—Rf 43; system TF—Rf 65; system TAD—Rf 51; system TAJ—Rf 51; system TAK—Rf 48; system TAL—Rf 91. (Marquis reagent, positive.)

Gas Chromatography. System GA—RI 2578.

Ultraviolet Spectrum. Aqueous acid—253, 304 nm (A_1^1=96a).

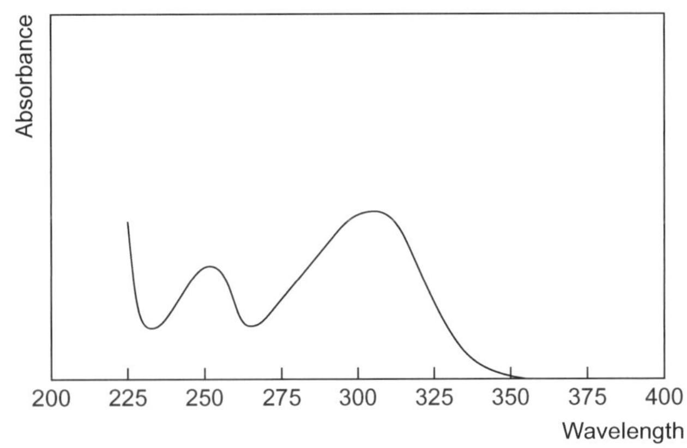

Infra-red Spectrum. Principal peaks at wavenumbers 1170, 1490, 1263, 824, 1224, 1036 cm^{-1} (KBr disk).

Dose. In the treatment of glaucoma, 250 to 500 mg daily.

Ethyl Acetate

Flavouring Agent/Solvent

Synonym. Acetic Ether
$C_4H_8O_2$=88.10
CAS—141-78-6

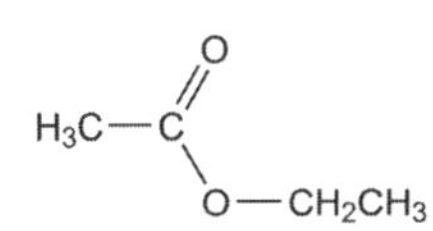

A colourless flammable liquid. Sp. gr. 0.894 to 0.898. B.p. 77°.
Soluble 1 in 15 of water; miscible with acetone, ethanol, chloroform and ether.

Partition Coefficient. Log *P* (octanol/water), 0.7.

Gas Chromatography. System GA—RI 596; system GI—Retention time 9.4 min.

Mass Spectrum. Principal ions at *m/z* 43, 61, 45, 70, 29, 27, 73, 42.

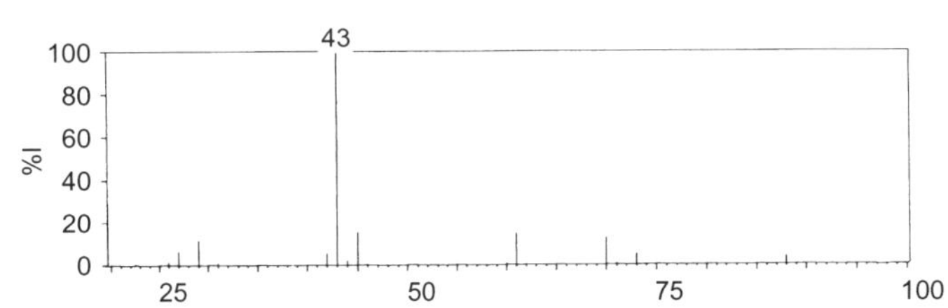

Ethyl Biscoumacetate

Anticoagulant

Synonyms. Aethylis Biscoumacetas; BOEA; Ethyldicoumarol; Neodicumarinum.

Proprietary names. Pelentan; Stabilène; Tromexan.
Ethyl-4-hydroxy-α-(4-hydroxy-2-oxo-2*H*-1-benzopyran-3-yl)-2-oxo-2*H*-1-benzopyran-3-acetate
$C_{22}H_{16}O_8$=408.4
CAS—548-00-5

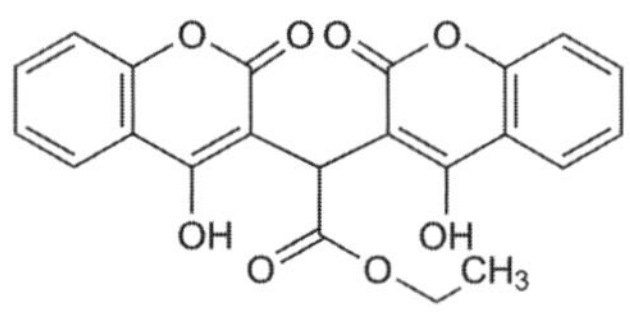

A white to yellowish-white, fine crystalline powder. There are two forms, one melts at 154° to 157° and the other at 177° to 182°.
Practically insoluble in water; soluble 1 in 20 of acetone; slightly soluble in alcohol and ether; soluble in chloroform.

Dissociation Constant. pK_a 3.1.

Partition Coefficient. Log *P* (octanol/water), 1.9.

Colour Test. Sulfuric Acid—orange-yellow.

Thin-layer Chromatography. System TD—Rf 04; system TE—Rf 24; system TF—Rf 32; system TAD—Rf 21. (Acidified potassium permanganate solution, positive.)

Ultraviolet Spectrum. Water—275 nm (A_1^1=449b), 303 nm; aqueous alkali—311 nm (A_1^1=622b).

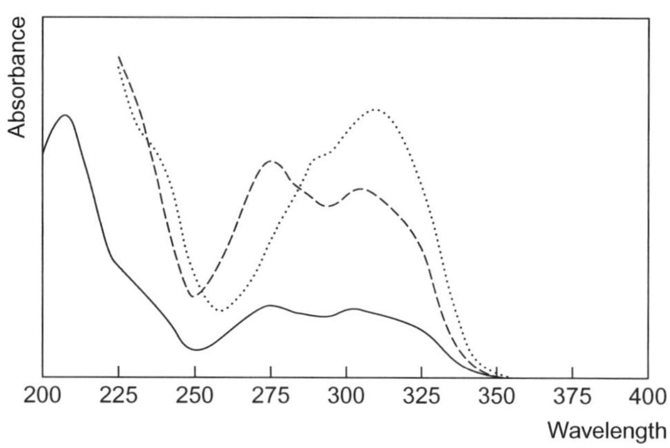

Infra-red Spectrum. Principal peaks at wavenumbers 1653, 1600, 768, 1560, 754, 1730 cm^{-1}.

Mass Spectrum. Principal ions at *m/z* 121, 318, 317, 173, 120, 362, 44, 31.

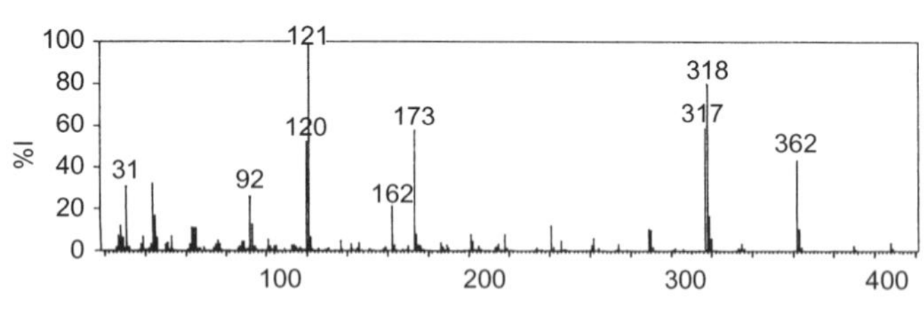

Quantification
High performance liquid chromatography. In plasma: limit of detection 100 µg/L, UV detection—M. Arman and F. Jamali, *J. Chromatogr.*, 1983, *272*; *Biomed. Appl.*, *23*, 406–410.

High performance liquid chromatography–mass spectrometry. In serum: ethyl biscoumacetate and its metabolite 7-hydroxyethyl bicoumacetate—J. Pospisil *et al.*, *J. Chromatogr.*, 1992, *574*, 71–75.

Disposition in the Body. Readily absorbed after oral administration and extensively metabolised. About 5 to 15% of a dose is excreted in the urine as hydroxyethyl biscoumacetate and only traces are excreted unchanged.

Therapeutic concentration
Following a single oral dose of 300 mg to 4 subjects, peak plasma concentrations of 10.2 to 12.4 mg/L (mean 11.2) were attained in 1 to 1.5 h [M. Arman and F. Jamali, *J. Chromatogr.*, 1983, *272*; *Biomed. Appl.*, *23*, 406–410].

After a single 300 mg oral dose of ethyl biscoumacetate to 10 subjects, peak plasma concentrations of 4.46 mg/L were reached in 1.62 h; equivalent values for the main metabolite, 7-hydroxyethyl biscoumacetate, were 12.74 mg/L in 3.29 h [F. Perlik and V. Patzelova, *Int. J. Clin. Pharmacol. Ther.*, 1994, *32*, 622–624].

Half-life. Plasma half-life, about 1 to 2 h.

Protein binding. In plasma, about 90%.

Dose. Maintenance, 300 to 600 mg daily.

Ethyl Gallate

Antoxidant

Proprietary name. Progallin A
Ethyl-3,4,5-trihydroxybenzoate
$C_9H_{10}O_5$=198.2
CAS—831-61-8

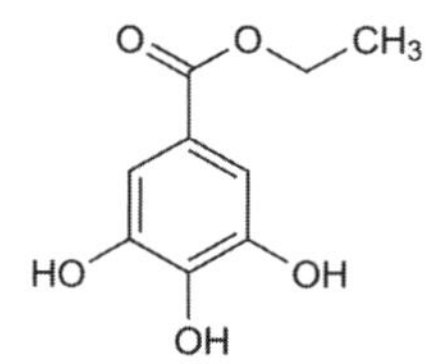

A white to creamy-white crystalline powder. M.p. 151° to 154°.
Soluble 1 in 500 of water, 1 in 3 of ethanol, 1 in 3 of ether and 1 in 3 of propylene glycol.

Partition Coefficient. Log *P* (octanol/water), 1.3.

Colour Test. Ferric Chloride—violet-black→blue-black.

Ultraviolet Spectrum. Methanol—275 nm (A_1^1=540b).

Ethyl Hydroxybenzoate

Preservative

Synonyms. Aethylum Hydroxybenzoicum; Ethylis Paraoxybenzoas; Ethylparaben.
Proprietary names. Nipagin A; Solbrol A.
Ethyl-4-hydroxybenzoate
$C_9H_{10}O_3$=166.2
CAS—120-47-8

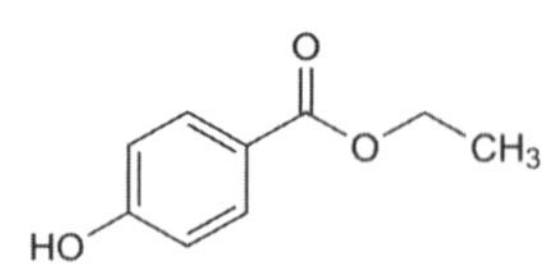

Colourless crystals or white crystalline powder. M.p. 116°.
Soluble 1 in 1500 of water, 1 in 2 of ethanol, 1 in 1.2 of acetone, 1 in 10 of chloroform and 1 in 3.5 of ether.

Sodium Ethyl Hydroxybenzoate
Proprietary name. Nipagin A Sodium.
$C_9H_9NaO_3$=188.2
CAS—35285-68-8
A white hygroscopic crystalline powder.
Soluble 1 in 2 of water and 1 in 3 of ethanol (50%).

Dissociation Constant. pK_a 8.3 (25°).

Partition Coefficient. Log *P* (octanol/water), 2.5.

Colour Test. Millon's Reagent—red

Thin-layer Chromatography. System TD—Rf 64; system TE—Rf 46; system TF—Rf 66; system TAD—Rf 57; system TAE—Rf 88.

Gas Chromatography. System GA—RI 1580.

Ultraviolet Spectrum. Aqueous acid—254 nm (A_1^1=956b); aqueous alkali—295 nm (A_1^1=1390b).

Infra-red Spectrum. Principal peaks at wavenumbers 1290, 1673, 1170, 1240, 1610, 1590 cm^{-1} (KBr disk).

Ethyl Nicotinate

Topical Vasodilator

Proprietary names. It is an ingredient of PR Heat Spray, Thermal, Thermocutan, Transvane and Transvasin.
$C_8H_9NO_2$=151.2
CAS—614-18-6

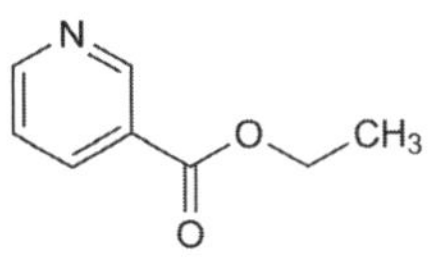

A liquid. M.p. 8° to 9°. B.p. 225°.
Very soluble in water, ethanol and ether.

Dissociation Constant. pK_a 3.4 (20°).

Partition Coefficient. Log *P* (octanol/water), 1.3.

Thin-layer Chromatography. System TA—Rf 00. (Acidified potassium permanganate solution, positive.)

Ultraviolet Spectrum. Aqueous acid—261 nm (A_1^1=341a).

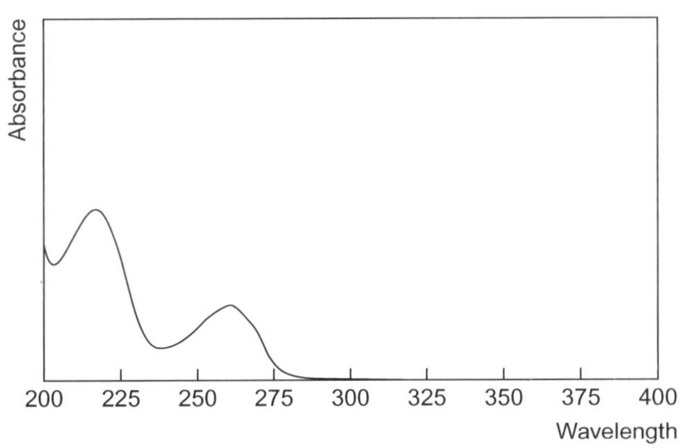

Infra-red Spectrum. Principal peaks at wavenumbers 1286, 1724, 1110, 740, 1591, 1025 cm^{-1} (KBr disk).

Use. Topically in concentrations of 1 to 2%.

Ethylene Glycol

Antifreeze/Solvent

Synonyms. Ethylene Alcohol; Glycol.
1,2-Ethanediol
$C_2H_6O_2$=62.1
CAS—107-21-1

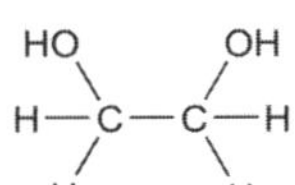

A colourless, hygroscopic, syrupy liquid. Mass per mL about 1.114 g. F.p. about −13°. B.p. about 197°.
Miscible with water, glycerol, acetic acid, ethanol and acetone; slightly soluble in ether; practically insoluble in benzene.

Dissociation Constant. pK_a 15.0.

Partition Coefficient. Log *P* (octanol/water), −1.4.

Gas Chromatography. System GA—RI 798; system GI—Retention time 17.0 min (tailing peak).

Mass Spectrum. Principal ions at *m/z* 31, 33, 29, 32, 43, 28, 27, 42.

Quantification
Spectrofluorimetry. In serum: limit of detection 50 mg/L—J. M. Meola *et al.*, *Clin. Chem.*, 1980, *26*, 1709.

Gas chromatography. In plasma: ethylene glycol, methanol, ethanol, acetone and isopropanol—S. T. Cheung and W. N. Lin, *J. Chromatogr.*, 1987, *414*, 248–250. In plasma: limit of detection 50 mg/L, FID—D. W. Robinson and D. S. Reive, *J. Anal. Toxicol.*, 1981, *5*, 69–72.

Gas chromatography–mass spectrometry. In serum: ethylene glycol and other glycols, limit of detection 0.7 mg/L—V. Gembus *et al.*, *J. Anal. Toxicol.*, 2002, *26*, 280–285. In plasma: limit of detection 0.01 g/L and limit of quantification 0.1 g/L for ethylene glycol and diethylene glycol—H.H. Maurer *et al.*, *J. Chromatogr. B Biomed. Sci. Appl.*, 2001, *254*, 401–409.

Review. For a review of assay methods see D. J. Doedens, *Vet. Hum. Toxicol.*, 1983, 25, 96–101.

Disposition in the Body. Ethylene glycol is metabolised initially to glycoaldehyde and subsequently to lactic acid and oxalic acid. Calcium oxalate crystals are deposited in the kidneys and some oxalate may be excreted in the urine together with unchanged ethylene glycol.

Toxicity. Ethylene glycol itself is probably non-toxic and the serious toxic effects are due to the metabolites. In adults the minimum lethal dose is about 100 mL although survival has been reported after ingestion of 250 mL. Toxic effects are usually associated with plasma concentrations greater than 500 mg/L. The maximum permissible atmospheric concentration of ethylene glycol vapour is 100 ppm.

A 51-year-old man ingested 600 mL of antifreeze solution but recovered after treatment. A blood concentration of 6500 mg/L of ethylene glycol was reported 2½ h after ingestion; pharmacokinetic studies indicated that the volume of distribution of ethylene glycol was about 0.8 L/kg and the plasma half-life was about 3 h [C. D. Peterson *et al.*, *N. Engl. J. Med.*, 1981, *304*, 21–23].

A 36-year-old man was admitted to hospital 6 h after ingesting 500 mL of an antifreeze mixture containing ethylene glycol and methanol; initial serum concentrations were 1900 mg/L for ethylene glycol and 1130 mg/L for methanol; the subject recovered after treatment with ethanol and haemodialysis [N. P. Vites *et al.*, *Lancet*, 1984, *1*, 562].

The plasma ethylene glycol concentration in a 36-year-old man who ingested approx. 3 L of ethylene glycol antifreeze in a suicide attempt was 18.89 g/L. Despite this very high level, the man survived after haemodialysis and ethanol infusion [B. Johnson *et al.*, *Ann. Emerg. Med.*, 1999, *33*, 108–110].

5 h after ingesting an unknown amount of ethylene glycol, the plasma concentration in a 23-year-old man was 1162 mg/L. The man died 27 h after ingestion. Just before death the plasma ethylene glycol concentration was 359 mg/L and concentrations in postmortem tissue homogenates 70 h after death were: right and left kidney 227.6 and 258.5 mg/L, right and left lung 310 and 281.7 mg/L, heart 57.6 mg/L, liver 299.8 mg/L, spleen 310 mg/L, brain 134.5 mg/L, pancreas not detected, gastric contents 859.2 mg/L, bile 785.6 mg/L, pleural fluid 700.7 mg/L [P. Hantson *et al.*, *Am. J. Forensic Med. Pathol.*, 2002, *23*, 159–161].

Note. For a review of the management of ethylene glycol poisoning see J. Brent, *Drugs*, 2001, *61*, 979–988.

Ethylenediamine Hydrate

Pharmaceutical Adjuvant

$C_2H_8N_2,H_2O$=78.1
CAS—107-15-3 (anhydrous); 6780-13-8 (monohydrate)

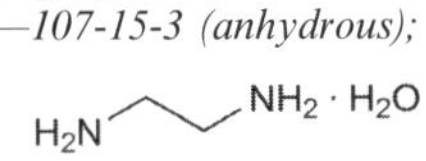

A clear, colourless or slightly yellow, strongly alkaline liquid. It is hygroscopic and absorbs carbon dioxide from the air. It solidifies on cooling to a crystalline mass (M.p. 10°). Mass per mL about 0.96 g. B.p. about 120°.

Miscible with water and ethanol; soluble 1 in 130 of chloroform; slightly soluble in ether.
Caution. It is irritant to the skin and mucous membranes.

Dissociation Constant. pK_a 7.2, 10.0 (20°).

Partition Coefficient. Log *P* (octanol/water), −2.0 (anhydrous).

Colour Test. Dissolve 1 mL in 5 mL of water and to 3 drops of this solution add 2 mL of a 1% solution of copper sulfate and shake—violet-blue.

Mass Spectrum. Principal ions at *m/z* 30, 42, 43, 27, 44, 29, 31, 41.

Quantification
High performance liquid chromatography. In plasma or urine: limit of detection 50 µg/L in plasma, UV detection—I. A. Cotgreave and J. Caldwell, *Biopharm. Drug Dispos.*, 1983, *4*, 53–62.

Disposition in the Body. Absorbed after oral administration and rapidly metabolised.

Toxicity. The maximum permissible atmospheric concentration is 10 ppm.

Half-life. Plasma half-life, about 0.5 to 1 h.

Use. Ethylenediamine hydrate is used in the manufacture of aminophylline and in the preparation of aminophylline injections.

Ethylestrenol

Anabolic Steroid

Synonym. Ethyloestrenol
Proprietary names. Durabolin-O; Maxibolin; Orabolin; Orgabolin; Orgaboral.
(17α)-19-Norpregn-4-en-17-ol
$C_{20}H_{32}O$=288.5
CAS—965-90-2

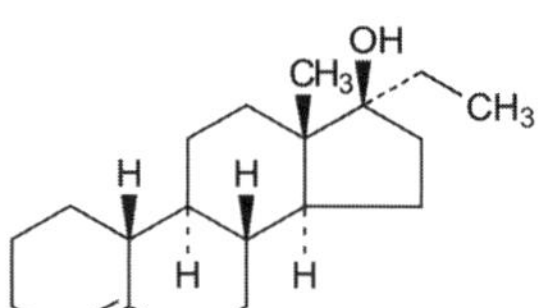

A white crystalline powder. M.p. 76° to 78°.
Practically insoluble in water; soluble 1 in 9 of ethanol, 1 in 2 of chloroform and 1 in 6 of ether.

Partition Coefficient. Log *P* (octanol/water), 5.5.

Thin-layer Chromatography. System TP—Rf 79; system TQ—Rf 50; system TR—Rf 94; system TS—Rf 99.

Ultraviolet Spectrum. No significant absorption, 230 to 360 nm.

Infra-red Spectrum. Principal peaks at wavenumbers 975, 994, 964, 1299, 1142, 1165 cm^{-1} (Nujol mull).

Dose. Usually 2 to 4 mg daily.

Ethylmorphine

Narcotic Analgesic

7,8-Didehydro-4,5-epoxy-3-ethoxy-17-methylmorphinan-6-ol
$C_{19}H_{23}NO_3$=313.4
CAS—76-58-4

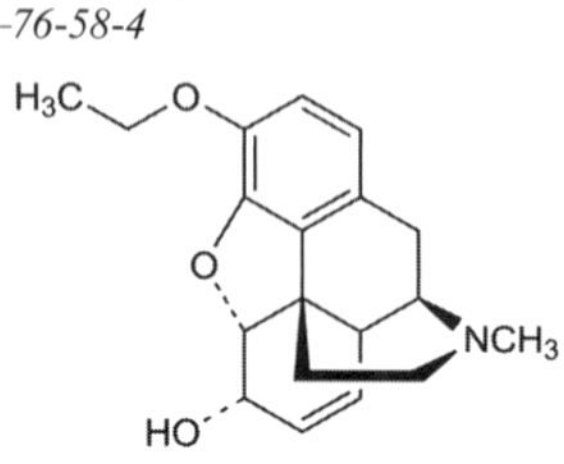

Crystals. M.p. 199° to 201°.

Ethylmorphine Hydrochloride

Synonym. Chlorhydrate de Codéthyline
Proprietary name. It is an ingredient of Natirose.
$C_{19}H_{23}NO_3,HCl,2H_2O$=385.9
CAS—125-30-4 (anhydrous); 6746-59-4 (dihydrate)
A white crystalline powder. M.p. about 123°, with decomposition.
Soluble 1 in 10 of water, 1 in 25 of ethanol, 1 in 1 of warm ethanol and 1 in 250 of chloroform; slightly soluble in ether.

Dissociation Constant. pK_a 8.2 (20°).

Partition Coefficient. Log *P* (octanol/water), 1.8.

Colour Test. Marquis Test—yellow→violet→black.

Thin-layer Chromatography. System TA—Rf 40; system TB—Rf 07; system TC—Rf 22; system TE—Rf 36; system TL—Rf 6; system TAE—Rf 21; system TAF—Rf 26; system TAJ—Rf 13; system TAK—Rf 04; system TAL—Rf 54. (Dragendorff spray, positive; acidified iodoplatinate solution, positive; Marquis reagent, blue-violet.)

Gas Chromatography. System GA—ethylmorphine RI 2420, ethylmorphine-AC RI 2530, ethylmorphine-PFP RI 2430, ethylmorphine-TFA RI 2320, ethylmorphine-TMS RI 2540, M (nor-)-AC_2 RI 2930.

High Performance Liquid Chromatography. System HA—*k* 3.7 (tailing peak); system HC—*k* 1.06; system HS—*k* 1.45; system HX—RI 291; system HY—RI 244; system HAX—Retention time 6.7 min; system HAY—Retention time 3.6 min.

Ultraviolet Spectrum. Aqueous acid—284 nm (A^1_1=48a); aqueous alkali—281 nm.

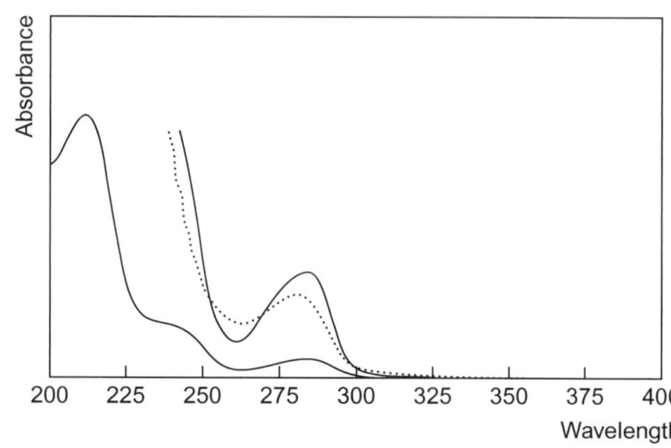

Infra-red Spectrum. Principal peaks at wavenumbers 1064, 1045, 1129, 1499, 1185, 1264 cm^{-1} (ethylmorphine hydrochloride, Nujol mull).

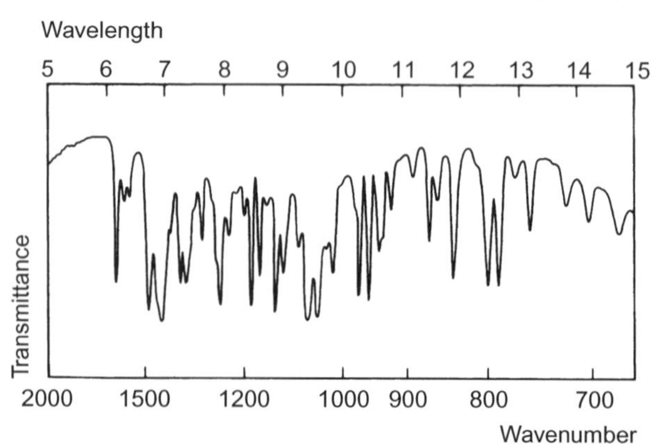

Mass Spectrum. Principal ions at *m/z* 313, 162, 314, 124, 284, 59, 42, 243; ethylmorphine-AC *m/z* 355, 296, 327, 234, 268, 204; ethylmorphine-PFP *m/z* 296, 459, 280, 266, 402, 430; ethylmorphine-TFA *m/z* 296, 409, 380, 280, 352, 266; ethylmorphine-TMS *m/z* 385, 192, 146, 196, 234, 357; M (nor-)-AC_2 *m/z* 87, 209, 237, 383, 341, 181.

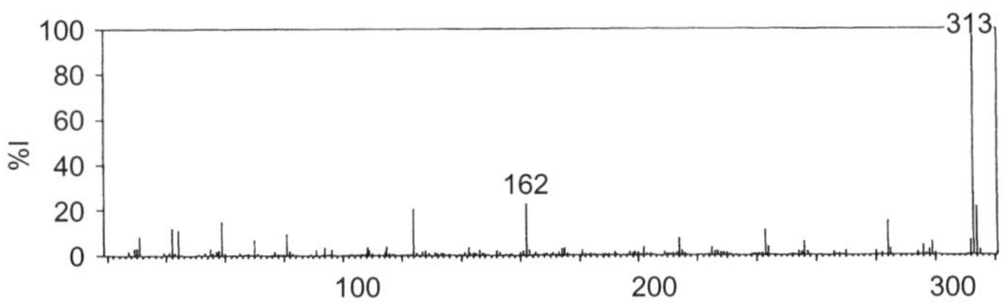

Quantification

Gas chromatography. In blood, urine or postmortem tissues: AFID—P. Demedts *et al.*, *J. Anal. Toxicol.*, 1983, *7*, 113–115. In plasma, urine or tissue: ethylmorphine and other opioids, nitrogen selective detection—P. Kintz *et al.*, *Z. Rechtsmed.*, 1989, *103*, 57–62. In blood: ethylmorphine and other opioids, limit of detection 10 µg/L, electron ionisation—S. Mykkanen *et al.*, *J. Anal. Toxicol.*, 2000, *24*, 122–126.

Gas chromatography–mass spectrometry. In blood: ethylmorphine, morphine and codeine, limit of detection for ethylmorphine 0.025 µmol/L—H. Gjerde *et al.*, *Forensic Sci. Int.*, 1991, *51*, 105–110. In hair: ethylmorphine and other opioids and their metabolites, limits of detection 0.1 to 0.8 µg/g—P. Kintz and P. Mangin, *Forensic Sci. Int.*, 1995, *73*, 93–100.

High performance liquid chromatography. In hair: ethylmorphine and other drugs including opioids, electrochemical detection—G. Achilli *et al.*, *J. Chromatogr. A*, 1996, *729*, 273–277.

Disposition in the Body. Absorbed after oral administration.

Toxicity. The estimated minimum lethal dose is 500 mg.

In a death attributed to oral ethylmorphine ingestion, the femoral blood concentration of the drug was 488 µg/L [P. Kintz *et al.*, *Arch. Toxicol.*, 1994, *68*, 210–211].

Ethylnoradrenaline

Sympathomimetic

Synonym. Ethylnorepinephrine

4-(2-Amino-1-hydroxybutyl)-1,2-benzenediol

$C_{10}H_{15}NO_3$=197.2

CAS—536-24-3

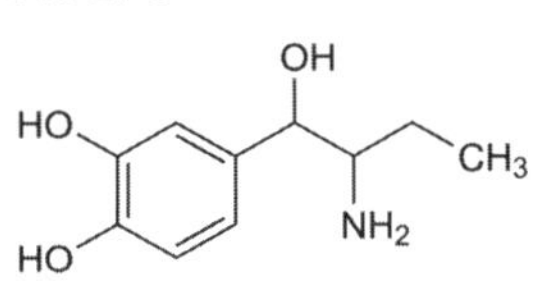

Ethylnoradrenaline Hydrochloride

Proprietary name. Bronkephrine

$C_{10}H_{15}NO_3$,HCl=233.7

CAS—3198-07-0

A crystalline solid. M.p. 199° to 200°, with decomposition.

Soluble in water.

Dissociation Constant. pK_a 8.4 (25°).

Colour Tests. Ferric Chloride—green; Mandelin's Test—orange; Marquis Test—orange→brown; Nessler's Reagent—black

Thin-layer Chromatography. System TA—Rf 42; system TB—Rf 01; system TC—Rf 02; system TE—Rf 15; system TL—Rf 24; system TAJ—Rf 00; system TAK—Rf 00; system TAL—Rf 15. (Acidified potassium permanganate solution, positive.)

Ultraviolet Spectrum. Aqueous acid—278 nm (A^1_1=154b).

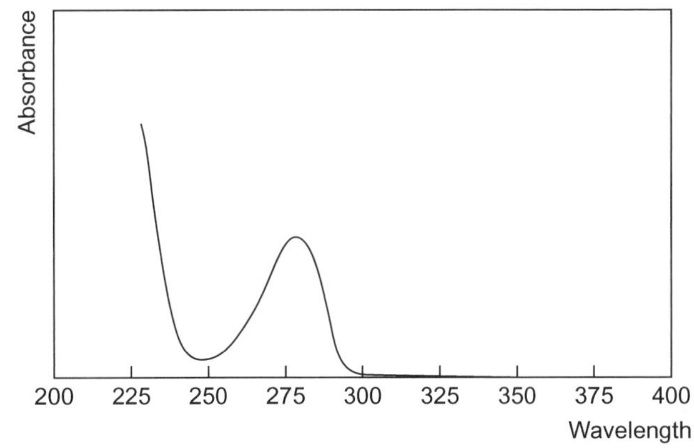

Infra-red Spectrum. Principal peaks at wavenumbers 1500, 1529, 1280, 1265, 1052, 1600 cm^{-1} (KBr disk).

Mass Spectrum. Principal ions at *m/z* 58, 41, 56, 30, 124, 65, 59, 93.

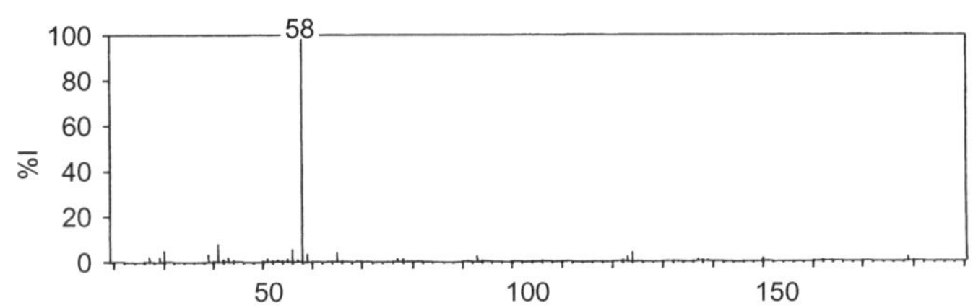

Dose. 1 to 2 mg of ethylnoradrenaline hydrochloride, subcutaneously or intramuscularly.

Etacrynic Acid

Diuretic

Synonyms. Ethacrynic Acid; Etacrynsäure.

Proprietary names. Edecril; Edecrin(e) (tablets); Hydromedin (tablets); Reomax; Uregyt.

[2,3-Dichloro-4-(2-methylene-1-oxobutyl)phenoxy]acetic acid

$C_{13}H_{12}Cl_2O_4$=303.1

CAS—58-54-8

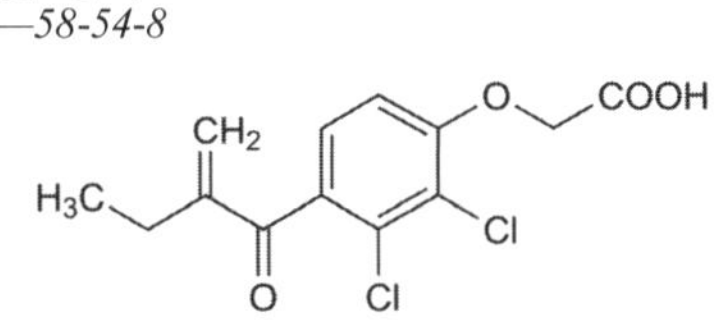

A white crystalline powder. M.p. about 121° to 122°.

Sparingly soluble in water and aqueous acids; soluble 1 in 1.6 of ethanol, 1 in 6 of chloroform and 1 in 3.5 of ether.

Caution. Etacrynic acid, especially in the form of dust, is irritating to the skin, eyes and mucous membranes.

Etacrynate Sodium

Synonyms. Etacrynate Sodium; Sodium Etacrynate.

Proprietary names. Edecrin(e) (injection); Hydromedin (injection); Reomax.

$C_{13}H_{11}Cl_2NaO_4$=325.1

CAS—6500-81-8

Dissociation Constant. pK_a 3.5 (20°).

Partition Coefficient. Log *P* (octanol/water), 3.7.

Thin-layer Chromatography. System TA—Rf 96; system TD—Rf 03; system TE—Rf 05; system TF—Rf 02; system TAD—Rf 05; system TAE—Rf 71; system TAJ—Rf 05; system TAK—Rf 42; system TAL—Rf 57.

Gas Chromatography. System GA—etacrynic acid, not eluted, etacrynic acid-Me RI 2195; system GX—etacrynic acid-Me, Retention time 4.0 min; system GY—etacrynic acid-Me, Retention time 3.3 min.

High Performance Liquid Chromatography. System HX—RI 521; system HY—RI 497.

Ultraviolet Spectrum. Acid methanol—270 nm (A_1^1=115a).

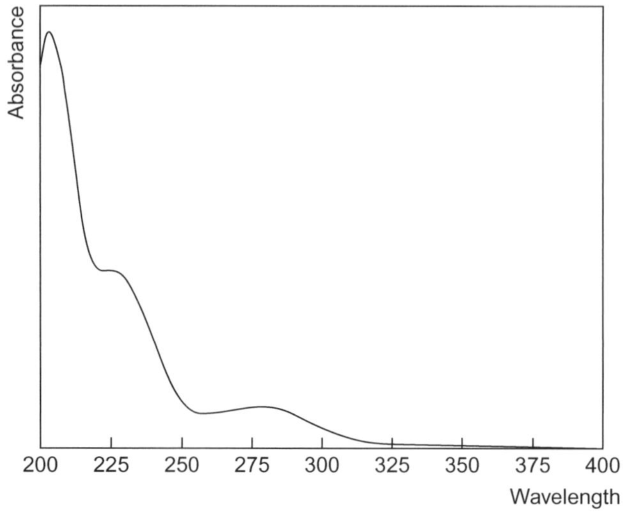

Infra-red Spectrum. Principal peaks at wavenumbers 1726, 1249, 1279, 1077, 1586, 1661 cm^{-1} (KBr disk).

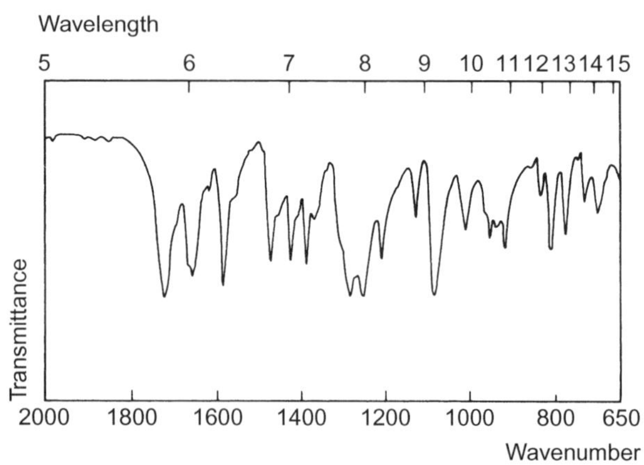

Mass Spectrum. Principal ions at *m/z* 247, 189, 249, 191, 243, 55, 29, 245; etacrynic acid-Me *m/z* 261, 263, 243, 245, 281, 316.

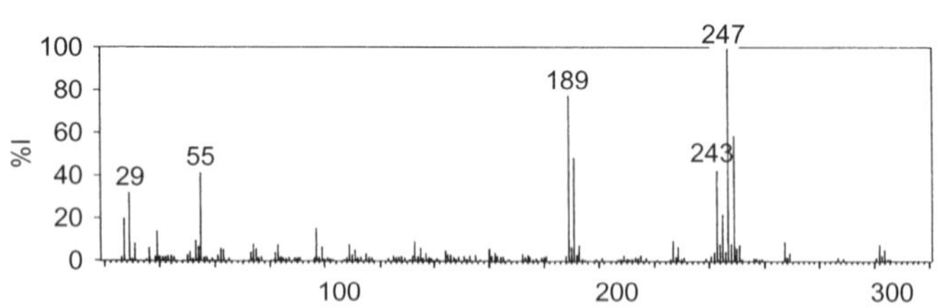

Quantification

Gas chromatography–mass spectrometry. In plasma: limit of detection 10 to 20 µg/L—W. Stuber *et al.*, *J. Chromatogr.*, 1982, *227*; *Biomed. Appl.*, *16*, 193–198.

High performance liquid chromatography. In plasma: limit of detection 0.1 mg/L, UV detection—F. P. LaCreta *et al.*, *J. Chromatogr.*, 1991, *571*, 271–276. In plasma or urine: etacrynic acid and its conjugated metabolite, limit of detection for etacrynic acid <20 µg/L, UV detection—B. Voith *et al.*, *J. Pharm. Biomed. Anal.*, 1995, *13*, 1373–1382.

Disposition in the Body. Readily absorbed after oral administration and distributed to the liver and kidneys. After intravenous administration, 60% is excreted in the urine and 30% in the bile in 24 h; urinary excretion is pH-dependent and the material excreted in the urine consists of unchanged drug, a cysteine conjugate and a third unstable metabolite, in approx. equal proportions.

Toxicity. Thrombocytopenia and fatal agranulocytosis have been reported during chronic treatment.

Half-life. Plasma half-life, 0.5 to 1 h.

Protein binding. In plasma, significantly bound.

Dose. Usually 50 to 150 mg daily; maximum of 400 mg daily.

Etidocaine

Local Anaesthetic

N-(2,6-Dimethylphenyl)-2-(ethylpropylamino)butanamide
$C_{17}H_{28}N_2O$=276.4
CAS—36637-18-0

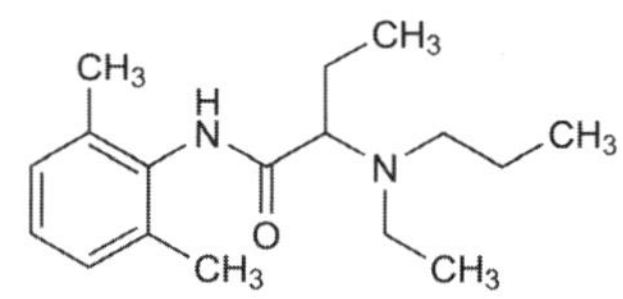

A white crystalline powder. M.p. 87° to 91°.
Soluble 1 in about 7000 of water; freely soluble in organic solvents.

Etidocaine Hydrochloride
Proprietary name. Duranest
$C_{17}H_{28}N_2O,HCl$=312.9
CAS—36637-19-1
A white crystalline powder. M.p. 202° to 205°, with decomposition.
Soluble 1 in 10 of water and 1 in 5 of chloroform; practically insoluble in ether.

Dissociation Constant. pK_a 7.9.

Partition Coefficient. Log *P* (octanol/water), 3.7.

Thin-layer Chromatography. System TA—Rf 91; system TE—Rf 75; system TAE—Rf 80; system TAJ—Rf 66; system TAK—Rf 19; system TAL—Rf 75.

Gas Chromatography. System GA—RI 2040.

Ultraviolet Spectrum. Aqueous acid—262 nm (A_1^1=17a), 271 nm (A_1^1=14a).

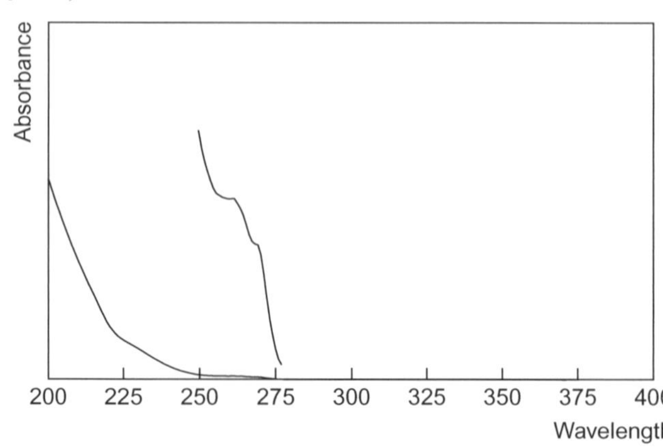

Infra-red Spectrum. Principal peaks at wavenumbers 1650, 1520, 765, 1235, 1272, 1180 cm^{-1} (KBr disk).

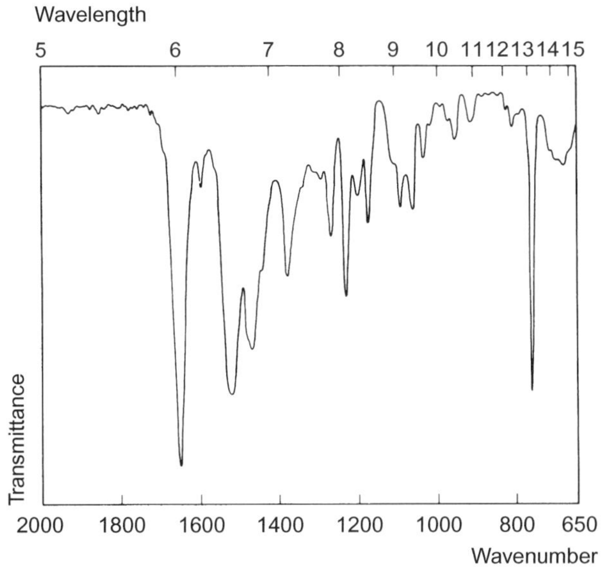

Quantification

Gas chromatography. In plasma or urine: etidocaine and *N*-desalkyl metabolites, limit of detection 20 µg/L, FID—D. J. Morgan *et al.*, *Eur. J. Clin. Pharmacol.*, 1977, *12*, 359–365. In serum: etidocaine and other drugs including local anaesthetics, limit of detection for etidocaine 10 µg/L, nitrogen–phosphorus detection—D. E. Coyle and D. D. Denson, *Ther. Drug Monit.*, 1986, *8*, 98–101. In biological samples: etidocaine and other local anaesthetics, nitrogen-sensitive detection—O. W. Lau *et al.*, *Methods Find. Exp. Clin. Pharmacol.*, 1991, *13*, 475–481.

High performance liquid chromatography. In plasma: etidocaine and other amide local anaesthetics, limit of detection about 30 µg/L, UV detection—H. A. Adams *et al.*, *Reg. Anesth.*, 1989, *12*, 53–57. In plasma: etidocaine and other local anaesthetics, UV detection—J. Drewe *et al.*, *J. Chromatogr. B. Biomed. Sci. Appl.*, 1997, *691*, 105–110.

Disposition in the Body. Rapidly absorbed into the circulation after epidural administration. Extensively metabolised by *N*-dealkylation, hydrolysis and ring hydroxylation. Desethyletidocaine and despropyletidocaine are detectable in plasma. Less than 1% of a dose is excreted in the urine unchanged in 48 h.

Toxicity. Plasma concentrations greater than 2 mg/L may be associated with toxic effects.

Half-life. Plasma half-life, after intravenous administration, about 2.5 h, increased to about 6 h after epidural administration.

Volume of distribution. About 2 L/kg.

Clearance. Plasma clearance, about 15 mL/min/kg.

Distribution in blood. Plasma:whole blood ratio, 1.7.

Protein binding. In plasma, about 94%.

Note. For a review of the pharmacokinetics of local anaesthetics see G. T. Tucker and L. E. Mather, *Clin. Pharmacokinet.*, 1979, *4*, 241–278.

Dose. Etidocaine hydrochloride is administered by injection as 0.5 to 1.5% solutions; maximum dose, 300 mg.

Etilefrine

Sympathomimetic

Synonyms. Ethyladrianol; Ethylnorphenylephrine.
α-[(Ethylamino)methyl]-3-hydroxybenzenemethanol
$C_{10}H_{15}NO_2$=181.2
CAS—709-55-7

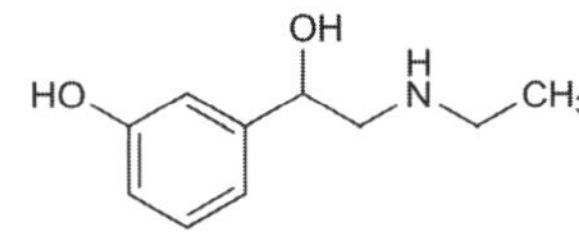

A white crystalline powder. M.p. 147° to 148°.
Soluble 1 in 25 of water and 1 in 15 of ethanol.

Etilefrine Hydrochloride

Proprietary names. Adrenam; Bioflutin-N; Cardanat; Cardialgine; Circupon RR; Circuvit-E; Effortil; Efortil; Efxine; Hyprosia; Thomasin; Tonus-forte-Tablinen; Tri-Effortil.
$C_{10}H_{15}NO_2$,HCl=217.7
CAS—534-87-2
A white crystalline powder. M.p. 121°.
Freely soluble in water; soluble in ethanol; practically insoluble in chloroform.

Dissociation Constant. pK_a 9.0, 10.2 (25°).

Partition Coefficient. Log *P* (octanol/water), 0.3.

Colour Tests. Folin–Ciocalteu Reagent—blue; Liebermann's Test—black; Mandelin's Test—grey→green→brown; Marquis Test—red

Thin-layer Chromatography. System TA—Rf 41; system TB—Rf 02; system TC—Rf 02; system TE—Rf 22; system TL—Rf 3; system TAE—Rf 15; system TAF—Rf 74. (Acidified potassium permanganate solution, positive.)

Gas Chromatography. System GA—etilefrine RI 1685, etilefrine-AC_3 RI 2150, etilefrine-Me_2-AC RI 2000.

High Performance Liquid Chromatography. System HX—RI 118; system HY—RI 142.

Ultraviolet Spectrum. Aqueous acid—272 nm (A^1_1=102a); aqueous alkali—237 nm (A^1_1=491b), 290 nm (A^1_1=167a).

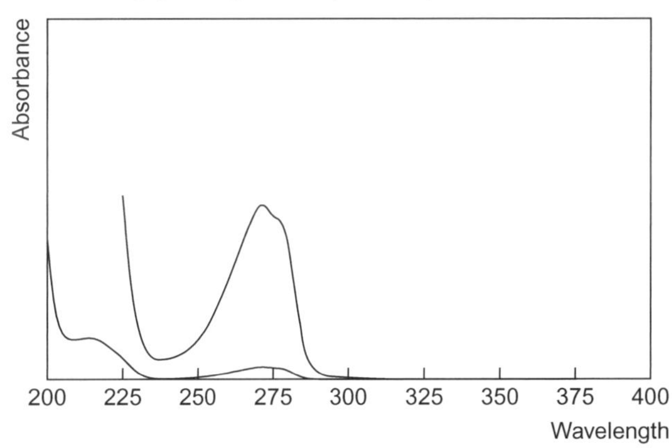

Infra-red Spectrum. Principal peaks at wavenumbers 1597, 1068, 797, 1305, 1279, 1222 cm^{-1} (etilefrine hydrochloride, KBr disk).

Mass Spectrum. Principal ions at *m/z* 58, 30, 59, 77, 29, 95, 65, 57.

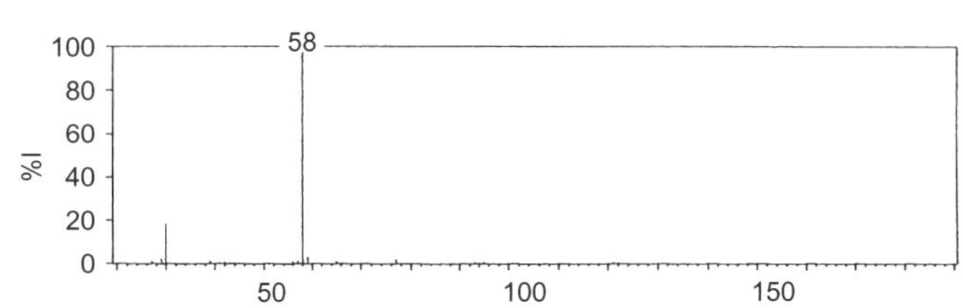

Dose. Etilefrine hydrochloride has been given in doses of 15 to 50 mg daily.

Etisazole

Antifungal (Veterinary)

N-Ethyl-1,2-benzisothiazol-3-ylamine
$C_9H_{10}N_2S$=178.3

CAS—7716-60-1

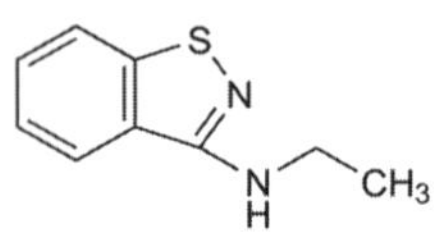

A white to slightly brown crystalline powder. M.p. 78°.

Etisazole Hydrochloride
Proprietary name. Netrosylla
$C_9H_{10}N_2S,HCl = 214.7$
CAS—7716-59-8
A crystalline powder. M.p. 182° to 186°.
Sparingly soluble in water; freely soluble in ethanol and methanol; slightly soluble in chloroform and ether.

Partition Coefficient. Log *P* (octanol/water), 2.3.

Colour Test. Liebermann's Test—red-brown.

Thin-layer Chromatography. System TA—Rf 74. (Acidified iodoplatinate solution, positive.)

Gas Chromatography. System GA—RI 1668.

Ultraviolet Spectrum. Aqueous acid—232 nm ($A_1^1 = 1200b$), 323 nm.

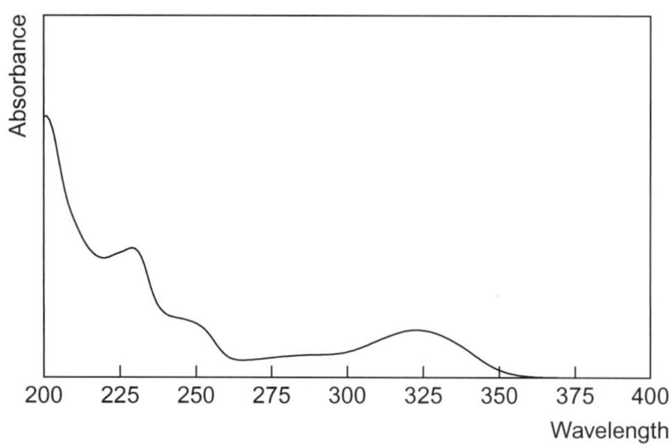

Infra-red Spectrum. Principal peaks at wavenumbers 1608, 1314, 1292, 772, 706, 1111 (KBr disk).

Etizolam

Anxiolytic

Synonyms. AHR-3219; Y-7131.
Proprietary names. Depas; Pasaden.
4-(2-Chlorophenyl)-2-ethyl-9-methyl-6*H*-thieno[3,2-*f*][1,2,4]triazolo-[4,3-*a*][1,4]diazepine
$C_{17}H_{15}ClN_4S = 342.9$
CAS—40054-69-1

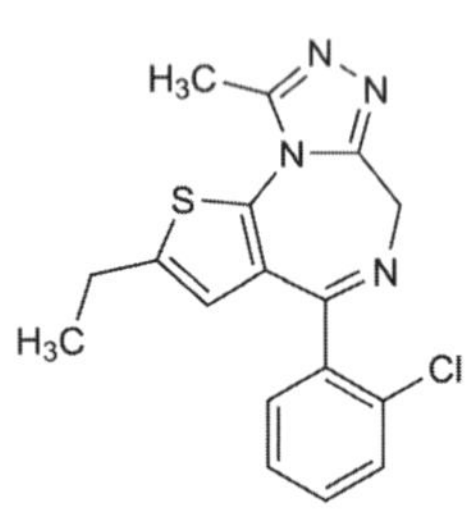

A white crystalline powder with M.p. 147° to 148°. It is insoluble in water; soluble in ethanol and chloroform.

Partition Coefficient. Log *P* (octanol/water), 3.1.

Thin-layer Chromatography. System TE—Rf 52; system TAE—Rf 72.

Plate: silica gel 60 F254 (10 × 10 cm). Mobile phase 1: cyclohexane: toluene:diethylamine (75:15:10); mobile phase 2: chloroform:methanol (90:10); mobile phase 3: chloroform:acetone (80:20). Dragendorff's reagent was used to visualise the spots. Rf 4 (mobile phase 1); Rf 45 (mobile phase 2); Rf 13 (mobile phase 3) [K. Otsubo *et al.*, *J. Chromatogr.*, 1995, *669*, *Biomed. Appl.*, 408–412].

Gas Chromatography. System GA—RI 2980.

High Performance Liquid Chromatography. System HAF—retention time 18.4 min.

Ultraviolet Spectrum. Aqueous acid (ethanol)—243 nm; aqueous acid—250, 294, 362 nm; aqueous alkali—243 nm.

Infra-red Spectrum. Principal peaks at wavenumbers 764, 1410, 1615, 1380, 1040, 1524 cm^{-1} (KBr disc).

Mass Spectrum. Principal ions at *m/z* 342, 18, 28, 266, 313, 224, 239, 45.

Quantification
High performance liquid chromatography. In plasma and urine: limits of detection are 2.5 µg/L and 1 µg/L, respectively—C. Fracasso *et al.*, *Eur. J. Clin. Pharmacol.*, 1991, *40(2)*, 181–185. In blood: limit of quantification 5 µg/L. UV detection (λ = 254 nm)—E. Tanaka *et al.*, *J. Chromatogr.*, 1996, *682, Biomed. Appl.*, 173–178.

Disposition in the Body. Etizolam is rapidly absorbed after oral administration and is almost entirely eliminated by non-renal pathways. Peak plasma concentrations are reached within 0.5 to 2 h. There is little accumulation of the drug in the body and elimination is by biotransformation of the drug; mainly microsomal oxidation to produce hydroxylated derivatives which are subsequently conjugated. The main metabolite is α-hydroxyetizolam (20% of which is in the unconjugated form) and is pharmacologically active as opposed to the other metabolites which are not.

Therapeutic concentration
6 healthy males, aged between 20 and 32 years (mean 26 years), were administered a 0.5 mg etizolam after an overnight fast. A peak plasma concentration of 8.3 µg/L was observed 0.9 h after dosing. Multiple dosing of 0.5 mg every 12 h for 1 week was also carried out. Peak plasma concentrations for the parent drug and its metabolite, α-hydroxyetizolam, were 9.3 µg/L and 9.9 µg/L, respectively observed at 1.2 and 2.5 h. [C. Fracasso *et al.*, *Eur. J. Clin. Pharmacol.*, 1991, *40(2)*, 181–185].

Half-life. Approx. 3.4 h.

Volume of distribution. 0.9 L (after a single 0.5 mg dose); usually referred to as 1.0 L/kg.

Clearance. Oral, between 10.4 and 19.3 (mean 13.8) L/h (after a single 0.5 mg dose).

Protein binding. Approx. 93%.

Dose. 1.5 to 3 mg daily.

Etodolac

Anti-inflammatory

Synonyms. AY-24236: CCRIS 3923; Etodolic Acid; NSC-282126.
Proprietary names. Edolan; Lodine; Ramoder; Tedolan; Ultradol; Zedolac.
1,8-Diethyl-1,3,4,9-tetrahydropyrano- [3,4-*b*]indole-1-acetic acid
$C_{17}H_{21}NO_3 = 287.4$
CAS—41340-25-4

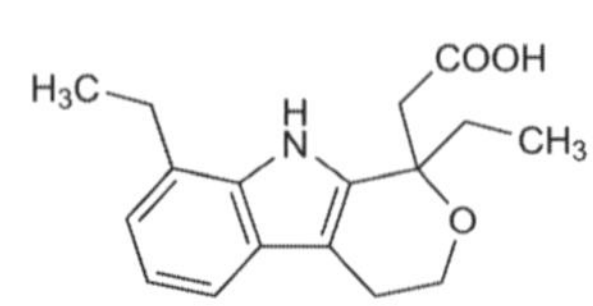

A white to almost white crystalline powder. It is practically insoluble in water; freely soluble in alcohol, chloroform, dimethyl sulfoxide and aqueous polyethylene glycol. M.p. 145° to 148°.

Dissociation Constant. pK_a 4.65.

Partition Coefficient. Log *P* (octanol/water), 3.93; (pH 7.4), 11.4.

Gas Chromatography. System GL—RI 2225 (etodolac-ME).

Column: methyl silicone (HP1, 0.2 mm i.d., 0.33 µm film thickness). Column temperature: 250°. Carrier gas: helium, 0.9 mL/min flow rate. Detection: mass spectrometer. Retention index: 2333 [T. Mills and J. C. Roberson, 1993. *Instrumental Data for Drug Analysis*, CRC Press, Boca Raton, USA, 2nd Edn,Vol. 6, pp. 80–81].

High Performance Liquid Chromatography. System HAA—retention time 21.5 min.

Column: (analytical) RP-18 (LiChrosorb, 250 × 4.0 mm i.d., 7 µm), (guard) (40 × 4.0 mm). Mobile phase: aqueous acetic acid (1%):acetonitrile (50:50), 1.3 mL/min flow rate. UV detection (λ=227 nm). Retention time: 8.5 min [M. R. Koupai-Abyazani *et al.*, *J. Anal. Toxicol.*, 1999, *23*, 200–209].

Column: (analytical) silica (Partisil 5 Silica, 5 µm, 250 × 4.6 mm i.d.), (guard) (5 cm, packed with 30 to 38 µm silica-coated glass beads). Mobile phase:hexane:ethyl acetate:isopropanol (85:15:0.2), 2 mL/min flow rate. UV detection (λ=280 nm). Retention time: *R*-enantiomer of etodolac, 21.9 min; *S*-enatiomer, 29.5 min [F. Jamali *et al.*, *J. Pharm. Sci.*, 1988, *77(11)*, 963–966].

Column: ODS Hypersil (100 × 4.6 mm i.d., 5 µm). Mobile phase: methanol, 1 mL/min flow rate. UV (λ=280 nm). Retention time: 2.8 min [T. Mills and J. C. Roberson, 1993. *Instrumental Data for Drug Analysis*, CRC Press, Boca Raton, USA, 2nd Edn, Vol. 6, pp. 80–81].

Ultraviolet Spectrum. Aqueous acid (0.2 M H_2SO_4)—272 nm; basic—274 nm.

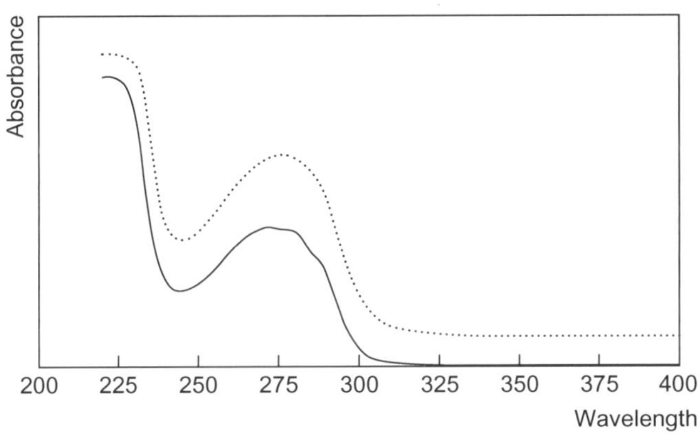

Infra-red Spectrum. Principal peaks at wavenumbers 1746, 1412, 1034, 748 cm^{-1} (KBr pellet).

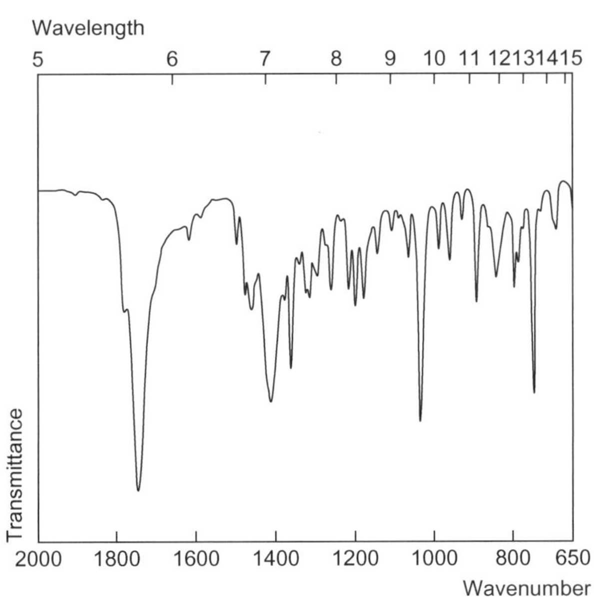

Mass Spectrum. Principal ions at *m/z* 228, 258, 287, 198, 57, 229, 259, 214.

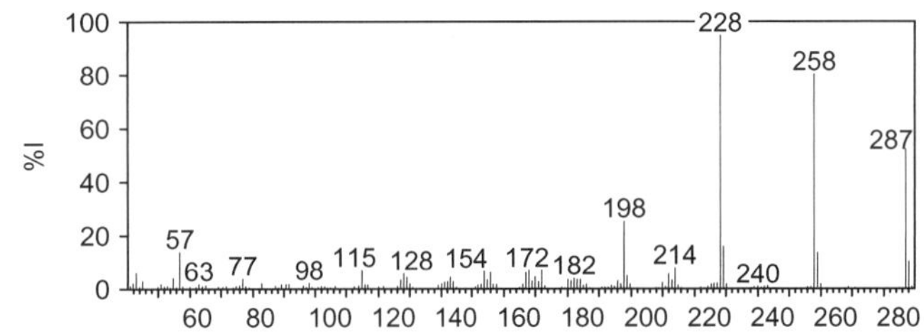

Quantification

High performance liquid chromatography. In serum and urine: limit of detection is 0.03 mg/L and 0.3 mg/L, respectively, limit of quantification is 0.04 mg/L and 0.4 mg/L, respectively. UV detection (λ=227 nm)—M. R. Koupai-Abyazani *et al.*, *J. Anal. Toxicol.*, 1999, *23*, 200–209.

Disposition in the Body. Etodolac is well absorbed after oral administration and extensively metabolised in the liver, via hydroxylation followed by conjugation and acyl glucuronidation. The drug is easily distributed into synovial fluid. Etodolac is primarily excreted in urine but also in faeces. 1% of a dose is detected unchanged in urine with hydroxylated etodolac (46%), glucuronidated etodolac (13%), hydroxylated metabolites (5%), hydroxylated glucuronide metabolites (20%) and 4-ureidoetodolac metabolite.

Therapeutic concentration. The serum therapeutic concentration range is 20 to 50 mg/L.

> 14 healthy male volunteers, with a mean age of 27 years, were administered a 400 mg dose of etodolac (in a solution and as the sustained release formulation). Peak plasma concentrations of 36.8 mg/L were reached within 0.55 h and 7.5 mg/L within 7.9 h, respectively [M. Dey *et al.*, *Int. J. Pharm.*, 1989, *49*, 121–128].

Toxicity. Gastro-intestinal toxicity including bleeding and perforation has been reported with overdosing as well as a case of coma.

Bioavailability. 80 to 100 %.

Half-life. 7 h.

Volume of distribution. 0.3 to 0.5 L/kg.

Clearance. 40 to 47 mL/h/kg.

Protein binding. 99%.

Dose. Patient with body weight >60 kg: a usual dose of 200 to 400 mg is administered every 6 to 8 h with a maximum of 1200 g daily. Patient <60 kg: maximum 20 mg/kg body weight daily.

Etofenamate

Analgesic

Proprietary names. Activon; Afrolate; Algesalona; Bayro; Etofen; Fenogel; Flexium; Flogoprofen; Reumon; Rheuma-Gel; Rheumon; Traumalix; Traumon; Zenavan.

2-[[3-(Trifluoromethyl)phenyl]amino]benzoic acid 2-(2-hydroxyethoxy)ethyl ester

$C_{18}H_{18}F_3NO_4$=369.3

CAS—30544-47-9

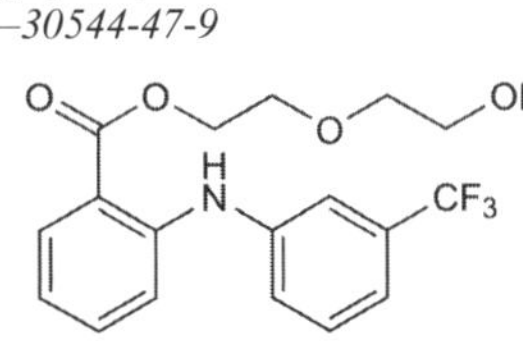

A pale yellow viscous liquid.

Practically insoluble in water; soluble in organic solvents.

Partition Coefficient. Log *P* (octanol/water), 4.2.

Thin-layer Chromatography. System TE—Rf 78; system TAE—Rf 89.

Ultraviolet Spectrum. Aqueous acid—284 nm (A^1_1=287b), 349 nm (A^1_1=165b).

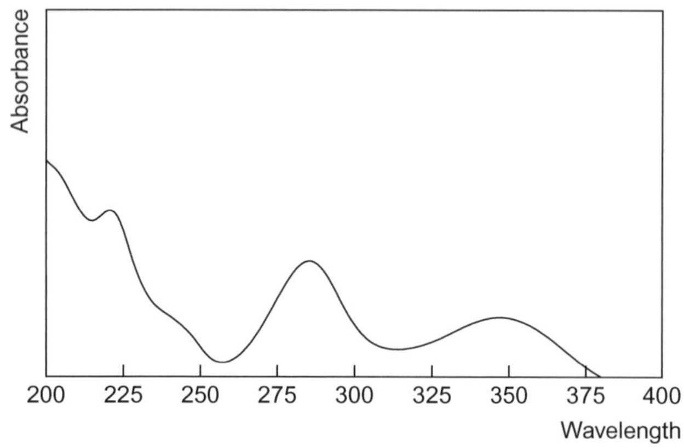

Quantification
Gas chromatography. In plasma, tissues or urine: FID—H.-D. Dell *et al.*, *Arzneimittelforschung.*, 1981, *31*, 17–21.

Disposition in the Body. Well absorbed from the gastro-intestinal tract and through the skin. The unchanged drug is found in small amounts in urine, together with hydroxylated derivatives of etofenamate and flufenamic acid.

Therapeutic concentration.
Following a single oral dose of 300 mg to 6 subjects, a mean peak plasma concentration of 10.0 mg/L was attained in 1 h; following topical administration of 6 g to 6 subjects, a mean peak plasma concentration of 0.15 mg/L was attained in 2 h [H.-D. Dell *et al.*, *Arzneimittelforschung.*, 1977, *27*, 1322–1325].

Half-life. Plasma half-life, about 1.6 h after ingestion and about 3.3 h after topical administration.

Use. Topically in a concentration of 5%.

Etofylline

Xanthine Bronchodilator

Synonyms. Aethophyllinum; Hydroxyethyltheophyllinum; Oxyetophylline.
Proprietary names. Actophlem; Alcophyllex; Apoplectal; Bio-Phyllin; Coroverlan; Dilinct; Flebo Stop; Instenon; Oxyphylline; Perphyllon; Solphyllex; Solphyllin; Theophen; Theo-Talusin.
3,7-Dihydro-7-(2-hydroxyethyl)-1,3-dimethyl-1*H*-purine-2,6-dione
$C_9H_{12}N_4O_3$=224.2
CAS—519-37-9

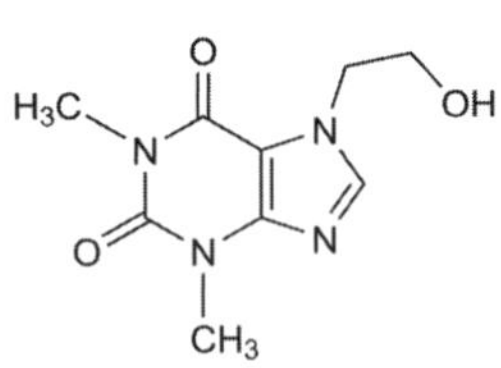

A white crystalline powder. M.p. 161° to 166°.
Freely soluble in water; moderately soluble in ethanol; sparingly soluble in chloroform; practically insoluble in ether.

Partition Coefficient. Log *P* (octanol/water), −0.8.

Thin-layer Chromatography. System TB—Rf 00; system TE—Rf 38; system TF—Rf 06; system TAE—Rf 66.

Gas Chromatography. System GA—etophylline RI 2125, etophylline-AC RI 2200, etophylline clofibrate RI 3125.

High Performance Liquid Chromatography. System HX—RI 289.

Ultraviolet Spectrum. Aqueous acid—270 nm (A_1^1=416b).

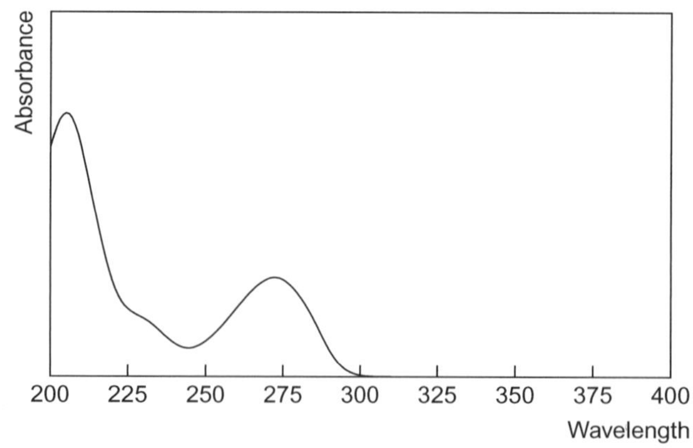

Dose. Up to 1.5 g daily.

Etomidate

General Anaesthetic

Proprietary names. Amidate; Hypnomidat(e); Radenarcon.
1-[(1*R*)-1-Phenylethyl]-1*H*-imidazole-5-carboxylic acid ethyl ester
$C_{14}H_{16}N_2O_2$=244.3
CAS—33125-97-2

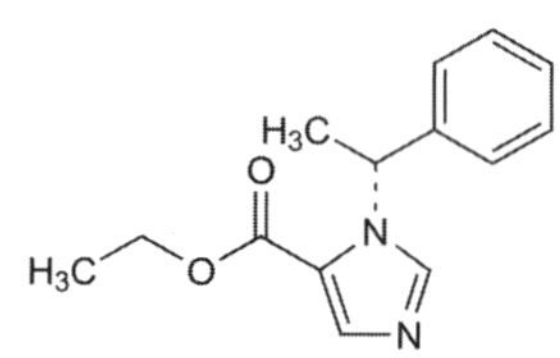

A white or yellowish crystalline or amorphous powder. M.p. about 67°.
Solubility in water at 25°, 0.0045 mg in 100 mL; soluble in chloroform, methanol, ethanol, propylene glycol and acetone.

Dissociation Constant. pK_a 4.2.

Partition Coefficient. Log *P* (octanol/water), 3.0.

Thin-layer Chromatography. System TA—Rf 67; system TB—Rf 26; system TC—Rf 71; system TE—Rf 73; system TL—Rf 52; system TAE—Rf 78; system TAF—Rf 85.

Gas Chromatography. System GA—etomidate RI 1870, M (COOH-)-Me RI 1840.

High Performance Liquid Chromatography. System HX—RI 475; system HY—RI 417.

Ultraviolet Spectrum. Water—242 nm (A_1^1=450b).

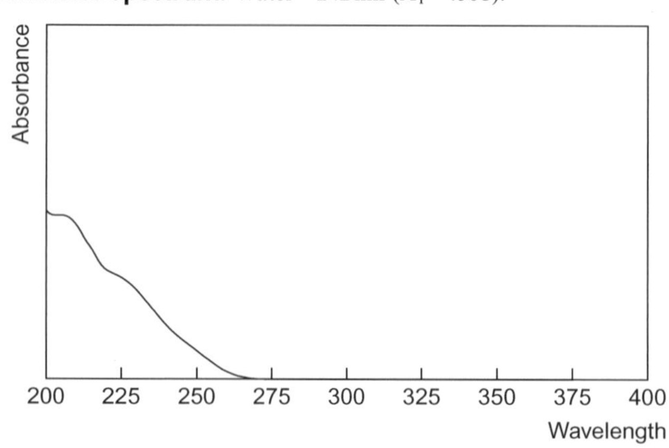

Infra-red Spectrum. Principal peaks at wavenumbers 1212, 1708, 712, 1112, 1132, 664 cm^{-1} (KBr disk).

Mass Spectrum. Principal ions at *m/z* 105, 104, 77, 79, 244, 106, 108, 27.

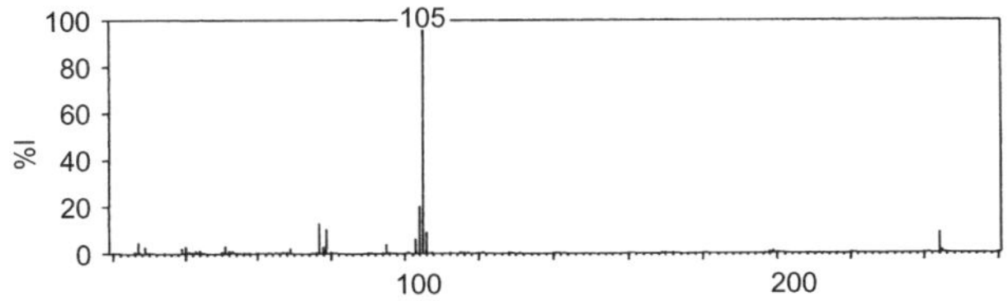

Quantification

Gas chromatography. In plasma: limit of detection 5 μg/L, AFID—A. G. de Boer *et al.*, *J. Chromatogr.*, 1979, *162*; *Biomed. Appl.*, *4*, 591–595.

Gas chromatography–mass spectrometry. In plasma: limit of detection 1 μg/L—M. J. Van Hamme *et al.*, *J. Pharm. Sci.*, 1977, *66*, 1344–1346.

High performance liquid chromatography. In plasma: limit of detection 2 μg/L, UV detection—E. O. Ellis and P. R. Beck, *J. Chromatogr.*, 1982, *232*; *Biomed. Appl.*, *21*, 207–211. In plasma—M. P. McIntosh and R. A. Rajewski, *J. Pharm. Biomed. Anal.*, 2001, *24*, 689–694.

Disposition in the Body. Rapidly distributed after intravenous injection. It is metabolised in the liver by hydrolysis and *N*-dealkylation to inactive metabolites. About 90% of a dose is excreted in the urine as the carboxylic acid derivative, together with mandelic acid and benzoic acid; less than 5% is excreted as unchanged drug.

Therapeutic concentration

After intravenous injection of 0.3 mg/kg to 8 subjects, plasma concentrations of 0.22 to 0.41 mg/L (mean 0.32) were reported at 4 min [M. J. Van Hamme *et al.*, *Anesthesiology*, 1978, *49*, 274–277].

Half-life. Plasma half-life, 2 to 11 h (mean 5).

Volume of distribution. About 4 to 5 L/kg.

Clearance. Plasma clearance, 9 to 18 mL/min/kg.

Distribution in blood. Plasma:whole blood ratio, 0.62.

Protein binding. In plasma, about 75%.

Dose. 300 μg/kg intravenously, with supplementary doses of 100 to 200 μg/kg, as required.

Etoposide

Antineoplastic

Synonyms. EPEG; NSC-141540; VP-16; VP-16-213.
Proprietary names. Celltop; Eposin; Exitop; Lastet; Toposar; Vepesid; Vepeside.
9-[(4,6-*O*-Ethylidene-β-D-glucopyranosyl)oxy]-5,8,8a,9-tetrahydro-5-(4-hydroxy-3,5-dimethoxyphenyl)furo[3',4':6,7]naphtho[2,3-*d*]-1,3-dioxol-6(5a*H*)-one
$C_{29}H_{32}O_{13}$=588.6
CAS—33419-42-0

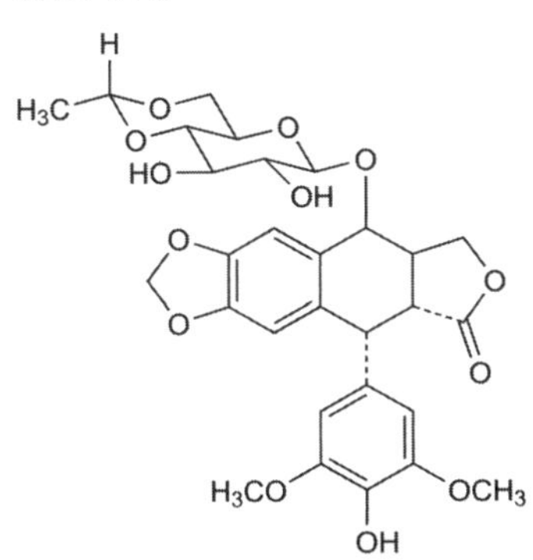

A fine white, or almost white, crystalline powder. M.p. 236° to 251°. It is practically insoluble or very slightly soluble in water; slightly soluble in ethanol, in chloroform, in dichloromethane, in ethyl acetate, and in methylene chloride; sparingly soluble in methanol.

Etoposide Phosphate
Proprietary name. Etopophos
$C_{29}H_{33}O_{16}P$=668.6

Dissociation Constant. pK_a 9.8.

Partition Coefficient. Log *P* (octanol/water), 0.60.

High Performance Liquid Chromatography. Column: phenyl (μBondapak, 300 × 3.9 mm, 10 μm). Mobile phase: acetonitrile:water:glacial acetic acid (35:64:1), 1.0 mL/min flow rate. Fluorescence detection (λ_{ex}=288 nm, λ_{em}=328 nm). Internal standard (IS): teniposide. Retention times: etoposide, 6.5 min; IS, 18 min [I. Robieux *et al.*, *J. Chromatogr.*, 1996, *686*, *Biomed. Appl.*, 35–41].

Column: ODS Hypersil Si-10 (300 × 4 mm i.d., 10 μm). Mobile phase: methanol with 1% NHOH: methylene chloride (2:98), flow rate 2 mL/min. UV detection (λ=254 nm). Retention time: 4.6 min [T. Mills and J. C. Roberson, 1993. *Instrumental Data for Drug Analysis*, CRC Press, Boca Raton, USA, 2nd Edn, Vol. 1, pp. 908–909].

Ultraviolet Spectrum. Methanol—283 nm (A_1^1=72.2); ethanol—284, 291 nm.

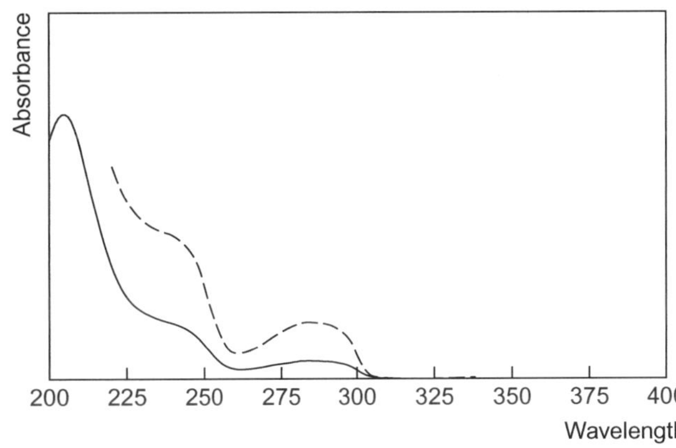

Infra-red Spectrum. Principal peaks at wavenumbers 1775, 1610, 1515, 1485, 1250 cm^{-1}.

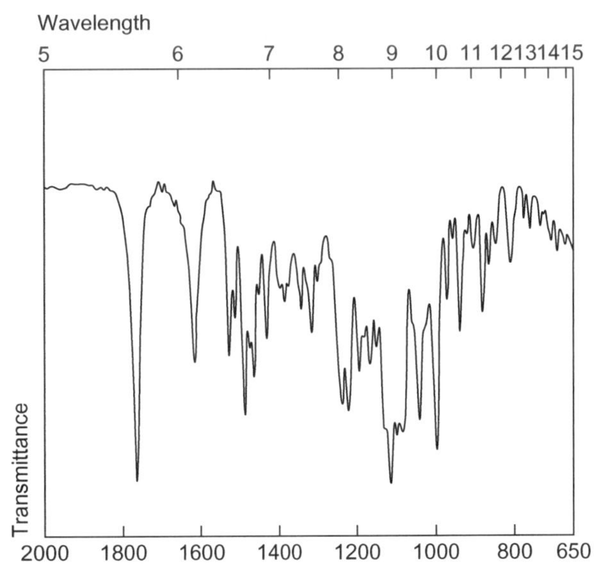

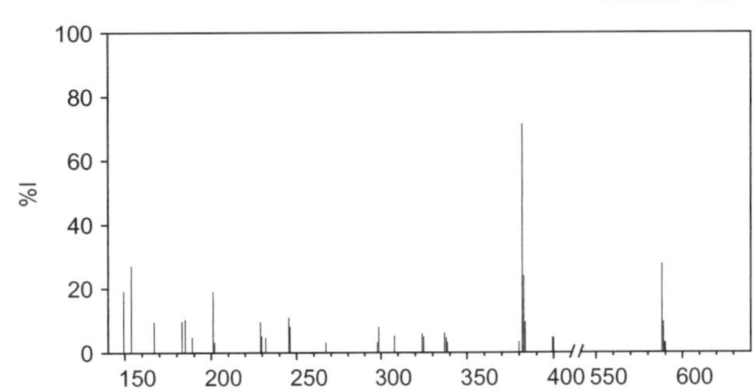

Quantification

High performance liquid chromatography. In plasma or urine: limit of detection 100 µg/L, UV detection—V. J. Harvey *et al.*, *J. Chromatogr.*, 1985, *339*, *Biomed. Appl.*, *40*, 419–423. In plasma: limit of detection 50 µg/L, fluorescence detection—I. Robieux *et al.*, *J. Chromatogr.*, 1996, *686*, *Biomed. Appl.*, 35–41. In serum, plasma, or urine: limit of detection 0.008 µg in plasma, fluorescence detection—C. E. Werkhoven-Goewie *et al.*, *J. Chromatogr.*, 1983, *276*, 349–57. In plasma: limit of detection 10 µg/L, electrochemical detection—G. F. Duncan *et al.*, *J. Chromatogr.*, 1986, *380*, *Biomed. Appl.*, *53*, 357–365. In plasma: limit of detection 5 µg/L, electrochemical detection—T. J. Littlewood *et al.*, *J. Chromatogr.*, 1984, *336*, *Biomed. Appl.*, *37*, 434–437. In plasma: limit of detection 0.01 µg/L, electrochemical detection—A. el-Yazigi and C. R. Martin, *Clin. Chem.*, 1987, *33*, 803–805.

Disposition in the Body. Pharmacokinetics show wide interindividual variation. Absorption is variable after oral administration, but on average about 50% of a dose is absorbed. Peak plasma concentrations occur 0.5 to 3 h after oral administration. Undergoes rapid distribution. It is metabolised to several metabolites, including a hydroxy acid metabolite, glucuronide and sulfate conjugates, and an *O*-demethylated compound. Excreted in urine and via bile in the faeces (a small amount) as unchanged drug and metabolites; 30 to 50% of a dose is excreted in urine over 72 h as the unchanged drug and 20% as metabolites. Crosses the blood–brain barrier poorly; concentrations in CSF about 1 to 10% of those in plasma. It is distributed into breast milk.

Therapeutic concentration. The trough serum therapeutic concentration range is 2 to 6 mg/L and peak, 8 to 14 mg/L.

12 patients with biopsy-proven cancer, less than 65 years old, were split into four groups and administered either 400, 500, 600 or 800 mg/m^2 daily via a 2- to 3-h infusion. The maximum plasma-etoposide concentration following infusion of 400 mg/m^2 for 3 consecutive days ranged from 26 to 53 mg/L, 27 to 73 mg/L for the 500 mg/m^2 dose, 42 to 114 mg/L for 600 mg/m^2 and 72 mg/L for the single patient administered 800 mg/m^2. These concentrations were observed during the infusion period [K. R. Hande *et al.*, *Cancer Res.*, 1984, *44*, 379–382].

15 adult patients with various malignancies, aged between 25 and 74 years, were administered 80 to 120 mg/m^2 etoposide over 30 to 60 min. All patients were receiving polychemotherapy as well. A mean peak concentration of 24.2 mg/L was observed [K-H. Pfluger *et al.*, *Cancer Chemother. Pharmacol.*, 1987, *20*, 59–66].

Toxicity. Etoposide doses of 2.4 to 3.5 mg/m^2 administered intravenously over 3 days caused severe mucositis and myelotoxicity. Metabolic acidosis and cases of severe hepatotoxicity have also been reported with doses above the recommended [Bristol Myers Squibb Pharmaceuticals Ltd., prescribing data].
The dose-limiting toxicity is dose-related myelosuppression.

Half-life. Plasma half-life, 3 to 19 h.

Volume of distribution. Adults, 7 to 17 L/m^2; children, 5 to 10 L/m^2.

Clearance. Plasma, adult, 15 to 35 mL/min/m^2 (0.9 to 2.1 L/h/m^2); children, 20 to 40 mL/min/m^2 (1.2 to 2.4 L/h/m^2).

Protein binding. In plasma, about 94%.

Note. For reviews of etoposide, see J. M. Henwood and R. N. Brogden, *Drugs*, 1990, *39*, 438–490 and P. I. Clark and M. L. Slevin, *Clin. Pharmacokinet.*, 1987, *12*, 223–252.

Dose. From 120 mg/m^2 up to 240 mg/m^2 of etoposide intravenously daily for five days. Oral dose is twice the intravenous dose.

Etorphine

Narcotic Analgesic (Veterinary)

Synonyms. 19-Propylorvinol; M-99
(−)-[5α,7α(*R*)]-4,5-Epoxy-3-hydroxy-6-methoxy-α,17-dimethyl-α-propyl-6,14-ethenomorphinan-7-methanol
$C_{25}H_{33}NO_4$=411.5
CAS—14521-96-1

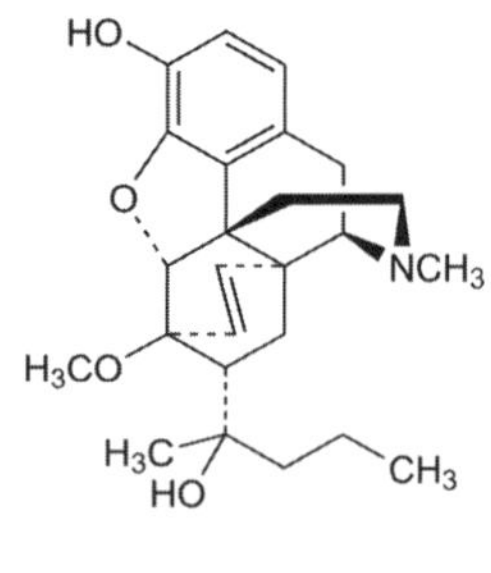

M.p. 214° to 217°.
Soluble 1 in 30 000 of water; freely soluble in ethanol, chloroform, and ether.
Caution. It is dangerous to smell or taste this material.

Etorphine Hydrochloride

Proprietary name. It is an ingredient of Immobilon.
$C_{25}H_{33}NO_4,HCl$=448.0
CAS—13764-49-3
A white microcrystalline powder. M.p. 266° to 267°.
Soluble 1 in 40 of water, 1 in 30 of ethanol, and 1 in 2200 of chloroform; practically insoluble in ether.

Partition Coefficient. Log *P* (octanol/pH 7.4), 1.9.

Colour Test. Marquis Test—blue-grey→yellow-brown.

Thin-layer Chromatography. System TA—Rf 73; system TB—Rf 08; system TC—Rf 61; system TE—Rf 72; system TL—Rf 63; system TAE—Rf 84; system TAJ—Rf 52; system TAK—Rf 00; system TAL—Rf 60. (Acidified iodoplatinate solution, positive; Marquis reagent, grey; acidified potassium permanganate solution, positive.)

Gas Chromatography. System GA—RI 3033; system GB—RI 3211; system GM—not eluted.

High Performance Liquid Chromatography. System HA—*k* 0.6; system HC—*k* 1.11; system HX—RI 344; system HY—RI 292.

Ultraviolet Spectrum. Aqueous acid—289 (A^1_1=37a); aqueous alkali—302 nm (A^1_1=65a).

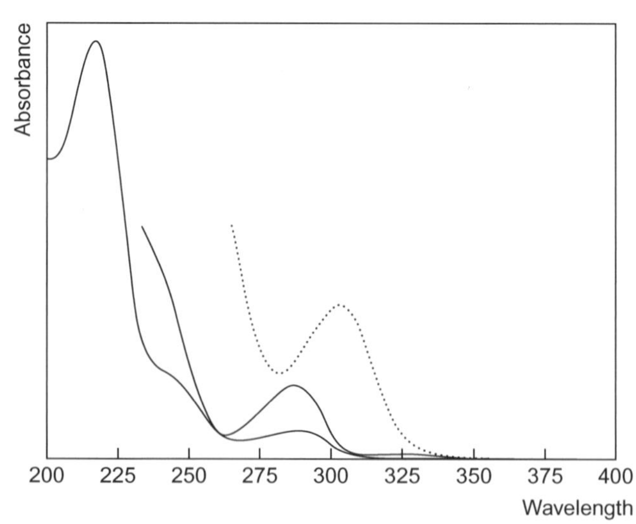

Infra-red Spectrum. Principal peaks at wavenumbers 1113, 1195, 1205, 1155, 1088, 1005 cm^{-1}.

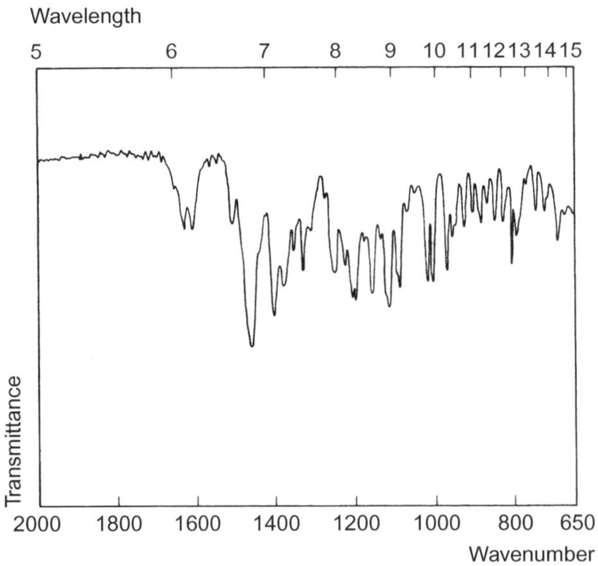

Mass Spectrum. Principal ions at m/z 44, 215, 411, 324, 45, 164, 42, 216.

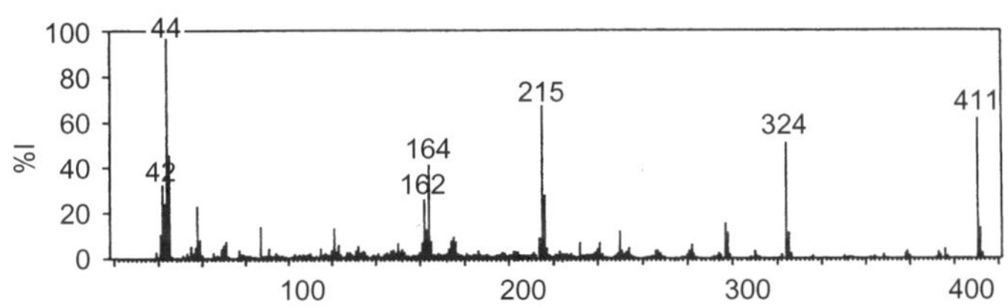

Quantification

Gas chromatography–mass spectrometry. In urine (equine): limit of detection 0.1 µg/L—Y. Bonnaire *et al.*, *J. Anal. Toxicol.*, 1989, *13*, 193–196.

High performance liquid chromatography. In postmortem blood: UV diode-array detection—S. P. Elliott and K. A. Hale, *Forensic Sci. Int.*, 1999, *101*, 9–16.

Disposition in the Body.

Toxicity. It is up to 400 times more potent than morphine; several cases of poisoning, including one fatality, have been reported after accidental pricking of the skin with an injection needle.

A 54-year-old vet whose death was suspected to be due to parenteral administration of etorphine had the following postmortem tissue concentrations: femoral blood 14.5 µg/L, heart blood 23.5 µg/L, urine 0 µg/L. [S. P. Elliott and K. A. Hale, *Forensic Sci. Int.*, 1999, *101*, 9–16.]

Use. With acepromazine as a sedative for the control of large animals, and with levomepromazine as a neuroleptanalgesic in small animals.

Etoxazene

Analgesic

Synonyms. *p*-Ethoxychrysoidine; Ethoxazene.
4-(4-Ethoxyphenylazo)benzene-1,3-diyldiamine
$C_{14}H_{16}N_4O$=256.3
CAS—94-10-0

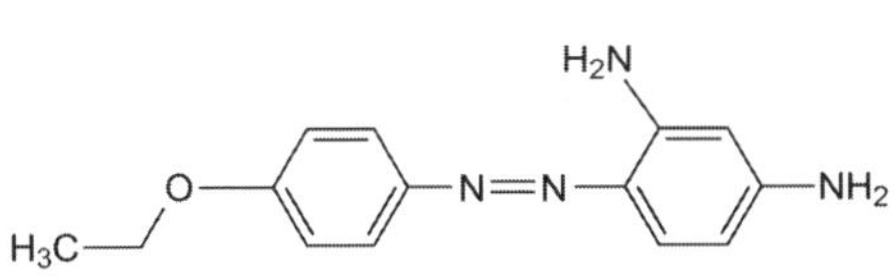

M.p. 117° to 120°.

Etoxazene Hydrochloride

Proprietary name. Serenium
$C_{14}H_{16}N_4O,HCl$=292.8
CAS—2313-87-3
A reddish powder.
Practically insoluble in water; soluble in boiling water and in ethanol.

Partition Coefficient. Log *P* (octanol/water), 2.7.

Colour Test. Marquis Test—violet

Thin-layer Chromatography. System TA—Rf 65; system TB—Rf 00; system TC—Rf 56; system TL—Rf 67; system TAJ—Rf 57; system TAK—Rf 02; system TAL—Rf 70. (Dragendorff spray, positive.)

Gas Chromatography. System GA—not eluted.

Ultraviolet Spectrum. Aqueous acid—261 nm (A^1_1=308b), 310 nm.

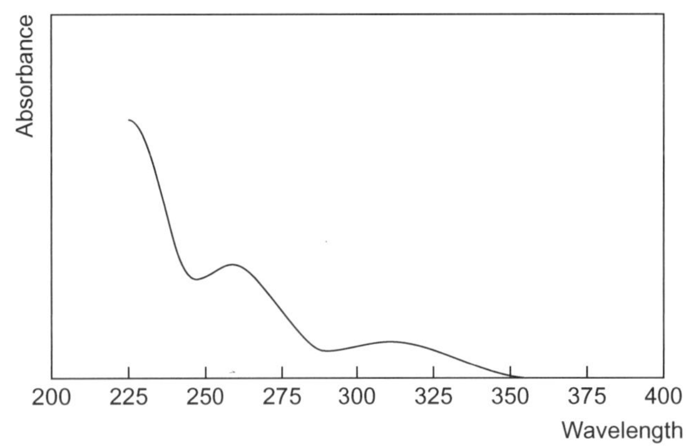

Infra-red Spectrum. Principal peaks at wavenumbers 1245, 1624, 1635, 1600, 1185, 1501 cm^{-1} (KBr disk).

Dose. Etoxazene hydrochloride has been given in doses of 300 mg daily.

Etretinate

Dermatological

Synonym. Ro-10-9359
Proprietary names. Tegison; Tigason.
(*all-E*)-9-(4-Methoxy-2,3,6-trimethylphenyl)-3,7-dimethyl-2,4,6,8-nonatetraenoic acid ethyl ester
$C_{23}H_{30}O_3$=354.5
CAS—54350-48-0

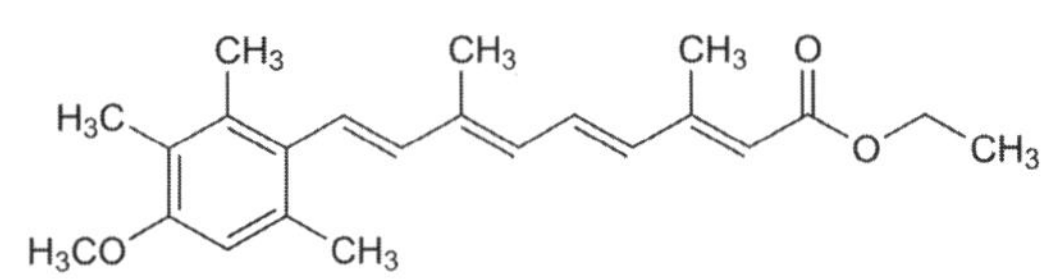

Crystals. M.p. 104° to 105°.

Gas Chromatography. Column: methyl silicone (HP1, 0.2 mm i.d., 0.33 µm film thickness). Column temperature: 280°. Carrier gas: helium, 0.9 mL/min flow rate. Detection: mass spectrometer. Retention index: 2761 [T. Mills and J. C. Roberson, 1993. *Instrumental Data for Drug Analysis*, CRC Press, Boca Raton, USA, 2nd Edn, Vol. 5, pp. 180–181].

High Performance Liquid Chromatography. Column: ODS Hypersil (100 × 4.6 mm i.d., 5 µm). Mobile phase: methanol, 1 mL/min flow rate. UV detection (λ=365 nm). Retention time: 3.4 min. [T. Mills and J. C. Roberson, *Instrumental Data for Drug Analysis*, CRC Press, 2nd Edn, Vol. 5, pp. 180–181].

Column: Nucleosil 5 C_{18} (250 × 4.6 mm), steel. Mobile phase: acetonitrile:0.1 M ammonium acetate (80:20), 2.5 mL/min flow rate. UV diode array detection. Retention time: 6.8 min [P. Jakobsen *et al.*, *J. Chromatogr.*, 1987, *415*; *Biomed. Appl.*, *59*, 413–418].

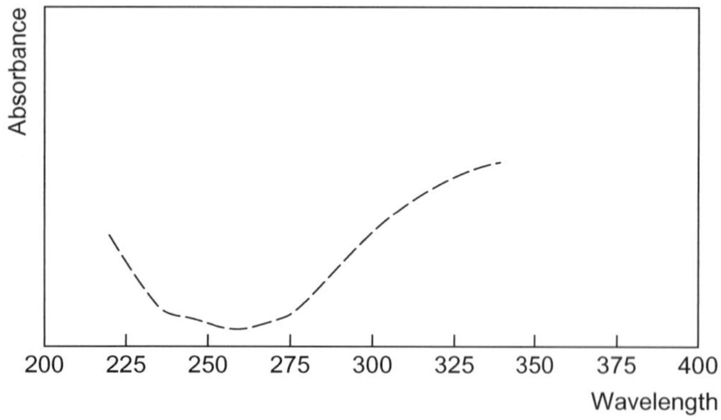

Infra-red Spectrum. Principal peaks at wavenumbers 1703, 1140, 957 cm^{-1} (KBr disk).

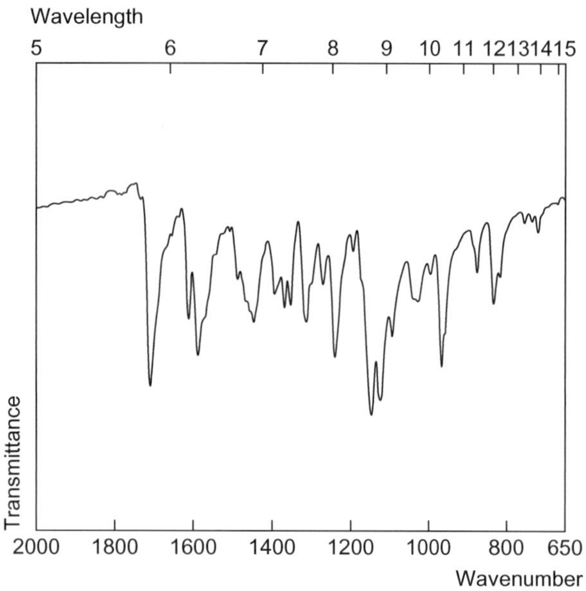

Quantification

High performance liquid chromatography. In plasma: limit of detection 1 µg/L, UV detection—P. Jakobsen *et al.*, *J. Chromatogr.*, 1987, *415*, *Biomed. Appl.*, *59*, 413–418. In plasma: limit of quantification 2 µg/L, UV detection (λ=360 nm)—R. Wyss and F. Bucheli, *J. Chromatogr.*, 1988, *431*, 297–307. In plasma: limit of detection 4 µg/L, UV detection—U. Paravicini and A. Busslinger, *J. Chromatogr.*, 1983, *276*, 359–366. In plasma: limit of detection 3 µg/L, UV detection (λ=350 nm)—A. P. De Leenheer *et al.*, *J. Chromatogr.*, 1990, *500*, 637–642. In plasma: limit of detection 25 µg/L, UV detection—J.-G. Besner *et al.*, *J. Chromatogr.*, 1982, *231*, 467–472.

Disposition in the Body. Etretinate is rapidly absorbed after an initial lag time of approx. 1 h following oral administration. Peak plasma concentrations occur after about 2 to 6 h. Absorption is increased by administration with milk or fatty food. The drug undergoes significant first-pass metabolism (hydrolysis) and the active metabolite is acitretin (the carboxyl acid, Ro 10-1670) which may itself be metabolised to etretinate. Subsequent metabolism occurs to inactive 13-*cis*-acitretin (Ro 13-7652, the major metabolite in blood following multiple dosing) and other metabolites. Etretinate accumulates in adipose tissue (especially in liver and subcutaneous fat) after repeated dosing; detectable concentrations have been found in serum up to 3 years after discontinuation of therapy. Up to 75% of a dose is excreted via bile in faeces mainly as the unchanged drug, acitretin, β-glucuronides and other minor metabolites (18 metabolites have been identified in total). It is also excreted in urine as metabolites. No intact drug is present in urine. It crosses the placenta and is distributed into breast milk.

Therapeutic concentration

Peak plasma concentrations of 180 to 353 µg/L (mean 238 µg/L) occurred after 3 to 3.5 h in patients with severe psoriasis (aged between 41 and 72 years) who had been taking 40 mg of etretinate daily for 3 months. The drug was administered after an overnight fast and also patients fasted for 3 h after dosing [F. G. Larsen *et al.*, *Pharmac. Toxicol.*, 1987, *61*, 85–88].

Toxicity. Etretinate is teratogenic at therapeutic doses.

Bioavailability. 40%.

Half-life. Plasma half-life, 120 days.

Volume of distribution. 40 L/kg (measured after oral administration).

Distribution in blood. Blood:plasma ratio, 0.60. Red blood cell:plasma, 0.11.

Protein binding. In plasma, >99% (mainly to lipoproteins).

Dose. Initially, 0.75 to 1 mg/kg per day with a maximum of 1.5 mg/kg, orally. 75 mg daily should not be exceeded.

Etynodiol Diacetate

Progestational Steroid

Proprietary names. Femulen; Lutométrodiol. It is an ingredient of Conova 30, Demulen, Normex, Ovulen and Zovia.

(3β,17α)-19-Norpregn-4-en-20-yne-3,17-diol diacetate

$C_{24}H_{32}O_4$=384.5

CAS—1231-93-2 (etynodiol); 297-76-7 (diacetate)

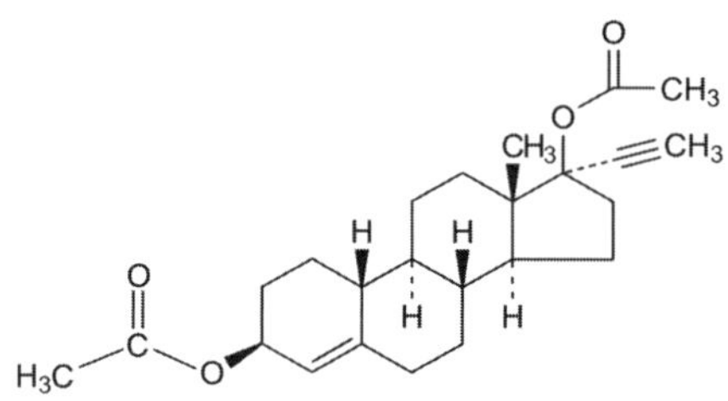

A white crystalline powder. M.p. 126° to 131°.

Very slightly soluble in water; soluble 1 in 15 of ethanol, 1 in 1 of chloroform and 1 in 3.5 of ether.

Partition Coefficient. Log *P* (octanol/water), 3.6 (etynodiol).

Thin-layer Chromatography. System TB—Rf 11; system TE—Rf 71; system TF—Rf 57; system TP—Rf 83; system TQ—Rf 61; system TR—Rf 95; system TS—Rf 99; system TAE—Rf 89.

Gas Chromatography. System GA—RI 2445 and 2779.

High Performance Liquid Chromatography. System HX—RI 549.

Infra-red Spectrum. Principal peaks at wavenumbers 1252, 1226, 1746, 1737, 1012, 1028 cm^{-1} (KBr disk).

Dose. 0.5 to 6 mg daily.

Eucatropine

Anticholinergic

α-Hydroxybenzeneacetic acid 1,2,2,6-tetramethyl-4-piperidinyl ester

$C_{17}H_{25}NO_3$=291.4

CAS—100-91-4

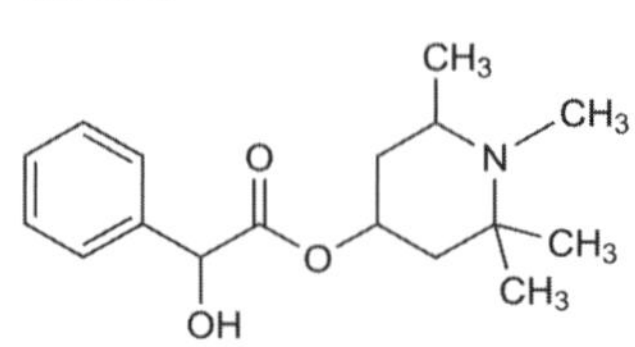

Eucatropine Hydrochloride

$C_{17}H_{25}NO_3,HCl$=327.9

CAS—536-93-6
A white granular powder. M.p. 183° to 186°.
Very soluble in water; freely soluble in ethanol and chloroform; practically insoluble in ether.

Partition Coefficient. Log *P* (octanol/water), 1.9.

Thin-layer Chromatography. System TA—Rf 46; system TB—Rf 18; system TC—Rf 13; system TE—Rf 60; system TL—Rf 12; system TAJ—Rf 03; system TAK—Rf 02; system TAL—Rf 33. (Acidified iodoplatinate solution, positive.)

Gas Chromatography. System GA—RI 2026.

Ultraviolet Spectrum. Aqueous acid—252, 258 nm (A^1_1=6.8a), 264 nm.

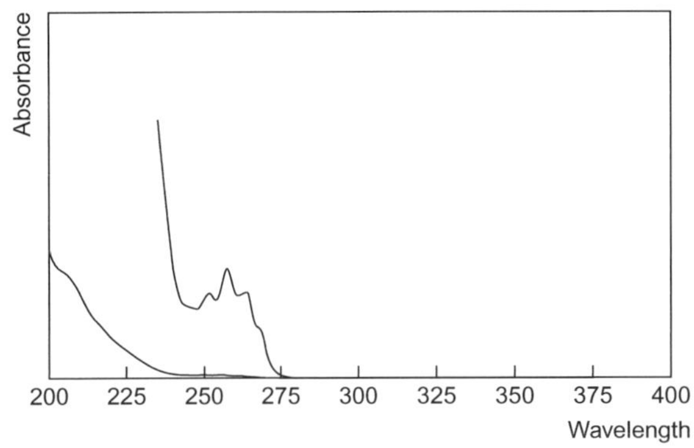

Infra-red Spectrum. Principal peaks at wavenumbers 1720, 1235, 1740, 1295, 1145, 1262 cm^{-1} (KBr disk).

Mass Spectrum. Principal ions at *m/z* 124, 276, 58, 140, 56, 72, 125, 41.

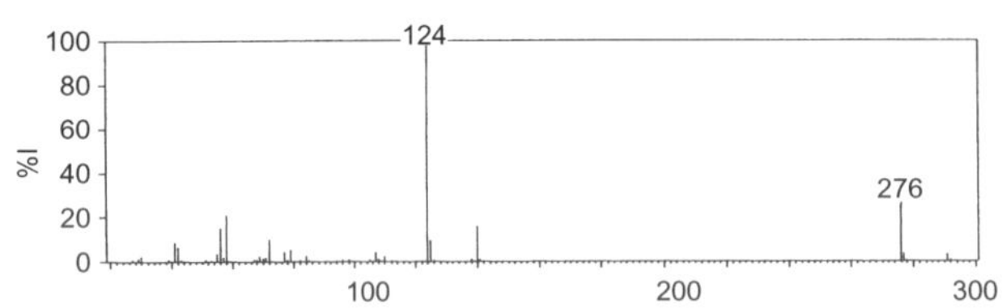

Use. Eucatropine hydrochloride is used as a 2 to 10% ophthalmic solution.

Eugenol

Essential Oil

Synonyms. 4-Allylguaiacol; Caryophyllic Acid; Eugenic Acid.
2-Methoxy-4-(2-propenyl)phenol
$C_{10}H_{12}O_2$=164.2
CAS—97-53-0

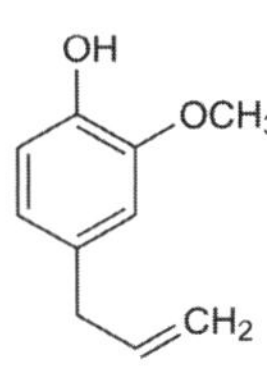

Eugenol is the principal constituent of clove oil.
A colourless or pale yellow liquid with an odour of clove. It darkens in colour with age or on exposure to air. Mass per mL 1.064 to 1.068 g. B.p. 255°. Refractive index, at 20°, 1.540 to 1.542.
Practically insoluble in water; soluble 1 in 2 of ethanol (70%); miscible with ethanol, chloroform and ether; soluble in glacial acetic acid and in aqueous fixed alkali hydroxide solutions.

Dissociation Constant. pK_a 9.8 (20°).

Partition Coefficient. Log *P* (octanol/water), 2.3.

Thin-layer Chromatography. System TA—Rf 95; system TE—Rf 87; system TAJ—Rf 85; system TAK—Rf 78; system TAL—Rf 96.

Gas Chromatography. System GA—RI 1368; system GB—RI 1380.

High Performance Liquid Chromatography. System HY—RI 430.

Ultraviolet Spectrum. Aqueous alkali—246 nm (A^1_1=552b), 296 nm (A^1_1=262b); ethanol—232 nm (A^1_1=406b), 282 nm (A^1_1=193b).

Mass Spectrum. Principal ions at *m/z* 164, 149, 131, 137, 103, 77, 133, 165.

Quantification

Gas chromatography–mass spectrometry. In urine: eugenol and other methoxyphenols—R. L. Dills *et al.*, *Environ. Res.*, 2001, *85*, 145–158.

High performance liquid chromatography. In serum, bile, or urine—I. U. Fischer and H. J. Dengler, *J. Chromatogr.*, 1990, *525*, 369–377.

Exemestane

Aromatase inhibitor/Antineoplastic

Synonym. FCE-24304
Proprietary name. Aromasin
6-Methylenandrosta-1,4-diene-3,17-dione
$C_{20}H_{24}O_2$=296.4
CAS—107868-30-4

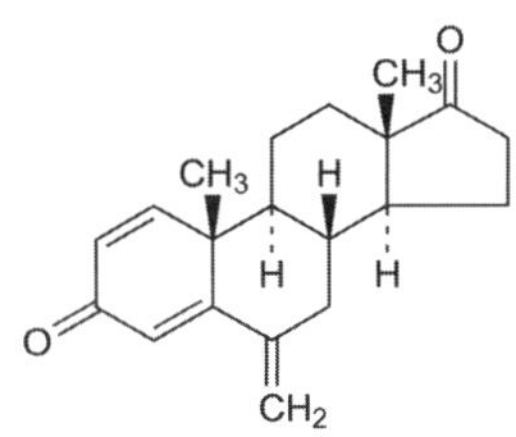

A white to slightly yellow crystalline powder. It is freely soluble in *N,N*-dimethylformamide; soluble in methanol; practically insoluble in water.

High Performance Liquid Chromatography. Column: (analytical) RP18 (Lichrocart, 125 × 4.6 mm i.d., 5 µm); (pre-column) Pellicular ODS (37 to 53 µm). Mobile phase: acetonitrile:potassium dihydrogen phosphate (0.05 M, pH 4.5) (35:65), 1.5 mL/min flow rate. UV detection (λ=247 nm). Retention time: exemestane, 14 min; 17-dihydroexemestane, 10 min [M. Breda *et al.*, *J. Chromatogr.*, 1993, *620, Biomed. Appl.*, 225–231].

Column: (analytical) Zorbax SB C_8 (150 × 4.6 mm i.d., 5 µm); (pre-column) New Guard RP 8 Aquapore Octyl (15 × 3.2 mm, 7 µm). Mobile phase: 100% acetonitrile, 1 mL/min flow rate. MS–MS detection. Retention time: 2.3 min [V. Cenacchi *et al.*, *J. Pharm. Biomed. Anal.*, 2000, *22*, 451–460].

Ultraviolet Spectrum. Aqueous acid (pH 4)—251 nm.

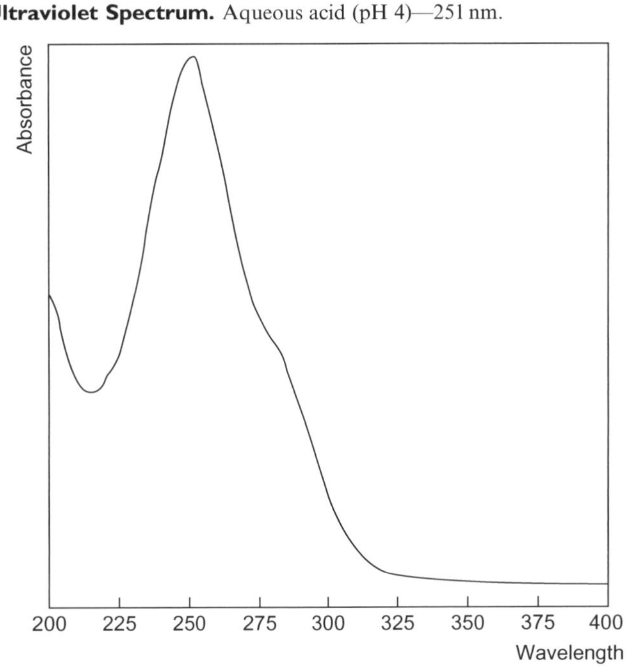

Quantification

High performance liquid chromatography. In plasma: limit of quantification 10 µg/L, UV detection (λ=247 nm)—M. Breda *et al.*, *J. Chromatogr.*, 1993, *620(2)*, 225–231. In plasma: limit of quantification 0.05 µg/L. MS–MS detection— V. Cenacchi *et al.*, *J. Pharm. Biomed. Anal.*, 2000, *22*, 451–460.

Disposition in the Body. Exemestane is rapidly absorbed after oral administration; more rapidly in women with breast cancer compared with those without. The presence of food can enhance absorption. It is extensively distributed into body tissues and is cleared from systemic circulation mainly by metabolism. The drug undergoes extensive metabolism, in the liver, by oxidation and reduction to inactive or active metabolites which are less active than the parent drug including the 17-dihydro metabolite. Plasma levels can increase, by up to 40%, when the drug is administered with a high-fat meal. Plasma levels of the metabolite, 17-hydroxyexemestane are less than one tenth of the corresponding unchanged drug level. Exemestane is excreted, equally, in both urine and faeces with less than 1% of the dose being detected unchanged in urine.

Therapeutic concentration

32 healthy post-menopausal women were administered multiple doses of 1.0, 2.5, 5.0 and 10.0 mg daily (8 volunteers each dose) for 7 days. Peak plasma concentrations were generally reached within 1 to 2 h and the concentrations measured on day 7 were 0.83, 2.18, 7.29 and 11.04 µg/L for the four doses, respectively [S. Persiani *et al.*, *Eur. J. Cancer*, 1995, *31 (Suppl.5)*, S198].

15 healthy post-menopausal women, with a mean age of 60 years (range 48 to 75 years) and a mean time from menopause of 12.3 years (2 to 36 years), were administered single doses of 50, 200, 400 and 800 mg exemestane 15 to 30 min after a high lipid breakfast. Subjects were observed for 2 weeks at each dose level before it was increased. Peak plasma concentrations, observed between 1 and 2 h, were 27, 221, 343 and 414 µg/L for the doses, respectively. [T. R. Evans *et al.*, *Cancer Res.*, 1992, *52*, 5933–5939].

Half-life. Approx. 24 to 27 h.

Clearance. Total, 517 L/h.

Distribution in blood. Distribution of the drug and its metabolites into blood cells is negligible.

Protein binding. 90% bound to plasma proteins, especially albumin and α_1-acid glycoprotein.

Dose. 25 mg once daily.

Exifone

Nootropic

Synonym. 4-Galloylpyrogallol
Proprietary name. Adlone
(2,3,4-Trihydroxyphenyl)(3,4,5-trihydroxyphenyl)methanone
$C_{13}H_{10}O_7$=278.2
CAS—52479-85-3

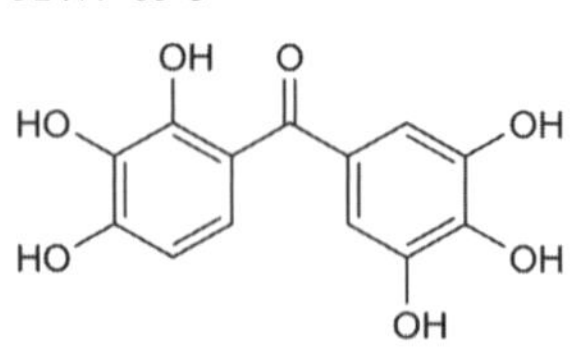

A pale yellow crystalline powder. M.p. 270°.

Partition Coefficient. Log *P* (octanol/water), 1.89.

High Performance Liquid Chromatography. Column: C_{18} RCM (NovaPak, 4 µm, 100 × 5 mm i.d.). Mobile phase: acetonitrile:orthophosphoric acid (300 mM, pH 2.2) (15:85), 0.9 mL/min flow rate. Electrochemical detection. Retention time: 8 min [J. J. Descombe *et al.*, *J. Chromatogr.*, 1989, *496*, 345–353].

Quantification

High performance liquid chromatography. In plasma and urine: limit of quantification 1.0 ng/L—J. J. Descombe *et al.*, *J. Chromatogr.*, 1989, *496*, 345–353.

Toxicity

In a reported fatality, a 74-year-old woman administered with 600 mg/day of exifone for memory loss developed hepatitis after 5 months of treatment [D. Pateron *et al.*, *Gastroenterol. Clin. Biol.*, 1990, *14*, 294–295].

Dose. 200 mg three times daily with a maximum of 1200 mg daily.

Famciclovir

Antiviral

Synonyms. BRL-42810; FCV.
Proprietary names. Famvir; Vectavir.
9-[4-Acetoxy-3-(acetoxymethyl)but-1-yl]-2-aminopurine
$C_{14}H_{19}H_5O_4$=321.3
CAS—104227-87-4

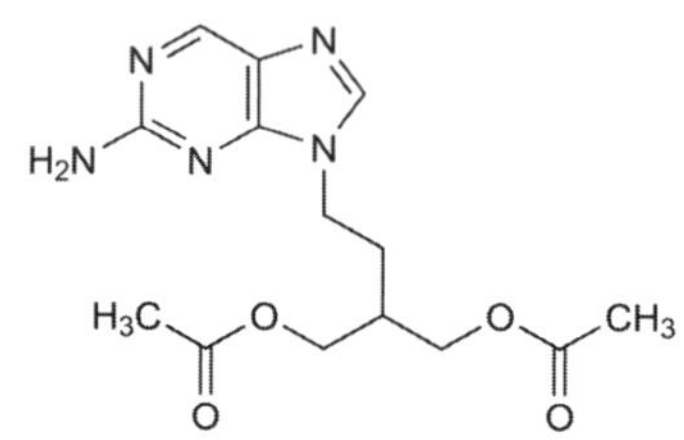

A white to pale yellow solid. M.p. 102° to 104°. It is soluble in water (>25% at 25°), acetone and methanol; sparingly soluble in ethanol and isopropanol.

Partition Coefficient. Log *P* (octanol/water, pH 4.8), 1.09; log *P* (octanol/buffer pH 7.4), 2.08.

Gas Chromatography. Column: methyl silicone (HP1, 0.2 mm i.d., 0.33 µm film thickness). Column temperature: 280°. Carrier gas: helium, 0.9 mL/min flow rate. MS detection. Retention index: 2552 [T. Mills and J. C. Roberson, 1993. *Instrumental Data for Drug Analysis*, CRC Press, Boca Raton, USA, 2nd Edn, Vol. 6, pp. 82–83].

High Performance Liquid Chromatography. Column: ODS (Apex 1, 100 × 4.6 mm i.d., 3 µm). Mobile phase: (A)-methanol:disodium hydrogen orthophosphate (0.01 M, pH 7.0) (7:93); (B)-methanol:disodium hydrogen orthophosphate (0.01 M, pH 7.0) (35:65). Elution programme: (A:B) (100:0) to (0:100) in 4 min, held for 1.5 min, back to initial conditions in 1 min, 2.0 mL/min flow rate. UV detection: dual wavelength (λ_1=254 nm, λ_2=305 nm). Retention time: penciclovir (metabolite), 1.6 min; 6-deoxyfamciclovir precursor, 2.6 min; famciclovir, 6.0 min [C. F. Winton *et al.*, *Anal. Proc.*, 1990, *27*, 181–182].

Column: ODS (Apex 1, 100 × 4.6 mm i.d., 3 µm). Mobile phase: methanol: sodium phosphate buffer (0.01 M, pH 7.0) (5:95), 1.0 mL/min flow rate. UV detection: dual wavelength (λ_1=254 nm, λ_2=305 nm). Retention time: penciclovir, 7.8 min; 6-deoxyfamciclovir precursor, 14.0 min [J. R. McMeekin *et al.*, *Anal. Proc.*, 1990, *29*, 178–180].

Ultraviolet Spectrum. Aqueous acid—224, 246, 310 nm; basic—304 nm.

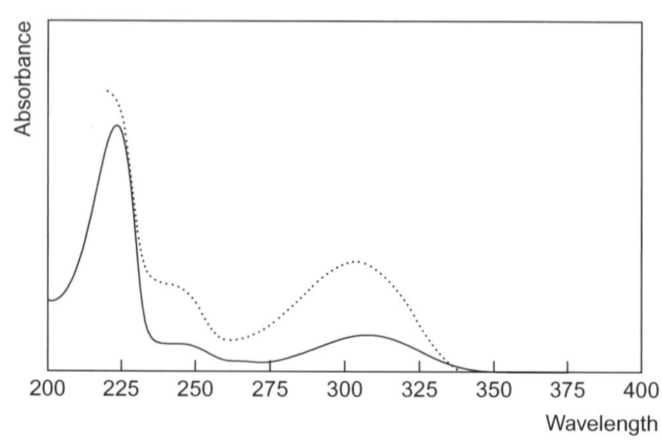

Infra-red Spectrum. Principal peaks at wavenumbers 1730, 1616, 1216 cm^{-1} (KBr disk).

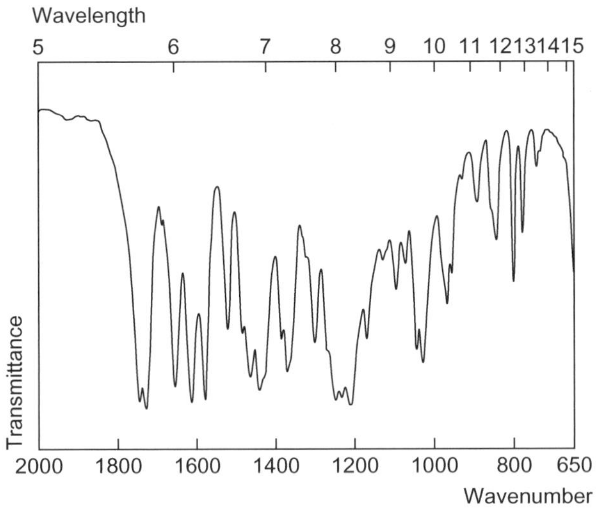

Mass Spectrum. Principal ions at *m/z* 43, 262, 136, 202, 135, 321, 83, 148.

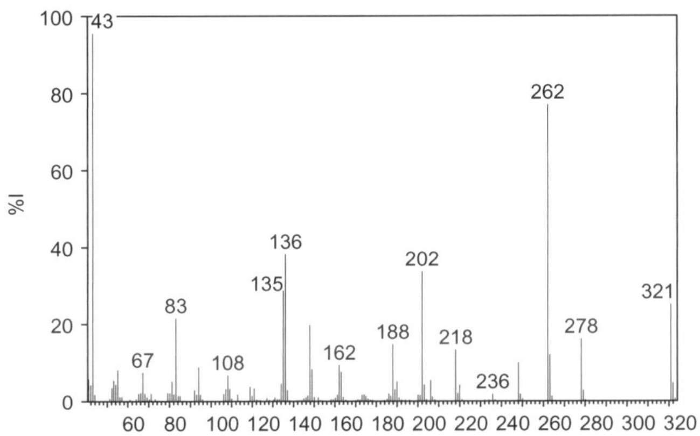

Quantification

High performance liquid chromatography. In plasma and urine: limit of quantification 0.2 and 10 mg/L, respectively. UV detection (λ_1=254 nm, λ_2=305 nm)—J. R. McMeekin *et al.*, *Anal. Proc.*, 1992, *29*, 178–180.

Disposition in the Body. Famciclovir is rapidly absorbed after oral administration and converted, by deacetylation, in blood, and oxidation (aldehyde oxidase), in the liver, to penciclovir (BR-39123) and several inactive metabolites. Virtually no famciclovir is detected in plasma or urine. Penciclovir is converted by intracellular virus-induced thymine kinase to penciclovir triphosphate which is responsible for the antiviral activity. The drug is excreted, primarily, in urine as the metabolite, penciclovir, and the 6-deoxy precursor, BRL-42359. 73% of penciclovir can be detected in urine over 24 h and the remainder appears in faeces. Elimination is reduced in patients with renal impairment.

Therapeutic concentration

20 healthy male volunteers, with a mean age of 36 years, were administered single oral doses of 125, 250, 500 and 750 mg famciclovir, after 10 h fasting. The peak plasma concentrations of penciclovir: 0.84, 1.59, 3.34 and 5.09 mg/L, respectively, were reached within 0.5 to 0.75 h. Concentrations reached below 0.2 mg/L within 6 h for the 125 and 250 mg doses, and within 10 h for the higher doses [M. A. Pue *et al.*, *J. Antimicrob. Chemother.*, 1994, *33*, 119–127].

Bioavailability. Approx. 77%.

Half-life. 2 to 3 h.

Volume of distribution. Steady state, 0.98 to 1.08 L/kg; metabolite, penciclovir, 1.5 L/kg.

Clearance. Approx. 0.48 L/h/kg.

Distribution in blood. The blood:plasma ratio for the metabolite, penciclovir is approx. 1.0.

Protein binding. The metabolite, penciclovir, is <20% bound.

Dose. The usual dose administered is between 250 and 500 mg every 8 h. Dosing interval is extended in patients with renal impairment.

Famotidine

H_2-receptor Antagonist/Antiulcerative

Synonyms. Famotidinum; L643341; MK-208; YM-11170.
Proprietary names. Amfamox; Brolin; Dispromil; Famodil; Famodine; Famosan; Famoxal; Ganor; Gastor; Gastropen; Ifada; Lecedil; Motiax; Pepcid; Pepcidac; Pepcidin; Pepcidine; Pepdine; Pepdul; Ulcusan; Ulfinol.
3-[[[2-[(Aminoiminomethyl)amino]-4-thiazolyl]methyl]thio]-*N*-(aminosulfonyl)propanimidamide
$C_8H_{15}N_7O_2S_3$ = 337.5
CAS—76824-35-6

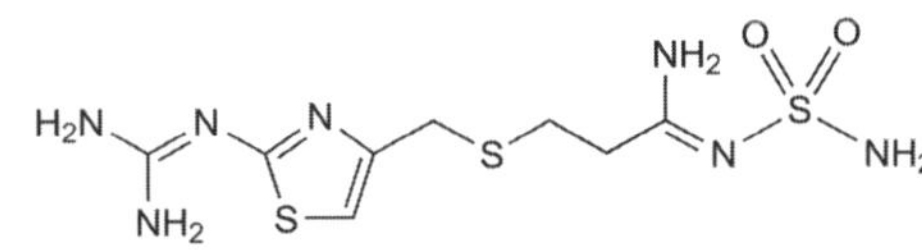

A white to pale yellowish white crystalline powder with M.p. 163° to 164°. Protect from light. It is very slightly soluble in water (0.1% at 20°) and dehydrated alcohol; practically insoluble in acetone, alcohol, chloroform (< 0.01%, 20°), ether and ethyl acetate (< 0.01%, 20°); slightly soluble in methyl alcohol; freely soluble in dimethylformamide (80%, 20°) and glacial acetic acid (50%, 20°). It dissolves in dilute mineral acids.

Dissociation Constant. pK_a 7.06.

Partition Coefficient. Log *P* (octanol/water), −0.64.

Thin-layer Chromatography. System TB—Rf 00; system TE—Rf 25; system TAE—Rf 53.

High Performance Liquid Chromatography. System HX—RI 233; system HY—RI 191; system HZ—retention time 1.8 min; system HAA—retention time 3.5 min.

Column: LC-8 (Supelcosyl, 250 × 4.6 mm i.d., 5 μm), protected by 2 cm guard column (40 μm, Pelliguard). Mobile phase: methanol:acetonitrile:phosphoric acid (0.016 M) (10:10:80), 1.0 mL/min flow rate. UV detection (λ=254 nm). Retention time: 9.5 min [G. Carlucci *et al.*, *J. Pharm. Biomed. Anal.*, 1988, *6(5)*, 515–519].

Column: (analytical) ODS-3 (Prodigy, 250 × 3.9 mm i.d., 5 μm), (guard) C_{18} (Bondapak/Corasil, 37 to 50 μm). Mobile phase: acetonitrile:heptanesulfonic acid (2.5 g/L) in sodium acetate buffer (20 mM, pH 4.7) (23:77), 1.0 mL/min flow rate. Internal standard (IS): cimetidine. UV detection (λ=267 nm). Retention time: 8.4 min; IS, 6.8 min [T. C. Dowling and R. F. Frye, *J. Chromatogr. B Biomed. Sci. Appl.*, 1999, *732*, 239–243].

Ultraviolet Spectrum. Aqueous acid—265 nm; basic—286 nm.

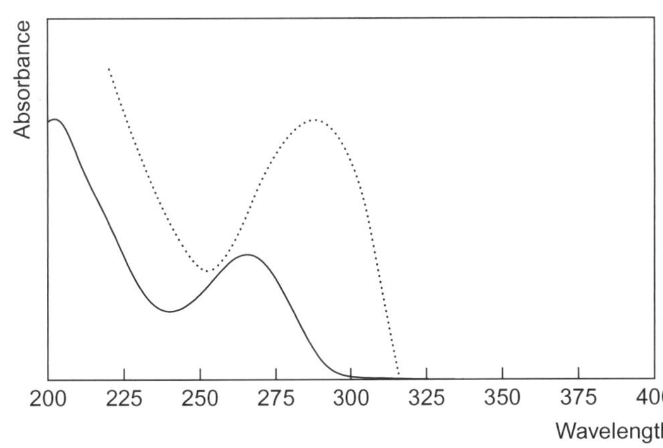

Infra-red Spectrum. Principal peaks at wavenumbers 1638, 1535, 1290, 781 cm^{-1}.

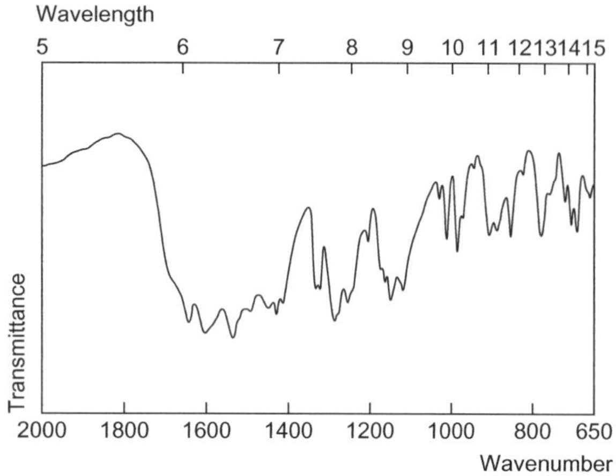

Mass Spectrum. Principal ions at *m/z* 188, 155, 113, 43, 45, 85, 69, 146.

Quantification
High performance liquid chromatography. In plasma: limit of quantification 1 µg/L. UV detection (λ=267 nm)—L. Zhong and K. C. Yeh, *J. Pharm. Biomed. Anal.*, 1998, *16*, 1051–1057. In plasma and urine: limit of quantification 0.005 and 0.5 mg/L, respectively. UV detection (λ=267 nm)—W. C. Vincek *et al.*, *J. Chromatogr.*, 1985, *338, Biomed. Appl.*, 438–443. In plasma and urine: limit of detection 0.075 mg/L and 1 mg/L, respectively. UV detection (λ=267 nm)—T. C. Dowling and R. F. Frye, *J. Chromatogr. B Biomed. Sci. Appl*, 1999, *732*, 239–243. In plasma: limit of quantification 5 µg/L. UV detection (λ=267 nm)—S. Wanwimolruk *et al.*, *J. Chromatogr.*, 1991, *572*, 227–238.

Disposition in the Body. After intravenous administration, the plasma famotidine concentration–time profile exhibits a biexponential decay. Famotidine is readily but incompletely absorbed after oral administration. There are three formulations available (tablet, capsule and suspension), which appear to be bioequivalent. Only a small amount of the drug is metabolised in the liver to famotidine *S*-oxide and the remainder is excreted unchanged in urine (approx. 67%). The drug is widely distributed in body tissues and can be detected in breast milk. Famotidine interacts neither with the hepatic oxidative drug metabolism nor with tubular secretion of other commonly used therapeutic agents such as theophylline, warfarin and procainamide. Coadministration of potent antacids reduces the oral absorption of famotidine by 20 to 30%. A prolongation of elimination half-life and a decrease in total body clearance and renal clearance are observed in patients with renal failure indicating that dosage adjustment may be necessary in patients who have renal insufficiency. No significant changes occur in famotidine disposition in patients with cirrhosis indicating that no reduction in drug dosage should be necessary in these patients. The pharmacokinetics and pharmacodynamics of intravenous famotidine appear to be similar in both children over the age of 1 year and adults.

Therapeutic concentration. The serum therapeutic concentration range is 0.02 to 0.06 mg/L.

8 healthy males, aged between 22 and 27 years, were administered a single 40 mg dose of famotidine, after an overnight fast. Peak plasma levels of 0.156 ± 0.022 mg/L were reached within 3 h [N. Barzaghi *et al.*, *J. Clin. Pharmacol.*, 1989, *29*, 670–672].

10 young patients, aged between 5 and 19 days, were administered a 0.5 mg/kg body weight infusion over 15 min. Peak concentrations of 0.641 mg/L were reached by the end of administration [L. P. James *et al.*, *J. Clin. Pharmacol.*, 1998, *38*, 1089–1095].

Plasma concentrations following intravenous continuous infusion of 40 (group A) or 20 (group B) mg/day over more than two days, were analysed in 10 adult patients. The mean age, dose and plasma concentration were 64.8 years, 0.81 mg/kg/day and 0.141 mg/L in group A, and 54.2 years, 0.34 mg/kg/day and 0.045 mg/L in group B, respectively [V. R. Espitia *et al.*, *Intern. Med.* (*Tokyo, Japan*), 1992, 31, 299–303].

Toxicity. Convulsions and mental deterioration have been reported in the elderly with renal failure owing to grossly elevated plasma and cerebrospinal fluid concentrations of the drug. Toxic epidermal necrolysis can also occur. Since 1992, there have been 60 reports of serious blood dyscrasias.

Bioavailability. 20 to 66%.

Half-life. Distribution half-life is approx. 0.18 to 0.5 h in adults. Elimination half-life is approx. 3 h in adults, which can increase to 24 h in patients with suppressed urine excretion. The elimination half-life for infants is approx. 10 h. Elimination half-life is 3.3 h in paediatric patients with normal kidney function, aged between 2 and 7 years.

Volume of distribution. In adults: 0.94 to 1.33 L/kg; in infants: 0.82 L/kg. In paediatric patients (aged between 2 and 7 years): 1.4 L/kg.

Clearance. 0.19 to 0.43 L/min. In patients with end-stage renal failure: 0.034 L/min. In paediatric patients with normal kidney function: 0.3 L/h/kg.

Protein binding. 15 to 22% in plasma.

Dose. A usual dose of 20 to 40 mg is administered once or twice daily. A paediatric dosage for intravenous famotidine is 0.3 to 0.5 mg/kg every 8 to 12 h similarly as adults. Patients with impaired renal function: dose is reduced or dose interval extended.

Famprofazone

Analgesic

Proprietary name. It is an ingredient of Gewodin.

4-Isopropyl-1-methyl-5-[*N*-methyl-*N*-(α-methylphenethyl)aminomethyl]-2-phenyl-4-pyrazolin-3-one

$C_{24}H_{31}N_3O$=377.5

CAS—22881-35-2

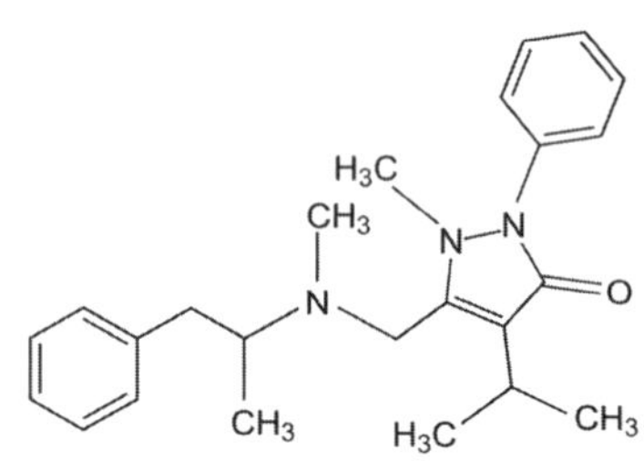

A white crystalline powder. M.p. 132° to 133°.

Practically insoluble in water; slightly soluble in dilute acetic acid.

Colour Tests. Liebermann's Test—red-orange; Marquis Test—orange

Thin-layer Chromatography. System TA—Rf 72; system TB—Rf 37; system TC—Rf 74; system TE—Rf 87; system TL—Rf 67; system TAE—Rf 90. (Acidified iodoplatinate solution, positive.)

Gas Chromatography. System GA—Famprofazone RI 2965, M (OH-propyphenazone) RI 2410, M (OH-propyphenazone)-AC RI 2240, M (metamfetamine) RI 1175.

High Performance Liquid Chromatography. System HD—*k* 2.5.

Ultraviolet Spectrum. Aqueous acid—243, 279 nm (A_1^1=248a).

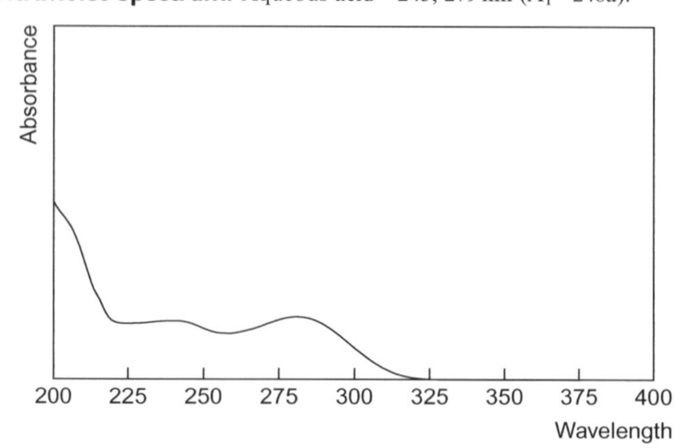

Mass Spectrum. Principal ions at *m/z* 286, 229, 91, 81, 287, 41, 77, 228.

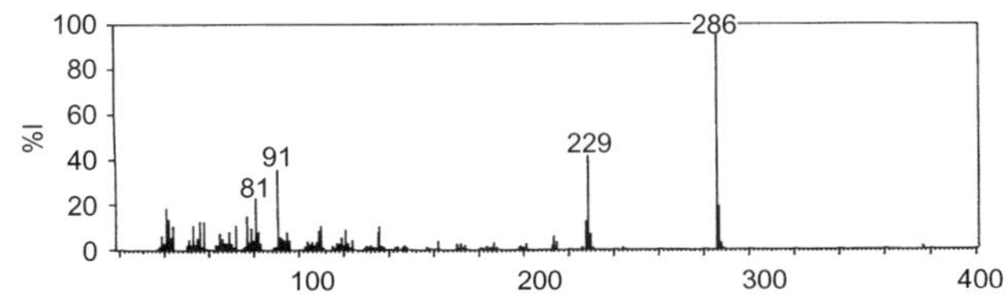

Disposition in the Body

Therapeutic concentration

After a single 100 mg dose of famprofazone to 2 subjects, the plasma concentration of metamfetamine was 24 to 44 µg/L over 2 to 12 h and declined to 10 µg/L in one subject and an undetectable level in the other after 24 h [E. S. Oh *et al.*, *Xenobiotica*, 1992, *22*, 377–384].

Dose. Famprofazone has been given in doses of up to 150 mg daily.

Fasudil

Vasodilator

Hexahydro-1-(5-isoquinolinylsulfonyl)-1*H*-1,4-diazepine
$C_{14}H_{17}N_3O_2S=291.4$
CAS—103745-39-7

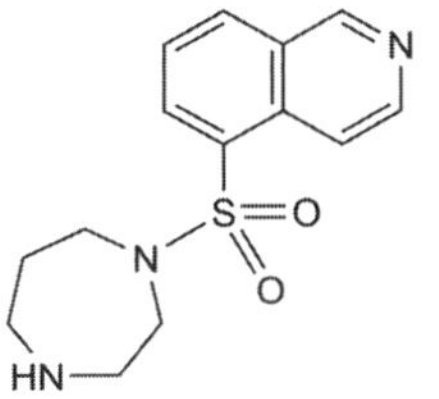

Fasudil Hydrochloride

Synonyms. AT-877; HA-1077.
Proprietary names. Eril; Fadil.
$C_{14}H_{17}N_3O_2S,HCl=327.8$
CAS—105628-07-7

A white crystalline powder with M.p. 219.3°. It is soluble in water up to 2×10^{-2} M at pH 5.0 to 7.0.

Fazadinium Bromide

Muscle Relaxant

Proprietary name. Fazadon
1,1′-Azobis[3-methyl-2-phenylimidazo[1,2-*a*]pyridinium] dibromide
$C_{28}H_{24}Br_2N_6=604.3$
CAS—36653-54-0 (fazadinium); 49564-56-9 (bromide)

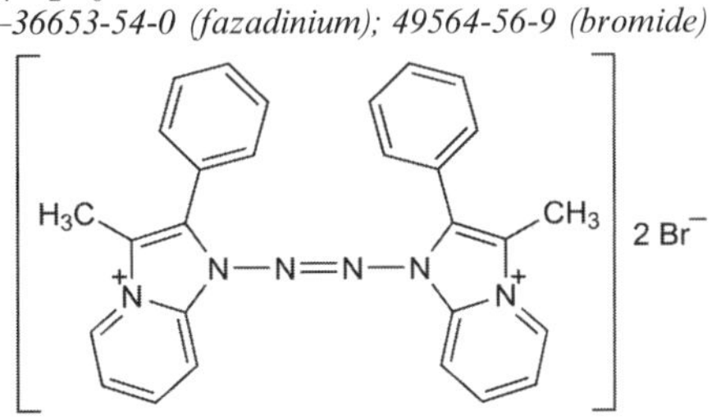

A yellow solid. M.p. 215°.
Soluble in water.

Ultraviolet Spectrum. Aqueous acid—283 nm ($A^1_1=188a$).

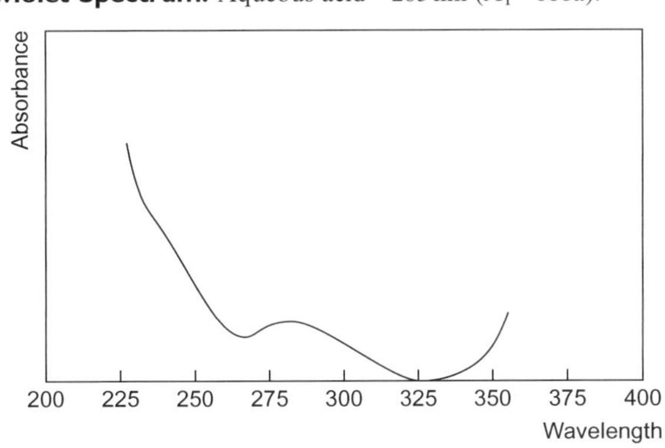

Infra-red Spectrum. Principal peaks at wavenumbers 1280, 1220, 1160, 1250, 760, 780 cm^{-1} (Nujol mull).

Quantification

Spectrofluorimetry. In plasma: limit of detection 50 µg/L—A. M. Pastorino, *Arzneimittelforschung.*, 1978, *28*, 1728–1730.

Disposition in the Body. About 50% of a dose is excreted in the urine in 24 h, mainly unchanged. Extensive biliary excretion has been reported.

Therapeutic concentration

Following an intravenous dose of 70 mg to 5 subjects, the mean plasma concentration was > 10 mg/L at 2 min and 2.2 mg/L at 1 h [J. D'Souza *et al.*, *J. Pharm. Pharmacol.*, 1979, *31*, 416–418].

Half-life. Plasma half-life, about 1 h.

Volume of distribution. About 0.3 L/kg.

Clearance. Plasma clearance, about 3 mL/min/kg.

Protein binding. In plasma, about 17%.

Dose. Initially, the equivalent of 0.75 to 1 mg/kg of fazadinium, intravenously.

Felbamate

Anticonvulsant

Synonyms. ADD-03055; W-554.
Proprietary names. Felbamyl; Felbatol; Taloxa; Taloxoral.
2-Phenyl-1,3-propanediol dicarbamate
$C_{11}H_{14}N_2O_4=238.2$
CAS—25451-15-4

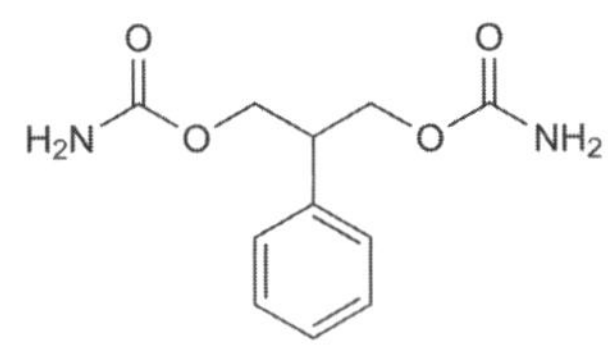

A white, odourless powder with M.p. 151° to 152°.
It is sparingly soluble in water, methanol, ethanol, acetone, and chloroform; freely soluble in dimethylsulfoxide, 1-methyl-2-pyrrolidinone, and dimethylformamide

Partition Coefficient. Log *P* (octanol/water), 0.76.

Gas Chromatography. System GB—RI 1475.

Column: methylsilicone (HP, 10 m × 0.53 mm i.d., 0.33 µm film thickness). Column temperature: 170°, held 0.1 min, increased to 280° at 10°/min, held 2 min. Injector and detector temperatures: 235° and 300°, respectively. Carrier gas: helium, flow rate 16.4 mL/min, hydrogen 4 mL/min, and air 75 mL/min. Detection: nitrogen selective. IS: methylfelbamate. Retention time(s): felbamate, 3.71 min; IS, 4.11 min. [P. Gur *et al.*, *J. Anal. Toxicol.*, 1995, *19*, 499–503.]

Column: DB-1 (30 m × 0.25 mm i.d., 0.25 µm film thickness). Column temperature: 240°. Injector and detector temperatures: 280° and 320°, respectively. Carrier gas: hydrogen, 15 psi inlet pressure. Detection: FID. IS: 2-methyl-2-phenyl-1,3-propanedioldicarbamate. Retention time(s): felbamate, 2.29 min; IS, 2.50 min. [M. A. Poquette, *Ther. Drug Monit.*, 1995, *17(2)*, 168–173.]

High Performance Liquid Chromatography. Column: C_{18} (Zorbax, 250 × 4.6 mm i.d.). Mobile phase: acetonitrile:methanol: tetrahydrofuran:phosphate buffer (210:410:500:2880), flow rate 1.5 mL/min. UV detection (λ=254 nm). IS: methylfelbamate. Retention time: felbamate, 5.0 min; IS, 7.0 min. [P. Gur *et al.*, *J. Anal. Toxicol.*, 1995, *19*, 499–503.]

Column: ODS-2 (Spherisorb, 150 × 4.6 mm i.d., 3 µm). Mobile phase: potassium dihydrogen phosphate (4.2 g in 850 mL water, adjusted to pH 4.0 with phosphoric acid) and 150 mL acetonitrile, flow rate 1.0 mL/min. IS: 2-methyl-2-phenyl-1,3-propanedioldicarbamate. Retention time: felbamate, 11.0 min; 2-hydroxyfelbamate, 4.5 min; *p*-hydroxyfelbamate, 3.2 min; monocarbamate derivative, 7.1 min; IS, 18.8 min. [L. A. Romanyshyn *et al.*, *Ther. Drug Monit.*, 1994, *16(1)*, 83–89.]

Ultraviolet Spectrum. Aqueous acid—251, 256, 262 nm; basic—246, 251, 256, 262 nm.

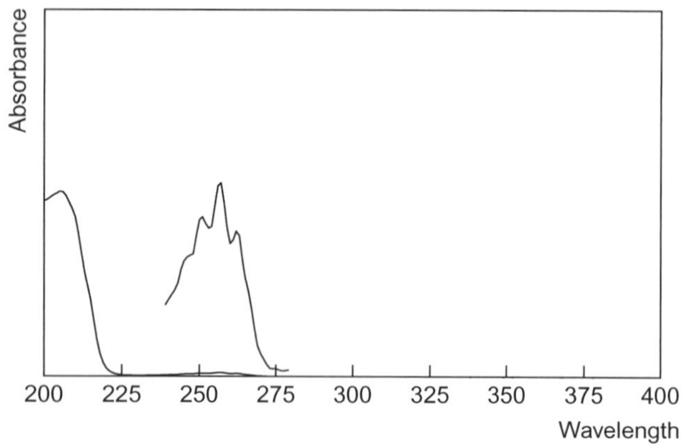

Infra-red Spectrum. Principal peaks at wavenumbers 1693, 1614, 1082 cm^{-1} (KBr disk).

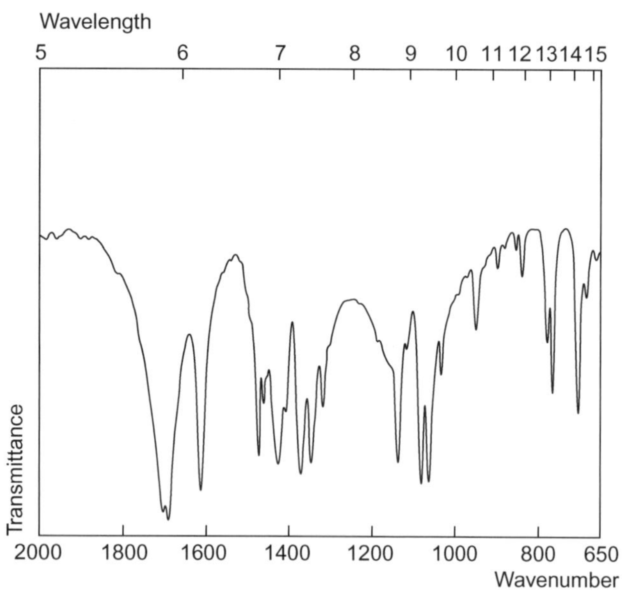

Mass Spectrum. Principal ions at *m*/*z*: 134, 104, 103, 91, 77, 78, 105, 44.

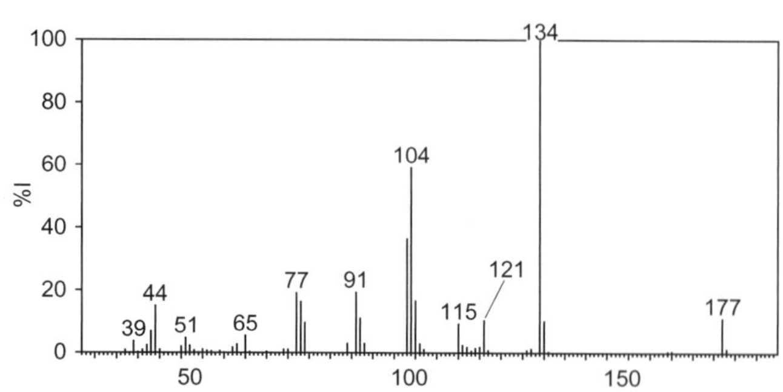

Quantification

Gas chromatography–mass spectrometry. In serum: limit of detection and quantification 5 mg/L—P. Gur *et al.*, *J. Anal. Toxicol.*, 1995, *19*, 499–503.

High performance liquid chromatography. In serum: limit of detection and quantification 5 mg/L—P. Gur *et al.*, *J. Anal. Toxicol.*, 1995, *19*, 499–503.

Disposition in the Body. Felbamate is well absorbed (approx. 90%) after oral administration and is partly metabolised in the liver by hydroxylation and conjugation, to produce active and inactive metabolites. The drug is excreted in urine unchanged (40 to 50%), as unidentified metabolites and conjugates (40%) and known active metabolites (15%), including 2-hydroxyfelbamate, *p*-hydroxyfelbamate, a monocarbamate derivative, and 3-carbamoyloxy-2-phenyl propionic acid. <5% of the dose is excreted in faeces.

Therapeutic concentration. The therapeutic plasma concentration is between 30 and 80 μg/L.

A study was carried out with 24 healthy, elderly volunteers (male and female), aged between 66 and 78 years, and 11 younger volunteers, 18 to 45 years. Low dosage regimen: a single dose of 600 mg felbamate was administered on day 1, followed by 600 mg every 12 h (days 6 to 7) and 600 mg every 12 h (days 8 to 14) for a multiple dosing study. High dosage regimen: a single 1200 mg dose was administered on day 1 followed by 600 mg every 12 h and 1200 mg every 12 h, on the respective days. For the elderly group, peak plasma concentrations of 13.0 and 22.0 μg/L were reached for the low and high single doses, respectively. For the younger volunteers, 8.9 and 19.6 μg/L were reached, respectively. All peak concentrations were reached within 2 h of administration. After multiple dosing, peak plasma concentrations reached 32.7 and 78.5 μg/L for the low and high doses, respectively (young) and 41.1 and 75.5 μg/L, respectively for the elderly. [A. Richens *et al.*, *Br. J. Clin. Pharmacol.*, 1997, *44*, 129–134.]

Toxicity

Acute liver failure has been reported with 4 fatalities out of 8 cases [Schering-Plough manufacturers report, 1994] and aplastic anaemia with 2 out of 10 cases resulting in death [US Food and Drug Administration report, 1994].

Half-life. Elimination half-life, 14 to 23 h.

Volume of distribution. 0.76 to 0.81 L/kg.

Clearance. 25 mL/min/kg (single dose), 41 mL/min/kg (repeated dose).

Distribution in blood. Equilibrates freely between plasma and whole blood.

Protein binding. 22 to 36%.

Dose. An initial dose of 1.2 g daily is administered to adults with a maximum 3.6 g daily. In children: an initial dose of 15 mg/kg body weight, maximum 45 mg/kg. Dose may be adjusted for patients with renal dysfunction.

Felodipine

Antihypertensive

Synonyms. H-154/82; Felodipinum.
Proprietary name. Agon; Feloday; Felodur; Fensil; Flodil; Hydac; Modip; Munobal; Perfudal; Plendil; Preslow; Prevex; Renedil; Spendil.
4-(2,3-Dichlorophenyl)-1,4-dihydro-2,6-dimethyl-3,5-pyridinedicarboxylic acid ethyl methyl ester
$C_{18}H_{19}Cl_2NO_4$=384.3
CAS—72509-76-3; 86189-69-7

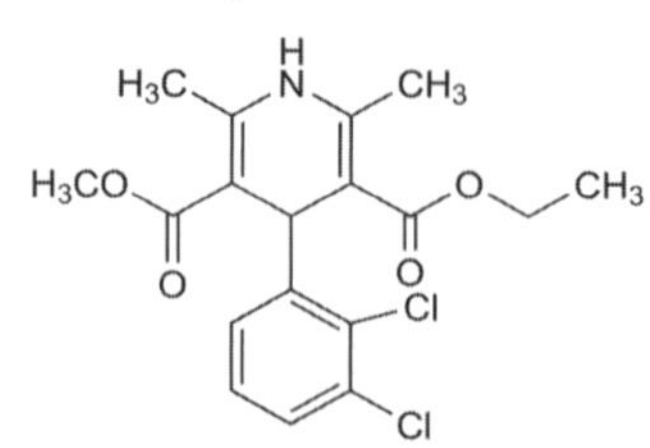

A white to light yellow crystalline powder. M.p. 145°. Protect from light. It is practically insoluble in water (19.17 mg/L at 25°); freely soluble in acetone, absolute alcohol, methyl alcohol and dichloromethane.

Partition Coefficient. Log *P* (octanol/water), 3.86.

Thin-layer Chromatography. System TB—Rf 02; system TE—Rf 77; system TF—Rf 60; system TAE—Rf 87.

Gas Chromatography. System GB—RI 2793; system GP— RI 2235 (M (dehydro-desethyl-)-ME); RI 2280 (M (dehydro-)).

Column: silica (25 m × 0.32 mm i.d.), silanised with diphenyltetramethyldisilazane. Column temperature: programmed at 8°/min to 270°. Injector and detector temperatures: 270° and 350°, respectively. Carrier gas: helium at 1.2 bar pressure. Detection: electron capture, ^{63}Ni. Retention time: 14.8 min [M. Ahnoff, *J. Pharm. Biomed. Anal.*, 1984, *2*, 519–526].

Column: methyl silicone (HP1, 0.2 mm i.d., 0.33 µm film thickness). Column temperature: 280°. Carrier gas: helium, 0.9 mL/min flow rate. Detection: mass spectrometer. Retention index: 2647. [T. Mills and J. C. Roberson, 1993. *Instrumental Data for Drug Analysis*, CRC Press, Boca Raton, USA, 2nd Edn, Vol. 6, pp. 86–87].

High Performance Liquid Chromatography. System HX—RI 690; system HZ—25.8 min; system HAA—retention time 24.4 min.

Column: (analytical) RP-select B (LiChrospher 60, 250 × 4.0 mm i.d., 5 µm), (guard) cyano (Brownlee, 15 × 3.2 mm i.d., 7 µm). Mobile phase: A-methanol:phosphate buffer (0.05 M, pH 3.5) (45:55); B-methanol:phosphate buffer (0.05 M, pH 3.5) (80:20), 1.15 mL/min flow rate. Elution program: (A:B) (100:0) for 17 min, to (0:100) in 5 min, held for 5 min. UV detection (λ=220 nm). Internal standard (IS): 3,5-pyridine dicarboxylic acid. Retention time: felodipine metabolites, M3, 10.4 min; M4, 17.4 min; M6, 9.4 min; M7, 15.1 min; IS, 13.2 min [M. Gabrielsson *et al.*, *J. Chromatogr.*, 1992, *573*, *Biomed. Appl.*, 265–274].

Ultraviolet Spectrum. Aqueous acid—237, 359 nm; basic—281 nm.

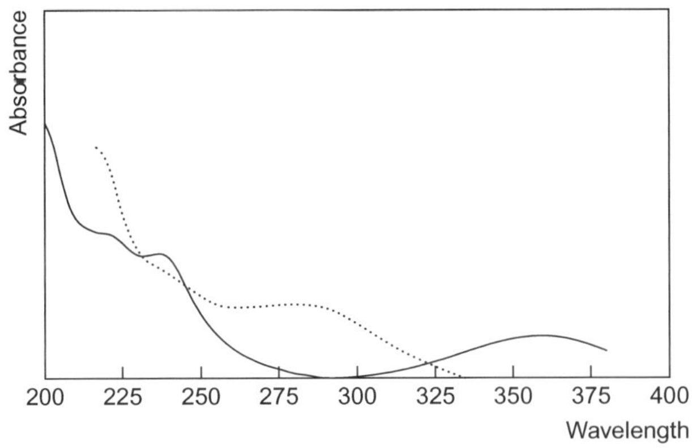

Infra-red Spectrum. Principal peaks at wavenumbers 1698, 1496, 1206, 1099 cm^{-1} (KBr pellet).

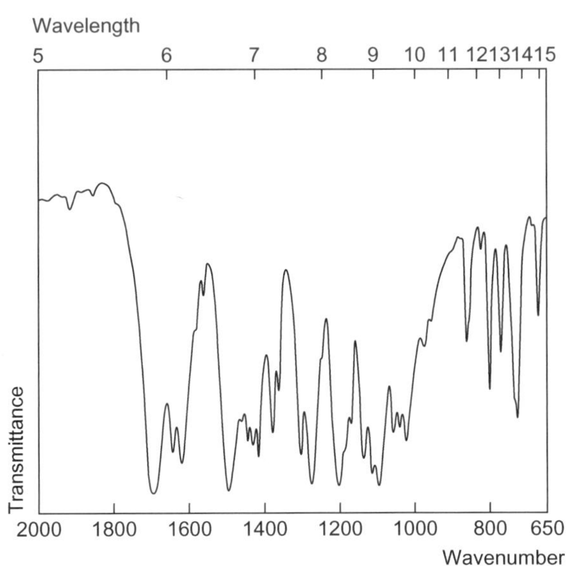

Mass Spectrum. Principal ions at *m/z* 238, 210, 239, 354, 383, 338, 178, 310.

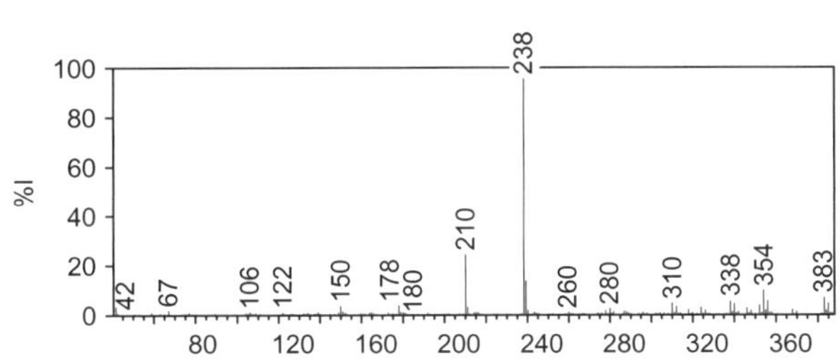

Quantification

Gas chromatography. In plasma: limit of detection 0.4 to 0.8 µg/L—M. Ahnoof, *J. Pharm. Biomed. Anal.*, 1984, *2*, 519–526. In plasma: limit of quantification 0.1 µg/L for felodipine and 0.3 µg/L for its metabolite—P. A. Soons *et al.*, *J. Chromatogr.*, 1990, *528, Biomed. Appl.*, 343–356.

High performance liquid chromatography. In plasma: limit of detection 8 µg/L. UV detection (λ=220 nm)—M. Gabrielsson *et al.*, *J. Chromatogr.*, 1992, *573*, *Biomed. Appl.*, 265–274. In plasma: limit of detection of each enantiomer 5 µg/L—P. A. Soons *et al.*, *J. Chromatogr.*, 1990, *528, Biomed. Appl.*, 343–356.

Disposition in the Body. Felodipine is almost completely absorbed after oral administration and undergoes extensive first-pass metabolism in the liver, by microsomal cytochrome P450 3A enzyme, to form a pyridine analogue (1,4-dihydropyridine goes to inactive dehydrofelodipine). Subsequent oxidation results in approx. 15 inactive metabolites. 70% of a dose is excreted in urine, with < 0.5% unchanged, and the rest in faeces, as metabolites.

Therapeutic concentration. The serum therapeutic concentration range is 1 to 8 µg/L.

A total of 140 volunteers: men and women, healthy and hypertensive (all women), aged between 20 and 39 years old (70 people), 40 and 59 (30 people) and 60 and 80 years (40 people) were administered doses of 5 mg twice daily and 10 mg twice daily. The duration of the treatment varied from 6 to 30 days. Peak plasma concentrations increased with age where levels of 0.019 ± 0.009, 0.023 ± 0.010, 0.030 ± 0.0129 nM were reached for the 20 to 39 years, 40 to 59, 60 to 80 age groups, respectively. All peak levels were reached within 2 h. [E. Blychert *et al.*, *Br. J. Clin. Pharm.*, 1991, *31*, 15–24].

12 healthy males, mean age 25 years (range 20 to 34 years) were administered with 20 mg (racemate) felodipine. Peak plasma concentrations for the racemate drug were 30.3 (13.6 to 47.6) µg/L; for (*S*)-felodipine, 20.4 (0.53 to 32.7) µg/L and (*R*)-felodipine, 9.77 (5.07 to 15.6) µg/L. All concentrations were observed at a mean of 58 min (range 19 to 180) [P. A. Soons *et al.*, *Eur. J. Clin. Pharmacol.*, 1993, *44(2)*, 163–169].

Toxicity. The serum toxic concentration range is 10 to 15 µg/L. Overdosing may cause excessive peripheral vasodilation with marked hypotension and possibly bradycardia.

Bioavailability. 15%.

Half-life. 11 to 16 h (oral administration in normal patients); 2 h (patients with renal failure).

Volume of distribution. Apparent volume of distribution, 10 L/kg (normal patients); 5.6 L/kg (patients with cirrhosis).

Clearance. Systemic plasma clearance, about 0.8 L/min.

Protein binding. Felodipine is approx. 99% bound to plasma proteins, mainly albumin.

Dose. An initial dose of 5 mg daily is given followed by a usual maintenance dose of 2.5 to 10 mg. Elderly and patients with impaired liver function: initial dose of 2.5 mg daily.

Fenamiphos

Nematicide

Synonyms. B-68138; Bay 68138; Bayer 68138; Phenamiphos; SRA-3886.
Proprietary name. Nemacur
(1-Methylethyl)phosphoramidic acid ethyl 3-methyl-4-(methylthio)phenyl ester
$C_{13}H_{22}NO_3PS$=303.4
CAS—22224-92-6

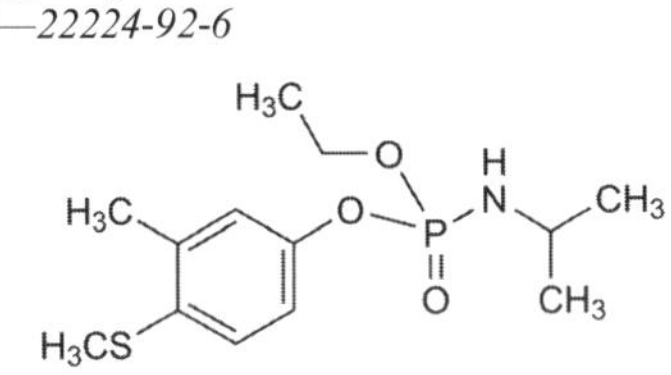

A colourless, crystalline solid or a tan, waxy solid (technical state). M.p. 49° (46° technical state).

It is soluble in water (329 mg/L at 20°), 2-propanol, dichloromethane, toluene, and isopropanol.

Dissociation Constant. pK_a 10.5 (25°).

Partition Coefficient. Log *P* (octanol/water), 3.25.

Gas Chromatography. System GA—RI 2020.

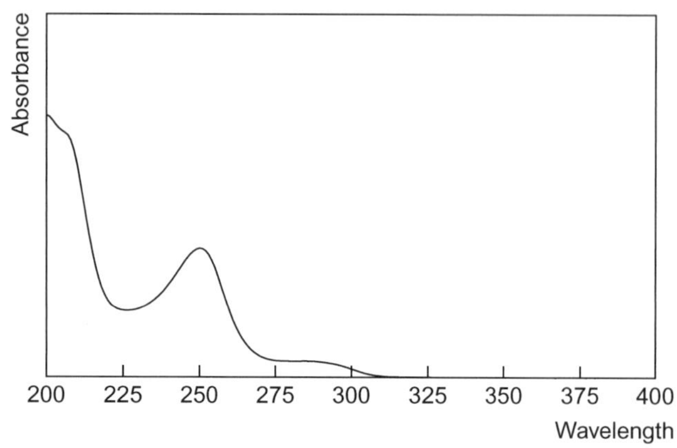

Infra-red Spectrum. Principal peaks at wavenumber 967, 1049, 1226, 1278, 1158, 1473 cm^{-1}.

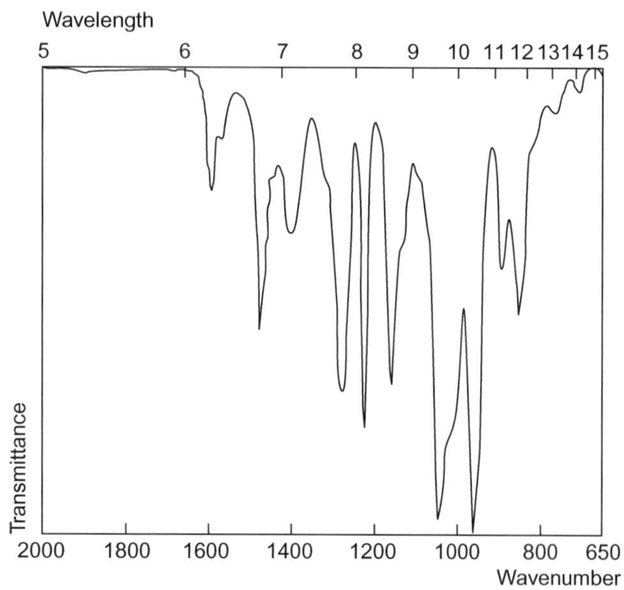

Mass Spectrum. Principal ions at *m/z* 303, 154, 217, 44, 288, 80, 260, 153.

Disposition in the Body. Fenamiphos is readily absorbed after oral ingestion (approx. 95%) and after inhalation, via the lungs. It is rapidly broken down within the body to produce the two major oxidative metabolites—fenamiphos sulfoxide and fenamiphos sulfone—which may be followed by subsequent hydrolysis and conjugation. These are excreted in urine. The majority of a dose is recovered in urine 15 h after exposure.

Toxicity. Fenamiphos is highly toxic if ingested orally and by inhalation. It can also cause acute dermal toxicity if exposed and significant eye damage at acute exposure levels. The allowed daily intake is 0.5 μg/kg body weight.

Fenbendazole

Anthelmintic

Proprietary names. Axilur; Curazole; Fencare; Fenzol; Flexadin; Forazole; Granofen; Multiwurma-F; Orazole; Panacur; Parazole; Safe-Guard; Wormaway Feben; Zerofen (all vet.).

[5-(Phenylthio)-1*H*-benzimidazol-2-yl]carbamic acid methyl ester

$C_{15}H_{13}N_3O_2S = 299.3$

CAS—43210-67-9

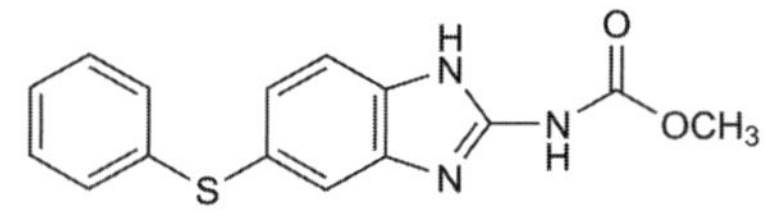

A light brownish-grey crystalline powder. M.p. 233°, with decomposition. Insoluble in water; freely soluble in dimethyl sulfoxide.

Partition Coefficient. Log *P* (octanol/water), 3.8.

High Performance Liquid Chromatography. System HY—RI 370.

Ultraviolet Spectrum. Aqueous acid—289, 302 nm; aqueous alkali—238, 312 nm; ethanol—296 nm (A^1_1=416b).

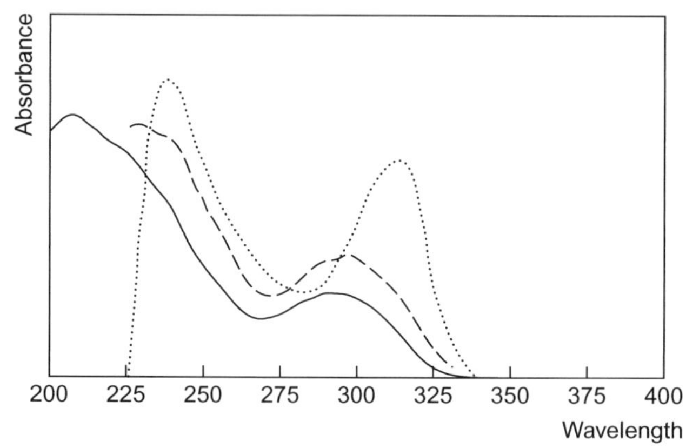

Mass Spectrum. Principal ions at *m/z* 267, 299, 266, 31, 51, 268, 29, 77.

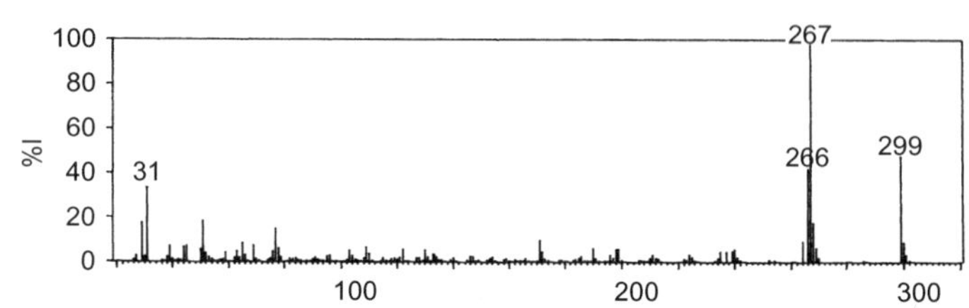

Dose. Fenbendazole has been given in doses of 1 to 1.5 g.

Fenbufen

Analgesic

Proprietary names. Cincopal; Cinopal; Lederfen; Reugast.

γ-Oxo-[1,1′-biphenyl]-4-butanoic acid

$C_{16}H_{14}O_3 = 254.3$

CAS—36330-85-5

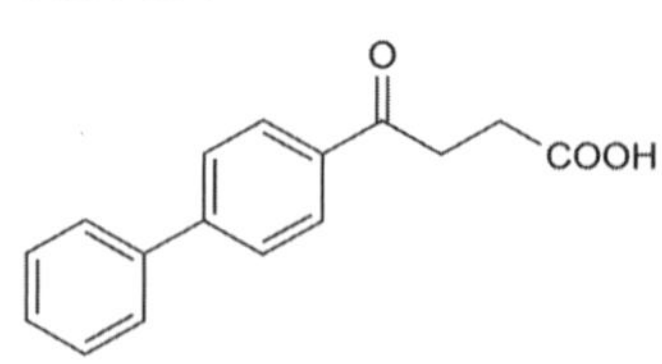

Crystals. M.p. about 180°.

Dissociation Constant. pK_a 4.5.

Partition Coefficient. Log *P* (octanol/water), 3.2.

Colour Tests. Liebermann's Test—red-brown; Marquis Test—orange→brown; Sulfuric Acid—yellow

Thin-layer Chromatography. System TA—Rf 92; system TD—Rf 18; system TE—Rf 04; system TF—Rf 30; system TG—Rf 09; system TAD—Rf 39; system TAJ—Rf 43; system TAK—Rf 68; system TAL—Rf 91.

Gas Chromatography. System GA—fenbufen RI 3078, fenbufen-Me RI 2315; System GD—RRT of methyl derivative 1.79 (relative to *n*-$C_{16}H_{34}$); system GL—fenbufen-Me RI 1975, M (acetic acid OH-)-Me_2 RI 2190.

High Performance Liquid Chromatography. System HD—*k* 4.0; system HV—RRT 0.81 (relative to meclofenamic acid); system HX—RI 520; system HY—RI 461; system HAA—Retention time, 19.3 min.

Ultraviolet Spectrum. Aqueous alkali—285 nm (A_1^1 = 835a).

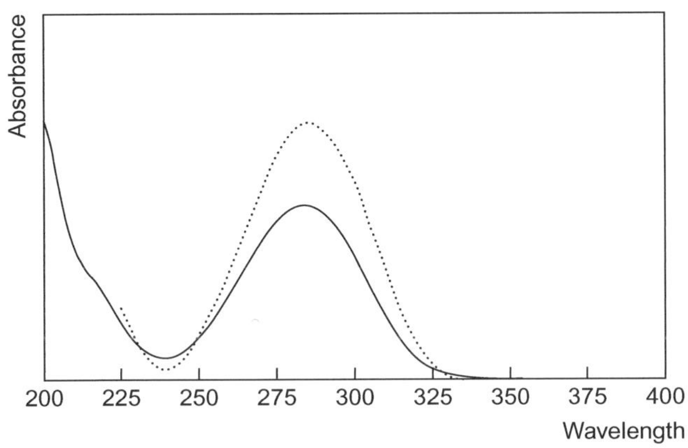

Infra-red Spectrum. Principal peaks at wavenumbers 764, 1674, 1708, 1242, 1268, 829 cm^{-1} (KBr disk).

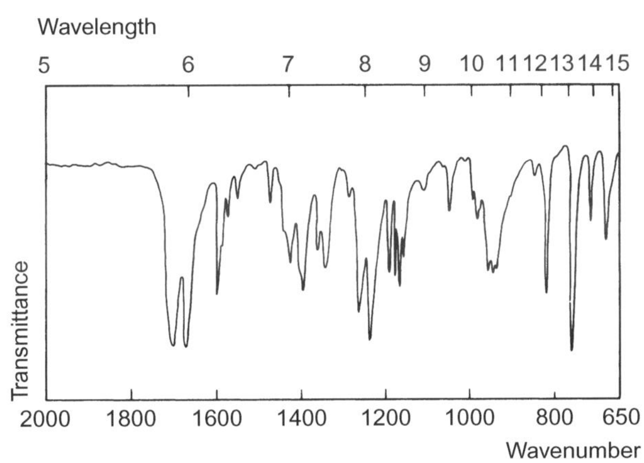

Mass Spectrum. Principal ions at *m/z* 181, 152, 153, 254, 182, 151, 76, 127; fenbufen-Me *m/z* 181, 152, 153, 182, 268, 237; M (acetic acid OH-)-Me_2 *m/z* 197, 256, 154, 128, 152, 198.

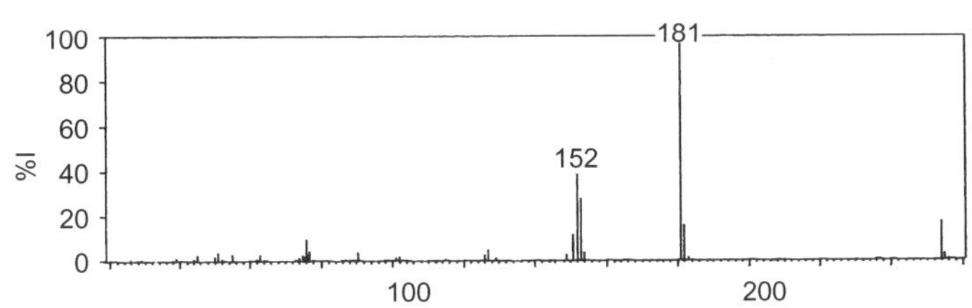

Quantification

Gas chromatography. In plasma: limit of detection, fenbufen 50 μg/L, metabolites (i) and (ii) (see under Disposition) 100 μg/L, FID—G. Cuisinaud *et al.*, *J. Chromatogr.*, 1978, *148*, 509–513.

High performance liquid chromatography. In serum or urine: fenbufen and metabolites, limit of detection 500 μg/L in serum, 1 μg/L in urine, UV detection—G. E. Van Lear *et al.*, *J. Pharm. Sci.*, 1978, *67*, 1662–1664. In serum: fenbufen and metabolites (i) and (ii), limit of detection 500 μg/L, UV detection—J. S. Fleitman *et al.*, *J. Chromatogr.*, 1982, *228*; *Biomed. Appl.*, *17*, 372–376. In plasma: fenbufen, rufloxacin and felbinac, limit of detection for fenbufen 0.3 mg/L, UV detection—G. Carlucci *et al.*, *J. Chromatogr.*, 1996, *682*, *Biomed Appl.*, 315–319. In serum: fenbufen and its metabolites, limit of detection 10 μg/L, fluorescence detection—M. Siluveru and J. T. Stewart, *J. Chromatogr.*, 1996, *682*, *Biomed. Appl.*, 89–94. In urine: fenbufen and other NSAIDs, limit of detection for fenbufen 0.05 mg/L, UV detection—T. Hirai *et al.*, *J. Chromatogr. B. Biomed. Sci. Appl.*, 1997, *692*, 375–388. In serum: fenbufen and other NSAIDs, limits of detection 300 to 800 μg/L—A. Haque and J. T. Stewart, *Biomed. Chromatogr.*, 1999, *13*, 51–56.

Disposition in the Body. Readily absorbed after oral administration, and extensively metabolised to active metabolites. A number of metabolites have been identified including (i) 4-(biphenyl-4-yl)-4-hydroxybutyric acid, (ii) biphenyl-4-ylacetic acid, (iii) (4′-hydroxybiphenyl-4-yl)acetic acid, and (iv) 4-hydroxy-(4′-hydroxybiphenyl-4-yl)butyric acid. About 40% of a dose is excreted in the urine in 24 h. The major urinary metabolites are metabolite (iii), about 11% of the dose, and metabolite (iv), about 17% of the dose; metabolites (i) and (ii) are excreted in amounts less than about 3% of the dose. Very little unchanged drug is excreted in the urine. Less than 2% of the dose is eliminated in the faeces in 24 h.

Therapeutic concentration

After a single oral dose of 600 mg administered to 3 subjects, mean peak serum concentrations of 8.1 mg/L of fenbufen and 64.9 mg/L of metabolite (i) were attained in about 2 h. A mean peak serum concentration of 13.2 mg/L of metabolite (ii) was attained in about 8 h [F. S. Chiccarelli *et al.*, *Arzneimittelforschung*, 1980, *30*, 728–735].

Half-life. Plasma half-life, fenbufen and metabolites (i) and (ii), about 10 h.

Protein binding. In plasma, fenbufen and metabolite (ii), more than 99%; metabolite (i), about 98%.

Note. For a review of the pharmacokinetics of fenbufen see R. N. Brogden *et al.*, *Drugs*, 1981, *21*, 1–22.

Dose. 600 to 900 mg daily.

Fenbutrazate

Anorectic

Synonym. Phenbutrazate

α-Ethylbenzeneacetic acid 2-(3-methyl-2-phenyl-4-morpholinyl)ethyl ester

$C_{23}H_{29}NO_3$ = 367.5

CAS—4378-36-3

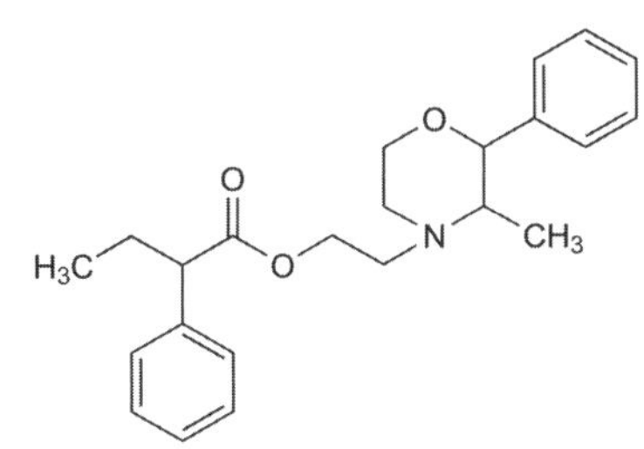

A viscous oil.

Soluble in methanol.

Fenbutrazate Hydrochloride

Synonym. Phenbutrazate Hydrochloride

$C_{23}H_{29}NO_3$,HCl = 403.9

CAS—6474-85-7

A fine white crystalline powder. M.p. 154°.

Slightly soluble in water; soluble in ethanol and acetone; practically insoluble in ether and benzene.

Partition Coefficient. Log *P* (octanol/water), 4.4.

Colour Tests. Liebermann's Test—red-orange; Marquis Test—yellow (slow).

Thin-layer Chromatography. System TA—Rf 72; system TB—Rf 47; system TC—Rf 78; system TE—Rf 86; system TL—Rf 67; system TAE—Rf 88. (Acidified iodoplatinate solution, positive.)

Gas Chromatography. System GA—RI 2670.

High Performance Liquid Chromatography. System HA—*k* 0.3.

Ultraviolet Spectrum. Aqueous acid—252, 257 nm (A_1^1=10b), 261, 267 nm.

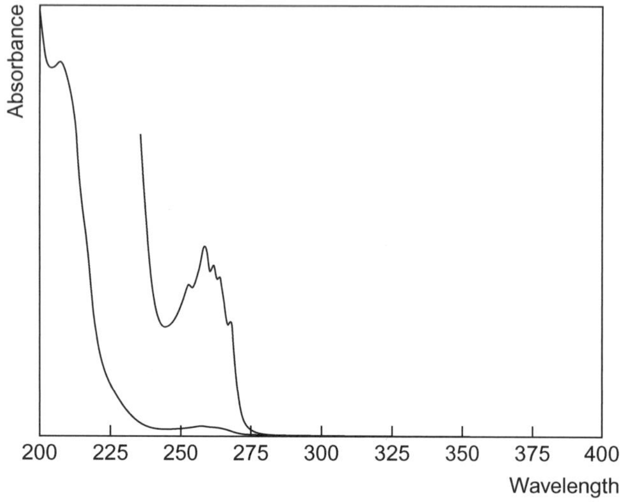

Infra-red Spectrum. Principal peaks at wavenumbers 1715, 1100, 1200, 690, 760, 1020 cm^{-1} (KBr disk).

Mass Spectrum. Principal ions at *m*/*z* 69, 56, 71, 91, 261, 84, 119, 70.

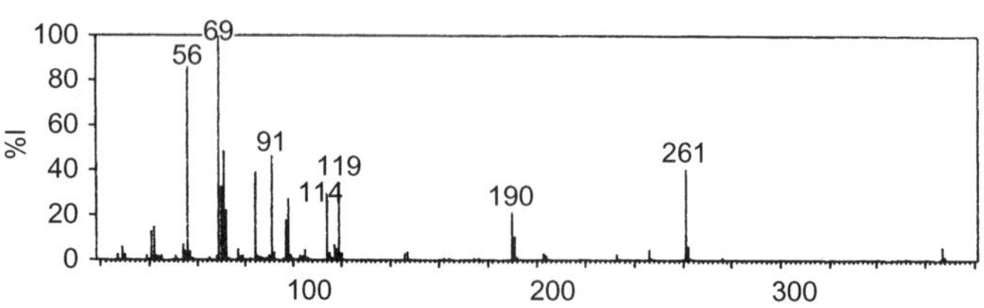

Dose. Fenbutrazate hydrochloride has been given in doses of 40 to 60 mg daily.

Fencamfamin

Central Stimulant

N-Ethyl-3-phenylbicyclo[2.2.1]heptan-2-amine
$C_{15}H_{21}N$=215.3
CAS—1209-98-9

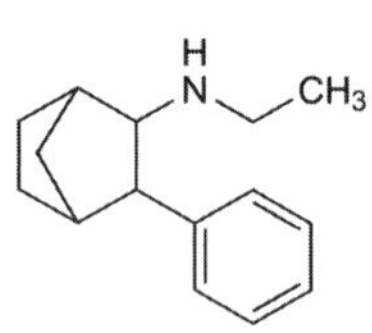

Practically insoluble in water; soluble in chloroform.

Fencamfamin Hydrochloride

Proprietary name. It is an ingredient of Reactivan.
$C_{15}H_{21}N,HCl$=251.8
CAS—2240-14-4
A white crystalline solid. M.p. 192°.
Freely soluble in water, ethanol, methanol and chloroform; slightly soluble in benzene; practically insoluble in ether.

Dissociation Constant. pK_a 8.7 (25°).

Partition Coefficient. Log *P* (octanol/water), 3.2.

Colour Tests. Liebermann's Test—red-orange; Marquis Test—orange

Thin-layer Chromatography. System TA—Rf 54; system TB—Rf 62; system TC—Rf 34; system TE—Rf 77; system TL—Rf 30; system TAE—Rf 21. (Acidified iodoplatinate solution, positive.)

Gas Chromatography. System GA—fencamfamin RI 1675, fencamfamin-AC RI 2085, fencamfamin-TFA RI 1970, fencamfamin-TMS RI 1780, fencamfamin-PFP RI 1755, M (desethyl-)-AC RI 2005, M (desethyl-OH-)-AC_2 RI 2305; system GB—RI 1737; system GC—RI 2180.

High Performance Liquid Chromatography. System HA—*k* 1.3; system HC—*k* 0.72; system HX—RI 354; system HY—RI 309.

Ultraviolet Spectrum. Aqueous acid—253, 259 nm (A_1^1=10a), 265, 269 nm.

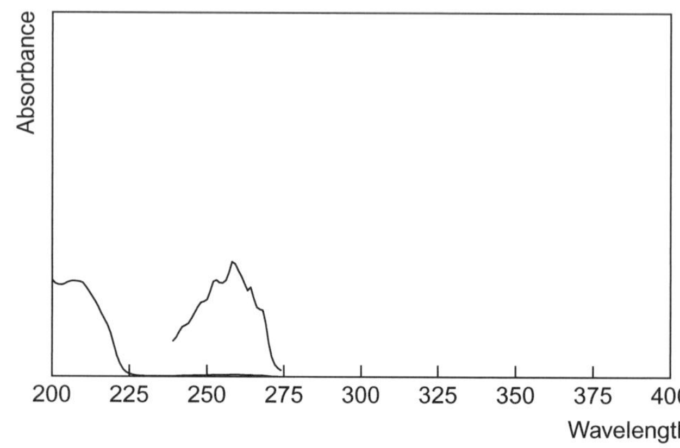

Infra-red Spectrum. Principal peaks at wavenumbers 708, 756, 1042, 797, 738, 1492 cm^{-1} (fencamfamin hydrochloride, Nujol mull).

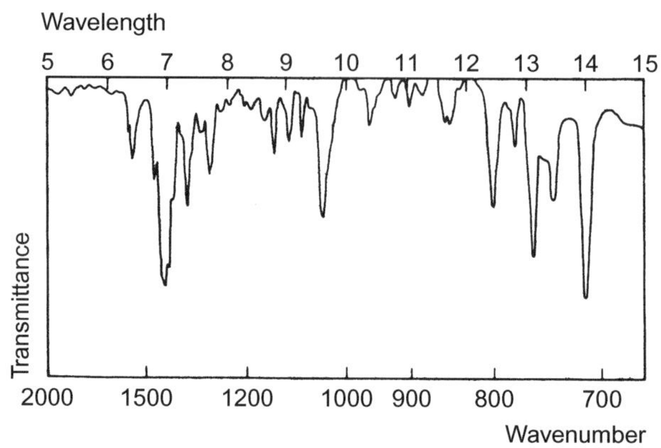

Mass Spectrum. Principal ions at *m*/*z* 98, 215, 58, 84, 91, 56, 71, 186; fencamfamin-AC *m*/*z* 170, 142, 58, 97, 91, 84; M (desethyl-)-AC *m*/*z* 170, 142, 91, 171, 115, 229; M (desethyl-OH-)-AC_2 *m*/*z* 142, 168, 228, 91, 119, 287.

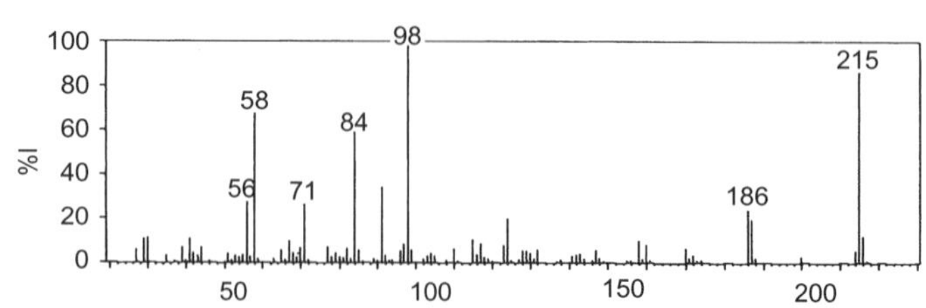

Quantification

Gas chromatography. In urine: limit of detection 40 µg/L for fencamfamin, 50 µg/L for the desethyl metabolite, ECD—F. T. Delbeke and M. Debackere, *Biopharm. Drug Dispos.*, 1981, *2*, 17–30.

Disposition in the Body. Absorbed after oral administration. Metabolised by de-ethylation. About 10 to 30% of a dose is excreted in the urine as unchanged drug and desethylfencamfamin in 3 days. The extent and rate of excretion is dependent on the urinary pH.

Half-life. Derived from urinary excretion data, about 16 h.

Dose. Usually 30 mg of fencamfamin hydrochloride daily.

Fenclofenac

Analgesic

[2-(2,4-Dichlorophenoxy)phenyl]acetic acid
$C_{14}H_{10}Cl_2O_3$=297.1
CAS—34645-84-6

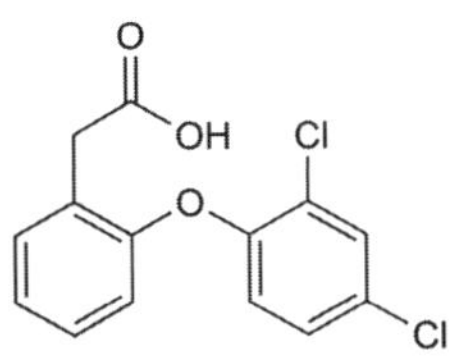

A white powder. M.p. about 136°.
Slightly soluble in water, but less soluble in acid solutions; freely soluble in most organic solvents.

Dissociation Constant. pK_a 5.5.

Partition Coefficient. Log *P* (octanol/water), 4.8.

Colour Tests. Liebermann's Test—orange (slow), (→brown at 100°); Marquis Test—red (slow).

Thin-layer Chromatography. System TG—Rf 20.

Gas Chromatography. System GD—RRTs of methyl derivative 1.55 and 1.26 (relative to n-$C_{16}H_{34}$).

High Performance Liquid Chromatography. System HV—RRT 0.91 (relative to meclofenamic acid).

Ultraviolet Spectrum. Methanol—270 nm (A^1_1=72b), 276 nm.

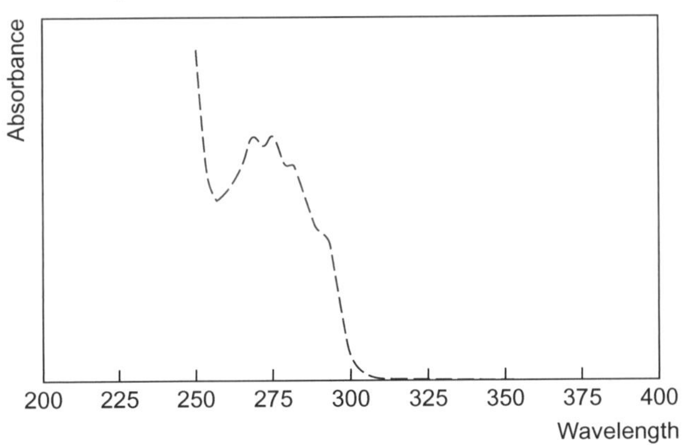

Infra-red Spectrum. Principal peaks at wavenumbers 1242, 1258, 1707, 1215, 1100, 772 cm^{-1} (KBr disk).

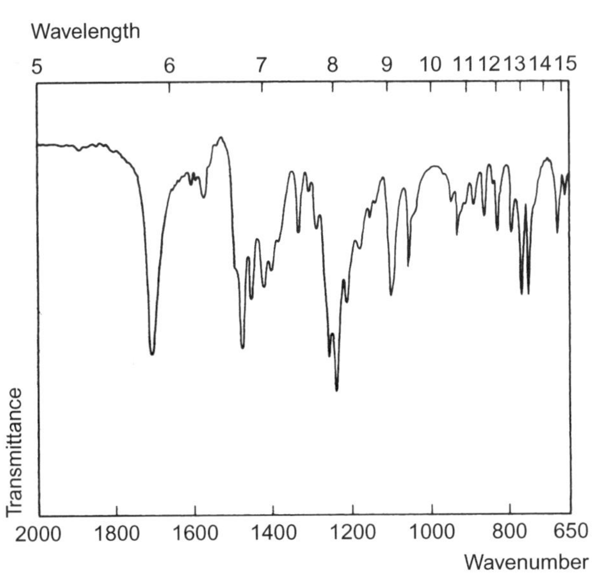

Mass Spectrum. Principal ions at *m/z* 296, 215, 217, 298, 216, 152, 181, 251.

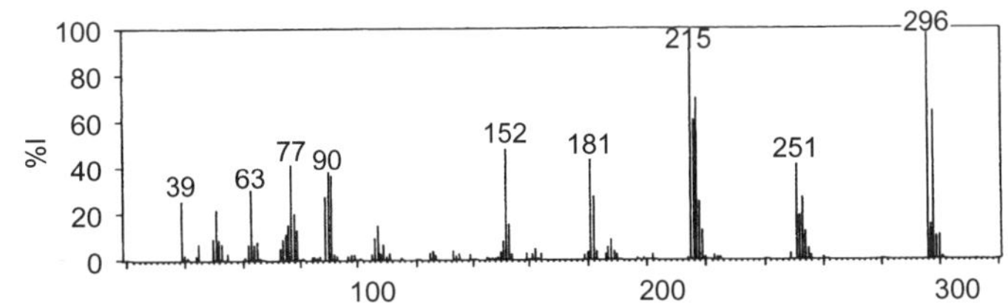

Quantification

Gas chromatography. In plasma: limit of detection 300 µg/L, ECD—R. Henson *et al.*, *Eur. J. Drug Met. Pharmacokinet.*, 1980, *5*, 217–223.

Disposition in the Body. Well absorbed after oral administration. More than 90% of a dose is excreted in the urine in the form of conjugates of the drug and hydroxylated metabolites.

Therapeutic concentration

A single oral dose of 600 mg to 9 subjects produced a mean peak plasma concentration of 63 mg/L in 3 to 4 h. Daily oral doses of 1200 mg to 5 subjects produced a mean steady-state plasma concentration of 87 mg/L [R. Henson *et al.*, *Eur. J. Drug Met. Pharmacokinet.*, 1980, *5*, 217–223].

Following daily oral doses of 10 to 25 mg/kg to 18 children for 3 weeks, maximum steady-state plasma concentrations of 52 to 372 mg/L (mean 120) were reported 2 to 8 h after a dose [A.-L. Makela *et al.*, *Eur. J. Clin. Pharmacol.*, 1983, *25*, 381–388].

Toxicity. Fenclofenac was used in rheumatic disorders but it had a high incidence of adverse effects, especially skin reactions, and was withdrawn from the market.

Half-life. Plasma half-life, 15 to 40 h (mean 26).

Volume of distribution. About 0.2 L/kg.

Distribution in blood. Plasma:whole blood ratio, about 1.7.

Protein binding. In plasma, about 99%.

Dose. 0.6 to 1.2 g daily.

Fendosal

Analgesic

Proprietary name. Alnovin
5-(4,5-Dihydro-2-phenyl-3*H*-benz[*e*]indol-3-yl)-2-hydroxybenzoic acid
$C_{25}H_{19}NO_3$=381.4
CAS—53597-27-6

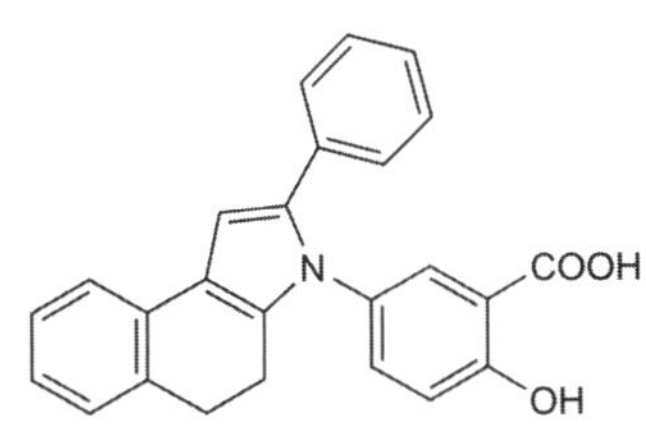

A yellow powder. M.p. 239° to 241°.
Practically insoluble in water; soluble 1 in 50 of ethanol; slightly soluble in alkaline solutions and in propylene glycol.

Dissociation Constant. pK_a 3.1.

Thin-layer Chromatography. System TA—Rf 95; system TE—Rf 22; system TAJ—Rf 05; system TAK—Rf 68; system TAL—Rf 83.

Ultraviolet Spectrum. Aqueous alkali—292 nm (A^1_1=564b).

Infra-red Spectrum. Principal peaks at wavenumbers 1675, 1242, 1500, 1615, 1298, 765 cm^{-1} (KBr disk).

Quantification

Fluorescence spectrophotometry. In plasma: limit of detection 0.1 mg/L—H. M. Hill *et al.*, *Biopharm. Drug Dispos.*, 1980, *1*, 97–102.

Dose. Fendosal has been given in doses of 200 to 400 mg.

Fenetylline

Xanthine Stimulant

Synonyms. Amfetyline; 7-Ethyltheophylline Amfetamine; Fenethylline.
3,7-Dihydro-1,3-dimethyl-7-[2-[(1-methyl-2-phenylethyl)amino]ethyl]-1*H*-purine-2,6-dione
$C_{18}H_{23}N_5O_2=341.4$
CAS—3736-08-1

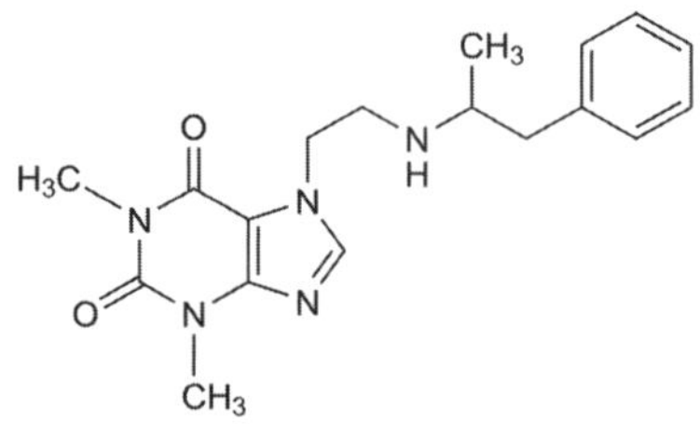

Practically insoluble in water; soluble in chloroform.

Fenetylline Hydrochloride

Synonyms. Fenethylline Hydrochloride; H814; R-720-11.
Proprietary names. Captagon; Fitton.
$C_{18}H_{23}N_5O_2,HCl=377.9$
CAS—1892-80-4
A white crystalline powder. M.p. 227° to 229° and 237° to 239°.
Soluble in water.

Colour Tests. Amalic Acid Test—pink-orange/violet; Marquis Test—orange.

Thin-layer Chromatography. System TA—Rf 55; system TB—Rf 03; system TC—Rf 45; system TE—Rf 54; system TL—Rf 14; system TAE—Rf 44. (Acidified iodoplatinate solution, positive.)

Gas Chromatography. System GA—fenetylline RI 2830, fenetylline-AC RI 3110, M (*N*-desalkyl-)-AC RI 2480, M (amfetamine) RI 1125, M (etofylline) RI 2125; system GB—fenetylline RI 2900.

High Performance Liquid Chromatography. System HC—*k* 0.27; system HX—RI 336; system HY—RI 277.

Ultraviolet Spectrum. Aqueous acid—275 nm (A_1^1=242a). No alkaline shift. (See below)

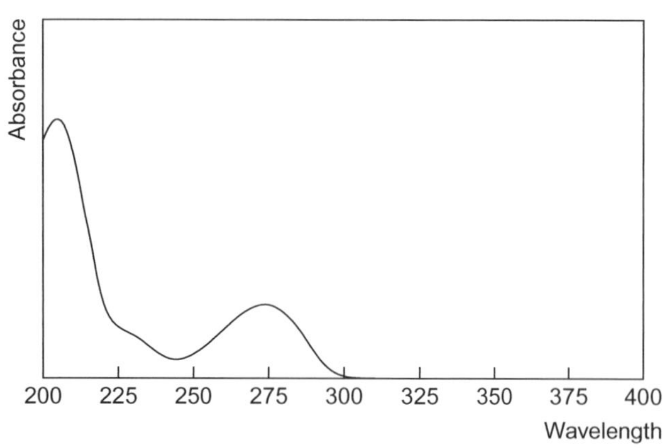

Infra-red Spectrum. Principal peaks at wavenumbers 1664, 1705, 1600, 1546, 746, 1219 cm^{-1} (KBr disk).

Mass Spectrum. Principal ions at *m/z* 250, 70, 207, 91, 251, 119, 148, 56.

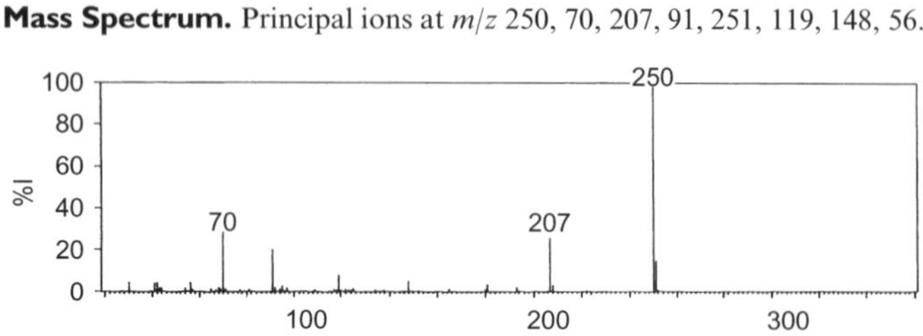

Quantification

Mass spectrometry–gas chromatography. In hair—R. Kikura and Y. Nakahara, *J. Anal. Toxicol.*, 1997, *21*, 291–296.

Dose. Fenetylline hydrochloride has been given in doses of 25 to 100 mg daily to treat narcolepsy.

Fenfluramine

Anorectic

N-Ethyl-α-methyl-3-(trifluoromethyl)benzeneethanamine
$C_{12}H_{16}F_3N=231.3$
CAS—458-24-2

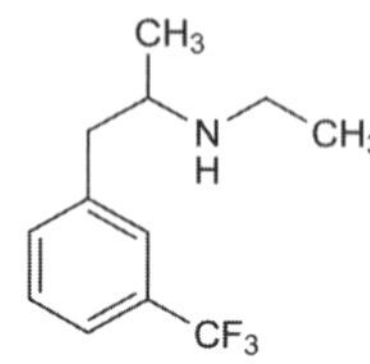

Practically insoluble in water; soluble in chloroform.

Fenfluramine Hydrochloride

Proprietary names. Dima-Fen; Pesos; Ponderal; Ponderax; Pondimin.
$C_{12}H_{16}F_3N,HCl=267.7$
CAS—404-82-0
A white crystalline powder. M.p. 168° to 172°.
Soluble 1 in 20 of water, 1 in 10 of ethanol and 1 in 10 of chloroform; practically insoluble in ether.

Dissociation Constant. pK_a 9.1 (25°).

Partition Coefficient. Log *P* (octanol/water), 3.4.

Colour Test. Liebermann's Test (at 100°)—yellow.

Thin-layer Chromatography. System TA—Rf 48; system TB—Rf 42; system TC—Rf 16; system TE—Rf 61; system TL—Rf 11; system TAE—Rf 20; system TAJ—Rf 07; system TAK—Rf 25; system TAL—Rf 68. (Acidified iodoplatinate solution, positive.)

Gas Chromatography. System GA—fenfluramine RI 1230, norfenfluramine RI 1133, fenfluramine-TFA RI 1455, fenfluramine-PFP RI 1455, fenfluramine-AC RI 1580, norfenfluramine-AC RI 1510; system GB—fenfluramine RI 1252, norfenfluramine RI 1157; system GC—fenfluramine RI 1621, norfenfluramine RI 1470.

High Performance Liquid Chromatography. System HA—fenfluramine *k* 1.3, norfenfluramine *k* 1.0; system HC—*k* 0.88; system HX—RI 371; system HY—RI 315; system HZ—Retention time, 3.9 min; system HAA—Retention time, 13.1 min.

Ultraviolet Spectrum. Aqueous acid—264 nm (A_1^1=22a), 271 nm.

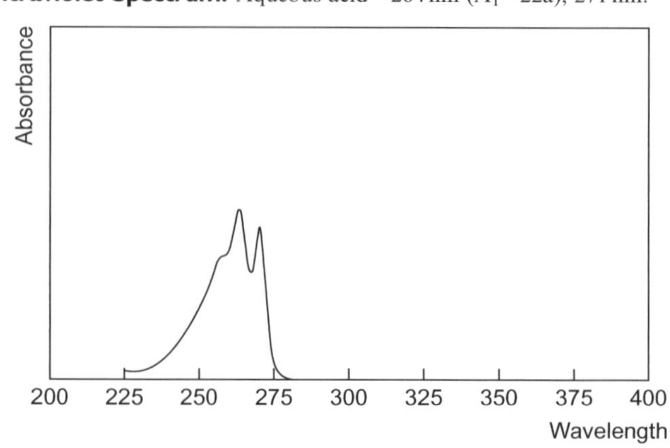

Infra-red Spectrum. Principal peaks at wavenumbers 1165, 1116, 1070, 698, 793, 1202 cm^{-1} (fenfluramine hydrochloride, KBr disk).

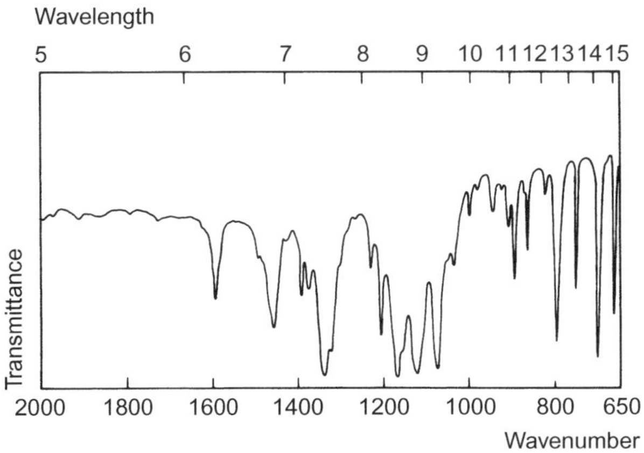

Mass Spectrum. Principal ions at m/z 72, 44, 159, 73, 58, 42, 109, 56; norfenfluramine 44, 42, 159, 43, 45, 184, 41, 109.

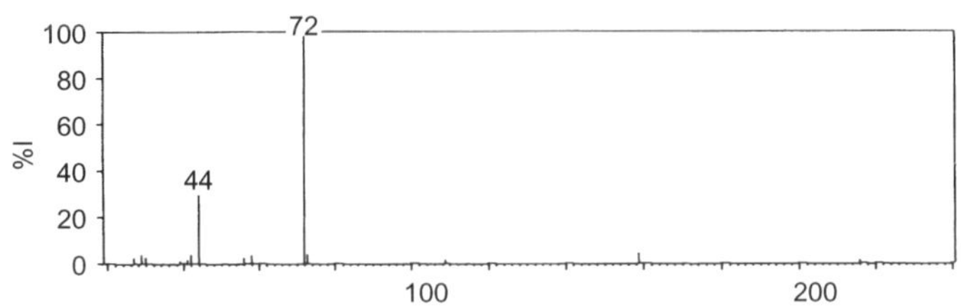

Quantification

Gas chromatography. In plasma or urine: fenfluramine and norfenfluramine, limits of detection fenfluramine 5 µg/L and norfenfluramine 100 ng/L in plasma, ECD—K. K. Midha *et al.*, *Can. J. Pharm. Sci.*, 1979, *14*, 18–21. In plasma: enantiomers of fenfluramine and norfenfluramine, ECD—N. R. Srinivas *et al.*, *J. Chromatogr.*, 1988, *433*, 105–117. In plasma or urine: D-fenfluramine and D-norfenfluramine, nitrogen-specific detection—R. P. Richards *et al.*, *Xenobiotica*, 1989, *19*, 547–553.

Gas chromatography–mass spectrometry. In blood: fenfluramine, amfetamine and metamfetamine, limit of detection for fenfluramine 5 µg/L—A. Namera *et al.*, *Forensic Sci. Int.*, 2000, *109*, 215–223. In urine: fenfluramine and amfetamine-related drugs—A. Namera *et al.*, *J. Chromatogr. Sci.*, 2002, *40*, 19–25.

High performance liquid chromatography. In plasma: DL-fenfluramine, DL-norfenfluramine and phentermine, fluorescence detection—A. Kaddoumi *et al.*, *J. Chromatogr. B. Biomed. Sci. Appl.*, 2001, *763*, 79–90.

Disposition in the Body. Readily absorbed after oral administration and accumulates in the tissues. The major metabolite in the blood is the *N*-desethyl derivative, norfenfluramine, which is active. It is also metabolised by oxidation to *m*-trifluoromethylbenzoic acid which is conjugated with glycine to form *m*-trifluoromethylhippuric acid. The rate of elimination is influenced by urinary pH and urinary flow. In acidic urine about 23% of a dose is excreted unchanged and about 17% as norfenfluramine in 48 h; the remainder consists of *m*-trifluoromethylhippuric acid; in alkaline urine about 2% is excreted as unchanged drug and norfenfluramine; when the urinary pH is not controlled, 3 to 10% may be excreted as unchanged drug and 3 to 14% as norfenfluramine. Up to 5% of a dose is eliminated in the faeces as fenfluramine and norfenfluramine.

Therapeutic concentration. In plasma, usually in the range 0.05 to 0.15 mg/L.

There is considerable intersubject variation in plasma concentrations and it has been reported that the therapeutic effect (weight loss) is greater in those patients who can tolerate higher plasma concentrations (more than 0.2 mg/L) [J. A. Innes *et al.*, *BMJ*, 1977, *2*, 1322–1325].

A single oral dose of 60 mg administered to 5 subjects, resulted in a mean plasma concentration of 0.06 mg/L of fenfluramine in 2 to 4 h and 0.016 mg/L of norfenfluramine in 4 to 6 h. Steady-state plasma concentrations of 0.04 to 0.12 mg/L of fenfluramine were attained in 3 to 4 days after daily administration of 60 mg, in divided doses, to 6 subjects; concentrations of norfenfluramine were similar [D. B. Campbell, *Br. J. Pharmacol.*, 1971, *43*, 465P–466P].

Toxicity. In adults the minimum lethal dose is probably in excess of 2 g but for young children as little as 200 mg may cause death. Toxic effects may be produced when the plasma concentration is greater than about 0.5 mg/L, and death has occurred at concentrations above 6 mg/L.

3 children aged 6 years, 3 years, and 1 year 9 months ingested between them about 4 g of fenfluramine hydrochloride. The youngest and the oldest child died; postmortem blood concentrations were 6.5 and 16 mg/L respectively and liver concentrations were 48 and 136 µg/g; a urine concentration of 60 mg/L was found in the younger child [R. G. Gold *et al.*, *Lancet*, 1969, *2*, 1306].

A 13-year-old boy died after ingesting 2 g of fenfluramine hydrochloride; postmortem concentrations, mg/L or µg/g, were:

	Fenfluramine	Norfenfluramine
Blood	6.5	0.75
Bile	64.5	10.2
Brain	42	5.3
Kidney	27.1	1.5
Liver	49	8.5
Urine	89	10

[M. R. Fleisher and D. B. Campbell, *Lancet*, 1969, *2*, 1306–1307.].

In a fatality involving the suicidal ingestion of fenfluramine, a blood concentration of 7.46 mg/L was reported. Chronic fenfluramine use was demonstrated by the presence of the drug in hair (14.1 µg/g) [P. Kintz and P. Mangin, *Hum. Exp. Toxicol.*, 1992, *11*, 51–52].

Half-life. Plasma half-life, 11 to 30 h (mean 20).

Distribution in blood. Plasma:whole blood ratio, about 0.74.

Protein binding. In plasma, about 30%.

Note. For reviews of fenfluramine see R. M. Pinder *et al.*, *Drugs*, 1975, *10*, 241–323 and L. E. Vivero *et al.*, *J. Emerg. Med.*, 1998, *16*, 197–205. For a review of fenfluramine poisoning see K. E. von Muhlendahl and E. G. Krienke, *Clin. Toxicol.*, 1979, *14*, 97–106.

Dose. Initially 40 mg of fenfluramine hydrochloride daily, increasing to 60 to 120 mg daily.

Fenitrothion

Insecticide

Synonyms. AC-47300; Bayer 41831; Bayer S 5660; ENT-25715; MEP; OMS-45; OMS-223; S-5660; S-1102-A; metathion.
Proprietary names. Accothion; Agrothion; Cyfen; Cytel; Cyten; Dicofen; Etalene; Fenitox; Folithion; Micromite; Novathion; Nuvanol; Pestroy; Sumithion; Verthion.
Phosphorothioic acid *O*,*O*-dimethyl *O*-(3-methyl-4-nitrophenyl) ester
$C_9H_{12}NO_5PS$ = 277.2
CAS—122-14-5

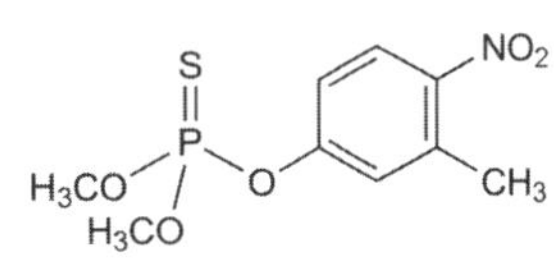

A yellow to brown oil. M.p. 3.4°. B.p. 118° at 0.05 mmHg.
It is practically insoluble in water (14 mg/L at 30°); has low solubility in aliphatic hydrocarbons; soluble in most organic solvents including alcohol esters, ketones, aromatic hydrocarbons, and chlorinated hydrocarbons. It has a solubility in hexane of 42 g/kg at 20 to 25°, dichloromethane, methanol, and xylene > 1000 g/kg, propan-2-ol 193 g/kg.

Partition Coefficient. Log P (octanol/water), 3.43.

Thin-layer Chromatography. System TX—Rf 32; system TY—Rf 76; system TZ—Rf 82; system TAA—Rf 65; system TAB—Rf 50; system TAC—Rf 17.

Gas Chromatography. System GA—RI 1905; system GK—RRT 1.01 (relative to caffeine); system GKA—RI 1944; system GKB—RI 2112; system GKC—RI 2278.

High Performance Liquid Chromatography. System HAP—*k* 2.86; system HAO—*k* 0.22.

Ultraviolet Spectrum. Aqueous acid—268 nm.

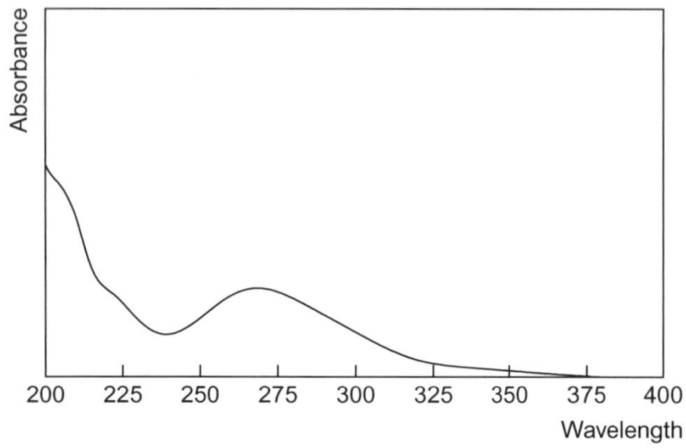

Infra-red Spectrum. Principal peaks at wavenumber 1055, 830, 971, 1243, 1359, 1539 cm^{-1}.

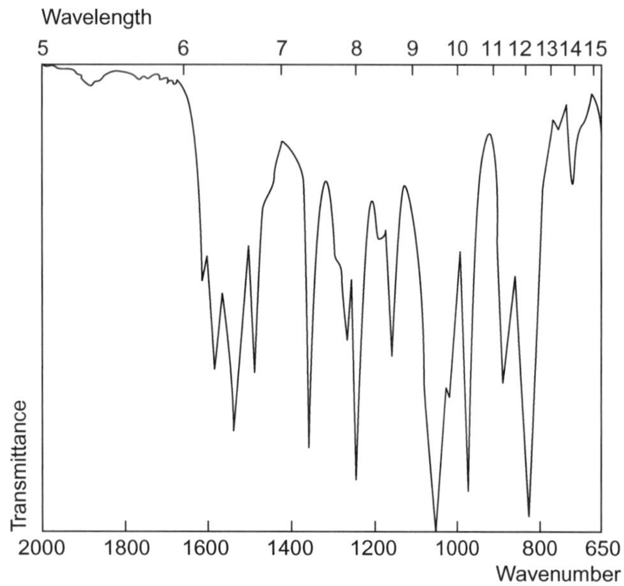

Mass Spectrum. Principal ions at *m/z* 125, 109, 79, 277, 47, 93, 63, 260.

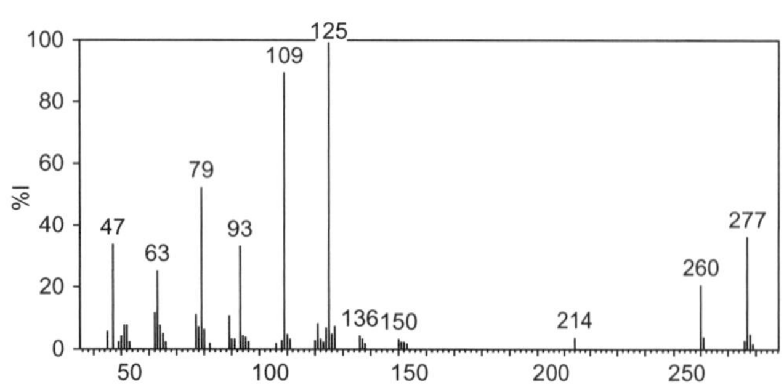

Quantification

High performance liquid chromatography. In urine: limit of detection 3.4 µg/L, UV detection (λ=315 nm)—M. J. W. Chang and R. S. Lin, *Bull. Envir. Contam. Toxicol.*, 1995, *55(1)*, 29–35.

Disposition in the Body. Fenitrothion is rapidly absorbed after ingestion and is metabolised to 3-methyl-4-nitrophenol, aminofenitrothion, aminofenitroxon, acetyl-aminofenitroxon, and *S*-methylfenitrothion. It is distributed among various tissues. All metabolites have been detected in urine and excretion mainly occurs within the first 12 h. 50 to 70% of a dose is excreted in urine within 24 h as the metabolites. No evidence exists to show that fenitrothion accumulates within the body but it is stored in fat tissues and possibly released under stress conditions.

Toxicity. Allowed daily intake is 0.003 mg/kg bodyweight. A blood concentration of 260 ng/g causes low to mild poisoning. The low toxic dose reported for acute oral toxicity in a female is 800 mg/kg.

A 23-year-old male was admitted to hospital after an attempted suicide. He had ingested 50 mL of fenitrothion emulsion (5%) but vomited soon after. A blood fenitrothion concentration of 169.5 ng/g was observed 3 h after ingestion. The male made a full recovery and was discharged from hospital 3 days after admission. [T. Kojima *et al.*, *Forensic Sci. Int.*, 1989, *41(3)*, 245–253.]

A 56-year-old male attempted suicide by ingesting 60 mL of 50% fenitrothion emulsion. 5 h later he was treated with haemodialysis and haemoperfusion. After 60 min his symptoms gradually improved but 4 days after the initial ingestion, cholinergic symptoms recurred and he died 2 days later despite immediate treatment. Toxicological analysis showed that tissue and organ distribution was high with the highest concentration in fat (59 mg/kg wet weight, which is ten times greater than in other organs, suggesting a slow release of the pesticide from fat). [M. Yoshida *et al.*, *Hum Toxicol.*, 1987, *6*, 403–406.]

Half-life. 4.5 h.

Fenoldopam

Antihypertensive

Synonym. SKF-82526
6-Chloro-2,3,4,5-tetrahydro-1-(4-hydroxyphenyl)-1*H*-3-benzazepine-7,8-diol
$C_{16}H_{16}ClNO_3$=305.8
CAS—*67227-56-9*

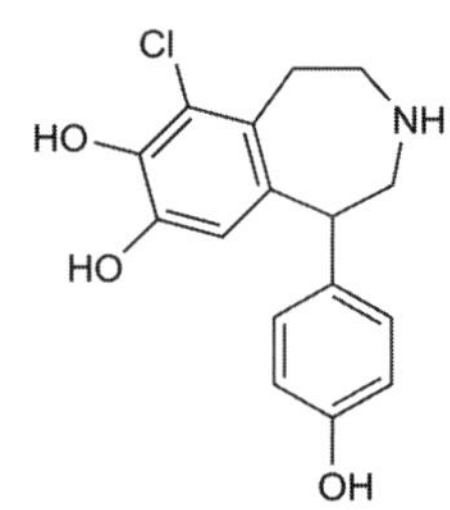

Fenoldopam Hydrobromide

$C_{16}H_{17}BrClNO_3$=386.7
M.p. 277°.

Fenoldopam Methanesulfonate

Synonyms. Fenoldopam mesylate; SKF-82526-J.
Proprietary name. Corlopam
$C_{17}H_{20}ClNO_6S$=401.9
CAS—67227-57-0
M.p. 274°, water solubility is 4003 mg/L at 25°.

Partition Coefficient. Log *P* (octanol/water), 2.39.

High Performance Liquid Chromatography. Column: octadecylsilica (Ultrasphere, 5 µm, 250 × 4.6 mm i.d.). Mobile phases: (A)-methanol: citrate-acetate buffer, pH 4.0 (20:80); B-methanol: monochloroacetate buffer, pH 3.2 (18:82), flow rate 1.0 mL/min. Electrochemical detection. Retention time: (A) fenoldopam, 8.7 min; (B) fenoldopam 8-sulfate metabolite, 14.8 min [V. K. Boppana *et al.*, *J. Chromatogr.*, 1984, *317*, *Biomed. Appl.*, 463–474].

Quantification

High performance liquid chromatography. In plasma: limit of detection 0.025 µg/L for fenoldopam, 2 µg/L sulfate metabolites and 0.5 µg/L methoxy metabolites. Electrochemical detection—V. K. Boppana *et al.*, *J. Chromatogr.*, 1989, *487(2)*, 385–399.

Disposition in the Body. Fenoldopam is extensively metabolised by conjugation: glucuronidation, sulfation and methylation. Metabolites include fenoldopam 7-sulfate and 8-sulfate which are excreted predominantly in urine (90%) and faeces (10%). Approx. 4% of a dose is excreted unchanged in urine. Less than 0.005% of the drug crosses the blood–brain barrier.

Therapeutic concentration

16 men and 2 women patients with New York Heart Association Class III heart failure, aged between 33 and 67 years, were administered 100 mg dose of fenoldopam. The dose was either administered with food or after a 12 h fast. Peak plasma concentrations of 26.5 and 10.9 μg/L fenoldopam were reached for the fasted and fed patients, respectively, within 1.3 to 2 h. Fenoldopam 7-sulfate and fenoldopam 8-sulfate were also detected at concentrations of 1357 and 689 μg/L, respectively, in the fasted patients and 1411 and 707 μg/L in the fed. These concentrations were reached between 2.4 and 3.6 h after administration [D. G. Blanchett *et al.*, *Clin. Pharmacol. Ther.*, 1991, *49*, 449–456].

Toxicity. Reported to be 6 times as potent as dopamine in causing vasodilation.

Bioavailability. Approx. 6% (oral).

Half-life. Approx. 5 to 10 min.

Volume of distribution. 0.23 L/kg (0.025 μg/kg body weight/min dose) to 0.66 L/kg (0.25 and 0.5 μg/kg body weight/min).

Clearance. 1.49 L/h/kg (0.025 μg/kg body weight/min dose) to 2.29 L/h/kg (0.5 μg/kg body weight/min dose).

Protein binding. Approx. 88%.

Dose. IV: usual dose of 0.1 to 1.6 μg/kg body weight/min is administered and adjusted in 0.05 to 1.0 μg/kg body weight increments. Oral: 100 mg two to four times daily.

Fenoprofen

Analgesic

α-Methyl-3-phenoxybenzeneacetic acid
$C_{15}H_{14}O_3 = 242.3$
CAS—31879-05-7

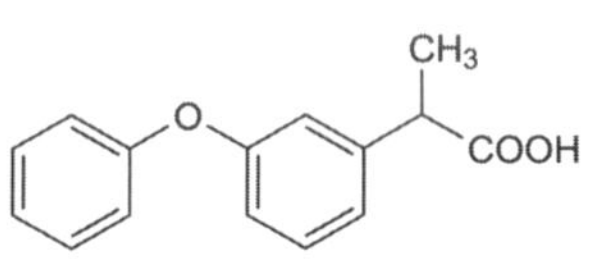

Fenoprofen Calcium

Proprietary names. Fenopron; Fepron; Nalfon; Nalgésic; Progesic; Trandor.
$(C_{15}H_{13}O_3)_2Ca,2H_2O = 558.6$
CAS—34597-40-5 (anhydrous); 53746-45-5 (dihydrate)
A white crystalline powder. M.p. 105° to 110°.
Soluble 1 in 400 to 1 in 500 of water, 1 in 15 of ethanol and 1 in 300 of chloroform.

Dissociation Constant. pK$_a$ 4.5 (25°).

Partition Coefficient. Log *P* (octanol/pH 7.4), 0.8.

Colour Tests. Liebermann's Test—red-brown; Marquis Test—pink

Thin-layer Chromatography. System TA—Rf 96; system TD—Rf 42; system TE—Rf 06; system TF—Rf 38; system TG—Rf 16; system TAD—Rf 50; system TAJ—Rf 58; system TAK—Rf 78; system TAL—Rf 76. (Ludy Tenger reagent, orange.)

Gas Chromatography. System GA—fenoprofen RI 2016, fenoprofen-Me RI 1906; system GD—RRT of methyl derivative 1.31 (relative to *n*-$C_{16}H_{34}$); system GL—fenoprofen-Me RI 1970, M (OH-)-Me$_2$ RI 2130.

High Performance Liquid Chromatography. System HD—*k* 7.9; system HX—RI 574; system HY—RI 524; system HZ—Retention time, 10.9 min; system HAA—Retention time, 21.2 min; system HAX—Retention time, 8.0 min; system HAY—Retention time, 8.9 min.

Ultraviolet Spectrum. Aqueous acid—272 nm (A^1_1 = 72a); methanol—273 nm (A^1_1 = 72a), 280 nm.

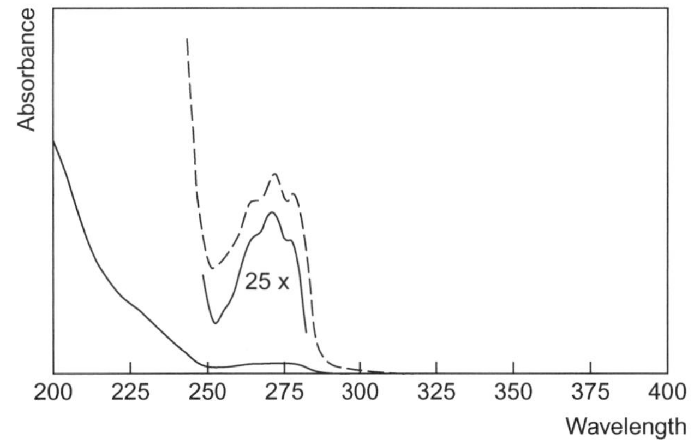

Infra-red Spectrum. Principal peaks at wavenumbers 1562, 1225, 696, 1211, 1268, 1248 cm^{-1} (fenoprofen calcium, KBr disk).

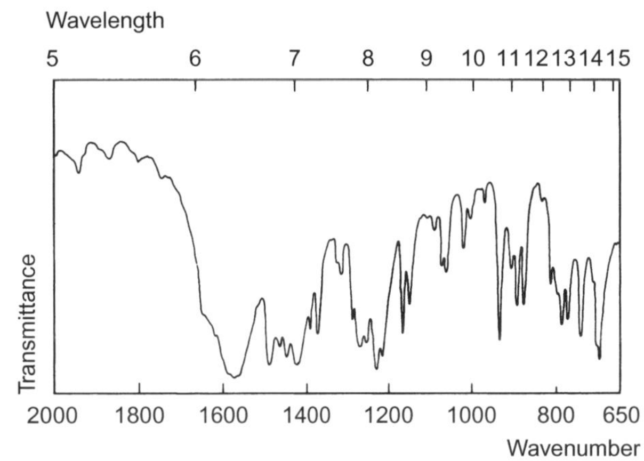

Mass Spectrum. Principal ions at *m/z* 197, 241, 198, 77, 242, 104, 91, 103; fenoprofen-Me *m/z* 197, 256, 198, 257, 91, 103; M (OH-)-Me$_2$ *m/z* 286, 227, 287, 123, 91, 152.

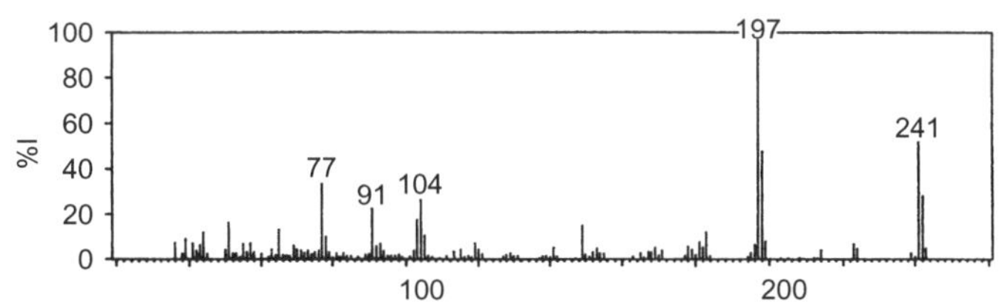

Quantification

Gas chromatography. In plasma: limit of detection 250 μg/L, FID—J. F. Nash *et al.*, *J. Pharm. Sci.*, 1971, *60*, 1062–1064.

High performance liquid chromatography. In plasma: limit of detection 500 μg/L, UV detection—R. J. Bopp *et al.*, *J. Pharm. Sci.*, 1981, *70*, 507–509. In plasma: fenoprofen and other NSAIDs, UV detection—S. G. Owen *et al.*, *J. Chromatogr.*, 1987, *416*, 293–302. In plasma or urine: fenoprofen enantiomers, UV detection—R. Mehvar and F. Jamali, *Pharm. Res.*, 1988, *5*, 53–56. In plasma: fenoprofen, ibuprofen and ketoprofen, limit of detection for fenoprofen 0.25 mg/L, UV detection—S. Menzel-Soglowek *et al.*, *J. Chromatogr.*, 1990, *532*, 295–303. In plasma or urine: fenoprofen enantiomers and metabolites, UV detection—C. Volland *et al.*, *J. Chromatogr.*, 1990, *534*, 127–138.

Disposition in the Body. Readily absorbed after oral administration. About 90% of a dose is excreted in the urine in 24 h, about 3% of the excreted material being unchanged drug, about 45% fenoprofen glucuronide, about 42% 4-hydroxyfenoprofen glucuronide and about 2% free 4-hydroxyfenoprofen. About 2% of a dose is eliminated in the faeces in 24 h.

Therapeutic concentration

After a single oral dose of 250 mg administered to 4 subjects, peak plasma concentrations of 23 to 31 mg/L (mean 27) were attained in 0.5 to 2 h [A. Rubin *et al.*, *J. Pharm. Sci.*, 1971, *60*, 1797–1801].

Toxicity. Recovery has been reported after the ingestion of about 60 g.

A 17-year-old girl presented with coma, metabolic acidosis, hypotension and respiratory depression within 4 h of ingesting 24 to 36 g of fenoprofen as a suicidal gesture; treatment led to recovery within 3 days [J. M. Kolodzik *et al.*, *Ann. Emerg. Med.*, 1990, *19*, 378–381].

Half-life. Plasma half-life, 2 to 3 h.

Volume of distribution. About 0.1 L/kg.

Protein binding. In plasma, about 99%.

Note. For a review of the pharmacological properties of fenoprofen see R. N. Brogden *et al.*, *Drugs*, 1977, *13*, 241–65.

Dose. The equivalent of 0.9 to 2.4 g of fenoprofen daily.

Fenoterol

Sympathomimetic

5-[1-Hydroxy-2-[[2-(4-hydroxyphenyl)-1-methylethyl]amino]ethyl]-1,3-benzenediol
$C_{17}H_{21}NO_4$=303.4
CAS—13392-18-2

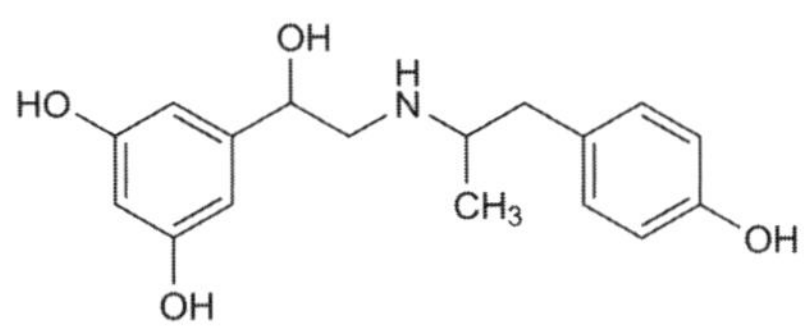

Fenoterol Hydrobromide

Proprietary names. Berotec; Dosberotec; Partusisten. It is an ingredient of Duovent.
$C_{17}H_{21}NO_4$,HBr=384.3
CAS—1944-12-3
A white crystalline powder. M.p. about 230°, with decomposition.
Soluble 1 in 10 of water and 1 in 11 of ethanol; practically insoluble in chloroform and ether.

Dissociation Constant. pK_a 8.5, 10.0.

Partition Coefficient. Log *P* (octanol/water), 1.2.

Thin-layer Chromatography. System TA—Rf 76; system TB—Rf 00; system TC—Rf 01; system TE—Rf 25; system TF—Rf 00; system TL—Rf 04; system TAE—Rf 38; system TAF—Rf 81.

Gas Chromatography. System GA—fenoterol RI 1416, fenoterol-H_2O-AC_4 RI 3440.

High Performance Liquid Chromatography. System HA—*k* 0.7; system HX—RI 287; system HY—RI 246; system HAX—Retention time 5.7 min; system HAY—Retention time 3.4 min.

Ultraviolet Spectrum. Aqueous acid—275 nm (A_1^1=107a); aqueous alkali—295 nm (A_1^1=190b).

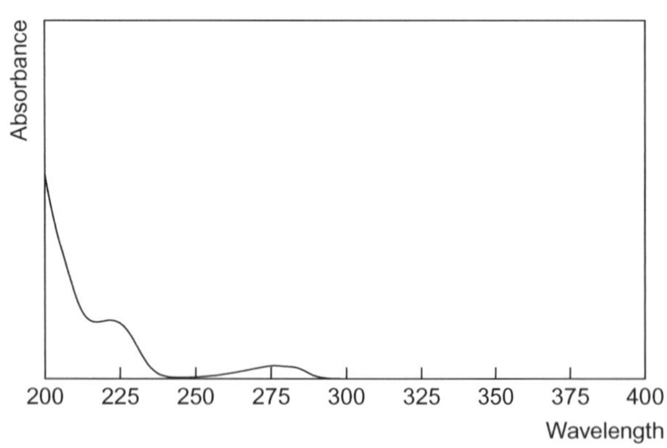

Infra-red Spectrum. Principal peaks at wavenumbers 1605, 1510, 700, 1160, 1575, 1200 cm^{-1} (fenoterol hydrobromide, KBr disk).

Quantification

Gas chromatography–mass spectrometry. In postmortem blood: fenoterol, salbutamol and terbutaline, limit of detection <1 µg/L—F. J. Couper and O. H. Drummer, *J. Chromatogr.* 1996, *685*, *Biomed Appl.*, 265–272.

High performance liquid chromatography. In plasma: limit of detection <376 ng/L, fluorescence detection—S. Kramer and G. Blaschke, *J. Chromat. B. Biomed. Sci. Appl.*, 2001, *751*, 169–175. In plasma: fluorescence detection—I. Meineke *et al.*, *J. Pharm. Biomed. Anal.*, 2002, *29*, 147–152.

Disposition in the Body. Rapidly but incompletely absorbed after inhalation or oral administration. It undergoes extensive first-pass metabolism by sulfate conjugation. About 35% of an oral dose is excreted in the urine in 24 h, mainly as the inactive sulfate conjugate, and less than 2% as unchanged drug; about 40% of an oral dose is eliminated in the faeces.

Therapeutic concentration

After oral administration of 5 mg of tritiated fenoterol to 8 subjects, peak plasma radioactivity equivalent to about 0.04 mg/L of fenoterol was attained in 2 h; most of the radioactivity was due to metabolites. Following inhalation of a 200 µg or 500 µg metered-dose by 3 subjects, peak plasma radioactivity equivalent to about 0.0003 to 0.0004 mg/L of fenoterol was reported [L. Buchelt and K. L. Rominger, *Med. Proc.*, 1972, *18*, 15–20].

Fenoterol was given by intravenous infusion to 5 subjects at a dose of 0.5, 1.0 or 2.0 µg/min over 3 h. Steady-state plasma concentrations of 385, 636 and 980 ng/L, respectively, were reached within 90 to 120 min [K. Warnke *et al*, *Eur. J. Clin. Pharmacol.*, 1992, *43*, 663–665].

In 20 healthy subjects receiving an intravenous infusion of fenoterol 1 µg/min for 4 h, steady-state plasma concentrations were reached by 2 h later (median 0.89 µg/L, range 0.72 to 1.16 µg/L). The maximum plasma concentration of fenoterol glucuronide was 0.88 µg/L (range 0.74 to 0.97) at the end of the infusion and that of fenoterol sulfate was 0.65 µg/L (0.49 to 0.70). A 10 mg oral dose every 20 min up to a total dose of 30 mg in the same subjects produced a median peak plasma-fenoterol level of 0.54 µg/L (range 0.25 to 0.69), with the concentrations of fenoterol glucuronide and sulfate reaching a maximum of 14.3 µg/L (range 8.7 to 17.9) and 92 µg/L (87 to 105), respectively, at about 2 h [R. Hildebrandt *et al.*, *Xenobiotica*, 1994, *24*, 71–77].

Half-life. Plasma half-life, about 6 to 7 h.

Note. For a review of fenoterol see N. Svedmyr, *Pharmacotherapy*, 1985, *5*, 109–126.

Dose. Up to 360 µg of fenoterol hydrobromide every 4 h, by aerosol inhalation; 15 to 20 mg daily has been given by mouth.

Fenpipramide

Antispasmodic (Veterinary)

Synonym. Fenpiverinium
2,2-Diphenyl-4-piperidinobutyramide
$C_{21}H_{26}N_2O$=322.4
CAS—77-01-0

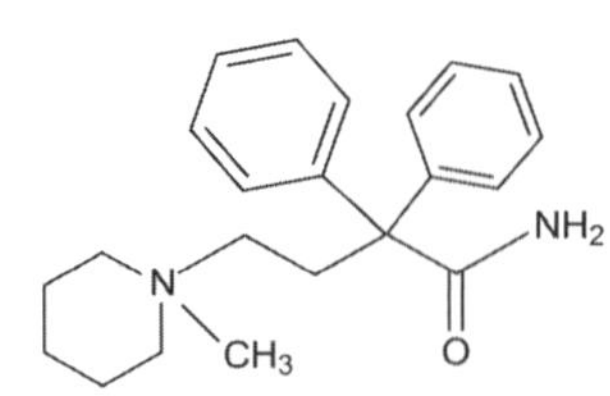

White crystals. M.p. 188°.
Practically insoluble in water; soluble in chloroform.

Fenpipramide Hydrochloride

Proprietary name. It is an ingredient of Efosin.
$C_{21}H_{26}N_2O$,HCl,H_2O=376.9
CAS—14007-53-5 (anhydrous)
A white crystalline powder.
Soluble in water, ethanol and chloroform.

Colour Test. Liebermann's Test—orange

Thin-layer Chromatography. System TA—Rf 54; system TB—Rf 03; system TC—Rf 16; system TE—Rf 48; system TL—Rf 15; system TAE—Rf 25. (Acidified iodoplatinate solution, positive.)

Gas Chromatography. System GA—RI 2690.

Ultraviolet Spectrum. Aqueous acid—253, 259 nm (A_1^1=12a), 265 nm.

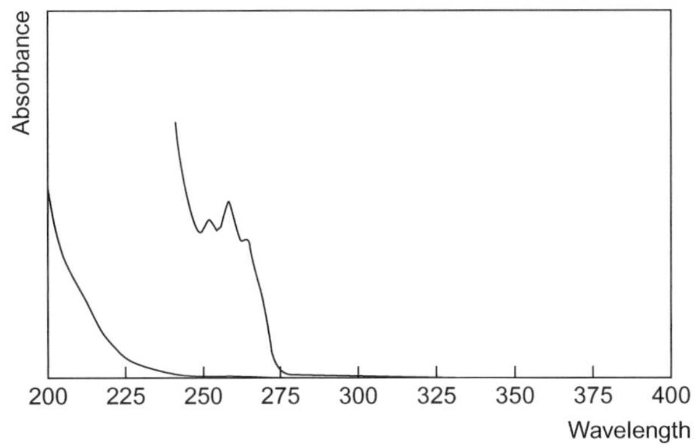

Infra-red Spectrum. Principal peaks at wavenumbers 1618, 1684, 695, 712, 702, 764 cm^{-1} (KBr disk).

Mass Spectrum. Principal ions at *m/z* 98, 112, 99, 55, 42, 41, 211, 84.

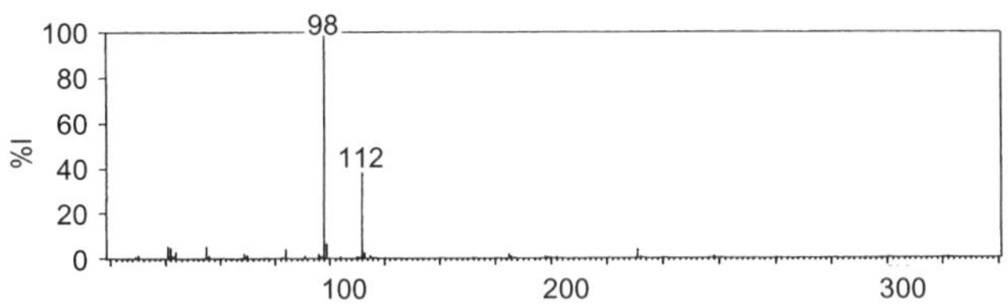

Fenpiprane

Antispasmodic (Veterinary)

1-(3,3-Diphenylpropyl)piperidine
$C_{20}H_{25}N=279.4$
CAS—3540-95-2

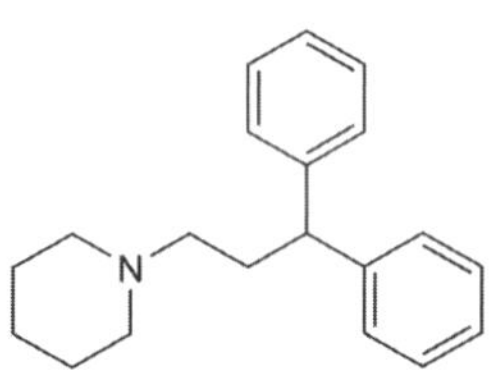

Crystals. M.p. 41° to 42.5°.
Practically insoluble in water; soluble in chloroform.

Fenpiprane Hydrochloride
Proprietary names. Aspasan. It is an ingredient of Efosin.
$C_{20}H_{25}N,HCl=315.9$
CAS—3329-14-4
A white crystalline powder. M.p. 216° to 217°.
Soluble in water and chloroform.

Colour Tests. Liebermann's Test—brown; Mandelin's Test—green; Marquis Test—red

Thin-layer Chromatography. System TA—Rf 61. (Acidified iodoplatinate solution, positive.)

Ultraviolet Spectrum. Aqueous acid—259 nm ($A_1^1=16.7a$), 268 nm.

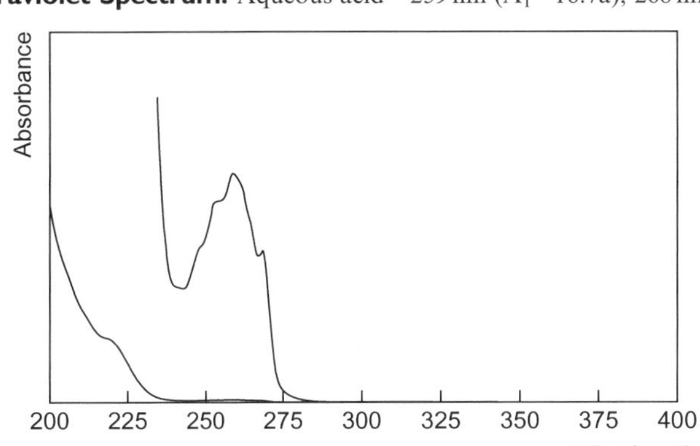

Infra-red Spectrum. Principal peaks at wavenumbers 1492, 1631, 1092, 698, 1010, 1600 cm^{-1} (KBr disk).

Fenproporex

Anorectic

Synonym. *N*-2-Cyanoethylamphetamine
Proprietary names. Fenoproporex and Fenoproporex Hydrochloride; Antiobes; Delgafen; Desobesi-M; Dicel; Drenur; Fenisec; Gacilin; Igrasmin; Ifa Dex; Ifa Diety; Inobesin; Lipomax; Nobese; Obisin; Pesex-R; Solvolip; Tegisec (includes proprietary names of the hydrochloride salt).
3-[(1-Methyl-2-phenylethyl)amino]propanenitrile
$C_{12}H_{16}N_2=188.3$
CAS—15686-61-0; 18305-29-8 (hydrochloride)

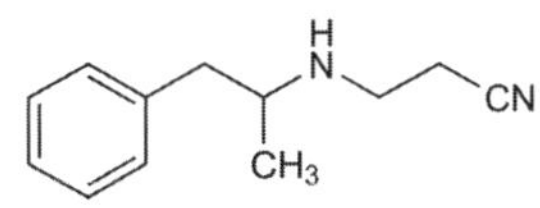

Partition Coefficient. Log *P* (octanol/water), 1.7.

Thin-layer Chromatography. System TE—Rf 77.

Gas Chromatography. System GA—Fenproporex RI 1585, fenproporex-TFA RI 1705, fenproporex-PFP RI 1685, fenproporex-AC RI 1915; system GB—fenproporex RI 1648.

High Performance Liquid Chromatography. System HY—RI 226; system HAA—Retention time, 19.3 min.

Ultraviolet Spectrum. Aqueous acid—252, 257, 263 nm.

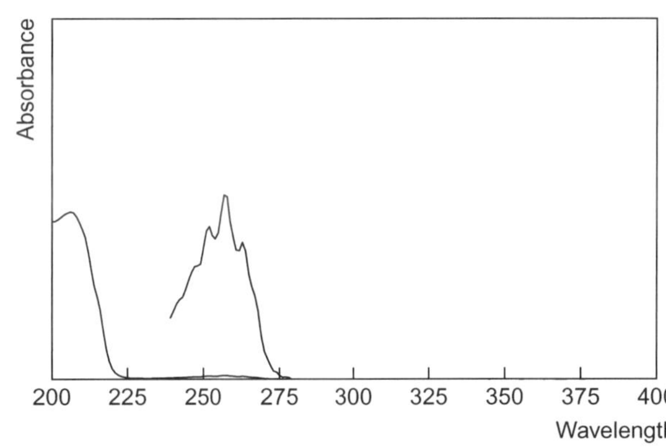

Infra-red Spectrum. Principal peaks at wavenumbers 745, 1583, 697, 1019, 707, 1139 cm^{-1} (fenproporex hydrochloride, KBr disk).

Mass Spectrum. Principal ions at *m/z* 97, 56, 91, 68, 132, 173; fenproporex-AC *m/z* 97, 56, 139, 91, 118, 65; fenproporex-PFP *m/z* 243, 118, 190, 56, 91, 202; fenproporex-TFA *m/z* 193, 118, 140, 91, 56, 152.

Disposition in the Body
Toxicity
In a fatality attributed to fenproporex in a young adult, the following tissue concentrations were found for fenproporex and amfetamine, respectively: inferior vena cava blood 0.90 and 0.084 mg/L, urine 1.2 and 0.94 mg/L, total gastric content 120 and 0.14 mg; other drugs detected in the blood included diazepam (0.54 mg/L), nordazepam (0.46 mg/L), diphenhydramine (0.12 mg/L) and gamma-hydroxybutyric acid (1100 mg/L) [R. R. Bell *et al., J. Anal. Toxicol.*, 2001, *25*, 652–656.]

Dose. Fenproporex has been given as the hydrochloride in usual doses equivalent to 20 mg of the base daily.

Fentanyl

Narcotic Analgesic

Synonyms. Fentanylum; Phentanyl.
N-Phenyl-*N*-[1-(2-phenylethyl)-4-piperidinyl]propanamide
$C_{22}H_{28}N_2O=336.5$
CAS—437-38-7

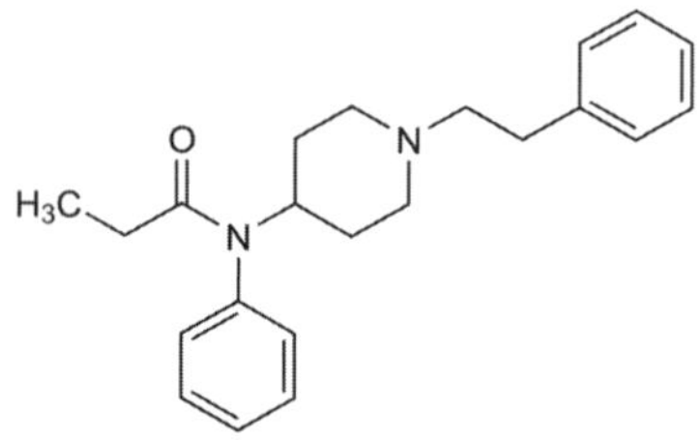

Crystals. M.p. 83° to 84°.
Sparingly soluble in water.

Fentanyl Citrate
Synonyms. Fentanyli Citras; McN-JR-4263-49; R-4263.
Proprietary names. Actiq; Durogesic; Fentanest; Haldid; Leptanal; Sintenyl; Sublimaze; Tanyl. It is an ingredient of Fentazin (vet.), Hypnorm (vet.), Inoval, Innovar, Leptofen, Marcain with Fentanyl, and Thalamonal.
$C_{22}H_{28}N_2O,C_6H_8O_7=528.6$
CAS—990-73-8
White granules or a white glistening crystalline powder. M.p. 149° to 151°. Soluble 1 in 40 of water, 1 in 140 of ethanol, 1 in 350 of chloroform, and 1 in 10 of methanol; slightly soluble in ether.
Caution. Avoid contact with skin and the inhalation of particles of fentanyl citrate.

Partition Coefficient Log *P* (octanol/pH 7.4), 2.3.

Colour Test. Marquis Test—orange.

Thin-layer Chromatography. System TA—Rf 70; system TB—Rf 43; system TC—Rf 74; system TE—Rf 78; system TL—Rf 58; system TAE—Rf 70; system TAF—Rf 77; system TAJ—Rf 59; system TAK—Rf 08; system TAL—Rf 84. (Acidified iodoplatinate solution, positive.)

Gas Chromatography. System GA—RI 2720; system GB—RI 2833.

High Performance Liquid Chromatography. System HA—*k* 0.8; system HC—*k* 1.11; system HX—RI 373; system HY—RI 299; system HAA—retention time 14.2 min; system HAX—retention time 11.4 min; system HAY—retention time 6.0 min.

Ultraviolet Spectrum. Aqueous acid—251, 257 (A_1^1=13a), 263 nm.

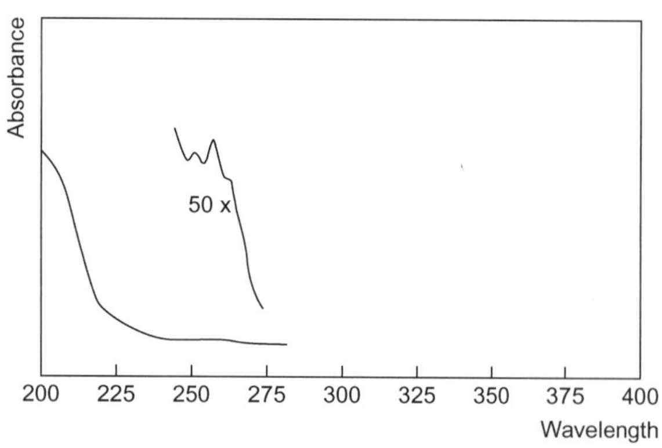

Infra-red Spectrum. Principal peaks at wavenumbers 1660, 701, 1493, 1263, 1273, 1236 cm^{-1} (KBr disk). (See below)

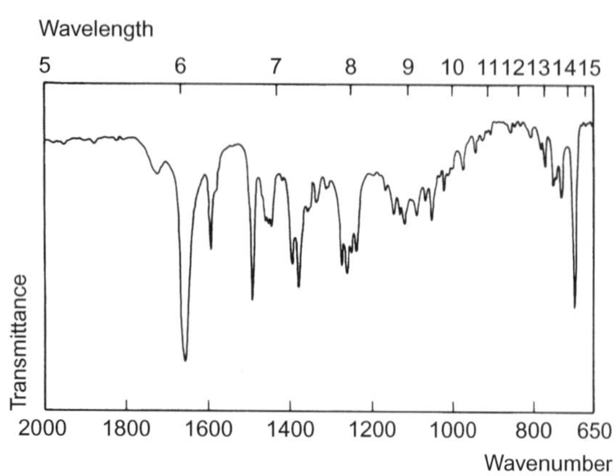

Mass Spectrum. Principal ions at *m/z* 245, 146, 42, 189, 44, 105, 29, 43.

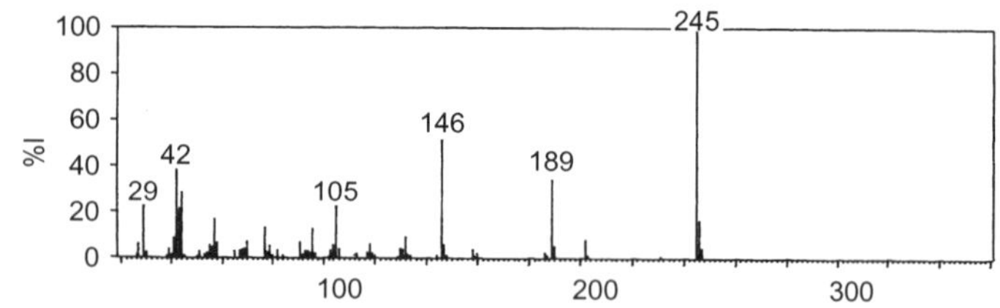

Quantification
Gas chromatography. In plasma: limit of detection 20 ng/L, AFID—J. A. Phipps *et al.*, *J. Chromatogr.*, 1983, *272* (23) *B Biomed. Appl.*, 392–395.

Gas chromatography–mass spectrometry. In hair: fentanyl and sufentanil—H. Sachs *et al.*, *Int. J. Legal Med.*, 1996, *109*, 213–215. In plasma: limit of detection 20 ng/L (comparison with RIA)—B. Fryirs *et al.*, *J. Chromatogr. B Biomed. Sci. Appl.*, 1997, *688*, 79–85.

High performance liquid chromatography. In plasma: fentanyl and alfentanil—K. Kumar *et al.*, *J. Pharm. Biomed. Anal.*, 1996, *14*, 667–673. In plasma: fentanyl in presence of midazolam, limit of detection for fentanyl 200 ng/L, UV detection—E. J. Portier *et al.*, *J. Chromatogr. B Biomed. Sci. Appl.*, 1999, *723*, 313–318.

Radioimmunoassay. In plasma: limit of detection 60 ng/L—M. Michiels *et al.*, *Eur. J. Clin. Pharmacol.*, 1977, *12*, 153–158.

Disposition in the Body. Rapidly metabolised in the liver. Two metabolites, norfentanyl and despropionylfentanyl, have been detected in plasma at concentrations similar to those of fentanyl. About 70% of a dose is excreted in the urine in 72 h, mostly as metabolites, with about 10 to 20% of a dose being excreted as unchanged drug in 48 h. About 9% of a dose is eliminated in the faeces. It crosses the placenta and small amounts may be found in breast milk.

Therapeutic concentration

After 10 subjects received 200 μg fentanyl by IV injection or 2000 μg of 50% free and 50% liposome-encapsulated fentanyl by aerosol inhalation, the mean peak plasma fentanyl level was significantly greater for the IV route (4.67 ± 1.87 at 3.6 min vs 1.15 ± 0.36 μg/L at 22.7 min); but at 8 and 24 h after administration the plasma levels were greater following inhalation (0.16 ± 0.10 vs 0.25 ± 0.14 μg/L at 8 h and 0.05 ± 0.06 vs 0.12 ± 0.16 μg/L at 24 h, for IV and inhalation, respectively). [O. R. Hung *et al.*, *Anesthesiology*, 1995, *83*, 277–284.]

In 10 children receiving treatment with fentanyl transdermal patches, the time to reach peak plasma concentration was 18 to >66 h for patches releasing 25 μg/h fentanyl. Peak plasma concentrations of 0.91 μg/L were obtained with 25-μg/h patches and 39.3 μg/L with 200-μg/h patches. [J. J. Collins *et al.*, *J. Pediatr.*, 1999, *134*, 319–323.]

Administration of fentanyl (10 to 15 μg/kg) via an oral transmucosal delivery system to 17 children resulted in peak plasma concentrations of 1.03 ± 0.31 μg/L. The children were thought to have swallowed a large fraction of the dose, leading to a relatively late and variable peak concentration time of 53 ± 40 min. [M. Wheeler *et al.*, *Pediatr. Anaesth.*, 2002, *12*, 594–599.]

Toxicity. The estimated minimum lethal dose is 2 mg.

The following postmortem tissue concentrations were reported in a fatality resulting from the self-administration of fentanyl (in μg/L or μg/g): serum 17.7, blood 27.5, urine 92.7, bile 58.2, liver 0.0775, kidney 0.0415, brain 0.0302, lung 0.0834, stomach 31.6. A partly filled syringe containing 2.8 mg/L fentanyl was found near the scene of death. [A. K. Chaturvedi *et al.*, *J. Anal. Toxicol.*, 1990, *14*, 385–387.]

In a review of 25 fatalities involving fentanyl transdermal patches, the following postmortem tissue concentrations were reported (in μg/L or μg/g): heart blood 1.89 to 139 (23 cases), femoral blood 3.1 to 43 13 cases), vitreous 2 to 20 (4 cases), liver 0.0058 to 0.613 (22 cases), bile 3.5 to 262 (15 cases), urine 2.9 to 895 (19 cases), gastric 0 to 122 μg total (17 cases), spleen 0.0078 to 0.079 (3 cases), kidney 0.011 (1 case), lung 0.031 (1 case). [D. T. Anderson and J. J. Muto, *J. Anal. Toxicol.*, 2000, *24*, 627–634.]

An 83-year-old female who was found dead with three 100 μg/h fentanyl patches on her chest, had the following tissue concentrations at postmortem: blood 25 μg/L, brain 0.054 μg/g, heart 0.094 μg/g, kidney 0.069 μg/g, liver 0.104 μg/g. [L. E. Edinboro *et al.*, *J. Forensic Sci.*, 1997, *42*, 741–743.]

A postmortem serum fentanyl concentration of 2 µg/L was reported in a 35-year-old woman who had injected the contents of a transdermal fentanyl patch (5 mg, shared with another person who survived); 0.16 g/L ethanol was also found in the serum [M. D. Reeves and C. J. Ginifer, *Med. J. Aust.*, 2002, *177*, 552–554.]

Half-life. Plasma half-life, about 3.7 h (dose-dependent; also increased in the elderly and premature infants and during cardiopulmonary by-pass surgery).

Volume of distribution. About 4 L/kg.

Clearance. Plasma clearance, about 13 mL/min/kg.

Distribution in blood. Plasma:whole blood ratio, 1.0.

Protein binding. In plasma, about 80%.

Note. For a review of the pharmacokinetics of fentanyl, see L. E. Mather, *Clin. Pharmacokinet.*, 1983, *8*, 422–446.

Dose. For analgesia in surgery, initially, the equivalent of 50 to 200 µg of fentanyl, IV; supplementary doses of 50 µg. With assisted ventilation, an initial dose of 300 to 3500 µg may be given.

Fenthion

Acaricide, Insecticide

Synonyms. Bay 29493; Bayer 29493; DMTP; ENT25540; MPP; Mercaptophos; OMS2; S-1752.
Proprietary names. Baycid; Baytex; Entex; Lebaycid; Lysoff; Queletox; Spotten; Talodex; Tiguvon.
Phosphorothioic acid *O*,*O*-dimethyl *O*-[3-methyl-4-(methylthio)phenyl] ester
$C_{10}H_{15}O_3PS_2$=278.3
CAS—55-38-9

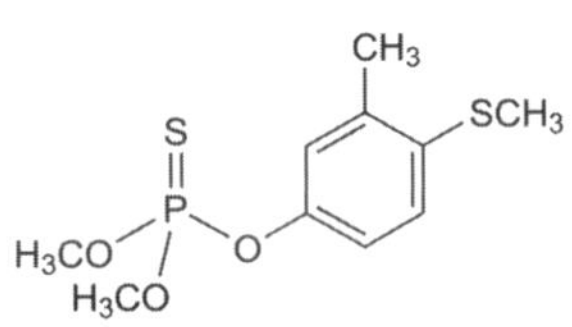

Pure fenthion is a colourless liquid. The technical form is a yellowish-brown oily liquid. M.p. 7.5°. B.p. 87° at 0.01 mmHg.
It is practically insoluble in water; readily soluble in methanol, ethanol, acetone, 2-propanol, dichloromethane, toluene, and most organic solvents including alcohol, ethers, esters, and halogenated aromatics; slightly soluble in hexane.

Partition Coefficient. Log *P* (octanol/ water), 4.09.

Thin-layer Chromatography. System TX—Rf 41; system TY—Rf 81; system TZ—Rf 90; system TAA—Rf 68.

Plate: silica gel. Mobile phase: benzene: methanol (9:1). Developed by spraying with 0.2% palladium chloride solution. Rf 0.9. [E. Meyer *et al.*, *J. Anal. Toxicol.*, 1998, *22*, 248–252.]

Gas Chromatography. System GA—RI 1938.

Column: SGE BPX5 (25 m × 0.22 mm i.d., 0.25 µm film thickness). Column temperature: 60°; to 120° at 30°/min; to 220° at 10°/min; to 290° at 5°/min and to 300°, held for 3 min. Carrier gas: helium, 0.8 mL/min. IS: fenitrothion. MS detection (EI, SIM). Retention time: 14.25 min. [E. Meyer *et al.*, *J. Anal. Toxicol.*, 1998, *22(3)*, 248–252.]

High Performance Liquid Chromatography. Column: (analytical) RP-select B (Alusphere, 125 × 4.0 mm i.d., 5 µm), (guard) 60 RP-select B (Alusphere, 4 × 4.0 mm i.d., 30 µm). Mobile phase: (A)-sodium hydroxide (0.0125 M) in methanol; (B)-sodium hydroxide (0.0125 M) in water. Elution programme: (A:B) (10:90) for 5 min to (90:10) over 15 min, held 5 min, flow rate 1.0 mL/min. Retention time: 18.3 min. [E. Meyer *et al.*, *J. Anal. Toxicol.*, 1998, *22(3)*, 248–252.]

Ultraviolet Spectrum. Methanol—229 nm; aqueous acid—252 nm.

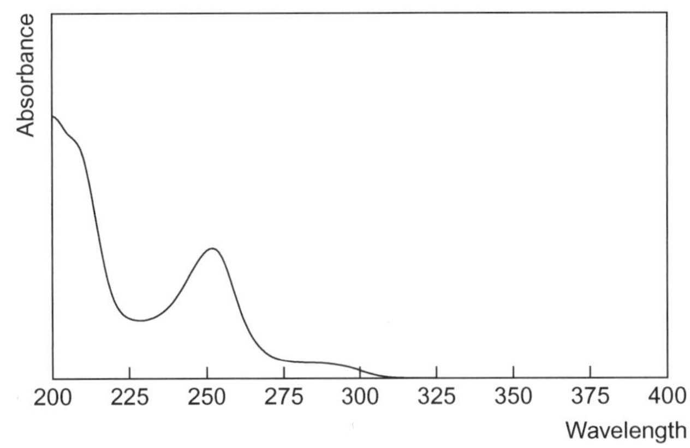

Mass Spectrum. Principal ions at *m/z* 278, 125, 109, 169, 79, 93.

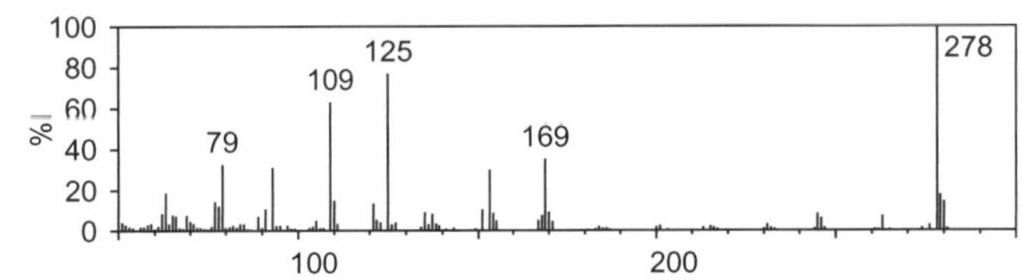

Quantification

Gas chromatography–mass spectrometry. In blood: limit of quantification 0.1 mg/L—E. Meyer *et al.*, *J. Anal. Toxicol.*, 1998, *22(3)*, 248–252.

High performance liquid chromatography. In blood: limit of quantification 0.25 mg/L—E. Meyer *et al.*, *J. Anal. Toxicol.*, 1998, *22(3)*, 248–252.

Disposition in the Body. Fenthion is readily absorbed into the blood stream via the digestive tract, lungs, and skin, and is systematically distributed. It is rapidly metabolised to weak active products by a number of pathways, the major being by hepatic hydrolysis. It is eliminated through urine and faeces as the hydrolysis products. Fenthion is stored in fat and its release is delayed for metabolism.

Toxicity. Fenthion is moderately toxic after ingestion and dermal exposure, and is slightly toxic if inhaled. The allowed daily intake is 0.001 mg/kg. A lethal dose of 50 mg/kg has been established but the route of administration is not known.

A 66-year-old woman was found dead in her bathroom: a suicide case which was not suspected to be fenthion poisoning. After toxicological analysis, a fenthion blood concentration of 3.8 mg/L was detected and it was determined that fenthion ingestion was the cause of death. A total amount of 17 g fenthion was found in the stomach and 203 g/g in the liver. [E. Meyer *et al.*, *J. Anal. Toxicol.*, 1998, *22(3)*, 248–252.]

Fenticlor

Antifungal

Proprietary names. Novex. It is an ingredient of Dermisdin.
2,2′-Thiobis[4-chlorophenol]
$C_{12}H_8Cl_2O_2S$=287.2
CAS—97-24-5

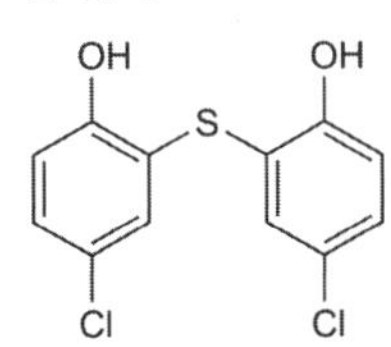

A white crystalline powder. M.p. 176°.
Practically insoluble in water; freely soluble in ethanol; soluble in aqueous solutions of sodium hydroxide.

Partition Coefficient. Log *P* (octanol/water), 4.6.

Thin-layer Chromatography. System TAE—Rf 91.

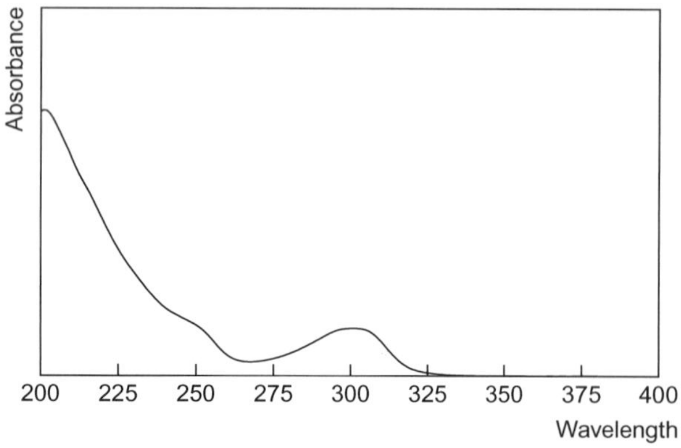

Infra-red Spectrum. Principal peaks at wavenumbers 1269, 825, 1209, 818, 889, 1104 cm^{-1}.

Use. Fenticlor has been applied topically in concentrations of up to 2%.

Fenyramidol

Analgesic/Muscle Relaxant

Synonym. Phenyramidol
α-[(2-Pyridinylamino)methyl]benzenemethanol
$C_{13}H_{14}N_2O=214.3$
CAS—553-69-5

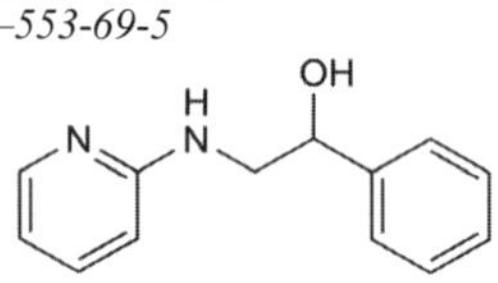

Crystals. M.p. 82° to 85°.

Fenyramidol Hydrochloride

Synonyms. Phenyramidol Hydrochloride IN-511; MJ-505; NSC-17777.
Proprietary name. Cabral
$C_{13}H_{14}N_2O,HCl=250.7$
CAS—326-43-2
A white crystalline powder. M.p. 140° to 142°.
Freely soluble in water; soluble in ethanol.

Dissociation Constant. pK_a 5.9.

Partition Coefficient. Log *P* (octanol/water), 1.7.

Colour Tests. Cyanogen Bromide—orange-pink; Mandelin's Test—blue; Marquis Test—yellow.

Thin-layer Chromatography. System TA—Rf 69; system TB—Rf 08; system TC—Rf 52; system TE—Rf 76; system TL—Rf 59; system TAE—Rf 80; system TAF—Rf 86. (Dragendorff spray, positive; acidified iodoplatinate solution, positive; acidified potassium permanganate solution, positive.)

Gas Chromatography. System GA—RI 1960.

High Performance Liquid Chromatography. System HX—RI 282.

Ultraviolet Spectrum. Aqueous acid—237 ($A_1^1=666a$), 309 nm.

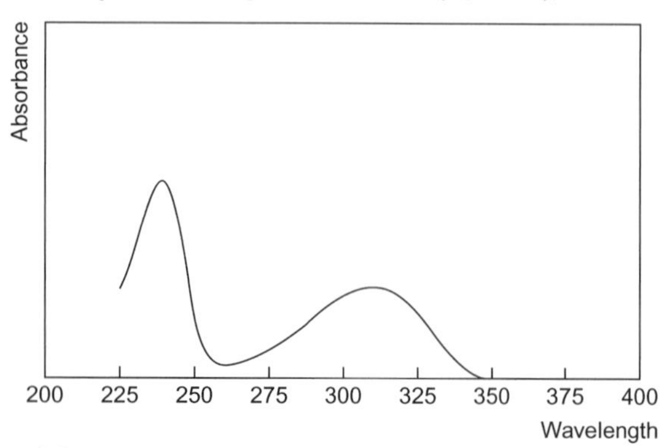

Infra-red Spectrum. Principal peaks at wavenumbers 1613, 1524, 700, 768, 1058, 752 cm^{-1} (KBr disk).

Mass Spectrum. Principal ions at *m/z* 107, 108, 78, 79, 80, 77, 51, 52.

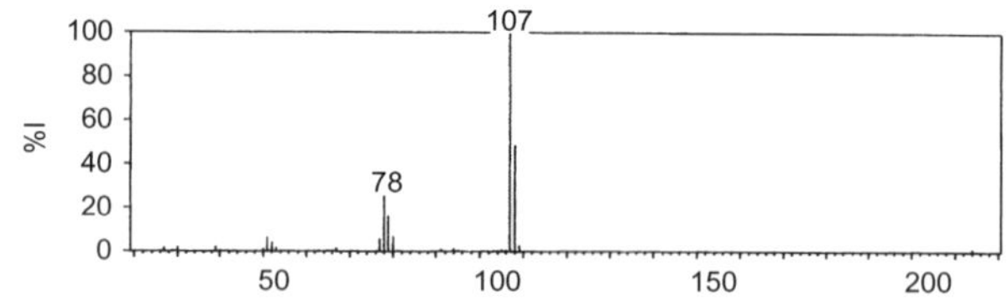

Dose. Up to 3.2 g of fenyramidol hydrochloride daily.

Feprazone

Analgesic

Synonyms. Phenylprenazone; Prenazone.
Proprietary names. Brotazona; Methrazone; Reuflodol; Zepelan; Zepelin.
4-(3-Methyl-2-butenyl)-1,2-diphenyl-3,5-pyrazolidinedione
$C_{20}H_{20}N_2O_2=320.4$
CAS—30748-29-9

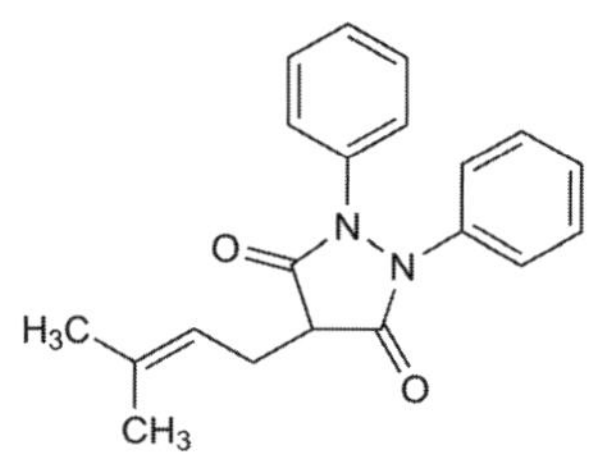

A white crystalline powder. M.p. about 157°.
Practically insoluble in water; slightly soluble in cyclohexane, ethanol and ether; very soluble in acetone and chloroform; sparingly soluble in acetonitrile and benzene.

Partition Coefficient. Log *P* (octanol/water), 3.9.

Colour Tests. *p*-Dimethylaminobenzaldehyde—red; Liebermann's Test—brown-orange (→brown at 100°).

Thin-layer Chromatography. System TE—Rf 19; system TG—Rf 45; system TAE—Rf 92. (Chromic acid solution, yellow; Ludy Tenger reagent, orange; mercurous nitrate spray, positive.)

Gas Chromatography. System GA—RI 2380; system GD—RRT of methyl derivative 1.81 (relative to $n\text{-}C_{16}H_{34}$); system GF—RI 2800.

High Performance Liquid Chromatography. System HV—RRT 0.92 (relative to meclofenamic acid).

Ultraviolet Spectrum. Methanolic alkali—266 nm ($A_1^1=700b$).

Infra-red Spectrum. Principal peaks at wavenumbers 1715, 1300, 767, 1745, 715, 703 cm^{-1} (KBr disk).

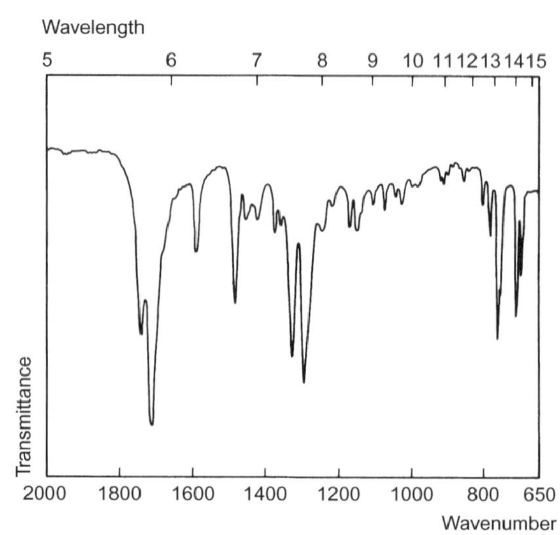

Mass Spectrum. Principal ions at *m/z* 183, 77, 252, 320, 184, 41, 69, 51.

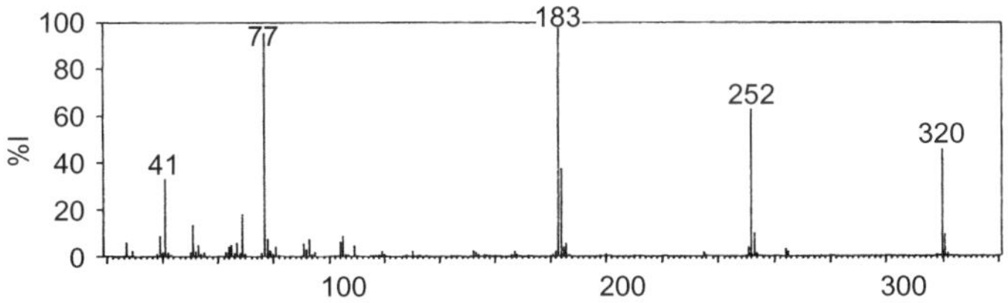

Quantification

High performance liquid chromatography. In plasma: limit of detection, feprazone 100 µg/L, 4-(3-hydroxymethyl)feprazone 200 µg/L, UV detection—H. Spahn and E. Mutschler, *J. Chromatogr.*, 1982, *232*; *Biomed. Appl.*, *21*, 145–153.

Disposition in the Body. Absorbed after oral administration. Metabolised by hydroxylation to 4-(3-hydroxymethyl)feprazone. Less than 1% of a dose is excreted unchanged in the urine.

Therapeutic concentration

Following a single oral dose of 400 mg to 8 subjects, peak plasma concentrations of 30.2 to 54.7 mg/L (mean 40.6) were attained in 4 to 8 h; peak plasma concentrations of 1.09 to 3.60 mg/L (mean 1.9) of the 4-(3-hydroxymethyl) metabolite were reported at about 27 h [H. Spahn and E. Mutschler, *Arzneimittelforschung.*, 1985, *35*, 167–169].

Half-life. Plasma half-life, 6 to 30 h (mean 20).

Protein binding. In plasma, 90 to 99%.

Dose. 200 to 600 mg daily.

Fexofenadine

Antihistamine

Synonyms. Carboxyterfenadine; MDL-16455 M-I; Terfenadine carboxylate.

α,α-Dimethyl-4-[1-hydroxy-4-[4-(hydroxydiphenylmethyl)-1-piperidinyl]butyl]benzene acetic acid

$C_{32}H_{39}NO_4$ = 501.7

CAS—*83799-24-0*

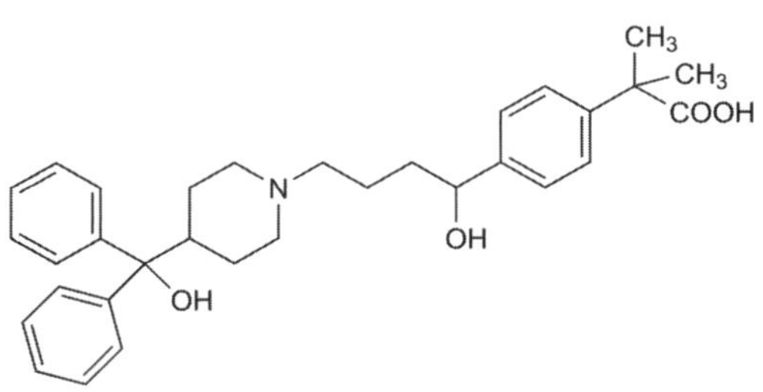

A white to off-white crystalline powder with M.p. 142° to 143°.

Fexofenadine Hydrochloride

Synonym. Terfenadine Carboxylate Hydrochloride

Proprietary names. Allegra; Telfast.

$C_{32}H_{39}NO_4$, HCl = 538.1

CAS—138452-21-8

A white to off-white crystalline powder which is freely soluble in methanol, ethanol; slightly soluble in chloroform and water; insoluble in hexane.

Partition Coefficient. Log *P* (octanol/ water), 2.81.

High Performance Liquid Chromatography. Column: BSA-7 (Resolvosil, 150 × 4 mm i.d., 5 µm). Mobile phase: 2-propanol:sodium phosphate (0.08 M, pH 8.0) (1.5:98.5), 0.4 mL/min flow rate. UV detection (λ = 210 or 254 nm). Retention time(s): (*S*)-fexofenadine, 10.2 min; (*R*)-fexofenadine, 14.4 min [K. Y. Chan *et al.*, *J. Chromatogr.*, 1991, *571*, 291–297].

Ultraviolet Spectrum. Aqueous acid—259 nm.

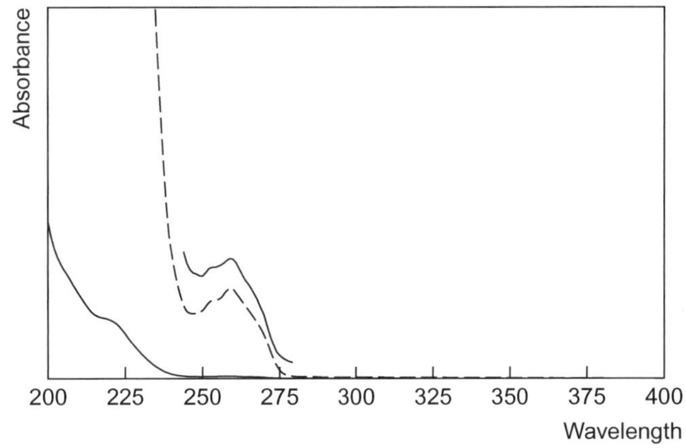

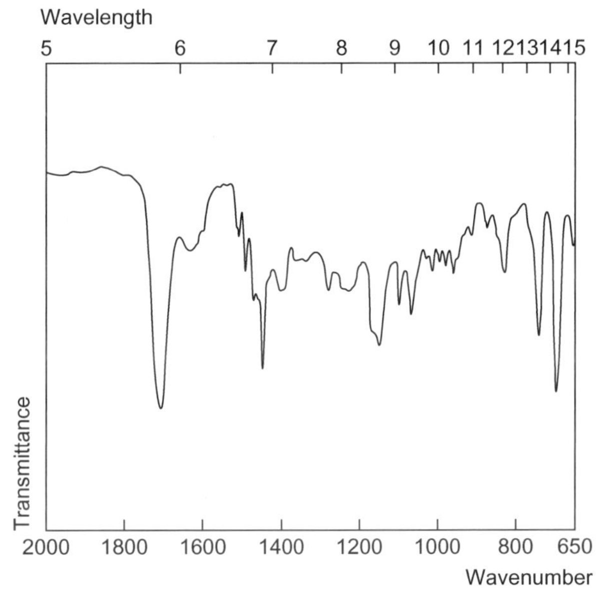

Mass Spectrum. Principal ions at *m/z* 280, 105, 281, 501, 77, 183, 85, 147.

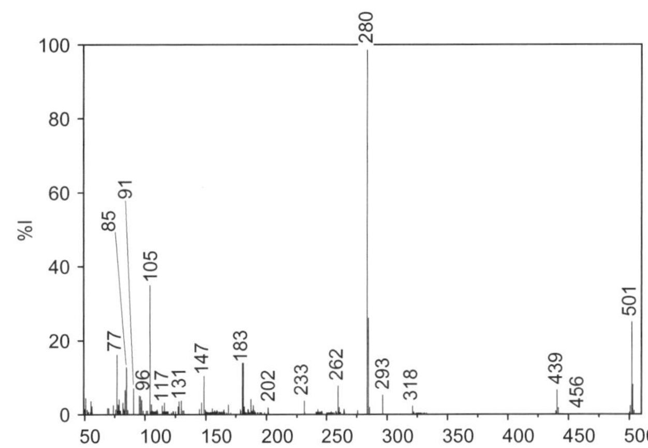

Disposition in the Body. Fexofenadine is rapidly absorbed after oral administration and only 5% of a dose is metabolised by intestinal mucosa, 0.5 to 1.5 % undergoes hepatic biotransformation. The drug is mainly excreted in faeces unchanged (80%) and 10% in urine. Fexofenadine is a metabolite of terfenadine and therefore has been detected in breast milk after administration of terfenadine. Fexofenadine does not cross the blood–brain barrier.

Therapeutic concentration

24 healthy adult volunteers were administered a single oral dose every 12 h for 7 days. A 60 mg dose produced peak plasma concentrations of 0.29 mg/L, 120 mg dose 0.6 mg/L and 240 mg dose 1.53 mg/L. All levels were reached within 1.02 to 1.33 h [D. K. Robbins *et al.*, *Biopharm. Drug Dispos.*, 1998, *19(7)*, 455–463].

Toxicity

A 67-year-old man was admitted to hospital after fainting and an abnormally long QT time was seen on the electrocardiogram (ECG). He had started taking 180 mg daily fexofenadine two months earlier. Fexofenadine treatment was stopped on admission to hospital and the QTc time shortened. 180 mg daily was restarted and the QTc time was seen to increase again. After 11 days of treatment with fexofenadine, he suffered tachycardia and fibrillation. He was successfully defibrillated and treatment was stopped for good. QT time decreased [Y. M. Pinto *et al.*, *Lancet*, 1999, *353*, 980].

Half-life. 14 to 18 h.

Volume of distribution. 5.4 to 5.8 L/kg.

Clearance. 14 to 18 mL/min/kg.

Protein binding. 60 to 70%.

Dose. A usual dose of 120 mg daily is administered but is reduced to 60 mg in patients with renal impairment. The maximum dose is 180 mg daily.

Finasteride

Azasteroid/5-α-Reductase Inhibitor

Synonyms. MK-906; MK-0906.
Proprietary names. Andozac; Chibro-Proscar; Finastid; Proscar; Prostide; Propecia; Urprosan.
(5α,17β)-*N*-(1,1-Dimethylethyl)-3-oxo-4-aza-androst-1-ene-17-carboxamide
$C_{23}H_{36}N_2O_2$=372.6
CAS—98319-26-7

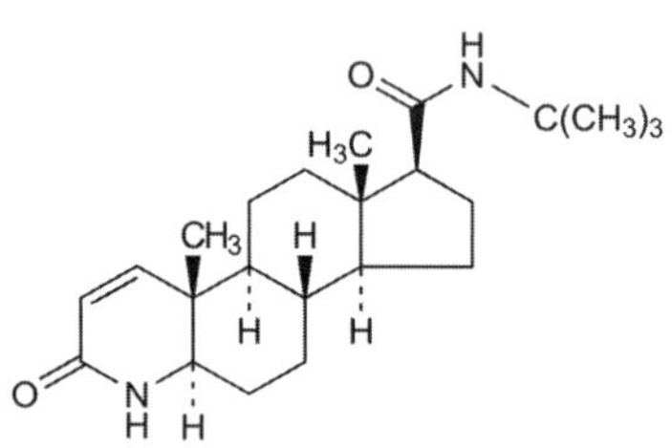

A white to off-white crystalline solid with M.p. 252° to 254°, also reported as 257°.
It is freely soluble in chloroform, dimethylsulfoxide, ethanol, methanol, and *n*-propanol; sparingly soluble in propylene glycol and polyethylene glycol 400; very slightly soluble in hydrochloric acid (0.1 M) and sodium hydroxide (0.1 M); practically insoluble in water (11.68 mg/L at 25°).

Partition Coefficient. Log *P* (octanol/water), 3.03.

Thin-layer Chromatography. Plate: silica. Mobile phase: chloroform:methanol:water:ammonium hydroxide (55:35:6:4). Finasteride ω-oic acid Rf 0.58.

Plate: silica. Mobile phase: ethyl acetate:2-butanol:formic acid (90:8:2). Finasteride ω-oic acid Rf 0.43. [J. R. Carlin *et al.*, *Drug Metab. Dispos.*, 1992, *20(2)*, 148–155.]

Gas Chromatography. Column: methylsilicone (12 m × 0.22 mm i.d., 0.33 μm film thickness). Column temperature: 70° for 1 min, ramp to 200° at 30°/min, hold 1 min; ramp to 280° at 10°/min, hold for 10 min; ramp to 300° at 20°/min, hold for 5 min. Injector temperature: 280°, splitless. Carrier gas: helium (35 kPa inlet pressure). MS detection (SIM at *m/z* 372.2). Retention time: 19.7 min. [A. Guarna *et al.*, *J. Chromatogr.* 1995, *674 B Biomed. Appl.*, 197–204].

High Performance Liquid Chromatography. Column: C_8 (Zorbax, 250 × 4.6 mm i.d., 5 μm). Mobile phase: acetonitrile:methanol:water (26:39:35), flow rate 0.9 to 1.0 mL/min. UV detection (λ=210 nm). Retention time: ω-hydroxyfinasteride, 6.5 min; finasteride, 13.4 min; 4-*n*-methylfinasteride, 21.0 min. [J. R. Carlin *et al.*, *Drug Met. Dispos.*, 1992, *20(2)*, 148-155.]

Column: RP symmetry (250 × 4.6 mm i.d., 5 μm), with pre-column (Pelliguard, 20 × 4.6 mm i.d., 40 μm). Mobile phase: acetonitrile: orthophosphoric acid (0.04 M, pH 4.0) (45:55), flow rate 1.2 mL/min. UV detection (λ=215 nm). IS: 4-androstene-3,17-dione. Retention time: 14.6 min. [G. Carlucci *et al.*, *J. Chromatogr. B Biomed. Sci. Appl.*, 1997, *693*, 245–248.]

Column: 100-3 C_{18} (Nucleosil, 150 × 3.2 mm i.d., 3 μm) with pre-column 120-5 C_{18} (Nucleosil, 10 × 4 mm i.d., 5 μm). Mobile phase: acetonitrile:potassium dihydrogen phosphate buffer (15 mM) (40:60), flow rate 0.6 mL/min at 30°. UV detection (λ=210 nm). IS: clobazam. Retention time(s): finasteride, 17 min; IS, 10 min. [P. Ptacek *et al.*, *J. Chromatogr. B Biomed. Sci. Appl.*, 2000, *738*, 305–310.]

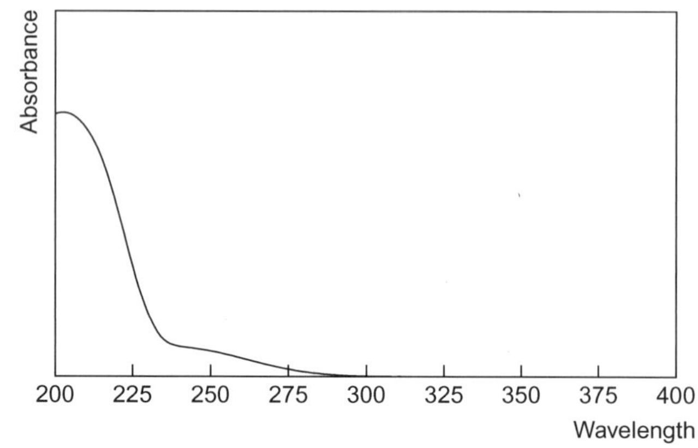

Mass Spectrum. Principal ions at *m/z*: 372, 58, 110, 357, 272, 57, 373, 72.

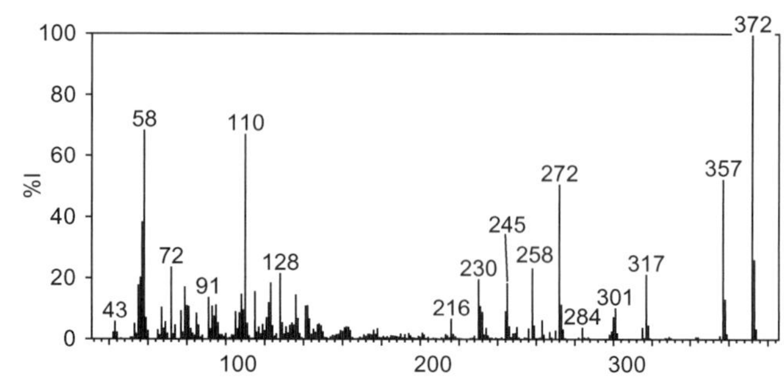

Quantification

Gas chromatography–mass spectrometry. In plasma: limit of detection 0.05 μg/L—A. Guarna *et al.*, *J. Chromatogr.* 1995, *674(2) B Biomed. Appl.*, 197–204.

High performance liquid chromatography. In plasma: limit of quantification 1 μg/L—T. Takano and S. Hata, *J. Chromatogr.* 1996, *676(1) B Biomed. Appl.*, 141–146. In plasma: limit of quantification 4 μg/L—P. Ptacek *et al.*, *J. Chromatogr. B Biomed. Sci. Appl.*, 2000, *738(2)*, 305–310.

Disposition in the Body. Finasteride is well absorbed after oral administration and metabolised in the liver by oxidation to a (17)-monocarboxylic acid metabolite (18.5% of the dose) and ω-hydroxylated finasteride. There is virtually no unchanged drug. The metabolites are excreted in urine (approx. 40%) and faeces (50 to 65%). The drug is widely distributed throughout the body and crosses the blood–brain barrier.

Therapeutic concentration

32 healthy males, aged between 28 and 53 years, were administered with single doses of 5, 10, 20, 50, and 100 mg finasteride after an overnight fast. Peak plasma concentrations increased with dose: 38.1, 81.5, 147.1, 442.0, and 835.5 μg/L, respectively and time to reach this peak also increased from 1.8 to 2.8 h. The same volunteers were also administered with multiple doses of 10 mg daily for 7 days. On day 1 peak plasma concentrations of 82.5 μg/L were reached followed by 88.7 and 96.2 μg/L for days 4 and 7, respectively. Peak concentrations were reached between 3.7 and 4.5 h after administration. [M. Ohtawa *et al.*, *Eur. J. Drug Metab. Pharmacokinet.*, 1991, *16*, 15–21.]

Bioavailability. Reported as 63 and also 80%.

Half-life. Approx. 6 h (individuals <60 years old); 8 h (>70 years).

Volume of distribution. 44 to 96 L.

Clearance. 165 mL/min.

Protein binding. 90%.

Dose. A usual dose of 1 mg daily is recommended with a maximum dose of 5 mg.

Flavoxate

Antispasmodic

3-Methyl-4-oxo-2-phenyl-4*H*-1-benzopyran-8-carboxylic acid 2-(1-piperidinyl)ethyl ester
$C_{24}H_{25}NO_4$=391.5
CAS—15301-69-6

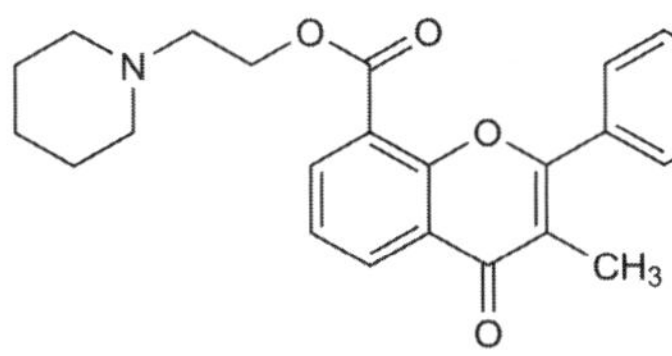

Soluble in ethanol and chloroform.

Flavoxate Hydrochloride

Proprietary names. Bladderon; Bladuril; Cleanxate; Flavorin; Genurin; Spasuret; Spasuri; Urispadol; Urispas; Uronid; Uroxate.
$C_{24}H_{25}NO_4$,HCl=427.9
CAS—3717-88-2
A creamy-white crystalline powder. M.p. 230° to 236°.
Soluble 1 in 150 of water, 1 in 500 of ethanol, 1 in 40 of chloroform and 1 in 120 of methanol; practically insoluble in ether.

Dissociation Constant. pK_a 7.3.

Partition Coefficient. Log *P* (octanol/water), 4.9.

Colour Test. Liebermann's Test—yellow.

Thin-layer Chromatography. System TA—Rf 62; system TB—Rf 36; system TC—Rf 67; system TE—Rf 77; system TL—Rf 45; system TAE—Rf 48; system TAJ—Rf 52; system TAK—Rf 71; system TAL—Rf 92. (Acidified iodoplatinate solution, strong reaction.)

Gas Chromatography. System GA—not eluted.

High Performance Liquid Chromatography. System HA—*k* 2.2; system HAX—Retention time 11.3 min; system HAY—Retention time 6.0 min.

Ultraviolet Spectrum. Aqueous acid—241 nm (A^1_1=360b), 293, 320 nm.

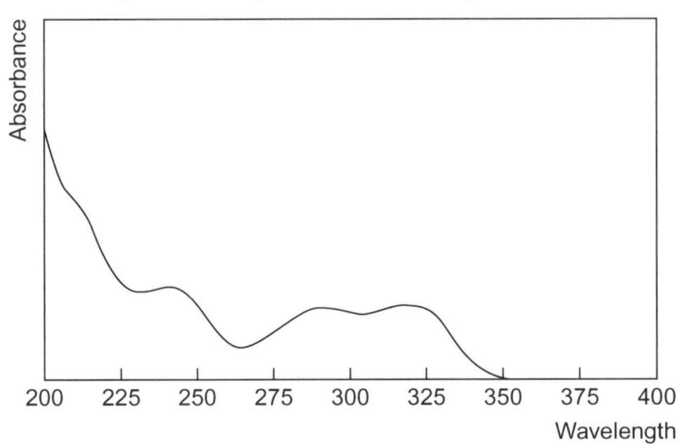

Infra-red Spectrum. Principal peaks at wavenumbers 1633, 1121, 1718, 1255, 759, 1272 cm^{-1} (KBr disk).

Mass Spectrum. Principal ions at *m/z* 98, 111, 99, 147, 55, 41, 42, 96.

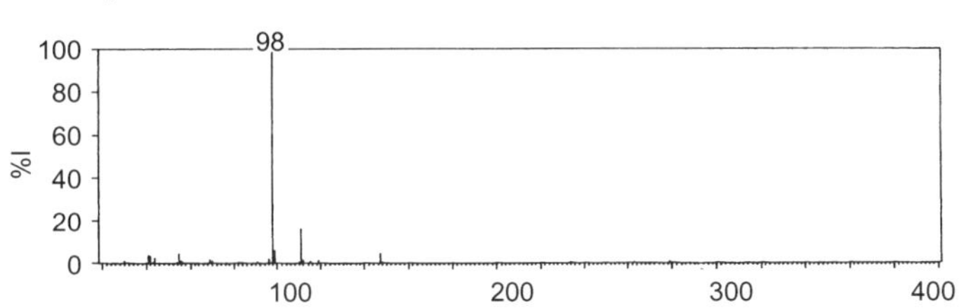

Dose. 300 to 800 mg of flavoxate hydrochloride daily.

Flecainide

Anti-arrhythmic

N-(2-Piperidinylmethyl)-2,5-bis(2,2,2-trifluoroethoxy)benzamide
$C_{17}H_{20}F_6N_2O_3$=414.3
CAS—54143-55-4; 99495-87-1 (±)

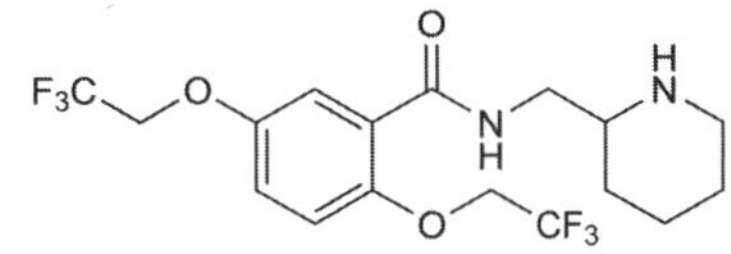

A white, granular solid. M.p. 105° to 107°.

Flecainide Acetate

Synonym. R-818
Proprietary names. Almarytm; Apocard; Aristocor; Corflene; Flecaine; Tambocor.
$C_{17}H_{20}F_6N_2O_3,C_2H_4O_2$=474.4
CAS—54143-56-5
A white to slightly off-white granular solid. M.p. 145° to 147°. It is soluble in water (48.4 g/L at 37°) and ethanol (300 g/L at 37°); freely soluble in dilute acetic acid; practically insoluble in dilute hydrochloric acid.

Dissociation Constant. pK_a 9.3 (flecainide acetate).

Partition Coefficient. Log *P* (octanol/water), 3.8.

Thin-layer Chromatography. System TB—Rf 06; system TE—Rf 49; system TAE—Rf 28.

Gas Chromatography. System GA—RI 2250 (flecainide); RI 2500 (Art (formyl)); system GB—RI 2351 (flecainide); RI 2240 (Art (formyl)).

High Performance Liquid Chromatography. System HX—RI 419; system HY—RI 355; system HZ—retention time 5.2 min.

Column: RP C_6 (Spherisorb, 150 × 4.6 mm i.d., 5 µm). Mobile phase: acetonitrile:potassium dihydrogen phosphate (15 mM, pH 3) (60:40), 1.5 mL/min flow rate. Internal standard (IS): S-15277. UV detection (λ=300 nm) or fluorescence detection (λ_{ex}=300 nm, λ_{em}=370 nm). Retention time: flecainide, 8.39 min; IS, 6.17 min [R. Verbesselt *et al.*, *Ther. Drug Monit.*, 1991, *13*, 157–165].

Column: (analytical) RP C_{18} (Radial-Pak, 100 × 8 mm, 5 µm); (guard) C_{18} (Bondapak/Corasil, 37 to 50 µm). Mobile phase: methanol:25% ammonia (99.9:0.1), 0.7 mL/min flow rate. IS: *N*-(2-piperidinylmethyl)-2,3-bis(2,2,2-trifluoroethoxy)benzamide hydrochloride. Fluorescence detection (λ_{ex}=293 nm, λ_{em}=340 nm). Retention time: flecainide, 7.2 min; IS, 8.3 min [T. A. Plomp *et al.*, *J. Anal. Toxicol.*, 1986, *10*, 102–106].

Ultraviolet Spectrum. Ethanol—205 (A^1_1=521), 230 (A^1_1=219), 300 (A^1_1=59) nm.

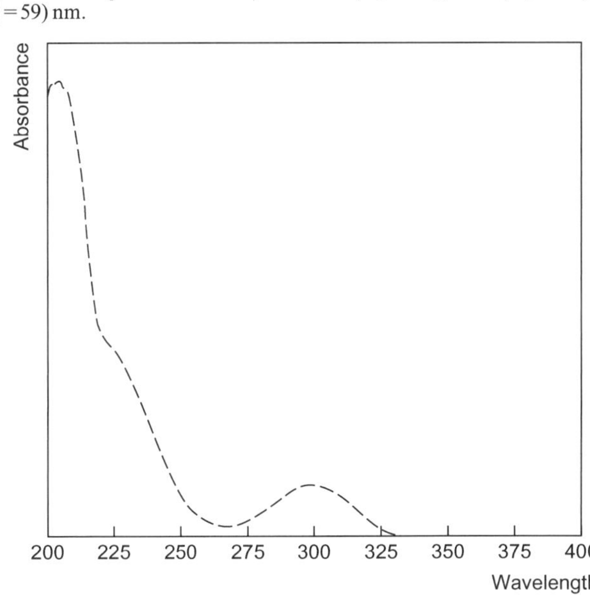

Infra-red Spectrum. Principal peaks at wavenumbers 1169, 1221, 1291, 1637, 1083, 1549 cm^{-1} (KBr disk).

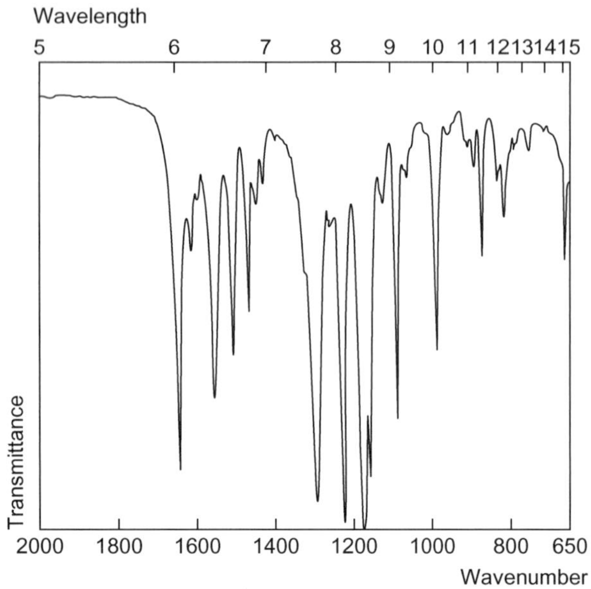

Mass Spectrum. Principal ions at *m/z* 84, 97, 301, 56, 85, 96, 218, 82.

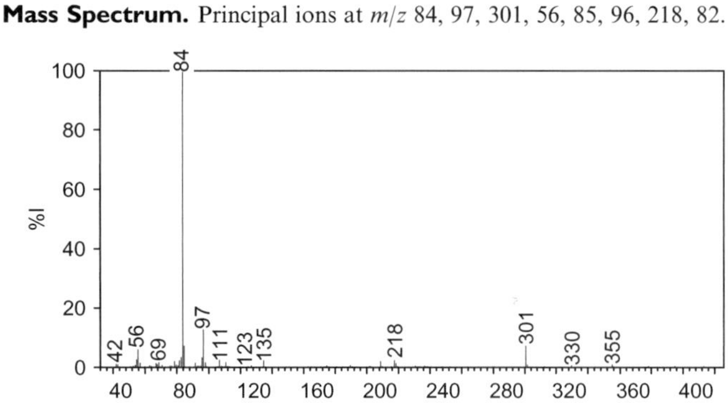

Quantification

High performance liquid chromatography. In blood, plasma, or serum: limit of detection 20 µg/L, fluorescence detection—R. K. Bhamra *et al.*, *J. Chromatogr.*, 1984, *307*, *Biomed. Appl.*, *32*, 439–444. In plasma: limit of detection 3 µg/L with fluorescence detection and 50 µg/L with UV detection—S. F. Chang *et al.*, *Ther. Drug Monit.*, 1984, *6*, 105–111. In plasma: limit of detection 10 µg/L—T. A. Plomp *et al.*, *J. Anal. Toxicol.*, 1986, *10(3)*, 102–106. In plasma: limit of detection 50 µg/L, UV or fluorescence detection—R. Verbesselt *et al.*, *Ther. Drug Monit.*, 1991, *13*, 157–165.

Disposition in the Body. Flecainide is rapidly and almost completely absorbed after oral administration and peak plasma concentrations occur after 0.5 to 6 h. It is extensively metabolised (subject to genetic polymorphism) mainly to *m*-O-dealkylated flecainide and the *m*-O-dealkylated lactam of flecainide, which both have some activity. *m*-O-dealkylated flecainide makes up to 20% of the drug's anti-arrhythmic activity. CYP2D6 is involved in its metabolism. Flecainide is excreted mainly in urine (about 10 to 50% as the unchanged drug and the remainder as metabolites, depending on type of administration). About 5% is excreted in faeces. Excretion of flecainide is decreased in alkaline urine. Haemodialysis removes only about 1% of unchanged flecainide. It crosses the placenta and is distributed into breast milk.

Therapeutic concentration. The trough serum therapeutic concentration range is 0.45 to 0.9 mg/L and peak, 0.75 to 1.25 mg/L.

Trough plasma-flecainide concentrations at steady state in 13 individuals, aged between 28 and 72 years (average 53.7 years), taking 100, 200 and 250 mg of flecainide orally twice a day were 0.295 and 0.314 mg/L (2 subjects), 0.390 to 0.814 mg/L (5 subjects), and 0.753 and 1.387 mg/L, respectively. All participants suffered from coronary artery disease, heart disease or primary rhythm disorder [J. L. Anderson *et al.*, *N. Engl. J. Med.*, 1981, *305*, 473–477].

Normal, healthy volunteers were administered 200 mg and peak concentrations of 0.341 mg/L were observed at 2.4 h [T. B. Tjandramaga *et al.*, *Eur. Heart J.*, 1984, *5 (Suppl. B)*, 135].

20 men and 1 woman, aged 33 to 74 years, with impaired renal function (10 of whom had end-stage renal disease requiring haemodialysis) were administered a single, oral dose of 200 mg flecainide acetate. 7 to 14 days after this single dose, each patient received 100 mg flecainide acetate every 12 or 24 h for 10 days. Mean peak flecainide acetate concentrations were 0.33 mg/L, after 3.3 h, following the single dose and 0.687 mg/L, after 2.7 h, for the multiple dosing regimen [S. C. Forland *et al.*, *J. Clin. Pharmacol.*, 1988, *28(8)*, 727–735].

Toxicity. Overdosing with flecainide is potentially life threatening and can cause or worsen supraventricular or ventricular arrhythmias and heart failure. Plasma levels above 0.7 to 1.0 mg/L are associated with increased likelihood of adverse experiences; the toxic concentration range is 1.5 to 3.0 mg/L.

Three subjects receiving flecainide developed dose-related blurring of vision at plasma concentrations of 0.713 to 0.906 mg/L (mean 0.802 mg/L). Three other subjects who required plasma concentrations > 0.7 mg/L for efficacy reported no adverse effects [H. J. Duff *et al.*, *Am. J. Cardiol.*, 1981, *48*, 1133–1140].

A young woman attempted to commit suicide and was found with no effective blood pressure and in extreme cardiac suffering. A flecainide concentration of 5.4 mg/L was observed (therapeutic range 0.2 to 1.0 mg/L) and during 10 h of cardiopulmonary bypass support, this reduced to 1.4 mg/L. Blood pressure and effective cardiac rhythm eventually returned and treatment was continued until drug levels decreased further. Unfortunately, the woman died, however, owing to severe neurological damage which occurred at the time of overdose [R. K. Yasui *et al.*, *Ann. Emer. Med.*, 1997, *29(5)*, 680–682].

Bioavailability. 90 to 95%.

Half-life. Plasma half-life, 7 to 23 h; 19 h (patients with arrhythmia); 26 to 49 h (patients with renal/hepatic dysfunction); 50 h (patients with congestive heart failure).

Volume of distribution. Steady state, 5 to 13.4 L/kg; average 5.5 to 8.7 L/kg for intravenous administration and 10 L/kg for oral.

Clearance. Plasma, 4.6 to 12.1 mL/min/kg after an intravenous dose of 0.6 to 1.7 mg/kg; 4.1 to 17 mL/min/kg after an oral dose of 60 to 240 mg.

Protein binding. In plasma, 32 to 58%.

Note. For reviews of flecainide, see B. Holmes and R. C. Heel, *Drugs*, 1985, *29*, 1–33 and G. J. Conard and R. E. Ober, *Am. J. Cardiol.*, 1984, *53*, 41B–51B.

Dose. Intravenous administration: initially 2 mg/kg body weight is administered for the first 30 min, followed by 1.5 mg/kg/h for the first hour and maintained at 0.1 to 0.25 mg/kg/h for subsequent hours. The infusion period should not exceed 24 h and the maximum dose is 600 mg. For patients with severe renal impairment (creatinine clearance < 35 mL/min/ 1.73 m^2). Oral administration: initial dose is 50 to 100 mg twice daily, with a maximum of 300 to 400 mg daily. Flecainide is not recommended to children under 12 years old.

Floctafenine

Analgesic

Proprietary names. Idalon; Idarac.

2-[[8-(Trifluoromethyl)-4-quinolinyl]amino]benzoic acid 2,3-dihydroxypropyl ester

$C_{20}H_{17}F_3N_2O_4$=406.4

CAS—23779-99-9

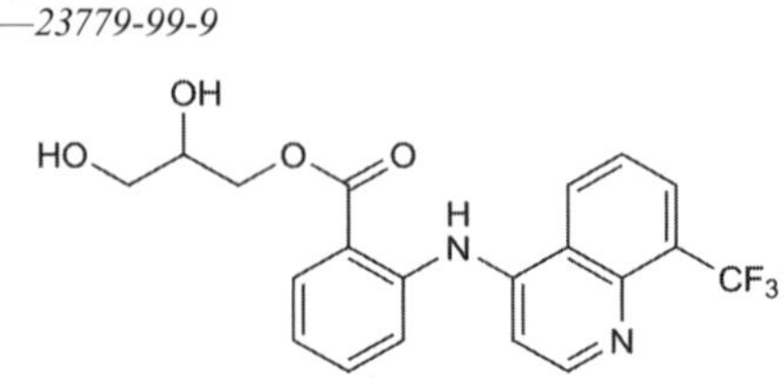

A yellowish-white powder. M.p. 175° to 179°.

Insoluble in water; soluble in ethanol and acetone; very slightly soluble in chloroform, ether and methylene chloride; freely soluble in dimethylformamide and pyridine.

Partition Coefficient. Log *P* (octanol/water), 4.0.

Thin-layer Chromatography. System TE—Rf 85; system TAE—Rf 85.

Gas Chromatography. System GA—floctafenine RI 3132, floctafenine-Me RI 2433.

High Performance Liquid Chromatography. System HZ—Retention time, 4.4 min; system HAA—Retention time, 17.2 min; system HAX—Retention time, 6.6 min; system HAY—Retention time, 5.8 min.

Ultraviolet Spectrum. Aqueous acid—233 nm (A^1_1=547a), 348 nm (A^1_1=450a); aqueous alkali—249 nm (A^1_1=392b), 359 nm (A^1_1=390b).

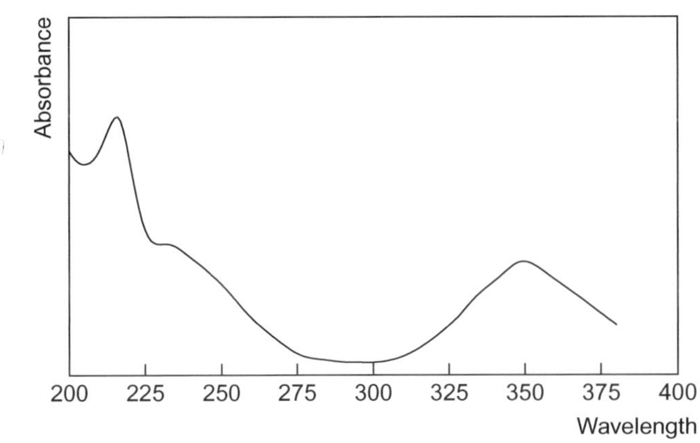

Infra-red Spectrum. Principal peaks at wavenumbers 1585, 1305, 1252, 1131, 1605, 1070 cm^{-1} (KBr disk). (See below.)

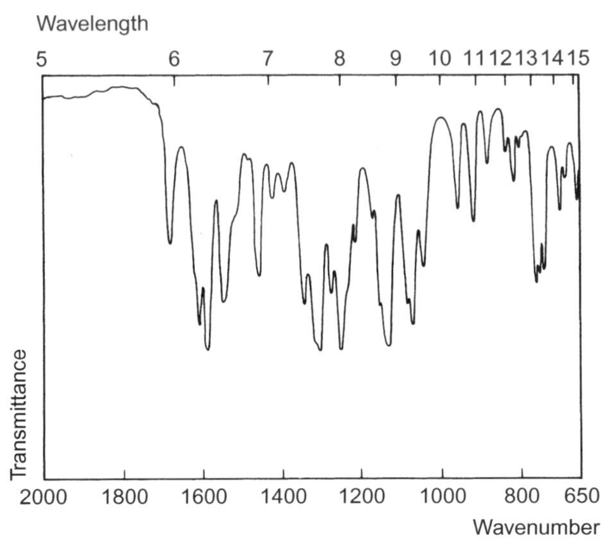

Quantification

High performance liquid chromatography. In plasma: floctafenine and glafenine, limit of detection for floctafenine about 3.2 μmol/L, UV detection—A. Tracqui *et al.*, *Ann. Biol. Clin. (Paris)*, 1988, *46*, 665–667. In plasma: floctafenine and its metabolite floctafenic acid, limits of detection 100 μg/L and 50 μg/L respectively, UV detection—M. H. Abdel-Hay and A. M. Gharaibeh. *J. Clin. Pharm. Ther.*, 1992, *17*, 31–35.

Thin-layer chromatography–spectrophotometry. In blood or urine: floctafenic acid and hydroxyfloctafenic acid—R. K. Lynn *et al.*, *J. Clin. Pharmacol.*, 1979, *19*, 20–30.

Disposition in the Body. Absorbed after oral administration. It is rapidly metabolised to floctafenic acid which is thought to be responsible for most of the analgesic activity. About 25% of a dose is excreted in the urine as floctafenic acid and hydroxyfloctafenic acid in 48 h.

Therapeutic concentration
A single oral dose of 400 mg administered to 7 subjects produced peak blood concentrations of floctafenic acid of 0.9 to 3.8 mg/L (mean 2.0) in 0.5 to 2.5 h [R. K. Lynn *et al.*, *J. Clin. Pharmacol.*, 1979, *19*, 20–30].

Protein binding. In plasma, floctafenic acid, extensively bound.

Dose. 0.8 to 1.6 g daily.

Fluanisone

Tranquilliser

Synonym. Haloanisone
Proprietary names. Sedalande. It is an ingredient of Hypnorm (vet.).
1-(4-Fluorophenyl)-4-[4-(2-methoxyphenyl)-1-piperazinyl]-1-butanone
$C_{21}H_{25}FN_2O_2$=356.4
CAS—1480-19-9

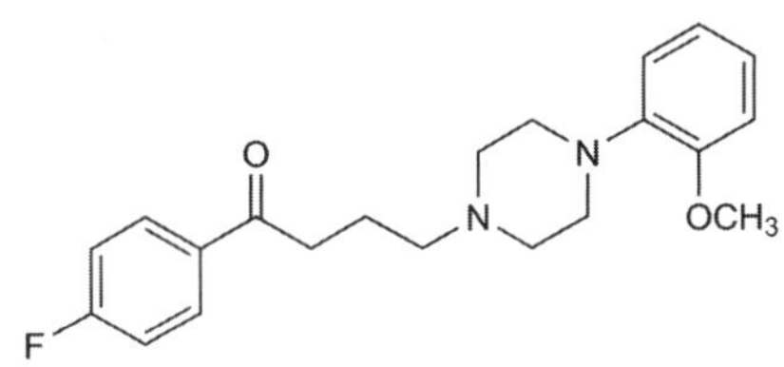

An almost white to buff-coloured crystalline powder. M.p. 67.5° to 68.5°. Practically insoluble in water; soluble 1 in 12 of ethanol, 1 in 1 of chloroform and 1 in 22 of ether.

Partition Coefficient. Log *P* (octanol/water), 3.6.

Colour Test. Mandelin's Test—brown

Thin-layer Chromatography. System TA—Rf 73; system TB—Rf 39; system TC—Rf 68; system TE—Rf 82; system TF—Rf 23; system TL—Rf 60; system TAE—Rf 67; system TAF—Rf 75. (Acidified potassium permanganate solution, positive.)

Gas Chromatography. System GA—fluanisone RI 2785, M (*O*-desmethyl-) RI 2715.

High Performance Liquid Chromatography. System HX—RI 423; system HY—RI 349.

Ultraviolet Spectrum. Acid isopropyl alcohol—243 nm (A^1_1=550a).

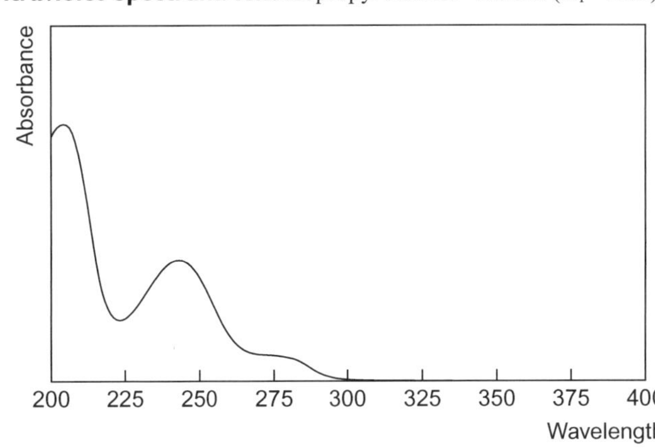

Infra-red Spectrum. Principal peaks at wavenumbers 1690, 1235, 1497, 1598, 1155, 750 cm^{-1} (KBr disk).

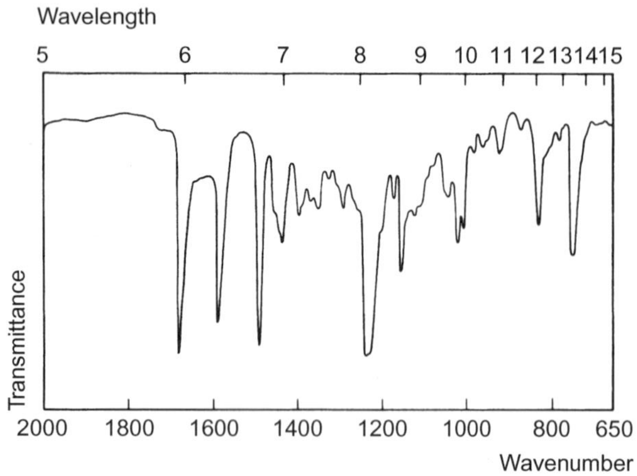

Mass Spectrum. Principal ions at *m/z* 205, 218, 123, 356, 219, 162, 95, 190; M (*O*-desmethyl-) *m/z* 194, 165, 123, 342, 338, 134.

Dose. Fluanisone has been given in doses of 5 to 7.5 mg daily.

Fluclorolone Acetonide

Corticosteroid

Synonym. Flucloronide
Proprietary names. Cutanit; Topilar.
(6α,11β,16α)-9,11-Dichloro-6-fluoro-21-hydroxy-16,17-[(1-methylethylidine)bis(oxy)]-pregna-1,4-diene-3,20-dione
$C_{24}H_{29}Cl_2FO_5$=487.4
CAS—3693-39-8

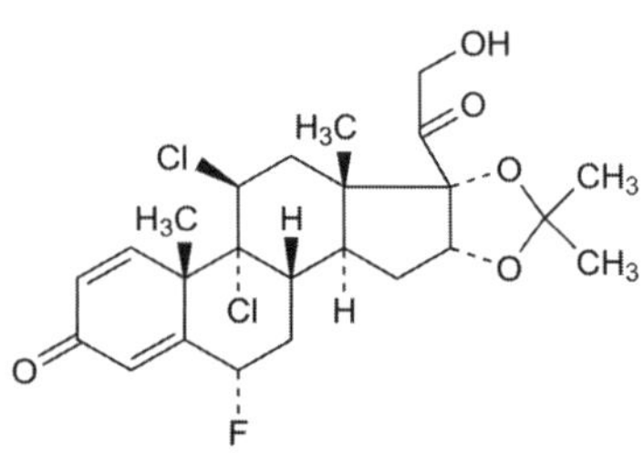

A white crystalline powder. M.p. about 245°, with decomposition. Practically insoluble in water; soluble in ethanol, chloroform and methanol.

Partition Coefficient. Log *P* (octanol/water), 4.2.

Ultraviolet Spectrum. Methanol—236 nm (A^1_1=242b).

Infra-red Spectrum. Principal peaks at wavenumbers 1666, 1086, 1052, 1063, 1724, 1639 cm^{-1}.

Use. Topically as a 0.025% cream or ointment.

Flucloxacillin

Antibiotic

Synonym. Floxacillin
Proprietary names. Flucloxil; Staphlex.
(2*S*,5*R*,6*R*)-6-[[[3-(2-Chloro-6-fluorophenyl)-5-methyl-4-isoxazolyl]-carbonyl]amino]-3,3-dimethyl-7-oxo-4-thia-1-azabicyclo[3.2.0]heptane-2-carboxylic acid
$C_{19}H_{17}ClFN_3O_5S$=453.9
CAS—5250-39-5

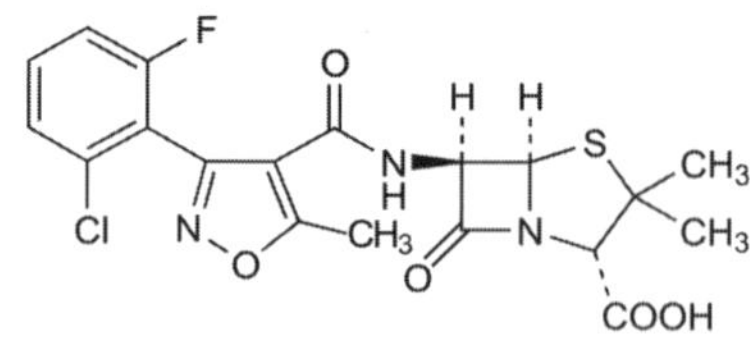

Flucloxacillin Sodium
Proprietary names. Betabiotic; Cloxillin; Evercid; Flopen; Floxapen (also as the magnesium salt); Flucil; Flucillin; Flucinal; Fluclomix; Fluclon; Flucloxin; Fluoclox; Galfloxin; Geriflox; Heracillin; Ladropen; Stafoxil; Staphlex; Staphycid (also as the magnesium salt); Staphylex; Zoxin. It is an ingredient of Magnapen.
$C_{19}H_{16}ClFN_3NaO_5S,H_2O$=493.9
CAS—1847-24-1 (anhydrous); 34214-51-2 (monohydrate)
A white, hygroscopic, crystalline powder.
Soluble 1 in 1 of water, 1 in 8 of ethanol, 1 in 8 of acetone and 1 in 2 of methanol.

Dissociation Constant. pK_a 2.7.

Partition Coefficient. Log *P* (octanol/water), 2.6.

High Performance Liquid Chromatography. System HY—RI 469.

Ultraviolet Spectrum. Aqueous acid—268, 274, 344 nm; aqueous alkali—268, 274, 318 nm.

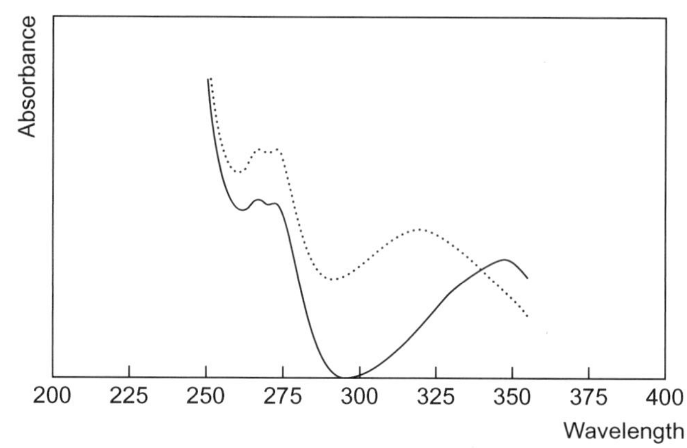

Infra-red Spectrum. Principal peaks at wavenumbers 1603, 1767, 1622, 1495, 1660, 794 cm^{-1} (flucloxacillin sodium, KBr disk).

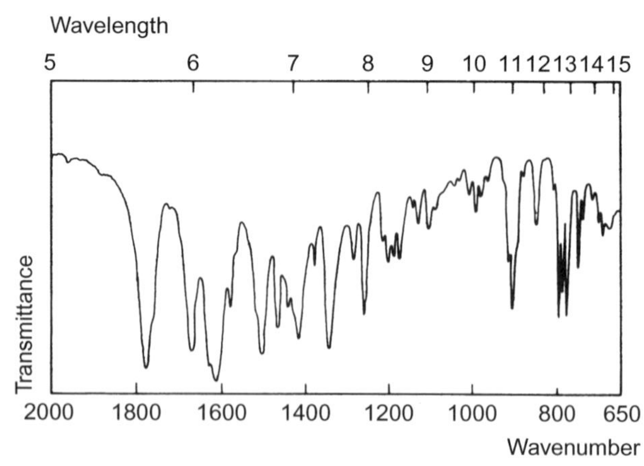

Quantification

High performance liquid chromatography. In plasma: flucloxacillin, cloxacillin and dicloxacillin, limit of detection for flucloxacillin 0.1 mg/L—C. T. Hung *et al.*, *J. Chromatogr.*, 1988, *425*, 3310–3341. In plasma: limit of detection 50 μg/L—B. G. Charles *et al.*, *J. Chromatogr.*, 1994, *660*, *Biomed. Appl.*, 186–190.

Disposition in the Body

Therapeutic concentration

After a single oral dose of flucloxacillin sodium (500 mg) to 7 elderly subjects, the time to reach a mean peak plasma concentration of 15.3 mg/L (range ± 5.9) was 1.2 h; corresponding values for the 5-hydroxymethyl metabolite were 2.58 mg/L (±2.20) at 2.17 h. Intravenous administration of the same dose to the same subjects produced mean maximum plasma concentrations of flucloxacillin and its 5-hydroxymethyl metabolite, of 69.0 mg/L (±21.2) at 0.14 h and 3.36 mg/L (±2.72) at 1.77 h, respectively. [J. Gath *et al*, *J. Clin. Pharmacol.*, 1995, *35*, 31–36].

Dose. The equivalent of 1 to 2 g of flucloxacillin daily.

Fluconazole

Antifungal

Synonym. UK-49858.
Proprietary names. Biozolene; Diflucan; Elazor; Fungata; Lavisa; Loitin; Solacap; Triflucan.
α-(2,4-Difluorophenyl)-α-(1*H*-1,2,4-triazol-1-ylmethyl)-1*H*-1,2,4-triazole-1-ethanol
$C_{13}H_{12}F_2N_6O = 306.3$
CAS—86386-73-4

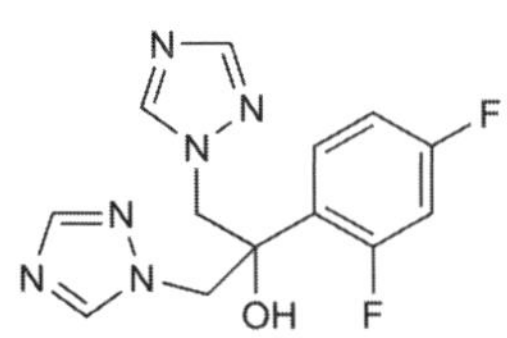

A white crystalline solid. M.p. 138° to 140°. It is slightly soluble in water and saline.

Dissociation Constant. pK_a 2.03 (37°).

Partition Coefficient. Log *P* (octanol/pH 7.4), 1.0.

Thin-layer Chromatography. System TB—Rf 00; system TE—Rf 35; system TAE—Rf 67.

Gas Chromatography. Column: 5% methylphenyl:95% dimethylpolysiloxane, silica DB5 (15 m × 0.32 mm i.d., 0.25 μm film thickness). Column temperature: 230°. Injector and detector temperatures: 280° and 285°, respectively. Carrier gas: hydrogen, 25 mL/min flow rate. Detection: nitrogen-selective. Internal standard (IS): medazepam. Retention time: fluconazole, 1.5 min; IS, 3.2 min [D. Debruyne *et al.*, *J. Pharm. Sci.*, 1988, *77*, 534–535].

Column: 1-methylsilicone gum (10 m × 0.53 mm i.d.). Column temperature: 220°. Injector and detector temperatures: 250° and 300°, respectively. Carrier gas: argon:methane (95:5), 5 mL/min flow rate. Detection: electron capture. IS: medazepam. Retention time: fluconazole, 4.35 min; IS, 6.40 min [J. H. Beijnen *et al.*, *J. Pharm. Biomed. Anal.*, 1991, *9*, 1173–1175].

High Performance Liquid Chromatography. System HAA—retention time 11.4 min; system HX—RI 340; system HY—RI 289.

Column: analytical: C_{18} (Adsorbosphere, 250 × 4.6 mm i.d., 5 μm); guard: identical packing. Mobile phase: tris(hydroxymethyl)aminomethane phosphate (25 mM, pH 7):acetonitrile (75:25), 1.0 mL/min flow rate. UV detection (λ=210 nm). IS: UK-48134. Retention time: fluconazole, 6.6 min; IS, 9.0 min [K. Inagaki *et al.*, *Ther. Drug Monit.*, 1992, *14*, 306–311].

Column: analytical: C_{18} (Genesis, 150 × 4.6 mm i.d., 4 μm), guard: identical packing. Column temperature: 40°. Mobile phase: water:acetonitrile (60:40) with acetic acid (5 mM), pH 3.7, 0.9 mL/min flow rate. IS: metronidazole. MS detection (APCI (atmospheric pressure chemical ionisation), MRM (multiple reaction monitoring) at *m/z* 306.9 to 219.8 for fluconazole and 171.8 to 127.7 for IS.). Retention time: fluconazole, 3.1 min; IS, 2.8 min [L. A. Moraes *et al.*, *Ther. Drug Monit.*, 1999, *21*, 200–207].

Ultraviolet Spectrum. Aqueous acid—261, 266 nm; basic—261, 267 nm.

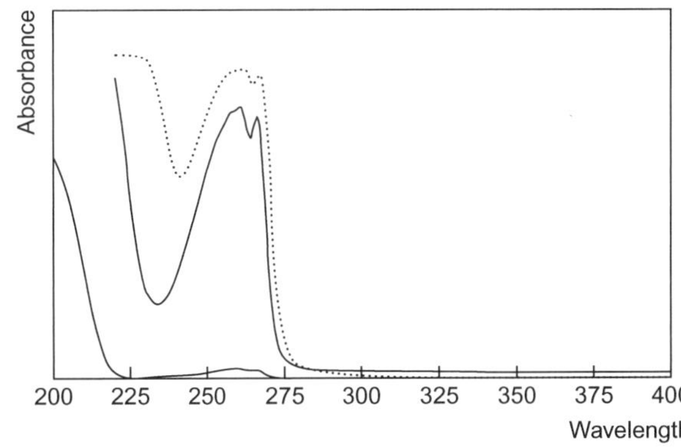

Infra-red Spectrum. Principal peaks at wavenumbers 1507, 1279, 1144, 680, 1620, 966 cm^{-1}.

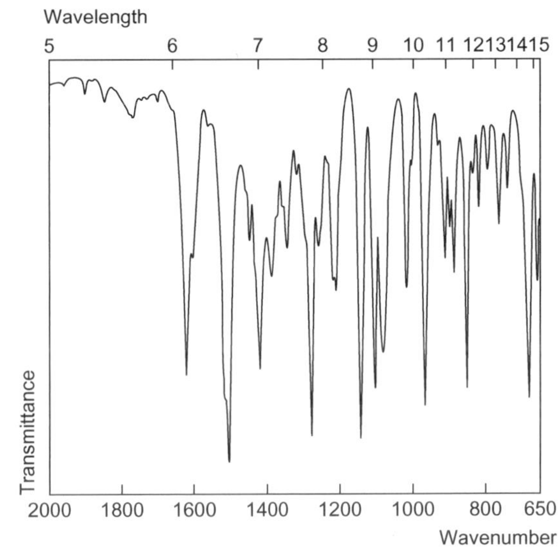

Mass Spectrum. Principal ions at *m/z* 224, 82, 127, 55, 83, 141, 125, 113.

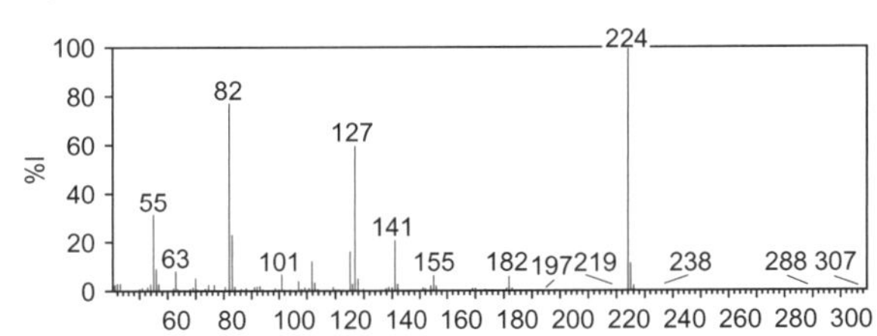

Quantification

Gas chromatography. In serum: limit of detection 0.05 mg/L, nitrogen-selective detector—D. Debruyne *et al.*, *J. Pharm. Sci.*, 1988, *77* 534–535. In plasma: limit of detection 0.003 mg/L, ECD—J. H. Beijnen *et al.*, *J. Pharm. Biomed. Anal.*, 1991, *9*, 1173–1175.

High performance liquid chromatography. In serum: limit of detection 0.1 mg/L, UV detection (λ=210 nm)—K. Inagaki *et al.*, *Ther. Drug. Monit.*, 1992, *14*, 306–311. In plasma: limit of quantification 0.005 mg/L. MS detection—L. A. Moraes *et al.*, *Ther. Drug Monit.*, 1999, *21*, 200–207.

Bioassay. In plasma and serum: limit of detection 0.2 mg/L—J. W. Van't Wout *et al.*, *J. Antimicrob. Chemother.*, 1988, *21*, 665–672. In plasma: limit of detection 2 mg/L—J. H. Rex *et al.*, *Antimicrob. Agents Chemother.*, 1991, *35*, 846–850.

Disposition in the Body. Fluconazole is well absorbed after oral administration and is widely distributed throughout the body. It penetrates all body fluids and has been detected in breast milk, joint fluid, saliva, sputum, vaginal fluid and peritoneal fluid. 80% of the parent drug is excreted unchanged in urine and 11% as metabolites.

Therapeutic concentration. Multiple dosing increases peak plasma concentrations and steady state concentrations are reached between 6 and 10 days. The serum therapeutic concentration range is 5 to 15 mg/L.

10 AIDS patients and 10 healthy volunteers were administered, intravenously, over 20 min with 100 mg fluconazole. Peak plasma concentrations reached 2.9 ± 0.9 and 2.8 ± 0.4 mg/L for the AIDS and healthy patients, respectively [R. A. Yeates *et al.*, *Br. J. Clin. Pharmacol.*, 1994, *38*, 77–79].

Toxicity. The toxic serum concentration is 20 mg/L.

Case: A 56-year-old woman was found dead at home. Toxicological investigation of her blood found a fluconazole concentration of 29.18 mg/L and an acenocoumarol concentration of 0.72 mg/L. Fluconazole inhibited the cytochrome P450 enzymes and thus decreased the clearance of acenocoumarol, resulting in death owing to the haemorrhaging effects of the drug [P. Kintz *et al.*, *TIAFT Bulletin Case Notes*, 1995, *25(4)*].

Half-life. Approx. 30 h (range from 20 to 50 h); increased in patients with impaired renal function.

Bioavailability Approx. 90%.

Volume of distribution. Apparent volume of distribution, 0.7 to 1.0 L/kg.

Clearance. In adults: approx. 0.23 mL/min/kg; 5 to 15 years old: 0.58 mL/min/kg; 9 months to 13 years old: 0.455 mL/min/kg.

Protein binding. Fluconazole binds plasma proteins approx. 12%.

Dose. Doses range from 50 to 400 mg daily, depending on symptoms and severity. Patients with renal impairment: reduced doses. Children: 3 mg/kg to 12 mg/kg daily (> 4 weeks old), every 72 h (< 2 weeks) and every 48 h (between 2 and 4 weeks).

Flucytosine

Antifungal

Synonym. 5-Fluorocytosine
Proprietary names. Alcobon; Ancobon; Ancotil.
4-Amino-5-fluoro-2(1*H*)-pyrimidinone
$C_4H_4FN_3O$=129.1
CAS—2022-85-7

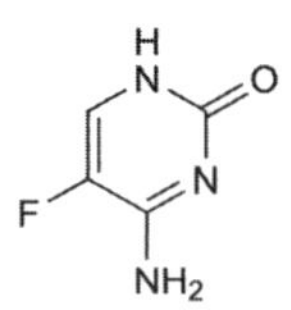

A white crystalline powder. M.p. 295° to 297°, with decomposition. Soluble 1 in 67 of water; slightly soluble in ethanol; practically insoluble in chloroform and ether.

Dissociation Constant. pK_a 2.9, 10.7.

Partition Coefficient. Log *P* (octanol/water), −1.4.

Thin-layer Chromatography. System TB—Rf 00; system TE—Rf 09; system TAE—Rf 57.

High Performance Liquid Chromatography. System HX—RI 72; system HZ—Retention time, 1.5 min; system HAA—Retention time, 3.1 min.

Ultraviolet Spectrum. Aqueous acid—286 nm (A^1_1=709a); aqueous alkali—293 nm.

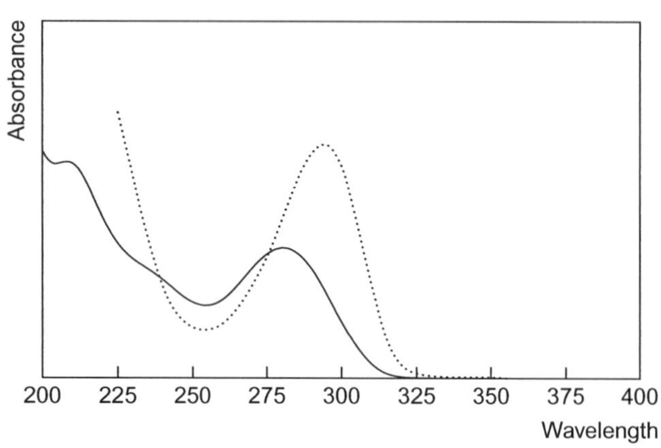

Infra-red Spectrum. Principal peaks at wavenumbers 1676, 1638, 1548, 1230, 1516, 1211 cm^{-1} (KBr disk).

Quantification

High performance liquid chromatography. In serum: comparison with bioassays—G. St-Germain *et al.*, *Antimicrob. Agents Chemother.*, 1989, *33*, 1403–1405; J. W. Hulsewede, *Zentralbl. Bakteriol.*, 1994, *281*, 513–518. In serum: flucytosine and other antifungal drugs, limits of detection 80 to 625 µg/L—T. K. Ng *et al.*, *J. Antimicrob. Chemother.*, 1996, *37*, 465–472. In plasma: flucytosine and fluorouracil, diode-array detection—J. S. Torano *et al.*, *Biomed. Chromatogr.*, 2001, *15*, 89–94.

Dose. 350 to 200 mg/kg daily.

Fludarabine

Antineoplastic

Synonyms. 2-F-ara-A; 2-Fluorovidarabine; NSC-118218; NSC-118218-H.
9-*β*-D-Arabino-furanosyl-2-fluoro-9*H*-purin-6-amine
$C_{10}H_{12}FN_5O_4$=285.2
CAS—*21679-14-1*

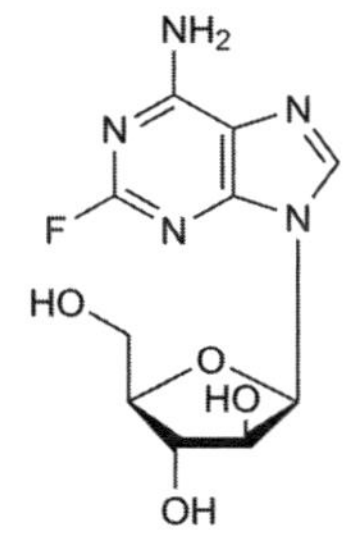

Crystals from ethanol and water. M.p. 260°. It is sparingly soluble in water and organic solvents.

Fludarabine Phosphate

Synonyms. Fludarabine-5′-monophosphate; 2-F-ara-AMP; 2-Fluoro-AMP; NSC-312887; NSC-328002.
Proprietary names. Beneflur; Fludara.
$C_{10}H_{13}FN_5O_7P$=365.2
CAS—75607-67-9

Partition Coefficient. Log *P* (octanol/water), −1.18.

High Performance Liquid Chromatography. Column: RP-18 (LiChrosorb, 200 × 4 mm i.d., 7 µm). Mobile phase: methanol:phosphate buffer (pH 4.15) (20:80), 1.0 mL/min flow rate. Internal standard (IS): mercaptopurine. UV detection (λ=254 nm). Retention time: fludarabine, 6.3 min; IS, 3.3 min [G. Misztal *et al.*, *Pharmazie*, 1996, *51*, 733–734].

Column: C-18 (Ultrasphere, 5 µm, 250 × 4.6 mm). Mobile phase: methanol:$(NH_4)H_2PO_4$ (10 mM, pH 4.15) (6:94), 1.0 to 1.2 mL/min flow rate. UV detection (λ=254 nm). Retention time: 55 min [M. R. Hersh *et al.*, *Cancer Chemother. Pharmacol.*, 1986, *17*, 277–280].

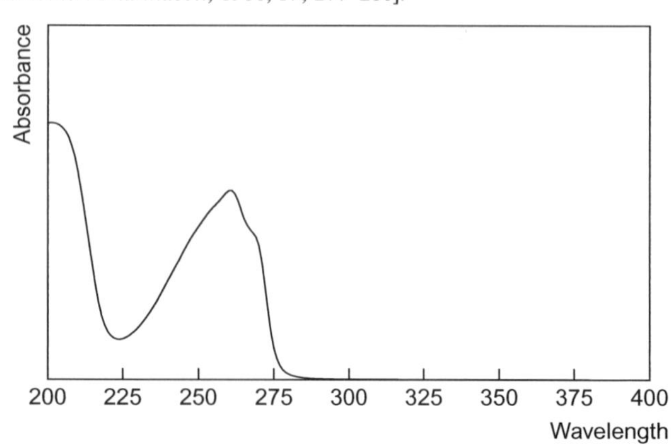

Quantification

High performance liquid chromatography. In plasma: limit of quantification 0.6 µg/L. Fluorescence detection—A. Kemena *et al.*, *Clin. Chim. Acta*,

1991, *200*, 95–106. In plasma: limit of detection 50 µg/L, UV detection (λ=254 nm)—G. Misztal *et al.*, *Pharmazie*, 1996, *51*, 733–734. In urine: limit of detection 0.0125 ng/L, UV detection (λ=254 nm)—M. R. Hersh *et al.*, *Cancer Chemother. Pharmacol.*, 1986, *17*, 277–280.

Disposition in the Body. Fludarabine phosphate is rapidly dephosphorylated to fludarabine, after intravenous administration, and is taken up by lymphocytes where it is rephosphorylated, by kinase, to active fludarabine triphosphate (2-F-ara-ATP). Peak plasma concentrations of 2-F-ara-ATP are observed approx. 4 h after administration and then undergo triphasic clearance. Excretion is mainly via the kidneys with approx. 60% of a dose being excreted in urine within 24 h. Considerable variations in pharmacokinetics have been observed between individuals.

Therapeutic concentration

A single dose of 25 mg 2-F-ara-AMP/m^2 was administered, by infusion, over 30 min, to a number of cancer patients. Maximum plasma concentrations of 2-F-ara-A reached 3.5 to 3.7 µg/L by the end of the infusion. Moderate accumulation was observed after the fifth dose to 4.4 to 4.8 µg/L. [Data as supplied by Schering Health Care Limited]

Toxicity. High doses of fludarabine phosphate are associated with irreversible central nervous system toxicity with symptoms such as blindness, coma and even death. Also, myelosuppression, pulmonary toxicity, ototoxicity, severe thrombocytopenia and neutropenia, owing to bone marrow suppression, have also been observed. The main intracellular metabolite, 2-F-ara-ATP, has cytotoxicity activity.

Overdose case: the usual dose of fludarabine phosphate, for chronic lymphocytic leukaemia, was administered and six months into treatment, progressive cerebral dysfunction due to leucoencephalopathy developed. The patient slipped into a coma and died 8 weeks later [A. Zabernigg *et al.*, *Lancet*, 1994, *344*, 1780].

Bioavailability. Systemic bioavailability of 2-F-ara-ATP, 50 to 65%.

Half-life. Initial half-life is 1 to 2 h and terminal half-life ranges from 10 to 30 h.

Volume of distribution. Steady state, 2.4 ± 1.6 L/kg (83 ± 55 L/m^2).

Clearance. Plasma clearance, 2.2 ± 1.2 mL/min/kg (79 ± 40 mL/min/kg).

Protein binding. No tendency to bind proteins.

Dose. A usual dose of 25 to 40 mg fludarabine phosphate/m^2 body surface is administered over 30 min, intravenously, daily for 5 days and courses repeated every 28 days. Dosage is reduced with severe or persistent myelosuppression and mild to moderate renal impairment (by up to 50%).

Fludrocortisone

Corticosteroid

Synonym. 9α-Fluorohydrocortisone
Proprietary name. Astonin-H
(11β)-9-Fluoro-11,17,21-trihydroxypregn-4-ene-3,20-dione
$C_{21}H_{29}FO_5$=380.5
CAS—127-31-1

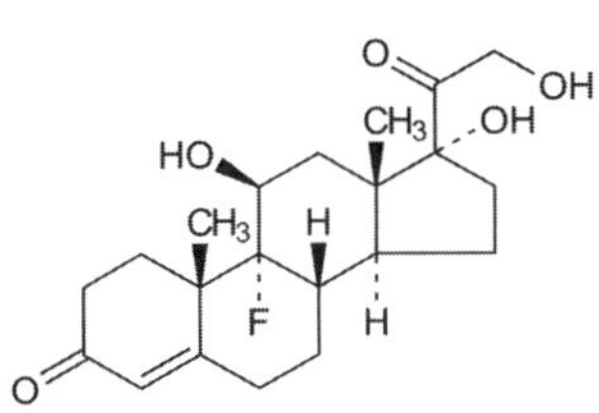

Crystals which decompose between 260° and 262°.
Very soluble in water.

Fludrocortisone Acetate

Synonym. 9α-Fluorohydrocortisone 21-acetate
Proprietary names. Florinef. It is an ingredient of Panotile.
$C_{23}H_{31}FO_6$=422.5
CAS—514-36-3
A white to pale yellow, hygroscopic, crystalline powder. M.p. 233° to 234° (occasionally 205° to 208° with resolidification on further heating then M.p. 226° to 228°). A solution in dioxan is dextrorotatory.
Practically insoluble in water; soluble 1 in 50 of ethanol, 1 in 50 of chloroform and 1 in 250 of ether.

Colour Tests. Antimony Pentachloride—orange; Naphthol–Sulfuric Acid—violet/brown; Sulfuric Acid—orange. (Green fluorescence under ultraviolet light.)

Partition Coefficient. Log *P* (octanol/water), 1.7.

Thin-layer Chromatography. Fludrocortisone acetate: system TA—Rf 90; system TE—Rf 86; system TP—Rf 58; system TQ—Rf 12; system TR—Rf 30; system TS—Rf 00. Fludrocortisone: system TAJ—Rf 55; system TAK—Rf 35; system TAL—Rf 91; system TAM—Rf 90. (DPST solution.)

Ultraviolet Spectrum. Fludrocortisone acetate: dehydrated alcohol—240 nm (A^{1}_{1}=405a).

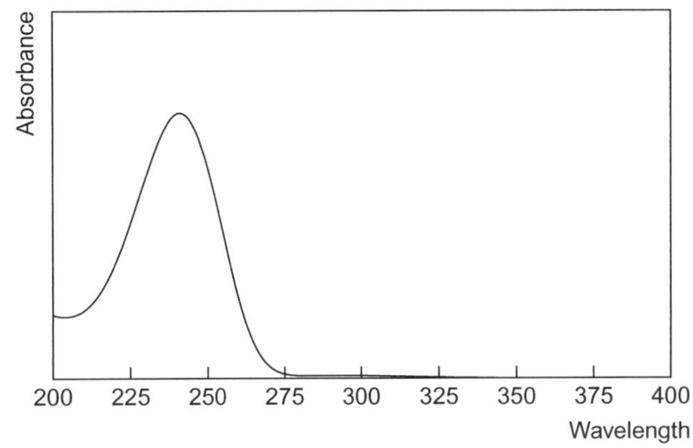

Infra-red Spectrum. Principal peaks at wavenumbers 1651, 1271, 1714, 1736, 1246, 1041 cm^{-1} (fludrocortisone acetate, KBr disk).

Dose. Usually 100 to 300 µg of fludrocortisone acetate daily.

Fludroxycortide

Corticosteroid

Synonyms. Fluorandrenolone; 6α-Fluoro-16α-hydroxyhydrocortisone 16,17-acetonide; Flurandrenolide; Flurandrenolone.
Proprietary names. Cordran; Drenison; Haelan; Sermaka.
(6α,11β,16α)-6-Fluoro-11,21-dihydroxy-16,17-[(1-methylethylidene)bis(oxy)]pregn-4-ene-3,20-dione
$C_{24}H_{33}FO_6$=436.5
CAS—1524-88-5

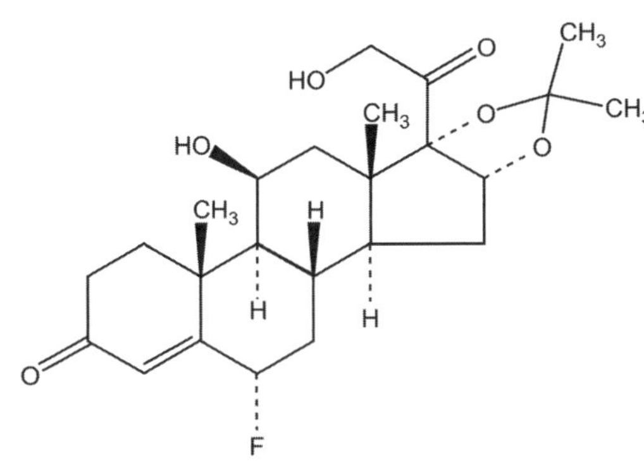

A white, fluffy, crystalline powder. M.p. 247° to 255°.
Practically insoluble in water and ether; soluble 1 in 72 of ethanol, 1 in 10 of chloroform and 1 in 25 of methanol.

Partition Coefficient. Log *P* (octanol/water), 3.0.

Colour Tests. Naphthol–Sulfuric Acid—green, brown dichroism/yellow; Sulfuric Acid—yellow (green fluorescence under ultraviolet light).

Ultraviolet Spectrum. Methanol–235 nm (A^{1}_{1} = 324a).

Infra-red Spectrum. Principal peaks at wavenumbers 1675, 1701, 1059, 1045, 1095, 1079 cm^{-1} (KBr disk).

Use. Topically in concentrations of 0.0125 to 0.05%.

Flufenamic Acid

Analgesic

Proprietary names. Achless; Ansatin; Arlef; Dignodolin; Fullsafe; Meralen; Paraflu; Parlef; Rheuma Lindofluid; Sastridex; Surika; Tecramine.
2-[[3-(Trifluoromethyl)phenyl]amino]benzoic acid
$C_{14}H_{10}F_3NO_2$=281.2
CAS—530-78-9

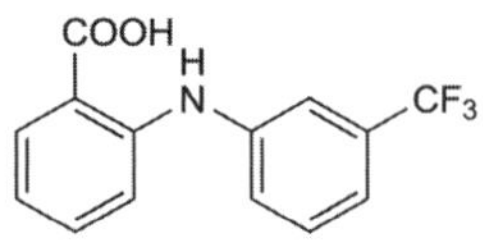

A pale yellow crystalline powder. M.p. 124° to 125°, with resolidification and remelting at 134° to 136°.
Practically insoluble in water; soluble 1 in 4 of ethanol, 1 in 7 of chloroform and 1 in 3 of ether.

Dissociation Constant. pK_a 3.9.

Partition Coefficient. Log *P* (octanol/water), 5.2.

Thin-layer Chromatography. System TA—Rf 96; system TE—Rf 18; system TG—Rf 37; system TAE—Rf 84; system TAJ—Rf 55; system TAK—Rf 78; system TAL—Rf 95. (Chromic acid solution, blue.)

Gas Chromatography. System GA—RI 1950; system GD—RRT of methyl derivative 1.26 (relative to n-$C_{16}H_{34}$); system GL—flufenamic acid-Me RI 1875, M (OH-)-Me_2 RI 2115.

High Performance Liquid Chromatography. System HD—*k* 19.7; system HV—RRT 1.00 (relative to meclofenamic acid); system HX—RI 671; system HY—RI 667.

Ultraviolet Spectrum. Methanol—288 nm (A_1^1=593a), 339 nm.

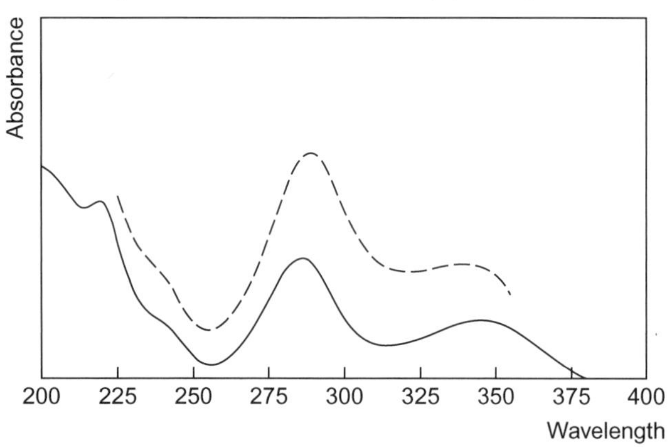

Infra-red Spectrum. Principal peaks at wavenumbers 1115, 1176, 1653, 1284, 1265, 1600 cm^{-1} (KBr disk). Five polymorphic forms occur.

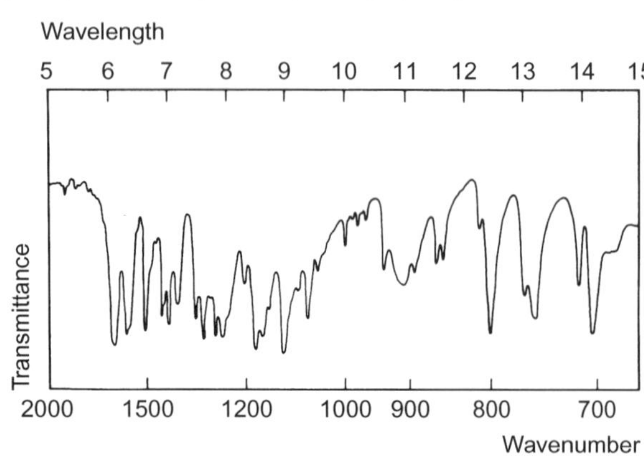

Mass Spectrum. Principal ions at *m/z* 263, 281, 166, 92, 145, 167, 235, 139; flufenamic acid-Me *m/z* 263, 295, 235, 166, 264, 92; M (OH-)-Me_2 *m/z* 325, 293, 278, 250, 223, 202.

Quantification

High performance liquid chromatography. In plasma: flufenamic acid and mefenamic acid, limit of detection 1 mg/L, UV detection—C. K. Lin *et al.*, *J. Pharm. Sci.*, 1980, *69*, 95–97. In urine: flufenamic acid, mefenamic acid and tolfenamic acid, limit of detection for flufenamic acid about 3.5 ng, UV detection—E. Mikami *et al.*, *J. Chromatogr. B. Biomed. Sci. Appl.*, 2000, *744*, 81–89.

Disposition in the Body. Readily absorbed after oral administration. Metabolised by hydroxylation and glucuronic acid conjugation. About 50% of a dose is excreted in the urine in 72 h and about 36% is eliminated in the faeces. The material excreted in the urine consists mainly of conjugated flufenamic acid and free and conjugated 4′-hydroxyflufenamic acid with smaller amounts of the 5′-hydroxy and dihydroxy derivatives.

Therapeutic concentration

Following oral administration of 200 mg three times daily for 4 days to 10 subjects, plasma concentrations of 0.3 to 17 mg/L (mean 6.4) were reported 2 h after the morning dose [R. A. Buchanan *et al.*, *Curr. Ther. Res.*, 1969, *11*, 533–538].

Half-life. Plasma half-life, about 3 h.

Protein binding. In plasma, extensively bound.

Dose. 400 to 600 mg daily.

Flugestone

Progestational Steroid (Veterinary)

Synonym. Flurogestone
9α-Fluoro-11β,17α-dihydroxypregn-4-ene-3,20-dione
$C_{21}H_{29}FO_4$=364.5
CAS—337-03-1

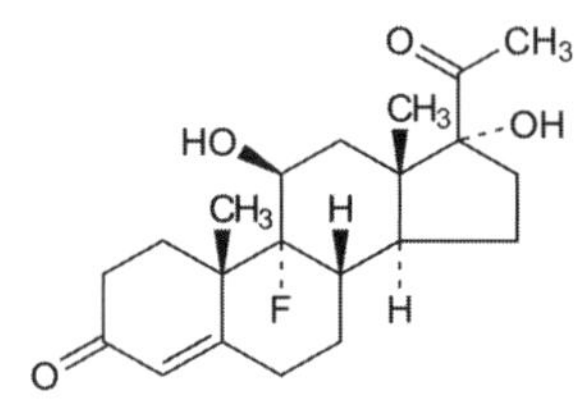

Flugestone Acetate

Proprietary names. Chronogest; Ovakron.
$C_{23}H_{31}FO_5$=406.5
CAS—2529-45-5
A white or creamy-white powder. M.p. 266° to 269°.
Very slightly soluble in water; soluble 1 in 23 of ethanol, 1 in 2.5 of chloroform and 1 in 100 of methanol.

Partition Coefficient. Log *P* (octanol/water), 2.0 (flugestone acetate).

Ultraviolet Spectrum. Flugestone acetate: methanol—238 nm (A_1^1=425b).

Flumazenil

Benzodiazepine Antagonist

Synonyms. Flumazepil; Ro-15-1788.
Proprietary names. Anexate; Lanexat; Mazicon; Romazicon.
8-Fluoro-5,6-dihydro-5-methyl-6-oxo-4*H*-imidazo[1,5-*a*][1,4]-benzodiazepine-3-carboxylic acid ethyl ester
$C_{15}H_{14}FN_3O_3$=303.3
CAS—*78755-81-4*

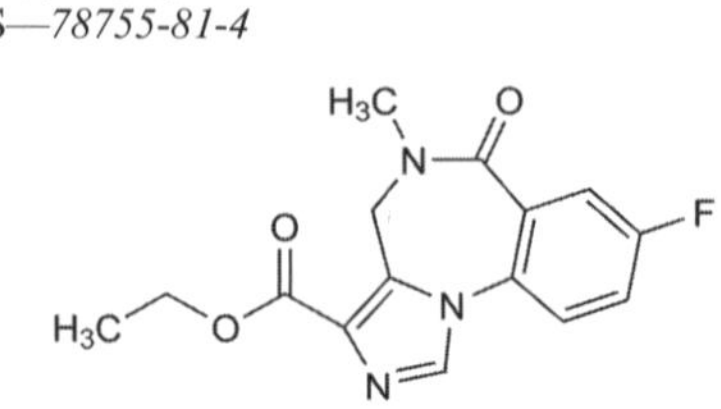

A white to off-white crystalline compound. M.p. 201° to 203°. It is insoluble in water; slightly soluble in dilute acidic solutions.

Dissociation Constant. pK_a 1.8.

Partition Coefficient. Log *P* (octanol/water): 1.0.

Thin-layer Chromatography. System TA—Rf 71; system TB—Rf 03; system TC—Rf 63; system TD—Rf 30; system TE—Rf 61; system TF—Rf 14; system TL—Rf 44; system TAD—Rf 61; system TAE—Rf 76; system TAF—Rf 72.

Gas Chromatography. Column: RTX-5 capillary (30 m × 0.32 mm i.d., 0.25 μm film thickness). Column temperature: 260°. Injector and detector temperature: 260° and 300°, respectively. Carrier gas: helium, 103 kPa inlet pressure. Internal standard (IS): clinazolam. Detection: nitrogen–phosphorus. Retention time: flumazenil, 7 min; IS, 12 min [L. E. Fisher *et al.*, *J. Chromatogr.*, 1995, *665*, *Biomed. Appl.*, 217–221].

High Performance Liquid Chromatography. System HX—RI 387; system HY—RI 327; system HZ—retention time 2.6 min.

Column: CP-microsphere C_{18} (100 × 4.6 mm i.d., 3 μm). Mobile phase: methanol:aqueous sodium dihydrogen phosphate monohydrate (0.3%, pH 3.9) (34.75:65.25), 1.5 mL/min flow rate. IS: Ro 15-3505. UV detection (λ=245 nm). Retention time: flumazenil, 4.86 min; IS, 6.17 min [L. T. Breimer *et al.*, *Clin. Pharmacokinet.*, 1991, *20*, 491–496].

Column: (analytical) C_{18} RP cartridge (NovaPak, 100 × 8 mm, 4 μm); (precolumn) C_8 (30 × 4.6 mm, 30 μm). Mobile phase: 32% acetonitrile:sodium hydrogen phosphate buffer (0.04 M with 1 mL/L TEA (triethylamine), pH 7.2) (32:68), 1.5 mL/min flow rate. UV detection (λ=220 nm). IS: flurazepam. Retention time: flumazenil, 3.8 min; IS, 18.5 min [K. Chan and R. D. Jones, *J. Chromatogr.*, 1993, *619*, *Biomed. Appl.*, *130*, 154–60].

Ultraviolet Spectrum. Aqueous base—244 nm.

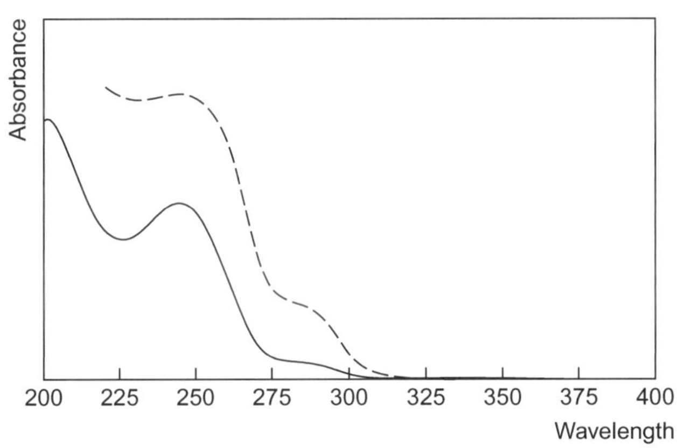

Infra-red Spectrum. Principal peaks at wavenumbers 1724, 1652, 1161 cm^{-1} (KBr pellet).

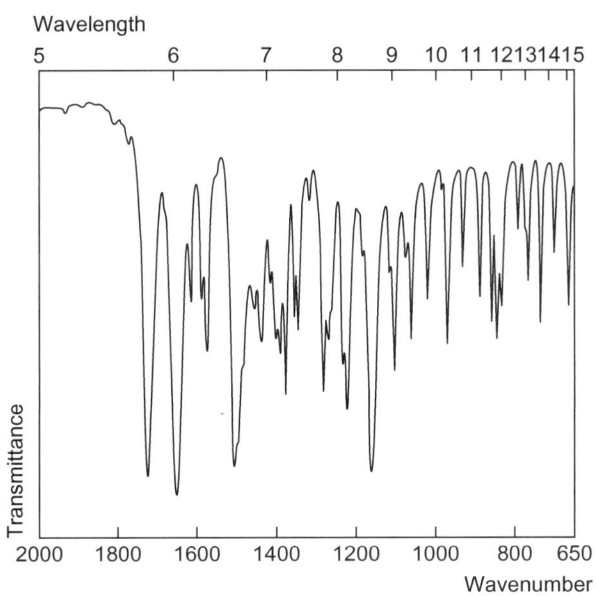

Mass Spectrum. Principal ions at *m*/*z* 229, 257, 303, 42, 230, 258, 201, 215.

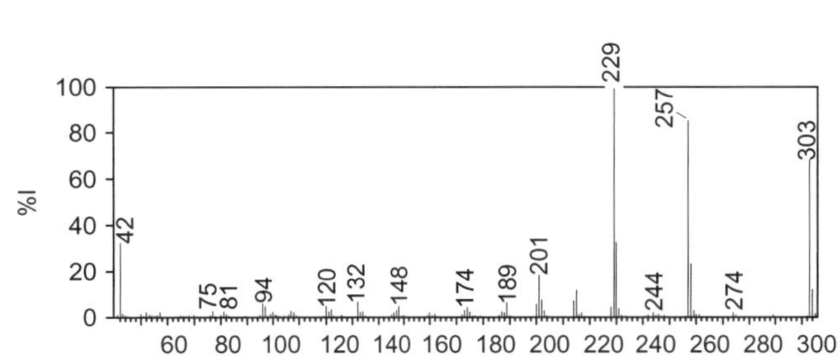

Quantification

Gas chromatography. In plasma: limit of detection 3 μg/L, nitrogen–phosphorus detection—L. E. Fisher *et al.*, *J. Chromatogr.*, 1995, *665*, *Biomed. Appl.*, 217–221. In plasma: limit of detection 0.05 μg/L, nitrogen-selective detection—M. Zell and U. Timm, *J. Chromatogr.*, 1986, *382*, *Biomed. Appl.*, *55*, 175–188.

Gas chromatography–mass spectrometry. In plasma: limit of quantification 1 μg/L—D. Song *et al.*, *J. Chromatogr.*, 1995, *663*, *Biomed. Appl.*, 263–273. In plasma: limit of quantification, 0.5 μg/L—E. K. Fukuda *et al.*, *J. Chromatogr.*, 1989, *491*, *Biomed. Appl.*, *83*, 97–106.

High performance liquid chromatography. In plasma or urine: flumazenil and metabolites, limit of detection 4 μg/L, UV detection (λ=220 nm)—K. Chan and R. D. Jones, *J. Chromatogr.*, 1993, *619*, *Biomed. Appl.*, *130*, 154–60. In plasma: limit of detection 0.3 μg/L, limit of quantification 2 μg/L, UV detection (λ=220 nm)—A. A. Vletter *et al.*, *J. Chromatogr.*, 1990, *530*; *Biomed. Appl.*, *95*, 177–185. In plasma: limit of quantification 0.5 μg/L, UV detection (λ=245 nm)—L. T. Breimer *et al.*, *Clin. Pharmacokinet.*, 1991, *20*, 491–496.

Disposition in the Body. Flumazenil is rapidly and well absorbed after oral administration, but undergoes extensive first-pass hepatic metabolism. It is therefore given by intravenous administration. It is rapidly distributed into the brain. Flumazenil is extensively metabolised in the liver to an inactive carboxylic acid form and excreted predominantly in urine (less than 1% is excreted unchanged). Metabolites include *N*-desmethylflumazenil, *N*-desmethylflumazenil acid and flumazenil acid. Some (5 to 10%) is excreted via bile in faeces.

Therapeutic concentration. The trough serum therapeutic concentration range is 10 to 50 μg/L and peak, 200 to 300 μg/L.

6 healthy male volunteers, aged between 28 and 42 years, were administered intravenously a dose of 2.5 mg over 30 s. The effective plasma concentration was 60 μg/L during the infusion which stayed constant until 5 min after infusion had ended. It then rapidly declined to 3 μg/L over a 3 h period [U. Klotz *et al.*, *Eur. J. Clin. Pharmacol.*, 1984, *27*, 115–117].

Bioavailability. Approx. 16%.

Half-life. Plasma half-life, 0.7 to 1.3 h.

Volume of distribution. 0.9 to 1.1 L/kg.

Clearance. Plasma clearance, 0.8 to 1.0 L/h/kg; 31 to 78 L/h. Blood, 43 L/h.

Distribution in blood. Blood:plasma ratio is 0.8 to 1.3.

Protein binding. In plasma, 50% (of which about two-thirds is bound to albumin).

Note. For a review of the pharmacokinetics of flumazenil, see U. Klotz and J. Kanto, *Clin. Pharmacokinet.*, 1988, *14*, 1–12.

Dose. Usually, 300 to 600 μg as an intravenous injection; 100 to 400 μg/h may be given by intravenous infusion.

Flumetasone

Corticosteroid

Synonyms. Flumethasone; 6α-dexamethasone
Proprietary name. Flucort (vet.)
(6α,11β,16α)-6,9-Difluoro-11,17,21-trihydroxy-16-methylpregna-1,4-diene-3,20-dione
$C_{22}H_{28}F_2O_5$=410.5
CAS—2135-17-3

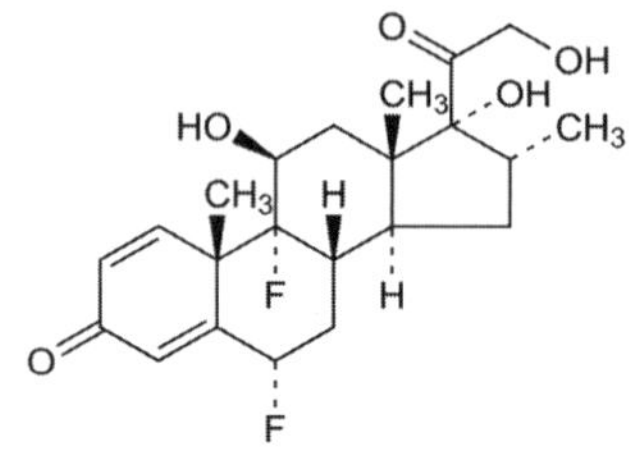

Flumetasone Pivalate
Synonym. Flumetasone Trimethylacetate.
Proprietary names. Cerson; Locacorten; Locorten(e).
$C_{27}H_{36}F_2O_6$=494.6
CAS—2002-29-1
A white crystalline powder.
Practically insoluble in water; soluble 1 in 89 of ethanol, 1 in 350 of chloroform and 1 in 2800 of ether.

Partition Coefficient. Log *P* (octanol/water), 1.9.

Thin-layer Chromatography. System TAM—Rf 64.

Ultraviolet Spectrum. Methanol—238 nm (A_1^1=438a).

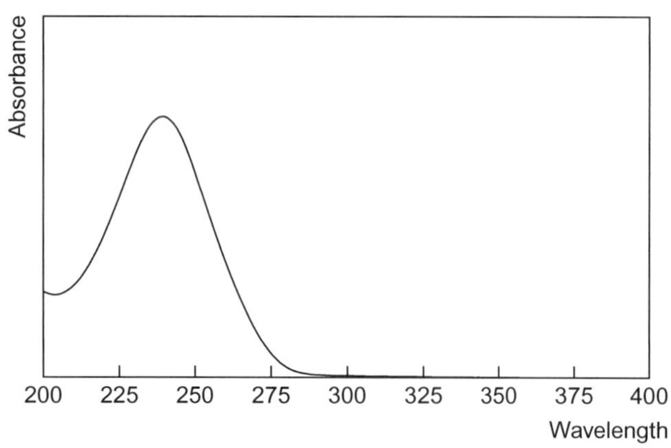

Infra-red Spectrum. Principal peaks at wavenumbers 1664, 1623, 901, 1733, 1139, 1160 cm^{-1} (flumetasone pivalate, KBr disk).

Use. Flumetasone pivalate is used topically in a concentration of 0.02%.

Flunitrazepam

Hypnotic

Synonyms. Flunitrazepamum; Ro-5-4200.
Proprietary names. Absint; Darkene; Flunimerck; Fluninoc; Flunipam; Flupam; Fluscand; Fluserin; Flutraz; Hypnodorm; Hypnor; Insom; Narcozep; Rohipnol; Rohypnol; Roipnol; Ronal; Somnubene; Valsera.
5-(2-Fluorophenyl)-1,3-dihydro-1-methyl-7-nitro-2*H*-1,4-benzodiazepin-2-one
$C_{16}H_{12}FN_3O_3$=313.3
CAS—1622-62-4

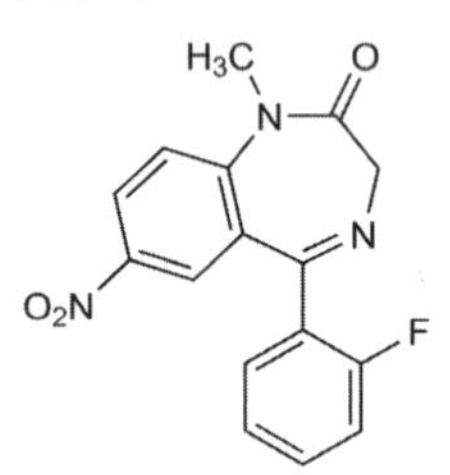

An almost white to pale yellow crystalline solid. M.p. about 170°.
Sparingly soluble in water; soluble 1 in 172 of ethanol, 1 in 3 of chloroform, 1 in 300 of ether, and 1 in 100 of methanol.

Dissociation Constant. pK_a 1.8.

Partition Coefficient. Log *P* (octanol/water), 2.1.

Colour Test. Formaldehyde–Sulfuric Acid—orange.

Thin-layer Chromatography. System TA—Rf 63; system TB—Rf 10; system TC—Rf 72; system TD—Rf 54; system TE—Rf 74; system TF—Rf 47; system TL—Rf 63; system TAD—Rf 72; system TAE—Rf 80; system TAF—Rf 82; system TAJ—Rf 69; system TAK—Rf 59; system TAL—Rf 95.

Gas Chromatography. System GA—flunitrazepam RI 2600, M (nor-) RI 2720, M (7-amino-) RI 2723, M (nor-amino-) RI 2825; system GB—flunitrazepam RI 2744, M (nor-) RI 2816, M (nor-)-TMS RI 2622, M (7-amino-) RI 2804, M (7-amino-)-TMS RI 2836; system GG—flunitrazepam RI 3190.

High Performance Liquid Chromatography. System HI—*k* 3.15; system HK—*k* 0.47; system HX—RI 483; system HY—RI 305; system HZ—retention time 5.6 min; system HAA—retention time 18.6 min; system HAL—flunitrazepam retention time 6.2 min, M (nor) retention time 3.7 min; system HAZ—flunitrazepam *k* 0.86, M (nor-) *k* 0.65, M (7-amino) *k* 0.22; system HBH—flunitrazepam *k* 3.34; system HBI—flunitrazepam *k* 0.86.

Ultraviolet Spectrum. Methanol—252 (A_1^1=516a), 308 nm (A_1^1=332a).

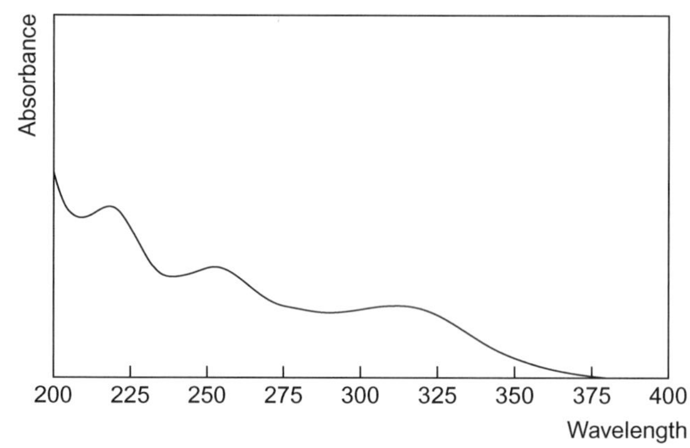

Infra-red Spectrum. Principal peaks at wavenumbers 1697, 1620, 1490, 1528, 1107, 783 cm^{-1} (KBr disk). (See below)

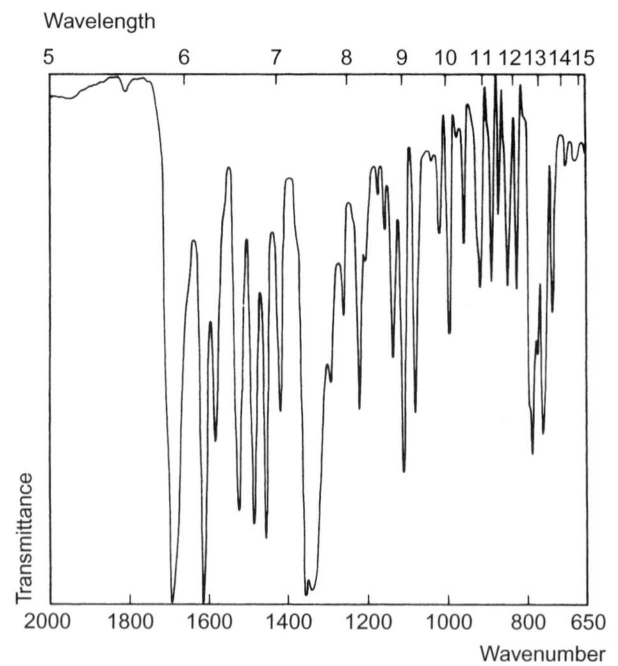

Mass Spectrum. Principal ions at *m/z* 285, 312, 313, 286, 266, 238, 294, 284; 7-amino-1-desmethylflunitrazepam 269, 240, 241, 268, 270, 107, 121, 213; 7-aminoflunitrazepam 283, 44, 255, 282, 254, 284, 264, 256; desmethylflunitrazepam 298, 271, 299, 224, 272, 270, 252, 280.

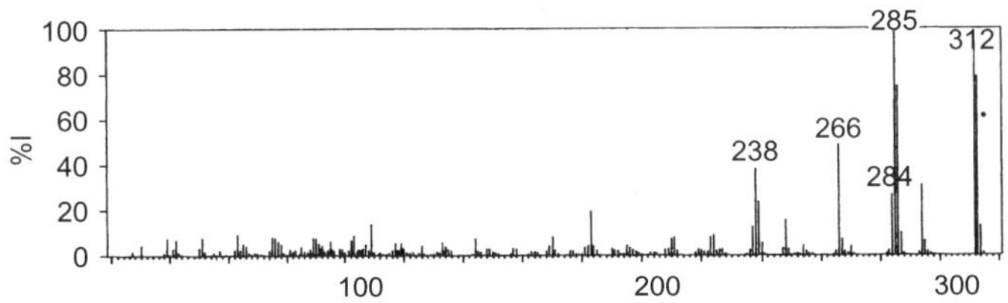

Quantification

Gas chromatography. In plasma: limit of detection 0.5 μg/L, ECD—Y. C. Sumirtapura *et al.*, *Arzneimittelforschung*, 1982, *32*, 252–257. In plasma and whole blood: flunitrazepam and other benzodiazepines, ECD and nitrogen–phosphorus detection—P. Lillsunde and T. Seppala, *J. Chromatogr.*, 1990, *533*, 97–110. In blood: flunitrazepam and other benzodiazepines, ECD—H. Gjerde *et al.*, *J. Pharm. Biomed. Anal.*, 1992, *10*, 317–322. In plasma or urine: flunitrazepam and other benzodiazepines—K. J. Reubsaet *et al.*, *J. Pharm. Biomed. Anal.*, 1998, *18*, 667–680.

Gas chromatography–mass spectrometry. In serum or urine: flunitrazepam and other benzodiazepines, limit of quantification 2 μg/L—M. Kleinschnitz *et al.*, *J. Chromatogr. B Biomed. Appl.*, 1996, *676*, 61–67. In hair: NCI detection—V. Cirimele *et al.*, *J. Anal. Toxicol.*, 1996, *20*, 596–598. In urine: flunitrazepam and its metabolites, limit of detection for metabolites < 1 μg/L—M. A. ElSohly *et al.*, *J. Anal. Toxicol.*, 1997, *21*, 335–340. In blood and bloodstains: flunitrazepam and its metabolites, limit of detection 1 μg/L—A. A. Elian, *Forensic Sci. Int.*, 1999, *101*, 107–111. In whole blood or plasma: flunitrazepam and its metabolites—M. A. ElSohly *et al.*, *J. Anal. Toxicol.*, 1999, *23*, 486–489. In urine: 7-aminoflunitrazepam—J. Feely *et al.*, *Ir. J. Med. Sci.*, 1999, *168*, 189–192. In urine: flunitrazepam and its major metabolites—H. Nguyen and D. R. Nau, *J. Anal. Toxicol.*, 2000, *24*, 37–45. In urine: flunitrazepam and other benzodiazepines, limits of detection 13 to 30 μg/L (scan mode) and 1 to 1.7 μg/L (SIM)—D. Borrey *et al.*, *J. Chromatogr. B Biomed. Sci. Appl.*, 2001, *765*, 187–197. Limit of quantification is 2.5 to 5 μg/L (full scan) and 0.1 to 0.5 μg/L (SIM, *m/z* 312)—D. Borrey *et al.*, *J. Chromatogr. A*, 2001, *910*, 105–118. In oral liquid: flunitrazepam and 7-aminoflunitrazepam, limits of detection 0.05 μg/L and 0.1 μg/L respectively—N. Samyn *et al.*, *J. Anal. Toxicol.*, 2002, *26*, 211–215.

High performance liquid chromatography. In plasma: limit of detection 1 μg/L, UV detection—T. B. Vree *et al.*, *J. Chromatogr.*, 1977, *143(1) B Biomed. Appl.*, 530–534. In plasma: flunitrazepam and droperidol, limit of detection for flunitrazepam 10 μg/L—J. Guichard *et al.*, *J. Chromatogr.*, 1993, *612*, 269–275. In plasma: limit of detection 5 μg/L—F. Benhamou-Batut *et al.*, *J. Pharm. Biomed. Anal.*, 1994, *12*, 931–936. In postmortem blood: flunitrazepam and other nitrobenzodiazepines and their 7-amino metabolites, limits of detection 1 to 8 μg/L, UV detection—M. D. Robertson and O. H. Drummer, *J. Chromatogr. B Biomed. Appl.*, 1995, *667*, 179–184. In plasma or urine: flunitrazepam and its metabolites, diode-array detection—W. He and N. Parissis, *J. Pharm. Biomed. Anal.*, 1997, *16*, 707–715. In urine: flunitrazepam and its metabolites, limit of detection <2 μg/L, UV detection—I. Deinl *et al.*, *J. Chromatogr. B Biomed. Sci. Appl.*, 1997, *704*, 251–258. In plasma, serum, or urine: flunitrazepam and metabolites, limit of detection in plasma or serum 1 μg/L, UV detection—I. Deinl *et al.*, *J. Anal. Toxicol.*, 1998, *22*, 197–202. In plasma or serum: flunitrazepam and its metabolites, limit of detection 1 μg/L, UV detection—I. Deinl *et al.*, *J. Anal. Toxicol.*, 1999, *23*, 598–602. In serum: flunitrazepam and other benzodiazepines, photodiode-array detection—B. Ahrens *et al.*, *Arzneimittelforschung*, 2000, *50*, 1057–1062. In whole blood: flunitrazepam and other benzodiazepines, diode-array detection—A. El Mahjoub and C. Staub, *J. Anal. Toxicol.*, 2001, *25*, 209–214. In hair: flunitrazepam and other benzodiazepines, photodiode-array detection—A. El Mahjoub and C. Staub, *Forensic Sci. Int.*, 2001, *123*, 17–25.

High performance liquid chromatography–mass spectrometry. In serum, blood, or urine: flunitrazepam and its metabolites, SID—M. J. Bogusz *et al.*, *J. Chromatogr. B Biomed. Sci. Appl.*, 1998, *713*, 361–369. In serum: limit of quantification 0.5 μg/L, ion trap detection—J. Darius and P. Banditt, *J. Chromatogr. B Biomed. Sci. Appl.*, 2000, *738*, 437–441. In plasma: flunitrazepam and its major metabolites, limit of detection for flunitrazepam 0.25 μg/L—M. Kollroser and C. Schober, *J. Pharm. Biomed. Anal.*, 2002, *28*, 1173–1182.

Note. For GC/MS screening of acetylated benzodiazepines, see D. Borrey *et al.*, *J. Chromatogr. A*, 2001, *910*, 115–118.

Disposition in the Body. Readily absorbed after oral administration. It is extensively metabolised in the liver to desmethylflunitrazepam, which has some activity, and 7-aminoflunitrazepam, which is inactive; other metabolites include 3-hydroxyflunitrazepam, 3-hydroxy-7-acetamidoflunitrazepam, and 7-amino-1-desmethylflunitrazepam. Flunitrazepam is excreted in the urine almost entirely as metabolites, both free and conjugated, with less than 1% as unchanged drug. About 10% of a dose is eliminated in the faeces. Flunitrazepam crosses the placental barrier and it is excreted in breast milk.

Therapeutic concentration

After single oral doses of 1 mg and 2 mg given to 11 and 5 subjects, mean peak plasma concentrations of 2.5 and 1.5 μg/L, respectively, were attained in about 1 h. [R. S. J. Clarke *et al.*, *Br. J. Anaesth.*, 1980, *52*, 437–445.]

Following oral doses of 2 mg daily for 28 days given to 7 subjects, a mean peak plasma concentration of about 20 μg/L was reported 3 h after the last dose. [E. Wickstrom *et al.*, *Eur. J. Clin. Pharmacol.*, 1980, *17*, 189–196.]

Infusion of flunitrazepam over 20 min (0.2 mg/kg) to 25 neonates and 6 infants; produced peak plasma concentrations of 0.077 to 1.028 mg/L (mean 243). [A. Pariente-Khayat *et al.*, *Clin. Pharmacol. Ther.*, 1999, *66*, 136–139.]

Toxicity

Of 8 deaths involving flunitrazepam, 4 had 7-aminoflunitrazepam levels of 0.45 mg/L (where the fatality involved flunitrazepam alone) and 4 had 7-aminoflunitrazepam levels of 0.16 mg/L (where the fatality involved flunitrazepam and ethanol); in the latter group the mean ethanol concentration was 1600 mg/L. Levels of flunitrazepam were low, suggesting that 7-aminoflunitrazepam was produced postmortem [O. H. Drummer *et al.*, *Am. J. Forensic Med. Pathol.*, 1993, *14*, 238–243.]

Bioavailability. About 80% to 90%.

Half-life. Plasma half-life, 3 h (distribution); 16 to 35 h (elimination).

Volume of distribution. About 3.5 to 5.5 L/kg.

Clearance. Plasma clearance, about 2 mL/min/kg.

Distribution in blood. Plasma:whole blood ratio, about 0.75.

Protein binding. In plasma, about 77 to 80%.

Note. For a review of flunitrazepam, see M. A. K. Mattila and H. M. Larni, *Drugs*, 1980, *20*, 353–374. For a review of flunitrazepam, use, abuse, and toxicity, see H. Druid *et al.*, *Forensic Sci. Int.*, 2001, *122*, 136–141.

Dose. 0.5 to 2 mg, as a hypnotic. There is evidence that flunitrazepam has been misused as a drug-facilitated sexual assault (DFSA) agent.

Flunixin

Analgesic

2-[[2-Methyl-3-(trifluoromethyl)phenyl]amino]-3-pyridinecarboxylic acid

$C_{14}H_{11}F_3N_2O_2$=296.2

CAS—38677-85-9

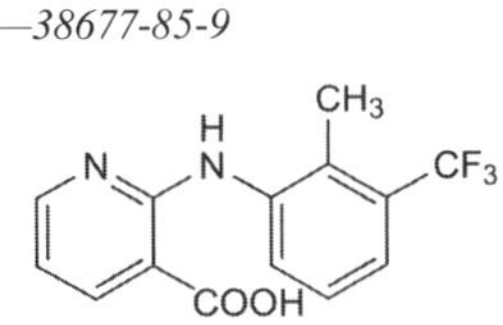

Crystals. M.p. 226° to 228°.

Flunixin Meglumine

Proprietary names. Banamine; Binixin; Cronyxin; Equileve; Equi-Phar Equigesic; Finadyne; Flumeglumine; Flu-Nix; Flunixamine; Meflosyl; Resprixin; Suppressor (all veterinary).

$C_{14}H_{11}F_3N_2O_2,C_7H_{17}NO_5$=491.5

CAS—42461-84-7

Colourless crystals. M.p. 135° to 139°.

Soluble in water.

Thin-layer Chromatography. System TA—Rf 96; system TE—Rf 12; system TG—Rf 33; system TAJ—Rf 37; system TAK—Rf 20; system TAL—Rf 83. (Ludy Tenger reagent, orange.)

Gas Chromatography. System GD—RRT of methyl derivative 1.39 (relative to n-$C_{16}H_{34}$).

High Performance Liquid Chromatography. System HV—RRT 0.99 (relative to meclofenamic acid); system HY—RI 414.

Ultraviolet Spectrum. Aqueous acid—252, 327 nm; aqueous alkali—281 nm (A_1^1=490b).

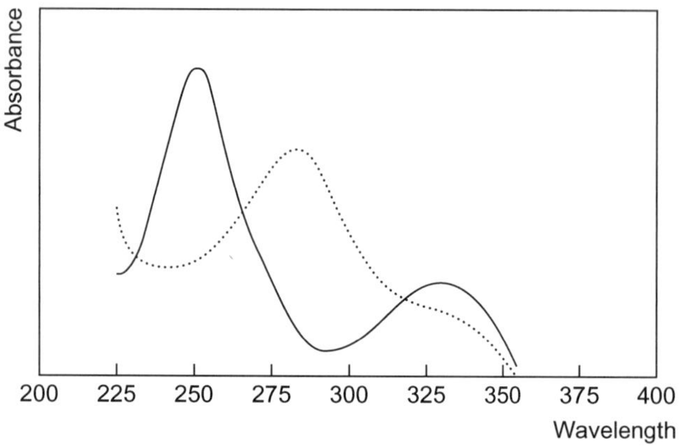

Infra-red Spectrum. Principal peaks at wavenumbers 1122, 1315, 1572, 1237, 1142, 1165 cm^{-1}.

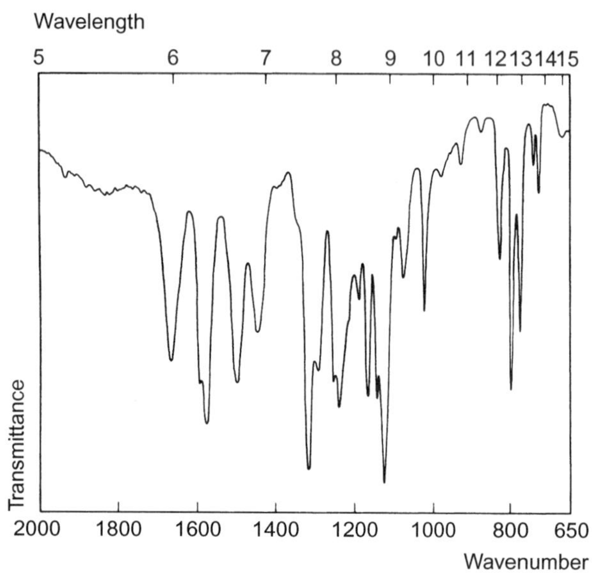

Quantification

Gas chromatography. In equine urine: limit of detection 74 µg/L, nitrogen–phosphorus detection—M. Johansson and E. L. Anler, *J. Chromatogr.*, 1988, *427*, 55–66.

High performance liquid chromatography. In equine plasma: limit of detection 50 µg/L, UV detection—G. E. Hardee *et al.*, *J. Liq. Chromatogr.*, 1982, *5*, 1991–2003. In equine plasma or inflammatory exudates: limit of detection 50 µg/L, UV detection—A. J. Higgins *et al.*, *Equine Vet. J.* 1987, *19*, 303–306. In bovine plasma: limit of detection <7 µg/L—K. Odensvik and I. M. Johansson, *Am. J. Vet. Res.*, 1995, *56*, 489–495.

Fluocinolone Acetonide

Corticosteroid

Synonym. 6α,9α-Difluoro-16α-hydroxyprednisolone Acetonide

Proprietary names. Alfa-Fluorone; Boniderma; Capex; Cortamide; Cortoderm; Dermalar; DermaSmoothe/FS; Dermobeta; Dermoline; Flucinar; Flunolone-V; Fluocortan; Fluoderm; Fluonid; Flurosyn; Gelidina; Jellin; Jellisoft; Synalar; Synamol; Synandone; Synemol.

(6α,11β,16α)-6,9-Difluoro-11,21-dihydroxy-16,17-[(1-methylethylidene)bis(oxy)]-pregna-1,4-diene-3,20-dione

$C_{24}H_{30}F_2O_6$=452.5

CAS—67-73-2

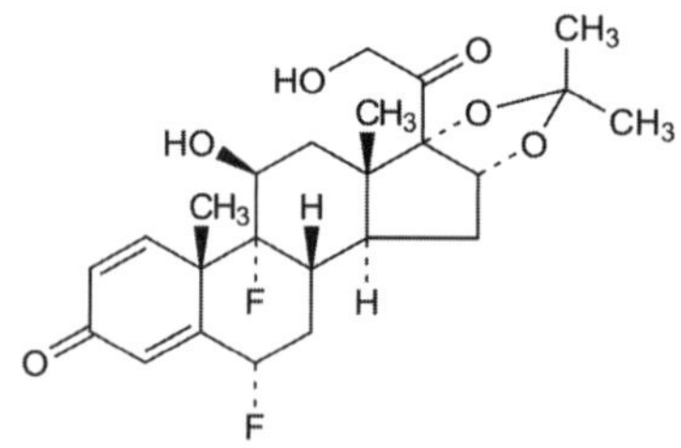

A white crystalline powder. M.p. about 270°, with decomposition. A solution in dioxan is dextrorotatory.

Practically insoluble in water; soluble 1 in 26 of dehydrated alcohol, 1 in 10 of acetone, 1 in 15 to 1 in 25 of chloroform, and 1 in 350 of ether; soluble in methanol.

Partition Coefficient. Log *P* (octanol/water), 2.5.

Colour Tests. Naphthol–Sulfuric Acid—green/yellow; Sulfuric Acid—yellow (green fluorescence under ultraviolet light).

Thin-layer Chromatography. System TP—Rf 42; system TQ—Rf 08; system TR—Rf 10; system TS—Rf 01; system TAM—Rf 68. (DPST solution.)

High Performance Liquid Chromatography. System HY—RI 491 (fluocinolone).

Ultraviolet Spectrum. Ethanol—240 nm (A_1^1=360a).

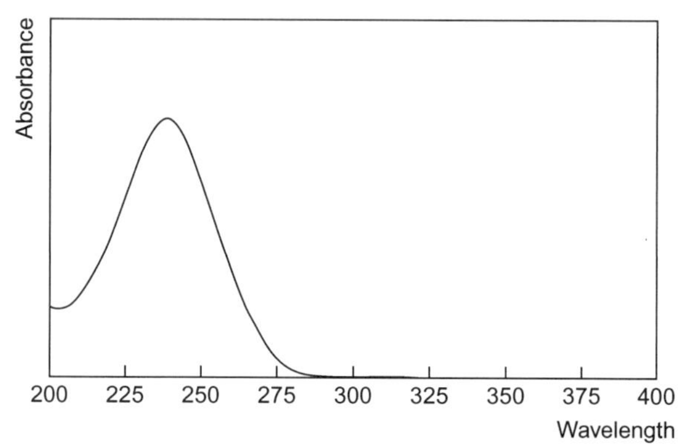

Infra-red Spectrum. Principal peaks at wavenumbers 1669, 1074, 1629, 910, 1056, 1615 cm^{-1} (KBr disk).

Use. Topically in concentrations of 0.01 to 0.2%.

Fluocinonide

Corticosteroid

Synonym. Fluocinolone Acetonide 21-Acetate

Proprietary names. Cusigel; Flu-21; Fluonex; Gelisyn; Klariderm; Korticoid; Lidemol; Lidex; Lyderm; Lydonide; Metosyn; Novoter; Tiamol; Topsym; Topsymin; Topsyn(e); Vasoderm.

(6α,11β,16α)-21-(Acetyloxy)-6,9-difluoro-11-hydroxy-16,17-[(1-methylethylidene)bis(oxy)]pregna-1,4-diene-3,20-dione

$C_{26}H_{32}F_2O_7$=494.5

CAS—356-12-7

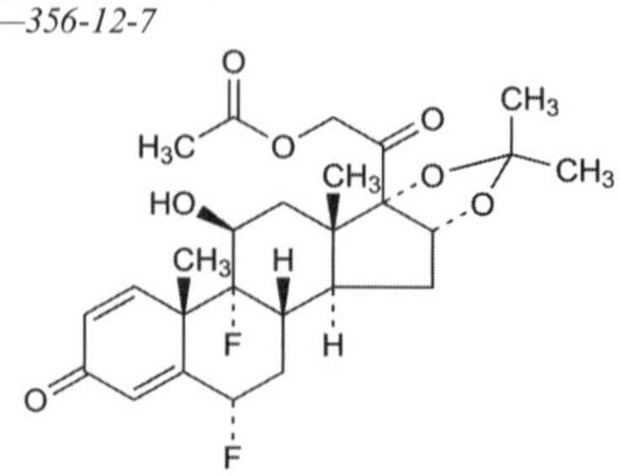

A white to cream-coloured crystalline powder. M.p. about 300°, with decomposition.

Practically insoluble in water; soluble 1 in 70 of ethanol, 1 in 10 of acetone, and 1 in 10 of chloroform; very slightly soluble in ether.

Partition Coefficient. Log *P* (octanol/water), 3.2.

Ultraviolet Spectrum. Methanol—240 nm (A_1^1=360a).

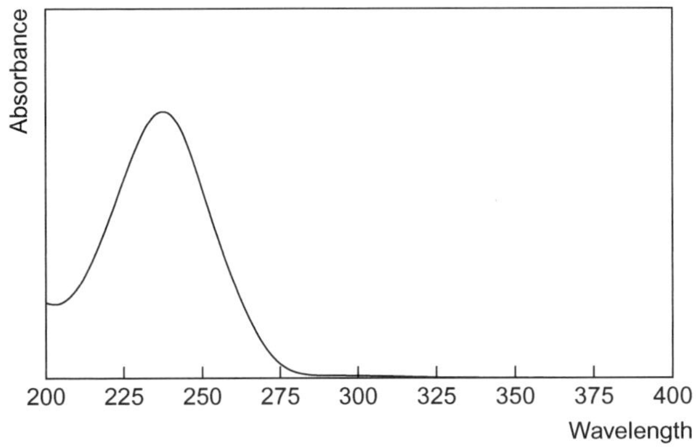

Infra-red Spectrum. Principal peaks at wavenumbers 1670, 1240, 1730, 1750, 1070, 1635 cm^{-1}(KBr disk).

Use. Topically in a concentration of 0.05%.

Fluocortolone

Corticosteroid

Synonym. 6α-Fluoro-16α-methyldehydrocorticosterone
Proprietary names. Ultralan (tablets). It is an ingredient of Ultralanum.
(6α,11β,16α)-6-Fluoro-11,21-dihydroxy-16-methylpregna-1,4-diene-3,20-dione
$C_{22}H_{29}FO_4$=376.5
CAS—152-97-6

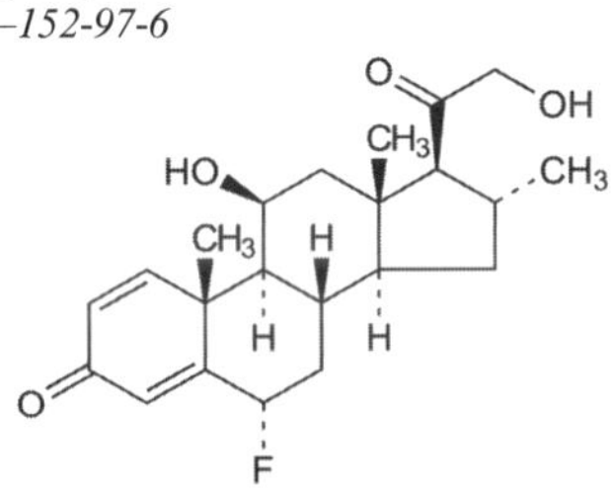

A white crystalline powder. M.p. 188° to 190.5°.
Practically insoluble in water; soluble 1 in 120 of ethanol; soluble in chloroform and ether.

Fluocortolone Hexanoate

Synonym. Fluocortolone Caproate
Proprietary names. It is an ingredient of Ultradil Plain, Ultralan (cream and lotion), and Ultralanum.
$C_{28}H_{39}FO_5$=474.6
CAS—303-40-2
A white to creamy-white crystalline powder. M.p. 242° to 245°.
Practically insoluble in water and ether; very slightly soluble in ethanol and methanol; soluble 1 in 18 of chloroform.

Fluocortolone Pivalate

Synonym. Fluocortolone Trimethylacetate
Proprietary names. It is an ingredient of Ultradil Plain, Ultralan (cream and lotion), and Ultralanum Plain (cream).
$C_{27}H_{37}FO_5$=460.6
CAS—29205-06-9
A white to creamy-white crystalline powder. M.p. 187°.
Almost insoluble in water; soluble 1 in 36 of ethanol and 1 in 3 of chloroform; freely soluble in dioxan; slightly soluble in ether.

Partition Coefficient. Log *P* (octanol/water), 2.1.

Colour Tests. Antimony Pentachloride—green-yellow; Naphthol–Sulfuric Acid—red-brown/red-brown; Sulfuric Acid—orange-yellow.

Thin-layer Chromatography. Fluocortolone: system TE—Rf 50; system TF—Rf 28. Fluocortolone hexanoate: system TP—Rf 79; system TQ—Rf 39; system TR—Rf 88; system TS—Rf 00. (*p*-Toluenesulfonic acid solution, positive.) Fluocortolone pivalate: system TP—Rf 78; system TQ—Rf 35; system TR—Rf 89; system TS—Rf 58.

Gas Chromatography. System GA—fluocortolone RI 3225, fluocortolone-AC_2 RI 3400, fluocortolone-AC RI 3420.

Ultraviolet Spectrum. Methanol—242 nm (A_1^1=429a).

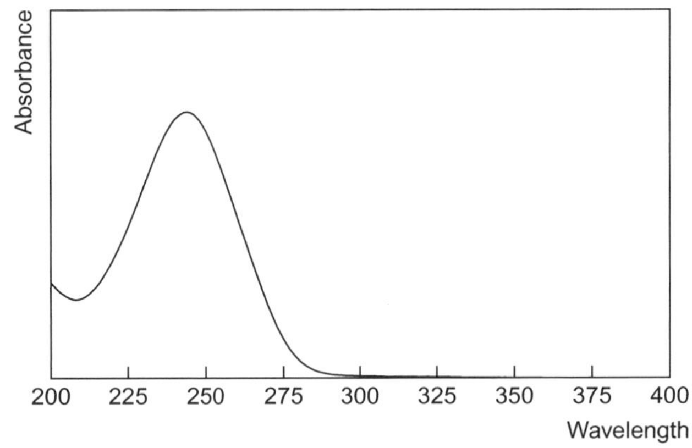

Infra-red Spectrum. Principal peaks at wavenumbers 1658, 1163, 1622, 1722, 1176, 1747 cm^{-1} (fluocortolone hexanoate, KBr disk); 1662, 1159, 1725, 1619, 1605, 1285 cm^{-1} (fluocortolone pivalate, KBr disk).

Disposition in the Body

Therapeutic concentration

Administration of 20, 50, and 100 mg oral doses of fluocortolone to 9 subjects at weekly intervals resulted in mean maximum plasma concentrations of 199, 419, and 812 mg/L, respectively, 1 to 2 h after dosing. [U. Tauber *et al.*, *Eur. J. Clin. Pharmacol.*, 1986, *30*, 433–438.]

Dose. Fluocortolone has been given by mouth in doses of 5 to 60 mg daily.

Fluoroacetamide

Rodenticide

Synonym. Compound 1081
Fluoroacetic acid amide
FCH_2CONH_2=77.1
CAS—640-19-7

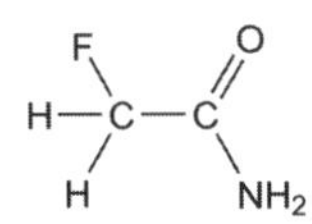

A fine fluffy white powder which decomposes if heated appreciably above 100°.
Freely soluble in water; soluble in acetone; sparingly soluble in chloroform; relatively insoluble in organic solvents.

Partition Coefficient. Log *P* (octanol/water), −1.0.

Colour Test. Nessler's Reagent—brown-orange.

Infra-red Spectrum. Principal peaks at wavenumbers 1667, 1036, 1117, 1020, 810, 1239 cm^{-1} (Nujol mull).

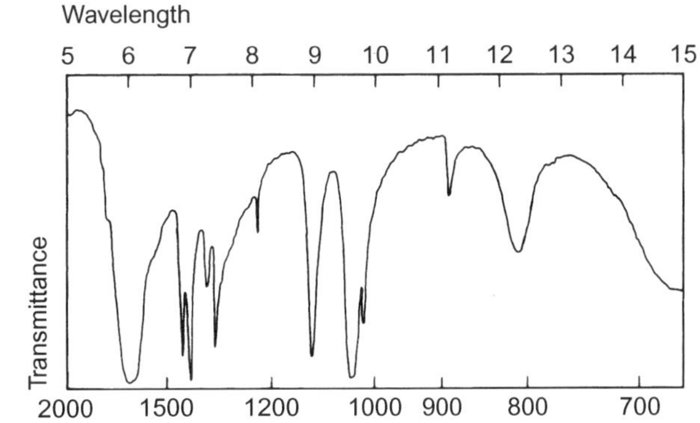

Quantification. See under Fluoroacetic Acid.

Disposition in the Body. Rapidly absorbed after ingestion or through cuts and abrasions. It is converted to fluoroacetic acid and then to fluorocitric acid.

Toxicity. Fluoroacetamide is extremely toxic to animals and man but its lethal action is slower than sodium fluoroacetate.

Fluoroacetic Acid

Rodenticide

Synonyms. Fluoroethanoic Acid; Gifblaar Poison; Monofluoroacetic Acid.
$C_2H_3FO_2$=78.0
CAS—144-49-0

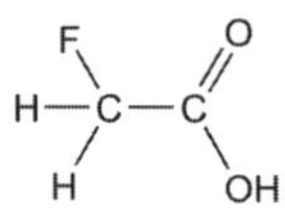

Fluoroacetic acid is the toxic principle of the South African plant gifblaar, *Dichapetalum cymosum* (= *Chailletia cymosa*) (Dichapetalaceae). Crystals. M.p. 33°. B.p. 165°.
Soluble in water and ethanol; practically insoluble in most common organic solvents.

Sodium Fluoroacetate

Synonyms. Compound 1080; Sodium Monofluoroacetate.
$C_2H_2FNaO_2$=100.0
CAS—62-74-8
A white hygroscopic powder which decomposes at 200° to 202°.
Very soluble in water; relatively insoluble in organic solvents.

Dissociation Constant. pK_a 2.6 (25°).

Partition Coefficient. Log *P* (octanol/water), 0.03.

Quantification

Gas chromatography. In tissues: limit of detection 100 ng/g, ECD—I. Okuno *et al.*, *J. Assoc. Off. Anal. Chem.*, 1982, *65*, 1102–1105.

Gas chromatography–mass spectrometry. In tissues: limits of detection 700 ng/g for fluoroacetamide, 100 ng/g for fluoroacetic acid—H. M. Stevens *et al.*, *Forensic Sci.*, 1976, *8*, 131–137. In serum: limit of detection 0.02 mg/L—F. Sporkert *et al.*, *J. Chromatogr. B Anal. Technol. Biomed. Life Sci.*, 2002, *772*, 45–51.

Disposition in the Body. Fluoroacetic acid and sodium fluoroacetate are absorbed rapidly through cuts and abrasions but less rapidly from intact skin. Sodium fluoroacetate is converted to fluorocitric acid which inhibits the citric acid cycle and leads to accumulation of citrate.

Toxicity. Fluoroacetic acid and sodium fluoroacetate are extremely toxic to animals and man; the minimum lethal dose is about 5 mg/kg. Toxic effects are delayed for several hours following ingestion or absorption through the skin. The maximum permissible atmospheric concentration is 50 μg/m^3.

Fluorometholone

Corticosteroid

Proprietary names. Delmeson; Efflumidex; Eflone; Flarex; Flu Oph; Fluaton; Flucon; Fluforte; Flumetol; Fluor-Op; Fluoropos; FML; Oxylone; Semplice.
(6α,11*β*)-9-Fluoro-11,17-dihydroxy-6-methylpregna-1,4-diene-3,20-dione
$C_{22}H_{29}FO_4$=376.5
CAS—426-13-1

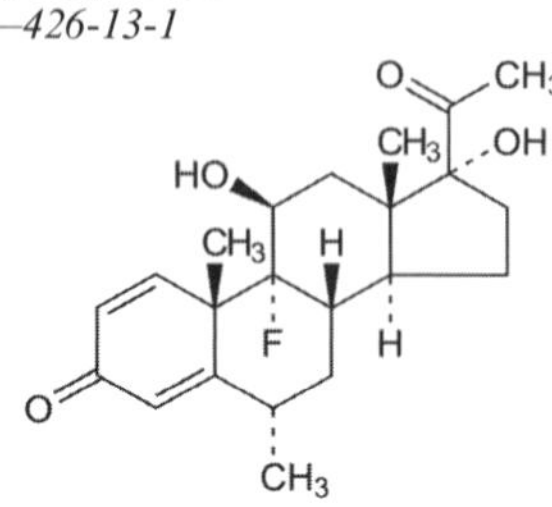

A white to yellowish-white crystalline powder. M.p. about 280°, with decomposition.
Practically insoluble in water; soluble 1 in 200 of ethanol and 1 in 2200 of chloroform; very slightly soluble in ether.

Partition Coefficient. Log *P* (octanol/water), 2.0.

Thin-layer Chromatography. System TB—Rf 00; system TE—Rf 68; system TF—Rf 52; system TAE—Rf 91; system TAJ—Rf 46; system TAK—Rf 26; system TAL—Rf 90; system TAM—Rf 86.

High Performance Liquid Chromatography. System HX—RI 470.

Ultraviolet Spectrum. Methanol—241 nm (A^1_1=375a).

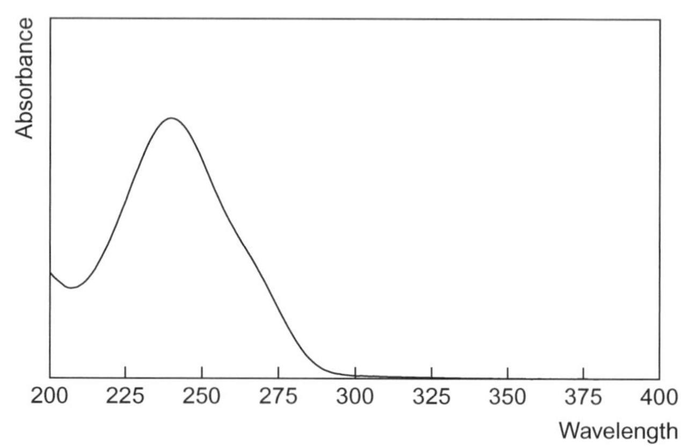

Use. Usually applied as a 0.025% cream or ointment and is also available as a 0.1% ophthalmic suspension.

Fluorouracil

Antineoplastic

Synonyms. 5-Fluorouracil; 5-FU.
Proprietary names. AccuSite; Adrucil; Cinkef-U; Effluderm; Efudex; Efudix; Fiverocil; Fivoflu; Flurablastin; Fluracedyl; Fluroblastin(e); Fluoroplex; Flurox; O-fluor; Rhonuracil; Ribofluor.
5-Fluoro-2,4(1*H*,3*H*)-pyrimidinedione
$C_4H_3FN_2O_2$=130.1
CAS—51-21-8

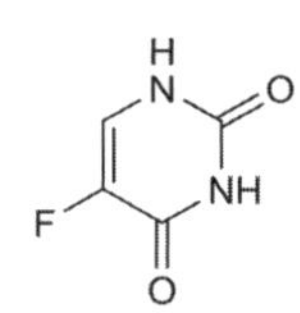

A white crystalline powder which decomposes at about 282°.
Sparingly soluble in water; slightly soluble in ethanol; practically insoluble in chloroform and ether. Solutions discolour on storage.
Caution. Fluorouracil is an irritant; avoid contact with skin and mucous membranes.

Dissociation Constant. pK_a 8.0, 13.0.

Partition Coefficient. Log *P* (octanol/pH 7.4), -1.0.

Thin-layer Chromatography. System TE—Rf 4; system TF—Rf 20.

Gas Chromatography. System GA—RI 2090.

High Performance Liquid Chromatography. System HX—RI 70; system HY—RI 96; system HAA—Retention time, 3.4 min.

Ultraviolet Spectrum. Aqueous acid—266 nm (A^1_1=552a).

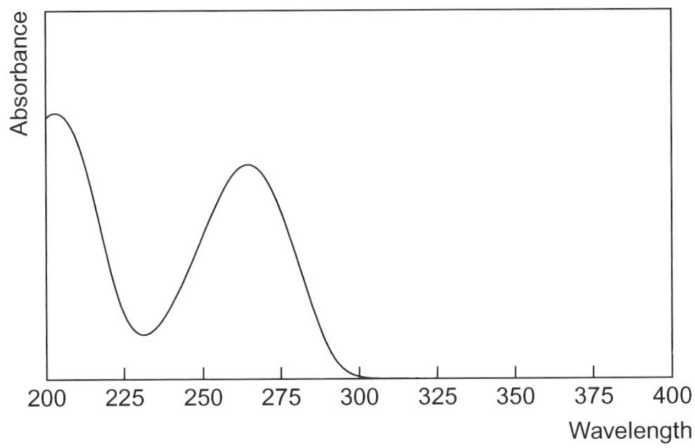

Infra-red Spectrum. Principal peaks at wavenumbers 1653, 1242, 1718, 816, 1220, 1495 cm^{-1} (KBr disk).

Quantification

Gas chromatography–mass spectrometry. In plasma: limit of detection 0.4 µg/L, selected-ion monitoring—C. D. Bates *et al., J. Pharm. Biomed. Anal.*, 1991, *9*, 19–21. In plasma: limit of detection <0.5 µg/L—L. W. Anderson *et al., J. Chromatogr.*, 1992, *581*, 195–201. In plasma: fluorouracil and α-fluoro-β-alanine, limit of detection <1 µg/L for fluorouracil—D. Anderson *et al., J. Chromatogr. B Biomed. Sci. Appl.*, 1997, *688*, 87–93.

High performance liquid chromatography. In plasma: fluorouracil and folinic acid—C. Vandenbosch *et al., J. Chromatogr.*, 1993, *612*, 77–85. In tissue: limit of detection 3 ng/g, fluorescence detection—C. Jochheim *et al., Anal. Biochem.*, 1994, *217*, 285–291. In plasma: limit of detection 25 µg/L, UV detection—P. Compagnon *et al., J. Chromatogr. B Biomed. Appl.*, 1996, *677*, 380–383; R. A. Coe *et al., J. Pharm. Biomed. Anal.*, 1996, *14*, 1733–1741. In plasma: fluorouracil and dihydrofluorouracil, limit of detection 26 µg/L, UV detection—S.P. Ackland *et al., Anal. Biochem.*, 1997, *246*, 79–85. In plasma, erythrocytes or whole blood: limit of detection 10 µg/L—W. Wattanatorn *et al., J. Chromatogr. B Biomed. Sci. Appl.*, 1997, *692*, 233–237. In plasma: fluorouracil and its major metabolites, limit of detection 10 µg/L, UV detection—J. M. Joulia *et al., J. Chromatogr. B Biomed. Sci. Appl.*, 1997, *692*, 427–435. In plasma: fluorouracil and uracil, UV detection—L. K. House *et al., J. Chromatogr. B Biomed. Sci. Appl.*, 1998, *720*, 245–250. In plasma: limit of detection <26 µg/L, UV detection—W. J. Loos *et al., J. Chromatogr. B Biomed. Sci. Appl.*, 1999, *735*, 293–297. In plasma: limit of detection <2 µg/L—J. Escoriaza *et al., J. Chromatogr. B Biomed. Sci. Appl.*, 1999, *736*, 97–102. In plasma: fluorouracil and flucytosine, diode-array detection—J. S. Torano *et al., Biomed. Chromatogr.*, 2001, *15*, 89–94. In plasma: limit of detection 5 µg/L, UV detection—M. A. Nassim *et al., Int. J. Mol. Med.*, 2002, *10*, 513–516.

High performance liquid chromatography–mass spectrometry. In plasma: limit of detection <1 µg/L—K. Wang *et al., J. Am. Soc. Mass Spectrom.*, 1998, *9*, 970–976.

Disposition in the Body

Therapeutic concentration

Seventeen subjects received fluorouracil, either 1 mg/m^2 orally (combined with eniluracil) twice daily or 300 mg/m^2 by continuous IV infusion, for 7 days. The mean steady-state plasma concentration during IV infusion was 104 µg/L compared with 38.1 µg/L for oral fluorouracil [A. A. Adjei *et al., J. Clin. Oncol.*, 2002, *20*, 1683–1691.]

Dose. Initially 12 mg/kg daily IV, to a maximum of 1 g daily, for 3 or 4 days.

Fluoxetine

Antidepressant

N-Methyl-γ-[4-(trifluoromethyl)phenoxy]benzenepropanamine
$C_{17}H_{18}F_3NO$=309.3
CAS—54910-89-3

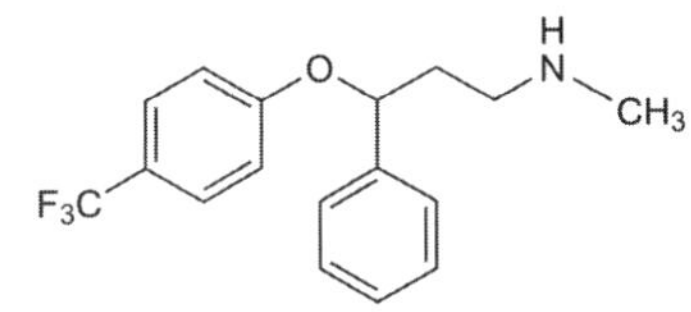

Solubility in water 78.24 mg/L (25°).

Fluoxetine Hydrochloride

Synonym. LY-110140
Proprietary names. Adofen; Docutrix; Erocap; Fluctin; Fluctine; Fluoxeren; Fontex; Foxetin; Lorien; Lovan; Mutan; Prozac; Prozyn; Reneuron; Sanzur; Zactin.
$C_{17}H_{18}F_3NO.HCl$=345.8
CAS—59333-67-4
A white to off-white crystalline solid. M.p. 138°. It is soluble in methanol, ethanol, acetonitrile, chloroform and acetone; slightly soluble in ethyl acetate, dichloromethane and water (maximum 14 g/L); insoluble in toluene, cyclohexane and hexane.

Fluoxetine Oxalate

$C_{17}H_{18}F_3NO.C_2H_4$=397.4
Crystals from ethylacetate–methanol. M.p. 179° to 182°.

Partition Coefficient. Log *P* (octanol/water), 4.05; (octanol/pH 7.4), 1.82.

Thin-layer Chromatography. System TB—Rf 13 (fluoxetine); Rf 12 (M-nor); system TE—Rf 47 (fluoxetine); Rf 47 (M-nor); system TAE—Rf 11 (fluoxetine); Rf 11 (M-nor).

Plate: silica gel 60 F_{254}. Mobile phase: methanol:concentrated ammonium hydroxide (90:10). Fluoxetine hydrochloride Rf 0.58 [D. S. Risley and R. J. Bopp, in *Analytical Profiles of Drug Substances and Excipients*, Vol. 19, H. G. Brittain (ed), New York, Academic Press, 1990, p. 193–219].

Gas Chromatography. System GA—RI 1859 (fluoxetine); RI 1851 (norfluoxetine), RI 2250 (acetylfluoxetine), RI 2190 (noracetylfluoxetine); system GB—RI 1903 (fluoxetine), RI 1888 (norfluoxetine), RI 2319 (acetylfluoxetine), RI 2278 (noracetylfluoxetine); system GM—RRT 0.304 (fluoxetine); 0.284 (norfluoxetine relative to iprindole).

Column: DB-5 MS 5% phenylmethyl silicone (25 m × 0.2 mm i.d., 0.33 mm film thickness). Column temperature: 100° held 2 min, 15°/min to 210°, 210° to 280° at 20°/min, held 5 min. Carrier gas: helium, 0.7 mL/min flow rate. MS detection (EI (electron ionisation) SIM (selected-ion monitoring) at *m/z* 117 and 294 for fluoxetine-pentafluoropropionic anhydride (PFPA), *m/z* 117, 176 and 280 for norfluoxetine-PFPA). Internal standard (IS): fluoxetine-d_5-PFPA. Retention time: fluoxetine-PFPA, 13.36 min; norfluoxetine-PFPA, 12.89 min; IS, 13.34 min [J. A. Crifasi *et al., J. Anal. Toxicol.*, 1997, *21*, 415–419].

Column: HP-5 MS 5% PH ME siloxane film (30 m x 0.25 mm i.d., 0.25 µm film thickness). Column temperature: 150° for 0.5 min then 10°/min to 270°, held 2.5 min. Carrier gas: helium, 1.0 mL/min flow rate. MS detection (EI, SIM at *m/z* 309.3 for fluoxetine and 295.3 for norfluoxetine). IS: clomipramine (*m/z* 314.3). Retention time: fluoxetine, 7.25 min; norfluoxetine, 6.99 min; IS, 12.34 [K. E. Ferslew *et al., J. Forensic Sci.*, 1998, *43*, 1082–1085].

High Performance Liquid Chromatography. System HY—RI 400; system HZ—retention time 7.6 min (fluoxetine); retention time 6.7 min (desmethylfluoxetine); system HAA—retention time 16.2 min; system HAX—retention time 12.2 min; system HAY—retention time 7.07 min.

Ultraviolet Spectrum. Methanol—227, 264, 268, 275 nm (fluoxetine); (0.025 M sulfuric acid)—226.5 nm (fluoxetine); (0.2 M H_2SO_4)—226, 263, 275 nm (norfluoxetine); basic—264, 275 nm (norfluoxetine).

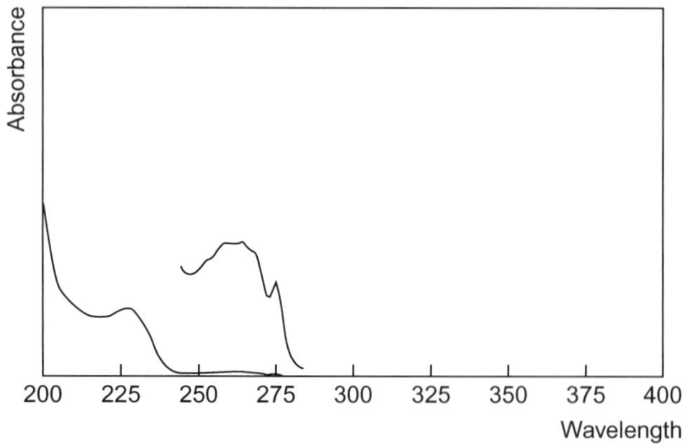

Infra-red Spectrum. Principal peaks at wavenumbers 2986, 2772, 1614, 1329, 1257, 1122 cm^{-1}; (norfluoxetine) 1335, 1240, 1110 cm^{-1} (KBr disk).

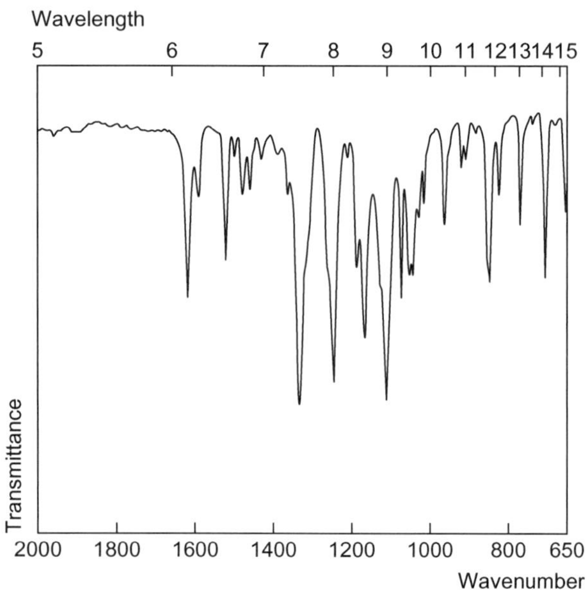

Mass Spectrum. Principal ions at *m/z* 44, 309, 183, 104, 251, 91, 197, 242 (fluoxetine); *m/z* 134, 104, 191, 143, 162, 77 (norfluoxetine).

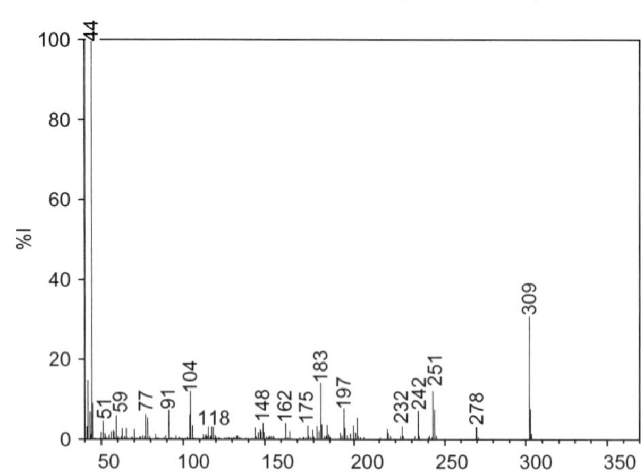

Quantification

Gas chromatography. In plasma: fluoxetine and norfluoxetine, limit of detection 0.3 μg/L, nitrogen–phosphorus detection—P. Fontanille *et al.*, *J. Chromatogr. B Biomed. Sci. Appl.*, 1997, *692*, 337–343. In plasma: fluoxetine and norfluoxetine, limit of detection 5 μg/L, ECD—R. J. Lantz *et al.*, *J. Chromatogr.*, 1993, *614*, *Biomed. Appl.*, *125*, 175–179.

Gas chromatography–mass spectrometry. In blood, urine, vitreous and other tissue samples: limit of quantification 25.0 μg/L and limit of detection 12.5 μg/L—J. A. Crifasi *et al.*, *J. Anal. Toxicol.*, 1997, *21*, 415–419. In plasma: fluoxetine and norfluoxetine, limit of detection 1 μg/L—C. B. Eap *et al.*, *J. Chromatogr.*, 1996, *682*, *Biomed. Appl.*, 265–272.

High performance liquid chromatography. In serum: limit of detection 25 μg/L. UV detection (λ=226 nm)—P. J. Orsulak *et al.*, *Clin. Chem.*, 1988, *34(9)*, 1875–1878. In plasma or brain tissue: limit of detection 0.7 μg/L in plasma, fluorescence detection (λ_{ex}=345 nm, λ_{em}=470 nm)—P. Clausing *et al.*, *J. Chromatogr. B Biomed. Sci. Appl.*, 1997, *692*, 419–426. In plasma: fluoxetine and norfluoxetine, limit of detection 6 μg/L, UV detection (λ=214 nm)—S. H. Wong *et al.*, *J. Chromatogr.*, 1990, *499*, 601–608. In plasma: fluoxetine and norfluoxetine, limit of detection 2 μg/L, UV detection (λ=226 nm)—P. Thomare *et al.*, *J. Chromatogr.*, 1992, *583*; *Biomed. Appl.*, *121*, 217–221. In plasma: fluoxetine and norfluoxetine, limit of detection 5 μg/L, UV detection (λ=226, 254, 400 nm)—G. Aymard *et al.*, *J. Chromatogr. B Biomed. Sci. Appl.*, 1997, *700*, 183–189. In plasma: fluoxetine and norfluoxetine, limit of detection 3 μg/L, fluorescence detection (λ_{ex}=235 nm, λ_{em}=470 nm)—R. F. Suckow *et al.*, *Clin. Chem.*, 1992, *38*, 1756–1761.

Disposition in the Body. Fluoxetine is readily absorbed after oral administration and is extensively metabolised in the liver by demethylation. The primary active metabolite is norfluoxetine, which is excreted via the kidneys. Further metabolism can occur by O-dealkylation producing *p*-trifluoromethylphenol and hippuric acid. 80% of a drug dose is excreted in urine with less than 10% as the unchanged parent drug and 15% excreted in faeces. Fluoxetine is widely distributed throughout the body and secreted into breast milk.

Therapeutic concentration

Therapeutic serum concentrations are 0.15 to 0.5 mg/L (fluoxetine) and for norfluoxetine 0.1 to 0.5 mg/L.

Single doses of fluoxetine 40 mg given to 6 subjects produced maximum plasma concentrations of fluoxetine of 0.03 to 0.055 mg/L after 4 to 8 h; maximum plasma-norfluoxetine concentrations were 0.006 to 0.036 mg/L after 48 to 96 h [G. R. Aronoff *et al.*, *Clin. Pharmacol. Ther.*, 1984, *36*, 138–144].

Toxicity. Blood concentrations of 1.3 to 6.8 mg/L fluoxetine and 0.9 to 5.0 mg/L norfluoxetine have been associated with fatalities. Serum levels of 1.96 mg/L fluoxetine (0.42 mg/L norfluoxetine) have been associated with seizures.

Overdose case: a 46-year-old man with a history of drug abuse was found dead in a chair and toxicological analysis showed blood levels of 1.3 mg/L fluoxetine and 1.2 mg/L norfluoxetine [A. D. Fraser *et al.*, *TIAFT Bulletin Case Notes*, 1991, *21(3)*].

A 44-year-old man was found dead and medication at the scene included clozapine (Clorazil) and fluoxetine (Prozac). Toxicological analysis showed 0.7 mg/L of fluoxetine and 0.6 mg/L norfluoxetine in the man's blood, as well as 4.9 mg/L clozapine and 350 mg/L ethanol. Death was due to an overdose of fluoxetine and clozapine, which resulted in a fatal drug interaction [K. E. Ferslew *et al.*, *J. Forensic Sci.*, 1998, *43*, 1082–1085].

A 13-year-old boy who claimed to have taken 1880 mg of fluoxetine suffered abdominal pain and nausea, and, about 3.5 h after ingestion, a generalised tonic-clonic seizure. The serum fluoxetine concentration about 90 min after ingestion was 0.428 mg/L; serum-norfluoxetine concentration was 0.211 mg/L [M. A. Riddle *et al.*, *J. Am. Acad. Child Adolesc. Psychiatry*, 1989, *28*, 587–588].

Bioavailability. Approx. 60%.

Half-life. 4 to 6 days (fluoxetine); 4 to16 days (norfluoxetine).

Volume of distribution. 27 L/kg (between 20 and 42 L/kg for both fluoxetine and norfluoxetine).

Clearance. Renal clearance, 0.6 L/kg/h; also reported as 20.8 L/h for fluoxetine and 8.7 L/h for norfluoxetine.

Protein binding. Approx. 94.5%.

Dose. A usual dose of 20 mg daily is administered for depression and 60 mg daily for bulimia nervosa. A maximum dose of 80 mg may be given daily. Dose is reduced for patients with renal and hepatic impairment. Not recommended for children.

Fluoxymesterone

Androgen

Synonym. Fluorohydroxymethyltestosterone
Proprietary names. Halotestin; Oratestin; Ora-Testryl; Stenox; Testoral; Ultandren.
Note. Testoral is also used as a proprietary name for testosterone.
(11β,17β)-9-Fluoro-11,17-dihydroxy-17-methylandrost-4-en-3-one
$C_{20}H_{29}FO_3$=336.4
CAS—76-43-7

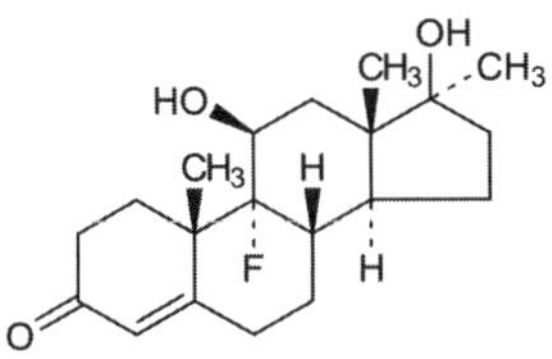

A white or creamy-white crystalline powder. M.p. 270° with decomposition.
Practically insoluble in water; soluble 1 in 70 of ethanol and 1 in 200 of chloroform; soluble in pyridine; slightly soluble in acetone; practically insoluble in ether, benzene, and hexanes.

Partition Coefficient. Log *P* (octanol/water), 2.4.

Colour Tests. Antimony Pentachloride—brown; Naphthol–Sulfuric Acid—green-yellow/yellow; Sulfuric Acid—yellow (green fluorescence under UV light).

Thin-layer Chromatography. System TP—Rf 51; system TQ—Rf 09; system TR—Rf 38; system TS—Rf 16, streaking may occur; system TAJ—Rf 41; system TAK—Rf 35; system TAL—Rf 91; system TAM—Rf 74.

Gas Chromatography. System GA—RI 2835; system GAG—RRT 1.50 (relative to testosterone); system GAI—RRT 1.155 (relative to 17α-methyl-5α-androstan-3β,17β-diol); system GAR—Retention time 14.6 min.

High Performance Liquid Chromatography. System HY—RI 427; system HATb—RRT 0.70 (relative to testosterone); system HAR—RRT 0.78 (relative to testosterone).

Ultraviolet Spectrum. Dehydrated alcohol—240 nm (A_1^1=495a).

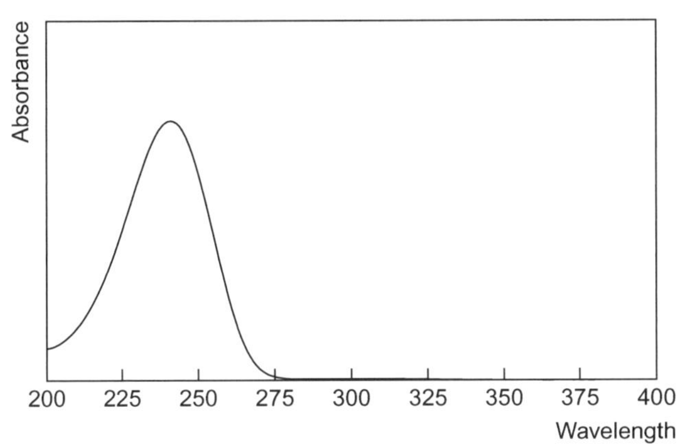

Infra-red Spectrum. Principal peaks at wavenumbers 1654, 867, 1036, 1247, 926, 1282 cm^{-1} (KBr disk).

Mass Spectrum. Principal ions at *m/z* 43, 71, 55, 79, 91, 109, 123, 336.

Quantification

Gas chromatography–mass spectrometry. In hair: fluoxymesterone and other anabolic steroids—X. S. Deng *et al.*, *J. Forensic Sci.*, 1999, *44*, 343–346.

High performance liquid chromatography. In serum: UV detection—V. J. Capponi *et al.*, *J. Pharm. Sci.*, 1985, *74*, 308–311.

Dose. 2 to 10 mg daily; up to 30 mg daily may be given.

Flupentixol

Tranquilliser

Synonyms. Flupenthixol; LC-44; N-7009.
4-[3-[2-(Trifluoromethyl)-9*H*-thioxanthen-9-ylidene]propyl]-1-piperazine ethanol
$C_{23}H_{25}F_3N_2OS$=434.5
CAS—2709-56-0

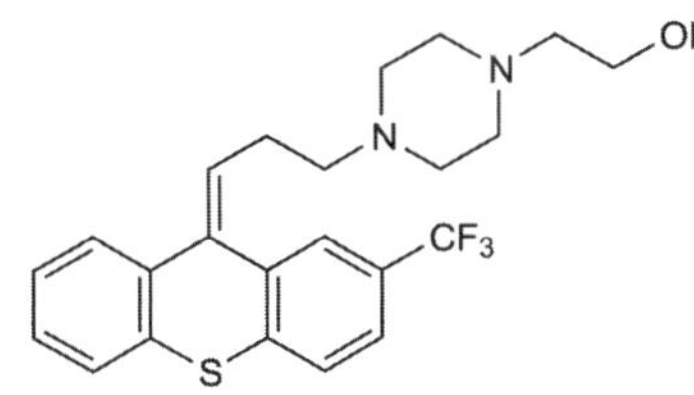

cis-form

Flupentixol Decanoate

Synonyms. (*Z*)-Flupenthixol Decanoate; *cis*-Flupenthixol Decanoate.
Proprietary names. Depixol (injection); Fluanxol Depot.
$C_{33}H_{43}F_3N_2O_2S$=588.8
CAS—30909-51-4
A yellow oil.
Very slightly soluble in water; soluble in ethanol; freely soluble in chloroform and ether.

Flupentixol Hydrochloride

Synonyms. Flupenthixol Dihydrochloride; Flupenthixol Hydrochloride.
Proprietary names. Depixol (tablets); Fluanxol (tablets). It is an ingredient of Deanxit.
$C_{23}H_{25}F_3N_2OS$,2HCl=507.4
CAS-2413-38-9
A white or yellowish-white powder. M.p. 230° to 240°.
Soluble in water and ethanol; very slightly soluble in chloroform; practically insoluble in ether.

Partition Coefficient. Log *P* (octanol/buffer pH 7.0), 3.0.

Colour Tests. Formaldehyde–Sulfuric Acid—red (orange fluorescence under UV light); Liebermann's Test—red; Mandelin's Test—red; Marquis Test—orange-red; Sulfuric Acid—orange (fluoresces under UV light).

Thin-layer Chromatography. System TA—Rf 62; system TB—Rf 06; system TC—Rf 33; system TE—Rf 46; system TAE—Rf 50. (Acidified iodoplatinate solution, strong reaction.)

Gas Chromatography. System GA—flupentixol -*cis*-isomer RI 3058, M (ring) RI 2190, M (*N*-oxide) RI 2120, flupentixol-AC RI 3045, M (desalkyl-dihydro-)-AC RI 3055, M (dihydro-)-AC RI 3005; system GB—flupentixol -*cis*-isomer RI 3199, flupentixol -*trans*-isomer RI 3217, M (desalkyl-)-*cis* RI 2832, M (desalkyl-)-*trans* RI 2855.

High Performance Liquid Chromatography. System HA—flupentixol *k* 1.2, flupentixol sulfoxide *k* 1.3; system HX—RI 475; system HY—RI 435; system HZ—retention time 10.7 min; system HAA—retention time 17.4 min; system HAX—retention time 13.7 min; system HAY—retention time 7.5 min.

Ultraviolet Spectrum. Aqueous acid—230 nm.

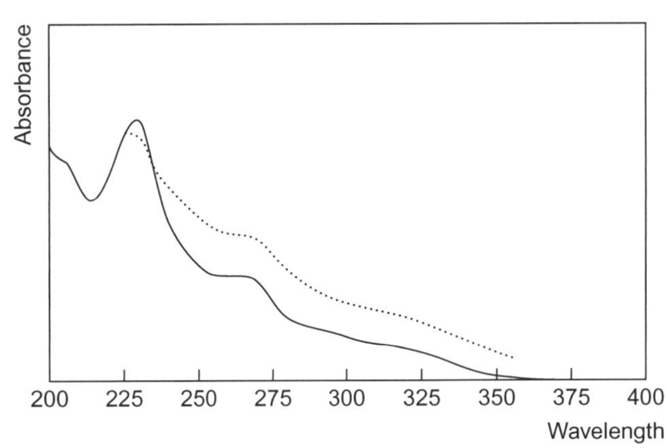

Infra-red Spectrum. Principal peaks at wavenumbers 1119, 1320, 1160, 1081, 1253, 1287 cm^{-1} (KBr disk).

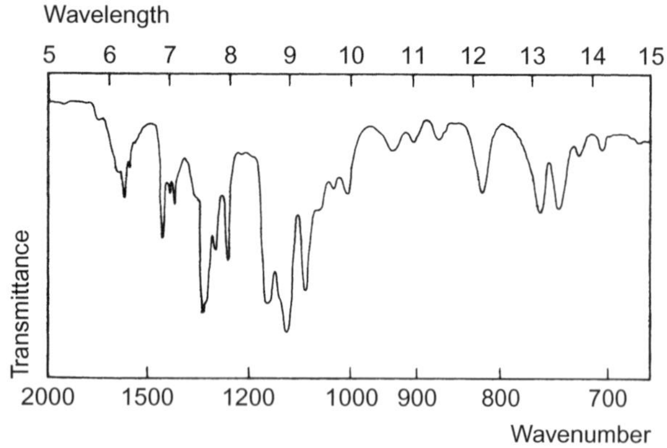

Mass Spectrum. Principal ions at *m/z* 143, 70, 100, 144, 42, 98, 58, 56.

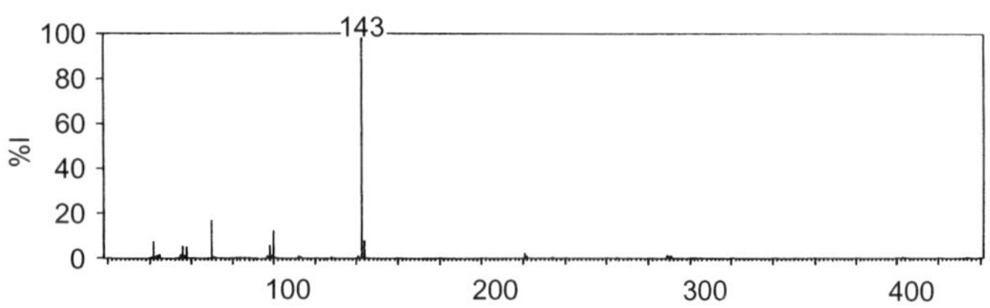

Quantification

Gas chromatography. In plasma: limit of detection <0.5 µg/L, nitrogen-phosphorus detection (comparison with radioimmunoassay)—A. E. Balant-Gorgia *et al., Ther. Drug Monit.*, 1985, 7, 229–235.

High performance liquid chromatography. In serum: flupentixol and haloperidol enantiomers, limit of detection for flupentixol <0.5 µg/L, UV detection—S. Walter *et al., J. Chromatogr. B Biomed. Sci. Appl.*, 1998, *720*, 231–237.

Radioimmunoassay. In serum: *cis*-flupentixol, limit of detection 300 ng/L—A. Jørgensen, *Life Sci.*, 1978, *23*, 1533–1542.

Disposition in the Body. Readily absorbed after oral administration. Flupentixol decanoate is very slowly absorbed from the site of IM injection. Peak plasma concentrations are attained about 3 to 6 h after oral administration and 3 to 7 days after IM injection. The main metabolic reactions are sulfoxidation, side-chain *N*-dealkylation, and glucuronic acid conjugation. *N*-Desalkylflupentixol and flupentixol sulfoxide are the major metabolites found in plasma (both are inactive). Numerous metabolites are excreted in the urine and faeces and there is evidence of enterohepatic circulation. Flupentixol crosses the placenta and it is found in small amounts in breast milk.

Bioavailability. About 55%.

Half-life. Biological half-life of flupentixol hydrochloride, about 35 h.

Note. For information on the pharmacokinetics of flupentixol, see A. Jørgensen, *Eur. J. Clin. Pharmacol.*, 1980, *18*, 355–360.

Dose. For psychoses, the equivalent of 6 to 18 mg of flupentixol daily, by mouth.

Fluphenazine

Tranquilliser

Synonym. Triflumethazine

4-[3-[2-(Trifluoromethyl)-10*H*-phenothiazin-10-yl]propyl]-1-piperazine-ethanol

$C_{22}H_{26}F_3N_3OS = 437.5$

CAS—69-23-8

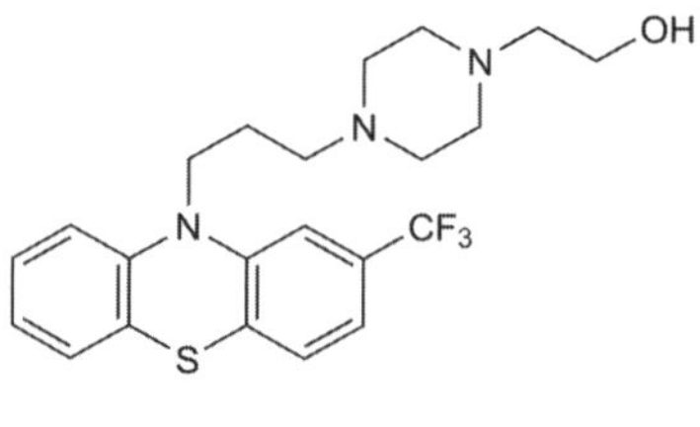

Fluphenazine Decanoate

Synonym. Fluphenazini Decanoas

Proprietary names. Anatensol; Dapotum; Lyogen; Lyorodin; Modecate; Moditen Depot; Prolixin; Siqualone.

$C_{32}H_{44}F_3N_3O_2S = 591.8$

CAS—5002-47-1

A pale yellow viscous liquid or a yellow crystalline oily solid. M.p. 30° to 32°. Insoluble in water; very soluble in alcohol, chloroform, cyclohexane, and ether.

Fluphenazine Enantate

Synonyms. Fluphenazini Enantas; Fluphenazine Enanthate; Fluphenazine Heptanoate.

Proprietary names. Anatensol; Moditen (injection); Prolixin.

$C_{29}H_{38}F_3N_3O_2S = 549.7$

CAS—2746-81-8

A pale yellow to yellow-orange, clear to slightly turbid, viscous liquid or a yellow crystalline oily solid.

Practically insoluble in water; soluble 1 in less than 1 of ethanol and of chloroform, and 1 in 2 of ether.

Fluphenazine Hydrochloride

Synonym. Fluphenazini Hydrochloridum.

Proprietary names. Anatensol; Cenilene; Dapotum; Lyogen; Lyorodin; Moditen (tablets); Omca; Pacinol; Permitil; Phenazin; Prolixin; Sevinol; Siqualone. It is an ingredient of Dominans, Motipress, and Motival.

$C_{22}H_{26}F_3N_3OS{,}2HCl = 510.4$

CAS—146-56-5

A white crystalline powder. M.p. about 230°.

Soluble 1 in 10 or less of water; slightly soluble in ethanol, acetone, and chloroform; practically insoluble in ether.

Dissociation Constant. pK_a 3.9, 8.1.

Partition Coefficient. Log *P* (octanol/buffer pH 7.0), 3.5.

Colour Tests. Formaldehyde–Sulfuric Acid—red; Forrest Reagent—orange; FPN Reagent—orange; Mandelin's Test—brown; Marquis Test—red.

Thin-layer Chromatography. System TA—Rf 63; system TB—Rf 05; system TC—Rf 23; system TE—Rf 45; system TL—Rf 10; system TAE—Rf 45; system TAF—Rf 49; system TAJ—Rf 06; system TAK—Rf 00; system TAL—Rf 41. (Dragendorff spray, positive; FPN reagent, pink; acidified iodoplatinate solution, positive; Marquis reagent, brown; ninhydrin spray, positive.)

Gas Chromatography. System GA—fluphenazine RI 3050, M (ring) RI 2190, fluphenazine-AC RI 3170, M (amino-)-AC RI 2765, M (desalkyl-)-AC RI 3145; system GB—fluphenazine RI 3194.

High Performance Liquid Chromatography. System HA—*k* 1.2; system HX—RI 462; system HY—RI 471; system HZ—retention time 10.1 min; system HAA—retention time 17.4 min; system HAX—retention time 13.6 min; system HAY—retention time 7.2 min.

Ultraviolet Spectrum Aqueous acid—256 (A^1_1 = 690a), 306 nm.

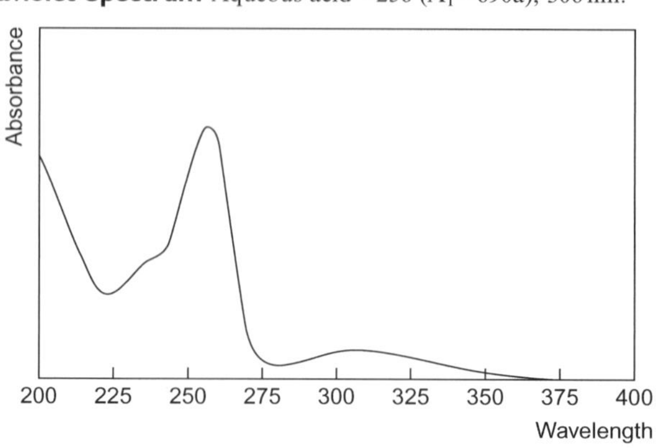

Infra-red Spectrum. Principal peaks at wavenumbers 1116, 767, 1245, 1144, 1084, 836 cm^{-1} (fluphenazine hydrochloride, KBr disk).

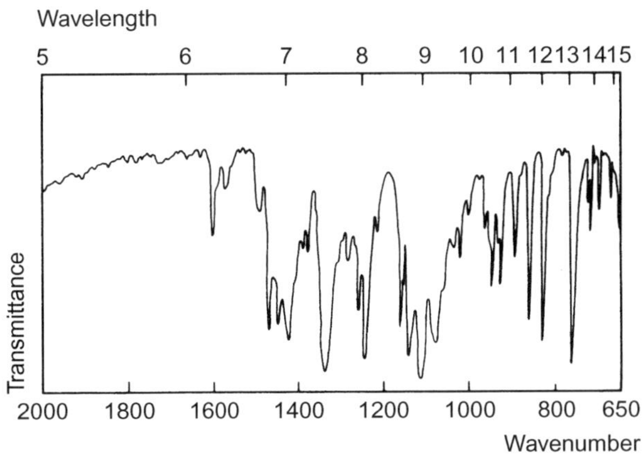

Mass Spectrum. Principal ions at *m/z* 280, 143, 42, 70, 437, 406, 113, 56.

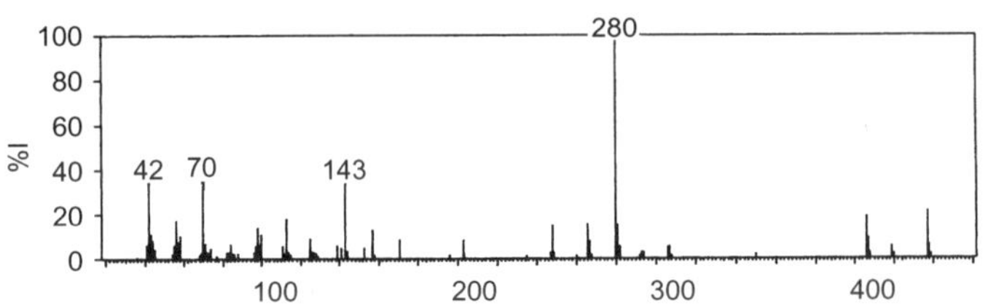

Quantification

Gas chromatography. In plasma: limit of detection 500 ng/L, AFID—J. I. Javaid *et al.*, *J. Chromatogr. Sci.*, 1981, *19*, 439–443. In urine: free and conjugated fluphenazine, limit of detection 2 µg/L, AFID—R. Whelpton and S. H. Curry, *J. Pharm. Pharmacol.*, 1976, *28*, 869–873.

Gas chromatography-mass spectrometry. In plasma: limit of detection 80 ng/L—G. McKay *et al.*, *Biomed. Mass Spectrom.*, 1983, *10*, 550–555. In plasma: limit of detection <50 ng/L—M. Jemal *et al.*, *Biomed. Environ. Mass Spectrom.*, 1987, *14*, 699–704. In serum: fluphenazine decanoate—W. M. Glazer *et al.*, *Schizophr. Res.*, 1992, *8*, 111–117.

High performance liquid chromatography. In plasma: fluphenazine and fluphenazine decanoate, limit of detection 0.1 µg/L, coulometric detection—J. P. Luo *et al.*, *J. Chromatogr. B Biomed. Sci. Appl.*, 1997, *688*, 303–308.

High performance liquid chromatography–radioimmunoassay. In plasma: fluphenazine, related phenothiazines, and metabolites, limit of detection 160 pg for fluphenazine—S. A. Goldstein and H. Van Vunakis, *J. Pharmacol. Exp. Ther.*, 1981, *217*, 36–43.

Radioimmunoassay. In plasma: 7-hydroxyfluphenazine, limit of detection 0.1 µg/L—M. Aravagiri *et al.*, *Ther. Drug Monit.*, 1994, *16*, 21–29.

Disposition in the Body. The hydrochloride is well absorbed after oral administration; the decanoate and enantate are slowly absorbed from sites of injection. Fluphenazine is metabolised by sulfoxidation, hydroxylation, and conjugation with glucuronic acid or sulfate. Fluphenazine sulfoxide and 7-hydroxyfluphenazine have been detected in urine and faeces. After an oral dose of the hydrochloride, 20% is excreted in the urine and 60% is eliminated in the faeces in 7 days; after an IM dose of the enantate, 26% is eliminated in the faeces and 14% excreted in the urine in 14 days; after an IM dose of the decanoate, 17% is eliminated in the faeces and 6% excreted in the urine in 30 days.

Therapeutic concentration

Following a single oral dose of 5 mg of fluphenazine hydrochloride to 6 subjects, peak plasma concentrations of 0.3 to 1.0 µg/L (mean 0.6) were attained in 2.8 h. [K. K. Midha *et al.*, *Eur. J. Clin. Pharmacol.*, 1983, *25*, 709–711.]

Following daily oral doses of 20 mg of fluphenazine hydrochloride to 18 subjects, steady-state plasma concentrations of 0.2 to 4.0 µg/L were reported. [J. I. Javaid *et al.*, *J. Chromatogr. Sci.*, 1981, *19*, 439–443.]

In 24 subjects receiving continuous treatment with depot IM fluphenazine, steady-state plasma concentrations were <0.1 to 27.9 µg/L (median 0.5 µg/L). [R. S. Miller *et al.*, *J. Clin. Pharm. Ther.*, 1995, *20*, 55–62.]

Of 12 subjects given a single oral dose of 12 mg fluphenazine hydrochloride, those given an immediate-release formulation had peak plasma concentrations of 2.3 µg/L at 2.8 h and those given a slow-release formulation had a peak plasma concentration of 1.2 µg/L at 4.6 h. The plasma level in the same subjects 10 min after being given an IV bolus dose of 2.5 mg was 0.261 mg/L. [R. Koytchev *et al.*, *Eur. J. Clin. Pharmacol.*, 1996, *51*, 183–187.]

Half-life. Plasma half-life, fluphenazine hydrochloride about 15 h; fluphenazine decanoate about 5 to 12 days and fluphenazine enantate about 3 to 4 days, following IM injection.

Protein binding. In plasma, about 99%.

Dose. Usually 1 to 5 mg of fluphenazine hydrochloride daily; up to 20 mg daily has been given.

Flupirtine

Analgesic

Synonym. D-9998

[2-Amino-6-[[(4-fluorophenyl)methyl]amino]-3-pyridinyl]carbamic acid ethyl ester

$C_{15}H_{17}FN_4O_2$=304.3

CAS—56995-20-1

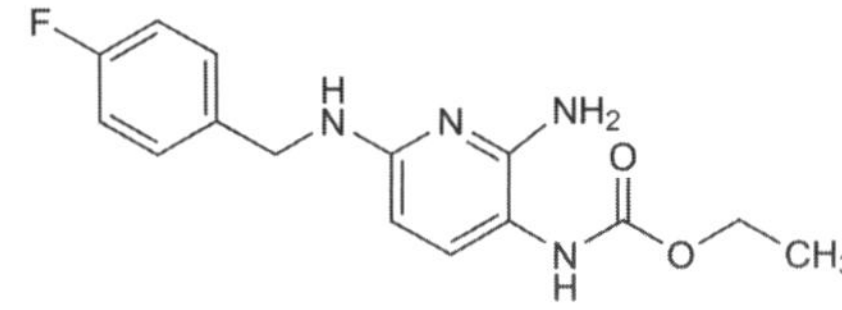

A crystalline powder. M.p. 115° to 116°. In 5% ethanol solution, is colourless turning green on exposure to air for 20 h.

Flupirtine Hydrochloride

$C_{15}H_{17}FN_4O_2.HCl$=340.8

A crystalline powder with M.p. 214° to 215°.

Flupirtine Maleate

Synonym. W-2964M

Proprietary names. Katadolon; Trancopal Dolo.

$C_{15}H_{17}FN_4O_2.C_4H_4O_4$=420.4

CAS—75507-68-5

A colourless, crystalline powder with M.p. 175.5° to 176°. It is freely soluble in water.

Partition Coefficient. Log *P* (octanol/water), 2.66.

Gas Chromatography. System GA—RI 2603.

High Performance Liquid Chromatography. Column: ODS (Hypersil, 250 × 4.6 mm i.d., 5 µm). Mobile phase: (A)-phosphate buffer (10 mM, pH 3), (B)-acetonitrile:methanol (50:50). Elution programme: (A:B) (40:60) to (30:70) over 8 min, held 3 min, 1.4 mL/min flow rate. Internal standard (IS): D-09925. Fluorescence detection (λ_{ex}=323 nm, λ_{em}=380 nm). Retention time: flupirtine, 6.0 min; flupirtine acetylated metabolite, 4.4 min; IS, 9.38 min [G. Niebch *et al.*, *Arzneimittelforshung*, 1992, *42*, 1343–1345].

Column: (analytical) ODS (Ultrasphere, 250 × 4.6 mm i.d., 5 µm), (guard) Co:Pell ODS (70 × 2.3 mm i.d., 30 to 38 µm). Mobile phase: acetonitrile:methanol:phosphate buffer (5 mM) (32:32:36), pH 6.7, flow rate 1.4 mL/min. IS: flupirtine dimethyl derivative. Fluorescence detection (λ_{ex}=323 mn, λ_{em}=370 nm). Retention time: flupirtine, 3.73 min; IS, 6.08 min [P. K. Narang *et al.*, *J. Chromatogr.*, 1984, *305*, 135–143].

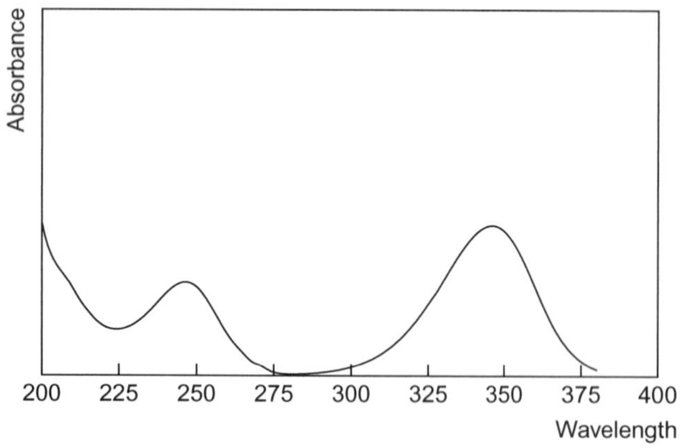

Mass Spectrum. Principal ions at *m/z* 109, 304, 231, 124, 258, 110, 83, 123.

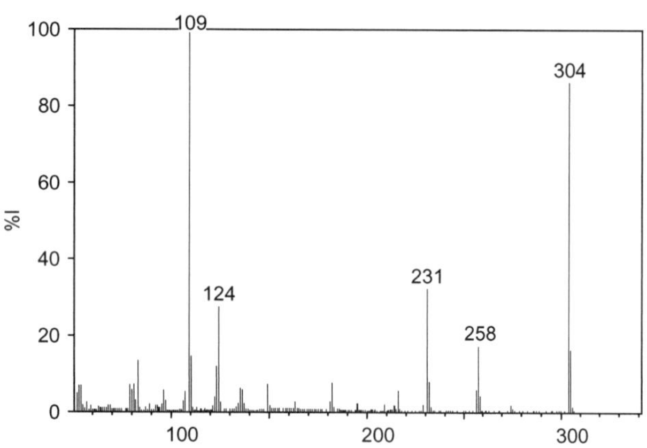

Quantification

High performance liquid chromatography. In plasma and urine: limit of detection, flupirtine 0.03 mg/L and acetylated metabolite 0.5 mg/L. Fluorescence detection (λ_{ex}=323 nm, λ_{em}=370 nm)—P. K. Narang *et al.*, *J. Chromatogr.*, 1984, *305(1)*, *Biomed. Appl.*, 135–143. In blood: limit of quantification is 0.025 mg/L. Fluorescence detection (λ_{ex}=323 nm, λ_{em}=380 nm)—G. Niebch *et al.*, *Arzneimittelforschung*, 1992, *42*, 1343–1345.

Disposition in the Body. Flupirtine is almost completely absorbed and undergoes oxidative degradation and acetylation of the hydrolysis product, in the liver, to two major metabolites; *p*-fluorohippuric acid and an acteylated metabolite, respectively. 72% of a dose is excreted in urine as the parent drug and as metabolites, and 18% in faeces. It is known to cross the blood–brain barrier and appears quickly in cerebrospinal fluid. Less than 0.005% of a dose is secreted in breast milk.

Therapeutic concentration

Healthy subjects aged between 18 and 35 years, and 66 and 83 years and patients with renal impairment (creatine clearance 44 to 99 mL/min) were administered a single 100 mg dose of flupirtine. Peak plasma concentrations of 0.77, 1.12 and 0.72 mg/L were reached within 1.6 to 1.8 h [S. M. L. Abrams *et al.*, *Postgrad. Med. J.*, 1988, *64*, 361–363].

Toxicity. Moderately toxic by ingestion and subcutaneous routes.

Half-life. 8.5 to 10.7 h, depending on type of administration.

Bioavailability. Approx. 90% (oral administration); 73% (suppositories).

Volume of distribution. 1.15 to 1.16 L/kg.

Clearance. 16.5 L/h.

Protein binding. 80 to 90% bound to albumin proteins.

Dose. Usual oral dose of 100 mg three or four times a day is administered in the maleate form with doses up to 600 or 900 mg daily.

Fluquinconazole

Insecticide

Synonym. SN-597265
Proprietary names. Aventis; Castellan; Diablo; Flamenco; Jockey F: Jockey Flexi; Vista.
3-(2,4-Dichlorophenyl)-6-fluoro-2-(1*H*-1,2,4-triazol-1-yl)-4-(3*H*)-quinazolinone
$C_{16}H_8Cl_2FN_5O$=376.2
CAS—136426-54-5

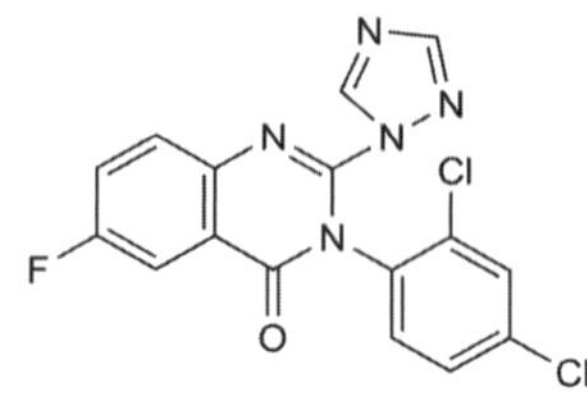

An off-white particulate solid. M.p. 191.5° to 193°.
Its solubility in water is 1 mg/L at 20°. It is also soluble in dimethyl sulfoxide (150 g/L at 20°), acetone (44 g/L at 20°), xylene (10 g/L at 20°), and ethanol (3 g/L at 20°).

Partition Coefficient. Log *P* (octanol/water), 3.2.

Flurazepam

Hypnotic

7-Chloro-1-[2-(diethylamino)ethyl]-5-(2-fluorophenyl)-1,3-dihydro-2*H*-1,4-benzodiazepin-2-one
$C_{21}H_{23}ClFN_3O$=387.9
CAS—17617-23-1

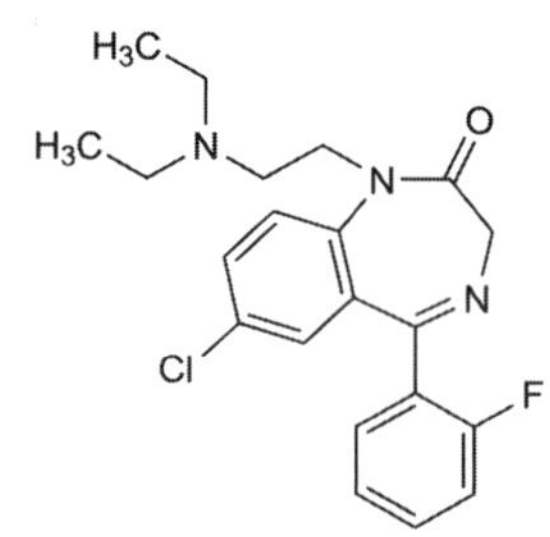

White crystals. M.p. 77° to 82°.
Soluble in chloroform.

Flurazepam Hydrochloride

Synonyms. Flurazepam Dihydrochloride; NSC-78559; Ro-5-6901.
Proprietary names. Dalmadorm; Dalmane; Dormodor; Felison; Felmane; Flunox; Morfex; Remdue; Somnol; Staurodorm; Valdorm. Includes proprietary names of flurazepam monohydrochloride.
$C_{21}H_{23}ClFN_3O,2HCl$=460.8
CAS—1172-18-5
An off-white to yellow crystalline powder. M.p. 190° to 220°.
Soluble 1 in 2 of water, 1 in 4 of ethanol, 1 in 90 of chloroform, and 1 in 3 of methanol; very slightly soluble in ether.

Flurazepam Monohydrochloride

Proprietary names. See above under flurazepam hydrochloride.
$C_{21}H_{23}ClFN_3O,HCl$=424.3
CAS—36105-20-1
A white crystalline powder.
Very soluble in water; freely soluble in ethanol; practically insoluble in ether.

Dissociation Constant. pK_a 1.9, 8.2.

Partition Coefficient. Log *P* (octanol/buffer pH 7.4), 2.3.

Colour Test. Formaldehyde–Sulfuric Acid—pink.

Thin-layer Chromatography. System TA—Rf 62; system TB—Rf 30; system TC—Rf 48; system TD—Rf 03; system TE—Rf 71; system TF—Rf 03; system TL—Rf 40; system TAD—Rf 41; system TAE—Rf 52; system TAF—Rf 45; system TAJ—Rf 32; system TAK—Rf 08; system TAL—Rf 73. (Acidified iodoplatinate solution, positive.)

Gas Chromatography. System GA—flurazepam RI 2780, M (2-OH-ethyl-) RI 2675, M (desalkyl-) RI 2470, M (desalkyl-OH-) RI 2255, M (didesethyl-) RI 2694; system GB—flurazepam RI 2896, M (desalkyl-) RI 2559, M (desalkyl-)-TMS RI 2350, M (2-OH-ethyl-) RI 2805, M (2-OH-ethyl-)-TMS RI 2778, M (bis-desethyl-) RI 2739, M (desalkyl-OH-) RI 2373; system GF—flurazepam RI 3210; system GG—flurazepam RI 3220.

High Performance Liquid Chromatography. System HA—flurazepam *k* 1.3, M (desalkyl-) *k* 0.1; system HI—M (desalkyl-) *k* 5.19, M (OH-ethyl-) *k* 4.27; system HJ—flurazepam *k* 3.19; system HK—flurazepam *k* 6.50, M (desalkyl-) *k* 1.52, M (2-OH-ethyl-) *k* 1.43; system HX—flurazepam RI 397; system HY—flurazepam RI 305; system HZ—flurazepam retention time 4.2 min; system HAX—flurazepam retention time 10.5 min; system HAY—flurazepam retention time 5.5 min; system HAZ—flurazepam *k* 0.73; system HBH—flurazepam *k* 12.98; system HBI—flurazepam *k* 3.12.

Ultraviolet Spectrum. Aqueous acid—236 (A^1_1=620b), 284; aqueous alkali—231 (A^1_1=856b), 312 nm (A^1_1=53b).

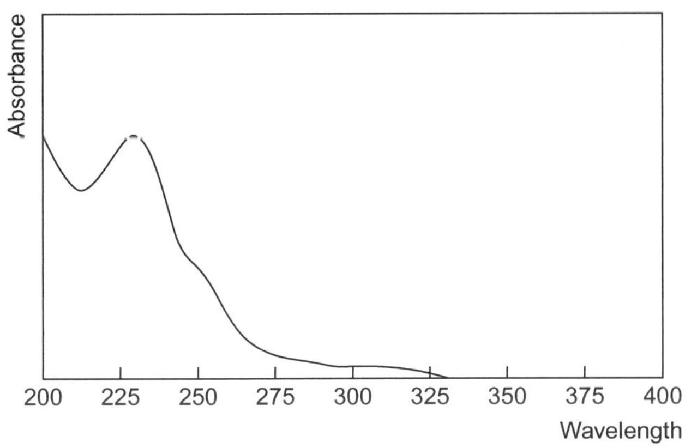

Infra-red Spectrum. Principal peaks at wavenumbers 1672, 1613, 1316, 1211, 1171, 1100 cm^{-1} (KBr disk).

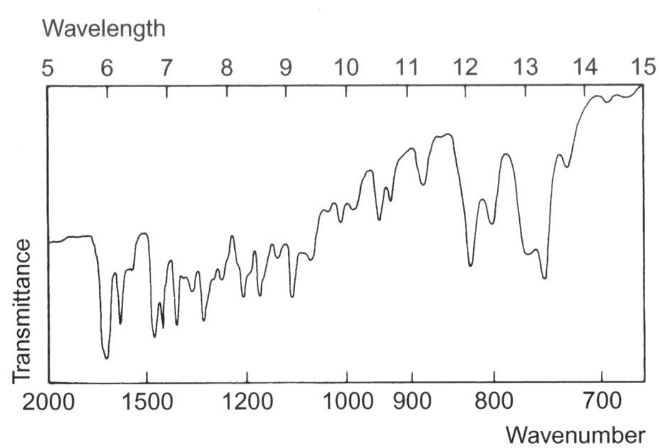

Mass Spectrum. Principal ions at *m/z* 86, 87, 99, 58, 84, 387, 315, 56; N^1-desalkylflurazepam 260, 259, 288, 287, 261, 289, 262, 290; didesethylflurazepam 30, 313, 246, 211, 273, 274, 302, 183; N^1-(2-hydroxyethyl)flurazepam 288, 273, 331, 287, 304, 290, 289, 275.

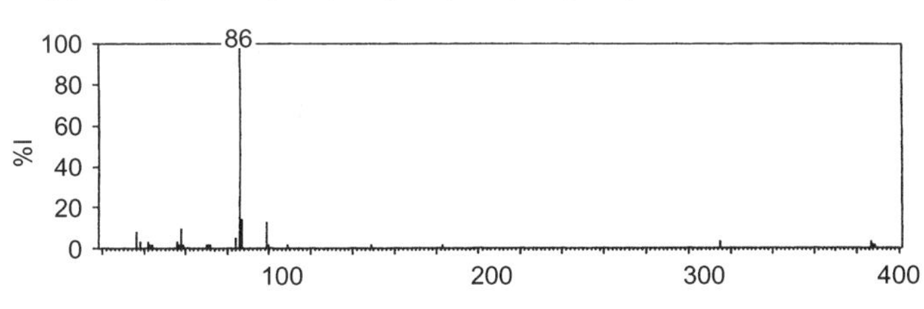

Quantification

Gas chromatography. In blood or urine: limits of detection, N^1-(2-hydroxyethyl)flurazepam and flurazepam-N^1-ylacetic acid 0.3 μg/L, flurazepam 0.5 μg/L, N^1-desalkylflurazepam and N^1-desalkyl-3-hydroxyflurazepam 2 μg/L, ECD—M. Hasegawa *et al.*, *Chem. Pharm. Bull.*, 1975, *23*, 1826–1833. In plasma: limits of detection, flurazepam 3 μg/L, N^1-(2-hydroxyethyl)flurazepam 1 μg/L, N^1-desalkylflurazepam 0.6 μg/L, ECD—S. F. Cooper and D. Drolet, *J. Chromatogr.* 1982, *231*(20) *B Biomed. Appl.*, 321–331. In biological samples: flurazepam and its metabolites, ECD—E. S. Burstein *et al.*, *J. Anal. Toxicol.*, 1988, *12*, 122–125. In blood: flurazepam and its metabolites, limit of quantification for flurazepam 1 μg/L, ECD—Z. Salama *et al.*, *Arzneimittelforschung*, 1988, *38*, 400–403.

Gas chromatography–mass spectrometry. Limit of quantification 2.5 to 5 μg/L (full scan) and 0.1 to 0.5 μg/L (SIM, *m/z* 86)—D. Borrey *et al.*, *J. Chromatogr. A*, 2001, *910*, 105–118.

High performance liquid chromatography. In urine: N^1-(2-hydroxyethyl)flurazepam, limit of detection 500 μg/L, UV detection—R. E. Weinfeld and K. F. Miller, *J. Chromatogr.* 1981, *223*(12) *B Biomed. Appl.*, 123–130.

Note. For GC/MS screening of acetylated benzodiazepines, see D. Borrey *et al.*, *J. Chromatogr. A*, 2001, *910*, 105–118.

Disposition in the Body. Readily absorbed after oral administration; about 70% of a dose is metabolised during the first pass through the liver. The major metabolites in blood are N^1-desalkylflurazepam and N^1-(2-hydroxyethyl)flurazepam which are both pharmacologically active and accumulate on daily administration; 7-chloro-5-(2-fluorophenyl)-1,3-dihydro-2-oxo-2*H*-1,4-benzodiazepin-1-acetaldehyde has also been detected in plasma. Other active metabolites found in urine include monodesethyl- and didesethylflurazepam and N^1-desalkyl-3-hydroxyflurazepam, but these are not detectable in blood. Up to 60% of a dose may be excreted in the urine in 48 h, with about 40% of the dose as a glucuronide/sulfate conjugate of N^1-(2-hydroxyethyl)flurazepam and about 4% as conjugated N^1-desalkyl-3-hydroxyflurazepam and conjugated flurazepam-N^1-ylacetic acid; only trace amounts of unchanged flurazepam and the unconjugated metabolites are present. N^1-(Hydroxyethyl)-3-hydroxyflurazepam has also been detected. About 9% of a dose is eliminated in the faeces.

Therapeutic concentration. Flurazepam is rapidly metabolised and hence blood concentrations of the unchanged drug are low and quickly decrease; for normal doses the peak concentration is usually in the range 0.0005 to 0.03 mg/L. The blood concentration of N^1-desalkylflurazepam is usually in the range 0.04 to 0.06 mg/L.

Following a single oral dose of 30 mg of flurazepam hydrochloride to 2 subjects, peak blood concentrations were attained as follows: flurazepam, 0.001 and 0.005 mg/L at 3 h; N^1-(2-hydroxyethyl)flurazepam 0.005 and 0.01 mg/L at 3 h; N^1-desalkylflurazepam, 0.010 and 0.012 mg/L at 24 h. [J. A. F. de Silva *et al.*, *J. Pharm. Sci.*, 1974, *63*, 1837–1841.]

Following daily oral doses of 15 mg to 18 subjects, steady-state plasma concentrations of N^1-desalkylflurazepam of 0.03 to 0.15 mg/L (mean 0.08) were reported. [D. J. Greenblatt *et al.*, *Clin. Pharmacol. Ther.*, 1981, *30*, 475–486.]

Toxicity. Blood concentrations greater than 0.2 mg/L of flurazepam or 0.5 mg/L of N^1-desalkylflurazepam may be toxic, and blood concentrations greater than 0.5 mg/L of flurazepam may be fatal.

In a fatality attributed to flurazepam overdose, the following postmortem concentrations (mg/L or μg/g) were reported for flurazepam, N^1-desalkylflurazepam, and N^1-(2-hydroxyethyl)flurazepam, respectively: blood 0.51, 0.14, 9; urine 7, 3.9, 98. The amount ingested was estimated to be more than 2.4 g. [R. Aderjan and R. Mattern, *Arch. Toxicol.*, 1979, *43*, 69–75.]

In a 5-year-old child who died following the ingestion of flurazepam and phenobarbital, the following postmortem tissue concentrations were reported for flurazepam, N^1-desalkylflurazepam, and N^1-(2-hydroxyethyl)-flurazepam, respectively: blood 3.2, 1.8, and 2.5 mg/L; brain 0.8, 0.7, and 0.7 μg/g, kidney 0.9, 0.6, and 1.1 μg/g, liver 2.7, 3.1, and 3.5 μg/g. Phenobarbital concentrations were consistent with a therapeutic dose and low concentrations of phenytoin were also detected. [S. D. Ferrara *et al.*, *J. Forensic Sci.*, 1979, *24*, 61–69.]

In a 52-year-old female whose death was attributed to suicidal ingestion of up to 2.2 g flurazepam, the following postmortem tissue concentrations were reported (in mg/L or μg/g): femoral blood 5.5, liver 130, bile 33, vitreous humour 1.3, urine 3.3, gastric contents 600 mg (total); desalkylfurazepam was also detected in blood, liver, bile, and vitreous humour, but at concentrations much lower than the parent compound. [I. M. McIntyre *et al.*, *J. Forensic Sci.*, 1994, *39*, 1571–1574.]

Half-life. Plasma half-life, flurazepam 2 to 3 h, N^1-desalkylflurazepam 2 to 5 days, N^1-(2-hydroxyethyl)flurazepam 10 to 20 h.

Protein binding. In plasma, flurazepam about 97%, N^1-desalkylflurazepam about 98% and N^1-(2-hydroxyethyl)flurazepam about 90%.

Note. For a review of the pharmacokinetics of flurazepam, see D. J. Greenblatt *et al.*, *Clin. Pharmacol. Ther.*, 1975, *17*, 1–14.

Dose. The equivalent of 15 to 30 mg of flurazepam, as a hypnotic.

Flurbiprofen

Analgesic

Proprietary names. Ansaid; Antadys; Benactiv; Cebutid; Edolfene; Evril; Fenomel; Flurofen; Froben; Ocufen; Ocuflur; Reupax; Strefen; Strepfen; Transact.

2-Fluoro-α-methyl-[1,1′-biphenyl]-4-acetic acid

$C_{15}H_{13}FO_2$=244.3

CAS—5104-49-4

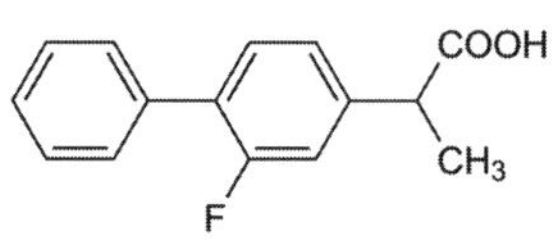

A colourless crystalline solid. M.p. about 110°.

Slightly soluble in water; freely soluble in most organic solvents.

Partition Coefficient. Log *P* (octanol/water), 4.2.

Colour Tests. Liebermann's Test—brown; Marquis Test—red.

Thin-layer Chromatography. System TD—Rf 30; system TE—Rf 06; system TF—Rf 30; system TG—Rf 16; system TAD—Rf 45; system TAJ—Rf 47; system TAK—Rf 69; system TAL—Rf 91. (Ludy Tenger reagent, orange.)

Gas Chromatography. System GA—flurbiprofen RI 1900; flurbiprofen-Me RI 1885; M (OH-)-Me_2 RI 2180; M (OH-methoxy)-Me_2 RI 2310; system GD—RRT of methyl derivative 1.30 (relative to n-$C_{16}H_{34}$); system GL—flurbiprofen-Me RI 1880; M (OH-)-Me_2 RI 2180.

High Performance Liquid Chromatography. System HV—RRT 0.89 (relative to meclofenamic acid); system HX—RI 585; system HZ—Retention time, 11.8 min; system HAA—Retention time, 21.3 min; system HAX—Retention time 8.0 min; system HAY—Retention time 8.9 min.

Ultraviolet Spectrum. Aqueous acid—247 nm (A^1_1=787b). No alkaline shift.

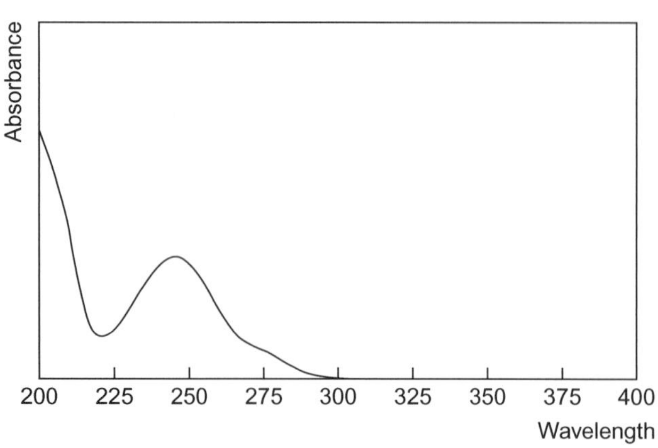

Infra-red Spectrum. Principal peaks at wavenumbers 1695, 1220, 707, 930, 773, 960 cm^{-1} (KBr disk).

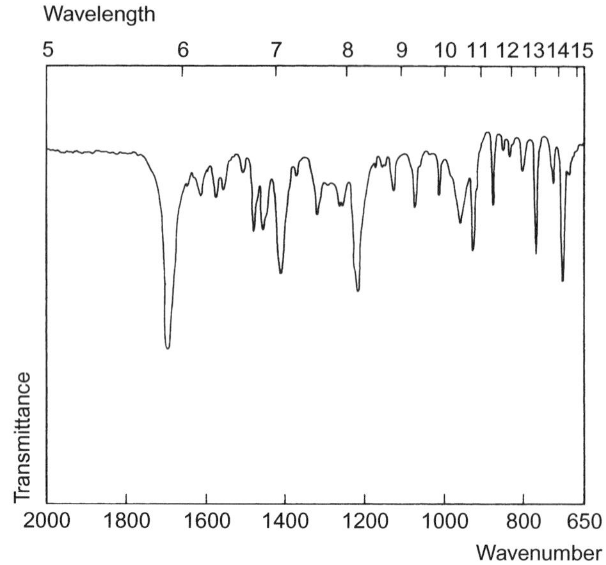

Mass Spectrum. Principal ions at *m/z* 199, 244, 200, 178, 179, 184, 183, 245.

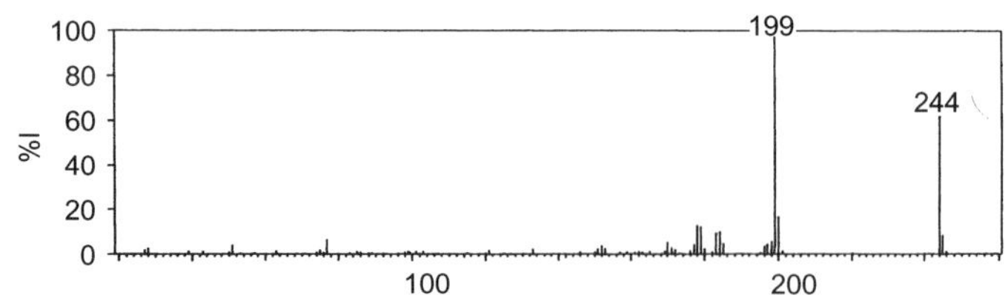

Quantification

Gas chromatography. In plasma: limit of detection 50 μg/L, ECD—D. G. Kaiser *et al.*, *J. Pharm. Sci.*, 1974, *63*, 567–570.

Gas chromatography–mass spectrometry. In plasma: limit of detection 1 μg/L—K. Kawahara *et al.*, *J. Chromatogr.* 1981, *223 B Biomed. Appl.*, *12*, 202–207. In plasma: limit of detection <0.5 mg/L—M. Satomoto *et al.*, *Masui*, 2002, *51*, 431–434.

High performance liquid chromatography. In serum: limit of detection 40 μg/L, UV detection—B. G. Snider *et al.*, *J. Pharm. Sci.*, 1981, *70*, 1347–1349. In plasma: flurbiprofen and ibuprofen, limit of detection 200 μg/L, UV detection—J. Askholt and F. Nielsen-Kudsk, *Acta Pharmacol. Toxicol. (Copenh.)*, 1986, *59*, 382–386. In plasma or urine: flurbiprofen enantiomers and metabolites, fluorescence detection—M. P. Knadler and S. D. Hall, *J. Chromatogr.*, 1989, *494*, 173–182. In crevicular fluid—P. A. Heasman *et al.*, *J. Periodontal Res.*, 1990, *25*, 88–92. In plasma: flurbiprofen enantiomers, limit of detection <50 μg/L, UV detection—G. Geisslinger *et al.*, *J. Chromatogr.*, 1992, *573*, 163–167. In ocular fluids: flurbiprofen and diclofenac, limit of detection 3 to 4 μg/L, UV detection—M. Riegel and P. P. Ellis, *J. Chromatogr. B Biomed. Appl.*, 1994, *654*, 140–145. In urine: flurbiprofen and other NSAIDs, limit of detection 0.05 mg/L, UV detection—T. Hirai *et al.*, *J. Chromatogr. B Biomed. Sci. Appl.*, 1997, *692*, 375–388. In plasma or urine: flurbiprofen and 4′-hydroxyflurbiprofen, limit of detection <0.25 mg/L for flurbiprofen, fluorescence detection—J. M. Hutzler *et al.*, *J. Chromatogr. B Biomed. Sci. Appl.*, 2000, *749*, 119–125.

Disposition in the Body. Readily absorbed after oral administration. About 95% of a dose is excreted in the urine in 24 h, mainly as the 4′-hydroxy, 3′,4′-dihydroxy, and 4′-methoxy metabolites, which are excreted partly as conjugates; about 25% of a dose is excreted as unchanged drug.

Therapeutic concentration

After a single oral dose of 100 mg, administered to 6 subjects, peak serum concentrations of 9.1 to 16.6 mg/L (mean 12) were attained in about 1.5 h [N. Cardoe *et al.*, *Curr. Med. Res. Opin.*, 1977, *5*, 21–25.]

A single oral dose of 200 mg administered as a sustained-release capsule produced peak plasma concentrations of 4 to 10 mg/L and 4 to 8 mg/L, respectively, in 10 young and 9 elderly subjects at approximately 6 and 9 h. On continuing the same dosage once daily, a mean steady-state level of approximately 6 mg/L was achieved in all subjects [R. C. Hamdy *et al.*, *Eur. J. Clin. Pharmacol.*, 1990, *39*, 267–270.]

Half-life. Plasma half-life, 2 to 6 h (mean 3.5).

Volume of distribution. About 0.1 L/kg.

Clearance. Plasma clearance, about 0.3 mL/min/kg.

Protein binding. In plasma, about 99%.

Note. For a review of the pharmacokinetics of flurbiprofen see R. N. Brogden *et al.*, *Drugs*, 1979, *18*, 417–438 and N. M. Davies, *Clin. Pharmacokinet.*, 1995, *28*, 100–114.

Dose. 150 to 300 mg daily.

Fluspirilene

Tranquilliser

Proprietary names. Fluspi; Imap; Kivat; Redeptin.
8-[4,4-Bis(4-fluorophenyl)butyl]-1-phenyl-1,3,8-triazaspiro[4.5]decan-4-one
$C_{29}H_{31}F_2N_3O$=475.6
CAS—1841-19-6

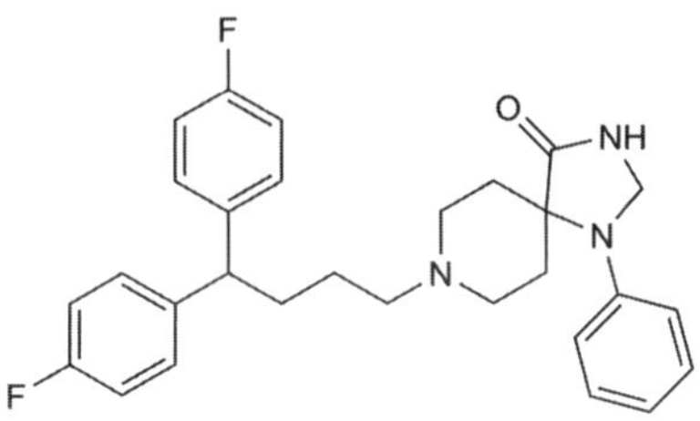

A white to yellowish, amorphous or crystalline powder. M.p. 187.5° to 190°.
Practically insoluble in water; slightly soluble in ethanol and ether; sparingly soluble in acetone; freely soluble in chloroform.

Partition Coefficient. Log *P* (octanol/water), 5.9.

Thin-layer Chromatography. System TA—Rf 69; system TB—Rf 04; system TC—Rf 59; system TE—Rf 71; system TL—Rf 49; system TAE—Rf 63; system TAF—Rf 78.

Gas Chromatography. System GA—fluspirilene RI 1017; M (*N*-desalkyl-oxo-) RI 2405; M (desamino-OH-) RI 2120; M (desamino-carboxy-) RI 2230.

High Performance Liquid Chromatography. System HX—RI 538; system HAX—Retention time 18.3 min; system HAY—Retention time 9.8 min.

Ultraviolet Spectrum. Methanol—252 (A_1^1=295a), 273, 293 nm.

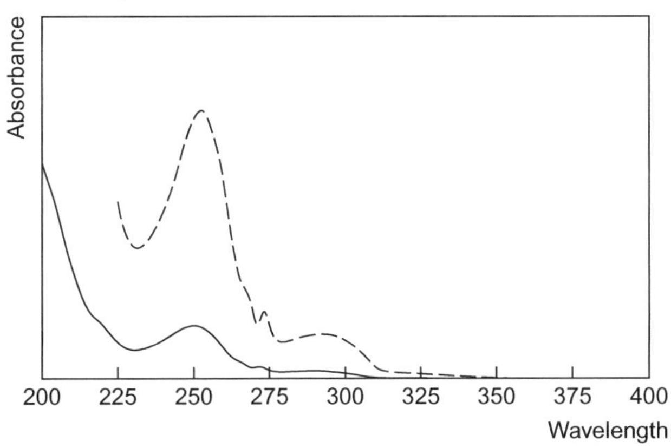

Infra-red Spectrum. Principal peaks at wavenumbers 1710, 1505, 1596, 1220, 743, 1230 cm^{-1} (KBr disk). Polymorphism may occur.

Mass Spectrum. Principal ions at *m/z* 244, 42, 72, 475, 109, 245, 85, 476.

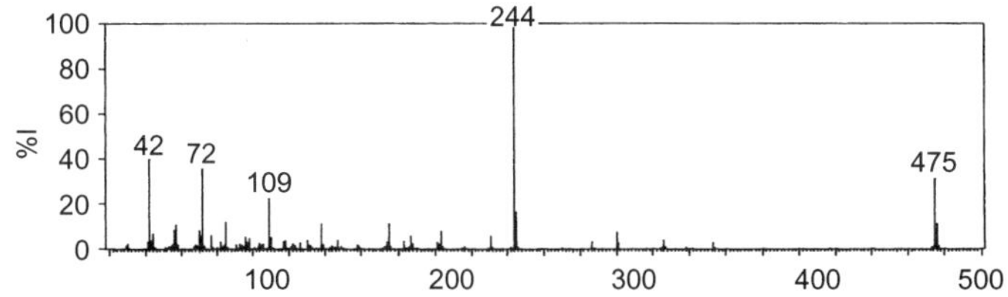

Quantification

High performance liquid chromatography–mass spectrometry. In plasma: limit of detection <21 ng/L—K. J. Swart *et al.*, *J. Chromatogr. A.*, 1998, *828*, 219-227.

Dose. Usually 2 to 8 mg weekly, by deep IM injection; maximum of 20 mg weekly.

Flutazolam

Anxiolytic

Synonyms. MS-4101: Ro-7-6102.
Proprietary name. Coreminal
10-Chloro-11b-(2-fluorophenyl)-2,3-7,11b-tetrahydro-7-(2-hydroxy-ethyl)oxazolo[3,2-*d*][1,4]benzodiazepin-6-(5*H*)-one
$C_{19}H_{18}ClFN_2O_3$=376.8
CAS—27060-91-9

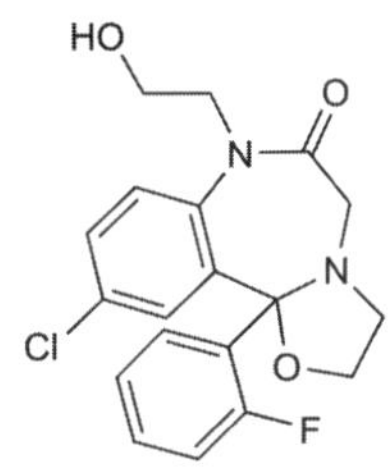

White prisms from toluene with M.p. 142° to 147°. It is freely soluble in chloroform and ethanol; moderately soluble in acetone, benzene and methanol; practically insoluble in water.

Dissociation Constant. pK_a 5.4.

Thin-layer Chromatography. System TE—Rf 68; system TAE—Rf 84.

Gas Chromatography. System GA—RI 2460.

High Performance Liquid Chromatography. System HAF—retention time 32.2 min.

Mass Spectrum. Principal ions at *m/z* 289, 245, 246, 210, 259, 211, 183, 291.

Quantification

High performance liquid chromatography. In serum: limit of quantification 0.01 mg/L—E. Tanaka *et al.*, *J. Chromatogr.*, 1996, *682, Biomed. Appl.*, 173–178.

Fluticasone Propionate

Anti-inflammatory

Synonym. CCI-18781
Proprietary names. Atemur; Axotide; Cutivate; Flixonase; Flixotide; Flonase; Flovent; Flunase; Flutide; Flutivate.
(6α,11β,16α,17α)-6,9-Difluoro-11-hydroxy-16-methyl-3-oxo-17-(1-oxo-propoxy)androsta-1,4-diene-17-carbothioic acid *S*-(fluoromethyl) ester
$C_{25}H_{31}F_3O_5S$=500.6
CAS—80474-14-2

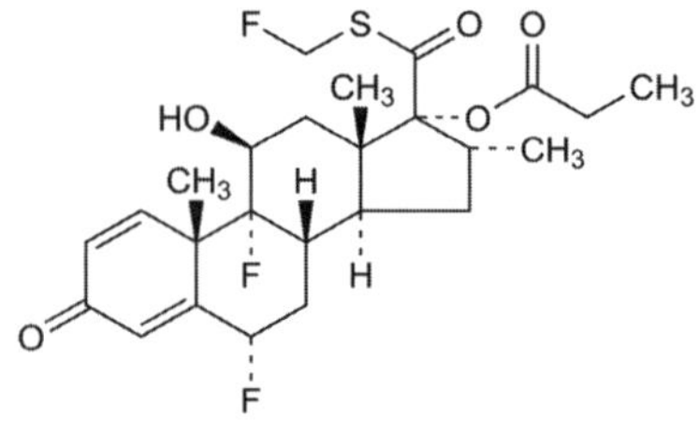

A white to almost white crystalline powder. M.p. 272° to 273°. It is practically insoluble in water; slightly soluble in methanol and ethanol (95%); freely soluble in diemethylformamide and dimethylsulfoxide; sparingly soluble in acetone and dichloromethane.

High Performance Liquid Chromatography. Column: (analytical) ODS Hypersil (100 × 2.1 mm i.d., 5 μm), (guard) C_{18} ODS (20 × 2.1 mm i.d., 5 μm). Mobile phase: ethanol:water (50:50), 0.45 mL/min flow rate. MS detection (APCI, SIM at *m/z* 501.2 for fluticasone propionate and 473.2 for internal standard (IS)). IS: 22*R* epimer of budesonide acetate. Retention time: fluticasone propionate, 3.09 min; IS, 3.35 min [Y. N. Li *et al.*, *J. Pharm. Biomed. Anal.*, 1997, *16*, 447–452.].

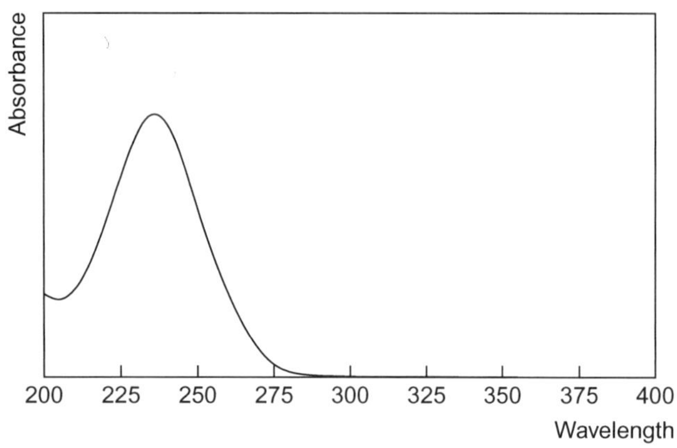

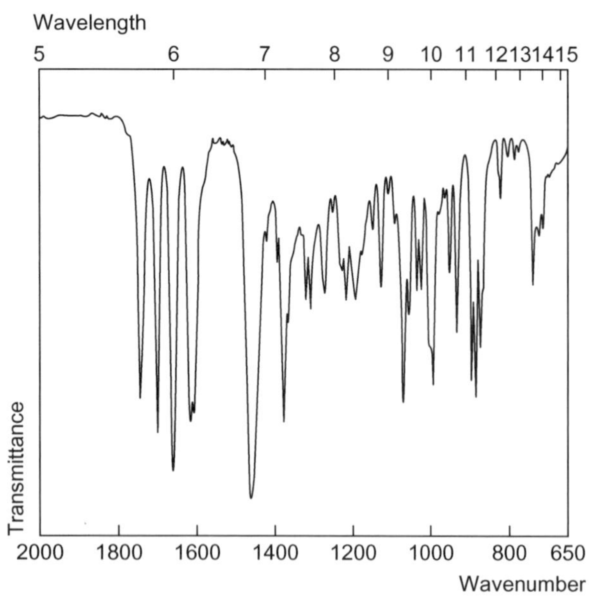

Mass Spectrum. Fluticasone propionate, principal ions at *m/z* 57, 139, 351, 134, 121, 333, 313, 109.

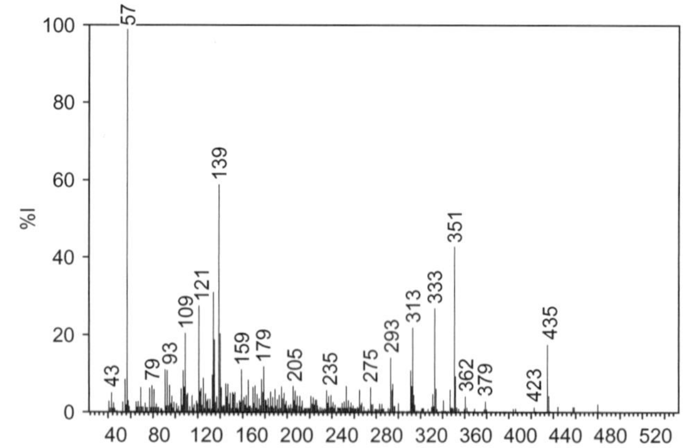

Quantification

High performance liquid chromatography. In plasma: limit of quantification is 0.025 μg/L. MS–MS detection—L. Laugher *et al.*, *J. Pharm. Biomed. Anal*, 1999, *21(4)*, 749–758. In plasma: limit of detection 0.01 μg/L—S. Krishnaswami *et al.*, *J. Pharm. Biomed. Anal.*, 2000, *22*, 123–129.

Disposition in the Body. Fluticasone is poorly absorbed and undergoes extensive first-pass metabolism. The only known metabolite in humans is a 17β-carboxylic acid metabolite. Less than 5% of a dose is excreted in urine as the metabolite with the remainder being excreted in faeces as the parent drug (up to 75%) and the metabolite. Oral bioavailability is approx. 1%. After intravenous administration, the drug is extensively administered in the body.

Therapeutic concentration

6 healthy subjects were administered single doses of 0.25, 0.5, 1.0 and 3.0 mg fluticasone propionate. Maximum serum concentrations of 0.09 μg/L for the 0.25 mg dose and 0.40 μg/L for the 3.0 mg dose were reached within 0.5 to 1.0 h [H. Mollman *et al.*, *Eur. J. Clin. Pharmacol.*, 1998, *53(6)*, 459–467].

12 healthy males, aged between 21 and 38 years, were administered 250, 500 and 1000 μg fluticasone propionate intravenously over 3 min. Peak plasma concentrations were rapidly reached after administration was completed, 12.8, 32.8 and 63.7 μg/L, respectively [A. E. Mackie *et al.*, *Br. J. Clin. Pharmacol.*, 1996, *41*, 539–542].

Toxicity. Acute overdosing in excess of the recommended dose and chronic overdosing of > 2 mg, over a prolonged period of time, leads to temporary adrenal suppression.

Half-life. 7.8 h.

Volume of distribution. 4.2 L/kg (range 2.3 to 16.7 L/kg), also reported as 318 L.

Clearance. Total blood clearance, 0.0182 L/h (range 0.0103 to 0.0284 L/h). Plasma clearance, 1.1 L/min.

Protein binding 91% plasma bound.

Dose. Adults (by inhalation): usual dose of 100 to 250 μg twice a day up to 500 to 1000 μg twice a day. Children > 4 years old: 50 to 100 μg twice a day. Oral dose: 5 mg four times a day.

Flutoprazepam

Anxiolytic

Synonyms. KB-509; ID-1937.
Proprietary names. Restar; Restas.
7-Chloro-1-(cyclopropylmethyl)-5-(2-fluorophenyl)-1,3-dihydro-2*H*-1,4-benzodiazepin-2-one
$C_{19}H_{16}ClFN_2O$=342.8
CAS—25967-29-7

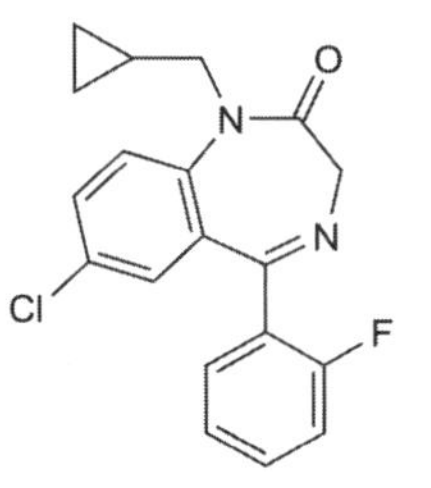

Crystals. M.p. 118° to 122°.

Gas Chromatography. Column: cross-linked methylsilicone (12 × 0.2 m i.d.). Column temperature: 170° (1 min), increased to 270° at 8°/min, held for 10 min. Carrier gas: helium, 14.4 psi (99.3 kPa). Detection: mass spectrometer (SIM, *m/z* 313 for flutoprazepam and 256 for internal standard (IS)). IS: diazepam. Retention time: flutoprazepam, 10.6 min; IS, 8.6 min. [N. Barzaghi *et al.*, *Eur. J. Drug Metab. Pharmacokinet.*, 1989, *14*, 293–298].

High Performance Liquid Chromatography. Column: C_{18} (µBondapak, 10 µm, 300 × 3.9 mm i.d.). Mobile phase: potassium dihydrogen phosphate (0.01 M):acetonitrile (50:50), adjusted to pH 4.5 with orthophosphoric acid, 1.2 mL/min flow rate. UV detection (λ=235 nm). Retention times: flutoprazepam, 16 min; norflutoprazepam, 6 min; 3-hydroxynorflutoprazepam, 4 min; 3-hydroxyflutoprazepam, 12 min [I. Conti *et al.*, *Eur. J. Drug Metab. Pharamcokinet.*, 1991, *16*, 53–58].

Quantification

Gas chromatography–mass spectrometry. In serum: limit of detection 1 µg/L— N. Barzaghi *et al.*, *Eur. J. Drug Metab. Pharmacokinet.*, 1989, *14*, 293–298.

High performance liquid chromatography. In serum: limit of detection of norflutoprazepam, 3-hydroxyflutoprazepam and *N*-desalkyl-3-hydroxyflutoprazepam 2 µg/L, UV detection (λ=235 nm)—N. Barzaghi *et al.*, *Eur. J. Drug Metab. Pharmacokinet.*, 1989, *14*, 293–298. In plasma: limit of detection of flutoprazepam 25 µg/L and 10 µg/L for norflutoprazepam. UV detection (λ=235 nm)—I. Conti *et al.*, *Eur. J. Drug Metab. Pharmacokinet.*, 1991, *16*, 53–58.

Disposition in the Body. Flutoprazepam is well absorbed after oral administration and undergoes extensive hepatic metabolism, by *N*-dealkylation, to an active metabolite, norflutoprazepam. Other possible metabolites include 3-hydroxyflutoprazepam and *N*-desalkyl-3-hydroxyflutoprazepam (both found in urine), and glucuronic acid conjugates of these. Extremely low bioavailability.

Therapeutic concentration

8 young, healthy males between 20 and 28 years old were administered a single oral dose of flutoprazepam (2 mg), after overnight fasting. Peak plasma concentrations of norflutoprazepam ranged between 10.6 and 32.4 µg/L and were reached within 2 to 12 h [N. Barzaghi *et al.*, *Eur. J. Drug Metab. Pharmacokinet.*, 1989, *14*, 293–298].

Toxicity. Flutoprazepam is moderately toxic by ingestion and intraperitoneal routes.

Half-life. Norflutoprazepam, approx. 87 ± 22 h.

Dose. Usual dose of 2 to 4 mg flutoprazepam once daily.

Fluvastatin

Antihyperlipoproteinaemic

(3*R*,5*S*,6*E*)-*rel*-7-[3-(4-Fluorophenyl)-1-(1-methylethyl)-1*H*-indol-2-yl]-3,5-dihydroxy-6-heptenoic acid
$C_{24}H_{26}FNO_4$=411.5
CAS—93957-54-1

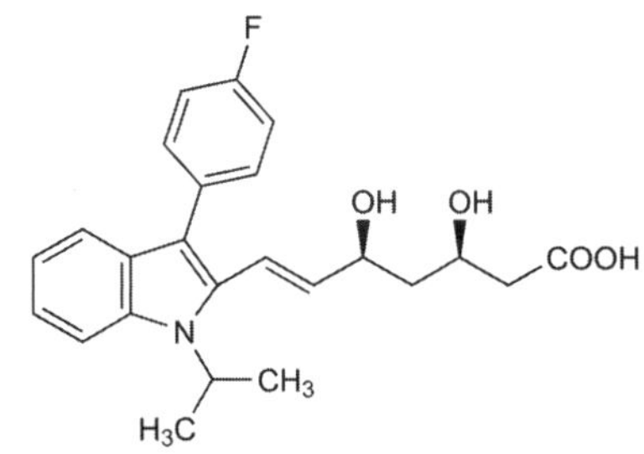

Fluvastatin Sodium
Synonyms. XU-62-320; Fluidostatin.
Proprietary names. Canef; Cranoc; Fractal; Lescol; Lipaxan; LOCOL; Lymetel; Primesin; Vastin.
$C_{24}H_{25}FNNaO_4$=433.5
CAS—93957-55-2
A white to pale yellow, hygroscopic powder, M.p. 194° to 197°. It is soluble in water, ethanol and methanol.

Dissociation Constant. pK_a 4.6.

Partition Coefficient. Log *P* (octanol/water), 4.85.

High Performance Liquid Chromatography. Column: (analytical) Rx-C8 (Zorbax, 150 × 4.6 mm i.d., 5 µm), (guard) CN (Brownlee, 15 × 3.2 mm i.d., 7 µm). Column temperature: 40°. Mobile phase: aqueous TBAF (tetrabutylammonium fluoride): phosphate buffer (0.1 M, pH 6.0):methanol (15:25:60), flow rate 1.0 mL/min. Fluorescence detection (λ_{ex}=305 nm, λ_{em}=390 nm). Retention time: 15 min. [H. Toreson and B-M. Eriksson, *J. Chromatogr. A*, 1996, *729*, 13–18].

Ultraviolet Spectrum. Aqueous acid—235, 305 nm.

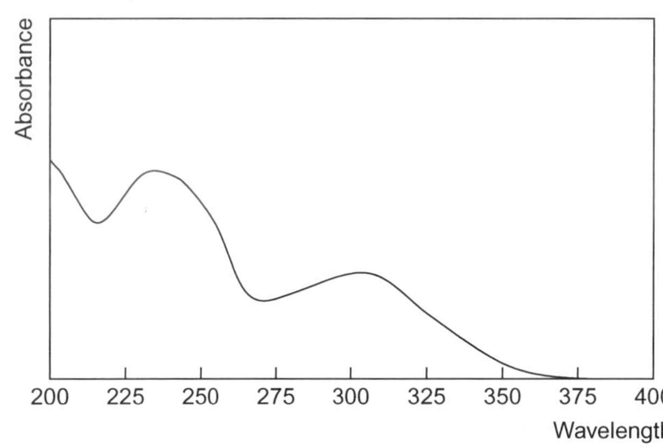

Mass Spectrum. Principal ions at *m/z* 236, 235, 264, 235, 307, 278, 321, 248, 207.

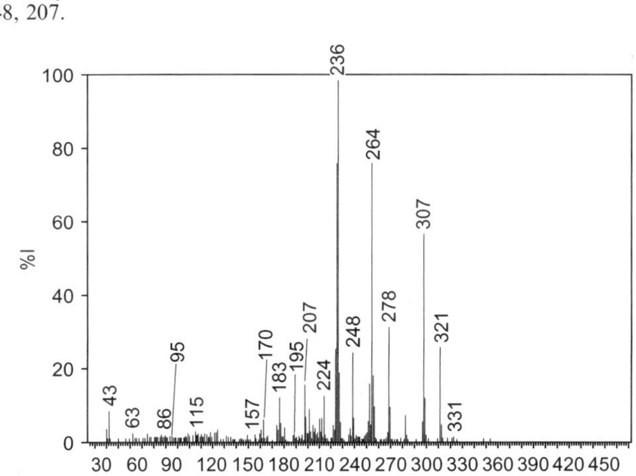

Quantification

High performance liquid chromatography. In plasma: limit of detection is 1.0 µg/L, fluorescence detection (λ_{ex}=305 nm, λ_{em}=390 nm)—G. Kalafsky and H. T. Smith, *J. Chromatogr.*, 1993, *614*, *Biomed. Appl.*, 307–313.

Disposition in the Body. Fluvastatin is rapidly and completely absorbed after oral administration and undergoes extensive first pass metabolism in the liver, the primary site of action. Hydroxylation of the indole rings at the 5- and 6- positions as well as N-dealkylation and β-oxidation of the side chains occurs. The main metabolite, *N*-desisopropylpropionic acid metabolite, is inactive. The active metabolite, fluvastatin lactone is rapidly eliminated and not in significant amounts in plasma. Excretion is mainly via faeces, approx. 90% (< 2% unchanged drug) and 6% in urine. Fluvastatin is secreted in breast milk.

Therapeutic concentration

12 healthy males, aged between 18 and 32 years, were administered a single 2 or 10 mg dose of fluvastatin sodium. Peak plasma concentrations of 5.6 ± 1.8 and 23 ± 4.5 μg/L, respectively were reached within 0.5 h. 6 healthy males, between 22 and 44 years, were administered a daily dose of 40 mg for 6 days in a multiple dose study. Peak concentrations of 438 ± 92 μg/L were observed [L. S. Francis *et al.*, *J. Clin. Pharmacol.*, 1992, *32*, 630–638].

Toxicity. There are no clinically significant adverse reactions with a 60 mg dose of fluvastatin sodium (the maximum dose used in healthy volunteers). Potential hazards to the fetus.

Bioavailability. Approx. 24%.

Half-life. 0.5 to 1.0 h, also reported as 2.3 ± 0.9 h.

Volume of distribution. Steady state, 0.35 to 0.42 L/kg, also reported as 34.4 L.

Clearance. Plasma clearance, 36.6 L/h; body clearance, 0.97 L/h/kg.

Distribution in blood. Plasma:blood ratio is 1.8.

Protein binding. > 98% bound to plasma proteins.

Dose. A usual dose of 20 to 40 mg fluvastatin sodium is taken once daily and can be increased at intervals of up to 4 weeks, to a maximum of 40 mg twice daily.

Fluvoxamine

Antidepressant

(*E*)-5-Methoxy-1-[4-(trifluoromethyl)phenyl]-1-pentanone *O*-(2-aminoethyl)oxime
$C_{15}H_{21}F_3N_2O_2$=318.3
CAS—54739-18-3

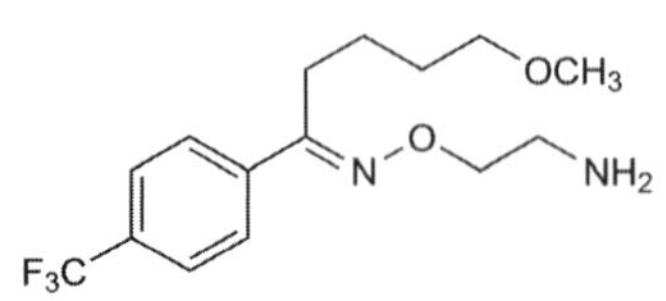

Fluvoxamine Maleate

Synonyms. DU-23000; MK-264.
Proprietary names. Avoxin; Depromel; Dumirox; Dumyrox; Faverin; Fevarin; Floxyfral; Luvoxe; Maveral; Servox.
$C_{15}H_{21}F_3N_2O_2,C_4H_4O_4$=434.4
CAS—61718-82-9
A white or off-white odourless crystalline powder. M.p. 120° to 121.5°. It is sparingly soluble in water; freely soluble in ethanol, methanol and in chloroform; practically insoluble in diethyl ether.

Dissociation Constant. pK_a 8.7 (fluvoxamine maleate)

Partition Coefficient. Log *P* (*n*-heptane/water), 0.04.

Thin-layer Chromatography. System TB—Rf 12; system TE—Rf 46; system TAE—Rf 18.

Gas Chromatography. System GA—RI 1885; system GB—RI 1911; system GM—RRT 0.295.

Column: fused-silica Optima 5 capillary (15 m × 0.25 mm i.d., 0.25 μm film thickness). Column temperature: 145°, held 0.5 min; increased to 207° at 30°/min (during 7 min); 1°/min to 221°; 30°/min to 290°. Injector temperature: 250°. Carrier gas: helium, 50 mL/min flow rate. Internal standard (IS): clovoxamine fumarate. MS detection (EI, SIM mode, *m/z*: 166). Retention time: fluvoxamine, 20.0 min; IS, clovoxamine 25.9 min [C. B. Eap *et al.*, *J. Chromatogr.*, 1996, *682*, *Biomed. Appl.*, 265–272].

High Performance Liquid Chromatography. System HX—RI 430; system HY——RI 363; system HZ—retention time 5.6 min; system HAA—retention time 15.3 min; system HAX—retention time 10.0 min; system HAY—retention time 5.9 min.

Column: (analytical) Nucleosil 100 CN (250 × 4.6 mm i.d., 5 μm); (guard) Hypersil CPS CN (20 × 4.6 mm i.d., 5 μm). Mobile phase: methanol:acetonitrile:0.01 mol/L potassium phosphate buffer, pH 6.8 (188:578:235), 1.5 mL/min flow rate. IS: oxaprotiline. UV detection (λ=214 nm). Retention time: fluvoxamine, 6.2 min; IS, 10.2 min [S. Härtter *et al.*, *Clin. Chem.*, 1992, *38*, 2082–2086].

Column: (analytical) Supelcosil LC-18-DB (250 × 4.6 mm i.d., 5 μm); (guard) NewGuard RP-8 (15 × 3.2 mm, 7 μm). Mobile phase: acetonitrile:potassium phosphate (10 mM), pH 7.2 (85:15). IS: nortriptyline hydrochloride. Fluorescence detection. Retention time: fluvoxamine, 5.3 min; IS, 9.7 min [R. H. Pullen and A. A. Fatmi, *J. Chromatogr.*, 1992, *574*, *Biomed. Appl.*, *112*, 101–107].

Ultraviolet Spectrum. Aqueous acid—254 nm (A_1^1=0.310).

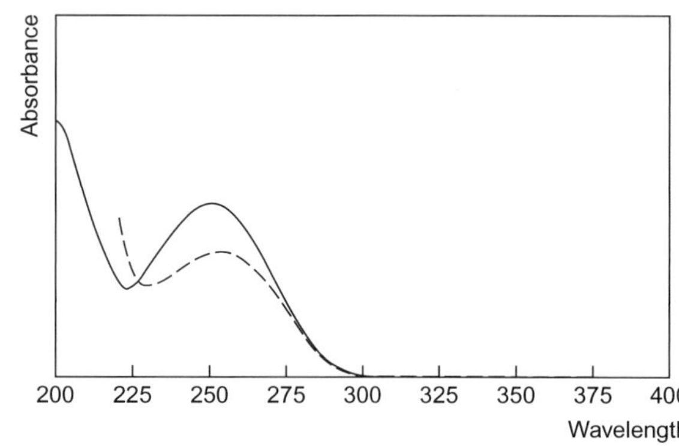

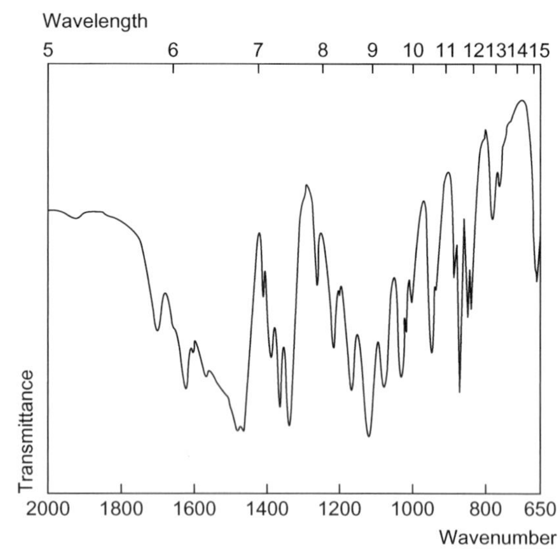

Mass Spectrum. Principal ions at *m/z* 187, 71, 45, 276, 43, 172, 145, 200.

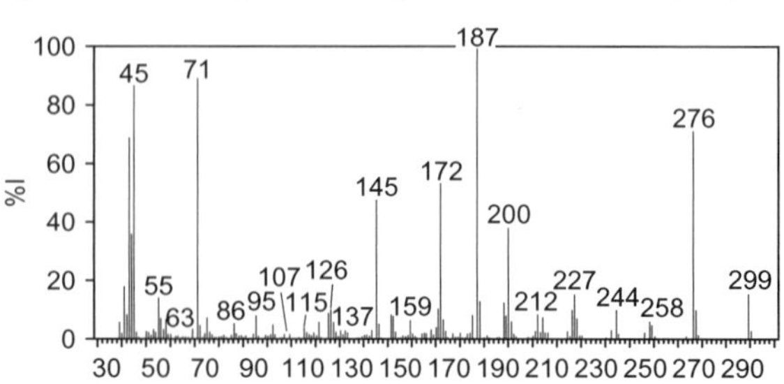

Quantification

Thin-layer chromatography. In plasma: limit of detection < 2 μg/L, fluorescence detection—C. Schweitzer *et al.*, *J. Chromatogr.*, 1986, *382*, *Biomed. Appl.*, *55*, 405–411.

Gas chromatography–mass spectrometry. In plasma: limit of quantification 2 µg/L—C. B. Eap *et al.*, *J. Chromatogr.*, 1996, *682*, *Biomed. Appl.*, 265–272.

High performance liquid chromatography. In plasma: limit of quantification 10 µg/L, fluorescence detection—R. H. Pullen and A. A. Fatmi, *J. Chromatogr.*, 1992, *574*, *Biomed. Appl.*, *112*, 101–107. In plasma: limit of detection 25 µg/L, UV detection (λ=215 nm)—J. P. Foglia *et al.*, *J. Chromatogr.*, 1989, *495*, *Biomed. Appl.*, *87*, 295–302. In plasma: limit of detection 0.5 µg/L, UV detection (λ=254 nm)—V. Van der Meersch-Mougeot and B. Diquet, *J. Chromatogr.*, 1991, *567*; *Biomed. Appl.*, *105*, 441–449. In plasma: limit of detection < 0.5 µg/L, fluorescence detection—C. Schweitzer *et al.*, *J. Chromatogr.*, 1986, *382*; *Biomed. Appl.*, *55*, 405–411. In plasma: limit of detection 10 µg/L, UV detection—S. Härtter *et al.*, *Clin. Chem.*, 1992, *38*, 2082–2086.

Disposition in the Body. Fluvoxamine is readily and completely absorbed after oral administration with peak plasma concentrations occurring after about 2 to 8 h (prolonged with enteric-coated tablets to 4 to 12 h). However, it undergoes significant first-pass metabolism and bioavailability is about 53%. It is widely distributed. Fluvoxamine undergoes extensive metabolism in the liver mainly by oxidative deamination, oxidative demethylation and N-acetylation to produce a number of inactive metabolites. The parent and its metabolites (11 in total detected) have been recovered in urine; less than 4% as the parent drug. Fluvoxamine appears to inhibit the following cytochrome P450 isoenzymes; 1A2, 2C9, 3A4. It is distributed into breast milk.

Therapeutic concentration. The therapeutic serum concentration is 50 to 250 µg/L.

6 healthy, young volunteers, 25 to 31 years old, and 13 elderly individuals, aged 63 to 77 years, were administered single and multiple doses (twice daily) of 50 mg fluvoxamine, after an overnight fast. The mean plasma concentration after the single dose was 30 µg/L (range 18 to 48 µg/L) for the younger individuals and a concentration of 93 (range 32 to 300) µg/L was observed for the multiple dosing regimen. These concentrations were observed at 6 (4 to 8) h and 5 (0 to 12) h, respectively. For the elderly individuals, after multiple dosing for 31 days, the mean concentration was 62 (range 32 to 225) µg/L at 5 h (range 4 to 12) [M. H. De Vries *et al.*, *Ther. Drug Monit.*, 1992, *14*, 493–498].

Toxicity. 12 g of fluvoxamine maleate has been ingested with no sequelae.

A 74-year-old female who had ingested 3 g fluvoxamine and 250 mg of temazepam was admitted to hospital unconscious. She remained unconscious for 5 days. On admission serum-fluvoxamine concentration was 160 µg/L. This increased to more than 1400 µg/L on day 3 [A. K. Banerjee, *Br. Med. J.* (Clinical research ed.), 1988, *296*, 1774].

Half-life. Plasma half-life, 17 to 22 h, after repeated dosing.

Volume of distribution. 25 L/kg.

Clearance. Plasma clearance, 3 L/min (oral); 1.5 L/min (intravenous).

Protein binding. In plasma, 77%, mostly to albumin.

Note. For a review of fluvoxamine, see P. Benfield and A. Ward, *Drugs*, 1986, *32*, 313–334 (correction *Drugs*, *33* (no. 2 contents page)). For a review of the pharmacokinetics of fluvoxamine, see E. Perucca *et al.*, *Clin. Pharmacokinet.*, 1994, *27*, 175–190 and J. van Harten, *Clin. Pharmacokinet.*, 1995, *29*, (*Suppl 1*), 1–9. For reviews of the pharmacokinetics of selective serotonin reuptake inhibitors, see M. L. Catterson and S. H. Preskorn, *Pharmacol. Toxicol.*, 1996, *78*, 203–208, S. H. Preskorn, *Clin. Pharmacokinet.*, 1997, *32*, (*Suppl.*), 1–21 and P. Baumann, *Clin. Pharmacokinet.*, 1996, *31*, 444–469.

Dose. 100 to 300 mg daily of fluvoxamine maleate.

Folic Acid

Vitamin

Synonyms. Folacin; Folinsyre; Pteroylglutamic Acid; Pteroylmonoglutamic Acid.
Proprietary names. Acfol; Endofolin; Folacin; Folarell; Folasic; Fol-Asmedic; Folatine; Folavit; Folicare; Foldine; Folettes; Folsan; Folverlan; Folvite; Lafol; Lexpec; Megafol; Novo-Folacid; Preconceive; RubieFol; Specifoldine. It is an ingredient of many proprietary preparations—see Martindale, *The complete drug reference*, 33rd Edn.

N-[4-[[(2-Amino-1,4-dihydro-4-oxo-6-pteridinyl)methyl]amino]benzoyl]-L-glutamic acid
$C_{19}H_{19}N_7O_6$=441.4
CAS—59-30-3

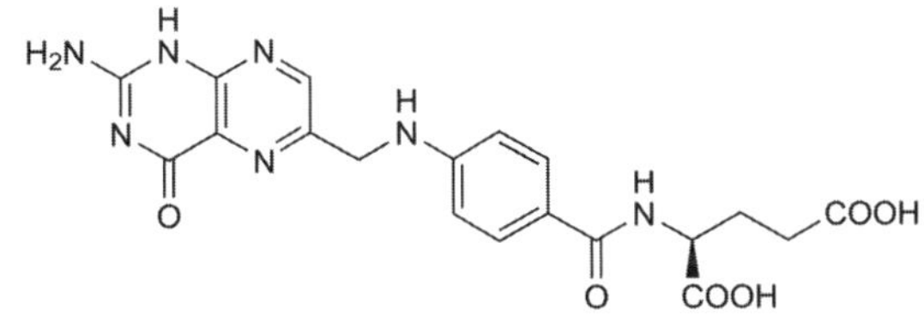

A yellow to orange microcrystalline powder.
Very slightly soluble in cold water; relatively soluble in acetic acid, phenol, and pyridine; slightly soluble in methanol, appreciably less soluble in ethanol and butanol; insoluble in acetone, benzene, chloroform, and ether. Soluble in dilute solutions of alkali hydroxides and carbonates, yielding a clear orange-brown solution; soluble in hydrochloric acid and in sulfuric acid, yielding very pale yellow solutions. Solutions are inactivated by UV light; alkaline solutions are sensitive to oxidation and acid solutions are sensitive to heat.

Dissociation Constant. pK_a 4.7, 6.8, 9.0 (30°).

Partition Coefficient. Log *P* (octanol/water), −2.8.

High Performance Liquid Chromatography. System HZ—Retention time, 1.5 min (folate); system HAA—Retention time, 3.6 min.

Ultraviolet Spectrum. Aqueous alkali—256 (A^1_1=549a), 283 nm (A^1_1=539a).

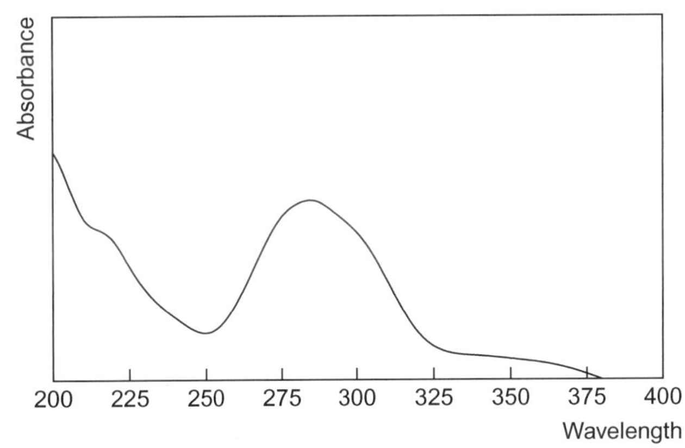

Infra-red Spectrum. Principal peaks at wavenumbers 1686, 1602, 1636, 1191, 1567, 1225 cm^{-1} (KBr disk).

Dose. 2.5 to 20 mg daily.

Fomepizole

Alcohol Dehydrogenase Inhibitor

Synonym. 4-MP
Proprietary name. Antizol
4-Methyl-1*H*-pyrazole
$C_4H_6N_2$=82.1
CAS—7554-65-6

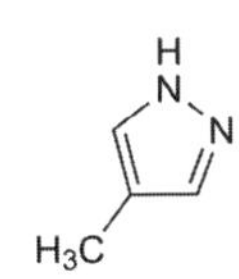

M.p. 15.5° to 18.5°. It is soluble in water and alcohol.

Dissociation Constant. pK_a 2.91.

Partition Coefficient. Log *P* (octanol/water), 0.61.

Gas Chromatography. Column: 5% carbowax (20 M) and 2% potassium hydroxide on 80 to 100 mesh Chromosorb G (HP-5) (1.22 m × 2 mm i.d.). Column, injector and detector temperature: 135°, 250° and 300°, respectively. Carrier gas: helium, 30 mL/min flow rate. Detection: nitrogen–phosphorus. Internal standard (IS): 3-methylpyrazole. Retention time: fomepizole, 10 min; IS, 8 min [R. Achari and M. Mayersohn, *J. Pharm. Sci.*, 1984, *73(5)*, 690–692].

High Performance Liquid Chromatography. Column: 100 RP-18 (Lichrospher, 125 × 4 mm i.d., 5 μm) with RP-select B (Lichrospher 60, 4 × 4 mm, 5 μm) precolumn. Column temperature: 40°. Mobile phase: acetonitrile:potassium phosphate buffer (5 mM, pH 6) (7.5:92.5), 1.5 mL/min flow rate. UV detection (λ=220 nm). IS: 3-methylpyrazole. Retention time: fomepizole, 4.9 min; IS, 4.1 min [E. Jobard *et al.*, *J. Chromatogr. B, Biomed. Sci. Appl.*, 1997, *695*, 444–447].

Ultraviolet Spectrum. Ethanol—220 nm; acid (6 M hydrochloric acid)—226 nm.

Mass Spectrum. Principal ions at *m/z* 82, 81, 54, 28, 52, 55, 53, 51.

Quantification

Gas chromatography. In plasma (and urine): limit of detection 0.1 mg/L and limit of quantification 0.025 mg/L—R. Achari and M. Mayersohn, *J. Pharm. Sci.*, 1984, *73(5)*, 690–692.

High performance liquid chromatography. In plasma: limit of quantification 0.3 mg/L—E. Jobard *et al.*, *J. Chromatogr. B Biomed. Sci. Appl.*, 1997, *695*, 444–447.

Disposition in the Body. Fomepizole is rapidly distributed to total body water. It is metabolised to the primary metabolite, 4-carboxypyrazole (80 to 85% of the dose), 4-hydroxymethylpyrazole and the *N*-glucuronide conjugates of these. Fomepizole is mainly eliminated via urine with 1 to 3.5% as the unchanged drug.

Therapeutic concentration

15 healthy male volunteers, aged between 20 and 40 years, were administered 10, 20, 50 and 100 mg/kg body weight doses. Mean peak plasma concentrations of 132, 326, 759 and 1425 μmol/L were reached for the doses, respectively. All peaks were observed between 0.5 and 2 h. Each mg/kg increase in dose resulted in an increase of 13 to 16 mg/L to the peak plasma concentration [D. Jacobsen *et al.*, *Eur. J. Clin. Pharmacol.*, 1989, *37(6)*, 599–604].

Half-life. Approx. 5.2 h.

Volume of distribution. 0.6 to 0.7 L/kg.

Protein binding. Negligible.

Dose. The usual dose is 5 to 15 mg/kg body weight every 12 h.

Formaldehyde

Disinfectant

Synonyms. Formic Aldehyde; Methanal; Methylene Oxide; Oxomethane.
CH_2O=30.0
A colourless inflammable gas.
Very soluble in water; soluble in ethanol and ether.

Formaldehyde Solution

Synonyms. Formalin; Formol.
Proprietary names. Diformil; Emoform; Formadon; Formitrol; Lazerformaldehyde; Lysoform; Veracur.
CAS—50-00-0
An aqueous solution containing 34 to 38% w/w of CH_2O, with methanol as a stabilising agent.
A colourless liquid. Mass per mL about 1.08 g.
Miscible with water, ethanol, and acetone; immiscible with chloroform and ether.

Dissociation Constant. pK_a 13.3 (25°).

Partition Coefficient. Log *P* (octanol/water), 0.4.

Colour Tests. Chromotropic Acid—red.
Add a little resorcinol to a solution containing formaldehyde, shake, then carefully add sulfuric acid to form a layer under the solution—red-violet ring at the junction of the two layers.

Mass Spectrum. Principal ions at *m/z* 29, 30, 28, 31, 32, -, -, -.

Quantification

High performance liquid chromatography. In plasma: limit of detection 0.46 mg/L, fluorescence detection—W. Luo *et al.*, *J. Chromatogr. B Biomed. Sci. Appl.*, 2001, *753*, 253–257.

Disposition in the Body. Rapidly metabolised in the body tissues to formic acid and methanol, especially in the liver and erythrocytes; the formic acid may then be excreted in the urine as formates, or metabolised to labile methyl groups.
Formaldehyde is a metabolite of methanol.

Toxicity. Formaldehyde is very irritant to mucous membranes and inhalation of the vapour causes intense irritation of the respiratory tract which may lead to bronchitis and pneumonia. Atmospheric concentrations of 2 to 3 ppm may cause mild irritation of the mucous membranes and exposure to concentrations of 10 to 20 ppm for only a few minutes may cause moderate to severe irritation. Adverse effects have been reported as a result of release of formaldehyde fumes from synthetic foam insulation. Few fatalities have been recorded but 30 mL of Formaldehyde Solution may be fatal in an adult. The maximum permissible atmospheric concentration is 2 ppm or 3 mg/m^3.

In a fatality due to the ingestion of 120 mL of Formaldehyde Solution, the following blood concentrations were reported 0.5 h after ingestion: formic acid 500 mg/L, formaldehyde 4.8 mg/L, methanol 420 mg/L; after 17 h they had declined to 300, 2 and 70 mg/L respectively; death occurred approximately 28 h after ingestion [J. T. Eells *et al.*, *J. Am. Med. Assoc.*, 1981, *246*, 1237–1238.]

In 2 fatalities occurring 3 and 8 weeks after the ingestion of an unknown amount of formaldehyde, formic acid plasma levels of 280 and 210 mg/L were reported on admission to hospital. In the second case formic acid levels declined to 70 mg/L 6 h after admission [C. Koppel *et al.*, *Intensive Care Med.*, 1990, *16*, 212–214.]

A 58-year-old male died 12 h after ingesting approximately 4 ounces of a formaldehyde solution in a suicide attempt. The plasma levels of formaldehyde, formate, and methanol 1.5 h after ingestion were, respectively, 0.16, 16.0, and 5.8 mmol/L; at 5.5 h post ingestion these levels were 0.32, 29.6, and 7.4 mmol/L. After this time, formaldehyde levels declined and methanol levels continued to increase, reaching 0.14 and 10.6 mmol/L at 12 h post ingestion [K. K. Burkhart *et al.*, *Vet. Hum. Toxicol.*, 1990, *32*, 135–137.]

Formestane

Antineoplastic Aromatase Inhibitor

Synonyms. BRN 1889793; CCRIS 7483; CGP-32349: 4-OHA; 4-OHAD.
Proprietary names. Lentare; Lentaron.
4-Hydroxyandrost-4-ene-3,17-dione
$C_{19}H_{26}O_3$=302.4
CAS—566-48-3

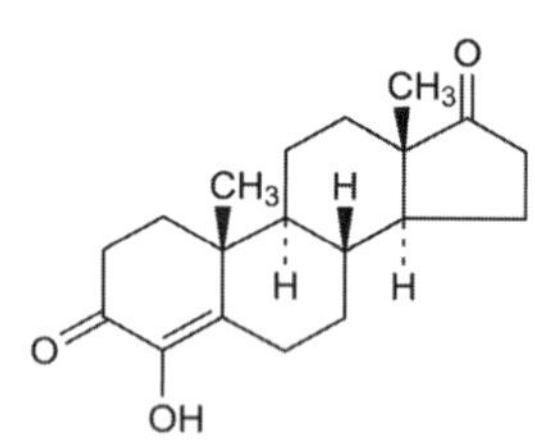

A white to slightly yellow lyophilised solid, which is poorly soluble in aqueous media. Needles from aqueous methanol, M.p. 199° to 202°; also reported as crystals from ethyl acetate, M.p. 203.5° to 206°.

Thin-layer Chromatography. Plate: kiesel gel 60 F_{254} (Merck 5714, 0.2 mm layer). Mobile phase (A): chloroform:methanol:water (6:4:1); (B): chloroform:methanol (19:1). Rf (formestane glucuronide metabolite) 0.5 (mobile phase (A)) and 0.71 (mobile phase (B)) [P. E. Goss *et al.*, *J. Steroid Biochem.*, 1986, *24(2)*, 619–622].

Gas Chromatography. Column: 3% OV-225 on Supelcoport, 80 to 100 mesh (1.5 m × 2 mm), Pyrex glass. Column temperature: 275°. Injector and detector temperatures: 250° and 350°, respectively. Carrier gas: nitrogen, flow rate 40 mL/min. IS: 17α-ethinylestradiol. Detection: electron capture, ^{63}Ni. Retention time(s): 4-OHA PFB-derivative, 3 min; IS, 2 min [P. H. Degen and W. Schneider, *J. Chromatogr.*, 1991, *565*; *Biomed. Appl.*, 67–73].

High Performance Liquid Chromatography. Column: C_{18} (Supelco, 3 µm, 250 × 2.1 mm i.d.). Mobile phase: acetonitrile (20%) in NH_4OAc (10 mM), 5 min, up to 100% acetonitrile in 15 min, 0.2 mL/min flow rate. MS–MS detection. Retention time(s): formestane glucuronide, 10.6 min; sulfate, 12.0 min [G. K. Poon *et al.*, *Drug Metab. Dispos.*, 1992, *20*, 941–947.]

Column: ODS (APEX II, 150 × 4.6 mm i.d., 5 µm). Mobile phase: methanol:water (60:40) containing formic acid (0.1%), flow rate 1.2 mL/min. MS detection. Retention time: formestane, 8.1 min [G. K. Poon *et al.*, *J. Chromatogr.*, 1992, *576 Biomed. Appl.*, 235–244].

Ultraviolet Spectrum. Ethanol—278 nm.

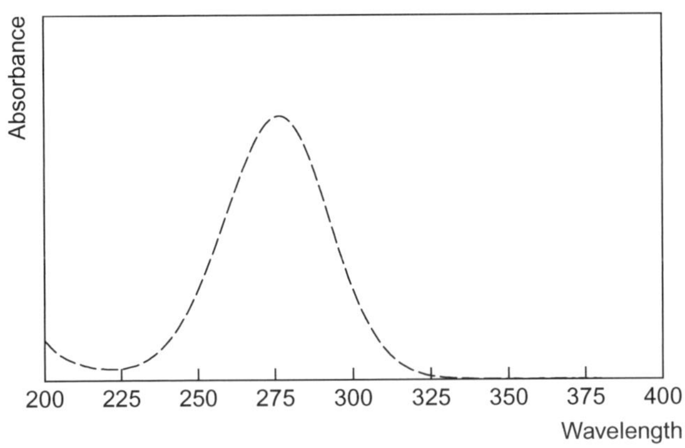

Quantification

Gas chromatography. In plasma: limit of detection 0.02 nmol per sample (6 ng). ECD—P. H. Degen and W. Schneider, *J. Chromatogr.*, 1991, *565 Biomed. Appl.*, 67–73.

Gas chromatography–mass spectrometry. In plasma: limit of detection 65 pg—A. Guerna *et al.*, *J. Steroid Biochem.*, 1989, *32(5)*, 699–702.

Disposition in the Body. After intramuscular injection, there is a slow release of the active drug into systemic circulation, with systemic uptake of 20 to 25% of the dose, taking place over 14 days. Formestane is metabolised in the liver by conjugation into an inactive glucuronide metabolite and, also, by sulfation. Metabolites include 4-hydroxytestosterone (4-OHT), 3-*β*-hydroxy-5-*α*-androstan-4,17-dione (3-*α*-OHA)-sulfate, 4-hydroxyandrosta-4,6-diene-3,17-dione and 3-*α*-17-dihydroxy-5-*β*-androstan-4-one (3,17-OHA)-sulfate. Less than 1% of the dose is detected in urine unchanged.

Therapeutic concentration

Healthy volunteers were administered with single oral doses of formestane, 250 and 500 mg. Peak plasma concentrations were reached within 0.5 to 4 h and the drug was detected in serum 5 min after administration. Plasma levels peaked at 79.2 and 119.7 µg/L, respectively [M. Doursett *et al.*, *Eur. J. Cancer*, 1992, 415–420.]

Toxicity. Clinical trials with doses up to 1000 mg/week only showed an increase in the frequency of the adverse reactions, for example rash, hot flushes, nausea, sore throat and vomiting.

Half-life. 5 to 6 days.

Protein binding. About 85%.

Dose. Usual dose, 250 mg every two weeks.

Formic Acid

Synonym. Aminic Acid
Proprietary names. It is an ingredient of Aciforin, Berggeist, Discmigon, Euphon, Fortalis, Rubistenol, Rubjovit, and Step 2.
CH_2O_2=46.0
CAS—64-18-6

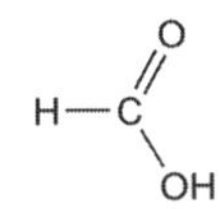

A colourless liquid containing about 25% w/w of CH_2O_2. Mass per mL about 1.05 g. B.p. about 101°.
Miscible with water, acetone, ethyl acetate, ethanol, and ether; partially soluble in benzene, toluene, and xylenes.

Dissociation Constant. pK_a 3.8 (25°).

Partition Coefficient. Log *P* (octanol/water), −0.5.

Colour Test. Warm with sulfuric acid in a tube—carbon monoxide is evolved; the gas can be ignited at the mouth of the tube and burns with a blue flame.

Mass Spectrum. Principal ions at *m/z* 29, 46, 45, 28, 44, 30, 47, -.

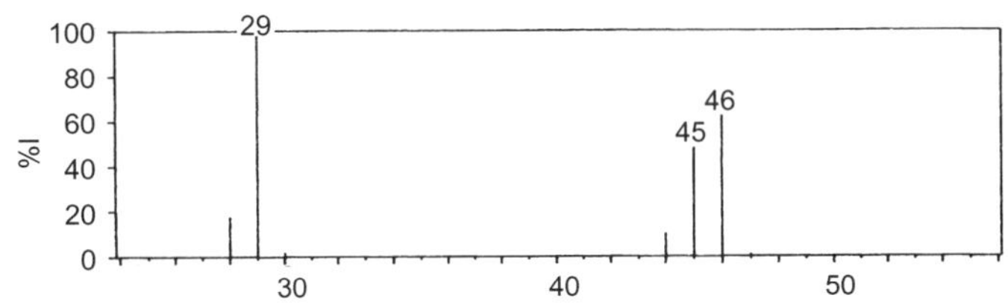

Quantification

Ultraviolet spectrophotometry. In urine: determination at 340 nm before and after treatment with formate dehydrogenase, limit of detection 500 µg/L—G. Triebig and K. H. Schaller, *Clinica Chim. Acta*, 1980, *108*, 355–360.

Gas chromatography. In blood or urine: head-space analysis, limit of detection 5 mg/L, FID—C. Abolin *et al.*, *Biochem. Med.*, 1980, *15*, 209–218.

Disposition in the Body. Formic acid is an intermediate in normal metabolism; when administered it probably takes part in the metabolism of 1-carbon compounds to produce methyl groups; it is excreted in the urine and also undergoes oxidation to carbon dioxide. Together with formaldehyde, it is a metabolite of methanol and the two are probably mainly responsible for the effect of methanol on vision.

Formic acid concentrations of 2 to 30 mg/L (mean 13) were reported in the urine of normal subjects [G. Triebig and K. H. Schaller, *Clinica Chim. Acta*, 1980, *108*, 355–360.]

Toxicity. The minimum lethal dose is about 30 mL. Formic acid is dangerously caustic to the skin. The maximum permissible atmospheric concentration is 5 ppm or 9 mg/m^3; the estimated acceptable daily intake is up to 3 mg/kg.

Ingestion of more than 45 g was fatal in 14 out of 16 subjects [D. B. Jefferys and H. M. Wiseman, *Hum. Toxicol.*, 1983, *2*, 423.]

In a fatality involving ingestion of formic acid, the blood concentration on admission was 348 mg/L [A. G. Verstraete *et al.*, *Am. J. Emerg. Med.*, 1989, *7*, 286–290.]

In a fatality due to intentional ingestion of a decalcifying agent containing formic acid, the blood concentration on admission to hospital was 370.3 mg/L and declined to 13.9 mg/L after 6.5 h of haemodialysis. Postmortem concentrations were: heart blood 855.4 mg/L, gastric contents 2712 mg/L, haemorrhagic fluid from abdominal cavity 1128 mg/L, bile 3051 mg/L, contents of small intestine 2664 mg/L, liver 442.7 µg/g, kidney 542.3 g/g [F. Westphal *et al.*, *Int. J. Legal Med.*, 2001, *114*, 181–185.]

Note. Formic acid is the principal ingredient (about 60%) of several proprietary preparations used for descaling kettles.

Formoterol

Anti-asthmatic

Synonym. Eformoterol
rel-N-[2-Hydroxy-5-[(1*R*)-1-hydroxy-2-[[(1*R*)-2-(4-methoxyphenyl)-1-methylethyl]amino]ethyl]phenyl]formamide
$C_{19}H_{24}N_2O_4$=344.4

CAS 73573-87-2

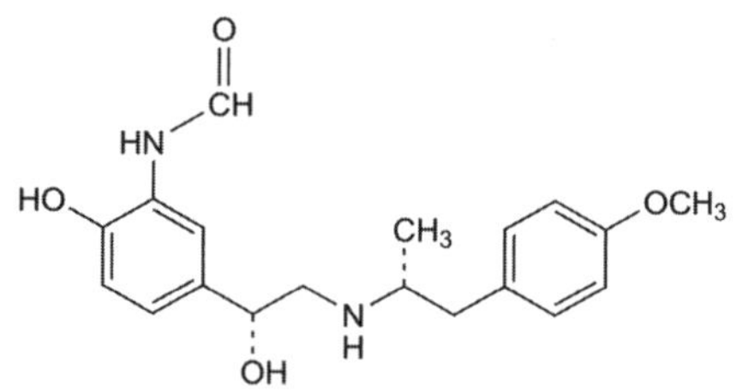

Formoterol Fumarate Dihydrate
Synonyms. Eformoterol Fumerate; BD-40A; CGP-25827A.
Proprietary names. Atock; Eolus; Foradil; Foradile; Neblik; Oxis; Oxeze.
$(C_{19}H_{24}N_2O_4)_2.C_4H_4O_4.2H_2O$=804.9
CAS—43229-80-7
Crystals from 95% isopropyl alcohol. M.p. 138° to 140°.

Dissociation Constant. pKa, 7.82; 8.53.

Partition Coefficient. Log *P* (octanol/pH 7), 0.10; (octanol/pH7.4), 0.4.

High Performance Liquid Chromatography. Column: C_8 (Alltech, 100 × 4.6 mm i.d., 3 µm), C_8 (1 cm, 5 µm) pre-column. Mobile phase: citrate buffer (0.031 M sodium acetate, 0.012 M citric acid, 0.033 M sodium hydroxide, pH 6.0):methanol (61.5:38.5), 1 mL/min flow rate. Internal standard (IS): bromoformoterol. Electrochemical detection. Retention time: formoterol, 5.6 min; IS, 10.0 min [B. T. J. van den Berg *et al., Ther. Drug Monit.*, 1994, *16*, 196–199].

Ultraviolet Spectrum. Aqueous acid—212, 283 nm.

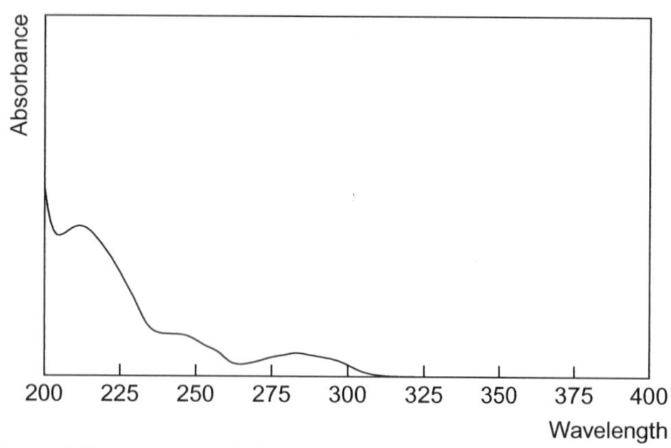

Infra-red Spectrum. Principal peaks at wavenumbers 1690, 1515, 1370, 1250 cm^{-1}.

Mass Spectrum. (Formoterol glucuronide) Principal ions at *m/z* 122, 119, 77, 78, 91, 107, 65, 63.

Quantification
Gas chromatography–mass spectrometry. In urine: limit of detection 5 µg/L—H. Kamimura *et al., J. Chromatogr.*, 1982, *229*, 337–345.

High performance liquid chromatography. In plasma: limit of detection is 0.02 µg/L, electrochemical detection—B. T. J. van der Berg *et al., Ther. Drug Monit.*, 1994, *16*, 196–199. In plasma: limit of detection is 0.004 µg/L, electrochemical detection—J. Campestrini *et al., J Chromatogr. B Biomed. Sci. Appl.*, 1997, *704*, 221–229.

Disposition in the Body. After inhalation of formoterol, there is rapid absorption. Metabolism is mainly via direct glucuronidation and O-demethylation, and this is the main route of elimination. Formoterol is also sulfated to some extent to a sulfate conjugate. 8 to 13% of an oral dose is excreted unmetabolised in urine (20% for intravenous administration and 24% for an inhaled dose). 62% of a total dose is recovered in urine with 24% as faeces.

Therapeutic concentration
12 healthy volunteers (8 male and 4 female) were administered a single 120 µg dose of formoterol fumarate (by inhalation). In 9 of the volunteers, peak plasma concentrations were reached within 5 min after inhalation, with a mean peak of 266 pmol/L [J. B. Lecaillon *et al., Eur. J. Clin. Pharmacol.*, 1999, *55*, 131–138].

Toxicity. Possible side effects include tremors, headaches, palpitations, tachycardia, hypotension and hyperglycaemia. It is a poison by intraperitoneal and intravenous routes and moderately toxic by ingestion and subcutaneous routes.

Half-life. Elimination half-life is approx. 10 h.

Protein binding. Plasma protein binding is approx. 50%.

Dose. A usual dose of formoterol fumarate is 12 or 24 µg twice daily (inhalation or aerosol), or 80 µg twice daily by mouth.

Foscarnet Sodium

Antiviral

Synonyms. A-29622; EHB-776; Phosphonatoformate Trisodium; Phosphonoformate Trisodium; Trisodium Carboxyphosphate.
Proprietary Names. Foscavir; Triapten; Virudin.
Dihydroxyphosphinecarboxylic acid oxide trisodium salt
CNa_3O_5P=192.0
CAS—63585-09-1; 34156-56-4 (hexahydrate)

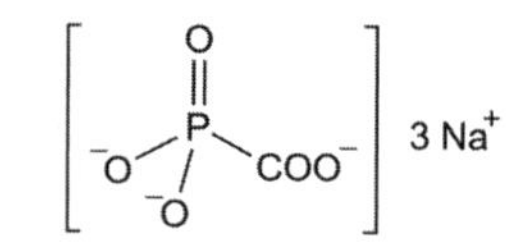

A white crystalline powder. M.p. > 25° (hexahydrate). It is soluble in water; practically insoluble in alcohol.

Dissociation Constant. pK_a 0.5, 3.4, 7.3.

High Performance Liquid Chromatography. Column: Kromasil 100 C_{18} (150 × 4.6 mm i.d., 5 µm), polyether ether ketone (PEEK) column. Mobile phase: methanol:disodium phosphate buffer (40 mM, pH 7.6, containing 0.25 mM tetrahexylammonium sulfate) ($THAHO_4$) (25:75), 1.0 mL/min flow rate. Amperometric detection (glassy carbon at + 1.125 V). Retention time: 6.06 min. [B. B. Ba *et al., J. Chromatogr. B, Biomed. Sci. Appl.*, 1999, *724*, 127–136].

Column: C_{18} (Novapak, 4 µm). Mobile phase: methanol containing 0.001 M $THAHO_4$ (ion pairing agent):phosphate buffer (60 mM, pH 5.8) (30:70), also 0.0002 M pyrophosphoric acid was added and final pH adjusted to 5.8, 0.7 mL/min flow rate. Electrochemical detection. Internal standard (IS): hydrochlorothiazide. Retention time: foscarnet sodium, 12.0 min; IS, 18.9 min [M. K. Hassanzadeh *et al., J. Chromatogr.*, 1990, *525, Biomed. Appl., 90*, 133–140].

Ultraviolet Spectrum. Aqueous acid—236 nm.

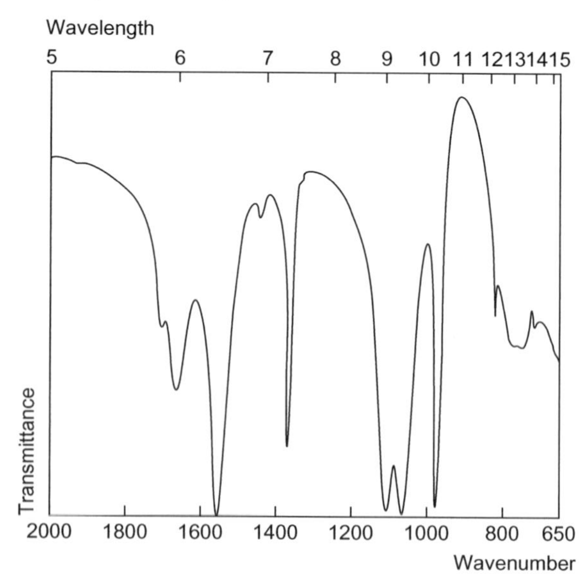

Quantification
High performance liquid chromatography. In plasma or urine: limit of quantification, 0.033 mg/L, electrochemical detection—M. K. Hassanzadeh *et al., J. Chromatogr.*, 1990, *525, Biomed. Appl., 90*, 133–140. In serum:

limit of quantification, 0.015 mg/L, electrochemical detection—B. B. Ba *et al.*, *J. Chromatogr., Biomed. Sci. Appl.*, 1999, *724*, 127–136.

Note. For a review of chromatographic methods for the determination of antivirals in biological fluids see C. M. Riley *et al.*, *J. Chromatogr.*, 1990, *531, Biomed. Appl.*, *96*, 295–368.

Disposition in the Body. The pharmacokinetics of foscarnet are complicated by the high incidence of renal function impairment during therapy and by the deposition and subsequent gradual release of foscarnet from bone. The estimation of half-life thus depends on duration of foscarnet therapy. Foscarnet is poorly absorbed after oral administration and not metabolised to a great extent. It crosses the blood–brain barrier in variable amounts; CSF concentrations of between 0 and 300% of plasma concentrations have been reported. The drug is excreted mostly unchanged in the urine by glomerular filtration and tubular secretion, and is also cleared by uptake into bones (14 to 22%). It is removed by haemodialysis.

Therapeutic concentration

Administration of 90 mg/kg (infused over 2 h) every 12 h to 10 patients, with AIDS and disease of the GI tract (aged between 34 and 45 years), produced mean peak plasma concentrations of 0.621 mg/L on day 1 and 0.687 mg/L at steady state (after 17 to 21 days) at the end of the infusion [D. T. Dieterich *et al.*, *Antimicrob. Agents Chemother.*, 1997, *41*, 1226–1230].

Administration of 60 mg/kg (infused over 2 h) every 8 h to 8 AIDS patients (aged between 25 and 43 years, mean 34) for 14 days, produced mean peak and trough concentrations of 0.509 mg/L (range 0.306 to 0.876) and 0.098 mg/L (0.062 to 0.147 mg/L), respectively, on day 3 and 0.495 (range 0.272 to 0.699) mg/L and 0.126 (0.057 to 0.225) mg/L, respectively, on day 14 [F. Aweeka *et al.*, *Antimicrob. Agents Chemother.*, 1989, *33*, 742–745].

Toxicity. Renal impairment is the major toxicity. Seizures related to alterations in plasma minerals and electrolytes have also been associated with foscarnet therapy.

Overdosing has been reported in 33 patients with the highest approx. 10 times the prescribed dose. 28 of these experienced adverse effects, 5 had no ill effects connected with overdose and 4 died owing to respiratory and cardiac arrest with organ failure [Data as supplied by Astra Pharmaceuticals Limited].

Half-life. Plasma half-life, 4.5 h.

Volume of distribution. 0.3L to 0.74 L/kg.

Clearance. Plasma clearance, 6 to 13 L/h/1.73 m^2; 1.7 to 1.9 mL/min/kg (101 to 106 mL/min/1.73 m^2).

Protein binding. In plasma, 14 to 17%.

Note. For reviews of foscarnet see P. Chrisp and S. P. Clissold, *Drugs*, 1991, *41*, 104–129 and A. J. Wagstaff and H. M. Bryson, *Drugs*, 1994, *48*, 199–226.

Dose. The usual dose is 60 mg/kg intravenously (over 1 to 2 h) every 8 h for 2 to 3 weeks, followed by 60 to 120 mg/kg daily.

Fosinopril

ACE inhibitor/Antihypertensive

Synonym. Fosenopril

(4*S*)-4-Cyclohexyl-1-[[(*R*)-[(1*S*)-2-methyl-1-(1-oxopropoxy)-propoxy](4-phenylbutyl)phosphinyl]acetyl]-L-proline

$C_{30}H_{46}NO_7P$=563.7

CAS—98048-97-6

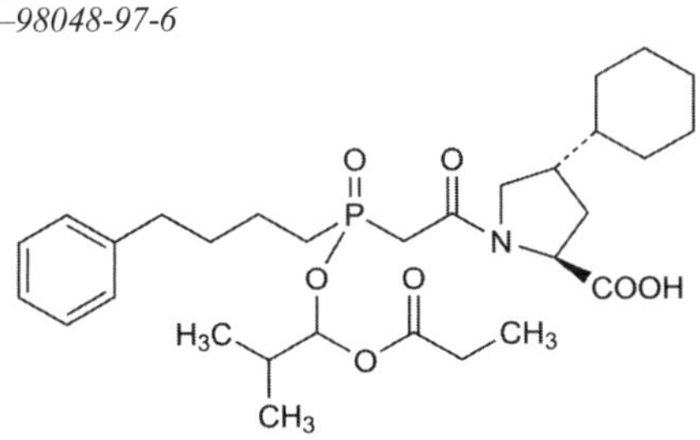

Fosinopril Sodium

Synonyms. Fosenopril Sodium; SQ-28555.

Proprietary names. Acecor; Dynacil; Eliten; Fosinorm; Fosipres; Fositens; Fozitec; Hiperlix; Monopril; New Ace; Secorvas; Staril; Tensogard; Tenso Stop; Tensozide.

$C_{30}H_{45}NNaO_7P$=585.6

CAS—88889-14-9

A white to off white crystalline powder. It is soluble in water (100 g/L), methanol and ethanol; slightly soluble in hexane.

Fosinopril Diacid

Synonym. SQ-27519

$C_{23}H_{34}NO_5P$=435.5

M.p. 149° to 153°.

Partition Coefficient. Log *P* (octanol/water), 6.61.

High Performance Liquid Chromatography. Column: alkylphenyl (300 × 4.0 mm i.d., 10 μm). Mobile phase: methanol:phosphoric acid (0.2%) (72:28), 2 mL/min flow rate. UV detection (λ=215 nm). Retention time: 10.5 min [R. Lozano *et al.*, *J. Pharm. Biomed. Anal.*, 1995, *13*, 139–148].

Column: Resolve (Waters, 150 × 3.9 mm, 5 μm). Column temperature: 32°. Mobile phase: acetonitrile:water:orthophosphoric acid (4000:15:2), 1 mL/min flow rate. UV detection (λ=205 nm). Retention time: 5.13 min [J. Kirschbaum *et al.*, *J. Chromatogr.*, 1990, *507, Biomed. Appl.*, 165–170].

Ultraviolet Spectrum. Aqueous base—252, 258, 268 nm.

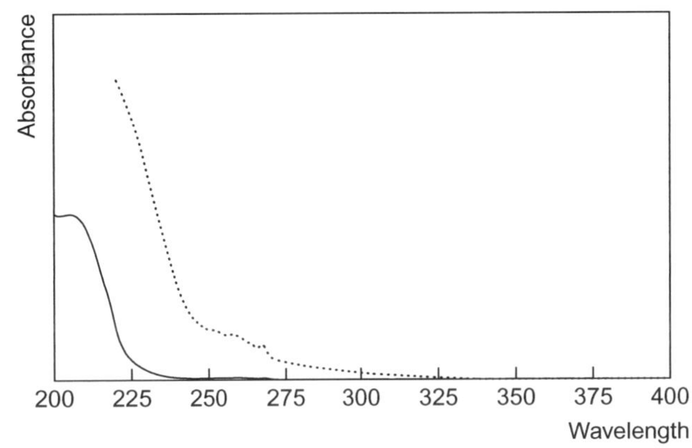

Infra-red Spectrum. Principal peaks at wavenumbers 1600, 1759, 1409, 1064 cm^{-1} (KBr pellet).

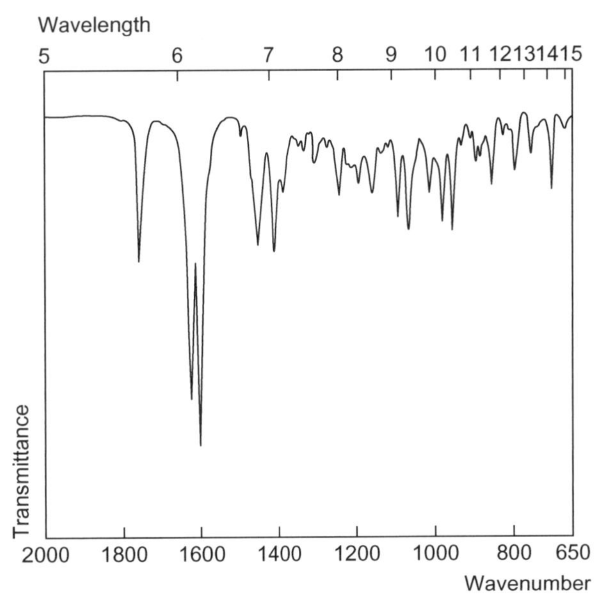

Quantification

Gas chromatography. In serum: limit of detection 10 μg/L. Detection: nitrogen–phosphorus—M. Jemal *et al.*, *J. Chromatogr.*, 1985, *345*, *Biomed. Appl.*, 299–307.

High performance liquid chromatography—mass spectrometry. In serum: limit of quantification 1.17 μg/L—M. Jemal *et al.*, *J. Chromatogr. B Biomed. Sci. Appl.*, 2000, *739*, 255–271.

Disposition in the Body. 36% of an orally administered dose of fosinopril is absorbed. It is rapidly and completely hydrolysed to fosinoprilat, a *p*-hydroxy metabolite and a glucuronide conjugate of fosinoprilat. Metabolism occurs by esterases in gastro-intestinal mucosa and in the liver. The metabolites are excreted in urine and faeces via bile. During 96 h post-intravenous administration, 90% of a dose is recovered, 44% in urine and 46% in faeces. For oral administration, however, 13 to 16% is recovered in urine and 73 to 78% in faeces. The drug has also been detected in breast milk.

Therapeutic concentration

13 patients with renal impairment (mean creatine clearance 55.7 mL/min) and 13 healthy volunteers (mean creatine clearance 102.5 mL/min) were administered 20 mg fosinopril sodium daily for 5 days. On day 1: the renally impaired patients reached peak plasma concentrations of 3870.2 μg/L within 3.5 h, and the healthy volunteers 3240.3 μg/L in 3 h. On day 5: the patients with renal impairment had peak plasma concentrations of 5170.4 μg/L and the healthy volunteers 3570.2 μg/L, both reached within 3 h [P. O'Grady *et al.*, *Br. J. Clin. Pharmacol.*, 1999, *48(3)*, 375–381].

Toxicity. Hypotension.

Half-life. Approx. 11.5 h in healthy volunteers; 14 h in patients with renal impairment.

Volume of distribution. Steady state, 1.525 L/kg (Caucasian); 0.074 L/kg (Chinese).

Clearance. Fosinopril, body clearance, 1.55 to 2.35 L/h; fosinoprilat, 26 to 39 mL/min.

Protein binding. Fosinopril is bound >95% and fosinoprilat 89 to 99.8 %.

Dose. An initial dose of 10 mg daily is administered. Maintenance dose: 10 to 40 mg daily.

Fosphenytoin

Anticonvulsant

5,5-Diphenyl-3-[(phosphonooxy)methyl]-2,4-imidazolidinedione
$C_{16}H_{15}N_2O_6P$=362.3
CAS—93390-81-9

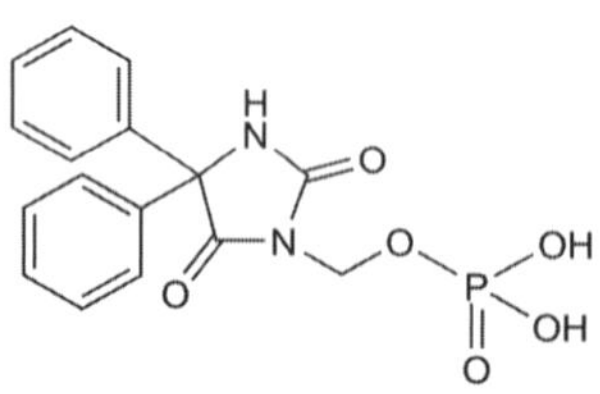

Fosphenytoin Sodium

Synonyms. ACC-9653; Acc-9653-010; CI-982; PD-135711-15B.
Proprietary names. Cerebyx; Pro-Epanutin.
$C_{16}H_{13}N_2Na_2O_6P$=406.2
CAS—92134-98-0
It is freely soluble in aqueous solutions.

High Performance Liquid Chromatography. Column: C_{18} (μBondapak, 150 × 3.9 mm i.d., 10 μm). Mobile phase: tetrabutylammonium dihydrogen phosphate (0.01 M):methanol (53:43%), flow rate 1.7 mL/min. Retention time: fosphenytoin sodium, 4.5 min [N. Gerber *et al.*, *J. Clin. Pharmacol.*, 1988, *28*, 1023–1032.]

Column: (analytical) C_{18} (Resolve, 150 × 3.9 mm i.d., 5 μm), (guard) C_{18} (Guard-Pak insert, Resolve, 5 μm, 5 × 6 mm). Mobile phase: acetonitrile:water:phosphoric acid (85%) (57:75:0.09) containing tetrabutylammonium sulfate (5 mM), flow rate 2 mL/min. Retention time: fosphenytoin, 9.1 min [J. H. Fischer *et al.*, *Ann. Pharmacother.*, 1997, *31*, 553–559.]

Column: (analytical) C_{18} (150 × 3.9 mm i.d., 5 μm), (guard) C_{18} (Resolve). Mobile phase: acetonitrile (20%) in deionised water containing TBA (0.005 M), pH adjusted to 2.2 to 2.5 with phosphoric acid (85%), flow rate 2.0 mL/min. Retention time: 8.8 min [M. J. Cwik *et al.*, *J. Chromatogr. Biomed. Sci. Appl.*, 1997, *693*, 407–414.]

Ultraviolet Spectrum. Ethanol—258 nm.

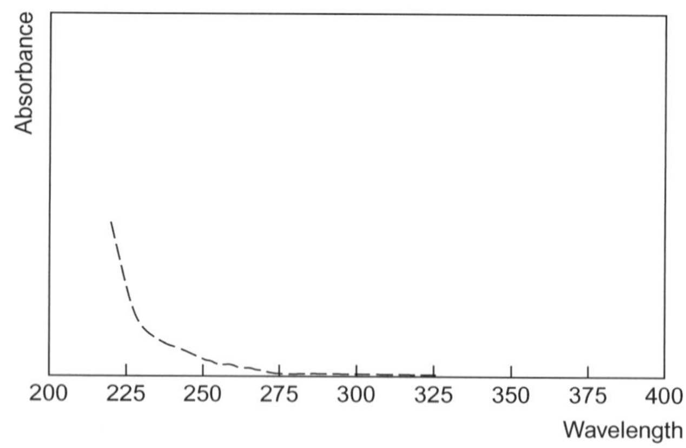

Quantification

High performance liquid chromatography. In formulations: limit of quantification 15 mg/L—J. H. Fischer *et al.*, *Ann. Pharmacother.*, 1997, *31*, 553–559. In plasma: limit of detection 0.1 mg/L and limit of quantification 0.4 mg/L—M. J. Cwik *et al.*, *J. Chromatogr. Biomed. Sci. Appl.*, 1997, *693*, 407–414.

Disposition in the Body. Fosphenytoin sodium is rapidly and completely metabolised to phenytoin and other metabolites including phosphate and formaldehyde which are subsequently converted to formate and further metabolites. Phenytoin is metabolised to 5-(*p*-hydroxyphenyl)-5-phenylhydantoin. The metabolites are excreted in urine. It is distributed in cerebrospinal fluid, saliva, semen, gastro-intestinal fluids, bile and breast milk.

Therapeutic concentration

20 healthy, male volunteers (Caucasian, Black, Hispanic and Asian) were administered with a single intravenous dose of 150, 300, 600 and 1200 mg fosphenytoin sodium over 30 min. Peak plasma concentrations of fosphenytoin were observed half an hour after the beginning of the infusion and reached mean levels of 20, 36, 75 and 129 mg/L, respectively. Peak phenytoin plasma concentrations were reached at 2.2, 4.0, 7.4 and 17.2 mg/L, respectively, approx. 51 to 109 min from the end of infusion [N. Gerber *et al.*, *J. Clin. Pharmacol.*, 1988, *28*, 1023–1032.]

Toxicity. The blood toxic range is 30 to 50 mg/L and a concentration of >100 mg/L has been associated with fatalities. Acute hepatotoxicity and hypersensitivity reactions have been observed and phenytoin and the other metabolites may result in toxicity after overdosing, including hypotension, coma and respiratory or circularity depression which may be fatal.

Bioavailability. About 90%.

Half-life. (Intramuscular administration) 33 min, (intravenous administration) 8 min.

Volume of distribution. Adults and children: 0.6 to 0.7 L/kg, infants: 0.7 to 0.7 L/kg, full term neonates: 0.8 to 0.9 L/kg and premature neonates: 1 to 1.2 L/kg.

Clearance. 19.8 L/h.

Protein binding. About 90 to 99%.

Dose. An initial dose of 10 to 15 mg phenytoin sodium equivalent (PSE)/kg body weight is administered at a rate of 50 to 150 mg/min. A daily maintenance dose of 4 to 5 mg/kg body weight is then administered. The dose is reduced in the elderly and patients with renal or hepatic impairment. Up to 450 mg has been administered intramuscularly in adults and intravenous doses of up to 3000 mg (38 mg/kg body weight).

Furaltadone

Antibacterial (Veterinary)

Synonyms. Furmethonol; Nitrofurmethonum.
Proprietary names. Altafur; Altabactina; Furazolin; Ibifur; Medifuran; Nitraldone; Otifuril; Sepsinol; Ultrafur; Unifur; Valsyn. It is an ingredient of Panotile (furaltadone hydrochloride).
5-(4-Morpholinylmethyl)-3-[[(5-nitro-2-furanyl)methylene]amino]-2-oxazolidinone
$C_{13}H_{16}N_4O_6$=324.3

CAS—139-91-3; 59302-14-6 (±)

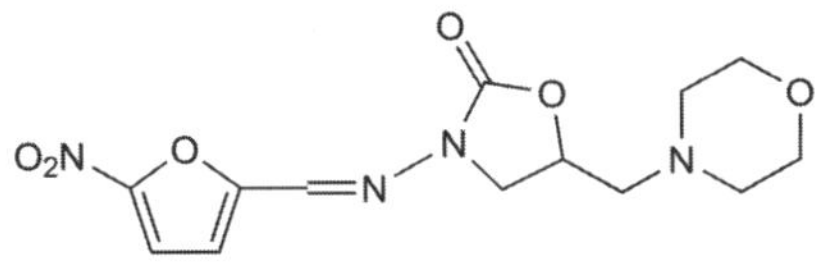

A yellow crystalline powder. M.p. about 205°.
Soluble 1 in 2000 of water, 1 in 1000 of ethanol, and 1 in 300 of chloroform; practically insoluble in ether.

Partition Coefficient. Log *P* (octanol/water), 0.2.

Colour Test. Marquis Test—yellow.

Thin-layer Chromatography. System TA—Rf 43; system TB—Rf 00; system TC—Rf 40; system TL—Rf 40; system TAJ—Rf 35; system TAK—Rf 00; system TAL—Rf 62. (Acidified iodoplatinate solution, positive.)

High Performance Liquid Chromatography. System HAA—Retention time, 8.9 min.

Ultraviolet Spectrum. Aqueous acid—255, 362 nm.

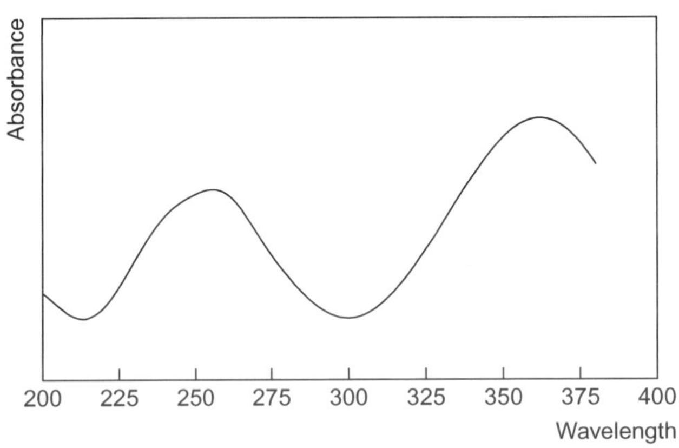

Infra-red Spectrum. Principal peaks at wavenumbers 1755, 1226, 1250, 1110, 1020, 1315 cm^{-1} (KBr disk).

Mass Spectrum. Principal ions at *m/z* 100, 56, 101, 42, 185, 184, 41, 128.

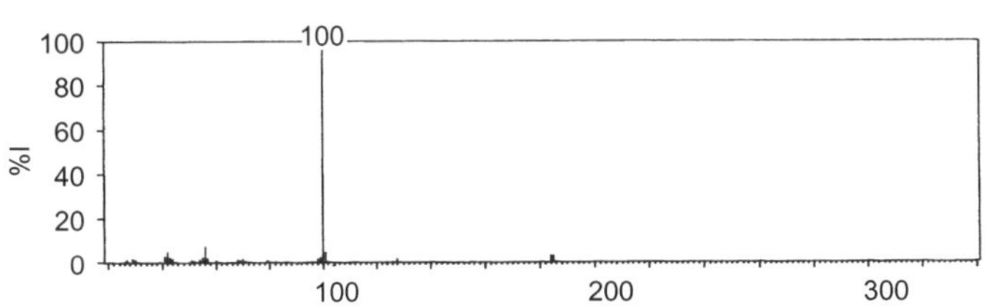

Disposition in the Body

Toxicity. It was formerly administered by mouth, but preparations were withdrawn owing to its toxic effects It is used in preparations for ear disorders.

Furazolidone

Antimicrobial

Synonym. Nifurazolidonum
Proprietary names. Coryzium (vet.); Exofur; Furasian; Furion; Furovag; Furoxane; Furoxona; Furoxone; Fuxol; Giardil; Giarlam; Medaron; Neftin (vet.); Nicolen; Nifulidone; Nifuran; Novafur; Ortazol; Quimefuran; Roptazol; Salmocide; Seforman; Tikofuran; Topazone; Tricofuron.
3-[[(5-Nitro-2-furanyl)methylene]amino]-2-oxazolidinone
$C_8H_7N_3O_5$=225.2
CAS—67-45-8

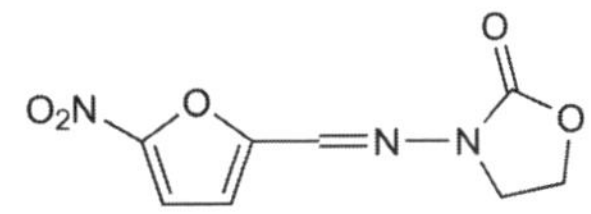

A yellow crystalline powder. M.p. about 259°, with decomposition.
Very slightly soluble in water and ethanol; slightly soluble in chloroform; practically insoluble in ether.

Partition Coefficient. Log *P* (octanol/water), −0.04.

Colour Test. Dissolve 1 mg in 1 mL of dimethylformamide with 0.05 mL of M ethanolic potassium hydroxide—deep blue.

Thin-layer Chromatography. System TA—Rf 44; system TB—Rf 00; system TC—Rf 47; system TE—Rf 46; system TF—Rf 18; system TL—Rf 59; system TAE—Rf 56.

High Performance Liquid Chromatography. System HAA—Retention time 12.2 min; system HX—RI 336.

Ultraviolet Spectrum. After solution in dimethylformamide and dilution with water—259, 367 nm (A_1^1=754a).

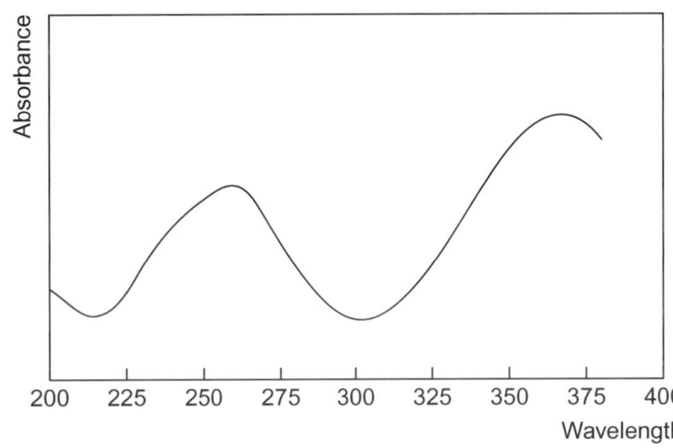

Infra-red Spectrum. Principal peaks at wavenumbers 1227, 1739, 1015, 1250, 1101, 738 cm^{-1} (Nujol mull). (See below.)

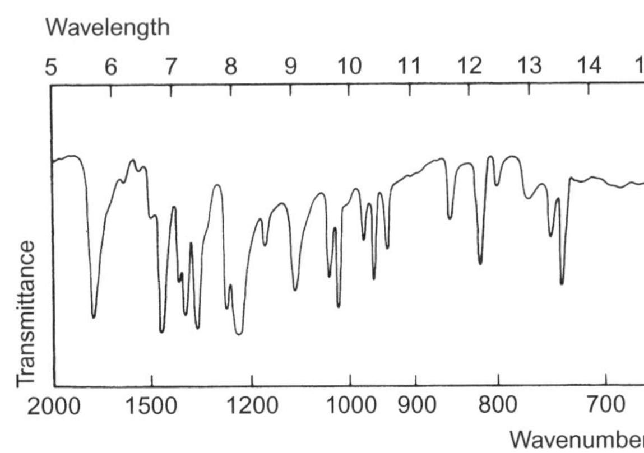

Mass Spectrum. Principal ions at *m/z* 87, 79, 51, 225, 42, 50, 86, 80.

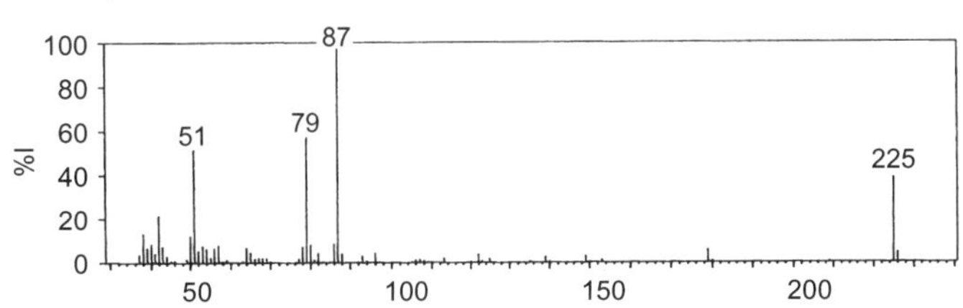

Quantification

High performance liquid chromatography. In biological fluids: limit of detection 50 µg/L—A. Valadez-Salazar *et al.*, *J. Antimicrob. Chemother.*, 1989, *23*, 589–595.

Dose. 400 mg daily.

Furosemide

Diuretic

Synonyms. Furosemidum; Fursemide; Frusemide; LB-502.
Proprietary names. Dryptal; Froop; Frumax; Frusid; Frusol; Lasix; Rusyde; Tenkafruse. See *Martindale, The complete drug reference*, 33rd Edn., London, Pharmaceutical Press, 2002 for further proprietary names. It is an ingredient of Aridil, Diumide-K, Frumil, Frusemek, Frusene, Lasikal, Lasilactone, and Lasoride.
5-(Aminosulfonyl)-4-chloro-2-[(2-furanylmethyl)amino]benzoic acid
$C_{12}H_{11}ClN_2O_5S=330.7$
CAS—54-31-9

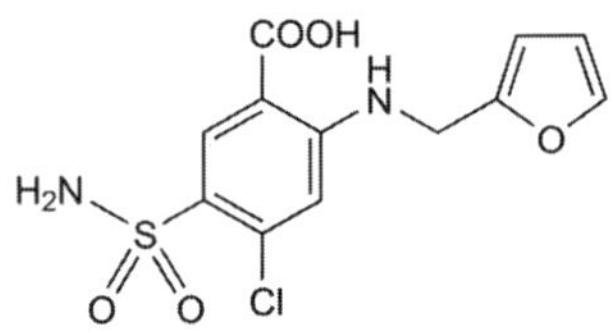

A white or slightly yellow crystalline powder. M.p. about 206°, with decomposition.
Slightly soluble in water and chloroform; soluble 1 in 75 of ethanol, 1 in 15 of acetone, and 1 in 850 of ether; soluble in dimethylformamide.

Dissociation Constant. pK_a 3.9 (20°).

Partition Coefficient. Log *P* (octanol/water), 2.0.

Colour Tests. Koppanyi–Zwikker Test—violet; Liebermann's Test—black; Sulfuric Acid—yellow.

Thin-layer Chromatography. System TB—Rf 00; system TD—Rf 01; system TE—Rf 06; system TF—Rf 07; system TG—Rf 19; system TAD—Rf 07; system TAE—Rf 86; system TAJ—Rf 10; system TAK—Rf 25; system TAL—Rf 70. (Mercurous nitrate spray, positive; acidified potassium permanganate solution, positive; Van Urk reagent, pink-brown.)

Gas Chromatography. System GA—furosemide not eluted, furosemide-Me RI 2890, furosemide-Me_2 RI 2850, furosemide-Me_3 RI 2800, art (-SO_2NH) RI 2040, art (-SO_2NH)-Me RI 2020, art (-SO_2NH)-Me_2 RI 2050, M (*N*-desalkyl-)-Me RI 2750, M (*N*-desalkyl-)-Me_2 RI 2450; system GD—RRT of methyl derivative 2.64 (relative to *n*-$C_{16}H_{34}$); system GX—furosemide-Me_3 retention time 7.0 min; system GY—furosemide-Me_3 retention time 4.7 min.

High Performance Liquid Chromatography. System HV—RRT 0.45 (relative to meclofenamic acid); system HX—RI 435; system HY—RI 380; system HZ—retention time 3.5 min; system HAA—retention time 15.2 min; system HAX—retention time 5.8 min; system HAY—retention time 5.0 min.

Ultraviolet Spectrum. Aqueous acid—235 (A^1_1=1333a), 274 (A^1_1=600a), 342; aqueous alkali—271 (A^1_1=580a), 333 nm.

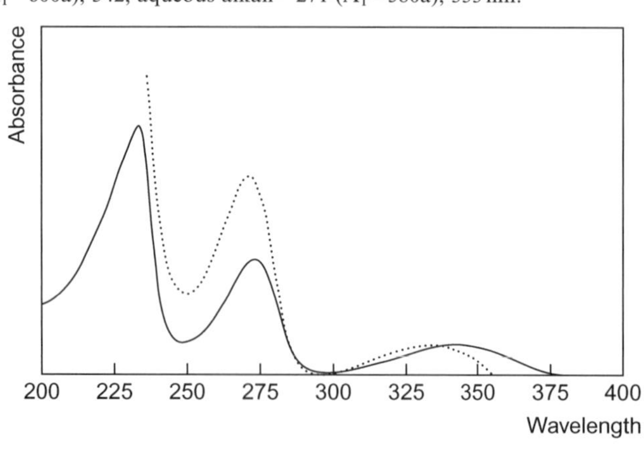

Infra-red Spectrum. Principal peaks at wavenumbers 1143, 1668, 1565, 1240, 1590, 1260 cm^{-1} (KBr disk).

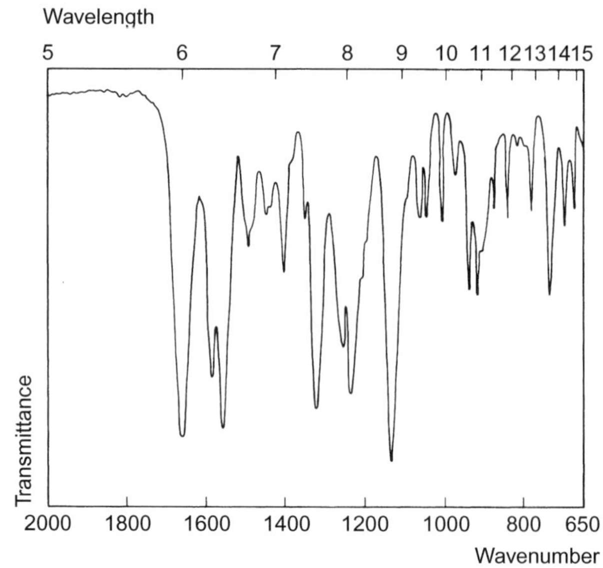

Mass Spectrum. Principal ions at *m/z* 81, 53, 330, 96, 82, 332, 64, 63.

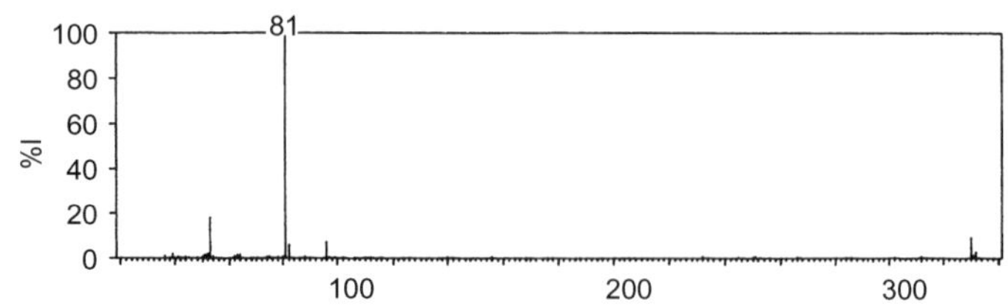

Quantification

Gas chromatography. In plasma or urine: limit of detection 20 µg/L, ECD—E. Keller *et al.*, *Eur. J. Clin. Pharmacol.*, 1981, *20*, 27–33.

Gas chromatography–mass spectrometry. In plasma or urine: selected ion monitoring—P. Ptacek *et al.*, *Arzneimittelforschung*, 1996, *46*, 277–283.

High performance liquid chromatography. In plasma or urine: limit of detection 100 µg/L in plasma and 500 µg/L in urine, fluorescence detection—A. L. M. Kerremans *et al.*, *J. Chromatogr.* 1982, *229*(18) *B Biomed. Appl.*, 129–139. In plasma or urine: furosemide and its glucuronide metabolite, limit of detection 8 µg/L for furosemide in plasma, fluorescence detection—D. E. Smith *et al.*, *Drug Met. Disp.*, 1980, *8*, 337–342. In plasma or urine: limit of detection 5 µg/L, fluorescence detection—M. Saugy *et al.*, *J. Chromatogr.*, 1991, *564*, 567–578. In plasma: furosemide and amiloride, limit of detection for furosemide 0.3 µg/L, fluorescence detection—H. J. Reeuwijk *et al.*, *J. Chromatogr.*, 1992, *575*, 269–274. In plasma: limit of detection 1.8 µg/L, fluorescence detection—D. Farthing *et al.*, *J. Pharm. Sci.*, 1992, *81*, 569–571. In neonatal plasma: fluorescence detection—J. S. Sidhu and B. G. Charles, *J. Chromatogr.*, 1993, *612*, 161–165. In plasma or urine: furosemide and its acyl glucuronide, fluorescence detection—T. B. Vree *et al.*, *J. Chromatogr. B Biomed. Appl.*, 1994, *655*, 53–62. In urine: furosemide and piretanide, amperometric detection—M. B. Barroso *et al.*, *J. Chromatogr.* 1996, *675*, *B Biomed. Appl.*, 303–312. In serum—T. Okuda *et al.*, *J. Chromatogr. B Biomed. Appl.*, 1996, *682*, 343–348. In plasma or urine: limit of detection 5 µg/L—H. S. Abou-Auda *et al.*, *J. Chromatogr. B Biomed. Sci. Appl.*, 1998, *710*, 121–128. In urine: UV detection—A. A. Nava-Ocampo *et al.*, *J. Chromatogr. B Biomed. Sci. Appl.*, 1999, *730*, 49–54.

High performance liquid chromatography–mass spectrometry. In plasma: limit of detection 10 µg/L—M. E. Abdel-Hamid, *Farmaco*, 2000, *55*, 448–454.

Disposition in the Body. Rapidly but incompletely absorbed after oral administration. Up to 90% of an IV dose is excreted in the urine, mainly as unchanged drug with up to 14% of the dose as a glucuronide conjugate. 2-Amino-4-chloro-5-sulfamoylanthranilic acid has been reported as a metabolite in several studies, but in other cases it has not been detected and it has been suggested that it is an analytical artefact produced during acid extraction procedures. In normal subjects, about 6 to 18% of a dose is eliminated in the faeces after IV administration; this may be increased to about 60% in renal failure. It crosses the placenta and is found in breast milk.

Therapeutic concentration

Following a single oral dose of 80 mg to 8 fasting subjects, peak serum concentrations of 1.8 to 4.9 mg/L (mean 2.3) were attained in 60 to 70 min. [M. R. Kelly *et al.*, *Clin. Pharmacol. Ther.*, 1974, *15*, 178–186.]

Plasma concentrations averaging 7.5 mg/L were reported 10 min after an IV dose of 40 mg to 9 subjects. [D. E. Smith *et al.*, *Drug Metab. Dispos.*, 1980, *8*, 337–342.]

Bioavailability. About 60 to 70%.

Half-life. Plasma half-life, about 1 to 3 h, increased in subjects with renal failure, congestive heart failure, liver disease, and in neonates (up to about 46 h).

Volume of distribution. About 0.1 to 0.2 L/kg, increased in subjects with liver disease, nephrotic syndrome, and in neonates.

Clearance. Plasma clearance, about 1 to 3 mL/min/kg, decreased in uraemia, heart failure, the elderly, and neonates.

Protein binding. In plasma, about 99%, decreased in patients with cirrhosis, the nephrotic syndrome, and uraemia.

Note. For reviews of furosemide pharmacokinetics, see L. Z. Benet, *J. Pharmacokinet. Biopharm.*, 1979, *7*, 1–27 and R. E. Cutler and A. D. Blair, *Clin. Pharmacokinet.*, 1979, *4*, 279–296.

Dose. Usually 20 to 80 mg daily; in oliguria, up to maximum single dose of 2 g.

Fusidic Acid

Antibiotic

Proprietary names. Fucidin (suspension); Fucithalmic; Futasole.
(3α,4α,8α,9β,11α,13α,14β,16β,17Z)-16-(Acetyloxy)-3,11-dihydroxy-29-nordammara-17(20),24-dien-21-oic acid hemihydrate
$C_{31}H_{48}O_6,½H_2O$=525.7
CAS—6990-06-3 (anhydrous)

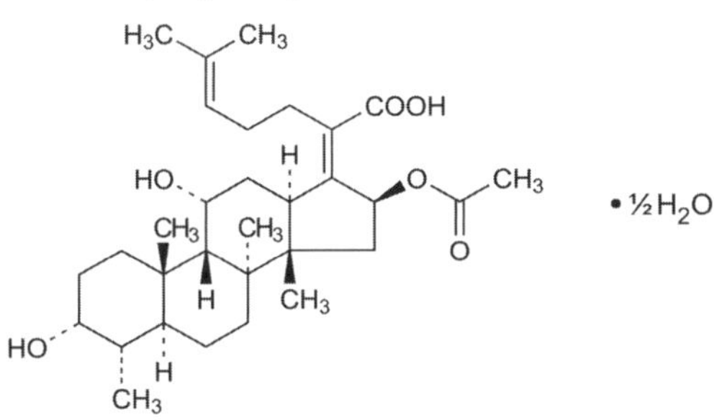

A white crystalline powder. M.p. about 193°.
Sparingly soluble in water and hexane; soluble 1 in 5 of ethanol, 1 in 4 of chloroform, and 1 in 60 of ether; soluble in acetone, pyridine, and dioxane.

Sodium Fusidate

Synonym. Fusidate Sodium
Proprietary names. Dermomycin; Fucidin(e) (tablets).
$C_{31}H_{47}NaO_6$=538.7
CAS—751-94-0
A white, slightly hygroscopic, crystalline powder.
Soluble 1 in 1 of water, 1 in 1 of ethanol, and 1 in 350 of chloroform; practically insoluble in ether.

Dissociation Constant. pK_a 5.4.

Partition Coefficient. Log *P* (octanol/water), 6.8.

High Performance Liquid Chromatography. System HAA—Retention time, 24.9 min.

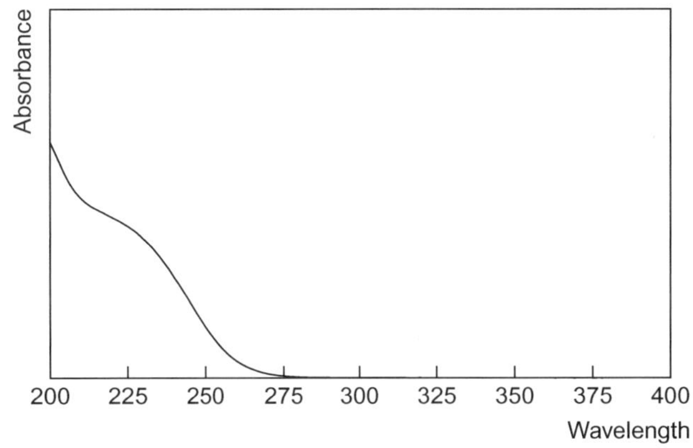

Infra-red Spectrum. Principal peaks at wavenumbers 1267, 1547, 1706, 1238, 1020, 966 cm^{-1} (sodium fusidate, KBr disk).

Quantification

High performance liquid chromatography. In plasma: limit of detection 500 µg/L, UV detection—A. H. Hikal, *Int. J. Pharmaceut.*, 1983, *13*, 297–301. In plasma: limit of detection 200 µg/L, UV detection—A. Rahman and N. E. Hoffman, *J. Chromatogr.*, 1988, *433*, 159–166.

Dose. 1.5 to 3 g of sodium fusidate daily.

Gabapentin

Anticonvulsant

Synonyms. CI-945; GOE-3450.
Proprietary names. Aclonium; Neurontin.
1-(Aminomethyl)cyclohexaneacetic acid
$C_9H_{17}NO_2$=171.2
CAS—60142-96-3

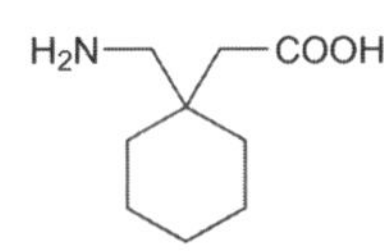

A white to off-white crystalline solid. M.p. 162° to 166°, also reported as 165° to 167°. It is freely soluble in water (4491 mg/L at 25°), basic and acidic aqueous solutions.

Dissociation Constant. pK_a 3.68, 10.7.

Partition Coefficient. Log *P* (octanol/water), −1.10.

Gas Chromatography. System GA—gabapentin-H_2O RI 1750, gabapentin-H_2O-Me RI 1560; system GB—gabapentin-H_2O RI 1633.

Column: capillary (Megabore DB-1, 30 m × 0.53 mm, i.d., 1.5 µm film thickness). Column temperature: 160°, hold 4 min, to 260° at 15°/min. Injector and detector temperature: 285°. Carrier gas: helium, flow rate 8 mL/min. IS: Go-3609A. Detection: FID. Retention time: gabapentin, 7.24 min; IS, 9.0 min [W. D. Hooper *et al.*, *J. Chromatogr.*, 1990, *529*; *Biomed. Appl.*, 167–174].

High Performance Liquid Chromatography. Column: (analytical) C_{18} (Ultrasphere, 250 × 4.6 mm i.d.), (guard) Permaphase ETH (20 × 2 mm i.d., 30 µm). Mobile phase: water:acetonitrile:acetic acid:*n*-butylamine, pH <4.5 (480:520:1.0:0.1), flow rate 1.2 mL/min. IS: 1-(aminomethyl)cycloheptaneacetic acid. UV detection (λ=340 nm). Retention time(s): gabapentin, 9.8 min; IS, 13.3 min [G. L. Lensmeyer *et al.*, *Ther. Drug Monit.*, 1995, *17*, 251–258.]

Column: (analytical) C_{18} (Hypersil BDS, 125 × 3 mm i.d., 3 µm), (guard) (Hypersil BDS, 4 × 4 mm i.d., 3 µm). Column temperature: 35°. Mobile phase: solvent A—phosphate buffer (250 mM):acetonitrile:water (32:9.5:58.5), solvent B—acetonitrile:methanol:water (28:24:48). Elution programme: A:B (42:58) for 7 min, then (35:65) for 6 min to (25:74) for 3 min, then to (0:100) for 7 min, flow rate 0.45 mL/min. Fluorescence detection (λ_{ex}=340 nm, λ_{em}=440 nm). Retention time: 16.7 min [N. Ratnaraj and P. N. Patsalos, *Ther. Drug Monit.*, 1998, *20*, 430–434.]

Mass Spectrum. Principal ions at *m/z* 81, 153, 67, 152, 55, 54, 68, 96 (gabapentin-H_2O).

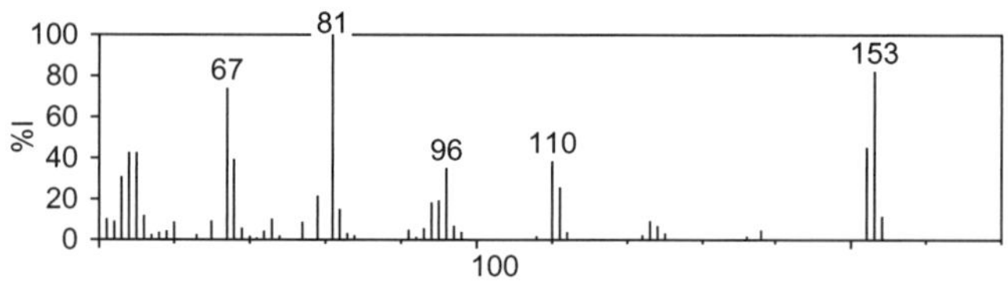

Quantification

Gas chromatography. In plasma: limit of quantification 0.2 mg/L, urine: 5 mg/L—W. D. Hooper *et al., J. Chromatogr.*, 1990, *529 Biomed. Appl.*, 167–174.

High performance liquid chromatography. In serum: limit of detection 0.03 to 0.05 mg/L, UV detection (λ=340 nm)—G. L. Lensmeyer *et al., Ther. Drug Monit.*, 1995, *17*, 251–258. In serum: limit of quantification 0.9 mg/L, limit of detection 0.2 mg/L, fluorescence detection (λ_{ex}=340 nm, λ_{em}=440 nm)—N. Ratnaraj and P. N. Patsalos, *Ther. Drug Monit.*, 1998, *20*, 430–434.

Disposition in the Body. Gabapentin is well absorbed after oral administration but is not metabolised within the body. 80% of a single dose is excreted unchanged in urine and the rest in faeces. It is widely distributed throughout the body and easily crosses the blood–brain barrier.

Therapeutic concentration

Healthy male volunteers were orally administered with single doses of 300, 600, 900, 1200, 1800, 2400, 3600 and 4800 mg gabapentin. Peak plasma concentrations increased with dose with 1.91, 3.29, 4.02, 5.50, 8.46, 7.65, 11.9 and 12.4 mg/L, respectively and were all reached between 1.8 and 2.8 h [*Eur. J. Clin. Pharmacol.*, 1989, *36*, *suppl.* A310.]

Toxicity. Up to 49 g of gabapentin has been reported in a single overdose with drowsiness, mild diarrhoea, dizziness, double vision, slurred speech and lethargy as symptoms. Full recovery was made.

Bioavailability. Absolute bioavailability is approx. 60% over the dose range 300 to 600 mg, but outside this, as dose increases, bioavailability decreases.

Half-life. 5 to 7 h.

Volume of distribution. 0.6 to 0.8 L/kg.

Distribution in blood. Drug penetrates red blood cells. Extravascular distribution.

Protein binding. <3%.

Dose. Initial adult dose is 300 mg/day, 300 mg twice a day (2nd day of treatment), 300 mg three times a day (third day), with a maximum of 2.4 g a day. Usual range is between 0.9 and 1.8 g a day. Reduced for elderly patients and those with reduced renal function.

Galantamine

Alzheimer's Disease/ Cholinesterase inhibitor

Synonyms. Galanthamine; Jilkon; Lycoremin; Lycoremine; NSC-100058.
(4a*S*,6*R*,8a*S*)-4a,5,9,10,11,12-Hexahydro-3-methoxy-11-methyl-6*H*-benzofuro[3a,3,2-e,f][2]benzazepin-6-ol
$C_{17}H_{21}NO_3$=287.4
CAS—357-70-0

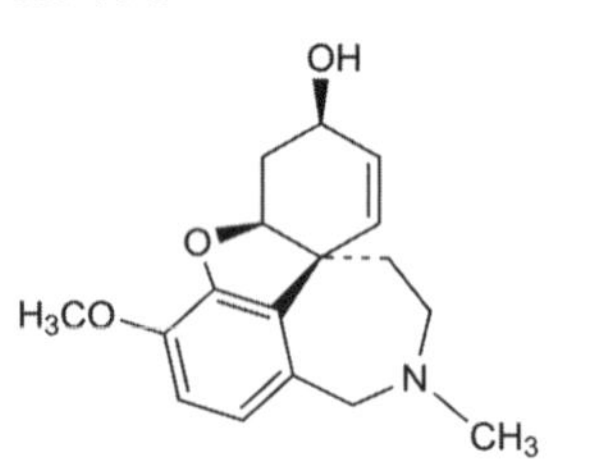

Crystals from benzene, M.p. 126° to 127°. It is fairly soluble in hot water; freely soluble in alcohol, acetone and chloroform; less soluble in benzene and ether. Solubility in water is 31 g/L (pH 6).

Galantamine Hydrochloride

$C_{17}H_{21}NO_3$, HCl=323.8
Crystals from water, M.p. 256° to 257° (dec.). It is sparingly soluble in cold water; more soluble in hot water; very sparingly soluble in alcohol and acetone.

Galantamine Hydrobromide

Proprietary names. Nivalin; Reminyl.
$C_{17}H_{21}NO_3$, HBr=368.3
CAS—1953-04-4
Crystals from water, M.p. 246° to 247° (dec.).

Dissociation Constant. pK_a 8.2.

Partition Coefficient. Log *P* (octanol/pH 12), 1.09.

Gas Chromatography. System GA—RI 2285.

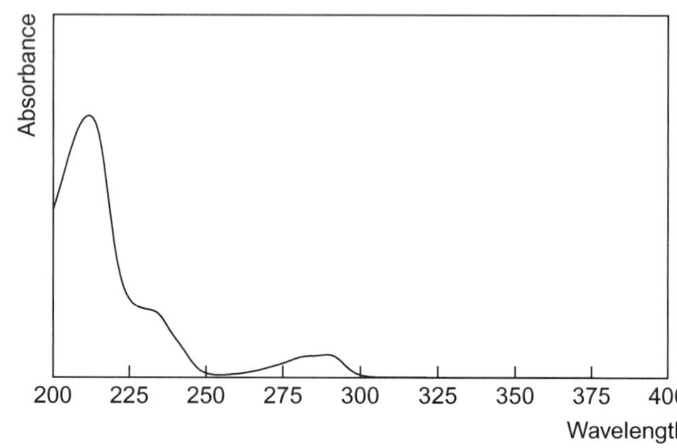

Quantification

High performance liquid chromatography. In plasma: limit of detection 1 µg/L for galantamine and epigalantamine and 15 µg/L for galantaminone, fluorescence detection (λ_{ex}=290, λ_{em}=320 nm)—U. Bickel *et al., Neuropharmacology*, 1991, *30*, 447–454.

Disposition in the Body. The presence of food delays the rate of absorption of galantamine but does not affect the extent. Patients with Alzheimer's disease tend to produce plasma drug concentrations 30 to 40% higher than healthy, young subjects. Galantamine is metabolised in the liver by the cytochrome P450 isoenzymes, CYP2D6 and CYP3A4, and approx. 75% of the dose is metabolised. Metabolites include norgalantamine (active), *N*-oxide-galantamine, *O*-desmethylgalantamine (active), *O*-desmethylnorgalantamine (active), epigalantamine and galantaminone. No active metabolites have been detected in the unconjugated forms in plasma. The majority of the dose is excreted in urine; 18 to 22% as the unchanged drug during the 24 h period after dosing. A minor amount is excreted in faeces. The drug does not appear to accumulate after multiple dosing.

Therapeutic concentration

8 healthy male volunteers, aged 21 to 35 years (mean age, 29.5 years), were fasted overnight and administered with 5 mg and 10 mg galantamine intravenously as a constant-rate infusion over 30 min. The same subjects were also administered with a 10 mg solution and tablet form orally. The peak plasma concentrations for the intravenous doses were 24.2 to 42.9 µg/L for the 5 mg dose and 50.7 to 97.4 µg/L for the 10 mg dose. For the oral doses, the peak concentrations were 28.7 to 57.9 µg/L for the tablet, observed at 0.5 to 2.0 h, and 28.9 to 56.5 µg/L for the oral solution at 0.5 to 1.25 h [U. Bickel *et al., Clin. Pharmacol. Ther.*, 1991, *50*, 420–428.]

8 female patients, aged 38 to 79 years, undergoing minor gynaecological operations were treated with 0.3 mg/kg galantamine hydrobromide (equivalent to 0.234 mg free base) intravenously by rapid infusion. The patients were already anaesthetically induced with althesin, fentanyl and nitrous oxide, and the galantamine dose was administered at the end of surgery. The peak serum concentrations obtained were 543 µg/L at 2 min and 128 µg/L after 30 min [P. Westra *et al., Br. J. Anaesth.*, 1986, *58*, 1303–1307.]

Toxicity

Significant overdosing of galantamine can lead to signs and symptoms similar to those observed with overdosing of other cholinomimetics; generally involving the central nervous system, the parasympathetic nervous system and the neuromuscular junction. Symptoms include muscle weakness or fasciculations, severe nausea, vomiting, gastro-intestinal cramping, salivation, lacrimation, urination, defecation, sweating, bradycardia, hypotension, collapse and convulsions. Increasing muscle weakness along with tracheal hypersecretions and bronchospasm, may result in vital airway compromise. [Patient information leaflet, Janssen-Cilag Ltd.]

Bioavailability. Absolute, 88.5%.

Half-life. 7 to 8 h.

Volume of distribution. 175 L; steady state, 2.64 L/kg (194.8 L).

Clearance. Plasma, 0.34 L/h/kg; serum, 5.37 mL/min. Clearance is approx. 20% lower in females than males and 25% lower in poor metabolisers of galantamine than extensive metabolisers.

Protein binding. 18%.

Dose. Initially 4 mg is administered twice daily for 4 weeks and can be increased to 8 mg twice daily for 4 weeks. The maintenance dose is 8 to 12 mg twice daily. For patients with moderate hepatic impairment, the dose is 4 mg once daily and should not exceed 8 mg.

Gallamine Triethiodide

Muscle Relaxant

Synonym. Bencurine Iodide
Proprietary names. Flaxedil; Miowas G; Relaxan.
2,2′,2″[1,2,3-Benzenetriyltris(oxy)]tris[*N*,*N*,*N*-triethylethanaminium] triiodide
$C_{30}H_{60}I_3N_3O_3$=891.5
CAS—153-76-4 (gallamine); 65-29-2 (triethiodide)

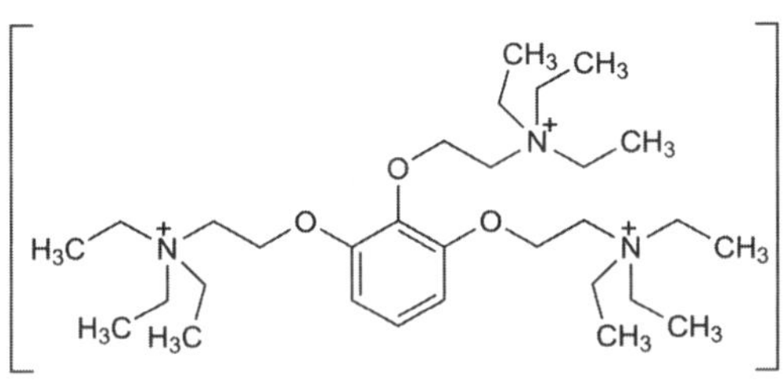

A white, or faintly cream-coloured, hygroscopic powder. M.p. about 235°, with decomposition.
Soluble 1 in 0.6 of water, 1 in 115 of ethanol, and 1 in 1500 of chloroform; freely soluble in dilute acetone; sparingly soluble in anhydrous acetone, ether, and benzene.

Partition Coefficient. Log *P* (octanol/water), −6.4.

Thin-layer Chromatography. System TA—Rf 00; system TN—Rf 34; system TO—Rf 05. (Acidified iodoplatinate solution, positive.)

Gas Chromatography. System GA—RI 2625.

Ultraviolet Spectrum. Aqueous acid—225 (A^1_1=525a), 266 nm (A^1_1 = 9a).

Infra-red Spectrum. Principal peaks at wavenumbers 1100, 1120, 1260, 1000, 780, 1600 cm^{-1} (KBr disk).

Quantification

Spectrofluorimetry. In plasma: limit of detection 50 ng—M. I. Ramzan *et al.*, *Eur. J. Clin. Pharmacol.*, 1980, *17*, 135–143.

Disposition in the Body. Slowly and incompletely absorbed after oral administration; absorbed after IM administration but is generally given by the IV route. Small amounts enter the CSF. Almost 100% of a dose is excreted unchanged in the urine in 24 to 30 h. Negligible amounts are excreted in the bile.

Half-life. Plasma half-life, 2 to 3 h; greatly increased in renal failure.

Volume of distribution. About 0.3 L/kg.

Clearance. Plasma clearance, about 1.4 mL/min/kg.

Dose. 40 to 120 mg IV.

Gallium Nitrate

Antihypercalcaemic

Synonyms. Gallium Trinitrate; Gallium (III) Nitrate; Gallium Salt:Nitric Acid; NSC-15200; WR-135675.
Proprietary name. Ganite
Gallium nitrate
GaN_3O_9=255.7
CAS—135886-70-3 (nonahydrate); 13494-90-1 (anhydrous)

A white crystalline powder with M.p. 110°. It is very soluble in water; soluble in warm and cold aqueous solutions and absolute alcohol; insoluble in ether.

Disposition in the Body. Up to 70% of a dose is excreted by the kidneys with approx. 50% of a dose excreted in urine within the first 48 h, mostly in the first 6 h.

Therapeutic concentration

25 patients (male and female) with non-small cell lung cancer, aged between 39 and 88 years old, were administered 700 mg/m^2 intravenous doses of gallium nitrate over 30 min. The mean peak plasma concentration was 15.2 mg/L, with a range from 9.5 to 21.2 mg/L. Most of the gallium remained ultrafilterable for the first 10 h but by 48 h, only 11% of the dose was present as ultrafilterable gallium. Total gallium present reached a peak at 1.9 mg/L within 8 to 12 h. Maximum urine concentration of gallium was 40 to 196 mg/L [L. K. Webster *et al.*, *Cancer Chemother. Pharmacol.*, 2000, *45(1)*, 55–58].

Toxicity. Gallium nitrate is a poison by intraperitoneal, intravenous and subcutaneous routes, and moderately toxic by ingestion. An intravenous dose of 7 mg/kg can result in gastro-intestinal tract toxicity and 144 mg/kg in blood toxicity. It can also cause severe skin and eye irritations, at doses > 500 mg. Serious nephrotoxicity can also occur.

Half-life. 25 to 111 h.

Dose. The usual dose is 100 to 200 mg/m^2 body surface administered once daily.

Gamma-butyrolactone

Depressant

Synonyms. γ-BL; 1,2-Butanolide; Butyrylactone; Dihydro-2(3*H*)-furanone; Gamma Hydroxybutyric Acid Lactone; Gamma Lactone; 2-Oxanolone; Tetrahydro-2-furanone.
Proprietary names. Blue Nitro; Blue Nitro Vitality; Firewater; Gamma G; GH Revitalizer; Insom-X; Invigorate; Longevity; Remforce; Renewtrient; Revivarant; Revivarant G.
Dihydro-2(3*H*)-furanone
$C_4H_6O_2$=86.1
CAS—96-48-0

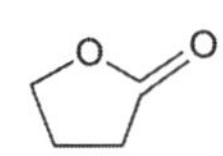

A colourless liquid. M.p. −43°; B.p. 204°. It is miscible with water, alcohol, ketones, esters and aromatic hydrocarbons; limited solubility in aliphatic and cycloaliphatic hydrocarbons.

(S)-3-Hydroxy-gamma-butyrolactone

Synonyms. HGB
$C_4H_6O_3$=102.0
CAS—7331-52-4
A pale yellow liquid with B.p. 98° to 100°.

Partition Coefficient. Log *P* (octanol/water), −0.64.

Colour Tests. Specific tests using mixtures of several common reagents are given in the Colour Tests chapter.

Gas Chromatography. System GAO—GBL Retention time 4.0 min; GHB-TMS$_2$ 5.6 min.

Column: Bonded phase capillary (HP Ultra 1, 12 m × 0.2 mm i.d., 0.33 µm film thickness). Column temperature: 50° for 0.6 min, 15°/min to 275°. Carrier gas: helium. IS: delta-valerolactone. MS detection. Retention time(s): gamma butyrolactone, 2.6 min; IS, 4.1 min [S. D. Ferrara *et al.*, *J. Pharm. Biomed. Anal.*, 1993, *11*, 483–487].

Column: DB-624 capillary (30 m × 0.25 mm i.d., 1.4 µm film thickness). Column temperature: 50°, held 3 min, 20°/min to 150°, held 7 min. Injector temperature: 150°. Carrier gas: nitrogen, linear velocity, 34 cm/s. IS: gamma-butyrolactone-d_6. MS detection. Retention time(s): gamma butyrolactone, 11.2 min; IS, 12.7 min [M. A. LeBeau *et al.*, *J. Anal. Toxicol.*, 2000, *24*, 421–428.]

Column: FFAP (acid-modified polyethylene glycol) capillary (25 m × 0.2 mm i.d., 0.3 µm film thickness). Column temperature: 50°, held 1.5 min; increased to 240° at 30°/min, held 2 min. Carrier gas: helium, flow rate 0.8 mL/min. IS: gamma butyrolactone-d_6. MS detection. Retention time(s): gamma-butyrolactone, 6.5 min; IS, 6.5 min [G. Frison *et al.*, *Rapid Commun. Mass Spectrom.*, 2000, *14*, 2401–2407.]

High Performance Liquid Chromatography. System HBG—GBL Retention time 4.0 min, GHB 3.5 min.

Column: C_{18} µBondapak (300 × 3.9 mm i.d., 10 µm). Mobile phase: potassium dihydrogen phosphate buffer (10 mM, pH 3.0):methanol (70:30), flow rate 1.0 mL/min. UV detection (λ=215 nm). Retention time: gamma-butyrolactone, 3.96 min; gamma-hydroxybutyric acid (GHB), 3.45 min [M. Z. Mesmer and R. D. Satzger, *J. Forensic Sci.*, 1998, *43*, 489–492.]

Infra-red Spectrum. Principal peaks at wavenumbers 1820, 1163, 1047, 2993, 2909, 874 cm^{-1}.

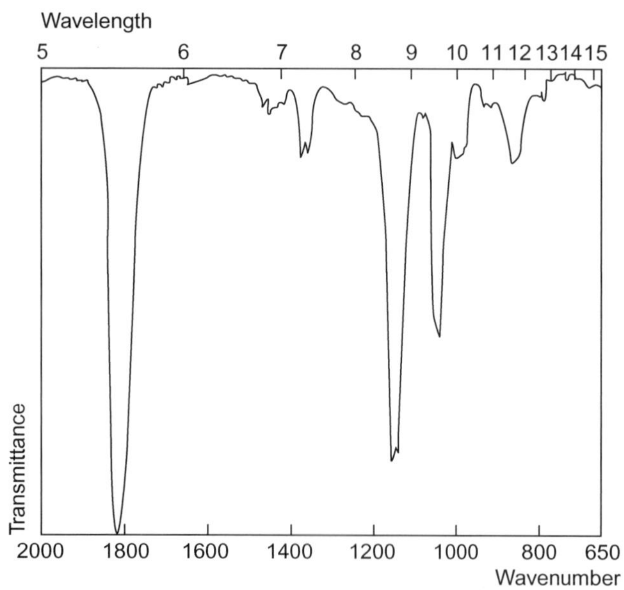

Mass Spectrum. Principal ions at *m/z* 42, 28, 41, 29, 27, 86, 56, 39.

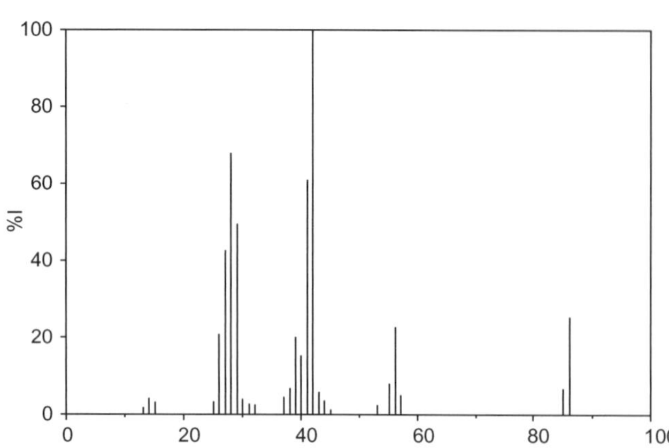

Quantification

Gas chromatography. In blood and urine: limit of detection for GHB 0.5 mg/L, FID—M. A. LeBeau *et al.*, *J. Anal. Toxicol.*, 2000, *24*, 421–428.

Gas chromatography–mass spectrometry. In blood and urine: limit of detection for GHB 0.5 mg/L—M. A. LeBeau *et al.*, *J. Anal. Toxicol.*, 2000, *24*, 421–428. In plasma and urine: limit of detection for GHB 0.05 mg/L and 0.1 mg/L, respectively—G. Frison *et al.*, *Rapid Commun. Mass Spectrom.*, 2000, *14*, 2401–2407.

Disposition in the Body. Gamma butyrolactone (GBL) is well absorbed after administration and is biotransformed in the body to gamma-hydroxybutyric acid (GHB) which is a potent central nervous system depressant. This conversion can occur very quickly, within a matter of minutes. GBL has a greater bioavailability than GHB.

Toxicity. Signs and symptoms of toxicity can include prolonged unconsciousness and coma, respiratory depression including respiratory arrest, nausea/vomiting, confusion, anxiety/nervousness, cardiac arrest and seizures.

A 19-year-old woman was offered a drink from a plastic container at a party. After drinking some, she had no recollection of the rest of the evening and her friends described her as being 'drunker than she should have been'. A sexual assault examination indicated that intercourse had occurred. 9 h after the drink was consumed, a urine sample revealed a concentration of GBL at 4.4 mg/L. GHB was only detected at concentrations consistent with endogenous levels.

A 25-year-old man was found sleeping behind the wheel of his car in the middle of a busy street. In the car there was a container of RenewTrient, a GBL-containing product. Blood analysis showed a concentration of GHB of 157 mg/L but GBL was not detected.

[M. A. LeBeau *et al.*, *J. Anal. Toxicol.*, 2000, *24*, 421–428.]

Note. GBL is used for the manufacture of GHB (gamma-hydroxybutyric acid).

Gamma-hydroxybutyric Acid

Anaesthetic Agent

Synonyms. BRN-1720582; GHB; Gamma Hydroxybutyrate.
Street names. Georgia Home Boy; Grievous Bodily Harm; Liquid Ecstasy; Scoop; Fantasy.
4-Hydroxybutanoic acid
$C_4H_8O_3$=104.1
CAS—591-81-1

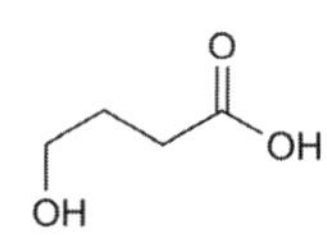

It is water soluble and produces solutions that are mildly saline.

Sodium Gamma-hydroxybutyrate

Synonyms. NSC-84223; Sodium Gamma-hydroxybutyric Acid; Sodium Oxybate: Sodium Oxybutyrate; Wy3478.
Proprietary names. Alcover; Gamma-OH; Somatomax PM; Somsanit; Xyrem.
Sodium-4-hydroxybutyrate
$C_4H_8NaO_3$=127.1
CAS—502-85-2
A colourless, odourless powder, capsules or liquid.

Colour Tests. Specific tests using mixtures of several common reagents are given in the Colour Tests chapter.

Gas Chromatography. System GAO—GHB-TMS_2 Retention time 5.6 min; GBL (gamma butyrolactone) 4.0 min.

Column: 100% polydimethylsiloxane (HP-1, 12 m × 0.2 mm i.d., 0.33 µm film thickness). Column temperature: 60°, held 2 min; increased to 260° at 30°/min, held 1 min. Injector and detector temperatures: 280° and 300°, respectively. Carrier gas: helium, flow rate 0.5 mL/min. IS: GHB-d_6. MS detection (SIM mode, *m/z*: 233, 234, 235 for GHB and 239, 240, 241 for IS). Retention time(s): GHB, 4.43 min; IS, 4.41 min [A. A. Elian *et al.*, *Forensic Sci. Int.*, 2000, *109*, 183–187].

Column: cross-linked methylsiloxane (HP-1MS, 12 m × 0.25 mm i.d., 0.25 µm film thickness). Column temperature: 65°, held for 0.5 min; increased to 105° at 15°/min; 25°/min to 300°. Injector temperature: 260°. Carrier gas: helium, flow rate 1.6 mL/min. MS detection (SIM mode, *m/z*:

as above). IS: GHB-d_6. Retention time: 3.7 min [R. R. McCusker *et al.*, *J. Anal. Toxicol.*, 1999, *23*, 301–305].

High Performance Liquid Chromatography. System HBG—GHB Retention time 3.5 min; GBL 4.0 min.

Column: C_{18} μBondapak (300 × 3.9 mm i.d., 10 μm). Mobile phase: potassium dihydrogen phosphate buffer (10 mM, pH 3.0):methanol (70:30), flow rate 1.0 mL/min. Retention time: GHB, 3.45 min; gamma butyrolactone, 3.96 min [M. Z. Mesmer and R. D. Satzger, *J. Forensic Sci.*, 1998, *43*, 489–492].

Mass Spectrum. Principal ions at *m/z* 147, 73, 75, 117, 233, 148, 45, 149 (GHB-TMS_2).

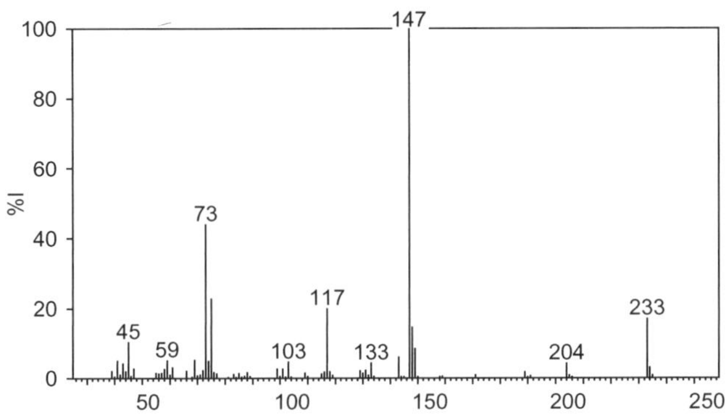

Quantification

Gas chromatography. In blood and urine: limit of detection 0.5 mg/L, FID—M. A. LeBeau *et al.*, *J. Anal. Toxicol.*, 2000, *24*, 421–428.

Gas chromatography–mass spectrometry. In urine: limit of detection 0.2 mg/L—P. V. Kavanagh *et al.*, *J. Pharm. Pharmacol.*, 2001, *53*, 399–402. In blood and urine: limit of detection 0.5 mg/L—M. A. LeBeau *et al.*, *J. Anal. Toxicol.*, 2000, *24*, 421–428. In urine: limit of detection 5 mg/L—R. R. McCusker *et al.*, *J. Anal. Toxicol.*, 1999, *23*, 301–305. In plasma and urine: limit of detection 0.2 mg/L and 0.1 mg/L, respectively—S. D. Ferrara *et al.*, *J. Pharm. Biomed. Anal.*, 1993, *11*, 483–487.

High performance liquid chromatography. In plasma and urine: limit of detection 1 mg/L and 0.2 mg/L, respectively—S. D. Ferrara *et al.*, *Br. J. Clin. Pharmacol.*, 1992, *34*, 231–235.

Disposition in the Body. Gamma-hydroxybutyric acid (GHB) is readily absorbed after oral administration and rapidly metabolised in the liver by oxidative enzymes. Conversion to gamma-butyrolactone (GBL) can occur and elimination is rapid, via the kidneys, with urine recovery virtually complete within 8 h of administration. Only negligible amounts of the parent drug are recovered unchanged in urine (<5%) and after 12 h, the drug is not detectable. It crosses the blood–brain barrier and the placental barrier.
Endogenous concentrations of GHB are thought to be up to 10 mg/L in urine and 4 mg/L in antemortem plasma of individuals not suffering from the genetic disorder gamma-hydroxybutyric aciduria. Endogenous concentrations appear to be increased postmortem, particularly in blood.

Therapeutic concentration

8 healthy non-smoker males, aged between 22 and 26 years, were administered 12.5, 25 and 50 mg/kg single doses, after an overnight fast. Peak plasma concentrations reached 23 ± 9, 23 ± 11, 20 ± 7 mg/L within 25 ± 20, 30 ± 20, 45 ± 30 min, respectively [P. Palatini *et al.*, *Eur. J. Clin. Pharmacol.*, 1993, *45*, 353–356].

Toxicity. Doses greater than 50 mg/kg can lead to a decrease in cardiac output, respiratory depression/arrest, seizure-like activity and, possibly, death. An intoxicating dose is 15 mg/kg and a dose of 4 g has been associated with death. It has also been reported that doses between 5 and 10 g can be toxic or fatal. Effects usually occur within 20 min post dose and are also associated with a steep dose–response curve that may result in accidental overdosage.

18-year-old male admitted to hospital unresponsive and in respiratory failure, died 30 min later. Toxicological postmortem analysis showed a 309.4 mg/L blood concentration of GHB along with alcohol, cocaine, cocaethylene and benzoylecgonine [A. Mozayani *et al.*, *TIAFT website* (www.tiaft.org), 1998].

22-year-old female who had taken a suspected single dose of liquid GHB revealed a postmortem femoral blood concentration of 330 mg/L and a frontal cortex brain tissue concentration of 221 μg/g. GHB was also detected in the hair. No other drugs were detected [K. Kalansinsky *et al.*, *J. Forensic Sci.*, 2001, *46(3)*, 728–730].

Half-life. Terminal half-life, 0.3 to 1.0 h.

Volume of distribution. 0.5 L/kg.

Clearance. Oral, 9.6 mL/min/kg (range, 4.7 to 15.3).

Protein binding. None.

Dose. Usual dose required for general anaesthesia is 50 mg/kg, for treatment of amnesia/as an analgesic is 10 to 20 mg. There is evidence that GHB has been misused as a drug-facilitated sexual assault (DFSA) agent.

Ganciclovir

Antiviral

Synonyms. BIOLF-62; BW-759; BW-B759U; BW-759U; DHPG; Dihydroxypropoxymethylguanine; 2′-NDG; 2′-Nor-2′-deoxyguanosine; RS-21592.
2-Amino-1,9-[[2-hydroxy-1-(hydroxymethyl)ethoxy]methyl]-6*H*-purin-6-one
$C_9H_{13}N_5O_4$=255.2
CAS—82410-32-0

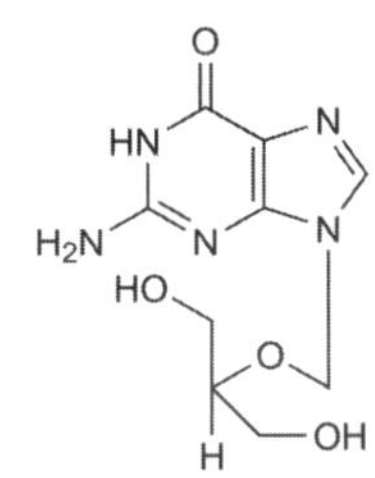

A white to off-white crystalline powder. M.p. 250° (decomposes). It is soluble 2.6 g/L in water at 25°; 4.3 g/L in solution at pH 7.

Ganciclovir Sodium

Proprietary names. Citovirax; Cymevan; Cymeven; Cymevene; Cytovene; Denosine; Virgan; Vitrasert.
$C_9H_{12}N_5NaO_4$=277.2
CAS—107910-75-8

Dissociation Constant. pK_a 2.2, 9.4.

Partition Coefficient. Log *P* (octanol/water), −1.66.

High Performance Liquid Chromatography. Column: Lichrospher RP8e (125 × 4 mm i.d., 5 μm). Mobile phase: methanol:1-octanesulfonic acid (50 mM) in phosphate buffer (0.1 M, pH 3), 1.0 mL/min flow rate. Internal standard (IS): guanosine. Fluorescence detection (λ_{ex}=285 nm, λ_{em}=380 nm). Retention time: ganciclovir, 4.71 min; IS, 7.35 min [M. Koel and P. Nebinger, *J. Pharm. Biomed. Anal.*, 1994, *12(3)*, 429–432].

Column: (analytical) RP Hypersil ODS (100 × 4.6 mm, 3 μm); (pre-column) (10 × 4.6 mm). Column temperature: 40°. Mobile phase: 0.1 M sodium hydrogen phosphate monohydrate:0.04 M triethylamine, pH 6.6, 1.0 mL/min flow rate. Internal standard: acyclovir. UV detection (λ=254 nm). Retention time: ganciclovir, 4.0 min; IS, 5.1 min [M. A. Campanero *et al.*, *J. Chromatogr. B Biomed. Sci. Appl.*, 1998, *706*, 311–317].

Ultraviolet Spectrum. Aqueous acid—255 nm: Methanol—254 nm; aqueous base—264 nm.

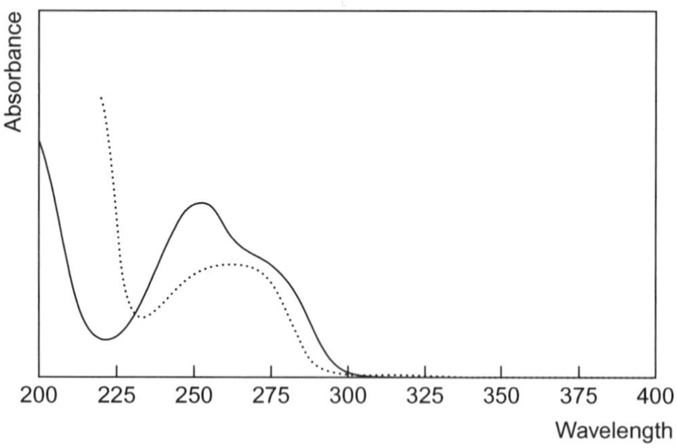

Infra-red Spectrum. Principal peaks at wavenumbers 1647, 1379, 1041 cm^{-1} (KBr disk).

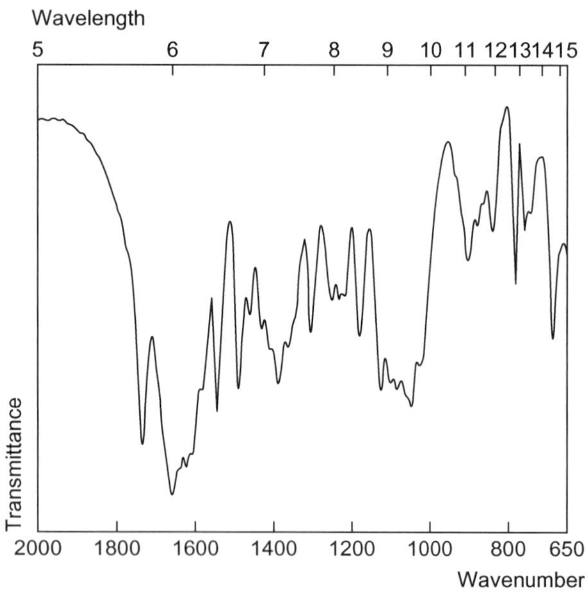

Quantification

High performance liquid chromatography. In plasma or CSF: limit of detection 0.25 mg/L, UV detection—C. Fletcher *et al., Clin. Pharmacol. Ther.*, 1986, *40*, 281–286. In plasma: limit of detection 0.5 μg/L, UV detection (λ=254 nm)—R. Boulieu *et al., J. Chromatogr.*, 1991, *571*, *Biomed. Appl.*, *109*, 331–333. In serum: limit of detection 50 μg/L with UV detection, 0.01 mg/L with fluorescence detection—M. Koel and P. Nebinger *J. Pharm. Biomed. Anal.*, 1994, *12*, 429–432. In serum or urine: limit of quantification 0.05 mg/L, UV detection (λ=254 nm)—T. Page *et al., J. Chromatogr.*, 1996, *675*, *Biomed. Appl.*, 342–346. In plasma: limit of detection 0.003 mg/L and quantification 0.01 mg/L, UV detection (λ=254 nm)—M. Cociglio *et al., J. Chromatogr. B Biomed. Sci. Appl.*, 1998, *705*, 79–85. In plasma: limit of detection is 0.01 mg/L, limit of quantification 0.05 mg/L, UV detection (λ=254 nm)—M. A. Campanero *et al., J. Chromatogr. B Biomed. Sci. Appl.*, 1998, *706*, 311–317.

Review. For a review of chromatographic methods for the determination of antiviral drugs in biological fluids see C. M. Riley *et al., J. Chromatogr.*, 1990, *531*, *Biomed. Appl.*, *96*, 295–368.

Disposition in the Body. Ganciclovir is poorly absorbed after oral administration; peak plasma concentrations are reached after about 2 to 4 h. Following intravenous administration, it is widely distributed to body tissues and fluids including intra-ocular fluid and CSF. It crosses the placenta. The drug is excreted unchanged in the urine by glomerular filtration and active tubular secretion; approx. 90% of an oral dose is excreted in urine within 24 h of administration. With an intravenous dose, on the other hand, the majority is excreted in faeces. Haemodialysis reduces plasma concentrations by about 50%. Ganciclovir does not accumulate in plasma after repeated dosing.

Therapeutic concentration. The trough serum therapeutic concentration is 0.2 to 1.0 mg/L and peak, 5.0 to 12.5 mg/L.

97 patients with AIDS and life-threatening or sight-threatening cytomegalovirus infections, mean age 36.2 years, were administered intravenously with doses of 1, 2.5 and 5 mg/kg (infused over 1 h) every 8 h. Mean peak steady-state plasma concentrations of 0.0094, 0.0203 and 0.0445 mg/L, respectively, were measured after the last dose [O. L. Laskin *et al., Am. J. Med.*, 1987, *83*, 201–207].

6 subjects (bone marrow recipients aged between 13 and 53 years) were administered intravenously with 2.5 mg/kg (infused over 1 h) every 8 h, for 10 days. Plasma concentrations between 3.93 and 4.45 mg/L 15 min after the end of the infusion were observed. The mean CSF concentration measured 2.75 h after intravenous administration was 0.51 mg/L [C. Fletcher *et al., Clin. Pharmacol. Ther*, 1986, *40*, 281–286].

20 mg/kg was orally administered, every 6 h, to 4 subjects with AIDS and CMV retinitis, after an overnight fast which was continued for 1 h after administration. 4 to 6 months prior to this treatment, the patients were also administered 2.5 mg/kg intravenously every 8 h, for 10 days, and 5 to 7.5 mg/kg daily 5 days a week. The 20 mg/kg dose produced mean peak and trough steady-state plasma concentrations of 2.96 μg/L and 1.05 μg/L, respectively, on day 3. The 2.5 mg/kg intravenous dose produced a peak concentration of 18.0 μg/L; the 5 mg/kg dose, 40.0 μg/L and a 10 mg/kg oral dose every 6 h produced a peak concentration of 2.01 μg/L. These were observed after approx. 1 h [M. A. Jacobson *et al., Antimicrob. Agents Chemother.*, 1987, *31*, 1251–1254].

Toxicity. The trough serum toxic concentration is 3 to 5 mg/L and peak, 20 mg/L.

Bioavailability. 5 to 8%; increases when administered with food.

Half-life. Plasma half-life, 2.5 to 4 h.

Volume of distribution. 0.5 to 2.0 L/kg; quoted as 0.74 L/kg. Also reported as 33 to 45 L.

Clearance. Plasma clearance, 200 mL/min/1.73 m^2; 0.1 L/h/kg.

Protein binding. In plasma, 1 to 2%.

Note. For reviews of ganciclovir see D. Faulds and R. C. Heel, *Drugs*, 1990, *39*, 597–638, A. Markham and D. Faulds, *Drugs*, 1994, *48*, 455–484, C. S. Crumpacker, *N. Engl. J. Med.*, 1996, *335*, 721–729 and S. Noble and D. Faulds, *Drugs*, 1998, *56*, 115–146. For a review of the pharmacokinetics of antiviral nucleosides see G. D. Morse *et al., Clin. Pharmacokinet.*, 1993, *24*, 101–123.

Dose. Initially, 5 mg/kg (of ganciclovir) intravenously over 1 h every 12 h for 14 to 21 days. Orally, 1 g (of ganciclovir) three times daily.

Gelsemine

Central Depressant

$C_{20}H_{22}N_2O_2$=322.4
CAS—509-15-9

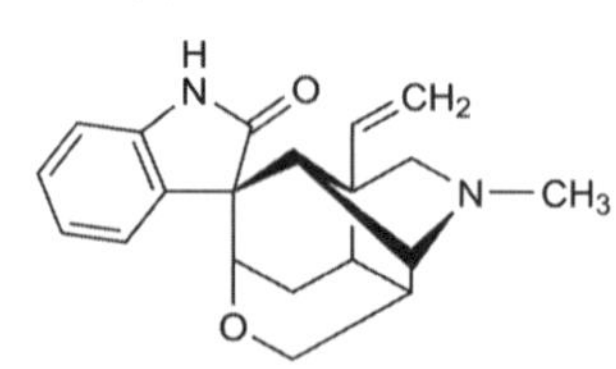

An alkaloid present in gelsemium, the dried rhizome and roots of *Gelsemium sempervirens* (Loganiaceae).
Crystals. M.p. 178°.
Slightly soluble in water; soluble in ethanol, chloroform, benzene, acetone, dilute acids, and ether.

Partition Coefficient. Log *P* (octanol/water), 1.4.

Colour Test. Mandelin's Test—red→green.

Thin-layer Chromatography. System TA—Rf 49; system TB—Rf 09; system TE—Rf 52; system TAE—Rf 25. (Acidified iodoplatinate solution, positive.)

Gas Chromatography. System GA—RI 2850.

High Performance Liquid Chromatography. System HX—RI 290.

Ultraviolet Spectrum. Aqueous acid—252 (A_1^1=220b); aqueous alkali—268 nm.

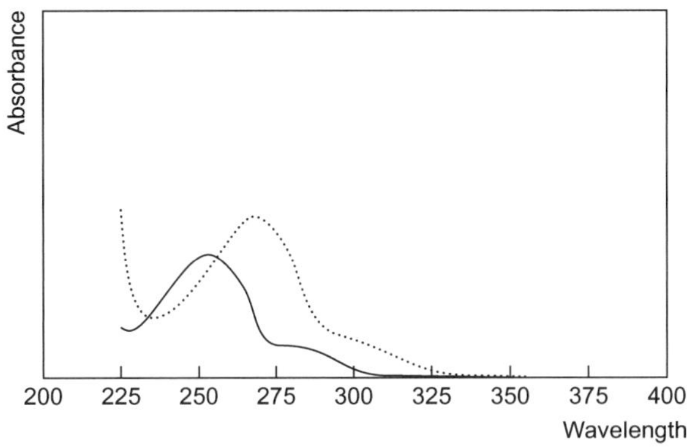

Infra-red Spectrum. Principal peaks at wavenumbers 1715, 1620, 1100, 747, 759, 1237 cm^{-1}.

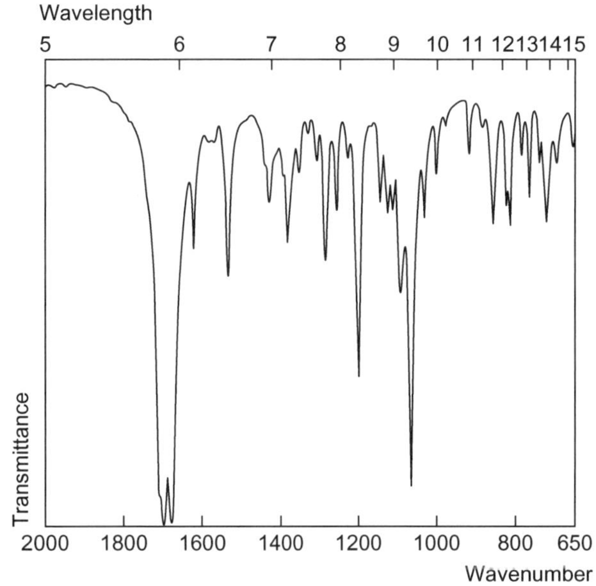

Disposition in the Body

Toxicity. Death has been caused by the ingestion of 4 mL of a 1:1 fluid extract.

Gemcitabine

Antineoplastic

Synonyms. dFdC; dFdCyd; LY-188011.
2′-Deoxy-2′,2′-difluorocytidine
$C_9H_{11}F_2N_3O_4$=263.2
CAS—95058-81-4

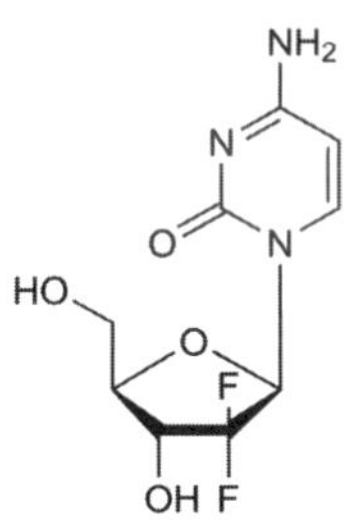

Gemcitabine Hydrochloride

Proprietary name. Gemzar
$C_9H_{11}F_2N_3O_4$,HCl=299.7
CAS—122111-03-9
A white to off-white solid. M.p. 287° to 292°. It is soluble in water; slightly soluble in methanol; practically insoluble in ethanol and in polar organic solvents.

Dissociation Constant. pK_a 3.6.

Ultraviolet Spectrum. Aqueous acid—204, 274 nm.

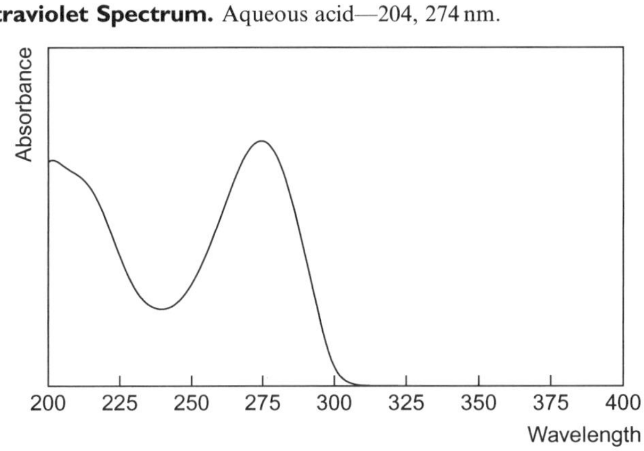

Quantification

High performance liquid chromatography. In plasma or urine: limit of quantification 0.05 mg/L and 20 mg/L, respectively, UV detection (λ=272 nm)—K. B. Freeman *et al.*, *J. Chromatogr.* 1995, *665*, *Biomed. Appl.*, 171–181.

Disposition in the Body. Following intravenous administration, gemcitabine is rapidly cleared from blood and is metabolised by cytidine deaminase in the liver, kidney, blood and other tissues. The pharmacokinetics of gemcitabine are significantly affected by gender and age of patient and length of time over which the drug is infused. Clearance is approx. 30% lower in women compared to men. It is not distributed extensively into tissues. Less than 10% of the drug is excreted in urine as the unchanged drug and the rest as metabolites. Approx. 1% of a dose is excreted in faeces. The primary, inactive metabolite is dFdU (2′-deoxy-2′,2′-difluorouridine) which has been observed in both plasma and urine. Other metabolites detected in plasma and urine include the gemcitabine mono, di and triphosphates, the latter are considered active.

Therapeutic concentration

In a total of seven studies, 121 women and 232 men, aged between 29 and 79 years, diagnosed with non-small cell lung cancer or pancreatic cancer, were administered doses of 500 to 1592 mg/m^2 over an infusion period of 0.4 to 1.2 h. Peak plasma concentrations of 3.2 to 45.5 mg/L were observed within 5 min of the end of the infusion. The peak plasma concentration for the metabolite, dFdU, is 28 to 52 mg/L observed 3 to 15 min after the end of a 30-min infusion of 1 g/m^2. [Data as supplied by Eli Lilly & Company Ltd.]

Toxicity. The most severe toxicity is possible life-threatening oesophagitis and pneumonitis observed in patients receiving radical radiotherapy to thorax in association with gemcitabine.

Half-life. Plasma half-life, 0.7 to 1.6 h, depending on age and gender; 0.18 to 0.43 (mean 0.28) h for gemcitabine triphosphate.

Volume of distribution. Steady state, 17 (range 9 to 30) L/m^2 (gemcitabine); 150 L/m^2 (range 96 to 228 L/m^2) (metabolite, dFdU).

Clearance. Systemic, ranges between 29.2 and 92.2 L/h/m^2 depending on age and gender. Total body, 90 (range 40 to 130) L/h/m^2.

Protein binding. In plasma, negligible.

Note. For reviews of gemcitabine, see W. Plunkett *et al.*, *Semin. Oncol.*, 1995, *22(Suppl. 11)*, 3–10 and S. Noble and K. L. Goa, *Drugs*, 1997, *54*, 447–472.

Dose. Usually 1 g/m^2 body surface is administered intravenously, over an hour, once a week; adjusted up to 1250 or 1500 mg/m^2 according to response and toxicity.

Gentamicin

Antibiotic

CAS—1403-66-3

A mixture of isomeric aminoglycoside antibiotics (gentamicin C_1, gentamicin C_{1A}, and gentamicin C_2) produced by *Micromonospora purpurea* or *M. echinospora*.

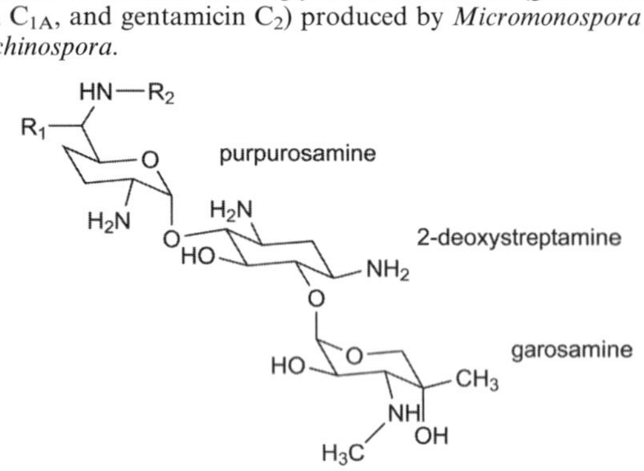

Gentamicin C_1 $R_1 = R_2 = CH_3$
Gentamicin C_2 $R_1 = CH_3$, $R_2 = H$
Gentamicin C_{1a} $R_1 = R_2 = H$

A white amorphous powder. M.p. 102° to 108°.

Freely soluble in water; soluble in pyridine; moderately soluble in methanol, ethanol, and acetone; sparingly soluble in chloroform; practically insoluble in benzene and halogenated hydrocarbons.

Gentamicin Sulfate

Proprietary names. Alcomicin; Cidomycin; Garamycin; Genoptic; Gentacidin; Gentak; Gentalline; Gentasol; Genticin; Gentigan; G-Myticin; Jenamicin; Lugacin; Ocu-Mycin; Refobacin; Sulmycin. It is an ingredient of many proprietary preparations—see Martindale, *The complete drug reference*, 33rd Edn.

CAS—1405-41-0

A white to buff-coloured powder. M.p. 218° to 237°.

Soluble in water, ethylene glycol and formamide; practically insoluble in ethanol, chloroform, and ether.

Partition Coefficient. Log *P* (octanol/water), −1.9.

Colour Tests. Nessler's Reagent (100°)—black; Ninhydrin (heat for 4 min)—violet.

High Performance Liquid Chromatography. System HAA—Retention time, 14.0 min.

Ultraviolet Spectrum. Aqueous acid—247; aqueous alkali—251 nm.

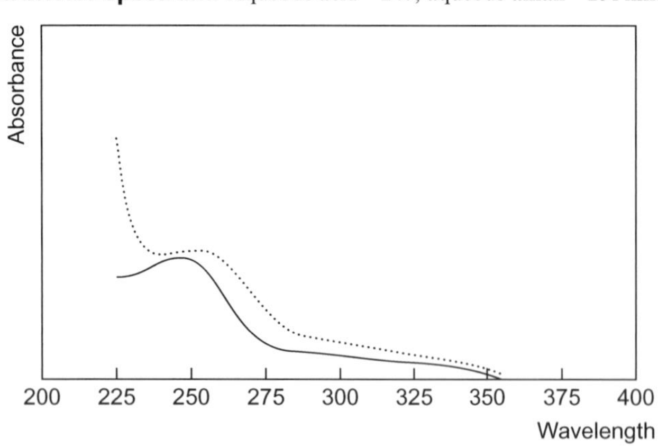

Infra-red Spectrum. Principal peaks at wavenumbers 1120, 1060, 1625, 1525, 1290, 880 cm^{-1} (KBr disk).

Quantification See also under Amikacin

High performance liquid chromatography. In plasma or urine: gentamicin components C_1, C_{1A} and C_2, limit of detection 500 µg/L, fluorescence detection—J. D'Souza and R. I. Ogilvie, *J. Chromatogr.*, 1982, *232*; *B Biomed. Appl.*, *21*, 212–218. In plasma: fluorescence detection (comparison with fluorescence polarisation immunoassay)—A. Yusuf *et al.*, *Ther. Drug Monit.*, 1999, *21*, 647–652. In plasma or urine: gentamicin isomers (C_1, C_{1A}, and C_2), UV detection—N. Isoherranen and S. Soback, *Clin. Chem.*, 2000, *46*, 837–842. In urine: limit of detection 75 µg/L, fluorescence detection—A. I. Al-Amoud *et al.*, *J. Chromatogr. B Anal. Technol. Biomed. Life Sci.*, 2002, *769*, 89–95.

Immunoassay. In serum: enzyme immunoassay, limit of detection 100 µg/L—P. J. Wills and R. Wise, *Antimicrob. Agents Chemother.*, 1979, *16*, 40–42. In serum: fluoroimmunoassay—A. J. Munro *et al.*, *J. Antimicrob. Chemother.*, 1982, *9*, 47–51.

Reviews. For a review of methods for the determination of gentamicin in serum, see W. Hospes *et al.*, *Pharm. Weekbl., Sci. Edn*, 1982, *4*, 32–37. For a review of HPLC methods for the determination of gentamicin and other aminoglycosides in biological fluids, see L. Soltes, *Biomed. Chromatogr.*, 1999, *13*, 3–10.

Disposition in the Body. Poorly absorbed after oral administration but rapidly absorbed after IM injection; it is also absorbed systemically following topical application to wounds. In normal subjects it is rapidly excreted in the urine as unchanged drug, up to 80% of a dose being excreted in 24 h. It accumulates in the tissues and there may be considerable intersubject variation in the pharmacokinetics. Gentamicin may be detected in serum and urine for several days after cessation of treatment.

Therapeutic concentration. During treatment the serum concentration should be in the range 4 to 12 mg/L and should be monitored regularly, especially in patients who have renal insufficiency. During multiple dosing, the trough concentration immediately preceding a dose should not exceed 2 mg/L.

A single IM dose of 1 mg/kg given to 10 subjects, produced a mean peak serum concentration of 5.8 mg/L in 0.5 to 1 h [M. Chung *et al.*, *Antimicrob. Agents Chemother.*, 1980, *17*, 184–187.]

In 11 subjects, a 30-min IV infusion of 6 or 2 mg/kg produced respective mean plasma concentrations of 35.0 and 10.1 mg/L at the end of the infusion, 17.0 and 5.4 mg/L 30 min after the end of the infusion, and 0.45 and 0.69 mg/L at the end of the dosing interval [K. S. Sangha *et al.*, *Ann. Pharmacother.*, 1995, *29*, 117–119.]

Toxicity. Toxic effects may be produced at serum concentrations of 12 mg/L or more, or during chronic treatment, if the trough serum concentration exceeds 2 mg/L.

Half-life. Plasma half-life, about 2 to 4 h, increased in renal failure; a very long terminal elimination phase of several days has also been reported.

Volume of distribution. About 0.2 L/kg.

Clearance. Plasma clearance, about 1 mL/min/kg.

Protein binding. In plasma, less than 30%.

Dose. The equivalent of 3 to 5 mg/kg of gentamicin daily, given parenterally.

Gestonorone Caproate

Progestational Steroid

Synonym. Gestronol Hexanoate

Proprietary names. Depostat; Primostat.

17-[(1-Oxohexyl)oxy]-19-norpregn-4-ene-3,20-dione

$C_{26}H_{38}O_4 = 414.6$

CAS—1253-28-7

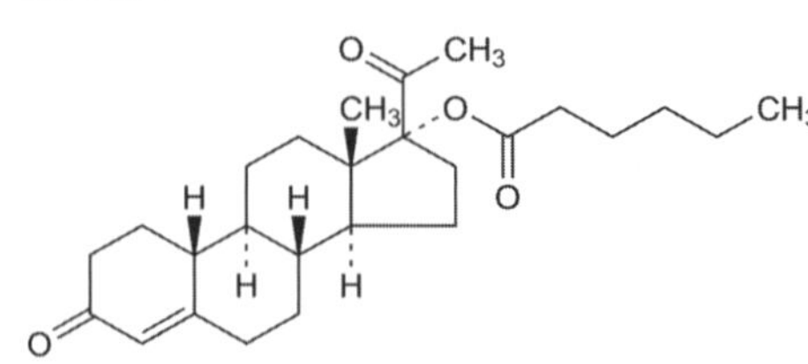

A white to creamy-white crystalline powder. M.p. 123° to 124°; a polymorph melting at 119° to 123° may also occur.

Soluble in ethanol and methanol; freely soluble in acetone and chloroform; sparingly soluble in ether.

Partition Coefficient. Log *P* (octanol/water), 5.2.

Thin-layer Chromatography. System TB—Rf 31; system TE—Rf 83; system TF—Rf 59.

Gas Chromatography. System GA—RI 3440.

Ultraviolet Spectrum. Methanol—240 nm (A_1^1=415b).

Infra-red Spectrum. Principal peaks at wavenumbers 1733, 1667, 1715, 1266, 1250, 1618 cm^{-1} (KBr disk).

Dose. 200 to 400 mg IM every 5 to 7 days.

Gestrinone

Anabolic Steroid/Beta$_2$-agonist

Synonyms. A46745; Ethylnorgestrienone; R2323; RU2323.
Proprietary names. Dimetriose; Dimetrose; Nemestran; Trodomose.
(17α)-13-Ethyl-17-hydroxy-18,19-dinorpregna-4,9,11-trien-20-yn-3-one
$C_{21}H_{24}O_2$=308.4
CAS—16320-04-0; 40542-65-2

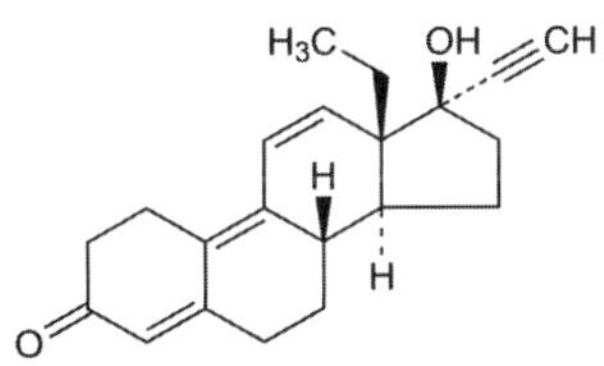

A white to slightly yellow powder. M.p. 154°.

High Performance Liquid Chromatography. Column: C_{18} UG120, (Capcell pack, 150 × 2.0 mm i.d., 5 μm). Column temperature: 40°. Mobile phase: acetonitrile:water (A:B). Elution programme: (5:95) to (30:70) in 3 min, to (52.5:47.5) in 14 min, to (100:0) in 3 min, held for 5 min. UV detection (λ=345 nm). Retention time(s): gestrinone, 16.3 min; metabolite 1, 11.3 min; metabolite 2, 12.2 min. [Y. Kim *et al.*, *Rapid Commun. Mass Spectrom.*, 2000, *14*, 1717–1726.]

Ultraviolet Spectrum. Neutral—235, 347 nm.

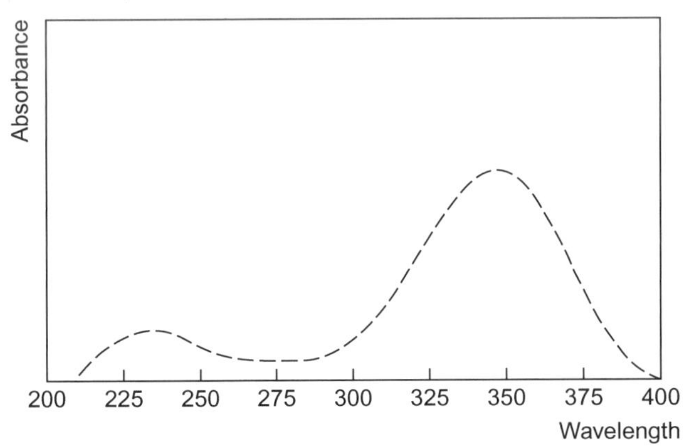

Disposition in the Body. Gestrinone is well absorbed after oral administration with negligible first-pass metabolism. It is metabolised in the liver by hydroxylation to two unknown metabolites and the conjugate forms. It is excreted as the latter.

Therapeutic concentration. Peak plasma concentrations are observed about 3 h after administration.

Half-life. Approx. 24 h.

Dose. A usual dose of 2.5 mg is administered twice weekly.

Glafenine

Analgesic

Synonym. Glaphenine
Proprietary names. Glifan; Glifanan; Privadol.
2,3-Dihydroxypropyl 2-[(7-chloro-4-quinolinyl)amino]benzoate
$C_{19}H_{17}ClN_2O_4$=372.8
CAS—3820-67-5

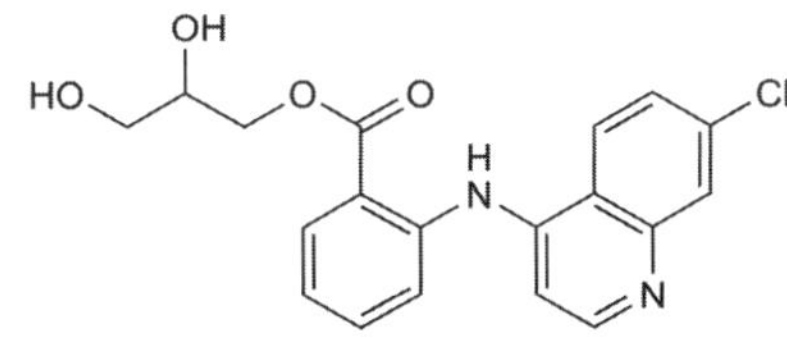

A white or slightly yellow crystalline powder. M.p. 169° to 170°. Practically insoluble in water; slightly soluble in absolute alcohol, acetone, ether, benzene, and chloroform; soluble in dilute aqueous alkalis and acids.

Partition Coefficient. Log *P* (octanol/water), 3.7.

Thin-layer Chromatography. System TA—Rf 67; system TB—Rf 01; system TC—Rf 38; system TE—Rf 46; system TF—Rf 03; system TL—Rf 40; system TAE—Rf 81; system TAF—Rf 78.

Gas Chromatography. System GA—glafenine, not eluted; glafenine-Me RI 2770.

High Performance Liquid Chromatography. System HX—RI 372; system HY—RI 276; system HZ—Retention time, 2.3 min.

Ultraviolet Spectrum. Aqueous acid—345 nm (A_1^1=467b).

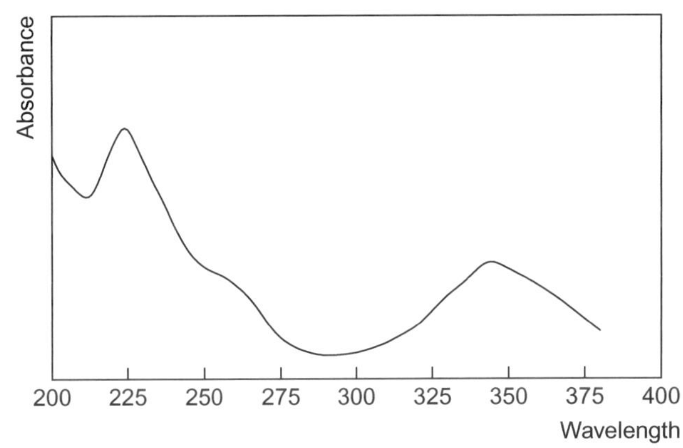

Quantification

High performance liquid chromatography. In plasma: glafenine and metabolites, limits of detection 500 μg/L for glafenine and hydroxyglafenic acid, 200 μg/L for glafenic acid, UV detection—M. C. Tournet *et al.*, *J. Chromatogr.*, 1981, *224*; *B Biomed. Appl.*, *13*, 348–352. In plasma: glafenine and glafenic acid, limits of detection 50 μg/L and 250 μg/L respectively, UV detection—A. Ennachachibi *et al.*, *J. Chromatogr.*, 1988, *427*, 307–314. In plasma: glafenine and floctafenine, limit of detection for glafenine about 2 μmol/L—A. Tracqui *et al.*, *Ann. Biol. Clin. (Paris)*, 1988, *46*, 665–667.

Disposition in the Body. Absorbed after oral administration with peak plasma concentrations occurring about 1 to 2 hours after ingestion. It is hydrolysed to glafenic acid which is excreted in the urine as an acylglucuronide conjugate; glafenic acid is found in plasma at concentrations greater than those of unchanged drug. Small amounts of unconjugated *N*-oxide of glafenic acid, and hydroxyglafenic acid which is mainly conjugated, have also been found in urine.

Therapeutic concentration

After a single 400-mg oral dose of glafenine, a mean peak plasma concentration of 0.7 mg/L was achieved in 1.5 h in 12 healthy subjects and 2.2 mg/L in 2.8 h in 12 cirrhotic subjects; the large hepatic first-pass effect observed in healthy subjects was markedly reduced in cirrhotic subjects (ratio of C_{max} glafenic acid to C_{max} glafenine=18.9 in healthy subjects and 3.6 in cirrhosis) [N. Vermerie *et al.*, *Fundam. Clin. Pharmacol.*, 1992, *6*, 197–203.]

Toxicity. Plasma concentrations greater than 75 mg/L may be associated with toxic effects.
It has a high incidence of anaphylactic reactions and has been withdrawn from the market in most countries.

Half-life. About 1 to 2 h.

Dose. Up to 1.2 g daily.

Glibenclamide

Antidiabetic

Synonyms. Glybenclamide; Glyburide; Glycbenzcyclamide.
Proprietary names. Azuglucon; Basstiverit; Calabren; Daonil; DiaBeta; Diabetamide; Diacon; Euglucan; Euglucon; Glib; Gliben; Glibenbeta; Gluconorm; Glucoremed; Glynase; Hemi-Doanil; Libanil; Malix; Maninil; Micronase; Miglucan; Semi-Daonil; Semi-Euglucon.
5-Chloro-*N*-[2-[4-[[[(cyclohexylamino)carbonyl]amino]sulfonyl]-phenyl]ethyl]-2-methoxybenzamide
$C_{23}H_{28}ClN_3O_5S$ = 494.0
CAS—10238-21-8

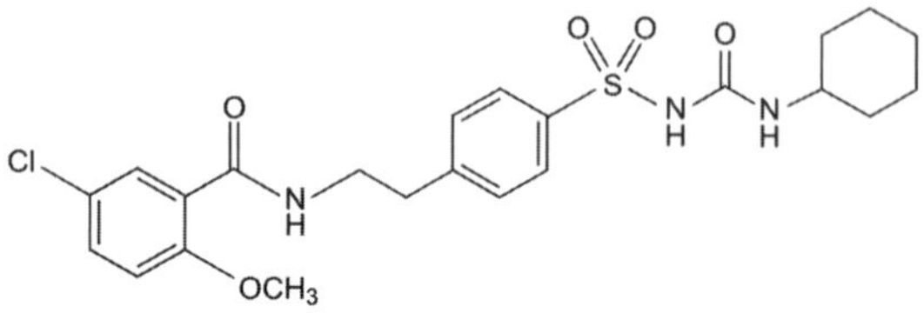

A white crystalline powder. M.p. 172° to 174°.
Sparingly soluble in water; practically insoluble in ether; soluble 1 in 330 of ethanol, 1 in 36 of chloroform, and 1 in 250 of methanol.

Dissociation Constant. pK_a 5.3.

Partition Coefficient. Log*P* (octanol/water), 4.8.

Colour Tests. Aromaticity (Method 2) —yellow/orange; Liebermann's Test (100°)—orange (15 s).

Thin-layer Chromatography. System TA—Rf 80; system TB—Rf 00; system TD—Rf 30; system TE—Rf 11; system TF—Rf 30; system TAD—Rf 57; system TAE—Rf 90. (Acidified iodoplatinate solution, positive.)

Gas Chromatography. System GA—glibenclamide-Me RI 3800; glibencamide-Me_2 RI 3840.

High Performance Liquid Chromatography. System HX—RI 637; system HY—RI 571; system HZ—Retention time, 14.4 min; system HAA—Retention time, 22.0 min; system HAX—Retention time, 8.5 min; system HAY—Retention time, 9.8 min.

Ultraviolet Spectrum. Methanol—275, 300 nm (A^1_1 = 63a).

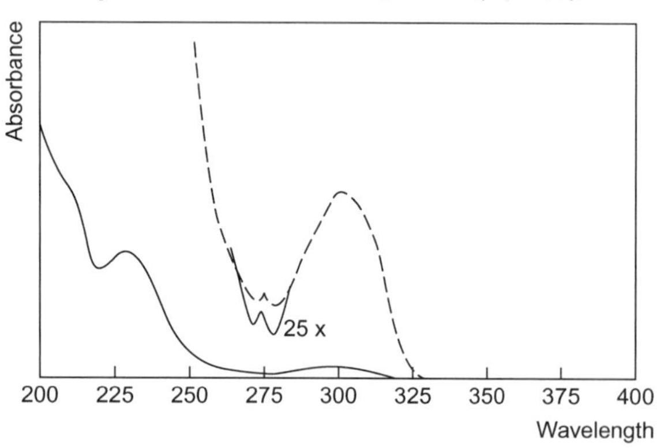

Infra-red Spectrum. Principal peaks at wavenumbers 1524, 1160, 1623, 1718, 1276, 823 cm^{-1} (KBr disk).

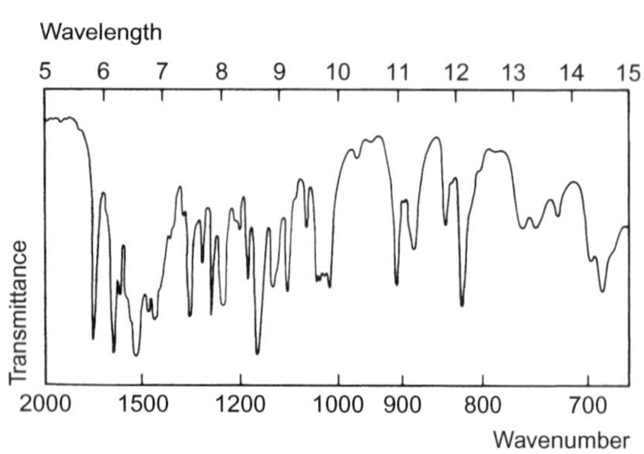

Quantification

Gas chromatography. In plasma: limit of detection 5 µg/L, ECD—D. Castoldi and O. Tofanetti, *Clinica Chim. Acta*, 1979, *93*, 195–198. In serum or urine: glibenclamide and its major metabolites; limit of detection for glibenclamide in serum 1 µg/L, UV detection—T. Rydberg *et al.*, *J. Chromatogr.*, 1991, 564, 223–233.

High performance liquid chromatography. In serum: limit of detection 10 µg/L, fluorescence detection—W. J. Adams *et al.*, *Anal. Chem.*, 1982, *54*, 1287–1291. In plasma or urine: limits of detection 5 to 10 µg/L—H. Emilsson *et al.*, *J. Chromatogr.*, 1986, *383*, 93–102. In serum: limit of detection 20 µg/L, UV detection—M. E. Abdel-Hamid *et al.*, *J. Clin. Pharm. Ther.*, 1989, *14*, 181–188. In plasma: glibenclamide and other sulfonylureas, limit of detection 10 to 40 µg/L—A. Sener *et al.*, *Acta Diabetol.*, 1995, *32*, 64–68. In plasma: limit of detection 5 µg/L, UV detection—J. R. Valdes Santurio and E. Gonzalez Porto, *J. Chromatogr. B Biomed. Appl.*, 1996, *682*, 364–370. In plasma: limit of detection 5 µg/L, fluorescence detection—J. Khatri *et al.*, *J. Pharm. Pharm. Sci.*, 2001, *4*, 201–206. In plasma: limit of detection $<$10 µg/L—I. Niopas and A. C. Daftsios, *J. Pharm. Biomed. Anal.*, 2002, *28*, 653–657.

Disposition in the Body. Readily absorbed after oral administration; widely distributed throughout the body and metabolised mainly by 4-*trans*- and 3-*cis*-hydroxylation of the cyclohexyl ring. About 20 to 50% of a dose is excreted in the urine in 24 h, mainly as metabolites; about 45 to 75% of a dose is eliminated in the faeces over a period of 5 days.

Therapeutic concentration
After a single oral dose of 5 mg to 2 subjects, peak plasma concentrations of 0.17 to 0.36 mg/L were attained in 3 h. [L. Balant *et al.*, *Eur. J. Clin. Pharmacol.*, 1975, *8*, 63–69.]

Toxicity
In a suicide attempt, a concentration of 0.6 mg/L was found in the serum initially. After 84 h the concentration had declined to $<$0.1 mg/L. [M. Berger *et al.*, *Dtsch. Med. Wochenschr.*, 1977, *102*, 586–587.]

Half-life. Plasma half-life, 5 to 16 h.

Volume of distribution. About 0.3 L/kg.

Distribution in blood. Plasma:whole blood ratio, 2.

Protein binding. In plasma, about 99%.

Note. For reviews of the pharmacokinetics of hypoglycaemic drugs see L. Balant, *Clin. Pharmacokinet.*, 1981, *6*, 215–241 and J. E. Jackson and R. Bressler, *Drugs*, 1981, *22*, 211–245.

Dose. 5 to 15 mg daily.

Glibornuride

Antidiabetic

Proprietary names. Gluborid; Glutril.
[1*S*-(*endo*,*endo*)]-*N*-[[(3-Hydroxy-4,7,7-trimethylbicyclo[2.2.1]hept-2-yl)amino]carbonyl]-4-methylbenzenesulfonamide
$C_{18}H_{26}N_2O_4S$ = 366.5
CAS—26944-48-9

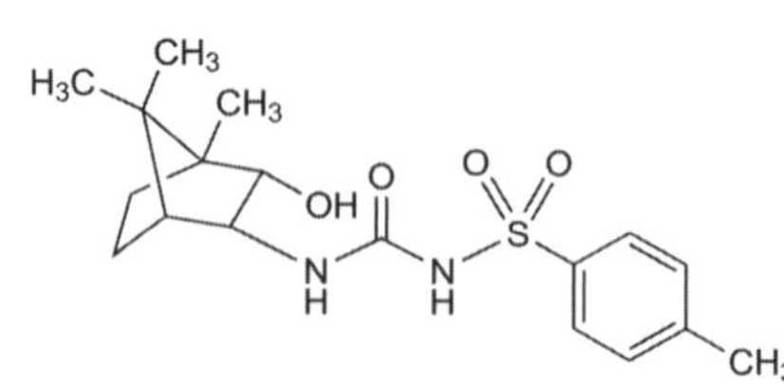

Crystals. M.p. 192° to 195°.

Colour Tests. Koppanyi–Zwikker Test—violet; Mercurous Nitrate—black.

Thin-layer Chromatography. System TD—Rf 40; system TE—Rf 05; system TF—Rf 60; system TAD—Rf 54; system TAE—Rf 92.

Gas Chromatography. System GA—Art (methylsulfonamide) RI 1730, art (methylsulfonamide)-Me RI 1740, art (amide) RI 1620, M (OH-)-art (sulfonamide)-Me RI 2265, M (OH-)-art (sulfonamide)-Me_2 RI 2030, M

(COOH-)-art (sulfonamide)-Me_3 RI 1955; system GB—glibornuride, not eluted, art (methylsulfonamide) RI 1660, art (amide) RI 1695.

Ultraviolet Spectrum. Ethanol—257, 264 (A^1_1=17a), 275 nm.

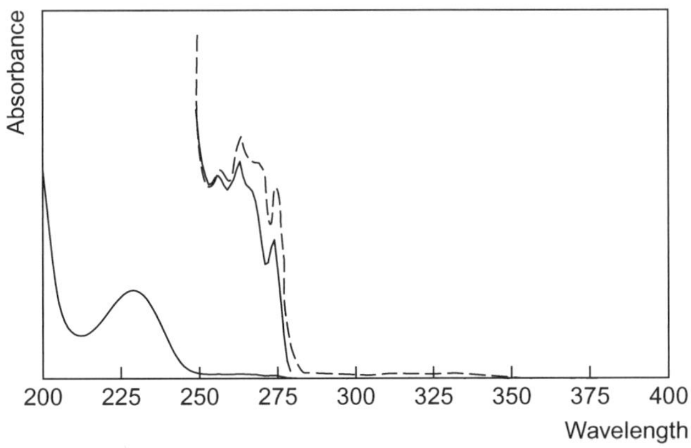

Infra-red Spectrum. Principal peaks at wavenumbers 1170, 1682, 1520, 1710, 1050, 1100 cm^{-1} (KBr disk).

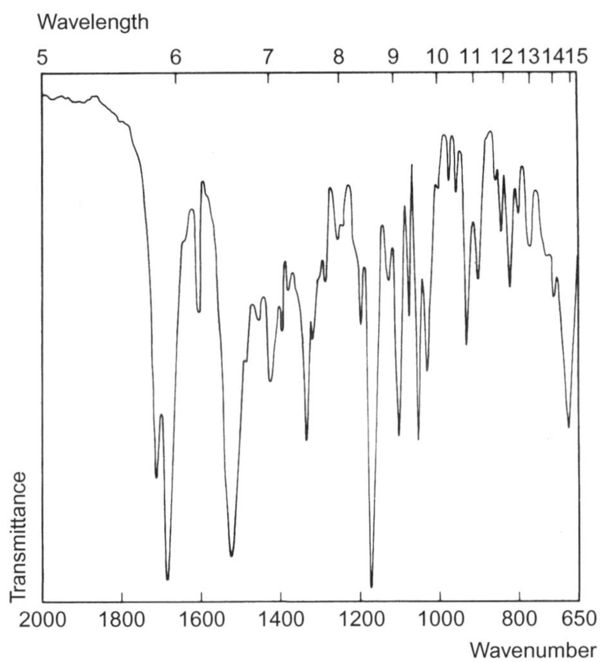

Mass Spectrum. Principal ions at *m*/*z* 91, 155, 197, 65, 84, 39, 95, 41.

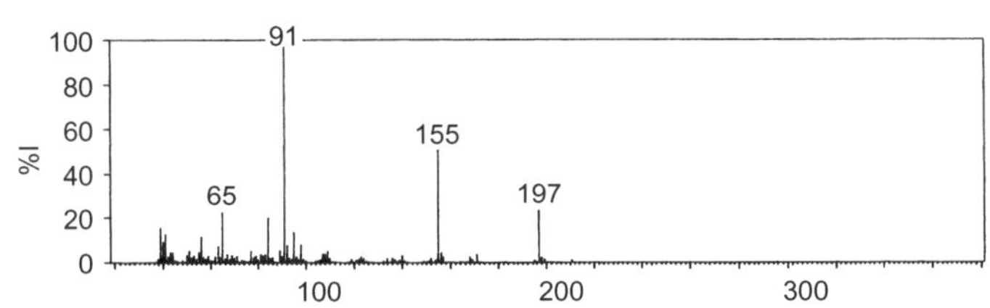

Quantification

Spectrofluorimetry. In plasma or serum: limit of detection 40 µg/L—R. Becker, *Arzneimittelforschung*, 1977, *27*, 102–104.

High performance liquid chromatography. In serum: limit of detection 500 µg/L, UV detection—K. Harzer, *J. Chromatogr.*, 1980, *183*; *B Biomed. Appl.*, *9*, 115–117.

Disposition in the Body. Readily absorbed after oral administration. Extensively metabolised by hydroxylation to a series of inactive or almost inactive compounds and by oxidation to a *p*-carboxy derivative. About 60 to 70% of a dose is excreted in the urine as metabolites; four hydroxylated derivatives account for about 75% of the urinary material, *p*-hydroxyglibornuride accounts for about 6%, and *p*-carboxyglibornuride for about 7%; the remainder of a dose is eliminated in the faeces.

Therapeutic concentration

After an oral dose of 50 mg to 7 subjects, peak plasma concentrations of 1.6 to 3.4 mg/L were attained in about 3 to 4 h [G. Rentsch *et al.*, *Arzneimittelforschung.*, 1972, *22*, 2209–2212.]

Half-life. Plasma half-life, 5 to 11 h (mean 8).

Volume of distribution. 0.15 to 0.35 L/kg.

Protein binding. In plasma, about 95%.

Note. For reviews of the pharmacokinetics of sulfonylurea hypoglycaemic drugs, see L. Balant, *Clin. Pharmacokinet.*, 1981, *6*, 215–241 and J. E. Jackson and R. Bressler, *Drugs*, 1981, *22*, 211–245.

Dose. 12.5 to 75 mg daily.

Gliclazide

Antidiabetic

Proprietary names. Cadicon; Diabeside; Diabrezide; Diaclaron; Diaglyk; Dialoc; Diamexon; Diamicron; Dramion; Glicron; Glimicron; Glucozide; Glyade; Glycemirex; Glycon; Glycron; Medoclazide; Serviclazide; Sun-Glizide; Ziclin.

N-[[(Hexahydrocyclopenta[*c*]pyrrol-2(1*H*)-yl)amino]carbonyl]-4-methylbenzenesulfonamide

$C_{15}H_{21}N_3O_3S$=323.4

CAS—21187-98-4

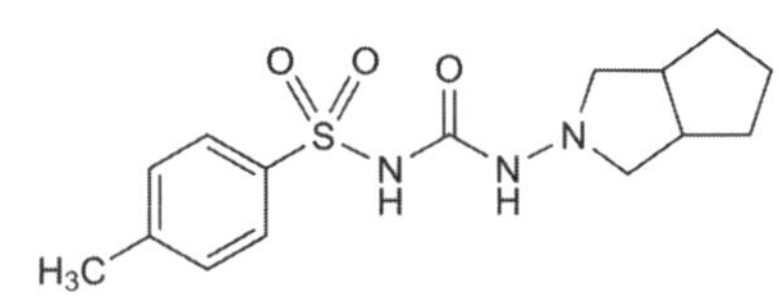

A crystalline solid. M.p. about 181°.

Dissociation Constant. pK_a 5.8.

Partition Coefficient. Log *P* (octanol/water), 2.1.

Colour Tests. Liebermann's Test—yellow; Mercurous Nitrate—black.

Thin-layer Chromatography. System TB—Rf 00; system TE—Rf 09; system TAE—Rf 84.

Gas Chromatography. System GA—Art 1-Me RI 1545; art (amide) RI 1620; art 3 RI 1670; art (methylsulfonamide) RI 1730; art (methylsulfonamide)-Me RI 1740; M (OH-)-art (sulfonamide)-Me RI 2265; M (OH-)-art (sulfonamide)-Me_2 RI 2030; M (HOOC-)-art (sulfonamide)-Me_3 RI 1955; system GB—art (methylsulfonamide) RI 1660.

High Performance Liquid Chromatography. System HX—RI 536; system HY—RI 483; system HZ—Retention time, 8.8 min; system HAA—Retention time, 20.5 min.

Ultraviolet Spectrum. Aqueous acid—230 nm (A^1_1=440b); aqueous alkali—263 nm (A^1_1=20b).

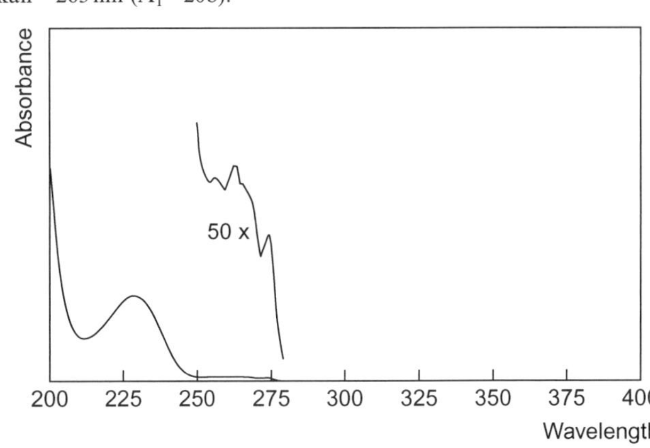

Infra-red Spectrum. Principal peaks at wavenumbers 1707, 1162, 920, 667, 1089, 997 cm^{-1} (KBr disk).

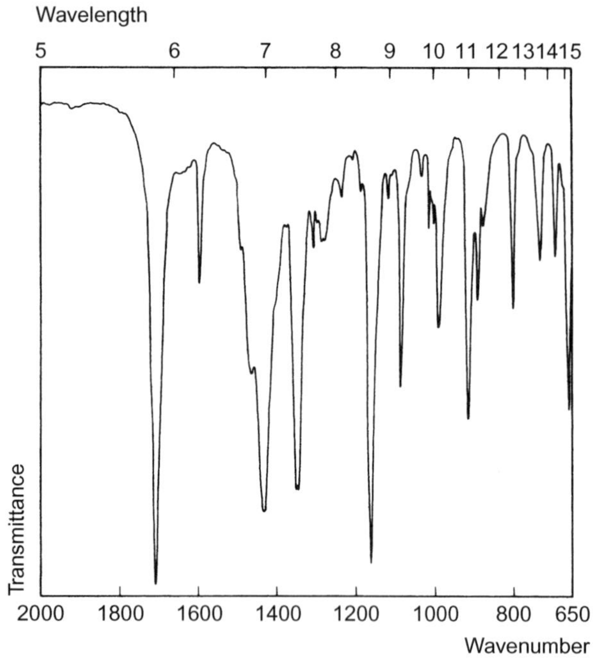

Quantification

High performance liquid chromatography. In serum: limit of detection 200 µg/L, UV detection—M. Kimura *et al.*, *J. Chromatogr.*, 1980, *183 Biomed. Appl.*, *9*, 467–473. In plasma: limit of detection 300 µg/L, UV detection—M. Kimura *et al.*, *Chem. Pharm. Bull.*, 1980, *28*, 344–346. In serum: limit of detection 20 µg/L, UV detection—H. Noguchi *et al.*, *J. Chromatogr.*, 1992, *583*, 266–269. In plasma: gliclazide and other sulfonylureas, limit of detection 10 to 40 µg/L—A. Sener *et al.*, *Acta Diabetol.*, 1995, *32*, 64–68.

Disposition in the Body. Absorbed after oral administration. It is extensively metabolised by hydroxylation, *N*-oxidation and oxidation to several inactive metabolites; the *p*-carboxy metabolite, which accounts for about 1% of the plasma concentration, has no hypoglycaemic activity but has some antithrombotic activity. About 60 to 70% of a dose is excreted in the urine with less than 5% as unchanged drug. The *p*-carboxy and *N*-oxide metabolites account for about 40% of the dose. About 10 to 20% of the dose is eliminated in the faeces as metabolites.

Therapeutic concentration

After a single oral dose of 80 mg to 23 subjects, peak plasma concentrations of 0.7 to 4.9 mg/L were attained in about 4 h. Following daily oral administration of 80 mg to 144 subjects, steady-state plasma concentrations of 0.3 to 8.2 mg/L (mean 2.5) were reported [D. B. Campbell *et al.*, Pharmacokinetics and metabolism of gliclazide, in *Gliclazide and the Treatment of Diabetes*, H. Keen *et al.* (eds), London, Royal Society of Medicine, 1980, pp. 71–82].

Half-life. Plasma half-life, 6 to 14 h (mean 10).

Protein binding. In plasma, 85 to 95%.

Dose. 40 to 320 mg daily.

Glimepiride

Antidiabetic

Synonym. HOE-490
Proprietary name. Amaryl
3-Ethyl-2,5-dihydro-4-methyl-*N*-[2-[4-[[[[(*trans*-4-methylcyclohexyl)-amino]carbonyl]amino]sulfonyl]phenyl]ethyl]2-oxo-1*H*-pyrrole-1-carboxamide
$C_{24}H_{34}N_4O_5S = 490.6$
CAS—93479-97-1

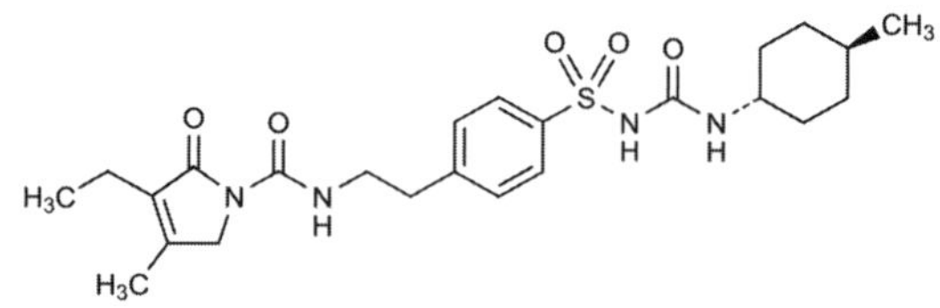

A white to yellowish-white crystalline almost odourless powder. M.p. 207°. It is practically insoluble in water.

High Performance Liquid Chromatography. In serum—column: ODS (Spherisorb, 125 × 4.6 mm i.d., 5 µm). Mobile phase: (A)-0.05 M perchloric acid:acetonitrile (60:40); after 6 min, switched to (B)-0.05 M perchloric acid:acetonitrile (42:58); after 8 min, (A), 2 mL/min flow rate. Retention time: (derivatives) glimepiride, 11.3 min; metabolites, 4.3 and 5.2 min. In urine—column: ODS (Spherisorb, 125 × 4.6 mm i.d., 5 µm). Mobile phase: 0.05 M perchloric acid:acetonitrile (60:40), 2 mL/min flow rate. UV detection (λ=350 nm). Retention time: (derivatives) metabolites, 4.8 and 5.6 min [K. H. Lehr and P. Damm, *J. Chromatogr.*, 1990, *526*, *Biomed. Appl.*, *91*, 497–505].

Ultraviolet Spectrum. Methanol—226, 273 nm.

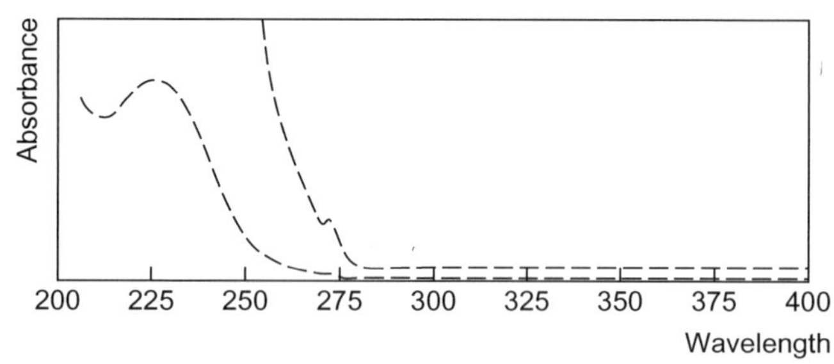

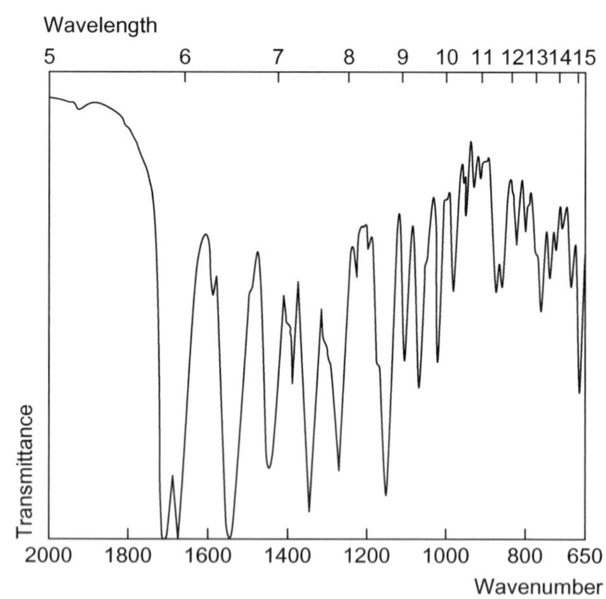

Quantification

High performance liquid chromatography. In serum or urine: limit of detection 5 µg/L, UV detection (λ=350 nm)—K. H. Lehr and P. Damm, *J. Chromatogr.*, 1990, *526*, *Biomed. Appl.*, *91*, 497–505.

Disposition in the Body. Glimepiride is completely absorbed after oral administration. Peak plasma concentrations are attained within about 2 to 3 h. It is completely metabolised principally in the liver, mainly to the cyclohexyl hydroxy methyl derivative that has about a third the pharmacological activity of glimepiride, and the carboxyl derivative. These metabolites appear rapidly after administration of the parent drug.

Cytochrome P450 isoenzyme 2C9 is involved in the formation of the cyclohexyl hydroxy methyl derivative. Glimepiride is distributed into breast milk and crosses the placenta. About 40% of a dose is eliminated in faeces as metabolites and about 60% of a dose is eliminated in urine as metabolites.

Therapeutic concentration

42 healthy volunteers, with a mean age of 27 years, were administered a single dose of 0.25 to 1.5 mg after an overnight, 10 to 12 h fast. The serum concentration measured 30 min after administration was 54 to 247 µg/L and after 180 min, 17 to 72 µg/L [K. Ratheiser *et al.*, *Arzneimittelforschung*, 1993, *43*, 856–858].

12 healthy volunteers were administered single doses of 1, 2, 4 or 8 mg glimepiride. Mean drug concentrations were 103.2, 176.8, 307.8 and 550.8 µg/L for the doses at 2.3, 2.4, 2.1 and 2.8 h, respectively [V. Malerczyk *et al.*, *Drug Metab. Drug Interact.*, 1994, *11(4)*, 341–357].

Half-life. Plasma half-life, 5 h after single dose; 9 h after multiple doses.

Volume of distribution. Approx. 113 mL/kg; 8.8 L.

Clearance. Total body, 2.7 to 3.4 L/h.

Protein binding. In plasma, more than 99.5%.

Note. For a review of glimepiride see H. D. Langtry and J. A. Balfour, *Drugs*, 1998, *55*, 563–584.

Dose. Usually up to 4 mg daily.

Glipizide

Antidiabetic

Synonyms. Glipizidum; Glydiazinamide; K-4024; CP-28720.
Proprietary names. Apamid; Diasef; Dipazide; Glibenese; Glidiab; Glipid; Glipiscand; Gluco-Rite; Glucotrol; Glupital; Glygen; Melizid(e); Mindiab; Minidiab; Minodiab; Ozidia.
N-[2-[4-[[[(Cyclohexylamino)carbonyl]amino]sulfonyl]phenyl]ethyl]-5-methylpyrazinecarboxamide
$C_{21}H_{27}N_5O_4S = 445.5$
CAS—29094-61-9

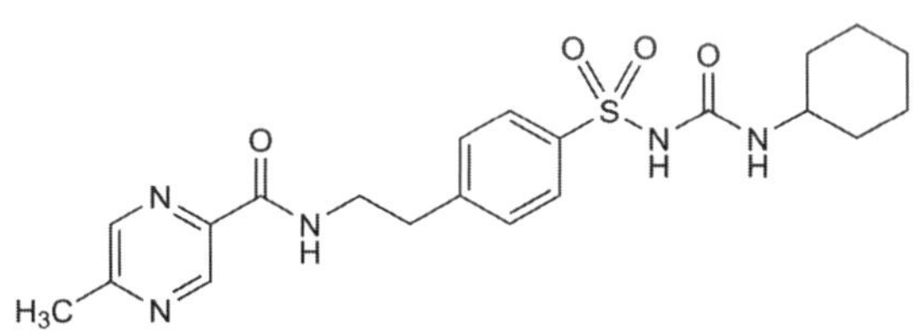

A white powder. M.p. about 205°.
Practically insoluble in water and ethanol; soluble in chloroform, dimethylformamide, and dilute solutions of alkali hydroxides; sparingly soluble in acetone.

Dissociation Constant. pK_a 5.9.

Partition Coefficient. Log *P* (octanol/water), 1.9.

Colour Test. Mercurous Nitrate—black.

Thin-layer Chromatography. System TA—Rf 87; system TB—Rf 00; system TC—Rf 41; system TE—Rf 07; system TL—Rf 05; system TAE—Rf 86.

Gas Chromatography. System GA—glipizide-Me RI 3420; glipizide-Me_2 RI 3455.

High Performance Liquid Chromatography. System HX—RI 478; system HY—RI 423; system HZ—retention time 4.5 min; system HAA—retention time 17.6 min.

Ultraviolet Spectrum. Aqueous acid—276 nm (A^1_1 = 231a). No alkaline shift.

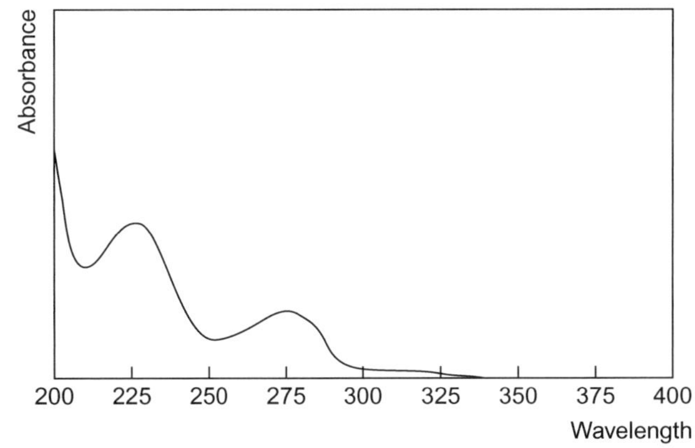

Infra-red Spectrum. Principal peaks at wavenumbers 1528, 1690, 1650, 1159, 1032, 900 cm^{-1} (KBr disk).

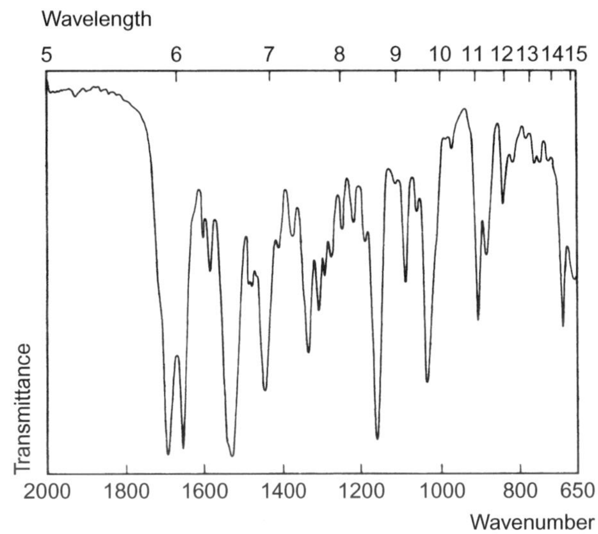

Mass Spectrum. Principal ions at *m/z* 150, 121, 56, 93, 39, 151, 66, 94.

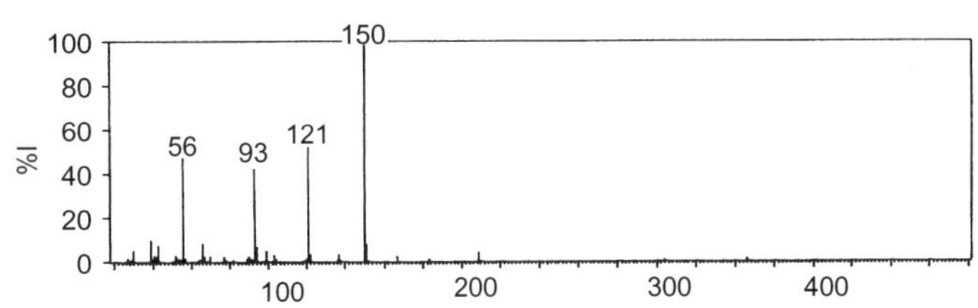

Quantification

High performance liquid chromatography. In serum: limit of detection 20 µg/L, UV detection—E. Wåhlin-Boll and A. Melander, *J. Chromatogr.* 1979, *164*(6) *B Biomed. Appl.*, 541–546. In plasma or urine: limits of detection 5 to 10 µg/L, UV detection—H. Emilsson, *J. Chromatogr.*, 1987, *421*, 319–326. In plasma: glipizide and other sulfonylureas, limits of detection 10 to 40 µg/L—A. Sener *et al.*, *Acta Diabetol.*, 1995, *32*, 64–68.

Radioimmunoassay. In plasma: limit of detection 1 µg/L—E. Maggi *et al.*, *Eur. J. Clin. Pharmacol.*, 1981, *21*, 251–255.

Disposition in the Body. Readily absorbed after oral administration. Metabolised by hydroxylation to form a number of inactive metabolites, principally the 4-*trans*-hydroxycyclohexyl and 3-*cis*-hydroxycyclohexyl derivatives. About 65 to 85% of a dose is excreted in the urine in 24 h, with about 3 to 10% as unchanged drug, up to 80% as hydroxylated metabolites, mainly the 4-*trans*-hydroxycyclohexyl derivative, and about 1 to 2% as an *N*-acetamido metabolite; about 11% of a dose is eliminated in the faeces.

Therapeutic concentration
After a single oral dose of 5 mg given to 6 subjects, peak serum concentrations of 0.11 to 0.49 mg/L (mean 0.33) were attained in about 1.6 h. [E. Wåhlin-Boll *et al.*, *Clin. Pharmacokinet.*, 1982, *7*, 363–372.]

Bioavailability. Almost 100%.

Half-life. Plasma half-life, 2 to 4 h.

Volume of distribution. About 0.2 L/kg.

Clearance. Plasma clearance, about 0.6 mL/min/kg.

Protein binding. In plasma, about 98%.

Note. For a review of the pharmacokinetics of glipizide, see R. N. Brogden *et al.*, *Drugs*, 1979, *18*, 329–353.

Dose. Usually 2.5 to 20 mg daily; up to 40 mg have been used.

Gliquidone

Antidiabetic

Proprietary names. Glurenor; Glurenorm.
N-[(Cyclohexylamino)carbonyl]-4-[2-(3,4-dihydro-7-methoxy-4,4-dimethyl-1,3-dioxo-2(1*H*)-isoquinolinyl)ethyl]benzenesulfonamide
$C_{27}H_{33}N_3O_6S = 527.6$
CAS—33342-05-1

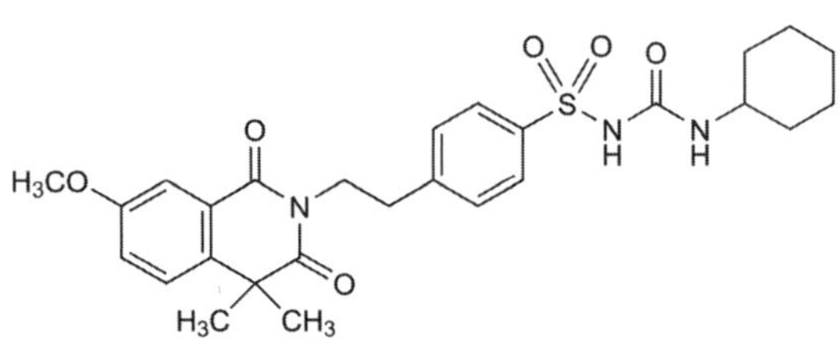

A white or slightly yellow crystalline substance. M.p. about 178°.
Practically insoluble in water; slightly soluble in ethanol and methanol; soluble in acetone and chloroform.

Partition Coefficient. Log *P* (octanol/water), 4.6.

Colour Test. Koppanyi–Zwikker Test—violet.

Thin-layer Chromatography. System TAE—Rf 93.

Gas Chromatography. System GA—gliquidone RI 2024, gliquidone-Me RI 3850.

High Performance Liquid Chromatography. System HY—RI 667.

Ultraviolet Spectrum. Methanol—311 ($A_1^1 = 50a$); aqueous alkali—276 nm.

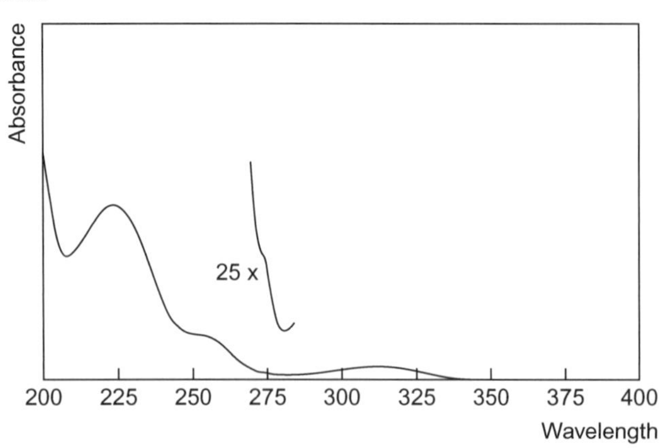

Infra-red Spectrum. Principal peaks at wavenumbers 1700, 1652, 1160, 1285, 1295, 1530 cm^{-1} (KBr disk).

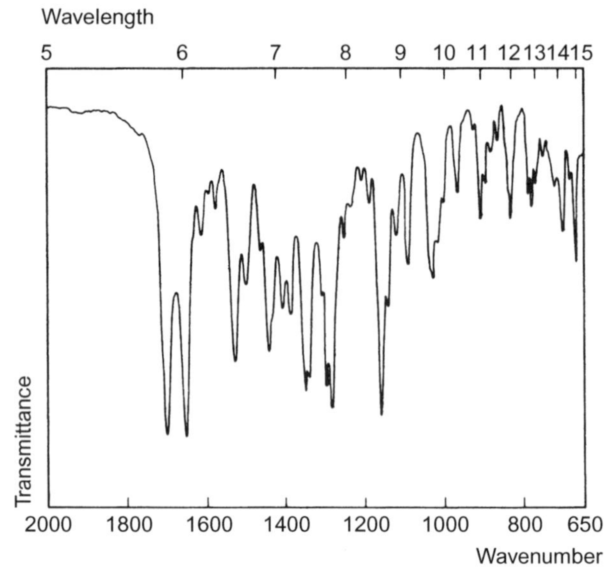

Quantification
High performance liquid chromatography. In plasma: limit of detection 30 µg/L, UV detection—P. Guo *et al.*, *Yao Xue Xue Bao*, 1992, *27*, 452–455. In plasma: gliquidone and other sulfonylureas, limit of detection 10 to 40 µg/L—A. Sener *et al.*, *Acta Diabetol.*, 1995, *32*, 64–68.

Radioimmunoassay. In plasma: limit of detection 1 µg/L—Z. Kopitar and H. E. Kompa, *Arzneimittelforschung*, 1975, *25*, 1469–1472.

Disposition in the Body. Readily absorbed after oral administration. Extensively metabolised by hydroxylation and demethylation to inactive metabolites. Less than 5% of a dose is excreted in the urine and about 95% is eliminated in the faeces, via the bile.

Therapeutic concentration
After a single oral dose of 15 mg to 10 subjects, peak plasma concentrations of about 0.7 mg/L, and peak blood concentrations of about 0.37 mg/L were reported [Z. Kopitar, *Arzneimittelforschung*, 1975, *25*, 1455–1460.]

In 20 subjects, a single 30-mg oral dose produced peak plasma concentrations of 0.12 to 2.14 mg/L (mean 0.65) at 1.25 to 4.75 h (2.25) [H. von Nicholai *et al*, *Arzneimittelforschung.*, 1997, *47*, 247–252.]

Half-life. Plasma half-life, about 1.5 h.

Distribution in blood. Plasma:whole blood ratio, about 1.9.

Protein binding. In plasma, about 99%.

Dose. 15 to 180 mg daily.

Gloxazone

Anaplasmodastat (Veterinary)

2,2′-[1-(1-Ethoxyethyl)-1,2-ethanediylidene]bishydrazinecarbothioamide
$C_8H_{16}N_6OS_2 = 276.4$
CAS—2507-91-7

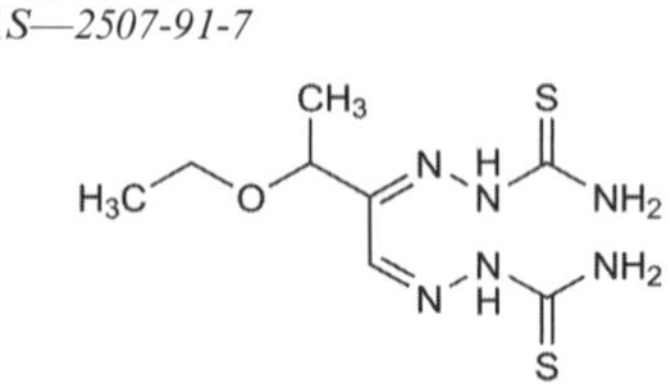

A yellow powder.
Practically insoluble in water and ether; slightly soluble in chloroform.

Colour Test. Palladium Chloride—red.

Thin-layer Chromatography. System TA—Rf 77. (Acidified iodoplatinate solution, positive.)

Ultraviolet Spectrum. Aqueous acid—329 nm; aqueous alkali—303 nm. (See below.)

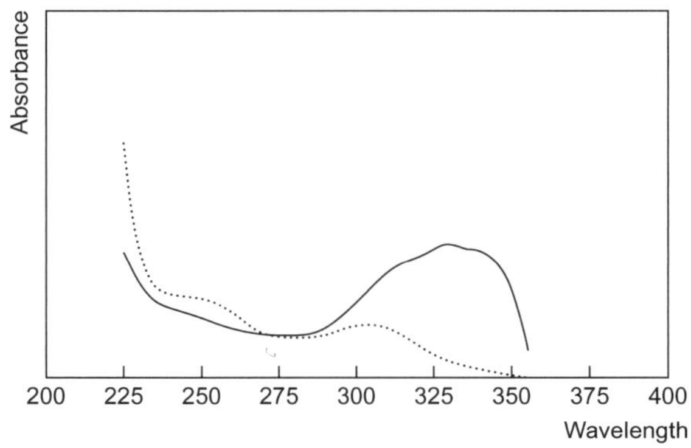

Infra-red Spectrum. Principal peaks at wavenumbers 1587, 1079, 1228, 1259, 1575, 1022 cm^{-1} (KBr disk).

Glutethimide

Hypnotic

Synonyms. Glutethimidum; Glutetimide.
Proprietary name. Doriden(e)
3-Ethyl-3-phenyl-2,6-piperidinedione
$C_{13}H_{15}NO_2$=217.3
CAS—77-21-4

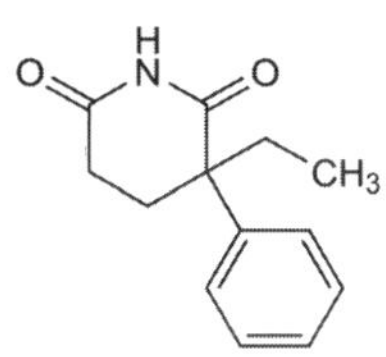

Colourless crystals or white crystalline powder. M.p. 85° to 89°. Practically insoluble in water; soluble 1 in 5 of ethanol, 1 in less than 1 of chloroform, and 1 in 12 of ether; freely soluble in acetone.

Dissociation Constant. pK_a 9.2.

Partition Coefficient. Log *P* (octanol/water), 1.9.

Colour Tests. Koppanyi–Zwikker Test—violet; Liebermann's Test—red-orange; Mercurous Nitrate—black.

Thin-layer Chromatography. System TA—Rf 75; system TB—Rf 31; system TD—Rf 63; system TE—Rf 80; system TF—Rf 62; system TAD—Rf 70; system TAE—Rf 86; system TAF—Rf 89. (Dragendorff spray, weak reaction; acidified iodoplatinate solution, positive; mercuric chloride–diphenylcarbazone reagent, positive; mercurous nitrate spray, black.)

Gas Chromatography. System GA—glutethimide RI 1830, M (OH-ethyl-) RI 1865, M (OH-phenyl-) RI 1875, M (OH-ethyl-)-AC RI 2060, M (OH-phenyl-)-AC RI 2250; system GB—glutethimide RI 1910, M (OH-ethyl-) RI 1958, M (OH-phenyl-) RI 2040; system GF—RI 2315.

High Performance Liquid Chromatography. System HE—*k* 7.97; system HX—RI 436; system HY—RI 401; system HZ—retention time 4.8 min; system HAX—retention time 6.6 min; system HAY—retention time 6.2 min.

Ultraviolet Spectrum. Ethanol—252, 258 (A_1^1=18a), 264 nm.

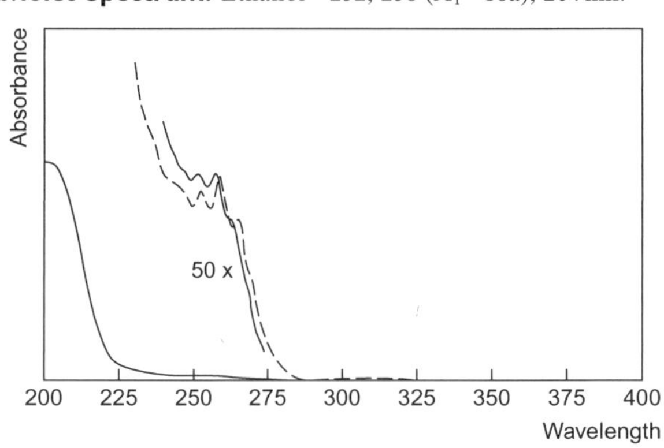

Infra-red Spectrum. Principal peaks at wavenumbers 1686, 1710, 1200, 1270, 1281, 704 cm^{-1} (KBr disk).

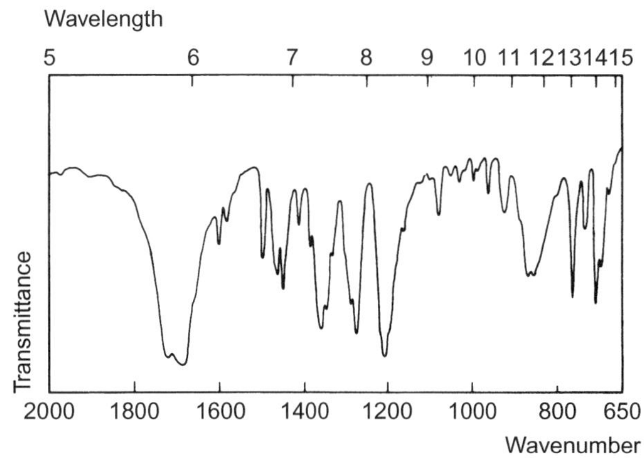

Mass Spectrum. Principal ions at *m/z* 189, 132, 117, 160, 91, 115, 103, 77; 4-hydroxyglutethimide 146, 233, 103, 133, 91, 117, 115, 77; 2-phenylglutarimide 104, 189, 103, 117, 78, 91, 51, 146.

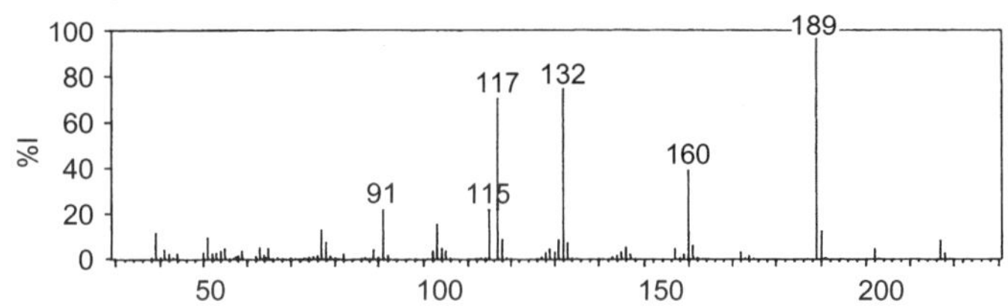

Quantification

Gas chromatography. In plasma, tissues or urine: glutethimide and 4-hydroxyglutethimide, limit of detection 200 μg/L for glutethimide and 500 μg/L for 4-hydroxyglutethimide in plasma, FID—A. R. Hansen and L. J. Fischer, *Clin. Chem.*, 1974, *20*, 236–242. In serum: limit of detection 250 μg/L, FID—D. Kadar and W. Kalow, *J. Chromatogr.*, 1972, *72*, 21–27.

Gas chromatography–mass spectrometry. In plasma or urine: glutethimide and six metabolites, limit of detection 50 μg/L—K. A. Kennedy *et al.*, *Biomed. Mass Spectrom.*, 1978, *5*, 679–685.

Disposition in the Body. Irregularly absorbed from the gastro-intestinal tract; absorption is enhanced if alcohol is taken concomitantly. Widely distributed in body tissues and fat. Glutethimide is a racemate; the (+)-isomer is metabolised in the liver to 4-hydroxyglutethimide and the (−)-isomer to 2-(1-hydroxyethyl)-2-phenylglutarimide. 4-Hydroxyglutethimide is twice as active as glutethimide in animals but does not appear to contribute to the effects of single therapeutic doses in man; however it tends to accumulate in the plasma during intoxication and may contribute to the central nervous depression in overdose cases. Both hydroxylated metabolites are converted to glucuronides and undergo enterohepatic circulation; they are still being excreted in the urine after more than 48 h. 2-Ethyl-2-(4-hydroxyphenyl)glutarimide is a major metabolite during chronic administration. Other metabolites include 2-phenylglutarimide, α-phenyl-γ-butyrolactone, and 2-ethyl-2-phenylglutaconimide which are pharmacologically active; numerous other mono- and dihydroxyphenyl metabolites have been isolated from human urine. Less than 2% of a dose is excreted unchanged in the urine in 24 h. 2-Phenylglutarimide and 2-ethyl-2-phenylglutaconimide each account for about 2 to 4% of the dose as urinary excretion products and the remainder consists largely of glucuronide conjugates of the hydroxylated metabolites. It crosses the placenta and traces are found in breast milk.

Therapeutic concentration

Following single oral doses of 500 mg to 6 subjects, peak plasma concentrations of 2.8 to 7.1 mg/L (mean 4.3) were attained in 1 to 6 h (mean 2). [S. Curry *et al.*, *Clin. Pharmacol. Ther.*, 1971, *12*, 849–857.]

Toxicity. The estimated minimum lethal dose is 5 g although recoveries have occurred after the ingestion of up to 10 g. Blood concentrations of 3.4 to 27 to 48 mg/L of glutethimide have been associated with toxic effects and concentrations of 25 to 48 to 90 mg/L have been associated with fatalities.

Postmortem blood concentrations of about 10 mg/L may be indicative of poisoning if the survival time has been prolonged.

In a review of 11 fatalities, blood concentrations of glutethimide were reported to range from 10 to 97 mg/L (mean 45) and liver concentrations from 63 to 141 µg/g (mean 89). [R. C. Baselt and R. H. Cravey, *J. Anal. Toxicol.*, 1977, *1*, 81–103.]

In a suicide attempt involving the ingestion of a glutethimide preparation that had been stored for 20 years, a blood concentration of 5 mg/L and a urinary concentration of 11 mg/L were reported. [W. Mankowski *et al.*, *Przegl. Lek.*, 2002, *59*, 390–391.]

Half-life. Plasma half-life, biphasic with a half-life of up to 22 h for the terminal phase; in acute intoxication the plasma half-life has an average value of about 40 h but may exceed 100 h.

Volume of distribution. About 3 L/kg.

Protein binding. In plasma, about 50%.

Dose. Usually 250 to 500 mg, has been given as a hypnotic.

Glyceryl Trinitrate

Anti-anginal Vasodilator

Synonyms. Glonoin; Nitroglycerin; Nitroglycerol; Trinitrin; Trinitroglycerin.

Proprietary names. Coro-Nitro; Deponit; Glytrin; Minitran; Nitrek; Nitro-Bid; Nitrocine; Nitro-Derm; Nitrodisc; Nitro-Dur; Nitrogard; Nitroglyn; Nitrol; Nitrolingual; Nitromin; Nitrotime; Nitronal; Nitrong; NitroQuick; Nitrostat; NitroTab; NTS; Percutol; Suscard; Sustac; Transdermal-NTG; Transderm-Nitro;Transiderm-Nitro; Tridil.

1,2,3-Propanetriol trinitrate

$C_3H_5N_3O_9$=227.1

CAS—55-63-0

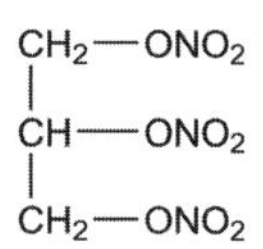

A colourless, slightly volatile, oily liquid. It explodes on rapid heating or on percussion. Mass per mL about 1.6 g.

Soluble 1 in 800 of water and 1 in 4 of ethanol; miscible with acetone, glacial acetic acid, ethyl acetate, benzene, pyridine, chloroform, and ether; sparingly soluble in petroleum ether, liquid petrolatum, and glycerol.

Caution. In fatty or oily solution it is safe and stable but in alcoholic solution the substance must be handled with the utmost caution.

Partition Coefficient. Log *P* (octanol/water), 1.6.

Colour Test. Ferrous Sulfate—red.

Thin-layer Chromatography. System TD—Rf 71; system TE—Rf 86; system TF—Rf 72.

High Performance Liquid Chromatography. System HY—RI 499.

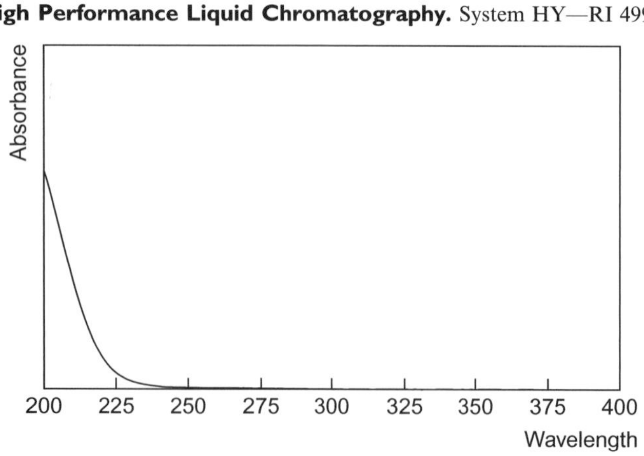

Infra-red Spectrum. Principal peaks at wavenumbers 1647, 1279, 843, 1013, 903, 754 cm^{-1}.

Quantification

Gas chromatography. In plasma: limit of detection 25 ng/L, ECD—P. K. Noonan *et al.*, *J. Pharm. Sci.*, 1984, *73*, 923–927. In biological samples: glycerol 1-nitrate and glycerol 2-nitrate, ECD—F. Scharpf *et al.*, *J. Chromatogr.*, 1987, *413*, 91–99. In plasma: 1,2- and 1,3- glyceryl dinitrates, limit of detection 250 ng/L, ECD—A. Sioufi *et al.*, *J. Chromatogr.*, 1987, *413*, 101–108. In plasma: limit of detection 0.1 µg/L, ECD—B. Hennig and R. Benecke, *Pharmazie*, 1987, *42*, 507–510. In plasma: glyceryl trinitrate and its dinitrate metabolites, limits of detection 0.025 µg/L and 0.1 µg/L respectively, ECD—F. W. Lee *et al.*, *J. Chromatogr.*, 1988, *426*, 259–266. In serum: glyceryl trinitrate and dinitrate metabolites, limit of detection 50 ng/L for glyceryl trinitrate, ECD—J. J. Janssens *et al.*, *J. Pharm. Biomed. Anal.*, 1989, *7*, 1631–1634. In plasma: glyceryl trinitrate, isosorbide dinitrate and their metabolites, limit of detection for glyceryl trinitrate 0.75 nmol—B. P. Booth *et al.*, *Biopharm. Drug Dispos.*, 1990, *11*, 663–677. In plasma: glyceryl trinitrate and its dinitrate metabolites, limit of detection about 0.2 nmol, ECD—M. Jorgensen *et al.*, *J. Chromatogr.*, 1992, *577*, 167–170. In plasma: glyceryl trinitrate and its mono- and di-nitrate metabolites, limit of detection <0.4 µg/L, ECD—C. Han *et al.*, *J. Chromatogr.*, *579*, 237–245.

High performance liquid chromatography. In plasma: limit of detection 500 ng/L—R. J. Spanggord and R. G. Keck, *J. Pharm. Sci.*, 1980, *69*, 444–446. In plasma: glyceryl trinitrate and its dinitrate metabolites, limit of detection 0.05 µg/L, thermal energy analyser detection—A. J. Woodward *et al.*, *J. Pharm. Sci.*, 1984, *73*, 1838–1840.

Disposition in the Body. Readily absorbed from the skin and mucous membranes; less readily absorbed after oral administration. It is rapidly metabolised in the body to dinitrates, which are active, and to inactive mononitrates. About 20% of a sublingual dose is excreted in the urine in 24 h, mainly as the mononitrate.

Therapeutic concentration

After sublingual administration of 0.3 mg to 1 subject, a blood concentration of about 0.001 mg/L was attained in 3 min; following an oral dose of 6.5 mg or application of an ointment containing 16 mg of glyceryl trinitrate to the same subject, peak blood concentrations of about 0.0002 to 0.0003 mg/L were reported, 20 to 60 min after the dose [H. P. Blumenthal *et al.*, *Br. J. Clin. Pharmacol.*, 1977, *4*, 241–242.]

Following sublingual administration of 0.5 mg to 6 subjects, a mean peak plasma concentration of 0.0014 mg/L was attained in 3 min; after oral administration of 6.4 mg, a peak plasma concentration of 0.0026 mg/L was reported at 2 to 4 h, and after topical administration of 35 mg, a mean peak plasma concentration of 0.0025 mg/L was attained in 1 h. Plasma nitrate and nitrite concentrations were undetectable after sublingual administration; after oral administration peak plasma concentrations of about 0.5 mg/L of nitrate and nitrite were attained in 5 and 2 h respectively, and following topical administration, peak concentrations of about 0.7 mg/L were reported at 5 h and 1 h respectively [A. Bashir *et al.*, *Br. J. Clin. Pharmacol.*, 1982, *14*, 779–784.]

Toxicity. The estimated minimum oral lethal dose is 2 g and the maximum permissible atmospheric concentration is 0.2 ppm.

Half-life. Plasma half-life, after IV administration about 2 to 5 min; after sublingual administration about 5 min.

Volume of distribution. About 3 L/kg.

Note. For a review of the pharmacokinetics of organic nitrates, see M. G. Bogaert, *Clin. Pharmacokinet.*, 1983, *8*, 410–421. For a review of IV glyceryl trinitrate see E. M. Sorkin *et al.*, *Drugs*, 1984, *27*, 45–80.

Dose. Usually the equivalent of 0.5 to 1 mg of glyceryl trinitrate sublingually, repeated as required; doses of 5.2 to 38.4 mg daily are given by mouth as sustained-release tablets.

Glycopyrronium Bromide

Anticholinergic

Synonym. Glycopyrrolate

Proprietary names. Gastrodyn; Nodapton; Ronanul; Robinul; Tarodyl; Tarodyn.

3-[(Cyclopentylhydroxyphenylacetyl)oxy]-1,1-dimethylpyrrolidinium bromide

$C_{19}H_{28}BrNO_3$=398.3

CAS—596-51-0

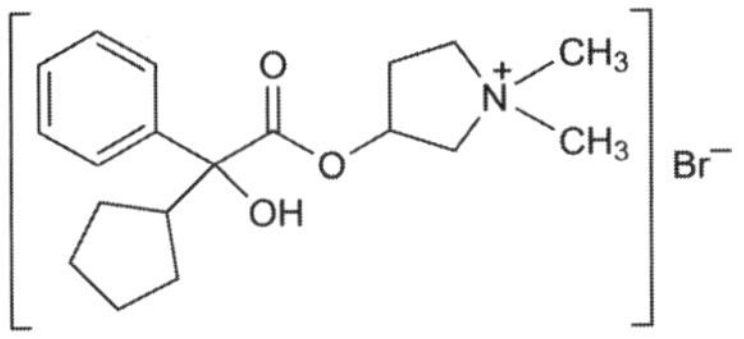

A white crystalline powder. M.p. 193° to 198°.
Soluble 1 in about 5 of water and 1 in 10 of ethanol; practically insoluble in chloroform and ether.

Partition Coefficient. Log *P* (octanol/water), −1.0.

Colour Test. The following test is performed on glycopyrronium nitrate (see Chapter 19): Liebermann's Test—black.

Thin-layer Chromatography. System TA—Rf 03; system TE—Rf 01; system TAE—Rf 03. (Acidified iodoplatinate solution, positive.)

Gas Chromatography. System GA—RI 2120.

High Performance Liquid Chromatography. System HA—*k* 3.2 (tailing peak).

Ultraviolet Spectrum. Aqueous acid—252, 258 (A^1_1=7.1a), 264 nm.

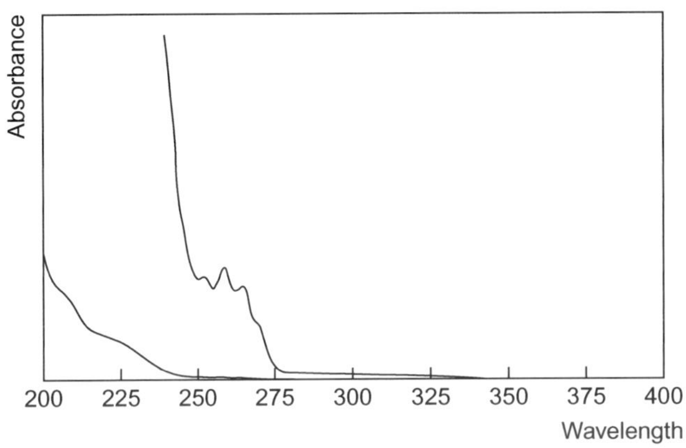

Infra-red Spectrum. Principal peaks at wavenumbers 1738, 1225, 1164, 1178, 1115, 1192 cm^{-1}.

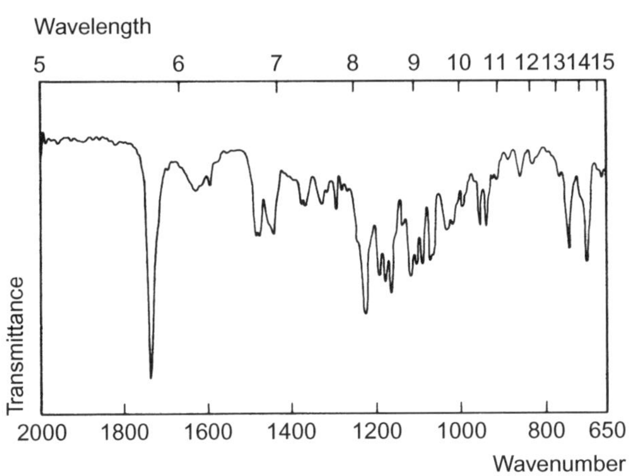

Quantification

Gas chromatography. In plasma: nitrogen-sensitive detection—G. R. Murray *et al.*, *J. Chromatogr.*, 1984, *308*, 143–151.

Disposition in the Body

Therapeutic concentration

Following a single IM injection of glycopyrronium at a dose of 8 µg/kg to 9 subjects, peak plasma concentrations of 5.03 to 26.55 µg/L (mean 15.79) were achieved in 16.11 min [T. M. Ali-Melkkila *et al.*, *Br. J. Anaesth.*, 1990, *64*, 667–669.]

Dose. 2 to 12 mg daily.

Glymidine Sodium

Antidiabetic

Synonyms. Glidiazine Sodique; Glycodiazine Sodium; Sodium Glymidine.

Proprietary names. Glyconormal; Gondafon; Lycanol; Redul.

The sodium salt of *N*-[5-(2-methoxyethoxy)-2-pyrimidinyl]-benzenesulfonamide.

$C_{13}H_{14}N_3NaO_4S$=331.3

CAS—3459-20-9

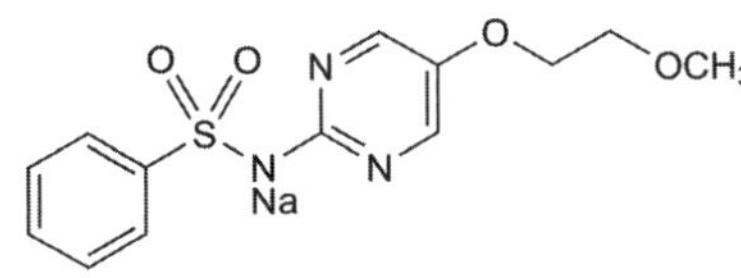

A white crystalline powder. M.p. 221° to 226°.
Soluble in water; sparingly soluble in ethanol.

Colour Tests. Koppanyi–Zwikker Test—pink-violet; Mercurous Nitrate—black.

Thin-layer Chromatography. System TA—Rf 76; system TB—Rf 00; system TC—Rf 65; system TE—Rf 05.

Gas Chromatography. System GA—RI 1632; system GB—RI 2750; system GJ—RRT of methyl derivative 0.53 (relative to griseofulvin).

Ultraviolet Spectrum. Aqueous acid—273, 299; aqueous alkali—243, 317 nm.

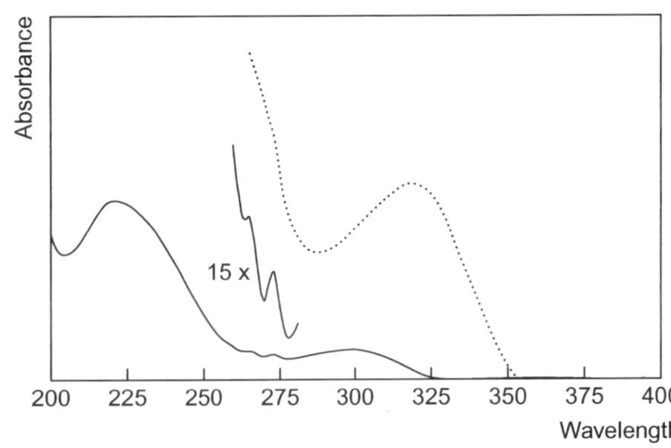

Infra-red Spectrum. Principal peaks at wavenumbers 1130, 1092, 1267, 1247, 691, 1220 cm^{-1} (KBr disk).

Mass Spectrum. Principal ions at *m*/*z* 244, 59, 77, 29, 43, 31, 45, 55.

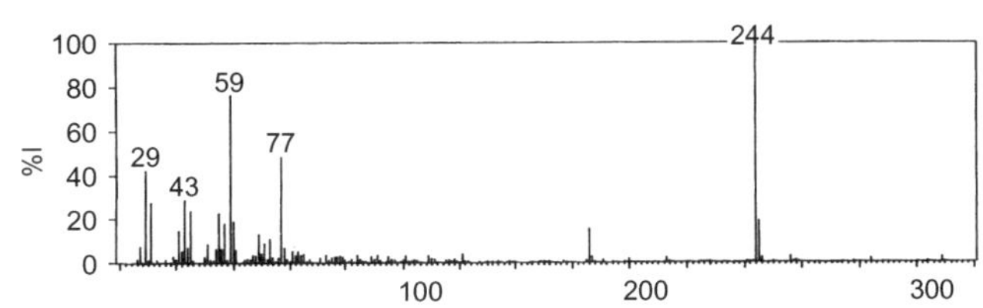

Quantification

Spectrofluorimetry. In plasma (glymidine sodium) or urine (desmethyl and carboxy metabolites): limit of detection, 1 mg/L for glymidine sodium in plasma—H. Held *et al.*, *Arzneimittelforschung*, 1970, *20*, 1927–1929.

Gas chromatography. In blood: limit of detection 1.5 mg/L, ECD—H. J. Schlicht *et al.*, *J. Chromatogr.*, 1978, *155*, 178–181.

Thin-layer chromatography-spectrophotometry. In plasma: glymidine sodium and metabolites, limit of detection 2.5 mg/L—J. C. Soyfer *et al.*, *Chim. Ther.*, 1969, *4*, 131–135.

Disposition in the Body. Almost completely absorbed after oral administration. Metabolised by demethylation to an active metabolite and oxidation to an inactive carboxy derivative. About 85 to 95% of a dose is excreted in the urine in 48 h, with less than 1% of the urinary material as unchanged drug, 20 to 40% as the desmethyl metabolite, and 60 to 80% as the carboxy metabolite; about 6% of a dose is eliminated in the faeces.

Half-life. Plasma half-life, about 2 to 6 h, increased in subjects with hepatic disease.

Protein binding. In plasma, about 80%.

Dose. 0.5 to 2 g daily.

Glyphosate

Herbicide

Proprietary names. Acrion; Agriguard; Bronco; Gallup; Gliakla; Landmaster; MON 0573; MON 2139; MON 6000; Pondmaster; Ranger; Rattler 4AS; Sonic; Spasor; Sting; Tumbleweed.
N-(Phosphoromethyl)glycine
$C_3H_8NO_5P$=169.1
CAS—1071-83-6

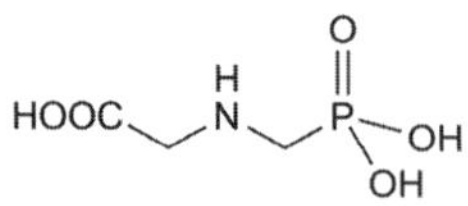

A white solid/ colourless crystals (pure state) or light amber to brown liquid (technical state). M.p. 230°.
It is soluble in water (12 g/L at 25°); insoluble in most common organic solvents.

Glyphosate Isopropylammonium

Synonym. MON-2139
Proprietary names. Drat; Glifonox; Glycel; Liphadione; Quick; Revoke; Rodeo; Rondo; Roundup.
$C_6H_{17}N_2O_5P$=228.2
CAS—38641-94-0
It is very soluble in water.

Glyphosate Sesquisodium Salt

Synonym. Sodium glyphosate
Proprietary names. MON-8000; Polado.
$C_3H_5NNaO_5P$=235.0
CAS—70393-85-0

Glyphosate Trimesium

Synonyms. SC-0224; Sulfosate.
Proprietary name. Touchdown
$C_{12}H_{32}NO_5PS_3$=245.2
CAS—81591-81-3

Dissociation Constant. pK_a 0.8 (also reported as 5.6).

Partition Coefficient. Log *P* (octanol/water), −4.00.

Thin-layer Chromatography. System TAB—Rf 00 (glyphosate acid); system TAC—Rf 00 (glyphosate acid).

Gas Chromatography. System GA—glyphosate-Me_3 RI 1410; glyphosate-Me_4 RI 1390.

Ultraviolet Spectrum. Acetonitrile—257 nm.

Mass Spectrum. (*tert*-Butyldimethylsilyl (BDMS) derivative) principal ions at *m/z* 73, 352, 454, 253, 144, 42, 212, 455.

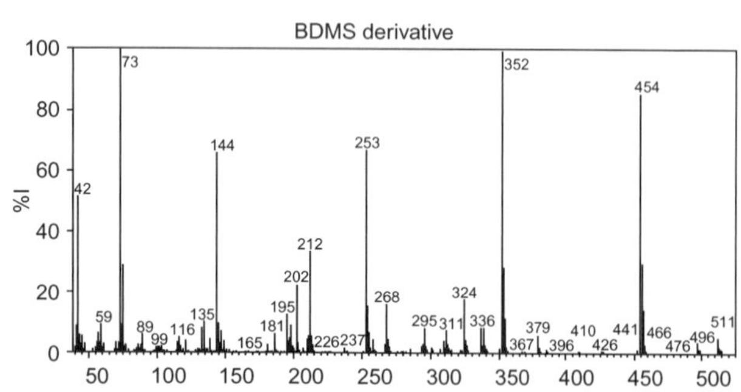

Quantification

Gas chromatography. Limit of detection 100 mg/L—N. Tsunoda, *J. Chromatogr.*, 1993, *637(2)*, 167–173.

Gas chromatography–mass spectrometry. Limit of detection 10 mg/L—N. Tsunoda, *J. Chromatogr.*, 1993, *637(2)*, 167–173.

High performance liquid chromatography. In serum: limit of detection of glyphosate 0.3 mg/L and the metabolite, AMPA 0.2 mg/L—M. Tomita *et al.*, *J. Chromatogr.* 1991, *566(1)*, *B Biomed. Sci. Appl.*, 239–243.

Disposition in the Body. Glyphosate is poorly absorbed through the skin and from the digestive tract after ingestion. It is mostly excreted unchanged but one metabolite identified is (aminomethyl)phosphonic acid (AMPA). There is no significant evidence that glyphosate accumulates in tissue.

Toxicity. Glyphosate is practically non-toxic by ingestion. The allowed daily intake is 0.3 mg/kg body weight. Minimum lethal dose is 60 mL (84-year-old man). Individuals over 40 years old who ingest over 150 mL of glyphosate are at a higher risk of death than those who are younger.

A 58-year-old man was found collapsed by his wife at home but was pronounced dead by the emergency services on arrival. Postmortem analysis discovered a dark greenish-brown fluid material in his stomach. Toxicological analysis determined that there were glyphosate concentrations of 0.30 g/L, 1.03 g/L, and 92.6 g/L in his blood, urine, and stomach contents, respectively. It was concluded that the man had consumed the Touchdown found by the side of his body. [Y. Sato *et al.*, *XXXV TIAFT Annual Meeting*, 1997, *Abstract 145*.]

Granisetron

Anti-emetic

Synonym. BRL-43694
1-Methyl-*N*-[(3-*endo*)-9-methyl-9-azabicyclo[3.3.1]non-3-yl]-1*H*-indazole-3-carboxamide
$C_{18}H_{24}N_4O$=312.4
CAS—109889-09-0

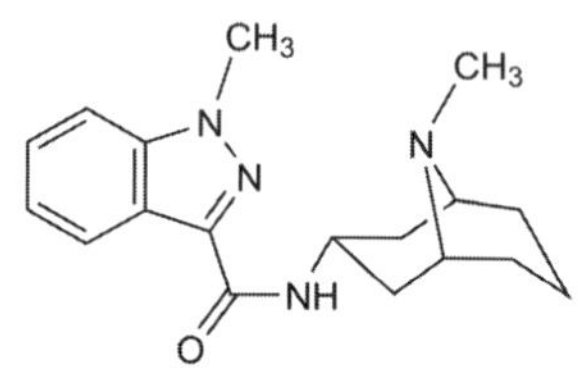

Granisetron Hydrochloride

Synonym. BRL-43694A
Proprietary name. Kytril
$C_{18}H_{24}N_4O.HCl$=348.9
CAS—107007-99-8
A white to off-white solid with M.p. 290° to 292°. It is readily soluble in water and normal saline at 20°.

Thin-layer Chromatography. System TB—Rf 18; system TE—Rf 51; system TAE—Rf 14.

High Performance Liquid Chromatography. System HX—RI 359.

Column: Apex CN (250 × 4.5 mm i.d., 10 μm), 5 cm guard column. Mobile phase: sodium acetate buffer (3%, 0.05 M) adjusted to pH 6.0 with triethylamine (0.25%) and methanol (97%). Internal standard (IS): BRL-43704. Fluorescence detection (λ_{ex}=305 nm, λ_{em}=360 nm). Retention time: granisetron, 13.5 min; IS, 19.2 min [A. Clarkson *et al.*, *Br. J. Pharmacol.*, 1987, *90*, 136P].

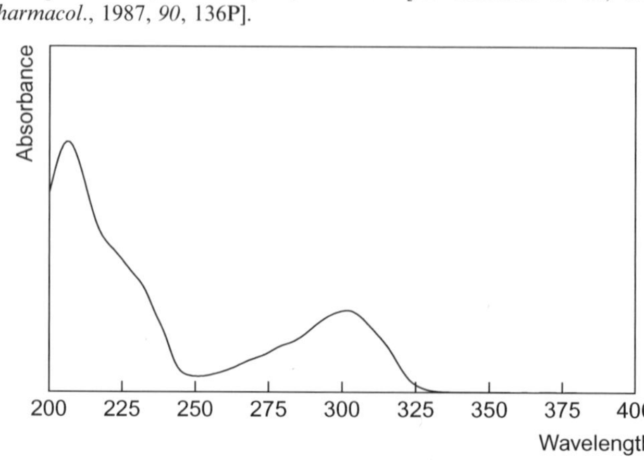

Mass Spectrum. Principal ions at *m/z* 96, 94, 159, 110, 97, 98, 136, 137.

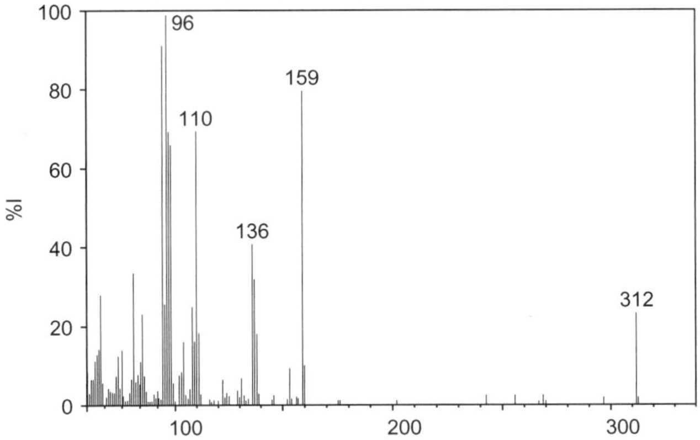

Quantification

High performance liquid chromatography. In plasma: limit of detection, 0.019 μg/L. UV detection (λ=305 nm)—B. R. Capacio *et al., J. Anal. Toxicol.*, 1993, *17(3)*, 151–155. In plasma: limit of quantification for granisetron 0.1 μg/L and for 7-hydroxygranisteron 0.25 μg/L. Fluorescence detection—V. K. Boppana, *J. Chromatogr. A*, 1995, *692(1-2)*, 195–202.

Disposition in the Body. Granisetron is rapidly and completely absorbed after oral administration and is metabolised in the liver by 7-hydroxylation, N-demethylation, aromatic ring oxidation and conjugation. Its active metabolite is 7-hydroxygranisetron. < 20% of a dose is recovered in urine unchanged and the rest is excreted in urine and faeces as its metabolites.

Therapeutic concentration

In clinical trials, 27 cancer patients and 39 healthy volunteers were administered a single dose of 1.0 mg. Mean peak plasma concentrations of 3.63 μg/L (range of 0.27 to 9.14 μg/L) were reached. Receiving 1.0 mg doses daily for 7 days, peak concentrations were 5.99 μg/L (range 0.63 to 30.9 μg/L). Peak plasma concentrations can increase up to 30% in fasted states [SmithKline Beecham, data on file].

Toxicity. During clinical trials, one patient received over 10 times the recommended dose (total of 38.5 mg) and complained of a headache only. Acute overdose: somnolence and myalgia.

Bioavailability. Oral, 60%.

Half-life. In healthy volunteers: 3 to 4 h; in patients with cancer: 9 to 12 h.

Volume of distribution. 2 to 3 L/kg, also reported as 200 L.

Clearance. 0.2 to 0.5 L/h/kg.

Distribution in blood. Distributed freely between plasma and red blood cells.

Protein binding. 65% bound.

Dose. Adults: intravenously: a single 3 mg dose of granisetron is administered, repeated if necessary with a maximum daily dose of 9 mg. Oral dose of 2 mg daily can be administered. Children: the usual dose is 10 to 40 μg/kg body weight intravenously with a maximum of 3 mg daily.

Griseofulvin

Antifungal

Synonym. Curling Factor

Proprietary names. Erlivin; Fulcin; Fulvicin; Fulvina; Grifulvin V; Grisactin; Grisaltin; Grisefuline; Griseo; Griseomed; Griseostatin; Grisovin; Gris-PEG; Grivin; Krisovin; Lamoryl; Likuden M; Medofulvin; Microcidal; Neo-Fulcin; neofulvin; Polygris; Polcyl-FP; Spirofulvin; Sporostatin; Trivanex.

(1′*S*,6′*R*)-7-Chloro-2′,4,6-trimethoxy-6′-methylspiro[benzofuran-2-(3*H*),1′-[2]-cyclohexene]-3,4′-dione

$C_{17}H_{17}ClO_6$=352.8

CAS—126-07-8

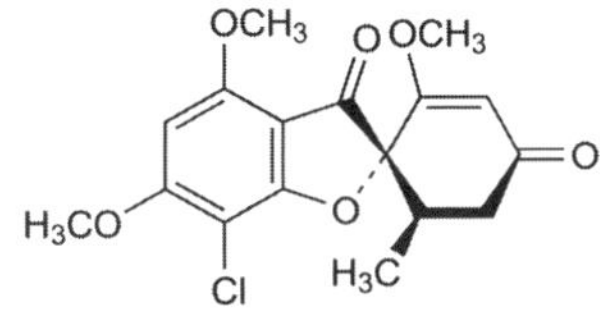

A white to pale cream-coloured powder. M.p. 217° to 224°.

Practically insoluble in water and petroleum ether; soluble 1 in 300 of dehydrated alcohol, 1 in 20 of acetone, and 1 in 25 of chloroform; soluble in dimethylformamide; slightly soluble in benzene, ethyl acetate, and acetic acid.

Partition Coefficient. Log *P* (octanol/water), 2.2.

Colour Test. Dissolve 5 mg in 1 mL of sulfuric acid and add 5 mg of powdered potassium dichromate—red.

Thin-layer Chromatography. System TD—Rf 52; system TE—Rf 69; system TF—Rf 37; system TAD—Rf 68; system TAE—Rf 78; system TAJ—Rf 68; system TAK—Rf 48; system TAL—Rf 96.

Gas Chromatography. System GA—RI 2700.

High Performance Liquid Chromatography. System HY—RI 488; system HAA—Retention time, 18.4 min.

Ultraviolet Spectrum. Dehydrated alcohol—236, 291 nm (A_1^1=686a).

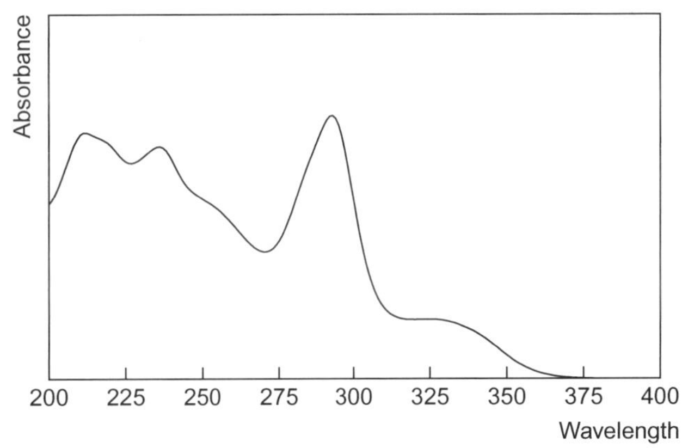

Infra-red Spectrum. Principal peaks at wavenumbers 1220, 1611, 1210, 1583, 1135, 800 cm^{-1} (KBr disk).

Mass Spectrum. Principal ions at *m/z* 138, 352, 215, 310, 214, 69, 321, 354.

Dose. 0.5 to 1 g daily.

Guaifenesin

Expectorant

Synonyms. Glyceryl Guaiacolate; Glycerylguayacolum; Guaiacol Glycerol Ether; Guaiacyl Glyceryl Ether; Guaiphenesin; Guajacolum Glycerolatum.

Proprietary names. Anti-Tuss; Benylin Children's Chesty Coughs; Breonesin; Duratuss G; Expulin Chesty Cough; Famel Expectorant; Fenesin; Genatuss; Glyate; Glycotuss; Glytuss; Hill's Balsam Chesty Cough; Jackson's All Fours; Hytuss; Jackson's Bronchial Balsam; Owbridges for Chesty Coughs; Robitussin for Chesty Coughs; Tixylix Chesty Cough; Vicks Vaposyrup for Chesty Coughs.

It is an ingredient of many proprietary preparations—see Martindale, *The complete drug reference* , 33rd Edn.

3-(2-Methoxyphenoxy)-1,2-propanediol

$C_{10}H_{14}O_4$=198.2

CAS—93-14-1

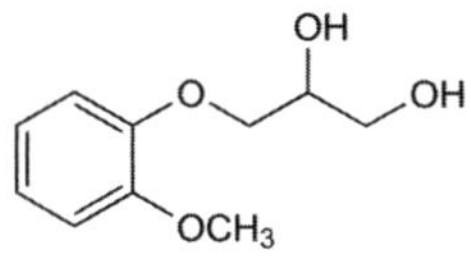

White or slightly grey crystals or crystalline aggregates. M.p. 78° to 82°. Soluble 1 in 33 of water, 1 in 11 of ethanol, 1 in 11 of chloroform, and 1 in 100 of ether; soluble in glycerol and propylene glycol; moderately soluble in benzene; practically insoluble in petroleum ether.

Partition Coefficient. Log *P* (octanol/water), 1.4.

Colour Tests. Liebermann's Test—black; Mandelin's Test—grey-green; Marquis Test—violet.

Thin-layer Chromatography. System TB—Rf 02; system TD—Rf 11; system TE—Rf 39; system TF—Rf 17; system TAD—Rf 40; system TAE—Rf 81; system TAJ—Rf 42; system TAK—Rf 27; system TAL—Rf 74.

Gas Chromatography. System GA—guaifenesin RI 1650; M (*O*-desmethyl-) RI 1700; guaifenesin-AC_2 RI 1865; M (OH-methoxy-)-AC_2 RI 2290.

High Performance Liquid Chromatography. System HX—RI 328; system HY—RI 262; system HAA—Retention time, 11.4 min; system HAX—Retention time 4.9 min; system HAY—Retention time 3.9 min.

Ultraviolet Spectrum. Aqueous acid—273 nm (A_1^1=125a). No alkaline shift.

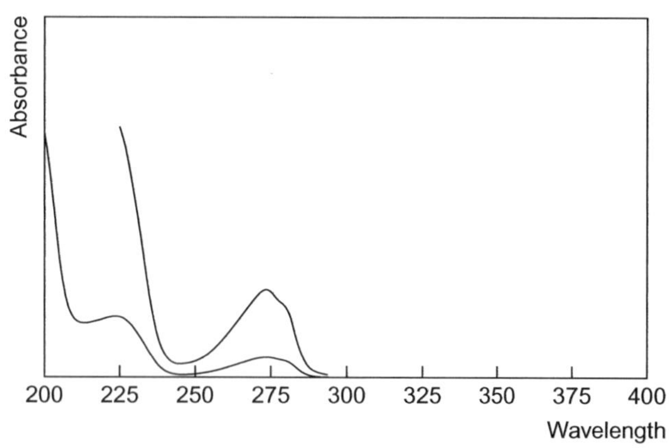

Infra-red Spectrum. Principal peaks at wavenumbers 1255, 1510, 740, 1230, 1125, 1020 cm^{-1} (KBr disk).

Mass Spectrum. Principal ions at *m/z* 124, 109, 198, 81, 77, 125, 52, 31.

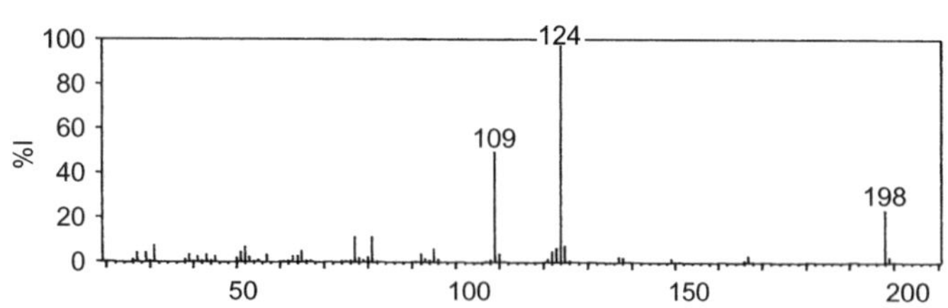

Quantification

Gas chromatography. In plasma: limit of detection 15 µg/L, ECD—S. Singhawangcha *et al.*, *J. Chromatogr.*, 1980, *183*; *B Biomed. Appl.*, *9*, 433–439. In blood: ECD—W. R. Maynard, and R. B. Bruce, *J. Pharm. Sci.*, 1970, *59*, 1346–1348.

Disposition in the Body. Readily absorbed after oral administration. It is rapidly metabolised by oxidation to *β*-(2-methoxyphenoxy)lactic acid; about 40% of a dose is excreted as this metabolite in the urine in 3 h.

Therapeutic concentration

After a single oral dose of 600 mg given to 3 subjects, a mean peak blood concentration of about 1.4 mg/L was attained in 15 min [W. R. Maynard, and R. B. Bruce, *J. Pharm. Sci.*, 1970, *59*, 1346–1348.]

Toxicity

In a fatality due to ingestion of cough syrup containing guaifenesin and hydrocodone, postmortem blood concentrations of 14 and 3 mg/L respectively were reported [R. H. Cravey per R. C. Baselt, *Disposition of Toxic Drugs and Chemicals in Man*, 5th Edn, Davis, California, Biomedical Publications, 2000, pp 397–398.]

In a suicide involving the ingestion of guaifenesin, diphenhydramine, and chlorphenamine by a 48-year-old female, the following postmortem tissue concentrations were reported, respectively: heart blood 27.4, 8.8, and 0.2 mg/L; urine 21, 29, and 3.6 mg/L, bile 222, 89, and 3 mg/L, gastric content 7700, 635, and 56 mg/L, vitreous humour 7, 1, and 0.1 mg/L, CSF 13, 2.7, and 0.32 mg/L [H. Wogoman *et al.*, *Am. J. Forensic Med. Pathol.*, 1999, *20*, 199–202.]

Half-life. Blood half-life, about 1 h.

Volume of distribution. About 1 L/kg.

Dose. 100 to 200 mg every 2 to 4 h.

Guanethidine

Antihypertensive

[2-(Hexahydro-1(2*H*)-azocinyl)ethyl]guanidine
$C_{10}H_{22}N_4$=198.3
CAS—55-65-2

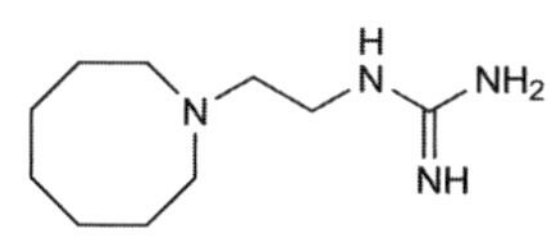

Guanethidine Monosulfate
Synonym. Guanethidine Sulfate
Proprietary names. Ismelin(e); Sanotensin; Vitutensil. It is an ingredient of Esimil, Ganda, and Suprexon.
$C_{10}H_{22}N_4,H_2SO_4$=296.4
CAS—645-43-2
A colourless crystalline powder. M.p. about 250°, with decomposition.
Soluble 1 in 1.5 of water; very slightly soluble in alcohol; practically insoluble in chloroform and ether.

Dissociation Constant. pK_a 8.3, 11.4 (20°).

Partition Coefficient. Log *P* (octanol/water), 0.9.

Thin-layer Chromatography. System TA—Rf 01; system TB—Rf 00; system TC—Rf 02; system TE—Rf 01; system TL—Rf 00; system TN—Rf 56; system TO—Rf 50; system TAE—Rf 03; system TAF—Rf 30; system TAJ—Rf 00; system TAK—Rf 00; system TAL—Rf 16. (Dragendorff spray, positive; acidified iodoplatinate solution, positive.)

Gas Chromatography. System GA—not eluted.

Ultraviolet Spectrum. No significant absorption, 230 to 360 nm.

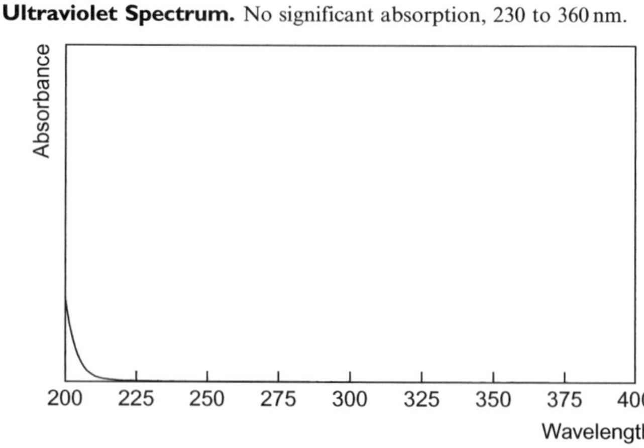

Infra-red Spectrum. Principal peaks at wavenumbers 1030, 1143, 1127, 1070, 1050, 1630 cm^{-1} (guanethidine sulfate, KBr disk).

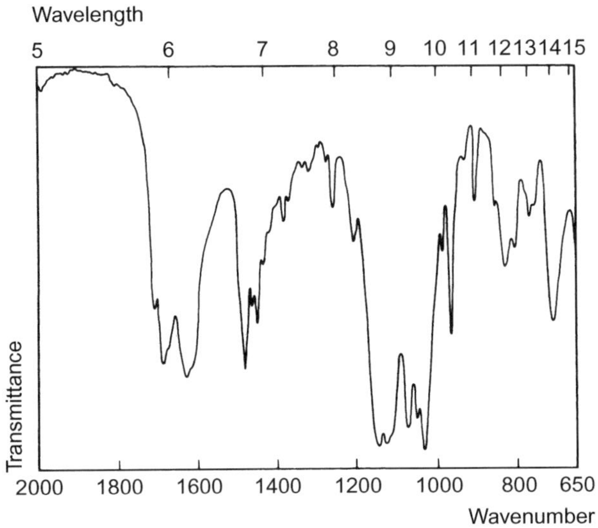

Mass Spectrum. Principal ions at *m*/*z* 126, 44, 30, 42, 41, 55, 43, 58.

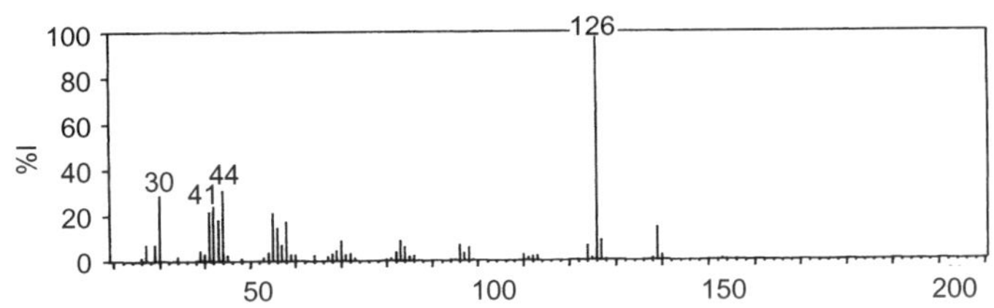

Quantification

Gas chromatography–mass spectrometry. In plasma or urine: guanethidine and other guanido-containing drugs, limit of detection 100 μg/L using FID and 1 μg/L using MID—J. H. Hengstmann *et al.*, *Anal. Chem.*, 1974, *46*, 34–39.

Radioimmunoassay. In plasma: limit of detection 4 μg/L—L. J. Loeffler and A. W. Pittman, *J. Pharm. Sci.*, 1979, *68*, 1419–1423.

Disposition in the Body. Incompletely absorbed after oral administration. Up to about 25% of an oral dose is excreted in the urine in 24 h as unchanged drug and two metabolites, guanethidine *N*-oxide and 2-(6-carboxyhexylamino)ethylguanidine; the proportion of metabolites to unchanged drug is variable. A total of about 40% of an oral dose is excreted in the urine in 9 days and about 40 to 47% is eliminated in the faeces as unchanged drug in 6 days.

Therapeutic concentration. In plasma, usually in the range 0.008 to 0.017 mg/L.

After a single oral ^{3}H-labelled dose of 50 mg to 1 subject, a peak plasma-guanethidine concentration of 0.009 mg/L was attained in 3 h and was almost constant over the period 1 to 12 h, declining slowly to about 0.003 mg/L at 24 h; a peak total metabolite concentration of about 0.04 mg/L was reported at 2 to 4 h [C. McMartin *et al.*, *Clin. Pharmacol. Ther.*, 1970, *11*, 423–431.]

Following daily oral doses of 25 mg to 8 subjects, steady-state plasma-guanethidine concentrations of 0.003 to 0.016 mg/L (mean 0.009) were reported; after oral doses of 37.5 mg daily to 8 subjects, the steady-state plasma-guanethidine concentrations ranged from 0.008 to 0.015 mg/L (mean 0.011) [I. E. Walter *et al.*, *Clin. Pharmacol. Ther.*, 1975, *18*, 571–580.]

Bioavailability. About 20%.

Half-life. Plasma half-life, about 4 to 8 days.

Protein binding. In plasma, not significantly bound.

Note. For a review of guanethidine disposition, see G. Lukas, *Drug Metab. Rev.*, 1973, *2*, 101–116.

Dose. Usually 10 to 100 mg of guanethidine monosulfate daily; up to 300 mg daily may be given.

Guanoclor

Antihypertensive

1-[2-(2,6-Dichlorophenoxy)ethylamino]guanidine
$C_9H_{12}Cl_2N_4O$=263.1
CAS—5001-32-1

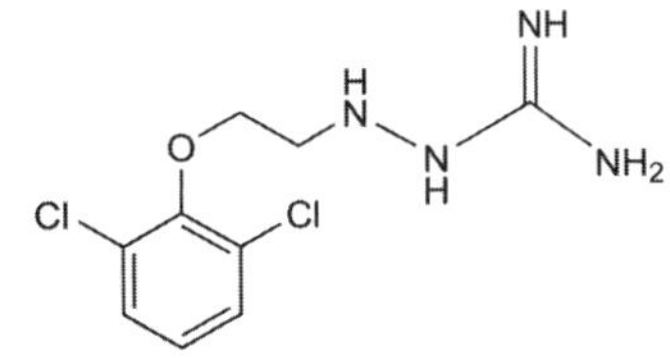

Guanoclor Sulfate

Proprietary name. Vatensol
$(C_9H_{12}Cl_2N_4O)_2,H_2SO_4$=624.3
CAS—551-48-4
A white crystalline powder. M.p. about 208°.
Soluble 1 in about 400 of water.

Partition Coefficient. Log *P* (octanol/water), 1.5.

Colour Test. Mandelin's Test—violet→orange→brown-yellow.

Thin-layer Chromatography. System TA—Rf 03; system TB—Rf 00; system TC—Rf 00; system TL—Rf 00. (Acidified iodoplatinate solution, positive.)

Ultraviolet Spectrum. Aqueous acid—272 (A^1_1=14b), 278 nm.

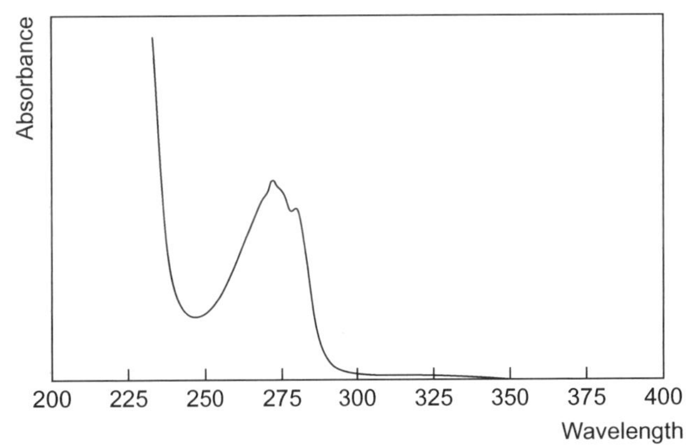

Infra-red Spectrum. Principal peaks at wavenumbers 1672, 1134, 1652, 1050, 765, 1243 cm^{-1} (KBr disk).

Mass Spectrum. Principal ions at *m*/*z* 162, 43, 63, 164, 30, 44, 98, 42.

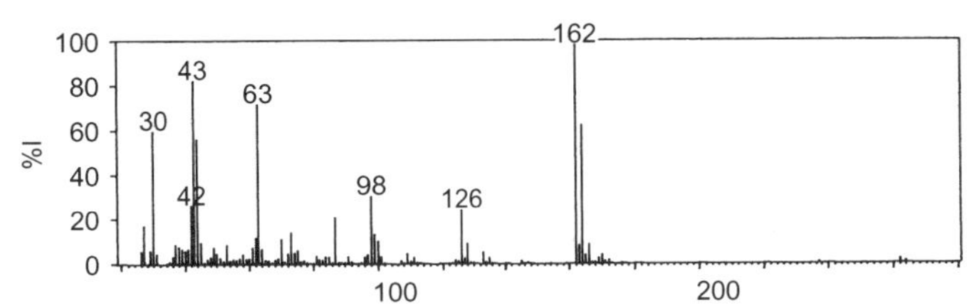

Dose. 10 to 120 mg of guanoclor sulfate daily; doses of 200 mg or more daily have been given.

Guanoxan

Antihypertensive

[(2,3-Dihydro-1,4-benzodioxin-2-yl)methyl]guanidine
$C_{10}H_{13}N_3O_2$=207.2
CAS—2165-19-7

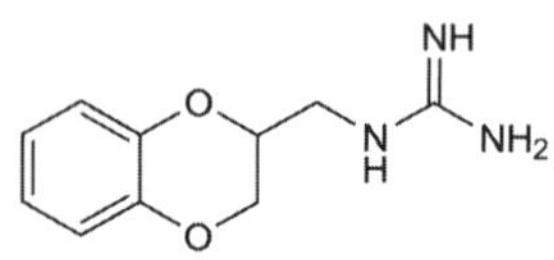

Crystals. M.p. 164° to 165°.

Guanoxan Sulfate
Proprietary name. Envacar
$(C_{10}H_{13}N_3O_2)_2,H_2SO_4$=512.5
CAS—5714-04-5
A white crystalline powder. M.p. about 206°.
Soluble 1 in 50 of water.

Dissociation Constant. pK_a 12.3.

Colour Tests. Mandelin's Test—green, sometimes violet, depending on relative proportions of test material and reagent; Marquis Test—violet.

Thin-layer Chromatography. System TA—Rf 01; system TB—Rf 00; system TC—Rf 00; system TE—Rf 00; system TL—Rf 00; system TAE—Rf 03; system TAF—Rf 76. (Acidified potassium permanganate solution, positive.)

High Performance Liquid Chromatography. System HX—RI 295.

Ultraviolet Spectrum. Aqueous acid—275 nm (A^1_1=104b).

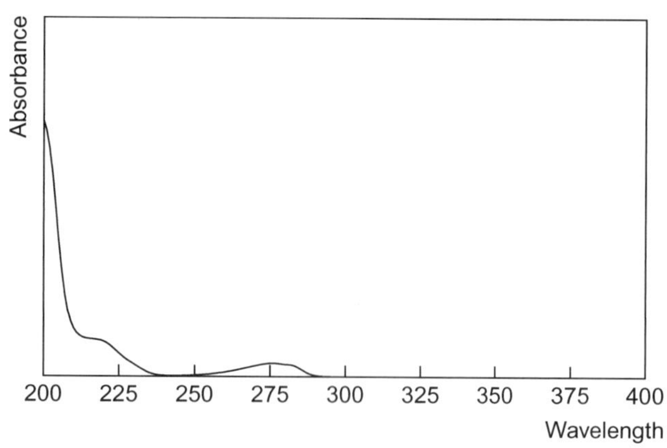

Infra-red Spectrum. Principal peaks at wavenumbers 1115, 1495, 1264, 1665, 1592, 748 cm^{-1} (KBr disk).

Mass Spectrum. Principal ions at *m/z* 30, 72, 43, 135, 121, 148, 52, 56.

Dose. 10 to 50 mg of guanoxan sulfate daily; doses of 120 mg or more daily have been given.

Halazone

Disinfectant

Synonym. Pantocide
Proprietary names. Clordispenser; Speton; Steridrolo a rapida idrolisi.
4-[(Dichloroamino)sulfonyl]benzoic acid
$C_7H_5Cl_2NO_4S$=270.1
CAS—80-13-7

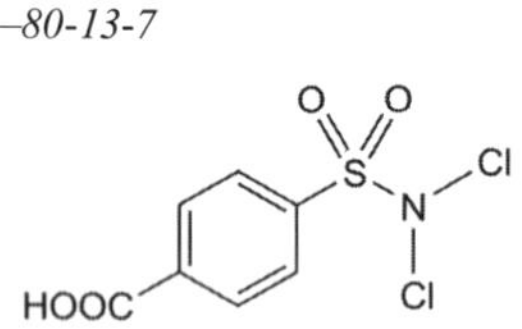

A white crystalline powder containing about 52% of 'available chlorine'. M.p. about 195°, with decomposition.
Slightly soluble in water, chloroform, and ether; soluble 1 in 140 of ethanol; soluble in glacial acetic acid, and in aqueous solutions of alkali hydroxides and carbonates.

Partition Coefficient. Log *P* (octanol/water), −0.2.

Ultraviolet Spectrum. Aqueous acid—237; aqueous alkali—229 nm (A^1_1=382b).

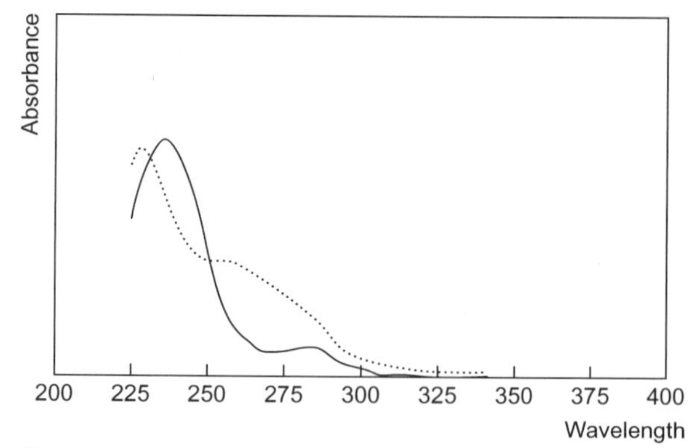

Mass Spectrum. Principal ions at *m/z* 121, 65, 36, 185, 50, 38, 76, 39.

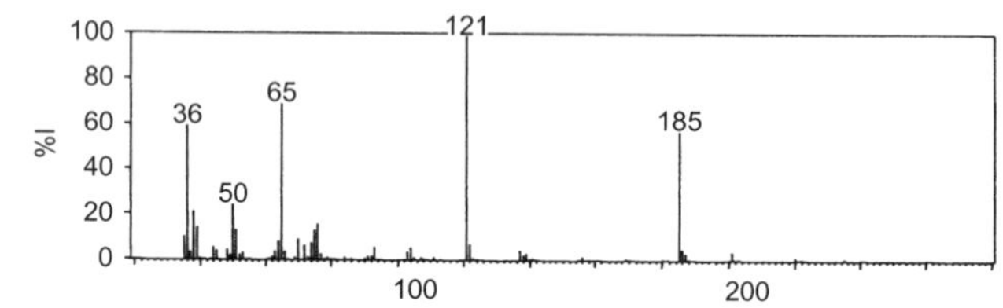

Halcinonide

Corticosteroid

Proprietary names. Betacortone; Dermalog; Halciderm; Halcimat; Halog.
(11β,16α)-21-Chloro-9-fluoro-11-hydroxy-16,17-[(1-methylethylidene)-bis(oxy)]pregn-4-ene-3,20-dione
$C_{24}H_{32}ClFO_5$=455.0
CAS—3093-35-4

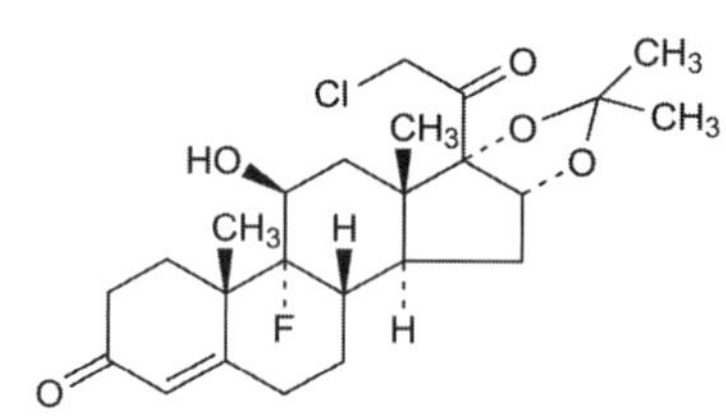

Crystals. M.p. 264° to 265°, with decomposition.
Insoluble in water and hexanes; soluble in acetone and chloroform; slightly soluble in benzene, ethanol, ethyl ether, and methanol.

Partition Coefficient. Log *P* (octanol/water), 2.9.

Thin-layer Chromatography. System TAJ—Rf 62; system TAK—Rf 58; system TAL—Rf 91

Ultraviolet Spectrum. Methanolic acid—238 nm (A^1_1=370b). No alkaline shift.

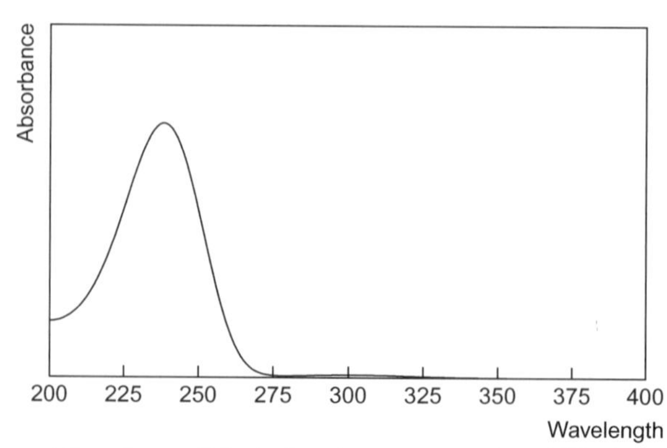

Infra-red Spectrum. Principal peaks at wavenumbers 1660, 1060, 1730, 1080, 1250, 1175 cm^{-1} (KBr disk).

Mass Spectrum. Principal ions at *m/z* 377, 43, 55, 246, 278, 59, 378, 41.

Use. Topically in concentrations of 0.025 to 0.1%.

Halofantrine

Antimalarial

1,3-Dichloro-α-[2-(dibutylamino)ethyl]-6-(trifluoromethyl)-9-phenanthrenemethanol
$C_{26}H_{30}Cl_2F_3NO = 500.4$
CAS—69756-53-2 (halofantrine); 66051-63-6 (racemic halofantrine)

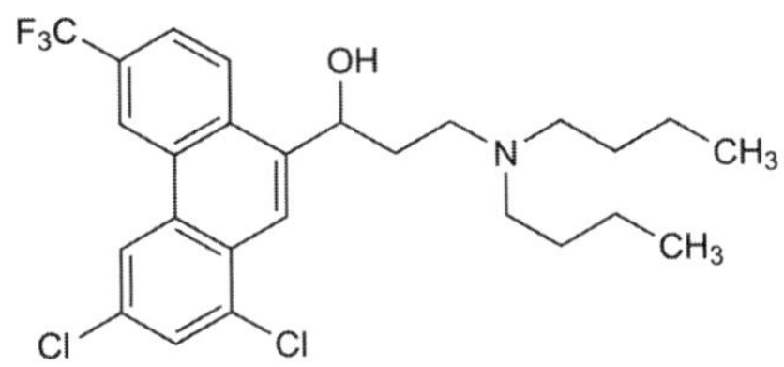

Halofantrine Hydrochloride

Synonyms. SKF-102886; WR-171669.
Proprietary name. Halfan
$C_{26}H_{30}Cl_2F_3NO,HCl = 536.9$
CAS—36167-63-2
Two crystalline forms of the hydrochloride with M.p. 93° to 96° and 203° to 204°.

Halofantrine β-Glycerophosphate

$C_{29}H_{39}Cl_2F_3NO_7P = 672.5$
White crystals with M.p. 60° to 65°.

Thin-layer Chromatography. System TB—Rf 50 (halofantrine); Rf 12 (desbutylhalofantrine); system TE—Rf 88 (halofantrine); Rf 61 (desbutylhalofantrine); system TAE—Rf 56 (halofantrine); Rf 19 (desbutylhalofantrine).

High Performance Liquid Chromatography. System HX—RI 800 (halofantrine); RI 618 (desbutylhalofantrine); system HAA—retention time 23.0 min (halofantrine); retention time 20.5 min (desbutylhalofantrine).

Column: Lichrosorb RP-18 (200 × 4.6 mm i.d., 10 μm). Mobile phase: methanol:0.05 M potassium dihydrogen phosphate (70:30) with 55 mM/L perchloric acid, pH 3.1, 1.3 mL/min flow rate. UV detection (λ=254 nm). Retention time: halofantrine, 7.5 min; desbutylhalofantrine, 5.3 min [C. O. Onyeji and S. O. Aideloje, *Ther. Drug Monit.*, 1997, *19*, 682–687].

Column: (analytical) Hypersil 5 ODS (250 × 4.6 mm i.d.), stainless steel; (guard) CN RP-18 end-capped (10 × 4.6 mm, 5 μm). Mobile phase: water:acetonitrile (35:65) containing triethylamine (1%), adjusted to pH 4 with orthophosphoric acid, 2.0 mL/min flow rate. Internal standard (IS): BL-22312. UV detection (λ=254 nm). Retention times: halofantrine, 8.5 min; *N*-desbutylhalofantrine, 4.5 min; IS, 11.0 min [E. K. Mberu *et al.*, *J. Chromatogr.*, 1992, *581*, *Biomed. Appl.*, *119*,156–160].

Column: Ultrasphere C_8 bonded-phase (250 × 4.6 mm i.d., 5 μm). Mobile phase: acetonitrile:water (75:25) with 0.2% SDS (sodium dodecyl sulfate) and 0.2% glacial acetic acid, 1.5 mL/min flow rate. IS: BL-22312. UV detection (λ=257 nm). Retention time: halofantrine, 8.3 min; desbutylhalofantrine, 5.5 min; IS, 11.5 min [D. Keeratithakul *et al.*, *Ther. Drug Monit.*, 1991, *13*, 64–68].

Ultraviolet Spectrum. Aqueous acid—258, 215, 230, 298 nm.

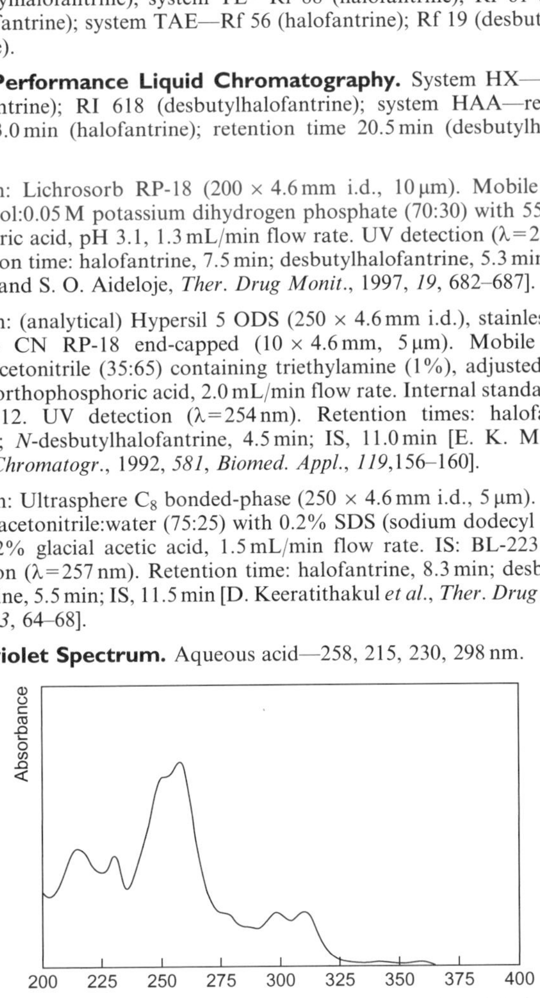

Mass Spectrum. Principal ions at *m/z* 100, 142, 280, 456, 116, 58, 458, 42.

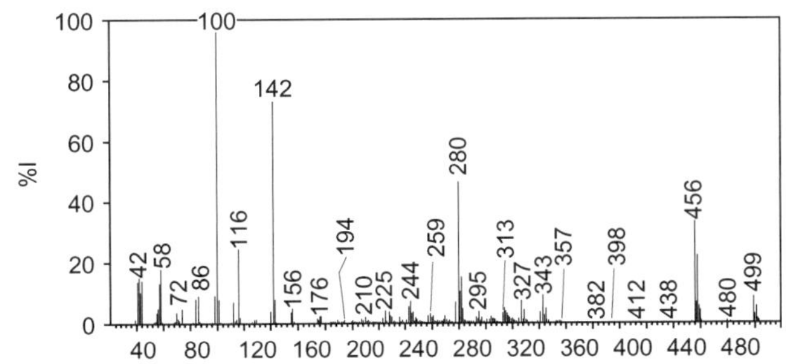

Quantification

High performance liquid chromatography. In plasma or blood: halofantrine and metabolite, limit of quantification 10 μg/L, UV detection (λ=254 nm)—E. K. Mberu *et al.*, *J. Chromatogr.*, 1992, *581*, *Biomed. Appl.*, *119*,156–160. In plasma: halofantrine and metabolite, limit of quantification 6 μg/L, fluorescence detection (λ_{ex}=300 nm, λ_{em}=380 nm)—H. Terefe and G. Blaschke, *J. Chromatogr.*, 1994, *657*, *Biomed. Appl.*, 238–242. In plasma, packed red blood cells, or urine: halofantrine and metabolite, limit of detection 1 μg/L in plasma and 2 μg/L in red blood cells, UV detection (λ=254 nm)—K. A. Milton *et al.*, *J. Chromatogr.*, 1988, *433*, *Biomed. Appl.*, *77*, 339–344. In plasma or blood: halofantrine and metabolite, limit of detection 0.9 μg/L in plasma and blood, fluorescence detection—M. Gawienowski *et al.*, *J. Chromatogr.*, 1988, *430*, 412–419. In serum: halofantrine and metabolite, limit of detection 5 and 3 μg/L, respectively, UV detection (λ=257 nm)—D. Keeratithakul *et al.*, *Ther. Drug Monit.*, 1991, *13*, 64–68. In plasma: halofantrine and metabolite, limit of detection 2.5 μg/L, UV detection (λ=254 nm)—C. O. Onyeji and S. O. Aideloje, *Ther. Drug Monit.*, 1997, *19*, 682–687.

Disposition in the Body. After oral administration, halofantrine is slowly and erratically absorbed and the drug enters systemic circulation within 1 h. The rate and extent of absorption are increased in the presence of food. Peak concentrations are observed 3 to 6 h after administration. There is wide and unpredictable interindividual variability of peak plasma concentrations. The major metabolite is *N*-desbutylhalofantrine which is active and has a longer half-life than halofantrine. Peak concentrations of the metabolite are observed after 12 to 20 h and are 2 to 4 times lower than the drug levels. The main route of elimination is in faeces as the unchanged drug.

Therapeutic concentration

6 adult volunteers, aged between 23 and 54 years, were administered 250 mg at 6-h intervals and after the last of 3 doses, the drug concentrations were measured. Mean maximum plasma concentrations were halofantrine 621.4 μg/L at 16.2 h and *N*-desbutylhalofantrine 114.9 μg/L at 43.2 h [F. Gimenez *et al.*, *Eur. J. Clin. Pharmacol.*, 1994, *46*, 561–562].

6 male adult patients of Melanesian origin with uncomplicated falciparum malaria (most severe form), mean age 22.7 years, were treated with 500 mg of halofantrine hydrochloride every 6 h for a total of 1.5 g. The mean concentration for halofantrine was 896 μg/L after 15 h and 491 μg/L after 56 h for the metabolite, *N*-desbutylhalofantrine [J. R. Veenendaal *et al.*, *Eur. J. Clin. Pharmacol.*, 1991, *41*, 161–164].

Half-life. Plasma half-life, 38 h in healthy volunteers and 91 to 113 h in patients with malaria (halofantrine); 103 h in healthy individuals and 79 to 118 h in those with malaria (*N*-desbutylhalofantrine).

Volume of distribution. 73 L/kg (patients with malaria); 8572 L (healthy individuals).

Clearance. Plasma clearance, 0.58 L/h/kg.

Note. For a review of halofantrine, see H. M. Bryson and K. L. Goa, *Drugs*, 1992, *43*, 236–258. For a review of the pharmacokinetics of halofantrine, see J. Karbwang and K. Na Bangchang, *Clin. Pharmacokinet.*, 1994, *27*, 104–119.

Dose. Three doses of 500 mg at 6-h intervals.

Haloperidol

Tranquilliser

Synonyms. Aloperidolo; Haloperidolum; McN-JR-1625; R-1625.
Proprietary names. Bioperidolo; Buteridol; Cereen; Dozic Haldol; Haloneural; Haloper; Haloperil; Kepsidol; Novo-Peridol; Pericate; Peridol; Peridor; Pulsit; Serenace; Serenase; Serenelfi; Sigaperidol.
4-[4-(4-Chlorophenyl)-4-hydroxy-1-piperidinyl]-1-(4-fluorophenyl)-1-butanone
$C_{21}H_{23}ClFNO_2$=375.9
CAS—52-86-8

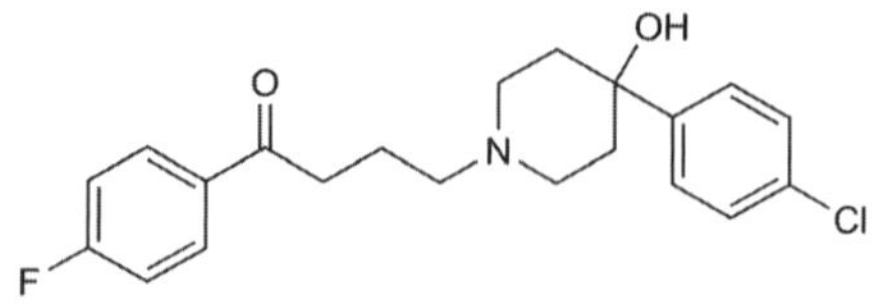

A white to faintly yellowish, amorphous or microcrystalline powder. M.p. 148.0° to 149.4°.
Practically insoluble in water; soluble 1 in 50 to 1 in 60 of ethanol, 1 in 15 to 1 in 20 of chloroform, 1 in 200 of ether, and 1 in 55 of methanol.

Dissociation Constant. pK_a 8.3.

Partition Coefficient. Log *P* (octanol/water), 3.23.

Colour Tests. Aromaticity (Method 2)—yellow/orange-red; Liebermann's Test—brown.

Thin-layer Chromatography. System TA—Rf 67; system TB—Rf 11; system TC—Rf 27; system TE—Rf 76; system TL—Rf 33; system TAE—Rf 51; system TAF—Rf 75; system TAJ—Rf 06; system TAK—Rf 02; system TAL—Rf 61. (Acidified iodoplatinate solution, positive.)

Gas Chromatography. System GA—haloperidol RI 2930, haloperidol-H_2O RI 2965, M (reduced) RI 3152, M (*N*-desalkyl-oxo-)-$2H_2O$ RI 1650, M (*N*-desalkyl-) RI 1800; system GB—haloperidol RI 3094, M (reduced) RI 3152, M (*N*-desalkyl-oxo-)-$2H_2O$ RI 1707; system GV—retention time 23.3 min.

High Performance Liquid Chromatography. System HA—*k* 1.2; system HX—RI 421; system HY—RI 316; system HZ—retention time 5.8 min; system HAA—retention time 14.4 min; system HAX—retention time 11.1 min; system HAY—retention time 6.2 min; system HAZ—*k* 0.72.

Ultraviolet Spectrum. Methanolic acid—245 nm (A_1^1=340a). No alkaline shift.

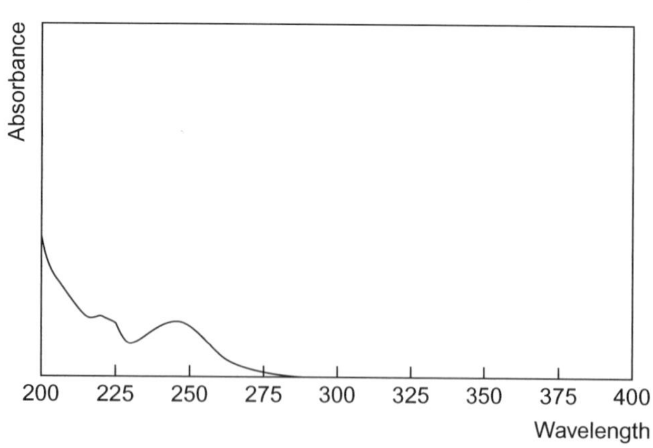

Infra-red Spectrum. Principal peaks at wavenumbers 832, 1151, 1673, 1217, 1136, 1598 cm^{-1} (KBr disk).

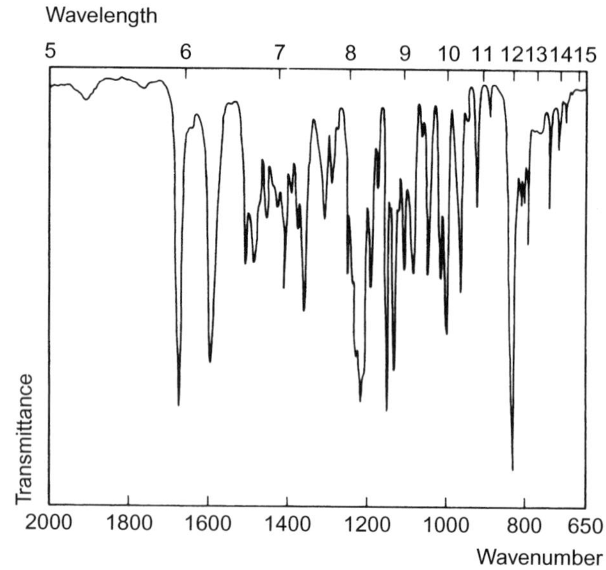

Mass Spectrum. Principal ions at *m/z* 224, 42, 237, 226, 123, 206, 239, 56 (no peaks above 240).

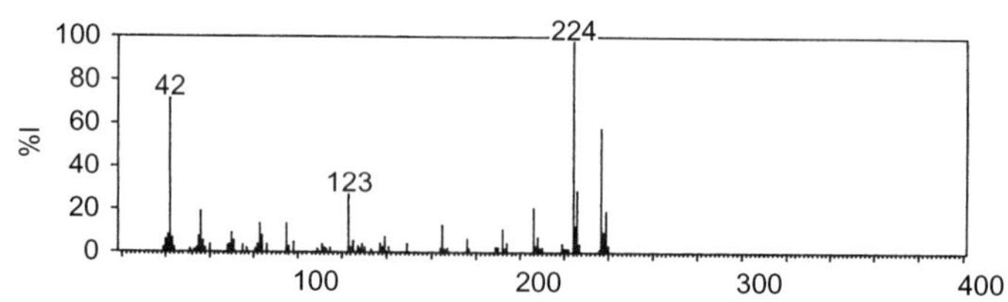

Quantification

Gas chromatography. In serum or CSF: limit of detection 0.5 µg/L, AFID—D. R. Abernethy *et al.*, *J. Chromatogr.* 1984, *307*(32) *B Biomed. Appl.*, 194–199. In blood or urine: haloperidol and other butyrophenones, limit of detection 0.1 pmol, SID—H. Seno *et al.*, *Nippon Hoigaku Zasshi*, 1993, *47*, 367–371. In serum: limit of detection 1.1 µg/L, SID, (comparison with GC/MS)—T. Fujii *et al.*, *J. Chromatogr. B Biomed. Appl.*, 1996, *687*, 395–403.

Gas chromatography–mass spectrometry. In urine: limit of detection 10 µg/L (*m/z* 206, 237, 224)—M. L. Olmos-Carmona and M. Hernandez-Carrazquilla, *J. Chromatogr. B Biomed. Sci. Appl.*, 1999, *734(1)*, 113–120.

High performance liquid chromatography. In plasma or serum: haloperidol and reduced metabolite, limit of detection 1 µg/L, electrochemical detection—E. R. Korpi *et al.*, *Clin. Chem.*, 1983, *29*, 624–628. In breast milk: limit of detection 5 µg/L, UV detection—T. Ohkubo *et al.*, *J. Pharm. Sci.*, 1992, *81*, 947–949. In serum: limit of detection 0.5 µg/L—D. W. Hoffman and R. D. Edkins, *Ther. Drug Monit.*, 1994, *16*, 504–508. In urine: pyridinium metabolites of haloperidol, fluorescence detection—D. W. Eyles *et al.*, *Clin. Pharmacol. Ther.*, 1994, *56*, 512–520. In serum or plasma: haloperidol and reduced haloperidol, limit of detection for haloperidol 0.4 µg/L, nitrogen-phosphorus detection—S. Ulrich *et al.*, *J. Chromatogr.* 1995, *663*, *B Biomed. Appl.*, 289–296. In plasma: haloperidol and its reduced metabolite, limits of quantification 2 µg/L with UV detection and 0.5 µg/L with electrochemical detection—L. Pan *et al.*, *Ther. Drug Monit.*, 1998, *20*, 224–230. In serum: haloperidol and flupentixol, limit of quantification for haloperidol 0.3 µg/L, UV detection—S. Walter *et al.*, *J. Chromatogr. B Biomed. Sci. Appl.*, 1998, *720*, 231–237. In serum: haloperidol and other antipsychotic drugs, limit of quantification for haloperidol 4 µg/L, UV detection—H. R. Angelo and A. Petersen, *Ther. Drug Monit.*, 2001, *23*, 157–162.

High performance liquid chromatography–mass spectrometry. In plasma: haloperidol and reduced haloperidol—H. Hoja *et al.*, *J. Chromatogr. B Biomed. Sci. Appl.*, 1997, *688*, 275–280. In blood: haloperidol and other butyrophenones, limit of detection 0.1 µg/L—H. Seno *et al.*, *J. Chromatogr. B Biomed. Sci. Appl.*, 2000, *746*, 3–9. In plasma or urine: haloperidol and metabolites, limit of detection for haloperidol 5 µg/L—T. Arinobu *et* al., *J. Chromatogr. B. Analyt. Technol. Biomed. Life Sci.*, 2002, *776*, 107–113.

Radioimmunoassay. In serum: limit of quantification 0.3 µg/L—Y. Terauchi *et al.*, *J. Pharm. Sci.*, 1990, *79*, 432–436.

Disposition in the Body. Readily absorbed after oral administration. Haloperidol is localised in the tissues and rapidly taken up by the brain. It is slowly excreted in the urine, about 40% of a dose being eliminated in 5 days with only about 1% of the dose as unchanged drug; about 15% of a dose is excreted in the bile. It is metabolised by oxidative *N*-dealkylation. Metabolites which have been identified in urine are 4-fluorobenzoylpropionic acid and 4-fluorophenylaceturic acid (the glycine conjugate of 4-fluorophenylacetic acid), both of which are inactive. Haloperidol is also metabolised by reduction of the ketone group to a secondary alcohol (reduced haloperidol). Haloperidol is excreted in breast milk.

Therapeutic concentration. There is considerable inter-subject variation in steady-state blood concentrations. However, for normal doses (up to 15 mg per day), the serum concentration is usually below 0.05 mg/L.

Steady-state serum concentrations of 0.8 to 33 µg/L (mean 6.5) were attained after daily oral administration of 1 to 14 mg (mean 6) to 34 patients. [A. O. Forsman and R. Öhman, *Curr. Ther. Res.*, 1977, *21*, 396–411.]

There has been much discussion regarding the relationship between serum concentrations and the therapeutic effect of haloperidol in schizophrenia and related disorders. A review of about 50 clinical studies concluded that the therapeutic window for haloperidol was in the range 5.6 to 16.9 µg/L. [S. Ulrich *et al.*, *Clin. Pharmacokinet.*, 1998, *34*, 227–263.]

In a study of the effect of CYP2D6 polymorphism on haloperidol pharmacokinetics in 172 patients, the mean haloperidol and reduced haloperidol serum trough concentration was 7.0 and 7.2 µg/L, respectively, in patients with ultrafast CYP2D activity (daily dose 14 mg), 7.3 and 2.0 µg/L in those with extensive CYP2D6 activity (daily dose 12 mg), 8.6 and 4.2 µg/L in those with intermediate CYP2D6 activity (daily dose 12 mg), and 6.9 and 9.5 µg/L in those with poor CYP2D6 activity (daily dose 13 mg). [J. Frockmoller *et al.*, *Clin. Pharmacol. Ther.*, 2002, *72*, 438–452.]

Toxicity. The minimum lethal dose is probably in excess of 3 g. Toxic effects may appear with blood concentrations greater than about 0.05 mg/L but there is considerable inter-subject variation.

A psychiatric patient who committed suicide by running into traffic had haloperidol concentrations of 1.2 mg/L in heart blood, 2.7 mg/g in brain, and 10.8 mg/g in liver. [G. R., Johnson, *J. Forensic Sci.*, 1988, *33*, 823–825.]

In a fatality attributed to a suicidal overdose of haloperidol, the following postmortem tissue concentrations were reported for haloperidol and reduced haloperidol, respectively: blood 1.9 and 1.4 mg/L, bile 3.4 and 1.6 mg/L, liver 44 and 43 µg/g, urine 6.6 and 5.7 mg/L. In a second case believed to be a natural cardiac death, the postmortem tissue concentrations of haloperidol and reduced haloperidol were: blood 0.6 mg/L and not reported, bile 0.4 and 0.5 mg/L, kidney 0.7 and 2.3 µg/g, liver 5.0 and 13 µg/g, urine 0.4 and 2.3 mg/L. [B. S. Levine *et al.*, *J. Anal. Toxicol.*, 1991, *15*, 282–284.]

In 24 children who received an accidental overdosage of haloperidol at the same hospital, the maximum blood level measured within 4 days of the final administration was 28.9 µg/L (dosage unknown); symptoms of acute toxicity were evident (disturbances in consciousness, tremor, oculogyric crisis, dysarthria, drooling, akathisia, hyperreflexia, opisthotonos, elevated liver enzyme values, abnormal ECG). [I. Yoshida *et al.*, *Acta Paediatr.*, 1993, *82*, 877–880.]

Bioavailability. 38 to 86% (mean 58%).

Half-life. Plasma half-life, 10 to 40 h (mean 20).

Volume of distribution. 10 to 30 L/kg (mean 18).

Clearance. Plasma clearance, 8 to 17 mL/min/kg (mean 12).

Distribution in blood. Plasma:whole blood ratio, about 0.93.

Protein binding. In plasma, about 92%.

Dose. 1 to 15 mg daily by mouth; up to 100 mg daily may be required; rarely, higher doses have been used.

Halothane

General Anaesthetic

Synonyms. Alotano; Phthorothanum.
Proprietary names. Fluothane; Rhodialothan.
2-Bromo-2-chloro-1,1,1-trifluoroethane
$C_2HBrClF_3 = 197.4$
CAS—151-67-7

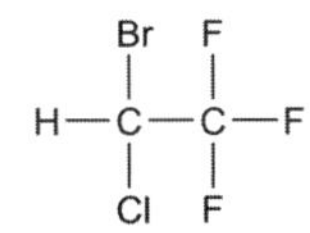

A colourless, mobile, heavy, non-flammable liquid. B.p. 49° to 51°. Refractive index, at 20°, 1.3695 to 1.3705.
Halothane contains thymol 0.01% w/w as a preservative.
Soluble 1 in 400 of water; miscible with dehydrated alcohol, chloroform, and ether.

Partition Coefficient. Log *P* (octanol/water), 2.3.

Gas Chromatography. System GA—RI 533; system GI—Retention time 8.5 min; system GR—Retention time 4.2 min.

Mass Spectrum. Principal ions at *m/z* 117, 198, 196, 119, 129, 67, 127, 98.

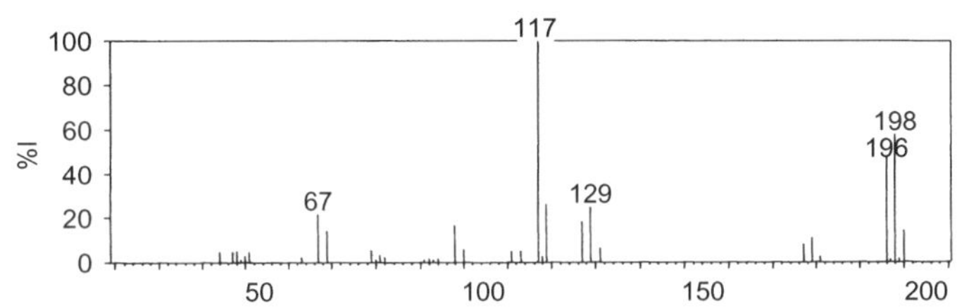

Quantification

Gas chromatography. In whole blood: direct injection, FID—W. J. Cole *et al.*, *Br. J. Anaesth.*, 1975, *47*, 1043–1047. In blood: FID—M. K. Tham *et al.*, *Anesthesiology*, 1972, *37*, 647–649. In plasma, serum or urine: trifluoroacetic acid (TFA) and bromide, limit of detection, TFA 300 µg/L in plasma, 1 mg/L in urine, FID—R. M. Maiorino *et al.*, *J. Anal. Toxicol.*, 1980, *4*, 250–254. In blood or tissues: 2-chloro-1,1-difluoroethylene and 2-chloro-1,1,1-trifluoroethane, limit of detection 200 and 300 ng/L, respectively, in blood, FID—R. M. Maiorino *et al.*, *J. Chromatogr.*, 1979, *164*; *B Biomed. Appl.*, *6*, 63–72. In blood: halothane, enflurane, and isoflurane, FID—J. Flynn *et al.*, *Analyst*, 1989, *114*, 1207–1210 and J. Flynn *et al.*, *Analyst*, 1989, *114*, 1211–1213. In blood: halothane, isoflurane, enflurane, and sevoflurane, limits of detection 10 to 100 µg/L, FID—T. Kojima *et al.*, *J. Chromatogr. B Biomed. Sci. Appl.*, 2001, *762*, 103–108.

Gas chromatography–mass spectrometry. In blood: halothane, enflurane, isoflurane, and sevoflurane—K. Saito *et al.*, *J Anal. Toxicol.*, 1995, *19*, 115–119. In urine: halothane, isoflurane and nitrous oxide, limit of detection <30 ng/L for halothane—D. Poli *et al.*, *J. Chromatogr. B Biomed. Sci. Appl.*, 1999, *732*, 115–125. In postmortem blood, liver, kidney, brain, urine, bile or stomach contents: limit of detection 0.004 mg/kg in blood—F. Musshoff *et al.*, *J. Anal. Toxicol.*, 2000, *24*, 372–376. In blood: halothane and other fluorinated inhalation anaesthetics—N. C. Yang *et al.*, *J. Chromatogr. B Biomed. Sci. Appl.*, 2001, *759*, 307–318.

High performance liquid chromatography–ion chromatography. In plasma or urine: TFA and bromide—D. C. Hankins and E. D. Kharasch, *J. Chromatogr. B Biomed. Sci. Appl.*, 1997, *692*, 413–418.

Disposition in the Body. Rapidly absorbed upon inhalation; blood:gas partition coefficient about 2.4. It accumulates in adipose tissue. About 60 to 80% of an absorbed dose is exhaled unchanged from the lungs in 24 h and smaller amounts continue to be exhaled for several days or weeks. A variable amount is metabolised in the liver by debromination and dechlorination; replacement of a fluorine atom by a methoxy group followed by glucuronic acid conjugation occurs to a limited extent. Other metabolites which have been detected in expired air and in blood are 2-chloro-1,1,1-trifluoroethane and 2-chloro-1,1-difluoroethylene. Up to about 20% of a dose may be excreted in the urine as trifluoroacetic acid and its salts. Bromide ion is slowly excreted in the urine.

Therapeutic concentration. During surgical anaesthesia, concentrations in blood are usually in the range 22 to 84 mg/L. Venous blood concentrations lag behind arterial concentrations during induction and decline less rapidly during recovery.

Blood concentrations ranging from 50.5 to 106.5 mg/L were reported in 8 patients following anaesthesia with 1.5% halothane for 20 min. At recovery 10 min later the range was 22 to 30 mg/L; traces were still detectable after 44 h; bromide concentrations increased during the post-anaesthetic period [M. M. Atallah and I. C. Geddes, *Br. J. Anaesth.*, 1973, *45*, 464–470.]

Peak plasma-bromide concentrations occurred in surgical patients 2 to 3 days after anaesthesia and ranged from 52 to 180 mg/L [J. H. Tinker *et al.*, *Anesthesiology*, 1976, *44*, 194–196.]

Toxicity. The minimum lethal dose by ingestion or inhalation is about 10 mL although one case of recovery after the ingestion of 250 mL has been reported. Blood concentrations of 7 to 40 to 310 mg/L have been associated with fatalities.

In one fatality involving the ingestion of 35 mL of halothane, the following postmortem tissue concentrations were reported: blood 650 mg/L, brain 1560 µg/g, lung 500 µg/g, liver 880 µg/g, spleen 230 µg/g, urine 20 mg/L; salicylate and an unidentified barbiturate were also present [J. A. E. Spencer and N. M. Green, *J. Am. Med. Assoc.*, 1968, *205*, 702–703.]

Dose. For induction of anaesthesia, 2 to 3% of the vapour by inhalation; maintenance, 0.5 to 1.5%.

Haloxon

Anthelmintic (Veterinary)

Proprietary names. Galloxon; Loxon; Luxon; Ruby Horse Wormer.
Bis(2-chloroethyl) 3-chloro-4-methyl-2-oxo-2*H*-1-benzopyran-7-yl phosphate
$C_{14}H_{14}Cl_3O_6P$=415.6
CAS—321-55-1

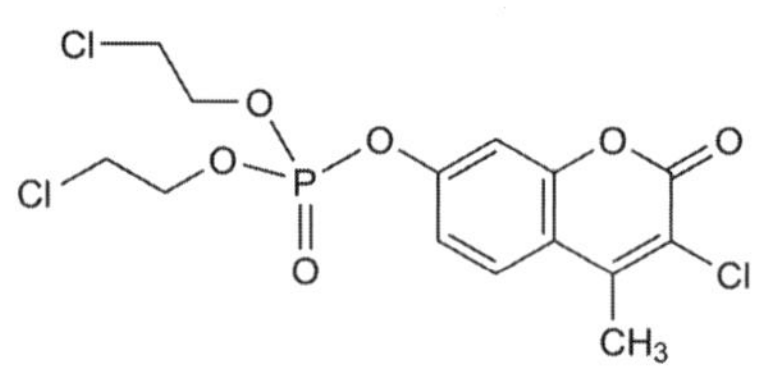

A white powder. M.p. 88° to 93°.
Practically insoluble in water; soluble 1 in 9 of ethanol, 1 in 4 of acetone, and 1 in 2 of chloroform.

Partition Coefficient. Log *P* (octanol/water), 3.2.

Ultraviolet Spectrum. After solution in dioxan and dilution with acid methanol—290, 312 nm.

Infra-red Spectrum. Principal peaks at wavenumbers 1738, 1010, 1070, 1036, 1277, 1605 cm^{-1} (KBr disk).

Halquinol

Antimicrobial

Synonyms. Chlorhydroxyquinoline; Chlorquinol.
Proprietary names. Capitrol (chloroxine); Valpeda.
A mixture of the chlorinated products of quinolin-8-ol containing 57 to 74% of 5,7-dichloroquinolin-8-ol (chloroxine), 23 to 40% of 5-chloroquinolin-8-ol, and not more than 4% of 7-chloroquinolin-8-ol.
CAS—8067-69-4
A yellowish-white to yellowish-grey, voluminous powder.
Practically insoluble in water; soluble 1 in 250 of ethanol, 1 in 50 of chloroform, and 1 in 130 of ether; soluble in acids.

Colour Tests. Mandelin's Test—yellow; Marquis Test—yellow; Sulfuric Acid—yellow.

Thin-layer Chromatography. System TA—Rf 19, streaking. (Acidified iodoplatinate solution, positive.)

Gas Chromatography. System GA—RI 1743.

Ultraviolet Spectrum. Aqueous acid—258 (A^1_1=2187a); aqueous alkali—259, 343; methanol—248, 263, 334 nm.

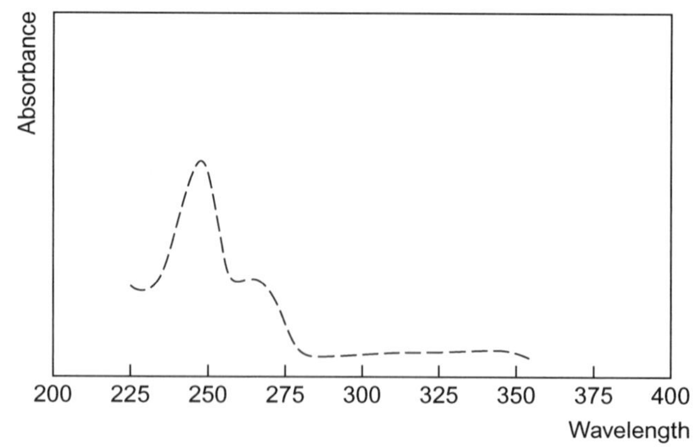

Infra-red Spectrum. Principal peaks at wavenumbers 1512, 1282, 812, 1200, 950, 785 cm^{-1} (KBr disk).

Dose. 3 to 4 g daily for 5 days.

Harmaline

Hallucinogen

4,9-Dihydro-7-methoxy-1-methyl-3*H*-pyrido[3,4-*b*]indole
$C_{13}H_{14}N_2O$=214.3
CAS—304-21-2

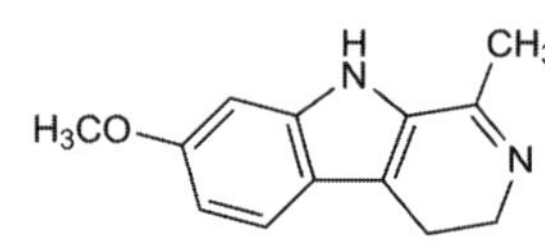

An alkaloid obtained from peganum, the dried seeds of *Peganum harmala* (Zygophyllaceae). It is also found, together with harmine, in the South American hallucinogenic drink *caapi*, also known as *Yagé* and *ayahuasca*.
M.p. 249° to 250°, with decomposition.
Slightly soluble in water, ethanol, and ether.

Partition Coefficient. Log *P* (octanol/water), 4.6.

Colour Tests. Mandelin's Test—green-brown; Marquis Test—brown-green.

Thin-layer Chromatography. System TA—Rf 38; system TE—Rf 49; system TAJ—Rf 00; system TAK—Rf 02; system TAL—Rf 38. (Acidified iodoplatinate solution, positive.)

Gas Chromatography. System GA—harmaline RI 2430; harmaline-2H (harmine) RI 2291; M (*O*-desmethyl-)-2H RI 2550; art (dihydro-) RI 2375.

Ultraviolet Spectrum. Aqueous acid—256; aqueous alkali—330; methanol—260 (A^1_1=288b), 344 nm (A^1_1=468b).

Mass Spectrum. Principal ions at *m/z* 213, 214, 170, 198, 169, 115, 63, 143.

Quantification

High performance liquid chromatography. In plasma: harmine, harmaline, tetrahydroharmine, and *N,N*-dimethyltryptamine, limit of detection <2 µg/L, fluorescence detection—J. C. Callaway *et al.*, *J. Anal. Toxicol.*, 1996, *20*, 492–497.

Harman

Alkaloid

Synonyms. Aribine; Harmane; Loturine.
1-Methyl-9*H*-pyrido[3,4-*b*]indole
$C_{12}H_{10}N_2$=182.2
CAS—486-84-0

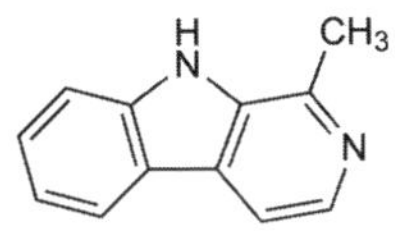

An alkaloid present in passion flower, the dried flowering and fruiting tops of *Passiflora incarnata* (Passifloraceae).
Crystals. M.p. about 238°.
Sparingly soluble in hot water; soluble in ethanol, chloroform, dilute acids, and ether.
Note. Harman may be found in tobacco smoke and in home-made wine. It may also be found as a putrefactive base, particularly in cases where embalming has taken place. It is a condensation product of tryptophan and acetaldehyde.

Partition Coefficient. Log *P* (octanol/water), 3.1.

Colour Tests. Mandelin's Test—green; Marquis Test—green.

Thin-layer Chromatography. System TA—Rf 70; system TB—Rf 02; system TC—Rf 40; system TE—Rf 57; system TL—Rf 33; system TAE—Rf 72; system TAF—Rf 76; system TAJ—Rf 24; system TAK—Rf 03; system TAL—Rf 50. (Acidified iodoplatinate solution, positive.)

Gas Chromatography. System GA—harman RI 1952; M (1-OH) RI 1920, 2015, and 2290.

High Performance Liquid Chromatography. System HX—RI 319.

Ultraviolet Spectrum. Aqueous acid—245 (A_1^1=1987a), 300; aqueous alkali—232, 284 nm.

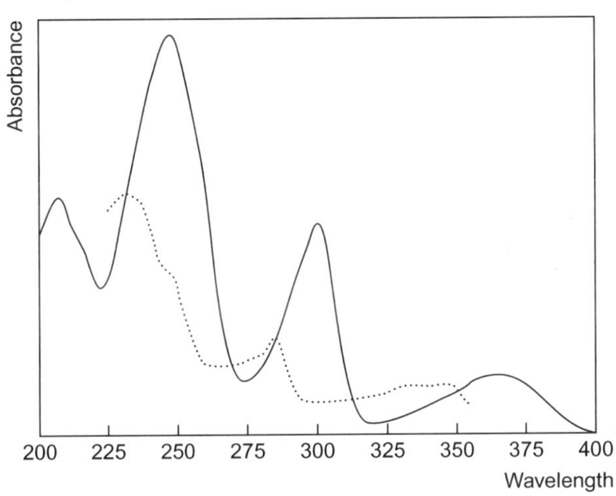

Infra-red Spectrum. Principal peaks at wavenumbers 751, 1317, 1235, 1504, 1245, 1567 cm^{-1}.

Mass Spectrum. Principal ions at *m/z* 182, 57, 43, 55, 40, 69, 41, 181.

Quantification
High performance liquid chromatography. In blood: harmine and harman, limits of detection 81 ng/L and 206 ng/L respectively, fluorescence detection—W. Zheng *et al.*, *Anal. Biochem.*, 2000, *279*, 125–129. In plasma: harman and norharman, fluorescence detection—U. Breyer-Pfaff *et al.*, *Life Sci.*, 1996, *58*, 1425–1432.

Harmine

Hallucinogen

7-Methoxy-1-methyl-9*H*-pyrido[3,4-*b*]indole
$C_{13}H_{12}N_2O$=212.3
CAS—442-51-3

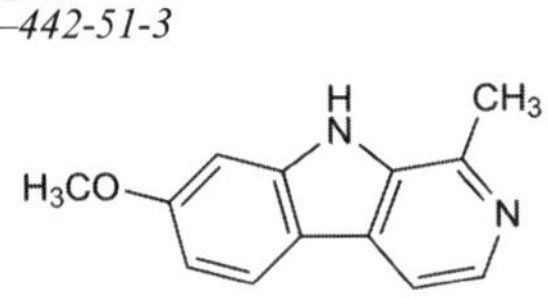

An alkaloid obtained from peganum, the dried seeds of *Peganum harmala* (Zygophyllaceae). Harmine is identical with an alkaloid known as banisterine or telepathine obtained from *Banisteria caapi* (Malpighiaceae) and with the alkaloid, yageine, from *Haemadictyon amazonicum* (Apocynaceae). It is also found, together with harmaline, in the South American hallucinogenic drink *caapi*, also known as *Yagé* and *ayahuasca*.
Crystals. M.p. 261°, with decomposition or sublimation.
Slightly soluble in water, ethanol, chloroform, and ether.

Dissociation Constant. pK_a 7.6 (20°).

Partition Coefficient. Log *P* (octanol/water), 3.6.

Colour Tests. *p*-Dimethylaminobenzaldehyde—red; Mandelin's Test—blue→green; Marquis Test—orange.

Thin-layer Chromatography. System TA—Rf 63; system TB—Rf 00; system TC—Rf 22; system TE—Rf 52; system TL—Rf 28; system TAE—Rf 65; system TAF—Rf 68; system TAJ—Rf 12; system TAK—Rf 03; system TAL—Rf 48. (Acidified iodoplatinate solution, positive.)

Gas Chromatography. System GA—harmine RI 2291; harmine-AC RI 2545; M (*O*-desmethyl-) RI 2550; M (*O*-desmethyl-)-AC RI 2600; system GB—harmine RI 2322.

High Performance Liquid Chromatography. System HA—*k* 0.8; system HX—RI 339; system HY—RI 271.

Ultraviolet Spectrum. Aqueous acid—247 (A_1^1 = 1927a), 319; aqueous alkali—243, 275, 300 nm.

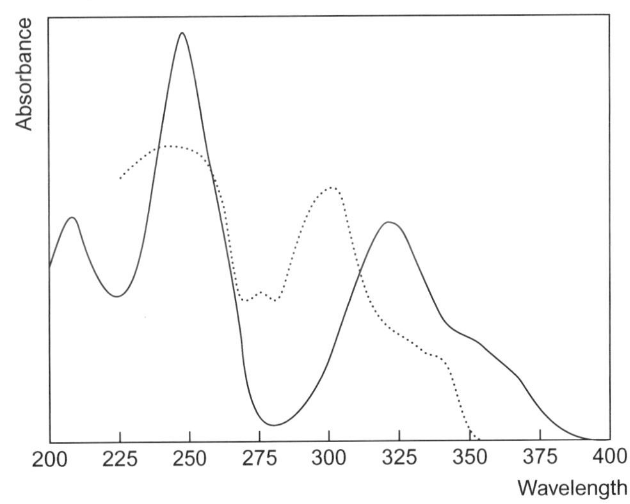

Infra-red Spectrum. Principal peaks at wavenumbers 1165, 817, 1629, 1200, 1282, 1239 cm^{-1} (KBr disk).

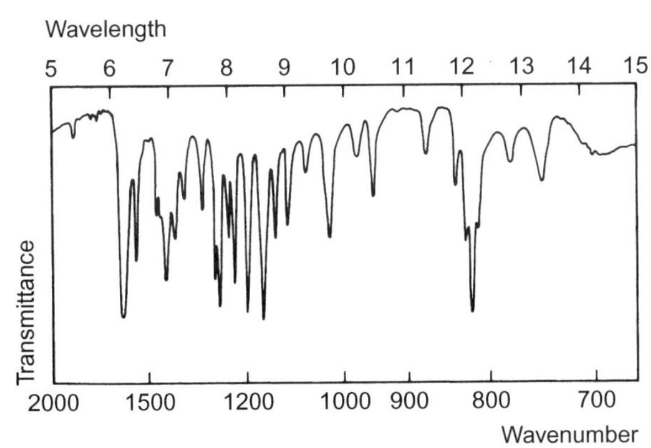

Mass Spectrum. Principal ions at *m/z* 212, 169, 197, 213, 106, 211, 170, 168.

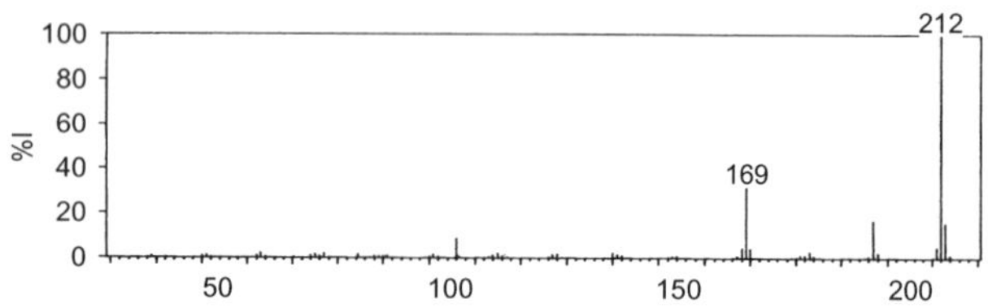

Quantification

High performance liquid chromatography. In plasma: harmine, harmaline, tetrahydroharmine, and *N,N*-dimethyltryptamine, limit of detection <2 µg/L, fluorescence detection—J. C. Callaway *et al.*, *J. Anal. Toxicol.*, 1996, *20*, 492–497. In blood: harmine and harman, limits of detection 81 ng/L and 206 ng/L respectively, fluorescence detection—W. Zheng *et al.*, *Anal. Biochem.*, 2000, *279*, 125–129.

Heptabarb

Sedative/Barbiturate

Synonym. Heptabarbital (distinguish from Heptobarbitalum); Heptabarbitone

Proprietary names. Heptadorm; Medomin(e).

5-(1-Cyclohepten-1-yl)-5-ethyl-2,4,6(1*H*,3*H*,5*H*)-pyrimidinetrione

$C_{13}H_{18}N_2O_3$=250.3

CAS—509-86-4

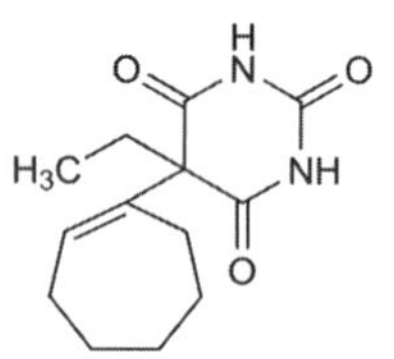

A white crystalline powder. M.p. 174°.

Very sparingly soluble in water; soluble 1 in 30 of ethanol, 1 in 20 of acetone, and 1 in 75 of chloroform; soluble in solutions of alkali hydroxides.

Dissociation Constant. pK_a 7.5 (20°).

Partition Coefficient. Log *P* (octanol/pH 7.4), 2.2.

Colour Tests. Koppanyi–Zwikker Test—violet; Mercurous Nitrate—black; Vanillin Reagent—violet-red/colourless.

Thin-layer Chromatography. System TD—Rf 50; system TE—Rf 38; system TF—Rf 64; system TH—Rf 62; system TAD—Rf 59; system TAE—Rf 88. (Mercuric chloride–diphenylcarbazone reagent, positive; mercurous nitrate spray, black; acidified potassium permanganate solution, yellow-brown; Zwikker's reagent, pink.)

Gas Chromatography. System GA—heptabarb RI 2055, 3′-hydroxyheptabarbital RI 2275, 3′-oxoheptabarbitone RI 2320; system GB—heptabarb RI 2110; system GF—RI 2940; system GAJ—heptabarb RRT 1.282 (relative to methylphenobarbital).

High Performance Liquid Chromatography. System HG—*k* 9.90; system HH—*k* 4.93; system HX—RI 416; system HY—RI 377; system HZ—Retention time, 3.9 min.

Ultraviolet Spectrum. Borax buffer 0.05 M (pH 9.2)—239 (A^1_1=413a); 1 M sodium hydroxide (pH 13)—255 nm (A^1_1=326b). (See below.)

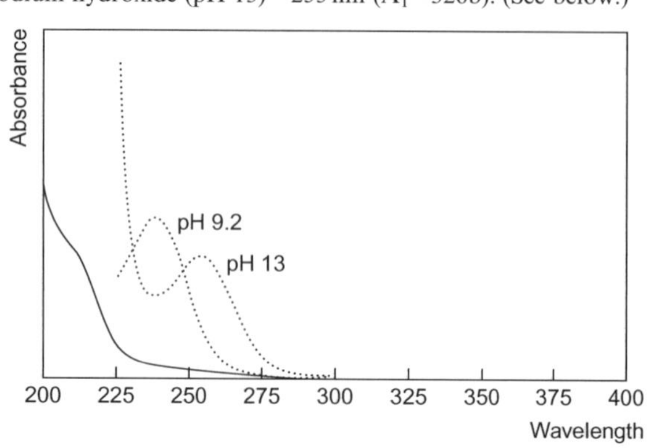

Infra-red Spectrum. Principal peaks at wavenumbers 1673, 1761, 1718, 1237, 1292, 1303 cm^{-1} (KBr disk). (See below.)

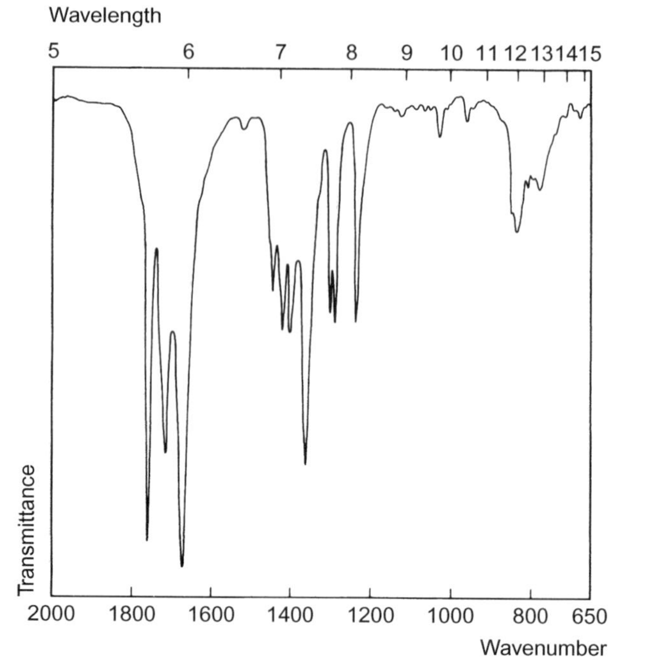

Mass Spectrum. Principal ions at *m/z* 221, 43, 78, 93, 80, 41, 141, 39.

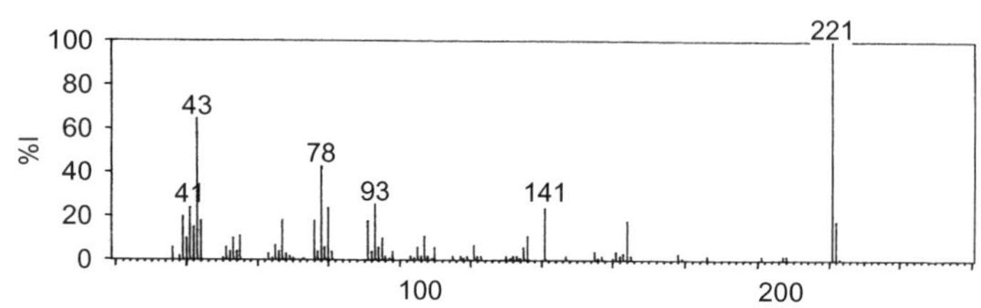

Quantification. See under Amylobarbital.

Disposition in the Body. Readily absorbed after oral administration. Less than 1% of a dose is excreted unchanged in the urine. Major metabolites which have been identified in the urine are 3′-oxoheptabarbitone and 3′-hydroxyheptabarbitone.

Therapeutic concentration. In plasma, usually in the range 1 to 4 mg/L.

After a single oral dose of 200 mg administered to 7 subjects, peak plasma concentrations of 1.3 to 2.4 mg/L (mean 1.9) were attained in 1.5 to 4 h [D. D. Breimer *et al.*, *Eur. J. Clin. Pharmacol.*, 1975, *9*, 169–178.]

Toxicity. The estimated minimum lethal dose is 2 g. Plasma concentrations greater than about 8 mg/L may produce toxic effects.

Half-life. Plasma half-life, 6 to 11 h.

Volume of distribution. About 1 L/kg.

Note. For a review of the clinical pharmacokinetics of barbiturates, see D. D. Breimer, *Clin. Pharmacokinet.*, 1977, *2*, 93–109.

Dose. 150 to 400 mg daily.

Heptachlor

Insecticide

Proprietary names. Drinox; Heptamul; Velsicol 104.

1*H*-1,4,5,6,7,8,8-Heptachloro-3a,4,7,7a-tetrahydro-4,7-methanoindene

$C_{10}H_5Cl_7$=373.3

CAS—76-44-8

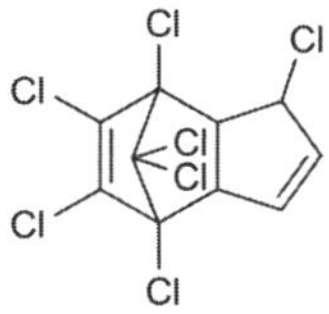

The pure substance is a white crystalline solid and the technical grade is a soft, waxy solid which contains about 72% of heptachlor and 28% of related compounds. Heptachlor may be found as an impurity in chlordane.
M.p. 95° to 96° (pure substance), 46° to 74° (technical grade).
Practically insoluble in water; soluble 1 in 22 of ethanol.

Partition Coefficient. Log *P* (octanol/water), 6.1.

Thin-layer Chromatography. System TB—Rf 74; system TE—Rf 89; system TF—Rf 75; system TX—Rf 84; system TY—Rf 97; system TAB—Rf 69; system TAC—Rf 51.

Gas Chromatography. System GA—RI 1880; system GK—RRT 0.85 (relative to caffeine).

High Performance Liquid Chromatography. System HX—RI 1072; system HAO—*k* 0.0; system HAP—*k* 20.8.

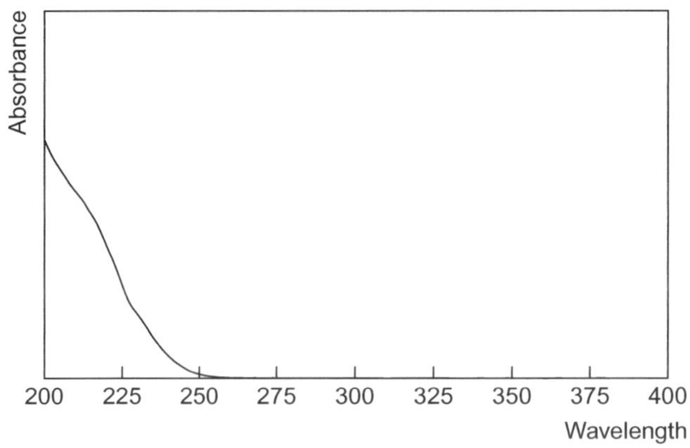

Mass Spectrum. Principal ions at *m/z* 100, 272, 274, 270, 237, 102, 65, 276.

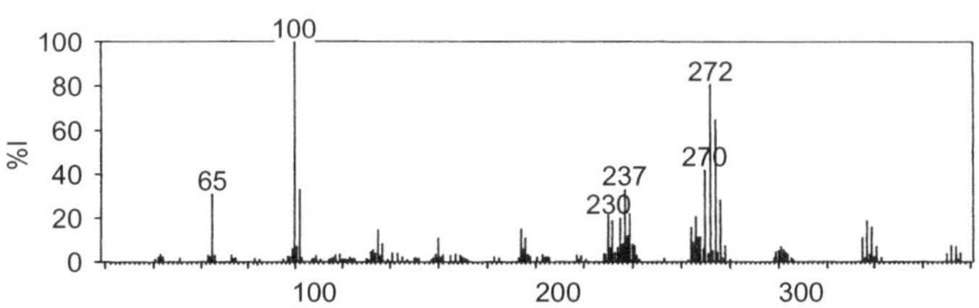

Quantification

Gas chromatography. In serum: heptachlor and other chlorinated hydrocarbon pesticides, ECD—J. J. Saady and A. Poklis, *J. Anal. Toxicol.*, 1990, *14*, 301–304.

Gas chromatography–mass spectrometry. In serum: heptachlor and other polychlorinated biphenyl congeners, selected ion monitoring—J. Dmitrovic *et al.*, *Toxicol. Lett.*, 2002, *134*, 253–258.

Heptaminol

Cardiac Stimulant/Vasodilator

6-Amino-2-methyl-2-heptanol
$C_8H_{19}NO = 145.2$
CAS—372-66-7

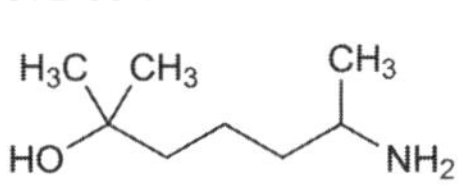

Heptaminol Hydrochloride

Proprietary names. Ampecyclal; Coreptil; Cortensor; Eoden; Hept-a-myl; Heptylon.

$C_8H_{19}NO,HCl = 181.7$
CAS—543-15-7
A white crystalline powder. M.p. 150°.
Freely soluble in water; soluble in ethanol; practically insoluble in acetone, benzene, and ether.

Partition Coefficient. Log *P* (octanol/water), 1.2.

Thin-layer Chromatography. System TA—Rf 23; system TB—Rf 01; system TC—Rf 02; system TE—Rf 22; system TL—Rf 05; system TAE—Rf 14. (Acidified potassium permanganate solution, positive.)

Gas Chromatography. System GA—heptaminol RI 1120; heptaminol-AC_2 RI 1530.

Ultraviolet Spectrum. No significant absorption, 230 to 360 nm.

Infra-red Spectrum. Principal peaks at wavenumbers 1529, 1537, 896, 1622, 1153, 1614 cm^{-1} (KBr disk).

Mass Spectrum. Principal ions at *m/z* 44, 43, 59, 56, 69, 55, 41, 113.

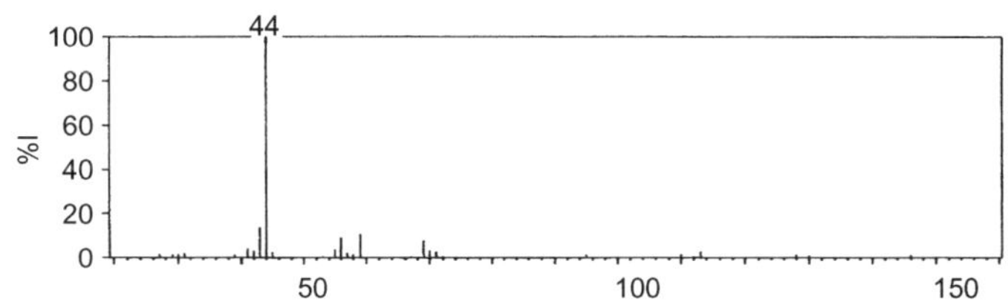

Quantification

High performance liquid chromatography. In plasma or urine: limit of detection 100 µg/L in plasma, fluorescence detection—R. R. Brodie *et al.*, *J. Chromatogr.*, 1983, *274*; *B Biomed. Appl.*, *25*, 179–186.

Dose. Heptaminol hydrochloride has been given in doses of 0.3 to 1.6 g daily.

Heteronium Bromide

Anticholinergic

1,1-Dimethyl-3-(α-2-thienylmandeloyloxy)pyrrolidinium bromide
$C_{18}H_{22}BrNO_3S = 412.3$
CAS—7247-57-6

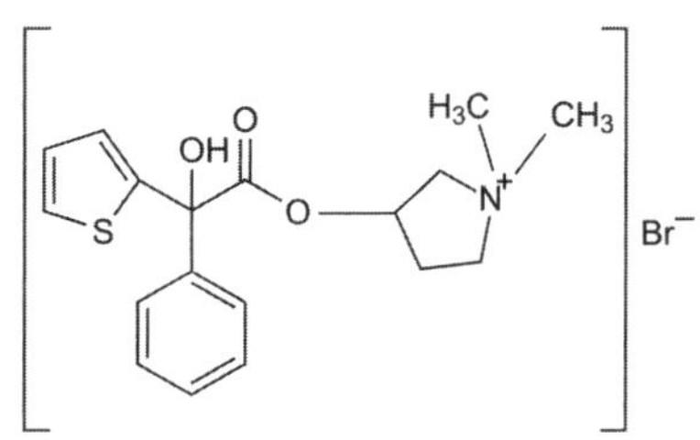

A white crystalline powder. M.p. 182° to 184°.
Very soluble in water and ethanol.

Partition Coefficient. Log *P* (octanol/water), −1.5.

Thin-layer Chromatography. System TA—Rf 03. (Acidified iodoplatinate solution, positive.)

Ultraviolet Spectrum. Aqueous acid—234 nm ($A_1^1 = 235b$).

Infra-red Spectrum. Principal peaks at wavenumbers 1735, 1219, 1085, 1234, 1063, 700 cm^{-1}.

Hexachlorophene

Disinfectant

Synonym. Hexachlorophane
Proprietary names. Aknefug simplex; Dermalex; Hexaphenyl; Lotocreme; Phaisohex; pHisoHex; Sapoderm; Ster-Zac. It is an ingredient of Anacal.
2,2′-Methylenebis[3,4,6-trichlorophenol]
$C_{13}H_6Cl_6O_2 = 406.9$
CAS—70-30-4

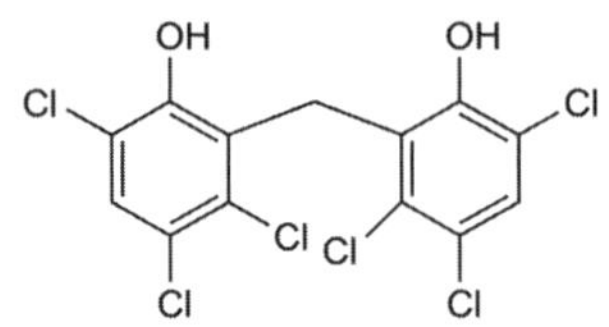

A white or pale buff, crystalline powder. M.p. 161° to 167°.
Practically insoluble in water; soluble 1 in 3.5 of ethanol, 1 in less than 1 of acetone, and 1 in less than 1 of ether; soluble in chloroform (possibly with turbidity) and propylene glycol.

Dissociation Constant. pK_a 5.7.

Partition Coefficient. Log *P* (octanol/water), 7.5.

Colour Tests. Ferric Chloride—violet (transient); Fuming Nitric Acid—orange-red/orange/orange-brown.

Thin-layer Chromatography. System TB—Rf 00; system TD—Rf 32; system TE—Rf 30; system TF—Rf 34; system TAD—Rf 44; system TAE—Rf 94; system TAF—Rf 98; system TAJ—Rf 56; system TAK—Rf 71; system TAL—Rf 91.

Gas Chromatography. System GA—RI 2795.

High Performance Liquid Chromatography. System HX—RI 936.

Ultraviolet Spectrum. Ethanol—299 (A_1^1=155a); aqueous alkali—249 (A_1^1=400b), 320 nm (A_1^1=312a).

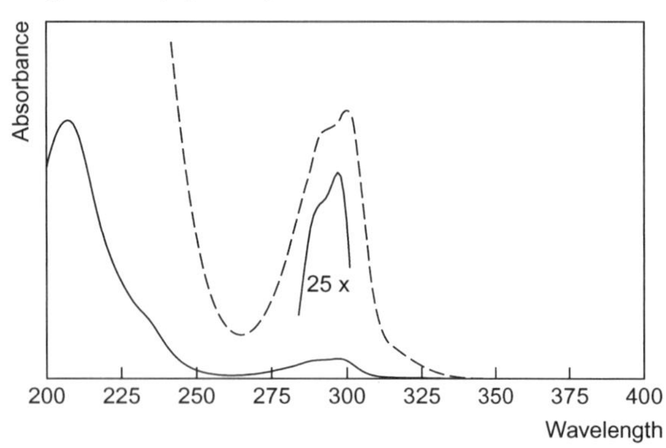

Infra-red Spectrum. Principal peaks at wavenumbers 1276, 1182, 737, 1139, 960, 1213 cm^{-1} (KBr disk).

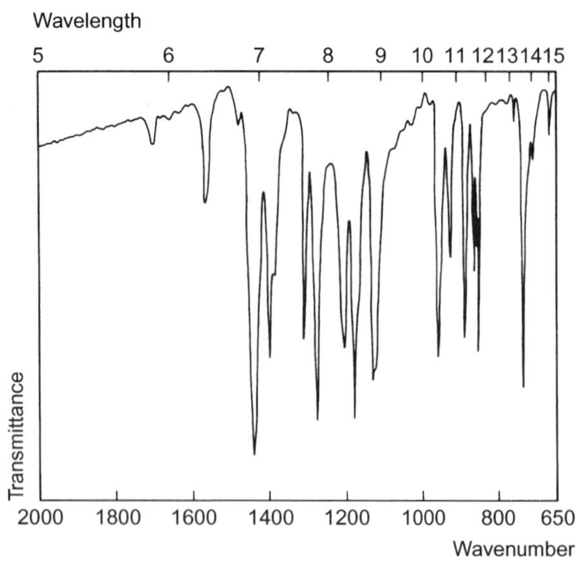

Quantification

Gas chromatography. In blood: ECD—W. Dodson *et al.*, *Clin. Chem.*, 1977, *23*, 944–947. In blood or urine: ECD—R. S. Browning *et al.*, *J. Pharm. Sci.*, 1968, *57*, 2165–2166.

Disposition in the Body. Absorbed after oral administration and through the skin. Percutaneous absorption may be significant in premature infants and through damaged skin. After topical application, up to about 10% may be excreted in the urine over a period of 4 to 5 days.

Blood concentration

Cord-blood concentrations of 0.003 to 0.18 mg/L (mean 0.02) were reported in 50 neonates at birth. After washing once daily for 1 to 11 days with a 3% solution of hexachlorophene diluted with 50 to 100 mL of water, whole blood concentrations of 0.009 to 0.65 mg/L (mean 0.11) were attained [A. Curley *et al.*, *Lancet*, 1971, *2*, 296–297.]

After whole-body washing with 30 mL of a 3% skin-cleansing product once daily, blood concentrations in 36 adults reached a plateau of about 0.6 mg/L after 3 to 5 weeks and decreased to about 0.3 to 0.4 mg/L after 7 to 8 weeks [B. Calesnick *et al.*, *Toxicol. Appl. Pharmacol.*, 1975, *32*, 204–211.]

Toxicity. The estimated minimum lethal dose is 5 g. A number of deaths have occurred after accidental ingestion and also after chronic application for the treatment of burns. Repeated exposure of neonates and infants to high concentrations of hexachlorophene has been associated with spongy lesions of the brain. Fatalities have been associated with blood concentrations greater than 2 mg/L, although recovery has occurred after development of plasma concentrations up to 90 mg/L.

In an epidemic of percutaneous poisoning which occurred in 1972 in infants and children due to exposure to a talcum powder accidentally contaminated with 6% of hexachlorophene, 36 children died. An antemortem serum concentration of 1.15 mg/L was reported in 1 child and the following postmortem tissue concentrations were reported: brain 1 to 149 µg/g (mean 21, 23 cases), kidney 17 to 43 µg/g (mean 26, 4 cases), liver 12.5 to 1080 µg/g (mean 133, 25 cases), lung 10 to 67 µg/g (mean 30, 17 cases), and skin 1 to 392 µg/g (mean 52, 30 cases) [G. Martin-Bouyer *et al.*, *Lancet*, 1982, *1*, 91–95.]

Use. In soaps and creams at a concentration of 0.25 to 3%.

Hexaconazole

Fungicide

Synonyms. R154523; PP 523; ICIA-0523.
Proprietary names. Anvil; Planete.
α-Butyl-α-(2,4-dichlorophenyl)-1*H*-1,2,4-triazole-1-ethanol
$C_{14}H_{17}Cl_2N_3O$=314.2
CAS—79983-71-4

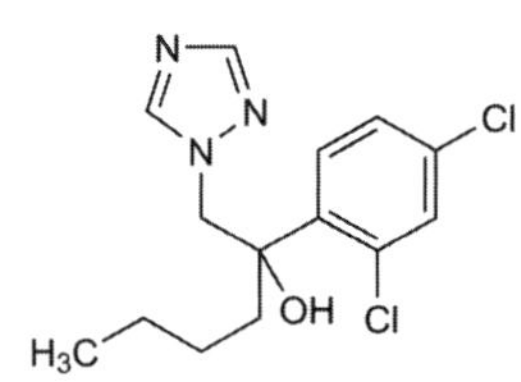

White crystalline solid. M.p. 111°.
It is soluble in water at 17 mg/L (20°), methanol (246 g/L at 20°), acetone (164 g/L at 20°), toluene (59 g/L at 20°), and hexane (0.8 g/L at 20°).

Partition Coefficient. Log *P* (octanol/water), 3.90.

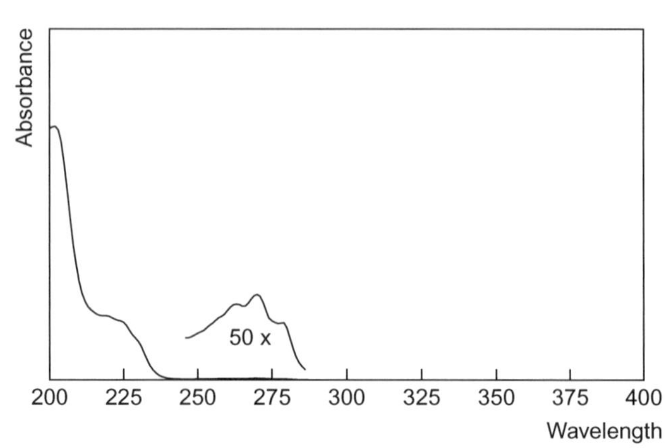

Disposition in the Body. Hexaconazole is rapidly excreted from the body with no significant retention of the substance in the body.

Toxicity. Hexaconazole is moderately toxic by ingestion and via skin exposure.

Hexamethonium Bromide

Antihypertensive

Synonyms. Hexamethone Bromide; Hexonium Bromide.
Proprietary names. Esametina; Gangliostat; Simpatoblock; Vegolysen; Vegolysin.
N,N,N,N′,N′,N′-Hexamethyl-1,6-hexanediaminium dibromide
$C_{12}H_{30}Br_2N_2=362.2$
CAS—60-26-4 (hexamethonium); 55-97-0 (dibromide)

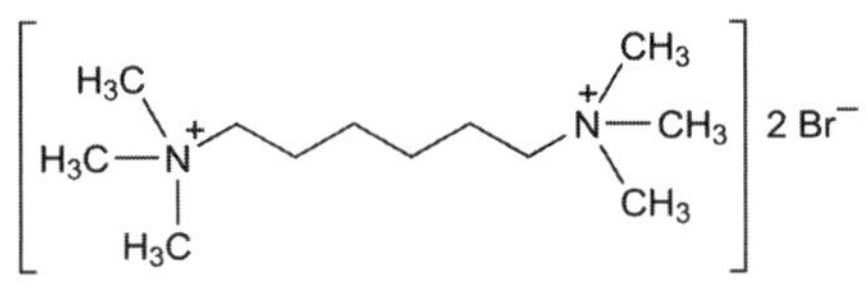

A white or creamy-white hygroscopic powder. M.p. 274° to 276°.
Soluble 1 in less than 1 of water and 1 in 60 of ethanol; insoluble in acetone, chloroform, and ether.

Hexamethonium Iodide

Synonym. Hexonium Iodide
Proprietary name. Hexathide
$C_{12}H_{30}I_2N_2=456.2$
CAS—870-62-2
A white, slightly hygroscopic, crystalline powder.
Soluble 1 in 2 of water; practically insoluble in ethanol.

Thin-layer Chromatography. System TA—Rf 00; system TN—Rf 36; system TO—Rf 10. (Acidified iodoplatinate solution, positive.)

Gas Chromatography. System GA—not eluted.

Ultraviolet Spectrum. No significant absorption, 230 to 360 nm.

Infra-red Spectrum. Principal peaks at wavenumbers 913, 970, 1630, 945, 1063, 1000 cm^{-1} (KBr disk).

Disposition in the Body

Toxicity

A healthy subject taking part in a pharmacological trial died after receiving about 1 g of hexamethonium by inhalation (a non-standard route of administration) [S. Ramsay, *Lancet*, 2001, *358*, 213.]

Dose. Hexamethonium bromide has been given parenterally in doses of up to 500 mg daily.

Hexestrol

Estrogen

Synonyms. Dihydrostilboestrol; Hexanoestrol; Hexoestrol; Synestrol; Synoestrol.
Proprietary names. Cycloestrol; Hormoestrol (tablets); Synthovo; Syntrogene.
4,4′-(1,2-Diethyl-1,2-ethanediyl)bisphenol
$C_{18}H_{22}O_2=270.4$
CAS—5635-50-7; 84-16-2 (meso)

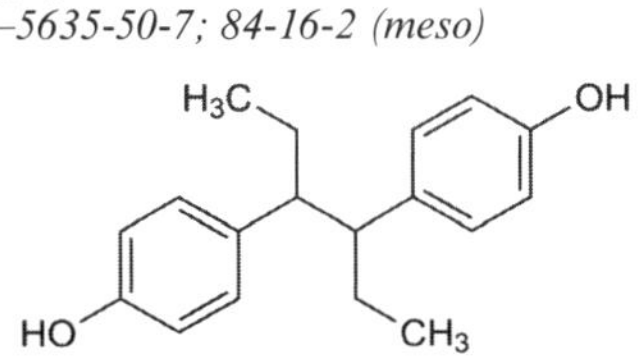

Colourless crystals or white crystalline powder. M.p. 185° to 188°.
Practically insoluble in water and dilute mineral acids; freely soluble in ether; soluble in ethanol and acetone; slightly soluble in benzene and chloroform.

Hexestrol Dipropionate

Proprietary names. Hormoestrol (injection); Retalon Oleosum.
$C_{24}H_{30}O_4=382.5$
CAS—4825-53-0
A white crystalline powder. M.p. 127° to 128°.
Sparingly soluble in water; soluble in warm ethanol and ether.

Partition Coefficient. Log *P* (octanol/water), 5.6.

Thin-layer Chromatography. System TB—Rf 02; system TE—Rf 73; system TF—Rf 70; system TAE—Rf 88.

Gas Chromatography. System GA—RI 2402.

High Performance Liquid Chromatography. System HX—RI 618.

Ultraviolet Spectrum. Ethanol—230 nm ($A^1_1=775$b), 280 nm ($A^1_1=135$a); aqueous alkali—242 nm ($A^1_1=965$b), 297 nm ($A^1_1=175$b). (See below)

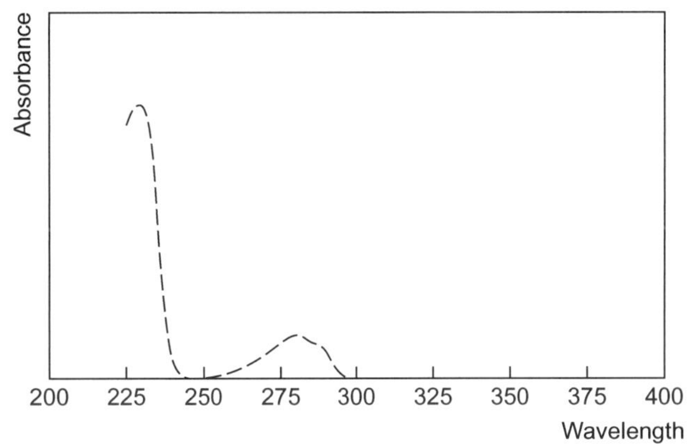

Infra-red Spectrum. Principal peaks at wavenumbers 1175, 1523, 1220, 840, 857, 1615 cm^{-1} (KBr disk).

Dose. Hexestrol has been given in doses of 1 to 5 mg daily.

Hexethal

Barbiturate

5-Ethyl-5-hexyl-2,4,6(1*H*,3*H*,5*H*)-pyrimidinetrione
$C_{12}H_{20}N_2O_3=240.3$
CAS—77-30-5

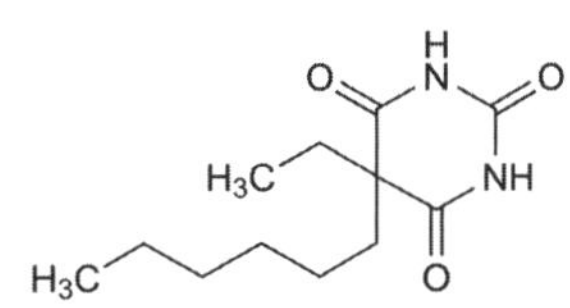

Hexethal Sodium

Proprietary names. Hebarel; Ortal Sodium.
$C_{12}H_{19}N_2NaO_3=262.3$
CAS—144-00-3
A white or slightly yellowish powder. M.p. 126°.
Very soluble in water; soluble in ethanol; insoluble in ether and benzene. Aqueous solutions are unstable and decompose on standing.

Dissociation Constant. pK_a 8.0.

Partition Coefficient. Log *P* (octanol/water), 2.5.

Thin-layer Chromatography. System TD—Rf 53; system TE—Rf 44; system TF—Rf 67; system TH—Rf 74; system TAD—Rf 60.

Gas Chromatography. System GA—hexethal RI 1850; hexethal-Me_2 RI 1745.

High Performance Liquid Chromatography. System HG—*k* 34.28; system HH—*k* 20.39; system HY—RI 451.

Ultraviolet Spectrum. Borax buffer 0.05 M (pH 9.2)—238 ($A^1_1=423$b); 1 M sodium hydroxide (pH 13)—253 nm ($A^1_1=323$b).

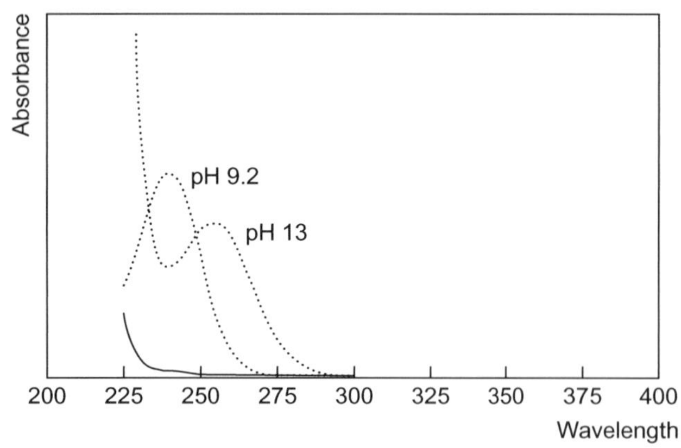

Infra-red Spectrum. Principal peaks at wavenumbers 1698, 1720, 1757, 1316, 1230, 850 cm^{-1} (hexethal sodium).

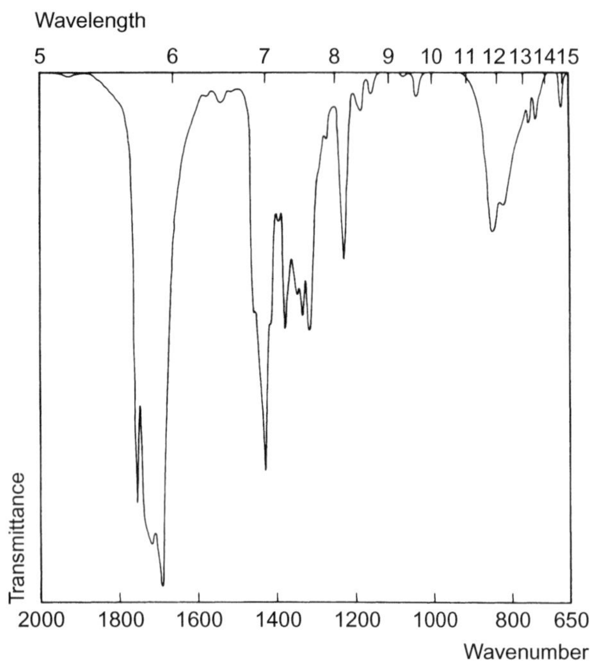

Mass Spectrum. Principal ions at *m*/*z* 156, 141, 55, 41, 157, 43, 98, 39.

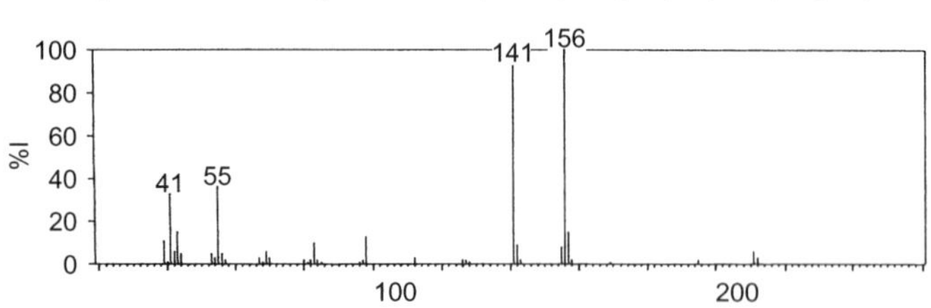

Hexetidine

Antimicrobial

Proprietary names. Bactidol; Collu-Hextril; Doreperol N; Drossadin; Gurfix; Hexatin; Hexifluor; Hexigel; Hexoral; Hextril; Isozid-H; Kleenosept; Oraldene; Oraldine; Oraseptic; Oralspray; Steri/Sol; Vagi-Hex.
1,3-Bis(2-ethylhexyl)hexahydro-5-methyl-5-pyrimidinamine
$C_{21}H_{45}N_3$=339.6
CAS—141-94-6

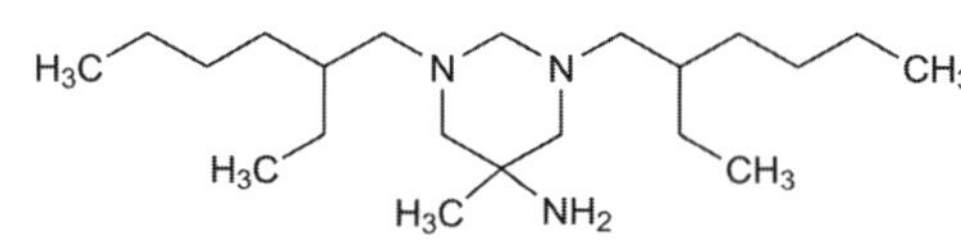

A viscous oil. Mass per mL about 0.87 g. Refractive index 1.466. Practically insoluble in water; soluble in ethanol, acetone, chloroform, petroleum ether, and benzene.

Dissociation Constant. pK_a 8.3.

Partition Coefficient. Log *P* (octanol/water), 5.3.

Thin-layer Chromatography System TA—Rf 70; system TB—Rf 48; system TC—Rf 40; system TE—Rf 79; system TL—Rf 20; system TAE—Rf 30; system TAF—Rf 91. (Acidified iodoplatinate solution, positive.)

Gas Chromatography. System GA—RI 2093.

Ultraviolet Spectrum. No significant absorption, 230 to 360 nm.

Infra-red Spectrum. Principal peaks at wavenumbers 1093, 854, 1300, 910, 1176, 1234 cm^{-1} (thin film).

Mass Spectrum. Principal ions at *m*/*z* 142, 57, 42, 197, 185, 339, 240, 226.

Quantification
High performance liquid chromatography. In saliva—C. P. McCoy *et al.*, *J. Pharm. Pharmacol.*, 2000, *52*, 1355–1359.

Use. As a 0.1% solution.

Hexobarbital

Sedative/Barbiturate

Synonyms. Ciclobarbital; Enhexymalum; Enimal; Hexobarbitalum; Hexobarbitone; Methexenyl; Methyl-cyclohexenylmethyl-barbitursäure; Methylhexabarbital.
Proprietary names. Noctivane; Sombulex.
5-(1-Cyclohexen-1-yl)-1,5-dimethyl-2,4,6(1*H*,3*H*,5*H*)-pyrimidinetrione
$C_{12}H_{16}N_2O_3$=236.3
CAS—56-29-1

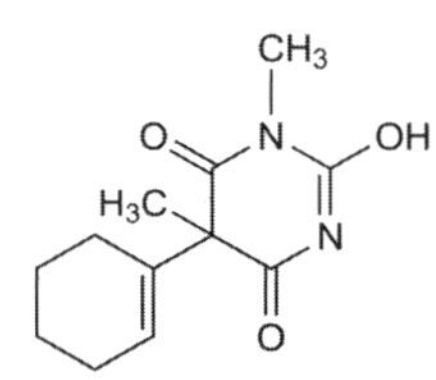

Colourless crystals or a white crystalline powder. M.p. 145° to 147°. Practically insoluble in water; soluble 1 in 45 of ethanol, 1 in 4 of chloroform, and 1 in 80 of ether; soluble in acetone, benzene, and methanol.

Hexobarbital Sodium
Synonyms. Enhexymalnatrium; Hexenalum; Sodium Hexobarbitone; Soluble Hexobarbital.
Proprietary names. Evipan-Natrium; Noctivane Sodium.
$C_{12}H_{15}N_2NaO_3$=258.3
CAS—50-09-9
A white, very hygroscopic powder. It discolours on exposure to air.
Very soluble in water; freely soluble in ethanol, acetone, and methanol; practically insoluble in chloroform, ether, and benzene. A solution in water slowly decomposes.

Dissociation Constant. pK_a 8.2 (20°).

Partition Coefficient. Log *P* (octanol/water), 2.0.

Colour Tests. Koppanyi–Zwikker Test—violet; Mercurous Nitrate—black; Vanillin Reagent—brown/violet.

Thin-layer Chromatography. System TD—Rf 65; system TE—Rf 53; system TF—Rf 65; system TH—Rf 85; system TAD—Rf 69; system TAE—Rf 85. (Mercuric chloride–diphenylcarbazone reagent, positive; mercurous nitrate spray, black; acidified potassium permanganate solution, yellow-brown on violet.)

Gas Chromatography. System GA—hexobarbital RI 1855, M (1,5-dimethyl-5-(3-oxo-1-cyclohexen-1-yl)barbituric acid) RI 2050, M (nor-) RI

1980, M (3′-oxo) RI 2055, M (OH-)-H_2O RI 1970, hexobarbital-Me RI 1800, M (oxo-)-Me RI 2020; system GF—RI 2380; system GAJ—hexobarbital RRT 0.940 (relative to methylphenobarbital).

High Performance Liquid Chromatography. System HG—*k* 7.37; system HH—*k* 5.67; system HX—RI 419; system HY—RI 242; system HZ—retention time 4.3 min; system HAL—retention time 2.4 min.

Ultraviolet Spectrum. Borax buffer 0.05 M (pH 9.2)—243 (A^1_1=331a); 1 M sodium hydroxide (pH 13) —243 nm (A^1_1=301b).

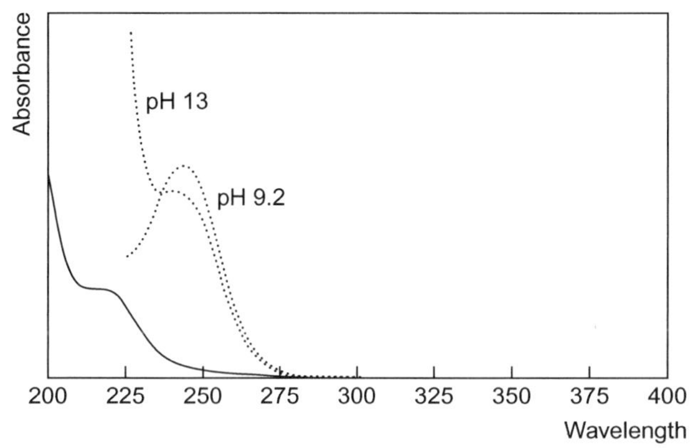

Infra-red Spectrum. Principal peaks at wavenumbers 1720, 1665, 1748, 1200, 1275, 1045 cm^{-1} (KBr disk).

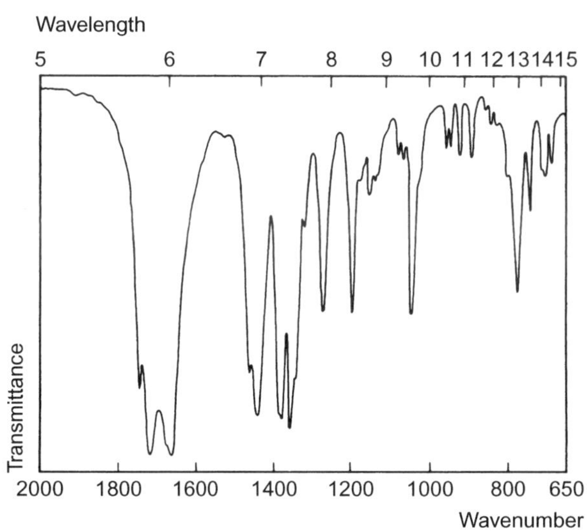

Mass Spectrum. Principal ions at *m/z* 221, 81, 157, 80, 79, 155, 41, 77; 3′-oxohexobarbital 250, 95, 39, 235, 66, 207, 41, 193.

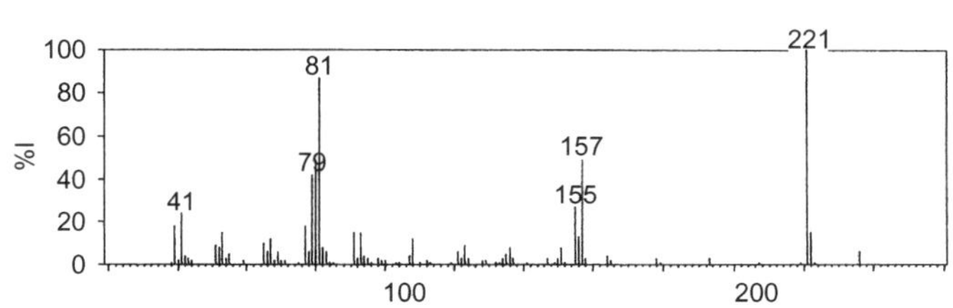

Quantification. See also under Amylobarbital.

Gas chromatography–mass spectrometry. In plasma or urine: hexobarbital enantiomers and metabolites—C. Prakash *et al.*, *Biol. Mass Spectrom.*, 1991, *20*, 559–564.

Disposition in the Body. Readily absorbed after oral administration. The sodium salt has a very short duration of action and is usually administered intravenously. Hexobarbital is inactivated in the liver by *N*-demethylation and oxidation. About 32% of a dose is excreted in the urine in 24 h as 3′-oxohexobarbital, 5% as 3′-hydroxyhexobarbital, and 18% as 1,5-dimethylbarbituric acid; less than 1% of a dose is excreted unchanged in the urine in 24 h.

Therapeutic concentration. In plasma, usually in the range 1 to 5 mg/L.

Following a single oral dose of 500 mg to 6 subjects, peak plasma concentrations of 4.9 to 10.9 mg/L (mean 7) were attained in about 1 h. [N. P. E. Vermeulen *et al.*, *Br. J. Clin. Pharmacol.*, 1983, *15*, 459–464.]

Toxicity. The estimated minimum lethal dose is 2 g. Plasma concentrations greater than about 8 mg/L may produce toxic effects.

Half-life. Plasma half-life, 3 to 7 h.

Volume of distribution. About 1 L/kg.

Clearance. Plasma clearance, about 3.5 mL/min/kg.

Protein binding. In plasma, 42 to 52%.

Note. For a review of the pharmacokinetics of barbiturates, see D. D. Breimer, *Clin. Pharmacokinet.*, 1977, *2*, 93–109.

Dose. 250 to 500 mg, as a hypnotic; up to 750 mg daily in divided doses, as a sedative.

Hexobendine

Anti-anginal Vasodilator

1,2-Ethanediylbis[(methylimino)-3,1-propanediyl]-3,4,5-trimethoxybenzoate
$C_{30}H_{44}N_2O_{10}$=592.7
CAS—54-03-5

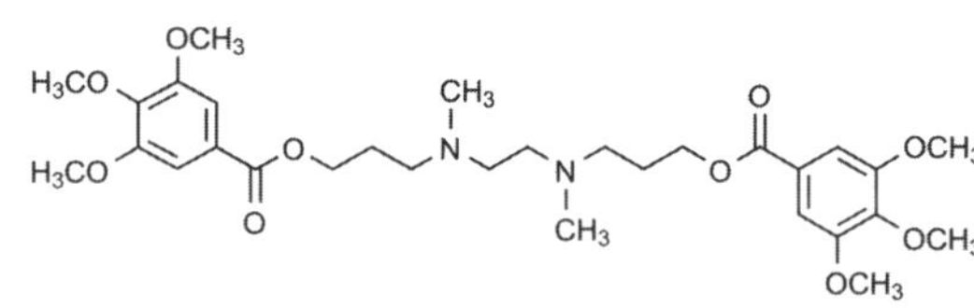

M.p. 75° to 77°.

Hexobendine Hydrochloride

Proprietary names. Reoxyl; Ustimon.
$C_{30}H_{44}N_2O_{10}$,2HCl=665.6
CAS—50-62-4
A white crystalline powder. M.p. 170° to 174°.
Freely soluble in water; soluble in chloroform; slightly soluble in ethanol; practically insoluble in ether.

Partition Coefficient. Log *P* (octanol/water), 2.7.

Colour Tests. Liebermann's Test—black; Mandelin's Test—violet.

Thin-layer Chromatography. System TA—Rf 47; system TB—Rf 10; system TC—Rf 44; system TE—Rf 16; system TL—Rf 06; system TAE—Rf 12. (Acidified iodoplatinate solution, positive.)

Gas Chromatography. System GA—not eluted.

Ultraviolet Spectrum. Aqueous acid—265 nm (A^1_1=311a).

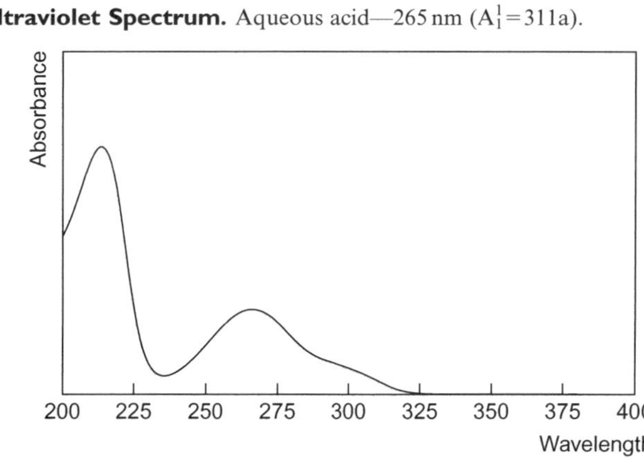

Infra-red Spectrum. Principal peaks at wavenumbers 1123, 1219, 1703, 1585, 1497, 1171 cm^{-1} (KBr disk).

Mass Spectrum. Principal ions at *m/z* 296, 195, 58, 297, 253, 196, 212, 84.

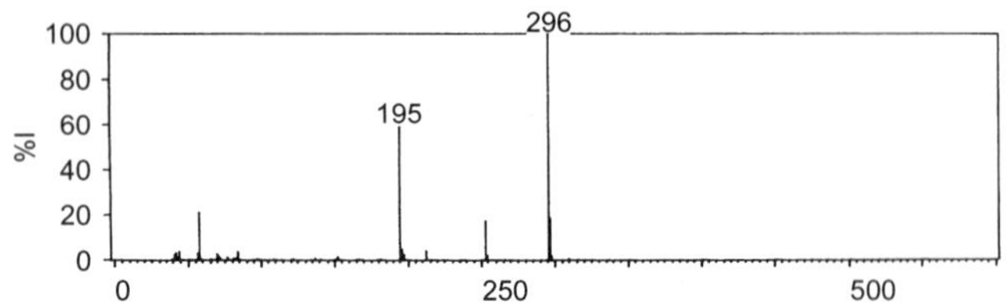

Dose. Hexobendine hydrochloride has been given in doses of 60 to 180 mg daily.

Hexocyclium Metilsulfate *Anticholinergic/Antispasmodic*

Proprietary names. Tral; Tralin.
4-(2-Cyclohexyl-2-hydroxy-2-phenylethyl)-1,1-dimethylpiperazinium methylsulfate
$C_{20}H_{33}N_2O,CH_3SO_4$=428.6
CAS—6004-98-4 (hexocyclium); 115-63-9 (metilsulfate)

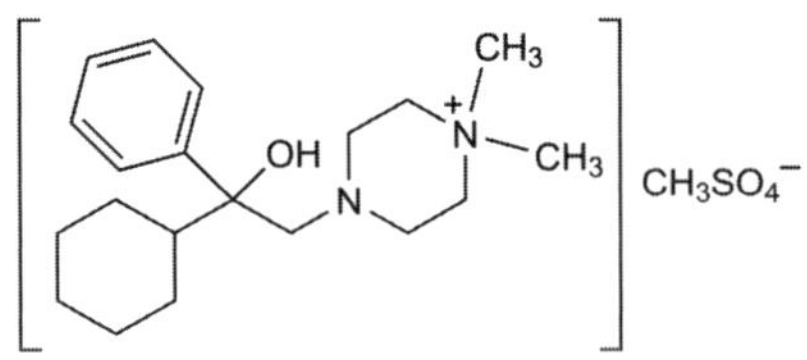

A white powder. M.p. 200° to 210°.
Soluble 1 in 2 of water; slightly soluble in chloroform; practically insoluble in ether.

Partition Coefficient. Log *P* (octanol/water), 1.0.

Colour Tests. Mandelin's Test—blue-violet; Marquis Test—violet.

Thin-layer Chromatography. System TA—Rf 02; system TE—Rf 01; system TAE—Rf 03. (Acidified iodoplatinate solution, positive.)

Ultraviolet Spectrum. Aqueous acid—252, 257 (A^1_1=5.3b), 264 nm.

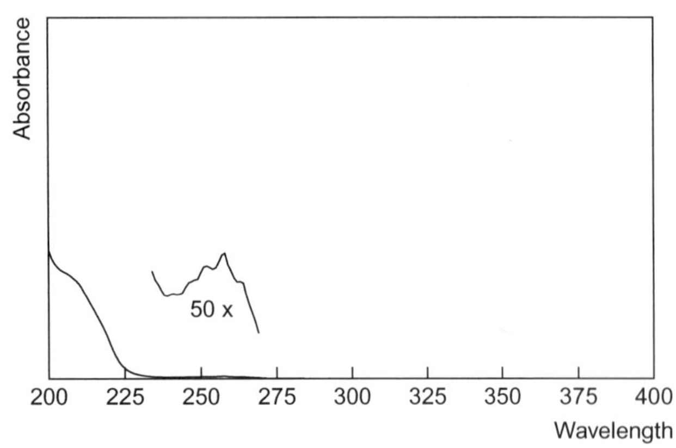

Infra-red Spectrum. Principal peaks at wavenumbers 1224, 1005, 748, 1052, 700, 770 cm^{-1} (KBr disk).

Dose. Initially, 100 mg daily.

Hexoprenaline *Sympathomimetic*

Proprietary name. Ipradol
4,4′-[1,6-Hexanediylbis[imino(1-hydroxy-2,1-ethanediyl)]]bis-1,2-benzenediol
$C_{22}H_{32}N_2O_6$=420.5
CAS—3215-70-1

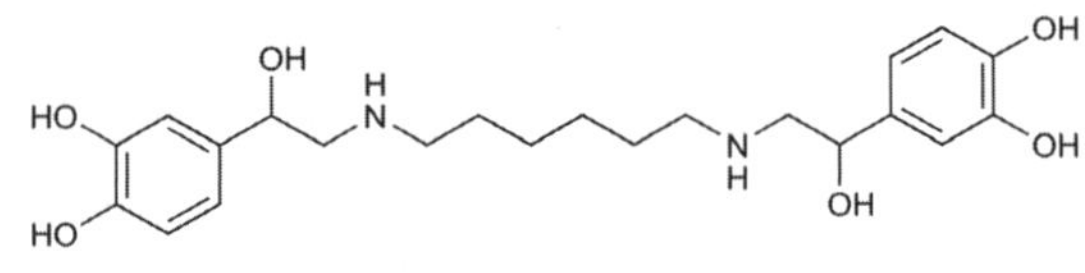

Crystals. M.p. 162° to 165° (hemihydrate).

Hexoprenaline Hydrochloride
Proprietary name. Ipradol
$C_{22}H_{32}N_2O_6$,2HCl=493.4
CAS—4323-43-7
Crystals. M.p. 197° to 198°.

Hexoprenaline Sulfate
Proprietary names. Bronalin; Delaprem; Etoscol; Gynipral; Ipradol; Leanol.
$C_{22}H_{32}N_2O_6,H_2SO_4$=518.6
CAS—32266-10-7
A white crystalline powder. M.p. 214°, with decomposition.
Soluble in water and dilute hydrochloric acid; practically insoluble in ethanol.

Colour Tests. Ammoniacal Silver Nitrate—red→brown→black/-; Ferric Chloride—orange; Folin–Ciocalteu Reagent—blue; Mandelin's Test—orange-yellow; Marquis Test—red; Methanolic Potassium Hydroxide—orange→brown; Nessler's Reagent—black; Potassium Dichromate (Method 1)—green→brown (30 s); Sulfuric Acid—orange-yellow.

Thin-layer Chromatography. System TA—Rf 03; system TB—Rf 01; system TC—Rf 00; system TE—Rf 71; system TL—Rf 01; system TAE—Rf 12. (Acidified iodoplatinate solution, positive.)

Ultraviolet Spectrum. Aqueous acid—280 nm (A^1_1=129a).

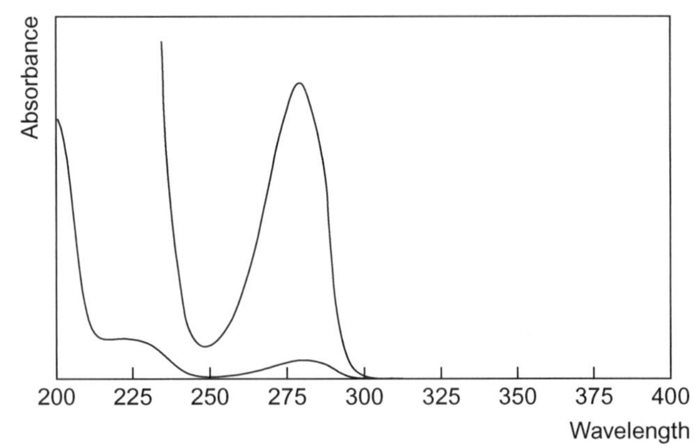

Infra-red Spectrum. Principal peaks at wavenumbers 1102, 1242, 1190, 1605, 1517, 1280 cm^{-1} (hexoprenaline sulfate, KBr disk).

Mass Spectrum. Principal ions at *m/z* 30, 27, 124, 56, 123, 87, 78, 41.

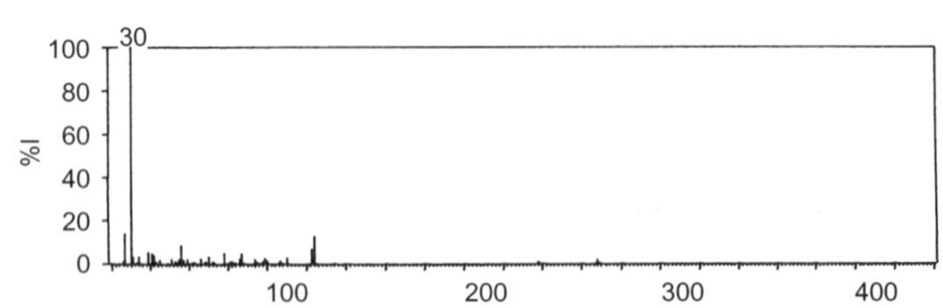

Dose. Hexoprenaline sulfate has been given in doses of 0.75 to 1.5 mg daily.

Hexyl Nicotinate *Topical Vasodilator*

Proprietary names. It is an ingredient of Hipodor, Transvane, and Transvasin.
n-Hexyl nicotinate

$C_{12}H_{17}NO_2$=207.3
CAS—23597-82-2

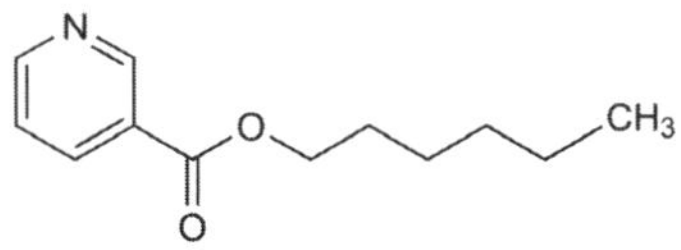

A pale yellow liquid.
Practically insoluble in water; soluble in ethanol, chloroform, and methanol.

Partition Coefficient. Log *P* (octanol/water), 3.5.

Thin-layer Chromatography. System TA—Rf 70. (Acidified iodoplatinate solution, positive.)

Ultraviolet Spectrum. Aqueous acid—260 nm (A_1^1=268b).

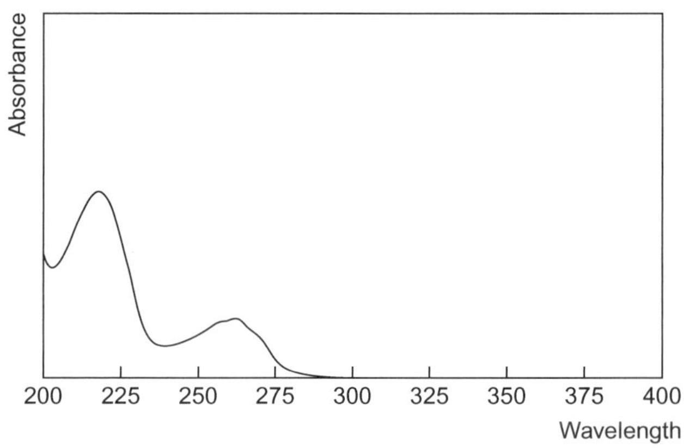

Infra-red Spectrum. Principal peaks at wavenumbers 1724, 1276, 1111, 741, 1022, 1590 cm^{-1} (KBr disk).

Use. Topically in a concentration of 2%.

Hexylcaine

Local Anaesthetic

1-(Cyclohexylamino)-2-propanol benzoate
$C_{16}H_{23}NO_2$=261.4
CAS—532-77-4

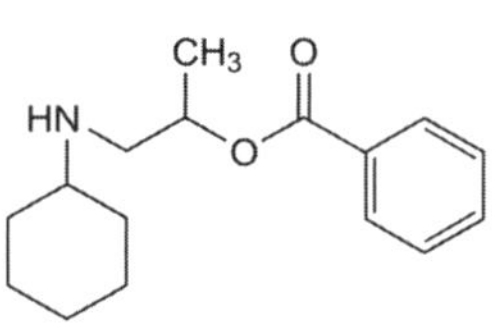

Hexylcaine Hydrochloride

Proprietary name. Cyclaine
$C_{16}H_{23}NO_2$,HCl=297.8
CAS—532-76-3
A white powder. M.p. 182° to 184°.
Soluble 1 in 17 of water; freely soluble in ethanol and chloroform; practically insoluble in ether.

Dissociation Constant. pK_a 9.1.

Partition Coefficient. Log *P* (octanol/water), 0.9 (hydrochloride).

Thin-layer Chromatography. System TA—Rf 01; system TE—Rf 80; system TAJ—Rf 29; system TAK—Rf 15; system TAL—Rf 70. (Acidified iodoplatinate solution, positive.)

Gas Chromatography. System GA—RI 1965.

Ultraviolet Spectrum. Aqueous acid—232 nm (A_1^1=485a), 275 nm (A_1^1=43a).

Infra-red Spectrum. Principal peaks at wavenumbers 1270, 1718, 1105, 710, 1068, 1022 cm^{-1} (KBr disk).

Mass Spectrum. Principal ions at *m/z* 112, 77, 105, 139, 55, 41, 96, 56.

Use. Hexylcaine hydrochloride has been used in concentrations of up to 5%.

Hexylresorcinol

Anthelmintic

Proprietary names. Ascaryl; Benylin Sore Throat Lozenge; Caprokol; Crystoids; Gelovermin; Lemsip Sore Throat; Mac Dual Action; Strepsils Extra; Sucrets; Worm-Agen
4-Hexyl-1,3-benzenediol
$C_{12}H_{18}O_2$=194.3
CAS—136-77-6

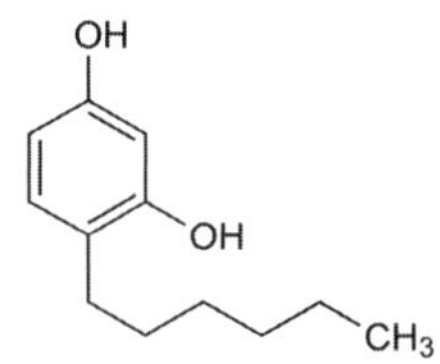

White or yellowish-white acicular crystals, crystalline plates or crystalline powder. It acquires a brownish-pink tint on exposure to light and air. M.p. 62° to 68°.
Soluble 1 in 2000 of water; soluble in acetone, ethanol, chloroform, and ether; slightly soluble in petroleum ether.
Caution. Hexylresorcinol is irritating to the oral mucosa, to the respiratory tract and to the skin; ethanolic solutions have vesicant properties.

Partition Coefficient. Log *P* (octanol/water), 3.4.

Colour Test. Ferric Chloride—green

Thin-layer Chromatography. System TB—Rf 00; system TE—Rf 60; system TF—Rf 65; system TAE—Rf 88.

Gas Chromatography. System GA—RI 1830.

High Performance Liquid Chromatography. System HX—RI 579; system HY—RI 528.

Ultraviolet Spectrum. Methanol—282 nm (A_1^1=160c).

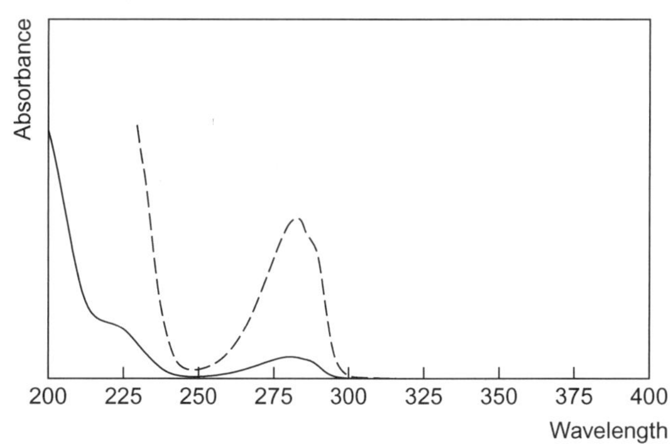

Infra-red Spectrum. Principal peaks at wavenumbers 970, 980, 1185, 1616, 1150, 1205 cm^{-1} (KBr disk).

Disposition in the Body. Partly absorbed after oral administration. About 20 to 30% of a dose is rapidly excreted unchanged in the urine and the remainder is eliminated in the faeces.

Dose. 1 g as a single dose.

Histamine

Diagnostic Agent (Gastric Secretion)

Synonym. Ergotidine
Proprietary name. Destamin
1*H*-Imidazole-4-ethanamine

$C_5H_9N_3$=111.1
CAS—51-45-6

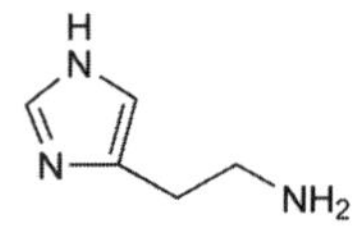

Deliquescent acicular crystals. M.p. 83° to 84°.
Freely soluble in water, ethanol, and hot chloroform; practically insoluble in ether.

Histamine Acid Phosphate

Synonyms. Histamine Diphosphate; Histamine Phosphate.
$C_5H_9N_3,2H_3PO_4$=307.1
CAS—51-74-1
Colourless crystals. M.p. 130° to 133°.
Soluble 1 in 4 of water; slightly soluble in ethanol; practically insoluble in ether.

Histamine Hydrochloride

Synonym. Histamine Dihydrochloride
Proprietary name. Maxamine. It is an ingredient of Histadestil, Histaglobin, Midalgan, and Radalgin.
$C_5H_9N_3,2HCl$=184.1
CAS—56-92-8
Hygroscopic colourless crystals or white crystalline powder. M.p. about 245°, with decomposition.
Freely soluble in water and methanol; soluble in ethanol and acetone; practically insoluble in chloroform and ether.

Dissociation Constant. pK_a 5.9, 9.7 (25°).

Partition Coefficient. Log *P* (octanol/water), −0.7.

Thin-layer Chromatography. System TA—Rf 13; system TB—Rf 00; system TC—Rf 00; system TE—Rf 07; system TL—Rf 00; system TAE—Rf 00; system TAF—Rf 03. (Acidified iodoplatinate solution, positive.)

Gas Chromatography. System GA—RI 1497.

Ultraviolet Spectrum. No significant absorption, 230 to 360 nm.

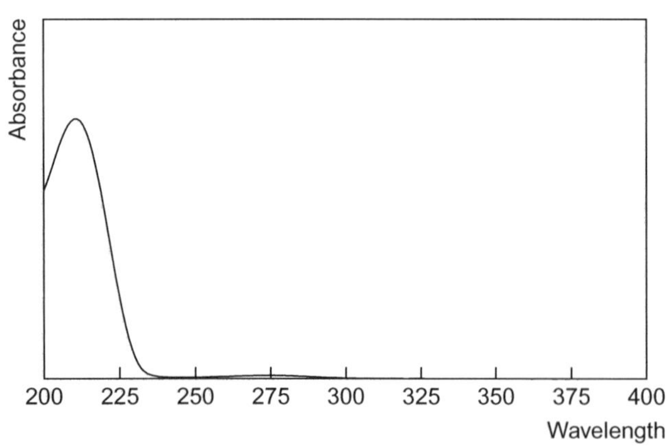

Infra-red Spectrum. Principal peaks at wavenumbers 840, 1622, 1522, 1084, 802, 1577 cm^{-1} (histamine hydrochloride, KBr disk).

Mass Spectrum. Principal ions at *m/z* 82, 30, 81, 54, 28, 55, 83, 41.

Quantification

High performance liquid chromatography. In biological fluids: histamine and *N*-methylhistamine, electrochemical detection—A. A. Houdi *et al.*, *J. Pharm. Sci.*, 1987, *76*, 398–401. In biological fluids or tissues: fluorescence detection—D. Tsikas *et al.*, *J. Chromatogr.*, 1993, *614*, 37–41.

Disposition in the Body

Toxicity

Harbour workers experienced allergy-like symptoms of toxicity after handling bags containing fish flour contaminated with histamine (510 mg/100 g). [J. Macan *et al.*, *Occup. Med. (Lond.)*, 2000, *50*, 22–24.]

Dose. Histamine acid phosphate is given subcutaneously, in a dose of 40 µg/kg, following administration of a large dose of an antihistamine.

Histapyrrodine

Antihistamine

N-Phenyl-*N*-(phenylmethyl)-1-pyrrolidineethanamine
$C_{19}H_{24}N_2$=280.4
CAS—493-80-1

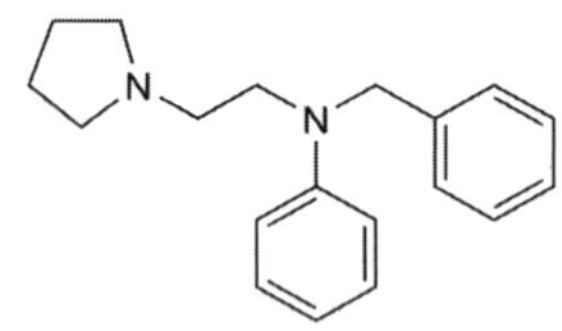

An oil.

Histapyrrodine Hydrochloride

Proprietary names. Calcistin; Domistan; Luvistin.
$C_{19}H_{24}N_2,HCl$=316.9
CAS—6113-17-3
A white powder. M.p. 196°.
Solubility in water (at 18°), 2 g in 100 mL.

Partition Coefficient. Log *P* (octanol/water), 4.2.

Colour Test. Mandelin's Test—red-violet.

Thin-layer Chromatography. System TA—Rf 60; system TE—Rf 75; system TAE—Rf 32. (Acidified iodoplatinate solution, positive.)

Gas Chromatography. System GA—histapyrrodine RI 2240, M (OH-) RI 2500, M (oxo-) RI 2570, M (*N*-desbenzyl-) RI 1800, M (*N*-desbenzyl-oxo-) RI 2120, M (*N*-desphenyl-oxo-)-H_2O RI 2100.

High Performance Liquid Chromatography. System HA—*k* 3.0.

Ultraviolet Spectrum. Aqueous acid—250 nm (A_1^1=141a), 295 nm.

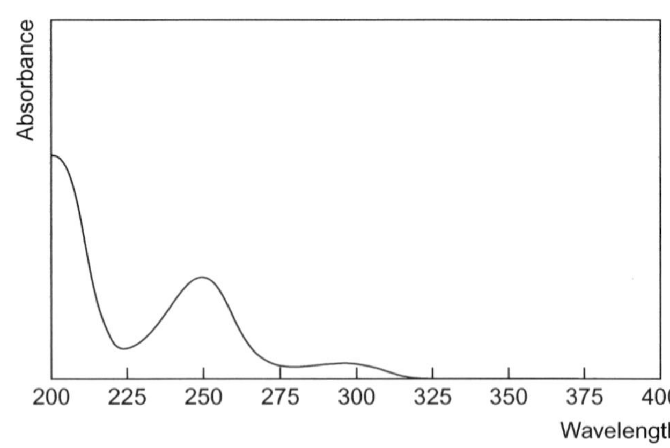

Infra-red Spectrum. Principal peaks at wavenumbers 1513, 1604, 750, 698, 1500, 732 cm^{-1}.

Mass Spectrum. Principal ions at *m/z*: M (OH-) 84, 91, 212, 296, 213, 297; M (oxo-) 91, 196, 209, 197, 275, 294; M (*N*-desbenzyl-) 84, 190, 106, 111, 122, 77; M (*N*-desbenzyl-oxo-) 106, 119, 118, 98, 77, 204; M (*N*-desphenyl-oxo-)-H_2O 91, 159, 216, 160, 215, 84.

Dose. Histapyrrodine hydrochloride has been given in doses of 50 to 150 mg daily.

Homatropine

Anticholinergic

Proprietary names. Homasedin; Homatropil; Homo; Pasmolit.
8-Methyl-8-azabicyclo[3.2.1]oct-3-yl-*endo*-α-hydroxybenzeneacetate
$C_{16}H_{21}NO_3$=275.3
CAS—87-00-3

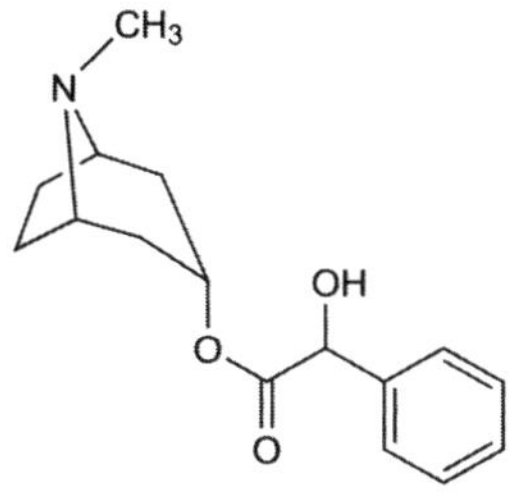

Small white prismatic crystals or coarse crystalline powder. M.p. 99° to 100°.
Slightly soluble in water; soluble in ethanol, benzene, acetone, dilute acids, chloroform, and ether.

Homatropine Hydrobromide

Synonym. Tropyl Mandelate Hydrobromide
Proprietary names. Bufopto Homatrocel; Homat; Homatrisol; Homatrocil; Homatrop.
$C_{16}H_{21}NO_3$,HBr=356.3
CAS—51-56-9
Colourless crystals or a white crystalline powder. M.p. 214° to 217°, with decomposition.
Soluble 1 in 6 of water, 1 in 60 of ethanol, and 1 in 420 of chloroform; practically insoluble in ether.

Dissociation Constant. pK_a 9.9 (20°).

Partition Coefficient. Log *P* (octanol/water), 1.4.

Thin-layer Chromatography. System TA—Rf 01; system TB—Rf 05; system TC—Rf 01; system TE—Rf 23; system TL—Rf 01; system TAE—Rf 07; system TAF—Rf 27; system TAJ—Rf 00; system TAK—Rf 02; system TAL—Rf 34. (Acidified iodoplatinate solution, positive.)

Gas Chromatography. System GA—RI 2072; system GB—RI 2165.

High Performance Liquid Chromatography. System HA—*k* 4.2 (tailing peak); system HX—RI 272; system HY—RI 223; system HAX—retention time 6.8 min; system HAY—retention time 3.6 min.

Ultraviolet Spectrum. Aqueous acid—252, 258 nm (A_1^1=7.3a), 264 nm. No alkaline shift.

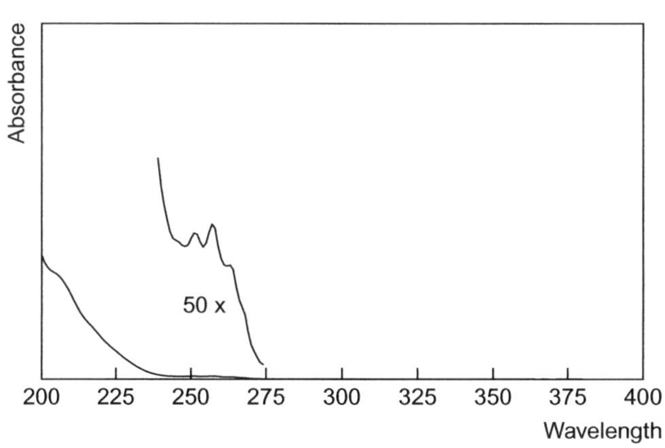

Infra-red Spectrum. Principal peaks at wavenumbers 1730, 1172, 1030, 735, 1063, 1125 cm^{-1} (KBr disk).

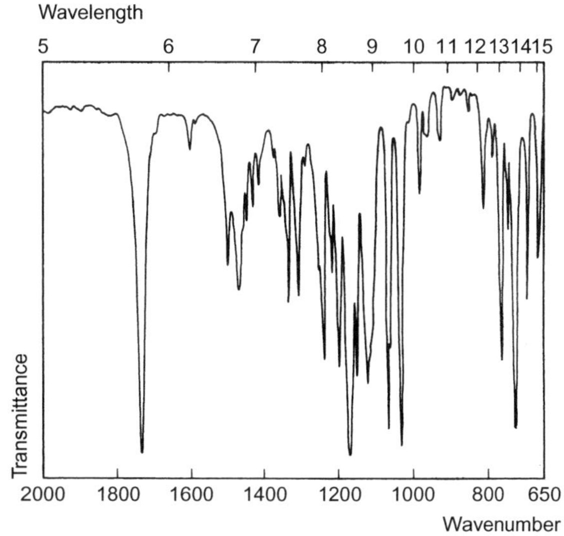

Mass Spectrum. Principal ions at *m/z* 124, 107, 82, 83, 42, 77, 79, 94.

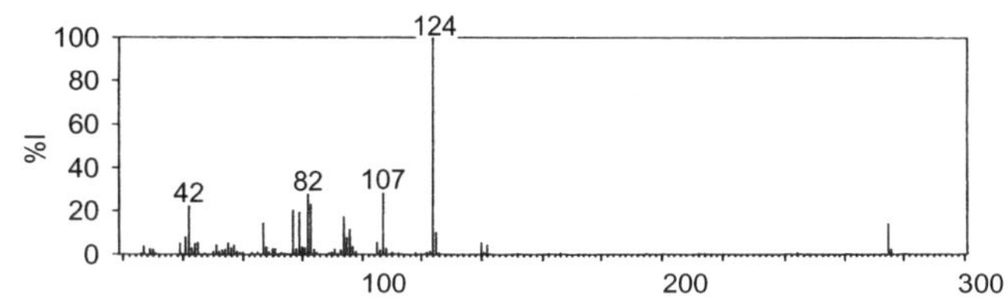

Use. Homatropine hydrobromide is used as a 2% ophthalmic solution.

Homatropine Methylbromide

Anticholinergic

Synonyms. Homatropine Methobromide; Methylhomatropinium Bromide.
Proprietary names. Arkitropin; Homapin; Malcotran; Mesopin; Novatrin; Novatropina; Sethyl.
8-Methyl-8-azabicyclo[3.2.1]oct-3-yl-*endo*-α-hydroxybenzeneacetate methylbromide
$C_{16}H_{21}NO_3$,CH_3Br=370.3
CAS—80-49-9
A white powder. M.p. about 190°.
Freely soluble in water and ethanol; practically insoluble in acetone and ether.

Thin-layer Chromatography. System TA—Rf 00; system TB—Rf 00; system TC—Rf 00; system TE—Rf 00; system TL—Rf 00; system TAE—Rf 00; system TAF—Rf 12. (Acidified iodoplatinate solution, positive.)

Gas Chromatography. System GA—not eluted.

High Performance Liquid Chromatography. System HX—RI 262.

Ultraviolet Spectrum. Aqueous acid—252, 258 nm (A_1^1=5.8b), 264 nm.

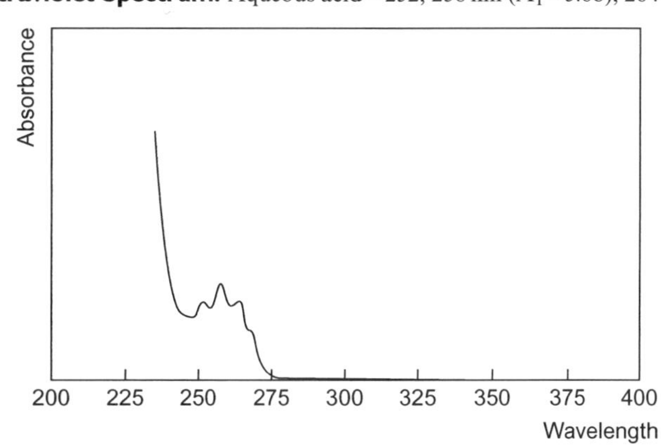

Infra-red Spectrum. Principal peaks at wavenumbers 1724, 1179, 1160, 1195, 1044, 935 cm^{-1} (KBr disk).

Dose. Usually 12 to 40 mg daily.

Homidium Bromide

Trypanocide (Veterinary)

Synonym. Ethidium Bromide
Proprietary name. Dromilac
3,8-Diamino-5-ethyl-6-phenylphenanthridinium bromide
$C_{21}H_{20}BrN_3$=394.3
CAS—1239-45-8

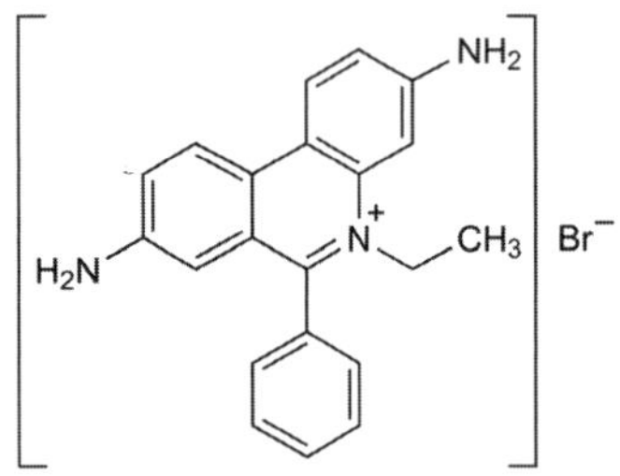

A dark purple crystalline or amorphous powder. M.p. 245°, with decomposition.
Soluble 1 in 20 of water and 1 in 750 of chloroform.

Colour Test. The test is performed on homidium nitrate (see Colour tests chapter): Mandelin's Test—yellow

Thin-layer Chromatography. System TA—Rf 55. (Acidified potassium permanganate solution, positive.)

Ultraviolet Spectrum. Aqueous acid—242, 283 nm (A^1_1=785a).

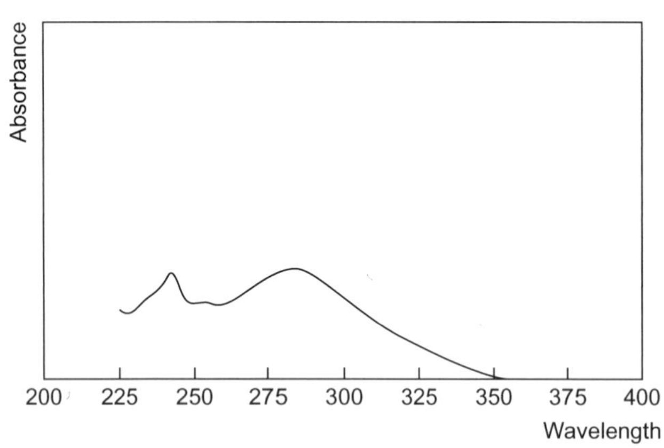

Infra-red Spectrum. Principal peaks at wavenumbers 1628, 1492, 1260, 1312, 836, 1077 cm^{-1} (KBr disk).

Homochlorcyclizine

Antihistamine

Proprietary name. Homoclomin (hydrochloride)
1-[(4-Chlorophenyl)phenylmethyl]hexahydro-4-methyl-1*H*-1,4-diazepine
$C_{19}H_{23}ClN_2$=314.9
CAS—848-53-3

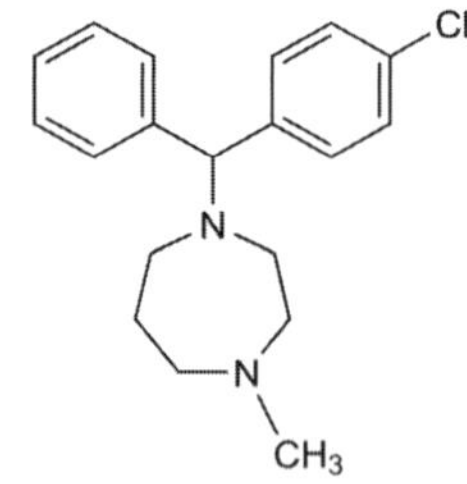

A white crystalline powder.
Soluble in dilute acetic acid.

Partition Coefficient. Log *P* (octanol/water), 4.1.

Thin-layer Chromatography. System TA—Rf 28. (Acidified iodoplatinate solution, positive.)

Ultraviolet Spectrum. Aqueous acid—233 (A^1_1=457b), 258, 263, 270 nm.

Infra-red Spectrum. Principal peaks at wavenumbers 1135, 1010, 1600, 1618, 1630, 720 cm^{-1} (KBr disk).

Quantification
High performance liquid chromatography. In urine: homochlorcyclizine enantiomers, limit of detection <50 µg/L, UV detection—M. Nishikata *et al.*, *J. Chromatogr.*, 1993, *612*, 239–244.

Dose. Homochlorcyclizine has been given in doses of 30 to 60 mg daily.

Hordenine

Sympathomimetic

4-[2-(Dimethylamino)ethyl]phenol
$C_{10}H_{15}NO$=165.2
CAS—539-15-1

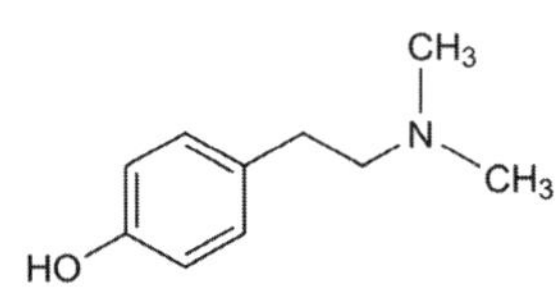

Hordenine occurs naturally in germinating barley and other Gramineae.
Crystals. M.p. 117° to 118°.
Slightly soluble in water; very soluble in ethanol, chloroform, and ether; sparingly soluble in benzene, toluene, and xylene; practically insoluble in petroleum ether.

Hordenine Sulfate
$(C_{10}H_{15}NO)_2,H_2SO_4,2H_2O$=464.6
CAS—622-64-0 (anhydrous); 6202-17-1 (dihydrate)
Crystals. M.p. 197°, and 210° after drying at 100°.
Soluble in water; slightly soluble in ethanol; practically insoluble in ether.

Partition Coefficient. Log *P* (octanol/water), 1.5.

Colour Tests. Mandelin's Test—grey-green; Marquis Test—brown→green.

Thin-layer Chromatography. System TA—Rf 40; system TB—Rf 05; system TC—Rf 06; system TE—Rf 52; system TL—Rf 05; system TAJ—Rf 03; system TAK—Rf 00; system TAL—Rf 20. (Acidified potassium permanganate solution, positive.)

Gas Chromatography. System GA—RI 1432.

High Performance Liquid Chromatography. System HB—*k* 2.00.

Ultraviolet Spectrum. Aqueous acid—274 nm.

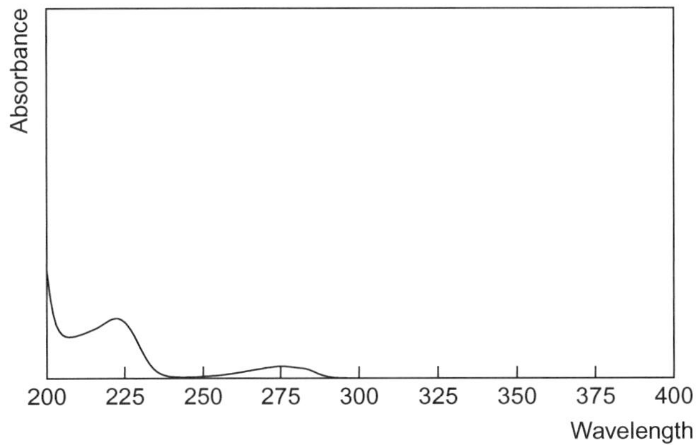

Infra-red Spectrum. Principal peaks at wavenumbers 1252, 1512, 820, 1612, 1270, 869 cm^{-1} (KBr disk).

Mass Spectrum. Principal ions at *m*/*z* 58, 42, 59, 30, 77, 107, 57, 51.

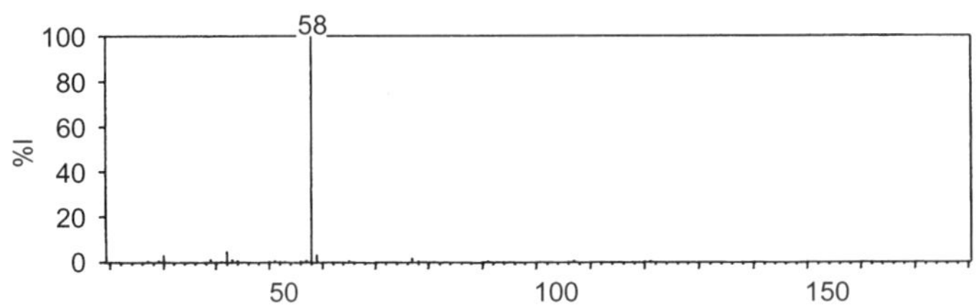

Hydralazine

Antihypertensive

Synonym. Hydrallazine
1(2*H*)-Phthalazinone hydrazone
$C_8H_8N_4$=160.2
CAS—86-54-4

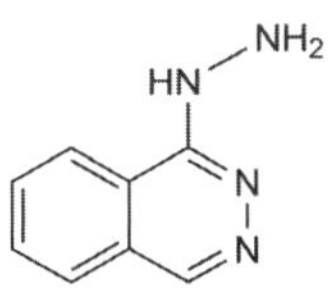

Yellow crystals. M.p. 172° to 173°.
Soluble 1 in 12 of warm methanol.

Hydralazine Hydrochloride

Synonym. Apressinum
Proprietary names. Alphapress; Apresolina; Apresolin(e); Cesoline; Hydrapres; Hyperphen; Novo-Hylazin; Nu-Hydral; Rolazine.
$C_8H_8N_4$,HCl=196.6
CAS—304-20-1
A white crystalline powder. M.p. 273°, with decomposition.
Soluble 1 in 25 of water and 1 in 500 of ethanol; very slightly soluble in ether; practically insoluble in chloroform.

Dissociation Constant. pK_a 0.5, 7.1.

Partition Coefficient. Log *P* (octanol/water), 1.0.

Colour Test. Nessler's Reagent—black

Thin-layer Chromatography. System TA—Rf 51; system TB—Rf 41; system TC—Rf 11; system TE—Rf 80; system TL—Rf 64; system TAE—Rf 73; system TAJ—Rf 01; system TAK—Rf 01; system TAL—Rf 25. (Acidified iodoplatinate solution, positive.)

Gas Chromatography. System GA—RI 1528; system GB—RI 1914.

High Performance Liquid Chromatography. System HX—RI 193; system HY—RI 132; system HZ—retention time 1.9 min; system HAX—retention time 6.5 min; system HAY—retention time 3.5 min.

Ultraviolet Spectrum. Water—240 nm (A_1^1=675a), 260 nm (A_1^1=675a), 304, 315 nm.

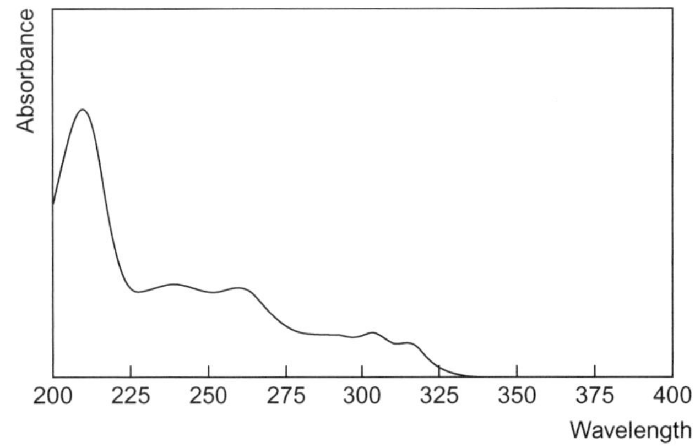

Infra-red Spectrum. Principal peaks at wavenumbers 1665, 790, 1582, 1000, 810, 1175 cm^{-1} (hydralazine hydrochloride, KBr disk).

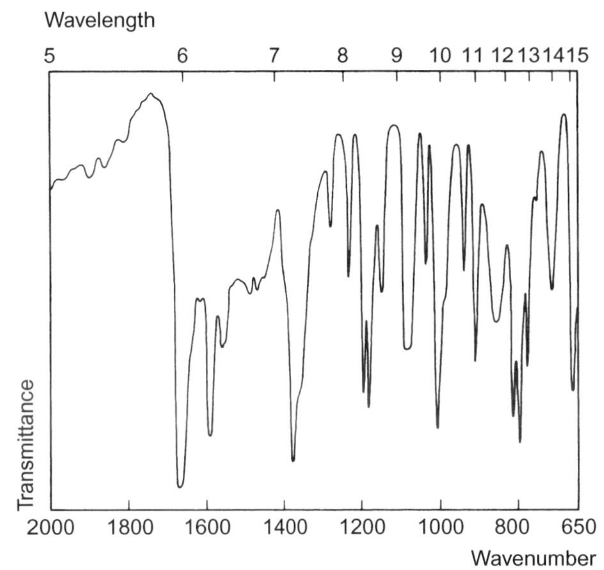

Mass Spectrum. Principal ions at *m*/*z* 160, 103, 89, 131, 115, 76, 161, 104.

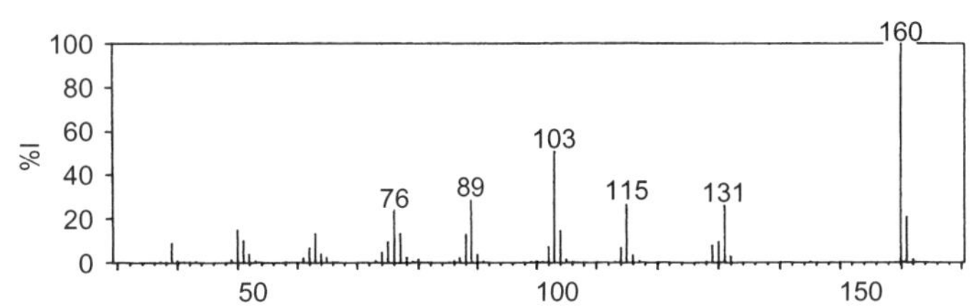

Quantification

High performance liquid chromatography. In plasma: limit of detection 1 µg/L for hydralazine and 200 ng/L for hydralazine pyruvic acid hydrazone, fluorescence detection—P. A. Reece *et al.*, *J. Chromatogr.* 1980, *181(7) B Biomed. Appl.*, 427–440. In blood: limit of detection 1 µg/L, UV detection—T. M. Ludden *et al.*, *J. Pharm. Sci.*, 1983, *72*, 693–695. In plasma: electrochemical detection—J. K. Wong *et al.*, *J. Chromatogr.*, 1987, *385*, 261–266. In blood: limit of detection 300 ng/L—H. A. Semple *et al.*, *Pharm. Res.*, 1988, *5*, 383–386.

Note. Spectrophotometric and gas chromatographic assays have been shown to be non-selective owing to interference from acid-labile hydrazones—see P. A. Reece *et al.*, *J. Pharm. Sci.*, 1978, *67*, 1150–1153 and T. M. Ludden *et al.*, *Clin. Pharmacokinet.*, 1982, *7*, 185–205.

Disposition in the Body. Readily absorbed after oral administration. It undergoes first-pass acetylation, the extent of which is genetically determined. The major metabolites are: 3-methyl-1,2,4-triazolo[3,4-*a*]phthalazine (MTP—the acetylation product); hydralazine pyruvic acid hydrazone (HPH) which is the major plasma metabolite; 4-(2-acetylhydrazino)phthalazin-1-one (*N*-AcHPZ) which is the major urinary metabolite; 3-hydroxymethyl-1,2,4-triazolo[3,4-*a*]phthalazine (3-OHMTP). About 65% of a dose is excreted in the urine in 24 h. In rapid acetylators, about 30% is excreted as *N*-AcHPZ and 10 to 30% as conjugated 3-OHMTP; in slow acetylators, about 15 to 20% is excreted as *N*-AcHPZ and up to 10% as conjugated 3-OHMTP. Other metabolites include phthalazin-1-one (PZ), 1,2,4-triazolo[3,4-*a*]phthalazine (TP), 9-hydroxy-MTP, phthalazine, tetrazolo[5,1-*a*]phthalazine and hydrazones of hydralazine formed with acetone and α-ketoglutaric acid. About 10% of a dose is eliminated in the faeces.

Therapeutic concentration

Following a single oral dose of 1 mg/kg to 4 rapid acetylators, a mean peak plasma hydralazine concentration of 0.05 mg/L was attained in 0.4 h and a mean peak plasma HPH concentration of 0.26 mg/L was attained in 0.6 h; after the same dose was given to 4 slow acetylators the corresponding peak plasma concentrations were 0.17 mg/L of hydralazine and 0.54 mg/L of HPH in 0.3 h and 1 h, respectively. [A. Shepherd *et al.*, *Clin. Pharmacol. Ther.*, 1980, *28*, 804–811.]

Bioavailability. About 30 to 35% in slow acetylators, 10 to 16% in rapid acetylators.

Half-life. Plasma half-life, hydralazine 0.4 to 2 h, HPH about 4 h, MTP about 1.5 to 2 h.

Volume of distribution. About 3 to 8 L/kg.

Note. For a review of the pharmacokinetics of hydralazine see T. M. Ludden *et al.*, *Clin. Pharmacokinet.*, 1982, *7*, 185–205.

Dose. 50 to 200 mg of hydralazine hydrochloride daily.

Hydrastine

Alkaloid

(3*S*)-6,7-Dimethoxy-3-[(5*R*)-5,6,7,8-tetrahydro-6-methyl-1,3-dioxolo[4,5-*g*]isoquinolin-5-yl]-1(3*H*)-isobenzofuranone
$C_{21}H_{21}NO_6$=383.4
CAS—118-08-1

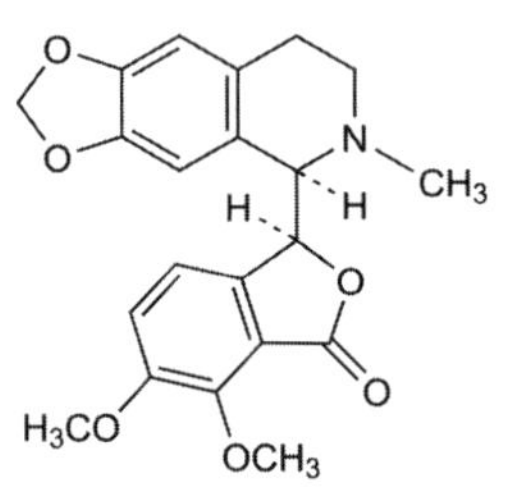

An alkaloid obtained from hydrastis, the dried rhizome and roots of golden seal, *Hydrastis canadensis* (Ranunculaceae).
Crystals. M.p. 132°.
Insoluble in water; soluble 1 in 210 of ethanol, 1 in 1 of chloroform, and 1 in 245 of ether; freely soluble in acetone and benzene.

Hydrastine Hydrochloride

$C_{21}H_{21}NO_6$,HCl=419.9
CAS—5936-28-7
A white or creamy-white hygroscopic powder. M.p. 116°.
Very soluble in water and ethanol; slightly soluble in chloroform; very slightly soluble in ether.

Dissociation Constant. pK_a 6.2 (25°).

Partition Coefficient. Log *P* (octanol/water), 1.9.

Colour Tests. Liebermann's Test—green; Mandelin's Test—red-brown→red.

Thin-layer Chromatography. System TA—Rf 61; system TB—Rf 15; system TC—Rf 64; system TE—Rf 71; system TL—Rf 52; system TAE—Rf 59; system TAF—Rf 57. (Acidified iodoplatinate solution, positive.)

Gas Chromatography. System GA—RI 2988.

High Performance Liquid Chromatography. System HY—RI 280.

Ultraviolet Spectrum. Aqueous acid—294 nm (A_1^1=195b); aqueous alkali—292 nm.

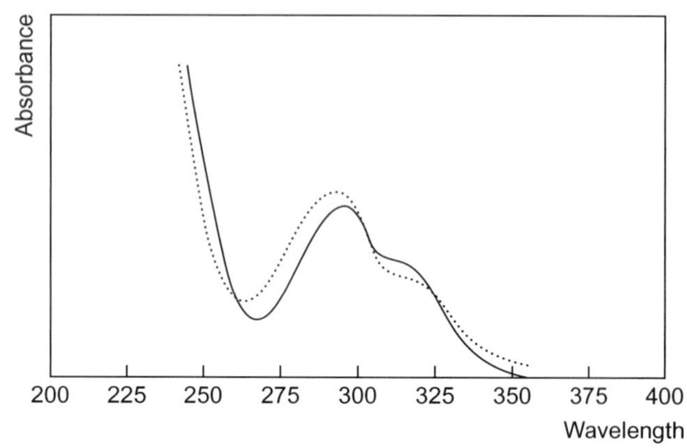

Infra-red Spectrum. Principal peaks at wavenumbers 1760, 1501, 1037, 1260, 1020, 1111 cm^{-1} (KBr disk).

Dose. Hydrastine hydrochloride was formerly given in doses of 15 to 60 mg.

Hydrastinine

Alkaloid

5,6,7,8-Tetrahydro-6-methyl-1,3-dioxolo[4,5-*g*]isoquinolin-5-ol
$C_{11}H_{13}NO_3$=207.2
CAS—6592-85-4

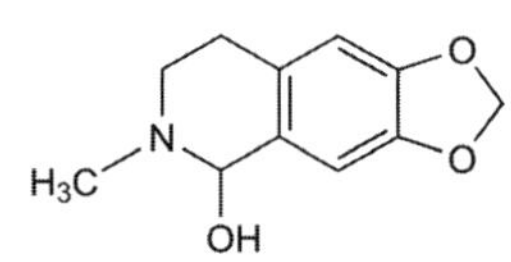

An alkaloid produced by oxidation of hydrastine.
A white crystalline substance. M.p. 117°.
Moderately soluble in hot water; freely soluble in ethanol, chloroform, dilute acids, and ether.

Hydrastinine Hydrochloride

$C_{11}H_{11}NO_2$,HCl=225.7
CAS—4884-68-8
Pale yellow crystals or crystalline powder. M.p. 212°, with decomposition.
Very soluble in water and ethanol; sparingly soluble in chloroform and ether.
Solutions in water show a blue fluorescence.

Partition Coefficient. Log *P* (octanol/water), 1.9.

Colour Test. Mandelin's Test—orange→green.

Thin-layer Chromatography. System TA—Rf 00; system TB—Rf 46; system TC—Rf 00; system TE—Rf 37; system TL—Rf 00; system TAE—Rf 01; system TAF—Rf 15. (Acidified iodoplatinate solution, positive.)

Gas Chromatography. System GA—RI 1590.

Ultraviolet Spectrum. Aqueous acid—249, 306, 363 nm.

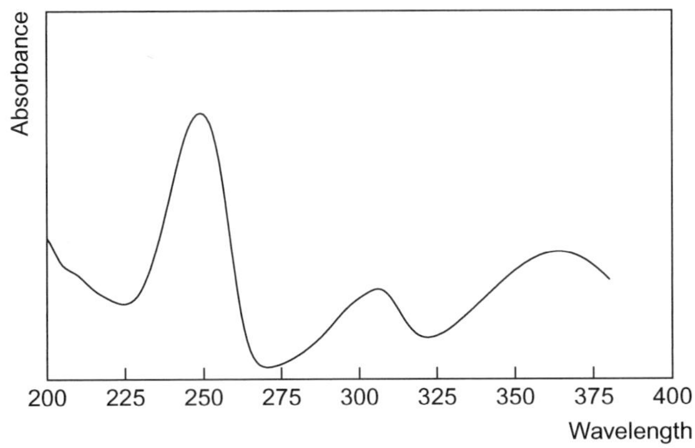

Infra-red Spectrum. Principal peaks at wavenumbers 1235, 1032, 1499, 925, 1075, 934 cm^{-1} (KBr disk).

Dose. Hydrastinine hydrochloride was formerly given in doses of 15 to 60 mg as a cardiotonic.

Hydrochlorothiazide

Diuretic

Synonyms. Chlorosulthiadil; Hidroclorotiazida; Hydrochlorothiazidum.
Proprietary names. Acuretic; Apo-Hydro; Clorana; Dichlotride; Diclotride; Didralin; Di-Ertride; Direma; Disalunil; Disothiazide; Dithiazid; Diuret-P; Diurezin; Drenol; Esidrex; Esidrix; Hidrosaluretil; Hydrex; Hydro-Aquil; HydroDiuril; HydroSaluric; Hydro-Z; Hydrozide; Novo-Hydrazide; Microzide; Mictrin; Oretic; Servithiazid; Thiuretic.
Hydrochlorothiazide is an ingredient of many proprietary preparations—see *Martindale*, *The complete drug reference*, 33rd Edn, London, Pharmaceutical Press, 2002.
6-Chloro-3,4-dihydro-2*H*-1,2,4-benzothiadiazine-7-sulfonamide 1, 1-dioxide
$C_7H_8ClN_3O_4S_2$=297.7
CAS—58-93-5

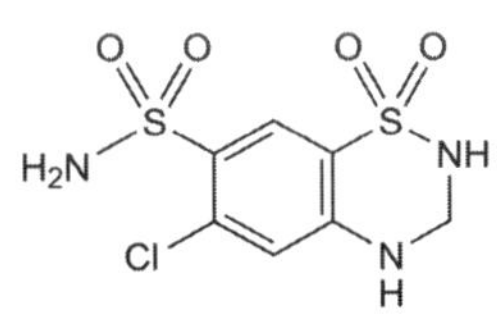

A white crystalline powder. M.p. 273° to 275°.
Practically insoluble in water, chloroform, and ether; soluble 1 in 200 of ethanol and 1 in 20 of acetone; freely soluble in dimethylformamide and solutions of alkali hydroxides.

Dissociation Constant. pK_a 7.0, 9.2.

Partition Coefficient. Log *P* (octanol/water), −0.1.

Colour Tests. Chromotropic Acid—violet, after dilution; Koppanyi-Zwikker Test—violet; Liebermann's Test—blue-green.

Thin-layer Chromatography. System TD—Rf 04; system TE—Rf 34; system TF—Rf 34; system TAD—Rf 11; system TAE—Rf 78; system TAJ—Rf 09; system TAK—Rf 00; system TAL—Rf 40. (Mercuric chloride–diphenylcarbazone reagent, positive.)

Gas Chromatography. System GA—hydrochlorothiazide, not eluted; hydrochlorothiazide-Me_4 RI 2966; art (-SO_2NH)-Me RI 2170; system GX—hydrochlorothiazide-Me_4 retention time 9.0 min; system GY—hydrochlorothiazide-Me_4 retention time 5.0 min.

High Performance Liquid Chromatography. System HN—*k* 0.70; system HX—RI 294; system HY—RI 255; system HZ—retention time 2.2 min; system HAX—retention time 5.1 min; system HAY—retention time 4.0 min.

Ultraviolet Spectrum. Aqueous acid—272 (A_1^1=644a), 318; aqueous alkali—274 (A_1^1=520a), 324 nm.

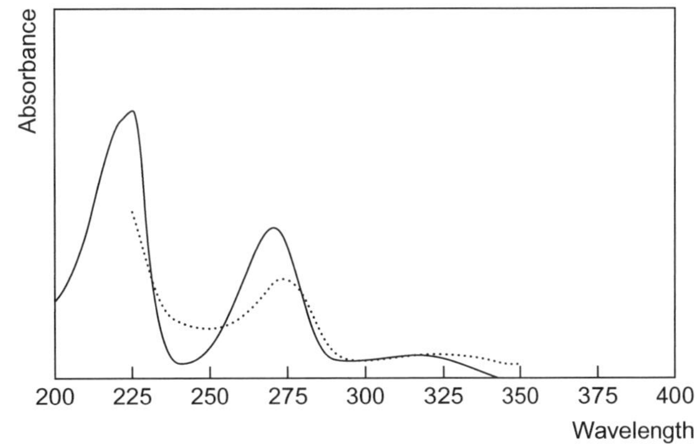

Infra-red Spectrum. Principal peaks at wavenumbers 1318, 1180, 1150, 1168, 1602, 1060 cm^{-1} (KBr disk).

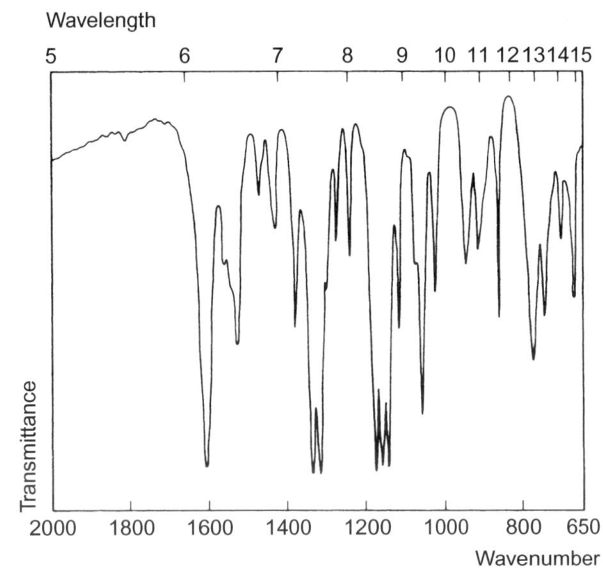

Mass Spectrum. Principal ions at *m/z* 269, 205, 221, 297, 271, 62, 285, 124.

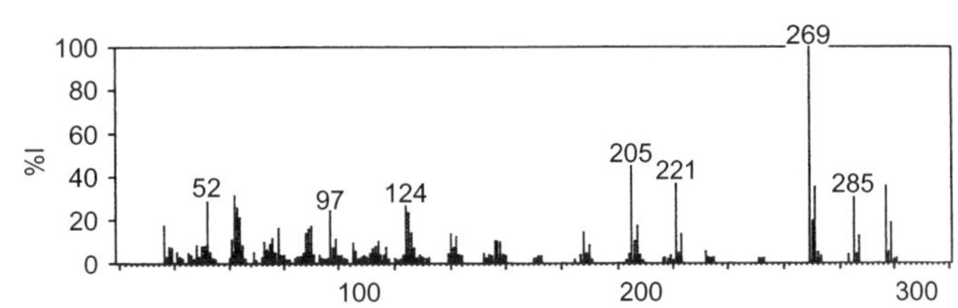

Quantification

Gas chromatography. In blood or plasma: limit of detection 5 µg/L, ECD—E. Redalieu *et al.*, *J. Pharm. Sci.*, 1978, *67*, 726–728. In plasma, erythrocytes, or urine: limit of detection 10 µg/L in plasma, ECD and FID—B. Lindström *et al.*, *J. Chromatogr.*, 1975, *114*, 459–462.

Gas chromatography–mass spectrometry. In urine: hydrochlorothiazide and other diuretics—D. Carreras *et al.*, *J. Chromatogr. A*, 1994, *683*, 195–202.

High performance liquid chromatography. In plasma or urine: hydrochlorothiazide and chlorothiazide, limits of detection 10 µg/L in plasma and 2 mg/L in urine, UV detection—R. H. Barbhaiya *et al.*, *J. Pharm. Sci.*, 1981, *70*, 291–295. In plasma—B. S. Kuo *et al.*, *Pharm. Res.*, 1990, *7*, 1257–1261. In plasma or urine: limits of detection 10 µg/L and 200 µg/L respectively—J. X. de Vries and A. Voss, *Biomed. Chromatogr.*, 1993, *7*, 12–14. In serum: limit of detection <5 µg/L, electrochemical detection—K. Richter *et al.*, *J. Chromatogr. A*, 1996, *729*, 293–296. In urine: limit of detection 1 mg/L, UV detection—D. Farthing *et al.*, *J. Pharm. Biomed. Anal.*, 1998, *17*, 1455–1459. In plasma—A. Medvedovici *et al.*, *Eur. J. Metab. Pharmacokinet.*, 2000, *25*, 91–96.

Disposition in the Body. Rapidly but incompletely absorbed after oral administration. More than 95% of an IV dose is excreted unchanged in the urine. About 65% of an oral dose is excreted in the urine unchanged in 24 h. It crosses the placenta and is distributed into breast milk.

Therapeutic concentration

Peak plasma concentrations of 0.18 to 0.43 mg/L (mean 0.26) were attained in 2 to 4 h, following a single oral dose of 50 mg given to 8 subjects. [B. Beerman *et al.*, *Eur. J. Clin. Pharmacol.*, 1977, *12*, 297–303.]

Steady-state plasma concentrations of 0.05 to 0.16 mg/L (mean 0.1) were achieved after daily oral doses of 75 mg to 8 subjects. [B. Beerman and M. Groschinsky-Grind, *Eur. J. Clin. Pharmacol.*, 1978, *13*, 195–201.]

Bioavailability. About 65 to 70%.

Half-life. Plasma half-life, 5 to 15 h.

Volume of distribution. About 0.8 L/kg.

Distribution in blood. Plasma:whole blood ratio, 0.41.

Protein binding. In plasma, about 60%.

Note. For a review of the pharmacokinetics of diuretics, see B. Beerman and M. Groschinsky-Grind, *Clin. Pharmacokinet.*, 1980, *5*, 221–245.

Dose. 25 to 200 mg daily.

Hydrocodone

Narcotic Analgesic/Antitussive

Synonym. Dihydrocodeinone
4,5-Epoxy-3-methoxy-17-methylmorphinan-6-one
$C_{18}H_{21}NO_3 = 299.4$
CAS—125-29-1

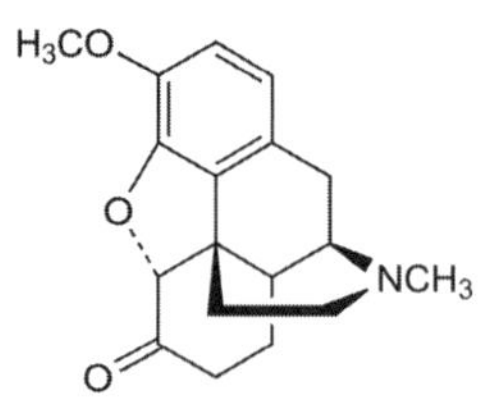

M.p. 198°.
Insoluble in water; soluble in ethanol and dilute acids.

Hydrocodone Hydrochloride

Synonym. Dihydrocodeinone Hydrochloride
Proprietary name. Dicodid (injection)
$C_{18}H_{21}NO_3,HCl,2\frac{1}{2}H_2O = 380.9$
CAS—25968-91-6 (anhydrous)
A white crystalline powder.
Soluble 1 in 2 of water; soluble in ethanol.

Hydrocodone Phosphate

$C_{18}H_{21}NO_3,1\frac{1}{2}H_3PO_4 = 446.4$
CAS—34366-67-1
A white or yellowish-white crystalline powder.
Soluble in water; practically insoluble in ethanol, chloroform, and ether.

Hydrocodone Tartrate

Synonyms. Dihydrocodeinone Acid Tartrate; Hydrocodone Acid Tartrate; Hydrocodone Bitartrate; Hydrocone Bitartrate.
Proprietary names. Biocodone; Dicodid (tablets); Hycodan; Robidone. It is an ingredient of many preparations, see *Martindale, The complete drug reference* 3rd Edn, London, Pharmaceutical Press, 2002.
$C_{18}H_{21}NO_3,C_4H_6O_6,2\frac{1}{2}H_2O = 494.5$
CAS—143-71-5 (anhydrous); 34195-34-1 (hemipentahydrate).
White crystals or crystalline powder. M.p. 118° to 128°.
Soluble 1 in 16 of water and 1 in 150 of ethanol; practically insoluble in chloroform and ether.

Dissociation Constant. pK_a 8.3 (20°).

Partition Coefficient. Log *P* (octanol/water), 2.2.

Colour Test. Marquis Test—yellow→brown→violet.

Thin-layer Chromatography. System TA—Rf 25; system TB—Rf 04; system TC—Rf 20; system TE—Rf 33; system TL—Rf 04; system TAE—Rf 11; system TAF—Rf 13; system TAJ—Rf 09; system TAK—Rf 03; system TAL—Rf 54. (Dragendorff spray, positive; acidified iodoplatinate solution, positive; Marquis reagent, violet.)

Gas Chromatography. System GA—hydrocodone RI 2440, M (dihydromorphine) RI 2400, M (nor-)-AC RI 2760, M (nor-dihydro-)-AC RI 2700; system GB—hydrocodone RI 2580, hydrocodone-TMS RI 2674, M (nor-) RI 2599; system GC—RI 3028; system GF—RI 2930.

High Performance Liquid Chromatography. System HA—*k* 7.1 (tailing peak); system HC—*k* 2.17; system HX—RI 286; system HY—RI 231; system HAX—retention time 6.9 min; system HAY—retention time 3.7 min.

Ultraviolet Spectrum. Aqueous acid—280 nm ($A_1^1 = 41a$). No alkaline shift.

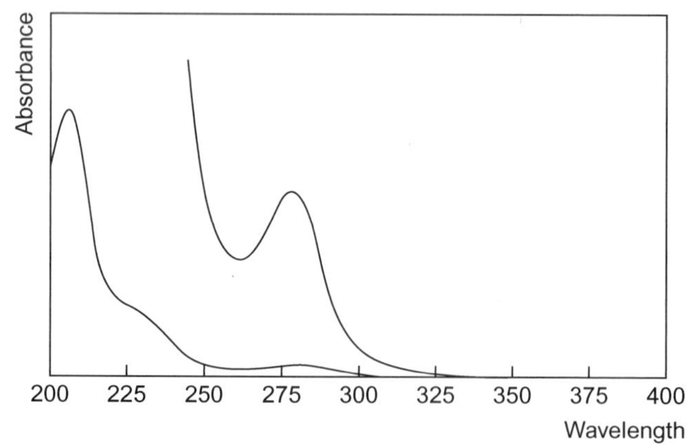

Infra-red Spectrum. Principal peaks at wavenumbers 1720, 1270, 1500, 959, 1055, 800 cm^{-1} (KBr disk).

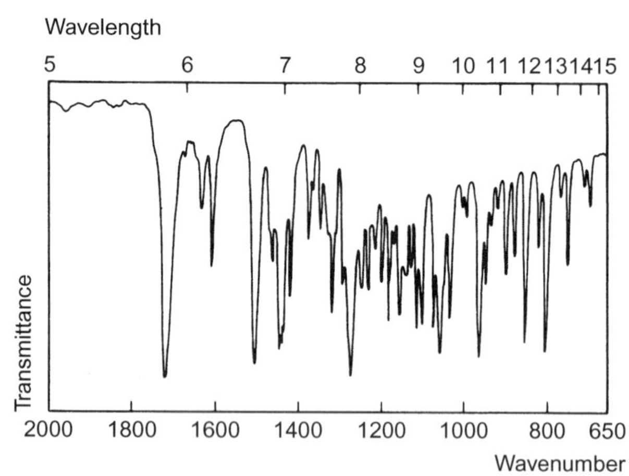

Mass Spectrum. Principal ions at *m/z* 299, 242, 59, 243, 42, 96, 70, 214.

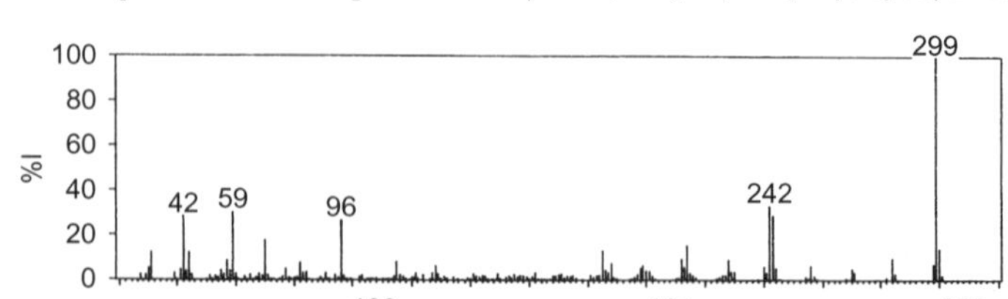

Quantification

Gas chromatography. In serum: limit of detection 1 µg/L, ECD—J. W. Barnhart and W. J. Caldwell, *J. Chromatogr.*, 1977, *130*, 243–249. In postmortem blood: limit of detection 100 µg/L, AFID—G. Cimbura and E. Koves, *J. Anal. Toxicol.*, 1981, *5*, 296–299.

Gas chromatography–mass spectrometry. In urine: hydrocodone and metabolites, limit of detection 10 µg/L—E. J. Cone and W. D. Darwin, *Biomed. Mass Spectrom.*, 1978, *5*, 291–295. In urine: hydrocodone and other opioids—L. A. Broussard *et al.*, *Clin. Chem.*, 1997, *43*, 1029–1032; R. Meatherall, *J. Anal. Toxicol.*, 1999, *23*, 177–186. In blood or urine: hydrocodone and hydromorphone—M. Balikova *et al.*, *Soud. Lek.*, 2000, *45*, 11–16. In hair or oral fluids: hydrocodone and other opioids—J. Jones *et al.*, *J. Anal. Toxicol.*, 2002, *26*, 171–175. In urine: hydrocodone and other opioids limit of quantification 25 µg/L—R. Meatherall, *J. Anal. Toxicol.*, 1999, *23*, 177–186.

Radioimmunoassay. In plasma: limit of detection 10 µg/L—I. L. Honigberg and J. T. Stewart, *J. Pharm. Sci.*, 1980, *69*, 1171–1173.

Disposition in the Body. Absorbed after oral administration. Metabolised by demethylation and reduction of the 6-keto group. About 26% of a dose is excreted in the urine in 72 h, with 12% of the dose as unchanged drug, 5% as norhydrocodone, 4% as conjugated hydromorphone, 3% as 6-hydrocodol, and 0.1% as conjugated 6-hydromorphol. Hydrocodol and hydromorphol exist as stereoisomers. The unconjugated metabolites are thought to be active.
Hydrocodone is a metabolite of codeine.

Therapeutic concentration

After a single oral dose of 10 mg of hydrocodone tartrate to 5 subjects, peak serum concentrations of 0.018 to 0.032 mg/L (mean 0.023) were attained in 1.5 h. [J. W. Barnhart and W. J. Caldwell, *J. Chromatogr.* 1977, *130*, 243–249.]

Toxicity. The estimated lethal dose is 200 mg. Fatalities have occurred at blood concentrations greater than 0.1 mg/L.

In 2 fatalities due to the ingestion of hydrocodone and phenyltoloxamine, the following postmortem concentrations were reported: blood, hydrocodone 0.3 mg/L (both cases), bile, hydrocodone 14.3, - mg/L, hydromorphone 98, 48 mg/L; in the first case phenyltoloxamine was present in bile at a concentration of 0.4 mg/L. [J. I. Park *et al.*, *J. Forensic Sci.*, 1982, *27*, 223–224.]

Half-life. Plasma half-life, about 4 h.

Dose. 5 to 10 mg of hydrocodone tartrate by mouth every 4 to 6 h.

Hydrocortisone

Corticosteroid

Synonyms. Compound F; Cortisol; 17-Hydroxycorticosterone.
Note. Cortisol is also used as a proprietary name for cortisone acetate.
Proprietary names. Hydrocortisone and its esters are ingredients of many proprietary preparations—see *Martindale, The complete drug reference*, 33rd Edn., Pharmaceutical Press, London, 2002.
(11*β*)-11,17,21-Trihydroxypregn-4-ene-3,20-dione
$C_{21}H_{30}O_5$=362.5
CAS—50-23-7

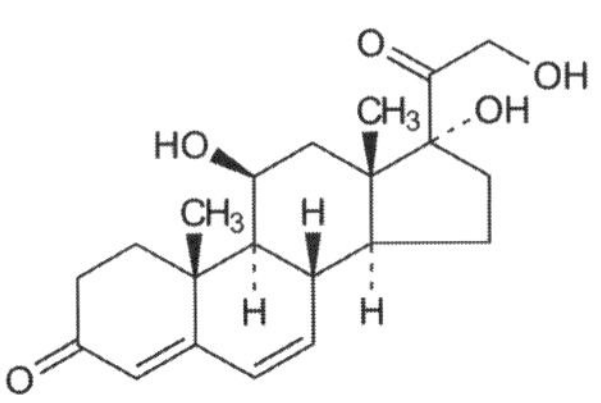

A white crystalline powder. M.p. about 214°, with decomposition. A solution in dioxan is dextrorotatory.
Practically insoluble in water and ether; soluble 1 in 40 of ethanol; slightly soluble in chloroform; very soluble in dioxan.

Hydrocortisone Acetate

Synonym. Hydrocortisone 21-Acetate
$C_{23}H_{32}O_6$=404.5
CAS—50-03-3
A white crystalline powder. M.p. about 220°, with decomposition.
Practically insoluble in water and ether; soluble 1 in 230 of ethanol; slightly soluble in chloroform; soluble in dioxane.

Hydrocortisone Butyrate

Synonym. Hydrocortisone 17-Butyrate
$C_{25}H_{36}O_6$=432.6
CAS—13609-67-1

Hydrocortisone Cipionate

Synonyms. Hydrocortisone Cypionate; Hydrocortisone Cyclopentylpropionate.
$C_{29}H_{42}O_6$=486.6
CAS—508-99-6
A white crystalline powder.
Practically insoluble in water; soluble in ethanol; very soluble in chloroform; slightly soluble in ether.

Hydrocortisone Hydrogen Succinate

Synonyms. Cortisol Hemisuccinate; Hydrocortisone Hemisuccinate.
$C_{25}H_{34}O_8$=462.5
CAS—2203-97-6
A white crystalline powder. M.p. 170° to 173° or 210° to 214°.
Practically insoluble in water; soluble 1 in 40 of ethanol and 1 in 7 of dehydrated alcohol.

Hydrocortisone Sodium Phosphate

$C_{21}H_{29}Na_2O_8P$=486.4
CAS—6000-74-4
A white or light yellow hygroscopic powder.
Soluble 1 in 4 of water; slightly soluble in ethanol; practically insoluble in chloroform and ether.

Hydrocortisone Sodium Succinate

Synonym. Hydrocortisone 21-Sodium Succinate
$C_{25}H_{35}NaO_8$=484.5
CAS—125-04-2
A white, hygroscopic, crystalline powder or amorphous solid. M.p. 169.0° to 171.2°.
Soluble 1 in 3 of water and 1 in 34 of ethanol; practically insoluble in chloroform and ether. It is unstable in aqueous solution.

Hydrocortisone Valerate

Synonym. Hydrocortisone 17-Valerate
$C_{26}H_{38}O_6$=446.6
CAS—57524-89-7

Dissociation Constant. Hydrocortisone sodium succinate, pK_a 5.1.

Partition Coefficient. Log *P* (octanol/water), 1.6.

Colour Tests. Antimony Pentachloride—orange; Naphthol–Sulfuric Acid—yellow-brown/yellow-brown; Sulfuric Acid—green, orange dichroism (green fluorescence under ultraviolet light).

Thin-layer Chromatography. Hydrocortisone: system TA—Rf 96; system TB—Rf 00; system TE—Rf 45; system TF—Rf 28; system TP—Rf 27; system TQ—Rf 02; system TR—Rf 08; system TS—Rf 00; system TAE—Rf 86; system TAJ—Rf 36; system TAK—Rf 05; system TAL—Rf 74; system TAM—Rf 58. Hydrocortisone acetate: system TP—Rf 51; system TQ—Rf 11; system TR—Rf 38; system TS—Rf 00. Hydrocortisone hydrogen succinate: system TP—Rf 08; system TQ—Rf 00; system TR—Rf 00; system TS—Rf 00. Hydrocortisone sodium phosphate: system TP—Rf 00; system TQ—Rf 00; system TR—Rf 00; system TS—Rf 00. (DPST solution.)

Gas Chromatography. System GA—RI 2740

High Performance Liquid Chromatography. System HT—*k* 5.8; system HX—RI 403; system HY—RI 349; system HAA—retention time 17.7 min.

Ultraviolet Spectrum. Ethanol—240 nm (A^1_1=435a).

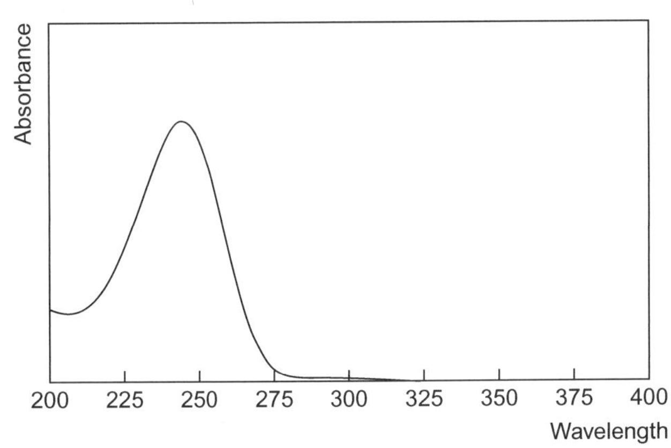

Infra-red Spectrum. Principal peaks at wavenumbers 1640, 1702, 1610, 1232, 1042, 1115 cm^{-1} (KBr disk).

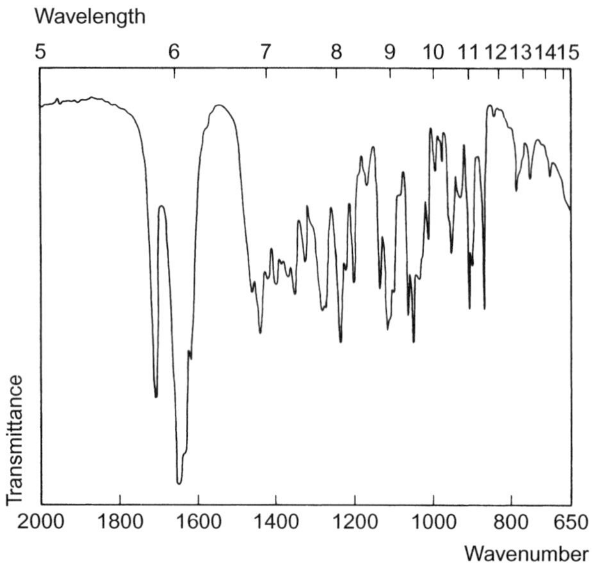

Quantification

High performance liquid chromatography. In plasma: limit of detection 5 µg/L, UV detection—R. D. Toothaker *et al.*, *J. Pharm. Sci.*, 1982, *71*, 573–576. In plasma: hydrocortisone and hydrocortisone succinate, limits of detection 0.2 mg/L and 0.5 mg/L, respectively, UV detection—E. Iwasaki, *Clin. Chem.*, 1987, *33*, 1412–1415. In plasma: limit of detection 300 ng/L, UV detection—M. Hariharan *et al.*, *Clin. Chem.*, 1992, *38*, 346–352. In plasma: hydrocortisone, prednisone and prednisolone, limit of detection <5 µg/L, UV detection—W. J. Jusko *et al.*, *J. Chromatogr.* 1994, *658 B Biomed Appl.*, 47–54. In plasma or urine: hydrocortisone and other glucocorticoids, limit of detection for hydrocortisone 0.1 µg/L, fluorescence—N. Shibata *et al.*, *J. Chromatogr. B. Biomed. Sci. Appl.*, 1998, *706*, 191–199.

Disposition in the Body. Hydrocortisone (cortisol) is the main glucocorticoid secreted by the adrenal cortex. It is administered parenterally as the sodium phosphate or sodium succinate ester in emergencies. Hydrocortisone is readily absorbed after oral administration and through the skin; hydrocortisone acetate is less well absorbed. It is metabolised in the liver and other tissues by reduction, hydroxylation, side-chain cleavage, and conjugation with glucuronic acid. About 90% of a dose is excreted in the urine in 24 h; less than 1% is excreted unchanged, 40% is the 5α- and 5β-forms of tetrahydrocortisol and the 5β-form of tetrahydrocortisone, 17% is a mixture of the 5α- and 5β- and 20α- and 20β-cortols and cortolones, and 6% is 11-hydroxy- and 11-keto-etiocholanolone; most of the metabolites are excreted as glucuronide conjugates; at plasma concentrations of greater than 0.2 mg/L, the amount of unchanged hydrocortisone excreted in the urine is increased.

Blood concentration. Endogenous hydrocortisone exhibits a diurnal variation in plasma concentrations; in the morning, concentrations are in the approximate range 0.08 to 0.20 mg/L and, in the evening, in the range 0.04 to 0.10 mg/L.

Following a single intravenous injection of 40 mg to 6 subjects, a mean plasma concentration of 1.85 mg/L was reported at 10 min. [R. D. Toothaker and P. G. Welling, *J. Pharmacokinet. Biopharm.*, 1982, *10*, 147–156.]

Half-life. Plasma half-life, about 1.5 h.

Volume of distribution. About 0.3 L/kg.

Protein binding. In plasma, more than 90%.

Dose. 10 to 30 mg daily, by mouth. In the treatment of certain medical emergencies, the equivalent of 100 to 500 mg of hydrocortisone by intravenous injection, 3 or 4 times daily.

Hydroflumethiazide

Diuretic

Synonym. Trifluoromethylhydrothiazide
Proprietary names. Diucardin; Elodrine; Finuret; Hydol; Hydrenox; Leodrine; Rodiuran; Rontyl; Saluron; Sisuril. It is an ingredient of Aldactide, Protensin-M, Rautrax, Salutensin, and Spio-Co.
3,4-Dihydro-6-(trifluoromethyl)-2*H*-1,2,4-benzothiadiazine-7-sulfonamide 1,1-dioxide
$C_8H_8F_3N_3O_4S_2 = 331.3$
CAS—135-09-1

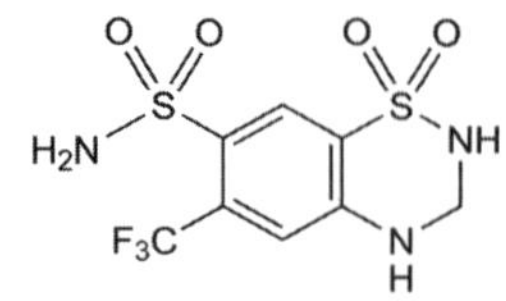

White or cream-coloured glistening crystals or crystalline powder. M.p. 272° to 273°.
Soluble 1 in 3000 of water, 1 in about 50 of ethanol, and 1 in 4 of acetone; practically insoluble in chloroform and ether.

Dissociation Constant. pK_a 8.5, 10.0 (20°).

Partition Coefficient. Log *P* (octanol/water), 0.4.

Colour Tests. Chromotropic Acid—violet, after dilution; Koppanyi–Zwikker Test—violet; Liebermann's Test—blue-green.

Thin-layer Chromatography. System TA—Rf 86; system TD—Rf 07; system TE—Rf 36; system TF—Rf 47; system TAD—Rf 13; system TAE—Rf 87; system TAJ—Rf 09; system TAK—Rf 00; system TAL—Rf 43. (Location under ultraviolet light, violet fluorescence; acidified potassium permanganate solution, faint reaction.)

Gas Chromatography. System GA—hydroflumethiazide, not eluted; hydroflumethiazide-Me_4 RI 2653; system GX—hydroflumethiazide-Me_4 retention time 6.3 min; hydroflumethiazide-Me_4 retention time 4.4 min.

High Performance Liquid Chromatography. System HN—*k* 1.30.

Ultraviolet Spectrum. Aqueous acid—273 nm (A_1^1=578a), 325 nm; aqueous alkali—274, 333 nm.

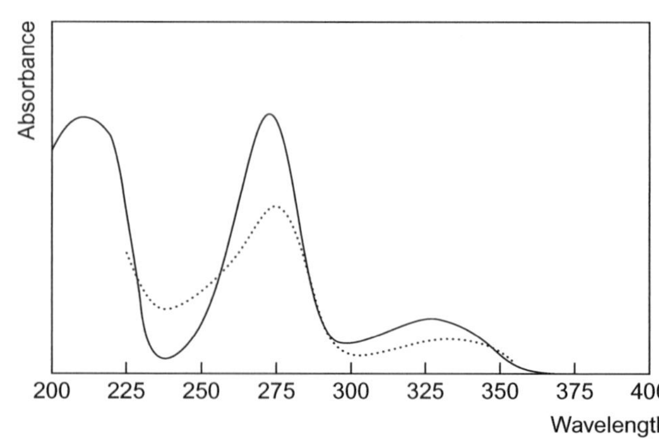

Infra-red Spectrum. Principal peaks at wavenumbers 1151, 1180, 1125, 1052, 1300, 1525 (KBr disk).

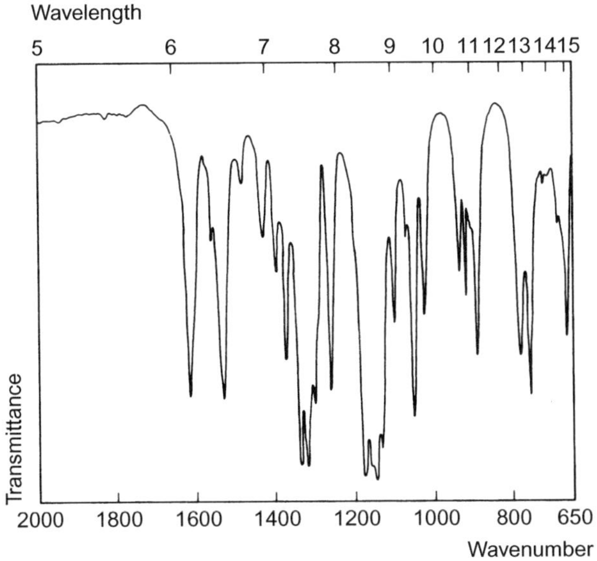

Mass Spectrum. Principal ions at m/z 303, 331, 239, 255, 30, 158, 64, 159.

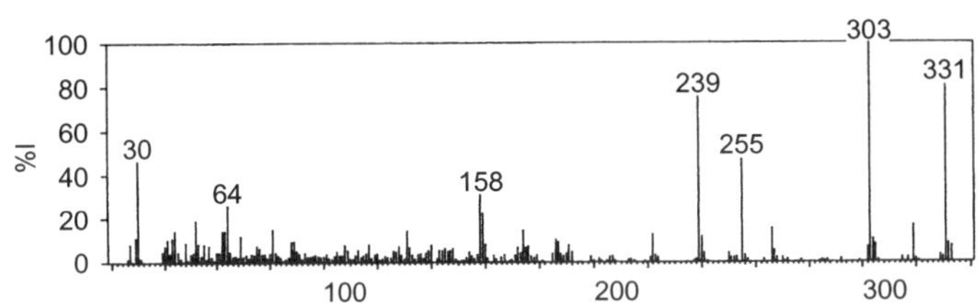

Quantification

Spectrofluorimetry. In plasma or urine: limit of detection 10 μg/L in plasma and 100 μg/L in urine—O. Brørs *et al.*, *Eur. J. Clin. Pharmacol.*, 1977, *11*, 149–154.

Thin-layer chromatography—spectrofluorimetry. In plasma or urine: limit of detection 10 μg/L in plasma and 500 μg/L in urine—Y. Garceau *et al.*, *J. Pharm. Sci.*, 1974, *63*, 1793–1795.

Disposition in the Body. Incompletely but fairly rapidly absorbed after oral administration. During daily dosing, 50 to 70% of a dose is excreted in the 24-h urine as unchanged drug and about 2% as 2,4-disulfamyl-5-trifluoromethylaniline (DTA).

Therapeutic concentration

Following single oral doses of 100 mg to 12 subjects, peak plasma concentrations of 0.17 to 0.6 mg/L (mean 0.4) were attained in 2 to 4 h. [G. Yakatan *et al.*, *J. Clin. Pharmacol.*, 1977, *17*, 37–47.]

Half-life. Derived from urinary excretion data, 5 to 18 h (dose-dependent).

Distribution in blood. Plasma:whole blood ratio, about 0.7.

Protein binding. In plasma, about 75%.

Dose. 25 to 200 mg daily.

Hydromorphone

Narcotic Analgesic

Synonyms. Dihydromorphinone; Dimorphone.

4,5-Epoxy-3-hydroxy-17-methylmorphinan-6-one

$C_{17}H_{19}NO_3$=285.3

CAS—466-99-9

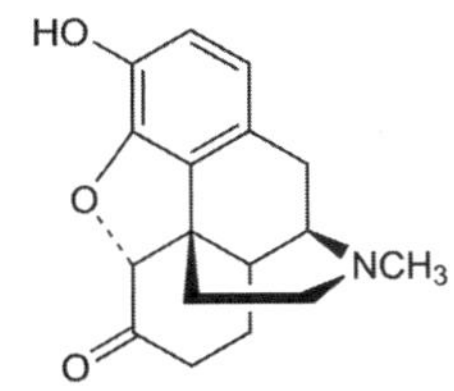

A fine, white, crystalline powder. M.p. 266° to 267° (crystals from ethanol). Slightly soluble in water; freely soluble in ethanol; very soluble in chloroform.

Hydromorphone Hydrochloride

Synonym. Dihydromorphinone Hydrochloride

Proprietary names. Dilaudid; Hydal; Hydromorph; Opidol; Palladon(e); Sophidone.

$C_{17}H_{19}NO_3$,HCl=321.8

CAS—71-68-1

A white crystalline powder, which is affected by light. M.p. 305° to 315°, with decomposition.

Soluble 1 in 3 of water and 1 in 100 of ethanol (90%); practically insoluble in chloroform and ether.

Dissociation Constant. pK_a 8.2 (20°).

Partition Coefficient. Log *P* (heptane/buffer pH 7.4), −4.0.

Colour Tests. Mandelin's Test—violet→orange; Marquis Test—yellow→red→violet.

Thin-layer Chromatography. System TA—Rf 23; system TB—Rf 03; system TC—Rf 09; system TE—Rf 18; system TL—Rf 02; system TAE—Rf 12; system TAF—Rf 14. (Dragendorff spray, positive; acidified iodoplatinate solution, positive; Marquis reagent, violet.)

Gas Chromatography. System GA—hydromorphone RI 2445, hydromorphone-AC RI 2595, hydromorphone-enol-AC_2 RI 2625, hydromorphone-PFP RI 2250, hydromorphone-enol-PFP_2 RI 2320, hydromorphone-enol-TFA_2 RI 2230, M (dihydromorphine) RI 2451; system GB—hydromorphone RI 2598, hydromorphone-TMS RI 2621, hydromorphone-enol-TMS_2 RI 2595, hydromorphone oxime-TMS_2 RI 2678.

High Performance Liquid Chromatography. System HA—*k* 7.9 (tailing peak); system HX—RI 240; system HY—RI 187; system HAX—Retention time 5.8 min; system HAY—Retention time 3.4 min.

Ultraviolet Spectrum. Aqueous acid—280 nm (A^1_1=50a); aqueous alkali—290 nm.

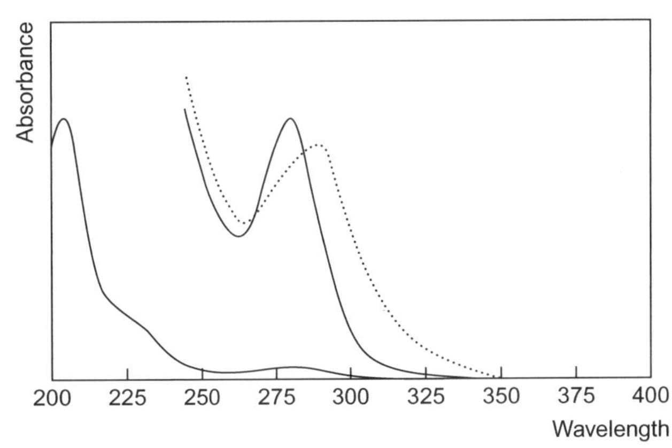

Infra-red Spectrum. Principal peaks at wavenumbers 1727, 1247, 1279, 1034, 757, 1500 cm^{-1} (KBr disk).

Mass Spectrum. Principal ions at m/z 285, 96, 229, 228, 70, 214, 115, 200.

Quantification

Gas chromatography. In urine: hydromorphone and metabolites, FID—E. J. Cone *et al.*, *J. Pharm. Sci.*, 1977, *66*, 1709–1713. In postmortem blood: limit of detection 100 μg/L, AFID—G. Cimbura and E. Koves, *J. Anal. Toxicol.*, 1981, *5*, 296–299.

Gas chromatography–mass spectrometry. In blood, serum or tissue homogenates: limit of detection 80 μg/L—J. J. Saady *et al.*, *J. Anal. Toxicol.*,

1982, *6*, 235–237. In urine: hydromorphone and other opioids—L. A. Broussard *et al.*, *Clin. Chem.*, 1997, *43*, 1029–1032; R. Meatherall, *J. Anal. Toxicol.*, 1999, *23*, 177–186. In blood or urine: hydromorphone and hydrocodone—M. Balikova *et al.*, *Soud. Lek.*, 2000, *45*, 11–16. In hair or oral fluids: hydromorphone and other opioids—J. Jones *et al.*, *J. Anal. Toxicol.*, 2002, *26*, 171–175.

High performance liquid chromatography. In postmortem tissues: hydromorphine, morphine and diamorphine, electrochemical detection—W. R. Sawyer *et al.*, *J. Forensic Sci.*, 1988, *33*, 1146–1155; W. R. Sawyer *et al.*, *J. Forensic Sci.*, 1990, *35*, 520–523. In plasma: hydromorphone and morphine, limit of detection for hydromorphone 2.5 µg/L, electrochemical detection—A. I. Bouquillon *et al.*, *J. Chromatogr.*, 1992, *577*, 354–357.

Radioimmunoassay. In plasma: limit of detection 2.5 µg/L—I. L. Honigberg and J. T. Stewart, *J. Pharm. Sci.*, 1980, *69*, 1171–1173. In plasma: hydromorphone and morphine, limit of detection for hydromorphone >50 ng/L—J. W. Lee *et al.*, *J. Pharm. Sci.*, 1991, *80*, 284–288.

Disposition in the Body. Rapidly but incompletely absorbed after oral administration. About 6% of a dose is excreted in the urine in 24 h as free hydromorphone with about 30% as conjugated hydromorphone and only traces of the active 6α- and 6β-hydroxy metabolites. It crosses the placenta. Hydromorphone is a metabolite of hydrocodone.

Therapeutic concentration

Following a single oral dose of 4 mg to 6 subjects, peak plasma concentrations of 0.018 to 0.027 mg/L (mean 0.022) were attained in about 1 h [J. J. Vallner *et al.*, *J. Clin. Pharmacol.*, 1981, *21*, 152–156].

In 43 patients with chronic severe pain receiving hydromorphone therapy, 7 achieved good pain control with doses of 24 to 96 mg daily (median 48) and had serum levels of ⩾0.004 mg/L [M. M. Reidenberg *et al.*, *Clin. Pharmacol. Ther.*, 1988, *44*, 376–313].

Following a single oral dose of 8, 16 or 32 mg hydromorphone as a sustained-release formulation or 8 mg as an immediate-release formulation to 12 subjects, the plasma concentration peaked later after the sustained-release oral preparation (9 to 13.5 h versus 0.8 to 1.0 h for the 8 mg dose). Peak plasma concentrations were 0.00474 ± 0.00176 mg/L for the 8 mg immediate-release formulation, 0.00077 ± 0.00033 mg/L for the 8 mg sustained-release formulation, 0.00145 ± 0.00043 mg/L for the 16 mg sustained-release formulation and 0.00241 ± 0.00085 mg/L for the 32 mg sustained-release formulation [M. S. Angst *et al.*, *Anesthesiology*, 2001, *94*, 63–73].

Toxicity. The estimated minimum lethal dose is 200 mg. Plasma concentrations greater than 0.1 mg/L may be toxic.

In a fatality attributed to hydromorphone overdose, the following tissue concentrations were reported: blood 1.2 mg/L, brain a trace, kidney 1.2 µg/g, liver 0.4 µg/g, urine 1.1 mg/L; diazepam was also detected [R. C. Baselt, *Bull. Int. Assoc. Forensic Toxicol.*, 1978, *14*(2), 20].

The following postmortem tissue concentrations were reported in a fatality caused by an injected overdose of hydromorphone: blood 0.17 mg/L, bile 8.6 mg/L, kidney 0.13 µg/g, liver 0.07 µg/g [H. C. Walls, *Bull. Int. Assoc. Forensic Toxicol.*, 1976, *12*(3), 7–8].

Bioavailability. About 50% but there is considerable intersubject variation.

Half-life. Plasma half-life, about 2.5 h.

Volume of distribution. About 3 L/kg.

Protein binding. In plasma, about 7%.

Dose. 1.3 to 4 mg of hydromorphone hydrochloride by mouth every 4 to 6 h.

Hydroquinidine

Anti-arrhythmic

Synonyms. Dihydrochinidin; Dihydroquinidine; Hydroconchinine.
(9*S*)-10,11-Dihydro-6′-methoxycinchonan-9-ol
$C_{20}H_{26}N_2O_2$=326.4
CAS—1435-55-8

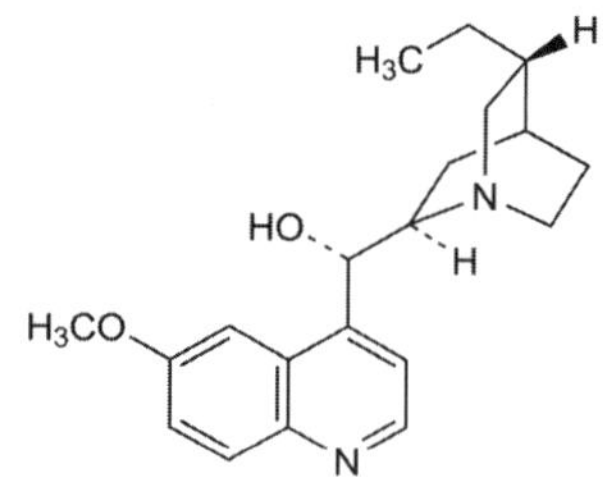

An alkaloid present in the bark of species of *Cinchona* (Rubiaceae).
Crystals. M.p. about 169°.
Slightly soluble in water and ether; readily soluble in hot alcohol.

Hydroquinidine Hydrochloride
Proprietary names. Lentoquine; Serecor.
$C_{20}H_{26}N_2O_2$,HCl=362.9
CAS—1476-98-8
Colourless crystals. M.p. 273° to 274°.
Freely soluble in chloroform and methanol; less readily soluble in water and ethanol.

Partition Coefficient. Log *P* (octanol/water), 3.4.

Colour Tests. Sulfuric Acid—yellow (fluoresces under ultraviolet light); Thalleioquin Test—green

Thin-layer Chromatography. System TA—Rf 45; system TB—Rf 03; system TC—Rf 08; system TE—Rf 43; system TL—Rf 05; system TAE—Rf 20; system TAF—Rf 70. (Acidified iodoplatinate solution, positive.)

Gas Chromatography. System GA—RI 2810.

Ultraviolet Spectrum. Aqueous acid—250 nm (A_1^1=1240b), 316, 345 nm (A_1^1=180b).

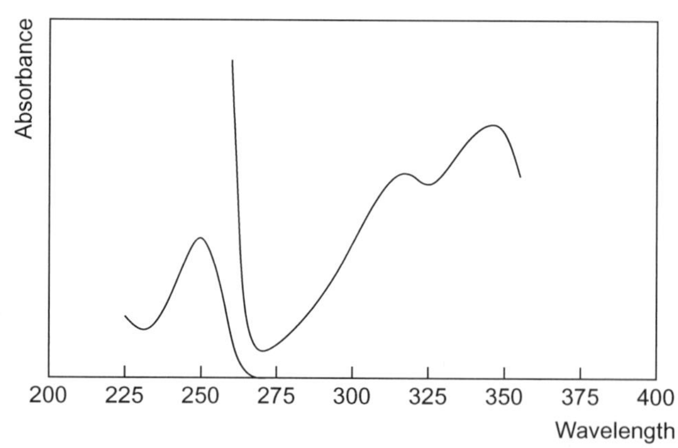

Infra-red Spectrum. Principal peaks at wavenumbers 1509, 1261, 1620, 1234, 854, 1030 cm^{-1}.

Mass Spectrum. Principal ions at *m/z* 138, 326, 55, 110, 189, 82, 160, 139.

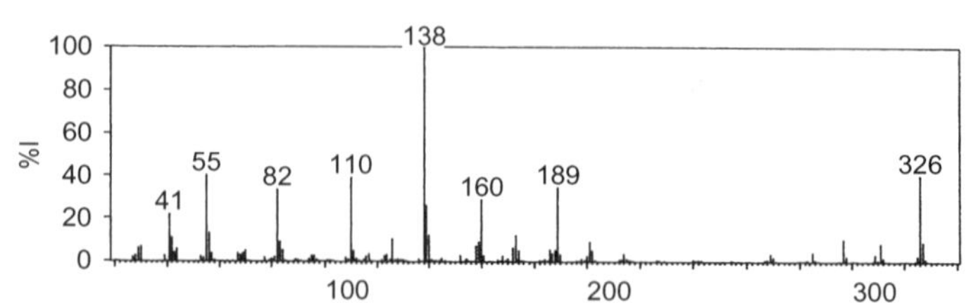

Quantification

High performance liquid chromatography. In serum: limit of detection 0.2 mg/L—R. Camsonne *et al.*, *Ther Drug Monit.*, 1984, *6*, 471–473. In plasma or urine: hydroquinidine, quinidine, hydroxyquinidine, and quinidine *N*-oxide, limits of detection <10 nM (plasma) and <25 nM (urine), fluorescence detection—F. Nielsen *et al.*, *J. Chromatogr.* 1994, *660 B Biomed. Appl.*, 103–110.

Dose. Usually 450 to 600 mg of hydroquinidine hydrochloride daily.

Hydroquinine

Alkaloid

Synonym. Dihydroquinine
(8α,9*R*)-10,11-Dihydro-6′-methoxycinchonan-9-ol
$C_{20}H_{26}N_2O_2$=326.4
CAS—522-66-7

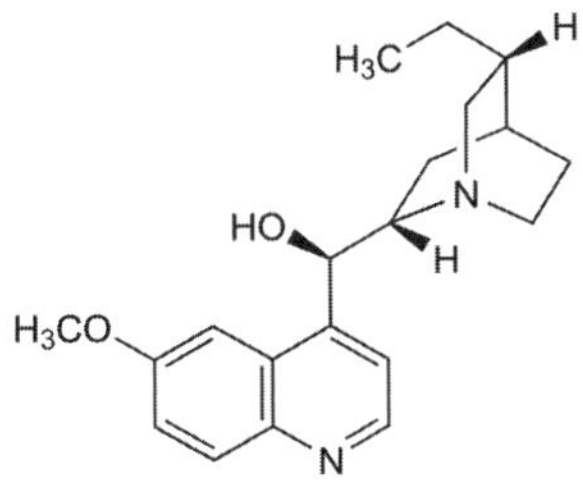

An alkaloid present in the bark of species of *Cinchona* (Rubiaceae). Crystals. M.p. 172°.
Almost insoluble in water; freely soluble in acetone, ethanol, chloroform, ether, and petroleum ether.

Dissociation Constant. pK_a, 5.33.

Partition Coefficient. Log *P* (octanol/water), 3.4.

Colour Tests. Sulfuric Acid—yellow (fluoresces under ultraviolet light); Thalleioquin Test—green

Thin-layer Chromatography. System TA—Rf 44; system TB—Rf 02; system TC—Rf 07; system TE—Rf 40; system TL—Rf 3; system TAE—Rf 21; system TAF—Rf 69. (Acidified iodoplatinate solution, positive.)

Gas Chromatography. System GA—RI 1450.

High Performance Liquid Chromatography. System HZ—retention time 2.8 min.

Ultraviolet Spectrum. Aqueous acid—250 nm (A^1_1=915b), 316, 345 nm (A^1_1=167b).

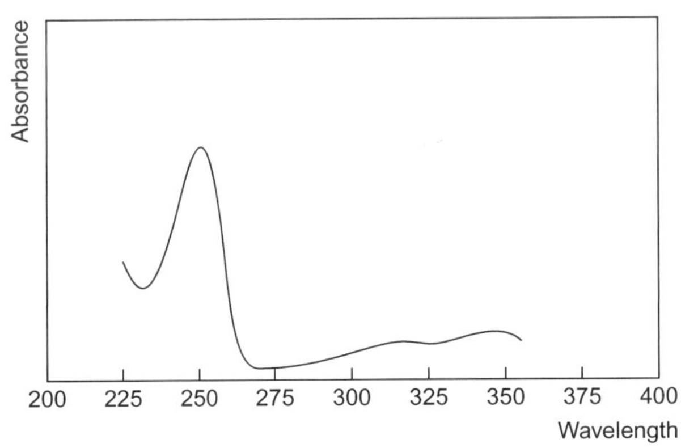

Infra-red Spectrum. Principal peaks at wavenumbers 1240, 1225, 1507, 1623, 1026, 1132 cm^{-1} (KBr disk).

Mass Spectrum. Principal ions at *m/z* 138, 55, 189, 82, 41, 110, 326, 42.

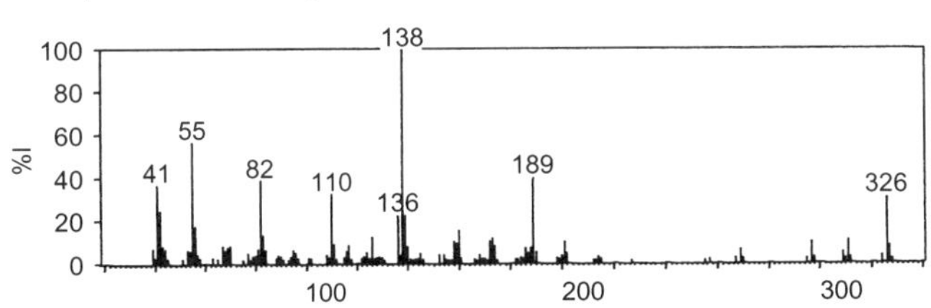

Hydroquinone

Depigmenting Agent/Antioxidant

Synonyms. Hydroquinol; Quinol.
Proprietary names. African Gold; Aida; Banishing Cream; Claripel; Discromil; Eldopaque; Eldoquin; Epocler; Esoteric; Hidroquin; Jouvence; Lustra; Melanex; Melanox; Melpaque HP; Melquin HP; Nadinola; Neostrata AHA; Porcelana; Solaquin; Tecquinol.
1,4-Benzenediol
$C_6H_6O_2$=110.1
CAS—123-31-9

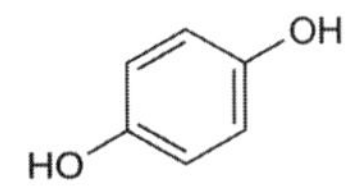

Fine white crystals, or white crystalline powder, which darken on exposure to light and air. M.p. 170° to 171°.
Soluble 1 in 14 of water, 1 in 4 of ethanol, 1 in 51 of chloroform, and 1 in 16 of ether; slightly soluble in benzene.

Dissociation Constant. pK_a 10.9 (25°).

Partition Coefficient. Log *P* (octanol/pH 7.4), 0.6.

Colour Tests. Ammoniacal Silver Nitrate—grey-yellow/brown; Benedict's Reagent—red; Ferric Chloride—green

Gas Chromatography. System GA—hydroquinone RI 1240; M (2-OH-) RI 1460; hydroquinone-AC_2 RI 1395.

Ultraviolet Spectrum. Ethanol—295 nm (A^1_1=282b).

Infra-red Spectrum. Principal peaks at wavenumbers 1210, 1192, 1520, 760, 1240, 813 cm^{-1} (KBr disk).

Quantification

Gas chromatography–mass spectrometry. In urine, liver, or kidney (postmortem)—T. Saito *et al.*, *J. Forensic Sci.*, 1994, *39*, 266–270.

High performance liquid chromatography. In urine: hydroquinone, catechol, and phenol, fluorescence detection—B. L. Lee *et al.*, *J. Chromatogr.*, 1993, *619*, 259–266. In urine: electrochemical detection—J. Wittig *et al.*, *J. Chromatogr. B. Biomed. Sci. Appl.*, 2001, *761*, 125–132.

Disposition in the Body

Toxicity

In a fatality involving the ingestion of photographic developer solution containing hydroquinone, tissue concentrations were: urine 3.4 mg/L, liver 0.5 µg/g, kidney 0.2 µg/g. [T. Saito *et al.*, *J. Forensic Sci.*, 1994, *39*, 266–270.]

Use. As a 2 to 5% ointment for depigmentation of the skin.

Hydroxocobalamin

Haemopoietic Vitamin

Synonyms. Vitamin B_{12a}; Vitamin B_{12b}.
Proprietary names. Alpha Cobione; Alpha Redisol; Alpha-Ruvite; Axlon; Cobalin-H; Codroxomin; Droxomin; Duradoc; Duralta-12; Hydroxo B_{12}; Neo-Betalin 12; Neo-Cytamen; Novobedouze; Redisol H; Rubesol-LA; Sytobex-H.
Coα-[α-(5,6-Dimethylbenzimidazol-1-yl)]-Coβ-hydroxocobamide
$C_{62}H_{89}CoN_{13}O_{15}P$=1346.4
CAS—13422-51-0

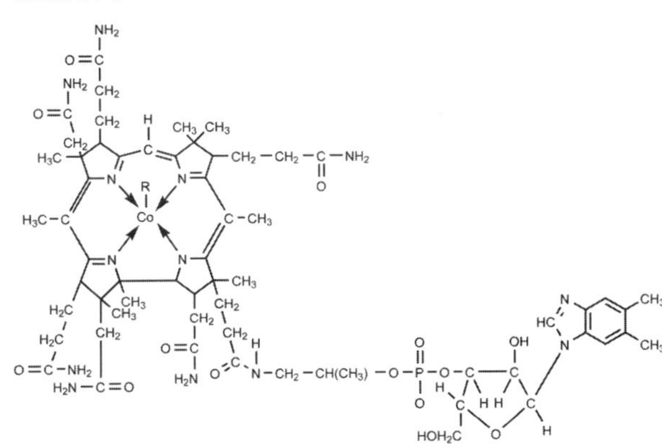

Hydroxocobalamin occurs either as aquocobalamin chloride [α-(5,6-dimethylbenzimidazol-1-yl)aquocobamide chloride], $C_{62}H_{90}ClCoN_{13}O_{15}P$, or as aquocobalamin sulfate, $C_{124}H_{180}Co_2N_{26}O_{34}P_2S$.

Note. In acid solutions, hydroxocobalamin takes up a hydrogen ion which converts the hydroxyl group to a co-ordinated water molecule, and in this form it is known as aquocobalamin, which is basic and forms salts with acids. In solution, aquocobalamin exists in equilibrium with hydroxocobalamin and, since it is more stable in acid solution, it usually occurs commercially in the form of aquocobalamin. [E. L. Smith *et al.*, *Analyst*, 1962, *87*, 183–186.]

Dark red crystals or crystalline powder.

Soluble 1 in 50 of water and 1 in 100 of ethanol; practically insoluble in acetone, benzene, chloroform, ether, and petroleum ether.

Ultraviolet Spectrum. Acetic acid—274, 351 nm.

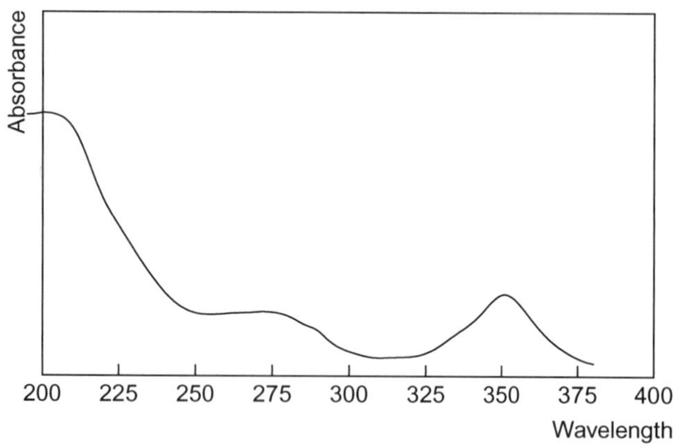

Quantification

High performance liquid chromatography. In plasma: hydroxocobalamin and cyanocobalamin, UV detection—A. Astier and F. J. Baud, *J. Chromatogr. B* 1995, *667*, *Biomed. Appl.*, 129–135.

Dose. Initially 0.25 to 1 mg, by intramuscular injection, daily or on alternate days.

Hydroxyamfetamine

Sympathomimetic

Synonym. Oxamfetamine; Oxamphetamine; PHA.

4-(2-Aminopropyl)phenol

$C_9H_{13}NO$=151.2

CAS—103-86-6; 1518-86-1 (±)

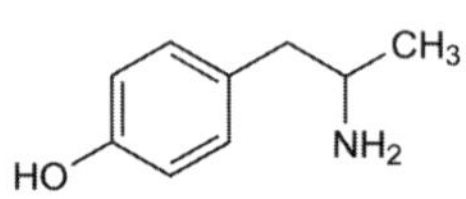

Crystals. M.p. 125° to 126°.

Soluble in water, ethanol, chloroform, and ethyl acetate.

Hydroxyamfetamine Hydrobromide

Proprietary name. Paredrine

$C_9H_{13}NO,HBr$=232.1

CAS—306-21-8; 140-36-3 (±)

A white crystalline powder. M.p. 189° to 192°.

Soluble 1 in 1 of water and 1 in 2.5 of ethanol; freely soluble in acetone; slightly soluble in chloroform; practically insoluble in ether.

Dissociation Constant. pK_a 9.3 (25°).

Partition Coefficient. Log *P* (octanol/water), 1.3.

Thin-layer Chromatography. System TA—Rf 35; system TB—Rf 02; system TC—Rf 02; system TE—Rf 00; system TL—Rf 11; system TAJ—Rf 00; system TAK—Rf 00; system TAL—Rf 19. (Acidified potassium permanganate solution, positive.)

Gas Chromatography. System GA—hydroxyamfetamine RI 1480; M (methoxy-) RI 1465; hydroxyamfetamine-AC RI 1890; hydroxyamfetamine-AC_2 RI 1900.

High Performance Liquid Chromatography. System HB—*k* 2.24; system HC—*k* 1.11; system HY—RI 166.

Ultraviolet Spectrum. Aqueous acid—275 nm (A_1^1=103a); aqueous alkali—238 nm (A_1^1=672b), 294 nm.

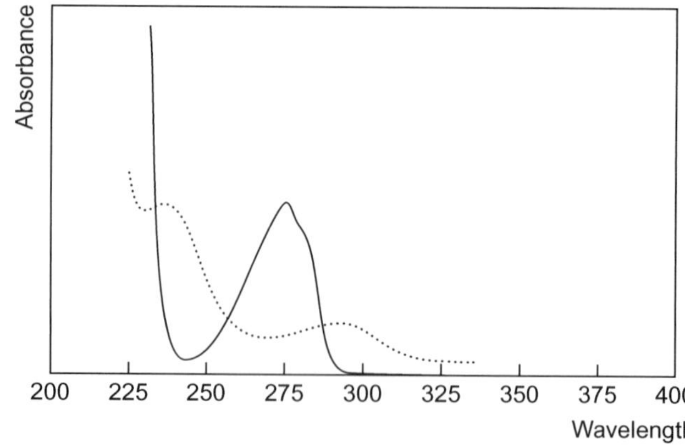

Infra-red Spectrum. Principal peaks at wavenumbers 1259, 1517, 1599, 1102, 813, 1111 cm^{-1} (KBr disk).

Mass Spectrum. Principal ions at *m*/*z* 44, 82, 80, 107, 77, 108, 81, 79.

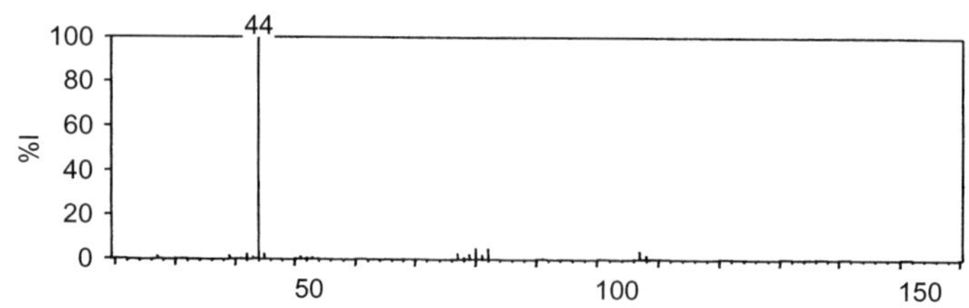

Quantification

Gas chromatography–mass spectrometry. In body fluids: hydroxyamfetamine and metamfetamine—K. Hara *et al.*, *Z. Rechtsmed.*, 1988, *100*, 231–236.

High performance liquid chromatography. In urine: hydroxyamfetamine and hydroxymetamfetamine, limit of detection about 50 pg, electrochemical detection—K. Shimosato *et al.*, *J. Chromatogr.*, 1986, *377*, 279–286; K. Shimosato *et al.*, *Arch. Toxicol.*, 1986, *59*, 135–140.

Disposition in the Body. Readily absorbed after oral administration. About 90% of a dose is excreted in the urine in 24 h as free and conjugated hydroxyamfetamine, with about 4% of the dose as free and conjugated 4′-hydroxynorephedrine.

Toxicity. The estimated minimum lethal dose, intranasally, in children up to 2 years of age is 200 mg, and in adults about 2 g.

Dose. Hydroxyamfetamine hydrobromide has been given in doses of 60 to 240 mg daily.

Hydroxycarbamide

Antineoplastic

Synonym. Hydroxyurea

Proprietary names. Droxia; Hydrea; Litalir; Mylocel; Onco-Carbide; Oxeron; Syrea.

$CH_4N_2O_2$=76.1

CAS—127-07-1

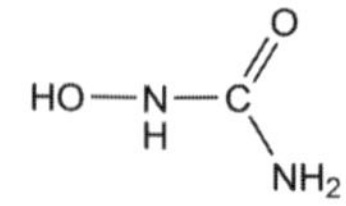

A white crystalline powder. It is hygroscopic and decomposes in the presence of moisture. M.p. above 133°, with decomposition.

Freely soluble in water and hot ethanol; slightly soluble in ethanol.

Partition Coefficient. Log *P* (octanol/water), −1.8.

Ultraviolet Spectrum. No significant absorption, 230 to 360 nm.

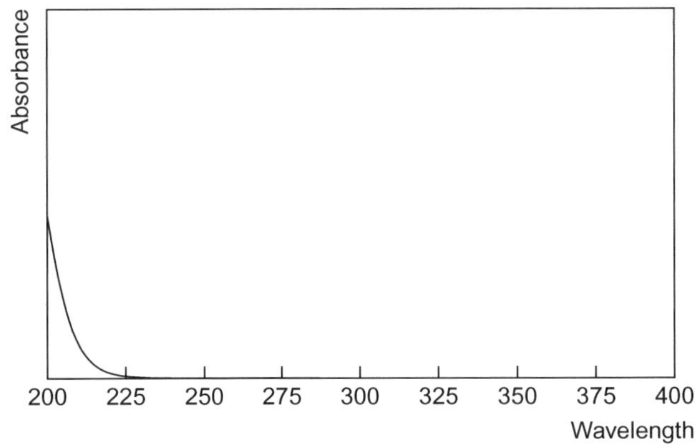

Infra-red Spectrum. Principal peaks at wavenumbers 1639, 1592, 1111, 1492, 812, 758 cm^{-1} (KBr disk).

Quantification

High performance liquid chromatography. In plasma: limit of detection 0.02 mmol/L, electrochemical detection—J. Havard *et al.*, *J. Chromatogr.*, 1992, *584*, 270–274. In serum: UV–Vis detection—K. K. Manouilov *et al.*, *J. Chromatogr. B. Biomed. Sci. Appl.*, 1998, *708*, 321–324. In plasma: UV detection—E. W. Iyamu *et al.*, *J. Chromatogr. B. Biomed. Sci. Appl.*, 1998, *709*, 119–126.

Disposition in the Body

Therapeutic concentration

In 30 subjects, the maximum tolerated dose of intravenous hydroxycarbamide given as a 24-h continuous infusion was 13.52 g/m^2 following a bolus of 1.69 g/m^2 and for a 48-h infusion the maximum tolerated dose was 17.576 g/m^2 following a bolus of 2.197 g/m^2; mean plasma steady-state concentrations were 146.8 mg/L and 108.8 mg/L, respectively. [C. D. Smith *et al.*, *Cancer Chemother. Pharmacol.*, 1993, *33*, 139–143.]

Note. For a review of the pharmacokinetics and pharmacodynamics of hydroxycarbamide, see P. R. Gwilt and W. G. Tracewell, *Clin. Pharmacokinet.*, 1998, *34*, 347–358.

Dose. 20 to 30 mg/kg daily or 80 mg/kg every third day, by mouth.

Hydroxychloroquine

Antimalarial

Synonym. Oxichlorochin

2-[[4-[(7-Chloro-4-quinolinyl)amino]pentyl]ethylamino]ethanol

$C_{18}H_{26}ClN_3O = 335.9$

CAS—118-42-3

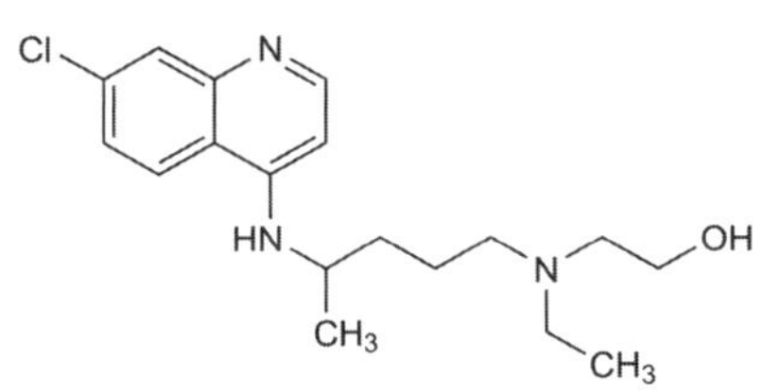

Crystals. M.p. 89° to 91°.

Hydroxychloroquine Sulfate

Proprietary names. Ercoquin; Plaquenil; Quensyl.

$C_{18}H_{26}ClN_3O,H_2SO_4 = 434.0$

CAS—747-36-4

A white crystalline powder. There are 2 forms, one melting at about 198° and the other at about 240°.

Soluble 1 in 5 of water; practically insoluble in ethanol, chloroform, and ether.

Partition Coefficient. Log *P* (octanol/water), 3.0.

Thin-layer Chromatography. System TA—Rf 45; system TB—Rf 02; system TC—Rf 02; system TE—Rf 37; system TL—Rf 03; system TAE—Rf 07; system TAJ—Rf 00; system TAK—Rf 00; system TAL—Rf 04. (Acidified iodoplatinate solution, positive.)

Gas Chromatography. System GA—RI 2872.

High Performance Liquid Chromatography. System HX—RI 280; system HZ—retention time 1.9 min; system HAX—retention time 9.6 min; system HAY—retention time 3.2 min.

Ultraviolet Spectrum. Aqueous acid—235 nm ($A_1^1 = 560a$), 256, 329, 343 nm; aqueous alkali—253, 330 nm.

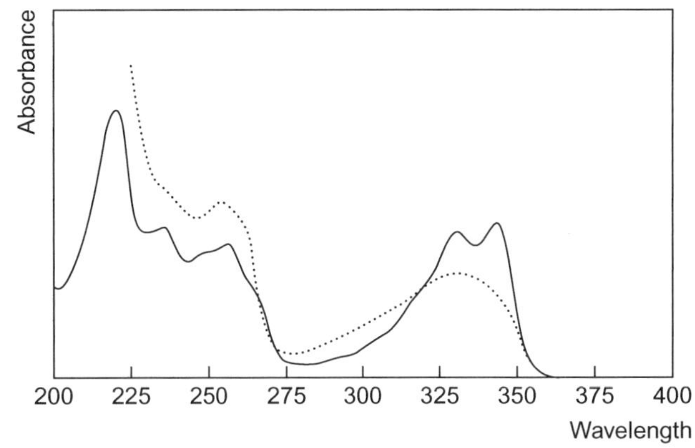

Infra-red Spectrum. Principal peaks at wavenumbers 1579, 1608, 1530, 1050, 1150, 810 cm^{-1} (KBr disk).

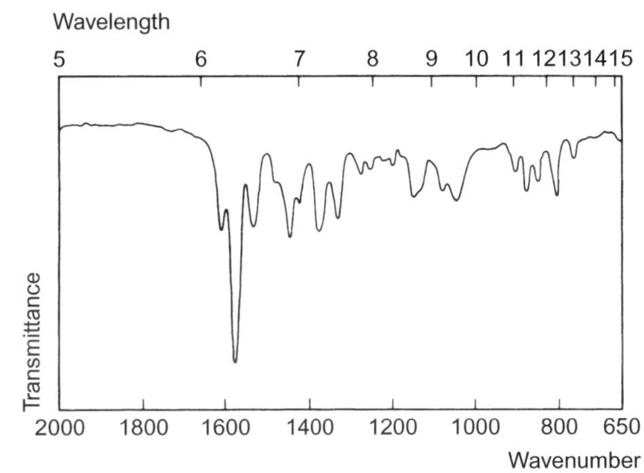

Mass Spectrum. Principal ions at *m/z* 102, 245, 247, 304, 305, 306, 58, 126.

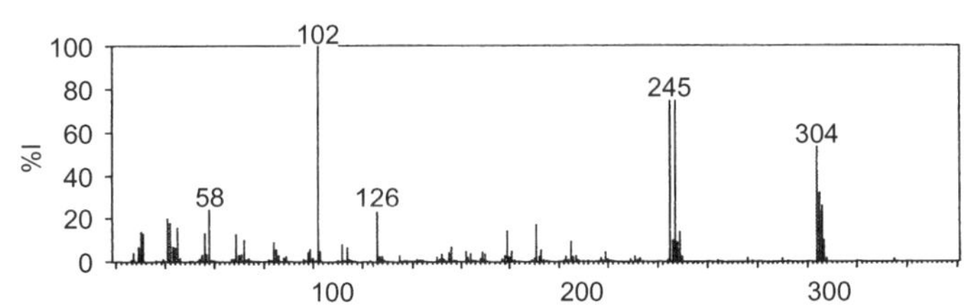

Quantification

High performance liquid chromatography. In blood or plasma: hydroxychloroquine and its major metabolites, limit of detection 1 μg/L, fluorescence detection—S. E. Tett *et al.*, *J. Chromatogr.*, 1985, *344*, 241–248. In blood or urine: hydroxychloroquine and its major metabolites, limit of detection for hydroxychloroquine 10 ppb, fluorescence detection—S. B. Williams *et al.*, *J. Chromatogr.*, 1988, *433*, 197–206. In plasma, serum, whole blood or urine: hydroxychloroquine enantiomers, UV detection—D. R. Brocks *et al.*, *J. Chromatogr.*, 1992, *581*, 83–92. In urine: hydroxychloroquine enantiomers and metabolites—H. Fieger *et al.*, *Chirality*, 1993, *5*, 65–70. In serum, whole blood or dried blood: hydroxychloroquine, chloroquine, quinine, and desethylchloroquine, limit of detection <5 μg/L, fluorescence detection—K. Croes *et al.*, *J. Anal. Toxicol.*, 1994, *18*, 255–260. In serum: hydroxychloroquine, chloroquine, and corticosteroids, diode-array detection—P. Volin, *J. Chromatogr.* 1995, *666 B Biomed. Appl.*, 347–353.

Ultraviolet spectrophotometry. In blood or urine—R. A. Dalley and D. Hainsworth, *J. Forensic Sci. Soc.*, 1965, *5*, 99–101.

Spectrofluorimetry. In plasma—E. W. McChesney *et al.*, *Antibiot. Chemother.*, 1962, *12*, 583–594.

Disposition in the Body. Rapidly and almost completely absorbed after oral administration. It is metabolised by de-ethylation. About 6% of a single dose is excreted in the urine over a period of 10 days and about 25% of a dose is eliminated in the faeces in 3 days as unchanged drug plus the de-ethylated metabolites. During daily therapy, less than 13% of a dose is excreted in the 24-h urine with 8% of the dose as unchanged drug, 2% as desethylchloroquine, 2% as desethylhydroxychloroquine, and 0.5% as didesethylchloroquine.

Therapeutic concentration

After an oral dose of hydroxychloroquine sulfate equivalent to 310 mg of the base to 6 subjects, peak plasma concentrations of 0.003 to 0.20 mg/L (mean 0.08) were attained in 3 h. Following oral administration of hydroxychloroquine diphosphate equivalent to 1264 mg of the base to 3 subjects, peak plasma concentrations of 0.29 to 1.0 mg/L (mean 0.64) were attained in 3 h and therapeutic concentrations greater than 0.01 mg/L were maintained for 240 h. [E. W. McChesney *et al.*, *Antibiot. Chemother.*, 1962, *12*, 583–594.]

In 23 subjects receiving 200 or 400 mg hydroxychloroquine sulfate orally daily, mean steady-state hydroxychloroquine concentrations at 6 months were 450.6 and 870.3 μg/L, respectively. [S. E. Tett *et al*, *J. Rheumatol.*, 2000, *27*, 1656–1660.]

Toxicity

In a fatality due to the ingestion of at least 12 g, the following postmortem tissue concentrations of hydroxychloroquine were reported: blood 48 mg/L, heart blood 61 mg/L, liver 71 μg/g, urine 970 mg/L. [R. A. Dalley and D. Hainsworth, *J. Forensic Sci. Soc.*, 1965, *5*, 99–101.]

Postmortem tissue concentrations in a 2½-year-old boy who died after ingesting an estimated 1800 mg of hydroxychloroquine were: blood 104 mg/L, stomach 1.2 mg in total, small intestine 75 mg in total, liver 500 μg/g. [A. V. Kemmenoe, *J. Anal. Toxicol.*, 1990, *14*, 186–188.]

An 18-year-old girl who survived after ingesting 20 g of hydroxychloroquine had a plasma level of 9.87 mg/L 2 h after ingestion [P. Jordan *et al.*, *J. Toxicol. Clin. Toxicol.*, 1999, *37*, 861–864.]

Half-life. Plasma half-life, about 3 days.

Dose. For an acute attack of malaria, 2 g of hydroxychloroquine sulfate given over 3 days (1.2 g on the first day). In rheumatoid arthritis, initially 400 to 800 mg daily.

Thin-layer Chromatography. System TA—Rf 35, streaking. (Acidified potassium permanganate solution, positive.)

Gas Chromatography. System GA—RI 1682.

High Performance Liquid Chromatography. System HB—*k* 0.73.

Ultraviolet Spectrum. Aqueous acid—273 nm (A^1_1=75b); aqueous alkali—242 nm (A^1_1=760b), 290 nm (A^1_1=131b).

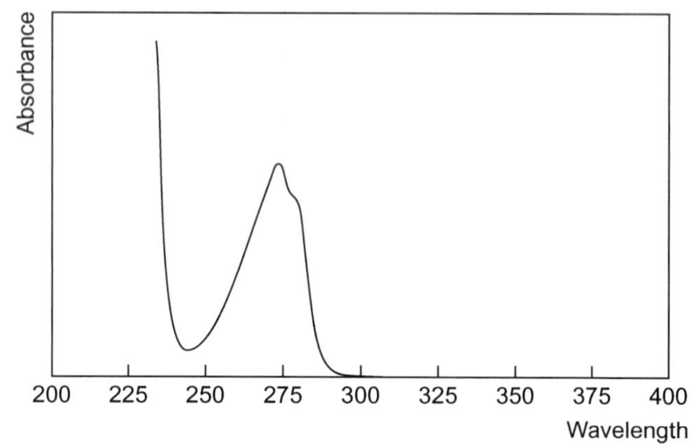

Infra-red Spectrum. Principal peaks at wavenumbers 980, 1238, 835, 1157, 1129, 792 cm^{-1} (KBr disk).

Mass Spectrum. Principal ions at *m/z* 58, 30, 59, 56, 77, –, –, –.

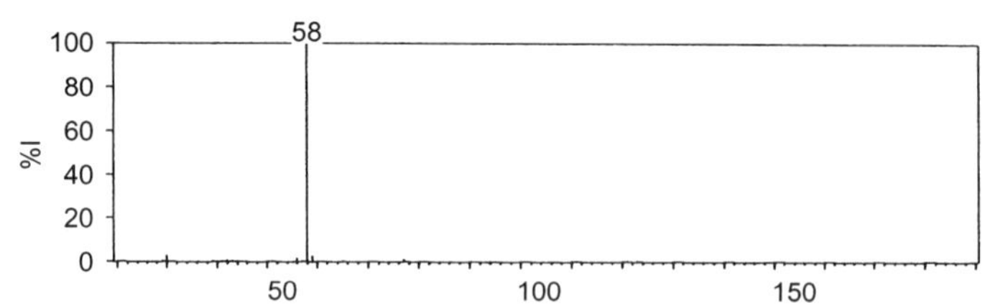

Dose. Hydroxyephedrine hydrochloride has been given in doses of 10 mg daily.

Hydroxyephedrine

Sympathomimetic

Synonyms. *p*-Hydroxyephedrine; Methylsynephrine; Oxyephedrine.
4-Hydroxy-α-[1-(methylamino)ethyl]benzenemethanol
$C_{10}H_{15}NO_2$=181.2
CAS—365-26-4

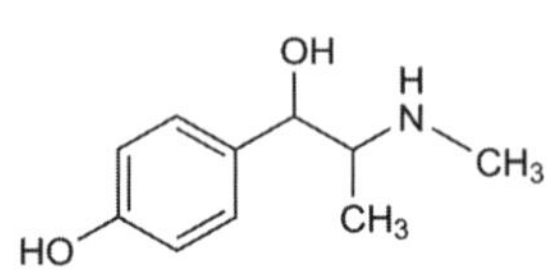

A crystalline powder. M.p. 152° to 154°.
Sparingly soluble in water, ethanol, and ether; readily soluble in dilute acids and sodium hydroxide solution.

Hydroxyephedrine Hydrochloride

Proprietary name. Carnigen
$C_{10}H_{15}NO_2$,HCl=217.7
CAS—942-51-8
A crystalline powder. M.p. 209° to 211°.
Soluble 1 in 3 of water, 1 in 5 of glycerol, and 1 in 10 of ethanol; sparingly soluble in acetone.

Partition Coefficient. Log *P* (octanol/water), 0.2.

Colour Tests. Liebermann's Test—black; Mandelin's Test—green; Marquis Test—yellow

Hydroxyphenamate

Tranquilliser

Synonym. Oxyfenamate
Proprietary name. Listica
2-Phenyl-1,2-butanediol 1-carbamate
$C_{11}H_{15}NO_3$=209.2
CAS—50-19-1

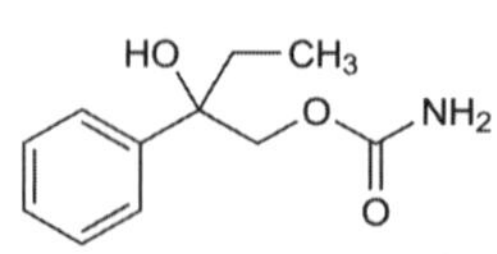

A white crystalline powder. M.p. 55° to 56.5°.
Soluble 1 in 40 of water; soluble in ethanol and chloroform.

Partition Coefficient. Log *P* (octanol/water), 1.1.

Thin-layer Chromatography. System TA—Rf 74. (Van Urk reagent, positive.)

Gas Chromatography. System GA—RI 1724.

Ultraviolet Spectrum. Aqueous acid—251, 257 nm (A^1_1=9.0a), 263 nm.

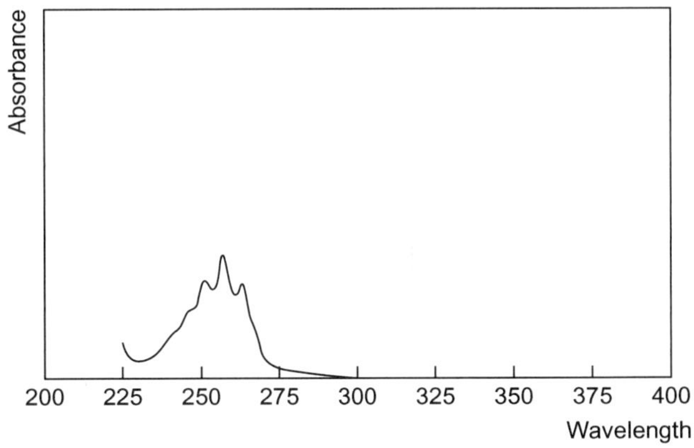

Infra-red Spectrum. Principal peaks at wavenumbers 1715, 1072, 700, 1603, 1110, 760 cm^{-1} (KBr disk).

Mass Spectrum. Principal ions at *m/z* 135, 57, 91, 77, 43, 119, 105, 180.

Dose. Hydroxyphenamate has been given in doses of 600 mg daily.

Hydroxyprogesterone

Progestational Steroid

17-Hydroxypregn-4-ene-3,20-dione
$C_{21}H_{30}O_3$=330.5
CAS—68-96-2

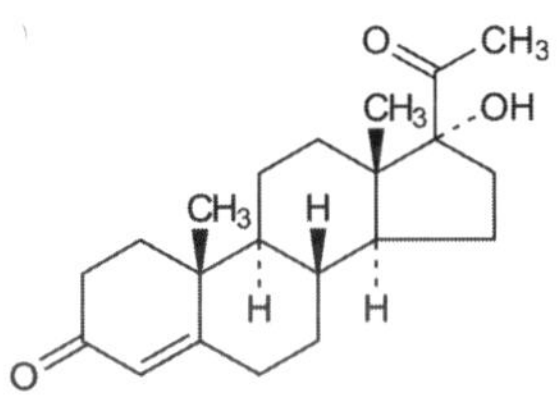

A crystalline powder. M.p. 222° to 223° with rapid heating; with slow heating it undergoes molecular rearrangement accompanied by partial resolidification and melts at 276°.

Hydroxyprogesterone Caproate

Synonyms. 17 AHPC; Hydroxyprogesterone Hexanoate.
Proprietary names. Caposten; Delalutin; Hylutin; Hyprogest; Hyproval PA; Lentogest; Primolut Depot; Proluton Depot; Relutin.
$C_{27}H_{40}O_4$=428.6
CAS—630-56-8
A white or creamy-white crystalline powder. M.p. 120° to 124°.
Practically insoluble in water; soluble 1 in 10 of ethanol, 1 in 0.4 of chloroform, and 1 in 10 of ether.

Partition Coefficient. Log *P* (octanol/water), 3.2.

Colour Tests. Antimony Pentachloride—orange; Naphthol–Sulfuric Acid—orange-red/blue, violet dichroism; Sulfuric Acid—yellow (green fluorescence under ultraviolet light).

Thin-layer Chromatography. Hydroxyprogesterone: system TB—Rf 38; system TE—Rf 85; system TF—Rf 63; system TAE—Rf 86. Hydroxyprogesterone caproate: system TP—Rf 81; system TQ—Rf 55; system TR—Rf 99; system TS—Rf 90. (*p*-Toluenesulfonic acid solution, positive.)

High Performance Liquid Chromatography. Hydroxyprogesterone: system HX—RI 1054.

Ultraviolet Spectrum. Hydroxyprogesterone caproate: dehydrated alcohol—240 nm (A^1_1=395a).

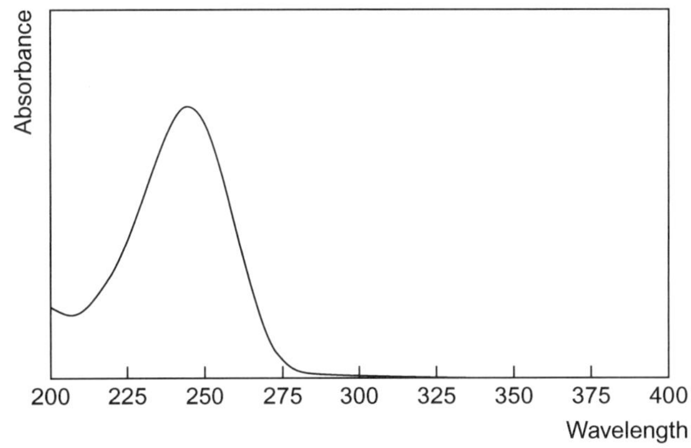

Infra-red Spectrum. Principal peaks at wavenumbers 1728, 1670, 1177, 1188, 1716, 1224 cm^{-1} (hydroxyprogesterone caproate, KBr disk).

Quantification
Gas chromatography–mass spectrometry. In plasma: limit of detection <1 pg—K. Shimizu *et al.*, *J. Chromatogr.*, 1988, *432*, 21–28. In dried blood: limit of detection 20 μg/L—C. C. Lai *et al.*, *J. Clin. Lab. Anal.*, 2002, *16*, 20–25. In plasma: hydroxyprogesterone, 4-androstenedione, and testosterone—S. A. Wudy *et al.*, *Pediatr. Res.*, 1995, *38*, 76–80.

Dose. Usually 250 to 500 mg of hydroxyprogesterone caproate weekly, by intramuscular injection.

Hydroxyquinoline

Antibacterial/Antifungal

Synonyms. Oxine; Oxyquinoline; 8-Quinolinol.
8-Quinolinol
C_9H_7NO=145.2
CAS—148-24-3

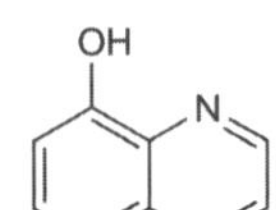

A white or faintly yellow crystalline powder. M.p. 76°.
Soluble 1 in 1500 of water; freely soluble in ethanol, acetone, benzene, aqueous mineral acids, and chloroform; almost insoluble in ether.

Hydroxyquinoline Sulfate

Synonyms. Chinosol; Chinosolum; Oxyquinol; Oxyquinoline Sulfate.
Proprietary name. Sérorhinol
$(C_9H_7NO)_2,H_2SO_4$=388.4
CAS—134-31-6
A light yellow powder. M.p. 175° to 178°.
Soluble 1 in 1 of water, 1 in 100 of ethanol, and 1 in 100 of glycerol; practically insoluble in chloroform and ether.

Potassium Hydroxyquinoline Sulfate

Synonyms. Oxyquinol Potassium; Potassium Oxyquinoline Sulfate.
Proprietary names. It is an ingredient of Auralgicin, Quinocaort, Quinoderm, Quinoped and Valderma.
An equimolecular mixture of potassium sulfate and 8-quinolinol sulfate, containing the equivalent of 50% of 8-quinolinol.
A pale yellow microcrystalline powder. It partly liquefies at 172° to 184°.
Soluble 1 in 2 of water; partly soluble in ethanol; practically insoluble in ether.

Dissociation Constant. pK_a 5.0, 9.9 (20°).

Partition Coefficient. Log *P* (octanol/water), 2.0.

Colour Test. Ferric Chloride—green

Thin-layer Chromatography. System TA—Rf 32, streaking. (Acidified iodoplatinate solution, positive.)

Ultraviolet Spectrum. Aqueous acid—251 nm (A^1_1=3930a), 308 nm (A^1_1=105a), 318, 356 nm.

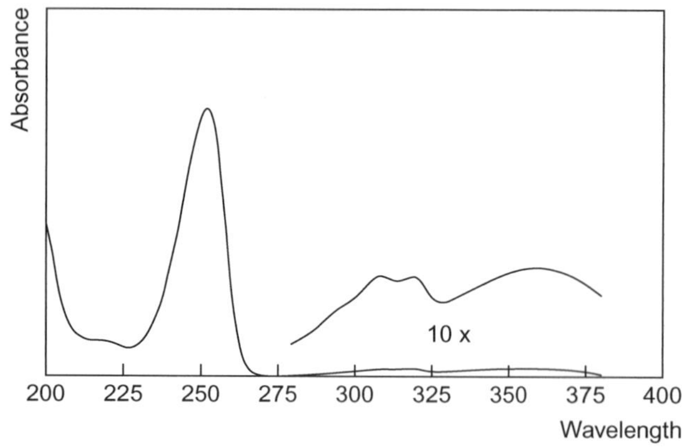

Infra-red Spectrum. Principal peaks at wavenumbers 1509, 779, 709, 1282, 1219, 1190 cm^{-1}.

Mass Spectrum. Principal ions at m/z 145, 117, 122, 89, 105, 90, 63, 146.

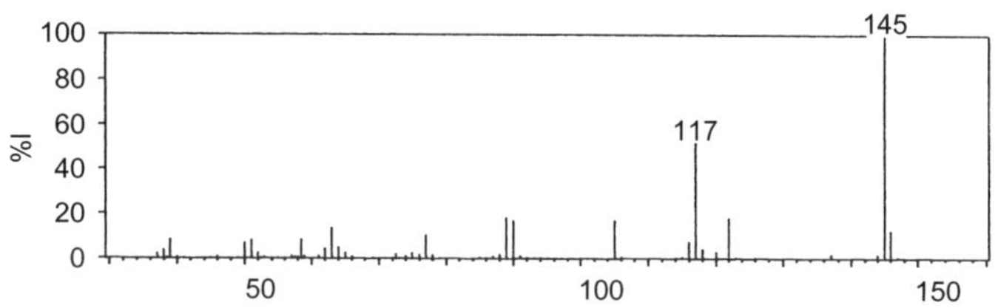

Use. Potassium hydroxyquinoline sulfate is used topically in concentrations of 0.05 to 0.5%.

Hydroxystilbamidine

Antifungal/Antiprotozoal

Synonym. Oxistilbamidine

4-[2-[4-(Aminoiminomethyl)phenyl]ethenyl]-3-hydroxybenzenecarboximidamide

$C_{16}H_{16}N_4O = 280.3$

CAS—495-99-8

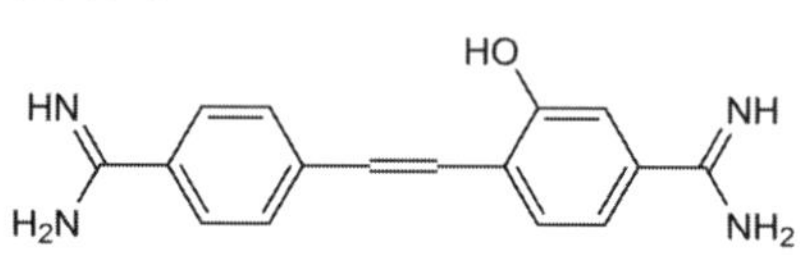

Yellow crystals. M.p. 235°.

Hydroxystilbamidine Isetionate

$C_{16}H_{16}N_4O,2C_2H_6O_4S = 532.6$

CAS—533-22-2

A fine, yellow, crystalline powder, which decomposes on exposure to light. M.p. 286°.

Freely soluble in water; slightly soluble in ethanol; practically insoluble in ether.

Partition Coefficient. Log *P* (octanol/water), 1.6.

Colour Tests. Folin–Ciocalteu Reagent—blue; Liebermann's Test—black; Mandelin's Test—blue-green.

Thin-layer Chromatography. System TA—Rf 01; system TB—Rf 00; system TC—Rf 00; system TL—Rf 00. (Acidified iodoplatinate solution, positive.)

Ultraviolet Spectrum. Aqueous acid—344 nm ($A^1_1 = 1093a$); aqueous alkali—310 nm ($A^1_1 = 811b$).

Infra-red Spectrum. Principal peaks at wavenumbers 1196, 1028, 1667, 1597, 742, 1053 cm^{-1} (hydroxystilbamidine isetionate, KBr disk).

Mass Spectrum. Principal ions at m/z 96, 44, 43, 31, 45, 27, 78, 264.

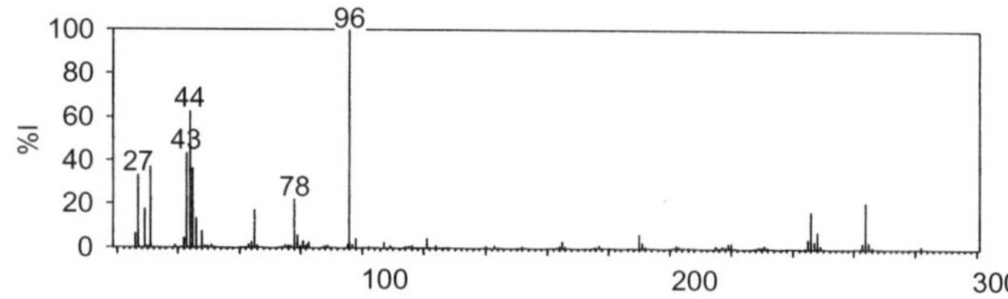

Dose. 225 or 250 mg of hydroxystilbamidine isetionate daily or on alternate days, by intravenous infusion.

Hydroxyzine

Antihistamine/Tranquilliser

2-[2-[4-[(4-Chlorophenyl)phenylmethyl]-1-piperazinyl]ethoxy]ethanol

$C_{21}H_{27}ClN_2O_2 = 374.9$

CAS—68-88-2

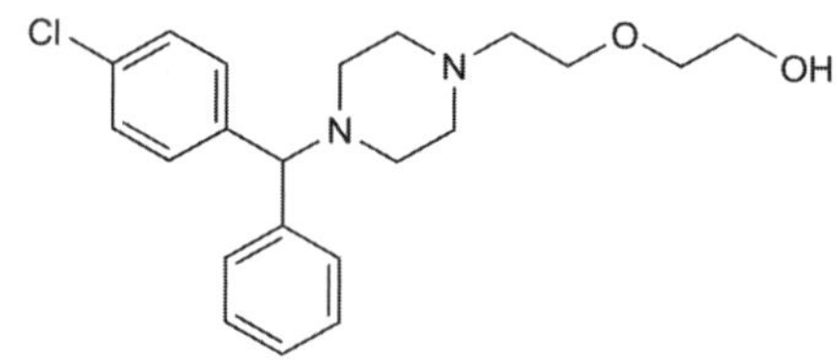

Hydroxyzine Embonate

Synonym. Hydroxyzine Pamoate

Proprietary names. Equipose; Masmoran; Paxistil; Vistaril (capsules and oral suspension).

$C_{21}H_{27}ClN_2O_2,C_{23}H_{16}O_6 = 763.3$

CAS—10246-75-0

A pale yellow powder.

Practically insoluble in water, chloroform, ether, and methanol; soluble 1 in 700 of ethanol and 1 in 10 of dimethylformamide.

Hydroxyzine Hydrochloride

Proprietary names. Alamon; Atarax; Atazina; Aterax; Durrax; Orgatrax; Quiess; Sedaril; Vistaril (injection).

$C_{21}H_{27}ClN_2O_2,2HCl = 447.8$

CAS—2192-20-3

A white crystalline powder. M.p. 193°.

Soluble 1 in 1 of water, 1 in 4.5 of ethanol, and 1 in 13 of chloroform; practically insoluble in ether.

Dissociation Constant. pK_a 2.1, 7.1.

Partition Coefficient. Log *P* (octanol/water), 2.4.

Thin-layer Chromatography. System TA—Rf 68; system TB—Rf 10; system TC—Rf 54; system TE—Rf 54; system TL—Rf 19; system TAE—Rf 57; system TAF—Rf 65; system TAJ—Rf 26; system TAK—Rf 00; system TAL—Rf 34. (Dragendorff spray, positive; acidified iodoplatinate solution, positive; Marquis reagent, green.)

Gas Chromatography. System GA—hydroxyzine RI 2880; M (4-chlorobenzophenone) RI 1850; M (4-chloromethylbiphenyl) RI 1600; M (OH-chlorobenzophenone) RI 2300; M (desalkyl-) RI 2520; system GB—hydroxyzine RI 3000; M (norchlorcyclizine) RI 2355; M (4-chlorobenzophenone) RI 1862; M (4-chloromethylbiphenyl) RI 1688; M (OH-chlorobenzophenone) RI 2230.

High Performance Liquid Chromatography. System HA—*k* 1.4; system HX—RI 437; system HY—RI 326; system HZ—retention time 5.7 min; system HAA—retention time 15.3 min; system HAX—retention time 11.4 min; system HAY—retention time 6.3 min.

Ultraviolet Spectrum. Aqueous acid—232 nm ($A^1_1 = 416a$), 258, 263, 270 nm. No alkaline shift.

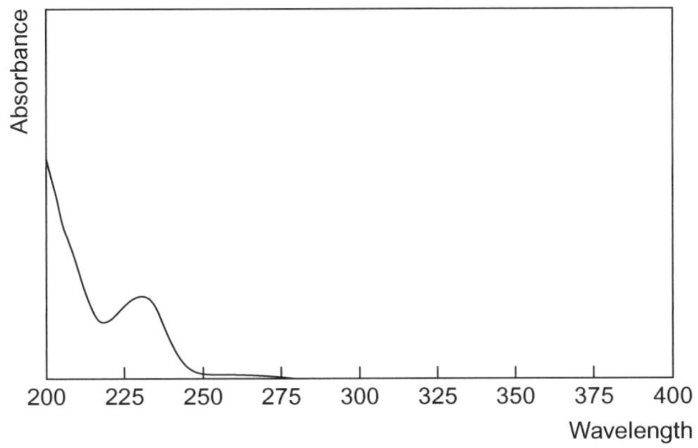

Infra-red Spectrum. Principal peaks at wavenumbers 1082, 1130, 1005, 1149, 1063, 800 cm^{-1} (KBr disk).

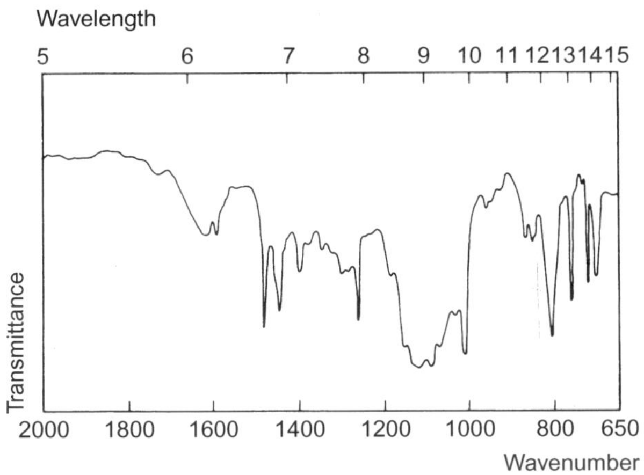

Mass Spectrum. Principal ions at *m/z* 201, 203, 165, 45, 299, 166, 202, 56.

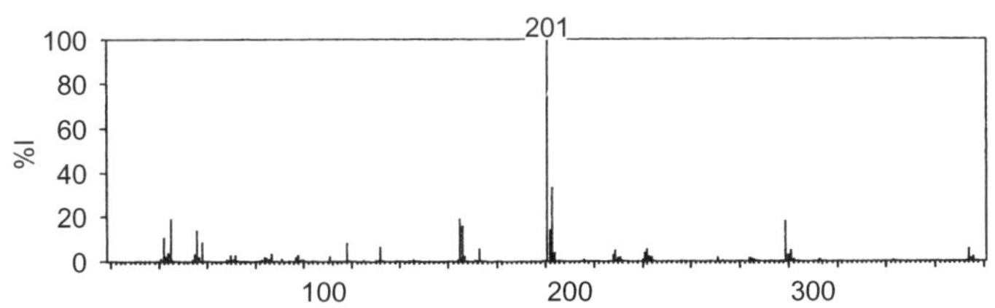

Quantification

Gas chromatography. In biological fluids: limit of detection in plasma 0.8 µg/L, NPD—P. Kintz *et al.*, *Forensic Sci. Int.*, 1990, *48*, 139–143.

Gas chromatography–mass spectrometry. In plasma: limit of detection 2 µg/L—H. G. Fouda *et al.*, *J. Pharm. Sci.*, 1979, *68*, 1456–1458.

Disposition in the Body

Therapeutic concentration

Following a single oral dose of 100 mg of the hydrochloride given to 4 subjects, peak plasma concentrations of 74 to 89 µg/L (mean 83) were attained in 2 to 4 h. [H. G. Fouda *et al.*, *J. Pharm. Sci.*, 1979, *68*, 1456–1458.]

Toxicity

A plasma concentration of 102.7 mg/L was reported 8.5 h after the ingestion of about 500 mg of hydroxyzine by a 13-month-old child; the child recovered within 72 h. [B. E. Magera, *Pediatrics*, 1981, *67*, 280–283.]

In a fatality due to hydroxyzine, the following postmortem tissue concentrations were reported: blood 39 mg/L, brain 163 µg/g, bile 122 mg/L, liver 414 µg/g, urine 19 mg/L. [G. R. Johnson, *J. Anal. Toxicol.*, 1982, *6*, 69–70.]

In a fatal self-poisoning attributed to hydroxyzine, postmortem tissue concentrations were: blood 4.18 mg/L, urine 1.43 mg/L, bile 23.24 mg/L, stomach content 78.23 mg/L. [P. Kintz *et al*, *Forensic Sci. Int.*, 1990, *48*, 139–143.]

Half-life. Plasma half-life, about 3 h.

Dose. 75 to 400 mg of hydroxyzine hydrochloride daily.

Hyoscine

Anticholinergic

Synonym. Scopolamine

Proprietary names. Scopoderm; Transcop; Transderm Scop.

Hyoscine and its salts are ingredients of many proprietary preparations—see *Martindale, The Complete Drug Reference*, 33rd Edn., London, Pharmaceutical Press, 2002.

(1α,2β,4β,5α,7β)-9-Methyl-3-oxa-9-azatricyclo[3.3.1.$0^{2,4}$]non-7-yl-(α-*S*)-α-(hydroxymethyl)benzene acetate

$C_{17}H_{21}NO_4$=303.4

CAS—51-34-3

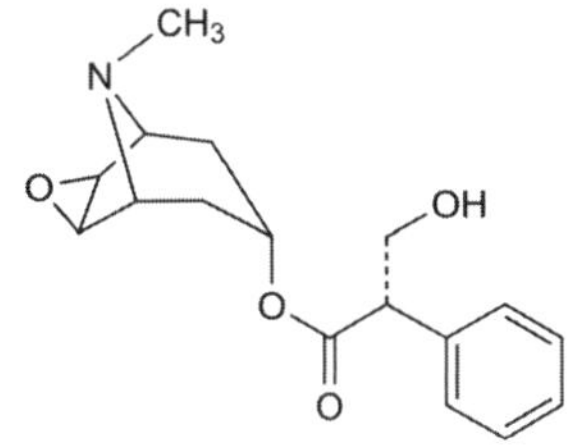

An alkaloid found in various solanaceous plants, particularly species of *Datura*, *Scopolia* and *Duboisia*.

A viscous liquid which forms a crystalline monohydrate with a M.p. of 59°.

Soluble 1 in 9.5 of water at 15°, freely soluble in hot water; freely soluble in ethanol, chloroform, acetone and ether; sparingly soluble in benzene and petroleum ether.

Hyoscine Hydrobromide

Synonyms. Scopolamine Bromhydrate; Scopolamine Hydrobromide.

Proprietary names. Joy-Rides; Kwells; Scopace; Travacalm HO; Travel Calm; Vorigeno.

$C_{17}H_{21}NO_4,HBr,3H_2O$=438.3

CAS—114-49-8 (anhydrous); 6533-68-2 (trihydrate)

Colourless transparent crystals or white crystalline powder; slightly efflorescent in dry air. M.p. 195°.

Soluble 1 in 1.5 of water and 1 in 20 of ethanol; practically insoluble in chloroform and ether.

Dissociation Constant. pK_a 7.6 (23°).

Partition Coefficient. Log *P* (octanol/buffer pH 7.4), 1.2.

Colour Test. Liebermann's Test—red-orange.

Thin-layer Chromatography. System TA—Rf 55; system TB—Rf 06; system TC—Rf 37; system TE—Rf 48; system TL—Rf 18; system TAE—Rf 49; system TAF—Rf 47; system TAJ—Rf 61; system TAK—Rf 49; system TAL—Rf 93. (Dragendorff spray, positive; acidified iodoplatinate solution, positive; Marquis reagent, pink.)

Gas Chromatography. System GA—hyoscine RI 2300, hyoscine-H_2O RI 2230, art (desacyl-) RI 1210; system GB—hyoscine RI 2427, hyoscine-H_2O RI 2255; system GF—RI 2885.

High Performance Liquid Chromatography. System HA—*k* 1.1; system HX—RI 270; system HY—RI 253; system HAA—Retention time, 7.4 min; system HAX—Retention time 7.0 min; system HAY—Retention time 3.7 min.

Ultraviolet Spectrum. Aqueous acid—251, 257 nm (A^1_1=6.3a), 263 nm.

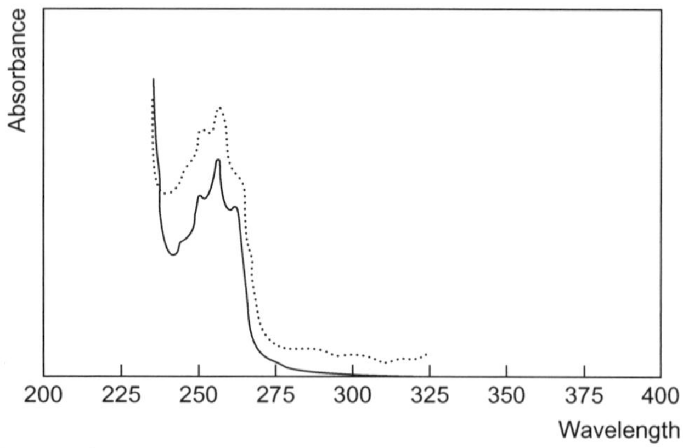

Infra-red Spectrum. Principal peaks at wavenumbers 1730, 853, 1166, 736, 705, 1047 cm^{-1} (hyoscine hydrobromide, KBr disk).

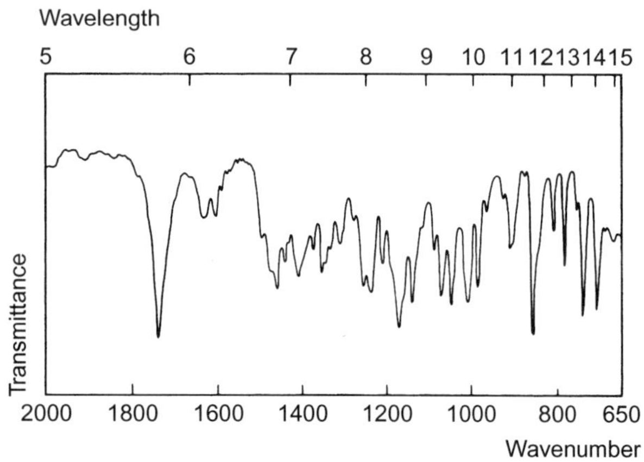

Mass Spectrum. Principal ions at *m/z* 94, 138, 42, 108, 136, 41, 96, 97.

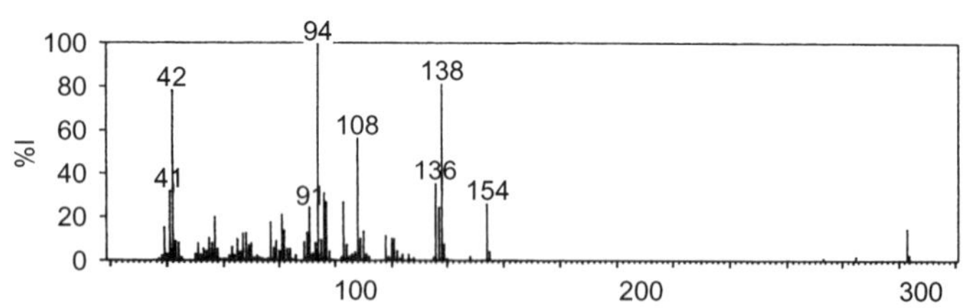

Quantification

Gas chromatography–mass spectrometry. In plasma or urine: limit of detection 50 ng/L—W. F. Bayne *et al.*, *J. Pharm. Sci.*, 1975, *64*, 288–291. In serum: limit of detection 50 ng/L—R. Oertel *et al.*, *J. Chromatogr.*, 1996, *682 Biomed. Appl.*, 259–264.

High performance liquid chromatography. In urine: limit of detection 5 ng, coulometric detection—R. Whelpton *et al.*, *Biomed. Chromatogr.*, 1992, *6*, 198–204.

Immunoassay. In serum: limit of detection 0.5 μg/L—K. Hagemann *et al.*, *Planta Med.*, 1992, *58*, 68–72.

Disposition in the Body. Readily absorbed after oral administration of the hydrobromide and extensively metabolised. About 5% of an oral dose is excreted in the urine as unchanged drug. Hyoscine is well absorbed following application to the skin. It crosses the blood–brain barrier and may cross the placenta.

Therapeutic concentration

Following a single oral dose equivalent to 415 μg of hyoscine to 10 subjects, a mean peak plasma concentration of 0.0003 mg/L was attained in 0.5 to 1 h, decreasing to 50% of the peak concentration in 2 to 4 h [C. Muir and R. Metcalfe, *J. Pharm. Biomed. Anal.*, 1983, *1*, 363–367].

A peak plasma concentration of 0.00055 ± 0.00006 mg/L was attained within 15 min in all but 2 of 8 subjects given 0.25% scopolamine eye drops unilaterally [K. Lahdes *et al.*, *J. Ocul. Pharmacol.*, 1990, *6*, 61–6].

Following administration of a single dose of 0.4 mg scopolamine bromide by the intranasal or oral route in 12 subjects (at least 2 weeks separated the doses), peak plasma concentrations of 0.00168 and 0.000164 mg/L were attained, respectively, within 1 h of dosing (0.37 h after intranasal dose and 0.78 h after oral dose) [L. Putcha *et al.*, *J. Pharm. Sci.*, 1996, *85*, 899–902].

Administration of scopolamine hydrobromide nasally at a dose of 0.2 g/0.05 L or 0.4 g/0.10 L in formulations of varying pH to 18 subjects produced average peak plasma concentrations of 0.000262, 0.000419 and 0.000488 mg/L after the 0.2 mg dose at pH 4, 7 and 9, respectively, and 0.000503, 0.000933 and 0.001308 mg/L after the 0.4 mg dose at the same pH values. At both doses, the average time to reach peak plasma concentration decreased linearly with a decrease in formulation pH (e.g. at the 0.4 g/L dose, the time to peak concentration was 26.7, 15.0 and 8.8 min at pH 4, 7 and 9, respectively) [S. Ahmed *et al.*, *Pharm. Res.*, 2000, *17*, 974–977].

Toxicity. The lethal dose in children may be as low as 10 mg but fatalities after hyoscine poisoning are rare.

Protein binding. Bound to plasma proteins.

Dose. 0.9 mg of hyoscine hydrobromide by mouth over 24 h; 1 mg of hyoscine over 72 h transdermally.

Hyoscine Butylbromide

Anticholinergic

Synonyms. Butylscopolamonii Bromidum; Hyoscine-*N*-Butyl Bromide; Scopolamine Butylbromide.
Proprietary name. Buscopan
[7(*S*)-(1α,2β,4β,5α,7β)]-9-Butyl-7-(3-hydroxy-1-oxo-2-phenylpropoxy)-9-methyl-3-oxa-9-azoniatricyclo[3.3.1.$0^{2,4}$]nonane bromide
$C_{21}H_{30}BrNO_4$=440.4
CAS—149-64-4

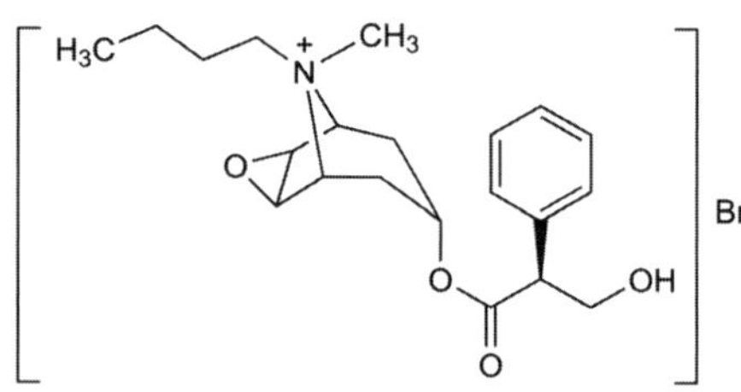

A white crystalline powder. M.p. 140° to 144°.
Soluble 1 in 1 of water, 1 in 50 of ethanol, and 1 in 5 of chloroform; practically insoluble in ether.

Partition Coefficient. Log *P* (octanol/water), −1.1.

Colour Tests. Aromaticity (Method 2)—colourless/yellow; Liebermann's Test—orange

Thin-layer Chromatography. System TA—Rf 08. (Acidified iodoplatinate solution, positive.)

High Performance Liquid Chromatography. System HY—RI 294.

Ultraviolet Spectrum. Aqueous acid—252 nm (A_1^1=3.7a), 258 nm (A_1^1=4.6a), 264 nm (A_1^1=3.6a).

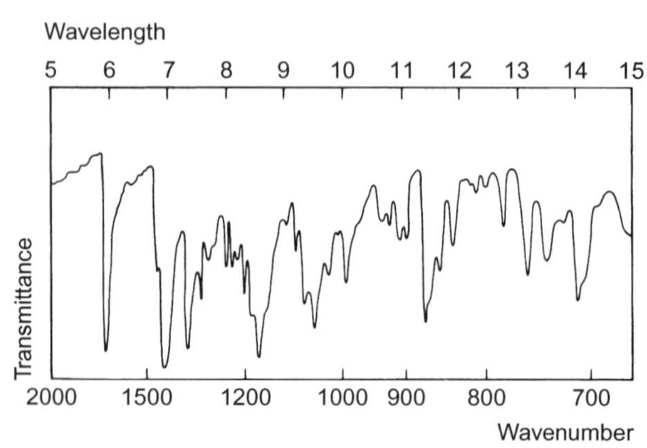

Infra-red Spectrum. Principal peaks at wavenumbers 1175, 1721, 1052, 874, 1072, 709 cm^{-1} (Nujol mull).

Disposition in the Body. Poorly absorbed after oral administration. About 90% of an oral dose is eliminated in the faeces and less than 10% is excreted in the urine. After intravenous administration, about 40% of a dose is excreted in the urine.

Half-life. Plasma half-life, about 8 h.

Protein binding. In plasma, about 10%.

Dose. 20 mg given parenterally, repeated if necessary; 80 mg daily, by mouth.

Hyoscine Methobromide

Anticholinergic

Synonyms. Epoxymethamine Bromide; Hyoscine Methylbromide; Methoscopolamine Bromide; Scopolamine Methylbromide.
Proprietary names. Holopon; Pamine.
(1α,2β,4β,5α,7β)-7-[(2*S*)-3-Hydroxy-1-oxo-2-phenylpropoxy]-9,9-dimethyl-3-oxa-9-azoniatricyclo[3.3.1.0^{2,4}]nonane bromide
$C_{18}H_{24}BrNO_4$=398.3
CAS—155-41-9

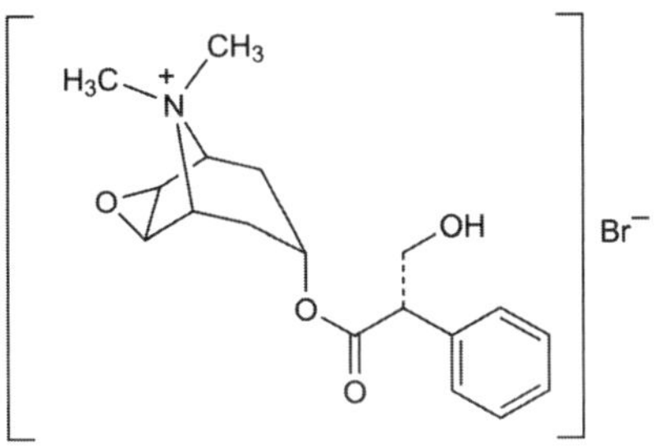

White crystals or crystalline powder. M.p. about 225°, with decomposition.
Soluble 1 in 3 of water, 1 in 100 of ethanol, and 1 in 40 of methanol; practically insoluble in chloroform.

Partition Coefficient. Log *P* (octanol/water), −2.6.

Colour Test. Aromaticity (Method 2)—colourless/yellow.

Ultraviolet Spectrum. Aqueous acid—253 nm (A^1_1=3.7b), 258 nm (A^1_1=4.4a), 264 nm (A^1_1=3.4b).

Infra-red Spectrum. Principal peaks at wavenumbers 1718, 1180, 1174, 1042, 923, 858 cm^{-1} (KBr disk).

Dose. 10 to 12.5 mg daily.

Hyoscine Methonitrate

Anticholinergic

Synonyms. Hyoscine Methylnitrate; Methscopolamine Nitrate; Methylhyoscini Nitras; Methylscopolamini Nitras; Scopolamine Methylnitrate.
Proprietary name. Skopyl
(1α,2β,4β,5α,7β-7-[(2*S*)-3-Hydroxy-1-oxo-2-phenylpropoxyl]-9,9-dimethyl-3-oxo-9-azoniatricyclo[3.3.1.0^{2,4}]nonane nitrate
$C_{18}H_{24}N_2O_7$=380.4
CAS—6106-46-3
Colourless hygroscopic crystals or a white crystalline powder. M.p. 194° to 199°.
Soluble 1 in 1.5 of water and 1 in 40 of ethanol; practically insoluble in chloroform and ether.

Partition Coefficient. Log *P* (octanol/water), 0.4.

Colour Tests. Aromaticity (Method 2)—colourless/violet (transient); Liebermann's Test—orange.

Thin-layer Chromatography. System TA—Rf 02. (Acidified iodoplatinate solution, positive.)

Ultraviolet Spectrum. Aqueous acid—251 nm (A^1_1=4.3a), 257 nm (A^1_1=5.1a), 263 nm (A^1_1=3.8a).

Infra-red Spectrum. Principal peaks at wavenumbers 1735, 1175, 1185, 1317, 860, 923 cm^{-1} (KBr disk).

Dose. Up to 12 mg daily.

Hyoscyamine

Anticholinergic

Synonym. L-Hyoscyamine
Proprietary name. Cystospaz
8-Methyl-8-azabicyclo[3.2.1]oct-3-yl [3(*S*)-*endo*]-α-(hydroxymethyl)-benzeneacetate
$C_{17}H_{23}NO_3$=289.4
CAS—101-31-5

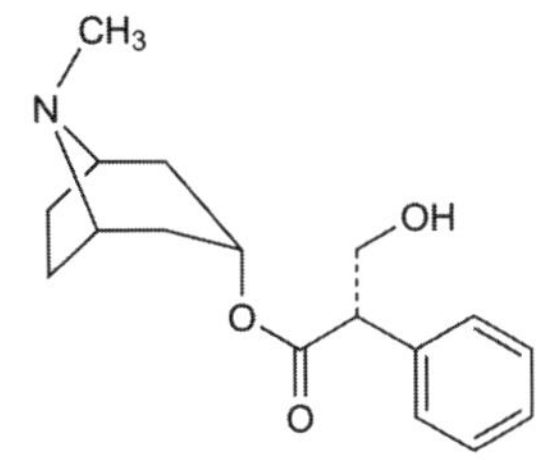

An alkaloid obtained from various solanaceous plants, *Hyoscyamus muticus* and *Duboisia myoporoides* being the best sources. It is the levo-isomer of atropine.
A white crystalline powder. M.p. 106° to 109°.
Soluble 1 in 280 of water, 1 in 1 of chloroform, 1 in 69 of ether, 1 in 150 of benzene; freely soluble in ethanol and dilute acids.

Hyoscyamine Hydrobromide
Synonym. Hyoscyamine Bromhydrate
$C_{17}H_{23}NO_3$,HBr=370.3
CAS—306-03-6
White prismatic crystals or crystalline powder. M.p. 152°.
Very soluble in water; soluble 1 in 3 of ethanol and 1 in 1.2 of chloroform; very slightly soluble in ether.

Hyoscyamine Sulfate
Proprietary names. Anaspaz; Cystospaz-M; Egacen(e); Egazil; Levsin; Levsinex; Peptard.
$(C_{17}H_{23}NO_3)_2,H_2SO_4,2H_2O$=712.9
CAS—620-61-1 (anhydrous); 6835-16-1 (dihydrate)
Colourless needles or a white deliquescent crystalline powder. M.p. about 203°, with decomposition.
Soluble 1 in 0.5 of water and 1 in 5 of ethanol; sparingly soluble in dehydrated alcohol; very slightly soluble in chloroform and ether.

Dissociation Constant. pK_a 9.7 (21°).

Partition Coefficient. Log *P* (octanol/water), 1.9.

Colour Test. Liebermann's Test—red-orange.

Thin-layer Chromatography. System TA—Rf 18; system TE—Rf 26; system TAJ—Rf 00; system TAK—Rf 01; system TAL—Rf 34. (Acidified iodoplatinate solution, positive.)

Gas Chromatography. System GA—RI 2190; system GB—RI 2293.

High Performance Liquid Chromatography. System HA—*k* 3.7 (tailing peak); system HAA—retention time 9.7 min.

Ultraviolet Spectrum. Aqueous acid—252 nm (A^1_1=6.2a), 258 nm (A^1_1=8.2a), 264 nm (A^1_1=6.2a).

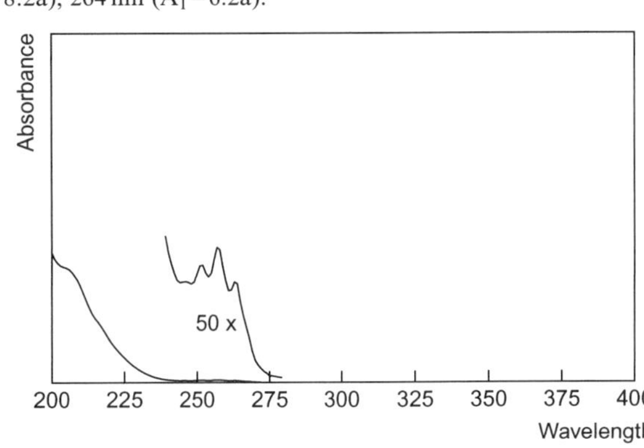

Infra-red Spectrum. Principal peaks at wavenumbers 1738, 1160, 1025, 1145, 1225, 1050 cm^{-1} (hyoscyamine hydrobromide, KBr disk).

Quantification. See under Atropine.

Dose. 0.6 to 1.2 mg daily.

Ibogaine

Alkaloid

12-Methoxyibogamine
$C_{20}H_{26}N_2O = 310.4$
CAS—83-74-9

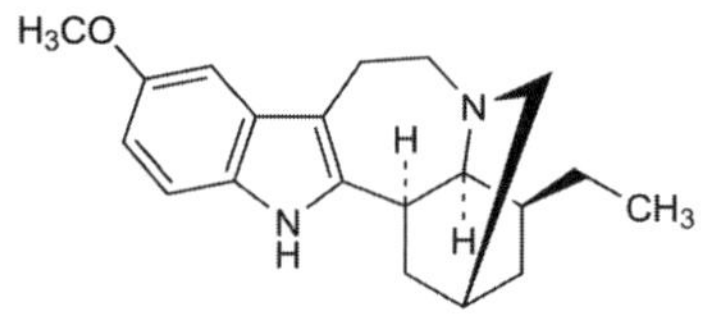

An alkaloid obtained from *Tabernanthe iboga* (Apocynaceae).
Crystals. M.p. 152° to 153°.
Practically insoluble in water; soluble in acetone, benzene, ethanol, chloroform, and ether.

Ibogaine Hydrochloride
$C_{20}H_{26}N_2O,HCl = 346.9$
CAS—5934-55-4
Crystals. M.p. 299° to 300°, with decomposition.
Soluble in water, ethanol, and methanol; slightly soluble in acetone and chloroform; practically insoluble in ether.

Partition Coefficient. Log *P* (octanol/water), 3.6.

Colour Tests. Liebermann's Test—black; Mandelin's Test—grey→violet; Marquis Test—grey→orange.

Thin-layer Chromatography. System TA—Rf 65; system TB—Rf 28; system TC—Rf 50; system TE—Rf 86; system TL—Rf 62; system TAE—Rf 39; system TAF—Rf 72; system TAJ—Rf 25; system TAK—Rf 05; system TAL—Rf 63. (Acidified iodoplatinate solution, positive.)

Gas Chromatography. System GA—RI 2885.

High Performance Liquid Chromatography. System HA—*k* 2.1; system HY—RI 321.

Ultraviolet Spectrum. Aqueous acid—278 nm ($A_1^1 = 212c$).

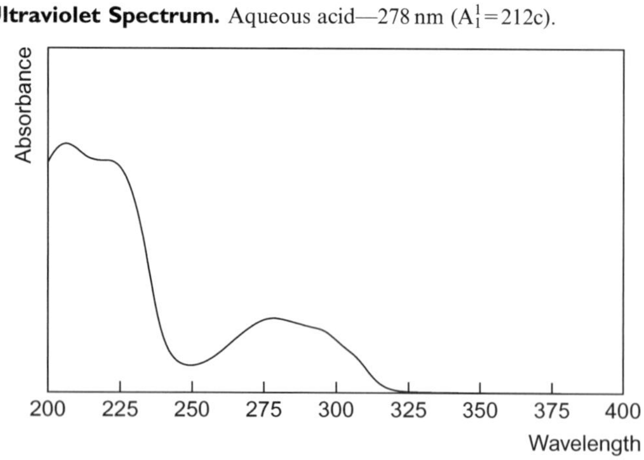

Infra-red Spectrum. Principal peaks at wavenumbers 1490, 1210, 1140, 810, 1020, 835 cm^{-1} (ibogaine hydrochloride, KBr disk).

Mass Spectrum. Principal ions at *m/z* 136, 310, 135, 225, 149, 122, 155, 311.

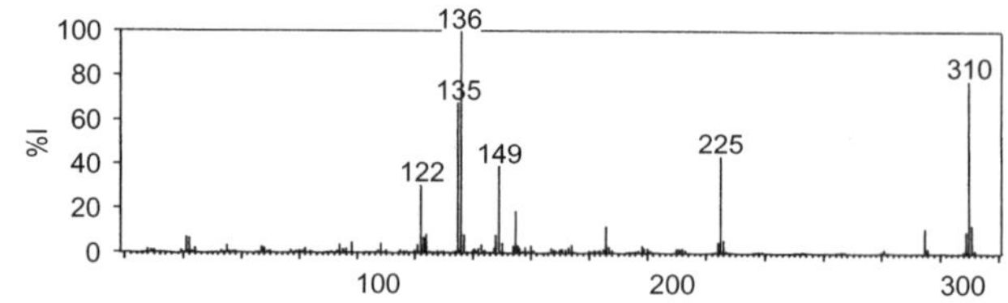

Quantification

Gas chromatography. In urine: limit of detection 5 ng, AFID—G. P. Cartoni and A. Giarusso, *J. Chromatogr.*, 1972, *71*, 154–158.

Gas chromatography–mass spectrometry. In biological samples: limit of detection 20 µg/L—C. A. Gallagher *et al.*, *Biochem. Pharmacol.*, 1995, *49*, 73–79. In plasma: ibogaine and 12-hydroxyibogamine, limit of detection 10 µg/L—M. E. Alburges *et al.*, *J. Anal. Toxicol.*, 1995, *19*, 381–386. In biological fluids and brain tissue: ibogaine and 12-hydroxyibogamine, limit of detection 5 µg/L—W. L. Hearn *et al.*, *J. Anal. Toxicol.*, 1995, *19*, 427–434. In plasma—F. R. Ley *et al.*, *J. Chromatogr. A*, 1996, *723*, 101–109.

Ibomal

Hypnotic/Barbiturate

Synonyms. Bromoaprobarbitone; Isopropyl-bromallyl-barbitursäure; Propallylonal.
Proprietary name. Noctal
5-(2-Bromo-2-propenyl)-5-(1-methylethyl)-2,4,6(1*H*,3*H*,5*H*)-pyrimidinetrione
$C_{10}H_{13}BrN_2O_3 = 289.1$
CAS—545-93-7

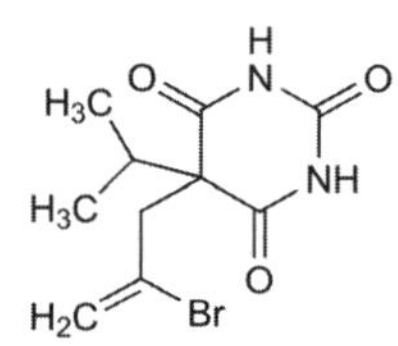

A white crystalline powder. M.p. 177° to 179°.
Slightly soluble in water; freely soluble in acetone, ethanol, and glacial acetic acid; sparingly soluble in benzene, chloroform, and ether.

Dissociation Constant. pK_a 7.7 (20°).

Partition Coefficient. Log *P* (octanol/water), 1.5.

Colour Test. Koppanyi–Zwikker Test—violet.

Thin-layer Chromatography. System TD—Rf 50; system TE—Rf 32; system TF—Rf 66; system TH—Rf 61; system TAD—Rf 56; system TAE—Rf 91.

Gas Chromatography. System GA—ibomal RI 1880, M (desbromo-OH-) RI 1770; ibomal-Me_2 RI 1745; M (desbromo-oxo-)-Me_2 RI 1720; M (desbromo-OH-)-Me_2 RI 1730. Also metabolised to aprobarbital RI 1618.

High Performance Liquid Chromatography. System HG—*k* 4.01; system HH—*k* 2.58; system HX—RI 379; system HY—RI 352.

Ultraviolet Spectrum. Borax buffer 0.05 M (pH 9.2)—240 nm ($A_1^1 = 307a$); 1 M sodium hydroxide (pH 13)—257 nm ($A_1^1 = 240b$).

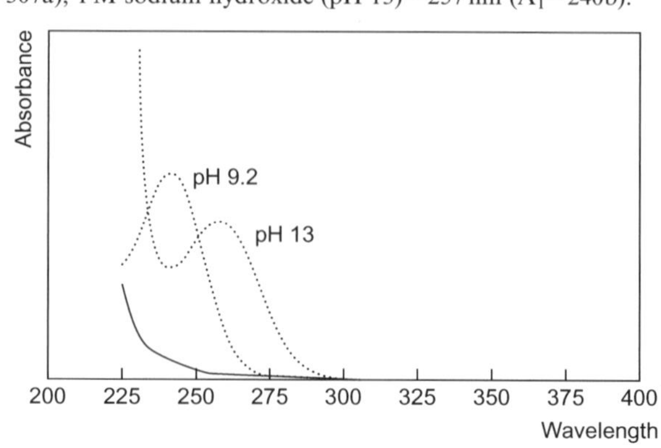

Infra-red Spectrum. Principal peaks at wavenumbers 1700, 1722, 1210, 1300, 830, 1622 cm^{-1}.

Mass Spectrum. Principal ions at *m/z* 167, 209, 43, 124, 39, 41, 53, 140.

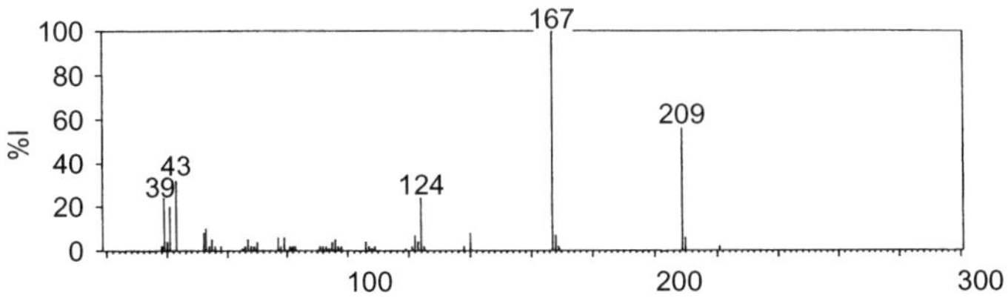

Disposition in the Body. Metabolised by side-chain oxidation to 5-(2-acetonyl)-5-isopropylbarbituric acid. About 6 to 16% of a dose is slowly excreted in the urine as the metabolite with about 1 to 3% as unchanged drug; the metabolite is still detectable in urine 9 days after a single dose.

Therapeutic concentration. In plasma, usually in the range 0.3 to 10 mg/L.

Toxicity. Blood concentrations greater than about 10 mg/L may be toxic or lethal.

Protein binding. In plasma, about 34%.

Dose. 100 to 400 mg, as a hypnotic.

Ibuprofen

Analgesic

Synonyms. Ibuprofenum; RD-13621; U-18573
Proprietary names. Advil; Apsifen; Arthrofen; Brufen; Cuprofen; Ebufac; Fenbid; Galprofen; Genpril; Haltran; Ibrufhalal; Ibu; Ibufac; Ibufem; Ibugel; Ibular; Ibuleve; Ibumousse; Ibuspray; Inoven; Isisfen; Junifen; Librofem; Lidifen; Manorfen; Menadol; Migrafen; Motrin; Novaprin; Nuprin; Nurofen; Obifen; Orbifen; Pacifene; PhorPain; Proflex; Relcofen; Rimafen; Saleto-200; Seclodin; Uniprofen.
Ibuprofen is an ingredient of many proprietary preparations—see *Martindale, The Complete Drug Reference*, 33rd Edn., London, Pharmaceutical Press, 2002.
α-Methyl-4-(2-methylpropyl)benzeneacetic acid
$C_{13}H_{18}O_2 = 206.3$
CAS—15687-27-1

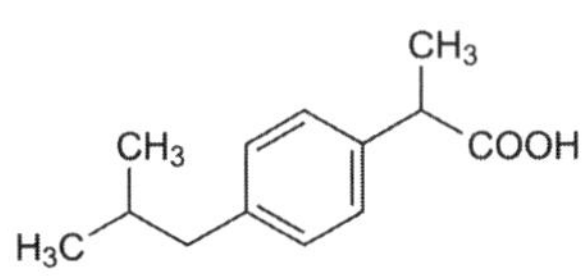

A white powder or crystals. M.p. 75° to 77°.
Practically insoluble in water; soluble 1 in 1.5 of ethanol, 1 in 1 of chloroform and 1 in 2 of ether.

Dissociation Constant. pK_a 4.4, 5.2.

Partition Coefficient. Log *P* (octanol/water), 4.0.

Colour Tests. Liebermann's Test—brown-orange; Marquis Test—brown(→orange at 100°).

Thin-layer Chromatography. System TD—Rf 46; system TE—Rf 06; system TF—Rf 57; system TG—Rf 18; system TAD—Rf 54; system TAE—Rf 75; system TAJ—Rf 59; system TAK—Rf 76; system TAL—Rf 93.

Gas Chromatography. System GA—ibuprofen RI 1615, ibuprofen-Me RI 1510, M (3-OH-)-Me RI 1630, M (OH-)-Me RI 1750; M (HOOC-)-Me_2 RI 1765; system GB—ibuprofen RI 1637, M (2-OH-) RI 2096; system GD—ibuprofen-Me RRT 0.89 (relative to *n*-$C_{16}H_{34}$); system GL—ibuprofen-Me RI 1505, M (3-OH-)-Me RI 1680.

High Performance Liquid Chromatography. System HD—*k* 15.1; system HX—RI 616; system HY—RI 598; system HZ—Retention time, 16.5 min; system HAA—Retention time, 23.8 min; system HAX—Retention time 8.1 min; system HAY—Retention time 10.5 min.

Ultraviolet Spectrum. Aqueous alkali—265 nm ($A^1_1 = 18.5a$), 273 nm.

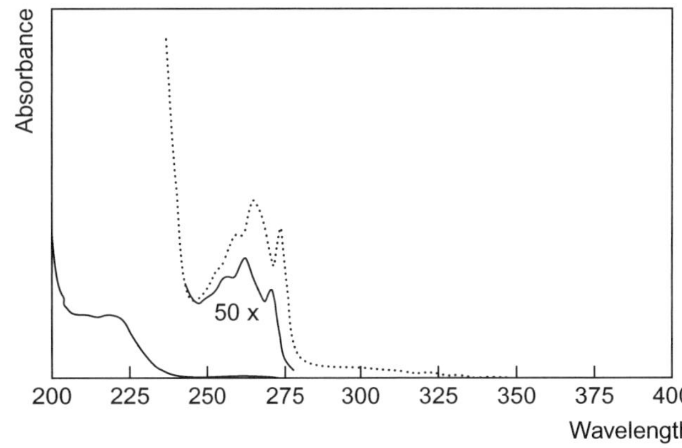

Infra-red Spectrum. Principal peaks at wavenumbers 1721, 1232, 779, 1185, 1273, 870 cm^{-1} (KBr disk). (See below.)

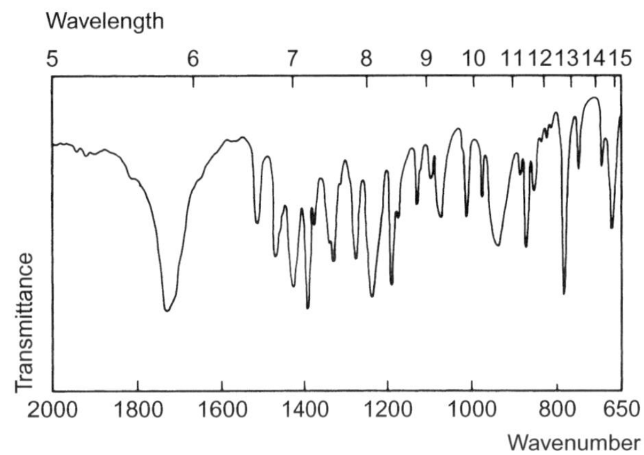

Mass Spectrum. Principal ions at *m/z* 163, 161, 119, 91, 206, 117, 107, 164.

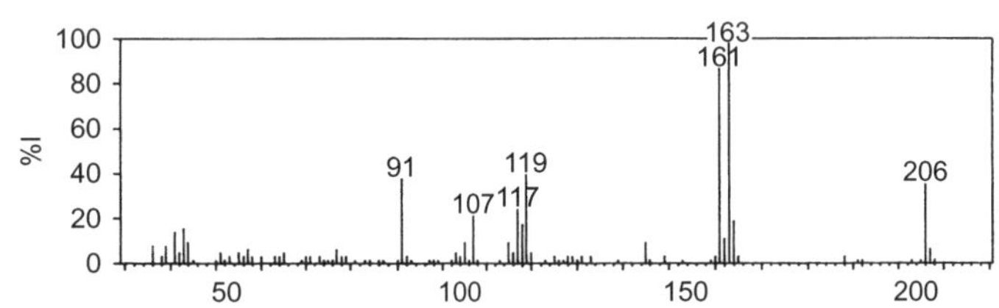

Quantification

Gas chromatography. In serum: limit of detection 500 µg/L, FID—D. J. Hoffman, *J. Pharm. Sci.*, 1977, *66*, 749–750. In serum: limit of detection 100 µg/L, ECD—D. G. Kaiser and R. S. Martin, *J. Pharm. Sci.*, 1978, *67*, 627–630.

Gas chromatography–mass spectrometry. In biological fluids: limit of detection 1 ng—J. B. Whitlam and J. H. Vine, *J. Chromatogr.*, 1980, *181*; *Biomed. Appl.*, *7*, 463–468. In plasma or synovial fluid: ibuprofen and ketoprofen enantiomers, limit of detection for ibuprofen <3 µg/L—D. S. Jack *et al.*, *J. Chromatogr.*, 1992, *584*, 189–197. In plasma: ibuprofen enantiomers—M. J. Zhao *et al.*, *J. Chromatogr.*, 1994, *656 Biomed. Appl.*, 441–446. In plasma: limit of detection 5 mg/L—B. A. Way *et al.*, *J. Clin. Lab. Anal.*, 1997, *11*, 336–339.

High performance liquid chromatography. In biological fluids: limit of detection, 1 mg/L for ibuprofen in plasma, 5 mg/L for ibuprofen or the hydroxy or carboxy metabolites in urine, UV detection—G. F. Lockwood and J. G. Wagner, *J. Chromatogr.*, 1982, *232 Biomed. Appl.*, *21*, 335–343. In plasma: limit of detection 25 µg/L, UV detection—A. M. Rustum, *J. Chromatogr. Sci.*, 1991, *29*, 16–20. In serum: ibuprofen and mefenamic acid, limit of detection 0.5 µg/L for ibuprofen, UV detection—K. Yamashita *et al.*, *J. Chromatogr.*, 1991, *570*, 329–338. In plasma or synovial fluid: ibuprofen, naproxen and diclofenac—I. S. Blagbrough *et al.*, *J.*

Chromatogr., 1992, *578*, 251–257. In biological fluids: ibuprofen enantiomers—M. R. Wright *et al.*, *J. Chromatogr.* 1992, *583*, 259–265. In plasma: ibuprofen and ibuprofen acyl glucuronide, UV detection—M. Castillo and P. C. Smith, *J. Chromatogr.*, 1993, *614*, 109–116. In plasma: fluorescence detection—C. H. Lemko *et al.*, *J. Chromatogr.*, 1993, *619*, 330–335. In plasma—N. Rifai *et al.*, *Clin. Chem.*, 1996, *42*, 1812–1816. In plasma: limit of detection 50 ng—T. K. Save *et al.*, *J. Chromatogr. B. Biomed. Sci. Appl.*, 1997, *690*, 315–319. In urine: ibuprofen and other NSAIDs, limit of detection for ibuprofen 50 μg/L—T. Hirai *et al.*, *J. Chromatogr. B. Biomed. Sci. Appl.*, 1997, *692*, 375–388. In urine: ibuprofen metabolites—D. R. Kepp *et al.*, *J. Chromatogr. B. Biomed. Sci. Appl.*, 1997, *696*, 235–241. In urine: hydroxyibuprofen and carboxyibuprofen, UV detection—S. C. Tan *et al.*, *J. Chromatogr. B. Biomed. Sci. Appl.*, 1997, *701*, 53–63. In plasma: ibuprofen enantiomers, spectrofluorometric detection—R. Canaparo *et al.*, *Biomed. Chromatogr.*, 2000, *14*, 219–226. In plasma: UV detection—H. Farrar *et al.*, *J. Chromatogr. B. Anal. Technol. Biomed. Life Sci.*, 2002, *780*, 341–348.

Disposition in the Body. Readily and almost completely absorbed after oral administration. More than 60% of a dose is excreted in the urine in 24 h, including about 9% of the dose as the 2-hydroxy metabolite, 2-[4-(2-hydroxy-2-methylpropyl)phenyl]propionic acid, about 17% as the conjugated hydroxy metabolite, about 16% as the 2-carboxy metabolite, 2-[4-(carboxypropyl)phenyl]propionic acid, and about 19% as the conjugated carboxy metabolite (both metabolites are inactive); less than 10% of a dose is excreted unchanged. The remainder of the dose is probably eliminated in the faeces after excretion in the bile; excretion is virtually complete within 24 h. It is found in breast milk in very low concentrations.
Ibuprofen's disposition is stereoselective and there is some metabolic conversion of the inactive *R*-(−)-enantiomer to the active *S*-(+)-form (dexibuprofen).

Therapeutic concentration. In plasma, usually in the range 20 to 30 mg/L.

Percutaneous application of ibuprofen 500 mg (10 g of a 5% gel under occlusion for 2 h, on the back 20 × 20 cm) produced a peak plasma concentration of 7.1 (±4.4) mg/L at 2.4 (±0.8) h in 18 subjects. In the same subjects, a single oral dose of 400 mg produced a peak plasma concentration of 36.7 (±7.5) mg/L at 1.1 (±0.8) h [C. H. Kleinbloesem *et al.*, *Arzneimittelforschung*, 1995, *45*, 1117–1121].

Ibuprofen lysine (10 mg/kg) given as an intravenous bolus within the first 3 h after birth to 21 premature neonates produced an ibuprofen plasma concentration of 180.6 (±11.1) mg/L after 1 h. In 5 of the neonates, maintenance doses of 5 mg/kg once daily on days 2 and 3 resulted in mean plasma concentrations of 116.6 (±54.5) mg/L and 113.6 (±58.2) mg/L, respectively [J. V. Aranda *et al.*, *Acta Paediatr.*, 1997, *86*, 289–293].

In 98 patients receiving high doses of ibuprofen (20 to 30 mg/kg intravenously as a single dose), plasma concentrations of 21 to 150 mg/L (mean 83) were attained in 1 to 3 h (mean 1.77) [D. J. Murry *et al.*, *Pharmacotherapy*, 1999, *19*, 340–345].

Toxicity

In an attempted suicide involving the ingestion of 12 g of ibuprofen, an initial serum concentration of 840 mg/L was reported; this declined to 220 mg/L at 3 h; chlorphenamine was also detected in the urine. The subject was comatose but recovered within 24 h [D. P. Hunt and R. J. Leigh, *BMJ*, 1980, *281*, 1458–1459].

In 2 overdoses caused by ibuprofen, plasma concentrations of 400 and 711 mg/L were reported about 1.5 h after ingestion. In the first case, the estimated dose was 14 to 16 g; both subjects recovered [H. Court *et al.*, *BMJ*, 1981, *282*, 1073].

A 26-year-old male with a history of ibuprofen overdose was found dead after having recently been issued with a prescription for ibuprofen. The following postmortem tissue concentrations were reported: heart blood 518.0 mg/L, femoral blood 348.3 mg/L, liver 942 μg/g, brain 283.9 μg/g, gastric contents 131 mg total [G. W. Kunsman and T. P. Rohrig, *Am. J. Forensic Med. Pathol.*, 1993, *14*, 48–50].

Half-life. Plasma half-life, about 2 h.

Volume of distribution. About 0.1 L/kg.

Protein binding. In plasma, about 99%.

Note. For a review of the clinical pharmacokinetics of ibuprofen, see N. M. Davies, *Clin. Pharmacokinet.*, 1998, *34*, 101–154.

Dose. 0.6 to 2.4 g daily.

Ibutilide

Anti-arrhythmic

N-[4-[4-(Ethylheptylamino)-1-hydroxybutyl]phenyl]methanesulfonamide
$C_{20}H_{36}N_2O_3S$=384.6
CAS—122647-31-8

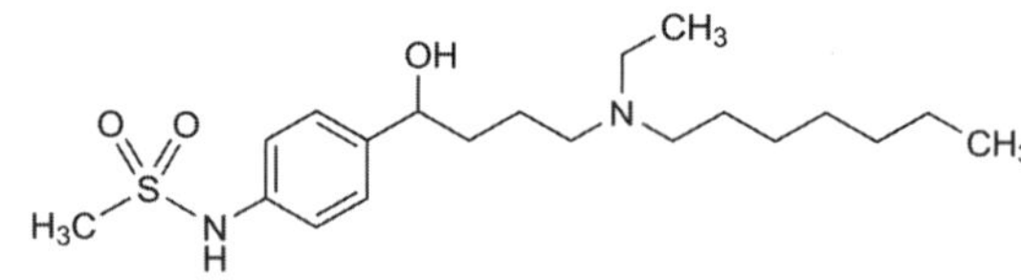

Ibutilide Fumarate
Synonym. U-70226E
Proprietary name. Corvert
$(C_{20}H_{36}N_2O_3S)_2$, $C_4H_4O_4$=885.2
CAS—122647-32-9
A white to off-white powder. M.p. 117° to 119°. Soluble (> 100 g/L) in solutions at pH 7 or less.

Dissociation Constant. pK_a 10.5 (pH < 6); 8.36 (pH > 6).

Quantification

High performance liquid chromatography. In plasma: limit of detection < 0.018 μg/L. Fluorescence detection (λ_{ex}=224 nm, λ_{em}=340 nm)—C. L. Hsu and R. R. Walters, *J. Chromat.* 1995, *667*, *Biomed. Appl.*, 115–128.

Ultraviolet Spectrum. Aqueous acid (ethanol)—228 , 267 nm.

Disposition in the Body. After intravenous administration, ibutilide is widely distributed in the body and extensively metabolised in the liver, to produce eight metabolites, by *O*-oxidation followed by sequential β-oxidation of the heptyl side chain. Approx. 82% of a dose may be excreted in urine with 7% as the unchanged drug, and up to 19% in excreted in faeces.

Therapeutic concentration. The peak serum concentration, after a 0.01 mg/kg infusion, is approx. 10 μg/L. Ibutilide has a low therapeutic dosage of 0.01 to 0.03 mg/kg, with peak plasma concentrations not reaching greater than 20 μg/L.

Toxicity. Acute toxicity can cause potentially fatal arrhythmias, also tachycardia, hypotension, congestive heart failure, myocardial depression, third degree atrioventricular (AV) block and renal failure. Poison by intravenous route. Moderately toxic by ingestion.

Half-life. 2 to 12 h, with an average of 6 h.

Volume of distribution. 9 to 13 L/kg.

Clearance. Plasma clearance, 29 mL/min/kg.

Protein binding. Ibutilide binds plasma proteins approx. 40%.

Dose. In patients with a body weight greater than 60 kg, a 1 mg dose of ibutilide fumarate is suggested. For those weighing less than 60 kg, 0.01 mg/kg body weight is administered. Usual dose between 0.01 and 0.10 mg/kg body weight.

Idarubicin

Antineoplastic

Synonyms. 4-Demethoxydaunomycin; 4-DMDR; IMI 30; NSC-256439.
(7*S*,9*S*)-9-Acetyl-7-[(3-amino-2,3,6-trideoxy-α-L-*lyxo*-hexopyranosyl)-oxy]-7,8,9,10-tetrahydro-6,9,11-trihydroxy-5,12-naphthacenedione
$C_{26}H_{27}NO_9$=497.5
CAS—58957-92-9

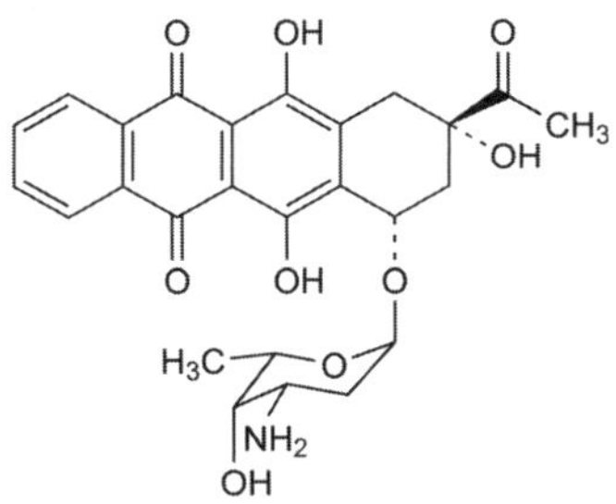

Idarubicin Hydrochloride
Proprietary names. Idamycin; Zavedos.
$C_{26}H_{27}NO_9.HCl=534.0$
CAS—57852-57-0
An orange crystalline powder. M.p. 183° to 185°, also reported as M.p. 172° to 174°.

Partition Coefficient. Log *P* (octanol/water), 2.10.

Thin-layer Chromatography. System TE—Rf 06; system TF—Rf 00.

High Performance Liquid Chromatography. System HX—RI 410.

Column: LC-CN5 (Supelcosil, 250 × 4.6 mm i.d., 5 μm). Mobile phase: monobasic sodium phosphate (50 mM):acetonitrile (65:35), adjusted to pH 4.0 with orthophosphoric acid, 1 mL/min flow rate. Fluorescence detection (λ_{ex}=480 nm, λ_{em}=560 nm). Retention time: idarubicin, 11.3 min; idarubicinol, 8.0 min [S. Fogli *et al.*, *Ther. Drug Monit.*, 1999, *21*, 367–375].

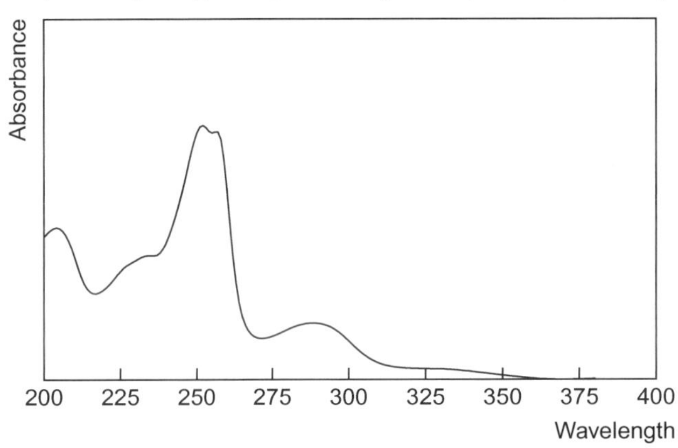

Quantification
High performance liquid chromatography. In plasma: limit of detection and quantification is 0.4 μg/L. Fluorescence detection (λ_{ex}= 480 nm, λ_{em}=560 nm)—S. Fogli *et al.*, *Ther. Drug Monit.*, 1999, *21*, 367–375. In serum: limit of quantification 5 μg/L. MS detection—F. Lachatre *et al.*, *J. Chromatogr. B Biomed. Sci. Appl.*, 2000, *738*, 281–291.

Disposition in the Body. After intravenous administration, idarubicin is rapidly distributed into body tissues and extensively tissue bound. After oral administration, idarubicin is rapidly absorbed. It is mostly metabolised in the liver, by aldoketoreductase, which reduces the ketone function at the C_{13} position to idarubicinol (1,3-dihydroidarubicin), the principal metabolite. The unchanged drug and metabolite are excreted mainly in bile but also in urine. Oral bioavailability is between 24 and 39% after oral administration.

Therapeutic concentration
13 male and 7 female patients with advanced malignant disease, for example, non-Hodgkins lymphoma, aged between 22 and 76 years, were administered 15 mg/m^2 over 1 min (intravenously). 11 patients were also administered 40 and 50 mg/m^2 oral doses of idarubicin. Peak plasma levels of idarubicin and idarubicinol ranged between 7.4 and 89.4 nmol/L and were reached 1.5 to 8 h after administration [H. C. Gillies *et al.*, *Br. J. Clin. Pharmacol.*, 1987, *23*, 303–310].

Toxicity. Acute/high doses of idarubicin (> 600 mg/m^2) can lead to myocardial toxicity, with potentially fatal congestive heart failure (CHF), life-threatening arrhythmias and serious gastro-intestinal events, for example, bleeding and preforations.

Half-life. 12 to 35 h (idarubicin); 50 to 70 h (idarubicinol).

Volume of distribution. Steady state, 1500 L/m^2.

Clearance. Plasma clearance, 60 L/h/m^2.

Protein binding. Idarubicin is 97% bound to plasma proteins and idarubicinol, 94%.

Dose. In adults: dose ranges from 8 to 12 mg/m^2/daily for 3 to 5 days (intravenously) and 15 to 45 mg/m^2/daily, alone or in combination, in a single dose or for 3 days (orally).
In children: 10 mg/m^2/daily for 3 days (intravenously). Maximum cumulative dose for all indications is 400 mg/m^2. Dose reduced if patient has impaired hepatic or renal function.

Idebenone

Nootropic

Synonym. CV-2619
Proprietary names. Avan; Daruma; Mneisis.
2-(10-Hydroxydecyl)-5,6-dimethoxy-3methyl-2,5-cyclohexadiene-1,4-dione
$C_{19}H_{30}O_5=338.4$
CAS—58186-27-9

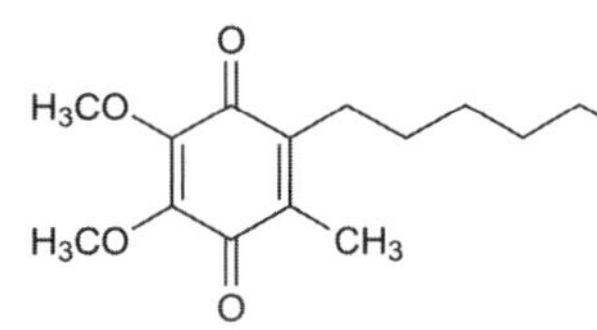

Orange needles from ligroin, M.p. 46° to 50°, also reported as crystals from hexane and ethylacetate, M.p. 52° to 53°.
It is soluble in organic solvents; practically insoluble in water.

High Performance Liquid Chromatography. Column: C_{18} (μBondapak, Waters). Mobile phase: isopropanol:dioxane:water (15:15:70) containing 0.05% acetic acid. UV detection (λ =280 nm). Retention time: 6.85 min [M. F. Backworth *et al.*, *Arzneimettelforscung.*, 1985, *35(2)*, 1704–1707].

Quantification
High performance liquid chromatography. In plasma: limit of quantification 0.02 mg/L. MS detection—P. Hu *et al.*, *Acta Pharmacol. Sin.*, 2000, *21(4)*, 306–308.

Disposition in the Body. Idebenone is metabolised by oxidation followed by β-oxidation, reduction and subsequent conjugation (sulfation and glucuronidation). Two of the main metabolites are QS-4 and QS-6. It is widely distributed in tissues and is excreted as the metabolites in urine and faeces. The ratio of idebenone:QS-4:QS-6 in urine is 2:89:9.

Therapeutic concentration
10 healthy males, aged between 21 and 30 years, were administered a single oral dose of 100 mg idebenone on days 1 and 35, in between doses of 300 mg daily were received. Peak serum concentrations of 0.65 and 0.85 mg/L were reached on days 1 and 35 within 4 to 5 h, respectively, for the parent drug. Peak concentrations for the two metabolites, QS-4 and QS-6, were 0.35 and 0.40 mg/L (days 1 and 35) and 0.035 and 0.045 mg/L, respectively, which were reached within 3 h for both metabolites [M. F. Backworth *et al.*, *Arzneimettelforsch.*, 1985, *35(2)*, 1704–1707].

Half-life. 18 h.

Protein binding. Approx. 90%.

Dose. 90 mg daily.

Idobutal

Hypnotic/Barbiturate

Synonym. *n*-Butylallylbarbituric Acid
5-Butyl-5-prop-2-enyl-2,4,6(1H,3H,5H)-pyrimidinetrione
$C_{11}H_{16}N_2O_3=224.3$
CAS—3146-66-5

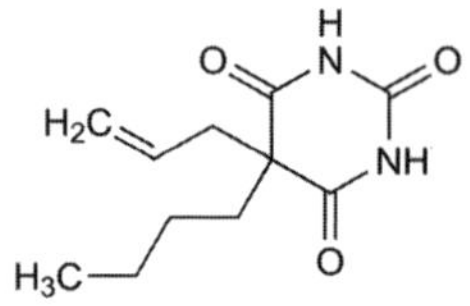

Crystals. M.p. 128°.
Slightly soluble in water; freely soluble in ethanol and ether.

Partition Coefficient. Log *P* (octanol/water), 2.3.

Thin-layer Chromatography. System TD—Rf 55; system TE—Rf 41; system TF—Rf 69; system TH—Rf 71; system TAD—Rf 59.

Gas Chromatography. System GA—idobutal RI 1700; idobutal-Me_2 RI 1610.

High Performance Liquid Chromatography. System HG—*k* 8.12; system HH—*k* 4.77; system HY—RI 357.

Ultraviolet Spectrum. Borax buffer 0.05 M (pH 9.2)—239 nm (A_1^1=434b); 1 M sodium hydroxide (pH 13)—254 nm (A_1^1=328b).

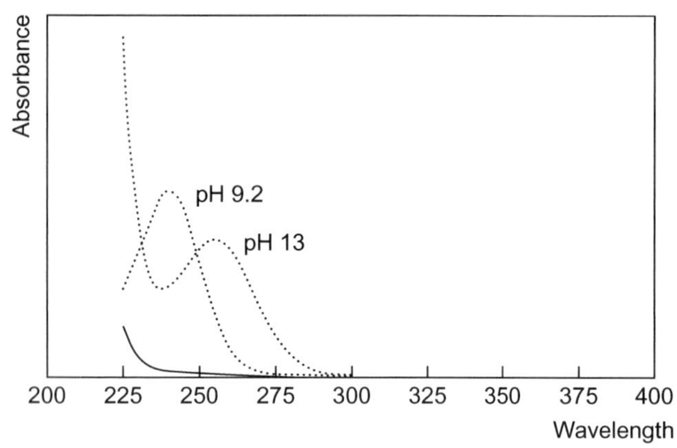

Infra-red Spectrum. Principal peaks at wavenumbers 1696, 1728, 1755, 835, 1290, 1207 cm^{-1}.

Mass Spectrum. Principal ions at *m/z* 167, 41, 168, 124, 39, 97, 141, 67.

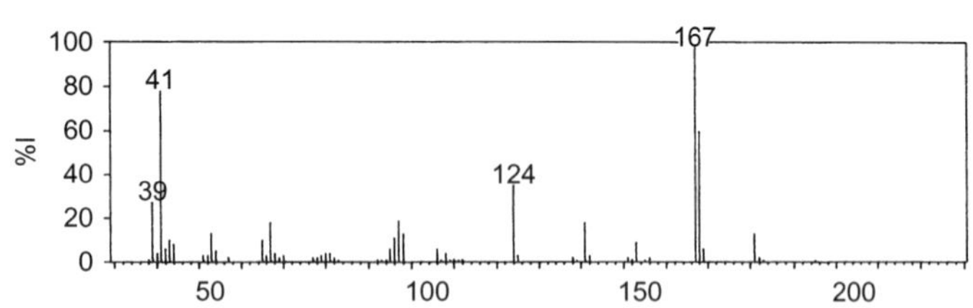

Idoxuridine

Antiviral

Synonyms. IDU; 5 IDUR.
Proprietary names. Herpid; Herpidu; Herplex; Iderpes; Idina; Idoxene; Iducher; Idulea; Iduridin; Idustatin; Iduviran; Kerecid; Ophthalmadine; Stoxil; Virexen; Virudox; Virunguent; Zostrum. It is an ingredient of Herpesine, Iducol, and Virasolve.
2′-Deoxy-5-iodouridine
$C_9H_{11}IN_2O_5$=354.1
CAS—54-42-2

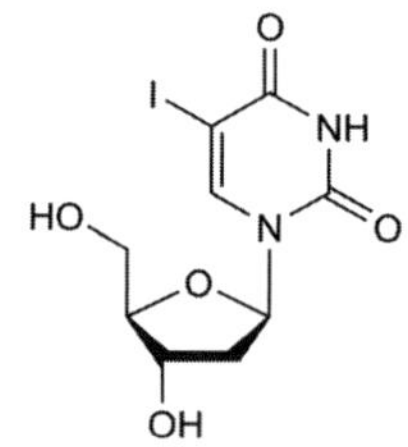

Colourless crystals or a white crystalline powder. It decomposes on heating with the liberation of iodine vapour.
Soluble 1 in 500 of water, 1 in 400 of ethanol, and 1 in 230 of methanol; practically insoluble in chloroform and ether.

Dissociation Constant. pK_a 8.3.

Partition Coefficient. Log *P* (octanol/water), −1.0.

Colour Test. Iodine Test—positive

Ultraviolet Spectrum. Aqueous acid—288 nm (A_1^1=220a); aqueous alkali—279 nm (A_1^1=162a).

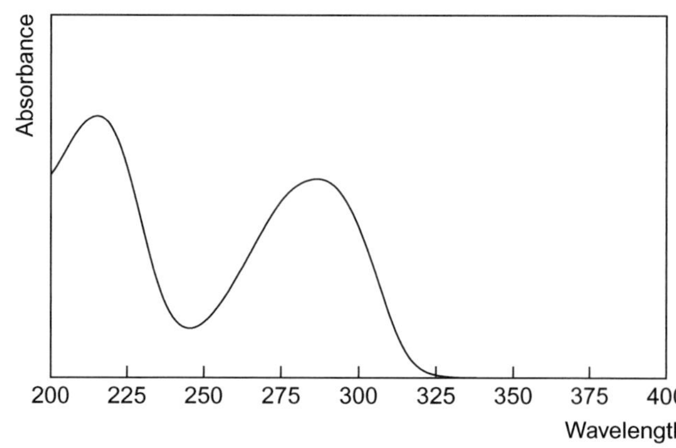

Infra-red Spectrum. Principal peaks at wavenumbers 1667, 1259, 1096, 1605, 1289, 1070 cm^{-1} (KBr disk).

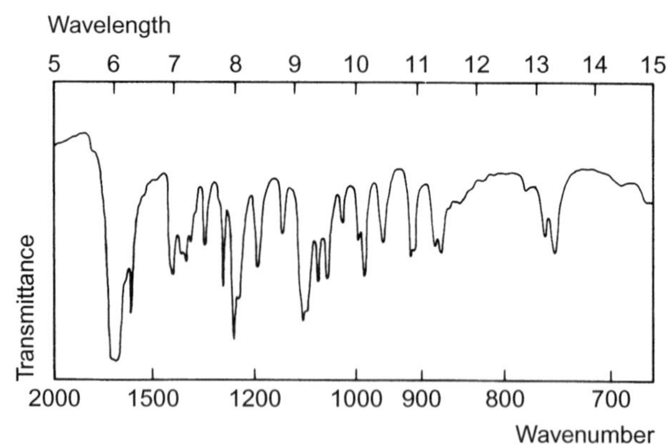

Quantification
High performance liquid chromatography. In serum: idoxuridine and its metabolite 5-iodouracil, UV detection—N. Belotto *et al.*, *J. Chromatogr.*, 1991, *572*, 327–332.

Use. Solutions of idoxuridine in dimethyl sulfoxide are used topically in concentrations of 5 to 40%.

Imidacloprid

Insecticide

Synonym. BAY-NTN 33893
Proprietary names. Admire; Confidor; Gaucho; Imazethepyr; Marathon; Merit; Premier; Premise; Provado.

1-[(6-Chloro-3-pyridinyl)methyl]-4,5-dihydro-*N*-nitro-1*H*-imidazol-2-amine
$C_9H_{10}ClN_5O_2$=255.7
CAS—138261-41-3; 105827-78-9

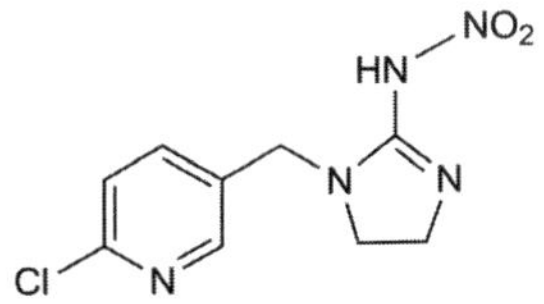

A colourless crystalline solid. M.p. 136° to 144°.
It is soluble in water (0.51 to 0.61 g/L), dichloromethane (50 to 100 g/L at 20°), isopropanol (1 to 2 g/L at 20°), toluene (0.5 to 1 g/L at 20°), and *n*-hexane (<0.1 g/L at 20°).

Partition Coefficient. Log *P* (octanol/water), 0.57 (22°).

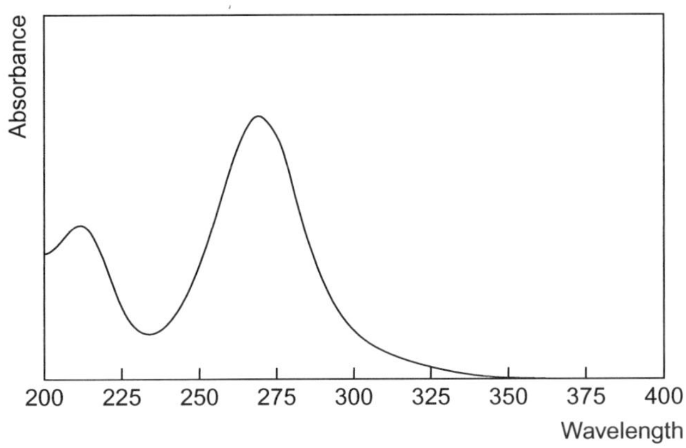

Disposition in the Body. Imidacloprid is quickly and almost completely absorbed after ingestion and degraded to 6-chloronicotinic acid which may be conjugated with glycine and then eliminated or reduced to guanidine. 70 to 80% of an administered dose may be excreted in urine with 20 to 30% in faeces.

Imidapril

Antihypertensive

Proprietary names. Novarok; Tanatril.
(4*S*)-3-[(2*S*)-2-[[(1*S*)-1-(Ethoxycarbonyl)-3-phenylpropyl]amino]-1-oxopropyl]-1-methyl-2-oxo-4-imidazolidinecarboxylic acid
$C_{20}H_{27}N_3O_6$=405.4
CAS—89371-37-9

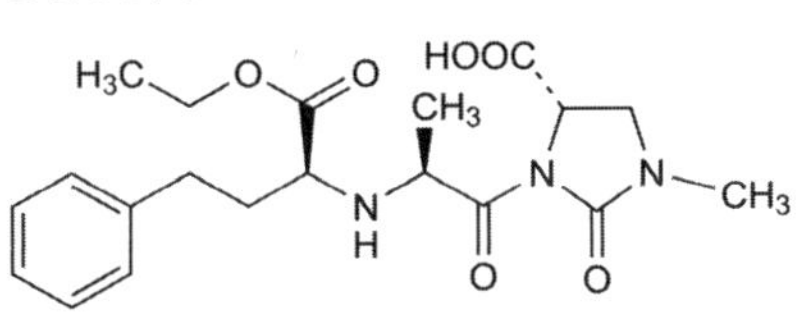

Colourless crystals (from ethyl acetate + *n*-hexane). M.p. 139° to 140°.

Imidaprilat
$C_{18}H_{23}N_3O_6$=377.4
CAS—89371-44-8
Crystals. M.p. 239° to 241°.

Imidapril Monohydrochloride
Synonym. TA-6366
Proprietary names. Novaloc; Tanatril.
$C_{20}H_{27}N_3O_6$.HCl=441.9
CAS—89396-94-1
Colourless crystals. M.p. 214° to 216° (dec).

High Performance Liquid Chromatography. Column: Symmetry C_{18} (100 × 2.1 mm i.d., 3.5 µm). Column temperature: 40°. Mobile phase: acetonitrile:0.05% formic acid (1:3), 0.2 mL/min flow rate. MS–MS detection (ESI, *m*/*z*: 406→234 for imidapril and 378→206 for imidaprilat). Retention time: imidapril, 3.06 min, imidaprilat, 4.39 min [M. Mabuchi *et al.*, *J. Chromatogr. B Biomed. Sci. Appl.*, 1999, *734*, 145–153].

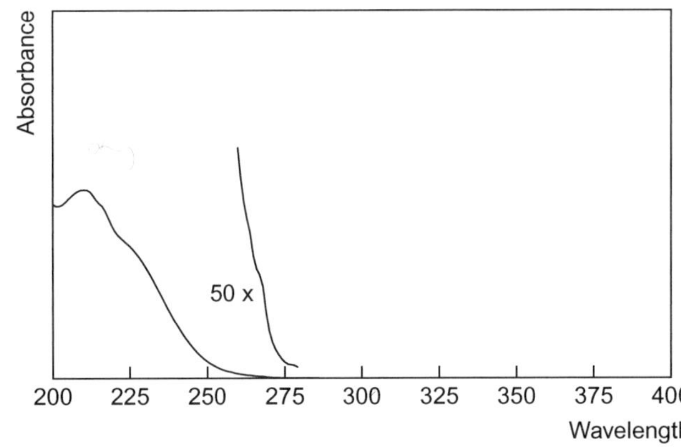

Mass Spectrum. Principal ions at *m*/*z* 234, 91, 74, 107, 70, 160, 55, 404 (TMS derivative).

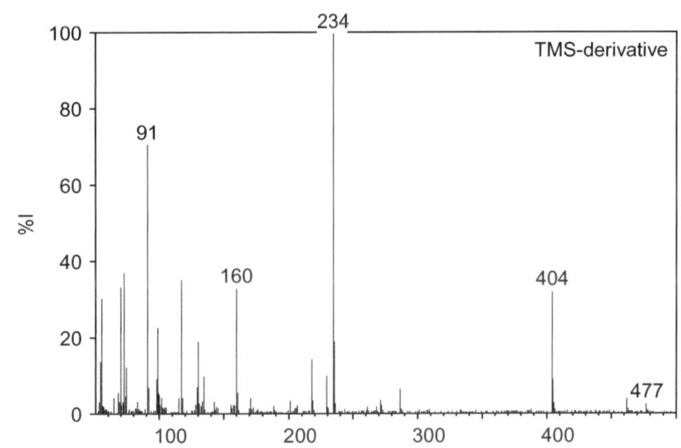

Quantification
Gas chromatography–mass spectrometry. In plasma and urine: limit of detection 1 µg/L and 5 µg/L, respectively for the metabolites—M. Matsuoka *et al.*, *J. Chromatogr.*, 1992, *581, Biomed. Appl.*, 65–73.

High performance liquid chromatography. In plasma and urine: limit of detection of imidapril and its active metabolite, imidaprilat, 0.2 µg/L and 10 µg/L, respectively—K. Tagawa *et al.*, *J. Chromatogr.*, 1993, *617(1)*, 95–103. In plasma: limit of determination 0.2 µg/L for imidapril and 0.5 µg/L for imidaprilat—S. Horimoto *et al.*, *Chem. Pharm. Bull.*, 1993, *41*, 699–702.

Disposition in the Body. Imidapril is rapidly absorbed and extensively metabolised in the liver, by de-esterification, to its pharmacologically active diacid metabolite, imidaprilat and a number of minor metabolites. Peak concentrations of the drug are seen after 2 h and the active metabolite, 7 to 8 h after administration. It is excreted in urine mainly as the metabolites.

Therapeutic concentration
10 hypertensive patients without renal or hepatic disease or diabetes, aged 37 to 72 years old, 3 males and 7 females, were administered a 10 mg single dose of imidapril and 10 mg daily for 4 weeks in a multiple dose study. Peak concentrations of 39.3 µg/L imidapril and 15.7 µg/L imidaprilat were observed 1 to 2 h and 5 to 10 h, respectively, after administration. In the multiple dosing study, levels reached 34.7 and 20.4 µg/L for the parent drug and its metabolite, respectively in 1 to 2 h and 3 to 6 h [S. Harder *et al.*, *Br. J. Clin. Pharmacol.*, 1998, *45(4)*, 377–380].

8 patients with normal liver function, with a mean age of 42 years, and 8 patients with liver dysfunction, mean age 55 years, were administered a 10 mg dose once daily for 7 days. The mean peak plasma concentration of imidapril was 33.9 µg/L, observed 1.1 to 2.5 h after administration, for the healthy individuals and 38.0 µg/L after 1.5 to 3.0 h for those with liver dysfunction. Mean concentrations for the metabolite, imidaprilat, were 12.0 µg/L and 5.2 µg/L, respectively for the two groups of patients observed

after 6.0 to 8.1 h, and 4.2 to 12.1 h [J. F. W. Hoogkamer *et al.*, *Eur. J. Clin. Pharmacol.*, 1997, *51*, 489–491].

Group 1: 8 volunteers with normal renal function, mean age 53 years. Group 2: 8 patients with moderate renal failure, mean age 58 years. Group 3: 8 patients with severe renal failure. All groups were administered 10 mg once daily for 7 days. The mean peak plasma concentrations of imidapril were 25.9, 37.8 and 75.8 μg/L, for the three groups, observed 1.0 to 3.5 h after administration. Mean concentrations for the metabolite, imidaprilat, were 8.6, 17.1 and 51.7 μg/L for groups 1, 2 and 3, respectively. These concentrations were seen 3.0 to 12.4 h after administration [J. F. W. Hoogkamer *et al.*, *Eur. J. Clin. Pharmacol.*, 1998, *54*, 59–61].

Bioavailability. About 20 %.

Half-life. 2 h (imidapril); 8 h (imidaprilat).

Protein binding. Plasma, 85%.

Dose. 5 to 10 mg daily, as the hydrochloride.

Imipramine

Antidepressant

Proprietary name. Topramine
10,11-Dihydro-*N*,*N*-dimethyl-5*H*-dibenz[*b*,*f*]azepine-5-propanamine
$C_{19}H_{24}N_2$=280.4
CAS—50-49-7

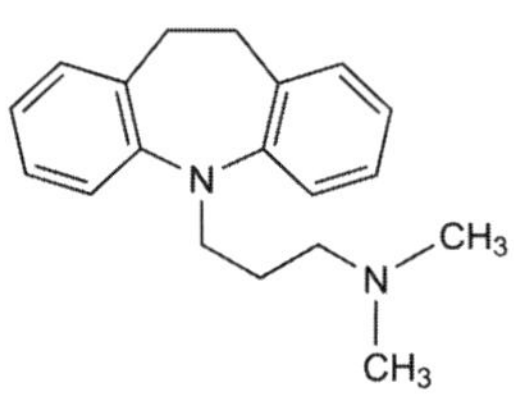

Imipramine Embonate

Synonym. Imipramine Pamoate
Proprietary name. Tofranil-PM
$(C_{19}H_{24}N_2)_2,C_{23}H_{16}O_6$=949.2
CAS—10075-24-8
A yellow powder.
Practically insoluble in water; soluble in ethanol, chloroform and ether.

Imipramine Hydrochloride

Synonym. Imizine
Proprietary names. Antidep; Berkomine; Celamine; Ethipramine; Imavate; Impril; Iramil; Janimine; Medipramine; Melipramine; Mipralin; Novo-Pramine; Presamine; Primonil; Pryleugan; Sermonil; Talpramin; Tofranil.
$C_{19}H_{24}N_2$,HCl=316.9
CAS—113-52-0
A white or slightly yellow crystalline powder. M.p. 174° to 175° (crystals from acetone).
Soluble 1 in 2 of water, 1 in 1.5 of ethanol and 1 in 1.5 of chloroform; sparingly soluble in acetone; practically insoluble in ether.

Dissociation Constant. pK_a 9.5 (24°).

Partition Coefficient. Log *P* (octanol/pH 7.4), 2.5.

Colour Tests. Forrest Reagent—blue; FPN Reagent—blue; Liebermann's Test—blue; Mandelin's Test—blue (add water).

Thin-layer Chromatography. System TA—Rf 48; system TB—Rf 48; system TC—Rf 23; system TE—Rf 67; system TL—Rf 13; system TAE—Rf 21; system TAF—Rf 47; system TAJ—Rf 07; system TAK—Rf 02; system TAL—Rf 52. (Dragendorff spray, positive; FPN reagent, blue; acidified iodoplatinate solution, positive; Marquis reagent, blue.)

Gas Chromatography. System GA—imipramine RI 2230; desipramine RI 2235; M (OH-) RI 2565; M (OH-methoxy-ring) RI 2390; M (OH-ring) RI 2240; M (di-OH-ring) RI 2600; M (ring) RI 1930; M (OH-)-AC RI 2610; M (OH-methoxy-ring)-AC RI 2370; M (OH-ring)-AC RI 2535; M (bis-nor-)-AC RI 2640; M (OH-)-Me RI 2480; system GB—imipramine RI 2314; M (2-OH-) RI 2636; M (10-OH-) RI 2494; M (di-OH-) RI 2962; M (OH-methoxy-) RI 2715; system GF—imipramine RI 2540; system GM—imipramine RRT 0.784 (relative to iprindole); system GS—imipramine Retention time, 17.1 min.

High Performance Liquid Chromatography. System HA—imipramine *k* 4.2, desipramine *k* 2.1, 2-hydroxydesipramine *k* 1.2, 2-hydroxyimipramine *k* 3.1; system HF—imipramine *k* 4.17, desipramine *k* 3.60; system HX—RI 437; system HY—RI 335; system HZ—Retention time, 6.7 min; system HAA—Retention time, 15.1 min; system HAM—imipramine Retention time 9.0 min; system HAV—imipramine *k* 6.4; system HAX—imipramine Retention time 14.7 min; system HAY—imipramine Retention time 6.8 min; system HAZ—imipramine *k* 1.62; M (10-OH-) *k* 0.39; M (2-OH-) *k* 0.39; M (*N*-oxide) *k* 1.85.

Ultraviolet Spectrum. Aqueous acid—251 nm (A^1_1=298a); aqueous alkali—252 nm. (See below.)

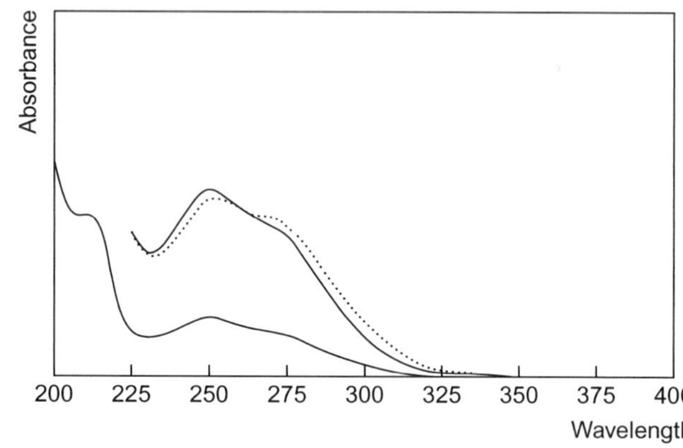

Infra-red Spectrum. Principal peaks at wavenumbers 740, 747, 765, 1230, 1110, 756 cm^{-1} (imipramine hydrochloride, KBr disk). (See below.)

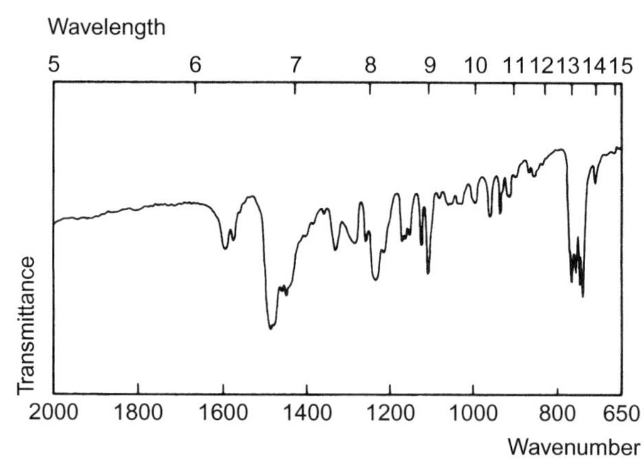

Mass Spectrum. Principal ions at *m*/*z* 58, 235, 85, 234, 236, 195, 193, 208; desipramine 235, 195, 208, 44, 234, 193, 194, 71; 2-hydroxyimipramine 58, 251, 250, 211, 85, 42, 209, 296; 2-hydroxydesipramine 44, 209, 211, 250, 210, 224, 42, 251.

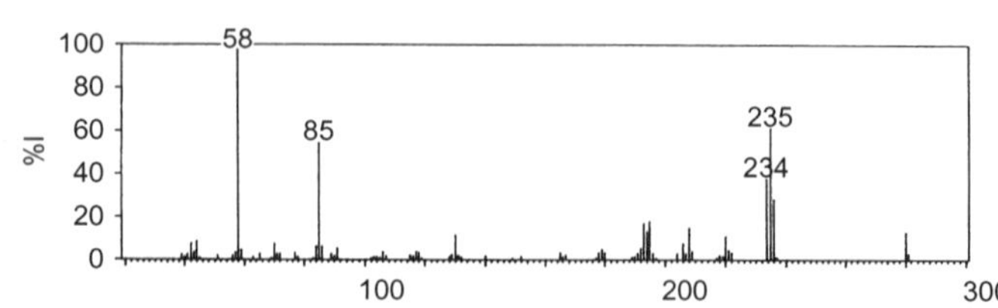

Quantification

Gas chromatography. In plasma: limit of quantification 90 μg/L, NPD—S. Ulrich and J. Martens, *J. Chromatogr. Biomed. Sci. Appl.*, 1997, *696(2)*, 217–234.

Gas chromatography–mass spectrometry. In serum or plasma: imipramine and desipramine, limit of detection 4 μg/L—D. Alkalay *et al.*, *Biomed. Mass Spectrom.*, 1979, *6*, 200–204. In plasma: imipramine and desipramine—F. Pommier *et al.*, *J. Chromatogr. B. Biomed. Sci. Appl.*, 1997, *703*, 147–158. In plasma: imipramine and other tricyclics, limit of quantification 25 μg/L—B. A. Way *et al.*, *J. Anal. Toxicol.*, 1998, *22*, 374–382. In blood: imipramine and other antidepressants, limits of detection 39 to 153 μg/L—M. A. Martinez *et al.*, *J. Anal. Toxicol.*, 2002, *26*, 296–302.

High performance liquid chromatography. In plasma: imipramine, desipramine and the 2-hydroxy metabolites, limit of detection 5 µg/L, electrochemical detection—R. F. Suckow and T. B. Cooper, *J. Pharm. Sci.*, 1981, *70*, 257–261. In plasma or serum: imipramine and desipramine, limit of detection 5 µg/L, UV detection—P. M. Kabra *et al.*, *Clin. Chim. Acta*, 1981, *111*, 123–132. In plasma: imipramine, desipramine and their hydroxy metabolites, UV and coulometric detection—J. P Foglia *et al.*, *J. Chromatogr.*, 1991, *572*, 247–258. In plasma or urine: imipramine and metabolites, UV detection—K. K. Nielsen and K. Brosen, *J. Chromatogr.*, 1993, *612*, 87–94. In plasma or urine: imipramine, desipramine and metabolites, limit of quantification for imipramine 0.5 µg/L, electrochemical detection—E. Koyama *et al.*, *Ther. Drug Monit.*, 1993, *15*, 224–235. In plasma or urine: imipramine, desipramine and metabolites, limit of quantification for imipramine and desipramine 3 µg/L, electrochemical detection—A. G. Chen *et al.*, *J. Chromatogr. B. Biomed. Sci. Appl.*, 1997, *693*, 153–158.

Disposition in the Body. Readily absorbed after oral administration and widely distributed throughout the tissues. Imipramine undergoes considerable first-pass metabolism, mainly by demethylation to the primary active metabolite desipramine. Other major metabolic reactions include hydroxylation at the 2- or 10-positions followed by conjugation. Both pathways are genetically determined. 2-Hydroxyimipramine and 2-hydroxydesipramine appear to be active. A large number of metabolites have been identified in the urine and less than 10% of a dose is excreted unchanged. A total of about 40% of a dose is excreted in the urine in 24 h and about 70% in 72 h. Of the urinary material, up to 40% consists of free and conjugated 2-hydroxydesipramine, up to about 25% is free and conjugated 2-hydroxyimipramine, and about 15% is free and conjugated 2-hydroxyiminodibenzyl; small amounts of didesmethylimipramine, free iminodibenzyl, and 10-hydroxydesipramine are also found. The excretion of unchanged drug and unconjugated metabolites is pH-dependent and is increased in acid urine. About 20% of a dose is eliminated in the faeces. Imipramine and desipramine cross the blood–brain barrier and placenta. They are excreted in breast milk in concentrations similar to those found in plasma.

Therapeutic concentration. Plasma concentrations vary considerably between individual subjects; therapeutic effect has been correlated with plasma concentrations of imipramine plus desipramine greater than 0.1 mg/L.

Following a single oral dose of 50 mg to 8 subjects, peak plasma concentrations of 0.010 to 0.083 mg/L (mean 0.03) of imipramine and 0.004 to 0.014 mg/L (mean 0.008) of desipramine were attained in about 3.4 h and 4.8 h, respectively [N. Sistovaris *et al.*, *J. Chromatogr.*, 1983, *277 Biomed. Appl.*, *28*, 273–281].

After daily oral doses of 50 to 300 mg (mean 100) to 24 subjects, the following steady-state plasma concentrations were reported: imipramine 0.01 to 0.11 mg/L (mean 0.05), desipramine 0.02 to 0.33 mg/L (mean 0.09), 2-hydroxyimipramine 0 to 0.02 mg/L (mean 0.01), 2-hydroxydesipramine 0 to 0.06 mg/L (mean 0.03), didesmethylimipramine 0 to 0.04 mg/L (mean 0.007) [L. F. Gram *et al.*, *Clin. Pharmacol. Ther.*, 1983, *33*, 335–342].

Toxicity. In adults the estimated minimum lethal dose is 1 g, although fatalities have occurred with less and patients have survived the ingestion of as much as 5 g. In children, as little as 350 mg may be fatal. Blood concentrations greater than 0.5 mg/L (imipramine and desipramine) may cause toxic effects and imipramine concentrations of 0.8 to 4.5 to 13 mg/L have been associated with fatalities.

In 5 fatalities attributed to overdosage with imipramine, the following postmortem concentrations were found: blood 0.3 to 4.1 mg/L (mean 2.7), bile 19.2 to 71.7 mg/L (mean 46, 4 cases), liver blood 0.2 to 9.6 mg/L (mean 4.6), urine 0.8 to 12.7 mg/L (mean 5.3, 3 cases) [A. E. Robinson *et al.*, *J. Anal. Toxicol.*, 1979, *3*, 3–13].

A 49-year-old female was found dead after having ingested 33 tablets equivalent to 925 mg of imipramine; blood and tissue concentrations were as follows: blood 14 mg/L, bile 88 mg/L, brain 25 µg/g, liver 75 µg/g [K. D. Singh *et al.*, *Bull. Int. Assoc. Forensic Toxicol.*, 1978, *14*(2), 21].

The following concentrations were reported in a fatality involving the ingestion of imipramine, paracetamol and ethanol (concentrations of imipramine, desipramine, 2-hydroxyimipramine and paracetamol, respectively): blood 9.0, 1.1, 3.9 and 11 mg/L; urine 92, 14, 42, not reported. The ethanol concentration in the blood and urine was < 100 mg/L and 1050 mg/L, respectively [A. D. Fraser *et al.*, *J. Forensic Sci.*, 1987, *32*, 543–549].

In 2 unrelated cases, a 7-year-old boy and a 21-year-old woman died suddenly while receiving chronic imipramine therapy—evidence indicated that neither had ingested an acute overdose. The following postmortem tissue concentrations were reported for imipramine and desipramine, respectively. In the boy: left femoral blood 0.5 and 6.7 mg/L, right femoral blood 1.2 and 9.9 mg/L, aorta blood 1.0 and 8.7 mg/L, liver 68 and 400 µg/g. In the female, the imipramine and desipramine concentrations were 0.6 and 3.74 mg/L in the femoral blood and 37 and 261 µg/g in the liver [J. R. Swanson *et al.*, *J. Forensic Sci.*, 1997, *42*, 335–339].

Bioavailability. About 50%, but there is considerable intersubject variation.

Half-life. Plasma half-life, imipramine 8 to 20 h, increased in children, elderly subjects, and after overdose; desipramine 10 to 35 h.

Volume of distribution. 10 to 20 L/kg.

Clearance. Plasma clearance, about 15 mL/min/kg, decreased in elderly subjects.

Distribution in blood. Plasma : whole blood ratio, 0.98.

Protein binding. In plasma, 85 to 95%.

Note. For a review of the pharmacokinetics of tricyclic antidepressants see G. Molnar and R. N. Gupta, *Biopharm. Drug Dispos.*, 1980, *1*, 283–305.

Dose. In the treatment of depression, 25 to 200 mg of imipramine hydrochloride daily; up to 300 mg daily has been given.

Imolamine

Anti-anginal Vasodilator

4-[2-(Diethylamino)ethyl]-5-imino-3-phenyl-Δ^2-1,2,4-oxadiazoline
$C_{14}H_{20}N_4O$=260.3
CAS—318-23-0

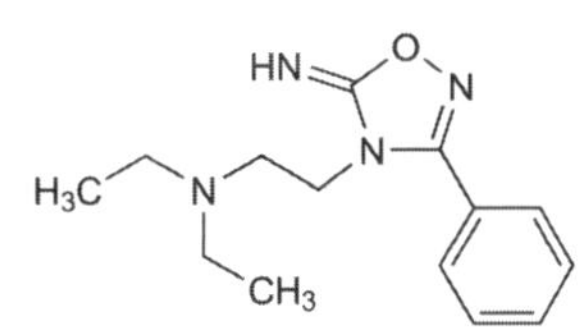

Imolamine Hydrochloride

Proprietary name. Irrigor
$C_{14}H_{20}N_4O,HCl$=296.8
CAS—15823-89-9
A white powder. M.p. 154° to 155°.
Soluble 1 in 1 of water and 1 in 500 of ethanol; slightly soluble in chloroform.

Partition Coefficient. Log *P* (octanol/water), 3.6.

Thin-layer Chromatography. System TA—Rf 56. (Acidified iodoplatinate solution, positive.)

Gas Chromatography. System GA—RI 2177.

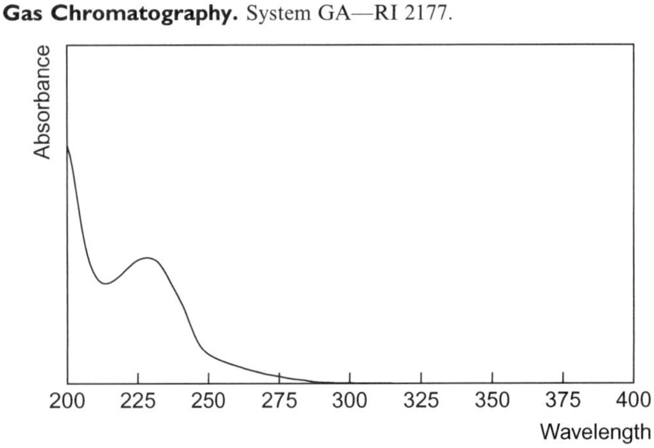

Infra-red Spectrum. Principal peaks at wavenumbers 1638, 698, 752, 1610, 1500, 1070 cm^{-1} (KBr disk).

Dose. Imolamine hydrochloride has been given in doses of 30 to 90 mg daily.

Indapamide

Diuretic

Proprietary names. Agelan; Clonilix; Dapamax; Dapa-Tabs; Daptril; Extur; Fludapamide; Fludex; Inamide; Indaflex; Indamol; Indanorm; Indolin; Lozol; Napamide; Naplin; Natramid; Natrilix; Nindaxa; Opumide; Pressural; Tandix; Tertensif.
3-(Aminosulfonyl)-4-chloro-*N*-(2,3-dihydro-2-methyl-1*H*-indol-1-yl)-benzamide
$C_{16}H_{16}ClN_3O_3S=365.8$
CAS—26807-65-8

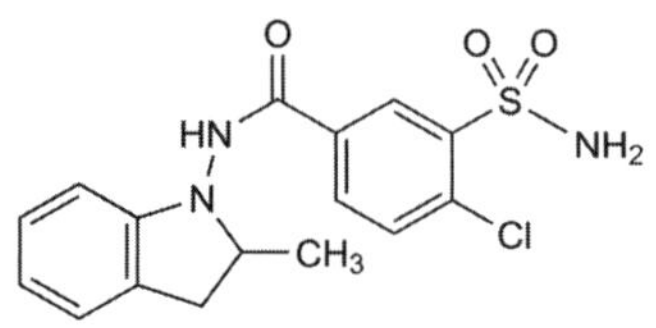

Partition Coefficient. Log *P* (octanol/water), 2.7.

Colour Tests. Koppanyi–Zwikker Test—violet; Liebermann's Test—violet-red; Mandelin's Test—red; Marquis Test—orange→violet; Mercurous Nitrate—black; Sulfuric Acid—pink (slow).

Thin-layer Chromatography. System TD—Rf 38; system TE—Rf 66; system TF—Rf 61; system TAD—Rf 46; system TAE—89; system TAJ—Rf 56; system TAK—Rf 22; system TAL—Rf 92.

Gas Chromatography. System GA—indapamide-Me_3 RI 3035; system GX—indapamide-Me_3 retention time 9.0 min.

High Performance Liquid Chromatography. System HA—*k* 0.1.

Ultraviolet Spectrum. Ethanol—242 nm (A^1_1=627b), 288 nm.

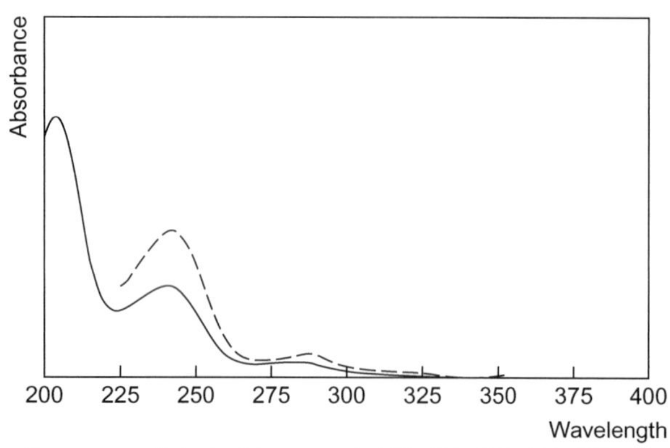

Mass Spectrum. Principal ions at *m/z* 147, 131, 130, 132, 119, 148, 365, 218.

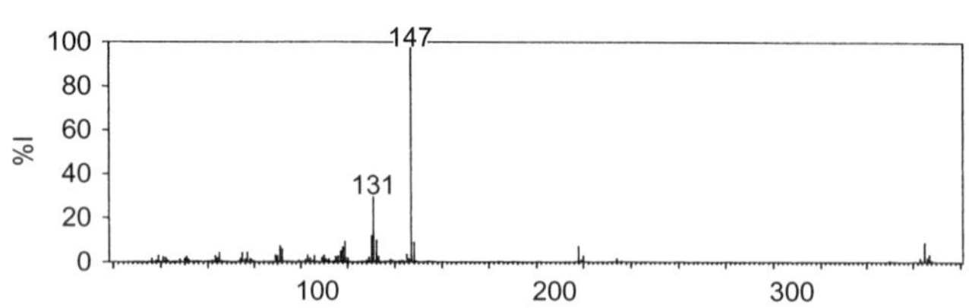

Quantification

High performance liquid chromatography. In blood, plasma or urine: limit of detection 25 µg/L in plasma, 50 µg/L in blood and urine, UV detection—R. L. Choi *et al.*, *J. Chromatogr.* 1982, *230(19) B Biomed. Appl.*, 181–187. In urine: indapamide and 4-chloro-3-sulfamoylbenzoic acid, limit of detection 25 µg/L, UV detection—P. Pietta *et al.*, *J. Chromatogr.*, 1982, *228(17) B Biomed. Appl.*, 377–381. In blood: UV detection—R. B. Miller *et al.*, *J. Chromatogr.*, 1993, *614*, 293–298. In urine: limit of detection < 1 µg/L, amperometric detection—M. J. Legorburu *et al.*, *J. Chromatogr. Sci.*, 1999, *37*, 283–287.

Disposition in the Body. Rapidly absorbed after oral administration. It is extensively metabolised and about 60% of a dose is slowly excreted in the urine over a period of 8 days with less than 5% as unchanged drug. About 20% of a dose is slowly eliminated in the faeces.

Therapeutic concentration

Following a single oral dose of 5 mg to 22 subjects, a mean peak plasma concentration of 0.26 mg/L was attained in about 2 to 3 h. [P. E. Grebow *et al.*, *Eur. J. Clin. Pharmacol.*, 1982, *22*, 295–299.]

Following daily oral doses of 2.5 mg to 6 subjects, steady-state plasma concentrations of 0.02 to 0.05 mg/L (mean 0.03) were attained in 3 days. [D. B. Campbell *et al.*, *Curr. Med. Res. Opin.*, 1977, *5*, Suppl. 1, 13–24.]

In 12 subjects, a single oral dose of indapamide as either a 2.5 mg immediate-release preparation or as a 1.5 mg sustained-release formulation produced a dose-normalised mean peak plasma concentration of 39.3 µg/L at 0.8 h and 17.6 µg/L at 12.3 h, respectively. [P. Schiavi *et al.*, *Fundam. Clin. Pharmacol.*, 2000, *14*, 139–146.]

Half-life. Plasma half-life, about 15 h.

Protein binding. In plasma, about 80%.

Note. For a review of indapamide see M. Chaffman *et al.*, *Drugs*, 1984, *28*, 189–235.

Dose. 2.5 to 5 mg daily.

Indeloxazine

Nootropic

Synonym. Indeloxacine
2-[(1H-Inden-7-yloxy)methyl]morpholine
$C_{14}H_{17}NO_2=231.3$
CAS—60929-23-9

Indeloxazine Hydrochloride

Synonyms. CI-874; YM-08054-1.
Proprietary Names. Elen; Noin.
$C_{14}H_{17}NO_2.HCl=267.8$
CAS—65043-22-3
(±)-form: pale yellow needles from methanol, M.p. 169° to 170°.Also reported as colourless acicular crystals from acetone, M.p. 155° to 156°. (+)-form: crystals from ethanol, M.p. 112° to 113°. (−)-form: crystals form isopropanol, M.p. 142° to 142.5°.

High Performance Liquid Chromatography. Column: SI-60 (LiChrosorb, 150 × 4 mm i.d., 5 µm). Mobile phase: *n*-heptane:ethyl acetate (20:3), 1.5 mL/min flow rate. Internal standard (IS): viloxazine. Fluorescence detection (λ_{ex}=350 nm, λ_{em}=505 nm). Retention time: indeloxazine, 3.4 min; IS, 4.2 min [H. Kamimura *et al.*, *J. Pharm. Sci.*, 1985, *74*, 559–561].

Mass Spectrum. Principal ions at *m/z* 100, 56, 231, 132, 103, 115, 57, 70.

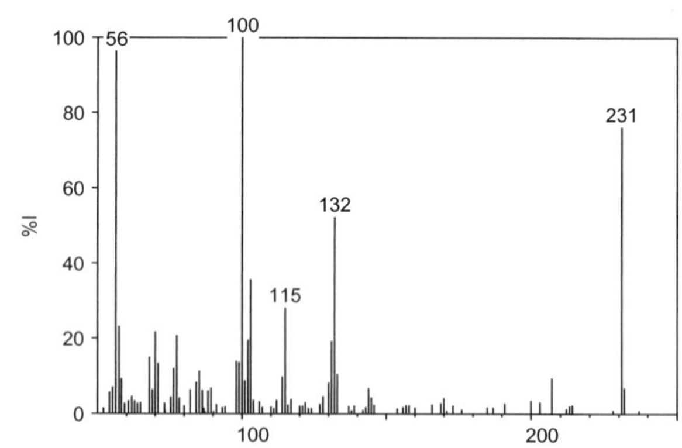

Quantification

Gas chromatography–mass spectrometry. In plasma: limit of detection 2 µg/L—H. Kamimura *et al.*, *J. Pharm. Sci.*, 1985, *74*, 559–561.

High performance liquid chromatography. In plasma: limit of detection 5 µg/L. Fluorescence detection (λ_{ex}=350 nm, λ_{em}=505 nm)—H. Kamimura *et al.*, *J. Pharm. Sci.*, 1985, *74*, 559–561.

Disposition in the Body. Indeloxazine is metabolised in the liver by glucuronidation and metabolites include *trans*-4-(2-morpholinylmethoxy)-1,2-indenediol and *trans*-6-[[(1,2-dihydroxy-4-indanyl)oxy]methyl]-3-morpholine.

Toxicity. Poison by subcutaneous and intravenous routes. Moderately toxic by ingestion.

Indinavir

Protease Inhibitor/Antiviral

2,3,5-Trideoxy-*N*-[(1*S*,2*R*)-2,3-dihydro-2-hydroxy-1*H*-inden-1-yl]-5-[(2*S*)-2-[[(1,1-dimethylethyl)amino]carbonyl]-4-(3-pyridinylmethyl)-1-piperazinyl]-2-(phenylmethyl)-D-*erythro*-pentonamide
$C_{36}H_{47}N_5O_4$=613.8
CAS—150378-17-9

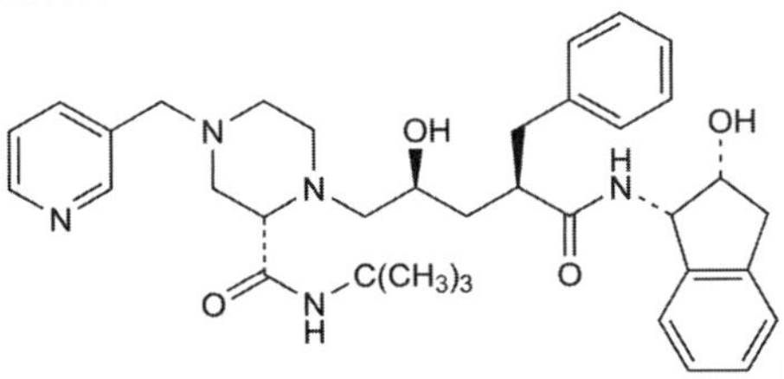

Crystalline two anhydrous forms, M.p. 153° to 154° (first anhydrous form), 167.5° to 168° (second anhydrous form). It is soluble in water: 0.015 g/L (unbuffered) and > 1.5 g/L (pH 4).

Indinavir Sulfate

Synonyms. L-735524; MK-639; MK-0639
Proprietary name. Crixivan
$C_{36}H_{47}N_5O_4.H_2SO_4$=711.9
CAS—157810-81-6
Crystals from absolute ethanol. M.p. 150° to 153° (softens 135°).

High Performance Liquid Chromatography. System HAB—retention time, 4.2 min; system HAC—k 2.0.

Ultraviolet Spectrum. Aqueous acid—210 (major band), 259 (minor) nm.

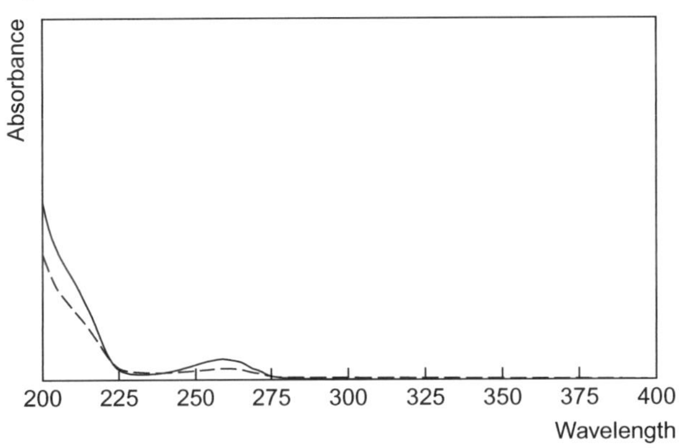

Infra-red Spectrum. Principal peaks at wavenumbers 3295, 1619, 1535, 1215, 1169, 1035 cm^{-1}.

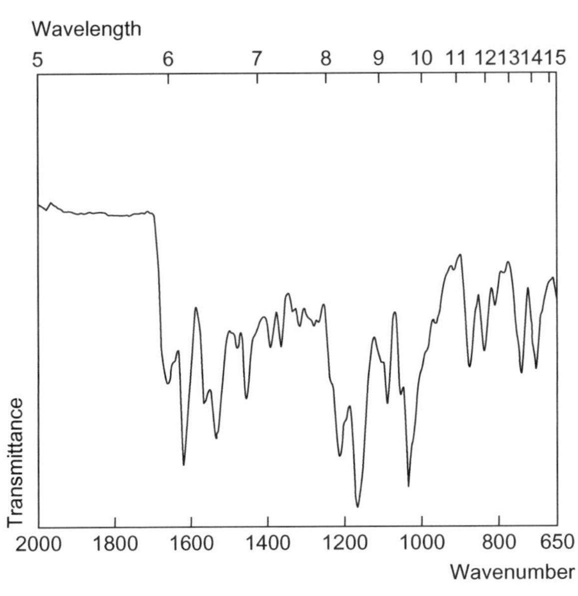

Mass Spectrum. Principal ions at *m/z* 596, 513, 465, 364, 338.

Quantification

High performance liquid chromatography. In plasma and urine: limit of quantification is 0.005 mg/L. UV detection (λ=210 nm)—E. Woolf *et al.*, *J. Chromatogr. A*, 1995, *692(1-2)*, 45–52. In plasma: limit of quantification is 0.05 mg/L. UV detection (λ=261 nm)—G. Aymard *et al.*, *J. Chromatogr. B Biomed. Sci. Appl.*, 2000, *744*, 227–240. In serum: limit of detection is 0.21 mg/L, UV detection (λ=250 nm)—V. A. Simon *et al.*, *J. Chromatogr. A*, 2001, *913(1-2)*, 447–453.

Disposition in the Body. Indinavir is rapidly absorbed after oral administration and peak plasma concentrations are reached within 0.8 h. Absorption is reduced when administration occurs with a high fat meal. The drug is metabolised by oxidation by the CYP3A4 isoenzyme in the liver and also glucuronidation, *para*-hydroxylation, 3′-hydroxylation and N-depyridomethylation. Seven metabolites have been isolated and identified; minor product identified as a 2′,3′-*trans*-dihydroxyindan analogue. Less than 20% of the absorbed dose is excreted in urine, with about half being the unchanged drug. The rest is excreted in faeces.

Therapeutic concentration

12 HIV-positive male patients, aged 40 to 49 years, were fasted overnight and administered indinavir as three dosing regimens. Group 1: 800 mg indinavir twice daily and 100 mg ritonavir twice daily. Group 2: 1200 mg indinavir twice daily. Group 3: 1200 mg indinavir twice daily and 100 mg ritonavir twice daily. The peak plasma indinavir concentration for group 1 was 8.7 mg/L (range 7.5 to 10.0 mg/L); group 2, 13.8 (range 9.5 to 18.0) mg/L; group 3, 15.4 mg/L. These levels were observed at 2.3 (0.5 to 4.0), 1.0 (0.5 to 1.5) and 1.0 to 1.5 h for the three groups, respectively [R. P. van Heeswijk *et al.*, *AIDS*, 1999, *13(14)*, F95–F99].

11 children, aged between 9.0 and 13.6 years (mean 11.0 years), infected with HIV-1 and previously treated with a nucleoside analogue reverse transcriptase inihibitor (zidovudine alone or in combination with dideoxyinosine) were included in the study. Indinavir was administered at 500 mg/m^2 every 8 h in combination with lamivudine and stavudine. The mean maximum plasma level observed was 12.3 mg/L (range 3.2 to 28.8 mg/L) at 1.9 h (1.0 to 4.0 h). The mean minimum level was 0.14 (0.05 to 0.13) mg/L [G. Gatti *et al.*, *Antimicrob. Agents Chemother.*, 2000, *44(3)*, 752–755].

Toxicity

In a study of 11 children undergoing treatment with 500 mg/m^2 indinavir every 8 h (with stavudine or lamivudine), toxicity was observed as renal side effects ranging from mild to severe. This included kidney stones, renal cholic and acute renal failure (serum creatinine level greater than 5 mg/L above the base-line) [G. Gatti *et al.*, *Antimicrob. Agents Chemother.*, 2000, *44(3)*, 752–755].

Bioavailability. 65%.

Half-life. 1.8 h; 0.77 h (children).

Volume of distribution. 195 L.

Clearance. Apparent, 110 L/h.

Protein binding. 61%.

Dose. A dose of 800 mg daily is administered as the sulfate. The dose is reduced to 600 mg in those with mild to moderate hepatic impairment.

Indometacin

Analgesic

Proprietary names. Amuno; Artracin; Confortid; Flexin Continus; Imbrilon; Indochron; Indocid; Indocin; Indoflex; Indolar; Indomax; Indotard; Maximet SR; Mobilan; Pardelprin; Rheumacin; Rimacid; Slo-Indo.
1-(4-Chlorobenzoyl)-5-methoxy-2-methyl-1*H*-indole-3-acetic acid
$C_{19}H_{16}ClNO_4$=357.8
CAS—53-86-1

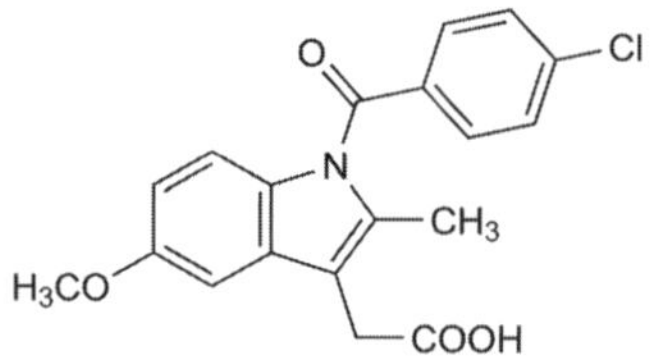

A white to yellow-tan, crystalline powder. M.p. about 155° to 162°. It exhibits polymorphism.

Practically insoluble in water; soluble 1 in 50 of ethanol, 1 in 30 of chloroform, and 1 in about 40 of ether; soluble in acetone.

Dissociation Constant. pK_a 4.5.

Partition Coefficient. Log *P* (octanol/pH 7.4), −1.0.

Colour Tests. Liebermann's Test—black; Mandelin's Test—grey; Marquis Test—orange; Sulfuric Acid—orange

Thin-layer Chromatography. System TA—Rf 94; system TD—Rf 16; system TE—Rf 05; system TF—Rf 13; system TG—Rf 20; system TAD—Rf 38; system TAE—Rf 83; system TAF—Rf 63; system TAJ—Rf 46; system TAK—Rf 90; system TAL—Rf 90. (Chromic acid solution, grey-brown; acidified potassium permanganate solution, positive.)

Gas Chromatography. System GA—indometacin RI 2550 (capillary), RI 2685 (packed); system GD—RRTs of methyl derivative 1.55 and 0.49 (relative to *n*-$C_{16}H_{34}$); system GL—indometacin-Me RI 2770, M (OH-)-Me_2 RI 2880.

High Performance Liquid Chromatography. System HD—*k* 6.95; system HV—RRT 0.87 (relative to meclofenamic acid); system HX—RI 607; system HY—RI 590; system HZ—retention time 14.4 min; system HAA—retention time 21.7 min; system HAX—retention time 8.5 min; system HAY—retention time 9.2 min.

Ultraviolet Spectrum. Methanolic acid—318 nm (A^1_1=180a); aqueous alkali—230, 279 nm (A^1_1=213a). (See below)

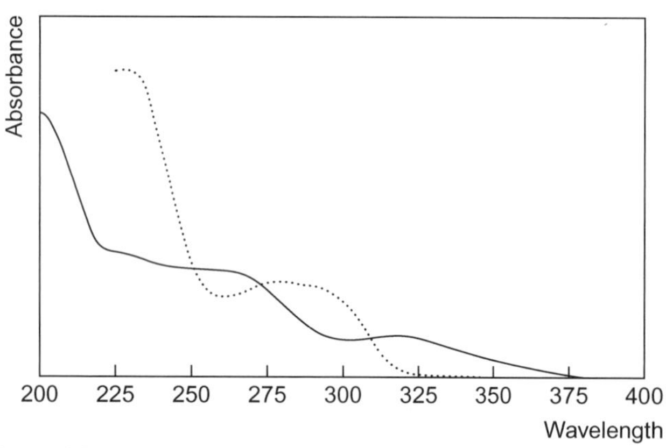

Infra-red Spectrum. Principal peaks at wavenumbers 1681, 1228, 1218, 1706, 1299, 1065 cm^{-1} (KBr disk).

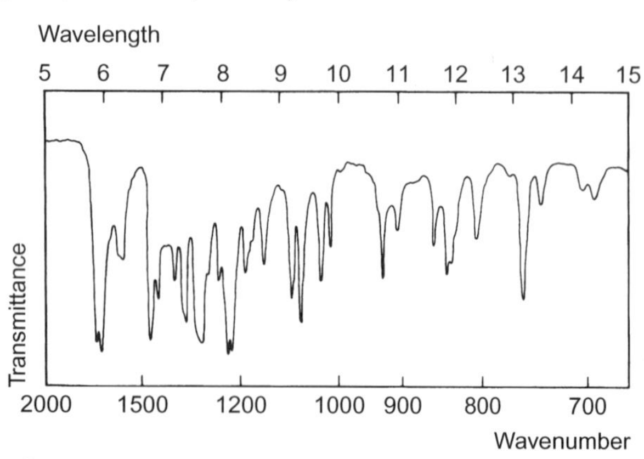

Mass Spectrum. Principal ions at *m/z* 139, 141, 357, 111, 359, 140, 113, 75; M (OH-)-Me_2 239, 298, 135, 191, 107, 103.

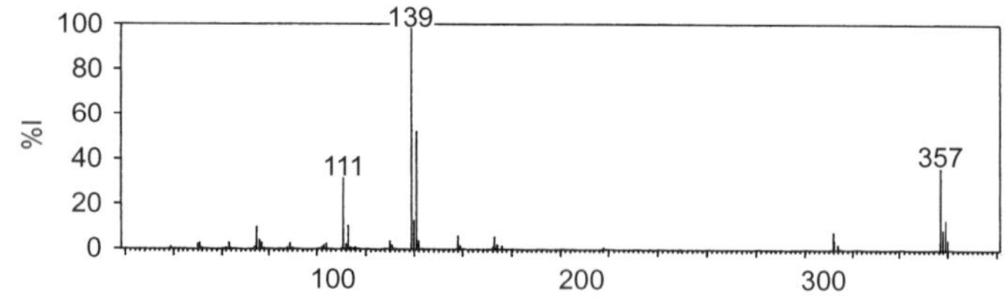

Quantification

Gas chromatography. In plasma or urine: indometacin and desmethylindometacin, limit of detection 10 µg/L, ECD—P. Guissou *et al.*, *J. Chromatogr.* 1983, *277(28) B Biomed. Appl.*, 368–373.

Gas chromatography–mass spectrometry. In plasma or synovial fluid, limit of detection <0.1 µg/L—M. Dawson *et al.*, *Biomed. Environ. Mass Spectrom.*, 1990, *19*, 453–458. In plasma or urine: indometacin and other NSAIDs—A. K. Singh *et al.*, *J. Chromatogr.*, 1991, *568*, 351–361.

High performance liquid chromatography. In plasma or urine: indometacin and desmethylindometacin, limit of detection 25 µg/L for indometacin in plasma, fluorescence detection—M. S. Bernstein and M. A. Evans, *J. Chromatogr.* 1982, *229(18) B Biomed. Appl.*, 179–187. In serum: limit of detection 20 µg/L—I. Roberts and I. M. Smith, *Ann. Clin. Biochem.*, 1987, *24*, 167–171. In plasma: limit of detection 10 µg/L, spectrophotometric detection—P. Hubert *et al.*, *J. Pharm. Biomed. Anal.*, 1989, *7*, 1819–1827. In plasma or urine: indometacin and other NSAIDs, limits of detection 50 to 500 µg/L, diode-array, UV, and fluorescence detection—A. K. Singh *et al.*, *J. Chromatogr.*, 1991, *568*, 351–361. In plasma: limit of detection <50 µg/L—A. G. Johnson and J. E. Ray, *Ther. Drug Monit.*, 1992, *14*, 61–65. In plasma or urine: indometacin and its metabolites, limit of detection for indometacin <60 µg/L—T. B. Vree *et al.*, *J. Chromatogr.*, 1993, *616*, 271–282. In plasma: indometacin and mefanamic acid, limit of detection for indometacin 60 µg/L, UV detection—I. Niopas and K. Mamzoridi, *J. Chromatogr.* 1994, *656 B Biomed. Appl.*, 447–450. In plasma: limit of detection about 50 µg/L, UV detection—J. Sato *et al.*, *J. Chromatogr. B. Biomed. Sci. Appl.*, 1997, *692*, 241–244.

High performance liquid chromatography–mass spectrometry. In plasma—P. J. Taylor *et al.*, *Ther. Drug Monit.*, 1998, *20*, 691–696.

Thin-layer chromatography. In plasma or urine: limit of detection 30 µg/L—I. Soendergaard and E. Steiness, *J. Chromatogr.* 1979, *162(4) B Biomed. Appl.*, 485–488.

Radioimmunoassay. In plasma or urine: limit of detection 50 µg/L—L. E. Hare *et al.*, *J. Pharm. Sci.*, 1977, *66*, 486–489.

Disposition in the Body. Readily and almost completely absorbed after oral administration. Indometacin is subject to considerable enterohepatic circulation. Metabolic reactions include *O*-demethylation, *N*-deacetylation, and glucuronic acid conjugation, the major metabolites being desmethylindometacin (DMI), deschlorobenzoylindometacin (DBI), and desmethyldeschlorobenzoylindometacin (DMBI) and their glucuronides. These substances, together with unchanged indometacin and its glucuronide, are excreted in both the urine (up to about 60% of the dose in 48 h) and the faeces (up to about 30% of the dose in 96 h) in variable amounts. Expressed as a percentage of the dose, the average amounts excreted in the urine in 48 h are: unchanged indometacin 5 to 20% (dependent on urinary pH), indometacin glucuronide 6 to 26%, DMI and its glucuronide 8 to 23%, DBI and its glucuronide 4 to 20%, DMBI and its glucuronide less than 3%; in the faeces the major metabolites found are DMBI (up to about 16%) and DMI (up to about 12%), with only small amounts of unchanged indometacin and DBI.

Therapeutic concentration. In plasma, usually in the range 0.5 to 3 mg/L.

After a single oral dose of 50 mg given to 20 subjects, peak plasma concentrations of 1.0 to 3.0 mg/L (mean 1.9) were attained in 1 to 4. [K. C. Kwan *et al.*, *J. Pharmacokinet. Biopharm.*, 1976, *4*, 255–280.]

Steady-state plasma concentrations of 0.31 to 0.63 mg/L (mean 0.49) were attained in about 6 days after oral doses of 25 mg three times a day to 5 subjects. [G. Alván *et al.*, *Clin. Pharmaol. Ther.*, 1975, *18*, 364–373.]

Toxicity. Toxic effects may be produced by plasma concentrations greater than 5 mg/L.

Half-life. Plasma half-life, 3 to 15 h.

Volume of distribution. About 1 L/kg.

Clearance. Plasma clearance, 1 to 2 mL/min/kg.

Distribution in blood. Plasma:whole blood ratio, 1.9.

Protein binding. In plasma, 90 to 99%.

Note. For a review of the pharmacokinetics of indometacin see L. Helleberg, *Clin. Pharmacokinet.*, 1981, *6*, 245–258.

Dose. 50 to 200 mg daily.

Indoprofen

Analgesic

Synonym. Isindone
Proprietary names. Bor-Ind; Flosin; Flosint; Isindone; Praxis; Reumofene.
4-(1,3-Dihydro-1-oxo-2*H*-isoindol-2-yl)-α-methylbenzeneacetic acid
$C_{17}H_{15}NO_3$=281.3
CAS—31842-01-0

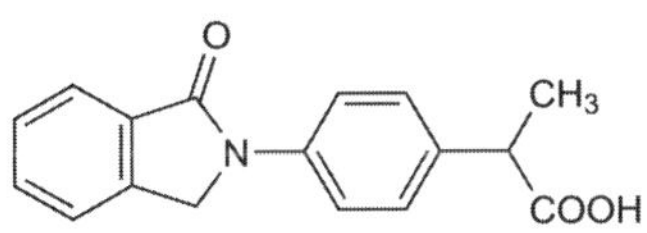

A white crystalline powder. M.p. 212°.
Practically insoluble in water; very slightly soluble in chloroform; freely soluble in dimethylformamide; slightly soluble in methanol; sparingly soluble in 0.1 M sodium hydroxide.

Dissociation Constant. pK_a 5.8.

Partition Coefficient. Log *P* (octanol/water), 2.8.

Thin-layer Chromatography. System TG—Rf 08. (Ludy Tenger reagent, brown-black.)

Gas Chromatography. System GA—indoprofen-Me RI 2708; system GD—RRTs of methyl derivative 2.27 and 2.07 (relative to *n*-$C_{16}H_{34}$).

High Performance Liquid Chromatography. System HD—*k* 1.2; system HV—RRT 0.52 (relative to meclofenamic acid); system HY—RI 406.

Ultraviolet Spectrum. Methanol—282 nm (A^1_1=505a).

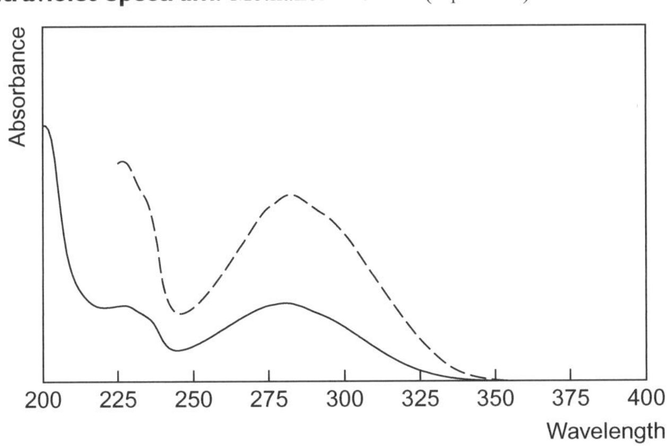

Infra-red Spectrum. Principal peaks at wavenumbers 1680, 1510, 730, 1300, 1220, 1605 cm^{-1} (KBr disk).

Quantification

Gas chromatography. In plasma: limit of detection 400 μg/L, FID—R. V. Smith *et al.*, *J.Pharm. Sci.*, 1977, *66*, 132–134.

High performance liquid chromatography. In plasma or urine: limit of detection 500 μg/L, UV detection—K. Lanbeck *et al.*, *J. Chromatogr.*, 1980, *182(8) B Biomed. Appl.*, 262–266. In plasma: indoprofen enantiomers—S. Bjorkman, *J. Chromatogr.*, 1985, *339*, 339–346.

Disposition in the Body. Rapidly and almost completely absorbed after oral administration. About 80 to 90% of a dose is excreted in the urine in 24 h as the glucuronide conjugate together with small amounts of unchanged drug and metabolites.

Therapeutic concentration
After a single oral dose of 100 mg given to 4 subjects, peak plasma concentrations of 6.9 to 14.3 mg/L were attained in 1 to 1.5 h; following a single oral dose of 200 mg, peak plasma concentrations of 14.2 to 26.1 mg/L were reported at 0.5 to 2 h. [V. Tamassia *et al.*, *Eur. J. Clin. Pharmacol.*, 1976, *10*, 257–262.]

Toxicity. Indoprofen was suspended from use in the United Kingdom in December 1983 because of reports of side-effects and fatalities.

Half-life. Plasma half-life, about 2 h.

Volume of distribution. About 0.1 L/kg.

Clearance. Plasma clearance, about 0.7 mL/min/kg.

Protein binding. In plasma, about 99%.

Dose. Indoprofen has been given in doses of 200 to 800 mg daily.

Indoramin

Antihypertensive

N-[1-[2-(1*H*-Indol-3-yl)ethyl]-4-piperidinyl]benzamide
$C_{22}H_{25}N_3O$=347.5
CAS—26844-12-2

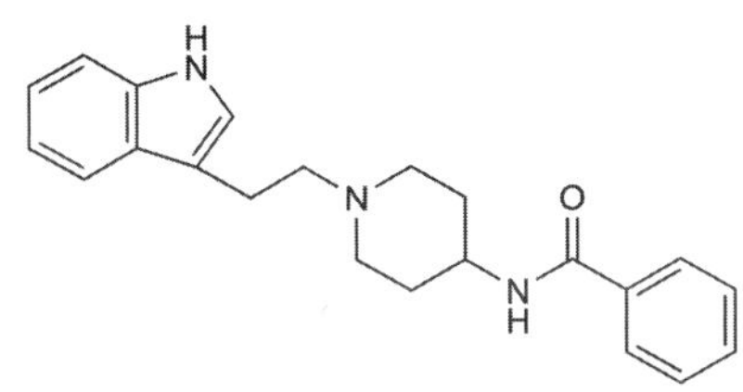

Indoramin Hydrochloride

Proprietary names. Baratol; Doralese; Orfidora; Vidora; Wypresin.
$C_{22}H_{25}N_3O,HCl$=383.9
CAS—33124-53-7 (xHCl)
Crystals. M.p. 230° to 232°.
Slightly soluble in water and chloroform; sparingly soluble in ethanol; soluble in methanol.

Dissociation Constant. pK_a 7.7.

Partition Coefficient. Log *P* (octanol/water), 3.6.

Thin-layer Chromatography. System TA—Rf 84; system TE—Rf 74; system TAJ—Rf 13; system TAK—Rf 10; system TAL—Rf 77.

High Performance Liquid Chromatography. System HAA—retention time 12.5 min.

Ultraviolet Spectrum. Ethanol—273 nm (A^1_1=187b), 279 nm (A^1_1=190b), 289 nm (A^1_1=159b).

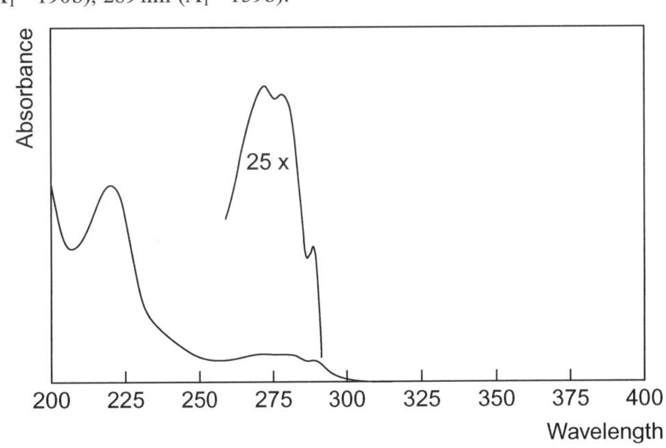

Infra-red Spectrum. Two major polymorphic forms exist. Principal peaks at wavenumbers 1640, 1535, 1316, 745, 1575, 715 cm^{-1} (indoramin hydrochloride form I, Nujol mull); 1620, 1630, 1540, 1560, 740, 1317 cm^{-1} (indoramin hydrochloride form II, Nujol mull).

Quantification

High performance liquid chromatography. In plasma: limit of detection 1 μg/L, fluorescence detection—A. J. Swaisland, *Analyst*, 1981, *106*, 717–719. In plasma: limit of detection 0.5 μg/L, electrochemical detection—D. E. Leelavathi *et al.*, *J. Pharm. Sci.*, 1986, *75*, 421–423.

Disposition in the Body. Readily absorbed after oral administration, but undergoes extensive first-pass metabolism to active metabolites. About 35% of a dose is excreted in the urine in 5 days, mainly as metabolites; less than 10% of a dose is excreted in the urine as unchanged drug; about 47% of a dose is eliminated in the faeces, mainly as metabolites; 6-hydroxyindoramin has been identified as a major metabolite. Other metabolites include acid-labile conjugates of indoramin and 6-hydroxyindoramin.

Therapeutic concentration

Following a single oral dose of 50 mg to 6 middle-aged female subjects, peak plasma concentrations of 4 to 90 μg/L (mean 20) were attained in about 3 h. After the same dose given to 5 elderly female subjects, peak plasma concentrations of 11 to 90 μg/L (mean 40) were attained after about 4 h. [H. M. Norbury *et al.*, *Eur. J. Clin. Pharmacol.*, 1984, *27*, 247–249.]

Following daily oral doses of 150 mg given to 5 subjects, steady-state plasma concentrations of 0.08 to 0.22 mg/L (mean 0.13) were reported. [G. H. Draffan *et al.*, *Br. J. Clin. Pharmacol.*, 1976, *3*, 489–495.]

Toxicity.

In a fatality attributed to indoramin overdose, an antemortem plasma concentration of 6.4 mg/L was reported together with an alcohol concentration of 2.25 g/L. [R. Hunter, *BMJ*, 1982, *285*, 1011.]

Half-life. Plasma half-life, 2 to 8 h (mean 5), increased in elderly subjects.

Volume of distribution. About 7 L/kg.

Clearance. Plasma clearance, about 20 mL/min/kg.

Protein binding. In plasma, about 70 to 90% (concentration-dependent).

Dose. The equivalent of 50 to 200 mg of indoramin daily.

Inositol Nicotinate

Vasodilator

Synonyms. Hexanicotinoyl Inositol; Inositol Niacinate.
Proprietary names. Dilcit; Dilexpal; Hamovannad; Hexanicit; Hexogen; Hexopal; Linodil; Mesonex; Mesotal; Nicolip; Palohex; Vasodil.
myo-Inositol hexa-3-pyridinecarboxylate
$C_{42}H_{30}N_6O_{12}$=810.7
CAS—6556-11-2

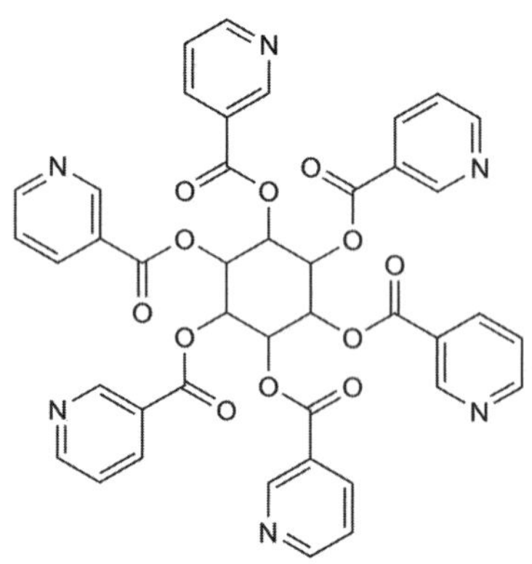

A white crystalline powder. M.p. 254.3° to 254.9°.
Practically insoluble in water and most organic solvents; soluble 1 in 100 of chloroform; soluble in dilute acids.

Partition Coefficient. Log *P* (octanol/water), 1.6.

Thin-layer Chromatography. System TA—Rf 57; system TB—Rf 01; system TC—Rf 43; system TL—Rf 16. (Acidified iodoplatinate solution, positive.)

Ultraviolet Spectrum. Aqueous acid—261 nm (A^1_1=352b).

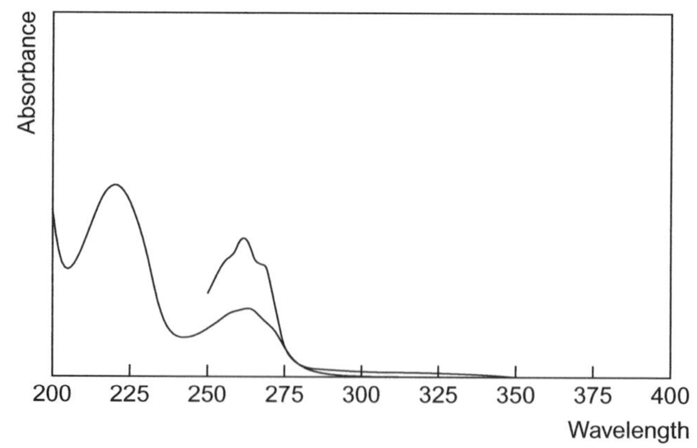

Infra-red Spectrum. Principal peaks at wavenumbers 1272, 1734, 1102, 1593, 1025, 718 cm^{-1} (KBr disk).

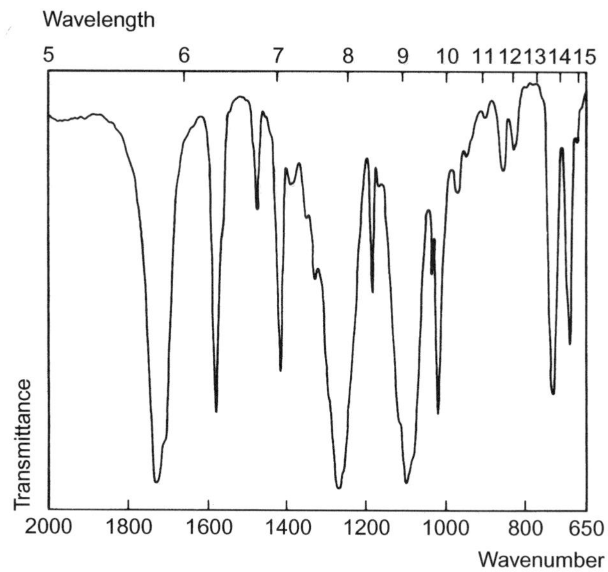

Dose. 1.5 to 4 g daily.

Insulin

Antidiabetic

Insulin is an amphoteric pancreatic protein which is extracted from beef or pork pancreas and purified by crystallisation. Insulin which is structurally identical with human insulin may be produced by chemical manipulation of animal insulin or by recombinant DNA technology.
CAS—9004-10-8; 11061-68-0 (human)

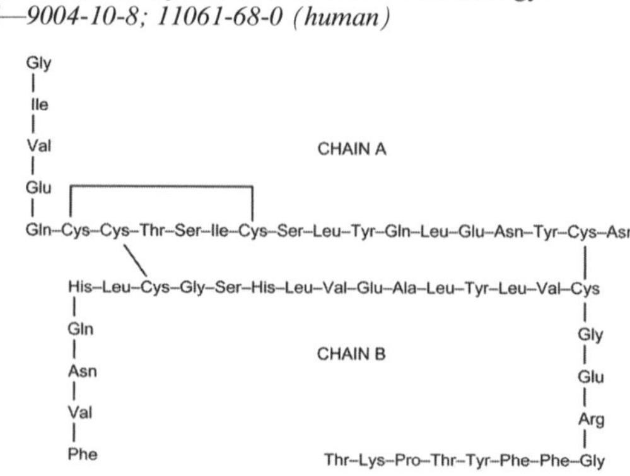

HUMAN INSULIN

A white crystalline powder.

Slightly soluble in water; practically insoluble in ethanol, chloroform and ether; soluble in dilute solutions of mineral acids and, with degradation, in solutions of alkali hydroxides.

Ultraviolet Spectrum. Aqueous acid—276 nm (A_1^1 = 10.3a).

Quantification

High performance liquid chromatography. In plasma: limit of detection 50 µU/mL, UV/visible detection—G. Khaksa *et al.*, *Anal. Biochem.*, 1998, *260*, 92–95.

Enzyme immunoassay. In serum: limit of detection 5 µU/mL—M. Yoshioka *et al.*, *Clin. Chem.*, 1979, *25*, 35–38.

Radioimmunoassay. In serum, subcutaneous fat, or tissues—S. J. Dickson *et al.*, *Forensic Sci.*, 1977, *9*, 37–42. In serum: free, total and antibody-bound insulin—W. D. Gennaro and J. D. Van Norman, *Clin. Chem.*, 1975, *21*, 873–879.

Disposition in the Body. Insulin is an endogenous hormone secreted by the beta cells of the islets of Langerhans of the pancreas; it consists of two linked polypeptide chains. Ineffective after oral administration owing to rapid inactivation by proteolytic enzymes, but well absorbed after subcutaneous or intramuscular injection. The rate of absorption from different sites depends on local blood flow; absorption from the abdomen being faster than that from the arm and that from the arm, faster than from either the thigh or buttock. Exercise may increase absorption. It circulates in the blood as a polymer with a molecular mass of 17 000 to 43 000 and is rapidly taken up by the tissues. About 50% of endogenous insulin in the portal vein is metabolised in a single passage through the liver. It is reduced to two separate chains by glutathione insulin transhydrogenase. The intact molecule or reduced chains may be metabolised by insulin-specific protease to peptides and amino acids. Insulin is filtered at the glomeruli but is reabsorbed and metabolised in the renal tubules, and only small amounts are excreted unchanged in the urine. It is also excreted in the bile.

Therapeutic concentration. In normal subjects, endogenous blood-insulin concentrations vary throughout the day. The fasting or basal concentration in the plasma is usually in the range of 5 to 40 mU/L (mean 17), with 50 to 100 mU/L in the portal vein. During absorption of food the peripheral blood concentration may increase by 10 to 15 times.

Serum-insulin concentrations were measured in 21 diabetics; the daily dose varied from 3 to 80 units (mean 36) and the treatment period from one month to 35 years. The concentration of free insulin in the serum was in the range 10 to 440 mU/L (mean 47) and total insulin (free and antibody-bound) varied from 67 to 17 020 mU/L (mean 2676) [W. D. Gennaro and J. D. Van Norman, *Clin. Chem.*, 1975, *21*, 873–879].

After subcutaneous administration of 0.4 units/kg neutral protamine insulin or neutral protamine lispro insulin to 8 subjects, plasma concentrations of 1.86 (±0.47) µg/L and 2.02 (±0.69) µg/L were attained in 394 (±166) min and 371 (±185) min, respectively [K. Rave *et al.*, *Diabetes Care*, 1999, *22*, 865–866 as reported by P. Roach and J. R. Woodworth, *Clin. Pharmacokinet.*, 2002, *41*, 1043–1057].

In 10 patients receiving two 240 unit doses of inhaled regular insulin via an inhaler and two 24 unit doses of subcutaneous regular insulin on 4 separate study days, a mean peak concentration of 96 mU/L occurred 76 min after the inhaled dose and 47 mU/L at 193 min after the subcutaneous dose [A. D. Perera *et al.*, *Diabetes Care*, 2002, *25*, 2276–2281].

Toxicity

In a 49-year-old diabetic man who intentionally injected himself intravenously with 150 to 250 units of NPH insulin (beef-pork species), a total insulin level of 1389 mU/L, with a free-insulin level of 378 mU/L, was reported; these levels had declined to 1105 and 123 mU/L, respectively, after 18 h [E. His and P. L. Werner, *Diabetes Care*, 1987, *10*, 255–256].

In 12 fatalities caused by insulin injection, the following postmortem tissue concentrations were reported 1 day to 6 weeks after death: blood 1 to 155 mU/L (mean 49), cerebrospinal fluid 62 to 64 mU/L (mean 63). In one case, selected as an example, in which a 43-year-old male was discovered next to empty insulin vials (1200 units in total), postmortem insulin levels were: heart blood 155 mU/L, femoral vein blood 78 mU/L [G. Kernbach-Wighton and K. Puschel, *Forensic Sci. Int.*, 1998, *93*, 61–73].

A 51-year-old non-diabetic woman who was found dead next to two empty insulin syringes (300 units of intermediate type human insulin) and one empty ampoule of 10 mg diazepam. Analysis of heart blood revealed an insulin concentration of 382 mU/L, a diazepam concentration of 210 µg/L, and a C-peptide concentration of 0.58 µg/L [E. Logemann *et al.*, *Arch. Kriminol.*, 1993, *191*, 28–36].

The body of a 68-year-old non-diabetic physician was discovered next to 3 used insulin syringes; a suicide note was found. At postmortem examination, the concentration of insulin was 1848.8 mU/L in serum and 0.4 mU/L in aqueous humour; C-peptide (0.5 mU/L), metoprolol (0.4 mg/L) and alcohol (1.22 g/L) were also present in the blood [M. Junge *et al.*, *Forensic Sci. Int.*, 2000, *113*, 457–460].

Half-life. Plasma half-life, about 5 to 6 min in normal subjects, but may be longer in diabetics who develop anti-insulin antibodies.

Protein binding. In plasma, about 5% in normal subjects, but in diabetics the binding capacity may be extremely high owing to formation of insulin-binding antibodies.

Note. For a review of the biochemistry and forensic aspects of insulin see S. M. Fletcher, *J. Forensic Sci. Soc.*, 1983, *23*, 5–17.

Dose. Usually 10 to 80 units a day, subcutaneously; a dose of more than 80 units would be unusual and may indicate insulin resistance.

Iprindole

Antidepressant

Synonym. Pramindole

6,7,8,9,10,11-Hexahydro-*N*,*N*-dimethyl-5*H*-cyclooct[*b*]indole-5-propanamine

$C_{19}H_{28}N_2$ = 284.4

CAS—5560-72-5

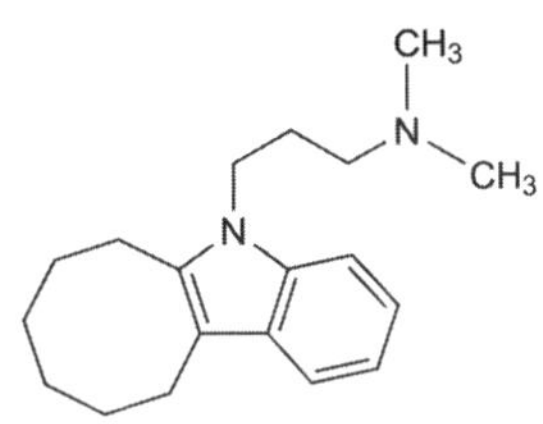

Iprindole Hydrochloride

Proprietary names. Galatur; Prondol.

$C_{19}H_{28}N_2$,HCl = 320.9

CAS—20432-64-8

A white powder. M.p. about 144°.

Soluble in water, ethanol, and chloroform.

Dissociation Constant. pK_a 8.2.

Partition Coefficient. Log *P* (octanol/water), 5.7.

Thin-layer Chromatography. System TA—Rf 47; system TB—Rf 49; system TC—Rf 34; system TL—Rf 16. (Acidified iodoplatinate solution, positive.)

Gas Chromatography. System GA—RI 2335; system GB—RI 2437; system GM—RRT 1.000 (relative to iprindole).

High Performance Liquid Chromatography. System HA—*k* 4.1; system HF—*k* 10.83.

Ultraviolet Spectrum. Aqueous acid—287 nm (A_1^1 = 248a), 293 nm; aqueous alkali—302 nm.

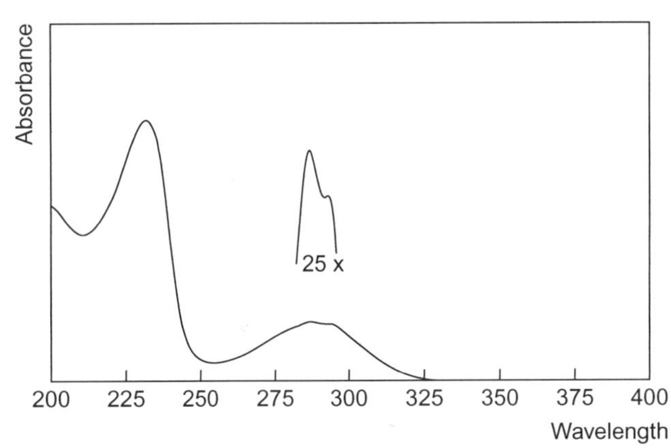

Infra-red Spectrum. Principal peaks at wavenumbers 738, 1650, 1612, 1145, 1173, 1040 cm^{-1} (KBr disk).

Mass Spectrum. Principal ions at *m/z* 58, 170, 284, 213, 145, 212, 159, 144.

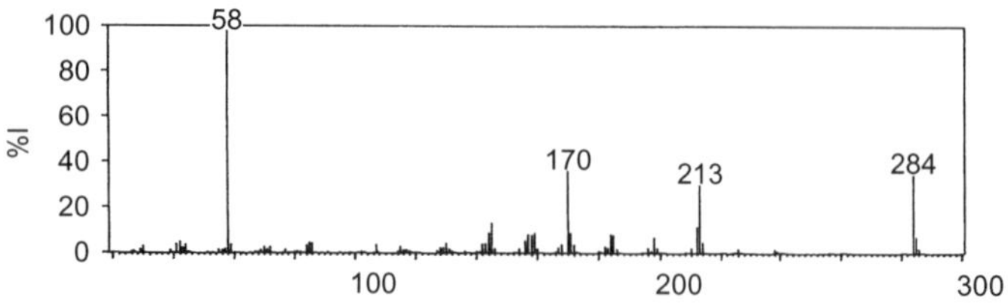

Quantification

Gas chromatography. In plasma: limit of detection 5 μg/L, AFID—G. Caillé *et al.*, *Biopharm. Drug Dispos.*, 1982, *3*, 11–17.

Disposition in the Body. Well absorbed after oral administration. It is slowly excreted in the urine, about 50% of a dose being eliminated in 3 days and it is still detectable 1 week after administration; only about 5% of a dose is excreted in the urine as unchanged drug.

Therapeutic concentration

After a single oral dose of 60 mg given to 5 subjects, peak plasma concentrations of 0.05 to 0.09 mg/L (mean 0.07) were attained in 2 to 4 h. Following oral administration of 30 mg three times daily to 4 subjects, plasma concentrations of 0.03 to 0.08 mg/L (mean 0.06) were reported 10 h after the final daily dose on day 21. [G. Caillé *et al.*, *Biopharm. Drug Dispos.*, 1982, *3*, 11–17.]

Half-life. Plasma half-life, about 35 to 70 h (mean 52).

Dose. The equivalent of 45 to 180 mg of iprindole daily.

Iproniazid

Antidepressant

4-Pyridinecarboxylic acid 2-(1-methylethyl)hydrazide
$C_9H_{13}N_3O = 179.2$
CAS—54-92-2

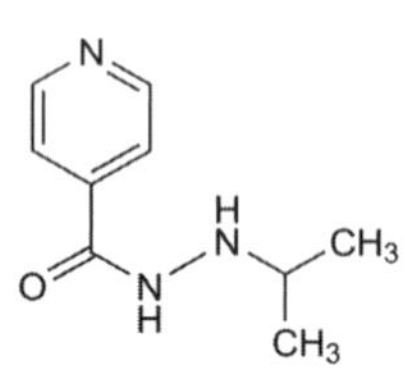

Crystals. M.p. 113°.
Freely soluble in water and ethanol.

Iproniazid Phosphate
Proprietary name. Marsilid
$C_9H_{13}N_3O,H_3PO_4 = 277.2$
CAS—305-33-9
A white crystalline powder. M.p. 175° to 184°.
Soluble 1 in 5 of water and 1 in 90 of ethanol; practically insoluble in chloroform and ether.

Partition Coefficient. Log *P* (chloroform/pH 7.4), 0.

Colour Tests. Cyanogen Bromide—orange-pink; Nessler's Reagent—black

Thin-layer Chromatography. System TA—Rf 69; system TB—Rf 01; system TC—Rf 23; system TE—Rf 41; system TL—Rf 17; system TAE—Rf 70; system TAF—Rf 69. (Dragendorff spray, positive; acidified iodoplatinate solution, positive; acidified potassium permanganate solution, positive.)

Gas Chromatography. System GA—RI 1593; system GB—RI1609

High Performance Liquid Chromatography. System HX—RI 249.

Ultraviolet Spectrum. Aqueous acid—266 nm ($A_1^1 = 235c$); aqueous alkali—242, 307 nm.

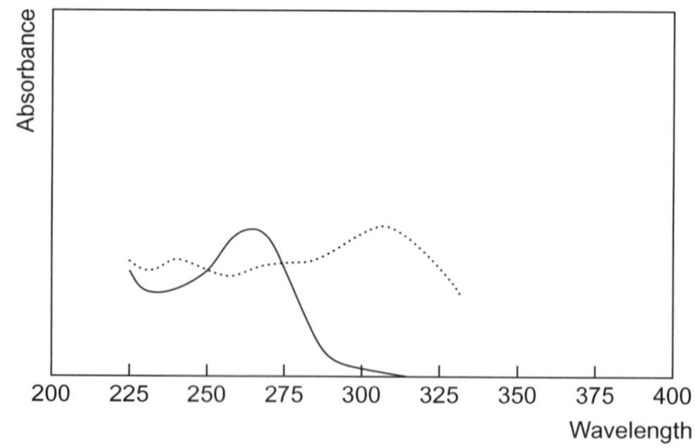

Infra-red Spectrum. Principal peaks at wavenumbers 975, 1090, 1672, 1110, 1065, 1025 cm^{-1} (KBr disk). (See below)

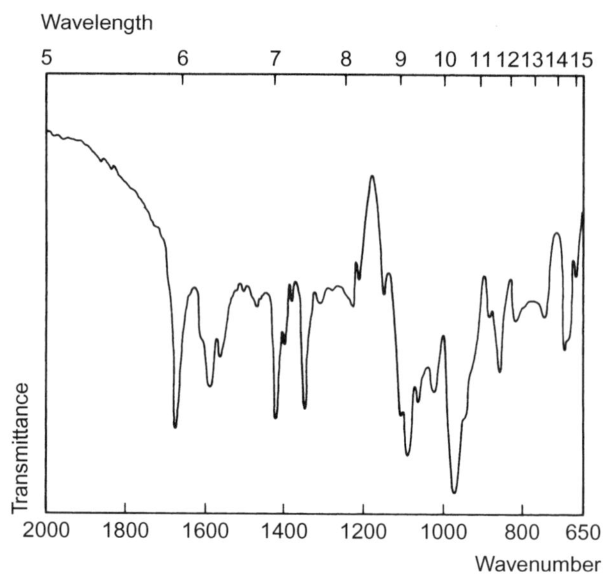

Mass Spectrum. Principal ions at *m/z* 123, 31, 58, 106, 79, 43, 78, 51; isonicotinic acid 123, 51, 78, 106, 50, 52, 105, 39.

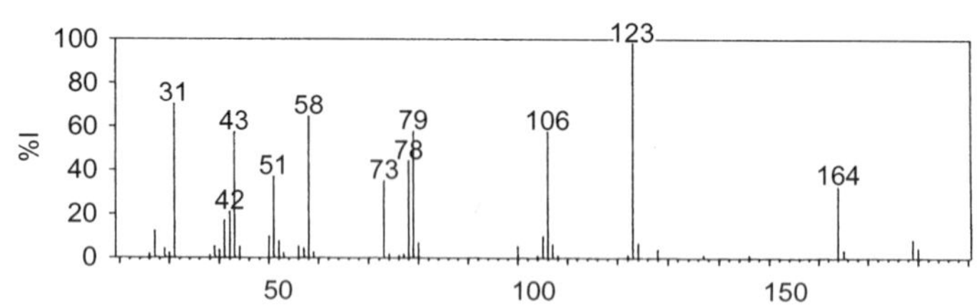

Quantification

Gas chromatography. In urine: FID—R. M. de Sagher *et al.*, *J. Pharm. Sci.*, 1976, *65*, 878–882.

Disposition in the Body. Readily absorbed after oral administration. It is excreted in the urine mainly as metabolites, principally isonicotinic acid, with up to 15% as unchanged drug.

Half-life. Plasma half-life, about 10 h.

Dose. The equivalent of 25 to 150 mg of iproniazid daily.

Irbesartan

Angiotensin II Receptor Antagonist

Synonyms. BMS-186295; SR-47436.
Proprietary names. Aprovel, Avapro.
2-Butyl-3-[[2′-(1*H*-tetrazol-5-yl)[1,1′-biphenyl]-4-yl]methyl]-1,3-diazaspiro[4.4]non-1-en-4-one

$C_{25}H_{28}N_6O$=428.5
CAS—138402-11-6

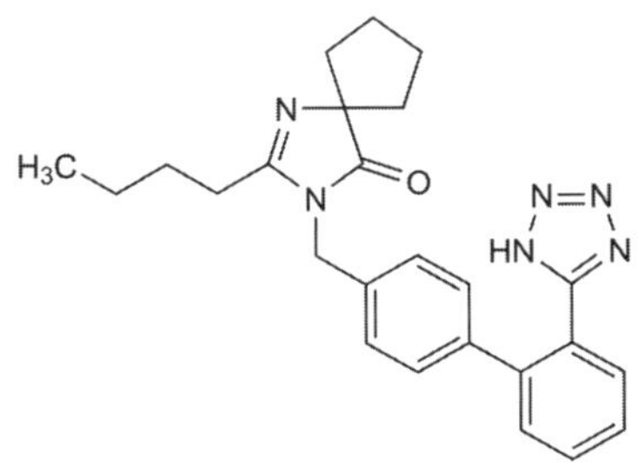

White to off-white crystals (from ethanol, 96%). M.p. 180° to 181°. It is slightly soluble in alcohol and methylene chloride. It is practically insoluble in water.

Dissociation Constant. pK_a 4.5.

Partition Coefficient. Log *P* (octanol/water), 10.1.

Ultraviolet Spectrum. Aqueous acid (0.2 M HCl)—224, 246 nm.

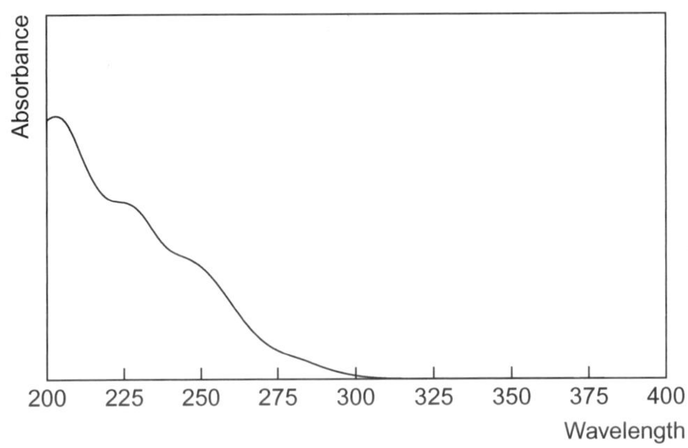

Mass Spectrum. Principal ions at *m/z* 192, 343, 342, 232, 190, 165, 193, 67.

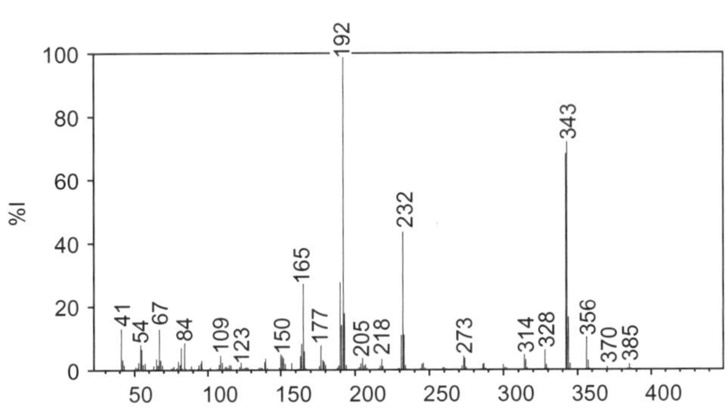

Quantification

High performance liquid chromatography. In plasma and urine: limit of quantification 1.0 µg/L. Fluorescence detection (λ_{ex}=250 nm, λ_{em}=371 nm)—S-Y. Chang *et al.*, *J. Chromatogr. B Biomed. Sci. Appl.*, 1997, *702*, 149–155.

Disposition in the Body. Irbesartan is almost completely absorbed after administration and steady state concentrations are reached within 3 to 4 days. No significant accumulation has been observed. Eight metabolites have been identified and are formed by either glucuronidation or oxidation, primarily by the cytochrome P450 CYP2C9. Excretion is mainly through faeces with less than 2% of an administered dose recovered unchanged in urine.

Therapeutic concentration

12 healthy male volunteers were administered a single oral dose of 50 mg. Peak plasma concentrations of 0.942 mg/L were reached within approx. 3 h [S-Y. Chang *et al.*, *J. Chromatogr. B Biomed. Sci. Appl.*, 1997, *702*, 149–155].

48 healthy men, aged between 18 and 45 years, were administered either a single oral dose of 150, 300, 600 or 900 mg irbesartan (9 in each group and 12 received placebo). Peak plasma concentrations after single doses were 1.9, 2.9, 4.9 and 5.3 mg/L, respectively, which were reached within 1.5 to 2 h. Peak concentrations were very similar after multiple dosing [M. R. Marino *et al.*, *J. Clin. Pharmacol.*, 1998, *38*, 246–255].

Bioavailability. 60 to 80%.

Half-life. 11 to 15 h.

Volume of distribution. 53 to 93 L.

Clearance. Plasma, 0.07 L/h/kg (healthy) and 0.12 L/h/kg (hepatic cirrhosis).

Protein binding. 90%.

Dose. 150 mg once daily which may be increased to 300 mg if necessary. In the elderly or those under haemodialysis, the dose may be reduced to 75 mg.

Irgarol

Insecticide

Proprietary names. Irgarol 1051; Irgarol 1071.
N-Cyclopropyl-*N'*-(1,1-dimethylethyl)-6-(methylthio)-1,3,5-triazine-2,4-diamine
$C_{11}H_{19}N_5S$=253.4
CAS—28159-98-0

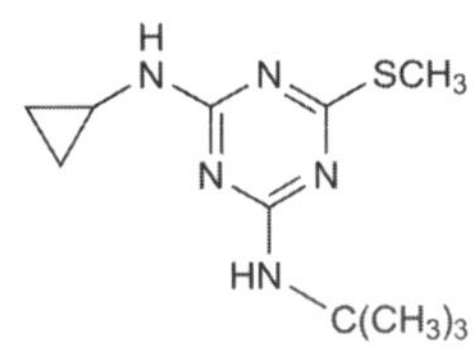

Crystals. M.p. 128° to 133°.
It is practically insoluble in water.

Partition Coefficient. Log *P* (octanol/water), 3.95.

Irinotecan

Antineoplastic

Synonym. CPT-11
[1,4'-Bipiperidine]-1'-carboxylic acid (4*S*)-4,11-diethyl-3,4,12,14-tetrahydro-4-hydroxy-3,14-dioxo-1*H*-pyrano[3',4':6,7]indolizino[1,2-*b*]quinolin-9-yl ester
$C_{33}H_{38}N_4O_6$=586.7
CAS—97682-44-5

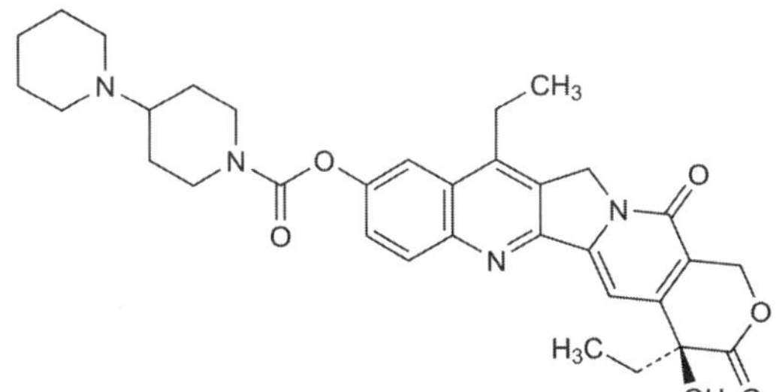

Pale yellow powder. M.p. 222° to 223°.

Irinotecan Hydrochloride

$C_{33}H_{39}ClN_4O_6$=623.2
CAS—100286-90-6

Irinotecan Hydrochloride Trihydrate
Synonyms. DQ-2805; U-101440E
Proprietary names. Campto; Camptosar; Topotectin.
$C_{33}H_{38}N_4P_6$, HCl, $3H_2O$=677.2
CAS—136572-09-3
A pale yellow to yellow crystalline powder. M.p. 256.5°. It is soluble in water and glacial acetic acid; partially soluble in chloroform; slightly soluble in methanol.

High Performance Liquid Chromatography. Columns: (analytical) ODS (Hypersil, 100 × 4.6 mm i.d., 5 µm), (guard) 100 RP-18 (LiChrospher, 4 × 4 mm, 5 µm). Column temperature: 50°. Mobile phase: (A) methanol:ammonium acetate (100 mM) containing tetrabutylammonium sulfate (10 mM) (35:65), adjusted to pH 5.5 with hydrochloric acid; (B) (30:70), adjusted to pH 5.3. Flow rate, 1 mL/min. Fluorescence detection (λ_{ex}=355 nm, λ_{em}=515 nm). Retention times: 8.3 min (A); 16.1 min (B) [P. de Bruijn *et al.*, *J. Chromatogr. B Biomed. Sci. Appl.*, 1997, *698*, 277–285 (A);A. Sparreboom *et al.*, *J. Chromatogr. B Biomed. Sci. Appl.*, 1998, *712*, 225–235 (B)].

Columns: (analytical) TSK gel ODS-80Ts (150 × 4.6 mm i.d., 5 µm), (guard) TSK guardgel ODS-120T (15 × 3.2 mm i.d.). Column temperature: 30°. Mobile phase: acetonitrile:sodium hydrogen phosphate (50 mM) (28:72) containing sodium 1-heptanesulfonate, adjusted to pH 3.0 with orthophosphoric acid. Flow rate, 1 mL/min. IS: camptothecin. Fluorescence detection (λ_{ex}=380 nm, λ_{em}=556 nm). Retention time: irinotecan, 5.4 min; IS, 8.8 min [H. Sumiyoshi *et al.*, *J. Chromatogr.*, 1995, *670*, *Biomed. Appl.*, 309–316].

Columns: (analytical) C_{18} (Zorbax SB, 150 × 4.6 mm, 3.5 µm), (guard) C_{18} (Chromapack, 10 × 3 mm). Mobile phase: acetonitrile:ammonium acetate (100 mM, pH 6.4):triethylamine (15.6:80:0.1) containing tetrabutylammonium phosphate (5 mM). Flow rate, 1.5 mL/min. Fluorescence detection (λ_{ex}=375 nm, λ_{em}=460 nm). Retention time: irinotecan (carboxylate form), 5.7 min; (lactone form), 11.2 min [V. M. M. Herben *et al.*, *J. Liq. Chromatogr. Relat. Technol.*, 1998, *21*, 1541–1558].

Column: (analytical) C_{18} (Nova-Pak, 100 × 5 mm, 4 µm), (guard) C_{18} (Nova-Pak, Guard-Pak). Mobile phase: acetonitrile:ammonium acetate (75 mM, pH 6.4) (22:78) containing tetrabutylammonium phosphate (5 mM). Fluorescence detection (λ_{ex}=355 nm, λ_{em}=515 nm). Retention time: irinotecan (carboxylate form), 4.2 min; (lactone form), 8.2 min [L. P. Rivory *et al.*, *J. Chromatogr.*, 1994, *661*, *Biomed. Appl.*, 133–141].

Ultraviolet Spectrum. Aqueous acid—221, 254, 359, 372 nm.

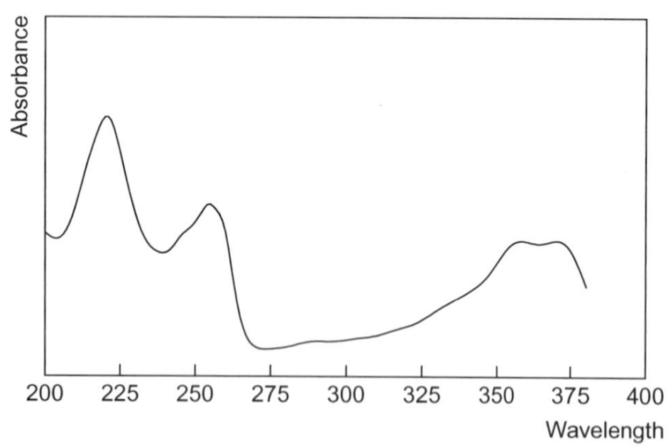

Quantification
High performance liquid chromatography. In plasma: limit of quantification of irinotecan 1.0 µg/L and 0.5 µg/L for the metabolite, SN-38—V. M. M. Herben *et al.*, *J. Liq. Chromatogr. Relat. Technol.*, 1998, *21*, 1541–1558. In faeces and urine: limit of quantification is 100 µg/L—A. Sparreboom *et al.*, *J. Chromatogr. B, Biomed. Sci. Appl.*, 1998, *712*, 225–235.

Disposition in the Body. After intravenous administration, irinotecan is metabolised, by carboxyesterase, in the liver to the active metabolite 7-ethyl-10-hydroxycamptothecin, SN-38 and carboxylic acid. SN-38 then undergoes conjugation, by UDP-glucuronyltransferase, to SN-38 glucuronide. Another metabolite 7-ethyl-10-[4-*N*-(5-aminopentanoic acid)-1-piperidino]-carbonyloxycamphothecin (APC) is produced by oxidative attack at the piperidine group. About 20% of the dose is excreted in urine within 24 h, <1% as SN-38 and approx. 3 to 6% as SN-38 glucuronide. Further excretion is via bile.

Therapeutic concentration
In phase I clinical studies, three patients were administered a dose of 100 mg/m^2, over 30 min, and peak plasma concentrations reached approx. 2800 µg/L by the end of infusion. Peak concentrations of the metabolite, SN-38, reached 35.5 ± 10.9 µg/L [I. Barilero *et al.*, *J. Chromatogr.*, 1992, 575; *Biomed. Appl.*, 275–280].

Toxicity. Diarrhoea if prolonged and over 24 h can be life threatening.

Half-life. 6 to 12 h; 10 to 20 h for the metabolite SN-38.

Volume of distribution. About 157 L/m^2.

Clearance. Body clearance, 15 L/m^2/h.

Protein binding. Irinotecan is approx. 65% (range between 30 and 68%) bound to plasma proteins and SN-38 metabolite 95%.

Dose. The usual dosage range is 40 mg/m^2 body surface to 250 mg/m^2 administered three times a week, once a week to once every 3 weeks. One suggested regimen is 125 mg/m^2 infused over 90 min, once a week for 4 weeks, followed by 2-week rest period. Dose is modified according to toxicity. The maximum dose is 750 mg/m^2/day.

Isoaminile

Cough Suppressant

α-[2-(Dimethylamino)propyl]-α-(1-methylethyl)benzeneacetonitrile
$C_{16}H_{24}N_2$=244.4
CAS—77-51-0

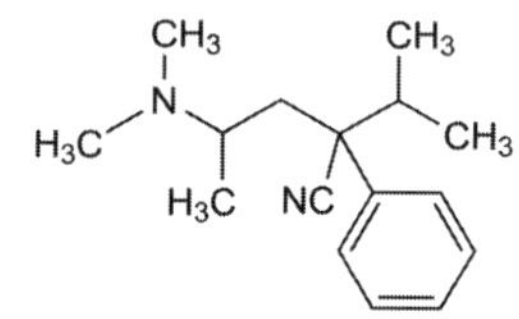

A liquid.

Isoaminile Citrate
Proprietary names. Dimyril; Perocan (citrate or cyclamate).
$C_{16}H_{24}N_2,C_6H_8O_7$=436.5
CAS—28416-66-2
Crystals. M.p. 63° to 64°.
Soluble in water.

Partition Coefficient. Log *P* (octanol/water), 3.5.

Colour Tests. Liebermann's Test—red-orange; Sodium Picrate—orange

Thin-layer Chromatography. System TA—Rf 68; system TB—Rf 58; system TC—Rf 54; system TE—Rf 81 system TL—Rf 55; system TAE—Rf 45.

Gas Chromatography. System GA—RI 1830.

Ultraviolet Spectrum. Aqueous acid—252, 258 nm (A_1^1=7.3a), 264 nm.

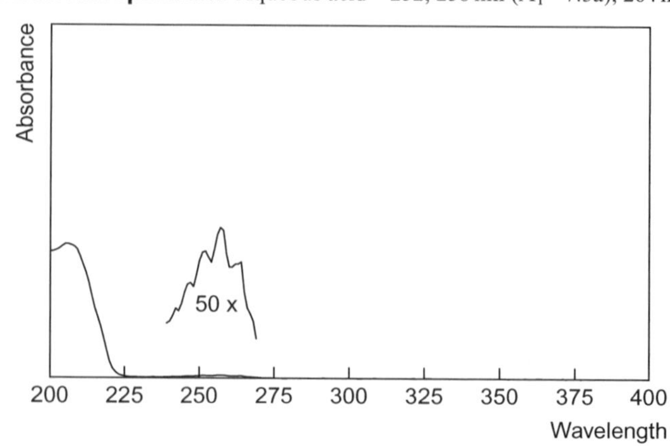

Mass Spectrum. Principal ions at *m/z* 72, 58, 71, 42, 73, 70, 56, 44.

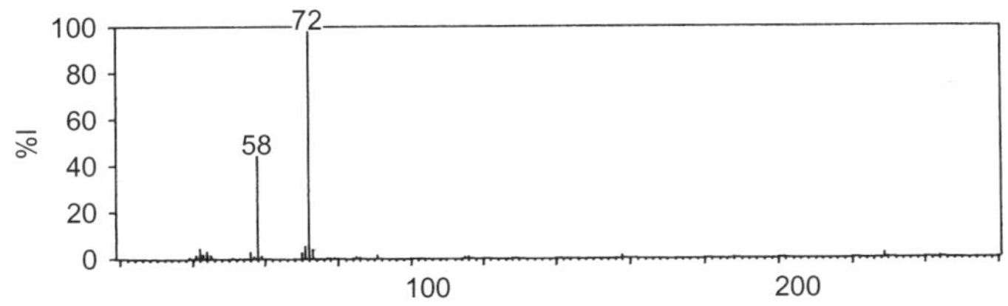

Dose. 40 mg of isoaminile citrate 3 to 5 times daily.

Isocarboxazid

Antidepressant

Proprietary name. Marplan
5-Methyl-3-isoxazolecarboxylic acid 2-benzylhydrazide
$C_{12}H_{13}N_3O_2$=231.3
CAS—59-63-2

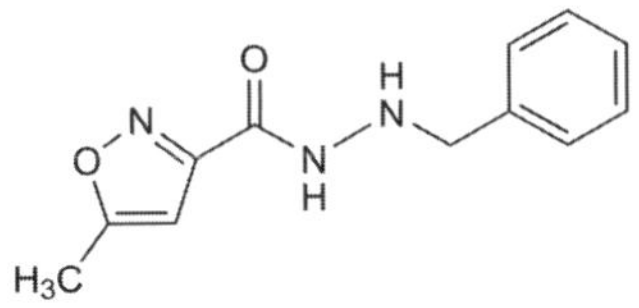

A white or creamy-white crystalline powder. M.p. 105° to 108°.
Very sparingly soluble in hot water; soluble 1 in 150 of ethanol, 1 in 3 of chloroform, and 1 in 50 of ether.

Dissociation Constant. pK_a 10.4.

Partition Coefficient. Log *P* (octanol/pH 7.4), 1.5.

Colour Tests. Liebermann's Test—red-orange; Nessler's Reagent—black

Thin-layer Chromatography. System TA—Rf 71; system TB—Rf 20; system TC—Rf 74; system TE—Rf 75; system TL—Rf 61; system TAE—Rf 84; system TAF—Rf 86; system TAJ—Rf 67; system TAK—Rf 67; system TAL—Rf 92. (Dragendorff spray, positive; FPN reagent, pink-yellow; acidified iodoplatinate solution, positive; Marquis reagent, brown; acidified potassium permanganate solution, positive.)

Gas Chromatography. System GA—RI 1949.

High Performance Liquid Chromatography. System HX—RI 392; system HY—RI 353.

Ultraviolet Spectrum. Aqueous alkali—274 nm (A_1^1=240b).

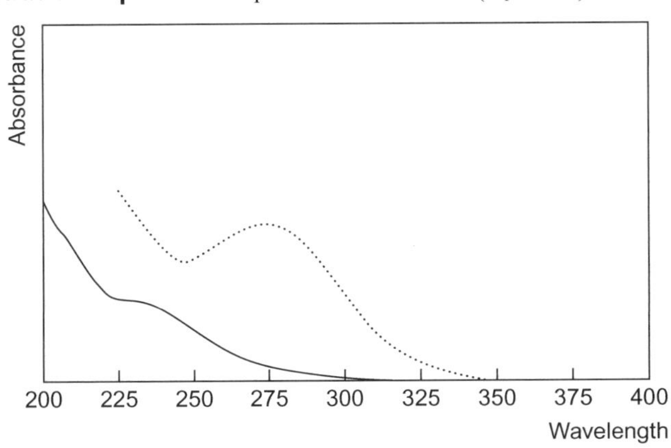

Infra-red Spectrum. Principal peaks at wavenumbers 1670, 750, 705, 870, 815, 1595 cm^{-1} (KBr disk).

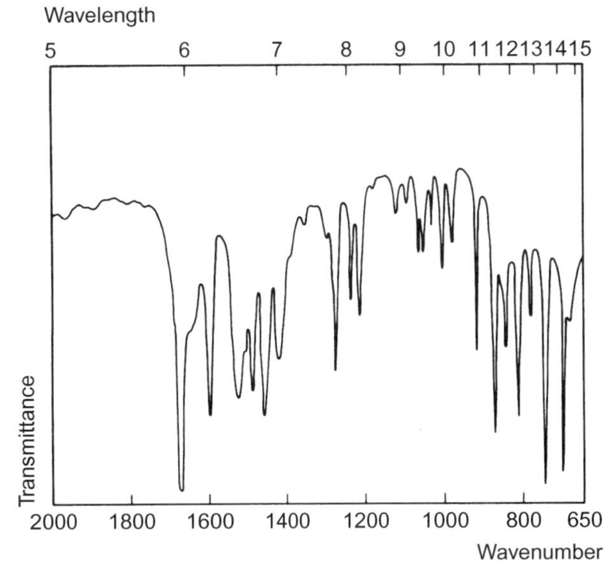

Mass Spectrum. Principal ions at *m/z* 91, 127, 106, 110, 43, 92, 65, 120; hippuric acid 105, 135, 51, 134, 77, 106, 50, 78.

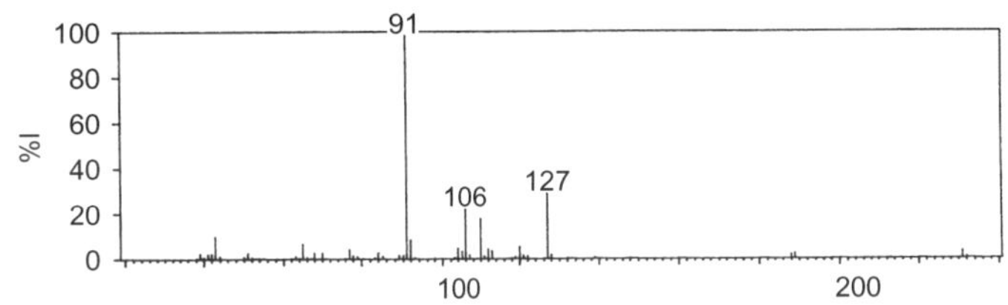

Disposition in the Body. Rapidly absorbed after oral administration. Metabolised by oxidation to benzoic acid followed by glycine conjugation to form hippuric acid; an active metabolite, benzhydrazine, has been detected in animal studies but its formation in man has not been confirmed. About 60% of a dose is excreted in the urine in 24 h and about 70% in 8 days; 90% of the excreted material is hippuric acid and about 2% is unchanged drug.

Therapeutic concentration. Peak plasma concentrations are attained about 4 h after oral administration. Maximal therapeutic effects are attained within 5 to 10 days after beginning treatment.

Toxicity. Toxic reactions from overdosage may occur in a matter of hours despite the long delay in onset of a therapeutic response. A fatality has been reported 24 h after ingestion of 400 mg.

Half-life. Plasma half-life, about 36 h.

Dose. 10 to 30 mg daily.

Isoetarine

Sympathomimetic

Synonyms. *N*-Isopropylethylnoradrenaline; Isoetharine; Win-3046.
Proprietary names. Dilabron; Neoisoprel.
4-[1-Hydroxy-2-[(1-methylethyl)amino]butyl]-1,2-benzenediol
$C_{13}H_{21}NO_3$=239.3
CAS—530-08-5

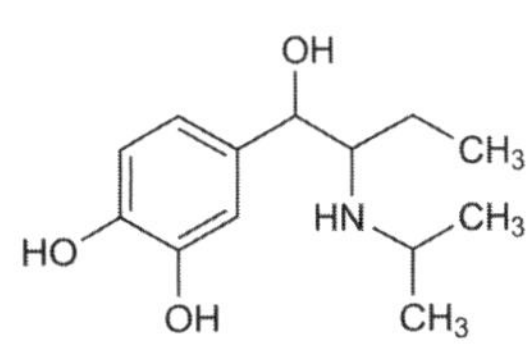

Isoetarine Hydrochloride

Synonym. Etyprenalinum Hydrochloridum
Proprietary names. Asthmalitan Depot; Beta-2; Bronkosol; Numotac.
$C_{13}H_{21}NO_3$,HCl=275.8

CAS—2576-92-3
A white crystalline solid. M.p. 196° to 208°, with decomposition.
Soluble in water; sparingly soluble in ethanol; practically insoluble in ether.

Isoetarine Mesilate
Synonym. Isoetarine Methanesulfonate
Proprietary name. Bronkometer
$C_{13}H_{21}NO_3,CH_4O_3S=335.4$
CAS—7279-75-6
White crystals. M.p. 162° to 168°.
Freely soluble in water; soluble in ethanol; practically insoluble in acetone and ether.

Partition Coefficient. Log *P* (octanol/water), 1.4.

Colour Tests. Ammoniacal Silver Nitrate—red/brown-orange; Ferric Chloride—green; Folin–Ciocalteu Reagent—blue; Mandelin's Test—brown; Marquis Test—yellow→orange; Methanolic Potassium Hydroxide—red→orange→yellow; Nessler's Reagent—black; Palladium Chloride—orange→brown; Potassium Dichromate (Method 1)—green→brown (30 s).

Thin-layer Chromatography. System TA—Rf 59; system TB—Rf 00; system TC—Rf 00; system TE—Rf 36; system TL—Rf 00; system TAE—Rf 73; system TAJ—Rf 00; system TAK—Rf 00; system TAL—Rf 26. (Acidified potassium permanganate solution, positive.)

High Performance Liquid Chromatography. System HX—RI 222.

Ultraviolet Spectrum. Aqueous acid—278 nm ($A_1^1=132a$).

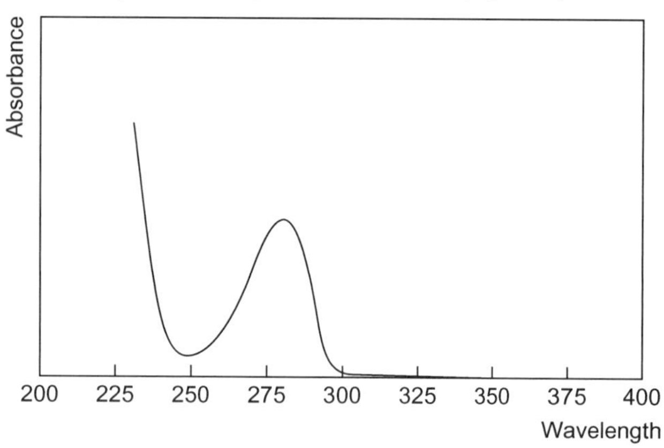

Infra-red Spectrum. Principal peaks at wavenumbers 1200, 1287, 1075, 1114, 1518, 1160 cm^{-1} (KBr disk).

Mass Spectrum. Principal ions at *m/z* 100, 58, 41, 101, 43, 56, 65, 30.

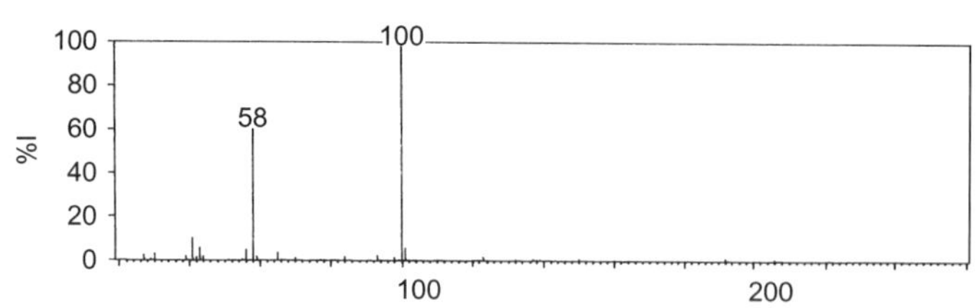

Quantification
High performance liquid chromatography. In plasma: limit of detection 500 µg/L, electrochemical detection—G. B. Park *et al., J. Pharm. Sci.*, 1982, *71*, 932–934.

Dose. 30 to 80 mg of isoetarine hydrochloride daily.

Isometheptene

Sympathomimetic

Synonym. Methyloctenylamine.
Proprietary names. Octin; Octon; Octanil.
N,6-Dimethyl-5-hepten-2-amine
$C_9H_{19}N=141.3$
CAS—503-01-5

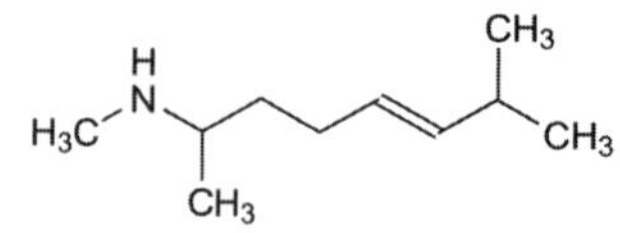

A colourless or slightly yellow oily liquid. B.p. 176° to 178°.
Practically insoluble in water; freely soluble in acetone, ethanol, chloroform and ether.

Isometheptene Hydrochloride
Proprietary name. Octinum (injection)
$C_9H_{19}N,HCl=177.7$
CAS—6168-86-1
An almost white, very hygroscopic, crystalline powder. M.p. 68° to 69°.
Soluble in water and ethanol.

Isometheptene Mucate
Synonym. Isometheptene Galactarate
Proprietary names. Octinum (tablets). It is an ingredient of Midrid.
$(C_9H_{19}N)_2,C_6H_{10}O_8=492.7$
CAS—7492-31-1
A white crystalline powder. M.p. about 152°.
Freely soluble in water; soluble in ethanol; almost insoluble in chloroform and ether.

Partition Coefficient. Log *P* (octanol/water), 3.0.

Colour Test. Mandelin's test—brown.

Thin-layer Chromatography. System TA—Rf 24; system TAJ—Rf 00; system TAK—Rf 04; system TAL—Rf 43. (Acidified potassium permanganate solution, positive.)

Gas Chromatography. System GA—RI 1052; system GB—RI 994.

Ultraviolet Spectrum. No significant absorption, 230 to 360 nm.

Mass Spectrum. Principal ions at *m/z* 58, 55, 41, 44, 43, 128, 59, 56.

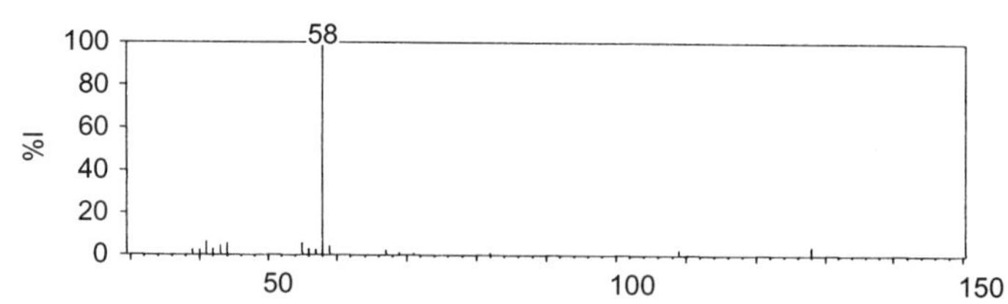

Dose. Isometheptene mucate has been given in doses of up to 520 mg daily.

Isoniazid

Tuberculostatic

Synonyms. INAH; INH; Isonicotinic Acid Hydrazide; Isonicotinoylhydrazine; Isonicotinylhydrazide; Isonicotinylhydrazine; Tubazid; RP-5015; FSR-3.
Proprietary names. Cemidon; Isotamine; Isotinyl; Laniazid; Neoteben; Nicizina; Niconyl; Nicotibine; Nicozid; Nydrazid; Panazid; Rimifon; Tebesium; Teebaconin; Trisofort; Tubilysin. It is an ingredient of Mynah, Rifinah, Rimactazid, Rimafate and Rifater.
4-Pyridinecarboxylic acid hydrazide
$C_6H_7N_3O=137.1$
CAS—54-85-3

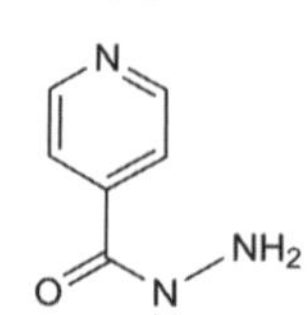

Colourless crystals or white crystalline powder. M.p. 170° to 174°.
Soluble 1 in 8 of water, 1 in about 45 of ethanol and 1 in 1000 of chloroform; practically insoluble in benzene and ether.

Isoniazid Aminosalicylate

Synonyms. Pasiniazid; GEWO-399.
Proprietary names. Dipasic; Paraniazide.
$C_6H_7N_3O,C_7H_7NO_3 = 290.3$
CAS—2066-89-9
Yellow crystals. M.p. 140° to 142°.
Sparingly soluble in water.

Dissociation Constant. pK_a 1.8, 3.5, 10.8 (20°).

Partition Coefficient. Log *P* (octanol/pH 7.4), −1.1.

Colour Tests. Cyanogen bromide—orange; Nessler's reagent—black.

Thin-layer Chromatography. System TA—Rf 47; system TAD—Rf 18; system TAE—Rf 55; system TAF—Rf 49; system TL—Rf 20; system TB—Rf 01; system TC—Rf 11; system TE—Rf 29; system TAJ—Rf 09; system TAK—Rf 03; system TAL—Rf 47. (Acidified iodoplatinate solution, positive.)

Gas Chromatography. System GA—RI 1670.

High Performance Liquid Chromatography. System HY—RI 246; system HZ—Retention time(s) 1.6 min.

Ultraviolet Spectrum. Aqueous acid—266 ($A_1^1 = 390a$); aqueous alkali—298 nm.

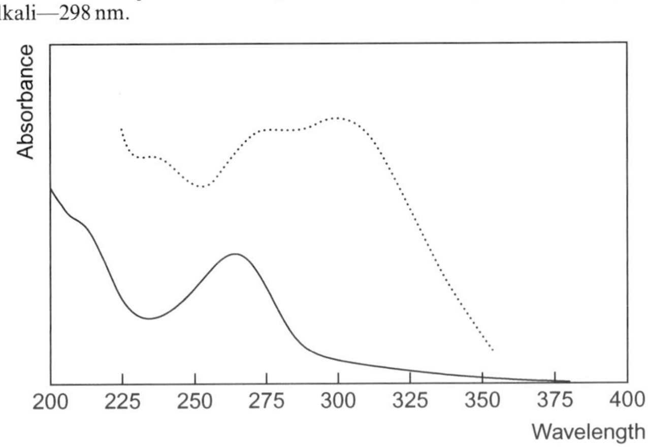

Infra-red Spectrum. Principal peaks at wavenumbers 1653, 1541, 1621, 676, 992, 845 cm^{-1} (KBr disk).

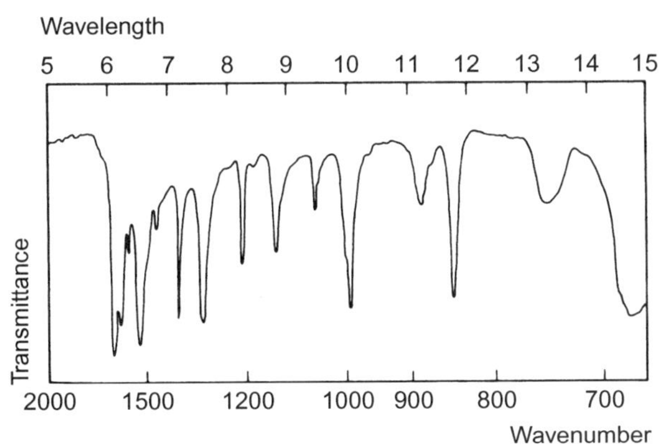

Mass Spectrum. Principal ions at *m/z* 106, 78, 51, 137, 50, 79, 107, 31; isonicotinic acid 123, 51, 78, 106, 50, 52, 105, 39.

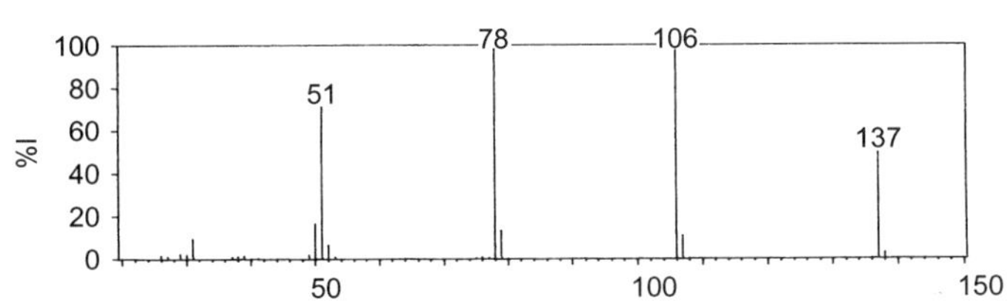

Quantification

Spectrofluorimetry. In plasma: isoniazid and acetylisoniazid—W. A. Olson *et al.*, *Clin. Chem.*, 1977, *23*, 745–748.

Gas chromatography. In urine: limit of detection 2 mg/L for isoniazid and acetylisoniazid, 400 µg/L for hydrazine, monoacetylhydrazine and diacetylhydrazine, AFID—J. A. Timbrell *et al.*, *J. Chromatogr.*, 1977, *138*, 165–172.

Gas chromatography–mass spectrometry. In plasma: limit of detection 100 µg/L for isoniazid and acetylisoniazid, 50 µg/L for hydrazine metabolites—B. H. Lauterburg *et al.*, *J. Chromatogr.*, 1981, *224*; *B Biomed. Appl.*, *13*, 431–438.

High performance liquid chromatography. In plasma: isoniazid and acetylisoniazid, limit of detection 100 µg/L, UV detection—M. R. Holdiness, *J. Liq. Chromatogr.*, 1982, *5*, 707–714. In urine: limit of detection 0.2 mg/L; fluorimetric detection—H. Kohno *et al.*, *Ther. Drug Monit.*, 1991, *13*, 428–432. In plasma: isoniazid and other antitubercular drugs—A. Walubo *et al.*, *J. Chromatogr. B Biomed. Appl.*, 1994, *658*, 391–396. In biological fluids: isoniazid, acetylisoniazid, and hydrazine, limit of detection for isoniazid <1 mg/L, UV detection—H. I. Seifart *et al.*, *J. Chromatogr. B Biomed. Appl.*, 1995, *674*, 269–275. In serum: UV detection—N. Sadeg *et al.*, *J. Chromatogr. B Biomed. Appl.*, 1996, *675*, 113–117. In plasma, alveolar cells, or bronchoalveolar lavage: coulometric detection—T. Delahunty *et al.*, *J. Chromatogr. B Biomed. Sci. Appl.*, 1998, *705*, 323–329. In plasma: isoniazid, rifampicin and pyrazinamide—P. J. Smith *et al.*, *Int. J. Tuberc. Lung Dis.*, 1999, *3*(11Suppl 3) S325–S328 and S351–S352. In serum: isoniazid and other antitubercular drugs, limits of detection <82 µg/L—M. C. Gennaro *et al.*, *J. Chromatogr. B Biomed. Sci. Appl.*, 2001, *754*, 477–486. In plasma: isoniazid and acetylisoniazid, UV detection—L. A. Moussa *et al.*, *J. Chromatogr. B. Analyt. Technol. Biomed. Life Sci.*, 2002, *766*, 181–187. In blood: isoniazid and other antitubercular drugs—M. Y. Khuhawar and F. M. Rind, *J. Chromatogr. B. Analyt. Technol. Biomed. Life Sci.*, 2002, *766*, 357–363.

Disposition in the Body. Isoniazid is readily absorbed after oral administration. The main metabolic reaction is acetylation and the rate at which this occurs shows genetic variation, approximately 40% of the population being rapid acetylators and the remainder slow acetylators. Other metabolic reactions which occur are hydrolysis, glycine conjugation, hydrazone formation and *N*-methylation. Metabolites include acetylisoniazid, isonicotinic acid, isonicotinylglycine, and mono- and diacetylhydrazine. All the metabolites are inactive with the exception of monoacetylhydrazine which is a reactive metabolite and is hepatotoxic. Up to about 70% of a dose is excreted in the urine in 24 h, most being excreted in the first 12 h. In slow acetylators, about 30% of the dose is excreted in the urine as unchanged drug, up to about 25% as acetylisoniazid, about 10% as isonicotinic acid and about 8% as diacetylhydrazine. In rapid acetylators, about 10% of a dose is excreted as unchanged drug, up to 45% as acetylisoniazid, about 20% as isonicotinic acid and about 25% as diacetylhydrazine. Small amounts of monoacetylhydrazine are also excreted in the urine. Less than 10% of a dose is eliminated in the faeces.

Therapeutic concentration. In plasma, usually in the range 3 to 10 mg/L.

Following a single oral dose of 300 mg to 6 fasting subjects classified as slow acetylators, mean peak serum concentrations of 7.2 mg/L of isoniazid and 1.7 mg/L of acetylisoniazid were attained in 0.6 and 3.7 h, respectively. Following a single oral dose of 300 mg given to 4 rapid acetylators, mean peak serum concentrations of 7.2 mg/L of isoniazid and 4.5 mg/L of acetylisoniazid were attained in 0.4 h and 2.6 h, respectively [P. Männistö *et al.*, *J. Antimicrob. Chemother.*, 1982, *10*, 427–434].

In 94 subjects, aged 1 to 13 years, with tuberculosis given rifampicin and isoniazid at a dose of 12 and 10 mg/kg/day, respectively, for 10 to 12 days, mean serum-rifampicin concentrations of 3.38 to 3.88 mg/L were achieved in 2 h and mean serum-isoniazid concentrations of 4.38 to 8.17 mg/L were achieved in 1 h; concentrations of both drugs were still much above those required for therapeutic efficacy at 7 to 8 h [V. Seth *et al.*, *Indian Pediatr.*, 1993, *30*, 1091–1098].

Toxicity. Serious toxic symptoms may occur with doses of 3 g or more. In children, toxic effects have occurred after ingestion of 0.9 g or more but a child has recovered after taking as much as 20 g. Toxic effects have been associated with plasma concentrations greater than 20 mg/L.

A 16-year-old girl who had ingested an unknown quantity of isoniazid had a serum concentration of 127 mg/L on admission to hospital and died 7 h later. Two children aged 1½ and 2½ years had serum concentrations of 103 mg/L and 35 mg/L, respectively, on admission to hospital following ingestion of isoniazid and subsequently recovered [J. Miller *et al.*, *Am. J. Dis. Childh.*, 1980, *134*, 290–292].

In a fatality due to the ingestion of isoniazid, the tissue distribution was as follows: heart blood 43 mg/L, subclavian blood 94 mg/L, urine 470 mg/L, bile 900 mg/L, liver 650 μg/g, kidney 110 μg/g, stomach contents 4 mg [C. P. LoDico *et al.*, *J. Anal. Toxicol.*, 1992, *16*, 57–59].

A 7-year-old boy who ingested 3 g (125 mg/kg) of isoniazid had blood levels of 250 mg/L approximately 6 h later (gastric content 450 mg/L and urine 760 mg/L); haemodialysis resulted in recovery [J. P. Orlowski *et al.*, *Ann. Emerg. Med.*, 1988, *17*, 73–76].

Bioavailability. About 80%.

Half-life. Plasma half-life, about 1 h in rapid acetylators and 3 to 5 h in slow acetylators.

Volume of distribution. About 0.8 L/kg.

Clearance. Plasma clearance, about 2.5 and about 7 mL/min/kg in slow and rapid acetylators, respectively.

Protein binding. In plasma, not significantly bound.

Note. For a review of the pharmacokinetics of isoniazid, see W. W. Weber and D. W. Hein, *Clin. Pharmacokinet.*, 1979, *4*, 401–422. For a review of isoniazid overdose, see J. A. Romero and F. J. Kuczler, *Am. Fam. Physician*, 1998, *57*, 749–752.

Dose. Usually 4 to 5 mg/kg daily, by mouth, to a maximum of 300 mg daily.

Isoprenaline

Sympathomimetic

Synonyms. Isopropylarterenol; Isopropylnoradrenaline; Isoproterenol; A-21.

Proprietary names. Aludrine; Asmalar; Bellasthman; Isoprel; Novodrin; Respifral; Saventrine.

4-[1-Hydroxy-2-[(1-methylethyl)amino]ethyl]-1,2-benzenediol

$C_{11}H_{17}NO_3 = 211.3$

CAS—7683-59-2

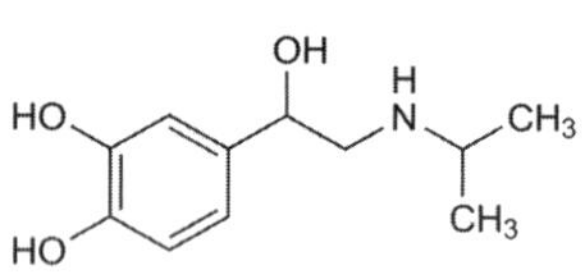

Crystals. M.p. 155°.

Isoprenaline Hydrochloride

Synonym. Isoproterenol Hydrochloride

Proprietary names. Aerolone; Imuprel; Isuprel; Lenoprel; Proternol; Saventrine.

$C_{11}H_{17}NO_3,HCl = 247.7$

CAS—51-30-9

A white crystalline powder. It gradually darkens on exposure to air and light. M.p. 165° to 170°, with decomposition.

Soluble 1 in less than 1 of water and 1 in about 50 of ethanol; practically insoluble in chloroform and ether. Aqueous solutions become pink to brownish-pink on standing exposed to air, and almost immediately so when made alkaline.

Isoprenaline Sulfate

Synonym. Isoproterenol Sulfate

Proprietary names. Aleudrina; Ingelan; Kattwilon N; Medihaler Iso; Norisodrine.

$(C_{11}H_{17}NO_3)_2,H_2SO_4,2H_2O = 556.6$

CAS—299-95-6 (anhydrous); 6700-39-6 (dihydrate)

A white crystalline powder. It gradually darkens on exposure to light and air. M.p. about 128°, with decomposition.

Soluble 1 in 4 of water; slightly soluble in ethanol; practically insoluble in benzene, chloroform and ether. Aqueous solutions become pink to brownish-pink on standing exposed to air, and almost immediately so when made alkaline.

Dissociation Constant. pK_a 8.6, 10.1, 12.0 (20°).

Partition Coefficient. Log *P* (octanol/water), 0.2.

Colour Tests. Ammoniacal Silver Nitrate—red→red-brown/brown; Ferric Chloride—green; Folin–Ciocalteu Reagent—blue; Mandelin's Test—brown; Marquis Test—brown→violet; Methanolic Potassium Hydroxide—orange→yellow; Nessler's Reagent—black; Potassium Dichromate—green→brown (30 s).

Thin-layer Chromatography. System TA—Rf 40; system TB—Rf 00; system TC—Rf 01; system TE—Rf 21; system TL—Rf 03; system TAE—Rf 14; system TAF—Rf 69. (Acidified potassium permanganate solution, positive.)

Gas Chromatography. System GA—RI 1730.

High Performance Liquid Chromatography. System HX—RI 79.

Ultraviolet Spectrum. Aqueous acid—279 ($A^1_1 = 134a$); aqueous alkali—297 nm.

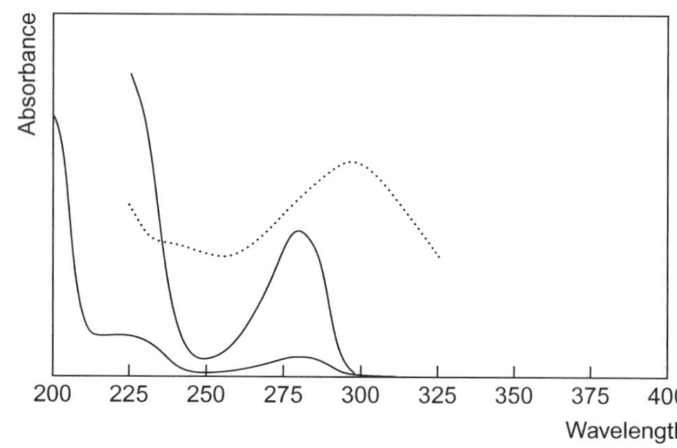

Infra-red Spectrum. Principal peaks at wavenumbers 1246, 1293, 1535, 1230, 1040, 1607 cm^{-1} (isoprenaline hydrochloride, KCl disk).

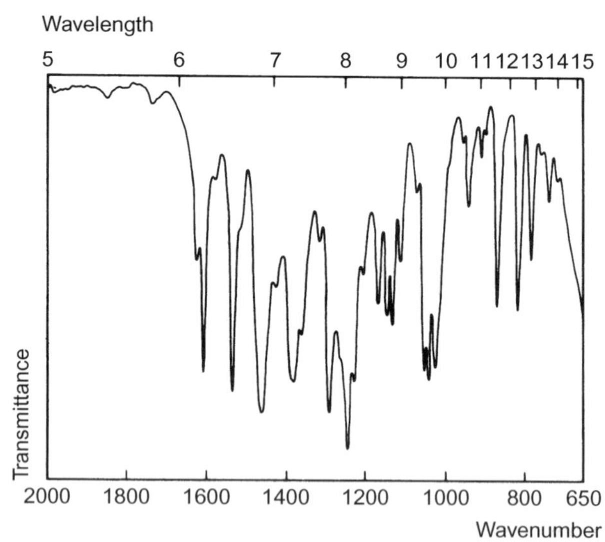

Mass Spectrum. Principal ions at *m/z* 72, 44, 43, 124, 123, 30, 42, 41.

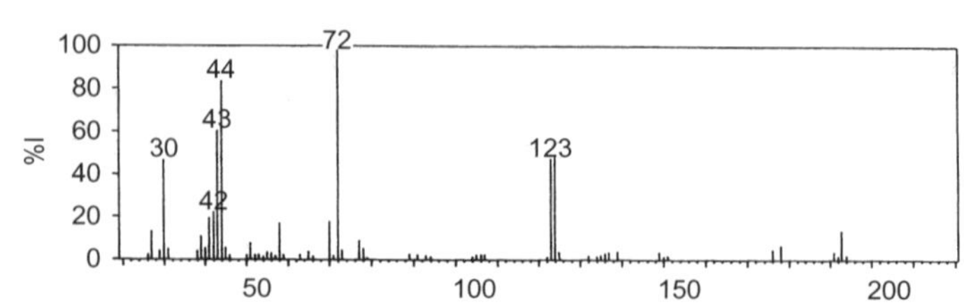

Quantification

High performance liquid chromatography. In plasma or urine: limit of detection 40 pg, fluorescence detection—Y. Kishimoto *et al.*, *J. Chromatogr.*, 1982, *231*; *B Biomed. Appl.*, *20*, 121–127. In plasma or urine: limit of detection 1 µg/L, electrochemical detection—R. C. Causon *et al.*, *J. Chromatogr.*, 1984, *306*; *B Biomed. Appl.*, *31*, 257–268.

Disposition in the Body. Isoprenaline is irregularly absorbed after oral or sublingual administration with extensive metabolism and conjugation occurring in the gut. Only about 10% of an inhaled dose reaches the lungs. It is rapidly metabolised by 3-*O*-methylation and sulfate conjugation; 3-*O*-methylisoprenaline exhibits weak activity. After IV administration, about 90% of a dose is excreted in the urine in 24 h, mostly as the conjugated 3-*O*-methyl metabolite, with up to about 15% of the dose as unchanged drug; after inhalation or oral administration, 68 to 94% of a dose is excreted as conjugated isoprenaline, with about 2 to 8% of a dose as the 3-*O*-methyl conjugate and less than 5% as unchanged drug or free 3-*O*-methylisoprenaline; small amounts of a dose are excreted in the bile, mainly as metabolites.

Therapeutic concentration

After a dose of 500 µg administered by aerosol inhalation, plasma concentrations of about 0.0003 mg/L were attained in 5 min in 2 subjects [E. W. Blackwell *et al.*, *Br. J. Pharmacol.*, 1970, *39*, 194P–195P].

After an oral dose of 0.2 mg/kg, plasma concentrations of about 0.5 mg/L of isoprenaline plus metabolites were attained within 90 min; in blood the major component was the sulfate ester together with small amounts of the methylated metabolite [M. E. Conolly *et al.*, *Br. J. Pharmacol.*, 1972, *46*, 458–472].

Toxicity. Estimated minimum lethal dose for children, applied to mucous membranes, 100 mg.

Half-life. Plasma half-life, 3 to 7 h.

Volume of distribution. About 0.5 L/kg.

Protein binding. In plasma, about 68%.

Dose. 90 to 840 mg of isoprenaline hydrochloride daily, by mouth, as sustained-release tablets.

Isopropamide Iodide

Anticholinergic

Proprietary names. Priamide. It is an ingredient of Combid, Ornade, and Stelabid.

γ-(Aminocarbonyl)-*N*-methyl-*N*,*N*-bis(1-methylethyl)-γ-phenylbenzenepropanaminium iodide

$C_{23}H_{33}IN_2O$=480.4

CAS—7492-32-2 (isopropamide); 71-81-8 (iodide)

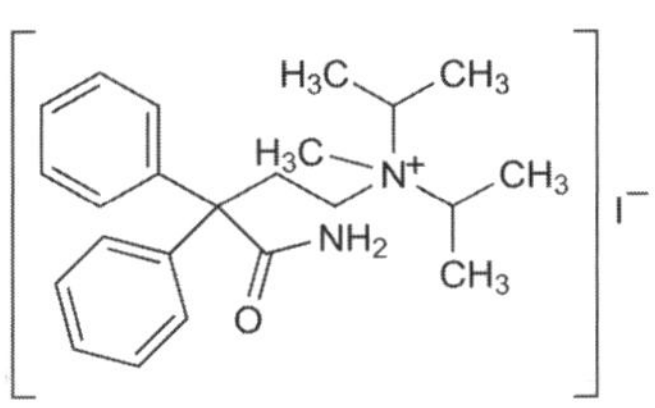

A white to pale yellow crystalline powder. M.p. 198° to 201°, with decomposition.

Soluble 1 in 50 of water, 1 in 10 of ethanol, and 1 in 5 of chloroform; practically insoluble in ether.

Partition Coefficient. Log *P* (octanol/water), 1.2.

Colour Tests. Aromaticity (Method 2)—colourless/brown; Liebermann's Test—grey

Thin-layer Chromatography. System TA—Rf 05; system TB—Rf 00; system TC—Rf 05; system TE—Rf 03; system TL—Rf 00; system TAE—Rf 03; system TAF—Rf 41; system TAJ—Rf 00; system TAK—Rf 00; system TAL—Rf 19. (Acidified iodoplatinate solution, positive.)

Gas Chromatography. System GA—RI 2022 and 2670.

High Performance Liquid Chromatography. System HA—*k* 2.4 (tailing peak); system HX—RI 379.

Ultraviolet Spectrum. Methanol—259 nm (A^1_1=9.1a), 265 nm.

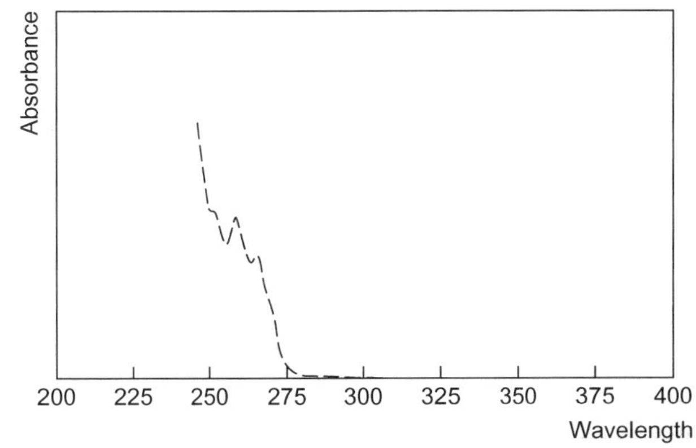

Infra-red Spectrum. Principal peaks at wavenumbers 1650, 1576, 705, 769, 757, 1500 cm^{-1} (KBr disk).

Mass Spectrum. Principal ions at *m/z* 86, 114, 100, 44, 238, 115, 56, 72.

Dose. The equivalent of 5 to 10 mg of isopropamide every 12 h.

Isopropyl Alcohol

Solvent

Synonyms. Alcohol Isopropylicus; Dimethyl Carbinol; Isopropanol; 2-Propanol; Secondary Propyl Alcohol.

Proprietary names. Alcojel; Alcowipe; Alko Isol; Avitracid; Clearasil Daily Face; Duonale; Medi-Swab; Mundisept; Sterets; Steriwipe.

2-Propanol

C_3H_8O=60.10

CAS—67-63-0

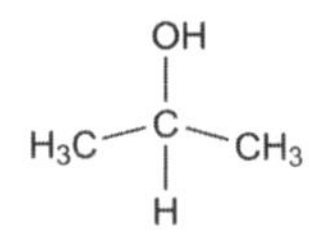

A clear, colourless, mobile, volatile, inflammable liquid. Macs per mL 0.784 to 0.786 g. B.p. 81° to 83°. Refractive index, at 20°, 1.377 to 1.380. Miscible with water, ethanol, chloroform and ether.

Dissociation Constant. pK_a 17.1.

Partition Coefficient. Log *P* (octanol/water), 0.

Colour Test. Potassium Dichromate (Method 2) —green.

Gas Chromatography. System GA—RI 530; system GI—Retention time(s) 4.0 min.

Infra-red Spectrum. Principal peaks at wavenumbers 952, 1123, 1162, 819, 1111, 1298 cm^{-1}.

Mass Spectrum. Principal ions at *m/z* 45, 43, 27, 41, 39, 29, 59, 44; acetone 43, 58, 59, 27, 42, 26, 39, 29.

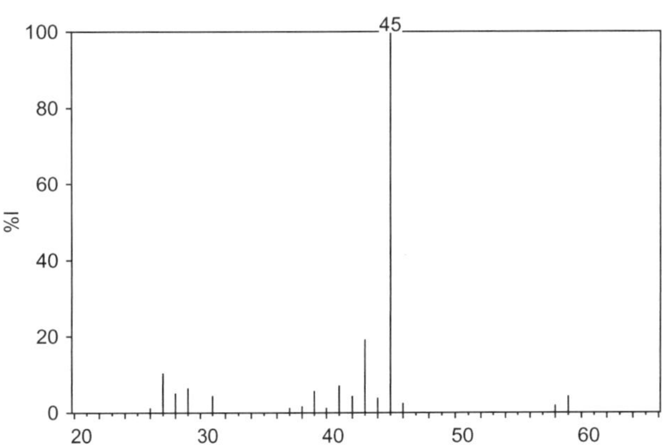

Quantification

Gas Chromatography. In blood—D. R. Daniel *et al.*, *J. Anal. Toxicol.*, 1981, *5*, 110–112. In serum: isopropyl alcohol and other alcohols and glycols, limits of detection 10 mg/L to 25 mg/L—R. H. Williams *et al.*, *J. Anal. Toxicol.*, 2000, *24*, 621–626.

Disposition in the Body. Isopropyl alcohol is readily absorbed after oral administration and slowly absorbed through intact skin. It is metabolised more slowly than ethanol; it is largely converted to acetone which is slowly excreted from the lungs and in the urine; acetone may be further metabolised to acetate, formate and carbon dioxide; some unchanged isopropyl alcohol may be excreted in the urine together with its glucuronide conjugate, particularly after large doses.

Toxicity. The estimated minimum lethal dose is 240 mL. Isopropyl alcohol is about twice as toxic as ethanol and the symptoms of intoxication are similar. Fatalities have been associated with blood concentrations greater than 1000 mg/L. The maximum permissible atmospheric concentration is 400 ppm. A dose of 16 mL has been ingested daily for 3 days without discomfort but marked depression has been observed following a dose of 23 mL. Recovery has followed treatment by haemodialysis in subjects with initial blood concentrations of up to 4400 mg/L of isopropyl alcohol.

In a review of 31 fatalities attributed solely to isopropyl alcohol poisoning, postmortem blood concentrations ranged from 100 to 2500 (mean 1400) mg/L for isopropyl alcohol and 400 to 3000 (mean 1700) mg/L for acetone [C. B. Alexander *et al.*, *J. Forensic Sci.*, 1982, *27*, 541–548].

A woman who died about 3 h after ingesting isopropyl alcohol was reported to have the following postmortem tissue concentrations: isopropyl alcohol, blood 3300 mg/L, brain 1800 µg/g, urine 2000 mg/L; acetone, blood 1200 mg/L, brain 600 µg/g, urine 700 mg/L [R. H. Cravey, in R. C. Baselt (Ed.), *Disposition of Toxic Drugs and Chemicals in Man*, 5th Edn, Davis, California, Biomedical Publications, 2000, pp 449–450].

In 4 fatalities due to the ingestion of isopropyl alcohol, the following antemortem or postmortem tissue concentrations were reported: blood 200 to 2000 mg/L (mean 1300 mg/L, 4 cases), brain 1000 µg/g (1 case), liver 1000 µg/g (1 case), spleen 1300 µg/g (1 case), urine 1500 and 1800 mg/L (2 cases) [L. Adelson, *Am. J. Clin. Pathol.*, 1962, *38*, 144–151].

Half-life. Blood half-life, about 3 h in subjects with acute intoxication.

Isopropylaminophenazone

Analgesic (Veterinary)

Synonyms. Isopyrin; Ramifenazone.
Proprietary names. It is an ingredient of Tomanol.
Note. The name Isopyrin has also been applied to isoniazid.
1,2-Dihydro-1,5-dimethyl-4-[(1-methylethyl)amino]-2-phenyl-3*H*-pyrazol-3-one
$C_{14}H_{19}N_3O = 245.3$
CAS—3615-24-5

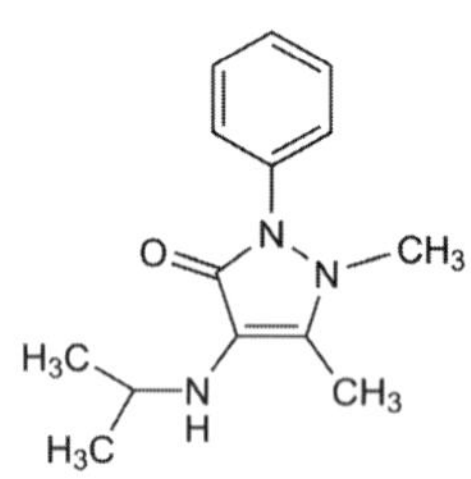

Crystals. M.p. 80°.

Partition Coefficient. Log *P* (octanol/water), 1.3.

Thin-layer Chromatography. System TE—Rf 63; system TAE—Rf 78.

Gas Chromatography. System GA—RI 2033.

Ultraviolet Spectrum. Aqueous acid—260 ($A_1^1 = 377b$); aqueous alkali—271 ($A_1^1 = 334b$); methanol—243 ($A_1^1 = 310b$), 269 nm ($A_1^1 = 381b$).

Isoproturon

Herbicide

Synonyms. CGA-18731; DPX 6774; HOE-16410; IP 50; IP Flo; I.P.U.
Proprietary names. Alon; Arelon; Augur; Avanon; Belgran; Graminon; Hytane; Isotop; Nocilon; Protugan; Sabre; Swing; Tolkan.
N,*N*-dimethyl-*N*′-[4-(1-methylethyl)phenyl]urea
$C_{12}H_{18}N_2O = 206.3$
CAS—34123-59-6

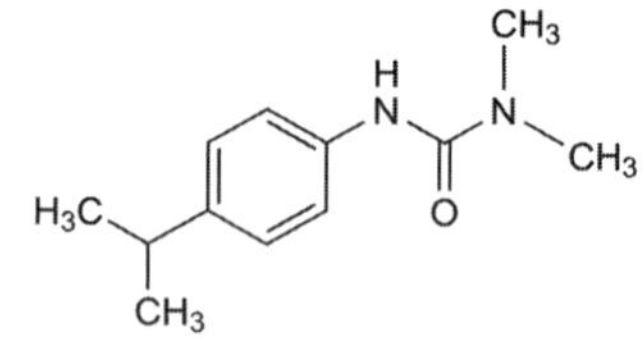

A colourless to white crystalline solid. M.p. 158°.
It is soluble in water (72 mg/L at 20°); readily soluble in common organic solvents, e.g. alcohol, ketones, esters, aromatic hydrocarbons, chlorinated hydrocarbons, methanol (56 g/L at 20°), dichloromethane (63 g/L at 20°), benzene (5 g/L at 20°), and hexane (0.1 g/L at 20°).

Partition Coefficient. Log *P* (octanol/water), 2.87.

Gas Chromatography. System GA—isoproturon-Me RI 1685.

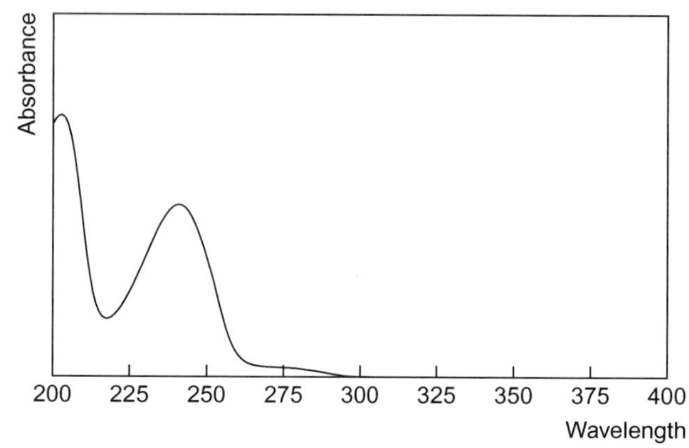

Mass Spectrum. Principal ions at *m*/*z* 72, 220, 148, 132, 205, -, -, - (methyl derivative).

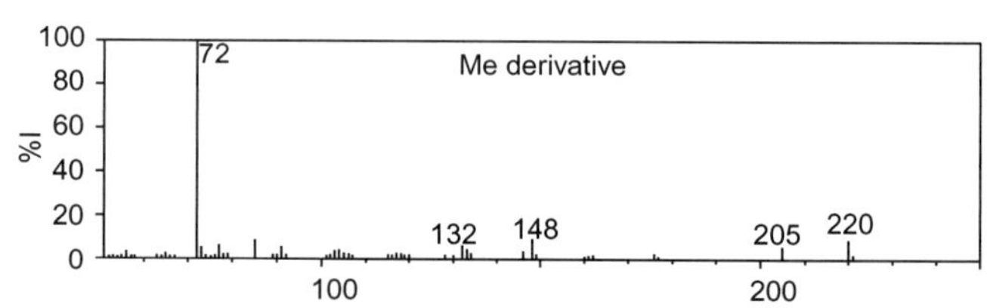

Disposition in the Body. Isoproturon is excreted in urine with approximately 50% of an administered dose being excreted within the first 8 h.

Isosorbide Dinitrate

Anti-anginal Vasodilator

Synonym. Sorbide Nitrate; Dinitrosorbide.
Proprietary names. Angitak; Cedocard; Corovliss; Dilatrate; Dinit; Disorlon; Imtack; Iso Mack; Isocard; Isodinit; Isoket; Isordil; Isotrate; Jeridin; Langoran; Nitrosid; Risordan; Soni-Slo; Sorbichew; Sorbid; Sorbidilat; Sorbitrate; Sorquad; Vascardin; Vasorbate; Vasotrate.
1,4:3,6-Dianhydro-D-glucitol dinitrate
$C_6H_8N_2O_8 = 236.1$
CAS—87-33-2

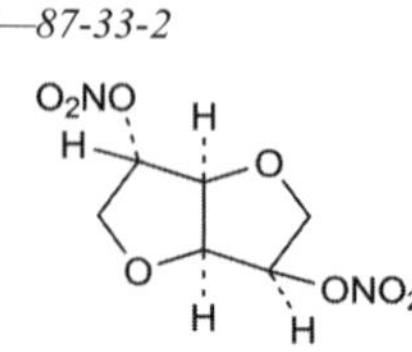

A white crystalline powder. M.p. 70°.

Sparingly soluble in water; freely soluble in acetone, ethanol and chloroform; soluble in methanol.
Caution. Isosorbide dinitrate may explode if subjected to percussion or excessive heat.

Partition Coefficient. Log *P* (octanol/water), 1.3.

High Performance Liquid Chromatography. System HY—RI 396.

Ultraviolet Spectrum. No significant absorption, 230 to 360 nm.

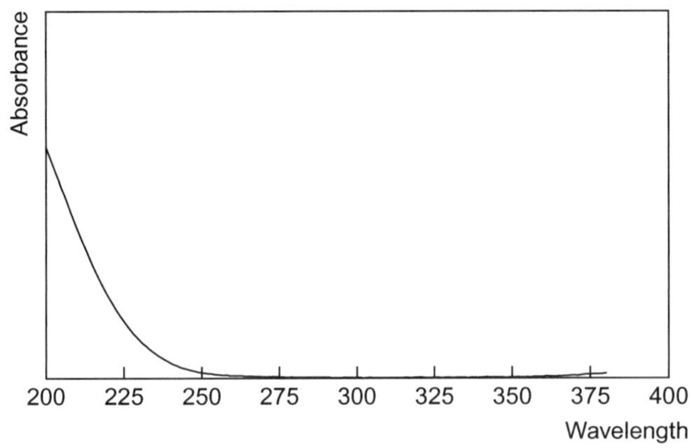

Infra-red Spectrum. Principal peaks at wavenumbers 1062, 1618, 862, 1266, 1653, 1089 cm^{-1} (isosorbide, Nujol mull).

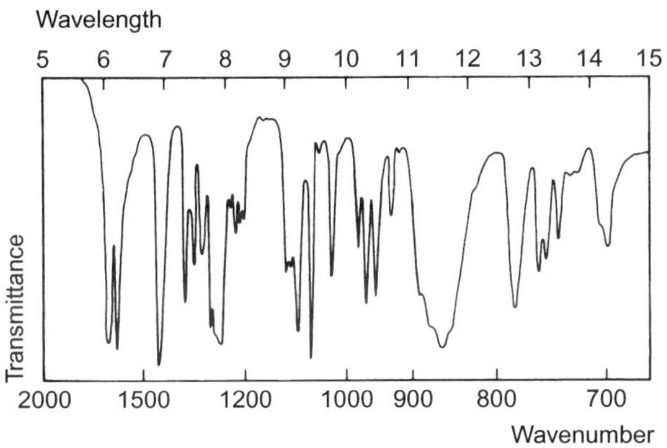

Mass Spectrum. Principal ions at *m/z* 43, 31, 29, 61, 60, 85, 73, 44.

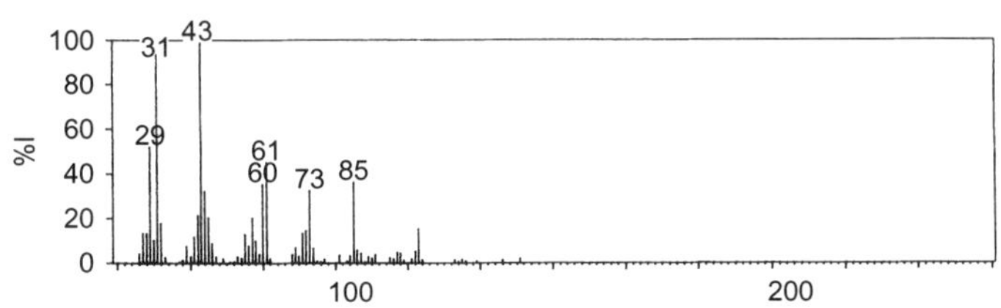

Quantification

Gas chromatography. In plasma or urine: limit of detection 0.5 µg/L, ECD—A. Sioufi and F. Pommier, *J. Chromatogr.*, 1982, *229*; *B Biomed. Appl.*, *18*, 347–353. In plasma: isosorbide dinitrate, glyceryl trinitrate and their metabolites, limit of detection for isosorbide dinitrate 20 µg/L—B. P. Booth *et al.*, *Biopharm. Drug Dispos.*, 1990, *11*, 663–677. In plasma: limits of detection 0.5 µg/L for isosorbide dinitrate, 2 µg/L for isosorbide 2-mononitrate and 10 µg/L for isosorbide 5-mononitrate, ECD—Y. Santoni *et al.*, *J. Chromatogr.*, 1984, *306*; *B Biomed Appl.*, *31*, 165–172. In plasma: isosorbide dinitrate and its metabolites, limit of detection 2.5 µg/L, ECD—F. Pommier *et al.*, *J. Chromatogr. B Biomed. Appl.*, 1996, *678*, 354–359.

High performance liquid chromatography. In plasma: limit of detection 200 pg—W. C. Yu and E. U. Goff, *Anal. Chem.*, 1983, *55*, 29–32.

Disposition in the Body. Isosorbide dinitrate is readily absorbed after sublingual or oral administration. It is metabolised by enzymatic denitration followed by glucuronide conjugation. Isosorbide 2-mononitrate and isosorbide 5-mononitrate have some pharmacological activity. About 80% of a dose is excreted in the urine in 24 h, of which about 50% is isosorbide glucuronide, up to 15% is free and conjugated isosorbide 5-mononitrate, about 1% is free isosorbide 2-mononitrate, and less than 1% is unchanged drug.

Therapeutic concentration. Isosorbide 5-mononitrate accumulates in the plasma during chronic treatment.

Following a single oral dose of 20 mg of isosorbide dinitrate to 8 subjects, peak plasma concentrations of 0.02 to 0.09 (mean 0.05) mg/L of isosorbide dinitrate, 0.02 to 0.06 (mean 0.04) mg/L of isosorbide 2-mononitrate, and 0.10 to 0.22 (mean 0.14) mg/L of isosorbide 5-mononitrate, were attained in 0.25, 0.7, and 1 h, respectively. [H. Laufen *et al.*, *Arzneimittelforschung*, 1983, *33*, 980–984].

After a single sublingual dose of 5 mg to 6 subjects, peak plasma concentrations of 0.007 to 0.015 (mean 0.009) mg/L were attained in 10 to 15 min. [D. F. Assinder *et al.*, *J. Pharm. Sci.*, 1977, *66*, 775–778].

Bioavailability. About 60% after sublingual administration and about 20% orally, but there is considerable intersubject variation.

Half-life. Plasma half-life, isosorbide dinitrate about 0.5 to 1.5 h, isosorbide 2-mononitrate about 2 h, isosorbide5-mononitrate 3 to 7 h. A longer terminal elimination half-life of about 8 h has been reported for isosorbide dinitrate.

Saliva. Plasma:saliva ratio, about 1.5.

Protein binding. In plasma, about 30%.

Note. For a review of the pharmacokinetics of organic nitrates, see M. G. Bogaert, *Clin. Pharmacokinet.*, 1983, *8*, 410–421.

Dose. 10 to 240 mg daily, by mouth.

Isosorbide Mononitrate

Anti-anginal Vasodilator

Synonym. Isosorbide 5-Mononitrate
Proprietary names. Angeze; Chemydur; Coleb; Conpin; Corangin; Duride; Dynamin; Elantan; Imdur; Imtrate; Isib; Ismo; Isodur; Isomonit; Isotard; Isotrate; MCR-50; Monicor; Modisal; Monit; Mono-Cedocard; Monoket; Monomax; Monosorb; Xismox.
1,4:3,6-Dianhydro-D-glucitol 5-nitrate
$C_6H_9NO_6$=191.1
CAS—16051-77-7

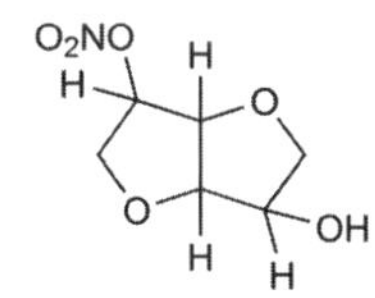

Colourless prismatic crystals. M.p. 89° to 91°.
Soluble in water, ethanol, acetone and methanol; slightly soluble in chloroform and ether.
Caution. Isosorbide mononitrate may explode if subjected to percussion or excessive heat.

Partition Coefficient. Log *P* (octanol/water), −0.2.

Ultraviolet Spectrum. No significant absorption, 230 to 360 nm.

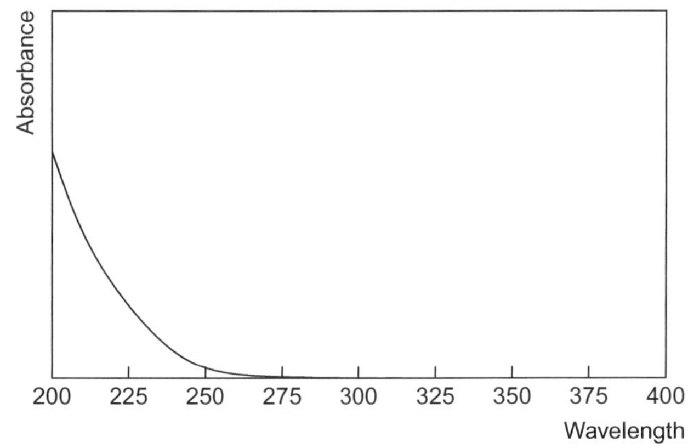

Infra-red Spectrum. Principal peaks at wavenumbers 1280, 1650, 1635, 852, 1090, 968 cm^{-1} (KBr disk).

Quantification

Gas chromatography (capillary column). In plasma: limit of detection 1 µg/L, ECD—P. Straehl and R. L. Galeazzi, *J. Pharm. Sci.*, 1984, *73*, 1317–1319. In plasma: limit of detection 2 µg/L, ECD—L. L. Yang *et al.*, *Yao Xue Xue Bao*, 1997, *32*, 773–776.

Gas chromatography–mass spectrometry. In plasma—C. Lauro-Marty *et al.*, *J. Chromatogr. B Biomed. Appl.*, 1995, *663*, 153–159.

Disposition in the Body. Isosorbide mononitrate is rapidly and almost completely absorbed after oral or sublingual administration. It is metabolised by enzymatic denitration and by glucuronide conjugation. About 80% of a dose is excreted in the urine in 24 h.

Therapeutic concentration Following a single oral dose of 20 mg given to 19 subjects, peak plasma concentrations of 0.34 to 0.68 (mean 0.48) mg/L were attained in 1 h [U. Abshagen *et al.*, *Eur. J. Clin. Pharmacol.*, 1981, *20*, 269–275.].

Toxicity.

A 15-year-old girl survived after ingesting 1.6 g of isosorbide mononitrate and 20 mg of glyceryl trinitrate in a suicide attempt. Plasma levels of isosorbide mononitrate measured 4 and 6 h after gastric lavage (performed 2 h after ingestion) were 2.993 and 3.140 mg/L, respectively; glyceryl trinitrate was not detected [J. M. Sobrino *et al.*, *Eur. Heart J.*, 1992, *13*, 145].

Bioavailability. Almost 100%.

Half-life. Plasma half-life, 3 to 7 h.

Volume of distribution. About 0.6 L/kg.

Clearance. Plasma clearance, about 1 to 2 mL/min/kg.

Saliva. Plasma : saliva ratio, about 0.8.

Protein binding. In plasma, less than 5%.

Dose. 20 to 120 mg daily.

Isothipendyl

Antihistamine

Synonym. D-201.

N,*N*,α-Trimethyl-10*H*-pyrido[3,2-*b*][1,4]benzothiazine-10-ethanamine

$C_{16}H_{19}N_3S = 285.4$

CAS—482-15-5

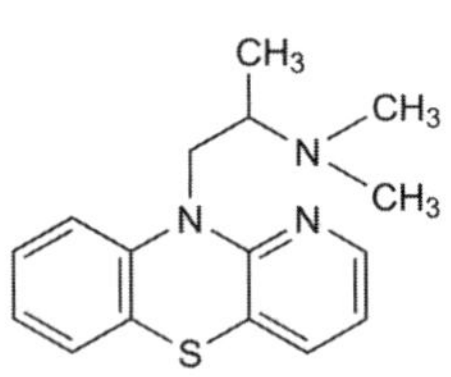

Isothipendyl Hydrochloride

Proprietary names. Andantol; Apaisyl; Calmogel; Istamyl; Nilergex; Sedermyl; Thiodantyl.

$C_{16}H_{19}N_3S,HCl = 321.9$

CAS—1225-60-1

A fine white crystalline powder. M.p. about 212°, with decomposition.

Soluble 1 in 5 of water, 1 in 60 of ethanol and 1 in 10 of chloroform; practically insoluble in ether.

Partition Coefficient. Log *P* (octanol/water), 3.9.

Colour Test. Marquis Test—orange.

Thin-layer Chromatography. System TA—Rf 52; system TB—Rf 41; system TC—Rf 30; system TE—Rf 64; system TL—Rf 14; system TAE—Rf 22; system TAF—Rf 35. (Dragendorff spray, positive; FPN reagent, yellow-pink; Acidified iodoplatinate solution, positive; Marquis reagent, pink; Ninhydrin spray, positive.)

Gas Chromatography. System GA—isothipendyl RI 2225; M(nor-) RI 2220; M(OH-) RI 2450; M(bis-nor-) RI 2230.

High Performance Liquid Chromatography. System HA—*k* 3.8; system HX—RI 390; system HAA—Retention time(s) 13.5 min.

Ultraviolet Spectrum. Aqueous acid—245 (A^1_1=860a); aqueous alkali—250 nm.

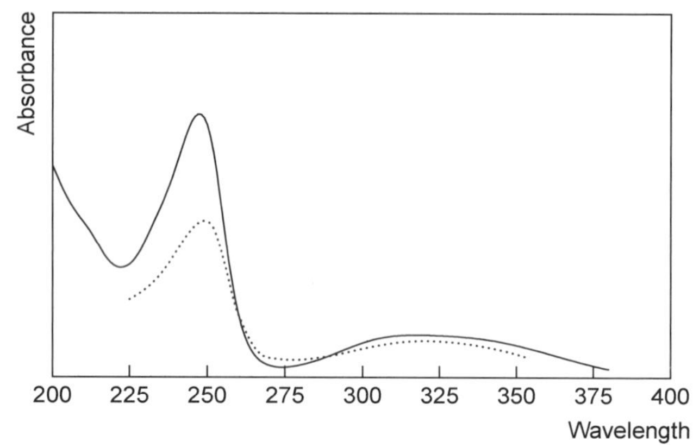

Infra-red Spectrum. Principal peaks at wavenumbers 1017, 1030, 1070, 987, 1090, 1080 cm^{-1} (KBr disk).

Mass Spectrum. Principal ions at *m/z* 72, 73, 214, 200, 44, 285, 86, 56.

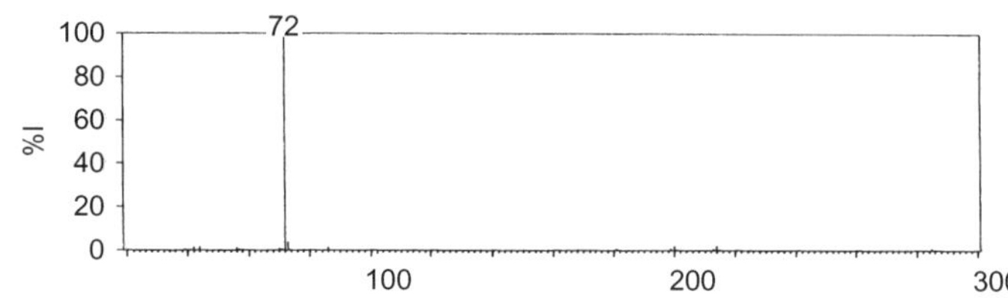

Dose. 12 to 32 mg of isothipendyl hydrochloride daily.

Isotretinoin

Dermatological

Synonyms. 13-*cis*-Retinoic Acid; 13-RA; 2-*cis*-Vitamin A Acid; Neovitamin A Acid; Ro-4-3780.

Proprietary names. Accure; Accutane; Isotrex; Isotrexin (multi-ingredient); Roaccutan; Roaccutane.

(2*Z*,4*E*,6*E*,8*E*)-3,7-Dimethyl-9-(2,6,6-trimethyl-1-cyclohexen-1-yl)nona-2,4,6,8-tetraenoic acid; (13*Z*)-15-Apo-β-caroten-15-oic acid

$C_{20}H_{28}O_2 = 300.4$

CAS—4759-48-2

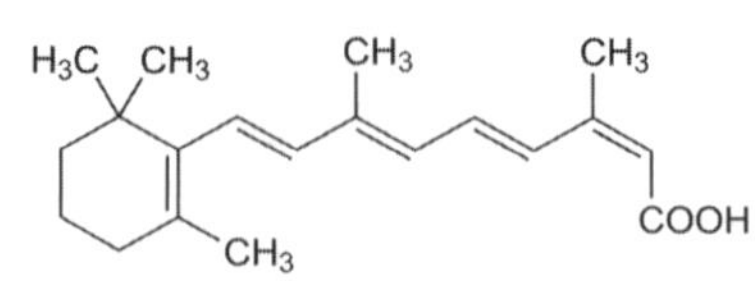

Reddish-orange plates from isopropyl alcohol. M.p. 174° to 175°. It is practically insoluble in water; sparingly soluble to slightly soluble in alcohol; sparingly soluble in ether and isopropyl alcohol; soluble in chloroform and dichloromethane.

Partition Coefficient. Log *P* (octanol/water), 2.8; also reported as 6.0.

Thin-layer Chromatography. System TF—Rf 45.

High Performance Liquid Chromatography. System HX—RI 939.

Column: RP C_{18} (Nova-Pak, 150 × 3.9 mm i.d.) and RP C_{18} (Nova-Pak, 75 × 3.9 mm). Column temperature: 40°. Mobile phase: (A)-acetonitrile; (B)-0.1 M ammonium acetate, pH 5 with acetic acid. (A):(B) (80:20) for 10 min, increased to (A):(B) (90:10). Internal standard (IS): acitretin. MS detection, SIM mode (*m/z* 414). Retention time: isotretinoin, 25.5 min; IS, 16.2 min [P. A. Lehman and T. J. Franz, *J. Pharm. Sci.*, 1996, *85(3)*, 287–290].

Column: μC_{18} RP (300 × 4.6 mm); guard, inert Corasil type II (37 to 50 μm). Mobile phase: methanol:water (80:20), 1.0 mL/min flow rate. IS: Ro-11-5036. UV detection (λ=350 nm). Retention time: isotretinoin, 6.3 min; IS, 5.6 min [A. A. Khan *et al.*, *Cancer Chemother. Pharmacol.*, 1996, *39*, 34–41].

Ultraviolet Spectrum. Aqueous acid—243, 359 nm.

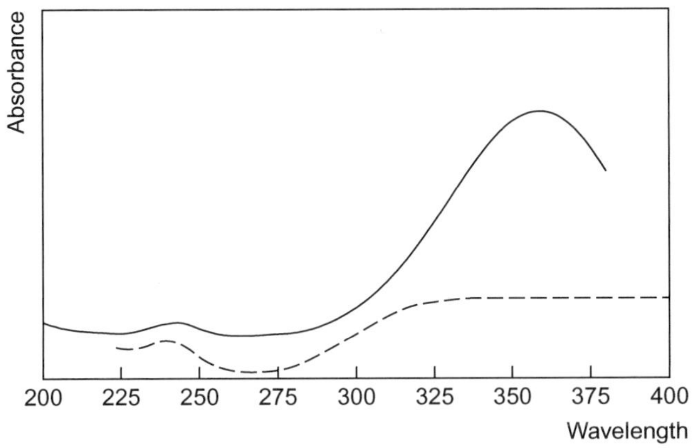

Quantification

High performance liquid chromatography. In plasma: limit of quantification 0.3 μg/L, UV detection (λ=360 nm)—R. Wyss and F. Bucheli, *J. Chromatogr. B Biomed. Sci. Appl.*, 1997, *700(1-2)*, 31–47. In serum: limit of detection 1.85 μg/L for isotretinoin and 1.05 μg/L for 4-oxo-isotretinoin and limit of quantification is 6.17 and 3.48 μg/L, respectively, UV detection (λ=360 nm)—T. E. Gundersen *et al.*, *J. Chromatogr. B Biomed. Sci. Appl.*, 1997, *691(1)*, 43–58. In plasma: limit of detection is 25 pg, MS detection—P. A. Lehman and T. J. Franz, *J. Pharm. Sci.*, 1996, *85(3)*, 287–290. In plasma: limit of quantification 0.3 μg/L, MS detection—U. B. Ranalder *et al.*, *J. Chromatogr.*, 1993, *617(1)*, 129–135. In serum: limit of detection 12 μg/L, UV detection (λ=365 nm)—R. R. Gadde and F. W. Burton, *J. Chromatogr.*, 1992, *593(1-2)*, 41–46.

Disposition in the Body. Isotretinoin is rapidly absorbed after oral administration; the extent of which is increased in the presence of food. Bioavailability of the drug is low as first pass metabolism occurs in the liver and also metabolism occurs in the gut wall. The major metabolite identified in blood is 4-oxo-isotretinoin; tretinoin and 4-oxo-tretinoin can also be detected. Both the drug and metabolites undergo enterohepatic recycling. Equal amounts of the absorbed drug are excreted in faeces, mainly as the unchanged drug, and in urine, as the metabolites. Isotretinoin crosses the placenta.

Therapeutic concentration

38 patients with high-risk neuroblastoma, aged 2 to 12 years, were administered 100, 125, 160 or 200 mg/m^2 daily for 2 weeks, followed by a 2-week rest period. The peak concentrations were 4.9, 5.7, 7.2 and 8.9 μg/L for the 4 doses observed at 3.7, 3.8, 4.1 and 4.0 h, respectively. The minimum concentrations observed at 2.8, 4.2, 4.1 and 3.9 μg/L for the 100, 125, 160 and 200 mg doses [A. A. Khan *et al.*, *Cancer Chemother. Pharmacol.*, 1996, *39*, 34–41].

Toxicity. Overdosing with isotretinoin has been associated with vomiting, facial flushing, abdominal pain, headache, dizziness and problems with muscle co-ordination/regularity.

A 29-year-old male ingested 900 mg isotretinoin (equivalent to 12.5 mg (/kg/day); 30 times the prescribed dose) and 1 day later he complained of a mild headache which was easily controlled with aspirin. 5 days after the overdose he was admitted to hospital with a persistent headache and eczema. The serum isotretinoin concentrations were 12, 5, 3 and less than 2 μg/L at 4, 5, 6 and 11 days after ingestion, respectively. The corresponding 4-oxo-isotretinoin concentrations were 562, 290, 114 and 22 μg/L, respectively [S. Aubin *et al.*, *Clin. Exp. Dermatol.*, 1995, *20(4)*, 348–350].

Half-life. 10 to 20 h.

Clearance. Total body, mean 5.64 L/m^2/h (children aged 2 to 12 years old).

Volume of distribution. Apparent, 29.45 L/m^2.

Protein binding. 99.9%.

Dose. The initial dose is 0.5 to 1.0 mg/kg daily with a maximum dose up to 2.0 mg/kg daily for 15 to 20 weeks. The dose may be adjusted according to the response of the disease and any clinical toxic effects observed.

Isoxsuprine

Vasodilator

4-Hydroxy-α-[1-[(1-methyl-2-phenoxyethyl)amino]ethyl]benzenemethanol
$C_{18}H_{23}NO_3$=301.4
CAS—395-28-8

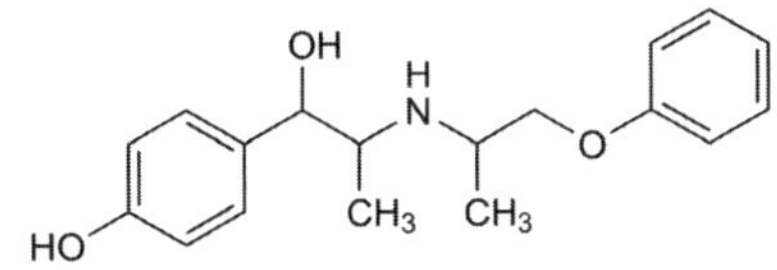

Crystals. M.p. 102.5° to 103.5°.

Isoxsuprine Hydrochloride
Synonym. Phenoxyisopropylnorsuprifen
Proprietary names. Dilavase; Dilum; Duvadilan; Duviculine; Fenam; Inibina; Vadosilan; Vasodilan; Vasolan; Vasoplex; Vasotran; Voxsuprine; Xuptin.
$C_{18}H_{23}NO_3$,HCl=337.8
CAS—579-56-6
A white crystalline powder. M.p. about 200°, with decomposition.
Soluble 1 in 500 of water, 1 in 100 of ethanol and dilute sodium hydroxide solution, and 1 in 2500 of dilute hydrochloric acid; practically insoluble in chloroform and ether.

Dissociation Constant. pK_a 8.0, 9.8.

Partition Coefficient. Log *P* (octanol/water), 2.4.

Colour Tests. Mandelin's Test—green; Marquis Test—red-violet.

Thin-layer Chromatography. System TA—Rf 78; system TB—Rf 03; system TC—Rf 32; system TE—Rf 62; system TL—Rf 53; system TAE—Rf 62; system TAF—Rf 81; system TAJ—Rf 13; system TAK—Rf 05; system TAL—Rf 60. (Acidified potassium permanganate solution, positive.)

Gas Chromatography. System GA—RI 2300.

High Performance Liquid Chromatography. System HA—*k* 0.8; system HX—RI 353; system HY—RI 301.

Ultraviolet Spectrum. Aqueous acid—269, 274 (A^1_1=82a); aqueous alkali—243 (A^1_1=450a), 270, 277, 292 nm (A^1_1=78b).

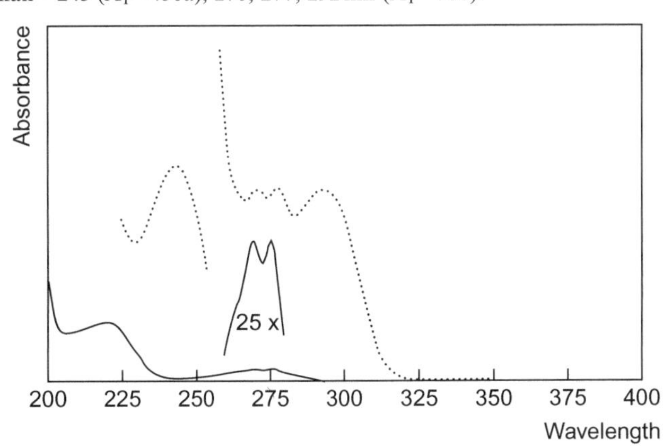

Infra-red Spectrum. Principal peaks at wavenumbers 1514, 1240, 745, 1220, 1043, 1500 cm^{-1}.

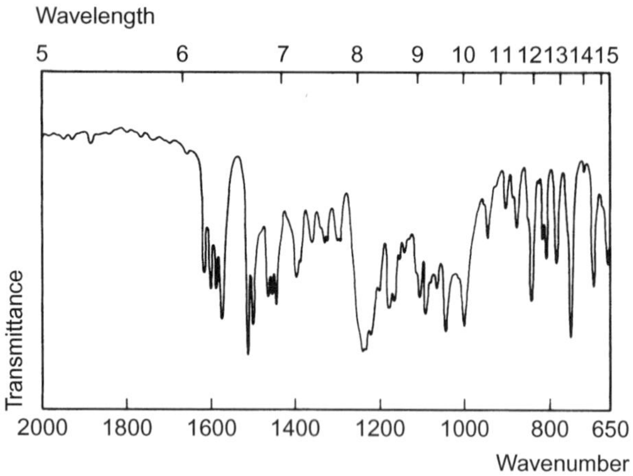

Mass Spectrum. Principal ions at m/z 178, 44, 135, 179, 77, 84, 107, 41.

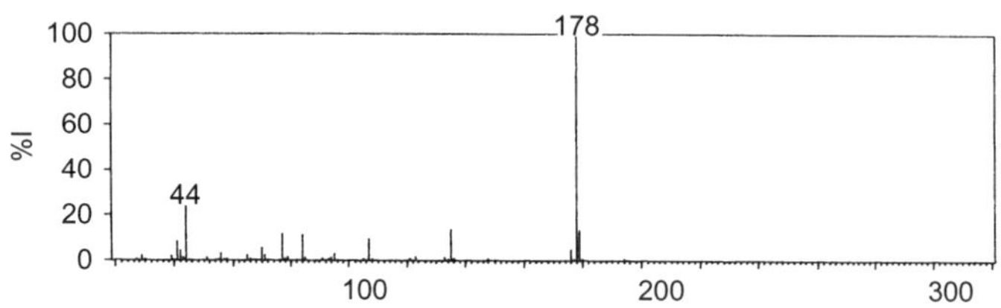

Quantification

Gas chromatography. In plasma: limit of detection 0.5 μg/L, ECD—D. Cova *et al.*, *Pharmacology*, 1983, *27*, 117–124.

Disposition in the Body. Isoxsuprine is absorbed after oral administration; peak blood concentrations are attained within 1 h of a dose. It is excreted in the urine partly unchanged and partly as a conjugate.

Dose. Up to 80 mg of isoxsuprine hydrochloride daily.

Isradipine

Calcium antagonist

Synonyms. Isrodipine; PN-200-110.
Proprietary names. Clivoten; DynaCirc; Esradin; Icaz; Lomir; Prescal; Rebriden; Vascal; Vaslan.
4-(4-Benzofurazanyl)-1,4-dihydro-2,6-dimethyl-3,5-pyridinedicarboxylic acid methyl 1-methylethyl ester
$C_{19}H_{21}N_3O_5$=371.4
CAS—75695-93-1

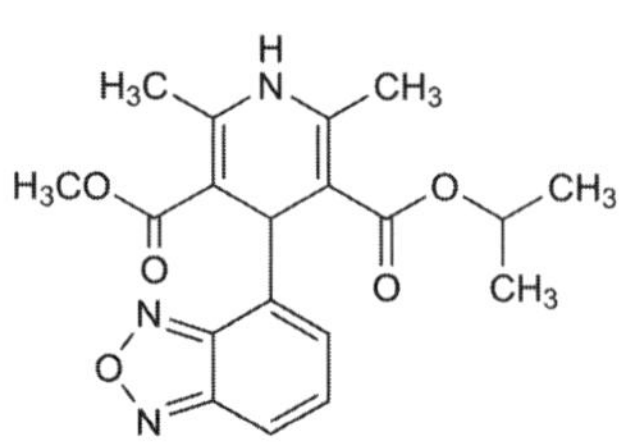

A yellow crystalline powder with M.p. 168° to 170°. Freely soluble in acetone, chloroform, methylene chloride; soluble in ethanol; practically insoluble in water (< 10 mg/L at 37°).

Partition Coefficient. Log P (octanol/water), 4.28.

Thin-layer Chromatography. System TB—Rf 04; system TE—Rf 74; system TF—Rf 59; system TAE—Rf 88.

Gas Chromatography. System GP—RI 2270 M (dehydro-deisopropyl)-ME; RI 2360 M (dehydro).

Column: methyl silicone HP1 (0.2 mm i.d., 0.33 μm film thickness). Column temperature: 280°. Carrier gas: helium, 0.9 mL/min flow rate. Detection: mass spectrometer. Retention index: 2619 [T. Mills and J. C. Roberson, 1993. *Instrumental Data for Drug Analysis*, CRC Press, Boca Raton, USA, 2nd Edn, Vol. 6, pp. 20–21].

Column: cross-linked methylsilicone (10 m × 0.53 mm i.d., 2.65 μm). Column and injector temperature: 230° and 350°, respectively. Carrier gas: methane, 10 mL/min flow rate. Detection: mass spectrometer (CI, SIM at m/z 311). Retention time: isradipine, 2.5 min; pyridinic metabolite, 1.3 min [C. Jean and R. Laplanche, *J. Chromatogr.*, 1988, *428*, 61–69].

High Performance Liquid Chromatography. System HAA—22.4 min; system HX—RI 632; system HZ—14.9 min.

Column: ODS (Hypersil, 100 × 4.6 mm i.d., 5 μm). Mobile phase: methanol, 0.5 mL/min flow rate. UV diode array detection. Retention time: 3.7 min [T. Mills and J. C. Roberson, 1993. *Instrumental Data for Drug Analysis*, CRC Press, Boca Raton, USA, 2nd Edn, Vol. 6, pp. 126–127].

Ultraviolet Spectrum. Aqueous base—266, 278, 291, 326 nm.

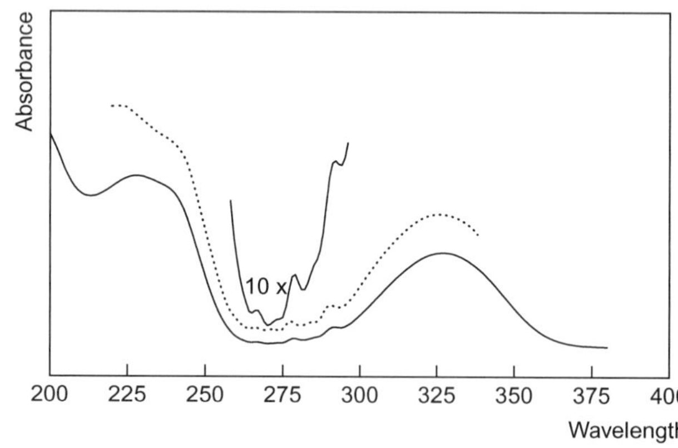

Infra-red Spectrum. Principal peaks at wavenumbers 1648, 1225, 1702, 1491 cm^{-1} (KBr pellet).

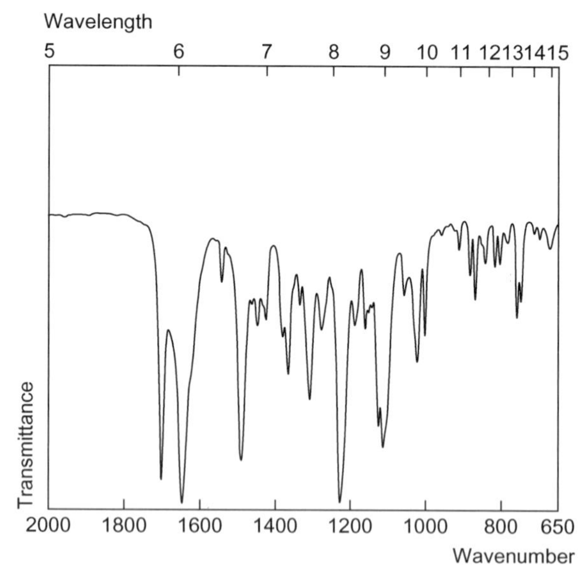

Mass Spectrum. Principal ions at m/z 210, 252, 371, 284, 312, 43, 178, 240.

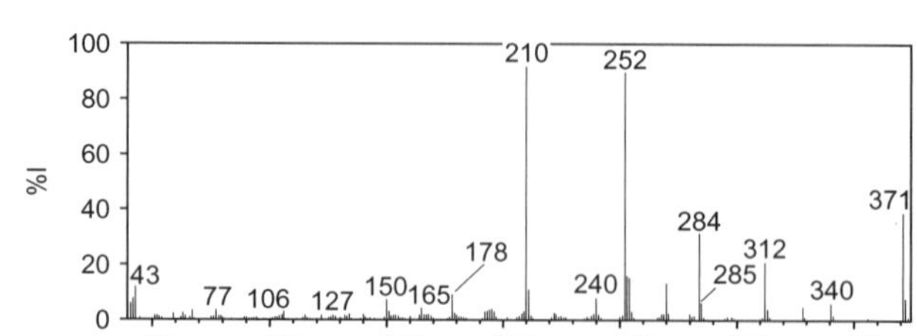

Quantification

Gas chromatography. In plasma: limit of detection 0.2 μg/L, ECD—M. C. Chellingsworth *et al.*, *Am. J. Med.*, 1988, *84 (Suppl. 3B)*, 72–79.

Gas chromatography–mass spectrometry. In plasma: limit of detection 0.04 μg/L—C. Jean and R. Laplanche, *J. Chromatogr.*, 1988, *428*, 61–69.

High performance liquid chromatography. In plasma: limit of detection 0.1 to 0.6 μg/L. UV detection (λ=325 nm)—J. Boutagy *et al.*, *J. Chromatogr.*, 1989, *487*, 483–488.

Disposition in the Body. Isradipine is rapidly and almost completely absorbed (90 to 95%) after oral administration with peak plasma concentrations after 2 h. It undergoes rapid and extensive first-pass hepatic metabolism to produce inactive pyridine and carboxylic acid derivatives. Four major metabolites have been isolated but only one has considerable pharmacological activity. The drug is excreted as metabolites in urine (70% of the dose) and the remainder in faeces (mostly as the unchanged drug). No unchanged drug is detected in urine. Excretion is virtually complete within 120 h. The pharmacokinetics of isradipine, especially the peak concentrations, half-lives and bioavailability, are increased in the elderly and those with hepatic dysfunction.

Therapeutic concentration

9 patients with hypertension (6 males and 3 females), aged between 38 and 68 years, were administered a single dose of 5 mg isradipine after an overnight fast. The mean peak concentration was 6 μg/L (range 1.6 to 18.4) which was observed after 1.5 h (range 0.5 to 4.0). Under steady state conditions, a peak plasma concentration of 3.2 (1.2 to 6.1) μg/L was observed after 1.2 h (range 0.5 to 2.0) [G. M. Shenfield *et al.*, *Eur. J. Clin. Pharmacol.*, 1990, *38*, 209–11].

12 healthy males, aged 20 to 39 years, were administered a single 5 or 20 mg dose or a 5 mg multiple dose after an 8-h fast. The mean peak plasma concentration was 2.1 μg/L after the 5 mg single isradipine dose and 9.1 μg/L after the 20 mg dose, and both were observed between 2 and 3 h. A peak concentration of 2.2 μg/L was detected after about 1 h for the multiple dosing study [F. L. S. Tse *et al.*, *Eur. J. Clin. Pharmacol.*, 1987, *32*, 361–365].

Bioavailability. 15 to 24% (varies between poor and extensive metabolisers).

Half-life. 8 h (< 4 h also reported).

Volume of distribution. 2.9 L/kg (283 L).

Clearance. Plasma, 40 L/h.

Distribution in blood. Erythrocyte:plasma ratio is 0.24.

Protein binding. Approx. 97%, mainly to α-1-glycoprotein acids.
For a general review of isradipine, see R. H. Grimm *et al.*, *Drugs*, 1990, *40 (Suppl. 2)*, 31–74.

Dose. 2.5 to 20 mg daily.

Itraconazole

Triazole Antifungal

Synonyms. Oriconazole; R-51211.
Proprietary names. Canadiol ;Hongoseril; Itrizole; Sempera; Siros; Sporanox; Triasporin.
4-[4-[4-[4-[[2-(2,4-Dichlorophenyl)-2-(1*H*-1,2,4-triazol-1-ylmethyl)-1,3-dioxolan-4-yl]methoxy]phenyl]-1-piperazinyl]phenyl]-2,4-dihydro-2-(1-methylpropyl)-3*H*-1,2,4-triazol-3-one
$C_{35}H_{38}Cl_2N_8O_4$=705.6
CAS—84625-61-6

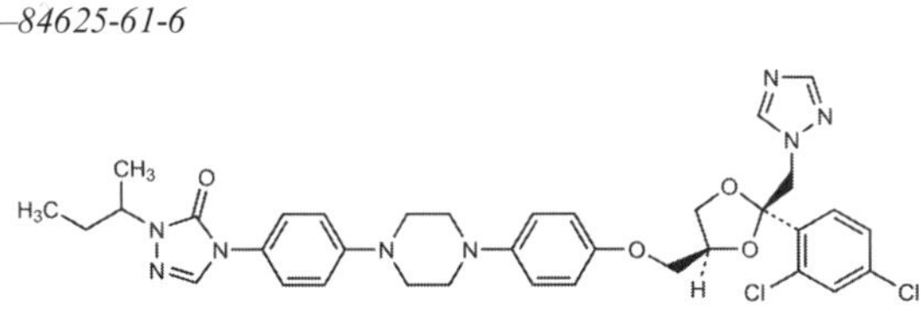

A white to off-white powder; crystals from toluene. M.p.166.2°. It is soluble in dichloromethane; sparingly soluble in tetrahydrofuran; practically insoluble in water and dilute acidic solutions.

Dissociation Constant. pK_a 3.7.

Partition Coefficient. Log *P* (*n*-octanol/buffer pH 8.1), 5.66.

Thin-layer Chromatography. System TB—Rf 01; system TE—Rf 79; system TF—Rf 11; system TAE—Rf 87.

High Performance Liquid Chromatography. System HX—RI 725.

Column: RP C_{18} (RsiL C18HL, 150 × 2.1 mm i.d., 5 μm). Mobile phase: water:acetonitrile (40:60), 0.5 mL/min flow rate. Internal standard (IS): R-51012. UV detection (λ=254 nm). Retention time: itraconazole, 4.3 min; IS, 5.8 min [R. Woestenborgh *et al.*, *J. Chromatogr.*, 1987, *413, Biomed. Appl.*, 332–337].
Column: RP C_{18} (Hypersil, 100 × 4.5 mm i.d., 3 μm). Mobile phase: water:acetonitrile (40:60) containing 0.03% diethylamine, pH 7.8 with dilute orthophosphoric acid, 1 mL/min flow rate. IS: R-51012. UV detection (λ=254 nm). k value: itraconazole, 7.4; hydroxyitraconazole, 2.7; IS, 10.8, [D. Law *et al.*, *Antimicrob. Agents Chemother.*, 1994, *38(7)*, 1561–1566].

Ultraviolet Spectrum. Aqueous acid—263 nm.

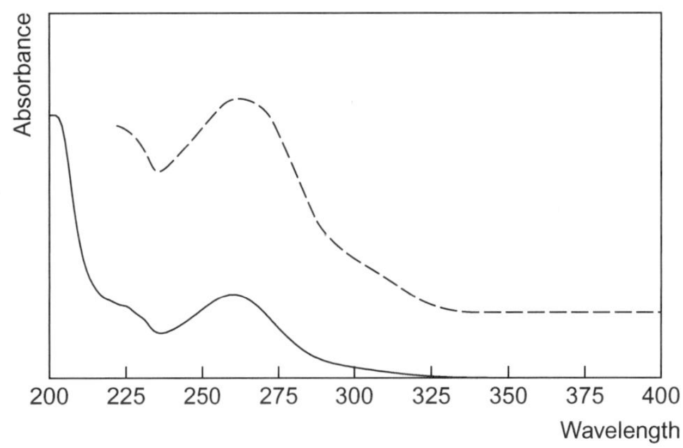

Quantification

High performance liquid chromatography. In plasma: lower limit of detection is 0.001 mg/L. UV detection (λ=254 nm)—R. Woestenborgh *et al.*, *J. Chromatogr.*, 1987, *413*, 332–337. In serum: limit of quantification 0.02 mg/L for the drug and its metabolites. UV detection (λ=254 nm)—D. Law *et al.*, *Antimicrob. Agents Chemother.*, 1994, *38*, 1561–1566. In serum: limit of detection 0.01 mg/L. UV detection (λ=263 nm)—P. O. Gubbins *et al.*, *J. Pharm. Biomed. Anal.*, 1998, *16*, 1005–1012.

Bioassay. In serum—D. Law *et al.*, *Antimicrob. Agents Chemother.*, 1994, *38*, 1561–1566.

Disposition in the Body. Itraconazole is slowly but well absorbed after oral administration with peak concentrations reached in approx. 4 h. Absorption is enhanced in the presence of food and in an acidic intragastric environment. It is metabolised, mainly via oxidative pathways, to inactive metabolites which are excreted via bile and in urine. Over 30 metabolites have been isolated and most are biologically inactive including a hydroxy metabolite (bioactive) and hydroxyitraconazole. Both the drug and hydroxyitraconazole are inhibitors of the CYP3A4 enzyme system. The drug is widely distributed throughout the body with small amounts detected in most body fluids and accumulation occurring in tissues. Itraconazole has also been detected in skin, hair and nail but it does not easily redistribute in these tissues. 3 to 18 % is excreted in the faeces as unchanged drug.

Therapeutic concentration. The trough serum therapeutic concentration is greater than 0.25 mg/L and for the sum of the parent drug and hydroxyitraconazole metabolite, 1 to 4 g/L.

7 healthy males and 5 females with a mean age of 34 years (range 22 to 51) were administered a 100 mg dose of itraconazole either after a 12-h fast (group 1), after a light breakfast (group 2) or after a full breakfast (group 3). Group 1: a mean peak plasma concentration of 0.11 mg/L was observed 3.33 h after ingestion. Group 2: 0.21 mg/L at 3.67 h. Group 3: peak concentration of 0.23 mg/L after 4.17 h [T. Zimmermann *et al.*, *Eur. J. Clin. Pharmacol.*, 1994, *46*, 147–150].

Toxicity. The serum toxic concentration is 6 mg/L (sum of itraconazole and its hydroxy metabolite).

Bioavailability. Dose dependent, increases with increasing dosage; 55% after a 100 mg dose (as solution).

Half-life. 20 h (following a 100 mg single dose); increases to 30 h on multiple dosing.

Volume of distribution. 10.7 L/kg; also reported as 561 L.

Clearance. Plasma, 22.9 L/h; also reported as 18.7 L/h.

Protein binding. Approx. 99.8 %, albumin.

Dose. 100 to 400 mg daily depending on indications and severity.

Kanamycin

Antibiotic

Synonym Kanamycin A
Proprietary names. Kanapat; Kanibel.
O-3-Amino-3-deoxy-α-D–glucopyranosyl-(1→6)-*O*–[6-amino-6-deoxy-α-D–glucopyranosyl-(1→4)]-2-deoxy-D-streptamine
$C_{18}H_{36}N_4O_{11}$=484.5
CAS—59-01-8

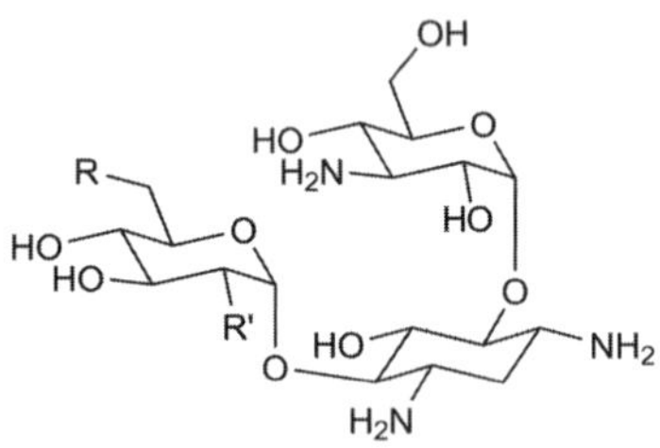

	R	R'
Kanamycin A	NH_2	OH
Kanamycin B	NH_2	NH_2
Kanamycin C	OH	NH_2

An antimicrobial substance produced by the growth of *Streptomyces kanamyceticus*.
A whitish powder.

Kanamycin Acid Sulfate

Proprietary names. Kangen; Kannasyn.
$C_{18}H_{36}N_4O_{11}$,1.7H_2SO_4=651.2
A white hygroscopic powder.
Soluble 1 in 1 of water; practically insoluble in ethanol, acetone, chloroform and ether.

Kanamycin Sulfate

Synonym. Kanamycin A Sulfate
Proprietary names. Kamycine; Kanacolirio; Kanamytrex; Kanasig; Kana-Stulln; Kancin; Kanescin; Kan-Ophtal; Kantrex.
$C_{18}H_{36}N_4O_{11}$,H_2SO_4=582.6
CAS—25389-94-0
A white crystalline powder.
Soluble 1 in 8 of water; practically insoluble in ethanol, acetone, chloroform and ether.

Dissociation Constant. pK_a 7.2.

Partition Coefficient. Log *P* (octanol/water), −6.7.

Thin-layer Chromatography System TA—Rf 01; system TAE—Rf 00. (Acidified potassium permanganate solution, positive.)

Ultraviolet Spectrum. Aqueous acid—249 (A_1^1=about 3b), 306 nm.

Infra-red Spectrum. Principal peaks at wavenumbers 1033, 1068, 1143, 1123, 980, 1516 cm^{-1} (kanamycin sulfate, KBr disk).

Quantification

Spectrofluorimetry. In serum or urine: limit of detection 50 μg/L—A. Csiba, *J. Pharm. Pharmacol.*, 1979, *31*, 115–116.

High performance liquid chromatography. In serum: kanamycin and dibekacin; fluorescence detection—H. Kubo *et al., Antimicrob. Agents Chemother.*, 1985, *28*, 521–523.

Bioassay. Aminoglycoside antibiotics in biological fluids—J. M. Broughall, Aminoglycosides, in *Laboratory Methods in Antimicrobial Chemotherapy*, D. S. Reeves *et al.* (Ed.), Edinburgh, Churchill Livingstone, 1978, pp. 194–207.

Immunoassay. In serum: fluorescence detection—A. F. DeCastro *et al., Antimicrob. Agents Chemother.*, 1986, *29*, 961–964.

Disposition in the Body. Kanamycin is poorly absorbed after oral administration, but rapidly and completely absorbed after IM injection. Up to 95% of a dose is excreted unchanged in the urine in 24 h, most being excreted within the first 6 h. A small amount is excreted in the bile.

Therapeutic concentration. During treatment, the serum concentration should be in the range 20 to 25 mg/L and should be monitored regularly, especially in patients who have renal insufficiency. During multiple dosing, the trough concentration immediately preceding a dose should not exceed 10 mg/L.

Toxicity. Toxic effects may be produced at serum concentrations of 30 mg/L or more, or during chronic treatment if the trough serum concentration exceeds 10 mg/L.

Half-life. Plasma half-life, about 2 to 4 h; increased to 4 to 5 days in renal failure.

Volume of distribution. About 0.3 L/kg.

Clearance. Plasma clearance, about 1.4 mL/min/kg.

Protein binding. In plasma, not significantly bound.

Dose. The equivalent of up to 1.5 g of kanamycin daily, by IM injection.

Ketamine

General Anaesthetic

2-(2-Chlorophenyl)-2-(methylamino)cyclohexanone
$C_{13}H_{16}ClNO$=237.7
CAS—6740-88-1

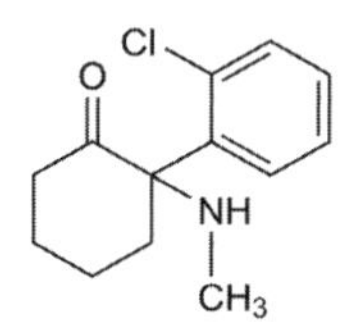

Crystals. M.p. 92° to 93°.

Ketamine Hydrochloride

Proprietary names. Brevinaze; Calypsol; Ketaject; Ketalar; Ketalin; Ketanarkon; Ketanest; Ketaset; Ketavet; Ketina; Ketolar; Velonarcan; Vetalar.
$C_{13}H_{16}ClNO$,HCl=274.2
CAS—1867-66-9
A white crystalline powder. M.p. 262° to 263°.
Soluble 1 in 4 of water, 1 in 14 of ethanol and 1 in 6 of methanol; sparingly soluble in chloroform; practically insoluble in ether.

Dissociation Constant. pK_a 7.5.

Partition Coefficient. Log *P* (octanol/water), 3.1.

Thin-layer Chromatography. System TA—Rf 63; system TB—Rf 37; system TC—Rf 63; system TE—Rf 79; system TL—Rf 64; system TAE—Rf 68; system TAF—Rf 72; system TAJ—Rf 47; system TAK—Rf 04; system TAL—Rf 43. (Acidified iodoplatinate solution, positive.)

Gas Chromatography. System GA—ketamine RI 1840, M (nor-) RI 1810, M (nor-OH-)-H_2O RI 1960, M (nor-OH-)-NH_3 RI 1740, M (nor-di-OH-)-2H_2O RI 1920; system GB—ketamine RI 1939, M (nor-) RI 1907, M (nor-OH-)-H_2O RI 2058, M (nor-OH-)-NH_3 RI 1840, M (nor-di-OH-)-2H_2O RI 2009, M (nor-)-H_2O RI 1931; system GM—ketamine RRT 0.427, M (nor-) RRT 0.423 (both relative to iprindole); system GV—Retention time, 10.4 min.

High Performance Liquid Chromatography. System HX—RI 311; system HY—RI 262; system HZ—Retention time, 2.4 min; system HAA—Retention time, 9.6 min.

Ultraviolet Spectrum. Aqueous acid—269 nm (A_1^1=25a), 276 nm.

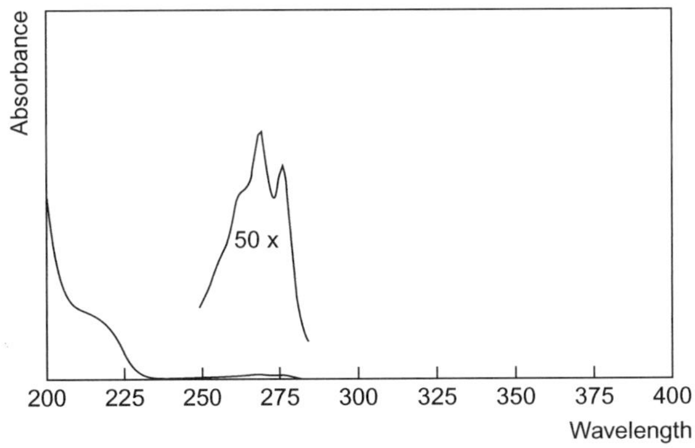

Infra-red Spectrum. Principal peaks at wavenumbers 1696, 747, 1142, 1120, 712, 1027 cm^{-1} (KBr disk).

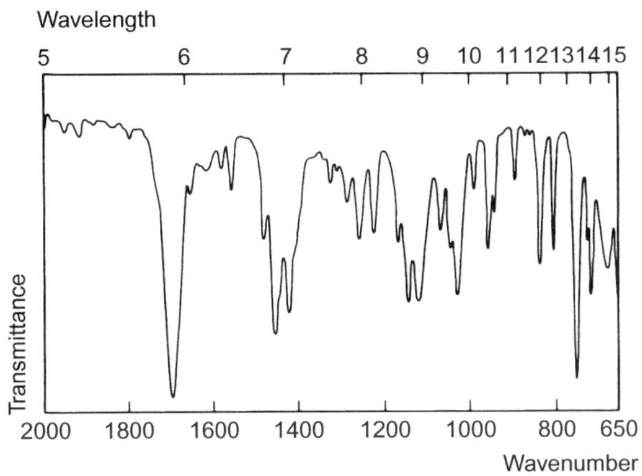

Mass Spectrum. Principal ions at *m/z* 180, 209, 182, 152, 181, 30, 211, 138.

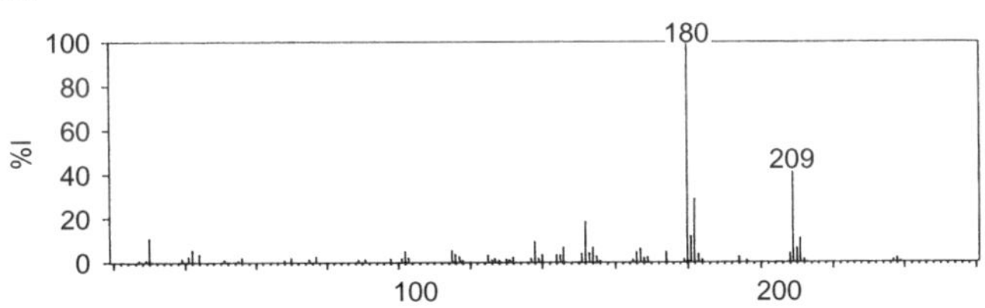

Quantification

Gas chromatography. In serum or urine: ketamine and metabolites, limit of detection 25 μg/L for ketamine in serum, FID—J. Wieber *et al.*, *Anaesthesist*, 1975, *24*, 260–263. In plasma or urine: ketamine and norketamine, limit of detection 10 μg/L, AFID—R. L. Stiller *et al.*, *J. Chromatogr.*, 1982, *232*; *Biomed. Appl.*, *21*, 305–314.

Gas chromatography–mass spectrometry. In plasma: limit of detection 10 μg/L—N. Feng *et al.*, *Ther. Drug Monit.*, 1995, *17*, 95–100. In urine: limit of detection is 5 μg/L—M. L. Olmos-Carmona and M. Hernandez-Carrazquilla, *J. Chromatogr. Biomed. Sci. Appl.*, 1999, *734(1)*, 113–120.

High performance liquid chromatography. In plasma: ketamine and norketamine, limit of quantification 40 μg/L, UV detection—G. Geisslinger *et al.*, *J. Chromatogr.*, 1991, *568*, 165–176. In plasma: ketamine and midazolam, limit of detection < 5 μg/L, UV detection—H. A. Adams *et al.*, *Anaesthetist*, 1992, *41*, 619–624. In plasma: ketamine and norketamine enantiomers, limit of detection about 2 μg/L, UV detection—J. O. Svensson and L. L. Gustafsson, *J. Chromatogr.*, 1996, *678 Biomed. Appl.*, 373–376. In plasma: ketamine, norketamine and dehydronorketamine, limit of quantification for ketamine and norketamine 5 μg/L—S. Bolze and R. Boulieu, *Clin. Chem.*, 1998, *44*, 560–564. In plasma: ketamine and bupivacaine, UV detection—A. S. Gross *et al.*, *J. Chromatogr. B. Biomed. Sci. Appl.*, 1999, *728*, 107–115. In plasma: ketamine and norketamine, limits of detection 5 μg/L and 10 μg/L respectively, UV detection—Y. Yanagihara *et al.*, *J. Chromatogr. B. Biomed. Sci. Appl.*, 2000, *746*, 227–231.

Disposition in the Body. Rapidly distributed in the tissues including the brain following parenteral administration. Ketamine crosses the placenta. It has a bi- or triexponential elimination pattern. In the first phase, ketamine exerts its anaesthetic effects in the CNS and it is then redistributed into peripheral tissues and metabolised in the liver. About 90% of a dose is excreted in the urine in 72 h, with about 2% of the dose as unchanged drug, 2% as norketamine, 16% as dehydronorketamine and 80% as conjugates of hydroxylated metabolites. Norketamine (which has about one-sixth of the potency of ketamine) and dehydronorketamine are found in the serum in concentrations similar to those of ketamine. It has been suggested that dehydronorketamine may be an analytical artefact rather than a metabolite.

Therapeutic concentration

Following single intravenous injections of 2.5 mg/kg to 5 subjects, serum concentrations of about 1 mg/L were reported after 15 min [J. Wieber *et al.*, *Anaesthesist*, 1975, *24*, 260–263].

During continuous intravenous infusion at an average rate of 41 μg/kg/min to 31 subjects, a mean steady-state plasma concentration of 2.2 mg/L was reported; norketamine and dehydronorketamine attained mean peak plasma concentrations of 1.1 mg/L and 0.7 mg/L, respectively, in about 3 h; the subjects awoke at an average plasma concentration of 0.64 mg/L [J. Idvall *et al.*, *Br. J. Anaesth.*, 1979, *51*, 1167–1173].

Following an intramuscular injection of 0.5 mg/kg to 6 subjects, peak plasma concentrations of 0.10 to 0.43 mg/L (mean 0.24) were attained in about 0.3 h; norketamine attained a mean peak plasma concentration of 0.09 mg/L at about 1 h [J. A. Clements *et al.*, *J. Pharm. Sci.*, 1982, *71*, 539–542].

Toxicity. Ketamine produces hallucinogenic effects similar to those of phencyclidine and may be subject to abuse.

The following postmortem tissue concentrations were reported in a fatality involving ketamine: blood 1.8 mg/L, urine 2.0 mg/L, brain 4.3 mg/kg, spleen 6.1 mg/kg, liver 4.9 mg/kg, kidney 3.6 mg/kg; ethanol was also detected at a blood concentration of 1700 mg/L [K. A. Moore *et al.*, *J. Forensic Sci.*, 1997, *42*, 1183–1185].

In a fatality caused by homicidal overdose of ketamine, tissue concentrations at postmortem examination were as follows: blood 27.4 mg/L, urine 8.51 mg/L, bile 15.2 mg/L, brain 3.24 mg/L, liver 6.6 mg/L, kidney 3.38 mg/L; norketamine was also detected in all samples but not quantified [M. Licata *et al.*, *J. Forensic Sci.*, 1994, *39*, 1314–1320].

Half-life. Plasma half-life, about 2 to 3 h.

Volume of distribution. About 4 L/kg.

Clearance. Plasma clearance, about 17 mL/min/kg.

Distribution in blood. Plasma : whole blood ratio, about 0.6.

Protein binding. In plasma, about 20 to 50%.

Note. For a study of the stability of ketamine and its metabolites in human biological samples, see Y. Hijazi *et al.*, *Clin. Chem.*, 2001, *47*, 1713–1715. For a review of the recent trend of ketamine misuse in the USA, see K. A. Moore *et al.*, *J. Anal. Toxicol.*, 2001, *25*, 583–588.

Dose. The equivalent of 1 to 4.5 mg/kg of ketamine, by slow intravenous injection or 6.5 to 13 mg/kg, intramuscularly.

Ketazolam

Tranquilliser

Synonym. U-28774

Proprietary names. Anseren; Contamex; Loftran; Marcen; Sedotime; Solatran; Unakalm.

11-Chloro-8,12b-dihydro-2,8-dimethyl-12b-phenyl-4*H*-[1,3]oxazino[3,2-*d*][1,4]benzodiazepine-4,7(6*H*)-dione

$C_{20}H_{17}ClN_2O_3 = 368.8$

CAS—27223-35-4

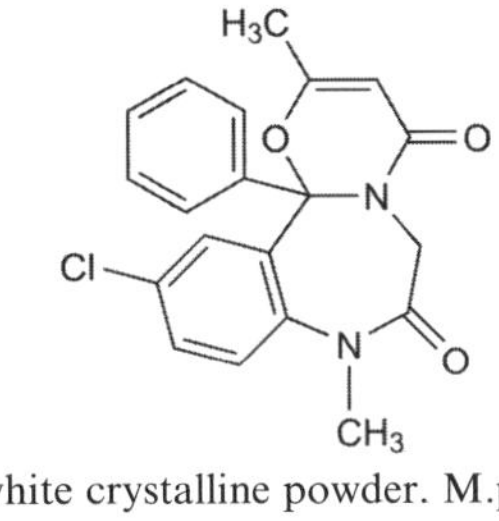

A white crystalline powder. M.p. 183°.

Slightly soluble in water.

Colour Test. Formaldehyde–Sulfuric Acid—orange.

Thin-layer Chromatography. System TA—Rf 66; system TB—Rf 14; system TC—Rf 64; system TD—Rf 45; system TE—Rf 74; system TF—Rf 45; system TL—Rf 66; system TAD—Rf 62; system TAE—Rf 83; system TAF—Rf 80. (Dragendorff spray, positive; furfuraldehyde reagent, dark grey; acidified iodoplatinate solution, positive; mercuric chloride–diphenylcarbazone reagent, pale blue; ninhydrin spray, pale yellow; acidified potassium permanganate solution, positive.)

Gas Chromatography. System GA—ketazolam RI 2444; diazepam RI 2428; oxazepam RI 2325; system GB—ketazolam RI 2552; diazepam RI 2556; oxazepam RI 2438; system GG—diazepam RI 2940; oxazepam RI 2803 (rearrangement can occur on-column to form diazepam).

High Performance Liquid Chromatography. System HI—*k* 12.81; system HJ—*k* 2.45; system HK—*k* 0.04; system HX—RI 577; system HY—RI 522; system HZ—Retention time 10.3 min; system HAX—Retention time 7.7 min; system HAY—Retention time 9.2 min; system HBH—*k* 10.78; system HBI—*k* 2.22.

Ultraviolet Spectrum. Ethanol—242 nm (A^1_1 = 492a).

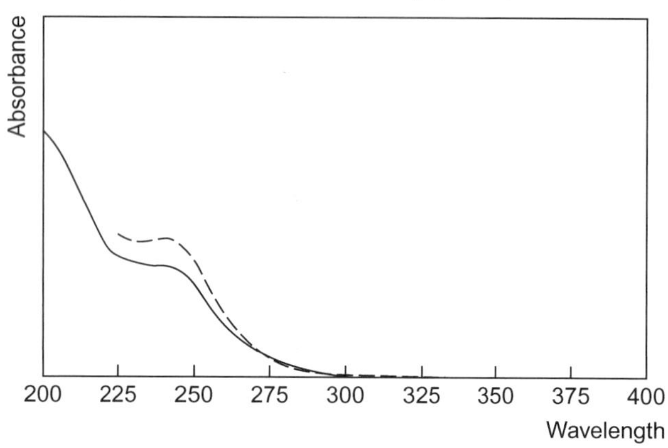

Infra-red Spectrum. Principal peaks at wavenumbers 1675, 820, 1105, 1195, 1308, 1242 cm^{-1} (KBr disk).

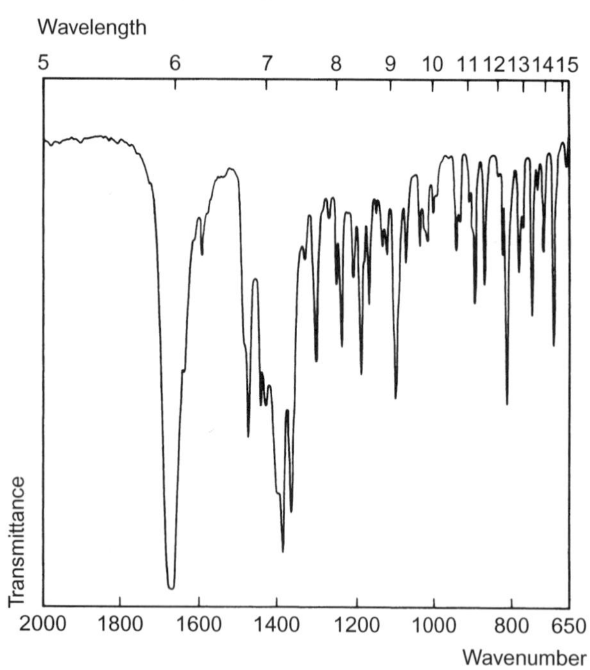

Mass Spectrum. Principal ions at *m/z* 256, 284, 283, 285, 84, 257, 258, 255; oxazepam 257, 77, 268, 239, 205, 267, 233, 259.

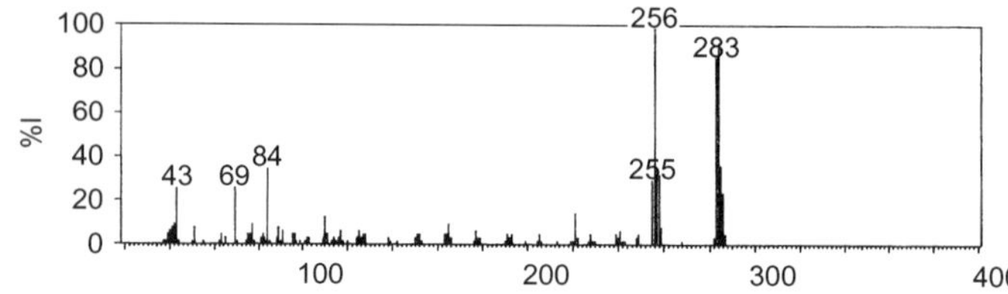

Quantification

Gas chromatography–mass spectrometry. Limit of quantification is 2.5 to 5 µg/L (full scan) and 0.1 to 0.5 µg/L (SIM, *m/z* 256)—D. Borrey *et al.*, *J. Chromatogr. A*, 2001, *910*, 105–118. In urine: ketazolam and other benzodiazepines, limits of detection 1 to 1.7 µg/L (scan mode) and 50 to 1000 µg/L (SIM mode)—D. Borrey *et al.*, *J. Chromatogr. B Biomed. Sci. Appl.*, 2001, *765*, 187–197.

Disposition in the Body. Readily absorbed after oral administration. Rapidly metabolised by *N*-demethylation to desmethylketazolam and desmethyldiazepam (nordazepam). About 80% of a dose is excreted in the urine as metabolites with only traces of unchanged drug. Of the material excreted in the urine, about 56% is oxazepam and the remainder is a mixture of minor metabolites including diazepam, desmethyldiazepam, temazepam, and other unidentified metabolites. About 20% of a dose is eliminated in the faeces, mainly as metabolites.

Therapeutic concentration

Following a single oral dose of 30 mg of ^{14}C-labelled ketazolam, peak plasma concentrations of about 0.004 mg/L of ketazolam, 0.017 µg/L of diazepam, and 0.127 mg/L of *N*-demethylated metabolites were attained in 2, 10, and 14 h, respectively [F. S. Eberts jun. *et al.*, *Pharmacologist*, 1977, *19*, 165].

Toxicity. Overdoses of up to 0.5 g have been ingested without serious toxic effects.

Half-life. Plasma half-life, ketazolam about 1.5 h, oxazepam 4 to 25 h (mean 8), diazepam 20 to 100 h (mean 48).

Dose. 15 to 60 mg daily.

Ketobemidone

Narcotic Analgesic

Synonym. Cetobemidone

1-[4-(3-Hydroxyphenyl)-1-methyl-4-piperidyl]-1-propanone

$C_{15}H_{21}NO_2$ = 247.3

CAS—469-79-4

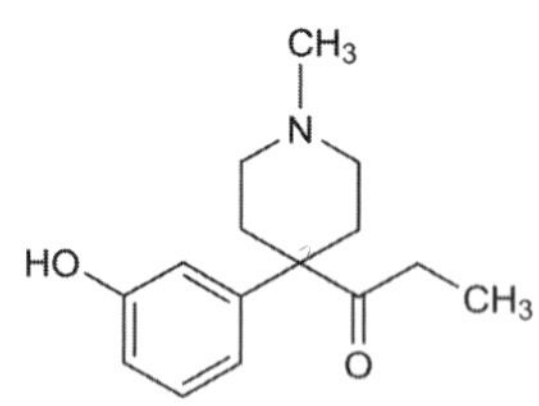

Crystals. M.p. 156° to 157°.

Ketobemidone Hydrochloride

Synonyms. Hoechst 10720; Win-1539.

Proprietary names. Cliradon; Cymidon; Ketogan; Ketogin; Ketodur; Ketorax.

$C_{15}H_{21}NO_2$,HCl = 283.8

CAS—5965-49-1

Crystals. M.p. 201° to 202°. Soluble in water, slightly soluble in alcohol.

Dissociation Constant. pK_a 8.7 (20°).

Partition Coefficient. Log *P* (heptane/pH 7.4), −3.0.

Colour Tests. Mandelin's Test—blue-green; Marquis Test—orange.

Thin-layer Chromatography. System TA—Rf 47; system TB—Rf 02; system TC—Rf 09; system TE—Rf 37; system TL—Rf 06; system TAE—Rf 26; system TAJ—Rf 03; system TAK—Rf 01; system TAL—Rf 40. (Acidified iodoplatinate solution, positive.)

Gas Chromatography. System GA—RI 2040.

High Performance Liquid Chromatography. System HA—*k* 2.8 (tailing peak); system HX—RI 294; system HY—RI 245.

Ultraviolet Spectrum. Aqueous acid—280 (A^1_1=81a); aqueous alkali—300 nm (A^1_1=126b).

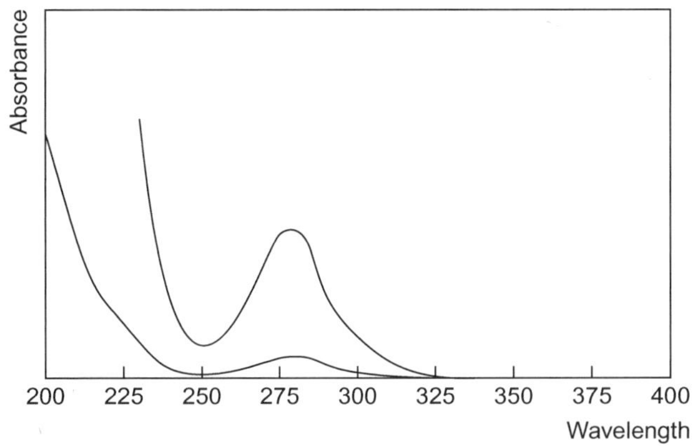

Infra-red Spectrum. Principal peaks at wavenumbers 1705, 1597, 1248, 777, 699, 1285 cm^{-1} (KBr disk).

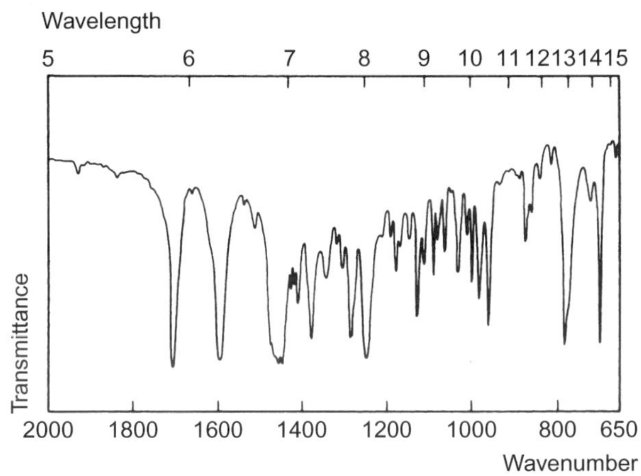

Mass Spectrum. Principal ions at *m/z* 70, 71, 42, 44, 57, 190, 29, 247.

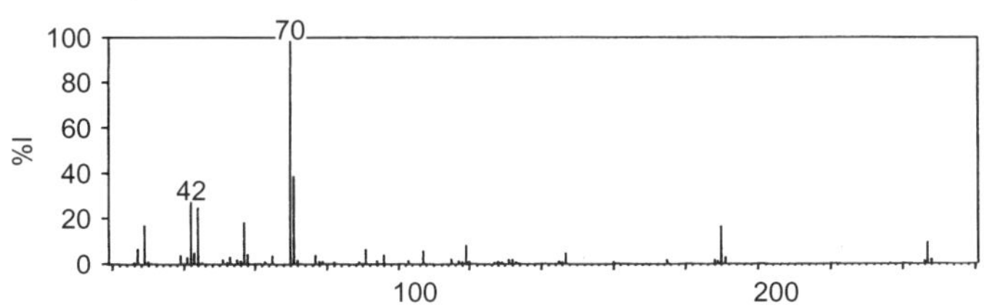

Quantification

Gas chromatography–mass spectrometry. In plasma: ketobemidone and desmethylketobemidone, limit of detection 5 µg/L—U. Bondesson *et al.*, *Biomed. Mass Spectrom.*, 1983, *10*, 283–286. In plasma or urine: ketobemidone and its major metabolites, limit of detection 0.8 µg/L—J. O. Svensson *et al.*, *Ther. Drug Monit.*, 2001, *23*, 399–405.

Disposition in the Body. Ketobemidone is poorly absorbed after oral or rectal administration. It is metabolised by *N*-demethylation.

Toxicity

In 76 fatalities attributed to ketobemidone (23 also involving alcohol and 26 also involving other drugs), tissue concentrations were as follows: blood 0.2 to 3.2 (median 0.5) µg/g after oral administration and 0.1 to 1.5 (median 0.3) µg/g after injection; liver 0.2 to 6.2 (median 1.3) µg/g after oral administration and 0.2 to 1.3 (median 0.5) µg/g after injection; muscle 0.2 to 0.5 (median 0.4) µg/g after oral administration and 0.1 to 1.1 (median 0.2) µg/g after injection. Where the blood alcohol concentration was >1 mg/g, the median ketobemidone concentrations were: blood 0.1 µg/g; liver 0.4 µg/g (after both oral and IV injection) [A. Steentoft and K. Worm, *J. Forensic Sci. Soc.*, 1994, *34*, 181–185].

Bioavailability. About 40%.

Half-life. Plasma half-life, about 2 h.

Volume of distribution. About 2 to 3 L/kg.

Clearance. Plasma clearance, about 10 mL/min/kg.

Dose. Ketobemidone has been given in doses of 5 to 10 mg.

Ketoconazole

Antifungal

Synonym. R-41400
Proprietary names. Daktarin Gold; Fungarest; Fungoral; Ketoderm; Ketoisdin; Nizoral; Orifungal M; Panfungol; Sebizole; Terzolin.
cis-1-Acetyl-4-[4-[[2-(2,4-dichlorophenyl)-2-(1*H*-imidazol-1-ylmethyl)-1,3-dioxolan-4-yl]methoxy]phenyl]piperazine
$C_{26}H_{28}Cl_2N_4O_4$=531.4
CAS—65277-42-1

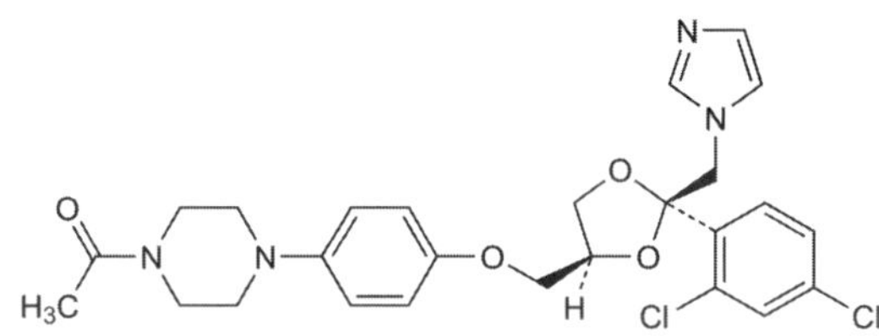

Crystals. M.p. 146°.
Practically insoluble in water; soluble 1 in 54 of ethanol, 1 in about 2 of chloroform and 1 in 9 of methanol; very slightly soluble in ether.

Partition Coefficient. Log *P* (octanol/water), 4.4.

Thin-layer Chromatography. System TB—Rf 00; system TE—Rf 50; system TAE—Rf 68.

High Performance Liquid Chromatography. System HX—RI 439; system HY—RI 464; system HZ—Retention time(s) 5.2 min; system HAA—Retention time(s) 15.7 min.

Ultraviolet Spectrum. Aqueous acid—269 (A^1_1=26a); aqueous alkali—287 (A^1_1=29b); methanol—244 (A^1_1=280b), 296 nm (A^1_1=32b).

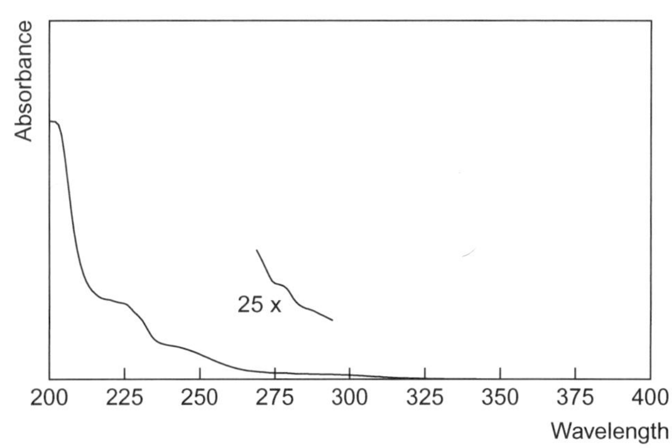

Infra-red Spectrum. Principal peaks at wavenumbers 1507, 1640, 1240, 1258, 1200, 1221 cm^{-1} (KBr disk).

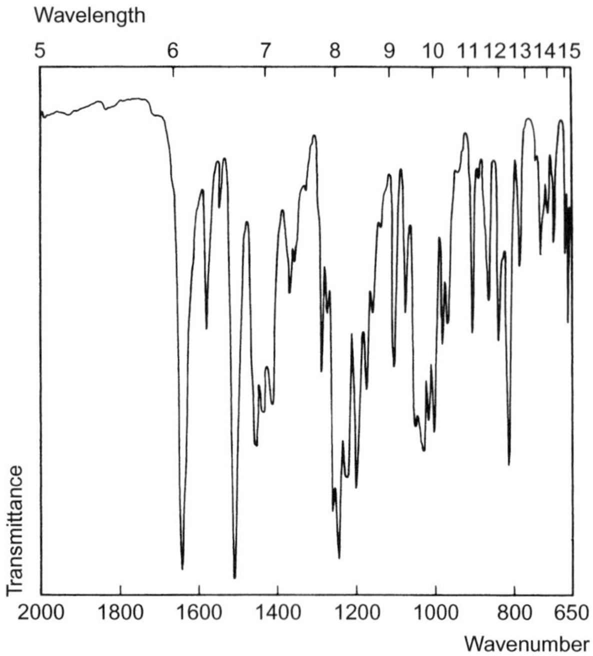

Quantification

High performance liquid chromatography. In plasma: limit of detection <100 µg/L, UV detection—K. B. Alton, *J. Chromatogr.*, 1980, *221*; *B Biomed. Appl.*, *10*, 337–344. In serum, plasma, cerebrospinal fluid or synovial fluid: limit of detection 40 µg/L, fluorescence detection—V. L. Pascucci *et al.*, *J. Pharm. Sci.*, 1983, *72*, 1467–1469. In plasma or saliva: electrochemical detection—D. W. Hoffman *et al.*, *Anal. Biochem.*, 1988, *172*, 495–498. In plasma: limit of detection 40 µg/L, fluorescence detection—K. H. Yuen and K. K. Peh, *J. Chromatogr. B Biomed. Sci. Appl.*, 1998, *715*, 436–440.

High performance liquid chromatography–mass spectrometry. In plasma: limit of detection <20 µg/L—Y. L. Chen *et al.*, *J. Chromatogr. B Analyt. Technol. Biomed. Life Sci.*, 2002, *774*, 67–78.

Disposition in the Body. Ketoconazole is readily but incompletely absorbed after oral administration and extensively metabolised to inactive metabolites. About 13% of a dose is excreted in the urine in 4 days and 57% is eliminated in the faeces in the same period.

Therapeutic concentration

Following single oral doses of 200 and 400 mg to 6 subjects, mean peak serum concentrations of 3.6 and 6.5 mg/L were attained in 2 and 3 h, respectively [T. K. Daneshmend *et al.*, *J. Antimicrob. Chemother.*, 1981, *8*, 299–304].

Half-life. Plasma half-life, about 6 to 10 h.

Distribution in blood. Plasma : whole blood ratio, 1.6.

Protein Binding. In plasma, about 99%.

Note. For a review of the pharmacokinetics of systemic antifungal drugs, see T. K. Daneshmend and D. W. Warnock, *Clin. Pharmacokinet.*, 1983, *8*, 17–42.

Dose. 200 to 400 mg daily.

Ketoprofen

Analgesic

Synonym. RP-19583.
Proprietary names. Actron; Actroneffix; Alrheumat; Alrheumun; Apo-Keto; Fastum; Fenoket; Gabrilen; Jomethid; Keral; Ketil; Ketocid; Ketofen; Ketolist; Ketotard; Ketovail; Ketozip; Ketum; Larafen; Orudis; Oruvail; Powergel; Profenid; Solpaflex; Topfena; Toprec.
3-Benzoyl-α-methylbenzeneacetic acid
$C_{16}H_{14}O_3$=254.3
CAS—22071-15-4

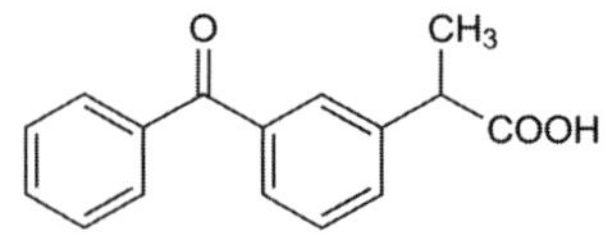

A white crystalline powder. M.p. 93° to 96°.
Slightly soluble in water; soluble in acetone, ethyl acetate, ethanol, chloroform and ether.

Dissociation Constant. pK_a 4.5.

Partition Coefficient. Log *P* (octanol/buffer pH 7.4), 0.

Colour Tests. Aromaticity (Method 2)—colourless/yellow; Koppanyi–Zwikker Test—violet.

Thin-layer Chromatography. System TD—Rf 27; system TE—Rf 06; system TF—Rf 25; system TG—Rf 14; system TAD—Rf 41; system TAE—Rf 85; system TAJ—Rf 54; system TAK—Rf 82; system TAL—Rf 98. (Ludy Tenger reagent, orange.)

Gas Chromatography. System GA—ketoprofen RI 2245; ketoprofen-Me RI 2090; system GD—Retention time of methyl derivative 1.45 relative to *n*-$C_{16}H_{34}$; system GL—ketoprofen-Me RI 2090; M(OH-)-Me_2 RI 2250.

High Performance Liquid Chromatography. System HAA—Retention time(s) 19.6 min; system HD—*k* 2.4; system HV—Retention time 0.66 relative to meclofenamic acid; system HX—RI 495; system HZ—Retention time(s) 6.4 min.

Ultraviolet Spectrum. Aqueous acid—260 (A_1^1=665a); aqueous alkali—262 nm (A_1^1=647a).

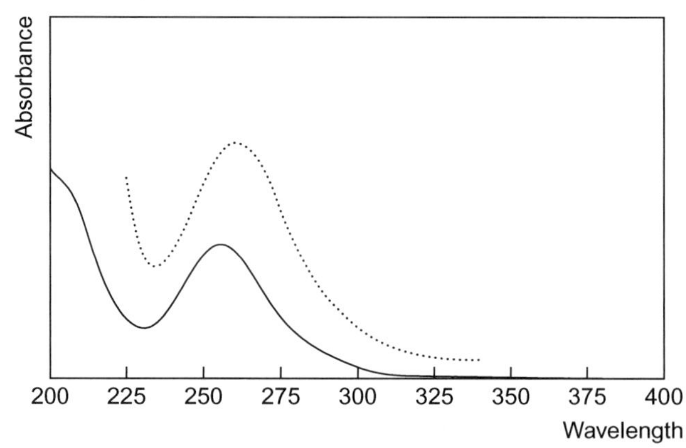

Infra-red Spectrum. Principal peaks at wavenumbers 1656, 1693, 1284, 714, 690, 1226 cm^{-1} (KBr disk). Two polymorphic forms may occur.

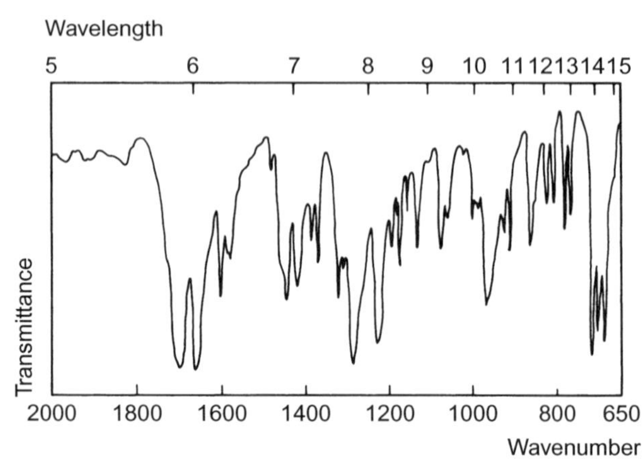

Mass Spectrum. Principal ions at *m*/*z* 105, 177, 77, 209, 254, 210, 103, 181.

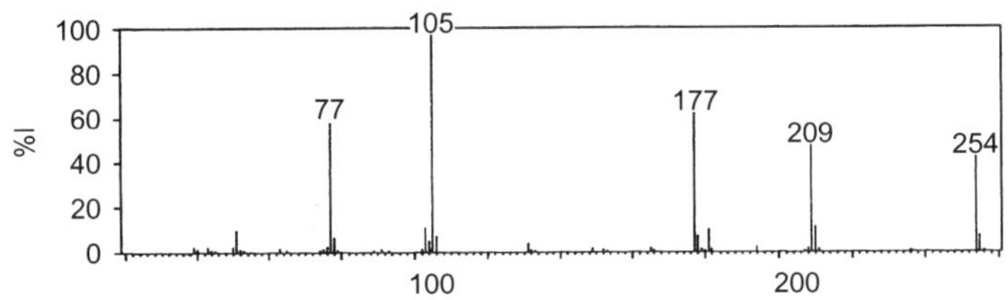

Quantification

Gas chromatography. In plasma: limit of detection 130 µg/L, ECD—P. Stenberg *et al.*, *J. Chromatogr.*, 1979, *177*, 145–148.

Gas chromatography–mass spectrometry. In plasma or synovial fluid: ketoprofen and ibuprofen, limit of detection for ketoprofen <2 µg/L, SIM—D. S. Rumble *et al.*, *J. Chromatogr.*, 1992, *584*, 189–197.

High performance liquid chromatography. In plasma or urine: limit of detection 50 µg/L, UV detection—C. M. Kaye *et al.*, *Br. J. Clin. Pharmacol.*, 1981, *11*, 395–398. In plasma or serum: ketoprofen and other NSAIDs, UV detection—P. J. Streete, *J. Chromatogr.*, 1989, *495*, 179–193. In plasma: ketoprofen enantiomers, limit of detection 20 µg/L, UV detection—M. Yagi *et al.*, *Chem. Pharm. Bull.*, 1990, *38*, 2513–2517. In plasma: enantiomers of ketoprofen, ibuprofen and fenoprofen, limit of detection for ketoprofen 0.1 mg/L, UV detection—S. Menzel-Soglowek *et al.*, *J. Chromatogr.*, 1990, *532*, 295–303. In plasma: ketoprofen enantiomers, limit of detection 150 µg/L—P. J. Hayball *et al.*, *J. Chromatogr.*, 1991, *570*, 446–452. In plasma: ketoprofen enantiomers—Y. Oda *et al.*, *J. Pharm. Biomed. Anal.*, 1992, *10*, 81–87; A. Shibukawa *et al.*, *J. Pharm. Sci.*, 1992, *81*, 710–715; R. Lovlin *et al.*, *J. Chromatogr. B Biomed. Appl.*, 1996, *679*, 196–198; J. Boisvert *et al.*, *J. Chromatogr. B Biomed. Sci. Appl.*, 1997, *690*, 189–193. In plasma or urine: UV detection—R. A. Carr *et al.*, *J. Chromatogr. B Biomed. Appl.*, 1995, *668*, 175–181. In plasma or dialysate: ketoprofen and its acyl glucuronides—N. G. Grubb *et al.*, *J. Chromatogr. B Biomed. Appl.*, 1996, *678*, 237–244. In plasma: limit of detection 1 mg/L—N. Rifai *et al.*, *Ther. Drug Monit.*, 1997, *19*, 175–178. In plasma or cerebrospinal fluid: limit of detection 20 µg/L—H. Kokki *et al.*, *Paediatr. Anaesth.*, 2002, *12*, 313–316.

Disposition in the Body. Ketoprofen is readily absorbed after oral, rectal, or IM administration. About 75% of a single oral dose is excreted in the urine in 24 h, mostly in the first 6 h, about 90% of which is the glucuronide conjugate; hydroxylation may also occur.

Therapeutic concentration

After oral administration of 100 mg as capsules, to 7 subjects, peak plasma concentrations of 6.0 to 14.3 (mean 10) mg/L were attained in 0.45 to 2.5 h; a single rectal dose of 100 mg produced peak plasma concentrations of 4.7 to 10.5 (mean 7.5) mg/L in 0.75 to 1.5 h, and an IM dose of 100 mg produced peak concentrations of 8.3 to 13.2 (mean 10.4) mg/L in 0.33 to 0.5 h. After oral doses of 50 mg four times a day to 7 subjects, mean maximum steady-state concentrations of 5.6 mg/L were reported [T. Ishizaki *et al.*, *Eur. J. Clin. Pharmacol.*, 1980, *18*, 407–414].

After administration of a single oral dose of 200 mg (as sustained-release granules) to 12 subjects, mean peak plasma ketoprofen levels of 4.51 mg/L were attained in 2 h and remained practically constant for at least 12 h. The same dose of a conventional sustained-release capsule resulted in a mean peak concentration of 5.91 mg/L at 4.17 h and administration of 100 mg ketoprofen, twice at a 12-h interval, as a prompt-release capsule produced mean peak plasma concentrations of 10.52 mg/L 1.38 h after the first dose and 12.80 mg/L 1.46 h after the second dose [A. Roda *et al.*, *Int. J. Pharm.*, 2002, *241*, 165–172].

Half-life. Plasma half-life, 1 to 4 h.

Volume of distribution. About 0.1 to 0.2 L/kg.

Clearance. Plasma clearance, about 1 to 2 mL/min/kg.

Protein binding. In plasma, about 95%.

Note. For a review of the pharmacokinetics of ketoprofen, see F. Jamali and D. R. Brocks, *Clin. Pharmacokinet.*, 1990, *19*, 197–217.

Dose. 100 to 200 mg daily.

Ketorolac

NSAID/Analgesic

Synonym. RS-37619

5-Benzoyl-2,3-dihydro-1*H*-pyrrolizine-1-carboxylic acid

$C_{15}H_{13}NO_3$=255.3

CAS—74103-06-3

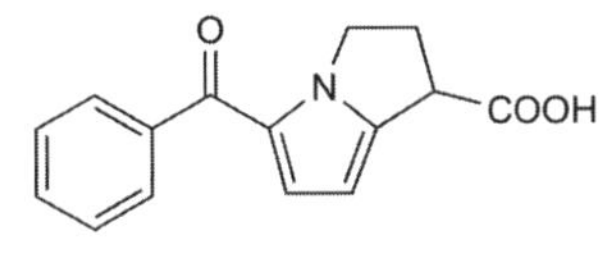

Crystals from ethyl acetate/ether. M.p. 160° to 161°.

Ketorolac Trometamol

Synonyms. RS-37619-00-31-3

Proprietary names. Acular; Dolac; Droal; Lixidol; Tarasyn; Tonum; Toradol; Toratex.

(±)-5-Benzoyl-2,3-dehydro-1*H*-pyrrolizine-1-carboxylic acid compound with 2-amino-2-(hydroxymethyl)-1,3-propanediol (1:1)

$C_{19}H_{24}N_2O_6$=376.4

CAS—74103-07-4

(+)-isomer: crystals from ethyl acetate/hexane, M.p. 174° (M.p. 154° to 156° also reported).

(−)-isomer: crystals from ethyl acetate/hexane, M.p. 169° to 170° (M.p. 153° to 155° also reported).

Dissociation Constant. pK_a 3.49.

Partition Coefficient. Log *P* (octanol/water), 2.32.

High Performance Liquid Chromatography. System HAX—retention time 6.3 min; system HAY—retention time 5.6 min; system HZ—retention time 4.1 min.

Column: (analytical) RCM 100 radial compression module with C_{18} (Radialpak, 100 × 8 mm i.d., 10 µm); (guard) C_{18} (Corasil, 35 to 50 µm). Mobile phase: water:acetonitrile:dibutylamine phosphate (pH 2.5) (30:20:1), 1.8 mL/min flow rate. Internal standard (IS): tolmetin sodium. UV detection (λ=313 nm). Retention time: ketorolac, 6.5 min; IS, 9.4 min [Z. Wang *et al.*, *J. Chromatogr. B Biomed Sci. Appl.*, 2001, *755*, 383–386].

Column: RP C_{18} Nucleosil (250 × 4.6 mm i.d., 5 µm). Mobile phase: acetonitrile:water (with sodium dihydrogen orthophosphate, 10 mM, and sodium lauryl sulfate, 1 mM; adjusted to pH 2.8) (35:65), 1.5 mL/min flow rate. UV detection (λ=355 nm). Retention time: 10.3 min [J. L. Mason and G. J. Hobbs, *J. Chromatogr.*, 1995, *665*, *Biomed. Appl.*, 410–415].

Ultraviolet Spectrum. Methanol—245, 312 nm.

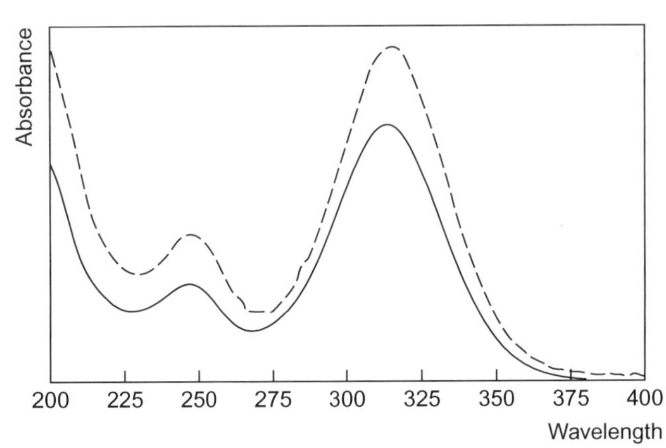

Mass Spectrum. Principal ions at *m/z* 105, 210, 255, 77, 51, 78, 132, 91.

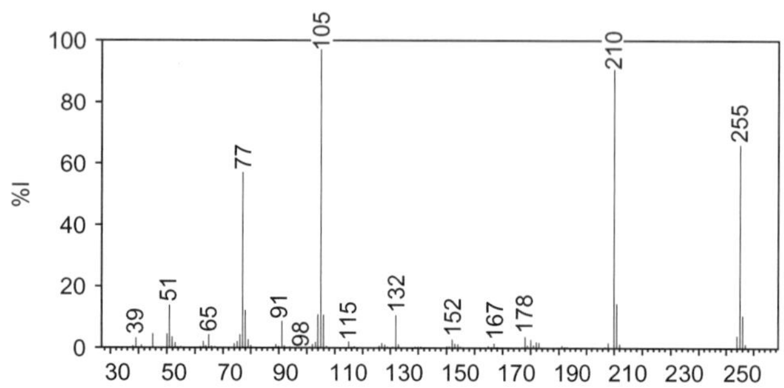

Quantification

High performance liquid chromatography. In plasma: limit of detection 5 μg/L (both enantiomers). UV detection (λ = 320 nm)—D. J. Jones and A. R. Bjorksten, *J. Chromatogr.*, 1994, *661*, *Biomed. Appl.*, 165–167. In plasma: limit of detection 35 μg/L. UV detection (λ = 325 nm)—M. H. Mills *et al.*, *J. Chromatogr.*, 1994, *658*, *Biomed. Appl.*, 177–182.

Disposition in the Body. Ketorolac trometamol is more hydrophilic than ketorolac and is rapidly absorbed after both oral and intramuscular administration. Peak plasma concentrations are reached between 30 and 60 min. The presence of food reduces the rate of absorption but not the extent. It is metabolised via conjugation and hydroxylation but does not undergo a significant degree of presystemic metabolism. The major metabolites are the acyl glucuronide and *p*-hydroxyketorolac which represent 77% and 12%, respectively, of an oral dose as urinary excretion products. However, the glucuronic acid conjugates are not detected in plasma. *p*-Hydroxyketorolac has about 20% of the anti-inflammatory activity and 1% of the analgesic activity of ketorolac. A small amount is distributed in breast milk. It does not readily penetrate the blood–brain barrier but crosses the placenta.

Therapeutic concentration. The serum therapeutic concentration is 0.22 to 3.50 mg/L.

13 healthy men and women, aged between 65 and 78 years (mean 72 years), and 16 young male volunteers, aged between 20 and 39 years (mean 30 years) were administered either an oral dose of 10 mg ketorolac or 30 mg intramuscularly (IM). Mean peak plasma levels of 2.99 (range 1.60 to 4.78) mg/L and 2.52 (1.45 to 3.82) mg/L were obtained for the young and elderly, respectively, after the IM dose. The times to peak concentrations were 0.75 and 0.97 h (range 0.33 to 2.0 h). Mean peak plasma concentrations of 0.86 (range 0.55 to 1.10) mg/L and 0.90 (0.57 to 1.44) mg/L were reached with the oral dose in the elderly and young, respectively. The times to peak concentrations were 0.33 and 0.72 (range 0.33 to 1.0) h, respectively [N. S. Jallad, *J. Clin. Pharmacol.*, 1990, *30*, 76–81].

Toxicity. Adverse effects include nausea, rash oedema, headache and hypertension, occurring at ketorolac plasma concentration above 5 mg/L.

A 30-year-old white woman was administered with an intramuscular injection of 60 mg of ketorolac trometamol after complaining of acute lower back pain. Shortly afterwards she suffered an apparent cardiac arrest. Blood postmortem examination revealed the presence of phenytoin, 31.1 mg/L, diazepam, 0.1 mg/L, lidocaine, 4.0 mg/L, procainamide, 9.8 mg/L and *N*-acetyl procainamide, 11.3 mg/L. All these drugs were administered during attempts at resuscitation. The ketorolac concentration was 2.9 mg/L and although this is within the therapeutic range and consistent with the administered dose of 60 mg, the cause of death was ruled as an acute anaphylactic drug reaction to ketorolac.

Bioavailability. 81 to 100% after administration of an oral solution.

Half-life. 3 to 6 h; 4 to 7 h (elderly); 9 to 10 h (renal impairment).

Volume of distribution. 0.15 to 0.33 L/kg.

Clearance. Oral dose: 0.39 mL/min/kg (elderly); 0.55 mL/min/kg (young). Intramuscular dose: 0.21 to 0.57 mL/min/kg (mean 0.32); 0.28 to 0.76 mL/min/kg (mean 0.44).

Protein binding. > 99%.

Dose. Orally: 10 mg every 4 to 6 h (6 to 8 h for the elderly) with a maximum of 40 mg daily. Intravenously: initial dose of 10 mg followed by 10 to 30 mg every 4 to 6 h. Maximum daily dose is 90 mg and 60 mg for the elderly and patients weighing less than 50 kg.

Ketotifen

Anti-allergic

4,9-Dihydro-4-(1-methyl-4-piperidinylidene)-10*H*-benzo[4,5]cyclohepta-[1,2-*b*]thiophen-10-one
$C_{19}H_{19}NOS = 309.4$
CAS—34580-13-7

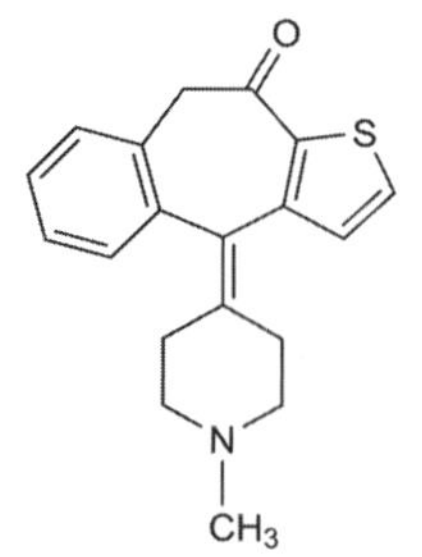

Crystals. M.p. 151° to 153°.

Ketotifen Fumarate

Proprietary names. Airvitess; Asdron; Asmafen; Asmalergin; Asmax; Asmen; Astifat; Broncoten; Cipanfeno; Ketasma; Ketof; Nemesil; Padiatifen; Profilasmin; Profiten; Quefeno; Zaditen; Zaditor; Zatofug.
$C_{19}H_{19}NOS,C_4H_4O_4 = 425.5$
CAS—34580-14-8
A white crystalline powder. M.p. 192°, with decomposition.
Slightly soluble in water; soluble in ethanol; sparingly soluble in chloroform.

Thin-layer Chromatography. System TB—Rf 24; system TE—Rf 52; system TAE—Rf 24.

Gas Chromatography. System GA—RI 2607.

High Performance Liquid Chromatography. System HX—RI 373; system HY—RI 315.

Ultraviolet Spectrum. Aqueous acid—297 (A^1_1 = 475a); aqueous alkali—237, 302 nm.

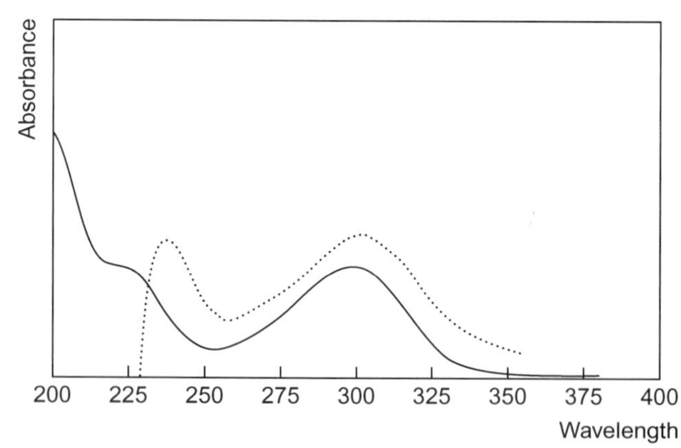

Infra-red Spectrum. Principal peaks at wavenumbers 1650, 1280, 1255, 1302, 1720, 1180 cm^{-1} (ketotifen fumarate, KBr disk).

Mass Spectrum. Principal ions at *m/z* 309, 96, 42, 58, 98, 70, 57, 44.

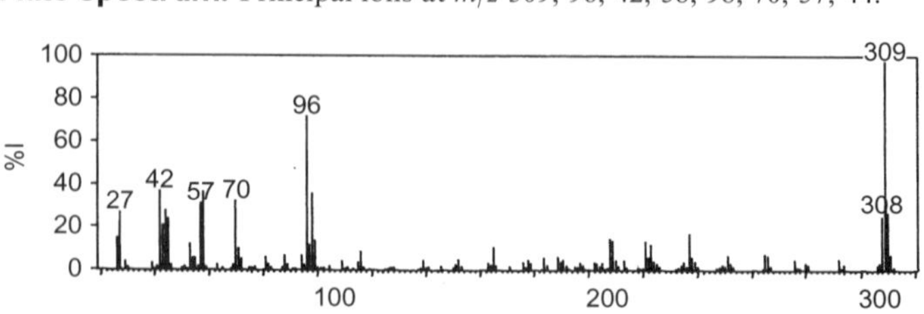

Quantification

Gas chromatography–mass spectrometry. In plasma: limit of detection 0.05 μg/L for ketotifen and the desmethyl metabolite, 0.3 μg/L for 10-hydroxyketotifen—C. Julien-Larose *et al.*, *Biomed. Mass Spectrom.*,

1983, *10*, 136–142. In plasma: limit of detection 0.01 μg/L—S. Tzvetanov *et al.*, *J. Chromatogr. B Biomed. Sci. Appl.*, 1999, *732*, 251–256.

Disposition in the Body. Ketotifen is absorbed after oral administration. It is metabolised by 10-hydroxylation, *N*-demethylation, and glucuronic acid conjugation. It is excreted in the urine and faeces as unchanged drug and metabolites.

Therapeutic concentration

Following a single oral dose of 2 mg to 3 subjects, a peak plasma concentration of about 0.0006 mg/L was attained in 2 h; a peak plasma concentration of about 0.015 mg/L of ketotifen glucuronide was attained in about 4 h [C. Julien-Larose *et al.*, *Biomed. Mass Spectrom.*, 1983, *10*, 136–142].

Toxicity

In 8 cases of overdose involving ingestion of up to 120 mg, drowsiness and other toxic effects were reported but in each case full recovery occurred within 12 h. In 3 cases involving the ingestion of 10, 50 and 120 mg, plasma concentrations were 0.016, 0.054 and 0.122 mg/L, respectively, at 5, 3 and 20 h after ingestion [D. B. Jefferys and G. N. Volans, *Br. Med. J.*, 1981, *282*, 1755–1756 and 2014].

In a fatality involving ketotifen, a postmortem blood concentration of 1.2 mg/L was reported [A. H. Stead and A. C. Moffat, personal communication].

Dose. The equivalent of 2 to 4 mg of ketotifen daily.

Labetalol

Antihypertensive

Synonym. Ibidomide

2-Hydroxy-5-[1-hydroxy-2-[(1-methyl-3–phenylpropyl)amino]ethyl]-benzamide

$C_{19}H_{24}N_2O_3=328.4$

CAS—36894-69-6

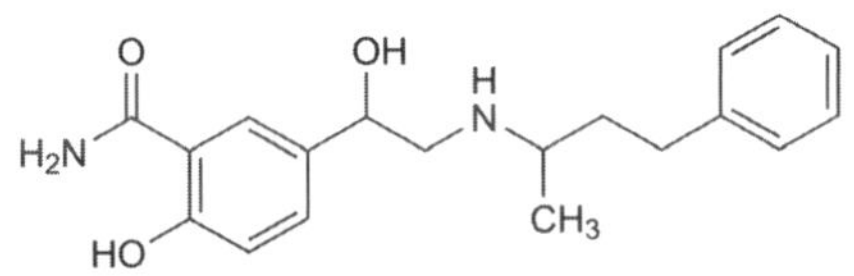

Labetalol Hydrochloride

Synonym. Sch-15719W

Proprietary names. Abetol; Albetol; Alfabetal; Amipress; Hybloc; Ipolab; Labrocol; Normodyne; Presolol; Pressalolo; Trandate.

$C_{19}H_{24}N_2O_3,HCl=364.9$

CAS—32780-64-6

A white crystalline solid. M.p. about 180°.

Soluble in water and ethanol; practically insoluble in chloroform and ether.

Dissociation Constant. pK_a 7.4 (phenol), 8.7 (-NH_2).

Partition Coefficient. Log *P* (octanol/water), 3.1.

Colour Tests. Ferric Chloride—violet; Folin–Ciocalteu Reagent—blue; Liebermann's Test—brown-orange; Mandelin's Test—green-blue; Marquis Test—red→brown-red; Nessler's Reagent (100°)—black.

Thin-layer Chromatography. System TB—Rf 00; system TE—Rf 29; system TF—Rf 01; system TAE—Rf 32.

Gas Chromatography. System GA—Art RI 1320; system GB—Art RI 1270.

High Performance Liquid Chromatography. System HA—*k* 1.7 (tailing peak); system HX—RI 365; system HY—RI 290; system HZ—Retention time(s) 3.0 min.

Ultraviolet Spectrum. Aqueous acid—302 (A^1_1=95a); aqueous alkali—246 (A^1_1=267a), 333 nm (A^1_1=161a).

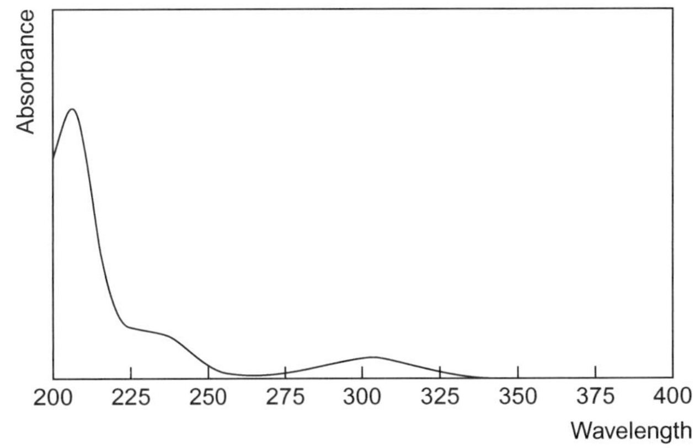

Infra-red Spectrum. Principal peaks at wavenumbers 1680, 1643, 1502, 1270, 820, 1250 cm^{-1} (labetalol hydrochloride, Nujol mull).

Quantification

Gas chromatography–mass spectrometry. In urine: enantiomers of labetalol metabolite 3-amino-1-phenylbutane, SIM—A. Changchit *et al.*, *Biol. Mass Spectrom.*, 1991, *20*, 751–758.

High performance liquid chromatography. In plasma, serum or whole blood: limit of detection 10 μg/L, UV detection—I. J. Hidalgo and K. T. Muir, *J. Chromatogr.*, 1984, *305*; *Biomed. Appl.*, *30*, 222–227. In postmortem tissues: UV detection—L. K. Panell *et al.*, *J. Anal. Toxicol.*, 1982, *6*, 193–195. In plasma: fluorescence detection—D. R. Luke *et al.*, *Clin. Chem.*, 1987, *33*, 1450–1452. In plasma: limit of detection 1 μg/L, fluorescence detection—V. Ostrovska *et al.*, *J. Chromatogr.*, 1988, *446*, 323–327. In biological samples: limits of detection 1.5 to 1.8 μg/L, fluorescence detection—J. M. Dakers *et al.*, *J. Chromatogr. B Biomed. Sci. Appl.*, 1997, *704*, 215–220. In urine: limit of detection 10 μg/L, amperometric detection—C. Ceniceros *et al.*, *J. Chromatogr. B Biomed. Sci. Appl.*, 1998, *705*, 97–103.

Radioreceptor assay. In plasma: limit of detection 5 μg/L—J. G. Kelly *et al.*, *Br. J. Clin. Pharmacol.*, 1981, *12*, 258–260.

Disposition in the Body. Labetalol is well absorbed after oral administration but undergoes extensive first-pass metabolism. The major metabolites are glucuronides of labetalol. Up to about 60% of a dose is excreted in the urine in 24 h as conjugates, one of which has been identified as the *O*-phenylglucuronide; about 5% of a dose is excreted as unchanged drug.

Therapeutic concentration

After a single oral dose of 100 mg given to 6 subjects, peak plasma concentrations of 0.09 to 0.25 (mean 0.16) mg/L were attained in about 0.5 h; following a single oral dose of 200 mg to the same subjects, peak plasma concentrations of 0.09 to 0.27 (mean 0.19) mg/L were reported at about 1 h [J. J. McNeil *et al.*, *Br. J. Clin. Pharmacol.*, 1979, *8*, Suppl. 2, 157S–161S].

Following oral administration of 200 mg twice daily to 9 subjects, average steady-state plasma concentrations of 0.04 to 0.18 (mean 0.09) mg/L were reported [J. J. McNeil *et al.*, *Br. J. Clin. Pharmacol.*, 1982, *13*, Suppl. 1, 75S–80S].

Continuous IV infusion of labetolol (1.5 mg/kg over 5 min, followed 30 min later by 0.2 mg/kg/h for 5.5 h) administered to 6 subjects resulted in a mean steady-state plasma concentration of 264 μg/L being achieved within 2 h [M. Chauvin *et al.*, *Br. J. Anaesth.*, 1987, *59*, 1250–1256].

Toxicity

A 68-year-old subject suffering from chronic respiratory disease died about 1 h after inadvertently being given 200 mg of labetalol. Postmortem kidney and liver concentrations of 10.6 and 20.5 μg/g, respectively, were reported and were considered to be consistent with a therapeutic dose; death was attributed to respiratory disease [L. K. Panell *et al.*, *J. Anal. Toxicol.*, 1982, *6*, 193–195].

A 25-year-old man suffered acute renal failure about 3 days after deliberately ingesting 6 g of labetalol plus 7 pints of lager; haemodialysis for 16 days was necessary to bring about recovery. [A. Korzets *et al.*, *Postgrad. Med. J.*, 1990. *66*. 66–67].

Bioavailability. 10 to 80% (mean 30%).

Half-life. Plasma half-life, 3 to 6 h.

Volume of distribution. About 3 to 10 (mean 7) L/kg.

Clearance. Plasma clearance, 10 to 40 (mean 25) mL/min/kg.

Protein binding. In plasma, about 50%.

Note. For a review of the pharmacokinetics of labetalol, see J. J. McNeil and W. J. Louis, *Clin. Pharmacokinet.*, 1984, *9*, 157–167.

Dose. 200 to 800 mg of labetalol hydrochloride daily; doses of 2.4 g daily have been given.

Lachesine Chloride

Anticholinergic

N-Ethyl-2-[(hydroxydiphenylacetyl)oxy]-*N*,*N*-dimethylethanaminium chloride
$C_{20}H_{26}ClNO_3$=363.9
CAS—1164-38-1

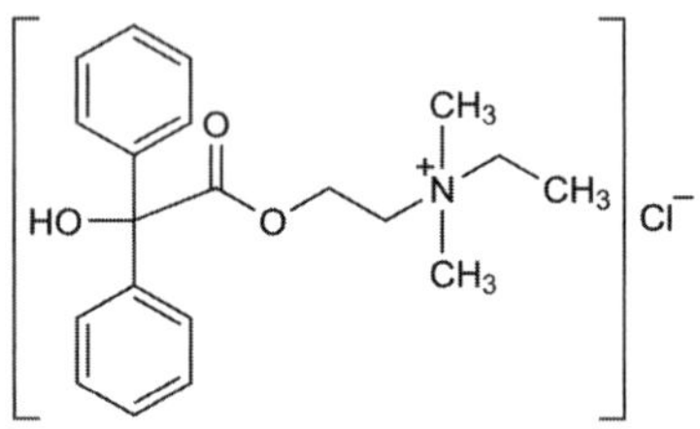

A white amorphous powder. M.p. 212° to 214°.
Soluble 1 in 3 of water and 1 in 10 of ethanol (90%); very slightly soluble in chloroform and ether.

Partition Coefficient. Log *P* (octanol/water), −1.1.

Colour Tests. Mandelin's Test—orange→green; Marquis Test—orange→green→blue.

Thin-layer Chromatography. System TA—Rf 02. (Acidified iodoplatinate solution, positive.)

Gas Chromatography. System GA—RI 1852.

Ultraviolet Spectrum. Aqueous acid—252, 258 (A^1_1=12b), 264 nm. No alkaline shift.

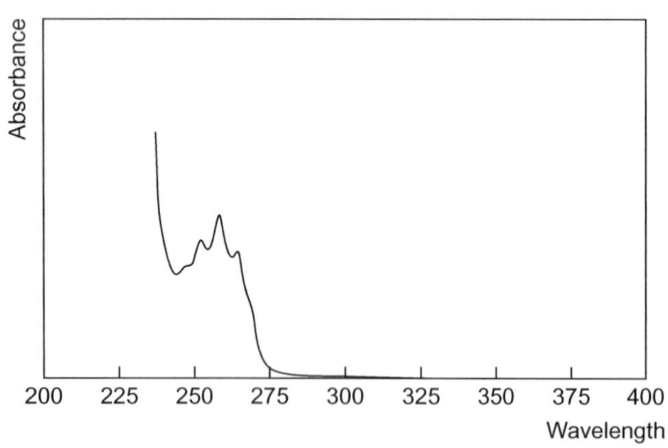

Infra-red Spectrum. Principal peaks at wavenumbers 1739, 1241, 699, 743, 1176, 1191 cm^{-1} (KBr disk).

Use. As a 1% ophthalmic solution.

Lacidipine

Calcium Antagonist

Synonyms. GR-43659X; GX-1048.
Proprietary names. Aponil; Caldine; Lacimen; Lacipil; Lacirex; Midotens; Motens; Viapres; Zascal.
(*E*)-4-[2-[3-(1,1-Dimethylethoxy)-3-oxo-1-propenyl]phenyl]-1,4-dihydro-2,6-dimethyl-3,5-pyridinedicarboxylic acid diethyl ester
$C_{26}H_{33}NO_6$=455.5
CAS—103890-78-4

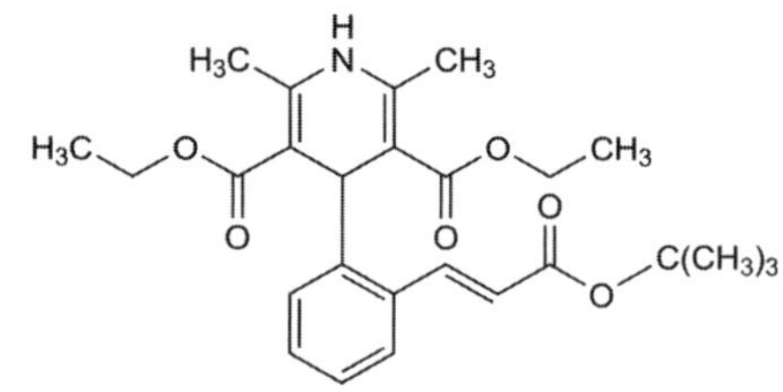

A crystalline solid with M.p. 174° to 175°.

Partition Coefficient. Log *P* (octanol/water), 5.20.

Thin-layer Chromatography. System TE—Rf 81; system TF—Rf 65.

High Performance Liquid Chromatography. System HX—RI 900; system HAA—retention time 27.2 min.

Column: (analytical) RP C_{18} (250 × 4.6 mm i.d., 5 µm) (guard) C_{18} µBondapak. Column temperature: 30°. Mobile phase: methanol:water (70:30), containing acetate buffer (2 mM, pH 5.0), 1 mL/min flow rate. Detection: ECD. Retention time: 15.7 min [J. A. Lopez *et al.*, *J. Chromatogr. A*, 2000, *870*, 105–114].

Column: (analytical) RP C_{18} (Novapak, 100 × 4.6 mm i.d.) (guard) RP C_{18} (30 × 4.6 mm i.d., 30 to 40 µm). Column temperature: 50°. Mobile phase: methanol:acetonitrile:water (35:10:55), containing ammonium acetate (0.05 M, pH 5.0), 1.2 mL/min flow rate. Elution programme: (35:10:55) for 7 min, to (60:10:30) in 23 min, to (80:10:10) in 5 min and held for 10 min. UV detection (λ=282 nm). Retention time not specified [M. Scandola, *J. Chromatogr.*, 1993, *647*, 155–166].

Ultraviolet Spectrum. Aqueous acid—239, 209, 282, 366 nm.

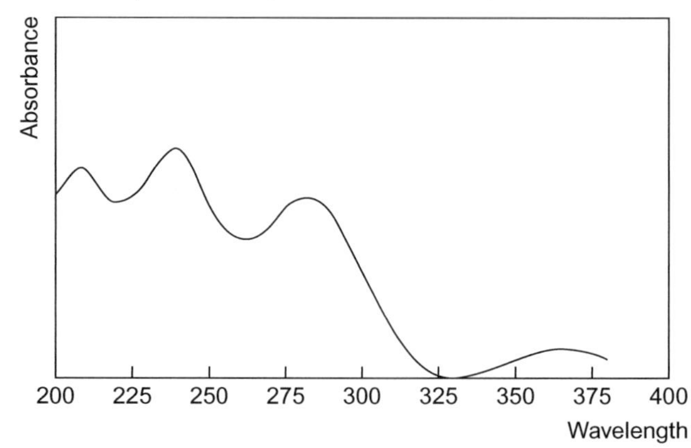

Mass Spectrum. Principal ions at *m*/*z* 252, 196, 326, 169, 119, 382, 69, 150.

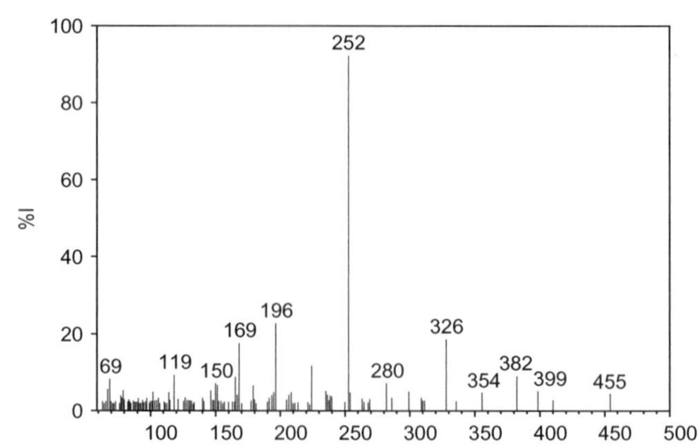

Quantification

High performance liquid chromatography. In plasma: limit of detection 0.5 µg/L—G. L. Evans *et al.*, *Methodol. Surv. Biochem. Anal.*, 1990, *20*, 285–290. In plasma: limit of detection 0.02 µg/L, in conjunction with radioimmunoassay—M. Pellegatti *et al.*, *J. Chromatogr.*, 1992, *573*, *Biomed. Appl.*, 105–111.

Disposition in the Body. Lacidipine is rapidly but poorly absorbed after oral administration and undergoes extensive first-pass metabolism. Two main metabolites have been identified as a pyridine analogue and a carboxylic acid analogue. It is eliminated by metabolism in the liver and the metabolites are excreted mainly via bile. Approx. 70% of an oral dose is eliminated in faeces and the remainder in urine. No parent drug has been detected in urine or faeces.

Therapeutic concentration

2 healthy volunteers were administered 4 mg lacidipine orally after an overnight fast. The peak plasma concentrations observed were 1.918 μg/L and 3.392 μg/L, 1 h after administration of the dose [M. Pellegatti *et al.*, *J. Chromatogr.*, 1992, *573*, *Biomed. Appl.*, 105–111].

17 healthy young volunteers were administered with oral doses of 4, 6 and 8 mg lacidipine. Peak concentrations of 2.8, 6.1 and 8.6 μg/L were observed about 1 h after administration [L. Squassante *et al.*, *J. Cardiovasc. Pharmacol.*, 1994, *23 (Suppl. 5)*, S94–S97].

Bioavailability. 18.5% (range 4 to 52%).

Half-life. 13 to 19 h.

Volume of distribution. 0.9 to 2.3 L/kg also reported as 537 L with high inter-subject variation.

Protein binding. > 95% (mainly albumin).

Dose. The usual initial dose is 2 mg once daily which may be increased to 4 or 6 mg if necessary after 3 to 4 weeks.

Lamivudine

Nucleoside Reverse Transcriptase Inhibitor/Antiviral

Synonyms. 3TC; GR-109714X; (–)-BCH-189.
Proprietary names. Epivir; Zeffix.
(2*R-cis*)-4-Amino-1-[2-(hydroxymethyl)-1,3-oxathiolan-5-yl]-2(1*H*)-pyrimidinone
$C_8H_{11}N_3O_3S$=229.3
CAS—134678-17-4

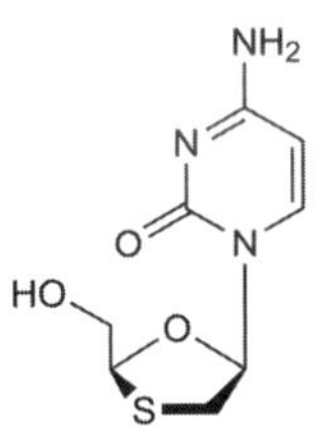

White crystals from boiling ethanol or white solid from methanol/ethyl acetate. M.p.160° to 162°. Solubility in water at 20°, 70 mg/mL.

High Performance Liquid Chromatography. System HAD—*k* 2.7.

Column: C_{18} (Keystone Aquasil, 150 × 2.1 mm i.d., 5 μm). Mobile phase: acetonitrile:water (15:85), 0.3 mL/min flow rate. MS–MS detection (*m/z* 230 to 112). Retention time: 2.5 min [K. B. Kenney *et al.*, *J. Pharm. Biomed. Anal.*, 2000, *22*, 967–983].

Ultraviolet Spectrum. Aqueous acid—212, 279 nm.

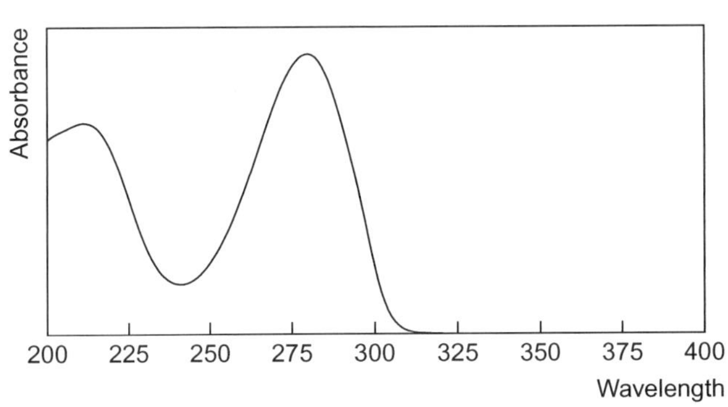

Quantification

High performance liquid chromatography. In urine: limit of quantification 0.5 mg/L—D. M. Morris and K. Selinger, *J. Pharm. Biomed. Anal.*, 1994, *12*, 255. In plasma: limit of quantification 0.02 mg/L. UV detection (λ=260 nm)—G. Aymard *et al.*, *J. Chromatogr. B Biomed. Sci. Appl.*, 2000, *744*, 227–240. In serum: limit of quantification 3 μg/L. Detection: MS–MS—K. B. Kenney *et al.*, *J. Chromatogr. B Biomed. Sci. Appl.*, 2000, *742*, 173–183. In serum: limit of detection 0.26 mg/L. UV detection (λ=250 nm)—V. A. Simon *et al.*, *J. Chromatogr. A*, 2001, *913(1-2)*, 447–453.

Disposition in the Body. In healthy volunteers lamivudine is rapidly absorbed following an oral administration, reaching peak plasma concentrations within 1 to 1.5 h. About 70% of the total dose is excreted unchanged in urine and between 5 and 10% undergoes hepatic metabolism to form a *trans*-sulfoxide metabolite.

Therapeutic concentration

Group 1: 6 HIV-infected males, aged between 29 and 41 years, with creatinine clearance ⩾ 60 mL/min. Group 2: 4 HIV-infected males and females, 29 to 68 years old, with creatinine clearance between 10 and 40 mL/min. Group 3: 6 males and females (31 to 51 years old), creatinine clearance < 10 mL/min. Each group was administered a single oral dose of 300 mg after an overnight fast. The mean peak plasma concentration for group 1 was 2.524 mg/L, group 2, 3.538 mg/L and group 3, 5.684 mg/L and these levels were reached within 1, 1 and 2 h, respectively [A. E. Heald *et al.*, *Antimicrob. Agents Chemother.*, 1996, *40*, 1514–1519].

Bioavailability. 80 to 87%.

Half-life. 5 to 7 h (after a single dose) and 11 h (when sampling for 48 h), which may increase in presence of renal impairment.

Volume of distribution. Approx. 100 L.

Protein binding. < 36%.

Dose. Adults: 100 mg daily to 150 mg every 12 h. Children (3 months to 12 years): 4 mg/kg every 12 h with a maximum of 300 mg daily.

Lamotrigine

Anticonvulsant/Anti-epileptic

Synonyms. BW-430C; LTG.
Proprietary name. Lamictal
6-(2,3-Dichlorophenyl)-1,2,4-triazine-3,5-diamine
$C_9H_7Cl_2N_5$=256.1
CAS—84057-84-1

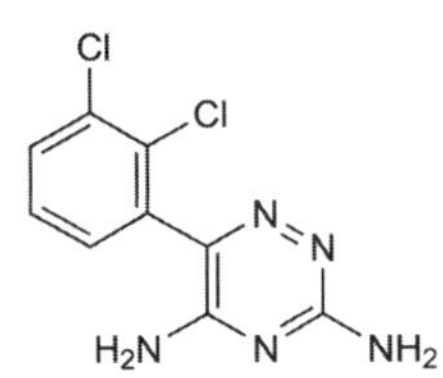

White to pale cream crystals from isopropanol, M.p. 216° to 218°. Solubility at 25° (mg/mL); water, 0.17; HCl (0.1 M), 4.1. It is practically insoluble in ethanol.

Dissociation Constant. pK_a 5.7.

Gas Chromatography. System GB—RI 2562; system GAJ—RRT 1.941 (relative to methylphenobarbital).

High Performance Liquid Chromatography. System HY—RI 272; system HZ—Retention time 2.3 min.

Ultraviolet Spectrum. Aqueous acid (0.025 M sulfuric acid)—208, 265 nm; (0.1 M $HCOONH_4$, pH 3)—267 nm; ethanol—307.5 nm.

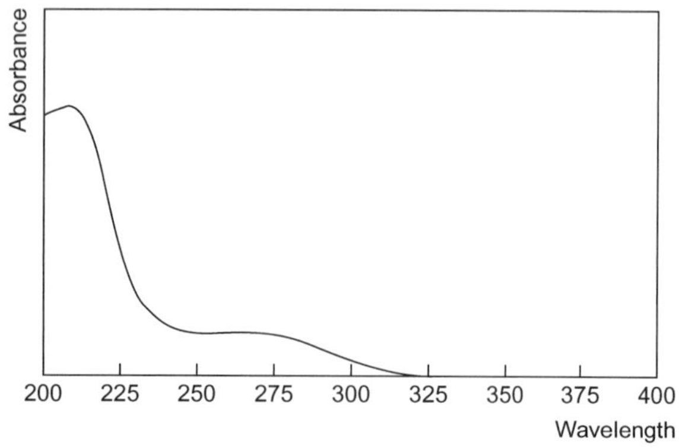

Infra-red Spectrum. Principal peaks at wavenumbers 1614, 1488, 1429, 1404 cm^{-1}.

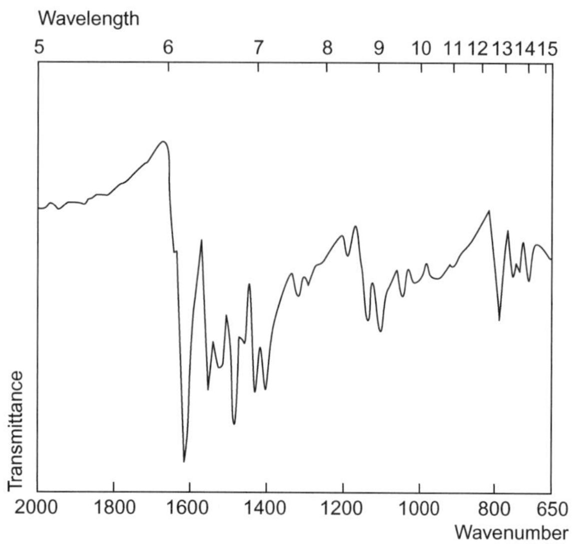

Mass Spectrum. Principal ions at *m/z* 185, 187, 255, 257, 123, 115, 157, 150.

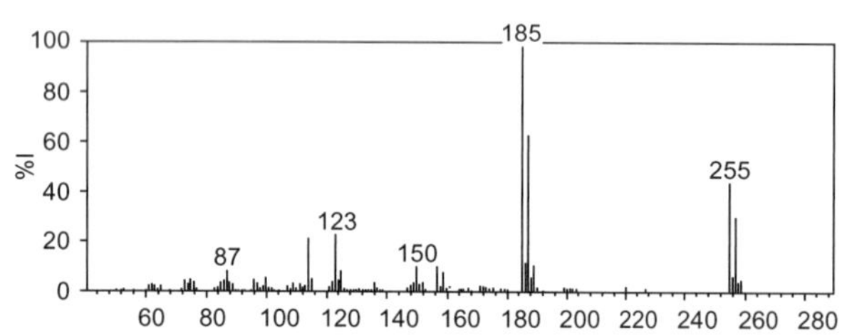

Quantification

High performance liquid chromatography. In plasma: limit of detection 0.05 mg/L, UV detection (λ=306 nm)—J. Posner *et al.*, *Br. J. Clin. Pharmacol.*, 1989, *28*, 117–120. In plasma: the limit of quantification 0.5 mg/L, limit of detection 0.1 mg/L, UV detection (λ=280 nm)—B. Sallustio and R. Morris, *Ther. Drug Monit.*, 1997, *19*, 688–693. In urine: limit of detection (for full spectra) 100 ng. MS detection—M. V. Doig and R. A. Clare, *J. Chromatogr.*, 1991, *554*, 181–189.

Disposition in the Body. Lamotrigine is readily and virtually completely absorbed, reaching peak concentrations in approx. 1.5 to 5 h. The presence of food does not affect absorption of the drug. A second peak may be seen 4 to 6 h after administration. Elimination is mainly via the kidneys (70% of dose in urine) with 10% as the unchanged drug: approx. 75 to 90% as glucuronide conjugate, trace amounts as the 2-*N*-methyl metabolite and less than 5% as the other metabolites. Approx. 2% is eliminated in faeces. The amount of unchanged drug excreted is 30% greater in Gilbert's Syndrome.

Therapeutic concentration. The serum therapeutic concentration is 4 to 10 mg/L and trough, 2 to 5 mg/L.

Group 1: 5 healthy males, aged between 27 and 49 years, were administered with a weekly doubling dose between 7.5 and 240 mg. Group 2: 10 healthy male and females, 19 to 61 years old, received a single dose of 120 mg lamotrigine. The mean peak plasma concentrations for group 1 were 0.40, 0.80, 1.60 and 3.16 mg/L for a 30, 60, 120 and 240 mg dose observed approx. 1.9, 1.7, 2.1 and 3.1 h after administration, respectively. Group 2 showed a mean peak concentration of 1.56 mg/L with a range between 1.19 and 1.93 mg/L which was reached 0.5 to 4 h (mean, 2.8 h) after dosing [E. Kilpatrick *et al.*, *Epilepsia*, 1996, *37*, 534–538].

Toxicity

No serious toxicity in a patient who took 1.35 g of lamotrogine and was subsequently treated with gastric lavage and activated charcoal [N.A. Buckley *et al.*, *Lancet*, 1993, *342*, 1552–1553]. Similarly a patient who ingested between 4 and 5 g was admitted to hospital with coma which lasted 8 to 12 h followed by recovery over the next 2 to 3 days. Another patient who ingested 5.6 g was found unconscious and recovered after treatment with activated charcoal and sleeping for 16 h.

Bioavailability. Oral formulation, 98%.

Half-life. Mean range (administration with no other medication) is 25 ± 10 h. Single dose, healthy volunteers is 24.1 ± 5.7 h. Multiple doses over 7 days, healthy volunteers, 25.5 ± 10.2 h. In the elderly (mean age 71 years, healthy volunteers), 31.2 ± 5.4 h.
Adults with epilepsy: 13.5 h; single dose co-administration with carbamazepine and phenytoin, mean is 15 h (range 7.8 to 33.3 h). Single dose co-administration with valproic acid, mean 59 h (range 30.5 to 88.8 h).
Gilbert's syndrome: plasma elimination half-life lower (37%).
Chronic renal failure (creatinine clearance approx. 18 mL/min): 36 h.

Volume of distribution. 1 to 1.4 L/kg for healthy volunteers administered with a single 120 mg dose. 0.77 to 1.04 L/kg for healthy males administered with a weekly doubling dose of 30 to 240 mg. The mean apparent volume of distribution is 12% lower in elderly (mean age 71 years, healthy volunteers).

Clearance. 20.7 to 52.3 (mean, 41.7) mL/min for healthy volunteers receiving a 120 mg single dose. 22.4 to 37.7 (mean 29.6) mL/min for those administered with a weekly doubling dose between 30 and 240 mg. The mean apparent clearance is 37% lower in the elderly (mean age 71 years, healthy volunteers). The mean oral clearance is 32% lower in Gilbert's syndrome and reduced by 9-fold in chronic renal failure.

Protein binding. Plasma, 56%.

Dose. 50 to 400 mg per day.

Lanatoside C

Cardiac Glycoside

Synonym. Celanide
Proprietary names. Allocor; Cedilanid; Ceglunat; Celadigal; Cetosanol; Lanimerck.
Note. The name Cedilanid is also applied to a preparation of deslanoside.
(3*β*,5*β*,12*β*)-3-[(*O*-*β*-D-Glucopyranosyl-(1→4)-*O*-3-*O*-acetyl-2,6-dideoxy-*β*-D-*ribo*-hexopyranosyl-(1→4)-*O*-2,6-dideoxy-*β*-D-*ribo*-hexopyranosyl-(1→4)-2,6-dideoxy-*β*-D-*ribo*-hexopyranosyl)oxy]-12,14-dihydroxycard-20(22)-enolide
$C_{49}H_{76}O_{20}$=985.1
CAS—17575-22-3

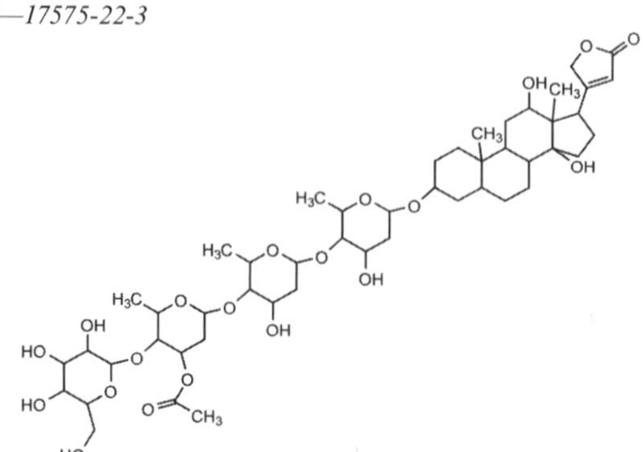

A glycoside obtained from the leaves of the woolly foxglove, *Digitalis lanata* (Scrophulariaceae).
Colourless or white hygroscopic crystals or white crystalline powder. It melts above 240°, indistinctly and with decomposition.

Practically insoluble in water and ether; sparingly soluble in ethanol; soluble 1 in 2000 of chloroform and 1 in 20,000 of methanol; freely soluble in dioxane and pyridine.

Partition Coefficient. Log *P* (octanol/water), 0.1.

Colour Tests. Antimony Pentachloride—yellow→brown→black-violet. Dissolve 2 to 3 mg in 5 mL of a solution containing 0.5 mL of 9% ferric chloride solution and 100 mL of acetic acid; underlay with 5 mL of sulfuric acid—an intense blue colour forms in the acetic acid layer and a brown ring free from red at the junction of the two liquids (see also Deslanoside).

Thin-layer Chromatography. System TE—Rf 06; system TAE—Rf 89. (Perchloric acid solution, followed by examination under UV light, blue fluorescence; *p*-Anisaldehyde reagent, blue.)

High Performance Liquid Chromatography. System HM—lanatoside C *k* 39.5, digoxin *k* 11.3.

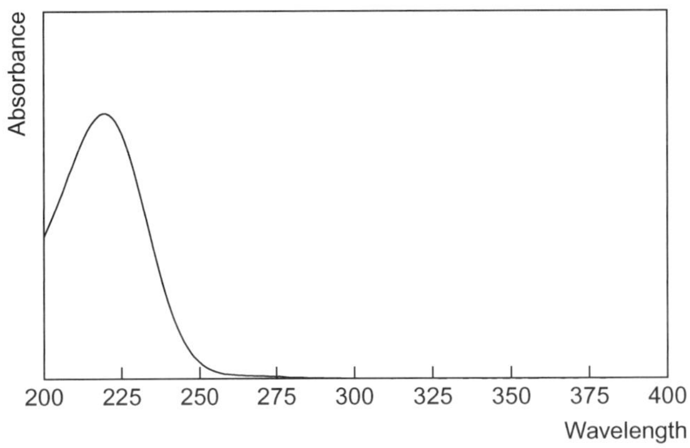

Mass Spectrum. Principal ions at *m*/*z* 41, 43, 29, 55, 39, 57, 73, 81; digoxin 73, 58, 57, 43, 41, 39, 29, 45 (no peaks above 360).

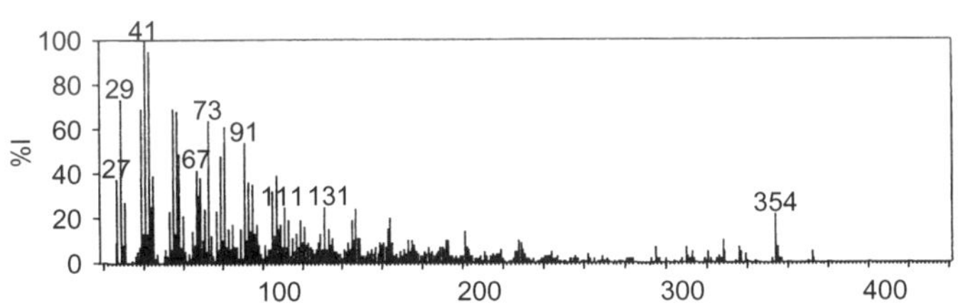

Quantification

High performance liquid chromatography–mass spectrometry. In plasma: lanatocide C and other cardiac glycosides, limit of detection 0.6 μg/L for lanatocide C—A. Traqui *et al.*, *J. Chromatogr. B Biomed. Sci. Appl.*, 1997, *692*, 101–109.

Radioimmunoassay. In serum—A. C. Moffat, *Acta Pharmacol. Toxicol.*, 1974, *35*, 386–394.

Disposition in the Body. Lanatoside C is poorly absorbed after oral administration; it is converted to digoxin in the gastro-intestinal tract and very little unchanged drug is found in the plasma or urine after oral administration. Hydrolysis to derivatives of digoxigenin and deacetylation to deslanoside also occur. After an oral dose, about 18% is excreted in the urine in 24 h, mostly as digoxin and metabolites of digoxigenin; after IV administration, about 30% of a dose is excreted in the urine in 24 h with about 70% of the urinary material consisting of unchanged drug and the remainder being digoxin and deslanoside. A total of about 60% of an IV dose is excreted in the urine in 5 days.

Therapeutic concentration. In serum, usually in the range 0.0004 to 0.001 mg/L.

Following a single oral dose of 0.5 mg of ^{3}H-lanatoside C to 9 subjects, peak plasma concentrations of unchanged drug plus metabolites of about 0.002 mg/L were attained after about 1 h and a second peak of approximately the same concentration was reported in each subject after 5 to 8 h. [S. Aldous *et al.*, *Aust. J. Pharm. Sci.*, 1972, *1*, 35–41].

Toxicity

A postmortem blood concentration of 0.047 mg/L was reported in a fatality involving an overdose of lanatoside C; death occurred 48 h after ingestion. [A. C. Moffat, *Acta Pharmacol. Toxicol.*, 1974, *35*, 386–394].

Distribution in blood. Plasma : whole blood ratio, 1.2.

Protein binding. In plasma, about 25%.

Dose. For slow digitalisation, 1.5 to 2 mg daily for 3 to 5 days; maintenance, 0.25 to 1.5 mg daily.

Lanreotide

Antineoplastic

Synonyms. Angiopeptin; DC 13-116; BIM-23014

3-(2-Naphthalenyl)-D-alanyl-L-cysteinyl-L-tyrosyl-D-tryptophyl-L-lysyl-L-valyl-L-cysteinyl-L-threoninamide cyclic (2→7)-disulfide

$C_{54}H_{69}N_{11}O_{10}S_2 = 1096.3$

CAS—108736-35-2

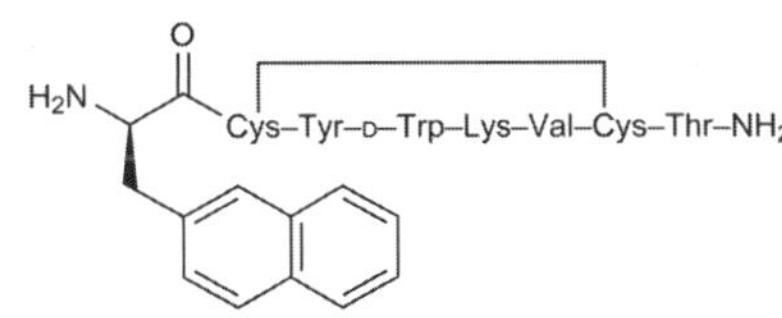

Lanreotide Acetate

Proprietary name. Somatuline LP

$C_{54}H_{69}N_{11}O_{10}S_2$, $xC_2H_4O_2$

CAS—127984-74-1

Disposition in the Body. Following the IM administration of sustained-release lanreotide, an initial rapid liberation of the drug is followed by more prolonged release.

Therapeutic concentration

8 healthy males were administered 30 mg lanreotide intramuscularly. Peak plasma concentration rose to 38.8 μg/L after 2 h, then decreasing progressively to 1.5 μg/L 11 days later and finally reaching 0.92 μg/L 2 weeks after injection. [J. M. Kuhn *et al.*, *Br. J. Clin. Pharmacol.*, 1994, *38*, 213–219.]

Bioavailability. About 50%.

Half-life. Approx. 5 days.

Dose. Given as a long-acting IM depot in the treatment of acromegaly.

Lansoprazole

Proton Pump Inhibitor

Synonyms. A-65006; AG-1749; Lanzoprazole.

Proprietary names. Agopton; Bamalite; Dakar; Lansox; Lanzor; Limpidex; Ogast; Opiren; Prevacid; Takepron; Zoton. It is also an ingredient of Prevpac.

2-[[[3-Methyl-4-(2,2,2-trifluoro-ethoxy)-2-pyridinyl]methyl]sulfinyl]-1*H*-benzimidazole

$C_{16}H_{14}F_3N_3O_2S = 369.4$

CAS—103577-45-3

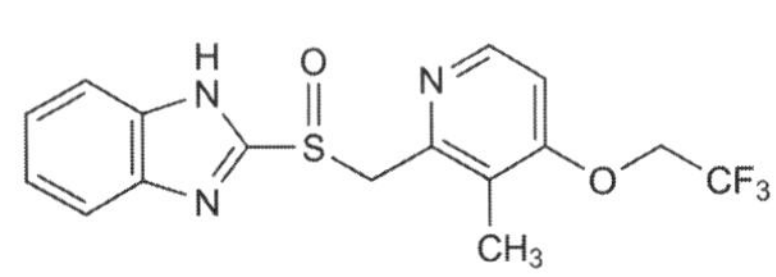

White to brownish-white odourless crystalline powder. M.p. 166° (dec). Freely soluble in dimethylformamide; soluble in methanol; sparingly soluble in ethanol; slightly soluble in ethylacetate, dichloromethane and acetonitrile; very slightly soluble in ether and practically insoluble in water and hexane.

High Performance Liquid Chromatography. System HAA—retention time 16.6 min.

Column: Chiralcel OD-R (250 × 4.6 mm i.d., 5 μm). Column temperature 30°. Mobile phase: methanol:water (75:25), 0.5 mL/min flow rate. Internal standard (IS): isobutyl 4-hydroxybenzoate. UV detection (λ=285 nm). Retention time(s): (+)-lansoprazole, 15.7 min; (−)-lansoprazole, 18.1 min; 5-hydroxylansoprazole, 10.7 min; lansoprazole sulfone, 13.6 min; IS, 12.3 min. [H. Katsuki *et al.*, *J. Chromatogr. B, Biomed. Sci. Appl.*, 2001, *757*, 127–133].

Column: C_{18} ODS (250 × 4.6 mm i.d., 5 μm). Column temperature: 40° to 43°. Mobile phase (premix): 35% aqueous acetonitrile solution with 1 mL/L *n*-octylamine and *N*-acetohydroxamic acid (5 mM), adjusted to pH 7. Flow rate, 1.0 mL/min for 15 min then 2.5 mL/min. IS: omeprazole. UV detection (λ=285 nm). Retention time(s): lansoprazole, 13.2 min; metabolites: sulfide, 22.4 min, hydroxylated sulfide, 12.0 min, hydroxylated sulfinyl, 6.5 min, sulfone, 16.4 min; IS, 7.6 min. [M. Karol *et al.*, *J. Chromatogr.*, 1995, *668*, *Biomed. Appl.*, 182–186].

Ultraviolet Spectrum. Aqueous acid—284 nm.

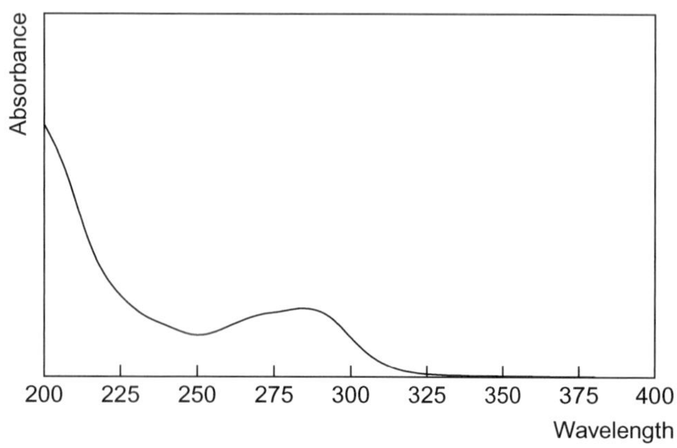

Quantification

High performance liquid chromatography. In serum and urine: limit of quantification 5 μg/L and 0.05 mg/L, respectively. UV detection (λ=285 nm)—I. Aoki *et al.*, *J. Chromatogr.*, 1991, *571*, 283–290. In plasma: limit of quantification 2 μg/L for lansoprazole and 3 to 5 μg/L for its metabolites. UV detection (λ=285 and 303 nm)—B. D. Landes *et al.*, *J. Chromatogr.*, 1992, *577*, 117–122.

Disposition in the Body. Lansoprazole is rapidly absorbed after oral administration and peak plasma concentrations are reached within approx. 1.5 h. The drug is extensively metabolised in the liver to its sulfide and sulfone metabolites, and the 5-hydroxy metabolites of these. The drug and its metabolites, in the form of glucuronides, are excreted mainly in faeces via bile with 15 to 30% of an administered dose in urine. No unchanged drug has been detected. Clearance is reduced in elderly patients and in those with liver disease.

Therapeutic concentration

10 healthy male volunteers were administered an oral 30 mg dose of the enteric coated formulation in a fasted state. The maximum serum concentration was approx. 0.8 mg/L and was reached within 2 to 3 h. [I. Aoki *et al.*, *J. Chromatogr.*, 1991, *571*, 283–290].

Group 1: 6 patients with mild renal dysfunction (creatinine clearance 40 to 60 mL/min). Group 2: 6 patients with moderate dysfunction (creatinine clearance 20 to 40 mL/min). Group 3: 5 patients with severe dysfunction (creatinine clearance < 20 mL/min). Group 4: 8 patients with hepatitis. Group 5: 8 patients with compensated cirrhosis. Group 6: 8 patients uncompensated cirrhosis. All patients were aged between 34 and 74 years, male and female, and administered a 30 mg dose of lansoprazole, as were a control group of 18 healthy volunteers aged between 20 and 32 years. Peak plasma concentrations for the groups of individuals were 1.279, 0.94, 0.942, 1.08, 1.44 and 1.14 mg/L, respectively, which were reached in 1.6, 1.7, 1.4, 1.4, 2.1 and 2.1 h, respectively. The healthy individuals reached peak concentrations of 1.033 mg/L in 1.5 h. [D. Delhotal-Landes *et al.*, *Eur. J. Clin. Pharmacol.*, 1993, *45*, 367–371].

Bioavailability. 80 to 90%; may be reduced by antacids and sucralfate if taken within an hour of taking lansoprazole.

Half-life. 1.4 to 2 h.

Volume of distribution. 0.45 L/kg.

Clearance. Oral, 0.26 L/h/kg.

Protein binding. 97%.

Note. For an update of the pharmacological properties of lansoprazole, see H. D. Langtry and M. I. Wilde, *Drugs*, 1997, *54*, 473–500.

Dose. 15 to 60 mg daily.

Leflunomide

Antirheumatic

Synonym. HWA-486
Proprietary name. Arava
5-Methyl-*N*-[4-(trifluoromethyl)phenyl]-4-isoxazolecarboxamide
$C_{12}H_9F_3N_2O_2$=270.2
CAS—75706-12-6

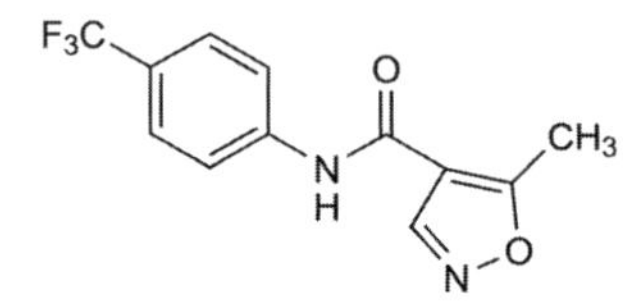

White crystalline powder (two polymorphic forms). M.p. 165° to 167°.

Dissociation Constant. pK_a (23°) 10.8.

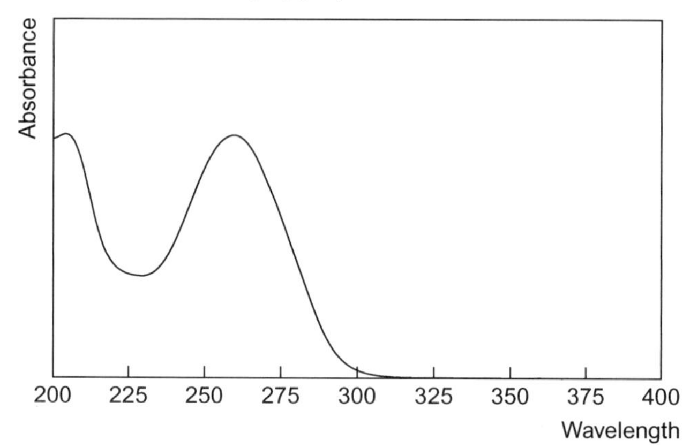

Quantification

High performance liquid chromatography. In whole blood or plasma: limit of detection 400 μg/L (0.25 mL sample); 40 μg/L (1.0 mL sample). UV detection (λ=280 nm)—V. C. Dias *et al.*, *Ther. Drug Monit.*, 1995, *17(1)*, 84–88.

Disposition in the Body. Leflunomide is rapidly and extensively metabolised, after absorption, to an active metabolite, A771726, responsible for the majority of the drug's immunosuppressive activity. The exact site of metabolism is not known, but is possibly the gut wall, plasma and the liver. The metabolite undergoes enterohepatic circulation and biliary recycling. The parent drug is not detected in plasma, only the metabolite. Peak plasma concentrations of the metabolite are observed 6 to 12 weeks after administration and bioavailability is not affected by the presence of food. Elimination of the metabolite is very slow (6 to 40 days) and approx. 90% of the dose is recovered in faeces and urine. In faeces, leflunomide is primarily excreted as the metabolite, and in urine as leflunomide glucuronides and the oxanilic acid derivative of the metabolite. Small amounts are distributed into breast milk. Steady state concentrations are reached after approx. 20 weeks of leflunomide dosing.

Therapeutic concentration

54 patients with rheumatoid arthiritis were administered 10 or 25 mg leflunomide daily. Steady state metabolite concentrations were 18 and 63 mg/L, respectively, after 24 days. [Hoecht Marion Roussel (Kansas City), 1998, data on file].

Bioavailability. About 80%.

Half-life. 7 to 8 days (after a single dose); average, 11.1 days (range, 3.7 to 28.4 days) (after multiple dosing for 14 days).

Volume of distribution. 0.13 L/kg (metabolite).

Clearance. 0.031 L/h (metabolite).

Protein binding. 99.4%, mainly to albumin (metabolite).

Note. For a review of leflunomide, see A. Prakash and B. Jarvis, *Drugs*, 1999, *58*, 1137–1164.

Dose. 100 mg once daily for the first 3 days and then a maintenance dose of 10 to 20 mg once daily.

Lepirudin

Anticoagulant/Thrombolytic

Synonyms. Recombinant Hirudin; HBW-0.23.
Proprietary name. Refludan
1-L-Leucine-2-L-threonine-63-desulfohirudin (Hirudo medicinalis isoform HV1)
$C_{287}H_{440}N_{80}O_{111}S_6$=6979.4
CAS—138068-37-8

A white powder.

Disposition in the Body. Lepirudin is rapidly distributed and essentially confined to extracellular fluids. Metabolism and excretion mainly take place in the kidneys with little in the liver. Approx. 48% of an administered dose is detected in urine with 35% as the unchanged drug. Metabolic pathways are not fully established. It is thought that catabolic hydrolysis of the parent drug causes a release of amino acids. Plasma concentrations increase proportionally with the dose and there is no evidence of accumulation.

Therapeutic concentration. The maximum plasma concentration after a single intravenous dose is 0.6 to 1 mg/L.

Half-life. 1.3 h.

Volume of distribution. 12.2 L (young and healthy); 18.7 L (healthy elderly); 18.0 L (renally impaired); 32.1 L (patients with heparin induced thrombocytopenia).

Clearance. Mean, 164 mL/min (young and healthy); 139 mL/min (elderly and healthy); 61 mL/min (patients with renal impairment); 114 mL/min (patients with heparin induced thrombocytopenia). In female patients, systemic clearance is approx. 25% lower compared to male patients.

Protein binding. <10%.

Dose. The initial dose administered is 0.4 mg/kg (maximum 44 mg) with a maintenance dose of 0.15 mg/kg/h (maximum 16.5 mg).

Letrozole

Antineoplastic

Synonym. CGS-20267
Proprietary names. Femar; Femara.
4, 4′-(1*H*-1,2,4-Triazol-1-ylmethylene)bisbenzonitrile
$C_{17}H_{11}N_5$=285.3
CAS—112809-51-5

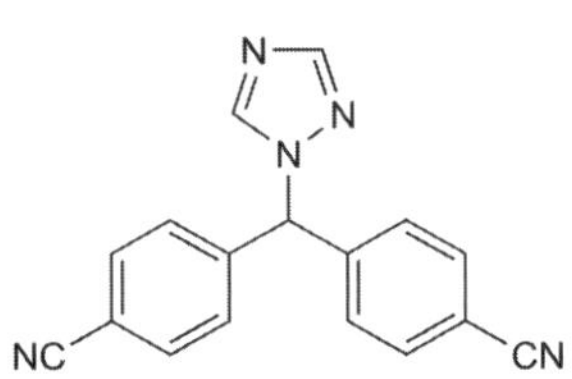

A white to yellowish crystalline powder. M.p. 181° to 183°, also reported as 184° to 185°. It is freely soluble in dichloromethane; slightly soluble in ethanol; practically insoluble in water.

High Performance Liquid Chromatography. Column: (analytical) ODS Hypersil C_{18} (200 × 4.6 mm i.d., 5 μm); (guard) Supelguard LC 18 (20 × 4.6 mm i.d., 5 μm). Mobile phase: phosphate buffer (0.01 M, pH 7):acetonitrile (70:30), 1.5 mL/min flow rate. Internal standard (IS): CGP-47645. Fluorescence detection (λ_{ex}=230 nm, λ_{em}=295 nm). Retention time(s): letrozole, 11.3 min; metabolite 1 (CGP-44645), 13.3 min; IS, 16.7 min. [F. Marfil *et al.*, *J. Chromatogr.*, 1996, *683*; *Biomed. Appl.*, 251–258].

Column: RP-8 (Lichrospher 100, 250 × 4.0 mm i.d., 5 μm); precolumn: RP-8 (Lichrospher 100, 4 × 4 mm i.d., 5 μm). Mobile phase: acetonitrile:methanol:60 mM phosphate buffer, pH 7 (39:6:55), 0.8 mL/min flow rate. IS: CGS-18320. UV detection (λ=234 nm). Retention time(s): letrozole, 8.9 min; IS, 10.7 min. [C. U. Pfister *et al.*, *J. Pharm. Sci.*, 1994, *83(4)*, 520–524].

Ultraviolet Spectrum. Aqueous acid—240, 273, 281 nm.

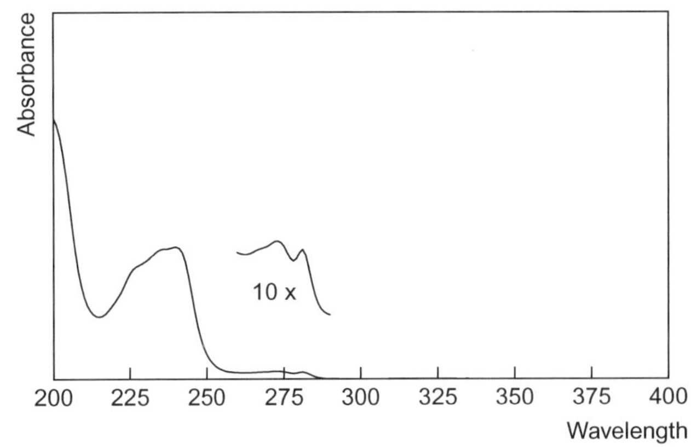

Mass Spectrum. Principal ions at *m/z* 217, 190, 285, 215, 216, 284, 102, 218.

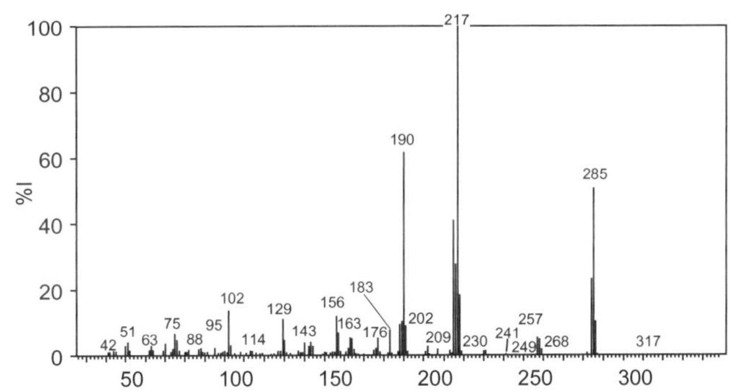

Quantification

High performance liquid chromatography. In plasma: limit of quantification 8.9 nmol/L. UV detection (λ=234 nm)—A. Sioufi *et al.*, *Biopharm. Drug Dispos.*, 1997, *18(6)*, 489–497. In plasma and urine: limit of quantification 0.4 and 0.8 μg/L, respectively. Fluorescence detection (λ_{ex}=230 nm, λ_{em}=295 nm)—F. Marfil *et al.*, *J. Chromatogr.*, 1996, *683*; *Biomed. Appl.*, 251–258. In plasma and urine: limit of quantification 8 μg/L in plasma and 52 μg/L in urine. UV detection (λ=234 nm)—C. U. Pfister *et al.*, *J. Pharm. Sci.*, 1994, *83(4)*, 520–524.

Bioassay. In plasma and urine: limit of detection 0.1 mg—C. U. Pfister *et al.*, *J. Pharm. Sci.*, 1994, *83(4)*, 520–524.

Disposition in the Body. Letrozole is rapidly and completely absorbed after oral administration which can be affected by the presence of food. Peak concentrations tend to be larger when the drug is administered without food and these concentrations are reached in about half the time compared with individuals who are administered letrozole with food. It is rapidly and extensively distributed to cells. It is metabolised slowly in the liver to an inactive carbinol metabolite, 4,4′-methanol-bisbenzonitrile, which undergoes subsequent glucuronidation, and the conjugates are excreted by the renal route. Approx. 90% of the dose is excreted in urine; 75% as the glucuronide of the metabolite, 9% unidentified metabolites and 6% unchanged drug. Steady state plasma concentrations are reached within 2 to 6 weeks and remain constant over time without accumulation of the drug.

Therapeutic concentration

12 healthy male volunteers, 28 to 44 years old, were fasted overnight and administered 2.5 mg letrozole with or without a standard high-fat

breakfast. Those administered the drug in the fasting state were fasted for an additional hour after dosing. The peak plasma concentrations for the fasted volunteers were 129 (range 94 to 164) nmol/L observed at 0.5 to 1.5 h and for the fed volunteers, 98.7 (74.5 to 146.0) nmol/L at 0.5 to 3.5 h. [A. Sioufi *et al.*, *Biopharm. Drug Dispos.*, 1997, *18(6)*, 489–497].

12 healthy, post-menopausal women and 22 patients with breast cancer were administered 2.5 mg letrozole. Peak concentrations reached 115 nmol/L at approx. 1.0 h. The trough steady state concentration observed was approx. 400 nmol/L. [H. M. Lamb *et al.*, *Drugs*, 1998, *56(6)*, 1125–1140].

Bioavailability. 99.9%.

Half-life. Approx. 2 days.

Volume of distribution. 1.9 L/kg.

Clearance. Body clearance, 2.21 L/h.

Distribution in blood. The concentration of letrozole in erythrocytes is approx. 80% of that found in plasma.

Protein binding. 60% (mainly albumin).

Note. For a review of letrozole see H. M. Lamb and J. C. Atkins, *Drugs*, 1998, *56*, 1125–1140. For a general review of aromatase inhibitors see V. C. Njar and A. M. H. Brodie, *Drugs*, 1999, *58*, 233–255.

Dose. 2.5 mg daily until tumour progression is evident.

Levacetylmethadol

Narcotic Analgesic/Treatment of Narcotic Addiction

Synonyms. l-Acetylmethadol; LAAM; LAM; Levomethadyl Acetate.
(αS)-β-[(2S)-2-(Dimethylamino)propyl]-α-ethyl-β-phenylbenzene-ethanol acetate
$C_{23}H_{31}NO_2$=353.5
CAS—1477-40-3

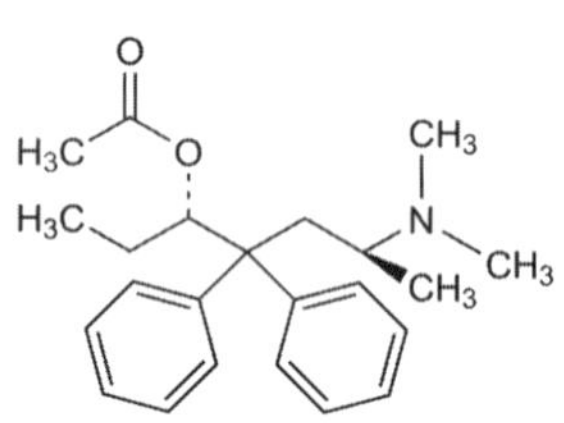

M.p. about 70°.

Levacetylmethadol Hydrochloride

Proprietary name. ORLAAM
$C_{23}H_{31}NO_2,HCl$=390.0
CAS—43033-72-3
Crystals. M.p. 215°.
Soluble in water.

Dissociation Constant. pK_a 8.3.

Colour Tests. Mandelin's Test—grey-green; Marquis Test—violet-brown→grey-green.

Thin-layer Chromatography. System TA—Rf 57; system TB—Rf 62; system TC—Rf 39. (Acidified iodoplatinate solution, positive.)

Gas Chromatography. System GB—levacetylmethadol RI 2267; M(nor-) RI 2262; M(di-nor-) RI 2255.

High Performance Liquid Chromatography. System HA—*k* 1.7.

Ultraviolet Spectrum. Aqueous acid—253, 258 nm.

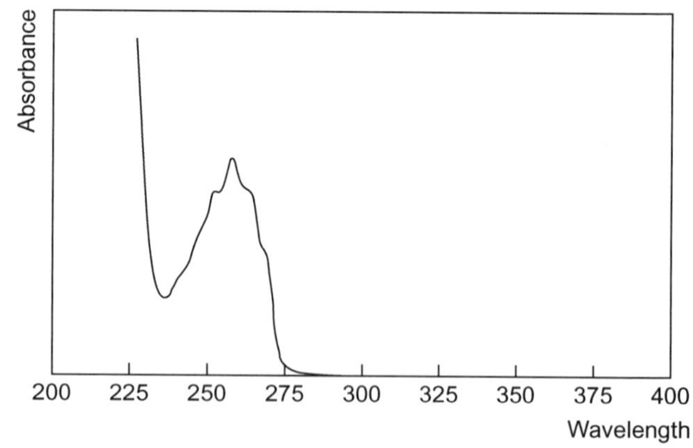

Infra-red Spectrum. Principal peaks at wavenumbers 1240, 1735, 702, 1496, 1015, 1031 cm^{-1}.

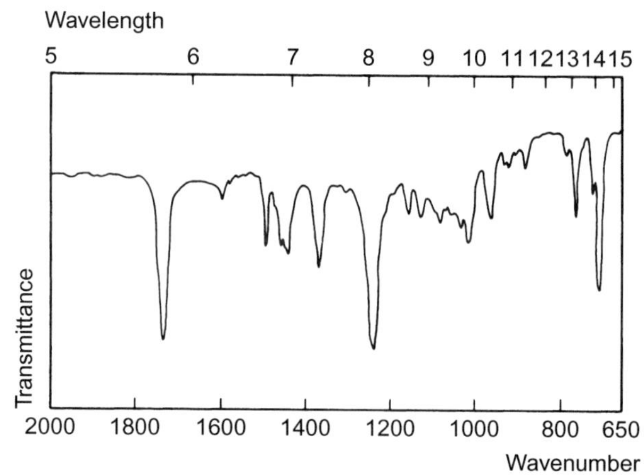

Mass Spectrum. Principal ions at *m/z* 72, 73, 43, 91, 224, 56, 71, 129.

Quantification

Gas chromatography. In plasma: limit of detection 10 µg/L for levacetylmethadol using FID, 5 µg/L and 25 µg/L for L-α-noracetylmethadol and L-α-dinoracetylmethadol, respectively, using ECD—F. L. S. Tse and P. G. Welling, *Biopharm. Drug Disp.*, 1980, *1*, 203–209.

Gas chromatography–mass spectrometry. In plasma, whole blood or tissues: levacetylmethadol and demethylated metabolites, limit of detection 5 µg/L—T. A. Jennison *et al.*, *J. Chromatogr. Sci.*, 1979, *17*, 64–74.

High performance liquid chromatography. In plasma or urine: levacetylmethadol and metabolites, limit of detection 6 µg/L for levacetylmethadol, L-α-noracetylmethadol and methadol, 10 µg/L for L-α-dinoracetylmethadol, normethadol and dinormethadol—C.-H. Kiang *et al.*, *J. Chromatogr.*, 1981, *222*; *B Biomed. Appl.*, *11*, 81–93.

Radioimmunoassay. In biological fluids: limit of detection 50 pg—K. L. McGilliard and G. D. Olsen, *J. Pharmacol. Exp. Ther.*, 1980, *215*, 205–212.

Disposition in the Body. Levacetylmethadol is absorbed after oral administration. It is metabolised principally by *N*-demethylation to L-α-noracetylmethadol and L-α-dinoracetylmethadol which are active narcotics, and also by deacetylation to methadol which is also active; further demethylation to normethadol and dinormethadol also occurs. L-α-Noracetylmethadol, L-α-dinoracetylmethadol and, in some subjects, unchanged drug accumulate during chronic oral administration, but there is considerable intersubject variation. About 20 to 25% of a dose is excreted in the urine as unchanged drug and demethylated metabolites, and about 2% as methadol and normethadol.

Therapeutic concentration

After a single oral dose of 60 mg given to 5 subjects, peak plasma concentrations of 0.09 to 0.16 (mean 0.13) mg/L of levacetylmethadol and 0.04 to 0.05 mg/L of L-α-noracetylmethadol were attained in about 2 to 4 h and 2 to 6 h, respectively; following chronic oral treatment with 85 mg three times a week for three months to 3 subjects, peak plasma concentrations were: levacetylmethadol 0.16 to 0.23 (mean 0.20) mg/L, L-α-noracetylmethadol 0.15 to 0.30 (mean 0.24) mg/L, and L-α-dinoracetylmethadol, mean 0.27 mg/L [G. L. Henderson *et al.*, *Clin. Pharmacol. Ther.*, 1977, *21*, 16–25].

Toxicity. The following postmortem tissue concentrations, mg/L (mean, *n*), were reported in 9 heroin addicts who died unexpectedly during treatment with levacetylmethadol:

	Levacetylmethadol	L-α-Noracetyl-methadol	L-α-Dinoracetyl-methadol
Blood	0.01–0.12 (0.05, 7)	0.01–0.22 (0.08, 7)	0.01–0.17 (0.05,7)
Brain	0.04, 0.24 (2)	0.07, 0.42 (2)	0.14, 0.34 (2)
Kidney	0.01–0.69 (0.28, 6)	0.01–1.2 (0.5, 6)	0.04–1.1 (0.66, 6)
Liver	0.01–0.7 (0.31, 7)	0.01–1.43 (0.70, 7)	0.03–2.08 (1.0, 7)
Lung	0.03–2.49 (0.95, 3)	0.04–6.0 (2.3, 3)	0.21–8.52 (3.8, 3)
Urine	0.05–1.76 (0.72, 4)	0.22–3.04 (1.1, 4)	0.46–2.0 (1.0, 4)

Other drugs (mainly diazepam, methadone or morphine) were detected in all subjects except one in which the cause of death was multiple stab wounds [D. M. Chinn *et al.*, *J. Anal. Toxicol.*, 1979, *3*, 143–149].

Half-life. Plasma half-life, levacetylmethadol about 50 h, L-α-noracetylmethadol 30 to 65 h, L-α-dinoracetylmethadol about 170 h.

Dose. Usually up to 80 mg three times a week.

Levallorphan

Narcotic Antagonist

17-(2-Propenyl)morphinan-3-ol
$C_{19}H_{25}NO = 283.4$
CAS—152-02-3

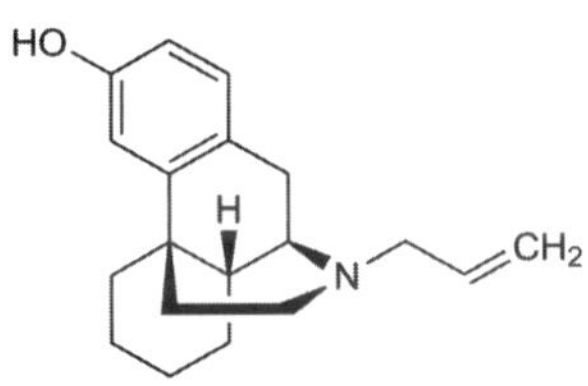

White crystals. M.p. 180° to 182°.

Levallorphan Tartrate

Proprietary names. Lorfan. It is an ingredient of Pethilorfan.
$C_{19}H_{25}NO,C_4H_6O_6 = 433.5$
CAS—71-82-9
A white crystalline powder. M.p. 174° to 177°.
Soluble 1 in about 20 of water, 1 in 100 of ethanol, 1 in 3300 of chloroform, 1 in 5000 of ether and 1 in 13 of methanol.

Dissociation Constant. pK_a 4.5, 6.9.

Partition Coefficient. Log *P* (octanol/buffer pH 7.4), 2.3.

Colour Tests. Aromaticity (Method 2) —yellow/orange; Liebermann's Test—black.

Thin-layer Chromatography. System TA—Rf 67; system TB—Rf 19; system TC—Rf 24; system TE—Rf 74; system TL—Rf 45; system TAE—Rf 42; system TAF—Rf 73; system TAJ—Rf 10; system TAK—Rf 06; system TAL—Rf 66. (Dragendorff spray, positive; FPN reagent, yellow; Acidified iodoplatinate solution, positive; Marquis reagent, grey.)

Gas Chromatography. System GA—levallorphan RI 2355; levallorphan-AC RI 2390; system GB—levallorphan RI 2460.

High Performance Liquid Chromatography. System HA—*k* 1.9 (tailing peak); system HC—*k* 1.46; system HX—RI 356; system HY—RI 291.

Ultraviolet Spectrum. Aqueous acid—279 (A^1_1=71a); aqueous alkali—240 (A^1_1=312a), 299 nm.

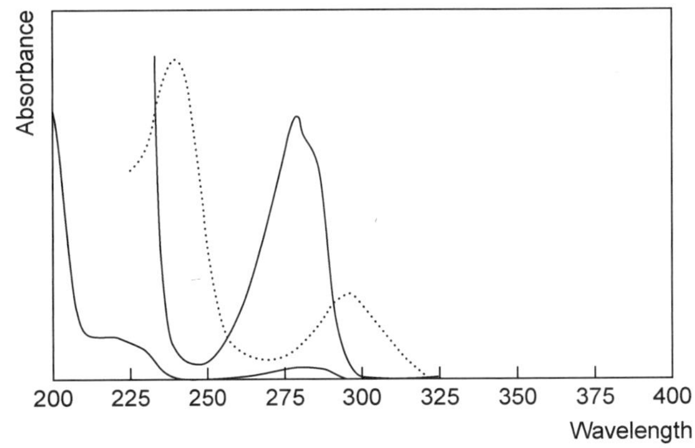

Infra-red Spectrum. Principal peaks at wavenumbers 759, 1271, 747, 1575, 1242, 932 cm^{-1} (Nujol mull).

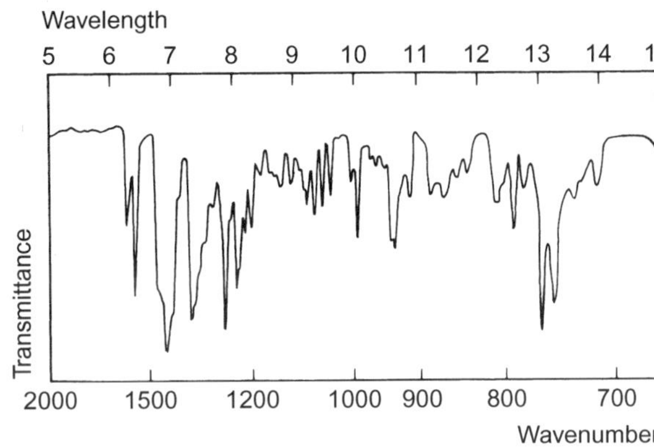

Mass Spectrum. Principal ions at *m/z* 283, 282, 256, 176, 157, 43, 41, 57.

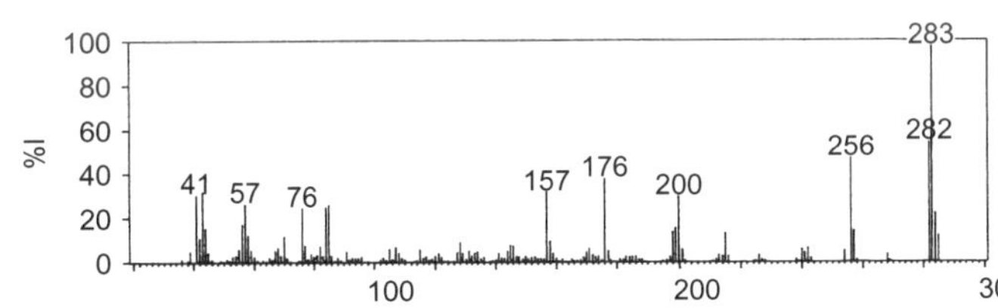

Disposition in the Body. Levallorphan is effective within 1 min of IV injection and the effects may last up to 4 h. It is metabolised by *N*-dealkylation and glucuronic acid conjugation.

Toxicity. The estimated minimum lethal dose is 0.2 g or 2 g for an addict.

Dose. 0.5 to 1 mg of levallorphan tartrate intravenously, repeated if necessary.

Levamfetamine

Central Stimulant

Synonyms. (−)-Amfetamine; Laevo-amfetamine; Levamphetamine.
(−)-α-Methylbenzeneethanamine
$C_9H_{13}N = 135.2$
CAS—156-34-3

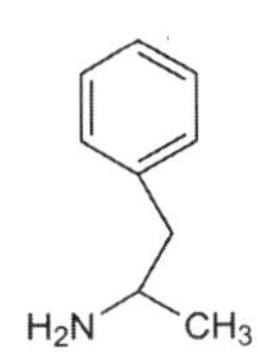

Dissociation Constant. pK_a 10.1 (20°).

Partition Coefficient Log *P* (octanol/water), 1.8.
For analytical data see under Amfetamine.

Levamisole

Anthelmintic

Synonym. l-Tetramisole
Proprietary names. Anthelpor (vet.); Levadin (vet.).
(6*S*)-2,3,5,6-Tetrahydro-6-phenylimidazo[2,1-*b*]thiazole
$C_{11}H_{12}N_2S$=204.3
CAS—14769-73-4

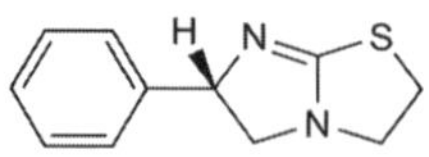

A white crystalline powder. M.p. 60° to 61.5°.
Soluble in dilute acetic acid and in chloroform.

Levamisole Hydrochloride

Proprietary names. Armadose (vet.); Ascaridil; Chanaverm (vet.); Decaris; Decazole (vet.); Ergamisol; Ketrax; Levacide (vet.); Levacur (vet.); Levasole (vet.); Nemicide (vet.); Nilverm (vet.); Ripercol (vet.); Solaskil; Spartakon (vet.); Sure (vet.); Tramisole (vet.); Vermisole (vet.); Wormaway (vet.).
$C_{11}H_{12}N_2S,HCl$=240.8
CAS—16595-80-5
A white to pale cream-coloured crystalline powder. M.p. 227° to 229°.
Soluble 1 in 2 of water and 1 in 5 of methanol; practically insoluble in ether.

Dissociation Constant. pK_a 8.0.

Partition Coefficient. Log *P* (octanol/water), 1.8.

Colour Tests. Liebermann's test—red-orange; Mandelin's test—orange→grey-green.

Thin-layer Chromatography. System TA—Rf 62; system TB—Rf 18; system TC—Rf 48; system TE—Rf 65; system TL—Rf 42; system TAE—Rf 53; system TAF—Rf 52. (Acidified iodoplatinate solution, positive.)

Gas Chromatography. System GA—RI 1928.

High Performance Liquid Chromatography. System HY—RI 238; system HAA—Retention time(s) 7.0 min.

Infra-red Spectrum. Principal peaks at wavenumbers 1587, 1575, 1197, 699, 1150, 1248 cm^{-1} (KBr disk).

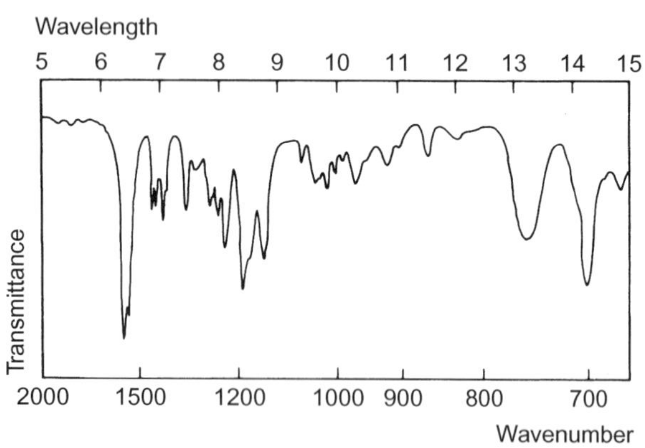

Mass Spectrum. Principal ions at *m/z* 204, 148, 73, 101, 203, 127, 104, 205.

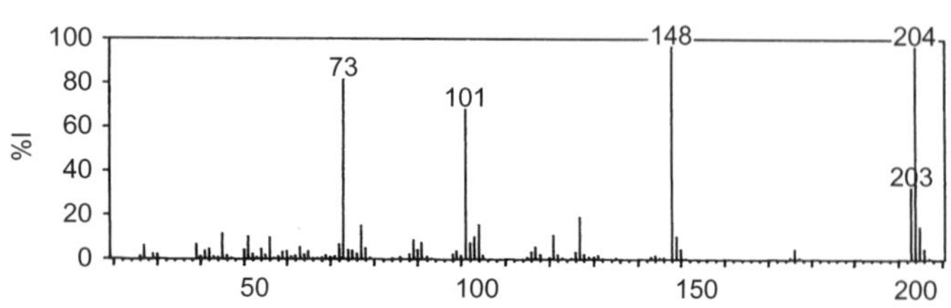

Quantification

Gas chromatography. In plasma: limit of detection 4 µg/L, AFID—F. Rousseau *et al.*, *Eur. J. Drug Metab. Pharmacokinet.*, 1981, *6*, 281–288. In plasma or urine: limit of detection in plasma 2 µg/L, FID—E. Kouassi *et al.*, *Biopharm. Drug Dispos.*, 1986, *7*, 71–89.

High performance liquid chromatography. In sheep or cattle plasma: limit of detection 20 µg/L, UV detection—S. Marriner *et al.*, *Analyst, Lond.*, 1980, *105*, 993–996. In urine: *p*-hydroxylevamisole, limit of detection 0.5 mg/L, UV detection—E. Kouassi *et al.*, *Biopharm. Drug Dispos.*, 1986, *7*, 71–89. In plasma: limit of detection 21 µg/L, UV detection—T. F. Vandamme *et al.*, *Eur. J. Metab. Pharmacokinet.*, 1995, *20*, 145–149.

Disposition in the Body. Levamisole is readily absorbed after oral administration, but extensively metabolised. It is almost completely excreted in the urine and faeces within 48 h.

Therapeutic concentration

Following single oral doses of 2.5 mg/kg and 5 mg/kg to 11 subjects, mean peak plasma concentrations of 0.7 and 1.5 mg/L, respectively, were attained within 2 h. [M. Luyckx *et al.*, *Eur. J. Drug Metab. Pharmacokinet.*, 1982, *7*, 247–254].

Half-life. Plasma half-life, about 4 h.

Dose. The equivalent of 2.5 to 5 mg/kg of levamisole daily, for 2 or 3 days.

Levetiracetam

Anti-epileptic

Synonyms. SIB-S1; UCB-L059.
Proprietary name. Keppra
(α*S*)-α-Ethyl-2-oxo-1-pyrrolidineacetamide
$C_8H_{14}N_2O_2$=170.2
CAS—102767-28-2

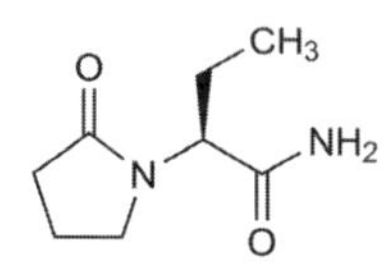

A white to off-white crystalline powder with a faint odour and bitter taste. Crystals from ethyl acetate, M.p. 117°. It is very soluble in water (104 g/100 mL); freely soluble in chloroform (65.3 g/100 mL) and methanol (53.6 g/100 mL); soluble in ethanol (16.5 g/100 mL); sparingly soluble in acetonitrile (5.7 g/100 mL); practically insoluble in *n*-hexane.

Gas Chromatography. System GB—RI 1629.

Column: (analytical) DB-FFAP megabore (30 m × 0.53 mm i.d., 1 µm film thickness); (pre-column) deactivated fused silica (1 m × 0.53 mm i.d.). Column temperature: 70° to 190° (40°/min); 190° to 250° (5°/min), held 2 min. Carrier gas: helium, flow rate 30 mL/min. IS: UCB -G025,. Detection: nitrogen–phosphorus. Retention time(s): levetiracetam, 14.0 min; IS, 11.5 min [T. A. C. Vermeij and P. M. Edelbroek, *J. Chromatogr.*, 1994, *662; Biomed. Appl.*, 134–139].

Column: 6-TBDMS-2,3-perme-β-cyclodextrin (20% w/w) in SE52 fused-silica capillary (10 m × 0.25 mm i.d., 0.5 µm film thickness). Column temperature: 110°, held 2 min; to 170° (10°/min), held 5 min. Injector temperature: 210°. Carrier gas: helium, linear velocity, 40 cm/s. IS: *N*-dimethylvalproyl glycinamide. Detection: tandem mass spectrometry (SIM, *m/z*: 69, 98, 126 for levetiracetam; *m/z*: 129, 157, 186 for IS). Retention time(s): (*S*)-levetiracetam, 8.6 min; (*R*)-levetiracetam, 8.8 min; IS, 10.3 min [N. Isoherranen *et al.*, *J. Chromatogr. Biomed. Sci. Appl.*, 2000, *745*, 325–332].

High Performance Liquid Chromatography. Column: (analytical) 60 RP-select B (LiChrospher, 250 × 4 mm i.d., 5 µm); (pre-column) 60 RP-select B (4 × 4 mm i.d., 5 µm). Mobile phase: acetonitrile:phosphate buffer (50 mM, pH 5.6) (15:85), flow rate 0.8 mL/min. IS: UCB-17025. UV detection (λ=220 nm). Retention time(s): levetiracetam, 5.4 min; IS, 6.8 min [N. Ratnaraj *et al.*, *Ther. Drug Monit.*, 1996, *18*, 154–157].

Column: RP 3ODS2 (Spherisorb, 150 × 4.6 mm i.d.). Mobile phase: (A)—acetonitrile; (B)—water. Elution programme: (A:B) (6:94) initial, to (20:80) in 5 min, to (40:60) in 1 min, hold for 10 min, to (6:94) in 1 min, hold for 4 min, flow rate 1.0 mL/min. IS: UCB-G025,. Diode-array detection (λ=205 nm). Retention time(s): levetiracetam, 6.4 min; IS, 7.8 min [T. A. C. Vermeij and P. M. Edelbroek, *J. Chromatogr.*, 1994, *662; Biomed. Appl.*, 134–139].

Mass Spectrum. Principal ions at m/z 126, 98, 41, 69, 58, 55, 127, 44.

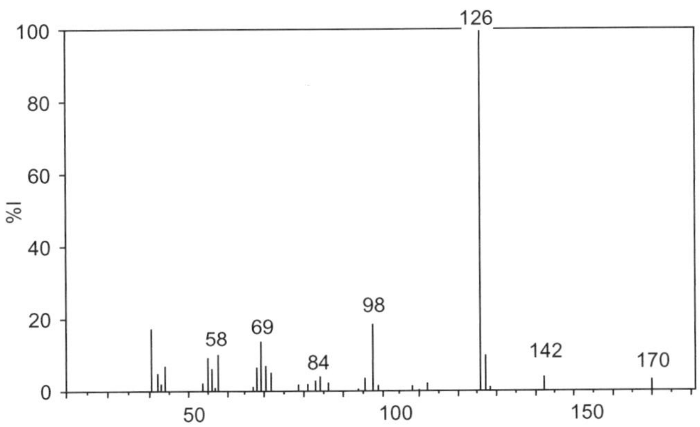

Quantification

Gas chromatography. In serum: limit of quantification 0.29 mg/L, nitrogen–phosphorous detection—T. A. C. Vermeij and P. M. Edelbroek, *J. Chromatogr.*, 1994, *662; Biomed. Appl.*, 134–139.

Gas chromatography–mass spectrometry. In plasma: limit of detection 0.94 pg/L and limit of quantification 2.35 pg/L (15 pg/L in urine), MS detection—N. Isoherranen *et al., J. Chromatogr. Biomed. Sci. Appl.*, 2000, *745*, 325–332.

High performance liquid chromatography. In plasma: limit of quantification 5 µmol/L—N. Ratnaraj *et al., Ther. Drug Monit.*, 1996, *18*, 154–157. In serum: limit of quantification 0.36 mg/L, diode-array detection—T. A. C. Vermeij and P. M. Edelbroek, *J. Chromatogr.*, 1994, *662; Biomed. Appl.*, 134–139.

Disposition in the Body. Levetiracetam is rapidly and almost completely absorbed after oral administration. The extent of absorption is not affected by the presence of food but peak plasma concentrations may be reduced by approx. 20%, and time to reach these concentrations may be prolonged by approx. 1.5 h. Peak plasma concentrations are reached, generally, within one hour and steady state is achieved after two days of multiple twice daily dosing. The major metabolic pathway is enzymatic hydrolysis which is not extensive and occurs in a number of tissues including blood cells. A carboxylic acid metabolite is produced. Two other minor metabolites have been detected; products of hydroxylation. The drug and its metabolites are excreted renally, with 66% of a dose excreted unchanged in urine.

Therapeutic concentration. In serum, 10 to 37 mg/L.

7 male patients with intractable epilepsy, mean age 41 years (range, 24 to 71 years) and having epilepsy for a period of 2 days to 19 years (mean, 9.7 years) with one or more seizures a week, participated in the study. The patients were administered with ascending doses of levetiracetam between 0.5 and 2.0 g daily; increased by 0.5 g every 4 weeks according to its tolerability and safety as determined by an initial trial period. The actual doses administered varied between 5.4 mg/kg and 32.2 mg/kg (mean, 15.96 mg/kg) and these produced peak plasma concentrations of 6.29 and 38.17 mg/L (mean, 22.25 mg/L) [M. K. Sharief *et al., J. Epilepsy*, 1996, *9*, 106–112].

Toxicity.

A 38-year-old woman was admitted into hospital 6 hours after ingesting 60 tablets of 500 mg levetiracetam. Her serum concentrations were 400 mg/L, 72 mg/L, 60 mg/L at 6, 18, and 20.5 hours, respectively. No other drugs were detected and she recovered the next day without sequelae [F. Barrueto, Jr *et al., J. Toxicol. Clin. Toxicol.*, 2002, *40*, 881–884].

Bioavailability. Oral, almost 100%.

Half-life. 6 to 8 h; increased in the elderly and in subjects with renal impairment.

Volume of distribution. 0.5 to 0.7 L/kg.

Clearance. Total body, 0.96 mL/min/kg; reduced in the elderly and those with renal impairment—40% in patients with mild impairment, 50% moderate impairment and 60% for those with severe impairment; increased in paediatric patients by approx. 40%.

Protein binding. Less than 10%.

Note. For a review of the pharmacokinetic profile of levetiracetam see P. N. Patsalas, *Pharmacol. Ther.*, 2000, *85*, 77–85; for a safety profile of levetiracetam see C. Harden, *Epilepsia*, 2001, *42* (*suppl. 4*), 36–39.

Dose. The usual dose is 500 mg twice daily which may be increased in increments of 1 g daily every 2 weeks; maximum 3 g daily. The dose may be adjusted for patients with renal impairment.

Levobunolol

Beta-blocker

Synonyms. *l*-Bunolol; W-6421A.
5-[(2*S*)-3-[(1,1-Dimethylethyl)amino]-2-hydroxypropoxy]-3,4-dihydro-1(2*H*)-naphthalenone
$C_{17}H_{25}NO_3 = 291.4$
CAS—47141-42-4

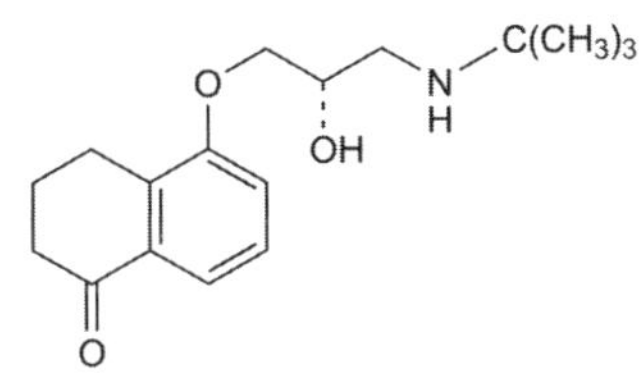

Levobunolol Hydrochloride

Synonyms. (–)-Bunolol Hydrochloride; *l*-Bunolol Hydrochloride; W-7000A;
Proprietary names. Betagan; Gotensian; Vistagan.
$C_{17}H_{25}NO_3,HCl = 327.9$
CAS—27912-14-7
A white or pinkish white, odourless crystalline powder. M.p. 209° to 211°. It is soluble to freely soluble in water; slightly to sparingly soluble in alcohol; soluble in methyl alcohol; slightly soluble in chloroform.

Dissociation Constant. pK_a 9.4.

Partition Coefficient. Log *P* (octanol/water), 2.40.

Gas Chromatography. Column: HP capillary cross-linked methylsilicone (12 m × 0.2 mm i.d., 0.33 µm film thickness). Column temperature: 100° to 310° at 30°/min. Carrier gas: helium, flow rate 2 mL/min. MS detection (EI). Retention index: 2460. [H. Maurer and K. Pfleger. *J. Chromatogr.*, 1986, *382*, 147–165].

High Performance Liquid Chromatography. Column: µBondapak C_{18} (250 × 4.6 mm i.d., 10 µm). Mobile phase: methanol:water (48:52), flow rate 2 mL/min. Internal standard (IS): metoprolol. Fluorescence detection (λ_{ex} = 225 nm, λ_{em} = 295 nm). Retention time(s): dihydrolevobunolol, 3.8 min; IS, 4.6 min. [H. Hengy *et al., J. Chromatogr.*, 1985, *338*, 444–449].

Ultraviolet Spectrum. Aqueous acid—223, 209, 256, 313 nm.

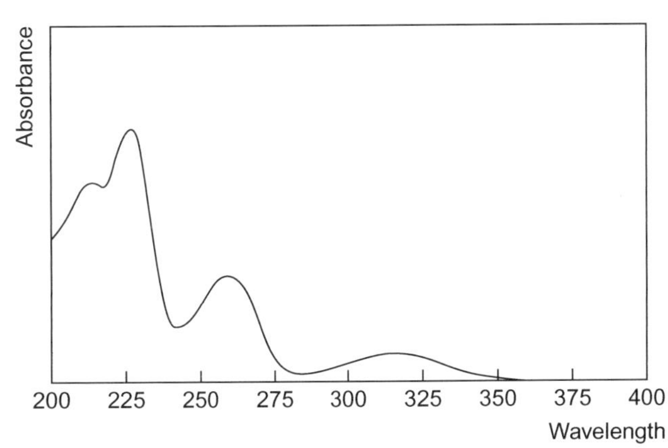

Mass Spectrum. Principal ions at m/z 86, 57, 318, 259, 99, 112, 200, 333 (levobunolol acetylated derivative).

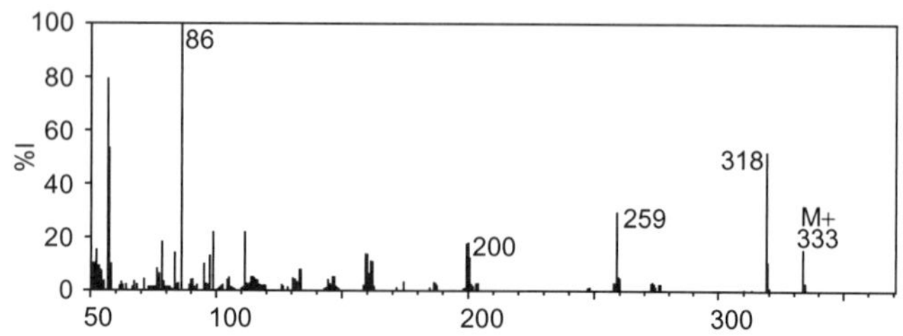

Quantification

High performance liquid chromatography. In blood and urine: limit of detection 0.5 to 1 µg/L. Fluorescence detection (λ_{ex}=225 nm, λ_{em}=295 nm)—H. Hengy *et al.*, *J. Chromatogr.*, 1985, *338*, 444–449.

Disposition in the Body. Some systemic absorption occurs following topical application, but after oral administration levobunolol is rapidly and almost completely absorbed from the gastro-intestinal tract. It is extensively metabolised in the liver and the principal metabolite is dihydrolevobunolol, which possesses β-blocking activity, approx. 65% of that of the parent drug. Other metabolites include bunolol glucuronide, bunolol sulfate and dihydrobunolol glucuronide. Levobunolol and its metabolites are subsequently glucuronidated. Metabolites and some of the unchanged drug are excreted in urine (78%) and in faeces (3%), in 4 days. The metabolism of levobunolol following ophthalmic application has not been clearly determined. Peak levels of the drug and metabolite are reached within 1 h and the duration of action is 12 to 14 h. Distribution has not been determined.

Therapeutic concentration

After oral administration to 6 healthy volunteers, the peak plasma concentration reached was 22.9 µg/L after approx. 3 h. [E. U. Kolle *et al.*, *Naunyn Schmiedebergs Arch. Pharmacol.*, 1983, *322*, *Suppl. R9/34*].

Toxicity. Respiratory and cardiac reactions have been reported, rarely resulting in death caused by bronchospasm or associated with cardiac failure. No data available on human overdose.

Bioavailability. 75%.

Half-life. Mean, (levobunolol) 6.1 h; (metabolite, dihydrolevobunolol) between 5.7 and 7.1 h.

Volume of distribution. 5.5 L/kg.

Clearance. Total plasma clearance, 0.66 L/h/kg.

Dose. Eye drops applied once or twice daily.

Levobupivacaine

Anaesthetic

(*S*)-1-Butyl-*N*-(2,6-dimethylphenyl)-2-piperidinecarboxamide
$C_{18}H_{28}N_2O$=288.4
CAS—*27262-47-1*

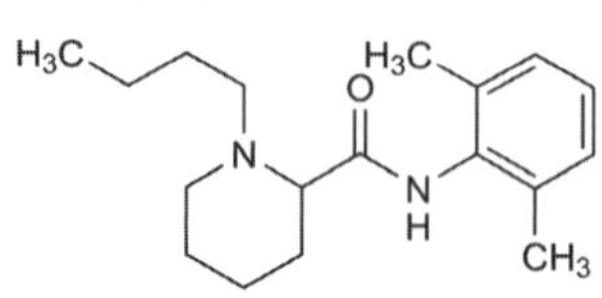

Crystals from isopropanol. M.p. 135° to 137°.

Levobupivacaine Hydrochloride

Proprietary name. Chirocaine
$C_{18}H_{28}N_2O$,HCl=324.9
CAS—27262-48-2
M.p. 255° to 257°. Solubility in water (20°): 100 mg/mL.

Dissociation Constant. pKa 8.09.

Partition Coefficient. Log *P* (oleyl alcohol/water), 1624.

Quantification

High performance liquid chromatography. In plasma, limit of quantification 0.3 mg/L. UV detection (λ=210 nm)—H. Bardsley *et al.*, *Br. J. Clin. Pharmacol.*, 1998, *46(3)*, 245–249.

Disposition in the Body. Levobupivacaine is extensively metabolised (NADPH dependent) in the liver, by the cytochrome P450 system. The major metabolite is 3-hydroxylevobupivacaine which may be subsequently converted to glucuronic acid and sulfate ester conjugates. Approx. 70% of a dose is excreted in urine as its metabolites and a little in faeces. No parent drug has been detected in urine or faeces. Approx. 95% of a dose is recovered within 48 h of dosing. Levobupivacaine crosses the placenta.

Therapeutic concentration

14 healthy male volunteers, aged 19 to 40 years (mean 29.5 years) were fasted overnight and intravenously administered a maximum of 150 mg at an infusion rate of 10 mg/min for 2 to 15 min. The mean dose administered was 56.1 mg which produced a mean maximum plasma concentration of 2.62 mg/L shortly after the end of infusion. At 5 and 10 min after infusion, the mean maximum concentration was 1.93 mg/L before decreasing to a range of 0.3 to 0.6 mg/L, 45 to 120 min after infusion. [H. Bardsley *et al.*, *Br. J. Clin. Pharmacol.*, 1998, *46(3)*, 245–249].

10 patients, aged 18 to 80 years old, were scheduled to undergo elective lower abdominal surgery, with epidural anaesthesia. They were premedicated with midazolam and 1% lidocaine, and subsequently administered an epidural injection of 0.75% concentration (total dose 150 mg) levobupivacaine. The peak plasma concentration was 0.84 mg/L at 0.04 h. The concentration of the (*S*)-isomer was larger than that observed for the (*R*)-isomer. [D. J. Kopacz *et al.*, *Anesth. Analg.*, 2000, *90*, 642–648].

18 patients scheduled for varicose vein surgery, under extradural anaesthesia, were administered 15 mL 0.5% levobupivacaine (total dose of 75 mg) and 0.75% (total dose 112.5 mg) as an epidural injection. The peak plasma concentrations for the two doses were 0.58 and 0.81 mg/L observed at 0.37 and 0.29 h, respectively. [K. A. Faccenda *et al.*, *Reg. Anesth. Pain Med.*, 1998, *23(3)*, *Suppl. 52*].

Toxicity. Intravenous administration of levobupivacaine can be associated with cardiac arrest.

Half-life. 1.3 h.

Volume of distribution. 66.9 L.

Clearance. Plasma, 39.1 L/h.

Protein binding. > 97%.

Dose. For surgical anaesthesia, the maximum dose is 150 mg depending on the type of surgery undertaken. For acute pain, 15 to 25 mg (as a 2.5 mg/mL solution).

Levocabastine

Antihistamine (topical)

Synonym. (−)-Cabastine
[3*S*-[1(*cis*),3α,4β]]-1-[4-Cyano-4-(4-fluorophenyl)cyclohexyl]-3-methyl-4-phenyl-4-piperidinecarboxylic acid
$C_{26}H_{29}FN_2O_2$=420.5
CAS—79516-68-0

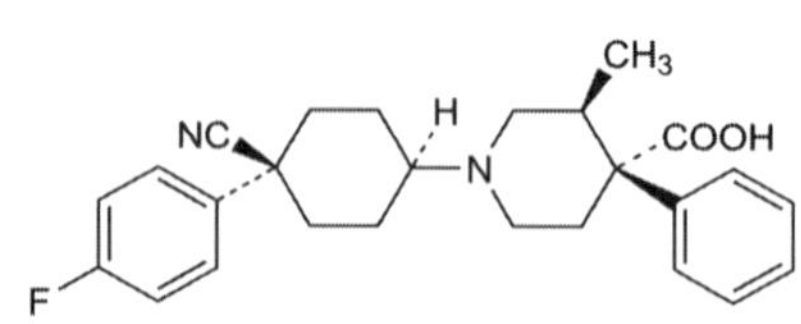

Cabastine (racemate of Levocabastine)

CAS—79449-98-2

Levocabastine Hydrochloride

Synonym. R-50547
Proprietary names. Levophta; Livostin.
$C_{26}H_{29}FN_2O_2$,HCl=457.0
CAS—79547-78-7

Thin-layer Chromatography. System TB—Rf 00; system TE—Rf 12; system TF—Rf 2; system TAE—Rf 76.

High Performance Liquid Chromatography. System HX—RI 431.

Ultraviolet Spectrum. Aqueous acid—258, 263, 269 nm.

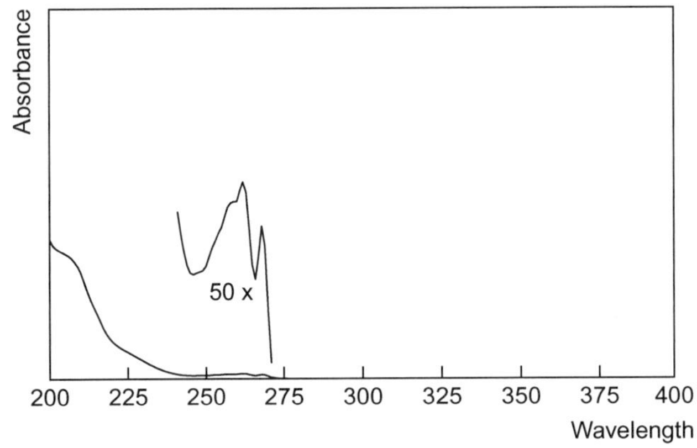

Disposition in the Body. Levocabastine is rapidly and completely absorbed after intranasal, ocular and oral administration, but peak plasma concentrations are low. First-pass metabolism is negligible and it is excreted in urine as the unchanged drug (70%) and as an acetylglucuronide metabolite which is biologically inactive (10%). The remaining proportion of the unchanged drug is excreted in faeces (20%). Trace amounts of the drug are found in breast milk.

Therapeutic concentration

Healthy volunteers were administered single doses of 0.5, 1.0 and 2.0 mg. Peak plasma concentrations of 7.3, 12.1 and 22.2 µg/L, respectively, were observed within 2 h of administration. Volunteers administered with a 0.2 mg dose of levocabastine by nasal administration gave peak concentrations between 1.4 and 2.2 µg/L within 1 to 2 h. A 0.04 mg dose, administered as eye drops, produced a concentration of 0.26 to 0.29 µg/L within 1 to 2 h. [J. Heykents *et al.*, unpublished reports, *Janssen Research Foundation, Beerse*, 1984].

Bioavailability. 60 to 80% (intranasal); 30 to 60% (ocular); 100% (oral).

Half-life. 33 to 40 h.

Volume of distribution. 1.14 L/kg (82 L).

Clearance. Plasma, 1.8 L/h.

Protein binding. 55%

Note. For a review of levocabastine, see S. Noble and D. McTavish, *Drugs*, 1995, *50*, 1032–1049.

Dose. 0.5 mg/mL suspension: two sprays per nostril or one drop per eye twice daily. Three to four times daily if necessary.

Levodopa

Antiparkinsonian

Synonyms. Dihydroxyphenylalanine; Dopa; L-Dopa; Laevo-dopa.
Proprietary names. Bendopa; Cidanopa; Deadopa, Dopaflex; Dopar; Doparl; Dopasol; Dopaston; Dopastral; Doprin; Eldopal; Eurodopa; Larodopa; Ledopa; Levopa; Levomet; Syndopa; Veldopa. It is an ingredient of Atamet, Madopar, Prolopa and Sinemet.
3-Hydroxy-L-tyrosine
$C_9H_{11}NO_4$=197.2
CAS—59-92-7

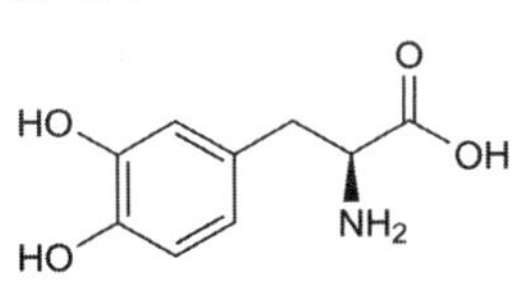

A white or slightly cream-coloured crystalline powder, which darkens on exposure to air and light. M.p. about 275°, with decomposition.
Soluble 1 in 300 of water; practically insoluble in benzene, ethyl acetate, ethanol, chloroform and ether; soluble in aqueous solutions of mineral acids and alkali carbonates.

Dissociation Constant. pK_a 2.3, 8.7, 9.7, 13.4 (25°).

Partition Coefficient. Log *P* (octanol/water), −2.4.

Colour Tests. Ammoniacal Silver Nitrate—yellow→brown/black; Ferric Chloride—green; Folin–Ciocalteu Reagent—blue; Methanolic Potassium Hydroxide—pink→red-brown; Millon's Reagent (cold)—brown-red; Nessler's Reagent—black; Palladium Chloride—orange (→brown); Potassium Dichromate (Method 1)—green→brown.

Thin-layer Chromatography. System TD—Rf 00; system TE—Rf 00; system TF—Rf 00; system TAD—Rf 00; system TAE—Rf 11; system TAJ—Rf 00; system TAK—Rf 00; system TAL—Rf 00.

High Performance Liquid Chromatography. System HX—RI 65; system HAA—Retention time(s) 3.6 min.

Ultraviolet Spectrum. Aqueous acid—280 nm (A^1_1 = 141a).

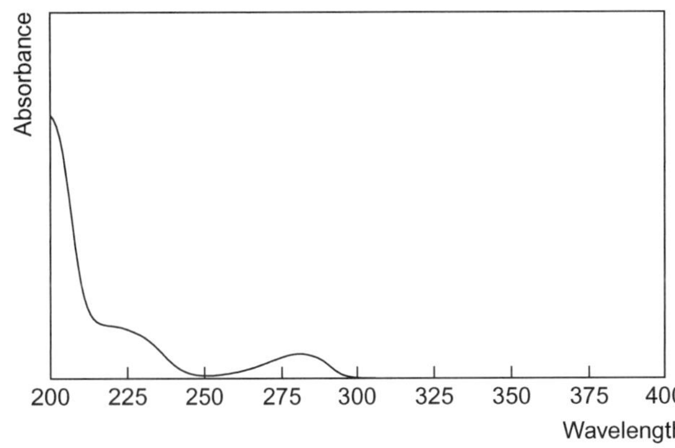

Infra-red Spectrum. Principal peaks at wavenumbers 1647, 1562, 1117, 1241, 1274, 1520 cm^{-1} (KBr disk).

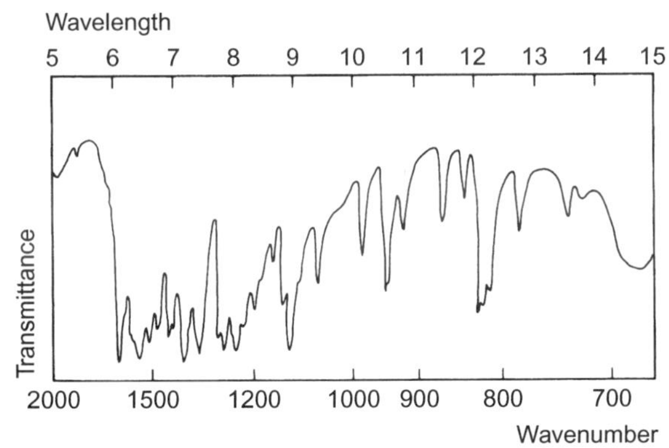

Mass Spectrum. Principal ions at *m/z* 123, 124, 77, 44, 51, 74, 53, 39.

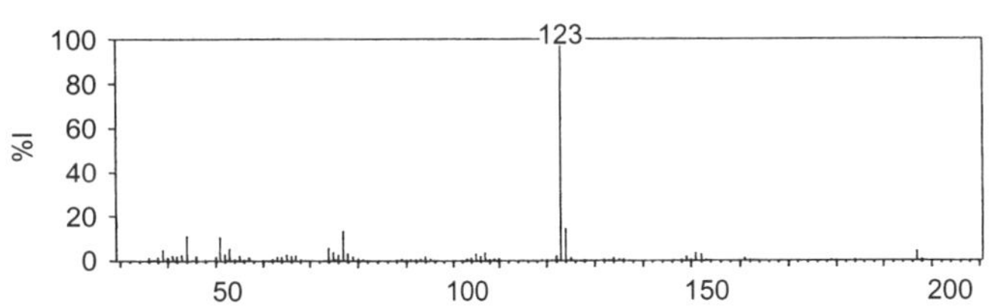

Quantification

Gas chromatography In plasma: levodopa and dopamine, ECD—Y. Mizuno, *Clinica Chim. Acta*, 1977, *74*, 11–19.

High performance liquid chromatography. In plasma: levodopa and 3,4-dihydroxyphenylacetic acid, limit of detection 1 µg/L, electrochemical detection—E. Nissinen and J. Taskinen, *J. Chromatogr.*, 1982, *231*; *Biomed. Appl.*, *20*, 459–462. In urine: levodopa and metabolites, UV and fluorescence detection—J. Seki *et al.*, *Chem. Pharm. Bull.*, 1981, *29*, 789–795. In plasma—H. Tsuchiya and T. Hayashi, *J. Chromatogr.*, 1989, *491*, 291–298. In plasma: levodopa, its metabolites and carbidopa, coulometric detection—C. Lucarelli *et al.*, *J. Chromatogr.*, 1990, *511*, 167–176. In plasma or urine: levodopa, carbidopa, 3-*O*-methyldopa and dopamine, electrochemical detection—D. C. Titus *et al.*, *J. Chromatogr.*, 1990, *534*, 87–100. In plasma: levodopa, its main metabolites and carbidopa, amperometric detection—T. Wikberg, *J. Pharm. Biomed. Anal.*, 1991, *9*, 167–176. In plasma: levodopa and its metabolites—S. Dethy *et al.*, *Clin. Chem.*,

1997, *43*, 740–744. In plasma: electrochemical detection (also L-tyrosine with fluorescence detection—S. Letellier *et al.*, *J. Chromatogr. B, Biomed. Sci. Appl.*, 1997, *696*, 9–17. In plasma or platelets: levodopa and its metabolite 3-*O*-methyldopa, limits of detection 1 µg/L and 3 µg/L, respectively, electrochemical detection—F. Blandini *et al.*, *J. Chromatogr. B, Biomed. Sci. Appl.*, 1997, *700*, 278–282. In plasma or urine: levodopa, carbidopa and their metabolites, limit of detection 5 µg/L for levodopa, amperometric detection—K. A. Sagar and M. R. Smyth, *J. Pharm. Biomed. Anal.*, 2000, *22*, 613–624.

Disposition in the Body. Levodopa is rapidly absorbed from the small bowel after oral administration and widely distributed in the tissues; less than 1% of a dose reaches the brain. It is extensively metabolised, mainly by decarboxylation to dopamine which is further metabolised, and also by methylation to 3-*O*-methyldopa which accumulates in the central nervous system; most of a dose is decarboxylated by the gastric mucosa before entering the systemic circulation; the decarboxylase activity is inhibited by carbidopa and benserazide. Dopamine is further metabolised to noradrenaline [norepinephrine], 3-methoxytyramine, and to the two major excretory metabolites, 3,4-dihydroxyphenylacetic acid (DOPAC) and 3-methoxy-4-hydroxyphenylacetic acid (homovanillic acid, HVA). During prolonged therapy, the rate of levodopa metabolism appears to increase, possibly due to enzyme induction. About 70 to 80% of a dose is excreted in the urine in 24 h. Of the material excreted in the urine, about 50% is DOPAC and HVA, 10% is dopamine, up to 30% is 3-*O*-methyldopa, and less than 1% is unchanged drug. Less than 1% of a dose is eliminated in the faeces. During prolonged therapy the ratio of the amount of DOPAC produced to that of HVA may be increased.

Therapeutic concentration. There is considerable intersubject variation in plasma concentrations and there appears to be no significant correlation between plasma concentrations of levodopa or its metabolites and therapeutic effect.

Following single oral doses of 1.5 g to 42 subjects, peak plasma-levodopa concentrations averaged about 1 mg/L at 1 to 2 h but there was a tenfold variation in peak concentrations. Peak plasma concentrations of 3-*O*-methyldopa of about 1.5 mg/L were attained in about 4 h and concentrations of HVA in the cerebrospinal fluid reached a maximum of about 0.15 mg/L in 8 h [S. Bergmann *et al.*, *Br. J. Clin. Pharmacol.*, 1974, *1*, 417–424].

Ten subjects receiving 300 to 1500 mg levodopa by mouth daily (treatment duration 3 to 25 years) were studied during daily activity at home and work. Steady-state plasma concentrations varied widely (0.5 to 7.1 (mean 2.0) mg/L for levodopa and 2.4 to 20.8 (mean 7.1) mg/L for 3-*O*-methyldopa) [D. Nyholm *et al.*, *Clin. Neuropharmacol.*, 2002, *25*, 89–96].

Bioavailability. About 33%.

Half-life. Plasma half-life, about 1 h which may be increased by concomitant administration of peripheral decarboxylase inhibitors; 3-*O*-methyldopa about 13 h.

Clearance. Plasma clearance, about 23 mL/min/kg.

Dose. Initially, 0.25 to 1 g daily; maintenance, up to 8 g daily.

Levofloxacin

Antibacterial

Synonyms. DR-3355; HR-355; RWJ-25213; *S*-(−)-Ofloxacin.
Proprietary names. Cravit; Levaquin; Quixin; Tavanic.
(−)-(*S*)-9-Fluoro-2,3-dihydro-3-methyl-10-(4-methyl-1-piperazinyl)-7-oxo-7*H*-pyrido[1,2,3-*de*]-1,4-benzoxazine-6-carboxylic acid
$C_{18}H_{20}FN_3O_4$=361.4
CAS—100986-85-4

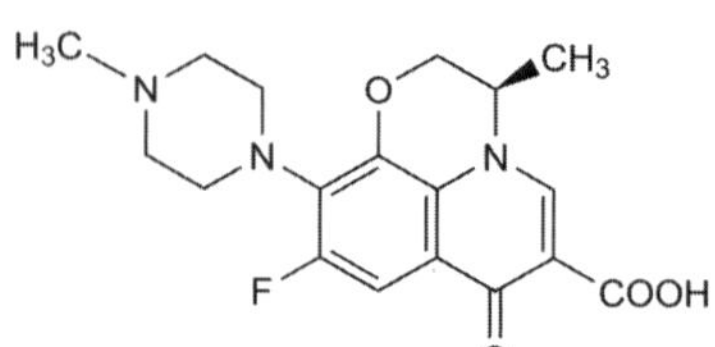

Light yellow to yellow-white crystals. It is freely soluble in glacial acetic acid and chloroform; sparingly soluble in water.

Levofloxacin Hemihydrate
$C_{18}H_{20}FN_3O_4.{}^1/_2H_2O$=370.4
CAS—138199-71-0
Needle-like crystals from ethanol/ethyl ether with M.p. 225° to 227° (dec).

High Performance Liquid Chromatography. Column: RP ODS-2 (Inertsil, 250 × 4.6 mm i.d., 5 µm). Column temperature: 35°. Mobile phase: methanol:copper (II) sulfate pentahydrate (5 mM, containing 10 mM L-isoleucine) (12.5:87.5), flow rate 1 mL/min. Internal standard (IS): ciprofloxacin. UV detection (λ=330 nm). Retention time(s): levofloxacin, 8 min; IS, 13 min. [F. A. Wong *et al.*, *J. Pharm. Biomed. Anal.*, 1997, *15(6)*, 765–771].

Ultraviolet Spectrum. Ethanol—226, 300 nm.

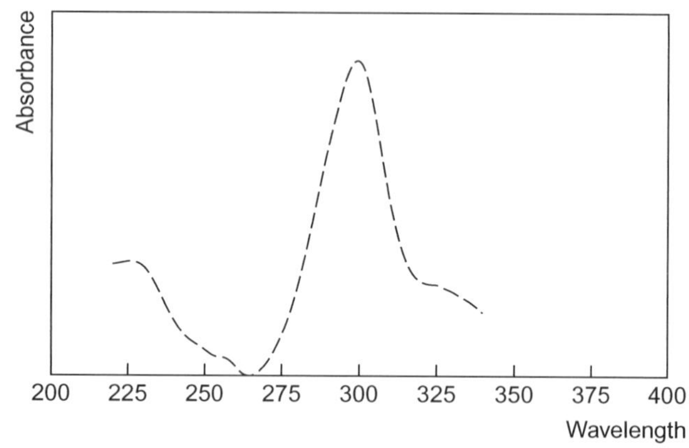

Quantification

High performance liquid chromatography. In plasma and urine: limit of quantification 80 µg/L. UV detection (λ=330 nm)—F. A. Wong *et al.*, *J. Pharm. Biomed. Anal.*, 1997, *15(6)*, 765–771. In plasma and urine: limit of detection 3 µg/L and 80 µg/L, respectively. Fluorescence detection (λ_{ex}=298 nm, λ_{em}=458 nm)—K. Lehr and P. Damm, *J. Chromatogr.*, 1988, *425*, 153–161.

Disposition in the Body. Levofloxacin is rapidly absorbed after oral administration with maximum plasma concentrations being reached approx. 1 h after a dose. The absorption of levofloxacin is little affected by the presence of food in the gastro-intestinal tract but administration with a high fat meal may slightly prolong the time to peak concentration. It is widely distributed throughout the body, crosses the placenta and has been detected in breast milk. Levofloxacin undergoes limited metabolism and is excreted mainly as the unchanged drug in urine (80 to 85%) and faeces (2%) within 24 h. The major urinary metabolites are desmethyllevofloxacin and levofloxacin *N*-oxide, each accounting for only 2% of a dose.

Therapeutic concentration

5 non-fasting, healthy male volunteers, aged between 27 and 36 years, were administered a 100 mg dose of levofloxacin. The mean peak plasma concentration was 1.35 mg/L and was observed about 1.8 h after ingestion. [O. Okazaki *et al.*, *Antimicrob. Agents Chemother.*, 1991, *35*, 2106–2109].

Bioavailability. 100%.

Half-life. 6 to 8 h; may be prolonged in renal impairment.

Volume of distribution. 1.0 to 1.25 L/kg (following single doses healthy subjects). Also reported as 89 to 112 L.

Clearance. 8.51 L/h/1.73 m^2 or 144 to 226 mL/min (mean body clearance); 7.14 L/h/1.73 m^2 or 96 to 142 mL/min (mean renal clearance).

Protein binding. 30 to 40% (mainly to albumin); a figure of 47 to 52% has been reported (assessed by measuring the *S*(−)-enantiomer of ofloxacin at a drug concentration of 1 mg/L).

Dose. The usual dose is 250 to 500 mg daily.

Levomepromazine

Tranquilliser

Synonyms. Methotrimeprazine; CL-36467; CL-39743; RP-7044; SKF-5116.

Proprietary names. Levium; Levocina; Levoprome; Levozin(e); Methozane; Minozinan; Neozine; Neurocil; Novo-Meprazine; Nozinan; Sinogan. Levomepromazine is an ingredient of Immobilon (for small animals). (Includes proprietary names of salts levomepromazine.)

(βR)-2-Methoxy-*N*,*N*,β-trimethyl-10*H*-phenothiazine-10-propanamine

$C_{19}H_{24}N_2OS = 328.5$

CAS—60-99-1

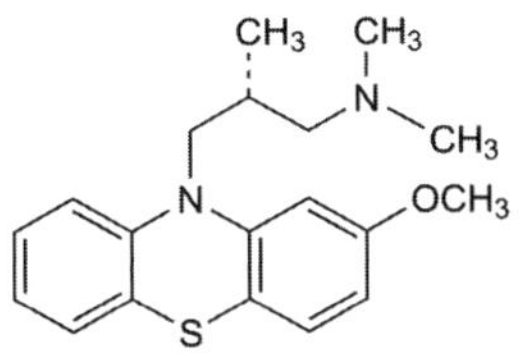

A fine, white, crystalline powder. M.p. about 126°.

Practically insoluble in water; sparingly soluble in ethanol; soluble 1 in 2 of chloroform and 1 in 10 of methanol; freely soluble in ether.

Levomepromazine Hydrochloride

$C_{19}H_{24}N_2OS,HCl = 364.9$

CAS—4185-80-2

Very soluble in water and ethanol.

Levomepromazine Maleate

Synonyms. Levomepromazine Hydrogen Maleate

$C_{19}H_{24}N_2OS,C_4H_4O_4 = 444.5$

CAS—7104-38-3; 17086-29-2

A white crystalline powder. M.p. about 190°, with decomposition.

Sparingly soluble in water and ethanol.

Dissociation Constant. pK_a 9.2.

Partition Coefficient. Log *P* (octanol/water), 4.7.

Colour Tests. Formaldehyde–Sulfuric Acid—blue; Forrest Reagent—violet; FPN Reagent—violet; Mandelin's Test—blue-violet; Marquis Test—blue-violet.

Thin-layer Chromatography. System TA—Rf 57; system TB—Rf 47; system TC—Rf 38; system TE—Rf 76; system TL—Rf 46; system TAE—Rf 32; system TAF—Rf 49; system TAJ—Rf 27; system TAK—Rf 19; system TAL—Rf 81. (Dragendorff spray, positive; FPN reagent, violet; acidified iodoplatinate solution, positive; Marquis reagent, violet.)

Gas Chromatography. System GA—RI 2514; system GB—levomepromazine RI 2641, M (norsulfoxide) RI 3088, M (sulfoxide) RI 3114; system GF—RI 2965; system GW—retention time 23.6 min.

High Performance Liquid Chromatography. System HA—*k* 3.2; system HX—RI 435; system HY—RI 381; system HZ—retention time 7.5 min; system HAX—retention time 15.2 min; system HAY—retention time 7.2 min; system HAM—not detected; system HAZ—*k* 1.82.

Ultraviolet Spectrum. Aqueous acid—250 ($A^1_1 = 783a$), 302; aqueous alkali—259, 323 nm.

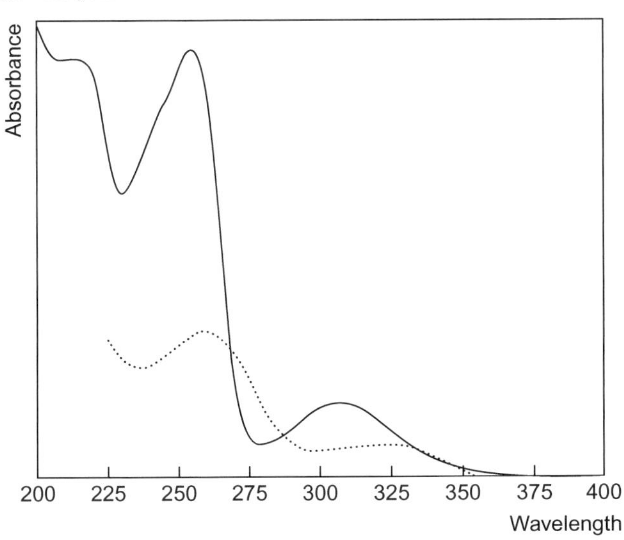

Infra-red Spectrum. Principal peaks at wavenumbers 1580, 1270, 1175, 1030, 1205, 752 cm^{-1} (KBr disk).

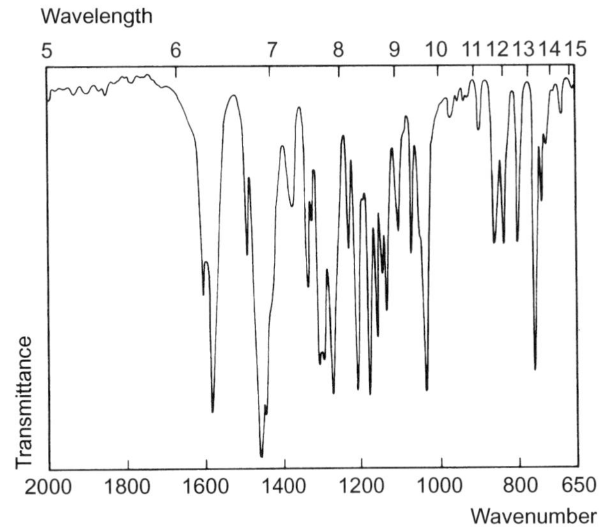

Mass Spectrum. Principal ions at *m/z* 58, 328, 100, 228, 185, 329, 242, 229.

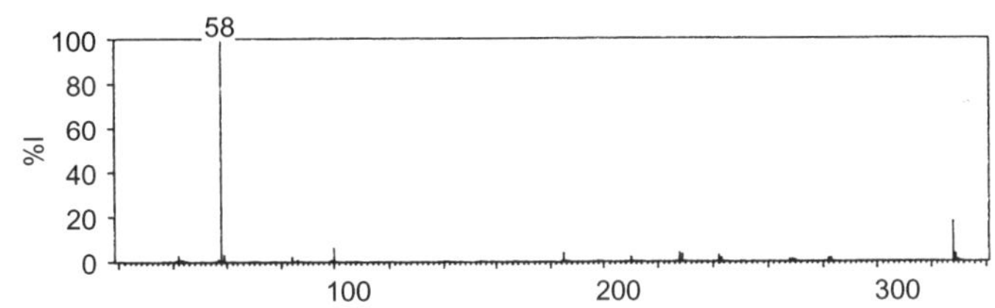

Quantification

Gas chromatography. In plasma or erythrocytes: levomepromazine and metabolites, AFID—S. G. Dahl *et al.*, *Ther. Drug Monit.*, 1982, *4*, 81–87. In plasma: limit of detection 5 µg/L, nitrogen-phosphorus detection—S. Kruggel and S. Ulrich, *Ther. Drug Monit.*, 2000, *22*, 723–728.

Gas chromatography–mass spectrometry. In plasma or urine: levomepromazine and metabolites—S. G. Dahl and M. Garle, *J. Pharm. Sci.*, 1977, *66*, 190–193.

High performance liquid chromatography. In plasma: limit of detection 2 µg/L, UV detection—J. E. Holt *et al.*, *Br. J. Clin. Pharmacol.*, 1982, *13*, 282P. In serum or urine: levomepromazine and its metabolites, limit of detection for levomepromazine 15 nmol/L—T. Loennechen *et al.*, *Ther. Drug Monit.*, 1990, *12*, 574–581. In serum or breast milk: UV detection—T. Ohkubo *et al.*, *Biomed Chromatogr.*, 1993, *7*, 227–228. In serum: levomepromazine, promethazine and chlorprothixene, limit of detection for levomepromazine 0.2 µg/L, electrochemical detection—M. Bagli *et al.*, *J. Chromatogr.* 1994, *657 B Biomed. Appl.*, 141–148.

Disposition in the Body. Readily absorbed after oral administration and widely distributed throughout the body. About 50% of an oral dose may reach the systemic circulation. The major metabolites are the sulfoxide and *N*-monodesmethyl derivative (active); hydroxylation also occurs. Less than 1% of a dose is excreted in the urine as unchanged drug in 24 h. About 10% of a dose is excreted in the urine as the sulfoxide.

Therapeutic concentration

After a single oral dose of 50 mg to 5 subjects, peak plasma concentrations of 0.016 to 0.04 mg/L were attained in 1 to 4 h; concentrations of the sulfoxide metabolite exceeded those of unchanged drug in each case. [S. G. Dahl, *Clin. Pharmacol. Ther.*, 1976, *19*, 435–442.]

Following daily oral doses of 300 to 400 mg to 4 subjects, steady-state plasma concentrations of 0.05 to 0.14 mg/L (mean 0.08) were reported; steady-state plasma concentrations of the sulfoxide metabolite ranged from 0.26 to 0.39 mg/L (mean 0.33); the *N*-monodesmethyl metabolite was also detected. [S. G. Dahl and M. Garle, *J. Pharm. Sci.*, 1977, *66*, 190–193.]

Toxicity
In a 42-year-old male who committed suicide by ingesting levomepromazine, the following postmortem body-fluid concentrations of levomepromazine, desmethyllevomepromazine and levomepromazine sulfoxide were reported, respectively: blood 4.1, 2.0, and 1.8 mg/L, urine 0.80, 1.2, and 8.9 mg/L, bile 70, 35, and 26 mg/L, vitreous humour 0.25, 0.20, and 0.90 mg/L. No other drugs were detected. [S. P. Avis and M. D. Holzbecher, *J. Forensic Sci.*, 1996, *41*, 1080–1081.]

The following postmortem concentrations were reported in a fatality attributed to levomepromazine overdose: blood 8 mg/L, liver 160 µg/g. [R. Bonnichsen *et al.*, *Z. Rechtsmed.*, 1970, *67*, 158–169.]

Half-life. Plasma half-life, levomepromazine 16 to 78 h (mean 27), sulfoxide metabolite 10 to 30 h (mean 20).

Volume of distribution. About 30 L/kg.

Distribution in blood. Plasma:whole blood ratio, about 1.2 but there is considerable intersubject variation.

Dose. Usually 25 to 50 mg of levomepromazine maleate daily; up to 1 g daily has been given.

Levopropoxyphene

Antitussive

α-[2-(Dimethylamino)-1-methylethyl]-α-phenylbenzeneethanol propanoate
$C_{22}H_{29}NO_2$=339.5
CAS—2338-37-6

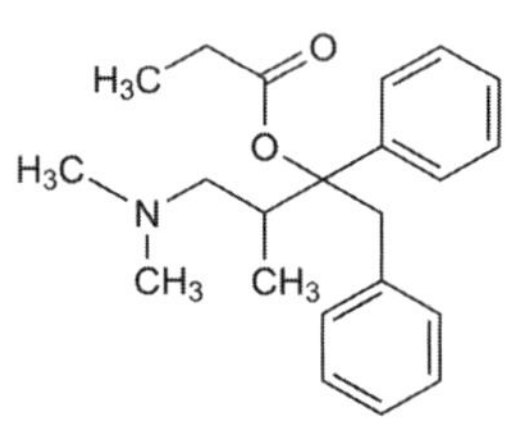

Crystals. M.p. 75° to 76°.

Levopropoxyphene Napsilate
Synonym. Levopropoxyphene Naphthalene-2-sulfonate
Proprietary names. Contratuss; Letusin; Novrad.
$C_{22}H_{29}NO_2,C_{10}H_8O_3S,H_2O$=565.7
CAS—5714-90-9 (anhydrous); 55557-30-7 (monohydrate)
A white powder. M.p. 158° to 165°.
Very slightly soluble in water; soluble 1 in 17 of ethanol and 1 in 2 of chloroform; soluble in acetone and methanol.

Partition Coefficient. Log *P* (octanol/water), 4.2.
For analytical data see under Dextropropoxyphene.

Dose. The equivalent of 50 to 100 mg of levopropoxyphene every 4 h.

Levorphanol

Narcotic Analgesic

Synonyms. Levorphan; Methorphinan; Ro-1-5431.
17-Methylmorphinan-3-ol
$C_{17}H_{23}NO$=257.4
CAS—77-07-6

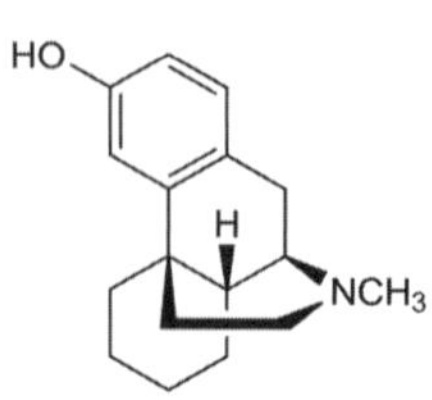

Crystals. M.p. 198° to 199°.

Levorphanol Tartrate
Synonym. Levorphanol Bitartrate
Proprietary names. Dromoran; Levo-Dromoran.
$C_{17}H_{23}NO,C_4H_6O_6,2H_2O$=443.5
CAS—125-72-4 (anhydrous); 5985-38-6 (dihydrate)
A white crystalline powder. M.p. 113° to 115° (dihydrate), m.p. 206° to 208° (anhydrous).
Soluble 1 in about 45 of water, 1 in about 110 of ethanol and 1 in 50 of ether; practically insoluble in chloroform.

Dissociation Constant. pK_a 8.2 (20°).

Partition Coefficient. Log *P* (octanol/buffer pH 7.4), 1.1.

Thin-layer Chromatography System TA—Rf 35; system TB—Rf 13; system TC—Rf 07. (Dragendorff spray, positive; Acidified iodoplatinate solution, positive.)

Gas Chromatography. System GA—RI 2230; system GC—RI 2230. (Metabolised to dextrorphan.)

High Performance Liquid Chromatography. System HA—*k* 4.4 (tailing peak); system HC—*k* 3.20; system HY—RI 265.

Ultraviolet Spectrum. Aqueous acid—279 (A^1_1=79a); aqueous alkali—240 (A^1_1=339a), 299 nm (A^1_1=119a).

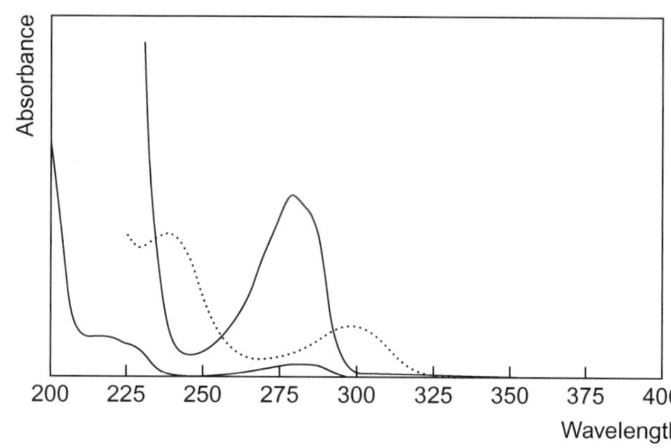

Infra-red Spectrum. Principal peaks at wavenumbers 1238, 1495, 753, 1278, 1578, 1608 cm^{-1} (KBr disk).

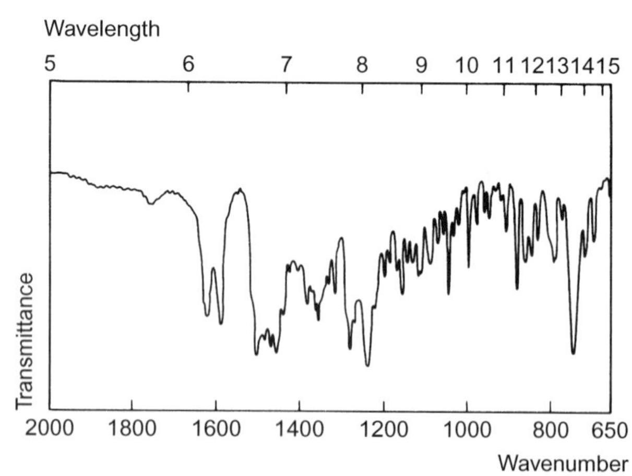

Mass Spectrum. Principal ions at *m*/*z* 59, 257, 150, 256, 44, 31, 200, 157.

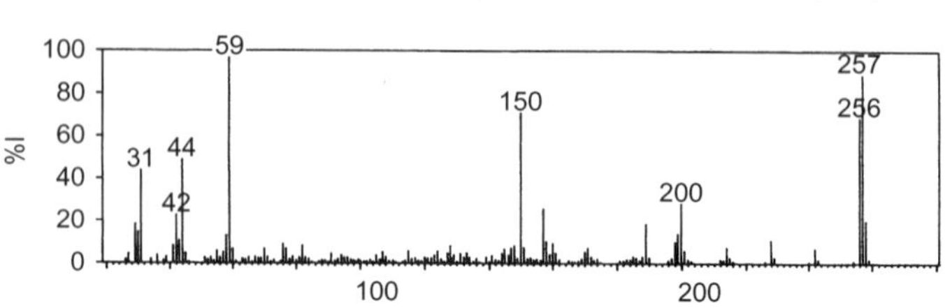

Quantification

Gas chromatography. In plasma: limit of detection <0.25 µg/L, ECD—E. T. Everhart *et al.*, *J. Chromatogr. B Biomed. Sci. Appl.*, 1999, *729*, 173–181.

Gas chromatography–mass spectrometry. In plasma: limit of detection 1 µg/L—B. H. Min *et al.*, *J. Chromatogr.*, 1982, *231*; *B Biomed. Appl.*, *20*, 194–199.

Radioimmunoassay. In plasma: limit of detection 1 µg/L—R. Dixon *et al.*, *Res. Commun. Chem. Path. Pharmacol.*, 1981, *32*, 545–548.

Disposition in the Body. Levorphanol is absorbed after oral administration. It is metabolised by 3-glucuronidation.

Toxicity

Postmortem concentrations in a 41-year-old female found dead after having ingested an unknown quantity of levorphanol were: blood 2.7 mg/L, bile 24 mg/L, brain 1.8 µg/g, kidney 3.4 µg/g, liver 5.4 µg/g, lung 17 µg/g, urine 2.3 mg/L [J. E. Turner *et al.*, *J. Anal. Toxicol.*, 1977, *1*, 103–104].

A 61-year-old man ingested 30 mg of levorphanol and died about 18 h later. The antemortem blood concentration was 0.8 mg/L. Concentrations in other fluids and tissues (samples taken after the body had been embalmed) were: bile 15 mg/L, kidney 1 µg/g, liver 11 µg/g [L. R. Bednarczyk, *J. Anal. Toxicol.*, 1979, *3*, 217–219].

Half-life. Plasma half-life, about 13 h.

Dose. 1.5 to 9 mg of levorphanol tartrate daily.

Levosimendan

Cardiotonic

Synonyms. (*R*)-Simendan; OR-1259.
Proprietary name. Simdax
[[4-[(4*R*)-1,4,5,6-Tetrahydro-4-methyl-6-oxo-3-pyridazinyl]phenyl]-hydrazono]propanedinitrile
$C_{14}H_{12}N_6O$=280.3
CAS—141505-33-1

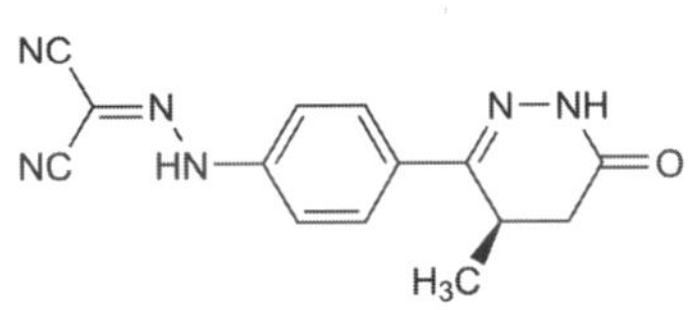

Yellow crystalline powder. M.p. 210° to 214°. Soluble in water.

Dissociation Constant. pK_a 6.3.

High Performance Liquid Chromatography. Column: RP-18 (LiChrosorb, 250 × 4 mm i.d., 10 µm). Mobile phase: monosodium dihydrogen phosphate buffer (32 mM):methanol:tetrahydrofuran (45:65:1), adjusted to pH 3.5 with phosphoric acid. 1.0 mL/min flow rate. Internal standard (IS): OR-1097. UV detection (λ=380 nm). Retention time(s): levosimendan, 6.4 min; IS, 5.4 min. [M. Karlsson *et al.*, *Biomed. Chromatogr.*, 1997, *11(1)*, 54–58].

Quantification

High performance liquid chromatography. In plasma: limit of quantification and limit of detection 5 µg/L. UV detection (λ=380 nm)—M. Karlsson *et al.*, *Biomed. Chromatogr.*, 1997, *11(1)*, 54–58. In plasma: limit of detection 10 µg/L. UV detection (λ=380 nm)—T. Wikberg *et al.*, *Chirality*, 1996, *8(7)*, 511–517.

Disposition in the Body. Levosimendan is rapidly absorbed after administration and distributed quickly around the body. It is completely metabolised with negligible amounts of the unchanged drug being detected in urine and faeces. The main metabolites are conjugates of the glutathione pathway and cyclic, *N*-acetylated cysteine or cysteinylglycine derivatives. These metabolites are biologically inactive and are slowly formed.

Therapeutic concentration

10 healthy subjects, aged 21 to 27 years (mean 24 years), were administered a single dose of levosimendan (2 mg) as an intravenous infusion (5 min infusion) and orally in the form of a conventional tablet; conventional capsule and a slow-release tablet. Doses were administered after an overnight fast and a washout period of 1 week was allowed between treatments. After the intravenous dose, the maximum plasma concentration was 180 µg/L at the end of the infusion. For oral administration, the conventional tablet and capsule gave maxima of 72 and 76 µg/L at 0.9 and 1.2 h, respectively; the slow release formulation produced lower concentrations of 14 µg/L at 2.8 h. Metabolites were detected up to 24 h after the slow release tablet but only up to 8 h for the other formulations. At 8 h, the metabolite concentrations were 93, 79, 53 and 1074 ng/L for the conventional tablet, conventional capsule, after the intravenous dose and after the slow release tablet, respectively. [S. Sundberg *et al.*, *Int. J. Clin. Pharmacol. Ther.*, 1998, *36(12)*, 629–635].

Bioavailability. Oral, 85%.

Half-life. 0.96 h (healthy individuals); 1.03 h (patients with mild congestive heart failure).

Volume of distribution. Steady state, 21.9 L (healthy); 19.5 L (patients with mild congestive heart failure). Also reported as 14.7 L.

Clearance. 359 mL/min (healthy); 296 mL/min (patients with mild congestive heart failure). Also reported as 246 mL/min.

Protein binding. 97 to 98%.

Dose. The usual dose (used in clinical trials) is a 6 to 12 µg/kg loading dose over 10 min followed by 0.05 to 0.2 µg/kg/min as a continuous intravenous infusion.

Levothyroxine

Thyroid Agent

Synonyms. Thyroxine; L-Thyroxine. The abbreviation T_4 is often used for thyroxine in medical and biochemical reports.
(−)-3-[4-(4-hydroxy-3,5-diiodophenoxy)-3,5-diiodophenyl]alanine
$C_{15}H_{11}I_4NO_4$=776.9
CAS—51-48-9

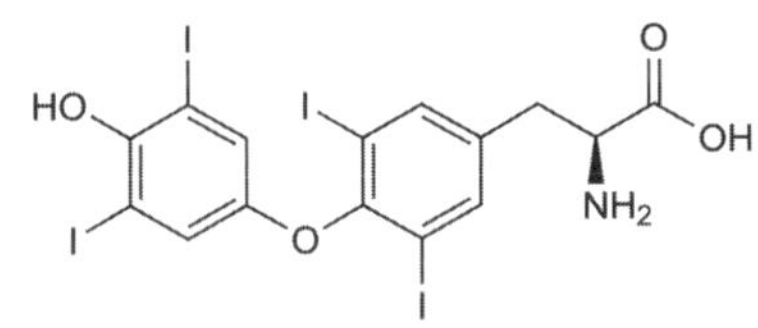

Crystals. M.p. 235° to 236°, with decomposition.

Levothyroxine Sodium

Synonyms. Thyroxine Sodium; Levothyroxinnatrium; Lexothyroxinum Natricum; Thyroxinum Natricum; Tirossina; Tiroxina Sodica.
Proprietary names. Dexnon; Elthyrone; Eltroxin; Euthyrox; Eutirox; Levaxin; Levotec; Levo-T; Levothroid; Levothyrox; Levoxyl; Oroxine; Synthroid; Thyrax; Thyrex; Tiracrin; Tirosint; Unithroid. It is an ingredient of Thyrolar.
$C_{15}H_{10}I_4NNaO_4$,xH_2O=798.9 (anhydrous)
CAS—55-03-8 (anhydrous); 25416-65-3 (hydrate)
A white to pale brownish-yellow, hygroscopic, amorphous, or crystalline powder. It may assume a slight pink colour on exposure to light.
Soluble 1 in 700 of water and 1 in 300 of ethanol; practically insoluble in acetone, chloroform, and ether; soluble in solutions of alkali hydroxides. Alkaline solutions are unstable.

Dissociation Constant. pK_a 2.2, 6.7, 10.1.

Partition Coefficient. Log *P* (octanol/water), 4.12.

Ultraviolet Spectrum. Aqueous alkali—325 nm (A^1_1=78a).

Infra-red Spectrum. Principal peaks at wavenumbers 1628, 1585, 1308, 1185, 1240, 1148 cm^{-1} (KBr disk).

Quantification

Gas chromatography. In serum: levothyroxine and liothyronine, limit of detection 10 µg/L and 2.7 µg/L, respectively, ECD—N. N. Nihei *et al.*, *Anal. Biochem.*, 1971, *43*, 433–445.

High performance liquid chromatography–mass spectrometry. In serum: limit of detection 6 pg, tandem MS detection (SIM)—V. I. De Brabandere *et al.*, *Rapid Commun. Mass. Spectrom.*, 1998, *12(16)*, 1099–1103.

High pressure liquid chromatography–radioimmunoassay. In hair—F. Tagliaro *et al.*, *J. Chromatogr. B Biomed. Sci. Appl.*, 1998, *716*, 77–82.

Enzyme immunoassay. In serum: limit of detection, 4 nmol/L—S. Akman *et al.*, *J. Immunoassay*, 1995, *16(3)*, 325–341.

Disposition in the Body. Incompletely and variably absorbed after oral administration. 48 to 80% of an administered dose may be absorbed. The extent of absorption increases in the fasted state and the degree of absorption may be affected by the formulation of the drug used. It is metabolised, in the liver and kidney, by de-iodination to liothyronine (tri-iodothyronine) which is the principal active form of levothyroxine; further de-iodination to thyroacetic acid (4-*p*-hydroxyphenoxy-phenylacetic acid), and conjugation with glucuronic acid and sulfate also occur. Deamination and decarboxylation of levothyroxine to the tetrone is a further metabolic pathway. Elimination from the body is slow. About 30 to 55% of a dose is excreted in the urine and 20 to 40% is eliminated in the faeces; of the urinary material about 40% is thyroacetic acid and 20% is liothyronine. Endogenous serum-levothyroxine concentrations range from 50 to 120 µg/L in normal subjects. A minimum amount of the drug crosses the placenta and can be detected in breast milk.

Therapeutic concentration

24 patients with hypothyroidism, receiving treatment with levothyroxine 100 µg daily in the form of a test or a reference preparation, had a mean peak plasma concentration of 98.4 and 108 µg/L at 3 and 2 h, respectively. [M. Vaisman *et al.*, *Arzneimittelforschung*, 2001, *51*, 246–252.]

14 euthyroid goitrous patients were orally administered 150 µg levothyroxine after an overnight fast, as a tablet or in solution. The mean levothyroxine basal concentration was 90.7 µg/L for the solution administration day and 89.0 µg/L for the tablet day. The maximum serum levothyroxine concentration was reached at the 2nd hour after administration for the solution, at 111.5 µg/L and at the 3rd hour for the tablet formulation, maximum 118.1 µg/L. [A. Carpi *et al.*, *Thyroidology*, 1993, *5(1)*, 9–12.]

30 healthy females (mean age, 34 years) were administered a single dose of 600 µg levothyroxine as 2 different formulations, Synthroid (A) or Levoxine (B), after an overnight fast. Fasting continued for 5 h after dosing and a wash-out period of 35 days was allowed between doses. The mean maximum plasma concentrations of levothyroxine were 59.1 and 71.2 µg/L for the 2 formulations, respectively, at 3.67 and 3.03 h. [J. A. Berg and G. H. Mayor, *J. Clin. Pharmacol.*, 1992, *32(12)*, 1135–1140.]

Toxicity

A 34-year-old male ingested approx. 900 tablets (a total of 720 mg) levothyroxine. He became lethargic 2 to 3 days after administration, had vomiting and insomnia on day 4; was agitated, aggressive, and incoherent on day 5 and was confused when he returned to hospital on day 6. While in hospital for 6 days, he was tachycardic. Free levothyroxine concentrations were >130 µg/L on day 6 and 12 µg/L on day 12. By day 15 he had lost 20 kg in weight. [J. B. Hack *et al.*, *Vet. Hum. Toxicol.*, 1999, *41(5)*, 323–326.]

The following peak serum concentrations were reported in a thyroidectomised patient who had attempted suicide by taking 2000 µg levothyroxine: levothyroxine (on 2nd day) 315 µg/L, FT_4 0.048 µg/L, reverse triiodothyronine 0.80 µg/L, triiodothyronine (on 3rd day) 1.92 µg/L; levothyroxine and reverse triiodothyronine levels returned to their normal range 13 to 17 days after the suicide attempt. [T. Ishihara *et al.*, *Endocr. J.*, 1998, *45*, 371–375.]

Over a 1-year period, 15 cases of acute levothyroxine overdose were studied; all patients were less than 5 years old and the majority were male. The estimated dose ingested by 10 patients was 1.5 to 8.8 mg (0.1 to 0.73 mg/kg) and all were examined 1 to 6 h after administration. Three patients had initial serum levothyroxine concentrations >750 µg/L and developed signs of toxicity within 12 to 48 h, including tachycardia, hypertension and agitation, which had disappeared within 24 to 60 h. [W. J. Lewander *et al.*, *Pediatrics*, 1989, *84(2)*, 262–265.]

Half-life. Plasma half-life, 6 to 7 days which may be increased in pregnancy or myxoedema and decreased in hyperthyroidism.

Protein binding. In plasma, more than 99.9%.

Dose. Adult, 50 to 100 µg of anhydrous levothyroxine sodium daily; increased by increments of 50 µg until desired result (usually, 100 to 200 µg daily). Children, (up to 1 month old) 5 to 10 µg/kg daily (>1 month old); 5 µg/kg daily initially and then increased by 25 µg every 2 to 4 weeks until desired result.

Lidocaine

Local Anaesthetic/Anti-arrhythmic

Synonym. Lignocaine

Proprietary names. Dentipatch; ELA-Max; Lidoderm; Vagisil; Zilactin-L. Lidocaine and Lidocaine Hydrochloride are ingredients of many proprietary preparations—see Martindale, *The complete drug reference*, 33rd Edn, London, Pharmaceutical Press, 2002.

2-(Diethylamino)-*N*-(2,6-dimethylphenyl)acetamide

$C_{14}H_{22}N_2O$=234.3

CAS—137-58-6

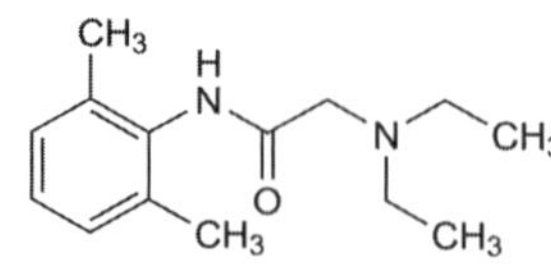

A white to slightly yellow crystalline powder. M.p. 68° to 69° (needles from benzene or alcohol).

Insoluble in water; soluble in ethanol, chloroform, benzene and ether.

Lidocaine Hydrochloride

Synonym. Lignocaine Hydrochloride

Proprietary names. Anestacon; Dilocaine; Duo-Trach Kit; Laryng-O-Jet; Lidocard; Lidocation; Lidocaton; Lidocord; Lidoject; LidoPen; Lidosen; Lignostab-A; Nervocaine; Octocaine; Rinstead (contact pastilles); Ultracaine; Uro-Jet; Xylocaine; Xylocard; Xylotox.

$C_{14}H_{22}N_2O,HCl,H_2O$=288.8

CAS—73-78-9 (anhydrous); 6108-05-0 (monohydrate)

A white crystalline powder. M.p. 77° to 78°.

Soluble 1 in 0.7 of water, 1 in 1.5 of ethanol, and 1 in 40 of chloroform; practically insoluble in ether.

Dissociation Constant. pK_a 7.9 (25°).

Partition Coefficient. Log *P* (octanol/water), 2.4.

Colour Test. To a 2% solution in water, add 1 mL dilute nitric acid and 3 mL mercuric nitrate solution and heat to boiling—yellow or yellow-green.

Thin-layer Chromatography. System TA—Rf 70; system TB—Rf 35; system TC—Rf 71; system TE—Rf 80; system TL—Rf 63; system TAE—Rf 72; system TAF—Rf 69; system TAJ—Rf 55; system TAK—Rf 00; system TAL—Rf 28. (Dragendorff spray, positive; acidified iodoplatinate solution, positive; Marquis reagent, pink.)

Gas Chromatography. System GA—lidocaine RI 1870, M (2,6-dimethylaniline) RI 1180, M (OH-) RI 2350, M (monoethylglycinexylidide) RI 1800, M (desethyl-) RI 1790, M (dimethylhydroxyaniline) RI 1460; system GF—lidocaine RI 2240; system GQ—lidocaine Retention time 6.0 min M (monoethylglycinexylidide) 5.5 min.

High Performance Liquid Chromatography. System HA—lidocaine *k* 0.6, M (monoethylglycinexylidide) *k* 1.2; system HQ—*k* 0.79; system HX—RI 288; system HY—RI 258; system HZ—Retention time 2.6 min; system HAA—Retention time 9.9 min; system HAM—lidocaine not detected; system HAX—Retention time 8.0 min; system HAY—Retention time 4.5 min.

Ultraviolet Spectrum. Aqueous acid—263 nm (A^1_1=19a), 272 nm. (See below.)

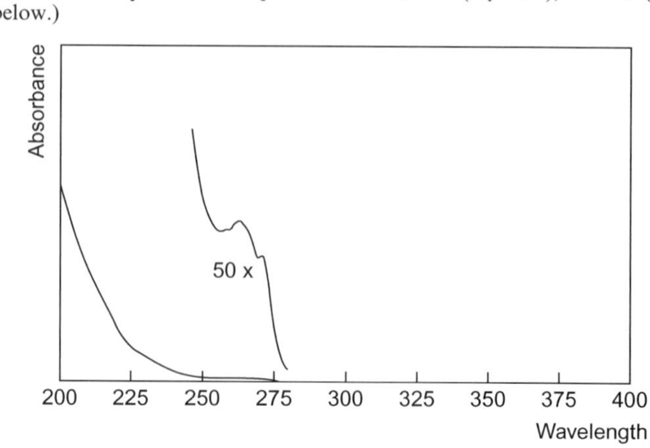

Infra-red Spectrum. Principal peaks at wavenumbers 1662, 1495, 762, 1204, 1290, 1086 cm^{-1} (KBr disk). (See below.)

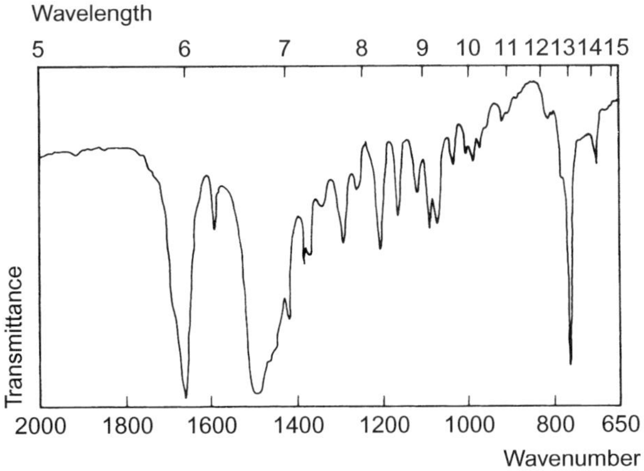

Mass Spectrum. Principal ions at *m*/*z* 86, 87, 58, 44, 72, 42, 120, 85.

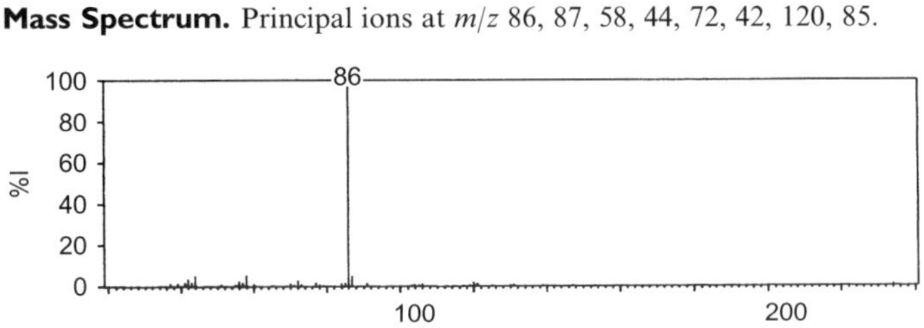

Quantification

Gas chromatography. In blood, serum or tissues: limit of detection 100 µg/L, AFID—B. Levine *et al.*, *J. Anal. Toxicol.*, 1983, *7*, 123–124. In plasma: lidocaine and monoethylglycinexylidide, limit of detection 300 µg/L, AFID—J. D. Hawkins *et al.*, *Ther. Drug Monit.*, 1982, *4*, 103–106. In blood or CSF: lidocaine, mepivacaine and bupivacaine, limits of detection 5 to 10 pg, SID—H. Hattori *et al.*, *J. Chromatogr.*, 1991, *564*, 278–282. In biological samples: lidocaine and other local anaesthetics, nitrogen-sensitive detection—O. W. Lau *et al.*, *Methods Find. Exp. Clin. Pharmacol.*, 1991, *13*, 475–481. In serum: lidocaine and bupivacaine and their metabolites, limit of detection 15 µg/L, nitrogen–phosphorus detection—A. M. Lorec *et al.*, *Ther. Drug Monit.*, 1994, *16*, 592–595. In plasma: lidocaine and *n*-butyl-*p*-aminobenzoate, nitrogen-selective detection—R. J. Grouls *et al.*, *J. Chromatogr. B Biomed. Appl.*, 1995, *673*, 51–57. In plasma: lidocaine and monoethylglycinexylidide, limit of detection 1 µg/L, nitrogen–phosphorus detection—N. Laroche *et al.*, *J. Chromatogr. B Biomed. Sci. Appl.*, 1998, *716*, 375–381. In plasma: limit of detection 5 µg/L—E. H. Koster *et al.*, *J. Chromatogr. B Biomed. Sci. Appl.*, 2000, *739*, 175–182.

Gas chromatography–mass spectrometry. In blood: lidocaine and other local anaesthetics, SIM—T. Watanabe *et al.*, *J. Chromatogr. B Biomed. Sci. Appl.*, 1998, *709*, 225–232. In postmortem hair: limit of detection 0.1 µg/g—F. Sporkert and F. Pragst, *J. Anal. Toxicol.*, 2000, *24*, 316–322. In breast milk: 2, 6-dimethylaniline, limit of detection 0.2 ppb—N. W. Puente and P. D. Josephy, *J. Anal. Toxicol.*, 2001, *25*, 711–715.

High performance liquid chromatography. In serum: limit of detection 100 µg/L for lidocaine, 50 µg/L for monoethylglycinexylidide and glycinexylidide, UV detection—R. Lindberg *et al.*, *Clin. Chem.*, 1983, *29*, 1572–1573. In plasma or serum: lidocaine and monoethylglycinexylidide, UV detection—Y. Chen *et al.*, *J. Chromatogr.*, 1992, *574*, 361–364; Y. Chen *et al.*, *Ther. Drug Monit.*, 1992, *14*, 317–321. In plasma: lidocaine and bupivacaine, UV detection—A. Sattler *et al.*, *Pharmazie*, 1995, *50*, 741–744; H. Lofti *et al.*, *Ther. Drug Monit.*, 1997, *19*, 160–164. In plasma: lidocaine and bupivacaine enantiomers, limits of detection 4 µg/L and 10 µg/L respectively, UV detection—I. Abraham *et al.*, *J. Chromatogr. B Biomed. Sci. Appl.*, 1997, *703*, 203–208. In aqueous humour: limit of detection 200 µg/L, UV detection—L. Manna *et al.*, *J. Pharm. Biomed. Anal.*, 2002, *29*, 1121–1126.

High performance liquid chromatography–mass spectrometry. In plasma: limit of quantitation 0.2 µg/L—L. D. Bo *et al.*, *J. Chromatogr. A*, 1999, *854*, 3–11. In plasma or urine: lidocaine and its metabolites, limits of quantitation 1.6 to 5 nmol/L—M. Abdel-Rehim *et al.*, *J. Chromatogr. B Biomed. Sci. Appl.*, 2000, *741*, 175–188.

Disposition in the Body. Readily absorbed from the gastro-intestinal tract, mucous membranes, damaged skin (poor absorption from intact skin), and after IM injection; poorly absorbed orally due to first-pass metabolism. Metabolism in the liver is rapid with about 90% of a dose being dealkylated to form monoethylglycinexylidide which is 60 to 80% as potent as lidocaine and glycinexylidide which is also active. Both have longer half-lives than lidocaine. Further metabolism occurs and metabolic reactions also include hydrolysis, and ring hydroxylation. Less than 10% of a dose is excreted in the urine as unchanged drug in 24 h, 40 to 70% as 4-hydroxy-2,6-xylidine, and about 4% as the active monoethylglycinexylidide; excretion of unchanged drug is increased if the urine is acid. Other metabolites include 2,6-xylidine, 3′-hydroxylignocaine, and 3′-hydroxymonoethylglycinexylidide. Glycinexylidide and the hydroxy metabolites are excreted as acid-hydrolysable conjugates. Glycinexylidide has also been detected in plasma after prolonged IV infusion. Lidocaine crosses the placenta and the blood–brain barrier and it is excreted in breast milk.

Therapeutic concentration. In plasma, usually in the range 2 to 5 mg/L.

Following topical administration of lidocaine patches (4 × 5% patches) to 20 subjects on each of 3 consecutive days, mean peak plasma concentrations of 0.1451, 0.1530, and 0.1538 mg/L (occurring at 18, 16.5, and 16.5 h) were reported on days 1, 2, and 3, respectively [A. R. Gammaitoni and M. W. Davis, *Ann. Pharmacother.*, 2002, *36*, 236–240].

In 15 patients with mild asthma, inhalation of lidocaine 10% (total dose: 5.0 mg/kg) produced a mean peak plasma concentration of 1.4 mg/L at about 13 min [H. Groeben *et al.*, *Eur. J. Anaesthesiol.*, 2000, *17*, 672–679].

A mean peak plasma concentration of 0.4 mg/L lidocaine was attained at 3 h in 24 subjects who received instillation of 200 mg lidocaine in adrenaline 1:500 000 into the intraperitoneal cavity after total abdominal hysterectomy. The highest concentration in any patient was 0.87 mg/L [K. M. Williamson *et al.*, *Br. J. Anaesth.*, 1997, *78*, 675–677].

Following IV infusions at rates varying between 20 and 50 µg/min/kg to 24 subjects, the following steady-state serum concentrations were reported: lidocaine 1.7 to 11.4 mg/L (mean 5.7), monoethylglycinexylidide 0.2 to 5.2 mg/L (mean 2.0), glycinexylidide 0 to 1.4 mg/L (mean 0.5) [D. E. Drayer *et al.*, *Clin. Pharmacol. Ther.*, 1983, *34*, 14–22].

Toxicity. Toxic effects are associated with plasma concentrations greater than 6 mg/L, and fatalities with blood concentrations greater than 14 mg/L.

Postmortem toxicological examination of a 32-year-old hospital patient whose death was attributed to an overdose of lidocaine (approx. 1500 mg) administered with homicidal intent revealed the following lidocaine tissue concentrations: blood, 22.2 mg/L, liver 43.6 µg/g, kidney 28.3 µg/g, brain 23.1 µg/g, heart 13.1 µg/g [J. R. Kalin and R. M. Brissie, *J. Forensic Sci.*, 2002, *47*, 1135–1138].

In 2 fatal cases of deliberate self-poisoning with lidocaine, the first by oral ingestion and the second by IV injection, postmortem blood analysis revealed concentrations of 40 and 53 mg/L, respectively; urine contained 49 mg/L lidocaine in the first victim [S. Dawling *et al.*, *Hum. Toxicol.*, 1989, *8*, 389–392].

In a fatality due to accidental IV injection of 2 g of lidocaine, the following postmortem tissue concentrations were reported: blood 30 mg/L, brain 135 µg/g, heart 106 µg/g, kidney 204 µg/g, lung 87 µg/g, skeletal muscle 20 µg/g [A. Poklis *et al.*, *J. Forensic Sci.*, 1984, *29*, 1229–1236].

Bioavailability. Oral, about 35%.

Half-life. Plasma half-life, lidocaine 1 to 2 h, increased in subjects with liver disease or after acute myocardial infarction; monoethylglycinexylidide about 1 to 2 h, glycinexylidide about 10 h.

Volume of distribution. About 1 to 2 L/kg.

Clearance. Plasma clearance, about 5 to 20 mL/min/kg.

Protein binding. In plasma, about 70% at therapeutic concentrations but there is considerable intersubject variation and binding appears to be concentration-dependent.

Note. For a review of the pharmacokinetics of lidocaine, see N. L. Benowitz and W. Meister, *Clin. Pharmacokinet.*, 1978, *3*, 177–201; for a review of the pharmacokinetics and pharmacodynamics of IV agents for ventricular arrhythmias, see P. E Nolan, *Pharmacotherapy*, 1997, *17*, 65S–75S; for a study of the pharmacokinetics of epidural lidocaine and bupivacaine during caesarean section, see J. W. Downing *et al.*, *Anesth. Analg.*, 1997, *84*, 527–532.

Dose. For local anaesthesia, the maximum single dose of lidocaine hydrochloride by injection should not exceed 300 mg (4.5 mg/kg), unless administered with adrenaline. For ventricular arrhythmias, initially 50 to 100 mg IV, followed by an infusion.

Lidoflazine

Anti-anginal

Synonyms. Ordiflazine; R-7904.
Proprietary names. Clinium; Corflazine; Klinium.
4-[4,4-Bis(4-fluorophenyl)butyl]-*N*-(2,6-dimethylphenyl)-1-piperazine-acetamide
$C_{30}H_{35}F_2N_3O$=491.6
CAS—3416-26-0

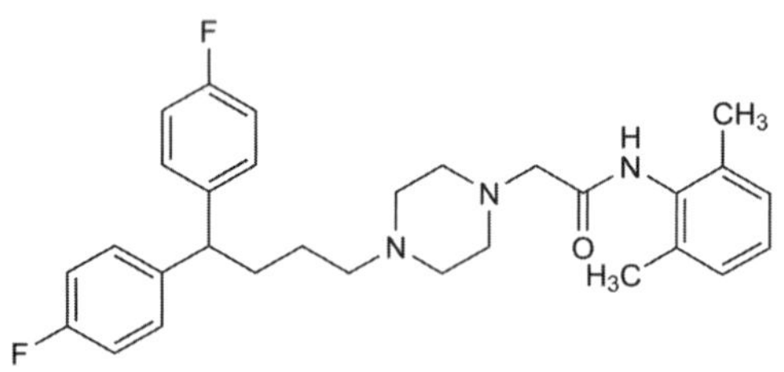

A white or slightly yellow amorphous powder. M.p. 159° to 161°.
Almost insoluble in water; soluble 1 in 90 of ethanol and 1 in 220 of ether; very soluble in chloroform.

Partition Coefficient. Log *P* (octanol/water), 5.6.

Colour Tests. Mandelin's Test—yellow; Marquis Test—yellow.

Thin-layer Chromatography. System TA—Rf 70; system TB—Rf 11; system TC—Rf 63; system TE—Rf 70; system TL—Rf 36; system TAE—Rf 70; system TAF—Rf 77. (Acidified iodoplatinate solution, positive.)

Gas Chromatography. System GA—lidoflazine RI 3870; M(desaminocarboxy-) RI 2230; M(desaminocarboxy-)-Me RI 2125; system GB—lidoflazine, not eluted.

High Performance Liquid Chromatography. System HA—*k* 0.6; system HX—RI 530.

Ultraviolet Spectrum. Acid isopropyl alcohol—266 (A_1^1=47b), 272 nm.

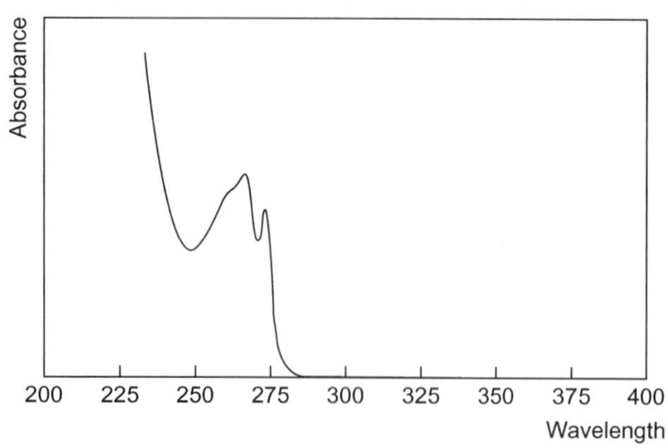

Infra-red Spectrum. Principal peaks at wavenumbers 1505, 1645, 1220, 1155, 835, 775 cm^{-1} (KBr disk).

Mass Spectrum. Principal ions at *m*/*z* 343, 70, 344, 109, 42, 113, 491, 56.

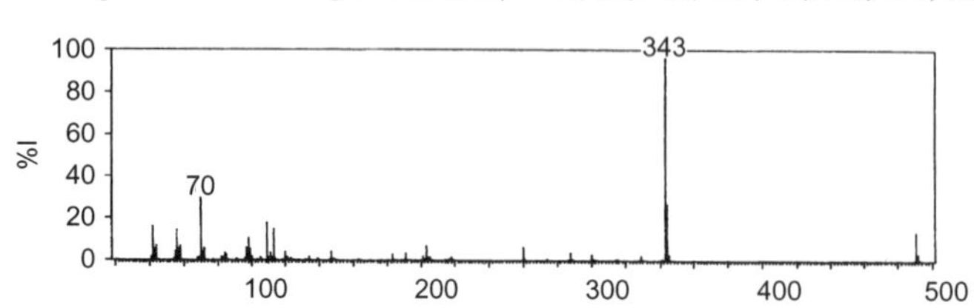

Disposition in the Body. Lidoflazine is well absorbed after oral administration. It is excreted mainly as metabolites, the major metabolites being bis(4-fluorophenyl)butyric acid and the glucuronide conjugate of bis(4-fluorophenyl)butan-1-ol. In 7 days, about 40% of an oral dose is excreted in the urine and about 40% is eliminated in the faeces.

Therapeutic concentration
After a single oral dose of 120 mg given with food, peak plasma concentrations of about 0.06 mg/L were attained in about 1 h. Following repeated oral administration of 120 mg three times a day, a mean steady-state plasma concentration of 0.12 mg/L was reported [P. M. Vanhoutte and J. M. Van Nueten, Lidoflazine, in *New Drugs Annual: Cardiovascular Drugs*, A. Scriabine (Ed.), New York, Raven Press, 1973, pp. 203–226].

Half-life. Plasma half-life, about 1 day.

Dose. 120 to 360 mg daily.

Lincomycin

Antibiotic

Synonym. NSC-70731.
(2*S*-*trans*)-Methyl 6,8-dideoxy-6-[[(1-methyl-4-propyl-2-pyrrolidinyl)carbonyl]amino]-1-thio-D-*erythro*-α-D-*galacto*-octopyranoside
$C_{18}H_{34}N_2O_6S$=406.5
CAS—154-21-2

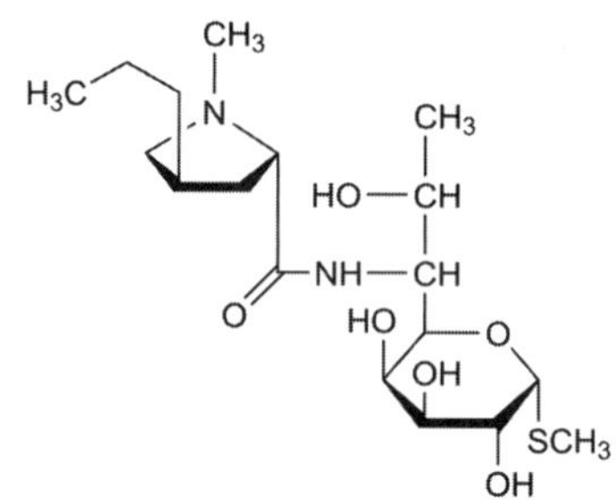

Slightly soluble in water; soluble in methanol, lower alcohols, ethyl acetate, acetone, and chloroform.

Lincomycin Hydrochloride

Proprietary names. Albiotic; Anbycin; Cillimicina; Frademicina; Fredcina; Linco; Lincocin(e); Lincocina; Lincogin; Lincolan; Lincomy; Linco-Plus; Lincorex; Lingo; Linmycin; Macrolin; Mycivin; Princol; Rimsalin.
$C_{18}H_{34}N_2O_6S,HCl,H_2O$=461.0
CAS—859-18-7 (anhydrous); 7179-49-9 (monohydrate)
A white crystalline powder.
Soluble 1 in 1 of water, 1 in 40 of ethanol and 1 in 20 of dimethylformamide; soluble in methanol; practically insoluble in chloroform and ether.

Dissociation Constant. pK_a 7.5.

Partition Coefficient. Log *P* (octanol/water), 0.6.

Colour Test. Sodium Nitroprusside (Method 3)—violet.

Thin-layer Chromatography. System TA—Rf 67; system TAE—Rf 75. (Acidified potassium permanganate solution, positive.)

Ultraviolet Spectrum. No significant absorption, 230 to 360 nm.

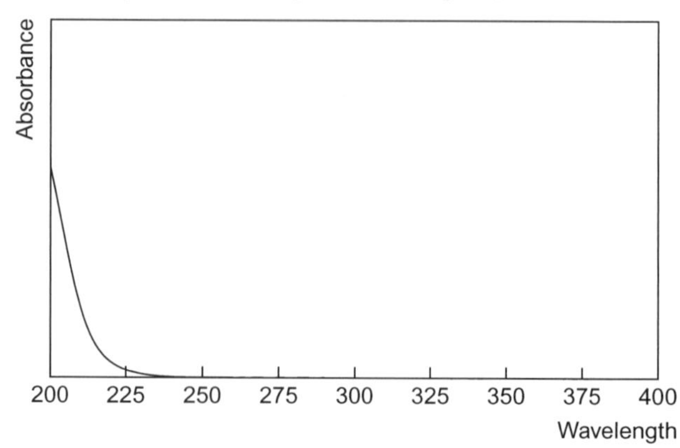

Infra-red Spectrum. Principal peaks at wavenumbers 1655, 1104, 1075, 1564, 1040, 1262 cm^{-1} (lincomycin hydrochloride, KBr disk).

Dose. The equivalent of 1.5 to 2 g of lincomycin daily.

Lindane

Pesticide

Synonyms. 666; Benhexachlor; Gamma Benzene Hexachloride; Gamma-BHC; Gamma-HCH; HCH; Hexicide.
Proprietary names. Aphtiria; Delitex N; Elentol; Escabin; Esoderm; Gambex; Gamene; GBH; G-Well; Hexicid; Hexit; Jacutin; Kwell; Kwellada; Lendianon; Lindanoxil; Lorexane; Pediletan; Pilensar; Piodrex; Pioletal; Pionax; Plurisan; Pruritrat; Quellada; Sarnapin; Sarpiol; Scabecid; Scabene.
(1α,2α,3β,4α,5α,6β)-1,2,3,4,5,6-Hexachlorocyclohexane
$C_6H_6Cl_6$=290.8
CAS—58-89-9

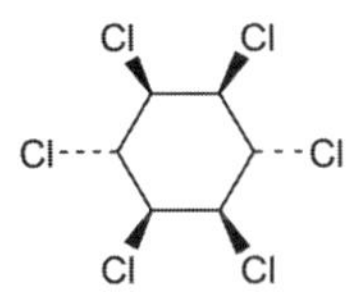

A white crystalline powder. M.p. 112.5°.
Practically insoluble in water; soluble 1 in 19 of dehydrated alcohol, 1 in 2 of acetone, 1 in 3.5 of chloroform, and 1 in 5.5 of ether.

Partition Coefficient. Log *P* (octanol/water), 3.7.

Thin-layer Chromatography. System TE—Rf 86; system TF—Rf 75; system TX—Rf 51; system TY—Rf 92.

Gas Chromatography. System GA—RI 1745; system GK—RRT 0.76 (relative to caffeine).

Infra-red Spectrum. Principal peaks at wavenumbers 680, 665, 695, 778, 840, 950 cm^{-1} (KBr disk).

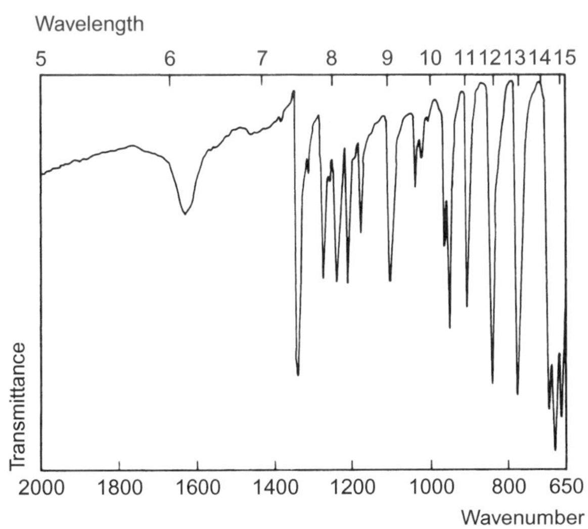

Mass Spectrum. Principal ions at *m/z* 181, 183, 109, 219, 111, 217, 51, 221.

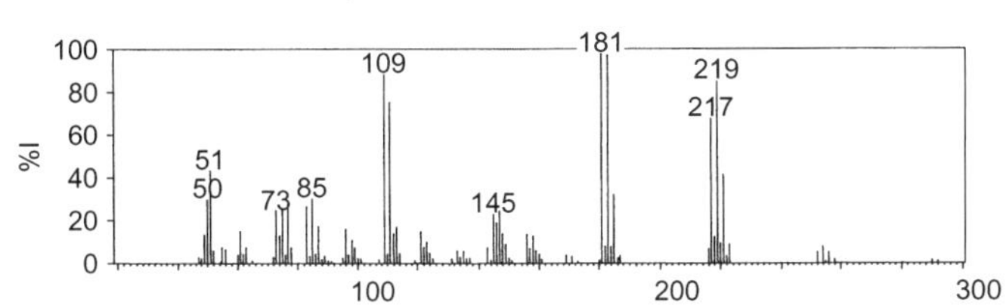

Quantification

Gas chromatography. In blood: ECD—N. Jain *et al.*, *J. Pharm. Pharmacol.*, 1965, *17*, 362–367. In blood or tissues: limit of detection 1 μg/L, ECD—J. L. Radomski and A. Ray, *J. Chromatogr. Sci.*, 1970, *8*, 108–114. In serum: limit of detection <7 μg/L, ECD—J. J. Saady and A. Poklis, *J. Anal. Toxicol.*, 1990, *14*, 301–401.

Disposition in the Body. Readily absorbed after ingestion, inhalation, or through the skin. It is stored in the body fat and adrenal glands. Metabolised by oxidation and dehydrohalogenation to a series of chlorinated phenols which are excreted mainly in the urine in free and conjugated form.

After intravenous administration, about 25% of the dose is excreted in the urine; after topical administration about 10% of the dose is recovered in the urine. [R. J. Feldmann and H. J. Maibach, *Toxicol. Appl. Pharmacol.*, 1974, *28*, 126–132.]

Blood concentration.

Blood-lindane concentrations in subjects with low occupational exposure ranged from 1 to 9 μg/L (mean 4), and concentrations in subjects with high dermal occupational exposure ranged from 6 to 93 μg/L (mean 31). [T. H. Milby *et al.*, *J. Occup. Med.*, 1968, *10*, 584–587.]

Average serum concentrations of 0.07, 0.19, and 0.04 mg/L of α-benzene hexachloride (α-BHC), β-BHC, and γ-BHC, respectively, were reported in 57 subjects who worked in a factory manufacturing lindane; β-BHC was the only isomer observed to accumulate on chronic exposure. A mean fat concentration of 45.6 μg/g of β-BHC was reported in 8 subjects. [K. Baumann *et al.*, *Int. Arch. Occup. Environ. Health*, 1980, *47*, 119–127.]

15 subjects with long-term (5 to 17 years) exposure to wood-preserving chemicals containing lindane and pentachlorophenol had mean serum levels of 0.085 and 43.6 μg/L, respectively. [M. Peper *et al.*, *Am. J. Ind. Med.*, 1999, *35*, 632–641.]

Toxicity. Lindane is not highly toxic when applied externally in the concentrations usually employed (0.1 to 1%), but when ingested it may cause convulsions; dusts may irritate the nose and throat when used in a confined space. Blood concentrations greater than 0.02 mg/L have been associated with toxic effects. The estimated minimum oral lethal dose is 200 mg/kg and the maximum permissible atmospheric concentration is 0.5 mg/m^3. Toxic doses or long-term exposure may cause liver necrosis. The maximum acceptable daily intake is 10 μg/kg.

A young girl who ingested about 1.6 g of lindane was found to have a serum concentration of 0.84 mg/L after 2 h, following convulsions; the concentration decreased to 0.49 mg/L after 4 h; urinary concentrations of individual free phenolic metabolites determined 5.5 h after ingestion ranged from 0.04 to 0.74 mg/L. [H. G. Starr and N. J. Clifford, *Arch. Environ. Health*, 1972, *25*, 374–375.]

A fat concentration of 343 μg/g was reported in a fatality caused by lindane. [W. J. Hayes and W. K. Vaughn, *Toxicol. Appl. Pharmacol.*, 1977, *42*, 235–252.]

Half-life. Derived from urinary excretion data, about 26 h.

Use. Topically in concentrations of 0.1 to 1%.

Linuron

Herbicide

Synonyms. Du Pont herbicide 326; HOE-2810.
Proprietary names. Afalon; Garnitan; Linex; Linorox; Linurex; Lorox; Premalin; Rotalin; Sarclex; Sinuron; Siolcid.
N′-(3,4-Dichlorophenyl)-*N*-methoxy-*N*-methylurea
$C_9H_{10}Cl_2N_2O_2$=249.1
CAS—330-55-2

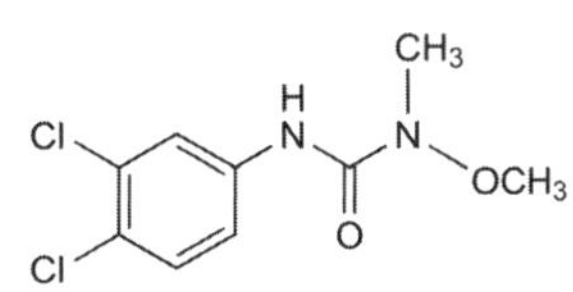

A white crystalline solid (fine flakes or coarse powder). M.p. 93° to 94°.
It is soluble in water (81 mg/L at 25°) and soluble in acetone (500 g/kg at 25°), ethanol (150 g/kg at 25°), benzene (150 g/kg at 25°), toluene, xylene (130 g/kg at 25°), and heptane (15 g/kg at 25°); readily soluble in dimethylformamide, chloroform, and diethyl ether; moderately soluble in aromatic hydrocarbons; sparingly soluble in aliphatic hydrocarbons.

Partition Coefficient. Log *P* (octanol/water), 3.00.

Thin-layer Chromatography. System TX—Rf 22; system TY—Rf 31.

Gas Chromatography. System GA—linuron RI 1927; linuron-Me RI 1785; 3,4-dichloroaniline RI 1323; system GK—linuron RRT 0.97, 3,4-dichloroaniline RRT 0.36, 3,4-dichlorophenyl-isocyanate RRT 0.13 (all relative to caffeine).

High Performance Liquid Chromatography. System HY—RI 506; system HAA—retention time 21.3 min.

Infra-red Spectrum. Principal peaks at wavenumber 2269, 1507, 1729, 1594, 1132, 1282 cm^{-1}.

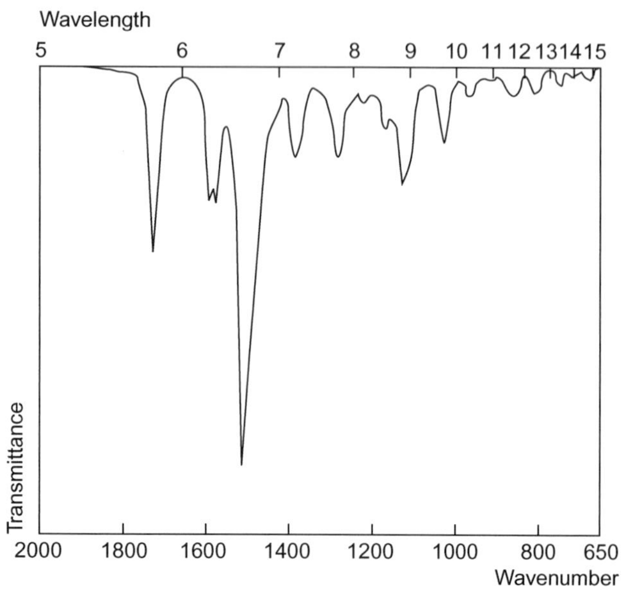

Mass Spectrum. Principal ions at *m/z* 61, 160, 132, 124, 46, 248, 73, 109.

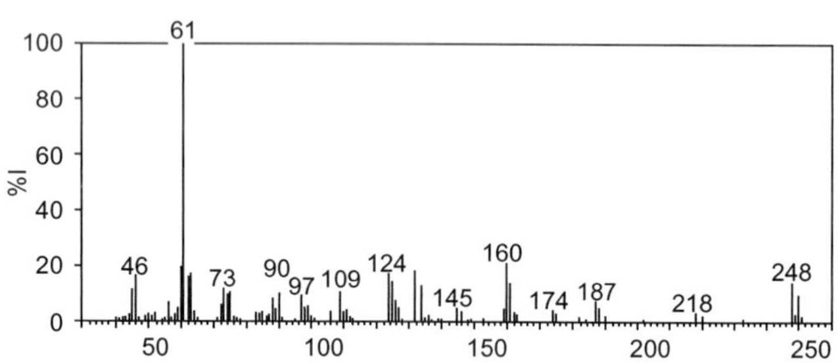

Disposition in the Body. Linuron is broken down completely after passing through the liver. It is unlikely to bioaccumulate. Metabolites include 3,4-dichloroaniline and 3,4-dichlorophenylisocyanate.

Liothyronine

Thyroid Agent

Synonyms. L-Tri-iodothyronine. The abbreviation T_3 is often used for tri-iodothyronine.
O-(4-Hydroxy-3-iodophenyl)-3,5-diiodo-L-tyrosine
$C_{15}H_{12}I_3NO_4$=651.0
CAS—6893-02-3

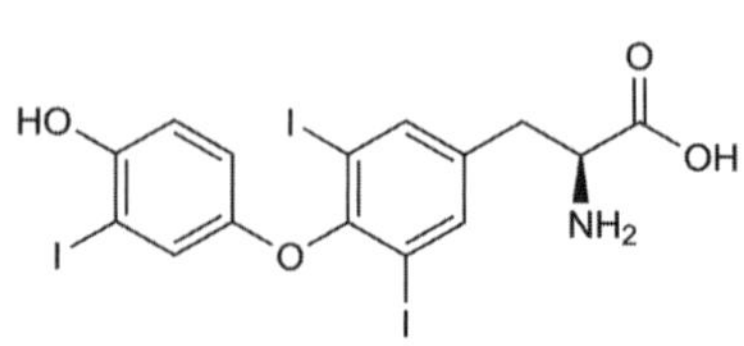

Crystals. M.p. 236° to 237°, with decomposition.

Insoluble in water, alcohol and propylene glycol; soluble in dilute alkalis.

Liothyronine Hydrochloride
Proprietary name. Thybon
$C_{15}H_{12}I_3NO_4,HCl$=687.4
CAS—6138-47-2
Long birefringent needles. M.p. 202° to 203° with decomposition.

Liothyronine Sodium
Synonym. Sodium Liothyronine
Proprietary names. Cynomel; Cytomel; Dispon; Neo-Tiroimade; Ro-Thyronine; Tertroxin; Thybon; Thyrotardin; Ti-Tre; Triostat; Triyodisan; Triyotex. It is an ingredient of Euthroid, Novothyral, and Thyrolar.
$C_{15}H_{11}I_3NNaO_4$=673.0
CAS—55-06-1
A white to buff-coloured solid or crystalline powder.
Practically insoluble in water, chloroform, ether and most other organic solvents; soluble 1 in 500 of ethanol; soluble in solutions of alkali hydroxides.

Dissociation Constant. pK_a 8.5.

Partition Coefficient. Log *P* (octanol/water), 3.0.

Ultraviolet Spectrum. Liothyronine sodium: aqueous alkali—319 nm (A_1^1=65a).

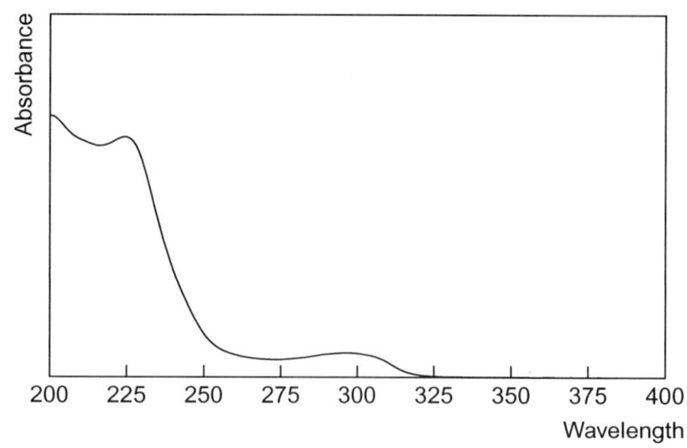

Infra-red Spectrum. Principal peaks at wavenumbers 1608, 1180, 1493, 1250, 1535, 1320 cm^{-1} (KBr disk).

Quantification See under Levothyroxine.

Disposition in the Body. Liothyronine is absorbed after oral or IM administration. It is metabolised by conjugation with glucuronic acid or sulfate, de-iodination oxidative deamination and decarboxylation. It is excreted mainly in the bile and faeces, and is subject to enterohepatic circulation; some iodide is excreted in the urine.
Endogenous serum concentrations range from 0.0010 to 0.0016 mg/L, in normal subjects.

Half-life. Plasma half-life, about 2 days.

Protein binding. In plasma, more than 99%.

Dose. Up to 100 μg of liothyronine sodium daily.

Lisinopril

Antihypertensive

Synonyms. L-154,826-000T; Lisinoprilum; MK-521.
(*S*)-1-[N^2-(1-Carboxy-3-phenylpropyl]-L-lysyl]-L-proline
$C_{21}H_{31}N_3O_5$=405.5
CAS—76547-98-3

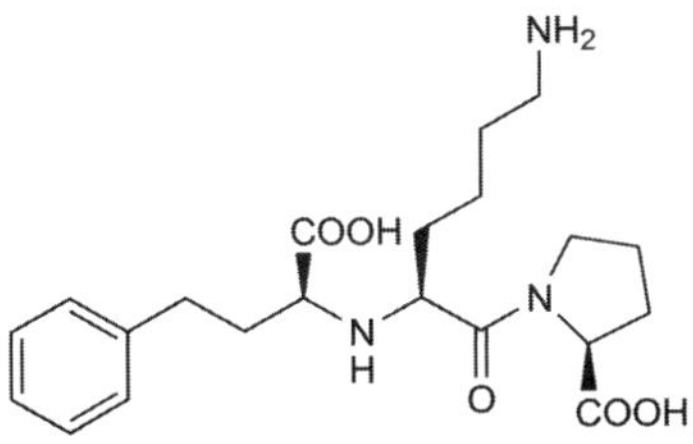

A white to off-white crystalline powder. It is soluble in water (1 in 10), methyl alcohol (1 in 70); practically insoluble in alcohol, acetone, chloroform and in ether.

Lisinopril Dihydrate

Proprietary names. Acemin; Acerbon; Alapril; Carace; Coric; Doneka; Prinil; Prinivil; Novatec; Tensopril; Vivatec; Zestril. Also an ingredient of Novazyd; Prinzide; Zestoretic.

$C_{21}H_{31}N_3O_3,2H_2O = 441.5$

CAS—83915-83-7

An off-white crystalline powder. Solubility: water (97 g/L), methanol (14 g/L), ethanol , acetone, acetonitrile, chloroform and *N,N*-dimethylformamide (<0.1 g/L).

Dissociation Constant. pK_a 2.5, 4.0, 6.7, 10.1 (25°).

Partition Coefficient. Log *P* (octanol/water), −1.22; log *P* (phosphate buffer (0.1 M, pH 7)/octanol), 10.2 ± 0.5 (room temperature).

Thin-layer Liquid Chromatography. System TB—Rf 00; system TE—Rf 00; system TF—Rf 00; system TAE—Rf 27.

High Performance Liquid Chromatography. System HX—RI 271; system HY—RI 250; system HZ—retention time 1.5 min.

Column: ILS (Hypersil, 250 × 4.6 mm i.d., 5 μm). Mobile phase: methanol:water:TEA (triethylamine) (50:50:0.1), adjusted to pH 2.6, 1 mL/min flow rate. UV detection (λ=210 nm); fluorescence detection (λ_{ex}=340 nm, λ_{em}=455 nm). Retention time(s): 2.9 min. [A. El-Gindy *et al.*, *J. Pharm. Biomed. Anal.*, 2001, *25*, 913–922].

Column: ODS (Hypersil, 250 × 4.5 mm i.d., 5 μm). Mobile phase: sodium heptanesulfonate (20 mM, pH 2.5):ACN (acetonitrile) (with 5% THF, tetrahydrofuran) (63:37), 1 mL/min flow rate. UV detection (λ= 215 nm). Retention time(s): 5.0 min. [D. Bonazzi *et al.*, *J. Pharm. Biomed. Anal.*, 1998, *16*, 431–438].

Column: C_{18} (μBondapak, 300 × 3.9 i.d., 10 μm). Column temperature: 40°. Mobile phase: potassium dihydrogen phosphate (15 mM, pH 2.9):ACN:methanol:THF (92:6:1:1), 1.5 mL/min flow rate. Internal standard (IS): enalaprilat. UV detection (λ=206 nm). Retention time(s): lisinopril, 7.5 min; IS, 10.5 min. [Y. Wong and B. Charles, *J. Chromatogr.* 1995, *673*, *Biomed. Appl.*, 306–310].

Ultraviolet Spectrum. Aqueous alkali (0.1 M sodium hydroxide)—246, 254, 258, 261, 267 nm; aqueous acid (0.1 M hydrochloric acid)—246, 253, 258, 264, 267 nm.

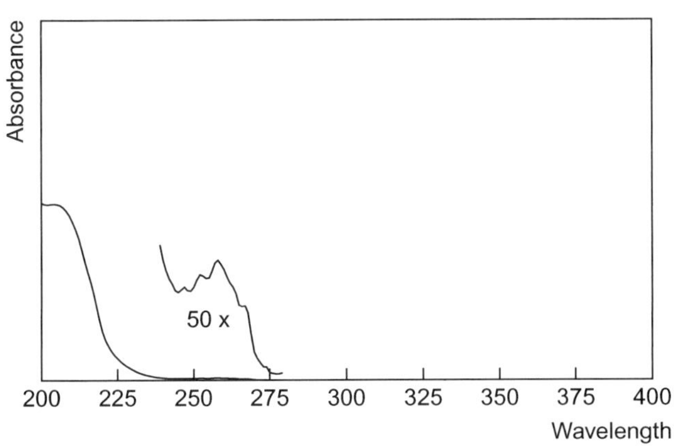

Infra-red Spectrum. Principal peaks at wavenumbers 1655, 1570, 1388, 741, 732 cm^{-1} (broad peak around 3000 cm^{-1}) (KBr).

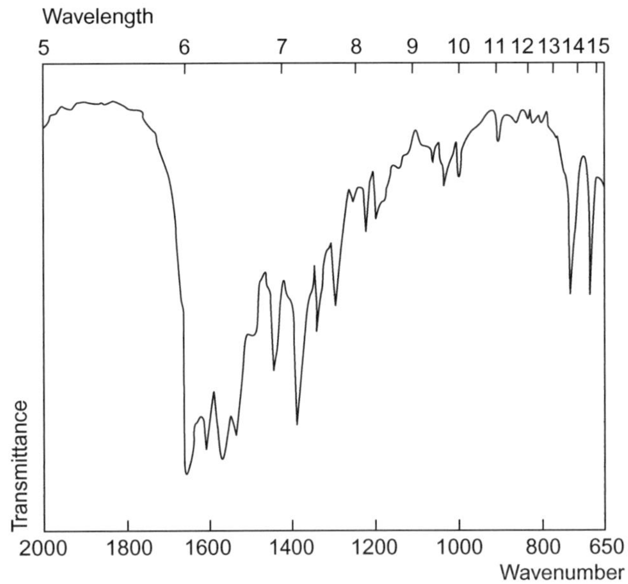

Mass Spectrum. Principal peaks at *m/z* 70, 91, 84, 113, 245, 41, 28, 224.

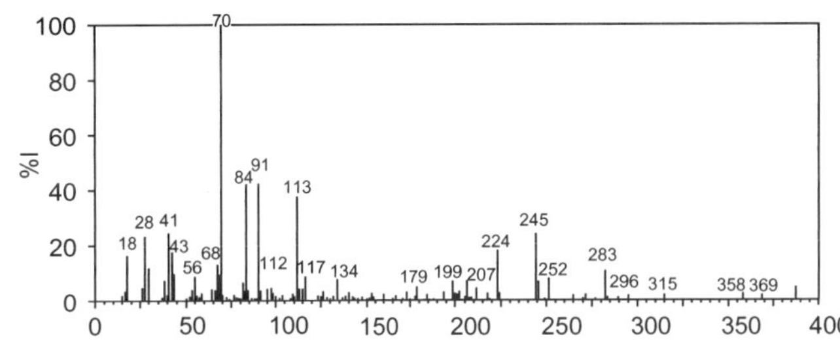

Quantification

Gas chromatography–mass spectrometry. In plasma and urine: limit of detection 0.5 μg/L in plasma and 5 μg/L in urine—H. Shioya *et al.*, *J. Chromatogr.*, 1989, *496*, 129–135.

Disposition in the Body. Lisinopril is slowly and incompletely absorbed after oral administration. Absorption varies between 6 and 60% depending on the individual, but on average is 25% of the dose. Metabolism does not occur as it is already an active diacid (a lysine derivative of enalaprilat). The absorbed drug is excreted unchanged in urine via the kidneys and the unabsorbed drug is excreted in faeces.

Therapeutic concentration. The serum therapeutic concentration is 20 to 70 μg/L.

12 healthy male volunteers were administered with an oral dose of 10 mg lisinopril. Peak serum concentrations of 0.095 ± 0.055 μg/L were observed in 7 ± 1 h. [E. H. Ulm *et al.*, *Br. J. Clin. Pharmacol.*, 1982, *14*, 357–362].

Bioavailability. 25 to 50%.

Half-life. 12 h.

Volume of distribution. Mean 124 L.

Clearance. 6.36 L/h (following a 10 mg oral dose in healthy subjects); reduced in renal impairment and the elderly. Clearance reduced in impaired renal function (glomerular filtration rate < 30 mL/min).

Protein binding. Negligible.

Note. For a review of lisinopril see K. Simpson and B. Jarvis, *Drugs*, 2000, *59*, 1149–1167. For a general review of the pharmacokinetics of ACE inhibitors see J. G. Kelly and K. O'Malley, *Clin. Pharmacokinet.*, 1990, *19*, 177–196.

Dose. 2.5 to 20 mg daily with a maximum of 40 mg daily.

Lithium Carbonate

Tranquilliser

Synonyms. CP-15467-61; Lithii Carbonas; Lithium Carb.; NSC-16895.
Proprietary names. Camcolit; Carbolit; Carbolith; Carbolithium; Eskalith; Hypnorex; Leukominerase; Li 450; Liskonum; Lithane; Litheum; Lithicarb; Lithizine; Lithobid; Lithonate; Lithosun; Lithotabs; Litiocar; Lito; Neurolepsin; Phasal; Plenur; Priadel; Quilonorm; Quilonum retard; Teralithe.
Li_2CO_3=73.9
CAS—554-13-2
A white granular powder. M.p. about 720°.
Soluble 1 in 78 of cold water and 1 in 140 of boiling water; practically insoluble in ethanol; soluble, with effervescence, in dilute mineral acids.

Lithium Citrate

Synonym. Lithii Citras
Proprietary names. Li-Liquid; Litarex; Lithonate-S.
$C_6H_5Li_3O_7,4H_2O$=282.0
CAS—919-16-4 (anhydrous); 6080-58-6 (tetrahydrate)
A white, somewhat deliquescent, crystalline powder.
Soluble 1 in 2 of water; practically insoluble in ethanol and ether.

Partition Coefficient. Log *P* (octanol/water), −6.2.

Quantification

Atomic absorption spectrophotometry. In postmortem blood: limit of detection 145 nmol/L—I. M. B. Scott, *J. Forens. Sci. Soc.*, 1982, *22*, 41–42.

Emission flame photometry. In blood or urine: limit of detection 2 nmol/L in blood, 30 nmol/L in urine—R. Robertson *et al.*, *Clinica Chim. Acta.*, 1973, *45*, 25–31. In serum: limit of detection 50 nmol/L (comparison with atomic absorption spectrophotometry) —A. L. Levi and E. M. Katz, *Clin. Chem.*, 1970, *16*, 840–842.

Disposition in the Body. Readily absorbed after oral administration. About 97% of a dose is excreted unchanged in the urine in 10 days with 50 to 60% in the first 24 h with only small amounts being found in the faeces, saliva and sweat. The urinary excretion of lithium appears to be slower in the elderly than the young and also appears to occur more slowly at night, resulting in a diurnal rhythm in excretion rate; its excretion is also markedly influenced by sodium and, possibly, potassium status; in subjects where the sodium intake is reduced, lithium is reabsorbed by the renal tubules and in subjects who have a high sodium intake the excretion of lithium is increased. Lithium is widely distributed throughout the body and higher concentrations may be found in bones, the thyroid gland and parts of the brain, than in plasma. It crosses the placenta and is excreted in breast milk.

Therapeutic concentration. Lithium plasma concentrations should be monitored 12 h after a dose to ensure that they are within the range 0.5 to 1.2 mmol/L.

Following a single oral dose of 600 mg to 10 subjects, peak plasma concentrations of 0.45 to 0.80 mmol/L (mean 0.64) were attained in about 2 h [J. M. Meinhold *et al.*, *J. Clin. Pharmacol.*, 1979, *19*, 701–703].

After daily oral doses of 1.5 to 1.7 g to 16 subjects, steady-state serum concentrations were in the range 0.7 to 0.9 mmol/L [J. L. Marini and M. H. Sheard, *J. Clin. Pharmacol.*, 1976, *16*, 276–283].

Administration of lithium 600 mg once daily as a slow-release capsule formulation to 18 subjects resulted in mean plasma concentrations (over 96 h) of 0.252 mmol/L as compared with 0.214 mmol/L following twice daily dosing with 300 mg of a standard-release preparation. Corresponding values for the first 24 h were 0.303 vs 0.264 mmol/L [P. Castrogiovanni, *Clin. Ter.*, 2002, *153*, 107–115].

Toxicity. Toxic effects may be produced by serum concentrations greater than 2 mmol/L. Blood concentrations of about 5 mmol/L or more are usually fatal, although in one instance of survival which occurred after the ingestion of 22.5 g of lithium carbonate, the maximum serum concentration was 8.2 mmol/L; a fatality due to the acute ingestion of lithium carbonate in which the serum concentration was 2.43 mmol/L on admission to hospital and 1.93 mmol/L at the time of death has also been reported.

Acute lithium intoxication followed a suicide attempt in a 51-year-old woman on chronic lithium therapy, in which she ingested 50 × 450 mg slow-release lithium carbonate tablets. Serum levels were reported to be 10.6 mmol/L 13 h after the ingestion and 5.8 mmol/L at 24 h [R. Nagappan *et al.*, *Anaesth. Intensive Care*, 2002, *30*, 90–92].

A 29-year-old male who ingested 8 g of lithium in the form of a sustained-release preparation had a plasma concentration of 2.38 mmol/L 15 h after the ingestion and 3.12 mmol/L at 25 h. Following 4 h of haemodialysis, the lithium level was 2.16 mmol/L [B. Astruc *et al.*, *Eur. Psychiatry*, 1999, *14*, 172–174].

A 48-year-old woman was admitted to hospital having ingested 97 tablets of immediate-release lithium carbonate (300 mg each) 60 min earlier. Her serum lithium concentration was 4.3 mmol/L. After stabilisation and transfer to the intensive care unit, the patient's serum lithium level was 3.1 mmol/L, and decreased to 1.5 mmol/L after haemodialysis. However, 9 h later the level had risen to 2.1 mmol/L. After the patient complained of vaginal burning sensation, she admitted to having inserted 80 lithium carbonate tablets (300 mg) intravaginally. Vaginal irrigation with 3 L normal saline resulted in the lithium level dropping to 1.3 mmol/L by the next morning and to 0.5 mmol/L after 24 h [J. L. Temte *et* al., *JAMA*, 1994, *272*, 1723–1724].

In 3 fatalities due to lithium intoxication, the following postmortem tissue concentrations were reported: blood 1.9, 3.0, and 4.6 mmol/L, brain 1.4, 5.2, and 4.2 mmol/kg, kidney 1.9, 5.9, and 9.6 mmol/kg, liver 1.9, 2.9, and 6.7 mmol/kg, urine 4.9, -, and 6.7 mmol/L [Z. Kosa and A. Benko, *Bull. Int. Assoc. Forenic. Toxicol.*, 1981, *16(2)*, 19–20; A. Alha *et al.*, *Bull. Int. Assoc. Forenic. Toxicol.*, 1981, *16(2)*, 20–21].

Half-life. Plasma half-life, about 20 to 24 h after a single dose but appears to be dependent on the duration of treatment. In patients on their first course of treatment a plasma half-life averaging 31 h has been reported; this increased to 40 h in subjects receiving lithium for less than one year and 58 h in those taking the drug for longer than one year. Half-life is increased in the elderly and in renal impairment.

Volume of distribution. About 0.7 L/kg.

Clearance. Apparent plasma clearance after a single dose, about 0.4 mL/min/kg, decreased in uraemia and in the elderly.

Distribution in blood. Lithium is taken up by erythrocytes to a variable extent which appears to be partly genetically determined.

The erythrocyte:plasma ratio was reported to range from 0.19 to 1.0 (mean 0.5), in 42 subjects [J. A. Smith *et al.*, *Med. J. Aust.*, 1979, *1*, 631–632].

Saliva. Plasma : saliva ratio, about 0.4 but there is considerable intersubject variation.

Protein binding. Lithium is not bound to plasma proteins.

Note. For a review of the pharmacokinetics of lithium, see M. E. Ward *et al.*, *J. Clin. Pharmacol.*, 1994, *34*, 280–285, and for a discussion on target serum lithium concentrations, see B. Sproule, *Clin. Pharmacokinet.*, 2002, *41*, 639–660. For a study of the effect of acute alcohol consumption on lithium kinetics, see R. F. Anton *et al.*, *Clin. Pharmacol. Ther.*, 1985, *38*, 52–55.

Dose. The dose of lithium depends on the preparation given since different preparations vary widely in bioavailability. Dosage is usually adjusted to provide a serum concentration of 0.4 to 1.0 mmol/L, with maintenance doses at lower end of the range.

Lobeline

Respiratory Stimulant

Synonym. Alpha-lobeline
Proprietary name. Butt-Out
[2*R*-[2α,6α(*S**)]]-2-[6-(2-Hydroxy-2-phenylethyl)-1-methyl-2-piperidinyl]-1-phenylethanone
$C_{22}H_{27}NO_2$=337.5
CAS—90-69-7

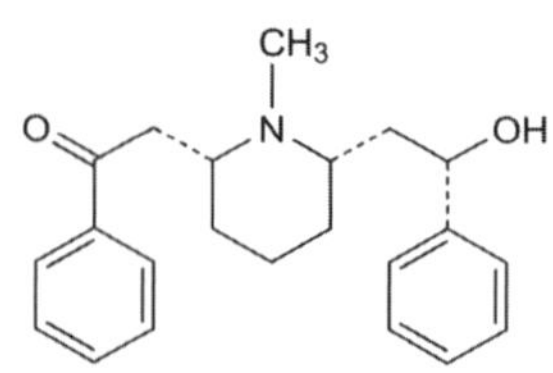

An alkaloid obtained from *Lobelia inflata* (Lobeliaceae).
Crystals.
M.p. 130° to 131°.

Very slightly soluble in water and petroleum ether; soluble in hot ethanol, benzene, chloroform and ether.

Lobeline Hydrochloride
Proprietary names. Cig-Ridettes; Lobron; Zoolobelin.
$C_{22}H_{27}NO_2,HCl$=373.9
CAS—134-63-4
A white crystalline or granular powder. M.p. 178° to 180°.
Soluble 1 in 40 of water and 1 in 12 of ethanol; very soluble in chloroform; very slightly soluble in ether.

Lobeline Sulfate
Proprietary names. Bantron; Lobatox; Lobeton; Lobidan; Nikoban; Nofum; Smokeless; Toban; Unilobin.
$(C_{22}H_{27}NO_2)_2,H_2SO_4$=773.0
CAS—134-64-5
Soluble 1 in about 30 of water; slightly soluble in alcohol.

Partition Coefficient. Log *P* (octanol/water), 3.7.

Colour Tests. Mandelin's Test—grey; Marquis Test—red-violet.

Thin-layer Chromatography. System TA—Rf 61; system TB—Rf 17; system TC—Rf 35; system TE—Rf 75; system TL—Rf 29; system TAE—Rf 23; system TAJ—Rf 11; system TAK—Rf 00; system TAL—Rf 35. (Acidified iodoplatinate solution, positive.)

Gas Chromatography. System GA—RI 1820.

High Performance Liquid Chromatography. System HAA—Retention time(s) 14.6 min.

Ultraviolet Spectrum. Aqueous acid—248 nm (A^1_1=416a).

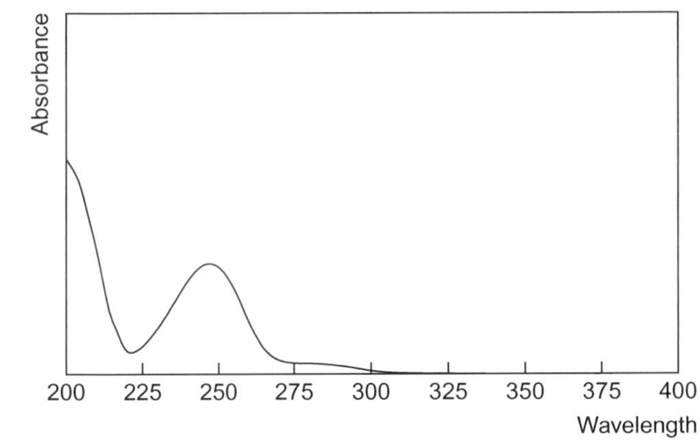

Infra-red Spectrum. Principal peaks at wavenumbers 1687, 700, 1211, 1115, 1052, 769 cm^{-1} (KBr disk).

Mass Spectrum. Principal ions at *m/z* 96, 105, 77, 97, 216, 42, 218, 51.

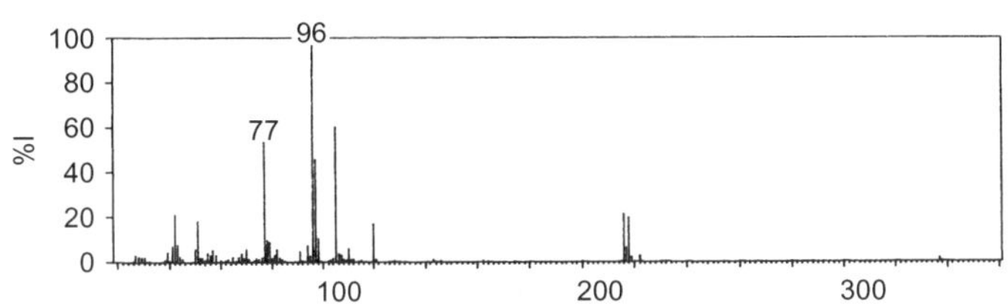

Dose. Lobeline hydrochloride was formerly given intramuscularly in doses of 3 to 10 mg.

Lofepramine

Antidepressant

Synonym. Lopramine
1-(4-Chlorophenyl)-2-[[3-(10,11-dihydro-5*H*-dibenz[*b,f*]azepin-5-yl)-propyl]methylamino]ethanone
$C_{26}H_{27}ClN_2O$=419.0
CAS—23047-25-8

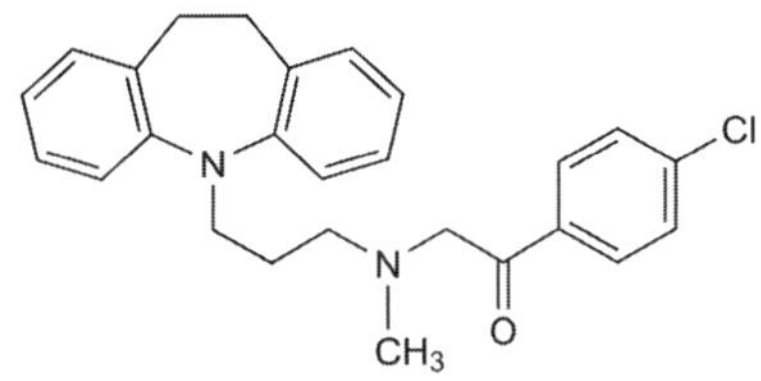

Colourless crystals, which become discoloured in air. M.p. 106°.
Practically insoluble in water; slightly soluble in ethanol; soluble in chloroform.

Lofepramine Hydrochloride
Proprietary names. Deprimil; Feprapax; Gamanil; Gamonil; Lomont; Timelit; Tymelyt.
$C_{26}H_{27}ClN_2O,HCl$=455.4
CAS—26786-32-3
Colourless crystals or yellowish-white microcrystalline powder. M.p. 152° to 154°.
Practically insoluble in water; soluble in ethanol, methanol and chloroform.

Partition Coefficient. Log *P* (octanol/water), 7.3.

Thin-layer Chromatography. System TAE—Rf 82; system TE—Rf 90.

Gas Chromatography. System GA—lofepramine, not eluted. (Metabolised to desipramine.)

High Performance Liquid Chromatography. System HA—lofepramine *k* 0.6, desipramine *k* 2.1, 2-hydroxydesipramine *k* 1.2.

Ultraviolet Spectrum. Methanol—255 nm (A^1_1=596a).

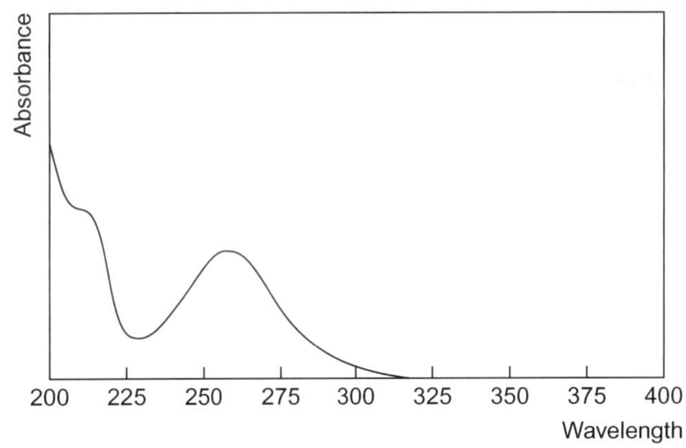

Infra-red Spectrum. Principal peaks at wavenumbers 1700, 1235, 1495, 1590, 1100, 763 cm^{-1} (lofepramine hydrochloride, KBr disk).

Mass Spectrum. Principal ions at *m/z* 58, 234, 193, 192, 42, 235, 194, 59; desipramine 235, 195, 208, 44, 234, 193, 194, 71; 2-hydroxydesipramine 44, 209, 211, 250, 210, 224, 42, 251.

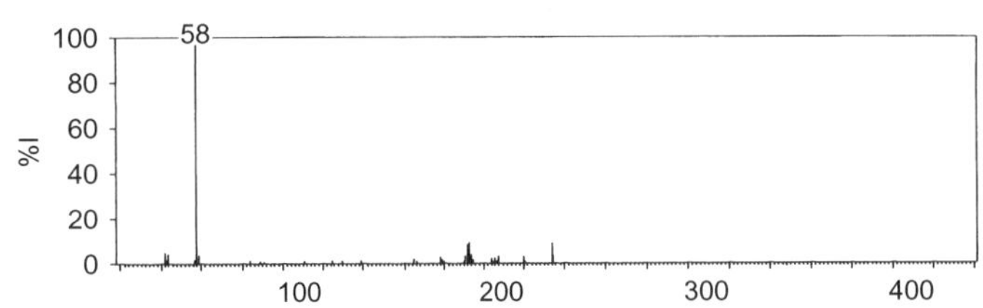

Quantification
Gas chromatography. In plasma: limit of detection, lofepramine 1 µg/L, desipramine 2 µg/L, FID—R. Lundgren *et al.*, *Acta Pharm. Suec.*, 1977, *14*, 81–94.

Gas chromatography–mass spectrometry. In plasma or urine: limit of detection 2 µg/L for lofepramine and desipramine, and 20 µg/L for 2-hydroxydesipramine—K. Matsubayashi *et al.*, *J. Chromatogr.*, 1977, *143*; *B Biomed. Appl.*, *1*, 571–580.

High performance liquid chromatography. In plasma: lofepramine and desipramine, limit of detection for lofepramine <10.5 µg/L, UV detection—T.

Elm and E. L. Hansen, *J. Chromatogr. B Biomed. Appl.*, 1995, *665*, 355–361.

Disposition in the Body. Lofepramine is readily absorbed after oral administration but undergoes extensive first-pass demethylation to desipramine which is the principal active metabolite. It is also metabolised by *N*-oxidation, hydroxylation, and conjugation and is excreted in the urine mainly as metabolites; a second active metabolite, 2-hydroxydesipramine, has been reported to be the major unconjugated urinary metabolite.

Therapeutic concentration

After a single oral dose of 2 mg/kg given to 6 subjects, peak plasma-lofepramine concentrations of 0.04 to 0.14 (mean 0.09) mg/L were attained in about 1 h; peak plasma-desipramine concentrations of 0.01 to 0.02 mg/L were attained in 3 to 8 h in 4 subjects. When a similar dose was given to the same subjects on a second occasion some weeks later, peak plasma-lofepramine concentrations of 0.05 to 0.27 (mean 0.13) mg/L were reported. Following oral doses of 70 mg three times a day for 10 days to 3 subjects, plasma concentrations of about 0.003 mg/L of lofepramine and 0.01 to 0.05 (mean 0.025) mg/L of desipramine were reported, determined immediately prior to a dose. [G. P. Forshell et al., *Eur. J. Clin. Pharmacol.*, 1976, *9*, 291–298].

Protein binding. About 99%.

Note. For a review of the pharmacokinetics of lofepramine and its efficacy in depression, see S. G. Lancaster and J. P. Gonzalez, *Drugs*, 1989, *37*, 123–140.

Dose. 70 to 210 mg daily.

Lofexidine *Antihypertensive*

Proprietary names. Almide; BritLofex.
2-[1-(2,6-Dichlorophenoxy)ethyl]-4,5-dihydro-1*H*-imidazole
$C_{11}H_{12}Cl_2N_2O=259.1$
CAS—31036-80-3

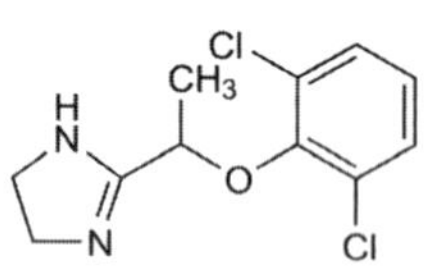

A colourless, crystalline substance with m.p. 126° to 128°.

Lofexidine Hydrochloride

Synonyms. MDL-14042A; Ba-168; RMI-14042A.
Proprietary names. BritLofex; Lofetensin; Loxacor.
$C_{11}H_{12}Cl_2N_2O,HCl=295.6$
CAS—21498-08-8
Crystals from ethanol/ether or propan-2-ol, m.p. 221° to 223°; also reported as 230° to 232°. It is very soluble in water and ethanol; slightly soluble in 2-propanol; poorly soluble in chloroform; practically insoluble in ether.

Partition Coefficient. Log *P* (water/octanol), 3.58.

Thin-layer Chromatography. System TE—Rf 53; system TAE—Rf 17.

Plate: silica gel plates 60 F_{254}. Mobile phase: chloroform: methanol:ammonia (25%) (70:26:4). Spray reagent bromocresol green (0.05%). Rf 0.85.

Plate: silica gel plates 60 F_{254}. Mobile phase: butan-1-ol:acetic acid:water (80:20:20). Spray reagent bromocresol green (0.05%). Rf 0.49. [H. Betzing *et al.*, *Arzneimittelforschung*, 1982, *32(8a)*, 916–918].

High Performance Liquid Chromatography. Column: C_{18} (μBondapak, 300 × 4 mm i.d., 10 μm). Mobile phase: (A:B) methanol:aqueous potassium dihydrogen phosphate (0.05 M, pH 2.5). Elution programme: (A:B) (30:70) to (70:30) in 20 min and back to initial conditions over 5 min, 2 mL/min flow rate. UV detection (λ=254 nm). Retention time(s): lofexidine, 11.2 min; glucuronide conjugate metabolites, 3.5 and 6.3 min. [I. Midgley *et al.*, *Xenobiotica*, 1983, *13(2)*, 87–95].

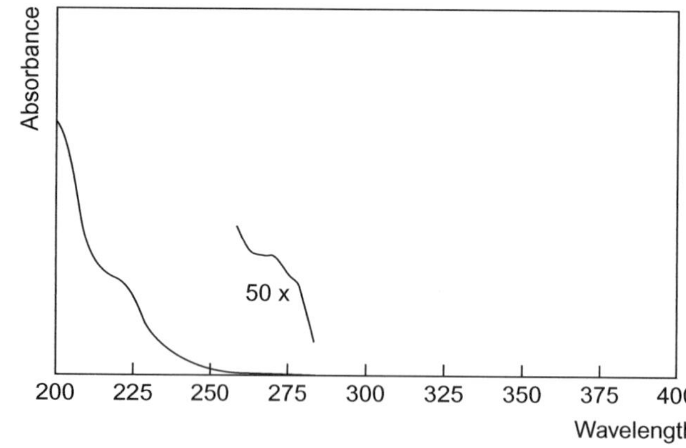

Infra-red Spectrum. Principal peaks at wavenumber 1610, 1445, 1240, 1095, 780 cm^{-1}.

Mass Spectrum. Principal ions at *m/z* 258, 260, 262.

Disposition in the Body. Lofexidine is rapidly absorbed after administration, extensively biotransformed and excreted mainly in urine (87%) and faeces (5%). The principal metabolite is 2,6-dichlorophenol, and minor metabolites have been detected including glucuronic acid conjugates. Renal excretion is rapid and is the most important route of elimination. 73 to 94.4% (mean 85%) of the drug is excreted in urine and 0.4 to 4.2% (mean 1.5%) in faeces. Peak plasma concentration occurs 2 to 5 h after administration. The rate of bioavailability is rapid and subject dependent.

Toxicity. Overdosage may cause hypotension, bradycardia and sedation.

Half-life. Lofexidine undergoes biphasic elimination with half-lives 1.3 to 3.7 h and 9.0 to 18.3 h; also reported as 11 h.

Protein binding. Approx. 40% at nominal concentration (2 and 4 μg/L) and 80 to 90% at peak concentration.

Dose. An initial oral dose of 200 μg is administered twice daily which may increase in steps of 200 to 400 μg daily to a maximum of 2.4 mg daily for a duration of 7 to 10 days.

Loperamide *Antidiarrhoeal*

4-(4-Chlorophenyl)-4-hydroxy-*N*,*N*-dimethyl-α,α-diphenyl-1-piperidine-butanamide
$C_{29}H_{33}ClN_2O_2=477.0$
CAS—53179-11-6

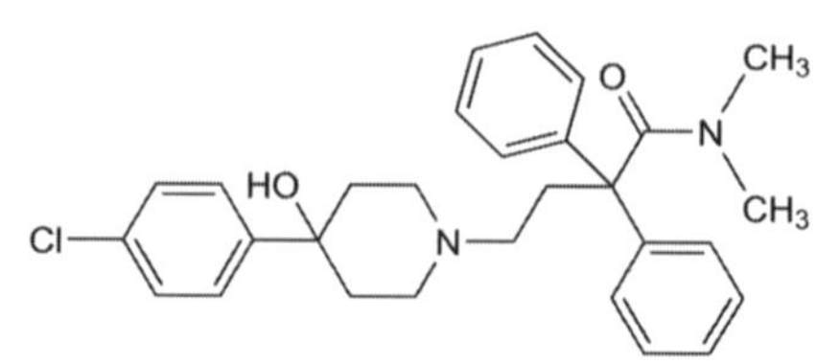

Loperamide Hydrochloride

Proprietary names. Altocel; Arestal; Arret; Blox; Celkalm; Diar-Limit; Diareze; Diasorb; Diocalm Ultra; Diocaps; Endiaron; Entrocalm; Imodium; Kaopectate II; Lodiar; Lopemid; LoperaGen; Maalox Anti-Diarrheal; Neo-Diarel; Norimode; Normaloe; Pepto Diarrhea Control.
$C_{29}H_{33}ClN_2O_2,HCl=513.5$
CAS—34552-83-5
A white or yellowish-white, amorphous or microcrystalline powder. M.p. about 225°, with some decomposition.
Slightly soluble in water; freely soluble in chloroform and methanol.

Partition Coefficient. Log *P* (octanol/water), 5.2.

Thin-layer Chromatography. System TA—Rf 70; system TB—Rf 09; system TC—Rf 32; system TE—Rf 74; system TL—Rf 22; system TAE—Rf 52; system TAF—Rf 81. (Dragendorff spray.)

High Performance Liquid Chromatography. System HX—RI 510; system HZ—Retention time(s), 14.0 min.

Ultraviolet Spectrum. Acid isopropyl alcohol—254, 260 (A_1^1=14b), 266 nm.

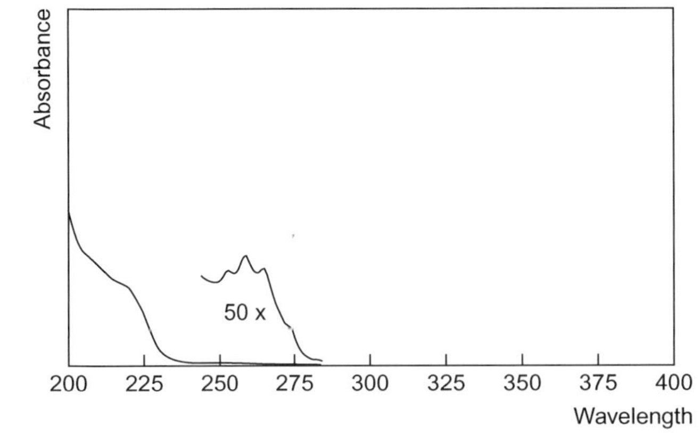

Infra-red Spectrum. Principal peaks at wavenumbers 1600, 700, 830, 765, 964, 986 cm^{-1} (loperamide hydrochloride, KBr disk).

Mass Spectrum. Principal ions at *m/z* 238, 42, 239, 224, 240, 56, 72, 226.

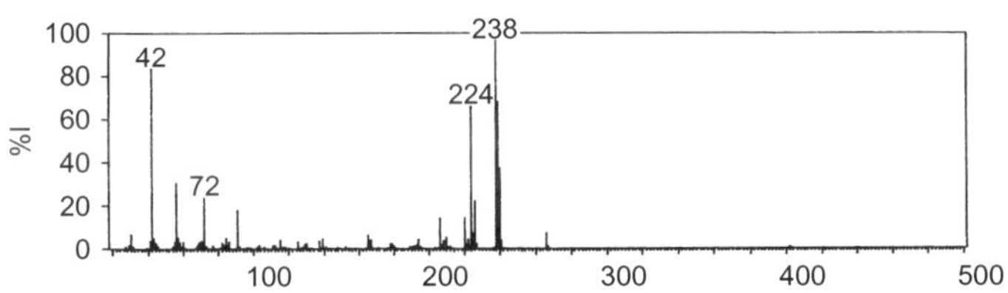

Quantification

Radioimmunoassay. In serum or urine—H. S. Weintraub *et al., Curr. Ther. Res.*, 1977, *21*, 867–876.

High performance liquid chromatography–mass spectrometry. In plasma: loperamide and *N*-demethylloperamide, limit of detection <0.12 µg/L, selected-ion monitoring—H. He *et al., J. Chromatogr. B. Biomed. Sci. Appl.*, 2000, *744*, 323–331.

Disposition in the Body. Loperamide is poorly absorbed after oral administration. About 1 to 2% of a dose is excreted in the urine as free or conjugated loperamide in 48 h. Up to 10% of a dose may be excreted in the urine in 8 days and about 40% is eliminated in the faeces over the same period.

Therapeutic concentration

Following oral administration of capsules containing 8 mg of loperamide hydrochloride to 6 subjects, peak serum concentrations of about 0.002 mg/L were attained in about 4 to 5 h [J. M. Killinger *et al., J. Clin. Pharmacol.*, 1979, *19*, 211–218].

24 subjects in a cross-over study received a single 16 mg dose of loperamide, either as tablets or in capsules, on two days. A mean peak plasma concentration of 3.35 µg/L occurred at 4.08 h after the tablets and 3.98 µg/L at 4.38 h after the capsules [K. Doser *et al., Int. J. Clin. Pharmacol. Ther.*, 1995, *33*, 431–436].

Half-life. Plasma half-life, 7 to 15 (mean 11) h.

Protein binding. In plasma, about 97%.

Note. For a review of the pharmacokinetics of loperamide, see R. C. Heel *et al., Drugs*, 1978, *15*, 33–52.

Dose. Up to 16 mg of loperamide hydrochloride daily.

Loprazolam

Sedative/Hypnotic

(*Z*)-6-(2-Chlorophenyl)-2,4-dihydro-2-[(4-methyl-1-piperazinyl)methylene]-8-nitro-1*H*-imidazo[1,2-*a*][1,4]benzodiazepin-1-one

$C_{23}H_{21}ClN_6O_3$=464.9

CAS—61197-73-7

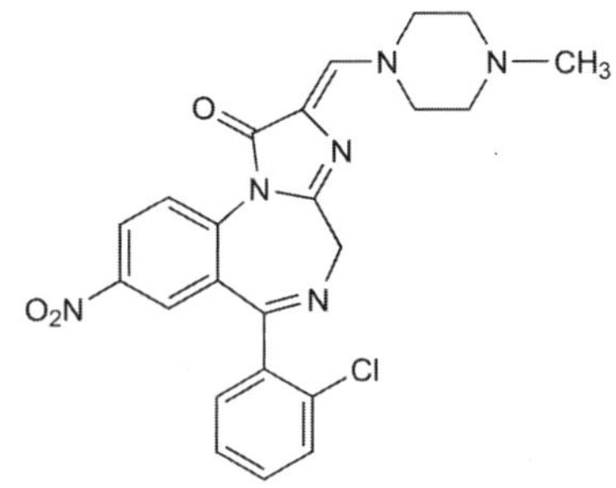

Crystals. M.p. 214° to 215°.

Loprazolam Mesilate

Proprietary names. Dormonoct; Havlane; Somnovit; Sonin.

$C_{23}H_{21}ClN_6O_3,CH_4SO_3,H_2O$=579.0

CAS—70111-54-5 (anhydrous)

A yellow powder. M.p. 242° to 245°, with decomposition.

Soluble 1 in about 100 of water, 1 in about 200 of ethanol and 1 in about 500 of chloroform; practically insoluble in ether.

Dissociation Constant. pK_a 6.0 (24°).

Thin-layer Chromatography. System TA—Rf 40; system TB—Rf 01; system TC—Rf 48; system TD—Rf 03; system TE—Rf 40; system TF—Rf 01; system TL—Rf 05; system TAD—Rf 36; system TAE—Rf 26; system TAF—Rf 15.

Gas Chromatography. System GA—not eluted; system GB—not eluted.

High Performance Liquid Chromatography. System HAA—Retention time(s), 13.4 min; system HX—RI 388.

Ultraviolet Spectrum. Ethanol—330 nm (A_1^1=884b).

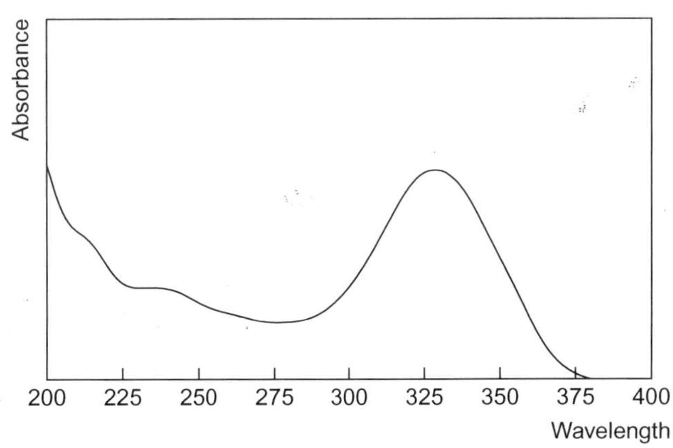

Infra-red Spectrum. Principal peaks at wavenumbers 1628, 1610, 1045, 1182, 1192, 1518 cm^{-1} (loprazolam mesilate, KBr disk).

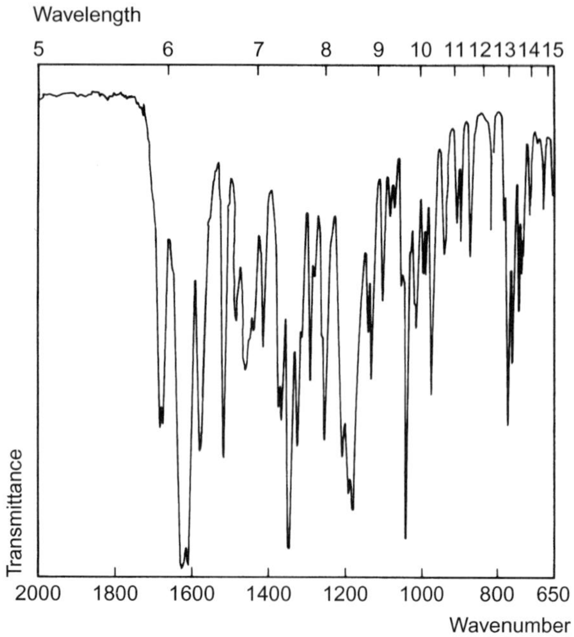

Quantification

Gas chromatography. In plasma: limit of detection 1 µg/L, ECD—F. A. Levasseur *et al.*, *Biopharm. Drug Dispos.*, 1985, *6*, 381–387.

Disposition in the Body. Loprazolam is readily absorbed after oral administration.

Therapeutic concentration

Following a single oral dose of 2 mg to 8 subjects, a mean peak serum concentration of 0.0097 mg/L was attained in 2.4 h. Following repeated oral doses of 2 mg daily for 8 days, a mean peak serum concentration of 0.012 mg/L was reported 2.2 h after the last dose [L. A. Stevens *et al.*, *Eur. J. Clin. Pharmacol.*, 1983, *25*, 651–655].

Half-life. Plasma half-life, 4 to 11 (mean 7) h.

Dose. The equivalent of 1 to 2 mg of loprazolam, as a hypnotic.

Loratadine

Antihistamine (non-sedating)

Synonyms. SCH-29851

Proprietary names. Allerfre; Civeran; Claritin; Clarityn; Fristamin; Lisino; Lorastyne; Optimin; Polaratyne; Sanelor; Velodan; Versal; Via-tin. It is also an ingredient of Loractin.

4-(8-Chloro-5,6-dihydro-11*H*-benzo[5,6]cyclohepta[1,2-*b*]pyridin-11-ylidene)-1-piperidinecarboxylic acid ethyl ester

$C_{22}H_{23}ClN_2O_2 = 382.9$

CAS—79794-75-5

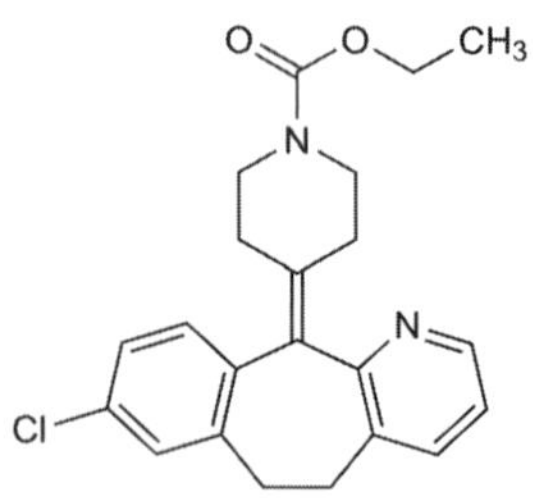

Crystals from acetonitrile. M.p. 134° to 136°. Soluble in alcohol (1 in 10); insoluble in water.

Dissociation Constant. pK_a 5.0.

Partition Coefficient. Log *P* (octanol/water), 5.20.

Thin-layer Chromatography. System TB—Rf 20; system TE—Rf 78; system TF—Rf 29; system TAE—Rf 86.

Gas Chromatography. System GB—RI 3236.

Column: HP-Ultra 1 capillary (25 m × 0.2 mm i.d.). Column temperature: 100°, held 2 min, increased to 310° at 15°/min, held 2.5 min. Carrier gas: helium, 1 mL/min flow rate. Internal standard (IS): etoloxamine. Detection: mass spectrometer (EI, SIM mode, *m/z*: 382.1 for loratadine; *m/z*: 86.2, 283.2 for IS). Retention time(s): loratadine, 17.2 min; IS, 11.9 min. [J. Martens, *J. Chromatogr.* 1995, *673(2)*; *Biomed. Appl.*, 183–188].

High Performance Liquid Chromatography. System HX—RI 523; system HY—RI 362; system HZ—retention time 14.6 min; system HAA—retention time 22.9 min; system HAX—retention time 10.9 min; system HAY—retention time 13.3 min.

Column: (analytical) LC-18-DB (250 × 4.6 mm i.d., 5 µm) (guard) LC-18-DB (20 × 4.6 i.d., 5 µm). Mobile phase: acetonitrile:water:potassium dihydrogen phosphate (0.5 M):orthophosphoric acid (440:480:80:1), pH 3.0, 1.8 mL/min flow rate. IS: diazepam. UV detection (λ = 200 nm). Retention time(s): loratadine, 4.1 min; IS, 4.7 min. [P. Kunicki, *J. Chromatogr. B, Biomed. Sci. Appl.*, 2001, *755*, 331–335].

Ultraviolet Spectrum. Aqueous acid—280 nm; Aqueous base—252 nm.

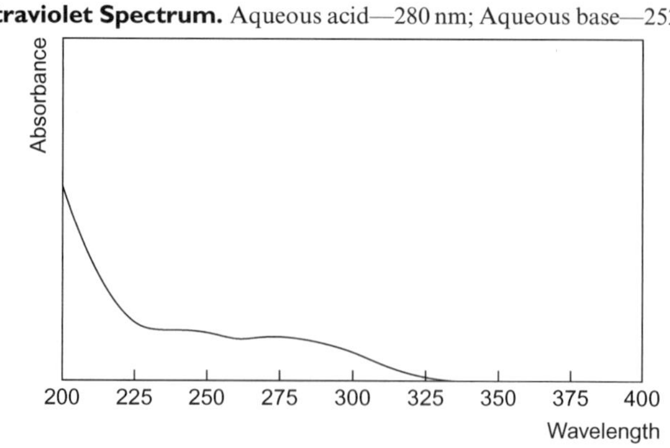

Infra-red Spectrum. Principal peaks at wavenumbers 1709, 1435, 1226, 997 cm^{-1} (KBr pellet).

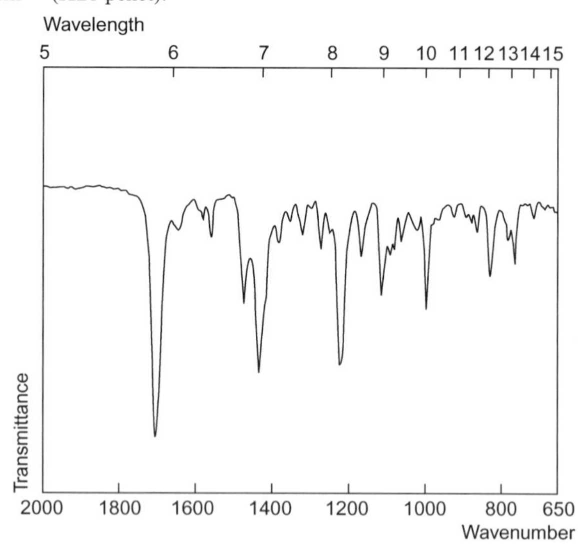

Mass spectrum. Principal ions at *m/z* 382, 266, 245, 280, 292, 384, 383, 294.

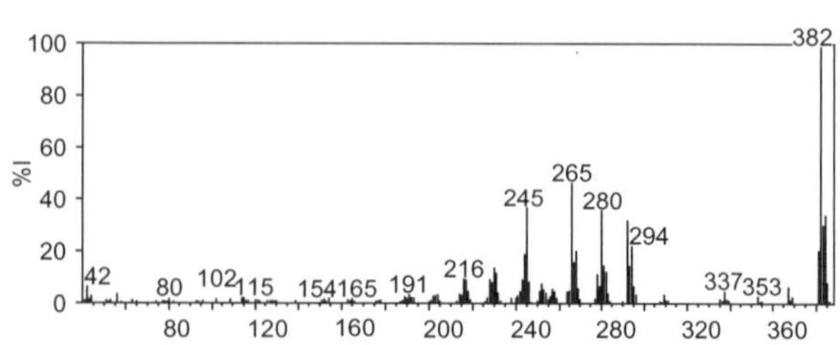

Quantification

Gas chromatography. In plasma: limit of quantification for loratadine and its metabolite 0.1 µg/L, NPD (nitrogen–phosphorus detection)—R. Johnson *et al.*, *J. Chromatogr.* 1994, *657*; *Biomed. Appl.*, 125–131.

Gas chromatography–mass spectrometry. In serum: limit of detection 0.5 μg/L; limit of quantification 1.5 μg/L—J. Martens, *J. Chromatogr.* 1995, *673(2)*; *Biomed. Appl.*, 183–188.

High performance liquid chromatography. In plasma: loratadine and metabolite, limit of detection 0.1 μg/L. MS detection (ESI, MRM (multiple reaction monitoring) mode)—F. Sutherland *et al.*, *J. Chromatogr. A*, 2001, *914*, 37–43. In plasma: limit of quantification 0.6 μg/L—E. Radwanski *et al.*, *J. Clin. Pharmacol.*, 1987, *27*, 530–533.

Disposition in the Body. Loratadine is rapidly absorbed after oral administration and undergoes extensive metabolism. Peak plasma concentrations are observed 1 to 1.5 h after administration. Steady state concentrations are achieved after 5 days. The major metabolite desloratadine (descarboethoxyloratadine) is rapidly formed and has antihistamine activity. It undergoes further oxidation and hydroxylation to several products. Excretion, in the form of metabolites, is via urine and faeces. 27% of a dose is excreted in urine within 24 h and 40% is excreted in urine and 42% in faeces over 10 days. Loratadine and its metabolites are also distributed in breast milk but do not appear to cross the blood–brain barrier to a significant extent.

Therapeutic concentration. The serum therapeutic concentration is 15 to 27 μg/L and descarboethoxyloratadine, 7 to 28 μg/L.

> 18 men and women, aged between 29 and 60 years (mean 22 years old), selected with a creatinine clearance >80 mL/min (group 1), ⩽30 mL/min (group 2) and with end-stage renal disease (group 3) (6 volunteers in each group) were administered a single 40 mg dose in the fasted state. Mean peak plasma concentrations of 24.3 (range 6.2 to 44.7) μg/L, 35.8 (10.7 to 61.9) μg/L and 42.2 (12.6 to 81.7) μg/L were reached for the three groups, respectively, between 1 and 2 h. Mean peak plasma concentrations of the metabolite desloratidine were 14.8 (11.3 to 19.0), 32.2 (19.7 to 56.6) and 26.3 (18.6 to 43.4) μg/L for groups 1, 2 and 3, respectively. These levels were observed between 1 and 10 h with a mean of 2.6 h for each group. [G. R. Matzke *et al.*, *J. Clin. Pharmacol.*, 1990, *30*, 364–371].

Half-life. Loratadine, 8 to 11 h; desloratadine, 17 to 28 h (37 h for patients with chronic alcohol liver disease).

Volume of distribution. 119 L/kg (range 32 to 261) for patients with creatinine clearance >80 mL/min; 50 (27 to 64) L/kg for patients with ⩽30 mL/min creatinine clearance; 92 L/kg (range 36 to 190) for patients with end stage renal disease.

Clearance. 239 mL/kg/min (range 88 to 585) for patients with creatinine clearance >80 mL/min; 109 (36 to 164) mL/kg/min for patients with ⩽30 mL/min creatinine clearance; 137 mL/kg/min (range 48 to 339) for patients with end-stage renal disease.

Protein binding. Loratadine, 97 to 99%; desloratadine, 73 to 76%.

Dose. 10 mg daily. Children (2 to 5 years): 5 mg daily.

Lorazepam

Tranquilliser

Synonyms. Lorazepamum; Wy-4036.
Proprietary names. Almazine; Ansilor; Ativan; Control; Equitam; Ergocalm; Laubeel; Lorabenz; Lorans; Lorapam; Lorenin; Loridem; Lorivan; Lorsedal; Lorzem; Merlit; Punktyl; Serenase; Sinestron; Somagerol; Tavor; Temesta; Tolid; Vigiten.
7-Chloro-5-(2-chlorophenyl)-1,3-dihydro-3-hydroxy-2*H*-1,4-benzodiazepin-2-one
$C_{15}H_{10}Cl_2N_2O_2 = 321.2$
CAS—846-49-1

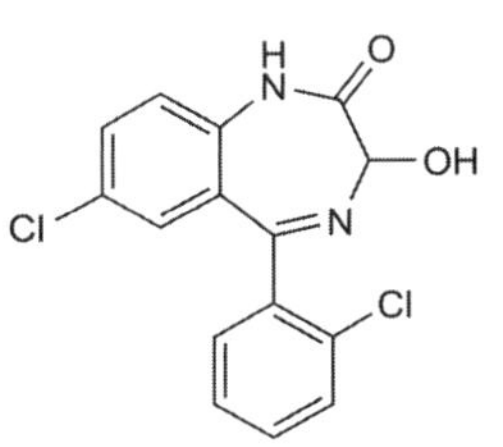

A white powder. M.p. 166° to 168°.
Solubility (mg/mL): water 0.08; chloroform 3; alcohol 14; propylene glycol 16; ethyl acetate 30.

Dissociation Constant. pK_a 1.3, 11.5 (20°).

Partition Coefficient. Log *P* (octanol/pH 7.4), 2.4.

Colour Tests. Formaldehyde–Sulfuric Acid—orange; Marquis Test—yellow; Sulfuric Acid—yellow.

Thin-layer Chromatography. System TA—Rf 52; system TB—Rf 01; system TC—Rf 36; system TD—Rf 23; system TE—Rf 43; system TF—Rf 41; system TL—Rf 28; system TAD—Rf 42; system TAE—Rf 82; system TAF—Rf 82; system TAJ—Rf 46; system TAK—Rf 42; system TAL—Rf 86. (Acidified iodoplatinate solution, positive; acidified potassium permanganate solution, positive.)

Gas Chromatography. System GA—RI 2410; system GB—lorazepam RI 2528, lorazepam-TMS_2 RI 2566; system GG—lorazepam RI 2910.

High Performance Liquid Chromatography. System HA—*k* 0.1; system HI—k 4.60; system HK—*k* 0.14; system HX—RI 444; system HY—RI 400; system HZ—Retention time 4.1 min; system HAA—Retention time 17.2 min; system HAF—Retention time 15.0 min; system HAL—Retention time 5.1 min; system HAM—Retention time 4.2 min; system HAX—Retention time 6.1 min; system HAY—Retention time 5.8 min; system HBH—*k* 5.16; system HBI—*k* 1.14.

Ultraviolet Spectrum. Ethanol—230 (A_1^1=1100b), 316 nm.

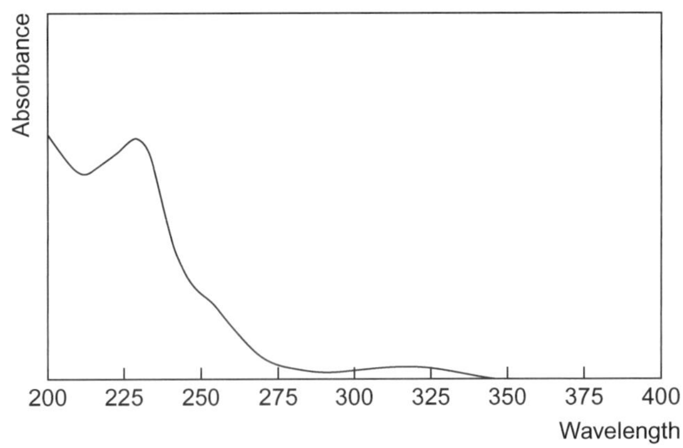

Infra-red Spectrum. Principal peaks at wavenumbers 1685, 1149, 1317, 1120, 1605, 826 cm^{-1} (KBr disk).

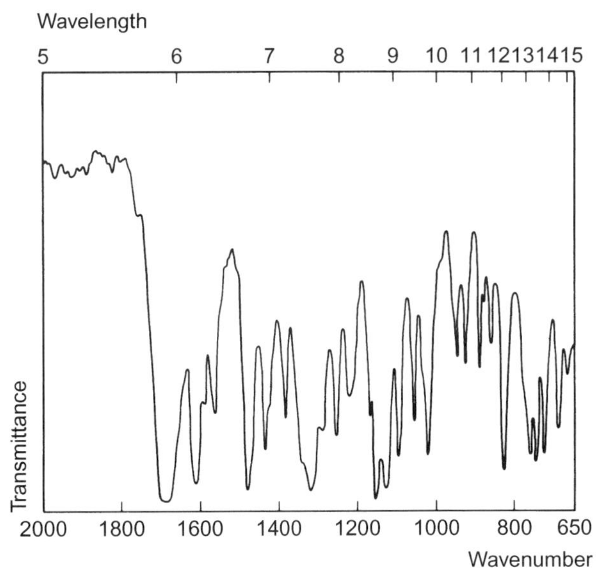

Mass Spectrum. Principal ions at *m/z* 291, 239, 274, 293, 75, 302, 276, 138.

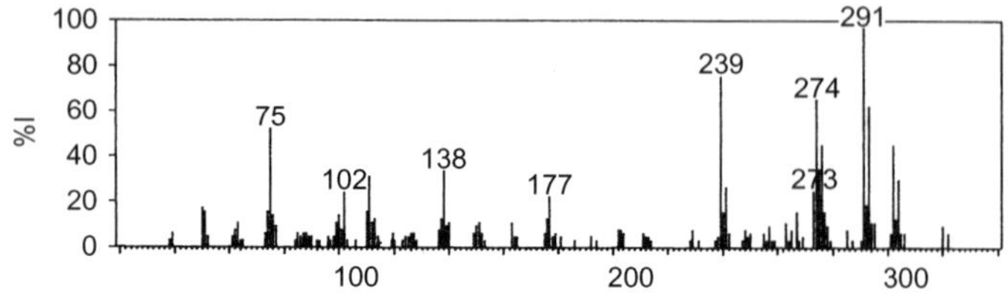

Quantification

Gas chromatography. In plasma or urine: lorazepam and lorazepam glucuronide, limit of detection 1 μg/L, ECD—D. J. Greenblatt *et al.*, *J. Chromatogr.*, 1978, *146*; *B Biomed. Appl.*, *3*, 311–320. In plasma or whole blood: lorazepam and other benzodiazepines, ECD and nitrogen–phosphorus detection—P. Lillsunde and T. Seppala, *J. Chromatogr.*, 1990, *533*, 97–110. In urine: nitrogen–phosphorus detection—Z. L. Jiang *et al.*, *Se Pu*, 2001, *19*, 341–343.

Gas chromatography–mass spectrometry. In plasma or urine: lorazepam and lorazepam glucuronide, limit of detection 2 μg/L—S. Higuchi *et al.*, *J. Chromatogr.*, 1979, *164*; *B Biomed. Appl.*, *6*, 55–61. In urine: lorazepam and other benzodiazepines, limit of quantification <10 μg/L—P. H. Dickson *et al.*, *J.Anal. Toxicol.*, 1992, *16*, 67–71. In urine: lorazepam and other benzodiazepines—R. L. Fitzgerald *et al.*, *J. Anal. Toxicol.*, 1993, *17*, 342–347; D. A. Black *et al.*, *J. Anal. Toxicol.*, 1994, *18*, 185–188; D. A. Black *et al.*, *J. Anal. Toxicol.*,1995, *19*, 58–59. In hair—V. Cirimele *et al.*, *Int. J. Legal Med.*, 1996, *108*, 265–267. In hair: lorazepam, other benzodiazepines and psychotropic drugs—M. Yegles *et al.*, *Forensic Sci. Int.*, 1997, *84*, 211–218. In plasma or urine: limit of quantification 0.1 μg/L—S. Pichini *et al.*, *J. Chromatogr. B Biomed. Sci. Appl.*, 1999, *732*, 509–514. In urine: lorazepam and other benzodiazepines, SIM—D. Borrey *et al.*, *J. Chromatogr. B Biomed. Sci. Appl.*, 2001, *765*, 187–197. Limit of quantification is 2.5 to 5 μg/L (full scan) and 0.1 to 0.5 μg/L (SIM, *m/z* 291)—D. Borrey *et al.*, *J. Chromatogr. A*, 2001, *910*, 105–118.

High performance liquid chromatography. In plasma: lorazepam and its glucuronide metabolite, limit of detection for lorazepam 0.5 μg/L—T. Kondo *et al.*, *Ther. Drug Monit.*, 1993, *15*, 35–38. In plasma or urine: lorazepam glucuronides and those of other benzodiazepines, limits of detection 5 to 10 μg/L—C. Franzelius and K. Besserer, *J. Chromatogr.*, 1993, *613*, 162–167. In serum: lorazepam and other benzodiazepines, UV detection—E. Tanaka *et al.*, *J. Chromatogr. B Biomed. Appl.*, 1996, *682*, 173–178; E. Tanaka *et al.*, *J. Chromatogr. B Biomed. Appl.*, 1998, *709*, 324.

Disposition in the Body. Readily absorbed after oral administration. Lorazepam crosses the blood–brain barrier and the placenta. It is found in breast milk. About 75% of a dose is excreted in the urine as the inactive glucuronide conjugate within 5 days (up to about 50% in the first 24 h) and 14% is excreted as conjugates of minor metabolites which include ring-hydroxylation products and quinazoline derivatives; only negligible amounts are excreted as free lorazepam; about 7% of a dose is eliminated in the faeces.
Lorazepam is a metabolite of lormetazepam.

Therapeutic concentration. In plasma, usually in the range 0.05 to 0.24 mg/L. Lorazepam glucuronide accumulates in plasma achieving concentrations greater than those of unchanged drug.

After a single oral dose of 0.05 mg/kg given to 9 subjects, peak plasma concentrations of 0.04 to 0.06 mg/L (mean 0.05) were attained in about 0.5 to 1.5 h; the maximum therapeutic effect was associated with plasma concentrations of 0.03 to 0.05 mg/L and concentrations below 0.01 mg/L were ineffective [E. G. Bradshaw *et al.*, *Br. J. Anaesth.*, 1981, *53*, 517–522].

Following daily oral doses of 6 mg to 8 subjects, mean steady-state plasma concentrations of 0.09 mg/L of lorazepam and 0.17 mg/L of lorazepam glucuronide were reported; in 7 subjects receiving 10 mg daily, the mean steady-state plasma concentrations were 0.16 and 0.27 mg/L respectively [D. J. Greenblatt *et al.*, *J. Clin. Pharmacol.*, 1977, *17*, 495–500].

Toxicity
Plasma concentrations of 0.3 to 0.6 mg/L were reported in 3 subjects suffering toxic effects after the ingestion of overdoses of lorazepam; the estimated amounts ingested were 100 and 120 mg in 2 of the cases. The subjects recovered within 24 to 30 h [M. D. Allen *et al.*, *Am. J. Psychiatry*, 1980, *137*, 1414–1415].

Bioavailability. About 95%.

Half-life. Plasma half-life, lorazepam 9 to 24 h (mean 14), lorazepam glucuronide about 16 h.

Volume of distribution. About 1 to 2 L/kg.

Clearance. Plasma clearance, about 1 mL/min/kg.

Protein binding. In plasma, about 90%; decreased in patients with cirrhosis.

Note. For reviews of the clinical pharmacokinetics of lorazepam see A. A. Kyriakopoulos *et al.*, *J. Clin. Psychiat.*, 1978, *39*, 16–23, and D. J. Greenblatt, *Clin. Pharmacokinet.*, 1981, *6*, 89–105.

Dose. 1 to 10 mg daily.

Lorcainide

Anti-arrhythmic

Synonyms. Isocainide; Socainide.
N-(4-Chlorophenyl)-*N*-[1-(1-methylethyl)-4-piperidinyl]-benzeneacetamide
$C_{22}H_{27}ClN_2O$ = 370.9
CAS—*59729-31-6*

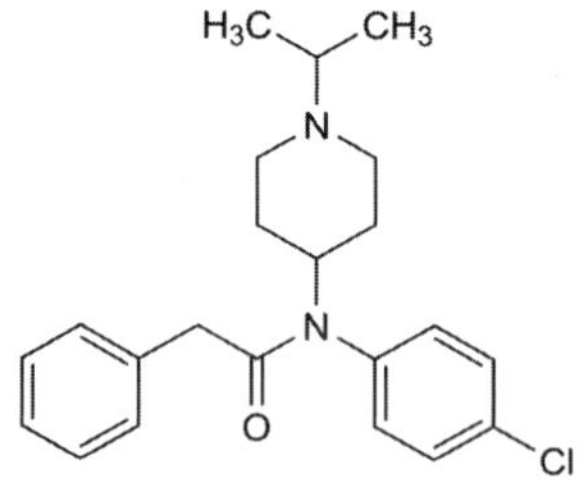

Lorcainide Hydrochloride

Proprietary name. Remivox
$C_{22}H_{27}ClN_2O,HCl$ = 407.4
CAS—*58934-46-6*
Crystals. M.p. 263°.
Freely soluble in water, ethanol, chloroform and methanol.

Partition Coefficient. Log *P* (octanol/water), 4.9.

Thin-layer Chromatography. System TB—Rf 48; system TE—Rf 80; system TAE—Rf 41.

Gas Chromatography. System GA—lorcainide RI 2810, M (nor-) RI 2660, M (OH-)-AC RI 2880, M (OH-dimethoxy-)-AC RI 3010, M (OH-methoxy-)-AC RI 2940, M (*N*-desalkyl-desacyl-)-AC_2 RI 2490, M (desacyl-) RI 2100, M (desacyl-)-AC RI 2200; system GB—lorcainide RI 2923, M (nor-) RI 2789.

High Performance Liquid Chromatography. System HA—*k* 1.8; system HX—RI 425; system HZ—Retention time, 6.6 min.

Ultraviolet Spectrum. Water—257 nm (A^1_1 = 14.3b), 263 nm (A^1_1 = 12.1b).

Infra-red Spectrum. Principal peaks at wavenumbers 1649, 716, 1094, 1298, 1153, 1016 cm^{-1} (lorcainide hydrochloride, KBr disk).

Quantification

Gas chromatography. In plasma or urine: limit of detection 10 μg/L for lorcainide and norlorcainide, ECD—U. Klotz *et al.*, *Clin. Pharmacokinet.*, 1978, *3*, 407–418. In plasma, urine or tissues: limit of detection 5 μg/L for lorcainide, 10 μg/L for norlorcainide, 10 to 15 μg/L for hydroxylated metabolites, ECD—R. Woestenborgh *et al.*, *J. Chromatogr.*, 1979, *164 Biomed. Appl.*, *6*, 169–176.
For a GC–MS screening method of antiarrhythmic drugs and their metabolites in urine, see H. H. Maurer, *Arch. Toxicol.*, 1990, *64*, 218–230.

High performance liquid chromatography. In serum: limit of detection 5 μg/L UV detection (λ = 226 nm)—X. Luo and F. D. Zeng, *Yao Xue Xue Bao*, 1995, *30*, 605–609. In plasma: limit of detection 5 μg/L for lorcainide and norlorcainide, UV detection—Y. G. Yee and R. E. Kates, *J. Chromatogr.*, 1981, *223 Biomed. Appl.*, *12*, 453–459.
For an HPLC screening method of antiarrhythmic drugs in plasma, see R. Verbesselt *et al.*, *Ther. Drug Monit.*, 1991, *13*, 157–165.

Disposition in the Body. Well absorbed after oral administration but undergoes extensive, saturable, first-pass metabolism. The principal active metabolite, norlorcainide, is found in high concentrations in plasma during chronic oral dosing. Other major metabolites include a 4-hydroxyphenyl derivative and a 4-hydroxy-3-methoxyphenyl compound. After intravenous administration, less than 2% of a dose is excreted in the urine as unchanged drug in 48 h; a total of about 60% of a dose is excreted in the urine as metabolites in 4 days and 35% is eliminated in the faeces.

Therapeutic concentration
Following oral doses of 100 mg twice a day to 8 subjects for 2 weeks, mean steady-state plasma concentrations of 0.05 to 0.50 mg/L (mean 0.19) of lorcainide and 0.16 to 0.68 mg/L (mean 0.32) of norlorcainide were reported [R. E. Kates *et al.*, *Clin. Pharmacol. Ther.*, 1983, *33*, 28–34].

Toxicity
A 15-year-old girl died 3 h after ingesting at least 2.5 g of lorcainide; the lorcainide concentration in a blood sample taken 30 to 60 min post ingestion was 1.82 mg/L [J. Evers and U. Buttner-Belz, *J. Toxicol. Clin. Toxicol.*, 1995, *33*, 157–159].

Bioavailability. About 30% after a single dose of 150 mg but almost 100% during chronic oral dosing.

Half-life. Plasma half-life, lorcainide 3 to 15 h (mean 8), increased in subjects with cirrhosis of the liver and during chronic oral dosing; norlorcainide 20 to 40 h (mean 27).

Volume of distribution. About 8 L/kg but there is considerable intersubject variation.

Clearance. Plasma clearance, 10 to 25 mL/min/kg.

Distribution in blood. Plasma : whole blood ratio, about 1.3.

Protein binding. In plasma, 80 to 85%.

Note. For a review of lorcainide see C. E. Eiriksson and R. N. Brogden, *Drugs*, 1984, *27*, 279–300.

Dose. The equivalent of 200 to 300 mg of lorcainide daily.

Lormetazepam

Hypnotic

Synonym. Wy-4082
Proprietary names. Aldosomnil; Ergocalm; Loramet; Loretam; Minias; Noctamid(e); Octonox; Pronoctan; Stilaze.
7-Chloro-5-(2-chlorophenyl)-1,3-dihydro-3-hydroxy-1-methyl-2*H*-1,4-benzodiazepin-2-one
$C_{16}H_{12}Cl_2N_2O_2$=335.2
CAS—848-75-9

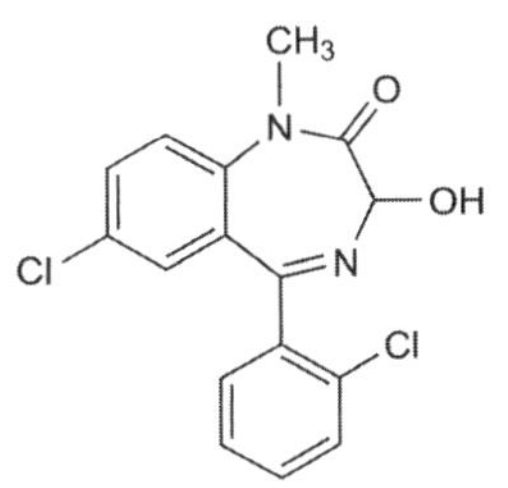

A white crystalline powder. M.p. 209° to 211°, with decomposition.
Practically insoluble in water; slightly soluble in ethanol and methanol; freely soluble in chloroform.

Partition Coefficient. Log *P* (octanol/water), 2.2.

Colour Test. Formaldehyde–Sulfuric Acid—orange.

Thin-layer Chromatography. System TA—Rf 52; system TB—Rf 06; system TC—Rf 61; system TD—Rf 46; system TE—Rf 59; system TF—Rf 45; system TL—Rf 50; system TAD—Rf 60; system TAE—Rf 82; system TAF—Rf 82. (Dragendorff spray, positive; FPN reagent, pale yellow; Marquis reagent, very weak pale yellow; mercuric chloride–diphenylcarbazone reagent, blue, on heating turns pale pink; acidified potassium permanganate solution, positive.)

Gas Chromatography. System GA—lormetazepam RI 2660, lorazepam RI 2410, decomposition product RI 2727; system GB—lormetazepam RI 2770, lorazepam RI 2528, lormetazepam-TMS_2 RI 2799, lorazepam-TMS_2 RI 2566.

High Performance Liquid Chromatography. System HI—*k* 6.32; system HK—*k* 0.08; system HX—RI 487; system HY—RI 463; system HZ—Retention time 6.2 min; system HBH—*k* 7.19; system HBI—*k* 1.46.

Ultraviolet Spectrum. Aqueous acid—231 (A^1_1=1030b), 311 nm (A^1_1=59b).

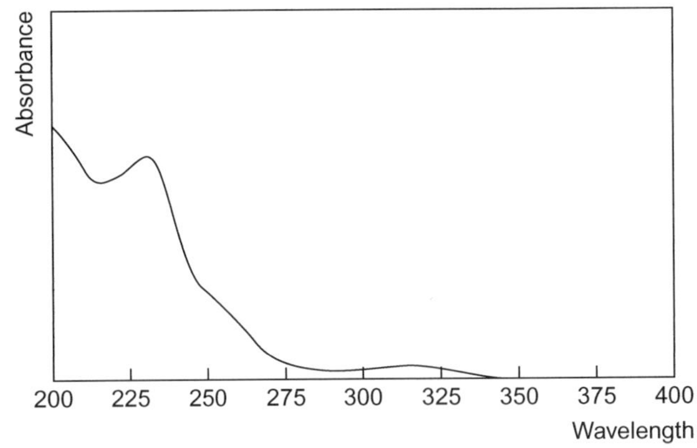

Infra-red Spectrum. Principal peaks at wavenumbers 1682, 1153, 1121, 1315, 1610, 843 cm^{-1} (KBr disk).

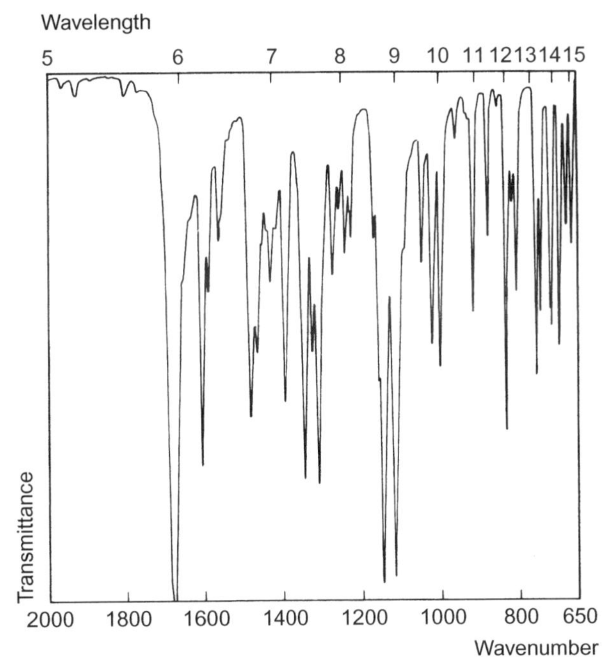

Mass Spectrum. Principal ions at *m/z* 305, 307, 306, 309, 308, 334, 102, 75; lorazepam 291, 239, 274, 293, 75, 302, 276, 138.

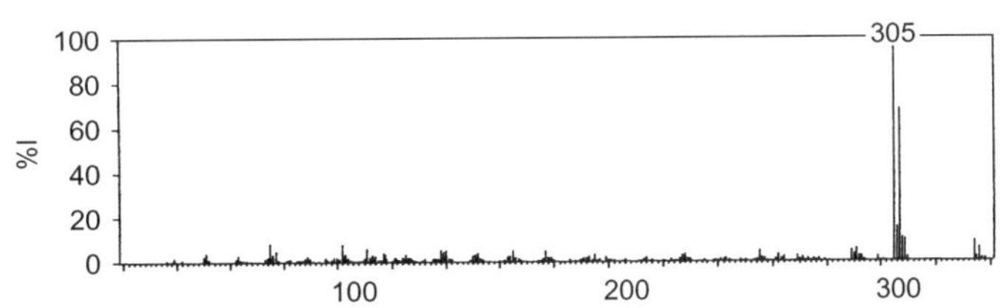

Quantification
Gas chromatography. In plasma: limit of detection 200 ng/L, ECD—D. M. Pierce *et al.*, *Br. J. Clin. Pharmacol.*, 1984, *18*, 31–35.

Gas chromatography–mass spectrometry. In urine: lormetazepam and other benzodiazepines, limits of detection 13 to 30 µg/L (scan mode) and 1 to 1.7

μg/L (SIM)—D. Borrey *et al.*, *J. Chromatogr. B Biomed. Sci. Appl.*, 2001, *765*, 187–197.

Radioimmunoassay. In plasma: limit of detection 30 ng/L—M. Hümpel *et al.*, *Clin. Pharmacol. Ther.*, 1980, *28*, 673–679.

Disposition in the Body. Well absorbed after oral administration. Metabolised to some extent by *N*-demethylation to lorazepam. About 80% of a dose is excreted in the urine as lormetazepam glucuronide in 72 h, and about 6% as lorazepam glucuronide.

Therapeutic concentration

Single oral doses of 1 mg and 3 mg given to 6 subjects, produced mean peak plasma concentrations of 0.006 and 0.016 mg/L, respectively, in 2 to 3 h [M. Hümpel *et al.*, *Clin. Pharmacol. Ther.*, 1980, *28*, 673–679].

Bioavailability. About 80%

Half-life. Plasma half-life, lormetazepam about 10 h, appears to be increased in elderly subjects; lormetazepam glucuronide about 13 h.

Volume of distribution. About 5 L/kg.

Clearance. Plasma clearance, about 4 mL/min/kg.

Protein binding. In plasma, about 90%.

Dose. 0.5 to 1.5 mg, as a hypnotic.

Losartan

Angiotensin II Receptor Antagonist

2-Butyl-4-chloro-1-[[2′-(1*H*-tetrazol-5-yl)[1,1′-biphenyl]-4-yl]methyl]-1*H*-imidazole-5-methanol

$C_{22}H_{23}ClN_6O$=422.9

CAS—114798-26-4

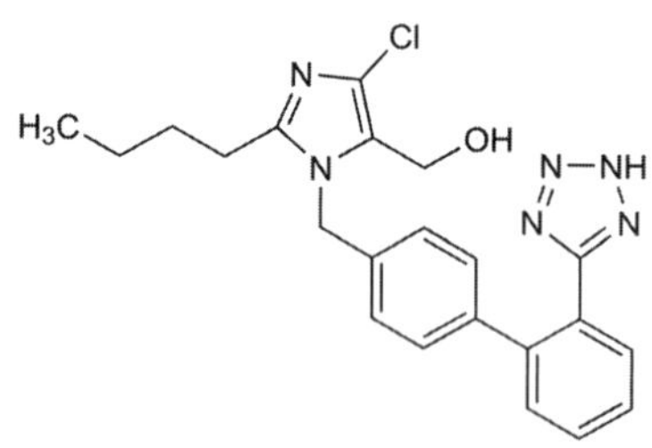

A light yellow solid. M.p. 183.5° to 184.5°.

Losartan Potassium

Synonyms. DUP-753; E-3340; MK-954.

Proprietary names. Cozaar; Lortaan; Losaprex; Neo-Lotan; Oscaar. It is also an ingredient of Hyzaar and Losazid.

$C_{22}H_{22}ClKN_6O$=461.0

CAS—124750-99-8

Dissociation Constant. pK_a 5 to 6.

Partition Coefficient. Log *P* (octanol/water), 4.01.

Gas Chromatography. System GP—RI 3555 (losartan-2ME).

High Performance Liquid Chromatography. Column: (analytical) RP C_{18} (250 × 2.0 mm i.d., 5 μm), (guard) C_{18} (40 × 4.0 mm i.d.). Mobile phase: ammonium phosphate (10 mM, with 0.02% sodium azide):acetonitrile:methanol:TEA pH 3.2 (60:30:10:0.04), 0.3 mL/min flow rate. Internal standard (IS): L-158809. UV detection (λ=254 nm). Retention time: losartan, 12.0 min; E-3174, 20.0 min; IS, 8.4 min. [P. Yeung *et al.*, *Int. J. Pharm.*, 2000, *204*, 17–22].

Column: RP C_8 (Spherisorb, 250 × 4.6 mm i.d.). Column temperature: 40°. Mobile phase: (A:B) acetonitrile:phosphate buffer (1 mM, pH 2.3). Elution programme: (40:60) to (75:25) in 25 min, hold for 5 min, 1.5 mL/min flow rate. UV detection (λ=230 nm). Retention time(s): not specified. [Z. Zhao *et al.*, *J. Pharm. Biomed. Anal.*, 1999, *20*, 129–136].

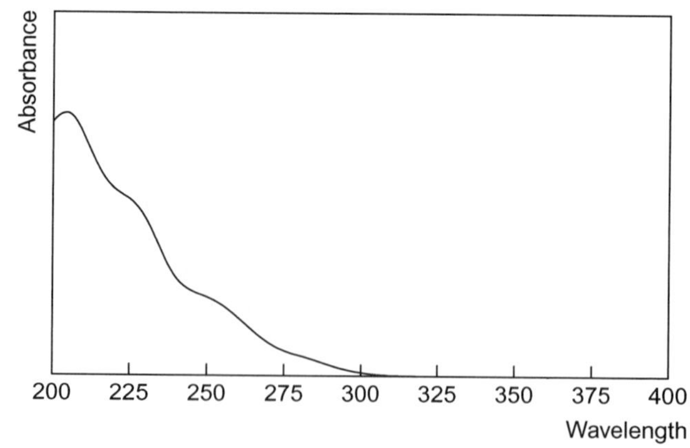

Mass Spectrum Principal ions at *m/z* 192, 201, 249, 165, 450 (losartan-2ME).

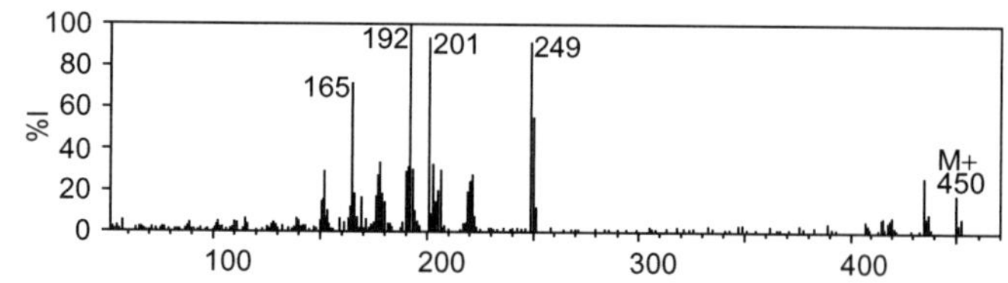

Quantification

High performance liquid chromatography. In plasma, urine and dialysate: limit of detection 1 μg/L. Fluorescence detection (λ_{ex}=250 nm, λ_{em}=375 nm)—D. Farthing *et al.*, *J. Chromatogr. B, Biomed. Sci. Appl.*, 1997, *704*, 374–378. In plasma: limit of quantification 0.02 mg/L for losartan and 0.017 mg/L for the metabolite, E-3174, UV detection (λ=254 nm)—A. Munafo *et al.*, *Clin. Pharmacol. Ther.*, 1992, *51*, 513–521. In plasma and urine: limit of quantification 0.01 mg/L and 0.02 mg/L, respectively, for both the drug and metabolite, UV detection (λ=254 nm)—M. Ohtawa *et al.*, *Br. J. Clin. Pharmacol.*, 1993, *35*, 290–297.

Disposition in the Body. Losartan is readily absorbed after oral administration. The drug undergoes extensive first-pass metabolism to form the active carboxylic acid metabolite, E-3174, as well as a number of inactive metabolites. After administration, peak plasma concentrations of losartan and E-3174 occur at about 1 h and 3 to 4 h, respectively. It is excreted in urine (35%) and in faeces (60%) via bile as the unchanged drug and as its metabolites. There is no evidence for accumulation of the drug.

Therapeutic concentration

6 young, healthy male volunteers, aged 20 to 30 years (mean 26 years) old were administered single doses of 40, 80 and 120 mg. The peak plasma concentrations of the parent drug, losartan, were 0.104, 0.244 and 0.544 mg/L, respectively and were reached about 1 h after administration. The peak concentrations for the metabolite, E-3174, were 0.164, 0.504 and 0.821 mg/L for the doses, respectively, and were observed at 3.7, 3.0 and 2.3 h after dosing. [A. Munafo *et al.*, *Clin. Pharmacol. Ther.*, 1992, *51*, 513–521].

Healthy males (23 to 48 years old) were administered either 25, 50, 100 or 200 mg after an overnight fast. Mean peak plasma concentrations were 84.5, 197.6, 800.5 and 1394.9 μg/L for losartan and 188.9, 462.5, 1210.8 and 2219.0 μg/L for the metabolite, respectively. These concentrations were observed 0.7 and 1.3 h for the drug and 2 to 4 h for the metabolite. [M. Ohtawa *et al.*, *Br. J. Clin. Pharmacol.*, 1993, *35*, 290–297].

Toxicity. Generally well tolerated but fetal toxicity has been observed.

Bioavailability. Around 33%.

Half-life. Losartan: 1.5 to 2.5 h; active metabolite: 3 to 9 h.

Volume of distribution. 34 L; active metabolite:12 L.

Clearance. Plasma clearance: losartan, 600 mL/min; active metabolite, 50 mL/min.

Protein binding. ⩾98%, mainly to albumin (both losartan and active metabolite).

Dose. 50 to100 mg daily.

Lovastatin

HMG-CoA Reductase Inhibitor/ Antihyperlipoproteinaemic

Synonyms. L-154803; MB-530B; MK-803; MSD-803; Monacolin K; 6α-Methylcompactin; Mevinolin.
Proprietary names. Lipofren; Lovalip; Mevacor; Mevinacor; Mevlor; Nergadan; Sivlor; Taucor.
(2*S*)-2-Methylbutanoic acid (1*S*,3*R*,7*S*,8*S*,8a*R*)-1,2,3,7,8,8a-hexahydro-3,7-dimethyl-8-[2-[(2*R*,4*R*)-tetrahydro-4-hydroxy-6-oxo-2*H*-pyran-2-yl]ethyl]-1-naphthalenyl ester
$C_{24}H_{36}O_5$=404.5
CAS—75330-75-5

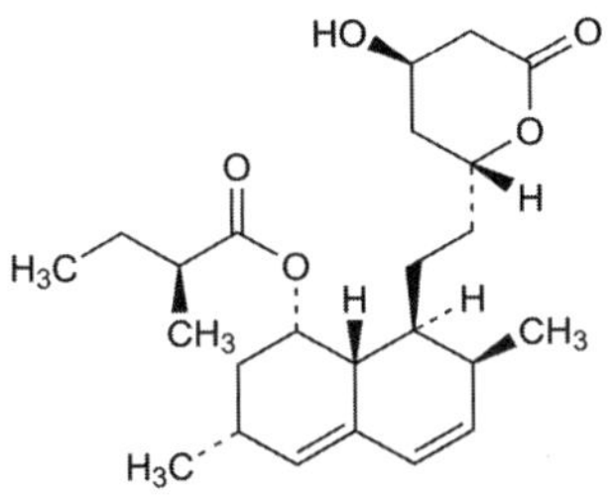

A white crystalline powder. M.p. 174.5°. It is practically insoluble in water (0.4×10^{-3}g/L) and petroleum spirit; sparingly soluble in low molecular weight alcohols (methanol, 28 g/L, ethanol, 16 g/L, isopropanol 20 g/L); soluble in acetone and acetonitrile; freely soluble in chloroform.

Partition Coefficient. Log *P* (octanol/water), 4.26; hydroxyacid derivative, 1.2×10^4; Log *P* (octanol/phosphate buffer pH 7.4), hydroxyacid derivative, 14.1.

Gas Chromatography. Column: DB-1701 (10 m × 0.25 mm i.d., 0.15 µm film thickness). Column temperature: 210°, held for 0.75 min after injection; ramped to 290° at 30°/min, held 2 min. Carrier gas: helium. Internal standard (IS): compactin. MS detection (NICI, SIM at *m/z* 565 for lovastatin and *m/z* 551 for IS). Retention time: lovastatin, 3.3 min; IS, 3.2 min. [D. Wang-Iverson *et al.*, *Rapid Commun. Mass Spectrom.*, 1989, *3(5)*, 132–134].

High Performance Liquid Chromatography. System HAX—retention time 13.8 min; system HAY—retention time 14.8 min.

Column: RP C_{18} (250 × 4.6 i.d., 5 µm). Mobile phase: methanol:sodium dihydrogen phosphate (25 mM, pH 4.5) (82:18), 1 mL/min flow rate. IS: Bay W 62230. UV detection (λ=236 nm). Retention time(s): lovastatin, 8.9 min; lovastatin acid, 6.4 min; IS, 5.6 min. [L. Y. Ye *et al.*, *Ther. Drug Monit.*, 2000, *22*, 737–741].

Ultraviolet Spectrum. Aqueous acid—231, 238, 247 nm.

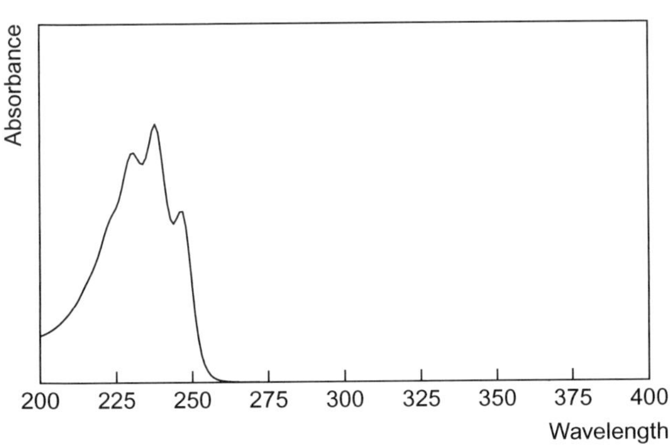

Infra-red Spectrum. Principal peaks at wavenumbers 1725, 1260, 1072, 1460 cm^{-1} (KBr disk).

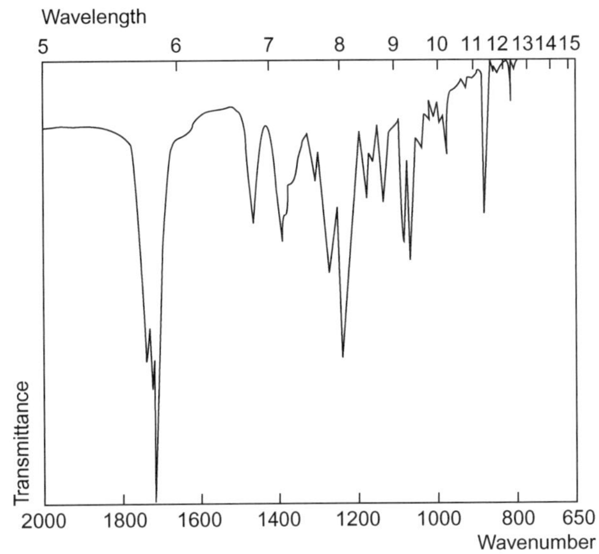

Mass Spectrum. Principal ions at *m/z* 159, 157, 64, 198, 172, 143, 105, 73.

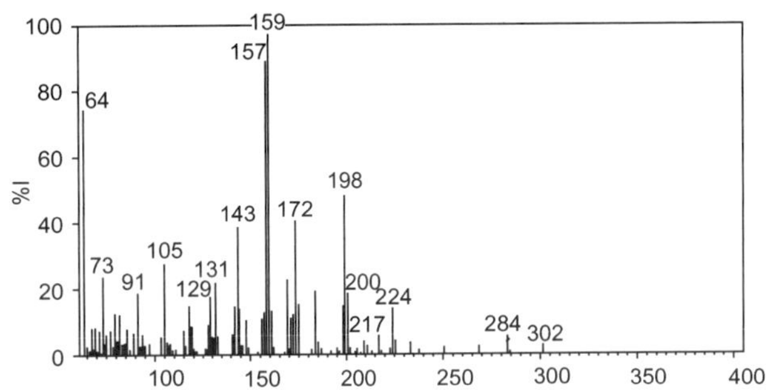

Quantification

Gas chromatography–mass spectrometry. In serum: limit of detection 0.5 µg/L—D. Wang-Iverson *et al.*, *Rapid Commun. Mass Spectrom.*, 1989, *3(5)*, 132–134.

High performance liquid chromatography. In plasma: limit of detection 25 µg/L. UV detection (λ=238 nm)—R. J. Stubbs *et al.*, *J. Chromatogr.*, 1986, *383*, 438–443.

Disposition in the Body. Lovastatin is absorbed after oral administration (30%) and is hydrolysed in the liver to the active β-hydroxyacid form. Three other metabolites have also been detected: 3-hydroxy, 3-hydroxymethyl and 3-exomethylene derivatives. The drug undergoes extensive first-pass metabolism with less than 5% of a dose reaching circulation. Peak plasma concentrations are reached within 2 to 4 h and steady state within 2 to 3 days. Lovastatin is mainly excreted in faeces (85% of an administered dose) and 10% in urine over 72 h. It crosses the blood–brain and placental barriers.

Therapeutic concentration

17 healthy male volunteers, aged between 19 and 27 years, were administered a 20 mg single dose of lovastatin. The peak plasma concentration of the active inhibitors was 14.5 µg(equivalent)/L which was reached in 2.4 h. The peak concentration for the total inhibitors was 27.1 µg(equivalent)/L in 2.1 h. [H. Y. Pan *et al.*, *Br. J. Clin. Pharmacol.*, 1991, *31*, 665–670].

12 healthy males, aged between 22 and 29 years, were administered a single 40 mg dose. The peak plasma concentration of the active inhibitors was 9.5 µg(equivalent)/L and total inhibitors 19.9 µg(equivalent)/L, reached in 2.9 and 2.6 h, respectively. [P. J. Pentikeinen *et al.*, *J. Clin. Pharmacol.*, 1992, *32*, 136–140].

Half-life. 1 to 2 h (active metabolite).

Clearance. Has been quoted as 30 to 1248 mL/min.

Protein binding. Both the parent drug and metabolite are >95% bound to plasma proteins.

Note. For a general review of statins, see I. Hu, *Ann. Pharmacother.*, 1995, *29*, 743–759.

Dose. An initial dose of 10 to 20 mg daily is administered and increased to 80 mg daily if necessary over a period of 4 weeks. In patients taking immunosuppressants the initial daily dose is 10 mg and the overall dose should not exceed 20 mg daily.

Loxapine

Tranquilliser

Synonyms. Oxilapine; SUM-3170.
Proprietary name. Loxapac (solution)
2-Chloro-11-(4-methyl-1-piperazinyl)dibenz[*b,f*][1,4]oxazepine
$C_{18}H_{18}ClN_3O = 327.8$
CAS—1977-10-2

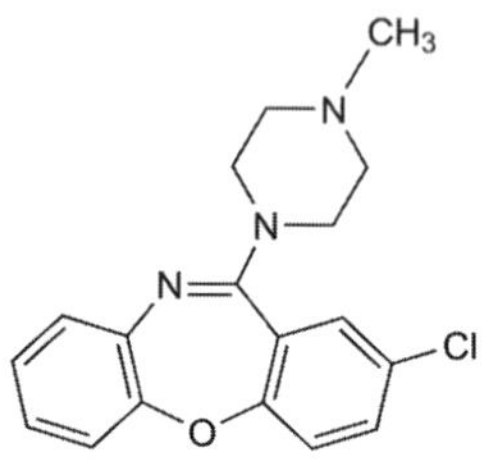

Pale yellowish crystals. M.p. 109° to 110°.

Loxapine Succinate
Proprietary names. Loxapac (capsules); Loxitane (capsules).
$C_{18}H_{18}ClN_3O,C_4H_6O_4 = 445.9$
CAS—27833-64-3
A white crystalline solid.

Laxapine Hydrochloride
Proprietary names. Laxapac; Loxitane (oral solution; injection)
$C_{18}H_{18}ClN_3O, HCl = 364.3$

Dissociation Constant. pK_a 6.6.

Partition Coefficient. Log *P* (octanol/water), 3.6.

Colour Tests. Liebermann's Test (50 to 60°)—orange.
Heat with nitric acid for 3 min at 100° and then dilute tenfold with water—yellow precipitate.

Thin-layer Chromatography. System TB—Rf 36; system TE—Rf 54; system TAE—Rf 49; system TAJ—Rf 45; system TAK—Rf 09; system TAL—Rf 78.

Gas Chromatography. System GA—loxapine RI 2555; M(8-OH-) RI 2931; M(amoxapine) RI 2638; M(7-OH-amoxapine) RI 2951; M(8-OH-amoxapine) RI 2959; system GB—loxapine RI 2717; M(8-OH-) RI 3077; M(7-OH-) RI 3068; M(amoxapine) RI 2746; M(7-OH-amoxapine) RI 3525; M(8-OH-amoxapine) RI 3546.

High Performance Liquid Chromatography. System HA—*k* 1.1; system HX—RI 407; system HY—RI 336; system HAA—Retention time(s), 14.6 min.

Ultraviolet Spectrum. Aqueous acid—251 (A^1_1=346b), 292 nm; aqueous alkali—248 (A^1_1=374b), 298 nm.

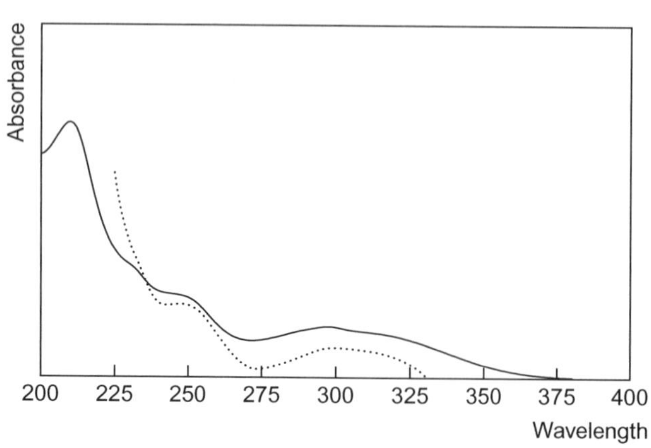

Infra-red Spectrum. Principal peaks at wavenumbers 1590, 1603, 1564, 1109, 1188, 1248 cm^{-1}.

Mass Spectrum. Principal ions at *m/z* 70, 83, 42, 257, 193, 56, 228, 164; amoxapine 245, 257, 247, 193, 56, 246, 228, 259.

Quantification
Gas chromatography. In serum: limit of detection 2 μg/L, AFID—J. Vasiliades *et al.*, *J. Chromatogr.*, 1979, *164*; *Biomed. Appl.*, *6*, 457–470. In plasma or urine: limit of detection 140 ng/L, ECD—S. F. Cooper *et al.*, *Xenobiotica*, 1979, *9*, 405–414. In serum or urine: loxapine and metabolites, ECD (serum) or FID (urine)—T. B. Cooper and R. G. Kelly, *J. Pharm. Sci.*, 1979, *68*, 216–219.

High performance liquid chromatography. In plasma: loxapine, amoxapine and hydroxylated metabolites—S. W. Cheung *et al.*, *J. Chromatogr.*, 1991, *564*, 213–221. In plasma: loxapine, amoxapine and hydroxylated metabolites, limits of detection 3.5 to 6.3 μg/L, UV detection—B. Hue *et al.*, *Ther. Drug Monit.*, 1998, *20*, 335–339.

Disposition in the Body. Loxapine is readily absorbed after oral administration. The major urinary metabolite appears to be 8-hydroxyloxapine; other metabolites which have been identified include 7-hydroxyloxapine, desmethyl-loxapine (amoxapine) and its 7-hydroxy and 8-hydroxy derivatives, loxapine *N*-oxide and 8-methoxyloxapine. Some unchanged drug is also excreted in the urine.

Therapeutic concentration. There is considerable intersubject variation in plasma concentrations.

After a single oral dose of 25 mg to 25 subjects, mean peak serum concentrations of 0.02 mg/L of loxapine, 0.05 mg/L of 8-hydroxyloxapine and 0.006 mg/L of 8-hydroxyamoxapine were attained in 1 to 2 h [M. A. Khan *et al.*, *Curr. Ther. Res.*, 1980, *28*, 277–283].

Two subjects receiving 100 mg daily were found to have serum concentrations, respectively, of 0.031 mg/L and 0.006 mg/L of loxapine, 0.072 mg/L and 0.041 mg/L of 8-hydroxyloxapine and 0.064 mg/L and 0.031 mg/L of 8-hydroxyamoxapine immediately prior to a morning dose [T. B. Cooper and R. G. Kelly, *J. Pharm. Sci.*, 1979, *68*, 216–219].

Toxicity
In a fatality attributed to loxapine overdose, the following postmortem tissue concentrations, mg/L or μg/g, were reported:

	Blood	Brain	Liver	Lung	Spleen
Loxapine	1.22	4.46	11.88	4.98	3.96
8-Hydroxyloxapine (conjugated)	1.51	–	7.98	1.59	0.93
8-Hydroxyloxapine (unconjugated)	0.76	3.80	4.38	3.28	3.26
Amoxapine	1.01	4.84	10.00	3.80	6.30
8-Hydroxyamoxapine (conjugated)	1.92	–	1.89	1.32	–
8-Hydroxyamoxapine (unconjugated)	1.98	3.71	25.47	9.44	14.17

[T. B Cooper *et al.*, *J. Anal. Toxicol.*, 1981, *5*, 99–100].

A 22-year-old female ingested about 2.5 g of loxapine and died after 12 days in coma. Concentrations on admission to hospital were: blood 1.9 mg/L, urine 0.4 mg/L; 24 h later the urine concentration was 8 mg/L; in a second fatality, postmortem blood and liver concentrations of 7.7 mg/L and 150 μg/g were reported [P. Reynolds *et al.*, *Clin. Toxicol.*, 1979, *14*, 181–185].

In a 69-year-old female who died after ingesting loxapine tablets, the loxapine and amoxapine concentrations in postmortem tissues were, respectively: heart blood 9.5 and 0.6 mg/L, bile 28.8 and 4.7 mg/L, gastric contents 278 mg/L and negative, vitreous humour 1.5 mg/L and negative [C. D. Mazzola *et al.*, *J. Anal. Toxicol.*, 2000, *24*, 638–641].

Half-life. Plasma half-life, loxapine 1 to 4 h, 8-hydroxyloxapine about 8 h, 8-hydroxyamoxapine about 36 to 48 h.

Dose. Usually the equivalent of 20 to 100 mg of loxapine daily; maximum of 250 mg daily.

Lymecycline

Antibacterial

Synonyms. Limeciclina; Tetracycline-L-methylenelysine.
Proprietary names. Armyl; Ciclolysal; Mucomycin;Tetralysal; Tetramyl.
A water-soluble combination of tetracycline, lysine and formaldehyde with a molecular weight of approximately 603.
[4S-(4a,4aα,5aα,6β,12aα)]-N^6-[[[[4-(Dimethylamino)-1,4,4a,5,5a,6,11,12a-octahydro-3,6,10,12,12a-pentahydroxy-6-methyl-1,11-dioxo-2-naphthacenyl]-carbonyl]amino]methyl]-L-lysine
$C_{29}H_{38}N_4O_{10}$=602.6
CAS—992-21-2

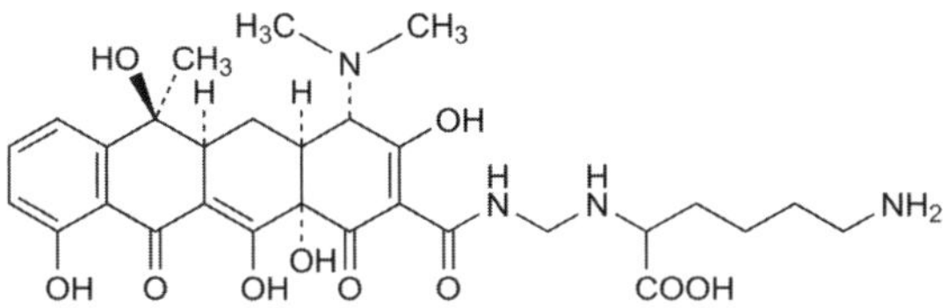

A yellow, very hygroscopic powder which darkens on exposure to light and air. M.p. above 200°, with slow decomposition.
Soluble 1 in less than 1 of water; slightly soluble in ethanol and methanol; practically insoluble in chloroform and ether.

Partition Coefficient. Log *P* (octanol/water), −3.2.

Colour Tests. Benedict's Reagent—red; Formaldehyde–Sulfuric Acid—brown-red; Mandelin's Test—violet-brown→yellow; Marquis Test—orange; Sulfuric Acid—red-brown.

Thin-layer Chromatography. System TA—Rf 05, streaking. (Location under ultraviolet light, orange fluorescence; Acidified potassium permanganate solution, positive.)

Ultraviolet Spectrum. Aqueous acid—269 (A^1_1=292a), 356 nm; aqueous alkali—239, 267 nm.

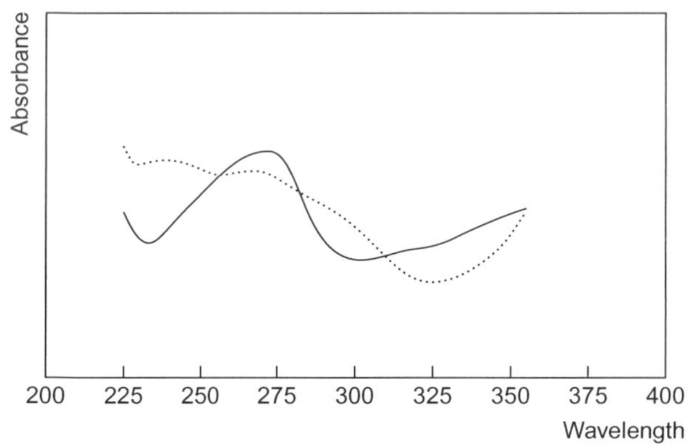

Dose. Usually 816 mg (the equivalent of 600 mg of tetracycline) daily.

Lynestrenol

Progestational Steroid

Synonyms. Lynenol; Lynoestrenol.
Proprietary names. Exlutena; Exluton(a); Orgametil; Orgametril.
It is an ingredient of many oral contraceptives, see *Martindale, The complete drug reference*, 33rd Edn., Pharmaceutical Press, London, 2002.
(17α)-19-Norpregn-4-en-20-yn-17-ol
$C_{20}H_{28}O$=284.4
CAS—52-76-6

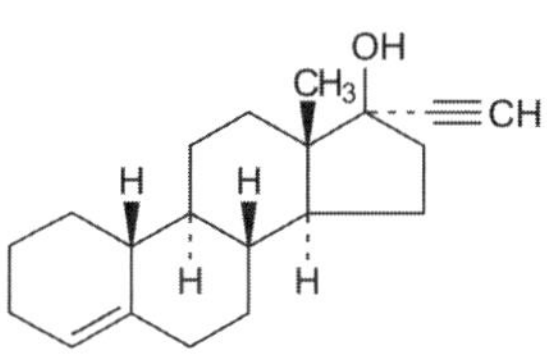

A white crystalline powder. M.p. 158° to 160°.

Practically insoluble in water; soluble 1 in 15 of ethanol, 1 in 8 of chloroform and 1 in 12 of ether.

Partition Coefficient. Log *P* (octanol/water), 4.8.

Thin-layer Chromatography. System TP—Rf 77; system TQ—Rf 55; system TR—Rf 99; system TS—Rf 97.

Ultraviolet Spectrum. No significant absorption, 230 to 360 nm.

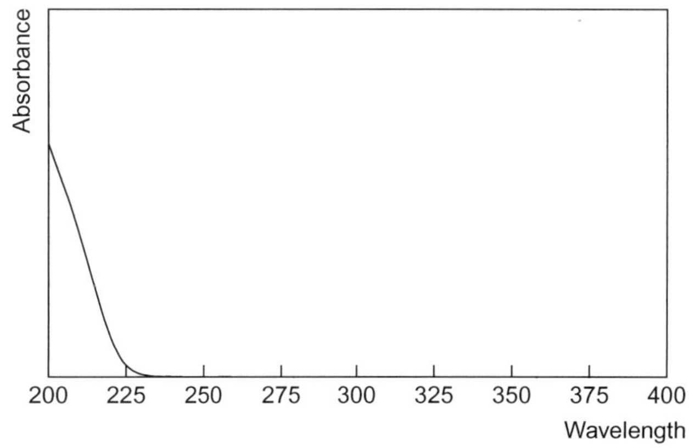

Infra-red Spectrum. Principal peaks at wavenumbers 683, 1040, 1014, 1053, 813, 1266 cm^{-1} (KBr disk).

Mass Spectrum. Principal ions at *m/z* 91, 79, 67, 201, 77, 105, 93, 120.

Dose. 2.5 mg daily, for courses of 22 days.

Lysergamide

Hallucinogen

Synonyms. Ergine; Lysergic Acid Amide.
9,10-Didehydro-6-methylergoline-8β-carboxamide
$C_{16}H_{17}N_3O$=267.3
CAS—478-94-4

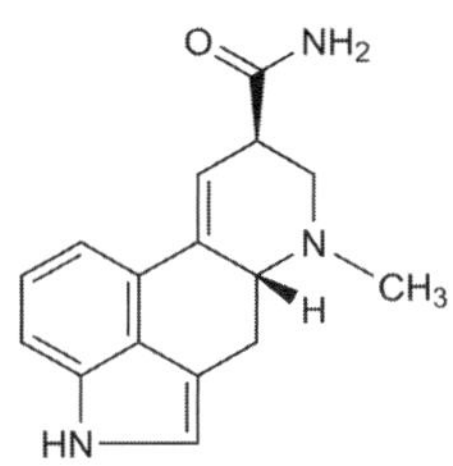

Lysergamide is found in *Rivea corymbosa*, *Ipomoea* spp. (Convolvulaceae) and ergot.
Crystals. It decomposes at 242°.

Colour Test. Marquis Test—brown.

Thin-layer Chromatography. System TA—Rf 60; system TB—Rf 00; system TC—Rf 19; system TE—Rf 36; system TL—Rf 06; system TM—Rf 27; system TAE—Rf 57; system TAF—Rf 51. (Van Urk reagent, blue.)

High Performance Liquid Chromatography. System HA—*k* 0.5; system HP—*k* 0.33.

Ultraviolet Spectrum. Aqueous acid—313 nm; aqueous alkali—309 nm.

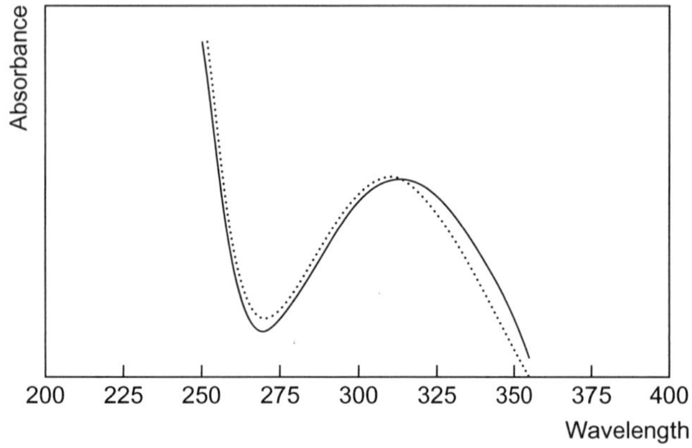

Infra-red Spectrum. Principal peaks at wavenumbers 1670, 760, 783, 1618, 1158, 1270 cm^{-1} (KBr disk).

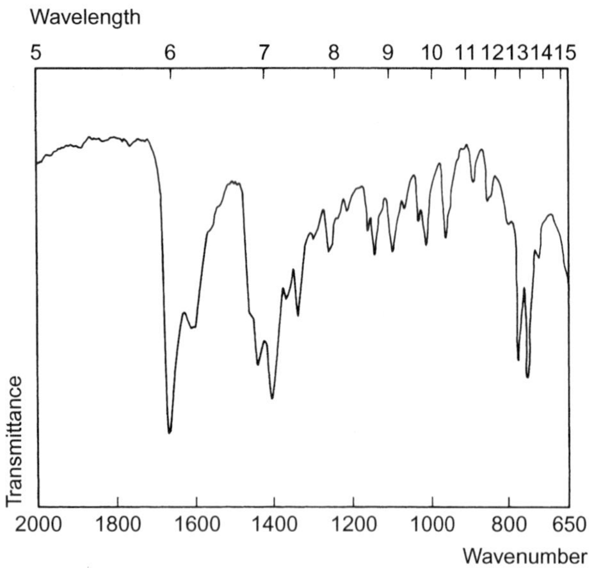

Mass Spectrum. Principal ions at *m/z* 267, 221, 207, 180, 223, 154, 196, 268.

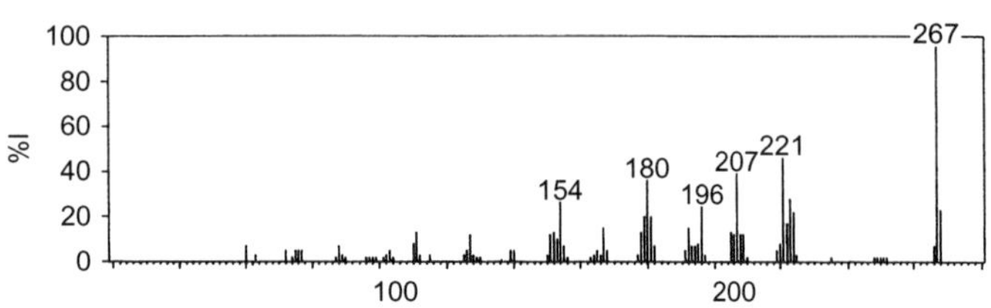

Lysergic Acid

Hallucinogen

9,10-Didehydro-6-methylergoline-8-carboxylic acid
$C_{16}H_{16}N_2O_2$=268.3
CAS—82-58-6

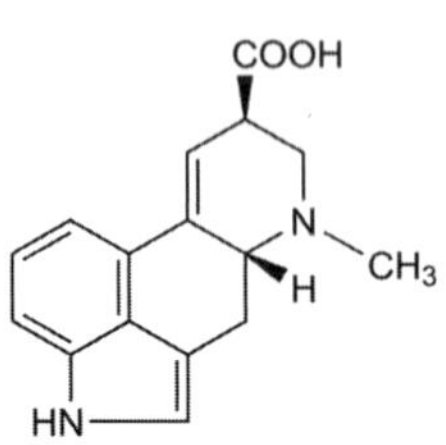

A white crystalline powder. M.p. 240°, with decomposition.

Sparingly soluble in water; soluble in dilute acids and alkalis; moderately soluble in pyridine.

Dissociation Constant. pK_a 3.4, 6.3.

Colour Tests. Mandelin's Test—green-brown; Marquis Test—brown.

Thin-layer Chromatography. System TA—Rf 58; system TB—Rf 00; system TC—Rf 00; system TD—Rf 00; system TE—Rf 00; system TF—Rf 00; system TL—Rf 00; system TM—Rf 00; system TAD—Rf 00; system TAE—Rf 70; system TAF—Rf 16; system TAJ—Rf 48; system TAK—Rf 07; system TAL—Rf 79. (Location under UV light, violet fluorescence; mercuric chloride–diphenylcarbazone reagent, blue; acidified potassium permanganate solution, positive; Van Urk reagent, blue.)

High Performance Liquid Chromatography. System HA—*k* 0.8 (tailing peak); system HP—*k* 0.00; system HY—RI 236.

Ultraviolet Spectrum. Aqueous acid—305 nm; aqueous alkali—308 nm.

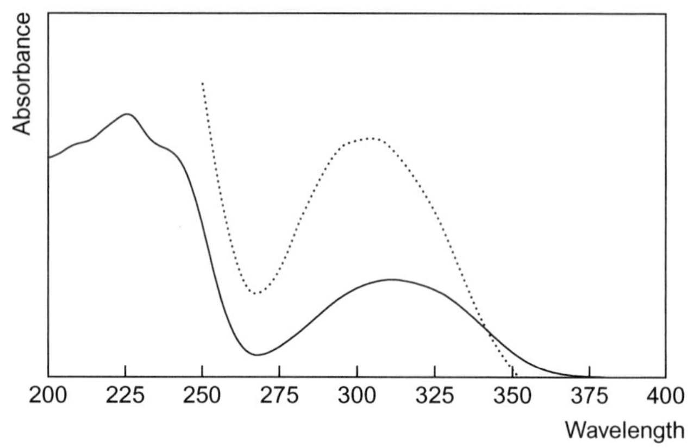

Infra-red Spectrum. Principal peaks at wavenumbers 1592, 787, 758, 1308, 691, 1015 cm^{-1}.

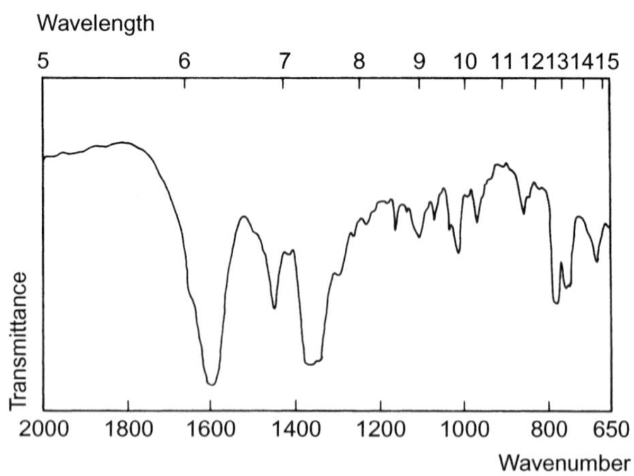

Mass Spectrum. Principal ions at *m/z* 268, 224, 154, 180, 207, 223, 192, 179.

Lysergide

Hallucinogen

Synonyms. LSD; LSD-25; Lysergic Acid Diethylamide.
9,10-Didehydro-*N*,*N*-diethyl-6-methylergoline-8β-carboxamide
$C_{20}H_{25}N_3O$=323.4
CAS—50-37-3

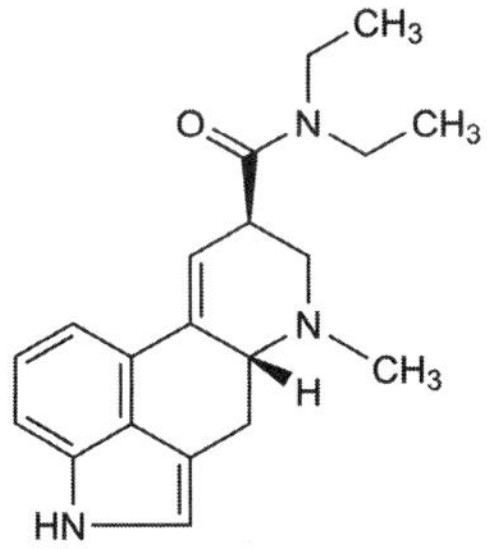

A colourless crystalline substance. M.p. 80° to 85°.
Soluble in water.
Note. There is evidence that LSD degrades readily in biological specimens when exposed to light or elevated temperatures. LSD may also bind to glass containers in acidic solutions.

Dissociation Constant. pK_a 7.5.

Partition Coefficient. Log *P* (octanol/water), 2.9.

Colour Tests. *p*-Dimethylaminobenzaldehyde—violet; Mandelin's Test—grey; Marquis Test—grey.

Thin-layer Chromatography. System TA—Rf 60; system TB—Rf 03; system TC—Rf 39; system TD—Rf 3; system TE—Rf 56; system TL—Rf 24; system TM—Rf 70; system TAE—Rf 60; system TAF—Rf 59; system TAJ—Rf 33; system TAK—Rf 02; system TAL—Rf 59. (Dragendorff spray, positive; acidified iodoplatinate solution, positive; Marquis reagent, grey; Van Urk reagent, blue.)

Gas Chromatography. System GA—LSD RI 3445, LSD-TMS RI 3595, iso-LSD-TMS RI 3515, M (nor-)-TMS RI 3705, M (nor-)-TMS_2 RI 3515, M (2-oxo-3-OH-)-TMS_2 RI 3430; system GB—LSD RI 3332; system GAL—LSD retention time 7.3 min.

High Performance Liquid Chromatography. System HA—lysergide *k* 0.7; system HP—lysergide *k* 1.83, 2-oxylysergide *k* 0.92; system HX—RI 362; system HAA—retention time 12.0 min; system HBE—retention time 5.3 min.

Ultraviolet Spectrum. Aqueous acid—315 (A^1_1=225a); aqueous alkali—310 nm.

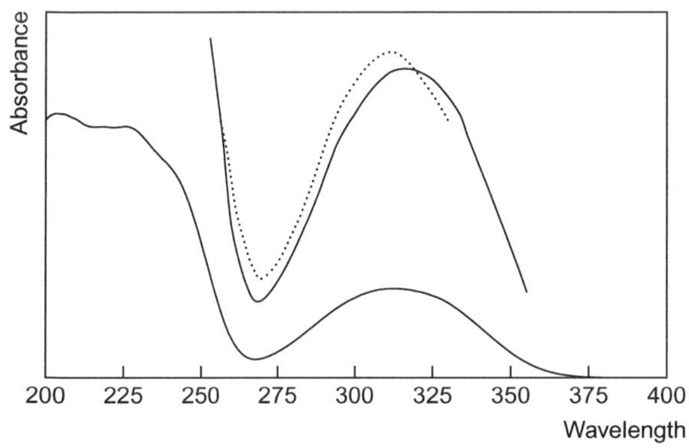

Infra-red Spectrum. Principal peaks at wavenumbers 1626, 1307, 1136, 1066, 1212, 749 cm^{-1} (KBr disk).

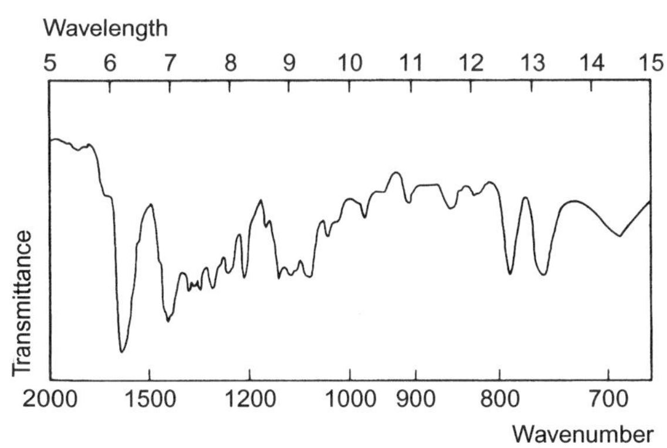

Mass Spectrum. Principal ions at *m/z* 323, 221, 181, 222, 207, 72, 223, 324.

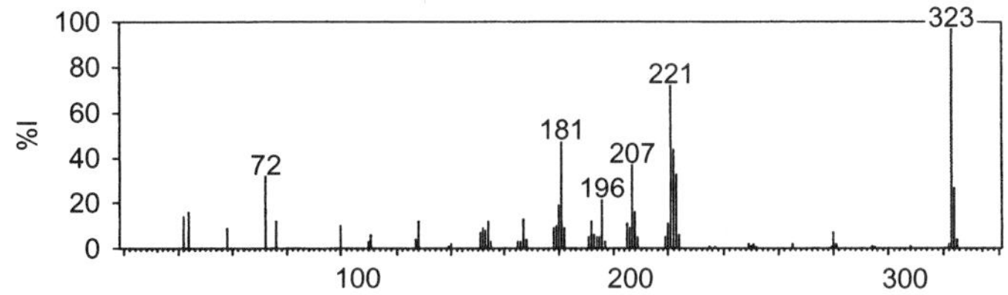

Quantification

Gas chromatography–mass spectrometry In urine: limit of detection 29 ng/L—B. D. Paul *et al.*, *J. Chromatogr.*, 1990, *529*, 103–112. In biological fluids: lysergide and its metabolites—C. C. Nelson and R. L. Foltz, *Anal. Chem.*, 1992, *64*, 1578–1585. In serum—F. Musshoff and T. Daldrup, *Forensic Sci. Int.*, 1997, *88*, 133–140. In urine: lysergide and its major metabolite, limit of detection 10 ng/L—S. A. Reuschel *et al.*, *J. Anal. Toxicol.*, 1999, *23*, 306–312.

High performance liquid chromatography. In whole blood or serum: limit of detection <0.05 µg/L—D. Bergemann *et al.*, *J. Forensic Sci.*, 1999, *44*, 372–374. In serum or hair: limit of detection 1 ng/g, fluorescence detection—J. Rohrich *et al.*, *Forensic Sci. Int.*, 2000, *107*, 181–190.

High performance liquid chromatography–mass spectrometry. In urine: limit of detection 0.5 µg/L—K. S. Webb *et al.*, *J. Forensic Sci.*, 1996, *41*, 938–946. In urine: limit of quantification 0.5 µg/L, SIM—S. A. White *et al.*, *J. Chromatogr. B Biomed. Sci. Appl.*, 1997, *689*, 335–340. In urine: limit of quantification 0.1 to 10 µg/L—S. A. White *et al.*, *J. Forensic Sci.*, 1999, *44*, 375–379. In urine: 2-oxo-3-hydroxy-lysergic acid, limit of detection 0.4 µg/L—G. K. Poch *et al.*, *J. Anal. Toxicol.*, 2000, *24*, 170–179. In blood or urine: lysergide and its metabolites—J. Canezin *et al.*, *J. Chromatogr. B Biomed. Sci. Appl.*, 2001, *765*, 15–27.

High performance liquid chromatography–radioimmunoassay. In biological fluids: limit of detection 1 µg/L, fluorescence detection—P. W. Twitchett *et al.*, *J. Chromatogr.*, 1978, *150*, 73–84.

Thin-layer chromatography (high performance). In illicit dosage forms: limit of detection 2 ng—L. Kraus *et al.*, *Bull. Narcot.*, 1980, *32*, 67–71.

Fluoroimmunoassay. In biological fluids: limit of detection 4 µg/L—A. R. Hubbard *et al.*, *Anal. Proc.*, 1983, *20*, 606–608.

Review. Methods for the determination of lysergide in body fluids—S. Schneider *et al.*, *J. Chromatogr. B Biomed. Sci. Appl.*, 1998, *13*, 189–200; S. A. Reuschel *et al.*, *J. Chromatogr. B Biomed. Sci. Appl.*, 1999, *733*, 145–159.

Note. Known interferences to LSD detection include: ergometrine, ergonovine, methylergometrine, dihydroergotamine, ergocornine, ergocristine, methysergide, and ergotamine. Several of these agents are used clinically for various medical conditions.

Disposition in the Body. Readily absorbed after oral administration. It is believed to undergo extensive biotransformation in the liver (hydroxylation and glucuronide conjugation) to inactive metabolites. A very small percentage crosses the blood–brain barrier and it is extensively bound to plasma proteins. About 1% of a dose is excreted unchanged in the urine in 24 h. 2-Oxylysergide is a major metabolite although 13-hydroxy- and 14-hydroxylysergide also appear.
As little as 0.5 to 1.5 µg/kg body weight is known to produce hallucinations. LSD is thought to produce its effects by binding to and activating the 5-hydroxytryptamine subtype 2 (5-HT_2) receptor.

Blood concentration

A single oral dose of 160 µg was administered to 13 subjects; plasma concentrations measured at intervals over a period of 2.5 h varied considerably but were in the range 0 to 9 µg/L. [D. G. Upshall and D. G. Wailling, *Clin. Chim. Acta*, 1972, *36*, 67–73.]

Single doses of 200 to 400 µg were administered to 8 subjects; the urinary concentration of lysergide or a closely related metabolite ranged from 1 to 55 µg/L in the 24 h after ingestion. [A. Taunton-Rigby *et al.*, *Science*, 1973, *181*, 165–166.]

Toxicity. Hallucinatory effects are produced with doses of 200 to 400 µg but recovery has occurred after much larger doses (up to 10 mg). Plasma concentrations greater than 1 µg/L have been associated with toxic effects.

A 25-year-old male died 16 h after being admitted to hospital. Post-mortem toxicological analysis by radioimmunoassay (RIA) and HPLC revealed the following LSD concentrations (μg/L):

Sample	RIA	HPLC
Antemortem serum	14.4	-
Antemortem plasma	14.8	8
Postmortem blood	4.8	-
Stomach content	55.2	60
Liver blood	7.2	-

[R. R. Fysh *et al.*, *Forensic Sci. Int.*, 1985, *28*, 109–113.]

Following a dinner party, 4 men and 4 women (age range 19 to 39 years) were admitted to hospital after 'snorting' 2 lines of white powder believed to be cocaine. Analysis of the white powder identified it as almost pure (80 to 90%) LSD tartrate. Emesis and collapse occurred along with signs of sympathetic overactivity, hyperthermia, coma, and respiratory arrest. Serum and gastric concetrations of LSD tartrate ranged from 2.1 to 26 μg/L and 1000 to 7000 μg/100 mL, respectively. All patients recovered with supportive care. [J. C. Klock *et al.*, *Clin. Toxicol.*, 1975, *8*, 191–203.]

Half-life. Plasma half-life, about 2.5 h.

Volume of distribution. About 0.3 L/kg.

Protein binding. In plasma, about 90%, decreasing to about 65% in overdose subjects.

Dose. In psychotherapy, doses of 100 to 750 μg have been given.

Mafenide

Sulfonamide/Antibacterial

Synonyms. Bensulfamide; Benzamsulfonamide; 4-Homosulfanilamide; Sulfabenzamine.
4-(Aminomethyl)benzenesulfonamide
$C_7H_{10}N_2O_2S = 186.2$
CAS—138-39-6

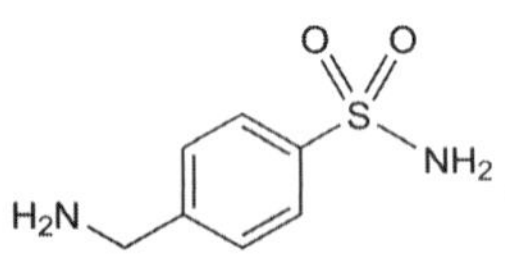

A white powder. M.p. 151° to 154°.
Sparingly soluble in water; soluble in methanol and in dilute acids and alkalis.

Mafenide Acetate

Proprietary names. Mafatate; Sulfamylon.
$C_7H_{10}N_2O_2S,C_2H_4O_2 = 246.3$
CAS—13009-99-9
A white crystalline powder. M.p. 151° to 152°.
Freely soluble in water and methanol; sparingly soluble in ethanol.

Mafenide Hydrochloride

Synonyms. Homosulfaminum; Maphenide.
$C_7H_{10}N_2O_2S,HCl = 222.7$
CAS—138-37-4
A colourless or white crystalline powder. M.p. about 260°.
Soluble 1 in 1.7 of water and 1 in 100 of ethanol; practically insoluble in chloroform and ether.

Mafenide Propionate

Proprietary name. Sulfomyl
$C_7H_{10}N_2O_2S,C_3H_6O_2 = 260.3$
CAS—12001-72-8
Colourless crystals. M.p. 158°.
Readily soluble in water.

Partition Coefficient. Log *P* (octanol/water), −0.6.

Colour Test. Koppanyi–Zwikker Test—violet.

Thin-layer Chromatography. System TA—Rf 49; system TD—Rf 01; system TE—Rf 27; system TF—Rf 01; system TAD—Rf 02; system TAE—Rf 22; system TAJ—Rf 00; system TAK—Rf 72; system TAL—Rf 93. (Acidified iodoplatinate solution, positive.)

Gas Chromatography. System GA—mafenide RI 2340; mafenide-Me_2 RI 1920; mafenide-Me_3 RI 1900; mafenide-Me_4 RI 1870; M(acetyl-) RI 2425; M(acetyl-)-Me RI 2300.

Ultraviolet Spectrum. Aqueous acid—267 (A^1_1 = 41a), 274 nm.

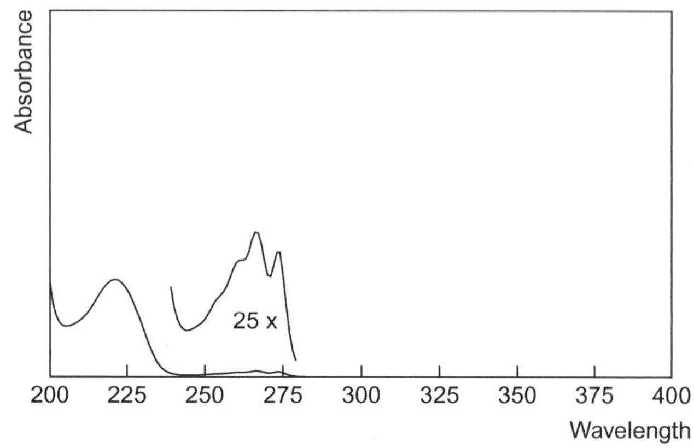

Infra-red Spectrum. Principal peaks at wavenumbers 1151, 1316, 1299, 897, 1089, 1592 cm^{-1} (KBr disk).

Mass Spectrum. Principal ions at *m/z* 106, 30, 77, 185, 105, 104, 89, 141.

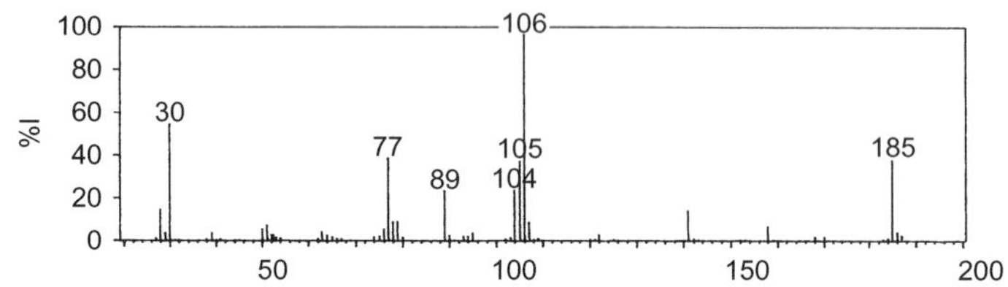

Quantification.
Thin-layer chromatography. In serum: limit of detection 1 mg/L—J. M. Steyn, *J. Chromatogr.*, 1977, *143*; *B Biomed. Appl.*, *1*, 210–213.

Disposition in the Body. Mafenide is absorbed from wounds into the circulation and metabolised to *p*-carboxybenzenesulfonamide which is excreted in the urine.

Use. Topically as a cream containing 8.5% mafenide (as the acetate).

Malathion

Pesticide

Synonyms. Carbofos; Compound 4047; OMS-1.
Proprietary names. Derbac (liquid); Prioderm; Suleo-M.
[(Dimethoxyphosphinothioyl)thio]butanedioic acid diethyl ester
$C_{10}H_{19}O_6PS_2 = 330.4$
CAS—121-75-5

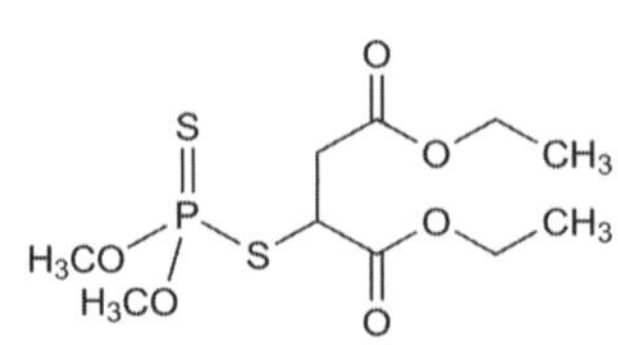

A colourless to light amber liquid which decomposes in strong acid or high humidity. Although stable in light, it decomposes at high temperatures. F.p. 2.85°. Refractive index 1.4985.
Slightly soluble in water; miscible with many organic solvents.

Partition Coefficient. Log *P* (octanol/water), 2.4.

Colour Tests. Palladium Chloride—brown; Phosphorus Test—yellow; Sodium Nitroprusside (Method 2)—violet.

Thin-layer Chromatography. System TE—Rf 99; system TW—Rf 74; system TX—Rf 31; system TY—Rf 53; system TZ—Rf 82; system TAA—Rf 33; system TAB—Rf 24; system TAC—Rf 14; system TAE—Rf 84.

Gas Chromatography. System GA—malathion RI 1925; M (malaoxon) RI 1890; system GK—RRT 1.03 (relative to caffeine).

High Performance Liquid Chromatography. System HZ—retention time, 5.4 min.

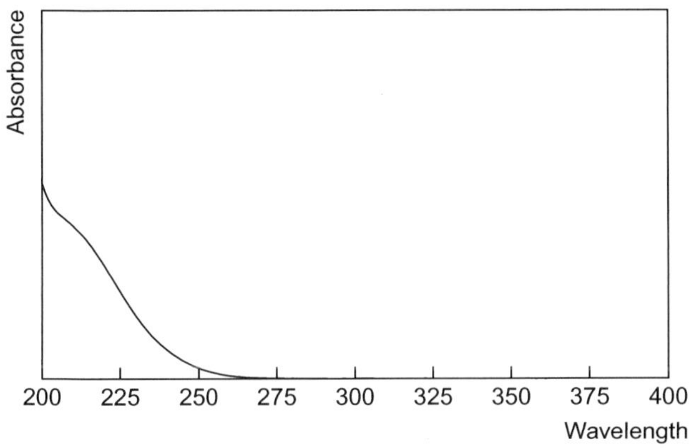

Infra-red Spectrum. Principal peaks at wavenumbers 1018, 1748, 1174, 1209, 824, 1250 cm^{-1} (thin film).

Mass Spectrum. Principal ions at *m/z* 125, 93, 127, 173, 158, 99, 55, 79.

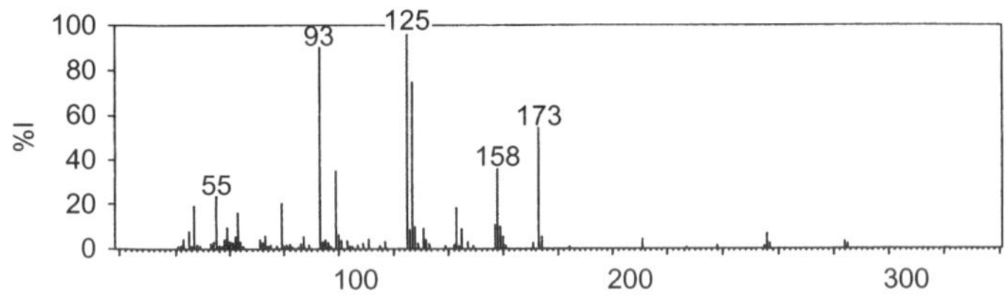

Quantification

Colorimetry. In blood or tissues—A. Faragó, *Arch. Toxicol.*, 1967, *23*, 11–16.

Gas chromatography. In urine: dialkyl phosphate residues, limits of detection 40 µg/L to 130 µg/L, FID—S. J. Reid and R. R. Watts, *J. Anal. Toxicol.*, 1981, *5*, 126–132. In urine: malathion α-mono- and dicarboxylic acid and alkyl phosphate metabolites, limit of detection 2 µg/L for the dicarboxylic acid and 5 µg/L for the α-monocarboxylic acid, FID—D. E. Bradway and T. M. Shafik, *J. Agric. Food Chem.*, 1977, *25*, 1342–1344.

For screening organophosphorus pesticides in blood using GC–MS, see F. Musshoff *et al.*, *J. Chromatogr. Sci.*, 2002, *40*, 29–34.

High performance liquid chromatography. In urine: malathion and other pesticides, limit of detection 0.05 mg/L to 6.8 mg/L, UV detection (λ=230 nm)—Y. Cho *et al.*, *Chem. Pharm. Bull. (Tokyo)*, 1997, *45*, 737–740.

High performance liquid chromatography–mass spectrometry. In urine: malathion and other pesticides, limit of detection 20 to 500 ng/L—S. E. Baker *et al.*, *J. Expo. Anal. Environ. Epidemiol.*, 2000, *10*, 789–798. In urine: malathion and metabolites, limit of detection 5 µg/L—M. D. Beeson *et al.*, *Anal. Chem.*, 1999, *71*, 3526–3530.

Thin-layer chromatography. In serum: limit of detection 0.12 mg/L. Derivatisation and UV detection—K. Futagami *et al.*, *J. Chromatogr. B Biomed. Sci. Appl.*, 1997, *704*, 369–373.

Disposition in the Body. Absorbed after oral ingestion but absorbed only slowly and to a small extent through intact skin. It is metabolised by conversion to malaoxon, the toxic keto analogue, and by hydrolysis to malathion α-mono- and dicarboxylic acids which are the major metabolites. Other hydrolysis products include dimethylthiophosphoric acid (DMTP) and dimethyldithiophosphoric acid (DMDTP) which have been detected in the urine of subjects exposed to malathion. After ingestion, up to 25% is excreted in the 24 h urine as ether-extractable phosphates, mostly in the first 8 h.

Toxicity. Malathion is less toxic than most other organophosphorus pesticides; the estimated minimum lethal dose is 25 g; the maximum permissible atmospheric concentration is 10 mg/m^3 and the maximum acceptable daily intake is 20 µg/kg.

In 6 cases of suspected poisoning caused by malathion, postmortem tissue concentrations were as follows: blood, 175 to 517 mg/L, lungs 77 to 330 µg/g, liver 198 to 383 µg/g, kidneys 280 to 616 µg/g, spleen 175 to 475 µg/g, brain 84 to 387 µg/g, heart 160 to 315 µg/g, muscles 8 to 40 µg/g, urine 33 to 189 mg/L, gastric contents 452 to 989 mg/L [R. K. Jadhav *et al.*, *Forensic Sci. Int.*, 1992, *52*, 223–229].

An 80-year-old woman who committed suicide by ingesting malathion mixed with a fruit drink had an antemortem blood concentration of 23.9 mg/L [U. Zivot *et al.*, *Am. J. Forensic Med. Pathol.*, 1993, *14*, 51–53].

In a fatality involving a 40-year-old woman who ingested a malathion-based pesticide (up to 350 to 400 mL), postmortem tissue concentrations were as follows: blood 1.7 to 1.9 mg/L, gastric contents 975 to 981 mg/L, liver not detected [T. S. Thompson *et al.*, *Forensic Sci. Int.*, 1998, *95*, 989–98].

Half-life. Derived from urinary excretion data, about 3 h.

Use. Topically in concentrations of 0.5 or 1% in the treatment of pediculosis.

Mandelic Acid

Antibacterial (Urinary)

Synonyms. Amygdalic Acid; Phenylglycollic Acid; Racemic Mandelic Acid.
Proprietary name. Uromaline
α-Hydroxybenzeneacetic acid
$C_8H_8O_3$=152.1
CAS—90-64-2; 611-72-3 (±)

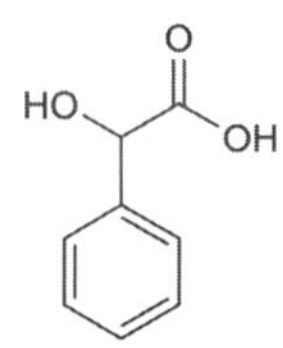

White crystals, which turn yellow on exposure to light. M.p. 119° to 121°. Soluble 1 in 6 of water, 1 in 1 of ethanol, 1 in 45 of chloroform and 1 in 6 of ether.

Ammonium Mandelate

$C_8H_7O_3NH_4$=169.2
CAS—530-31-4
A white, very hygroscopic, crystalline powder, which discolours on exposure to light.
Very soluble in water; sparingly soluble in ethanol.

Calcium Mandelate

Synonym. Calcium Amygdalate
$(C_8H_7O_3)_2Ca$=342.4
CAS—134-95-2
A white crystalline powder.
Soluble 1 in 100 of water and 1 in 4500 of ethanol (90%).

Dissociation Constant. pK_a 3.4 (25°).

Partition Coefficient. Log *P* (octanol/water), 0.6.

Thin-layer Chromatography. System TE—Rf 00; system TF—Rf 00.

Gas Chromatography. System GA—RI 1487.

Ultraviolet Spectrum. Aqueous acid—251 (A^1_1=10.9b), 257 (A^1_1=13.7b), 262 nm (A^1_1=11.2b). No alkaline shift.

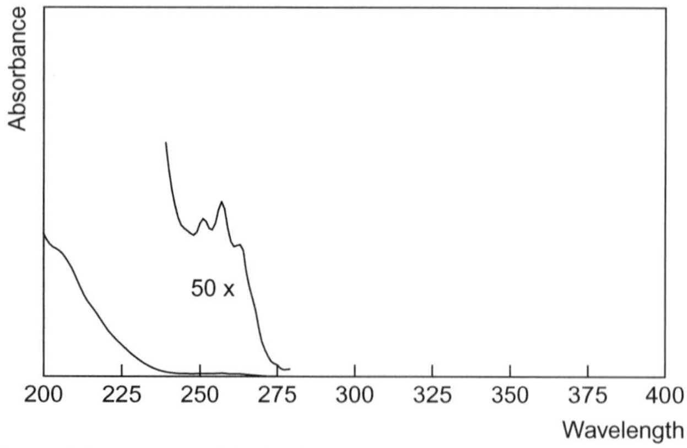

Infra-red Spectrum. Principal peaks at wavenumbers 1710, 1060, 1245, 1185, 690, 720 cm^{-1} (KBr disk).

Mass Spectrum. Principal ions at *m/z* 107, 79, 77, 51, 152, 105, 50, 78.

Quantification

Gas chromatography. In urine: mandelic and phenylglycoxylic acids, limit of detection 1 mg/L—R. L. Dills *et al.*, *Int. Arch. Occup. Environ. Health*, 1991, *62*, 603–606. In urine: mandelic and phenylglycoxylic acids, limit of detection 30 mg/L—V. L. Lanchote *et al.*, *J. Anal. Toxicol.*, 1994, *18*, 143–146. In urine: mandelic acid enantiomers, limits of detection 1 mg/L and 5 to 8 mg/L, ECD or FID—S. Kezic *et al.*, *J. Chromatogr. B. Biomed. Sci. Appl.*, 2000, *738*, 39–46.

High performance liquid chromatography. In urine: mandelic and phenylglycoxylic acids, limit of detection 5 mg/L, UV detection—S. C. Chua *et al.*, *J. Anal. Toxicol.*, 1993, *17*, 129–132. In urine: mandelic acid and other aromatic hydrocarbon metabolites—C. Burrini, *Med. Lav.*, 1998, *89*, 404–411.

Disposition in the Body. Mandelic acid is a urinary metabolite of several drugs and toxic chemicals, and is also found endogenously in normal urine at concentrations of up to 5 mg/L.

Dose. Mandelic acid has been given in doses of 12 g daily, usually as the calcium or ammonium salt.

Mannitol

Diuretic

Synonyms. NCI-C50362; Cordycepic Acid; E421; NCI-C50362; Manita; Manitol; Manna Sugar; Mannite; D-Mannitol; Mannitolum.

Proprietary names. Diosmol; Manicol; Mannidex; Osmitrol; Osmosal; Resectisol.

1,2,3,4,5,6-Hexanehexol

$C_6H_{14}O_6 = 182.2$

CAS—69-65-8

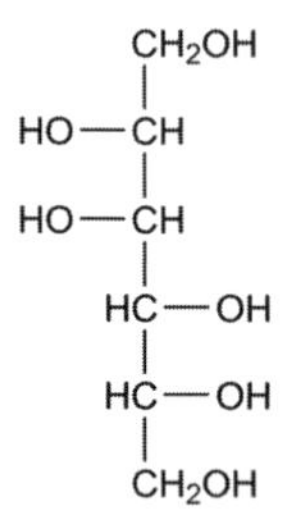

A white odourless crystalline powder or granules with a sweet taste. It is freely soluble in water (182 g/L at 25°); slightly soluble in pyridine, aniline, glycerol (1 g in 18 mL); very slightly soluble in alcohol; practically insoluble in ether. M.p. 166° to 168°. B.p. 290° to 295° at 3 to 5 mmHg.

Dissociation Constant. pK_a 13.5 (25°).

Partition Coefficient. Log *P* (octanol/water), −3.10.

Colour Test. 3 mL of 100 g/L solution of pyrocatechol with 6 mL sulfuric acid. Add 0.3 mL of a 5 g of carbon dioxide free water diluted to 50 mL with solvent. Heat for 30 s. Pink colour.

High Performance Liquid Chromatography. Column: (analytical) $LiNH_2$ (Lichrosorb NH_2, 130 × 4 mm i.d.), (guard) Co:Pell ODS (50 mm). Mobile phase: acetonitrile:deionised water (70:30), 2 mL/min flow rate. Detection: refractive index. Retention time(s): 6.8 min. [T. Mills and J. C. Roberson, *Instrumental Data for Drug Analysis*, 1993, CRC Press, Boca Raton, US. 2nd Edn, Vol. 2, pp. 1304–1305].

Column: sulfonated styrene–divinylbenzene copolymer with zinc ions (Gelpack, GL-C64Z, 150 × 6 mm i.d., 10 μm). Column temperature: 80°. Mobile phase: acetonitrile:water (80:20), flow rate 1 mL/min. MS detection (APCI (atmospheric pressure chemical ionisation), SIM at *m/z* 217 for chloride ion). Retention time(s): 12.5 min. [T. Niwa *et al.*, *J. Chromatogr.*, 1993, *613*, 9–14].

Column: (analytical) carbohydrate (Alltech 700 CH, 300 × 6.5 mm, 10 μm); (guard) carbohydrate (Alltech BC-100 Ca^{2+}). Column temperature: 85°. Mobile phase: water, 0.5 mL/min flow rate. Internal standard (IS): cellbiose. ELS detection. Retention time(s): mannitol, 13.3 min; IS, 7.6 min. [R. Marsilio *et al.*, *Clin. Chem.*, 1998, *44*, 1685–1691].

Column: HPIC-AS6 (Dionex, 250 × 40 mm). Mobile phase: 150 mM sodium hydroxide, 1.0 mL/min flow rate. Electrochemical detection. Retention time(s): 3 min. [S. C. Fleming *et al.*, *Clin. Chem.*, 1990, *36*, 797–799].

Infra-red Spectrum. Principal peaks at wavenumbers 1019, 1083, 1421, 1280 cm^{-1} (KBr pellet).

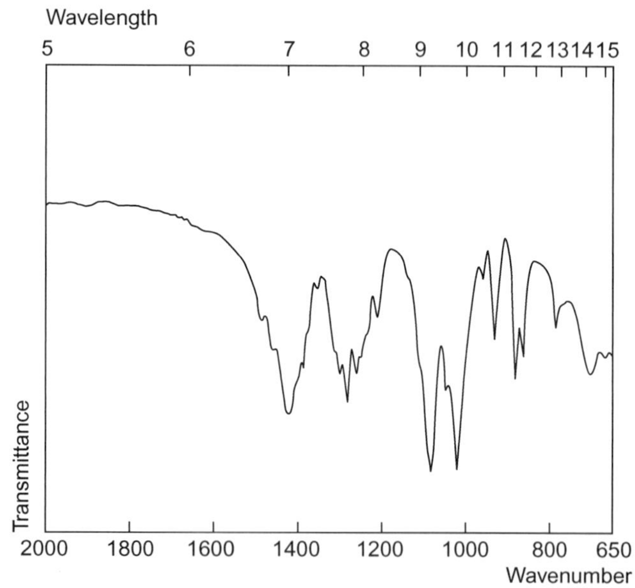

Mass Spectrum. Principal ions at *m/z* 73, 61, 103, 74, 43, 56, 45, 31 (mannitol); *m/z* 115, 187, 139, 145, 157, 170, 259, 289 (mannitol hexa-acetate).

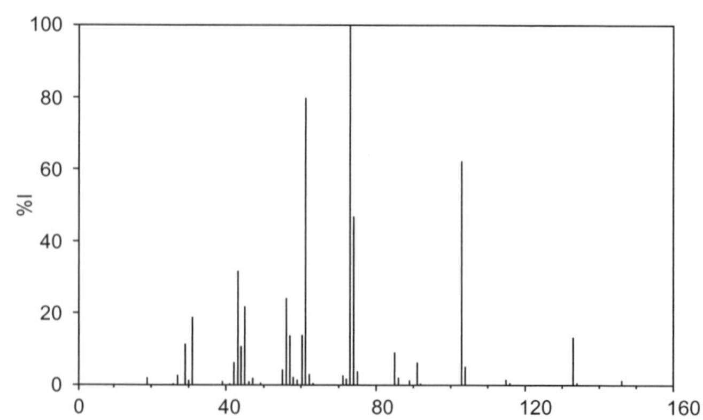

Quantification

Gas chromatography. In urine: limit of detection 0.9 μg/L. FID—R. Shippee *et al.*, *Clin. Chem.*, 1992, *38(3)*, 343–345.

High performance liquid chromatography. In urine: limit of detection 0.3 mg/L. Amperometric detection—S. C. Fleming *et al.*, *Clin. Chem.*, 1990, *36(5)*, 797–799. In urine: limit of detection 0.65 mg/L. ELS detection—R. Marsilio *et al.*, *Clin. Chem.*, 1998, *44*, 1685–1691. In blood: limit of detection 1 to 5 pg/L (benzoyl derivatives). UV detection (λ=228 nm)—J. Oehlke *et al.*, *J. Chromatogr.* 1994, *665*; *Biomed. Appl.*, 105–111.

Disposition in the Body. Only a small amount of mannitol is absorbed from the gastro-intestinal tract after ingestion and is eliminated unchanged in urine (80% within 3 h). It is metabolised only very slightly to glycogen in the liver. Following (IV) intravenous injection it is excreted rapidly by the kidneys before metabolism can take place in the liver. It is freely filtered by the glomeruli and undergoes tubular reabsorption. It does not cross the blood–brain barrier, unless in very high concentrations, or penetrate the eye. Distributed in the extracellular fluid.

Toxicity. Mannitol is mildly toxic by ingestion, intraperitoneal and intravenous routes. It may cause blood pressure elevation, bladder tubule changes, nausea or vomiting. When heated to decomposition it emits acrid smoke and fumes.

Bioavailability. Negligible oral bioavailability.

Half-life. In healthy volunteers the plasma half-life is 0.25 to 1.7 h and in those with renal failure, 6 to 36 h.

Clearance. Approx. 125 mL/h/kg in men and 116 mL/h/kg in women.

Dose. Adult: range from 50 to 100 g by intravenous infusion of a 5 to 25% solution. Children: 0.25 to 2 g/kg body weight.

Mannomustine

Antineoplastic

Synonyms. BCM; Mannitol Mustard.
Proprietary name. Degranol
1,6-Bis(2-chloroethylamino)-1,6-dideoxy-D-mannitol dihydrochloride
$C_{10}H_{22}Cl_2N_2O_4,2HCl=378.1$
CAS—551-74-6

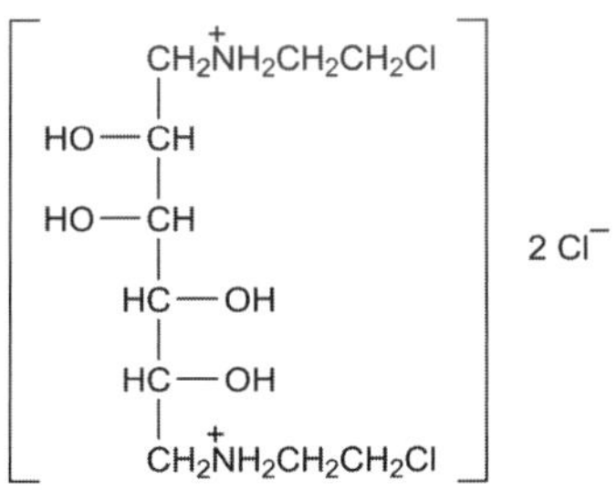

A white crystalline powder. M.p. 241°, with decomposition.
Soluble 1 in 2 of water; slightly soluble in ethanol; practically insoluble in chloroform and ether.

Partition Coefficient. Log *P* (octanol/water), −1.8.

Ultraviolet Spectrum. No significant absorption, 230 to 360 nm.

Infra-red Spectrum. Principal peaks at wavenumbers 1065, 1013, 1298, 1284, 1102, 1581 cm^{-1} (mannomustine hydrochloride, KBr disk).

Dose. Mannomustine hydrochloride has been given in doses of 50 to 100 mg daily, by intravenous injection.

Maprotiline

Antidepressant

N-Methyl-9,10-ethanoanthracene-9(10*H*)-propanamine
$C_{20}H_{23}N=277.4$
CAS—10262-69-8

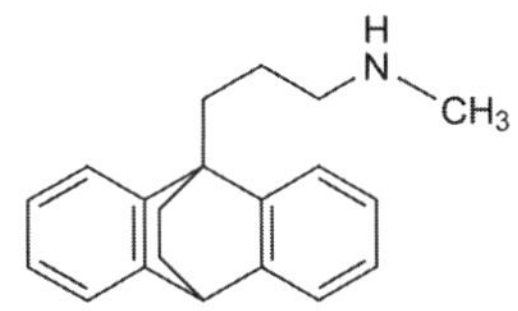

M.p. 92° to 94°.

Maprotiline Hydrochloride
Synonyms. Ba-34276; Maprotilini Hydrochloridum.
Proprietary names. Aneural; Deprilept; Ludiomil; Maludil; Maprolu; Melodil; Mirpan; Psymion.
$C_{20}H_{23}N,HCl=313.9$
CAS—10347-81-6
A white crystalline powder. M.p. 230° to 232° (from propan-2-ol).
Slightly soluble in water; freely soluble in methanol and chloroform; practically insoluble in isooctane.

Partition Coefficient. Log *P* (octanol/water), 4.5.

Colour Tests. Liebermann's Test—orange-brown; Mandelin's Test—blue; Marquis Test—red.

Thin-layer Chromatography. System TA—Rf 15; system TB—Rf 18; system TC—Rf 05; system TE—Rf 36; system TL—Rf 02; system TAE—Rf 6; system TAF—Rf 71; system TAL—Rf 50.

Gas Chromatography. System GA—maprotiline RI 2390; M (nor-) RI 2293; M (desamino-di-OH-) RI 2570; system GB—maprotiline RI 2440; M (nor-) RI 2404; M (desamino-di-OH-) RI 2603; system GM—maprotiline RRT 1.0861; M (nor-) RRT 1.107 (both relative to iprindole); system GS—maprotiline Retention time 21.0 min.

High Performance Liquid Chromatography. System HA—maprotiline *k* 2.2, desmethylmaprotiline *k* 1.1; system HF—*k* 4.92; system HX—RI 438; system HY—RI 389; system HZ—Retention time 6.6 min; system HAA—Retention time 15.5 min; system HAZ—*k* 1.44.

Ultraviolet Spectrum. Aqueous acid—265, 272 nm (A^1_1=52b).

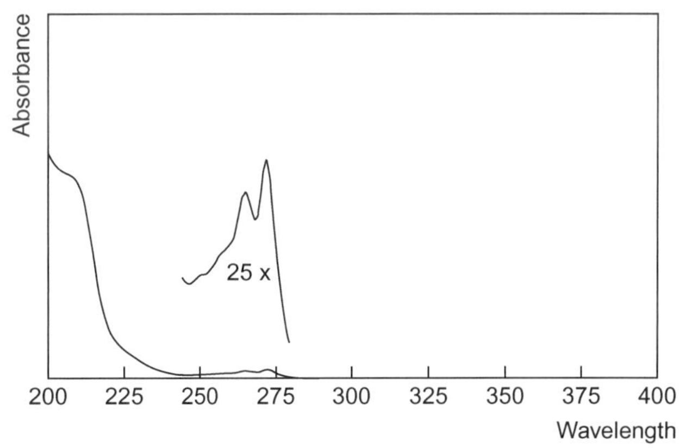

Infra-red Spectrum. Principal peaks at wavenumbers 759, 1140, 1592, 1032, 1308, 935 cm^{-1} (maprotiline hydrochloride, KBr disk).

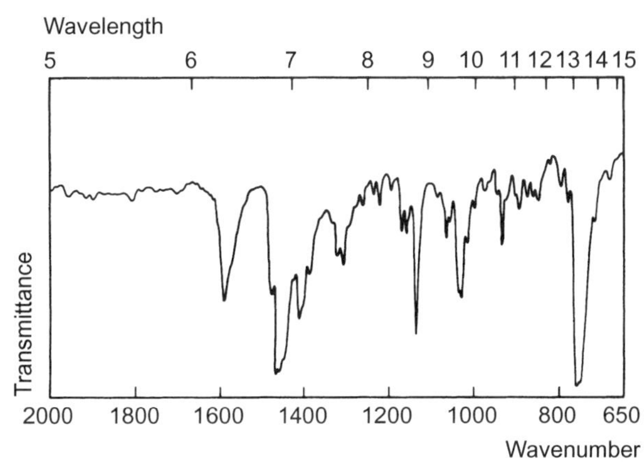

Mass Spectrum. Principal ions at *m/z* 44, 70, 59, 277, 71, 191, 278, 203.

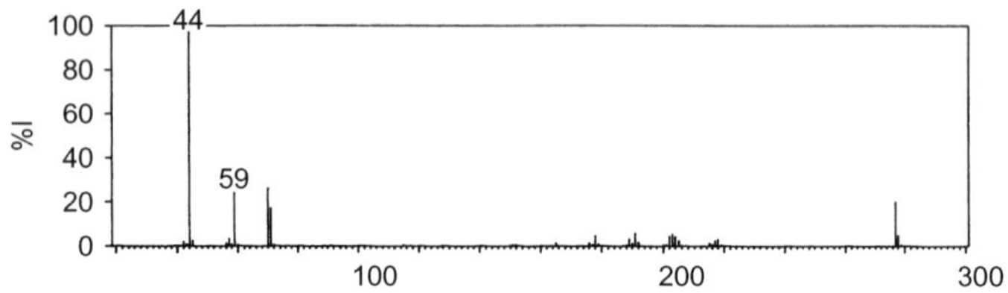

Quantification

Gas chromatography. In blood: limit of detection 20 µg/L for maprotiline and 50 µg/L for desmethylmaprotiline, AFID—A. Sioufi and A. Richard, *J. Chromatogr.*, 1980, *221*; *B Biomed. Appl.*, *10*, 393–398. In blood: limit of detection 10 µg/L, ECD—D. Alkalay *et al.*, *Anal. Lett. (Part B)*, 1982, *15*, 1493–1503. In plasma or urine: nitrogen–phosphorus detection—R. Drebit *et al.*, *J. Chromatogr.*, 1988, *432*, 334–339. In postmortem specimens: NPD—T. Keller and U. Zollinger, *Forensic Sci. Int.*, 1997, *88*, 117–123. In plasma: limit of quantification 200 µg/L, NPD—S. Ulrich and J. Martens, *J. Chromatogr. B Biomed. Sci. Appl.*, 1997, *696(2)*, 217–234.

Gas chromatography–mass spectrometry. In plasma: maprotiline and desmethylmaprotiline, limit of detection 2 µg/L—S. P. Jindal *et al., J. Pharm. Sci.*, 1980, *69*, 684–687. In whole blood: maprotiline and other tetracyclic antidepressants—A. Namera *et al.*, *J. Anal. Toxicol.*, 1998, *22*, 396–400.

High performance liquid chromatography. In plasma: maprotiline and desmethylmaprotiline, limit of detection 2 µg/L, UV detection—H. J. Kuss and E. Festenauer, *J. Chromatogr.*, 1981, *204*, 349–353. In plasma: limit of detection 0.1 µg/L, chemiluminescence detection—J. Ishida *et al.*, *J. Chromatogr. B Biomed. Appl.*, 1995, *669*, 390–396. In biological samples: maprotiline and other antidepressants, UV detection—E. Tanaka *et al.*, *J. Chromatogr. B Biomed. Sci. Appl.*, 1997, *692*, 405–412. In plasma: maprotiline and other antidepressants and their metabolites, UV detection—G. Aymard *et al.*, *J. Chromatogr. B Biomed. Sci. Appl.*, 1997, *700*, 183–189. In serum: maprotiline and other antidepressants, fluorescence detection—R. Waschgler *et al.*, *Int. J. Clin. Pharmacol. Ther.*, 2002, *40*, 554–559.

Disposition in the Body. Slowly but completely absorbed following oral administration. Concentrations in the CSF are 2 to 13% of those in serum. It is found in breast milk. It appears to undergo significant first-pass metabolism. After oral administration, about 66% of a dose is excreted in the urine and 30% in the faeces over a period of 21 days; less than 10% of the dose is excreted as unchanged drug. The principal metabolite is the desmethyl derivative, which has been shown to be active in animals, but hydroxylation also occurs to form phenolic derivatives which may be further converted to aromatic methoxy ethers or excreted as glucuronide conjugates; *N*-oxidation also occurs and maprotiline *N*-oxide has been reported to be active; numerous minor metabolites have been identified in urine.

Therapeutic concentration. Blood concentrations vary considerably between subjects and there appears to be no clear correlation between clinical response, dose, side-effects, and blood or plasma concentrations. Peak blood concentrations are usually attained 3 to 8 h after a single dose.

After a single oral dose of 75 mg to 6 subjects, peak blood concentrations of 0.012 to 0.037 mg/L (mean 0.023) and peak plasma concentrations of 0.016 to 0.031 mg/L (mean 0.024) were attained in 4 to 8 h [K. P. Maguire *et al.*, *Eur. J. Clin. Pharmacol.*, 1980, *18*, 249–254].

After daily oral doses of 50, 100, and 150 mg to 7 subjects, steady-state blood concentrations were: 0.02 to 0.15 mg/L (mean 0.07), 0.07 to 0.25 mg/L (mean 0.14), and 0.14 to 0.32 mg/L (mean 0.22) [W. Riess *et al.*, *J. Int. Med. Res.*, 1975, *3*, *Suppl. 2*, 16–41].

Following daily oral doses of 150 mg to 4 subjects for 22 days, steady-state serum concentrations of 0.05 to 0.24 mg/L of maprotiline and 0.02 to 0.13 mg/L of desmethylmaprotiline were reported [R. N. Gupta *et al.*, *Clin. Chem.*, 1977, *23*, 1849–1852].

Toxicity

The following postmortem tissue distribution was reported in a suicide case: axillary blood 6.2 mg/L, cardiac blood 2.0 mg/L, bile 161 mg/L, kidney 34.0 µg/g, liver 82.0 µg/g [A. E. Robinson *et al.*, *J. Anal. Toxicol.*, 1979, *3*, 3–13].

In a fatality due to the ingestion of 4.5 to 6 g of maprotiline, the following postmortem tissue concentrations were reported: blood 44.5 mg/L, brain 158 µg/g, liver 605 µg/g, urine 12.6 mg/L [T. A. Rejent and R. E. Doyle, *J. Anal. Toxicol.*, 1982, *6*, 199–201].

Bioavailability. About 70%.

Half-life. Plasma half-life, 20 to 70 h (mean 45).

Volume of distribution. 23 to 70 L/kg (mean 52).

Clearance. Plasma clearance, 6 to 20 mL/min/kg (mean 15).

Distribution in blood. Blood : plasma ratio, 1.7. However, the plasma:whole blood ratio has been reported to vary between individuals and may also vary between single and multiple dosing [K. P. Maguire *et al.*, *Eur. J. Clin. Pharmacol.*, 1980, *18*, 249–254].

Protein binding. In plasma, about 90%.

Note. For a review of the pharmacokinetics of maprotiline see R. M. Pinder *et al.*, *Drugs*, 1977, *13*, 321–352; for a review of the metabolism of some 'second' and 'fourth' generation antidepressants, see S. Rotzinger *et al.*, *Cell. Mol. Neurobiol.*, 1999, *19*, 427–442.

Dose. 30 to 150 mg of maprotiline hydrochloride daily; doses of up to 225 mg daily may be required in severely depressed hospitalised patients.

Mazindol

Anorectic

Proprietary names. Absten S; Dasten; Diestet; Fagolipo; Liofindol; Magrilon; Magrinex; Mazanor; Mazildene; Sanorex; Teronac.

5-(4-Chlorophenyl)-2,5-dihydro-3*H*-imidazo[2,1-*a*]isoindol-5-ol

$C_{16}H_{13}ClN_2O = 284.7$

CAS—22232-71-9

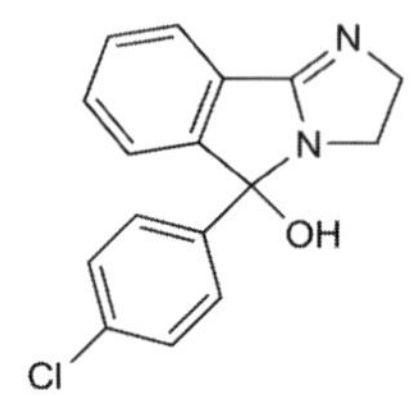

Crystals. M.p. 198° to 199°.
Insoluble in water; soluble in ethanol.

Dissociation Constant. pK_a 8.6.

Partition Coefficient. Log *P* (octanol/water), 4.1.

Colour Test. Sulfuric Acid—orange.

Thin-layer Chromatography. System TA—Rf 63; system TB—Rf 07; system TC—Rf 13; system TE—Rf 53; system TL—Rf 13; system TAE—Rf 46; system TAF—Rf 65; system TAJ—Rf 04; system TAK—Rf 00; system TAL—Rf 24.

Gas Chromatography. System GA—mazindol RI 2325; mazindol-AC RI 2705; system GB—mazindol RI 2504.

High Performance Liquid Chromatography. System HA—*k* 1.8; system HC—*k* 0.20; system HX—RI 357; system HY—RI 286; system HZ—Retention time(s), 3.6 min.

Ultraviolet Spectrum. Aqueous acid—271 nm (A^1_1 = 509a); aqueous alkali—269 (A^1_1 = 170b), 275 nm (A^1_1 = 173b).

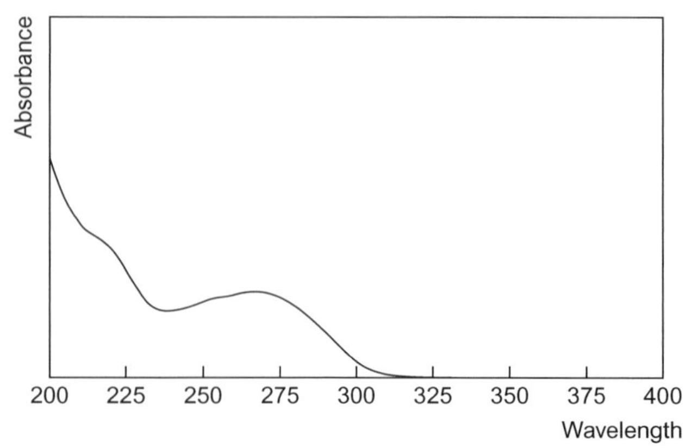

Infra-red Spectrum. Principal peaks at wavenumbers 763, 1656, 1063, 1175, 674, 1093 cm^{-1} (KBr disk).

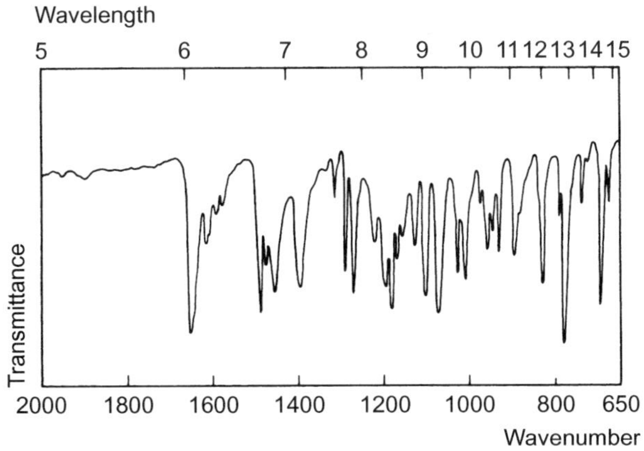

Mass Spectrum. Principal ions at *m/z* 266, 268, 267, 255, 231, 102, 88, 176.

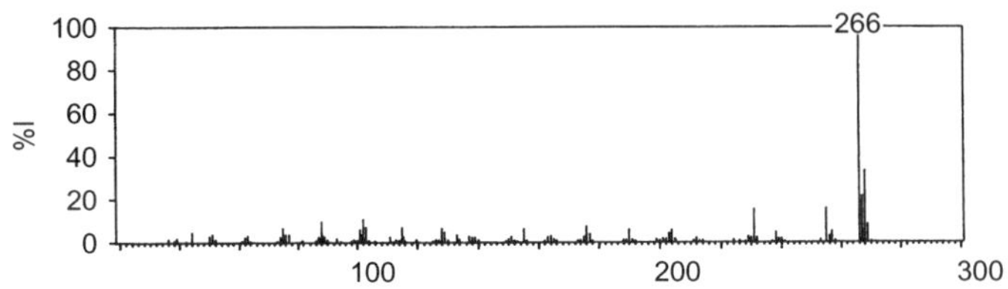

Quantification

High performance liquid chromatography. In plasma: mazindol and its major metabolite, limit of detection for mazindol 0.07 µg/L, UV detection—A. Kaddoumi *et al.*, *Analyst*, 2001, *126*, 1963–1968.

Disposition in the Body. Mazindol is absorbed after oral administration and slowly excreted in the urine, partly unchanged and partly as metabolites.

Half-life. About 12 to 24 h.

Dose. 2 to 3 mg daily.

Mebanazine

Antidepressant

α-Methylbenzylhydrazine
$C_8H_{12}N_2$ = 136.2
CAS—65-64-5

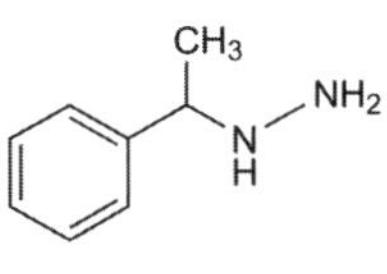

Practically insoluble in water, ethanol and ether; soluble in chloroform.

Colour Tests. Nessler's Reagent—black; Palladium Chloride—black; Sulfuric Acid—orange.

Thin-layer Chromatography. System TA—Rf 70; system TB—Rf 48; system TC—Rf 69; system TL—Rf 63.

Gas Chromatography. System GA—RI 1240.

High Performance Liquid Chromatography. System HA—*k* 0.2.

Ultraviolet Spectrum. Aqueous acid—251, 257, 261, 267 nm.

Infra-red Spectrum. Principal peaks at wavenumbers 699, 1175, 760, 1199, 1292, 1070 cm^{-1} (Nujol mull).

Dose. Mebanazine has been given in doses of 5 to 30 mg daily.

Mebendazole

Anthelmintic

Synonym. R-17635
Proprietary names. Anthex; Bantenol; Chanazole (vet.); Cipex; D-Worm; Lomper; Madicure; Menbandan; Mindol; Ovex; Ovitelmin (vet.); Oxitover; Pantelmin; Pharmamin (vet.); Pripsen; Sufil; Surfont; Telmin (vet.); Toloxim; Vermox; Wormgo; Wormstop.
Methyl-(5-benzoyl-1*H*-benzimidazol-2-yl)carbamate
$C_{16}H_{13}N_3O_3$ = 295.3
CAS—31431-39-7

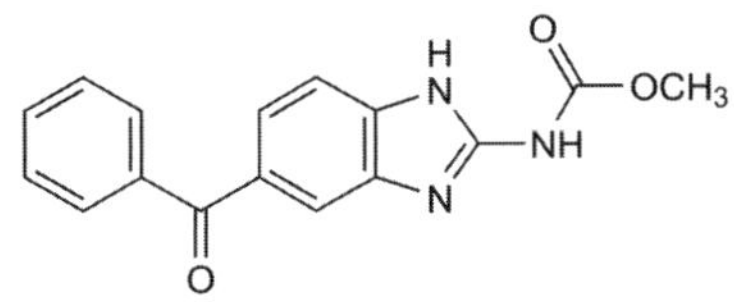

A white to slightly yellow amorphous powder. M.p. about 290°.
Practically insoluble in water, ethanol, chloroform, ether and dilute mineral acids; soluble in formic acid.

Partition Coefficient. Log *P* (octanol/water), 2.8.

Thin-layer Chromatography. System TA—Rf 65; system TB—Rf 00; system TC—Rf 59; system TE—Rf 60; system TL—Rf 49; system TAE—Rf 80; system TAF—Rf 84; system TAJ—Rf 58; system TAK—Rf 57; system TAL—Rf 93. (Dragendorff spray.)

High Performance Liquid Chromatography. System HX—RI 438; system HY—RI 322; system HAA—Retention time(s), 16.1 min.

Ultraviolet Spectrum. Acid isopropyl alcohol—234 (A^1_1 = 1000b), 288 nm (A^1_1 = 524b); alkaline isopropyl alcohol—270 (A^1_1 = 802b), 355 nm (A^1_1 = 653b).

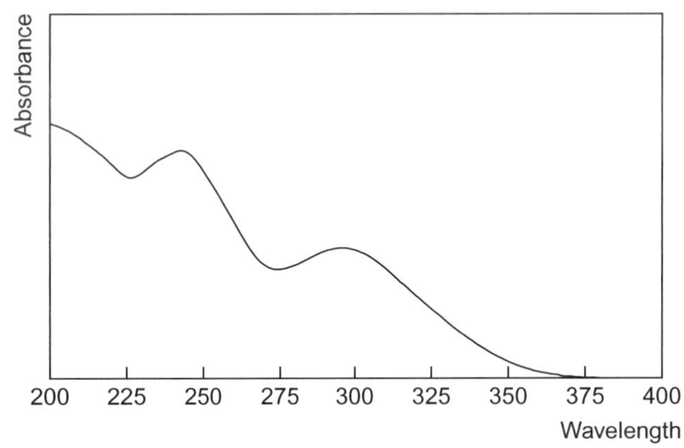

Infra-red Spectrum. Principal peaks at wavenumbers 1635, 1260, 1590, 1730, 1230, 705 cm^{-1} (KBr disk).

Mass Spectrum. Principal ions at *m/z* 186, 218, 77, 295, 263, 105, 51, 158.

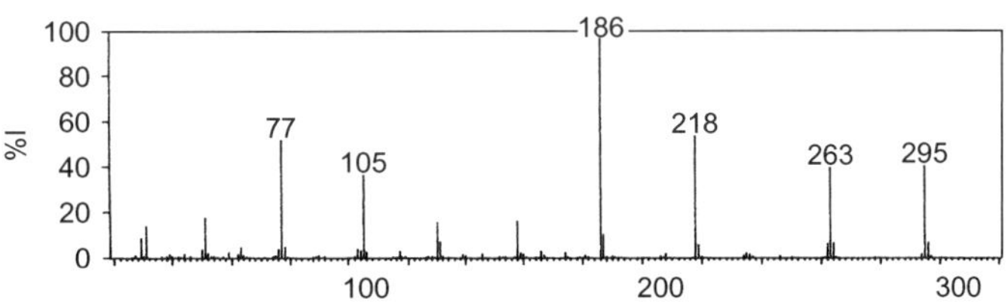

Quantification

High performance liquid chromatography. In plasma: limit of detection 10 µg/L for mebendazole, 60 µg/L for the 5-(α-hydroxy) metabolite and 30 µg/L for the 2-amino metabolite, UV detection—R. J. Allan *et al.*, *J. Chromatogr.*, 1980, *183*; *Biomed. Appl.*, *9*, 311–319. In serum: mebendazole and its metabolites, coulometric detection—P. Betto *et al.*, *J. Chromatogr.*, 1991, *563*, 115–123.

Disposition in the Body. Mebendazole is poorly absorbed after oral administration. It is metabolised to the 5-(α-hydroxy) derivative and by decarboxylation to the 2-amino metabolite, both of which are detectable in plasma at concentrations higher than those of unchanged mebendazole. Less than 10% of a dose is excreted in the urine; the major urinary metabolite is the 2-amino-5-(α-hydroxy) derivative. Biliary excretion and enterohepatic circulation have been reported.

Therapeutic concentration

Following single oral doses of 10 mg/kg to 5 subjects, peak plasma concentrations of 0.018 to 0.116 (mean 0.07) mg/L were attained in 2.5 to 7 (mean 5) h. [P. A. Braithwaite *et al.*, *Eur. J. Clin. Pharmacol.*, 1982, *22*, 161–169].

Half-life. Plasma half-life, 1.5 to 9 h.

Volume of distribution. About 2 L/kg.

Distribution in Blood. Plasma : whole blood ratio, about 1.2.

Protein binding. In plasma, about 95%.

Dose. Usually 200 mg daily for 3 days.

Mebeverine

Antispasmodic

3,4-Dimethoxybenzoic acid 4-[ethyl[2-(4-methoxyphenyl)-1-methylethyl]amino]-butyl ester

$C_{25}H_{35}NO_5=429.6$

CAS—3625-06-7

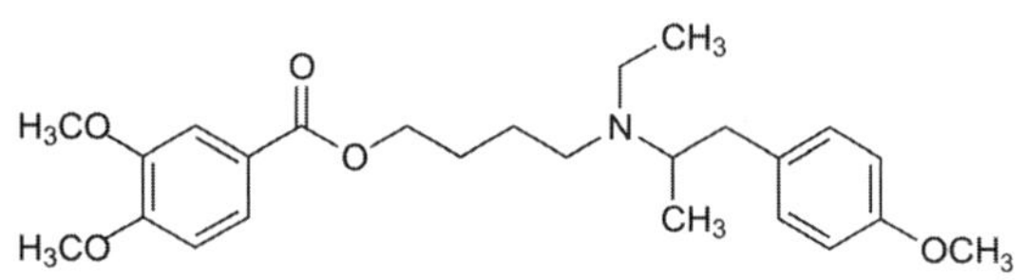

Soluble in chloroform.

Mebeverine Hydrochloride

Synonym. CSAG 144

Proprietary names. Bevispas; Colese; Colofac; Colopriv; Colotal; Duspatal; Duspatalin; Equilon; Mebemerck; Mebetin; Monosor; Spasmonal; Spasmopriv.

$C_{25}H_{35}NO_5,HCl=466.0$

CAS-2753-45-9

A white crystalline powder. M.p. 131° to 136°.

Soluble in water and ethanol; sparingly soluble in ether.

Partition Coefficient. Log *P* (octanol/water), 5.1.

Colour Test. Liebermann's Test—black.

Thin-layer Chromatography. System TA—Rf 63; system TB—Rf 40; system TC—Rf 53; system TE—Rf 86; system TL—Rf 49; system TAE—Rf 32. (Acidified iodoplatinate solution, positive.)

Gas Chromatography. System GA—RI 3045.

High Performance Liquid Chromatography. System HA—*k* 1.9; system HX—RI 448; system HZ—Retention time(s), 7.1 min.

Ultraviolet Spectrum. Aqueous acid—262 nm ($A_1^1=307b$); aqueous alkali—269, 290 nm.

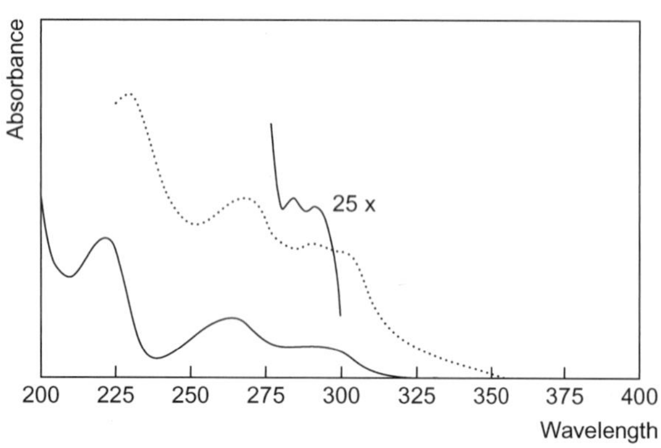

Infra-red Spectrum. Principal peaks at wavenumbers 1216, 1266, 1132, 1510, 1715, 1174 cm^{-1} (mebeverine hydrochloride, KBr disk).

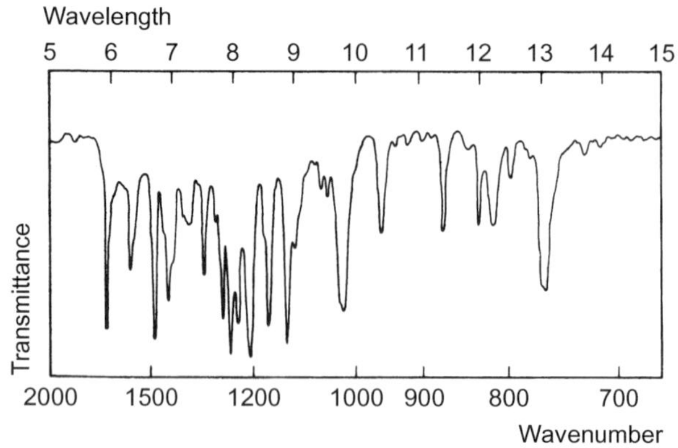

Mass Spectrum. Principal ions at *m/z* 308, 165, 309, 121, 55, 154, 98, 56.

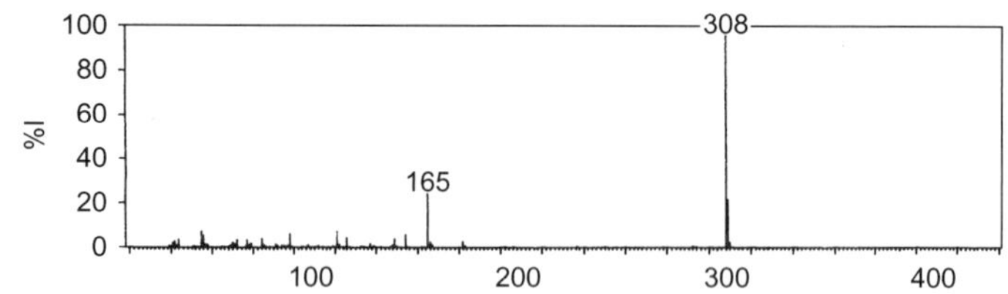

Quantification

Gas chromatography–mass spectrometry. In plasma: mebeverine alcohol and desmethylmebeverine alcohol, limit of detection 0.5 μg/L, SIM—L. J. Tulich *et al.*, *J. Chromatogr.* 1996, *682*; *Biomed. Appl.*, 273–281.

Disposition in the Body. Mebeverine is metabolised to 4-methoxyethylamfetamine.

Toxicity

In a fatality attributed to the ingestion of mebeverine and thioridazine, the following postmortem concentrations were reported: mebeverine, blood 36 mg/L, liver 15 μg/g, urine 24 mg/L; thioridazine, not detected in blood and urine, liver 2 μg/g [G. del Villar, *Bull. Int. Assoc. Forensic Toxicol.*, 1977, *13*(1&2), 23–24].

Dose. 405 mg of mebeverine hydrochloride daily.

Mebezonium Iodide

Muscle Relaxant

Proprietary name. It is an ingredient of Tanax (vet.).

4,4′-Methylenebis(cyclohexyltrimethylammonium)diiodide

$C_{19}H_{40}I_2N_2=550.3$

CAS—7681-78-9

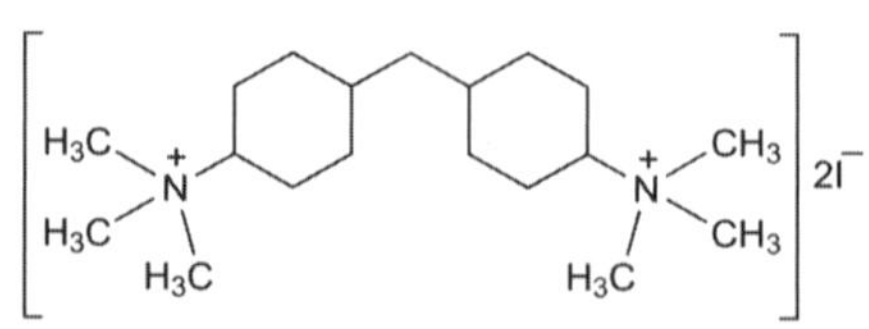

A white crystalline powder. M.p. 260°, with decomposition.

Soluble in water.

Thin-layer Chromatography. System TA—Rf 00. (Acidified iodoplatinate solution, positive.)

Infra-red Spectrum. Principal peaks at wavenumbers 961, 888, 831, 1621, 985, 1020 cm^{-1} (KBr disk).

Quantification

Thin-layer chromatography–ultraviolet spectrophotometry. In blood or urine—E. Bertol *et al.*, *J. Pharm. Biomed. Anal.*, 1983, 1, 373–377.

Disposition in the Body

Toxicity

In 3 fatalities due to the injection of a preparation containing mebezonium iodide and embutramide, the following postmortem concentrations (mg/L) were reported:

	Mebezonium iodide	Embutramide
Blood	4.5, 6.0, 7.5	3.0, 15.5, 12.1
Urine	0.8, 2.0, 1.8	2.0, 6.3, 4.5

[E. Bertol *et al.*, *J. Pharm. Biomed. Anal.*, 1983, *1*, 373–377].

Mebhydrolin

Antihistamine

2,3,4,5-Tetrahydro-2-methyl-5-(phenylmethyl)-1*H*-pyrido[4,3-*b*]indole
$C_{19}H_{20}N_2$=276.4
CAS—524-81-2

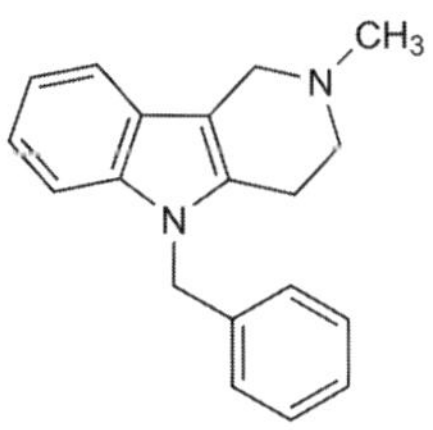

A white crystalline powder. M.p. 95°.
Practically insoluble in water; freely soluble in ethanol, methanol, chloroform and acetone; slightly soluble in ether.

Mebhydrolin Napadisilate

Synonyms. Diazolinum; Mebhydrolin Naphthalenedisulphonate.
Proprietary names. Dayhist; Fabahistin; Incidal; Omeril; Posidol.
$(C_{19}H_{20}N_2)_2,C_{10}H_8O_6S_2$=841.1
CAS—6153-33-9
A white powder. M.p. 280°, with decomposition.
Practically insoluble in water; sparingly soluble in hot glacial acetic acid; soluble in hot formamide.

Dissociation Constant. pK_a 6.7.

Partition Coefficient. Log *P* (octanol/water), 3.8.

Colour Tests. Mandelin's test—blue; Marquis test—grey-blue.

Thin-layer Chromatography. System TA—Rf 57; system TB—Rf 27; system TC—Rf 45; system TE—Rf 65; system TL—Rf 20; system TAE—Rf 36; system TAF—Rf 46. (Acidified iodoplatinate solution, positive.)

Gas Chromatography. System GA—RI 2450; system GB—RI 2575; system GC—RI 2739; system GF—RI 2920.

High Performance Liquid Chromatography. System HA—*k* 3.0 (tailing peak); system HX—RI 411; system HZ—Retention time(s), 5.3 min.

Ultraviolet Spectrum. Aqueous acid—286 (A_1^1=409b), 320 nm.

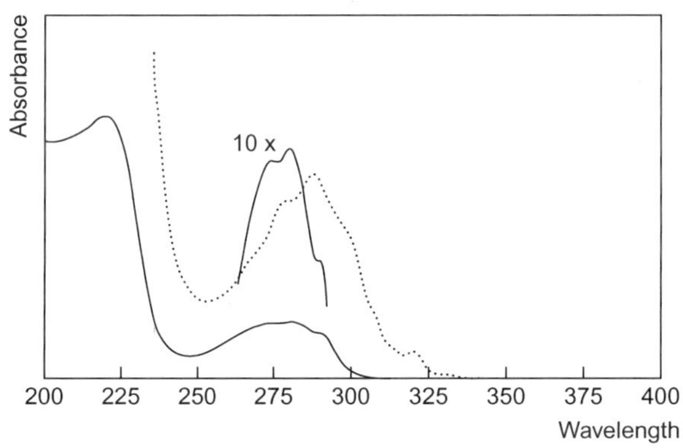

Infra-red Spectrum. Principal peaks at wavenumbers 737, 1134, 1316, 695, 1122, 1212 cm^{-1} (thin film).

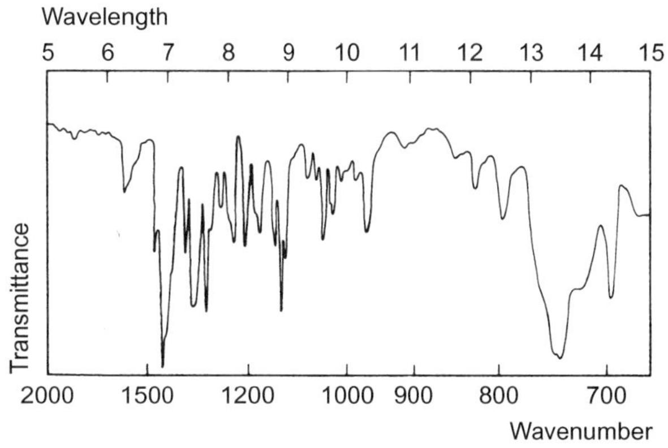

Mass Spectrum. Principal ions at *m/z* 91, 233, 30, 232, 31, 276, 275, 65.

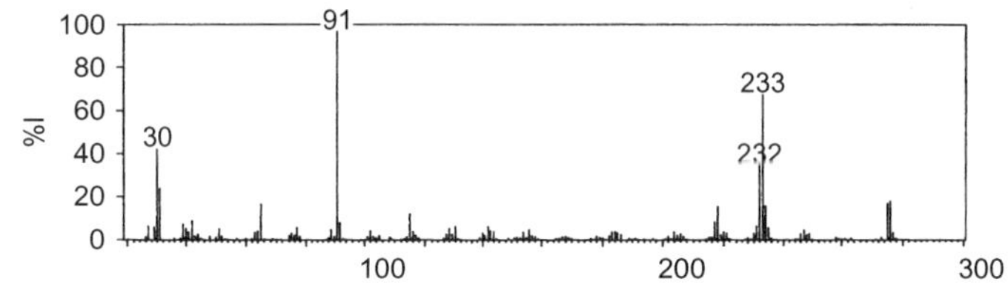

Dose. 150 to 300 mg daily.

Mebutamate

Tranquilliser

Proprietary names. Axiten; Butatensin; Capla; Carbuten; Dormate; Ipotensivo; Mebutina; No-Press; Prean; Sigmafon; Vallene.
2-Methyl-2-(1-methylpropyl)-1,3-propanediol dicarbamate
$C_{10}H_{20}N_2O_4$=232.3
CAS—64-55-1

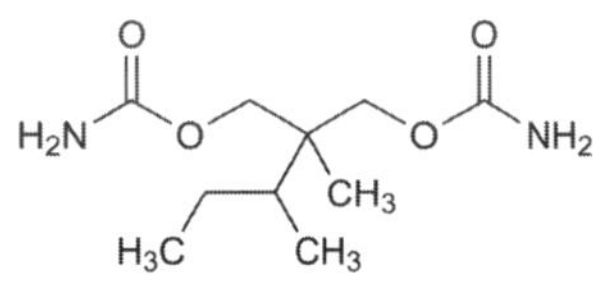

A white crystalline powder. M.p. 77° to 79°.
Slightly soluble in water; soluble in most organic solvents.

Partition Coefficient. Log *P* (octanol/water), 1.4.

Colour Tests. Furfuraldehyde—black; Nessler's Reagent—brown (slow).

Thin-layer Chromatography. System TB—Rf 00; system TC—Rf 33; system TD—Rf 10; system TE—Rf 60; system TF—Rf 35; system TL—Rf 56; system TAD—Rf 35; system TAE—Rf 82; system TAF—Rf 85; system TAJ—Rf 35; system TAK—Rf 47; system TAL—Rf 87.

Gas Chromatography. System GA—RI 1889.

Ultraviolet Spectrum. No significant absorption, 230 to 360 nm.

Infra-red Spectrum. Principal peaks at wavenumbers 1682, 1070, 1710, 1601, 1140, 788 cm^{-1} (KBr disk).

Mass Spectrum. Principal ions at *m/z* 97, 55, 69, 72, 71, 98, 43, 62.

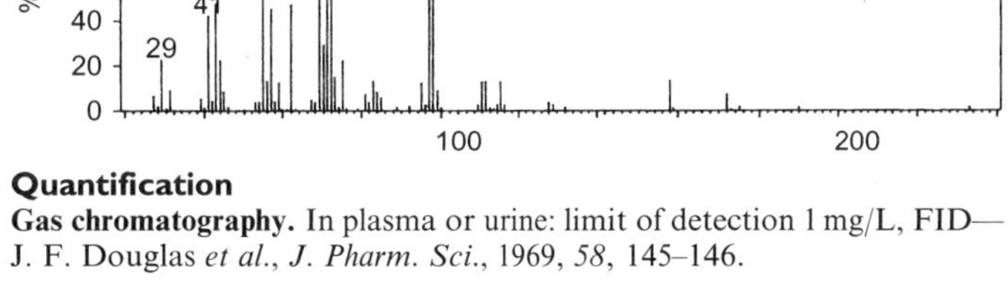

Quantification

Gas chromatography. In plasma or urine: limit of detection 1 mg/L, FID—J. F. Douglas *et al.*, *J. Pharm. Sci.*, 1969, *58*, 145–146.

Dose. 0.9 to 1.2 g daily.

Mecamylamine

Antihypertensive

N-2,3,3-Tetramethylbicyclo[2.2.1]heptan-2-amine
$C_{11}H_{21}N$=167.3
CAS—60-40-2

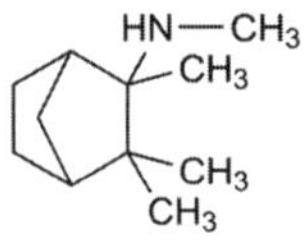

An oily liquid.
Slightly soluble in water.

Mecamylamine Hydrochloride
Proprietary names. Inversine; Mevasine.
$C_{11}H_{21}N,HCl$=203.8
CAS—826-39-1
A white crystalline powder. M.p. about 245°, with decomposition.
Soluble 1 in 5 of water and 1 in 12 of ethanol; freely soluble in chloroform; practically insoluble in ether.

Dissociation Constant. pK_a 11.3.

Partition Coefficient. Log *P* (octanol/water), 3.3.

Thin-layer Chromatography. System TA—Rf 16; system TB—Rf 51; system TC—Rf 02; system TL—Rf 04; system TAJ—Rf 00; system TAK—Rf 16; system TAL—Rf 58.

High Performance Liquid Chromatography. System HA—*k* 1.7.

Ultraviolet Spectrum. No significant absorption, 230 to 360 nm.

Infra-red Spectrum. Principal peaks at wavenumbers 1111, 1068, 1078, 1592, 1098, 890 cm^{-1} (mecamylamine hydrochloride, Nujol mull).

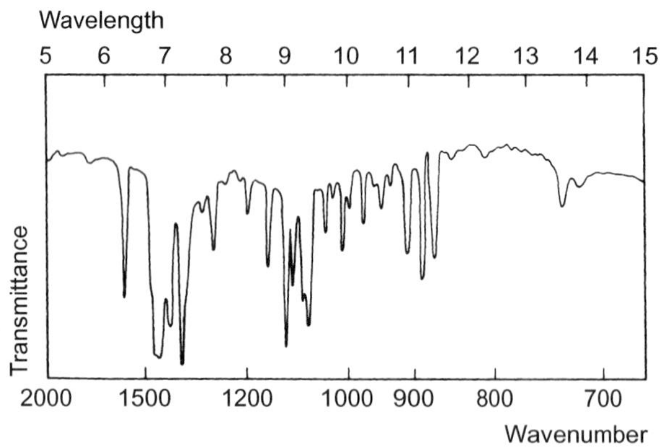

Mass Spectrum. Principal ions at *m*/*z* 98, 84, 71, 56, 41, 42, 99, 124.

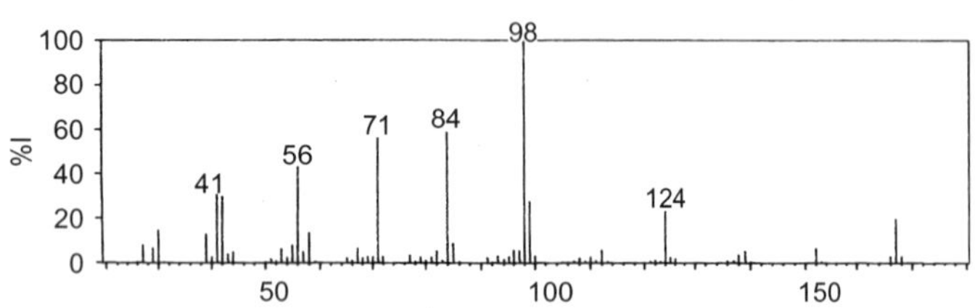

Quantification
Gas chromatography–mass spectrometry. In plasma: mecamylamine, nicotine and cotinine, limit of detection for mecamylamine <2 µg/L—P. Jacob *et al.*, *J. Pharm. Biomed. Anal.*, 2000, *23*, 653–661.

Disposition in the Body. Mecamylamine is almost completely absorbed after oral administration; high concentrations are found in the liver and kidney. More than 50% of a dose is excreted in 24 h as unchanged drug in acid urine; the excretion is reduced if the urine is alkaline.

Dose. 5 to 30 mg of mecamylamine hydrochloride daily.

Meclofenamic Acid

Analgesic

Synonyms. CI-583; INF-4668.
Proprietary names. Arquel (vet.); Lenidolor; Movens.
2-[(2,6-Dichloro-3-methylphenyl)amino]benzoic acid
$C_{14}H_{11}Cl_2NO_2$=296.2
CAS—644-62-2

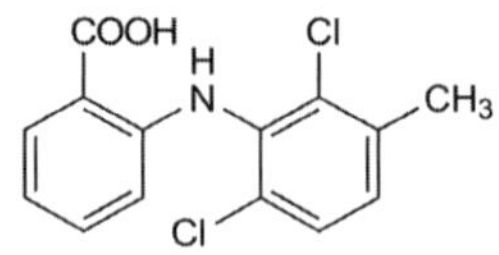

White crystals. M.p. 257° to 259° also reported as 248° to 250°.
Practically insoluble in water.

Meclofenamate Sodium
Proprietary names. Lenidolor; Meclodol; Meclomen; Movens.
$C_{14}H_{10}Cl_2NNaO_2$=318.1
CAS—6385-02-0
M.p. 289° to 291°.
Sparingly soluble in water.

Partition Coefficient. Log *P* (octanol/water), 6.0.

Thin-layer Chromatography. System TE—Rf 12; system TF—Rf 43; system TG—Rf 38; system TAJ—Rf 59; system TAK—Rf 77; system TAL—Rf 92. (Chromic acid solution, violet.)

Gas Chromatography. System GA—RI 2420; system GD—Retention time of methyl derivative 1.62 relative to *n*-$C_{16}H_{34}$; system GL—meclofenamic acid-Me RI 2240.

High Performance Liquid Chromatography. Meclofenamic acid is used as a reference substance in System HV. System HX—RI 653; system HY—RI 690.

Ultraviolet Spectrum. Aqueous alkali—275 (A_1^1= 240b), 319 nm (A_1^1=180b); methanol—242 (A_1^1=342b), 282 (A_1^1=235b), 331 nm (A_1^1=235b).

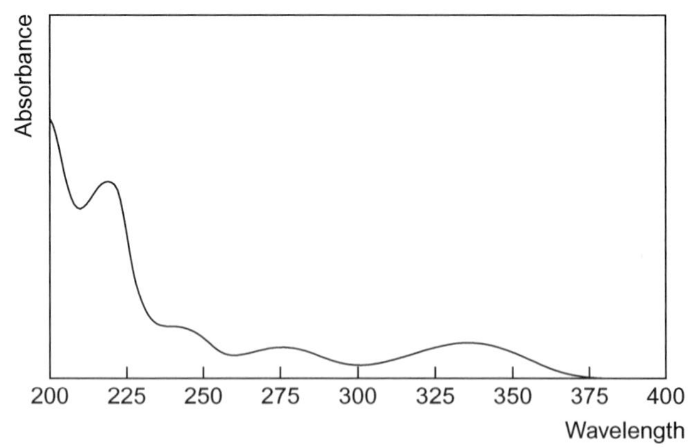

Dose. The equivalent of 200 to 400 mg of meclofenamic acid daily.

Meclofenoxate

Central Stimulant

Synonyms. Centrophenoxine; Clofenoxine; Clophenoxate; Deanol 4-Chlorophenoxyacetate; Meclofenoxane; ANP-235.
(4-Chlorophenoxy)-acetic acid 2-(dimethylamino)-ethyl ester
$C_{12}H_{16}ClNO_3$=257.7
CAS—51-68-3

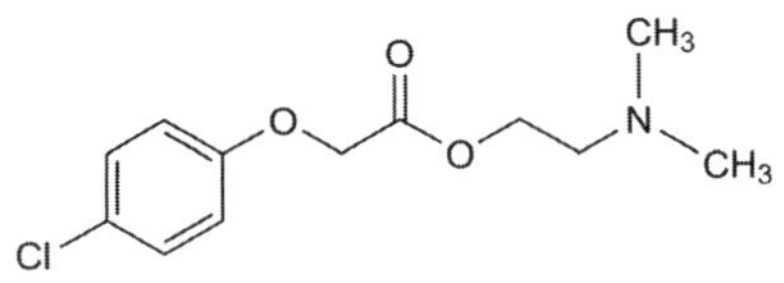

Meclofenoxate Hydrochloride

Proprietary names. Cerutil; Helfergin; Lucidril.
$C_{12}H_{16}ClNO_3,HCl$=294.2
CAS—3685-84-5
A white powder. M.p. 136°.
Soluble in cold water; sparingly soluble in cold isopropyl alcohol and acetone; practically insoluble in benzene, ether and chloroform. It rapidly hydrolyses in aqueous solution.

Partition Coefficient. Log *P* (octanol/water), 2.0.

Thin-layer Chromatography. System TA—Rf 77; system TB—Rf 26; system TC—Rf 42; system TE—Rf 67; system TL—Rf 22; system TAE—Rf 46. (Acidified potassium permanganate solution, positive.)

Gas Chromatography. System GA—RI 1770, system GB—RI 1804; system GC—RI 2200.

High Performance Liquid Chromatography. System HA—*k* 1.7.

Ultraviolet Spectrum. Aqueous acid—277 nm (A^1_1 = 44a).

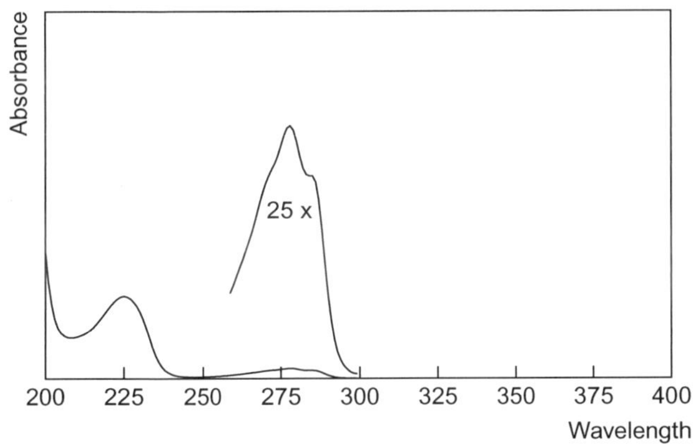

Infra-red Spectrum. Principal peaks at wavenumbers 1167, 1183, 1742, 1080, 833, 1768 cm^{-1} (KBr disk).

Mass Spectrum. Principal ions at *m/z* 58, 111, 71, 42, 75, 59, 141, 113.

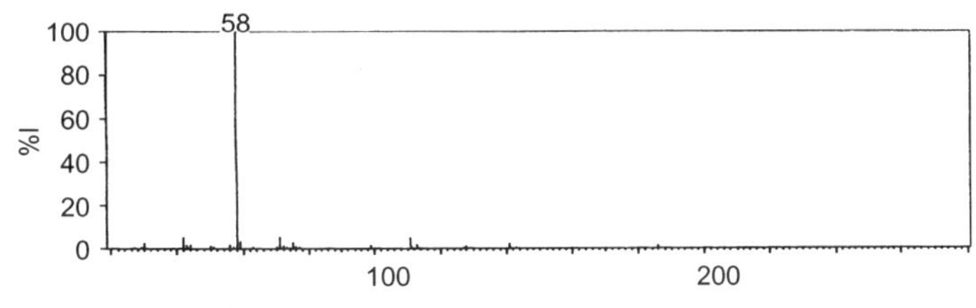

Dose. 0.9 to 1.5 g of meclofenoxate hydrochloride daily.

Mecloqualone

Hypnotic

Proprietary name. Nubarene
3-(2-Chlorophenyl)-2-methyl-4(3*H*)-quinazolinone
$C_{15}H_{11}ClN_2O$=270.7
CAS—340-57-8

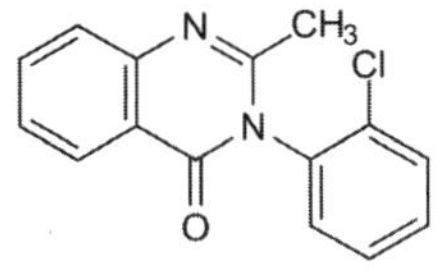

Crystals. M.p. 126° to 128°.

Partition Coefficient. Log *P* (octanol/water), 4.4.

Thin-layer Chromatography. System TB—Rf 25; system TE—Rf 76; system TAE—Rf 80; system TAJ—Rf 77; system TAK—Rf 68; system TAL—Rf 96.

Gas Chromatography. System GA—RI 2255.

High Performance Liquid Chromatography. System HX—RI 482.

Infra-red Spectrum. Principal peaks at wavenumbers 1682, 1605, 768, 782, 1282, 1583 cm^{-1}.

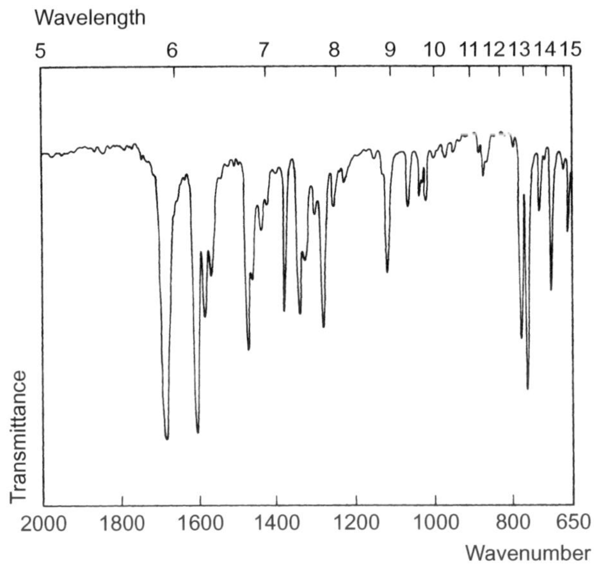

Dose. 150 to 300 mg, as a hypnotic.

Meclozine

Antihistamine

Synonyms. Histamethizine; Meclizine; Parachloramine.
1-[(4-Chlorophenyl)phenylmethyl]-4-[(3-methylphenyl)methyl]piperazine
$C_{25}H_{27}ClN_2$=391.0
CAS—569-65-3

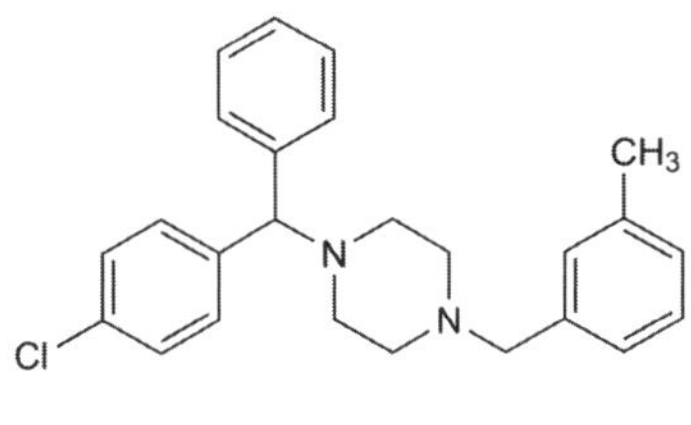

Meclozine Hydrochloride

Synonyms. Meclizine Hydrochloride; Meclizinium Chloride; Parachloramine Hydrochloride.
Proprietary names. Agyrax; Ancolan; Antivert; Antrizine; Bonamine; Bonine; Calmonal; Chiclida; Dizmiss; Dramamine II; Dramine; Duremesan; Marevit; Meni-D; Navicalm; Peremesin; Postafen(e); Sea-legs; Suprimal; Vergon; Vertin.
$C_{25}H_{27}ClN_2,2HCl,H_2O$=481.9
CAS—1104-22-9 (anhydrous); 31884-77-2 (monohydrate)
A white or slightly yellowish crystalline powder. M.p. 217° to 224°, with decomposition.
Soluble 1 in 1000 of water, 1 in 25 of ethanol, and 1 in 5 of chloroform; practically insoluble in ether; freely soluble in pyridine.

Dissociation Constant. pK_a 3.1, 6.2 (25°).

Partition Coefficient. Log *P* (octanol/water), 5.9.

Colour Test. Liebermann's Test—red-orange.

Thin-layer Chromatography. System TA—Rf 76; system TB—Rf 61; system TC—Rf 79; system TE—Rf 87; system TL—Rf 70; system TAE—Rf 80; system TAF—Rf 88; system TAJ—Rf 65; system TAK—Rf 24; system TAL—Rf 95. (Dragendorff spray, positive; acidified iodoplatinate solution, positive; Marquis reagent, brown-yellow; ninhydrin spray, positive.)

Gas Chromatography. System GA—meclozine RI 3035, M (*N*-desalkyl-) RI 2520; system GB—RI 3193.

High Performance Liquid Chromatography. System HA—*k* 0.7; system HX—RI 587; system HY—RI 398; system HAA—Retention time 20.0 min.

Ultraviolet Spectrum. Ethanol—230 (A^1_1=391a), 266 (A^1_1=27b), 273 nm.

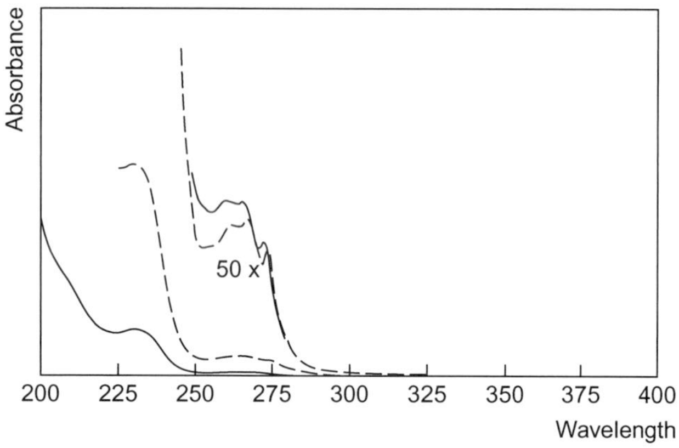

Infra-red Spectrum. Principal peaks at wavenumbers 700, 720, 760, 940, 805, 1491 cm^{-1} (meclozine hydrochloride, KBr disk).

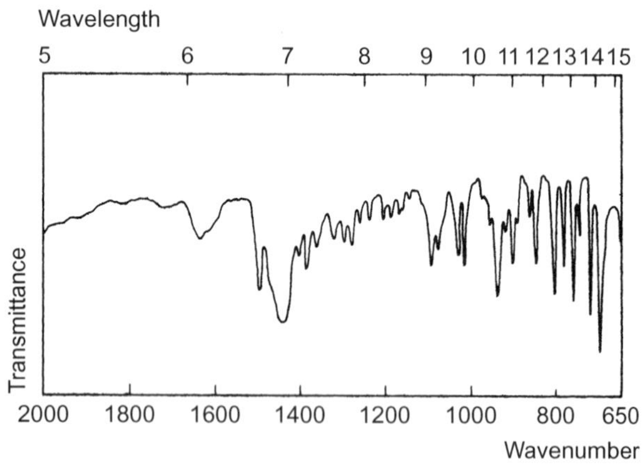

Mass Spectrum. Principal ions at *m*/*z* 189, 105, 201, 285, 165, 166, 190, 134.

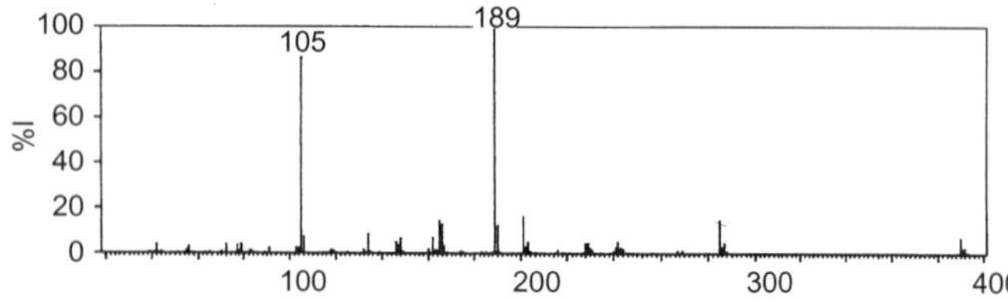

Quantification

Gas chromatography–mass spectrometry. In plasma: limit of detection 5 μg/L—H. G. Fouda *et al.*, *Biomed. Mass Spectrom.*, 1978, *5*, 491–494.

Dose. Usually 25 to 100 mg of meclozine hydrochloride daily.

Medazepam

Tranquilliser

Proprietary names. Nobrium; Rudotel.

7-Chloro-2,3-dihydro-1-methyl-5-phenyl-1*H*-1,4-benzodiazepine

$C_{16}H_{15}ClN_2$=270.8

CAS—2898-12-6

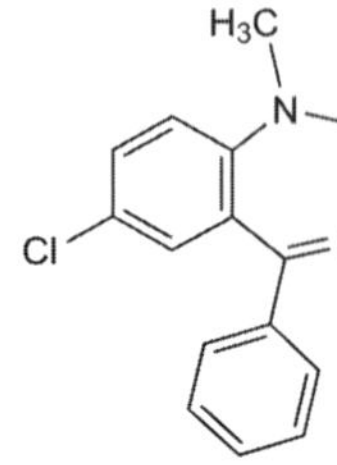

A white to greenish-yellow crystalline powder. M.p. 95° to 97° (crystals from ether and petroleum ether).

Practically insoluble in water; soluble 1 in 8 of ethanol, 1 in 1 of chloroform, and 1 in 5 of ether.

Dissociation Constant. pKa 6.2 (37°).

Partition Coefficient. Log *P* (octanol/pH 7.4), 4.0.

Colour Tests. Formaldehyde–Sulfuric Acid—orange (add water). Cold nitric acid—red colour.

Thin-layer Chromatography. System TA—Rf 67; system TB—Rf 41; system TC—Rf 74; system TD—Rf 54; system TE—Rf 78; system TF—Rf 40; system TL—Rf 62; system TAD—Rf 73; system TAE—Rf 79; system TAF—Rf 83; system TAJ—Rf 70; system TAK—Rf 12; system TAL—Rf 95. (Acidified iodoplatinate solution, positive.)

Gas Chromatography. System GA—medazepam RI 2235, M (nor-) RI 2280, nordazepam RI 2490, diazepam RI 2428; system GB—medazepam RI 2340, nordazepam RI 2625, diazepam RI 2556; system GF—medazepam RI 2640, diazepam RI 3045; system GG—medazepam RI 2620, nordazepam RI 3041, diazepam RI 2940.

High Performance Liquid Chromatography. System HA—*k* 0.2; system HJ—*k* 7.05; system HK—*k* 4.44; system HX—RI 405; system HY—RI 334; system HZ—Retention time 5.4 min; system HAA—Retention time 15.8 min; system HAL—Retention time 8.2 min; system HAM—not detected; system HBH—*k* 41.46; system HBI—*k* 6.31.

Ultraviolet Spectrum. Aqueous acid—253 nm (A^1_1=860a).

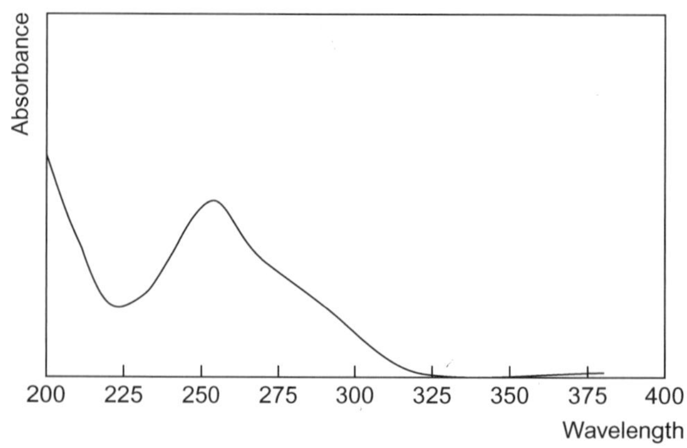

Infra-red Spectrum. Principal peaks at wavenumbers 1610, 1178, 1298, 700, 1255, 815 cm^{-1} (KBr disk).

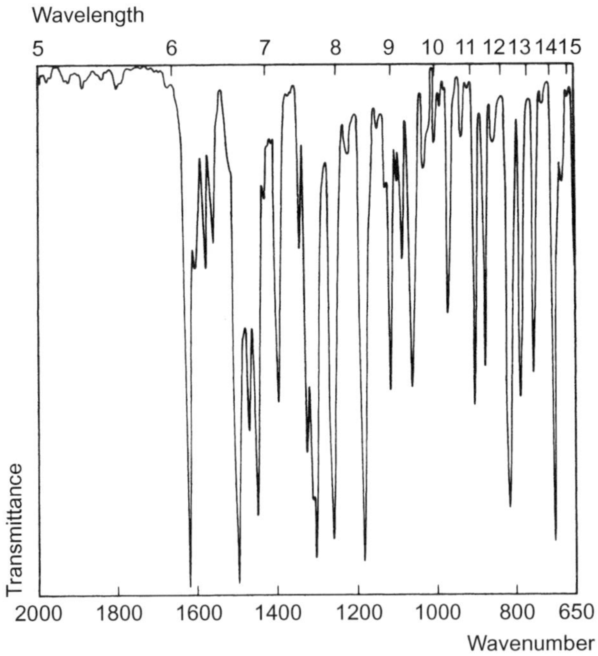

Mass Spectrum. Principal ions at *m/z* 242, 207, 244, 270, 243, 271, 269, 165; nordazepam 242, 269, 270, 241, 243, 271, 244, 272; desmethylmedazepam 193, 255, 228, 256, 257, 165, 230, 258; diazepam 256, 283, 284, 285, 257, 255, 258, 286.

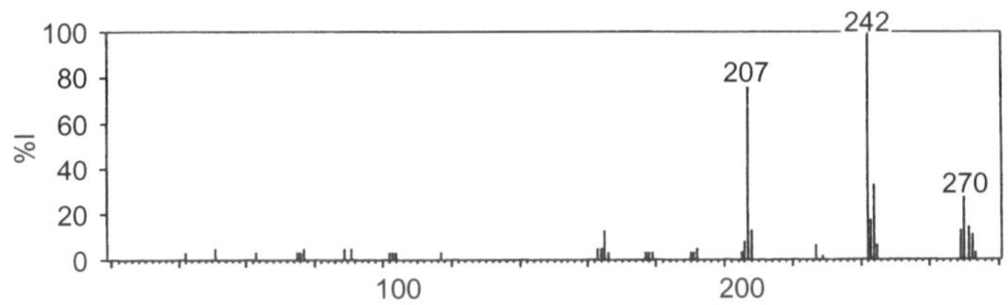

Quantification

Gas chromatography. In plasma or urine: limit of detection 40 µg/L, ECD—J. A. F. de Silva and C. V. Puglisi, *Anal. Chem.*, 1970, *42*, 1725–1736. In whole blood: limit of detection 80 µg/L, FID—M. S. Greaves, *Clin. Chem.*, 1974, *20*, 141–147.

High performance liquid chromatography–mass spectrometry. In serum or urine: medazepam and other benzodiazepines, limit of quantification 2 µg/L—M. Kleinschnitz *et al.*, *J. Chromatogr. B Biomed. Appl.*, 1996, *676*, 61–67.

Disposition in the Body. Readily absorbed after oral administration. The active metabolites desmethyldiazepam (nordazepam) and diazepam may be detected in the blood shortly after dosing; desmethyldiazepam accumulates during chronic treatment. Desmethylmedazepam has also been detected in plasma. A total of up to about 75% of a dose is excreted in the urine and about 20% is eliminated in the faeces. The major urinary metabolite is oxazepam glucuronide, 2 to 3% of a dose being excreted in this form in 72 h; other urinary metabolites include desmethyldiazepam and temazepam.

Therapeutic concentration

Following single oral doses of 10 mg given to 4 subjects, peak plasma concentrations of 0.14 to 0.26 g/L (mean 0.21) of medazepam were attained in about 1 h [D. M. Hailey and E. S. Baird, *Br. J. Anaesth.*, 1979, *51*, 493–496].

Doses of 10 to 50 mg given daily to 20 subjects, resulted in the following steady-state plasma concentrations: medazepam 0.01 to 0.16 g/L (mean 0.06), diazepam 0 to 0.12 g/L (mean 0.03), desmethyldiazepam 0.2 to 1.7 g/L (mean 0.7) [A. J. Bond *et al.*, *Br. J. Clin. Pharmacol.*, 1977, *4*, 51–56].

Half-life. Plasma half-life, medazepam 1 to 2 h, desmethyldiazepam about 40 to 100 h, but there is considerable intersubject variation—see under nordazepam.

Distribution in blood. Plasma : whole blood ratio, 1.9.

Protein binding. In plasma, almost completely bound.

Dose. Usually 10 to 20 mg daily, but doses of up to 60 mg daily have been given.

Medroxyprogesterone Acetate

Progestational Steroid

Synonyms. Methylacetoxyprogesterone; Metipregnone.
Proprietary names. Adgyn Medro; Alti-MPA; Amen; Cycrin; Cykrina; Depocon; Depo-Prodasone; Depo-Provera; Depo-Ralovera; Farlutal; Gen-Medroxy; Gestoral; Novo-Medrone; Perlutex; Proclim; Prodafem; Prodasone; Progevera; Provera; Ralovera.
17α-Acetoxy-6α-methylprogesterone
$C_{24}H_{34}O_4$=386.5
CAS—520-85-4 (medroxyprogesterone); 71-58-9 (acetate)

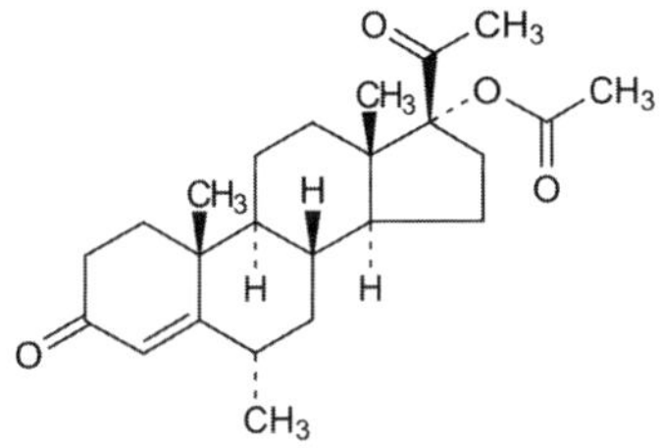

A white crystalline powder. M.p. about 204°. A solution in dioxan is dextrorotatory.
Practically insoluble in water; soluble 1 in 800 of ethanol, 1 in 50 of acetone and 1 in 10 of chloroform; slightly soluble in ether.

Partition Coefficient. Log *P* (octanol/water), 3.5 (medroxyprogesterone).

Thin-layer Chromatography. System TP—Rf 80; system TQ—Rf 50; system TR—Rf 98; system TS—Rf 85, streaking may occur.

Ultraviolet Spectrum. Ethanol—241 nm (A_1^1=426 a).

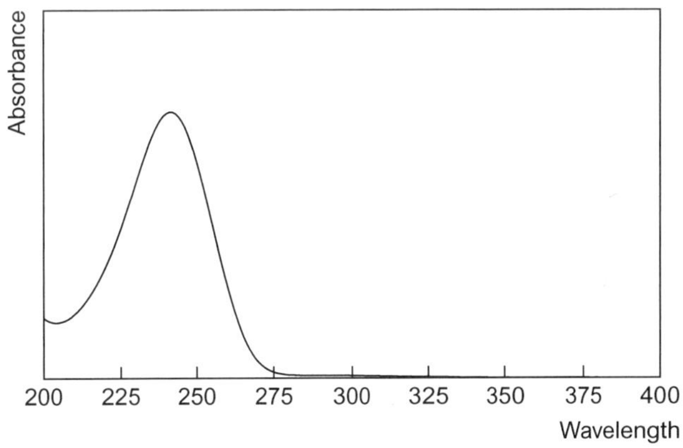

Infra-red Spectrum. Principal peaks at wavenumbers 1727, 1669, 1258, 1608, 967, 1188 cm^{-1} (medroxyprogesterone, KBr disk).

Quantification

Gas chromatography. In plasma: limit of detection 5 µg/L, ECD—E. Rossi *et al.*, *J. Chromatogr.*, 1979, *169*, 416–421.

Gas chromatography–mass spectrometry. In plasma: limit of detection 1 ng—G. Phillipou and R. G. Frith, *Clin. Chim. Acta*, 1980, *103*, 129–133. In serum: limit of detection <0.5 µg/L—T. Jarvinen *et al.*, *J. Chromatogr.*, 1989, *495*, 13–20.

High performance liquid chromatography. In plasma: limit of detection 4 µg/L, UV detection—G. Milano *et al.*, *J. Chromatogr.*, 1982, *232*; *Biomed. Appl.*, *21*, 413–417. In serum: limit of detection 9 µg/L, chemiluminescence detection—S. Uzu *et al.*, *J. Pharm. Biomed. Anal.*, 1992, *10*, 979–984.

High performance liquid chromatography–mass spectrometry. In plasma: limit of detection <0.05 µg/L—S. M. Kim and D. H. Kim, *Rapid Commun. Mass Spectrom.*, 2001, *15*, 2041–2045.

Dose. 2.5 to 10 mg daily, by mouth; up to 1 g daily may be given.

Mefenamic Acid

Analgesic

Synonyms. Acidum Mefenamicum; CI-473; CN-35355; INF-3355.
Proprietary names. Artriden; Contraflam; Coslan; Dysman; Dyspen; Fenamin; Lysalgo; Medicap; Mefacap; Mefalgic; Mefanacide; Mefenix; Mefic; Meflam; Namifen; Napan; Opustan; Parkemed; Pinalgesic; Ponac; Ponalar; Ponalgic; Ponmel; Ponstan; Ponstel; Ponstyl; Pontyl; Spiralgin.
2-[(2,3-Dimethylphenyl)amino]benzoic acid
$C_{15}H_{15}NO_2$=241.3
CAS—61-68-7

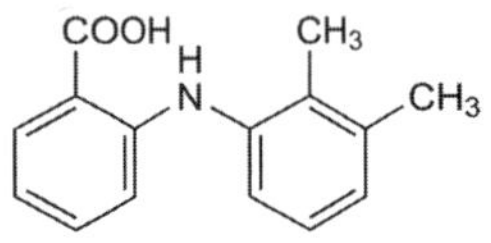

A white to greyish-white microcrystalline powder. M.p. 230° to 231°, with effervescence.
Practically insoluble in water; soluble 1 in 185 of ethanol, 1 in 150 of chloroform, and 1 in 80 of ether; soluble in solutions of alkali hydroxides.

Dissociation Constant. pK_a 4.2.

Partition Coefficient. Log *P* (octanol/water), 5.1.

Colour Test. Liebermann's Test—blue.

Thin-layer Chromatography. System TA—Rf 96; system TD—Rf 41; system TE—Rf 11; system TF—Rf 48; system TG—Rf 32; system TAD—Rf 54; system TAE—Rf 87; system TAJ—Rf 68; system TAK—Rf 86; system TAL—Rf 95. (Chromic acid solution, green.)

Gas Chromatography. System GA—mefenamic acid RI 2201, mefenamic acid-Me RI 2069; system GB—RI 2370; system GD—mefenamic acid-Me RRT 1.45 (relative to *n*-$C_{16}H_{34}$).

High Performance Liquid Chromatography. System HD—*k* 21.1; system HV—RRT 0.95 (relative to meclofenamic acid); system HX—RI 661; system HY—RI 686; system HAY—Retention time 9.8 min; system HAX—Retention time 13.1 min.

Ultraviolet Spectrum. Acid methanol—279 (A^1_1=357a), 350; aqueous alkali—285 (A^1_1=420a, 322 nm).

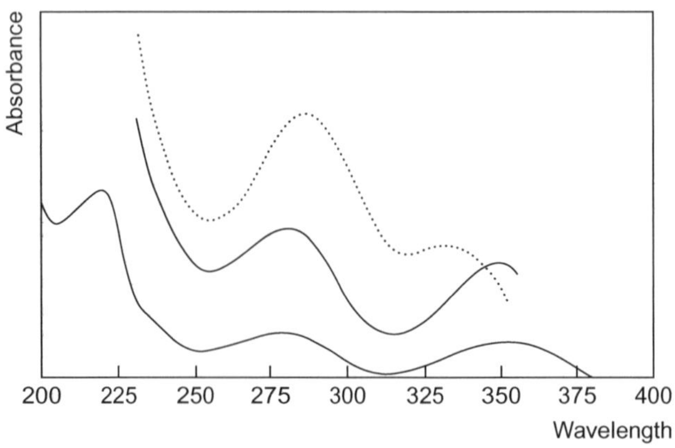

Infra-red Spectrum. Principal peaks at wavenumbers 1255, 1647, 1572, 1504, 757, 1163 cm^{-1} (KBr disk).

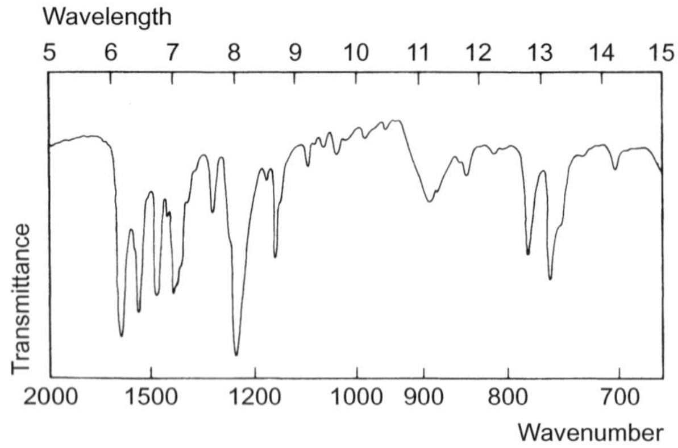

Mass Spectrum. Principal ions at *m/z* 223, 241, 208, 222, 194, 180, 77, 224; 3′-carboxymefenamic acid 44, 180, 209, 227, 223, 77, 208, 179; 3′-hydroxymethylmefenamic acid 209, 257, 180, 208, 210, 77, 44, 194.

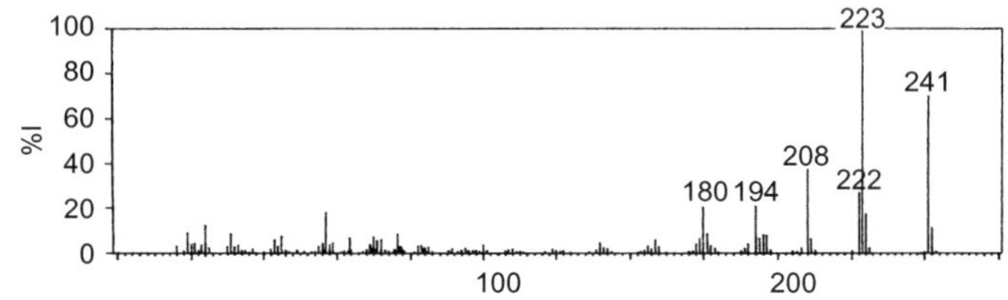

Quantification

Gas chromatography. In serum: limit of detection 1 g/L, FID—L. J. Dusci and L. P. Hackett, *J. Chromatogr.*, 1978, *161*, 340–342.

High performance liquid chromatography. In plasma: mefenamic acid and flufenamic acid, UV detection—C. K. Lin *et al.*, *J. Pharm. Sci.*, 1980, *69*, 95–97. In plasma or serum: mefenamic acid and other NSAIDs, UV detection—P. J. Streete, *J. Chromatogr.*, 1989, *495*, 179–193. In serum: mefenamic acid and ibuprofen, limit of detection for mefenamic acid 0.1 µg/L, UV detection—K. Yamashita *et al.*, *J. Chromatogr.*, 1991, *570*, 329–338. In plasma: mefenamic acid and indometacin, limit of detection for mefenamic acid 80 µg/L, UV detection—I. Niopas and K. Mamzoridi, *J. Chromatogr. B Biomed. Appl.*, 1994, *656*, 447–450. In urine: mefenamic acid and other NSAIDs, limit of quantification for mefenamic acid 50 µg/L, UV detection—T. Hirai *et al.*, *J. Chromatogr. B Biomed. Sci. Appl.*, 1997, *692*, 375–388. In urine: mefenamic acid and other anthranilic acid derivatives, limit of detection for mefenamic acid about 2 µg/L, UV detection—E. Mikami *et al.*, *J. Chromatogr. B Biomed. Sci. Appl.*, 2000, *744*, 81–89.

Disposition in the Body. Readily absorbed after oral administration. Metabolised by hydroxylation of the 3′-methyl group followed by oxidation to produce the 3′-carboxy metabolite; glucuronide conjugation also occurs. About 52% of a dose is excreted in the urine in 48 h, 6% as mefenamic acid and the other 46% as conjugated metabolites; about 20% of a dose is eliminated in the faeces, mostly as unconjugated 3′-carboxymefenamic acid. Trace amounts of mefenamic acid may be present in breast milk.

Therapeutic concentration

Following a single oral dose of 1 g to 6 subjects, a mean peak plasma concentration of 10 g/L was attained in about 2 h; the free and conjugated 3′-hydroxymethyl and 3′-carboxy metabolites attained similar concentrations after about 3 h, and 6 to 8 h respectively [A. J. Glazko, *Ann. Phys. Med.*, 1966, *9*, *Suppl.*, 23–26].

After oral administration of 250 mg 3 times a day for four days to 10 subjects, peak plasma concentrations of 0.3 to 2.4 g/L (mean 0.9) were reported 2 h after the morning dose [R. A. Buchanan *et al.*, *Curr. Ther. Res.*, 1968, *10*, 592–596].

Administration of mefenamic acid at an oral dose of 2 mg/kg at 24-h intervals to 17 preterm infants with patent *ductus arteriosus* resulted in a peak plasma concentration of 1.2 to 6.1 mg/L (mean 3.8) at 2 to 18 h after the first dose. For closure of ductus to take place, plasma concentrations above 2 mg/L needed to be maintained for at least 12 h [K. Ito *et al.*, *Acta Paediari. Jpn.*, 1994, *36*, 387–391].

Toxicity. Toxic effects are usually associated with plasma concentrations greater than 10 g/L.

In a survey of 29 cases of mefenamic acid overdose, plasma concentrations were in the range 11 to 148 g/L; in 11 of the cases convulsions occurred (mean plasma concentration 73 g/L). All the patients recovered [M. Balali-Mood *et al.*, *Lancet*, 1981, *1*, 1354–1356].

Half-life. Plasma half-life, about 2 to 4 h.

Protein binding. In plasma, about 99%.

Dose. Up to 1.5 g daily.

Mefruside

Diuretic

Proprietary name. Baycaron

4-Chloro-*N*[1]-methyl-*N*[1]-[(tetrahydro-2-methyl-2-furanyl)methyl]-1,3-benzenedisulfonamide

$C_{13}H_{19}ClN_2O_5S_2$=382.9

CAS—7195-27-9

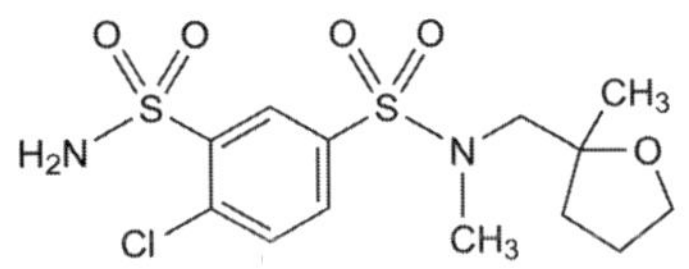

A white powder. M.p. 148° to 149°.

Practically insoluble in water; soluble in dilute solutions of sodium hydroxide.

Partition Coefficient. Log *P* (octanol/water), 1.5.

Colour Tests. Koppanyi–Zwikker Test—violet; Liebermann's Test—blue; Mercurous Nitrate—black.

Thin-layer Chromatography. System TD—Rf 45; system TE—Rf 67; system TF—Rf 58; system TAD—Rf 55.

Gas Chromatography. System GA—mefruside-Me_2 RI 2860; system GX—mefruside-Me_2 Retention time 7.4 min; M (5-oxo-)-Me_2 Retention time 9.8 min; system GY—mefruside-Me_2 Retention time 4.7 min; M (5-oxo-)-Me_2 Retention time 5.1 min.

High Performance Liquid Chromatography. System HN—*k* 8.67; system HY—RI 417.

Ultraviolet Spectrum. Methanol—276 nm (A^1_1 = 44a), 284 nm.

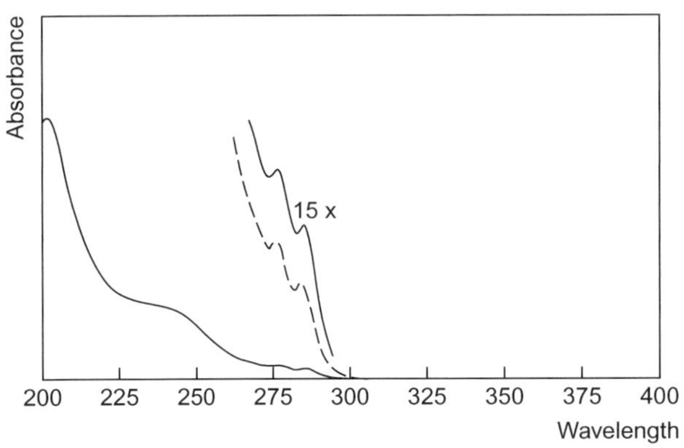

Infra-red Spectrum. Principal peaks at wavenumbers 1162, 1176, 819, 1041, 746, 909 cm^{-1}.

Mass Spectrum. Principal ions at *m*/*z* 85, 43, 42, 86, 44, 41, 75, 110.

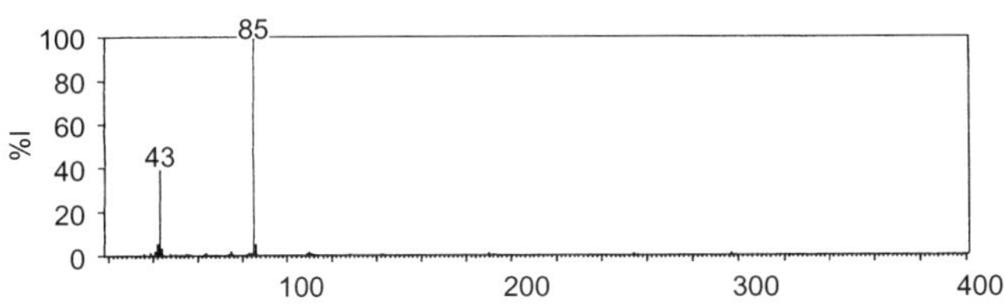

Quantification

Gas chromatography. In blood, plasma, erythrocytes or urine: limit of detection 5 µg/L in plasma, AFID—H. L. J. Fleuren *et al.*, *Arzneimittelforschung*, 1979, *29*, 1041–1047. In plasma, erythrocytes or urine: 5-oxomefruside and its hydroxycarboxylic acid analogue, limit of detection 25 ng, AFID—H. L. J. Fleuren *et al.*, *J. Chromatogr.*, 1980, *182*; *Biomed. Appl.*, *8*, 179–190.

High performance liquid chromatography. In urine: mefruside and its metabolites, UV detection—C. J. Little *et al.*, *Anal. Chem.*, 1977, *49*, 1311–1313.

Disposition in the Body. Readily absorbed after oral administration. About 13% of a dose is excreted in the urine as 5-oxomefruside, about 35 to 55% as the hydroxycarboxylic acid analogue of 5-oxomefruside and up to about 15% as a conjugate of this acid analogue. Both of these metabolites appear to be active. Less than 1% of the dose is excreted as unchanged drug.

Therapeutic concentration. There is considerable intersubject variation in plasma concentrations after therapeutic doses.

Peak plasma concentrations of 0.07 to 0.13 mg/L were attained 2 to 5 h after a single oral dose of 50 mg to 6 subjects [H. L. J. Fleuren *et al.*, *Eur. J. Clin. Pharmacol.*, 1980, *17*, 59–69].

Half-life. Plasma half-life, mefruside 3 to 12 h (mean 7), 5-oxomefruside 10 to 14 h, hydroxycarboxylic acid analogue 8 to 12 h.

Volume of distribution. About 6 L/kg.

Clearance. Plasma clearance, 5 to 30 mL/min/kg (mean 13).

Distribution in blood. Plasma : whole blood ratio, about 0.03.

Dose. 25 to 100 mg daily.

Megestrol Acetate

Progestational Steroid

Proprietary names. Acestrol; Borea; Maygace; Megace; Megefren; Megestat; Megestil; Megestin; Megostat; Nia; Niagestin; Prazoken.

17-Hydroxy-6-methylpregna-4,6-diene-3,20-dione acetate

$C_{24}H_{32}O_4$=384.5

CAS—3562-63-8 (megestrol); 595-33-5 (acetate)

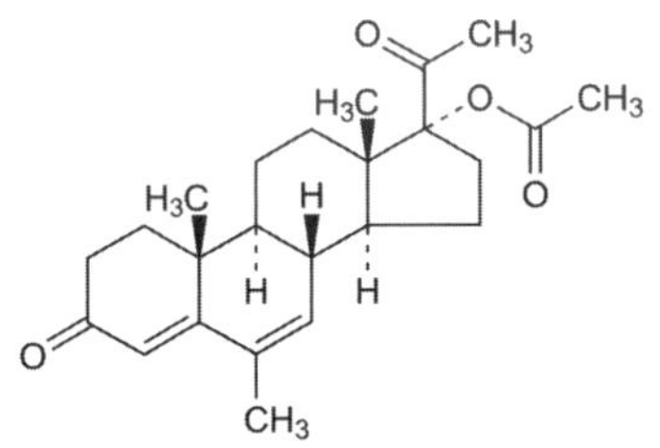

A white to creamy-white crystalline powder. M.p. about 217°. A solution in chloroform is dextrorotatory.

Practically insoluble in water; soluble 1 in 55 of ethanol, 1 in 0.8 of chloroform and 1 in 130 of ether; soluble in acetone.

Partition Coefficient. Log *P* (octanol/water), 4.0.

Thin-layer Chromatography. System TP—Rf 80; system TQ—Rf 50; system TR—Rf 98; system TS—Rf 85, streaking may occur.

Ultraviolet Spectrum. Dehydrated alcohol—287 nm (A^1_1=630a).

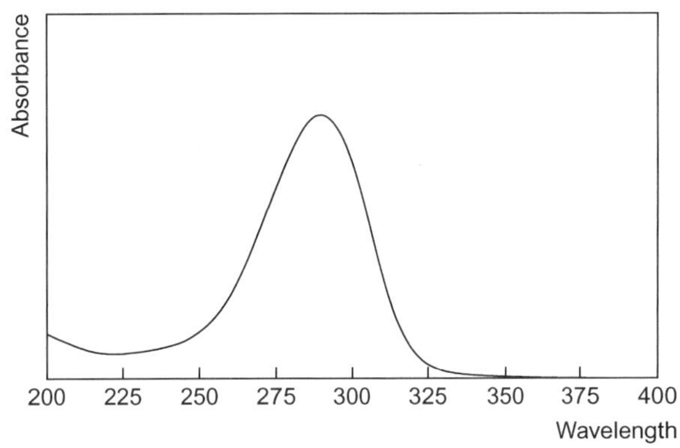

Infra-red Spectrum. Principal peaks at wavenumbers 1263, 1249, 1733, 1662, 1712, 1630 cm^{-1} (KBr disk).

Mass Spectrum. Principal ions at *m/z* 281, 43, 282, 187, 107, 91, 55, 105.

Quantification
High performance liquid chromatography. In plasma: limit of detection 5 µg/L, UV detection—R. C. Gaver *et al.*, *J. Pharm Sci.*, 1985, *74*, 664–667. In serum: megestrol acetate and cyproterone acetate, limit of detection 5 µg/L, UV detection—L. D. Dikkeschei *et al.*, *J. Chromatogr.*, 1990, *529*, 145–154.

Dose. 40 to 320 mg daily.

Meloxicam

COX-2 Inhibitor/NSAID

Synonym. UH-AC-62
Proprietary names. Metacam; Mobic.
4-Hydroxy-2-methyl-*N*-(5-methyl-2-thiazolyl)-2*H*-1,2-benzothiazine-3-carboxamide-1,1-dioxide
$C_{14}H_{13}N_3O_4S_2$=351.4
CAS—71125-38-7

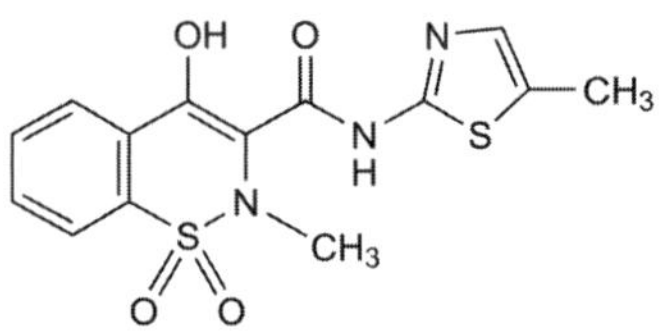

Crystals from ethylene chloride with m.p. 254°.

Dissociation Constant. pK_{a1} 1.1; pK_{a2} 4.2.

Partition Coefficient. Log *P* (octanol/water), 3.43.

High Performance Liquid Chromatography. System HZ—retention time 6.8 min.

Column: (analytical) RP C_{18} (Lichrocart, 125 × 4.0 mm i.d., 5 µm) (guard) RP C_{18} (Lichrocart, 40 × 4.0 mm i.d., 5 µm). Column temperature: 30°. Mobile phase: diammonium hydrogen phosphate (50 mM): methanol:acetonitrile (50:40:10), 1 mL/min flow rate. Internal standard (IS): piroxicam. Retention time(s): meloxicam, 2.7 min; IS, 1.9 min. [T. Velpandian *et al.*, *J. Chromatogr. B, Biomed. Sci. Appl.*, 2000, *738*, 431–436].

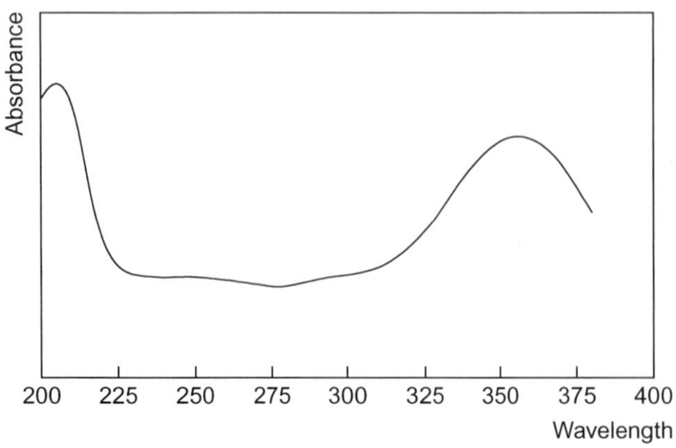

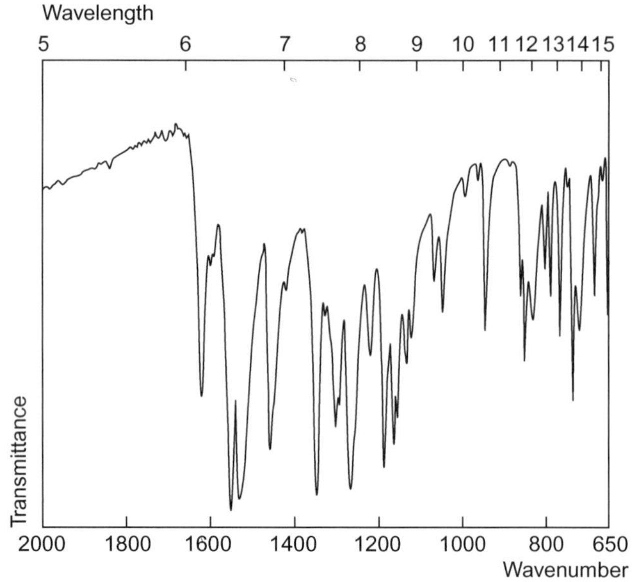

Quantification
High performance liquid chromatography. In plasma: limit of quantification 0.05 mg/L. UV detection (λ=355 nm)—D. Türck *et al. Clin. Drug Invest.*, 1995, *9*, 270–276. In plasma: limit of detection 0.03 mg/L. UV detection (λ=364 nm)—T. Velpandian *et al.*, *J. Chromatogr. B Biomed. Sci. Appl.*, 2000, *738*, 431–436.

Disposition in the Body. Meloxicam is well absorbed after oral administration reaching maximum concentration 5 to 6 h after once daily dose of 15 mg. After a single 15 mg intramuscular dose, the mean maximum plasma concentration is only about twice that observed after oral administration. Intravenous (IV) administration is associated with a markedly higher initial concentration (intravenous/oral ratio 2.99/0.93) followed by a rapid decline. Meloxicam is extensively metabolised via oxidation and the metabolites (four isolated in total) (approx. 97% of the dose) are excreted via urine and faeces in equal proportions. Less than 0.5% appears as the unchanged drug in urine. The pharmacokinetics of meloxicam are altered in renal impairment with lower total plasma meloxicam concentration and higher free fractions being observed at creatinine clearance 20 to 40 mL/min. However, there is no apparent risk of increased toxicity.

Therapeutic concentration

Study 1: 6 healthy volunteers, aged between 27 and 49 years, were administered a single oral 30 mg dose after an overnight fast or 10 to 20 min after a continental (light) breakfast. Study 2: 16 healthy volunteers, 24 to 47 years old, were administered a 15 mg dose after a 12 h fast or immediately after a high fat breakfast. The fasting individuals in study 1 reached peak plasma concentrations of 1.51 mg/L at about 10.7 h compared with the fed volunteers who showed peak concentrations of 1.43 mg/L at 9.7 h. In study 2, those given the dose after the 12-h fast showed peak concentrations of 0.928 mg/L at 8.8 h and those co-administered with a high fat meal reached 1.14 mg/L about 6.1 h after ingestion. [D. Türck *et al.*, *Clin. Drug Invest.*, 1995, *9*, 270–276].

4 healthy males were administered an IV 30 mg dose (over 15 min) or a single oral 30 mg dose, 2 h after a light breakfast. Peak plasma concentrations were 5.35 mg/L and 3.09 mg/L for the IV and oral doses, respectively, 2 h after administration. [J. Schmid *et al.*, *Drug Metab. Dispos.*, 1995, *23*, 1206–1213].

Bioavailability. Approx. 89%.

Half-life. 25 to 20 h.

Volume of distribution. 11.5 to 16.5 L (decreased by co-administration with a high fat meal); also reported as 10 L.

Clearance. Plasma, 7.25 to 8.5 mL/min.

Distribution in blood. <10% in red blood cells.

Protein binding. 99.4%, mainly to albumin.

Dose. Orally and via suppositories: usual dose is 7.5 to 15 mg daily. A lower daily dose of 7.5 mg is recommended in the elderly and those on renal dialysis.

Melphalan

Antineoplastic

Synonyms. PAM; Phenylalanine Nitrogen Mustard.
Note. Merphalan is the racemic form of melphalan; medphalan is the D-isomer of melphalan.
Proprietary name. Alkeran
4-[Bis(2-chloroethyl)amino]-L-phenylalanine
$C_{13}H_{18}Cl_2N_2O_2 = 305.2$
CAS—148-82-3

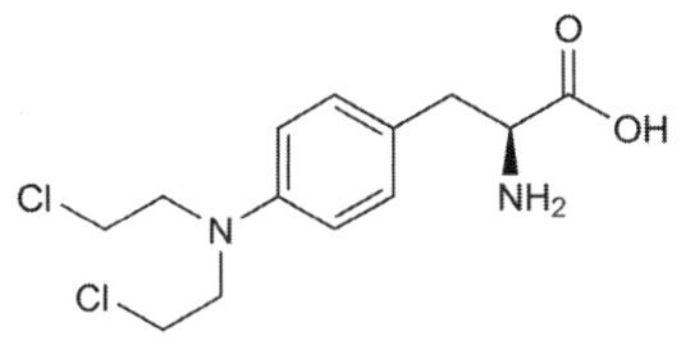

A white to buff-coloured powder. M.p. about 177° to 180°, with decomposition.
Practically insoluble in water, chloroform and ether; soluble in ethanol and propylene glycol; soluble in dilute mineral acids.

Partition Coefficient. Log *P* (octanol/water), −0.5.

High Performance Liquid Chromatography. System HAA—Retention time, 12.9 min.

Ultraviolet Spectrum. Methanol—260 nm (A^1_1 = 707a), 301 nm.

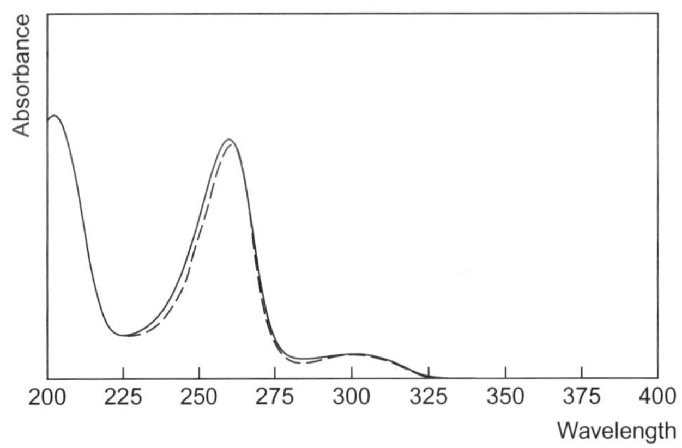

Infra-red Spectrum. Principal peaks at wavenumbers 1621, 1513, 1186, 1160, 1250, 1205 cm^{-1} (KBr disk).

Quantification

High performance liquid chromatography. In plasma: limit of detection 10 µg/L, fluorescence detection—K. W. Woodhouse and D. B. Henderson, *Br. J. Clin. Pharmacol.*, 1982, *13*, 605P. In plasma: limit of detection 50 µg/L, UV detection—S. Y. Chang *et al.*, *J. Pharm. Sci.*, 1978, *67*, 679–682. In blood or plasma: limit of detection < 30 µg/L, fluorescence detection—H. K. Osterheld *et al.*, *Cancer Chemother. Pharmacol.*, 1988, *21*, 156–162. In plasma: electrochemical detection—L. Silvestro *et al.*, *J. Chromatogr.*, 1991, *563*, 443–450. In plasma: melphalan and other nitrogen mustard anticancer drugs, limit of detection for melphalan 1 ng—J. Cummings *et al.*, *Anal. Chem.*, 1991, *63*, 1514–1519. In plasma: limit of detection 10 µg/L—Y. Kato *et al.*, *Ther. Drug Monit.*, 1992, *14*, 66–71. In plasma, perfusate or tissue: melphalan and metabolites, limit of detection for melphalan < 1.4 ng in plasma or perfusate and < 7.2 ng in tissue—Z. Y. Wu *et al.*, *J. Chromatogr.*, 1995, *673*, *Biomed. Appl.*, 267–279. In plasma: UV detection—F. Pinguet *et al.*, *J. Chromatogr.*, 1996, *686*, *Biomed. Appl.*, 43–49.

Therapeutic concentration

When administered as a 24 h continuous intravenous infusion to 21 subjects at a dose of 20, 30 and 40 mg/m^2, steady-state melphalan concentrations of 0.080, 0.121 and 0.206 mg/L were obtained; the maximum tolerated dose was 30 mg/m^2 [F. Pinguet *et al.*, *Clin. Cancer Res.*, 2000, *6*, 57–63].

Dose. 200 to 300 µg/kg daily, by mouth, for 4 to 6 days.

Menadione

Vitamin K Analogue

Synonyms. Menaphthene; Menaphthone; Methylnaphthochinonum; Vitamin K_3.
Proprietary names. Kappaxin; Kayquinone; Thyloquinone. It is an ingredient of Bilkaby.
2-Methyl-1,4-naphthalenedione
$C_{11}H_8O_2 = 172.2$
CAS—58-27-5

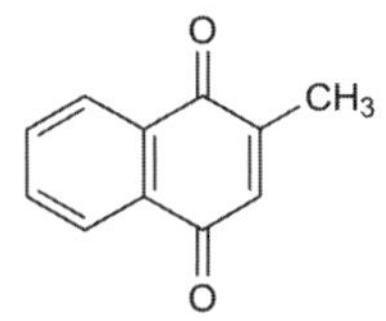

A bright yellow crystalline powder. On exposure to light it decomposes and darkens to light brown. M.p. 105° to 107°.
Insoluble in water; soluble 1 in 60 of ethanol and 1 in 10 of benzene; moderately soluble in chloroform and carbon tetrachloride; soluble in ether.

Caution. The powder is irritating to the respiratory tract and to the skin. The ethanolic solution has vesicant properties.

Menadione Sodium Bisulfite

Synonyms. Kavitanum; Vikasolum.
Proprietary names. Hykinone; Klotogen; K-Thrombin.
$C_{11}H_8O_2NaHSO_3,3H_2O = 330.3$
CAS—130-37-0 (anhydrous); 6147-37-1 (trihydrate)
A white, hygroscopic, crystalline powder.
Soluble 1 in about 2 of water; slightly soluble in ethanol; almost insoluble in ether and benzene.

Partition Coefficient. Log *P* (octanol/water), 2.2.

Colour Test. Dissolve about 0.5 mg in 5 mL of ethanol and add 2 mL of strong ammonia solution and a few drops of ethyl cyanoacetate—violet; add 5 mL of sodium hydroxide solution—brown-yellow. The violet colour is destroyed on the addition of acid or on exposure to sunlight.

Ultraviolet Spectrum. Aqueous acid—244 nm (A^1_1 = 1052b), 249 nm (A^1_1 = 1133b), 261 nm (A^1_1 = 990b), 340 nm (A^1_1 = 159b).

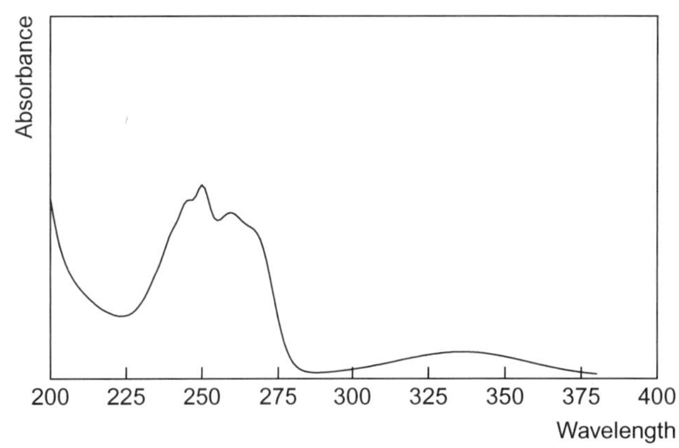

Quantification

High performance liquid chromatography. In plasma: limit of detection < 10 µg/L—O. Y. Hu *et al.*, *J. Chromatogr.*, 1995, *666*, *Biomed. Appl.*, 299–305.

Dose. Menadione is usually administered by intramuscular injection as a 0.5% solution in oil.

Menthol

Decongestant/Antipruritic

Synonym. Mentol
(1α,2β,5α)-5-Methyl-2-(1-methylethyl)cyclohexanol
$C_{10}H_{20}O$=156.3
CAS—89-78-1; 1490-04-6; 2216-51-5 (−); 15356-70-4 (±)

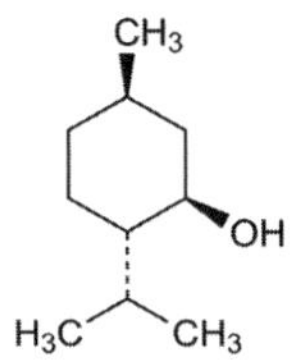

Menthol is natural laevo-menthol, obtained from the volatile oils of various species of *Mentha* (Labiatae), or synthetic laevo-menthol, or racemic menthol.
Colourless crystals or crystalline powder. M.p. of natural or synthetic (−)-menthol, 41° to 43° and of (±)-menthol, 27° to 28° (rising on prolonged stirring to 30° to 32°).
Slightly soluble in water; soluble 1 in 0.2 of ethanol, 1 in 0.25 of chloroform and 1 in 0.4 of ether; freely soluble in glacial acetic acid and liquid petrolatum.

Partition Coefficient. Log *P* (octanol/water), 3.4.

Gas Chromatography. System GA—RI 1206; system GB—RI 1194.

Ultraviolet Spectrum. No significant absorption, 230 to 360 nm.

Infra-red Spectrum. Principal peaks at wavenumbers 1046, 1026, 995, 1102, 1078, 979 cm^{-1} (Nujol mull).

Mass Spectrum. Principal ions at *m/z* 81, 95, 71, 41, 67, 55, 138, 123.

Quantification
Gas chromatography. In urine: menthol and its glucuronide, limit of detection 250 μg/L, FID—R. M. Kaffenberger and M. J. Doyle, *J. Chromatogr.*, 1990, *527*, 59–66. In plasma: menthol, camphor and methyl-salicylate, limit of detection 1 μg/L, FID—J. S. Valdez *et al.*, *J. Chromatogr. B. Biomed. Sci. Appl.*, 1999, *729*, 163–171.

Disposition in the Body. Menthol is excreted in the bile and urine as a glucuronide conjugate; the various stereoisomers differ quantitatively in the extent to which they conjugate with glucuronic acid. Menthol may occur in the conjugated form as a metabolite of pulagone which is a constituent of pulegium oil.

Toxicity. The minimum lethal dose has been estimated to be about 2 g. The application of drops or ointments containing menthol to the nostrils of infants is dangerous and may cause instant collapse. Ingestion of excess menthol may cause severe abdominal pain and coma.

Mepacrine

Antimalarial/Antiprotozoal

Synonyms. Acrichinum; Acrinamine; Atebrine; Chinacrina; Quinacrine.
N^4-(6-Chloro-2-methoxy-9-acridinyl)-N^1,N^1-diethyl-1,4-pentane-diamine
$C_{23}H_{30}ClN_3O$=400.0
CAS—83-89-6

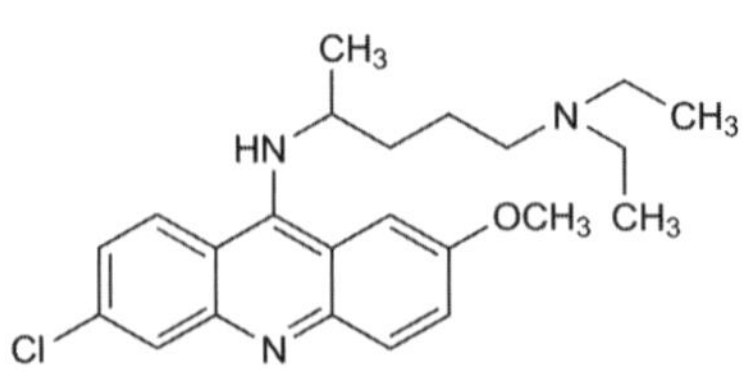

Mepacrine Hydrochloride
Synonyms. Antimalarinae Chlorhydras; Erion; Quinacrine Hydrochloride.
Proprietary name. Atabrine
$C_{23}H_{30}ClN_3O,2HCl,2H_2O$=508.9
CAS—69-05-6 (anhydrous); 6151-30-0 (dihydrate)
A bright yellow crystalline powder. M.p. 248° to 250°, with decomposition.
Soluble 1 in about 35 of water, more soluble in hot water; slightly soluble in ethanol; very slightly soluble in chloroform; insoluble in ether, benzene and acetone.

Mepacrine Mesilate
Synonym. Mepacrine Methanesulphonate
$C_{23}H_{30}ClN_3O,2CH_3SO_3H,H_2O$=610.2
CAS—316-05-2 (anhydrous)
Bright yellow crystals.
Soluble 1 in 3 of water and 1 in 36 of ethanol.

Dissociation Constant. pK_a 7.7, 10.3 (20°).

Partition Coefficient. Log *P* (octanol/water), 5.8.

Colour Tests. Mandelin's Test—violet→yellow; Marquis Test—yellow.

Thin-layer Chromatography. System TA—Rf 43; system TB—Rf 15; system TC—Rf 05; system TL—Rf 09. (Acidified iodoplatinate solution, positive.)

High Performance Liquid Chromatography. System HX—RI 345; system HY—RI 299.

Ultraviolet Spectrum. Aqueous acid—279 nm (A^1_1=1706a), 343 nm; aqueous alkali—270, 345 nm.

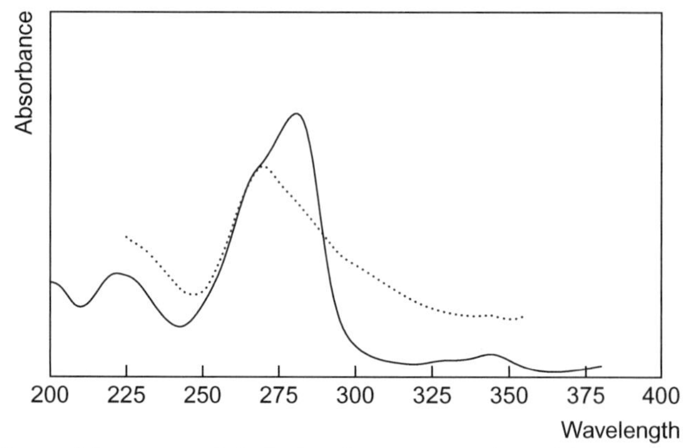

Infra-red Spectrum. Principal peaks at wavenumbers 1245, 1627, 1587, 1500, 1560, 1522 cm^{-1} (mepacrine hydrochloride, KBr disk).

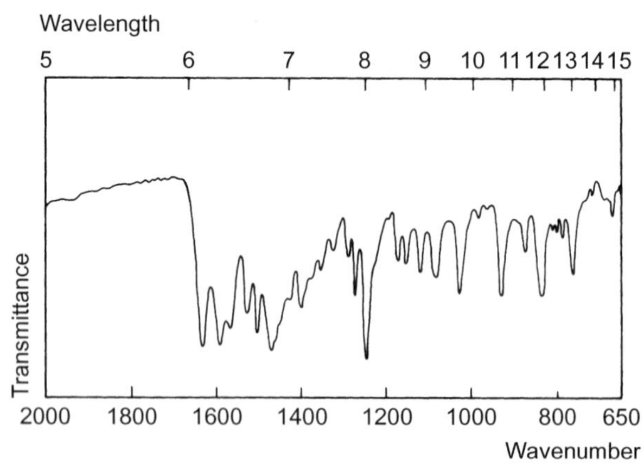

Mass Spectrum. Principal ions at *m/z* 86, 36, 126, 30, 58, 38, 112, 99.

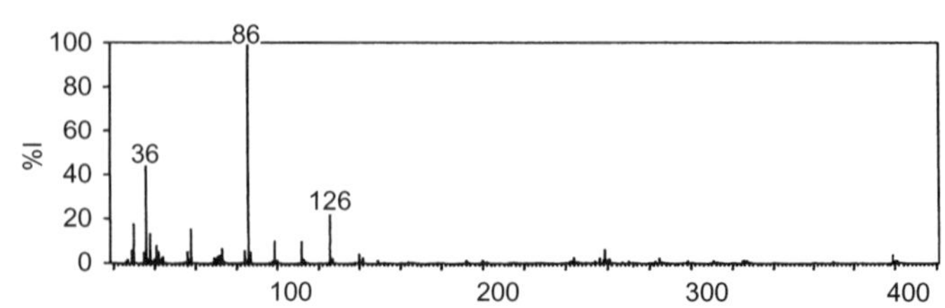

Quantification
High performance liquid chromatography. In plasma: fluorescence detection—S. Bjorkman and L. O. Elisson, *J. Chromatogr.*, 1987, *420*, 341–348.

Disposition in the Body. Readily absorbed after oral administration; it appears in the blood within 2 h, peak concentrations being attained in 8 h. Mepacrine accumulates in the body during chronic administration and is widely distributed, high concentrations being found in the liver, lungs and spleen; it also persists in the skin and finger-nails. The urine and skin may become yellow. It is excreted very slowly in the urine and bile with significant amounts detectable in the urine for at least 2 months after the discontinuation of therapy. Several metabolites are excreted but these account for not more than 5% of the dose.

Toxicity. Large doses may give rise to nausea and vomiting and occasionally to transient mental disturbances. Attempts at suicide with massive doses have not been successful.

Half-life. About 5 days.

Distribution in blood. Concentrated in the erythrocytes.

Protein binding. In plasma, about 90%.

Dose. 300 to 900 mg daily.

Mepenzolate Bromide

Anticholinergic

Proprietary names. Cantil; Cantril; Gastropidil; Trancolan.
3-[(Hydroxydiphenylacetyl)oxy]-1,1-dimethylpiperidinium bromide
$C_{21}H_{26}BrNO_3$=420.3
CAS—25990-43-6 (mepenzolate); 76-90-4 (bromide)

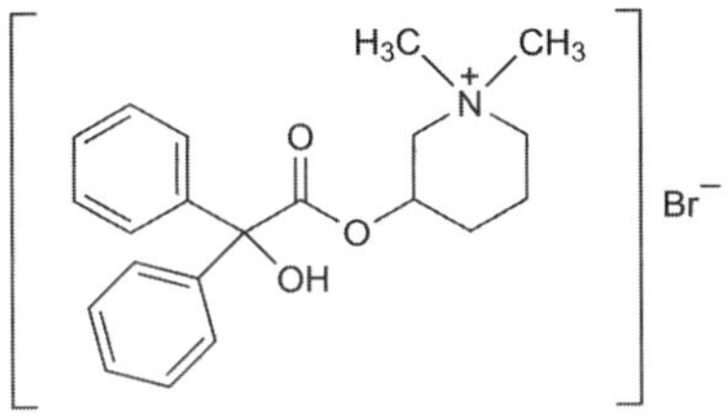

A white or light cream-coloured powder. M.p. 228° to 229°, with decomposition.
Soluble 1 in 110 of water, 1 in 120 of dehydrated alcohol, 1 in about 630 of chloroform and 1 in about 8 of methanol; practically insoluble in ether.

Partition Coefficient. Log *P* (octanol/water), −0.8.

Colour Tests. The following tests are performed on mepenzolate nitrate (see Chapter 19): Liebermann's Test—brown; Marquis Test—orange (transient).

Thin-layer Chromatography. System TA—Rf 01; system TAJ—Rf 42; system TAK—Rf 04; system TAL—Rf 52. (Acidified iodoplatinate solution, positive.)

Gas Chromatography. System GA—RI 2327.

High Performance Liquid Chromatography. System HA—*k* 4.1 (tailing peak).

Ultraviolet Spectrum. Aqueous acid—252, 258 nm (A^{1}_{1}=11b), 261, 263 nm.

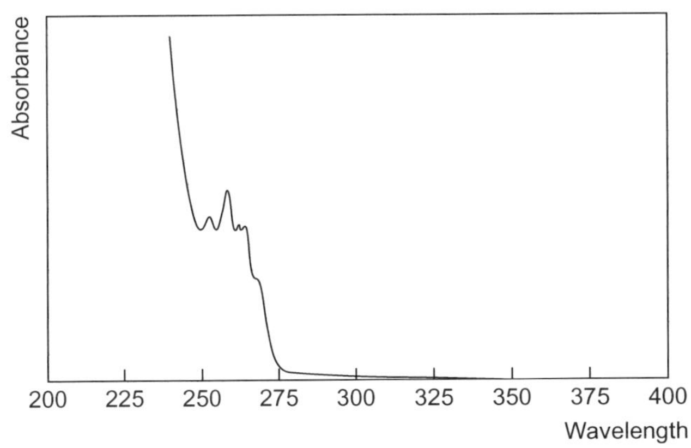

Infra-red Spectrum. Principal peaks at wavenumbers 1220, 1727, 1163, 763, 1062, 1093 cm^{-1} (KBr disk).

Mass Spectrum. Principal ions at *m/z* 97, 105, 77, 96, 42, 183, 98, 82.

Dose. 75 to 200 mg daily.

Mephenesin

Muscle Relaxant

Synonyms. Cresoxydiol; Glykresin.
Proprietary names. Decontractyl; DoloVisano M.
3-(2-Methylphenoxy)-1,2-propanediol
$C_{10}H_{14}O_3$=182.2
CAS—59-47-2

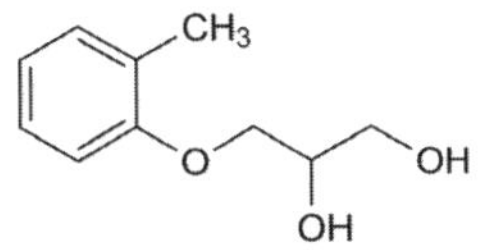

White crystals or crystalline aggregates. M.p. 70° to 71°.
Soluble 1 in 100 of water, 1 in 8 of ethanol and 1 in 12 of chloroform; soluble in ether; freely soluble in propylene glycol.

Mephenesin Carbamate
$C_{11}H_{15}NO_4$=225.2
CAS—533-06-2
White crystals. M.p. 93°.
Slightly soluble in water; freely soluble in ethanol; soluble 1 in 50 of chloroform.

Partition Coefficient. Log *P* (octanol/water), 1.4.

Colour Tests. Mephenesin carbamate: Mandelin's Test—grey-brown; Marquis Test—red.

Thin-layer Chromatography. System TA—Rf 64; system TB—Rf 02; system TC—Rf 43; system TL—Rf 57; system TAE—Rf 87; system TAF—Rf 89; system TAJ—Rf 45; system TAK—Rf 29; system TAL—Rf 78. (Marquis reagent, positive.)
Mephenesin carbamate: System TD—Rf 14; system TE—Rf 55; system TF—Rf 36; system TAD—Rf 35. (Furfuraldehyde reagent, positive.)

Gas Chromatography. System GA—RI 1568.

High Performance Liquid Chromatography. System HA—*k* 0.2; system HX—RI 364; system HY—RI 322.

Ultraviolet Spectrum. Aqueous acid—270 nm (A^{1}_{1}=87a), 276 nm. No alkaline shift.

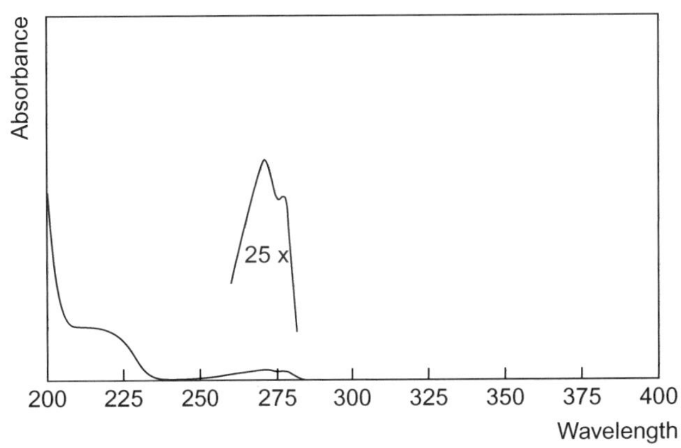

Infra-red Spectrum. Principal peaks at wavenumbers 1047, 1248, 1124, 1493, 756, 748 cm^{-1} (Nujol mull).

Mass Spectrum. Principal ions at *m/z* 108, 107, 91, 182, 109, 77, 79, 31; mephenesin carbamate 118, 108, 182, 91, 225, 107, 57, 75.

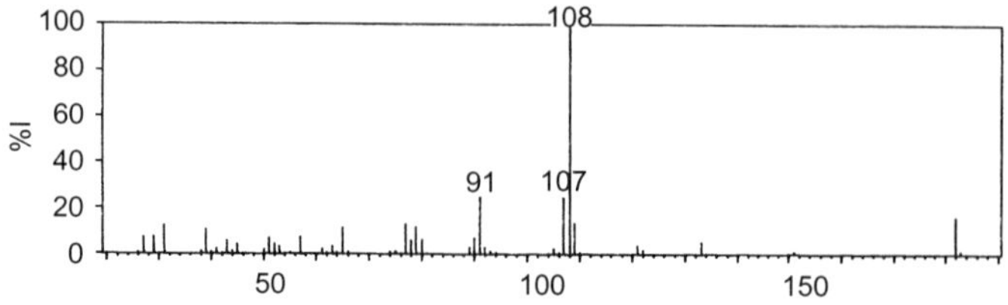

Disposition in the Body. Readily absorbed after oral administration and widely distributed throughout the tissues. It is rapidly metabolised to the inactive metabolites, β-(*o*-methylbenzoyloxy)lactic acid and β-(2-methyl-4-hydroxyphenoxy)lactic acid. Less than 2% of a dose is excreted in the urine as unchanged drug.

Therapeutic concentration

Following a single oral dose of 3 g to 4 subjects, a mean peak plasma concentration of about 10 mg/L was attained in 0.5 h [I. London and R. B. Poet, *Proc. Soc. Exp. Biol. Med.*, 1957, *94*, 191].

Toxicity

A 43-year-old woman, who ingested between 5.5 and 11 g of mephenesin recovered within about 10 h following treatment [D. W. Barron and T. G. Milliken, *Lancet*, 1960, *1*, 262].

Dose. 0.5 to 6 g of mephenesin daily.

Mephentermine

Sympathomimetic

Synonyms. Mephenterdrine; Mephetedrine.
N,α,α-Trimethylbenzeneethanamine
$C_{11}H_{17}N = 163.3$
CAS-100-92-5

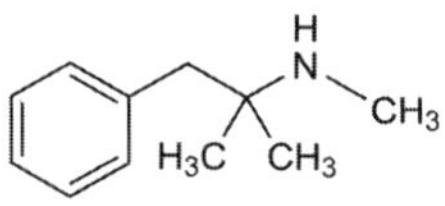

A clear, colourless to pale yellow liquid.
Practically insoluble in water; freely soluble in ethanol; soluble in ether.

Mephentermine Sulfate

Proprietary names. Wyamine It is an ingredient of Emergent-Ez.
$(C_{11}H_{17}N)_2,H_2SO_4,2H_2O = 460.6$
CAS-1212-72-2 (anhydrous); 6190-60-9 (dihydrate)
Colourless crystals or white crystalline powder. M.p. 215° to 217°, with decomposition.
Soluble 1 in about 20 of water and 1 in 150 of ethanol; practically insoluble in chloroform and ether.

Dissociation Constant. pK_a 10.4.

Partition Coefficient. Log *P* (octanol/water), 2.7.

Colour Tests. Liebermann's Test—red-orange; Marquis Test—orange→brown.

Thin-layer Chromatography. System TA—Rf 25; system TB—Rf 34; system TC—Rf 08; system TE—Rf 40; system TL—Rf 02; system TAE—Rf 06; system TAJ—Rf 00; system TAK—Rf 03; system TAL—Rf 36. (Dragendorff spray, positive; acidified iodoplatinate solution, positive; Marquis reagent, brown.)

Gas Chromatography. System GA—mephentermine RI 1240, mephentermine-TFA RI 1335, mephentermine-AC RI 1501, phentermine RI 1155; system GB—mephentermine RI 1250, phentermine RI 1191; system GC—mephentermine RI 1668, phentermine RI 1450.

High Performance Liquid Chromatography. System HA—mephentermine *k* 1.5, phentermine *k* 0.6; system HC—*k* 2.48; system HX—RI 294; system HY—RI 246.

Ultraviolet Spectrum. Aqueous acid—251, 257 nm ($A_1^1 = 10c$), 263 nm.

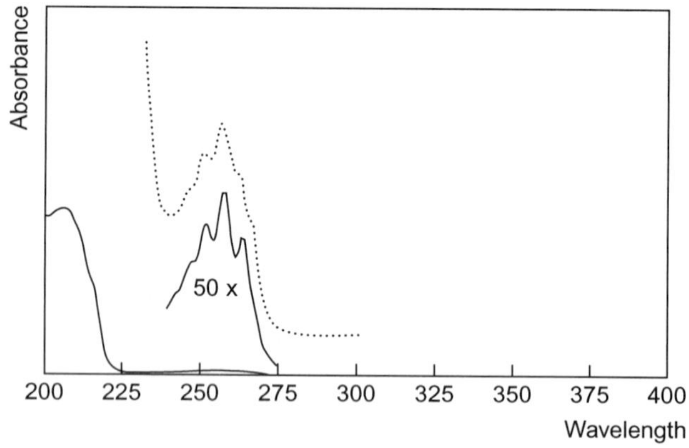

Infra-red Spectrum. Principal peaks at wavenumbers 1111, 711, 1162, 696, 763, 1587 cm^{-1}.

Mass Spectrum. Principal ions at *m/z* 72, 91, 73, 56, 148, 65, 57, 42; phentermine 58, 91, 42, 41, 134, 65, 59, 40.

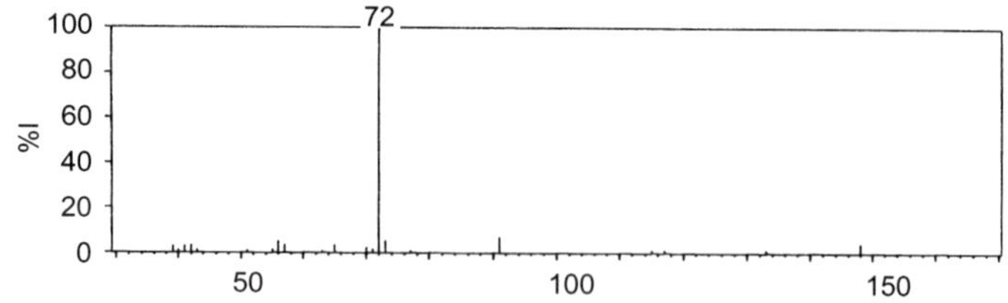

Quantification

Gas chromatography. In urine: mephentermine, chlorphentermine and phentermine, FID—A. H. Beckett and L. G. Brookes, *J. Pharm. Pharmacol.*, 1971, *23*, 288–294.

Disposition in the Body. Readily absorbed after oral or parenteral administration and rapidly metabolised by demethylation and hydroxylation. About 50 to 85% of a dose is excreted in the urine unchanged, together with 15 to 20% as phentermine. Conjugated *N*-hydroxymephentermine has also been detected in the urine in small quantities.

Toxicity. The estimated minimum lethal dose in children up to 2 years of age is 200 mg, and in adults is 2 g.

Half-life. Derived from urinary excretion data, about 6 to 20 h.

Dose. The equivalent of 15 to 80 mg of mephentermine has been given parenterally.

Mephenytoin

Anticonvulsant

Synonyms. Mephenetoin; Methoin; Methantoin; Phenantoin.
Proprietary names. Epilan; Insulton; Mesantoin; Phenantoin; Sacerno.
5-Ethyl-3-methyl-5-phenyl-2,4-imidazolidinedione
$C_{12}H_{14}N_2O_2 = 218.3$
CAS—50-12-4

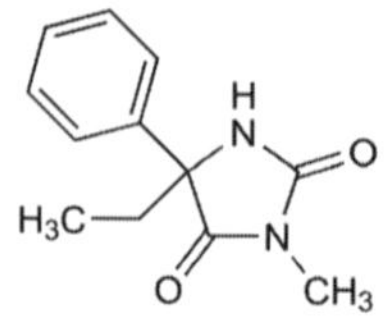

Colourless lustrous crystals or white crystalline powder. M.p. 136° to 137°. Soluble 1 in 1400 of water, 1 in 15 of ethanol, 1 in 3 of chloroform, and 1 in 90 of ether.

Dissociation Constant. pK_a 8.1.

Partition Coefficient. Log *P* (octanol/water), 1.7.

Colour Tests. Koppanyi–Zwikker Test—violet; Liebermann's Test—red-orange; Mercurous Nitrate—black.

Thin-layer Chromatography. System TD—Rf 62; system TE—Rf 74; system TF—Rf 58; system TAD—Rf 66; system TAJ—Rf 64; system TAK—Rf 70; system TAL—Rf 91.

Gas Chromatography. System GA—mephenytoin RI 1785, M (4-OH-) RI 2400, M (OH-methoxy-) RI 2380, M (nor-) RI 1950; system GE—mephenytoin RRT 0.55 and 0.73 for 5-ethyl-5-phenylhydantoin (both relative to phenytoin); system GAJ—RRT 0.918 (relative to methylphenobarbital).

High Performance Liquid Chromatography. System HY—RI 366; system HZ—retention time 3.7 min; system HAX—retention time 6.0 min; system HAY—retention time 5.4 min.

Ultraviolet Spectrum. Ethanol—257 ($A_1^1=11a$), 264 nm.

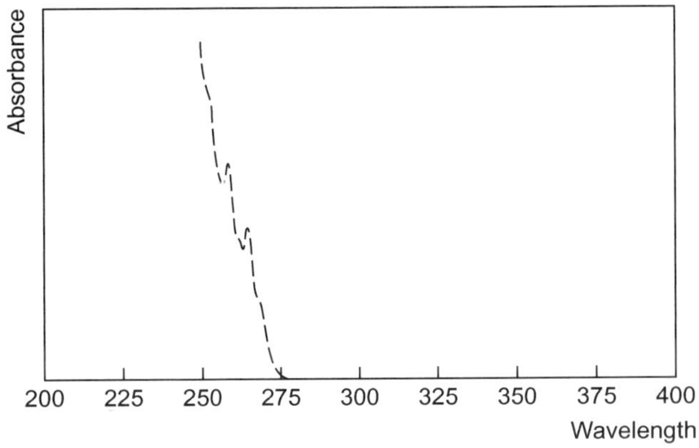

Infra-red Spectrum. Principal peaks at wavenumbers 1704, 1754, 733, 1052, 1302, 702 cm^{-1} (KBr disk).

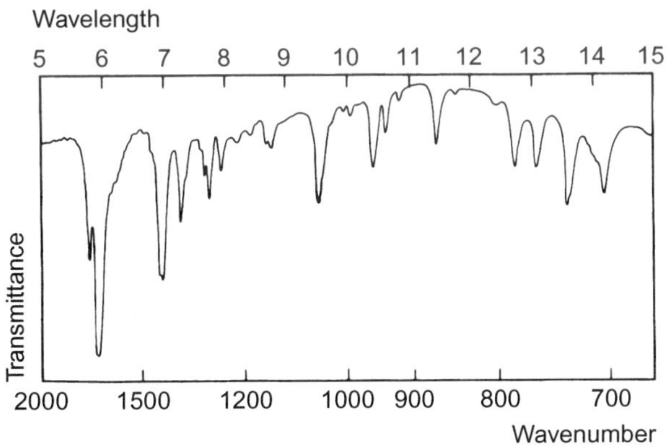

Mass Spectrum. Principal ions at *m/z* 189, 104, 190, 77, 44, 105, 132, 103.

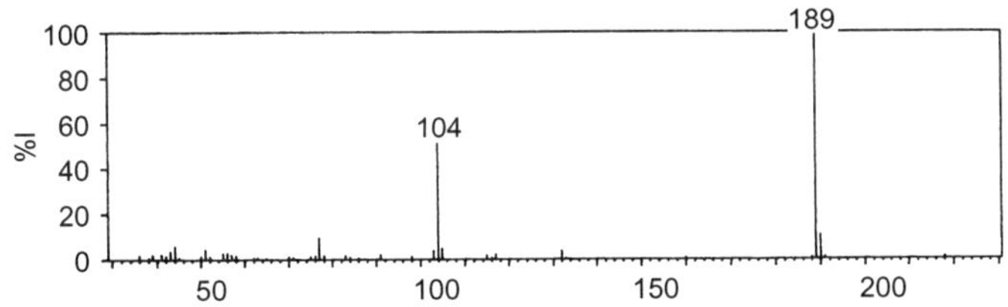

Quantification

Gas chromatography. In serum: limit of detection 5 mg/L for mephenytoin and 10 mg/L for 5-ethyl-5-phenylhydantoin, FID—V. A. Raisys *et al.*, *Clin. Chem.*, 1979, *25*, 172–175.

Gas chromatography–mass spectrometry. In plasma: limit of detection 10 µg/L for mephenytoin and 50 µg/L for 5-ethyl-5-phenylhydantoin—W. Yonekawa and H. J. Kupferberg, *J. Chromatogr.* 1979, *163*(5) *B Biomed. Appl.*, 161–167.

High performance liquid chromatography. In serum: mephenytoin and 5-ethyl-5-phenylhydantoin, limit of detection 1 mg/L, UV detection—P. M. Kabra *et al.*, *J. Anal. Toxicol.*, 1978, *2*, 127–133. In urine: mephenytoin and metabolites, UV detection—A. Küpfer *et al.*, *J. Chromatogr.* 1982, *232*(22) *B Biomed. Appl.*, 93–100. In urine: mephenytoin and 4′-hydroxymephenytoin, limits of detection 25 µg/L and 50 µg/L respectively, UV detection—Z. R. Ruan *et al.*, *Yao Xue Xue Bao*, 1994, *29*, 624–628. In urine: 4′-hydroxymephenytoin, UV detection—H. G. Xie *et al.*, *J. Chromatogr.* 1995, *668 B Biomed. Appl.*, 125–131. In urine: 4-hydroxymephenytoin, limit of detection <0.76 mg/L, electrochemical detection—M. Tanaka *et al.*, *J. Chromatogr.* 1996, *676 B Biomed. Appl.*, 87–94. In urine: mephenytoin enantiomers, limit of detection 12.5 µg/L, UV detection (comparison with GC) —S. L. Huang *et al.*, *Zhongguo Yao Li Xue Bao*, 1998, *19*, 548–550.

Disposition in the Body. Rapidly absorbed after oral administration. During chronic administration, the major metabolite is 5-ethyl-5-phenylhydantoin (nirvanol) which is a more active anticonvulsant than mephenytoin and accounts for at least 22% of the daily dose in the 24-h urine. After a single dose, the major metabolite is 4′-hydroxymethoin which is excreted in the urine as a glucuronide conjugate and accounts for 43% of a dose in 24 h; only about 1% of a single dose is excreted in the urine as 5-ethyl-5-phenylhydantoin; 5-ethyl-5-(4-hydroxyphenyl)-hydantoin has also been detected in the urine in both free and conjugated forms, together with minor amounts of other conjugated hydroxy metabolites; very little unchanged drug is excreted in the urine.

Therapeutic concentration. In plasma, mephenytoin plus metabolites, usually in the range 15 to 40 mg/L.

Following a single oral dose of 7 mg/kg to 5 subjects, peak serum concentrations of about 3 mg/L each of mephenytoin and 5-ethyl-5-phenylhydantoin were attained in about 1 h and 27 h respectively. [A. S. Troupin, *Ann. Neurol.*, 1979, *6*, 410–414.]

A mean steady-state serum concentration of 26 mg/L of total hydantoin was reported for 173 subjects receiving daily oral doses averaging 6.8 mg/kg; mephenytoin concentrations averaged 8% of the total hydantoin concentration. [A. S. Troupin *et al.*, *Epilepsia*, 1976, *17*, 403–414.]

Toxicity. The estimated minimum lethal dose is 5 g. Mephenytoin gives rise to toxic symptoms more frequently than phenytoin and cases of fatal aplastic anaemia have been reported; the toxicity of the drug is attributed to the proven toxicity of 5-ethyl-5-phenylhydantoin. Acute overdosage may result in coma.

Half-life. Plasma half-life, after a single dose, mephenytoin about 7 h, 5-ethyl-5-phenylhydantoin about 95 h; the half-life of the metabolite decreases to about 72 h during chronic treatment.

Saliva. Plasma:saliva ratio, about 1.6.

Protein binding. In plasma, about 40%.

Dose. Initially, 50 to 100 mg daily; maintenance, 200 to 600 mg daily.

Mepivacaine

Local Anaesthetic

N-(2,6-Dimethylphenyl)-1-methyl-2-piperidinecarboxamide
$C_{15}H_{22}N_2O=246.4$
CAS—96-88-8

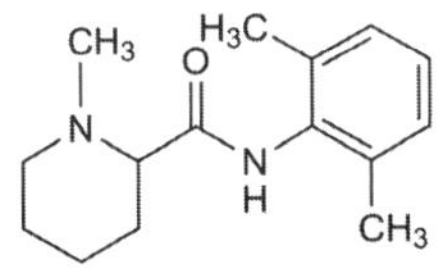

Yellow-white crystals. M.p. 150° to 151° (crystals from ether).

Mepivacaine Hydrochloride

Synonyms. Mepivacaini Chloridum; Mepivacaini Hydrochloridum.
Proprietary names. Carbocain(e); Chlorocain; Isocaine; Isogaine; Mecain; Meaverin; Mepi-Mynol; Mepicain; Mepident; Mepiforan; Mepyl; Optocain; Pericaina; Polocaine; Scandicain(e); Scandinibsa; Scandonest; Tevacaine.
$C_{15}H_{22}N_2O,HCl=282.8$
CAS—1722-62-9
A white crystalline powder. M.p. 262° to 264°.

Freely soluble in water and methanol; soluble 1 in 10 of ethanol; very slightly soluble in chloroform; practically insoluble in ether.

Dissociation Constant. pK_a 7.7 (20°).

Partition Coefficient. Log *P* (octanol/water), 1.9.

Colour Test. Liebermann's Test—brown-orange.

Thin-layer Chromatography. System TA—Rf 65; system TB—Rf 31; system TC—Rf 62; system TE—Rf 66; system TL—Rf 48; system TAE—Rf 63; system TAF—Rf 60; system TAJ—Rf 28; system TAK—Rf 02; system TAL—Rf 40. (Dragendorff spray, positive; acidified iodoplatinate solution, positive; Marquis reagent, brown; ninhydrin spray, positive.)

Gas Chromatography. System GA—mepivacaine RI 2065, M (OH-) RI 2410, M (oxo-) RI 2400; system GF—RI 2345; system GQ—Retention time 7.2 min.

High Performance Liquid Chromatography. System HA—*k* 0.9; system HQ—*k* 1.09; system HX—RI 296; system HY—RI 260; system HZ—Retention time 2.6 min; system HAX—Retention time 7.7 min; system HAY—Retention time 4.2 min.

Ultraviolet Spectrum. Aqueous acid—263 (A_1^1 = 18a), 271 nm.

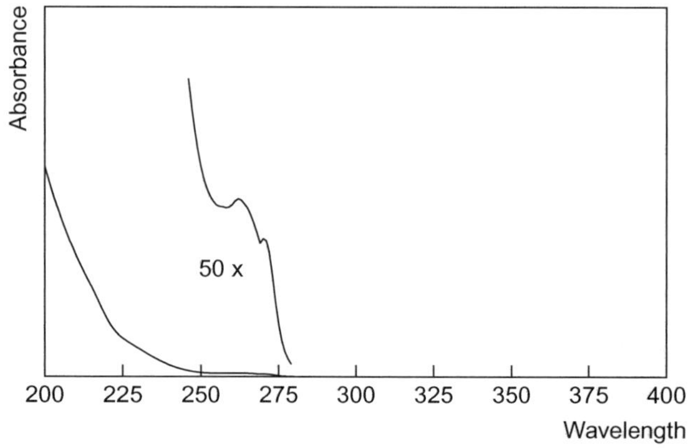

Infra-red Spectrum. Principal peaks at wavenumbers 1650, 1523, 760, 1220, 1123, 1265 cm^{-1} (KBr disk).

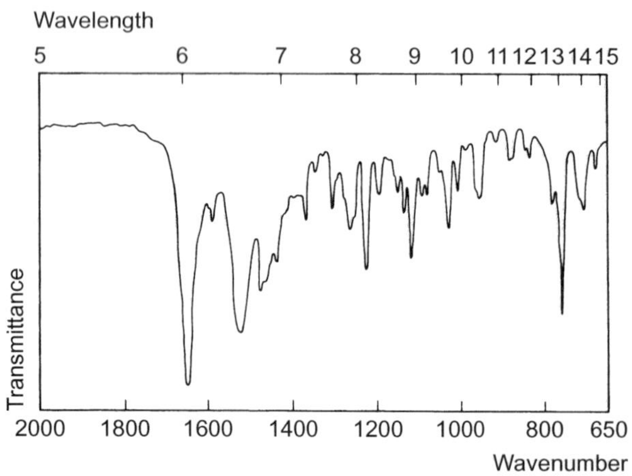

Mass Spectrum. Principal ions at *m/z* 98, 99, 70, 42, 96, 55, 41, 40 (no peaks above 100).

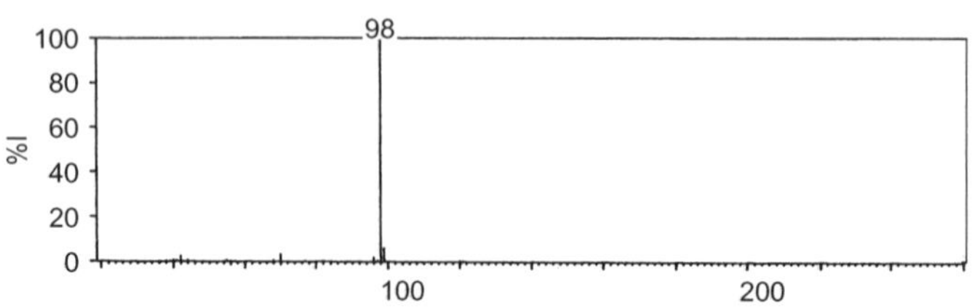

Quantification

Gas chromatography. In blood: limit of detection 40 ng, FID—J. H. Asling *et al.*, *Anesthesiology*, 1969, *31*, 458–461. In urine: mepivacaine and 3 metabolites, FID—J. Thomas and P. Meffin, *J. Med. Chem.*, 1972, *15*, 1046–1049. In biological samples: mepivacaine and other local anaesthetics, nitrogen-sensitive detection—O. W. Lau *et al.*, *Methods Find. Exp. Clin. Pharmacol.*, 1991, *13*, 475–481. In body fluids: mepivacaine and other local anaesthetics, limits of detection 5 to 10 pg, SID—H. Hattori *et al.*, *J. Chromatogr.*, 1991, *564*, 278–282.

Gas chromatography–mass spectrometry. In blood: mepivacaine and other local anaesthetics—T. Watanabe *et al.*, *J. Chromatogr. B Biomed. Sci. Appl.*, 1998, *709*, 225–232. In plasma and urine: mepivacaine and other local anaesthetics, limit of quantification 40 µg/L and limit of detection 50 µg/L (SIM, *m/z* 82)—T. Ohshima and T. Takayasu, *J. Chromatogr. B Biomed. Sci. Appl.*, 1999, *726(1–2)*, 185–194.

High performance liquid chromatography. In plasma: mepivacaine enantiomers, limit of detection 3 µg/L, UV detection—A. A. Vletter *et al.*, *J. Chromatogr. B Biomed. Appl.*, 1996, *678*, 369–372. In serum: mepivacaine enantiomers, limit of detection 100 to 150 µg/L, UV detection—M. Siluveru and J. T. Stewart, *J. Chromatogr. B Biomed. Sci. Appl.*, 1997, *690*, 359–362; M. Siluveru and J. T. Stewart, *J. Pharm. Biomed. Anal.*, 1997, *15*, 1751–1756. In plasma: limit of detection 100 µg/L, UV detection—R. Murtaza *et al.*, *J. Pharmacol. Toxicol. Methods*, 2001, *46*, 131–136.

Disposition in the Body. Rapidly absorbed into the circulation following epidural and paracervical injection. Mepivacaine crosses the placenta and the ratio of fetal to maternal concentrations has been reported to be about 0.7. Rapidly metabolised by hydroxylation to the 3′- and 4′-hydroxy metabolites and by *N*-demethylation to 2′,6′-pipecoloxylidide (PPX). Over 50% is excreted as metabolites into the bile but only small amounts are eliminated in the faeces; this may be due to enterohepatic circulation. Less than 10% of a dose is excreted in the urine as unchanged drug in 24 h; about 16% of a dose is excreted in the 24-h urine as 3′-hydroxymepivacaine, 12% as 4′-hydroxymepivacaine, and 2% as 2′,6′-pipecoloxylidide; the excretion of unchanged drug is increased in acid urine and in neonates.

Therapeutic concentration. In plasma, usually in the range 2 to 5 mg/L.

Following epidural administration of 250 to 580 mg to 8 subjects, plasma concentrations at delivery were 3.7 to 5.5 mg/L (mean 4.7) for mepivacaine and < 0.1 to 0.38 mg/L for 2′,6′-pipecoloxylidide [P. Meffin *et al.*, *Clin. Pharmacol. Ther.*, 1973, *14*, 218–225].

Following paracervical injection of 200 mg to 5 subjects, peak plasma concentrations of 1.4 to 4.0 mg/L (mean 2.3) were attained in about 30 min [K. Teramo and A. Rajamaki, *Br. J. Anaesth.*, 1971, *43*, 300–312].

Toxicity.

Mepivacaine had been given as a local anaesthetic (between 75 and 150 mL of a 2% solution) to a young woman who died while undergoing cosmetic surgery. Postmortem concentrations were: blood 50 mg/L, bile 50 mg/L, brain 51 µg/g, kidney 51 µg/g, liver 75 µg/g, spleen 72 µg/g. Salicylate and glutethimide were also found in the blood and urine [I. Sunshine and W. W. Fike, *N. Engl. J. Med.*, 1964, *271*, 487–490].

Half-life. Plasma half-life, about 2 to 3 h.

Volume of distribution. About 1 L/kg.

Clearance. Plasma clearance, about 5 mL/min/kg.

Distribution in blood. Plasma : whole blood ratio, 1.1.

Protein binding. In plasma, about 77%.

Note. For a review of the pharmacokinetics of local anaesthetics see G. T. Tucker and L. E. Mather, *Clin. Pharmacokinet.*, 1979, *4*, 241–278.

Dose. Mepivacaine hydrochloride is given by injection in doses of up to 400 mg; maximum of 1 g in 24 h.

Meprobamate

Tranquilliser

Synonyms. Meprobamatum; Meprotanum.

Proprietary names. Cyrpon; Dapaz; Epikur; Equanil; Meprate; Mepro; Meprodil; Meprospan; Miltaun; Miltown; Neuramate; Norgagil; Novalm; Novo-Mepro; Pertranquil; Procalmadiol; Quanil; Reposo-Mono; Restenil; anobamat; Visano N; Visano-mini. It is an ingredient of Deprol, Epromate, Equagesic, Equazine M, Micrainin, and Paxidal.

2-Methyl-2-propyl-1,3-propanediol dicarbamate

$C_9H_{18}N_2O_4$=218.3
CAS—57-53-4

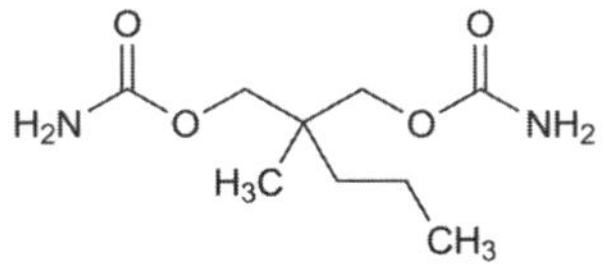

Colourless crystals or white crystalline powder. M.p. 104° to 106°.
Soluble 1 in 240 of water, 1 in 7 of ethanol, 1 in 80 of chloroform, and 1 in 70 of ether; freely soluble in acetone.

Partition Coefficient. Log *P* (octanol/water), 0.7.

Colour Tests. Furfuraldehyde—black; Nessler's Reagent (100°)—grey-black.

Thin-layer Chromatography. System TA—Rf 75; system TB—Rf 00; system TC—Rf 32; system TD—Rf 09; system TE—Rf 56; system TF—Rf 36; system TL—Rf 58; system TAD—Rf 32; system TAE—Rf 63; system TAF—Rf 87; system TAJ—Rf 35; system TAK—Rf 29; system TAL—Rf 78. (Furfuraldehyde reagent, positive; Van Urk reagent, yellow.)

Gas Chromatography. System GA—RI 1785; system GB—RI 1854; system GF—RI 2460.

High Performance Liquid Chromatography. System HZ—Retention time 2.4 min.

Ultraviolet Spectrum. No significant absorption, 230 to 360 nm.

Infra-red Spectrum. Principal peaks at wavenumbers 1688, 1069, 1090, 1590, 1310, 1140 cm^{-1} (KBr disk).

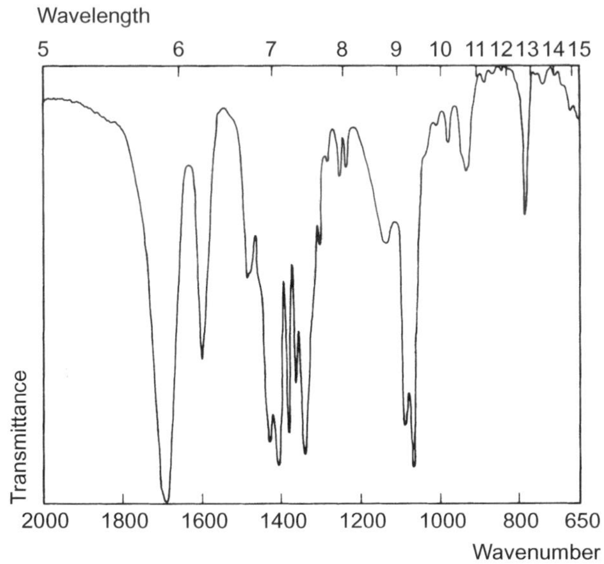

Mass Spectrum. Principal ions at *m/z* 83, 84, 55, 56, 43, 71, 41, 62 (no peaks above 160).

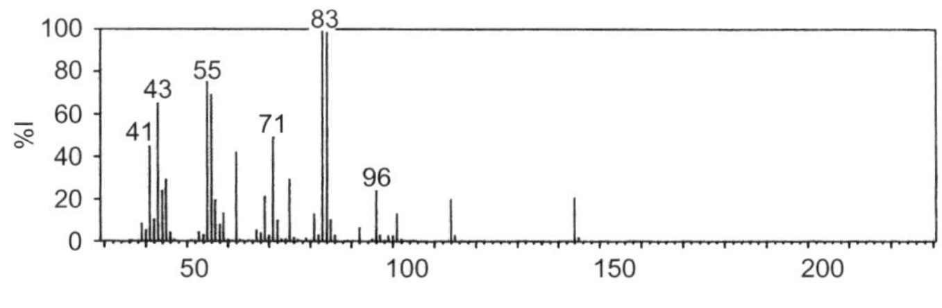

Quantification

Gas chromatography. In plasma or urine: FID—L. Martis and R. H. Levy, *J. Pharm. Sci.*, 1974, *63*, 834–837. In plasma or serum—Y. Gaillard *et al.*, *J. Chromatogr.*, 1992, *577*, 171–173. In plasma: FID—T. Trenque *et al.*, *J. Chromatogr.*, 1993, *615*, 343–346.

Gas chromatography–mass spectrometry. In plasma, urine, or hair—P. Kintz and P. Mangin, *J. Anal. Toxicol.*, 1993, *17*, 408–410. In postmortem blood—Y. Gaillard *et al.*, *Forensic Sci. Int.*, 1997, *86*, 173–180.

High performance liquid chromatography. In plasma: UV detection, comparison with a GC method—R. N. Gupta and F. Eng, *J. High Resolut. Chromatogr. Chromatogr. Commun.*, 1980, *3*, 419–420.

Disposition in the Body. Readily absorbed after oral administration. It is widely distributed and mainly metabolised in the liver. About 90% of a dose is excreted in the urine in 24 h, with about 10 to 20% of the dose as unchanged drug and the remainder as metabolites, mainly 2-hydroxypropylmeprobamate and meprobamate *N*-glucuronide. About 10% of the dose is eliminated in the faeces. Meprobamate crosses the placenta. Levels in breast milk may be up to 4 times higher than those found in plasma. Meprobamate is a minor metabolite of tybamate and is a metabolite of carisoprodol.

Therapeutic concentration. In plasma, usually in the range 5 to 20 g/L.

Following two oral doses of 800 mg, given to 5 subjects over a period of 1.5 h, peak blood concentrations of 18.6 to 26.6 g/L (mean 23.8) were attained in about 3.5 h [K. D. Parker *et al.*, *Clin. Toxicol.*, 1970, *3*, 131–145].

Toxicity. The estimated minimum lethal dose is 12 g, although recovery has occurred after much larger doses. Blood concentrations greater than about 50 mg/L may cause coma and fatalities have usually been associated with blood concentrations greater than about 70 mg/L.

In 19 fatalities involving meprobamate overdose, postmortem blood concentrations of 41 to 397 mg/L (mean 182) were reported [Y. Gaillard *et al.*, *Forensic Sci. Int.*, 1997, *86*, 173–180].

A postmortem blood concentration of 204.6 mg/L was reported in a fatality resulting from the deliberate ingestion of 90 tablets (400 mg) of meprobamate; the highest tissue concentration was found in the heart (708 µg/g) [P. Kintz *et al.*, *Am. J. Forensic Med. Pathol.*, 1988, *9*, 139–140].

In 4 cases of severe meprobamate intoxication, maximum plasma concentrations of 176, 180, 190, and 203 mg/L were reported; all patients survived (one was resuscitated from cardiac arrest), with 3 being treated by charcoal haemoperfusion [D. Jacobsen *et al.*, *J. Toxicol. Clin. Toxicol.*, 1987, *25*, 317–331].

Half-life. Plasma half-life, 6 to 17 h (mean 11); it may be much longer after chronic administration and may be dose-dependent.

Volume of distribution. About 0.7 L/kg.

Distribution in blood. Plasma : whole blood ratio, about 0.2 to 0.3.

Protein binding. In plasma, about 20%.

Dose. 1.2 to 2.4 g daily.

Meprylcaine

Local Anaesthetic

2-Methyl-2-propylaminopropyl benzoate
$C_{14}H_{21}NO_2$=235.3
CAS—495-70-5

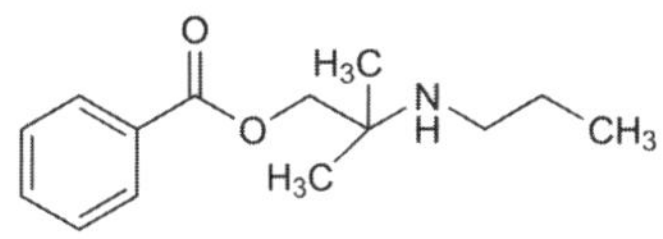

An oil.
Practically insoluble in water; soluble in ethanol and ether.

Meprylcaine Hydrochloride

$C_{14}H_{21}NO_2,HCl$=271.8
CAS-956-03-6
A white crystalline powder. M.p. 150° to 153°.
Soluble 1 in 6 of water, 1 in 5 of ethanol, 1 in 3 of chloroform and 1 in 12 of ether.

Ultraviolet Spectrum. Aqueous acid—232 nm (A^1_1=422b).

Mass Spectrum. Principal ions at *m/z* 100, 58, 105, 77, 56, 101, 41, 70.

Meptazinol

Narcotic Analgesic

Proprietary name. Meptid (tablets)
3-(3-Ethylhexahydro-1-methyl-1*H*-azepin-3-yl)phenol
$C_{15}H_{23}NO = 233.4$
CAS—54340-58-8

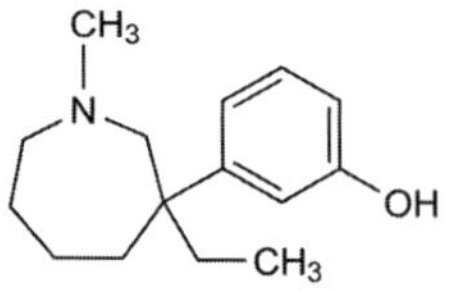

Crystals. M.p. 127° to 133°.
Very slightly soluble in water; soluble in ethanol; sparingly soluble in chloroform and ether.

Meptazinol Hydrochloride

Proprietary names. Meptid (injection); Meptidol.
$C_{15}H_{23}NO,HCl = 269.8$
CAS–59263-76-2; 34154-59-1 (±)
A white crystalline powder. M.p. 183° to 187°.
Soluble 1 in about 4 of water and 1 in 12 of ethanol; very slightly soluble in chloroform; practically insoluble in ether.

Dissociation Constant. pK_a 8.7 (-NH_2), 11.9 (phenol).

Gas Chromatography. System GA—meptazinol RI 1920, M (nor-) RI 1995, M (oxo-) RI 2410; system GB—meptazinol RI 1980, M (nor-) RI 2069, M (oxo-) RI 2600; system GM—meptazinol RRT 0.429, M (nor-) RRT 0.428 (all relative to iprindole).

High Performance Liquid Chromatography. System HA—*k* 3.1; system HY—RI 269.

Ultraviolet Spectrum. Ethanol—277 nm ($A^1_1 = 91b$).

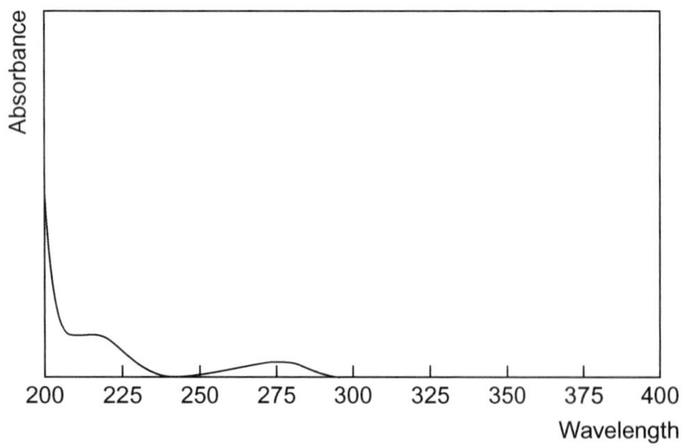

Infra-red Spectrum. Principal peaks at wavenumbers 1580, 708, 795, 1225, 1205, 1300 cm^{-1} (meptazinol hydrochloride, KBr disk).

Quantification

High performance liquid chromatography. In plasma: limit of detection 3 μg/L, fluorescence detection—T. Frost, *Analyst*, *Lond.*, 1981, *106*, 999–1001. In biological samples—C. Rudolphi and G. Blaschke, *J. Chromatogr.*, 1995, *663*, *Biomed. Appl.*, 315–326.

Disposition in the Body. Readily and almost completely absorbed after oral administration. Rapidly absorbed after intramuscular or rectal administration. It is excreted rapidly in the urine, mainly as the glucuronide conjugate, with less than 5% of a dose as unchanged drug, and about 5 to 10% as 7-oxomeptazinol. Both metabolites are inactive. Over 50% of a dose is excreted in the urine in 9 h and over 60% in 24 h. Less than 10% of an oral dose is eliminated in the faeces.

Therapeutic concentration

Following a single oral dose of 200 mg to 9 subjects, peak plasma concentrations of 0.01 to 0.11 mg/L (mean 0.06) were attained in 0.25 to 2 h; accumulation in plasma did not occur after repeated oral administration [H. M. Norbury *et al.*, *Eur. J. Clin. Pharmacol.*, 1983, *25*, 77–80].

After a single intramuscular dose of 50 mg to 4 subjects, peak plasma concentrations of 0.19 to 0.26 mg/L (mean 0.22) were attained in 10 min [G. Davies *et al.*, *Eur. J. Clin. Pharmacol.*, 1982, *23*, 535–538].

Toxicity

A 61-year-old woman who recovered after intentionally ingesting 200 mg meptazinol with whisky had serum meptazinol and alcohol levels of 20.1 and 210 mg/L, respectively, approx. 2½ h after the overdose [A. G. Davison *et al.*, *Hum. Toxicol.*, 1987, *6*, 331].

Bioavailability. 2 to 19% (mean 9) owing to extensive first-pass metabolism.

Half-life. Plasma half-life, about 2 h.

Volume of distribution. About 5 L/kg.

Clearance. Plasma clearance, about 30 mL/min/kg.

Protein binding. In plasma, about 27%.

Dose. 200 mg, by mouth, every 4 h; the equivalent of 50 to 100 mg of meptazinol parenterally.

Mepyramine

Antihistamine

Synonyms. Pyranisamine; Pyrilamine; RP-2786.
N-[(4-Methoxyphenyl)methyl]-*N*′,*N*′-dimethyl-*N*-2-pyridinyl-1,2-ethanediamine
$C_{17}H_{23}N_3O = 285.4$
CAS—91-84-9

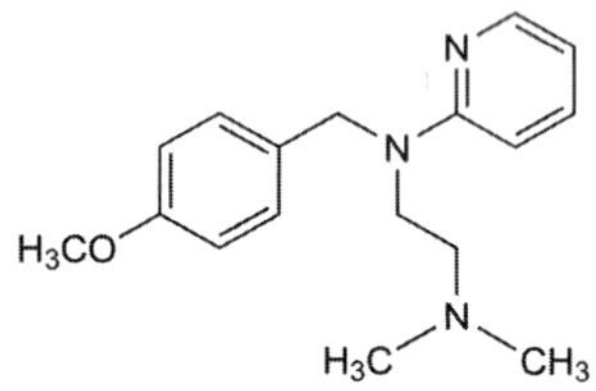

An oily liquid.

Mepyramine Maleate

Proprietary names. Anthisan. It is an ingredient of many proprietary preparations—see *Martindale, The complete drug reference*, 33rd Edn., Pharmaceutical Press, London, 2002.
$C_{17}H_{23}N_3O,C_4H_4O_4 = 401.5$
CAS-59-33-6
A white or creamy-white crystalline powder. M.p. 100° to 101°.
Soluble 1 in 0.4 of water, 1 in 2.5 of ethanol and 1 in 1.5 of chloroform; slightly soluble in ether and benzene.

Dissociation Constant. pK_a 4.0, 8.9 (25°).

Partition Coefficient. Log *P* (octanol/water), 2.8.

Colour Tests. Cyanogen Bromide—yellow; Mandelin's Test—violet; Marquis Test—violet.

Thin-layer Chromatography. System TA—Rf 51; system TB—Rf 39; system TC—Rf 25; system TE—Rf 58; system TL—Rf 14; system TAE—Rf 22; system TAF—Rf 33. (Dragendorff spray, positive; acidified iodoplatinate solution, positive; Marquis reagent, red.)

Gas Chromatography. System GA—mepyramine RI 2220, M (*N*-desalkyl-) RI 2120, M (*N*-desmethoxybenzyl-) RI 1580; system GB—RI 2328; system GF—RI 2560.

High Performance Liquid Chromatography. System HA—*k* 3.9; system HX—RI 448; system HY—RI 257.

Ultraviolet Spectrum. Aqueous acid—239 nm ($A^1_1 = 633a$), 316 nm; aqueous alkali—248, 312 nm.

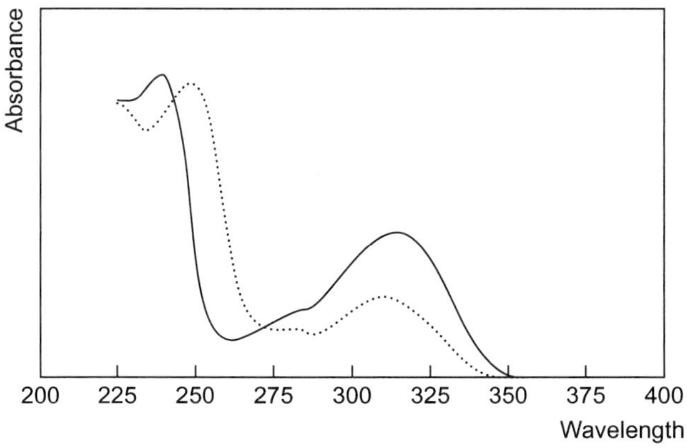

Infra-red Spectrum. Principal peaks at wavenumbers 1492, 1512, 1598, 1247, 1175, 1035 cm^{-1} (KBr disk).

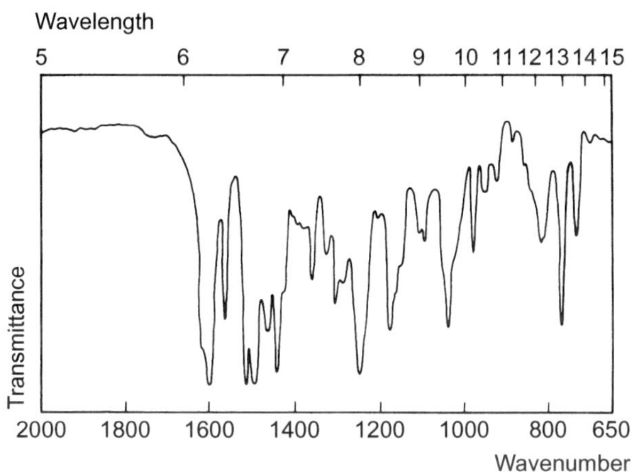

Mass Spectrum. Principal ions at *m/z* 121, 58, 72, 71, 214, 122, 215, 78.

Quantification

Gas chromatography. In postmortem tissues: FID—G. R. Johnson, *Clin. Toxicol.*, 1981, *18*, 907–909.

High performance liquid chromatography. In urine: limit of detection 1 ng/g, fluorescence detection—H. C. Thompson and C. L. Holder, *J. Chromatogr.*, 1984, *283*, 251–264.

Disposition in the Body. Absorbed after oral administration.

Toxicity

In a fatality due to mepyramine ingestion, the following postmortem tissue concentrations were reported: blood 11 mg/L, brain 71 μg/g, liver 18 μg/g [G. R. Johnson, *Clin. Toxicol.*, 1981, *18*, 907–909].

Dose. 0.3 to 1 g of mepyramine maleate daily.

Mequitazine

Antihistamine

Synonym. LM-209.

Proprietary names. Metaplexan; Mircol; Primalan; Primasone; Quitadrill.

10-(1-Azabicyclo[2.2.2]oct-3-ylmethyl)-10*H*-phenothiazine

$C_{20}H_{22}N_2S = 322.5$

CAS—29216-28-2

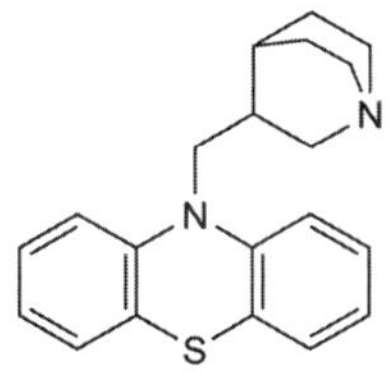

M.p. about 143°.

Practically insoluble in water; soluble in ethanol and chloroform.

Partition Coefficient. Log *P* (octanol/water), 5.7.

Colour Tests. Formaldehyde–Sulfuric Acid—red-violet; Forrest Reagent—red; FPN Reagent—orange-red; Liebermann's Test—green; Mandelin's Test—red; Marquis Test—red (slow); Sulfuric Acid (100°)—red (slow).

Thin-layer Chromatography. System TA—Rf 10; system TB—Rf 06; system TC—Rf 06; system TE—Rf 27; system TL—Rf 00; system TAE—Rf 03.

Gas Chromatography. System GA—mequitazine RI 2780, M (phenothiazine) RI 2020, M (sulfoxide) RI 3120, M (sulfone) RI 3250; system GB—mequitazine RI 2939, M (phenothiazine) RI 2130.

High Performance Liquid Chromatography. System HA—*k* 8.3 (tailing peak).

Ultraviolet Spectrum. Aqueous acid—256 nm (A^1_1 = 1060a), 307 nm. No alkaline shift. (See below)

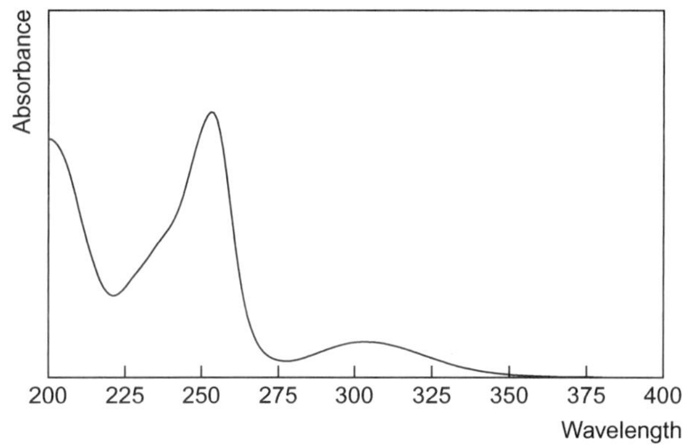

Infra-red Spectrum. Principal peaks at wavenumbers 751, 1250, 742, 1220, 729, 1042 cm^{-1} (KBr disk). (See below)

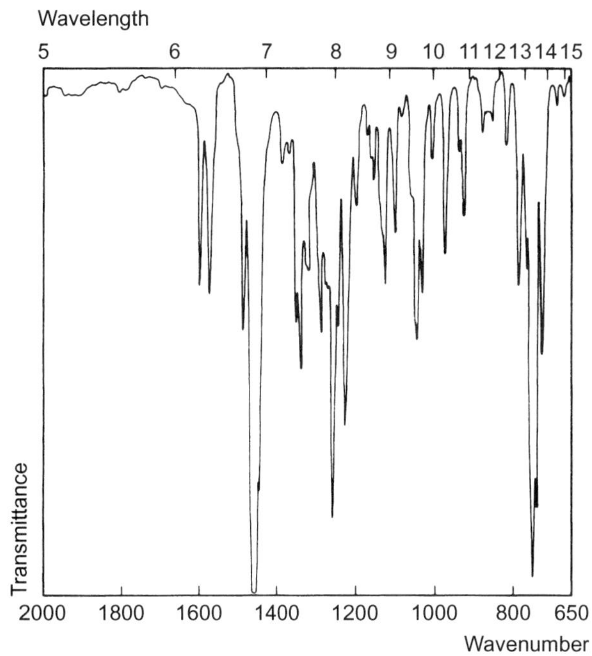

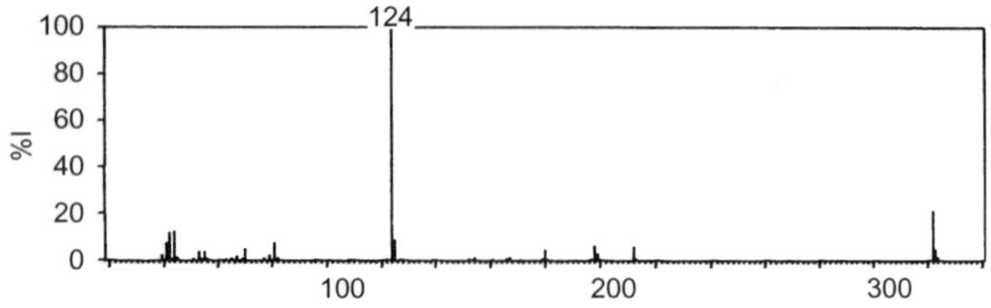

Dose. 10 mg daily.

Mercaptopurine

Antineoplastic

Synonym. 6MP
Proprietary names. Ismipur; Mercaptina; Puri-Nethol.
1,7-Dihydro-6*H*-purine-6-thione monohydrate
$C_5H_4N_4S,H_2O = 170.2$
CAS—50-44-2 (anhydrous); 6112-76-1 (monohydrate)

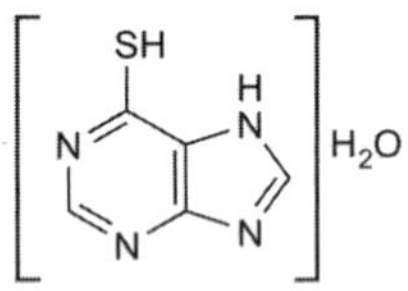

A yellow crystalline powder which darkens on exposure to air and light. M.p. above 308° with decomposition.
Insoluble in water, acetone, chloroform and ether; soluble in hot ethanol; soluble in solutions of alkali hydroxides.

Dissociation Constant. pK_a 7.7, 11.0 (20°).

Partition Coefficient. Log *P* (octanol/water), 0.0

Thin-layer Chromatography. System TB—Rf 00; system TE—Rf 02; system TF—Rf 00; system TAE—Rf 77.

Gas Chromatography. System GA—RI 1517.

High Performance Liquid Chromatography. System HX—RI 187.

Ultraviolet Spectrum. Mercaptopurine monohydrate: aqueous acid—325 nm ($A_1^1 = 1165a$); aqueous alkali—231 nm ($A_1^1 = 831a$), 310 nm ($A_1^1 = 1160a$).

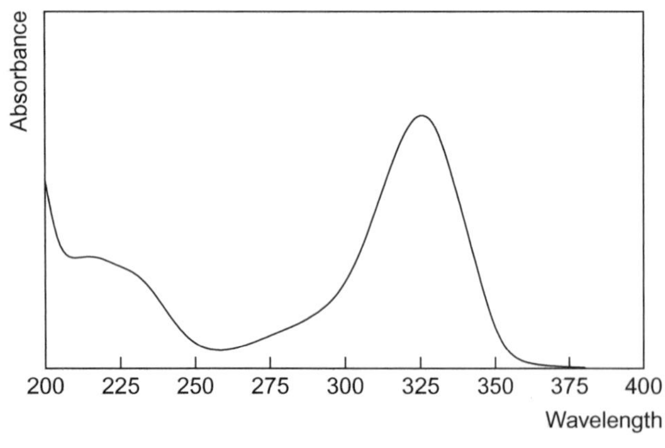

Infra-red Spectrum. Principal peaks at wavenumbers 1610, 1220, 1570, 1010, 865, 780 cm^{-1} (KBr disk).

Quantification

Gas chromatography–mass spectrometry. In plasma: limit of detection 2 µg/L—S. Floberg *et al.*, *J. Chromatogr.*, 1981, *225*; *Biomed. Appl.*, *14*, 73–81.

High performance liquid chromatography. In plasma: limit of detection <2 µg/L, fluorescence detection—R. E. Jonkers *et al.*, *J. Chromatogr.*, 1982, *233*; *Biomed. Appl.*, *22*, 249–255. In plasma or urine: mercaptopurine and metabolites, limits of detection for mercaptopurine 3.5 µg/L in plasma and 1.7 µg/L in urine, UV detection—I. Bruunshuus and K. Schmiegelow, *Scand. J. Lab. Invest.*, 1989, *49*, 779–784.

Disposition in the Body. Readily absorbed after oral administration. It is distributed throughout the body water and diffuses into the cerebrospinal fluid. Mercaptopurine is activated in the body by intracellular conversion to nucleotide forms including the ribonucleotide thioinosinic acid. It is metabolised by xanthine oxidase to inactive 6-thiouric acid which is excreted in the urine; inorganic sulfate may also be present. About 50% of an oral dose is excreted in the urine in 24 h, up to 8% as unchanged drug. Small amounts are excreted for up to 17 days. Mercaptopurine is a metabolite of azathioprine.

Therapeutic concentration

After a single oral dose of 75 mg/m^2 to 14 children (mean age 13 years) with acute lymphoblastic leukaemia, peak plasma concentrations of 0.04 to 0.28 mg/L (mean 0.14) were attained in 0.5 to 4 h (mean 2) [S. Zimm *et al.*, *N. Engl. J. Med.*, 1983, *308*, 1005–1009].

Daily oral doses of 75 mg/m^2 to 89 children with acute lymphoblastic leukaemia produced mean peak plasma concentrations of 0.10 (range 0.02 to 0.39) mg/L occurring at 0.5 to 3 h [F. M. Balis *et al.*, *Blood*, 1998, *92*, 3569–3577].

5 children with acute lymphoblastic leukaemia or malignant lymphoma were treated with 50 mg/m^2 oral mercaptopurine daily and 5 were treated with the same dose administered by rapid intravenous injection. The plasma concentrations were 0.23 to 0.42 mg/L (median 0.26) 5 min after intravenous infusion and 0.005 to 0.18 mg/L (median 0.06) one hour after oral administration; the time to peak plasma concentration following oral administration varied (1 h in 4 children, 2 h in 4 children and 3 h in 2 children) [H. Mawatari *et al.*, *Pediatr. Int.*, 2001, *43*, 673–677].

Toxicity

A 64-year-old woman took 200 mg of mercaptopurine every 8 h for about 2 weeks, because of an error in dispensing. She died 3 days later and the following postmortem concentrations were reported: blood 110 mg/L, bile 16 mg/L, brain 10 µg/g, kidney 33 µg/g [R.-L. Lin *et al.*, *J. Forensic Sci.*, 1982, *27*, 454–460].

Bioavailability. About 16% and very variable.

Half-life. Plasma half-life, about 0.5 to 1.5 h.

Protein binding. In plasma, about 20%.

Dose. Initially 2.5 mg/kg daily, by mouth.

Mersalyl Acid

Diuretic

A mixture of {3-[2-(carboxymethoxy)benzamido]-2-methoxypropyl}-hydroxymercury ($C_{13}H_{17}HgNO_6 = 483.9$) and its anhydrides.
CAS—486-67-9

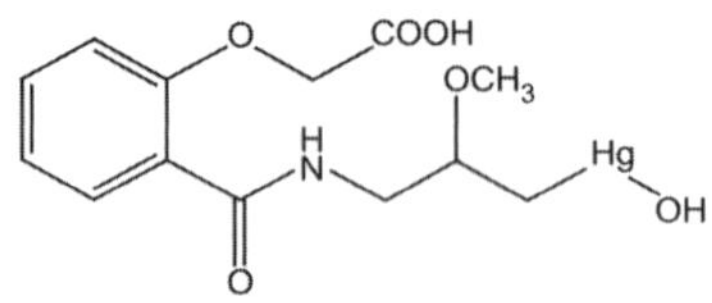

A white, slightly hygroscopic powder.
Slightly soluble in water and dilute mineral acids; soluble in solutions of alkali hydroxides.

Mersalyl Sodium

Synonym. Mersalyl
$C_{13}H_{16}HgNNaO_6 = 505.9$
CAS—492-18-2
A white deliquescent powder.
Soluble 1 in 1 of water, 1 in 3 of ethanol and 1 in 2 of methanol; practically insoluble in chloroform and ether.

Partition Coefficient. Log *P* (octanol/water), −1.5 (mersalyl sodium)

Thin-layer Chromatography. System TA—Rf 24.

Ultraviolet Spectrum. Aqueous acid—286 nm; aqueous alkali—290 nm ($A_1^1 = 63b$).

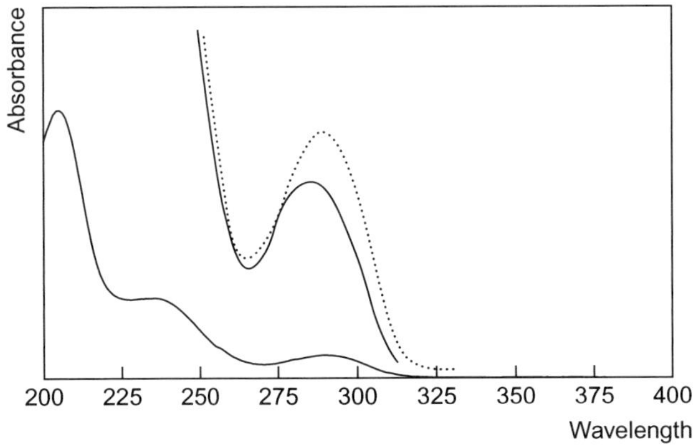

Dose. 50 to 200 mg of mersalyl sodium, intramuscularly.

Mescaline

Hallucinogen

Synonym. Mezcaline
3,4,5-Trimethoxybenzeneethanamine
$C_{11}H_{17}NO_3$=211.3
CAS—54-04-6

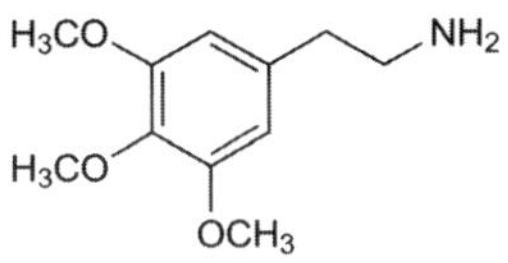

An alkaloid obtained from the cactus *Lophophora williamsii* (=*Anhalonium williamsii*=*A. lewinii*) (Cactaceae), which grows in the northern regions of Mexico. The cactus is also known by the names 'peyote' or 'peyotl' and dried slices of the cactus are called 'mescal buttons'.
Crystals which take up carbon dioxide from the air. M.p. 35° to 36°.
Moderately soluble in water; soluble in ethanol, chloroform and benzene; practically insoluble in ether and petroleum ether.

Mescaline Hydrochloride

$C_{11}H_{17}NO_3$, HCl=247.8
Needles. M.p. 181°. Soluble in water and alcohol.

Mescaline Sulfate Dihydrate

$(C_{11}H_{17}NO_3)_2$, H_2SO_4, $2H_2O$=540.7
Prisms. M.p. 183° to 186°. Soluble in hot water and methanol; sparingly soluble in cold water and ethanol.

Mescaline Acid Sulfate

$C_{11}H_{17}NO_3$, H_2SO_4=309.4
Crystals. M.p. 158°.

N-Benzoylmescaline

$C_{17}H_{21}NO_3$=287.4
Needles. M.p. 121°. Very soluble in alcohol and ether.

N-Methylmescaline

$C_{12}H_{19}NO_3$=225.3
Occurs naturally. B.p. 130° to 140°.

N-Acetylmescaline

$C_{13}H_{19}NO_4$=253.3
Occurs naturally. M.p. 94°.

Dissociation Constant. pK_a 9.6.

Partition Coefficient. Log *P* (octanol/water), 0.8.

Colour Tests. Liebermann's Test—black; Marquis Test—orange.

Thin-layer Chromatography. System TA—Rf 20; system TB—Rf 03; system TC—Rf 10; system TE—Rf 24; system TL—Rf 12; system TAE—Rf 06; system TAF—Rf 63; system TAJ—Rf 02; system TAK—Rf 09; system TAL—Rf 51. (Dragendorff spray, positive; FPN reagent, positive; acidified iodoplatinate solution, positive; Marquis reagent, yellow; ninhydrin spray, positive.)

Gas Chromatography. System GA—mescaline RI 1680, mescaline-AC RI 2160, mescaline precursor (trimethoxyphenylacetonitrile) RI 1610.

High Performance Liquid Chromatography. System HA—*k* 1.3; system HB—*k* 16.82; system HC—*k* 2.17; system HX—RI 272; system HY—RI 243.

Ultraviolet Spectrum. Aqueous acid—268 nm (A_1^1=34c). No alkaline shift.

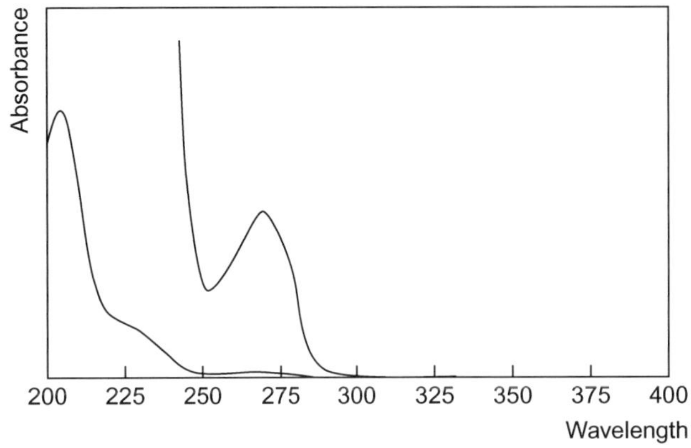

Infra-red Spectrum. Principal peaks at wavenumbers 1127, 1242, 1592, 996, 1513, 834 cm^{-1} (mescaline hydrochloride, KBr disk).

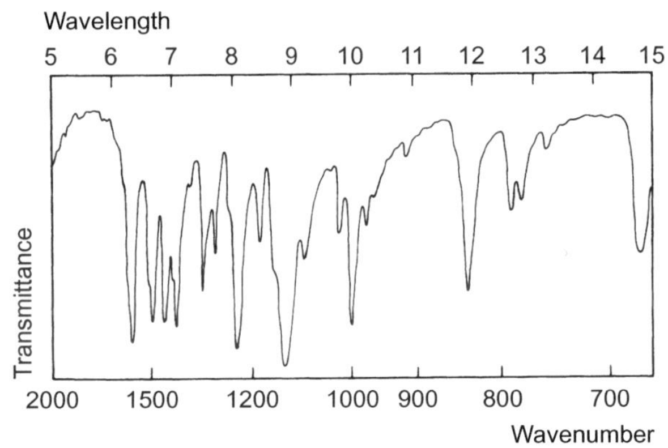

Mass Spectrum. Principal ions at *m/z* 182, 30, 181, 167, 211, 183, 151, 148.

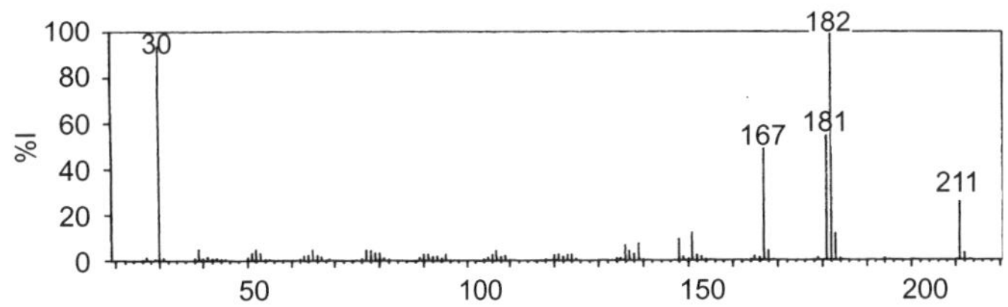

Quantification

Gas chromatography–mass spectrometry. In plasma—C. Van Peteghem *et al.*, *J. Pharm. Sci.*, 1980, *69*, 118–120.

High performance liquid chromatography. In urine: phenylalkylamine derivatives, limit of detection 26 to 56 μg/L, UV detection—H. J. Helmlin and R. Brenneisen, *J. Chromatogr.*, 1992, *593*, 87–94.

Disposition in the Body. Readily absorbed after oral administration. It is concentrated in the kidneys, liver, and spleen. About 90% of a dose is excreted in the urine in 24 h with about 30% as 3,4,5-trimethoxyphenylacetic acid, which is inactive; the remainder is mostly unchanged drug, together with 3,4-dihydroxy-5-methoxyphenylacetic acid which is excreted as a glutamine conjugate. Other metabolites include *N*-acetylmescaline and *N*-acetyl-3,4-dimethoxy-5-hydroxyphenethylamine.

Toxicity. Mescaline induces psychotic changes similar to those produced by lysergide, but it is less potent. The effects of a single dose may persist for about 12 h.

In a mescaline-related fatality, where the individual ran off a cliff and plunged 600 feet to his death, the concentrations were reported to be 9.7 mg/L, 70.8 mg/kg, and 1163 mg/L in the blood, liver, and urine, respectively [P. C. Reynolds and E. J. Jindrich, *J. Anal. Toxicol.*, 1985, *9*, 183–184].

Protein binding. In plasma, partly bound.

Note. For a historical article on mescaline use, see J. G. Bruhn *et al.*, *Lancet*, 2002, *359*, 1866. For a report of a fatal peyote ingestion, see K. B. Nolte and R. E. Zumwalt, *West. J. Med.*, 1999, *170*, 328.

Mesocarb

CNS Stimulant

Synonyms. Sidnocarb; Sydnocarbum; Synocarb.
3-(α-Methylphenethyl)-*N*-(phenylcarbamoyl)sydnone imine
$C_{18}H_{18}N_4O_2$=322.4
CAS—34262-84-5

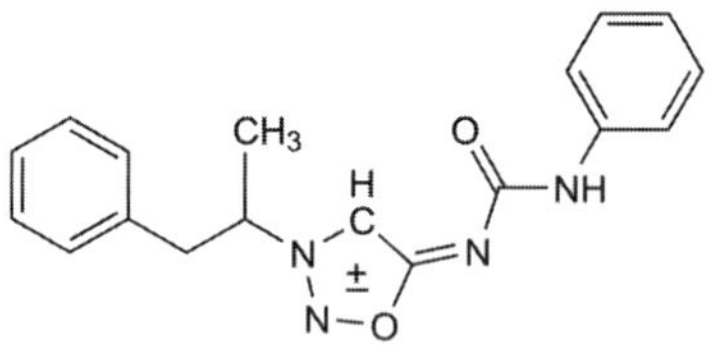

High Performance Liquid Chromatography. Column: C_{18} ODS (Ultrasphere, 75 × 4.6 mm i.d., 3 μm). Mobile phase: ammonium acetate (0.1 M, pH 3):acetonitrile (A:B), flow rate 1 mL/min. Elution programme: (90:10) to (85:15) in 2 min, to (55:45) in 3 min, to (40:60) in 3 min, held for 1 min. UV detection (diode array). Retention time: 7.8 min [R. Ventura *et al.*, *J. Chromatogr.*, 1993, *647*, 203–210].

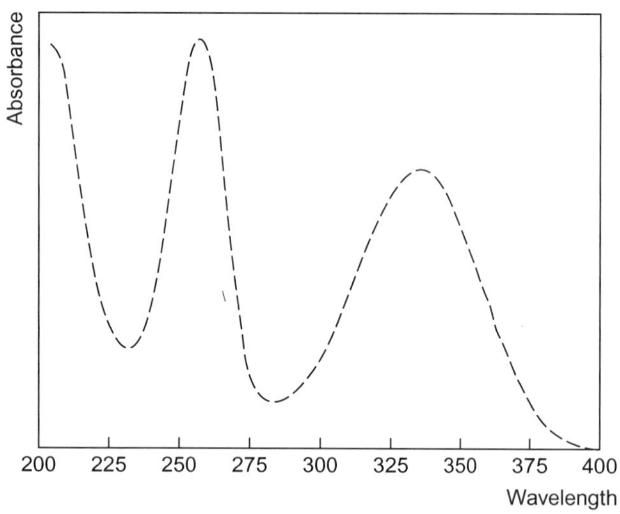

Note. Mesocarb is used as a psychostimulant in clinical practice in Russia as a primary and adjunct therapy for several psychiatric disorders. It is a stimulant with an addiction liability and toxicity less than that of amfetamines.
For a literature review of the toxicokinetics of amfetamines and their *N*-alkyl derivatives (including mesocarb), see T. Kraemer and H. H. Maurer, *Ther. Drug Monit.*, 2002, *24*, 277–289.

Mesoridazine

Tranquilliser

Synonym. Mesuridazine
10-[2-(1-Methyl-2-piperidinyl)ethyl]-2-(methylsulfinyl)-10*H*-phenothiazine
$C_{21}H_{26}N_2OS_2$=386.6
CAS—5588-33-0

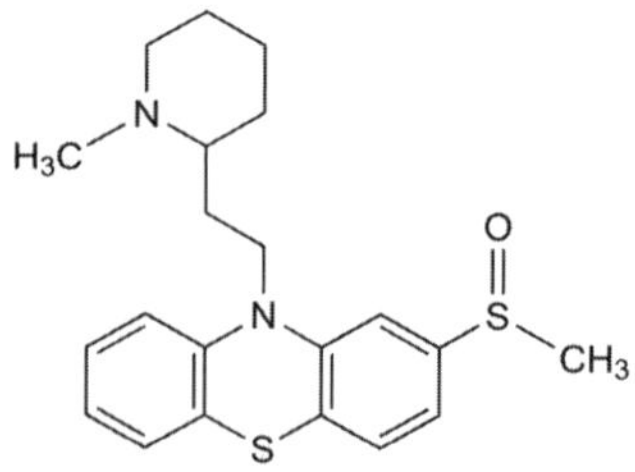

Soluble in chloroform.

Mesoridazine Benzenesulfonate
Synonym. Mesoridazine Besilate
Proprietary name. Serentil
$C_{21}H_{26}N_2OS_2,C_6H_6O_3S$=544.7
CAS—32672-69-8
A white to pale yellow, crystalline, powder. M.p. about 178°, with decomposition.
Soluble 1 in 1 of water, 1 in 11 of ethanol, 1 in 3 of chloroform and 1 in 6300 of ether; freely soluble in methanol.

Partition Coefficient. Log *P* (octanol/water), 5.6.

Colour Tests. Formaldehyde–Sulfuric Acid—violet; Forrest Reagent—red; FPN Reagent—red; Mandelin's Test—green-brown; Marquis Test—red→violet; Sulfuric Acid—violet→blue.

Thin-layer Chromatography. System TA—Rf 38; system TB—Rf 03; system TC—Rf 06; system TE—Rf 30; system TL—Rf 01; system TAE—Rf 11; system TAJ—Rf 02; system TAK—Rf 02; system TAL—Rf 52. (Acidified iodoplatinate solution, positive.)

Gas Chromatography. System GA—RI 3380; system GB—RI 3629.

High Performance Liquid Chromatography. System HA—*k* 5.0; system HY—RI 337; system HZ—Retention time, 3.4 min; system HAX—Retention time, 10.1 min; system HAY—Retention time 5.0 min.

Ultraviolet Spectrum. Aqueous acid—238, 262 nm (A^1_1= 773b), 310 nm.

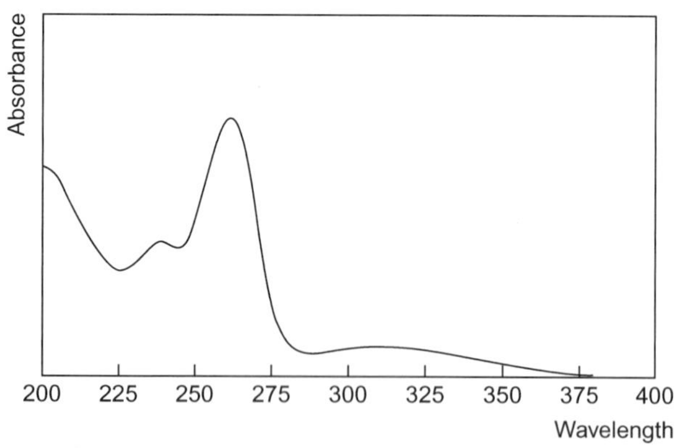

Infra-red Spectrum. Principal peaks at wavenumbers 1050, 752, 1239, 1282, 1562, 1091 cm^{-1} (KBr disk).

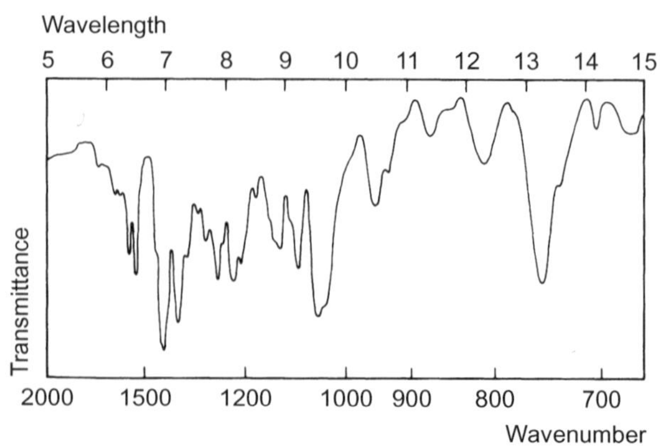

Mass Spectrum. Principal ions at *m*/*z* 98, 70, 99, 42, 386, 126, 55, 41.

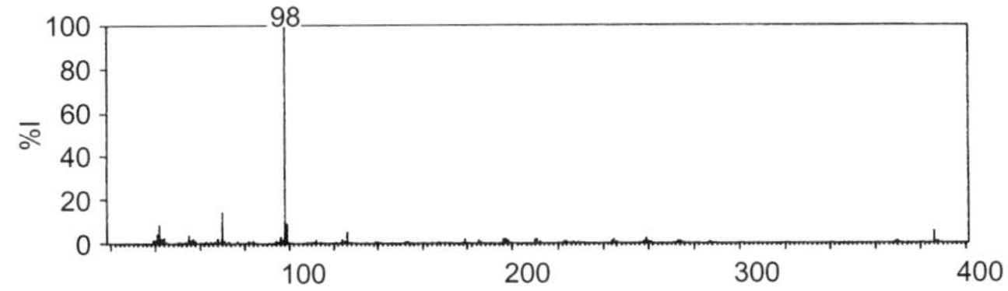

Quantification

Gas chromatography. In plasma: limit of detection 50 µg/L, FID—E. C. Dinovo *et al.*, *J. Pharm. Sci.*, 1976, *65*, 667–669.

High performance liquid chromatography. In whole blood: UV detection—J. R. McCutcheon, *J. Anal. Toxicol.*, 1979, *3*, 105–107.

Radioimmunoassay. In plasma—B. S. Chakraborty *et al.*, *Ther. Drug Monit.*, 1987, *9*, 464–471.

Disposition in the Body. Readily absorbed after oral administration. The major metabolite is sulforidazine which is pharmacologically active. Mesoridazine is a major metabolite of thioridazine.

Therapeutic concentration

Following a single intramuscular injection of 2 mg/kg to 6 subjects, peak plasma concentrations of 0.1 to 1.1 mg/L (mean 0.5) for mesoridazine, and 0.1 to 0.6 mg/L (mean 0.3) for sulforidazine, were attained in about 4 h [L. A. Gottschalk *et al.*, Plasma levels of mesoridazine and its metabolites, in *Pharmacokinetics of Psychoactive Drugs*, L. A. Gottschalk and S. Merlis (Eds), New York, Spectrum Publications, 1976, pp. 171–189].

Toxicity

In a fatality attributed to the ingestion of 2.5 g, the following postmortem tissue concentrations were reported: blood 3 mg/L, kidney 17 µg/g, liver 114 µg/g; in a second case in which 8 g had been ingested, the postmortem blood concentration was 4 mg/L [P. T. Donlon and J. P. Tupin, *Arch. Gen. Psychiatry*, 1977, *34*, 955–957].

A 23-year-old female died approx. 6 to 6½ h after ingesting an unknown quantity of mesoridazine. Her antemortem blood level of mesoridazine was 16 mg/L [J. E. Vertrees and G. Siebel, *Vet. Hum. Toxicol.*, 1987, *29*, 65–67].

Half-life. Plasma half-life, mesoridazine 2 to 9 h (mean 5), sulforidazine 6 to 25 h (mean 13).

Dose. The equivalent of 150 mg of mesoridazine daily; up to 400 mg daily has been given.

Mesterolone

Androgen

Proprietary names. Mestoranum; Pro-Viron.

(1α,5α,17β)-17-Hydroxy-1-methylandrostan-3-one

$C_{20}H_{32}O_2$=304.5

CAS—1424-00-6

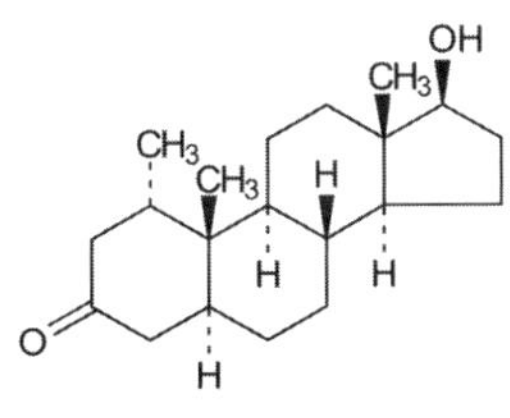

A white crystalline powder. M.p. about 210°.

Practically insoluble in water; soluble 1 in 50 of ethanol, 1 in 6 of chloroform and 1 in 150 of ether.

Partition Coefficient. Log *P* (octanol/water), 3.5.

High Performance Liquid Chromatography. System HATb—RRT 1.52 (relative to testosterone).

Ultraviolet Spectrum. No significant absorption, 230 to 360 nm.

Infra-red Spectrum. Principal peaks at wavenumbers 1706, 1068, 1055, 1252, 1238, 1032 cm^{-1} (KBr disk).

Quantification

Gas chromatography–mass spectrometry. In urine: mesterolone and other anabolic steroids, limits of detection 5 to 20 ppb—M. H. Choi *et al.*, *Rapid Commun. Mass Spectrom.*, 1999, *13*, 376–380. In hair: mesterolone and other anabolic steroids, limits of detection 0.002 to 0.05 µg/L—X. S. Deng *et al.*, *J. Forensic Sci.*, 1999, *44*, 343–346.

Dose. 50 to 100 mg daily.

Mestranol

Oestrogen

Synonyms. EE3ME; Ethinyloestradiol-3-methyl Ether.

Proprietary names. It is an ingredient of Enovid, Genora, Menophase, Necon, Nelova, Norethin, Norinyl and Ortho-Novin.

(17α)-3-Methoxy-19-norpregna-1,3,5(10)-trien-20-yn-17-ol

$C_{21}H_{26}O_2$=310.4

CAS—72-33-3

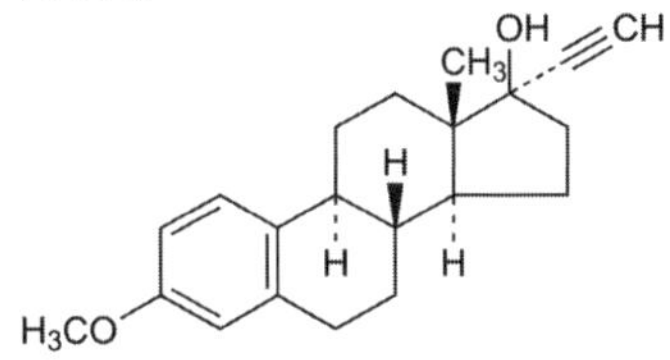

A white to creamy-white, crystalline powder. M.p. 146° to 154°.

Practically insoluble in water; soluble 1 in 44 of ethanol, 1 in 4.5 of chloroform and 1 in 23 of ether; soluble in dioxane and acetone; slightly soluble in methanol.

Caution. Mestranol is a powerful oestrogen. Contact with the skin or inhalation should be avoided.

Partition Coefficient. Log *P* (octanol/water), 4.7.

Colour Tests. Antimony Pentachloride—green; Liebermann's Test—red; Naphthol–Sulfuric Acid—red/red; Sulfuric Acid—orange-red (yellow fluorescence under ultraviolet light).

Thin-layer Chromatography. System TP—Rf 86; system TQ—Rf 52; system TR—Rf 90; system TS—Rf 90.

Gas Chromatography. System GA—RI 2612.

Ultraviolet Spectrum. Methanol—278 nm (A^1_1=61a), 287 nm.

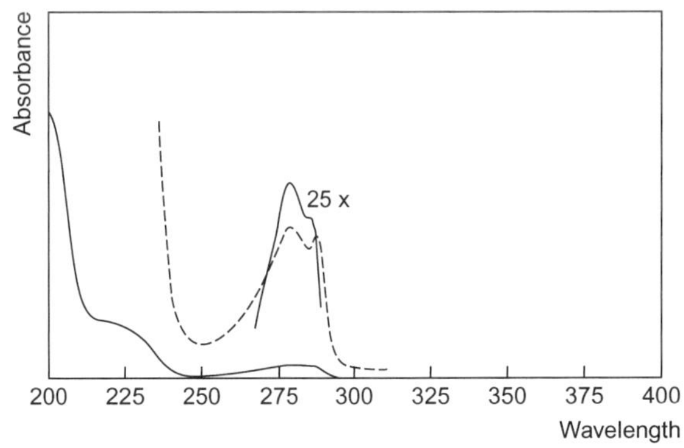

Infra-red Spectrum. Principal peaks at wavenumbers 1255, 1060, 1035, 1612, 1291, 1241 cm^{-1} (KBr disk).

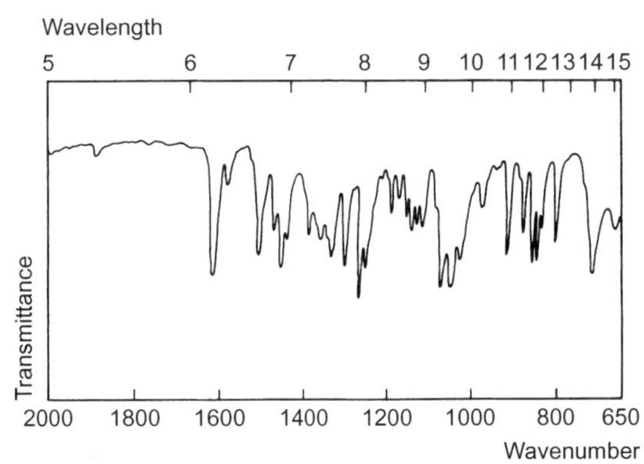

Mass Spectrum. Principal ions at m/z 227, 310, 174, 284, 147, 160, 173, 199.

Dose. Up to 100 µg daily.

Mesuximide

Anticonvulsant

Synonym. Methsuximide
Proprietary names. Celontin; Petinutin.
1,3-Dimethyl-3-phenyl-2,5-pyrrolidinedione
$C_{12}H_{13}NO_2$=203.2
CAS—77-41-8

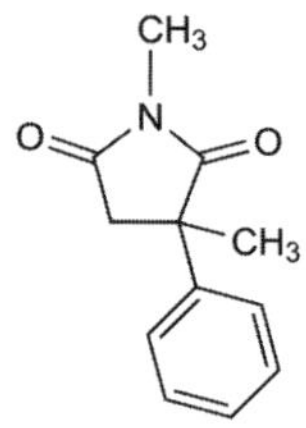

A white to greyish-white crystalline powder. M.p. 50° to 56°.
Soluble 1 in 350 of water, 1 in 3 of ethanol, 1 in less than 1 of chloroform, and 1 in 2 of ether.

Partition Coefficient. Log P (octanol/water), 1.4.

Thin-layer Chromatography. System TA—Rf 76; system TE—Rf 86; system TAE—Rf 90; system TAJ—Rf 85; system TAK—Rf 70; system TAL—Rf 98.

Gas Chromatography. System GA—mesuximide RI 1705; M (nor-) RI 1750; M (OH-) RI 2220; M (nor-OH-) RI 2300; system GE—RRT 0.35 for mesuximide and 0.50 for *N*-desmethylmesuximide (relative to phenytoin); system GAJ—RRT 0.689 for mesuximide and 0.779 for *N*-desmethylmesuximide (relative to methylphenobarbital).

High Performance Liquid Chromatography. System HE—k 6.02; system HY—RI 387; system HZ—Retention time 4.8 min.

Ultraviolet Spectrum. Methanol—247 (A_1^1=21a), 252, 258, 264 nm.

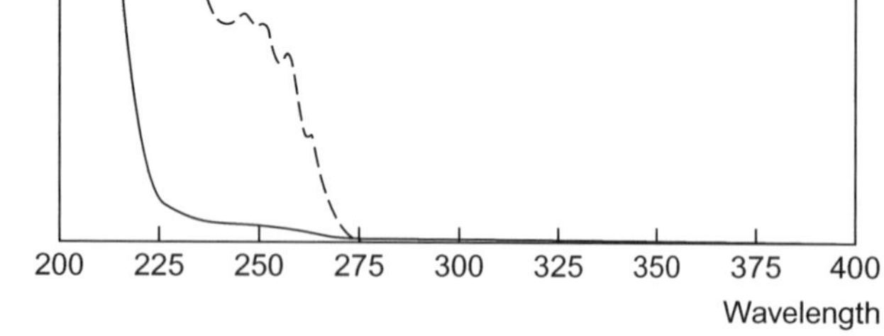

Infra-red Spectrum. Principal peaks at wavenumbers 1705, 1282, 1030, 699, 1775, 1086 cm^{-1} (KBr disk).

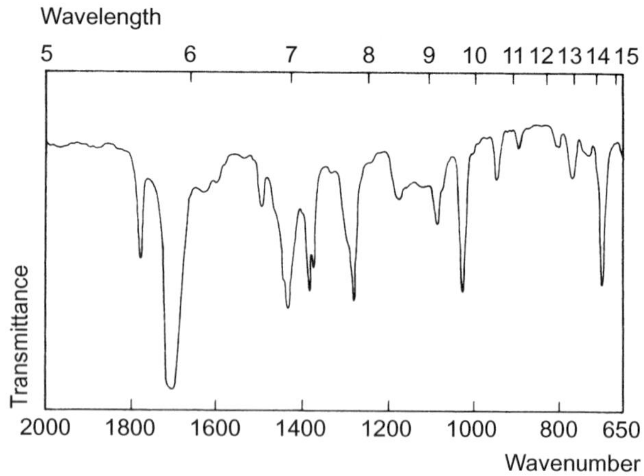

Mass Spectrum. Principal ions at m/z 118, 117, 203, 103, 77, 78, 119, 91.

Quantification

Gas chromatography. In serum: limit of detection 1 mg/L, FID—J. Bonitati, *Clin. Chem.*, 1976, *22*, 341–345. In plasma or serum: *N*-desmethylmesuximide, limit of detection 500 µg/L, ECD—J. E. Wallace *et al.*, *Clin. Chem.*, 1979, *25*, 252–255. In body fluids: mesuximide and *N*-desmethylsuximide, limits of detection 0.5 mg/L and 5 mg/L respectively, FID—D. S. Cardella *et al.*, *Clin. Biochem.*, 1988, *21*, 329–331.

High performance liquid chromatography. In serum: limit of detection 1 mg/L, UV detection—P. M. Kabra *et al.*, *J. Anal. Toxicol.*, 1978, *2*, 127–133.

Disposition in the Body. Rapidly absorbed after oral administration and metabolised to the active *N*-desmethyl derivative. Less than 1% of a dose is excreted in the urine as unchanged drug. The major urinary metabolites are conjugated 4-hydroxyphenyl derivatives; minor metabolites include the 3-hydroxy, 2-hydroxymethyl and 2-dihydrodihydroxyphenyl derivatives. Mesuximide increases its own rate of metabolism on chronic dosing.

Therapeutic concentration. In plasma, *N*-desmethylmesuximide, usually in the range 10 to 40 mg/L.

Following daily oral doses of 600 to 1200 mg to 8 subjects experiencing good seizure control, steady-state plasma concentrations of 0.01 to 0.11 mg/L (mean 0.04) and 16 to 37 mg/L (mean 25) for mesuximide and the *N*-desmethyl metabolite, respectively, were reported [J. M. Strong *et al.*, *Neurology*, 1974, *24*, 250–255.]

Toxicity. The estimated minimum lethal dose is 5 g. Toxic effects are usually associated with plasma *N*-desmethylmesuximide concentrations of more than 40 mg/L.

In a case of severe coma, which began several hours after the ingestion of nearly 10 g mesuximide in a suicide attempt, blood concentrations of 18 mg/L of mesuximide and 44 mg/L of the *N*-desmethyl metabolite were reported 14 h after ingestion; the coma persisted for about 80 h and correlated with the presence of the *N*-desmethyl metabolite in the blood [S. B. Karch, *J. Am. Med. Assoc.*, 1973, *223*, 1463–1465.]

Half-life. Plasma half-life, mesuximide about 3 h, but may reduce to one quarter of this value on chronic dosing; *N*-desmethylmesuximide about 30 to 40 h.

Protein binding. In plasma, not significantly bound.

Dose. 0.3 to 1.2 g daily; up to 3.6 g daily has been given.

Metaclazepam

Anxiolytic

Synonyms. Ka-2547; KC-2547; Brometazepam; Metuclazepam.
7-Bromo-5-(2-chlorophenyl)-2,3-dihydro-2-(methoxymethyl)-1-methyl-1*H*-1,4-benzodiazepine
$C_{18}H_{18}BrClN_2O$=393.7
CAS—84031-17-4

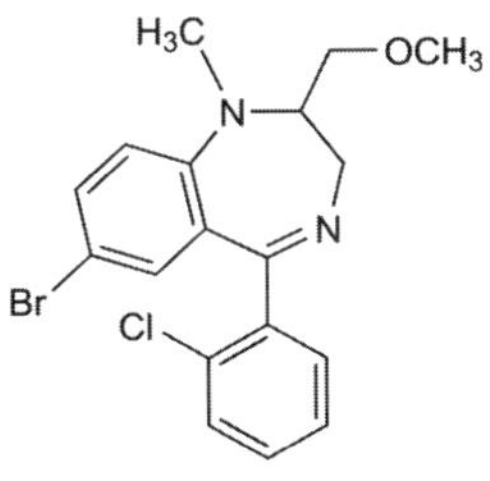

Yellow, odourless crystals. M.p. 88° to 90°.

Metaclazepam Hydrochloride
Synonym. Brometazepam Hydrochloride
Proprietary name. Talis
$C_{18}H_{18}BrClN_2O,HCl=430.2$
CAS—61802-93-5
A bright orange, crystalline powder with a slightly bitter taste. M.p. 193° to 196°. Solubility: 43 g/100 mL water; 73 g/100 mL methanol; 14 g/100 mL ethanol; 29 g/100 mL chloroform; 0.02 g/100 mL benzene.

Dissociation Constant. pK_a 5.9.

Partition Coefficient. Log *P* (octanol/phosphate buffer pH 7), 2000; (octanol/phosphate buffer pH 2), 3.

Thin-layer Chromatography. System TA—Rf 77 (metaclazepam); Rf 76 (M-nor); system TB—Rf 40 (metaclazepam); Rf 0 (M-dinor); Rf 15 (M-nor); system TC—Rf 73 (metaclazepam); Rf 68 (M-nor); system TD—Rf 47 (metaclazepam); Rf 33 (M-nor); system TE—Rf 79 (metaclazepam); Rf 46 (M-dinor); Rf 73 (M-nor); system TF—Rf 35 (metaclazepam); Rf 9 (M-dinor); Rf 25 (M-nor); system TL—Rf 62 (metaclazepam); Rf 58 (M-nor); system TAD—Rf 71 (metaclazepam); Rf 65 (M-nor); system TAE—Rf 82 (metaclazepam); Rf 81 (M-dinor); Rf 81 (M-nor); system TAF—Rf 84 (metaclazepam); Rf 84 (M-nor).

Plate: silica gel $60F_{254}$. Mobile phase: toluene:acetone (85:15). Fluorescence quenching detection at 254 nm. Rf 0.48. [W. Althaus *et al.*, *Arzneimittelforschung/Drug Res.* 1985, *36(9)*, 1302–1306].

Gas Chromatography. System GA—metaclazepam, RI 2640; M(O-desmethyl-), RI 2730; M(nor-), RI 2690.

Column: chromopack WCOT fused silica CP-Sil 5CB (25 m × 0.32 mm i.d.). Column temperature: 200° to 300° at 4°/min. Carrier gas: helium, linear velocity 30 cm/s. Detection: nitrogen specific. Retention time(s): approx. 15 min. [W. Althaus *et al.*, *Arzneimittelforschung/Drug Res.* 1985, *36(9)*, 1302–1306].

High Performance Liquid Chromatography. System HX—RI 451 (metaclazepam); RI 393 (M-dinor); RI 425 (M-nor).

Column: ODS Hypersil (Knauer cartridge, 30 + 100 × 4.0 mm i.d., 5 µm). Mobile phase: water:methanol:40% methylamine (350:650:1), flow rate 1.2 mL/min. UV detection (λ=230 nm). Retention time(s): 11.6 min. [W. Althaus *et al.*, *Arzneimittelforschung/Drug Res.*, 1985, *36(9)*, 1302–1306].

Ultraviolet Spectrum. Aqueous acid—252 nm.

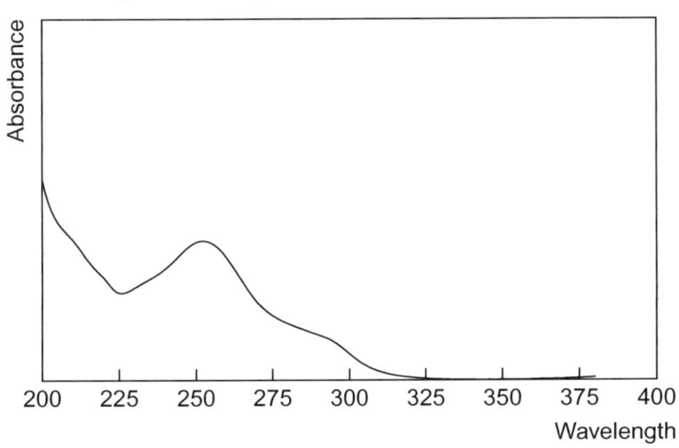

Infra-red Spectrum. Principal peaks at wavenumbers 1646, 1482, 1590, 772, 735, 819 cm^{-1}.

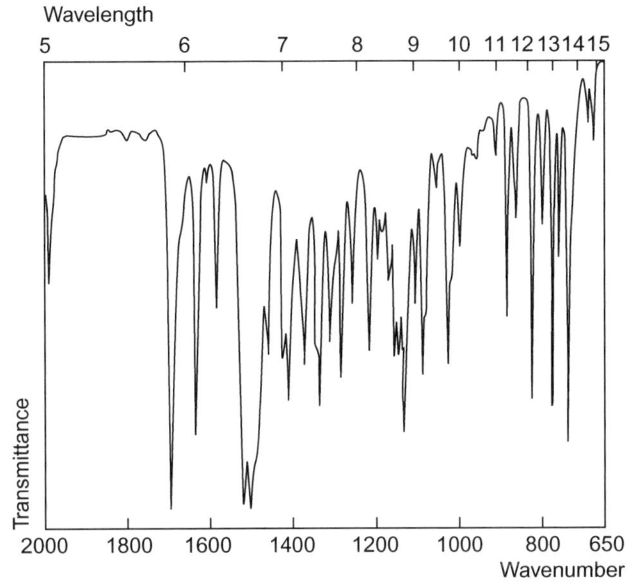

Mass Spectrum. Principal ions at *m/z* 335, 333, 349, 305, 378 (nor-metaclazepam).

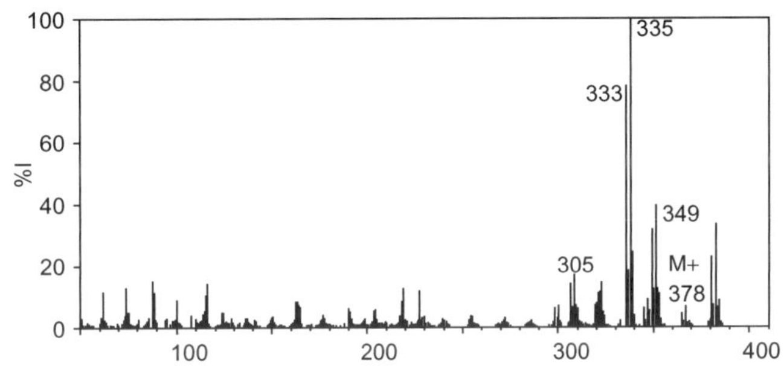

Quantification
Thin-layer chromatography. Limit of detection 0.1 µg—W. Althaus *et al.* *Arzneimforschung/Drug Res.*, 1985, *36(9)*, 1302–1306.

Disposition in the Body. Metaclazepam is rapidly metabolised yielding N^1-desmethyl and *O*-desmethyl benzapines as the main active products. No accumulation after repetitive administration is observed. Small amounts are distributed in breast milk.

Dose. The oral daily dose is 15 mg.

Metadoxine

Treatment of Alcohol Poisoning

Synonyms. Pyridoxine Pyrrolidonecarboxylate; Pyridoxol L, 2-Pyrrolidone-5-carboxlate.
Proprietary name. Metadoxil
3-Hydroxy-4,5-di(hydroxymethyl)-2-methylpyridine-5-oxo-2-pyrrolidinecarboxylaten
$C_{13}H_{18}N_2O_6=298.3$
CAS—74536-44-0

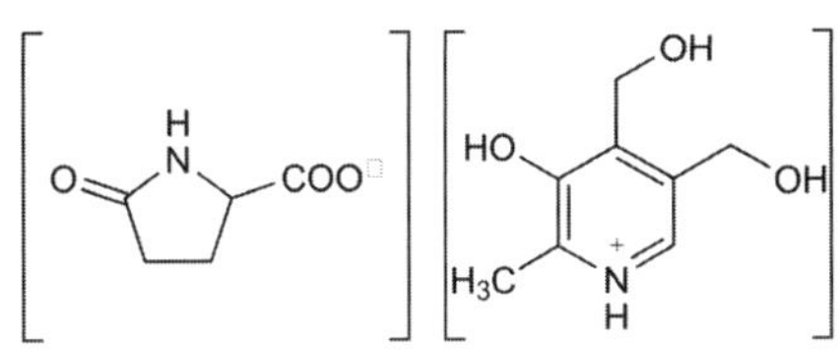

A white, odourless, crystalline powder with acidic taste. M.p 96° to 98°. It is soluble in water.

Dose. Two 500 mg tablets daily; 300 to 600 mg daily by intramuscular or intravenous administration.

Metadrenaline

Synonym. Metanephrine
4-Hydroxy-3-methoxy-α-(methylaminomethyl)benzenemethanol
$C_{10}H_{15}NO_3$=197.2
CAS—5001-33-2

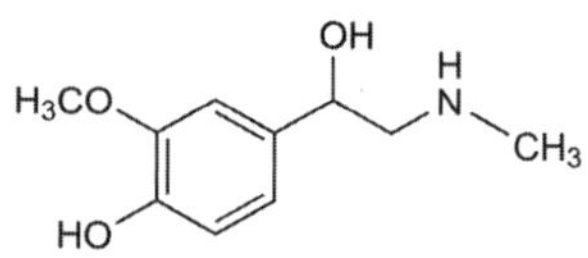

Partition Coefficient. Log *P* (octanol/water), −0.6.

Colour Tests. Mandelin's Test—green; Marquis Test—orange→violet-brown.

Thin-layer Chromatography. System TA—Rf 21. (Acidified potassium permanganate solution, positive.)

Ultraviolet Spectrum. Aqueous acid—277 nm; aqueous alkali—245, 291 nm.

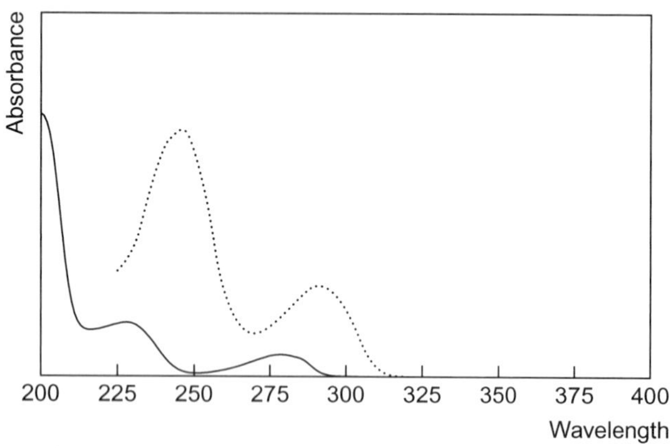

Quantification. See Normetadrenaline.

Disposition in the Body. Metadrenaline is a metabolite of adrenaline.

Metaldehyde

Molluscicide

Proprietary names. It is an ingredient of many proprietary preparations used for the destruction of slugs. As a compressed fuel, it is known as 'Meta'.
A polymer of acetaldehyde.
$(C_2H_4O)_x$
CAS—9002-91-9
A white crystalline solid which burns readily with a non-luminous carbon-free flame and sublimes at 112°. In the presence of acids it decomposes slowly to acetaldehyde.
Practically insoluble in water; soluble in benzene and chloroform; sparingly soluble in alcohol and ether.

Colour Test. Add 1 drop of sulfuric acid to a small amount of solid, then add a trace of pyrocatechol—violet-red.

Gas Chromatography. System GA—RI 1020.

Infra-red Spectrum. Principal peaks at wavenumbers 1094, 1113, 1163, 1074, 975, 1205 cm^{-1} (KBr disk).

Quantification
Gas chromatography. In plasma or urine—T. F. Booze and F. W. Oehme, *J. Anal. Toxicol.*, 1985, *9*, 172–173.

Disposition in the Body.
Toxicity. Metaldehyde probably decomposes slowly in the body to acetaldehyde which is further oxidised. Fatalities have occurred after the ingestion of about 3 g.

Metallibure

Hypothalamus and Pituitary Suppressant

N-Methyl-*N′*-(1-methyl-2-propenyl)-1,2-hydrazinedicarbothioamide
$C_7H_{14}N_4S_2$=218.3
CAS—926-93-2

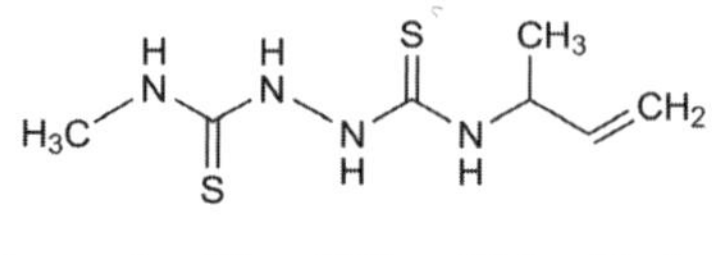

A white powder. M.p. 198° to 200°, with decomposition.
Practically insoluble in water and chloroform; soluble 1 in 100 of acetone and 1 in 200 of methanol; soluble in pyridine.
Caution. Protective gloves should be worn when handling metallibure.

Partition Coefficient. Log *P* (octanol/water), 0.3.

Colour Tests. Nessler's Reagent (100°)—black; Palladium Chloride—orange

Thin-layer Chromatography. System TA—Rf 79. (Acidified iodoplatinate solution, positive.)

Gas Chromatography. System GA—not eluted.

Ultraviolet Spectrum. Aqueous acid—243 nm (A_1^1=1340b); aqueous alkali—293 nm.

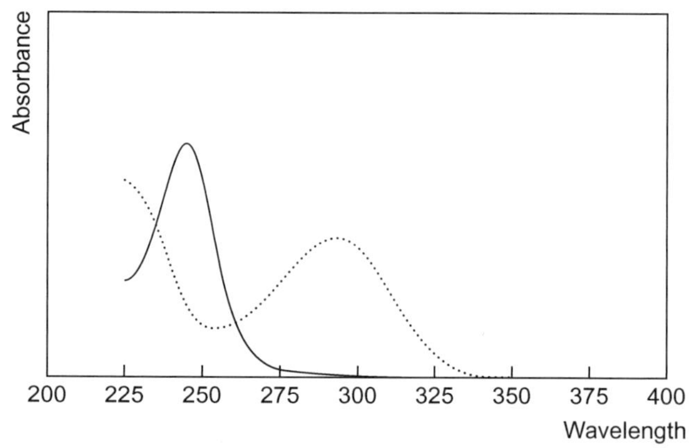

Infra-red Spectrum. Principal peaks at wavenumbers 1524, 1577, 1209, 1025, 1147, 1258 cm^{-1} (KBr disk).

Metamfetamine

Central Stimulant

Synonyms. *d*-Deoxyephedrine; Desoxyephedrine; Methamphetamine; Methylamfetamine; methylamphetamine; Phenylmethylaminopropane.
Note. Metamfetamine in a smokeable form has been known as Crank, Crystal, Crystal meth, Ice, meth, and Speed.
Proprietary name. Norodin
(α*S*)-*N*,α-Dimethylbenzeneethanamine
$C_{10}H_{15}N$=149.2
CAS—537-46-2

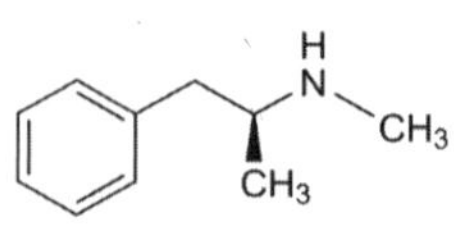

A clear, colourless, slowly volatile, mobile liquid. Mass per mL 0.921 to 0.922 g. B.p. about 214°.
Slightly soluble in water; miscible with ethanol, chloroform, and ether.

Metamfetamine Hydrochloride

Proprietary names. Amphedroxyn; Desfedrin; Desoxyfed; Desoxyn; Destim; Doxephrin; Drinalfa; Gerobit; Hiropon; Isophen; Madrine; Methampex; Methedrine; Methylisomyn; Pervitin; Soxysympamine; Syndrox; Tonedron.

$C_{10}H_{15}N,HCl = 185.7$

CAS—51-57-0

White crystals or crystalline powder. M.p. 170° to 175°.

Soluble 1 in 2 of water, 1 in 4 of ethanol, and 1 in 5 of chloroform; practically insoluble in ether.

Dissociation Constant. pK_a 10.1.

Partition Coefficient. Log *P* (octanol/water), 2.1.

Colour Test. Marquis Test—orange.

Thin-layer Chromatography. System TA—Rf 31; system TB—Rf 28; system TC—Rf 13; system TE—Rf 42; system TL—Rf 05; system TAE—Rf 09; system TAF—Rf 63; system TAJ—Rf 00; system TAK—Rf 03; system TAL—Rf 45. (Dragendorff spray, positive; acidified iodoplatinate solution, positive; Marquis reagent, brown; ninhydrin spray, positive; acidified potassium permanganate solution, positive.)

Gas Chromatography. System GA—metamfetamine RI 1175, amfetamine RI 1125, M (4-OH-, pholedrine) RI 1885, M (OH-methoxy-) RI 1810; system GB—metamfetamine RI 1200, amfetamine RI 1150; system GC—metamfetamine RI 1722, amfetamine RI 1536; system GF—metamfetamine RI 1335, amfetamine RI 1315.

High Performance Liquid Chromatography. System HA—metamfetamine *k* 2.0, amfetamine *k* 0.9; system HB—metamfetamine *k* 10.52, amfetamine k 8.48; system HC—metamfetamine *k* 2.07, amfetamine *k* 0.98; system HX—metamfetamine RI 262; system HY—metamfetamine RI 216; system HZ—metamfetamine Retention time 2.4 min; system HAA—metamfetamine Retention time 8.4 min.

Ultraviolet Spectrum. Aqueous acid—252, 257 ($A_1^1 = 12.1a$), 263 nm.

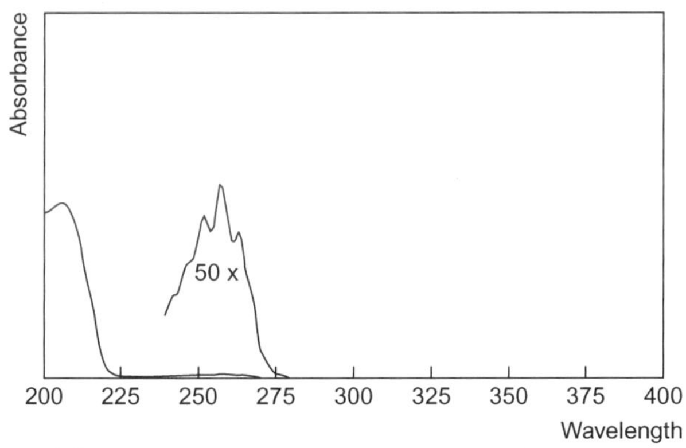

Infra-red Spectrum. Principal peaks at wavenumbers 747, 698, 1060, 1491, 1590, 1085 cm^{-1} (metamfetamine hydrochloride, KBr disk). (See below.)

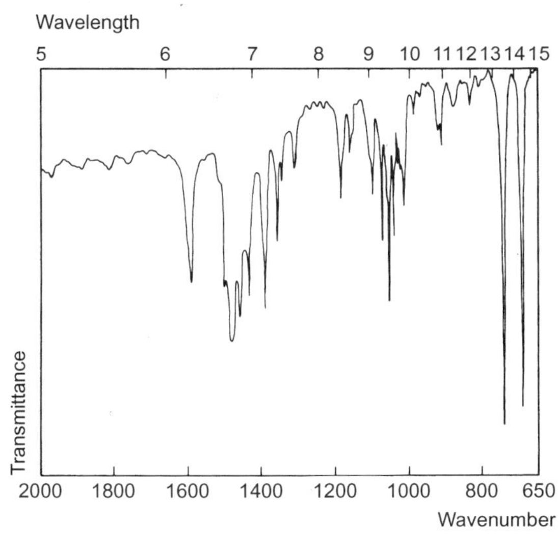

Mass Spectrum. Principal ions at *m/z* 58, 91, 59, 134, 65, 56, 42, 57; amfetamine 44, 91, 40, 42, 65, 45, 39, 43.

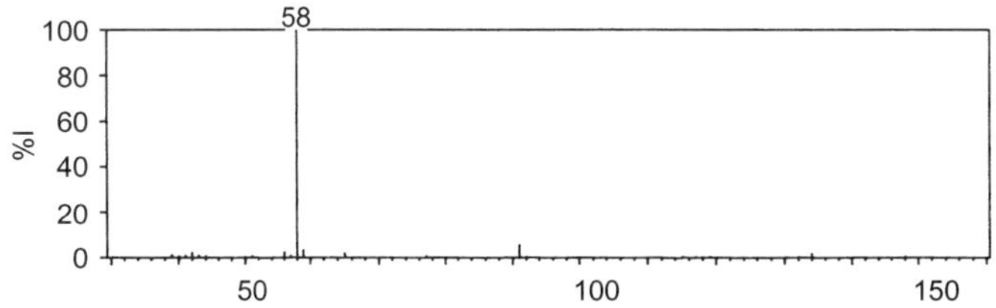

Quantification

Gas chromatography. In urine: metamfetamine and amfetamine, limit of detection 10 µg/L, ECD—M. Terada *et al., J. Chromatogr.*, 1982, *237*, 285–292. In urine: metamfetamine and amfetamine, limit of detection < 10 µg/L—P. Jacob *et al., J. Chromatogr. B Biomed. Appl.*, 1995, *664*, 449–457. In plasma or urine: metamfetamine and its metabolites, limit of detection 1 µg/L, NPD—S. Cheung *et al., J. Chromatogr. B Biomed. Sci. Appl.*, 1997, *690*, 77–87. In hair: metamfetamine and amfetamine, limits of detection 0.4 µg/g and 0.1 µg/g, NPD—I. Koide *et al., J. Chromatogr. B Biomed. Sci. Appl.*, 1998, *707*, 99–104.

Gas chromatography–mass spectrometry. In hair: metamfetamine and metabolites, limit of detection 0.05 µg/g—P. Kintz *et al., J. Chromatogr. B Biomed. Appl.*, 1995, *670*, 162–166. In urine: metamfetamine and amfetamine, limit of detection 5 µg/L—R. Meatherall, *J. Anal. Toxicol.*, 1995, *19*, 316–322. In blood: metamfetamine and amfetamine—N. Nagasawa *et al., Forensic Sci. Int.*, 1996, *78*, 95–102. In urine: metamfetamine and amfetamine, limit of detection for metamfetamine 90 µg/L—P. Dallakian *et al., J. Anal. Toxicol.*, 1996, *20*, 255–261. In sweat: comparison with enzyme immunoassay—J. Fay *et al., J. Anal. Toxicol.*, 1996, *20*, 398–403. In blood: metamfetamine and amfetamine—M. Sato and T. Mitsui, *J. Pharm. Biomed. Anal.*, 1997, *16*, 139–145. In urine: metamfetamine and amfetamine, limit of detection 100 µg/L—A. Dasgupta and J. Spies, *Am. J. Clin. Pathol.*, 1998, *109*, 527–532. In urine: metamfetamine, dimetamfetamine, and amfetamine, limit of detection < 1 to 10 µg/L—S. W. Myung *et al., J. Chromatogr. B Biomed. Sci. Appl.*, 1998, *716*, 359–365. In urine: metamfetamine and other amfetamines, limit of quantification for metamfetamine 10 µg/L—D. Hensley and J. T. Cody, *J. Anal. Toxicol.*, 1999, *23*, 518–523; C. Jurado *et al., J. Anal. Toxicol.*, 2000, *24*, 11–16. In blood: metamfetamine and amfetamine, limit of detection 5 ng/g—A. Namera *et al., Forensic Sci. Int.*, 2000, *109*, 215–223. In serum: metamfetamine and amfetamine—M. R. Lee *et al., J. Chromatogr. A*, 2000, *896*, 265–273. In serum: metamfetamine and other amfetamines—W. Weinmann *et al., Int. J. Legal Med.*, 2000, *113*, 229–235. In whole blood: metamfetamine and amfetamine—K. Okajima *et al., Forensic Sci. Int.*, 2001, *116*, 15–22. In hair: metamfetamine and other drugs of abuse, limit of detection 0.05 to 3 µg/g—L. Skender *et al., Forensic Sci. Int.*, 2002, *125*, 120–126. In blood: metamfetamine and amfetamine—M. Nishida *et al., Forensic Sci. Int.*, 2002, *125*, 156–162. In urine: metamfetamine and other amfetamines, limit of detection for metamfetamine about 16 µg/L—P. R. Stout *et al., J. Anal. Toxicol.*, 2002, *26*, 253–261. In blood: metamfetamine and amfetamine enantiomers—F. T. Peters *et al., Clin. Chem.*, 2002, *48*, 1472–1485. In urine: comparison with HPLC—H. Yamada *et al., J. Anal. Toxicol.*, 2002, *26*, 17–22. In urine: metamfetamine and related drugs—A. Namera *et al., J. Chromatogr. Sci.*, 2002, *40*, 19–25.

High performance liquid chromatography. In urine: metamfetamine and its metabolites, chemiluminescence detection—K. Hayakawa *et al., Biol. Pharm. Bull.*, 1993, *16*, 817–821. In urine: metamfetamine and amfetamine—P. Campins Falco *et al., J. Chromatogr. B Biomed. Appl.*, 1995, *663*, 235–245; P. Campins Falco *et al., J. Chromatogr. B Biomed. Appl.*, 1996, *687*, 239–246. In urine: metamfetamine and amfetamine, limits of detection 2 µg/L and 4 µg/L respectively, UV detection—C. Molins Legua *et al., J. Chromatogr. B Biomed. Appl.*, 1995, *672*, 81–88. In urine: metamfetamine and related compounds, limits of detection 0.2 to 0.3 µg/L, fluorescence detection—O. Al-Dirbashi *et al., J. Chromatogr. B Biomed. Sci. Appl.*, 1997, *695*, 251–258. In urine: metamfetamine and amfetamine, limit of detection 0.16 mg/L, UV detection—B. S. Foster *et al., J. Anal. Toxicol.*, 1998, *22*, 265–269. In urine: metamfetamine and metabolites, limits of detection 1.8 to 26.3 ng/L, fluorescence detection—O. Al-Dirbashi *et al., J. Chromatogr. B Biomed. Sci. Appl.*, 1998, *712*, 105–112; O. Al-Dirbashi *et al., Analyst*, 1998, *123*, 2333–2337. In urine: metamfetamine enantiomers, limit of detection 100 µg/L—Y. Makino *et al., J. Chromatogr. B Biomed. Sci. Appl.*, 1999, *729*, 97–101. In urine or hair: metamfetamine and its metabolites, fluorescence detection—O. Al-Dirbashi *et al., Biomed.*

Chromatogr., 1999, *13*, 543–547. In hair: metamfetamine and amfetamine enantiomers, limits of detection 3.0 ng/L to 14.0 ng/L, fluorescence detection—O. Y. Al-Dirbashi *et al.*, *Biomed. Chromatogr.*, 2000, *14*, 293–300. In urine: metamfetamine and amfetamine, fluorescence detection—O. Y. Al-Dirbashi *et al.*, *J. Forensic Sci.*, 2000, *45*, 708–714.

High performance liquid chromatography–mass spectrometry. In urine: metamfetamine and its metabolites, limits of detection 10 to 20 μg/L (scan mode) and 0.5 to 1 μg/L (SIM) —M. Katagi *et al.*, *J. Chromatogr. B Biomed. Appl.*, 1996, *676*, 35–43. In urine: metamfetamine and dimetamfetamine, limits of detection for metamfetamine 10 μg/L—M. Katagi *et al.*, *J. Anal. Toxicol.*, 2000, *24*, 354–358.

Radioimmunoassay. In urine: limit of detection 1 ng—S. Inayama *et al.*, *Chem. Pharm. Bull.*, 1980, *28*, 2779–2782.

Note. For a review of the determination of metamfetamine enantiomers—D. Jirovsky *et al.*, *Forensic Sci. Int.*, 1998, *96*, 61–70.

Disposition in the Body. Readily absorbed after oral administration. About 70% of a dose is excreted in the urine in 24 h. Under normal conditions, up to 43% of a dose is excreted as unchanged drug, up to 15% as 4-hydroxymetamfetamine, and about 5% as amfetamine, the major active metabolite. A number of other metabolites have been identified. Excretion of unchanged drug is dependent on the urinary pH, being increased in acidic urine and greatly reduced (to about 2% of a dose) if the urine is alkaline.
Metamfetamine is a metabolite of benzfetamine and selegiline.

Therapeutic concentration. In plasma, usually in the range 0.01 to 0.05 mg/L.

Following a single oral dose of 12.5 mg of metamfetamine hydrochloride to 10 subjects, a mean peak blood concentration of about 0.02 mg/L was attained in about 2 h [R. C. Driscoll *et al.*, *J. Pharm. Sci.*, 1971, *60*, 1492–1495].

Toxicity. The estimated minimum lethal dose is 1 g, but fatalities attributed to metamfetamine are rare.

Of 146 deaths in which metamfetamine was detected in the blood, 52 were directly attributed to the drug and 92 were classified as drug-related; a large proportion of the deaths resulted from homicidal (27%) or suicidal (15%) violence. The metamfetamine blood concentration in the 92 drug-related deaths was reported to be in the range 0.05 to 9.30 mg/L (median 0.42), with 90% of the population having concentrations $<$2.20 mg/L. In metamfetamine-related traffic deaths (n = 17), the blood concentration was reported to be 0.05 to 2.60 mg/L, with most deaths occurring at concentrations greater than 0.5 mg/L [B. K. Logan *et al.*, *J. Forensic Sci.*, 1998, *43*, 28–34].

A 37-year-old man who died following mixed drug abuse had the following postmortem metamfetamine concentrations: blood 0.7 mg/L, bile 21.7 mg/L, urine 32.0 mg/L, gastric contents 2.9 mg/L, liver 2.2 mg/kg, brain 2.7 mg/kg [K. A. Moore *et al.*, *J. Forensic Sci.*, 1996, *41*, 524–526].

The following postmortem tissue concentrations, mg/L or mg/kg, were reported in a 25-year-old female found dead after the IV abuse of metamfetamine followed by ingestion of about 1.5 g:

	Metamfetamine	Amfetamine
Blood	43	0.35
Brain	101.8	0.86
Kidney	75.5	0.72
Liver	174.6	1.30
Urine	277.5	10.0

[T. Kojima *et al.*, *Forens. Sci. Int.*, 1984, *24*, 87–93].

Half-life. Plasma half-life, about 9 h.

Dose. 2.5 to 25 mg of metamfetamine hydrochloride daily, by mouth; 15 to 20 mg IM, or 10 to 15 mg IV.

Metaraminol

Sympathomimetic

Synonym. Hydroxynorephedrine
(αR)-α-[(1*S*)-1-Aminoethyl]-3-hydroxybenzenemethanol
$C_9H_{13}NO_2$ = 167.2
CAS—54-49-9

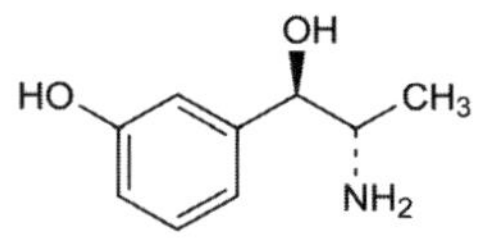

Metaraminol Tartrate

Synonyms. Metaradrini Bitartras; Metaraminol Acid Tartrate; Metaraminol Bitartrate.
Proprietary names. Aramin(e); Levicor.
$C_9H_{13}NO_2,C_4H_6O_6$ = 317.3
CAS—33402-03-8
A white crystalline powder. M.p. 176° to 177°.
Soluble 1 in 3 of water and 1 in 100 of ethanol; practically insoluble in chloroform and ether.

Dissociation Constant. pK_a 8.6.

Partition Coefficient. Log *P* (octanol/water), −0.3.

Colour Tests. Folin–Ciocalteu Reagent—blue; Mandelin's Test—blue

Thin-layer Chromatography. System TA—Rf 42; system TB—Rf 01; system TC—Rf 01; system TE—Rf 18; system TL—Rf 24; system TAE—Rf 13; system TAF—Rf 76; system TAJ—Rf 00; system TAK—Rf 00; system TAL—Rf 20. (Acidified potassium permanganate solution, positive.)

Gas Chromatography. System GA—metaraminol-AC_3 RI 2065.

High Performance Liquid Chromatography. System HA—*k* 0.9; system HX—RI 84.

Ultraviolet Spectrum. Aqueous acid—272 nm (A^1_1 = 110a); aqueous alkali—238 nm (A^1_1 = 533b), 292 nm (A^1_1 = 180b).

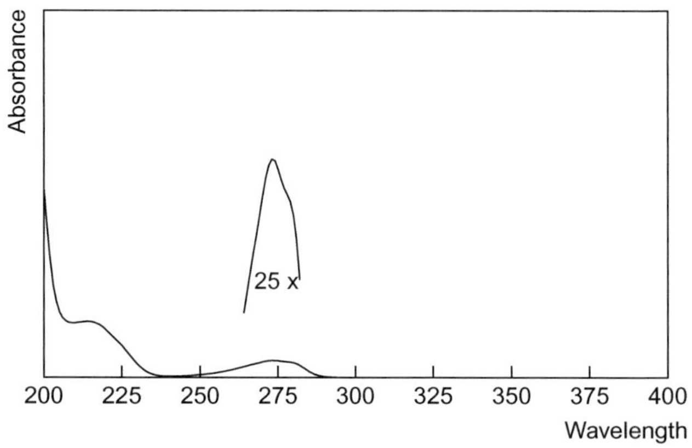

Infra-red Spectrum. Principal peaks at wavenumbers 1263, 1304, 1216, 1591, 1136, 1063 cm^{-1} (KBr disk).

Mass Spectrum. Principal ions at *m/z* 44, 77, 76, 29, 95, 39, 58, 42.

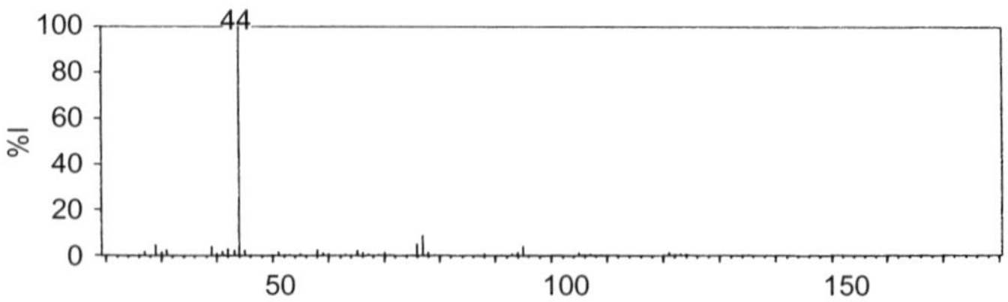

Dose. The equivalent of 2 to 10 mg of metaraminol, subcutaneously or intramuscularly.

Metenolone

Anabolic Steroid

Synonym. Methenolone
(5α,17β)-17-Hydroxy-1-methylandrost-1-en-3-one

$C_{20}H_{30}O_2$=302.5
CAS—153-00-4

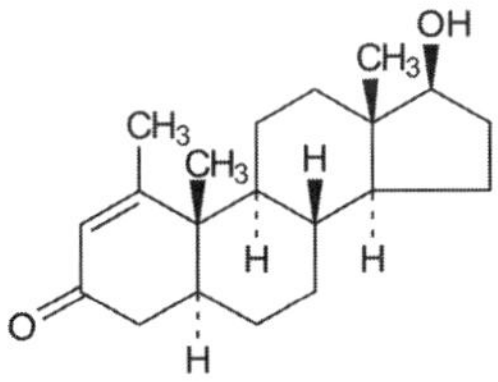

A crystalline powder with M.p. 149.5° to 152°, also reported as 160° to 161°.

Metenolone Acetate
Synonyms. NSC-74226; SH-567; SQ-16496.
Proprietary names. Primobolan; Primonabol.
$C_{22}H_{32}O_3$=344.5
CAS—434-05-9
M.p 138° to139°. It is soluble in methanol, ether and chloroform.

Metenolone Enantate
Synonyms. Methenolone Anantate; Metenolone Enanthate; Methenolone Oenanthate; NSC-64967; SH-601; SQ-16374.
Proprietary names. Primobolan-Depot; Primonabol-Depot
$C_{27}H_{42}O_3$=414.6
CAS—303-42-4

Partition Coefficient. Log *P* (octanol/water), 3.69.

Thin-layer Chromatography. System TE—Rf 87; system TF—Rf 62; system TAE—Rf 92.

System 1: plate: silica gel IB2-F (Baker-flex with a fluorescent indicator). Mobile phase: *n*-hexane:ethylacetate (6:4). Rf 0.35.

System 2: plate: silica gel 60 F_{254} (silanised pre-coated). Mobile phase: acetone:water (3:1). Rf 0.62. UV detection (λ = 254 nm) or 2,4-dinitrophenylhydrazine reagent [V. Cavrini *et al., Int. J. Pharm.*, 1983, *13*, 333–343].

Gas Chromatography. System GAI—metenolone RRT 0.993; 1-methylen-5α-androstan-3α-ol-17-one RRT 0.905 (both relative to 17α-methyl-5α-androstan-3β,17β-diol).

Column: 5% phenylmethylpolysiloxane cross-linked capillary (30 m × 0.2 mm i.d., 0.33 µm film thickness). Column temperature: 150° for 2 min, to 300° at 20°/min, held for 2 min. Injector temperature: 280°. IS: 1,2-d_2-testosterone. MS detection (NCI, precursor ion *m/z* 428). Retention time: metenolone metabolite (PFP derivative), Retention time 9.1 min [M. Choi *et al., Rapid Commun. Mass Spectrom.*, 1998, *12*, 1749–1755].

High Performance Liquid Chromatography. System HX—RI 809; system HATa—metenolone acetate RRT 1.26, metenolone enantate RRT 1.87 (both relative to testosterone); system HATb—metenolone acetate RRT 3.54 (relative to testosterone).

Column: RP monomeric C_{18} (MicroPack MCH-10, 300 × 4.0 mm i.d., 10 µm). Mobile phase: acetonitrile:water (92:8), flow rate 2 mL/min. UV detection (λ=240 nm). Retention time(s): metenolone, 2.9 min; metenolone acetate, 3.5 min; metenolone enantate, 9.1 min [V. Cavrini *et al., Int. J. Pharm.*, 1983, *13*, 333–343].

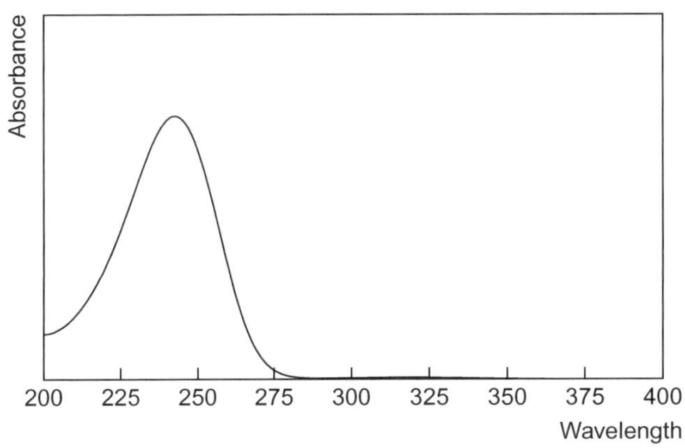

Infra-red Spectrum. Principal peaks at wavenumbers 1655, 1600, 1290, 1210, 1125, 1075 cm^{-1}.

Mass Spectrum. Principal ions at *m/z* 136, 123, 148, 83, 93, 107, 161, 67 (acetate); 136, 43, 123, 148, 161, 113, 83, 414.

Disposition in the Body. Metenolone is metabolised and excreted in urine as the parent drug and its metabolites including, 1-methylen-5α-androstan-3α-ol-17-one.

Toxicity. Moderately toxic by ingestion and intraperitoneal routes.

Dose. A usual dose of 10 to 20 mg daily is administered orally as the acetate and intramuscularly as the enanthate in doses of 100 mg every 2 to 4 weeks.

Metformin

Antidiabetic

N,N-Dimethylimidodicarbonimidic diamide
$C_4H_{11}N_5$=129.2
CAS—657-24-9

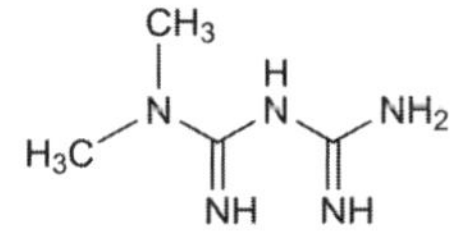

Metformin Hydrochloride
Proprietary names. Biocos; Diabesin; Diabetase; Diabetex; Diabex; Diaformin; Diformin; Glifage; Glucamet; Glucinan; Glucobon; Glucoformin; Glucohexal; Glucomet; Glucophage; Glycon; Glymax; Mediabet; Meglucon; Mescorit; Met; Metfirex; Metforem; Metiguanide; Novomet; Orabet; Stagid.
$C_4H_{11}N_5$,HCl=165.6
CAS—1115-70-4
A white, hygroscopic, crystalline powder. M.p. about 225°.
Soluble 1 in 2 of water and 1 in 100 of ethanol; practically insoluble in chloroform and ether.

Dissociation Constant. pK_a 2.8, 11.5 (32°).

Partition Coefficient. Log *P* (octanol/water), −2.6.

Thin-layer Chromatography. System TA—Rf 01; system TB—Rf 00; system TC—Rf 00; system TE—Rf 00, 80; system TL—Rf 00; system TAD—Rf 00; system TAE—Rf 03, 93; system TAF—Rf 48. (Acidified iodoplatinate solution, positive.)

Gas Chromatography. System GA—metformin, not eluted; system GB—metformin, not eluted; metformin-nitrobenzoyltriazine RI 3050.

High Performance Liquid Chromatography. System HX—RI 60; system HZ—retention time 1.7 min; system HAA—retention time 2.8 min; system HAX—retention time 5.7 min; system HAY—retention time 3.3 min.

Ultraviolet Spectrum. Methanol—236 nm (A^{1}_{1}=1163b).

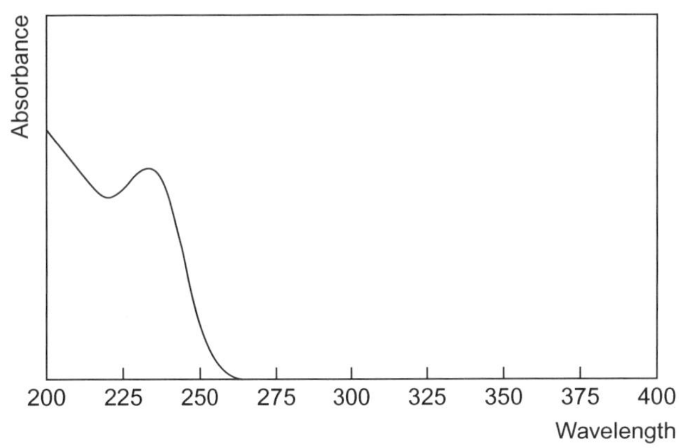

Infra-red Spectrum. Principal peaks at wavenumbers 1580, 1620, 1063, 1075, 935, 740 cm^{-1} (KBr disk).

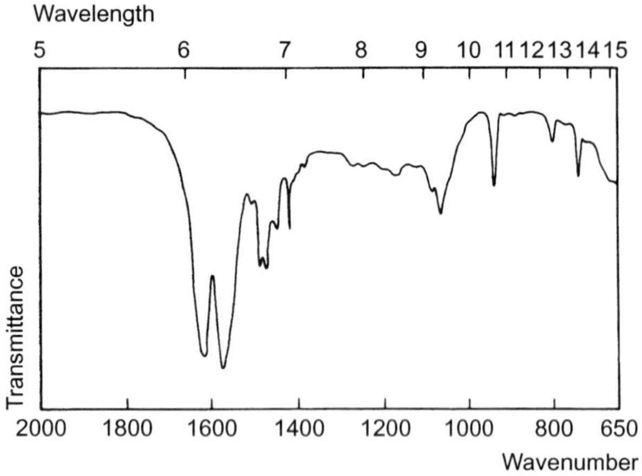

Mass Spectrum. Principal ions at *m/z* 43, 44, 85, 86, 42, 129, 68, 30.

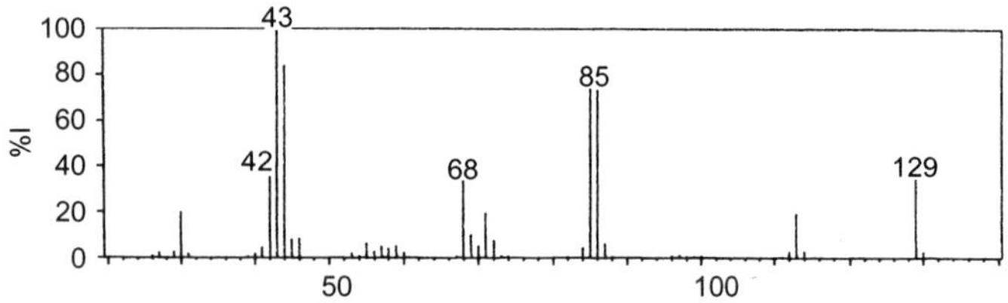

Quantification

Gas chromatography. In plasma or urine: limit of detection 25 μg/L, AFID—J. Brohon and M. Noel, *J. Chromatogr.* 1978, *146(3) B Biomed. Appl.*, 148–151.

High performance liquid chromatography. In plasma or urine: limit of detection 100 μg/L, UV detection—B. G. Charles *et al.*, *Clin. Chem.*, 1981, *27*, 434–436. In plasma: UV detection—R. Huupponen *et al.*, *J. Chromatogr.*, 1992, *583*, 270–273. In plasma: limit of detection 15 μg/L, UV detection—H. Y. Kah and K. P. Kok, *J. Chromatogr. B. Biomed. Sci. Appl.*, 1998, *710*, 243–246. In plasma: limit of detection <50 μg/L, UV detection—O. Vesterqvist *et al.*, *J. Chromatogr. B. Biomed. Sci. Appl.*, 1998, *716*, 299–304. In plasma: UV detection—A. R. Bonfigli *et al.*, *Ther. Drug Monit.*, 1999, *21*, 330–334. In plasma or breast milk: limit of detection <20 μg/L, UV detection—M. Zhang *et al.*, *J. Chromatogr. B. Analyt. Technol. Biomed. Life Sci.*, 2002, *766*, 175–179.

High performance liquid chromatography–mass spectrometry. In plasma: limit of detection 2.5 μg/L—C. L. Cheng and C. H. Chou, *J. Chromatogr. B. Biomed. Sci. Appl.*, 2001, *762*, 51–58.

Disposition in the Body. Slowly absorbed after oral administration;. About 30 to 50% of an oral dose is excreted in the urine as unchanged drug in 24 h, and about 30% of the dose is eliminated unchanged in the faeces.

Therapeutic concentration

Following single oral doses of 0.5 g and 1.5 g to 4 subjects, peak plasma concentrations of 0.59 to 1.3 mg/L (mean 1.0) and 1.8 to 4.0 mg/L (mean 3.1), respectively, were attained in about 2 h. [G. T. Tucker *et al.*, *Br. J. Clin. Pharmacol.*, 1981, *12*, 235–246.]

Following daily oral doses of 0.5 g, 1.7 g, and 2.5 g to 6, 13, and 12 subjects, mean steady-state plasma concentrations of 0.16, 0.38, and 1.0 mg/L, respectively, were reported. [C. R. Sirtori *et al.*, *Clin. Pharmacol. Ther.*, 1978, *24*, 683–693.]

Toxicity

Plasma and urine concentrations of 85 and 389 mg/L, respectively, were reported in 1 subject, 12 h after the ingestion of 25.5 g; death occurred after 2 weeks. [A. Larcan *et al.*, *Vet. Hum. Toxicol.*, 1979, *21*, Suppl., 19–22.]

A 58-year-old man who died after ingesting approx. 20 g metformin plus 4.8 g diltiazem had an initial metformin level of 110 mg/L. [F. Barrueto *et al.*, *J. Toxicol. Clin. Toxicol.*, 2002, *40*, 177–180.]

Bioavailability. About 50 to 60%

Half-life. Plasma half-life, after intravenous administration, about 1.5 to 4 h; half-life derived from urinary excretion data, about 16 h.

Volume of distribution. Variously reported as about 1 to 4 L/kg.

Clearance. Plasma clearance, about 7 to 10 mL/min/kg.

Protein binding. In plasma, not significantly bound.

Note. For a review of the clinical pharmacokinetics of metformin, see A. J. Scheen, *Clin. Pharmacokinet.*, 1996, *30*, 359–371.

Dose. 1.5 to 3 g of metformin hydrochloride daily.

Methacholine Chloride

Parasympathomimetic

Synonym. Acetyl-β-methylcholine Chloride
Proprietary names. Amechol; Mecholyl; Provocholine.
2-(Acetyloxy)-*N*,*N*,*N*-trimethyl-1-propanaminium chloride
$C_8H_{18}ClNO_2$=195.7
CAS—55-92-5 (methacholine); 62-51-1 (chloride)

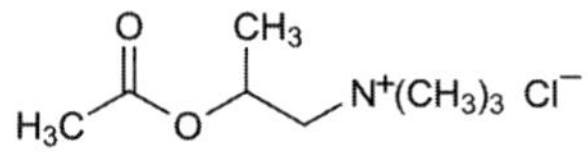

Colourless, very hygroscopic crystals, or a white crystalline powder. M.p. 170° to 173°.
Soluble 1 in 0.4 of water, 1 in 1.2 of ethanol, and 1 in 2.1 of chloroform; insoluble in ether.

Methacholine Bromide

$C_8H_{18}BrNO_2$=240.1
CAS—333-31-3
A white, very hygroscopic, crystalline powder. M.p. about 148°.
Soluble 1 in 0.3 of water, 1 in 0.8 of ethanol (90%), and 1 in 1.3 of chloroform; practically insoluble in ether.

Partition Coefficient. Log *P* (octanol/water), −3.0.

Thin-layer Chromatography. System TA—Rf 02. (Acidified iodoplatinate solution, positive.)

Infra-red Spectrum. Principal peaks at wavenumbers 1739, 1248, 1066, 1632, 972, 1128 cm^{-1} (KBr disk).

Dose. Methacholine has been given subcutaneously in doses of 10 to 25 mg (chloride), or orally in doses of 200 to 600 mg daily (bromide).

Methacycline

Antibiotic

Synonyms. Méthylènecycline; 6-Methyleneoxytetracycline.
[4*S*-(4α,4aα,5α,5aα,12aα)-4-Dimethylamino-1,4,4a,5,5a,6,11,12a-octahydro-3,5,10,12,12a-pentahydroxy-6-methylene-1,11-dioxo-2-naphthacenecarboxamide
$C_{22}H_{22}N_2O_8$=442.4
CAS—914-00-1

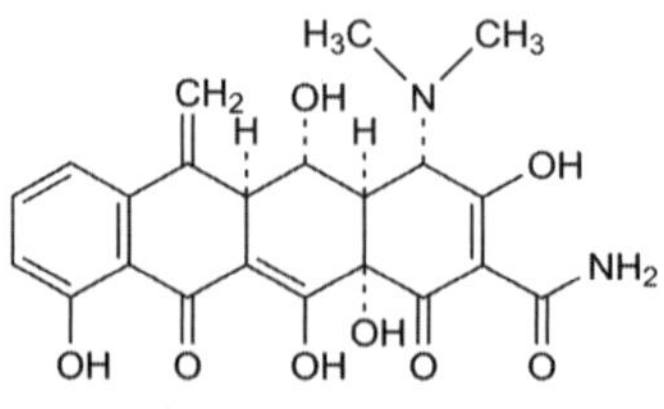

Methacycline Hydrochloride

Proprietary names. Esarondil; Lysocline; Optimycin; Physiomycine; Rondomycin(e); Rotilen; Stafilon.
$C_{22}H_{22}N_2O_8$,HCl=478.9
CAS—3963-95-9
A yellow crystalline powder. M.p. about 205°, with decomposition.
Soluble 1 in 65 to 1 in 100 of water, 1 in 80 to 1 in 300 of ethanol, and 1 in 30 of methanol; practically insoluble in chloroform and ether.

Dissociation Constant. pK_a 3.1, 7.6, 9.5 (20°).

Partition Coefficient. Log *P* (octanol/pH 7.5), −0.4.

Colour Tests. Benedict's Reagent—red; Formaldehyde–Sulfuric Acid—red-orange; Mandelin's Test—yellow→orange→violet; Marquis Test—orange; Sulfuric Acid—red

Thin-layer Chromatography. System TA—Rf 05, streaking. (Location under ultraviolet light, orange fluorescence; acidified potassium permanganate solution, positive.)

Ultraviolet Spectrum. Aqueous acid—243 nm (A_1^1 = 524a), 340 nm. (See below)

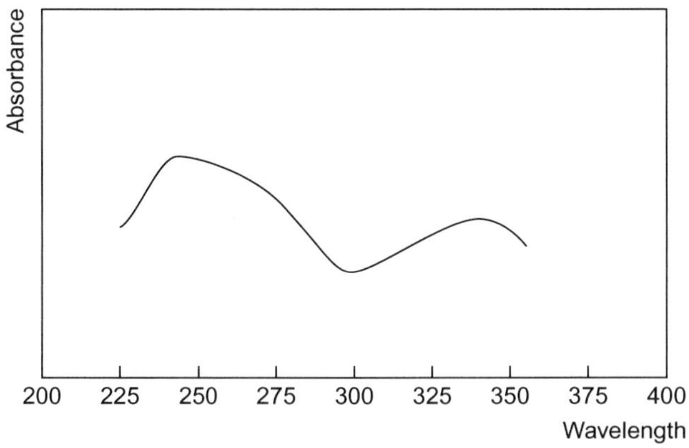

Infra-red Spectrum. Principal peaks at wavenumbers 1615, 1575, 1658, 1224, 1258, 1206 cm^{-1} (KBr disk).

Dose. Usually 600 mg of methacycline hydrochloride daily.

Methadone

Narcotic Analgesic

Synonyms. Amidine; Amidone.
6-Dimethylamino-4,4-diphenyl-3-heptanone
$C_{21}H_{27}NO$ = 309.4
CAS—76-99-3; 297-88-1 (±)

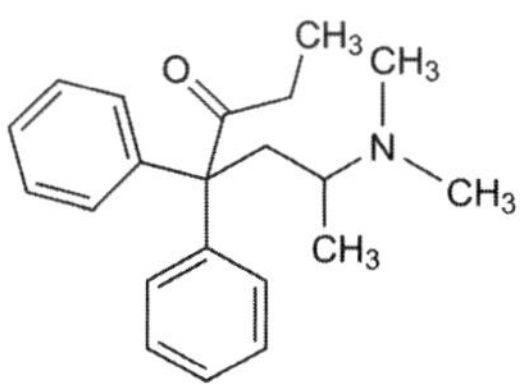

M.p. 78°.
It is soluble in water at 48.5 mg/L (25°).

Methadone Hydrochloride

Synonyms. Methadoni Hydrochloridum; Phenadone.
Proprietary names. Adolan; Biodone; Dolmed; Dolophine; Eptadone; Heptadon; Ketalgine; Mephenon; Metasedin; Methaddict; Methadose; Methex; Pallidone; Phymet DTF; Physeptone; Pinadone DTF; Symoron; Synastone.
$C_{21}H_{27}NO,HCl$ = 345.9
CAS—1095-90-5; 125-56-4 (±)
Colourless crystals or white crystalline powder. M.p. 235° (platelets from alcohol and ether).
Solubility (g/100 mL): water 12; alcohol 8; chloroform 3; isopropanol 2.4; practically insoluble in ether and glycerol.

Dissociation Constant. pK_a 8.3 (20°); 8.94 (25°).

Partition Coefficient. Log *P* (octanol/pH 7.4), 2.1; (octanol/water), 3.93.

Colour Tests. Liebermann's Test—brown-orange; Mandelin's Test—green→blue.

Thin-layer Chromatography. System TA—Rf 48; system TB—Rf 59; system TC—Rf 20; system TE—Rf 77; system TL—Rf 27; system TAE—Rf 16; system TAF—Rf 60; system TAJ—Rf 08; system TAK—Rf 00; system TAL—Rf 45. (Dragendorff spray, positive; acidified iodoplatinate solution, positive.)

Gas Chromatography. System GA—methadone RI 2145; 2-ethylidene-1,5-dimethyl-3,3-diphenylpyrrolidine (EDDP) RI 2040, 2-ethyl-5-methyl-3,3-diphenyl-1-pyrroline (EMDP) RI 2021, M (nor-) RI 2095; system GB—methadone RI 2228, M (EDDP) RI 2120, M (EMDP) RI 2069; system GC—RI 2470; system GF—methadone RI 2370, EDDP RI 2280, EMDP RI 2190; system GM—methadone RRT 0.606, M (EDDP) RRT 0.520 (both relative to iprindole).

High Performance Liquid Chromatography. System HA—methadone *k* 2.2; M (EDDP) *k* 2.8; M (EMDP) *k* 0.2; system HC—*k* 1.03; system HX—RI 440; system HY—RI 343; system HZ—Retention time 8.5 min; system HAA—Retention time 15.8 min; system HAX—Retention time 16.5 min; system HAY—Retention time 8.4 min.

Ultraviolet Spectrum. Aqueous acid—253, 259, 264, 292 nm (A_1^1 = 18a).

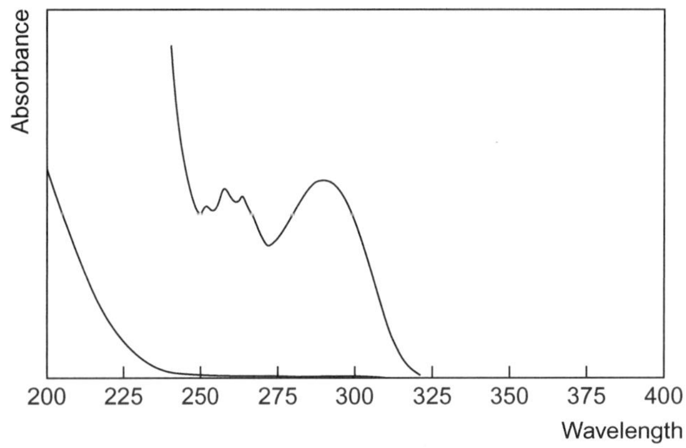

Infra-red Spectrum. Principal peaks at wavenumbers 710, 1709, 769, 1107, 943, 1133 cm^{-1} (methadone hydrochloride, Nujol mull).

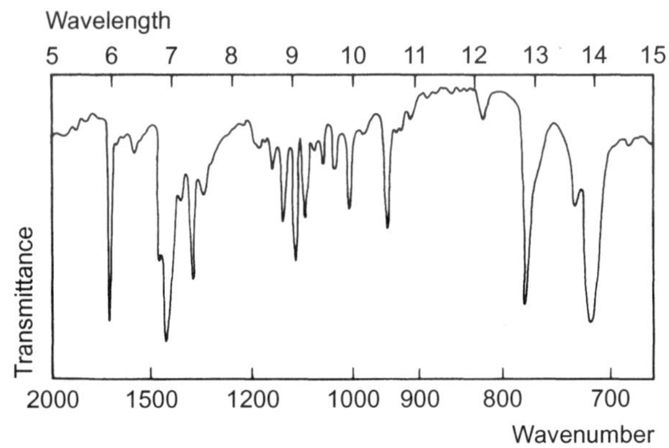

Mass Spectrum. Principal ions at *m/z* 72, 73, 91, 293, 223, 165, 85, 71; EMDP 208, 193, 130, 115, 91, 165, 179, 207.

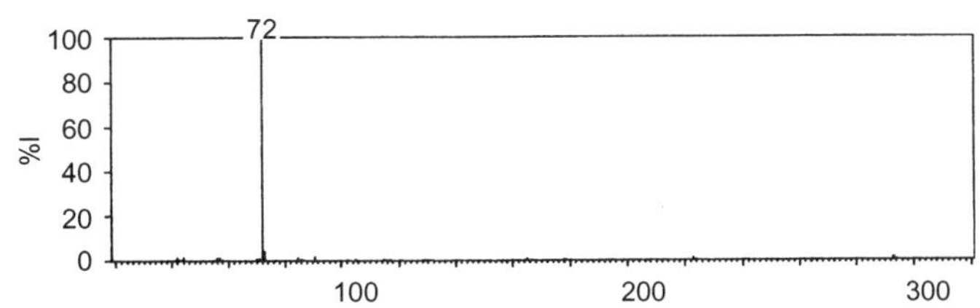

Quantification

Gas chromatography. In blood, plasma or urine: methadone and EDDP, limit of detection < 5 μg/L, AFID—P. Jacob *et al.*, *J. Anal. Toxicol.*, 1981, *5*, 292–295. In blood, urine or tissues: methadone and metabolites, detection limit 20 μg/L for methadone, FID—B. C. Thompson and Y. H. Caplan, *J. Anal. Toxicol.*, 1977, *1*, 66–69. In plasma, CSF and urine: limit of quantification 500 μg/L—N. Schmidt *et al.*, *Pharm. Research*, 1993, *10(3)*, 441–444. In serum, saliva or urine: methadone and its major metabolite, thermionic detection—N. Chikhi-Chorfi *et al.*, *J. Chromatogr. B*

Biomed. Sci. Appl., 1998, *718*, 278–284. In urine: limit of detection is <1 µg/L—S. W. Myung *et al.*, *Analyst*, 1999, *124(9)*, 1283–1286.

Gas chromatography–mass spectrometry. In plasma, saliva or urine: methadone and metabolites, limit of detection 20 µg/L for methadone in plasma or saliva—G. I. Kang and F. S. Abbott, *J. Chromatogr.*, 1982, *231; B Biomed. Appl.*, *20*, 311–319. In plasma, urine, or liver microsomes: methadone and its metabolites—M. E. Alburges *et al.*, *J. Anal. Toxicol.*, 1996, *20*, 362–368. In sweat: methadone enantiomers—P. Kintz et al., *Ther. Drug Monit.*, 1998, *20*, 35–40. In plasma: methadone and its metabolite EDDP, limit of quantification 50 µg/L—A. M. Bermejo *et al.*, *J. Anal. Toxicol.*, 2000, *24*, 66–69. In hair: limit of detection 30 mg/g for methadone and 50 mg/g for the metabolites, EDDP and EMDP—F. Sporkert and F. Pragst, *J. Chromatogr. B Biomed. Sci. Appl.*, 2000, *746(2)*, 255–264. In hair: limit of detection 500 mg/g—F. Sporkert and F. Pragst, *Forensic Sci. Int.*, 2000, *107*, 129–148. In saliva: limit of detection 40 µg/L for methadone and 8 µg/L for EDDP—A. C. dos Santos Lucas *et al.*, *J. Anal. Toxicol.*, 2000, *24*, 93–96. In hair: limit of quantification 1 µg/g—A. C. Lucas *et al.*, *Forensic Sci. Int.*, 2000, *107*, 225–232. In nail clippings—N. P. Lemos *et al.*, *J. Anal. Toxicol.*, 2000, *24*, 656–660. In meconium: methadone and its metabolites, limit of detection for methadone 10 ng/g—M. A. ElSohly *et al.*, *J. Anal. Toxicol.*, 2001, *25*, 40–44. In urine—C. Moore *et al.*, *Forensic Sci. Int.*, 2001, *119*, 155–160. In hair: methadone and EDDP, limits of quantification 0.05 µg/g and 0.2 µg/g respectively—C. Girod and C. Staub, *Forensic Sci. Int.*, 2001, *117*, 175–184.

High performance liquid chromatography. In plasma: limit of detection 200 µg/L, UV detection—R. G. Buice *et al.*, *Res. Commun. Subst. Abuse*, 1982, *3*, 97–107. In plasma: methadone enantiomers, limit of quantification 2.5 µg/L, UV detection—N. Schmidt *et al.*, *J. Chromatogr.*, 1992, *583*, 195–200. In serum: methadone enantiomers, limit of quantification 1.6 µg/L, UV detection—K. Kristensen *et al.*, *J. Chromatogr. A.*, 1994, *666*, 283–287. In plasma: methadone enantiomers, limit of quantification 5 µg/L, UV detection—R. L. Norris *et al.*, *J. Chromatogr. B Biomed. Appl.*, 1994, *661*, 346–350. In serum: limit of quantification 25 µg/L, UV detection—S. Rudaz and J. L. Veuthey *et al.*, *J. Pharm. Biomed. Anal.*, 1996, *14*, 1271–1279. In meconium: methadone and EDDP, diode-array detection (comparison with FPIA)—L. M. Stolk *et al.*, *J. Anal. Toxicol.*, 1997, *21*, 154–159. In serum or urine: methadone enantiomers and EDDP—C. Pham-Huy *et al.*, *J. Chromatogr. B Biomed. Sci. Appl.*, 1997, *700*, 155–163. In urine: methadone and EDDP, limit of quantification 9.3 µg/L, UV detection—H. R. Angelo *et al.*, *J. Chromatogr. B Biomed. Sci. Appl.*, 1999, *724*, 35–40. In urine: methadone and EDDP—Y. F. Cheng *et al.*, *J. Chromatogr. B Biomed. Sci. Appl.*, 1999, *729*, 19–31. In serum or urine: methadone enantiomers and EDDP, limits of quantification 2.5 µg/L and 5 µg/L respectively, UV detection—D. W. Boulton and C. L. Devane, *Chirality*, 2000, *12*, 681–687. In urine: methadone and EDDP, UV detection—D. J. Foster *et al.*, *J. Chromatogr. B Biomed. Sci. Appl.*, 2000, *744*, 165–176.

Fluorescence polarisation immunoassay. In plasma: limit of detection 50 µg/L—O. Beck *et al.*, *Ther. Drug Monit.*, 1990, *12(5)*, 473–477. In plasma: limit of quantification 25 µg/L—M. J. Kell and T. Techman, *J. Addict. Dis.*, 1996, *15*, 69–83.

Disposition in the Body. Rapidly absorbed after oral administration, and widely distributed in the tissues, with higher concentrations in the liver, lungs and kidneys than in the blood. It crosses the placental barrier and is also found in breast milk. Metabolism is mainly catalysed by the cytochrome P450 isoenzyme CYP3A4, but other isoenzymes may be involved. The main metabolic reaction is *N*-demethylation resulting in a substance which spontaneously cyclises to form the major metabolites, 2-ethylidene-1,5-dimethyl-3,3-diphenylpyrrolidine (EDDP) and 2-ethyl-5-methyl-3,3-diphenyl-1-pyrroline (EMDP), neither of which is active. Hydroxylation to methadol followed by *N*-demethylation to normethadol also occurs to some extent. Other metabolic reactions occur and there are at least eight known metabolites. In subjects on methadone maintenance, about 20 to 60% of a dose is excreted in the urine in 24 h, with up to about 33% of the dose as unchanged drug and up to about 43% as EDDP; EMDP accounts for about 5 to 10% of the dose. The ratio of EDDP to unchanged methadone is usually very much higher in the urine of patients on methadone maintenance treatment than in simple overdose cases. Urinary excretion of unchanged drug is pH-dependent, being increased in acid urine. Up to 30% of a dose may be eliminated in the faeces, but this appears to decrease with increasing dosage. About 75% of the total excreted material is unconjugated.

Therapeutic concentration. In plasma, usually in the range 0.05 to 1.0 mg/L. During methadone maintenance treatment, there are often considerable fluctuations in plasma concentrations from day to day, and there appears to be a decrease in concentration as dispositional tolerance develops.

Two regimens of epidural administration of methadone were compared in 90 patients requiring postoperative analgesia: one group (*n*=60) received initial doses of 3 to 6 mg followed by 6 to 12 mg every 24 h by continuous infusion for 72 h, the other group (*n*=30) received repeated epidural boluses of 3 to 6 mg every 8 h for 72 h. The mean plasma methadone concentrations were as follows (mg/L):

	Continuous infusion	Bolus infusion
After 24 h	0.078	0.112
After 48 h	0.050	0.071
After 72 h	0.049	0.078

Both regimens provided satisfactory post-operative analgesia [P. Prieto-Alvarez *et al.*, *Can. J. Anesth.*, 2002, *49*, 25–31].

In 180 patients receiving methadone maintenance therapy (10 to 350 mg daily), satisfactory abstinence from illicit opiates was obtained with an (*R*)-methadone plasma concentration of 0.25 mg/L and a racemic methadone concentration of 0.4 mg/L, with a higher specificity being calculated for (*R*)-methadone; doses required to produce the required concentration could theoretically range from 55 to 921 mg daily in a 70-kg patient [C. B. Eap *et al.*, *Drug Alcohol Depend.*, 2000, *61*, 47–54].

In 18 patients maintained on methadone 7.5 to 130 mg (0.12 to 1.9 mg/kg) daily for at least 2 months, opioid responses were strongly correlated with changes in plasma racemic methadone concentrations; peak plasma concentrations of 0.069 to 0.98 mg/L were achieved in about 3 h and pre-dose concentrations were 0.044 to 0.614 mg/L. Small changes in plasma concentrations had a relatively large effect on withdrawal severity [K. R. Dyer *et al.*, *Clin. Pharmacol. Ther.*, 1999, *65*, 685–694].

20 long-term opiate addicts were administered a mean oral dose of 60 mg methadone hydrochloride (range, 10 to 225 mg). The peak plasma methadone concentrations varied from 0.124 to 1.255 mg/L and 0.01 to 0.301 mg/L for EDDP and the steady-state concentrations, 0.065 to 0.63 mg/L and 0.005 to 0.055 mg/L, respectively [J. W. de Vos *et al.*, *Eur. J. Clin. Pharmacol.*, 1995, *48(5)*, 361–366].

Toxicity. The estimated minimum lethal dose is 50 mg but addicts on maintenance treatment may tolerate doses of 200 mg or more. In non-addicted subjects, toxic reactions are associated with plasma concentrations in the region of 1 to 2 mg/L and concentrations above 2 mg/L may be lethal. With serious overdose, respiratory depression, extreme somnolence including stupor or coma, skeletal muscle flaccidity, cold and clammy skin, bradycardia and hypotension may occur and with severe overdose, circulatory collapse, cardiac arrest and death.

In 3 cases in which death was attributed to methadone overdose, liver concentrations of 1.9, 1.3, and 0.7 µg/g and urine concentrations of 13, 25, and 4 µg/L, respectively, were reported [P. E. Nelson and R. C. Selkirk, *Forensic Sci.*, 1975, *6*, 175–186].

In 23 fatalities in which methadone was involved, the following postmortem tissue concentrations, mg/L or µg/g (mean, *n*), were reported:

	Methadone	EDDP
Blood	0–3 (1.2, *21*)	0–0.4 (0.1, *10*)
Bile	1.1–75 (13, *18*)	0.2–315 (41, *18*)
Brain	0.23–2.2 (0.9, *7*)	—
Kidney	0.51–18.3 (3.5, *19*)	0.5–3.1 (1.2, *14*)
Liver	0.05–49.5 (6, *23*)	0.02–2.7 (0.6, *16*)
Lung	1.6–110 (16, *17*)	0.01–0.98 (0.2, *10*)
Spleen	1.6–20.9 (5.3, *7*)	0–0.98 (0.7, *4*)
Urine	0.52–76.2 (21, *22*)	0.4–46.2 (11, *17*)

[J. C. Garriott *et al.*, *Clin. Toxicol.*, 1973, *6*, 163–173; A. E. Robinson and F. M. Williams, *J. Pharm. Pharmacol.*, 1971, *23*, 353–358; A. E. Robinson and A. T. Holder, *J. Chromatogr. Sci.*, 1974, *12*, 281–284; A. E. Robinson and A. T. Holder, *Z. Rechtsmed.*, 1973, *72*, 306–311; G. Norheim, *Z. Rechtsmed.*, 1973, *73*, 219–224].

Methadone was held to be the sole cause of death in 55 out of 111 fatalities involving methadone. 50 of these victims were aged between 17 and 51 years and 5 were under 14. For the adult deaths, the mean methadone concentration was 0.584 mg/L (range, 0.084 to 2.7 mg/L). For those aged 15 to 49 years, death was due to a combination of methadone and other drugs in 56 cases (mean methadone concentration 0.576 mg/L (range, 0.049 to 2.44 mg/L)) [C. M. Milroy and A. R. Forrest, *J. Clin. Pathol.*, 2000, *53(4)*, 277–281].

From 1997 to 1998, in 38 out of 3317 reported deaths in San Francisco, USA, methadone was detected. 17 of these cases were deemed as being due to methadone toxicity. The mean blood methadone concentration was 0.957 mg/L and the mean EDDP concentration was 0.253 mg/L. The mean ratio of methadone:EDDP in blood was 13.6:1.0 [S. B. Karch and B. G. Stephens, *West J. Med.*, 2000, *172(1)*, 11–14].

Half-life. Plasma half-life, after a single dose, 10 to 25 h (mean, 15); increased during long-term maintenance therapy to 13 to 55 h (mean, 30).

Volume of distribution. About 4 L/kg.

Clearance. Plasma clearance, about 2 mL/min/kg.

Distribution in blood. Plasma:whole blood ratio, about 1.3.

Protein binding. In plasma, about 92%, but there is considerable inter-subject variation.

Note. For a study of the disposition of nasal, IV and oral methadone in healthy volunteers, see O. Dale *et al.*, *Clin. Pharmacol. Ther.*, 2002, *72*, 536–545; for a review of interindividual variability of the clinical pharmacokinetics of methadone, see C. B. Eap *et al.*, *Clin. Pharmacokinet.*, 2002, *41*, 1153–1193; for a review of methadone use in cancer patients with pain, see E. Bruera and C. Sweeney, *J. Palliat. Med.*, 2002, *5*, 127–138.

Dose. For pain, initially, 2.5 to 10 mg of methadone hydrochloride every 3 to 8 h; doses of 30 mg have been given. In treatment of opioid dependence, initially 10 to 20 mg daily, increased to achieve stabilisation to a usual dose of 40 to 60 mg daily.

Methallenestril

Estrogen

Synonym. Methallenoestrol
Proprietary name. Vallestril
3-(6-Methoxy-2-naphthyl)-2,2-dimethylvaleric acid
$C_{18}H_{22}O_3$=286.4
CAS—517-18-0

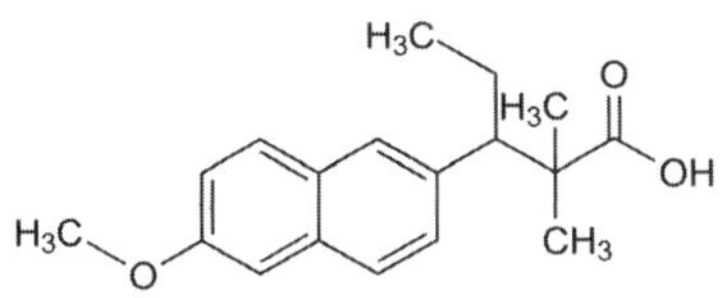

A white crystalline powder. M.p. about 138°.
Very slightly soluble in water; soluble 1 in 10 of ethanol, 1 in 2 of chloroform, and 1 in 8 of ether.

Partition Coefficient. Log *P* (octanol/water), 5.3.

Thin-layer Chromatography. System TP—Rf 79; system TQ—Rf 18; system TR—Rf 70; system TS—Rf 54, streaking may occur.

Ultraviolet Spectrum. Methanol—253, 264 nm (A_1^1=180a), 273 nm (A_1^1=180a), 317, 332 nm.

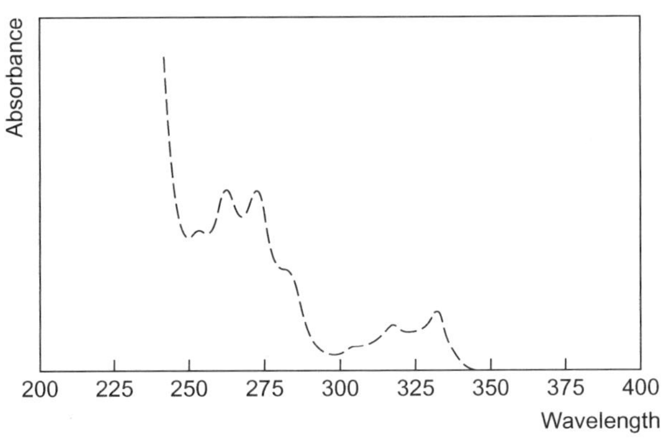

Infra-red Spectrum. Principal peaks at wavenumbers 1689, 1232, 1270, 857, 1606, 1149 cm^{-1} (KBr disk).

Dose. 3 to 9 mg daily.

Methamidophos

Acaricide, Insecticide

Synonyms. Acephate-met; Bayer 71628; ENT 27396; Ortho 9006; SRA 5172.
Proprietary names. Filitox; Metikar; Monitor; Nitofol; Nuratron; Patrole; Pillaron; Swipe; Tam; Tamanox; Tamaron; Vetaron.
Phosphoramidothioc acid *O,S*-dimethyl ester
$C_2H_8NO_2PS$=141.1
CAS—10265-92-6

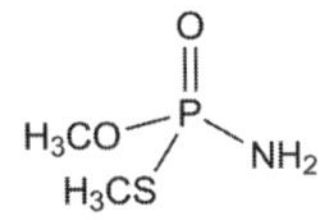

A colourless, crystalline solid with M.p. 54°.
It is readily soluble in water (90 g/L at 20°), ethanol, isopropanol (1400 g/L at 20°), xylene (<100 g/L at 20°), benzene (<100 g/L at 20°), dichloromethane (<25 g/L at 20°), toluene, diethyl ether (<25 g/L at 20°), kerosene (<10 g/L at 20°) and hexane (<10 g/L at 20°).

Partition Coefficient. Log *P* (octanol/water), −0.80.

Thin-layer Chromatography. System TX—Rf 01; system TY—Rf 00.

Gas Chromatography. System GA—RI 1190.
Column DB1 or DB1701 (30 m × 0.32 mm i.d., 0.25 μm film thickness), column temperature programmed from 130° (held 1 min) to 250° (held 2 min) at 10°/min. Carrier gas: helium. TSD. Retention time 4 min (DB1), 7.1 min (DB1701). [J. F. Lewin *et al.*, *TIAFT Bulletin Case Notes*, 1993, *23*(1)].

Mass Spectrometry. Principal ions at *m/z* 94, 95, 141, 64, 79, 80, 111, 110.

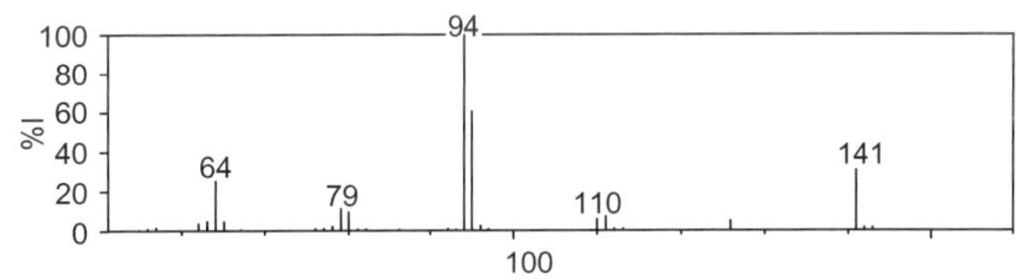

Quantification
Gas chromatography. In blood and liver: limit of detection 45 μg/L, TSD—J. F. Lewin *et al.*, *TIAFT Bulletin Case Notes*, 1993, *23*(1).

Disposition in the Body. Methamidophos is rapidly absorbed through the stomach, lungs and skin after exposure and is eliminated primarily via urine.

Toxicity. Methamidophos is highly toxic via oral, dermal and inhalation administration. The allowed daily intake is 0.0006 mg/kg.

A 61-year-old male plantation worker collapsed and was admitted to hospital. A bottle of Nitofol (methamidophos) was found on the floor beside him. He died 11 h after ingestion. Toxicological analysis showed that there was a concentration of 130 mg/L methamidophos in his blood and 240 mg/L in his liver. The cause of death was due to an overdose of methamidophos [J. F. Lewin *et al.*, *TIAFT Bulletin Case Notes*, 1993, *23*(1)].

Methandienone

Anabolic Steroid

Synonym. Methandrostenolone
Proprietary names. Anabol; Danabol; Dianabol; Melic; Metastenol; Nerobol; Vetanabol (vet.).

(17β)-17-Hydroxy-17-methylandrosta-1,4-dien-3-one
$C_{20}H_{28}O_2$=300.4
CAS—72-63-9

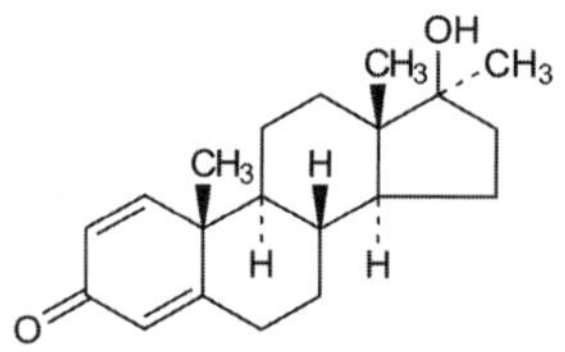

A white or faintly yellowish-white, crystalline powder. M.p. 163° to 167°. Practically insoluble in water; soluble 1 in 2 of ethanol, 1 in less than 1 of chloroform, and 1 in 70 of ether.

Partition Coefficient. Log *P* (octanol/water), 3.5.

Thin-layer Chromatography. System TA—Rf 86; system TE—Rf 80; system TP—Rf 65; system TQ—Rf 10; system TR—Rf 87; system TS—Rf 61; system TAJ—Rf 44; system TAK—Rf 61; system TAL—Rf 92; system TAM—Rf 88.

Gas Chromatography. System GA—RI 2672; system GAG—RRT 1.2 (relative to testosterone); system GAI—RRT of urinary metabolites: 17α-methyl-5β, (α)-androstan-3α,17β-diol 0.925; 17α-methyl-5β-androst-1-en-3α,17β-diol 0.921; 17α-methyl-1,4-androstadien-6β,17β-diol-3-one 1.117 (relative to 17α-methyl-5α-androstan-3β,17β-diol); system GAR—retention time 13.2 min.

High Performance Liquid Chromatography. System HAR—RRT 0.86 (relative to testosterone); system HATb—RRT 0.87 (relative to testosterone).

Ultraviolet Spectrum. Dehydrated alcohol—245 nm (A_1^1=516a).

Infra-red Spectrum. Principal peaks at wavenumbers 1660, 1620, 886, 1601, 1160, 1240 cm^{-1} (KBr disk).

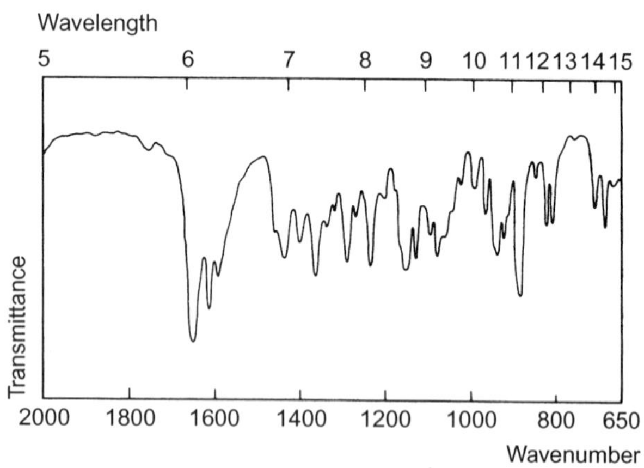

Quantification

Gas chromatography. In urine: limit of detection 30 ng for methandienone, 10 ng for 17-epimethandienone, and 6β-hydroxy-17-epimethandienone—H. H. Dürbeck *et al.*, *J. Chromatogr.*, 1978, *167*, 117–124.

Gas chromatography–mass spectrometry. In urine: methandienone metabolites—J. Kokkonen *et al.*, *J. Chromatogr. B. Biomed. Sci. Appl.*, 1999, *734*, 179–189.

High performance liquid chromatography. In urine: limit of detection 5 ng, UV detection—C. G. B. Frischkorn and H. E. Frischkorn, *J. Chromatogr.*, 1978, *151*, 331–338.

Dose. Initially 2.5 to 5 mg daily.

Methandriol

Anabolic Steroid

Synonyms. MAD; Mestenediol; Methylandrostenediol.
Proprietary names. Androdiol; Androteston-M; Crestabolic; Diolostene; Masdiol; Megabion; Methanabol; Methandiol; Methosten; Metisione; Metocryst; Nabadial; Neostene; Neutrirmone; Neutrosteron; Notandron; Protandren; Sinasex; Troformone.
(3β,17β)-17-Methylandrost-5-ene-3,17-diol
$C_{20}H_{32}O_2$=304.5
CAS—521-10-8

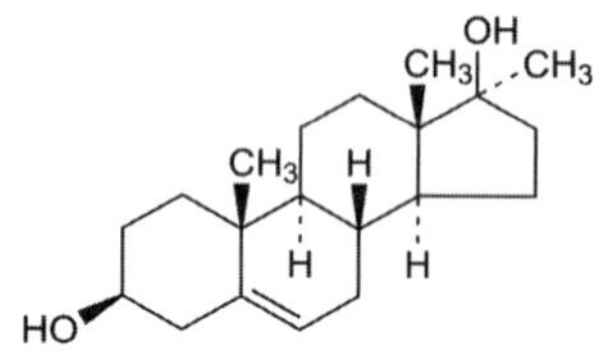

A crystalline powder with M.p 205.5° to 206.5°. It is insoluble in water; slightly soluble in some organic solvents.

Methandriol Diacetate

$C_{24}H_{36}O_4$=388.5
CAS—2061-86-1
M.p., 145° to 146° (Crystals from hexane).

Methandriol Dipropionate

Synonym. Methylandrostendiol Dipropionate
Proprietary name. Probolin
$C_{26}H_{40}O_4$=416.6
CAS—3593-85-9

Partition Coefficient. Log *P* (octanol/water), 4.35.

Gas Chromatography. System GAG—methandriol RRT 0.89, methandriol dipropionate RRT 1.70 (both relative to testosterone); system GAI—urine metabolite: 17α-methyl-5β-androstan-3α,17β-diol RRT 0.925 (relative to 17α-methyl-5α-androstan-3β,17β-diol); system GAR—methandriol Retention time 12.3 min; methandriol dipropionate Retention time 15.2 min.

Column: 3% OV-1 Chromosorb WHP 80/100 mesh (4′ × ¼″). Column temperature: 280°. Carrier gas: nitrogen, flow rate 32 mL/min. Detection: flame ionisation. RI: 2637 [T. Mills and J. C. Roberson, *Instrumental Data for Drug Analysis*, Vol. 2, 2nd Edn., CRC Press, Boca Raton, 1993, pp. 1384–1385].

High Performance Liquid Chromatography. System HAR—methandriol RRT 1.25, methandriol dipropionate (both relative to testosterone); system HATb—methandriol RRT 1.29 (relative to testosterone); system HATb—methandriol dipropionate RRT 2.75 (relative to testosterone).

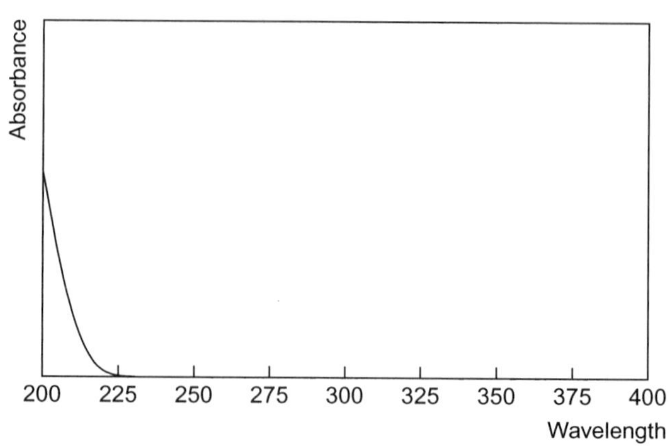

Infra-red Spectrum. Principal peaks at wavenumbers 1449, 1372, 1054, 942 cm^{-1}; (methandriol dipropionate) 1725, 1189, 1075 cm^{-1} (KBr disks).

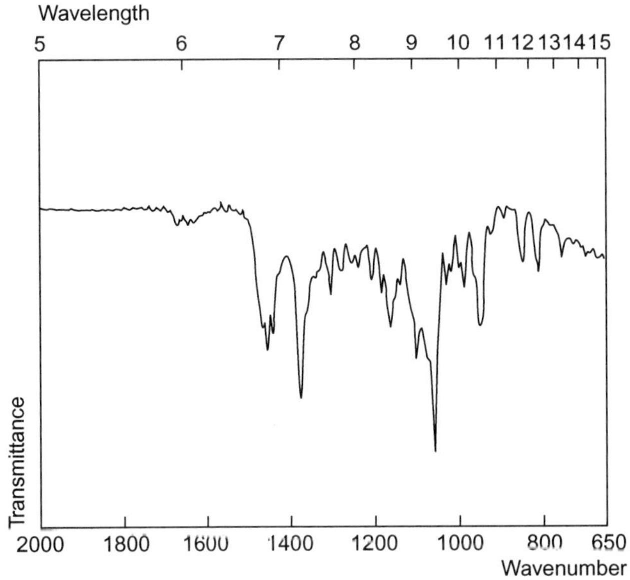

Mass Spectrum. Principal ions at *m*/*z* 253, 91, 213, 43, 105, 271, 79, 145; *m*/*z* 57, 342, 253, 268, 145, 147, 81, 91 (dipropionate).

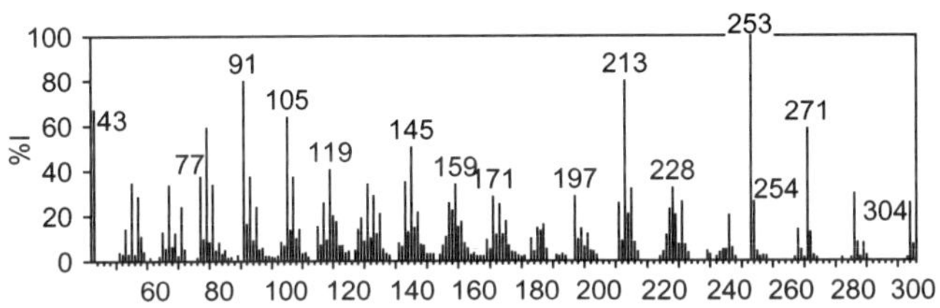

Disposition in the Body. Methandriol is excreted in urine as metabolites, one of which is 17α-methyl-5β-androstan-3α,17β-diol.

Methanol

Solvent

Synonym. Methyl Alcohol
$CH_3OH = 32.04$
CAS—67-56-1

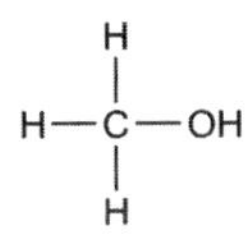

A clear, colourless, highly flammable liquid. B.p. 63.5° to 65.7°. Refractive index 1.328 to 1.329.
Miscible with water, ethanol, benzene, chloroform, ether, ketones, and most other organic solvents.
Note. The commercial substance known as 'wood naphtha', 'pyroxylic spirit', or 'wood spirit' contains 60 to 90% of methanol, together with acetone and other empyreumatic impurities. The variety used for denaturing ethanol (see under Ethanol) contains not less than 72% of methanol.

Dissociation Constant. pK_a 15.3.

Partition Coefficient. Log *P* (octanol/water), 0.8.

Colour Test. Potassium Dichromate (Method 2)—green.

Gas Chromatography. System GA—RI 491; system GI—retention time 0.7 min.

Mass Spectrum. Principal ions at *m*/*z* 31, 32, 29, 30, 28, 33, 34, 27; formic acid 29, 46, 45, 28, 44, 30, 47, –.

Quantification

Gas chromatography. In blood or urine: direct injection, FID—B. R. Manno and J. E. Manno, *J. Anal. Toxicol.*, 1978, *2*, 257–261.

Disposition in the Body. Readily absorbed after oral administration and distributed in the body according to the water content of the tissues; it may also be absorbed by inhalation or through intact skin. It is metabolised, much more slowly than ethanol, by oxidation to formaldehyde, formic acid, and possibly other products. Oxidation to formaldehyde is probably accomplished by alcohol dehydrogenase since the metabolism is inhibited by ethanol. Maximum concentrations of formic acid in the blood and urine occur 2 to 3 days after ingestion. Small amounts of methanol are excreted unchanged in the urine and expired air and about 10% of a dose is excreted in the urine as formic acid.

Blood concentration. Endogenous blood-methanol concentrations are approx. 1.5 mg/L, and urinary formic acid concentrations are usually about 12 to 17 mg/L.

Toxicity. The initial effects of methanol are much milder than those of ethanol and toxic effects are not usually seen until after a latent period of 8 to 36 h; the symptoms may include severe upper abdominal pain, visual disturbance often proceeding to incurable blindness, severe metabolic acidosis, and prolonged coma which may terminate in death from respiratory failure. The fatal dose varies greatly but is usually between 100 and 200 mL in adults, although ingestion of 30 mL is potentially lethal; permanent blindness has been caused by as little as 10 mL. Toxic effects are usually associated with blood concentrations greater than 100 mg/L and blood concentrations greater than 200 mg/L are indicative of severe poisoning and may be lethal. The maximum permissible atmospheric concentration is 200 ppm.

A 44-year-old man suffering from methanol intoxication was found comatose and had a serum concentration of 5.83 g/L on admission. The subject died 40 h later and the following postmortem concentrations were found (g/L or mg/g): blood 1.42, bile 1.75, brain 1.59, heart 0.93, kidney 1.30, liver, 1.07, lung 1.27, vitreous humour 1.73. [N. B. Wu Chen *et al.*, *J. Forensic Sci.*, 1985, *30*, 213–216.]

The following postmortem tissue concentrations were reported in a 41-year-old man who died after ingesting a large quantity of methanol: kidney 5.13 mg/g, liver 4.18 mg/g, vitreous humour 3.96 g/L, heart 3.45 mg/g, urine 3.43 g/L, pericardial fluid 3.29 g/L, blood 2.84 g/L, stomach content 2.21 g/L. [A. Pla *et al.*, *Forensic Sci. Int.*, 1991, *49*, 193–196.]

In 2 fatalities caused by ingestion of methanol (about 100 g), femoral blood concentrations of methanol and formic acid were 2.19 and 0.41 g/L, respectively, in the first subject and 1.96 and 0.38 g/L in the second. [H. Kinoshita *et al.*, *Int. J. Legal Med.*, 1998, *111*, 334–335.]

Volume of distribution. About 0.6 L/kg.

Note. For a review of methanol poisoning and its treatment, see D. G. Barceloux *et al.*, *J. Toxicol. Clin. Toxicol.*, 2002, *40*, 415–446.

Protein binding. In plasma, not significantly bound.

Methanthelinium Bromide

Anticholinergic

Synonyms. Bromuro de Metantelina; Dixamonum Bromidum; Methantheline Bromide; Methanthine Bromide.
Proprietary names. Asabaine; Avagal; Banthine; Bronerg; Doladene; Evogal; Gastron; Gastrosedan; Metanyl; Metaxan; Methanide; Uldumont; Vagamin; Vagantin; Xanteline; Xantenol.
N,*N*-Diethyl-*N*-methyl-2-[(9*H*-xanthen-9-ylcarbonyl)oxy]-ethanaminium bromide
$C_{21}H_{26}BrNO_3 = 420.3$
CAS—5818-17-7 (methanthelinium); 53-46-3 (bromide)

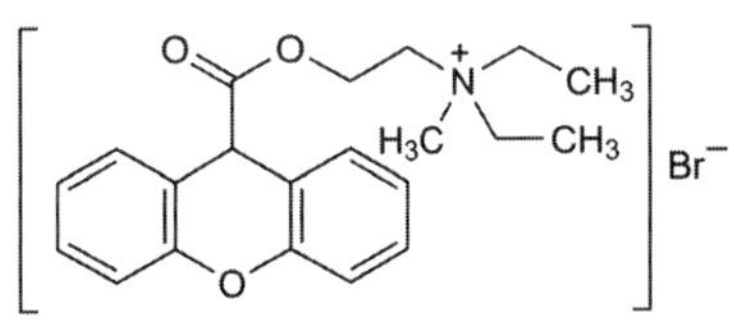

A white crystalline powder. M.p. 171° to 177°.
Soluble 1 in less than 5 of water, ethanol, and chloroform; practically insoluble in ether. Aqueous solutions decompose on standing.

Partition Coefficient. Log *P* (octanol/water), 1.7.

Colour Tests. Mandelin's Test—orange; Marquis Test—orange

Thin-layer Chromatography. System TA—Rf 02; system TB—Rf 00; system TE—Rf 76; system TAE—Rf 03. (Acidified iodoplatinate solution, positive.)

High Performance Liquid Chromatography. System HX—RI 418.

Ultraviolet Spectrum. Aqueous acid—282 nm (A_1^1=65a).

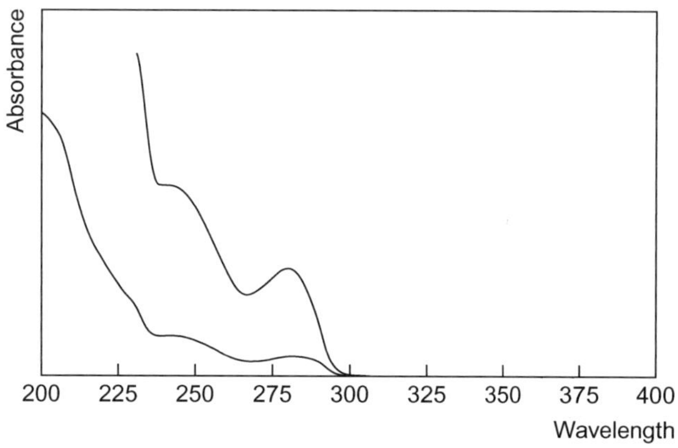

Infra-red Spectrum. Principal peaks at wavenumbers 1155, 1248, 1724, 761, 1200, 755 cm^{-1} (KBr disk).

Mass Spectrum. Principal ions at *m/z* 72, 181, 85, 152, 42, 44, 58, 43.

Dose. Methanthelinium bromide has been given in doses of 200 to 400 mg daily.

Methapyrilene

Antihistamine

Synonym. Thenylpyramine

N,*N*-Dimethyl-*N'*-2-pyridinyl-*N'*-(2-thienylmethyl)-1,2-ethanediamine

$C_{14}H_{19}N_3S$=261.4

CAS—91-80-5

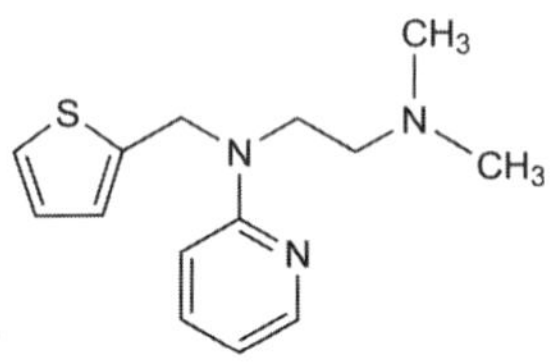

A liquid.

Methapyrilene Fumarate

$(C_{14}H_{19}N_3S)_2,3C_4H_4O_4$=871.0

CAS—33032-12-1

A white crystalline powder. M.p. 135° to 136°.

Soluble 1 in 20 of water and 1 in 30 of ethanol.

Methapyrilene Hydrochloride

Synonym. Methapyrilenium Chloride

$C_{14}H_{19}N_3S,HCl$=297.8

CAS—135-23-9

A white crystalline powder. M.p. 162°.

Soluble 1 in 0.5 of water, 1 in 5 of ethanol, and 1 in 3 of chloroform; practically insoluble in ether and benzene.

Dissociation Constant. pK_a 3.7, 8.9 (25°).

Partition Coefficient. Log *P* (octanol/water), 2.9.

Colour Tests. Liebermann's Test—red-brown; Mandelin's Test—black-violet; Marquis Test—black-violet; Sulfuric Acid—orange.

Thin-layer Chromatography. System TA—Rf 52; system TB—Rf 41; system TC—Rf 26; system TE—Rf 66; system TL—Rf 13; system TAE—Rf 21; system TAF—Rf 24; system TAJ—Rf 20; system TAK—Rf 00; system TAL—Rf 48. (Dragendorff spray, positive; acidified iodoplatinate solution, positive; Marquis reagent, violet.)

Gas Chromatography. System GA—RI 1981; system GF—RI 2305.

High Performance Liquid Chromatography. System HA—*k* 4.1; system HX—RI 342; system HY—RI 197.

Ultraviolet Spectrum. Aqueous acid—237 (A_1^1=720a), 314; aqueous alkali—241, 312 nm.

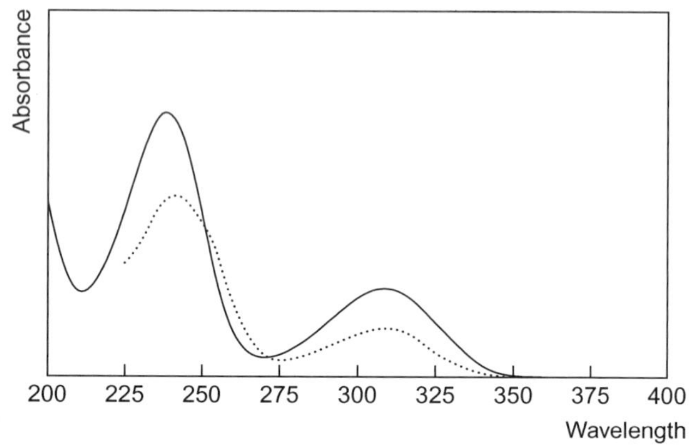

Infra-red Spectrum. Principal peaks at wavenumbers 1592, 765, 1558, 1250, 1158, 1316 cm^{-1} (KBr disk).

Mass Spectrum. Principal ions at *m/z* 58, 97, 72, 71, 42, 191, 79, 78.

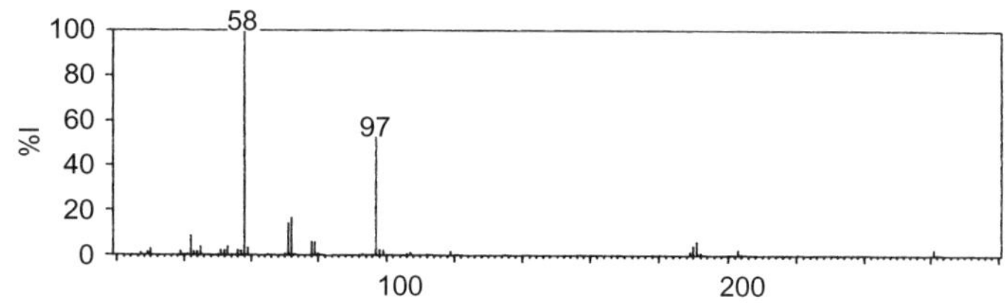

Quantification

Gas chromatography. In plasma or urine: limit of detection 10 μg/L in plasma, 50 μg/L in urine, AFID—R. C. Baselt and S. Franch, *J. Chromatogr.*, 1980, *183*; *B Biomed. Appl.*, *9*, 234–238. In blood, urine or tissues: FID—C. L. Winek *et al.*, *Clin. Toxicol.*, 1977, *11*, 287–294.

Disposition in the Body. Variably and incompletely absorbed after oral administration. Less than 2% of a dose is excreted in the urine as unchanged drug in 24 h.

Therapeutic concentration

After a single oral dose of 50 mg to 8 subjects, peak plasma concentrations of 0.006 to 0.05 mg/L (mean 0.024) were attained in about 1.5 h [E. P. Calandre *et al.*, *Clin. Pharmacol. Ther.*, 1981, *29*, 527–532.]

Toxicity. Methapyrilene has been shown to be carcinogenic in rats and is little used. Fatalities have occurred after ingestion of 7 g or more and toxic effects have been associated with plasma concentrations greater than 30 mg/L. In 13 fatalities attributed to methapyrilene overdose, reported blood concentrations ranged from 2 to 380 mg/L (mean 50) (salicylamide and ethanol were also detected in several cases).

The following postmortem tissue concentrations were reported in one fatality: blood 9 mg/L, kidney 52 μg/g, liver 82 μg/g, lung 119 μg/g, urine 200 mg/L [C. A. Ainsworth and J. D. Biggs, *Clin. Toxicol.*, 1977, *11*, 281–286.]

Half-life. Plasma half-life, about 1 to 2 h.

Volume of distribution. About 4 L/kg.

Clearance. Plasma clearance, about 30 mL/min/kg.

Distribution in blood. Plasma:whole blood ratio, about 1.0.

Dose. Methapyrilene hydrochloride has been given in doses of up to 200 mg daily.

Methaqualone

Hypnotic/Sedative

Synonyms. Methachalonum; Methaqualonum; QZ-2; R-148; TR-495; CI-705; CN-38703.
Proprietary names. Mequin; Normi-Nox; Pallidan; Quaalude. It is an ingredient of Toquilone Compositum.
A preparation containing methaqualone and diphenhydramine hydrochloride was formerly marketed under the proprietary name Mandrax.
Methaqualone has been withdrawn from the market in many countries because of problems with abuse.
2-Methyl-3-(2-methylphenyl)-4(3*H*)-quinazolinone
$C_{16}H_{14}N_2O$=250.3
CAS—72-44-6

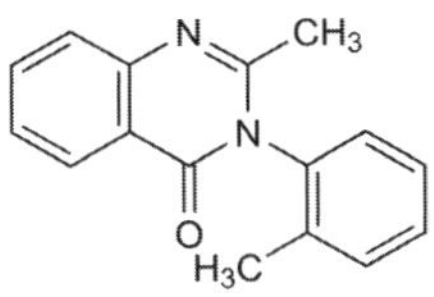

A white crystalline powder. M.p. 120°, also given as 114° to 116°.
Practically insoluble in water; soluble 1 in 12 of ethanol, 1 in 1 of chloroform, and 1 in 50 of ether.

Methaqualone Hydrochloride
$C_{16}H_{14}N_2O,HCl$=286.8
CAS—340-56-7
A white crystalline powder. M.p. 255° to 265°.
Practically insoluble in water; soluble in ether and ethanol.

Dissociation Constant. pK_a 2.5.

Partition Coefficient. Log *P* (octanol/water), 4.3.

Thin-layer Chromatography. System TA—Rf 70; system TB—Rf 36; system TC—Rf 80; system TD—Rf 63; system TE—Rf 78; system TL—Rf 56; system TAE—Rf 79; system TAF—Rf 84. (Dragendorff spray, positive; acidified iodoplatinate solution, positive.)

Gas Chromatography. System GA—methaqualone RI 2135, M (2-formyl-) RI 2240, M (2-OH-methyl-) RI 2360, M (2-carboxy-) RI 2400, M (2′-OH-methyl-) RI 2410, M (3′-OH-) RI 2490, M (4′-OH-) RI 2510, M (6-OH-) RI 2525, M (OH-methoxy-) RI 2560; system GB—methaqualone RI 2256, M (2-formyl-) RI 2370, M (2-OH-methyl-) RI 2437, M (2′-OH-methyl-) RI 2500, M (OH-methoxy-) RI 2698; system GF—methaqualone RI 2580.

High Performance Liquid Chromatography. System HA—*k* 0.2; system HX—RI 459; system HY—RI 400; system HZ—Retention time 5.4 min; system HAX—Retention time 6.8 min; system HAY—Retention time 7.4 min.

Ultraviolet Spectrum. Aqueous acid—234 (A^1_1=1320a), 269; aqueous alkali—265 (A^1_1=347b), 306 nm.

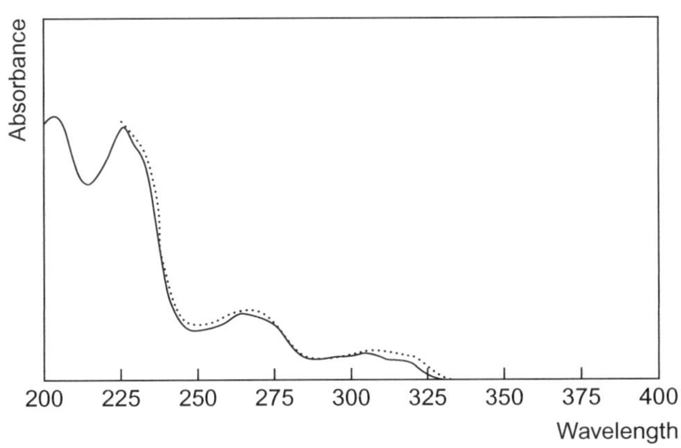

Infra-red Spectrum. Principal peaks at wavenumbers 1682, 1599, 1565, 770, 1265, 697 cm^{-1} (KBr disk).

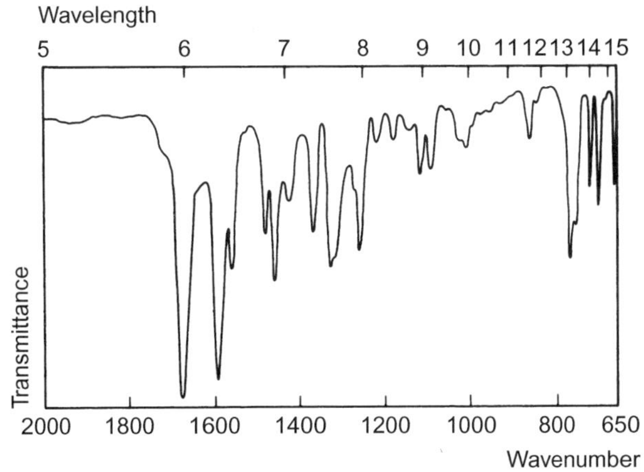

Mass Spectrum. Principal ions at *m/z* 235, 250, 91, 233, 236, 65, 76, 132; 4′-hydroxymethaqualone 251, 266, 249, 77, 143, 76, 252, 39.

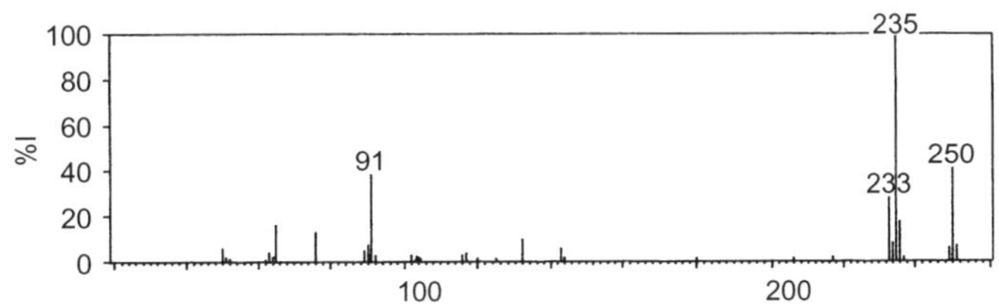

Quantification
Gas chromatography. In plasma or saliva: methaqualone and the 2′-hydroxymethyl metabolite, limit of detection 20 µg/L, AFID—M. A. Peat and B. S. Finkle, *J. Anal. Toxicol.*, 1980, *4*, 114–118. In blood or urine: total amount of methaqualone and its metabolites (UV detection), methaqualone (FID) —F. Liu *et al.*, *Yao Xue Xue Bao*, 1994, *29*, 610–616.

Gas chromatography–mass spectrometry. In urine: methaqualone and metabolites—L. Kazyak *et al.*, *Clin. Chem.*, 1977, *23*, 2001–2006. In urine: comparison with immunoassays—C. Brenner *et al.*, *Forensic Sci. Int.*, 1996, *79*, 31–41. In blood, urine, gastric content, or hair: limit of detection in urine about 0.1 mg/L—O. Plaut *et al.*, *Forensic Sci. Int.*, 1998, *92*, 219–227.

High performance liquid chromatography. In plasma: limit of detection 1 µg/L, UV detection—R. A. Hux *et al.*, *Anal. Chem.*, 1982, *54*, 113–117.

Radioimmunoassay–thin-layer chromatography. In urine: methaqualone and metabolites, limit of detection 1 mg/L—R. D. Budd *et al.*, *J. Chromatogr.*, 1980, *190*, 129–132.

Disposition in the Body. Readily absorbed after oral administration and widely distributed throughout the body. The major metabolites are 4′-hydroxymethaqualone, 2′-hydroxymethylmethaqualone and their *O*-glucuronides or *O*-methyl ethers, and methaqualone *N*-oxide. A large number of metabolites are known and there is considerable intersubject variation in the relative amounts produced. About 40 to 50% of a dose is excreted in the urine in 72 h, mostly as conjugated metabolites, with less than 2% of a dose as unchanged drug. In 24 h, about 10% of a dose is excreted in the urine as the conjugated 4′-hydroxy metabolite, 7% as the *N*-oxide, 5% as the conjugated 2′-hydroxymethyl derivative, and about 3% each as the conjugated 2-hydroxymethyl, 3′-hydroxy, and 6-hydroxy metabolites. Up to 4% of a dose may be eliminated unchanged in the faeces.

Therapeutic concentration. In plasma, usually in the range 0.4 to 5 mg/L.

After a single oral dose of 250 mg of the base to 7 subjects, peak plasma concentrations of 1.0 to 4.0 mg/L (mean 2.2) were attained in 2 h; following an equivalent dose of the hydrochloride, peak plasma concentrations of 2.0 to 4.9 mg/L (mean 3.7) were attained in 1 h [S. Goenechea *et al.*, *Arch. Toxicol.*, 1973, *31*, 25–30].

After daily oral doses of 300 mg to 8 subjects, a mean maximum steady-state plasma concentration of 3.7 mg/L was reported [R. K. Nayak *et al.*, *J. Pharmacokinet. Biopharm.*, 1974, *2*, 107–121].

Toxicity. The estimated minimum lethal dose is 5 g in non-tolerant subjects. Drug accumulation is likely in chronic dosing because of the

long half-life. Toxic effects may be associated with plasma concentrations greater than 2 mg/L, and plasma concentrations greater than about 8 mg/L are likely to produce coma and may be lethal. The 2′-hydroxymethyl metabolite, which has been found unconjugated in both blood and urine in overdose cases, may contribute to the degree of intoxication.
Abuse of methaqualone, particularly when taken in conjunction with diphenhydramine, has been reported.

The following postmortem concentrations were reported in a 62-year-old man who died after ingesting methaqualone and diphenhydramine with suicidal intent: blood 800 mg/L and 20 mg/L, bile 30 and 13 mg/L, gastric contents 12 000 and 7 mg/L, respectively [N. Fucci, *Am. J. Forensic Med. Pathol.*, 1996, *17*, 231–232].

In 6 fatal cases, postmortem blood concentrations of 5 to 42 mg/L (mean 22) and liver concentrations of 26 to 89 µg/g (mean 55) were reported [R. C. Baselt and R. H. Cravey, *J. Anal. Toxicol.*, 1977, *1*, 81–102].

In 19 mildly poisoned patients the plasma concentration on admission to hospital ranged from 2 to 20 mg/L (mean 9). In 9 more severe cases, a mean peak concentration of 27 mg/L was reached within 12 h of admission to hospital [A. A. H. Lawson and S. S. Brown, *BMJ*, 1966, *2*, 1455–1456].

Half-life. Plasma half-life, about 20 to 60 h (mean 35); a slower terminal elimination half-life of up to about 72 h has also been reported.

Volume of distribution. About 6 L/kg.

Distribution in blood. Plasma:whole blood ratio about 1.1 at therapeutic concentrations decreasing to about 0.5 at concentrations of 20 mg/L.

Saliva. Plasma:saliva ratio, about 9.

Protein binding. In plasma, about 75 to 95% (concentration-dependent).

Note. For a review of the pharmacokinetics of hypnotic drugs see D. D. Breimer, *Clin. Pharmacokinet.*, 1977, *2*, 93–109.

Dose. Usually up to 300 mg daily.

Metharbital

Anticonvulsant/Barbiturate

Synonyms. Endiemal; Metharbitone.
Proprietary name. Gemonil
5,5-Diethyl-1-methyl-2,4,6(1*H*,3*H*,5*H*)-pyrimidinetrione
$C_9H_{14}N_2O_3$ = 198.2
CAS—50-11-3

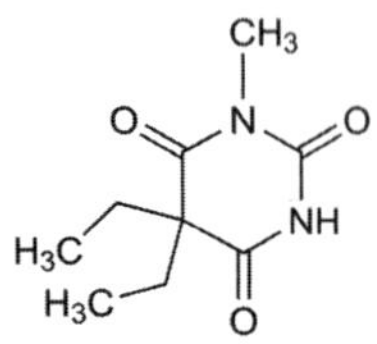

A white crystalline powder. M.p. 151° to 155°.
Soluble 1 in 830 of water, 1 in 23 of ethanol, and 1 in 40 of ether.

Dissociation Constant. pK_a 8.3 (20°).

Partition Coefficient. Log *P* (octanol/water), 1.2.

Colour Tests. Koppanyi–Zwikker Test—violet; Mercurous Nitrate—black.

Thin-layer Chromatography. System TD—Rf 66; system TE—Rf 54; system TF—Rf 65; system TH—Rf 86; system TAD—Rf 69; system TAE—Rf 87. (Mercurous nitrate spray, black; Zwikker's reagent, faint pink.)

Gas Chromatography. System GA—metharbital RI 1470, M (OH-) RI 1800; barbital RI 1489.

High Performance Liquid Chromatography. System HG—metharbital *k* 2.69, barbital *k* 1.11; system HH—metharbital *k* 1.99, barbital *k* 0.63; system HX—RI 435; system HY—RI 324.

Ultraviolet Spectrum. Borax buffer 0.05 M (pH 9.2)—244 (A^1_1 = 433a); 1 M sodium hydroxide (pH 13)—244 nm (A^1_1 = 458b).

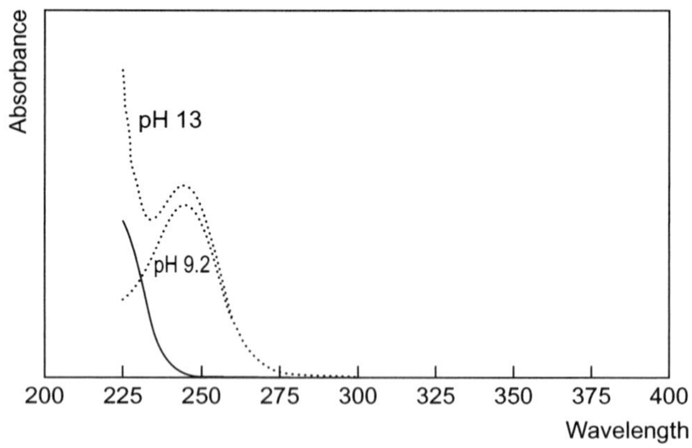

Infra-red Spectrum. Principal peaks at wavenumbers 1655, 1699, 1755, 1275, 1205, 815 cm^{-1} (KBr disk).

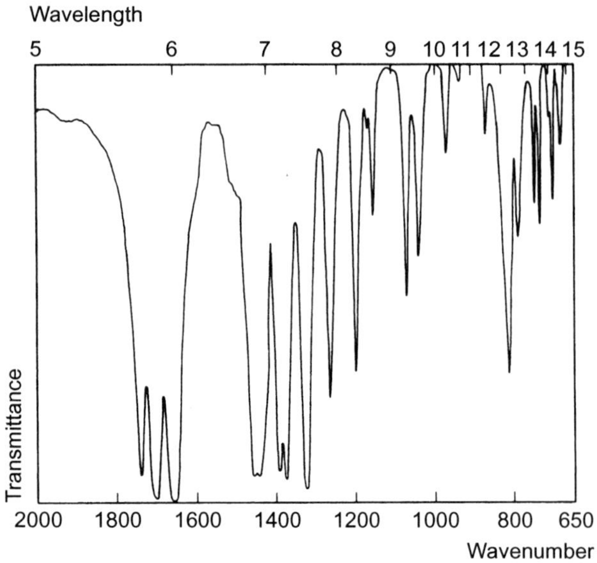

Mass Spectrum. Principal ions at *m/z* 155, 170, 112, 169, 55, 82, 41, 39; barbital 156, 141, 55, 155, 98, 39, 82, 43.

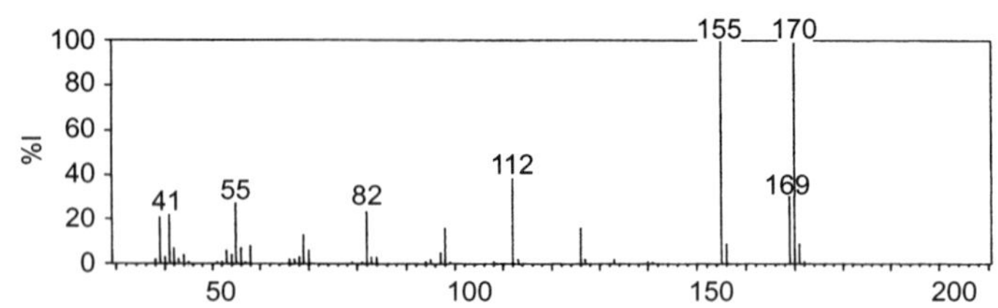

Quantification. See under Amylobarbital.

Disposition in the Body. About 1% of a dose is excreted in the urine in 48 h as unchanged drug and about 10% as the active metabolite, barbital; the remainder is thought to be slowly excreted in the urine as barbital over a period of 2 to 3 weeks.

Therapeutic concentration

Following daily oral doses of 300 mg for 14 days to 1 subject, metharbital reached a peak plasma concentration of 5 mg/L shortly after a dose, but was undetectable 8 h later when the plasma concentration of barbital was 26 mg/L [T. C. Butler and W. J. Waddell, *Neurology, Minneap.*, 1958, *8*, 106–112.]

Toxicity. The estimated minimum lethal dose is 2 g.

Dose. 100 to 300 mg daily.

Methazolamide

Carbonic Anhydrase Inhibitor

Proprietary names. GlaucTabs; MZM; Neptazane.
N-[5-(Aminosulfonyl)-3-methyl-1,3,4-thiadiazol-2(3*H*)-ylidene]-acetamide
$C_5H_8N_4O_3S_2=236.3$
CAS—554-57-4

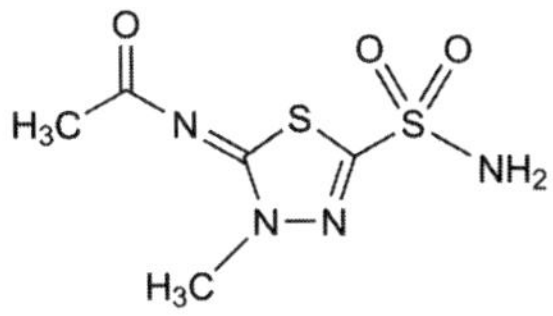

A white or faintly yellow, crystalline powder. M.p. about 213°.
Very slightly soluble in water and ethanol; slightly soluble in acetone; soluble in dimethylformamide.

Dissociation Constant. pK_a 7.3.

Partition Coefficient. Log *P* (ether/pH 7.4), −0.2.

Colour Test. Koppanyi–Zwikker Test—violet.

Thin-layer Chromatography. System TA—Rf 72; system TB—Rf 00; system TE—Rf 19; system TAE—Rf 84; system TAJ—Rf 44; system TAK—Rf 15; system TAL—Rf 78. (Acidified iodoplatinate solution, positive.)

Gas Chromatography. System GA—RI 2187.

High Performance Liquid Chromatography. System HX—RI 304; system HY—RI 265.

Ultraviolet Spectrum. Aqueous acid—255, 290 ($A^1_1=396a$); aqueous alkali—288 nm ($A^1_1=568a$).

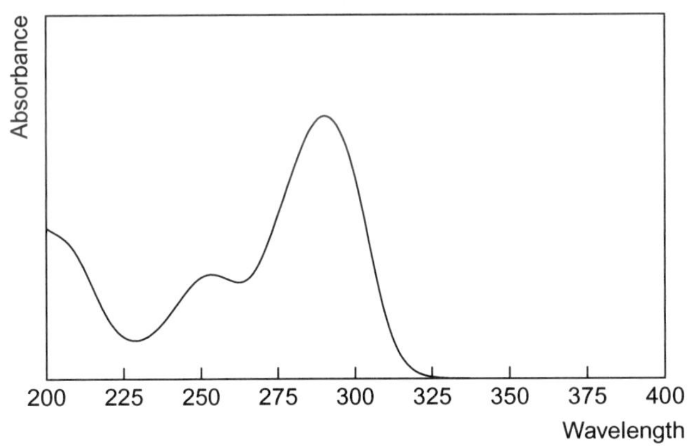

Mass Spectrum. Principal ions at *m/z* 43, 221, 83, 236, 56, 223, 222, 55.

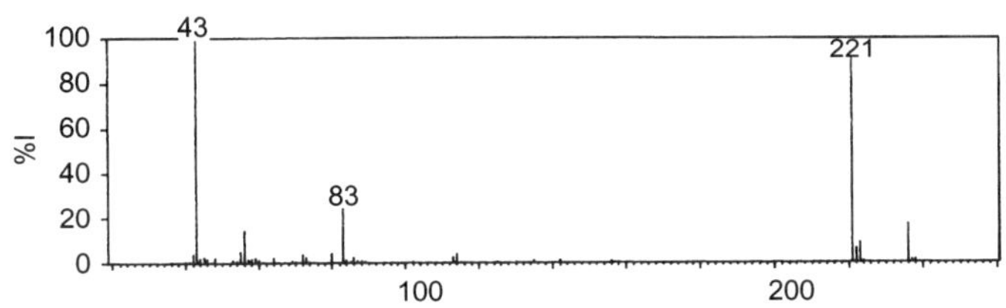

Quantification

Gas chromatography–mass spectrometry. In blood, plasma or urine: limit of detection <1 µg/L in plasma—W. F. Bayne *et al.*, *J. Pharm. Sci.*, 1981, *70*, 75–81. In blood, plasma, or urine: UV detection—G. R. Iyer and D. R. Taft, *J. Pharm. Biomed. Anal.*, 1998, *16*, 1021–1027.

Disposition in the Body. Well absorbed after oral administration. About 15 to 20% of a dose may be excreted in the urine in 24 h, of which about half is unchanged drug.

Therapeutic concentration

After a single oral dose of 50 mg to 1 subject, peak concentrations of 19.1 and 0.08 mg/L in blood and plasma respectively were reported at 3 h; the corresponding concentrations, 3 h after a dose of 150 mg to a different subject were 36.1 and 1.4 mg/L. Following oral doses of 100 mg three times a day to 1 subject, steady-state concentrations of about 40 mg/L and about 9.5 mg/L were reported for blood and plasma, respectively [W. F. Bayne *et al.*, *J. Pharm. Sci.*, 1981, *70*, 75–81.]

Distribution in blood. Plasma:erythrocyte ratio appears to be concentration-dependent, saturation of the carbonic anhydrase in the erythrocytes occurring at about 40 mg/L.

Protein binding. In plasma, about 55%.

Dose. In the treatment of glaucoma, 100 to 300 mg daily.

Methcathinone

Stimulant

Synonyms. α-Methylaminopropiophenone; Monomethylproprion.
Street names. Bathtub speed; Cadillac express; Catt; Cosmos; Ephedrone; Gagers; Gaggers; Goob; Jee cocktail; Jeff; Mulka; Speed; The C; Wild cat; Wonder star.
2-(Methylamino)-1-phenyl-1-propanone
$C_{10}H_{13}NO=163.2$
CAS—5650-44-2

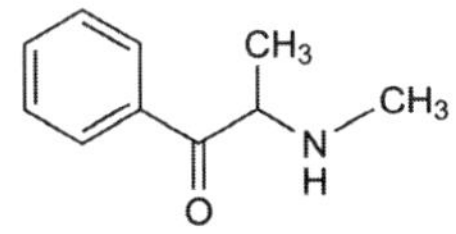

Methcathinone is derived from *S*-(−)-cathinone, a natural compound found in young leaves of the Khat shrub, *Catha edulis* (cathine).
It is a white to off white powder or colourless crystals. M.p. 182° to184°. Soluble in hydrochloric acid.

Methcathinone Hydrochloride

$C_{10}H_{13}NO, HCl=199.7$
CAS—49656-78-2
Crystals from alcohol acetone. M.p. 176° to 177°.
It is freely soluble in water and has a pungent taste.

Colour Tests. Cobalt Thiocyanate—faint blue; Chen's test—purple; Lieberman's Test—red/orange.

Gas Chromatography. Column: DB-5 (15 m × 0.25 mm i.d.). Column temperature: 140° for 1 min, to 220° at 20°/mins, held for 0.5 min, to 250° at 30°/min, held for 2.5 min. Injector and detector temperatures: 160° and 250°, respectively. Internal standard: amphetamine-d_6. Detection: MS. Retention time: methcathinone, 4.56 min; cathinone, 4.6 min; IS, 3.9 min; all as 4-carboethoxyhexafluorobutyryl derivatives. [B. Paul and K. Cole, *J. Anal. Toxicol.*, 2001, *25*, 525–530.]

Column: methyl silicone HP1 (0.2 mm i.d., 0.33 µm film thickness). Column temperature: 140°. Carrier gas: helium, flow rate 0.9 mL/min. MS detection. RI: 1323. [T. Mills and J. C. Roberson, *Instrumental data for drug analysis*, CRC Press, Boca Raton, Florida, 2nd Edn., Vol. 6, 1993, pp. 142–143.]

Ultraviolet Spectrum. Aqueous acid—251; basic—247 nm.

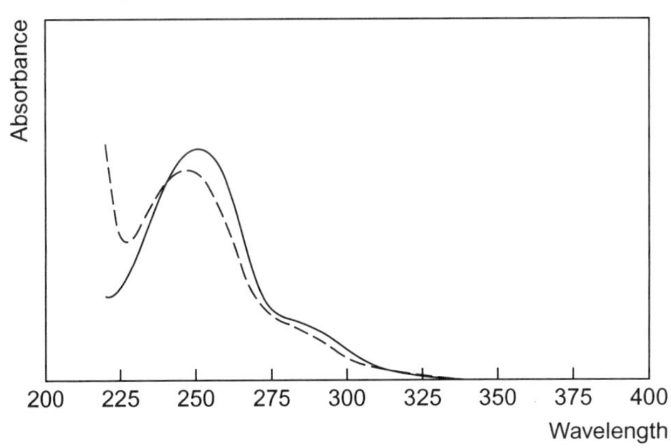

Infra-red Spectrum. Principal peaks at wavenumber 1691, 705, 1245, 1469 cm^{-1} (KBr disk).

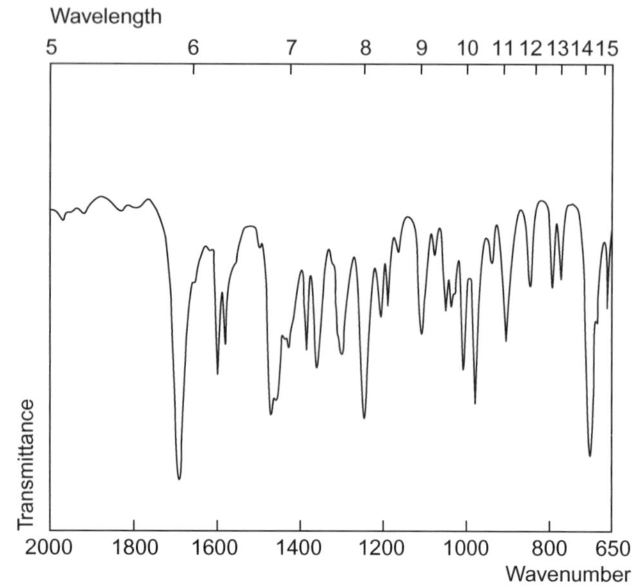

Mass Spectrum. Principal ions at *m*/*z* 58, 77, 51, 56, 42, 105, 50, 43.

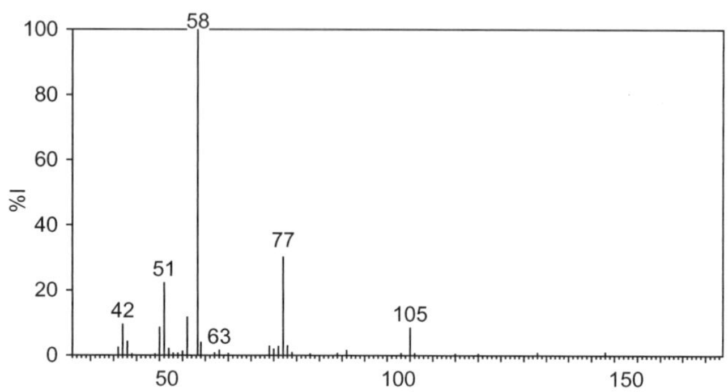

Quantification

Gas chromatography–mass spectrometry. In urine: limit of quantification 12.5 µg/L—B. Paul and K. Cole, *J. Anal. Toxicol.*, 2001, *25*, 525–530.

High performance liquid chromatography. In urine: UV Detection (λ=210 nm and 250 nm) —D. E. Bodrina *et al.*, *Sud. Med. Ekspert*, 1994, *37*, 23–26.

Disposition in the Body. 10 minutes after intranasal administration of an 80 to 250 mg dose, the onset of effects occurs and persists for a 5 to 8 h period. Both cathinone and methcathinone show activities similar to amfetamines.

Toxicity. Dose-related neurotoxic and locomotor stimulant effects that are species- and enantiomer-dependent have been observed. It shows a neurotoxic potential towards brain dopamine and/or serotonin neurons. Tolerance, craving, and addiction have also been reported.
The toxic dosage is estimated to be 80 to 250 mg by intranasal use.

Note. For neurotoxic and pharmacological studies of methcathinone in mice, see M. Sparago *et al.*, *J. Pharmacol. Exp. Ther.*, 1996, *279*, 1043–1052; also R. A. Glennon *et al.*, *Pharmacol. Biochem. Behav.*, 1987, *26*, 547–551.

Dose. 500 to 1000 mg a day intranasal and IV routes. Can be taken orally and by smoking.

Methdilazine

Antihistamine

Proprietary names. Tacaryl (chewable tablets); Tacryl.
10-[(1-Methyl-3-pyrrolidinyl)methyl]-10*H*-phenothiazine
$C_{18}H_{20}N_2S$=296.4
CAS—1982-37-2

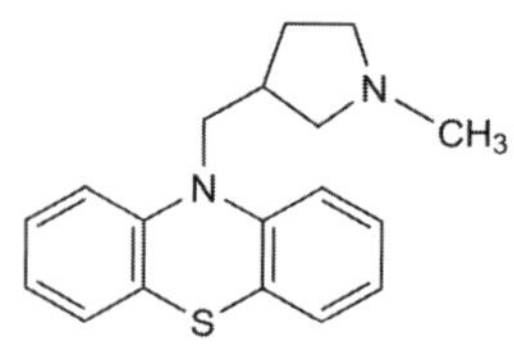

A light tan, crystalline powder. M.p. 87° to 88°.
Practically insoluble in water; soluble 1 in 2 of ethanol, 1 in 1 of chloroform, and 1 in 8 of ether.

Methdilazine Hydrochloride

Proprietary names. Dilosyn; Tacaryl (syrup and tablets).
$C_{18}H_{20}N_2S,HCl$=332.9
CAS—1229-35-2
A light tan, crystalline powder, which darkens on exposure to light. M.p. 184° to 190°.
Soluble 1 in 2 of water, 1 in 2 of ethanol, and 1 in 6 of chloroform; practically insoluble in ether.

Dissociation Constant. pK_a 7.5.

Partition Coefficient. Log *P* (octanol/water), 5.2.

Colour Tests. Formaldehyde–Sulfuric Acid—red-violet; Forrest Reagent—red-orange; FPN Reagent—red; Liebermann's Test—green-brown; Mandelin's Test—green→violet; Marquis Test—red-violet.

Thin-layer Chromatography. System TA—Rf 29; system TB—Rf 32; system TC—Rf 15; system TE—Rf 63; system TL—Rf 06; system TAJ—Rf 12; system TAK—Rf 19; system TAL—Rf 72. (Acidified iodoplatinate solution, positive.)

Gas Chromatography. System GA—RI 2467; system GF—RI 2920.

High Performance Liquid Chromatography. System HA—*k* 6.0; system HAX—Retention time 15.2 min; system HAY—Retention time 6.7 min.

Ultraviolet Spectrum. Aqueous acid—253 (A_1^1=982a), 302; aqueous alkali—255, 308 nm.

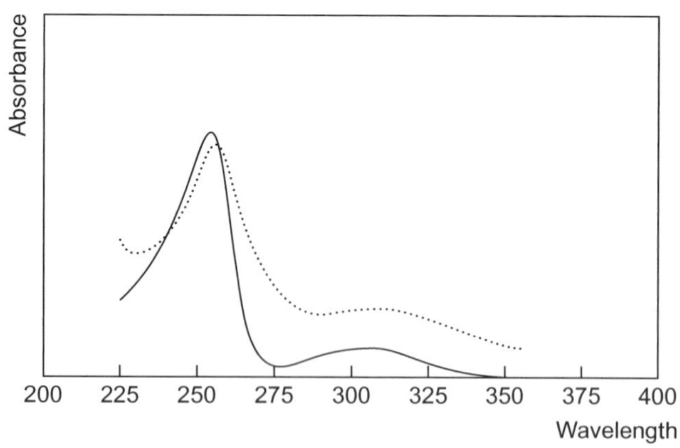

Infra-red Spectrum. Principal peaks at wavenumbers 753, 1242, 1319, 1222, 1277, 1031 cm^{-1} (methdilazine hydrochloride, KBr disk).

Mass Spectrum. Principal ions at *m*/*z* 97, 98, 296, 199, 55, 212, 96, 198.

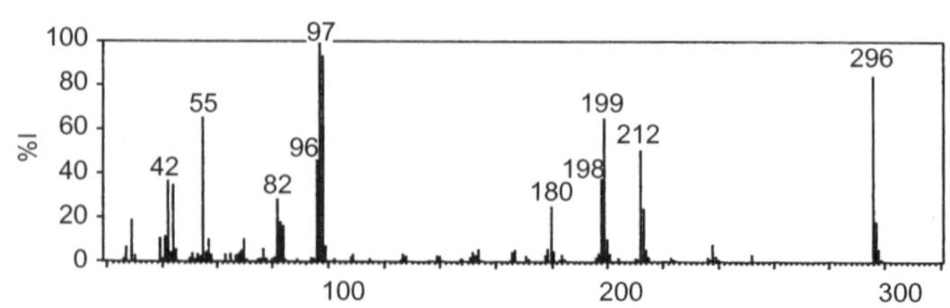

Dose. Usually 14.4 to 28.8 mg daily.

Methenamine

Antibacterial (Urinary)

Synonyms. Aminoform; Esammina; Formine; Hexamethylenamine; Hexamethylenetetramine; Hexamine; Urotropine.
Proprietary names. Antihydral; Uritone; Urotropina.
1,3,5,7-Tetraazatricyclo[3.3.1.1^{3,7}]decane
$C_6H_{12}N_4$=140.2
CAS—100-97-0

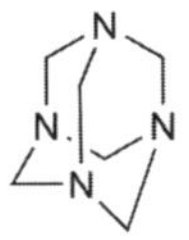

Colourless lustrous crystals or white crystalline powder. It sublimes at about 263° without melting.
Soluble 1 in 1.5 of water, 1 in 8 of ethanol (90%), 1 in 12 of chloroform, and 1 in 320 of ether.

Methenamine Hippurate

Synonym. Hexamine Hippurate
Proprietary names. Haiprex; Hiprex; Urex; Urotractan; Viapta.
$C_6H_{12}N_4,C_9H_9NO_3$=319.4
CAS—5714-73-8
A white crystalline powder. M.p. 105° to 110°.
Freely soluble in water and ethanol.

Methenamine Mandelate

Synonym. Hexamine Mandelate
Proprietary names. Mandelamine; Purerin; Uromandelin; Uronamin.
$C_6H_{12}N_4,C_8H_8O_3$=292.3
CAS—587-23-5
A white crystalline powder. M.p. 128° to 130°.
Very soluble in water; soluble 1 in 10 of ethanol, 1 in 20 of chloroform, and 1 in 350 of ether; slightly soluble in acetone.

Partition Coefficient. Log *P* (octanol/water), −4.2.

Colour Test. Mix 100 mg with an equal amount of salicylic acid and heat with 1 mL of sulfuric acid—a red colour is produced.

Thin-layer Chromatography. System TA—Rf 30; system TB—Rf 04; system TC—Rf 13; system TL—Rf 03; system TAE—Rf 12; system TAF—Rf 12. (Acidified iodoplatinate solution, positive.)

Gas Chromatography. System GA—RI 1210.

Ultraviolet Spectrum. Aqueous acid—251, 257 (A^1_1=15.5b), 263 nm.

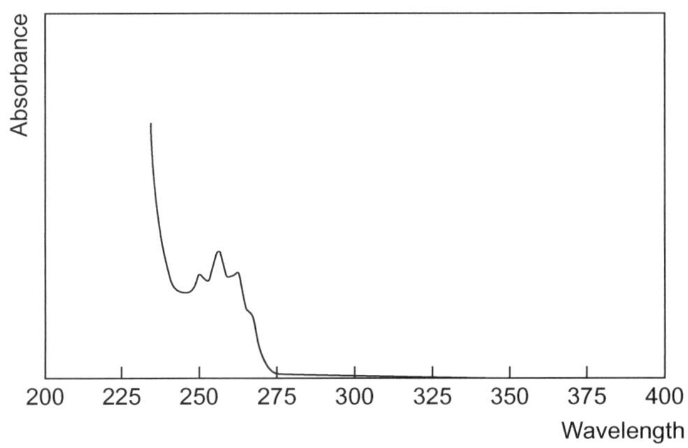

Infra-red Spectrum. Principal peaks at wavenumbers 1232, 812, 671, 1010, 1044, 724 cm^{-1} (Nujol mull).

Mass Spectrum. Principal ions at *m/z* 42, 140, 112, 41, 85, 43, 71, 141.

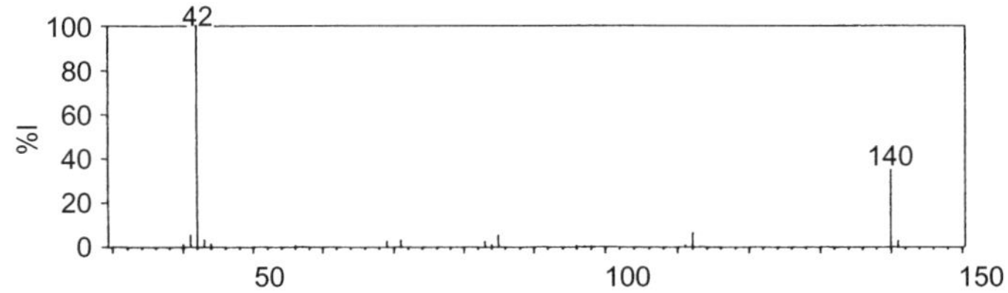

Quantification
Colorimetry. In urine: methenamine and formaldehyde, limit of detection 25 mg/L for methenamine, 5 mg/L for formaldehyde—R. Gollamudi *et al., Biopharm. Drug Disp.*, 1979, *1*,27–36.

Gas chromatography. In serum or urine: limit of detection <5 mg/L in serum—A.-L. Nieminen *et al., J. Chromatogr.*, 1980, *181*; *B Biomed. Appl.*, *7*, 11–16.

Disposition in the Body. Readily absorbed after oral administration and rapidly excreted unchanged in the urine. In acidic urine it is slowly hydrolysed, with the liberation of formaldehyde; this may also occur in the acid gastric secretions and 10 to 30% of a dose may be hydrolysed in the stomach.

Dose. Usually 2 g of methenamine hippurate or 4 g of methenamine mandelate daily.

Methocarbamol

Muscle Relaxant

Synonym. Guaifenesin Carbamate
Proprietary names. Delaxin; Labycarbol; Laxan; Lumirelax; Mebaxin; Musxan; Myosin; Myomethol; Ortoton; Robamol; Robaxin; Traumacut. It is an ingredient of Robaxisal.
3-(2-Methoxyphenoxy)-1,2-propanediol 1-carbamate
$C_{11}H_{15}NO_5$=241.2
CAS—532-03-6

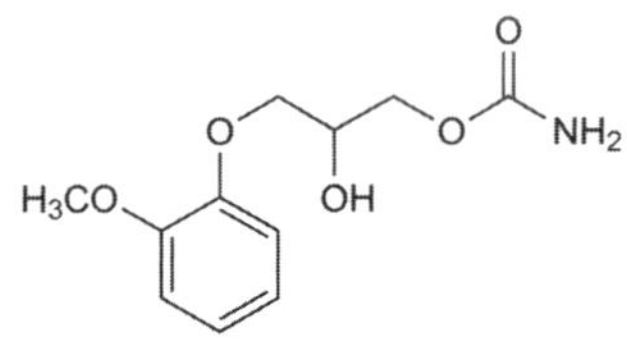

A white powder. M.p. about 94° or, if previously ground to a fine powder, about 90°.
Soluble 1 in 40 of water; soluble in ethanol only with heating; sparingly soluble in chloroform; soluble in propylene glycol; practically insoluble in *n*-hexane.

Partition Coefficient. Log *P* (octanol/water), 0.6.

Colour Tests. Liebermann's Test—violet; Mandelin's Test—green; Marquis Test—blue-violet.

Thin-layer Chromatography. System TA—Rf 70; system TB—Rf 00; system TD—Rf 07; system TE—Rf 47; system TF—Rf 23; system TAD—Rf 38; system TAE—Rf 83; system TAJ—Rf 41; system TAK—Rf 12; system TAL—Rf 72. (Furfuraldehyde reagent, positive; acidified potassium permanganate solution, positive.)

Gas Chromatography. System GA—methocarbamol RI 2050; methocarbamol-AC RI 2145; M (guaifenesin) RI 1620.

High Performance Liquid Chromatography. System HA—*k* 0.1; system HX—RI 345; system HY—RI 297; system HAX—Retention time 5.0 min; system HAY—Retention time 3.9 min.

Ultraviolet Spectrum. Methanol—275 nm (A^1_1=101a).

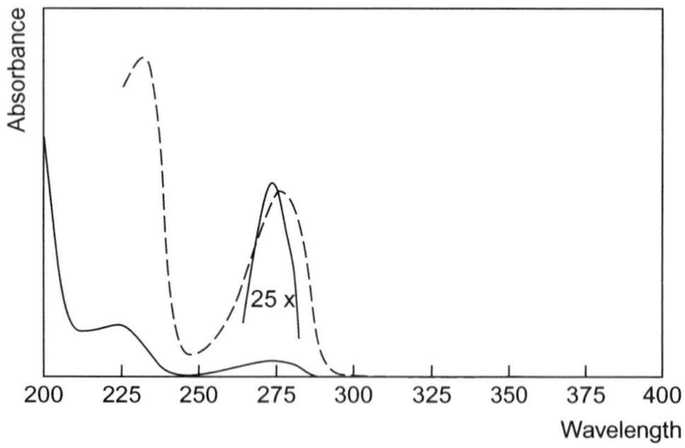

Infra-red Spectrum. Principal peaks at wavenumbers 1667, 1248, 1119, 1215, 1010, 1080 cm^{-1} (KBr disk).

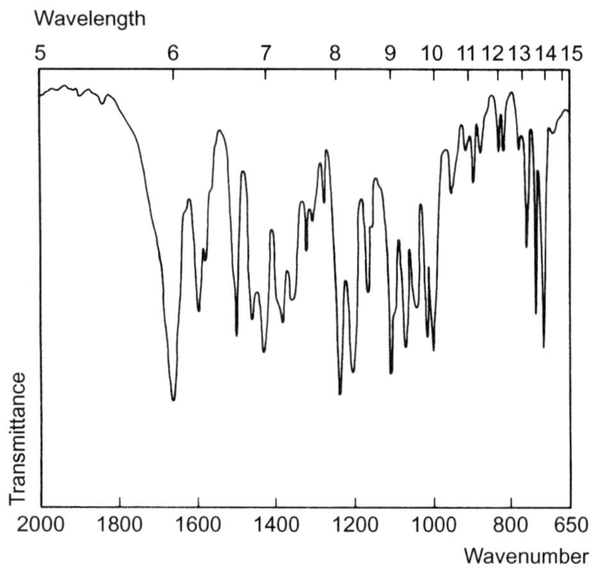

Mass Spectrum. Principal ions at *m/z* 124, 118, 198, 109, 43, 57, 125, 77.

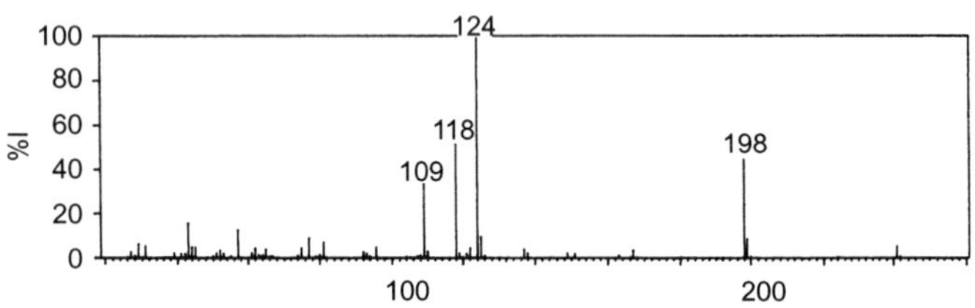

Quantification

Colorimetry. In serum—A. A. Forist and R. W. Judy, *J. Pharm. Sci.*, 1971, *60*, 1686–1688.

High performance liquid chromatography. In blood: UV detection—K. Sprague and A. Poklis, *J. Can. Soc. Forens. Sci.*, 1980, *13*, 31–36. In plasma: limit of detection <1 mg/L, UV detection—N. Weng *et al.*, *J. Chromatogr. B Biomed. Appl.*, 1994, *654*, 287–292.

Disposition in the Body. Absorbed after oral administration. Metabolised by demethylation and *p*-hydroxylation followed by conjugation with glucuronic acid or sulfate. About 98% of a dose is excreted in the urine in 72 h, with less than 1% as unchanged drug and the remainder as free and conjugated metabolites; most of the excretion occurs in the first 8 h.

Therapeutic concentration

Following a single oral dose of 2 g to 1 subject, a peak serum concentration of 25.8 mg/L was attained in 1 h [A. A. Forist and R. W. Judy, *J. Pharm. Sci.*, 1971, *60*, 1686–1688.]

Toxicity

In a fatality due to ingestion of methocarbamol and alcohol, the following postmortem tissue concentrations were reported: blood, methocarbamol 525 mg/L, alcohol 1400 mg/L, salicylate 20 mg/L; urine, methocarbamol 575 mg/L [M. Kemal *et al.*, *J. Forensic Sci.*, 1982, *27*, 217–222.]

The following postmortem tissue concentrations of methocarbamol were reported in a fatality due to the ingestion of methocarbamol and ethanol: blood 257 mg/L, bile 927 mg/L. urine 255 mg/L, gastric content 3.7 g, liver 459 μg/g, kidney 83 μg/g; blood and urine ethanol concentrations were 1350 and 2490 mg/L respectively [K. E. Ferslew *et al.*, *J. Forensic Sci.*, 1990, *35*, 477–482.]

Half-life. Plasma half-life, about 1 to 2 h.

Dose. 4 to 6 g daily.

Methohexital

Anaesthetic/Barbiturate

Synonym. Methohexitone

1-Methyl-5-(1-methyl-2-pentynyl)-5-(2-propenyl)-2,4,6(1*H*,3*H*,5*H*)-pyrimidinetrione

$C_{14}H_{18}N_2O_3$=262.3

CAS—151-83-7; 18652-93-2

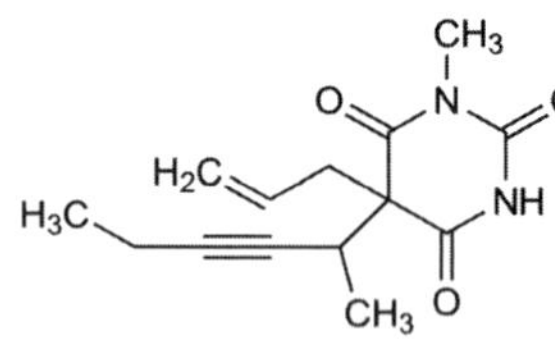

A white to faintly yellowish-white, crystalline powder. M.p. 92° to 96°. Very slightly soluble in water; slightly soluble in ethanol and chloroform.

Methohexital Sodium

Synonyms. Enallynymalnatrium; Sodium Methohexitone.

Proprietary names. Brevital Sodium; Brietal Sodium.

$C_{14}H_{17}N_2NaO_3$=284.3

CAS—309-36-4

A white crystalline substance.

Soluble in water.

Dissociation Constant. pK_a 8.3.

Colour Tests. Koppanyi–Zwikker Test—violet; Mercurous Nitrate—black; Vanillin Reagent—violet-brown/colourless.

Thin-layer Chromatography. System TD—Rf 73; system TE—Rf 58; system TF—Rf 72; system TH—Rf 93; system TAD—Rf 71; system TAE—Rf 85. (Mercuric chloride–diphenylcarbazone reagent, positive; mercurous nitrate spray, black; acidified potassium permanganate solution, yellow-brown; Zwikker's reagent, faint pink.)

Gas Chromatography. System GA—methohexital RI 1770; methohexital-Me RI 1735; M (OH-) RI 1880; system GB—methohexital RI 1827; methohexital-Me RI 1797; system GAJ—methohexital RRT 0.798 (relative to methylphenobarbital).

High Performance Liquid Chromatography. System HG—*k* 27.61; system HH—*k* 20.48; system HX—RI 503; system HY—RI 484.

Ultraviolet Spectrum. Borax buffer 0.05 M (pH 9.2)—246 (A^1_1=276a); 1 M sodium hydroxide (pH 13)—246 nm (A^1_1=308b).

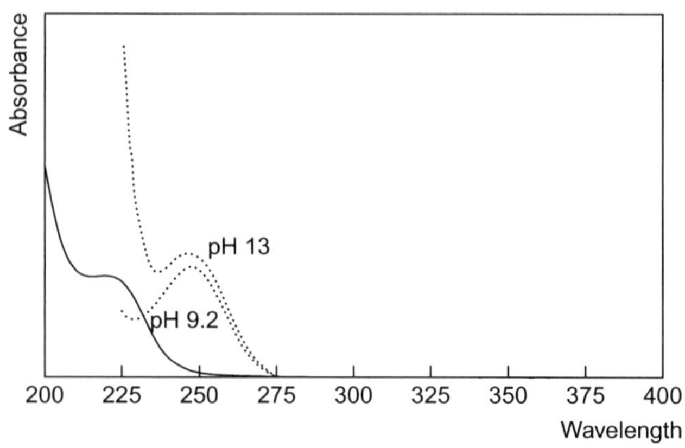

Infra-red Spectrum. Principal peaks at wavenumbers 1680, 1709, 1316, 1193, 1253, 1040 cm^{-1} (methohexital sodium).

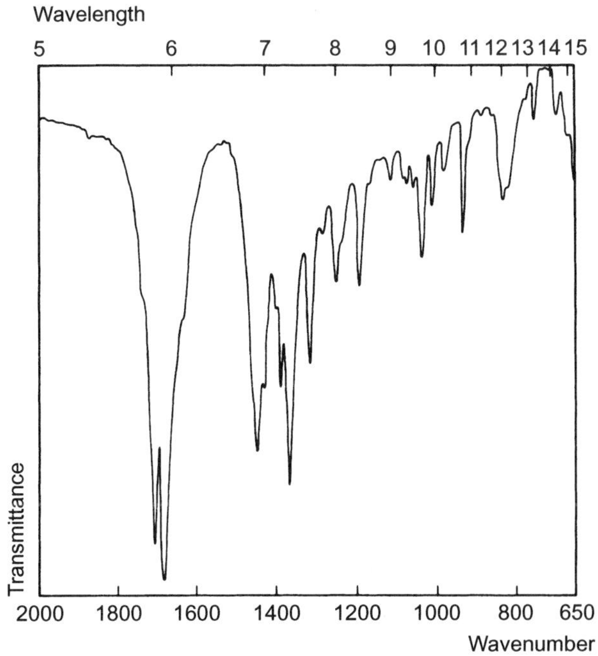

Mass Spectrum. Principal ions at *m/z* 41, 81, 53, 221, 79, 39, 178, 233.

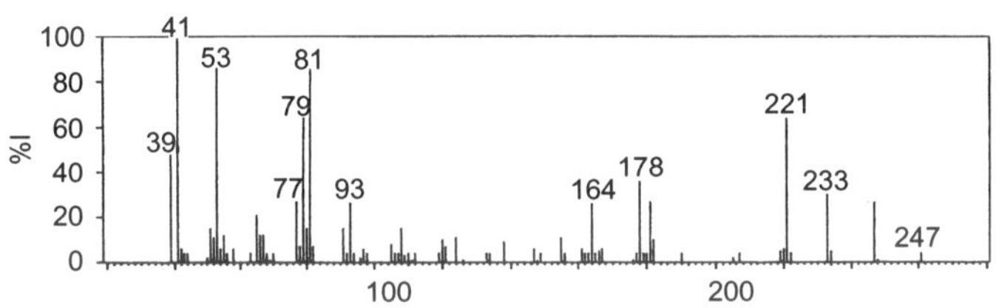

Quantification. See also under Amylobarbital.

Gas chromatography. In blood or plasma: methohexital and 4′-hydroxymethohexital, limit of detection 50 µg/L in plasma and 100 µg/L in blood, AFID—H. Heusler *et al.*, *J. Chromatogr.*, 1981, *226*; *B Biomed. Appl.*, *15*, 403–412. In serum: limit of detection 6 µg/L, nitrogen-selective detection—Y Le Normand *et al.*, *Fundam. Clin. Pharmacol.*, 1988, *2*, 551–558.

Disposition in the Body. Methohexital has a very short duration of action. It rapidly enters the brain and upon redistribution is localised in body fat but to a lesser extent than thiopental. Less than 1% of a dose is excreted unchanged in the urine in 24 h; the major metabolite is 4′-hydroxymethohexital.

Therapeutic concentration

Following an IV dose of 2 mg/kg of methohexital to 6 subjects, venous blood concentrations of 3.9 to 8.6 mg/L were reported at 1 to 3 min [I. Sunshine *et al.*, *Br. J. Anaesth.*, 1966, *38*, 23–28.]

After a slow IV infusion of 3 mg/kg of methohexital sodium over a period of 60 min to 1 subject, a peak plasma concentration of about 3 mg/L was reported [D. D. Breimer, *Br. J. Anaesth.*, 1976, *48*, 643–649.]

Following a rectal dose of 25 mg/kg methohexital as a 1% or 10% solution, the mean plasma concentration in 85 children was 6.5 and 4.7 µg/L, respectively, at 20 min and 4.9 and 4.1 µg/L at 30 min [S. N. Khalil *et al.*, *Anesth. Analg.*, 1990, *70*, 645–649.]

Toxicity. The estimated minimum lethal dose is 1 g.

The following postmortem tissue concentrations were reported in a fatal case involving the IV self-administration of methohexital: blood 103 mg/L, kidney 45 µg/g, liver 41 µg/g, spleen 41 µg/g; alcohol was also found in the blood [B. Finkle, 1967: personal communication.]

In a fatality due to the injection of about 300 mg of methohexital, postmortem blood and liver concentrations of 2 mg/L and 17 µg/g, respectively, were reported [J. E. Ryall, *Bull. Int. Assoc. Forensic Toxicol.*, 1981, *16*(2), 36–37.]

Half-life. Plasma half-life, about 1 to 2 h.

Volume of distribution. About 1 L/kg.

Clearance. Plasma clearance, about 12 mL/min/kg.

Distribution in blood. Plasma:whole blood ratio, about 1.5.

Protein binding. In plasma, about 73%.

Dose. For induction of anaesthesia, 50 to 120 mg of methohexital sodium, by slow IV injection.

Methoprotryne *Herbicide*

2-Isopropylamino-4-(3-methoxypropylamino)-6-methylthio-1,3,5-triazine
$C_{11}H_{21}N_5OS$=271.4
CAS—841-06-5

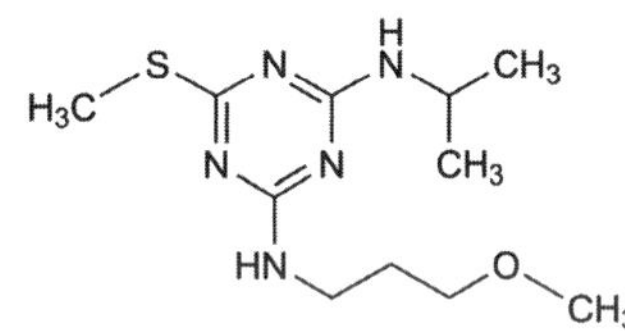

A crystalline solid. M.p. 68° to 70°.
Soluble 1 in 3000 of water; soluble in most organic solvents.

Partition Coefficient. Log *P* (octanol/water), 2.8.

Thin-layer Chromatography. System TA—Rf 74; system TX—Rf 19; system TY—Rf 11. (Dragendorff spray, positive.)

Gas Chromatography. System GA—RI 2098.

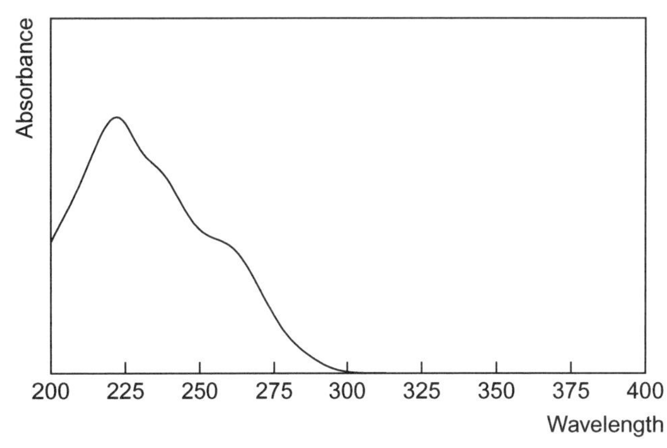

Infra-red Spectrum. Principal peaks at wavenumbers 1538, 811, 1304, 1121, 1272, 1175 cm^{-1} (KBr disk).

Methoserpidine *Antihypertensive*

Synonym. 10-Methoxydeserpidine
Proprietary name. Decaserpyl
Methyl 11-demethoxy-10-methoxy-18-*O*-(3,4,5-trimethoxybenzoyl) reserpate
$C_{33}H_{40}N_2O_9$=608.7
CAS—865-04-3

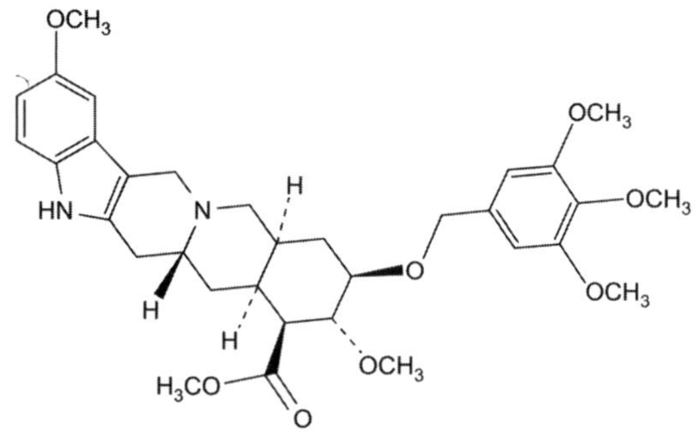

A cream-coloured, hygroscopic, microcrystalline powder, which darkens on exposure to light. M.p. about 171°, with decomposition.

Practically insoluble in water; soluble 1 in 60 of ethanol, 1 in 5 of chloroform, and 1 in 8 of dioxan.

Colour Tests. Mandelin's Test—grey-violet; Marquis Test—grey.

Thin-layer Chromatography. System TA—Rf 72; system TB—Rf 04; system TC—Rf 77; system TL—Rf 64. (Acidified iodoplatinate solution, positive.)

High Performance Liquid Chromatography. System HA—*k* 0.5.

Ultraviolet Spectrum. Dehydrated alcohol—273 nm (A^1_1=300a). (See below.)

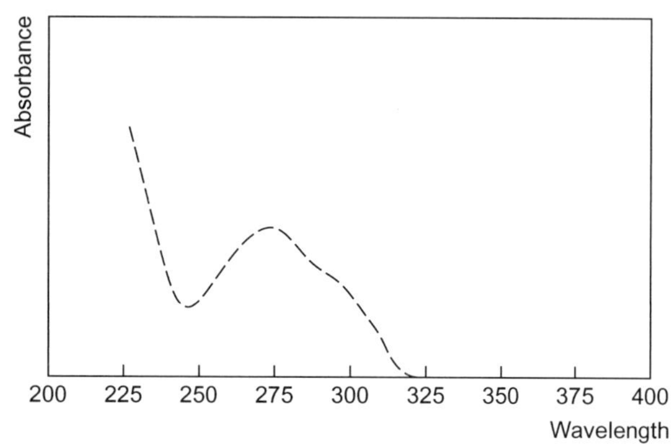

Infra-red Spectrum. Principal peaks at wavenumbers 1120, 1220, 1710, 1088, 1180, 1740 cm^{-1} (KBr disk). (See below.)

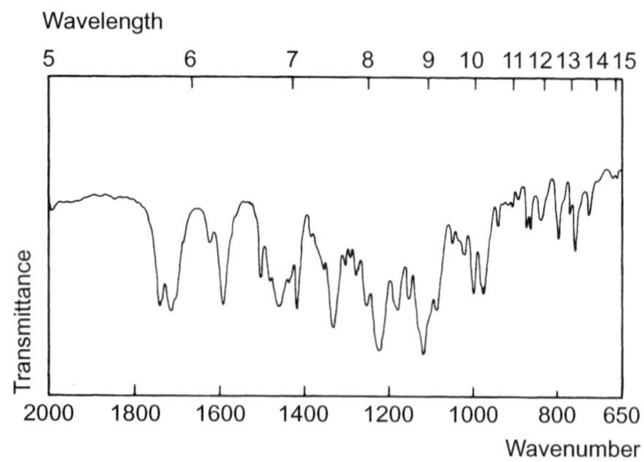

Mass Spectrum. Principal ions at *m/z* 608, 195, 607, 397, 609, 395, 381, 396.

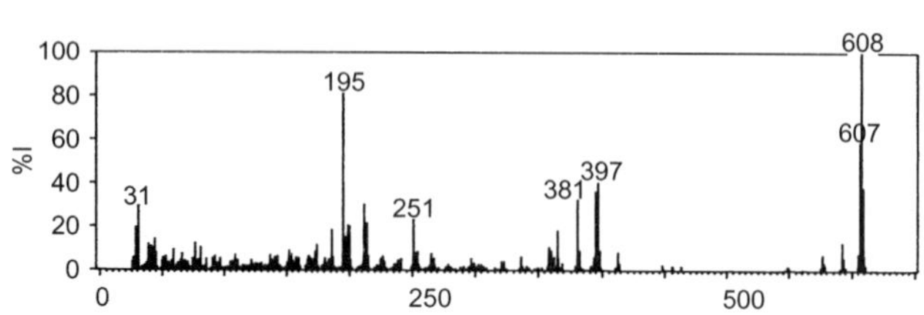

Dose. 15 to 50 mg daily.

Methotrexate

Antineoplastic

Synonyms. Amethopterin; 4-Amino-10-methylfolic Acid; α-Methopterin.
Proprietary names. Abitrexate; Emthexat(e); Farmitrexat; Folex; Lantarel; Ledertrexate; Maxtrex; Medsatrexate; Metex; Methoblastin(e); Metrotex; Mexate; Novatrex; O-trexat; Rheumatrex; Rhodamer; Texate; Trexall; Trexan; Trexeron; Trixilem; Xaken.

N-[4-[[(2,4-Diamino-6-pteridinyl)methyl]methylamino]benzoyl]-L-glutamic acid

$C_{20}H_{22}N_8O_5$=454.4

CAS—59-05-2

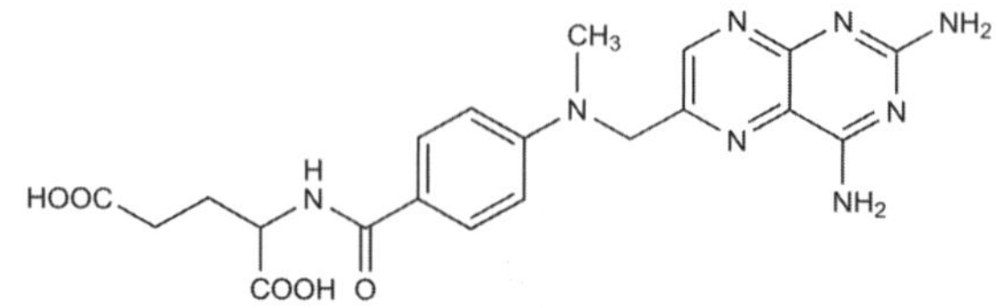

A yellow to orange-brown, crystalline powder. M.p. 182° to 189°.

Practically insoluble in water, ethanol, chloroform, and ether; very soluble in dilute solutions of alkali hydroxides and carbonates.

Caution. Methotrexate is an irritant; avoid contact with skin and mucous membranes.

Dissociation Constant. pK_a 3.8, 4.8, 5.6.

Partition Coefficient. Log *P* (octanol/water), −1.8.

Colour Tests. Mandelin's Test—red; Mercurous Nitrate—black; Nessler's Reagent—orange.

Thin-layer Chromatography. System TE—Rf 00; system TF—Rf 00.

High Performance Liquid Chromatography. System HX—RI 292; system HAX—Retention time 4.7 min; system HAY—Retention time 2.9 min.

Ultraviolet Spectrum. Aqueous acid—243 (A^1_1=372a), 307 (A^1_1=430a); aqueous alkali—258 (A^1_1=500a), 303 nm (A^1_1=500a).

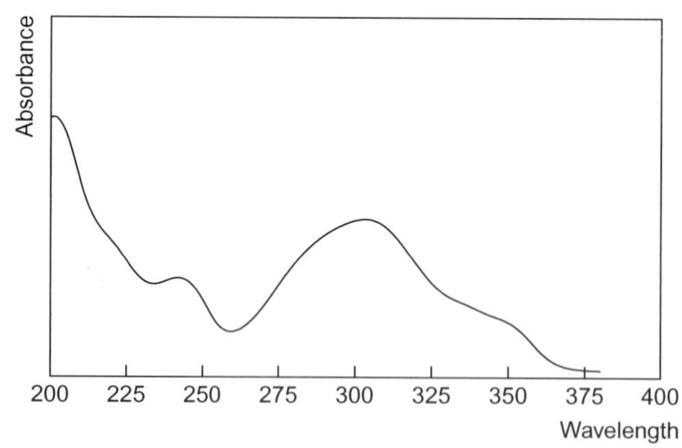

Infra-red Spectrum. Principal peaks at wavenumbers 1600, 1511, 1634, 1305, 1200, 1538 cm^{-1} (Nujol mull).

Quantification

High performance liquid chromatography. In serum or urine: methotrexate and 3 metabolites, limit of detection 12.5 μg/L for methotrexate in serum, UV detection—Y. Y. Z. Farid *et al.*, *J. Pharm. Biomed. Anal.*, 1983, *1*, 55–63. In plasma, urine or CSF: methotrexate and 2 metabolites, limit of detection 50 μg/L, UV detection—H. Breithaupt *et al.*, *Anal. Biochem.*, 1982, *121*, 103–113. In serum: methotrexate and 7-hydroxymethotrexate, limit of detection 100 μg/L for methotrexate, UV detection—G. J. Lawson *et al.*, *J. Chromatogr.*, 1981, *223*; *B Biomed. Appl.*, *12*, 225–231. In plasma, urine, or ascitic fluid: limit of detection 2×10^{-8} M, fluorescence detection—J. Salamoun and J. Frantisek, *J. Chromatogr.*, 1986, *378*, 173–181. In biological fluids including plasma: methotrexate, 7-hydroxymethotrexate, folinic acid and N^5-methyltetrahydrofolate—O. van Tellingen *et al.*, *J. Chromatogr.*, 1989, *488*, 379–388. In plasma: comparison with fluorescence polarisation immunoassay—T. A. Najjar *et al.*, *Ther. Drug Monit.*, 1992,

14, 142–146. In plasma, urine, or saliva: methotrexate and metabolites, limits of detection 0.1 nmol/L in plasma and saliva and 10 nmol/L in urine—F. Albertioni *et al.*, *J. Chromatogr. B Biomed. Appl.*, 1995, *665*, 163–170. In plasma: methotrexate and 7-hydroxymethotrexate, limit of detection 10 μg/L, UV detection—A. Sparreboom *et al.*, *J. Chromatogr. B Biomed. Sci. Appl.*, 1999, *735*, 111–119.

High performance liquid chromatography–mass spectrometry. In urine: limit of detection 0.2 μg/L—R. Turci *et al.*, *Rapid Commun. Mass Spectrom.*, 2000, *14*, 173–179.

Radioimmunoassay. In serum, urine or CSF: limit of detection 450 ng/L—G. W. Aherne *et al.*, *Br. J. Cancer*, 1977, *36*, 608–617.

Disposition in the Body. When given in low doses, it is rapidly absorbed after oral administration to give plasma concentrations equivalent to those obtained by IV administration; higher doses may be less well absorbed. It is distributed mainly in the extracellular spaces but a proportion penetrates cell membranes and is strongly bound to dihydrofolate reductase. Small amounts of methotrexate diffuse into the CSF, higher concentrations being achieved with high doses. The major metabolite appears to be 4-amino-10-methylpteroic acid; 7-hydroxymethotrexate has been detected after high doses; 7-hydroxy-4-amino-10-methylpteroic acid has also been reported to be a metabolite. About 50 to 95% of a dose is excreted unchanged in the urine in 24 h (dose-dependent); after oral administration, about 30% of a dose may be excreted as metabolites as a result of the action of intestinal bacteria prior to absorption; after IV administration, up to about 10% of a dose is excreted in the urine as metabolites and up to about 15% of a dose may be excreted in the bile.

Therapeutic concentration

After single oral doses of 15 mg/m^2 to 10 fasting subjects (children), peak serum concentrations of 0.18 to 0.73 mg/L (mean 0.41) were attained in 1 to 2 h [C. R. Pinkerton *et al.*, *Lancet*, 1980, *2*, 944–946.]

In 89 children receiving weekly oral methotrexate (20 mg/m^2) and daily oral mercaptopurine (75 mg/m^2), peak plasma concentrations ranged from 0.21 to 3.1 μmol/L (mean 1.2) for methotrexate and from 0.13 to 2.3 μmol/L (mean 0.56) for mercaptopurine [F. M. Balis *et al.*, *Blood*, 1998, *92*, 3569–3577.]

Low-dose oral methotrexate (7.5 or 15 mg weekly, divided into 3 doses given at 12-hour intervals) was given to 24 subjects. In the first week, peak plasma concentrations were 94 to 137 nmol/L (mean 117) 1 to 2 h after the third dose of 2.5 mg and 161 to 215 nmol/L (mean 172) 1 to 2 h after the third dose of 5 mg. In week 13, peak plasma concentrations 1 to 2 h after the third dose of 2.5 mg or 5 mg were 88 to 152 nmol/L (mean 95) and 142 to 200 nmol/L (mean 157) [J. Chladek *et al.*, *Br J. Clin. Pharmacol.*, 2002, *54*, 147–156.]

Toxicity. Toxic effects are usually associated with plasma concentrations greater than 4.5 mg/L, 24 h after a dose, or 0.45 mg/L, 48 h after a dose.

Half-life. Plasma half-life, about 4 to 10 h; a longer terminal elimination phase of 10 to 70 h (mean 27) has also been reported.

Volume of distribution. About 0.8 L/kg.

Distribution in blood. Plasma:whole blood ratio, 0.9.

Protein binding. In plasma, variously reported as 50 to 95%.

Note. For reviews of the clinical pharmacokinetics of methotrexate see D. D. Shen and D. L. Azarnoff, *Clin. Pharmacokinet.*, 1978, *3*, 1–13; F. M. Balis *et al.*, *Clin. Pharmacokinet.*, 1983, *8*, 202–232; and Y.-M. Wang and T. Fujimoto, *Clin. Pharmacokinet.*, 1984, *9*, 335–348.

Dose. 10 to 25 mg weekly, by mouth.

Methoxamine

Sympathomimetic

Synonym. Methoxamedrine
α-(1-Aminoethyl)-2,5-dimethoxybenzenemethanol
$C_{11}H_{17}NO_3$=211.3
CAS—390-28-3

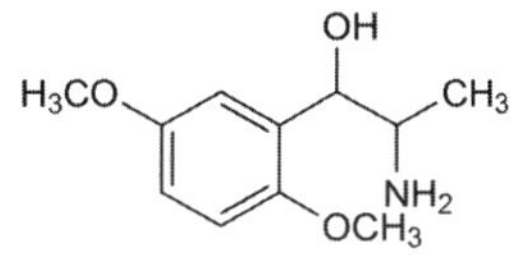

Methoxamine Hydrochloride
Proprietary names. Vasoxine; Vasoxyl.
$C_{11}H_{17}NO_3$,HCl=247.7
CAS—61-16-5
Colourless or white plate-like crystals or white crystalline powder. M.p. 212° to 216°.
Soluble 1 in 2.5 of water and 1 in 12 of ethanol; practically insoluble in benzene, chloroform and ether.

Dissociation Constant. pK_a 9.2 (25°).

Partition Coefficient. Log *P* (octanol/water), 0.4.

Colour Tests. Mandelin's Test—green-yellow; Marquis Test—violet-brown→green.

Thin-layer Chromatography. System TA—Rf 55; system TB—Rf 24; system TC—Rf 4; system TE—Rf 11; system TL—Rf 38; system TAE—Rf 12; system TAF—Rf 73; system TAJ—Rf 00; system TAK—Rf 12; system TAL—Rf 50. (Acidified potassium permanganate solution, positive.)

Gas Chromatography. System GA—RI 1726.

High Performance Liquid Chromatography. System HA—*k* 0.9; system HY—RI 228; system HAX—Retention time 6.4 min; system HAY—Retention time 3.6 min.

Ultraviolet Spectrum. Aqueous acid—290; water—290 nm (A_1^1=161a). No alkaline shift.

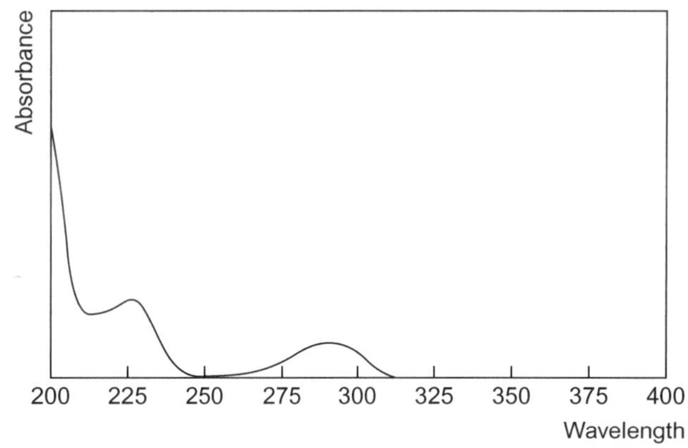

Infra-red Spectrum. Principal peaks at wavenumbers 1496, 1219, 1022, 1276, 1179, 1050 cm^{-1} (methoxamine hydrochloride, KBr disk).

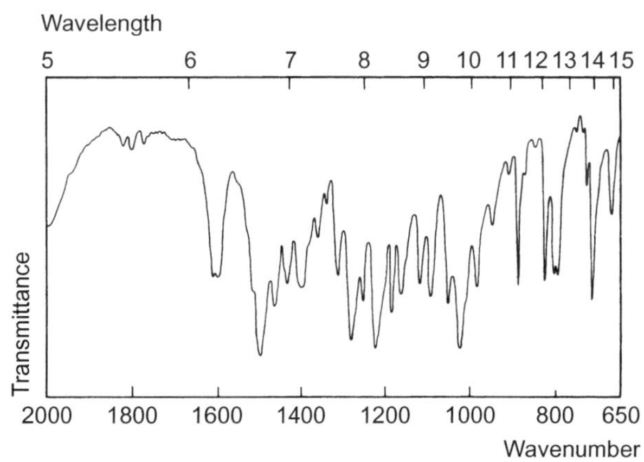

Mass Spectrum. Principal ions at *m/z* 168, 137, 44, 139, 43, 152, 124, 167.

Dose. 5 to 20 mg of methoxamine hydrochloride IM.

Methoxsalen

Pigmenting Agent

Synonyms. Ammoidin; 8-Methoxypsoralen; Metoxaleno; Xanthotoxin.
Proprietary names. Deltasoralen; Dermox; Geroxsalen; Meladinina; Meladinine; Mopsoralen; Oxsoralen; Puvasoralen; Ultramop; Uvadex.
9-Methoxy-7*H*-furo[3,2-*g*][1]benzopyran-7-one
$C_{12}H_8O_4$=216.2
CAS—298-81-7

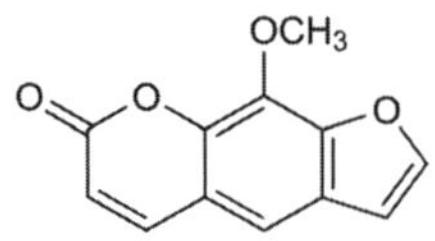

A constituent of the fruits of *Ammi majus*.
White to cream-coloured fluffy crystals. M.p. 143° to 148°.
Practically insoluble in cold water; sparingly soluble in boiling water and ether; soluble in boiling ethanol, acetic acid, propylene glycol, benzene, and acetone; freely soluble in chloroform.

Partition Coefficient. Log *P* (octanol/water), 2.1.

Thin-layer Chromatography. System TA—Rf 82; system TB—Rf 13; system TE—Rf 76; system TF—Rf 58; system TAE—Rf 82; system TAJ—Rf 82; system TAK—Rf 68; system TAL—Rf 96.

Gas Chromatography. System GA—RI 1980.

High Performance Liquid Chromatography. System HX—RI 457; system HZ—Retention time, 5.2 min.

Ultraviolet Spectrum. Aqueous acid—247, 304 nm.

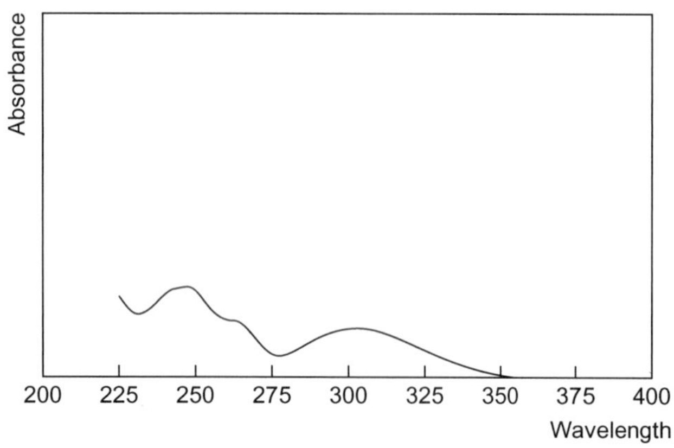

Infra-red Spectrum. Principal peaks at wavenumbers 1705, 1150, 1100, 1580, 1020, 1000 cm^{-1} (Nujol mull).

Quantification

Gas chromatography–mass spectrometry. In plasma: selected-ion monitoring—A. T. Cracco *et al.*, *J. Chromatogr.*, 1992, *574*, 156–160.

High performance liquid chromatography. In plasma: limit of detection 10 µg/L—F. P. Gasparro *et al.*, *J. Invest. Derm.*, 1988, *90*, 234–236. In plasma: limit of detection 1.5 µg/L—C. H. Ketchem *et al.*, *Clin. Chem.*, 1990, *36*, 1956–1957. In plasma: limit of detection 15 µg/L, UV detection—D. Kucova *et al.*, *J. Chromatogr.*, 1993, *614*, 340–344. In plasma: limit of detection about 0.4 µg/L, fluorescence detection—S. Vielhauer *et al.*, *J. Chromatogr. B Biomed. Appl.*, 1995, *666*, 315–322.

Disposition in the Body

Therapeutic concentration

After oral administration of 0.4 to 0.6 mg methoxsalen to 8 subjects, peak serum concentrations averaged 420 ± 80 µg/L within 40 min; during extracorporeal photophoresis, the concentration in the photoactivation chamber (so-called buffy coat fraction) was 134 µg/L [S. E. Shephard *et al.*, *Photodermatol. Photoimmunol. Photomed.*, 1999, *15*, 64–74.]

Plasma concentrations of methoxsalen after administration via various routes to 8 subjects were as follows: about 175 to 300 µg/L at 1 to 4 h after 0.6 or 1 mg/kg orally; about 5.5 µg/L 2 h after topical administration of a 0.1% cream; and about 1.2 µg/L 3 h after topical administration of a 3 mg/L bath [I. Tegeder *et al.*, *Clin. Pharmacol. Ther.*, 2002, *71*, 153–161.]

In 10 subjects given 3 oral doses of 0.46 to 0.56 mg/kg methoxsalen in a liquid formulation, peak serum levels were about 650 µg/L in the fasted state, about 200 µg/L after a low-fat breakfast, and about 150 µg/L after a fat-rich breakfast; food delayed the time to reach peak plasma levels (30 min in the fasted state vs 1.5 to 3 h following a fat-rich meal) [N. Bech-Thomsen *et al.*, *Br. J. Dermatol.*, 1992, *127*, 620–624.]

Dose. 20 mg daily; doses of up to 50 mg have been given.

Methoxyamfetamine

Hallucinogen

Synonym. *p*-Methoxyamphetamine; PMA; 4-methoxyamphetamine; 4-MA; α-Methyl-4-methoxyphenethylamine. Usually presented as "Ecstasy".
4-methoxy-α-methylbenzeneethanamine.
$C_{10}H_{15}NO$=165.2
CAS—23239-32-9

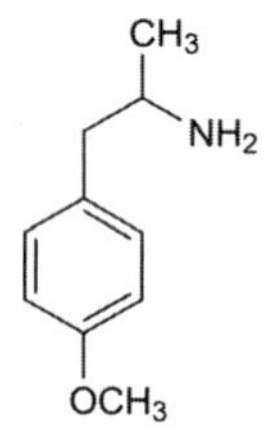

A colourless oil.
Practically insoluble in water; soluble in chloroform and dilute acids.

Methoxyamfetamine Hydrochloride

$C_{10}H_{15}NO,HCl$=201.7
CAS—3706-26-1
White crystals. Soluble in water.

Colour Test. Mandelin's Test—green; Marquis Test—no colour change.

Thin-layer Chromatography. System TA—Rf 73; system TB—Rf 23; system TC—Rf 77; system TE—Rf 43; system TL—Rf 69; system TAE—Rf 09; system TAF—Rf 74; system TAJ—Rf 04; system TAK—Rf 18; system TAL—Rf 58. (Acidified iodoplatinate solution, positive.)

Gas Chromatography. System GA—RI 1412; system GB—RI 1410.

Column: HP-5MS (15 m × 0.25 mm i.d., 0.25 µm film thickness). Column temperature: held at 60° for 2 min then increased to 280° at 15°/min and held for 3 min. Injector and detector temperatures: 250° and 300°, respectively. MS detection. Pentafluoropropionic anhydride derivative retention time: 9.0 min [H. E. Felgate *et al.*, *J. Anal. Toxicol.*, 1998, *22*, 169–172.]

High Performance Liquid Chromatography. System HB—*k* 14.95; system HX—RI 274; system HY—RI 228.

Columns: (analytical) C_{18} (µBondapack, 300 × 3.9 mm i.d.); or C_{18} (Ultracarb 5, 150 × 4.6 mm i.d.); or Phenyl (Hypersil 5, 150 × 4.6 mm i.d.); (guard) ODS (Co:Pell, 7 × 2.1 mm i.d.). Mobile phase: 0.05 M pH 3.0 phosphate buffer–acetonitrile (6:1), 1.5 mL/min flow rate for µBondapack and Ultracarb columns and 1.2 mL/min flow rate for Hypersil column (all separate analyses). UV detection (λ=254 and 280 nm). Retention time: PMA, 6.5 min (µBondapack) and 4.5 min (Ultracarb and Hypersil) [F. T. Noggle *et al.*, *J. Chromatogr. Sci.*, 1989, *27*, 607–611.]

Ultraviolet Spectrum. Aqueous acid—274 nm (A_1^1=80b). No alkaline shift.

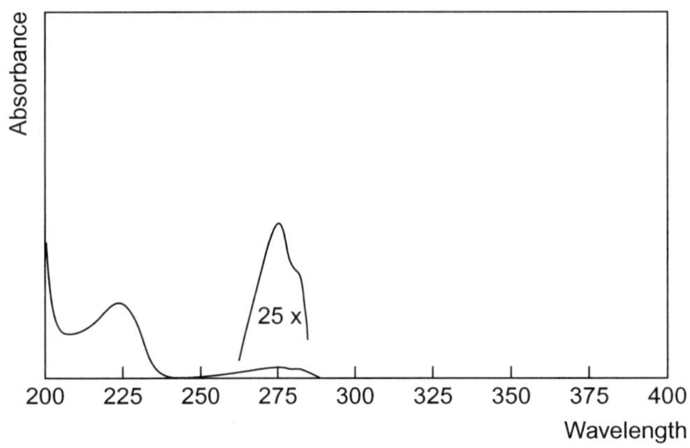

Infra-red Spectrum. Principal peaks at wavenumbers 1512, 1259, 1033, 808, 1190, 1623 cm^{-1} (methoxyamfetamine hydrochloride).

Mass Spectrum. Principal ions at *m/z* 44, 122, 78, 121, 65, 107, 91, 134.

Disposition in the Body. Absorbed after oral administration. About 80% of a dose is excreted in the urine in 24 h with up to 15% of the dose as unchanged drug, about 25% as free 4-hydroxyamfetamine, 50% as conjugated 4-hydroxyamfetamine, and 5% each as 4-hydroxynorephedrine and a conjugated *N*-oxidation product. The extent of *O*-demethylation appears to be genetically determined being decreased in poor metabolisers.

Toxicity. Methoxyamfetamine is about 3 times as potent as methylenedioxyamfetamine and appears to be more toxic. At least 20 deaths worldwide have been reported to be due to PMA toxicity, some involving other drugs. PMA can produce both CNS stimulation and hallucinogenic effects. Acute toxicity primarily results in hyperthermia but there may also be "serotonin syndrome" related symptoms and some respiratory depression. Such symptoms may be produced at blood concentrations over 0.5 mg/L.

PMA concentrations in postmortem femoral blood ranged from 0.24 to 4.9 mg/L (mean 2.3 mg/L) in 6 fatalities related to PMA poisoning. Corresponding liver concentrations ranged from 1.4 to 21 mg/kg (mean 8.9 mg/kg). Other amfetamines (including metamfetamine and MDMA) were detected in 5 of the 6 cases. All cases involved hyperthermia; in some cases rhabdomyolysis and haemorrhaging were also observed [H. E. Felgate *et al.*, *J. Anal. Toxicol.*, 1998, *22*, 169–172.]

In 5 instances of fatal PMA intoxication in Canada and the USA, PMA concentrations in the postmortem blood were found to be 0.6 mg/L and 1.3 mg/L [T. L. Martin, *J. Anal. Toxicol.*, 2001, *25*, 649–651]; and 1.9 mg/L, 0.6 mg/L and 1.07 mg/L [J. C. Kramer *et al.*, *J. Anal. Toxicol.*, 2001, *25*, 645–648], respectively. Other drugs of abuse were detected in 3 of the 5 cases.

In 9 fatalities due to the ingestion or IV administration of methoxyamfetamine, the following postmortem tissue concentrations were reported: blood 0.3 to 1.9 mg/L, bile 0.4 to 3 mg/L, liver 0.5 to 10.3 μg/g, urine 6 to 175 mg/L; alcohol was also detected in 4 cases [G. Cimbura, *Can. Med. Assoc. J.*, 1974, *110*, 1263–1264.]

Methoxychlor

Pesticide

Synonyms. Dimethoxy-DT; DMDT; Methoxy-DDT.
Proprietary name. Marlate
1,1′-(2,2,2-Trichloroethylidene)bis[4-methoxybenzene]
$C_{16}H_{15}Cl_3O_2 = 345.7$
CAS—72-43-5

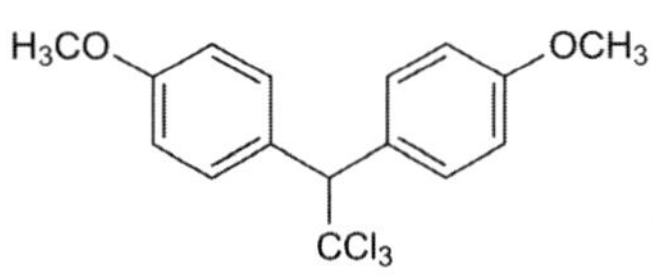

The technical product contains about 88% of methoxychlor and about 12% of related isomers.
The pure *pp*′-isomer occurs as colourless crystals; the technical product is a grey powder. M.p. pure isomer, about 89°; technical product, 77°.

Practically insoluble in water; soluble in ethanol and aromatic solvents; very soluble in ether.

Partition Coefficient. Log *P* (octanol/water), 5.1.

Colour Test. Liebermann's Test—black-violet.

Thin-layer Chromatography. System TE—Rf 87; system TF—Rf 72; system TX—Rf 43; system TY—Rf 84; system TAA—Rf 65.

Gas Chromatography. System GA—*op*′-methoxychlor RI 2417; methoxychlor RI 2445; system GK—*pp*′-methoxychlor RRT 1.46, *op*′-methoxychlor RRT 1.40 (both relative to caffeine).

High Performance Liquid Chromatography. System HX—RI 900; system HAA—Retention time, 27.4 min.

Ultraviolet Spectrum. Hexane—276 ($A_1^1 = 100b$), shoulder at 283 nm.

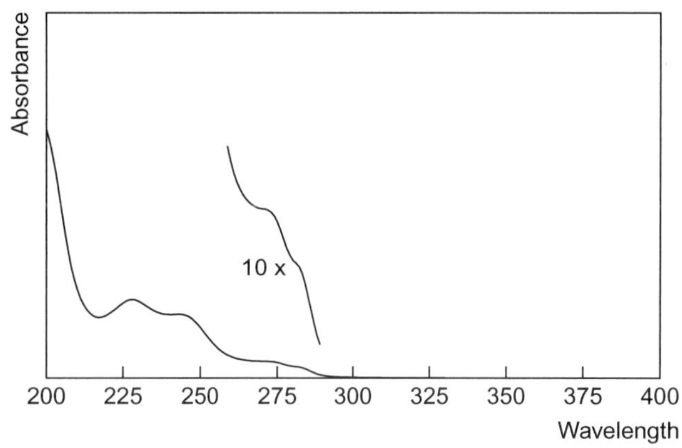

Mass Spectrum. Principal ions at *m/z* 121, 227, 228, 114, 152, 122, 63, 165 (*op*′-methoxychlor); 227, 228, 114, 152, 212, 63, 169, 115 (*pp*′-methoxychlor).

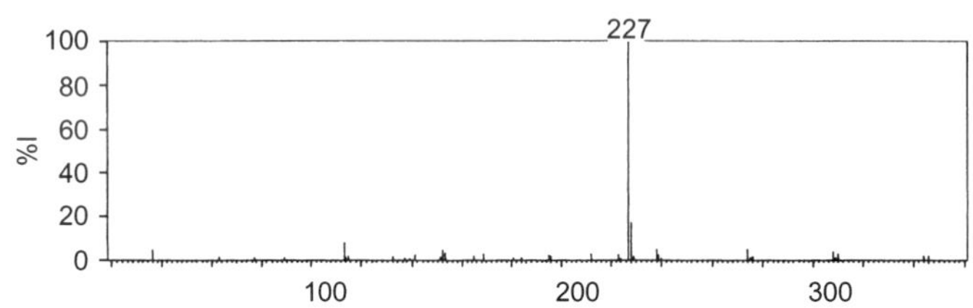

Quantification

Gas chromatography–mass spectrometry. In serum: methoxychlor and other pesticides—J. Dmitrovic *et al.*, *Toxicol. Lett.*, 2002, *134*, 253–258.

Disposition in the Body. Methoxychlor is less persistent than clofenotane. It is stored in the fat to a limited extent and disappears in 2 to 4 weeks after cessation of exposure. It is eliminated mainly in the faeces; small amounts are excreted in the urine.

Toxicity. Methoxychlor is the least toxic of the chlorinated hydrocarbon insecticides. The maximum permissible atmospheric concentration is 10 mg/m^3 and the maximum permissible concentration in food is 14 μg/g.

In a case of attempted suicide by ingestion of a product containing methoxychlor, a serum concentration of 0.67 mg/L was detected upon admission to hospital [T. S. Thompson and S. J. Vorster, *J. Anal. Toxicol.*, 2000, *24*, 377–380.]

Methoxyflurane

General Anaesthetic

Proprietary names. Metofane; Penthrane; Pentrane.
2,2-Dichloro-1,1-difluoro-1-methoxyethane
$C_3H_4Cl_2F_2O = 165.0$
CAS—76-38-0
A clear, almost colourless, non-flammable mobile liquid. Mass per mL 1.423 to 1.427 g. B.p. 103° to 108°.
Methoxyflurane (B.P.) contains butylated hydroxytoluene 0.01% w/w.

Soluble 1 in 500 of water; miscible with ethanol, chloroform, and ether.

Partition Coefficient. Log *P* (octanol/water), 2.2.

Gas Chromatography. System GA—RI 701; system GI—Retention time 17.6 min.

Ultraviolet Spectrum. No significant absorption, 230 to 360 nm.

Infra-red Spectrum. Principal peaks at wavenumbers 1315, 1063, 1136, 833, 1204, 1234 cm^{-1}.

Quantification

Gas chromatography. In blood: FID—W. J. Cole *et al.*, *Br. J. Anaesth.*, 1975, *47*, 1043–1047. In blood: limit of detection 10 mg/L, FID—P. L. Jones *et al.*, *Br. J. Anaesth.*, 1972, *44*, 124–130.

Dose. For maintenance of anaesthesia, 0.2 to 0.5% of the vapour by inhalation.

Methoxymetamfetamine

Serotonin Releasing Agent

Synonyms. 4-Methoxymethylamphetamine; 4-Methoxy-*N*-methylamphetamine; *p*-Methoxymethylamphetamine; 1-(4-Methoxyphenyl)-2-aminopropane; 2-Methylamino-1-(*p*-methoxyphenyl)propane; PMMA; 4-MMA. Usually presented as 'Ecstasy'.
(αS)-*N*,α-Dimethyl-4-methoxy-benzeneethanamine
$C_{11}H_{17}NO$=179.3

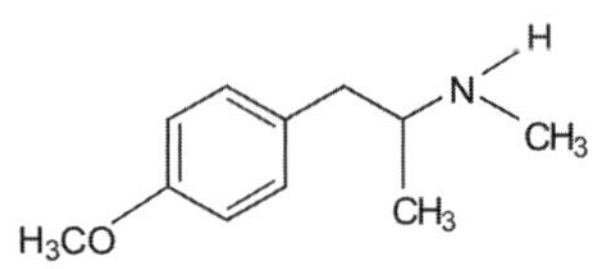

A white powder. M.p. 177° to 178°

Colour Test. Marquis—no colour change.

Gas Chromatography. Column: OV-1 (12 m × 0.31 mm i.d., 0.52 µm film thickness). Column temperature: 70° to 150°C at 15°C/min then from 150°C to 250°C at 25°C/min. MS detection. Retention time: within 7 min [F. T. Noggle *et al.*, *J. Chromatogr. Sci.*, 1989, *27*, 607–611].

High Performance Liquid Chromatography. Columns: (analytical) C_{18} (µBondapack, 300 × 3.9 mm i.d.); or C_{18} (Ultracarb 5, 150 × 4.6 mm i.d.); or phenyl (Hypersil 5, 150 × 4.6 mm i.d.); (guard) ODS (Co:Pell, 7 × 2.1 mm i.d.). Mobile phase: phosphate buffer (0.05 M, pH 3.0):acetonitrile (6:1), flow rate 1.5 mL/min for µBondapack and Ultracarb columns and 1.2 mL/min for Hypersil column (all separate analyses). UV detection (λ=254 and 280 nm). Retention time: 8.0 min (µBondapack) and 5.0 min (Ultracarb and Hypersil) [F. T. Noggle *et al.*, *J. Chromatogr. Sci.*, 1989, *27*, 607–611].

Ultraviolet Spectrum. Aqueous acid (0.1 M sulfuric acid)—274 nm.

Mass Spectrum. Principal ions at *m/z* 58, 121, 78, 91, 106, 148, 134, 164.

Toxicity. There are limited data regarding non-fatal and fatal PMMA intoxication. However, a few deaths related to PMMA toxicity have been reported in Europe, which also involved other amfetamine derivatives. PMMA can produce both CNS stimulation and hallucinogenic effects. Like PMA, acute PMMA toxicity can result in hyperthermia and possibly 'serotonin syndrome' related symptoms and some respiratory depression.

A PMMA concentration of 1.51 mg/L was measured in the postmortem blood of a 17-year-old male who felt ill when dancing. 3,4-Methylenedioxyethylamfetamine (MDEA) and 3,4-methylenedioxyamfetamine (MDA) were also detected in the blood (2.00 mg/L and 0.30 mg/L, respectively) along with ethanol (200 mg/L) [C. Lora-Tamayo *et al.*, *Forensic Sci. Int.*, 1997, *85*, 149–157].

Methoxyphenamine

Sympathomimetic

Synonyms. Methoxiphenadrin; Mexyphamine.
2-Methoxy-*N*,α-dimethylbenzeneethanamine
$C_{11}H_{17}NO$=179.3
CAS—93-30-1

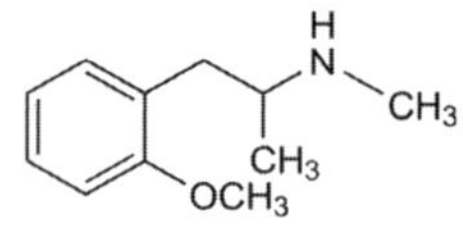

An oil.

Methoxyphenamine Hydrochloride
Synonyms. Methoxiphenadrin Hydrochloride; Mexyphamine Hydrochloride.
Proprietary names. Orthoxine; Proasma. It is an ingredient of Asmeton, Casacol, Cheracap, Orthoxicol, and Sedagripe.
$C_{11}H_{17}NO,HCl$=215.7
CAS—5588-10-3
White crystals or powder. M.p. 129° to 131° (crystals from ether and alcohol). Freely soluble in water, ethanol, and chloroform; slightly soluble in ether and benzene.

Dissociation Constant. pK_a 10.1.

Partition Coefficient. Log *P* (octanol/water), 2.3.

Colour Tests. Mandelin's Test—blue-green; Marquis Test—red.

Thin-layer Chromatography. System TA—Rf 23; system TB—Rf 26; system TC—Rf 04; system TE—Rf 32; system TL—Rf 02; system TAE—Rf 07; system TAJ—Rf 05; system TAK—Rf 20; system TAL—Rf 64. (Acidified iodoplatinate solution, positive.)

Gas Chromatography. System GA—RI 1361; system GB—RI 1416; system GC—RI 1670.

High Performance Liquid Chromatography. System HA—*k* 1.7; system HB—*k* 32.17; system HX—RI 303.

Ultraviolet Spectrum. Aqueous acid—271 nm (A^1_1=92a). No alkaline shift.

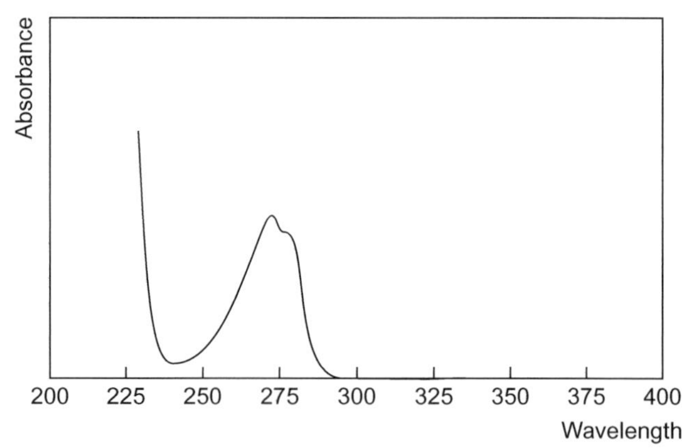

Infra-red Spectrum. Principal peaks at wavenumbers 1236, 749, 1047, 1125, 1026, 1175 cm^{-1} (Nujol mull).

Mass Spectrum. Principal ions at *m/z* 58, 91, 59, 56, 30, 42, 121, 78.

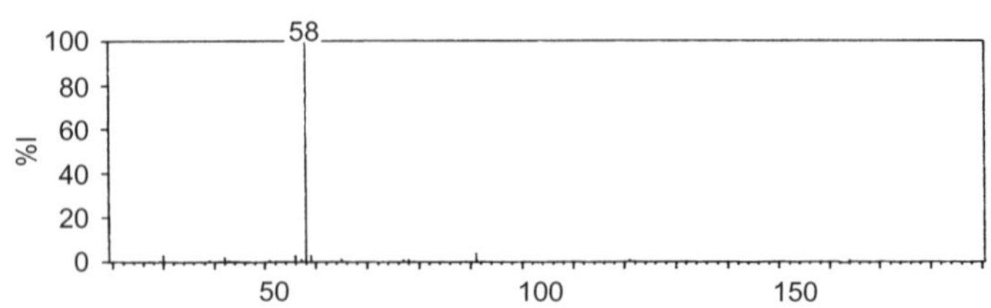

Quantification

Gas chromatography. In urine: methoxyphenamine enantiomers and metabolites, ECD—N. R. Srinivas *et al.*, *J. Chromatogr.*, 1989, *487*, 61–72.

Gas chromatography–mass spectrometry. In beard hair—Y. Nakahara *et al.*, *Forensic Sci. Int.*, 1993, *63*, 109–119.

Disposition in the Body. Readily absorbed after oral administration. Metabolites identified in urine include the *N*-desmethyl, *O*-desmethyl, and

5-hydroxy derivatives and their glucuronide and/or sulfate conjugates. Unchanged drug is also excreted in the urine.

Toxicity. The estimated minimum lethal dose for children up to 2 years of age is 200 mg and for adults is 2 g.

Dose. 50 to 100 mg of methoxyphenamine hydrochloride every 4 h.

Methyclothiazide *Diuretic*

Proprietary names. Aquatensen; Duretic; Enduron; Naturon. It is an ingredient of Enduronil, Enduronyl, and Isobar.
6-Chloro-3-(chloromethyl)-3,4-dihydro-2-methyl-2*H*-1,2,4-benzothiadiazine-7-sulfonamide 1,1-dioxide
$C_9H_{11}Cl_2N_3O_4S_2$=360.2
CAS—135-07-9

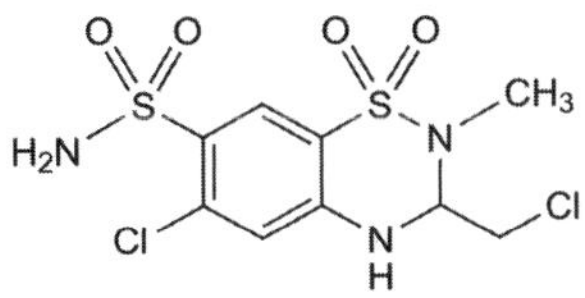

A white crystalline powder. M.p. 216°.
Almost insoluble in water, chloroform, and benzene; soluble 1 in about 90 of ethanol; very soluble in acetone and pyridine; soluble in solutions of alkali hydroxides and carbonates.

Dissociation Constant. pK_a 9.4.

Partition Coefficient. Log *P* (octanol/water), 1.4.

Colour Tests. Koppanyi–Zwikker Test—violet; Sulfuric Acid—orange.

Thin-layer Chromatography. System TA—Rf 87; system TD—Rf 19; system TE—Rf 53; system TF—Rf 50; system TAD—Rf 27; system TAJ—Rf 30; system TAK—Rf 08; system TAL—Rf 69.

Gas Chromatography. System GA—methyclothiazide, not eluted; system GX—methyclothiazide-Me₃, Retention time 9.9 min.

High Performance Liquid Chromatography. System HN—*k* 3.82; system HY—RI 364; system HAA—Retention time 15.4 min.

Ultraviolet Spectrum. Aqueous acid—270 (A^1_1=525b), 314; aqueous alkali—264, 300 nm.

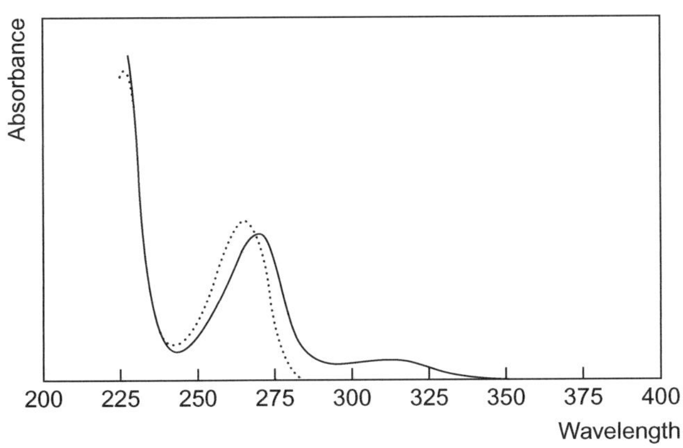

Infra-red Spectrum. Principal peaks at wavenumbers 1158, 1595, 715, 1063, 1515, 1300 cm^{-1} (KBr disk). (See below.)

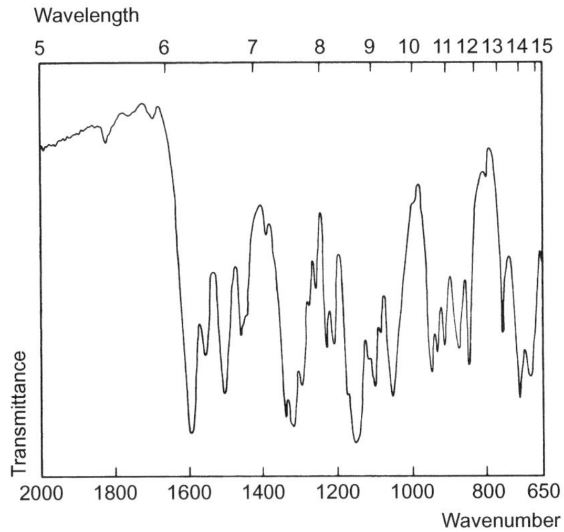

Mass Spectrum. Principal ions at *m*/*z* 310, 64, 36, 312, 42, 43, 62, 63.

Quantification
High performance liquid chromatography. In plasma: limit of detection 1.5 µg/L, UV detection—C. A. Hartman *et al., J. Chromatogr.*, 1981, *226*; *B Biomed. Appl.*, *15*, 510–513.

Dose. 2.5 to 10 mg daily.

Methyl Benzoquate *Coccidiostat (Veterinary)*

Synonym. Nequinate
Proprietary name. Statyl
Methyl 6-butyl-1,4-dihydro-4-oxo-7-(phenylmethoxy)-3-quinolinecarboxylate
$C_{22}H_{23}NO_4$=365.4
CAS—13997-19-8

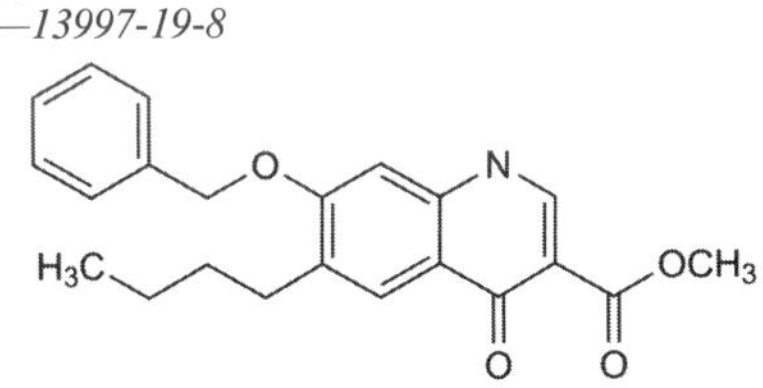

A white or creamy-white, amorphous powder. M.p. 287° to 288°.
Practically insoluble in water; very slightly soluble in ethanol, chloroform, and methanol.

Partition Coefficient. Log *P* (octanol/water), 6.6.

Colour Tests. Liebermann's Test—red-orange; Mandelin's Test—brown; Marquis Test—red-brown; Sulfuric Acid—yellow.

Ultraviolet Spectrum. Methanolic acid—261 nm (A^1_1=1955a).

Infra-red Spectrum. Principal peaks at wavenumbers 1621, 1689, 1250, 1089, 1211, 1550 $^{-1}$ (KBr disk).

Methyl Bromide *Insect fumigant*

Synonyms. MB; MeBr.
Proprietary names. Brom-o-Gas; Celfume; Embafume; Haltox; Methogas; Profume; Terr-o-Gas; Zytox.
Bromomethane
CH_3Br=94.9
CAS—74-83-9

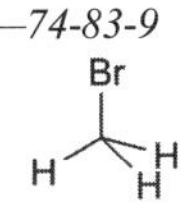

A colourless gas or liquid with M.p. −93.7° and B.p. 3.56°. It is soluble in water (1.75 g/100 g solution) and most organic solvents.

Crystal hydrate
$CH_3Br.20H_2O$=375.3
It is freely soluble in alcohol, chloroform, ether, carbon disulfide, carbon tetrachloride and benzene.

Partition Coefficient. Log *P* (octanol/water), 1.19.

Infra-red Spectrum. Principal peaks at wavenumbers 1319, 1295, 622, 594 cm^{-1}.

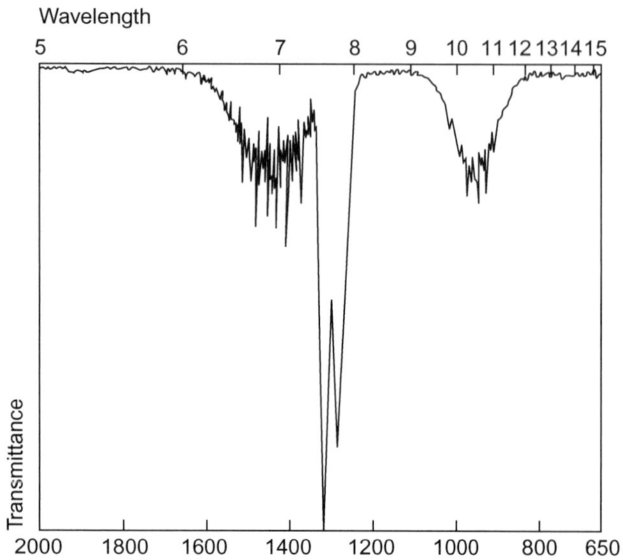

Mass Spectrum. Principal ions at *m/z* 94, 96, 15, 79, 81, 93, 95, 14.

Quantification
Gas chromatography. In urine: limit of detection 0.4 mg/L—M. Koga *et al.*, *J. Univ. Occup. Environ. Health*, 1991, *13(1)*, 19–24.

Disposition in the Body. Methyl bromide is readily absorbed through the skin and lung alveoli. It is excreted through the lungs unchanged but a significant amount can also be excreted in urine and faeces, after metabolic decomposition. It is decomposed to a bromide ion and methanol which can be detected in blood, stomach fluids, mucus and tissue. Organic bromides have also been detected, when the bromide ion reacts with the molecular carbons of the biomolecules.

Toxicity
A 6 mg/L dose for 10 to 20 h or 30 mg/L for 1.5 h is associated with fatalities. The allowed daily intake is 1.0 mg/kg (as the bromide ion).

A newborn infant died 12 to 13 h after exposure to methyl bromide which was used as a fumigant in the neighbouring house and had leaked through the sewage. The concentration of bromide ions in the infant's blood was 170 mg/L. The parents had also suffered from clinical intoxication as a result of the leakage. Bromide ions were found in their blood at concentrations of 130 and 110 mg/L. [S. Langard *et al.*, *J. Appl. Toxicol.*, 1996, *16(5)*, 445–448.]

Half-life. Approx. 12 days.

Methyl Ethyl Ketone

Solvent

Synonym. Ethyl Methyl Ketone
2-Butanone
C_4H_8O=72.1
CAS—78-93-3

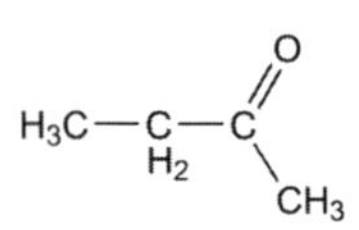

A flammable liquid. B.p. 80°.

Soluble 1 in about 4 of water, less soluble at higher temperatures; miscible with benzene, ethanol and ether.

Dissociation Constant pK_a 14.7 (25°).

Partition Coefficient. Log *P* (octanol/water), 0.3.

Gas Chromatography. System GA—RI 579; system GI—Retention time 7.3 min.

Mass Spectrum. Principal ions at *m/z* 43, 29, 27, 72, 57, 42, 44, 41.

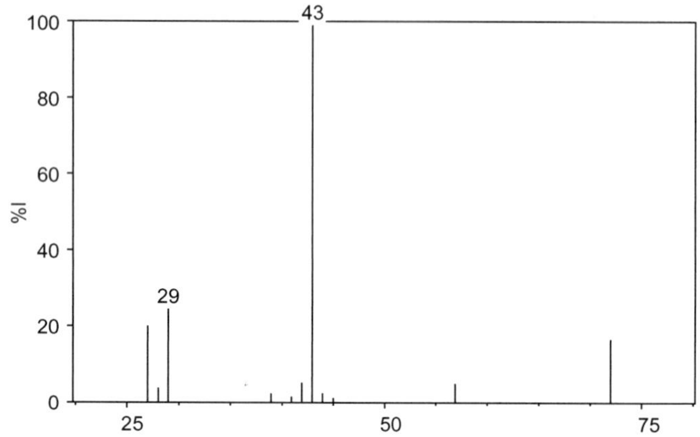

Quantification
Gas chromatography. In urine: methyl ethyl ketone and its metabolites, limits of detection 0.1 to 1.4 mg/L—S. Kezic and A. C. Monster, *J. Chromatogr.*, 1988, *428*, 275–280. In urine: limit of detection about 6 µg/L—H. Michitsuji *et al.*, *Sangyo Igaku*, 1992, *34*, 243–252. In urine: limit of detection about 4 µg/L, FID—J. S. Chou *et al.*, *J. Occup. Environ. Med.*, 1999, *41*, 1042–1047.

Methyl Hydroxybenzoate

Preservative

Synonyms. Metagin; Methyl Parahydroxybenzoate; Methylis Oxybenzoas; Methylparaben.
Proprietary Names. Methyl Chemosept; Methyl Parasept; Nipagin M; Tegosept M.
Methyl 4-hydroxybenzoate
$C_8H_8O_3$=152.1
CAS—99-76-3

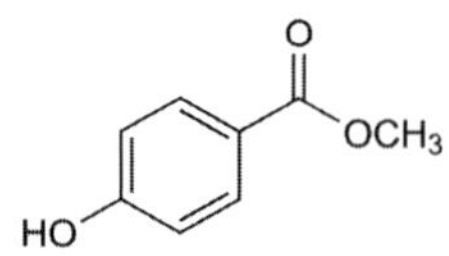

Colourless crystals or a fine, white, crystalline powder. M.p. 131°.
Soluble 1 in 400 to 1 in 500 of water, 1 in 20 of boiling water, 1 in 3 to 1 in 3.5 of ethanol, 1 in 40 of chloroform, and 1 in 10 of ether.

Sodium Methyl Hydroxybenzoate
Synonyms. Sodium Methylparaben; Soluble Methyl Hydroxybenzoate.
Proprietary name. Nipagin M Sodium
$C_8H_7NaO_3$=174.1
CAS—5026-62-0
A white, hygroscopic, crystalline powder.
Soluble 1 in 2 of water and 1 in 50 of ethanol.

Dissociation Constant. pK_a 8.4 (22°).

Partition Coefficient. Log *P* (octanol/water), 2.0.

Thin-layer Chromatography. System TA—Rf 95; system TD—Rf 62; system TE—Rf 44; system TF—Rf 65; system TAD—Rf 55; system TAE—Rf 81; system TAJ—Rf 61; system TAK—Rf 52; system TAL—Rf 91.

Gas Chromatography. System GA—methyl hydroxybenzoate RI 1432; M (OH-)-AC RI 1570; M (methoxy-) RI 1480; M (*p*-hydroxyhippuric acid)-Me RI 1820.

High Performance Liquid Chromatography. System HZ—Retention time 3.2 min.

Ultraviolet Spectrum. Ethanol—257 nm (A^1_1 = 1075a).

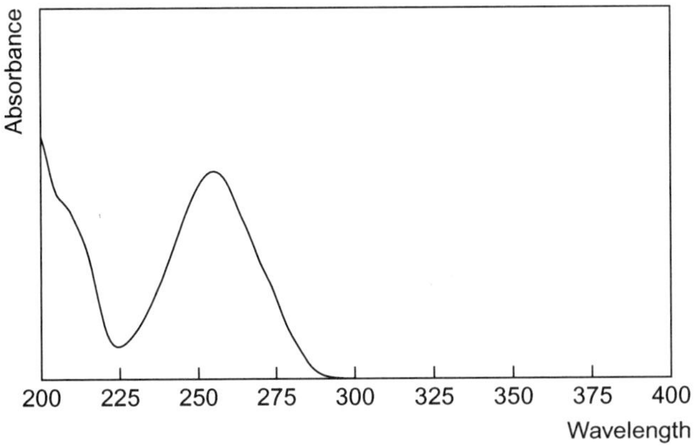

Mass Spectrum. Principal ions at *m/z* 121, 152, 40, 93, 65, -, -, -.

Methyl Nicotinate

Topical Vasodilator

Proprietary names. Pickles Chilblain Cream; Vas. It is an ingredient of Algipan, Arthricare, Cremalgin, Deep Heat Spray, Dubam, Fiery Jack, Musterole, Ralgex, Red Oil, and Transvasin.
Methyl 3-pyridinecarboxylate
$C_7H_7NO_2$ = 137.1
CAS—93-60-7

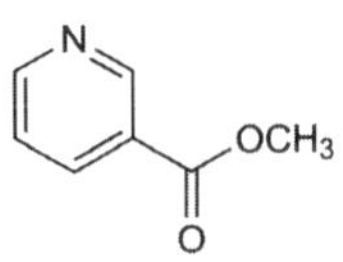

White crystals or crystalline powder; it darkens to a reddish colour on storage. M.p. 39°.
Soluble 1 in 0.7 of water and ethanol, 1 in 0.4 of chloroform, and 1 in 1 of ether; soluble in benzene.

Dissociation Constant. pK_a 3.1 (22°).

Partition Coefficient. Log *P* (octanol/water), 0.8.

Thin-layer Chromatography. System TA—Rf 61; system TB—Rf 37; system TC—Rf 66; system TE—Rf 72; system TL—Rf 59; system TAE—Rf 74; system TAF—Rf 77.

Gas Chromatography. System GA—RI 1100.

Ultraviolet Spectrum. Water—264 nm (A^1_1 = 230b).

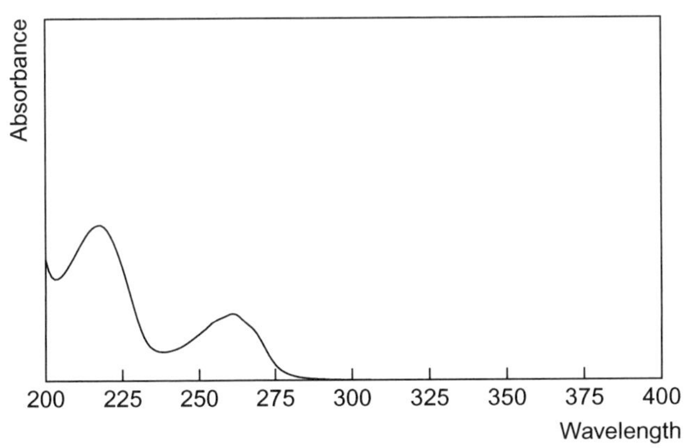

Infra-red Spectrum. Principal peaks at wavenumbers 1282, 1718, 1111, 741, 1022, 703 cm^{-1} (KBr disk).

Mass Spectrum. Principal ions at *m/z* 78, 106, 51, 137, 50, 136, 107, 79.

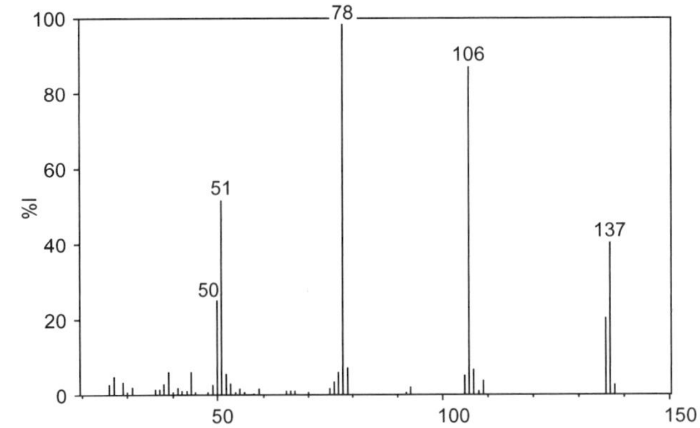

Use. Topically in a concentration of 1%.

Methyl Salicylate

Analgesic

Synonym. Wintergreen Oil
Proprietary names. It is an ingredient of many proprietary preparations—see Martindale, *The complete drug reference*, 33rd Edn, London, Pharmaceutical Press, 2002.
Methyl 2-hydroxybenzoate
$C_8H_8O_3$ = 152.1
CAS—119-36-8

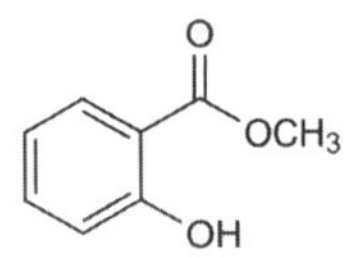

A colourless or pale yellow liquid. Relative density 1.182 to 1.187. B.p. about 221°, with some decomposition. Refractive index 1.535 to 1.538.
Slightly soluble in water; soluble in chloroform and ether; miscible with ethanol (90%) and with most organic solvents.

Dissociation Constant. pK_a 9.9 (20°).

Partition Coefficient. Log *P* (octanol/water), 2.6.

Thin-layer Chromatography. System TA—Rf 96; system TE—Rf 84; system TF—Rf 68; system TAF—Rf 90; system TAJ—Rf 95; system TAK—Rf 86.

Gas Chromatography. System GA—methyl salicylate RI 1195, salicylic acid RI 1308; system GB—methyl salicylate RI 1228; system GL—methyl salicylate RI 1210.

High Performance Liquid Chromatography. System HD—methyl salicylate *k* 3.9, salicylic acid *k* 0.7; system HX—RI 480; system HY—RI 449.

Ultraviolet Spectrum. Ethanol—238 (A^1_1 = 581a), 306 nm (A^1_1 = 280a).

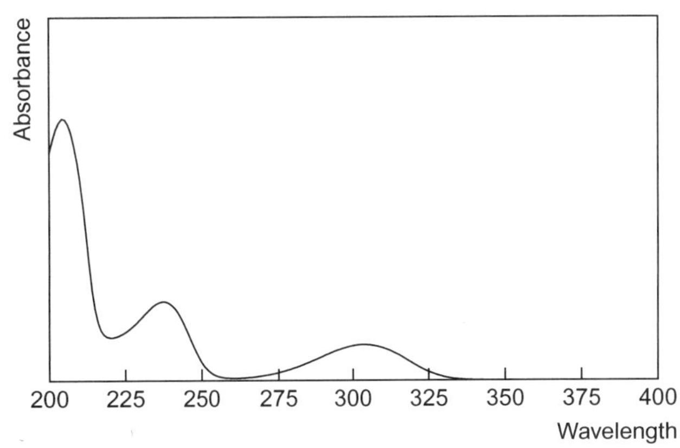

Infra-red Spectrum. Principal peaks at wavenumbers 1680, 705, 1310, 1220, 760, 1255 cm^{-1} (thin film).

Mass Spectrum. Principal ions at *m/z* 120, 92, 152, 121, 65, 64, 93, 63; salicylic acid 120, 92, 138, 64, 39, 63, 121, 65.

Disposition in the Body. Poorly absorbed through intact skin; absorbed after oral ingestion. It is incompletely hydrolysed to salicylic acid.

Therapeutic concentration

Following application of 5 g of an ointment containing 12.5% methyl salicylate twice daily for 4 days to 12 subjects, serum levels of 0.31 to 0.91 mg/L were reported within 1 h of the first application and peak levels of 2 to 6 mg/L were observed following the seventh application on day 4 [P. Morra *et al.*, *Ann. Pharmacother.*, 1996, *30*, 935–940.]

Toxicity. Methyl salicylate is more toxic than salicylic acid. Deaths have occurred in children after ingestion of as little as 4 mL and doses of 30 mL are usually fatal in adults.

In a fatality due to the ingestion of about 120 mL of methyl salicylate, postmortem salicylic acid concentrations were, blood 615 mg/L and liver 455 μg/g [J. Ryall, *Bull. Int. Assoc. Forensic Toxicol.*, 1974, *10*(1), 10.]

Use. Topically in liniments and ointments or in undiluted form.

Methylchlorophenoxyacetic Acid *Herbicide*

Synonym. MCPA

(4-Chloro-2-methylphenoxy)acetic acid

$C_9H_9ClO_3=200.6$

CAS—94-74-6

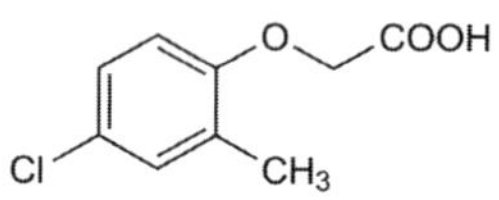

A white crystalline solid. M.p. pure compound, 118° to 119°; technical product, 100° to 115°.

Practically insoluble in water; soluble 1 in 160 of ethanol and 1 in 80 of ether.

Colour Test. Liebermann's Test—black.

Thin-layer Chromatography. System TD—Rf 09; system TE—Rf 05; system TF—Rf 11; system TX—Rf 00; system TY—Rf 00; system TAB—Rf 04; system TAC—Rf 02; system TAD—Rf 15.

Gas Chromatography. Methylchlorophenoxyacetic acid methyl ester: system GK—RRT 0.54 (relative to caffeine).

Ultraviolet Spectrum. Methanol—280 ($A^1_1=80a$), 287 nm.

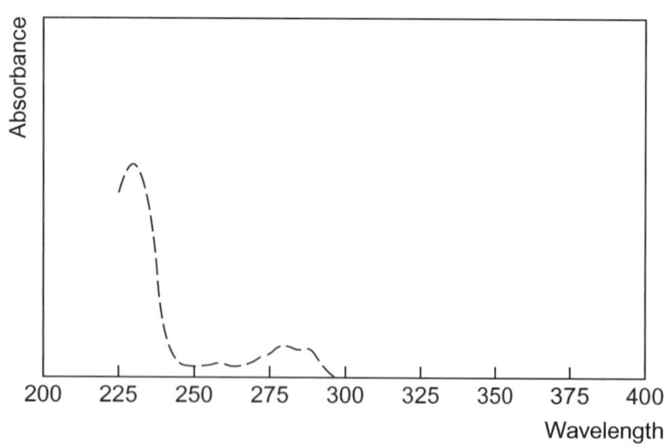

Infra-red Spectrum. Principal peaks at wavenumbers 1247, 1198, 1748, 1499, 1143, 806 cm^{-1} (Nujol mull).

Mass Spectrum. Principal ions at *m/z* 214, 141, 155, 125, 46, 77, 89, 143 (methylchlorophenoxyacetic acid methyl ester).

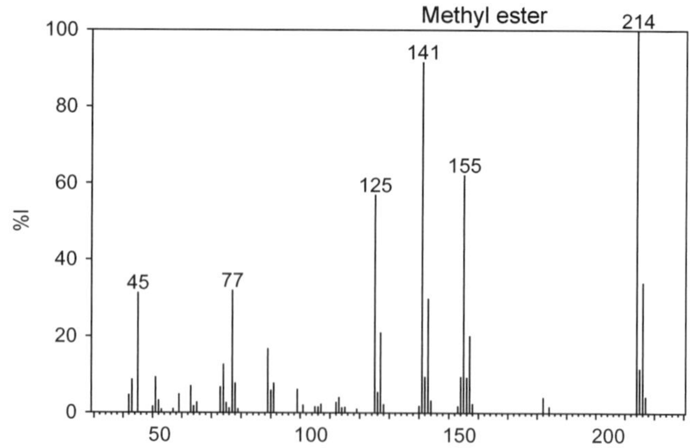

Disposition in the Body

Toxicity

After intentional ingestion of methylchlorophenoxyacetic acid, a man suffered burning in his mouth, spasmodic pain in the extremities and a severe hypotensive crisis; a plasma concentration of 546 mg/L was reported 2 h after ingestion, which rapidly declined to 6 mg/L following forced diuresis and alkalinisation of the urine on day 4 [A. Schmoldt *et al.*, *J. Toxicol. Clin. Toxicol.*, 1997, *35*, 405–408.]

Methyldopa *Antihypertensive*

Synonyms. Alpha-methyldopa; Methyldopum Hydratum; Metildopa.

Proprietary names. Aldomet; Aldometil; Aldomin; Aldopren; Amender; Cardin; Dopamet; Dopegyt; Hipten; Hydopa; Isomet; Medimet-250; Medomet; Medopren; Meldopa; MetalphaNovo-Medopa; Nudopa; Nu-Medopa; Presinol; Prodop; Pulsoton; Selm; Sembrina; Tenzone.

3-Hydroxy-α-methyl-L-tyrosine sesquihydrate

$C_{10}H_{13}NO_4,1\frac{1}{2}H_2O=238.2$

CAS—555-30-6 (anhydrous); 41372-08-1 (sesquihydrate)

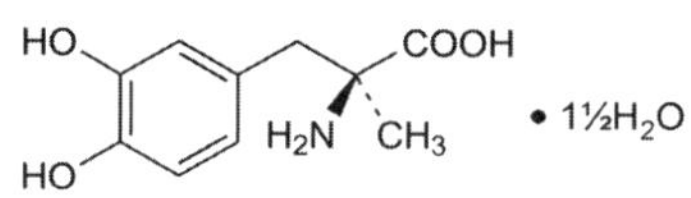

Colourless crystals or a white to yellowish-white, fine powder. M.p. about 310°.

Soluble 1 in 100 of water, 1 in 400 of ethanol, and 1 in 0.5 of dilute hydrochloric acid; practically insoluble in chloroform and ether.

Dissociation Constant. pK_a 2.2 (-COOH), 9.2 (-OH), 10.6(-NH_2), 12.0 (-OH), (25°).

Partition Coefficient. Log *P* (octanol/water), −1.8.

Colour Tests. Ammoniacal Silver Nitrate—red-brown/black; Ferric Chloride—green; Folin–Ciocalteu Reagent—blue; Mandelin's Test—orange; Marquis Test—yellow→violet; Methanolic Potassium Hydroxide—yellow→orange; Nessler's Reagent—black; Potassium Dichromate (Method 1)—green→brown (30 s).

Thin-layer Chromatography. System TA—Rf 49; system TB—Rf 01; system TC—Rf 01; system TE—Rf 02; system TL—Rf 01; system TAE—Rf 60; system TAF—Rf 75; system TAJ—Rf 00; system TAK—Rf 00; system TAL—Rf 06. (Mercuric chloride–diphenylcarbazone reagent, white-blue; acidified potassium permanganate solution, positive; Van Urk reagent, violet.)

Gas Chromatography. System GA—not eluted.

High Performance Liquid Chromatography. System HX—RI 69; system HZ—Retention time 1.4 min; system HAA—Retention time 3.0 min; system HAX—Retention time 4.1 min; system HAY—Retention time 2.8 min.

Ultraviolet Spectrum. Aqueous acid—279 ($A^1_1=130a$); aqueous alkali—302 nm.

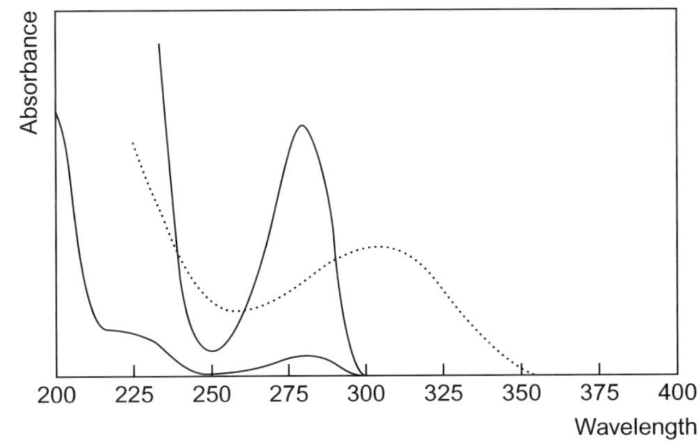

Infra-red Spectrum. Principal peaks at wavenumbers 1600, 1288, 1261, 1530, 1123, 1219 cm^{-1} (KBr disk).

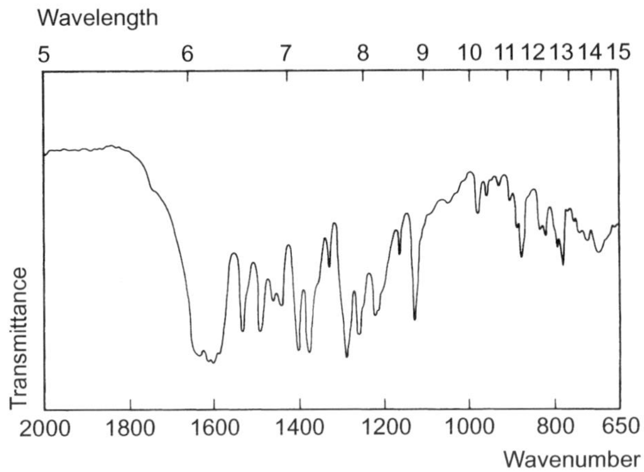

Mass Spectrum. Principal ions at *m/z* 88, 42, 123, 124, 89, 77, 51, 44.

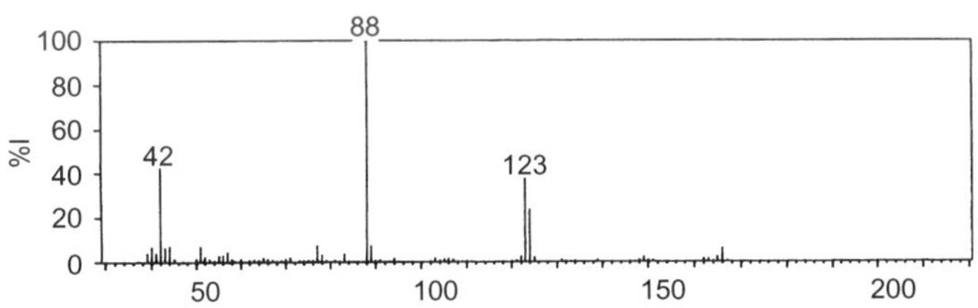

Quantification

Spectrofluorimetry. In plasma or urine: limit of detection 100 μg/L—B. K. Kim and R. T. Koda, *J. Pharm. Sci.*, 1977, *66*, 1632–1634.

High performance liquid chromatography. In plasma or breast milk: electrochemical detection—J. A. Hoskins and S. B. Holliday, *J. Chromatogr.*, 1982, *230*; *B Biomed. Appl.*, *19*, 162–167. In urine: limit of detection 5 mg/L, electrochemical detection—G. M. Kochak and W. D. Mason, *Anal. Lett.* (Part B), 1981, *14*, 439–449. In plasma: limit of detection 50 μg/L, electrochemical detection—C. Dilger *et al.*, *Arzneimittelforschung*, 1987, *37*, 1399–1401. In plasma or urine: methyldopa and its metabolite, electrode coulometric detection—C. Lucarelli *et al.*, *J. Chromatogr.*, 1991, *541*, 285–296. In plasma: limit of detection < 10 μg/L, fluorescence detection—K. Rona *et al.*, *J. Chromatogr. A.*, 1996, *730*, 125–131.

High performance liquid chromatography–mass spectrometry. In plasma: limit of detection <20 μg/L—C. H. Oliveira *et al.*, *J. Chromatogr. B Anal. Technol. Biomed. Life Sci.*, 2002, *768*, 341–348.

Disposition in the Body. Poorly absorbed after oral administration. It is mainly excreted as unchanged drug and as the mono-*O*-sulfate conjugate. After oral dosage, about 40% of the dose is excreted in the urine in 48 h, of which about 40% is the conjugate. A considerable amount of unchanged drug is eliminated in the faeces. After IV administration, the amount of conjugate excreted is much less than after oral dosage; a total of 52 to 82% of an IV dose is excreted in the urine in 36 h, only about 2% of which is the conjugate. Other metabolites and their conjugates which have been identified in the urine in small amounts (each less than 5% of the dose) include 3-*O*-methyl-α-methyldopa, α-methyldopamine, 3-*O*-methyl-α-methyldopamine, and 3,4-dihydroxyphenylacetone.
Methyldopa is a metabolite of methyldopate.

Therapeutic concentration. In plasma, usually in the range 1 to 5 mg/L.

After a single oral dose of 750 mg administered to 12 subjects, mean peak plasma concentrations of 2.6 mg/L of unchanged drug and 1.3 mg/L of the conjugate were attained in 3 h. An IV infusion of 250 mg given over 90 min to 12 subjects produced, at the end of the infusion period, a mean peak plasma concentration of 7.5 mg/L; no conjugate was found in the plasma [K. C. Kwan *et al.*, *J. Pharmacol. Exp. Ther.*, 1976, *198*, 264–277.]

Toxicity
In a fatality involving the ingestion of methyldopa, postmortem blood and urine concentrations of 9 and 1400 mg/L, respectively, were reported [V. Tamminen and A. Alha, *Bull. Int. Assoc. Forensic Toxicol.*, 1970, *7*(2), 2–3.]

Half-life. Plasma half-life, about 2 h; a longer terminal elimination half-life has also been reported.

Volume of distribution. About 0.6 L/kg.

Clearance. Plasma clearance, about 3 mL/min/kg.

Protein binding. In plasma, less than 20%.

Note. For a review of the pharmacokinetics of methyldopa see E. Myhre *et al.*, *Clin. Pharmacokinet.*, 1982, *7*, 221–233.

Dose. The equivalent of 0.5 to 3 g of anhydrous methyldopa daily.

Methyldopate

Antihypertensive

3-Hydroxy-α-methyl-L-tyrosine ethyl ester
$C_{12}H_{17}NO_4$=239.3
CAS—2544-09-4

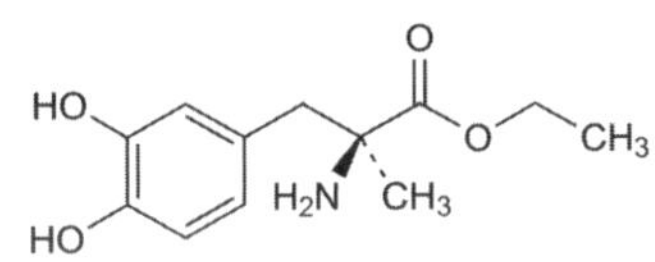

Methyldopate Hydrochloride

Proprietary name. Aldomet (injection)
$C_{12}H_{17}NO_4$,HCl=275.7
CAS—2508-79-4
A white crystalline powder.
Soluble 1 in 1 of water, 1 in 3 of ethanol, and 1 in 2 of methanol; slightly soluble in chloroform; practically insoluble in ether.

Colour Tests. Ammoniacal Silver Nitrate—orange-brown/orange-brown; Ferric Chloride—green; Folin–Ciocalteu Reagent—blue; Mandelin's Test—orange; Marquis Test—yellow→violet; Methanolic Potassium Hydroxide—blue→orange; Nessler's Reagent—black; Potassium Dichromate (Method 1)—green→brown (30 s).

Thin-layer Chromatography. System TA—Rf 65. (Acidified potassium permanganate solution, positive.)

Ultraviolet Spectrum. Aqueous acid—280 nm (A_1^1=115a).

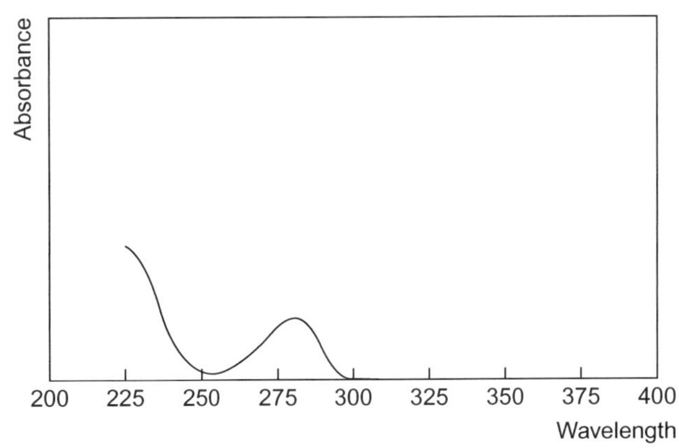

Infra-red Spectrum. Principal peaks at wavenumbers 1527, 1726, 1516, 1290, 1240, $1215\,cm^{-1}$ (KBr disk).

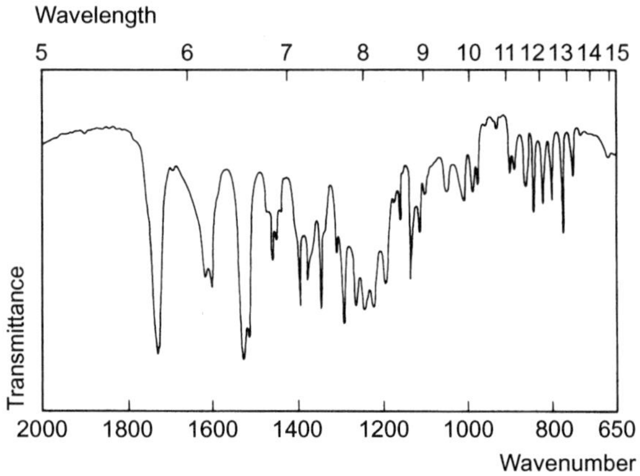

Quantification

High performance liquid chromatography. In plasma or breast milk: electrochemical detection—J. A. Hoskins and S. B. Holliday, *J. Chromatogr.*, 1982, *230*; *B Biomed. Appl.*, *19*, 162–167.

Disposition in the Body. Metabolised by de-esterification to methyldopa; a small amount of sulfate conjugation also occurs.

Therapeutic concentration

After an IV dose of 250 mg to 5 subjects, peak plasma concentrations of 0.8 to 2.2 mg/L (mean 1.6) of free and esterified methyldopa, and 1.0 to 2.2 mg/L (mean 1.5) of conjugated methyldopa were attained in about 1 h [J. A. Saavedra *et al.*, *Eur. J. Clin. Pharmacol.*, 1975, *8*, 381–386.]

Half-life. Plasma half-life, about 4 h.

Volume of distribution. About 2 L/kg.

Dose. Usually 250 to 500 mg of methyldopate hydrochloride, by IV infusion, every 6 h.

Methylene Chloride

Solvent

Dichloromethane
CH_2Cl_2=84.93
CAS—75-09-2

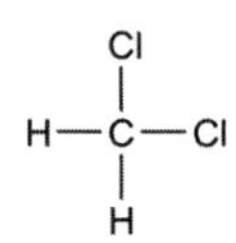

A clear, colourless, volatile liquid. Mass per mL about 1.32 g. B.p. 39° to 41°.
Soluble 1 in 50 of water; miscible with ethanol and ether.

Partition Coefficient. Log *P* (octanol/water), 1.2.

Gas Chromatography. System GA—RI 515; system GI—Retention time 1.9 min.

Mass Spectrum. Principal ions at *m*/*z* 49, 84, 86, 51, 47, 35, 88, 41.

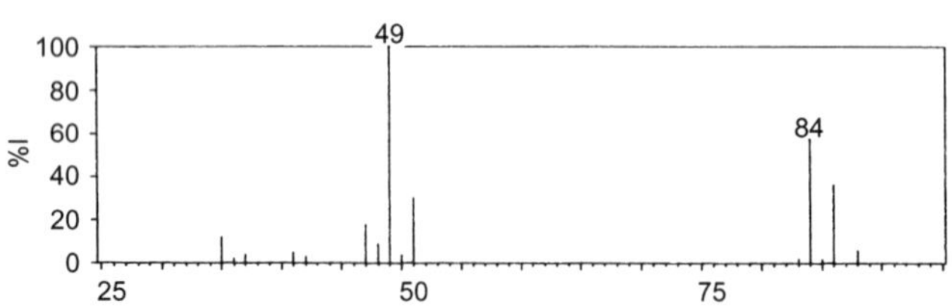

Quantification

Gas chromatography. In blood or urine: methylene chloride and chloroform, limits of detection 0.3 mg/L in blood and 0.2 mg/L in urine, FID—H. Seno *et al.*, *Med. Sci. Law*, 1999, *39*, 332–336.

Disposition in the Body

Toxicity. Methylene chloride is widely used in paint strippers and several non-fatal and fatal cases of accidental inhalation have been reported. The maximum permissible atmospheric concentration is 200 ppm and the temporary estimated acceptable daily intake is up to 500 μg/kg.

The following tissue concentrations were reported in a fatality due to accidental methylene chloride poisoning: blood 252 mg/L, brain 75 μg/g, heart 30 μg/g [N. Y. Kim *et al.*, *J. Forensic Sci.*, 1996, *41*, 527–529.]

Blood concentrations collected at autopsy in 2 cases of fatal methylene chloride poisoning were 572 and 601 mg/L; air concentrations a few hours after discovery of the bodies were up to 168 000 ppm [M. Manno *et al.*, *Hum. Exp. Toxicol.*, 1992, *11*, 540–545.]

The following postmortem tissue concentrations were reported in a 47-year-old factory worker who died while making an inventory of the annual stock of methylene chloride contained in several tanks, one of which overflowed: blood 150 mg/L, urine 2.0 mg/L, gastric content 5.6 mg/L, brain 122 μg/g, fat 99 μg/g, liver 44 μg/g, lung 20 μg/g, kidney 15 μg/g [J. P. Goulle *et al.*, *J. Anal. Toxicol.*, 1999, *23*, 380–383.]

Methylenedioxyamfetamine

Hallucinogen

Synonyms. MDA; Methylenedioxyamphetamine; Tenamfetamine; SKF-5.
α-Methyl-1,3-benzodioxole-5-ethanamine
$C_{10}H_{13}NO_2$=179.2
CAS—4764-17-4

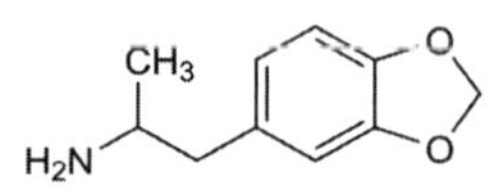

Almost colourless oil.

Methylenedioxyamfetamine Hydrochloride
$C_{10}H_{13}NO_2$, HCl=215.7
CAS—6292-91-7

Dissociation Constant. pK_a 9.67 (25°).

Partition Coefficient. Log *P* (octanol/water), 1.64.

Colour Tests. Liebermann's Test—black; Mandelin's Test—green→blue; Marquis Test—blue-black; Sulfuric Acid—violet.

Thin-layer Chromatography. System TA—Rf 39; system TB—Rf 18; system TC—Rf 12; system TE—Rf 42; system TL—Rf 17; system TAE—Rf 10; system TAF—Rf 76. (Acidified potassium permanganate solution, positive.)

Gas Chromatography. System GA—MDA RI 1480, MDA-TFA RI 1615, MDA-PFP RI 1605, MDA-AC RI 1860, art (formyl) RI 1520; system GB—MDA RI 1512, art (formyl) RI 1689.

High Performance Liquid Chromatography. System HC—*k* 0.98; system HX—RI 266; system HY—RI 248; system HZ—Retention time 2.1 min; system HAA—Retention time 8.1 min; system HAX—Retention time 6.9 min; system HAY—Retention time 3.8 min.

Ultraviolet Spectrum. Aqueous acid—233 nm (A_1^1=216b), 285 nm.

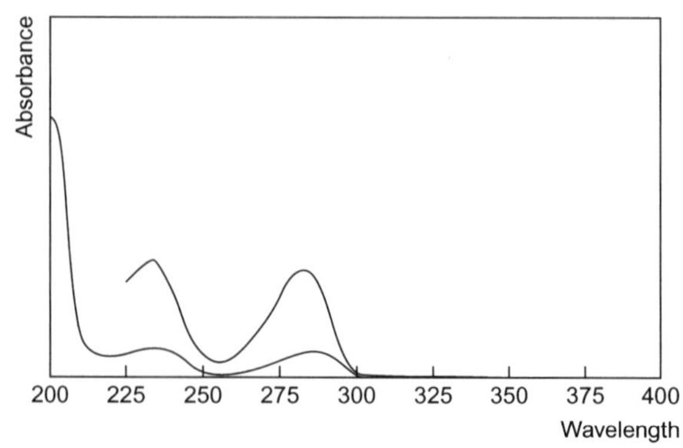

Infra-red Spectrum. Principal peaks at wavenumbers 1490, 1257, 1038, 1504, 799, $1188\,cm^{-1}$ (KBr disk).

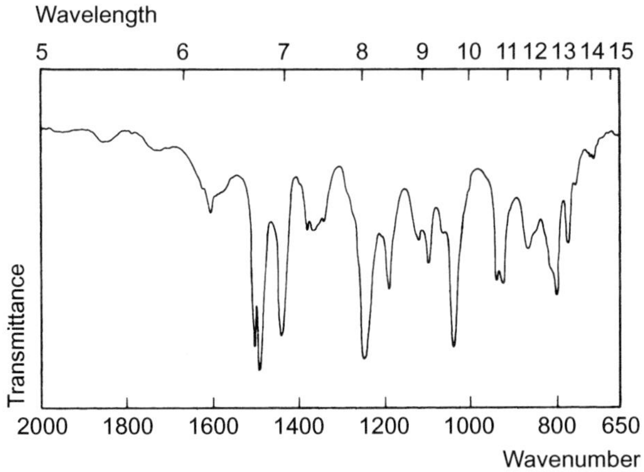

Mass Spectrum. Principal ions at *m/z* 44, 136, 51, 135, 77, 42, 78, 45.

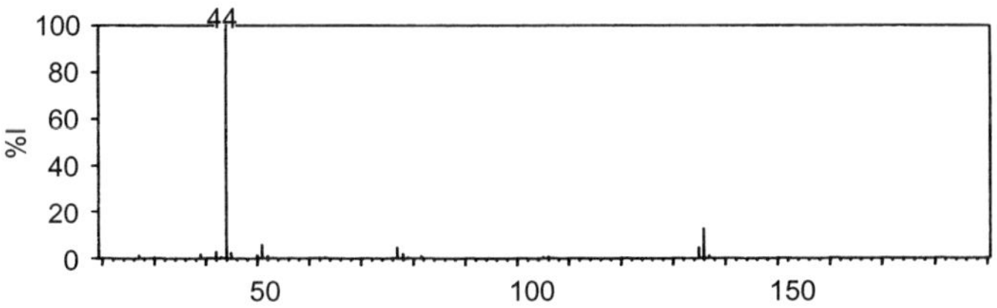

Quantification

Gas chromatography. In urine: limit of detection 15 μg/L, NPD—H. G. Ugland *et al.*, *J. Pharm. Biomed. Anal.*, 1999, *19(3-4)*, 463–475. In plasma and urine: limit of detection <1.6 μg/L and 47 μg/L, respectively—J. Ortuno *et al.*, *J. Chromatogr. B Biomed. Sci. Appl.*, 1999, *723(1–2)*, 221–232.

Gas chromatography–mass spectrometry. In hair: limit of detection 0.05 μg/g—P. Kintz *et al.*, *J. Chromatogr. B Biomed. Sci. Appl.*, 1995, *670*, 162–166. In hair: limit of detection 0.01 μg/g—J. Rohrich and G. Kauert, *Forensic Sci. Int.*, 1997, *84*, 179–188. In urine: limit of detection is 15 μg/L—H. G. Ugland *et al.*, *J. Pharm. Biomed. Analysis*, 1999, *19*, 463–475. In urine: methylenedioxyamfetamine and other amfetamines, limit of detection about 10 μg/L—D. Hensley and J. T. Cody, *J. Anal. Toxicol.*, 1999, *23*, 518–523. In urine: limit of quantification 20 μg/L—C. Jurado *et al.*, *J. Anal. Toxicol.*, 2000, *24*, 11–16. In serum: methylenedioxyamfetamine and other drugs of abuse—W. Weinmann *et al.*, *Int, J. Legal Med.*, 2000, *113*, 229–235. In hair: methylenedioxyamfetamine and other drugs of abuse, limits of detection 0.05 to 0.3 μg/g—L. Skender *et al.*, *Forensic Sci. Int.*, 2002, *125*, 120–126. In urine: methylenedioxyamfetamine and related drugs, limit of detection for MDA about 31 μg/L—P. R. Stout *et al.*, *J. Anal. Toxicol.*, 2002, *26*, 253–261.

High performance liquid chromatography. In whole blood and other biological tissues: limit of detection 1 μg/L, ECD—R. E. Michel *et al.*, *J. Neurosci. Methods*, 1993, *50(1)*, 61–66. In hair: limit of detection <1 μg/L (0.1 μg/g)—F. Tagliaro *et al.*, *J. Chromatogr. B Biomed. Sci. Appl.*, 1999, *723(1–2)*, 195–202. In whole blood, serum, urine and vitreous humour: limit of quantification 2 μg/L in whole blood, serum and vitreous humour and in urine 100 μg/L—K. M. Clauwaert *et al.*, *Clin. Chem.*, 2000, *46(12)*, 1968–1977. In plasma and urine: limit of detection 10 μg/L—R. Herraez-Hernandez *et al.*, *Analyst*, 2001, *126(5)*, 581–586.

Toxicity. The estimated lethal dose is 0.5 g.

A 21-year-old man was found dead in bed 7 h after being last seen in a 'normal' state. Temazepam tablets as well as two types of white tablets were found by his bedside. Toxicological analysis revealed the presence of the following drugs:

	Blood (mg/L)	Stomach content (mg/L)	Urine
Amfetamine	0.256	Less than 0.1	Present
MDA	8.5	299	Present
MDMA	2.1	96	Present
MDEA	3.5	324	Present

[R. Forrest *et al.*, *Forensic Sci. Int.*, 1994, *64*, 57–59].

In 5 fatalities due to the ingestion of methylenedioxyamfetamine, the following postmortem tissue concentrations were reported: blood 6 to 26 mg/L (mean 14, 5 cases), bile 5 to 9 mg/L (mean 6, 3 cases), liver 8 to 17 μg/g (mean 11, 3 cases), urine 46 to 160 mg/L (mean 102, 3 cases) [G. Cimbura, *J. Forensic Sci.*, 1972, *17*, 329–333].

In a fatality in which death occurred shortly after the ingestion of methylenedioxyamfetamine, the following postmortem concentrations were reported: blood 2.3 mg/L, bile 7 mg/L, liver 11 μg/g, urine 175 mg/L [T. Lukabzewski, *Clin. Toxicol.*, 1979, *15*, 405–409].

Note. For a review of the pharmacology of MDA see D. L. Simpson and B. H. Rumack, *Arch. Intern. Med.*, 1981, *141*, 1507–1509; for a distribution study of MDMA and MDA in a fatal overdose see E. A. De Letter *et al.*, *J. Anal. Toxicol.*, 2002, *26*, 113–118.

Methylenedioxyethylamfetamine

Stimulant/Hallucinogen

Synonyms. *N*-Ethyl-3,4-methylenedioxyphenylisopropylamine; Eve; MDE; MDEA; 3,4-Methylenedioxyethamphetamine; 3,4-Methylenedioxyethylamphetamine. Usually presented as Ecstasy.
N-ethyl-α-methyl-1,3-benzodioxole-5-ethanamine
$C_{12}H_{17}NO_2$=207.3
CAS—82801-81-8

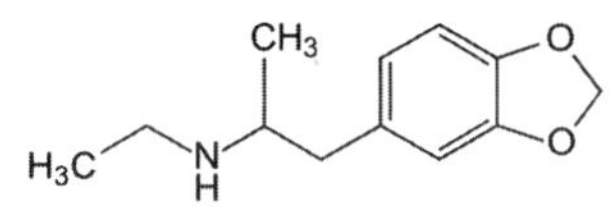

A viscous, colourless oil. B.p. 0.2, 85° to 95°.

Methylenedioxyethylamfetamine Hydrochloride

$C_{12}H_{17}NO_2$, HCl=243.8
CAS—74341-78-9
A white to off-white crystalline powder with a bitter taste.

Gas Chromatography. System GA—MDEA RI 1560, methylenedioxyamfetamine (MDA) RI 1480, MDEA-TFA RI 1770, MDEA-PFP RI 1755, MDEA-TMS RI 1825, MDEA-AC RI 1985; system GB—MDEA RI 1630, MDA RI 1512.

High Performance Liquid Chromatography. Column: C_{18} BDS (Hypersil, 100 × 2.1 mm i.d., 3 μm). Mobile phase: (A)-ammonium acetate (0.1 M):methanol:acetonitrile (90:10:10); (B)-methanol:acetonitrile:water (45:45:10), flow rate 1 mL/min. Elution programme: (A:B) (100:0) for 6 min to (30:70) in 14 min. IS: methylenedioxymethylpropylamfetamine (MDMPA). Fluorescence detection (λ_{ex} = 288 nm, λ_{em} = 324 nm). Retention time(s): MDMA, 14.1 min; MDA, 13.1 min; MDEA, 15.1 min; IS, 17.1 min [K. Clauwaert *et al.*, *Clin. Chem.*, 2000, *46*, 1968–1977].

Quantification

Gas chromatography–mass spectrometry. In whole blood: limits of quantification 10 μg/L for amfetamine, MDMA and MDEA—P. Marquet *et al.*, *J. Chromatogr. B Biomed. Sci. Appl.*, 1997, *700*, 77–82.

High pressure liquid chromatography. In whole blood, serum and vitreous humour: limit of detection 0.8 μg/L; in urine 2.5 μg/L—K. Clauwaert *et al.*, *Clin. Chem.*, 2000, *46*, 1968–1977.

Disposition in the Body. It is absorbed into the blood stream after ingestion and excreted in urine, mainly as the parent drug (19%), methylenedioxyamfetamine (MDA, 28%) and also 4-hydroxy-3-methoxyethylamfetamine (HMEA, 32%). Metabolism occurs by a number of routes: *N*-de-ethylation, catalysed by CYP3A4 to MDA and demethylation to 3,4-dihydroxyethylamfetamine catalysed by CYP2D6 and CYP3A2.

Toxicity

In a 20-year-old male whose death was attributed to injection of MDMA and MDEA, postmortem blood concentrations of 2.0 and 0.7 mg/L, respectively, were reported [N. Raikos *et al.*, *Forensic Sci. Int.*, 2002, *128*, 31–34].

A 19-year-old man died after ingesting 10 tablets of Ecstasy (containing MDEA as the main active ingredient, approximately 130 mg/tablet) over a period of 8 hours. Postmortem analysis carried out 29 hours after death revealed the following tissue concentrations of MDEA (mg/L or µg/g): femoral vein serum 12, heart serum 22, urine 201, gastric content 52, liver 30, kidney 15, bile 19, cerebrum 28, cerebellum 18, hair 17. Trace amounts of MDMA were found in urine and blood [W. Weinmann and M. Bohnert, *Forensic Sci. Int.*, 1998, *91*, 91–101].

The following postmortem tissue concentrations were reported in a 27-year-old woman with a history of depression who committed suicide by ingesting a large dose of MDEA: blood 1.2 mg/L, urine 1.9 mg/L, bile 3.6 mg/L; the patient had attempted suicide several days earlier by ingesting benzodiazepines and these were also detected in the blood [J. Arimany *et al.*, *Am. J. Forensic Med. Pathol.*, 1998, *19*, 148–151].

A 31-year-old male whose death was attributed to MDEA ingestion had a blood concentration of 3.1 mg/L; the respective concentrations in the liver, lung, and kidney were 4.8, 5.2, and 4.8 µg/g [A. M. Tsatsakis *et al.*, *Vet. Hum. Toxicol.*, 1997, *39*, 241–244].

A 22-year-old male died following ingestion of alcohol and 2½ Ecstasy tablets at a rave. On admission to hospital he had blood concentrations of 0.24 mg/L MDA, 0.55 mg/L MDMA, and 0.49 mg/L MDEA. The respective concentrations in gastric aspirate were 0.11, 2.09, and 0.25 mg/L and the respective urine concentrations were 1.75, 14.3, and 68.0 mg/L. At postmortem, carried out approximately 36 hours after death, concentrations in the femoral blood were 0.25, 0.43, and 0.30 mg/L [D. E. Cox and K. R. Williams, *Forensic Sci. Int.*, 1996, *77*, 101–108].

In 2 fatal cases associated with the ingestion of unknown amounts of MDEA with suicidal intent, the first (a 19-year-old male) had plasma levels of 20.2 mg/L upon admission to hospital; postmortem concentrations of 45 mg/L in the blood and 40.6 mg/L in the cerebrospinal fluid were reported (no other drugs were detected). In the second case (a 24-year-old male, who also stabbed himself to death), blood concentrations of 0.22 mg/L MDEA and 0.75 mg/L amfetamine were detected (alcohol was also present) [S. Iwersen and A. Schmoldt, *J. Toxicol. Clin. Toxicol.*, 1996, *34*, 241–244].

In 2 deaths associated with the use of MDEA, the first was a 25-year-old man who was involved in a fatal traffic accident the day after complaining of pleuritic chest pain. At postmortem, the only injury was a 4-cm laceration on his forehead but toxicological analysis revealed the presence of MDEA (0.95 mg/L) and butalbital (0.8 mg/L) in the blood; no alcohol was detected. The second case involved a 21-year-old man who was found unconscious after ingesting 3 Ecstasy capsules (approx. 300 mg), one propoxyphene 65-mg capsule, and several drinks over a period of 10 to 11 hours. Resuscitation was unsuccessful. Postmortem tissue concentrations of MDEA were: blood, 2.0 mg/L, liver 4.51 µg/g, kidney 2.55 µg/g, heart 1.68 µg/g, lung 4.54 µg/g, spleen 3.33 µg/g. Propoxyphene was present in the blood at a concentration of 0.26 mg/L and norpropoxyphene at 1.0 mg/L. No MDMA (the drug the man thought he was taking) or alcohol was detected [G. P. Dowling *et al.*, *JAMA*, 1987, *257*, 1615–1617].

Note. For a review of the metabolism and toxicokinetic data of designer drugs, see T. Kraemer and H. H. Maurer, *Ther. Drug Monit.*, 2002, *24*, 277–289.

Dose. The usual dose is between 30 and 100 mg in the form of tablets or capsules, however, these usually also contain varying amounts of MDA or MDMA.

Methylenedioxymethamfetamine

Stimulant/ Hallucinogen

Synonyms. Adam; Clarity; E; Ecstasy; Elaine; Essence; Euphoria; MDM; MDMA; 3,4-Methylenedioxymetamfetamine; 3,4-methylenedioxymethylamphetamine; *N*-methyl-3, 4-methylenedioxyphenylisopropylamine; (2-Benzol[1,3]dioxol-5-yl-1-methyl-ethyl)methylamine; Stacy; X; XTC.

Street names. Several tablets and capsules have been in circulation over the years, containing varying amounts of MDMA and other phenethylamines, recognisable by logos on tablets or colours of capsules. Some examples of tablets or capsules include: Apples; Beans; Baby slits; Brownies; Burgers; Crowns; Dennis the Menaces; Diamond Whites; Disco biscuits; Dollars; Doves; Love Doves; Mitsubishis; Mitsies; New Yorkers; Pink Calis; Rhubarb & Custards; Tangos; White Doves.

N,α-Dimethyl-1,3,benzodioxole-5-ethanamine

$C_{11}H_{15}NO_2$=193.2

CAS—42542-10-9

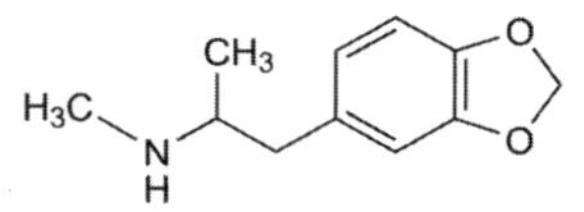

A viscous, colourless oil. B.p. 100° to 110°.

Methylenedioxymethamfetamine Hydrochloride

$C_{11}H_{15}NO_2$,HCl=229.75

CAS—64057-70-1

A white to off-white crystalline powder with a bitter taste. M.p. 147° to 148° for crystals from isopropanol/*n*-hexane; M.p. 152° to 153° for crystals from isopropan-2-ol/ether.

Dissociation Constant. pK_a (pH 9.0), (benzene) 9.41, (hexane) 8.69, (ethyl acetate) 8.84.

Colour Test. Marquis Reagent—black with dark purple halo.

Thin-layer Chromatography. System TA—Rf 33; system TB—Rf 24; system TE—Rf 39; system TF—Rf 20; system TAE—Rf 08; system TAJ—Rf 03; system TAK—Rf 17; system TAL—Rf 57.

Gas Chromatography. System GA—MDMA RI 1585, methylenedioxyamfetamine (MDA) RI 1480, MDMA-TFA RI 1720, MDMA-PFP RI 1830, MDMA-TMS RI 1710, MDMA-AC RI 2140; system GB—MDMA RI 1572, MDA RI 1512; system GAK—MDMA retention time 8.7 min.

Column: 3% OV-1 Chromosorb WHP 80/100 mesh (4′ × ¼″). Column temperature: 200°. Carrier gas: nitrogen, flow rate 32 mL/min. Detection: flame ionisation. RI: 1559. [T. Mills and J. C. Roberson, *Instrumental data for drug analysis*, CRC Press, Boca Raton, FL, 2nd Edn., 2, 1993, pp. 1464–1465.]

High Performance Liquid Chromatography. System HX—RI 278; system HY—RI 252; system HZ—retention time 2.2 min; system HAA—retention time 9.1 min; system HBC—retention time 2.42 min; system HBD—retention time 5.31 min.

Column: C_{18} BDS (Hypersil, 100 × 2.1 mm i.d., 3 µm). Mobile phase: (A)—ammonium acetate (0.1 M):methanol:acetonitrile (90:10:10); (B)—methanol:acetonitrile:water (45:45:10), 1 mL/min flow rate. Elution programme: (A:B) (100:0) for 6 min to (30:70) in 14 min. Internal standard: methylenedioxymethylpropylamfetamine (MDMPA). Fluorescence detection (λ_{ex}=288 nm; λ_{em}=324 nm). Retention time: MDMA, 14.1 min; MDA, 13.1 min; MDEA, 15.1 min; IS, 17.1 min. [K. Clauwaert *et al.*, *Clin. Chem.*, 2000, *46*, 1968–1977.]

Column: ODS Hypersil Si-10 (300 × 4.0 mm i.d., 10 µm). Mobile phase: methanol with 1% NHOH:methylene chloride (10:90), flow rate 2 mL/min. UV detection (λ=254 nm). Retention time: 4.4 min. [T. Mills and J. C. Roberson, *Instrumental data for drug analysis*, CRC Press, Boca Raton, FL, 2nd Edn., 2, 1993, pp. 1464–1465.]

Column: Zorbax CN (150 × 4.6 mm i.d., 5 µm). Mobile phase: methanol:acetate buffer (0.1 M, pH 4.56) (50:50). UV detection (λ=280 and 284 nm). Retention time(s): MDMA, 6.69 min; MDA, 5.83 min. [E. Garrett *et al.*, *Acta Pharm. Nord.*, 1991, *3(1)*, 9–14.]

Ultraviolet Spectrum. Aqueous acid—234, 285; (0.1 M $HCOONH_4$, pH 3)—285; basic—232, 285 nm.

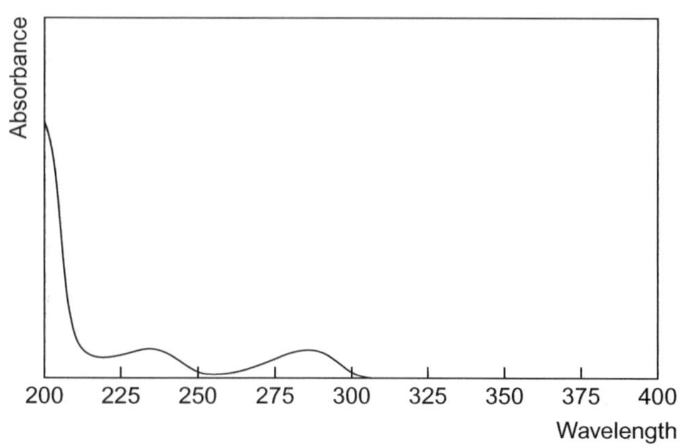

Infra-red Spectrum. Principal peaks at wavenumber 1033, 930, 805, 1489, 1442, 1189 cm^{-1} (hydrochloride).

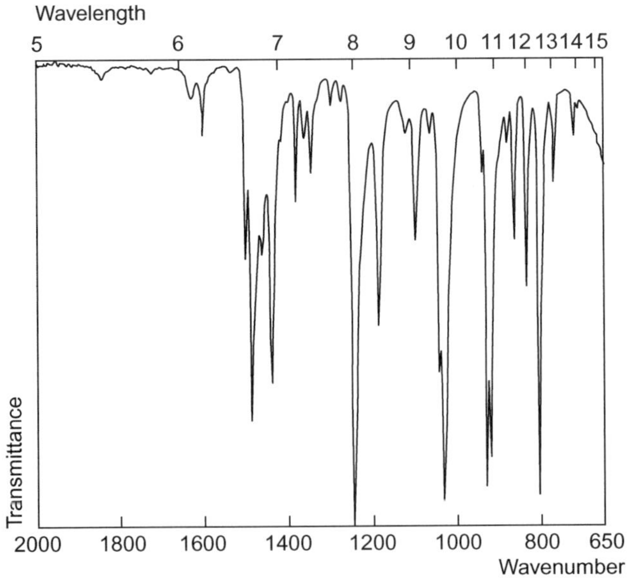

Mass Spectrum. Principal peaks at *m/z* 58, 135, 77, 51, 55, 136, 105, 63.

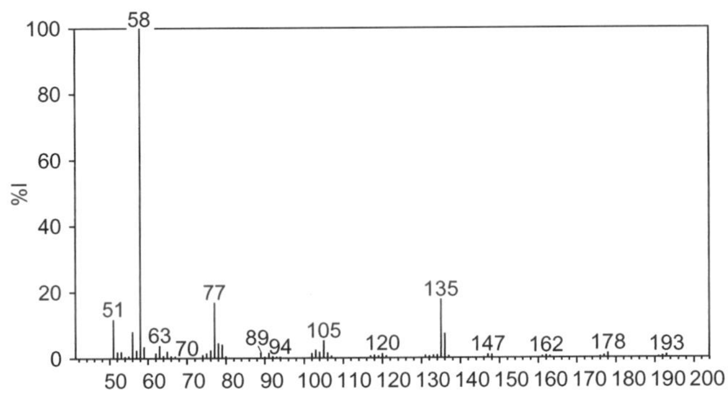

Quantification

Gas chromatography. In plasma and urine: limits of detection 1.6 µg/L and 47 µg/L respectively for MDMA and MDA NPD—J. Ortuno *et al.*, *J. Chromatogr. B Biomed Sci. Appl.*, 1999, *723*, 221–232.

Gas chromatography–mass spectrometry. In urine: MDMA and MDA, limit of quantification 20 µg/L—C. Jurado *et al.*, *J. Anal. Toxicol.*, 2000, *24*, 11–16. In urine: MDMA enantiomers limit of quantification 25 µg/L—D. Hensley and J. T. Cody, *J. Anal. Toxicol.*, 1999, *23*, 518–523. In whole blood: limits of quantification 10 µg/L for amfetamine, MDMA, and methylenedioxyethylamfetamine (MDEA); 20 µg/L for metamfetamine and 50 µg/L for MDA—P. Marquet *et al.*, *J. Chromatogr. B Biomed. Sci. Appl.*, 1997, *700*, 77–82.

High performance liquid chromatography. In whole blood, serum, and vitreous humour: limit of detection 0.8 µg/L; in urine 2.5 µg/L—K. Clauwaert *et al.*, *Clin. Chem.*, 2000, *46*, 1968–1977. In hair: limit of detection $<$1.0 µg/L—F. Tagliaro *et al.*, *J. Chromatogr. B Biomed. Sci. Appl.*, 1999, *723*, 195–202. In plasma: limit of detection 3.68 µg/L—E. Garrett *et al.*, *Acta Pharm. Nord.*, 1991, *3(1)*, 9–14.

Capillary electrophoresis. Limit of detection 0.5 µg/L—C. Fang *et al.*, *Forensic Sci. Int.*, 2002, *125*, 142–148.

Disposition in the Body. It is absorbed into the blood stream after ingestion and excreted in urine, the majority of the dose unchanged (65% within 3 days). Metabolism occurs by a number of routes: *N*-demethylation of the parent compound to 3,4-methylenedioxyamfetamine (MDA) (7%) with further *O*-demethylation to 3,4-dihydroxymetamfetamine (HHMA) and 3,4-dihydroxyamfetamine (HHA). Both HHMA and HHA are subsequently *O*-methylated by catechol-*O*-methyltransferase (COMT) mainly to 4-hydroxy-3-methoxymetamfetamine (HMMA) and 4-hydroxy-3-methoxyamfetamine (HMA). These four metabolites are excreted in the urine as the conjugated glucuronide or sulfate metabolites.

Therapeutic concentration

8 healthy male volunteers, aged between 21 and 31 years old, were administered a 75 mg dose of MDMA. The mean peak plasma concentration was 0.13 mg/L after 1.8 h. Mean peak plasma concentrations of the metabolite, MDA, were 7.8 µg/L approximately 5 h after administration. [R. de la Torre *et al.*, *Br. J. Clin. Pharmacol.*, 2000, 49, 104–109.]

After the administration of a single oral dose of 1.5 mg/kg body weight MDMA to 2 patients, plasma and urine samples were collected over periods of 9 and 22 h, respectively. Peak plasma concentrations of MDMA and MDA were 331 µg/L after 2 h and 15 µg/L after 6.3 h, respectively. Peak concentrations of 28.1 µg/L MDMA in urine appeared after 21.5 h. Up to 2.3 µg/L MDA, 35.1 µg/L HMMA, and 2.1 µg/L HMA were measured within 16 to 21.5 h, also in urine. [H. J. HelmLin *et al.*, *J. Anal. Toxicol.*, 1996, *20*, 432–440.]

Toxicity. Fatalities with doses of 300 mg have been reported. Risk of adverse reaction is high but the pattern is varied. Severe acute toxic effects and morbidity are noted. Capable of causing severe toxicity and the pattern of acute toxicity is due to the circumstances in which it is misused. Circumstances associated with ingestion and direct effects of the drug are thought to influence toxicity. Amount of MDMA ingested is difficult to determine because the concentration of the tablets is unknown and it may be mixed with other substances. A lethal concentration of 0.35 to 0.50 mg/L in serum has been noted although some overdose cases report concentrations 10 times this amount, without fatality.

A 28-year-old male was found unconscious in a bar. A postmortem examination was carried out roughly 28 h later which revealed the following MDMA and MDA concentrations:

Sample	MDMA (mg/L or µg/g)	MDA (mg/L or µg/g)
Subclavian blood	3.5	0.09
Femoral blood	3.1	0.093
Serum (subclavian blood)	4.2	0.1
Vitreous humour	3.4	0.06
Urine	170.9	4
Bile	14.2	0.32
Liver	26.2	1.203
Stomach content	118.1	0.448
Spleen	10	0.264
Brain (frontal lobe)	17.4	0.296
Brain (parietal lobe)	17.1	0.362
Brainstem	13.2	0.22
Cerebellum	11.7	0.225

Cotinine, caffeine, and trace amounts of benzoylecgonine were also detected. [E.A. De Letter *et al.*, *J. Anal. Toxicol.*, 2002, *26*, 113–118.]

A 30-year-old man was admitted to hospital after taking 50 ecstasy tablets, 10 oxazepam tablets (10 mg), and 5 units of alcohol over a period of 4 to 5 h. Presenting features were unconciousness, apnoea, and convulsions. Toxicological analysis revealed the following MDMA and MDA concentrations:

		MDMA (mg/L)		MDA (mg/L)	
Time after ingestion (h)	Sample	R-(−)	S-(+)	R-(−)	S-(+)
4	Urine	44	42	nd	0.4
	Gastric lavage	70	72	nd	nd
36	Urine	36	17	3	7
60	Urine	18	10	5	4
	Serum	0.8	0.2	nd	nd

The individual recovered after a few days without sequelae. [S. Ramcharan *et al.*, *J. Toxicol. Clin. Toxicol.*, 1998, *36*, 727–731.]

After 12 h of ingesting a maximum of 40 ecstasy tablets, a 19-year-old man was admitted to an intensive care unit. Toxicological analysis revealed the following MDMA concentrations:

Time after ingestion (h)	Serum MDMA (mg/L)	Urine MDMA (mg/L)
13	4.3	630
24	1.4	180
30	0.75	105

The individual recovered after a few days without sequelae. [R. Regenthal *et al.*, *Intensive Care Med.*, 1999, *25*, 640-641.]

An 18-year-old male ingested 3 tablets and collapsed. He was unconscious on the floor for 60 min and died 2.5 h after admission to hospital. A plasma concentration of 0.36 mg/L MDMA was detected.

A 16-year-old female ingested 1 tablet and suffered from seizures and experienced hallucinations. The MDMA plasma concentration was 0.424 mg/L. She died 36 h after admission to hospital.

A 21-year-old female ingested an unknown number of tablets and suffered from hyperactivity leading to convulsions and repeated seizures. Plasma concentration of MDMA was 0.11 mg/L. She underwent a liver transplantation after 4 days but died after 18 days.

An 18-year-old male ingested 3 tablets and suffered from seizures and sweating. The MDMA concentration was 1.26 mg/L in plasma. He died 6.5 h after admission.

A 23-year-old male ingested 3 tablets and suffered from convulsions and agitation. The MDMA plasma concentration was 0.2 mg/L. He was hospitalised for 33 days.

A 19-year-old female ingested 2 tablets and suffered from vomiting, and watery diarrhoea, and was in a coma. Plasma concentrations were MDMA 0.24, MDA 0.02, and amfetamine 0.02 mg/L. She recovered. [J. Henry *et al.*, *Lancet*, 1992, *340*, 384–387.]

Half-life. About 6 to 7 h.

Clearance. The mean total clearance of MDMA for a 75 mg dose is 86.9 L/h.

Protein binding. About 65%

Note. For a solid-phase extraction method and its use in profiling ecstasy tablets, see A. M. Rashed *et al.*, *J. Forensic Sci.*, 2000, *45*, 413–417. For a review of Ecstasy: history, neurochemistry and toxicology, see J. A. Rochester and J. T. Kirchner, *J. Am. Board Fam. Pract.*, 1999, *12*, 137–142; see also G.A. Ricaurte *et al.*, *Toxicol. Lett.*, 2000, vol. 112–113, 143–146; and H. H. Maurer, *Ther. Drug Monit.*, 1996, *18*, 465–470. For a review of MDMA deaths in New York City, see J. R. Gill *et al.*, *J. Forensic. Sci.*, 2002, *47*, 121–126. For a report on MDMA and driving impairment, see B. K. Logan and F. J. Couper, *J. Forensic Sci.*, 2001, *46*, 1426–1433; see also M. R. Moeller and M. Hartung, *J. Anal. Toxicol.*, 1997, *21*, 591.

Dose. The usual dose is between 80 and 200 mg (more often 100 to 150 mg).

Methylephedrine

Sympathomimetic

Synonyms. *l*-Methylephedrine; *l*-*N*-Methylephedrine.
α-[1-(Dimethylamino)ethyl]benzenemethanol
$C_{11}H_{17}NO=179.3$
CAS—552-79-4

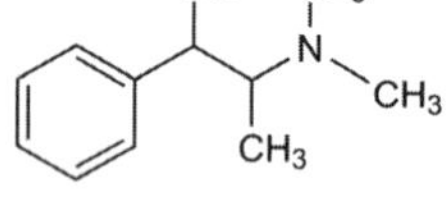

Soluble in chloroform and ether.

Methylephedrine Hydrochloride

Proprietary names. It is an ingredient of Coughmin, Hustazol-C, Ilvico, Methorcon, Tossamine plus, and Tussoretardin.
$C_{11}H_{17}NO,HCl=215.7$
CAS—38455-90-2
A white crystalline powder. M.p. 207° to 208° (crystals from acetone). Freely soluble in water; soluble in ethanol; practically insoluble in ether.

Dissociation Constant. pK_a 9.3 (25°).

Partition Coefficient. Log *P* (octanol/water), 0.9.

Thin-layer Chromatography. System TA—Rf 32; system TE—Rf 35; system TAE—Rf 12. (Acidified iodoplatinate solution, positive.)

Gas Chromatography. System GA—methylephedrine RI 1405, ephedrine RI 1365; system GB—methylephedrine RI 1451, ephedrine RI 1410; system GC—methylephedrine RI 1480, ephedrine RI 1467.

High Performance Liquid Chromatography. System HA—methylephedrine *k* 2.3, ephedrine *k* 1.0; system HC—methylephedrine *k* 1.83, ephedrine *k* 1.79.

Ultraviolet Spectrum. Aqueous acid—251, 257 ($A_1^1=11a$), 263 nm. (See below)

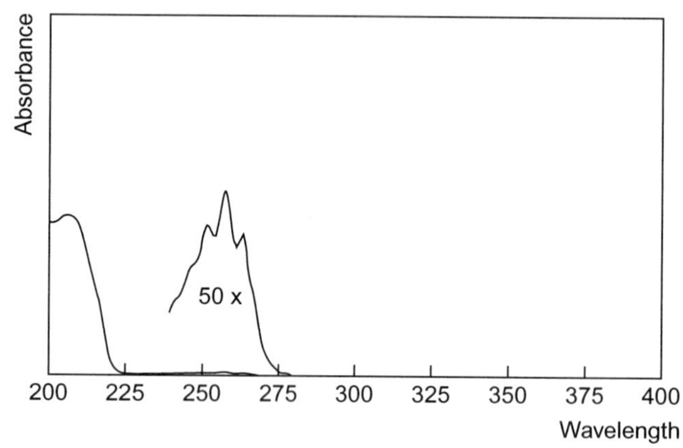

Infra-red Spectrum. Principal peaks at wavenumbers 742, 1039, 702, 1052, 990, 1162 cm^{-1} (KBr disk). (See below)

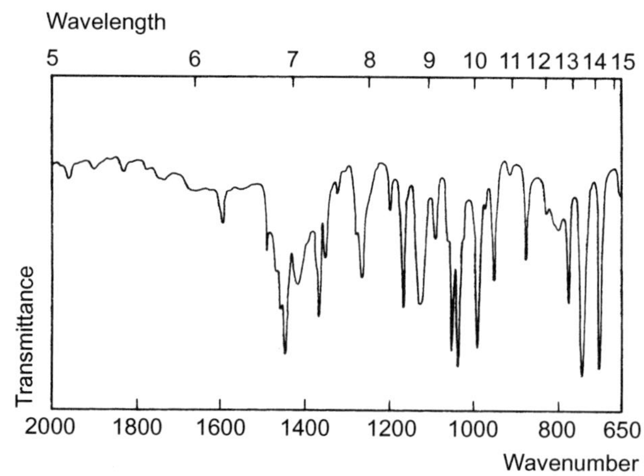

Mass Spectrum. Principal ions at *m/z* 58, 72, 30, 77, 56, 44, 42, 73; ephedrine 58, 146, 56, 105, 77, 42, 106, 40.

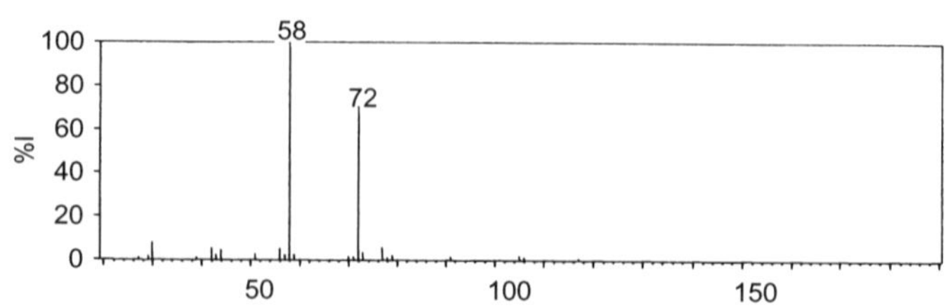

Quantification

Gas chromatography. In blood or urine: nitrogen–phosphorus detection—G. W. Kunsman *et al.*, *J. Anal. Toxicol.*, 1998, *22*, 310–313. In urine: methylephedrine and other ephedrines, nitrogen–phosphorus detection—P. Van Eenoo *et al.*, *J. Chromatogr. B Biomed. Sci. Appl.*, 2001, *760*, 255–261.

Gas chromatography–mass spectrometry. In hair: methylephedrine, ephedrine, and phenylpropanolamine, limit of quantification 0.5 ng/mg—Y.

Nakahara and R. Kikura, *J. Chromatogr. B Biomed. Sci. Appl.*, 1997, *700*, 83–91.

High performance liquid chromatography. In urine: methylephedrine and other ephedrines, UV detection—C. Imaz *et al.*, *J. Chromatogr.*, 1993, *631*, 201–205; P. J. van der Merwe *et al.*, *J. Chromatogr. B Biomed. Appl.*, 1994, *661*, 357–361.

Disposition in the Body. Absorbed after oral administration. About 32% of a dose is excreted in the urine unchanged and 8% is excreted as the demethylated metabolite, ephedrine; the rate of excretion is dependent on the urinary pH.

Toxicity

Although methylephedrine is not available in the USA, it was identified in 15 cases received by the Armed Forces Institute of Pathology, Rockville, Maryland. Blood methylephedrine concentrations ranged from less than 0.05 to 0.28 mg/L whilst the mean methylephedrine urine concentration was 1.6 mg/L (range 0.15 to 6.8 mg/L). As no evidence suggested that methylephedrine was present at toxic concentrations, it appears that blood methylephedrine concentrations of less than 0.3 mg/L are not associated with significant toxicity [G. W. Kunsman *et al.*, *J. Anal. Toxicol.*, 1998, *22*, 310–313].

A 19-year-old white male was found dead in his family's home. Postmortem examination revealed the following drug concentrations (mg/L): methylephedrine (5.6), dihydrocodeine (4.7), chlorphenamine (2.6), salicylate (150.0) and verapamil (6.0). The first three drugs listed appear in an over-the-counter cold medication, in Japan, under the trade name Bron. The cause of death was multiple drug intoxication [B. Levine *et al.*, *J. Anal. Toxicol.*, 1993, *17*, 381–383].

Note. For a study of the metabolism of methylephedrine in rat and man see T. Inoue and S. Suzuki, *Xenobiotica*, 1990, *20*, 99–106.

Dose. Methylephedrine hydrochloride has been given in doses of up to 200 mg daily in divided doses.

Methylergometrine

Uterine Stimulant

Synonyms. Methylergobasine; Methylergonovine.
(8*β*)-9,10-Didehydro-*N*-[(1*S*)-1-(hydroxymethyl)propyl]-6-methylergoline-8-carboxamide
$C_{20}H_{25}N_3O_2$=339.4
CAS—113-42-8

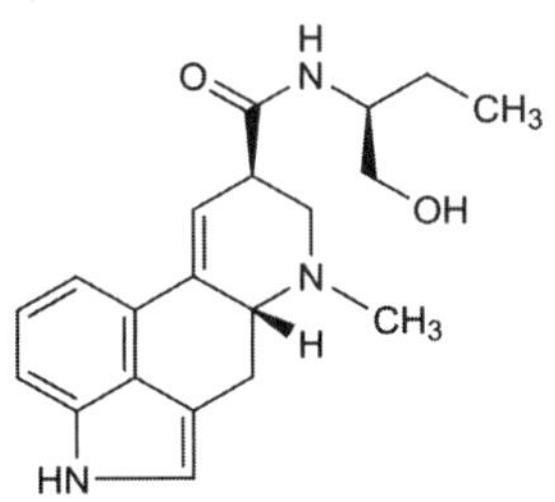

Crystals. M.p. 172°, with decomposition.
Sparingly soluble in water; freely soluble in ethanol and acetone.

Methylergometrine Maleate

Proprietary names. Basofortina; Ergotyl; Metenerin; Methergin(e); Methylergobrevin; Metrine; Nathergen; Ryegonovin; Spametrin-M.
$C_{20}H_{25}N_3O_2,C_4H_4O_4$=455.5
CAS—57432-61-8
A white or pinkish-tan, crystalline powder, which darkens on exposure to light.
M.p. 185° to 195°, with decomposition.
Soluble 1 in 200 of water and 1 in 140 of ethanol giving a blue fluorescence; very slightly soluble in chloroform and ether.

Dissociation Constant. pK_a 6.7 (24°).

Partition Coefficient. Log *P* (octanol/water), 1.0.

Colour Tests. Mandelin's Test—violet-brown; Marquis Test—grey-brown.

Thin-layer Chromatography. System TA—Rf 62; system TB—Rf 00; system TC—Rf 14; system TE—Rf 41; system TL—Rf 12; system TM—Rf 31; system TAE—Rf 69. (Van Urk reagent, blue.)

Gas Chromatography. System GA—not eluted.

High Performance Liquid Chromatography. System HA—*k* 0.4; system HP—*k* 0.83; system HX—RI 320; system HZ—Retention time 2.1 min.

Ultraviolet Spectrum. Aqueous acid—313 (A_1^1=255a); aqueous alkali—310 nm.

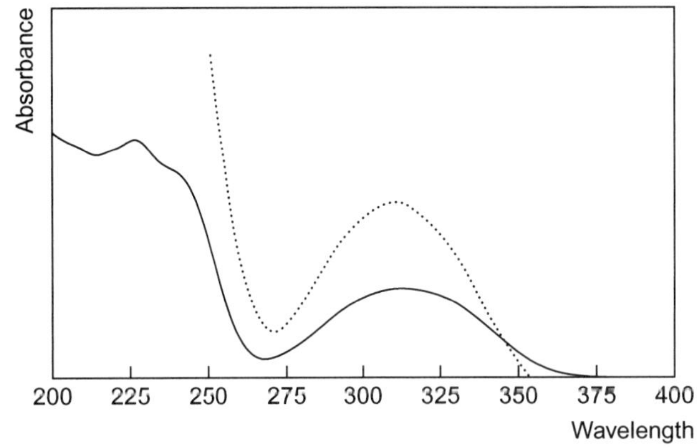

Infra-red Spectrum. Principal peaks at wavenumbers 1580, 1490, 1650, 1620, 1065, 1103 cm^{-1} (KBr disk).

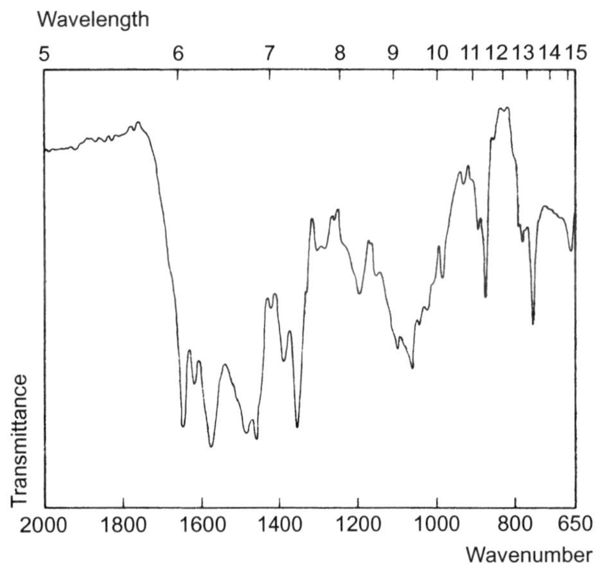

Mass Spectrum. Principal ions at *m/z* 339, 221, 196, 181, 207, 223, 222, 72.

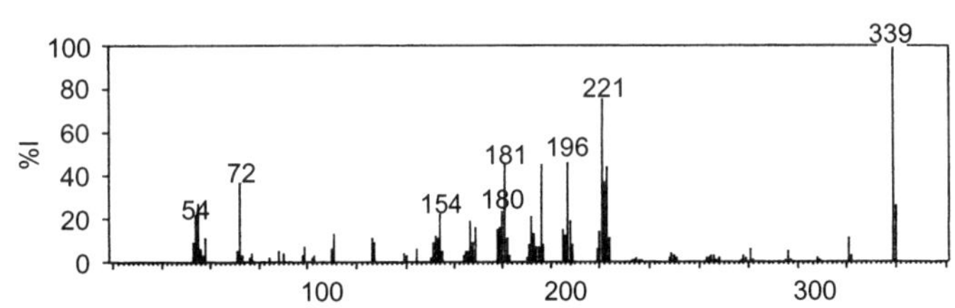

Quantification

High performance liquid chromatography. In plasma or serum: methylergometrine and ergotamine, limit of detection 100 ng/L, fluorescence detection—P. O. Edlund, *J. Chromatogr.*, 1981, *226*; *B Biomed. Appl.*, *15*, 107–115.

Disposition in the Body. Rapidly absorbed after oral administration. About 2 to 3% of a dose is excreted in the urine as unchanged drug in 24 h.

Therapeutic concentration

After a single oral dose of 0.25 mg to 6 subjects, peak plasma concentrations of about 0.003 mg/L were attained in 0.5 h [R. Mantyla *et al.*, *Int. J. Clin. Pharmacol. Biopharm.*, 1978, *16*, 254–257.]

Half-life. Plasma half-life, about 2 h.

Volume of distribution. About 0.5 L/kg.

Protein binding. In plasma, about 35%.

Dose. 0.375 to 1 mg of methylergometrine maleate daily, for up to 7 days.

Methylpentynol

Hypnotic/Sedative

Synonyms. Meparfynol; Methylparafynol.
Proprietary names. Allotopral; Oblivon.
3-Methyl-1-pentyn-3-ol
$C_6H_{10}O$=98.14
CAS—77-75-8

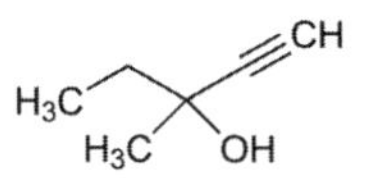

A colourless or pale yellow liquid. Mass per mL 0.865 to 0.873 g. B.p. about 120°. Refractive index, at 20°, 1.430 to 1.432.
Soluble 1 in 10 of water; soluble in ether; miscible with organic solvents.

Methylpentynol Carbamate

Synonym. Mepentamate
Proprietary names. Oblivon C; N-Oblivon.
$C_7H_{11}NO_2$=141.2
CAS—302-66-9
A white powder. M.p. 53° to 56°.
Soluble 1 in less than 200 of water, 1 in 1 of ethanol, and 1 in 2 of chloroform.

Partition Coefficient. Log *P* (octanol/water), 0.9.

Thin-layer Chromatography. Methylpentynol carbamate: system TD—Rf 49; system TE—Rf 74; system TF—Rf 62; system TAD—Rf 57. (Furfuraldehyde reagent, positive; acidified potassium permanganate solution, positive.)

Gas Chromatography. System GA—RI 715; system GI—Retention time 20.1 min.

Infra-red Spectrum. Principal peaks at wavenumbers 917, 1126, 1156, 995, 1030, 1050 cm^{-1} (thin film).

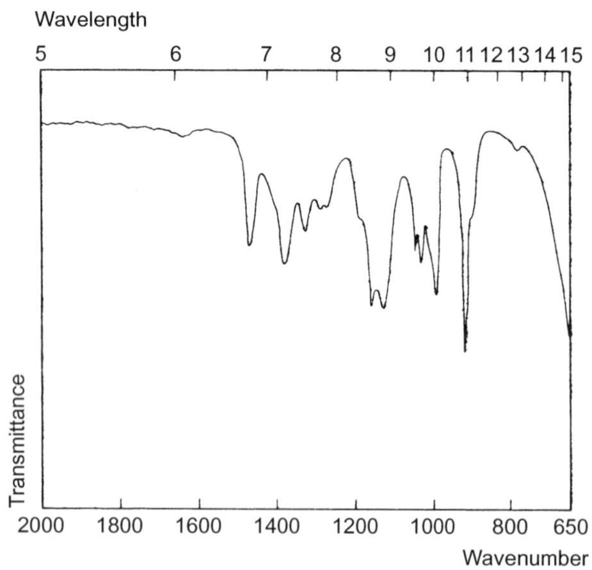

Mass Spectrum. Principal ions at *m/z* 69, 83, 43, 79, 41, 81, 53, 80 (methylpentynol carbamate).

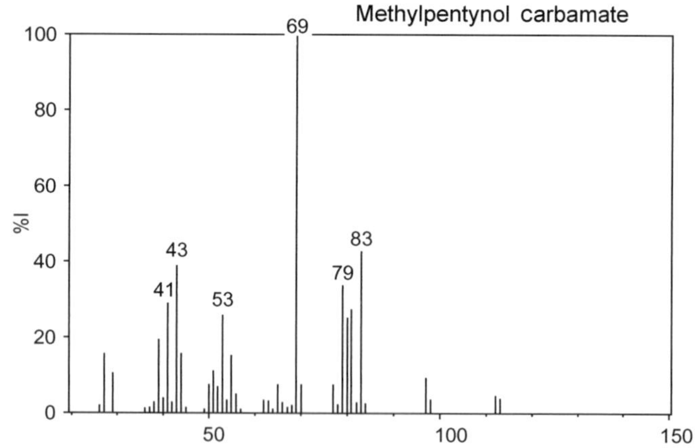

Quantification

Gas chromatography. In serum (methylpentynol) or urine (4-hydroxymethylpentynol): FID—J. Grove and B. K. Martin, *J. Chromatogr.*, 1977, *133*, 267–272.

Disposition in the Body. Absorbed after oral administration. It is almost completely metabolised with less than 1% being excreted in the urine as unchanged drug in 7 days; higher amounts of unchanged drug may be excreted after large doses. The major metabolite is the *N*-glucuronide which accounts for about 80% of the dose; the 4-hydroxy metabolite accounts for about 13% of a dose.

Toxicity. A fatality has been reported after a dose of 5 g although recoveries have occurred after ingestion of up to 10 g. Repeated medication may cause toxic reactions in the liver and skin.

A liver concentration of 1100 µg/g and a urine concentration of 410 mg/L were reported in one fatal poisoning case [J. V. Jackson, 1967-personal communication.]

Dose. 0.5 to 1 g daily.

Methylphenidate

Central Stimulant

Synonyms. Methyl Phenidate; Methyl Phenidylacetate; Methylphenidan.
α-Phenyl-2-piperidineacetic acid methyl ester
$C_{14}H_{19}NO_2$=233.3
CAS—113-45-1

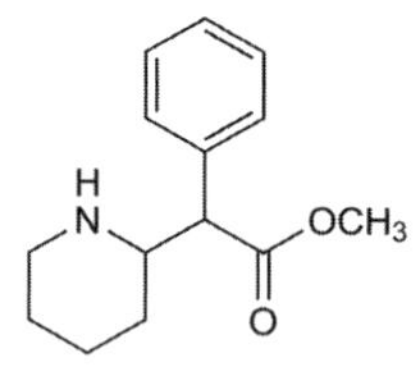

Crystals. M.p. 74° to 75°.
Practically insoluble in water and petroleum ether; soluble in ethanol, ethyl acetate and ether.

Methylphenidate Hydrochloride

Synonym. Ciba 4311b
Proprietary names. Attenta; Centedrin; Concerta; Equasym; Focalin; Metadate; Methidate; Methylin; Riphenidate; Ritalin(a); Ritaline; Rubifen.
$C_{14}H_{19}NO_2$,HCl=269.8
CAS—298-59-9
Fine, white, crystalline powder or acicular crystals. M.p. 224° to 226°.
Soluble in water, alcohol, and chloroform.

Dissociation Constant. pK_a 8.9.

Partition Coefficient. Log *P* (octanol/water), 0.2.

Colour Test. Liebermann's Test—orange.

Thin-layer Chromatography. System TA—Rf 57; system TB—Rf 35; system TC—Rf 41; system TE—Rf 66; system TL—Rf 23; system TAE—Rf 40; system TAF—Rf 70; system TAJ—Rf 11; system TAK—Rf 04;

system TAL—Rf 70. (Dragendorff spray, positive; acidified iodoplatinate solution, positive; ninhydrin spray, positive; acidified potassium permanganate solution, positive.)

Gas Chromatography. System GA—methylphenidate RI 1725, methylphenidate-AC RI 2085, methylphenidate-TFA RI 1730; system GB—methylphenidate RI 1793; system GC—methylphenidate RI 2200; system GF—methylphenidate RI 1935.

High Performance Liquid Chromatography. System HA—*k* 1.7; system HC—*k* 0.36; system HY—RI 277; system HAX—Retention time 8.6 min; system HAY—Retention time 4.7 min.

Ultraviolet Spectrum. Aqueous acid—251, 257 (A^1_1=9.0a), 264 nm. No alkaline shift.

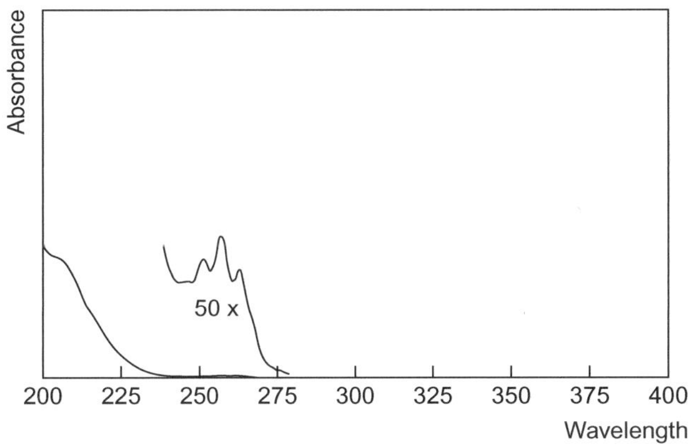

Infra-red Spectrum. Principal peaks at wavenumbers 1735, 1175, 1210, 1150, 705, 740 cm^{-1} (methylphenidate hydrochloride, KCl disk).

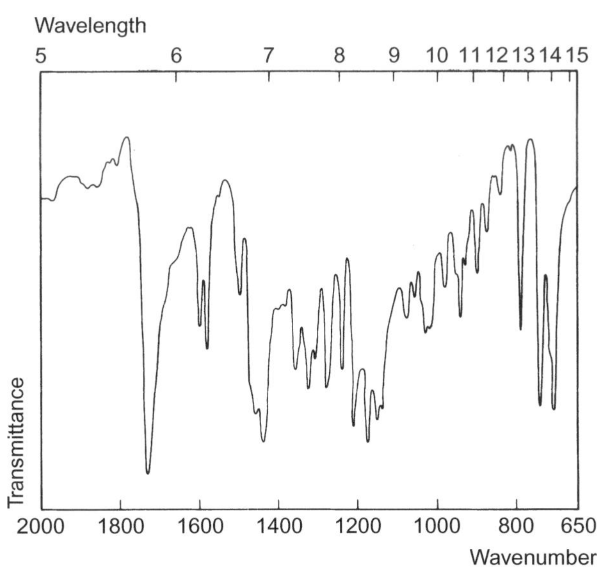

Mass Spectrum. Principal ions at *m*/*z* 84, 91, 85, 56, 55, 150, 41, 118 (no peaks above 150).

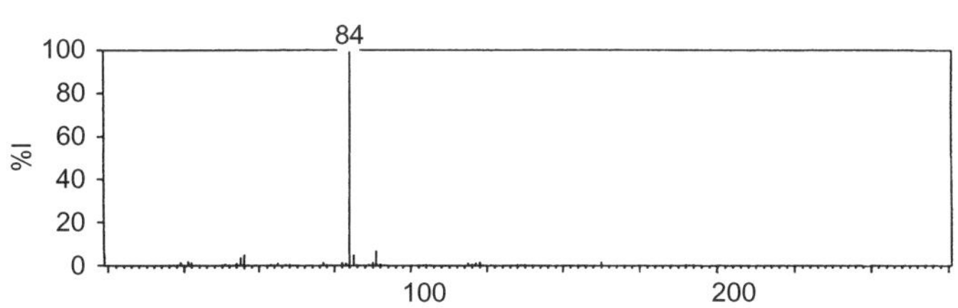

Quantification

Gas chromatography. In urine: limit of detection 30 µg/L, AFID—R. Dugal *et al.*, *J. Anal. Toxicol.*, 1978, *2*, 101–106. In urine: ritalinic acid, limit of detection about 1 mg/L, FID—H. W. Allen and B. Sedgwick, *J. Anal. Toxicol.*, 1984, *8*, 61–62. In plasma: methylphenidate and ritalinic acid, ECD—N. R. Srinivas *et al.*, *J. Chromatogr.*, 1990, *530*, 327–336. In urine: ritalinic acid, limit of detection 50 µg/L, NPD—T. Vu-Duc and A. Vernay, *J. Pharm. Biomed. Anal.*, 1992, *10*, 187–191.

Gas chromatography–mass spectrometry. In blood or urine: methylphenidate and ritalinic acid, limit of detection about 2 µg/L and 60 µg/L respectively—R. M. Milberg *et al.*, *Biomed. Mass Spectrom.*, 1975, *2*, 2–8. In urine: methylphenidate and ritalinic acid—A. Solans *et al.*, *J. Chromatogr. B Biomed. Appl.*, 1994, *658*, 380–384. In plasma: limit of quantification 0.75 µg/L—S. N. Lin *et al.*, *J. Anal. Toxicol.*, 1999, *23*, 524–530. In plasma: limit of quantification about 0.15 µg/L—H. J. Leis *et al.*, *J. Mass Spectrom.*, 2000, *35*, 1100–1104.

High performance liquid chromatography. In serum: methylphenidate and ritalinic acid, limit of detection 20 µg/L, UV detection—S. J. Soldin *et al.*, *Clin. Chem.*, 1979, *25*, 401–404.

Disposition in the Body. Readily absorbed after oral administration. The rate but not the amount absorbed is increased by the presence of food in the stomach. About 80% of a dose is excreted in the urine in 24 h, of which 60 to 80% is ritalinic acid and 5 to 12% is 6-oxo-α-phenylpiperidine-2-acetic acid; only a small amount is excreted as unchanged drug.

Therapeutic concentration

Following a single oral dose of 20 mg to 2 subjects, peak plasma concentrations of 0.013 and 0.058 mg/L were attained in 3 h; ritalinic acid concentrations averaged 0.22 mg/L at the same time [R. M. Milberg *et al.*, *Biomed. Mass Spectrom.*, 1975, *2*, 2–8].

Following oral doses of 10 to 30 mg daily, administered to 4 hyperkinetic children, peak plasma concentrations of 0.008 to 0.023 mg/L (mean 0.018) were reported [B. L. Hungund *et al.*, *Br. J. Clin. Pharmacol.*, 1979, *8*, 571–576].

35 subjects were given methylphenidate hydrochloride in single oral doses of 18, 36, or 54 mg, in the form of one, two, or three 18-mg OROS (oral, osmotic, controlled-release) systems. Mean peak plasma concentrations of D-methylphenidate and L-methylphenidate after the 18-, 36-, and 54-mg doses were 0.00387 and 0.000095 mg/L (at 7.9 and 7.1 h), 0.00728 and 0.00017 mg/L (at 7.5 and 7.0 h), and 0.0106 and 0.00036 mg/L (at 7.2 and 6.1 h); corresponding mean peak plasma concentrations of D-ritalinic acid and L-ritalinic acid were 0.053 and 0.069 mg/L (at 8.8 and 8.1 h), 0.105 and 0.132 mg/L (at 8.8 and 7.6 h), and 0.155 and 0.192 mg/L (at 8.5 and 7.8 h) [N. B. Modi *et al.*, *J. Clin. Pharmacol.*, 2000, *40*, 1141–1149].

Toxicity. The estimated minimum lethal dose for adults is 2 g but few instances of serious toxicity due to overdosage have been reported. Abuse and dependence of the amfetamine type is not uncommon.

In 2 suicide victims who had overdosed on methylphenidate (co-ingested with ethanol), the following concentrations were reported at postmortem (mg/L or µg/g):

	Methylphenidate	Ritalinic acid	Ethylphenidate
Case 1			
Peripheral blood	0.310	2.8	0.008
Case 2			
Peripheral blood	1.6	2.0	0.001
Liver	0.310	1.2	0.002

[J. S. Markowitz *et al.*, *J. Clin. Psychopharmacol.*, 1999, *19*, 362–366].

The following postmortem tissue concentrations were reported in an accidental overdose fatality involving the IV injection of crushed methylphenidate tablets: blood 2.8 mg/L, bile 5.7 mg/L, kidney 3.0 µg/g, liver 2.1 µg/g, stomach contents 1.6 mg (total); other drugs were not detected [B. Levine, *J. Anal. Toxicol.*, 1986, *10*, 209–210].

Urine concentrations of 0.8 to 40 mg/L (mean 16) were reported in six arrested drivers who showed signs of drowsiness or hyperactivity [B. Schubert, *Acta Chem. Scand.*, 1970, *24*, 433–438].

Bioavailability. About 30% (11 to 51%) because it undergoes extensive first-pass metabolism.

Half-life. Plasma half-life, about 2 h, ritalinic acid about 8 h.

Volume of distribution. About 2.6 L/kg.

Clearance. Plasma, about 6.5 mg/min/kg

Protein binding. In plasma, about 15%.

Note. For a review of the pharmacokinetics and clinical effectiveness of methylphenidate, see H. C. Kimko *et al.*, *Clin. Pharmacokinet.*, 1999, *37*, 457–470 and for a review of its toxicity and abuse, see W. Klein-Schwartz, *Curr. Opin. Pediatr.*, 2002, *14*, 219–223.

Dose. Usually up to 60 mg of methylphenidate hydrochloride daily.

Methylphenobarbital

Sedative/Barbiturate

Synonyms. Enphenemalum; Mephobarbital; Methylphenobarbitone; Phemitone.
Proprietary names. Mebaral; Prominal.
5-Ethyl-1-methyl-5-phenyl-2,4,6(1*H*,3*H*,5*H*)-pyrimidinetrione
$C_{13}H_{14}N_2O_3$=246.3
CAS—115-38-8

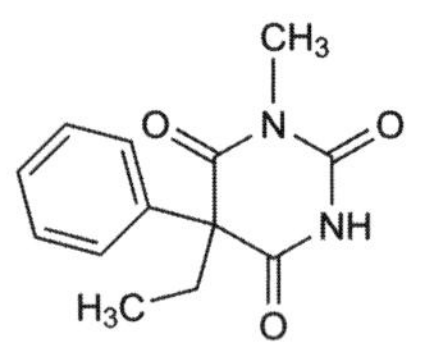

Colourless crystals or white crystalline powder. M.p. 176°.
Slightly soluble in cold water, freely soluble in hot water; soluble 1 in 240 of ethanol, 1 in 40 of chloroform, and 1 in 200 of ether; soluble in solutions of ammonia, alkali hydroxides, and carbonates.

Dissociation Constant. pK_a 7.8 (20°).

Partition Coefficient. Log *P* (octanol/water), 1.8.

Colour Tests. Koppanyi–Zwikker Test—violet; Liebermann's Test—red-orange; Mercurous Nitrate—black.

Thin-layer Chromatography. System TD—Rf 70; system TE—Rf 41; system TF—Rf 67; system TH—Rf 72; system TAD—Rf 70; system TAE—Rf 86. (Mercurous nitrate spray, black; Zwikker's reagent, faint pink.)

Gas Chromatography. System GA—methylphenobarbital RI 1890; phenobarbital RI 1953; methylphenobarbital-Me RI 1855; M (OH-) RI 2370; M (OH-methoxy-) RI 2310; M (nor-OH-) RI 2295; system GB—methylphenobarbital RI 2222; system GAJ—methylphenobarbital RRT 1.000.

High Performance Liquid Chromatography. System HG—*k* 7.27; system HH—*k* 3.84; system HX—RI 435; system HY—RI 395; system HZ—Retention time 4.6 min.

Ultraviolet Spectrum. Borax buffer 0.05 M (pH 9.2)—244 (A^1_1=355c); 1 M sodium hydroxide (pH 13)—243 nm (A^1_1=329b).

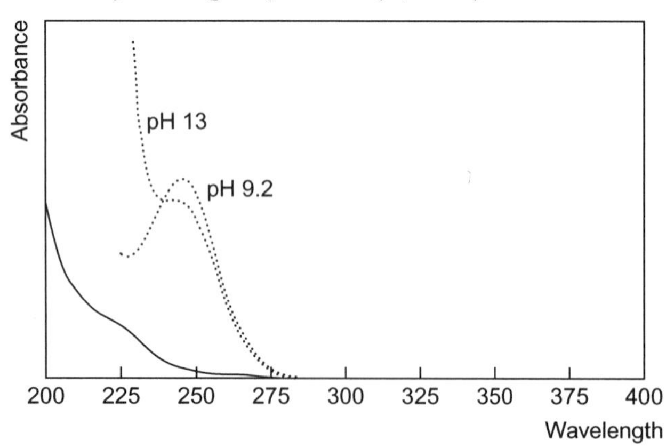

Infra-red Spectrum. Principal peaks at wavenumbers 1707, 1684, 1754, 720, 1298, 1050 cm^{-1} (KBr disk).

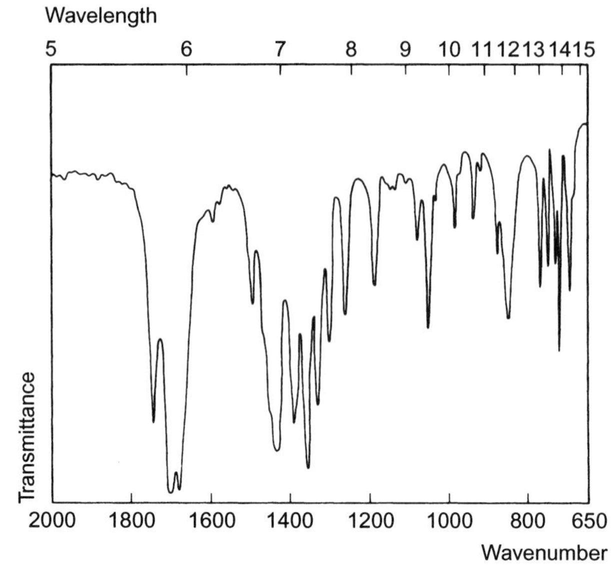

Mass Spectrum. Principal ions at *m/z* 218, 117, 118, 146, 103, 77, 91, 115; phenobarbital 204, 117, 146, 161, 77, 103, 115, 118.

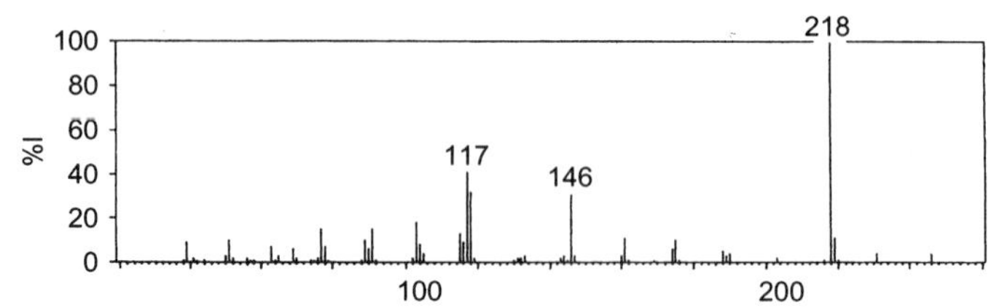

Quantification. See also under Amylobarbital.

Gas chromatography. In plasma or serum: methylphenobarbital and phenobarbital, FID—W. D. Hooper *et al.*, *J. Chromatogr.*, 1975, *110*, 206–209.

Gas chromatography–mass spectrometry. In plasma: methylphenobarbital and phenobarbital, limit of detection 20 µg/L for both compounds—W. D. Hooper *et al.*, *J. Chromatogr.*, 1981, *223*; *Biomed. Appl.*, *12*, 426–431.

High performance liquid chromatography. In serum: methylphenobarbital, phenobarbital and other anticonvulsants, limit of detection 500 µg/L, UV detection—P. M. Kabra *et al.*, *J. Anal. Toxicol.*, 1978, *2*, 127–133. In urine: the metabolites phenobarbital, *p*-hydroxyphenobarbital and *p*-hydroxymethylphenobarbital, limit of detection 500 µg/L for each compound, UV detection—H. E. Kunze *et al.*, *Ther. Drug Monit.*, 1981, *3*, 45–49.

Disposition in the Body. Incompletely absorbed after oral administration. Metabolised by *N*-demethylation to the active metabolite, phenobarbital, and by *p*-hydroxylation. Over a period of 10 days, less than 2% of a dose is excreted in the urine as unchanged drug, about 30 to 35% is excreted as *p*-hydroxymethylphenobarbital both free and conjugated, and up to 10% may be excreted as phenobarbital. Small amounts of *p*-hydroxyphenobarbital, 5-ethyl-5-(4-hydroxy-3-methoxyphenyl)barbituric acid, and 5-ethyl-5-(4-hydroxy-3-methoxyphenyl)-1-methylbarbituric acid have also been detected in the urine.

Therapeutic concentration

Following a single oral dose of 800 mg to 2 subjects, peak plasma concentrations of about 3 mg/L were attained in 3 to 6 h; peak phenobarbital plasma concentrations of 2 to 3 mg/L were attained in 4 to 6 days [W. D. Hooper *et al.*, *Ther. Drug Monit.*, 1981, *3*, 39–44.]

Following daily oral doses of 60 to 600 mg to 11 subjects, steady-state plasma concentrations of 0.2 to 1.7 mg/L (mean 0.9) of methylphenobarbital and 4 to 32 mg/L (mean 15) of phenobarbital were reported [H. J. Kupferberg and J. Longacre-Shaw, *Ther. Drug Monit.*, 1979, *1*, 117–122.]

Toxicity. The estimated minimum lethal dose is 2 g.

Bioavailability. About 70%.

Half-life. Plasma half-life, methylphenobarbital about 50 to 60 h, phenobarbital about 100 h.

Volume of distribution. About 2 to 3 L/kg.

Clearance. Plasma clearance, about 0.5 mL/min/kg.

Protein binding. In plasma, about 40 to 60%.

Dose. 90 to 600 mg daily.

Methylpiperidyl Benzilate *Hallucinogen*

1-Methyl-3-piperidyl benzilate
$C_{20}H_{23}NO_3$=325.4
CAS—3321-80-0

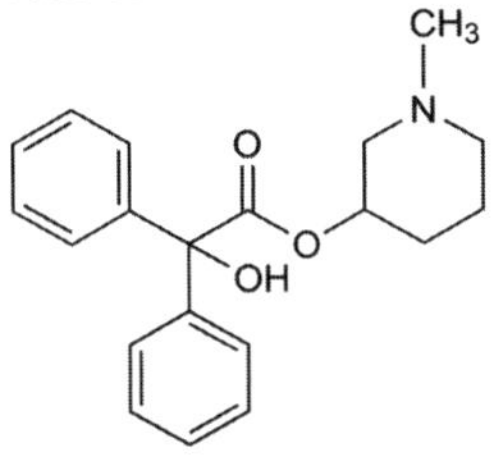

A clear liquid.
Practically insoluble in water; soluble in chloroform and most organic solvents.

Methylpiperidyl Benzilate Hydrochloride
A white powder. M.p. 212° to 218°, with decomposition.
Soluble in water; practically insoluble in chloroform.

Colour Tests. Liebermann's Test—brown; Mandelin's Test—orange→brown→green; Marquis Test—orange→green→blue; Sulfuric Acid—orange.

Thin-layer Chromatography. System TA—Rf 60; system TB—Rf 30; system TC—Rf 58; system TE—Rf 73; system TL—Rf 33; system TAE—Rf 58; system TAF—Rf 50. (Acidified iodoplatinate solution, positive.)

High Performance Liquid Chromatography. System HX—RI 377.

Ultraviolet Spectrum. Aqueous acid—251 (A_1^1=18b), 257 nm (A_1^1=20b).

Infra-red Spectrum. Principal peaks at wavenumbers 1734, 1195, 965, 685, 1160, 720 cm^{-1} (methylpiperidyl benzilate hydrochloride, KBr disk).

Mass Spectrum. Principal ions at *m/z* 97, 105, 77, 183, 84, 36, 42, 51.

Methylprednisolone *Corticosteroid*

Synonym. 6α-Methylprednisolone
Proprietary names. Esametone; Firmacort; Medrol; Medrone; Metilpren; Metisona; Metypred; Metysolon; Radilem; Urbason.
(6α,11β)-11,17,21-Trihydroxy-6-methylpregna-1,4-diene-3,20-dione
$C_{22}H_{30}O_5$=374.5
CAS—83-43-2

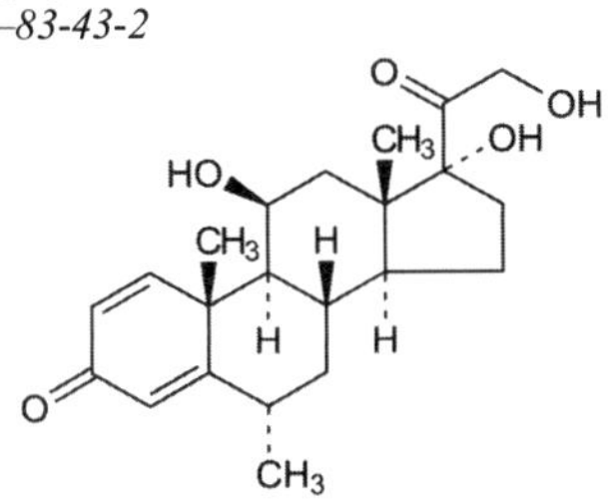

A white crystalline powder. M.p. about 228° to 237°. A solution in dioxan is dextrorotatory.
Practically insoluble in water; soluble 1 in 100 of dehydrated alcohol; slightly soluble in acetone and chloroform; very slightly soluble in ether; sparingly soluble in dioxan and methanol.

Methylprednisolone Acetate
Synonym. 6α-Methylprednisolone 21-Acetate
Proprietary names. Adlone; Depoject; depMedalone; Depo Moderin; Depomedrate; Depo-Medrol; Depo-Medrone; Depo-Nisolone; Depopred; D-Med; Duralone; Medralone; Medrate; Medrone; Metypred; M-Prednisol; Solsolona.
$C_{24}H_{32}O_6$=416.5
CAS—53-36-1
A white crystalline powder. M.p. 205° to 208°.
Practically insoluble in water; sparingly soluble in ethanol and acetone; soluble 1 in 250 of chloroform and 1 in 1500 of ether; soluble in dioxan.

Methylprednisolone Hemisuccinate
Synonym. Methylprednisolone Hydrogen Succinate
Proprietary name. Asmacortone
$C_{26}H_{34}O_8$=474.5
CAS—2921-57-5
A white hygroscopic solid.
Very slightly soluble in water; freely soluble in ethanol; soluble in acetone.

Methylprednisolone Sodium Succinate
Synonym. Sodium 6α-Methylprednisolone 21-Succinate
Proprietary names. A-methapred; Emmetipi; Firmacort; Metypred; Metypresol; Solu-Medrol; Solu-Medrone; Solu-Moderin; Urbason.
$C_{26}H_{33}NaO_8$=496.5
CAS—2375-03-3
A white, hygroscopic, amorphous powder.
Soluble 1 in 1.5 of water and 1 in 12 of ethanol; practically insoluble in chloroform and ether; very slightly soluble in acetone.

Partition Coefficient. Log *P* (octanol/water), 1.8.

Thin-layer Chromatography. System TA—Rf 87; system TB—Rf 00; system TE—Rf 41; system TF—Rf 27; system TP—Rf 23; system TQ—Rf 80; system TR—Rf 03; system TS—Rf 00; system TAE—Rf 87; system TAJ—Rf 31; system TAK—Rf 13; system TAL—Rf 78; system TAM—Rf 56.

High Performance Liquid Chromatography. System HT—*k* 7.5; system HX—RI 426; system HY—RI 390; system HAA—Retention time 18.9 min.

Ultraviolet Spectrum. Dehydrated alcohol—240 nm (A_1^1=400a).

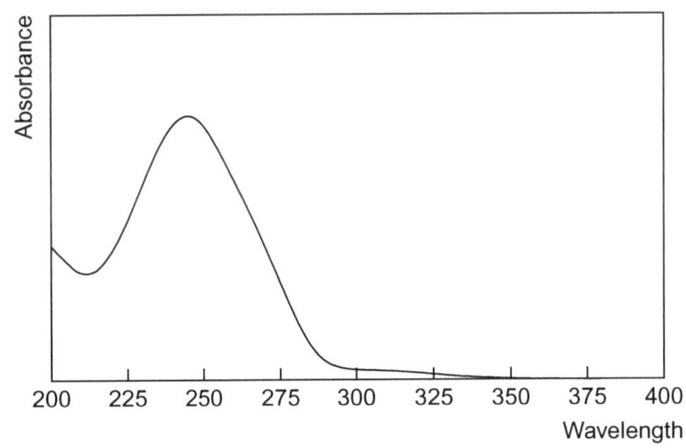

Infra-red Spectrum. Principal peaks at wavenumbers 1595, 1650, 1114, 914, 1313, 1248 cm^{-1} (KBr disk).

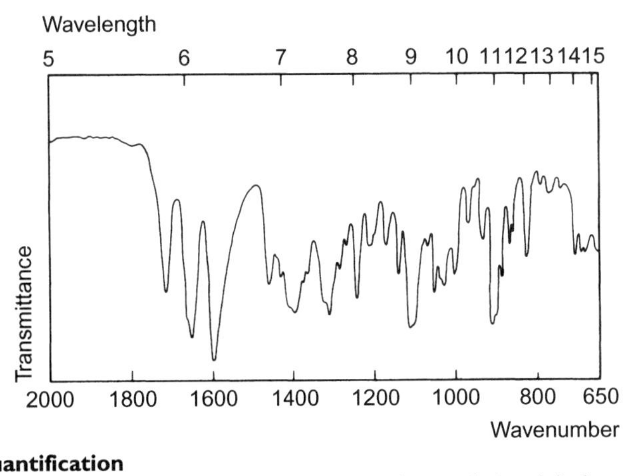

Quantification

Gas chromatography–mass spectrometry. In urine: methylprednisolone and its metabolites—G. M. Rodchenkov *et al.*, *J. Chromatogr.*, 1987, *423*, 15–22.

High performance liquid chromatography. In plasma: limit of detection about 7 µg/L, UV detection—J. A. Shah *et al.*, *J. Chromatogr.*, 1987, *414*, 1–10. In urine: limit of detection about 8 µg/L, UV detection—J. A. Shah and D. J. Weber, *J. Chromatogr.*, 1989, *496*, 245–254.

Dose. Usually 4 to 48 mg daily.

Methyltestosterone *Androgen*

Proprietary names. Android; Metandren; Neohombreol M; Oreton Methyl; Testotonic B; Testovis; Testred; Virilon. It is an ingredient of Prowess, Estratest, and Menogen.
(17*β*)-17-Hydroxy-17-methylandrost-4-en-3-one
$C_{20}H_{30}O_2$=302.5
CAS—58-18-4

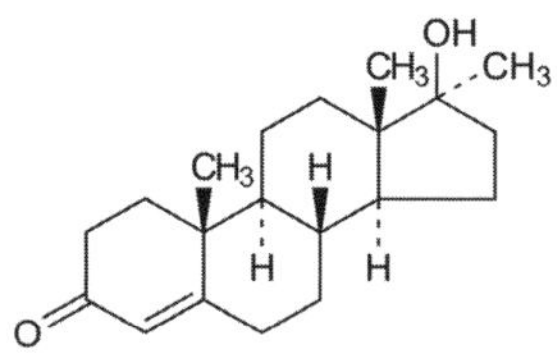

A white or slightly yellowish-white, slightly hygroscopic, crystalline powder. M.p. 162° to 168°. A solution in ethanol is dextrorotatory.
Practically insoluble in water; soluble 1 in 5 of ethanol; freely soluble in chloroform; soluble in ether.

Partition Coefficient. Log *P* (octanol/water), 3.4.

Thin-layer Chromatography. System TA—Rf 89; system TB—Rf 17; system TE—Rf 73; system TF—Rf 47; system TP—Rf 70; system TQ—Rf 16; system TR—Rf 91; system TS—Rf 71; system TAE—Rf 86; system TAF—Rf 86; system TAJ—Rf 60; system TAK—Rf 65; system TAL—Rf 92; system TAM—Rf 92.

Gas Chromatography. System GA—methyltestosterone RI 2645; methyltestosterone-AC RI 2770; methyltestosterone-TMS RI 2590; methyltestosterone enol-TMS_2 RI 2665; system GAG—RRT 1.05 (relative to testosterone); system GAI—urinary metabolite: 17α-methyl-5*β*, (α)-androstan-3α,17*β*-diol RRT 0.925 (relative to 17α-methyl-5α-androstan-3*β*,17*β*-diol); system GAR—methyltestosterone Retention time 13.1 min.

High Performance Liquid Chromatography. System HY—RI 587; system HATb—RRT 1.27 (relative to testosterone); system HAR—RRT 1.17 (relative to testosterone).

Ultraviolet Spectrum. Ethanol—241 nm (A^1_1=540a).

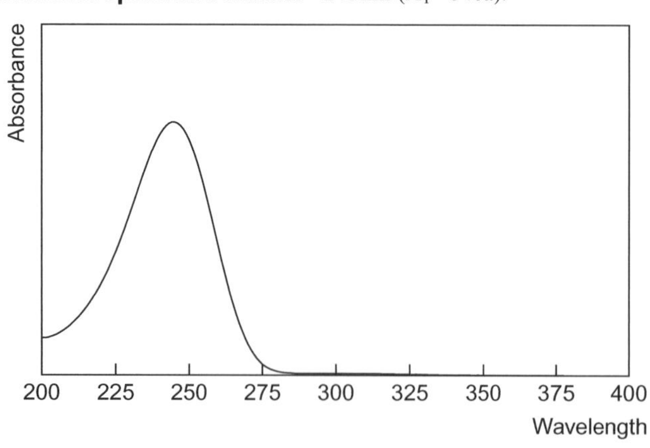

Infra-red Spectrum. Principal peaks at wavenumbers 1660, 1160, 1239, 950, 1612, 1090 cm^{-1} (KBr disk).

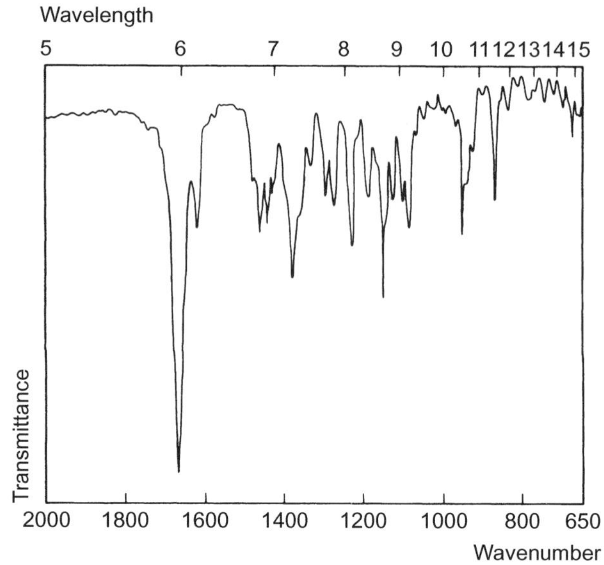

Mass Spectrum. Principal ions at *m/z* 302, 124, 43, 91, 79, 121, 105, 122.

Quantification
Spectrofluorimetry. In plasma or serum: limit of detection 1 µg/L—D. Alkalay *et al.*, *J. Pharm. Sci.*, 1972, *61*, 1746–1749.

Dose. 5 to 80 mg daily, by mouth; up to 200 mg daily has been given.

Methylthioamfetamine *Serotonin-Releasing Agent*

Synonyms. MTA; 4-MTA; *p*-methylthioamphetamine; α-methyl-4-methylthiophenethylamine.
Street names. Flatliners; Golden Eagle; MK; S-5.
α-Methyl-4-methylthiobenzeneethanamine
$C_{10}H_{15}NS$=181.3
CAS—14116-06-4

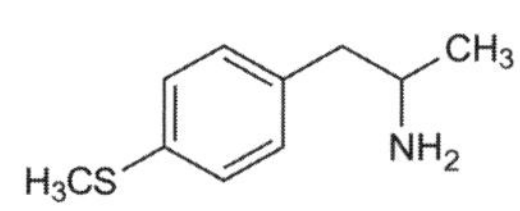

A white to off-white powder.

Colour Test. Marquis Test—no colour change; Cobalt Thiocyanate—blue.

Gas Chromatography. Column: DB5 (25 m x 0.32 mm i.d., 0.52 µm film thickness). Column temperature: 140°. Detection: nitrogen-phosphorus. Retention time: 4.3 min. [S. P. Elliott, *J. Anal. Toxicol.*, 2000, *24(2)*, 85–89.]

Column: HP Ultra-1 (12 m × 0.22 mm i.d., 0.25 µm film thickness). Column temperature: increased from 100° to 280° at 10°/min. Injector and detector temperature: 275° and 280°, respectively. MS detection, split ratio 50:1. Retention time: 5.1 min. [A. J. Poortman and E. Lock, *Forensic Sci. Int.*, 1999, *100*, 221–223.]

High Performance Liquid Chromatography. Column: (analytical) S5OD/CN (Spherisorb, 150 × 4.6 mm i.d.); (guard) S5ODS2 (Spherisorb, 10 × 4 mm i.d.). Mobile phase: acetonitrile:water (20:80), flow rate 2 mL/min. Internal standard: fenfluramine. UV detection (diode array, λ=205 and 255 nm). Retention time: MTA, 2.5 min; IS, 5.37 min. [S. P. Elliott, *J. Anal. Toxicol.*, 2000, *24(2)*, 85–89.]

Ultraviolet Spectrum. Acetonitrile—205, 255 nm; (0.025 M sulfuric acid)—254.5 nm.

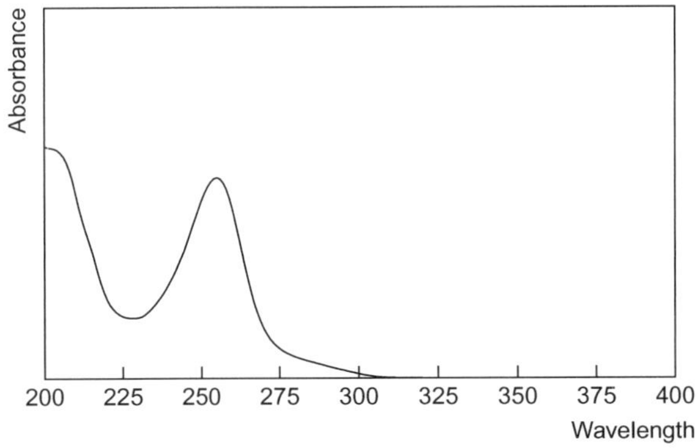

Infra-red Spectrum. Principal peaks at wavenumber 793, 1080, 1492, 1508, 1385, 843 cm^{-1} (hydrochloride).

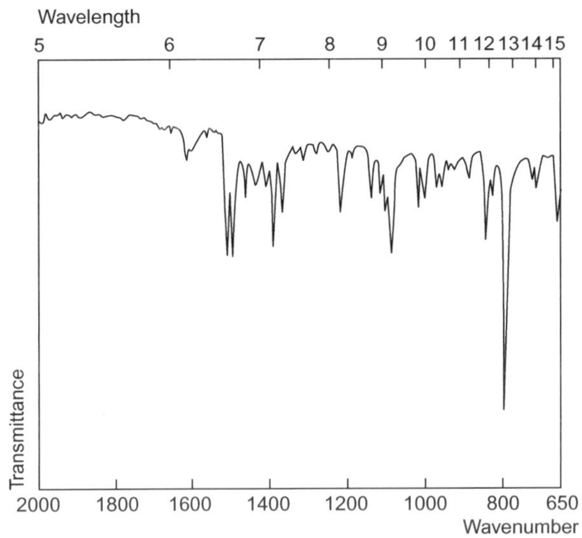

Mass Spectrum. Principal ions at *m/z* 44, 138, 122, 137, 121, 91, 78, 45.

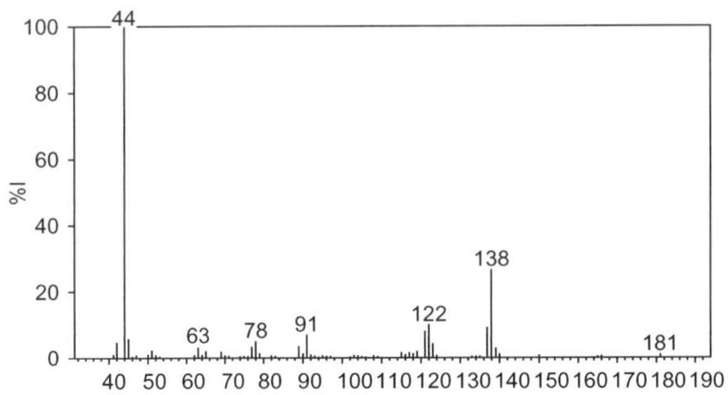

Toxicity. 4-MTA is thought to be responsible for at least eight deaths worldwide (mainly in Europe) on its own or in association with other drugs. Toxic symptoms may include 'serotonin syndrome', convulsions and respiratory depression. Such symptoms may be produced at plasma concentrations over 1 mg/L. A blood concentration over 4 mg/L could indicate an overdose or at least excessive usage.

The postmortem of a male death (22 years old and in previously good health) which implicated 3,4-methylenedioxymethamfetamine (MDMA) poisoning actually revealed the presence of 4-methylthioamfetamine (MTA) in femoral blood, perimortem blood and urine at concentrations of 4.6 mg/L, 4.2 mg/L, and 87.2 mg/L, respectively. This was the first reported death involving 4-MTA in the United Kingdom and the first case involving 4-MTA only. [S. P. Elliott, *J. Anal. Toxicol.*, 2000, *24(2)*, 85–89.]

A 27-year-old male died suddenly after a collapse and an intensive reanimation attempt. Postmortem toxicological analysis revealed the following 4-MTA concentrations: femoral vein blood, 5.23 mg/L; urine, 95.5 mg/L; vitreous humour, 1.31 mg/L; bile, 36.4 mg/L; liver 30.8 mg/kg; spleen 4.10 mg/kg and frontal lobe 31.7 mg/kg. MDMA was also found but at much lower concentrations and the cause of death was attributed to poisoning with 4-MTA. [T. Decaestecker *et al.*, *J. Anal. Toxicol.*, 2001, *25*, 705–710.]

Note. For a case report on the analytical profile of 4-MTA, see A. J. Poortman and E. Lock, *Forensic Sci. Int.*, 1999, *100*, 221–233.

Methylthiouracil

Antithyroid Agent

Proprietary names. Alkiron; Antibason; Basecil; Basethyrin; Methiacil; Methicil; Methiocil; Muracil; Prostrumyl; Strumacil; Thimecil; Thyreostat.

2,3-Dihydro-6-methyl-2-thioxo-4(1*H*)-pyrimidinone

$C_5H_6N_2OS = 142.2$

CAS—56-04-2

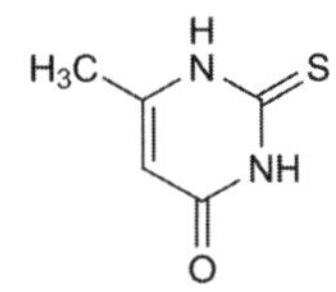

A white crystalline powder. M.p. 326° to 331°, with decomposition.

Soluble 1 in 2000 of water, 1 in 150 of boiling water, and 1 in 800 of ethanol; slightly soluble in acetone; very slightly soluble in ether; practically insoluble in benzene and chloroform; freely soluble in solutions of ammonium hydroxide and sodium hydroxide.

Dissociation Constant. pK_a 8.2 (20°).

Partition Coefficient. Log *P* (octanol/water), 1.4.

Ultraviolet Spectrum. Aqueous acid—276 ($A^1_1 = 1190b$); aqueous alkali—256 nm ($A^1_1 = 850b$).

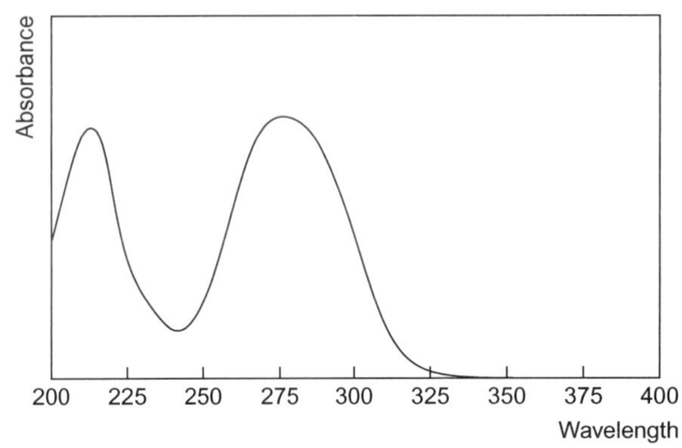

Infra-red Spectrum. Principal peaks at wavenumbers 1645, 1170, 1564, 1198, 850, 1240 cm^{-1}.

Dose. Initially, 200 to 400 mg daily; maintenance, 50 to 150 mg daily.

5-Methyltryptamine

Hallucinogen

5-Methyl-1*H*-indole-3-ethanamine

$C_{11}H_{14}N_2 = 174.2$

CAS—1821-47-2

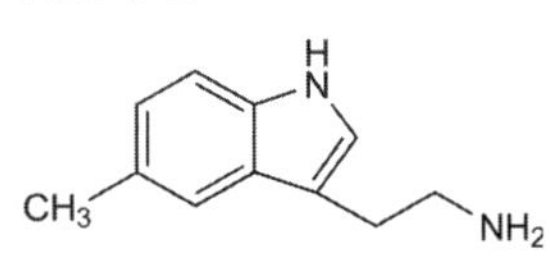

5-Methyltryptamine Hydrochloride

$C_{11}H_{14}N_2,HCl = 210.7$

CAS—1010-95-3

M.p. 289° to 292°.

Colour Tests. Mandelin's Test—green-orange; Marquis Test—orange→brown; Sulfuric Acid—yellow.

Thin-layer Chromatography. System TA—Rf 56. (Acidified iodoplatinate solution, positive.)

Gas Chromatography. System GA—RI 1795.

Infra-red Spectrum. Principal peaks at wavenumbers 800, 1515, 1612, 1587, 1234, 1315 cm^{-1} (5-methyltryptamine hydrochloride).

α-Methyltryptamine

Hallucinogen

3-(2-Aminopropyl)indole
$C_{11}H_{14}N_2$=174.2
CAS—299-26-3

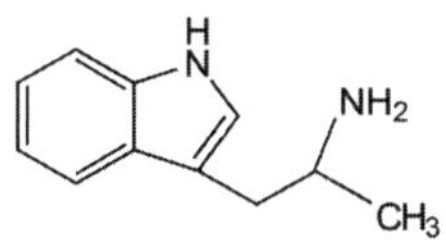

A white crystalline powder. M.p. 98° to 108°.
Soluble in chloroform and dilute acetic acid.

Colour Tests. Mandelin's Test—green→orange; Marquis Test—orange→brown; Sulfuric Acid—yellow

Thin-layer Chromatography. System TA—Rf 58. (Acidified iodoplatinate solution, positive.)

Gas Chromatography. System GA—RI 1740.

Ultraviolet Spectrum. Aqueous acid—279, 288 nm.

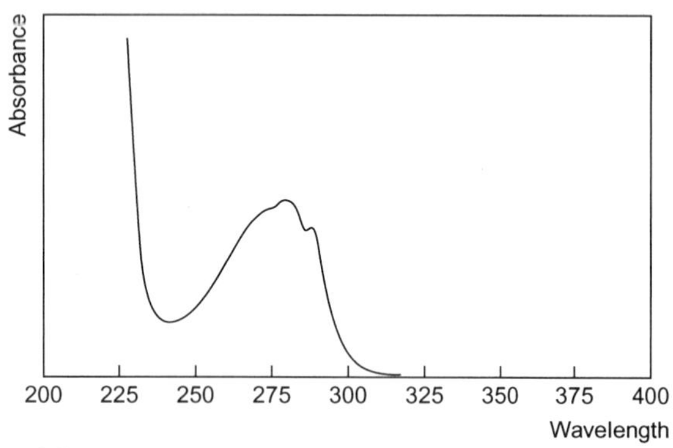

Infra-red Spectrum. Principal peaks at wavenumbers 1215, 1170, 1050, 750, 1520, 790 cm^{-1} (α-methyltryptamine esilate, KBr disk).

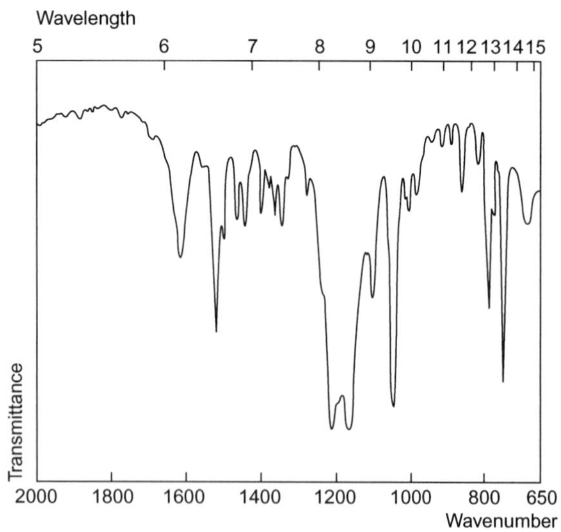

N-Methyltryptamine

Hallucinogen

N-Methyl-1*H*-indole-3-ethanamine
$C_{11}H_{14}N_2$=174.2
CAS—61-49-4

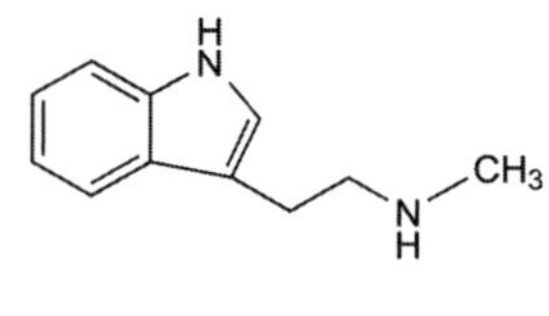

Colour Tests. Marquis Test—orange; Sulfuric Acid—yellow.

Thin-layer Chromatography. System TA—Rf 18. (Acidified iodoplatinate solution, positive.)

Gas Chromatography. System GA—RI 1770.

Infra-red Spectrum. Principal peaks at wavenumbers 700, 1040, 762, 1025, 1605, 1200 cm^{-1} (KBr disk).

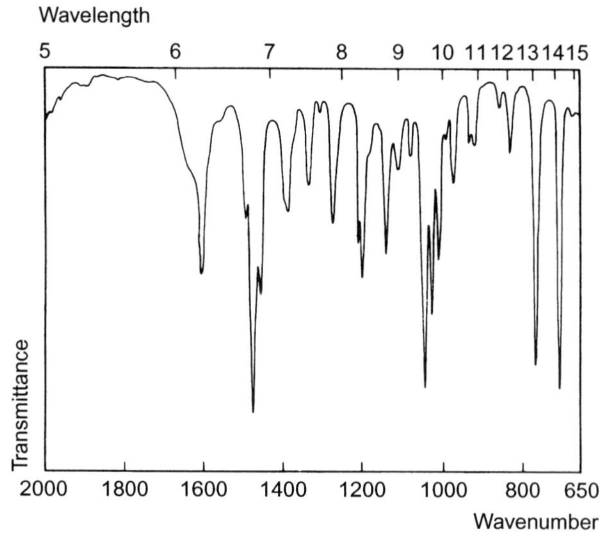

Quantification

Gas chromatography–mass spectrometry. In urine: *N*-methyltryptamine and other *N* -demethylated indoleamines—T. Forsstrom *et al.*, *Scand. J. Clin. Lab. Invest.*, 2001, *61*, 547–556. In urine: limit of detection 0.1 μg/L—R. W. Walker *et al.*, *J. Chromatogr.*, 1984, *289*, 223–229.

Methyprylon

Hypnotic

Synonym. Methyprylone
Proprietary names. Dimerin; Noctan; Noludar.
3,3-Diethyl-5-methyl-2,4-piperidinedione
$C_{10}H_{17}NO_2$=183.2
CAS—125-64-4

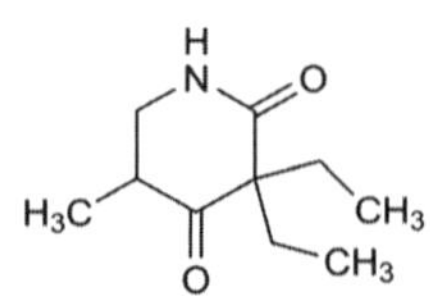

A white crystalline powder. M.p. 74° to 77°.
Soluble 1 in 14 of water, 1 in 0.7 of ethanol, 1 in 0.6 of chloroform, and 1 in 3.5 of ether.

Dissociation Constant. pK_a 12.0.

Partition Coefficient. Log *P* (octanol/water), 0.8.

Thin-layer Chromatography. System TA—Rf 58; system TD—Rf 31; system TE—Rf 63; system TF—Rf 25; system TAD—Rf 55; system TAE—Rf 78. (Acidified potassium permanganate solution, positive.)

Gas Chromatography. System GA—methyprylone RI 1527; M (OH-)-H_2O RI 1540; M (oxo-) RI 1870; methyprylone enol-AC RI 1610; system

GB—methyprylone RI 1581; M (OH-)-H_2O RI 1601; M (oxo-) RI 1870; system GF—RI 2090.

High Performance Liquid Chromatography. System HX—RI 347; system HY—RI 302.

Infra-red Spectrum. Principal peaks at wavenumbers 1660, 1693, 1085, 1310, 750, 869 cm^{-1} (KBr disk).

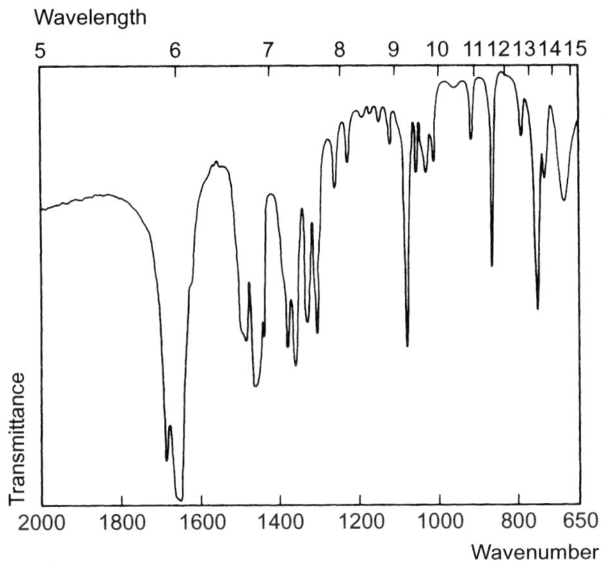

Mass Spectrum. Principal ions at *m/z* 155, 140, 83, 98, 55, 41, 84, 69.

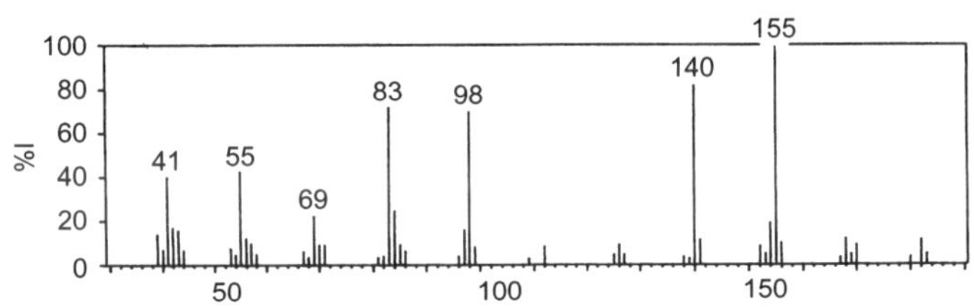

Quantification

Gas chromatography. In blood, plasma or urine: methyprylon and methylpersedon, limit of detection 1 mg/L, FID—R. R. Bridges and M. A. Peat, *J. Anal. Toxicol.*, 1979, *3*, 21–25. In blood, urine or tissues: methyprylon and metabolites, FID—M. Van Boven and I. Sunshine, *J. Anal. Toxicol.*, 1979, *3*, 174–176.

Disposition in the Body. Absorbed after oral administration. The principal metabolites are 2,4-dioxo-3,3-diethyl-5-methyltetrahydropyridine (methylpersedon) which is active, 6-oxomethyprylone, 5-hydroxymethyprylone, and 5-carboxymethyprylone. About 60% of a dose is excreted in the urine in 24 h as free and conjugated metabolites together with 3% of the dose as unchanged drug.

Therapeutic concentration. In plasma, usually in the range 10 to 20 mg/L.

Following a single oral dose of 300 mg to 10 subjects, peak plasma concentrations of 3.51 to 8.38 mg/L (mean 5.62) were obtained in 1.03 to 2.17 h (mean 1.59) [P. R. Gwilt *et al.*, *J. Pharm. Sci.*, 1985, *74*, 1001–1003.]

Following a single oral dose of 650 mg to 6 subjects, peak plasma concentrations averaging 10.2 mg/L were attained in 2 h [L. O. Randell *et al.*, *Arch. Int. Pharmacodyn. Thér.*, 1956, *106*, 388–394.]

Toxicity. Prolonged use of methyprylon may lead to dependence of the barbiturate–alcohol type. Numerous cases of overdose have been reported but there have been few fatalities; death has occurred after the ingestion of 6 g but at least two recoveries following doses of 30 g have been reported. Plasma concentrations of 12 to 75 to 128 mg/L have been associated with toxic effects and concentrations greater than 50 mg/L may be lethal.

In one fatality attributed to methyprylon overdose, the following postmortem tissue concentrations, mg/L or µg/g, were reported:

	Blood	Brain	Kidney	Liver	Spleen	Urine
Methyprylon	158	176	87	90	121	61
Methylpersedon	36	73	21	40	29	123
5-Hydroxymethyprylone	–	–	–	–	–	16
5-Carboxymethyprylone	2	–	10	7	16	80
6-Oxomethyprylone	16	18	9	8	3	68

[M. Van Boven and I. Sunshine, *J. Anal. Toxicol.*, 1979, *3*, 174–176.]

In 4 cases of fatal overdose, the following tissue disposition was reported: blood 53 to 66 mg/L (mean 59), kidney 10 to 108 µg/g (mean 62), liver 62 to 260 µg/g (mean 118), urine 17 to 166 mg/L (mean 86) [R. C. Baselt, *Disposition of Toxic Drugs and Chemicals in Man*, 5th Edn, Davis, California, Biomedical Publications, 2000, pp. 569–571.]

Half-life. Plasma half-life following a single oral dose, about 4 h, increased to about 50 h in acute intoxication.

Dose. 200 to 400 mg, as a hypnotic.

Methysergide

Migraine Prophylactic

(8*β*)-9,10-Didehydro-*N*-[(1*S*)-1-(hydroxymethyl)propyl]-1,6-dimethylergoline-8-carboxamide
$C_{21}H_{27}N_3O_2$=353.5
CAS—361-37-5

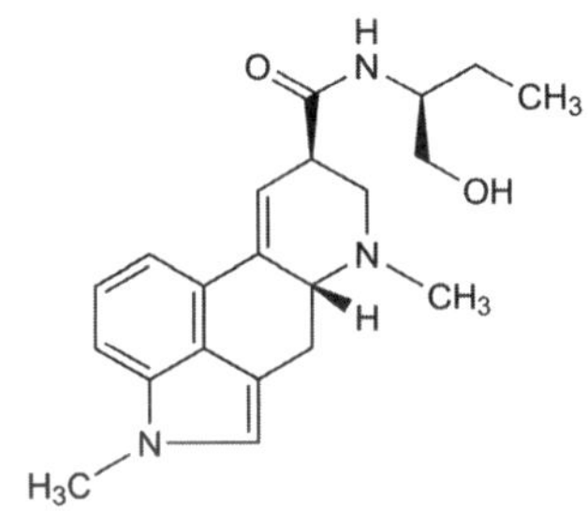

Crystals. M.p. 194° to 196°.

Methysergide Maleate
Synonym. 1-Methyl-D-lysergic Acid Butanolamide Maleate
Proprietary names. Deseril(a); Désernil; Sansert.
$C_{21}H_{27}N_3O_2,C_4H_4O_4$=469.5
CAS—129-49-7
A white to yellowish-white or reddish-white, crystalline powder.
Soluble 1 in 500 of water, 1 in 165 of ethanol, and 1 in 125 of methanol; practically insoluble in chloroform and ether.

Dissociation Constant. pK_a 6.6 (24°).

Partition Coefficient. Log *P* (octanol/water), 1.6.

Colour Tests. *p*-Dimethylaminobenzaldehyde—violet; Mandelin's Test—brown; Marquis Test—grey.

Thin-layer Chromatography. System TA—Rf 65; system TB—Rf 01; system TC—Rf 21; system TE—Rf 45; system TL—Rf 15; system TM—Rf 33; system TAJ—Rf 23; system TAK—Rf 04; system TAL—Rf 66. (Van Urk reagent, blue.)

Gas Chromatography. System GA—RI 3089.

High Performance Liquid Chromatography. System HA—*k* 0.4; system HP—*k* 2.33; system HZ—Retention time 2.4 min.

Ultraviolet Spectrum. Aqueous acid—230, 322 (A_1^1=223a); aqueous alkali—243, 320 nm.

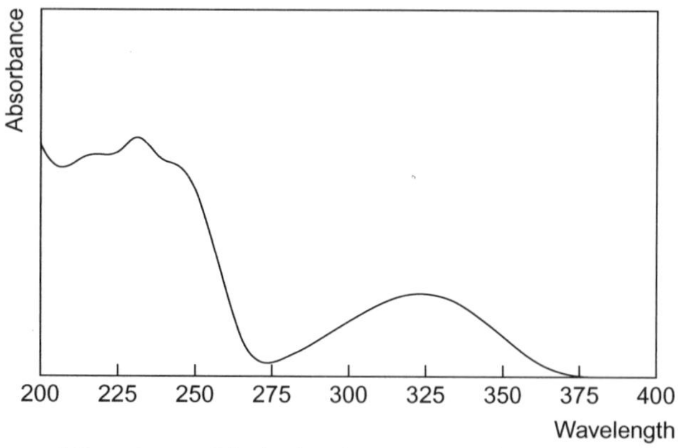

Infra-red Spectrum. Principal peaks at wavenumbers 1566, 1650, 863, 1615, 1190, 740 cm^{-1} (methysergide maleate, KBr disk). (See below.)

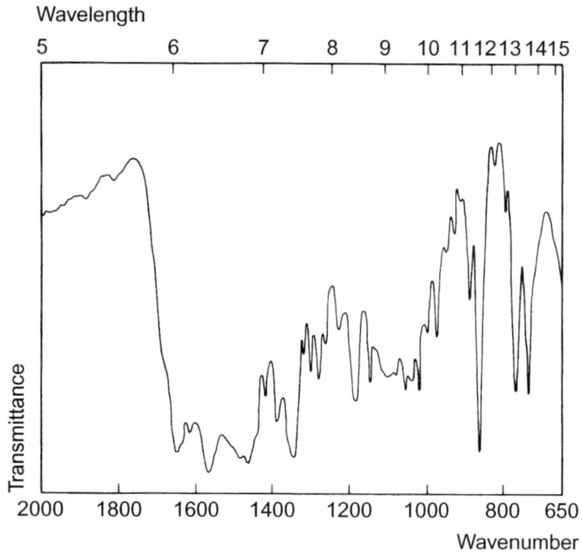

Mass Spectrum. Principal ions at m/z 353, 210, 235, 336, 72, 54, 236, 195.

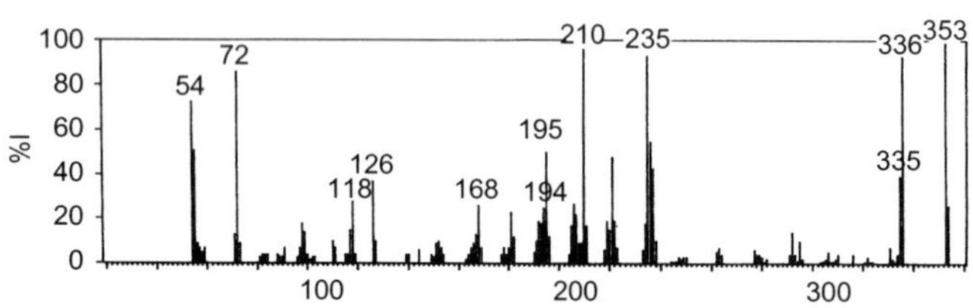

Dose. The equivalent of 2 to 6 mg of methysergide daily.

Meticillin

Antibiotic

Synonyms. Dimethoxyphenecillin; Dimethoxyphenyl Penicillin.
(2*S*,5*R*,6*R*)-6-[(2,6-Dimethoxybenzoyl)amino]-3,3-dimethyl-7-oxo-4-thia-1-azabicyclo[3.2.0]heptane-2-carboxylic acid
$C_{17}H_{20}N_2O_6S$=380.4
CAS—61-32-5

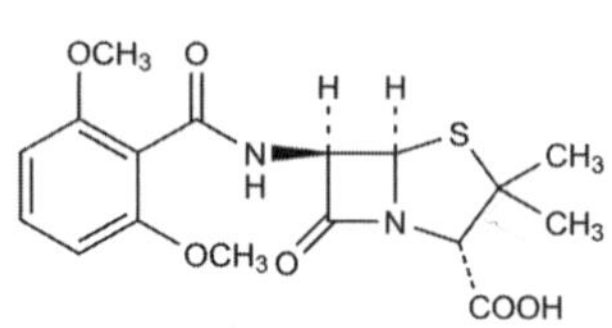

Meticillin Sodium
Synonym. Meticillinum Natricum

Proprietary names. Azapen; Belfacillin; Celbenin; Celpillina; Cinopenil; Flabelline; Pénistaph; Staficyn; Staphcillin.
$C_{17}H_{19}N_2NaO_6S,H_2O$=420.4
CAS—132-92-3 (anhydrous); 7246-14-2 (monohydrate)
A fine white crystalline powder. M.p. 196° to 197°, with decomposition. Soluble 1 in 0.6 of water and 1 in 35 of ethanol; slightly soluble in chloroform; practically insoluble in ether; freely soluble in methanol.

Dissociation Constant. pK_a 2.8 (25°).

Partition Coefficient. Log *P* (octanol/water), 1.2.

Ultraviolet Spectrum. Water—280 nm (A_1^1=61a). (See below.)

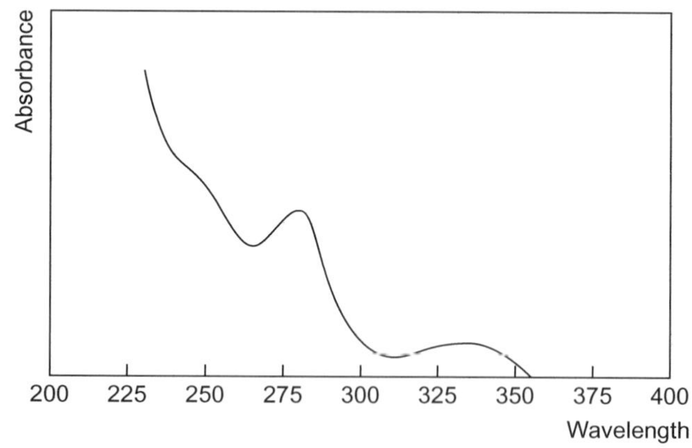

Infra-red Spectrum. Principal peaks at wavenumbers 1607, 1766, 1673, 1500, 1093, 1260 cm^{-1} (meticillin sodium, KBr disk). (See below.)

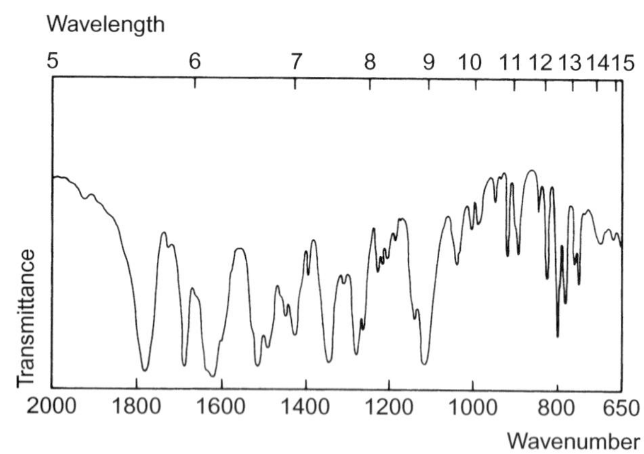

Dose. Up to 12 g of meticillin sodium daily, by slow IV injection.

Metildigoxin

Cardiac Glycoside

Synonyms. Medigoxin; β-Methyl Digoxin; β-Methyldigoxin.
Proprietary names. Cardiolan; Lanirapid; Lanitop; Miopat.
3β,12β,14β-Trihydroxy-5β-card-20(22)-enolide-3-(4‴-*O*-methyltridigitoxoside)
$C_{42}H_{66}O_{14}$=795.0
CAS—30685-43-9

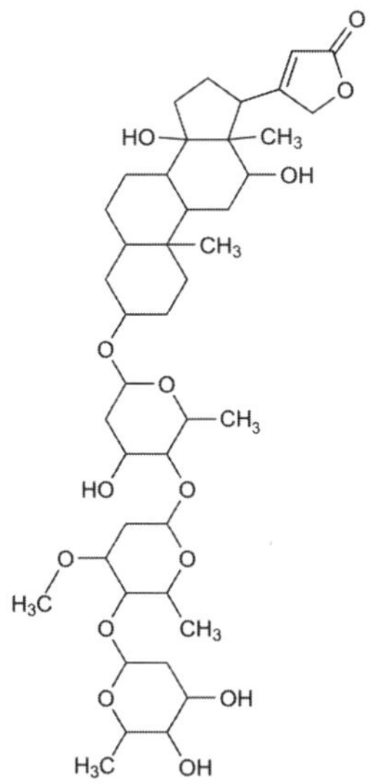

A white crystalline powder. M.p. 227° to 231°.
Very slightly soluble in water; soluble in ethanol and chloroform.

Partition Coefficient. Log *P* (octanol/water), 1.8.

Infra-red Spectrum. Principal peaks at wavenumbers 1085, 1014, 1730, 1163, 1130, 864 cm^{-1} (KBr disk).

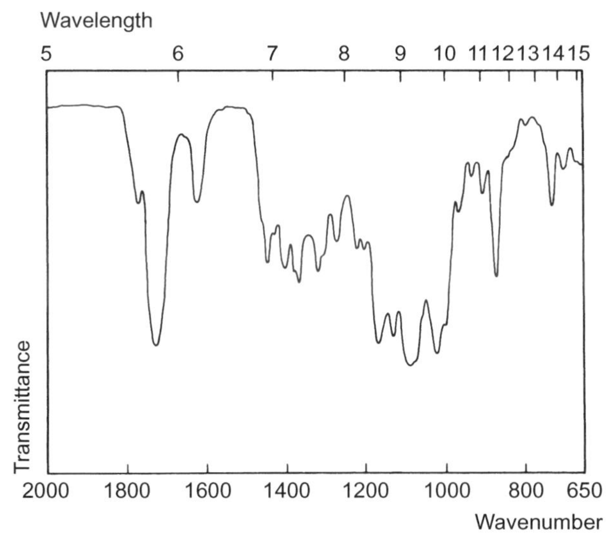

Quantification

Radioimmunoassay. In plasma: limit of detection 200 ng/L (comparison with methods using radiolabelled drug)—E. R. Garrett and P. H. Hinderling, *J. Pharm. Sci.*, 1977, *66*, 806–810.

Disposition in the Body. Rapidly and almost completely absorbed after oral administration. Metabolised by demethylation to digoxin and by hydrolysis to the bis- and mono-glycosides. About 75% of a dose is excreted in the urine over a period of several days with about 25 to 30% being excreted in the first 24 h. Of the material excreted in the urine, about 30 to 50% is unchanged drug, 15% consists of conjugated bis- and mono-glycosides, and the remainder is digoxin. About 15 to 30% of a dose is eliminated in the faeces over a period of 7 days.

Therapeutic concentration

Following a single oral dose of 0.4 mg to 17 subjects, a mean peak plasma concentration of 0.003 mg/L was attained in about 1 h. Following daily oral doses of 0.15 to 0.2 mg to 18 subjects, steady-state plasma concentrations of 0.0006 to 0.002 mg/L (mean 0.001) were reported [D. Boerner *et al.*, *Eur. J. Clin. Pharmacol.*, 1976, *9*, 307–314].

Toxicity

In a fatality in which death occurred about 1 h after ingestion of a metildigoxinmedigoxin overdose, the following postmortem tissue concentrations of glycosides were reported: blood 0.075 mg/L, bile 2.4 mg/L, kidney 0.237 μg/g, liver 0.047 μg/g, left ventricular myocardium 0.14 μg/g, right ventricular myocardium 0.16 μg/g, urine 0.91 mg/L [N. Rietbrock *et al.*, *Dtsch. Med. Wochenschr.*, 1978, *103*, 1841–1844].

Half-life. Plasma half-life, 40 to 70 h.

Volume of distribution. About 6 to 10 L/kg.

Clearance. Plasma clearance, about 2 mL/min/kg.

Distribution in blood. Plasma : whole blood ratio, 1.1.

Protein binding. In plasma, about 10 to 30%.

Dose. For rapid digitalisation, 600 μg daily for 2 to 4 days; maintenance, 200 to 300 μg daily.

Metindizate

Antispasmodic (Veterinary)

2-(1-Methylperhydroindol-3-yl)ethyl benzilate
$C_{25}H_{31}NO_3$=393.5
CAS—15687-33-9

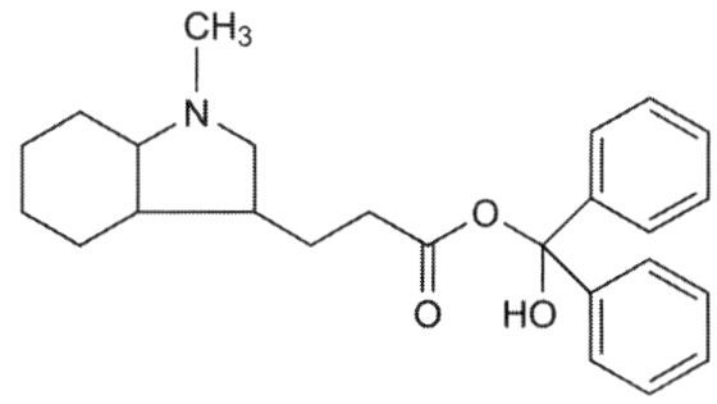

Metindizate Hydrochloride

Proprietary name. It is an ingredient of Isaverin.
$C_{25}H_{31}NO_3$,HCl=430.0
A fine, white, crystalline powder. M.p. 159° to 160°.
Freely soluble in water and ethanol; practically insoluble in chloroform and ether.

Colour Tests. Liebermann's Test—orange→brown; Mandelin's Test—brown; Marquis Test—orange→green; Sulfuric Acid—orange.

Thin-layer Chromatography. System TA—Rf 36. (Acidified iodoplatinate solution, positive.)

Ultraviolet Spectrum. Aqueous acid—251, 257 nm (A^1_1=10.3b).

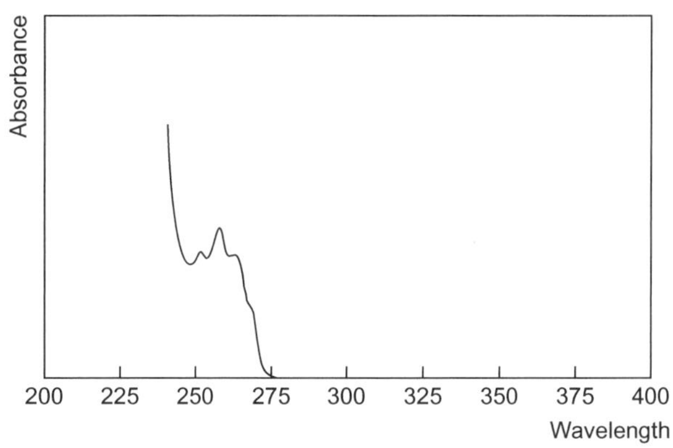

Infra-red Spectrum. Principal peaks at wavenumbers 1739, 1238, 1227, 702, 1058, 1093 cm^{-1} (KBr disk).

Metipranolol

Beta-adrenoceptor Blocking Agent

Synonyms. Methypranolum; Trimepranol.
Proprietary names. Betamann; Betanol; Beta-Ophtiole; Disorat; Glauline; Glausyn; OptiPranolol; Turoptin.
4-[2-Hydroxy-3-[(1-methylethyl)amino]propoxy]-2,3,6-trimethylphenol 1-acetate
$C_{17}H_{27}NO_4$=309.4
CAS—22664-55-7

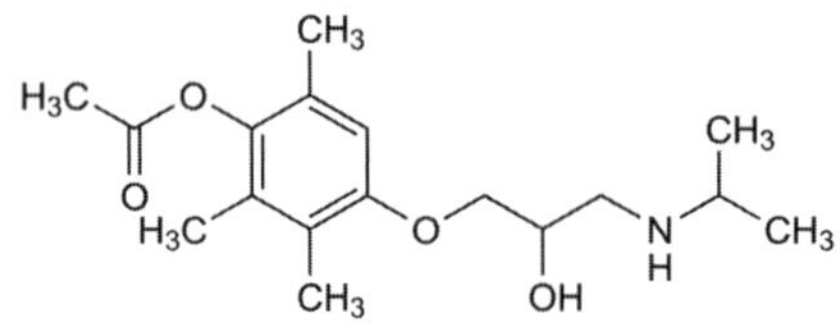

A white crystalline powder. M.p. 105° to 109°.
Practically insoluble in water; freely soluble in ethanol, chloroform, and benzene; slightly soluble in ether.

Partition Coefficient. Log *P* (octanol/water), 2.7.

Thin-layer Chromatography. System TB—Rf 08; system TE—Rf 47; system TF—Rf 00; system TAE—Rf 21.

Gas Chromatography. System GA—metipranolol RI 2241; metipranolol-AC RI 2260; M (desamino-OH-)-AC_2 RI 2240; M art (phenol)-AC RI 1610; system GB—metipranolol RI 2320.

High Performance Liquid Chromatography. System HX—RI 379; system HZ—Retention time 3.5 min.

Ultraviolet Spectrum. Aqueous acid—278 nm (A_1^1=44b).

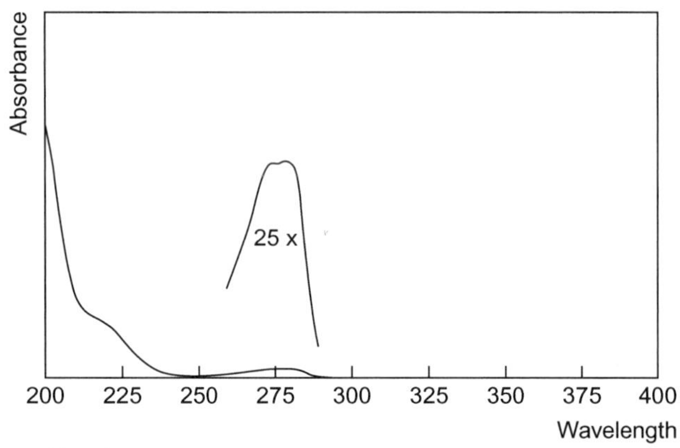

Quantification

High performance liquid chromatography. In plasma or urine: metipranolol and other topically applied beta blockers, limits of detection 4–27 µg/L—A. Tracqui *et al.*, *Forensic Sci. Int.*, 1988, *38*, 37–41. In plasma: desacetylmetipranolol, limit of detection 2 µg/L, electrochemical detection—M. Tkaczykova and L. Safarik, *J. Pharm. Biomed. Anal.*, 1989, *7*, 1805–1810.

Disposition in the Body. Readily absorbed after oral administration and rapidly metabolised to the active metabolite, desacetylmetipranolol. About 20% of a dose is excreted in the urine as unchanged drug.

Therapeutic concentration

After a single oral dose of 40 mg to 13 subjects, peak plasma concentrations of the desacetyl metabolite of 0.034 to 0.214 mg/L (mean 0.14) were attained in about 1 h. Oral administration of 20 mg twice daily to 6 subjects, produced mean steady-state plasma concentrations (desacetyl derivative) of 0.06 to 0.08 mg/L determined on the 6th to 8th day; considerable intersubject variation was reported [O. Mayer, *Int. J. Clin. Pharmacol. Ther. Toxicol.*, 1980, *18*, 113–120.]

Following administration of metipranolol 40 mg to 6 subjects as either a conventional- or a controlled-release preparation, mean peak plasma concentrations of 22 µg/L (at 1 h) and 11 µg/L (at 3 h), respectively, were reported [R. Lapka *et al.*, *Eur. J. Clin. Pharmacol.*, 1990, *38*, 243–247.]

Half-life. Plasma half-life, desacetylmetipranolol about 2 to 4 h but there is considerable intersubject variation.

Dose. Metipranolol has been given in doses of 10 to 120 mg daily.

Metisazone

Antiviral

Synonyms. *N*-Methylisatin *β*-Thiosemicarbazone; Methisazone.
Proprietary names. Marboran; Viruzona.
2-(1,2-Dihydro-1-methyl-2-oxo-3*H*-indol-3-ylidene)-hydrazinecarbothioamide
$C_{10}H_{10}N_4OS$=234.3
CAS—1910-68-5

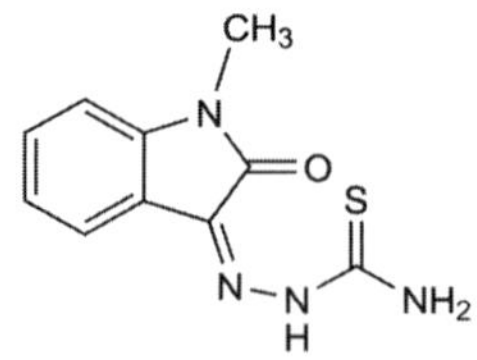

A very fine, orange-yellow powder. M.p. about 248°, with decomposition. Practically insoluble in water; soluble 1 in 25 of acetone and 1 in 800 of chloroform; soluble in warm dilute solutions of alkali hydroxides.

Partition Coefficient. Log *P* (octanol/water), 1.0.

Colour Tests. Mandelin's Test—violet→yellow; Palladium Chloride—yellow→orange→brown.

Thin-layer Chromatography. System TA—Rf 65; system TB—Rf 03; system TC—Rf 68; system TL—Rf 69. (Acidified iodoplatinate solution, positive.)

Ultraviolet Spectrum. Ethanol—241, 274 nm (A_1^1=588b).

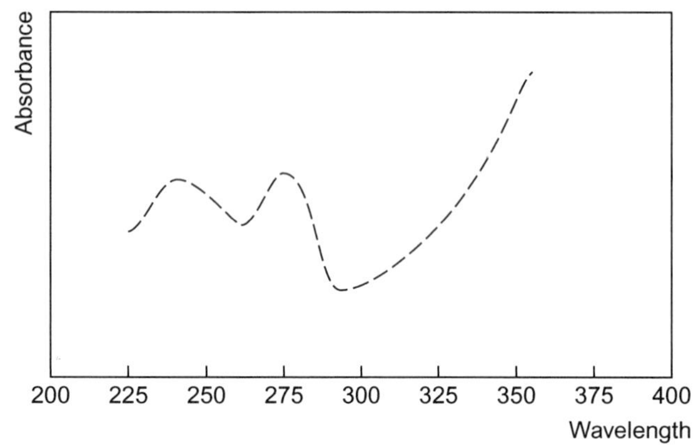

Infra-red Spectrum. Principal peaks at wavenumbers 1605, 1493, 1097, 1673, 1040, 826 cm^{-1} (KBr disk).

Mass Spectrum. Principal ions at *m/z* 234, 146, 179, 206, 131, 91, 117, 118.

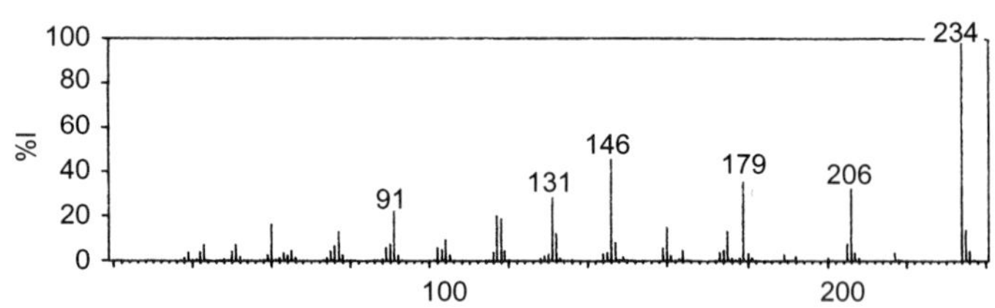

Dose. Usually 6 g daily (prophylactic dose).

Metixene

Anticholinergic

Synonym. Methixene
1-Methyl-3-(9*H*-thioxanthen-9-ylmethyl)piperidine
$C_{20}H_{23}NS$=309.5
CAS—4969-02-2

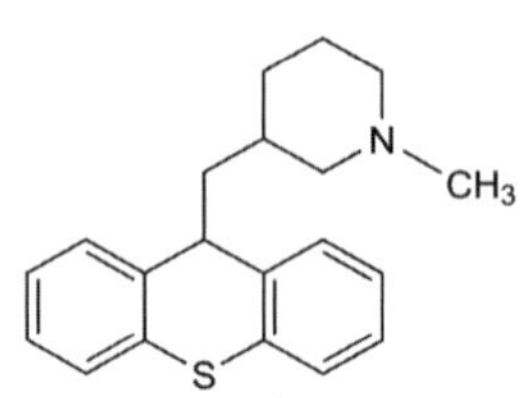

A pale yellow viscous liquid.

Insoluble in water.

Metixene Hydrochloride
Synonyms. Methixene Hydrochloride; Metixeni Hydrochloridum; NSC-78194; SJ-1977.
Proprietary names. Metixen; Tremaril; Tremarit; Tremonil; Tremoquil; Trest.
$C_{20}H_{23}NS,HCl=345.9$
CAS—1553-34-0 (anhydrous); 7081-40-5 (monohydrate)
A white crystalline powder. M.p. about 216°.
Soluble in water, ethanol, and chloroform.

Partition Coefficient. Log *P* (octanol/water), 5.7.

Colour Tests. Formaldehyde–Sulfuric Acid—orange; Liebermann's Test—red-orange; Mandelin's Test—orange; Sulfuric Acid—orange (fluoresces under UV light).

Thin-layer Chromatography. System TA—Rf 50; system TB—Rf 45; system TC—Rf 25; system TE—Rf 61; system TL—Rf 12; system TAE—Rf 21; system TAJ—Rf 16; system TAK—Rf 22; system TAL—Rf 73. (Acidified iodoplatinate solution, positive.)

Gas Chromatography. System GA—RI 2480; system GB—RI 2592; system GF—RI 2895.

High Performance Liquid Chromatography. System HA—*k* 3.6; system HX—RI 451.

Ultraviolet Spectrum. Aqueous acid—268 nm ($A_1^1=324a$).

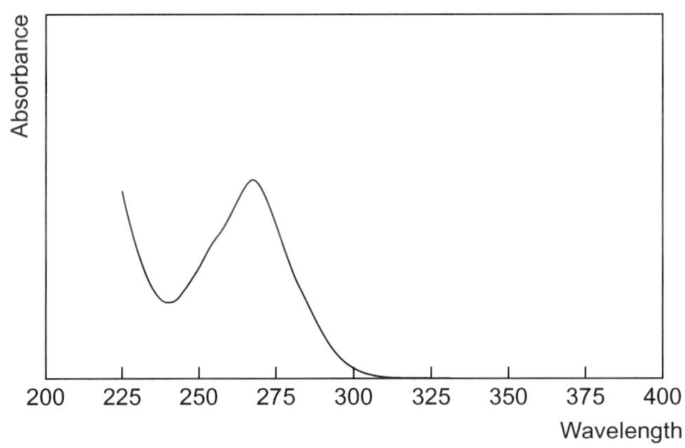

Infra-red Spectrum. Principal peaks at wavenumbers 750, 729, 1052, 1162, 1086, 1280 cm^{-1} (KBr disk).

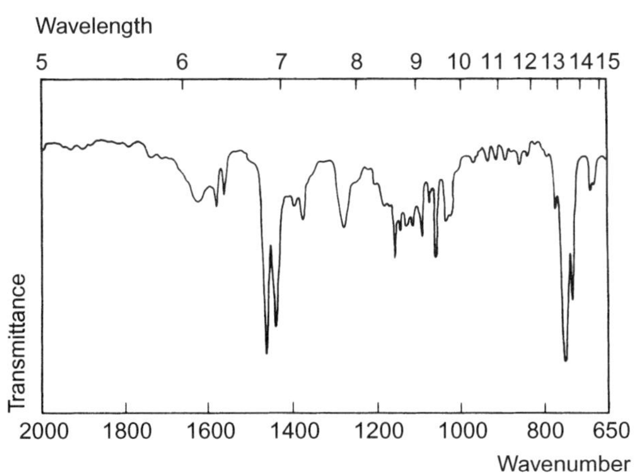

Mass Spectrum. Principal ions at *m/z* 99, 197, 44, 58, 112, 309, 41, 42.

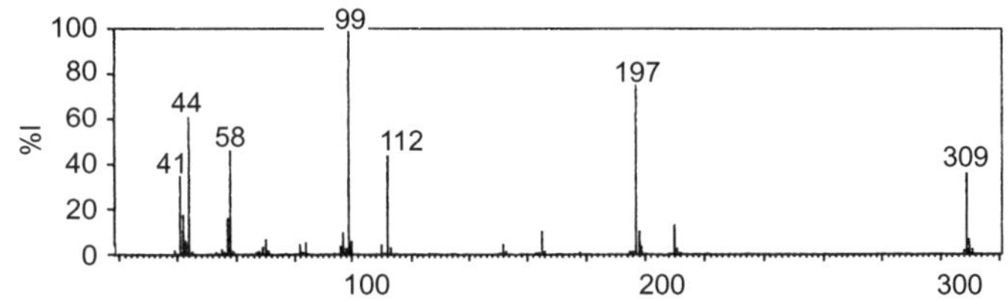

Disposition in the Body. Absorbed after oral administration. It is excreted in the urine, partly unchanged, partly as its two isomeric sulfoxides, and partly as the stereoisomeric sulfoxides of *N*-demethylated metixene.

Dose. 7.5 to 60 mg of metixene hydrochloride daily in divided doses.

Metoclopramide

Anti-emetic

4-Amino-5-chloro-*N*-[(2-diethylamino)ethyl]-2-methoxybenzamide
$C_{14}H_{22}ClN_3O_2=299.8$
CAS—364-62-5

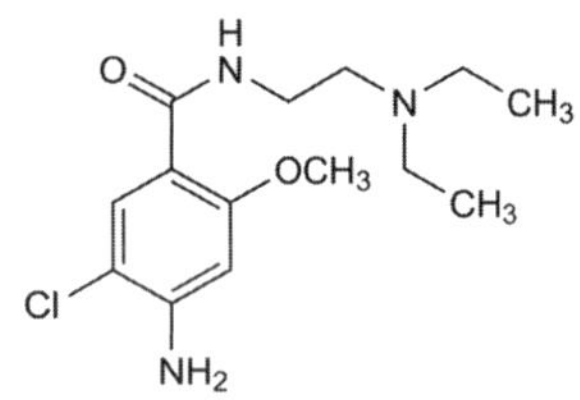

A white crystalline powder. M.p. 146.5° to 148.0°.
Practically insoluble in water; soluble 1 in 45 of ethanol and 1 in 15 of chloroform.

Metoclopramide Dihydrochloride
Proprietary names. Emetid; Gastronerton.
$C_{14}H_{22}ClN_3O_2,2HCl,H_2O=390.7$
Crystals. M.p. 45° with decomposition.

Metoclopramide Hydrochloride
Synonyms. AHR-3070-C; DEL-1267; Metoclopramidi Hydrochloridum; MK-745.
Proprietary names. Anausin; Clopra; Gastrobid Continus; Gastroflux; Gastromax; Intensol; Maxeran; Maxolon; Metalon; Metamide; Metopram; Mygdalon; Octamide; Parmid; Paspertin; Primperan; Reclomide; Reglan. It is an ingredient of Migramax, Migravess and Paramax.
$C_{14}H_{22}ClN_3O_2,HCl,H_2O=354.3$
CAS—7232-21-5 (anhydrous); 54143-57-6 (monohydrate)
A white crystalline powder. M.p. 182.5° to 184.0°.
Soluble 1 in 0.7 of water, 1 in 3 of ethanol, and 1 in 55 of chloroform; practically insoluble in ether.

Dissociation Constant. pK_a 9.3 (25°).

Partition Coefficient. Log *P* (octanol/water), 2.6.

Colour Tests. Coniferyl Alcohol—orange; Liebermann's Test—yellow; Mandelin's Test—brown.

Thin-layer Chromatography. System TA—Rf 47; system TB—Rf 01; system TC—Rf 07; system TE—Rf 51; system TL—Rf 13; system TAE—Rf 17. (Acidified iodoplatinate solution, positive.)

Gas Chromatography. System GA—metoclopramide RI 2620, metoclopramide-AC RI 2735, M (desethyl-) RI 2095, M (desethyl-)-AC2 RI 2900.

High Performance Liquid Chromatography. System HA—*k* 5.0; system HX—RI 324; system HY—RI 263; system HZ—Retention time 2.6 min; system HAA—Retention time 9.9 min; system HAX—Retention time 7.9 min; system HAY—Retention time 4.3 min.

Ultraviolet Spectrum. Aqueous acid—273 nm ($A_1^1=467b$), 309 nm.

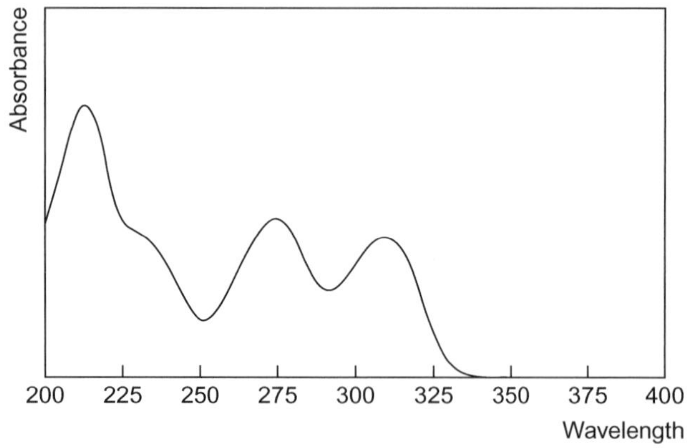

Infra-red Spectrum. Principal peaks at wavenumbers 1590, 1614, 1530, 1496, 1254, 1311 cm^{-1} (metoclopramide hydrochloride, KBr disk).

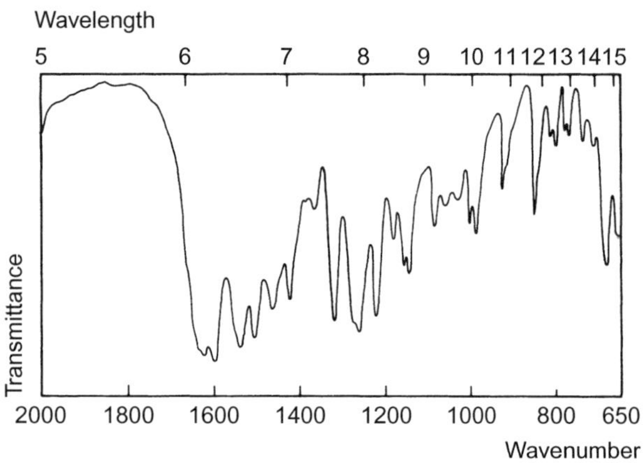

Mass Spectrum. Principal ions at m/z 86, 99, 184, 58, 30, 87, 201, 186.

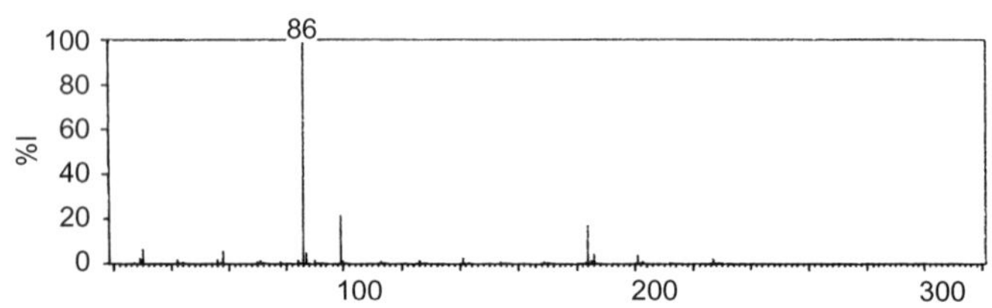

Quantification

Gas chromatography. In plasma: limit of detection 5 µg/L, ECD—L. M. Ross-Lee *et al.*, *J. Chromatogr.*, 1980, *183*; *B Biomed. Appl.*, *9*, 175–184.

High performance liquid chromatography. In plasma: limit of detection 10 µg/L, UV detection—G. Bishop-Freudling and H. Vergin, *J. Chromatogr.*, 1983, *273*; *B Biomed. Appl.*, *24*, 453–457. In serum, saliva or urine: limit of detection 4.5 µg/L for serum and saliva, 900 µg/L for urine, UV detection—J. Popović, *Ther. Drug Monit.*, 1984, *6*, 77–82. In plasma: limit of detection 3 µg/L, UV detection—D. C. Buss *et al.*, *Ther. Drug Monit.*, 1990, *12*, 293–296. In serum: limit of quantification 2 µg/L, electrochemical detection—H. Lamparczyk *et al.*, *Biomed. Chromat.*, 2001, *15*, 513–517.

Disposition in the Body. Rapidly and almost completely absorbed after oral administration. Up to about 60% of an oral dose undergoes first-pass metabolism but there is considerable intersubject variation. Metoclopramide crosses the blood–brain barrier. It crosses the placenta and concentrations in fetal plasma may be 60 to 70% of those in maternal plasma. It is found in breast milk in concentrations which may be higher than those found in plasma. Up to about 80% of a dose is excreted in the urine in 24 h with about 10 to 20% as unchanged drug, up to 50% as conjugated metoclopramide (mainly the *N*-4-sulfate), and a small amount as 2-(4-amino-5-chloro-2-methoxybenzamido)acetic acid. About 5% of a dose is excreted in the faeces via the bile.

Therapeutic concentration

After a single oral dose of 10 mg given to 6 subjects, peak plasma concentrations of 0.04 to 0.06 mg/L (mean 0.05) were attained in 0.5 to 2 h; following IV administration of 10 mg to 6 subjects, plasma concentrations of 0.07 to 0.13 mg/L were reported after 5 min [L. M. Ross-Lee *et al.*, *Eur. J. Clin. Pharmacol.*, 1981, *20*, 465–471].

The mean plasma concentration at the end of an infusion of metoclopramide to 14 patients was 1.01 mg/L in those patients in whom the dose had been adjusted to individual pharmacokinetic parameters (mean loading dose 2.22 mg/kg, mean maintenance dose 1.96 mg/kg/4 h) and 0.54 mg/L in those patients in whom the dose had been adjusted as usual to body weight (mean loading dose 1.40 mg/kg, mean maintenance dose 0.52 mg/kg/4 h) [J. M. Brechot *et al.*, *Eur. J. Clin. Pharmacol.*, 1991, *40*, 283–286].

Following subcutaneous administration of metoclopamide 10 mg every 6 h for 3 days to 10 patients with gastroparesis, a peak plasma concentration of 0.0997 mg/L was attained 30 min after the last dose; at 60 min, the concentration was 0.0939 mg/L [R. W. McCallum et al., *J. Pharmacol. Exp. Ther.*, 1991, *258*, 136–142].

Toxicity. Ingestion by adults of up to 0.8 g without serious adverse effects has been reported.

In a 25-year-old female who died 4 days after ingesting metoclopramide and diltiazem with suicidal intent, the blood levels 1 h after admission to hospital were 4.4 mg/L metoclopramide and 8.49 mg/L diltiazem [J. M. Beno and D. R. Nemeth, *J. Anal. Toxicol.*, 1991, *15*, 285–287].

Bioavailability. About 75%, with a wide intersubject variation of between 30 and 100%.

Half-life. Plasma half-life, 4 to 6 h, increased in renal impairment.

Volume of distribution. About 3.5 L/kg but there is considerable intersubject variation.

Clearance. Plasma clearance, 7 to 17 mL/min/kg (mean 11).

Distribution in blood. Plasma : whole blood ratio, 0.93.

Protein binding. In plasma, about 40%.

Note. For reviews of metoclopramide, see R. A. Harrington *et al.*, *Drugs*, 1983, *25*, 451–494 ; D. N. Bateman, *Clin. Pharmacokinet.*, 1983, *8*, 523–529; K. Lauritsen *et al.*, *Clin. Pharmacokinet.*, 1990, *19*, 11–31; H. H. Rotmensch *et al.*, *J. Clin. Pharmacol.*, 1997, *37*, 222–228, and G. L. Kearns *et al.*, *J. Clin Pharmacol.*, 1998, *38*, 12–138.

Dose. The equivalent of 30 mg of anhydrous metoclopramide hydrochloride daily.

Metocurine Iodide

Muscle Relaxant

Synonyms. Dimethyl Tubocurarine Iodide; Dimethyltubocurarine Iodide.
Note. The name dimethyltubocurarine iodide was based on the old empirical formula for tubocurarine.
Proprietary name. Metubine Iodide
6,6′,7′,12′-Tetramethoxy-2,2,2′,2′-tetramethyltubocuraranium diiodide
$C_{40}H_{48}I_2N_2O_6$=906.6
CAS—5152-30-7 (metocurine); 7601-55-0 (iodide)

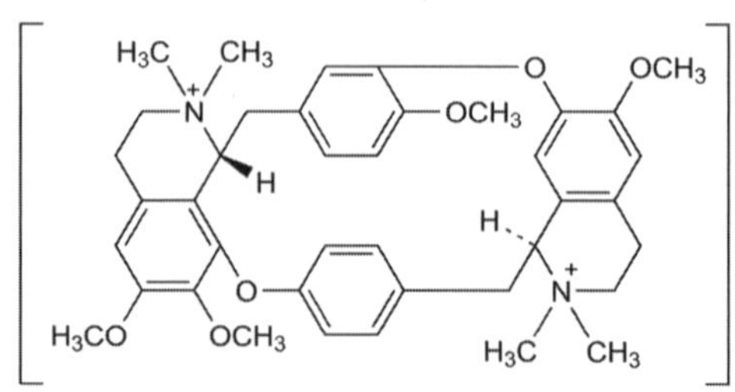

A white to pale yellow, crystalline powder. When heated to 257° to 267°, it decomposes with the evolution of gas.
Soluble 1 in 400 of water; very slightly soluble in ethanol; practically insoluble in benzene, chloroform, and ether; slightly soluble in dilute acids and alkalis.

Colour Tests. Aromaticity (Method 2)—yellow/orange.

Cold nitric acid gives a brown colour.

Ultraviolet Spectrum. Aqueous acid—280 nm (A_1^1=74b).

Infra-red Spectrum. Principal peaks at wavenumbers 1510, 1220, 1265, 1280, 1125, 1240 cm^{-1} (KBr disk).

Disposition in the Body. About 50% of a dose is excreted in the urine unchanged in 48 h, and about 2% of the dose is excreted in the bile in the same period.

Half-life. Plasma half-life, about 3 to 4 h.

Volume of distribution. About 0.4 L/kg.

Clearance. Plasma clearance, about 1.3 mL/min/kg.

Protein binding. In plasma, about 35%.

Dose. Initially, 1.5 to 8 mg intravenously.

Metolachlor

Herbicide

Synonyms. CGA 24705; Matelilachlor; Metolachlore.
Proprietary names. Bicep; Codal; Cotoran multi; Dual; Ontrack; Pace; Pennant; Pimagram; Primextra.
2-Chloro-*N*-(2-ethyl-6-methylphenyl)-*N*-(2-methoxy-1-methylethyl) acetamide
$C_{15}H_{22}ClNO_2$=283.8
CAS—51218-45-2

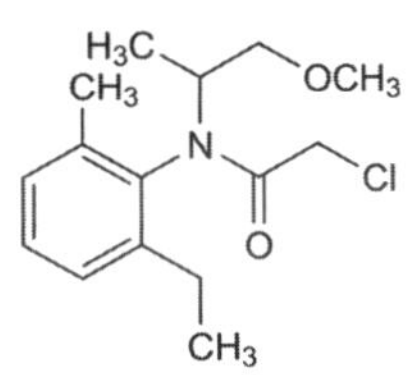

An off-white to colourless liquid at room temperature with B.p. 100° at 0.001 mm Hg. Formulations are opaque white to tan in colour. It is soluble in water (530 ppm at 20°) and miscible with benzene, dichloromethane, hexane, methanol, octanol, xylene, toluene, dimethylformamide, ethylene dichloride and cyclohexane; insoluble in ethylene glycol and propylene glycol.

Partition Coefficient. Log *P* (octanol/water), 3.13.

High Performance Liquid Chromatography. System HY—RI 562.

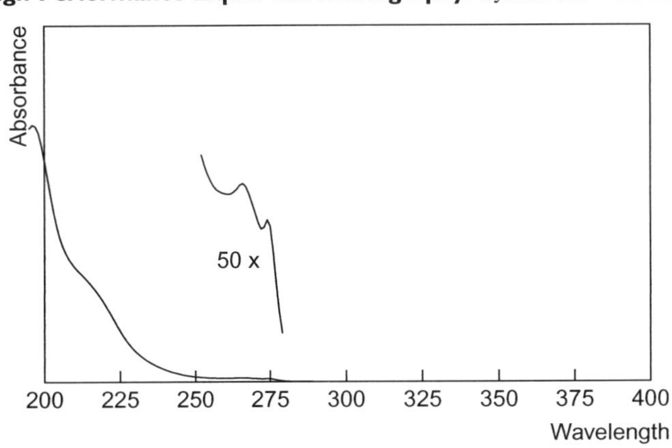

Infra-red Spectrum. Principal peaks at wavenumbers 1691, 1113, 1342, 1346, 1237, 1458 cm^{-1}.

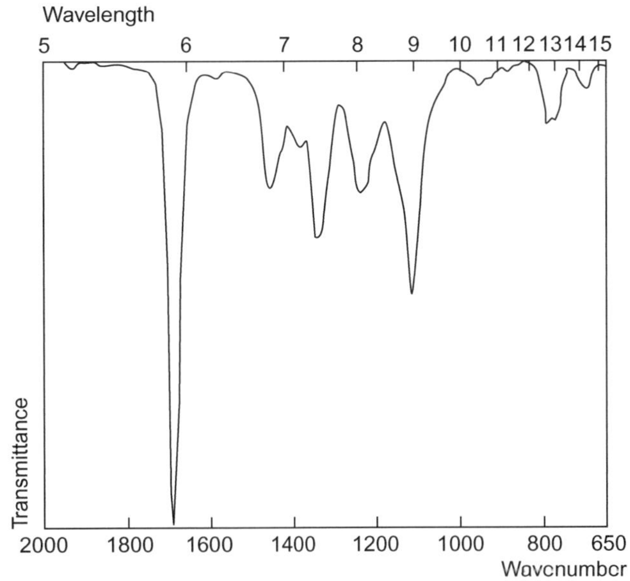

Mass Spectrum. Principal ions at *m/z* 162, 238, 45, 146, 240, 163, 91, 77.

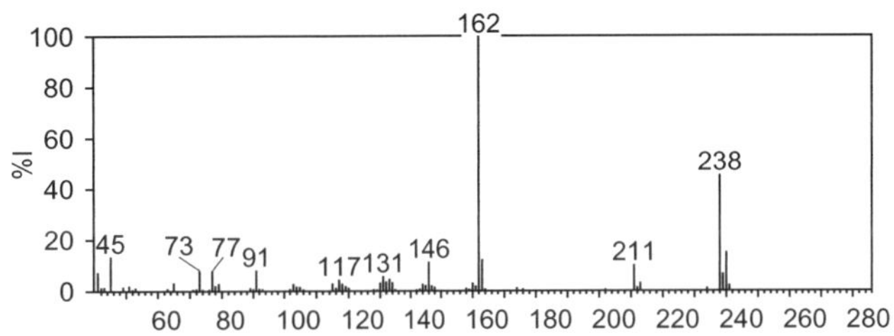

Disposition in the Body. Metolachlor is quickly broken down into its metabolites after ingestion. It is totally eliminated via urine and faeces. Metolachlor is not detected in urine, faeces or tissues.

Toxicity. Metolachlor is toxic by ingestion, although less so than other herbicides.

Metolazone

Diuretic

Proprietary names. Birobin; Diondel; Diulo; Metenix; Mykrox; Xuret; Zaroxolyn(e).
7-Chloro-1,2,3,4-tetrahydro-2-methyl–3-(2-methylphenyl)-4-oxo–6-quinazoline sulfonamide
$C_{16}H_{16}ClN_3O_3S$=365.8
CAS—17560-51-9

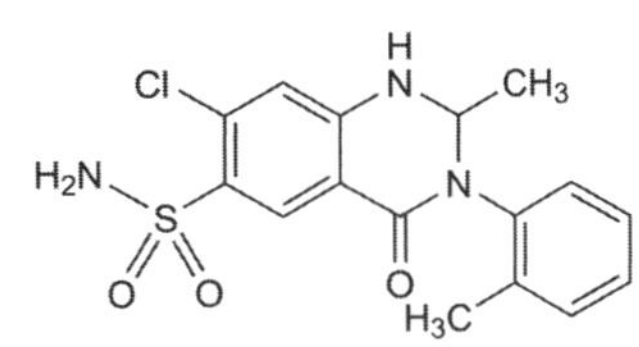

Colourless crystals. It may occur in two polymorphic forms which melt at 227° and 270°.
Sparingly soluble in water; more soluble in alkalis and organic solvents.

Dissociation Constant. pK_a 9.7.

Partition Coefficient. Log *P* (octanol/water), 1.8.

Colour Tests. Koppanyi–Zwikker test—violet; Liebermann's test—orange→green-brown; Methanolic potassium hydroxide—yellow; Sulfuric acid—yellow.

Thin-layer Chromatography. System TD—Rf 23; system TE—Rf 57; system TF—Rf 51; system TAD—Rf 33; system TAJ—Rf 34; system TAK—Rf 08; system TAL—Rf 75; system TAM—Rf 75.

Gas Chromatography. System GA—metolazone, not eluted; metolazone—Me_3 RI 3910.

High Performance Liquid Chromatography. System HN—*k* 4.89; system HY—RI 371.

Ultraviolet Spectrum. Aqueous acid—237 (A^1_1=1470b), 271, 344 nm.

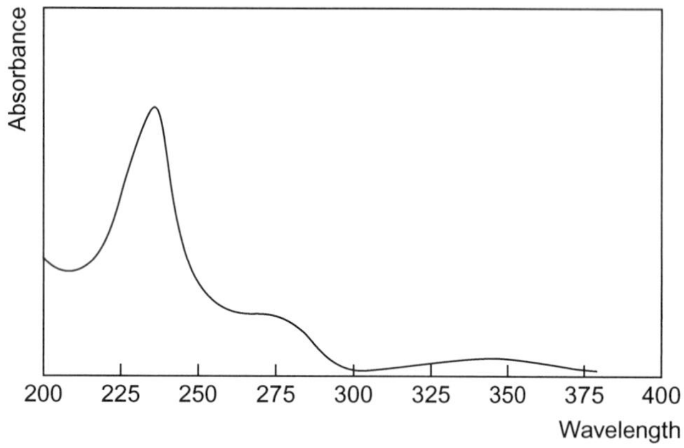

Infra-red Spectrum. Principal peaks at wavenumbers 1610, 1660, 1165, 1145, 962, 1012 cm^{-1}.

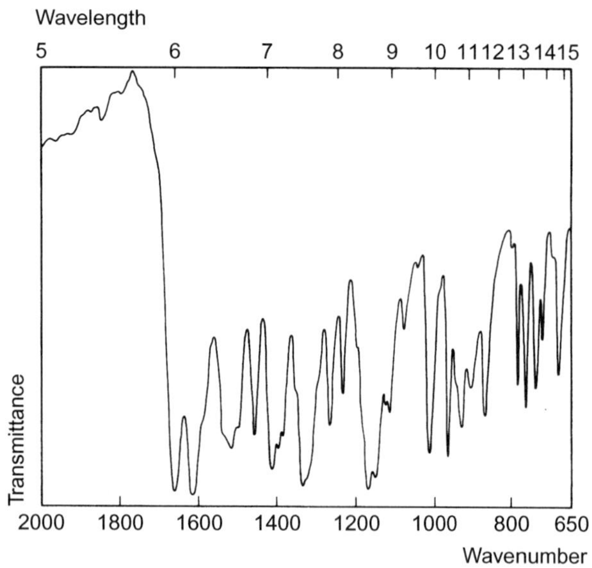

Mass Spectrum. Principal ions at *m/z* 350, 91, 259, 352, 348, 65, 351, 107.

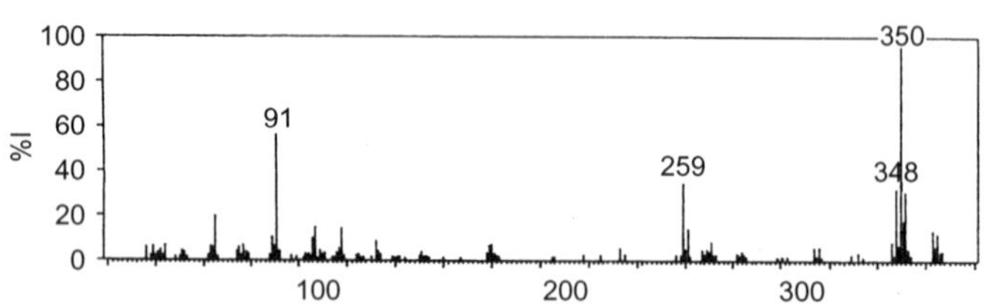

Quantification

Gas chromatography–mass spectrometry. In urine: metolazone and other diuretics, limits of detection 10 to 50 μg/L—A. M. Lisi *et al.*, *J. Chromatogr.*, 1992, *581*, 57–63.

High performance liquid chromatography. In plasma: limit of detection 2 μg/L, UV detection—R. R. Brodie *et al.*, *J. Chromatogr.*, 1981, *226*; *Biomed. Appl.*, *15*, 526–532. In plasma or urine: limit of detection 1 μg/L in plasma and 5 μg/L in urine, fluorescence detection—C. W. Vose *et al.*, *J. Chromatogr.*, 1981, *222*; *Biomed. Appl.*, *11*, 311–315. In urine: fluorescence detection—D. Farthing *et al.*, *J. Chromatogr.*, 1990, *534*, 228–232. In plasma or whole blood: limit of detection 1 μg/L, UV detection—D. Farthing *et al.*, *J. Chromatogr.*, 1994, *653*; *Biomed. Appl.*, 171–176.

Disposition in the Body. Metolazone is incompletely but fairly readily absorbed after oral administration. About 80% of a dose is excreted in the urine as unchanged drug in 48 h; about 10% is excreted in the bile.

Therapeutic concentration

After a single oral dose of 2.5 mg given to 3 subjects, a mean peak plasma concentration of about 0.01 mg/L was attained in 5 h. [W. J. Tilstone *et al.*, *Clin. Pharmacol. Ther.*, 1974, *16*, 322–329].

Half-life. Plasma half-life, about 18 h.

Volume of distribution. About 1.6 L/kg.

Clearance. Plasma clearance, about 1.4 mL/min/kg.

Distribution in blood. Plasma : whole blood ratio, 0.84.

Protein binding. In plasma, 95%.

Dose. Usually 2.5 to 10 mg daily; maximum of 80 mg daily.

Metomidate

Sedative (Veterinary)

Synonyms. Methoxymol; Methomidate.
1-(1-Phenylethyl)-1*H*-imidazole-5-carboxylic acid methyl ester
$C_{13}H_{14}N_2O_2$=230.3
CAS—5377-20-8

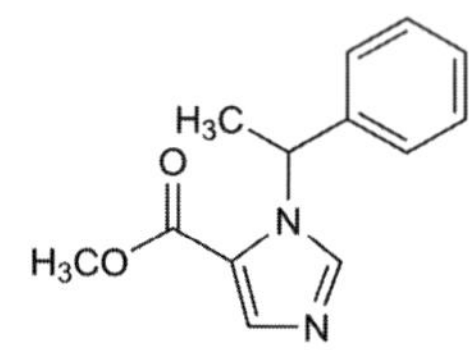

Metomidate Hydrochloride
Proprietary name. Hypnodil
$C_{13}H_{14}N_2O_2$,HCl=266.7
CAS—35944-74-2
An off-white crystalline powder. M.p. about 172°.
Very soluble in water.

Partition Coefficient. Log *P* (octanol/water), 2.6.

Colour Test. Liebermann's test—red-orange.

Thin-layer Chromatography. System TA—Rf 71; system TAE—Rf 77; system TAF—Rf 81; system TL—Rf 48; system TB—Rf 23; system TC—Rf 65; system TE—Rf 74. (Acidified iodoplatinate solution, positive.)

High Performance Liquid Chromatography. System HX—RI 424.

Ultraviolet Spectrum. Water—240 nm (A^1_1=408b).

Infra-red Spectrum. Principal peaks at wavenumbers 1730, 1230, 725, 770, 1288, 1200 cm^{-1} (metomidate hydrochloride, KBr disk).

Metopimazine

Anti-emetic

Synonyms. Exp-999; RP-9965.
Proprietary name. Vogalene
1-[3-[2-(Methylsulfonyl)-10*H*-phenothiazin-10-yl]propyl]-4-piperidine-carboxamide
$C_{22}H_{27}N_3O_3S_2$=445.6
CAS—14008-44-7

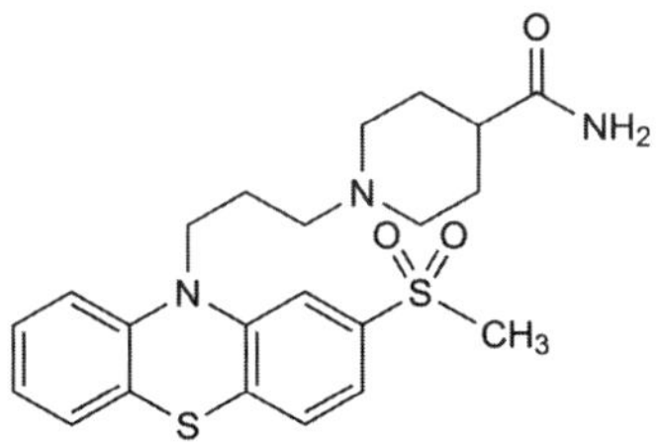

A white crystalline powder. M.p. 170° to 171°.
Soluble in chloroform and dilute acetic acid.

Partition Coefficient. Log *P* (octanol/water), 2.4.

Colour Tests. Formaldehyde–Sulfuric Acid—red; Forrest Reagent—brown; FPN Reagent—orange; Mandelin's Test—green; Marquis Test—red; Sulfuric Acid—red.

Thin-layer Chromatography. System TA—Rf 56; system TB—Rf 00; system TC—Rf 11; system TL—Rf 12. (Acidified iodoplatinate solution, positive.)

High Performance Liquid Chromatography. System HA—*k* 1.4.

Ultraviolet Spectrum. Aqueous acid—264 nm (A_1^1=922b), 310 nm.

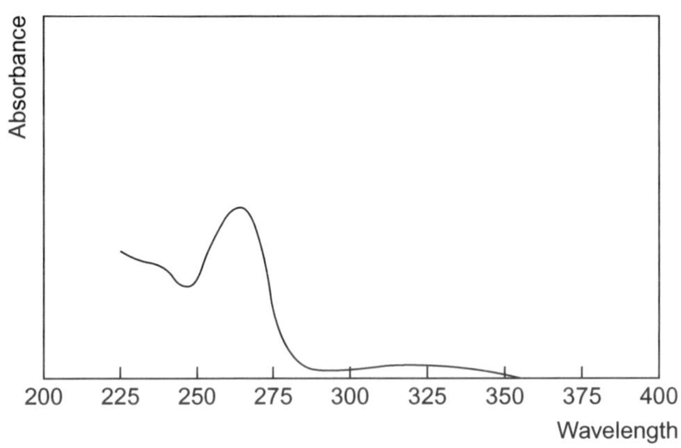

Infra-red Spectrum. Principal peaks at wavenumbers 1150, 1310, 750, 1665, 1102, 1248 cm^{-1} (KBr disk).

Mass Spectrum. Principal ions at *m/z* 141, 445, 169, 123, 155, 96, 42, 317.

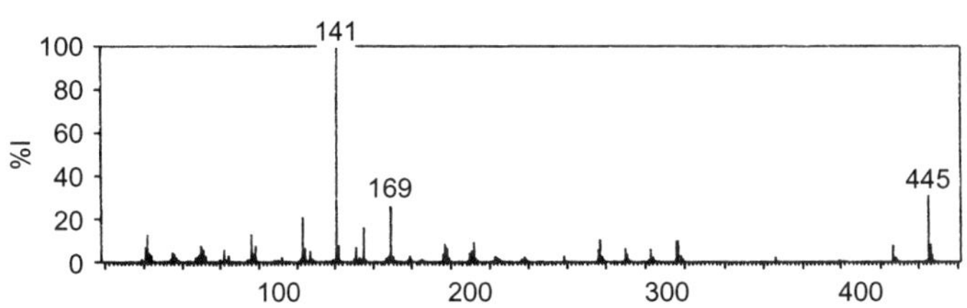

Quantification

High performance liquid chromatography. In serum: metopimazine and its acid metabolite, fluorescence detection—H. R. Angelo *et al.*, *J. Chromatogr.*, 1989, *496*, 472–477.

Therapeutic concentration

Administration of a single oral 20 or 50 mg dose of metopimazine before food in 6 subjects produced median peak plasma concentrations of 43 or 83 µg/L at 52 and 60 min, respectively. When the same doses were administered postprandially, the corresponding values were 22 or 51 µg/L, both at 90 min [J. Herrstedt *et al.*, *Br. J. Clin. Pharmacol.*, 1990, *30*, 237–243].

6 subjects were given 40 mg of metopimazine either as a single microenema or as a single oral dose or were given 10 mg metopimazine as a 60 min continuous intravenous infusion. The median peak plasma concentration was 59 µg/L (range 28 to 182) 53 min (25 to 90) after oral administration, 128 µg/L (69 to 218) 10 min (10 to 10) after rectal administration and 108 µg/L (74 to 193) 60 min (45 to 60) after intravenous administration [J. Herrstedt *et al.*, *Br. J. Clin. Pharmacol.*, 1996, *41*, 613–615].

Metopimazine 20, 30, 40, 50 or 60 mg was given orally every 4 h for 11 doses to 36 subjects. For the 50 mg dose, median peak plasma concentrations of 115, 108, 96, 183 and 109 µg/L were obtained at 1.5, 12, 24, 36 and 48 h after the first dose, respectively; the corresponding values for the 60 mg dose were 73, 52, 105, 96 and 70 µg/L. 6 doses of 30 mg were found to be safe [J. Herrstedt *et al.*, *Support Care Cancer*, 1997, *5*, 38–43].

Dose. 5 to 15 mg daily.

Metoprolol

Beta-adrenoceptor Blocking Agent

1-[4-(2-Methoxyethyl)phenoxy]-3-[(1-methylethyl)amino]-2-propanol
$C_{15}H_{25}NO_3$=267.4
CAS—37350-58-6

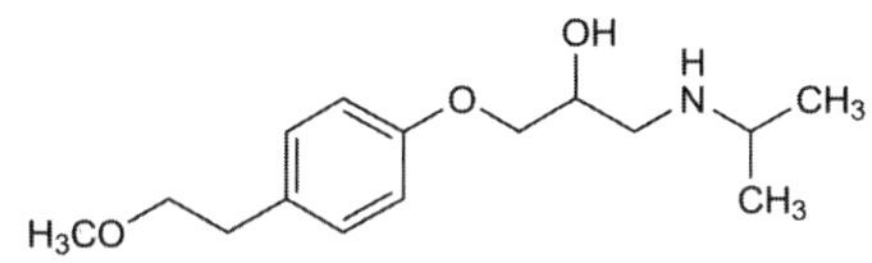

Metoprolol Tartrate

Synonyms. CGP-2175E; H-93/26; Metoprololi Tartras.
Proprietary names. Abralene; Azumetop; Beloc; Betaloc; Betazok; Jeprolol; Lanoc; Lopresor; Lopressor; Mepranix; Meprolol; Meto; Metocor; Metolol; Nu-Metop; Seloken; Toprol XL. It is an ingredient of Co-Betaloc, Logimax, Logroton, and Lopresor HCT.
$(C_{15}H_{25}NO_3)_2,C_4H_6O_6$=684.8
CAS—56392-17-7
A white crystalline powder. M.p. about 120°.
Very soluble in water; soluble in ethanol and chloroform; practically insoluble in ether.

Dissociation Constant. pK_a 9.7.

Partition Coefficient. Log *P* (octanol/water), 1.9.

Colour Tests. Liebermann's Test—pink-brown; Mandelin's Test—pink-brown; Marquis Test—pink.

Thin-layer Chromatography. System TA—Rf 49; system TB—Rf 10; system TC—Rf 08; system TE—Rf 44; system TL—Rf 09; system TAE—Rf 20; system TAF—Rf 74; system TAJ—Rf 02; system TAK—Rf 12; system TAL—Rf 70.

Gas Chromatography. System GA—metoprolol RI 2035, M (OH-)-AC$_3$ RI 2730, M (*O*-desmethyl-)-AC$_3$ RI 2620; system GB—RI 2090.

High Performance Liquid Chromatography. System HA—*k* 1.3; system HX—RI 326; system HY—RI 272; system HZ—retention time 2.5 min; system HAA—retention time 10.7 min; system HAX—retention time 7.1 min; system HAY—retention time 4.1 min.

Ultraviolet Spectrum. Aqueous acid—274 (A_1^1=52a), 280 nm (inflexion).

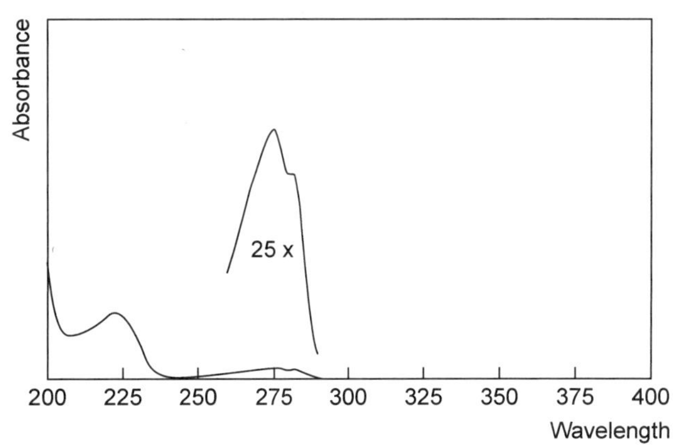

Infra-red Spectrum. Principal peaks at wavenumbers 1510, 1245, 1108, 1028, 1175, 810 cm^{-1} (KBr disk).

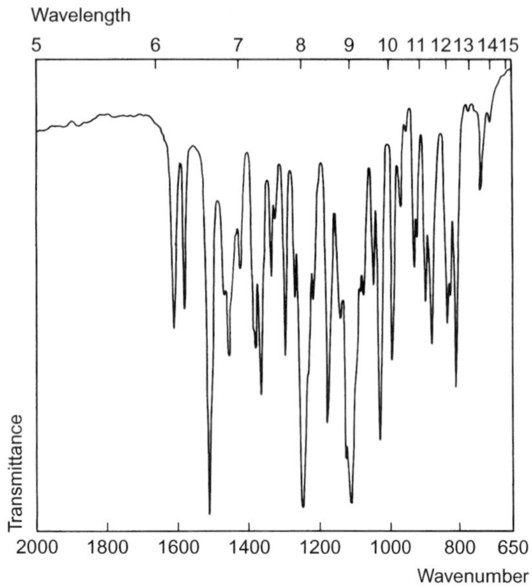

Mass Spectrum. Principal ions at m/z 72, 30, 107, 56, 45, 41, 44, 43.

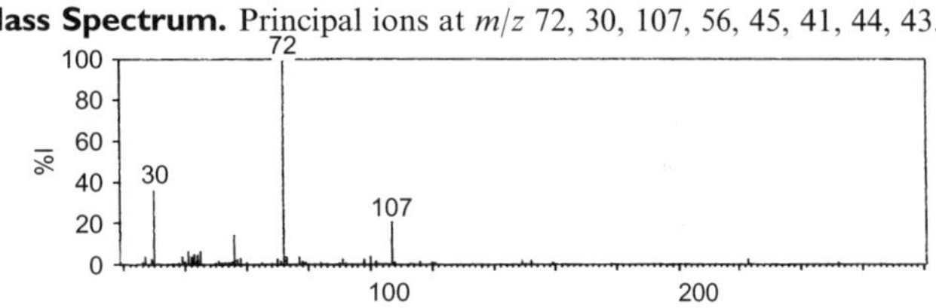

Quantification

Gas chromatography. In plasma or urine: limit of detection 3 μg/L, ECD—C. D. Kinney, *J. Chromatogr.* 1981, *225*(14) *B Biomed. Appl.*, 213–218. In plasma or urine: metoprolol metabolites, limit of detection 6 μg/L, ECD—C. P. Quarterman *et al.*, *J. Chromatogr.* 1980, *183*(9) *B Biomed. Appl.*, 92–98. In plasma: metoprolol and propranolol—M. P. Quaglio *et al.*, *Farmaco*, 1992, *47(Suppl 5)*, 799–809. In plasma: metoprolol and propranolol, limit of detection 50 μg/L, FID—M. P. Quaglio *et al.*, *J. Pharm. Sci.*, 1993, *82*, 87–90.

Gas chromatography–mass spectrometry. In plasma or urine: metoprolol and metabolites, limit of detection 300 ng/L—M. Ervik *et al.*, *Biomed. Mass Spectrom.*, 1981, *8*, 322–326. In plasma: metoprolol and propranolol, limit of detection 10 μg/L—M. P. Quaglio *et al.*, *J. Pharm. Sci.*, 1993, *82*, 87–90. In postmortem blood or urine: metoprolol and other beta-blockers, SID—S. B. Black *et al.*, *J. Chromatogr.* 1996, *685 B Biomed. Appl.*, 67–80. In urine: metoprolol and other beta-blockers, limit of detection for metoprolol 30 μg/L—K. Hartonen and M. L. Riekkola, *J. Chromatogr.* 1996, *676 B Biomed. Appl.*, 45–52.

High performance liquid chromatography. In plasma: limit of detection 3 μg/L for metoprolol and 12.5 μg/L for α-hydroxymetoprolol, fluorescence detection—D. B. Pautler and W. J. Jusko, *J. Chromatogr.* 1982, *228*(17) *B Biomed. Appl.*, 215–222. In plasma: metoprolol enantiomers, limit of detection 10 μg/L, fluorescence detection—V. L. Herring *et al.*, *J. Chromatogr.*, 1991, *567*, 221–227. In plasma or urine: metoprolol and α-hydroxy metabolite enantiomers, limit of detection for metoprolol 10 nmol/L in plasma, fluorescence detection—K. Balmer *et al.*, *J. Chromatogr.*, 1991, *553*, 391–397. In plasma: metoprolol enantiomers, fluorescence detection—M. M. Bhatti and R. T. Foster, *J. Chromatogr.*, 1992, *579*, 361–365. In urine: metoprolol and α-hydroxymetoprolol, fluorescence detection—H. G. Xie and H. H. Zhou, *Zhongguo Yao Li Xue Bao*, 1995, *16*, 32–35. In urine metoprolol enantiomers and major metabolite, fluorescence detection—F. Li *et al.*, *J. Chromatogr.* 1995, *668 B Biomed. Appl.*, 67–75. In urine: metoprolol and other beta-blockers, limits of quantification 15 to 500 ppb, amperometric detection—M. I. Maguregui *et al.*, *J. Chromatogr.* 1995, *674 B Biomed. Appl.*, 85–91. In urine: metoprolol and two metabolites, fluorescence detection—F. C. Chiu *et al.*, *J. Chromatogr. B Biomed. Sci. Appl.*, 1997, *696*, 69–74. In plasma: metoprolol and α-hydroxymetoprolol, fluorescence detection—B. Mistry *et al.*, *J. Pharm. Biomed. Anal.*, 1998, *16*, 1041–1049.

Review. HPLC methods for enantioselective analysis of metoprolol and other beta-blockers—G. Egginger *et al.*, *Biomed. Chromatogr.*, 1993, *7*, 277–295.

Disposition in the Body. Well absorbed after oral administration; although the bioavailibity is low because of extensive first-pass metabolism. Metoprolol crosses the blood–brain barrier and placental barrier; it is also excreted into breast milk. About 95% of a dose is excreted in the urine within 48 h, with about 65% of the dose as the inactive metabolite, 4-(2-hydroxy-3-isopropylaminopropoxy)phenylacetic acid, and about 10% as a further inactive metabolite, 2-hydroxy-3-[4-(2-methoxyethyl)-phenoxy]propionic acid. Two active metabolites, α-hydroxymetoprolol and *O*-desmethylmetoprolol are also excreted in the urine in amounts equivalent to about 10% and less than 1% of the dose, respectively. Up to about 10% of a dose is excreted as unchanged drug.

Therapeutic concentration

Following a single oral dose of 100 mg, given to 6 subjects, peak plasma concentrations of 0.03 to 0.28 mg/L (mean 0.13) were attained in about 2.5 h. [W. Kirch *et al.*, *Biopharm. Drug Dispos.*, 1983, *4*, 73–81.]

Following a single oral dose of 100 mg to 8 subjects, a mean peak plasma concentration of metoprolol of 0.12 mg/L was attained in 2 to 3 h; the α-hydroxy metabolite reached a mean peak of 0.07 mg/L in about 3 h. After repeated administration of 100 mg every 12 h, the mean peak plasma concentrations on the 8th day were 0.19 mg/L for metoprolol and 0.07 mg/L for the α-hydroxy metabolite. The concentration of the metabolite appears to be increased in elderly subjects. [C. P. Quarterman *et al.*, *Br. J. Clin. Pharmacol.*, 1981, *11*, 287–294.]

In 20 subjects receiving 100 mg metoprolol tartrate twice daily for a total of 9 doses by mouth, the reported peak plasma concentration of (*S*)-metoprolol was 0.0855 mg/L in men and 0.146 mg/L in women, and that of (*R*)-metoprolol was 0.0672 mg/L in men and 0.124 mg/L in women; peak concentrations occurred at 1.3 h in men and 1.6 h in women. [A. B. Luzier *et al.*, *Clin. Pharmacol. Ther.*, 1999, *66*, 594–601.]

Toxicity

In a massive fatal overdose of metoprolol, the following postmortem tissue concentrations of the active (*S*)-isomer were reported: blood, 33 mg/L, liver 224 μg/g, stomach contents 56 mg/61 g. Concentrations of the (R)-isomer were: blood 33 mg/L, liver 222 μg/g, stomach contents 55 mg/61 g. [A. Mozayani *et al.*, *J. Anal. Toxicol.*, 1995, *19*, 519–521.]

The following postmortem concentrations were reported in a death due to an intentional overdose of metoptolol: blood 19.8 mg/L, bile 83.1 mg/L, urine 1.6 mg/L, vitreous humour 15.1 mg/L; a blood ethanol concentration of 0.25 g/100 mL was also found. [T. P. Rohrig *et al.*, *J. Anal. Toxicol.*, 1987, *11*, 231–232.]

In a fatality due to the deliberate ingestion of metoprolol, the following postmortem tissue concentrations were reported: blood 4.7 mg/L, bile 254 mg/L, kidney 7.1 μg/g, liver 6.3 μg/g, urine 194 mg/L. [M. Stajić *et al.*, *J. Anal. Toxicol.*, 1984, *8*, 228–230.]

In a fatality due to metoprolol and salicylate, the following postmortem tissue concentrations were reported: blood, metoprolol 56 mg/L, salicylate 220 mg/L; bile, metoprolol 276 mg/L; liver, metoprolol 230 μg/g. [M. Holzbecher *et al.*, *J. Forensic Sci. Soc.*, 1982, *27*, 715–717.]

Bioavailability. About 40 to 50% (about 70% after modified-release preparations).

Half-life. Plasma half-life, metoprolol 3 to 4 h in fast hydroxylators and about 7 h in slow hydroxylators; α-hydroxymetoprolol 4 to 12 h (mean 6).

Volume of distribution. About 4 L/kg.

Clearance. Plasma clearance, about 15 mL/min/kg.

Distribution in blood. Plasma:whole blood ratio, 0.77.

Protein binding In plasma, about 11%.

Note. For a review of the clinical pharmacokinetics of metoprolol, see C.-G. Regardh and G. Johnsson, *Clin. Pharmacokinet.*, 1980, *5*, 557–569 and for a review of controlled-release metoprolol, see M. J. Kendall *et al.*, *Clin. Pharmacokinet.*, 1991, *21*, 319–330

Dose. In hypertension 100 to 400 mg of metoprolol tartrate daily.

Metronidazole

Antiprotozoal/Antibacterial

Synonyms. Bayer 5630; RP-8823.
Proprietary names. Anabact; Elyzol; Flagyl; Metizol; Metro; Metrocream; Metrogel; Metrogyl; Metrolyl; Metrotop; Metrozol(e); Metryl;

Norit(r)ate; Norzol; Protostat; Rozex; Trichozole; Vaginyl; Zadstat; Zidoval; Zyomet. It is an ingredient of Entamizole, Helidac and HeliMet.
2-Methyl-5-nitroimidazole-1-ethanol
$C_6H_9N_3O_3$=171.2
CAS—443-48-1

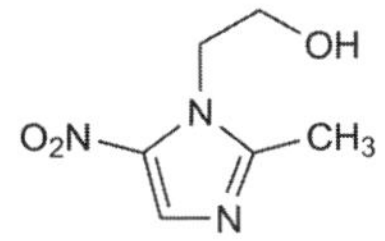

A white to pale yellow crystalline powder or crystals. It darkens on exposure to light. M.p. 158° to 160°.
Soluble 1 in 100 of water, 1 in 200 of ethanol, and 1 in 250 of chloroform; soluble in dilute acids; slightly soluble in ether.

Dissociation Constant. pK_a 2.5.

Partition Coefficient. Log *P* (octanol/buffer pH 7.4), −0.1.

Colour Test. Methanolic potassium hydroxide—red.

Thin-layer Chromatography. System TA—Rf 58; system TB—Rf 02; system TC—Rf 36; system TE—Rf 46; system TL—Rf 40; system TAD—Rf 32; system TAE—Rf 75; system TAF—Rf 70; system TAJ—Rf 32; system TAK—Rf 14; system TAL—Rf 75. (Acidified potassium permanganate solution, positive.)

Gas Chromatography. System GA—RI 1592.

High Performance Liquid Chromatography. System HX—RI 257; system HY—RI 226; system HAA—Retention time(s), 6.8 min.

Ultraviolet Spectrum. Aqueous acid—277 nm (A^1_1=377a); aqueous alkali—319 nm (A^1_1=520b).

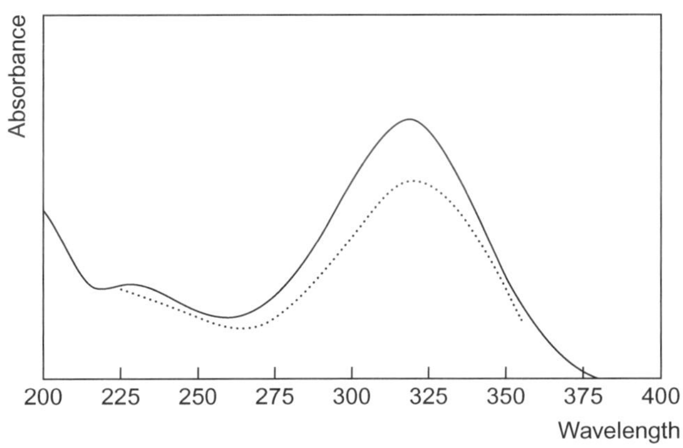

Infra-red Spectrum. Principal peaks at wavenumbers 1187, 1535, 1070, 1265, 745, 1160 cm^{-1} (KBr disk).

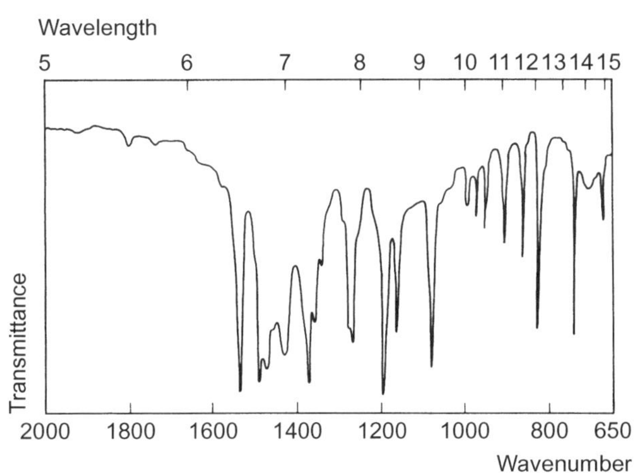

Mass Spectrum. Principal ions at *m/z* 81, 124, 54, 53, 125, 171, 45, 42.

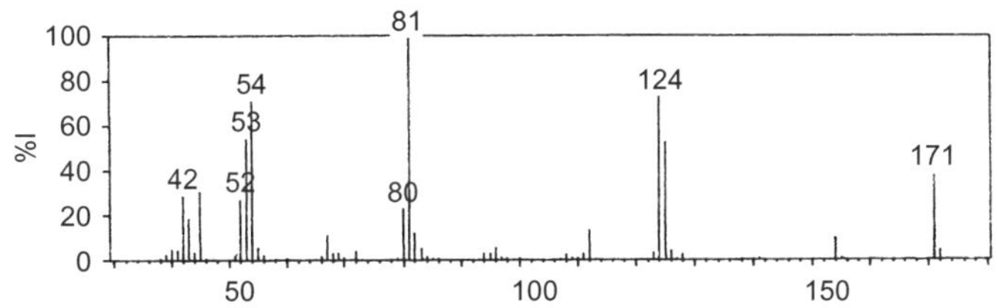

Quantification

High performance liquid chromatography. In plasma, serum, saliva, whole blood or urine: metronidazole and metabolites, UV detection—C. M. Kaye *et al., Br. J. Clin. Pharmacol.*, 1980, *9*, 528–529. In plasma: limit of detection 25 µg/L, UV detection—R. A. Gibson *et al., Clin. Chem.*, 1984, *30*, 784–787. In plasma or urine: metronidazole and chloroquine, UV detection—P. O. Okonkwo and E. I. Eta, *Life Sci.*, 1988, *42*, 539–545. In vaginal tissue: limit of detection about 100 ng/g, UV detection—T. G. Venkateshwaran and J. T. Stewart, *J. Chromatogr.*, 1995, *672*, *Biomed. Appl.*, 300–304. In plasma, saliva, or gastric juice: metronidazole and its hydroxy metabolite, limits of detection 0.25 mg/L and 0.2 mg/L respectively—M. J. Jessa *et al., J. Chromatogr.*, 1996, *677*, *Biomed. Appl.*, 374–379. In plasma or gastric fluid: metronidazole and omeprazole, limit of detection 0.1 mg/L, UV detection—P. K. Yeung *et al., J. Pharm. Biomed. Anal.*, 1998, *17*, 1393–1398. In serum: limit of detection 10 µg/L, UV detection—M. J. Galmier *et al., J. Chromatogr. B Biomed. Sci. Appl.*, 1998, *720*, 239–243. In plasma: metronidazole and amoxicillin, limit of detection 1 mg/L, photodiode array detection—A. Menelaou *et al., J. Chromatogr. B Biomed. Sci. Appl.*, 1999, *731*, 261–266.

Disposition in the Body. Metronidazole is readily and almost completely absorbed after oral administration and is widely distributed in the body. It is metabolised by oxidation to 2-hydroxymethylmetronidazole and 2-methyl-5-nitroimidazol-1-acetic acid, and by conjugation with glucuronic acid. About 70 to 80% of a dose is excreted in the urine in 48 h with less than 10% of the dose as unchanged drug, up to 10% as conjugated metronidazole, about 27% as 2-hydroxymethylmetronidazole, 10% as the conjugated 2-hydroxymethyl metabolite, and 20% as the acid metabolite.

Therapeutic concentration

Following a single oral dose of 400 mg to 7 subjects, peak plasma concentrations of 4.5 to 11.6 (mean 6.9) mg/L were attained in about 2 h; a mean peak plasma concentration of 1.6 mg/L of 2-hydroxymethylmetronidazole was attained in about 8 h. [J. C. Jensen and R. Gugler, *Clin. Pharmacol. Ther.*, 1983, *34*, 481–487].

54 subjects given IV metronidazole, 500 mg every 8 h, had mean peak and trough plasma concentrations of 28.9 and 18.0 mg/L, respectively. Mean peak and trough concentrations of the hydroxy metabolite were 6.6 and 4.2 mg/L. [T. Y. Ti *et al., Antimicrob. Agents Chemother.*, 1996, *40*, 2248–2251].

Toxicity

In a fatality attributed to an alcohol/metronidazole interaction, blood levels of 1620 mg/L alcohol, 46 mg/L acetaldehyde and 0.42 mg/L metronidazole were found. [S. J. Cina *et al., Am. J. Forensic Med. Pathol.* 1996, *17*, 343–346].

Half-life. Plasma half-life, about 8 h.

Volume of distribution. About 0.5 to 1 L/kg.

Clearance. Plasma clearance, about 1 mL/min/kg.

Protein binding. In plasma, less than 20%.

Note. For a review of the pharmacokinetics of metronidazole, see E. D. Ralph, *Clin. Pharmacokinet.*, 1983, *8*, 43–62.

Dose. Up to 2.4 g daily for 10 days.

Metyrapone

Diagnostic Agent (Pituitary Function)

Synonym. Methopyrapone; Su-4885.
Proprietary name. Metopiron(e)
2-Methyl-1,2-di-3-pyridyl-1-propanone
$C_{14}H_{14}N_2O$=226.3
CAS—54-36-4

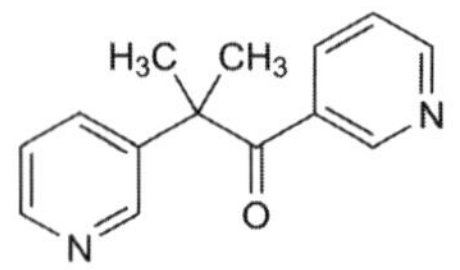

A white to light amber, fine, crystalline powder which darkens on exposure to light. M.p. 50° to 53°.
Soluble 1 in 100 of water, 1 in 3 of ethanol and chloroform; soluble in methanol.

Partition Coefficient. Log *P* (octanol/water), 1.9.

Colour Test. Cyanogen bromide—orange.

Thin-layer Chromatography. System TA—Rf 58; system TB—Rf 16; system TC—Rf 58; system TE—Rf 64; system TL—Rf 41; system TAE—Rf 66. (Acidified iodoplatinate solution, positive.)

Gas Chromatography. System GA—RI 1860.

Ultraviolet Spectrum. Aqueous acid—260 nm (A^1_1 = 500a), 233.

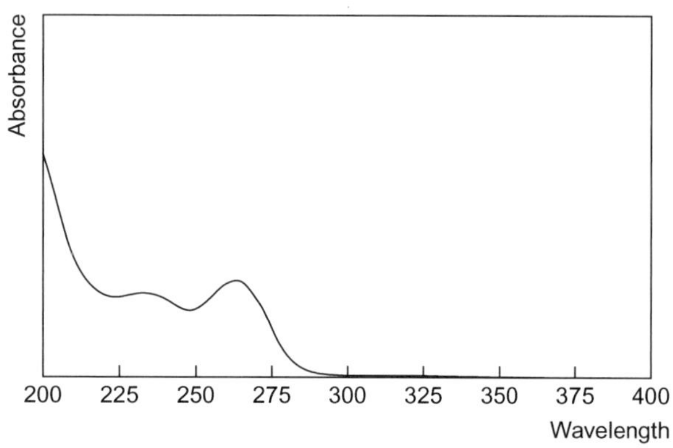

Infra-red Spectrum. Principal peaks at wavenumbers 1672, 1578, 1255, 714, 699, 970 cm^{-1} (KBr disk).

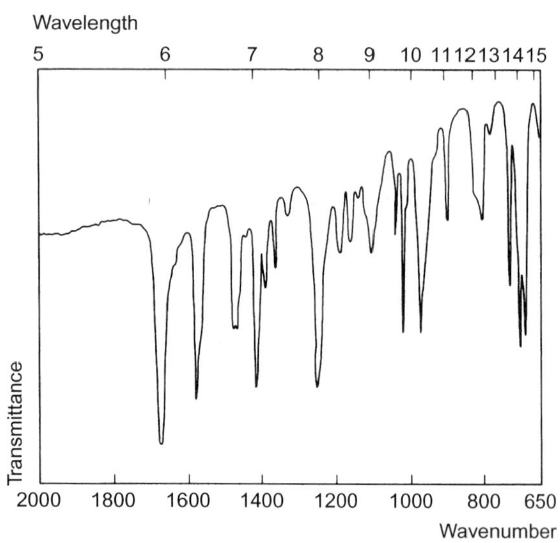

Mass Spectrum. Principal ions at *m*/*z* 120, 106, 78, 92, 51, 226, 41, 39.

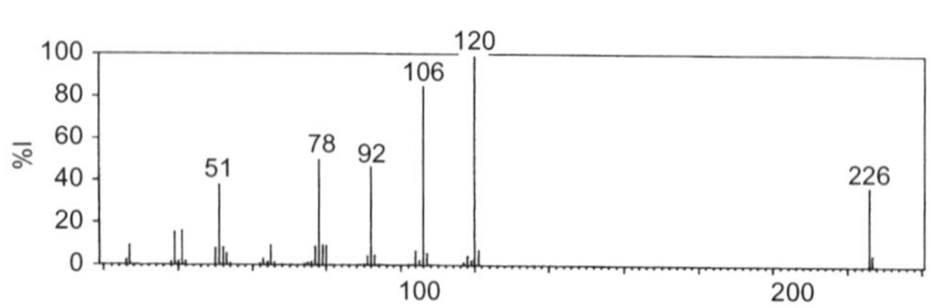

Quantification

Colorimetry. In plasma or tissues: limit of detection 5 mg/L for metyrapone, 2 mg/L for 1-hydroxymetyrapone—S. Szeberenyi *et al.*, *J. Chromatogr.*, 1969, *40*, 417–421.

Spectrofluorimetry. In plasma—A. W. Meikle *et al.*, *J. Lab. Clin. Med.*, 1969, *74*, 515–520.

Gas chromatography. In urine: metyrapone and 1-hydroxymetyrapone, FID—D. M. Hannah and J. G. Sprunt, *J. Pharm. Pharmacol.*, 1969, *21*, 877–878.

High performance liquid chromatography. In plasma: metyrapone and its enantiomeric metyrapol metabolites, limit of detection 0.045 mg/L, UV detection—N. M. Cassiano *et al.*, *Chirality*, 2002, *14*, 731–735.

Disposition in the Body. Metyrapone is metabolised by reduction to the 1-hydroxy derivative which is active. It is excreted in the urine mainly as the glucuronide conjugates of 1-hydroxymetyrapone and metyrapone. About 50% of a dose is excreted in the urine in 3 days.

Dose. Up to 4.5 g daily.

Mevinphos

Pesticide

Proprietary name. Phosdrin
3-[(Dimethoxyphosphinyl)oxy]-2-butenoic acid methyl ester
$C_7H_{13}O_6P = 224.1$
CAS—7786-34-7

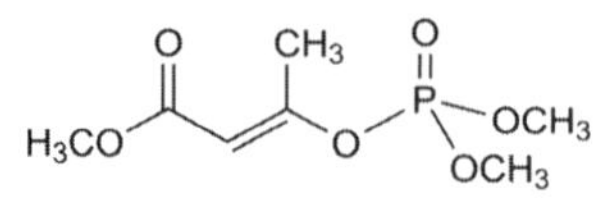

(*E*)- isomer

The technical product is a pale yellow to orange liquid.
Miscible with water, ethanol, acetone, benzene, carbon tetrachloride, toluene, xylene, and chloroform; soluble 1 in 20 of carbon disulfide; practically insoluble in hexane.

Partition Coefficient. Log *P* (octanol/water), 0.1.

Colour Test. Phosphorus Test—yellow.

Thin-layer Chromatography. System TE—Rf 75; system TW—Rf 23; system TX—Rf 12; system TY—Rf 10; system TAB—Rf 03; system TAC—Rf 02; system TAE—Rf 86.

Gas Chromatography. System GA—RI 1450; system GK—RRT 0.50 (relative to caffeine).

High Performance Liquid Chromatography. System HAO—*k* 1.37; system HAP—*k* 0.45.

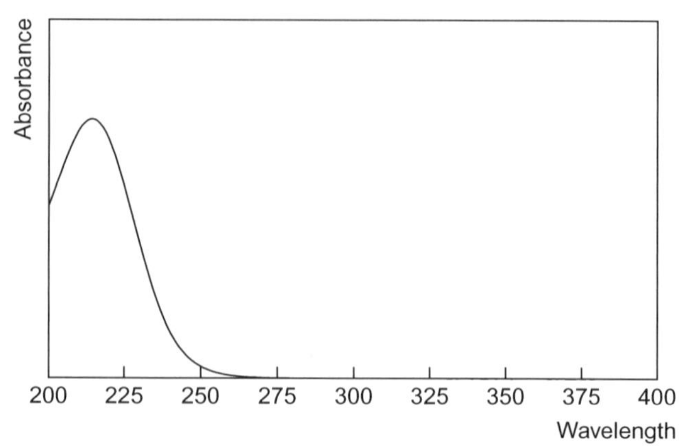

Mass Spectrum. Principal ions at *m*/*z* 127, 192, 109, 67, 43, 193, 39, 79.

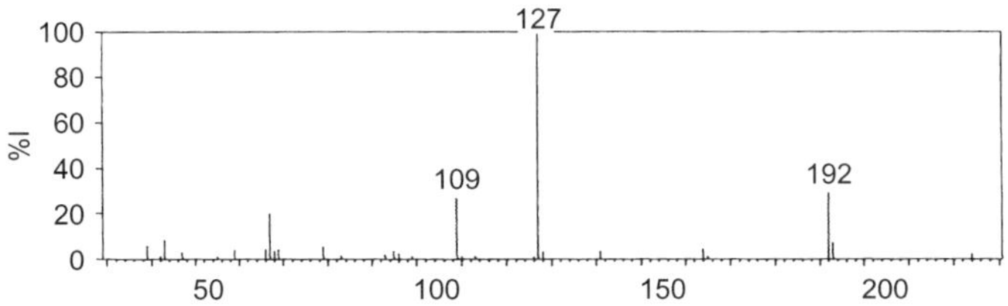

Quantification

Gas chromatography. In postmortem tissues and fluids: AFID—J. F. Lewin and J. L. Love, *Forens. Sci.*, 1974, *4*, 253–255.

Gas chromatography–mass spectrometry. In blood: mevinphos and other organophosphorus pesticides, limits of detection 0.01 to 0.3 µg/g—F. Musshoff *et al.*, *J. Chromatogr. Sci.*, 2002, *40*, 29–34.

Disposition in the Body

Toxicity. Mevinphos is extremely toxic by inhalation, ingestion, or percutaneous absorption and the estimated lethal dose is less than 500 mg. The maximum permissible atmospheric concentration is 0.1 mg/m^3.

The following postmortem tissue concentrations were reported in a fatality due to the ingestion of mevinphos: blood 360 mg/L, brain 3 µg/g, kidney 20 µg/g, liver 240 µg/g, skeletal muscle 86 µg/g, urine 8 mg/L; alcohol was detected in blood and urine at concentrations of 1250 mg/L and 1550 mg/L, respectively; death occurred within 45 min of ingestion [J. F. Lewin and J. L. Love, *Forensic Sci.*, 1974, *4*, 253–255.]

A 66-year-old man died about 1 min after ingesting 28 g of mevinphos [R. Lokan and R. James, *Forensic Sci. Int.*, 1983, *22*, 179–182.]

Mexazolam

Anxiolytic

Synonyms. CS-386; Methylcloxazolam.
Proprietary name. Melex
10-Chloro-11*b*-(2-chlorophenyl)-2,3,7,11b-tetrahydro-3-methyloxazolo-[3,2-*d*][1,4]-benzodiazepin-6(5*H*)-one
$C_{18}H_{16}Cl_2N_2O_2=363.2$
CAS—31868-18-5

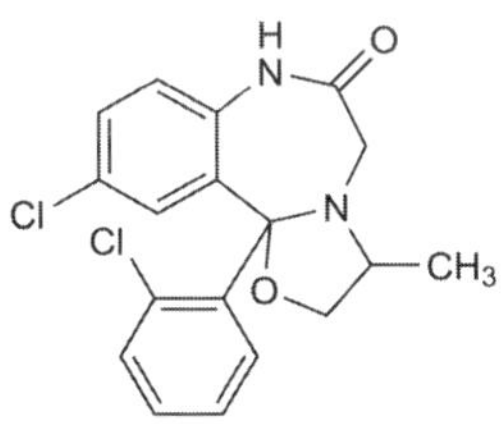

Crystalline powder. M.p. 172° to 175°.

Dissociation Constant. pK_a 6.7.

Thin-layer Chromatography. System TE—Rf 78; system TF—Rf 55; system TAE—Rf 86.

Gas Chromatography. System GA—RI 2600.

High Performance Liquid Chromatography. System HX—RI 345.

Ultraviolet Spectrum. Aqueous acid—241, 290, 373 nm; ethanol—244 nm; aqueous alkali—244 nm.

Infra-red Spectrum. Principal peaks at wavenumbers 1661, 1400, 1204, 1470, 1300, 1078 cm^{-1} (KBr disk).

Mass Spectrum. Principal ions at *m/z* 251, 70, 253, 28, 41, 42, 139, 18.

Mexenone

Sunscreen Agent

Synonym. Benzophenone-10
Proprietary name. It is an ungredient of Uvistat.
(2-Hydroxy-4-methoxyphenyl)(4-methylphenyl)methanone
$C_{15}H_{14}O_3=242.3$
CAS—1641-17-4

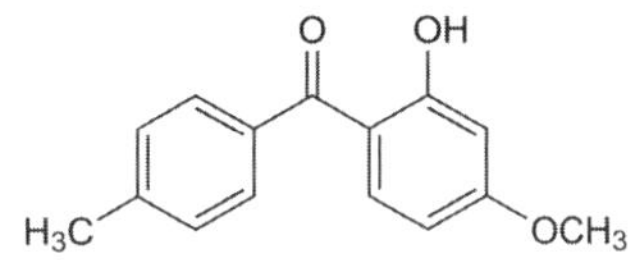

A pale yellow crystalline powder. M.p. 99° to 102°.
Practically insoluble in water; soluble 1 in 70 of ethanol and 1 in 7 of acetone.

Partition Coefficient. Log *P* (octanol/water), 4.1.

Ultraviolet Spectrum. Methanol—243 (A^1_1=353b), 287 (A^1_1=640a), 325 nm (A^1_1=440b).

Infra-red Spectrum. Principal peaks at wavenumbers 1260, 1598, 1637, 1211, 1613, 920 cm^{-1} (KBr disk).

Use. Topically in a concentration of 4% in a cream or a solid basis.

Mexiletine

Anti-arrhythmic

1-(2,6-Dimethylphenoxy)-2-propanamine
$C_{11}H_{17}NO=179.3$
CAS—31828-71-4

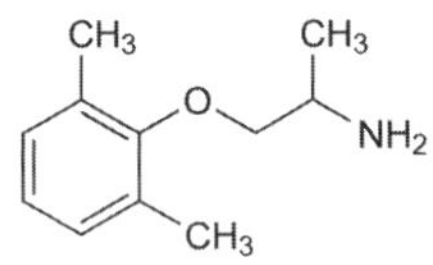

Mexiletine Hydrochloride

Synonym. Ko-1173
Proprietary name. Mexitil
$C_{11}H_{17}NO,HCl=215.7$
CAS—5370-01-4
A white crystalline powder. M.p. 198° to 204°.
Soluble 1 in 2 of water, 1 in 3 of ethanol, and 1 in 30 of chloroform; practically insoluble in ether.

Dissociation Constant. pK_a 9.0.

Partition Coefficient. Log *P* (octanol/water), 2.2.

Colour Tests. Liebermann's test—brown; Mandelin's test—brown-orange; Marquis test—red.

Thin-layer Chromatography. System TA—Rf 40; system TB—Rf 17; system TC—Rf 04; system TE—Rf 55; system TL—Rf 09; system TAE—Rf 25; system TAF—Rf 78.

Gas Chromatography. System GA—Mexiletene RI 1400; M(des amino-oxo-) RI 1350; system GB—mexiletene RI 1431; M (desamino-oxo-) RI 1395.

High Performance Liquid Chromatography. System HA—*k* 1.2; system HX—RI 329; system HY—RI 278; system HAA—Retention time(s) 11.5 min.

Ultraviolet Spectrum. Aqueous acid—260 nm (A^1_1=14a).

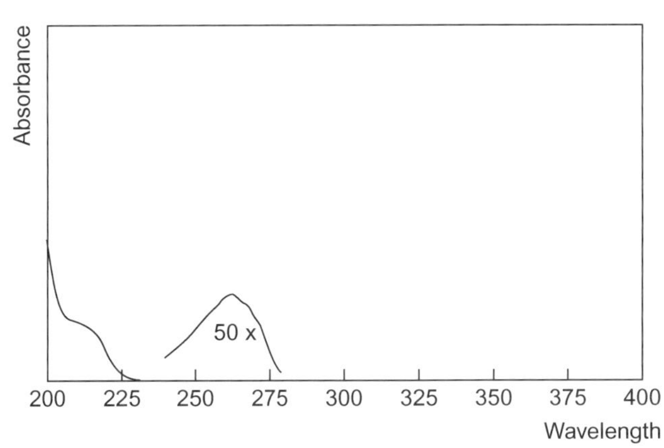

Infra-red Spectrum. Principal peaks at wavenumbers 1200, 1040, 770, 760, 1595, 1090 cm^{-1} (mexiletine hydrochloride, KBr disk).

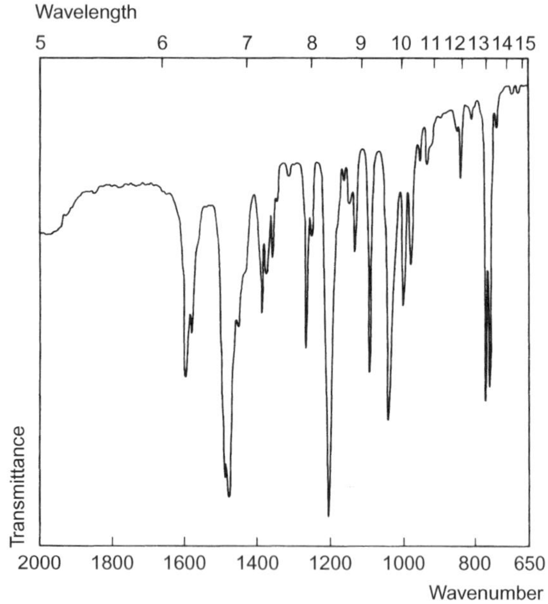

Mass Spectrum. Principal ions at *m/z* 58, 44, 41, 83, 77, 69, 85, 43.

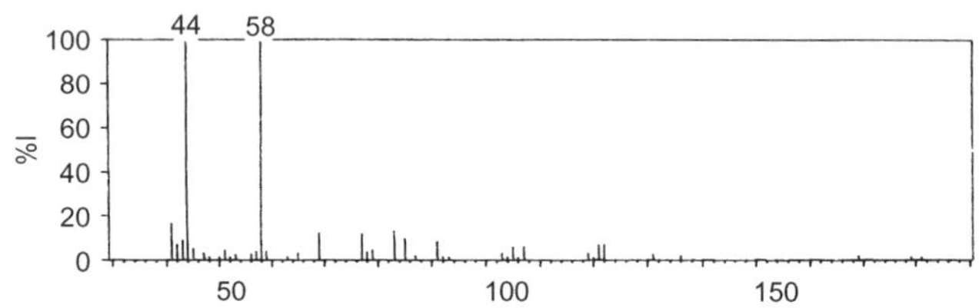

Quantification

Gas chromatography. In plasma or urine: limit of detection 50 µg/L, FID—K. Chan *et al.*, *J. Pharm. Pharmacol.*, 1980, *32*, *Suppl.*, 98P. In plasma: limits of detection 20 µg/L for mexiletine and 7 µg/L for the 2′-hydroxymethyl metabolite; ECD—A. Pachecus *et al.*, *Arzneimittelforschung*, 1982, *32*, 688–693. In blood or plasma: limit of detection 5 µg/L, AFID—K. J. Smith and P. J. Meffin, *J. Chromatogr.*, 1980, *181*; *Biomed. Appl.*, *7*, 469–472. In serum: FID—V. Marko, *Pharmazie*, 1987, *42*, 387–389. In plasma: limit of detection 10 ng, FID—S. G. Ji *et al.*, *Biomed. Chromatogr.*, 1993, *7*, 196–199. In urine: mexiletine enantiomers and hydroxylated metabolites—B. Knoche *et al.*, *Chirality*, 1996, *8*, 30–34.

Gas chromatography–mass spectrometry. In plasma: limit of detection 0.1 mg/L, selected-ion monitoring—M. B. Minnigh *et al.*, *J. Chromatogr. B Biomed. Appl.*, 1994, *662*, 118–122; A. Dasgupta *et al.*, *Ther. Drug Monit.*, 1998, *20*, 313–318; A Dasgupta and O. Yousef, *J. Chromatogr. B Biomed. Sci. Appl.*, 1998, *705*, 283–288.

High performance liquid chromatography. In plasma, urine or cerebrospinal fluid: limit of detection 10 µg/L, UV detection—H. Breithaupt and M. Wilfling, *J. Chromatogr.*, 1982, *230*; *B Biomed. Appl.*, *19*, 97–105. In plasma or urine: mexiletine enantiomers, limit of detection in plasma 5 µg/L, fluorescence detection—K. M. McErlane *et al.*, *J. Chromatogr.*, 1987, *415*, 335–346. In plasma or serum: limit of detection 0.02 mg/L, UV detection—D. Paczkowski *et al.*, *Pol. J. Pharmacol. Pharm.*, 1989, *41*, 459–467. In serum: mexiletine and other anti-arrhythmic drugs—E. vas-Binder and T. Annesley, *Biomed. Chromatogr.*, 1991, *5*, 19–22. In serum: limit of detection 5 µg/L, fluorescence detection—N. Shibata *et al.*, *J. Chromatogr.*, 1991, *566*, 187–194. In plasma: mexiletine and other anti-arrhythmic drugs, UV or fluorescence detection—R. Verbesselt *et al.*, *Ther. Drug Monit.*, 1991, *13*, 157–165. In serum: mexiletine and its hydroxylated metabolites, limit of detection 2 µg/L, UV detection—D. Paczkowski *et al.*, *J. Chromatogr.*, 1992, *573*, 235–246. In plasma: mexiletine enantiomers, fluorescence detection—Z. Abolfathi *et al.*, *J. Chromatogr.*, 1992, *579*, 366–370. In plasma or urine: mexiletine enantiomers and metabolites—H. Fieger and I. W. Wainer, *J. Pharm. Biomed. Anal.*, 1993, *11*, 1173–1179. In serum: mexiletine enantiomers, limit of detection 0.5 µg/L, fluorescence detection—D. K. Kowk *et al.*, *J. Chromatogr. B Biomed. Appl.*, 1994, *661*, 271–280. In plasma: mexiletine enantiomers, limit of detection 1 µg/L, fluorescence detection—V. L. Lanchote *et al.*, *J. Chromatogr. B Biomed. Appl.*, 1996, *685*, 281–289.

Disposition in the Body. Mexiletine is readily absorbed after oral administration. It is extensively metabolised; the major metabolites are the 4′-hydroxy and 2′-hydroxymethyl derivatives, which may be further metabolised by deamination to the corresponding alcohols. The rate and extent of renal excretion is dependent on the urinary pH. Under normal conditions, up to about 20% of a dose may be excreted in the urine as unchanged drug in 24 h, but this may be increased to about 50% if the urinary pH is maintained at about 5.

Therapeutic concentration. In plasma, usually in the range 0.5 to 2 mg/L.

Following a single oral dose of 400 mg to 6 subjects, peak plasma concentrations of 0.65 to 0.94 (mean 0.77) mg/L were attained in about 2 h. [V. Häselbarth *et al.*, *Clin. Pharmacol. Ther.*, 1981, *29*, 729–736].

Following daily oral doses of 450 mg to 10 subjects, steady-state plasma concentrations of 0.75 to 2.18 (mean 1.6) mg/L were reported. [K. Ohashi et al., *Arzneimittelforschung.*, 1984, *34*, 503–507].

In five subjects with painful alcoholic neuropathy, the minimum effective oral dose of mexiletine was 300 mg daily with an effective plasma concentration of 0.66 (±0.15) mg/L. [K. Nishiyama and M. Sakuta, *Intern. Med.*, 1995, *34*, 577–579].

Toxicity

In a fatality due to a mexiletine overdose, postmortem blood and liver concentrations of 44.3 mg/L and 636 µg/g, respectively, were reported. [R. C. Blackmore and M. D. Osselton, *Bull. Int. Assoc. Forensic Toxicol.*, 1983, *16*(3), 7–8].

In a fatality involving mexiletine, tissue distribution was as follows: heart blood 44.8 mg/L, femoral blood 10.0 mg/L, vitreous humour 8.6 mg/L, liver 171.6 µg/g, gastric contents 1464 mg. [T. P. Rohrig and L. E. Harty, *J. Anal. Toxicol.*, 1994, *18*, 354–356].

A 41-year-old woman survived after ingesting up to 1.8 g mexiletine in a suicide attempt; her serum level was 20 mg/L. [L. S. Nelson and R. S. Hoffman, *J. Toxicol. Clin. Toxicol.*, 1994, *32*, 731–736].

Bioavailability. 80 to 90%.

Half-life. There is considerable intersubject variation and the plasma half-life appears to vary with the urinary pH; it is usually in the range 7 to 25 h (mean 11 h in normal subjects, increased in subjects with arrhythmias).

Volume of distribution. About 8 L/kg but there is considerable intersubject variation.

Clearance. Plasma clearance, about 7 mL/min/kg with considerable inter-subject variation.

Protein binding. In plasma, about 70%.

Note. For a review of mexiletine, see B. G. Wulf, *Clin. Pharmacokinet.*, 1983, *2*, 34–346 and L. Labbe and J. Turgeon, *Clin. Pharmacokinet.*, 1999, *37*, 361–384.

Dose. 0.6 to 1 g of mexiletine hydrochloride daily.

Mianserin

Antidepressant

1,2,3,4,10,14b-Hexahydro-2-methyldibenzo[*c*,*f*]-pyrazino[1,2-*a*]azepine
$C_{18}H_{20}N_2 = 264.4$
CAS—24219-97-4

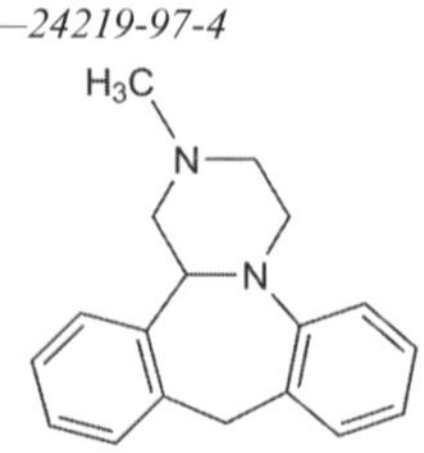

Mianserin Hydrochloride

Synonyms. Mianserini Hydrochloridum; Org-GB-94.

Proprietary names. Athymil; Bolvidon; Bonserin; Hopacem; Lantanon; Lerivon; Lumin; Miabene; Mianeurin; Miaxan; Norval; Prisma; Tolmin; Tolvin; Tolvon.

Note. The name Norval was formerly applied to a preparation containing docusate sodium.
$C_{18}H_{20}N_2,HCl=300.8$
CAS—21535-47-7
White crystals or crystalline powder. M.p. 282° to 284°.
Soluble 1 in 50 of water, 1 in 100 of ethanol, and 1 in 20 of chloroform.

Colour Tests. Liebermann's Test—violet; Mandelin's Test—violet.

Thin-layer Chromatography. System TA—Rf 58; system TB—Rf 39; system TC—Rf 58; system TE—Rf 68; system TL—Rf 23; system TAE—Rf 48; system TAF—Rf 50. (Acidified iodoplatinate solution, blue; Mandelin's reagent, violet.)

Gas Chromatography. System GA—mianserin RI 2210, M (nor-) RI 2235, M (8-OH-) RI 2495, M (*N*-oxide) RI 2202, M (OH-methoxy-) RI 2530; system GB—mianserin RI 2302, M (nor-) RI 2348, M (8-OH-) RI 2628; system GF—RI 2595; system GM—mianserin RRT 0.879, M (nor-) RRT 1.105 (both relative to iprindole); system GS—Retention time 18.1 min.

High Performance Liquid Chromatography. System HA—mianserin *k* 1.8, M(nor-) *k* 2.4; system HX—RI 391; system HY—RI 342; system HZ—Retention time 4.6 min; system HAA—Retention time 13.8 min; system HAZ—mianserin *k* 1.18, M (nor-) *k* 0.88, M (*N*-oxide) *k* 0.53, M (8-OH-) *k* 0.19.

Ultraviolet Spectrum. Aqueous acid—279 nm ($A_1^1=75a$). (See below.)

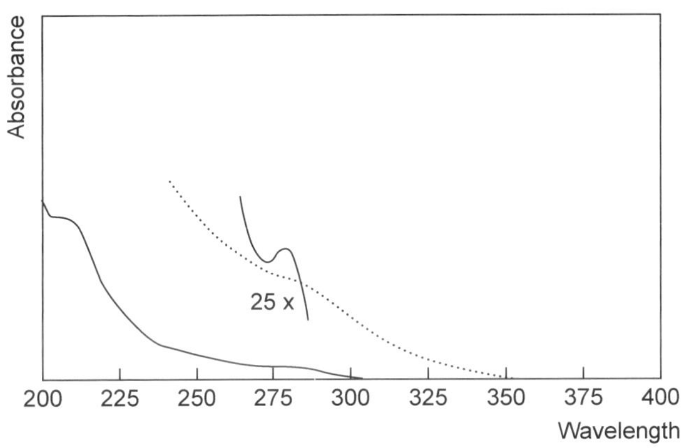

Infra-red Spectrum. Principal peaks at wavenumbers 787, 772, 1138, 1254, 1314, 742 cm^{-1} (mianserin hydrochloride, KBr disk).

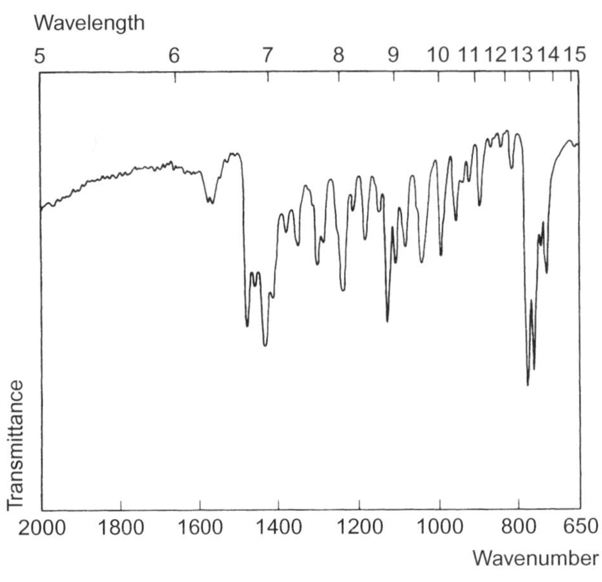

Mass Spectrum. Principal ions at *m/z* 193, 264, 43, 72, 71, 220, 192, 194; *N*-desmethylmianserin (M(nor)) 193, 208, 194, 250, 178, 192, 29, 179.

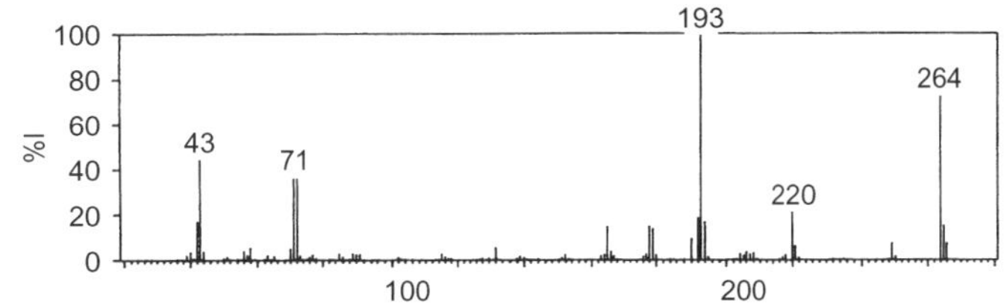

Quantification

Gas chromatography. In plasma: limit of detection 1 µg/L, AFID—G. F. Lachâtre *et al.*, *Ther. Drug Monit.*, 1982, *4*, 359–364. In plasma: limit of quantification 125 µg/L, NPD—S. Ulrich and J. Martens, *J. Chromatogr. B Biomed. Sci. Appl.*, 1997, *696(2)*, 217–234.

Gas chromatography–mass spectrometry. In plasma: limit of detection 5 µg/L—S. P. Jindal *et al.*, *J. Anal. Toxicol.*, 1982, *6*, 34–37. In whole blood: mianserin and other tetracyclic antidepressants—A. Namera *et al.*, *J. Anal. Toxicol.*, 1998, *22*, 396–400.

High performance liquid chromatography. In plasma: limit of detection 5 µg/L, electrochemical detection—R. F. Suckow *et al.*, *J. Pharm. Sci.*, 1982, *71*, 889–893. In plasma: limit of quantification 1.67 µg/L, electrochemical detection—L. W. Brown *et al.*, *J. Chromatogr.*, 1992, *582*, 268–272. In plasma or urine: enantiomers of mianserin and its metabolites, limits of quantification for mianserin enantiomers 2.5 µg/L and 4 µg/L—C. B. Eap *et al.*, *Chirality*, 1994, *6*, 555–563. In plasma: mianserin and desmethylmianserin, limit of detection < 10 nmol/L—G. Tybring *et al.*, *Ther. Drug Monit.*, 1995, *17*, 516–521. In postmortem scalp hair: mianserin and other antidepressant drugs (also GC–MS) —F. J. Couper *et al.*, *J. Forensic Sci.*, 1995, *40*, 87–90.

Disposition in the Body. Readily absorbed after oral administration; bioavailability is reduced by first-pass metabolism. The major metabolites are *N*-desmethylmianserin and 8-hydroxymianserin, which are both active, and mianserin *N*-oxide. About 30 to 40% of a dose is excreted in the urine in 24 h, and a total of about 70% is excreted over a period of several days, mainly as conjugated metabolites. About 5% of a dose is excreted in the urine unchanged. It crosses the blood–brain barrier and the placenta; it is found in breast milk.

Therapeutic concentration. In plasma, usually in the range 0.015 to 0.07 mg/L. *N*-desmethylmianserin is detectable in plasma at concentrations about one-third of those of mianserin.

Following a single oral dose of 60 mg given to 8 subjects, peak plasma concentrations of 0.05 to 0.14 mg/L (mean 0.10) and peak blood concentrations of 0.04 to 0.09 mg/L (mean 0.06) were attained in about 3 h [K. P. Maguire *et al.*, *Eur. J. Clin. Pharmacol.*, 1982, 21, 517–520].

Following oral doses of 20 mg three times a day to 10 subjects, minimum steady-state plasma concentrations of 0.03 to 0.09 mg/L (mean 0.06) were reported [G. F. Lachâtre *et al.*, *Ther. Drug Monit.*, 1982, *4*, 359–364].

Toxicity. Overdosage does not appear to cause the complications associated with overdose of tricyclic antidepressants. Toxic effects have been associated with plasma concentrations greater than 0.5 mg/L.

Plasma concentrations of 0.11 mg/L of mianserin and 0.5 mg/L of lorazepam were reported on admission to hospital in a comatose subject who had ingested 600 mg of mianserin plus an unknown amount of lorazepam; the patient died the following day [P. Crome and B. Newman, *BMJ*, 1977, *2*, 260].

Half-life. Plasma half-life, 6 to 40 h (mean 16), increased in elderly subjects.

Volume of distribution. About 13 L/kg.

Protein binding. In plasma, about 90%.

Note. For a review of the metabolism of some 'second' and 'fourth' generation antidepressants, see S. Rotzinger *et al.*, *Cell Mol. Neurobiol.*, 1999, *19*, 427–442; for a review of mianserin see R. Brogden *et al.*, *Drugs*, 1978, *16*, 273–301; for a review of the use of mianserin in acute cardiopathies, see P. Hourdebaigt-Larrusse and H. Perchet, *Ann. Cardiol. Angeiol.* (*Paris*), 1985, *34*, 637–641; for a report of mianserin and heart block, see K. K. Hla and O. Boyd, *Hum. Toxicol.*, 1997, *6*, 401–402.

Dose. 30 to 90 mg of mianserin hydrochloride daily; maximum of 200 mg daily.

Mibefradil

Calcium Antagonist

Synonyms. Mibefradilum; Ro-40-5967.
Methoxyacetic acid (1*S*,2*S*)-2-[2-[[3-(1*H*-benzimidazol-2-yl)-propyl]methylamino]ethyl]-6-fluoro-1,2,3,4-tetrahydro-1-(1-methylethyl)-2-naphthalenyl ester
$C_{29}H_{38}FN_3O_3$=495.6
CAS—116644-53-2

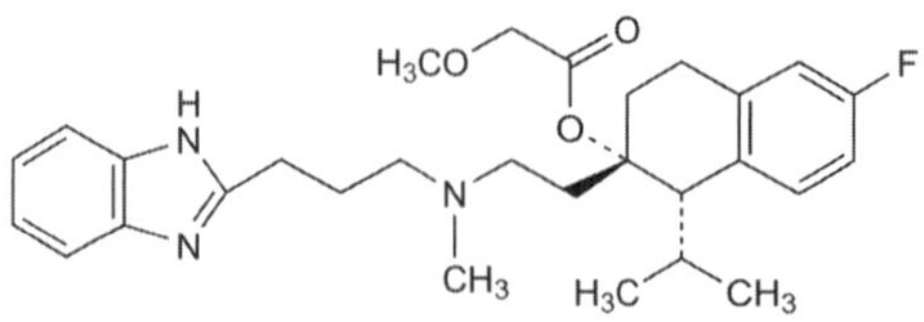

Mibefradil Dihydrochloride
Synonyms. Miberfradil Hydrochloride; Ro-40-5967/001.
Proprietary name. Posicor
$C_{29}H_{38}FN_3O_3$,2HCl=568.6
CAS—116666-63-8
A white crystalline powder. M.p. 128°. It is soluble in water.

Dissociation Constant. pK_a 4.8; 5.5 (Dihydrochloride).

High Performance Liquid Chromatography. Column: RP C_{18} (LiChrospher, RP Select-B). Mobile phase: acetonitrile:aqueous solution of potassium dihydrogen phosphate (39.3 mM) and sodium pentanesulfonic acid (8.2 mM) (38:62), flow rate 2 mL/min. Fluorescence detection (λ_{ex}=270 nm, λ_{em}=300 nm). Retention time(s): 10.7 min. [A. Skerjonec *et al.*, *J. Chromatogr.*, 1995, *669*, 377–382].

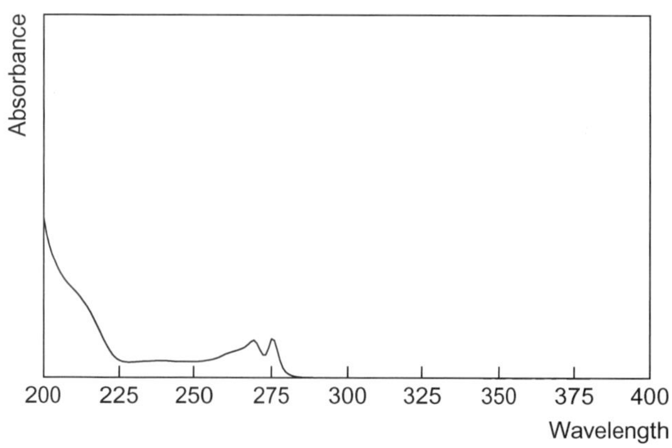

Quantification
High performance liquid chromatography. In plasma and urine: limit of detection 0.5 µg/L. Fluorescence detection (λ_{ex}=270 nm, λ_{em}=300 nm)—A. Skerjonec *et al.*, *J. Chromatogr.*, 1995, *669*, 377–382.

Disposition in the Body. Mibefradil is completely and rapidly absorbed with absorption unaffected by food. There is extensive distribution into peripheral tissues and it undergoes first-pass metabolism. The drug is metabolised via parallel pathways: esterase-catalysed hydrolysis and CYP3A4-mediated oxidation. The esterase pathway yields an alcohol metabolite, which has 10% of the pharmacological effect. After chronic dosing, the oxidative pathway becomes less important. The oxidation pathway leads to *O*-demethylation, *N*-demethylation and ring hydroxylation, yielding many identified metabolites. Elimination is via biliary (75%) and renal (25%) routes. 3% of the dose is excreted into urine as the unchanged drug. The drug displays zero order kinetics. Peak plasma level is reached within 1 to 2 h; steady state occurs within 3 to 4 days. Renal and mild-to-moderate hepatic dysfunction cause no change in pharmacokinetics.

Therapeutic concentration
In a study of 42 healthy males, aged 18 to 35 years, peak plasma concentrations were 26.7, 67.8, 115.0, 61.0, 495.0, 777.0 and 1490.0 µg/L following oral administration of mibefradil at doses of 10, 20, 40, 80, 120, 160 and 320 mg, respectively, after an overnight fast. These were observed at 1.00, 0.96, 0.86, 0.87, 1.38, 1.50 and 2.00 h, respectively.

3 to 5 healthy males, with a mean age of 32.4 years, were administered orally 100, 150 or 250 mg mibefradil once daily, after an overnight fast, for 28 days. Peak plasma concentrations on day 1 were 520, 739 and 1322 µg/L for the three doses observed at 2.33, 1.17 and 2.33 h, respectively. On day 28, peak concentrations reached 718, 914 and 1506 µg/L in the same time period.

12 hypertensive patients were administered for 8 days with doses of 50, 100, 150 or 200 mg daily, after an overnight fast. On day 1, plasma concentrations of 220, 478, 952 and 1116 µg/L were observed at 0.94, 1.09, 1.54 and 1.67 h, respectively. On day 8, however, peak concentrations were 402, 929, 1373 and 1538 µg/L for the four doses and were seen at 1.72, 1.62, 2.14 and 1.33 h post-dosing.

[H. A. Welker, *J. Pharm. Pharmacol.*, 1998, *50(9)*, 983–987].

Bioavailability. Approx. 80%.

Half-life. 17 to 25 h.

Volume of distribution. Steady state, 176 to 255 L; also reported as 3.5 to 5.7 L/kg.

Clearance. Plasma, 14.46 to 19.26 L/h; blood systemic, 26.16 L/h.

Distribution in blood. The blood:plasma ratio is 0.64.

Protein binding. Greater than 99%, mainly to α_1-acid glycoproteins.

Dose. 50 to 100 mg/day

Miconazole

Antifungal

Proprietary name. Daktarin
1-[2-(2,4-Dichlorophenyl)-2-[(2,4-dichlorophenyl)methoxy]ethyl]-1-*H*-imidazole
$C_{18}H_{14}Cl_4N_2O$=416.1
CAS—22916-47-8

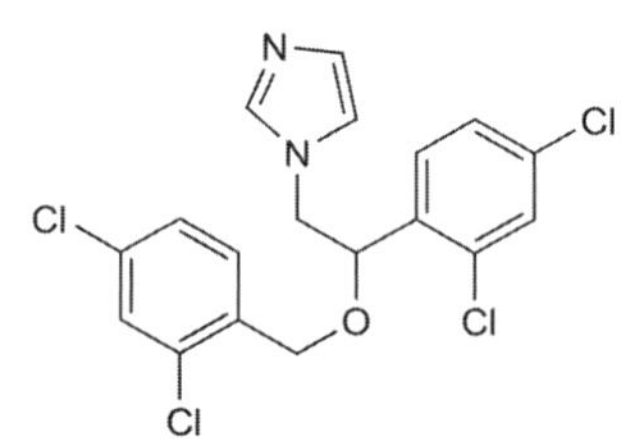

A white crystalline powder.
Very slightly soluble in water; very soluble in chloroform; soluble in most other organic solvents.

Miconazole Nitrate
Proprietary names. Albistat; Daktarin (cream); Dermonistat; Gyno-Daktarin; Micatin; Monistat.
$C_{18}H_{14}Cl_4N_2O,HNO_3$=479.1
CAS—22832-87-7
A white crystalline powder. M.p. about 182°.
Very slightly soluble in water and ether; soluble 1 in 140 of ethanol; slightly soluble in chloroform.

Dissociation Constant. pK_a 6.7.

Thin-layer Chromatography. System TA—Rf 73; system TB—Rf 11; system TC—Rf 67; system TE—Rf 80; system TF—Rf 07; system TL—Rf 37; system TAD—Rf 56; system TAE—Rf 77; system TAF—Rf 80. (Dragendorff spray.)

Gas Chromatography. System GA—RI 2965.

Ultraviolet Spectrum. Methanol—264, 272 (A_1^1=17a), 280 nm.

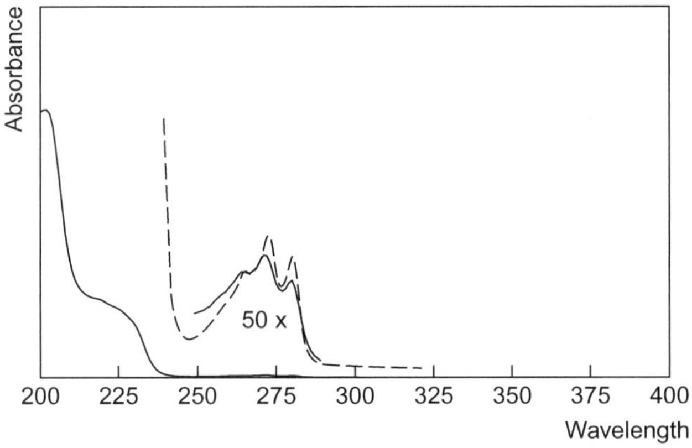

Infra-red Spectrum. Principal peaks at wavenumbers 1085, 1319, 827, 1302, 1038, 812 cm^{-1} (miconazole nitrate, KBr disk).

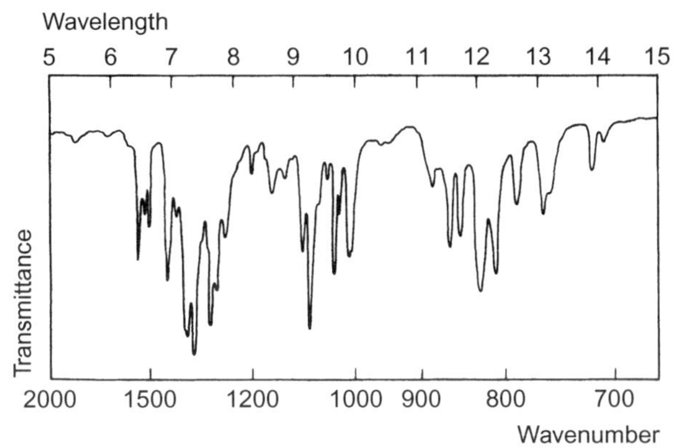

Mass Spectrum. Principal peaks at *m/z* 159, 161, 81, 335, 333, 163, 337, 205.

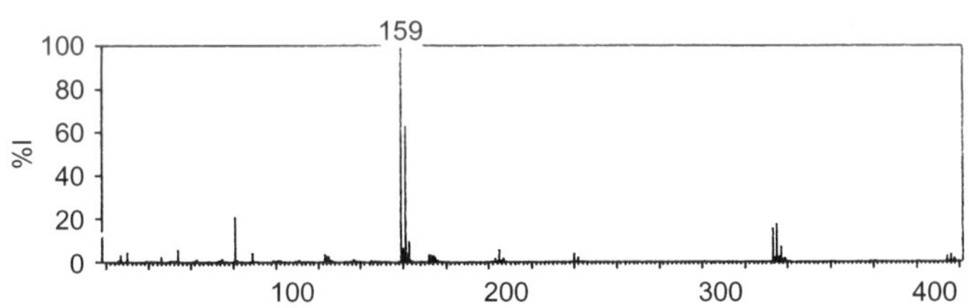

Quantification

Gas chromatography. In plasma: —S. C. Szathmary and I. Luhmann, *J. Chromatogr.*, 1988, *425*, 193–196. In serum: limit of detection 1 µg/L, ECD—P. T. Männistö *et al.*, *Antimicrob. Agents Chemother.*, 1982, 21, 730–733.

High performance liquid chromatography. In plasma: limit of detection 5 µg/L, UV detection (λ = 230 nm) —M. Kobylinska *et al.*, *J. Chromatogr. B Biomed. Appl.*, *685*, 191–195. In vaginal fluid: K. Selinger *et al.*, *J. Chromatogr.*, 1988, *434*, 259–264. In saliva: limit of detection 500 µg/L, UV detection—A. Turner and D. W. Warnock, *J. Chromatogr.*, 1982, *227*; *B Biomed. Appl.*, *16*, 229–232.

Bioassay. In serum—A. Espinel-Ingroff *et al.*, *Antimicrob. Agents Chemother.*, 1977, *11*, 365–368.

Note. For a rapid HPLC screen of antifungal agents in serum see T. K. Ng *et al.*, *J. Antimicrob. Chemother.*, 1996, *37*, 465–472.

Disposition in the Body. Incompletely absorbed after oral administration and poorly absorbed after topical administration. Metabolised by oxidation to 2,4-dichloromandelic acid and 2-(2,4-dichlorobenzyloxy)-2-(2,4-dichlorophenyl)acetic acid which are both inactive. About 10 to 20% of an oral or IV dose is excreted in the urine in 6 days, with only about 1% of the dose as unchanged drug. About 50% of an oral dose is eliminated in the faeces, mostly unchanged.

Therapeutic concentration

Following an IV infusion of 522 mg to 4 subjects, plasma concentrations of 2.0 to 9.1 µg/mL (mean 6.2) were reported at the end of the infusion [P. J. Lewi *et al.*, *Eur. J. Clin. Pharmacol.*, 1976, *10*, 49–54].

Toxicity. For a report of convulsions after miconazole overdose see K. Coulthard *et al.*, *Med. J. Aust.*, 1987, *146*, 57–58.

Half-life. Plasma half-life, about 24 h.

Volume of distribution. About 20 L/kg.

Protein binding. In plasma, about 92%.

Note. For a review of the pharmacokinetics of systemic antifungal drugs see T. K. Daneshmend and D. W. Warnock, *Clin. Pharmacokinet.*, 1983, *8*, 17–42.

Dose. 0.6 to 3.6 g daily by IV infusion; 1 g daily by mouth.

Midazolam

Hypnotic

Synonyms. Midazolamum; Ro-21-3971.
Proprietary names Dormicum; Dormonid; Hypnovel; Ipnovel; Midolam; Versed (includes proprietary names of salts of Midazolam).
8-Chloro-6-(2-fluorophenyl)-1-methyl-4*H*-imidazo[1,5-*a*][1,4]benzodiazepine
$C_{18}H_{13}ClFN_3 = 325.8$
CAS—59467-70-8

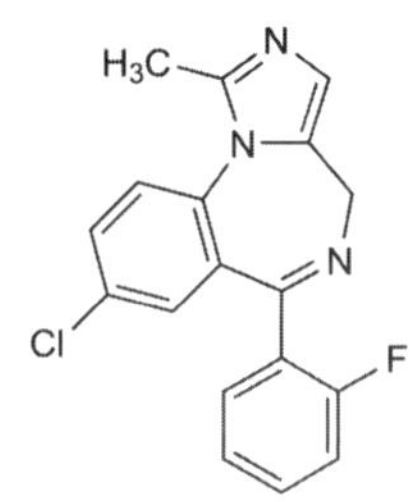

Colourless crystals. M.p. 158° to 160°.
Soluble in water.

Midazolam Hydrochloride

Synonym. Ro-21-3981-003
Proprietary name. Hypnovel
$C_{18}H_{13}ClFN_3,HCl = 362.2$
CAS—59467-96-8

Midazolam Maleate

Synonym. Ro-21-3981-001
Proprietary name. Dormicum
$C_{18}H_{13}ClFN_3,C_4H_4O_4 = 441.9$
CAS—59467-94-6

Dissociation Constant. pK_a 6.2.

Partition Coefficient. Log *P* (octanol/water), 4.3.

Thin-layer Chromatography. System TA—Rf 72; system TB—Rf 6; system TC—Rf 60; system TD—Rf 13; system TE—Rf 60; system TF—Rf 05; system TL—Rf 19; system TAD—Rf 53; system TAE—Rf 69; system TAF—Rf 70.

Gas Chromatography. System GA—midazolam RI 2575, M (α-OH-) RI 2830; system GB—midazolam RI 2722, M (α-OH-) RI 2901, M (α-OH-)-TMS RI 2866, M (4-OH-)-TMS RI 2775.

High Performance Liquid Chromatography. System HI—*k* 9.75; system HJ—*k* 2.10; system HK—*k* 5.90; system HX—RI 399; system HY—RI 306; system HZ—retention time 4.2 min; system HAA—retention time 14.9 min; system HAX—retention time 10.2 min; system HAY—retention time 6.3 min.

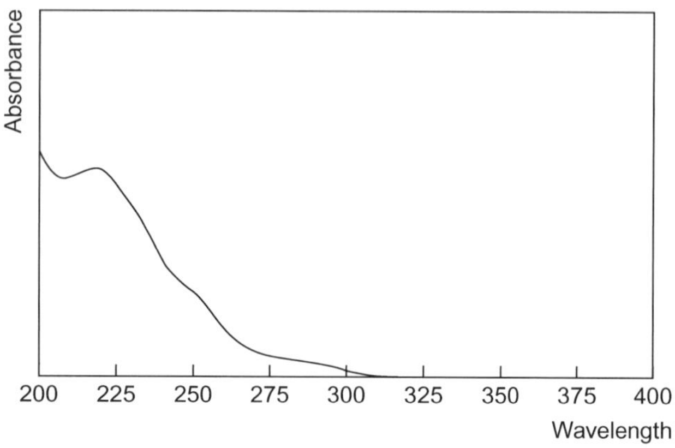

Infra-red Spectrum. Principal peaks at wavenumbers 1608, 820, 767, 1310, 1210, 995 cm^{-1} (KBr disk). (See below)

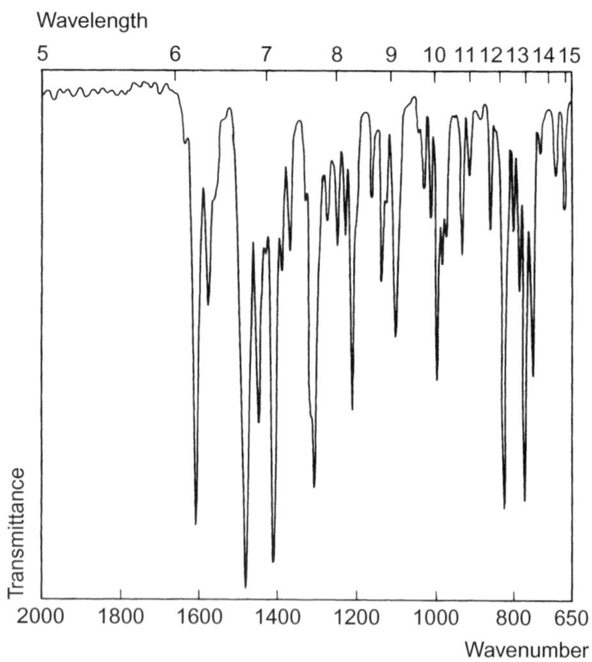

Mass Spectrum. Principal ions at *m*/*z* 310, 312, 311, 163, 325, 75, 39, 297.

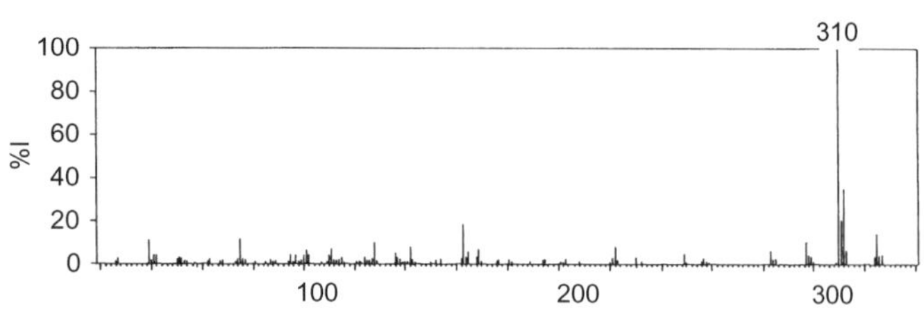

Quantification

Gas chromatography. In plasma: limit of detection 0.5 µg/L, ECD—M. T. Smith *et al.*, *Eur. J. Clin. Pharmacol.*, 1981, *19*, 271–278. In plasma: midazolam and flumazenil—L. E. Fisher *et al.*, *J. Chromatogr.* 1995, *665 B Biomed. Appl.*, 217–221.

Gas chromatography–mass spectrometry. In serum: midazolam and its metabolites, limit of detection for midazolam 0.2 µg/L—J. Martens and P. Banditt, *J. Chromatogr. B Biomed. Sci. Appl.*, 1997, *692*, 95–100. In plasma: limit of detection 1 µg/L—G. Frison *et al.*, *Rapid Commun. Mass Spectrom.*, 2001, *15*, 2497–2501.

High performance liquid chromatography. In plasma: midazolam and 1-hydroxymethylmidazolam, limit of detection 15 µg/L, UV detection—J. Vasiliades and T. H. Sahawneh, *J. Chromatogr.* 1981, *225*(14) *B Biomed. Appl.*, 266–271. In plasma: midazolam and its metabolite, limit of quantification 50 µg/L—V. Santou *et al.*, *J. Chromatogr.*, 1991, *571*, 298–304. In plasma: midazolam and ketamine, limit of detection < 5 µg/L, UV detection—H. A. Adams *et al.*, *Anaesthetist*, 1992, *41*, 619–624. In plasma or urine: midazolam and its α-hydroxy metabolite, limits of detection 2 µg/L and 4 µg/L respectively, UV detection—H. R. Ha *et al.*, *Ther. Drug Monit.*, 1993, *15*, 338–343. In plasma or urine: midazolam and metabolites and flumazenil, UV detection—K. Chan and R. D. Jones, *J. Chromatogr.*, 1993, *619*, 154–160. In plasma: limit of detection 2 µg/L, UV detection—R. Lauber *et al.*, *J. Chromatogr.* 1994, *654 B Biomed. Appl.*, 69–75. In plasma: midazolam and its metabolites, limit of quantification for midazolam 15 µg/L, UV detection—V. Mastey *et al.*, *J. Chromatogr.* 1994, *655 B Biomed. Appl.*, 305–310. In plasma: midazolam and its 1-hydroxy metabolite, limit of quantification 2 µg/L—B. Lehmann and R. Boulieu, *J. Chromatogr.* 1995, *674 B Biomed. Appl.*, 138–142. In plasma: midazolam and its 1-hydroxy metabolite, UV detection—T. C. Lee and B. Charles, *Biomed. Chromatogr.*, 1996, *10*, 65–68. In plasma: comparison with FPIA—P. Bourget *et al.*, *Ther. Drug Monit.*, 1996, *18*, 610–619. In serum: UV detection—P. Odou *et al.*, *Biomed. Chromatogr.*, 1997, *11*, 19–21. In plasma: UV detection—N. Van Brandt *et al.*, *Ther. Drug Monit.*, 1997, *19*, 352–357. In plasma: midazolam and metabolites, limit of detection 2.6 µg/L, UV detection—J. A. Carrillo *et al.*, *Ther. Drug Monit.*, 1998, *20*, 319–324. In plasma: midazolam and its 1-hydroxy metabolite, limits of quantification 1 µg/L and 0.5 µg/L respectively, UV detection—S. L. Eeckhoudt *et al.*, *J. Chromatogr. B Biomed. Sci. Appl.*, 1998, *710*, 165–171. In serum: 1-hydroxy midazolam glucuronide, UV detection—K. M. van Rij *et al.*, *Ther. Drug Monit.*, 1999, *21*, 416–420. In plasma: midazolam and fentanyl, limit of detection for midazolam 10 µg/L, UV detection—E. J. Portier *et al.*, *J. Chromatogr. B Biomed. Sci. Appl.*, 1999, *723*, 313–318. In hair: midazolam and other benzodiazepines, UV detection—A. El Mahjoub and C. Staub, *Forensic Sci. Int.*, 2001, *123*, 17–25. In whole blood: midazolam and other benzodiazepines, diode-array detection—A. El Mahjoub and C. Staub, *J. Anal. Toxicol.*, 2001, *25*, 209–214.

High performance liquid chromatography–mass spectrometry. In plasma: midazolam and other sedatives and anaesthetics—H. Kanazawa *et al.*, *J. Chromatogr. A.* 1998, *797*, 227–236.

Polarography. In urine: 1-hydroxymethylmidazolam, limit of detection 50 µg/L—C. V. Puglisi *et al.*, *J. Chromatogr.* 1978, *145*(2) *B Biomed. Appl.*, 81–96.

Note. For a comparison of various chromatographic methods see J. Vasiliades and T. H. Sahawneh, *J. Chromatogr.* 1982, *228*(17) *B Biomed. Appl.*, 195–203.

Disposition in the Body. Rapidly absorbed after oral administration and undergoes first-pass metabolism. Midazolam crosses the placenta. Small quantities are found in breast milk. Metabolised by hydroxylation to 1-hydroxymethylmidazolam (which is active), 4-hydroxymidazolam, and 4-hydroxy-1-hydroxymethylmidazolam; the hydroxy metabolites are then conjugated with glucuronic acid. Up to 90% of a dose is excreted in the urine in 24 h as the conjugated metabolites, mainly as conjugated 1-hydroxymethylmidazolam (60 to 70% of a dose). Less than 1% of a dose is excreted in the urine as unchanged drug.

Therapeutic concentration

Midazolam administered orally as a single dose (0.25 to 1.0 mg/kg) to 85 children aged 6 months to 15 years, provided maximal sedation at plasma concentrations of 0.138 (range 0.020 to 0.472) mg/L of midazolam and 0.090 (range 0.0048 to 0.180) mg/L α-hydroxymidazolam 30 min post dosing. [J. Marshall *et al.*, *J. Clin. Pharmacol.*, 2000, *40*, 578–589.]

Blood concentrations of 0.019 to 0.583 mg/L (mean 0.121) were attained 5 to 120 min after dosing in 60 mechanically ventilated pre-term infants administered midazolam 100 µg/kg (IV over 2 min) every 4 to 6 h. [T. C. Lee *et al.*, *Anesthesiology*, 1999, *90*, 451–457.]

The steady-state plasma concentration range was 0.010 to 0.147 mg/L (median 0.030) in 11 subjects receiving midazolam by continuous subcutaneous infusion at a rate 10 to 60 mg daily (median 20). [M. D. Bleasel *et al.*, *Palliat. Med.*, 1994, *8*, 231–236.]

In children given midazolam 0.2 mg/kg intranasally, 0.5 mg/kg orally, or 0.3 mg/kg rectally, blood concentrations of 0.146 mg/L were attained in 11.5 min by the intranasal route, 0.104 mg/L in 21 min by the rectal route, and 0.093 mg/L in 23.1 min by the oral route. [J. M. Malinovsky *et al.*, *Anaesthesia*, 1995, *50*, 351–354.]

Toxicity

In a 63-year-old man who developed cardiorespiratory depression approx. 5 min after receiving 10 mg midazolam during endoscopic retrograde cholangiopancreatography, blood and urine levels of 2.8 and 0.18 mg/L were reported approx. 40 min after the dose. Death occurred after 2 days and the postmortem midazolam blood concentration was 2.4 mg/L. [M. Michalodimitrakis *et al.*, *Am. J. Forensic. Med. Pathol.*, 1999, *20*, 93–97.]

The following postmortem tissue concentrations were reported in a death caused by self-injection of midazolam and sufentanil: blood 0.05 and 0.0011 mg/L for midazolam and sufentanil, respectively, urine 0.3 and 0.0013 mg/L, vitreous humour 0.0012 mg/L (sufentanil only), liver 930 and 1.75 µg/kg, kidney 290 and 5.5 µg/kg. [K. E. Ferslew *et al.*, *J. Forensic Sci.*, 1989, *34*, 249–257.]

Bioavailability. Reduced to 30 to 70% by first-pass metabolism. Bioavailability after IM administration is more than 90%.

Half-life. Plasma half-life, about 2 h, increased in elderly subjects, in obesity, and in cirrhosis.

Volume of distribution. 0.5 to 2 L/kg.

Clearance. Plasma clearance, 3 to 8 mL/min/kg (mean 5).

Protein binding. In plasma, about 95 to 98%.

Dose. As a sedative, the equivalent of 70 µg/kg of midazolam by slow IV injection; usual dose range 2.5 to 7.5 mg; for induction of anaesthesia, 200 µg/kg by slow IV injection.

Mifepristone

Antiprogestogenic Steroid

Synonyms. RU-486; RU-38486.
Proprietary name. Mifegyne
(11β,17β)-11-[4-(Dimethylamino)phenyl]-17-hydroxy-17-(1-propynyl)-estra-4,9-dien-3-one
$C_{29}H_{35}NO_2$=429.6
CAS—84371-65-3

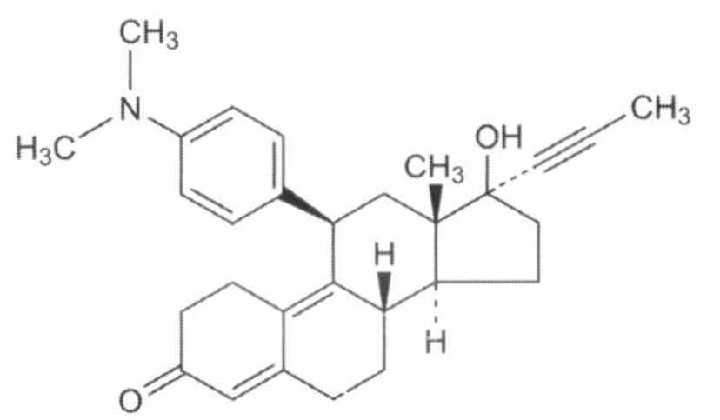

M.p. 150°.

High Performance Liquid Chromatography. Column: ODS RP (200 × 3.5 mm i.d.). Mobile phase: methanol:methylcyanide:water (42:28:30), 1 mL/min flow rate. Detection: not specified. Retention time(s): 10.37 min; monodemethylated metabolite, 6.92 min; didemethylated metabolite, 5.04 min; hydroxylated metabolite, 6.14 min. [Y. Shi *et al.*, *Contraception*, 1993, *48*, 133–149].

Ultraviolet Spectrum. Acid (0.1 M HCl in 95% ethanol)—302 nm; base (0.1 M NaOH in 95% ethanol)—256, 305 nm.

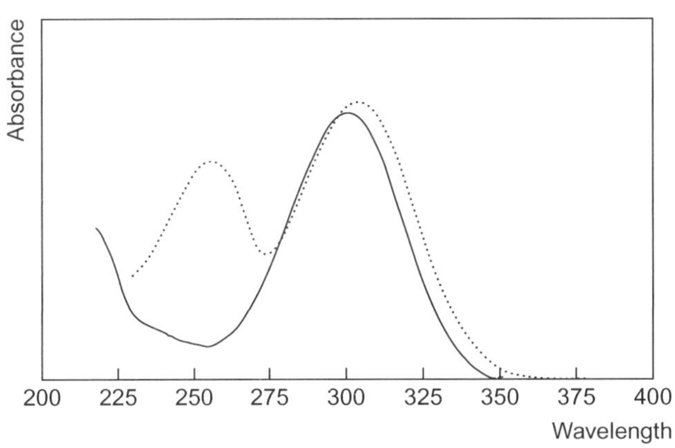

Infra-red Spectrum. Principal peaks at wavenumbers 1657, 1517, 1592, 1378, 1348, 1038 cm^{-1} (nujol).

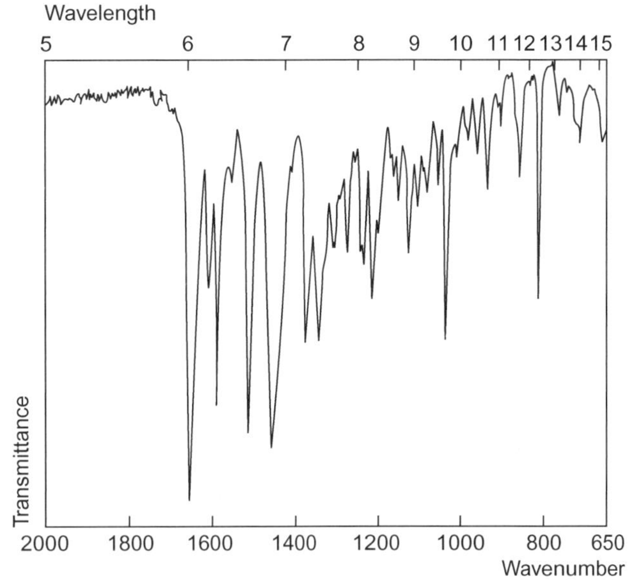

Mass Spectrum. Principal ions at *m/z* 121, 429, 280, 430, 389, 134, 122, 281.

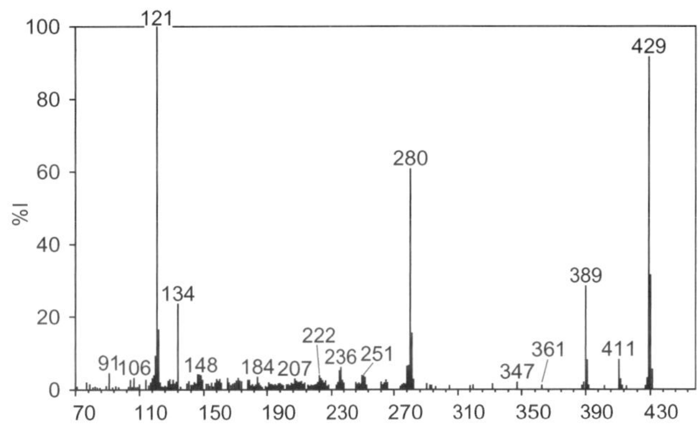

Quantification

High performance liquid chromatography. In plasma: limit of detection 0.01 mg/L—Y. Shi *et al.*, *Contraception*, 1993, *48*, 133–149.

Disposition in the Body. Mifepristone is rapidly absorbed after oral administration with peak plasma concentrations reached within 1 to 2 h. It undergoes metabolism in the liver, by rapid demethylation and hydroxylation, and its metabolites are excreted via the bile and eliminated in faeces. Metabolites include monodemethylated, didemethylated and hydroxylated derivatives which may undergo further metabolism before excretion. Only a small proportion of the parent drug is detected in urine.

Therapeutic concentration

Healthy female volunteers were administered with 12.5, 25, 50 or 100 mg mifepristone twice daily for 4 days. The peak plasma concentrations ranged between 1.4 and 1.7 mg/L for a dose ⩾50 mg twice daily. [O. Heikinheimo *et al.*, *J. Steroid. Biochem. Mol. Biol.*, 1989, *32*, 21–25].

9 non-pregnant and 36 pregnant healthy women, mean age 28.9 years, were administered doses of 25, 100, 400 and 600 mg mifepristone. For the non-pregnant women, mean peak plasma concentrations were 0.82, 1.66, 2.09 and 2.29 mg/L for the four doses observed at 1.7, 1.7, 1.4 and 1.6 h, respectively. The pregnant women produced concentrations of 0.75, 1.32, 1.73 and 1.91 mg/L, respectively, at 1.8, 2.1, 1.6 and 1.5 h. [Y. Shi *et al.*, *Contraception*, 1993, *48*, 133–149].

Bioavailability. 70% (also reported as 40% after a 100 mg oral dose).

Half-life. 18 h; also reported as 54 to 90 h, possibly due to cross-reacting of the metabolites.

Volume of distribution. Steady state, 25.7 L (8 L after 280 mg intravenous dose).

Clearance. Plasma, 3 L/h.

Protein binding. 98%.

Dose. The usual dose is 600 mg.

Milnacipran

Antidepressant

Synonym. Mildacipran
(1*R*,2*S*)-*rel*-2-(Aminomethyl)-*N*,*N*-diethyl-1-phenylcyclopropane-carboxamide
$C_{15}H_{22}N_2O$=246.4
CAS—92623-85-3

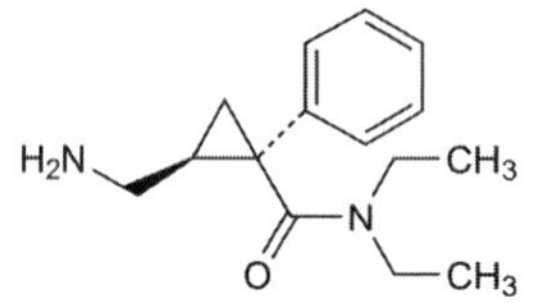

Milnacipran Hydrochloride

Synonym. F-2207
Proprietary names. Ixel; Toledomin.
$C_{15}H_{22}N_2O,HCl$=282.8
CAS— 101152-94-7
A white crystalline powder. M.p. 180°.

High Performance Liquid Chromatography. Column: ODS (Hypersil, 150 × 4.6 mm i.d., 3 μm). Mobile phase: methanol:sodium acetate (5 mM, pH 4.5) (70:30), flow rate 1 mL/min. Fluorescence detection (λ_{ex}=340 nm, λ_{em}=520 nm). Retention time(s): 11.1 min. [E. Lacassie *et al.*, *J. Chromatogr. B, Biomed. Sci. Appl.*, 2000, *742*, 229–238].

Disposition in the Body. Absorption of milnacipran is rapid and at least 90% is absorbed. First-pass metabolism is low. The drug shows linear pharmacokinetics and peak plasma concentrations are reached within 3 h of dosing. Steady state concentrations are rapidly achieved within 2 to 3 days of administration and the drug does not accumulate after multiple doses. The major metabolite is the glucuronide conjugate of the parent drug and no active metabolites has been identified. Urine is the main route of elimination with more than 90% of the dose recovered in this way and 5% in faeces over 96 h. 50 to 60% of the drug is excreted unchanged; 20 to 30% as the glucurono-conjugated drug and less than 20% as the glucurono-conjugated phase I metabolites including *N*-dealkylated milnacipran. Elimination is rapid and over 85% of the initial dose is recovered within the first 24 h. The metabolites are not pharmacologically active at clinically relevant doses. The liver and the kidney are both involved in the elimination of the drug.

Therapeutic concentration

6 healthy male and female volunteers aged between 37 and 64 years (mean, 51.2 years) and 11 patients with moderate to severe liver impairment (mean age 53.4 years; range 38 to 63 years) were administered a 50 mg single dose. The drug was administered after a 10 h overnight fast with a light breakfast. The peak plasma concentrations of unchanged milnacipran were 0.135 and 0.170 mg/L for the healthy individuals and patients observed at 2.0 and 2.7 h, respectively. The total drug concentrations were 0.323 and 0.242 mg/L at 2.5 and 3.6 h, respectively. [C. Puozzo *et al.*, *Eur. J. Drug Metab. Pharmacokinet.*, 1998, *23(2)*, 273–279].

6 healthy volunteers with a mean age of 30 years (range 25 to 36 years), creatinine clearance, 93 to 147 mL/min, and 8 patients with renal impairment (mean 51.5 years; range 27 to 65 years), creatinine clearance, 9 to 55.9 mL/min, were administered 50 mg milnacipran orally after an overnight fast and were fed a light breakfast 2 h after dosing. The peak plasma concentrations were 0.147 mg/L and 0.190 mg/L for the unchanged drug and 0.269 and 0.530 mg/L for total drug concentrations for the healthy individuals and patients, respectively. These concentrations were observed at 1.9 (unchanged concentration) and 1.7 (total) h for the healthy individuals and 1.9 (unchanged) and 4.9 (total) h for the patients. [C. Puozzo *et al.*, *Eur. J. Drug Metab. Pharmacokinet.*, 1998, *23(2)*, 280–286].

Bioavailability. 85%.

Half-life. 6.1 to 8.1 h

Volume of distribution. 5.5 L/kg (healthy); 6.3 L/kg (patients with liver impairment).

Clearance. Total apparent clearance, 40.0 L/h (healthy after oral administration), 34.3 L/h (intravenous administration); 27.6 L/h (patients with liver impairment after oral administration), 29.6 L/h (intravenous administration).

Protein binding. Low, non-saturable binding to plasma protein is approx. 13%.

Note. For a general review of milnacipran, see C. Spencer and M. Wilde, *Drugs*, 1998, *56*, 405–427.

Dose. The usual oral dose is 100 mg daily.

Milrinone

Cardiotonic

Synonym. Win-47203-2
Proprietary names. Corotrop; Corotrope; Milrila.
1,6-Dihydro-2-methyl-6-oxo-(3,4′-bipyridine)-5-carbonitrile
$C_{12}H_9N_3O$=211.2
CAS—78415-72-2

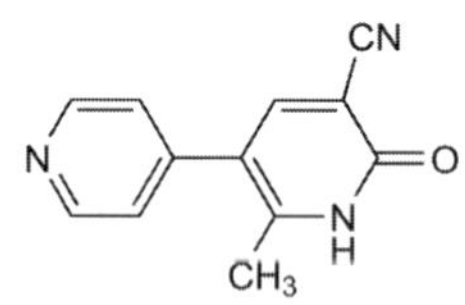

Off-white crystals from ethanol or dimethylformamide (DMF) and water. M.p. >300°. Very slightly soluble in water and chloroform, slightly soluble in methanol.

Milrinone Lactate

Proprietary name. Primacor
$C_{12}H_9N_3O,C_3H_6O_3$=301.3
CAS—100286-97-3

Partition Coefficient. Log *P* (octanol/water), 1.17.

High Performance Liquid Chromatography. Column: (analytical) RP Select B RT 250-4; (guard) RP-2 (10 × 3.0 mm i.d.). Mobile phase: methanol:ammonium acetate buffer (25 mM, pH 3.75) (25:75), flow rate 0.75 mL/min. UV detection (λ=331 nm). *k* value: 2.3. [R. Verrijk *et al.*, *J. Chromatogr.*, 1989, *491*, 265–268].

Column: ODS (Spherisorb, 250 × 4.0 mm i.d., 5 μm). Mobile phase: phosphate buffer (0.1 M, pH 6):tetrahydrofuran:acetonitrile (73:2:25), flow rate 1 mL/min. UV detection (λ=340 nm). Retention time(s): 4.3 min. [C. J. Oddie *et al.*, *J. Chromatogr.*, 1986, *374*, 209–214].

Ultraviolet Spectrum. Aqueous acid—218, 266, 327 nm; basic—282, 331 nm.

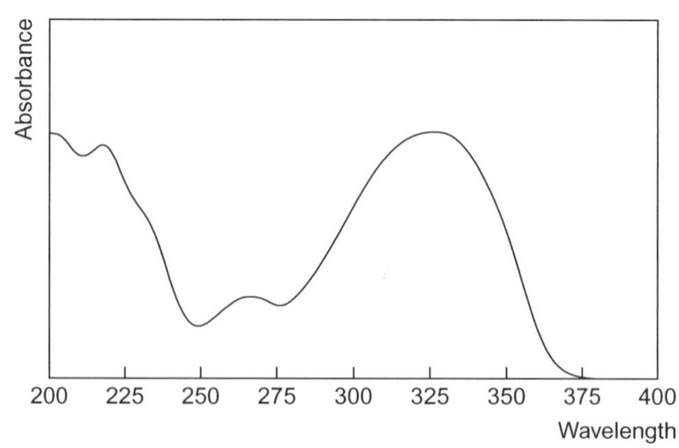

Infra-red Spectrum. Principal peaks at wavenumbers 1666, 1574, 590 cm^{-1} (KBr pellet).

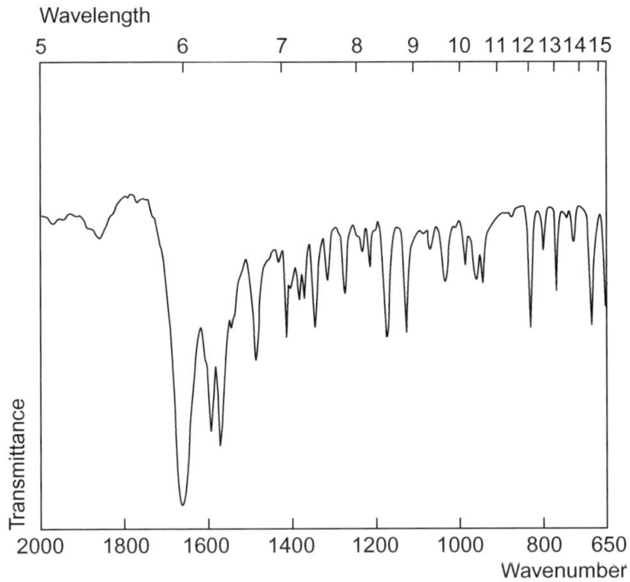

Mass Spectrum. Principal ions at *m/z* 211, 182, 184, 210, 212, 183, 155, 156.

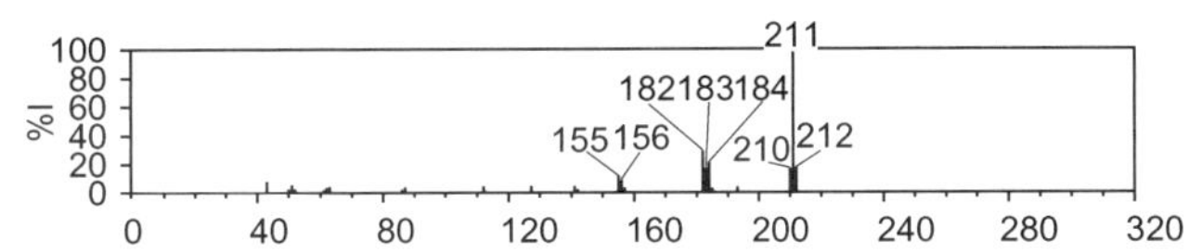

Quantification

High performance liquid chromatography. In plasma: limit of detection 5 μg/L. UV detection (λ = 331 nm)—R. Verrijk *et al.*, *J. Chromatogr.*, 1989, *491*, 265–268. In plasma: limit of detection 5 μg/L. UV detection (λ = 340 nm)—C. J. Oddie *et al.*, *J. Chromatogr.*, 1986, *374*, 209–214.

Disposition in the Body. Milrinone is rapidly and almost completely absorbed after oral administration but in practice it is given intravenously because of the association of a higher mortality rate with oral administration. It is eliminated mainly in urine with 80 to 85% of a dose detected as the unchanged drug and the remainder as its *O*-glucuronide metabolite. There are five metabolites but the *O*-glucuronide represents the major pathway of biotransformation.

Therapeutic concentration. The serum therapeutic concentration is 150 to 250 μg/L.

Group 1: 7 patients with stable chronic renal impairment (creatinine clearance 30 to 63 mL/min/1.73 m^2), aged between 19 and 65 years. Group 2: 7 patients with creatinine clearance 9 to 29 mL/min/1.73 m^2, aged 51 to 70 years (mean 63 years old). Both groups and 7 healthy males and females, aged between 41 and 58 years (mean of 48), were administered a single oral dose of 5 mg. A mean peak plasma concentration of 162 μg/L was reached for the healthy individuals in 0.64 h; for both groups with renal impairment, levels of 210 μg/L were observed at 1.19 h. [R. Larsson *et al.*, *Eur. J. Clin. Pharmacol.*, 1986, *29*, 549–553].

Toxicity. The toxic serum concentration is 0.3 mg/L.

In a study involving 1088 patients with severe chronic liver failure, 561 were treated with 40 mg milrinone and 527 received 40 mg placebo daily for 9 months. The study showed a 28% increase in mortality for those treated with milrinone compared with the placebo. An increase of 34% in cardiac mortality was also observed. [M. Packer *et al.*, *N. Engl. J. Med.*, 1991, *325*, 1468–1475].

Bioavailability. 92% (Healthy volunteers); 76% (patients with congestive heart failure). Also reported as 80%.

Half-life. 50 to 55 min (healthy individuals following oral and intravenous (IV) doses); 1.7 h (patients with congestive heart failure, IV dose) and 2.1 h (oral dose); 1.8 h (patients with moderate renal impairment) and 3.2 h (severe impairment). Also reported as 2.3 h.

Volume of distribution. 0.3 to 0.42 L/kg (after doses of 12.5 to 75 μg/kg administered to congestive heart failure patients intravenously) and 0.32 L/kg (after doses of 10 to 125 μg/kg administered to healthy individuals).

Clearance. 0.13 L/kg/h.

Protein binding. 70 to 80%.

Note. For a general review of phosphodiesterase inhibitors, see J. M. Arnold, *Pharmacol. Ther.*, 1993, *57*, 161–170.

Dose. An initial loading dose of 50 μg/kg body weight is administered over 10 min followed by a maintenance dose titrated between 0.375 and 0.75 μg/kg/min. The total daily dose should not exceed 1.13 mg/kg. Dosage may be reduced in patients with renal impairment.

Minocycline

Antibacterial

[4*S*-(4α,4aα,5aα,12aα)]-4,7-Bis(dimethylamino)-1,4,4a,5,5a,6,11,12a-octahydro-3,10,12,12a-tetrahydroxy-1,11-dioxo-2-napthacenecarboxamide

$C_{23}H_{27}N_3O_7 = 457.5$

CAS—10118-90-8

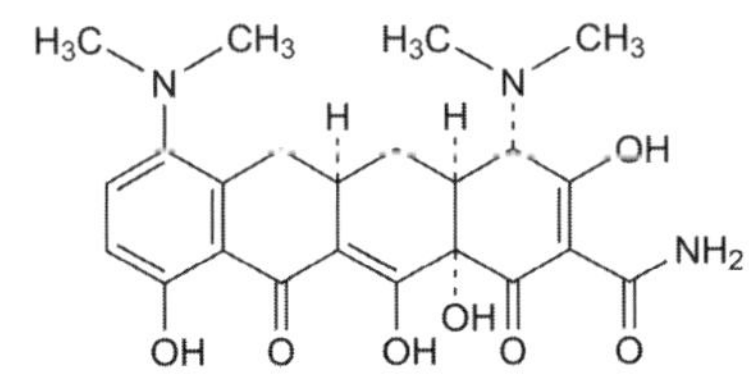

A bright yellow-orange amorphous solid.

Minocycline Hydrochloride

Proprietary names. Akamin; Aknemin; Aknin-N; Aknosan; Arestin; Blemix; Cyclomin; Dentomycin(e); Dermirex; Dynacin; Klinomycin; Klinotab; Logryx; Mino(x); Minocin; Minoclin; Minogal; Minomycin; Minotab(s); Mynocine; Udima; Ultramycin; Vectrin; Zacnan.

$C_{23}H_{27}N_3O_7,HCl = 493.9$

CAS—13614-98-7

A yellow crystalline powder.

Soluble in water and in solutions of alkali hydroxides and carbonates; slightly soluble in ethanol; practically insoluble in chloroform and ether.

Dissociation Constant. pK_a 2.8, 5.0, 7.8, 9.5.

Partition Coefficient. Log *P* (octanol/water), 0.1.

Colour Test. Sulfuric acid—yellow.

Thin-layer Chromatography. System TAE—Rf 88; System TAJ—Rf 02; System TAK—Rf 00; System TAL—Rf 08.

High Performance Liquid Chromatography. System HY—RI 240; system HAA—Retention time(s) 22.6 min.

Ultraviolet Spectrum. Aqueous acid—265 (A_1^1 = 400b), 354 nm; aqueous alkali—243 nm (A_1^1 = 414b).

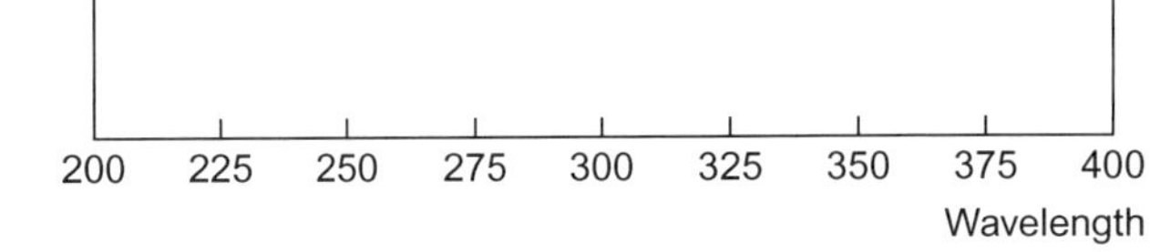

Infra-red Spectrum. Principal peaks at wavenumbers 1600, 1645, 1525, 1225, 1310, 1050 cm^{-1} (minocycline hydrochloride, KBr disk).

Quantitative

High performance liquid chromatography. In plasma: limit of detection 30 μg/L, UV detection—H. J. Mascher, *J. Chromatogr. A*, 1998, *812*,

339–342. In plasma or parotid saliva: limit of detection 100 µg/L, UV detection—V. Orti *et al.*, *J. Chromatogr. B Biomed Sci. Appl.*, 2000, *738*, 357–365.

High performance liquid chromatography–mass spectrometry. In plasma: limit of detection 5 µg/L—M. V. Araujo *et al.*, *J. Chromatogr. B Biomed. Sci. Appl.*, 2001, *755*, 1–7.

Therapeutic concentration

In 223 acne patients receiving minocycline at the recommended dose (100 mg daily) or a high dose (200 mg daily) in the form of a standard preparation or a modified-release formulation, mean serum levels were as follows: 0.15 to 3.51 mg/L (mean 1.20 mg/L for males and 1.68 mg/L for females) for 100 mg daily of the standard preparation; 0.42 to 5.15 mg/L (mean 2.18 for males and 2.58 for females) for 200 mg daily of the standard preparation; 0.16 to 3.77 mg/L (mean 1.38 for males, 1.56 for females) for 100 mg daily of the modified-release formulation; 0.36 to 6.81 mg/L (mean 2.62 for males, 2.83 for females) for 200 mg daily of the modified-release formulation (plasma concentrations were measured, at steady state, within 6 h of the previous dose). [K. J. Gardner *et al.*, *Clin. Exp. Dermatol.*, 1997, 22, 72–76].

Dose. The equivalent of 100 to 200 mg of minocycline daily.

Minoxidil

Antihypertensive

Synonyms. PDP; U-10858.
Proprietary names. Apo-Gain; Apohair; Alopexy; Alostil; Aloxidil; Folcress; Hairgain; Headway; Loniten; Lonnoten; Lonolox; Minona; Minovital; Minoxidine; Minox(i); Minoxigaine; Minoximen; Moxiral; Neoxidil; Normoxidil; Ralogaine; Regaine; Regro; Rogaine; Tricoxidil; Unipexil.
6-(1-Piperidinyl)-2,4-pyrimidinediamine 3-oxide
$C_9H_{15}N_5O = 209.3$
CAS—38304-91-5

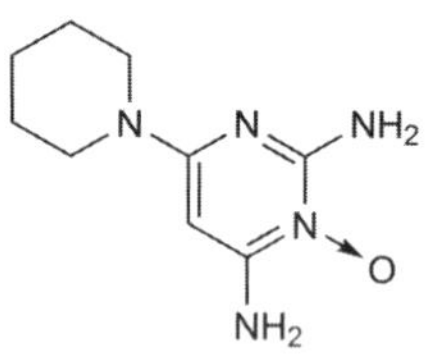

A white crystalline solid. M.p. about 225°, with decomposition.
Soluble 1 in about 500 of water; readily soluble in ethanol and propylene glycol; practically insoluble in chloroform.

Dissociation Constant. pK_a 4.6.

Partition Coefficient. Log *P* (octanol/water), 1.2.

Thin-layer Chromatography. System TA—Rf 51; system TB—Rf 00; system TC—Rf 03; system TE—Rf 18; system TL—Rf 00; system TAE—Rf 44.

High Performance Liquid Chromatography. System HX—RI 297; system HZ—Retention time(s) 2.4 min; system HAA—Retention time(s) 9.8 min.

Ultraviolet Spectrum. Aqueous acid—230, 281 nm ($A_1^1 = 547b$); aqueous alkali—262, 288 nm.

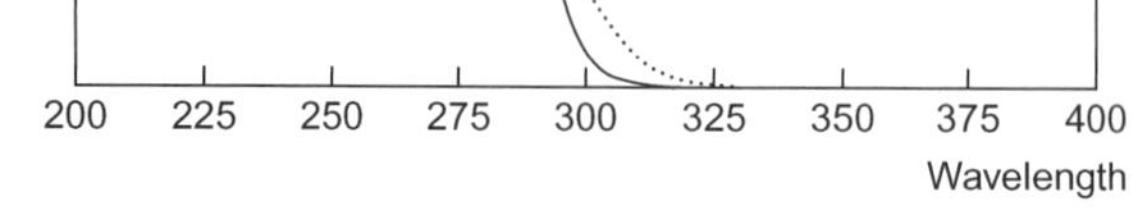

Infra-red Spectrum. Principal peaks at wavenumbers 1640, 1610, 1550, 1231, 1210, 758 (KBr disk).

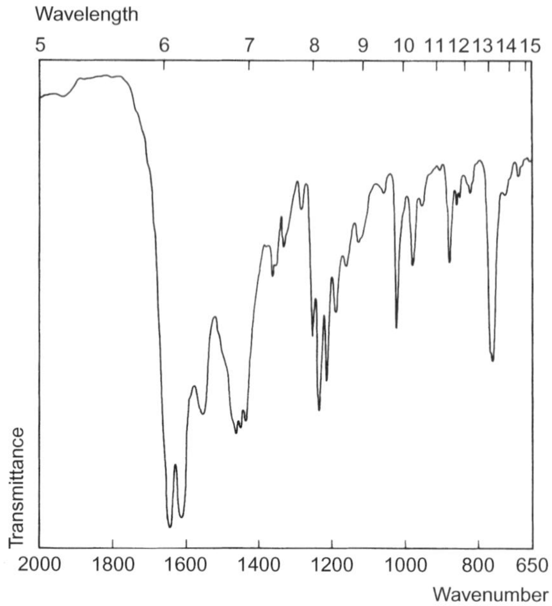

Mass Spectrum. Principal ions at *m/z* 84, 209, 67, 43, 110, 41, 192, 164.

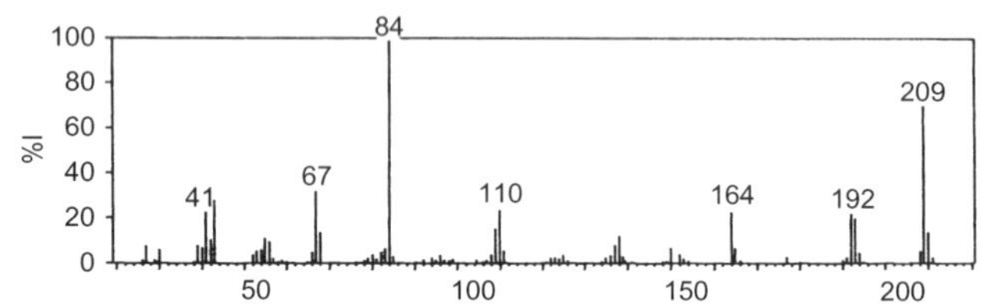

Quantification

High performance liquid chromatography. In plasma: limit of detection 500 ng/L, electrochemical detection—G. Carrum *et al.*, *J. Chromatogr.*, 1986, *381*, 127–135.

Radioimmunoassay. In serum: limit of detection 3 µg/L—M. E. Royer *et al.*, *J. Pharm. Sci.*, 1977, *66*, 1266–1269.

Disposition in the Body. Minoxidil is readily absorbed after oral administration. More than 80% of a dose is excreted in the urine in 24 h, mainly as glucuronide conjugates with less than 10% as unchanged drug; about 3% of a dose is eliminated in the faeces.

Therapeutic concentration

Following daily oral administration of 27 to 30 mg to 6 subjects, serum concentrations of 0.04 to 0.25 (mean 0.10) mg/L were reported 1 to 2 h after a dose. [D. T. Lowenthal *et al.*, *J. Clin. Pharmacol.*, 1978, *18*, 500–508].

Toxicity

The total serum-minoxidil concentration in a 20-year-old female who survived after ingesting an unknown quantity of minoxidil tablets in a suicide attempt was 3.14 mg/L. [S. W. Poff and S. R. Rose, *J. Emerg. Med.*, 1992, *10*, 53–57].

Half-life. Plasma half-life, about 3 to 4 h.

Protein binding. In plasma, not significantly bound.

Note. For a review of minoxidil, see V. M. Campese, *Drugs*, 1981, *22*, 257–278.

Dose. 5 to 50 mg daily; up to 100 mg daily has been given.

Mirtazapine

Antidepressant

Synonyms. 6-Azamianserin; Mirtazepine; Mepirzepine; Org-3770.
Proprietary names. Remergil; Remeron; Zispin.
1,2,3,4,10,14b-Hexahydro-2-methylpyrazino[2,1-*a*]pyrido[2,3-*c*][2]-benzazepine

$C_{17}H_{19}N_3 = 265.4$
CAS—61337-67-5

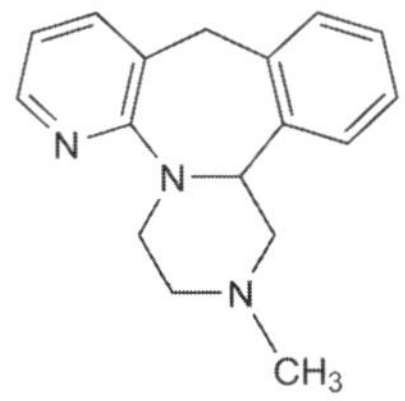

A white to creamy white crystalline powder with m.p. 114° to 116°. It is slightly soluble in water.

Partition Coefficient. Log *P* (octanol/water), 7.1.

Gas Chromatography. System GA—RI 2250; system GB—mirtazapine RI 2361; mirtazapine M(nor-) RI 2414; mirtazapine M(oxo-) RI 2665.

Column: HP-5 (15 m × 0.25 mm i.d., 0.25 μm film thickness) and HP-35 (15 m × 0.32 mm i.d., 0.32 μm). Column temperature: 140° for 0.50 min, to 300° at 10°/min, hold for 10.5 min. Injector and detector temperatures: 260° and 300°, respectively. Internal standard (IS): carbinoxamide maleate. Detection: nitrogen–phosphorus. Retention time(s): (HP-5 column) mirtazapine, 9.76 min; IS, 8.2 min; (HP-35) mirtazapine, 11.68 min; IS, 9.6 min. [D. Anderson *et al.*, *J. Anal. Toxicol.*, 1999, *23(6)*, 544–548].

High Performance Liquid Chromatography. System HZ—retention time(s): 2.8 min (mirtazapine), 2.3 min (desmethylmirtazapine).

Column: (analytical) Chiralpak AD (250 × 4.6 mm i.d., 10 μm); (guard) Chiralpak AD (50 × 4.6 mm i.d., 10 μm). Mobile phase: hexane: ethanol:isopropanol (98:1:1), flow rate 1.5 mL/min. IS: imipramine. UV detection (λ = 290 nm). Retention time(s): (+)-mirtazapine, 12.5 min; (−)-mirtazapine, 15.0 min. [S. Dodd *et al.*, *J. Chromatogrogr. B, Biomed. Sci. Appl.*, 2000, *748*, 439–443].

Ultraviolet Spectrum. Aqueous acid (0.025 M H_2SO_4)—314.5, 252.5 nm.

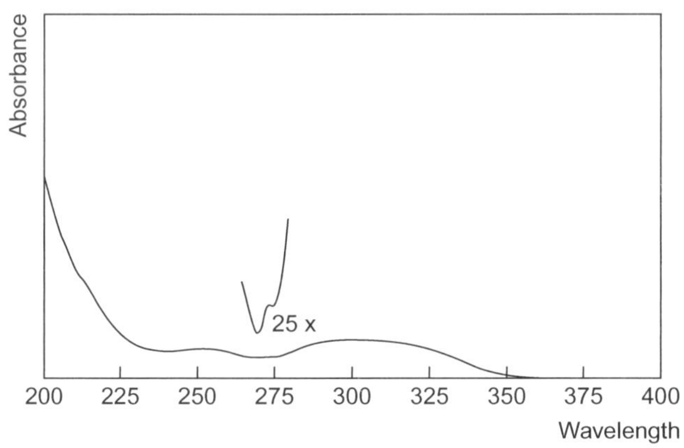

Mass Spectrum. Principal ions at *m/z* 195, 194, 42, 208, 196, 167, 180, 43 (mirtazapine); *m/z* 195, 194, 196, 209, 180, (desmethylmirtazapine).

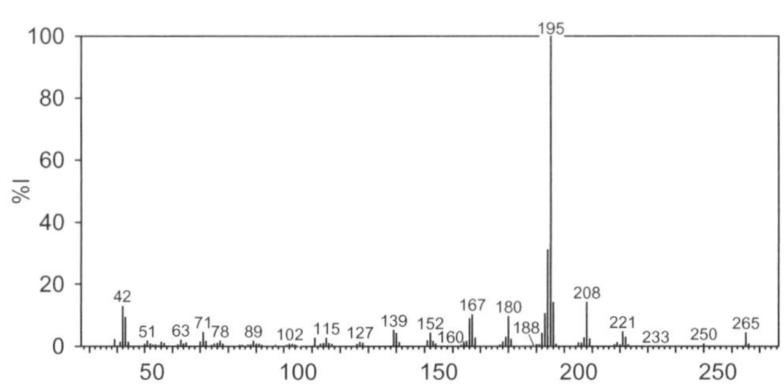

Quantification

Gas chromatography. In blood: limit of detection and limit of quantification are 25 μg/L. Nitrogen–phosphorus detection—D Anderson *et al.*, *J. Anal. Toxicol.*, 1999, *23*, 544–548. In plasma: limit of detection is 0.5 μg/L—J. E. Paanakker and H. J. M. Van Hal, *J. Chromatogr.*, 1987, *417*; *Biomed. Appl.*, 203–207.

Gas chromatography–mass spectrometry. In urine: limit of detection < 100 μg/L—J. Bickeboeller-Friedrich and H. H. Maurer, *Ther. Drug Monit.*, 2001, *23*, 61–70.

High performance liquid chromatography. In formulations: limit of detection 0.01 to 0.04%, limit of quantification 0.02 to 0.12%—G. Wynia *et al.*, *J. Chromatogr. A*, 1997, *773*, 339–350.

Disposition in the Body. Mirtazapine is rapidly and completely absorbed after oral administration from the gastro-intestinal tract. Peak plasma levels are reached after about 2 h. Steady state reached after 3 to 4 days. Linear pharmacokinetics with recommended dose range. Food intake has no influence on the pharmacokinetics. It is extensively metabolised in the liver and eliminated in urine (75%) and faeces (15%) within a few days. Metabolism occurs by the P450 cytochrome oxidase pathway into four metabolites via demethylation and hydroxylation followed by glucuronide conjugation. Cytochrome 2D6 and 1A2 are involved in the formation of 8-hydroxy metabolite and 3A in the *N*-desmethyl (active) and *N*-oxide metabolites. Elimination of the parent compound occurs via hepatic metabolism with demethylation and oxidation with subsequent conjugation of the metabolites.

Therapeutic concentration. The serum therapeutic concentration is 20 to 100 μg/L and the sum of the parent drug and desmethylmirtazepine, 50 to 300 μg/L.

After a 15 mg daily dose, peak plasma concentrations (steady state) of 27 to 51 μg/L are reached in approx. 5 days. After a 75 mg daily dose, peak plasma concentrations in the range of 137 to 225 μg/L are achieved. [E. S. Lavins *et al.*, *Joint SOFT /TIAFT International Meeting*, V. Spiehler (ed.), held at Albuquerque, New Mexico, 1998].

Toxicity. The toxic serum concentration (sum of the parent drug and metabolite) is 1 mg/L.

Bioavailability. Approx. 50%.

Half-life. 20 to 40 h. (The mean half-life for women is 37 h and for men is 26 h.)

Protein binding. Binding to protein plasma is approx. 85% over a concentration range of 0.01 to 10 mg/L.

Note. For a general review of mitarzapine, see K. Holm and A. Markham, *Drugs*, 1999, *57*, 607–631.

Dose. The usual dose is 15 to 45 mg daily.

Misoprostol

Prostaglandin Analogue/ Proton Pump Inhibitor

Synonym. SC-29333

Proprietary names. Cytotec; Arthrotec (with Diclofenac); Napratec (with Naproxen).

(11α,13*E*)-11,16-Dihydroxy-16-methyl-9-oxoprost-13-en-1-oic acid methyl ester

$C_{22}H_{38}O_5 = 382.5$
CAS—59122-46-2

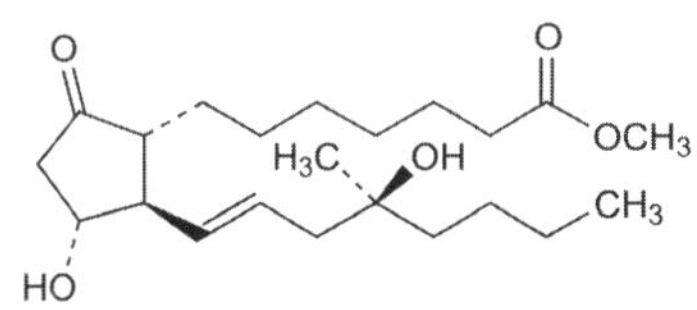

(11*R*, 16*S*)-Form

Light yellow oil. It is soluble in water.

Partition Coefficient. Log *P* (octanol/water), 4.96.

High Performance Liquid Chromatography. Column: C_8 (Zorbax, 250 × 4.6 mm i.d., 5 μm). Mobile phase: potassium phosphate buffer (0.02 M, pH 3):acetonitrile:methanol (46:30:24), flow rate 1.7 mL/min.

UV detection (λ=210 nm). Retention time(s): 18.5 min. [I. M. Womack *et al.*, *Prostaglandins*, 1996, *52*, 249–259].

Column: ODS (Supelco, 250 × 4.6 mm i.d.). Mobile phase: acetonitrile: methanol:water (45:20:35), flow rate 1.5 mL/min. UV detection (λ=280 nm). Retention time(s): 7.5 min. [D. A. Roston *et al.*, *J. Pharm. Biomed. Anal.*, *13*, 1513–1520].

Quantification

High performance liquid chromatography. In plasma: limit of quantification 0.6 µg, UV detection (λ=210 nm)—I. M. Womack *et al.*, *Prostaglandins*, 1996, *52*, 249–259.

Disposition in the Body. Misoprostol is rapidly absorbed after oral administration and metabolised to the active form misoprostol acid (SC-30695) which is further metabolised by oxidation and excreted mainly via urine as its dimer and tetramer (65%) and some in faeces (15%). Approx. 88% of a dose is absorbed. No unchanged drug has been detected in plasma or urine. Excretion is mainly in the form of metabolites but little as the unchanged drug. The rate of absorption from the gastro-intestinal tract is reduced by the presence of food but the extent of absorption appears to be unaffected. Peak plasma concentrations of the active metabolite have been observed after about 30 min. No accumulation of the metabolite occurs in plasma after repeated dosing of 400 µg twice daily.

Therapeutic concentration

6 healthy volunteers, with a mean age of 26 years, were administered a mean oral dose of 386 µg radiolabelled misoprostol. The mean peak plasma concentrations, observed at 30 and 12 min, were 6.08 µg/L for misoprostol.

24 healthy subjects (mean age 27 years) were administered a single oral dose of 200 or 400 µg misoprostol after an overnight fast. Peak plasma concentrations were 0.397 and 0.835 µg/L, respectively.

[Information supplied by Pharmacia Limited, UK].

Half-life. Misoprostol, less than 30 min; misoprostol acid, 20 min.

Volume of distribution. Approx. 6.6 L/kg.

Protein binding. 85% (the free acid of misoprostol).

Dose. The usual daily dose is between 400 and 800 µg.

Mitozantrone

Antineoplastic

Synonyms. DHAQ; Mitoxantrone; NSC-279836.
1,4-Dihydroxy-5,8-bis[[2-[(2-hydroxyethyl)amino]ethyl]amino]-9,10-anthracenedione
$C_{22}H_{28}N_4O_6$=444.5
CAS—65271-80-9

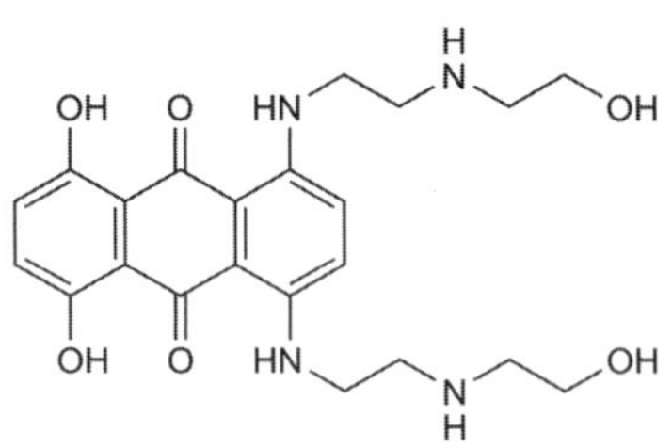

Crystals. M.p. 160° to 162°. It is sparingly soluble in water; slightly soluble in methanol; practically insoluble in acetone, acetonitrile and chloroform.

Mitozantrone Hydrochloride

Synonyms. CL-232315; DHAD; Dihydroxyanthracenedione Dihydrochloride; Mitoxantrone Hydrochloride; Mitoxantrani Hydrochloridum; NSC-301739.
Proprietary names. Novantron; Novantrone; Pralifan.
$C_{22}H_{28}N_4O_6$,2HCl=517.4
CAS—70476-82-3
A dark blue electrostatic, hygroscopic powder with m.p. 203° to 205°. It is sparingly soluble in water; slightly soluble in methanol; practically insoluble in acetone, acetonitrile and chloroform.

Dissociation Constant. pK_a 5.99 and 8.13.

Thin-layer Chromatography. (All these systems refer to mitozantrone hydrochloride.)

Plate: silica gel. Mobile phase: (A) methanol:ammonium solution (100:1.5); (B) chloroform:methanol:ammonia (9:3:1). Rf 0.04 (A); Rf 0.77 (B).

Plate: cellulose. Mobile phase: formic acid:water (4:96). Rf 0.33.

Plate: micropolyamide. Mobile phase: (A) methanol:strong ammonia solution (100:1.5); (B) formic acid:water (4:96). Rf 0.53 (A); Rf 0.92 (B).

Plate: reversed phase KC-18F. Mobile phase: dimethylformamide: 0.5 M sodium chloride solution:1 M ammonia:acetic acid (8:8:1:2). Rf 0.44.

[J. H. Beijnen *et al.*, in *Analytical Profiles of Drug Substances and Excipients*, 1991, Academic Press, New York; H. G. Brittain editor. Vol. 17, pp. 221–258].

High Performance Liquid Chromatography. Column: HIRPB (250 × 4.6 mm i.d.). Mobile phase: acetonitrile:ammonium formate buffer (0.05 M) (22:78), pH 3.6, flow rate 1.2 mL/min. UV detection (λ=242 and 612 nm). Retention time(s): 5 min. [P. M. Loadman and C. R. Calabrese, *J. Chromatogr. B, Biomed. Sci. Appl.*, 2001, *764*, 193–206].

Column: ODS (Nova-Pak, 75 × 3.9 mm i.d., 4 µm). Mobile phase: methanol:tetrahydrofuran:triethylamine phosphate:tetramethylammonium chloride (1 M):water (30:1:10:2:57), flow rate 1 mL/min. UV detection (λ= 658 nm). Retention time(s): 3.5 min. [K. Lin *et al.*, *J. Chromatogr.*, 1989, *465*, 75–86].

Column: (analytical) C_{18} (Nucleosil, 250 × 4.0 mm i.d., 5 µm); (guard) C_{18} (Nucleosil, 11 × 4.0 mm i.d., 5 µm). Mobile phase: acetonitrile:ammonium formate buffer (0.16 M, pH 2.7) (33:67), containing hexanesulfonic acid (0.25 M), flow rate 1 mL/min. UV detection (λ=658 nm). Retention time(s): 6.0 min. [K. Rentsch *et al.*, *J. Chromatogr.*, 1996, *679*, 185–192].

Ultraviolet Spectrum. Aqueous acid—242, 223, 276, 320 nm.

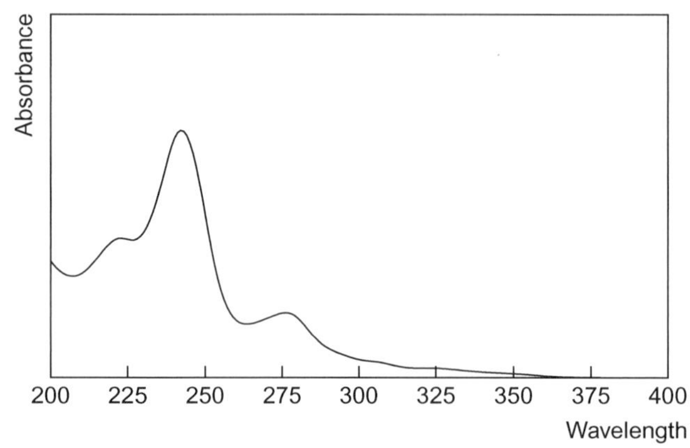

Infra-red Spectrum. Principal peaks at wavenumbers 1615, 1570, 1450, 1210, 825 cm^{-1} (KBr disc).

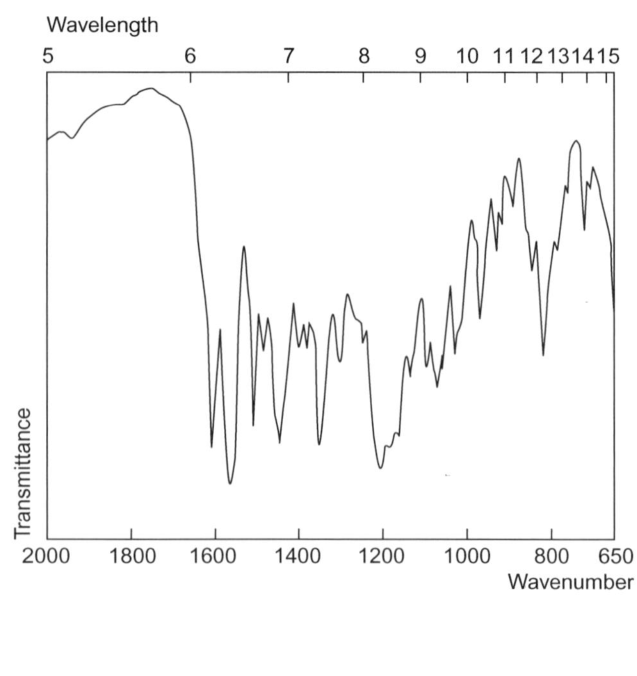

Mass Spectrum. Principal ions at m/z 74, 56, 44, 269, 41, 284, 239, 255.

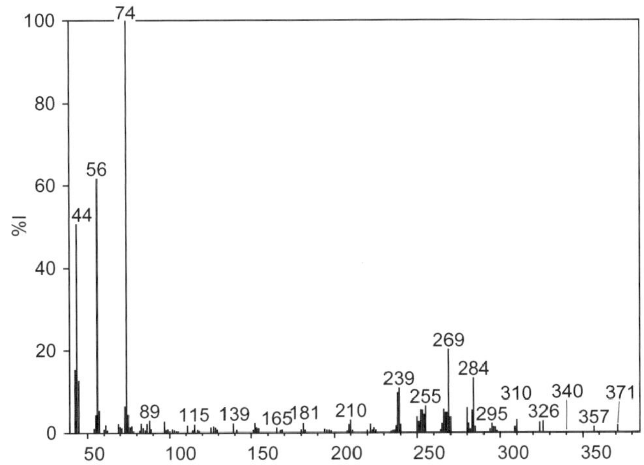

Quantification

High performance liquid chromatography. In blood: limit of detection 1.1 µg/L. UV detection (λ=658 nm)—L. Slordal *et al.*, *Ther. Drug Monit.*, 1993, *15*, 328–333. In blood: limit of quantification is 1 µg/L. UV detection (λ=658 nm)—K. Lin *et al.*, *J. Chromatogr.*, 1989, *465*, 75–86. In blood and tissues: limit of quantification 5 µg/L. UV detection (λ=658 nm)—K. Rentsch *et al.*, *J. Chromatogr.*, 1996, *679*, 185–192. In serum and urine: limit of quantification <1 µg/L and 0.2 µg/L, respectively. UV detection (λ=658 nm)—G. Ehninger *et al.*, *J. Chromatogr.*, 1985, *342*, 119–127.

Immunoassay. In serum: limit of detection 0.25 to 50 µg/L. Enzyme-linked immunosorbent assay (ELISA)—S. Flavell and D. Flavell, *J. Immunol. Methods*, 1988, *115*, 179–185.

Disposition in the Body. Mitozantrone is rapidly and extensively distributed in the body after intravenous administration. It is extensively tissue bound and undergoes very slow redistribution back into the plasma. It is slowly excreted in urine and bile as the unchanged drug and its metabolites: monocarboxylic and dicarboxylic acid derivatives. 20 to 32% of the dose is excreted within 5 days. Between 6 and 11% of the dose is recovered from urine and 13 to 25% in faeces. 65% of the unchanged drug is found in urine and 35% of the 2 inactive metabolites and their glucuronide conjugate. Two-thirds of excretion occurs during the first day. Tissue concentrations exceed those in blood during the terminal elimination phase. It does not appear to cross the blood–brain barrier.

Therapeutic concentration

5 patients with cancer of the peritoneal cavity were administered doses of between 20 and 50 mg/m^2 via the intraperitoneal route, as a 15 min infusion. The median peak plasma concentration was 1 µg/L and the peak peritoneal dialysate concentration, 490 µg/L. [J. D. Nagel *et al.*, *Cancer Chemother. Pharmacol.*, 1992, *29(6)*, 480–484].

Patients with liver metastasis were administered 12 mg/m^2 doses by intra-arterial infusions of 2 and 24 h. The peak plasma concentrations were 305 µg/L at 0.9 h during the 2 h infusion, and 244 µg/L at 5.5 h during the 24 h infusion. [M. J. Czejka *et al.*, *Eur. J. Drug Metab. Pharmacokinet.*, 1990, *15(3)*, 219–222].

Toxicity

Fatalities have occurred on rare occasions as a result of severe leucopenia with infection after accidental administration of a single bolus injection of mitozantrone at over 10 times the recommended dose. 4 patients received 140 to 180 mg/m^2 by single bolus injection and died owing to severe leucopenia. [APBI Compendium of data sheets and summaries of product characteristics 1999–2000. Epsom, Surrey: Datapharm Publications Ltd.].

Half-life. 5 to 18 days. Initial phase 3 to 10 min, intermediate phase 0.3 to 3.1 h, terminal phase 23 to 215 h (mean 75 h). Terminal phase also reported as 37.4 h.

Volume of distribution. 13.8 to14.4 L/kg or >2248 L/m^2. (Steady state >1000 L/m^2.)

Clearance. The mean body clearance is 238.7 mL/h/kg and is known to be reduced in hepatic impairment. Triphasic plasma clearance occurs.

Protein binding. Plasma binding approx. 95% and 78% (albumin).

Note. For a review of the pharmacokinetics of mitozantrone, see G. Ehninger *et al.*, *Clin. Pharmacokinet.*, 1990, *18*, 365–380. For a general review, see D. Faulds *et al.*, *Drugs*, 1991, *41*, 400–449.

Dose. The usual dose is 14 mg/m^2 body surface.

Mivacurium Chloride

Muscle Relaxant

Synonym. BW-B1090U
Proprietary name. Mivacron
(1*R*,1′*R*)-2,2′-[[(4*E*)-1,8-Dioxo-4-octene-1,8-diyl]bis(oxy-3,1-propanediyl)]bis[1,2,3,4-tetrahydro-6,7-dimethoxy-2-methyl-1-[(3,4,5-trimethoxyphenyl)methyl]]isoquinolinium dichloride
$C_{58}H_{80}Cl_2N_2O_{14}$=1100.2
CAS—106861-44-3

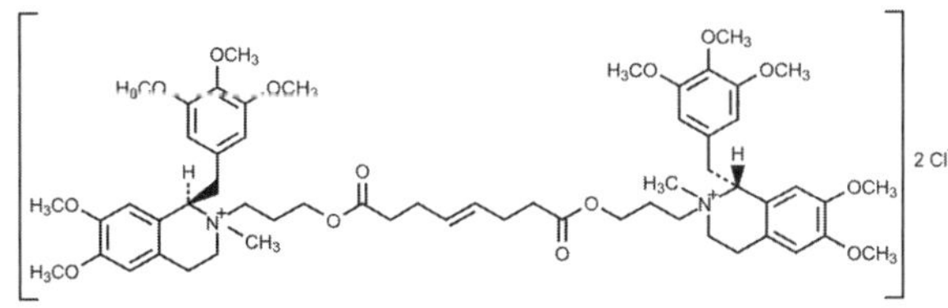

An amorphous solid.

Partition Coefficient. Log *P* (octanol/water), 0.015.

High Performance Liquid Chromatography. Column: C_1 (Spherisorb, 150 × 4.6 mm i.d., 5 µm). Mobile phase: (A) acetonitrile:potassium dihydrogen phosphate (10 mM, pH 3, containing 10% methanol) (70:30); (B) acetonitrile:potassium dihydrogen phosphate (50 mM, pH 3, containing 10% methanol) (70:30), flow rate 1 mL/min. Elution programme: (A:B) (100:0) for 3 min; to (0:100) in 2 min; hold for 4 min; to (100:0) in 2 min; hold for 2 min. Internal standard (IS): D-tubocurarine. Fluorescence detection (λ_{ex}=220 nm, λ_{em}=320 nm). Retention time(s): mivacurium chloride, 9.7 min; IS, 8.6 min. [M. Weindlmayr-Goettel *et al.*, *J. Chromatogr.*, 1996, *685(1)*; *Biomed. Appl.*, 123–127].

Column: SCX (Spherisorb, 250 × 4.6 mm, 10 µm). Mobile phase: acetonitrile:disodium sulfate (70 mM in 5 mM sulfuric acid) (60:40), flow rate 1 mL/min. IS: laudanosine. Fluorescence detection (λ_{ex}=220 nm, λ_{em}=320 nm). Retention time(s): mivacurium chloride: *cis–cis* isomer, 6.5 min; *cis–trans* isomer, 6.8 min; *trans–trans* isomer, 7.0 min; IS, 4.8 min. [M. Weindlmayr-Goettel *et al.*, *J. Chromatogr.*, 1996, *685*; *Biomed. Appl.*, 123–127].

Ultraviolet Spectrum. Aqueous acid—280 nm; Aqueous base—280 nm.

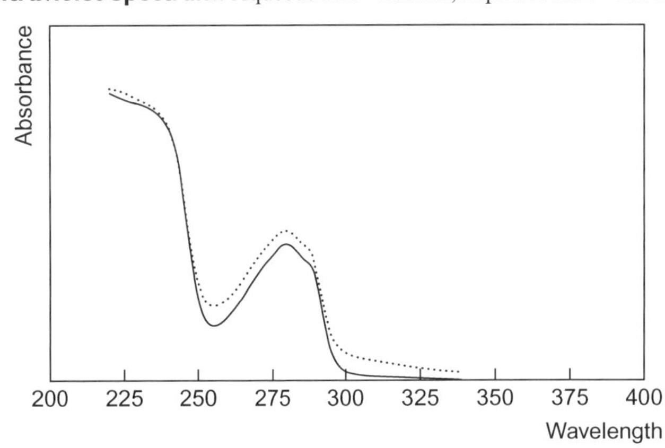

Infra-red Spectrum. Principal peaks at wavenumbers 1123, 1520, 1732, 1337 cm^{-1} (KBr disk).

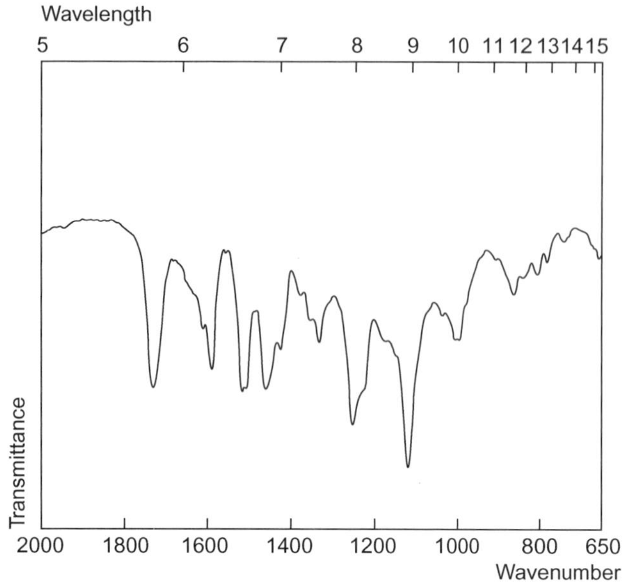

Quantification

High performance liquid chromatography. In plasma: limit of detection 1 µg/L. Fluororescence detection (λ_{ex}=220 nm, λ_{em}=320 nm)—M. Weindlmayr-Goettel *et al.*, *J. Chromatogr.*, 1996, *685(1)*; *Biomed. Appl.*, 123–127. In plasma: limit of quantification is 3.9, 4.1, 10.4 and 15.6 µg/L for the mivacurium isomers, *cis* monoester, *trans* monoester and the alcohol metabolites. Fluorescence detection (λ_{ex}=202 nm, λ_{em}=290 nm)—M. Lacroix *et al.*, *J. Chromatogr.*, 1995, *663(2)*; *Biomed. Appl.*, 297–307. In plasma: limit of quantification is 5 µg/L. Fluorescence detection (λ_{ex}=202 nm, λ_{em} = 320 nm)—A. R. Brown *et al.*, *J. Chromatogr.*, 1992, *578*, 302–308.

Disposition in the Body. Mivacurium undergoes enzymatic hydrolysis by plasma cholinesterases to inactivate the drug. Quaternary alcohol and monoester metabolites of the different isomers are produced. Peak concentrations of these can be observed approx. 25 s after an injection. Elimination of mivacurium occurs both in the kidneys and the liver with excretion in urine and bile, mostly as the metabolites (32 to 82% as the monoesters, 16 to 53% as the quaternary alcohols) and little unchanged drug (4 to 15% of a dose).

Therapeutic concentration

8 healthy patients (men and women) with a mean age of 33 years, were administered an intravenous dose of 0.15 mg/kg mivacurium chloride. Peak plasma concentrations of 4486, 2198 and 504 µg/L for the *trans–trans*, *cis–trans* and *cis–cis* isomers, respectively, were observed after 25 and 35 s. Plasma concentrations of the *trans–trans* and *cis–trans* isomers declined rapidly and could not be detected 10 to 20 min after administration. Peak concentrations of the *cis–cis* isomer declined less rapidly and it could still be detected up to 45 min after injection. [M. Lacroix *et al.*, *Anesthesiology*, 1997, *86(2)*, 322–330].

Toxicity. Prolonged muscle paralysis and its consequences are the main signs of overdosing.

Half-life. *Trans–trans* isomer, 2.4 min; *cis–trans* isomer, 2.0 min; *cis–cis* isomer, 28.5 min (mean values).

Volume of distribution. Drug in general, 0.2 L/kg. *Trans–trans* isomer, 0.047 L/kg; *cis–trans* isomer, 0.054 L/kg; *cis–cis* isomer, 0.189 L/kg.

Clearance. Plasma: *trans–trans* isomer, 29.2 mL/min/kg; *cis–trans* isomer, 45.7 mL/min/kg; *cis–cis* isomer, 6.7 mL/min/kg.

Note. For a general review of the pharmacology of mivacurium chloride, see J. E. Frampton and D. McTavish, *Drugs*, 1993, *45*, 1066–1089.

Dose. Initial dose is 70 to 250 µg/kg body weight intravenous injection and the maintenance dose is 100 µg/kg. Reduced doses may be necessary in the elderly. Continuous treatment may be at 8 to 10 µg/kg/min which can be increased in 1 µg/kg/min steps. Children 2 months to 12 years: 11 to 14 µg/kg/min.

Mizolastine

Antihistamine

Synonym. SL85-0324
Proprietary names. Mistamine; Mizollen; Zolim.
2-[[1-[1-[(4-Fluorophenyl)methyl]-1*H*-benzimidazol-2-yl]-4-piperidinyl]-methylamino]-4(1*H*)-pyrimidinone
$C_{24}H_{25}FN_6O$=432.5
CAS—108612-45-9

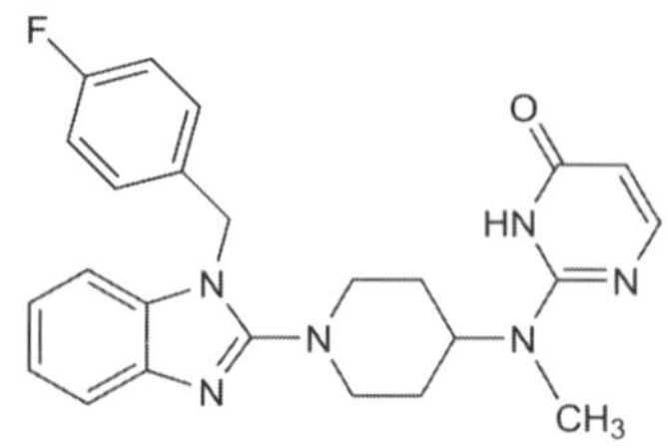

Crystals. M.p. 217°. Soluble in methanol.

High Performance Liquid Chromatography. Column: C_8 Ultra-base B5 (150 × 4.6 mm i.d., 5 µm). Mobile phase: potassium dihydrogen phosphate (25 mM, pH 2.5):acetonitrile (72:28), flow rate 1 mL/min. UV detection (λ=285 nm). Retention time(s): not specified. [O. Chosidow *et al.*, *Eur. J. Clin. Pharmacol.*, 1996, *50*, 327–333].

Ultraviolet Spectrum. Aqueous acid—208, 229, 281, 288 nm; Ethanol—214, 287 nm.

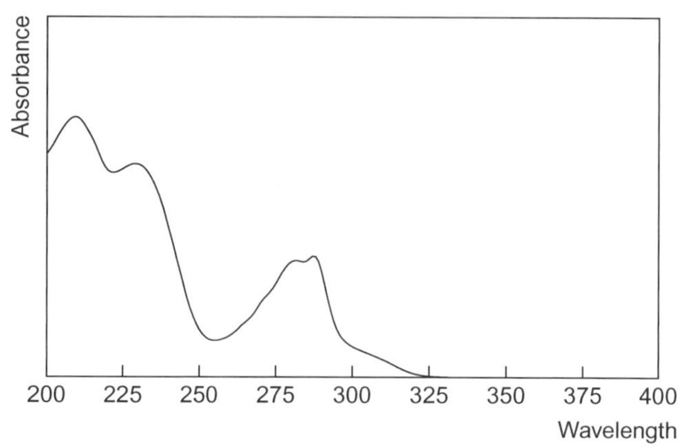

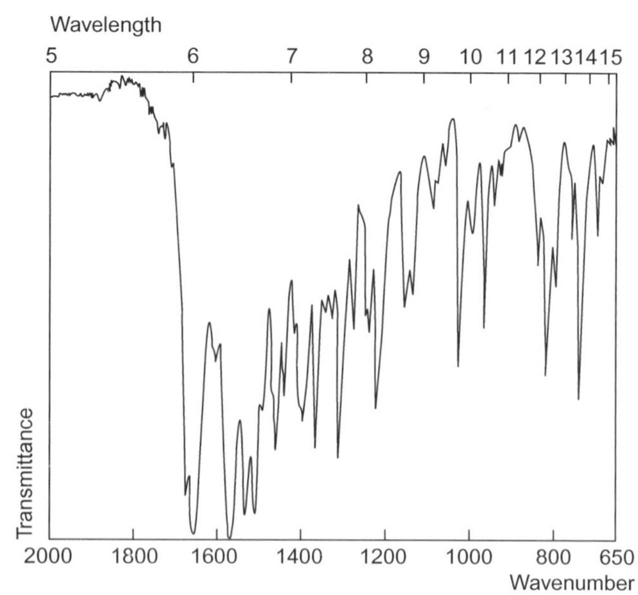

Mass Spectrum. Principal ions at *m/z*: 109, 27, 165, 198, 40, 55, 57, 288.

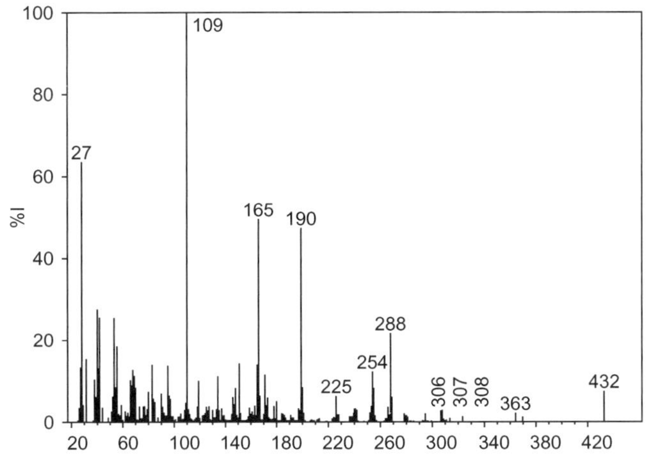

Quantification

High performance liquid chromatography. In plasma: limit of detection 0.5 µg/L—V. Ascalone and A. Rouchouse, *J. Chromatogr.*, 1993, *619*, 275–284.

Disposition in the Body. Mizolastine is rapidly absorbed from the gastro-intestinal tract and extensively metabolised. 0.5% of an administered dose is recovered from urine as the unchanged drug and 84 to 95% of the drug is excreted in faeces. 66% of the administered dose is metabolised by glucuronidation, and other metabolic pathways are also involved including metabolism by cytochrome P450 isoenzyme CYP3A4 with the formation of inactive metabolites. No active metabolites have been identified. Linear kinetics are observed. Steady state is reached on the third day of administration and accumulation does not occur.

Therapeutic concentration. Peak plasma concentrations of 276, 408 and 595 µg/L have been observed 1.5 h after oral doses of 5, 10 and 15 mg, respectively.

Bioavailability. Tablets: 65%. Capsules: 70%. Not influenced by food or alcohol.

Half-life. Approx. 13 h. In patients with hepatic impairment, 15.1 ± 1.7 h and renal impairment 19.2 ± 1.7 h.

Volume of distribution. 1.4 L/kg.

Clearance. A total clearance of 1.15 mL/min/kg and systemic plasma clearance of 0.69 L/h/kg.

Protein binding. Approx. 98.4%.

Dose. 10 mg daily.

Moclobemide

Antidepressant

Synonyms. Ro-11-1163; Ro-11-1163/000.
Proprietary names. Aurorix; Manerix; Moclamine.
4-Chloro-*N*-[2-(4-morpholinyl)ethyl]benzamide
$C_{13}H_{17}ClN_2O_2$ = 268.7
CAS—71320-77-9

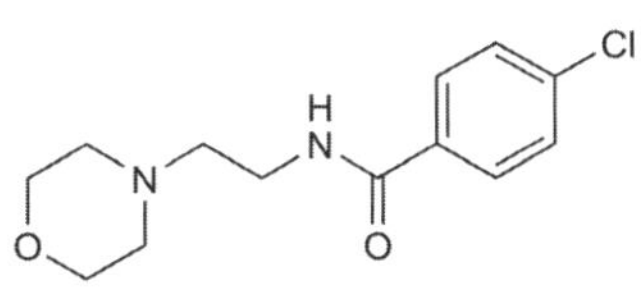

Crystals from isopropanol. M.p. 137°.

Moclobemide Hydrochloride

$C_{13}H_{17}ClN_2O_2$,HCl = 305.2
Crystals from isopropanol with m.p. 208°.

Dissociation Constant. pK_a 6.2.

Thin-layer Chromatography. System TB—Rf 01; system TE—Rf 52; system TAE—Rf 65.

Gas Chromatography. System GB—RI 2333; system GM—RRT 0.967.

Column: HP5 (0.32 mm i.d.). Column temperature: 140°, held for 0.5 min, ramped 20°/min, held at 300° for 2 min. Detection: nitrogen–phosphorous. Retention time(s): 3.0 min. [P. P. Singer and G. R. Jones, *J. Anal. Toxicol.*, 1997, *21*, 518–520].

High Performance Liquid Chromatography. System HX—RI 295; system HZ—retention time 2.4 min; system HAA—retention time 10.2 min; system HAX—retention time 6.9 min; system HAY—retention time 3.9 min.

Column: C_{18} (Kromasil, 150 × 4.6 mm i.d., 5 µm). Mobile phase: (A) methanol:water (90:10); (B) water:methanol (90:10); both (A) and (B) contain 0.0125 M sodium hydroxide. Elution programme: (A:B) (40:60) to (25:75) in 5 min, hold for 8 min, to (0:100) in 10 min, hold for 5 min. Internal standard (IS): Ro-11-9900. UV detection (λ = 237 nm). Retention time(s): moclobemide, 4.5 min; IS, 5.5 min. [G. K. Isbister *et al.*, *J. Anal. Toxicol.*, 2001, *25*, 716–717].

Column: S5 C_6 (Spherisorb, 125 × 4.0 mm i.d., 5 µm). Mobile phase: acetonitrile:potassium phosphate (67 mM) (30:320), pH 3.9, flow rate 1.3 mL/min. IS: Ro-11-9900. UV detection (λ = 240 nm). Retention time(s): moclobemide, 7.2 min; metabolite, 5.3 min; *N*-oxide metabolite, 8.6 min; lactam derivative metabolite, 15.1 min; IS, 12.7 min. [R. Geschke *et al.*, *J. Chromatogr.*, 1987, *420*, 111–120].

Ultraviolet Spectrum. Aqueous acid (pH 2.8)—238 nm.

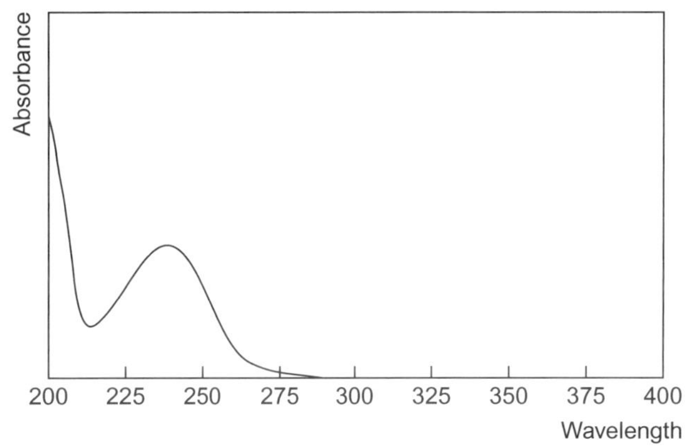

Mass Spectrum. Principal ions at *m/z* 100, 56, 113, 139, 111, 42, 70, 101.

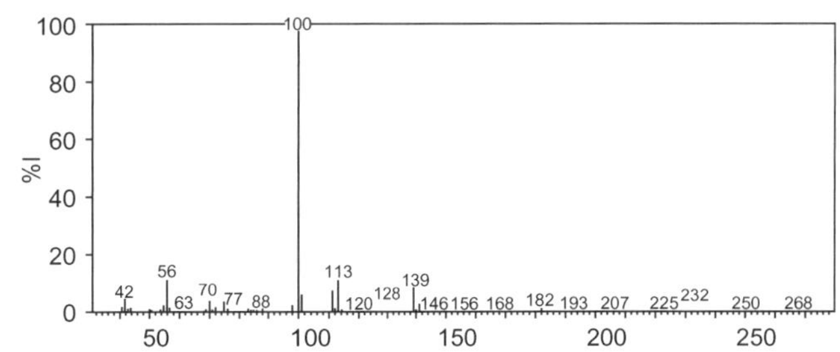

Quantification

Gas chromatography–mass spectrometry. In urine: limit of detection < 100 µg/L—J. Bickeboeller-Friedrich and H. H. Maurer, *Ther. Drug Monit.*, 2001, *23*, 61–70.

High performance liquid chromatography. In urine and plasma: limit of quantification for moclobemide and its *N*-oxide metabolite 75 and 150 µg/L, respectively, in urine; 20 and 30 µg/L in plasma. UV detection (λ = 240 nm)—R. Geschke *et al.*, *J. Chromatogr.*, 1987, *420*, 111–120. In blood: limit of detection 0.012 mg/L. UV detection (λ = 238 nm)—Y. Gaillard and G. Pepin, *Forensic Sci. Int.*, 1997, *87(3)*, 239–248.

Disposition in the Body. Moclobemide is readily absorbed after oral administration, with peak plasma concentrations observed after 1 to 2 h. The drug is almost completely absorbed and undergoes extensive and rapid hepatic metabolism to 19 metabolites, mostly by oxidation, deamination and aromatic hydroxylation. Absorption is delayed in the presence of food. The drug is almost entirely metabolised before it is eliminated from the body. Slow metabolisers and extensive metabolisers both exist. The main metabolite is the lactam derivative which is pharmacologically inactive but the other metabolites retain some activity, in particular the *N*-oxide of the drug. It is widely distributed throughout the body including breast milk and accumulation can occur. Moclobemide is excreted in urine mainly as the metabolites and a small amount as the unchanged drug (< 1%), and in faeces, less than 5%.

Therapeutic concentration. The trough serum therapeutic concentration is 0.4 to 1.0 mg/L and peak, 1.5 to 4.0 mg/L.

8 male volunteers, 29 to 37 years old (mean age of 33 years), were administered a single dose of 100 mg moclobemide. The mean peak plasma concentration was 575 μg/L with a range of 333 to 1076 μg/L which was observed at 0.9 h (0.3 to 1.5 h) post administration. [M. P. Schoerlin *et al.*, *Clin Pharmacol. Ther.*, 1991, *49*, 32–38].

Toxicity. Blood concentrations of 5 to 8 mg/L can be toxic and blood concentrations of 16 mg/L are sometimes associated with fatalities.

A 39-year-old woman was admitted to hospital with convulsions and a raised body temperature of 42.6°. The highest blood concentration measure was 36.5 mg/L and it was estimated that she had probably ingested 10 g of moclobemide. Her blood concentration was several-fold higher than the peak concentrations observed after a single oral dose of 1.2 g observed in tolerance studies (11 to 12 mg/L, 0.25 to 0.5 h after administration). The patient recovered after anticonvulsants had been administered and artificial respiration carried out. [M. P. Schoerlin *et al.*, *Hoffman-Roche Ltd.*, *Data on File*, 1987].

A 48-year-old woman with a history of depression and repeated suicide attempts was found dead at home. Postmortem toxicological analysis showed a blood-moclobemide concentration of 137 mg/L and a liver concentration of 432 mg/kg. Low levels of diazepam, nordiazepam and trifluoperazine were also detected. It was concluded that death was caused by acute poisoning by moclobemide (the first case to report death caused by the toxic effects of this drug on its own). [C. Camaris and D. Little, *J. Forensic Sci.*, 1997, *42(5)*, 954–955].

A 41-year old Caucasian man was found dead at his home; he had a history of depression and suicide attempts. Surrounding the man were a number of medication bottles and a bottle of whiskey. Toxicological analysis showed that the man had ethanol, lormetazepam, cotinine, caffeine, moclobemide and citalopram in his urine and blood. Moclobemide was detected in blood at a concentration of 5.62 mg/L and in urine, 204.0 mg/L. Its metabolite, 3-ketomoclobemide, was found at concentrations of 2.26 mg/L and 49.7 mg/L in the two fluids, respectively, and moclobemide *N'*-oxide at 424 mg/L in urine (this metabolite was not detected in blood). The cause of death was determined as the synergistic toxicity of moclobemide and citalopram; and death was ruled as multiple drug intoxication. [R. Dams *et al.*, *J. Anal. Toxicol.*, 2001, *25(2)*, 147–151].

Bioavailability. 55 to 95% (single dose); 80% (multiple dosing).

Half-life. 1 to 4 h.

Volume of distribution. 1.2 L/kg.

Clearance. Blood, 20 to 50 L/h.

Protein binding. 50%.

Note. For an update of the pharmacological properties and therapeutic use of moclobemide, see B. Fulton and P. Benfield, *Drugs*, 1996, *52*, 450–474.

Dose. The initial dose is 300 mg daily, divided in three doses, which may be adjusted if necessary. During therapy, the usual range is 150 to 600 mg daily.

Modafinil

CNS Stimulant/ Alpha$_1$-adrenergic Agonist

Synonyms. CEP-1538; CRL-40476.
Proprietary names. Modiodal; Provigil.
2-[(Diphenylmethyl)sulfinyl]acetamide
$C_{15}H_{15}NO_2S$=273.4
CAS—68693-11-8

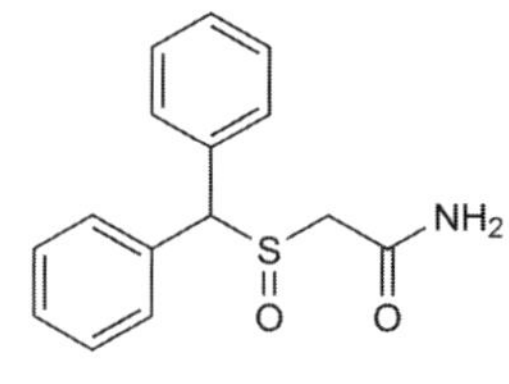

A white to off-white crystalline powder with m.p. 164° to 166°. It is practically insoluble in water and cyclohexane; sparingly to slightly soluble in methanol and acetone.

High Performance Liquid Chromatography. Column: μBondapak C_{18} (300 × 3.9 mm i.d., 10 μm). Mobile phase: acetonitrile:water:acetic acid (15:42:1.2), flow rate 1.4 mL/min. Internal standard (IS): [bis(4-fluorophenyl)methylsufinyl]acetic acid. UV detection (λ=236 nm). Retention time(s): modafinil, 11.0 min; IS, 24 min. [G. Moachon *et al.*, *J. Chromatogr.*, 1994, *654*; *Biomed. Appl.*, 91–96].

Column: β-Cyclodextrin (250 × 4.0 mm i.d., 5 μm). Column temperature: 12°. Mobile phase: phosphate buffer (0.02 M, adjusted to pH 3.0 with orthophosphoric acid):acetonitrile (84:16), flow rate 0.6 mL/min. IS: 3,3-diphenylpropylamine. UV detection (diode array, λ=225 nm). Retention time(s): *R*-modafinil, 19.0 min; *S*-modafinil, 22.0 min; IS, 9 min. [S. H. Gorman, *J. Chromatogr. B, Biomed. Sci. Appl.*, 1999, *730(1)*, 1–7].

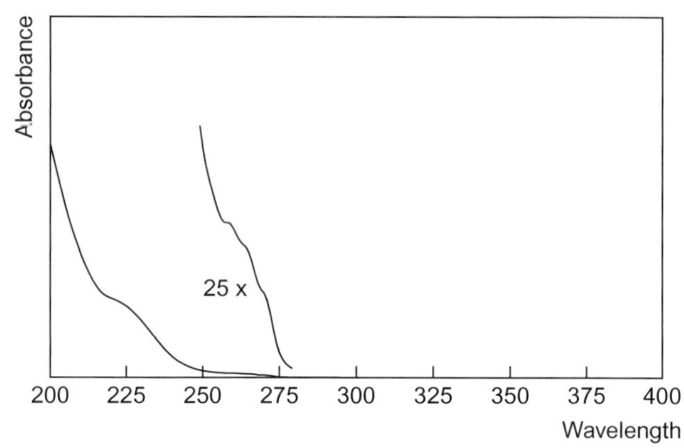

Quantification

High performance liquid chromatography. In plasma: limit of detection 0.04 mg/L (modafinil and acid metabolite), limit of quantification 0.13 mg/L (modafinil) and 0.14 mg/L (acid metabolite). UV detection (λ=236 nm)—G. Moachon and D. Matinier, *J. Chromatogr.*, 1994, *654*; *Biomed. Appl.*, 91–96. In plasma: limit of detection 0.01 mg/L and limit of quantification 0.10 mg/L. UV detection (λ=225 nm)—P. Burnat *et al.*, *J. Chromatogr. B, Biomed. Sci. Appl.*, 1998, *706*, 295–304. In plasma: limit of quantification is 0.1 mg/L. UV detection (λ=225 nm)—S. H. Gorman, *J. Chromatogr. B, Biomed. Sci. Appl.*, 1999, *730(1)*, 1–7.

Disposition in the Body. Modafinil is a racemic compound whose enantiomers have different pharmacokinetics. It is rapidly and well absorbed from the gastro-intestinal tract following oral administration. It is well distributed in tissues and metabolised in the liver by hydrolytic deamination, *S*-oxidation, aromatic ring hydroxylation and glucuronide conjugation. Modafinil shows a possible induction effect on its own metabolism after chronic administration of doses greater than 400 mg per day. The major metabolite is modafinil acid but there are at least 6 other metabolites present in much lower concentrations. The major route of elimination (about 90%) is metabolism, primarily by the liver, with subsequent renal elimination. < 10% of the dose is eliminated unchanged. Renal impairment does not effect pharmacokinetics. In hepatic impairment oral clearance is decreased by about 60% and steady state concentration is doubled. Steady state is achieved within 8 days.

Therapeutic concentration

12 healthy young males (aged 22 to 37 years; mean 29 years), 12 young females (19 to 40 years; mean 26 years) and 12 elderly males (mean 63 years; range 53 to 72 years) were administered a single oral dose of 200 mg modafinil after an overnight fast. The peak plasma mofafinil concentration was 4.21 mg/L for the young males which was observed at 2.0 h; 5.2 mg/L for the young females at 1.7 h and 4.81 mg/L at 1.7 h for the elderly males. For the metabolite, modafinil acid, concentrations were 2.06, 2.65 and

2.65 mg/L for the young males, females and elderly males observed at 2.8, 2.9 and 3.5 h, respectively. [Y. N. Wong *et al.*, *J. Clin. Pharmacol.*, 1999, *39(3)*, 281–288].

32 healthy male volunteers, aged between 20 and 39 years old (mean 26.2 years), were administered either a 200, 400, 600 or 800 mg dose of modafinil after breakfast for 7 consecutive days. Peak plasma concentrations of the parent drug were 4.8 and 6.4 mg/L for the 200 mg dose on days 1 and 7, respectively. For the 400 mg dose, concentrations reached 8.7 mg/L at 2.3 h on day 1 and 11.0 mg/L at 1.7 h on day 7. For the 600 mg dose, concentrations were 13.0 and 17.0 mg/L on days 1 and 7, respectively, observed at 2.5 and 2.3 h. On day 1, the 800 mg dose of modafinil produced concentrations of 15.0 mg/L at 2.3 h. [Y. N. Wong *et al.*, *J. Clin. Pharmacol.*, 1999, *39*, 30–40].

Toxicity. Doses of 4 g led to limited, expected and not life-threatening adverse experiences with patients making full recovery.

Half-life. 10 to 15 h.

Volume of distribution. Approx. 0.9 L/kg or 80 L.

Clearance. 3 to 5 L/h.

Protein binding. Approx. 62% (albumin).

Dose. 200 to 400 mg.

Moexipril

Antihypertensive

Synonym. RS-10085
(3*S*)-2-[(2*S*)-2-[[(1*S*)-1-(Ethoxycarbonyl)-3-phenylpropyl]amino]-1-oxopropyl]-1,2,3,4-tetrahydro-6,7-dimethoxy-3-isoquinolinecarboxylic acid
$C_{27}H_{34}N_2O_7$=498.6
CAS—103775-10-6

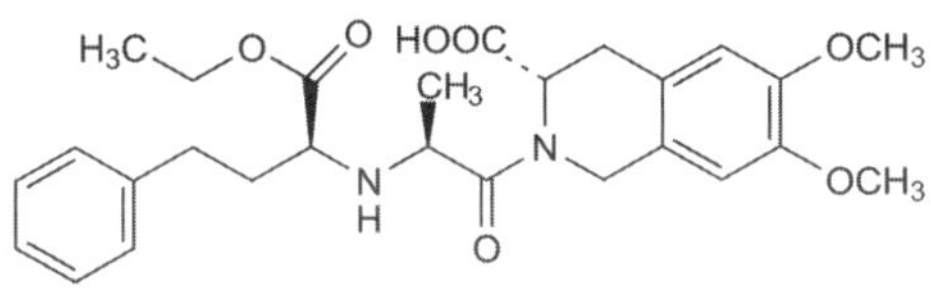

Moexipril Diacid Hydrochloride

Synonym. Moexiprilat Hydrochloride
$C_{27}H_{30}N_2O_7$,HCl=531.0
CAS—82586-57-0
Crystals from tetrahydrofuran and ethanol, m.p. 145° to 170°.

Moexipril Hydrochloride

Synonyms. CI-925; RS-10085-197; SPM-925.
Proprietary names. Femipres; Perdix; Univasc. It is also an ingredient of Uniretic.
$C_{27}H_{34}N_2O_7$,HCl=535.0
CAS—82586-52-5
A fine-white to off-white powder, m.p. 141° to 161°. It is soluble in distilled water at room temperature.

Dissociation Constant. pK_a 3.05 (25°); 5.40 (25°).

Partition Coefficient. Log *P* (pH 7.5), 0.25; (pH 1.0), 2.34.

Gas Chromatography. System GP—RI 3575 moexipril-ME, RI 3580 M(moexiprilate)-ME3, RI 3775 M(moexiprilate-H_2O)-ME3.

Column: DB-1 fused-silica capillary (10 m × 0.32 mm i.d., 0.25 μm film thickness). Column temperature: 150°, held 0.1 min, to 300° at 25°/min, held 1.5 min. Injector temperature: 70° to 300° at 10°/s, held for 5 min. Carrier gas: helium, inlet pressure 13.8 kPa. Internal standard (IS): quinapril hydrochloride. MS detection (NICI, SIM at *m/z*: 302 and 288 for moexipril and moexiprilat, respectively). Retention time(s): moexipril, 7.32 min; moexiprilat, 7.25 min; IS, 6.2 min. [W. Hammes *et al.*, *J. Chromatogr.*, 1995, *670(1)*; *Biomed. Appl.*, 81–89].

Ultraviolet Spectrum. Aqueous solution—283 nm (unaffected by pH).

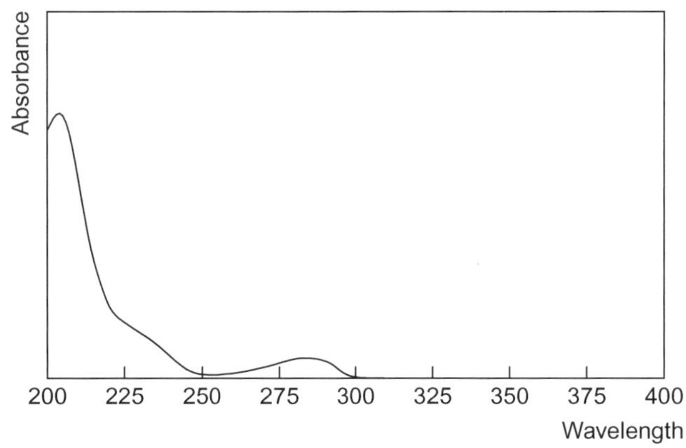

Infra-red Spectrum. Principal peaks at wavenumbers 702, 753, 858, 1115, 1215, 1256 cm^{-1}.

Quantification
Gas chromatography–mass spectrometry. In plasma: limit of quantification for moexipril and moexiprilat 0.5 μg/L—W. Hammes *et al.*, *J. Chromatogr.*, 1995, *670(1)*; *Biomed. Appl.*, 81–89.

Disposition in the Body. Moexipril is rapidly but incompletely absorbed after oral administration and de-esterified to its active metabolite, moexiprilat. Absorption is reduced with the presence of food, and peak plasma concentrations of the metabolite are reached within 1.5 h. Both the parent drug and the active metabolite are mainly eliminated in urine along with other minor metabolites including diketopiperazine, and some moexiprilat is excreted in faeces (20% of an intravenous dose and 52% of an oral dose). 40% of an intravenous dose is excreted as moexiprilat in urine (7% oral dose) and 26% as the unchanged drug (1% oral). The pharmacokinetics of moexipril are significantly altered in patients with severe renal impairment (creatinine clearance 40 mL/min) and those with liver cirrhosis.

Therapeutic concentration

Healthy volunteers were administered a 15 mg single dose of moexipril and peak plasma concentrations of 50 μg/L and 5 μg/L were respectively reached for the drug and its metabolite, moexiprilat, within 2 h. [M. Stimpel *et al.*, *Cardiovasc. Drug Rev.*, 1995, *13(3)*, 211–229].

Bioavailability. 22%.

Half-life. Approx. 10 h.

Volume of distribution. 183 L (moexipril and moexiprilat).

Clearance. Plasma, moexipril, 441 mL/min; moexiprilat, 232 mL/min.

Protein binding. Moexipril, 50%; moexiprilat 72%.

Note. For a review of the use of moexipril in the management of essential hypertension, see R. N. Brogden and L. R. Wiseman, *Drugs*, 1998, *55*, 845–860.

Dose. The usual initial dose is 7.5 mg and a maintenance dose of 7.5 to 15 mg daily is administered. Doses up to 30 mg may also be given. In the elderly, patients with renal failure or hepatic cirrhosis, and those being treated with a diuretic or nifedipine, the initial dose should be reduced by half.

Molgramostim

Antineoplastic/Antineutropenic

Synonym. Sch-39300
Proprietary names. Leucomax; Mielogen.
Colony-stimulating factor 2 (human clone pHG25, protein moiety reduced)
$C_{639}H_{1007}N_{171}O_{196}S_{18}$=14798.03
CAS—99283-10-0

Soluble in water.

Quantification
Enzyme immunoassay. In serum: limit of quantification is 0.1 μg/L—J. S. Cebon *et al.*, *Blood*, 1988, *72*, 1340–1347.

Disposition in the Body. Maximum serum concentrations increase with administered dose but appear larger with intravenous doses compared with subcutaneous administration. Concentrations reached with subcutaneous treatment, greater than 1 μg/L, are maintained longer than those with intravenous administration. Molgramostim has been detected in urine, but only in very small amounts, suggesting non-renal elimination.

Therapeutic concentration

33 male and female patients with advanced malignancy or neutropenia, aged between 30 and 74 years, were administered 0.3 to 30.0 μg/kg molgramostim per day as a subcutaneous bolus injection. Patients were also administered 0.3 to 20.0 μg/kg daily intravenously as a bolus injection or as a 2-h infusion. Molgramostim was detected within 30 min of the subcutaneous injection for those receiving 1.0 μg/kg and 5 to 15 min for the higher doses. The mean peak serum concentration was 22.1 μg/L for the patients receiving doses of 15.0 μg/kg and above. Serum concentrations were greater than 1.0 μg/L for those receiving 1.0 μg/kg molgramostim and above but not for doses below this. After the intravenous bolus injection, peak concentrations ranged from 6.9 to 95.7 μg/L as the dose increased. After the 2-h intravenous infusion, molgramostim was detected in serum after 15 min. The peak concentration ranged from 18.2 to 235.0 μg/L; not correlated to dose. [J. S. Cebon *et al.*, *Eur. J. Cancer*, 1990, *26*, 1064–1069].

Half-life. 0.24 to 1.18 h (after intravenous bolus dosing); mean 1.66 (range 1.33 to 1.88) h (intravenous infusion); mean 3.16 h (after subcutaneous dosing).

Clearance. Serum, 18.6 to 25.1 L/h (1.0 μg/kg subcutaneous dose of molgramostim); 33.3 L/h (3.0 μg/kg dose); 8.3 L/h at higher doses (10.0 to 30.0 μg/kg); and for doses 0.3 to 3.0 μg/kg, the clearance increased. After an intravenous bolus dose, 0.3 μg/kg, 16.0 L/h; intravenous infusion, 5.7 L/h.

Dose. For antineoplastic therapy: subcutaneous injection, 5 to 10 μg/kg body weight daily starting 24 h after the last dose of antineoplastic. Treatment for 7 to 10 days.

For bone marrow transplantation: intravenous infusion, 10 μg/kg body weight over 4 to 6 h. Up to 30 days' treatment starting the day after the transplant.

Molindone

Tranquilliser

3-Ethyl-1,5,6,7-tetrahydro-2-methyl-5-(4-morpholinylmethyl)-4*H*-indol-4-one

$C_{16}H_{24}N_2O_2$=276.4

CAS—7416-34-4

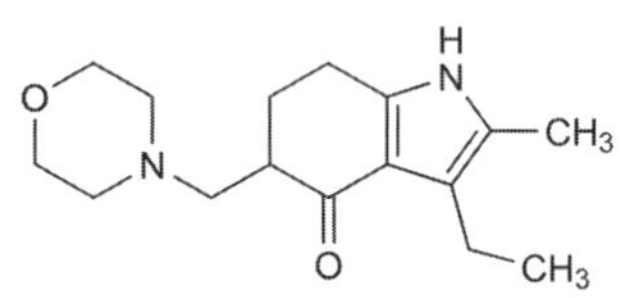

Crystals. M.p. 180° to 181°.

Molindone Hydrochloride

Synonym. EN-1733 A

Proprietary names. Lidone; Moban.

$C_{16}H_{24}N_2O_2$,HCl=312.8

CAS—15622-65-8

A white crystalline powder.

Freely soluble in water and ethanol.

Dissociation Constant. pK_a 6.9 (25°).

Partition Coefficient. Log *P* (octanol/water), 2.3.

Thin-layer Chromatography. System TAJ—Rf 24; system TAK—Rf 00; system TAL—Rf 37.

Gas Chromatography. System GA—RI 2465.

Ultraviolet Spectrum. Aqueous acid—255 (A_1^1=41b), 299 nm.

Mass Spectrum. Principal ions at *m/z* 100, 56, 42, 176, 98, 120, 70, 189.

Disposition in the Body. Molindone is readily absorbed after oral administration; peak plasma concentrations of unchanged drug are attained in 1 to 2 h. It is extensively metabolised and excreted in the urine and faeces almost entirely as metabolites.

Dose. 15 to 225 mg of molindone hydrochloride daily.

6-Monoacetylmorphine

Synonym. 6-MAM

6-*O*-Acetylmorphine

$C_{19}H_{21}NO_4$=327.4

CAS—2784-73-8

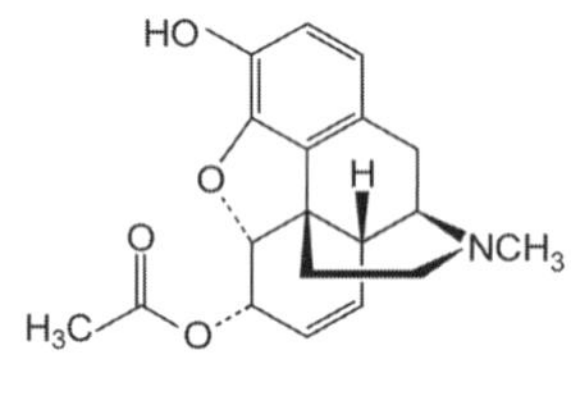

6-Monoacetylmorphine Hydrochloride

$C_{19}H_{21}NO_4$,HCl=363.8

CAS—36418-22-1

Crystals.

Soluble in water.

Colour Test. Marquis Test—violet.

Thin-layer Chromatography. System TA—Rf 46; system TB—Rf 06; system TC—Rf 19; system TAJ—Rf 13; system TAK—Rf 02; system TAL—Rf 51. (Acidified iodoplatinate solution, positive.)

Gas Chromatography. System GA—6-MAM RI 2525, 6-MAM-PFP RI 2650, 6-MAM-TMS RI 2590, diamorphine RI 2615; system GB—6-MAM RI 2646, 6-MAM-TMS RI 2688, diamorphine RI 2769.

Column: HP-5 capillary 95% dimethylsiloxane, 5% diphenylsiloxane (25 m × 0.25 mm i.d., 0.25 μm film thickness). Column temperature: 120°; held, 2 min; increased to 280° at 20°/min; held, 10 min. Carrier gas: helium, 1 mL/min flow rate. MS detection. Retention time: 13.5 min. [F. Pragst *et al.*, *J. Anal. Toxicol.*, 1999, *23*, 168–171.]

Column: fused silica capillary (25 m × 0.32 mm i.d., 0.12 μm film thickness). Column temperature: 120° to 200° at 10°/min and then 200° to 250° at 2°/min (purged by increasing to 280° at 30°/min, held 10 min, before cooling). Carrier gas: nitrogen, flow rate 1.3 mL/min. Detection: NSD or FID. Retention time: 22.4 min (NSD); 21.6 min (FID). [T. Vu-Duc and A. Vernay, *Biomed. Chromatogr.*, 1990, *4*, 65–69.]

High Performance Liquid Chromatography. System HA—*k* 3.6 (tailing peak); system HC—*k* 0.80; system HS—*k* 1.00; system HAA—retention time 7.3 min.

Column: (analytical) Phenyl (Nova-Pak, 150 mm × 3.9 mm i.d., 5 μm), (guard) Phenyl (Nova-Pak). Mobile phase: acetonitrile:sodium dihydrogen phosphate (10 mM, pH 6.6) (10:90), flow rate 1.2 mL/min. Detection: UV (λ=210 nm) and ECD. I.S.: nalorphine. Retention time: 6-monoacetylmorphine, 30.5 min; IS, 25.2 min. [J. Gerostamoulos *et al.*, *J. Chromatogr.*, 1993, *617(1)*, 152–156.]

Ultraviolet Spectrum. Aqueous acid—287 nm (A_1^1=45b).

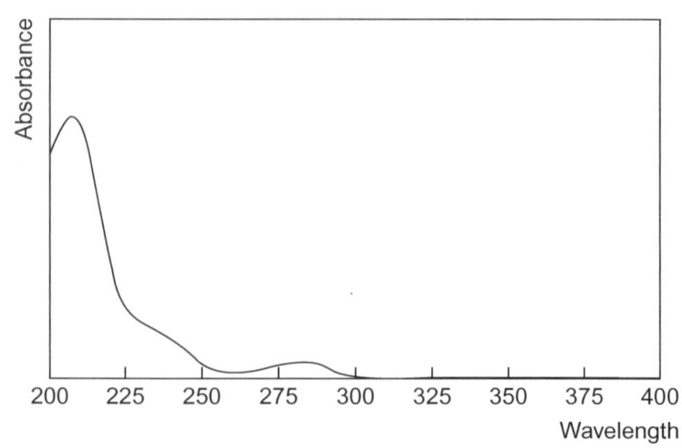

Infra-red Spectrum. Principal peaks at wavenumbers 1238, 1730, 1213, 1050, 1030, 1131 cm^{-1} (KBr disk).

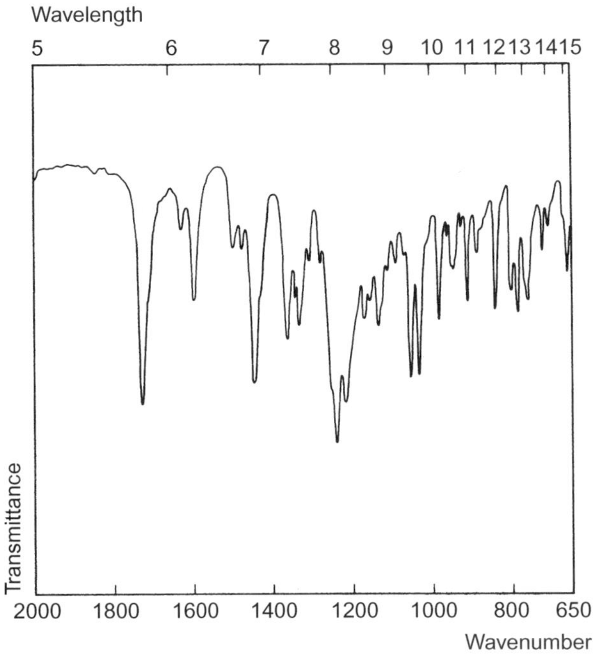

Mass Spectrum. Principal ions at *m/z* 327, 268, 42, 43, 215, 44, 328, 269.

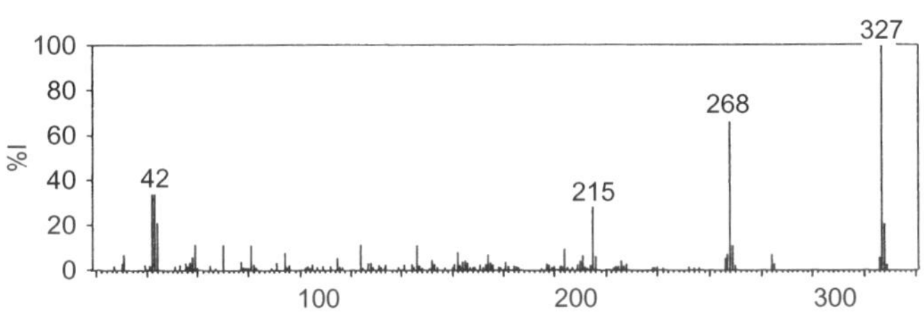

Quantification

Gas chromatography. In urine: limit of detection 2 µg/L with NPD and 4 µg/L with FID—T. Vu-Duc and A. Vernay, *Biomed. Chromatogr.*, 1990, *4(2)*, 65–69. In blood: 6-monoacetylmorphine (6-MAM) and other opioids, limit of quantification for 6-MAM 10 µg/L, electron ionisation detection—S. Mykkanen *et al.*, *J. Anal. Toxicol.*, 2000, *24*, 122–126.

Gas chromatography–mass spectrometry. In urine: limit of detection 0.1 µg/L—T. Vu-Duc and A. Vernay, *Biomed. Chromatogr.* 1990, *4*, 65–69. In urine: 6-MAM and morphine, limit of detection 0.81 µg/L—E. J. Cone *et al.*, *J. Anal. Toxicol.*, 1991, *15*, 1–7. In urine: 6-MAM, codeine, and morphine, limit of quantification 10 µg/L—D. C. Fuller and W. H. Anderson, *J. Anal. Toxicol.*, 1992, *16*, 315–318. In serum, blood, or postmortem blood: 6-MAM and other diamorphine metabolites, limit of detection 1 µg/L—F. Musshoff and T. Daldrup, *Int. J. Legal Med.*, 1993, *106*, 107–109. In plasma, blood, saliva, or urine: 6-MAM, diamorphine, and morphine, limit of detection 1 µg/L—B. A. Goldberger *et al.*, *Clin. Chem.*, 1993, *39*, 670–675. In plasma or whole blood: 6-MAM and other opioids—M. Krogh *et al.*, *J. Chromatogr.*, 1993, *621*, 41–48. In hair: 6-MAM and other opioids, cocaine and amfetamine, limit of detection 0.1 µg/g—M. R. Moeller *et al.*, *Forensic Sci. Int.*, 1993, *63*, 185–206. In hair: 6-MAM, diamorphine, and its other metabolites—A. Polettini *et al.*, *Forensic Sci. Int.*, 1993, *63*, 217–225. In hair: 6-MAM and morphine, limit of detection 0.2 µg/L—Y. Nakahara *et al.*, *J. Chromatogr.* 1994, *657 B Biomed. Appl.*, 93–101. In biological fluids: 6-MAM, codeine, and morphine—R. Wasels and F. Bellville, *J. Chromatogr. A*, 1994, *674*, 225–234. In serum, hair, or urine: comparison with radioimmunoassay—M. R. Moeller and C. Mueller, *Forensic Sci. Int.*, 1995, *70*, 125–133. In urine: 6-MAM and other diamorphine metabolites, limits of detection 4 to 20 µg/L, comparison with enzyme immunoassay—A. S. Low and R. B. Taylor, *J. Chromatogr.* 1995, *663 B Biomed. Appl.*, 225–233. In hair: 6-MAM, other opioids, and cocaine, limits of detection 0.1 to 0.8 µg/g, using a 30-mg hair sample, SIM—P. Kintz and P. Mangin, *Forensic Sci. Int.*, 1995, *73*, 93–100. In hair: 6-MAM and other opioids and cocaine—G. Kauert and J. Rohrich, *Int. J. Legal Med.*, 1996, *108*, 294–299. In plasma or whole blood: 6-MAM , morphine, codeine, and dihydrocodeine, limit of detection <5 µg/L—A. Geier *et al.*, *Int. J. Legal Med.*, 1996, *109*, 80–83. In urine: 6-MAM and other opioids, limit of detection and quantification 2 µg/L—C. L. O'Neal and A. Poklis, *J. Anal. Toxicol.*, 1997, *21*, 427–432. In vitreous humour: 6-MAM, codeine, and morphine, limit of detection for 6-MAM 10 µg/L—D. L. Lin *et al.*, *J. Anal. Toxicol.*, 1997, *21*, 258–261. In nails: 6-MAM and other drugs of abuse, limit of quantification 0.3 µg/g—D. A. Engelhart *et al.*, *J. Anal. Toxicol.*, 1998, *22*, 314–318. In hair: 6-MAM and morphine, limit of detection 0.5 µg/g—Z. Hong *et al.*, *Yao Xue Xue Bao*, 1998, *33*, 616–620. In hair: limit of quantification is 0.5 µg/g—K. M. Hold *et al.*, *J. Chromatogr. Sci.*, 1998, *36*, 125–130. In CSF, urine, and vitreous humour: 6-MAM and morphine, limit of quantification in urine 1 µg/L—F. Pragst *et al.*, *J. Anal. Toxicol.*, 1999, *23*, 168–172. In urine: 6-MAM and other opioids, limit of quantification 25 µg/L and limit of detection 10 µg/L—R. Meatherall, *J. Anal. Toxicol.*, 1999, *23*, 177–186. In urine: 6-MAM, codeine, and morphine, limit of detection for 6-MAM 0.5 µg/L—B. D. Paul *et al.*, *Clin. Chem.*, 1999, *45*, 510–519. In hair: 6-MAM, other opioids, and cocaine—S. Pichini *et al.*, *J. Anal. Toxicol.*, 1999, 23, 343–348. In urine: 6-MAM and other drugs of abuse, limits of detection 3 to 12 µg/L—V. Karacic and L. Skender, *Arh. Hig. Rada. Toksikol.*, 2000, *51*, 389–400. In hair or oral fluid: 6-MAM and other opioids—J. Jones *et al.*, *J. Anal. Toxicol.*, 2002, *26*, 171–175. In urine: 6-MAM and other opioids—C. Meadway *et al.*, *Forensic Sci. Int.*, 2002, *127*, 136–141.

High performance liquid chromatography. In plasma: 6-MAM and morphine, limit of quantification for 6-MAM 25 µg/L, fluorescence detection—D. A. Barrett *et al.*, *J. Chromatogr.*, 1991, *566*, 135–145. In urine: limit of detection 2 µg/L, electrochemical detection—W. Hanisch and L. V. Meyer, *J. Anal. Toxicol.*, 1993, *17*, 48–50. In urine: 6-MAM, morphine, and codeine, limit of detection for 6-MAM 40 µg/L, UV and ECD—J. Gerostamoulos *et al.*, *J. Chromatogr.*, 1993, *617*, 152–156. In plasma: 6-MAM and morphine, limit of detection for 6-MAM 4 µg/L, electrochemical detection—P. P. Rop *et al.*, *J. Chromatogr. Biomed. Sci. Appl.*, 1994, *661*, 245–253. In urine: 6-MAM and diamorphine and its other metabolites, limits of detection 4 to 20 µg/L—A. S. Low and R. B. Taylor, *J. Chromatogr. B Biomed. Appl.*, 1995, *663*, 225–233.

High performance liquid chromatography–mass spectrometry. In blood, CSF, serum, urine and vitreous humor: 2 µg/L—M. J. Bogusz *et al.*, *J. Chromatogr. B Biomed. Sci. Appl.*, 1997, *703*, 115–127. In serum: 4 µg/L—P. Zuccaro *et al.*, *J. Anal. Toxicol.*, 1997, *21*, 268–277. In blood: limit of quantification is 0.5 µg/L—A. Dienes-Nagy *et al.*, *J. Chromatogr. A*, 1999, *854*, 109–118.

Note. For a study of monitoring opiate use in substance abuse treatment patients with sweat and urine drug testing, see M. A Huestis *et al.*, *J. Anal. Toxicol.*, 2000, 24, 509–521.

Disposition in the Body. 6-Monoacetylmorphine is the first hydrolysis product of diamorphine. It is further metabolised to morphine.

Monocrotaline

Alkaloid

Synonyms. Crotaline; NSC-28693; NCI-C56462.

(13α,14α)-14,19-Dihydro-12,13-dihydroxy-20-norcrotolanan-11,15-dione

$C_{16}H_{23}NO_6$=325.4

CAS—315-22-0

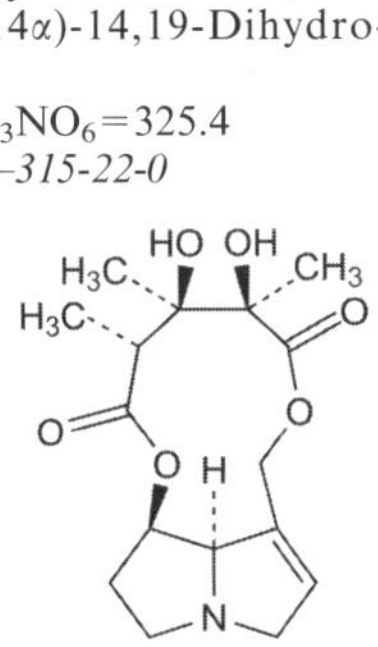

An alkaloid obtained from *Crotalaria spectabilis* and other species of *Crotalaria* (Leguminosae).

A white crystalline powder. M.p. 197° to 198°, with decomposition.

Soluble 1 in 80 of water; soluble in chloroform and dilute acetic acid.

Partition Coefficient. Log *P* (octanol/water), −1.2.

Colour Test. Mandelin's test—green.

Thin-layer Chromatography. System TA—Rf 36. (Acidified iodoplatinate solution, positive.)

Infra-red Spectrum. Principal peaks at wavenumbers 1736, 1064, 1110, 1183, 1242, 1174 cm^{-1} (KBr disk).

Monocrotophos

Acaricide, Insecticide

Synonyms. C-1414; ENT-27129; SD-9129.
Proprietary names. Azodrin; Bilobran; Crisodrin; Monocil; Monocron; Nuvacron; Pillardin; Plantdrin; Susvin.
(*E*)-Phosphoric acid dimethyl [1-methyl-3-(methylamino)-3-oxo-1-propenyl]ester
$C_7H_{14}NO_5P$=223.2
CAS—6923-22-4

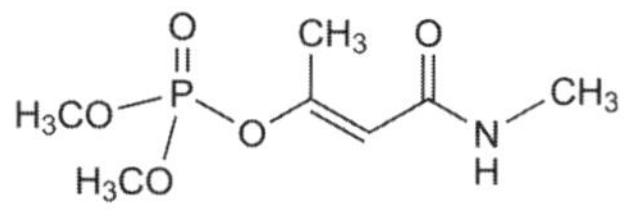

A reddish-brown crystalline solid (commercial product) with M.p. 25° to 30° or M.p. 54° to 55° (pure state). It is miscible with water (1 kg/kg at 20°) and soluble in acetone (700 g/kg at 20°), ethanol, diesel oils, kerosene, dichloromethane (800 g/kg at 20°), methanol (1000 g/kg at 20°), octan-1-ol (250 g/kg at 20°) and toluene (60 g/kg at 20°).

Partition Coefficient. Log *P* (octanol/water), −0.22.

Thin-layer Chromatography. System TX—Rf 01; system TY—Rf 01.

Gas Chromatography. System GA—monocrotophos RI 1665; monocrotophos-TFA RI 1540; system GK—monocrotophos RRT 0.9 (relative to caffeine).

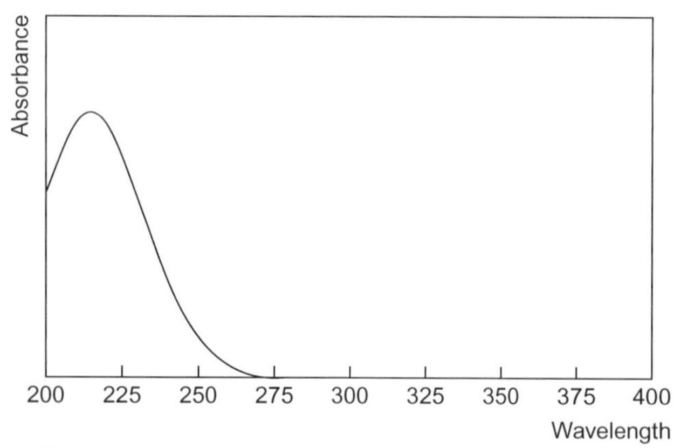

Mass Spectrometry. Principal ions at *m/z* 127, 67, 58, 97, 109, 192, 79, 223.

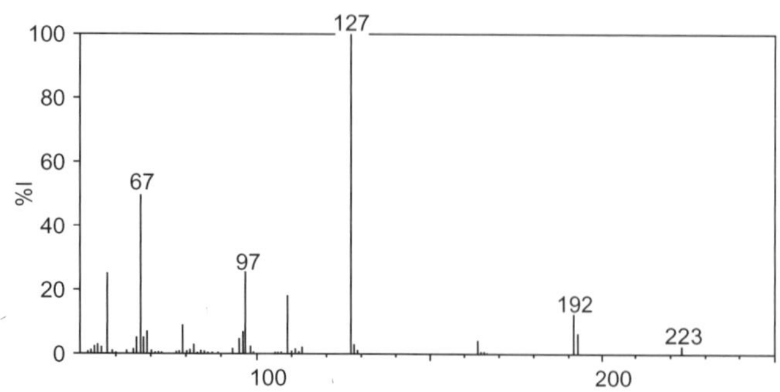

Quantification
Gas chromatography. In serum: limit of detection 0.03 mg/L, NPD—P. Papa *et al.*, *TIAFT Bulletin Case Notes*, 1998, *28(2)*.

Gas chromatography–mass spectrometry. In serum: limit of detection for dimethylphosphate 0.06 mg/L—F. A. Tarbah *et al.*, *TIAFT Poster Session*, 1998, *4*. In serum: limit of detection 0.03 mg/L, NPD—P. Papa *et al.*, *TIAFT Bulletin Case Notes*, 1998, *28(2)*.

Disposition in the Body. Monocrotophos is quickly metabolised by *N*-demethylation, *O*-demethylation and cleavage of the vinyl phosphate bond and excreted primarily in urine (70 to 90%). <10% can be found in faeces. One metabolite identified is dimethylphosphate (DMP). Some of the dose may also be excreted unchanged owing to its solubility in water, and is evenly distributed between tissues and organs. It does not appear to accumulate in the body and 60 to 65% of a dose is eliminated within the first 24 h. It is also readily absorbed through the skin.

Toxicity. The allowed daily intake is 0.6 μg/kg.

An adult female was found dead after ingesting a plant protective containing monocrotophos, dodine and dinocap. Monocrotophos could be detected in all tissues and in blood (at a concentration of 12 μg/g). Monocrotophos was found at concentrations of 13 μg/g in the lungs and brain, 11 μg/g in the kidneys, 1.8 μg/g in the liver and a total of 52 mg in the stomach. Small amounts of dodine and dinocap were only detected in the stomach. [H. P. Gelbke and H. J. Schlicht, *Toxicol. Eur. Res.*, 1978, *1(3)*, 181–184.]

A 55-year-old male floriculturist was found unconscious in his greenhouse and died 7 days later despite hospital treatment. The first blood sample received was 44 h after intoxication and toxicological analysis showed a serum monocrotophos concentration of 24.0 mg/L. The serum levels decreased with time and were less than 0.03 mg/L at the time of death but cholinesterase levels never recovered. It is believed that 1200 mg of the pesticide was ingested. [P. Papa *et al.*, *TIAFT Bulletin Case Notes*, 1998, *28(2)*].

Monoethanolamine

Sclerosing Agent

Synonyms. Aethanolaminum; Ethanolamine; Hydroxyethylamine; Olamine.
Proprietary names. Ethamolin (Oleate); Oldamin (Oleate).
2-Aminoethanol
C_2H_7NO=61.1
CAS—141-43-5

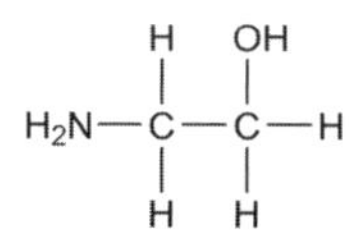

A clear, colourless or pale yellow, viscous liquid. Mass per mL 1.014 to 1.023 g. B.p. about 170°.
Miscible with water, acetone, ethanol, and chloroform; slightly soluble in ether.

Monoethanolamine Oleate

Synonyms. Aethanolaminum; Monoethanolamine Oleate; 2-Hydroxyethylamine Compound with Oleic Acid; 2-Aminoethanol Compound with Oleic Acid.
Proprietary names. Antivariz; Esclerosina; Ethamolin; Oldamin.
$C_2H_7NO,C_{18}H_{34}O_2$=343.5
CAS—2272-11-9
Miscible with water, alcohol, acetone, chloroform, and glycerol. Immiscible with petroleum spirit and fixed oils but will dissolve many essential oils.

Dissociation Constant. pK_a 9.4 (25°).

Partition Coefficient. Log *P* (octanol/water), −1.3.

Gas Chromatography. System GA—monoethanolamine RI 780.

Mass Spectrum. Principal ions at *m/z* 42, 31, 61, 43, 29, 27, 44, 41.

Disposition in the Body.
Toxicity. Overexposure to monoethanolamine oleate can lead to respiratory problems, skin and eye irritation, and lethargy.

Monoethanolamine oleate has been associated with acute renal failure (which did clear spontaneously within 3 weeks of treatment) in 2 obese women treated with injections of ethanolamine oleate. Injections of 15 to 20 mL containing 5% oleate and 2% benzyl alcohol were administered. [T. J. B. Maling and M. J. Cretney, *N. Z. Med. J.*, 1975, *82*, 269–270.]

Dose. Varicose veins, 2 to 5 mL 5% oleate solution; oesophageal varices, 1.5 to 5 mL 5% oleate solution per varix, maximum total of 20 mL per treatment.

Monolinuron

Herbicide

Synonym HOE 2747
Proprietary names. Aresin; Aresine; Arresin; Monorotox; Premalin.
Chlorophenyl-*N*′-methoxy-*N*′-methylurea
$C_9H_{11}ClN_2O_2$=214.6
CAS—1746-81-2

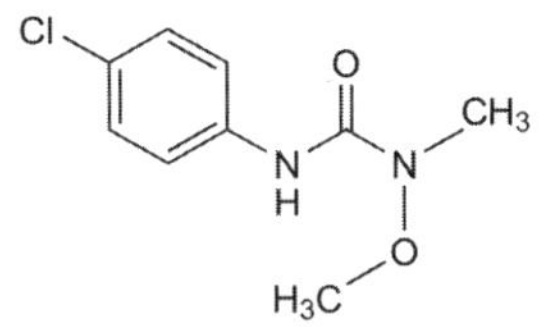

Solid with M.p. 80° to 83°. It is soluble in water (930 mg/L at 20°) and many organic solvents including alcohol, acetone, dioxane, xylene, chloroform and diethyl ether.

Partition Coefficient. Log *P* (octanol/water) 2.20.

Thin-layer Chromatography. System TX—Rf 23; system TY—Rf 30.

High Performance Liquid Chromatography. System HY—RI 411.

Gas Chromatography. System GA—monolinuron RI 1910; monolinuron-Me RI 1675; M art (HOOC-)-Me RI 1690; system GK—monolinuron RRT 0.78 (relative to caffeine).

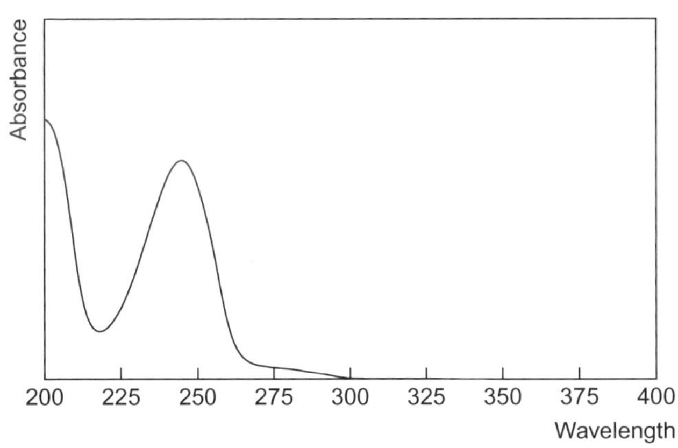

Mass Spectrometry. Principal ions at *m*/*z* 61, 46, 126, 214, 99, 60, 63, 153.

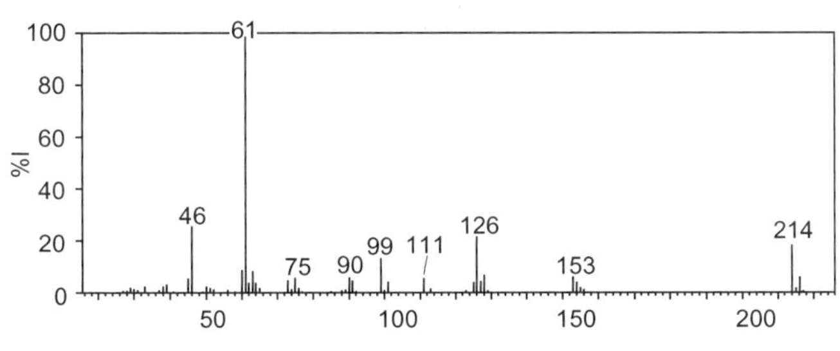

Disposition in the Body. Monolinuron is metabolised to methylated monolinuron.

Toxicity.
The allowed daily intake is 0.014 mg/kg. No toxic effect has been observed with levels of 250 mg/kg.

A 59-year-old male farmer attempted to commit suicide by ingesting Gramonol, containing paraquat and monolinuron. The plasma paraquat level was 1.1 mg/L (a fatal level) 8 h after ingestion but the man did not die until 10 days later due to renal, respiratory and liver failure. Methaemoglobinaemia also occurred 8 h after ingestion and this was a result of ingesting 40 mg/kg of monolinuron. [P. B. Casey *et al.*, *J. Toxicol. Clin. Toxicol.*, 1994, *32(2)*, 185–189.]

Montelukast

Antiasthmatic

Synonym. MK-0476
1-[[[(1*R*)-1-[3-[(1*E*)-2-(7-Chloro-2-quinolinyl)ethenyl]phenyl]-3-[2-(1-hydroxy-1-methylethyl)phenyl]propyl]thio]methyl]cyclopropaneacetic acid
$C_{35}H_{36}ClNO_3S$=586.2
CAS—158966-92-8

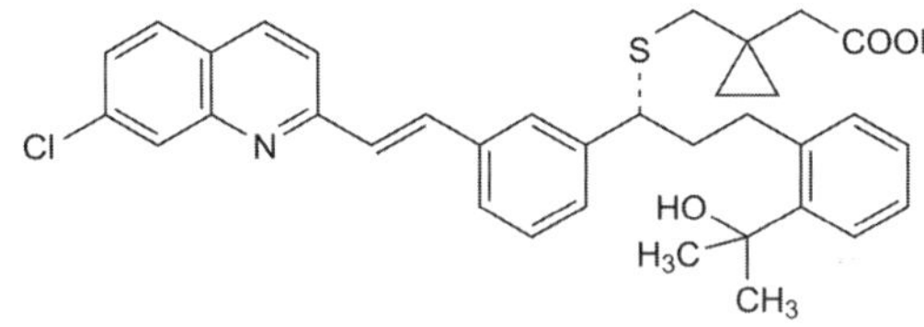

A white to off-white powder.

Montelukast Sodium
Synonym. MK-476
Proprietary name. Singulair
$C_{35}H_{35}ClNNaO_3S$=608.2
CAS—151767-02-1
A white to off-white powder. It is freely soluble in ethanol, methanol and water; practically insoluble in acetonitrile.

High Performance Liquid Chromatography. Column: (analytical) C_8 (Novapak, 100 × 8.0 mm i.d., 4 μm); (guard) Guard-Pak with C_8 NovaPak insert. Column temperature: 40°. Mobile phase: sodium acetate (25 mM, pH 4):acetonitrile (20:80), with 50 μL triethylamine, flow rate 1 mL/min. Internal standard (IS): quinine bisulfate. Fluorescence detection (λ_{ex}=350 nm, λ_{em}=400 nm). Retention time(s): montelukast sodium, 6.1 min; IS, 4.2 min. [S. Al-Rawithi *et al.*, *J. Chromatogr. B, Biomed. Sci. Appl.*, 2001, *754*, 527–531].

Column: Apex octadecyl (50 × 4.6 mm i.d., 3 μm). Mobile phase: acetonitrile:ammonium phosphate buffer (0.05 M, pH 3.5) (62:38). Fluorescence detection (λ_{ex}=350 nm, λ_{em}=400 nm). Retention time(s): 4.0 min. [R. Amin *et al.*, *J. Pharm. Biomed. Anal.*, 1995, *13*, 155–158].

Quantification
High performance liquid chromatography. In plasma: limit of detection 5 μg/L, limit of quantification 30 μg/L. Fluorescence detection (λ_{ex}=350 nm, λ_{em}=400 nm)—R. Amin *et al.*, *J. Pharm. Biomed. Anal.*, 1995, *13*, 155–158. In blood: limit of detection 9.6 μg/L. Fluorescence detection (λ_{ex}=350 nm, λ_{em}=400 nm)—L. Liu *et al.*, *J. Pharm. Biomed. Anal.*, 1997, *15*, 631–638.

Disposition in the Body. Montelukast is rapidly absorbed following oral administration. It is extensively metabolised by cytochromes P450 3A4, 2A6, 2C9. Montelukast and its metabolites are excreted almost exclusively via bile with less than 0.2% of the drug excreted in urine. Renal impairment and gender do not affect the pharmacokinetics of montelukast.

Therapeutic concentration. After a 10 mg tablet of montelukast, the mean peak plasma concentration is achieved within 3 h. After a 5 mg chewable tablet, mean peak plasma concentration is achieved within 2 h. At therapeutic doses, the plasma concentration of metabolites is undetectable at steady state in adults and children.

Bioavailability. With a 10 mg tablet, 64%; 5 mg chewable tablet, 73%, which is reduced to 63% by food.

Half-life. 2.7 to 5.5 h. In patients with mild–moderate hepatic insufficiency and clinical evidence of cirrhosis, the mean elimination half-life is prolonged to roughly 7.4 h.

Volume of distribution. 8 to 11 L at steady state.

Clearance. 45 mL/min in healthy adults. Montelukast clearance is only slightly decreased in the elderly compared to younger adults.

Protein binding. 99%.

Note. For a review of montelukast sodium and its therapeutic potential in persistent asthma, see B. Jarvis and A. Markham, *Drugs*, 2000, *59*, 891-928.

Dose. Adults, 10 mg; children, 5 mg.

Moracizine

Anti-arrhythmic

Synonyms. Moricizine; EN-313.
[10-[3-(4-Morpholinyl)-1-oxopropyl]-10*H*-phenothiazin-2-yl]carbamic acid ethyl ester
$C_{22}H_{25}N_3O_4S = 427.5$
CAS—31883-05-3

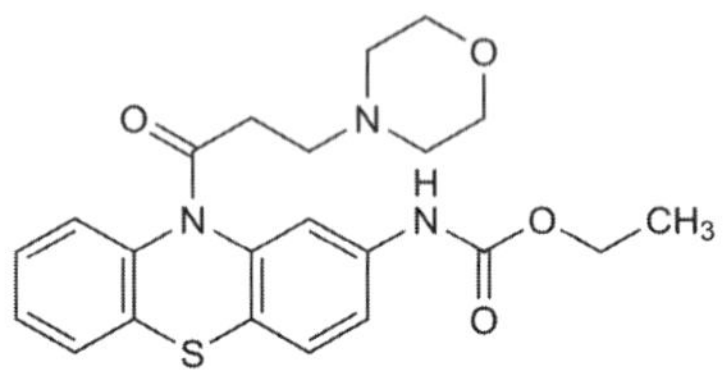

Crystals, m.p. 156° to 157°.

Moracizine Hydrochloride

Proprietary names. Ethmozin; Ethmozine.
$C_{22}H_{25}N_3O_4S,HCl = 464.0$
CAS—29560-58-5
A white to tan crystalline powder or crystals from dichloroethane with m.p. 189° (dec). It is freely soluble in water and in alcohol.

Dissociation Constant. pK_a 6.4.

Partition Coefficient. Log *P* (octanol/water), 2.98.

Gas Chromatography. Column: methyl silicone (HP1, 0.2 mm i.d., 0.33 μm film thickness). Column temperature: 280°. Carrier gas: helium, 0.9 mL/min flow rate. MS detection. Retention index: 3526. [T. Mills and J. C. Roberson, *Instrumental Data for Drug Analysis*, 1993, CRC Press, Boca Raton, US. 2nd Edn, Vol. 6, pp. 158–159].

High Performance Liquid Chromatography. Column: ODS Hypersil (100 × 4.6 mm i.d., 5 μm). Mobile phase: methanol, flow rate 0.5 mL/min. UV diode array detection. Retention time(s): 5.6 min. [T. Mills and J. C. Roberson, *Instrumental Data for Drug Analysis*, 1993, CRC Press, Boca Raton, US. 2nd Edn, Vol. 6, pp. 158–159].

Column: (analytical) C_{18} (μBondapak, 100 × 8.0 mm i.d., 10 μm); (guard) C_{18} (25 × 4.6 mm i.d., 30 μm). Mobile phase: methanol:water:triethylamine (65:35:0.5), flow rate 2.0 mL/min. Internal standard (IS): clozapine. UV detection (λ = 254 nm). Retention time(s): moracizine, 6.2 min; moracizine sulfoxide, 3.5 min; moracizine sulfone, 2.7 min; IS, 9.7 min. [J. M. Yang and K. Chan, *J. Chromatogr.*, 1995, *663*; *Biomed Appl.*, 172–176].

Ultraviolet Spectrum. Aqueous acid—267 nm; basic—259 nm.

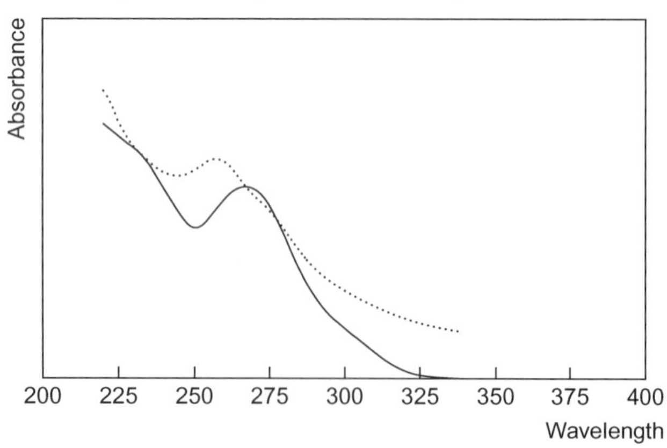

Infra-red Spectrum. Principal peaks at wavenumbers 1231, 1725, 1664, 1466 cm^{-1} (KBr disk).

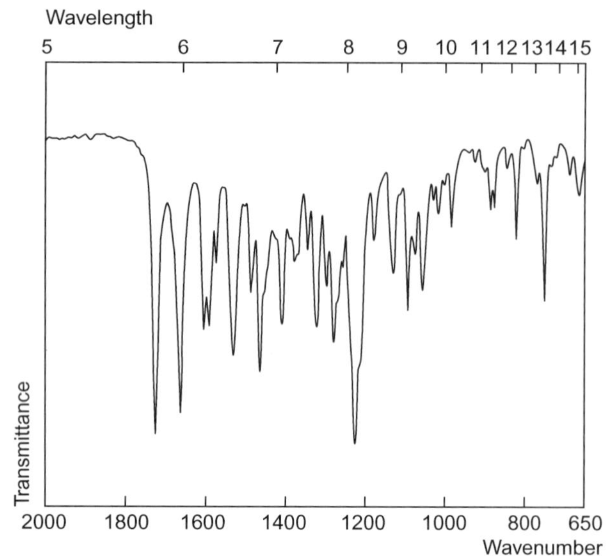

Mass Spectrum. Principal ions at *m/z* 100, 286, 142, 56, 42, 239, 70, 185.

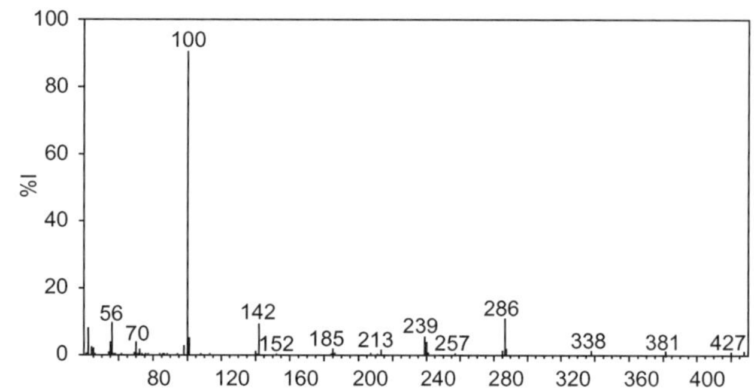

Quantification

High performance liquid chromatography. In plasma: limit of detection 10 μg/L. UV detection (λ = 268 nm)—C. C. Whitney *et al.*, *J. Pharm. Sci.*, 1981, *70*, 462–463. In plasma: limit of detection is 5 μg/L and limit of quantification 10 μg/L. UV detection (λ = 268 nm)—J. M. Poirier, *Ther. Drug Monit.*, 1985, *7(4)*, 439–441.

Disposition in the Body. Moracizine is readily and virtually completely absorbed after oral administration, with peak plasma concentrations being reached 0.5 to 2.0 h after administration. It undergoes hepatic metabolism to form many metabolites (approx. 26, 9 of which have been identified) at a concentration of less than 1% of the dose. Two metabolites, moracizine sulfoxide and phenothiazine-2-carbamic acid ethyl ester sulfoxide have anti-arrhythmic activity but represent <0.6% of the dose with a half-life of approx. 3 h. Moracizine is excreted mainly in faeces (56%) and urine (39%) with less than 1% as the unchanged drug. The drug appears in urine mainly as unconjugated metabolites and glucuronide-conjugated metabolites.

Therapeutic concentration. Therapeutic plasma concentration is 0.25 to 3.0 mg/L.

12 healthy males, aged between 19 and 36 years, non-smokers, were administered either 250 mg every 8 h for 14 days or 250 mg every 8 h for 7 days followed by placebo for 7 days. The mean peak concentrations were 0.64 mg/L after a single dose, 0.64 mg/L after 6 days and 0.55 mg/L after 13 days. These concentrations were observed after approx. 1 h (range 0.75 to 1.5 h) for both treatments. [I. H. Benedek *et al.*, *J. Clin. Pharmacol.*, 1994, *34*, 167–175].

Toxicity. In total 2 deaths have been attributed to moracizine overdose; 2.25 and 10 g. [DuPont Pharmaceuticals, data on file].

Bioavailability. 38%.

Half-life. 2 to 4 h (healthy individuals); 6 to 13 h (patients with arrhythmias).

Volume of distribution. 8.3 to 11.1 L/kg (oral administration); 185 to 210 L (intravenous (IV) administration).

Clearance. Plasma, 2.2 to 2.65 L/min (healthy, oral); 1.3 L/min (patients, IV).

Distribution in blood. 57% of a dose is associated with erythrocytes.

Protein binding. 81 to 95%.

Dose. The usual dose is 600 to 900 mg daily (in the hydrochloride form). Reduction may be required in patients with renal and hepatic impairment.

Morantel

Anthelmintic (Veterinary)

(*E*)-1,4,5,6-Tetrahydro-1-methyl-2-[2-(3-methyl-2-thienyl)ethenyl]-pyrimidine
$C_{12}H_{16}N_2S=220.3$
CAS—20574-50-9

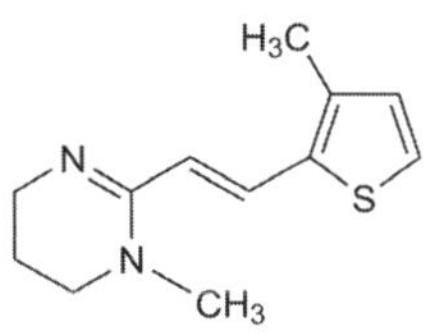

Crystals. M.p. 239° to 241°.

Morantel Citrate

Proprietary names. Exhelm; Wormtec.
$C_{12}H_{16}N_2S,C_6H_8O_7,H_2O=430.5$
CAS—69525-81-1

Morantel Tartrate

Synonym. CP-12009-18
Proprietary names. Equiban; Paratect; Rumatel.
$C_{12}H_{16}N_2S,C_4H_6O_6=370.4$
CAS—26155-31-7
Pale yellow to greenish-yellow crystals. M.p. 167° to 170°.
Readily soluble in water.

Partition Coefficient. Log *P* (octanol/water), 3.7.

Colour Tests. Liebermann's test—black; Mandelin's test—violet; Marquis test—blue-violet; Sulfuric acid—violet-red.

Thin-layer Chromatography. System TA—Rf 60. (Acidified iodoplatinate solution, positive.)

Gas Chromatography. System GA—not eluted.

Ultraviolet Spectrum. Methanol—322 nm ($A_1^1=864b$).

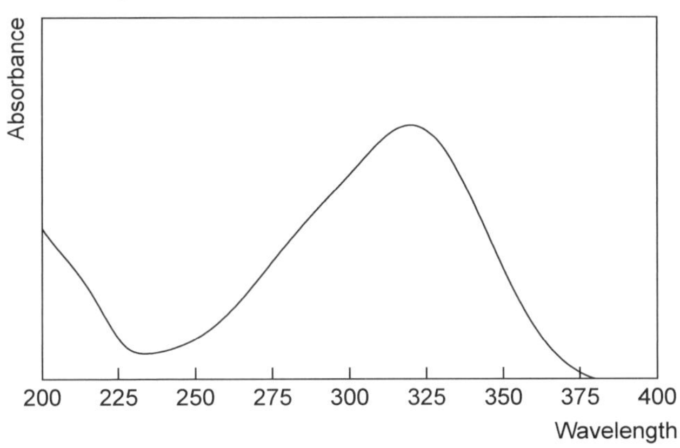

Infra-red Spectrum. Principal peaks at wavenumbers 1626, 1577, 1319, 1305, 1148, 955 cm^{-1} (KBr disk).

Morazone

Analgesic

Synonym. R-445
1,2-Dihydro-1,5-dimethyl-4–[(3-methyl-2–phenyl-4-morpholinyl)-methyl]-2-phenyl-3*H*-pyrazol-3-one
$C_{23}H_{27}N_3O_2=377.5$
CAS—6536-18-1

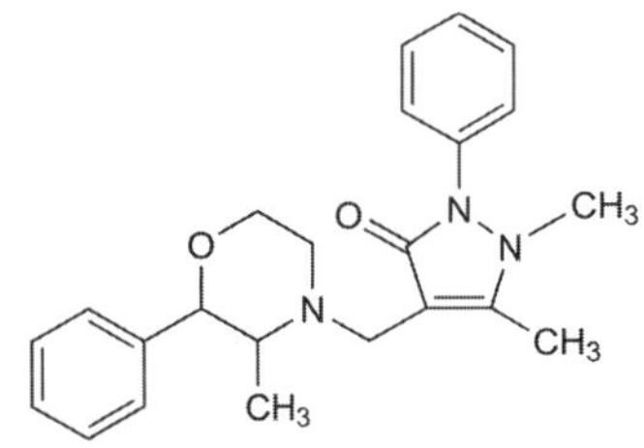

A white crystalline powder. M.p. 149° to 150°.
Freely soluble in chloroform; soluble in methanol and acetone; slightly soluble in ether.

Morazone Hydrochloride

Proprietary names. Rosimon-Neu; Tarugan.
$C_{23}H_{27}N_3O_2,HCl=413.9$
CAS—50321-35-2
Crystals. M.p. 171° to 172°, with decomposition.
Soluble in water.

Partition Coefficient. Log *P* (octanol/water), 2.0.

Colour Test. Liebermann's test—red-orange.

Thin-layer Chromatography. System TA—Rf 58; system TB—Rf 08; system TC—Rf 46; system TE—Rf 58; system TL—Rf 31; system TAE—Rf 61. (Acidified iodoplatinate solution, positive.)

Gas Chromatography. System GA—Morazone RI 3130; M(phenmetrazine) RI 1432; M(OH-phenmetrazine isomer 1) RI 1830; M(OH-phenmetrazine isomer 2) RI 1865; M(OH-MeO-phenmetrazine) RI 1900; system GB—M(phenmetrazine) RI 1483. Morazone is also metabolised to phenazone.

High Performance Liquid Chromatography. System HA—*k* 0.7; system HD—*k* 0.4; system HW—*k* 2.05; system HY—RI 294.

Ultraviolet Spectrum. Aqueous acid—258 nm ($A_1^1=212a$); aqueous alkali—244, 263 nm ($A_1^1=201b$).

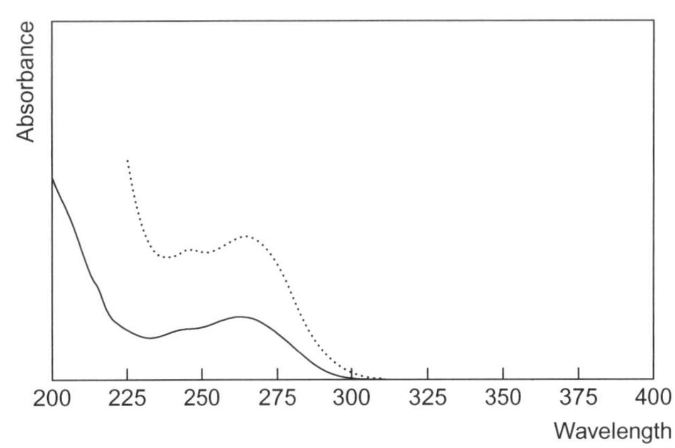

Infra-red Spectrum. Principal peaks at wavenumbers 754, 1656, 700, 1492, 1590, 1117 cm^{-1} (thin film).

Mass Spectrum. Principal ions at *m/z* 201, 176, 202, 56, 258, 70, 71, 42.

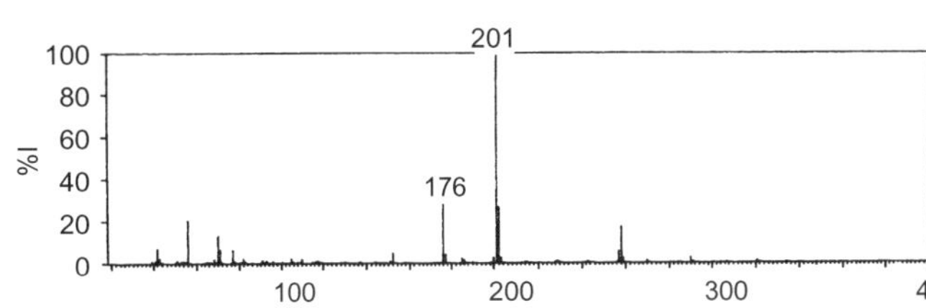

Dose. Morazone hydrochloride has been given in doses of 75 to 150 mg.

Morinamide

Tuberculostatic

Synonyms. Morphazinamide; B-2310.
N-(4-Morpholinylmethyl)pyrazinecarboxamide
$C_{10}H_{14}N_4O_2=222.2$
CAS—952-54-5

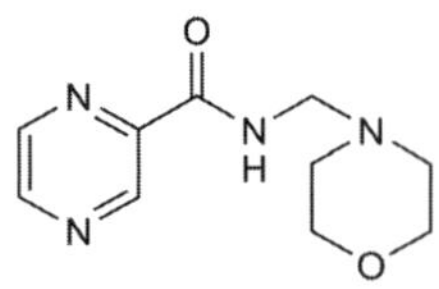

Crystals. M.p. 118.5° to 119.5°.
Soluble 1 in 3 of water, 1 in 30 of ethanol, 1 in 30 of benzene, and 1 in 2.5 of chloroform.

Morinamide Hydrochloride

Synonym. B-2311.
Proprietary name. Piazofolina
$C_{10}H_{14}N_4O_2,HCl=258.7$
CAS—1473-73-0
A white crystalline powder. M.p. 196°.
Soluble 1 in 2 of water, 1 in 350 of ethanol and 1 in 2000 of chloroform.

Partition Coefficient. Log *P* (octanol/water), −1.2.

Thin-layer Chromatography. System TA—Rf 54; system TB—Rf 08; system TC—Rf 49; system TL—Rf 32. (Acidified iodoplatinate solution, weak reaction; acidified potassium permanganate solution, positive.)

Gas Chromatography. System GA—RI 1906.

Ultraviolet Spectrum. Aqueous acid—269 ($A^1_1=340b$), 314 nm.

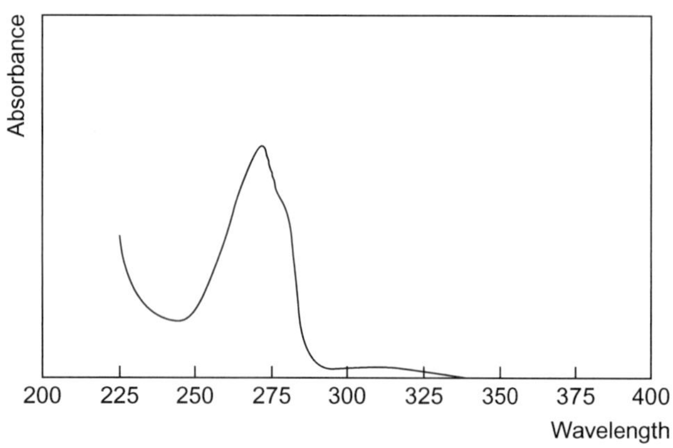

Infra-red Spectrum. Principal peaks at wavenumbers 1667, 1101, 1499, 1125, 1002, 1019 cm^{-1} (KBr disk).

Mass Spectrum. Principal ions at *m/z* 115, 86, 79, 57, 56, 107, 100, 52.

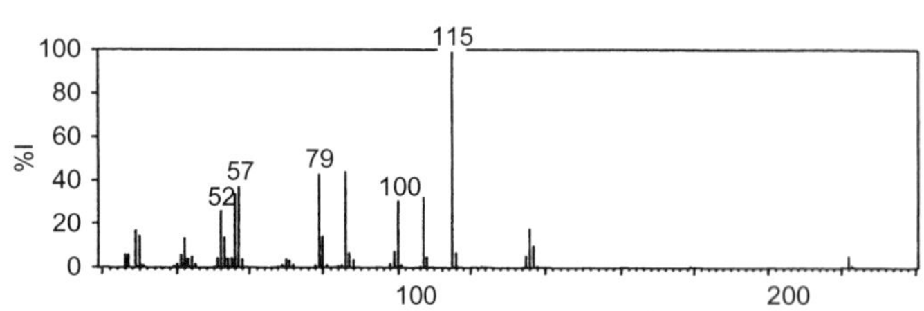

Dose. Morinamide has been given in doses of 3 g daily.

Morphine

Narcotic Analgesic

Synonym. Morphia
(5α,6α)-7,8-Didehydro-4,5-epoxy-17-methylmorphinan-3,6-diol monohydrate
$C_{17}H_{19}NO_3,H_2O=303.4$
CAS—57-27-2 (anhydrous); 6009-81-0 (monohydrate)

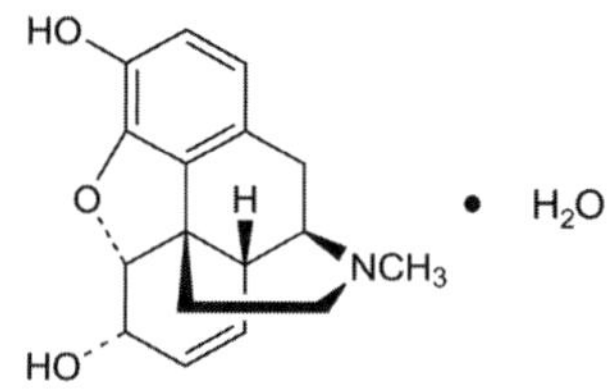

The principal alkaloid of opium. A white crystalline powder or colourless or white acicular crystals. M.p. 254° to 256°, with decomposition.
Soluble 1 in 5000 of water, 1 in 210 of ethanol, 1 in 1220 of chloroform, and 1 in 125 of glycerol; practically insoluble in ether. Note that the solubility can vary according to the method of preparation and the crystalline state.

Morphine Acetate

$C_{17}H_{19}NO_3,C_2H_4O_2,3H_2O=399.4$
CAS—596-15-6 (anhydrous); 5974-11-8 (trihydrate)
A white amorphous or crystalline powder.
Soluble 1 in 2.25 of water, 1 in 22 of ethanol, 1 in 4.75 of chloroform, and 1 in 4.5 of glycerol; practically insoluble in ether.

Morphine Hydrochloride

$C_{17}H_{19}NO_3,HCl,3H_2O=375.8$
CAS—52-26-6 (anhydrous); 6055-06-7 (trihydrate)
Colourless silky crystals or crystalline powder, or cubical white masses. A solution in water is laevorotatory.
Soluble 1 in 17.5 of water and 1 in 100 of ethanol; slowly soluble in glycerol; practically insoluble in chloroform and ether.

Morphine Sulfate

Proprietary names. Astramorph; Duramorph; Infumorph; Kadian; Moraxen; Morcap; MS Contin(us); MSIR; MST-Continus; MXL; Oramorph; RMS; Roxanol; Sevredol; Zomorph.
$(C_{17}H_{19}NO_3)_2,H_2SO_4,5H_2O=758.8$
CAS—64-31-3 (anhydrous); 6211-15-0 (pentahydrate)
White, acicular crystals, cubical masses, or crystalline powder. When exposed to air it gradually loses water of crystallisation. It darkens on prolonged exposure to light. M.p. 250°, with decomposition (anhydrous form). A solution in water is laevorotatory.
Soluble 1 in 15.5 of water and 1 in 1000 of ethanol; practically insoluble in chloroform and ether.

Morphine Tartrate

Proprietary name. It is an ingredient of Cyclimorph.
$(C_{17}H_{19}NO_3)_2,C_4H_6O_6,3H_2O=774.8$
CAS—302-31-8 (anhydrous); 6032-59-3 (trihydrate)
Minute, colourless, acicular, efflorescent crystals.
Soluble 1 in 11 of water and 1 in 1000 of ethanol; practically insoluble in chloroform, ether, and carbon disulfide.

Dissociation Constant. pK_a 8.0, 9.9 (20°).

Partition Coefficient. Log *P* (octanol/pH 7.4), –0.1.

Colour Tests. Ferric Chloride—blue; Liebermann's Test—black; Mandelin's Test—blue-grey; Marquis Test—violet.

Thin-layer Chromatography. System TA—Rf 37; system TB—Rf 00; system TC—Rf 09; system TE—Rf 20; system TL—Rf 01; system TAE—Rf 18; system TAF—Rf 23; system TAJ—Rf 00; system TAK—Rf 00; system TAL—Rf 15. (Dragendorff spray, positive; acidified iodoplatinate solution, positive; Marquis reagent, violet.)

Gas Chromatography. System GA—morphine RI 2445, morphine-AC_2 (diamorphine) RI 2615, morphine-PFP_2 RI 2360, morphine-TMS_2 RI 2560, morphine-TFA_2 RI 2250, M (nor-) RI 2459, M (nor-)-AC_3 RI 2955, M (nor-)-PFP_2 RI 2440, M (nor-) PFP_3 RI 2405, M (nor-)-TMS_3 RI 2605, codeine RI 2375, norcodeine RI 2388; system GB—morphine RI 2564, morphine-AC_2 (diamorphine) RI 2769, morphine-TMS_2 RI 2602, codeine RI 2511, norcodeine RI 2535; system GC—morphine RI 2542, codeine RI 2681; system GM—morphine, not eluted.

Column: 5% phenyl methyl siloxane capillary (30 m × 0.25 mm i.d., 0.25 μm film thickness). Column temperature: 150°, 1 min; increased to 250° at 40°/min, held for 21.5 min. Carrier gas: helium, 1.5 mL/min flow rate. MS detection. Retention time: 5.84 min. [B. Fryirs *et al.*, *J. Chromatogr. B Biomed. Sci. Appl.*, 1997, *693(1)*, 51–57.]

Column: HP-5 capillary 95% dimethylsiloxane, 5% diphenylsiloxane (25 m × 0.25 mm i.d., 0.25 μm film thickness). Column temperature: 120°; held 2 min; increased to 280° at 20°/min; held 10 min. Carrier gas helium:

1 mL/min flow rate. MS detection. Retention time: 12.88 min. [F. Pragst *et al.*, *J. Anal. Toxicol.*, 1999, *23*, 168–171.]

High Performance Liquid Chromatography. System HA—morphine *k* 3.8 (tailing peak), codeine *k* 4.8 (tailing peak), morphine *N*-oxide *k* 3.2 (tailing peak), norcodeine *k* 3.1 (tailing peak), normorphine *k* 2.9 (tailing peak); system HC—morphine *k* 1.30, codeine *k* 1.21, morphine-3-glucuronide *k* 1.56, norcodeine *k* 3.51, normorphine *k* 3.92; system HS—*k* 5.16; system HX—morphine RI 200, codeine RI 266; system HY—morphine RI 182, normorphine RI 237; system HZ—morphine retention time 1.8 min; system HAA—morphine retention time 3.3 min; system HAX—morphine retention time 5.6 min; system HAY—morphine retention time 3.2 min.

Column: C_{18} (Nucleosil, 250 × 8.4 mm i.d., 5 µm). Mobile phase: 1% acetonitrile in TEAP buffer, 0 to 8 min; 3% acetonitrile in TEAP buffer, 8 to 23 min, 1.0 mL/min flow rate. Fluorescence detection (λ_{ex} = 245 nm, λ_{em} = 345 nm). Retention time: morphine, 6.97 min; morphine-3-glucuronide, 4.91 min; morphine-6-glucuronide, 8.71 min. [R. Aderjan *et al.*, *J. Anal. Toxicol.*, 1995, *19(3)*, 163–168.]

Column: µPorasil (300 × 3.9 mm i.d., 10 µm): pre-column, silica (15 × 3.2 mm i.d., 7 µm). Mobile phase: sodium acetate buffer (5 mM, pH 3.75): acetonitrile (25:75), 1.2 mL/min flow rate. ECD. Retention time: 10.45 min (*k*, 5.04). [W. J. Liaw *et al.*, *J. Chromatogr. B Biomed. Sci. Appl.*, 1998, *714(2)*, 237–245.]

Column: Inertsil ODS-3 (150 × 3 mm i.d., 5 µm). Mobile phase: 1 mM ammonium formate (pH 3): acetonitrile (maintained at 5% for 5 min, increased to 20% in 5 min, held 5 min), 0.4 mL/min flow rate. MS detection. Retention time: morphine, 2.7 min; morphine-3-glucuronide, 2.2 min; morphine-6-glucuronide, 4.3 min. [A. Dienes-Nagy *et al.*, *J. Chromatogr. A*, 1999, *854(1–2)*, 109–118.]

Ultraviolet Spectrum. Aqueous acid—285 (A_1^1 = 52a); aqueous alkali—298 nm (A_1^1 = 92a).

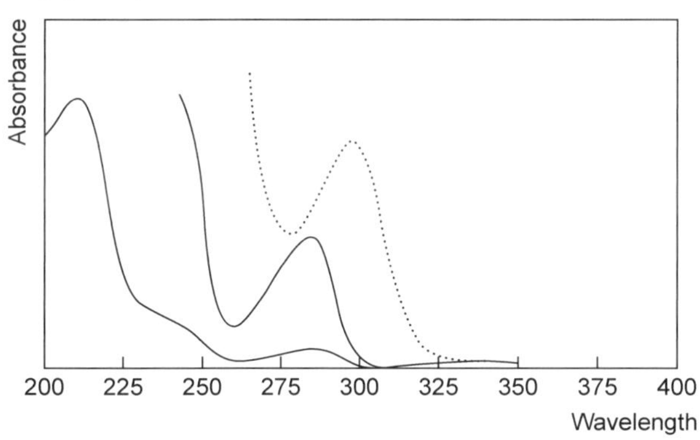

Infra-red Spectrum. Principal peaks at wavenumbers 805, 1243, 1118, 945, 1086, 833 cm^{-1} (Nujol).

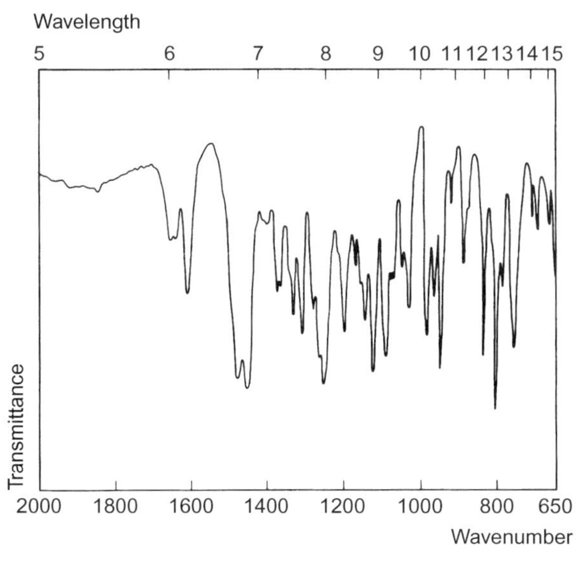

Mass Spectrum. Principal ions at *m/z* 285, 162, 42, 215, 286, 124, 44, 284; codeine 299, 42, 162, 124, 229, 59, 300, 69; norcodeine 285, 81, 215, 148, 286, 164, 110, 115; normorphine 271, 81, 150, 201, 148, 110, 272, 82.

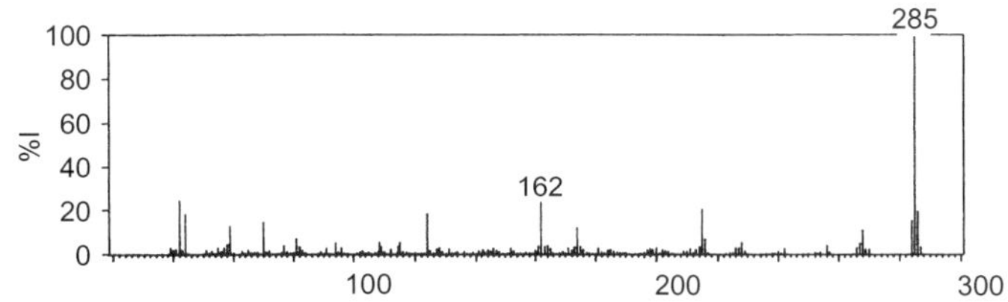

Quantification

Gas chromatography. In postmortem tissues: limit of detection 50 µg/L in blood, 300 ng/g in kidney and liver, 500 µg/L in urine, FID—G. R. Nakamura and E. L. Way, *Anal. Chem.*, 1975, *47*, 775–778. In whole blood: limit of detection 1 µg/L, ECD—S. Felby, *Forensic Sci. Int.*, 1979, *13*, 145–150. In raw opium and opium preparations—D. C. Garratt *et al.*, *Analyst, Lond.*, 1978, *103*, 268–283. In urine: NPD, FID—T. Vu-Duc and A. Vernay, *Biomed. Chromatogr.* 1990, *4(2)*, 65–69. In blood: morphine and other opioids, limit of quantification 10 µg/L, electron-ionisation detection—S. Mykkanen *et al.*, *J. Anal. Toxicol.*, 2000, *24*, 122–126. In postmortem bone and bone marrow: FID—N. Raikos *et al.*, *Forensic Sci. Int.*, 2001, *123*, 140–141.

Gas chromatography–mass spectrometry. In CSF, urine, and vitreous humor: limit of quantification 1 µg/L—F. Pragst *et al.*, *J. Anal. Toxicol.*, 1999, *23(3)*, 168–172. In serum and urine: limit of quantification 5.7 ng/L and 0.71 ng/L, respectively—U. Hofmann *et al.*, *J. Chromatogr. B Biomed. Sci. Appl.*, 1999, *727*, 81–88. In urine: limit of quantification 25 µg/L and limit of detection 10 µg/L—R. Meatherall, *J. Anal. Toxicol.*, 1999, *23(3)*, 177–186. In hair: limit of quantification is 0.5 mg/g—K. M. Hold *et al.*, *J. Chromatogr. Sci.*, 1998, *36(3)*, 125–130. In plasma: limit of quantification 0.75 µg/L and estimated limit of detection is 0.2 µg/L—B. Fryirs *et al.*, *J. Chromatogr. B Biomed. Sci. Appl.*, 1997, *693(1)*, 51–57. In urine: limit of detection is 2.0 µg/L and limit of quantification 10.0 µg/L—C. L. O'Neal and A. Poklis, *J. Anal. Toxicol.*, 1997, *21(6)*, 427–432. In hair: limit of detection 0.1 µg/g, using a 30-mg hair sample, SIM—P. Kintz and P. Mangin, *Forens. Sci. Int.*, 1995, *73(2)*, 93–100. In plasma or whole blood: morphine and other opioids, limit of detection <5 µg/L—A. Geier *et al.*, *Int. J. Legal Med.*, 1996, *109*, 80–83. In hair: morphine and other opioids, limits of detection 0.12 to 0.28 µg/L—Y. Gaillard and G. Pepin, *Forensic Sci. Int.*, 1997, *86*, 49–59. In urine: morphine and other opioids—L. A. Broussard *et al.*, *Clin. Chem.*, 1997, *43*, 1029–1032; M. Cremese *et al.*, *J. Forensic Sci.*, 1998, *43*, 1220–1224. In hair: morphine and other opioids—S. Pichini *et al.*, *J. Anal. Toxicol.*, 1999, *23*, 343–348. In plasma: limit of quantification about 0.8 µg/L—H. J. Leis *et al.*, *J. Chromatogr. B Biomed. Sci. Appl.*, 2000, *744*, 113–119. In urine: morphine and other drugs of abuse—S. P. Vorce *et al.*, *J. Anal. Toxicol.*, 2000, *24*, 595–601. In urine: morphine and other drugs of abuse, limits of detection 3 to 12 µg/L—V. Karacic and L. Skender, *Arh. Hig. Rada. Toksikol.*, 2000, *51*, 389–400. In hair: morphine, codeine, and cocaine—W. E. Brewer *et al.*, *Anal. Chem.*, 2001, *73*, 2371–2376. In serum, saliva, or hair: morphine and other opioids—W. Piekoszewski *et al.*, *Przegl. Lek.*, 2001, *58*, 287–289. In plasma: limit of quantification 0.38 µg/L—H. J. Leis *et al.*, *Rapid Commun. Mass Spectrom.*, 2002, *16*, 646–649. In plasma: morphine glucuronides—H. J. Leis *et al.*, *J. Mass Spectrom.* 2002, *37*, 395–400. In hair or oral fluid: morphine and other opioids—J. Jones *et al.*, *J. Anal. Toxicol.*, 2002, *26*, 171–175. In hair: morphine and other opioids—M. Montagna *et al.*, *Forensic Sci. Int.*, 2002, *128*, 79–83. In urine: morphine and other opioids—C. Meadway *et al.*, *Forensic Sci. Int.*, 2002, *127*, 136–141.

High performance liquid chromatography. In plasma: limit of detection is 0.1 µg/L, ECD—W. J. Liaw *et al.*, *J. Chromatogr. B Biomed. Sci. Appl.*, 1998, *714(2)*, 237–245. In serum: limit of detection 5 µg/L, fluorescence detection—R. Aderjan *et al.*, *J. Anal. Toxicol.*, 1995, *19(3)*, 163–168. In plasma: limit of detection is 1 µg/L morphine, ECD—P. P. Rop *et al.*, *J. Chromatogr. B Biomed. Sci. Appl.*, 1994, *661(2)*, 245–253. In urine: limit of detection 50 µg/L, UV and ECD—J. Gerostamoulos *et al.*, *J. Chromatogr.*, 1993, *617(1)*, 152–156. In plasma: limit of quantification 10 µg/L, fluorescence detection—D. A. Barrett *et al.*, *J. Chromatogr.*, 1991, *566(1)*, 135–145. In plasma: morphine and its glucuronides, limits of detection about 5 to 10 µg/L, fluorescence detection—R. Hartley *et al.*, *Biomed. Chromatogr.*, 1993, *7*, 34–37. In plasma: morphine and its metabolites, limit of quantification for morphine 1 µg/L, diode-array detection—D. Weilbo *et al.*, *J. Chromatogr.*, 1993, *615*, 164–168. In urine: morphine and other opioids, limit of detection for morphine 50 µg/L, UV and electrochemical detection—J. Gerostamoulos *et al.*, *J. Chromatogr.*, 1993, *617*, 152–156. In plasma and CSF: morphine and its glucuronides, limit of detection for morphine in plasma 6.1 µg/L, electrochemical detection—A. W. Wright *et al.*, *Ther. Drug Monit.*, 1994, *16*, 200–208; A. W. Wright *et al.*, *Ther. Drug Monit.*, 1998, *20*, 218. In blood or bile: morphine and codeine, limit of quantification in blood 100 µg/L, UV and fluorescence detection—K. L. Crump *et al.*, *J. Anal. Toxicol.*, 1994, *18*, 208–212. In plasma: morphine and its glucuronides, limit of detection for morphine 1 µg/L, fluorescence detection—J. Huwyler *et al.*, *J. Chromatogr.* 1995, *674 B Biomed. Appl.*, 57–63; Y. Rotshteyn and B. Weingarten, *Ther. Drug Monit.*, 1996, *18*, 179–188. In plasma: endogenous morphine, electrochemical detection—Y. Liu *et al.*, *Life Sci.*, 1997, *60*, 237–243. In blood: morphine and its glucuronides, fluorescence detection—J. Beike *et al.*, *Int. J. Legal Med.*, 1997, *110*, 226–229. In plasma: morphine and codeine, limit of quantification 50 µg/L, UV detection—M. Freiermuth and J. C. Plasse, *J. Pharm. Biomed. Anal.*, 1997, *15*, 759–764. In plasma: fluorescence detection—S. Emara, *Biomed. Chromatogr.*, 1998, *12*, 15–20. In plasma: morphine and its glucuronides, electrochemical detection—A. W. Wright and M. T. Smith, *Ther. Drug Monit.*, 1998, *20*, 215–218. In urine: electrochemical detection—B. A. Rashid *et al.*, *J. Chromatogr. A*, 1998, *797*, 245–250. In blood: morphine and its glucuronides, limit of detection 3 ng/g, fluorescence detection—J. Beike *et al.*, *J. Chromatogr. B Biomed. Sci. Appl.*, 1999, *726*, 111–119. In plasma: morphine and its glucuronides, limit of detection for morphine 0.1 µg/L, electrochemical and fluorescence detection—Q. C. Meng *et al.*, *J. Chromatogr. B Biomed. Sci. Appl.*, 2000, *742*, 115–123. In plasma: morphine and its glucuronides, limits of detection 0.5 µg/L and 10 µg/L respectively, UV detection—K. Ary and K. Rona, *J. Pharm. Biomed. Anal.*, 2001, *26*, 179–187.

High performance liquid chromatography–mass spectrometry. In serum: morphine and its glucuronides, limit of quantification for morphine 10 µg/L—R. Pacifini *et al.*, *J. Chromatogr.* 1995, *664 B Biomed. Appl.*, 329–334. In serum: morphine and its glucuronides, limit of quantification for morphine about 0.8 µg/L—N. Tyrefors *et al.*, *J. Chromatogr. A*, 1996, *729*, 279–285. In serum, urine, or CSF: morphine and its metabolites, limit of quantification for morphine in serum or CSF 0.4 µg/L and in urine 3.0 µg/L—G. Schanzle *et al.*, *J. Chromatogr. B Biomed. Sci. Appl.*, 1999, *721*, 55–65. In serum: morphine and its glucuronides, limit of quantification for morphine 1 µg/L—M. Blanchet *et al.*, *J. Chromatogr. A*, 1999, *854*, 93–108. In plasma: morphine and its glucuronides—M. H. Slawson *et al.*, *J. Anal. Toxicol.*, 1999, *23*, 468–473.

In blood: limit of quantification is 0.5 µg/L for morphine, 1.0 µg/L for its 6-glucuronide metabolite and 5 µg/L for the 3-glucuronide—A. Dienes-Nagy *et al.*, *J. Chromatogr. A*, 1999, *854(1–2)*, 109–118.

In serum: limit of quantification is 4.0 µg/L—P. Zuccaro *et al.*, *J. Anal. Toxicol.*, 1997, *21(4)*, 268–277. In blood, CSF fluid, serum, urine, and vitreous humour: 1 µg/L morphine, 5 µg/L for the 3-glucuronide and the 6-glucuronide metabolite—M. J. Bogusz *et al.*, *J. Chromatogr. B Biomed. Sci. Appl.*, 1997, *703(1–2)*, 115–127.

Note. For a study of monitoring opiate use in substance abuse treatment patients with sweat and urine drug testing, see M. A. Huestis *et al.*, *J. Anal. Toxicol.*, 2000, *24*, 509–521.

Disposition in the Body. Rapidly absorbed after subcutaneous, IV, or IM administration. Absorption after oral administration is variable and there is considerable first-pass metabolism. Enterohepatic circulation may occur. It is widely distributed, mainly in kidneys, liver, lungs, and spleen with lower concentrations in the brain and muscles, but does not accumulate in the tissues. Morphine crosses the blood–brain barrier and the placenta; it is found in breast milk and sweat. Approx. 90% of a dose is metabolised after administration. The major metabolic reaction is conjugation to form morphine-3- and 6-glucuronides; morphine 6-glucuronide probably contributes to the analgesic effect, but the 3-glucuronide may antagonise analgesia. Other reactions include *N*-demethylation, *O*-methylation, and *N*-oxide formation and other active metabolites include normorphine, codeine, and morphine ethereal sulfate. After a parenteral dose, up to 90% is excreted in the urine in 24 h, including about 10% of the dose as free morphine, 65 to 70% as conjugated morphine, up to 10% as morphine-3-ethereal sulfate, 1% as normorphine, and 3% as normorphine glucuronide. After an oral dose, about 60% is excreted in the urine in 24 h, and about 3% of the dose is excreted as free morphine in 48 h. The urinary excretion of morphine appears to be pH-dependent to some extent; as the urine becomes more acid, excretion of free morphine rises, and as the urine becomes more alkaline excretion of the glucuronide conjugate rises. Up to about 10% of a dose may be excreted in the bile.
Morphine is the major active metabolite of diamorphine, and is also a metabolite of codeine.

Note. Morphine may be slowly converted to pseudomorphine in cadavers and can be found as such on exhumation.

Therapeutic concentration. In plasma, usually in the range 0.01 to 0.07 mg/L.

4 healthy volunteers, aged 19 to 34 years, were administered 3 consecutive doses of 2.2, 4.4, and 8.8 mg morphine sulfate pentahydrate at 40-min intervals via an aerosol delivery system. Plasma morphine concentrations were proportional to the dose in this study. Additionally, 6 volunteers were administered 4.4 mg aerosolised morphine sulfate over a 2.1-min period on 3 occasions and IV infusions of 2 mg and 4 mg morphine sulfate over 3 min. The mean peak plasma morphine concentration for the aerosol dose was 0.109 mg/L (0.039 to 0.398) at 2.7 min, 0.165 mg/L for the 2 mg IV dose at 3.0 min, and 0.273 mg/L for the 4 mg IV dose at 3.2 min. [M. E. Ward *et al.*, *Clin. Pharmacol. Ther.*, 1997, *62(6)*, 596–609.]

12 patients with post-hepatic cirrhosis (mean age, 40.3 years; range, 35 to 45 years) and 10 healthy volunteers (mean, 39.3 years old) were administered 30 mg controlled-release morphine. The peak serum concentration was 0.035 mg/L in the cirrhotic patients and 0.013 mg/L in the healthy observed at 174.0 min and 142.5 min, respectively. [H. I. Kotb *et al.*, *Br. J. Anaesth.*, 1997, *79(6)*, 804–806.]

31 new-born infants (gestational age, 24 to 41 weeks) on ventilation were administered 140 µg/kg for 1 hour followed by 20 µg/kg/h, for 2 to 4 days. The mean serum morphine concentration during the constant infusion was 0.105 mg/L observed at 2 h. The mean steady state concentration was 0.167 mg/L which was achieved between 24 and 48 h of infusion. Steady-state concentrations of morphine-6-glucuronide and morphine-3-glucuronide were not reached within 60 h. [E. Saarenmaa *et al.*, *Clin. Pharmacol. Ther.*, 2000, *68(2)*, 160–166.]

In 10 patients receiving oral morphine as either a once-a-day extended-release formulation or a twice-a-day extended-release formulation for 7 days, plasma concentrations 30 min post-dose were reported as follows (mg/L):

	Twice daily	Once daily
Morphine	0.011	0.017
Morphine-3-glucuronide	0.592	0.709
Morphine-6-glucuronide	0.086	0.092

(normalised to a total daily dose of 100 mg). [R. K. Portenoy *et al.*, *Pain Symptom Manage.*, 2002, *23*, 292–300.]

In 8 patients receiving morphine, 60 to 3000 mg daily via chronic (8 to 160 days) subcutaneous infusion, for severe cancer pain, the normalised plasma concentrations of morphine, morphine-6-glucuronide, and morphine-3-glucuronide were 0.3 to 0.8 µg/L, 1.0 to 3.1 µg/L, and 6.8 to 24.3 µg/L, respectively. [A. Vermeire *et al.*, *Eur. J. Clin. Pharmacol.*, 1998, *53*, 325–330.]

Toxicity. The estimated minimum oral lethal dose for adults is 200 mg but addicts may be able to tolerate up to 10 times as much. Morphine is initially eliminated from the blood fairly quickly and blood concentrations are difficult to interpret, especially as toxic effects depend on the degree of tolerance that has been acquired.

An 8-year-old girl accidentally ingested morphine before going to bed and was found dead the next morning. Following a tonsillectomy, she was prescribed pethidine syrup at a dose of 100 mg every 4 h but the pharmacist accidentally dispensed Roxanol containing 20 mg/mL morphine sulfate. The girl took 1 to 2 teaspoons as prescribed. The blood morphine concentration was 0.128 mg/L, bile, 135 mg/L, and morphine was found in the stomach contents at a concentration of 16 mg/L (a total amount of 2.3 mg). The cause of death was determined as morphine poisoning which resulted in respiratory depression. [A. Poklis *et al.*, *Forens. Sci. Int.*, 1995, *76(1)*, 55–59.]

A 46-year-old woman who was admitted to hospital in a coma with severe respiratory failure later developed cardiovascular instability and convulsions but recovered sufficiently 2 days later to communicate in writing that she had ingested a large quantity of controlled-release morphine tablets. 60 hours after the presumed intake, the plasma concentrations of morphine, morphine-3-glucuronide, and morphine-6-glucuronide were 0.655, 6.504 and 1.157 mg/L, respectively; urinary recovery of morphine and its metabolites amounted to 6.8 mmol, equivalent to an oral intake of at least 2500 mg. [D. Westerling *et al.*, *Acta Anaesthesiol. Scand.*, 1998, *42*, 586–589.]

Bioavailability. About 20 to 30%.

Half-life. Plasma half-life, about 2 to 3 h.

Volume of distribution. About 3 to 5 L/kg.

Clearance. Plasma clearance, about 15 to 20 mL/min/kg; mean total body clearance for new-born infants (24 to 41 weeks' gestation age), 2.4 (range, 0.8 to 6.4) mL/min/kg.

Protein binding. In plasma, 20 to 35%.

Note. For a review of the metabolism of morphine, see L. L. Christrup, *Acta Anaesthesiol. Scand.*, 1997, *41*, 116–122 and for a review of the pharmacokinetics of sustained-release morphine, see G. K. Gourlay, *Clin. Pharmacokinet.*, 1998, *35*, 173–190.

Dose. 5 to 20 mg of morphine hydrochloride, sulfate, or tartrate, by mouth or parenterally, every 4 h.

Moxisylyte

Vasodilator

Synonym. Thymoxamine
4-[2-(Dimethylamino)ethoxy]-2-methyl-5-(1-methylethyl)phenol acetate
$C_{16}H_{25}NO_3 = 279.4$
CAS—54-32-0

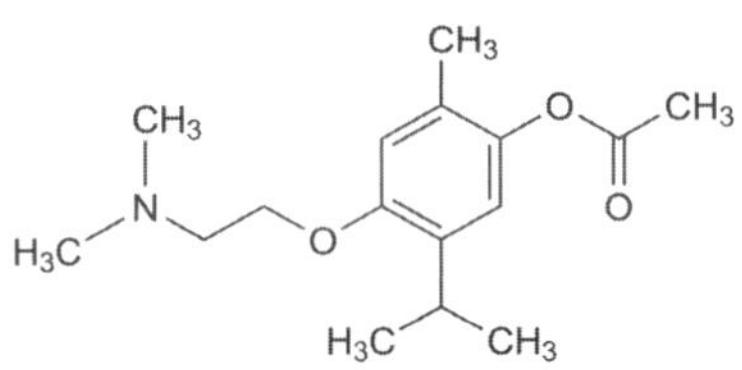

Practically insoluble in water; soluble in chloroform.

Moxisylyte Hydrochloride

Proprietary names. Arlitene; Carlytène; Icavex; Opilon; Vasoklin.
$C_{16}H_{25}NO_3,HCl = 315.8$
CAS—964-52-3
A white crystalline powder. M.p. 208° to 210°.
Soluble 1 in 2.5 of water, 1 in 11 of ethanol and 1 in 3 of chloroform; practically insoluble in ether.

Dissociation Constant. pK_a 8.7.

Partition Coefficient. Log *P* (octanol/water), 3.2.

Colour Test. Marquis test—yellow-brown.

Thin-layer Chromatography. System TA—Rf 52; system TL—Rf 19; system TB—Rf 31; system TC—Rf 44. (Acidified iodoplatinate solution, positive.)

Gas Chromatography. System GA—RI 1832.

High Performance Liquid Chromatography. System HA—Moxisylyte *k* 2.9, desacetylmoxisylyte *k* 2.3.

Ultraviolet Spectrum. Aqueous acid—275 ($A^1_1 = 80a$); aqueous alkali—235, 301 nm ($A^1_1 = 146b$).

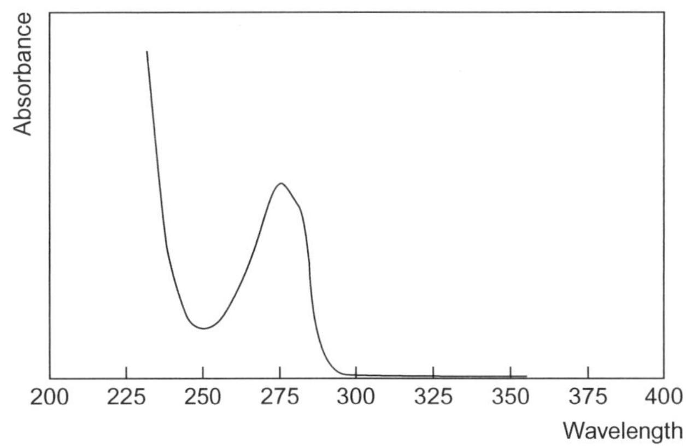

Infra-red Spectrum. Principal peaks at wavenumbers 1184, 1212, 1761, 1261, 1504, 931 cm^{-1} (moxisylyte hydrochloride, KBr disk).

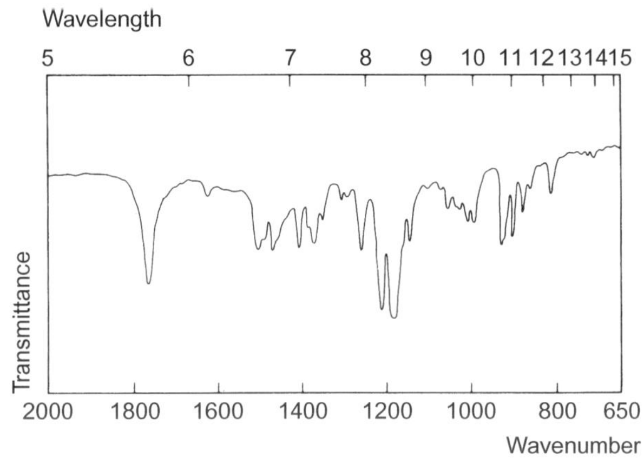

Mass Spectrum. Principal ions at *m/z* 58, 72, 279, 234, 151, 192, 166, 165.

Quantification

Spectrofluorimetry. In plasma—A. G. Arbab and P. Turner. *J. Pharm. Pharmacol.*, 1971, *23*, 719–721.

High performance liquid chromatography. In monkey plasma: metabolites of moxisylyte, limits of detection 2 ng for desacetylmoxisylyte and 4 ng for desmethyldesacetylmoxisylyte, fluorescence detection—A. E. Geahchan and P. L. Chambon, *Anal. Chem.*, 1980, *52*, 999–1001. In plasma or urine: metabolites of moxisylyte, fluorimetric detection—P. Costa *et al.*, *J. Pharm. Sci.*, 1993, *82*, 968–971. In plasma or urine: metabolites of moxisylyte, limits of detection 2.5 to 2.8 μg/L in plasma and 40 to 200 μg/L in urine for desacetyl and sulfate metabolites respectively, fluorescence detection—C. Marquer and F. Bressolle, *J. Chromatogr. B, Biomed. Sci. Appl.*, 1997, *691*, 389–396.

Disposition in the Body. Moxisylyte is poorly absorbed after oral administration. Deacetylation to give desacetylmoxisylyte and subsequent demethylation to give desmethyldesacetylmoxisylyte may occur.

Therapeutic concentration

After single oral doses of 150 mg to 4 female subjects, plasma concentrations of about 0.06 mg/L were achieved after 30 to 60 min in 2 subjects; the drug was not detected in the other 2 subjects. After an IV injection of 0.2 mg/kg over 2 min to 2 male subjects, plasma concentrations at 2, 7 and 15 min were 0.14, 0.08 and 0.05 mg/L in the first subject and 0.1, 0.04 and 0.03 mg/L in the other. [A. G. Arbab and P. Turner, *J. Pharm. Pharmacol.*, 1971, *23*, 719–721].

Dose. The equivalent of 160 mg of moxisylyte daily.

Moxonidine

Antihypertensive

Synonyms. BDF-5895, BE-5895.
Proprietary names. Cynt; Physiotens.
4-Chloro-*N*-(4,5-dihydro-1*H*-imidazol-2-yl)-6-methoxy-2-methyl-5-pyrimidinamine
$C_9H_{12}ClN_5O=241.7$
CAS—75438-57-2

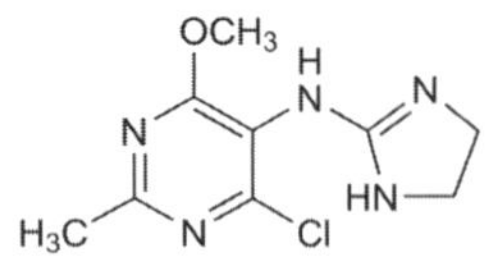

M.p. 217° to 219°.

Moxonidine Hydrochloride

$C_9H_{12}ClN_5O.xHCl$
CAS—75438-58-3
Crystals from isopropanol/ether with m.p. 189°.

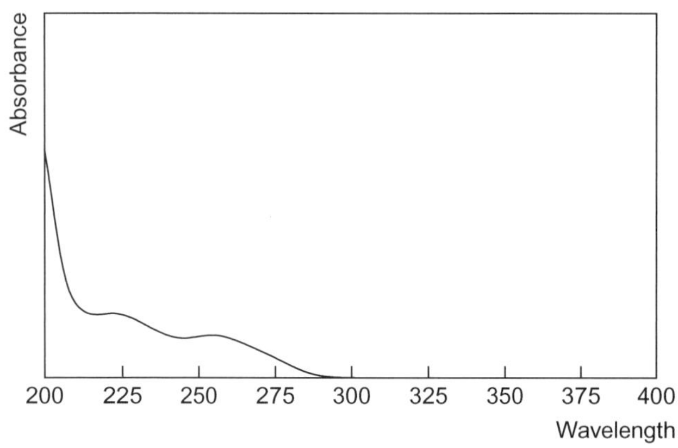

Quantification

Gas chromatography–mass spectrometry. In plasma: limit of quantification 0.1 µg/L, limit of detection 0.05 µg/L. MS detection (NICI, SIM at *m/z* 721)—W. Kirch, *J. Clin. Pharmacol.*, 1990, *30*, 1088–1095.

Disposition in the Body. Moxonidine is well absorbed after oral administration (peak plasma concentrations are reached between 0.5 and 3.0 h). It is not subject to first-pass metabolism and food does not interfere with its pharmacokinetics. It is metabolised mainly to 4,5-dehydromoxonidine and a guanine derivative. It is excreted in urine mainly as the unchanged drug (50 to 75%) and as its metabolites. Only 1% of a dose is excreted via faeces. The drug is detectable in breast milk.

Therapeutic concentration

8 hypertensive patients previously treated with antihypertensive therapy, aged between 32 and 69 years, were administered a single oral dose of 0.25 mg moxonidine. A mean peak concentration of 1.96 µg/L (range 1.16 to 3.06 µg/L) was observed at 1.07 h (0.29 to 2.55 h) after administration. [W. Kirch, *J. Clin. Pharmacol.*, 1990, *30*, 1088–1095].

Group 1: 8 individuals with normal renal function (creatinine clearance 6.4 L/h), group 2: 8 patients with moderately impaired renal function (creatinine clearance 3 L/h), group 3: 8 patients with severe renal dysfunction (creatinine clearance 1.4 L/h). Each group was administered 0.3 mg daily for 7 days. The peak plasma concentrations were 1.5, 2.1 and 2.3 µg/L for groups 1, 2 and 3, respectively, observed at 1.0, 1.3 and 1.1 h. [W. Kirch *et al.*, *Clin. Pharmacokinet.*, 1988, *15*, 245–253].

Toxicity

3 cases of overdose have been reported, two of which involved the children (2 to 3 years old) of 2 patients accidentally ingesting moxonidine. Full recoveries were made without any signs of cardiovascular disorder. A third case involved a 23-year-old man who intentionally ingested moxonidine, ranitidine and alcohol in a suicide attempt. Plasma concentrations were 70-fold higher than would be expected after ingestion of the recommended dose. Bradycardia, somnolence and hypotension were observed and treated, and the patient made a full recovery. [M. Schachter *et al.*, *Drug Safety*, 1998, *19*, 191–203].

Bioavailability. 88%.

Half-life. 2 to 3 h (prolonged in renal impairment).

Volume of distribution. 1.39 L/kg (0.85 to 1.75 L/kg).

Clearance. Plasma, 0.77 L/h/kg (43.6 to 69 L/h/kg; 32.9 L/h/kg for those with moderate renal impairment; 22.1 L/h/kg, severe renal impairment).

Protein binding. 5.8 to 7.9%.

Note. For a review of moxonidine, see B. N. Prichard *et al.*, *J. Hypertens.*, 1999, *17 Suppl. 3*, S41–S54.

Dose. The usual initial dose is 200 µg daily which may be increased to a maximum of 600 µg over a number of weeks. The dose may be reduced in those with renal impairment.

Mupirocin

Antibacterial (topical)

Synonyms. BRL-4910A, Pseudomonic Acid A; *trans*-Pseudomonic Acid.
Proprietary names. Bactoderm; Bactroban Ointment; Celefer; Plasimine; Eismycin; Turixin.
(2*E*)-5,9-Anhydro-2,3,4,8-tetradeoxy-8-[[(2*S*,3*S*)-3-[(1*S*,2*S*)-2-hydroxy-1-methylpropyl]oxiranyl]methyl]-3-methyl-L-*talo*-non-2-enonic acid, 8-carboxyoctyl ester
$C_{26}H_{44}O_9=500.6$
CAS—12650-69-0

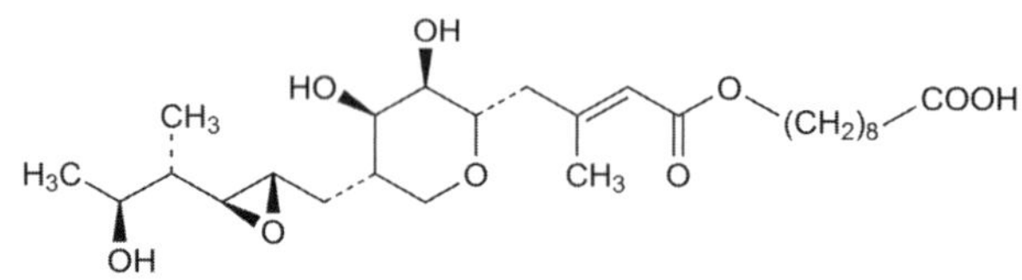

An off-white crystalline solid. M.p. 77° to 78°. It is soluble in dehydrated alcohol, acetone and chloroform; slightly soluble in water and ether.

Mupirocin Calcium

Proprietary names. Bactroban Nasal

Dissociation Constant. pKa (22°), 5.

Thin-layer Chromatography. System TE—Rf 1; system TF—Rf 00.

High Performance Liquid Chromatography. System HX—RI 459.

Ultraviolet Spectrum. Ethanol—222 nm; basic—287 nm.

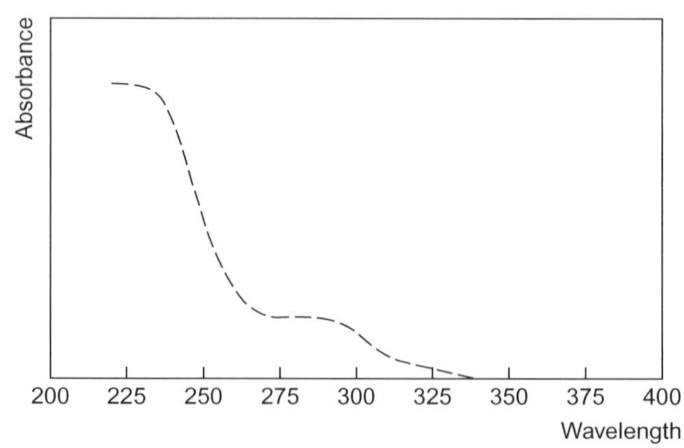

Infra-red Spectrum. Principal peaks at wavenumbers 1718, 1146, 1052 cm^{-1}.

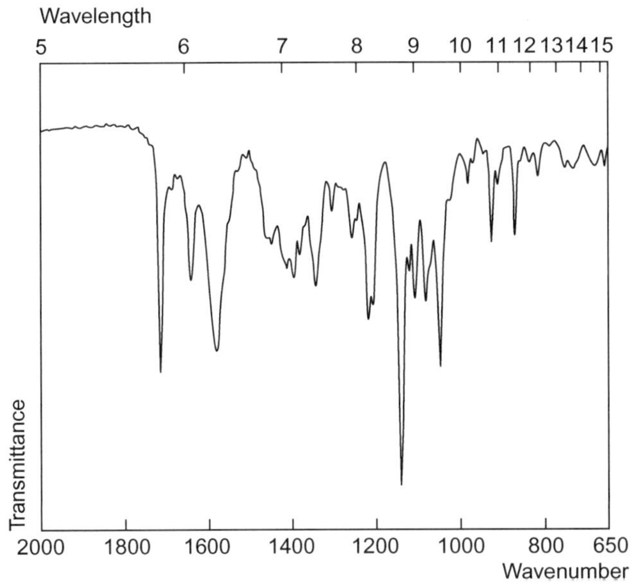

Disposition in the Body. Systemic absorption after topical application is very small. Mupirocin is rapidly metabolised to monic acid (microbiologically inactive) by de-esterification. Following IV administration of a single 125 mg mupirocin sodium salt dose, approx. 0.5% is excreted unchanged in urine, whereas 72% is excreted as monic acid within 12 h. Mupirocin does not appear to be inactivated by non-specific esterases present in blood.

Therapeutic concentration

Following IV infusions over 25 min, in healthy adult, of 31.3, 61.2, 125 and 252 mg mupirocin sodium salt, peak plasma concentrations reached were 1.9, 1.9, 7.1 and 14.1 μg/mL, respectively. Serum concentrations declined rapidly and mupirocin was undetectable within 3 h. [GlaxoSmithKline, Patient Information Leaflet, data on file].

Half-life. After IV administration, mupirocin, 15 to 30 min; monic acid, 32 to 78 min.

Protein binding. 95 to 97%.

Dose. Applied topically as a 2% ointment in macrogol bases for the treatment of various bacterial skin infections up to 3 times a day for up to 10 days.

Muzolimine

Diuretic

5-Amino-2-[1-(3,4-dichlorophenyl)ethyl]-2,4-dihydro-3*H*-pyrazol-3-one

$C_{11}H_{11}Cl_2N_3O$=272.1

CAS—55294-15-0

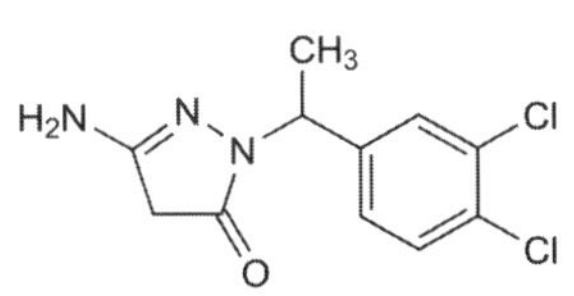

Crystals. M.p. 134° to 137°.

Practically insoluble in water; soluble 1 in 4 of ethanol, 1 in 9 of acetone and 1 in 3 of chloroform.

Dissociation Constant. pK_a 9.3.

Ultraviolet Spectrum. Methanolic acid—240 nm (A^1_1=489b).

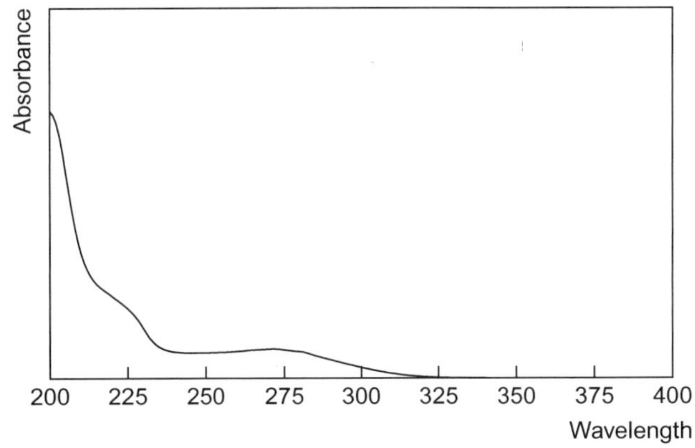

Infra-red Spectrum. Principal peaks at wavenumbers 1690, 1640, 1602, 835, 665, 880 cm^{-1} (KBr disk).

Quantification

Thin-layer chromatography. In plasma or urine: limit of detection 2 μg/L—W. Ritter, *J. Chromatogr.*, 1977, *142*, 431–440.

Disposition in the Body. Muzolimine is readily absorbed following oral administration. About 5% of a dose is excreted unchanged in the urine in 10 h.

Therapeutic concentration

After a single oral dose of 30 mg given to 6 subjects, peak plasma concentrations of 0.29 to 0.51 (mean 0.44) mg/L were attained in 1 to 3 h. [D. Loew *et al.*, *Eur. J. Clin. Pharmacol.*, 1977, *12*, 341–344].

Half-life. Plasma half-life, 10 to 17 h.

Dose. 40 to 80 mg daily.

Mycophenolate Mofetil

Immunosuppressant

Synonyms. RS-61443; Mycophenolate; Morpholinoethyl.

Proprietary name. CellCept

2-Morpholinoethyl-(*E*)-6-(4-hydroxy-6-methoxy-7-methyl-3-oxo-5-phthalanyl)-4-methyl-4-hexenoate

$C_{23}H_{31}NO_7$=433.5

CAS—115007-34-6; 128794-94-5

White to off-white crystalline powder. M.p. 93° to 94°. Slightly soluble in water; soluble in acetone and methanol; sparingly soluble in ethanol.

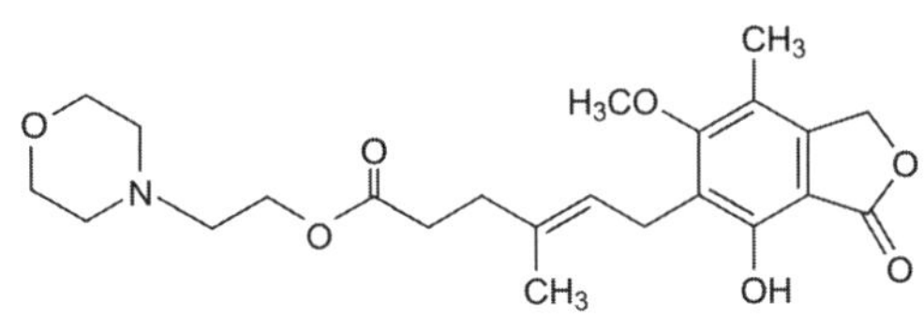

Mycophenolic Acid

6-(4-Hydroxy-6-methoxy-7-methyl-3-oxo-5-phthalanyl)-4-methyl-4-hexenoic acid

$C_{17}H_{20}O_6$=320.3

CAS—24280-93-1

Needles from hot water. M.p. 141°. It is soluble in alcohol; moderately soluble in ether and chloroform; sparingly soluble in toluene; almost insoluble in cold water.

Dissociation Constant. pK_a 5.6 (mycophenolate mofetil), 4.5 (acid).

Partition Coefficient. log *P* (octanol/phosphate buffer pH 2), 0.0085; (octanol/phosphate buffer pH 7.4), 238 (mycophenolate mofetil); log *P* (octanol/phosphate buffer pH 2), 570; (octanol/phosphate buffer pH 7.4), 1.6 (acid).

High Performance Liquid Chromatography. Column: (analytical) ODS (150 × 4.6 mm i.d., 5 μm); (guard) C_{18} (15 × 3.2 mm i.d., 7 μm). Mobile phase: methanol:trifluoroacetic acid (48:52), flow rate 1.5 mL/min. IS: suprofen. UV detection (λ=250 nm). Retention time(s): mycophenolic acid, 14.6 min; mycophenolate phenol glucuronide, 3.6 min; IS,

9.2 min. [K. Wiwattanawongsa *et al.*, *J. Chromatogr. B, Biomed. Sci. Appl.*, 2001, *763*, 35–45].

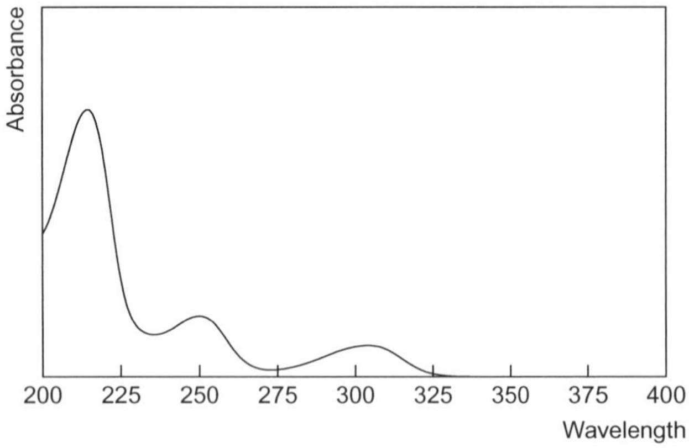

Quantification

High performance liquid chromatography. In skin: limit of detection 0.85 μg/L for mycophenolate mofetil, 1 μg/L for mycophenolic acid. MS detection—M. Platzer *et al.*, *J. Chromatogr. B, Biomed. Sci. Appl.*, 2001, *755*, 355–359. In body fluids: limit of detection 0.17 mg/L, UV detection (λ=215 nm and 304 nm)—N. Sugioka *et al.*, *J. Chromatogr.*, 1994, *654*; *Biomed. Appl.*, 249–256. In plasma: limit of quantification for mycophenolic acid 0.1 mg/L and its glucuronic conjugate 4.0 mg/L. UV detection (λ=254 nm)—I. Tsina *et al.*, *J. Chromatogr.*, 1996, *675*; *Biomed. Appl.*, 119–129.

Disposition in the Body. Mycophenolate mofetil is an ethyl ester prodrug. It is rapidly absorbed after oral administration and completely hydrolysed to form the active drug mycophenolic acid (MPA). Mycophenolic acid is further metabolised through glucuronidation to form an inactive metabolite (MPAG) which is excreted in urine. About 6% of the dose is excreted in faeces. The pharmacokinetics of MPA and MPAG are altered if mycophenolate mofetil is administered with a high fat content meal or antacids containing aluminium and magnesium hydroxides. Food has little effect on the bioavailability of mycophenolate mofetil but antacids reduce the peak plasma concentration by 40%.

Therapeutic concentration

10 patients with rheumatoid arthiritis, 6 females and 4 males, with a mean age of 55.6 years, were administered 2 g mycophenolate mofetil after an overnight fast. It was either administered on its own, with food, or with an antacid. The mean peak plasma concentrations of MPA were 23.8, 18 and 14.8 mg/L, respectively, and were observed between 0.5 and 3 h post-administration. Mean concentrations of MPAG at 52.7, 68.4 and 38.8 mg/L were reached in individuals in the fasting state, fed state and for those administered with an antacid, respectively. These levels were seen 2 to 4 h after administration. [R. Bullingham *et al.*, *Br. J. Clin. Pharmacol.*, 1996, *41*, 513–516].

Bioavailability. 94%.

Half-life. Mycophenolic acid, 18 h.

Volume of distribution. Mycophenolic acid, 3.6 L/kg.

Clearance. 11.6 L/h (193 mL/min).

Protein binding. Mycophenolic acid, 97%; MPAG (glucuronide metabolite), 82%.

Note. For a review of the pharmacokinetics of mycophenolate mofetil, see B. Fulton and A. Markham, *Drugs*, 1996, *51*, 278–298.

Dose. The initial dose is 2 g daily which may be increased to 3 g if necessary.

Myristicin

Hallucinogen

4-Methoxy-6-(2-propenyl)-1,3-benzodioxole
$C_{11}H_{12}O_3$=192.2
CAS—607-91-0

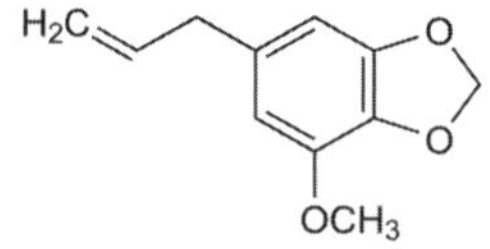

The most toxic principle of nutmeg and nutmeg oil. M.p. below −20°. B.p. 276° to 277°. Refractive index 1.5403.
Slightly soluble in ethanol; soluble in ether.

Nutmeg

Synonyms. Muscade; Myristica; Nux Moschata.
The dried kernels of the seeds of *Myristica fragrans* (Myristicaceae), containing not less than 5% of volatile oil.

Nutmeg Oil

Synonyms. *Essence de Muscade*; Myristica Oil; Oleum Myristicae.
CAS—8008-45-5
A volatile oil obtained by distillation from nutmeg. East Indian oil contains about 15% of myristicin and West Indian about 2%.
A colourless, pale yellow, or pale green liquid. Mass per mL, East Indian oil 0.885 to 0.915 g, West Indian oil 0.86 to 0.88 g. Refractive index 1.472 to 1.488. Freely soluble in ethanol (90%); soluble in glacial acetic acid.

Partition Coefficient. Log *P* (octanol/water), 3.5.

Disposition in the Body

Toxicity. Severe symptoms of poisoning have been caused by the ingestion of 1 to 1½ nutmegs, and doses of 5 g or more of nutmeg or nutmeg powder will produce a marked depressive action on the central nervous system.

A 28-year-old woman ingested 18.3 g of powdered nutmeg. Following a period of disorientation, delirium and excitement, the patient became semi-stuporous for 12 h. For some days she complained of numbness, dizziness and nausea and there were further periods of excitement. No specific therapy was given and she was discharged after 7 days. [R. C. Green, *J. Am. Med. Assoc.*, 1959, *171*, 1342–1344].

Two young women consumed 15 and 25 g respectively of ground nutmeg in order to experience its hallucinogenic action. Both became intoxicated but recovered. [H. O. Akesson and J. Walinder, *Lancet*, 1965, *1*, 1271–1272].

The cause of death in a 55-year-old woman was attributed to the ingestion of nutmeg. The concentration of myristicin in the postmortem blood was 4.0 mg/L (it was speculated that the ingested dose of nutmeg had been 560 to 840 mg/kg); flunitrazepam was also present (0.072 mg/L). In a 2-year period in which 7 cases of nutmeg poisoning had been recorded by the Erfurt Poison Information Centre, even where higher doses (20 to 80 g of powder; 280 to 1100 mg/kg) had been ingested, a life-threatening situation had never arisen; in one case a myristicin blood level of 2 mg/L was measured 8 h after ingestion of approximately 14 to 21 g (280 to 420 mg/kg) of nutmeg powder. [U. Stein *et al.*, *Forensic Sci. Int.*, 2001, *118*, 87–90].

Note. For a review of the toxic effects and uses of nutmeg, see A. T. Weil, *Bull. Narc.*, 1966, *18*(4), 15–23.

Nabilone

Anti-emetic

Synonym. LY-109514
Proprietary name. Cesamet
(6a*R*,10a*R*)-*rel*-3-(1,1-Dimethylheptyl)-6,6a,7,8,10,10a-hexahydro-1-hydroxy-6,6-dimethyl-9*H*-dibenzo[*b*,*d*]pyran-9-one
$C_{24}H_{36}O_3$=372.5
CAS—51022-71-0

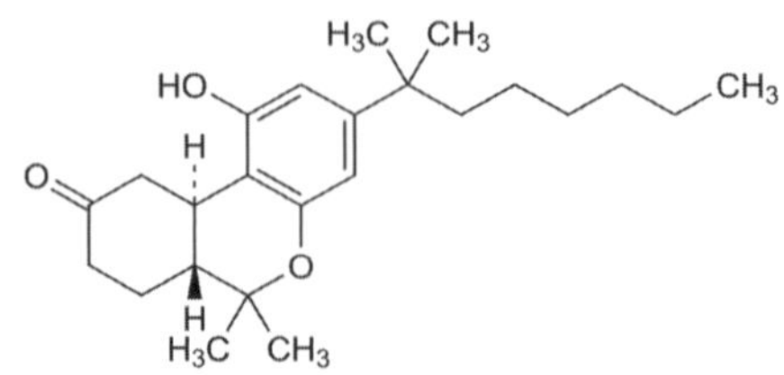

Nabilone is a synthetic cannabinoid.

Ultraviolet Spectrum. Methanol—275 (A^1_1=35b), 282 nm (A^1_1=35b).

Infra-red Spectrum. Principal peaks at wavenumbers 1696, 1619, 1574, 1260, 1100, 1038 cm^{-1} (KBr disk).

Mass Spectrum. Principal ions at m/z 288, 69, 178, 41, 287, 43, 289, 55.

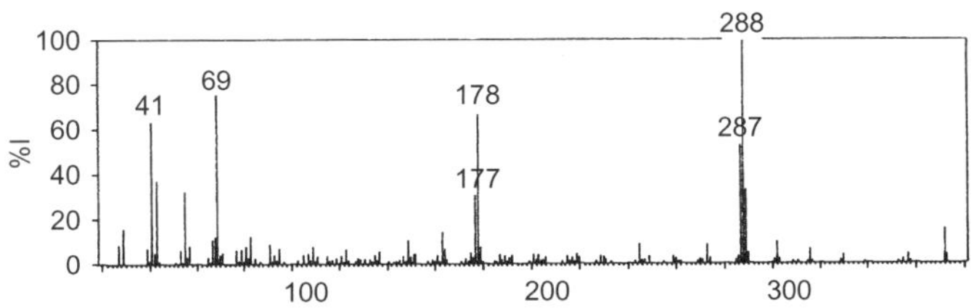

Disposition in the body. Nabilone is readily absorbed after oral administration; it is rapidly distributed into the tissues and metabolised by reduction of the 9-keto group, forming a mixture of isomeric alcohols (carbinols) together with several other unidentified metabolites. About 65% of a dose is eliminated in the faeces, and about 20% is excreted in the urine as polar acidic metabolites.

Half-life. Plasma half-life, about 2 h.

Dose. 2 to 4 mg daily; maximum of 6 mg daily.

Nabumetone

NSAID

Synonyms. BRL-14777, Nabumetonum.
Proprietary names. Arthaxan; Balmox; Consolan; Diosmal; Nabuser; Relafen; Relifen; Relifex.
4-(6-Methoxy-2-naphthalenyl)-2-butanone
$C_{15}H_{16}O_2$=228.3
CAS—42924-53-8

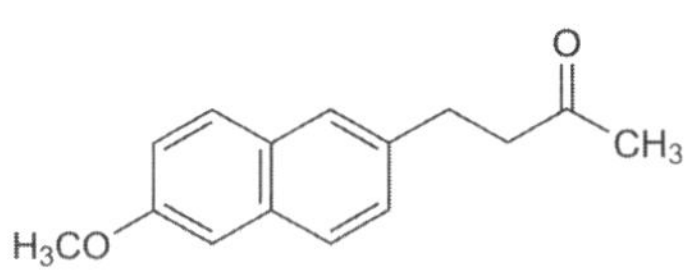

A white crystalline powder which is soluble in acetone and slightly soluble in methyl alcohol. M.p. 80°. Practically insoluble in water.

Partition Coefficient. Log P (octanol/phosphate buffer pH 7.4), 2400 for nabumetone; log P (octanol/water), 0.5 for 6-methoxy-2-naphthylacetic acid (6-MNA).

Gas Chromatography. System GB—RI 2084 (nabumatone); RI 2322 (M (6-MNA)); RI 2385 (M (*O*-desmethyl)).

Column: methyl silicone (HP1, 0.2 mm i.d., 0.33 µm film thickness). Column temperature: 250°. Carrier gas: helium, 0.9 mL/min flow rate. MS detection. Retention index: 2082. [T. Mills and J. C. Roberson, *Instrumental Data for Drug Analysis*, 1993, CRC Press, Boca Raton, US. 2nd Edn, Vol. 5, pp. 294–295].

High Performance Liquid Chromatography. System HZ—retention time 13.6 min.

Column: 5-C_{18} (Wakosil, 150 × 4.6 mm i.d., 5 µm). Mobile phase: acetonitrile:water:triethylamine (500:500:1), containing 0.5 g/L 1-heptane sulfonic acid, flow rate 1.0 mL/min. IS: methyl *p*-toluate. UV detection (λ=270 nm); fluorescence detection (λ_{ex}=280 nm; λ_{em}=350 nm). k values: nabumetone, 6.3; 6-methoxy-2-naphthylacetic acid, 1.9; IS, 4.6. [E. Mikami *et al.*, *J. Pharm. Biomed. Anal.*, 2000, *23*, 917–925].

Column: ODS Hypersil (100 × 4.6 mm i.d., 5 µm). Mobile phase: methanol:aqueous 0.01 M dihydrogen potassium phosphate buffer, adjusted to pH 3.5 with 85% phosphoric acid (70:30), flow rate 1 mL/min. UV diode array detection. Retention time: 3.4 min. [T. Mills and J. C. Roberson, *Instrumental Data for Drug Analysis*, 1993, CRC Press, Boca Raton, US. 2nd Edn, Vol. 5, pp. 294–295].

Ultraviolet Spectrum. Aqueous acid—230, 261, 270, 333 nm.

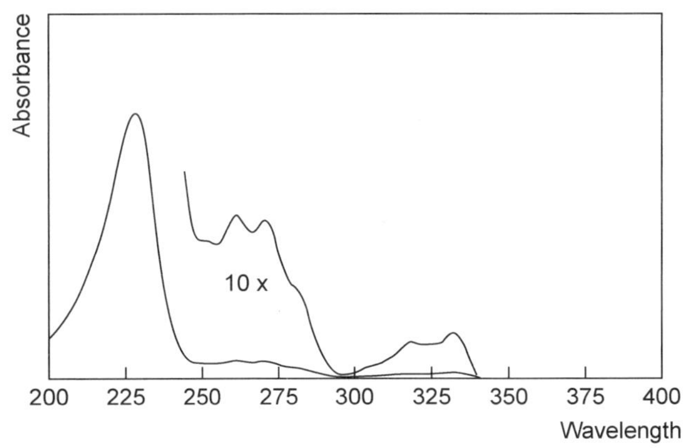

Infra-red Spectrum. Principal peaks at wavenumbers 1696, 1260, 1020 cm^{-1} (KBr disk).

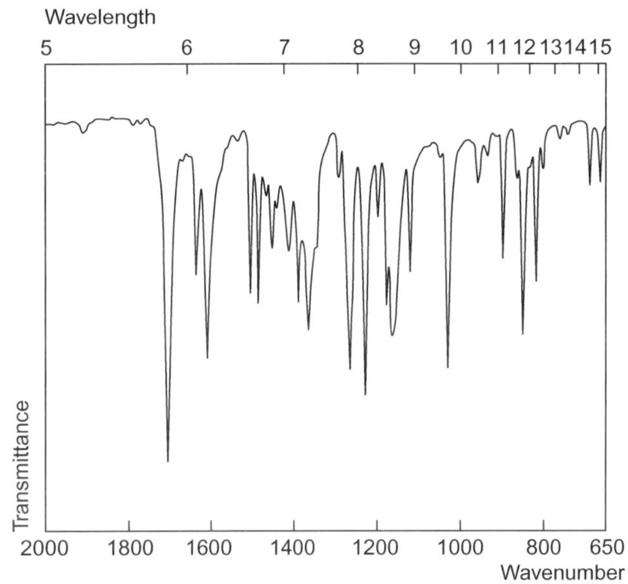

Mass Spectrum. Principal ions at m/z 171, 228, 172, 185, 128, 43, 115, 141, 158.

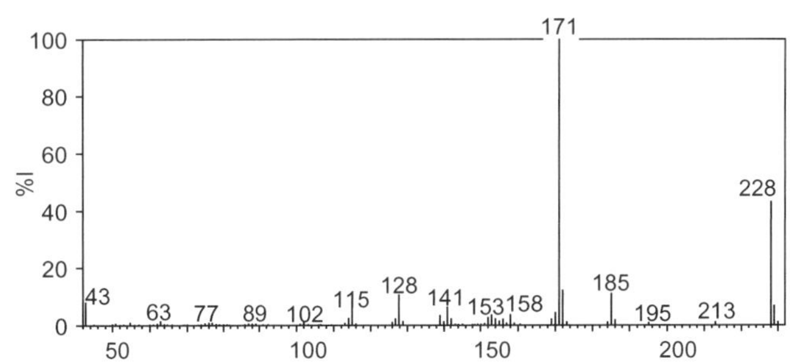

Quantification

High performance liquid chromatography. In plasma: limit of quantification 70 µg/L. UV detection (λ=280 nm)—A. D. Jager *et al.*, *J. Chromatogr. B, Biomed. Sci. Appl.*, 2000, *740*, 247–251. In pharmaceuticals and urine: limits of detection 120 and 16 µg for nabumetone and 6-methoxy-2-naphthylacetic acid, respectively. UV detection (λ=270 nm)—E. Mikami *et al.*, *J. Pharm. Biomed. Anal.*, 2000, *23(5)*, 917–925.

Disposition in the Body. Nabumetone is well absorbed from the gastrointestinal tract and rapidly converted to the active metabolite 6-methoxy-2-naphthylacetic acid (6-MNA) (BRL-10720) via hepatic metabolism. Peak plasma concentrations of 6-MNA are observed 2 to 8 h after administration with a possible secondary peak at 28 to 36 h. The active metabolite 6-MNA undergoes further metabolism via *O*-methylation and conjugation to

6-hydroxy-2-naphthylacetic acid which may also be conjugated. Alternative metabolic pathways are *O*-demethylation and reduction of the ketone to alcohol and esters. Other metabolites include 4-(6-hydroxy-2-naphthyl)-butan-2-one, 4-(6-hydroxy-2-naphthyl)-butan-2-ol and 6-hydroxy-2-naphthylacetic acid which may undergo further conjugation resulting in many metabolites detected in urine. Around 80% of the dose is excreted in urine as inactive metabolites with approx. 1% as unchanged 6-MNA. 10% is excreted in faeces. 6-MNA diffuses in synovial fluids.

Therapeutic concentration

12 healthy young male and female volunteers, aged between 18 and 21 years, were administered a 1 g single dose of nabumetone. 12 male and female elderly volunteers, 63 to 83 years old, were also administered with the same dose. This single dose study was followed by multiple dosing of 1 g daily. Mean peak plasma concentrations of 21.9 mg/L (range 11.3 to 34.0 mg/L) and 33.7 (range 6.7 to 64.1) mg/L were observed for the young and elderly individuals, respectively, for the single 1 g dose, and were observed between 3 and 24 h (mean 13 and 12.2 h, respectively). After multiple dosing, the plasma levels reached 52.3 (range 32.0 to 71.9) mg/L and 66.7 (between 15.1 and 103.0) mg/L for the young and elderly, respectively, approx. 5 h after administration (1 to 10 h). [M. J. Kendall *et al.*, *Eur. J. Clin. Pharmacol.*, 1989, *36*, 299–305].

Bioavailability. The absolute mean bioavailability is 38%.

Half-life. 6-MNA, 22 to 27 h (young healthy subjects), 25 to 34 h (elderly).

Volume of distribution. 7.5 L (steady state); ranges between 5 and 10 L (0.1 to 0.2 L/kg).

Clearance. The apparent clearance is 0.7 L/h (creatinine clearance 40 to >80 mL/min); 0.93 (creatinine clearance 10 to 39 mL/min); 1.41 (creatinine clearance <10 mL/min) after single oral doses.

Protein binding. 6-MNA, >99%.

Note. For a review of nabumetone, see H. A. Friedel *et al.*, *Drugs*, 1993, *45*, 131–156.

Dose. 1 g administered at night with 0.5 to 1 g extra in the morning if necessary. The elderly are administered 0.5 to 1 g.

Nadolol

Beta-blocker

Proprietary names. Apo-nadol; Corgard; Solgol. It is an ingredient of Corgaretic, Corzide and Solgeretik.

5-[3-[(1,1-Dimethylethyl)amino]-2-hydroxypropoxy]-1,2,3,4-tetrahydro-2,3-naphthalenediol

$C_7H_{27}NO_4$=309.4

CAS—42200-33-9

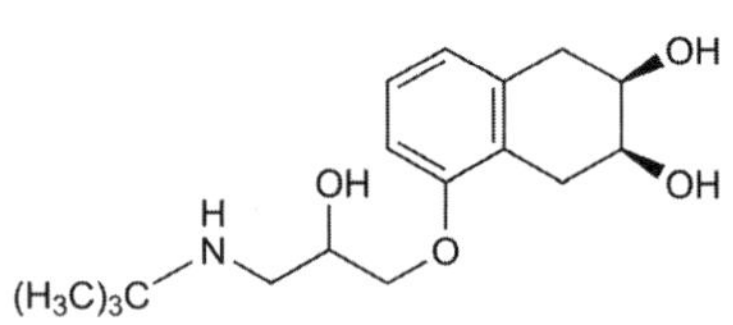

A white crystalline powder. M.p. 124° to 136°.

Soluble in water; freely soluble in ethanol and propylene glycol; slightly soluble in chloroform; insoluble in acetone, benzene, ether and hexane.

Partition Coefficient. Log *P* (octanol/water), 0.8.

Colour Tests. Liebermann's test—brown; Mandelin's test—brown-red; Marquis test—red; Nessler's reagent—brown.

Thin-layer Chromatography. System TA—Rf 42; system TB—Rf 01; system TC—Rf 01; system TE—Rf 20; system TL—Rf 1; system TAE—Rf 14.

Gas Chromatography. System GA—nadolol RI 2540; art RI 2560; system GB—nadolol RI 2658; art RI 2670.

High Performance Liquid Chromatography. System HA—*k* 1.2; system HX—RI 288; system HY—RI 249; system HAA—Retention time(s) 6.8 min.

Ultraviolet Spectrum. Aqueous acid—269, 276 nm; methanol—270, 278 nm (A_1^1=38a). No alkaline shift.

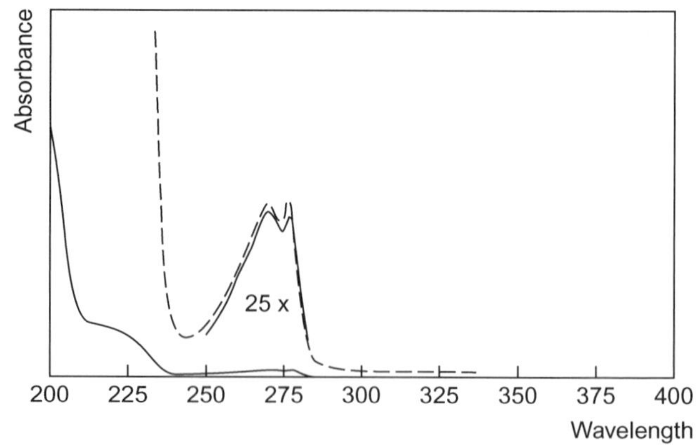

Infra-red Spectrum. Principal peaks at wavenumbers 1092, 1070, 1248, 1262, 1582, 1217 cm^{-1} (KBr disk).

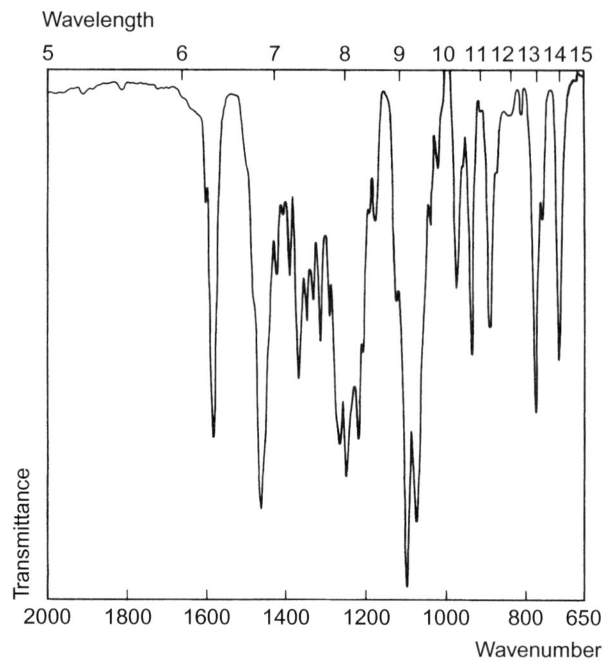

Mass Spectrum. Principal ions at *m/z* 30, 86, 57, 294, 71, 310, 70, 87.

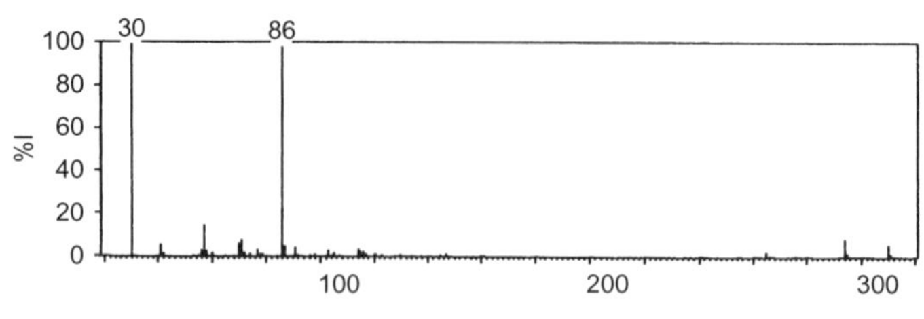

Quantification

Spectrofluorimetry. In serum or urine: limit of detection <10 µg/L—E. Ivashkiv, *J. Pharm. Sci.*, 1977, *66*, 1168–1172.

Gas chromatography–mass spectrometry. In serum: limit of detection 7 µg/L—P. T. Funke *et al.*, *J. Pharm. Sci.*, 1978, *67*, 653–657.

High performance liquid chromatography. In serum: electrochemical detection—P. Surmann, *Arch. Pharm. Berl.*, 1980, *313*, 1052–1054. In plasma: nadolol and other beta-blockers, UV or fluorescence detection—G. Musch *et al.*, *J. Pharm. Biomed. Anal.*, 1989, *7*, 484–497. In serum: limit of detection 1 µg/L, fluorescence detection—H. Noguchi *et al.*, *J. Chromatogr.*, 1992, *573*, 336–338. In plasma: limit of detection 5 µg/L, fluorescence detection—N. R. Srinivas *et al.*, *Biomed. Chromatogr.*, 1995, *9*, 75–79. In plasma: nadolol enantiomers, limit of detection 2.5 µg/L, fluorescence detection—F. J. Belas *et al.*, *Biomed. Chromatogr.*, 1995, *9*, 140–145. In plasma: nadolol enantiomers, limit of detection 2 µg/L, fluorescence detection—N. R. Srinivas *et al.*, *Biomed. Chromatogr.*, 1995, *9*, 226–228. In urine: nadolol and other beta-blockers, limits of detection 15 ppb to 500 ppb, amperometric detection—M. I. Maguregui *et al.*, *J. Chromatogr. B Biomed. Appl.*, 1995, *674*, 85–91.

Disposition in the Body. Nadolol is absorbed after oral administration. It is excreted almost entirely as unchanged drug; about 15 to 21% of the dose is excreted in the urine and 68 to 85% is eliminated in the faeces in 4 days, after oral administration. After IV administration, about 75% of a dose is excreted in the urine unchanged.

Therapeutic concentration

Following single oral doses of 60 and 120 mg to 7 subjects, peak plasma concentrations of 0.02 to 0.14 (mean 0.07) mg/L and 0.05 to 0.25 (mean 0.13) mg/L were attained in 1 to 4 h. [M. Schäfer-Korting *et al.*, *Eur. J. Clin. Pharmacol.*, 1984, *26*, 125–127].

Single oral doses of 80 mg to 4 subjects resulted in peak plasma concentrations of 0.04 to 0.21 (mean 0.14) mg/L in 1 to 4 h. During daily oral dosing of 4 subjects with 80 mg a day, peak plasma concentrations of 0.11 to 0.24 (mean 0.22) mg/L were observed 2 to 4 h after a morning dose. [J. Dreyfuss *et al.*, *J. Clin. Pharmacol.*, 1979, *19*, 712–720].

Toxicity

Following intentional overdose, a 57-year-old woman presented in a poorly responsive state with haemodynamic compromise and an elevated nadolol serum concentrations of 0.39 mg/L; other drugs were present within their normal therapeutic range (diltiazem, paracetamol, salicylate). [G. R. Ehgartner and M. S. Zelinka, *Arch. Intern. Med.*, 1988, *148*, 801–802].

Bioavailability. About 30%.

Half-life. Plasma half-life, 6 to 24 h.

Volume of distribution. About 2 L/kg.

Clearance. Plasma clearance, about 3 mL/min/kg.

Protein binding. In plasma, about 4 to 30% (mean 14%).

Note. For a review of the pharmacokinetics of nadolol, see R. C. Heel *et al.*, *Drugs*, 1980, *20*, 1–23.

Dose. 40 to 240 mg daily.

Nafarelin

Gonadorelin Analogue/ Treatment of Endometriosis

Synonyn. NAG

5-Oxo-L-prolyl-L-histidyl-L-tryptophyl-L-seryl-L-tyrosyl-3-(2-naphthyl)-D-alanyl-L-leucyl-L-arginyl-L-prolylglycinamide

$C_{66}H_{83}N_{17}O_{13}$=1322.5

CAS—76932-56-4

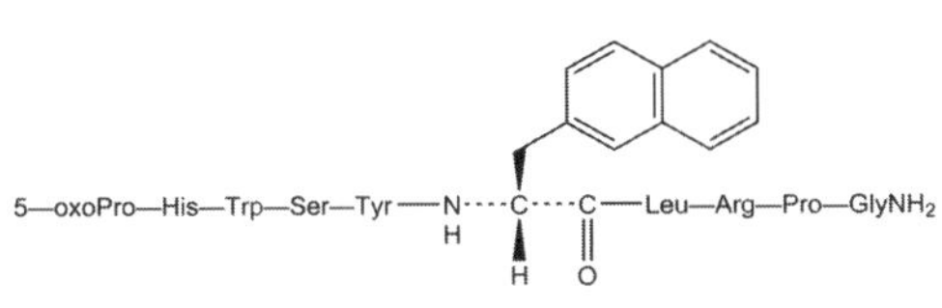

Nafarelin Monoacetate

$C_{66}H_{83}N_{17}O_{13},C_2H_4O_2$=1382.6

M.p. 188° to 190°.

Nafarelin Acetate Hydrate

Synonyms. RS-94991-298; D-Nal(2)[6]-LHRH Acetate Hydrate.

Proprietary names. Nacenyl; Nasanyl; Synarel; Synarela; Synrelina.

$C_{66}H_{83}N_{17}O_{13},xC_2H_4O_2,yH_2O$

CAS—86220-42-0

High Performance Liquid Chromatography. Column: silica (TSK 2000 SW, 300 × 7.5 mm i.d.). Mobile phase: acetonitrile (initially 100%; stepped to 30% in 0.15 mM phosphate buffer):$NaClO_4$ (13 mM) (85:15), flow rate 1.0 mL/min. UV detection (λ=225 nm). Retention time(s): 22 min. [R. A. Kenley *et al.*, *Anal. Chem.*, 1987, *59*, 2050–2054].

Disposition in the Body. Nafarelin is rapidly absorbed after intranasal administration, and peak plasma concentrations are reached within approx. 20 min. It is metabolised by peptidases in the body and is excreted in urine as the metabolites and a small amount as the unchanged drug. The most common metabolites are the (5–10) hexapeptide amine (the key intermediate for the other metabolites) and the naphthylalanine. Metabolites are excreted in urine (44 to 55%) and faeces (18.5 to 44.2%). Only about 3% of unchanged nafarelin is excreted in urine. The drug is rapidly distributed throughout the body and undergoes extensive extravascular distribution.

Therapeutic concentration

10 women, aged 32 to 59 years, were intranasally administered total doses of 84, 206 and 391 µg (4 women for each dosage). Peak plasma concentrations of 0.10, 0.35 and 1.59 µg/L were reached within 0.34, 0.46 and 0.28 h, respectively. 23 men, 20 to 54 years old, were administered a 400 µg dose of nafarelin subcutaneously and 304 µg intranasally. Mean peak concentrations of 13.66 µg/L were observed for the subcutaneous dose and 4.02 µg/L for the nasally administered dose. These levels were reached at 0.72 and 0.20 h, respectively. [R. L. Chan *et al.*, *Clin. Pharmacol. Ther.*, 1988, *44*, 275–282].

Bioavailability. 4 to 21% (intranasal administration).

Half-life. 3 to 4 h (intranasal administration). Also reported as 2.0 to 2.7 h after subcutaneous and intranasal administration.

Protein binding. 78 to 84%, mostly albumin.

Note. For a review of nafarelin, see P. Chrisp and K. L. Goa, *Drugs*, 1990, *39*, 523–551.

Dose. The usual dose is 200 to 800 µg twice daily intranasally.

Naftidrofuryl Oxalate

Vasodilator

Synonym. Nafronyl Oxalate

Proprietary names. Artocoron; Azunaftil; Di-Actane; Dusodril; Esedril; Gevatran; Luctor; Nafti; Naftilong; Naftilux; Naftodril; Praxilene; Sodipryl retard; StimLor.

Tetrahydro-α-(1-naphthalenylmethyl)-2-furanpropanoic acid 2-(diethylamino)ethyl ester acid oxalate

$C_{24}H_{33}NO_3,C_2H_2O_4$=473.6

CAS—31329-57-4 (naftidrofuryl); 3200-06-4 (oxalate)

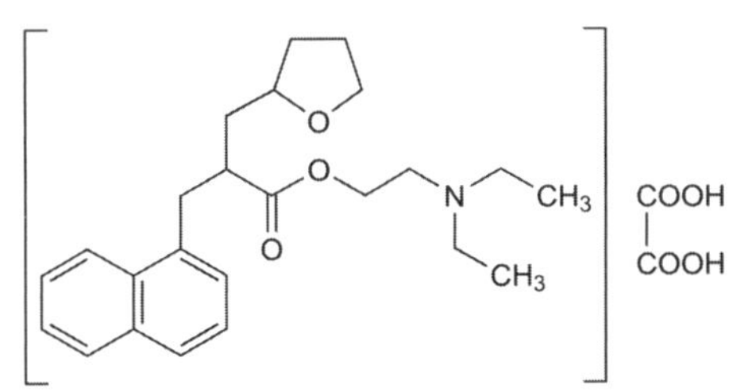

A white powder. M.p. about 108°.

Soluble in water.

Dissociation Constant. pK_a 8.2 (30°).

Partition Coefficient. Log *P* (octanol/water), 5.4 (naftidrofuryl).

Thin-layer Chromatography. Naftidrofuryl: system TA—Rf 64; system TB—Rf 52; system TC—Rf 41; system TE—Rf 78; system TL—Rf 35; system TAE—Rf 43.

Gas Chromatography. System GA—RI 2748.

High Performance Liquid Chromatography. Naftidrofuryl: system HY—RI 409; system HAA—Retention time(s) 15.8 min.

Ultraviolet Spectrum. Aqueous acid—273, 283 nm (A^1_1=141a). No alkaline shift.

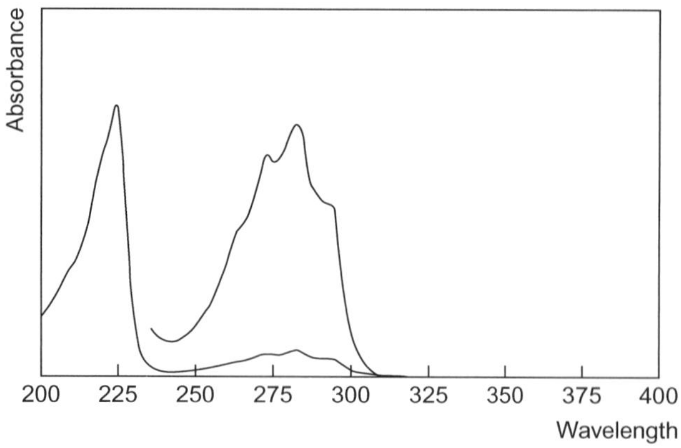

Infra-red Spectrum. Principal peaks at wavenumbers 1730, 1165, 722, 1280, 1620, 1070 cm^{-1} (KBr disk).

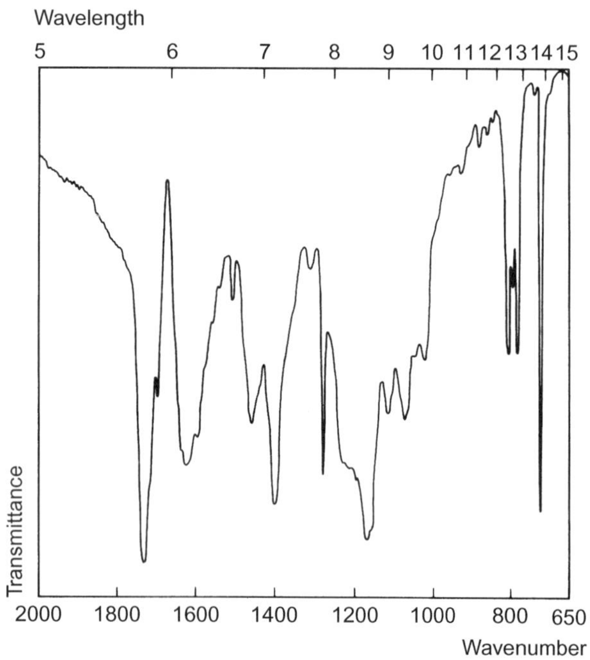

Mass Spectrum. Principal ions at *m/z* 86, 99, 100, 141, 87, 71, 44, 58 (naftidrofuryl).

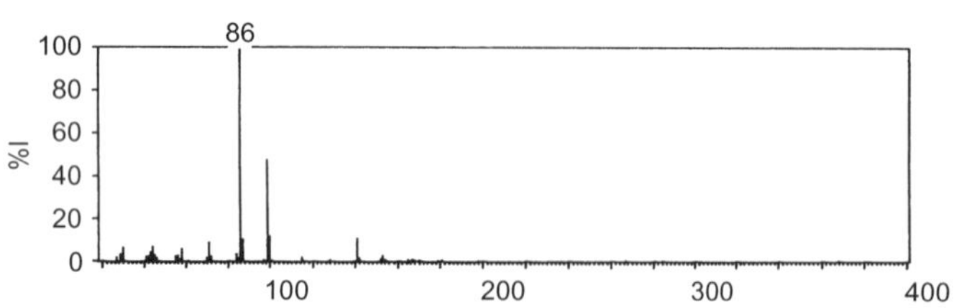

Quantification

High performance liquid chromatography. In plasma: limit of detection 20 µg/L, UV detection—R. R. Brodie *et al., J.Chromatogr.,* 1979, *164*; *Biomed. Appl.*, *6*, 534–540. In plasma: naftidrofuryl and its metabolite naftidrofuryl acid, limit of detection for naftidrofuryl 4 µg/L, fluorescence detection—P. Stehlik and H. Houbova, *Cesk. Farm.*, 1990, *39*, 394–399.

Disposition in the Body. Naftidrofuryl oxalate is absorbed after oral administration. It is metabolised by hydrolysis to the free acid, 3-(1-naphthyl)-2-tetrahydrofurfuryl propionic acid. Less than 1% of a dose is excreted in the urine in 48 h as free or conjugated naftidrofuryl. Most of a dose appears to be excreted in the bile.

Therapeutic concentration

After oral administration of 100 mg to 2 subjects, peak plasma concentrations averaging 0.21 mg/L were attained in 0.5 to 0.75 h. [R. R. Brodie *et al., J.Chromatogr.*, 1979, *164*; *Biomed. Appl.*, *6*, 534–540].

Dose. 300 to 600 mg daily.

Nalbuphine

Narcotic Analgesic

(5α,6α)-17-(Cyclobutylmethyl)-4,5-epoxymorphinan-3,6,14-triol
$C_{21}H_{27}NO_4$=357.4
CAS—20594-83-6

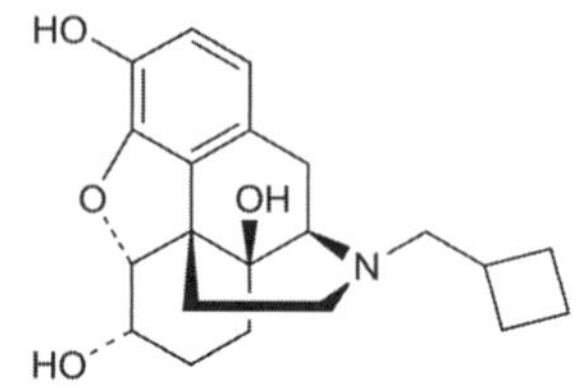

Crystals. M.p. about 231°.

Nalbuphine Hydrochloride
Synonym. EN-2234A
Proprietary names. Azerty; Bufigen; Bufilem; Intapan; Nalbu; Nubain.
$C_{21}H_{27}NO_4$,HCl=393.9
CAS—23277-43-2

Thin-layer Chromatography. System TB—Rf 00; system TE—Rf 34; system TAE—Rf 58; system TAJ—Rf 19; system TAK—Rf 00; system TAL—Rf 20.

Gas Chromatography. System GA—RI 2960; system GB—not eluted.

High Performance Liquid Chromatography. System HX—RI 295.

Ultraviolet Spectrum. Aqueous acid—284 nm (A_1^1=46b); aqueous alkali—297 nm.

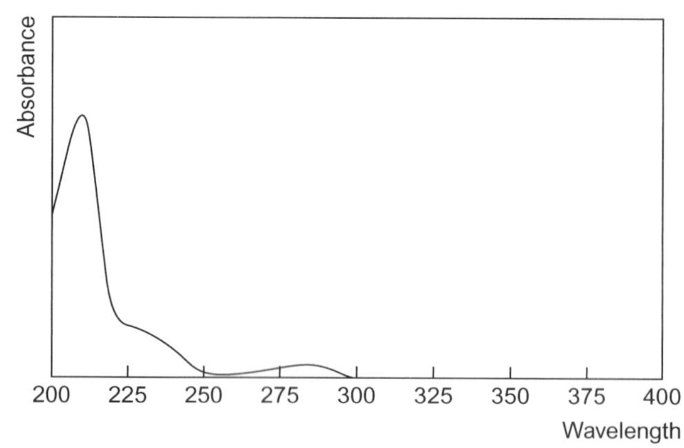

Infra-red Spectrum. Principal peaks at wavenumbers 970, 1080, 1033, 1060, 1115, 1495 cm^{-1}.

Quantification

Gas chromatography. In plasma: limit of detection 500 ng/L, ECD—S. H. Weinstein *et al., J. Pharm. Sci.*, 1978, *67*, 547–548.

Gas chromatography–mass spectrometry. In biological fluid: limit of detection 2 µg/g—P. Kintz *et al., J. Chromatogr.*, 1992, *579*, 172–176. In urine: nalbuphine and its metabolites nornalbuphine and 6-ketonalbuphine—Y. C. Yoo *et al., J. Anal. Toxicol.*, 1995, *19*, 120–123.

High performance liquid chromatography. In plasma: limit of detection 1 ng, electrochemical detection—C. L. Lake *et al., J. Chromatogr.*, 1982, *233*; *B Biomed. Appl.*, *22*, 410–416. In plasma: limit of detection 0.3 µg/L, electrochemical detection—L. M. Dube *et al., J. Chromatogr.*, 1988, *427*, 113–120. In plasma: limit of detection <50 ng/L, electrochemical detection—N. Wetzelsberger *et al., Arzneimittelforschung*, 1988, *38*, 1768–1771. In biological fluid: limit of detection 25 µg/g, diode-array detection—P.

Kintz *et al.*, *J. Chromatogr.*, 1992, *579*, 172–176. In plasma: limit of detection 0.1 µg/L, coulometric detection—E. Nicolle *et al.*, *J. Chromatogr.* 1995, *663*, *B Biomed. Appl.*, 111–117. In plasma: limit of detection <0.75 µg/L, UV detection—S. T. Ho *et al.*, *J. Chromatogr.* 1996, *678*, *B Biomed. Appl.*, 289–296. In plasma: limit of detection 0.1 µg/L, electrochemical detection—F. de Cazenove *et al.*, *J. Chromatogr. B Biomed. Sci. Appl.*, 1997, *690*, 203–210. In plasma: limit of detection 0.02 µg/L, electrochemical detection—E. Nicolle *et al.*, *J. Chromatogr. B, Biomed. Sci. Appl.*, 1997, *690*, 89–97.

Disposition in the Body. Nalbuphine is absorbed after oral administration, but there is thought to be considerable first-pass metabolism; it is rapidly absorbed after intramuscular or subcutaneous injection. The major metabolic reaction is conjugation to form nalbuphine glucuronide (inactive); oxidation to 6-oxonalbuphine occurs, and the desalkyl derivative, 7,8-dihydro-14-hydroxynormorphine, has also been identified as a metabolite. Unchanged nalbuphine, its conjugates and the two metabolites have been detected in the urine.

Therapeutic concentration

Following a single oral dose of 30 mg to 3 subjects, a peak plasma concentration of about 0.015 mg/L was attained in 1 h. Following a single IM dose of 10 mg to 6 subjects, peak plasma concentrations of 0.038 to 0.059 (mean 0.052) mg/L were attained in 15 to 30 min. [R. E. S. Bullingham, Pharmacokinetics of Nalbuphine, in *Opioid Agonist/Antagonist Drugs in Clinical Practice*, W. S. Nimmo and G. Smith (Ed.), Oxford, Excerpta Medica, 1984, pp 115–122].

Half-life. Plasma half-life, about 5 h.

Note. For a review of nalbuphine see J. K. Errick and R. C. Heel, *Drugs*, 1983, *26*, 191–211.

Dose. 10 to 20 mg of nalbuphine hydrochloride parenterally, every 3 to 6 h.

Nalidixic Acid

Antibacterial (Urinary)

Synonyms. Nalidixinic Acid; Win-18320.
Proprietary names. Acidex; Acinal; Betaxina; Fardixon; Labydon; Lidinal; Lidixin; Nadiwil; Nalidixan; Nalidixin; Nalidoid; Naligram; Nalissina; Nalix; NegGram; Negram; Puromylon; Seltomylon; Unidixina; Uralgin; Uriben; Uri-Flor; Urigram; Urlix; Urogram; Wintomilon; Winlomylon; Wintomylon. It is an ingredient of Mictral.
1-Ethyl-1,4-dihydro-7-methyl-4-oxo-1,8-naphthyridine-3-carboxylic acid
$C_{12}H_{12}N_2O_3$=232.2
CAS—389-08-2

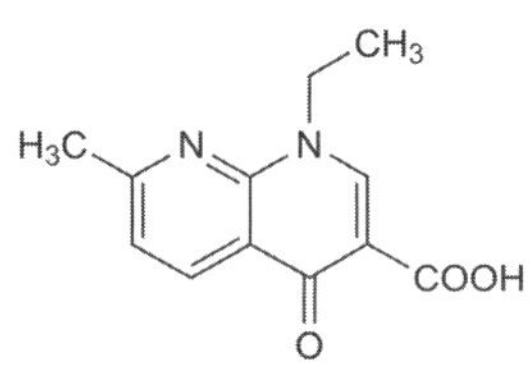

An almost white or very pale yellow crystalline powder. M.p. 229° to 230°. Practically insoluble in water; soluble 1 in 910 of ethanol and 1 in 35 of chloroform; very slightly soluble in ether; soluble in solutions of alkali hydroxides and carbonates.

Dissociation Constant. pK_a 6.0.

Partition Coefficient. Log *P* (octanol/water), 1.6.

Thin-layer Chromatography. System TD—Rf 39; system TE—Rf 02; system TF—Rf 31; system TAD—Rf 62; system TAE—Rf 63.

High Performance Liquid Chromatography. System HY—RI 380; system HAA—Retention time(s) 16.0 min.

Ultraviolet Spectrum. Aqueous acid—257 (A^1_1=1233b), 315 nm; aqueous alkali—258 (A^1_1=1120a), 334 nm.

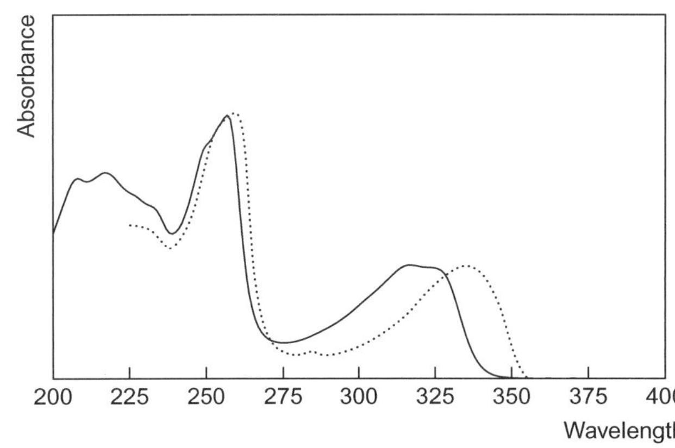

Infra-red Spectrum. Principal peaks at wavenumbers 1613, 1704, 809, 1250, 1225, 1515 cm^{-1} (KBr disk).

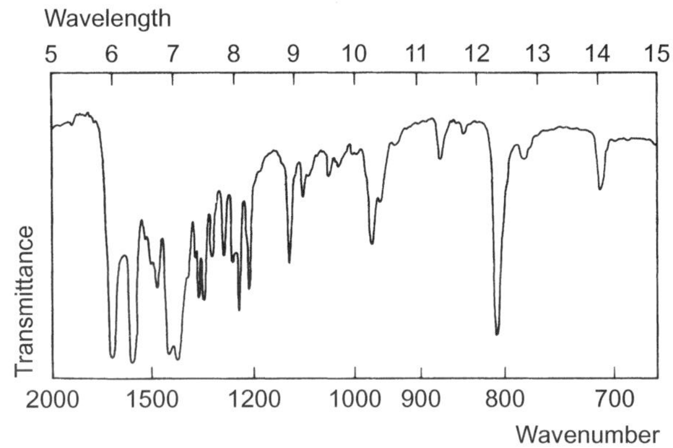

Mass Spectrum. Principal ions at *m/z* 188, 189, 159, 132, 53, 173, 131, 145.

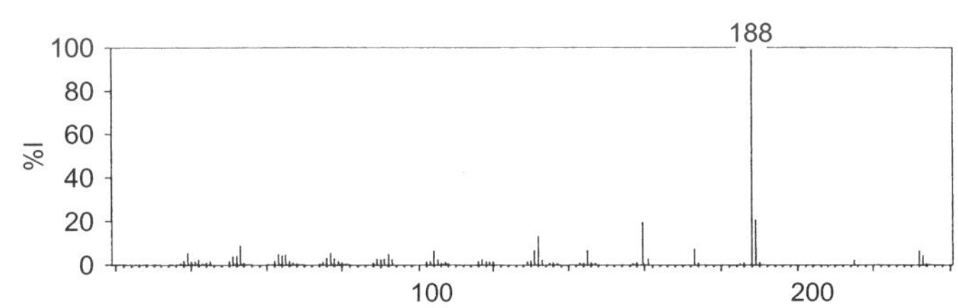

Quantification

Gas chromatography. In plasma: limit of detection 5 mg/L, FID—H. Roseboom *et al.*, *J. Chromatogr.*, 1979, *163*; *Biomed. Appl.*, *5*, 92–95. In urine: nalidixic acid and 3,7-dicarboxynalidixic acid, FID—S. M. Wu *et al.*, *Gaoxiong Yi Xue Ke Xue Za Zhi*, 1989, *5*, 630–636.

High performance liquid chromatography. In plasma or urine: nalidixic acid, 7-hydroxynalidixic acid and 7-carboxynalidixic acid, limit of detection 500 µg/L, UV detection—G. Cuisinaud *et al.*, *J. Chromatogr.*, 1980, *181*; *B Biomed. Appl.*, *7*, 399–406. In urine: nalidixic acid and other quinolone antibacterials, UV and fluorimetric detection—I. Duran Meras *et al.*, *J. Chromatogr. A*, 1997, *787*, 119–127. In plasma or urine: nalidixic acid and its metabolites—T. B. Vree *et al.*, *Pharm. World Sci.*, 1993, *15*, 98–104.

Thin-layer chromatography. In plasma: limit of detection 200 µg/L, fluorescence detection—H. K. L. Hundt and E. C. Barlow, *J.Chromatogr.*, 1981, *223*; *Biomed. Appl.*, *12*, 165–172.

Disposition in the Body. Nalidixic acid is readily absorbed after oral administration. The major metabolite, 7-hydroxynalidixic acid, is active; other metabolites include glucuronide conjugates of nalidixic acid and 7-hydroxynalidixic acid, and a 7-carboxy metabolite, all of which are inactive. About 80% of a dose is excreted in the urine in 8 h, mainly as glucuronide conjugates with about 2 to 3% as unchanged drug.

Therapeutic concentration

Following a single oral dose of 1 g to 11 female subjects, a mean peak plasma concentration of nalidixic acid of 27.3 mg/L was attained in 1.5 h; concentrations of 7-hydroxynalidixic acid reached a maximum of about 10 mg/L within 1 h. After repeated oral administration of 1 g twice daily to the same subjects, a peak plasma concentration of 33 mg/L of nalidixic acid was reported on the seventh day. Urinary concentrations of nalidixic acid plus 7-hydroxynalidixic acid following single or multiple dose administration were in excess of about 200 mg/L for 8 h in all subjects, and in some cases greater than 50 mg/L for 12 h. [N. Ferry *et al., Clin. Pharmacol. Ther.*, 1981, *29*, 695–698].

Toxicity. Toxic effects have been associated with plasma concentrations greater than 40 mg/L.

Half-life. Plasma half-life, nalidixic acid and the 7-hydroxy metabolite about 7 h; increased in renal failure to about 20 h.

Volume of distribution. About 0.4 L/kg.

Protein binding. In plasma, nalidixic acid about 93%, 7-hydroxynalidixic acid about 60%.

Dose. 2 to 4 g daily.

Nalmefene

Narcotic Antagonist

Synonyms. JF-1; ORF-11676.
(5α)-17-(Cyclopropylmethyl)-4,5-epoxy-6-methylenemorphinan-3,14-diol
$C_{21}H_{25}NO_3$=339.4
CAS—55096-26-9

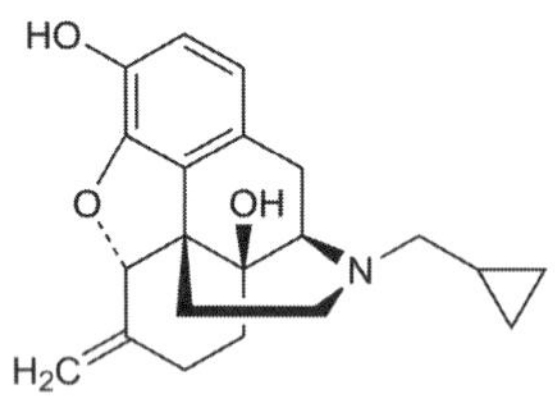

A white to off-white crystalline powder. M.p. 188° to 190°. It is soluble in water (140 mg/L at 25°).

Nalmefene Hydrochloride

Synonyms. Nalmetrene Hydrochloride; 6-Desoxy-6-methylene-naltrexone Hydrochloride.
Proprietary name. Revex
$C_{21}H_{25}NO_3$, HCl=375.9
CAS—58895-64-0
A white to off-white crystalline powder. M.p. 180° to 185° to a clear liquid. It is very soluble in water and methanol; soluble in ethanol (86.2 g/L), acetonitrile (1.07 g/L), acetone (0.23 g/L) and chloroform (0.13 g/L).

Dissociation Constant. pK_a 7.63 (hydrochloride).

Partition Coefficient. Log *P* (octanol/water), 2.66; −1.125 (hydrochloride).

Thin-layer Chromatography. Plate: silica gel 60 F_{254}. Mobile phase: cyclohexane:chloroform:diethylamine (10:75:15). UV detection (λ=254 nm). Rf values: nalmefen, Rf 0.41; bisnalmefene, Rf 0.07 [H. G. Brittain (Ed.), *Analytical Profiles of Drug Substances and Excipients,* Vol. 24, 1996, Academic Press, UK, pp. 351–395].

Gas Chromatography. Column: HP1 (0.2 mm i.d., 0.33 μm film thickness). Column temperature: 250°. Carrier gas: helium, flow rate 0.9 mL/min. Detection: flame ionisation. RI: 2700 [T. Mills and J. C. Roberson (Eds.), *Instrumental Data for Drug Analysis*, 2nd Edn., 1993, Boca Raton, CRC Press, Vol. 6, p. 162].

High Performance Liquid Chromatography. Column: phenyl (Nova-Pak Radial Pak, 100 × 8 mm i.d., 4 μm). Mobile phase: acetonitrile:water (containing sodium pentanesulfonic acid monohydrate (5 mM), pH 3.1 with orthophosphoric acid) (30:70), flow rate 1.2 mL/min. IS: nalbuphine. Electrochemical detection. Retention time(s): nalmefene, 12 min; IS, 7 min [J.Z Chou *et al., J.Chromatogr.*, 1993, *613*, 359–364].

Ultraviolet Spectrum. Methanol—211, 230, 285 nm; aqueous acid—284 nm; basic—298 nm.

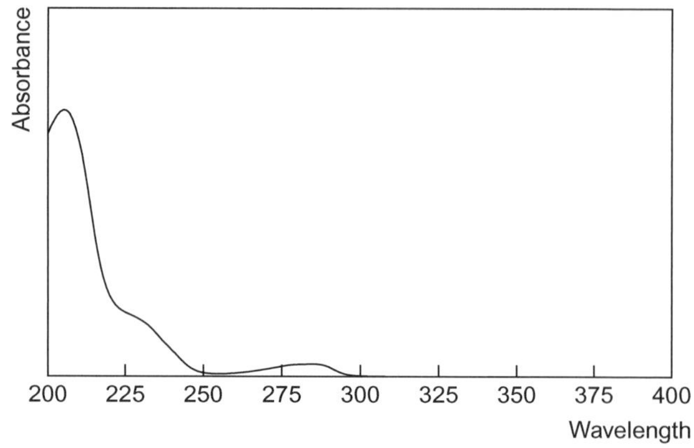

Infra-red Spectrum. Principal peaks at wavenumber 1170, 904, 814, 1619, 1638 cm^{-1}. (KBr disk).

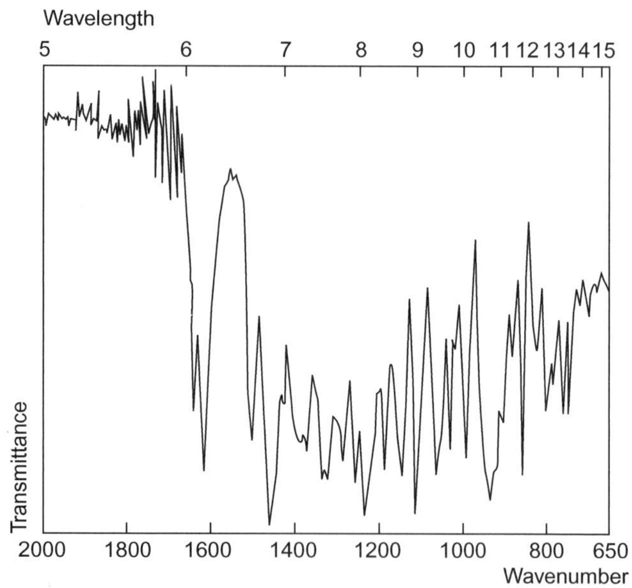

Mass Spectrum. Principal ions at *m/z* 55, 339, 110, 36, 298, 82, 242, 96.

Quantification

High performance liquid chromatography. In urine: limit of detection 80 μg/L. Electrochemical detection—R Dixon *et al., J. Clin. Pharmacol.*, 1987, *27,* 233–239. In plasma: limit of detection 3 μg/L. Electrochemical detection—J. Hiao and R. Dixon, *Res. Commun. Chem. Pathol. Pharmacol.*, 1983, *42*, 449–545.

Disposition in the Body. Nalmefene is rapidly and almost completely absorbed following oral administration, but absorption is delayed after intramuscular and subcutaneous injection. It is metabolised in the liver, mainly to the inactive glucuronide conjugate and trace amounts of *N*-dealkylated metabolite have been detected. It is mainly excreted in urine (83%) with some of the dose excreted in the faeces. It may undergo enterohepatic recycling. Less than 5% of a dose is excreted unchanged in urine and 17% in faeces.

Therapeutic concentration

24 healthy males, aged between 19 and 46 years, (average age 29 years), were administered with 2, 6, 12 and 24 mg doses of nalmefene hydrochloride after an overnight fast and continued 4 h after administration. The peak plasma concentrations were approx. 12, 36, 85 and 110 μg/L for the four doses, respectively, observed by the end of infusion [R. Dixon *et al., Clin. Pharmacol. Ther.*, 1986, *39(1)*, 49–53].

Young, healthy individuals, with a mean age of 23.8 years, and elderly individuals with a mean age of 70.7 years were administered with a 1 mg intravenous dose of nalmefene, and individuals, mean age 28.1 years and 68.3 years, a 2 mg dose. In the elderly, peak concentrations reached approx. 6.8, 3.8, 2.6, 1.2 and 0.4 μg/L at 0.08, 0.25, 0.5, 1.0 and 12.0 h after dosing. Peak concentrations of approx. 4.1, 3.1, 2.6, 1.2 and 0.38 μg/L were observed at the same time periods for the young individuals [R. F. Frye *et al.*, *Br. J. Clin. Pharmacol.*, 1996, *42(3)*, 301–306].

Half-life. Oral: 11 h, intravenous: 8 to 9 h.

Volume of distribution. 8.5 L/kg.

Clearance. 1.37 L/h/kg.

Protein binding. 45%.

Dose. The usual intravenous dose is 0.5 to 1 mg every 2 min up to 2 mg and orally 1 to 2 mg.

Nalorphine

Narcotic Antagonist

Synonyms. Allorphine; Autorphine; NANM.
(5α,6α)-7,8-Didehydro-4,5-epoxy-17-(2-propenyl)morphinan-3,6-diol
$C_{19}H_{21}NO_3$=311.4
CAS—62-67-9

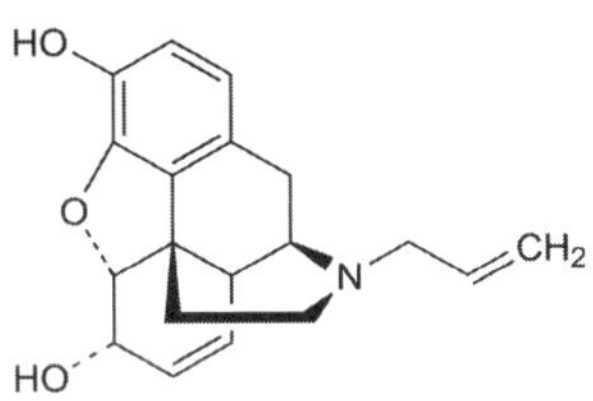

Crystals. M.p. 208°.
Sparingly soluble in water and ether; soluble in ethanol, acetone, dilute alkalis and chloroform.

Nalorphine Hydrobromide

Proprietary names. Lethidrone; Norfin.
$C_{19}H_{21}NO_3$,HBr=392.3
CAS—1041-90-3
A white to creamy-white crystalline powder. M.p. about 206°, with decomposition.
Soluble 1 in 24 of water and 1 in 35 of ethanol. Aqueous solutions may deposit crystals of the dihydrate; the dihydrate is readily soluble in dehydrated alcohol but the solution rapidly yields a deposit of the anhydrous salt.

Nalorphine Hydrochloride

Proprietary name. Nalline
$C_{19}H_{21}NO_3$,HCl=347.8
CAS—57-29-4
A white crystalline powder which slowly darkens on exposure to air and light. M.p. 260° to 263°.
Soluble 1 in 8 of water and 1 in 35 of ethanol; practically insoluble in chloroform and ether; soluble in dilute solutions of alkali hydroxides.

Dissociation Constant. pK_a 7.8 (20°).

Partition Coefficient. Log *P* (octanol/buffer pH 7.4), 1.5.

Colour Test. Marquis test—violet.

Thin-layer Chromatography. System TA—Rf 59; system TB—Rf 01; system TC—Rf 23; system TE—Rf 32; system TL—Rf 29; system TAE—Rf 57; system TAF—Rf 59; system TAJ—Rf 18; system TAK—Rf 01; system TAL—Rf 46. (Acidified iodoplatinate solution, positive.)

Gas Chromatography. System GA—RI 2620; system GB—not eluted.

High Performance Liquid Chromatography. System HA—*k* 1.0; system HAA—Retention time(s) 4.8 min; system HC—*k* 0.29; system HX—RI 260; system HY—RI 237.

Ultraviolet Spectrum. Aqueous acid—285 nm (A_1^1=49a); aqueous alkali—251 (A_1^1=190a), 298 nm (A_1^1=81a).

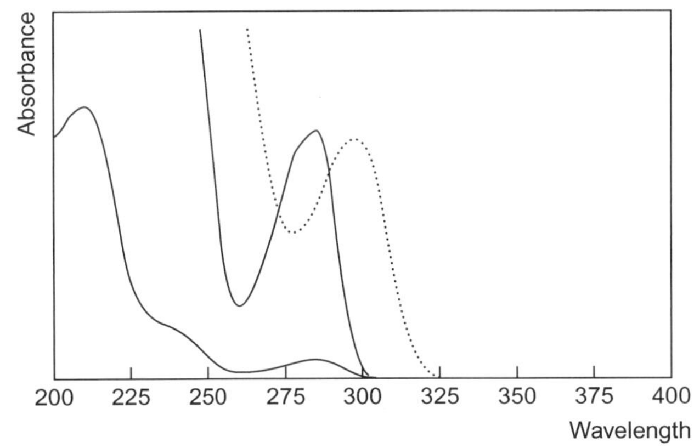

Infra-red Spectrum. Principal peaks at wavenumbers 1505, 1121, 1155, 1304, 805, 945 cm^{-1} (nalorphine hydrobromide, KBr disk).

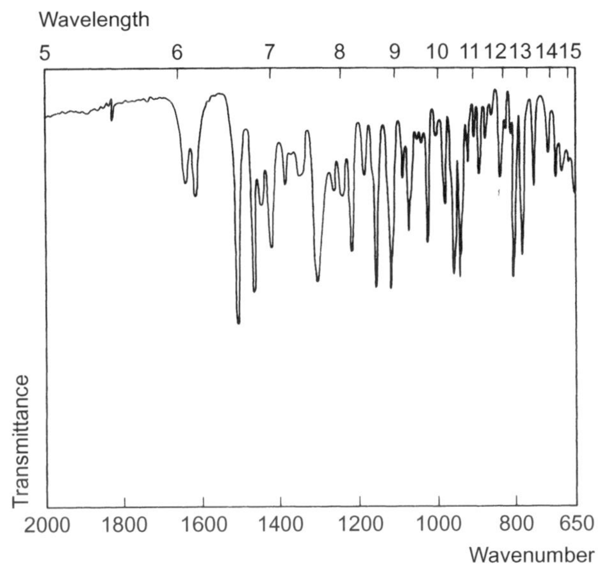

Mass Spectrum. Principal ions at *m/z* 311, 312, 41, 188, 80, 82, 81, 241.

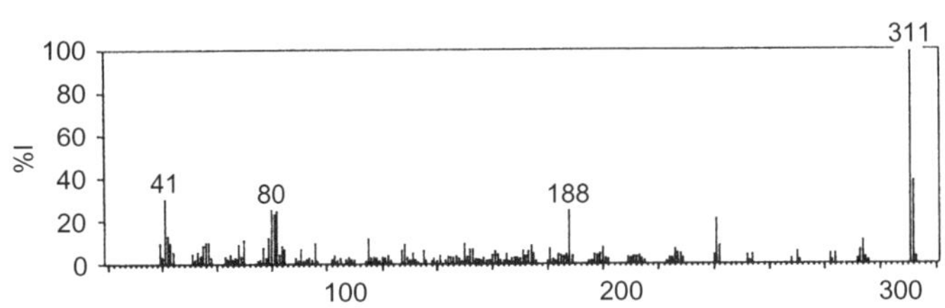

Disposition in the Body. Nalorphine is absorbed after oral administration but undergoes extensive first-pass metabolism. It is excreted in the urine mainly as metabolites and glucuronide conjugates with about 2 to 6% of a dose as unchanged drug.

Toxicity. The estimated minimum lethal dose is 200 mg. The administration of nalorphine to morphine addicts may be followed by a typical withdrawal syndrome.

Dose. 5 to 10 mg of nalorphine hydrobromide intravenously, repeated if necessary.

Naloxone

Narcotic Antagonist

Synonym. Allylnoroxymorphone
(5α)-4,5-Epoxy-3,14-dihydroxy-17-(2-propenyl)morphinan-6-one
$C_{19}H_{21}NO_4$=327.4
CAS—465-65-6

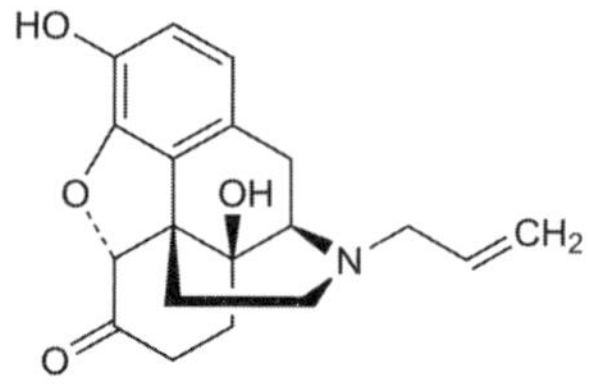

Crystals. M.p. 177° to 180°.
Soluble in chloroform; practically insoluble in petroleum ether.

Naloxone Hydrochloride

Synonym. EN-15304
Proprietary names. Nalone; Narcan; Narcanti; Naxolan; Zynox.
$C_{19}H_{21}NO_4$, HCl=363.8
CAS—357-08-4 (anhydrous); 51481-60-8 (dihydrate)
A white powder. M.p. 200° to 205°.
Soluble in water; slightly soluble in ethanol; practically insoluble in chloroform and ether.

Dissociation Constant. pK_a 7.9.

Partition Coefficient. Log *P* (octanol/buffer pH 7.4), 1.5.

Colour Tests. Folin–Ciocalteu reagent—blue; Liebermann's test—black; Mandelin's test—violet→brown; Marquis test—brown→violet.

Thin-layer Chromatography. System TA—Rf 65; system TB—Rf 09; system TC—Rf 66; system TE—Rf 47; system TL—Rf 63; system TAE—Rf 74; system TAJ—Rf 58; system TAK—Rf 01; system TAL—Rf 45. (Acidified iodoplatinate solution, positive.)

Gas Chromatography. System GA—RI 2715; system GB—not eluted.

High Performance Liquid Chromatography. System HA—*k* 1.4; system HC—*k* 0.17; system HY—RI 238; system HZ—Retention time(s) 2.0 min; system HAA—Retention time(s) 14.0 min.

Ultraviolet Spectrum. Aqueous acid—281 nm.

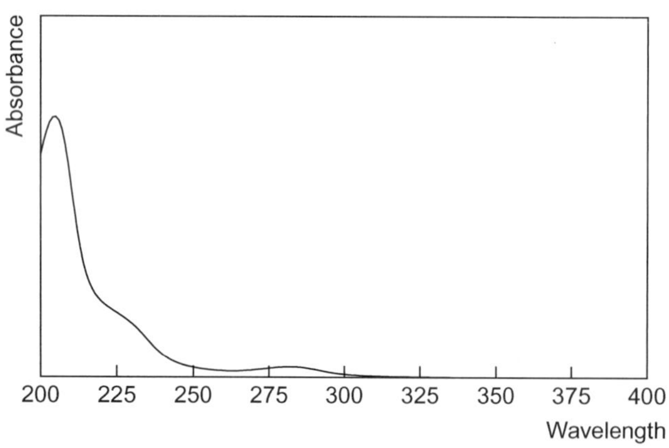

Infra-red Spectrum. Principal peaks at wavenumbers 1244, 1728, 940, 1230, 922, 1050 cm^{-1} (KBr disk).

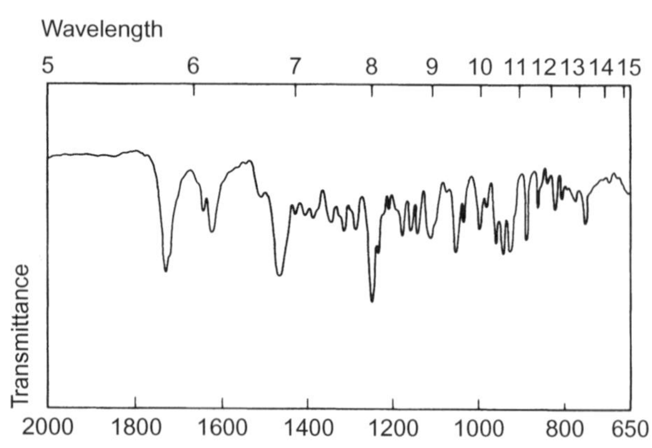

Mass Spectrum. Principal ions at *m*/*z* 327, 328, 41, 242, 286, 96, 229, 70.

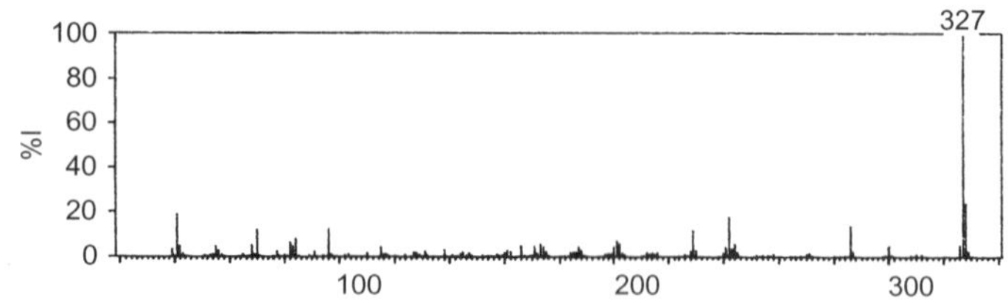

Quantification

Gas chromatography. In biological fluids: limit of detection 5 ng, ECD—P. J. Meffin and K. J. Smith, *J. Chromatogr.*, 1980, *183*; *Biomed. Appl.*, *9*, 352–356.

High performance liquid chromatography. In plasma or urine: naloxone and naltrexone, limit of detection 2 to 5 μg/L for plasma, 10 μg/L for urine, electrochemical detection—H. Derendorf *et al.*, *J. Pharm. Sci.*, 1984, *73*, 621–624. In biological fluids: naloxone, naltrexone and morphine, electrochemical detection—E. F. O'Connor *et al.*, *J. Chromatogr.*, 1989, *491*, 240–247. In plasma: limit of detection 3 μg/L, electrochemical detection—H. Albeck *et al.*, *J. Chromatogr.*, 1989, *488*, 435–445.

Radioimmunoassay. In plasma: limit of detection < 500 ng/L—E. F. Hahn *et al.*, *J. Pharm. Pharmacol.*, 1983, *35*, 833–836.

Disposition in the Body. Naloxone is rapidly absorbed after oral administration but undergoes extensive first-pass metabolism. It is rapidly but incompletely excreted in the urine, mainly as conjugated metabolites, with about 30% of a dose being excreted in 6 h but only 60% being excreted in 72 h. Metabolites which have been identified include naloxone-3-glucuronide and the *N*-desalkyl and 6-hydroxy derivatives together with their glucuronide conjugates.

Therapeutic concentration

Following intravenous administration of 0.4 mg to 9 subjects, mean serum concentrations of 0.01 mg/L were reported after 2 min. [S. H. Ngai *et al.*, *Anesthesiology*, 1976, *44*, 398–401].

During constant intravenous infusion of 0.02 mg/min to 3 subjects, steady-state plasma concentrations of 0.014, 0.015 and 0.030 mg/L were reported. [E. F. Hahn *et al.*, *J. Pharm. Pharmacol.*, 1983, *35*, 833–836].

3 subjects were given naloxone orally once daily. Peak plasma levels of 3.35 and 6.1 mg/L were achieved in the first subject with a dose of 12 and 16 mg, respectively; peak plasma levels for the second subject were 7.3 and 8.0 mg/L after doses of 12 and 16 mg, respectively, and less than 5 mg/L after a dose of 16 mg for the third subject. [J. A. Culpepper-Morgan *et al.*, *Clin. Pharmacol. Ther.*, 1992, *52*, 90–95].

Half-life. Plasma half-life, about 1 to 2 h.

Volume of distribution. About 3 L/kg.

Clearance. Plasma clearance, about 20 to 30 mL/min/kg.

Protein binding. In plasma, about 40%.

Dose. 0.4 to 2 mg of naloxone hydrochloride parenterally, repeated as necessary.

Naltrexone

Narcotic Antagonist

Synonym. UM-792
(5α)-17-(Cyclopropylmethyl)-4,5-epoxy-3,14-dihydroxymorphinan-6-one
$C_{20}H_{23}NO_4$=341.4
CAS-16590-41-3

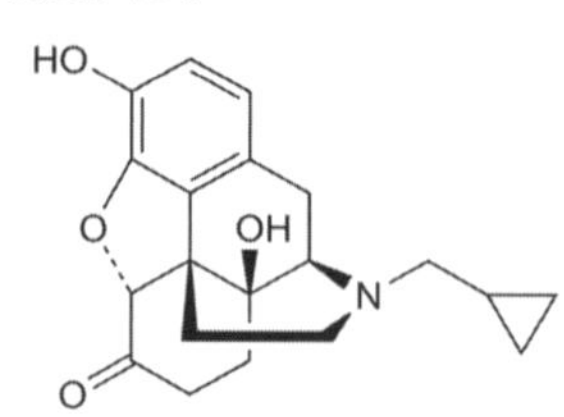

Crystals. M.p. 168° to 170°.

Naltrexone Hydrochloride
Proprietary names. Antaxone; Basinal; Celupan; Depade; Nalorex; Narcoral; Nemexin; Revia; Trexan.
$C_{20}H_{23}NO_4,HCl=377.9$
CAS-16676-29-2
A white powder. M.p. 274° to 276°.
Soluble in water, dilute acids and alkali.

Partition Coefficient. Log *P* (octanol/water), 1.9.

Thin-layer Chromatography. System TAJ—Rf 49; system TAK—Rf 01; system TAL—Rf 40.

Gas Chromatography. System GA—RI 2880; system GB—not eluted.

Ultraviolet Spectrum. Aqueous acid—281 nm (A_1^1=34b); aqueous alkali—293 nm.

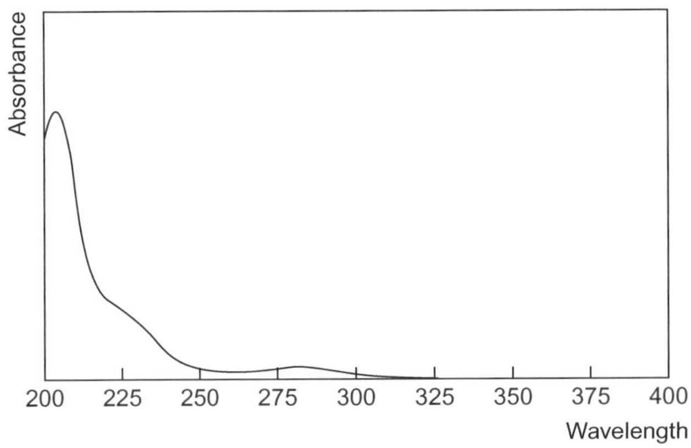

Infra-red Spectrum. Principal peaks at wavenumbers 1716, 1505, 1280, 1639, 1115, 909 cm^{-1} (naltrexone hydrochloride, KBr disk).

Mass Spectrum. Principal ions at *m/z* 341, 55, 36, 300, 342, 110, 243, 256.

Quantification

Gas chromatography. In plasma, erythrocytes, saliva or urine: naltrexone, 6*β*-naltrexol and 2-hydroxy-3-methoxy-6*β*-naltrexol, limit of detection 0.5 to 1 μg/L in plasma, ECD and FID—K. Verebey *et al., J. Anal. Toxicol.*, 1980, *4*, 33–37.

Gas chromatography–mass spectrometry. In plasma or milk: naltrexone and its metabolite 6*β*-naltrexol—C. F. Chan *et al., J. Chromatogr. B, Biomed. Sci. Appl.*, 2001, *761*, 85–92.

High performance liquid chromatography. In biological fluids: naltrexone, naloxone and morphine, electrochemical detection—E. F. O'Connor *et al., J. Chromatogr.*, 1989, *491*, 240–247.

Disposition in the Body. Naltrexone is rapidly and almost completely absorbed after oral administration. It is metabolised by reduction to 6*β*-naltrexol which has weak activity; both naltrexone and 6*β*-naltrexol are conjugated with glucuronic acid. About 40% of an oral dose is excreted in the urine in 24 h, with about 8% of the dose as naltrexone (mainly conjugated), 26% as 6*β*-naltrexol (mainly unconjugated), and about 4% as free 2-hydroxy-3-methoxy-6*β*-naltrexol. About 2% of a dose is eliminated in the faeces in 24 h, mainly as 6*β*-naltrexol.

Therapeutic concentration
After a single oral dose of 100 mg to 4 subjects, peak plasma concentrations of 0.01 to 0.06 (mean 0.04) mg/L of naltrexone and 0.08 to 0.13 (mean 0.10) mg/L of 6*β*-naltrexol were attained in 1 to 2 h and 1 to 4 h, respectively. [K. Verebey *et al., Clin. Pharmacol. Ther.*, 1976, *20*, 315–328].

Half-life. Plasma half-life, after oral administration, about 10 h for naltrexone and about 12 h for 6*β*-naltrexol; after intravenous administration, naltrexone about 3 h.

Volume of distribution. About 20 L/kg.

Clearance. Plasma clearance, about 70 mL/min/kg.

Protein binding. In plasma, about 20%.

Note. For a review of the pharmacokinetics of naltrexone, see B. L. Crabtree, *Clin. Pharm.*, 1984, *3*, 273–280.

Dose. Usually 50 mg of naltrexone hydrochloride daily.

Nandrolone

Anabolic Steroid

Synonym. Nortestosterone
(17*β*)-17-Hydroxyestr-4-en-3-one
$C_{18}H_{26}O_2=274.4$
CAS—434-22-0

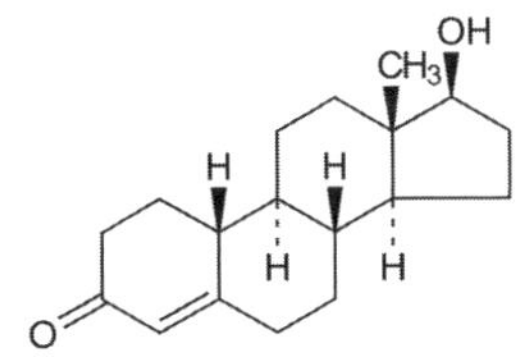

Crystals. Two polymorphic forms occur; m.p. 112°, and 124°.
Soluble in ethanol, chloroform, and ether.

Nandrolone Decanoate
Synonym. Nortestosterone Decylate
Proprietary names. Androlone-D; Deca-Durabol; Deca-Durabolin; Deca-Noralone; Hybolin Decanoate; Kabolin; Neo-Durabolic.
$C_{28}H_{44}O_3=428.7$
CAS—360-70-3
A white to creamy-white crystalline powder. M.p. 32° to 35°.
Practically insoluble in water; soluble 1 in 1 of ethanol; freely soluble in acetone, chloroform and ether.

Nandrolone Phenylpropionate
Synonyms. Nandrolone Phenpropionate; 19-Norandrostenolone Phenylpropionate; Nortestosteronum Phenylpropionicum.
Proprietary names. Activin; Androlone; Durabolin; Nandrolin; Noralone; Stenabolin.
$C_{27}H_{34}O_3=406.6$
CAS—62-90-8
A white crystalline powder. M.p. 95° to 96°.
Practically insoluble in water; soluble 1 in 20 of ethanol; soluble in chloroform.

Nandrolone Cyclohexanecarboxylate
Synonyms. 19-Nortestosterone Hexahydrobenzoate
Proprietary names. Norlongandron; Nor-Durandron.
$C_{25}H_{36}O_3=384.6$
CAS—18470-94-5

Nandrolone Propionate
Synonym. 19-Nortestosterone Propionate
Proprietary names. Norybol-19; Nortesto.
$C_{21}H_{30}O_3=330.5$

Partition Coefficient. Log *P* (octanol/water), 2.6.

Thin-layer Chromatography. Nandrolone decanoate: system TP—Rf 88; system TQ—Rf 49; system TR—Rf 97; system TS—Rf 95.
Nandrolone phenylpropionate: System TP—Rf 87; system TQ—Rf 48; system TR—Rf 97; system TS—Rf 95.

Gas Chromatography. System GA—nandrolone RI 2395; nandrolone-TMS RI 2760; system GAG—RRT 0.91 (relative to testosterone); system GAR—nandrolone, Retention time 12.5 min.

High Performance Liquid Chromatography. System HAR—RRT 0.84 (relative to testosterone); system HATb—RRT 0.92 (relative to testosterone).

Ultraviolet Spectrum. Nandrolone decanoate:dehydrated alcohol—240 nm (A_1^1=407a).
Nandrolone phenylpropionate:dehydrated alcohol—240 nm (A_1^1=430a).

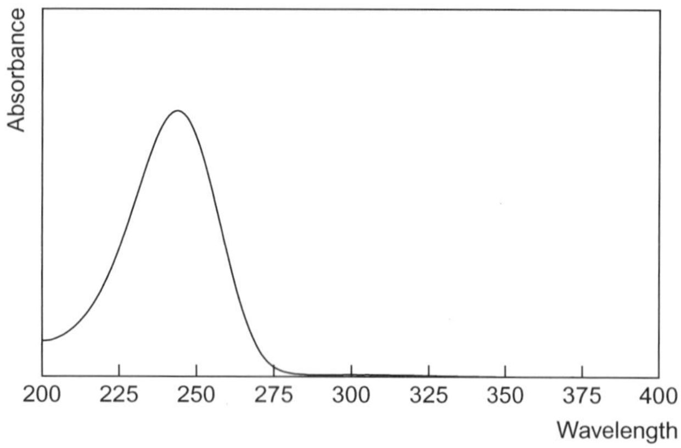

Infra-red Spectrum. Principal peaks at wavenumbers 1679, 1733, 1205, 1178, 1255, 692 cm^{-1} (nandrolone phenylpropionate).

Disposition in the body. In man, nandrolone is excreted in the urine mainly as the two metabolites, 19-norandrosterone and 19-noretiocholanolone. In the horse, the major metabolites are 5α-estrane-3β,17α-diol, excreted mainly as the glucuronide conjugate, and its 17β-epimer which is excreted as the sulfate conjugate.

Dose. By IM injection: 25 to 100 mg of nandrolone decanoate every 3 weeks; 25 to 50 mg of nandrolone phenylpropionate weekly.

Naphazoline

Sympathomimetic

4,5-Dihydro-2-(1-naphthalenylmethyl)-1*H*-imidazole
$C_{14}H_{14}N_2=210.3$
CAS—835-31-4

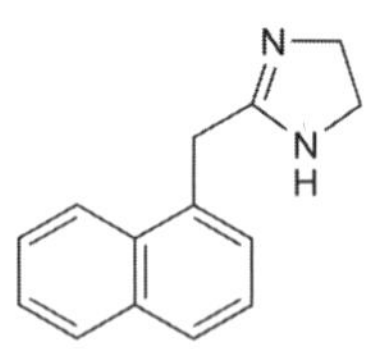

M.p. about 120°.

Naphazoline Hydrochloride

Proprietary names. Aconex; Ak-Con; Albalon; All Clear; Allerest; Allersol; Clear Eyes; Clera; Coldan; Degest; Isoftal; Murine; Nafazair; Napha Forte; Naphcon; Optazine; Privine; Rhino-Mex-N; Rhinon; Rhinoperd; Vasocon.
$C_{14}H_{14}N_2,HCl=246.7$
CAS—550-99-2
A white crystalline powder. M.p. about 255° to 260°.
Soluble 1 in 6 of water and 1 in 15 of ethanol; slightly soluble in chloroform; insoluble in benzene and ether.

Naphazoline Nitrate

Proprietary names. Deltarhinol-Mono; Imidazyl; Privin; Rinazina. It is an ingredient of Antistin-Privine.
$C_{14}H_{14}N_2,HNO_3=273.3$
CAS—5144-52-5
A white crystalline powder. M.p. about 168°.
Soluble 1 in 36 of water and 1 in 16 of ethanol; very slightly soluble in chloroform; practically insoluble in ether.

Dissociation Constant. pK_a 10.9 (20°).

Partition Coefficient. Log *P* (chloroform/pH 7.4), −0.3.

Colour Tests. Mandelin's Test—brown-violet; Marquis Test—grey-green.

Thin-layer Chromatography. System TA—Rf 14; system TB—Rf 03; system TC—Rf 06; system TE—Rf 27; system TAE—Rf 03; system TAF—Rf 52. (Dragendorff spray, positive; acidified iodoplatinate solution, positive; Marquis reagent, green.)

Gas Chromatography. System GA—RI 2100; system GC—RI 2457.

High Performance Liquid Chromatography. System HA—*k* 2.4; system HX—RI 320; system HY—RI 263; system HAX—Retention time, 9.1 min; system HAY—Retention time, 4.8 min.

Ultraviolet Spectrum. Aqueous acid—271, 281 nm (A^1_1=321a), 288, 291 nm. No alkaline shift.

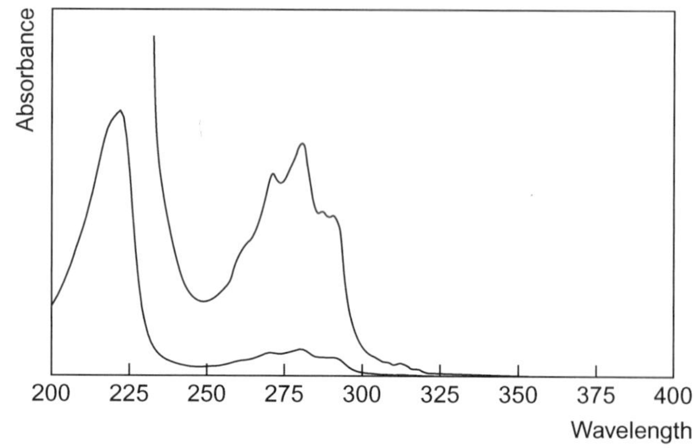

Infra-red Spectrum. Principal peaks at wavenumbers 1615, 780, 1499, 791, 1211, 800 cm^{-1} (KBr disk).

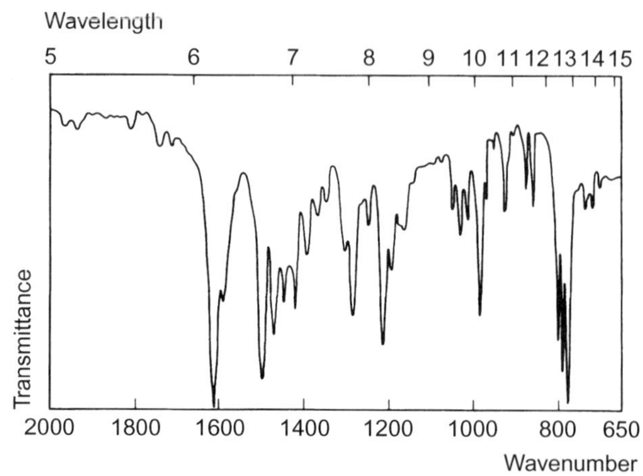

Mass Spectrum. Principal ions at *m*/*z* 209, 210, 141, 115, 153, 208, 46, 181.

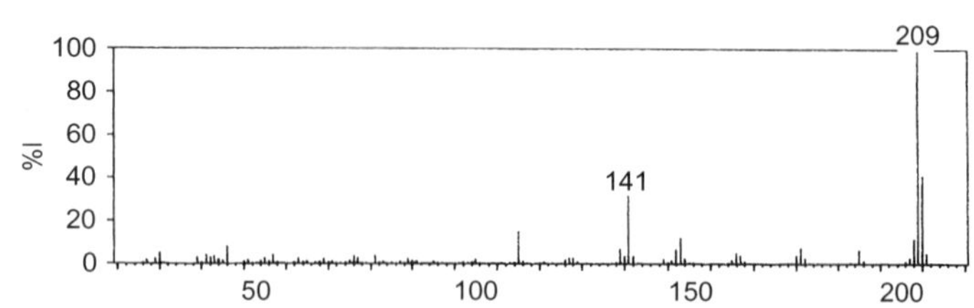

Disposition in the Body. Systemic absorption has been reported following topical application of solutions of naphazoline. It is not used systemically but is readily absorbed from the gastro-intestinal tract.

Toxicity. The estimated minimum lethal dose is 10 mg, intranasally.

Use. Naphazoline hydrochloride and nitrate are used as 0.05 to 0.1% aqueous solutions.

Naphthalene

Antiseptic/Anthelmintic

Synonym. Naphthalin
$C_{10}H_8=128.2$

CAS—91-20-3

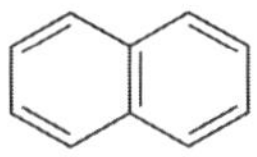

Colourless transparent scales. M.p. 80.2°. B.p. 218°.
Insoluble in water; soluble 1 in 13 of ethanol, 1 in 3.5 of benzene or toluene, 1 in 1.2 of carbon disulfide and 1 in 2 of chloroform or carbon tetrachloride; very soluble in ether.

Partition Coefficient. Log *P* (octanol/water), 3.3.

Gas Chromatography. System GA—RI 1186.

High Performance Liquid Chromatography. System HY—RI 558; system HAA—Retention time(s) 23.3 min.

Ultraviolet Spectrum. Ethanol—266 nm (A_1^1=411b), 275 (A_1^1=454b), 286 nm (A_1^1=307b).

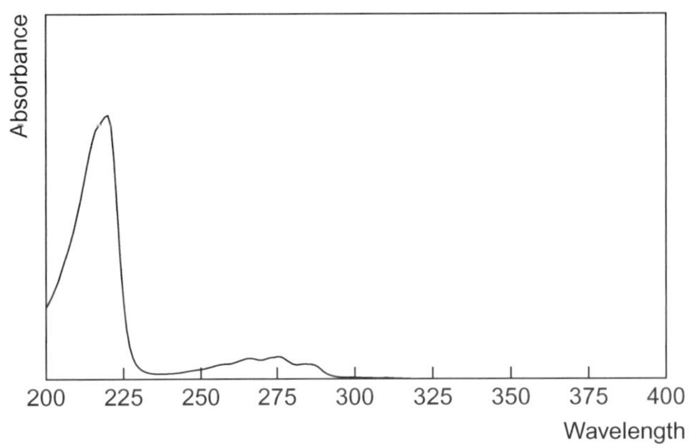

Naproxen

Analgesic

Synonyms. Naproxenum; RS-3540.
Proprietary names. Arthrosin; Arthroxen; Condrotex; Laraflex; Laser; Napratec; Naprel; Naprex; Naprius; Naprobene; Naprocoat; Naprodil; Naprometin; Napromex; Napronet; Naproscript; Naproaian; Naprosyn(e); Naproval; Naproxi; Napxen; Nycopren; Proxen; Rimoxyn; Timpron; Xenar.
(αS)-6-Methoxy-α-methyl-2-naphthaleneacetic acid
$C_{14}H_{14}O_3$=230.3
CAS—22204-53-1

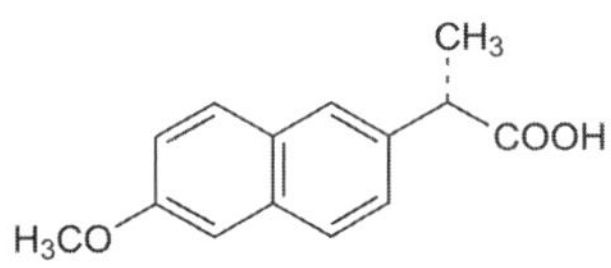

A white crystalline powder. M.p. 152° to 154° (crystals from acetone-hexane).
Practically insoluble in water; soluble 1 in 25 of ethanol, 1 in 15 of chloroform, and 1 in 40 of ether.

Naproxen Sodium

Synonym. RS-3650
Proprietary names. Aleve; Anaprox; Naprelan; Naprodil; Naprogesic; Naprorex; Naproso; Naprosyn; Naprovite; Synflex.
$C_{14}H_{13}NaO_3$=252.2
CAS—26159-34-2
M.p. 244° to 246° (crystals from acetone).

Dissociation Constant. pK_a 4.2 (25°).

Partition Coefficient. Log *P* (octanol/water), 3.2.

Colour Tests. Liebermann's Test—black-green; Marquis Test—brown; Sulfuric Acid—orange.

Thin-layer Chromatography. System TD—Rf 33; system TE—Rf 06; system TF—Rf 38; system TG—Rf 14; system TAD—Rf 44; system TAE—Rf 82; system TAJ—Rf 60; system TAK—Rf 75; system TAL—Rf 93. (Ludy Tenger reagent, orange.)

Gas Chromatography. System GA—naproxen RI 2045, naproxen-Me RI 1980, M (*O*-desmethyl-)-Me_2 RI 1980, M (OH-)-Me_2 RI 1800; system GB—naproxen RI 2337, M (*O*-desmethyl-) RI 2396; system GD—naproxen-Me RRTs 1.37 and 1.18 (relative to *n*-$C_{16}H_{34}$); system GL—naproxen-Me RI 2120, M (*O*-desmethyl-)-Me_2 RI 2120, M (OH-)-Me_2 RI 1800.

High Performance Liquid Chromatography. System HD—*k* 3.3; system HF—RRT 0.67 (relative to meclofenamic acid); system HX—RI 501; system HY—RI 468; system HZ—retention time 6.8 min; system HAX—retention time 7.0 min; system HAY—retention time 7.2 min.

Ultraviolet Spectrum. Aqueous acid—262 (A_1^1=208b), 272 (A_1^1=215b), 315 (A_1^1=52b), 328 (A_1^1=63b); aqueous alkali—261 (A_1^1=218b), 271 (A_1^1=218b), 316, 330 nm.

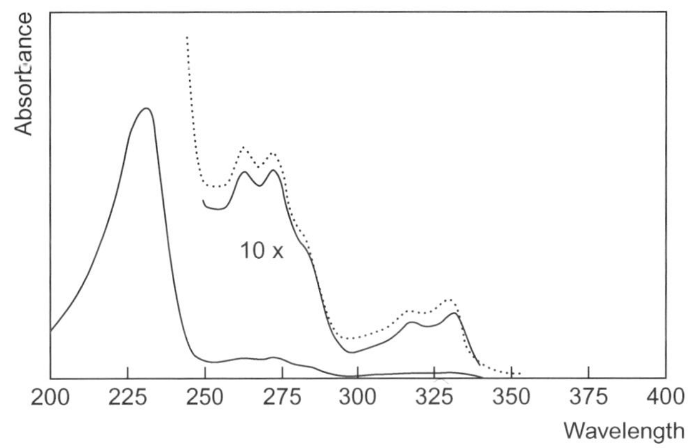

Infra-red Spectrum. Principal peaks at wavenumbers 1724, 1174, 1155, 1223, 1190, 1681 cm^{-1} (KBr disk).

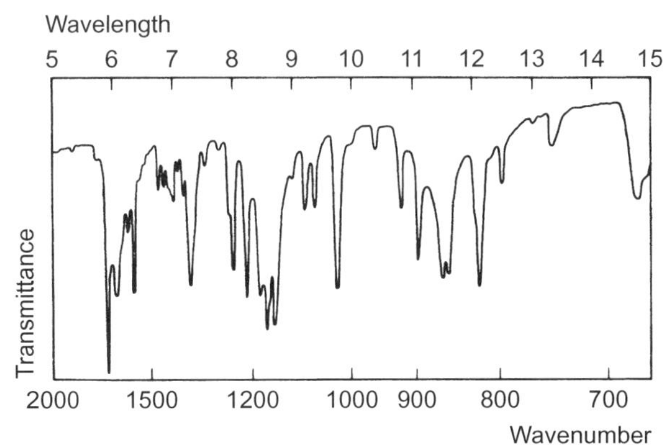

Mass Spectrum. Principal ions at *m/z* 185, 230, 141, 186, 184, 115, 170, 153.

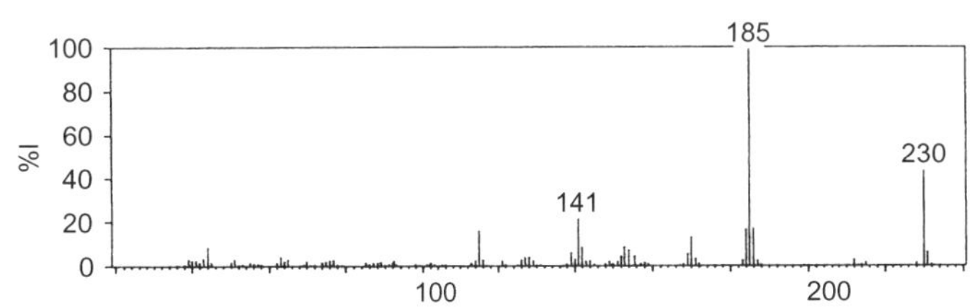

Quantification

Ultraviolet spectrophotometry. In serum—M. Holzbecher *et al.*, *Clin. Biochem.*, 1979, *12*, 66–67.

Spectrofluorimetry. In serum: limit of detection 500 µg/L—M. Anttila, *J. Pharm. Sci.*, 1977, *66*, 433–434.

Gas chromatography. In serum: limit of detection 2 mg/L, FID—S. S. Weber *et al.*, *Ther. Drug Monit.*, 1981, *3*, 75–83. In urine: naproxen and metabolites, FID—S. H. Wan and S. B. Matin, *J. Chromatogr.*, 1979, *170*, 473–478.

High performance liquid chromatography. In plasma or urine: naproxen and 6-*O*-desmethylnaproxen, limit of detection 100 µg/L, fluorescence detection—J. W. A. van Loenhout *et al.*, *J. Liq. Chromatogr.*, 1982, *5*, 549–561. In plasma or urine: naproxen and 6-*O*-desmethylnaproxen and conjugates—J. V. Andersen and S. H. Hansen, *J. Chromatogr.*, 1992, *577*, 325–333. In plasma or urine: naproxen and 6-*O*-desmethylnaproxen and conjugates, limit of quantification 1.5 mg/L—T. B. Vree *et al.*, *J. Chromatogr.*, 1992, *578*, 239–249. In plasma or synovial fluid, naproxen, ibuprofen and diclofenac—I.S. Blagbrough *et al.*, *J. Chromatogr.*, 1992, *578*, 251–257. In urine: naproxen and other NSAIDs, limit of detection 5 µg/L, UV detection—T. Hirai *et al.*, *J. Chromatogr. B Biomed. Sci. Appl.*, 1997, *692*, 375–388. In urine: naproxen and nabumetone and its metabolite, limit of detection for naproxen 3 ng, UV detection—E. Mikami *et al.*, *J. Pharm. Biomed. Anal.*, 2000, *23*, 917–925.

Disposition in the Body. Readily and almost completely absorbed after oral or rectal administration. Naproxen crosses the placenta and small amounts are found in breast milk; it also diffuses into synovial fluid. About 50% of a dose is excreted in the urine in 24 h and about 94% in 5 days together with about 1 to 2% in the faeces. Of the material excreted in the urine, approximately 60% is conjugated naproxen, 5% is 6-*O*-desmethylnaproxen, and 20% is conjugated desmethylnaproxen. Less than 10% of the excreted material is unchanged drug.

Hydrolysis of conjugated naproxen has been reported during storage of urine samples, and assays carried out immediately after collection suggested that only very small amounts of unchanged drug were excreted. [R. A. Upton *et al.*, *J. Pharm. Sci.*, 1980, *69*, 1254–1257.]

Therapeutic concentration. Plasma concentrations are dose-dependent at doses of up to 500 mg twice daily; at larger doses the increase in concentration is non-linear and renal clearance is accelerated.

Following single oral doses of 250 mg to 6 subjects, peak plasma concentrations of 26 to 51 mg/L (mean 38) were attained in 2 to 4 h; peak plasma concentrations of 49 to 69 mg/L (mean 60) were attained in 3 subjects, 2 h after a single oral dose of 500 mg; peak concentrations of the desmethyl metabolite were about 0.1 to 0.2 mg/L. [G. Tomson *et al.*, *Clin. Pharmacol. Ther.*, 1981, *29*, 168–173.]

Toxicity

A serum concentration of 414 mg/L was reported in one subject 15 h after the ingestion of 25 g of naproxen; the only toxic effect was mild gastro-intestinal distress. [E. W. Fredell and L. J. Strand, *JAMA*, 1977, *238*, 938.]

A 15-year-old girl who had rapidly developed severe metabolic acidosis and seizures after ingesting approx. 50 × 275 mg naproxen sodium tablets (each containing 250 mg naproxen and 25 mg sodium) had a serum naproxen concentration of 12.9 g/L 14.5 h after the ingestion; serum bicarbonate levels returned to normal after 12.5 h. [R. Martinez *et al.*, *Ann. Emerg. Med.*, 1989, *18*, 1102–1104.]

Half-life. Plasma half-life, 10 to 20 h (mean 14).

Volume of distribution. About 0.16 L/kg.

Clearance. Plasma clearance, 0.13 mL/min/kg.

Protein binding. In plasma, more than 99% at normal therapeutic concentrations; decreased at higher plasma concentrations and in subjects with liver disease.

Note. For a review of naproxen, see R. N. Brogden *et al.*, *Drugs*, 1979, *18*, 241–277 and for a review of its pharmacokinetics, see N. M. Davies and K. E. Anderson, *Clin. Pharmacokinet.*, 1997, *32*, 268–293.

Dose. Usually 0.5 to 1 g daily.

Naratriptan

Antimigraine

Synonym. GR-85548X
N-Methyl-3-(1-methyl-4-piperidinyl)-1*H*-indole-5-ethanesulfonamide
$C_{17}H_{25}N_3O_2S = 335.4$
CAS—121679-13-8

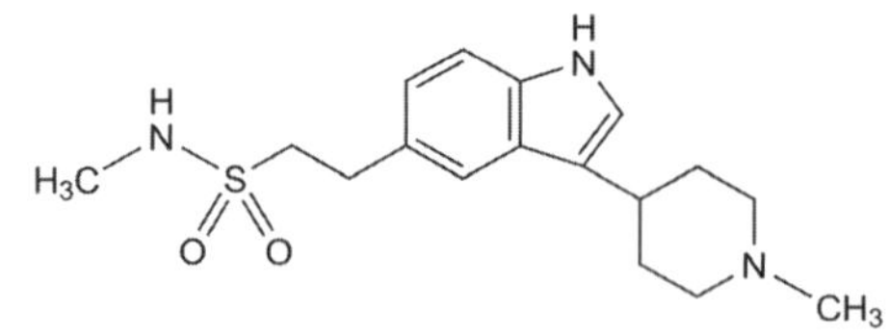

Crystals from ethyl acetate, m.p. 170° to 171°.

Naratriptan Hydrochloride

Synonym. GR-85548A
Proprietary names. Amerge; Naramig.
$C_{17}H_{25}N_3O_2S,HCl = 371.9$
CAS—121679-19-4; 143388-64-1
Microcrystals, m.p. 237 to 239°.

High Performance Liquid Chromatography. System HZ—retention time 2.1 min.

Column: (analytical) silica (Alltech, 150 × 2.1 mm i.d., 5 µm); (guard) C_8 (Optiguard, 1 mm). Mobile phase: ammonium acetate (20 mM, pH 4 with glacial acetic acid, to pH 2.7 with formic acid):methanol:acetonitrile (80:10:10), flow rate 300 µL/min. IS: bufotemine. MS–MS detection (ESI, MRM with *m/z*: 336 to 98 for naratriptan and 205 to 160 for IS). Retention time(s): naratriptan, 2.71 min; IS, 2.35 min. [K. Vishwanathan *et al.*, *Rapid Commun. Mass Spectrom.*, 2000, *14(3)*, 168–172].

Ultraviolet Spectrum. Aqueous acid (pH 2.38)—224, 278, 284, 295 nm; ethanol—285, 296 nm.

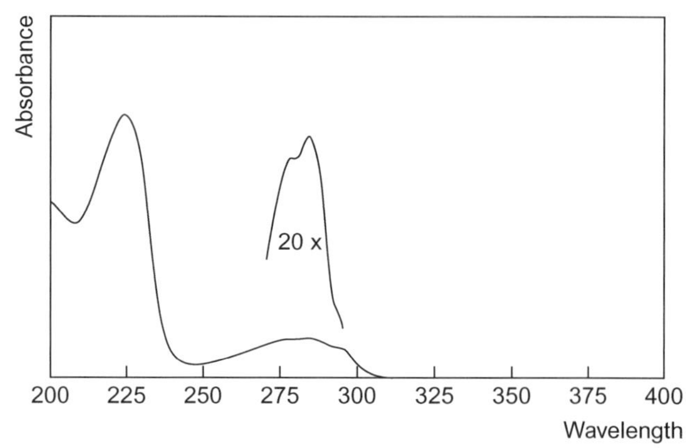

Mass Spectrum. Principal ions at *m/z* 70, 96, 97, 71, 42, 43, 44, 169.

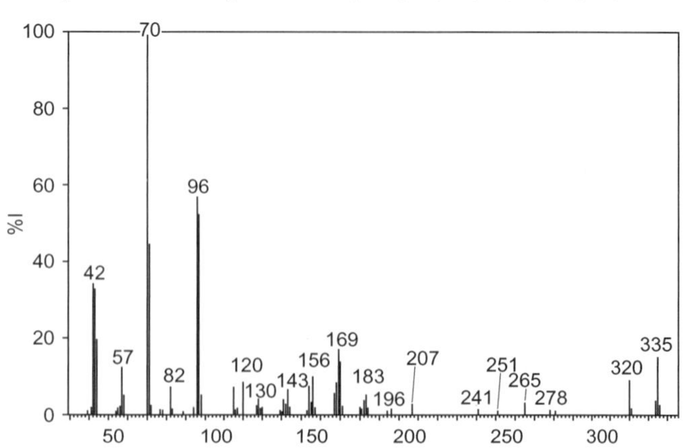

Quantification

High performance liquid chromatography–mass spectrometry. In serum: limit of detection 0.1 µg/L. MS–MS detection (ESI)—K. Vishwanathan *et al.*, *Rapid Commun. Mass Spectrom.*, 2000, *14(3)*, 168–172.

Disposition in the Body. Naratriptan is rapidly and well absorbed after administration and undergoes some hepatic metabolism by a wide range of cytochrome P450 isoenzymes. Renal excretion is the main route of elimination and the drug is predominately excreted in urine with 50% of the dose being recovered as the unchanged drug and 30% as the inactive metabolite. It displays linear pharmacokinetics over the therapeutic range and repeat administration does not lead to accumulation of the drug. Food does not alter the absorption.

Therapeutic concentration

7 Adolescent migraine patients, aged between 12 and 16 years, were administered a single dose of 2.5 mg naratriptan outside a migraine attack. The mean naratriptan plasma concentration was 8.0 µg/L (range 5.9 to 10.7) observed between 1.5 and 4 h after dosing. [M. L. Christensen *et al.*, *J. Clin. Pharmacol.*, 2001, *41(2)*, 170–175].

Bioavailability. Men, 63%; women, 74%.

Half-life. Approx. 4.5 to 5.5 h; prolonged in patients with renal and hepatic impairment.

Volume of distribution. 170 L.

Clearance. Systemic, 6.6 mL/min/kg; reduced by 26% in the elderly and by 50% in renal impaired individuals.

Protein binding. 28 to 31% (concentration range 50 to 1000 µg/L).

Note. For a review of naratriptan use in migraine treatment, see D. A. Dulli, *Ann. Pharmacother.*, 1999, *33*, 704–711.

Dose. Oral administration: initial dose is 2.5 mg in the UK; 1 to 2.5 mg in the US and a second dose if required. The maximum dose is 5 mg daily.

Narceine

Alkaloid

6-[[6-[2-(Dimethylamino)ethyl]-4-methoxy-1,3-benzodioxol-5-yl]-acetyl]-2,3-dimethoxybenzoic acid
$C_{23}H_{27}NO_8$=445.5
CAS—131-28-2 (anhydrous)

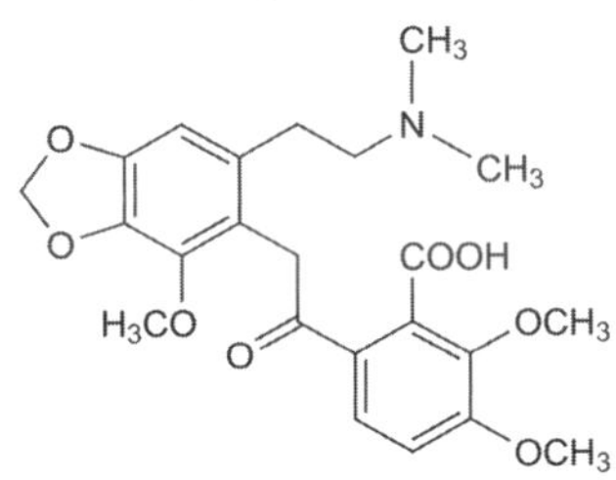

An alkaloid present in opium.
White silky crystals. M.p. 176°. The anhydrous substance melts at about 138° and is very hygroscopic.
Slightly soluble in water; soluble in ethanol; soluble in alkali hydroxide solutions and dilute mineral acids; practically insoluble in benzene, chloroform, ether and petroleum ether.

Narceine Hydrochloride

$C_{23}H_{27}NO_8$,HCl=481.9
CAS—4901-03-5
Prismatic crystals. M.p. 192° to 193°.
Slightly soluble in hot water and ether; soluble in hot ethanol.

Dissociation Constant. pK_a 3.8 (20°).

Partition Coefficient. Log *P* (octanol/water), 2.0.

Colour Tests. Liebermann's test—black; Mandelin's test—green-brown; Marquis test—brown→green.

Thin-layer Chromatography. System TA—Rf 52; system TB—Rf 00; system TC—Rf 03; system TE—Rf 00; system TL—Rf 00; system TAE—Rf 34; system TAF—Rf 14; system TAJ—Rf 02; system TAK—Rf 01; system TAL—Rf 36. (Acidified iodoplatinate solution, positive.)

High Performance Liquid Chromatography. System HA—*k* 0.7; system HX—RI 360.

Ultraviolet Spectrum. Aqueous acid—277 nm (A^1_1=306a). No alkaline shift.

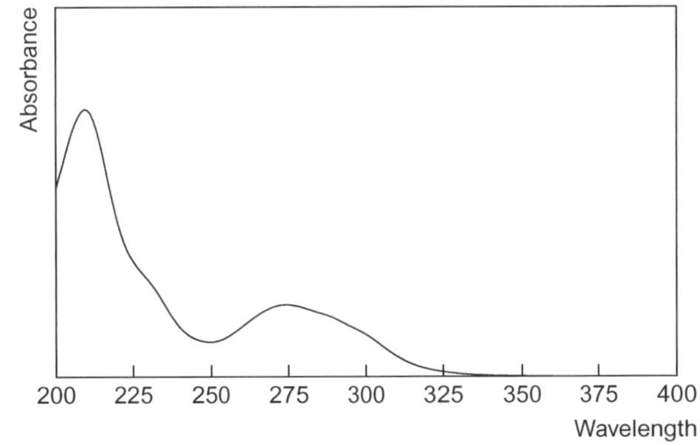

Infra-red Spectrum. Principal peaks at wavenumbers 1253, 1582, 1060, 1090, 1000, 1047 cm^{-1} (KCl disk).

Mass Spectrum. Principal ions at *m/z* 58, 427, 234, 59, 50, 42, 428, 91.

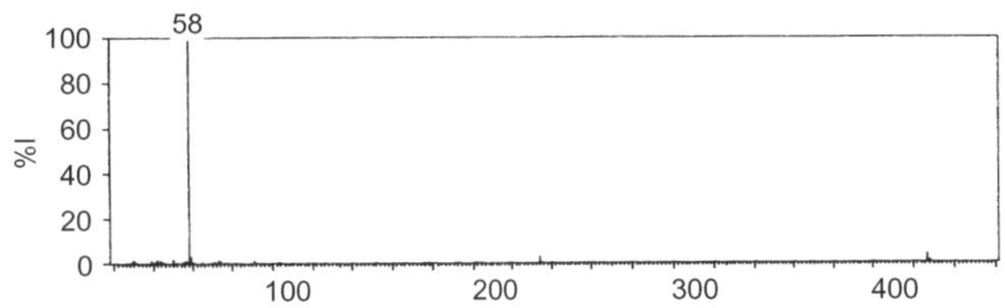

Natamycin

Antifungal

Synonyms. Pimaricin; CL-12625; Antibiotic A 5283; Tennecetin.
Proprietary names. Deronga Heilpaste; Natacyn; Natafucin; Pima Biciron N; Pimafucin(e).
$C_{33}H_{47}NO_{13}$=665.7
CAS—7681-93-8

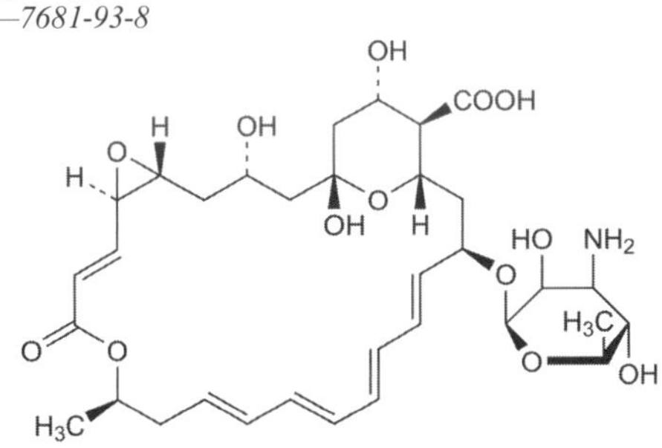

An antibiotic produced by the growth of *Streptomyces natalensis.*
A white crystalline powder, which may discolour slightly on storage.
Very slightly soluble in water and ethanol; practically insoluble in chloroform and ether; readily soluble in dilute acids and alkalis, forming salts.

Partition Coefficient. Log *P* (octanol/water), −3.7.

Ultraviolet Spectrum. Acid methanol—290 (A^1_1=795b), 303 (A^1_1=1250b), 318 nm (A^1_1=1145b).

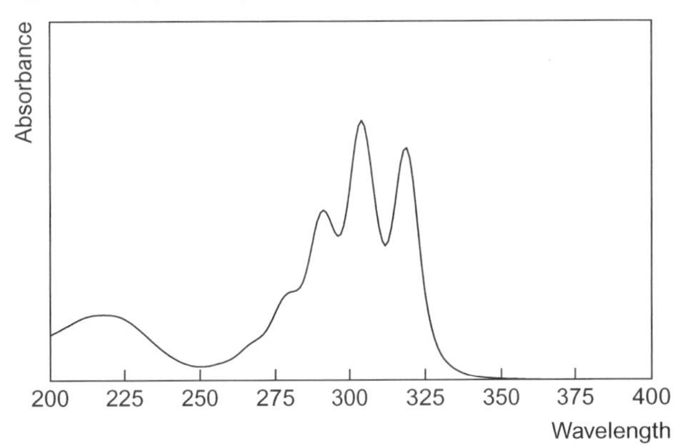

Infra-red Spectrum. Principal peaks at wavenumbers 1062, 1002, 1563, 1709, 1101, 1258 cm^{-1} (KBr disk).

Uses. Topically in concentrations of 2 to 5%; by inhalation in a dose of 7.5 mg daily.

Nealbarbital

Barbiturate/Sedative

Synonyms. Alneobarbital; Nealbarbitone; Neallymalum.
Proprietary names. Censedal; Nevental.
5-(2,2-Dimethylpropyl)-5-(2-propenyl)-2,4,6(1*H*,3*H*,5*H*)-pyrimidinetrione
$C_{12}H_{18}N_2O_3$=238.3
CAS—561-83-1

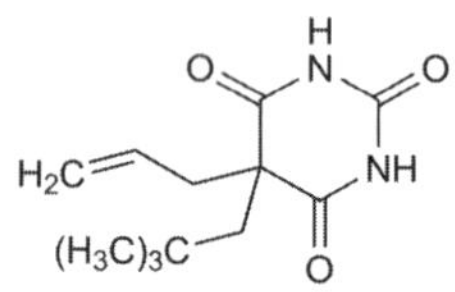

A white or slightly cream-coloured powder. M.p. 155° to 157°.
Soluble 1 in 5000 of water, 1 in 4 of ethanol, 1 in 80 of chloroform and 1 in 5 of ether; freely soluble in acetone; soluble in aqueous solutions of alkalis; practically insoluble in petroleum ether.

Dissociation Constant. pK_a 7.2 (20°).

Partition Coefficient. Log *P* (octanol/water), 2.1.

Thin-layer Chromatography. System TD—Rf 58; system TE—Rf 44; system TF—Rf 68; system TH—Rf 78; system TAD—Rf 60; system TAE—Rf 92. (Mercurous nitrate spray, black; acidified potassium permanganate solution, yellow-brown; Zwikker's reagent, pink.)

Gas Chromatography. System GA—Nealbarbital RI 1720; nealbarbital-Me_2 RI 1620; system GAJ—RRT 0.789 (relative to methylphenobarbital); system GF—RI 2460.

High Performance Liquid Chromatography. System HG—*k* 10.22; system HH—*k* 6.19; system HX—RI 417; system HY—RI 382.

Ultraviolet Spectrum. Borax buffer 0.05 M (pH 9.2)—240 nm (A_1^1=396b); 1 M sodium hydroxide (pH 13)—255 nm (A_1^1=303b).

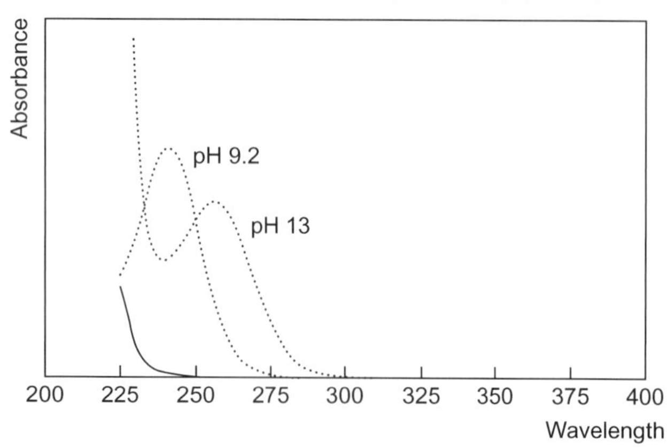

Infra-red Spectrum. Principal peaks at wavenumbers 1695, 1752, 1265, 833, 1205, 775 cm^{-1} (KBr disk).

Mass Spectrum. Principal ions at *m/z* 57, 41, 141, 167, 39, 83, 55, 182.

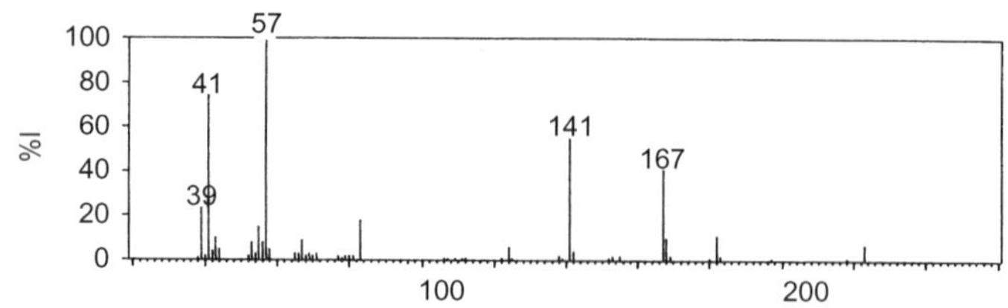

Dose. Nealbarbital has been given in doses of up to 200 mg as a hypnotic.

Nebivolol

Beta-blocker

Synonyms. R-65824; R-67555; Narbivolol.
Proprietary name. Nebilet
α,α′-[Iminobis(methylene)]bis[6-fluoro-3,4-dihydro-2*H*-1-benzopyran-2-methanol]
$C_{22}H_{25}F_2NO_4$=405.4
CAS—99200-09-6

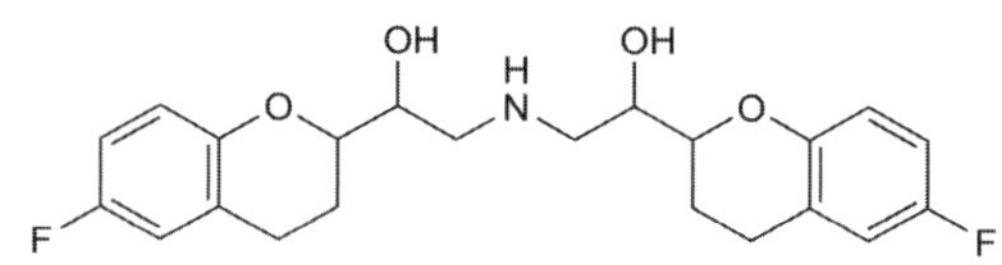

Crystals. M.p. 140.7°.

Nebivolol Hydrochloride
$C_{22}H_{26}ClF_2NO_4$=441.9

Dissociation Constant. pK_a (base), 8.22.

Partition Coefficient. Log *P* (octanol/water), 3.23; 4.03 (pH 11.8, 23°).

High Performance Liquid Chromatography. Column: Chiralpak AD-RH (150 × 4.6 mm i.d., 5 μm). Mobile phase: 1-propanol, flow rate 0.5 mL/min. UV detection (λ=220 nm). Retention time(s): (+)-nebivolol, 13.17 min; (−)-nebivolol, 17.45 min. [H. Y. Aboul-Enein and I. Ali, *Pharmazie*, 2001, *56*, 214–216].

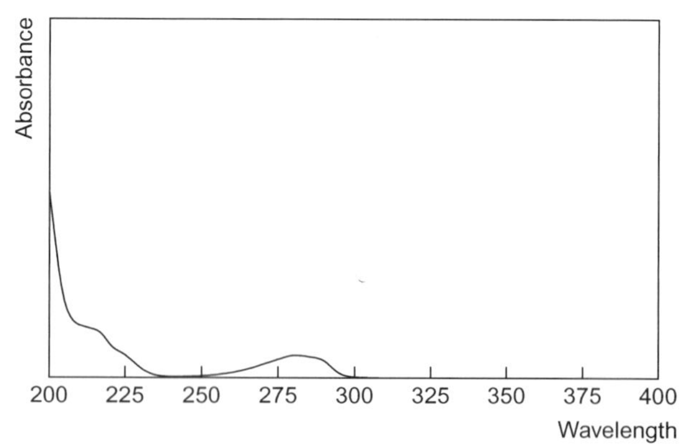

Mass Spectrum. Principal ions at *m/z* 428, 471, 82, 103, 233, 151, 472, 412 (tri-acetylated derivative).

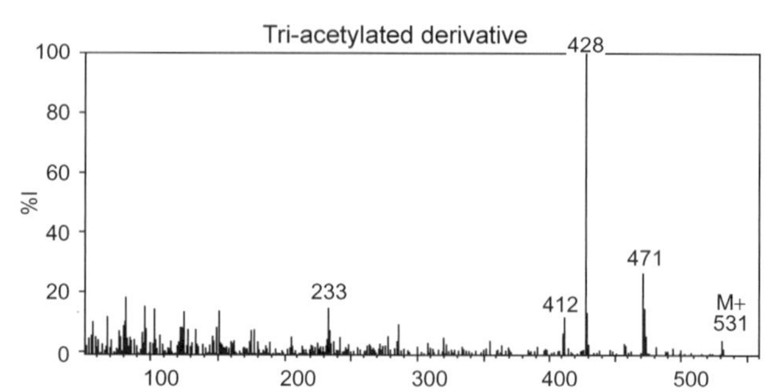

Quantification

High performance liquid chromatography. In plasma: limit of detection 0.1 μg/L, fluorescence detection—R. Woestenborgh *et al.*, in

Methodological Surveys in Biochemistry and Analysis, 1988, Plenum Press, US. Vol. 18, pp. 215–216.

Disposition in the Body. The metabolism of nebivolol is complex with formation of numerous metabolites, and varies between individuals; they may be fast or slow metabolisers. Aromatic hydroxylation is the major pathway and also involved are alicyclic hydroxylation and glucuronidation pathways. Urinary and faecal excretion of unconjugated parent drug are less than 0.5% of a dose.

Therapeutic concentration. Peak plasma levels of 1 μg/L in fast metabolisers and 3 μg/L in slow metabolisers following a 5 mg oral dose.

Bioavailability. 12% (fast metabolisers) and 96% (slow metabolisers).

Half-life. 8 (fast metabolisers) to 27 (slow metabolisers) h.

Volume of distribution. 10.1 to 39.4 L/kg.

Clearance. Total body, 51.6 L/h (healthy); 71.6 L/h (obese individuals).

Protein binding. 98%.

Dose. A daily oral dose of 5 mg.

Nedocromil

Anti-asthmatic

Synonym. FPL-59002

9-Ethyl-6,9-dihydro-4,6-dioxo-10-propyl-4*H*-pyranol[3,2-g]quinoline-2,8-dicarboxylic acid

$C_{19}H_{15}NO_7 = 371.3$

CAS—69049-73-6

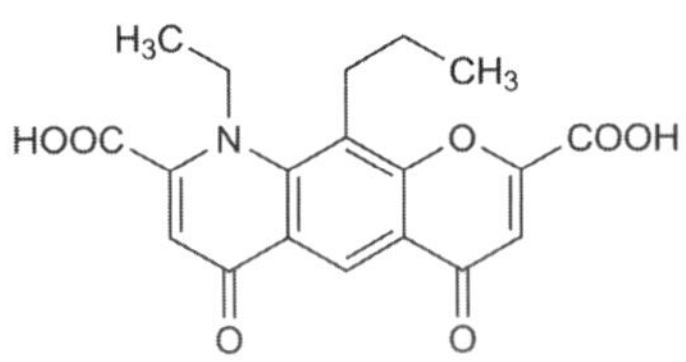

A yellow powder. M.p. 298° to 300° (dec).

Nedocromil Calcium

Synonym. FPL-59002KC

$C_{19}H_{15}CaNO_7 = 411.5$

CAS—101626-68-0

Nedocromil Sodium

Synonym. FPL-59002KP

Proprietary names. Alocril; Brionil; Cetimil; Halamid; Ildor; Irtan; Kovilen; Kovinal; Tilade; Tilarin; Tilavist; Rapitil.

$C_{19}H_{15}NO_7,Na_2 = 415.3$

CAS—69049-74-7

A yellow powder. Soluble in water.

Partition Coefficient. Log *P* (octanol/water), 2.22.

Thin-layer Chromatography. System TE—Rf 00; system TF—Rf 00.

High Performance Liquid Chromatography. System HX—RI 318.

Column: (analytical) C_8 (Spherisorb, 250 × 4.6 mm i.d., 5 μm); (guard) C_8 (Spherisorb, 10 × 4.6 mm i.d.). Mobile phase: methanol:phosphate buffer (45 mM):dodecyl triethyl ammonium phosphate (0.5 M) (550:447.6:2.4), adjusted to pH 2.3 with orthophosphoric acid, flow rate 0.85 mL/min. Internal standard: sodium cromoglycate. UV detection (λ=256 nm). *k* value: 13.3 (retention time, 43.1 min); I. S., *k* 8.5. [O. A. Aswania *et al.*, *J. Chromatogr. Biomed. Sci. Appl.*, 1998, *718*, 290–295].

Ultraviolet Spectrum. Water—255, 286, 345, 378 nm.

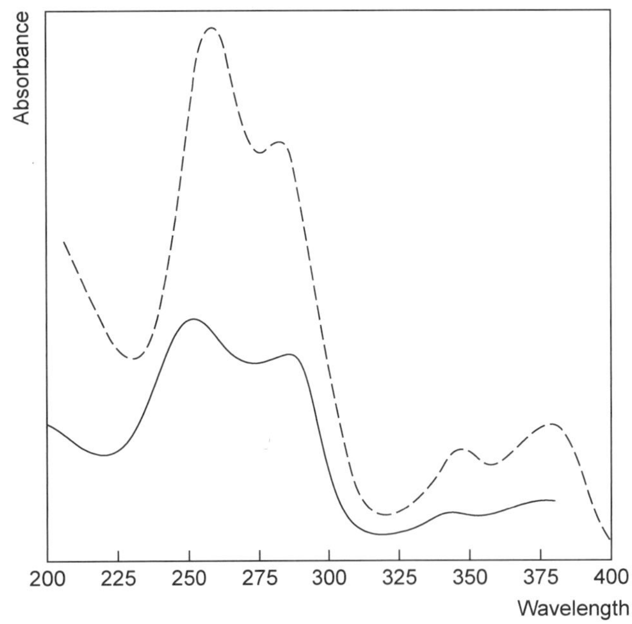

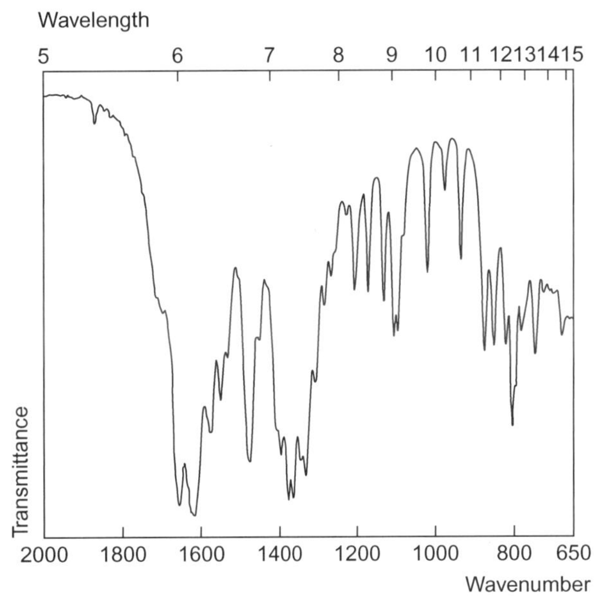

Quantification

High performance liquid chromatography. In urine: limit of quantification is 20 μg/L. UV detection (λ=253 nm)—P. R. Baker *et al.*, *J. Chromatogr.* 1995, *668(1)*; *Biomed. Appl.*, 59–65. In urine: limit of detection is 40 μg/L and limit of quantification 75 μg/L. UV detection (λ=256 nm)—O. A. Aswania *et al.*, *J. Chromatogr. Biomed. Sci. Appl.*, 1998, *718*, 290–295.

Disposition in the Body. A small amount of nedocromil (5% of dose) is absorbed after inhalation and excreted unchanged in urine and bile. Absorption is through the nasolacrimal duct rather than through the conjuctiva. It is reversibly bound to plasma proteins and therefore not metabolised. Accumulation does not occur. Approximately 80% of an intravenous dose is recovered in urine within 90 min. In healthy individuals, <10% of a dose is excreted in urine within 72 h.

Therapeutic concentration

Healthy volunteers (6 men and 7 women, aged between 22 and 54 years) and those suffering from asthma (4 men and 8 women, 22 to 59 years old) were administered with 4 mg nedocromil sodium (inhaled). The mean peak plasma concentrations were 3.3 μg/L and 2.8 μg/L, respectively, and were reached after approximately 20 and 40 min, respectively. [M. G. Neale *et al.*, *Br. J. Clin. Pharmacol.*, 1987, *24*, 493–501].

Bioavailability. 7 to 9% (2 to 3% oral; 5 to 6% respiratory).

Half-life. 1.5 to 3.3 h.

Volume of distribution. 0.43 L/kg (after a 6 μg/kg, 30 min intravenous dose).

Clearance. 10.2 ± 1.3 mL/min/kg (after a 6 μg/kg, 30 min intravenous dose).

Protein binding. About 89%.

Dose. The usual dose is 4 mg inhaled four times daily and may be decreased to twice daily.

Nefazodone

Antidepressant

2-[3-[4-(3-Chlorophenyl)-1-piperazinyl]propyl]-5-ethyl-2,4-dihydro-4-(2-phenoxyethyl)-3*H*-1,2,4-triazol-3-one
$C_{25}H_{32}ClN_5O_2 = 470.0$
CAS—83366-66-9

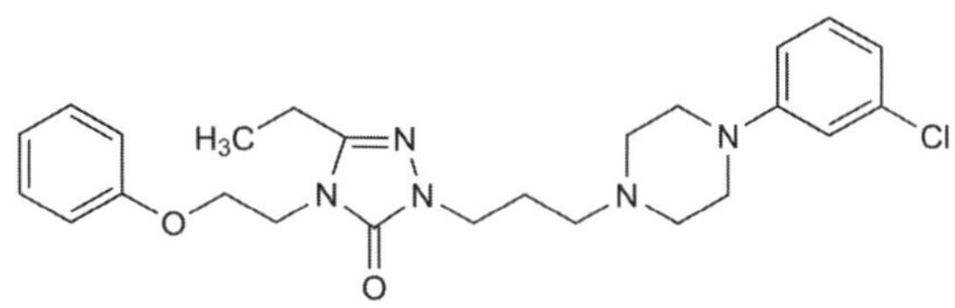

Non-hygroscopic white crystalline solid. M. p. 83° to 84°. Freely soluble in chloroform, soluble in propylene glycol, slightly soluble in polyethylene glycol and water.

Nefazodone Hydrochloride

Synonyms. BMY-13754; MJ-13754-1.
Proprietary names. Dutonin; Serzone.
$C_{25}H_{32}ClN_5O_2,HCl = 506.5$
CAS—82752-99-6
Crystals from ethanol. M.p. 175° to 177°.

Dissociation Constant. pK_a 6.6.

Partition Coefficient. Log *P* (octanol/water), 5.0.

Gas Chromatography. System GB—RI 1806, *m*-chlorophenylpiperazine (*m*CPP).

High Performance Liquid Chromatography. System HZ—retention time 7.7 min.

Column: ODS-3v (Inertsil, 250 × 4.6 mm i.d., 5 μm). Mobile phase: potassium dihydrogen phosphate (50 mM, pH 3.0):acetonitrile:methanol (50:40:10), flow rate 1 mL/min. UV detection (λ=220 nm). Retention time(s): 8.5 min. [D. Sreenivas Rao *et al.*, *J. Pharm. Biomed. Anal.*, 2001, *26*, 629–636].

Column: (analytical) C_{18} BDS (Hypersil, 100 × 2.0 mm i.d., 3 μm); (guard) C_{18} BDS (Hypersil, 10 × 2.0 mm i.d.). Mobile phase: acetonitrile:ammonium formate (10 mM, pH 4 with formic acid) (45:55), flow rate 0.3 mL/min. Internal standard: trazodone. MS detection [PIAPCI, SIM at *m/z*: 470.4 for nefazodone (NEF), 486.2 for hydroxynefazodone (OH-NEF), 458.1 for triazoledione (Dione), 197.0 for *m*-chlorophenylpiperazine (*m*CPP) and 372.0 for I. S.]. Retention time(s): NEF, 4.47 min; OH-NEF, 2.80 min; Dione, 2.34 min; *m*CPP, 1.48 min; I. S., 1.77 min. [M. Yao and N. Srinivas, *Biomed. Chromatogr.*, 2000, *14*, 106–112].

Column: (analytical) cyanopropyl (150 × 4.6 mm i.d., 5 μm); (guard) C_2 (5 μm). Mobile phase: potassium phosphate buffer (40 mM, pH 6.6):acetonitrile:methanol (600:225:175), flow rate 1.4 mL/min. Internal standard: aprindine. Coulometric detection. Retention time: NEF, 3.2 min; OH-NEF, 4.0 min; *m*CPP, 5.0 min; I. S., 5.6 min. [M. Franklin, *J. Pharm. Biomed. Anal.*, 1993, *11*, 1109–1113].

Ultraviolet Spectrum. Aqueous acid—210, 249, 276 nm.

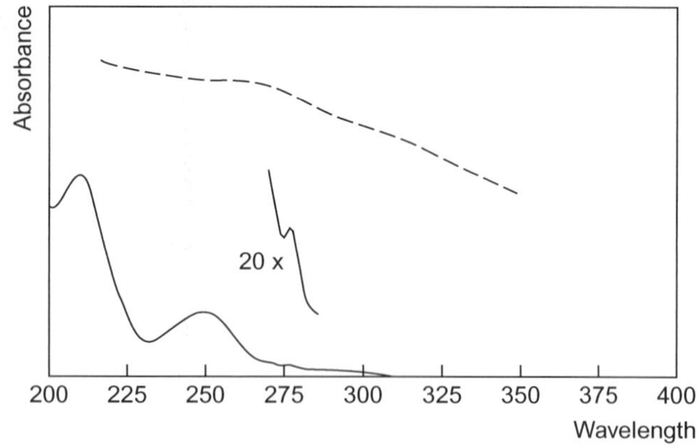

Infra-red Spectrum. Principal peaks at wavenumber 1699, 1594, 1242 cm^{-1} (KBr).

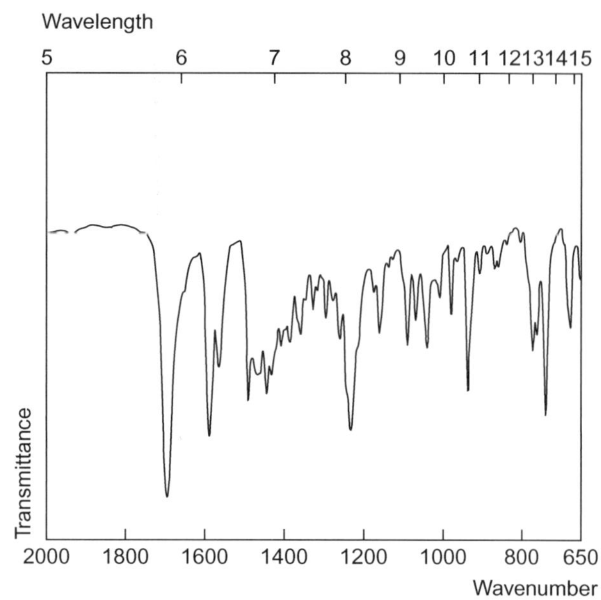

Mass Spectrum. Principal ions at *m/z* 303, 70, 274, 304, 260, 209, 96, 317.

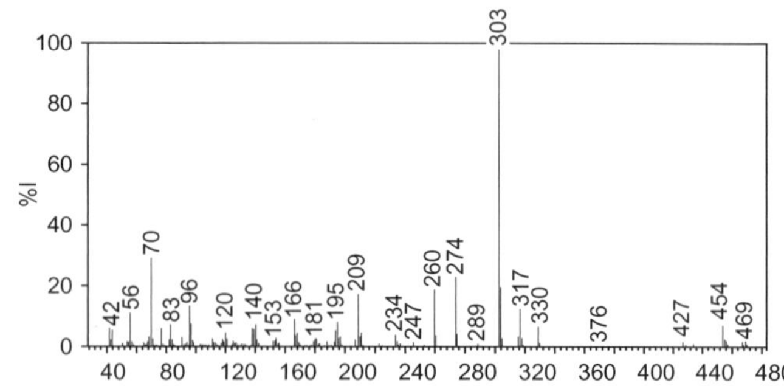

Quantification

Gas chromatography–mass spectrometry. In urine: limit of detection is <100 μg/L—J. Bickeboeller-Friedrich and H. H. Maurer, *Ther. Drug Monit.*, 2001, *23*, 61–70.

High performance liquid chromatography. In breast milk: limit of quantification 200 μg/L. UV detection (λ=205 nm)—S. Dodd *et al.*, *J. Chromatogr. B Biomed. Sci. Appl.*, 1999, *730*, 249–255. In plasma: limit of detection for NEF is 5 μg/L, *m*CPP 1 μg/L, *p*-hydroxynefazodone 10 μg/L and HO-NEF 5 μg/L. Limit of quantification of NEF and HO-NEF is 10 μg/L; *p*-hydroxynefazodone 20 μg/L and *m*CPP 2.5 μg/L. UV detection (λ=254 nm)—J. E. Franc *et al.*, *J. Chromatogr.*, 1991, *570*, 129–138. In plasma: limit of quantification for NEF, *m*CPP and HO-NEF is 0.9, 0.2

and 0.6 µg/L, respectively. Coulometric detection—M. Franklin, *J. Pharm. Biomed. Anal.*, 1993, *11*, 1109–1113.

Disposition in the Body. Nefazodone is rapidly and completely absorbed after oral administration with peak plasma concentration being reached within 0.5 to 2 h. The drug undergoes extensive first-pass hepatic metabolism with only 20% of a dose reaching systemic circulation. It is extensively metabolised via *N*-dealkylation and aromatic hydroxylation and excreted via urine (55%) and faeces (25%) after additional glucuronidation. Less than 10% of the drug is present in urine unchanged. Three active metabolites: hydroxynefazodone (the major metabolite, HO-NEF), *m*-chlorophenylpiperazine (*m*CPP) and desethylhydroxynefazodone have been identified.

Therapeutic concentration. The therapeutic concentration is variable and dose dependent.

18 healthy males, aged between 19 and 35 years, were administered with a single oral dose of 50, 100 or 200 mg nefazodone hydrochloride after an overnight fast. A steady state study was also carried out where a dose of 50, 100 or 200 mg was administered twice daily for 7 days after meals (final dose followed an overnight fast). Mean peak plasma concentrations of 84, 196 and 392 µg/L were observed for the single oral 50, 100 and 200 mg doses, respectively 0.9, 1.0 and 1.3 h after dosing. The steady state values were 72, 732 and 2047 µg/L for the 50, 100 and 200 mg doses reached 0.7, 0.9 and 1.2 h after administration. [S. Kaul *et al.*, *J. Clin. Pharmacol.*, 1995, *35*, 830–834].

Toxicity. Instances of overdosage with up to 11 g of the drug have been reported without fatalities. Victims have manifested nausea, vomiting and somnolence.

Nefazodone is safe and well tolerated at oral doses up to 450 mg three times daily. [M. F. D'Amico *et al.*, *Psychopharmacol. Bull.*, 1990, *26*, 147–150].

Clinical overdoses of 3400 and 3600 mg produced no significant clinical/life threatening symptoms. [R. Fontaine *et al.*, *Clin. Neuropharmacol.*, 1992, *15 (Suppl. 1)*, 99A].

Bioavailability. 15 to 23% oral, regular release; decreases by 18% when administered with food.

Half-life. Dose dependent; nefazodone, 2 to 5 h (at dose of 200 mg twice daily); hydroxynefazodone, 2 to 4 h; desethylhydroxynefazodone, 18 to 33 h; *m*-chlorophenylpiperazine, 4 to 9 h.

Volume of distribution. 0.22 to 0.87 L/kg.

Protein binding. 98.4 to 99.8% for the drug and its metabolite, HO-NEF; 66 to 74% for the metabolite, *m*CPP.

Note. For a review of nefazodone see R. Davis *et al.*, *Drugs*, 1997, *53*, 608–636.

Dose. Initially 50 to 100 mg twice daily which may be increased to a maximum of 300 mg twice daily. In the elderly, the maximum dose is 100 to 200 mg twice daily.

Nefopam

Analgesic

3,4,5,6-Tetrahydro-5-methyl-1-phenyl-1*H*-2,5-benzoxazocine
$C_{17}H_{19}NO$=253.3
CAS—13669-70-0

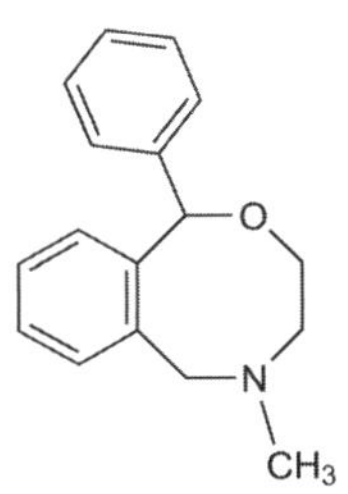

Nefopam Hydrochloride

Proprietary names. Acupan; Ajan; Nefadol; Nefam; Oxadol; Silentan.
$C_{17}H_{19}NO,HCl$=289.8
CAS—23327-57-3
A white crystalline powder. M.p. about 238° to 242°.
Soluble in water, chloroform and methanol.

Dissociation Constant. pK_a 9.2.

Partition Coefficient. Log *P* (octanol/water), 3.0.

Colour Tests. Liebermann's Test—brown-orange→brown; Marquis Test—orange→brown; Sulfuric Acid—orange.

Thin-layer Chromatography. System TA—Rf 50; system TB—Rf 33; system TC—Rf 32; system TE—Rf 59; system TL—Rf 17; system TAE—Rf 30; system TAJ—Rf 23; system TAK—Rf 17; system TAL—Rf 71.

Gas Chromatography. System GA—nefopam RI 2035; system GB—nefopam RI 2106, M (nor) RI 2116, M (OH-) RI 2266, M (nor-di-OH) RI 2649; system GF—RI 2380.

High Performance Liquid Chromatography. System HA—*k* 3.0; system HY—RI 313; system HAA—Retention time, 12.7 min.

Ultraviolet Spectrum. Aqueous acid—267 nm (A^1_1=29b), 275 nm.

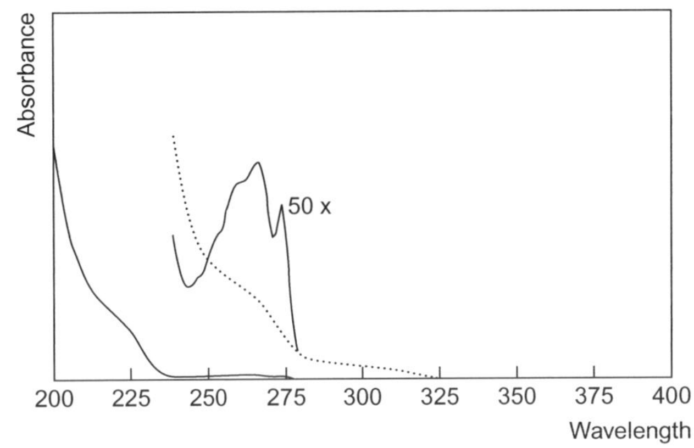

Infra-red Spectrum. Principal peaks at wavenumbers 720, 760, 775, 1112, 1130, 1038 cm^{-1} (nefopam hydrochloride).

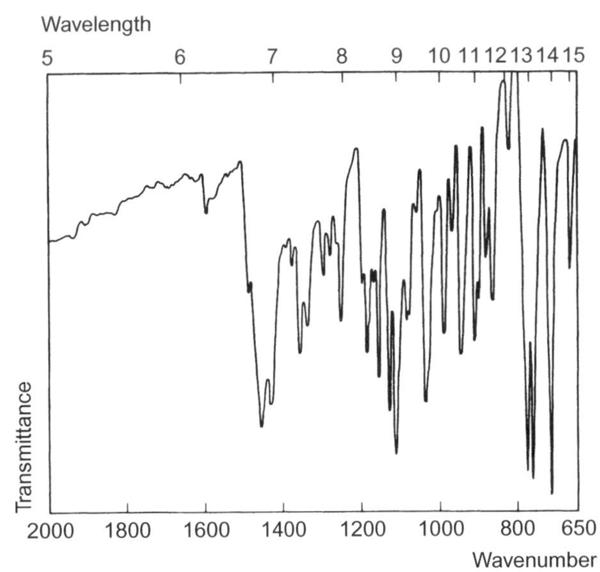

Mass Spectrum. Principal ions at *m/z* 58, 179, 180, 225, 178, 165, 42, 210.

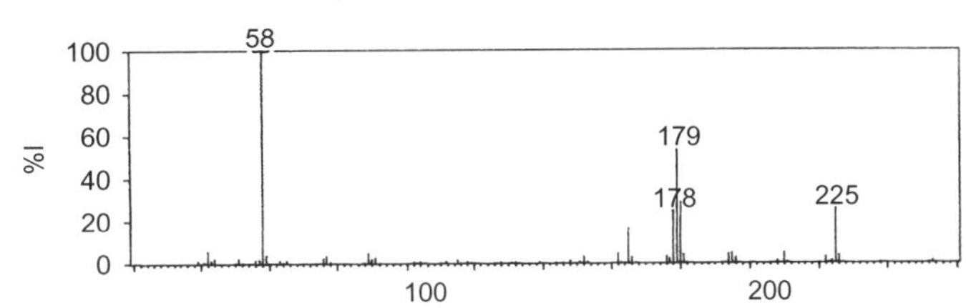

Quantification

Gas chromatography. In plasma, saliva, or cerebrospinal fluid: limit of detection 5 μg/L, AFID—S. F. Chang *et al.*, *J. Chromatogr.*, 1981, *226*; *Biomed. Appl.*, *15*, 79–89.

High performance liquid chromatography. In plasma or urine: nefopam and desmethylnefopam, limits of detection 1 μg/L and 5 μg/L for nefopam in plasma and urine, respectively, UV detection—G. Aymard *et al.*, *J. Pharm. Biomed. Anal.*, 2002, *30*, 1013–1021.

Disposition in the Body. Rapidly absorbed after oral administration. It is extensively metabolised, less than 5% of a dose being excreted unchanged in the urine; metabolites include desmethylnefopam and its *N*-glucuronide, and nefopam *N*-oxide. About 87% of a dose is excreted in the urine and about 8% in the faeces in 5 days.

Therapeutic concentration

Following a single oral dose of 90 mg, peak blood concentrations of 0.07 to 0.15 mg/L were reported at 1 to 3 h [R. C. Heel *et al.*, *Drugs*, 1980, *19*, 249–267].

Toxicity

A postmortem blood concentration of 11.9 mg/L was reported in a suicide due to nefopam overdose; in a second non-fatal overdose case, a plasma concentration of 3.8 mg/L was reported 3 h after ingestion, declining to 0.9 mg/L at 19 h [D. M. Piercy *et al.*, *Br. Med. J.*, 1981, *283*, 1508–1509].

In a fatality involving the intentional ingestion of an unknown quantity of nefopam and dihydrocodeine, the nefopam plasma concentration was 4.3 mg/L one hour after ingestion; the postmortem plasma concentration was 0.6 mg/L (corresponding dihydrocodeine concentrations were 5.9 and 1.7 mg/L) [S. C. Urwin and H. S. Smith, *Br. J. Anaesth.*, 1999, *83*, 501–502].

A 37-year-old woman died after self-administering a massive intravenous dose of nefopam (300 mg). Postmortem tissue concentrations, measured about 7 to 10 days after death, were as follows: heart blood 4.38 mg/L, liver 59.12 μg/g, kidney 14.57 μg/g, lung 44.07 μg/g, myocardium 14.87 μg/g [A. Tracqui *et al*, *J. Anal. Toxicol.*, 2002, *26*, 239–243].

Half-life. Plasma half-life, 3 to 8 h (mean 4).

Protein binding. In plasma, about 75%.

Note. For a review of nefopam see R. C. Heel *et al.*, *Drugs*, 1980, *19*, 249–267.

Dose. 90 to 270 mg of nefopam hydrochloride daily.

Nelfinavir

Protease Inhibitor/Antiviral (HIV)

Synonym. AG-1346

(3*S*,4a*S*,8a*S*)-*N*-(1,1-Dimethylethyl)decahydro-2-[(2*R*,3*R*)-2-hydroxy-3-[(3-hydroxy-2-methylbenzoyl)amino]-4-(phenylthio)butyl]-3-isoquinolinecarboxamide

$C_{32}H_{45}N_3O_4S = 567.8$

CAS—159989-64-7

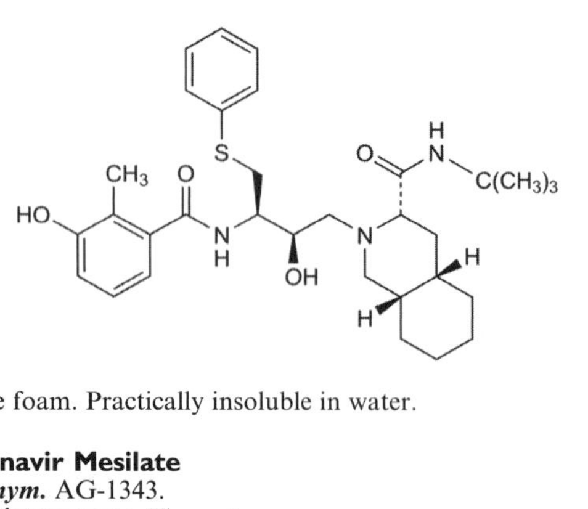

White foam. Practically insoluble in water.

Nelfinavir Mesilate

Synonym. AG-1343.

Proprietary name. Viracept

$C_{32}H_{45}N_3O_4S,CH_3SO_3H = 663.9$

CAS—159989-65-8

White powder. Solubility: 4.5 mg/mL in water, 2.6 mg/mL in 0.1 N HCl, 70 mg/g in glycerine, > 100 mg/g in propylene glycol, > 200 mg/g in PEG. Very soluble in methanol, ethanol, acetonitrile; practically insoluble in soybean oil and mineral oil.

Dissociation Constant. pK_{a1} 6.00; pK_{a2} 11.06; pK_a –1.20 (mesilate).

Partition Coefficient. Log *P* (octanol/water), 4.1.

High Performance Liquid Chromatography. System HAC—*k* 17.3; HAE—retention time, 8.0 min.

Column: ABZ-plus (Supelcosil, 250 × 4.6 mm i.d., 3 μm). Column temperature: 45°. Mobile phase: potassium dihydrogen phosphate (20 mM, with 10 mM octylsulfonic acid, pH 4):methanol:acetonitrile (45:30:25), flow rate 1.0 mL/min. Internal standard: ritonavir. UV detection (λ=240 nm). Retention times: nelfinavir, 16.7 min; hydroxy-*tert*-butylamide metabolite, 7.2 min; I. S., 12.7 min. [Y. Khaliq *et al.*, *Br. J. Clin. Pharmacol.*, 2000, *50*, 108–115].

Ultraviolet Spectrum. Aqueous acid 252 nm.

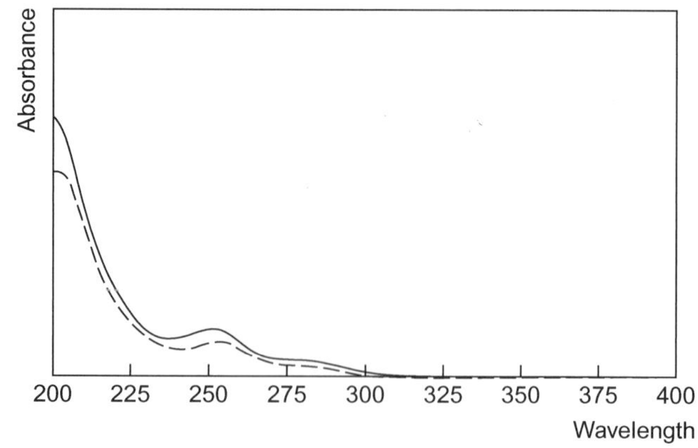

Infra-red Spectrum. Principal peaks at wavenumbers 1639, 1536, 1460, 1285, 1158, 1040 cm^{-1}.

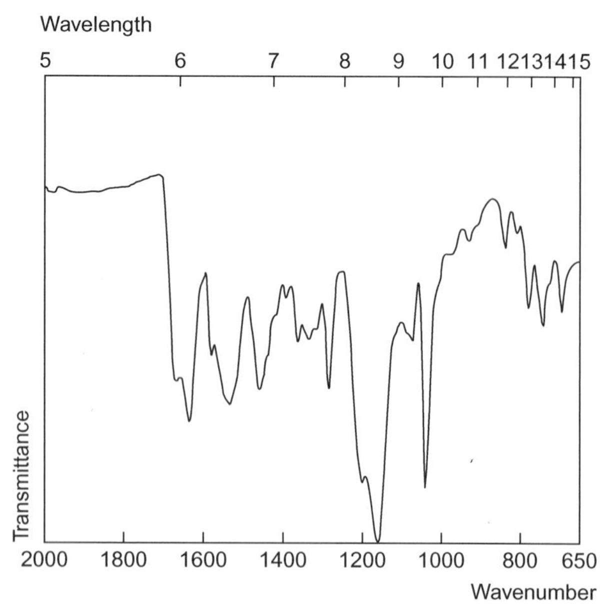

Quantification

High performance liquid chromatography. In plasma: limit of quantification 0.05 mg/L. UV detection (λ=215 nm)—H. Yamada *et al.*, *J. Chromatogr. B Biomed. Sci. Appl.*, 2001, *755*, 85–89. In plasma: limit of quantification 0.05 mg/L. UV detection (λ=254 nm)—G. Aymard *et al.*, *J. Chromatogr. Biomed. Sci. Appl.*, 2000, *744*, 227–240. In plasma: limit of quantification 0.03 mg/L. UV detection (λ=240 nm)—Y. Khaliq *et al.*, *Br. J. Clin. Pharmacol.*, 2000, *50*, 108–115. In plasma: limit of quantification 0.15 mg/L. UV detection (λ=260 nm)—V. Proust *et al.*, *J. Chromatogr. Biomed. Sci. Appl.*, 2000, *742*, 453–458. In serum: limit of detection 0.4 mg/

L. UV detection (λ=250 nm)—V. A. Simon *et al.*, *J. Chromatogr. A*, 2001, *913(1–2)*, 447–453.

Disposition in the Body. Nelfinavir is well absorbed after oral administration and this is enhanced by administration with food. It is oxidised by the cytochrome P450 isoenzymes CYP2C19 and CYP2D6, to a hydroxy-*tert*-butylamide metabolite with *in vitro* antiviral activity. Approximately 50% of the drug is eliminated by this means but the activity of CYP2C19 may be impaired in patients with reduced liver function or disease. Nelfinavir may induce its own metabolism. Elimination of the metabolite is predominantly controlled by the isoenzyme CYP3A4. 87% of a 750 mg dose is recovered in faeces, 22% as nelfinavir and 78% as the oxidative metabolites. It is distributed in breast milk.

Therapeutic concentration

8 Caucasian HIV-positive patients with liver disease, a mean age of 35 years (range, 29 to 42 years), participated in the study. Two of the patients had already been receiving nelfinavir for more than 8 weeks (750 mg every 8 h) and three others had been taking stavudine (40 mg) and lamivudine (150 mg) every 12 h for 12 weeks or longer. For the new patients starting treatment with nelfinavir, they were administered a single dose of 500 mg or 750 mg and then twice or three times daily for multiple dosing. During the multiple dosing, nelfinavir was co-administered with lamivudine (150 mg every 12 h) and either zidovudine (300 mg every 12 h) or stavudine (40 mg every 12 h). One patient also received 1000 mg saquinavir every 12 h. Steady state plasma concentrations were measured after 10 and 19 days of multiple dosing. After the 500 mg single dose, the mean peak plasma concentration was 1.72 mg/L; after the 750 mg single dose, 2.70 mg/L; 250 mg twice daily, 1.7 mg/L; 500 mg twice daily, 4.1 mg/L; 750 mg twice daily, 3.1 mg/L; 250 mg three times daily, 2.5 mg/L and 750 mg three times daily, 4.73 mg/L. [Y. Khaliq *et al.*, *Br. J. Clin. Pharmacol.*, 2000, *50*, 108–115].

Half-life. 3.5 to 5 h.

Volume of distribution. 2 to 7 L/kg.

Clearance. Plasma, mean, 24 L/h. Also reported as 24 to 33 L/h after a single dose and 26 to 61 L/h after multiple doses.

Protein binding. Greater than 98%.

Note. For an update on the use of Nelfinavir in HIV infection, see A. Bardsley-Elliot and G. L. Plosker, *Drugs*, 2000, *59*, 581–620.

Dose. Adult: 2.25 g daily in three divided doses. Children (2 to 13 years): 20 to 30 mg/kg body weight three times daily.

Nemonapride

Antipsychotic

Synonyms. YM-09151-2; emonapride.
Proprietary name. Emilace
cis-N-(1-Benzyl-2-methyl-3-pyrrolidinyl)-5-chloro-4-(methylamine)-*o*-anisamide
$C_{21}H_{26}ClN_3O_2$ = 387.9
CAS—93664-94-9; 75272-39-8

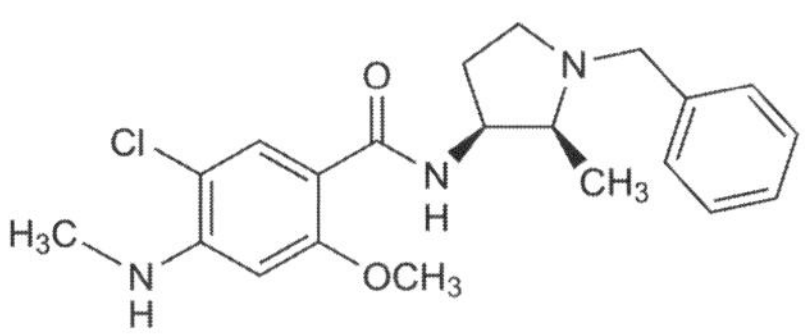

Odourless, non-hygroscopic white crystals or crystalline powder. M.p. 152° to 153°, also reported as 150°. It is practically insoluble in water; freely soluble in glacial acetic acid and chloroform; sparingly soluble in methanol and ethanol; slightly soluble in ether.

Dissociation Constant. pK_a 0.40; 8.18.

Partition Coefficient. Log *P* (octanol/buffer pH 7.0), 3.20.

High Performance Liquid Chromatography. System HAA—retention time 15.0 min.

Ultraviolet Spectrum. Aqueous acid—285, 314 nm.

Infra-red Spectrum. Principal peaks at wavenumber 1624, 1602, 1284, 1244 cm^{-1}.

Mass Spectrum. Principal ions at *m/z* 388, 310, 215, 198, 173, 91.

Quantification

High performance liquid chromatography. In plasma: limit of quantification for nemonapride and its active metabolite, desmethylnemonapride, 0.25 μg/L. Electrochemical detection—T. Nagasaki *et al.*, *J. Chromatogr. Biomed. Sci. Appl.*, 1998, *714*, 293–298.

Disposition in the Body. The plasma concentration of the unchanged drug reaches its peak 2 to 3 h after oral administration. No unchanged drug is detected in urine during the 24 h after oral administration. The major urinary metabolites are produced by *N*-demethylation, debenzylation and oxidation of the α-position of the pyrrolidine ring.

Half-life. 2.5 to 4.5 h.

Dose. Orally 9 to 36 mg daily. Maximum dose is 60 mg.

Neomycin

Antibiotic

$C_{23}H_{46}N_6O_{13}$ = 614.6 (neomycin B)
CAS—1404-04-2 (neomycin); 3947-65-7 (neomycin A); 119-04-0 (neomycin B); 66-86-4 (neomycin C)

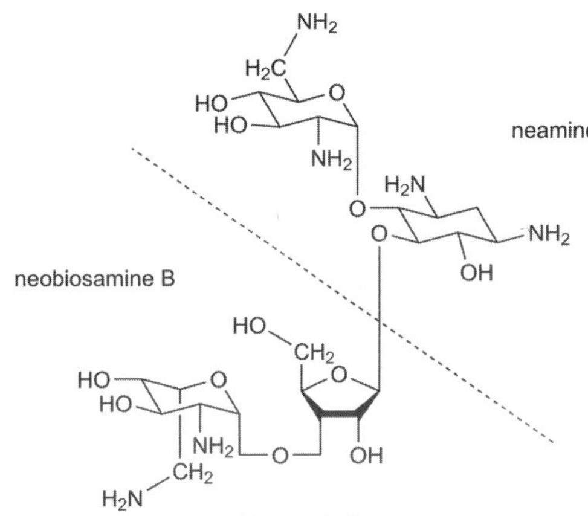

Neomycin B

A mixture of the 2 isomers, neomycins B and C, with neomycin A (neamine), an inactive component and degradation product of neomycins B and C.
Neomycin is obtained from certain selected strains of *Streptomyces fradiae*.

Neomycin Sulfate

Synonyms. Fradiomycin Sulfate; Neomycin.
Proprietary names. It is an ingredient of many proprietary preparations—see Martindale, *The Complete Drug Reference*, 33rd Edn., Pharmaceutical Press, London, 2002.
CAS—1405-10-3
A white to yellowish-white hygroscopic powder.
Slowly soluble 1 in 1 of water; very slightly soluble in ethanol; practically insoluble in chloroform and ether.

Neomycin Undecylenate

Synonym. Neomycin Undecenoate
Proprietary name. It is an ingredient of Audicort.
CAS—1406-04-8
A yellowish-white to pale yellow, waxy, unctuous powder.
Practically insoluble in water; very soluble in ethanol; soluble in chloroform.

Thin-layer Chromatography. System TA—Rf 00; system TAE—Rf 00. (Acidified potassium permanganate solution, positive.)

Ultraviolet Spectrum. No significant absorption, 230 to 360 nm.

Dose. As an intestinal antiseptic, up to 12 g of neomycin sulfate daily, by mouth; it is also applied topically.

Neopine

Alkaloid

Synonym. β-Codeine. It has been incorrectly called hydroxycodeine.
(5α,6α)-8,14-Didehydro-4,5-epoxy-3-methoxy-17-methylmorphinan-6-ol
$C_{18}H_{21}NO_3$=299.4
CAS—467-14-1

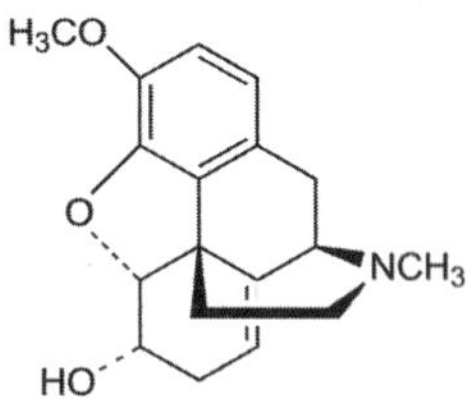

An alkaloid obtained from opium.
Crystals. M.p. about 127°.
Slightly soluble in water; soluble in chloroform.

Neopine Hydrobromide
$C_{18}H_{21}NO_3$,HBr=380.3
Crystals which darken at about 240° and decompose at about 283°.
Relatively insoluble in water, hence ease of separation from other opium alkaloids.

Partition Coefficient. Log *P* (octanol/water), 1.4.

Colour Test. Marquis test—blue-violet.

Thin-layer Chromatography. System TA—Rf 35; system TB—Rf 05; system TC—Rf 12; system TL—Rf 04. (Acidified iodoplatinate solution, positive.)

Gas Chromatography. System GA—RI 2395.

Ultraviolet Spectrum. Aqueous acid—285 nm (A^1_1=39b). No alkaline shift.

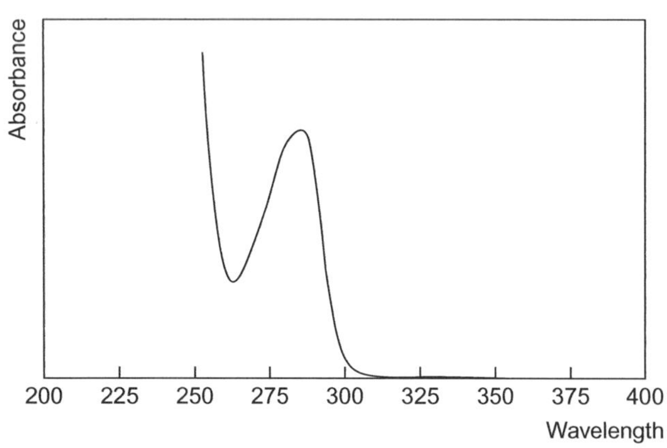

Infra-red Spectrum. Principal peaks at wavenumbers 1275, 1500, 1118, 1050, 1250, 782 cm^{-1} (KBr disk).

Mass Spectrum. Principal ions at *m/z* 299, 162, 229, 123, 59, 42, 44, 300.

Neostigmine Bromide

Anticholinesterase

Synonyms. Proserine Bromide; Synstigmine Bromide.
Proprietary names. Neoeserin; Normastigmin; Prostigmin(e) (tablets).
3-[[(Dimethylamino)carbonyl]oxy]-*N*,*N*,*N*-trimethylbenzenaminium bromide
$C_{12}H_{19}BrN_2O_2$=303.2
CAS—59-99-4 (neostigmine); 114-80-7 (bromide)

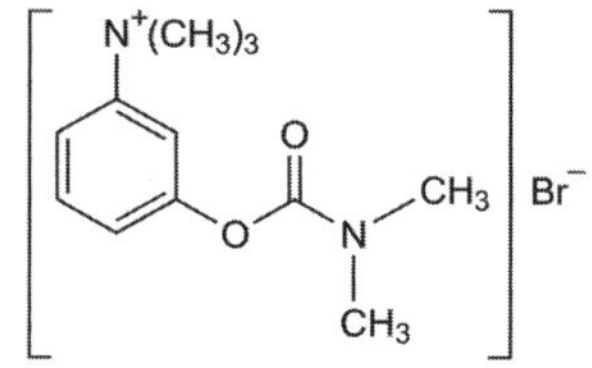

Colourless crystals or a white crystalline, slightly hygroscopic powder. M.p. 171° to 176°, with decomposition.
Soluble 1 in 0.5 of water, 1 in 8 of ethanol and 1 in 5 of chloroform; practically insoluble in ether.

Neostigmine Methylsulfate
Synonym. Proserinum
Proprietary name. Glycostigmin; Intrastigmina; Normastigmin; Prostigmin(e); Prostigmina; Robinul-Neostigmin(e) (injection).
$C_{13}H_{22}N_2O_6S$=334.4
CAS—51-60-5
Colourless crystals or a white crystalline powder. M.p. 144° to 149°.
Soluble 1 in 0.5 of water and 1 in 6 of ethanol.

Dissociation Constant. pK_a 12.0.

Thin-layer Chromatography. Neostigmine bromide: system TA—Rf 02. Neostigmine methylsulfate: system TB—Rf 00; system TE—Rf 00; system TF—Rf 00; system TAE—Rf 00. (Acidified iodoplatinate solution, positive.)

Gas Chromatography. System GA—RI 1770.

High Performance Liquid Chromatography. System HA—*k* 4.7 (tailing peak).

Ultraviolet Spectrum. Aqueous acid—260 (A^1_1=16a), 266 nm. No alkaline shift.

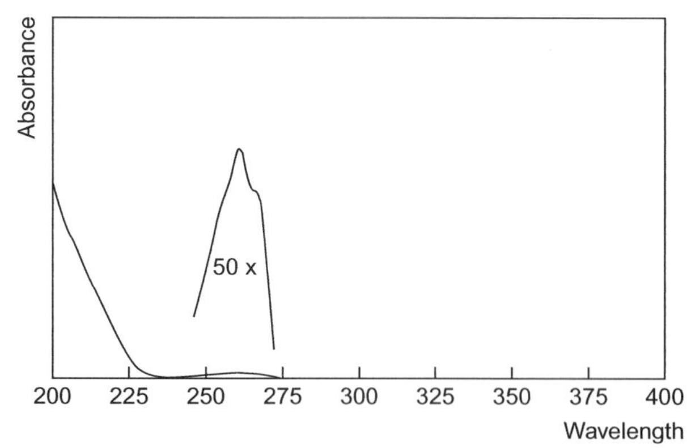

Infra-red Spectrum. Principal peaks at wavenumbers 1711, 1215, 1154, 1176, 948, 690 cm^{-1} (KBr disk).

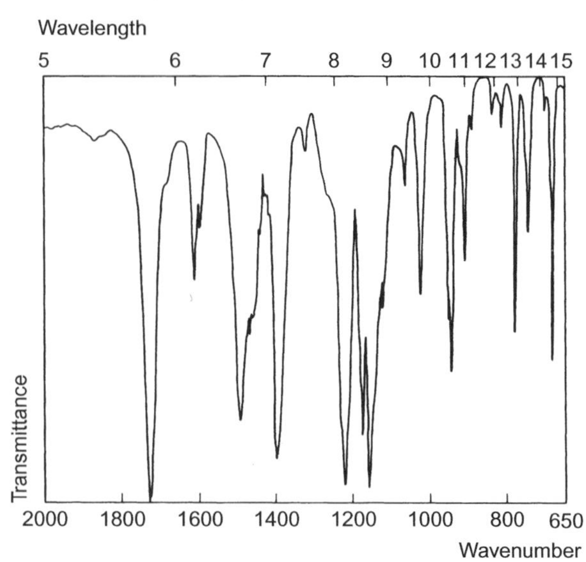

Mass Spectrum. Principal ions at *m/z* 72, 42, 208, 108, 65, 73, 66, 39.

Quantification

Gas chromatography. In plasma: limit of detection 50 μg/L, AFID—K. Chan *et al., J. Chromatogr.*, 1976, *120*, 349–358.

Gas chromatography–mass spectrometry. In plasma: limit of detection 1 μg/L—S.-M. Aquilonius *et al., Eur. J. Clin. Pharmacol.*, 1979, *15*, 367–371.

High performance liquid chromatography. In plasma or cerebrospinal fluid: limit of detection <2.6 μg/L, UV detection—F. Varin *et al., J. Chromatogr. B. Biomed. Sci. Appl.*, 1999, *723*, 319–323.

Mass spectrometry. In urine: neostigmine bromide and other quaternary ammonium compounds, limits of detection 20 to 150 μg/L—M. Nisikawa *et al., Forensic Sci. Int.*, 1991, *51*, 131–138.

Disposition in the Body. Neostigmine bromide is poorly absorbed after oral administration. It is metabolised by ester hydrolysis to form 3-hydroxytrimethylanilinium bromide which is active. About 20% of an oral dose is excreted in the urine with less than 5% as unchanged drug; about 50% of an oral dose is eliminated in the faeces. After intramuscular administration, about 80% of a dose is excreted in the urine in 24 h, with approx. 50% consisting of unchanged drug and 15% as the 3-hydroxytrimethylanilinium metabolite.

Therapeutic concentration

After a single oral dose of 30 mg to 3 subjects, peak plasma concentrations of 0.004 to 0.009 mg/L were attained in 1 to 2 h. [S.- M. Aquilonius *et al., Eur. J. Clin. Pharmacol.*, 1979, *15*, 367–371].

Following intravenous administration of 5 mg to 5 subjects, plasma concentrations of 0.84 to 6.25 mg/L were reported at 2 min. [N. E. Williams *et al., Br. J. Anaesth.*, 1978, *50*, 1065–1067].

Half-life. Plasma half-life, about 1 h.

Volume of distribution. About 1 L/kg.

Clearance. Plasma clearance, about 11 mL/min/kg.

Dose. Usually 75 to 300 mg of neostigmine bromide daily, by mouth; 1 to 2.5 mg of neostigmine methylsulfate daily, given parenterally.

Nevirapine

Non-nucleoside Reverse Transcriptase Inhibitor/Antiviral (HIV)

Synonyms. BI-RG-587; BIRG-0587.
Proprietary name. Viramune
11-Cyclopropyl-5,11-dihydro-4-methyl-6*H*-dipyrido[3,2-*b*:2′,3′-*e*]-[1,4]diazepin-6-one
$C_{15}H_{14}N_4O = 266.3$
CAS—129618-40-2

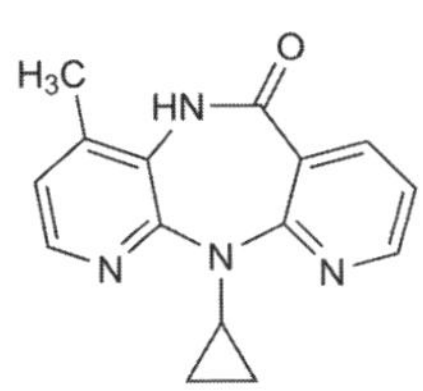

Crystals from pyridine/water. M.p. 247° to 249°. It is highly soluble in water at pH < 3 but solubility decreases to approximately, 0.1 g/L at neutral pH.

Dissociation Constant. pK_a 2.8.

Partition Coefficient. Log *P* (octanol/water), 83.

High Performance Liquid Chromatography. System HAD—*k* 11.1.

Column: C_{18} (Spherisorb, 300 × 4.6 mm i.d., 3 μm). Mobile phase: phosphate buffer (10 mM, pH 5):acetonitrile (82:18) with 10 mM triethylamine, flow rate 1.0 mL/min. UV detection (λ = 240 nm). Retention time: 2.0 min. [R. M. Lopez *et al., J. Chromatogr. B Biomed. Sci. Appl.*, 2001, *751*, 371–376].

Column: (analytical) RP LC-8 (Supelco, 150 × 4.6 mm i.d., 5 μm); (guard) LC-8. Mobile phase: phosphate buffer (25 mM, pH 6):methanol:acetonitrile (63:21.5:15.5) with 25 mM 1-butane-sulfonic acid, flow rate 1.0 mL/min. Internal standard: BIRH-414. UV detection (λ = 280 nm). Retention time(s): nevirapine, 5.5 min; I. S., 7.5 min. [J. W. Pav *et al., J. Pharm. Biomed. Anal.*, 1999, *20*, 91–98].

Column: (analytical) C_8 (150 × 4.6 mm i.d., 5 μm); (guard) C_{18} (10 × 3 mm i.d.). Mobile phase: phosphate buffer (25 mM, pH 5.5):methanol:acetonitrile (7:2:1) with 25 mM hexane-1-sulfonic acid, flow rate 1.0 mL/min. UV detection (λ = 282 nm). Retention time: 9.5 min. [R. P. van Heeswijk *et al., J. Chromatogr. Biomed. Sci. Appl.*, 1998, *713(2)*, 395–399].

Ultraviolet spectrum. Aqueous acid—205, 216, 280 nm.

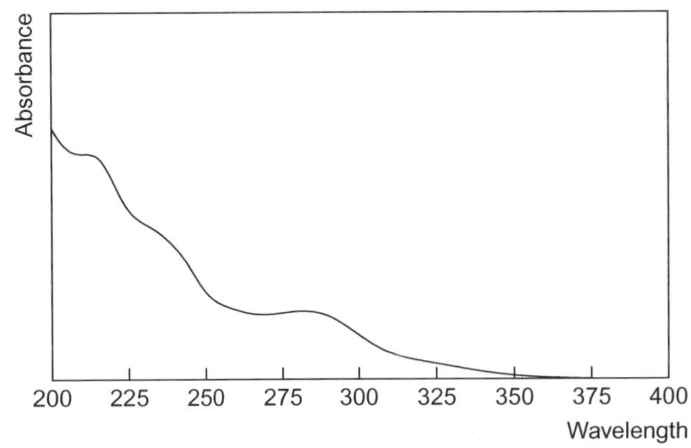

Mass Spectrum. Principal ions at *m/z* 265, 251, 267, 133, 237, 135, 78, 211.

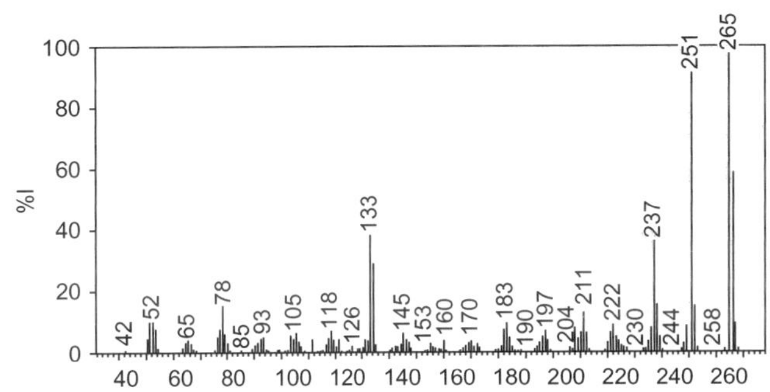

Quantification

High performance liquid chromatography. In plasma: limit of quantification is 0.01 mg/L. UV detection (λ = 245, 280 nm)—A. Jayaraj *et al., Pharm. Res.*, 1992, *9 (Suppl. S334)*. In plasma: limit of detection is 0.05 mg/L, limit of quantification 0.1 mg/L. UV detection (λ = 280 nm)—R. M. Hollanders *et al., J. Chromatogr. Biomed. Sci. Appl.*, 2000, *744(1)*, 65–71. In plasma: limit of quantification is 0.052 mg/L. UV detection (λ = 282 nm)—R. P. van Heeswijk *et al., J. Chromatogr. Biomed. Sci. Appl.*, 1998, *713(2)*, 395–399. In plasma, serum, milk and cerebrospinal fluid: limit of quantification 0.025 mg/L. UV detection (λ = 280 nm)—J. W. Pav *et al., J. Pharm. Biomed. Anal.*, 1999, *20*, 91–98. In plasma: limit of quantification is 0.1 mg/L. UV detection (λ = 260 nm)—G. Aymard *et al., J. Chromatogr. Biomed. Sci. Appl.*, 2000, *744*, 227–240. In serum: limit of detection is 0.084 mg/L, UV detection (λ = 250 nm)—V. A. Simon *et al., J. Chromatogr. A*, 2001, *913(1–2)*, 447–453.

Disposition in the Body. Nevirapine is readily absorbed after oral administration with a peak plasma concentration at 4 h. Absorption is not affected by food. The concentration of the drug in the CNS is 45% of that in plasma. It crosses the placenta and has been detected in breast milk. Nevirapine undergoes extensive metabolism in the liver mainly be the cytochrome P450 isoenzymes of the CYP3A family and the major metabolite is hydroxymethyl-nevirapine. It is excreted via urine as the glucuronide conjugates of the hydroxylated metabolites. The drug is widely distributed in body tissues and the CNS.

Therapeutic concentration. The therapeutic concentration is above 1 mg/L.

18 male and 3 HIV-1-infected female patients, aged between 19 and 46 years, with an absolute CD4 count <400/μL were administered with doses of 12.5, 25, 50, 100, 200 and 400 mg nevirapine after an overnight fast (3

patients for each dose). The mean peak plasma concentrations were 0.145, 0.416, 0.560, 1.215, 2.070 and 3.068 mg/L respectively to the doses, achieved after 1.0, 1.7, 3.7, 3.8, 2.0 and 2.25 h, respectively. [S. H. Cheeseman *et al.*, *Antimicrob. Agents Chemother.*, 1993, *37*, 178–182].

Bioavailability. Oral, about 93%.

Half-life. 45 h which decreases on multiple dosing to 20 to 30 h over a 2- to 4-week period.

Volume of distribution. Steady state, 1.2 to 1.5 L/kg. Reported as 1.54 L/kg in females and 1.38 L/kg in males.

Clearance. Oral, 0.27 to 0.52 mL/kg/min. Plasma, 3.96 L/h (after a 200 mg dose).

Protein binding. 60%.

Note. For a safety profile of nevirapine, see R. B. Pollard *et al.*, *Clin. Ther.*, 1998, *20*, 1071–1092.

Dose. Adult: 200 mg once daily which can be increased to 400 mg daily after 2 weeks. Children under 50 kg (2 months to 8 years): 4 mg/kg increased to 7 mg/kg twice daily (maximum 400 mg daily). (8 to 16 years): 4 mg/kg once daily increased to twice daily (maximum 400 mg).

Nialamide

Antidepressant

Proprietary names. Espril; Niamid(al); Niaquitil; Nuredal; Nyazin.

4-Pyridinecarboxylic acid 2-[3-oxo-3-[(phenylmethyl)amino]propyl]-hydrazide

$C_{16}H_{18}N_4O_2=298.3$

CAS—51-12-7

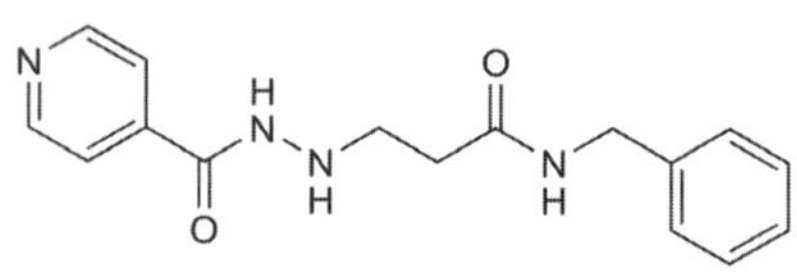

A white crystalline powder. M.p. 151° to 153°.

Soluble 1 in 400 of water, 1 in 40 of ethanol, 1 in 150 of chloroform and 1 in 10 of methanol; freely soluble in acidic solvents.

Partition Coefficient. Log *P* (octanol/buffer pH 7.4), 0.9.

Colour Tests. Liebermann's test—red-orange; Mandelin's test—red; Nessler's reagent—black.

Thin-layer Chromatography. System TA—Rf 70; system TB—Rf 02; system TC—Rf 25; system TL—Rf 04; system TAE—Rf 68; system TAF—Rf 64. (Dragendorff spray, positive; acidified iodoplatinate solution, positive; Marquis reagent, brown.)

Gas Chromatography. System GA—RI 1500.

High Performance Liquid Chromatography. System HA—*k* 1.2 (tailing peak); system HX—RI 334.

Ultraviolet Spectrum. Aqueous acid—266 nm (A_1^1=193a); aqueous alkali—307 nm.

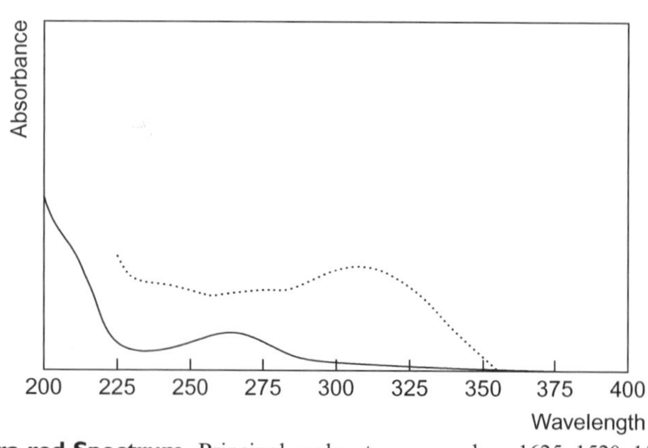

Infra-red Spectrum. Principal peaks at wavenumbers 1625, 1520, 1547, 698, 670, 1600 cm^{-1} (KBr disk).

Mass Spectrum. Principal ions at *m/z* 91, 177, 44, 106, 45, 78, 123, 51.

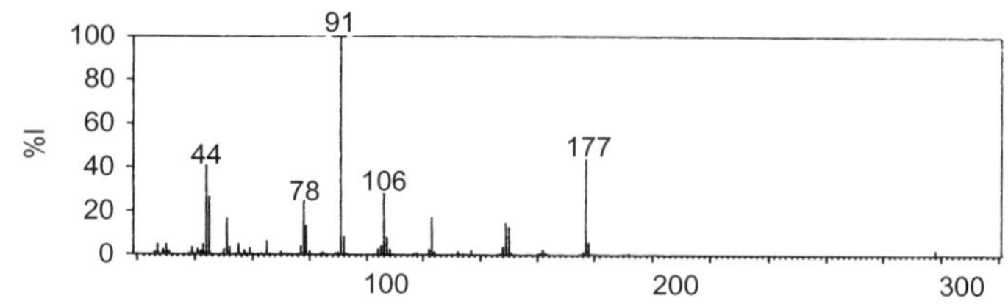

Dose. 75 to 150 mg daily.

Nicametate

Vasodilator

Proprietary name. Eucast

3-Pyridinecarboxylic acid 2-(diethylamino)ethyl ester

$C_{12}H_{18}N_2O_2=222.3$

CAS—3099-52-3

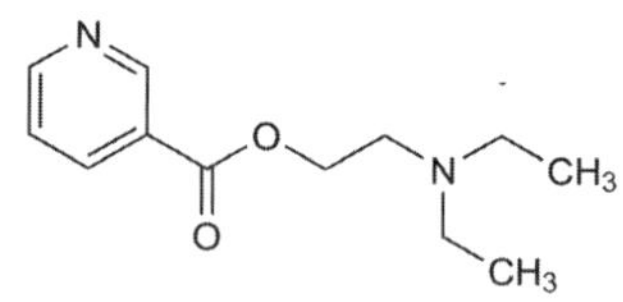

A liquid.

Nicametate Citrate

Proprietary names. Euclidan; Nurtin; Soclidan.

$C_{12}H_{18}N_2O_2,C_6H_8O_7,H_2O=432.4$

CAS—1641-74-3

A white crystalline powder.

Partition Coefficient. Log *P* (octanol/water), 1.3.

Colour Test. Cyanogen bromide—orange.

Thin-layer Chromatography. System TA—Rf 56; system TB—Rf 41; system TC—Rf 35; system TE—Rf 68; system TL—Rf 20; system TAE—Rf 35. (Acidified iodoplatinate solution, positive.)

Gas Chromatography. System GA—nicametate RI 1608, nicotinic acid—RI 1335.

Ultraviolet Spectrum. Aqueous acid—261 nm (A_1^1 =120b).

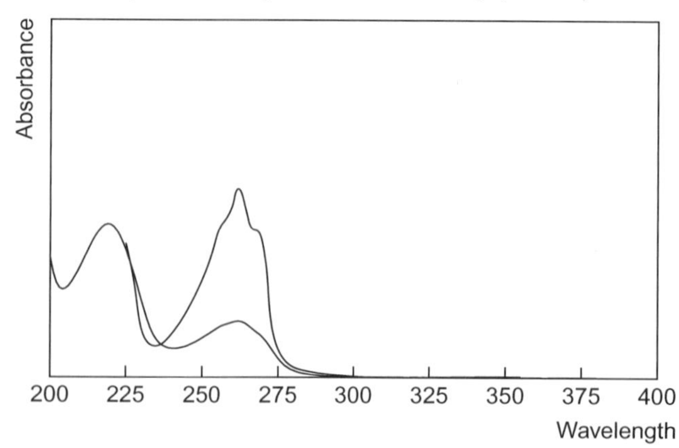

Infra-red Spectrum. Principal peaks at wavenumbers 1729, 1283, 1594, 1130, 1116, 743 cm^{-1} (KBr disk).

Mass Spectrum. Principal ions at *m/z* 86, 30, 58, 123, 78, 51, 29, 42; nicotinic acid 123, 105, 78, 51, 106, 77, 124, 50.

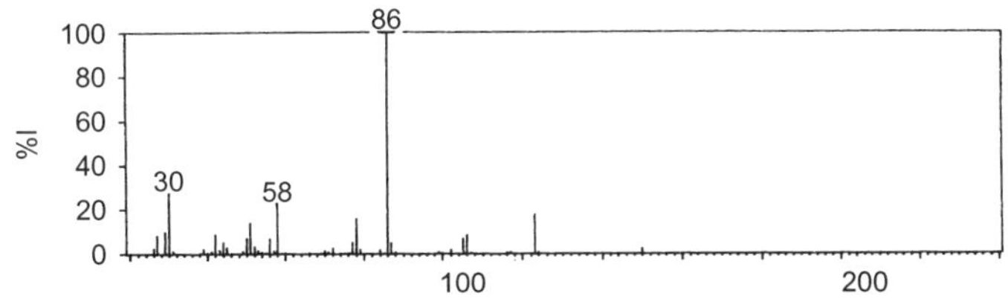

Disposition in the Body. Slowly hydrolysed to nicotinic acid and diethylaminoethanol.

Dose. 300 mg of nicametate citrate daily.

Nicergoline

Vasodilator

Synonyms. Nicotergoline; Nimergoline; FI-6714.
Proprietary names. Cebran; Circo-Maren; Duracebrol; Ergobel; Ergolin; Ergotop; Fisifax; Memoq; Neugen; Nicer; Nicergobeta; Nicerium; Sermion; Varson.
(8β)-10-Methoxy-1,6-dimethylergoline-8-methanol 5-bromo-3-pyridine-carboxylate
$C_{24}H_{26}BrN_3O_3$=484.4
CAS—27848-84-6

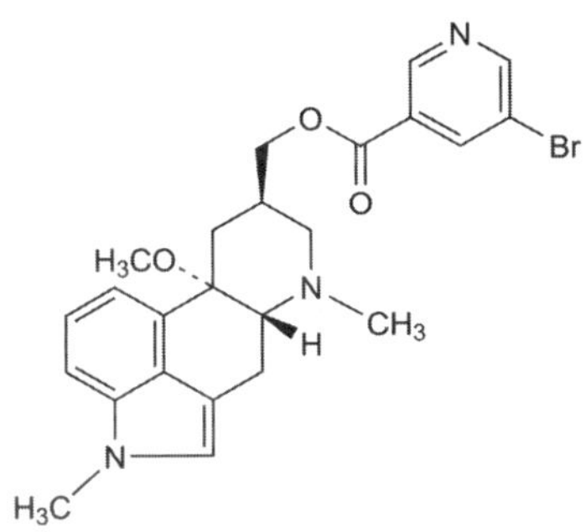

A yellowish-white crystalline powder.
M.p. 136° to 138°.
Practically insoluble in water; soluble in ethanol and chloroform; slightly soluble in ether.

Colour Tests. Liebermann's test—black; Mandelin's test—violet-brown→brown; Marquis test—blue→grey; Sulfuric acid—violet.

Thin-layer Chromatography. System TA—Rf 64; system TAE—Rf 43; system TE—Rf 73. (Acidified iodoplatinate solution, positive.)

Gas Chromatography. System GA—not eluted.

High Performance Liquid Chromatography. System HAA—Retention time(s), 15.5 min.

Ultraviolet Spectrum. Aqueous acid—286 nm; aqueous alkali—280 nm; ethanol—287 nm (A_1^1=200b).

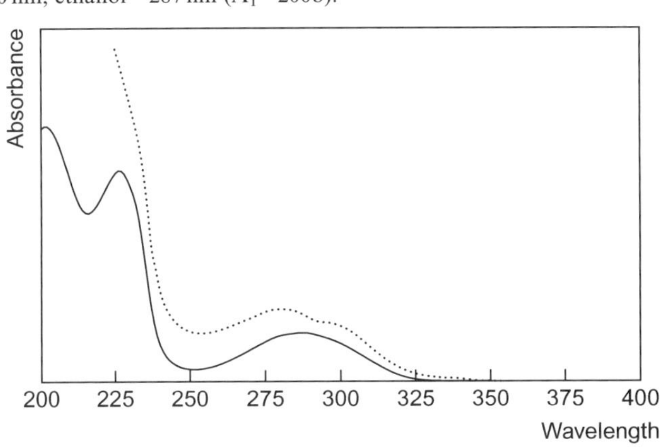

Infra-red Spectrum. Principal peaks at wavenumbers 1281, 751, 1718, 1306, 1075, 1103 cm^{-1} (KBr disk).

Quantification

High performance liquid chromatography. In urine: 10α-methoxy-9,10 dihydrolysergol, a metabolite of nicergoline, UV detection—A. Sioufi *et al., Biomed. Chromatogr.*, 1992, *6*, 9–11.

High performance liquid chromatography–mass spectrometry. In plasma or urine: nicergoline and its metabolites, limits of detection 2 μg/L in plasma and 10 μg/L in urine—K. Banna *et al., J. Chromatogr.*, 1991, *568*, 375–384.

Radioimmunoassay. In plasma or urine: limit of detection <60 ng/L—C. A. Bizollon *et al., Eur. J. Nucl. Med.*, 1982, *7*, 318–321.

Disposition in the Body. Nicergoline is extensively metabolised, mainly by hydrolysis and N^1-demethylation, and is excreted in the urine as free and conjugated (glucuronide) metabolites.

Dose. Usually 15 mg daily.

Niclosamide

Anthelmintic

Synonym. Phenasale
Proprietary names. Atenase; Kontal; Mansonil (vet.); Niclocide; Trédémine; Yomesan.
5-Chloro-*N*-(2-chloro-4-nitrophenyl)-2-hydroxybenzamide
$C_{13}H_8Cl_2N_2O_4$=327.1
CAS—50-65-7

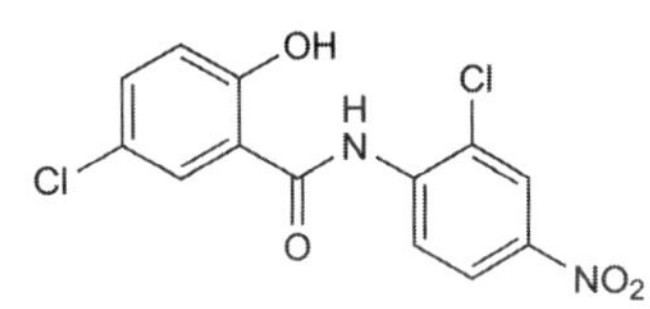

A cream-coloured powder. M.p. 225° to 230°.
Practically insoluble in water; soluble 1 in 150 of ethanol, 1 in 400 of chloroform and 1 in 350 of ether; soluble in acetone.

Partition Coefficient. Log *P* (octanol/water), 4.6.

Colour Tests. Mandelin's Test—green; Methanolic Potassium Hydroxide—yellow.

Thin-layer Chromatography. System TA—Rf 91; system TB—Rf 00; system TE—Rf 23; system TAE—Rf 93. (Acidified iodoplatinate solution, positive.)

High Performance Liquid Chromatography. System HX—RI 723; system HAA—Retention time, 23.9 min.

Ultraviolet Spectrum. Aqueous alkali—334, 377 nm; methanol—333 nm (A_1^1=527b).

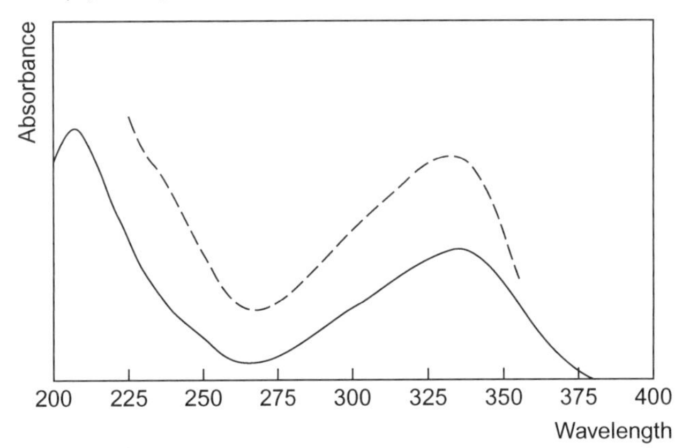

Infra-red Spectrum. Principal peaks at wavenumbers 1572, 1515, 1613, 1285, 1650, 1218 cm^{-1} (KBr disk).

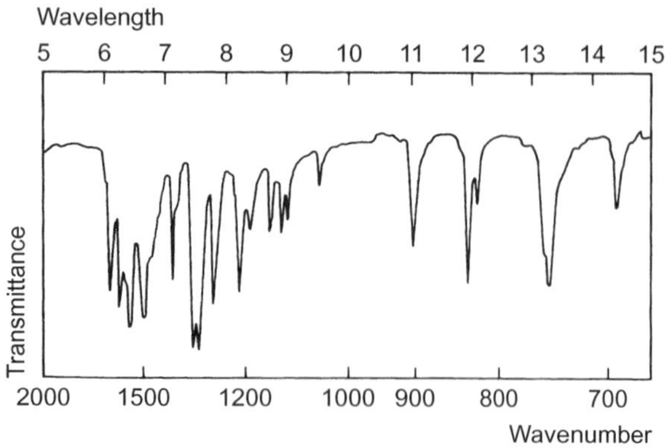

Dose. Usually 2 g as a single dose.

Nicofuranose

Vasodilator

Synonyms. Tetranicotinoylfructofuranose; Tetranicotinoylfructose.
Proprietary name. Bradilan
β-D-Fructofuranose-1,3,4,6-tetra-3-pyridinecarboxylate
$C_{30}H_{24}N_4O_{10}$=600.5
CAS—15351-13-0

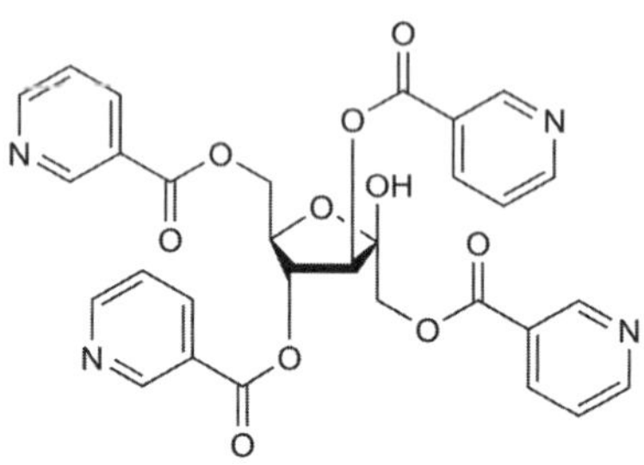

A creamy-white crystalline powder. M.p. 132° to 143°.
Practically insoluble in water; soluble 1 in 4 of chloroform and 1 in 70 of methanol; sparingly soluble in dilute solutions of hydrochloric acid and sodium hydroxide.

Partition Coefficient. Log *P* (octanol/water), 0.1.

Colour Tests. Add 50 mg to 5 mL of potassium cupritartrate solution and heat to boiling for 1 min—red precipitate.
Fuse 50 mg with 10 mg of 2,4-dinitrochlorobenzene, cool, add about 3 mL of ethanol and 1 mL of 1 M sodium hydroxide—intense red-violet colour.

Thin-layer Chromatography. System TA—Rf 61; system TB—Rf 42; system TC—Rf 70; system TL—Rf 61. (Acidified iodoplatinate solution, positive.)

Ultraviolet Spectrum. Aqueous acid—262 nm (A_1^1=380b); aqueous alkali—263 nm.

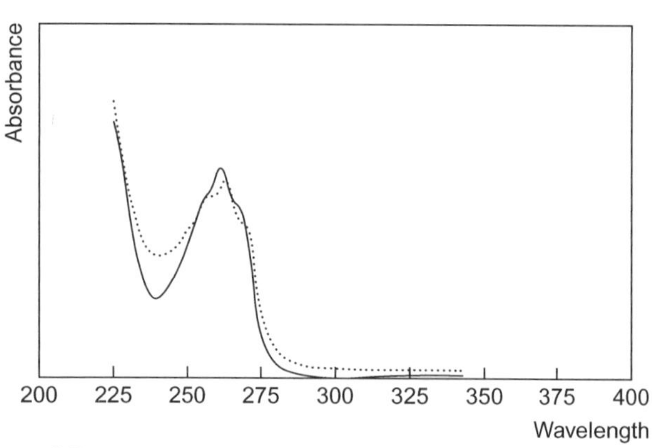

Infra-red Spectrum. Principal peaks at wavenumbers 1721, 1271, 1107, 737, 1587, 1022 cm^{-1} (KBr disk).

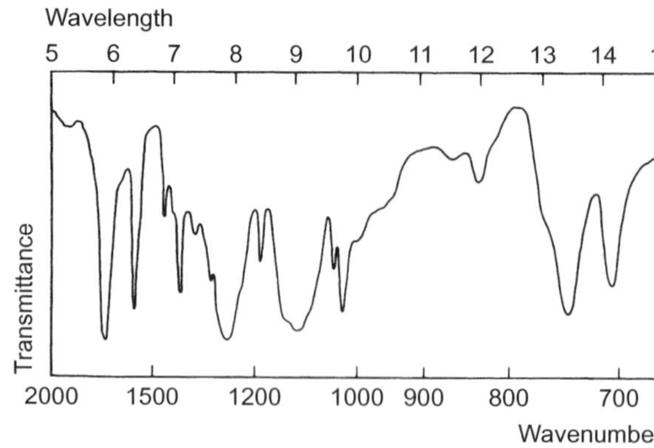

Mass Spectrum. Principal ions at *m/z* 123, 106, 78, 51, 105, 50, 77, 52; nicotinic acid 123, 105, 78, 51, 106, 77, 124, 50.

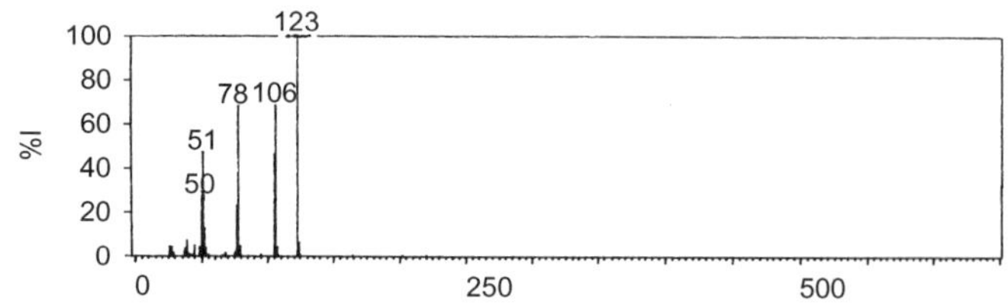

Disposition in the Body. Nicofuranose is slowly hydrolysed in the small intestine to nicotinic acid which is readily absorbed.

Therapeutic concentration

Following a single oral dose of 500 mg to 27 subjects, a mean peak plasma concentration of 0.72 mg/L was attained in 3 h. [H. A. Salmi and H. Frey, *Curr. Ther. Res.*, 1974, *16*, 669–674].

Dose. 1.5 to 3 g daily.

Nicorandil

Anti-anginal/ Nitrovasodilator/ Potassium-channel Activator

Synonym. SG-75
Proprietary names. Adancor; Dancor; Ikorel; Perisalol; Sigmart.
N-[2-(Nitrooxy)ethyl]-3-pyridine carboxamide
$C_8H_9N_3O_4$=211.2
CAS—65141-46-0

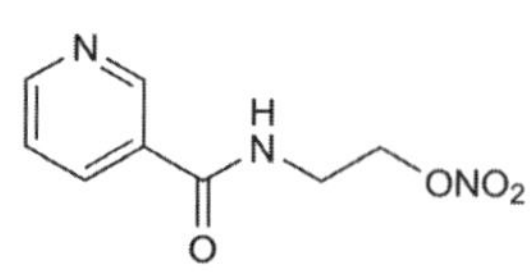

A colourless to off-white crystalline powder. M.p. 92° to 93°.

Partition Coefficient. Log *P* (octanol/water), 0.43.

High Performance Liquid Chromatography. System HZ—retention time, 2.2 min.

Column: (analytical) C_8 (Finepak SIL, 250 × 4.6 mm i.d., 5 μm); (guard) C_{18} Corasil. Column temperature: 30°. Mobile phase: methanol:water (15:85), flow rate 1.2 mL/min. Internal standard: (*N*-[2-(nitrooxy)propyl]-3-pyridine carboxamide) chlorohydrate. UV detection (λ=230 nm). Retention time: nicorandil, 35.3 min; (*N*-(2-hydroxyethyl)nicotinamide), 11.1 min; I. S., 59.7 min. [A. Ojha and A. Pargal, *J. Pharm. Biomed. Anal.*, 1999, *21*, 175–178].

Column: Phenyl (Nucleosil, 150 × 4.6 mm i.d., 5 μm). Mobile phase: ammonium acetate buffer (0.01 M, pH 6.2 with acetic acid):acetonitrile (10:3), flow rate 1.0 mL/min. MS detection (APCI, full scan). Retention time: 6 min. [S. Andrensek *et al.*, *J. Chromatogr. Biomed. Sci. Appl.*, 1999, *735(1)*, 103–109].

Column: C_{18} (μBondapak, 300 × 3.9 mm i.d., 10 μm). Mobile phase: acetonitrile:water:borate buffer (0.1 M, pH 8) (15:70:15), flow rate 1 mL/min. Internal standard: SG-89. UV detection (λ=220 nm). Retention time: 8 min. [M. Tanikawa *et al.*, *J. Chromatogr.*, 1993, *617*, 163–167].

Quantification

Gas chromatography–mass spectrometry. In plasma: limit of detection 0.1 to 0.25 µg/L—A. Frydman, *J. Cardiovasc. Pharmacol.*, 1992, *20 Suppl. 3*.

High performance liquid chromatography. In blood: limit of detection 3 µg/L. UV detection (λ=220 nm)—M. Tanikawa *et al.*, *J. Chromatogr.*, 1993, *617*, 163–167. In plasma: limit of quantification is 1.0 µg/L. MS and UV detection (λ=256 nm)—S. Andrensek *et al.*, *J. Chromatogr. Biomed. Sci. Appl.*, 1999, *735(1)*, 103–109.

Disposition in the Body. Nicorandil is rapidly and well absorbed from the gastro-intestinal tract, but food can decrease the rate of absorption. There is no significant first pass metabolism. It is extensively metabolised, mainly via denitration and there are two predominant biotransformation pathways: the formation of nicotamide through degradation of the side chain and the production of *N*-(2-hydroxyethyl)nicotinamide from denitration which eventually degrades to nicotinic acid. Further metabolism of these products leads to non-toxic water soluble vitamin B complex substances. The kidney is the major route of elimination with 20% of an administrated dose being excreted in urine mainly as metabolites. Less than 2% of the dose is excreted via the biliary route. 10% of the administered dose can be found in plasma but it is rapidly eliminated.

Therapeutic concentration. After a 5 mg dose, a plasma concentration of 64 µg/L is achieved; 10 mg dose, 107 µg/L; 20 mg dose, 261 µg/L; and a 40 mg dose, 490 µg/L. The maximum plasma concentration occurs 30 to 60 min after oral administration. 8 to 24 h after dosing, the mean plasma concentration remains in the range 0.8 to 1.5 µg/L. There is a linear relationship between dose and increase in maximum plasma concentration. Steady state is achieved 96 to 120 h after continuous dosing.

Bioavailability. 75% to 80%

Half-life. Approx. 1 h.

Volume of distribution. 1.0 to 1.4 L/kg; also reported as 100 L.

Clearance. The total body clearance is 0.87 to 1.15 L/min (52 to 69 L/h).

Protein binding. Weakly bound to albumin and other plasma proteins at approx. 25% (19% to albumin).

Dose. The initial dose is 10 mg twice daily; the usual dose is 10 to 20 mg twice daily with a maximum of 30 mg twice daily.

Nicotinamide

Vitamin

Synonyms. Niacinamide; Nicotinic Acid Amide; Nicotylamide; Vitamin PP.

Proprietary names. Nacro; Nicobion; Nicotinoid; Nicovital; Papulex; Ucemine PP.

3-Pyridinecarboxamide

$C_6H_6N_2O=122.1$

CAS—98-92-0

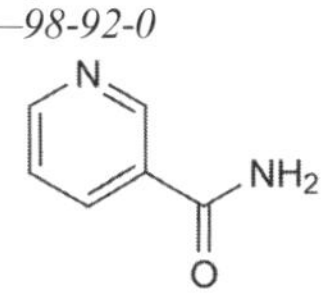

A white crystalline powder or colourless crystals. M.p. 128° to 131°. Soluble 1 in 1 of water, 1 in 1.5 of ethanol and 1 in 10 of glycerol; slightly soluble in chloroform and ether.

Dissociation Constant. pK_a 3.3 (20°).

Partition Coefficient. Log *P* (octanol/water), −0.4.

Colour Tests. Cyanogen Bromide—orange; Nessler's Reagent—brown-orange.

Thin-layer Chromatography. System TA—Rf 54, streaking; system TB—Rf 00; system TC—Rf 21; system TE—Rf 40; system TL—Rf 27; system TAE—Rf 68; system TAF—Rf 66.

Gas Chromatography. System GA—nicotinamide RI 1436, nicotinic acid RI 1335.

High Performance Liquid Chromatography. System HX—RI 168.

Ultraviolet Spectrum. Aqueous acid—261 nm ($A^1_1=451a$).

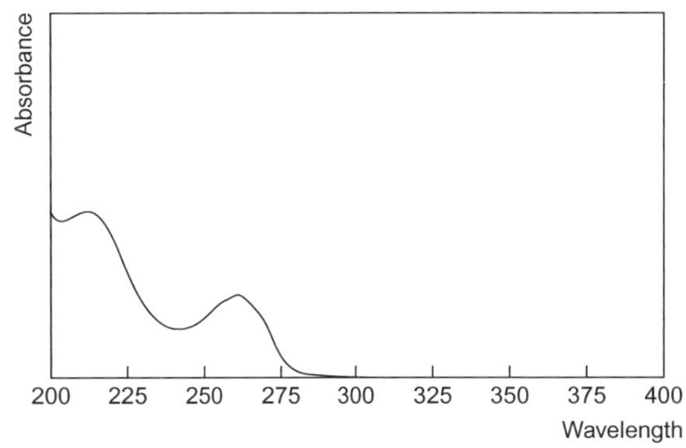

Infra-red Spectrum. Principal peaks at wavenumbers 1680, 1698, 703, 1618, 1594, 1026 cm^{-1} (KBr disk).

Mass Spectrum. Principal ions at *m/z* 122, 78, 106, 51, 50, 52, 44, 123; nicotinic acid 123, 105, 78, 51, 106, 77, 124, 50.

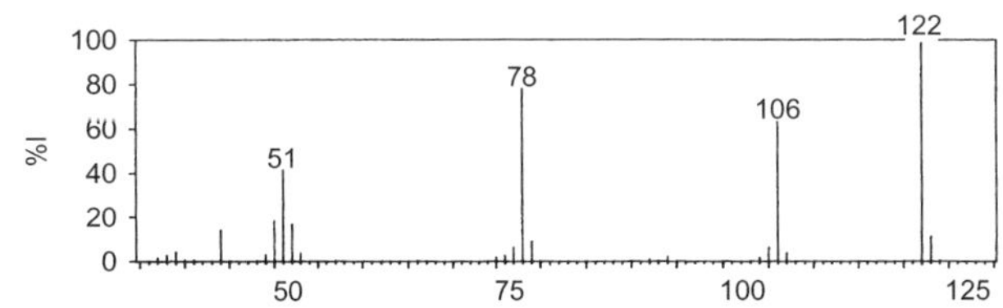

Quantification. See also Nicotinic Acid.

High performance liquid chromatography. In plasma or urine: *N*-methylnicotinamide, limit of detection <2 µg/L, fluorescence detection—A. Somogyi *et al.*, *Anal. Biochem.*, 1990, *187*, 160-165. In plasma or urine: nicotinamide and its metabolites—M. R. Stratford and M. F. Dennis, *J. Chromatogr.*, 1992, *582*, 145–151. In plasma: nicotinamide and *N*-methylnicotinamide—H. A. Gillmor *et al.*, *Biomed. Chromatogr.*, 1999, *13*, 360–362.

Disposition in the Body. It is excreted in the urine as unchanged drug, nicotinic acid, *N*-methylnicotinamide, and nicotinuric acid. Nicotinamide is a metabolite of nikethamide.

Therapeutic concentration

In 15 subjects given 6 g of nicotinamide daily by mouth, a mean maximum plasma concentration of 1.166 mmol/L (range 0.787 to 2.312) was achieved in 1 to 6 h (1 h in 54% of the subjects) [J. Bernier *et al.*, *Radiother. Oncol.*, 1998, *48*, 123–133].

22 subjects given nicotinamide orally at a dose of 60 mg/kg (maximum 6 g) daily, had a mean peak plasma concentration of 0.793 mmol/L (range 0.516 to 1.513) at 0.77 h (0.22 to 3.05); co-administration with domperidone did not significantly change these values [J. Bussink *et al.*, *Radiother. Oncol.*, 2002, *63*, 285–291].

Dose. Up to 250 mg daily.

Nicotine

Insecticide/Aid to Smoking Cessation

Proprietary names. Habitrol; Nicabate; Nicoderm; Nicogum; Nicolan; Nicomax; Niconil; Nicopatch; Nicorette; Nicotinell; Nicotrans; Nicotrol; Nikofrenon; Nikotugg; NiQuitin; Prostep; Quit; Stoppers; Stubit (anti-smoking preparations).

3-[(2*S*)-1-Methyl-2-pyrrolidinyl]pyridine

$C_{10}H_{14}N_2=162.2$

CAS—54-11-5

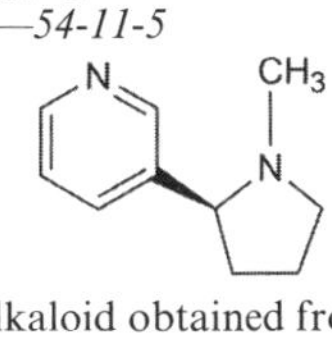

An alkaloid obtained from the dried leaves of the tobacco plant, *Nicotiana tabacum* (Solanaceae).

A colourless to pale yellow, very hygroscopic, oily liquid with an unpleasant pungent odour. It gradually becomes brown on exposure to air or

light. Mass per mL about 1.01 g. B.p. 247°, with decomposition. Refractive index 1.5280.
Miscible with water below 60°; very soluble in ethanol, chloroform, petroleum ether, kerosene, oils, and ether.

Dissociation Constant. pK_a 3.2, 7.9 (25°).

Partition Coefficient. Log *P* (octanol/water), 1.2.

Colour Test. Cyanogen Bromide—orange.

Thin-layer Chromatography. System TA—Rf 54; system TB—Rf 39; system TC—Rf 35; system TE—Rf 61; system TL—Rf 13; system TX—Rf 04; system TY—Rf 01; system TAE—Rf 39; system TAF—Rf 22; system TAJ—Rf 09; system TAK—Rf 00; system TAL—Rf 11. (Dragendorff spray, positive; acidified iodoplatinate solution, positive.)

Gas Chromatography. System GA—nicotine RI 1350, M (cotinine) RI 1715; system GB—nicotine RI 1380, M (cotinine) RI 1645; system GC—nicotine RI 1573, M (cotinine) RI 2111; system GF—nicotine RI 1525, M (cotinine) RI 2195.

High Performance Liquid Chromatography. System HA—nicotine *k* 1.1, M (cotinine) *k* 0.2; system HX—nicotine RI 69, M (cotinine) RI 215; system HZ—retention time nicotine 1.73 min, M (cotinine) 1.71 min.

Ultraviolet Spectrum. Aqueous acid—259 (A_1^1 = 338a); aqueous alkali—261 nm.

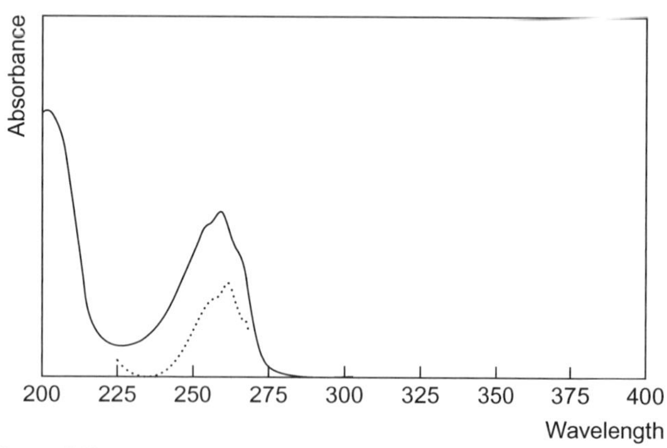

Infra-red Spectrum. Principal peaks at wavenumbers 712, 1022, 810, 1575, 1310, 1040 cm^{-1} (thin film).

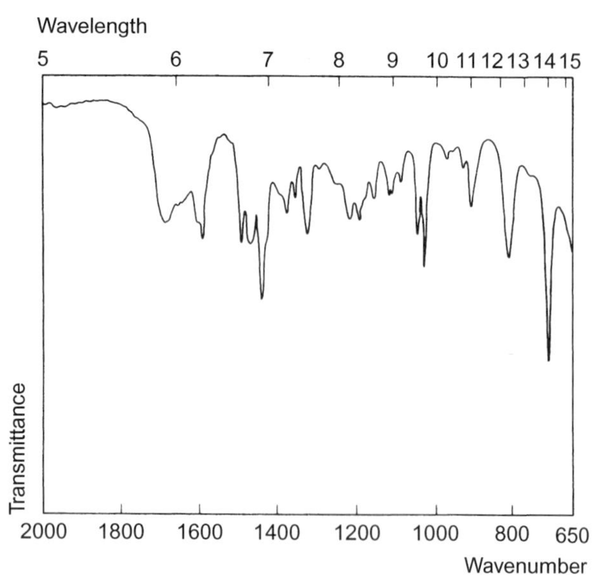

Mass Spectrum. Principal ions at *m/z* 84, 133, 42, 162, 161, 105, 77, 119; cotinine 98, 176, 42, 118, 41, 119, 51, 175; nicotine-1′-*N*-oxide 84, 178, 161, 133, 118, -, -, -.

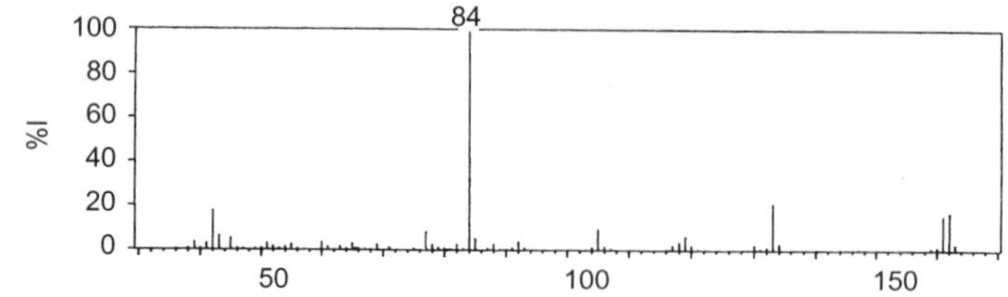

Quantification

Gas chromatography. In plasma or urine: limits of detection in plasma, 5 µg/L for nicotine and cotinine and 15 µg/L for the *N*-oxide; detection limits in urine, 30 µg/L for nicotine and cotinine and 100 µg/L for the *N*-oxide, FID—G. Stehlich *et al., J.Chromatogr.* 1982, *232*(21) *B Biomed. Appl.*, 295–303. In hair: nitrogen-phosphorus detection—A. Mizuno *et al., Ther. Drug Monit.*, 1993, *15*, 99–104. In plasma—L. Nystrom *et al., J. Chromatogr. B Biomed. Sci. Appl.*, 1997, *701*, 124–128.

Gas chromatography. In plasma: limits of detection 1 µg/L for nicotine, 5 µg/L for cotinine, AFID—K. G. Verebey *et al., J. Anal. Toxicol.*, 1982, *6*, 294–296. In urine: trans-3′-hydroxycotinine, nitrogen-phosphorus detection (or MS with SIM) —P. Jacob *et al., J. Chromatogr.*, 1992, *583*, *145*–154.

Gas chromatography–mass spectrometry. In biological tissues: nicotine and cotinine, limits of detection 5 ng/g and 10 ng/g respectively—N. Urakawa *et al., Int. J. Leg. Med.*, 1994, *106*, 232–236. In hair—K. Zahlsen and O. G. Nilsen, *Pharmacol. Toxicol.*, 1994, *75*, 143–149. In plasma: limit of quantification 0.5 µg/L—E. Davoli *et al., J. Chromatogr. B Biomed. Sci. Appl.*, 1998, *707*, 312–316. In plasma or urine: nicotine and cotinine, limits of detection 0.16 µg/L—H. James *et al., J. Chromatogr. B Biomed. Sci. Appl.*, 1998, *708*, 87–93. In serum or urine: limit of detection 2 µg/L, SIM—L. B. Baskin *et al., Ann. Clin. Biochem.*, 1998, *35*, 522–527. In urine: trans-3′-hydroxycotinine and cotinine, limits of quantification 50 µg/L and 20 µg/L respectively—A. J. Ji *et al., Clin. Chem.*, 1999, *45*, 85–91. In plasma: nicotine, cotinine, and mecamylamine, limits of quantification 1 µg/L, 2 µg/L, and 2 µg/L respectively—P. Jacob *et al., J. Pharm. Biomed. Anal.*, 2000, *23*, 653–661. In plasma, saliva, or urine: nicotine and cotinine, limits of detection 1 µg/L in plasma and saliva, and 0.2 µg/L in urine—H. S. Shin *et al., J. Chromatogr. B Analyt. Technol. Biomed. Life Sci.*, 2002, *769*, 177–183.

High performance liquid chromatography. In plasma or urine: limit of detection 2 µg/L for nicotine or cotinine in urine, UV detection—M. P. Maskarinec *et al., J. Anal. Toxicol.*, 1978, *2*, 124–126. In serum: nicotine and its metabolites, limits of detection 3 to 10 µg/L, UV detection—P Zuccaro *et al., J Chromatogr.*, 1993, *621*, 257–261. In urine: nicotine and its metabolites—P. Zuccaro *et al., J. Chromatogr. B Biomed. Sci. Appl.*, 1995, *668*, 187–188. In hair: nicotine and cotinine, UV detection—S. Pichini *et al., Forensic Sci. Int.*, 1997, *84*, 243–252. In meconium: nicotine and its metabolites and mecamylamine, diode-array detection—J. Baranowski *et al., J. Chromatogr. B Biomed. Sci. Appl.*, 1998, *707*, 317–321. In urine: nicotine and cotinine, limits of quantification 5 µg/L and 0.5 µg/L respectively, UV detection—C. Oddoze *et al., J. Chromatogr. B Biomed. Sci. Appl.*, 1998, *708*, 95–101. In plasma: nicotine and cotinine, limits of quantification 0.2 µg/L and 1 µg/L respectively, UV detection—M. Nakajima *et al., J. Chromatogr. B Biomed. Sci. Appl.*, 2000, *742*, 211–215. In plasma: nicotine metabolites, limits of detection 10 µg/L for cotinine and hydroxycotinine and 20 µg/L for total 3′-hydroxycotinine, UV detection—O. A. Ghosheh *et al., J. Pharm. Biomed. Anal.*, 2000, *23*, 543–549. In urine: cotinine, UV detection—F. Ceppa *et al., J. Chromatogr. B Biomed. Sci. Appl.*, 2000, *746*, 115–122. In hair: electrochemical detection—G. N. Mahoney and W. Al-Delaimy, *J. Chromatogr. B Biomed. Sci. Appl.*, 2001, *753*, 179–187.

High performance liquid chromatography–mass spectrometry. In urine: nicotine metabolites—S. S. Hecht *et al., Chem. Res. Toxicol.*, 1999, *12*, 172–179. In urine: nicotine and its metabolites and mecamylamine, limits of detection 10 µg/L for nicotine and 1 µg/L for its metabolites—T. Tuomi *et al., Clin. Chem.*, 1999, *45*, 2164–2172. In serum or urine: nicotine and its metabolites, limits of quantification 0.5 to 5 µg/L—T. P. Moyer *et al., Clin. Chem.*, 2002, *48*, 1460–1471. In urine: nicotine and its metabolites—M. Meger *et al., J. Chromatogr. B Analyt. Technol. Biomed. Life Sci.*, 2002, *778*, 251–261.

Disposition in the Body. Readily absorbed from the gastro-intestinal tract, the buccal mucosa, the respiratory tract, and intact skin, and widely distributed throughout the tissues. Nicotine undergoes first-pass metabolism when administered orally, thus reducing the bioavailability. It is widely distributed, crossing the placental barrier and it is also found in breast milk. It is metabolised by oxidation via cytochrome P450 enzyme CYP2A6 to cotinine and nicotine-1′-*N*-oxide followed by further degradation to produce hydroxycotinine, norcotinine, and a ring cleavage product. About 5% is excreted unchanged in the urine in 24 h and about 10% as cotinine; the excretion of unchanged drug is decreased if the urine is alkaline.

Blood concentration

6 smokers received a single dose of nicotine (1 mg nasal spray; average dose absorbed 0.8 mg; range 0.7 to 1.0) and 6 others smoked cigarettes (1 puff per min for 10 min; average dose absorbed 4.4 mg; range 1.5 to 3.2); all subjects also received a 30-min IV infusion of nicotine (average dose 5.1 mg; range 4.1 to 6.3) beginning 70 min after administration of the spray or commencement of smoking. In the subjects who received cigarettes, a mean peak plasma concentration of 0.0398 mg/L was attained at 8.2 min in arterial blood and 0.0186 mg/L at 11.9 min in venous blood. In the subjects who received nicotine intranasally, these values were 0.0104 mg/L in 4.7 min in arterial blood and 0.0054 mg/L in 24.8 min in venous blood. Mean peak plasma concentrations in arterial and venous blood after the IV infusion were 0.049 mg/L in 29 min and 0.0295 mg/L in 30 min, respectively. [S. G. Gourlay and N. L. Benowitz, *Clin. Pharmacol. Ther*., 1997, *62*, 453–463.]

After 25 subjects were administered nicotine via transdermal patches (15-mg 16-h patch or two different 21-mg 24-h patches; each patch applied for 3 consecutive days), mean minimum and maximum plasma nicotine concentrations of 0.00153 and 0.0123 mg/L were reported for the 15-mg 16-h patch, 0.013 and 0.0195 mg/L for the first 21-mg 24-h patch and 0.0119 and 0.0278 mg/L for the second 21-mg 24-h patch. The times taken to reach peak plasma concentration were 6.0, 8.0, and 2.8 h for the respective patches. [R. V. Fant *et al.*, *Pharmacol. Biochem. Behav*., 2000, *67*, 479–482.]

A heavy smoker who abused lozenges containing nicotine (approximately 240 × 0.4 mg daily) had saliva and blood cotinine levels of 1.154 and 0.947 mg/L, respectively. 20 min after his 70th 0.4-mg lozenge of the day, his plasma nicotine concentration was 0.0321 mg/L. In 8 non-smoking subjects who consumed 8 × 1.1-mg nicotine lozenges, mean nicotine levels increased from 0.0003 to 0.0064 mg/L. [J. Foulds *et al.*, *Addiction*, 1998, *93*, 1427–1431.]

10 non-smoking patients with ulcerative colitis received nicotine tartrate liquid enema at a dose of 3 mg nicotine base nightly for 1 week, then 6 mg for 3 weeks. Only one patient had a detectable peak nicotine concentration (0.0023mg/L) and none had a detectable trough concentration; the mean trough plasma cotinine concentration was 0.012 mg/L. [W. J. Sandborn *et al.*, *Aliment. Pharmacol. Ther*., 1997, *11*, 663–671.]

In a group of 150 habitual smokers, nicotine concentrations in samples of plasma withdrawn 2 min after smoking were in the range 0.003 to 0.063 mg/L (mean 0.019); corresponding cotinine concentrations ranged from 0.02 to 0.26 mg/L (mean 0.22). [M. J. Kogan *et al.*, *J. Forensic Sci.*, 1981, *26*, 6–11.]

Toxicity. Nicotine is highly toxic and, in acute poisoning, death may occur within a few minutes because respiratory failure arises from paralysis of the respiratory muscles. The lethal dose for an adult is between 40 and 60 mg. Blood concentrations greater than 5 mg/L may be fatal. The maximum permissible atmospheric concentration is 0.5 mg/m^3.

In 5 adults who ingested 20 to 25 g of nicotine and died within 1 h, postmortem blood concentrations were between 11 and 63 mg/L (mean 29). [R. C. Baselt and R. H. Cravey, *J. Anal. Toxicol.*, 1977, *1*, 81–103.]

Bioavailability. About 30% (oral).

Half-life. After inhalation or parenteral administration, plasma half-life, nicotine 0.5 to 2 h, cotinine 6 to 16 h (mean 11).

Volume of distribution. About 1 to 3 L/kg.

Clearance. Plasma clearance, 10 to 30 mL/min/kg.

Protein binding. In plasma, about 5%.

Note. For a review of the clinical pharmacokinetics of the nicotine inhaler, see N. G. Schneider *et al.*, *Clin. Pharmacokinet*., 2001, *40*, 661–684; for a review of the pharmacology of nicotine and its therapeutic use in smoking cessation and neurodegenerative disorders, see D. J. Balfour and K. O. *Fagerstrom, Pharmacol. Ther*., 1996, *72*, 51–81; for a review of the metabolism of nicotine, see G. A. Kyerematen and E. S. Vesell, *Drug Metab. Rev*., 1991, *23*, 3–41.

Dose. As an aid to smoking withdrawal, dose depends on the level of smoking and formulation of preparation used.

Nicotinic Acid

Vitamin/Vasodilator

Synonym. Niacin
Proprietary names. Hipocol; Natinate; Niacor; Niaspan; Nicangin; Nico-400; Nicobid; Nico-Span; Nicotinex; Pepevit; Slo-Niacin.
3-Pyridinecarboxylic acid
$C_6H_5NO_2$=123.1
CAS—59-67-6

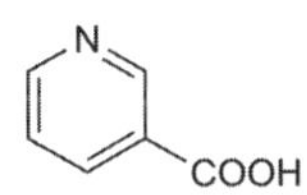

White or creamy-white crystals or crystalline powder. M.p. 234° to 237°. Soluble 1 in 60 of water and 1 in 100 of ethanol; very slightly soluble in chloroform; insoluble in ether; freely soluble in boiling water and alcohol and in solutions of alkali hydroxides and carbonates.

Dissociation Constant. pK_a 2.0 (-N=), 4.8 (-COOH), (25°).

Partition Coefficient. Log *P* (octanol/water), 0.4.

Colour Test. Cyanogen Bromide—orange.

Thin-layer Chromatography. System TA—Rf 58; system TC—Rf 17; system TD—Rf 01; system TE—Rf 00; system TF—Rf 00; system TAD—Rf 4; system TAE—Rf 72; system TAJ—Rf 04; system TAK—Rf 10; system TAL—Rf 56.

Gas Chromatography. System GA—nicotinic acid RI 1335, nicotinic acid-Me RI 1390.

High Performance Liquid Chromatography. System HAA—retention time 3.2 min.

Ultraviolet Spectrum. Methanol—263 nm (A_1^1=229a).

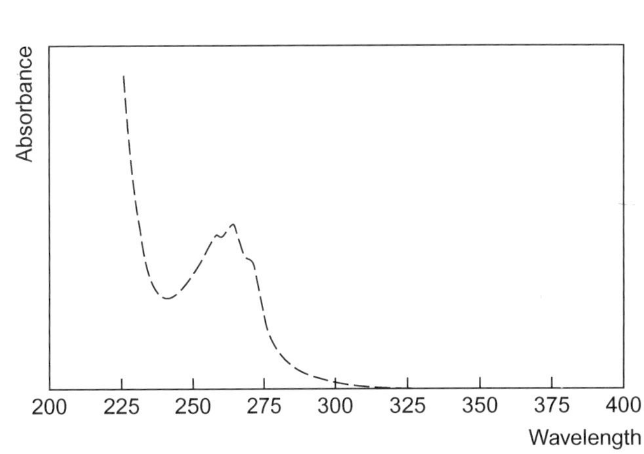

Infra-red Spectrum. Principal peaks at wavenumbers 1300, 744, 1710, 1042, 694, 1180 cm^{-1} (KBr disk).

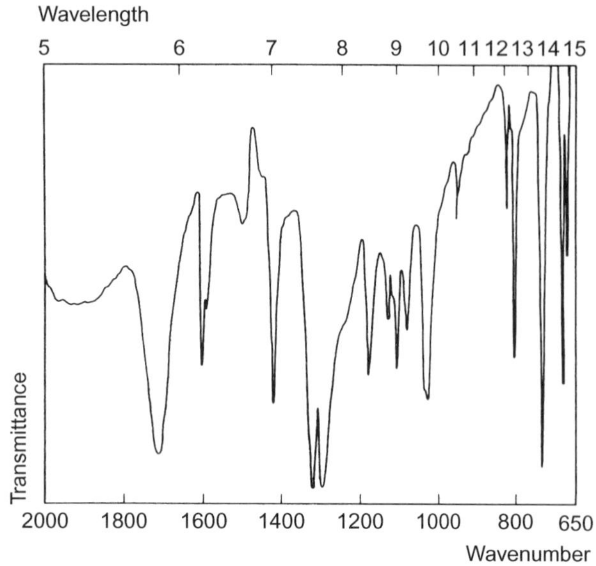

Mass Spectrum. Principal ions at *m/z* 123, 105, 78, 51, 106, 77, 124, 50; *N*-methylnicotinamide 78, 106, 135, 136, 51, 50, 79, 52.

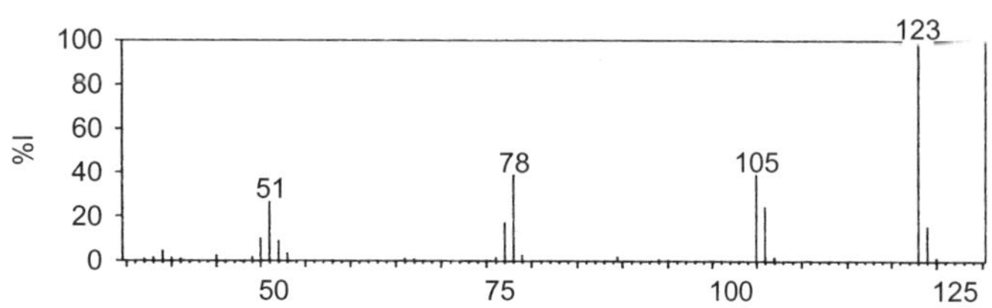

Quantification. See also Nicotinamide.

Gas chromatography–mass spectrometry. In tissues: nicotinic, quinolinic, and picolinic acids, limit of detection <1 fmol—G. A. Smythe *et al.*, *Anal. Biochem.*, 2002, *301*, 21–26.

High performance liquid chromatography. In plasma or urine: nicotinic acid and nicotinuric acid, limit of detection 500 µg/L, UV detection—N. Hengen *et al.*, *Clin. Chem.*, 1978, *24*, 1740–1743. In plasma: nicotinic acid, nicotinuric acid, and nicotinamide, limit of detection 100 µg/L, 500 µg/L, and 1 mg/L, respectively—K. Takikawa *et al.*, *J.Chromatogr.* 1982, *233*(22) *B Biomed. Appl.*, 343–348. In plasma: nicotinic acid, nicotinamide, and nicotinuric acid—Y. Miyauchi *et al.*, *Int. J. Vitam. Nutr. Res.*, 1993, *63*, 145–149.

Disposition in the Body. Readily absorbed after oral administration. Metabolised to *N*-methylnicotinamide, *N*-methyl-6-oxo-pyridine-3-carboxamide, *N*-methyl-4-oxopyridine-3-carboxamide, and by glycine conjugation to nicotinuric acid. It is rapidly excreted in the urine, and after administration of therapeutic doses about 34% is excreted unchanged in 6 h.
Nicotinic acid is a metabolite of nicergoline, nicotinamide, and nicotinyl tartrate.

Therapeutic concentration
After a single oral dose of 300 mg to 5 subjects, peak plasma concentrations of 3.5 to 18.4 mg/L (mean 9.3) were attained in about 40 min. [M. Lesne *et al.*, *Pharm. Acta Helv.*, 1976, *51*, 367–370.]

Half-life. Plasma half-life, about 0.3 to 0.8 h.

Distribution in blood. Plasma:whole blood ratio, 0.01.

Note. For a review of the clinical pharmacology and pharmacokinetics of nicotinic acid, see M. Weiner, *Drug Metab. Rev.*, 1979, *9*, 99–106; for a survey of nicotinic acid and its derivatives, see W. Hotz *Adv. Lipid Res.*, 1983, *20*, 195–217; for a review of the pharmacokinetics of nicotinic acid, see R. Gugler, *Clin. Pharmacokinet.*, 1978, *3*, 425–439.

Dose. Up to 500 mg daily.

Nicotinyl Alcohol

Vasodilator

Synonyms. 3-Hydroxymethylpyridine; Nicotinic Alcohol; 3-Pyridinemethanol; β-Pyridylcarbinol.
3-Pyridinemethanol
$C_6H_7NO = 109.1$
CAS—100-55-0

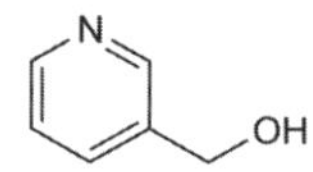

A very hygroscopic liquid. Refractive index 1.5425.
Freely soluble in water and ether; sparingly soluble in petroleum ether.

Nicotinyl Tartrate

Proprietary names. Niltuvin; Radecol; Roniacol; Ronicol.
$C_6H_7NO,C_4H_6O_6 = 259.2$
CAS—6164-87-0
A white crystalline powder. M.p. 147° to 148°.
Soluble in water, ethanol and ether.

Partition Coefficient. Log *P* (octanol/water), 0.0.

Thin-layer Chromatography. System TA—Rf 56; system TB—Rf 04; system TC—Rf 17; system TE—Rf 45; system TL—Rf 22; system TAE—Rf 74; system TAF—Rf 69. (Dragendorff spray, positive; acidified iodoplatinate solution, positive.)

Gas Chromatography. System GA—nicotinyl alcohol RI 1215, nicotinic acid RI 1335.

High Performance Liquid Chromatography. System HX—RI 55.

Ultraviolet Spectrum. Aqueous acid—260 nm. No alkaline shift. (See below.)

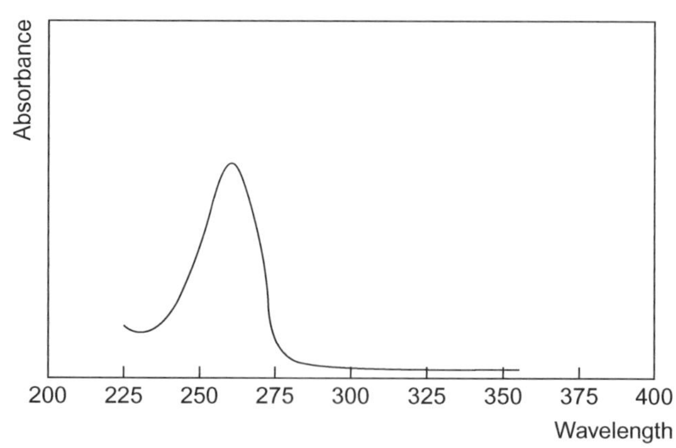

Infra-red Spectrum. Principal peaks at wavenumbers 675, 1262, 1305, 1556, 1215, 788 cm^{-1} (KBr disk).

Mass Spectrum. Principal ions at *m/z* 109, 108, 80, 53, 51, 39, 91, 27; nicotinic acid 123, 105, 78, 51, 106, 77, 124, 50.

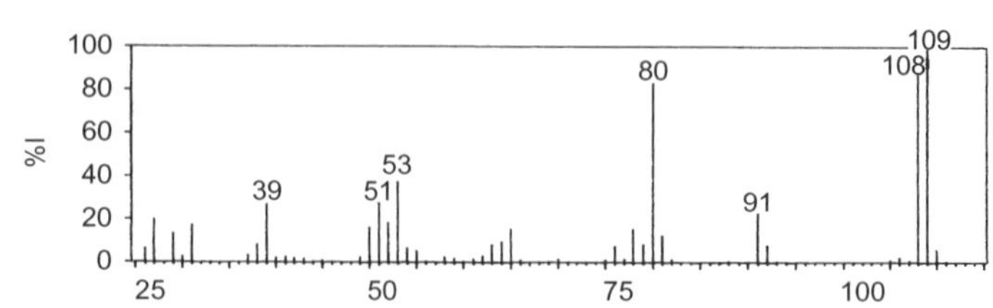

Disposition in the Body. Nicotinyl tartrate is absorbed after oral administration and partly metabolised to nicotinic acid. It is excreted in the urine.

Dose. The equivalent of 100 to 200 mg of nicotinyl alcohol daily; up to 600 mg daily given as a sustained-release preparation.

Nifedipine

Anti-anginal Vasodilator

Synonyms. Bay-a-1040; Nifedipina; Nifedipinum.
Proprietary names. Adalat(e); Adipine; Angiopine; Calanif; Calcilat; Cardilate MR; Coracten; Coroday; Fortipine; Hypolar Retard; Nifed; Nifedical; Nifedipress; Nifedotard; Nifelease; Nifopress; Nimodrel; Nivaten; Pinifed; Procardia; Slofedipine; Systepin; Tensipine; Unipine XL; Vasofed.
Dimethyl 1,4-dihydro-2,6-dimethyl-4-(2-nitrophenyl)pyridine-3,5-dicarboxylate
$C_{17}H_{18}N_2O_6$=346.3
CAS—21829-25-4

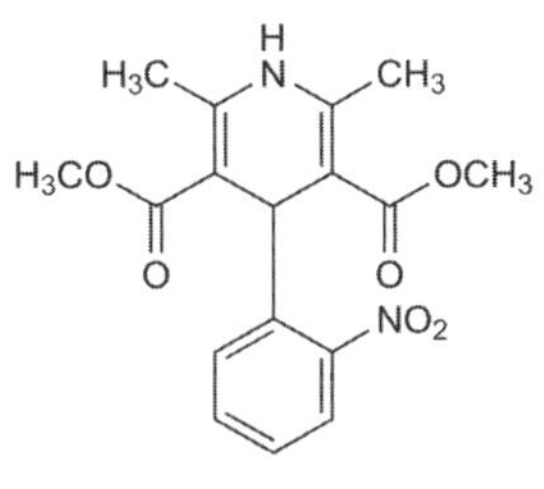

A yellow crystalline powder. M.p. 172° to 174°.
Practically insoluble in water; slightly soluble in ethanol; soluble in acetone and chloroform.

Partition Coefficient. Log *P* (octanol/water), 2.2.

Colour Tests. Methanolic Potassium Hydroxide—orange; Sulfuric Acid—orange.

Thin-layer Chromatography. System TA—Rf 68; system TB—Rf 01; system TC—Rf 65; system TE—Rf 71; system TL—Rf 68; system TAE—Rf 79.

Gas Chromatography. System GA—nifedipine RI 2545, M (dehydro-) RI 2250, M (dehydro-COOH-) RI 2290; system GB—nifedipine RI 2708, M (dehydro-) RI 2370; system GP—M (dehydro-) RI 2255, M (dehydro-2-COOH-)-Me RI 2695.

High Performance Liquid Chromatography. System HA—*k* 0.2; system HX—RI 527; system HY—RI 464; system HZ—Retention time 7.2 min; system HAA—Retention time 19.5 min; system HAX—Retention time 7.4 min; system HAY—Retention time 7.9 min.

Ultraviolet Spectrum. Aqueous acid—238 (A^1_1=595b), 338 nm (A^1_1=165b). No alkaline shift.

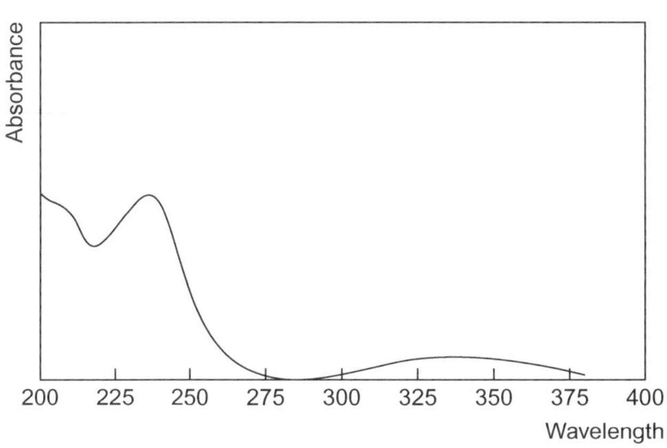

Infra-red Spectrum. Principal peaks at wavenumbers 1690, 1225, 1527, 1120, 1496, 1310 cm^{-1} (KBr disk).

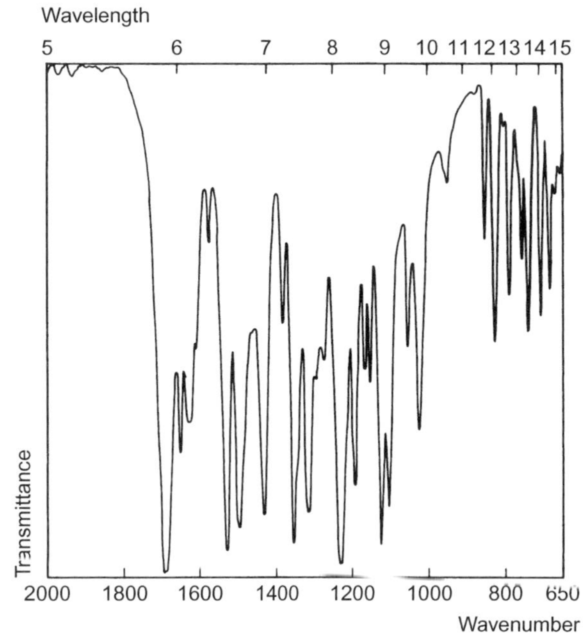

Mass Spectrum. Principal ions at *m/z* 329, 284, 224, 268, 330, 285, 225, 270.

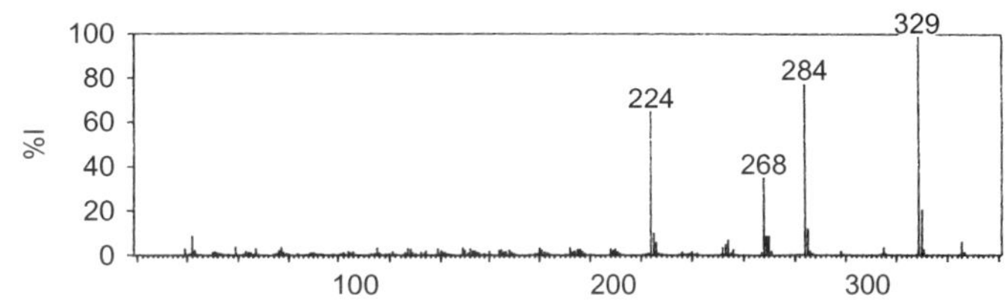

Quantification

Gas chromatography. In plasma: nifedipine and dimethyl 2,6-dimethyl-4-(2-nitrophenyl)pyridine-3,5-dicarboxylate, limit of detection 1 µg/L, ECD—J. Dokladalova *et al.*, *J.Chromatogr.*, 1982, *231*; *B Biomed. Appl.*, *20*, 451–458. In plasma: limit of detection 0.5 µg/L—C. Le Guellec *et al.*, *Biomed. Chromatogr.*, 1992, *6*, 20–23. In gingival crevicular fluid, ECD—J. S. Ellis *et al.*, *J. Chromatogr.*, 1993, *621*, 95–101.

Gas chromatography–mass spectrometry. In serum: limit of detection 2 µg/L—J. Martens *et al.*, *J. Chromatogr. B Biomed. Appl.*, 1994, *660*, 297–302.

High performance liquid chromatography. In plasma: UV detection—T. Sadanaga *et al.*, *Chem. Pharm. Bull.*, 1982, *30*, 3807–3809. In plasma: limit of quantification 7 µg/L—P. Thongnopnua and K. Viwatwongsa, *J. Pharm. Biomed. Anal.*, 1994, *12*, 119–125. In plasma: limit of detection 1 µg/L, UV detection—J. S. Grundy *et al.*, *J. Chromatogr. B Biomed. Appl.*, 1994, *654*, 146–151. In serum: limit of detection 5 µg/L, comparison with GC—A. Jankowski and H. Lamparczyk, *J. Chromatogr. A*, 1994, *668*, 469–473. In serum—A. Goldnik *et al.*, *Acta Pol. Pharm.*, 1996, *53*, 7–8. In plasma: limit of quantification 2 µg/L, UV detection—M. Yriti *et al.*, *J. Chromatogr. A.*, 2000, *870*, 115–119. In plasma: limit of detection 3 µg/L—H. S. Abou-Auda *et al.*, *J. Pharm. Biomed. Anal.*, 2000, *22*, 241–249. In serum: limit of detection 3 µg/L, UV detection—M. Zaater *et al.*, *Pol. J. Pharmacol.*, 2000, *52*, 307–312.

High performance liquid chromatography–mass spectrometry. In plasma: limit of quantification 0.5 µg/L—J. Dankers *et al.*, *J. Chromat. B Biomed. Sci. Appl.*, 1998, *710*, 115–120.

Disposition in the Body. Rapidly and almost completely absorbed after oral or sublingual administration. It is completely metabolised, undergoing first-pass metabolism. It is found in breast milk. Between 70 and 90% of a dose is excreted in the urine in 24 h as inactive metabolites including 5-methoxycarbonyl-2,6-dimethyl-4-(2-nitrophenyl)pyridine-3-carboxylic acid, dimethyl 2,6-dimethyl-4-(2-nitrophenyl)pyridine-3,5-dicarboxylate, and 2-hydroxymethyl-5-methoxycarbonyl-6-methyl-4-(2-nitrophenyl)pyridine-3-carboxylic acid, and its lactone derivative. Up to 15% of a dose is eliminated in the faeces as metabolites in 4 days.

Therapeutic concentration

Following a single oral dose of 10 mg to 9 subjects, a mean peak plasma concentration of 0.07 mg/L was attained in about 0.6 h; in a further 3 subjects, absorption was much slower with peak plasma concentrations reported at 2 to 6 h [T. S. Foster *et al.*, *J. Clin. Pharmacol.*, 1983, *23*, 161–170].

Following single oral doses of 20, 40, and 60 mg to 8 hypertensive subjects, mean peak plasma concentrations of 0.06, 0.11, and 0.17 mg/L were reported at 1.6, 2.1, and 1.8 h, respectively [O. Banzet, *Eur. J. Clin. Pharmacol.*, 1983, *24*, 145–150].

Toxicity

A 57-year-old man who took 30 × 20 mg nifedipine retarded-release tablets developed hypotension, tachycardia and flushing; 10 h after the overdose, the nifedipine plasma concentration was 0.604 mg/L and that of the M-I metabolite was 0.110 mg/L [R. E. Ferner *et al.*, *Hum. Exp. Toxicol.*, 1990, *9*, 309–311].

Bioavailability. Between 45 and 75% for liquid-filled capsules but less for longer-acting formulations.

Half-life. Plasma half-life, about 2 to 6 h.

Volume of distribution. About 0.8 L/kg.

Clearance. Plasma clearance, about 7 mL/min/kg.

Protein binding. In plasma, 92 to 98%.

Dose. As the long acting preparation, 10 to 90 mg daily; as liquid-filled capsules, 15 to 60 mg daily.

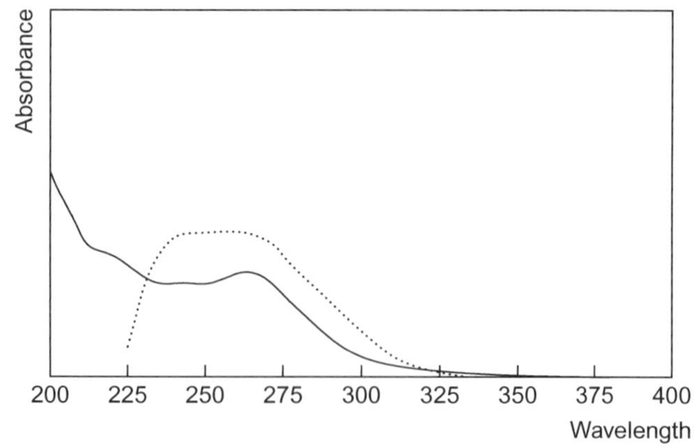

Infra-red Spectrum. Principal peaks at wavenumbers 1648, 1670, 1588, 1511, 1302, 1495 cm^{-1} (KBr disk).

Dose. 0.5 to 1.5 g daily.

Nifenazone

Analgesic

Synonym. Nicotinylamidoantipyrine

Proprietary names. Neopiran; Nicopyron; Nicoreumal; Reumatosil.

N-(2,3-Dimethyl-5-oxo-1-phenyl-3-pyrazolin-4-yl)nicotinamide

$C_{17}H_{16}N_4O_2$=308.3

CAS—2139-47-1

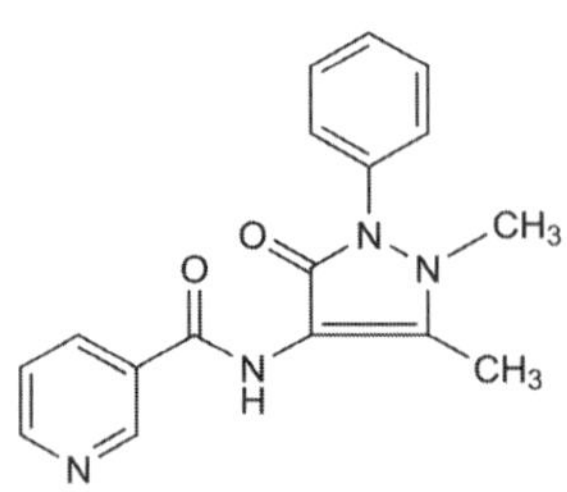

A pale yellow crystalline powder.

Slightly soluble in water and ether.

Partition Coefficient. Log *P* (octanol/water), 0.6.

Colour Tests. Cyanogen bromide—orange; Ferric chloride—brown-red; Liebermann's test (100°)—yellow.

Thin-layer Chromatography. System TA—Rf 57; system TB—Rf 00; system TE—Rf 36; system TAE—Rf 58. (Acidified potassium permanganate solution, positive.)

Gas Chromatography. System GA—nifenazone RI 3080; M(desacetyl) RI 1955.

High Performance Liquid Chromatography. System HD—*k* 0.1; system HW—*k* 0.45; system HX—RI 310.

Ultraviolet Spectrum. Aqueous acid—262 nm (A^1_1=502a).

Niflumic Acid

Analgesic

Synonym. UP-83

Proprietary names. Actol; Flaminon; Flunir; Niflactol; Niflam; Niflugel; Niflurıl.

2-[[3-(Trifluoromethyl)phenyl]amino]-3-pyridinecarboxylic acid

$C_{13}H_9F_3N_2O_2$=282.2

CAS—4394-00-7

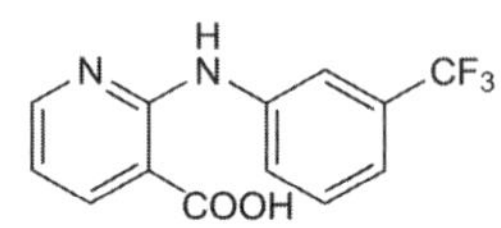

Crystals. M.p. 204°.

Partition Coefficient. Log *P* (octanol/water), 4.4.

Thin-layer Chromatography. System TD—Rf 03; system TE—Rf 11; system TF—Rf 03; system TG—Rf 28; system TAD—Rf 15; system TAE—Rf 88; system TAJ—Rf 27; system TAK—Rf 56; system TAL—Rf 90. (Ludy Tenger reagent, orange-brown.)

Gas Chromatography. System GA—Niflumic acid RI 2085; niflumic acid-Me RI 1955; System GD—Retention time of methyl derivative 1.38 relative to *n*-C_6H_{34}; system GL—niflumic acid-Me RI 1960; M(OH-) Me_2 RI 2140.

High Performance Liquid Chromatography. System HV—Retention time 0.93 relative to meclofenamic acid; system HX—RI 595; system HY—RI 530; system HAA—Retention time(s), 22.0 min.

Ultraviolet Spectrum. Aqueous acid—255 (A^1_1=471b), 329 nm (A^1_1=202b); aqueous alkali—288 nm (A^1_1=788b).

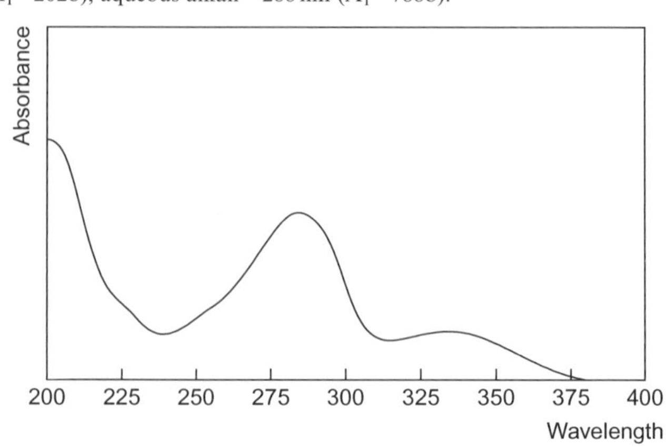

Mass Spectrum. Principal ions at *m/z* 282, 236, 237, 281, 263, 145, 44, 93.

Quantification

High performance liquid chromatography. In plasma or urine—A. Avgerinos and S. Malamataris, *J. Chromatogr.*, 1990, *533*, 271–274.

Dose. 0.5 to 1 g daily.

Nifuratel

Antimicrobial/Antiprotozoal

Synonyms. Methylmercadone; Thiodinone.
Proprietary names. Inimur; Macmiror; Magmilor; Omnes; Polmiror; Tydantil.
5-[(Methylthio)methyl]-3-[[(5-nitro-2-furanyl)methylene]amino]-2-oxazolidinone
$C_{10}H_{11}N_3O_5S = 285.3$
CAS—4936-47-4

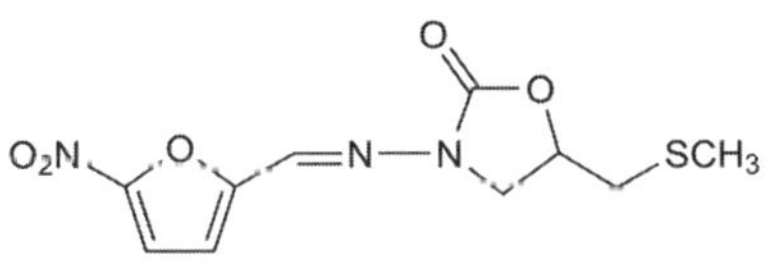

A yellow crystalline powder. M.p. 186° to 188°.
Practically insoluble in water; soluble 1 in 400 of chloroform; sparingly soluble in acetone; soluble in dimethylformamide.

Partition Coefficient. Log *P* (octanol/water), 1.5.

Colour Tests. Methanolic potassium hydroxide—orange; Palladium chloride—black.

Thin-layer Chromatography. System TA—Rf 73; system TB—Rf 00; system TE—Rf 67; system TF—Rf 43; system TAE—Rf 77. (Acidified iodoplatinate solution, positive.)

Gas Chromatography. System GA—RI 2590.

High Performance Liquid Chromatography. System HX—RI 432.

Ultraviolet Spectrum. Aqueous acid—259 ($A^1_1 = 452a$), 367 nm.

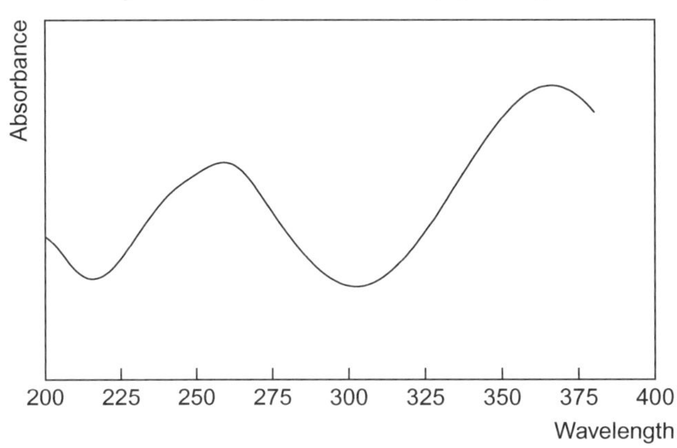

Infra-red Spectrum. Principal peaks at wavenumbers 1748, 1253, 1232, 1520, 1027, 1126 cm^{-1} (KBr disk).

Dose. 600 mg daily.

Nifursol

Antiprotozoal (Veterinary)

Proprietary name. Salfuride
3,5-Dinitro-2′-(5-nitrofurfurylidene)salicylohydrazide
$C_{12}H_7N_5O_9 = 365.2$
CAS—16915-70-1

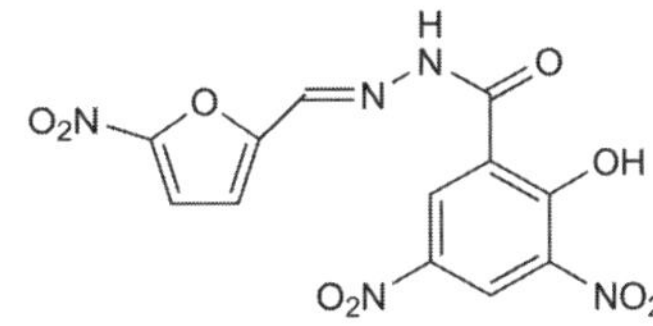

A bright yellow crystalline powder. M.p. 214° to 225°, with decomposition. Very slightly soluble in water, ethanol and chloroform; soluble 1 in 350 of acetone; practically insoluble in ether; slightly soluble in methanol.

Colour Test. Methanolic potassium hydroxide—orange.

Thin-layer Chromatography. System TA—Rf 86. (Visible yellow spot; acidified potassium permanganate solution, positive.)

Gas Chromatography. System GA—not eluted.

Infra-red Spectrum. Principal peaks at wavenumbers 1251, 1281, 1606, 1176, 1674, 1566 cm^{-1} (KBr disk).

Nikethamide

Respiratory Stimulant

Synonyms. Cardiamide; Diethylamide Nicotinic Acid; Nicethamidum; Nicorine; Nicotinoyldiaethylamidum; Nikethylamide.
Proprietary names. Coramin(e); Cormed; Juvacor; Kardonyl.
N,N-Diethyl-3-pyridinecarboxamide
$C_{10}H_{14}N_2O = 178.2$
CAS—59-26-7

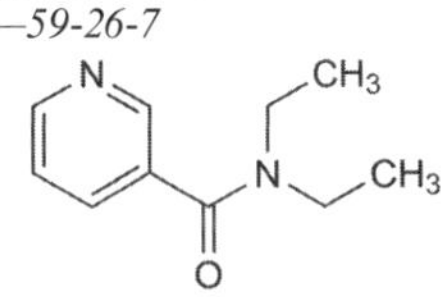

A colourless or slightly yellow, oily liquid or crystalline solid. Relative density 1.060 to 1.066. F.p. 23° to 25°. B.p. 280°. Refractive index 1.524 to 1.526.
Miscible with water, acetone, ethanol, chloroform, and ether.

Dissociation Constant. pK_a 3.5 (20°).

Partition Coefficient. Log *P* (octanol/water), 0.3.

Colour Test. Cyanogen Bromide—orange.

Thin-layer Chromatography. System TA—Rf 59; system TB—Rf 15; system TC—Rf 56; system TE—Rf 59; system TL—Rf 29; system TAE—Rf 71; system TAF—Rf 67; system TAJ—Rf 59; system TAK—Rf 19; system TAL—Rf 89. (Dragendorff spray, positive; acidified iodoplatinate solution, positive.)

Gas Chromatography. System GA—nikethamide RI 1525; M (nicotinamide) RI 1341, M (*N*-ethylnicotinamide) RI 1605; system GB—nikethamide RI 1569; M (nicotinamide) RI 1418; system GC—RI 1852; system GF—RI 1895.

High Performance Liquid Chromatography. System HX—RI 304; system HY—RI 239.

Ultraviolet Spectrum. Aqueous acid—264 ($A^1_1 = 280a$); aqueous alkali—256, 261 nm.

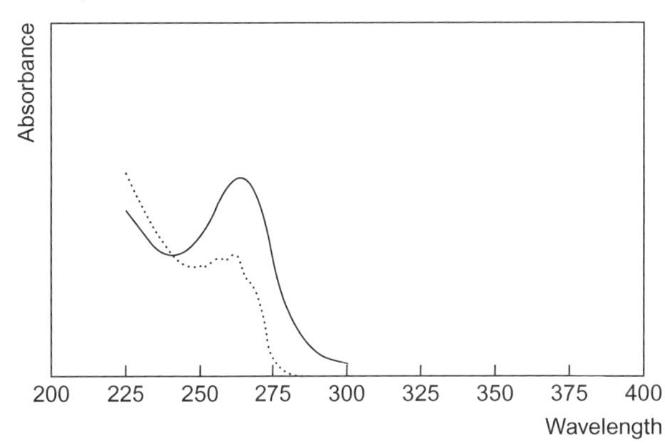

Infra-red Spectrum. Principal peaks at wavenumbers 1635, 1590, 1291, 1103, 1316, 712 cm^{-1} (KBr disk).

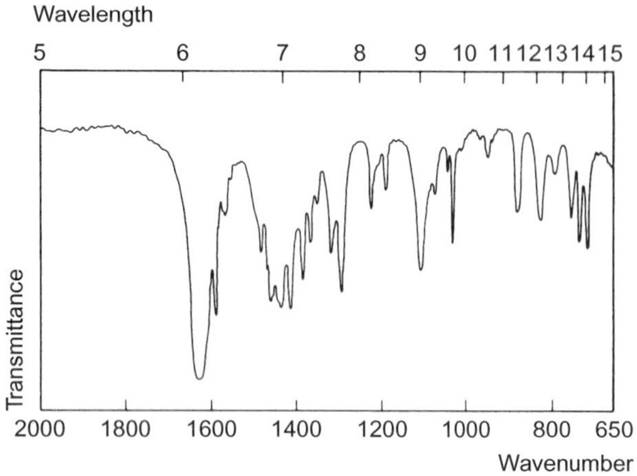

Mass Spectrum. Principal ions at *m/z* 106, 78, 177, 51, 178, 107, 149, 40; nicotinamide 122, 78, 106, 51, 50, 52, 44, 123.

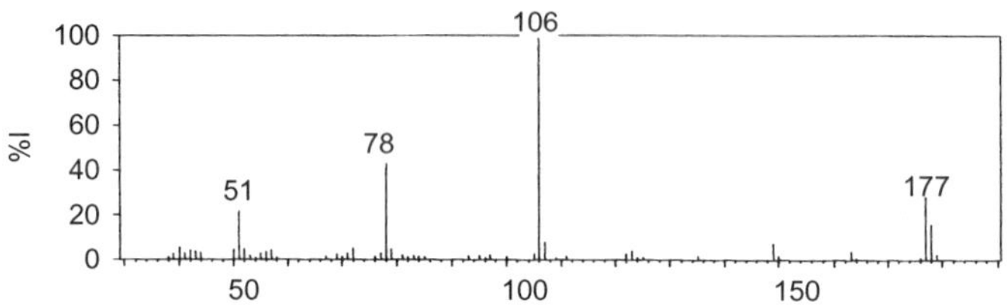

Quantification

Gas chromatography. In canine blood or urine: FID—J. H. Lewis, *J.Chromatogr.*, 1979, *172*, 295–302.

Disposition in the body. Rapidly absorbed after oral or parenteral administration and metabolised by *N*-dealkylation to *N*-ethylnicotinamide and nicotinamide; rapidly excreted in the urine; the major urinary metabolite is *N*-ethylnicotinamide.

Dose. 0.5 to 2 g IV, repeated if necessary.

Nimodipine

Calcium Antagonist/ Calcium-channel Blocker

Synonym. Bay-e-9736

Proprietary names. Admon; Brainal; Calnit; Kenesil; Modus; Nimotop; Remontal; Periplum.

1,4-Dihydro-2,6-dimethyl-4-(3-nitrophenyl)-3,5-pyridinedicarboxylic acid 2-methoxyethyl-1-methylethyl ester

$C_{21}H_{26}N_2O_7 = 418.4$

CAS—66085-59-4

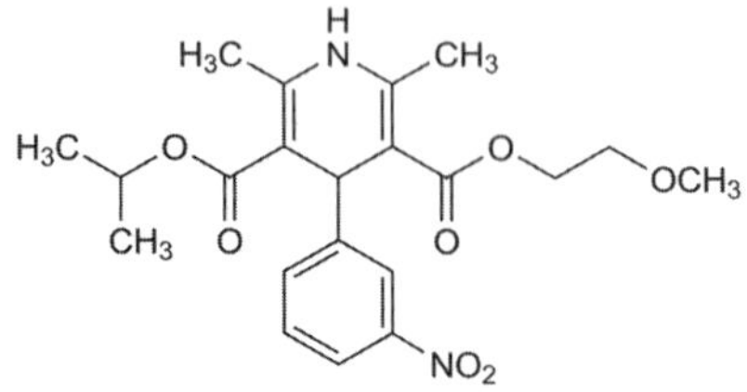

A yellow crystalline powder; crystals from petroleum ether/acetic ester. M.p. 125°. It is soluble in ethyl acetate, sparingly soluble in absolute alcohol and insoluble in water. Exposure to light leads to formation of nitrophenylpyridine derivatives.

Partition Coefficient. Log *P* (octanol/water), 3.05.

Thin-layer Chromatography. System TB—Rf 01; system TE—Rf 78; system TAE—Rf 87.

Gas Chromatography. System GA—RI 2929; system GB—RI 3096; system GP—RI 2300 M (dehydro-desisopropyl-desmethoxyethyl)-ME2; RI 2390 M (dehydro-desmethoxyethyl)-ME; RI 2645 M (dehydro-desisopropyl-*O*-desmethyl-HOOC)-ME; RI 2655 M (dehydro-); RI 2665 M (dehydro-desisopropyl-*O*-desmethyl)-ME; RI 2740 M (dehydro-*O*-desmethyl-HOOC-)-ME.

Column: HP1 methyl silicone (0.2 mm i.d., 0.33 μm film thickness). Column temperature: 280°. Carrier gas: helium, 0.9 mL/min flow rate. Detection: mass spectrometer. Retention index: 2961. [T. Mills and J. C. Roberson, *Instrumental Data for Drug Analysis*, 1993, CRC Press, Boca Raton, US. 2nd Edn., Vol. 5, pp. 308–309].

High Performance Liquid Chromatography. System HX—RI 668; system HY—RI 584; system HZ—17.7 min.

Column: ODS (Hypersil, 100 × 4.6 mm i.d., 5 μm). Mobile phase: methanol:potassium dihydrogen phosphate (10 mM, pH 3.5 with phosphoric acid) (70:30), flow rate 1 mL/min. UV detection (diode array). Retention time: 3.8 min. [T. Mills and J. C. Roberson, *Instrumental Data for Drug Analysis*, 1993, CRC Press, Boca Raton, US. 2nd Edn., Vol. 5, pp. 308–309].

Column: ODS (Spherisorb, 150 × 4.6 mm i.d., 3 μm). Mobile phase: (A) acetonitrile:water (57:43); (B) methanol:water (66:34), flow rate 0.5 mL/min. UV detection (λ = 238 nm). Retention times: solvent (A) nimodipine, 12.19 min; pyridine analogue, 13.02 min; solvent (B) nimodipine, 17.33 min; pyridine analogue, 19.89 min. [G.J. Krol *et al.*, *J. Chromatogr.*, 1984, *305*; *Biomed. Appl.*, 105–118].

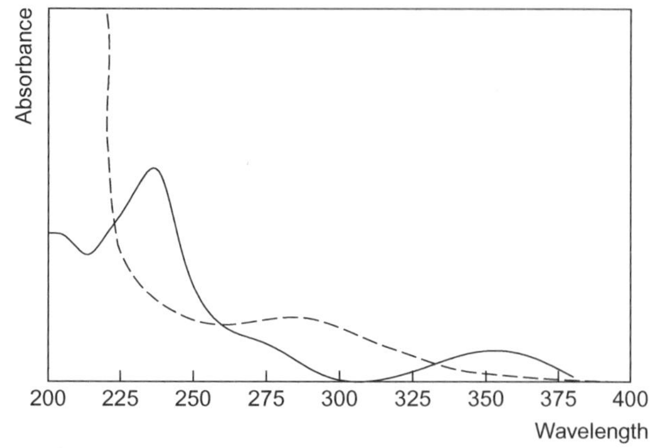

Infra-red spectrum. Principal peaks at wavenumber 1689, 1337, 1098 cm^{-1} (KBr pellet).

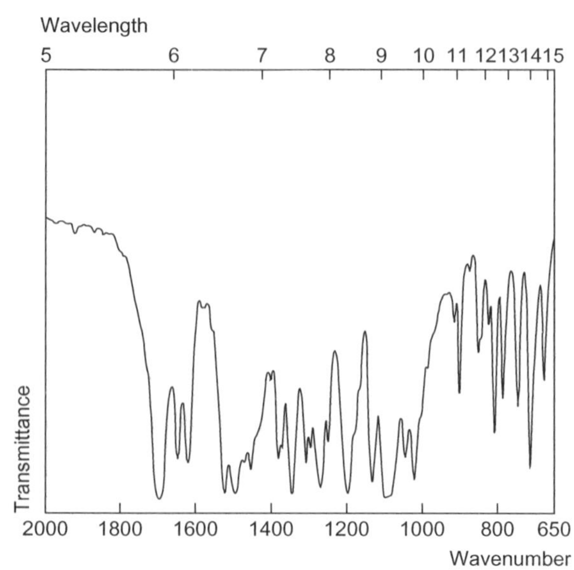

Mass spectrum. Principal ions at *m/z* 296, 254, 196, 273, 59, 67, 151, 178.

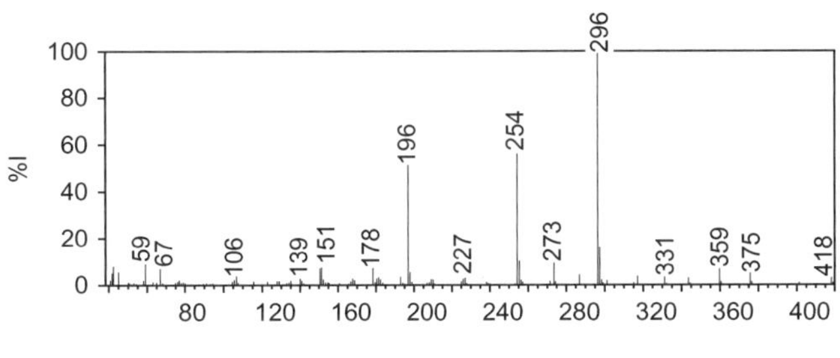

Quantification

Gas chromatography. In plasma and cerebrospinal fluid: limit of detection is 1 µg/L. ECD—G.J. Krol *et al.*, *J. Chromatogr*. 1984, *305*; *Biomed. Appl*., 105–118. In serum: limit of detection is 0.2 µg/L. ECD—F. M. Gengo *et al.*, *Br. J. Clin. Pharmacol*., 1987, *23*, 47–53.

Gas chromatography–mass spectrometry. In serum: limit of quantification is 0.1 µg/L—C. Fischer *et al.*, *J. Pharm. Sci*., 1993, *82(3)*, 244–250.

High performance liquid chromatography. In serum: limit of quantification is 0.038 µg/L. UV detection (λ=238 nm)—C. Fischer *et al.*, *J. Pharm. Sci*., 1993, *82(3)*, 244–250. In plasma and cerebrospinal fluid: limit of detection is 1 µg/L. UV detection (λ=238 nm)—G.J. Krol *et al.*, *J. Chromatogr*., 1984, *305*; *Biomed. Appl*., 105–118. In plasma and serum: limit of detection 3 µg/L—P. R. Bach, *Clin. Chem*., 1983, *29(7)*, 1344–1348.

Disposition in the Body. Nimodipine is rapidly and readily absorbed after oral administration and undergoes hepatic metabolism. It is rapidly distributed throughout the body to tissues and organs. Metabolism occurs entirely in the liver and includes dehydrogenation to produce a pyridine analogue, followed by subsequent demethylation, ester hydrolysis and hydroxylation. Three metabolites have been isolated, the *O*-desmethyl metabolite which has slight activity and the pyridine and *O*-desmethyl pyridine metabolites which are both inactive. It is excreted mainly as metabolites in urine (50% of a dose excreted over 4 days) and faeces (32%). Virtually no unchanged drug is present in urine.

Therapeutic concentration. The serum therapeutic concentration is 10 to 50 µg/L.

6 patients with biopsy-proven cirrhosis, 38 to 72 years old (mean 55.3 years) and 5 healthy volunteers, aged between 42 and 68 years (mean 52.4 years) were administered with a 60 mg oral dose after an overnight fast. The mean peak plasma concentration was 115.8 µg/L (range 25.3 to 250.9 µg/L) for the patients with liver disease and 80.2 (between 58.5 and 126.5) µg/L for the healthy individuals. These concentrations were reached by 1.75 h (0.5 to 5.0 h) and 0.7 (0.25 to 1.0) h, respectively. Additionally, they were asked to take a 30 mg oral dose by sublingual administration. This meant that the actual dose received ranged between 8 and 18 mg. Peak concentrations of 12.4 (7.7 to 17.9) µg/L and 19 (4.6 to 53.6) µg/L were observed at 2.5 h (range 1 to 10 h) and 1.3 (0.75 to 3.06) h for the patients and volunteers, respectively. [F. M. Gengo *et al*., *Br. J. Clin. Pharmacol*., 1987, *23*, 47–53].

Toxicity. No specific or general toxic effects with therapeutic treatment, but cardiovascular problems may arise with higher doses.

Bioavailability. 13%.

Half-life. 9 h (with initial rapid phase with half-life around 1 to 2 h).

Volume of distribution. Steady state, 0.9 to 2.3 L/kg.

Clearance. Plasma, 0.84 L/kg/h; 0.23 L/kg/h (patients with renal failure). Also, reported as 1.21 L/kg/h.

Distribution in blood. Erythrocytes:plasma ratio is unity.

Protein binding. 95 to 98%.

Note. For a review of nimodipine, see M. S. Langley and E. M. Sorkin, *Drugs*, 1989, *37*, 669–699. For a review of the pharmacokinetics of nimodipine, see L. Parnetti, *Clin. Pharmacokinet*., 1995, *29*, 110–129.

Dose. Oral, 360 mg daily; intravenous, 1 mg/h initially, increased to 2 mg/h after 2 h.

Nimorazole

Antiprotozoal

Synonym. Nitrimidazine
Proprietary names. Acterol Forte; Esclama; Naxogin.
4-[2-(5-Nitro-1*H*-imidazol-1-yl)ethyl]morpholine
$C_9H_{14}N_4O_3$=226.2
CAS—6506-37-2

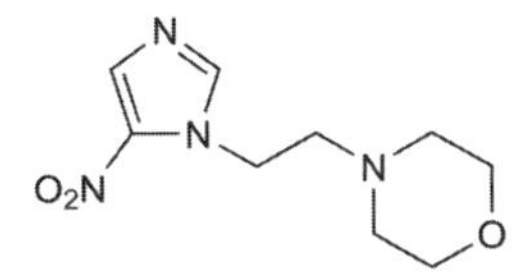

A whitish crystalline powder. M.p. about 110°.
Soluble 1 in 33 of water; soluble in acetone, alcohols, chloroform, and dilute acetic acid.

Colour Test. Dissolve 10 mg in 1 mL of methanol, add 10 mL of water, 10 mL of 6 M sodium hydroxide containing 20 mg of alpha-naphthol and 10 mL of 12 M sodium hydroxide, and heat for 30 min on a boiling water-bath—an intense brown colour develops.

Partition Coefficient. Log *P* (octanol/water), 0.1.

Thin-layer Chromatography. System TA—Rf 57; system TB—Rf 03; system TC—Rf 44; system TE—Rf 58; system TL—Rf 33; system TAE—Rf 60. (Acidified iodoplatinate solution, positive.)

Gas Chromatography. System GA—RI 1803.

Ultraviolet Spectrum. Aqueous acid—297 nm; aqueous alkali—305 nm.

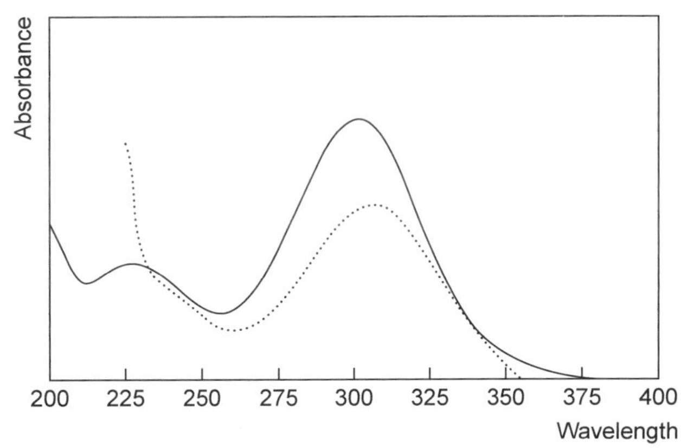

Mass Spectrum. Principal ions at *m/z* 100, 56, 42, 101, 55, 54, 41, 30.

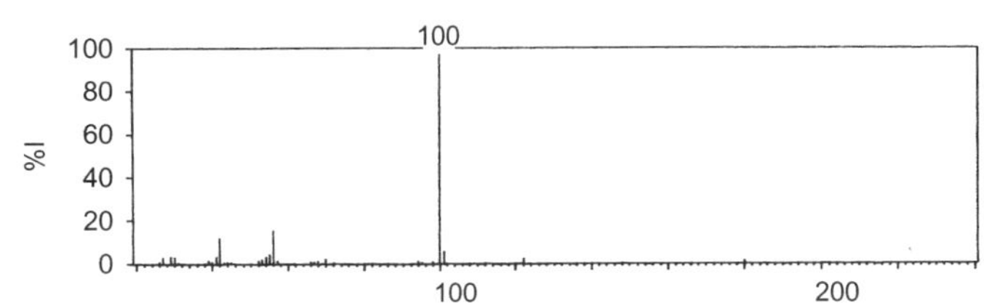

Note. For studies of the pharmacokinetic properties of nimorazole, see J. Overgaard *et al*., *Br. J. Cancer*, 1983, *48*, 27–34.

Dose. Usually 2 g as a single dose.

Niridazole

Anthelmintic

Synonym. Ba-32644
Proprietary name. Ambilhar
1-(5-Nitro-2-thiazolyl)-2-imidazolidinone
$C_6H_6N_4O_3S$=214.2

CAS—61-57-4

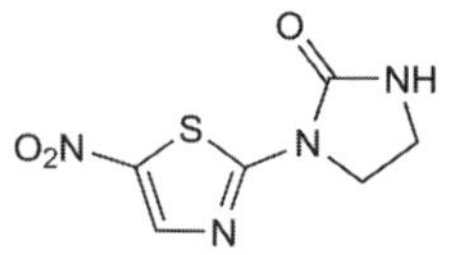

A yellow crystalline powder. M.p. 260° to 264°.
Practically insoluble in water, ethanol, acetone, chloroform and ether; soluble in dimethyl sulfoxide, dimethylformamide and pyridine.

Colour Test. Methanolic potassium hydroxide—yellow.

Partition Coefficient. Log *P* (octanol/water), 1.0.

Thin-layer Chromatography. System TA—Rf 54; system TB—Rf 01; system TC—Rf 44; system TL—Rf 53. (Visible yellow spot.)

Ultraviolet Spectrum. Aqueous acid—239 nm; aqueous alkali—233, 282 nm.

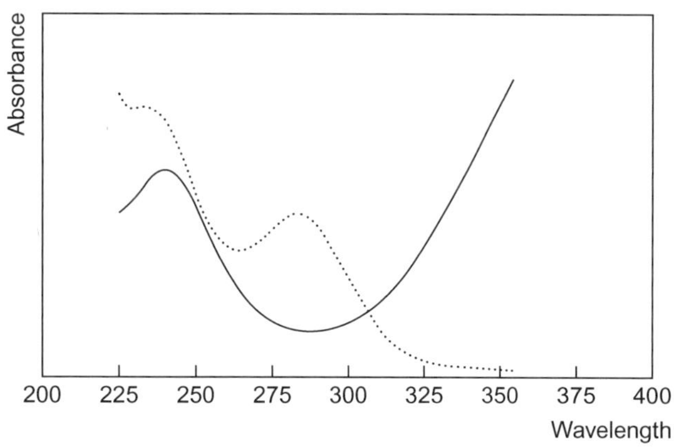

Mass Spectrum. Principal ions at *m/z* 158, 214, 57, 145, 124, 45, 70, 96.

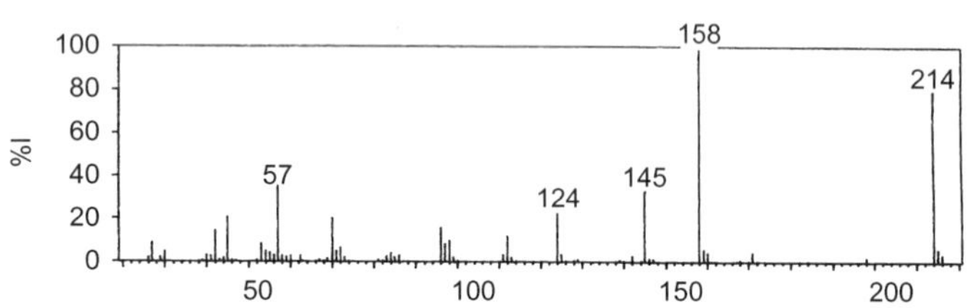

Quantification

Gas chromatography. In serum or urine: limit of detection 250 µg/L, FID—J. J. Miller and R. J. Oake, *J. Chromatogr.*, 1977, *131*, 442–443.

High performance liquid chromatography. In plasma or urine: limit of detection 50 µg/L, UV detection—J. J. Miller *et al., J. Chromatogr.*, 1978, *147*, 507–508.

Disposition in the Body. Niridazole is slowly absorbed after oral administration. It undergoes extensive first-pass metabolism in the liver to inactive metabolites. About 50% of a dose is excreted in the urine as metabolites in 48 h; niridazole is also excreted as metabolites in bile.

Therapeutic concentration

After a single oral dose of 25 mg/kg, peak blood concentrations of unchanged drug of about 0.2 mg/L were attained in about 3 h, and peak blood concentrations of metabolites of about 5 to 10 mg/L were reported after 6 to 9 h. [J. W. Faigle, *Acta Pharmacol. Toxicol.*, 1971, *29*, *Suppl.* 3, 233–239].

Half-life. Plasma half-life, 12 to 15 h.

Protein binding. In plasma, niridazole metabolites extensively bound.

Dose. 25 mg/kg daily, by mouth, up to a maximum of 1.5 g daily.

Nisoldipine

Calcium Antagonist/ Calcium-channel Blocker

Synonym. Bay-k-5552

Proprietary names. Baymycard; Cornel; Sular; Syscor; Zadipina.

1,4-Dihydro-2,6-dimethyl-4-(2-nitrophenyl)-3,5-pyridinedicarboxylic acid methyl 2-methylpropyl ester

$C_{20}H_{24}N_2O_6 = 388.4$

CAS—63675-72-9

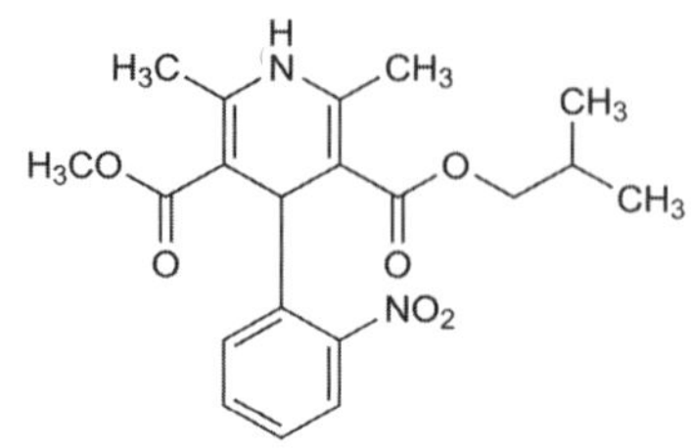

Yellow crystals. M.p. 151° to 152°. Practically insoluble in water; soluble in ethanol.

Partition Coefficient. Log *P* (octanol/water), 3.26.

Thin-layer Chromatography. System TAE—Rf 86; system TB—Rf 45; system TE—Rf 85; system TF—Rf 65.

Gas Chromatography. System GP—RI 2255 M (dehydro-desisobutyl-)-ME; RI 2450 M (dehydro-); RI 2615 M (dehydro-OH$^-$); RI 2695 M (dehydro-desisobutyl-2-HOOC$^-$)-ME2.

Column: Ultra 1 (12.5 m × 0.2 mm i.d., 0.33 µm film thickness). Column temperature: 100° for 1 min, to 280° at 35°/min, hold for 3 min. Injector and detector temperatures: 280° and 300°, respectively. Carrier gas: helium; flow rate, 1.9 mL/min. Internal standard: nitrendipine. MS detection (EI, SIM at *m/z* 270.2 and 371.35 for nisoldipine and *m/z* 360 for I. S.). Retention time: nisoldipine, 6.86 min; I. S., 6.77 min. [M. P. Marques *et al., J. Chromatogr. B Biomed. Sci. Appl.*, 2001, *762*, 87–95].

Column: methyl silicone (HP1, 0.2 mm i.d., 0.33 µm film thickness). Column temperature: 250°. Carrier gas: helium, 0.9 mL/min flow rate. MS detection. Retention index: 2139. [T. Mills and J. C. Roberson, *Instrumental Data for Drug Analysis*, 1993, CRC Press, Boca Raton, US. 2nd Edn. Vol. 5, pp. 310–311].

High Performance Liquid Chromatography. System HX—RI 690.

Column: (analytical) C_{18} (Supelcosil, 250 × 4.6 mm i.d., 5 µm); (guard) C_{18} µBondapak. Column temperature: 30°. Mobile phase: methanol:water (containing sodium acetate buffer (2 mM)), adjusted to pH 5.0, flow rate 1 mL/min. Electrochemical detection. *k* value: 2.27. [J. A. Lopez *et al., J. Chromatogr. A*, 2000, *870*, 105–114].

Column: ODS (Hypersil, 100 × 4.6 mm i.d., 5 µm). Mobile phase: methanol:potassium dihydrogen phosphate (10 mM), adjusted to pH 7.0 with 30 drops/L triethylamine (70:30), flow rate 1 mL/min. UV diode array detection. Retention time: 4.3 min. [T. Mills and J. C. Roberson, *Instrumental Data for Drug Analysis*, 1993, CRC Press, Boca Raton, US. 2nd Edn. Vol. 5, pp. 310–311].

Ultraviolet Spectrum. Aqueous acid—235, 331 nm; basic—324 nm.

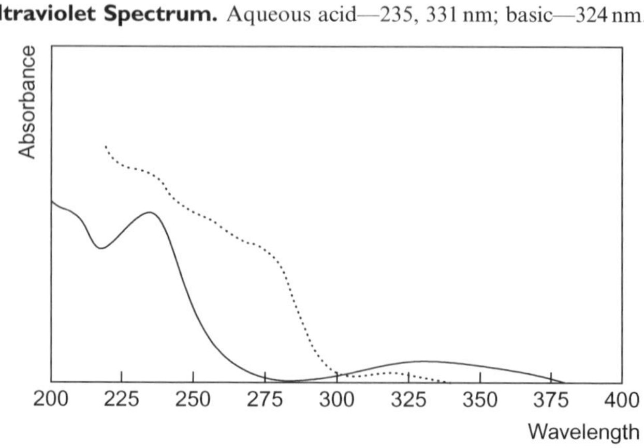

Infra-red Spectrum. Principal peaks at wavenumber 1647, 1485, 1210 cm^{-1} (KBr pellet).

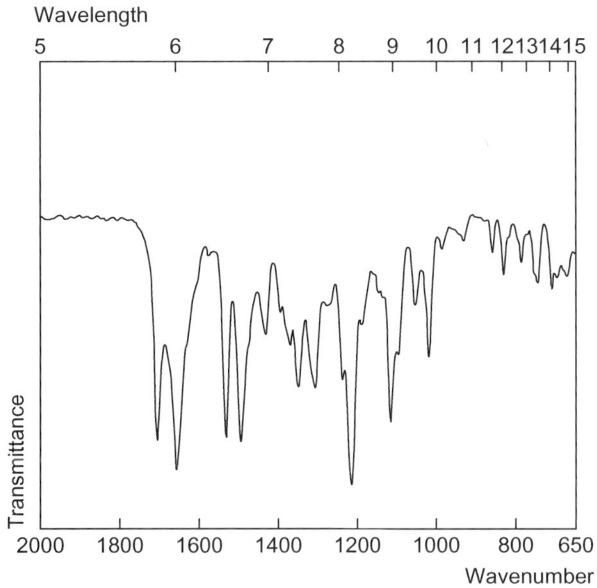

Mass Spectrum. Principal ions at *m/z* 371, 210, 270, 266, 284, 254, 268, 41.

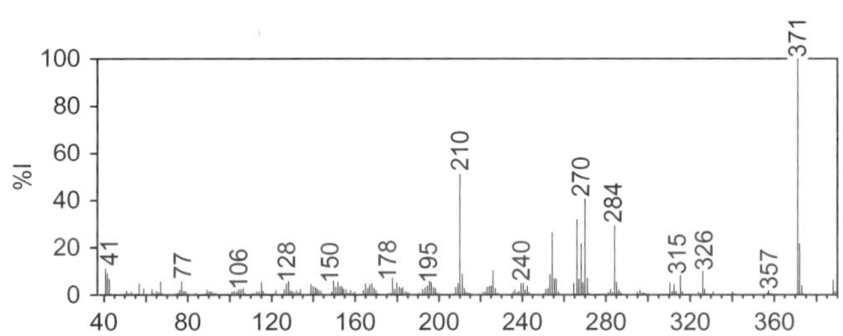

Quantification

Gas chromatography. In plasma: limit of detection 0.1 µg/L, ECD—P. A. Soons *et al.*, *J. Chromatogr.*, 1990, *528*, 343–356.

High performance liquid chromatography. In plasma: limit of quantification 0.1 µg/L. UV detection (λ=230 nm)—R. Heinig *et al.*, *J. Chromatogr.*, 1994, *655*; *Biomed. Appl.*, 286–292.

Disposition in the Body. Nisoldipine is well absorbed after oral administration from the gastrointestinal tract and the concentration of the active (+)-nisoldipine enantiomer is about 6 times higher than the inactive (–)-nisoldipine enantiomer. It extensively metabolised in the gut wall and liver to five major urinary metabolites which include BAYs-1869 and BAYs-4755. A hydroxylated derivative of the side chain appears to be the only active metabolite, having about 10% of the activity of the parent compound. Cytochrome P450 3A4 enzymes are believed to be involved. Between 60 and 80% of an administered dose is excreted in urine and the remainder in faeces, mostly as metabolites. Less than 1% of a single dose is excreted unchanged.

Therapeutic concentration.

4 healthy male volunteers, 22 to 38 years old, were administered with a 40 mg dose of the controlled release formulation. The mean peak plasma concentration was 3.40 µg/L for the (+)-formulation drug and 0.37 µg/L for the (–)-drug 3 h after administration. [R. Heinig *et al.*, *J. Chromatogr.*, 1994, *655*; *Biomed. Appl.*, 286–292].

Toxicity. Studies have revealed that, when administered with grapefruit juice, nisoldipine mean peak plasma concentrations increase three-fold.

A 72-year-old woman with a history of depression was admitted because of severe shock, hypothermia and renal insufficiency. Routine screening revealed therapeutic drug concentrations of clomipramine (177 µg/L) and desmethylclomipramine (173 µg/L), but a nisoldipine serum concentration of 1544 µg/L was found. The patient was discharged 4 days later without sequelae. [H. K Louagie *et al.*, *J. Toxicol. Clin. Toxicol.*, 1998, *36*, 125–127].

Bioavailability. 5.5% (oral, modified release formulation). Ranges between 4 and 8%.

Half-life. 2 h (beta phase) and 10 to 12 h (gamma phase). Terminal elimination half-life is 7 to 12 h.

Volume of distribution. 2.7 L/kg.

Protein binding. >99%.

Dose. 10 to 40 mg daily.

Nitrazepam

Hypnotic

Synonyms. Nitrazepamum; NSC-58775; Ro-4-5360; Ro-5-3059.
Proprietary names. Alodorm; Apodorm; Arem; Dima; Dormalon; Dormicum; DormoPuren; Dumolid; Eatan N; Imeson; Insoma; Insomin; Mogadon; Nitrados; Nitrazadon; Nitrazepol; Noctesed; Novanox; Numbon; Ormodon; Pacisyn; Paxadorm; Radedorm; Remnos; Serenade; Somnite; Sonebon; Sonotrat; Surem; Unisomnia.
1,3-Dihydro-7-nitro-5-phenyl-2*H*-1,4-benzodiazepin-2-one
$C_{15}H_{11}N_3O_3$=281.3
CAS—146-22-5

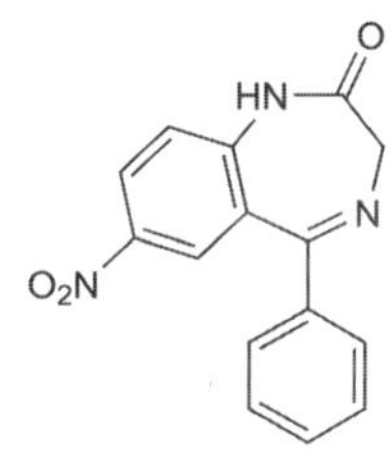

A yellow crystalline powder. M.p. 224° to 226° (crystals from ethanol). Practically insoluble in water, benzene, and hexane; soluble 1 in 120 of ethanol, 1 in 45 of chloroform, and 1 in 900 of ether; soluble in acetone and ethyl acetate.

Dissociation Constant. pK_a 3.2, 10.8 (20°).

Partition Coefficient. Log *P* (octanol/buffer pH 7.4), 2.1.

Colour Test. Formaldehyde–Sulfuric Acid—orange.

Thin-layer Chromatography. System TA—Rf 68; system TB—Rf 00; system TC—Rf 36; system TD—Rf 35; system TE—Rf 64; system TF—Rf 46; system TL—Rf 55; system TAD—Rf 53; system TAE—Rf 90; system TAF—Rf 86; system TAJ—Rf 53; system TAK—Rf 52; system TAL—Rf 92. (Dragendorff spray, positive; acidified iodoplatinate solution, positive.)

Gas Chromatography System GA—nitrazepam RI 2740, M (7-acetamido-) RI 3205, M (7-amino-) RI 2785, 2-amino-5-nitrobenzophenone RI 2388; system GB—nitrazepam RI 2915, nitrazepam-TMS RI 2642, M (7-amino-) RI 2878, M (7-amino-)-TMS_3 RI 2634; system GG—RI 3450.

High Performance Liquid Chromatography. System HA—*k* 0.1; system HI—nitrazepam *k* 2.96, M (7-acetamido-) *k* 0.68, M (7-amino-) *k* 0.46; system HK—nitrazepam *k* 1.49, M (7-acetamido-) *k* 1.93, M (7-amino-) *k* 0.00; system HX—RI 448; system HY—RI 370; system HZ—retention time 4.2 min; system HAA—retention time 16.9 min; system HAF—retention time 9.1 min; system HAL—retention time 4.6 min; system HAM—retention time 4.5 min; system HAX—retention time 6.3 min; system HAY—retention time 6.0 min; system HAZ—*k* 0.88; system HBH—*k* 3.22; system HBI—*k* 0.97.

Ultraviolet Spectrum. Methanolic acid—280 nm (A_1^1=910a).

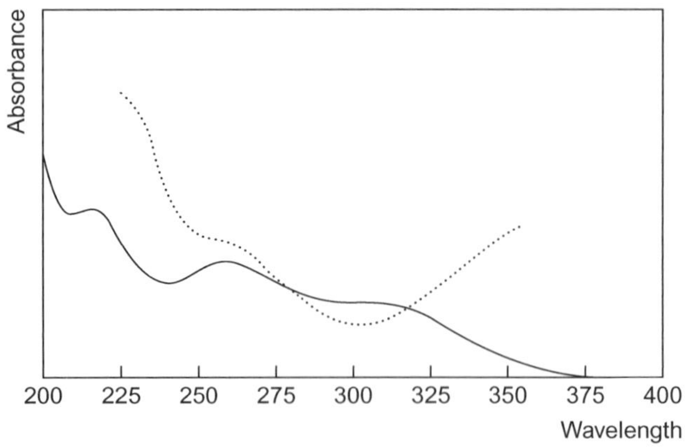

Infra-red Spectrum. Principal peaks at wavenumbers 1690, 1610, 698, 1536, 745, 784 cm^{-1} (KBr disk).

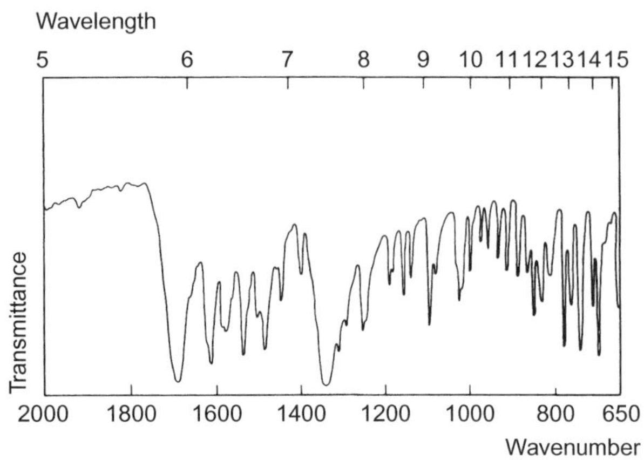

Mass Spectrum. Principal ions at *m/z* 280, 253, 281, 206, 234, 252, 254, 264; 7-acetamidonitrazepam 293, 265, 264, 292, 43, 222, 223, 294; 7-aminonitrazepam 251, 222, 223, 250, 252, 195, 110, 97; 2-amino-5-nitrobenzophenone 241, 77, 242, 105, 44, 43, 195, 57.

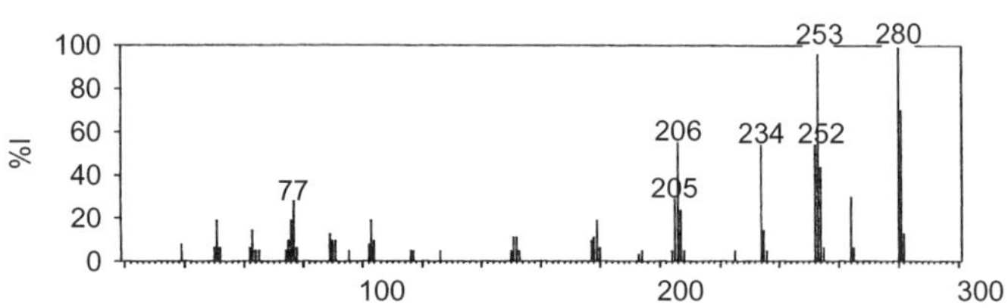

Quantification

Spectrofluorimetry. In plasma or urine: nitrazepam and metabolites, limit of detection about 10 µg/L for nitrazepam, 25 µg/L for the sum of the 7-amino and 7-acetamido metabolites—J. Rieder, *Arzneimittelforschung*, 1973, *23*, 207–211.

Gas chromatography. In urine: detection limits 200 ng/L for nitrazepam using ECD, and 50 µg/L for metabolites using AFID—L. Kangas, *J. Chromatogr.*, 1979, *172*, 273–278. In plasma: comparison of two procedures using the hydrolysis product and intact drug, limit of detection 200 ng/L and 1 µg/L respectively, ECD—L. Kangas, *J. Chromatogr.*, 1977, *136*, 259–270. In plasma or whole blood: nitrazepam and other benzodiazepines, nitrogen-phosphorus detection or ECD—P. Lillsunde and T. Seppala, *J. Chromatogr.*, 1990, *533*, 97–110. In blood: nitrazepam and other benzodiazepines—H. Gjerde *et al.*, *J. Pharm. Biomed. Anal.*, 1992, *10*, 317–322.

High performance liquid chromatography. In plasma, serum, or whole blood: limits of detection 5 µg/L for nitrazepam and 7-acetamidonitrazepam, 50 µg/L for 7-aminonitrazepam, UV detection—H. Kelly *et al.*, *Clin. Chem.*, 1982, *28*, 1478–1481. In plasma: nitrazepam and other benzodiazepines, UV detection—A. Boukhabza *et al.*, *J. Anal. Toxicol.*, 1991, *15*, 319–322. In postmortem blood: nitrazepam and other nitrobenzodiazepines and their 7-amino metabolites, limits of detection 1 to 8 µg/L, UV detection—M. D. Robertson and O. H. Drummer, *J. Chromatogr.* 1995, *667 B Biomed. Appl.*, 179–184. In plasma or serum: nitrazepam and other benzodiazepines, limit of detection 5 nmol/L—K. K. Akerman *et al.*, *Clin. Chem.*, 1996, *42*, 1412–1416. In serum: nitrazepam and diazepam—B. Welk, *Acta Pol. Pharm.*, 1996, *53*, 3–6. In serum: nitrazepam and other benzodiazepines, UV detection—E. Tanaka *et al.*, *J. Chromatogr.* 1996, *682 B Biomed. Appl.*, 173–178; E. Tanaka *et al.*, *J. Chromatogr. B Biomed. Sci. Appl.*, 1998, *709*, 324.

High performance liquid chromatography–mass spectrometry. In serum or urine: nitrazepam and other benzodiazepines, limit of quantification 2 µg/L—M. Kleinschnitz *et al.*, *J. Chromatogr.* 1996, *676 B Biomed. Appl.*, 61–67.

Radioimmunoassay. In plasma: limit of detection 4 µg/L—R. Dixon *et al.*, *Life Sci.*, 1979, *25*, 311–316.

Disposition in the Body. Readily absorbed after oral administration. It crosses the blood–brain barrier. Nitrazepam crosses the placenta and is found in breast milk. The major metabolites, 7-aminonitrazepam and the 7-acetamido derivative accumulate to some extent in plasma. Other metabolites include 2-amino-5-nitrobenzophenone and 2-amino-3-hydroxy-5-nitrobenzophenone; all the metabolites are inactive. After oral administration, about 50 to 70% of a dose is excreted in the urine in 120 h and up to 20% is eliminated in the faeces. Up to about 37% of a dose may be excreted in the first 24 h with about 5 to 10% of the dose as free 7-acetamidonitrazepam, 5% as 7-aminonitrazepam, 5% as conjugated 2-amino-3-hydroxy-5-nitrobenzophenone, and 20% as unknown acidic compounds. About 20% of an oral dose is found in the faeces. After IV administration, about 90% is excreted in the urine in 120 h and up to about 10% is eliminated in the faeces. Only a small amount (less than 4%) is excreted as unchanged nitrazepam after oral or IV administration.

Therapeutic concentration. In plasma, usually in the range 0.03 to 0.07 mg/L.

Following a single oral dose of 5 mg to 9 subjects, peak plasma concentrations of 0.028 to 0.045 mg/L (mean 0.04) were attained in 0.5 to 4 h. [D. D. Breimer *et al.*, *Br. J. Clin, Pharmacol.*, 1977, *4*, 709–711.]

Following daily oral doses of 5 mg to 4 subjects, steady-state plasma-nitrazepam concentrations of 0.035 to 0.044 mg/L (mean 0.04) were reported; combined steady-state concentrations of the 7-amino and 7-acetamido metabolites were in the range 0.018 to 0.053 mg/L (mean 0.03). [J. Rieder and G. Wendt, Pharmacokinetics and Metabolism of the Hypnotic Nitrazepam, in *The Benzodiazepines*, S. Garattini, E. Mussini and L. O. Randall (Ed.), New York, Raven Press, 1973, pp. 99–127.]

Toxicity. Blood concentrations greater than 0.2 mg/L may produce toxic effects.

The following postmortem tissue concentrations of nitrazepam and 7-aminonitrazepam, respectively, were reported in a 52-year-old woman who died due to drowning following nitrazepam overdose and cold exposure: (in mg/L or µg/g) aorta blood 0.741 and 0.498, femoral vein 0.450 and 1.56, CSF 0.074 and 0.098, vitreous humour 0.099 and 0.032, pericardial fluid 0.188 and 0.780, bile 4.08 and 1.67, urine 0.580 and 1.09, cerebral cortex 3.49 and 2.55, diencephalons 6.22 and 2.49, cerebellum 2.17 and 5.11, myocardium 2.77 and 0.816, left lung 0.656 and 0.717, right lung 1.27 and 1.01, spleen 0.458 and 0.329, liver 0.059 and 0.113, kidney 0.077 and 1.21, femoral muscle 2.12 and 1.04, stomach contents (total amount in mg) 201 and 20.9. [F. Moriya and Y. Hashimoto, *Forensic Sci. Int.*, 2003, *131*, 108–112.]

In 2 fatalities due to overdoses of nitrazepam, postmortem urine concentrations of 5.9 and 6.0 mg/L were reported; in the first case alcohol was also present at a blood concentration of 2100 mg/L. [J. S. Oliver and H. Smith, *Forensic Sci.*, 1974, *4*, 183–186.]

In a fatality due to ingestion of up to 250 mg of nitrazepam, postmortem blood and liver concentrations of 9 mg/L and 4 µg/g, respectively, were reported. [M. R. Loveland, *Bull. Int. Assoc. Forensic Toxicol.*, 1974, *10(1)*, 16–18.]

Half-life. Plasma half-life, 18 to 38 h (mean 28).

Volume of distribution. About 2 to 3 L/kg, increased in elderly subjects.

Clearance. Plasma clearance, about 1 mL/min/kg.

Protein binding. In plasma, 85 to 88%.

Note. For a review of the pharmacokinetics of nitrazepam see L. Kangas and D. D. Breimer, *Clin. Pharmacokinet.*, 1981, *6*, 346–366.

Dose. Usually 5 to 10 mg.

Nitrendipine

Calcium Antagonist/ Calcium-channel Blocker

Synonyms. Bay-e-5009; Nitrendipinum.
Proprietary names. Bayotensin; Baypresol; Baypress; Bylotensin; Deiten; Gericin; Monopress; Nidrel; Niprina; Nitrendepat; Nitrepress; Subtension; Tensogradal; Trendinol; Vastensium.
1,4-Dihydro-2,6-dimethyl-4-(3-nitrophenyl)-3,5-pyridinedicarboxylic ethyl methyl ester
$C_{18}H_{20}N_2O_6 = 360.4$
CAS—39562-70-4

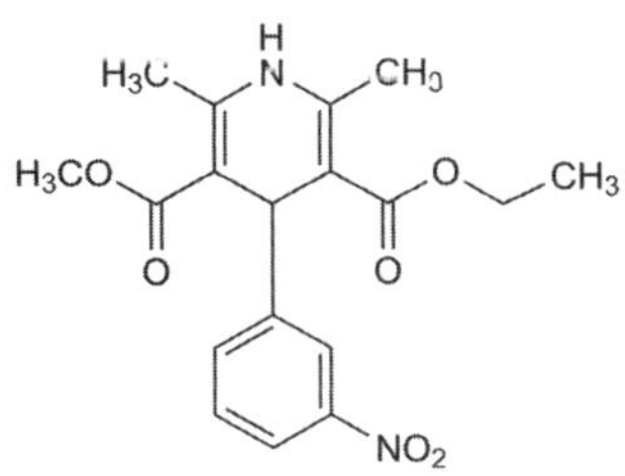

A yellow crystalline powder. M.p. 158°. It is practically insoluble in water; sparingly soluble in absolute alcohol and methanol; freely soluble in ethyl acetate. Exposure to light leads to formation of nitrophenylpyridine derivatives.

Partition Coefficient. Log *P* (octanol/water), 2.88.

Thin-layer Chromatography. System TB—Rf 02; system TE—Rf 80; system TAE—Rf 87.

Plate: silica gel 60 F_{254} (10 × 10 cm, 5 μm). Mobile phase: ethyl acetate:chloroform (1:9). UV detection (λ=254 nm). Rf 0.68. [D. N. Tipre and P. R. Vavia, *J. Pharm. Biomed. Anal.*, 2001, *24*, 705–714].

Gas Chromatography. System GA—RI 2635 nitrendipine; RI 2275 M (dehydro-desethyl-)-CO_2; RI 2330 M (dehydro-desmethyl-)-CO_2; RI 2650 M (dehydro-desethyl-OH-)-H_2O; RI 2690 M (dehydro-desethyl-OH-)-H_2O; system GP—RI 2300 M (dehydro-desethyl-)-ME; RI 2370 M (dehydro-).

Column: SE-52 fused silica capillary (25 m × 0.32 mm i.d., film thickness 0.26 μm). Column temperature: 110° for 1 min, to 320° at 30°/min. Carrier gas: methane. MS detection (NICI, SIM at *m/z*: 360). Retention time: 6.7 min. [C. Fischer *et al.*, *J. Pharm. Sci.*, 1993, *82(3)*, 244–250].

Column: (analytical) DB1 fused-silica (40 m × 0.25 mm i.d., 0.25 mm); (pre-column) DB1 fused-silica (7 m × 0.56 mm i.d., 0.15 mm). Column temperature: 250°. Carrier gas: hydrogen, 32 cm/s. Internal standard: amlodipine. Detection: ^{63}Ni electron-capture. Retention time(s): nitrendipine, 6.7 min; I. S., 9.9 min. [S. C. Monkman *et al.*, *J. Chromatogr.*, 1996, *678*; *Biomed. Appl.*, 360–364].

High Performance Liquid Chromatography. System HX—RI 625; system HY—RI 554; system HAA—retention time 22.1 min.

Column: Lichrocart (125 × 4.0 mm i.d., 5 μm). Mobile phase: methanol:water:acetonitrile (45:45:10), flow rate 1.2 mL/min. UV detection (λ=235 nm). Retention time: 5.94 min. [D. N. Tipre and P. R. Vavia, *J. Pharm. Biomed. Anal.*, 2001, *24*, 705–714].

Column: ODS (Jasco, 250 × 4.0 mm i.d., 5 μm). Mobile phase: acetonitrile:potassium dihydrogen phosphate (10 mM, pH 4.5), flow rate 1.5 mL/min. Internal standard: felodipine. UV detection (λ=250 nm). Retention time(s): nitrendipine, 6.93 min; I. S., 12.20 min. [Y. P. Patel *et al.*, *J. Chromatogr. A*, 1998, *28*, 283–286].

Ultraviolet Spectrum. Aqueous acid—236, 203, 350 nm.

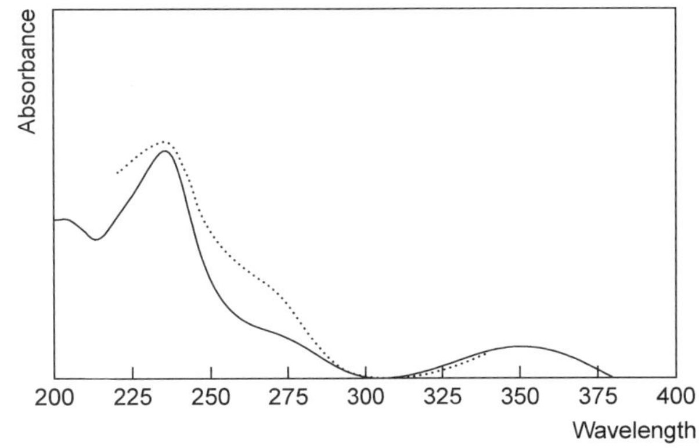

Infra-red Spectrum. Principal peaks at wavenumber 1640, 1203 and 896 cm^{-1} (KBr pellet).

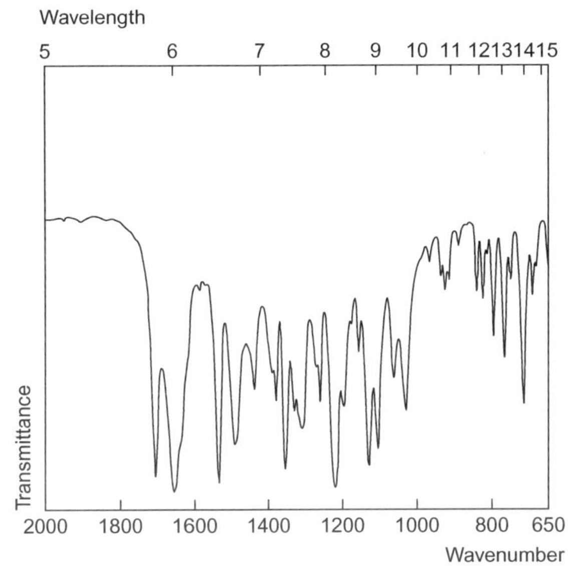

Mass Spectrum. Principal ions at *m/z* 238, 210, 239, 287, 360, 150, 178, 67, 315.

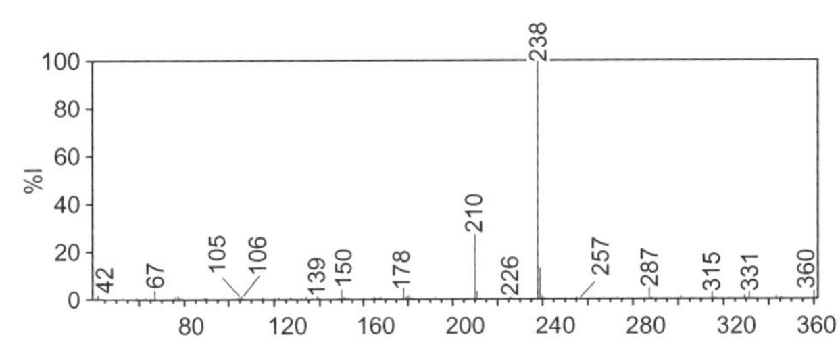

Quantification

Gas chromatography–mass spectrometry. In serum: limit of quantification 0.1 μg/L. MS detection—C. Fischer *et al.*, *J. Pharm. Sci.*, 1993, *82(3)*, 244–250. In plasma: limit of quantification <0.5 μg/L. MS detection—O. Beck and T. Ryman, *J. Chromatogr.*, 1985, *337*, 402–407.

High performance liquid chromatography. In plasma: limit of detection 15 μg/L. UV detection (λ=250 nm)—Y. P. Patel *et al.*, *J. Chromatogr. A*, 1998, *28*, 283–286. In blood: limit of detection 1 μg/L, UV detection—R. Janis *et al.*, *J. Clin. Pharmacol.*, 1983, *23*, 266–273.

Disposition in the Body. Nitrendipine is well absorbed following oral administration and undergoes extensive first pass metabolism in the liver to inactive metabolites. Major routes of metabolism are dehydrogenation to the pyridine analogue, cleavage of ester groups by hydrolysis to carboxylic acids and hydroxylation of methyl groups with subsequent glucuronide conjugation in the bile. All five known metabolites are 1000 times less potent than the parent drug; hence the dihydropyridine ring is thought to be essential for activity. It is excreted as inactive polar metabolites mainly in urine (80%) and a small amount in faeces (8%). Less than 0.1% of an oral dose appears as unchanged drug in the urine.

Therapeutic concentration

20 male and female patients with chronic renal failure and elevated diastolic blood pressure were involved in this study. 10 of the patients required maintenance haemodialysis, mean age of 63.7 years, and the other 10 were at the pre-dialysis stage, mean 55.6 years. All were administered with an oral dose of 5 mg nitrendipine as a solution. The peak plasma concentration for the patients undergoing dialysis was 17.3 (9.0 to 33.0) μg/L observed at 0.5 (0.25 to 3.0) h and for the non-dialysis patients, 12.4 (6.9 to 22.2) μg/L at 0.5 (0.25 to 2.5) h. [H. Kierdorf *et al., Eur. J. Clin. Pharmacol.*, 1993, *45(2)*, 129–134].

7 elderly hypertensive patients with chronic renal failure, mean age 72 years (range 56 to 87 years) and 6 control subjects with hypertension but normal renal function, mean age 67 years (range 48 to 85 years) were involved in the study. They were all administered with 20 mg nitrendipine, before breakfast, once daily for 7 days. For the patients, peak concentrations for the racemate drug were 39.1 (18.4 to 64.1) μg/L; for (*S*)-nitrendipine, 26.3 (12.5 to 40.4) μg/L; and for (*R*)-nitrendipine, 12.8 (5.9 to 23.7) μg/L. All were observed at 1.9 (0.5 to 3.0) h. In the control subjects, concentrations were 25.6 (10.9 to 36.4) μg/L, 16.7 (7.3 to 22.9) μg/L and 9.0 (3.6 to 13.5) μg/L for the racemate, (*S*)-nitrendipine and (*R*)-nitrendipine, respectively. Again all concentrations were observed at 1.7 (1.0 to 2.0) h. [P. A. Soons *et al., Eur. J. Clin. Pharmacol.*, 1992, *42(4)*, 423–427].

Toxicity. There is a potential for seizures precipitously following acute ingestion of large doses.

Bioavailability. 10 to 23%. Depends partly on dosage form. Bioavailability of tablet relative to solution is approx. 75%.

Half-life. 10 to 22 h.

Volume of distribution. 4 to 8 L/kg.

Clearance. The total oral clearance from plasma is 81 to 87 L/h.

Protein binding. 98%.

Note. For a general review of nitrendipine see K. L. Goa and E. M. Sorkin, *Drugs*, 1987, *33*, 123–155.

Dose. 20 mg daily with a maximum of 40 mg.

Nitrobenzene

Synonyms. Nitrobenzol; Oil of Mirbane.
$C_6H_5NO_2$=123.1
CAS—98-95-3

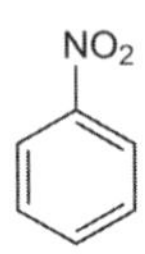

A pale yellow, oily liquid. Mass per mL about 1.203 g. B.p. 210° to 212°. Practically insoluble in water; freely soluble in alcohol, benzene, ether and oils.

Partition Coefficient. Log *P* (octanol/water), 1.8.

Ultraviolet Spectrum. Ethanol—258 nm (A_1^1=697b).

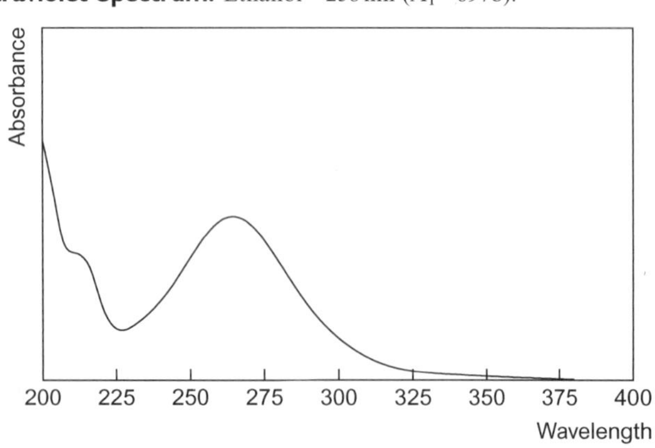

Mass Spectrum. Principal ions at *m/z* 77, 51, 123, 50, 65, 93, 30, 78.

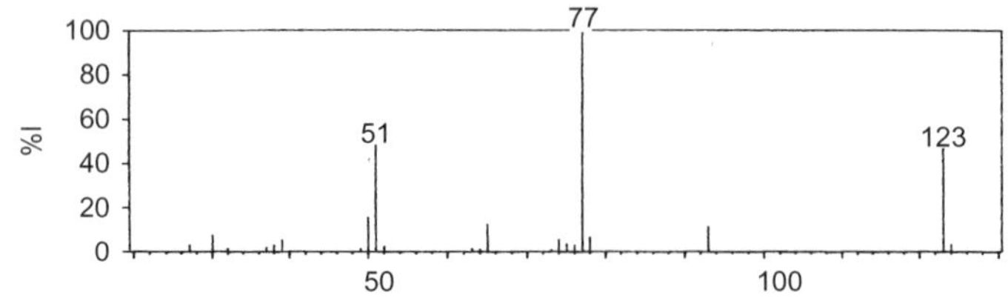

Quantification

Gas chromatography–mass spectrometry. In urine: nitrobenzene and other nitroaromatic compounds—M. Bader *et al., J. Chromatogr. B. Biomed. Sci. Appl.*, 1998, *710*, 91–99.

High performance liquid chromatography. In urine; metabolites of nitrobenzene and other aromatic compounds—A. Astier, *J. Chromatogr.*, 1992, *573*, 318–322.

Nitrofurantoin

Antibacterial (Urinary)

Synonym. Furadonium
Proprietary names. Berkfurin; Cyantin; Furadantin(e); Furadöine; Furan; Furatine; Ituran; Macrodantin; Nephronex; Nifuran; Nitrex; Novofuran; Trantoin; Urantoin; Urolong. It is an ingredient of Ceduran.
1-[[(5-Nitro-2-furanyl)methylene]amino]-2,4-imidazolidinedione
$C_8H_6N_4O_5$=238.2
CAS—67-20-9 (anhydrous); 17140-81-7 (monohydrate)

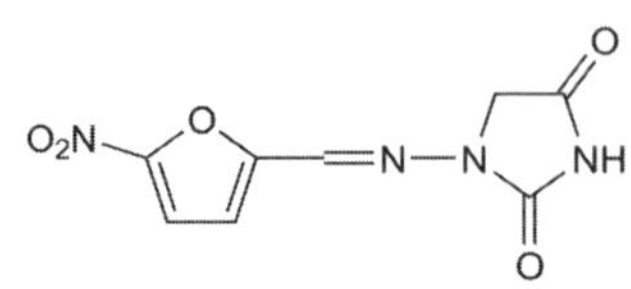

Yellow crystals or fine powder. It is discoloured by alkalis and by exposure to light. M.p. about 271°.
Soluble 1 in 5000 of water, 1 in 2000 of ethanol, 1 in 200 of acetone and 1 in 16 of dimethylformamide.

Nitrofurantoin Sodium
Proprietary name. Ivadantin
$C_8H_5N_4NaO_5$=260.1
CAS-54-87-5
A yellow to orange-coloured powder.

Dissociation Constant. pK_a 7.2 (25°).

Partition Coefficient. Log *P* (octanol/water), −0.5.

Colour Test. Methanolic potassium hydroxide—yellow-orange.

Thin-layer Chromatography. System TB—Rf 00; system TD—Rf 02; system TE—Rf 06; system TF—Rf 30; system TAD—Rf 33; system TAE—Rf 84; system TAJ—Rf 46; system TAK—Rf 09; system TAK—Rf 72.

High Performance Liquid Chromatography. System HX—RI 319; system HY—RI 288; system HZ—Retention time(s), 2.4 min.

Ultraviolet Spectrum. After solution in dimethylformamide and dilution with water—266, 367 nm (A_1^1=765a).

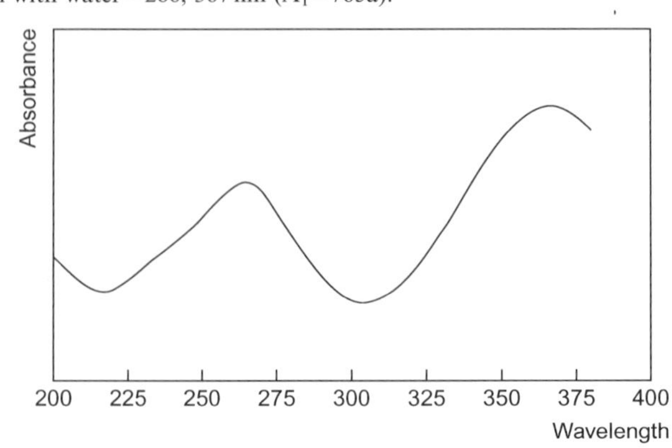

Infra-red Spectrum. Principal peaks at wavenumbers 1718, 1237, 1205, 1770, 1513, $1126\,cm^{-1}$ (KBr disk).

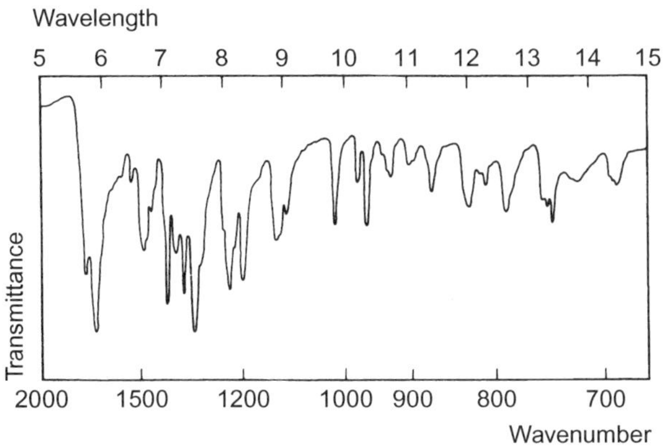

Quantification

Spectrofluorimetry. In plasma or urine—N. Watari *et al., J. Pharm. Sci.*, 1980, *69*, 106–107.

High performance liquid chromatography. In plasma or urine: limit of detection 20 μg/L, UV detection—T. B. Vree *et al., J. Chromatogr.*, 1979, *162*; *Biomed. Appl.*, *4*, 110–116. In plasma or urine: aminofurantoin and cyanofurantoin, limit of detection 4 mg/L in plasma, UV detection—B.-A. Hoener and J. L. Wolff, *J. Chromatogr.*, 1980, *182*; *Biomed. Appl.*, *8*, 246–251. In plasma or urine: limit of detection 0.01 mg/L and 0.38 mg/L respectively, UV detection—P. Muth *et al., J. Chromatogr. A*, 1996, *729*, 251–258.

Disposition in the Body. Nitrofurantoin is readily and almost completely absorbed after oral administration. About 40% of a dose is excreted in the urine unchanged in 24 h together with small amounts of the reduced metabolite, aminofurantoin.

Therapeutic concentration

Following a single oral dose of 50 mg to 6 fasting subjects, peak plasma concentrations of 0.29 to 0.66 (mean 0.43) mg/L were attained in 1 to 4 h. [B.-A. Hoener and S. E. Patterson, *Clin. Pharmacol. Ther.*, 1981, *29*, 808–816].

Half-life. Plasma half-life, about 0.5 to 1 h.

Volume of distribution. About 0.6 L/kg.

Clearance. Plasma clearance, about 10 mL/min/kg.

Distribution in blood. Plasma: whole blood ratio, 1.3.

Protein binding. In plasma, about 60%.

Dose. Usually 400 mg daily.

Nitrofurazone

Antibacterial

Synonyms. Furacilinum; Nitrofural.
Proprietary name. Furacin(e)
2-[(5-Nitro-2-furanyl)methylene]hydrazinecarboxamide
$C_6H_6N_4O_4$=198.1
CAS—59-87-0

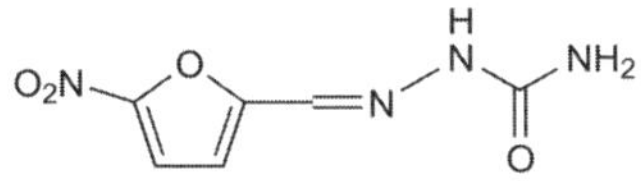

A lemon to brownish-yellow crystalline powder which slowly darkens on exposure to light and discolours in contact with alkalis. M.p. 236° to 240°, with decomposition.
Soluble 1 in 4200 of water, 1 in 590 of ethanol, 1 in 350 of propylene glycol; soluble in dimethylformamide; soluble in alkaline solutions; practically insoluble in chloroform and ether.

Dissociation Constant. pK_a 10.0.

Partition Coefficient. Log *P* (octanol/water), 0.2.

Colour Test. Methanolic potassium hydroxide—red.

Thin-layer Chromatography. System TB—Rf 00; system TE—Rf 41; system TF—Rf 11; system TAE—Rf 78; system TAJ—Rf 34; system TAK—Rf 36; system TAL—Rf 83.

High Performance Liquid Chromatography. System HX—RI 316.

Ultraviolet Spectrum. Aqueous acid—261 nm (A^1_1=610b); aqueous alkali—284 nm (A^1_1=475b).

Infra-red Spectrum. Principal peaks at wavenumbers 1023, 1250, 1200, 970, 1718, $1585\,cm^{-1}$ (Nujol mull).

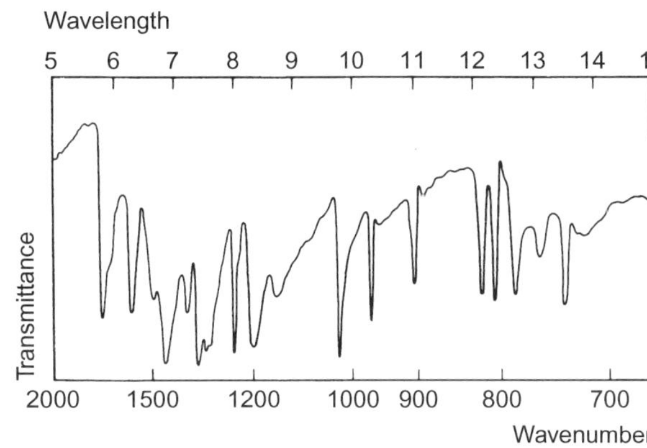

Uses. Topically in a concentration of 0.2%; doses of 0.4 to 2 g daily have been given orally.

Nitroxinil

Anthelmintic (Veterinary)

Synonym. Nitroxynil
4-Hydroxy-3-iodo-5-nitrobenzonitrile
$C_7H_3IN_2O_3$=290.0
CAS—1689-89-0

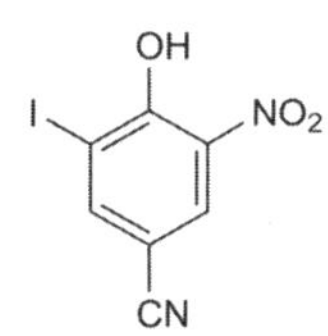

A yellow powder. M.p. 136° to 139°.
Sparingly soluble in water; soluble 1 in 120 of ethanol and 1 in 60 of ether; soluble in solutions of alkali hydroxides.

Nitroxinil Eglumine Salt
Proprietary name. Trodax
$C_7H_3IN_2O_3,C_8H_{19}NO_5$=499.3
CAS—27917-82-4
Readily soluble in water.

Partition Coefficient. Log *P* (octanol/water), 3.2.

Colour Tests. Iodine Test—positive; Methanolic Potassium Hydroxide—yellow.

Thin-layer Chromatography. System TA—Rf 83. (Acidified iodoplatinate solution, positive.)

Gas Chromatography. System GA—RI 1754.

Ultraviolet Spectrum. Aqueous acid—243, 350 nm; aqueous alkali—271 nm (A^1_1=660a).

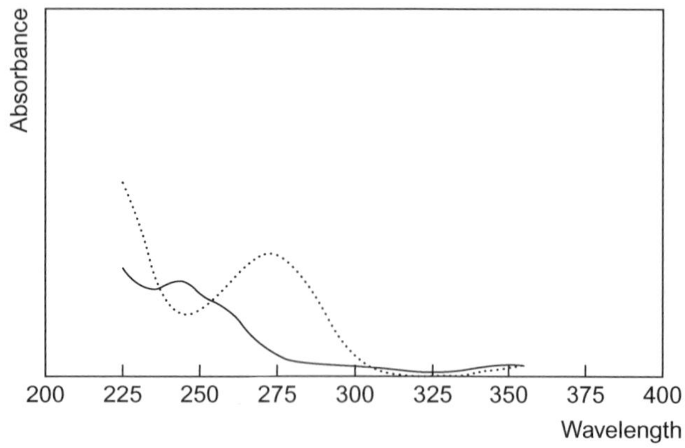

Infra-red Spectrum. Principal peaks at wavenumbers 1529, 1245, 1123, 730, 1309, 1600 cm^{-1} (KBr disk).

Nitroxoline

Antibacterial (Urinary)

Proprietary names. Nibiol; Uro-Coli.
5-Nitro-8-quinolinol
$C_9H_6N_2O_3 = 190.2$
CAS—4008-48-4

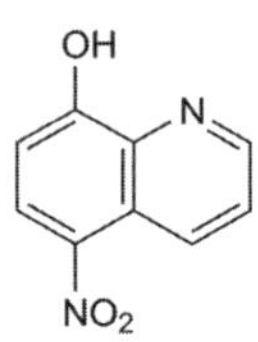

A yellow crystalline powder. M.p. 179° to 182°.
Sparingly soluble in ethanol and ether; freely soluble in alkalis and hot hydrochloric acid.

Partition Coefficient. Log *P* (octanol/water), 2.0.

Colour Tests. Mandelin's test—green; Methanolic potassium hydroxide—yellow.

Thin-layer Chromatography. System TA—Rf 13, streaking. (Visible yellow spot; acidified iodoplatinate solution, positive.)

Ultraviolet Spectrum. Aqueous acid—249 ($A_1^1 = 1914a$), 293 nm.

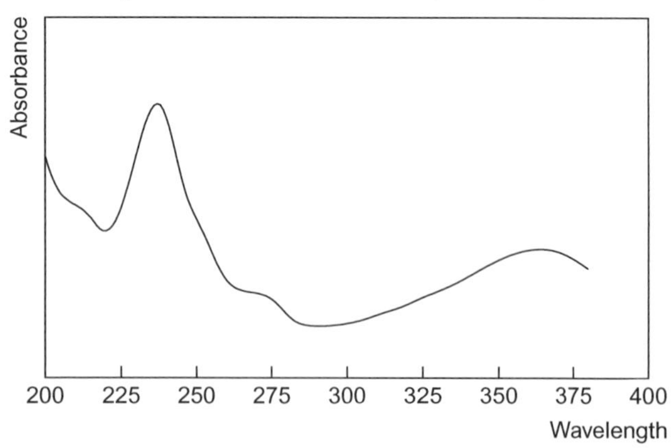

Infra-red Spectrum. Principal peaks at wavenumbers 1504, 1277, 1307, 1189, 1149, 1565 cm^{-1} (KBr disk).

Quantification

High performance liquid chromatography. In plasma or urine: absorbance detection (λ=436 nm)—R. H. A. Sorel *et al., J. Chromatogr.*, 1981, *222*; *Biomed. Appl.*, *11*, 241–248.

Disposition in the Body. Nitroxoline is readily and almost completely absorbed after oral administration. About 60% of a dose is excreted in the urine in 24 h, mainly as conjugated nitroxoline.

Dose. 300 to 500 mg daily.

Nizatidine

Histamine H_2-Receptor Antagonist/ Ulcer-healing Drug

Synonyms. LY-139037; ZE-101; ZL-101.
Proprietary names. Antizid; Axid; Calmaxid; Cronizat; Distaxid; Gastrax; Naxidine; Nizax; Nizaxid; Panaxid; Tazac; Ulcosal; Ulxit; Zanizal; Zinga.
N-[2-[[[2-[(Dimethylamino)methyl]-4-thiazolyl]methyl]thio]ethyl]-*N'*-methyl-2-nitro-1,1-ethenediamine
$C_{12}H_{21}N_5O_2S_2 = 331.5$
CAS—76963-41-2

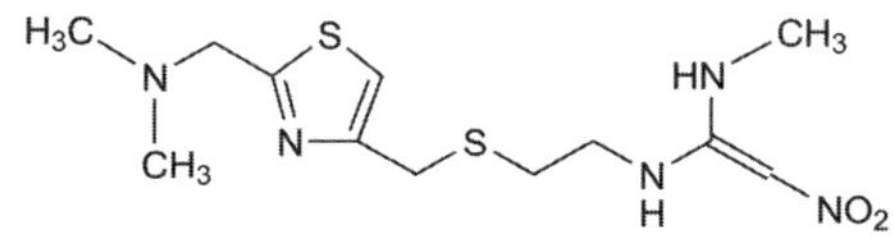

A white to off-white crystalline solid. It is freely soluble in chloroform; soluble in methanol; sparingly soluble in water and buffered solutions; slightly soluble in ethyl acetate and isopropane; essentially insoluble in benzene, diethyl ether and octanol. M.p.130° to 132°.

Dissociation Constant. pK_a 2.1, 6.8 (in aqueous media); 6.3, 8.4 (dimethylformamide).

Partition Coefficient. Log *P* (octanol/water), –0.43.

Thin-layer Chromatography. System TB—Rf 00; system TE—Rf 28; system TAE—Rf 45.

High Performance Liquid Chromatography System HY—RI 178; system HAA—retention time 3.3 min; system HAX—retention time 5.6 min; system HAY—3.1 min.

Column: ODS-2 (Inertsil, 150 × 4.6 mm i.d., 5 μm). Mobile phase: sodium dihydrogen phosphate (0.04 M):acetonitrile:methanol:triethylamine (345:20:35:0.7), flow rate 1 mL/min. Internal standard: procaine hydrochloride. UV detection (λ=230 nm). Retention time(s): nizatidine, 18.6 min; I. S., 10.7 min. [C. Ho *et al., Drug Dev. Ind. Pharm.*, 1999, *25*, 379–385].

Column: Si-60 (Lichrosorb, 150 × 4.6 mm i.d., 5 μm). Mobile phase: acetonitrile:methanol:water:25% ammonia solution (1000:200:20:5), flow rate 2.0 mL/min. Internal standard: ranitidine. UV detection (λ=320 nm). Retention time(s): nizatidine, 2.7 min; *N*-desmethylnizatidine, 4.2 min; nizatidine sulfoxide, 6.2 min; I. S., 5.1 min. [A. Tracqui *et al., J. Chromatogr.*, 1990, *529*, 369–376].

Ultraviolet spectrum. Aqueous acid (0.2 M H_2SO_4)—319, 254 nm; methanol—240, 325 nm; basic—313 nm; water—260, 314 nm.

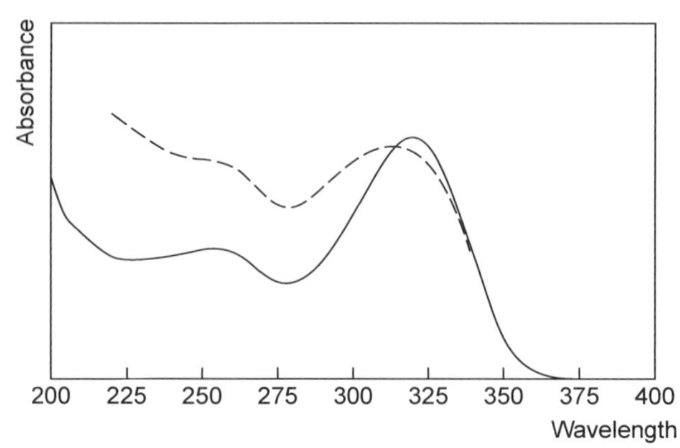

Infra-red spectrum. Principal peaks at wavenumber 1227, 1436, 1586 cm^{-1}.

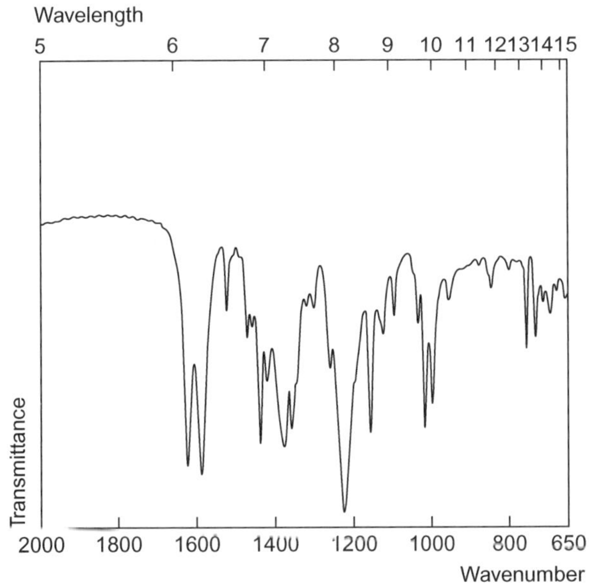

Mass spectrum. Principal ions at *m/z* 58, 254, 111, 227, 214, 45, 44, 71.

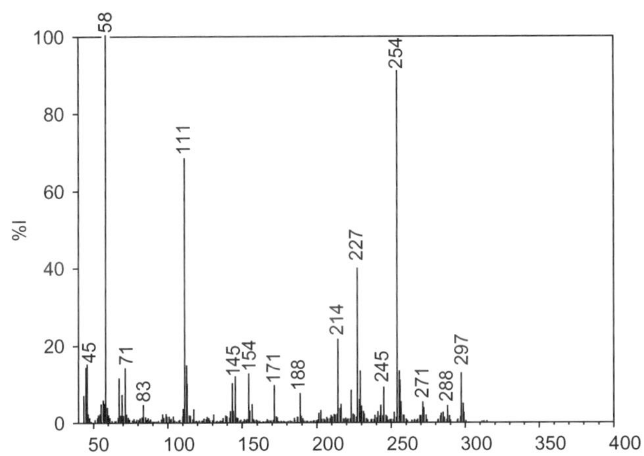

Quantification

High Performance Liquid Chromatography. In plasma, saliva and urine: limit of detection 0.01 mg/L. UV detection (λ=313 nm)—M. P. Knadler *et al., Drug Metab. Dispos.*, 1986, *14*, 175–182.

Disposition in the Body. Nizatidine is readily and almost completely absorbed after oral administration and peak plasma concentrations are reached within 1 to 3 h. Absorption is increased by the presence of food and decreased by 10% in the presence of antacids such as aluminium hydroxide gel and magnesium silicate. It is partially metabolised by the liver, but does not inhibit the hepatic mixed function oxidase system. Three metabolites have been identified, nizatidine *N*-2-oxide, nizatidine *S*-oxide and *N*-2-monodesmethylnizatidine (60% activity of nizatidine). Nizatidine is widely distributed throughout the body and has been detected in breast milk (0.1% of the administered dose). 90% of an administered dose is excreted in urine, partly by active tubular secretion, with 60% as the unchanged drug. Less than 6% of a dose is excreted in faeces.

Therapeutic concentration. The serum therapeutic concentration is 0.15 to 1.0 mg/L.

5 lactating and 5 non-lactating women, aged between 19 and 34 years, were administered with a single dose of 150 mg nizatidine and 150 mg every 12 h for a total of 5 doses (multiple dosing study). The mean peak plasma concentrations were 1.455 mg/L for the lactating women and 1.46 mg/L for the non-lactating women after the single dose. Both concentrations were reached at about 1.5 h. The multiple doses produced peak levels of 1.59 and 1.16 mg/L for the lactating and non-lactating women, respectively in 1.8 and 1.3 h. [B. D. Obermeyer *et al., Clin. Pharmacol. Ther.*, 1990, *47*, 724–730].

Toxicity. Little experience with human overdosing.

Bioavailability. Greater than 70%.

Half-life. 1.3 to 1.6 h (prolonged in renal impairment).

Volume of distribution. Approx. 1.2 to 1.6 L/kg (single 150 mg dose); 1.1 to 1.9 L/kg (multiple doses).

Clearance. Serum, 37.5 to 41.4 L/h (single 150 mg dose); 39.1 to 44.6 L/h (multiple doses). Plasma, 40 to 51 L/h.

Protein binding. 35%.

Distribution in blood. Plasma:blood cell ratio is 3:1.

Dose. Orally: the usual daily dose is 150 to 600 mg. The total intravenous daily dose should not exceed 480 mg. Patients with renal impairment: 150 mg once or twice daily, or alternate days (creatinine clearance 20 to 50 mL/min) and 150 mg daily, alternate days or every third day (creatinine clearance < 20 mL/min).

Nomifensine

Antidepressant

1,2,3,4-Tetrahydro-2-methyl-4-phenyl-8-isoquinolinamine
$C_{16}H_{18}N_2$=238.3
CAS—24526-64-5

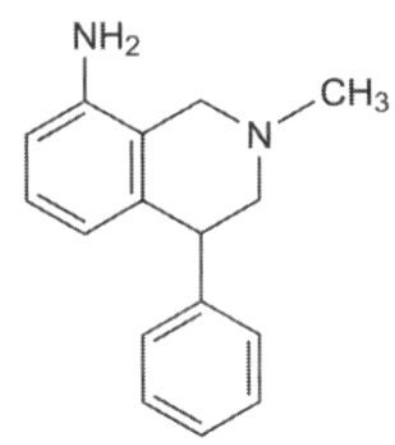

M.p. 179° to 181°.

Nomifensine Maleate

Synonym. HOE-984
Proprietary names. Alival; Merital; Psicronizer.
$C_{16}H_{18}N_2,C_4H_4O_4$=354.4
CAS—32795-47-4
A white or slightly yellowish powder. M.p. about 195°.
Soluble in dimethylformamide and methanol.

Partition Coefficient. Log *P* (octanol/water), 2.4.

Colour Tests. Coniferyl alcohol—yellow; Diazotisation—red; Liebermann's test—orange; Marquis test—orange (slow).

Thin-layer Chromatography. System TA—Rf 56; system TB—Rf 09; system TC—Rf 29; system TE—Rf 64; system TL—Rf 31; system TAE—Rf 53; system TAF—Rf 52; system TAJ—Rf 25; system TAK—Rf 06; system TAL—Rf 50.

Gas Chromatography. System GA—Nomifensine RI 2130; M(OH-) RI 2450; M(isomer 1) RI 2505; M(isomer 2) RI 2590; system GB—RI 2239; system GF—RI 2670; system GM—RRT 0.850 (relative to iprindole).

High Performance Liquid Chromatography. System HA—*k* 0.9; system HF—*k* 0.42; system HX—RI 349; system HY—RI 296.

Ultraviolet Spectrum. Aqueous alkali—284 nm (A_1^1=75b); methanol—241 (A_1^1=461b), 292 nm (A_1^1=124a).

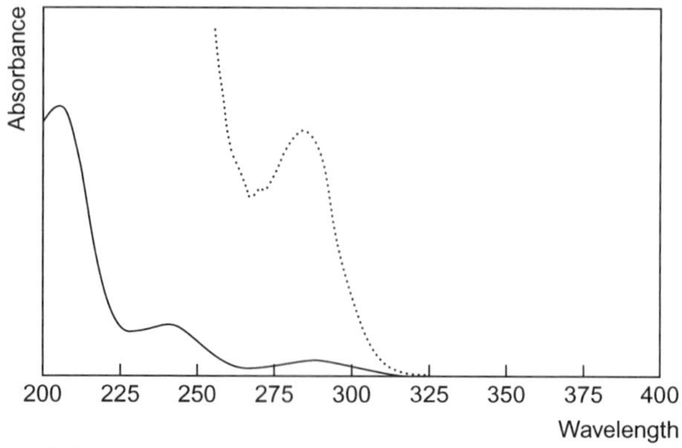

Infra-red Spectrum. Principal peaks at wavenumbers 1580, 877, 741, 1000, 708, 775 cm^{-1} (nomifensine maleate).

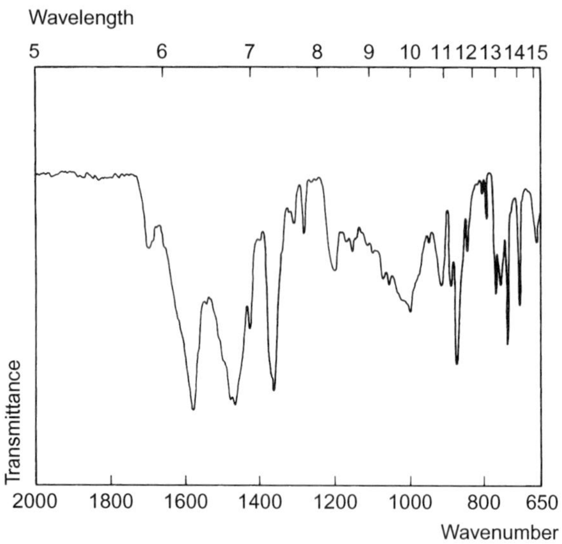

Mass Spectrum. Principal ions at *m/z* 194, 195, 238, 193, 72, 178, 45, 196.

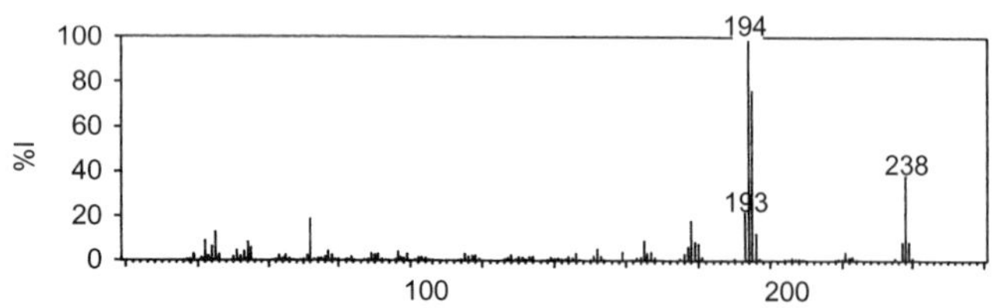

Quantification

Gas chromatography. In plasma: limit of detection 5 µg/L, AFID—I. M. McIntyre *et al.*, *Br. J. Clin, Pharmacol.*, 1981, *12*, 691–694.

Radioimmunoassay. In plasma: limit of detection 1 µg/L— I. M. McIntyre *et al.*, *Br. J. Clin, Pharmacol.*, 1981, *12*, 691–694.

Disposition in the Body. Nomifensine is readily absorbed after oral administration. More than 99% of the dose is excreted within 48 h, about 96% in the urine and about 3% in the faeces. Of the material excreted in the urine, about 60% is the glucuronide conjugate of nomifensine; the metabolites found in urine include 4′-hydroxynomifensine, which is active, 4′-hydroxy-3′-methoxy nomifensine, and 3′-hydroxy-4′-methoxynomifensine, each of which account for about 7% of the dose. A further four metabolites, accounting for less than 1% of the dose, have also been identified and the remaining material is present as unidentified stable conjugates. After a single dose, less than 5% is usually excreted as unchanged drug. The proportion of free nomifensine found in the urine is dependent on the urinary pH, the time and temperature of storage of the sample, and the extraction procedure, because the glucuronide is readily hydrolysed if the pH is below 7.1 and the sample is not frozen.

Therapeutic concentration. A relationship between plasma concentration and clinical effect has not been established. Nomifensine is present in plasma mainly as the glucuronide conjugate; when both free and conjugated nomifensine concentrations are required to be measured, plasma samples must be deep-frozen immediately after collection to prevent hydrolysis. Steady-state concentrations are usually achieved within 5 days.

Following a single oral dose of 100 mg to 6 male subjects, peak plasma concentrations of 0.09 to 0.18 (mean 0.13) mg/L of free nomifensine and 2.65 to 3.68 (mean 3.1) mg/L of total nomifensine were attained in 1 to 2 h; after a single oral dose of 100 mg to 6 female subjects, the corresponding peak plasma concentrations were 0.03 to 0.05 (mean 0.04) mg/L, and 1.95 to 3.32 (mean 2.6) mg/L, for free and total nomifensine, respectively. [I. M. McIntyre *et al.*, *Br. J. Clin. Pharmacol.*, 1982, *13*, 740–743].

Following oral administration of 25 mg three times a day to 9 subjects for 6 days, plasma concentrations of 0.005 to 0.017 (mean 0.011) mg/L were reported 6 h after a dose. [E. Bailey *et al.*, *J. Chromatogr.*, 1977, *131*, 347–355].

Toxicity. Ingestion of 3.5 g has been reported without serious toxic effects.

In 26 cases of suspected overdose where the estimated mean dose was 1.15 g, there were few serious toxic reactions; of the subjects who had ingested only nomifensine, only one became comatose and all eventually recovered. [S. Dawling *et al.*, *Lancet*, 1979, *1*, 56].

In a fatality involving the ingestion of alcohol and nomifensine, the following postmortem concentrations of nomifensine were reported: blood 17 mg/L, kidney 141 µg/g, liver 32 µg/g, urine 400 mg/L; a blood-alcohol concentration of 5000 mg/L was also reported. [A. F. Reyfer *et al.*, *Beitr. Gerichtl. Med.*, 1979, *37*, 313–318].

Half-life. Plasma half-life, 1.5 to 4 h, prolonged in severe renal impairment.

Protein binding. In plasma, 60 to 75%.

Note. For a review of nomifensine, see R. N. Brogden *et al.*, *Drugs*, 1979, *18*, 1–24.

Dose. 75 to 200 mg of nomifensine maleate daily.

Noradrenaline

Sympathomimetic

Synonyms. *l*-Arterenol; Levarterenol.
4-[(1*R*)-2-Amino-1-hydroxyethyl]-1,2-benzenediol
$C_8H_{11}NO_3$=169.2
CAS—51-41-2

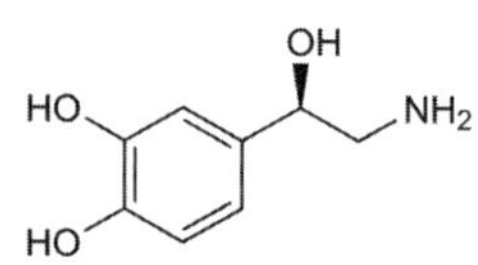

Microcrystals. M.p. 216.5° to 218°, with decomposition.
Slightly soluble in water, ethanol and ether.

Noradrenaline Acid Tartrate

Synonyms. Norepinephrine Tartrate.
Proprietary names. Levophed; Noradrec.
$C_8H_{11}NO_3,C_4H_6O_6,H_2O$=337.3
CAS—51-40-1 (anhydrous); 69815-49-2 (monohydrate)
A white or faintly grey, crystalline powder which darkens on exposure to air and light. M.p. 102° to 104°, with decomposition.
Soluble 1 in 2.5 of water and 1 in 300 of ethanol; practically insoluble in chloroform and ether.

Noradrenaline Hydrochloride

Proprietary name. Arterenol
$C_8H_{11}NO_3,HCl$=205.6
CAS—329-56-6
Crystals. M.p. about 145.2° to 146.4°.
Freely soluble in water.

Dissociation Constant. pK_a 8.6, 9.8, 12.0 (20°).

Partition Coefficient. Log *P* (octanol/water), −1.2.

Colour Tests. Ammoniacal silver nitrate (room temperature)—black; Ferric chloride—green; Folin–Ciocalteau reagent—blue; Mandelin's test—orange; Marquis test—brown; Methanolic potassium hydroxide—blue→orange; Nessler's reagent—black; Potassium dichromate (method 1)—green→brown (30 s).

Thin-layer Chromatography. System TA—Rf 00; system TB—Rf 00; system TC—Rf 00. (Acidified potassium permanganate solution, positive.)

High Performance Liquid Chromatography. System HB—*k* 0.10; system HY—RI 21; system HAA—Retention time(s), 2.8 min.

Ultraviolet Spectrum. Aqueous acid—279 nm (A_1^1 = 160a); aqueous alkali—296 nm.

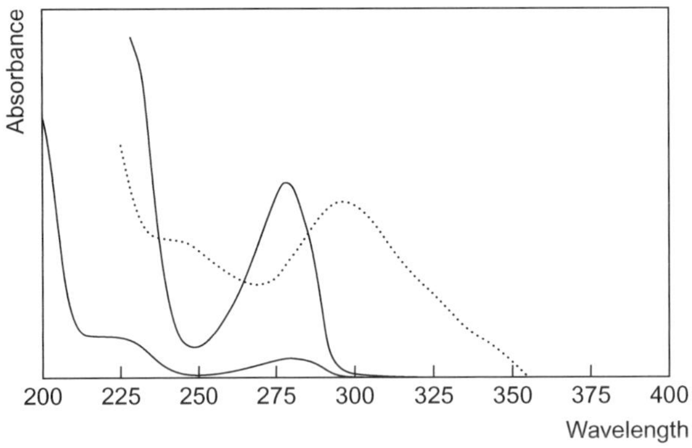

Infra-red Spectrum. Principal peaks at wavenumbers 1265, 1293, 1216, 1200, 1066, 1137 cm^{-1} (noradrenaline acid tartrate, KBr disk).

Mass Spectrum. Principal ions at *m/z* 44, 45, 58, 76, 60, 43, 42, 46 (no peaks above 90); normetanephrine 153, 93, 30, 65, 152, 154, 125, 110.

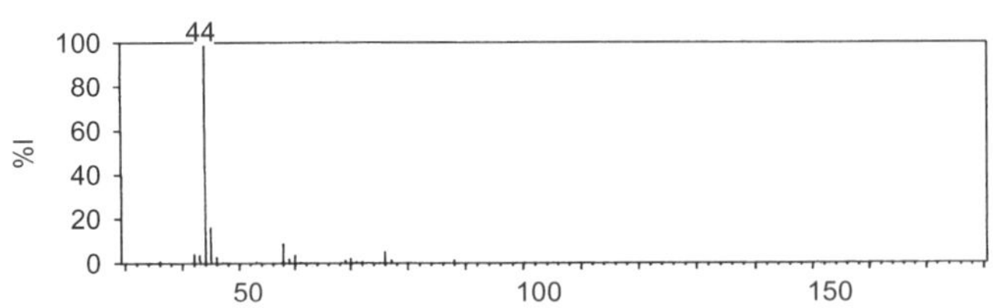

Quantification

Gas chromatography. In plasma, erythrocytes, serum or urine: FID—H. G. Lovelady and L. L. Foster, *J. Chromatogr.*, 1975, *108*, 43–52.

High performance liquid chromatography. In plasma: limit of detection 0.1 fmol, electrochemical detection—C. D. Forster and I. A. Macdonald, *Biomed. Chromatogr.*, 1999, *13*, 209–215. In plasma: noradrenaline, adrenaline, dopamine and 3,4-dihydroxyphenylacetic acid, limit of detection <10 pg, electrochemical detection—Y. Wang *et al.*, *J. Pharm. Biomed. Anal.*, 1999, *21*, 519–525. In urine: noradrenaline and adrenaline, electrochemical detection; comparison with GC–MS method—J. J. Willemsen *et al.*, *Ann. Clin. Biochem.*, 2001, *38*, 356–364 and 722–730.

High performance liquid chromatography–mass spectrometry. In urine: noradrenaline, adrenaline, dopamine and metanephrines, limits of detection 5 µg/L (catecholamines) and 2.5 µg/L (metanephrines)—E. C. Chan and P. C. Ho, *Rapid Commun. Mass Spectrom.*, 2000, *14*, 1959–1964.
In urine: noradrenaline and other catecholamines, limit of detection 10 µg/L for noradrenaline—M. M. Kushnir *et al.*, *Clin. Chem.*, 2002, *48*, 323–331.

Radioenzymatic assay. In plasma: limit of detection 30 ng/L—H. Hörtnagl *et al., Br. J. Clin. Pharmacol.*, 1977, *4*, 553–558.

Disposition in the Body. Noradrenaline is rapidly metabolised before reaching the systemic circulation and is therefore ineffective after oral administration; it is poorly absorbed after subcutaneous injection; it is widely distributed throughout the body. The principal metabolic reaction is *O*-methylation catalysed by catechol-*O*-methyltransferase to form normetanephrine; this is followed by oxidative deamination catalysed by monoamine oxidase, to form 4-hydroxy-3-methoxymandelic aldehyde which is converted to 4-hydroxy-3-methoxymandelic acid (vanillylmandelic acid) and to 4-hydroxy-3-methoxyphenyl glycol; the reaction sequence also occurs in reverse, producing 3,4-dihydroxymandelic acid which is methylated to 4-hydroxy-3-methoxymandelic acid; the metabolites are conjugated with glucuronic acid or sulfate or further metabolised. Up to about 16% of an intravenous dose is excreted unchanged in the urine together with methylated and deaminated metabolites in free and conjugated forms; negligible amounts of endogenous noradrenaline are excreted in the urine in normal subjects.
Noradrenaline is a metabolite of dopamine and levodopa.

Endogenous plasma concentrations are approximately in the range 0.1 to 0.3 µg/L.

Dose. Initially, the equivalent of 8 to 12 µg/min of noradrenaline by intravenous infusion.

Norandrostenediol

Anabolic Steroid

Disposition in the Body. Norandrostenediol is a hormone precursor and is metabolised in the liver to nortestosterone (nandrolone) after oral administration.

Norandrostenedione

Anabolic Steroid

Synonym. 19-Norandrostenedione
Proprietary names. Androbolic; Androdyne; Androstat Pro Six; CycloROID; MHP Nor-Stak; Nortesten.
4-Estrene-3,17-dione
An almost white powder with M.p. 165° (fine product) or almost yellow powder with M.p. 156° (crude product).

Disposition in the Body. Norandrostenedione is a hormone precursor and after administration and absorption is converted to nortestosterone (nandrolone), especially in the liver. Conversion can also occur in the placenta.

Dose. A dose of 100 to 250 mg 1 to 3 times daily is recommended for optimum effect.

Norbormide

Rodenticide

3a,4,7,7a-Tetrahydro-5-(hydroxyphenyl-2-pyridinylmethyl)-8-(phenyl-2-pyridinylmethylene)-4,7-methano-1*H*-isoindole-1,3(2*H*)-dione
$C_{33}H_{25}N_3O_3$ = 511.6
CAS—991-42-4

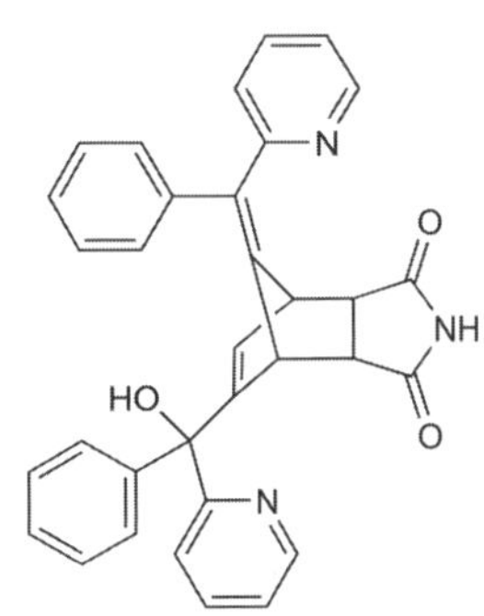

A white crystalline powder consisting of a mixture of stereoisomers. M.p. 190° to 198°.
Practically insoluble in water, ethanol, and ether; very slightly soluble in chloroform.

Partition Coefficient. Log *P* (octanol/water), 3.2.

Colour Tests. Koppanyi–Zwikker Test—violet; Liebermann's Test—green-brown.

Thin-layer Chromatography. System TA—Rf 70; system TB—Rf 00; system TC—Rf 62; system TL—Rf 64. (Acidified iodoplatinate solution, positive.)

Gas Chromatography. System GA—RI 2050.

Ultraviolet Spectrum. Methanolic acid—238, 300 nm (A_1^1 = 136b).

Infra-red Spectrum. Principal peaks at wavenumbers 1708, 701, 751, 1590, 1190, 1754 cm^{-1} (KBr disk).

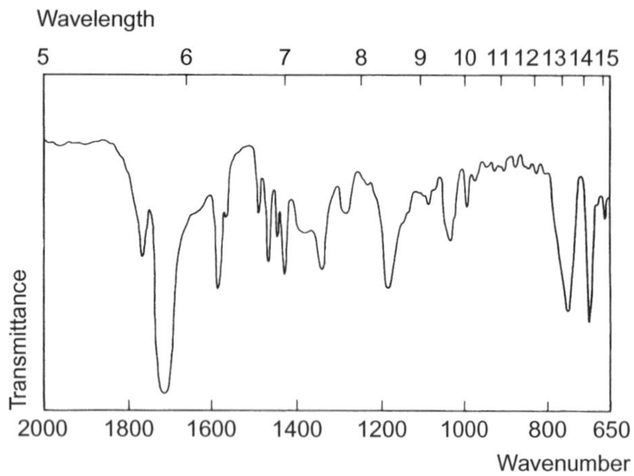

Mass Spectrum. Principal ions at m/z 91, 58, 86, 106, 231, 45, 77, 230.

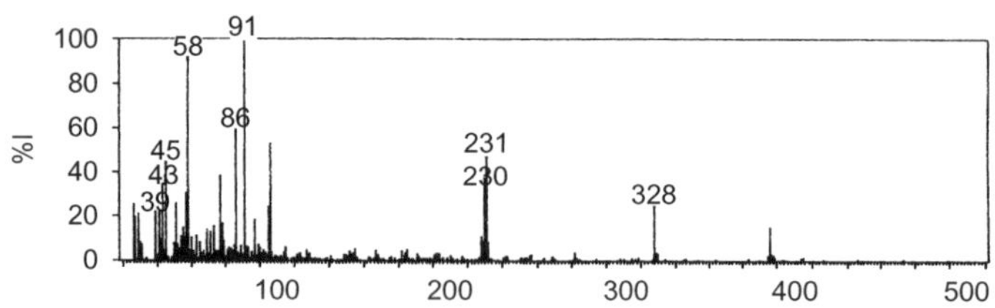

Norcodeine

Narcotic Analgesic

Synonyms. *N*-Demethylcodeine; Normorphine 3-Methyl Ether.
(5α,6α)-7,8-Didehydro-4,5-epoxy-3-methoxymorphinan-6-ol
$C_{17}H_{19}NO_3$=285.3
CAS—467-15-2

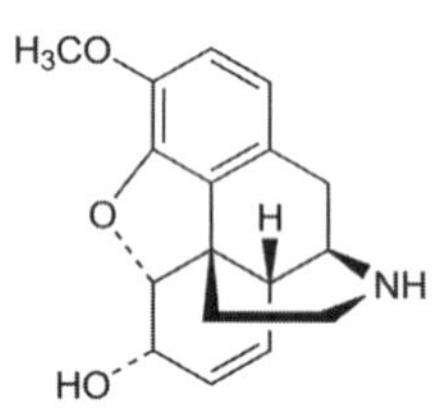

Crystals. M.p. 185°.
Sparingly soluble in water and ether; freely soluble in ethanol; moderately soluble in acetone.

Norcodeine Hydrochloride
$C_{17}H_{19}NO_3$,HCl,$3H_2O$=375.8
CAS—14648-14-7 (anhydrous)
Crystals. The anhydrous form decomposes at 309°.
Sparingly soluble in cold water, more soluble in hot water; freely soluble in ethanol; almost insoluble in acetone.

Dissociation Constant. pK_a 9.2 (25°).

Partition Coefficient. Log P (octanol/water), 0.7.

Colour Test. Marquis test—yellow→violet.

Thin-layer Chromatography. System TA—Rf 13; system TB—Rf 00; system TC—Rf 05. (Dragendorff spray, positive; acidified iodoplatinate solution, positive; Marquis reagent, blue-violet; ninhydrin spray, positive.)

Gas Chromatography. System GA—RI 2388; system GB—RI 2535.

High Performance Liquid Chromatography. System HA—k 3.1 (tailing peak); system HC—k 3.51; system HY—RI 235.

Ultraviolet Spectrum. Aqueous acid—284 nm. No alkaline shift.

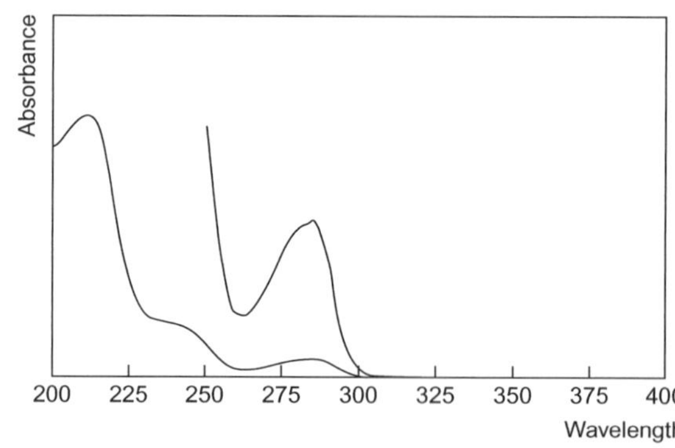

Infra-red Spectrum. Principal peaks at wavenumbers 800, 1515, 1065, 1130, 1290, 1205 cm^{-1} (KBr disk). Polymorphism may occur.

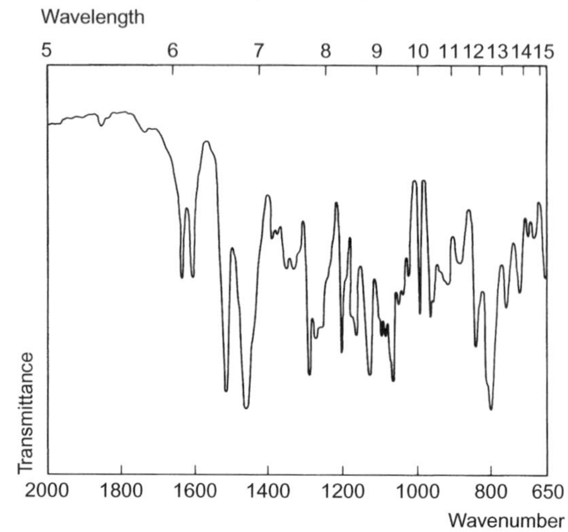

Mass Spectrum. Principal ions at m/z 285, 81, 215, 148, 286, 164, 110, 115.

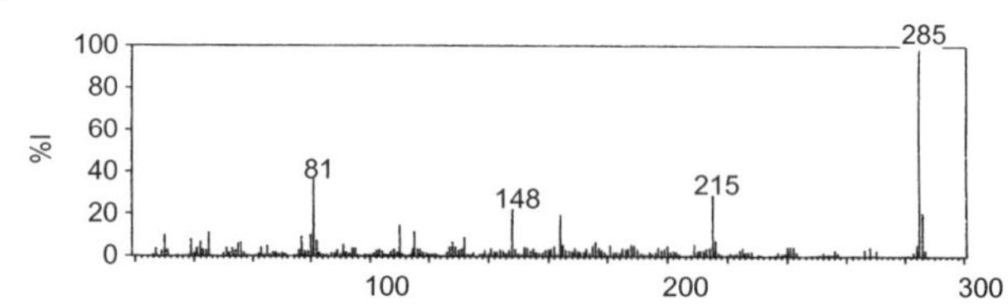

Quantification. See under Codeine.

Disposition in the Body. Norcodeine is a metabolite of codeine.

Nordazepam

Tranquilliser

Synonyms. A-101; Demethyldiazepam; Desmethyldiazepam; *N*-Desmethyldiazepam; Nordiazepam; Ro-5-2180.
Proprietary names. Calmday; Madar; Nordaz; Sopax; Stilny; Tranxilium N; Vegesan.
7-Chloro-1,3-dihydro-5-phenyl-2*H*-1,4-benzodiazepin-2-one
$C_{15}H_{11}ClN_2O$=270.7
CAS—1088-11-5

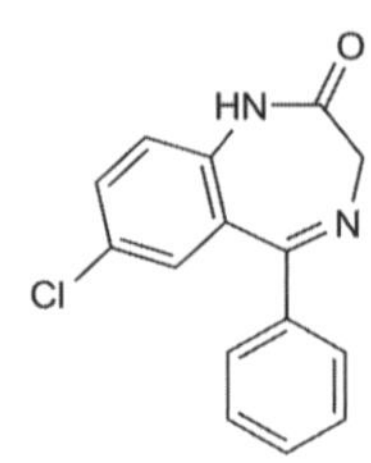

A white or pale yellow crystalline powder. M.p. 216° to 217° (crystals from acetone).
Practically insoluble in water; slightly soluble in ethanol and chloroform.

Dissociation Constant. pK_a 3.5, 12.0.

Partition Coefficient. Log *P* (octanol/water), 2.9.

Colour Test. Formaldehyde–Sulfuric Acid—orange.

Thin-layer Chromatography. System TA—Rf 62; system TB—Rf 03; system TC—Rf 55; system TD—Rf 34; system TE—Rf 67; system TF—Rf 45; system TL—Rf 60; system TAD—Rf 57; system TAE—Rf 82; system TAF—Rf 83; system TAJ—Rf 53; system TAK—Rf 60; system TAL—Rf 92. (Dragendorff spray, positive; acidified iodoplatinate solution, positive.)

Gas Chromatography. System GA—nordazepam RI 2490, oxazepam RI 2325; system GB—nordazepam RI 2625, oxazepam RI 2438; system GF—nordazepam RI 3041, oxazepam RI 2803.

High Performance Liquid Chromatography. System HA—*k* 0.2; system HI—nordazepam *k* 8.00, oxazepam *k* 4.62; system HK—nordazepam *k* 1.99, oxazepam *k* 0.73; system HX—nordazepam RI 470; system HY—nordazepam RI 372; system HAK—nordazepam retention time 7.6 min; system HAL—nordazepam retention time 7.9 min; oxazepam 4.4 min; system HAX—nordazepam retention time 6.7 min; oxazepam 6.0 min; system HAY—nordazepam retention time 6.8 min, oxazepam 4.5 min; system HAZ—nordazepam *k* 1.88; oxazepam *k* 1.23; system HBH—nordazepam *k* 8.97; oxazepam *k* 5.42; system HBI—nordazepam *k* 1.89; oxazepam *k* 1.25.

Ultraviolet Spectrum. Aqueous acid—238 (A^1_1=1140b), 283, 361; aqueous alkali—240, 340 nm.

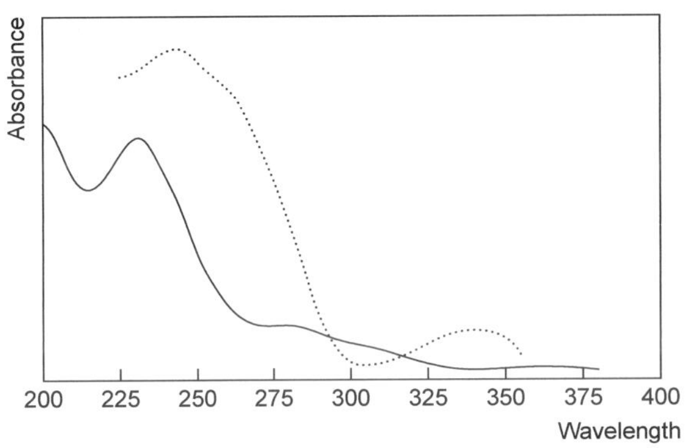

Infra-red Spectrum. Principal peaks at wavenumbers 1680, 700, 1602, 820, 738, 790 cm^{-1} (KBr disk).

Mass Spectrum. Principal ions at *m/z* 242, 269, 270, 241, 243, 271, 244, 272; oxazepam 257, 77, 268, 239, 205, 267, 233, 259.

Quantification. See also under Diazepam.

Gas chromatography. In plasma: limit of detection 1 μg/L, ECD—A. Viala *et al.*, *J.Chromatogr.*, 1978, *147*, 349–357.

Gas chromatography–mass spectrometry. In serum: nordazepam and oxazepam—J. M. Duthel *et al.*, *J. Chromatogr.*, 1992, *579*, 85–91. In hair: nordazepam and oxazepam—P. Kintz *et al.*, *J. Chromatogr.* 1996, *677 B Biomed. Appl.*, 241–244.

High performance liquid chromatography. In plasma: nordazepam and diazepam—J. Atta-Politou *et al.*, *J. Pharm. Biomed. Anal.*, 1999, *20*, 389–396. In serum: nordazepam and other benzodiazepines, photodiode-array detection—B. Ahrens *et al.*, *Arzneimittelforschung*, 2000, *50*, 1057–1062. In urine: nordazepam and other benzodiazepines, limit of detection for nordazepam 100 μg/L, UV detection—W. M. Mullett and J. Pawliszyn, *Anal. Chem.*, 2002, *74*, 1081–1087. In serum: nordazepam and other benzodiazepines, limit of detection for nordazepam 22 μg/L—W. M. Mullett *et al.*, *J. Chromatogr. A*, 2002, *963*, 325–334.

Radioimmunoassay. In serum: limit of detection 3 μg/L—R. Dixon *et al.*, *J. Pharm. Sci.*, 1979, *68*, 1471.

Disposition in the Body. Absorbed after oral administration, maximum blood concentrations being attained in 2 to 4 h. It is metabolised to oxazepam and then to oxazepam glucuronide.
Nordazepam is a metabolite of several benzodiazepines including chlordiazepoxide, clorazepate, diazepam, medazepam, and prazepam.

Therapeutic concentration

Following a single oral dose of 10 mg to 2 subjects, a mean peak plasma concentration of 0.17 mg/L was reported. [G. M. Pacifici *et al.*, *Eur. J. Drug Metab. Pharmacokinet.*, 1982, *7*, 69–72.]

Following daily oral doses of 20 to 30 mg to 9 subjects for 10 days, plasma concentrations of 0.63 to 1.84 mg/L (mean 1.1) were reported 10 h after a dose. [G. Tognoni *et al.*, *Br. J. Clin, Pharmacol.*, 1975, *2*, 227–232.]

Bioavailability. About 50%.

Half-life. The plasma half-life is very variable and values ranging from 25 to over 200 h have been reported. Mean values that have been reported are usually in the range 40 to 100 h in normal subjects. The plasma half-life is prolonged in elderly subjects and in subjects with liver disease.

Volume of distribution. 0.5 to 2.5 L/kg, increased in elderly subjects.

Clearance. Plasma clearance, about 0.1 to 0.3 mL/min/kg.

Distribution in blood. Plasma:whole blood ratio, 1.7.

Protein binding. In plasma, about 97%.

Dose. Nordazepam has been given in doses of 15 mg daily.

Norethandrolone

Anabolic Steroid

Synonym. 17α-Ethyl-19-nortestosterone
Proprietary name Nilevar
(17*α*)-17-Hydroxy-19-norpregn-4-en-3-one
$C_{20}H_{30}O_2$=302.5
CAS—52-78-8

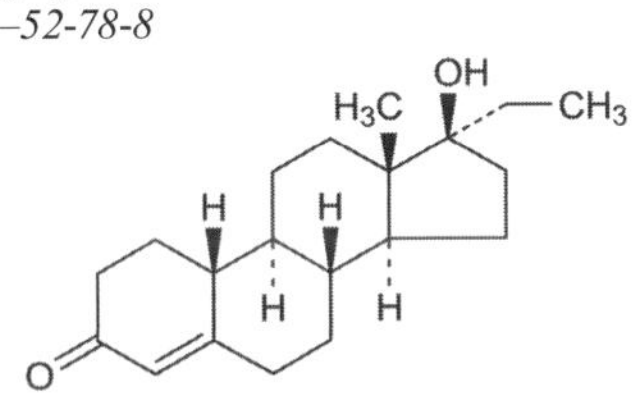

A white crystalline powder. M.p. about 135°.
Insoluble in water; soluble 1 in 8 of ethanol, 1 in 5 of chloroform, and 1 in 3 of methanol; very soluble in acetone; soluble in benzene, ether, and ethyl acetate.

Partition Coefficient. Log *P* (octanol/water), 3.8.

Colour Tests. Antimony Pentachloride—brown; Naphthol–Sulfuric Acid—orange, green dichroism/red-orange; Sulfuric Acid—orange (green-yellow fluorescence under UV light).

Thin-layer Chromatography. System TP—Rf 71; system TQ—Rf 20; system TR—Rf 95; system TS—Rf 78. (*p*-Toluenesulfonic acid solution, positive.)

Gas Chromatography. System GAI—Urinary metabolite: 17α-(2-hydroxyethyl)-5α-estran-3α,17*β*-diol RRT 1.078 (relative to 17α-methyl-5α-androstan-3*β*,17*β*-diol).

High Performance Liquid Chromatography. System HATb—RRT 1.55 (relative to testosterone).

Ultraviolet Spectrum. Methanol—240 nm (A^1_1=565a).

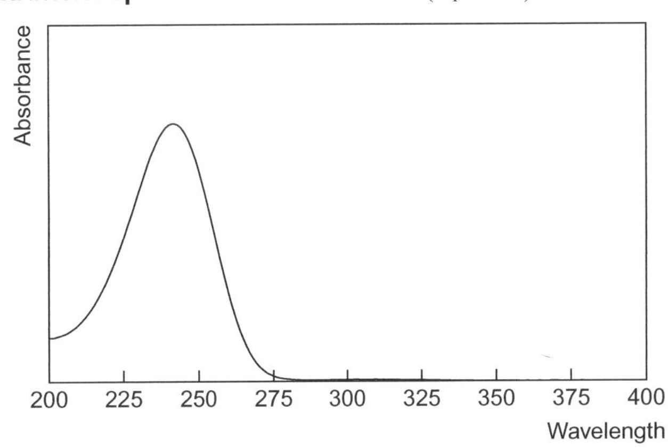

Infra-red Spectrum. Principal peaks at wavenumbers 1650, 1263, 1612, 1210, 894, 1185 cm^{-1} (KBr disk).

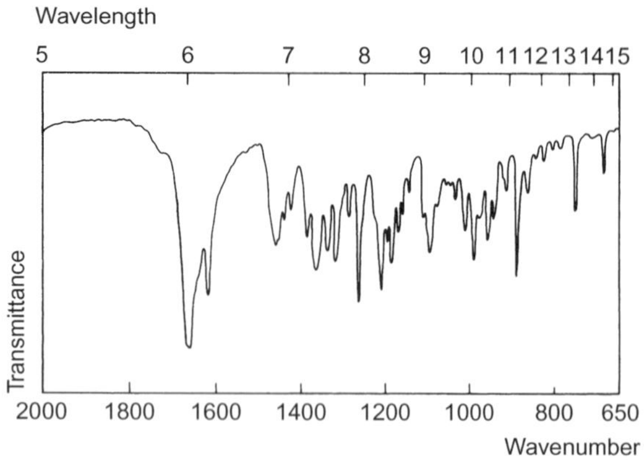

Mass Spectrum. Principal ions at *m/z* 302, 57, 85, 231, 91, 110, 79, 215.

Dose. 10 to 30 mg daily.

Norethisterone

Progestational Steroid

Synonyms. Ethinylnortestosterone; Norethindrone; Norpregneninolone.
Proprietary names. Micronor; Micronovum; Norfor; Noriday; Norlutin; Nor-QD; Primolut N; Utovlan.
Norethisterone is an ingredient of many proprietary preparations—see *Martindale, The Complete Drug Reference*, 33rd Edn., Pharmaceutical Press. London, 2002.
(17α)-17-Hydroxy-19-norpregn-4-en-20-yn-3-one
$C_{20}H_{26}O_2$=298.4
CAS—68-22-4

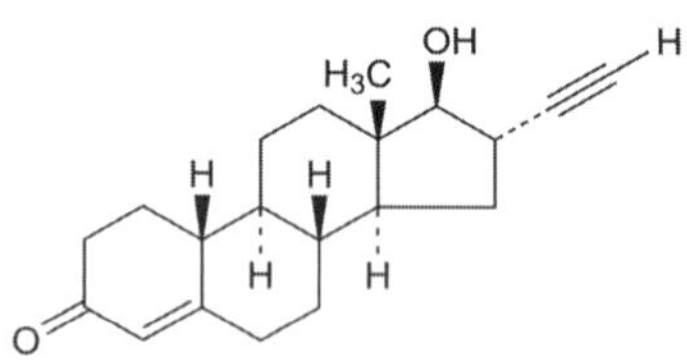

A white or creamy-white crystalline powder. M.p. 201° to 208°.
Practically insoluble in water; soluble 1 in 150 of ethanol, 1 in 30 of chloroform and 1 in 5 of pyridine; slightly soluble in ether.

Norethisterone Acetate

Synonym. Norethindrone Acetate
Proprietary names. Milligynon; Norlutate; Primolut Nor; SH 420.
Norethisterone acetate is an ingredient of many proprietary preparations—see *Martindale, The Complete Drug Reference*, 33rd Edn., Pharmaceutical Press, London, 2002.
$C_{22}H_{28}O_3$=340.5
CAS—51-98-9
A white or creamy-white crystalline powder. M.p. about 163°.
Practically insoluble in water; soluble 1 in about 12 of ethanol, 1 in 4 of acetone, 1 in less than 1 of chloroform, 1 in 2 of dioxan, and 1 in 18 of ether.

Partition Coefficient. Log *P* (octanol/water), 3.0.

Colour Tests. Antimony pentachloride—brown; Naphthol–sulfuric acid—orange/orange-brown; Sulfuric acid—orange (orange fluorescence under ultraviolet light).

Thin-layer Chromatography. Norethisterone: System TB—Rf 20; system TE—Rf 76; system TF—Rf 57; system TP—Rf 71; system TQ—Rf 22; system TR—Rf 87; system TS—Rf 63, streaking may occur; system TAE—Rf 86. Norethisterone acetate: System TP—Rf 87; system TQ—Rf 39; system TR—Rf 98; system TS—Rf 90.

Gas Chromatography. System GA—RI 2625.

High Performance Liquid Chromatography. System HX—RI 536; system HY—RI 676; system HAA—Retention time(s), 24.0 min.

Ultraviolet Spectrum. Ethanol—240 nm (A^1_1=570a).

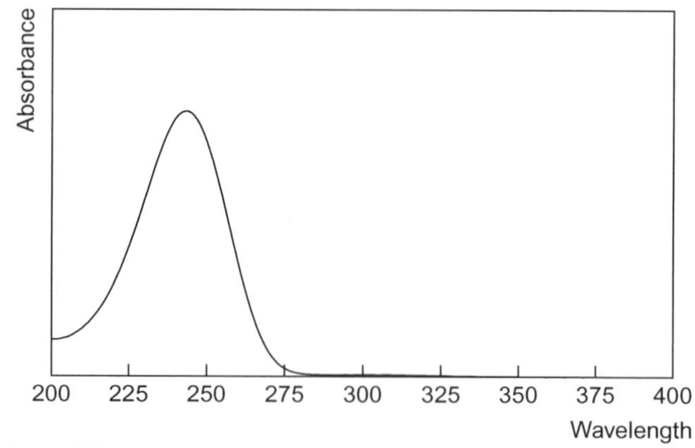

Infra-red Spectrum. Principal peaks at wavenumbers 1649, 1068, 1617, 689, 1272, 660 cm^{-1} (KBr disk).

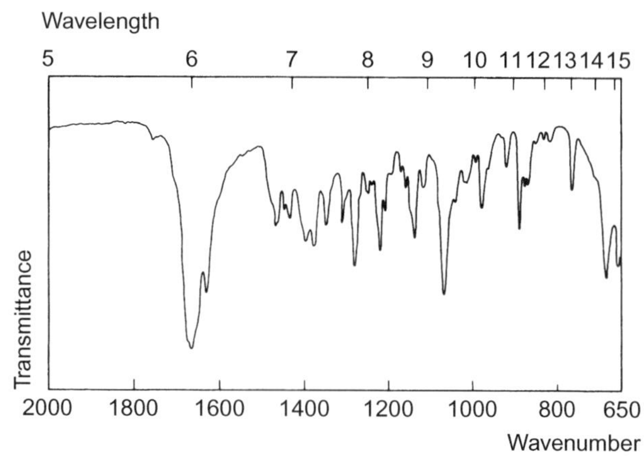

Mass Spectrum. Principal ions at *m/z* 43, 340, 298, 325, 91, 41, 231, 280 (norethisterone acetate).

Quantification

Gas chromatography–mass spectrometry. In plasma: norethisterone metabolites—M. S. Rizk *et al.*, *Acta Pharm. Nord.*, 1991, *3*, 205–210. In plasma: norethisterone and its metabolites, limits of detection <0.5 to 8 µg/L—F. Pommier *et al.*, *J. Chromatogr.*, 1995, *674*; *Biomed. Appl.*, 155–165. In plasma: limit of detection <0.1 µg/L—F. Pommier *et al.*, *J. Chromatogr. A*, 1996, *750*, 75–81.

Dose. 5 to 25 mg of norethisterone or 2.5 to 15 mg of norethisterone acetate daily; doses of up to 60 mg daily have been given.

Noretynodrel

Progestational Steroid

(17α)-17-Hydroxy-19-norpregn-5(10)-en-20-yn-3-one
$C_{20}H_{26}O_2$=298.4
CAS—68-23-5

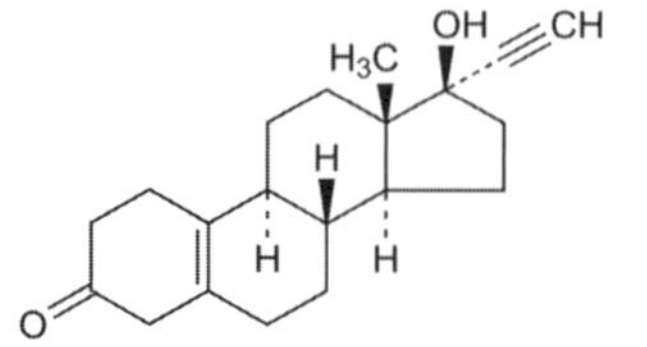

A white crystalline powder. M.p. about 174° to 184°.
Practically insoluble in water; soluble 1 in 30 of ethanol, 1 in 7 of chloroform, and 1 in 60 of ether; soluble in acetone.

Partition Coefficient. Log *P* (octanol/water), 3.5.

Colour Tests. Antimony pentachloride—green-brown; Naphthol–sulfuric acid—orange-red/brown-red; Sulfuric acid—orange (orange fluorescence under ultraviolet light).

Dissolve 2 mg in 0.3 mL of a 0.5% solution of dinitrobenzene in ethanol and add 2 drops of benzalkonium chloride solution. Mix, and add 2 mL of dilute ammonia solution—intense violet immediately, changing to red-brown in about 5 min.

Thin-layer Chromatography. System TP—Rf 79; system TQ—Rf 32; system TR—Rf 91; system TS—Rf 71.

Gas Chromatography. System GA—RI 2551.

Ultraviolet Spectrum. No significant absorption, 230 to 360 nm.

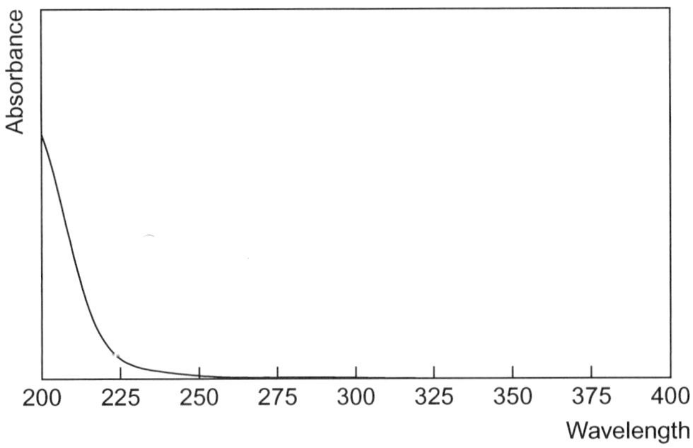

Infra-red Spectrum. Principal peaks at wavenumbers 1066, 1690, 1729, 1140, 1008, 1242 cm^{-1} (KBr disk).

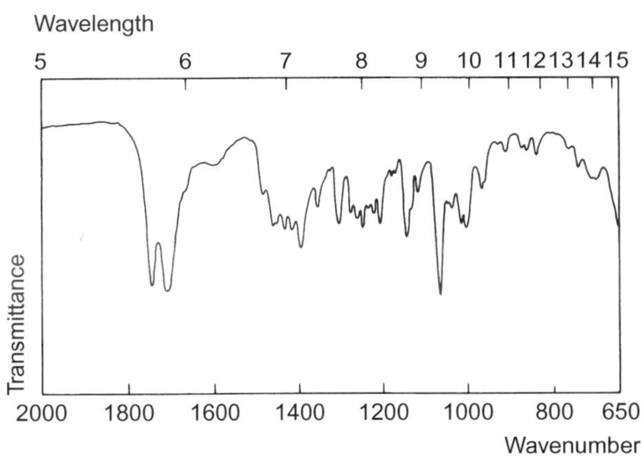

Mass Spectrum. Principal ions at *m/z* 91, 215, 79, 105, 77, 55, 41, 298.

Dose. 5 to 40 mg daily.

Norharman

Putrefactive Base

Synonym. β-Carboline
9*H*-Pyrido[3,4-*b*]indole
$C_{11}H_8N_2$ = 168.2
CAS—244-63-3

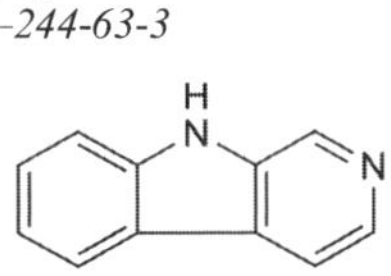

Colourless crystals. M.p. 199°.
Soluble in hot water, ethanol and ether.

Partition Coefficient. Log *P* (octanol/water), 3.2.

Colour Tests. Mandelin's test—green→yellow; Marquis test—green.

Thin-layer Chromatography. System TA—Rf 64; system TB—Rf 00; system TC—Rf 30; system TL—Rf 33. (Acidified iodoplatinate solution, positive.)

Ultraviolet Spectrum. Aqueous acid—247 (A^1_1 = 1723a), 300 nm.

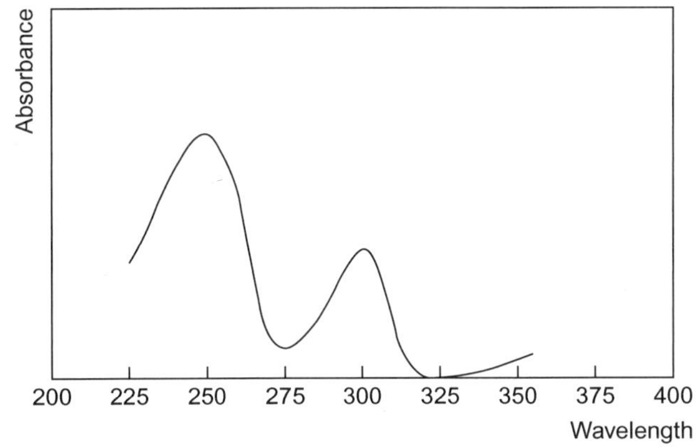

Infra-red Spectrum. Principal peaks at wavenumbers 1247, 731, 747, 1630, 813, 1280 cm^{-1} (KBr disk).

Mass Spectrum. Principal ions at *m/z* 168, 140, 169, 114, 141, 167, 113, 63.

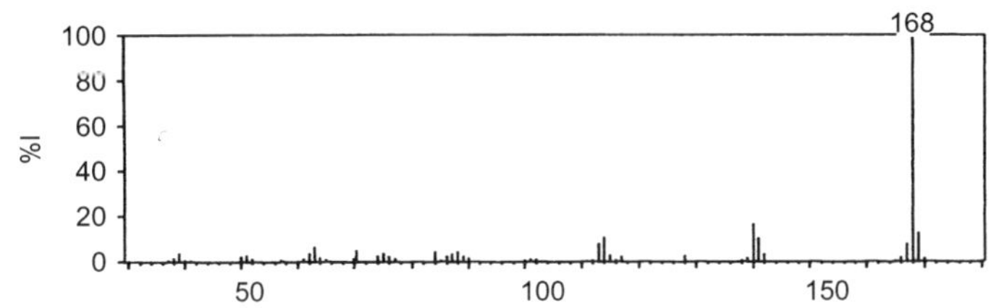

Normetadrenaline

Synonym. Normetanephrine
α-(Aminomethyl)-4-hydroxy-3-methoxybenzenemethanol
$C_9H_{13}NO_3$ = 183.2
CAS—97-31-4

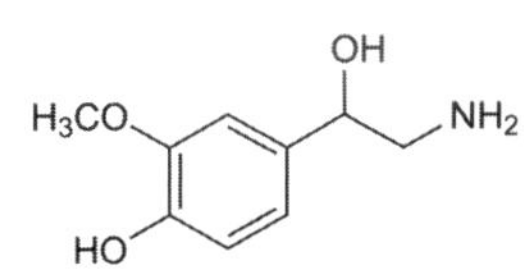

Dissociation Constant. pK_a 8.8.

Partition Coefficient. Log *P* (octanol/water), −1.0.

Colour Tests. Liebermann's test—black; Mandelin's test—green; Marquis test—orange→violet-brown.

Thin-layer Chromatography. System TA—Rf 33. (Acidified potassium permanganate solution, positive.)

High Performance Liquid Chromatography. System HC—*k* 1.08.

Ultraviolet Spectrum. Aqueous acid—278 nm (A^1_1 = 85b).

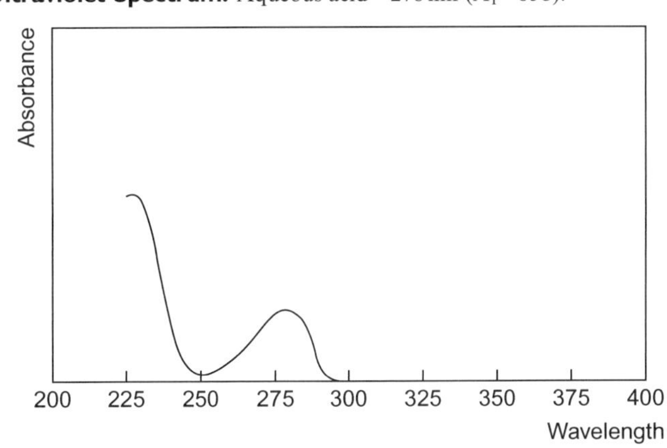

Infra-red Spectrum. Principal peaks at wavenumbers 1529, 1162, 1250, 1037, 1290, 1123 cm^{-1} (normetanephrine hydrochloride, KBr disk).

Mass Spectrum. Principal ions at *m/z* 153, 93, 30, 65, 152, 154, 125, 110.

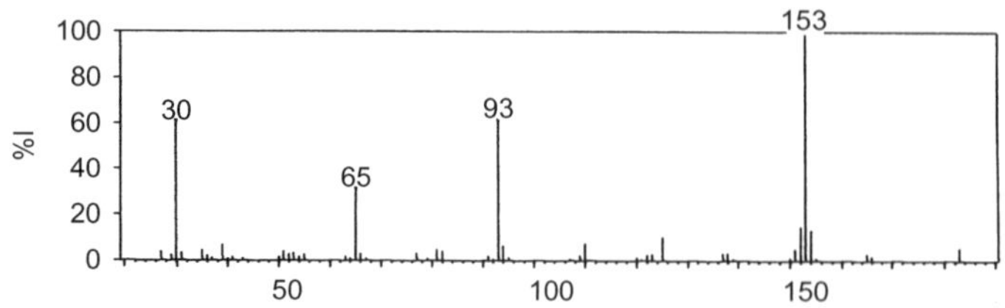

Quantification

High performance liquid chromatography. In plasma: normetadrenaline and metanephrine, electrochemical detection—R. Pagliari *et al.*, *J. Chromatogr.*, 1991, *563*, 23–36. In urine: normetadrenaline, metadrenaline and catecholamines, coulometric detection—G. Santagostino *et al.*, *Farmaco*, 1991, *46*, 1217–1223. In plasma or urine: catecholamines, their precursors and metabolites including normetadrenaline, limits of detection 0.1 to 17.5 μg/L, fluorescence detection—H. K. Jeon *et al.*, *Anal. Biochem.*, 1992, *200*, 332–338. In urine; normetadrenaline, metadrenaline and 3-methoxytyramine, electrochemical detection—P. Volin, *J. Chromatogr.*, 1992, *578*, 165–174. In plasma: normetadrenaline and metadrenaline, electrochemical detection—J. W. Lenders *et al.*, *Clin. Chem.*, 1993, *39*, 97–103. In urine: normetadrenaline and metadrenaline, limit of detection 2.6 μg/L, coulometric array detection—P. H. Gamache *et al.*, *Clin Chem.*, 1993, *39*, 1825–1830. In urine: catecholamines and their metabolites, normetadrenaline and metadrenaline, fluorimetric detection—E. C. Chan *et al.*, *J. Chromatogr. B. Biomed. Sci. Appl.*, 2000, *749*, 179–189. In urine: normetadrenaline and metadrenaline, electrochemical detection (comparison with GC–MS method)—J. J. Willemsen *et al.*, *Ann. Clin. Biochem.*, 2001, *38*, 356–364 and 722–730.

Gas chromatography–mass spectrometry. In urine: normetadrenaline and metadrenaline, limit of detection <25 μg/L—D. K. Crockett *et al.*, *Clin. Chem.*, 2002, *48*, 332–337. In urine: normetadrenaline and metadrenaline, limit of detection 10 μg/L—R. L. Taylor and R. J. Singh, *Clin. Chem.*, 2002, *48*, 533–539.

Disposition in the Body. Normetadrenaline is a metabolite of noradrenaline [norepinephrine].

Normethadone

Narcotic Analgesic

Synonyms. Desmethylmethadone; Phenyldimazone.
6-(Dimethylamino)-4,4-diphenyl-3-hexanone
$C_{20}H_{25}NO$=295.4
CAS—467-85-6

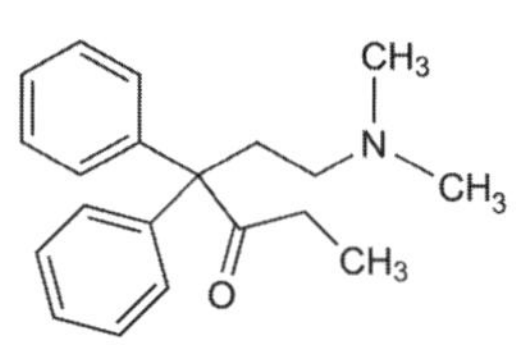

An oily liquid.

Normethadone Hydrochloride
Proprietary name. Ticarda
$C_{20}H_{25}NO,HCl$=331.9
CAS—847-84-7
Crystals. M.p. 174° to 175°.
Soluble in water and ethanol.

Dissociation Constant. pK_a 9.2.

Partition Coefficient. Log *P* (octanol/water), 3.8.

Colour Test. Mandelin's test—yellow-green.

Thin-layer Chromatography. System TA—Rf 56; system TB—Rf 40; system TC—Rf 34; system TAJ—Rf 19; system TAK—Rf 20; system TAL—Rf 78. (Acidified iodoplatinate solution, positive.)

Gas Chromatography. System GA—RI 2095.

High Performance Liquid Chromatography. System HC—*k* 0.53; system HY—RI 366.

Ultraviolet Spectrum. Aqueous acid—253, 259, 265, 292 nm (A^1_1=19a).

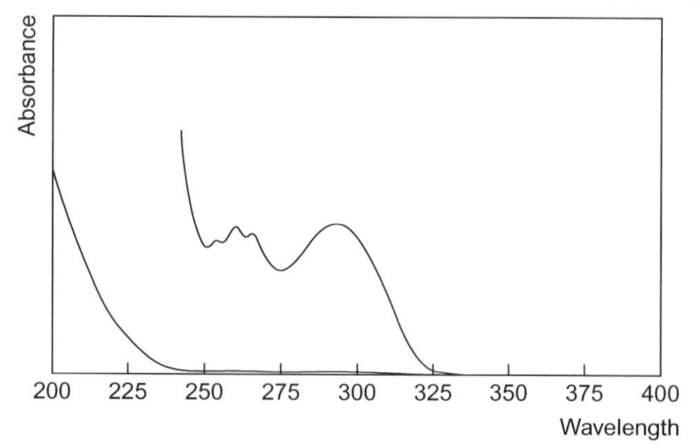

Infra-red Spectrum. Principal peaks at wavenumbers 1711, 701, 1495, 1122, 1032, 760 cm^{-1} (KBr disk).

Mass Spectrum. Principal ions at *m/z* 58, 72, 29, 42, 71, 57, 59, 224.

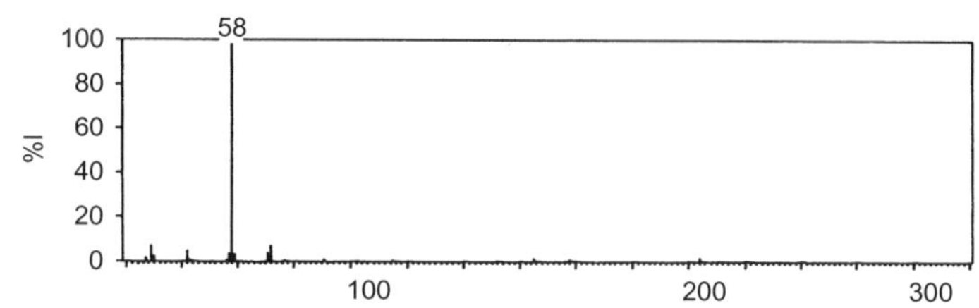

Normorphine

Narcotic Analgesic

Synonym. Desmethylmorphine
(5α,6α)-7,8-Didehydro-4,5-epoxymorphinan-3,6-diol
$C_{16}H_{17}NO_3$=271.3
CAS—466-97-7

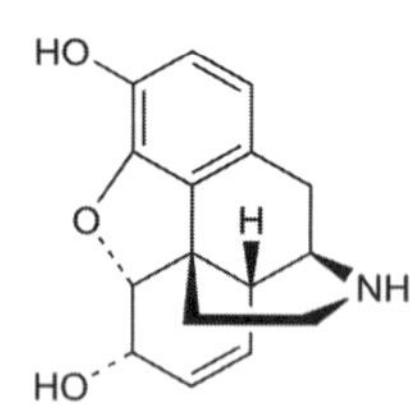

Crystals. M.p. 273° to 277°.
Slightly soluble in water and ethanol; practically insoluble in chloroform and ether.

Dissociation Constant. pK_a 9.8 (25°).

Partition Coefficient. Log *P* (ether/pH 7.0), −2.8.

Colour Tests. Mandelin's test—grey-green; Marquis test—violet.

Thin-layer Chromatography. System TA—Rf 17; system TAJ—Rf 00; system TAK—Rf 00; system TAL—Rf 28. (Acidified iodoplatinate solution, positive.)

Gas Chromatography. System GA—RI 2459.

High Performance Liquid Chromatography. System HA—*k* 2.9 (tailing peak); system HC—*k* 3.92; system HY—RI 133.

Ultraviolet Spectrum. Aqueous acid—285 nm (A^1_1=57b).

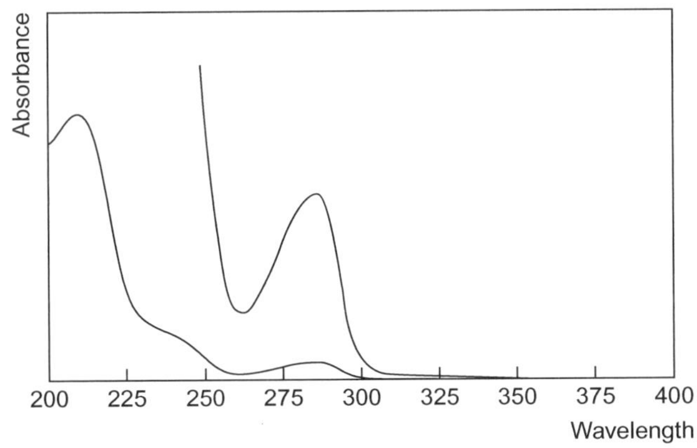

Infra-red Spectrum. Principal peaks at wavenumbers 1312, 790, 1258, 1066, 1275, 1030 cm^{-1} (KBr disk).

Mass Spectrum. Principal ions at *m/z* 271, 81, 150, 201, 148, 110, 272, 82.

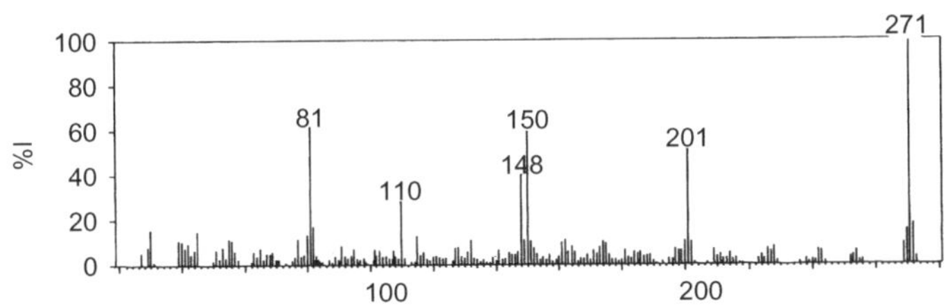

Quantification

High performance liquid chromatography. In serum, plasma or cerebrospinal fluid: morphine and its metabolites including normorphine, limit of detection <0.5 µg/L, fluorescence detection—R. F. Venn and A. Michalkiewicz, *J. Chromatogr.*, 1990, *525*, 379–388. In plasma: morphine and its metabolites including normorphine, fluorometric detection—P. A. Glare *et al.*, *Ther. Drug Monit.*, 1991, *13*, 226–232. In plasma: morphine and its metabolites including normorphine, limit of detection for normorphine 10 µg/L, diode-array detection—D. Wielbo *et al.*, *J. Chromatogr.*, 1993, *615*, 164–168.

High performance liquid chromatography–mass spectrometry. In plasma, serum or cerebrospinal fluid, morphine and its metabolites including normorphine, limit of detection 0.3 µg/L for normorphine—G. Schanzle *et al.*, *J. Chromatogr. B. Biomed. Sci. Appl.*, 1999, *721*, 55–65.

Disposition in the Body. Normorphine is a metabolite of codeine, diamorphine and morphine.

Norpipanone

Narcotic Analgesic

4,4-Diphenyl-6-(1-piperidinyl)-3-hexanone
$C_{23}H_{29}NO = 335.5$
CAS—561-48-8

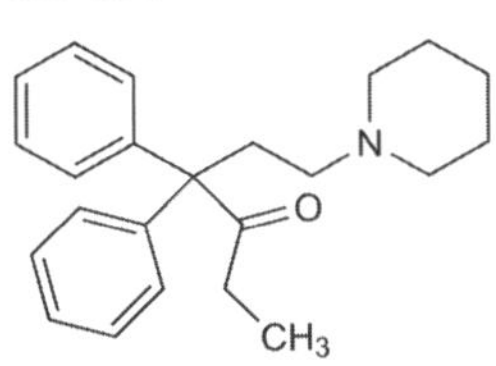

Norpipanone Hydrochloride

$C_{23}H_{29}NO,HCl = 371.9$
CAS—6033-41-6
Crystals. M.p. 181° to 182°.
Soluble in water and ethanol.

Norpipanone Hydrobromide

$C_{23}H_{29}NO,HBr = 415.4$
CAS—6033-42-7
Crystals. M.p. 192° to 193°.
Soluble in water and ethanol.

Partition Coefficient. Log *P* (octanol/water), 5.1.

Colour Test. Mandelin's test—brown→blue.

Thin-layer Chromatography. System TA—Rf 68; system TB—Rf 58; system TC—Rf 50; system TE—Rf 80; system TL—Rf 38; system TAE—Rf 43. (Dragendorff spray, positive; acidified iodoplatinate solution, positive; Marquis reagent, dull orange.)

Gas Chromatography. System GA—RI 2488.

High Performance Liquid Chromatography. System HC—*k* 0.35; system HX—RI 466.

Ultraviolet Spectrum. Aqueous acid—260 nm ($A_1^1 = 17b$), 294 nm.

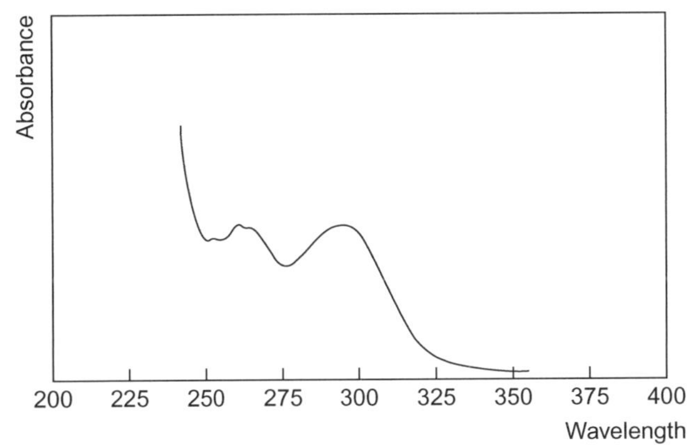

Infra-red Spectrum. Principal peaks at wavenumbers 1705, 700, 1115, 1492, 1600, 1157 cm^{-1} (KBr disk).

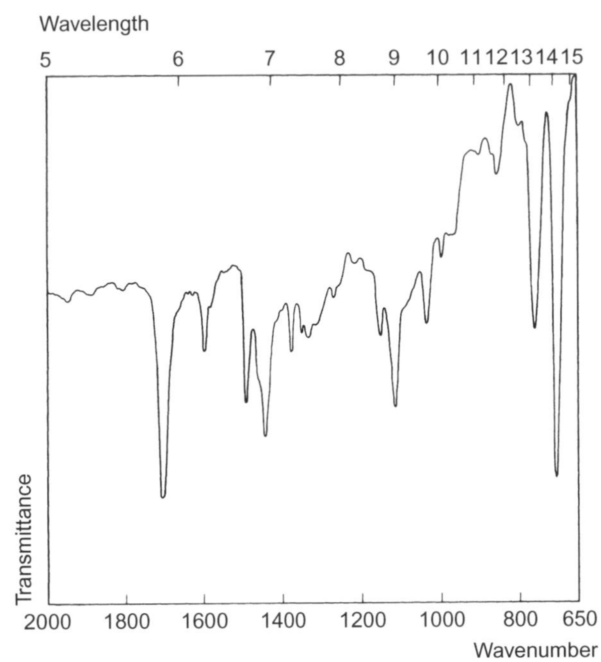

Mass Spectrum. Principal ions at *m/z* 98, 111, 99, 42, 55, 41, 29, 112.

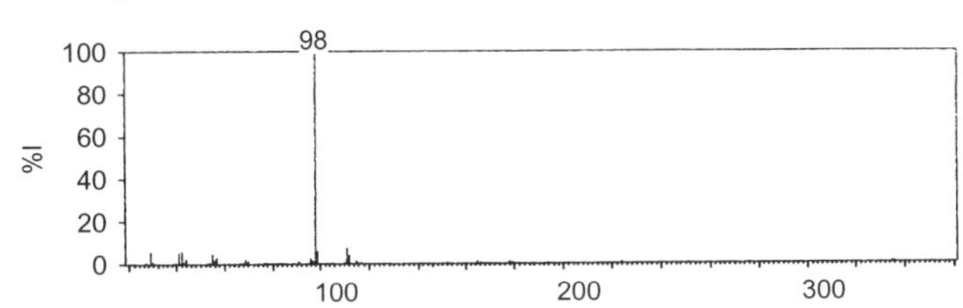

Dose. Norpipanone hydrochloride has been given in doses of 18 mg daily.

Nortriptyline

Antidepressant

3-(10,11-Dihydro-5*H*-dibenzo[*a*,*d*]cyclohepten-5-ylidene)-*N*-methyl-1-propanamine
$C_{19}H_{21}N$=263.4
CAS—72-69-5

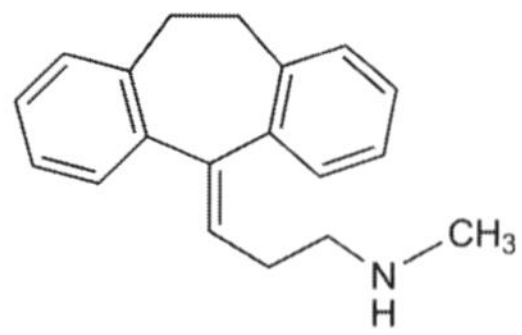

Nortriptyline Hydrochloride

Synonyms. 38489; Nortriptylini Hydrochloridum.
Proprietary names. Allegron; Altilev; Aventyl; Martimil; Norfenazin; Noritren; Norpress; Nortab; Norterol; Nortrilen; Ortrip; Pamelor; Paxtibi; Psychostyl; Sensaval; Vividyl. It is an ingredient of Motipress and Motival.
$C_{19}H_{21}N,HCl$=299.8
CAS—894-71-3
A white powder. M.p. 213° to 215° (crystals from ether and ethanol).
Soluble 1 in 50 of water, 1 in 10 of ethanol, and 1 in 5 of chloroform; practically insoluble in ether, acetone, and benzene.

Dissociation Constant. pK_a 9.7.

Partition Coefficient. Log *P* (octanol/buffer pH 7.4), 1.7.

Colour Tests. Mandelin's Test—brown→green; Marquis Test—orange-brown; Sulfuric Acid—orange.

Thin-layer Chromatography. System TA—Rf 34; system TB—Rf 27; system TC—Rf 16; system TAJ—Rf 01; system TAK—Rf 09; system TAL—Rf 68. (Dragendorff spray, positive; acidified iodoplatinate solution, positive; Marquis reagent, brown.)

Gas Chromatography. System GA—nortriptyline RI 2215, M (*cis*-10-OH-) RI 2375, M (*trans*-10-OH-) RI 2375, M (acetyl-) RI 2660; system GB—nortriptyline RI 2304, M (*cis*-10-OH-) RI 2480, M (*trans*-10-OH-) RI 2494, M (norcyclobenzaprine) RI 2343, M (acetyl-) RI 2774, M (norcyclobenzaprine)-AC RI 2949; system GM—nortriptyline RRT 0.816, M (*cis*-10-OH-) RRT 1.261, M (*trans*-10-OH-) RRT 1.323, M (norcyclobenzaprine) RRT 0.880 (all relative to iprindole); system GS—nortriptyline retention time 17.5 min.

High Performance Liquid Chromatography. System HA—nortriptyline *k* 2.0; 10-hydroxynortriptyline *k* 1.8; system HF—*k* 4.58; system HY—RI 338; system HZ—retention time 6.6 min; system HAA—retention time 15.6 min; system HAM—not detected; system HAX—retention time 13.7 min; system HAY—retention time 6.8 min; system HAZ—*k* 1.71.

Ultraviolet Spectrum. Aqueous acid—239 nm (A^1_1=517a). No alkaline shift.

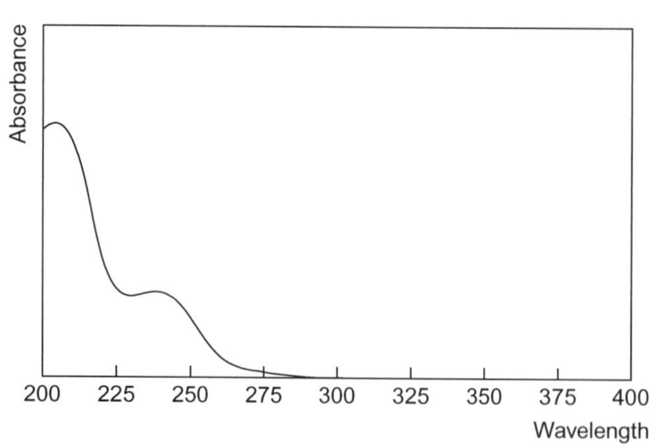

Infra-red Spectrum. Principal peaks at wavenumbers 756, 742, 768, 720, 775, 1590 cm^{-1} (nortriptyline hydrochloride, KBr disk).

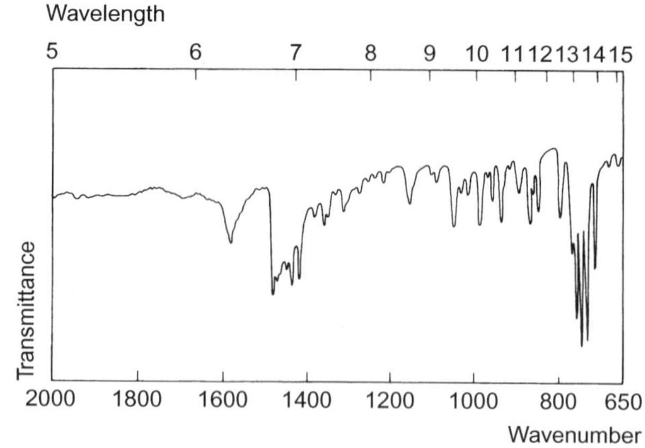

Mass Spectrum. Principal ions at *m/z* 44, 202, 45, 220, 218, 215, 91, –; 10-hydroxynortriptyline 44, 45, 26, 218, 215, 203, 202, 42.

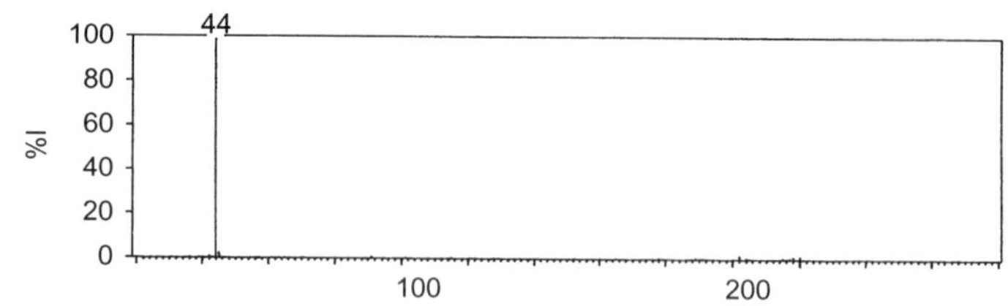

Quantification. See also under Amitriptyline.

Gas chromatography. In plasma: nortriptyline and 10-hydroxynortriptyline, limits of quantification 1 μg/L and 3 μg/L respectively, ECD—S. L. Anliker *et al.*, *J. Chromatogr.*, 1992, *573*, 141–145. In plasma: limit of quantification is 125 μg/L, NPD—S. Ulrich and J. Martens, *J. Chromatogr. B Biomed. Sci. Appl.*, 1997, *696(2)*, 217–234.

High performance liquid chromatography. In serum: UV detection—O. V. Olesen *et al.*, *J. Chromatogr. B Biomed. Sci. Appl.*, 2000, *746*, 233–239.

High performance liquid chromatography–mass spectrometry. In plasma: nortriptyline and 10-hydroxynortriptline, limit of quantification 0.8 μg/L—G. Tybring *et al.*, *J. Chromatogr. B Biomed. Sci. Appl.*, 1998, *716*, 382–386.

Disposition in the Body. Readily absorbed after oral administration and undergoes first-pass metabolism. The main metabolic reactions are *N*-demethylation and 10-hydroxylation; glucuronide conjugation of nortriptyline and its metabolites also occurs. Up to 60% of the daily dose is excreted in the urine within 24 h, with less than 5% as unchanged drug, 30 to 50% as free or conjugated 10-hydroxynortriptyline, 6 to 15% as free and conjugated 10-hydroxydinortriptyline, and about 1% as dinortriptyline. Nortriptyline is a metabolite of amitriptyline.

Therapeutic concentration. In plasma, usually in the range 0.05 to 0.15 mg/L. Plasma concentrations vary considerably between individuals and are influenced by exposure to other drugs.

Following a single oral dose of 100 mg to 10 subjects, peak plasma concentrations of 0.015 to 0.050 mg/L (mean 0.03) of nortriptyline and 0.039 to 0.172 mg/L (mean 0.10) of 10-hydroxynortriptyline were attained in 3 to 24 h. [S. Nakano and L. E. Hollister, *Clin. Pharmacol Ther.*, 1978, *23*, 199–203.]

Following average daily oral doses of 82 mg to 62 subjects, the following steady-state plasma concentrations were reported: nortriptyline 0.03 to 0.34 mg/L (mean 0.12), 10-hydroxynortriptyline 0.04 to 0.42 mg/L (mean 0.16), conjugated 10-hydroxynortriptyline 0.075 to 1.07 mg/L (mean 0.37). [S. Dawling *et al.*, *Clin. Pharmacol. Ther.*, 1982, *32*, 322–329.]

Toxicity. Relatively few cases of serious intoxication have been attributed to nortriptyline in comparison to the tertiary amine tricyclic antidepressants. Toxic effects are usually associated with blood concentrations greater than 0.25 mg/L and concentrations above 1 mg/L may produce coma. Recovery has occurred after the ingestion of 2.5 g.

The following distribution was reported in 9 fatal cases: blood 0 to 26 mg/L (mean 11, 3 cases), kidney 7 to 94 μg/g (mean 43, 5 cases), liver 8 to 220 μg/g (mean 90, 9 cases), urine 25 to 120 mg/L (mean 76, 4 cases). [R. Bonnichsen *et al.*, *Z. Rechtsmed.*, 1970, *67*, 190–200.]

A 62-year-old woman survived after an intentional overdose of nortriptyline despite having a peak plasma concentration of 2.29 mg/L; high levels (up to 2 mg/L) of E-10-hydroxynortriptyline were still detected for 4 to 5 days after drug intake. [E. J. Franssen *et al.*, *Ther. Drug Monit.*, 2003, *25*, 248–251.]

Bioavailability. About 50 to 60%.

Half-life. Plasma half-life, 15 to 90 h (mean 30).

Volume of distribution. 14 to 40 L/kg (mean 23).

Clearance. Plasma, 7.2 mL/min/kg.

Protein binding. In plasma, 90 to 95%.

Note. For a review of tricyclic antidepressants, see G. Molnar and R. N. Gupta, *Biopharm. Drug Disp.*, 1980, *1*, 283–305. For a review of E-10-hydroxynortriptyline, see L. Bertilsson *et al.*, *Psychopharmacol. Ser.*, 1989, *7*, 52–59. For a review of nortriptyline, see E. H. Rubin, *J. Clin Psychiatry*, 1985, *46*, 418–424.

Dose. Usually, the equivalent of 30 to 100 mg of nortriptyline daily; maximum 150 mg daily.

Noscapine

Cough Suppressant

Synonyms. Narcotine; l-α-Narcotine; Noscapinum; NSC-5366.
Proprietary names. Capval; Finipect; Nipaxon; Nitepax (resin complex).
(3*S*)-6,7-Dimethoxy-3-[(5*R*)-5,6,7,8-tetrahydro-4-methoxy-6-methyl-1,3-dioxolo[4,5-*g*]isoquinolin-5-yl]-1(3*H*)-isobenzofuranone
$C_{22}H_{23}NO_7 = 413.4$
CAS—128-62-1

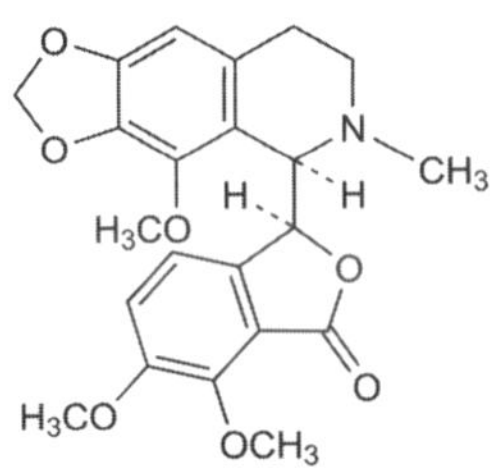

An alkaloid obtained from opium.
Colourless crystals or a fine white crystalline powder. M.p. 176°, with decomposition.
Practically insoluble in water; slightly soluble in ethanol and ether; soluble in acetone and chloroform.

Noscapine Hydrochloride

Proprietary names. Capval; Libronchin Prikkelhoest; Noscaflex; Roter Noscapect; Tuscalman; Tussanil N.
$C_{22}H_{23}NO_7,HCl,H_2O = 467.9$
CAS—912-60-7 (anhydrous)
Hygroscopic, colourless crystals or a fine white crystalline powder. M.p. about 200°, with decomposition.
Soluble 1 in 4 of water and 1 in 8 of ethanol; freely soluble in chloroform; practically insoluble in ether. Aqueous solutions may deposit the base on standing.

Dissociation Constant. pK_a 6.2 (20°).

Partition Coefficient. Log *P* (octanol/water), 2.0.

Colour Tests. Liebermann's Test—black; Marquis Test—blue-violet (fades).

Thin-layer Chromatography. System TA—Rf 64; system TB—Rf 21; system TC—Rf 74; system TE—Rf 78; system TL—Rf 64; system TAE—Rf 72; system TAF—Rf 75; system TAJ—Rf 65; system TAK—Rf 18; system TAL—Rf 93. (Acidified iodoplatinate solution, positive.)

Gas Chromatography. System GA—RI 3145; system GB—RI 3358.

High Performance Liquid Chromatography. System HA—*k* 0.3; system HC—*k* 0.15; system HS—*k* 0.01; system HX—RI 368; system HY—RI 289; system HAA—retention time 12.8 min.

Ultraviolet Spectrum. Aqueous acid—290, 312 ($A_1^1 = 84a$); aqueous alkali—281, 315 nm.

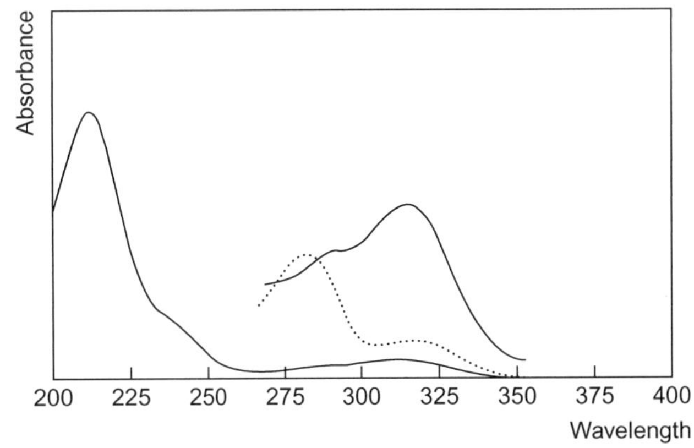

Infra-red Spectrum. Principal peaks at wavenumbers 1745, 1276, 1038, 1010, 1498, 1080 cm^{-1} (KBr disk).

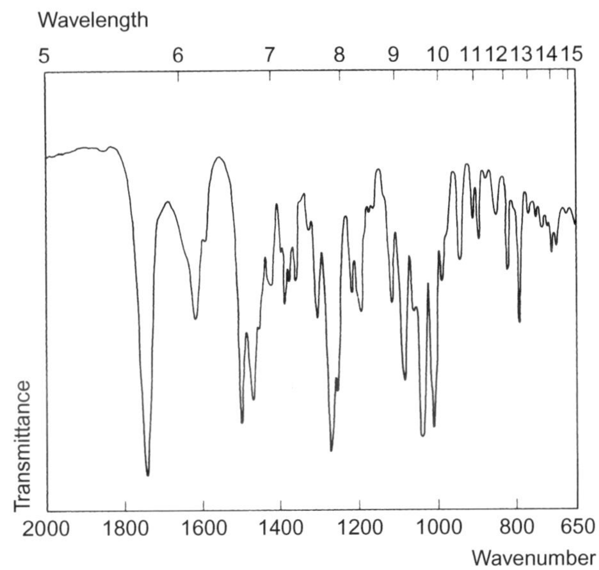

Mass Spectrum. Principal ions at *m/z* 220, 221, 205, 147, 42, 193, 77, 118.

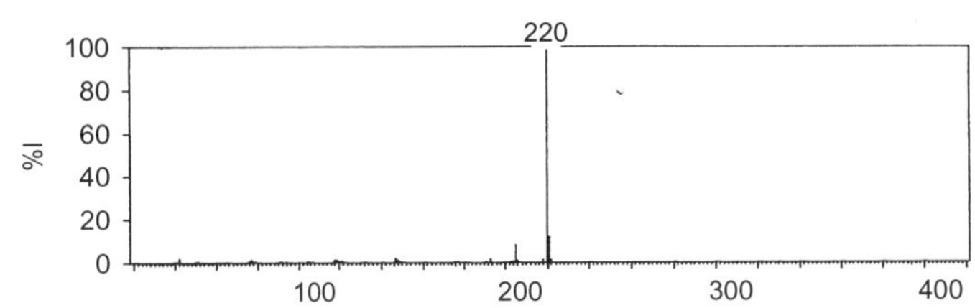

Quantification

Spectrofluorimetry. In plasma or urine: limit of detection 50 µg/L—S. Vedso, *Acta Pharmacol. Toxicol.*, 1961, *18*, 119–128.

High performance liquid chromatography. In plasma: noscapine and its metabolites, limit of quantification for noscapine 9 µg/L, UV detection—M. Johansson *et al.*, *J. Chromatogr.*, 1988, *459*, 301–311. In plasma: limit of quantification about 7 µg/L—D. F. Chollet *et al.*, *J. Chromatogr. B Biomed. Sci. Appl.*, 1997, *701*, 81–85.

Disposition in the Body. Rapidly absorbed after oral administration. About 1% of a dose is excreted in the urine in 6 h as free and conjugated noscapine.

Therapeutic concentration
Following a single oral dose of 150 mg to 5 subjects, peak plasma concentrations of 0.20 to 0.35 mg/L (mean 0.27) were attained in 0.5 to 2.5 h. [B. Dahlström *et al.*, *Eur. J. Clin. Pharmacol.*, 1982, *22*, 535–539.]

Bioavailability. About 30%.

Half-life. Plasma half-life, 1.5 to 4 h (mean 2.5).

Volume of distribution. 3 to 7 L/kg (mean 5).

Clearance. Plasma clearance, about 20 mL/min/kg.

Dose. Up to 150 mg daily in divided doses.

Noxiptiline

Antidepressant

Synonyms. Dibenzoxine; Noxiptyline.
10,11-Dihydro-5*H*-dibenzo[*a*,*d*]cyclohepten-5-one *O*-[2-(dimethylamino)ethyl]oxime
$C_{19}H_{22}N_2O = 294.4$
CAS—3362-45-6

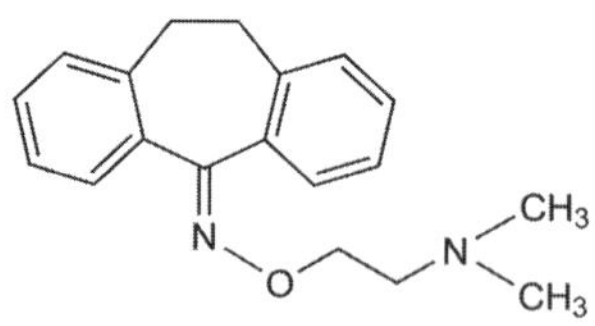

Soluble in chloroform.

Noxiptiline Hydrochloride

Synonym. Bay 1521
Proprietary names. Agedal; Nogédal.
$C_{19}H_{22}N_2O,HCl = 330.9$
CAS—4985-15-3
A white crystalline powder. M.p. 189° to 191°.
Soluble in water.

Partition Coefficient. Log *P* (octanol/water), 4.3.

Colour Test. Liebermann's test—black.

Thin-layer Chromatography. System TA—Rf 53; system TAE—Rf 29; system TB—Rf 43; system TC—Rf 35; system TE—Rf 66. (Acidified iodoplatinate solution, positive.)

Gas Chromatography. System GA—Noxiptyline RI 2270; M(dibenzocycloheptanone) RI 1850; system GB—M(OH-dibenzocycloheptanone)-H_2O RI 2200.

High Performance Liquid Chromatography. System HF—*k* 1.63; system HY—RI 330.

Ultraviolet Spectrum. Aqueous acid—250 nm (A_1^1=477a). No alkaline shift.

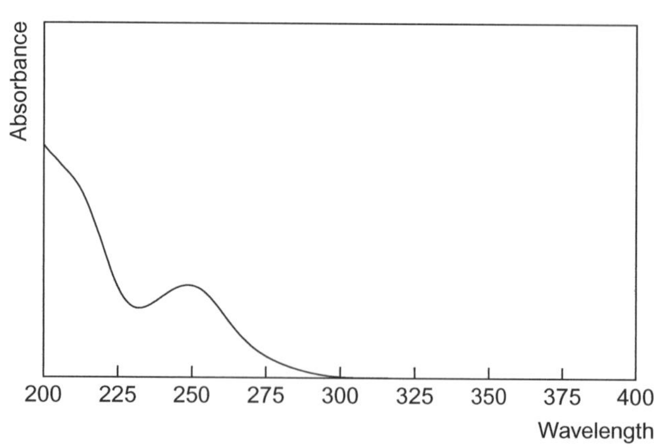

Mass Spectrum. Principal ions at *m/z* 58, 71, 208, 72, 59, 42, 89, 57.

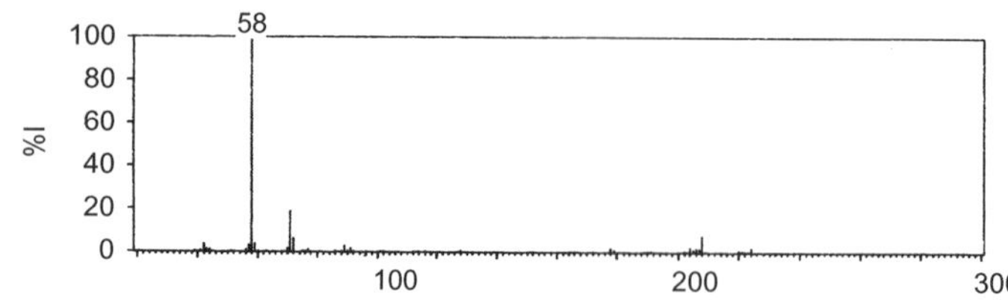

Quantification
Gas chromatography. In plasma, urine or tablets: limit of detection 100 µg/L, AFID—E. Szyszko and W. Wejman, *J. Chromatogr.*, 1981, *219*, 291–296.

Dose. The equivalent of 10 to 200 mg of noxiptiline daily.

Noxytiolin

Antibacterial/Antifungal

Synonym. Noxythiolin
Proprietary name. Noxyflex-S
N-(Hydroxymethyl)-*N*′-methylthiourea
$C_3H_8N_2OS = 120.2$
CAS—15599-39-0

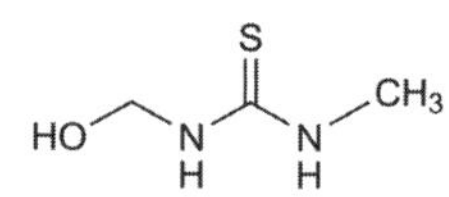

A white crystalline powder. M.p. 88° to 90°.
Soluble 1 in 10 of water; soluble in chloroform.

Partition Coefficient. Log *P* (octanol/water), −1.8.

Colour Test. Palladium chloride—brown.

Thin-layer Chromatography. System TA—Rf 74. (Acidified iodoplatinate solution, positive.)

Gas Chromatography. System GA—RI 2370.

Ultraviolet Spectrum. Methanol—244 nm (A_1^1=1180a).

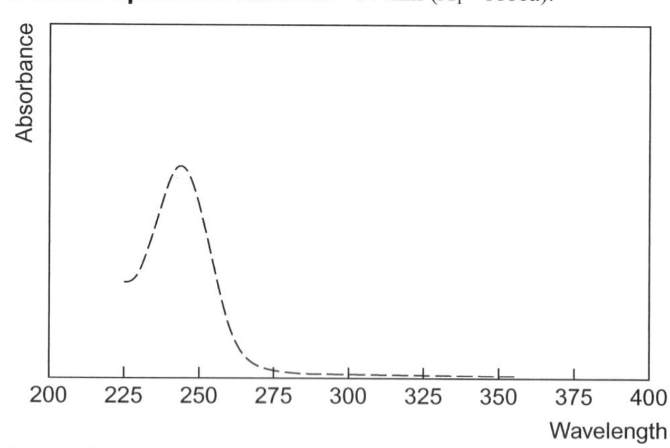

Infra-red Spectrum. Principal peaks at wavenumbers 1558, 1042, 1230, 987, 1026, 1517 cm^{-1} (KBr disk).

Quantification
High performance liquid chromatography. In serum—D. Debruyne *et al.*, *J. Pharm. Sci.*, 1985, *74*, 224–226.

Use. In concentrations of 1 to 2.5%.

Nystatin

Antifungal

Synonyms. Fungicidin; Nistatina.
Proprietary names. Nyspes; Nystan; Nystavescent.
Nystatin is an ingredient of many proprietary preparations—see *Martindale, The Complete Drug Reference*, 33rd Edn., Pharmaceutical Press, London, 2002.

CAS—1400-61-9

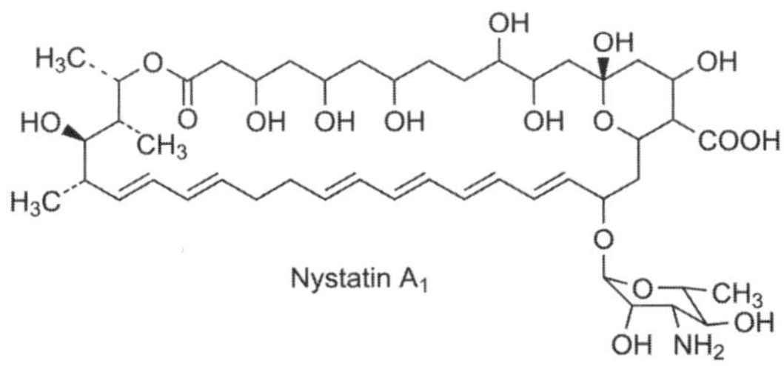

A mixture of antifungal polyenes produced by the growth of certain strains of *Streptomyces noursei*, or by any other means. It consists largely of nystatin A. Approximate molecular formula: $C_{47}H_{75}NO_{17}$=926.1.

A yellow to light brown, hygroscopic powder.

Very slightly soluble in water; sparingly soluble in ethanol; practically insoluble in chloroform and ether; freely soluble in dimethylformamide and formamide.

Partition Coefficient. Log *P* (octanol/water), 7.1.

Gas Chromatography. System GA—RI 1945.

Ultraviolet Spectrum. Aqueous alkali—291 (A_1^1=405b), 305 (A_1^1=600b), 319 nm (A_1^1=530b).

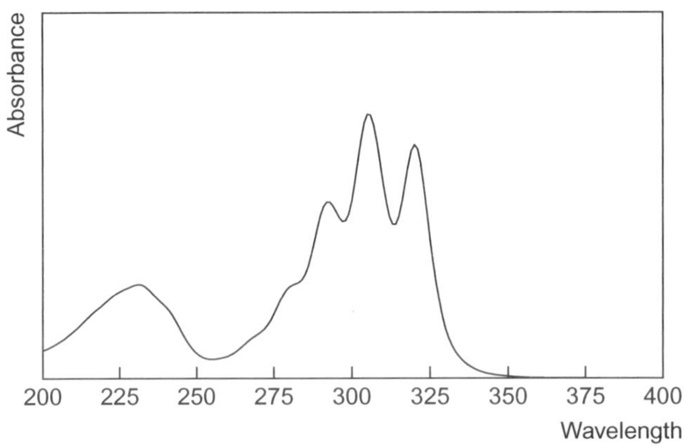

Infra-red Spectrum. Principal peaks at wavenumbers 1067, 1000, 1570, 1175, 1316, 847 cm^{-1} (Nujol mull).

Uses. Topically in preparations containing 100 000 units per g; orally in doses of 1500 000 to 4000 000 units daily.

Obidoxime Chloride

Antidote (Organophosphate Insecticide Poisoning)

Synonym. BH-6
Proprietary name. Toxogonin
1,1′-[Oxybis(methylene)]bis[4-(hydroxyimino)methyl]pyridinium dichloride
$C_{14}H_{16}Cl_2N_4O_3$=359.2
CAS—7683-36-5 (obidoxime); 114-90-9 (chloride)

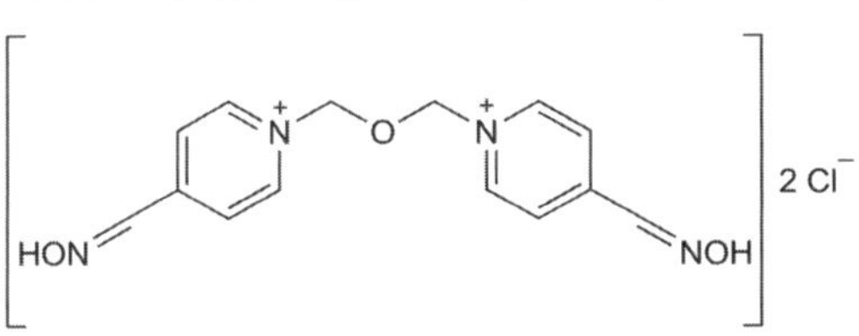

White crystals, occurring in two interchangeable isomeric forms. M.p. 225°, with decomposition.

Freely soluble in water; slightly soluble in ethanol and methanol; practically insoluble in chloroform and ether.

Dissociation Constant. pK_a 7.6, 8.3 (25°).

Partition Coefficient. Log *P* (octanol/water), −2.0.

Colour Tests. Mandelin's test—green→blue; Methanolic potassium hydroxide—orange

Thin-layer Chromatography. System TA—Rf 01; system TB—Rf 00; system TC—Rf 00; system TE—Rf 00; system TL—Rf 00; system TAE—Rf 53; system TAF—Rf 08. (Acidified iodoplatinate solution, positive.)

Ultraviolet Spectrum. Aqueous acid—285 nm (A_1^1=947a); aqueous alkali—353 nm (A_1^1=1440b).

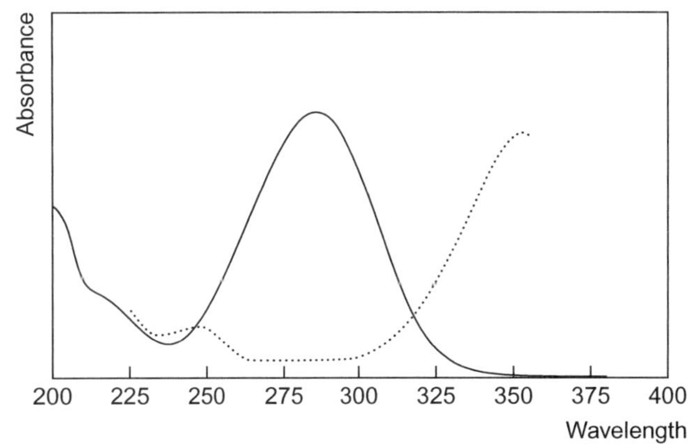

Infra-red Spectrum. Principal peaks at wavenumbers 996, 1090, 1637, 1600, 1282, 847 cm^{-1} (KBr disk).

Quantification

Polarography. In serum or urine: limit of detection 4 mg/L—Z. Korićanac *et al.*, *Acta Pharm. Jugoslav.*, 1982, *32*, 297–302.

High performance liquid chromatography. In urine: limit of detection 1.8 mg/L, UV detection (λ=288 nm)—C. Grasshoff *et al.*, *J. Chromatogr. B, Biomed. Sci. Appl.*, 2001, *753*, 203–208.

Disposition in the Body. Obidoxime chloride is poorly absorbed after oral administration. After intramuscular administration, more than 80% of a dose is excreted unchanged in the urine in 24 h.

Therapeutic concentration

Following intramuscular doses of 2.5 to 10 mg/kg to 10 subjects, peak plasma concentrations of 6.3 to 26.5 mg/L were attained in about 20 min. [F. R. Sidell and W. A. Groff, *J. Pharm. Sci.*, 1970, *59*, 793–797].

Obidoxime plasma levels of 35.9 to 71.8 mg/L were achieved when it was administered to 5 subjects as an intravenous bolus of 250 mg followed by continuous infusion of 750 mg/24 h. [H. Thiermann *et al.*, *Hum. Exp. Toxicol.*, 1997, *16*, 473–480].

Half-life. Plasma half-life, about 1.4 h.

Distribution in blood. Plasma : whole blood ratio, 1.9.

Dose. Obidoxime chloride has been given parenterally in doses of 250 mg.

Octafonium Chloride

Cationic Disinfectant

Synonym. Octaphonium Chloride; Phenoctide
Benzyldiethyl-{2-[4-(1,1,3,3-tetramethylbutyl)phenoxy]ethyl}ammonium chloride monohydrate
$C_{27}H_{42}ClNO,H_2O$=450.1
CAS—15687-40-8 (anhydrous)

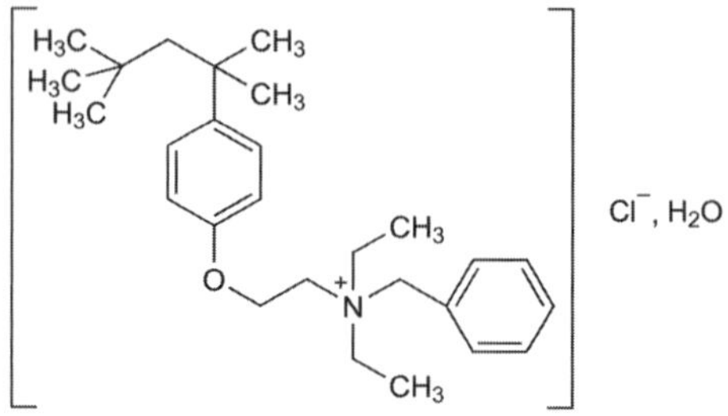

A white crystalline powder.
Soluble 1 in 5 of water; soluble in ethanol and chloroform.

Colour Tests. Liebermann's test—black; Mandelin's test—violet-brown; Marquis test—grey-brown; Sulfuric acid—grey-brown.

Thin-layer Chromatography. System TA—Rf 15, streaking. (Dragendorff spray, positive.)

Gas Chromatography. System GA—RI 2013.

Ultraviolet Spectrum. Aqueous acid—269 (A^1_1=32a), 274, 281 nm; ethanol—263 (A^1_1=25b), 269 (A^1_1=30b), 274 (A^1_1=29b), 282 nm (A^1_1=25b).

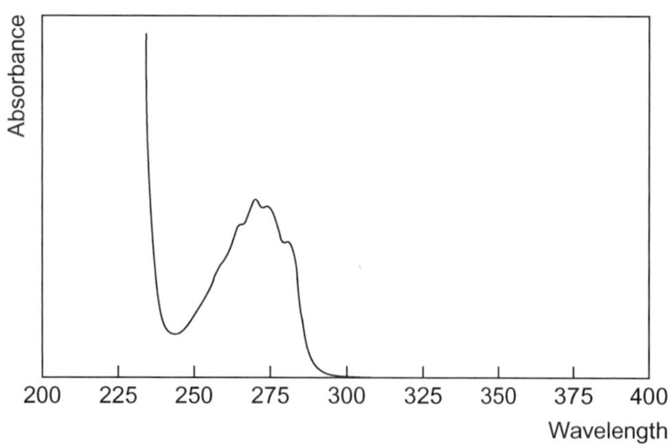

Infra-red Spectrum. Principal peaks at wavenumbers 1240, 840, 760, 1515, 708, 1185 cm^{-1} (Nujol mull).

Octamylamine

Antispasmodic

Synonym. Octisamyl
N-Isopentyl-1,5-dimethylhexylamine
$C_{13}H_{29}N$=199.4
CAS—502-59-0

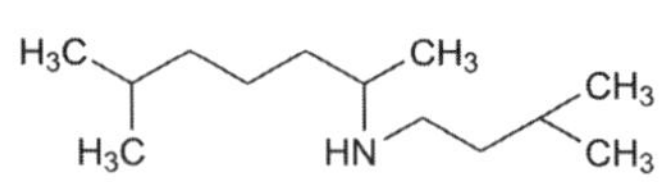

An oily liquid.

Octamylamine Hydrochloride

Proprietary name. Octometine
$C_{13}H_{29}N,HCl$=235.8
CAS—5964-56-7
White crystals. M.p. 121°.
Soluble in water, ethanol and ether.

Partition Coefficient. Log *P* (octanol/water), 5.0.

Thin-layer Chromatography. System TA—Rf 22; system TB—Rf 28; system TC—Rf 11; system TL—Rf 25. (Acidified iodoplatinate solution, positive.)

Gas Chromatography. System GA—RI 1303.

Mass Spectrum. Principal ions at *m*/*z* 30, 44, 41, 45, 86, 55, 43, 69.

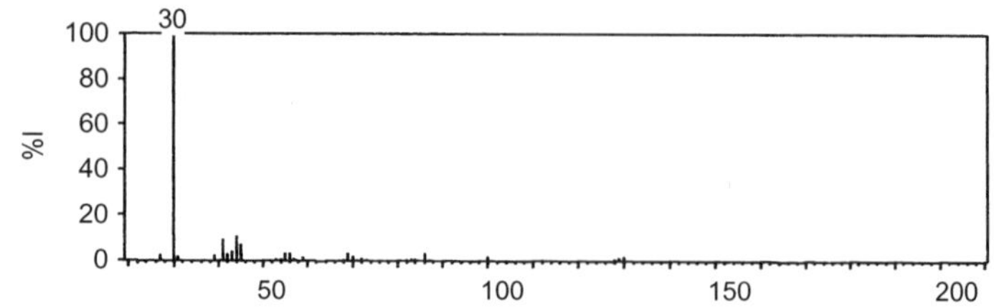

Dose. Octamylamine hydrochloride is given in doses of 100 to 200 mg.

Octatropine Methylbromide

Anticholinergic

Synonyms. Anisotropine Methobromide; Anisotropine Methylbromide.
Proprietary name. Valpin
endo-8,8-Dimethyl-3-[(1-oxo-2-propylpentyl)oxy]-8-azoniabicyclo-[3.2.1]octane bromide
$C_{17}H_{32}BrNO_2$=362.3
CAS—80-50-2

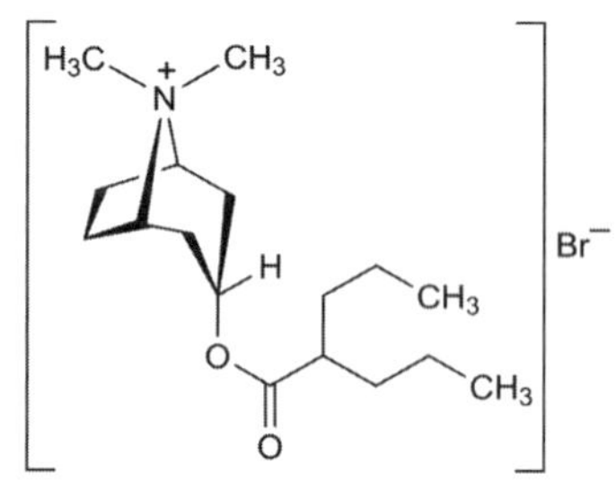

A white, glistening, hygroscopic powder. M.p. 329°.
Soluble in water; freely soluble in ethanol and chloroform; practically insoluble in ether.

Partition Coefficient. Log *P* (octanol/water), 0.6.

Thin-layer Chromatography. System TA—Rf 02. (Acidified iodoplatinate solution, positive.)

Infra-red Spectrum. Principal peaks at wavenumbers 1735, 1155, 1178, 1040, 1237, 1203 cm^{-1} (KBr disk).

Dose. 30 to 150 mg daily.

Octreotide

Somatostatin Analogue (Octopeptide)

Synonym. SMS-201-995
Proprietary name. Longastatin.
D-Phenylalanyl-L-cysteinyl-L-phenylalanyl-D-tryptophyl-L-lysyl-L-threonyl-*N*-[2-hydroxy-1-(hydroxymethyl)propyl]-L-cysteinamide cyclic (2→7)-disulfide
$C_{49}H_{66}N_{10}O_{10}S_2$ = 1019.3
CAS—83150-76-9

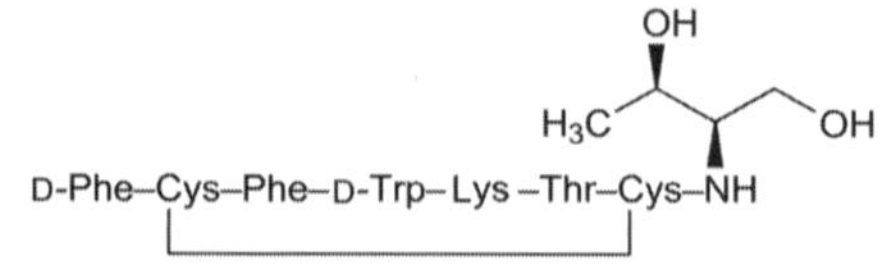

Octreotide Acetate

Synonym. SMS-201-995
Proprietary name. Sandostatin
$C_{49}H_{66}N_{10}O_{10}S_2.xC_2H_4O_2$
CAS—79517-01-4

High Performance Liquid Chromatography. Column: (analytical) Lichrospher-60 RP select B (125 × 4.0 mm i.d., 5 μm); (guard) C_8 (20 × 2 mm i.d., 30–40 μm). Mobile phase: acetonitrile:phosphate buffer (20 mM, pH 7.4) (35:65). UV detection (λ = 210 nm). Retention time: 5.5 min. [N. Kyaterekera *et al.*, *J. Pharm. Biomed. Anal.*, 1999, *21*, 327–330].

Ultraviolet Spectrum. Aqueous acid—280, 288 nm (no alkaline shift).

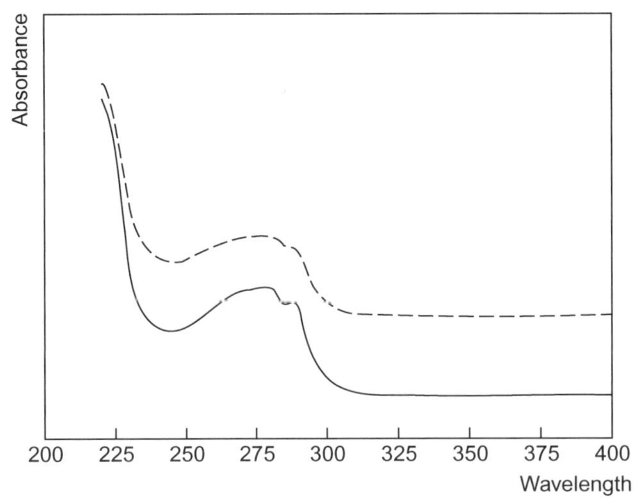

Disposition in the Body. Octreotide is rapidly and completely absorbed after subcutaneous administration and peak plasma concentrations are reached within 30 min. It undergoes considerable hepatic metabolism with 30 to 40% of a dose eliminated in this way. Between 11 and 33% of the dose is excreted unchanged in urine and less than 2% in faeces. It is distributed to body tissues.

Therapeutic concentration. The therapeutic range is 1 to 3 μg/L.

14 acromegalic patients, male and female, aged between 35 and 59 years, were administered with 100 μg of octreotide subcutaneously. Peak plasma concentrations of 3.5 μg/L were reached after 27.4 min. [J. Nicholls *et al.*, *Clin. Endocrinol.*, 1990, *32*, 545–550].

8 healthy male volunteers were administered with intravenous doses of 25, 50, 100 and 200 μg octreotide. Peak plasma concentrations of 5.7, 9.6, 24.2 and 27.8 μg/L, respectively, were reached within 3.7, 4.1, 3.4 and 7.3 min. Subcutaneous doses were also administered at doses of 50, 100, 200 and 400 μg to the same individuals. Peak levels were observed to be 2.4, 4.4, 10.6 and 23.5 μg/L at 26, 26, 35 and 28 min, respectively. [K. Kutz *et al.*, *Scand. J. Gastroenterol.*, 1986, *Suppl. 119*, 65–72].

Toxicity. It has been reported that one patient was accidentally overdosed with Sandostatin at a dose of 250 μg/h for 48 h instead of 25 μg/h, and no side-effects were experienced. [Sandostatin Ampoules and Multidose Vial in: *Medicines Compendium 2002*, Epsom, Surrey: Datapharm Communications Ltd, Virtual Health Network and Pharmaceutical Press, 2002, pp. 1762–1763.]

Half-life. 1.5 h (prolonged in the elderly and those with renal failure).

Volume of distribution. 0.27 L/kg; also reported as 13.6 L.

Clearance. Total body clearance, 9.6 L/h which may be increased to 18 L/h in patients with acromegaly and reduced to 4.5 L/h in those with chronic renal failure.

Protein binding. 65% (mainly to liprotein and to a lesser extent, albumin).

Distribution in blood. The drug is distributed mainly to the plasma component of blood. The amount of drug bound to blood cells is negligible.

Dose. The initial dose is 50 μg once or twice daily which is gradually increased to 200 μg three times daily, if necessary.

Ofloxacin

Quinolone Antibiotic/Antibacterial

Synonyms. DL-8280; HOE-280; ofloxacine.
Proprietary names. Apo-Oflox; Bactoflox; Bioquil; Exocin; Floxal; Floxstat; Inoflox; Konovid; Megasin; Monoflocet; Occidal; Oflovir; O-Flox; Ofloxcin; Qinolon; Seracin; Tarivid; Trafloxal.
9-Fluoro-2,3-dihydro-3-methyl-10-(4-methyl-1-piperazinyl)-7-oxo-7*H*-pyrido[1,2,3-*de*]-1,4-benzoxazine-6-carboxylic acid
$C_{18}H_{20}FN_3O_4$ = 361.4
CAS—82419-36-1; 83380-47-6

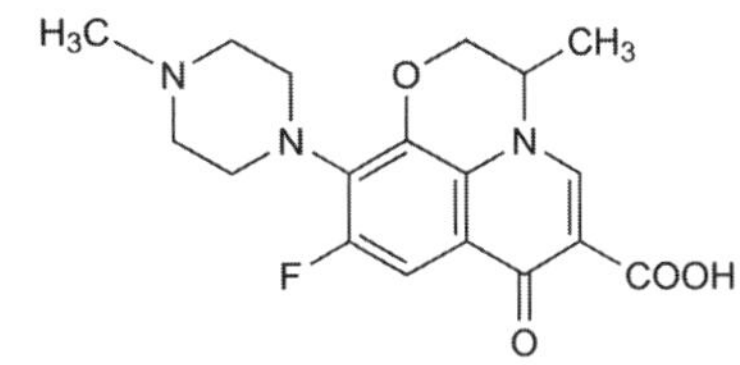

Colourless needles from ethanol. M.p. 250° to 257°.

Levofloxacin (Ofloxacin *S*-(−)-form)

Synonyms. DR-3355; HR-355; RWJ-25213; *S*-(−)-ofloxacin.
Proprietary names. Cravit; Quixin; Tavanic.
$C_{18}H_{20}FN_3O_4$ = 361.4
CAS—100986-85-4
Hemihydrate needles from ethanol/ethyl ether. M.p. 225° to 227°.

Ofloxacin Hydrochloride

Proprietary name. Tarivid intravenous infusion

Thin-layer Chromatography. System TE—Rf 00; system TF—Rf 00.

Plate: silica F_{254} (10 × 10 cm). Mobile phase: chloroform:methanol: triethylamine (3:1:1). Diastereometric L-leucinamide derivative of (−)-ofloxacin, Rf 0.57; (+)-ofloxacin derivative, 0.49. [K.-H. Lehr and P. Damm, *J. Chromatogr.*, 1988, *425*; *Biomed. Appl.*, 153–161].

High Performance Liquid Chromatography. System HX—RI 314; system HY—RI 260; system HZ—2.0 min; system HAA—retention time 8.6 min.

Column: ODS.A (YMC, 250 × 4.6 mm i.d., 5 μm). Mobile phase: phosphate buffer (50 mM, pH 2.6):acetonitrile (82:18), flow rate 1.5 mL/min. Fluorescence detection (λ_{ex} = 290 nm, λ_{em} = 460 nm). Retention time: 7 min. [C. Immanuel *et al.*, *J. Chromatogr. B Biomed. Sci. Appl.*, 2001, *760*, 91–95].

Column: ET Resolvosil-BSA-7 (150 × 4 mm i.d.). Mobile phase: phosphate buffer (0.2 M, pH 8):propan-2-ol (97:3), flow rate 1.0 mL/min. Fluorescence detection (λ_{ex} = 298 nm, λ_{em} = 458 nm). Retention times: (−)-ofloxacin, 5.2 min; (+)-ofloxacin, 7.5 min. [K.-H. Lehr and P. Damm, *J. Chromatogr.*, 1988, *425*; *Biomed. Appl.*, 153–161].

Ultraviolet Spectrum. Aqueous acid —225, 226, 256, 326 nm; basic—288, 332 nm.

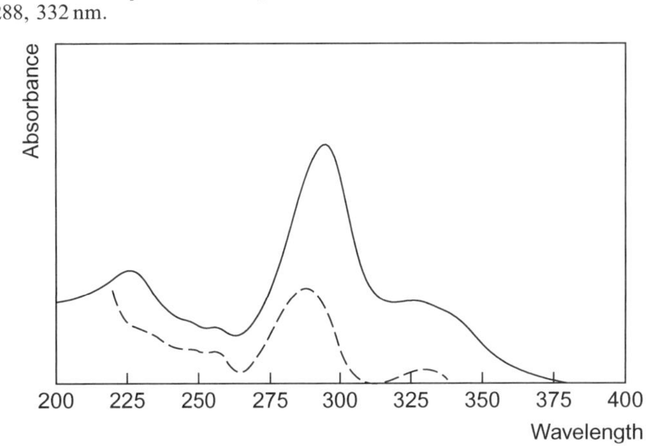

Infra-red Spectrum. Principal peaks at wavenumber 1459, 1621, 1713, 1086 cm^{-1} (KBr pellet).

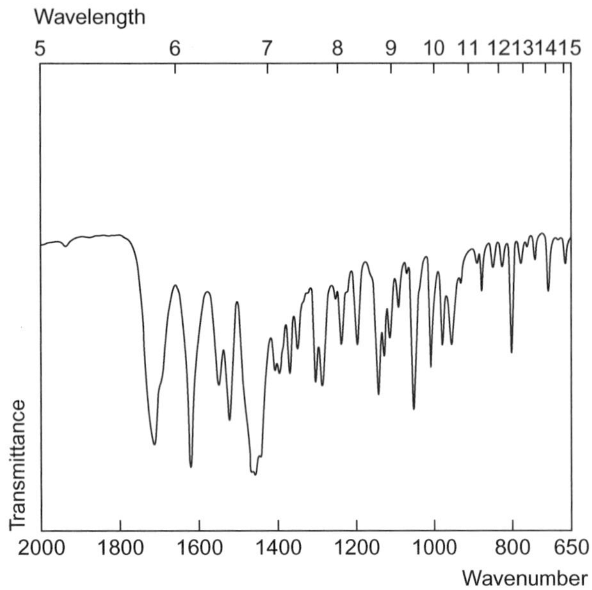

Mass Spectrum. Principal ions at *m/z* 71, 375, 70, 246, 305, 290 (ofloxacin-ME).

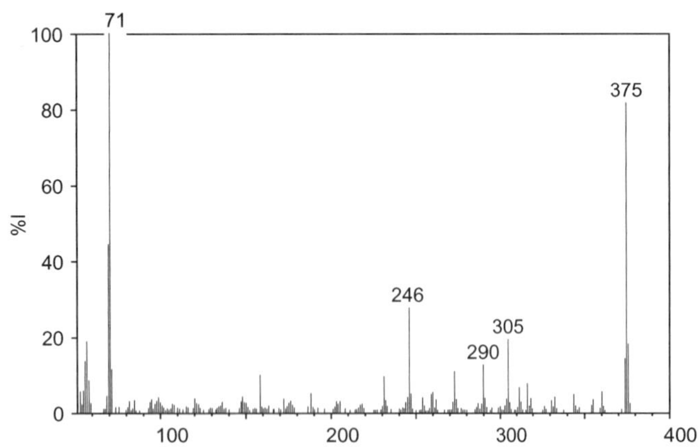

Quantification

High performance liquid chromatography. In serum and tissue: limit of detection 10 µg/mL. Fluorescence detection (λ_{ex} = 295 nm, λ_{em} = 490 nm)—S. Bottcher *et al., J. Pharm. Biomed. Anal.*, 2001, *25*, 197–203. In serum, plasma and urine: limit of detection is 0.01 mg/L—J. Knoller *et al., J. Chromatogr. Biomed. Sci. Appl.*, 1998, *427*, 257–267. In plasma and urine: limit of detection is 0.003 mg/L and 0.08 mg/L, respectively. Fluorescence detection (λ_{ex} = 298 nm, λ_{em} = 458 nm)—K.-H. Lehr and P. Damm, *J. Chromatogr.*, 1988, *425*; *Biomed. Appl.*, 153–161.

Disposition in the Body. Ofloxacin is absorbed rapidly after oral administration. The rate of absorption may be affected by food but not the extent. It is widely distributed in body fluids, including CSF, and tissue penetration is good. It also crosses the placenta and is distributed in breast milk. A small amount of the dose is metabolised to desmethyl ofloxacin (moderate activity) and *N*-oxide ofloxacin. Excretion is mainly via the kidneys with around 80% of the dose being excreted as the unchanged drug in urine over 24 to 48 h and between 4 to 8% being excreted in faeces.

Bioavailability. Approximately 100% after oral administration.

Therapeutic concentration. The serum therapeutic concentration range is 1.0 to 4.0 mg/L; trough, 0.05 to 5.0 mg/L and peak, 1.0 to 7.0 mg/L.

Half-life. 5 to 8 h; renal impairment 15 to 60 h.

Protein binding. 25%.

Dose. The dose varies between 200 and 400 mg daily, and may also be increased to 400 mg twice daily if necessary.

Olanzapine

Antipsychotic

Synonym. LY-170053
Proprietary name. Zyprexa
2-Methyl-4-(4-methyl-1-piperazinyl)-10*H*-thieno[2,3-*b*][1,5]-benzodiazepine
$C_{17}H_{20}N_4S = 312.4$
CAS—132539-06-1

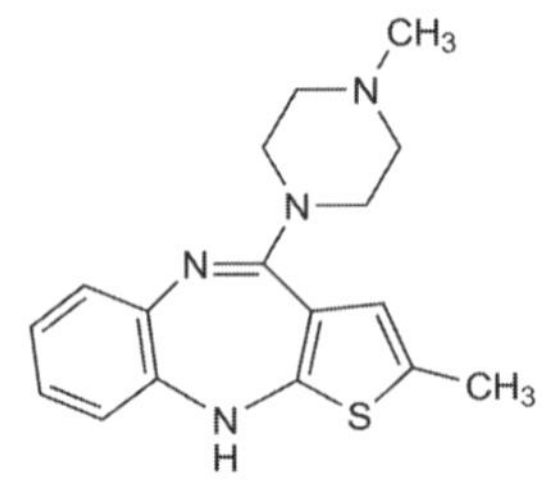

A yellow crystalline solid. It is practically insoluble in water.

Dissociation constant. pK_{a1}, 5.0; pK_{a2}, 7.4.

Gas Chromatography. System GB—RI 2861; RI 2911 M (nor-).

Columns (dual): RTx-50, 50% phenyl–50% methyl polysiloxane capillary column (30 m × 0.32 mm i.d., 0.25 µm film thickness); RTx-200, cross-bond trifluropropylmethyl polysiloxane capillary column (30 m × 0.32 mm i.d., 0.25 µm). Column temperature: 130° for 3 min, to 270° at 10°/min, held for 10 min; then to 295° at 10°/min and held for 5 min. Injector and detector temperature: 250° and 300°, respectively. Carrier gas: helium, flow rate 3 mL/min. Internal standard: promazine. Detection: nitrogen–phosphorus. Retention time(s): olanzapine, 20.3 min; I. S., 15.1 min (RTx-200); olanzapine, 20.0 min, I. S., 15.8 min (RTx-50). [A. Jenkins *et al. J. Anal. Toxicol.* 1998, 22, 605–609].

Column: 5% phenyl–95% methyl silicone (HP 5MS, 15 m × 0.25 mm i.d., 0.25 mm film thickness). Column temperature: 60° for 1 min, increased at 20°/min to 300° held for 3 min. Injector and detector temperature: 280° and 300°, respectively. Carrier gas: helium, flow rate 1.0 mL/min. Internal standard: ethyl morphine. Detection: nitrogen–phosphorus. Retention time: olanzapine, 12.1 min; I. S., 10.8 min. [A. A. Elian, *Forensic Sci. Int.*, 1998, *91*, 231–235].

High Performance Liquid Chromatography. System HZ—retention time 1.8 min.

Column: Microsorb CN (100 × 4.6 mm i.d.). Column temperature: 37°. Mobile phase: acetonitrile:methanol:sodium phosphate buffer (50 mM, pH 6.5) (5:28:67), flow rate 1.5 mL/min. Internal standard: clozapine. Retention time: olanzapine, 9.6 min; I. S., 12.5 min. [I. Prieto *et al. Ther. Drug Monit.* 1997, *19*, 580].

Column: YMC basic (150 × 4.6 mm i.d., 5 µm). Column temperature: 40°. Mobile phase: sodium phosphate (75 mM, pH 7):methanol:acetonitrile (48:26:26), flow rate 1.2 mL/min. Electrochemical detection. Retention time: 7.0 min. [J. Catlow *et al. J. Chromatogr.*, 1995, *668*; *Biomed. Appl.*, 85–90].

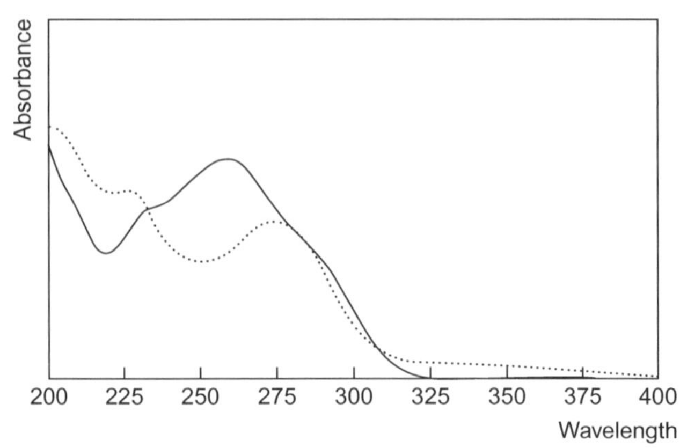

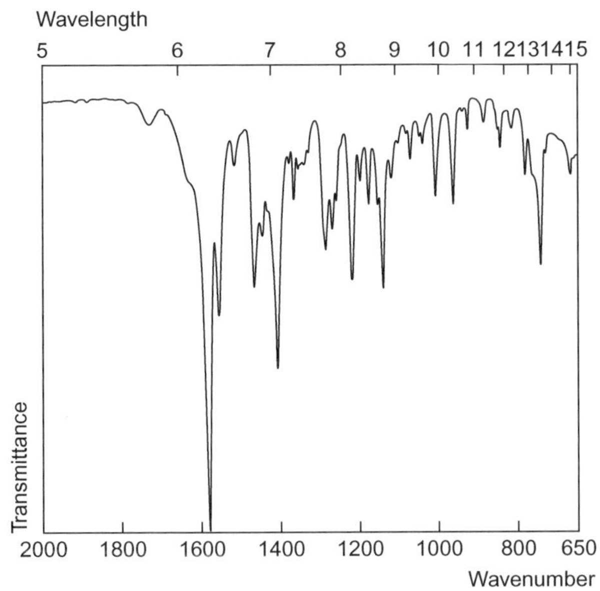

Mass Spectrum. Principal ions at *m/z* 242, 229, 213, 42, 56, 43, 198, 312.

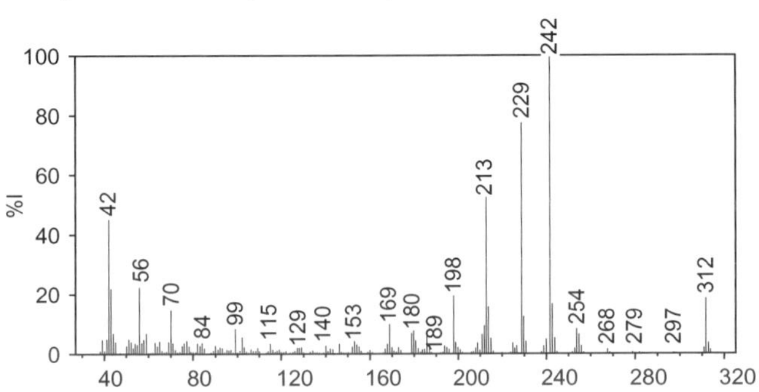

Quantification

Gas chromatography–mass spectrometry. In urine: limit of detection <100 µg/L—J. Bickeboeller-Friedrich and H. H. Maurer, *Ther. Drug Monit.*, 2001, *23*, 61–70. In blood, bile and gastric contents: limit of detection 50 µg/L and limit of quantification 100 µg/L—A. Jenkins *et al.*, *J. Anal. Toxicol.*, 1998, *22*, 605-609.

High performance liquid chromatography. In blood: limit of detection 1 µg/L—I. Prieto *et al.*, *Ther. Drug Monit.*, 1997, *19*, 580. In blood: limit of detection 0.25 µg/L. Electrochemical detection—M. Aravagiri *et al.*, *Ther. Drug Monit.*, 1997, *19*, 307–313. In plasma: limit of quantification 0.25 µg/L. ECD—J. Catlow *et al.*, *J. Chromatogr.*, 1995, *668*; *Biomed. Appl.*, 85–90.

Disposition in the Body. Olanzapine is well absorbed from the gastrointestinal tract and is eliminated extensively by first pass metabolism, mainly by conjugative and oxidative pathways. Approximately 40% of the dose is metabolised before reaching systemic circulation. Food does not affect the rate or extent of absorption. It is extensively distributed and metabolised throughout the body. 7% of the dose is recovered in urine as the unchanged drug indicating that it is highly metabolised. Approximately 57% of the dose is recovered in urine and 30% in faeces as metabolites. The main metabolites include the 10-*N*-glucuronide, *N*-desmethyl, 2-hydroxymethyl, 2-carboxy, *N*-desmethyl-2-carboxy and 4′-*N*-oxide derivatives of olanzapine and these lack pharmacological activity. Renal impairment has little effect on the pharmacokinetics.

Therapeutic concentration. The serum therapeutic concentration is 0.01 to 0.05 mg/L.

6 patients with hepatic impairment (creatinine clearance, >5.4 L/h/1.73 m^2); 6 patients with creatinine clearance <0.6 L/h/1.73 m^2 (drug given after haemodialysis); 6 patients with creatinine clearance <0.6 L/h/1.73 m^2 (drug given before haemodialysis). Each were given 5 mg olanzapine and peak plasma concentrations were 5.9, 8.2 and 9.5 µg/L for the three groups of individuals observed at 6.2, 5.2 and 4.2 h, respectively. [R. F. Bergstorm *et al.*, 1996, *Eli Lilly & Co., data on file*].

15 elderly healthy individuals and 5 young were administered with 10 mg olanzapine. Peak concentrations were 9.23 µg/L at 8 h and 12.6 µg/L at 6.1 h for the these two groups. [J. T. Calleghen *et al.*, 1995, *Eli Lilly & Co., data on file*].

4 healthy individuals were administered with 7.5 mg olanzapine along with 8 patients with cirrhosis. Peak plasma concentrations for the healthy individuals were 9.2 µg/L at 8 h and for the cirrhosis patients were 7.7 µg/L at 6.6 h. [H. R. Thomasson *et al.*, 1996, *Eli Lilly & Co., data on file*].

30 male non-smokers and 19 male smokers were administered with 9.5 mg and 10.5 mg, respectively. Peak concentrations were observed at 6.1 h for the non-smokers to be 12.9 µg/L and at 5.5 h for the smokers to be 13.2 µg/L. [J. C. Kisicki *et al.*, 1995, *Eli Lilly & Co., data on file*].

6 males were fasted overnight and administered with 15 mg olanzapine; concentrations reached 13.3 µg/L observed at 5.8 h. In comparison, 6 males administered the drug in a fed state produced levels of 13.8 µg/L approximately 4.7 h after dosing. [D. P. Henry *et al.*, 1995, *Eli Lilly & Co., data on file*].

Toxicity. The minimum toxic concentration in blood is 0.1 mg/L.

A 59-year-old woman was found unresponsive in a hotel room and later died. At the scene were two empty bottles of olanzapine tablets (each bottle containing 30 tablets at 10 mg each, filled only days earlier) and suicide notes. The blood concentration of the drug was 0.049 mg/L and 0.410 mg/L in the gastric contents. [A. A. Elian, *Forensic Sci. Int.*, 1998, *91*, 231–235].

A 43-year-old male psychiatric outpatient died after ingesting 600 mg of olanzapine. Analysis of postmortem blood and urine yielded olanzapine concentrations of 1.24 and 6.99 mg/L, respectively, which are far in excess of the therapeutic concentration. [B. G. Stephens *et al.*, *J. Forensic Sci.*, 1998, *43*, 1252–1253].

Bioavailability. Approx. 80%.

Half-life. A mean of 33.8 h (range 30 to 60 h) for young, healthy individuals and 51.8 h for elderly individuals. The half-life tends to be longer in female than in male patients.

Volume of distribution. Approximately 1150 L (660 to 1790 L); 22 L/kg; also reported as 10 to 20 L/kg.

Clearance. Plasma clearance ranges from 12 to 47 L/h with a mean of 25 L/h. Hepatic impairment may reduce clearance. It is generally 30% lower in women than men and 40% higher in smokers than non-smokers.

Protein binding. 93% bound to plasma proteins. Binding primarily to albumin and α_1-acid glycoprotein.

Dose. Adults: usual oral dose is 10 mg daily with a range between 5 and 20 mg. Elderly: possibly reduced to 5 mg daily to begin with. Patients with renal and/or hepatic impairment: starting dose of 5 mg daily and only increased with caution.

Oleandomycin

Antibiotic

Synonym. PA-105
Proprietary names. Triolmicina Romicil; Landomycin.
$C_{35}H_{61}NO_{12}$=687.9
CAS—3922-90-5

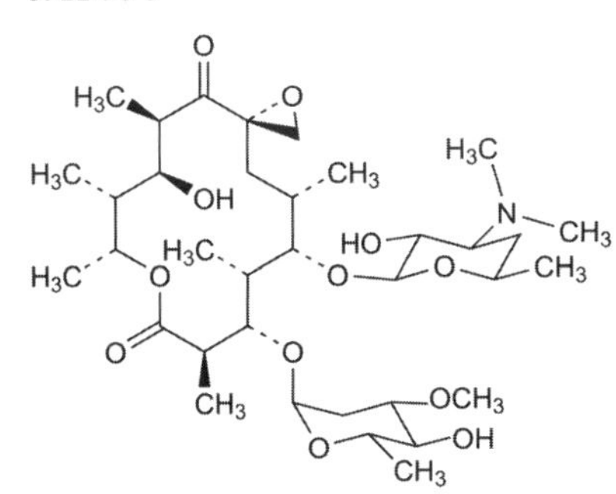

An antimicrobial substance produced by the growth of *Streptomyces antibioticus*.
A white amorphous powder.

Moderately soluble in water; freely soluble in butanol, ethanol, acetone and methanol; soluble in dilute acids; practically insoluble in hexane, carbon tetrachloride and dibutyl ether.

Oleandomycin Phosphate
$C_{35}H_{61}NO_{12},H_3PO_4$=785.9
CAS—7060-74-4
A white crystalline powder.
Soluble 1 in 2.5 of water and 1 in 3 of ethanol; slightly soluble in ether.

Dissociation Constant. pK_a 8.8 (25°).

Partition Coefficient. Log *P* (octanol/water), 1.7.

Colour Tests. Mandelin's Test—green; Marquis Test—green.

Thin-layer Chromatography. System TA—Rf 45. (Acidified potassium permanganate solution, positive.)

Ultraviolet Spectrum. Aqueous acid—242 nm (A_1^1=7b).

Infra-red Spectrum. Principal peaks at wavenumbers 1111, 1052, 1075, 1010, 1162, 1190 cm^{-1} (oleandomycin phosphate).

Quantification
High performance liquid chromatography. In serum or urine: limits of detection <0.25 mg/L and <1 mg/L respectively, UV detection—C. Stubbs *et al., J. Chromatogr.*, 1986, *353*, 33–38.

Dose. Oleandomycin phosphate has been given in doses of 1 to 2 g daily.

Olsalazine *Anti-inflammatory/Aminosalicylate*

Synonyms. Azodisal; CI mordant yellow 5; 5,5′-azobis(salicylic acid).
3,3′-Azobis(6-hydroxybenzoic acid)
$C_{14}H_{10}N_2O_6$=302.2
CAS—15722-48-2

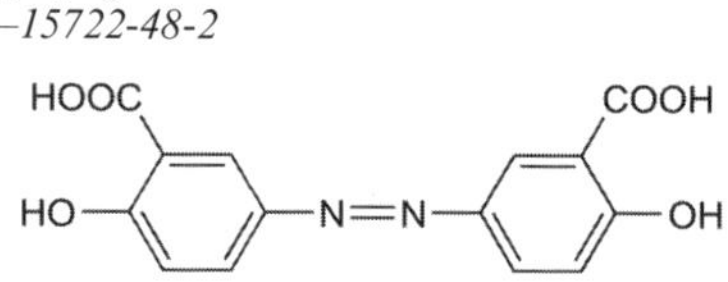

Olsalazine Sodium
Synonyms. Azodisal Sodium; CI mordant yellow 5 disodium salt; CL-14130; CJ-91B; sodium azodisalicylate.
Proprietary names. Dipentum
Disodium 5,5′-asodisalicylate
$C_{14}H_8N_2Na_2O_6$=364.2
CAS—6054-98-4
It is a yellow, fine, crystalline powder. M.p. 240°. It is sparingly soluble in water; soluble in dimethylsulfoxide; very slightly soluble in methanol; practically insoluble in ethanol, chloroform and ether.

High Performance Liquid Chromatography. Column: (analytical) C_{18} (Nucleosil, 250 4 mm i.d., 10 μm); (pre-column) RP-18 (Perisorb, 30 × 4 mm i.d., 30 to 40 μm). Mobile phase: methanol:phosphate buffer (pH 7.4), (52:48) with 0.02 M TBA (tetrabutylammonium hydrogen sulfate). UV detection (λ=365 nm); fluorescence detection (λ_{ex}=312 nm, λ_{em}=469 nm). *k* values: olsalazine, 5.2; olsalazine-sulfate, 1.2. [M. Ryde and N-O. Ahnfelt, *Eur. J. Clin. Pharmacol.*, 1988, *34(5)*, 481–488].

Ultraviolet Spectrum. Aqueous acid—358, 221, 249 nm.

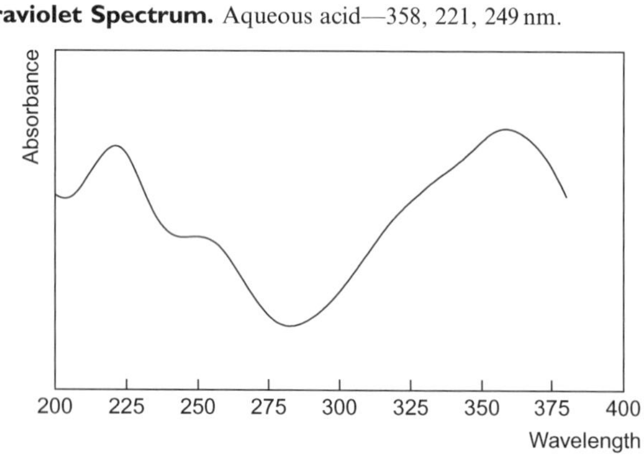

Quantification
High performance liquid chromatography. In serum and urine: limit of quantification 0.5 and 1 μg/L, respectively. UV detection (λ=365 nm); fluorescence detection (λ_{ex}=312 nm, λ_{em}=469 nm)—E. M. Ryde *et al. Eur. J. Clin. Pharmacol.*, 1988, *34*, 481–488.

Disposition in the Body. Olsalazine is not well absorbed after oral administration and almost the entire dose reaches its site of action in the colon intact. It is broken down by colonic bacteria flora into 5-aminosalicylic acid (mesalazine), some of which is absorbed and acetylated. Both mesalazine and its acetylated metabolite are absorbed from the colon. The presence of food has no significant effect on the absorption. 1 to 2% of the intact olsalazine absorbed is excreted, mainly in urine. A dose of olsalazine is almost completely metabolised by sulfate conjugate in the liver. Approx. 17 to 20% of the total dose is recovered in urine within 24 h of intravenous administration in patients with active inflammatory bowel disease, but this decreases for an oral dose. Less than 5% of the ingested dose is recovered in faeces as the unchanged drug. Steady state concentrations of conjugated olsalazine are achieved within days of the start of administration. Approx. 0.1% of an oral dose of olsalazine is metabolised in the liver to olsalazine-*O*-sulfate (olsalazine-*S*) and 22 to 33% appears in the urine almost all as acetyl 5-aminosalicylate. Olsalazine-*S* has a half-life of 7 days and accumulates to steady state within 2 to 3 weeks.

Therapeutic concentration

7 healthy males, aged 27 to 44 years, administered with a 10 mg intravenous dose of olsalazine showed peak serum concentrations of 7.5 μg/L (range 3.8 to 9.2 μg/L) by the end of the infusion.

8 healthy male volunteers were administered with 1 g olsalazine with or without food, and also 2 g and 4 g in the fasting state. Mean peak serum concentrations of the parent drug were 2.3 (range 1.1 to 4.6), 3.6, 5.9 (range 3.9 to 9.8) and 32 (range 14 to 47) μg/L, for the 1 g (with food), 1, 2 and 4 g (fasting) doses, respectively. Mean peak concentrations for olsalazine sulfate were 0.5, 1.2, 1.9 and 8.3 μg/L, respectively; 5-aminosalicyclic acid (5-ASA) 1.6, 1.2, 4.5 and 3.8 μg/L, respectively; *N*-acetyl-aminosalicyclic acid (ac-5-ASA) 3.2, 4.1, 10.0 and 9.1 μg/L, respectively. Peak olsalazine concentrations were observed approx. 1 h after administration of the parent drug, peak olsalazine sulfate concentrations after 4 h, and peak 5-ASA and ac-5-ASA at approx. 8 h. [E. M. Ryde and N. O. Ahnfelt, *Eur. J. Clin. Pharmacol.*, 1988, *34(5)*, 481–488].

Bioavailability. Varies from 2.4, 1.9 to 4.8% after 1, 2 and 4 g doses, respectively.

Half-life. Olsalazine, 0.9 to 1 h and the 5-aminosalicylic acid metabolite, 7 days.

Volume of distribution. Mean, 6.2 L.

Distribution in blood. Olsalazine does not enter the erythrocytes.

Protein binding. Olsalazine is bound >99% and the 5-aminosalicylic acid metabolite, 74%.

Dose. The usual dose is 1 g daily with a maximum of 3 g daily.

Omeprazole *Proton Pump Inhibitor*

Synonym. H-168/68
Proprietary names. Antra; Gastroguard; Gastroloc; Logastric; Losec; Mepral; Mopral; Omepral; Omeprazen; Parizac; Pepticum; Prilosec; Zoltum.
5-Methoxy-2-[[(4-methoxy-3,5-dimethyl-2-pyridinyl)methyl]sulfinyl]-1*H*-benzimidazole
$C_{17}H_{19}N_3O_3S$=345.4
CAS—73590-58-6

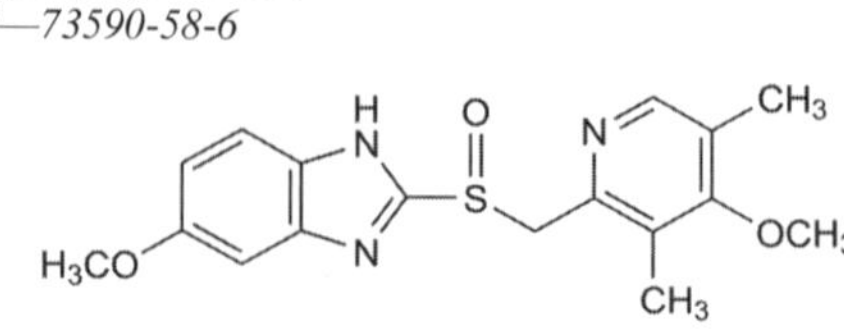

A white or almost white powder. M.p. 156°. It is very slightly soluble in water; soluble in alcohol, methyl alcohol and dichloromethane; very soluble in alkaline solutions.

Omeprazole Sodium
$C_{17}H_{18}N_3O_3S,Na = 367.4$
CAS—95510-70-6
A white or almost white hygroscopic powder. It is freely soluble in water and alcohol; soluble in propylene glycol; very slightly soluble in dichloromethane.

Dissociation Constant. pK_a, 4.0.

Partition Coefficient. Log *P* (octanol/water), 2.23.

High Performance Liquid Chromatography. System HZ—2.8 min; system HAA—retention time 14.1 min.

Column: (analytical) C_{18} (Crestpak, 150 × 4.6 mm i.d., 5 μm); (guard) C_{18} (Perisorb, 30–40 μm pellicular). Mobile phase: disodium hydrogen orthophosphate (0.05 M):acetonitrile (65:35), pH 6.5, flow rate 1 mL/min. Internal standard: chloramphenicol. UV detection (λ = 302 nm). Retention time(s): omeprazole, 6.3 min; I. S., 4.5 min. [K. H. Yuen *et al.*, *J. Pharm. Biomed. Anal.*, 2001, *24*, 715–719].

Column: C_{18} SG120, (Capcell pak), 250 × 4.6 mm i.d., 5 μm). Mobile phase: acetonitrile:phosphate buffer (0.05 M, pH 8.5) (25:75), flow rate 0.8 mL/min. Internal standard: phenacetin. UV detection (λ = 302 nm). Retention time(s): omeprazole, 16.8 min; hydroxyomeprazole, 6.6 min; omeprazole sulfone, 11.5 min; I. S., 13.6 min. [K. Kobayashi *et al.*, *J. Chromatogr.*, 1992, *579*, 299–305].

Ultraviolet Spectrum. Aqueous acid (0.2 M H_2SO_4)—277, 303 nm; basic—276, 305 nm.

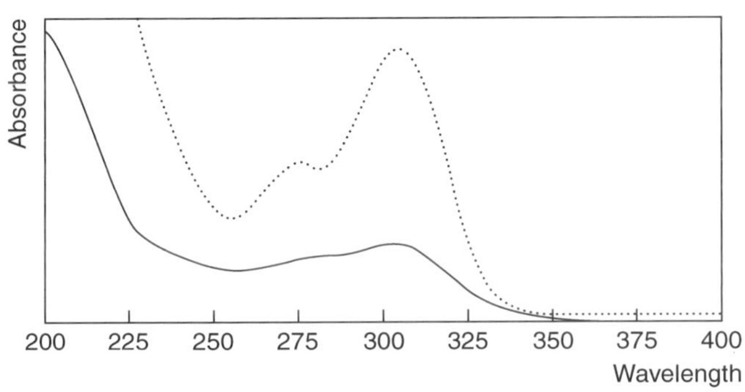

Infra-red Spectrum. Principal peaks at wavenumber 1628, 1205, 1015 cm^{-1} (KBr disk).

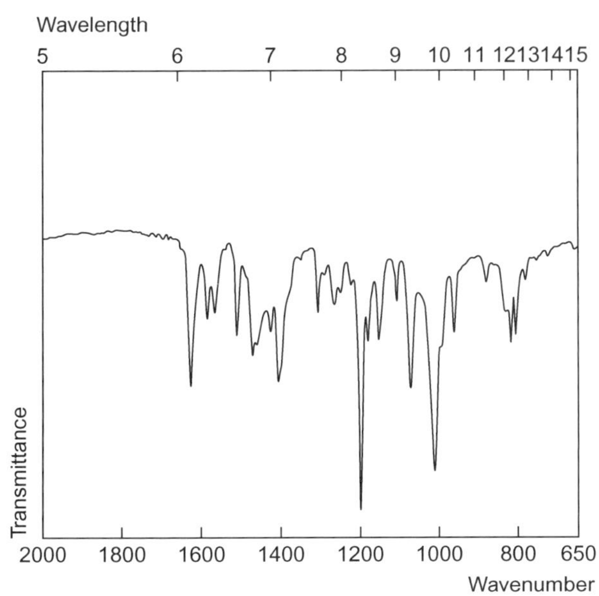

Mass Spectrum. Principal ions at *m/z*: 151, 136, 121, 120, 180, 297, 77, 93.

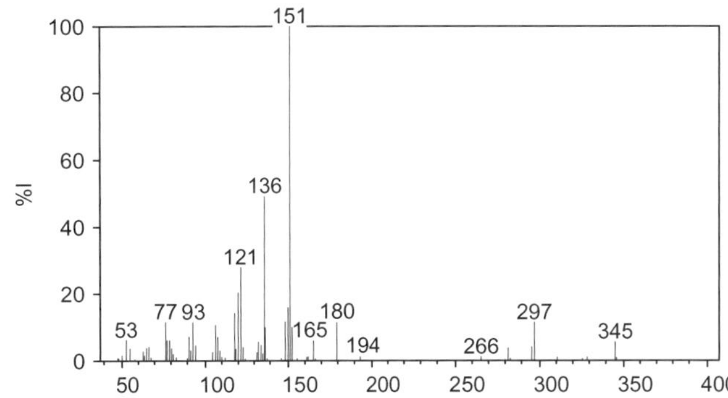

Quantification

High performance liquid chromatography. In plasma: limit of detection 2.5 μg/L. UV detection (λ = 302 nm)—K. H. Yuen *et al.*, *J. Pharm. Biomed. Anal.*, 2001, *24*, 715–719. In plasma: limit of quantification 5 μg/L. UV detection—G. Garcia-Encina *et al.*, *J. Pharm. Biomed. Anal.*, 1999, *21*, 371–382. In plasma: limit of quantification 10 μg/L. MS detection—E. J. Woolf and B. K. Matuszewski, *J. Chromatogr. A*, 1998, *828*, 229–238. Limit of detection, omeprazole sulfone 0.002 ng/L (2 ng/L in incubate), hydroxyomeprazole 0.025 ng/L (25 ng/L in incubate) —T. Andersson *et al.*, *J. Chromatogr.*, 1993, *619*, 291–297.

Disposition in the Body. Omeprazole is rapidly absorbed after oral administration and absorption is not affected by the presence of food. It is almost completely metabolised in the liver, mainly by the cytochrome P450 isoform, CYP2C19, and excreted in urine. Metabolites include omeprazole sulfone, 5-hydroxymethylomeprazole, 5-carboxyomeprazole and at least three other unidentified compounds. Distribution and elimination of the drug are both rapid. About 80% of metabolites are excreted in urine, the rest in faeces.

Therapeutic concentration

13 patients undergoing treatment for acute gastro-intestinal disease involving gastric acidity, mostly with normal hepatic and renal function, aged between 0.3 and 20 years old, were involved in the study. Doses were administered intravenously with a median of 22 mg (47.4 mg/1.73 m^2) and range 6 to 40 mg (36.9 to 60.2 mg/1.73 m^2). The mean maximum concentration observed was 0.58 (range 0.23 to 1.66) μg/L at 2.0 (1.0 to 4.4) h. [E. Jazqz-Aigrain *et al.*, *Eur. J. Clin. Pharmacol.*, 1994, *47*, 181–185].

10 healthy males, aged 23 to 40 years, were administered with 40 mg and 80 mg orally on two separate occasions. The mean maximum concentration was 3.6 μmol/L (range, 2.34 to 5.54 μmol/L) for the 40 mg dose and 7.99 μmol/L (5.02 to 12.71 μmol/L) for the 80 mg dose. These concentrations were observed at 0.2 h (0.12 to 0.32 h). For the sulfone metabolite, mean concentrations were 0.7 (0.54 to 0.9) μmol/L and 1.6 (1.09 to 2.37) μmol/L for 40 and 80 mg, respectively, at 0.38 (0.23 to 0.61) h and 0.52 (0.33 to 0.84) h. For the hydroxy-metabolite, mean concentrations were 2.13 (1.81 to 2.51) μmol/L and 2.95 (2.37 to 3.68) μmol/L for 40 and 80 mg, respectively, at 0.27 (0.18 to 0.41) h and 0.27 (0.20 to 0.36) h. [T. Andersson and C.-G. Regårdh *Drug Invest.*, 1990, *2*, 255–263].

Toxicity

A 26-year-old woman ingested 16 omeprazole capsules (20 mg enteric-coated granules) which she had been prescribed for abdominal pain. She became drowsy, sweaty and complained of a headache. She was admitted to hospital and it was noted she was flushed and tachycardic (110 beats/min). 6 h after administration, no more abnormal signs were observed and after 24 h, only abdominal pain was still present. The initial plasma concentration was 1.01 mg/L.

A 40-year-old lorry driver was admitted to hospital 20 h after overdosing on 20 capsules (20 mg enteric-coated granules). He complained of drowsiness, blurred vision, dry mouth and a throbbing headache. Clinical examination showed that total blood count, creatinine, urea and electrolytes were normal. All symptoms had gone 32 h after ingestion. [R. E. Ferner *et al.*, *Human Exp. Toxicol.*, 1993, *12*, 541–542].

Bioavailability. Oral bioavailability increases from about 35% after the first dose, to about 50% after several doses.

Half-life. 0.5 to 3 h.

Volume of distribution. 0.27 to 0.45 L/kg.

Clearance. Systemic clearance, 0.23 L/kg/h.

Protein binding. Approximately 95%.

Note. For a review of the pharmacokinetics of omeprazole, see C. W. Howden, *Clin. Pharmacokinet.*, 1991, *20*, 38–49.

Dose. A usual oral dose of 20 to 120 mg daily. Children >2 years: 0.7 to 1.4 mg/kg daily, with a maximum of 40 mg.

Omethoate

Acaricide, Insecticide

Synonym Dimethoate-met
Proprietary names. Bay-45432; Dimethoxon; Folimat; S-6876.
O,*O*-Dimethyl-*S*-methylcarbamoylmethylphosphorothioate
$C_5H_{12}NO_4PS = 213.2$
CAS—1113-02-6

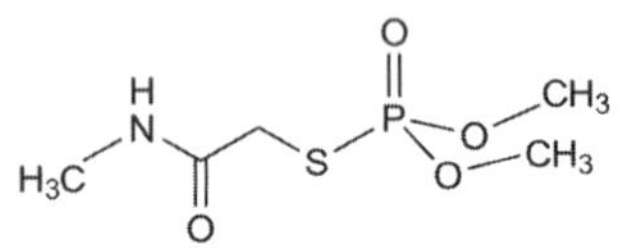

A colourless to yellow oil. M.p. −28°, decomposes at 135°. It is soluble in water, alcohol, acetone and many hydrocarbons; slightly soluble in diethyl ether; insoluble in petroleum ether.

Partition Coefficient. Log *P* (octanol/water), −0.74.

Thin-layer Chromatography. System TX—Rf 00; system TY—Rf 00.

Gas Chromatography. System GA—RI 1595; system GK—RRT 0.73 (relative to caffeine).

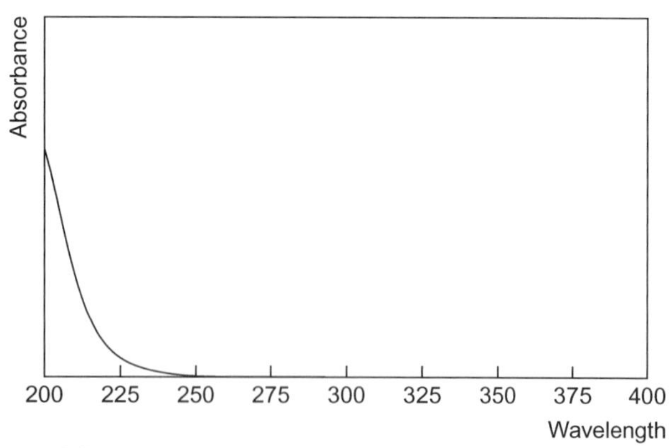

Infra-red Spectrum. Principal peaks at wavenumbers 1046, 1714, 1278, 775, 2964, 599 cm^{-1}.

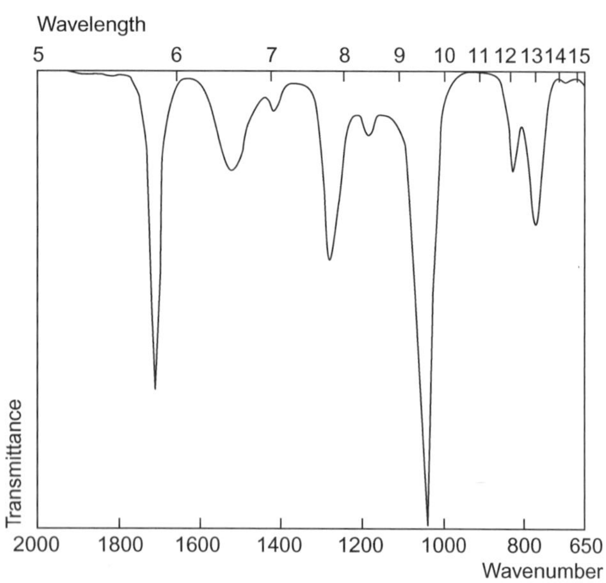

Mass Spectrum. Principal ions at *m/z* 110, 156, 109, 79, 58, 15, 47, 126.

Disposition in the Body. Omethoate is eliminated in urine, mostly within 48 h after ingestion.

Toxicity. The allowed daily intake is 0.3 μg/kg.

An adult female was admitted to hospital a few hours after ingestion of a pesticide. The omethoate blood level was determined on admission at 1.6 mg/L, fenthion was also detected at 2.9 mg/L. The patient remained clinically well and was discharged three days later. [A. M. Tsatsakis *et al.*, *J. Environ. Sci Health B*, 1998, *33(6)*, 657–670.]

Ondansetron

Serotonin Receptor (5HT$_3$) Antagonist/Anti-emetic

Synonym. GR-38032
1,2,3,9-Tetrahydro-9-methyl-3-[(2-methyl-1*H*-imidazol-1-yl)methyl]-4*H*-carbazol-4-one
$C_{18}H_{19}N_3O = 293.4$
CAS—99614-02-5

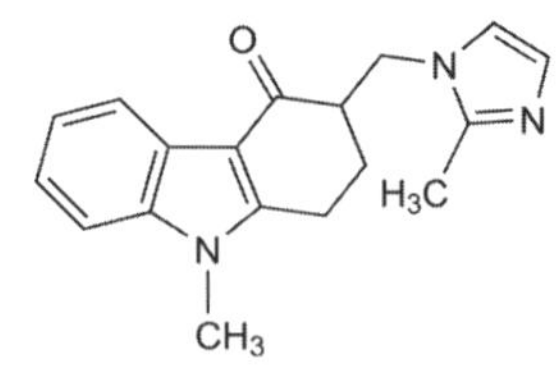

Crystals from methanol. M.p. 231° to 232°.

Ondansetron Hydrochloride Dihydrate

Synonyms. GR-38032F; GR-C507/75; SN-307.
Proprietary names. Zofran; Zophren.
1,2,3,9-Tetrahydro-9-methyl-3-[(2-methyl-1*H*-imidazol-1-yl)methyl]-4*H*-carbazol-4-one hydrochloride dihydrate
$C_{18}H_{19}N_3O,HCl,2H_2O = 365.9$
CAS—99614-01-4
A white crystalline solid from water/isopropanol with m.p. 178.5° to 179.5°. It is soluble in aqueous solutions but solubility decreases with pH >5.7.

Dissociation Constant. Hydrochloride dihydrate; pK_a 7.4.

High Performance Liquid Chromatography. System HZ—retention time 2.9 min.

Column: Spherisorb silica (S3W, 100 × 4.6 mm i.d., 3 μm). Column temperature: 35°. Mobile phase: sodium acetate buffer (25 mM, pH 4.2 with glacial acetic acid):acetonitrile (6:4), flow rate 1 mL/min. UV detection (λ=305 nm). Retention time: 4–5 min. [P. V. Colthup *et al.*, *J. Pharm. Sci.*, 1991, *80(9)*, 868–871].

Column: (analytical) Chiralcel OD (250 × 4.6 mm i.d., 10 μm); (guard) Chiralcel OD (50 × 4.6 mm i.d., 10 μm). Mobile phase: hexane:95% ethanol:2-propanol:acetonitrile (65:25:10:1), flow rate 1 mL/min. Internal standard: prazosin. UV detection (λ=216 nm). Retention times: *R*(−)-ondansetron, 10.0 min; *S*(+)-ondansetron, 11.6 min; I. S., 8.0 min. [J. W. Kelly *et al.*, *J. Chromatogr.*, 1993, *622*, 291–295].

Column: RP C_{18} (Spherisorb, 100 × 4.6 mm i.d., 10 μm). Mobile phase: acetonitrile:sodium phosphate monobasic buffer (20 mM, pH 3 with phosphoric acid) (60:40), flow rate 1.5 mL/min. Internal standard: loxapine. UV detection (λ=305 nm). Retention time: ondansetron, 3.9 min; I. S., 5.5 min. [M. Depot *et al.*, *J. Chromatogr. Biomed. Sci. Appl.*, 1997, *693*, 399–406].

Ultraviolet Spectrum. Aqueous acid (pH 2.8)—210, 248, 266, 310 nm.

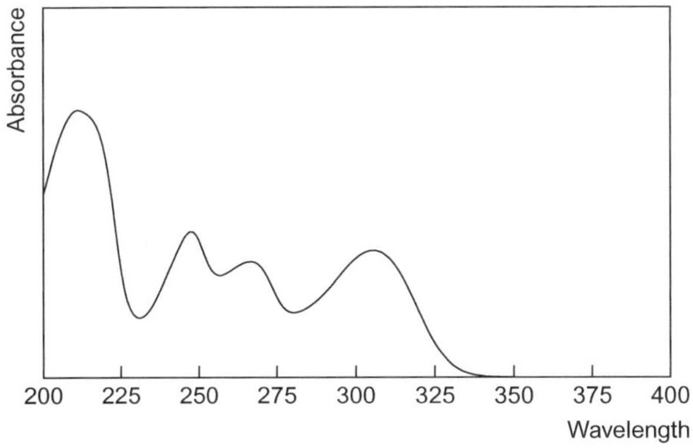

Mass Spectrum. Principal ions at *m/z*: 96, 293, 198, 211, 143, 183, 55, 115.

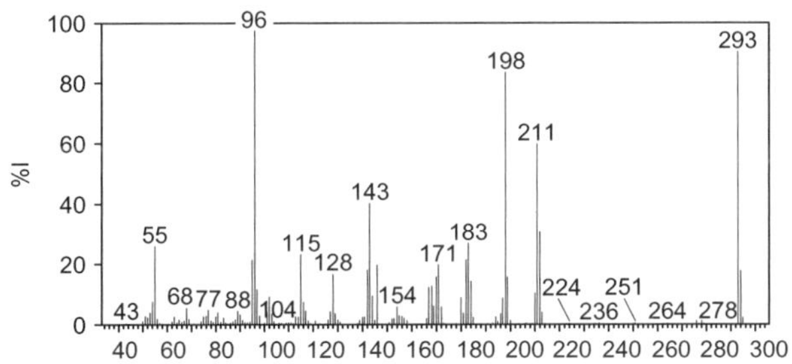

Quantification

High performance liquid chromatography. In serum: limit of detection 0.25 μg/L. MS detection—X. Xu *et al.*, *J. Mass Spectrom.*, 2000, *35(11)*, 1329–1334. In plasma: limit of detection, 1 μg/L. UV detection (λ=305 nm)—P. V. Colthup *et al.*, *J. Pharm. Sci.*, 1991, *80(9)*, 868–871. In serum: limit of quantification, 15 μg/L for each enantiomer and limit of detection, 7 μg/L, UV detection (λ=210 nm)—J. Liu and J. T. Stewart, *J. Chromatogr. Biomed. Sci. Appl.*, 1997, *694(1)*, 179–184. In serum: limit of quantification, 10 μg/L for each enantiomer and limit of detection, 2.5 μg/L, UV detection (λ=216 nm)—J. W. Kelly *et al.*, *J. Chromatogr.*, 1993, *622*, 291–295. In plasma: limit of quantification 0.5 μg/L. UV detection (λ=305 nm)—M. Depot *et al.*, *J. Chromatogr. Biomed. Sci. Appl.*, 1997, *693*, 399–406.

Disposition in the Body. Ondansetron is readily and completely absorbed after oral administration with peak plasma concentrations of 0.03 to 0.04 mg/L (after an 8 mg dose) being reached within 2 h. The drug is first detected in plasma after 30 min. It undergoes extensive hepatic metabolism with less than 5% being excreted via urine unchanged. At least 40% of a single dose is oxidised to 8-hydroxy-ondansetron in the liver, 20% to 7-hydroxy-ondansetron, <5% to 6-hydroxy-ondasetron and a little appears as *N*-demethyl-ondansetron. The metabolites have also been detected in faeces. These intermediates are glucuronide or sulfate conjugated before leaving the liver and being excreted in urine.

Therapeutic concentration. The serum therapeutic concentration range is 30 to 300 μg/L.

12 healthy male and female volunteers, aged between 26 and 69 years (mean age 44.8 years) and 12 patients with mild, moderate and severe liver disease (4 for each), aged between 31 and 65 years (mean, 47.3), were administered with an 8 mg oral dose or an 8 mg intravenous dose. Peak plasma concentrations for the oral dose were 38.6, 40.1 and 43.0 μg/L for the mild, moderate and severe hepatically impaired patients, respectively, and 27.9 μg/L for the healthy individuals. These concentrations were observed at 1.25, 1.07, 1.5 and 1.9 h, respectively. Peak concentrations for the intravenous dose were 97.8 μg/L for the patients with mild liver disease, 115.0 μg/L moderate liver disease and 64.5 μg/L for those with severe liver disease, observed at 0.38, 0.25 and 0.31 h, respectively. The healthy individuals reached a peak at 129 μg/L in 0.22 h. [W. D. Figg *et al.*, *J. Clin. Pharmacol.*, 1996, *36*, 206–215].

Bioavailability. 60% (young healthy subjects), 65% (elderly); 85% (patients with cancer) and 100% (severe hepatic impairment).

Half-life. 3 h (young healthy subjects), 5 h (elderly) and 15 to 32 h (severe hepatic impairment).

Volume of distribution. Approx. 140 to 160 L; also reported as 1.3 to 2.9 L/kg. 3.05 L/kg (mild liver disease); 3.36 L/kg (moderate); 3.86 L/kg (severe); 2.5 L/kg (healthy individuals).

Clearance. 16.6 L/h (patients with mild liver disease); 15.9 L/h (moderate liver disease); 11.6 L/h (severe); 28.3 L/h (healthy volunteers).

Distribution in blood. Blood:plasma ratio is 0.83. It distributes into erythrocytes and circulates bound within.

Protein binding. 70 to 75%.

Dose. Adult: 8 mg (orally) before treatment followed by 8 mg every 12 h. 16 mg daily (by rectum administration) or 32 mg (intravenously). Children: 5 mg/m^2 (intravenously) immediately before treatment and then 4 mg orally every 12 h. Alternatively, 100 μg/kg (maximum 4 mg) (over 2 years old).

Opipramol

Antidepressant

4-[3-(5*H*-Dibenz[*b,f*]azepin-5-yl)propyl]-1-piperazineethanol
$C_{23}H_{29}N_3O$=363.5
CAS—315-72-0

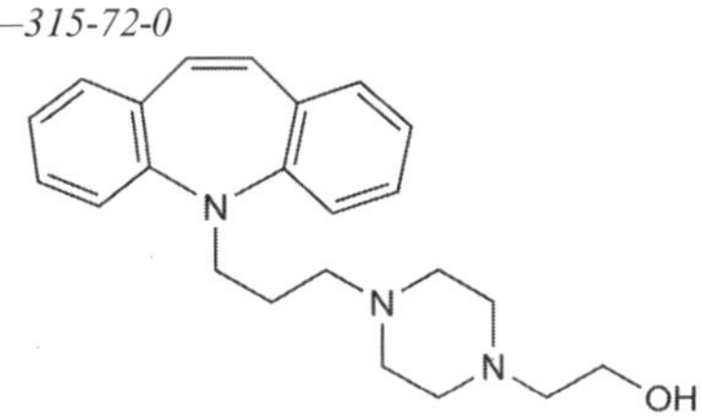

Crystals. M.p. 100° to 101°.

Opipramol Hydrochloride

Proprietary name. Insidon
$C_{23}H_{29}N_3O,2HCl$=436.4
CAS—909-39-7
A light yellow, crystalline powder which develops a reddish tinge on prolonged exposure to light. M.p. about 210°, with decomposition.
Soluble in water and ethanol; sparingly soluble in acetone.

Dissociation Constant. pK_a 3.8.

Partition Coefficient. Log *P* (octanol/water), 3.4.

Colour Tests. Forrest Reagent—blue; Mandelin's Test—yellow-green.

Thin-layer Chromatography. System TA—Rf 54; system TB—Rf 06; system TC—Rf 22; system TE—Rf 38; system TL—Rf 07; system TAE—Rf 35; system TAF—Rf 39; system TAJ—Rf 06; system TAK—Rf 05; system TAL—Rf 59. (Acidified iodoplatinate solution, positive.)

Gas Chromatography. System GA—opipramol RI 3050, M (ring) RI 1985; system GB—opipramol RI 3219.

High Performance Liquid Chromatography. System HA—*k* 2.2; system HF—*k* 1.63; system HX—RI 377; system HY—RI 340; system HZ—Retention time, 3.9 min; system HAA—Retention time, 14.2 min.

Ultraviolet Spectrum. Aqueous acid—253 (A_1^1=870a), 216, 338 nm. No alkaline shift.

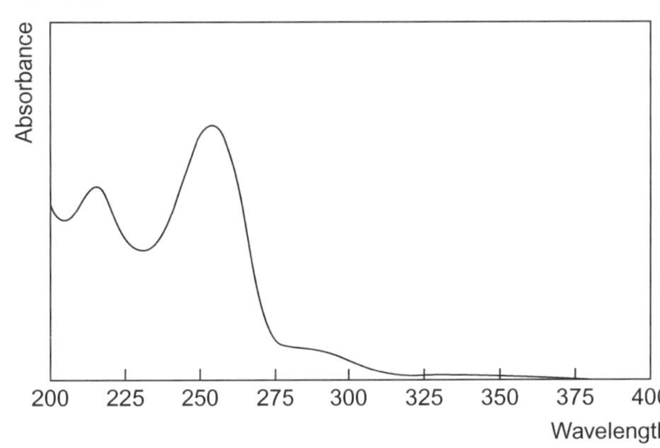

Infra-red Spectrum. Principal peaks at wavenumbers 755, 1155, 790, 1237, 1115, 1126 cm^{-1} (KBr disk).

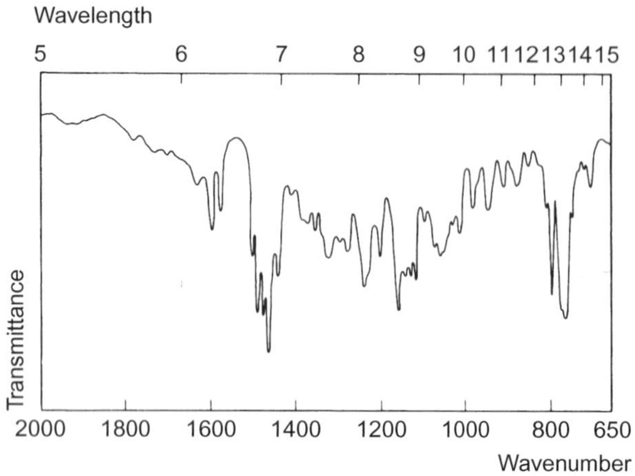

Mass Spectrum. Principal ions at *m/z* 363, 206, 143, 42, 70, 207, 218, 113.

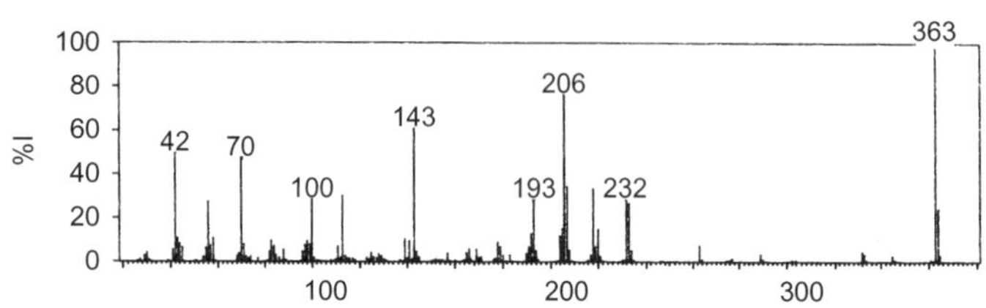

Quantification

Double radioisotope technique. In biological samples—W. Riess, *Anal. Chim. Acta*, 1977, *88*, 109–115.

High performance liquid chromatography. In plasma: limit of detection 250 µg/L, photometric detection—F. Kees *et al.*, *J. Chromatogr. B. Biomed. Sci. Appl.*, 2001, *753*, 337–342.

Disposition in the Body. Readily absorbed after oral administration.

Toxicity

Somnolence was reported in a 27-year-old subject following an overdose of opipramol; a maximum serum concentration of 0.115 mg/L was determined; ethanol was also detected [O. L. Pedersen *et al.*, *Eur. J. Clin. Pharmacol.*, 1982, *23*, 513–521].

In a fatality involving the intentional ingestion of an unknown quantity (up to 3 g) of opipramol dihydrochloride, postmortem tissue concentrations of opipramol dihydrochloride and deshydroxyethyl opipramol dihydrochloride, respectively, were: blood (heart) 29.6 and 5.2 mg/L; urine 19.1 and 4.7 mg/L; liver 260.7 and 50.6 µg/g; lung 68.9 and 24.0 µg/g; brain 113.5 and 5.1 µg/g; kidney 69.6 and 11.8 µg/g; muscle 9.1 and 1.5 µg/g [G. Skopp *et al.*, *Forensic Sci. Int.*, 1996, *77*, 45–51].

Dose. 150 to 300 mg of opipramol hydrochloride daily.

Orciprenaline

Sympathomimetic

Synonym. Metaproterenol
5-[1-Hydroxy-2-[(1-methylethyl)amino]ethyl]-1,3-benzenediol
$C_{11}H_{17}NO_3$=211.3
CAS—586-06-1

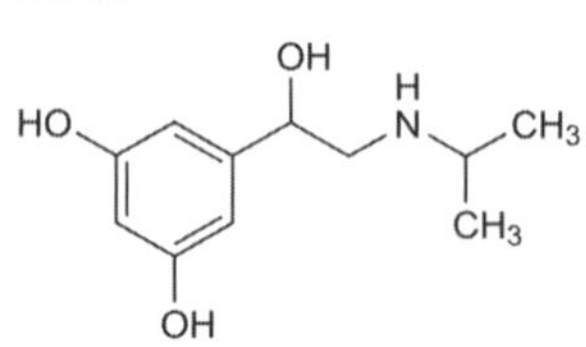

Crystals. M.p. 100°.

Orciprenaline Sulfate

Proprietary names. Alupent; Dosalupent; Metaprel.
$(C_{11}H_{17}NO_3)_2,H_2SO_4$=520.6
CAS—5874-97-5
A white crystalline powder. M.p. about 205°.
Soluble 1 in 2 of water and 1 in 1 of ethanol; practically insoluble in chloroform and ether.

Dissociation Constant. pK$_a$ 9.0 (—OH), 10.1 (—NH—), 11.4 (—OH), (25°).

Partition Coefficient. Log *P* (octanol/water), 0.2.

Colour Tests. *p*-Dimethylaminobenzaldehyde—orange/violet; Folin–Ciocalteu Reagent—blue; Marquis Test—yellow; Potassium Dichromate (Method 1)—brown (slow).

Thin-layer Chromatography. System TA—Rf 48; system TB—Rf 01; system TC—Rf 03; system TE—Rf 18; system TL—Rf 06; system TAE—Rf 21; system TAF—Rf 77. (Acidified potassium permanganate solution, positive.)

Gas Chromatography. System GA—not eluted.

High Performance Liquid Chromatography. System HX—RI 151; system HY—RI 131.

Ultraviolet Spectrum. Aqueous acid—276 nm (A^1_1=89a); aqueous alkali—297 nm (A^1_1=155a).

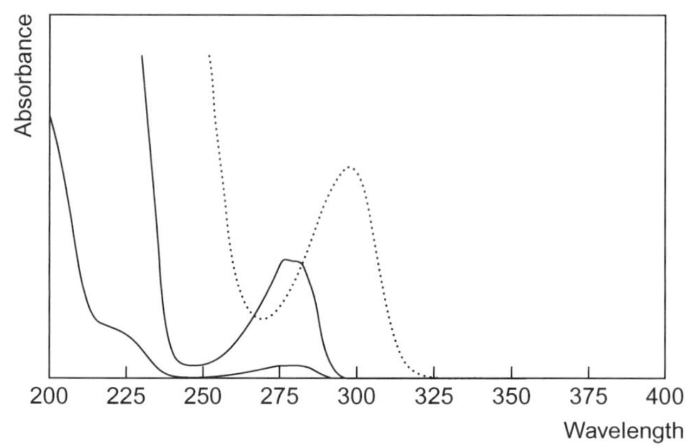

Infra-red Spectrum. Principal peaks at wavenumbers 1086, 1173, 1605, 1010, 1305, 995 cm^{-1} (orciprenaline sulfate, KBr disk).

Mass Spectrum. Principal ions at *m/z* 72, 43, 73, 41, 70, 65, 40, 39.

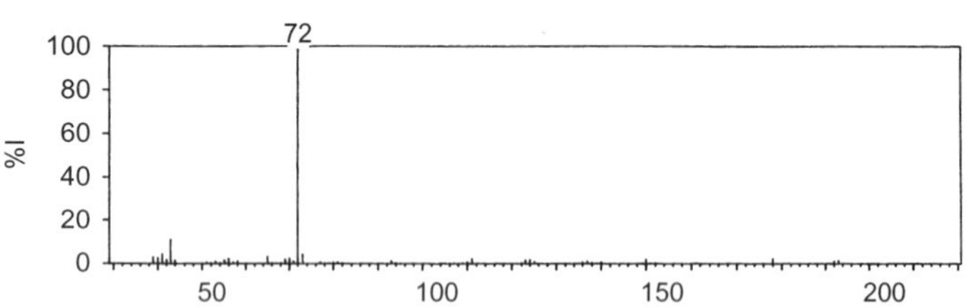

Quantification

Gas chromatography–mass spectrometry. In plasma: limit of detection 100 ng/L—H. J. Leis *et al.*, *Biomed. Environ. Mass Spectrom.*, 1990, *19*, 382–386.

Dose. 80 mg of orciprenaline sulfate daily.

Orlistat

Anti-obesity Agent/Gastric and Pancreatic Lipase Inhibitor

Synonyms. Orlipastat; Ro-18-0647; Ro-18-0647/002; (−)-Tetrahydrolipstatin.
Proprietary name. Xenical
N-Formyl-L-leucine (1*S*)-1-[[(2*S*,3*S*)-3-hexyl-4-oxo-2-oxetanyl]-methyl]dodecyl ester

$C_{29}H_{53}NO_5 = 495.7$
CAS—96829-58-2

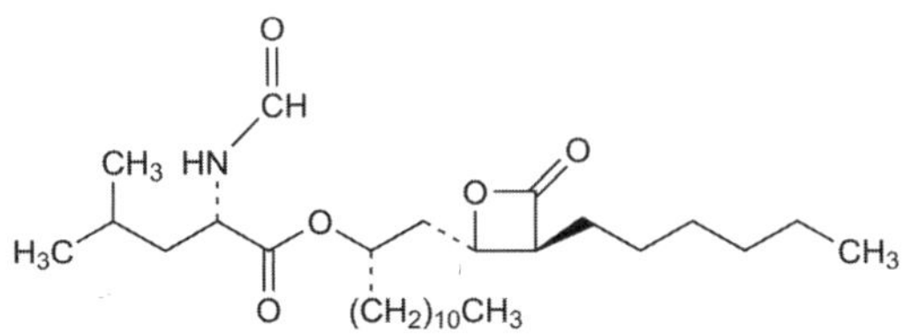

A white to off-white crystalline powder. M.p 40° to 43°. It is practically insoluble in water; freely soluble in chloroform; very soluble in methanol and ethanol.

Dissociation constant. pK_a out of physiological range.

High Performance Liquid Chromatography. Column: Spherisorb C_6 (100 × 2 mm, 2 µm). Mobile phase: (A) acetonitrile:0.1% formic acid (95:5), flow rate 150 µL/min; (B) methanol:water (85:15), flow rate 150 µL/min. Rapid change to 100% methanol at 300 µL/min for 3 min then re-equilibration with 85% methanol. MS–MS detection. Retention time: (A) 1.1 min; (B) 2.4 min. [R. Wieboldt *et al., J. Chromatogr. Biomed. Sci. Appl.*, 1998, *708*, 121–129].

Quantification.
High performance liquid chromatography–mass spectrometry. In plasma: limit of quantification 0.3 µg/L, MS–MS detection—R. Wieboldt *et al., J. Chromatogr. Biomed. Sci. Appl.*, 1998, *708*, 121–129. In plasma: limit of detection 0.2 µg/L, MS–MS detection—P. K. Bennett *et al., J. Mass Spectrom.*, 1997, *32*, 739–749. In serum: limit of detection 0.25 µg/L—X. Xu *et al., J. Mass Spectrom.*, 2000, *35*, 1329–1334.

Disposition in the Body. Orlistat is not absorbed following oral administration and plasma concentrations of intact orlistat are non-measurable. There is no evidence of accumulation and no defined systemic pharmacokinetics. Metabolism may occur within the gastro-intestinal wall. There are two metabolites M1 (4-member lactone ring hydrolysed) and M3 (M1 with *N*-formyl leucine moiety cleaved) which account for approximately, 42% of the total plasma concentration. Elimination is mainly by faecal excretion of the unabsorbed drug with approximately, 97% of the administered dose excreted in this way, 83% of which is the unchanged drug. Cumulative renal excretion of total orlistat related material was <2% of the dose. Complete excretion occurs within 3 to 5 days. Orlistat, M1 and M3 are all subject to biliary excretion.

Therapeutic concentration. With therapeutic doses, detection of intact orlistat in plasma is difficult and concentrations are extremely low, <10 µg/L. Low plasma levels of M1 (26 µg/L) and M3 (108 µg/L) are observed 2 to 4 h after a therapeutic dose. <5 µg/L 8 h following administration with 360 mg orlistat.

Half-life. Ranges between 1 and 2 h for the parent drug; for the metabolites approx. 2 h for M1 and 13.5 h for M3.

Volume of distribution. Cannot be determined since minimally absorbed and no definite systemic pharmacokinetics.

Distribution in blood. Minimally partitions into erythrocytes.

Protein binding. >99%. Mainly lipoprotein and albumin.

Dose. 120 mg three times a day.

Orphenadrine

Anticholinergic

Synonyms. Mephenamine; Orphenadin.
N,N-Dimethyl-2-[(2-methylphenyl)phenylmethoxy]ethanamine
$C_{18}H_{23}NO = 269.4$
CAS—83-98-7

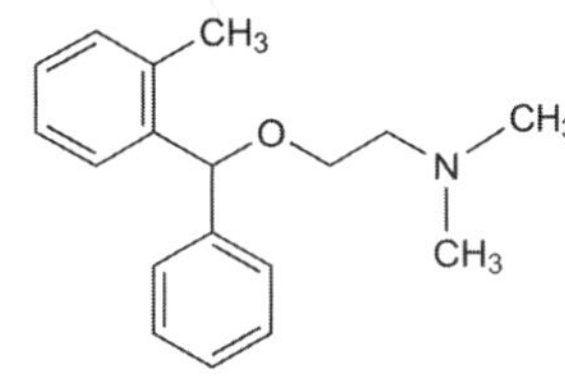

A liquid.

Orphenadrine Citrate

Proprietary names. Banflex; Flexoject; Flexon; Myolin; Norflex; Orfenace. It is an ingredient of Norgesic and Orphengesic.
$C_{18}H_{23}NO,C_6H_8O_7 = 461.5$
CAS—4682-36-4
A white crystalline powder. M.p. 134° to 138°.
Soluble 1 in 70 of water; slightly soluble in ethanol; practically insoluble in chloroform and ether.

Orphenadrine Hydrochloride

Synonym. BS-5930
Proprietary names. Biorphen; Disipal; Lysantin; Orfenal.
$C_{18}H_{23}NO,HCl = 305.8$
CAS—341-69-5
A white crystalline powder. M.p. 156° to 157°.
Soluble 1 in 1 of water, 1 in 1 of ethanol, and 1 in 2 of chloroform; sparingly soluble in acetone and benzene; practically insoluble in ether.

Dissociation Constant. pK_a 8.4.

Partition Coefficient. Log *P* (octanol/water), 3.8.

Colour Tests. Mandelin's Test—orange; Marquis Test—yellow-orange; Sulfuric Acid—orange.

Thin-layer Chromatography. System TA—Rf 55; system TB—Rf 48; system TC—Rf 33; system TE—Rf 68; system TL—Rf 16; system TAE—Rf 25; system TAF—Rf 49; system TAJ—Rf 14; system TAK—Rf 02; system TAL—Rf 47. (Dragendorff spray, positive; acidified iodoplatinate solution, positive; Marquis reagent, yellow.)

Gas Chromatography. System GA—orphenadrine RI 1935, M (nor-) RI 1900, M (methylbenzophenone) RI 1700; system GB—orphenadrine RI 2014, M (nor-) RI 2007, M (methylbenzophenone) RI 1700; system GF—RI 2185.

High Performance Liquid Chromatography. System HA—orphenadrine *k* 3.0, *N*-monodesmethylorphenadrine *k* 1.7, orphenadrine *N*-oxide *k* 1.1 (tailing peak); system HX—RI 418; system HY—RI 323; system HZ—retention time 6.0 min.

Ultraviolet Spectrum. Aqueous acid—258, 264 nm ($A^1_1 = 24a$). No alkaline shift. (See below)

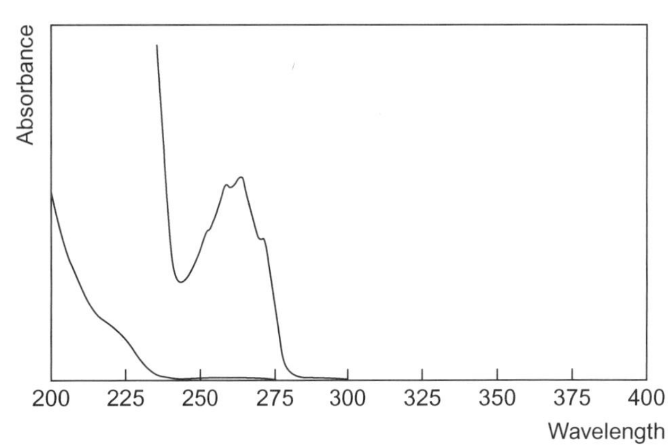

Infra-red Spectrum. Principal peaks at wavenumbers 1718, 1216, 1108, 1285, 1585, 1265 cm^{-1} (orphenadrine citrate, KBr disk). (See below)

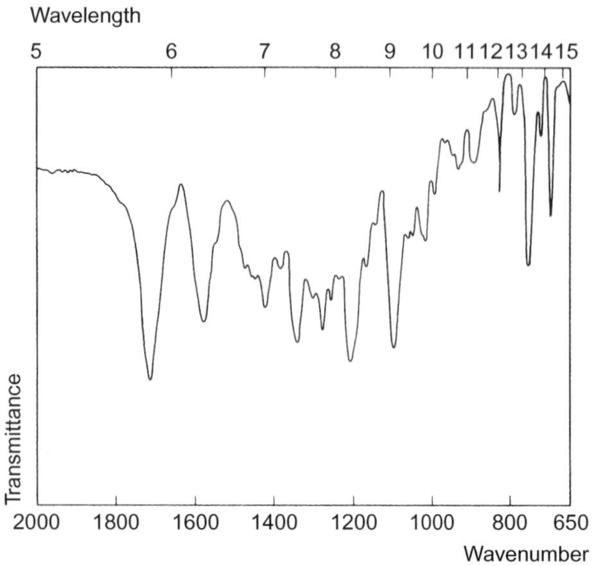

Mass Spectrum. Principal ions at *m/z* 58, 73, 44, 45, 165, 42, 40, 181 (no ions above 200); *N*-monodesmethylorphenadrine 44, 59, 165, 166, 181, 179, 178, 43; orphenadrine *N*-oxide 58, 181, 43, 45, 60, 44, 165, 73.

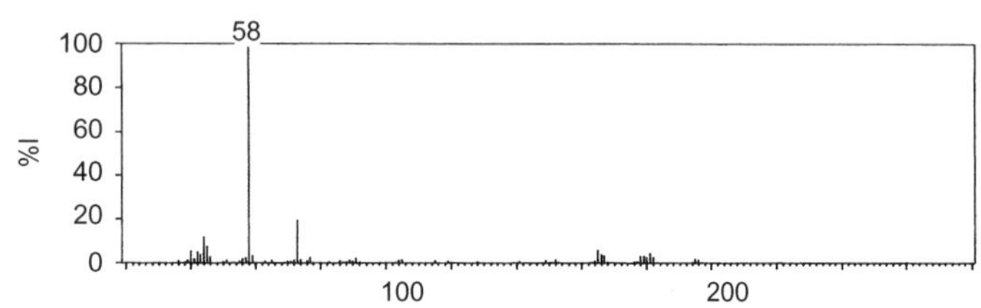

Quantification

Gas chromatography. In plasma or urine: orphenadrine and metabolites, limit of detection 10 µg/L, AFID—J. J. M. Labout *et al.*, *J. Chromatogr.*, 1977, *144*, 201–208. In postmortem tissues: FID—L. F. Wilkinson *et al.*, *J. Anal. Toxicol.*, 1983, *7*, 72–75. In plasma: nitrogen-phosphorus detection—M. Contin *et al.*, *Biomed. Chromatogr.*, 1987, *2*, 193–194. In whole blood or urine: orphenadrine and other diphenylmethane antihistamines, limits of detection 0.1 to 0.25 µg/L, SID—H. Hattori *et al.*, *J. Chromatogr.*, 1992, *581*, 213–218. In whole blood or urine: orphenadrine and other diphenylmethane antihistamines, limits of detection 76 to 473 µg/L in blood and 13 to 186 µg/L in urine—M. Nishikawa *et al.*, *J. Chromatogr. Sci.*, 1997, *35*, 275–279.

Disposition in the Body. Readily absorbed after oral administration and rapidly distributed. Up to about 60% of an oral dose is excreted in the urine in 3 days. During 24 h after dosage, under uncontrolled conditions, about 4% of a dose is excreted as unchanged drug, about 5% as *N*-monodesmethylorphenadrine (tofenacin), about 3% as *N,N*-didesmethylorphenadrine, about 3% as orphenadrine *N*-oxide, about 8% as a conjugate of 2-methylbenzhydryloxyacetic acid, and about 6% as a conjugate of 2-methylbenzhydrol. The urinary excretion appears to be dependent on urinary pH.

Therapeutic concentration. In plasma, usually in the range 0.1 to 0.2 mg/L.

Toxicity. The lethal dose is estimated to be in excess of about 2 g. Blood concentrations greater than about 0.5 mg/L may cause toxic reactions and concentrations greater than 5 mg/L may be lethal.

In a survey of 9 fatalities attributed to orphenadrine overdose, blood concentrations ranged from 1.1 to 37 mg/L (mean 15); in 5 cases the bile concentration was 85 to 234 mg/L (mean 150), and in 7 cases the urine concentration was 3 to 122 mg/L (mean 53). In one case in which a more complete analysis was reported, the concentrations were: blood 33 mg/L, bile 202 mg/L, brain 3.3 mg/kg, kidney 15 mg/kg, liver 23 mg/kg, lung 19.5 mg/kg, spleen 26.5 mg/kg. [A. E. Robinson *et al.*, *Forensic Sci.*, 1977, *9*, 53–62.]

In a fatality due to an orphenadrine overdose in which death occurred within 2.5 h of ingestion, the following postmortem concentrations were reported: blood 18.1 mg/L, liver 242 mg/kg, urine 7 mg/L. [L. F. Wilkinson *et al.*, *J. Anal. Toxicol.*, 1983, *7*, 72–75.]

A 38-year-old man whose death was attributed to massive ingestion of orphenadrine and clozapine with suicidal intent, had the following postmortem tissue concentrations: heart blood 183 and 44 mg/L (orphenadrine and clozapine, respectively), urine 331 and 245 mg/L, gastric content – and 859 mg/L; the heart blood concentration of orphenadrine (183 mg/L) was the highest reported thus far in an acute intoxication. [N. Fucci *et al.*, *Forensic Sci. Int.*, 2001, *123*, 13–16.]

Half-life. Plasma half-life, about 14 h.

Protein binding. In plasma, about 20%.

Dose. 150 to 400 mg of orphenadrine hydrochloride daily.

Ouabain

Cardiac Glycoside/Cardiotonic

Synonyms. G-Strophanthin; Strophanthin-G; Strophanthinum; Strophanthoside-G; Uabaina; Ubaína.
Proprietary names. Ouabaine Arnaud; Purostrophan; Strodival; Strophoperm.
(1β,3β,5β,11α)-3-[(6-Deoxy-α-L-mannopyranosyl)oxy]-1,5,11,14,19-pentahydroxycard-20(22)-enolide
$C_{29}H_{44}O_{12},8H_2O = 728.8$
CAS—630-60-4 (anhydrous); 11018-89-6 (octahydrate)

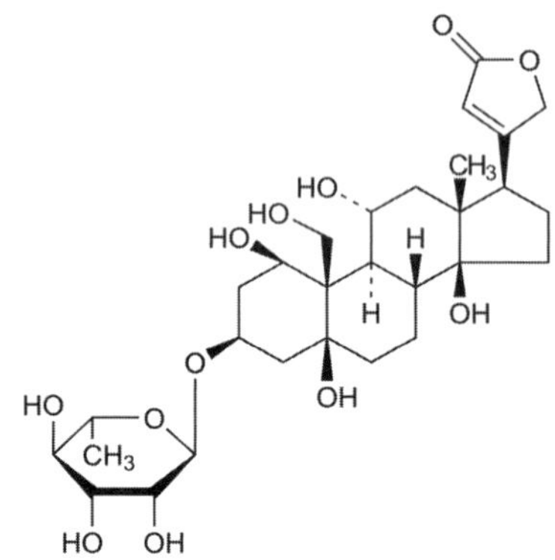

A glycoside obtained from the seeds of *Strophanthus gratus* or from the wood of *Acokanthera schimperi* or *A. ouabaio* (Apocynaceae).
Colourless crystals or white crystalline powder. M.p. about 190°, with decomposition.
Slowly soluble 1 in 75 of water, 1 in 5 of boiling water; soluble 1 in 100 of ethanol and 1 in 30 of methanol; soluble in amyl alcohol and dioxane; slightly soluble in chloroform, ether and ethyl acetate.

Partition Coefficient. Log *P* (octanol/water), −2.0.

Colour Test. Sulfuric Acid—orange-brown (slow). (Perchloric acid solution, followed by examination under ultraviolet light, yellow-green fluorescence; *p*-anisaldehyde reagent, yellow.)

Mass Spectrum. Principal ions at *m/z* 183, 43, 29, 60, 41, 129, 91, 73.

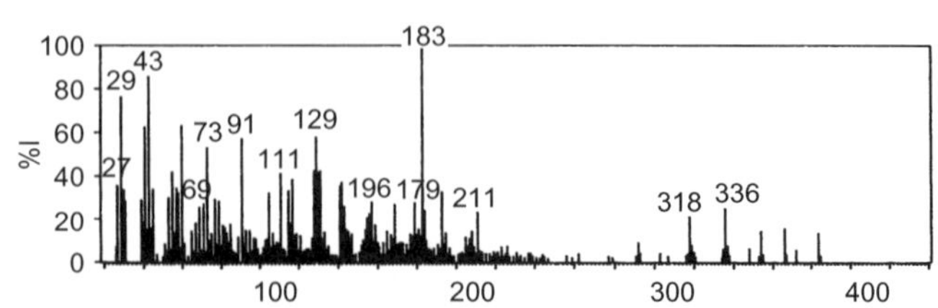

Quantification

Radioimmunoassay. In plasma or urine: limit of detection 50 ng/L—R. Selden and T. W. Smith, *Circulation*, 1972, *45*, 1176—1182. In plasma: limit of detection 5 ng/L—O. Vakkuri *et al.*, *J. Endocrinol.*, 2000, *165*, 669–677.

Disposition in the Body. Irregularly absorbed after oral administration. About 30 to 60% of a dose is excreted in the urine in 24 h and about 25% is eliminated in the faeces in 3 days. Under steady-state conditions about 40% of the daily dose is excreted in the 24-hour urine.

Therapeutic concentration

After a single intravenous dose of 0.5 mg to 3 subjects, a plasma concentration of about 0.012 mg/L was reported in 5 min; following daily intravenous administration of 0.25 mg to 3 subjects, steady-state plasma concentrations of about 0.0005 mg/L were attained on the 4th or 5th day [R. Selden and T. W. Smith, *Circulation*, 1972, *45*, 1176–1182].

Half-life. Plasma half-life, about 10 to 20 h.

Protein binding. In plasma, about 5 to 10%.

Dose. 250 to 500 µg intravenously; further injections of 100 µg may be given up to a total dose of 1 mg in 24 h.

Oxalic Acid

Ethanedioic acid
$C_2H_2O_4$ = 90.0
CAS—144-62-7 (anhydrous); 6153-56-6 (dihydrate)

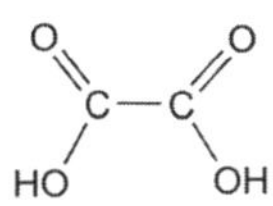

Colourless, transparent, efflorescent crystals. M.p. 101° to 102°.
Soluble 1 in about 7 of water, 1 in 2 of boiling water, 1 in 2.5 of ethanol and 1 in 100 of ether; practically insoluble in benzene, chloroform and petroleum ether.

Dissociation Constant. pK_a 1.2, 4.2 (25°).

Partition Coefficient. Log *P* (octanol/water), −2.2.

Colour Test. Add a few drops of a strong solution of ferrous sulfate to the acid or to a slightly acid solution of an oxalate—yellow.

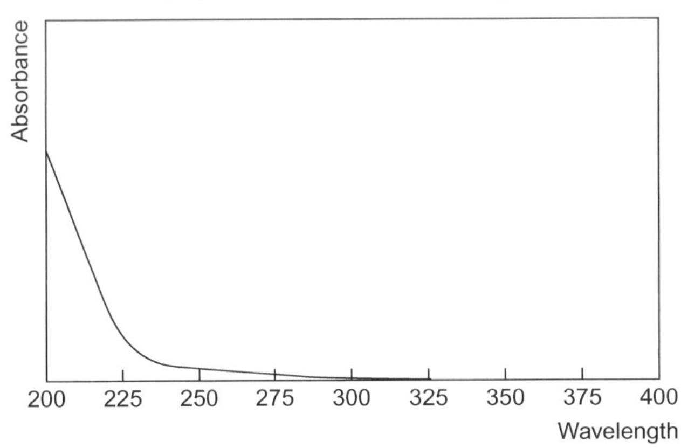

Infra-red Spectrum. Principal peaks at wavenumbers 1666, 1250, 1123, 724 cm^{-1}.

Quantification

Colorimetry. In urine—H. Baadenhuijsen and A. P. Jansen, *Clin. Chim. Acta*, 1975, *62*, 315–324.

Gas chromatography. In blood or serum: FID—P. Nuret and M. Offner, *Clin. Chim. Acta*, 1978, *82*, 9–12. In postmortem blood or urine: limit of detection 13 mg/L, AFID—G. Gauthier *et al.*, *J. Can. Soc. Forensic Sci.*, 1980, *13*(4), 1–9.

Gas chromatography–mass spectrometry. In blood and tissues: oxaloacetate, limit of detection 0.05 nmol per sample—A. Laplante *et al.*, *Anal. Biochem.*, 1995, *224*, 580–587.

High performance liquid chromatography. In urine: limit of detection 1 mg/L, electrochemical detection—W. J. Mayer *et al.*, *J. Chromatogr. Sci.*, 1979, *17*, 656–660. In plasma or urine: electrochemical detection—I. D. Fry and B. J. Starkey, *Ann. Clin. Biochem.*, 1991, *28*, 581–587. In urine: oxalic acid and citric acid, UV detection—M. H. Khaskhali *et al.*, *J. Chromatogr.*, 1996, *675*, *Biomed. Appl.*, 147–151.

Disposition in the Body. Less than 5% of ingested oxalic acid is absorbed in healthy adults. About 8 to 40 mg of oxalic acid is normally excreted in the urine daily; this is derived mainly from the metabolism of dietary ascorbic acid and glycine with small amounts from dietary oxalic acid and other minor metabolic sources. Calcium oxalate is a major constituent of kidney stones and is frequently found as crystals in freshly voided urine. In normal subjects, concentrations of oxalic acid in blood range from about 1 to 3 mg/L. Small amounts of oxalate are produced as a metabolite of ethylene glycol.
After intravenous administration of oxalic acid to normal subjects, more than 90% of the dose was excreted in the urine in 36 h [T. D. Elder and J. B. Wyngaarden, *J. Clin. Invest.*, 1960, *39*, 1337–1344].

Toxicity. In dilute solution, oxalic acid and its salts are toxic owing to withdrawal of ionisable calcium from the blood and tissues with resulting tetany. Strong solutions of oxalic acid are corrosive. The mean adult lethal dose is about 15 to 30 g, although a fatality has been reported after the intravenous injection of only 1.2 g. Blood concentrations greater than 10 mg/L are usually lethal. The maximum permissible atmospheric concentration is 1 mg/m^3.

In a fatal poisoning case, a blood concentration of 110 mg/L of oxalic acid was reported 6 h after the ingestion of potassium hydrogen oxalate; postmortem tissue concentrations of 21 µg/g in the brain and 382 µg/g in the liver were also reported; a second subject who survived the ingestion of potassium hydrogen oxalate had a blood concentration of 3.7 mg/L after 6 h. Postmortem blood concentrations of 18 and 77 mg/L were reported in 2 other fatalities [P. M. Zarembski and A. Hodgkinson, *J. Clin. Pathol.*, 1967, *20*, 283–285].

In a fatality caused by oxalic acid poisoning, a postmortem blood concentration of 370 mg/L was reported [G. Gauthier *et al.*, *J. Can. Soc. Forensic Sci.*, 1980, *13*, 1–9].

Distribution in blood. Plasma : whole blood ratio, about 0.8.

Protein binding. In plasma, not significantly bound at physiological pH values.

Note. For a review of oxalic acid metabolism in man, see A. Hodgkinson and P. M. Zarembski, *Calcif. Tissue Res.*, 1968, *2*, 115–132.

Oxaliplatin

Antineoplastic

Synonyms. Oxalatoplatin; oxalatoplatinum; l-OHP; RP-54780; NSC-266046.
Proprietary name. Eloxatin
(*SP*-4-2)-[(1*R*,2*R*)-1,2-Cyclohexanediamine-κ*N*,κ*N*′][ethanedioato-(2−)-κO^1,κO^2]platinum
$C_8H_{14}N_2O_4Pt$ = 397.3
CAS—61825-94-3

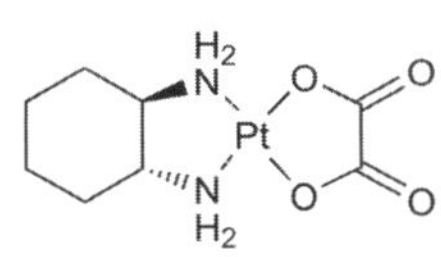

Colourless, thin triangular plates with truncated vertices. It is soluble in water at 7.9 g/L.

High Performance Liquid Chromatography. Column: ODS-2 (Inertsil, 250 × 4.6 mm i.d.). Column temperature: 40°. Mobile phase: acetonitrile:acetate buffer (10 mM, pH 5.5) (5:95), flow rate 1 mL/min. UV detection (λ = 290 nm). Retention time: 11.6 min. [R. Kizu *et al.*, *Chem. Pharm. Bull.*, 1995, *43(1)*, 108–114].

Quantification.

High performance liquid chromatography. In plasma and urine: limit of detection 0.1 µg/L. UV detection (λ = 290 nm)—R. Kizu *et al.*, *Chem. Pharm. Bull.*, 1995, *43(1)*, 108–114.

Disposition in the Body. Biotransformation is extensive and no intact drug is detectable in plasma ultrafiltrate at the end of a 2-h infusion. Renal elimination is the major pathway. 50% or more of the platinum administered was recovered in urine within 1 to 5 days following administration. Less than 5% is eliminated in faeces.

Therapeutic concentration
The maximum plasma concentration of platinum following a constant rate infusion of oxaliplatin at 20 mg/m^2/day for 5 days was 330 to 720 µg/L. [F. Levi *et al. Clin. Pharmacokinet.*, 2000, *38(1)*, 1–21].

Half-life. About 24 h.

Volume of distribution. Ranges between 582 and 812 L.

Clearance. About 17.6 L/h.

Distribution in blood. Maximum platinum uptake in erythrocytes was 37% of the total platinum. Plasma ultrafiltrate:total plasma:erythrocytes ratio is approx. 1:4:3 at the end of a 2-h infusion.

Dose. 130 mg/m^2 body surface.

Oxandrolone

Androgen/Anabolic Steroid

Synonyms. NSC-67068; SC-11585.
Proprietary names. Anavar; Lonavar; Oxandrin; Provitar; Vasorome.
(5α,17β)-17-Hydroxy-17-methyl-2-oxaandrostan-3-one
$C_{19}H_{30}O_3$=306.4
CAS—53-39-4

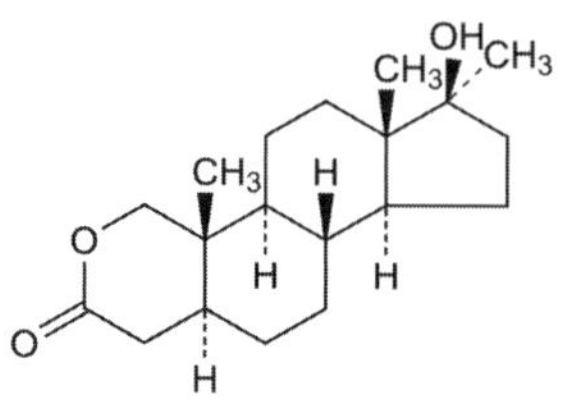

A white odourless crystalline powder with M.p. 235° to 238°. It is soluble in water (1 in 5200), alcohol (1 in 57), acetone (1 in 69), chloroform (1 in less than 5) and ether (1 in 860).

Partition Coefficient. Log *P* (octanol/water), 2.58.

Thin-layer Chromatography. Plate: silica gel HF_{254} (5 × 20 cm). Mobile phase: chloroform:methanol:glacial acetic acid (94:5:1). Visualisation by iodine vapour. Detection by zonal scraping method. Rf 0.5 [A. Karim, *Clin. Pharmacol. Ther.*, 1973, *14(5)*, 862–869].

Gas Chromatography. System GAG—RRT 1.17 (relative to testosterone); system GAI—RRT 1.111 (relative to 17α-methyl-5α-androstan-3β,17β-diol); system GAR—Retention time 13.7 min.

Column: 5% phenyl, methyl silicone (HP Ultra-2, 25 m × 0.2 mm i.d., 0.33 µm film thickness). Column temperature: 100°, 1 min hold, increased to 220° at 16°/min, then to 300° at 3.8°/min, with a 10 min hold. Carrier gas: helium. 0.6 mL/min flow rate. MS detection (EI, SIM at *m/z*: 143.1, 363.3, 378.3). RRT: (relative to oxandrolone TMS derivative, Retention time 27.97 min) δ-hydroxy acid metabolite, 0.90; 16α-hydroxyoxandrolone, 1.13; 16β-hydroxyoxandrolone, 1.16; 17-epioxandrolone, 0.93. (Relative to 5α-androstan-17-one-TMS-enol derivative, Retention time 17.95 min) oxandrolone, 1.56; δ-hydroxy acid metabolite, 1.40; 16-α-hydroxyoxandrolone, 1.77; 16-β-hydroxyoxandrolone, 1.81; 17-epioxandrolone, 1.44 [R. Masse *et al.*, *Biomed. Environ. Mass Spectrom.*, 1989, *18*, 429–438].

High Performance Liquid Chromatography. System HATb—RRT 0.75 (relative to testosterone).

Infra-red Spectrum. Principal peaks at wavenumbers 1717, 1202, 1231, 1258 cm^{-1}.

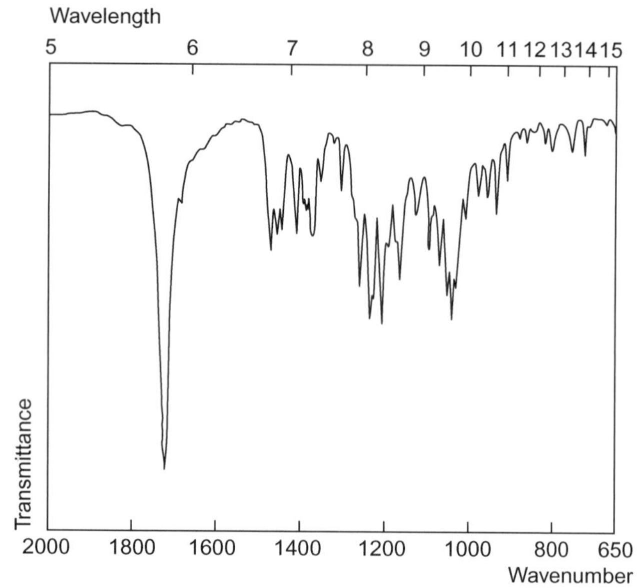

Mass Spectrum. Principal ions at *m/z* 291, 248, 43, 79, 91, 93, 107, 176.

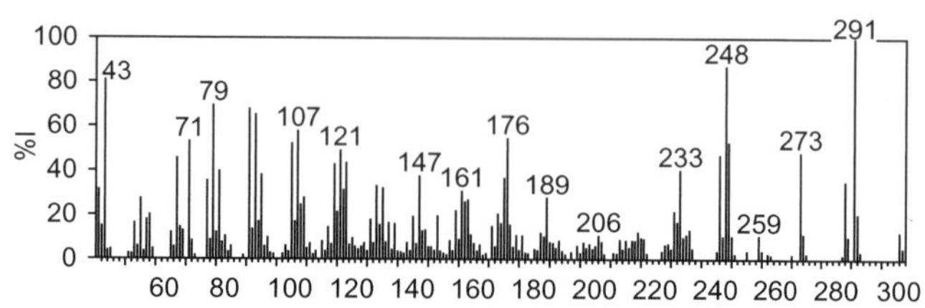

Quantification

Gas chromatography–mass spectrometry. In urine: limit of detection 0.005 mg/L—R. Masse *et al.*, *Biomed. Environ. Mass Spectrom.*, 1989, *18*, 429–438.

High performance liquid chromatography. In pharmaceutical preparations: limit of detection 5 mg/L. UV detection (λ=210 nm)—M. J. Walters *et al.*, *J. Assoc. Off. Anal. Chem.*, 1990, *73*, 904–926.

Disposition in the Body. Oxandrolone is rapidly absorbed from the gastro-intestinal tract and excreted mainly in urine as metabolites; 16-β-hydroxyoxandrolone and 16-α-hydroxyoxandrolone (total 3%), 17-epi-oxandrolone (8.4%) and a small amount as the δ-hydroxy acid metabolite, and the parent drug (35.8%). The drug is first detected in urine 2 h after dosing and can be detected for up to 72 h. A small amount is excreted in faeces (approx. 2.8%).

Therapeutic concentration. The maximum plasma concentration of 0.417 mg/L was observed between 30 and 90 min following oral ingestion of a 10 mg dose [A. Karim *et al*, *Clin. Pharmacol. Ther.*, 1973; *14*, 862–869].

Toxicity. Moderately toxic by ingestion and intraperitoneal routes. When heated to decomposition temperature will emit acrid smoke and fumes.

Bioavailability. 97%.

Half-life. Biphasic plasma elimination: from 90 min to 4 h, and 33 min, and from 4 to 48 h, and 9 h.

Volume of distribution. Approx. 578 mL/kg.

Clearance. Plasma clearance, 43 mL/h/kg.

Protein binding. 94 to 97%.

Dose. The usual dose is 2.5 to 20 mg by mouth. Usual dose 5 to 10 mg daily in divided doses for 2 to 4 weeks.

Oxazepam

Tranquilliser

Synonyms. Oxazepamum; Wy-3498.
Proprietary names. Adumbran; Alepam; Alopam; Anxiolit; Azutranquil; Benzotran; Isodin; Mirfudorm; Murelax; Opamox; Oxabenz; Oxahexal; Oxaline; Oxamin; Oxanid; Oxapax; Oxepam; Noctazepam; Praxiten; Sigacalm; Serax; Serenal; Serenid-D; Serepax; Seresta; Serpax; Sobril; Tranquo; Uskan.
7-Chloro-1,3-dihydro-3-hydroxy-5-phenyl-2*H*-1,4-benzodiazepin-2--one
$C_{15}H_{11}ClN_2O_2$=286.7
CAS—604-75-1

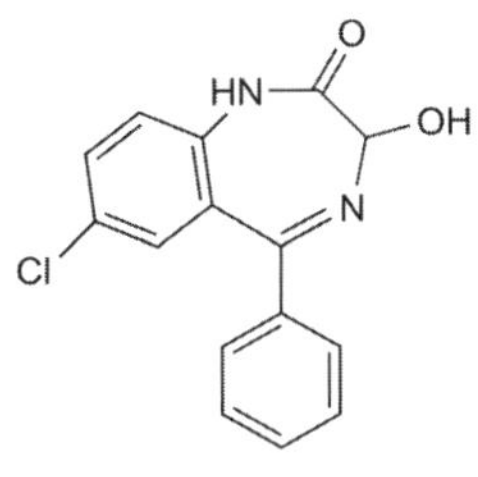

A white to pale yellow crystalline powder. M.p. 205° to 206° (crystals from alcohol).
Practically insoluble in water; soluble 1 in 220 of ethanol, 1 in 270 of chloroform, and 1 in 2200 of ether; soluble in dioxan.

Dissociation Constant. pK_a 1.7, 11.6 (20°).

Partition Coefficient. Log *P* (octanol/pH 7.4), 2.2.

Colour Test. Formaldehyde–Sulfuric Acid—orange.

Thin-layer Chromatography. System TA—Rf 56; system TB—Rf 00; system TC—Rf 40; system TD—Rf 22; system TE—Rf 45; system TF—Rf 35; system TL—Rf 51; system TAD—Rf 42; system TAE—Rf 82; system TAF—Rf 91; system TAJ—Rf 47; system TAK—Rf 47; system TAL—Rf 89. (Acidified iodoplatinate solution, positive; acidified potassium permanganate solution, positive.)

Gas Chromatography. System GA—RI 2325; system GB—oxazepam RI 2438, oxazepam-TMS_2 RI 2468; system GG—RI 2803.

High Performance Liquid Chromatography. System HI—*k* 4.62; system HK—*k* 0.73; system HX—RI 441; system HY—RI 390; system HZ—retention time 3.8 min; system HAL—retention time 4.4 min; system HAM—retention time 3.4 and 4.4 min; system HAX—retention time 6.0 min; system HAY—retention time 4.5 min; system HAZ—*k* 1.23; system HBH—*k* 5.42; system HBI—*k* 1.25.

Ultraviolet Spectrum. Aqueous acid—234, 280; aqueous alkali—233, 344; ethanol—230 (A^1_1=1235a), 315 nm (A^1_1=85a). (See below)

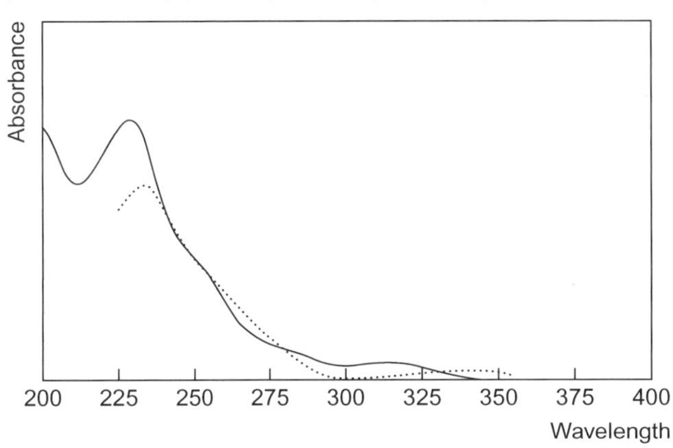

Infra-red Spectrum. Principal peaks at wavenumbers 1687, 1706, 693, 830, 1136, 1123 cm^{-1} (KBr disk). (See below)

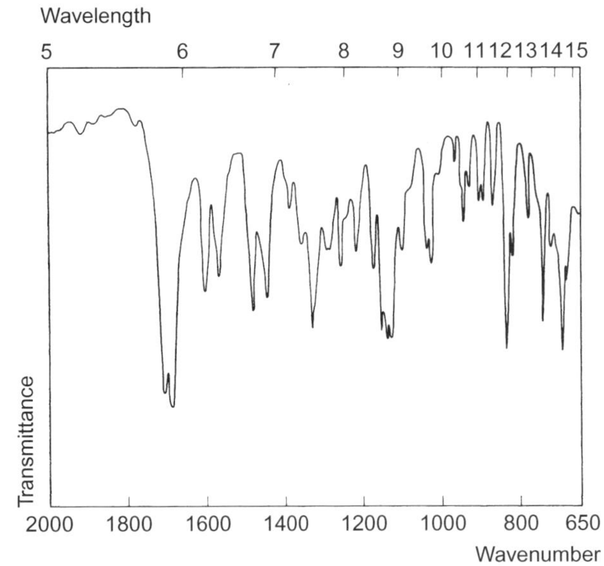

Mass Spectrum. Principal ions at *m/z* 257, 77, 268, 239, 205, 267, 233, 259.

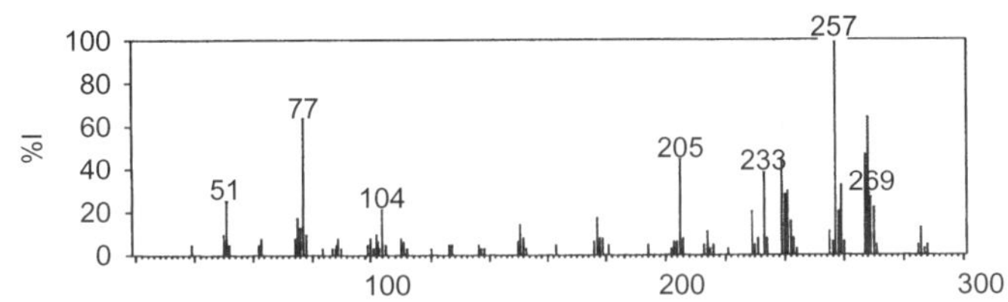

Quantification

Gas chromatography. In plasma: limit of detection 10 μg/L, ECD—H. G. Giles *et al*., *Can. J. Pharm. Sci*., 1978, *13*, 64–65. In plasma or whole blood: oxazepam and other benzodiazepines, NPD and ECD—P. Lillesunde and T. Seppala, *J. Chromatogr*., 1990, *533*, 97–110. In plasma or urine: oxazepam and other benzodiazepines, limits of detection 0.01 to 0.45 μg/L—K. J. Reubsaet *et al*., *J. Pharm. Biomed. Anal*., 1998, *18*, 667–680.

Gas chromatography–mass spectrometry. In serum: oxazepam and other 'natural' benzodiazepines, SIM—J. M. Duthel *et al*., *J. Chromatogr*., 1992, *579*, 85–91. In hair: oxazepam and nordazepam—P. Kintz *et al*., *J. Chromatogr*. 1996, *677 B Biomed. Appl*., 241–244. In serum: oxazepam and other benzodiazepines, limits of detection 13 to 30 μg/L (scan mode) and 1 to 1.7 μg/L (SIM)—D. Borrey *et al*., *J. Chromatogr. B Biomed. Sci. Appl*., 2001, *765*, 187–197. Limit of quantification 2.5 to 5 μg/L (full scan) and 0.1 to 0.5 μg/L (SIM, *m/z* 257)—D. Borrey *et al*., *J. Chromatogr. A*, 2001, *910*, 105–118.

High performance liquid chromatography. In plasma or urine: oxazepam and diazepam—A. Goldnik *et al*., *Acta Pol. Pharm*., 1993, *50*, 421–422. In plasma or urine: oxazepam and other benzodiazepine glucuronides, limits of detection 5 to 10 μg/L—C. Franzelius and K. Besserer, *J. Chromatogr*., 1993, *613*, 162–167. In urine: limit of detection 4 μg/L, fluorescence detection—L. A. Berrueta *et al*., *J. Chromatogr*., 1993, *616*, 344–348. In plasma and urine: limit of quantification and detection is 10 μg/L, UV detection (λ = 232 nm)—R. M. Azzam *et al*., *J. Chromatogr. B Biomed. Sci. Appl*., 1998, *708(1–2)*, 304–309. In serum: oxazepam and other benzodiazepines, photodiode-array detection—B. Ahrens *et al*., *Arzneimittelforschung*, 2000, *50*, 1057–1062. In blood: oxazepam and other benzodiazepines, limit of quantification for oxazepam 25 μg/L, diode-array detection—A. El Mahjoub and C. Staub, *J. Anal. Toxicol*., 2001, *25*, 209–214. In hair: oxazepam and other benzodiazepines, limit of quantification for oxazepam 100 μg/g, UV detection—A. El Mahjoub and C. Staub, *Forensic Sci. Int*., 2001, *123*, 17–25. In plasma: limit of detection 30 μg/L, UV detection—A. Zarghi and M. Jenabi, *Boll. Chim. Farm*., 2001, *140*, 455–457. In urine: oxazepam and other benzodiazepines, limit of detection for oxazepam 750 μg/L, UV detection—W. M. Mullett and J. Pawliszyn, *Anal. Chem*., 2002, *74*, 1081–1087.

Disposition in the Body. Readily absorbed after oral administration. It crosses the placenta and is found in breast milk. About 70 to 80% of a single dose is excreted in the urine in 72 h almost entirely as oxazepam glucuronide, with only traces of unchanged oxazepam and other minor metabolites. Up to 10% of a dose is eliminated in the faeces, mostly as unchanged drug.
Oxazepam is a metabolite of several benzodiazepines including chlordiazepoxide, clorazepate, demoxepam, desmethyldiazepam (nordazepam), diazepam, ketazolam, medazepam, prazepam, and temazepam.

Therapeutic concentration. In plasma, usually in the range 0.5 to 2 mg/L.

A single oral dose of 45 mg administered to 8 subjects, produced serum concentrations of 0.88 to 1.44 mg/L (mean 1.1) of oxazepam in about 2 h, and concentrations of 0.7 to 1.4 mg/L (mean 0.9) of oxazepam glucuronide in 2 to 4 h. Daily oral doses of 10 mg every 6 h administered to 6 subjects, produced serum concentrations of 0.14 to 0.56 mg/L (mean 0.3) of oxazepam 2 h after a dose, and concentrations of 0.22 to 0.40 mg/L (mean 0.3) of oxazepam glucuronide 4 h after a dose. [J. A. Knowles and H. W. Ruelius, *Arzneimittelforschung*, 1972, *22*, 687–692.]

Toxicity. Blood concentrations greater than 2 mg/L may produce toxic effects.

Half-life. Plasma half-life, 4 to 15 h (mean 8).

Volume of distribution. 0.5 to 2 L/kg.

Clearance. Plasma clearance, about 1 to 2 mL/min/kg.

Distribution in blood. Plasma:whole blood ratio, about 0.9.

Protein binding. In plasma, about 95%.

Note. For a review of the clinical pharmacokinetics of oxazepam, see D. J. Greenblatt, *Clin. Pharmacokinet.*, 1981, *6*, 89–105.

Dose. 30 to 120 mg daily.

Oxcarbazepine

Anticonvulsant

Synonyms. GP-47680; Oxacarbazepine.
Proprietary name. Trileptal
10,11-Dihydro-10-oxo-5*H*-dibenz[*b*,*f*]azepine-5-carboxamide
$C_{15}H_{12}N_2O_2$=252.3
CAS—28721-07-5

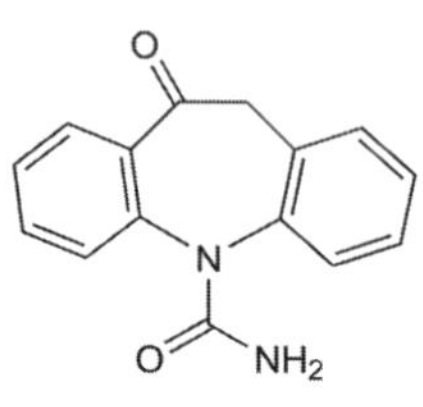

White to faintly orange crystalline powder. M.p. 215° to 216°. Practically insoluble in water, ether and ethanol; slightly soluble in chloroform, dichloromethane, acetone and methanol.

Partition Coefficient. Log *P* (octanol/water), 1.11.

Thin-layer Chromatography. System TB—Rf 00; system TE—Rf 54; system TF—Rf 20; system TAE—Rf 78.

Gas Chromatography. System GA—M (formylacridine) RI 2025, M (carbamazepine) RI 2285; system GB—oxcarbamazepine RI 2266, M (formylacridine) RI 2158, M (methylacridine) RI 2054, M (10-OH-) RI 2580, M (carbamazepine) RI 2435; system GAJ—M (carbamazepine) RRT 1.716 (relative to methylphenobarbital).

Column: cross-linked methyl silicone (30 m × 0.31 mm i.d., 1.0 μm). Column temperature: 140° to 240° at 30°/min. Carrier gas: hydrogen. Detection: FID. Retention time(s): 10-hydroxycarbazepine, 7.8 min; oxcarbazepine, 8.8 min; carbazepine-*trans*-diol, 10.4 min [G. E. von Unruh and W. D. Paar, *J. Chromatogr.*, 1985, *345(1)*, 67–76].

High Performance Liquid Chromatography. System HX—RI 396; HZ—oxcarbazepine Retention time 2.9 min, M (10-OH-) Retention time 2.2 min.

Column: Chiral OD (Diacel Chiralcel, 250 × 4.6 mm i.d.). Mobile phase: *n*-hexane:ethanol:2-propanol (18:2:1) with 0.1% glacial acetic acid, flow rate 1.0 mL/min. IS: oxcarbazepine oxime. UV detection (λ=215 nm). Retention time(s): oxcarbazepine, 18.3 min; *R*-(−)-10-hydroxycarbazepine, 10.6 min; *S*-(+)-10-hydroxycarbazepine, 13.3 min; IS, 14.9 min [A. Volosov *et al.*, *J. Chromatogr. Biomed. Sci. Appl.*, 2000, *738*, 419–425].

Column: C_{18} (Novapak, 150 × 3.9 mm i.d., 4 μm). Mobile phase: acetonitrile:water (20:80), flow rate 1.5 mL/min. IS: 10,11-epoxycarbamazepine. UV detection (λ=215 nm). Retention time(s): oxcarbazepine, 7.7 min; 10-hydroxycarbazepine, 3.6 min; IS, 6.0 min [K. M. Matar *et al.*, *J. Clin. Pharm. Ther.*, 1995, *20*, 229–234].

Ultraviolet Spectrum. Aqueous acid—256, 306 nm.

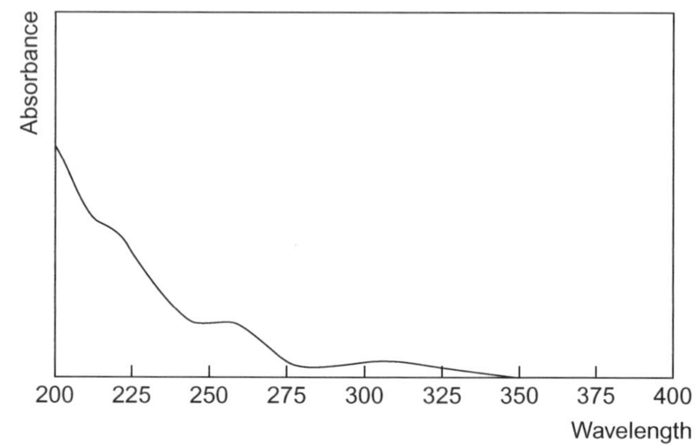

Mass Spectrum. Principal ions at *m/z* 180, 209, 252, 208, 152, 179, 181, 210.

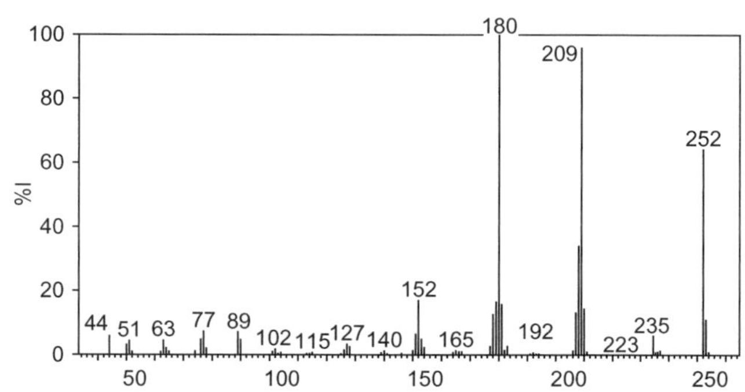

Quantification

Gas chromatography. In plasma: limit of detection 10 μg/L and 25 μg/L for 10-hydroxycarbazepine and 10,11-dihydro-10-hydroxycarbamazepine, respectively—G. E. von Unruh and W. D. Paar, *J. Chromatogr.*, 1985, *345*, 67–76.

Gas chromatography–mass spectrometry. In plasma: limit of detection 0.1 μg/L and 1 μg/L for 10-hydroxycarbazepine and 10,11-dihydro-10-hydroxycarbamazepine, respectively—G. E. von Unruh and W. D. Paar, *Biomed. Environ. Mass Spectrom.*, 1986, *13(12)*, 651–656.

High performance liquid chromatography. In urine: limit of quantification of 10-hydroxycarbazepine 200 μg/L and the 10,11-dihydro-10-hydroxycarbamazepine metabolite 400 μg/L, UV detection—A. Volosov *et al.*, *J. Chromatogr. Biomed. Sci. Appl.*, 2000, *738(2)*, 419–425. In plasma: limit of detection for oxcarbazepine 50 μg/L and 10,11-dihydro-10-hydroxycarbamazepine, 20 μg/L—K. M. Matar *et al.*, *J. Clin. Pharm. Ther.*, 1995, *20*, 229–234.

Disposition in the Body. Oxcarbazepine is rapidly and well absorbed after oral administration and is widely distributed in the body. It is rapidly and extensively metabolised in the liver to 10,11-dihydro-10-hydroxycarbamazepine which possesses anti-epileptic activity, and a monohydroxy derivative (MHD). The drug is mainly excreted in urine as the metabolites with less than 1% as the unchanged drug. Faecal excretion accounts for less then 4% of a dose. About 80% of a dose is excreted in urine either as glucuronides of MHD (49%) or as unchanged MHD (27%) whereas conjugates of oxcarbazepine account for 13% of the dose. Both the drug and the monohydroxy metabolite cross the placenta and are distributed into breast milk.

Therapeutic concentration. The serum therapeutic concentration range of hydroxycarbazepine is 12 to 30 mg/L.

12 young, healthy (30 to 31 years) and 12 elderly (61 to 82 years) males were administered with a single dose of 300 mg oxcarbazepine on day 1 and 300 mg twice daily on days 5 to 12. 12 young (18 to 32 years) and 12 elderly (60 to 79 years) females were administered with a single 600 mg dose on day 1, 150 mg twice daily on day 5 and 300 mg twice daily on days 6 to 11. The maximum plasma concentration after the single doses were 2.33 and 2.88 mg/L for the young and elderly males, respectively. These were observed at 4 (4 to 6) h and 5 (4 to 10) h, respectively. For the young females, concentrations were 5.17 mg/L at 4 (2 to 12) h and for the elderly, 7.20 mg/L at 5 (3 to 20) h. For the multiple dosing, the maximum concentrations were 8.49 and 12.03 mg/L at 2 (2 to 4) and 4 (2 to 8) h for the young and elderly males, respectively, and 9.34 and 11.72 mg/L at 3 (2 to 4) h for the young and elderly females [P. N. Van Heinigen *et al.*, *Clin Pharmacol. Ther.*, 1991, *50(4)*, 410–419].

Toxicity. The toxic serum concentration is 45 mg/L.

Half-life. Oxcarbazepine, 1 to 2.5 h; monohydroxy derivative, 8 to 14 h.

Volume of distribution. 3.94 L/kg; monohydroxy derivative, 49 L.

Clearance. Oral, 2.5 L/kg/h.

Protein binding. Approx. 40% (primarily to albumin).

Dose. The initial daily dose is 300 mg with a maintenance dose of 600 to 1200 mg. The dose may need to be reduced in those with moderate to severe renal impairment (dose halved).

Oxedrine

Sympathomimetic

Synonyms. Oxyphenylmethylaminoethanol; Sympaethaminum; Synephrine.
Note. *m*-Synephrine has been used as a synonym for phenylephrine.
4-Hydroxy-α-[(methylamino)methyl]benzenemethanol
$C_9H_{13}NO_2$=167.2
CAS—94-07-5

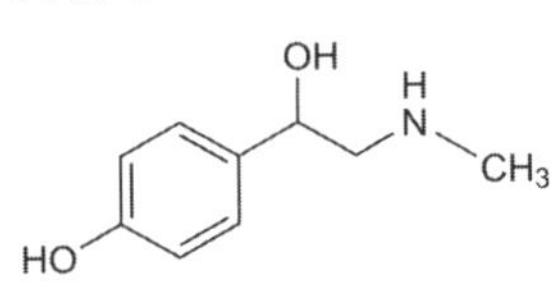

Crystals. M.p. 184° to 185°.

Oxedrine Tartrate

Synonym. Aethaphenum Tartaricum
Proprietary names. Dulcidrine; Sympatol.
$(C_9H_{13}NO_2)_2,C_4H_6O_6$=484.5
CAS—16589-24-5; 67-04-9 (±)
Colourless crystals or white crystalline powder. M.p. 188° to 190°, with some decomposition.
Soluble 1 in 2 of water and 1 in 400 of ethanol; practically insoluble in chloroform and ether.

Dissociation Constant. pK_a 9.3 (—OH), 10.2 (—NH—), (25°).

Partition Coefficient. Log *P* (octanol/water), −0.4.

Thin-layer Chromatography. System TA—Rf 25; system TB—Rf 04; system TC—Rf 01. (Acidified potassium permanganate solution, positive.)

High Performance Liquid Chromatography. System HB—*k* 0.27.

Ultraviolet Spectrum. Aqueous acid—273 nm (A^1_1=81a); aqueous alkali—241 nm (A^1_1=810b), 291 nm.

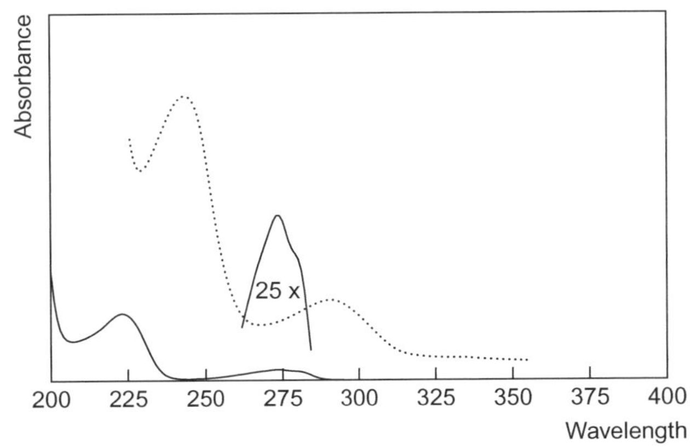

Infra-red Spectrum. Principal peaks at wavenumbers 835, 1510, 1054, 1271, 1098, 1611 cm^{-1} (KBr disk).

Mass Spectrum. Principal ions at *m/z* 44, 108, 42, 77, 107, 149, 95, 123.

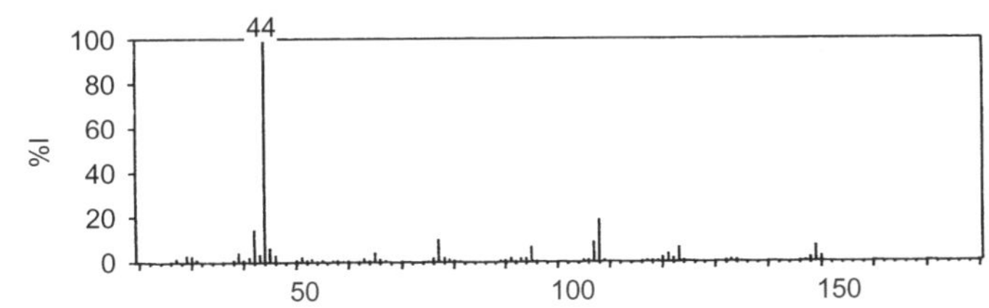

Dose. Oxedrine tartrate has been given in doses of about 300 mg daily.

Oxeladin

Antitussive

2-[2-(Diethylamino)ethoxy]ethyl-α,α-diethylbenzeneacetate
$C_{20}H_{33}NO_3$=335.5
CAS-468-61-1

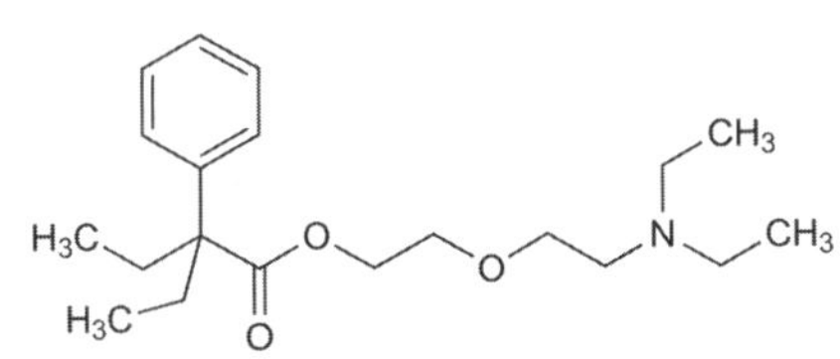

A yellow oil.
Practically insoluble in water; soluble in ethanol, acetone, toluene and ether.

Oxeladin Citrate

Proprietary names. Dorex-retard; Paxeladine.
$C_{20}H_{33}NO_3,C_6H_8O_7$=527.6
CAS—52432-72-1
A white crystalline powder. M.p. 90° to 91°.
Soluble in water.

Partition Coefficient. Log *P* (octanol/water), 4.3.

Colour Test. Marquis Test—orange.

Thin-layer Chromatography. System TA—Rf 50; system TB—Rf 51; system TC—Rf 22; system TE—Rf 67; system TL—Rf 19; system TAE—Rf 19. (Acidified iodoplatinate solution, positive.)

Gas Chromatography. System GA—RI 2190.

High Performance Liquid Chromatography. System HA—*k* 3.0.

Ultraviolet Spectrum. Aqueous acid—252, 258, 264 nm.

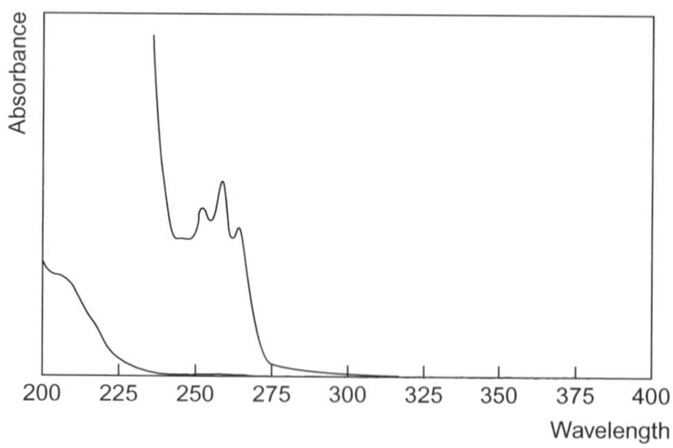

Infra-red Spectrum. Principal peaks at wavenumbers 1731, 1128, 1221, 1100, 700, 1080 cm^{-1} (KBr disk).

Mass Spectrum. Principal ions at *m/z* 86, 91, 105, 87, 144, 58, 100, 56.

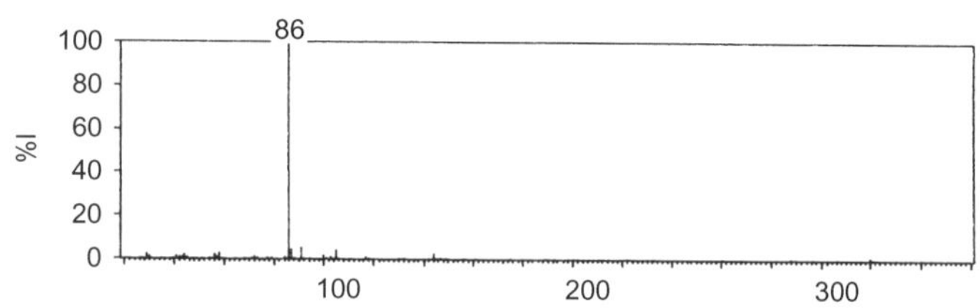

Dose. 80 to 120 mg of oxeladin citrate daily.

Oxetacaine

Local Anaesthetic

Synonym. Oxethazaine
Proprietary names. It is an ingredient of Mucaine, Mucoxin, Mutesa, Muthesa, Oxaine and Tepilta.
2,2′-[(2-Hydroxyethyl)imino]bis[*N*-(1,1-dimethyl-2-phenylethyl)-*N*-methylacetamide]
$C_{28}H_{41}N_3O_3$=467.6
CAS—126-27-2

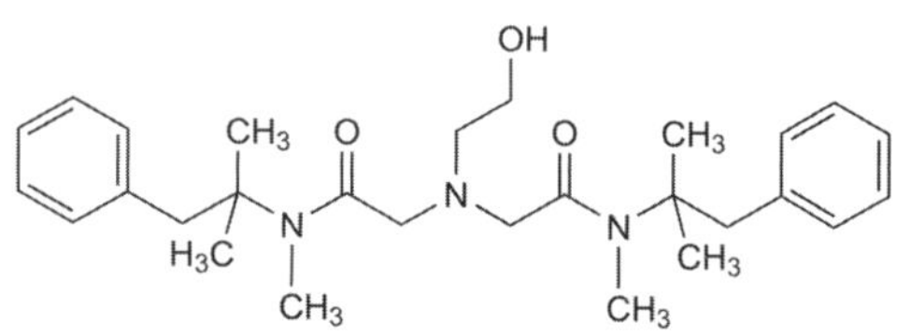

A white crystalline powder. M.p. about 104°.
Insoluble in water; soluble in ethanol and in dilute acids.

Oxetacaine Hydrochloride

Proprietary name. Emoren
CAS—13930-31-9 (xHCl)
M.p. 146° to 147°.
Soluble in water.

Partition Coefficient. Log *P* (octanol/water), 3.4.

Colour Tests. Mandelin's Test—violet-brown; Marquis Test—red-brown.

Thin-layer Chromatography. System TA—Rf 52; system TAE—Rf 61; system TB—Rf 10; system TC—Rf 07; system TE—Rf 38; system TL—Rf 15. (Acidified iodoplatinate solution, positive.)

Gas Chromatography. System GA—RI 2525.

High Performance Liquid Chromatography. System HR—*k* 4.14.

Ultraviolet Spectrum. Aqueous acid—248, 252, 258, 264 nm.

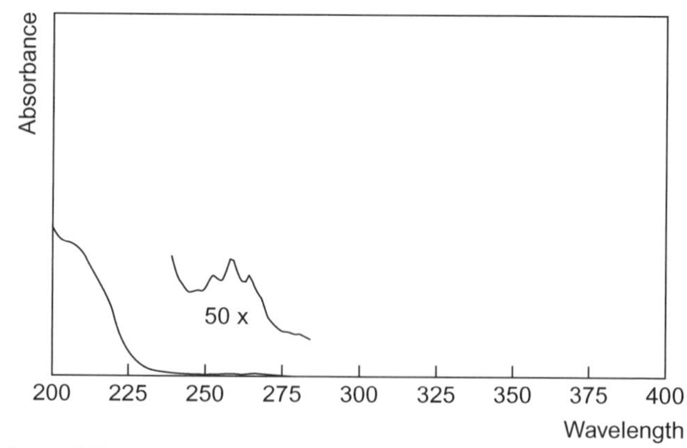

Infra-red Spectrum. Principal peaks at wavenumbers 1645, 756, 707, 1219, 1101, 1068 cm^{-1}.

Mass Spectrum. Principal ions at *m/z* 72, 91, 114, 145, 75, 160, 117, 92.

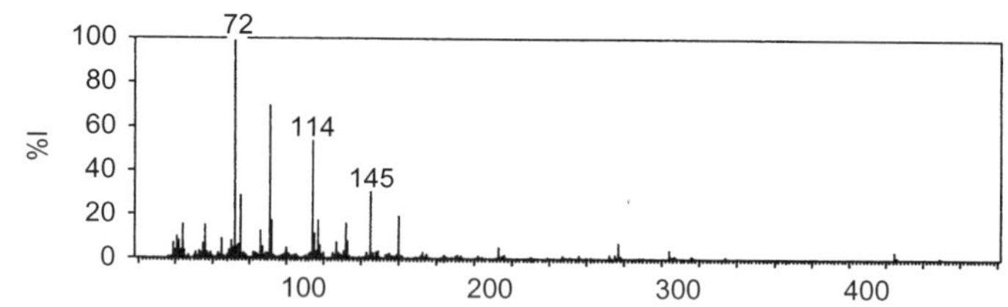

Dose. 30 to 80 mg daily, by mouth.

Oxprenolol

Beta-blocker

Synonym. Oxyprenolol
1-[(1-Methylethyl)amino]-3-[2-(2-propenyloxy)phenoxy]-2-propanol
$C_{15}H_{23}NO_3$=265.4
CAS—6452-71-7; 22972-98-1 (±)

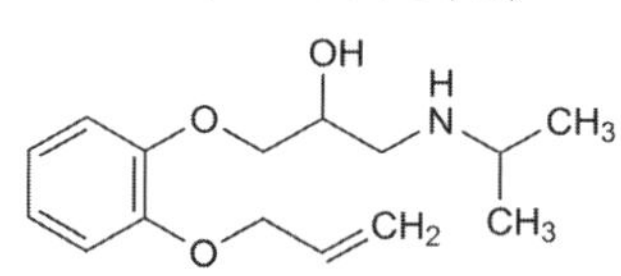

Crystals. M.p. 75° to 80°.

Oxprenolol Hydrochloride

Proprietary names. Apsolox; Laracor; Slow-Pren; Slow-Trasicor; Trasicor. It is an ingredient of Trasidrex.
$C_{15}H_{23}NO_3$,HCl=301.8
CAS—6452-73-9; 22972-97-0 (±)
A white to slightly cream-coloured crystalline powder. M.p. 107° to 109°.
Soluble 1 in less than 1 of water and 1 in 1.5 of ethanol; very slightly soluble in ether.

Dissociation Constant. pK_a 9.5.

Partition Coefficient. Log *P* (octanol/water), 2.1.

Colour Tests. Liebermann's Test—black; Mandelin's Test—grey-violet; Marquis Test—violet; Sulfuric Acid—orange-red (fluoresces under ultra-violet light at 350 nm).

Thin-layer Chromatography. System TA—Rf 48; system TB—Rf 11; system TC—Rf 11; system TE—Rf 45; system TL—Rf 13; system TAE—Rf 20; system TAF—Rf 78. (Acidified iodoplatinate solution, positive.)

Gas Chromatography. System GA—Oxprenolol RI 1870, Art RI 1985; M (desamino-OH-desalkyl-) RI 1700; system GB—oxprenolol RI 1972, Art RI 2062; system GF—RI 2270.

High Performance Liquid Chromatography. System HA—*k* 1.3; system HX—RI 354; system HY—RI 284; system HZ—Retention time, 3.0 min; system HAA—Retention time, 12.0 min.

Ultraviolet Spectrum. Aqueous acid—273 nm (A^1_1=85a). No alkaline shift.

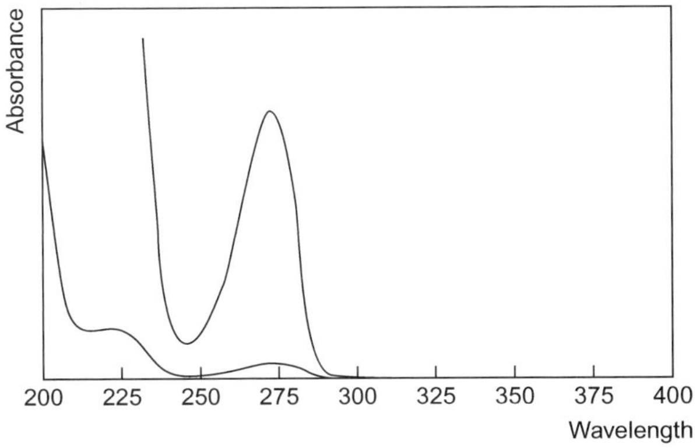

Infra-red Spectrum. Principal peaks at wavenumbers 1258, 750, 1500, 1120, 1092, 1037 cm^{-1} (oxprenolol hydrochloride, KBr disk).

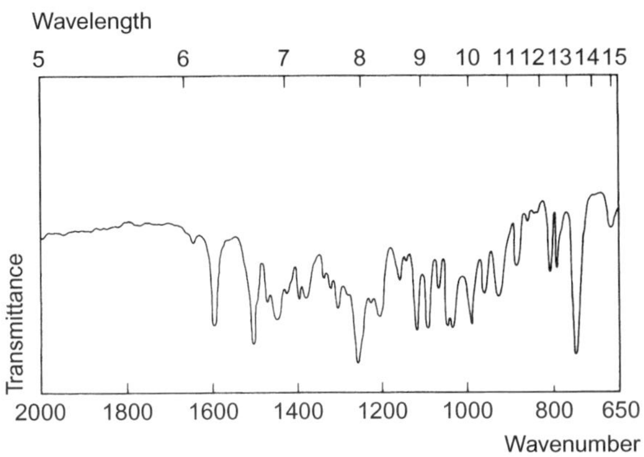

Mass Spectrum. Principal ions at *m/z* 72, 41, 56, 43, 221, 73, 57, 45.

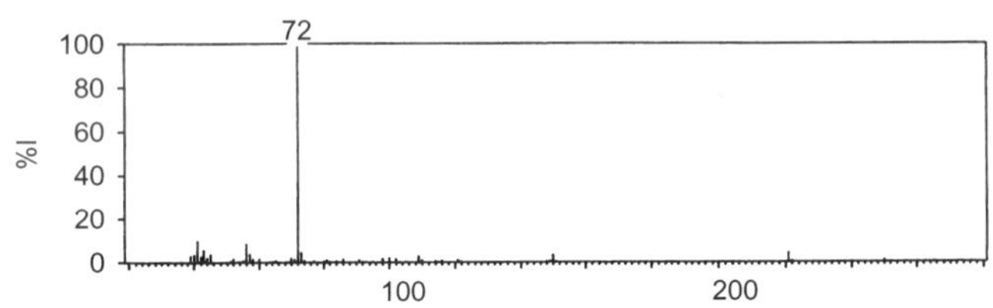

Quantification

Gas chromatography. In serum: limit of detection 2 pg, ECD—D. DeBruyne *et al., J. Pharm. Sci.*, 1979, *68*, 511–512.

Gas chromatography–mass spectrometry. In postmortem blood or urine: oxprenolol and other beta blockers—S. B. Black *et al., J. Chromatogr.*, 1996, *685*, *Biomed. Appl.*, 67–80.

High performance liquid chromatography. In plasma, blood or urine: limit of detection 10 μg/L, UV detection—S. Tsuei *et al., J. Chromatogr.*, 1980, *181*; *Biomed. Appl.*, *7*, 135–140. In plasma: limit of detection 20 μg/L, UV detection—J. Godbillon *et al., J. Chromatogr.*, 1985, *345*, 365–371. In plasma: oxprenolol and celiprolol, limit of detection <25 μg/L for oxprenolol, UV detection—A. J. Braza *et al., J. Chromatogr. B. Biomed. Sci. Appl.*, 1998, *718*, 267–272.

High performance liquid chromatography–gas chromatography. In serum or urine: oxprenolol and other beta blockers, limits of detection 18 to 44 μg/L—T. Hyotylainen *et al., J. Chromatogr. Sci.*, 1997, *35*, 280–286.

Thin-layer chromatography–spectrofluorimetry. In plasma: limit of detection 10 μg/L—M. Schäefer and E. Mutschler, *J. Chromatogr.*, 1979, *164*; *Biomed. Appl.*, *6*, 247–252.

Disposition in the Body. Readily absorbed after oral administration but subject to extensive first-pass metabolism. The major metabolite is oxprenolol glucuronide. About 70 to 90% of a dose is excreted in the urine in 24 h, with less than 5% as unchanged drug.

Therapeutic concentration

Following a single oral dose of 40 mg to 7 subjects, peak blood concentrations of 0.09 to 0.24 mg/L (mean 0.15) of oxprenolol and 0.11 to 0.35 mg/L (mean 0.24) of oxprenolol glucuronide were attained in 0.5 to 1.5 h and 1 to 2.5 h respectively [P. Dayer *et al., Eur. J. Drug Metab. Pharmacokinet.*, 1983, *8*, 181–188].

Following oral administration of 160 mg twice daily to 27 subjects, steady-state plasma concentrations of 0.1 to 1.8 mg/L (mean 0.9) were reported, determined 1 h after a dose [B. Silke *et al., Eur. J. Clin. Pharmacol.*, 1983, *24*, 7–14].

Toxicity

In a fatality attributed to oxprenolol overdose, a postmortem liver concentration of 58 μg/g was reported [J. S. Oliver and A. A. Watson, *Med. Sci. Law*, 1977, *17*, 279–281].

In a fatality in which death occurred 2 h after the ingestion of 4.5 g, the following postmortem concentrations were reported: blood 10 mg/L, brain 71 μg/g, liver 230 μg/g [A. Khan and J. M. Muscat-Baron, *BMJ*, 1977, *1*, 552].

Half-life. Plasma half-life, 1 to 3 h.

Volume of distribution. About 1 L/kg.

Protein binding. In plasma, about 80%.

Dose. 80 to 480 mg of oxprenolol hydrochloride daily.

Oxybuprocaine

Local Anaesthetic

Synonym. Benoxinate

2-(Diethylamino)ethyl-4-amino-3-butoxybenzoate

$C_{17}H_{28}N_2O_3 = 308.4$

CAS—99-43-4

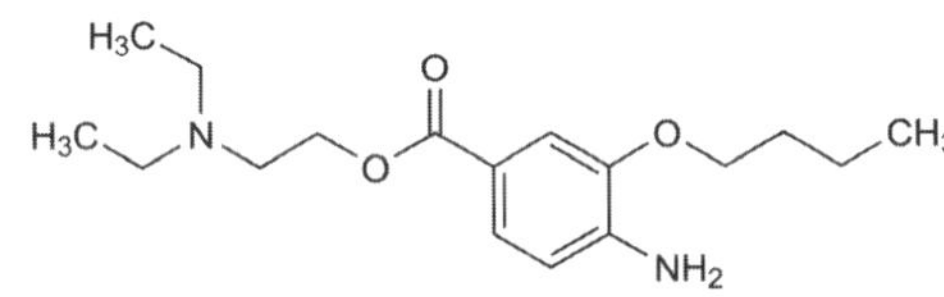

Oxybuprocaine Hydrochloride

Proprietary names. Cébésine; Conjuncain; Novesine.

$C_{17}H_{28}N_2O_3,HCl = 344.9$

CAS—5987-82-6

White crystals or crystalline powder. M.p. about 155° (also reported as 157° to 160°).

Soluble 1 in 0.8 of water, 1 in 2.6 of ethanol and 1 in 2.5 of chloroform; practically insoluble in ether.

Partition Coefficient. Log *P* (octanol/water), 3.5.

Colour Tests. Coniferyl Alcohol—orange; Diazotisation—red.

Thin-layer Chromatography. System TA—Rf 62; system TB—Rf 23; system TC—Rf 41; system TE—Rf 83; system TL—Rf 36; system TAE—Rf 54. (Acidified iodoplatinate solution, positive.)

Gas Chromatography. System GA—RI 2471.

High Performance Liquid Chromatography. System HQ—*k* 16.25; system HR—*k* 0.86; system HX—RI 405.

Ultraviolet Spectrum. Aqueous acid—235 nm (A_1^1=437b), 298 nm; aqueous alkali—231, 310 nm.

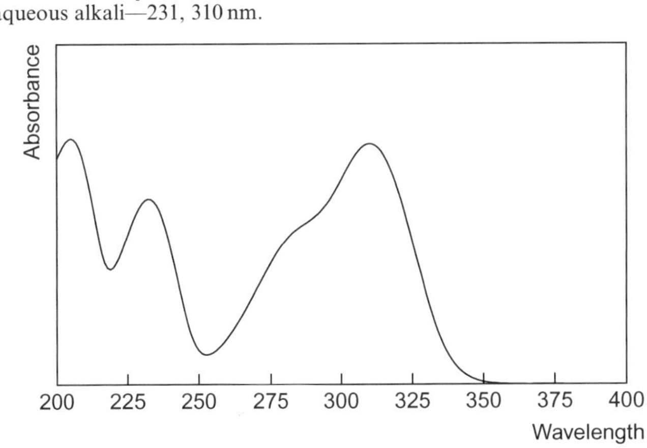

Infra-red Spectrum. Principal peaks at wavenumbers 1709, 1214, 1261, 1613, 1294, 1311 cm^{-1} (oxybuprocaine hydrochloride, KBr disk).

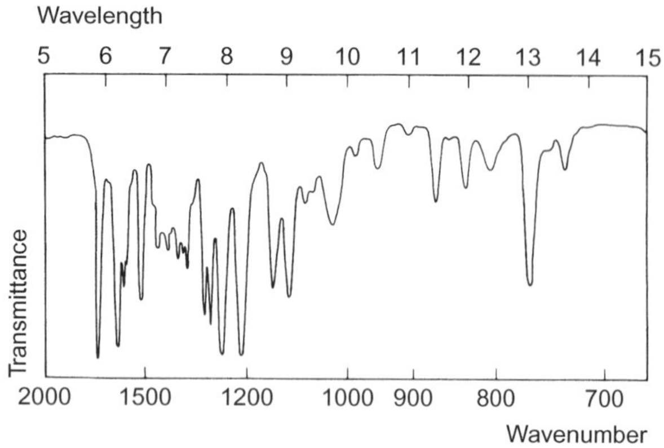

Mass Spectrum. Principal ions at m/z 86, 99, 29, 30, 100, 71, 87, 192.

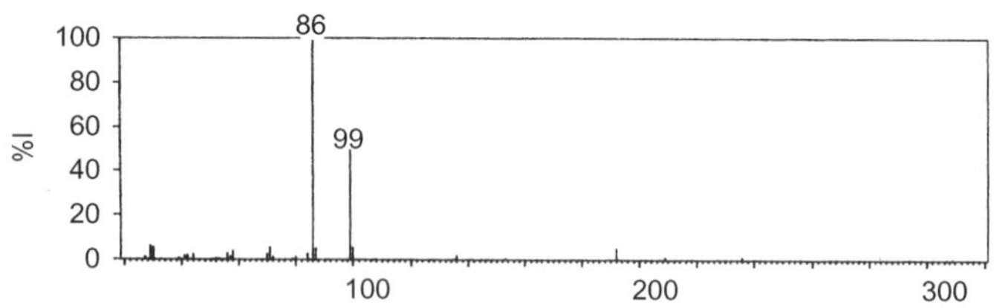

Quantification

Gas chromatography. In blood or cerebrospinal fluid: oxybuprocaine and other local anaesthetics, limit of detection 5 to 10 pg, surface ionisation detection—H. Hattori *et al.*, *J. Chromatogr.*, 1991, *564*, 278–282.

High performance liquid chromatography. In aqueous humour: oxybuprocaine and diclofenac, limit of detection 50 µg/L for oxybuprocaine, electrochemical detection—O. Kuhlmann *et al.*, *J. Pharm. Biomed. Anal.*, 1998, *17*, 1351–1356.

Use. Oxybuprocaine hydrochloride is used as a 0.4% solution.

Oxyclozanide

Anthelmintic (Veterinary)

Proprietary name. Zanil

2,3,5-Trichloro-*N*-(3,5-dichloro-2-hydroxyphenyl)-6-hydroxybenzamide

$C_{13}H_6Cl_5NO_3$=401.5

CAS—2277-92-1

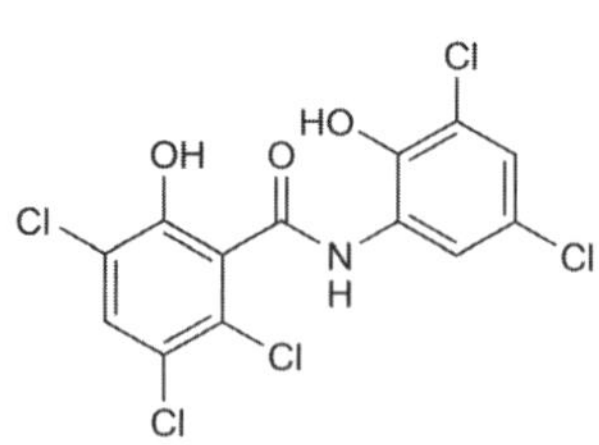

A cream-coloured powder. M.p. 209° to 211°.

Very slightly soluble in water; soluble 1 in 20 of ethanol, 1 in 5 of acetone and 1 in 600 of chloroform; soluble in solutions of alkali hydroxides and carbonates.

Partition Coefficient. Log *P* (octanol/water), 6.0.

Colour Test. Mandelin's Test—violet→orange.

Thin-layer Chromatography. System TA—Rf 87. (Acidified potassium permanganate solution, positive.)

Gas Chromatography. System GA—not eluted.

Ultraviolet Spectrum. Aqueous alkali—324 nm (A_1^1=338b); methanol—303 nm (A_1^1=188b).

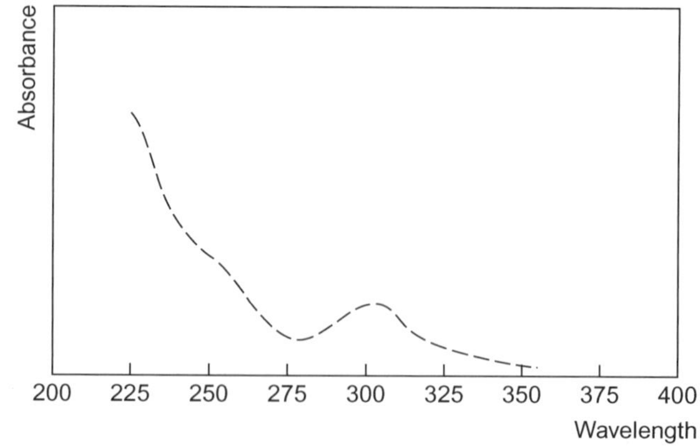

Infra-red Spectrum. Principal peaks at wavenumbers 1203, 1527, 1166, 1587, 1155, 1219 cm^{-1} (KBr disk).

Oxycodone

Narcotic Analgesic

Synonyms. 7,8-Dihydro-14-hydroxycodeinone; Dihydrone; Oxycone; NSC-19043.

(5α)-4,5-Epoxy-14-hydroxy-3-methoxy-17-methylmorphinan-6-one

$C_{18}H_{21}NO_4$=315.4

CAS—76-42-6

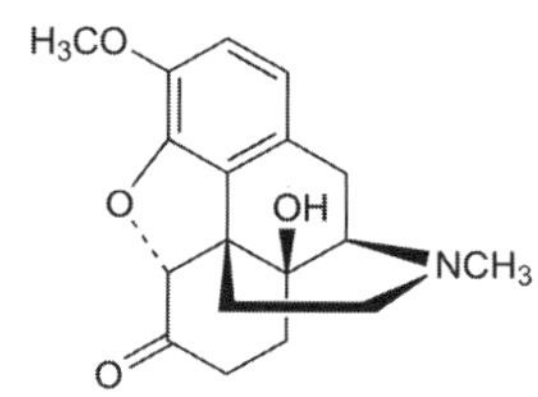

M.p. 218° to 220° (from alcohol).

It is practically insoluble in water and ether; soluble in ethanol and chloroform.

Oxycodone Hydrochloride

Synonym. Thecodine

Proprietary names. Endocodone; Endone; Eubine; Oxanest; Oxycod; Oxycontin; Oxyfast; Oxygesic; OxyIR; OxyNorm; Percolone; Roxicodone; Supeudol. It is an ingredient of Percocet, Percodan, Roxicet, Roxilox, Roxiprin, and Tylox.

$C_{18}H_{21}NO_4,HCl,3H_2O$=405.9

CAS—124-90-3 (anhydrous)

A white crystalline powder. M.p. 270° to 272° (rods from water), with decomposition.

It is soluble 1 in 10 of water, 1 in 60 of ethanol, and 1 in 600 of chloroform; practically insoluble in ether.

Dissociation Constant. pK_a 8.9 (20°).

Partition Coefficient. Log *P* (octanol/water), 0.7.

Colour Test. Marquis Test—yellow→brown→violet.

Thin-layer Chromatography. System TA—Rf 50; system TB—Rf 25; system TC—Rf 51; system TE—Rf 62; system TL—Rf 39; system TAE—Rf 30; system TAF—Rf 33; system TAJ—Rf 27; system TAK—Rf 01; system TAL—Rf 36. (Dragendorff spray, positive; acidified iodoplatinate solution, positive; Marquis reagent, violet.)

Plate: silica (10 × 20 cm). Mobile phase: propanol:acetic acid:water:25% ammonia:methanol (20:1:1:3:10). UV detection. Rf 0.6. [H. E. M. Salomies and P. K. Salo, *J. AOAC Int.*, 2000, *83(6)*, 1497–1501.]

Gas Chromatography. System GA—oxycodone RI 2524, oxycodone-AC RI 2555, oxycodone-enol-AC_2 RI 2560, oxycodone-TFA RI 2290, M (nor-)-enol-AC_3 RI 2680, M (dihydro-)-AC_2 RI 2570, M (nor-dihydro-)-AC_3 RI 2935, M (nor-dihydro-)-AC_2 RI 2900, oxymorphone RI 2538;

system GB—oxycodone RI 2671, oxycodone-TMS RI 2703, oxycodone-enol-TMS_2 RI 2602, oxycodone-oxime-TMS_2 RI 2740, M (nor-) RI 2703, M (nor-)-TMS_2 RI 2763, M (nor-)-enol-TMS_2 RI 2621, M (nor-)-enol-TMS_3 RI 2746, M (dihydro-) RI 2666, oxymorphone RI 2723.

Column: HP-Ultra-2 capillary (25 m × 0.2 mm i.d., 0.33 μm film thickness). Column temperature: 90°, held 2 min; increased to 310° at 15°/min, held at 310° for 15 min. Carrier gas: helium, 0.8 mL/min flow rate. MS detection, SIM (*m/z* 315, 230, 140). Retention time: 18.1 min. [O. H. Drummer *et al.*, *J. Forens. Sci.*, 1994, *39(4)*, 1069–1075.]

Column: fused silica capillary (HP-1, 25 m × 0.2 mm i.d., 0.33 μm film thickness). Column temperature: 150°, increased to 245° at 35°/min. Carrier gas: helium, flow rate 1.5 mL/min at 40° and 0.5 mL/min at 150°. Detection: NPD. Retention time: 12.8 min. [R. P. Kapil *et al.*, *J. Chromatogr.*, 1992, *577(2)*, 283–287.]

High Performance Liquid Chromatography. System HA—oxycodone *k* 6.9 (tailing peak), oxymorphone *k* 6.7 (tailing peak); system HC—*k* 0.85; system HX—RI 277; system HY—RI 246; system HAX—retention time 6.5 min; system HAY—retention time 5.8 min.

Column: Hypersil BDS C_{18} (100 × 46 mm i.d., 3 μm). Mobile phase: potassium dihydrogen phosphate (10 mM, pH 3):acetonitrile (93:7), 1.0 mL/min flow rate. UV detection, (λ = 212 nm). Retention time: 9.1 min. [J. A. Pascual and J. Sanagustin, *J. Chromatogr. B Biomed. Sci. Appl.*, 1999, *724(2)*, 295–302.]

Ultraviolet Spectrum. Aqueous acid—280 nm (A^1_1=44a). No alkaline shift.

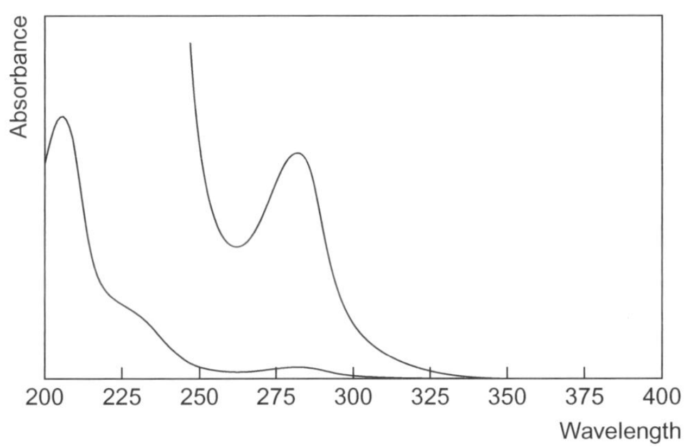

Infra-red Spectrum. Principal peaks at wavenumbers 1719, 1501, 1033, 1255, 934, 980 cm^{-1}(KBr disk).

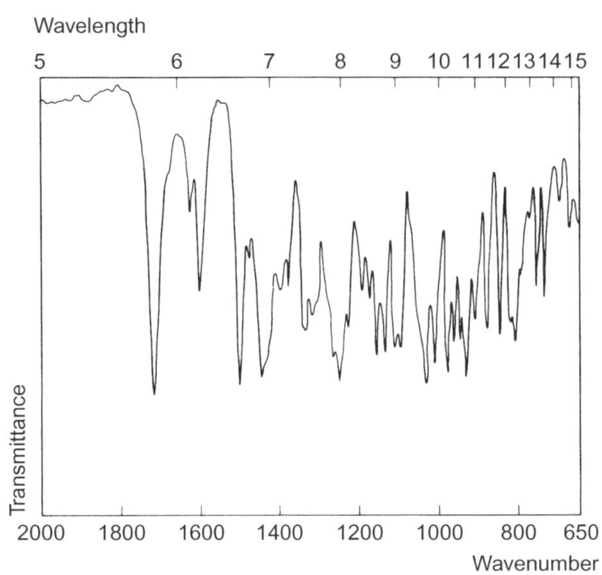

Mass Spectrum. Principal ions at *m/z* 315, 230, 316, 70, 44, 42, 258, 140; oxymorphone 301, 216, 44, 42, 70, 302, 203, 57.

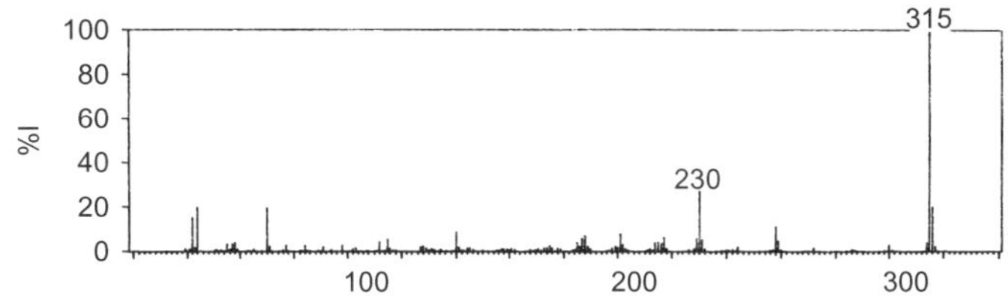

Quantification

Gas chromatography. In plasma: limit of quantification 1.8 μg/L, NPD—R. P. Kapil *et al.*, *J. Chromatogr.*, 1992, *577(2)*, 283–287.

Gas chromatography–mass spectrometry. In urine: oxycodone and other opioids, comparison with immunoassays—M. L. Smith *et al.*, *J. Anal. Toxicol.*, 1995, *19*, 18–26. In urine: oxycodone and other opioids, limit of quantification for oxycodone is 25 μg/L and limit of detection 10 μg/L (*m/z* 344)—R. Meatherall, *J. Anal. Toxicol.*, 1999, *23(3)*, 177–186. In hair or oral fluid: oxycodone and other opioids—J. Jones *et al.*, *J. Anal. Toxicol.*, 2002, *26*, 171–175.

High performance liquid chromatography. In plasma: limit of detection 10 μg/L, ECD—M. T. Smith *et al.*, *Ther. Drug Monit.*, 1991, *13*, 126–130. In plasma: limit of quantification 5.3 pmol, electrochemical detection—A. W. Wright *et al.*, *J. Chromatogr. B Biomed. Sci. Appl.*, 1998, *712*, 169–175.

High performance liquid chromatography—mass spectrometry. In plasma: limit of quantification 1 μg/L. MS detection (ESI)—M. Dawson *et al.*, *J. Chromatogr. Sci.*, 2002, *40*, 40–44.

Disposition in the Body. Absorbed after oral administration. Metabolised to some extent by *O*-demethylation to oxymorphone which is active, and by *N*-demethylation to noroxycodone. About 30 to 60% of a dose is excreted in the urine in 24 h as free and conjugated oxycodone, conjugated oxymorphone, and noroxycodone. Oxymorphone is excreted mainly in the conjugated form and noroxycodone as the unconjugated. After multiple dosing, accumulation of the drug does not occur. Oxycodone is secreted in breast milk.

Therapeutic concentration

24 healthy volunteers, aged 21 to 50 years (mean, 34.5 years old) were administered either a 10-mg controlled-release oxycodone hydrochloride tablet every 12 h for 4 days or 5 mg of immediate-release oxycodone hydrochloride solution every 6 h for 4 days. Volunteers were fasted 2 h before and after drug administration. Steady-state concentrations were observed after 1 day of dosing and maintained until day 4. The mean maximum plasma oxycodone concentration, after the controlled-release formulation, was 15.1 μg/L and after the immediate-release formulation, 15.6 μg/L. These concentrations were observed at 3.2 and 1.4 h, respectively. [R. F. Reder *et al.*, *Clin. Ther.*, 1996, *18(1)*, 95–105.]

In 28 subjects administered a single 20-mg oral controlled-release oxycodone tablet, mean maximum plasma concentrations of 23.2 μg/L for oxycodone, 15.2 μg/L for noroxycodone, and 0.8 μg/L for oxymorphone occurred at 3.2, 4.3, and 4.5 h after dosing, respectively. When compared for gender and age, young and elderly women (7 subjects in each group) had the highest oxycodone AUC values, the lowest oxymorphone AUC values, and the greatest drug effect. Young and elderly men (7 subjects in each group) had the lowest oxycodone AUC values, the highest oxymorphone AUC values, and the lowest drug effect. [R. F. Kaiko *et al.*, *Clin. Pharmacol. Ther.*, 1996, *59*, 52–61.]

9 healthy, young, male and female volunteers were administered 0.14 mg/kg oxycodone hydrochloride once IM (equivalent to 0.11 mg/kg free base) in the first study and 0.28 mg/kg oxycodone chloride orally (equivalent to 0.22 mg/kg free base) in two additional studies at intervals of 2 weeks. The mean maximum plasma oxycodone concentration was 34.0 μg/L for the IM dose and 38.0 μg/L for the oral doses, observed within an hour of administration. The peak noroxycodone concentration, after the IM dose, was 4.0 μg/L and after the oral doses, 14.8 μg/L. These were observed at 1.75 (0.75 to 5.0) h and 0.75 (0.25 to 2.0) h, respectively. [R. Poyhia *et al.*, *Br. J. Clin. Pharmacol.*, 1992, *33(6)*, 617–621.]

12 patients with moderate-to-severe cancer pain and a mean age of 58 years (23 to 71 years old) were administered 5 mL oxycodone hydrochloride (concentration 5 mg/mL, equivalent to 4.6 mg/mL base) as an IV infusion and 10 mg oxycodone hydrochloride every 4 h (equivalent to 9.1 mg base). A mean maximum plasma concentration of 34.6 (17.0 to 62.2) μg/L was observed at 1.6 h for the oral dose. A steady state concentration of 47.7 (26.8 to 68.9) μg/L was observed at 1.04 (0.25 to 2.0) h. The minimum

steady-state concentration was 23.5 (10.4 to 43.1) μg/L. [K. P. Leow *et al.*, *Clin. Pharmacol. Ther.*, 1992, *52(5)*, 487–495.]

Toxicity. The estimated minimum lethal dose is 500 mg. Prolonged use of oxycodone may lead to dependence of the morphine type. A toxic serum concentration is 0.2 mg/L and a probable lethal concentration 0.6 mg/L.

A review of postmortem and coroners' reports from 10 countries for 2000 and 2001 revealed 88 cases of death caused by oxycodone or hydrocodone exposure, 24 of which were attributed to oxycodone alone. Mean and median postmortem oxycodone blood concentrations of 1.23 and 0.43 mg/L, respectively, were reported (range 0.12 to 8.0 mg/L); in 13 cases the concentration was ⩾0.5 mg/L. In 7 cases in which death was attributed to a combination of oxycodone and hydrocodone, the mean concentrations were reported to be 0.34 and 0.14 mg/L, respectively. [H. A. Spiller, *J. Forensic Sci.*, 2003, *48*, 429–431.]

A 45-year-old woman who was admitted to hospital after suffering a generalised convulsion, had been discovered next to a nearly full bottle of controlled-release oxycodone tablets; unfortunately the bottle was left near her bedside and, approximately 20 min after her arrival, she ingested the remaining contents (when full, the bottle contained 100 × 40-mg tablets). The patient developed CNS and respiratory depression, and IV naloxone and oral activated charcoal were administered. Naloxone proved inadequate and mechanical ventilation was required for 3 days before the patient recovered completely. Three serum oxycodone levels were noted: the initial and highest was 2400 μg/L 10 h after admission; the level declined to approximately 1000 μg/L at 15 h and 100 μg/L at 70 h. [A. B. Scneir *et al.*, *Ann. Emerg. Med.*, 2002, *40*, 425–428.]

A 28-year-old male heroin addict with acquired immune deficiency syndrome (AIDS) died while in police custody. Toxic concentrations of oxycodone were found in femoral blood at a concentration of 1.2 mg/L and in his liver at 1.9 mg/kg. Traces of flunitrazepam were also detected in his blood. His death was determined to be caused by a combination of the toxic effects of both oxycodone and flunitrazepam. In a total of 9 cases investigated by the Victorian Institute of Forensic Pathology, Australia (one example as above), the mean femoral blood oxycodone concentration was 0.9 mg/L (range, 0.6 to 1.4 mg/L). Oxycodone was not detected very often in the gastric contents. It was shown that oxycodone femoral blood concentrations of 0.6 mg/L or higher may result in death. [O. H. Drummer *et al.*, *J. Forensic Sci.*, 1994, *39(4)*, 1069–1075.]

Half-life. Elimination, 2 to 3 h.

Note: for a review of the clinical pharmacokinetics and pharmacodynamics of oxycodone, see R. Poyhia *et al.*, *J. Pain Symptom. Manage.*, 1993, *8*, 63–67.

Dose. Oxycodone hydrochloride may be given by mouth in doses of 10 to 40 mg.

Oxymetazoline

Sympathomimetic

3-[(4,5-Dihydro-1*H*-imidazol-2-yl)methyl]-6-(1,1-dimethylethyl)-2,4-dimethylphenol
$C_{16}H_{24}N_2O$=260.4
CAS—1491-59-4

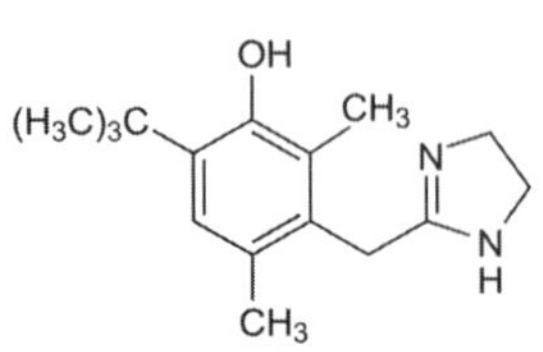

Crystals. M.p. 181° to 183°.

Oxymetazoline Hydrochloride

Proprietary names. Afrazine; Afrin; Drixine; Durazol; Hazol; Iliadin-Mini; Nafrine; Nasivin; Rhinolitan.
$C_{16}H_{24}N_2O,HCl$=296.8
CAS—2315-02-8
A white, hygroscopic, crystalline powder. M.p. 300° to 303°, with decomposition.
Soluble 1 in 6.7 of water and 1 in 3.6 of ethanol; practically insoluble in benzene, chloroform and ether.

Partition Coefficient. Log *P* (octanol/water), 4.9.

Colour Test. Mandelin's Test—green.

Thin-layer Chromatography. System TA—Rf 09; system TB—Rf 01; system TC—Rf 01; system TE—Rf 34; system TL—Rf 01; system TAE—Rf 80; system TAJ—Rf 00; system TAK—Rf 01; system TAL—Rf 25. (Acidified iodoplatinate solution, positive.)

Gas Chromatography. System GA—RI 2170.

High Performance Liquid Chromatography. System HA—*k* 1.7.

Ultraviolet Spectrum. Aqueous acid—280 nm (A^1_1=68a); aqueous alkali—303 nm (A^1_1=164b).

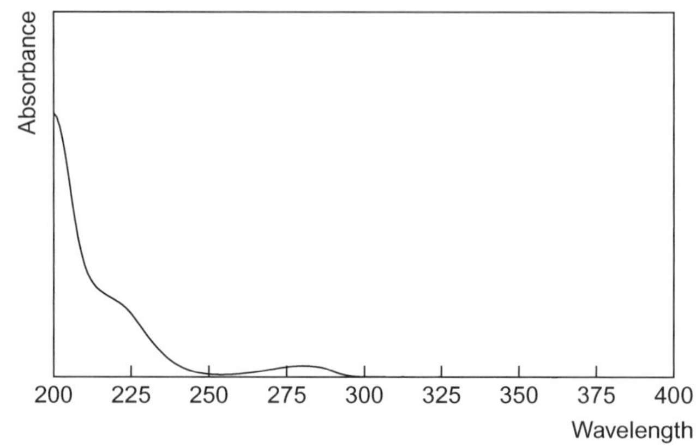

Infra-red Spectrum. Principal peaks at wavenumbers 1595, 1199, 1285, 1250, 1070, 765 cm^{-1} (oxymetazoline hydrochloride, KBr disk).

Mass Spectrum. Principal ions at *m/z* 245, 260, 44, 217, 218, 246, 261, 259.

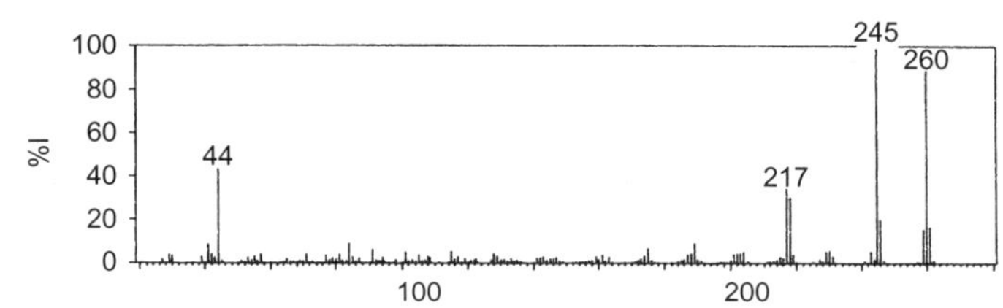

Use. Oxymetazoline hydrochloride is used as a 0.05% solution.

Oxymetholone

Anabolic Steroid

Proprietary names. Adroyd; Anadrol-50; Anapolon; Anasteron; Nastenon; Pardroyd; Plenastril.
(5α,17β)-17-Hydroxy-2-(hydroxymethylene)-17-methylandrostan-3-one
$C_{21}H_{32}O_3$=332.5
CAS—434-07-1

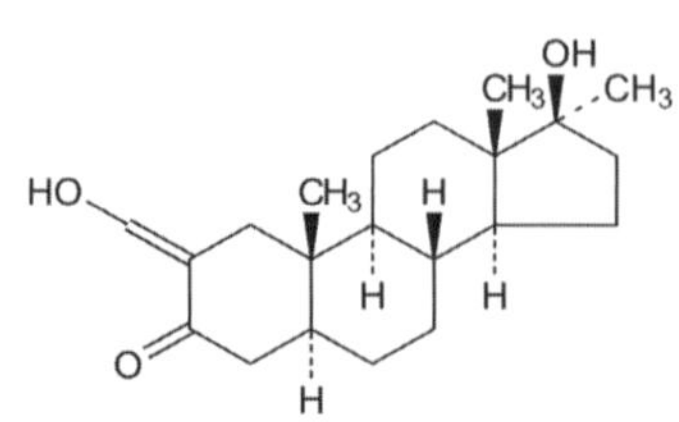

A white to creamy-white crystalline powder. M.p. 172° to 180°.
Practically insoluble in water; soluble 1 in 50 of ethanol; freely soluble in chloroform; soluble in dioxan; slightly soluble in ether.

Partition Coefficient. Log *P* (octanol/water), 3.6.

Colour Tests. Antimony Pentachloride—brown; Naphthol–Sulfuric Acid—brown/pink-orange; Sulfuric Acid—orange.

Thin-layer Chromatography. System TA—Rf 95; system TE—Rf 09; system TP—Rf 69; system TQ—Rf 23; system TR—Rf 85; system TS—Rf

82; system TAJ—Rf 70; system TAK—Rf 74; system TAL—Rf 94; system TAM—Rf 86. (*p*-Toluenesulfonic acid solution, positive.)

Gas Chromatography. System GA—oxymetholone RI 3005; oxymetholone enol-TMS_3 RI 2870; system GAI—urinary metabolites: 17α-methyl-5α-androstan-3α,17β-diol RRT 0.925, 2-hydroxymethyl-17α-methyl-5-androstan-3,17-diol RRT 1.106, 2-hydroxymethyl-17α-methyl-5-androstan-3, 6, 17-triol RRT 1.180 (relative to 17α-methyl-5α-androstan-3β,17β-diol); system GAG—RRT 1.28 (relative to testosterone); system GAR—oxymetholone, Retention time 13.7 min.

High Performance Liquid Chromatography. System HATb—RRT 2.64 (relative to testosterone).

Ultraviolet Spectrum. Methanolic acid—277 nm (A_1^1=300b); methanolic alkali—315 (A_1^1=547a).

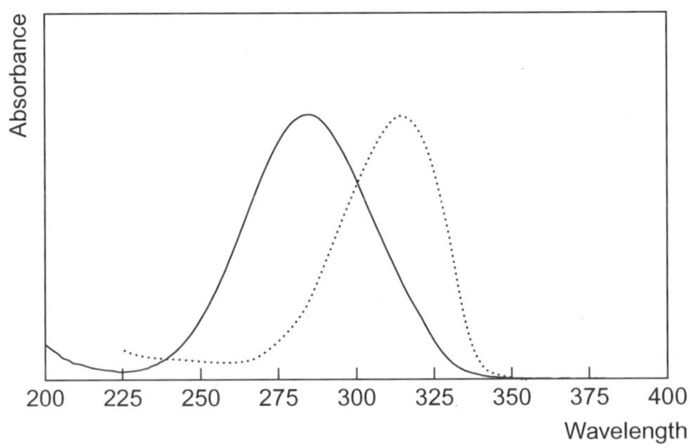

Infra-red Spectrum. Principal peaks at wavenumbers 1612, 1204, 1219, 1306, 1157, 935 cm^{-1} (KBr disk).

Quantification
Gas chromatography–mass spectrometry. In plasma—C. R. Cardoso *et al.*, *J. Chromatogr. B Anal. Technol. Biomed. Life Sci.*, 2002, *775*, 1–8.

Dose. Usually 5 to 10 mg daily; doses of 100 to 350 mg daily may be given.

Oxymorphone

Narcotic Analgesic

Synonyms. 7,8-Dihydro-14-hydroxymorphinone; Oximorphone; Oxydimorphone.
(5α)-4,5-Epoxy-3,14-dihydroxy-17-methylmorphinan-6-one
$C_{17}H_{19}NO_4$=301.3
CAS—76-41-5

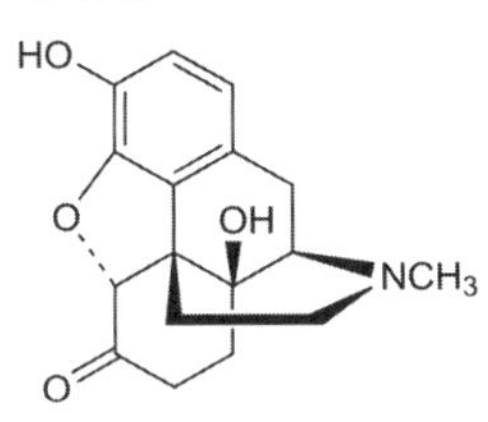

Crystals. M.p. 248° to 249°, with decomposition.
Soluble in boiling acetone and chloroform; readily soluble in aqueous alkalies; moderately soluble in boiling ethanol; sparingly soluble in benzene.

Oxymorphone Hydrochloride

Proprietary name. Numorphan
$C_{17}H_{19}NO_4$,HCl=337.8
CAS—357-07-3
A white powder which darkens on exposure to light.
Soluble 1 in 4 of water, 1 in 100 of ethanol, and 1 in 25 of methanol; very slightly soluble in chloroform and ether.

Dissociation Constant. pK_a 8.5, 9.3.

Partition Coefficient. Log *P* (octanol/pH 7.4), 0.

Colour Test. Marquis Test—grey-violet.

Thin-layer Chromatography. System TA—Rf 48; system TB—Rf 10; system TC—Rf 37; system TE—Rf 33; system TL—Rf 30; system TAE—Rf 27; system TAF—Rf 36; system TAJ—Rf 13; system TAK—Rf 00; system TAL—Rf 13. (Dragendorff spray, positive; acidified iodoplatinate solution, positive; Marquis reagent, grey.)

Gas Chromatography. System GA—oxymorphone RI 2723, oxymorphone-TMS RI 2715, oxymorphone-TMS_2 RI 2728, oxymorphone-TMS_3 RI 2641, oxymorphone-oxime-TMS_3 RI 2748, M (nor-) not eluted, M (nor-)-enol-TMS_2 RI 2788, M (nor-)-enol-TMS_3 RI 2662, M (nor-)-enol-TMS_4 RI 2773, M (dihydro-) RI 2690.

Column: DB-5 (30 m × 0.25 mm i.d., 0.25 μm film thickness). Column temperature: 130° for 1 min to 270° at 10°/min. Carrier gas: helium. MS detection (EI, FS). Retention time: 20.5 min. [W. Nowatzke *et al.*, *J. Pharm. Biomed. Anal.*, 1999, *20*, 815–828.]

High Performance Liquid Chromatography. System HA—*k* 6.7 (tailing peak); system HX—RI 217; system HY—RI 184.

Ultraviolet Spectrum. Aqueous acid—281 (A_1^1=34a); aqueous alkali—292 nm.

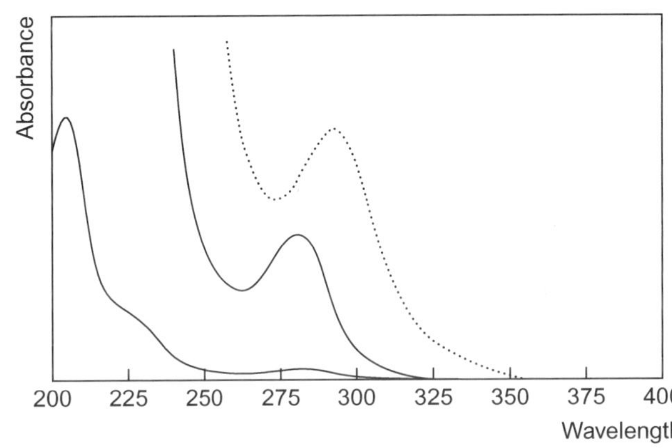

Infra-red Spectrum. Principal ions at wavenumbers 1730, 1240, 1225, 1145, 941, 953 cm^{-1} (KBr disk).

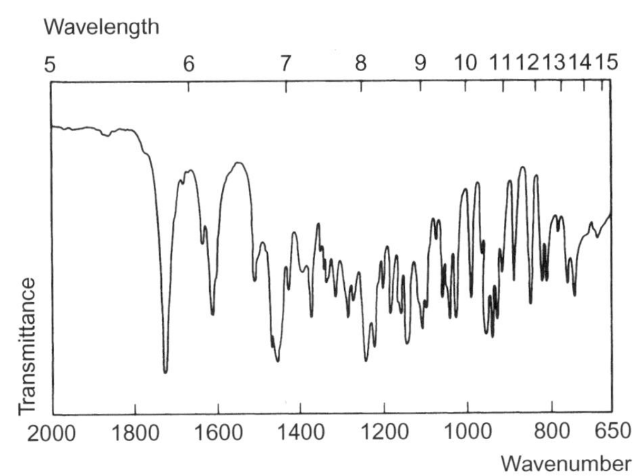

Mass Spectrum. Principal ions at *m*/*z* 301, 216, 44, 42, 70, 302, 203, 57.

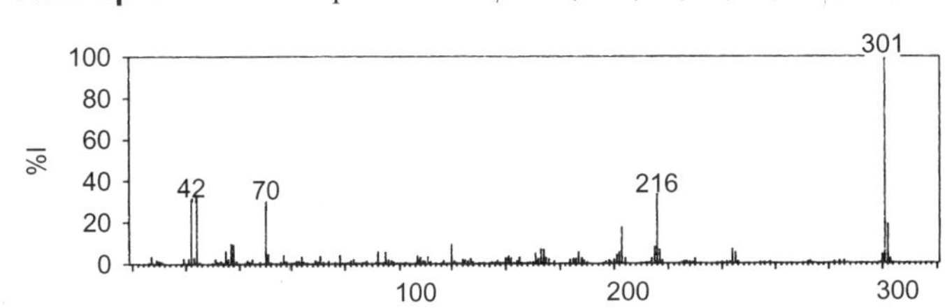

Quantification
Gas chromatography–mass spectrometry. In urine: oxymorphone and other opioids, comparison with immunoassays—M. L. Smith *et al.*, *J. Anal.*

Toxicol., 1995, *19*, 18–26. In urine: oxymorphone and other opioids, limit of quantification for oxymorphone is 25 μg/L and limit of detection 10 μg/L (*m/z* 330)—R. Meatherall, *J. Anal. Toxicol.*, 1999, *23(3)*, 177–186. In hair or oral fluid: oxymorphone and other opioids—J. Jones *et al.*, *J. Anal. Toxicol.*, 2002, *26*, 171–175.

Disposition in the Body. Absorbed after oral administration. About 50% of an oral dose is excreted in the urine in 5 days (mostly in the first 24 h), mainly as conjugated oxymorphone together with small quantities of unchanged drug and the conjugated 6α- and 6β-hydroxy metabolites. Oxymorphone is a metabolite of oxycodone.

Therapeutic concentration

2 healthy male volunteers with a history of heroin abuse participated in the study. Prior to the study, each subject was required to test negative for morphine in urine for 3 consecutive days. Each volunteer was administered 1.5 mg and 3 mg IM oxymorphone. Peak plasma concentrations for subject 1 after 24 and 36 h were 164 μg/L and 91 μg/L, respectively, for the 1.5-mg dose and 435 μg/L and 120 μg/L, respectively, for the 3-mg dose. For subject 2, the levels at 24 and 36 h were 434 μg/L and 381 μg/L, respectively, for the 1.5-mg dose and 654 μg/L and 129 μg/L, respectively, for the 3-mg dose. [M. L. Smith *et al.*, *J. Anal. Toxicol.*, 1995, *19*, 18–26.]

Toxicity. The estimated minimum lethal dose is 50 mg. Prolonged use of oxymorphone may lead to dependence of the morphine type.

Note. For a study of oxymorphone metabolism in human, rat, guinea pig, rabbit and dog, see E. J. Cone *et al.*, *Drug Met. Disp.*, 1983, *11*, 446–450.

Dose. 0.5 to 1.5 mg of oxymorphone hydrochloride given parenterally; doses of 5 to 10 mg have been given by mouth.

Oxypertine

Tranquilliser

Synonym. Win-18501-2

Proprietary names. Equipertine; Forit; Integrin; Opertil.

5,6-Dimethoxy-2-methyl-3-[2-(4-phenyl-1-piperazinyl)ethyl]-1*H*-indole

$C_{23}H_{29}N_3O_2$=379.5

CAS—153-87-7

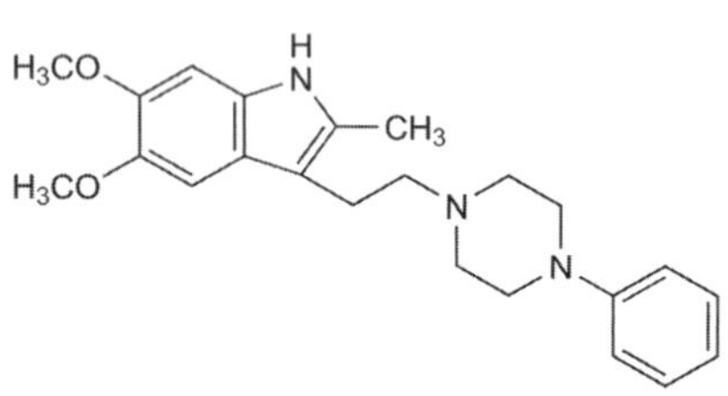

A white crystalline powder.

Slightly soluble in water and ethanol.

Partition Coefficient. Log *P* (octanol/water), 3.8.

Colour Tests. Liebermann's Test—blue; Mandelin's Test—grey; Marquis Test—grey-green.

Thin-layer Chromatography. System TA—Rf 68; system TB—Rf 04; system TC—Rf 65; system TE—Rf 78; system TL—Rf 58; system TAE—Rf 74. (Acidified iodoplatinate solution, positive.)

Gas Chromatography. System GA—RI 2355.

High Performance Liquid Chromatography. System HA—*k* 0.7; system HF—*k* 1.33; system HX—RI 402.

Ultraviolet Spectrum. Aqueous acid—301 nm (A^1_1=212b). No alkaline shift.

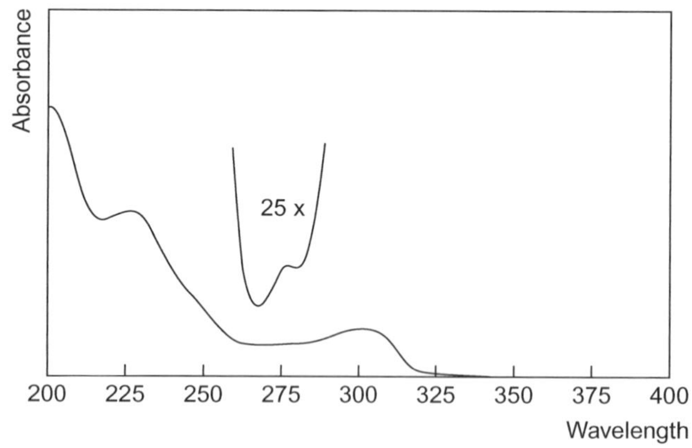

Infra-red Spectrum. Principal peaks at wavenumbers 1233, 1153, 1205, 1592, 762, 1003 cm^{-1} (KBr disk).

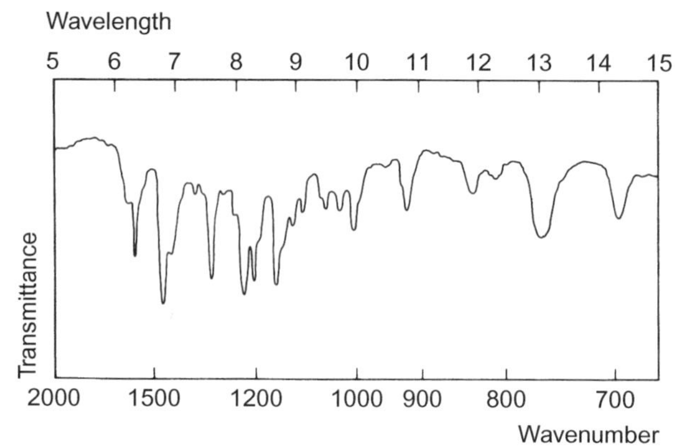

Mass Spectrum. Principal ions at *m/z* 175, 70, 176, 132, 379, 204, 56, 217.

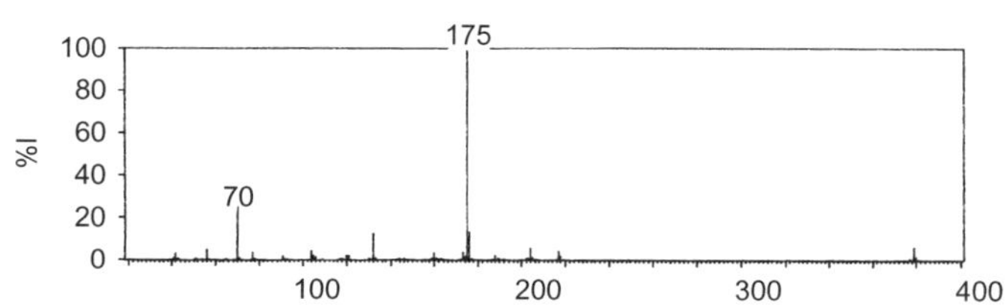

Quantification

Gas chromatography. In plasma: oxypertine and other antipsychotic drugs, limits of detection 5 to 200 μg/L, nitrogen–phosphorus detection—H. Tokunaga *et al.*, *Nippon Hoigaku Zasshi*, 1996, *50*, 196–202.

High performance liquid chromatography. In serum: limit of 20 μg/L, UV detection—Y. Minatogawa *et al.*, *J. Chromatogr.*, 1983, *274*; *Biomed. Appl.*, *25*, 413–416.

Dose. Usually up to 300 mg daily.

Oxyphenbutazone

Analgesic

Synonym. Hydroxyphenylbutazone; G-27202

Proprietary names. Imbun; Isobutil; Oxalid; Oxybutazone; Phlogase; Rheumapax; Tandearil; Tanderil.

4-Butyl-1-(4-hydroxyphenyl)-2-phenyl-3,5-pyrazolidinedione

$C_{19}H_{20}N_2O_3,H_2O$=342.4

CAS—129-20-4 (anhydrous); 7081-38-1 (monohydrate)

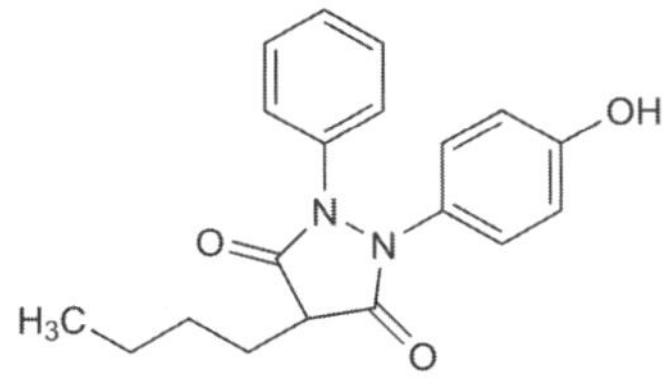

A white to yellowish-white crystalline powder. M.p. 96°. Monohydrate. Soluble in ethanol, methanol, chloroform, benzene and ether. Forms a water-soluble sodium salt.

Dissociation Constant. pK_a 4.7 (22°).

Partition Coefficient. Log *P* (octanol/water), 2.7.

Colour Test. Marquis Test—yellow.

Thin-layer Chromatography. System TA—Rf 77; system TB—Rf 00; system TD—Rf 52; system TE—Rf 09; system TF—Rf 62; system TG—Rf 25; system TAD—Rf 57; system TAE—Rf 90; system TAJ—Rf 56; system TAK—Rf 41; system TAL—Rf 92. (Chromic acid solution, yellow; Ludy Tenger reagent, orange; mercurous nitrate spray, positive; acidified potassium permanganate solution, positive.)

Gas Chromatography. System GA—oxyphenbutazone—not eluted; oxyphenbutazone-Me_2 (isomer 1) RI 2545; oxyphenbutazone-Me_2 (isomer 2) RI 2720; system GD—RRT of methyl derivative 2.11 (relative to *n*-$C_{16}H_{34}$.)

High Performance Liquid Chromatography. System HD—*k* 1.95; system HV—RRT 0.69 (relative to meclofenamic acid); system HX—RI 501; system HY—RI 459; system HZ—Retention time, 6.7 min.

Ultraviolet Spectrum. Aqueous acid—237 nm; aqueous alkali—254 nm (A^1_1=750a).

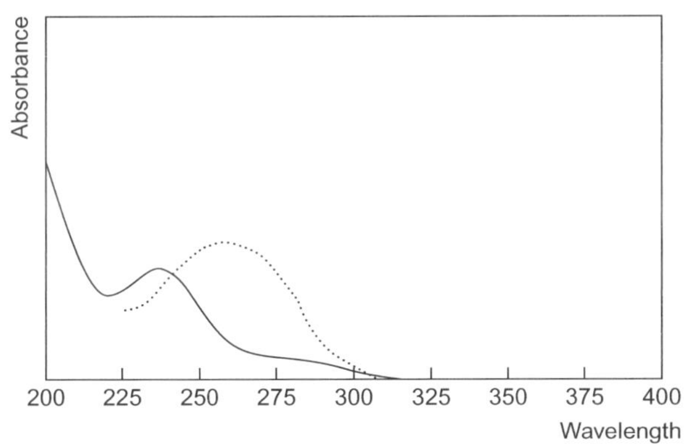

Infra-red Spectrum. Principal peaks at wavenumbers 1683, 1736, 1275, 1512, 765, 1600 cm^{-1} (KBr disk).

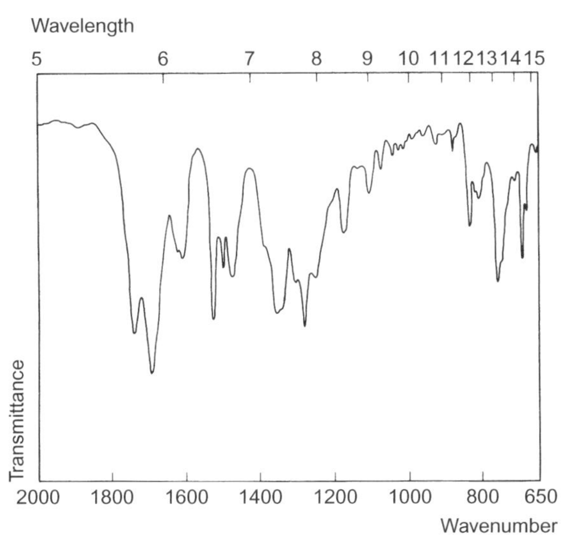

Mass Spectrum. Principal ions at *m/z* 199, 324, 93, 77, 65, 55, 121, 135.

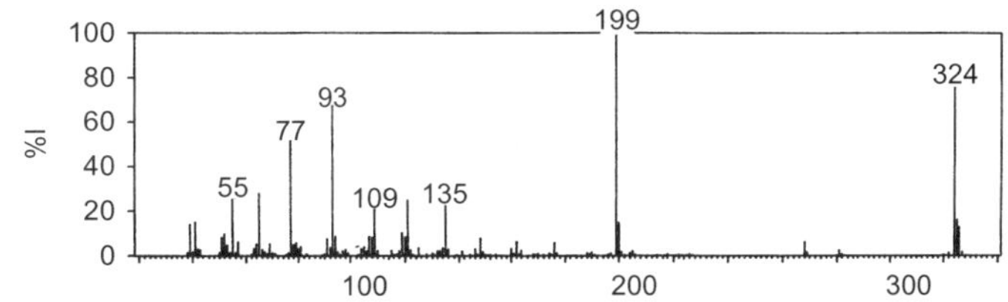

Quantification. See also Phenylbutazone.

Gas chromatography. In plasma: limit of detection 2.5 mg/L, AFID—M. Bertrand *et al.*, *J. Chromatogr.*, 1979, *171*, 377–383.

High performance liquid chromatography. In plasma: limit of detection 250 µg/L, UV detection—N. J. Pound and R. W. Sears, *J. Pharm. Sci.*, 1975, *64*, 284–287.

Disposition in the Body. Almost completely absorbed after oral administration. It is slowly metabolised by glucuronide conjugation and by hydroxylation; it is slowly excreted in the urine, less than 2% of a dose being excreted as unchanged drug and about 1 to 5% as the *O*-glucuronide conjugate in 24 h.

Oxyphenbutazone is a major metabolite of phenylbutazone.

Therapeutic concentration

Following a single oral dose of 200 mg to 10 subjects, peak plasma concentrations of 11.4 to 43.7 mg/L were attained in 2 to 12 h [M. Bertrand *et al.*, *J. Chromatogr.*, 1979, *171*, 377–383].

Following daily oral doses of 300 to 400 mg to 6 subjects, steady-state plasma concentrations determined immediately before a dose ranged from 27 to 95 mg/L (mean 62) [M. Weiner *et al.*, *Proc. Soc. Exp. Biol. Med.*, 1967, *124*, 1170–1173].

Toxicity. The estimated minimum lethal dose is 5 g.

Half-life. Plasma half-life, about 2 to 3 days.

Volume of distribution. About 0.1 L/kg.

Protein binding. In plasma, about 99%.

Dose. Oxyphenbutazone has been given in doses of 100 to 800 mg daily.

Oxyphencyclimine

Anticholinergic

Proprietary names. Antalcus; Zamanil.

α-Cyclohexyl-α-hydroxybenzeneacetic acid (1,4,5,6-tetrahydro-1-methyl-2-pyrimidinyl)methyl ester

$C_{20}H_{28}N_2O_3$=344.5

CAS—125-53-1

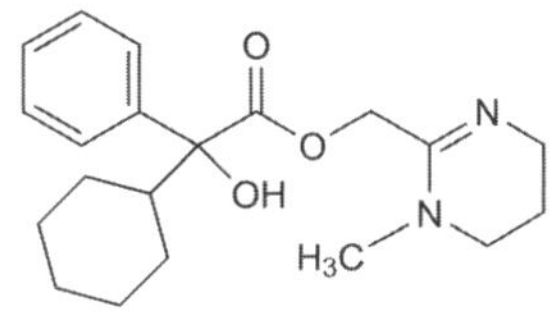

Oxyphencyclimine Hydrochloride

Proprietary names. Daricon; Manir; Vagogastrin. It is an ingredient of Enarax and Vistrax.

$C_{20}H_{28}N_2O_3$,HCl=380.9

CAS—125-52-0

A white crystalline powder. M.p. 231° to 232° with decomposition.

Soluble 1 in 100 of water, 1 in 75 of ethanol, 1 in 500 of chloroform, 1 in 3000 of ether and 1 in 20 of methanol.

Partition Coefficient. Log *P* (octanol/water), 3.5.

Colour Test. Mandelin's Test—grey-green.

Thin-layer Chromatography. System TA—Rf 02; system TB—Rf 01; system TC—Rf 03; system TE—Rf 06; system TL—Rf 00; system TAE—Rf 02; system TAF—Rf 18; system TAJ—Rf 00; system TAK—Rf 01; system TAL—Rf 24. (Acidified iodoplatinate solution, positive.)

Gas Chromatography. System GA—RI 1661 and 2250; system GF—RI 2900.

High Performance Liquid Chromatography. System HA—*k* 2.8; system HX—RI 424.

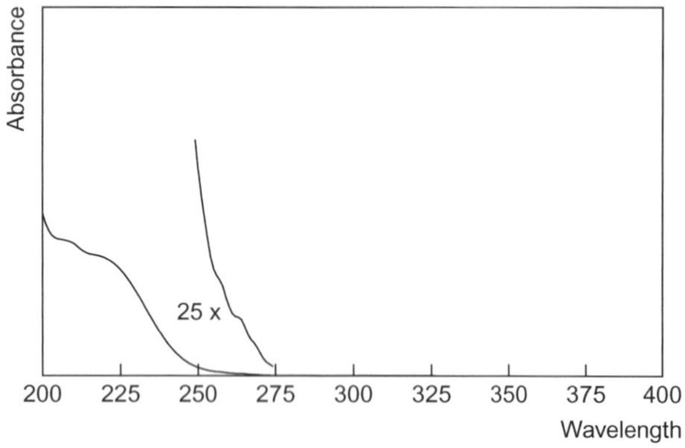

Infra-red Spectrum. Principal peaks at wavenumbers 1656, 1737, 1227, 705, 1201, 1211 cm^{-1} (oxyphencyclimine hydrochloride, KBr disk).

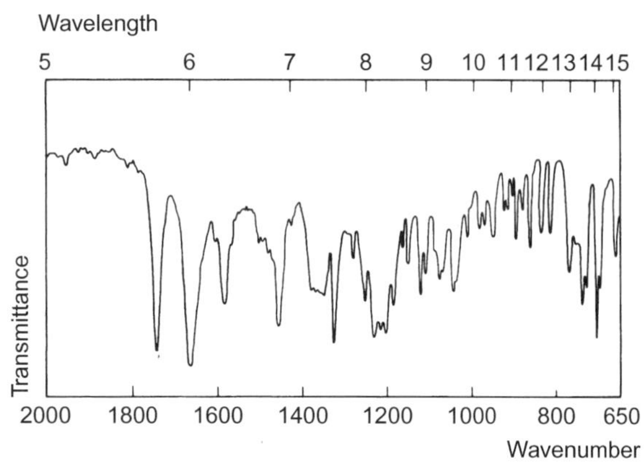

Mass Spectrum. Principal ions at *m/z* 105, 129, 112, 77, 42, 313, 41, 55.

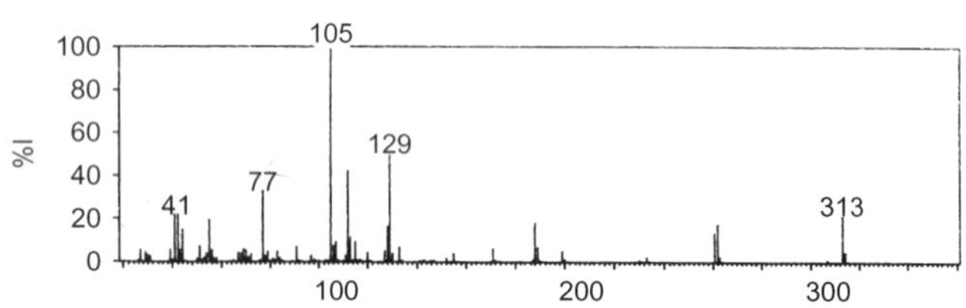

Dose. 10 to 20 mg of oxyphencyclimine hydrochloride daily; up to 50 mg daily has been given.

Oxyphenisatine

Purgative

Synonym. Dihydroxyphenylisatin
Proprietary name. Veripaque
3,3-Bis[4-hydroxyphenyl]-1,3-dihydro-2*H*-indol-2-one
$C_{20}H_{15}NO_3$=317.3
CAS—125-13-3

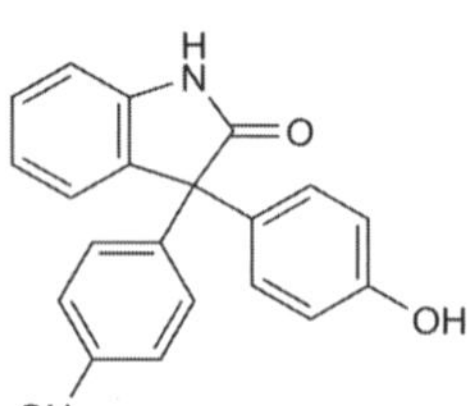

Oxyphenisatine Acetate

Synonyms. Acetphenolisatin; Bisatin; Diacetoxydiphenylisatin; Diacetyldiphenolisatin; Diasatin; Diphesatin; Isaphenin; Oxyphenisatin Acetate.
$C_{24}H_{19}NO_5$=401.4
CAS—115-33-3

A white crystalline powder. M.p. about 242°.
Practically insoluble in water, ether and dilute hydrochloric acid; soluble 1 in 70 of chloroform; slightly soluble in ethanol.

Partition Coefficient. Log *P* (octanol/water), 3.5 (acetate).

Colour Tests. Folin–Ciocalteu Reagent—blue; Koppanyi–Zwikker Test—violet; Liebermann's Test—black; Mandelin's Test—violet; Marquis Test—violet; Mercurous Nitrate—black.

Thin-layer Chromatography. System TA—Rf 82. (Acidified potassium permanganate solution, positive.)

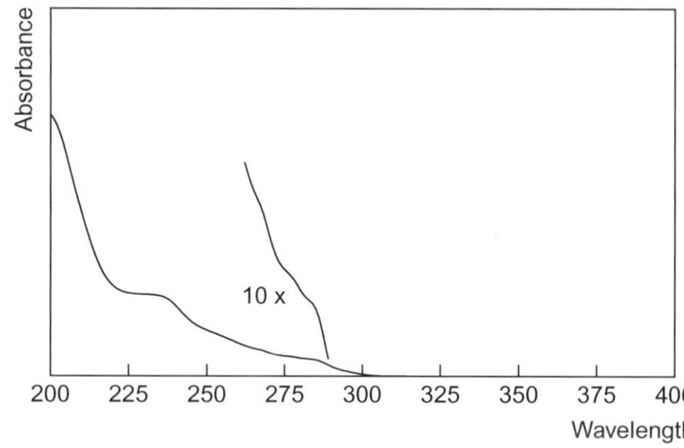

Infra-red Spectrum. Principal peaks at wavenumbers 1188, 1727, 1495, 1232, 1162, 1011 cm^{-1} (KBr disk).

Mass Spectrum. Principal ions at *m/z* 317, 288, 359, 401, 43, 318, 289, 196 (oxyphenisatine acetate).

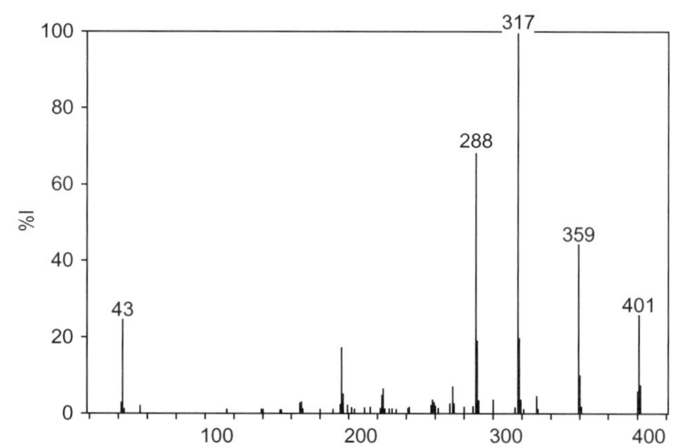

Dose. Oxyphenisatine acetate has been given in a dose of 5 to 20 mg.

Oxyphenonium Bromide

Anticholinergic

Synonyms. Ba-5473; C-5473; Spasmophen.
Proprietary names. Antrenil; Antrenyl.
2-[(Cyclohexylhydroxyphenylacetyl)oxy]-*N*,*N*-diethyl-*N*-methylethanaminium bromide
$C_{21}H_{34}BrNO_3$=428.4
CAS—14214-84-7 (oxyphenonium); 50-10-2 (bromide)

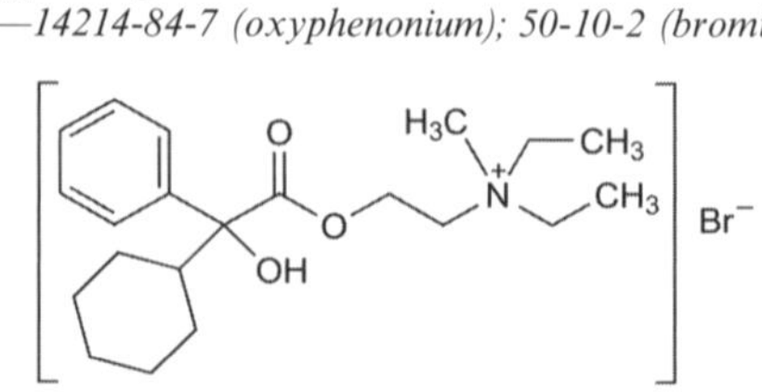

A white crystalline powder. M.p. about 190°.
Freely soluble in water; sparingly soluble in alcohol.

Partition Coefficient. Log P (octanol/water), 0.2.

Thin-layer Chromatography. System TA—Rf 03; system TB—Rf 00; system TC—Rf 01; system TE—Rf 01; system TL—Rf 00; system TAE—Rf 02; system TAF—Rf 36. (Acidified iodoplatinate solution, positive.)

Gas Chromatography. System GA—Art RI 2173 and 2243.

High Performance Liquid Chromatography. System HA—k 2.6 (tailing peak); system HX—RI 424.

Ultraviolet Spectrum. Aqueous acid—252, 258 nm (A_1^1=5.3a), 264 nm.

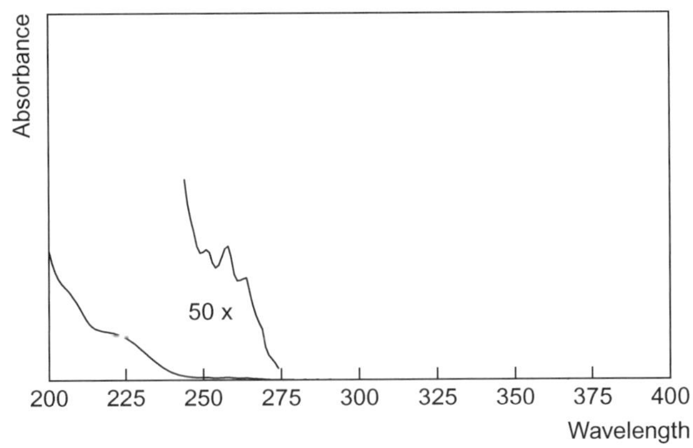

Infra-red Spectrum. Principal peaks at wavenumbers 1225, 1719, 729, 704, 1030, 1111 cm^{-1} (KBr disk).

Quantification

Gas chromatography. In plasma or urine: limits of detection 2 µg/L and 200 µg/L respectively, ECD—J. E. Greving *et al.*, *J. Chromatogr.*, 1977, *142*, 611–619.

Dose. 20 to 40 mg daily.

Oxytetracycline Dihydrate

Antibacterial

Synonyms. 5-Hydroxytetracycline; Oxytetracycline; Terrafungine.
Proprietary names. Abbocin; Chemocycline (tablets); Galenomycin; Imperacin; Oxymed; Oxymycin; Terramycin (tablets).
[4*S*-(4α,4aα,5α,5aα,6β,12aα,)]-4-(Dimethylamino)-1,4,4a,5,5a,6,11,12a-octahydro-3,5,6,10,12,12a,-hexahydroxy-6-methyl-1,11-dioxo-2-naphthacenecarboxamide dihydrate
$C_{22}H_{24}N_2O_9,2H_2O$=496.5
CAS—79-57-2 (anhydrous); 6153-64-6 (dihydrate)

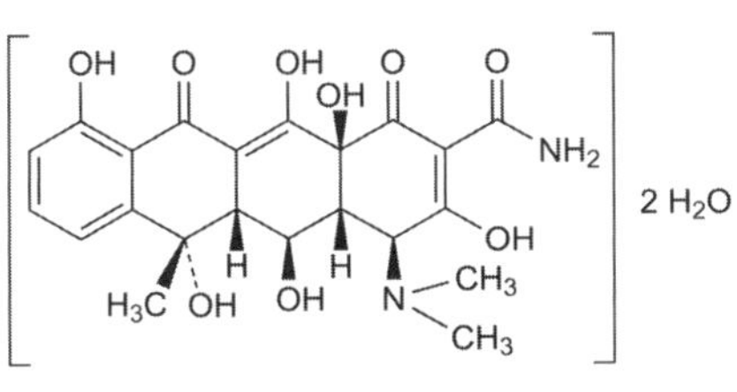

A yellow to tan-coloured crystalline powder. Stable in air but darkens on exposure to strong sunlight.
Soluble 1 in 4150 of water, 1 in 66 of dehydrated alcohol and 1 in 6250 of ether; sparingly soluble in ethanol; practically insoluble in chloroform; soluble in dilute acids and alkalis.

Oxytetracycline Calcium

Proprietary names. Chemocycline (syrup); Terramycin (syrup).
$C_{44}H_{46}CaN_4O_{18}$=958.9
CAS—15251-48-6 (xCa)
A yellow to light brown crystalline powder.
Practically insoluble in water; soluble in dilute solutions of sodium hydroxide.

Oxytetracycline Hydrochloride

Proprietary names. Macocyn; Terramycin (capsules); Unimycin. It is an ingredient of Bisolvomycin and Terra-Cortril.
$C_{22}H_{24}N_2O_9,HCl$=496.9
CAS—2058-46-0
A yellow, hygroscopic, crystalline powder, which darkens on exposure to sunlight or to moist air above 90°. It decomposes above 180°.
Soluble 1 in 2 of water, 1 in 45 of ethanol and 1 in 45 of methanol; less soluble in dehydrated alcohol; practically insoluble in chloroform and ether. Solutions in water become turbid on standing owing to precipitation of oxytetracycline base.

Dissociation Constant. pK_a 3.3, 7.3, 9.1 (25°).

Partition Coefficient. Log P (octanol/pH 7.5), −1.6.

Colour Tests. Benedict's Reagent—red; Formaldehyde–Sulfuric Acid—brown-red; Liebermann's Test—red; Mandelin's Test—violet→red→orange; Marquis Test—orange; Sulfuric Acid—violet-red.

Thin-layer Chromatography. System TA—Rf 05, streaking; system TB—Rf 00; system TE—Rf 00; system TAD—Rf 00; system TAE—Rf 08. (Location under ultraviolet light, orange fluorescence; acidified potassium permanganate solution, positive.)

High Performance Liquid Chromatography. System HX—RI 299; system HY—RI 260.

Ultraviolet Spectrum. Aqueous acid—268 nm (A_1^1=400a), 352 nm; aqueous alkali—246, 269 nm.

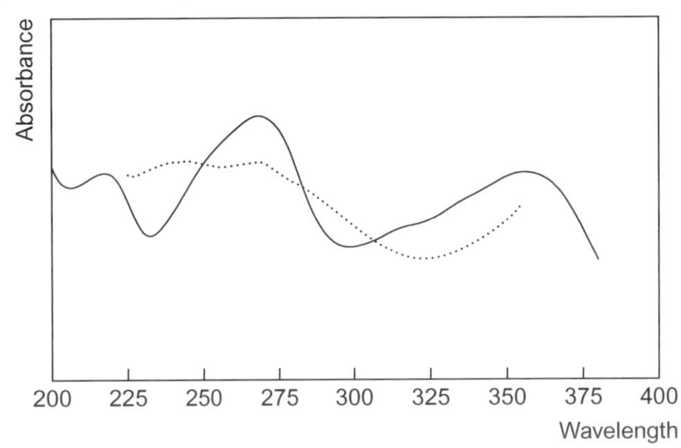

Infra-red Spectrum. Principal peaks at wavenumbers 1616, 1584, 1665, 1235, 1180, 1138 cm^{-1} (oxytetracycline hydrochloride, KBr disk).

Quantification

Spectrofluorimetry. In blood or plasma: limit of detection <100 µg/L—B. Scales and D. A. Assinder, *J. Pharm. Sci.*, 1973, *62*, 913–917.

Disposition in the Body. Incompletely and irregularly absorbed after oral administration and widely distributed throughout the body. About 70% of a dose is excreted in the urine; biliary excretion also occurs.

Therapeutic concentration

Following oral doses of 500 mg to 4 subjects, peak plasma concentrations of 1.2 to 3.4 mg/L (mean 2.1) were attained in 2 to 3 h [B. Scales and D. A. Assinder, *J. Pharm. Sci.*, 1973, *62*, 913–917].

Half-life. Plasma half-life, about 9 h, increased in renal impairment.

Protein binding. In plasma, about 20 to 35%.

Dose. Up to 3 g of oxytetracycline hydrochloride daily.

Paclitaxel

Taxane/Antineoplastic

Synonyms. BMS-181339-01; NSC-125973.
Proprietary names. Anzatax; Paxene; Taxol; Taxol A; Yewtaxan.
[2a*R*-[2aα,4β,4aβ,6β,9α(α*R**,β*S**),11α,12α,12aα,12bα]]-β-(Benzoylamino)-α-hydroxybenzenepropanoic acid 6,12b-bis(acetyloxy)-12-(benzoyloxy)-2a,3,4,4a,5,6,9,10,11,12,12a,12b-dodecahydro-4,11-dihydroxy-4a,8,13,13-tetramethyl-5-oxo-7,11-methano-1*H*-cyclodeca-[3,4]benz[1,2-*b*]oxet-9-yl ester
$C_{47}H_{51}NO_{14}$=853.9
CAS—33069-62-4

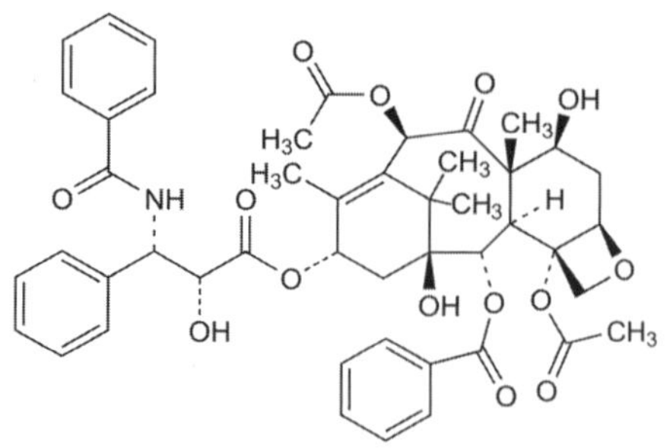

White to off-white crystalline powder. M.p.216° to 217°, with decomposition. It is virtually insoluble in water and shows poor solubility in most pharmaceutically approved solvents.

High Performance Liquid Chromatography. Column: C_8 (MOS Hypersil, 150 × 4.6 mm i.d., 5 µm). Mobile phase: methanol:acetate buffer (0.02 M, pH 4.5) (65:35), flow rate 2 mL/min. UV detection (λ=227 nm). *k* value: 5.5. [J. Rizzo *et al., J. Pharm. Biomed. Anal.*, 1990, *8(2)*, 159–164].

Column: (analytical) C_{18} Radial-Pak cartridge (100 × 8 mm i.d., 10 µm); (guard) C_{18} (Guard-Pak). Mobile phase: water:acetonitrile (65:35) to (0:100) exponentially over 20 min. Internal standard: *N*-cyclohexylbenzamide. UV detection (λ=227 nm). Retention time: paclitaxel, 19.5 min; I. S., 12.5 min. [S. M. Longnecker *et al., Cancer Treat. Rep.*, 1987, *71(1)*, 53–59].

Ultraviolet Spectrum. Aqueous acid—227, 273 nm.

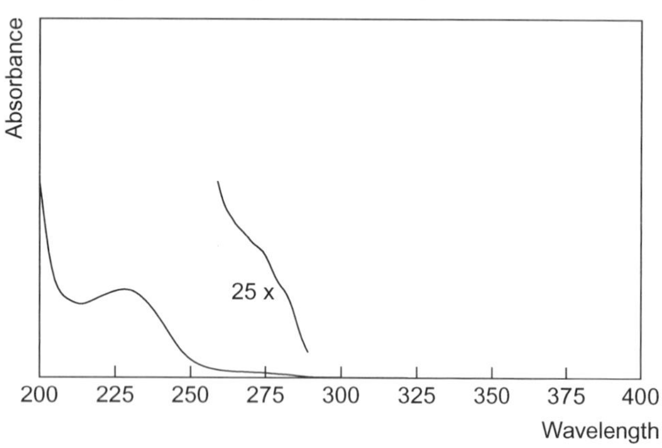

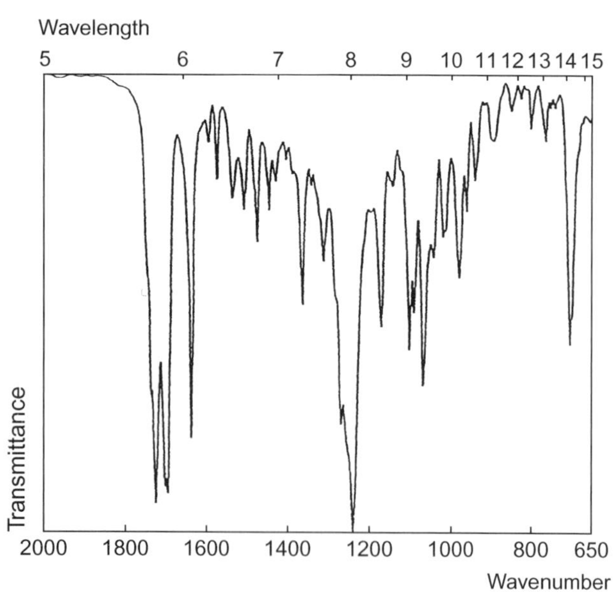

Quantification

High performance liquid chromatography. In plasma: limit of quantification 5 µg/L. UV detection (λ=227 nm)—J. G. Supko *et al., J. Pharm. Biomed. Anal.*, 1999, *21*, 1025–1036. In plasma and urine: limit of quantification 25 and 40 µg/L, respectively. UV detection (λ=227 nm)—N. Martin *et al., J. Chromatogr. B, Biomed. Sci. Appl.*, 1998, *709*, 281–288. In plasma: limit of quantification 10 µg/L. UV detection (λ=230 nm)—A. Sparreboom *et al., J. Chromatogr. B, Biomed. Sci. Appl.*, 1998, *705*, 159–164. In plasma: limit of detection 0.10 µg/L. UV detection (λ=227 nm)—J. Rizzo *et al., J. Pharm. Biomed. Anal.*, 1990, *8(2)*, 159–164. In serum: limit of detection is 0.25 µg/L. MS detection—X. Xu *et al., J. Mass Spectrom.*, 2000, *35(11)*, 1329–1334.

Enzyme-linked immunosorbent assay. In serum: limit of detection is 42 µg/L—J. G. Leu *et al., Cancer Res.*, 1993, *53(6)*, 1388–1391.

Competitive inhibition enzyme immunoassay. In plasma: limit of detection 0.3 µg/L—P. G. Grothaus *et al., J. Immunol. Methods*, 1993, *158(1)*, 5–15.

Disposition in the Body. Paclitaxel is not significantly absorbed after oral administration and is metabolised in the liver with the help of the cytochrome P450 isoforms CYP2C8 and CYP3A4. It undergoes extensive extravascular distribution and/or tissue binding, but does not cross the blood–brain barrier. Five metabolites including two mono-hydroxylated and one di-hydroxylated derivatives have been identified in humans. The major metabolite is 6α-hydroxytaxol; minor metabolites include 3′-*p*-hydroxypaclitaxel and 6α,3′-*p*-dihydroxypaclitaxel. Less than 5 to 10% of a dose is excreted in urine as the unchanged drug and it has also been detected in bile (75% of a dose; mainly as its metabolites and approximately, 20% unchanged).

Therapeutic concentration

30 patients with advanced cancer were administered with either a single intravenous dose of 210, 250 or 300 mg/m^2 over 3 h. Peak plasma concentrations were reached by the end of infusion at 6, 9.2 and 14.2 µmol/L, respectively. [J. Schiller *et al., J. Clin. Oncol.*, 1994, *12*, 532–538].

30 pediatric patients aged between 2.3 and 22.8 years, were administered with doses of 200, 250, 350 and 420 mg/m^2 paclitaxel over 24 h. Peak concentrations ranged between 1.06 and 1.26 µmol/L, 0.31 to 1.56, 0.54 to 2.61 and 1.18 to 6.77 µmol/L, respectively and were reached by the end of infusion. [P. Sonnichsen *et al., J. Clin. Oncol.*, 1994, *12*, 532–538].

Toxicity

The major clinical toxicity is myelosuppression which is dose-dependent and reversible. Dose-limiting myelosuppression without granulocyte colony-stimulating factor (G-CSF) was observed at 250 mg/m^2 and the dose-limiting toxicity for paclitaxel with G-CSF was neuropathy at 300 mg/m^2. Therefore, the maximum doses for paclitaxel when administered over a 3-h infusion with or without G-CSF support, are 250 and 210 mg/m^2, respectively. [J. H. Schiller *et al., J. Clin. Oncol.*, 1994, *12(2)*, 241–248].

Half-life. 3 to 50 h (non-linear pharmacokinetics, independent of dose and wide inter-patient variability).

Volume of distribution. 200 to about 700 L/m^2.

Clearance. Plasma, 11.6 to 24.0 L/h/m^2; mean, 0.42 L/m^2/day (from peritoneal cavity).

Protein binding. 88 to 98%.

Dose. The dose varies between 100 and 175 mg/m^2 body surface by intravenous infusion over 3 h every 2 to 3 weeks depending on condition and response. Dose may be reduced by 20% in some cases.

Padimate

Sunscreen Agent

Synonyms. Amyl Dimethylaminobenzoate; Isoamyl Dimethylaminobenzoate; Padimate A.

Proprietary names. Chapstick. It is an ingredient of Chapstick Sun Block, Filter OTC, and Vaseline Intensive Care Blockout.

A mixture of pentyl, isopentyl, and 2-methylbutyl 4-dimethylaminobenzoates.

$C_{14}H_{21}NO_2$=235.3

CAS—14779-78-3; 21245-01-2.

A yellow liquid.

Practically insoluble in water; soluble in ethanol, chloroform, and isopropyl alcohol.

Padimate O

Synonyms. 2-Ethylhexyl 4-(dimethylamino)benzoate; Octyl Dimethyl PABA.
Proprietary names. Banana Boat Dark Tanning; Chapstick; Escalol 507; Ice Lipbalm; Lipbalm with Sunscreen; Lip-Sed; Spectraban. It is an ingredient of many proprietary preparations—see Martindale, *The complete drug reference*, 2003 CD-ROM, London, Pharmaceutical Press, 2003.
$C_{17}H_{27}NO_2$=277.4
CAS—21245-02-3
A light yellow, mobile liquid.
Practically insoluble in water; soluble in ethanol and isopropyl alcohol.

Colour Tests. Aromaticity (Method 2)—yellow/orange; Liebermann's Test (100°)—blue.

Thin-layer Chromatography. System TA—Rf 75. (Acidified iodoplatinate solution, positive.)

Gas Chromatography. System GA—RI 1964.

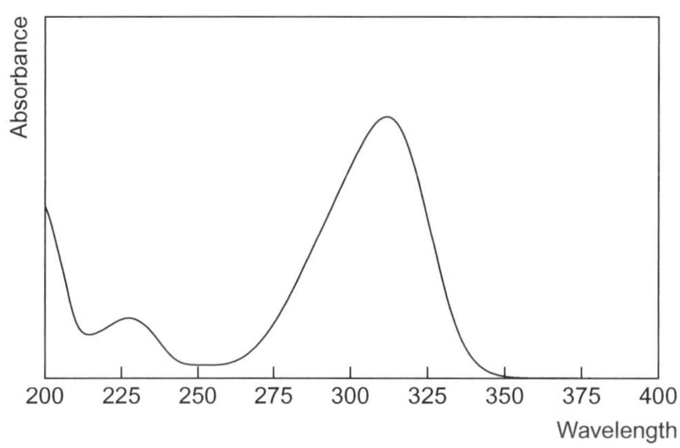

Quantification

High performance liquid chromatography. In plasma: padimate O and other sunscreen agents, limit of detection 50 µg/L for padimate O, UV detection—R. Jiang *et al., J. Chromatogr. B Biomed. Appl.*, 1996, *682*, 137–145.

Uses. Topically in a concentration of 2.5%.

Pancuronium Bromide

Muscle Relaxant

Synonym. Poncuronium Bromide
Proprietary names. Bromurex; Curon-B; Minopres; Pancuron; Pancurox; Panlem; Parulon; Pavulon.
1,1′-[(2β,3α,5α,16β,17β)-3,17-Bis(acetyloxy)androstane-2,16-diyl]bis-[1-methylpiperidinium] dibromide
$C_{35}H_{60}Br_2N_2O_4$=732.7
CAS—15500-66-0

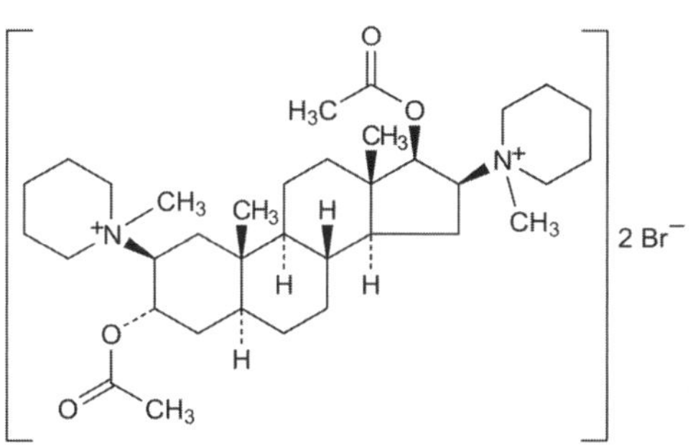

White, hygroscopic crystals or crystalline powder. M.p. 215°. A solution in water is dextrorotatory.
Soluble 1 in 1 of water, 1 in 5 of ethanol, 1 in 5 of chloroform, and 1 in 1 of methanol; practically insoluble in ether.

Partition Coefficient. Log *P* (octanol/water), –1.2.

Colour Test. Antimony Pentachloride—green.

Thin-layer Chromatography. System TA—Rf 01; system TB—Rf 00; system TC—Rf 00; system TE—Rf 00; system TL—Rf 00; system TN—Rf 80; system TAE—Rf 00; system TAF—Rf 15. (Acidified iodoplatinate solution, positive.)

Gas Chromatography. System GA—not eluted.

High Performance Liquid Chromatography. System HAA—Retention time 3.0 min.

Ultraviolet Spectrum. No significant absorption, 230 to 360 nm.

Infra-red Spectrum. Principal peaks at wavenumbers 1225, 1745, 1031, 1056, 1013, 907 cm^{-1} (KBr disk). (See below.)

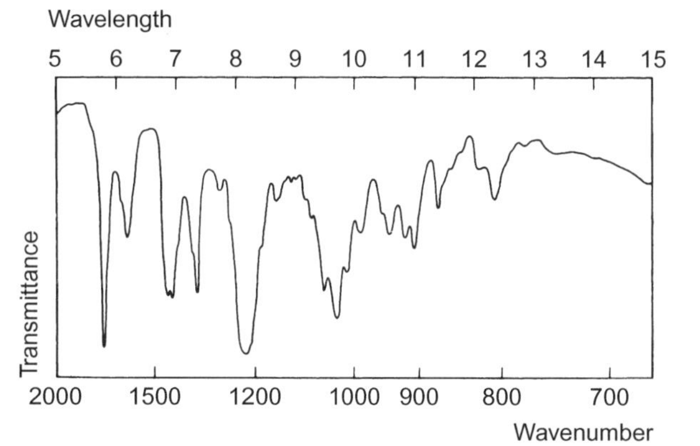

Quantification

Gas chromatography. In plasma, bile, or urine: pancuronium, its desacetyl metabolite, and other quaternary ammonium drugs, limit of detection 2 µg/L, nitrogen-sensitive detection—T. Furuta *et al., J. Chromatogr.*, 1988, *427*, 41–53.

Mass spectrometry. In urine: pancuronium and other quaternary ammonium compounds, limits of detection 20 to 150 µg/L—M. Nisikawa *et al., Forensic Sci. Int.*, 1991, *51*, 131–138.

Spectrofluorimetry. In serum: limit of detection 50 µg/L—L. B. Wingard *et al., J. Pharm. Sci.*, 1979, *68*, 914–916.

Disposition in the Body. Metabolised by hydroxylation to 3-hydroxypancuronium which is about half as active as pancuronium, and to a small extent to the 17-hydroxy and 3,17-dihydroxy derivatives which are virtually inactive. About 25% of a dose is excreted in the urine unchanged and 15% as the 3-hydroxy metabolite, in about 30 h; about 10% of a dose is excreted in the bile.

Therapeutic concentration

After an IV injection of 4 mg to 6 subjects, plasma concentrations of about 0.6 mg/L were reported at 5 min, decreasing to 0.07 mg/L at 4 h [K. McLeod *et al., Br. J. Anaesth.*, 1976, *48*, 341–345.]

Toxicity

In a suicide case due to the IV administration of pancuronium bromide, postmortem concentrations were: blood 1.6 mg/L, urine 1.5 mg/L; thiopental and thioridazine were also detected [A. Poklis and E. G. Melanson, *J. Anal. Toxicol.*, 1980, *4*, 275–280.]

The following postmortem concentrations of pancuronium and midazolam, respectively, were reported in a 25-year-old male anaesthesiologist who was found dead with an IV drip line connected to his leg and several empty ampoules of pancuronium, midazolam, and buprenorphine nearby: blood 0.3 and 0.1 µg/g, urine 0.9 and 0.05 µg/g; death was attributed to pancuronium [M. Yashiki *et al., Nippon Hoigaku Zasshi*, 1992, *46*, 282–285.]

A 79-year-old man died 6 days after receiving a total of 105 mg pancuronium bromide by continuous IV infusion over 4 days. The plasma concentration post-infusion was 400 µg/L of pancuronium and 400 µg/L of 3-desacetyl pancuronium; the next day these levels declined to 150 µg/L and 350 µg/L, respectively, and the level of 3-desacetyl pancuronium was 240 and 110 µg/L on the third and fourth days post-infusion. The following postmortem tissue concentrations of pancuronium plus its metabolite were reported: liver 6.38 µg/g, spleen 1.68 µg/g, kidneys 0.68 µg/g, lungs 0.40 µg/g, heart 0.60 µg/g, muscles 0.80 µg/g, gastro-intestinal contents 16.67 µg/g [R. H. Vandenbrom and J. M. Wierda, *Anesthesiology*, 1988, *69*, 996–997.]

Half-life. Plasma half-life, about 2 h.

Volume of distribution. 0.1 to 0.4 L/kg.

Clearance. Plasma clearance, about 1 to 2 mL/min/kg.

Protein binding. In plasma, about 87%.

Note. For a review of the pharmacokinetics of muscle relaxants see M. I. Ramzan *et al.*, *Clin. Pharmacokinet.*, 1981, *6*, 25–60.

Dose. Initially 40 to 100 μg/kg IV.

Pantoprazole

Proton Pump Inhibitor

Synonyms. B8510-029; SK&F-96022.
5-(Difluoromethoxy)-2-[[(3,4-dimethoxy-2-pyridinyl)methyl]sulfinyl]-1*H*-benzimidazole
$C_{16}H_{15}F_2N_3O_4S = 383.4$
CAS—102625-70-7

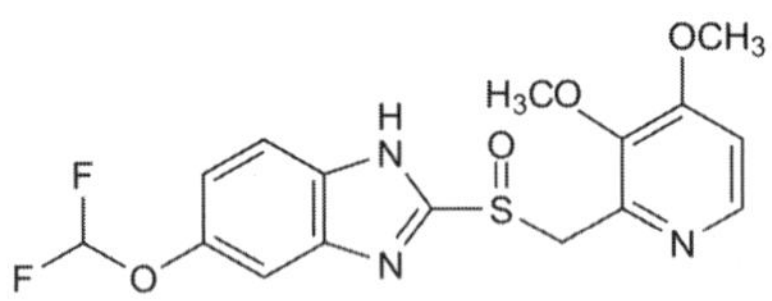

An off-white solid. M.p.139° to 140°. Freely soluble in water; practically insoluble in hexane; very slightly soluble in phosphate buffer (pH 7.4).

Pantoprazole Sodium Sesquihydrate

Synonyms. BY 1023; B8610-023; SK&F-96022-Z.
Proprietary names. Pantozol; Protium; Protonix.
$C_{16}H_{14}F_2N_3NaO_4S.{}^3/_2H_2O = 432.5$
CAS—164579-32-2
A white to off-white solid.

Dissociation Constant. pK_a 3.92; 8.19 (21° to 22°).

Partition Coefficient. Log *P* (octanol/buffer), 2.05 (pH 7.4); −0.26 (pH 11.4) (21–22°).

High Performance Liquid Chromatography. Column: (analytical) RP-18 (Hypersil, 125 × 4.6 mm i.d., 5 μm); (guard) RP-18 (12 × 4.6 mm i.d.). Mobile phase: (A:B) methanol:diammonium hydrogen phosphate buffer (10 mM, pH 6.5), flow rate 1 mL/min. Elution programme: (43:57) for 2 min, to (83:17) in 17 min, to (100:0) in 2 min; to (43:57) in 7 min. UV detection (λ=290 nm). Retention times: pantoprazole, 16.5 min; sulfone metabolite, 13 min. [R. Huber and W. Muller, *J. Chromatogr.*, 1990, *529*; *Biomed. Appl.*, 389–401].

Ultraviolet Spectrum. (Sodium Sesquihydrate) Aqueous acid—290 nm.

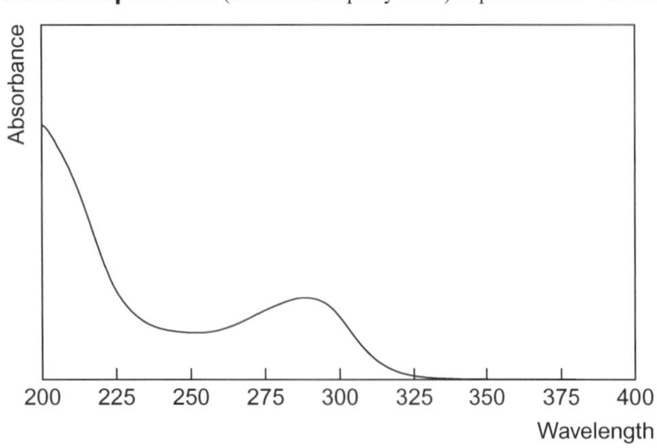

Infra-red Spectrum. Principal peaks at wavenumber 1590, 1493, 1277, 1170, 1122, 1041 cm^{-1}.

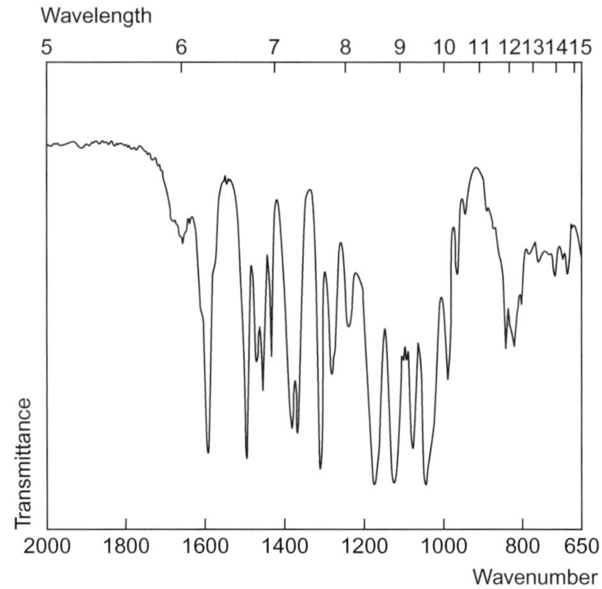

Quantification
High performance liquid chromatography. In serum: limit of detection is 0.004 mg/L—R. Huber *et al.*, *J Chromatogr.*, 1990, *529*, 389–401.

Disposition in the Body. Pantoprazole is rapidly absorbed after administration and almost exclusively metabolised in the liver. Co-administration with food delays absorption. It is extensively metabolised mainly via hepatic cytochrome P450 CYP2C19 isoenzyme. CYP34A, CYP2D6 and CYP2C9 metabolise the drug to a much lesser extent. The main metabolite is desmethylpantoprazole which is conjugated with sulfur and has been detected in plasma and urine. The metabolites are excreted primarily via renal elimination (approximately, 80%) and the remainder in faeces.

Therapeutic concentration

12 healthy males, aged between 19 and 29 years, were administered with a 40 mg intravenous dose over 15 min or a 40 mg oral dose, both after an overnight fast. The mean peak plasma concentrations were 4.62 mg/L (range 3.21 to 7.05) for the IV dose, observed at the end of the infusion and 2.09 (1.11 to 3.12) mg/L for the oral dose, observed 2 to 4 h after ingestion. [M. A. Pue *et al.*, *Eur. J. Clin. Pharmacol.*, 1993, *44*, 575–578].

Bioavailability. For the enteric coated tablet form, 77%.

Half-life. 1 to 2 h in good metabolisers (pantoprazole); 6 h in poor metabolisers (drug); 1.5 h (metabolites).

Volume of distribution. 0.15 L/kg; apparent volume of distribution also reported as 11.0 to 23.6 L.

Clearance. Plasma, 0.1 L/h/kg. Total, 7.6 to 14.0 L/h.

Distribution in blood. Pantoprazole and metabolites are essentially located in blood plasma with only negligible penetration in erythrocytes. Blood:plasma ratio is 0.55.

Protein binding. Approx. 98% (primarily to albumin).

Note. For a general review of proton pump inhibitors, see P. Richardson *et al.*, *Drugs*, 1998, *56*, 307–335.

Dose. 20 or 40 mg daily.

Papaverine

Antispasmodic

1-[(3,4-Dimethoxyphenyl)methyl]-6,7-dimethoxyisoquinoline
$C_{20}H_{21}NO_4 = 339.4$
CAS—58-74-2

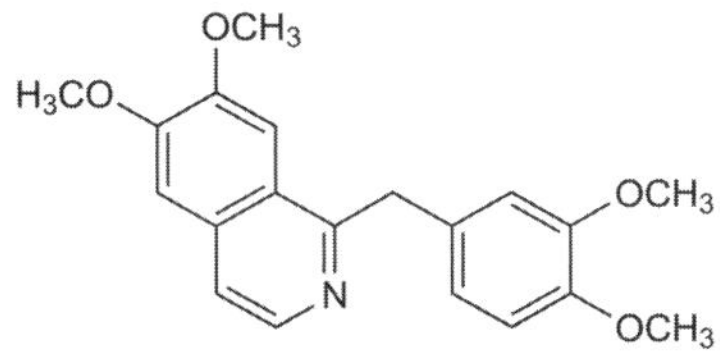

An alkaloid obtained from opium or prepared synthetically.
Crystals or white crystalline powder. M.p. 147° (from alcohol and ether).
Almost insoluble in water; soluble in hot benzene, glacial acetic acid, and acetone; slightly soluble in chloroform, carbon tetrachloride, and petroleum ether.

Papaverine Hydrochloride
Proprietary names. Albatran; Cerebid; Cerespan; Genabid; Oxadilene; Panergon; Pavabid; Pavacap; Pavacen; Pavakey; Pavarine; Pavased; Pavatine; Paverolan; Therapav; Vasal; Vasospan.
$C_{20}H_{21}NO_4,HCl = 375.9$
CAS—61-25-6
White crystals or crystalline powder. M.p. 220° to 225° (from water).
Soluble 1 in about 40 of water, 1 in 120 of ethanol, and 1 in 10 of chloroform; practically insoluble in ether.

Papaverine Sulfate
$(C_{20}H_{21}NO_4)_2,H_2SO_4,5H_2O = 866.9$
CAS—32808-09-6 (anhydrous)
White crystals or crystalline powder.
Soluble 1 in 2 of water, 1 in 20 of ethanol, and 1 in 5000 of ether; slightly soluble in chloroform.

Dissociation Constant. pK_a 6.4 (25°).

Partition Coefficient. Log *P* (ether), 0.5.

Colour Tests. Liebermann's Test—black; Mandelin's Test—grey-green.

Thin-layer Chromatography. System TA—Rf 61; system TB—Rf 08; system TC—Rf 65; system TE—Rf 69; system TL—Rf 47; system TAE—Rf 74; system TAF—Rf 74; system TAJ—Rf 66; system TAK—Rf 08; system TAL—Rf 93. (Dragendorff spray, positive; acidified iodoplatinate solution, positive.)

Gas Chromatography. System GA—RI 2825; system GB—RI 2973.

High Performance Liquid Chromatography. System HA—*k* 0.3; system HC—*k* 0.16; system HS—*k* 0.04; system HX—RI 363; system HY—RI 295; system HAA—retention time 12.1 min.

Ultraviolet Spectrum. Aqueous acid—250 ($A_1^1 = 1830a$); aqueous alkali—236 ($A_1^1 = 1994b$), 277, 326 nm.

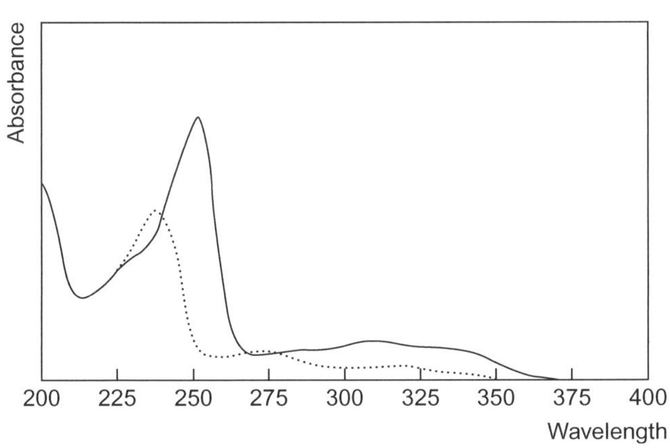

Infra-red Spectrum. Principal peaks at wavenumbers 1279, 1508, 1263, 1026, 1292, 1238 cm^{-1} (papaverine hydrochloride, KBr disk).

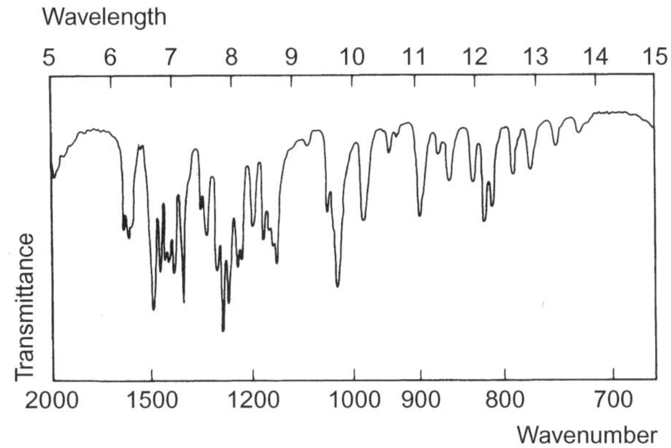

Mass Spectrum. Principal ions at *m/z* 339, 324, 338, 325, 340, 308, 154, 292.

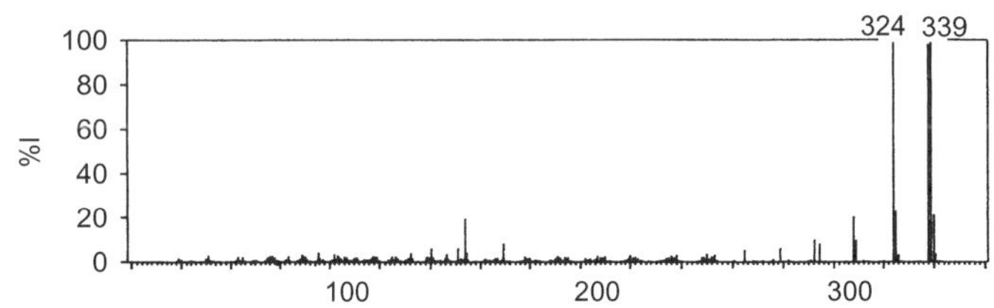

Quantification.
Gas chromatography. In blood: limit of detection 5 µg/L, AFID—V. Bellia *et al.*, *J. Chromatogr.*, 1978, *161*, 231–235.

Gas chromatography–mass spectrometry. In blood: limit of detection 5 µg/L—J. De Graeve *et al.*, *J. Chromatogr.*, 1977, *133*, 153–160.

High performance liquid chromatography. In plasma: limit of detection 2 µg/L, UV detection—S. L. Pierson *et al.*, *J. Pharm. Sci.*, 1979, *68*, 1550–1551. In blood: limit of detection 5 µg/L, UV detection—G. Hoogewijs *et al.*, *J. Chromatogr.* 1981, 226(15) *B Biomed. Appl.*, 423–430.

Disposition in the Body. Readily and completely absorbed after oral administration but undergoes extensive first-pass metabolism. Metabolised by demethylation and glucuronic acid and sulfate conjugation of the resulting phenolic groups. About 50 to 80% of a dose is excreted in the urine in 48 h as conjugated phenolic metabolites, mostly 6-hydroxypapaverine (37% of the dose) and 4′-hydroxypapaverine (about 8.5% of the dose). Less than 1% of a dose is excreted in the urine unchanged.

Therapeutic concentration
After oral administration of single doses of 150 mg given as an elixir and tablets, respectively, to 6 subjects, mean peak plasma concentrations of 0.58 and 0.53 mg/L were attained in about 1 h. [M. C. Meyer *et al.*, *J. Clin. Pharmacol.*, 1980, *19*, 435–444.]

Half-life. Plasma half-life, about 7 h, but there is wide variation and a biological half-life of 1 to 2 h is also reported.

Bioavailability. About 30%.

Protein binding. In plasma, about 90%.

Dose. Up to 600 mg of papaverine hydrochloride daily.

Paracetamol

Analgesic

Synonyms. Acetaminophen; *N*-Acetyl-*p*-aminophenol.
Proprietary names. Paracetamol is an ingredient of many proprietary preparations—see *Martindale, The complete drug reference*, 33rd Edn., Pharmaceutical Press, London, 2002.
N-(4-Hydroxyphenyl)acetamide
$C_8H_9NO_2 = 151.2$
CAS—103-90-2

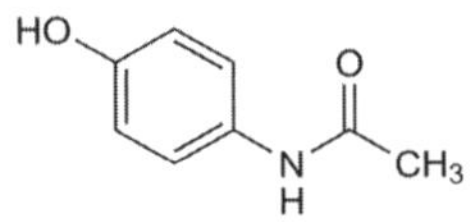

White crystals or crystalline powder. M.p. 169.0° to 170.5° (from water). Very slightly soluble in cold water, considerably more soluble in hot water; soluble in ethanol, methanol, dimethylformamide, ethylene dichloride, acetone, and ethyl acetate; very slightly soluble in chloroform; slightly soluble in ether; practically insoluble in petroleum ether, pentane, and benzene.

Dissociation Constant. pK_a 9.5 (25°).

Partition Coefficient. Log *P* (octanol/water), 0.5.

Colour Tests. Ferric Chloride—blue; Folin–Ciocalteu Reagent—blue; Liebermann's Test—violet; Nessler's Reagent—brown (slow).
Boil 0.1 g with 1 mL of hydrochloric acid for 3 min, add 10 mL of water, cool, and add 0.05 mL of 0.02 M potassium dichromate—violet, developing slowly (which in contrast to phenacetin does not become red).

Thin-layer Chromatography. System TA—Rf 95; system TB—Rf 00; system TD—Rf 15; system TE—Rf 45; system TF—Rf 32; system TAD—Rf 26; system TAE—Rf 77; system TAJ—Rf 30; system TAK—Rf 05; system TAL—Rf 73. (Ferric chloride solution, faint blue; acidified potassium permanganate solution, positive.)

Gas Chromatography. System GA—paracetamol RI 1665, art (*p*-aminophenol) RI 1253, paracetamol-Me RI 1512, art (*p*-aminophenol)-Me_2 RI 1220; system GB—paracetamol RI 1722, art (*p*-aminophenol) RI 1280; system GL—paracetamol-Me RI 1630.

High Performance Liquid Chromatography. System HD—*k* 0.1; system HW—*k* 0.32; system HX—RI 264; system HY—RI 241; system HZ—retention time 1.9 min; system HAA—retention time 5.6 min; system HAM—retention time 2.0 min; system HAX—retention time 4.8 min; system HAY—retention time 3.7 min.

Ultraviolet Spectrum. Aqueous acid—245 (A_1^1=668a); aqueous alkali—257 nm (A_1^1=715a).

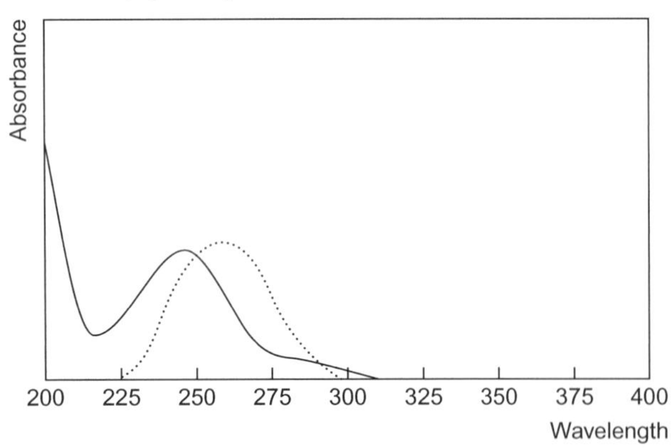

Infra-red Spectrum. Principal peaks at wavenumbers 1506, 1657, 1565, 1263, 1227, 1612 cm^{-1} (KBr disk). (See below)

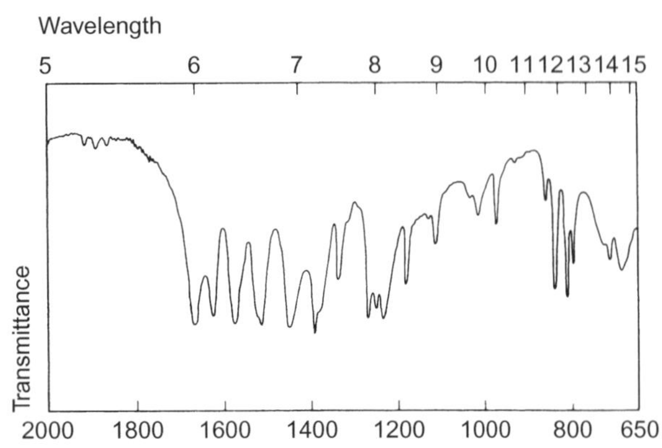

Mass Spectrum. Principal ions at *m/z* 109, 151, 43, 80, 108, 81, 53, 52; cysteine conjugate 141, 43, 183, 44, 140, 80, 108, 52; mercapturic acid conjugate 43, 141, 183, 42, 87, 41, 140, 165.

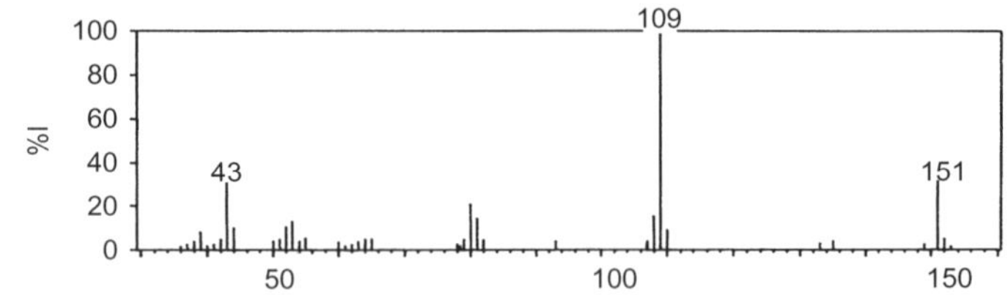

Quantification

Gas chromatography. In serum: limit of detection 7.5 mg/L, FID—E. Kaa, *J. Chromatogr.* 1980, *221(10) B Biomed. Appl.*, 414–418.

Gas chromatography–mass spectrometry. In whole blood or liver—J. Speed *et al.*, *J. Anal. Toxicol.*, 2001, *25*, 198–202.

High performance liquid chromatography. In plasma: limit of detection 50 µg/L, UV detection—J. N. Buskin *et al.*, *J. Chromatogr.* 1982, *230(19) B Biomed. Appl.*, 443–447. In urine: paracetamol and 7 metabolites, electrochemical and UV detection—J. M. Wilson *et al.*, *J. Chromatogr.* 1982, 227(16) *B Biomed. Appl.*, 453–462. In blood or postmortem tissues: UV detection—J. C. West, *J. Anal. Toxicol.*, 1981, *5*, 118–121. In blood or plasma: limit of detection 0.1 mg/L, electrochemical detection—R. Whelpton *et al.*, *Biomed. Chromatogr.*, 1993, *7*, 90–93. In plasma or urine: paracetamol and its major metabolites, UV detection—G. S. Lau and J. A. Critchley, *J. Pharm. Biomed. Anal.*, 1994, *12*, 1563–1572. In plasma, urine, or saliva—S. S. al-Obaidy *et al.*, *J. Pharm. Biomed. Anal.*, 1995, *13*, 1033–1039. In urine: paracetamol and its glucuronide and sulfate metabolites, UV detection—A. Di Girolamo *et al.*, *J. Pharm. Biomed. Anal.*, 1998, *17*, 1191–1197. In blood, urine, CSF, synovial fluid, vitreous humour, or tissue samples: UV detection—E. Pufal *et al.*, *Fresenius J. Anal. Chem.*, 2000, *367*, 596–599. In serum: paracetamol–protein adducts, electrochemical detection—K. L. Muldrew *et al.*, *Drug Metab. Dispos.*, 2002, *30*, 446–451. In blood (on spot card): limit of detection 600 pg, UV detection—E. J. Oliveira *et al.*, *J. Pharm. Biomed. Anal.*, 2002, *29*, 803–809.

Disposition in the Body. Small doses are readily absorbed but the absorption of larger doses varies considerably and is influenced by gastric emptying rate, the presence of food, and the time of day. Paracetamol is widely distributed throughout most body fluids and is present in the saliva at concentrations paralleling those in plasma. It crosses the placenta and is found in breast milk. It undergoes first-pass metabolism and is metabolised mainly by conjugation to form glucuronides and ethereal sulfates; 3-hydroxylation also occurs followed by conjugation or *O*-methylation of the hydroxy group. Oxidation to a reactive metabolite thought to be acetylimino-*p*-benzoquinone occurs to a small extent after therapeutic doses but becomes more significant after larger doses, and this metabolite appears to be responsible for hepatic necrosis in paracetamol overdosage; it is normally detoxified by glutathione conjugation to form mercapturic acid and cysteine conjugates but, once sources of glutathione are depleted, the free metabolite is available to bind covalently with liver cell protein; this binding occurs about 10 to 12 h after dosing. About 90% of a therapeutic dose is excreted in the urine in 24 h; of the excreted material, 1 to 4% is unchanged, 20 to 30% is conjugated with sulfate, 40 to 60% is conjugated with glucuronic acid, 5 to 10% consists of the 3-hydroxy-3-sulfate, the 3-methoxyglucuronide, and the 3-methoxy-3-sulfate metabolites, and about 5 to 10% consists of the mercapturic acid and cysteine conjugates; 3-methylthio-4-hydroxyacetanilide has also been identified at concentrations of less than 1%. Larger amounts of the mercapturic acid and cysteine conjugates are excreted in overdose.
Paracetamol is a metabolite of benorilate and phenacetin.

Therapeutic concentration. In plasma, usually in the range 10 to 20 mg/L. Plasma concentrations vary considerably between subjects. The glucuronide and sulfate conjugates accumulate in subjects with impaired renal function.

After a single oral dose of 1.5 g to 14 subjects, peak plasma paracetamol concentrations of 7.4 to 37 mg/L (mean 24) were attained in 0.5 to 3 h (mean 1.4). [R. C. Heading *et al.*, *Br. J. Pharmacol.*, 1973, *47*, 415–421.]

Of 24 children (over 25 kg) undergoing elective surgery, given paracetamol rectally at a dose of 1 or 40 mg/kg, most children in the 1-g group failed to attain therapeutic plasma levels whereas those in the 40 mg/kg group did (mean peak plasma concentration 7.8 vs 15.9 mg/L attained at 3.8 and 2.6 h, respectively). [T. K. Howell and D. Patel, *Anaesthesia*, 2003, *58*, 69–73.]

Following administration of 4 rectal doses of paracetamol, 20 mg/kg every 6 h, to 10 term neonates undergoing painful procedures or having painful conditions, mean peak serum concentrations were 10.79, 15.34, and 6.24 mg/L in the whole group, boys, and girls, respectively; the median time to peak serum concentration was 1.5 h after the first dose and 15 h for multiple doses. A starting dose of 30 mg/kg followed by 20 mg/kg rectally at intervals increasing from 6 to 8 h was proposed for neonates. [R. A. van Lingen *et al.*, *Clin. Pharmacol. Ther.*, 1999, *66*, 509–515.]

Toxicity. The minimum lethal dose is about 10 g. Symptoms of hepatic damage do not occur for at least 12 h after overdosage but may not appear until 4 to 6 days later. Plasma concentrations have been used to indicate possible hepatic necrosis; at 4 h, hepatic necrosis is possible at concentrations of paracetamol of 120 to 300 mg/L, probable at concentrations above 300 mg/L, and unlikely at concentrations below 120 mg/L. Similarly, at 12 h, concentrations above 120 mg/L indicate the probability of necrosis, concentrations of 50 to 120 mg/L indicate that it is possible, and concentrations below 50 mg/L indicate that it is unlikely.

Of 93 patients hospitalised for paracetamol toxicity, 80 were classified as suicidal and 13 had accidentally poisoned themselves in an attempt to relieve pain. Peak plasma levels were higher in the suicidal overdose group (mean 121.7 mg/L) than in the accidental overdose group (64.5 mg/L). [G. G. GyamLani and C. R. Parikh, *Crit. Care*, 2002, *6*, 155–159.]

A 6-year-old child died after receiving paracetamol overdosage over a period of 3 days. The prescribed dose for fever (associated with measles) had been 325 mg every 6 h, but the child's mother, believing paracetamol to be non-toxic, had progressively increased the dose firstly in response to the fever and subsequently for abdominal pain (500 mg every 4 h for 48 h followed by 500 mg every 2 to 3 h for 12 h had been given). On admission to hospital 11 h after the last dose, the child's serum paracetamol concentration was 163 mg/L. Despite appropriate treatment, the child died on the 11th day. [K. V. Blake *et al.*, *Clin. Pharm.*, 1988, *7*, 391–397.]

The following postmortem tissue concentrations were reported in 3 fatalities: blood 160, 200, and 387 mg/L, bile 180, -, 900 mg/L, liver -, -, 385 μg/g, liver blood 200, -, 475 mg/L, urine 180, 620, - mg/L. [A. E. Robinson *et al.*, *J. Forensic Sci.*, 1977, *22*, 708–717.]

Bioavailability. 70 to 90%.

Half-life. Plasma half-life after therapeutic doses, adults about 1 to 3 h, neonates, about 5 h; plasma half-lives greater than about 4 h in adults are indicative of possible liver damage.

Volume of distribution. About 1 L/kg.

Clearance. Plasma clearance, about 5 mL/min/kg.

Protein binding. In plasma, not bound at concentrations less than 60 mg/L. In poisoned subjects, protein binding has been reported to vary between about 8% and 40%.

Note. For a review of the pharmacokinetics of paracetamol, see J. A. H. Forrest *et al.*, *Clin. Pharmacokinet.*, 1982, *7*, 93–107. For a review of its use in infants, see A. Arana *et al.*, *Acta Anaesthesiol. Scand.*, 2001, *45*, 20–29. For a review of paracetamol overdosage, see American Academy of Pediatrics Committee on Drugs, *Pediatrics*, 2001, *108*, 1020–1024 and E. Kozer and G. Koren, *Drug Saf*, 2001, *24*, 503–512.

Dose. Up to maximum of 4 g daily.

Parachlorophenol

Disinfectant

Synonym. *p*-Chlorophenol
Proprietary names. It is an ingredient of the proprietary preparations Esofenol Ferri and Cresophene.
4-Chlorophenol
$C_6H_5ClO = 128.6$
CAS—106-48-9

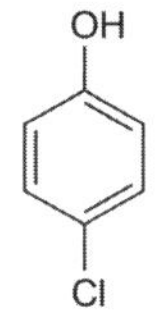

White or pink crystals. M.p. about 43°.
Soluble 1 in 60 of water; very soluble in ethanol, chloroform, and ether.

Dissociation Constant. pK_a 9.2 (20°).

Partition Coefficient. Log *P* (octanol/water), 2.4.

Colour Test. Ferric Chloride—blue.

Gas Chromatography. System GA—RI 1390.

Ultraviolet Spectrum. Aqueous alkali—298 ($A_1^1 = 194b$); ethanol—284 ($A_1^1 = 149b$), inflexion at 291 nm.

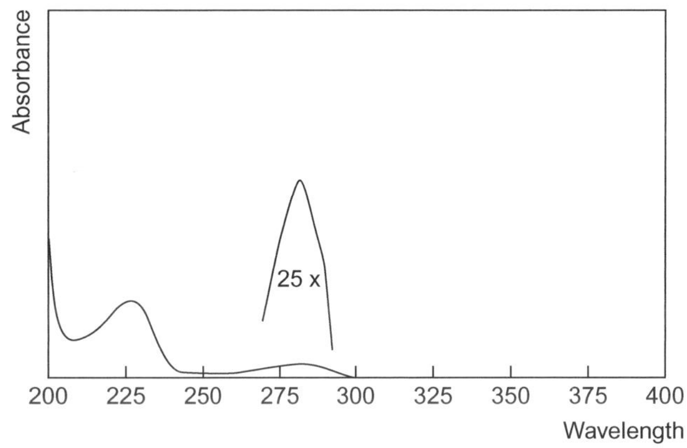

Mass Spectrum. Principal ions at *m/z* 128, 130, 65, 39, 64, 63, 129, 99.

Paradichlorobenzene

Insecticide

Synonym. Dichlorbenzol
Proprietary names. Paracide; Para-zene; Paramoth. It is an ingredient of Cerumol, Cerumenol, and Otoceril.
1,4-Dichlorobenzene
$C_6H_4Cl_2 = 147.0$
CAS—106-46-7

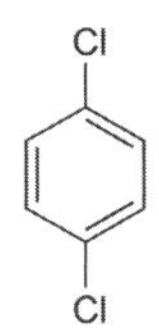

Colourless shining crystals; slowly volatile in air. M.p. 53° to 54°.
Practically insoluble in water; soluble in most organic solvents.

Partition Coefficient. Log *P* (octanol/water), 3.4.

Ultraviolet Spectrum. Ethanol—272 ($A_1^1 = 27b$), 265 ($A_1^1 = 20b$), 282 nm ($A_1^1 = 17b$).

Infra-red Spectrum. Principal peaks at wavenumbers 1012, 1091, 817, 1121, 951, 1000 cm^{-1}.

Mass Spectrum. Principal ions at *m/z* 146, 148, 111, 75, 50, 150, 113, 147.

Disposition in the Body

Toxicity. The estimated minimum lethal dose is 25 g and the maximum permissible atmospheric concentration is 75 ppm or 450 mg/m^3. Paradichlorobenzene is very irritant to the eyes, mucous membranes and skin, and it may cause narcosis.

Paraldehyde

Anticonvulsant/Hypnotic/Sedative

Synonym. Paracetaldehyde
Proprietary name. Paral
The trimer of acetaldehyde; 2,4,6-trimethyl-1,3,5-trioxane.
$(C_2H_4O)_3=132.2$
CAS—123-63-7

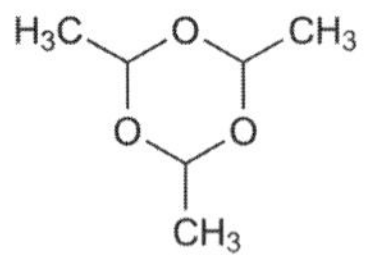

A clear colourless or pale yellow liquid which decomposes and increases in toxicity on storage. Relative density 0.991 to 0.996. F.p. 10° to 13°. B.p. 123° to 126°. At low temperatures it solidifies to form a crystalline mass. Soluble 1 in 10 of water, but only 1 in 17 of boiling water; miscible with ethanol, chloroform, and ether.

Partition Coefficient. Log *P* (octanol/water), 0.7.

Gas Chromatography. System GA—paraldehyde RI 786, acetaldehyde RI 372; system GI—paraldehyde Retention time 23.2 min, acetaldehyde Retention time 0.7 min.

Infra-red Spectrum. Principal peaks at wavenumbers 1095, 1170, 946, 860, 846, 763 cm^{-1} (thin film).

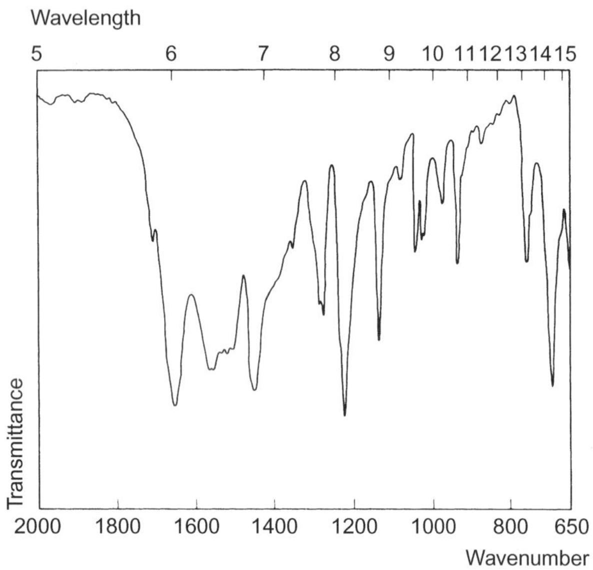

Mass Spectrum. Principal ions at *m/z* 43, 44, 87, 31, 45, 42, 131, 71; acetaldehyde 29, 44, 43, 42, 26, 41, 28, 27.

Quantification

Gas chromatography. In blood, plasma or urine: headspace analysis; limit of detection 2 mg/L—R. M. Anthony *et al.*, *J. Anal. Toxicol.*, 1978, *2*, 262–264. In blood or gastric fluid: headspace analysis after conversion to acetaldehyde—J. P. Hancock *et al.*, *J. Anal. Toxicol.*, 1977, *1*, 161–163. In serum—D. W. Hessel, *J. Anal. Toxicol.*, 1988, *12*, 350–353.

Disposition in the Body. Readily absorbed after oral, rectal or IM administration and distributed throughout the tissues. Probably metabolised by depolymerisation to acetaldehyde which is oxidised to acetic acid and ultimately to carbon dioxide. About 7% of an oral dose is exhaled unchanged in 4 h.

Therapeutic concentration. In plasma, usually in the range 30 to 100 mg/L. Concentrations in the CSF are about 70% of those in plasma.

After oral doses of 100 mg/kg, peak blood concentrations of 100 to 150 mg/L were attained in 0.5 h; following rectal administration of 100 mg/kg, peak blood concentrations of 50 to 100 mg/L were reported at 1.5 to 2 h [R. M. Anthony *et al.*, *J. Anal. Toxicol.*, 1978, *2*, 262–264.]

Following an IM injection of 10 mL to 1 subject, a peak plasma concentration of 77 mg/L was attained in 1.2 h [R. Maes *et al.*, *J. Forensic Sci.*, 1969, *14*, 235–254.]

Toxicity. The minimum lethal dose has been estimated as 25 mL orally and 12 mL rectally, although recovery has occurred after the ingestion of 125 mL. Toxic effects have been associated with blood concentrations of 200 to 400 mg/L. Blood concentrations of about 500 mg/L, or less if alcohol has also been ingested, may be lethal. On storage, paraldehyde may depolymerise to acetaldehyde and acetic acid; severe acidosis and fatalities may follow the use of partly depolymerised material.

In 15 fatalities attributed to paraldehyde overdose, blood concentrations of 490 to 1600 mg/L were reported [J. N. Hayward and B. R. Boshell, *Am. J. Med.*, 1957, *23*, 965–976.]

The following postmortem tissue concentrations were reported in 3 fatalities, 2 of which involved alcohol: blood 115, 480 and 140 mg/L, brain 150, 300 and 370 µg/g, kidney 190, 50 and 260 µg/g, liver 210, 200 and 600 µg/g, urine –, –, 130 mg/L [C. J. Rehling, Poison Residues in Human Tissues, in *Progress in Chemical Toxicology*, Vol. 3, A. Stolman (Ed.), New York, Academic Press Inc., 1967, pp. 363–386.]

Half-life. Plasma half-life, 4 to 10 h.

Volume of distribution. About 1 L/kg.

Clearance. Plasma clearance, about 2 mL/min/kg.

Dose. 5 to 10 mL by mouth or by IM injection.

Paramethadione

Anticonvulsant

Proprietary name. Paradione
5-Ethyl-3,5-dimethyl-2,4-oxazolidinedione
$C_7H_{11}NO_3=157.2$
CAS—115-67-3

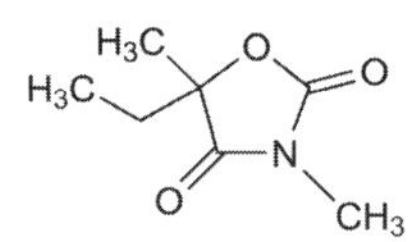

A clear colourless liquid. Refractive index, at 25°, 1.4485 to 1.4505. Sparingly soluble in water; freely soluble in ethanol, benzene, chloroform, and ether.

Partition Coefficient. Log *P* (octanol/water), 1.1.

Colour Test. Koppanyi–Zwikker Test—violet.

Thin-layer Chromatography. System TA—Rf 86; system TD—Rf 00; system TE—Rf 07; system TF—Rf 60; system TAD—Rf 56; system TAJ—Rf 87; system TAK—Rf 70; system TAL—Rf 94.

Gas Chromatography. System GA—RI 1115; system GE—paramethadione RRT 0.06, *N*-desmethylparamethadione RRT 0.22 (both relative to phenytoin).

Ultraviolet Spectrum. No significant absorption, 230 to 360 nm.

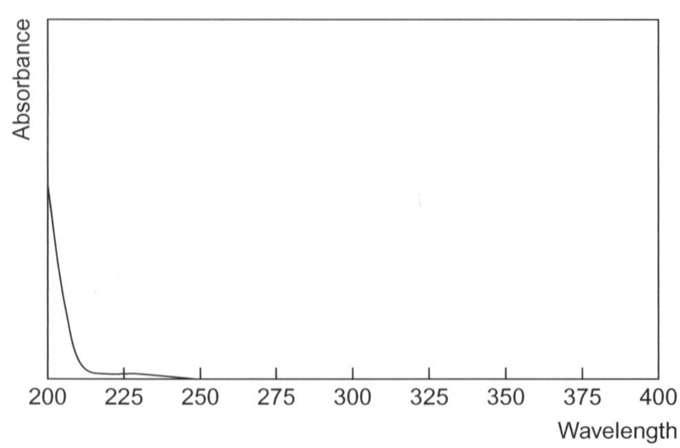

Infra-red Spectrum. Principal peaks at wavenumbers 1730, 1805, 1100, 1040, 1280, 1070 cm^{-1} (thin film).

Mass Spectrum. Principal ions at *m/z* 43, 129, 57, 56, 41, 72, 39, 58.

Quantification
Gas chromatography. In serum: paramethadione and 5-ethyl-5-methyloxazolidine-2,4-dione, limit of detection 200 µg/L, FID—D. J. Hoffman and A. H. C. Chun, *J. Pharm. Sci.*, 1975, *64*, 1702–1703.

Disposition in the Body. Readily absorbed after oral administration. Metabolised by *N*-demethylation to 5-ethyl-5-methyloxazolidine-2,4-dione which is active and accumulates during chronic administration; 30 to 80% of a dose is excreted slowly in the urine as the *N*-desmethyl metabolite with less than 1% as unchanged drug.

Therapeutic concentration
After a single oral dose of 300 mg to 3 subjects, peak serum concentrations of paramethadione of 5.4 to 7.6 mg/L (mean 6.3) were attained in 0.5 to 1 h; concentrations of the *N*-desmethyl metabolite gradually increased to a plateau of 8.1 to 8.6 mg/L (mean 8.4) at 32 h [D. J. Hoffman and A. H. C. Chun, *J. Pharm. Sci.*, 1975, *64*, 1702–1703.]

Following oral administration of 900 mg daily to 2 subjects for 14 days, peak plasma concentrations of the *N*-desmethyl metabolite of about 240 mg/L were reported [T. C. Butler, *J. Pharmacol. Exp. Ther.*, 1955, *113*, 178–185.]

Toxicity. The estimated minimum lethal dose is 5 g.

Half-life. Plasma half-life, paramethadione about 16 h after a single dose, *N*-desmethylparamethadione about 7 to 14 days during chronic administration.

Protein binding. In plasma, not significantly bound.

Dose. 0.9 to 1.8 g daily.

Paramethasone *Corticosteroid*

(6α,11β,16α)-6-Fluoro-11,17,21-trihydroxy-16-methylpregna-1,4-diene-3,20-dione
$C_{22}H_{29}FO_5$=392.5
CAS—53-33-8

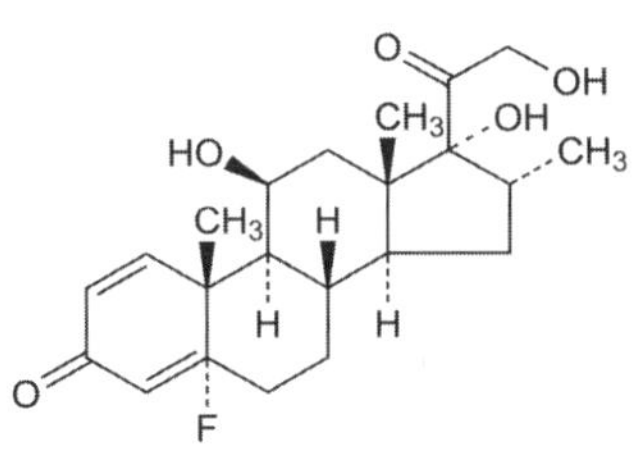

Paramethasone Acetate
Synonym. 6α-Fluoro-16α-methylprednisolone 21-acetate
Proprietary names. Cordidene; Depodillar; Dilar; Haldrone; Metilar; Monocortin; Paramezone.
$C_{24}H_{31}FO_6$=434.5
CAS—1597-82-6
A white to creamy-white, fluffy, crystalline powder. M.p. 228° to 241°, with decomposition.
Practically insoluble in water; soluble in ethanol, acetone, and ether; soluble 1 in 50 of chloroform.

Partition Coefficient. Log *P* (octanol/water), 1.7.

Thin-layer Chromatography. System TA—Rf 91; system TE—Rf 88; system TAJ—Rf 54; system TAK—Rf 39; system TAL—Rf 91; system TAM—Rf 91.

Ultraviolet Spectrum. Paramethasone acetate: methanol—241 nm (A_1^1=500b).

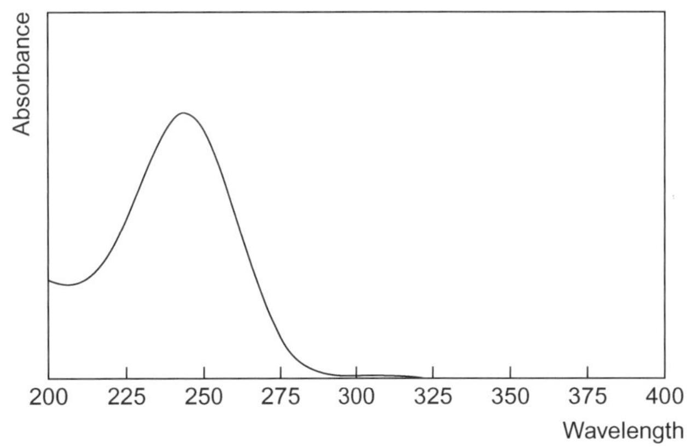

Infra-red Spectrum. Principal peaks at wavenumbers 1658, 1227, 1600, 905, 1745, 1034 cm^{-1} (Nujol mull).

Quantification
High performance liquid chromatography. In plasma or urine: paramethasone and other corticosteroids, UV detection—Z. Saito *et al.*, *Nippon Naibunpi Gakkai Zasshi*, 1979, *55*, 1296–1306.

Dose. Up to 12 mg of paramethasone acetate daily.

Paraphenylenediamine *Dye*

Synonyms. 'Para'; *p*-Phenylenediamine.
$C_6H_8N_2$=108.1
CAS—106-50-3

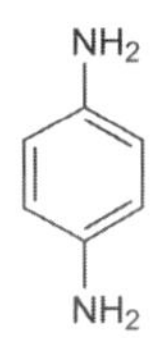

White or reddish crystals. M.p. 145° to 147°.
Soluble 1 in 100 of water; soluble in ethanol, chloroform, and ether.

Dissociation Constant. pK_a 6.2 (25°).

Partition Coefficient. Log *P* (octanol/water), –0.3.

Colour Tests. Ferric Chloride—green; Mandelin's Test—yellow.

Thin-layer Chromatography. System TA—Rf 61. (Acidified iodoplatinate solution, positive.)

Paraquat *Herbicide*

1,1′-Dimethyl-4,4′-bipyridinium
$[C_{12}H_{14}N_2]^{2+}$=186.3
CAS—4685-14-7

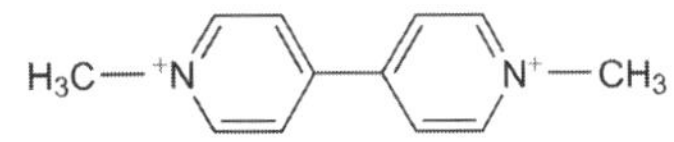

Paraquat Dichloride
Proprietary names. Dextrone X; Gramoxone. It is an ingredient of Dexuron, Pathclear and Weedol.
$C_{12}H_{14}Cl_2N_2$=257.2
CAS—1910-42-5
A white crystalline solid. M.p. about 300° with decomposition.
Very soluble in water. Hydrolysed by alkalis.

Partition Coefficient. Log *P* (octanol/water), −4.2.
Note. Unless otherwise stated, the analytical information given below refers to paraquat dichloride. For information on the monoene and diene

reduction products for GC–MS analysis, see under Quaternary Ammonium Herbicides, Chapter 14.

Colour Test. Sodium Dithionite—blue.

Thin-layer Chromatography. System TA—Rf 00; system TB—Rf 00; system TC—Rf 00; system TE—Rf 00; system TL—Rf 00; system TN—Rf 22; system TO—Rf 10; system TAB—Rf 00; system TAC—Rf 00; system TAE—Rf 00; system TAF—Rf 00. (Acidified iodoplatinate solution, positive.)

Gas Chromatography. System GK—monoene reduction product RRT 0.36, diene reduction product RRT 0.58 (both relative to caffeine).

High Performance Liquid Chromatography. System HX—RI 0.

Ultraviolet Spectrum. Aqueous acid—257 nm (A_1^1 = 693b).

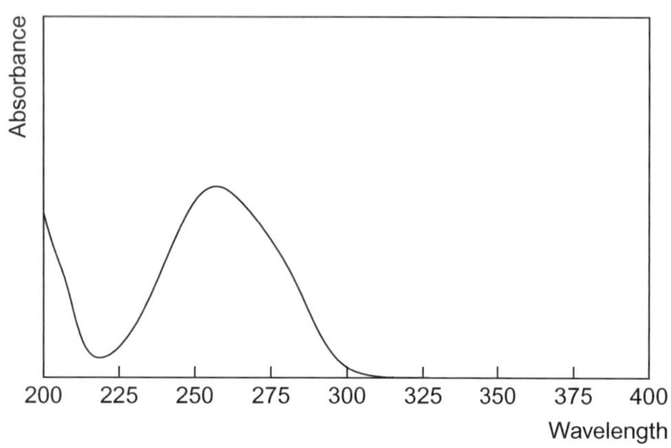

Infra-red Spectrum. Principal peaks at wavenumbers 1174, 1638, 1064, 1229, 1284, 850 cm^{-1} (KBr disk).

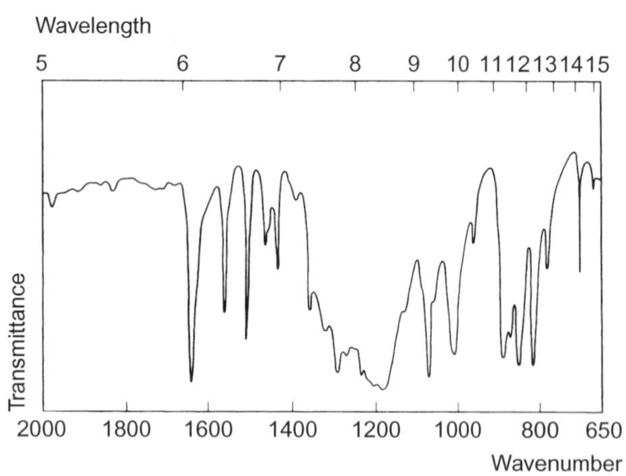

Mass Spectrum. Principal ions at *m/z* 156, 50, 155, 52, 157, 51, 75, 102 (paraquat); 96, 42, 70, 72, 150, 122, 194, 43 (monoene reduction product); 96, 42, 148, 192, 94, 122, 134, 44 (diene reduction product).

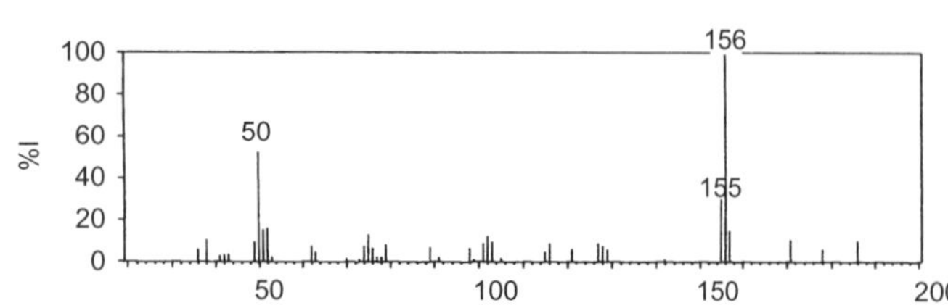

Quantification

Colorimetry. In plasma or serum: limit of detection 50 µg/L—D. R. Jarvie and M. J. Stewart, *Clin. Chim. Acta*, 1979, *94*, 241–251.

Gas chromatography. In plasma: limit of detection 30 µg/L, AFID—A. van Dijk *et al.*, *J. Anal. Toxicol.*, 1977, *1*, 151–154.

High performance liquid chromatography. In postmortem blood or liver: limit of detection 50 µg/L and 100 µg/L, respectively, UV detection—E. A. Querée *et al.*, *J. Anal. Toxicol.*, 1985, *9*, 10–14. In urine: paraquat and diquat, limit of detection <1 mg/L, UV detection—R. Gill *et al.*, *J. Chromatogr.*, 1983, *255*, 483–490. In human tissues: paraquat and diquat, limit of detection 0.05 µg/g, UV detection—S. Ito *et al.*, *J. Chromatogr.*, 1993, *617*, 119–123. In serum: limit of detection 25 µg/L—K. Croes *et al.*, *J. Anal. Toxicol.*, 1993, *17*, 310–312. In postmortem tissues, blood or urine: diode-array detection—K. Arys *et al.*, *J. Anal. Toxicol.*, 2000, *24*, 116–121. In plasma or serum: limit of detection 0.1 mg/L—P. Paixao *et al.*, *J. Chromatogr. B. Anal. Technol. Biomed. Life Sci.*, 2002, *775*, 109–113.

Thin-layer chromatography. In plasma or urine: limit of detection 50 ng, FID—J. Ikebuchi *et al.*, *J. Anal. Toxicol.*, 1988, *12*, 80–83.

Disposition in the Body. Less than 10% is absorbed after ingestion. It is slowly excreted unchanged in the urine and faeces, detectable concentrations have been found in the urine for up to 26 days after acute ingestion.

Toxicity. Several hundred fatalities caused by the accidental or suicidal ingestion of paraquat have occurred. The estimated minimum lethal dose is about 1 g. The maximum permissible atmospheric concentration is 0.1 mg/m^3 and the maximum acceptable daily intake is 2 µg/kg as the dichloride. Large amounts of paraquat produce death in a few hours or days owing to pulmonary oedema, haemorrhage and the toxic effects on the kidney, liver and heart. Smaller doses may result in later mortality by progressive respiratory failure and death may still ensue even after concentrations in blood or urine are almost undetectable. Tissue concentrations in fatal cases therefore vary considerably according to the length of survival after ingestion. Blood concentrations greater than about 2 mg/L at 4 h and 0.1 mg/L at 24 h are likely to be lethal in most subjects but individual response is variable and some subjects with much higher concentrations have recovered.

In a review of 26 fatalities attributed to paraquat poisoning, the following postmortem tissue concentrations, mg/L or µg/g (mean *n*) were reported:

	Death within 24 h	Death within 1 to 7 days	Death after 8 days or more
Blood	1.4–52 (14, 5)	0.2–4.4 (1.3, 8)	not detected
Kidney	22.5–279 (79, 6)	1.4–74 (16, 10)	0.6–2.8 (1.5, 5)
Liver	8.8–141 (41, 6)	0.3–57.6 (8, 10)	0.2, 1.4 (2)
Lung	12.8–186 (78, 3)	1.6–21.4 (7, 6)	–
Urine	1210 (1)	4–15.8 (9, 3)	trace, 2.2 (2)

[D. J. L. Carson and E. D. Carson, *Forensic Sci.*, 1976, *7*, 151–160].

A mother administered a paraquat solution to her 3 children (8 years, 6 years and 15 months) before taking an unknown amount of it herself. 30 h after the ingestions, the serum paraquat concentrations of the children were 0.06, <0.006 and 0.025 mg/L, respectively. The children recovered following haemoperfusion and, in 2 cases, plasmapheresis and erythroporesis but the mother died [P. Kalabalikis *et al.*, *Vet. Hum. Toxicol.*, 2001, *43*, 31–33].

A crop-dusting accident resulted in the death of a worker who absorbed paraquat through the skin after sustaining 37% TBSA burns. After 9.5 h cutaneous exposure, a paraquat level of 169 mg/L was obtained at 20 h [A. J. Gear *et al.*, *J. Burn Care Rehabil.*, 2001, *22*, 347–351].

In a fatality caused by massive ingestion of paraquat, the following postmortem concentrations were reported: blood 5.05 mg/L, urine 6.00 mg/L, stomach contents, 17.2 g/L, liver 4.86 µg/g, kidney 80.6 µg/g [K. Arys *et al.*, *J. Anal. Toxicol.*, 2000, *24*, 116–121].

A 71-year-old man who was admitted to hospital 2 days after ingesting Korean weed killer (and had ingested some more the evening before admission), died 6 days later after experiencing increasing respiratory distress. Serum paraquat measured on day 1 after admission was 0.7 mg/L; the quantity of paraquat ingested was about 90 mL of a 25% solution [T. Erickson *et al.*, *J. Emerg. Med.*, 1997, *15*, 649–652].

Note. For reviews of the toxicology of paraquat see J. A. Vale *et al.*, *Hum. Toxicol.*, 1987, *6*, 41–47 and C Bismuth *et al.*, *Drug Safety*, 1990, *5*, 243–251.

Parathion

Pesticide

Proprietary names. Alkron; Aphamite; Folidol; Fostex E; Fosferno 20; Niran; Nitrostigmine; Paraphos; Rhodiatox; Thiophos.
Phosphorothioic acid *O*,*O*-Diethyl *O*-(4-nitrophenyl) ester
$C_{10}H_{14}NO_5PS$=291.3
CAS—56-38-2

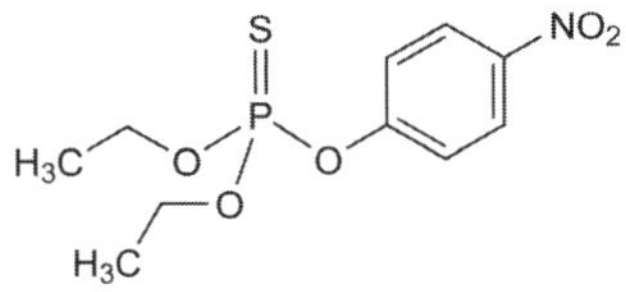

A pale yellow liquid which is decomposed by heat and darkens on exposure to light. M.p. 6°. B.p. 375°. Refractive index, at 25°, 1.5367.
Practically insoluble in water; miscible with most organic solvents. It is rapidly hydrolysed in alkaline solution.

Partition Coefficient. Log *P* (octanol/water), 3.8.

Colour Tests. Palladium Chloride—brown; Phosphorus Test—yellow.

Thin-layer Chromatography. System TW—parathion Rf 81; parathion methyl Rf 77; system TX—parathion ethyl Rf 41; parathion methyl Rf 30; system TY—parathion ethyl Rf 84; parathion methyl Rf 73.

Gas Chromatography. System GA—parathion ethyl RI 1950; parathion methyl RI 1855; M (amino-) RI 1892; M (*p*-nitrophenol) RI 1525; paraoxon RI 1895; system GK—parathion ethyl RRT 1.04; parathion methyl 0.96 (both relative to caffeine).

High Performance Liquid Chromatography. System HY—paraoxon RI 428; system HZ—parathion Retention time 35.5 min; paraoxon Retention time 6.5 min; paraoxon decomposition Retention time 3.7 min.

Ultraviolet Spectrum. Ethanol—274 nm (A^1_1=343b).

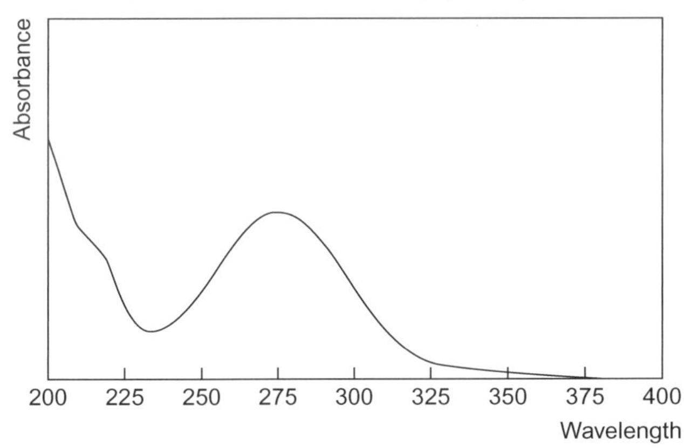

Infra-red Spectrum. Principal peaks at wavenumbers 1020, 925, 1515, 1219, 1587, 970 cm^{-1}.

Mass Spectrum. Principal ions at *m*/*z* 97, 109, 291, 139, 125, 137, 155, 123.

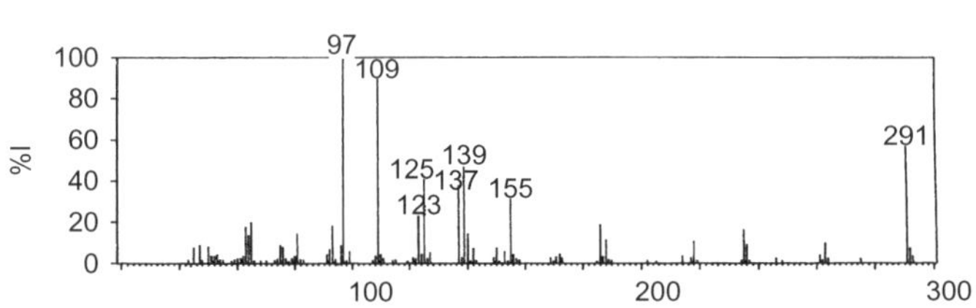

Quantification

Gas chromatography. In urine: 4-nitrophenol, limit of detection 20 µg/L, ECD—D. E. Bradway and T. M. Shafik, *Bull. Envir. Contam. Toxicol.*, 1973, *9*, 134–139.

Gas chromatography–mass spectrometry. In blood: limit of detection 0.02 to 0.05 µg/g—F. Musshoff *et al.*, *Clin. Chem. Lab. Med.*, 1999, *37*, 639–642. In blood: parathion and other pesticides, GC with electrochemical detection confirmed by GC–MS—R. Garcia-Repetto *et al.*, *JAOAC Int.*, 2001, *84*, 342–349. In blood: parathion-ethyl, parathion-methyl and other pesticides, limits of detection 0.01 to 0.03 µg/g—F. Musshoff *et al.*, *J. Chromatogr. Sci.*, 2002, *40*, 29–34.

High performance liquid chromatography–gas chromatography. In urine: paranitrophenyl sulfate—M. L. Oneto *et al.*, *Sci. Justice*, 1995, *35*, 207–211.

Radioimmunoassay. In plasma: limit of detection 100 µg/L—C. D. Ercegovich *et al.*, *J. Agric. Food Chem.*, 1981, *29*, 559–563.

Disposition in the Body. Parathion is activated in the liver by metabolism to paraoxon. Parathion and paraoxon are further metabolised to diethylthiophosphoric acid (DETP), diethylphosphoric acid (DEP), and 4-nitrophenol which are the major urinary excretion products although DETP and DEP are unstable in stored urine. Urinary 4-nitrophenol concentrations may be indicative of the extent of exposure to parathion. 4-Nitrophenol is rapidly excreted in the urine and is not detectable 48 h after exposure by inhalation or ingestion, but excretion is more prolonged after exposure of intact skin due to the much slower absorption of parathion by this route. Aminoparathion has been detected in postmortem blood and tissues.

Urinary 4-nitrophenol concentrations ranged from 0.4 to 13.2 mg/L in 23 occupationally-exposed asymptomatic workers and correlated well with serum-parathion concentrations which were in the range 0.003 to 0.20 mg/L [C. C. Roan *et al.*, *Bull. Environ. Contam. Toxicol.*, 1969, *4*, 362–369.]

Toxicity. The estimated minimum lethal dose by inhalation or ingestion is 20 mg and the maximum permissible atmospheric concentration is 0.1 mg/m^3. Urinary concentrations of about 2 mg/L or more of 4-nitrophenol may be associated with severe toxicity. Numerous fatalities have occurred due to contamination of food by parathion and also from suicidal ingestion.

The following postmortem tissue concentrations were reported in 19 fatalities due to parathion poisoning (determined by a bioassay based on cholinesterase inhibition): blood 0.5 to 34 mg/L (mean 9.0, 11 cases); brain 0.9 to 12.5 µg/g (mean 4.9, 4 cases); kidney 0.2 to 11.9 µg/g (mean 3.3, 9 cases); liver 0.08 to 120 µg/g (mean 11, 13 cases); urine 0.4 to 78 mg/L (mean 10, 10 cases) [A. Heyndrickx and F. De Clerc, *J. Pharm. Belg.*, 1977, *32*, 149–161.]

In 2 fatalities due to parathion, the following postmortem tissue concentrations, mg/L or µg/g, were reported:

	Parathion	Aminoparathion
Blood	0.01, 0.15	0.27, 6.7
Bile	—, 0.63,	—, 0.31
Liver	ND, ND	0.47, 32
Urine	ND, —	0.02, —

(ND=not detected)

[L. T. F. Chan *et al.*, *J. Forensic Sci.*, 1983, *28*, 122–127.]

Half-life. Derived from urinary excretion data, about 8 h.

Parbendazole

Anthelmintic (Veterinary)

Proprietary names. Helmatac; Verminum; WormGuard.
(5-Butyl-1*H*-benzimidazol-2-yl)carbamic acid methyl ester
$C_{13}H_{17}N_3O_2$=247.3
CAS—14255-87-9

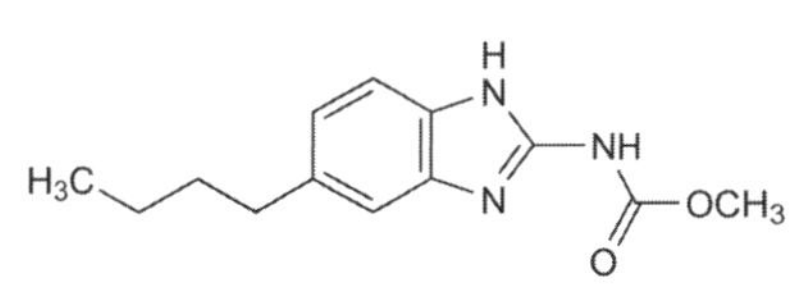

A white crystalline powder. M.p. 225° to 227°, with decomposition.
Practically insoluble in water; soluble 1 in 900 of ethanol and 1 in 300 of chloroform; very slightly soluble in ether; soluble in dilute mineral acids.

Partition Coefficient. Log *P* (octanol/water), 3.6.

Colour Test. Dissolve 5 mg in 5 mL of 0.1 M hydrochloric acid and add 3 mg of *p*-phenylenediamine dihydrochloride; shake to dissolve and add 0.1 g of zinc powder. After mixing, allow to stand for 2 min and add 10 mL of ferric ammonium sulfate solution—a blue or violet-blue colour develops.

Thin-layer Chromatography. System TA—Rf 70. (Acidified iodoplatinate solution, positive.)

Gas Chromatography. System GA—not eluted.

High Performance Liquid Chromatography. System HAA—Retention time 18.2 min.

Ultraviolet Spectrum. Aqueous acid—281, 288 (A^1_1=760a); aqueous alkali—254, 297 (A^1_1=816b), 303 nm.

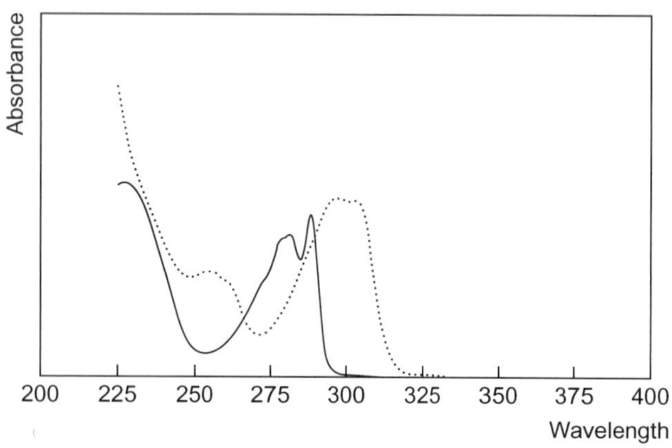

Infra-red Spectrum. Principal peaks at wavenumbers 1626, 1600, 1274, 1093, 1100, 1193 cm^{-1} (KBr disk).

Pargyline

Antihypertensive

N-Methyl-*N*-2-propynylbenzenemethanamine
$C_{11}H_{13}N$=159.2
CAS—555-57-7

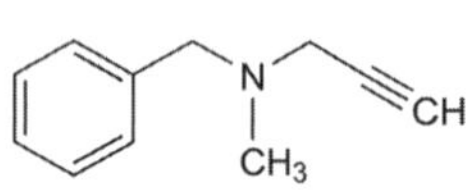

Pargyline Hydrochloride
Proprietary name. Eutonyl
$C_{11}H_{13}N,HCl$=195.7
CAS—306-07-0
A white crystalline powder. M.p. 154° to 155°; sublimation occurs when kept at raised temperatures.
Soluble 1 in 0.6 of water, 1 in 5 of ethanol, and 1 in about 7 of chloroform. Aqueous solutions are unstable.

Dissociation Constant. pK_a 6.9.

Partition Coefficient. Log *P* (octanol/water), 2.0.

Thin-layer Chromatography. System TA—Rf 70; system TE—Rf 60; system TAE—Rf 77; system TAJ—Rf 71; system TAK—Rf 20; system TAL—Rf 93. (Acidified iodoplatinate solution, positive.)

Gas Chromatography. System GA—RI 1214; system GB—RI 1257; system GC—RI 1440.

High Performance Liquid Chromatography. System HA—*k* 0.2; system HY—RI 203.

Ultraviolet Spectrum. Aqueous acid—251, 256, 261 (A^1_1=16a), 268; aqueous alkali—252, 257, 263 nm.

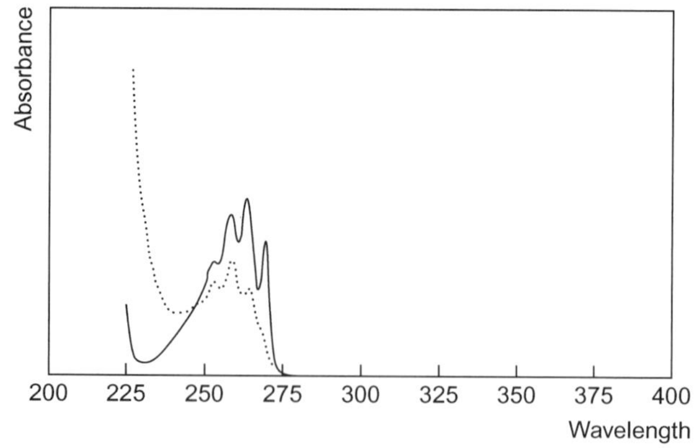

Infra-red Spectrum. Principal peaks at wavenumbers 697, 746, 714, 724, 1052, 1515 cm^{-1} (KBr disk).

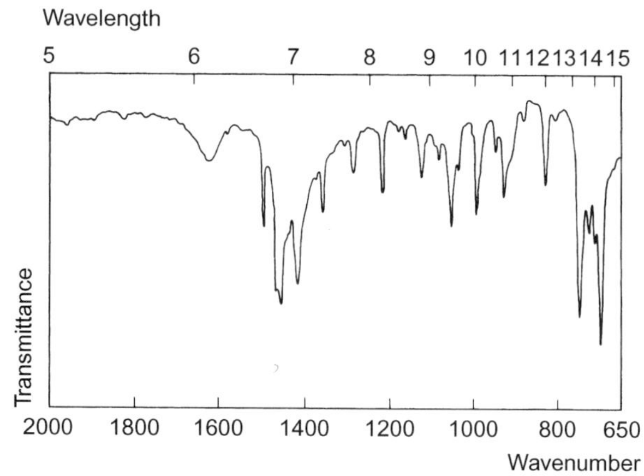

Mass Spectrum. Principal ions at *m/z* 82, 68, 91, 159, 42, 158, 92, 65.

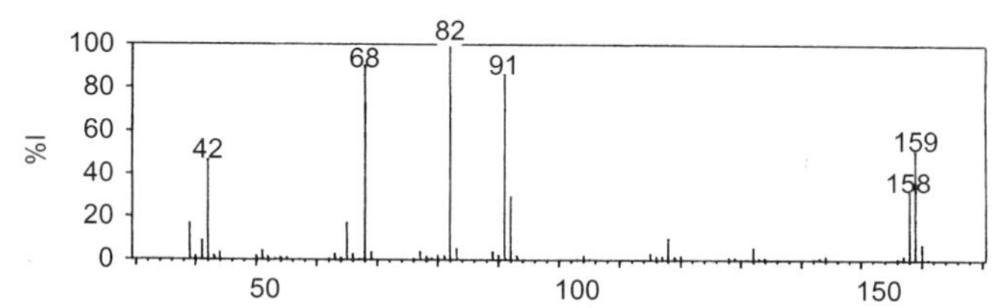

Dose. Usually 25 to 50 mg of pargyline hydrochloride daily; maximum of 200 mg daily.

Paroxetine

Antidepressant

Synonyms. BRL-29060; FG-7051.
(3*S*-*trans*)-3-[(1,3-Benzodioxol-5-yloxy)methyl]-4-(4-fluorophenyl)-piperidine
$C_{19}H_{20}FNO_3$=329.4
CAS—61869-08-7

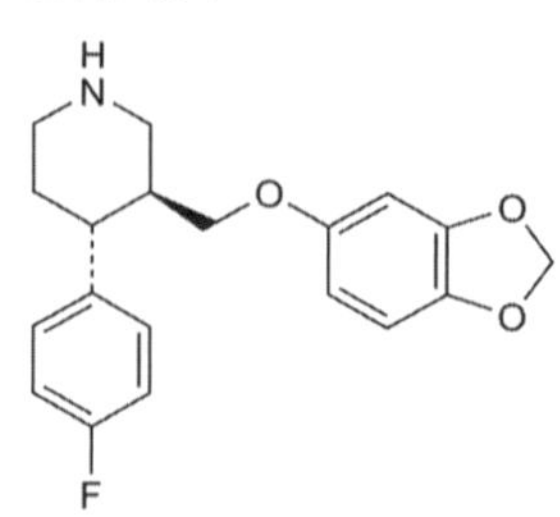

Paroxetine Hydrochloride Hemihydrate
Synonym. BRL-29060A
Proprietary names. Aropax; Deroxat; Frosinor; Motivan; Paxil; Sereupin; Seroxat; Tagonis.

$C_{19}H_{20}FNO_3,HCl.{}^1/_2H_2O=374.8$
CAS—78246-49-8; 110429-35-1
Crystals. M.p. 129° to 131°.

Dissociation Coefficient. pKa 9.9.

Partition Coefficient. Log *P* (octanol/water), 3.95.

Thin-layer Chromatography. System TB—Rf 04; system TE—Rf 40; system TAE—Rf 08; system TAJ—Rf 04; system TAK—Rf 04; system TAL—Rf 54.

Gas Chromatography. System GB—RI 2691 (paroxetine); RI 2734 M (desmethylenyl-3-methyl-); RI 2687 paroxetine M; system GM—RRT 2.047 (relative to iprindole).

Column: HP5 capillary (10 m × 0.25 mm i.d.). Column temperature: 140°, held 1 min, to 300° at 20°/min, held for 3 min. IS: clovoxamine. MS detection (EI, SIM at *m/z* 138 for paroxetine and 192 for IS). Retention time(s): trifluoroacetyl derivative of paroxetine, 7.9 min; IS, 6.0 min. [P. P. Singer and G. R. Jones, *J. Anal. Toxicol.*, 1997, *21*, 518–520].

Column: methyl silicone (HP1, 0.2 mm i.d., 0.33 μm film thickness). Column temperature: 250°. Carrier gas: helium, 0.9 mL/min flow rate. MS detection. Retention index: 2492. [T. Mills and J. C. Roberson, *Instrumental Data for Drug Analysis*, 1993, CRC Press, Boca Raton, US. 2nd Edn, Vol. 6, pp. 192–193].

High Performance Liquid Chromatography. System HX—RI 426; system HY—RI 337; system HZ—retention time 5.6 min; system HAA—retention time 15.3 min; system HAX—retention time 11.1 min; system HAY—retention time 5.8 min.

Ultraviolet Spectrum. Aqueous acid—233, 264, 270, 293 nm; basic—233, 264, 270, 292 nm.

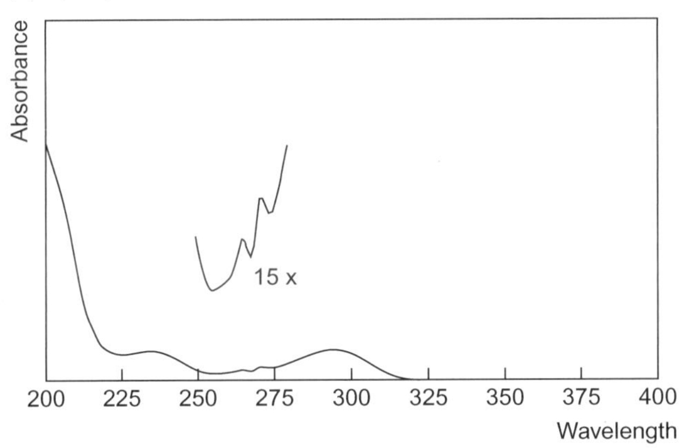

Infra-red Spectrum. Principal peaks at wavenumbers 1185, 1512, 1490 cm^{-1} (paroxetine hydrochloride) (KBr disk).

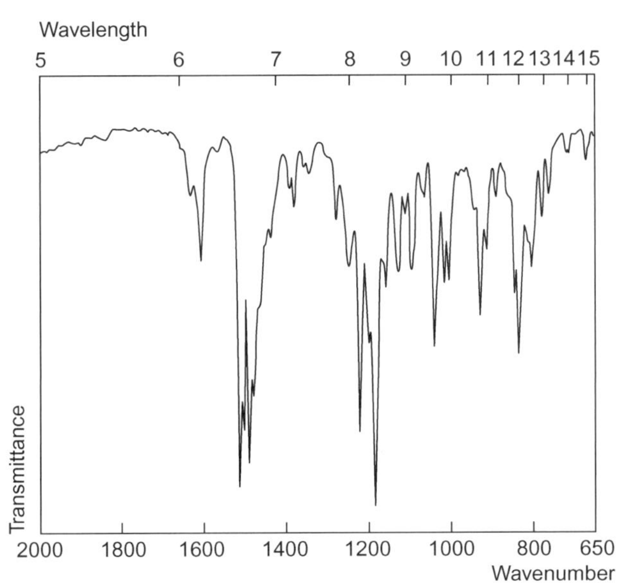

Mass Spectrum. Principal ions at *m/z* 44, 329, 192, 70, 138, 109, 42, 41.

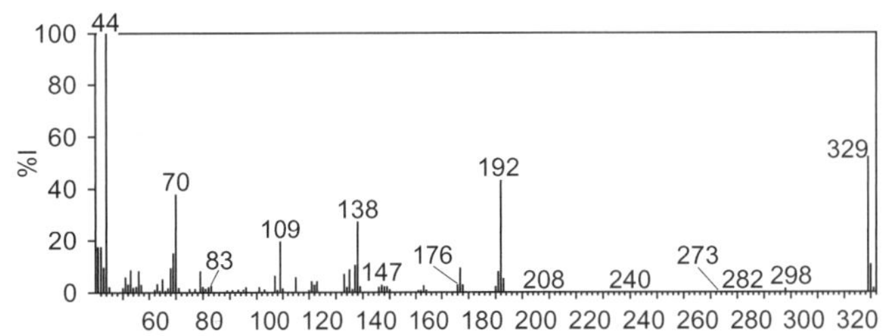

Quantification

High performance liquid chromatography. In serum—limit of detection 5 μg/L, fluorescence detection (λ_{ex}=295 nm, λ_{em}=365 nm)—R. N. Gupta, *J. Chromatogr.*, 1994, *661*; *Biomed. Appl.*, 362–365. In plasma: limit of detection 0.2 μg/L, fluorescence detection (λ_{ex}=300 nm, λ_{em}=350 nm)—M. A. Brett *et al.*, *J. Chromatogr.*, 1987, *419*, 438–444.

Disposition in the Body. Paroxetine is readily absorbed after oral administration and undergoes extensive first-pass hepatic metabolism: *O*-demethylenation in a reaction regulated by CYP2D6, giving rise to a catechol-type metabolite further *O*-methylated and conjugated with glucuronic acid and sulfate. Peak plasma concentrations can be observed about 5 h after administration. Paroxetine is distributed throughout the body, including the CNS, with only 1% remaining in the plasma. It is excreted mainly as metabolites in urine (approx. 64%) and faeces (approx. 36%). Less than 2% of a dose is found in urine as the parent drug. It is distributed in breast milk and widely distributed throughout the body.

Therapeutic concentration. The serum therapeutic concentration range is 10 to 75 μg/L.

12 patients, aged 28 to 69 years, with biopsy proven alcohol cirrhosis and 6 healthy individuals, 26 to 60 years, with no signs of liver disease were administered 30 mg paroxetine hydrochloride daily for 14 days. The maximum steady state concentration observed for the patients was 134.7 μg/L, measured on days 13 and 14, and the minimum was 102.9 μg/L. For the healthy subjects, the maximum was 74.4 μg/L and the minimum, 45.9 μg/L. [K. Dalhoff *et al.*, *Eur. J. Clin. Pharmacol.*, 1991, *41*, 351–354].

Toxicity. Toxic effects may occur with conc. greater than 400 μg/L.

A young man was found at home shivering and incoherent, after which he had numerous seizures. 4 h after he was found, he suffered from full cardiac arrest and it was impossible for the paramedics to resuscitate him because his jaw was unusually stiff and they could not open his mouth to intubate him. Toxicological analysis showed a paroxetine concentration of 1.58 mg/L in subclavian blood, 15.3 mg/kg in liver and 0.0101 mg/g in the gastric contents. His death was actually attributed to a combined toxicity of moclobemide and paroxetine. Moclobemide was found in his blood at a concentration of 18.5 mg/L, in liver at 28.5 mg/kg and in the gastric contents at 1.116 mg/g. [P. P. Singer and G. R. Jones, *J. Anal. Toxicol.*, 1997, *21(6)*, 518–520].

Half-life. 12 to 40 h.

Volume of distribution. 3 to 28 L/kg.

Protein binding. 95%.

Note. For a general review, see N. S. Gunasekara *et al.*, *Drugs*, 1998, *55*, 85–120.

Dose. The usual dose is 10 or 20 mg daily which may be increased to 50 or 60 mg in increments if necessary, with a maintenance dose of 40 mg daily. In the elderly and debilitated patients: maximum 40 mg daily. Those with severe renal or hepatic impairment: 20 mg.

Pecazine

Tranquilliser

Synonym. Mepazine
10-[(1-Methyl-3-piperidinyl)methyl]-10*H*-phenothiazine
$C_{19}H_{22}N_2S=310.5$
CAS—60-89-9

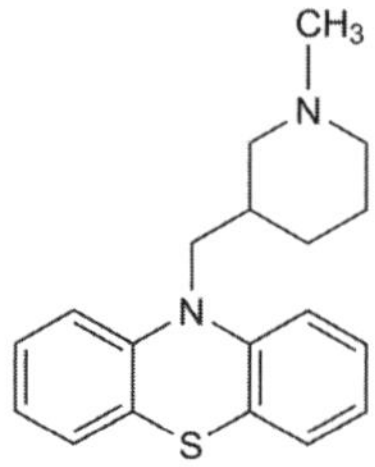

Pecazine Hydrochloride
$C_{19}H_{22}N_2S,HCl,H_2O=364.9$
CAS—2975-36-2
A white crystalline powder. M.p. 180° to 181°.
Very slightly soluble in water; freely soluble in dehydrated alcohol; soluble in chloroform; practically insoluble in ether and benzene.

Dissociation Constant. pK_a 9.7 (24°).

Partition Coefficient. Log *P* (octanol/water), 5.4.

Colour Tests. Mandelin's Test—green→violet; Marquis Test—violet.

Thin-layer Chromatography. System TA—Rf 53; system TB—Rf 47; system TC—Rf 44; system TE—Rf 65; system TF—Rf 01; system TL—Rf 16; system TAE—Rf 27. (Acidified iodoplatinate solution, positive.)

Gas Chromatography. System GA—RI 2540; system GB—RI 2669.

High Performance Liquid Chromatography. System HA—*k* 3.9; system HX—RI 443; system HY—RI 382; system HAX—Retention time 15.3 min; system HAY—Retention time 7.0 min.

Ultraviolet Spectrum. Aqueous acid—253 (A^1_1=892a), 300; aqueous alkali—265 nm.

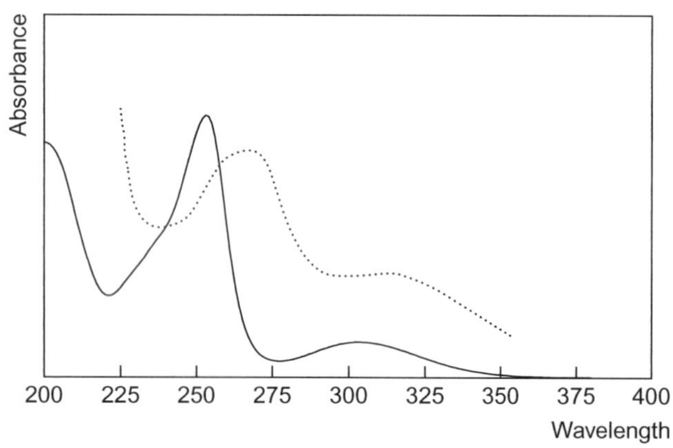

Infra-red Spectrum. Principal peaks at wavenumbers 750, 768, 1219, 1250, 1162, 1282 cm^{-1} (pecazine hydrochloride, KBr disk).

Mass Spectrum. Principal ions at *m/z* 310, 58, 199, 112, 311, 111, 212, 41.

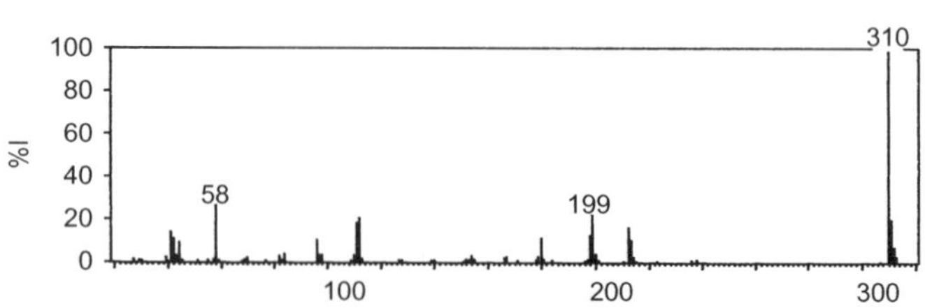

Dose. Pecazine hydrochloride has been given in doses equivalent to 37.5 to 75 mg of the base daily.

Pemoline

Central Stimulant

Synonyms. Phenilone; Phenoxazole; Phenylisohydantoin; Phenylpseudohydantoin.

Proprietary names. Cylert; Deltamine; Dynalert; Hyperilex; Nitan; PemADD; Sigmadyn; Senior; Stimul; Tradon; Volital.
2-Amino-5-phenyl-4(5*H*)-oxazolone
$C_9H_8N_2O_2=176.2$
CAS—2152-34-3

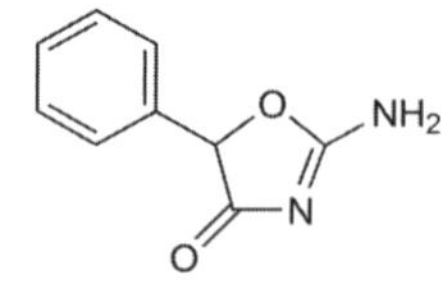

A white crystalline powder. M.p. 256° to 257°, with decomposition.
Practically insoluble in water, acetone, and ether; soluble 1 in 100 of propylene glycol.

Dissociation Constant. pK_a 10.5.

Partition Coefficient. Log *P* (octanol/water), 0.5.

Colour Test. Koppanyi–Zwikker Test—violet.

Thin-layer Chromatography. System TA—Rf 60; system TB—Rf 00; system TC—Rf 23; system TE—Rf 36; system TF—Rf 11; system TL—Rf 40; system TAE—Rf 81; system TAF—Rf 81; system TAJ—Rf 12; system TAK—Rf 14; system TAL—Rf 60. (Marquis reagent, yellow-brown; ninhydrin spray, positive; acidified potassium permanganate solution, positive.)

Gas Chromatography. System GA—pemoline RI 1969; pemoline-Me_2 RI 1590, mandelic acid RI 1485; system GB—pemoline RI 2081.

High Performance Liquid Chromatography. System HA—*k* 0.2; system HC—*k* 0.1; system HX—RI 307; system HY—RI 271.

Ultraviolet Spectrum. Aqueous acid—256 (A^1_1=20a), 262, 268 nm.

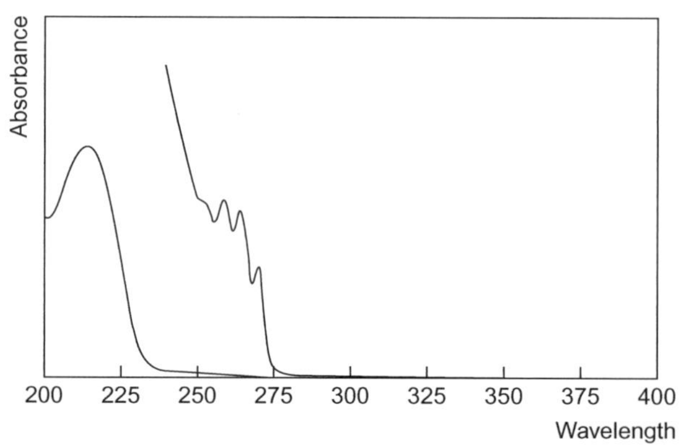

Infra-red Spectrum. Principal peaks at wavenumbers 1218, 1653, 695, 1560, 1137, 1275 cm^{-1} (KBr disk).

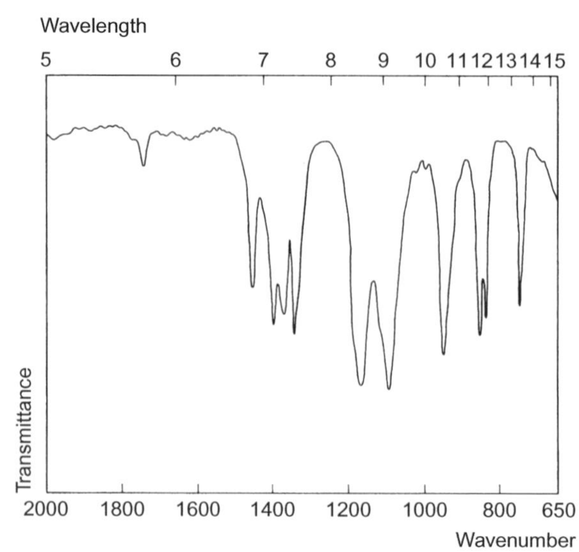

Mass Spectrum. Principal ions at *m/z* 107, 176, 90, 77, 70, 105, 42, 79; mandelic acid 107, 79, 77, 51, 152, 105, 50, 78; 5-phenyloxazolidine-2,4-dione 90, 177, 105, 77, 106, 51, 89, 50.

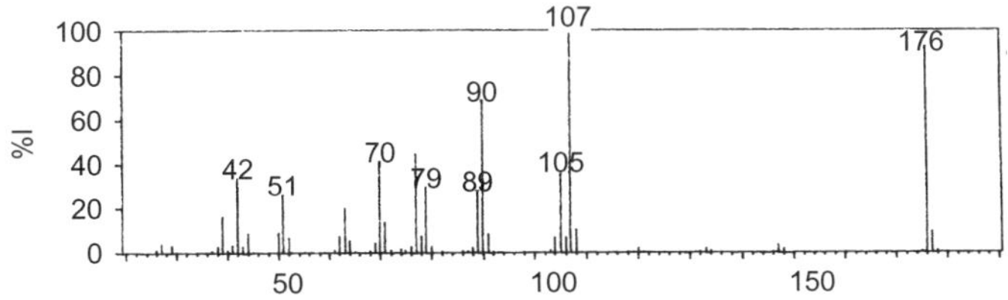

Quantification

Gas chromatography. In serum or urine: limit of detection 50 µg/L, AFID—D. J. Hoffman, *J. Pharm. Sci.*, 1979, *68*, 445–447. In horse plasma or urine: limit of detection 50 µg/L and 100 µg/L, respectively, ECD—O. J. Igwe and J. W. Blake, *J. Chromatogr. Sci.*, 1981, *19*, 617–624.

High performance liquid chromatography. In plasma, saliva, or urine: limit of detection 20 µg/L, UV detection—K. Nishihara *et al.*, *Ther. Drug Monit.*, 1984, *6*, 232–237.

Disposition in the Body. Slowly absorbed after oral administration. About 50% of a dose is excreted in the urine as unchanged drug in 48 h and about 4% as 5-phenyloxazolidine-2,4-dione; the remainder is excreted in the urine as conjugated pemoline and unidentified polar metabolites; mandelic acid is also a metabolite of pemoline. Less than 1% of a dose is eliminated in the faeces.

Therapeutic concentration

After a single oral dose of 50 mg given to 3 subjects, peak plasma concentrations of 0.77 to 1.22 mg/L (mean 1.0) were attained in about 2 to 3 h; peak concentrations in saliva of 0.47 to 0.75 mg/L (mean 0.59) were reported after 2 to 4 h; following administration of 37.5 mg to 1 subject, peak plasma and saliva concentrations of 0.89 and 0.58 mg/L, respectively, were attained in about 4 h [N. P. E. Vermeulen *et al.*, *Br. J. Clin. Pharmacol.*, 1979, *8*, 459–463.]

After daily oral doses of 37.5 and 75 mg to 28 hyperactive children for seven days, mean plasma concentrations of about 2 and 4 mg/L respectively, were reported 3 h after the last dose [C. P. Tomkins *et al.*, *Ther. Drug Monit.*, 1980, *2*, 255–260.]

Peak plasma concentrations of 4.3 (± 1.0) mg/L were attained in 2.8 (±1.8) h after a single 2 mg/kg oral dose of pemoline to 7 prepubescent boys [F. Sallee *et al.*, *Clin. Pharmacol. Ther.*, 1985, *37*, 606–609.]

Toxicity. Estimated minimum lethal dose, 2 g for an adult, 0.2 g for children up to 2 years, although recovery has occurred following the ingestion of up to 1.8 g by young children.

Half-life. Plasma half-life, about 10 to 18 h.

Protein binding. In plasma, about 30%.

Dose. Usually 40 mg daily; maximum of 120 mg daily.

Pempidine

Antihypertensive

1,2,2,6,6-Pentamethylpiperidine
$C_{10}H_{21}N = 155.3$
CAS—79-55-0

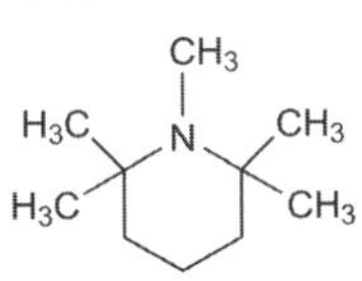

A liquid.

Pempidine Tartrate

Proprietary names. Pempidil; Pempiten; Perolysen; Tenormal; Tensinol; Tensoral.
$C_{10}H_{21}N,C_4H_6O_6 = 305.4$
CAS—546-48-5
A white crystalline powder. M.p. 160°.
Soluble 1 in 2 of water and 1 in 14 of ethanol; very slightly soluble in acetone; practically insoluble in chloroform and ether.

Thin-layer Chromatography. System TA—Rf 24; system TB—Rf 68; system TC—Rf 03; system TL—Rf 10. (Acidified iodoplatinate solution, positive.)

Infra-red Spectrum. Principal peaks at wavenumbers 1308, 1261, 1210, 1136, 1063, 675 cm^{-1} (pempidine tartrate, KBr disk).

Mass Spectrum. Principal ions at *m/z* 140, 84, 56, 41, 72, 69, 29, 39.

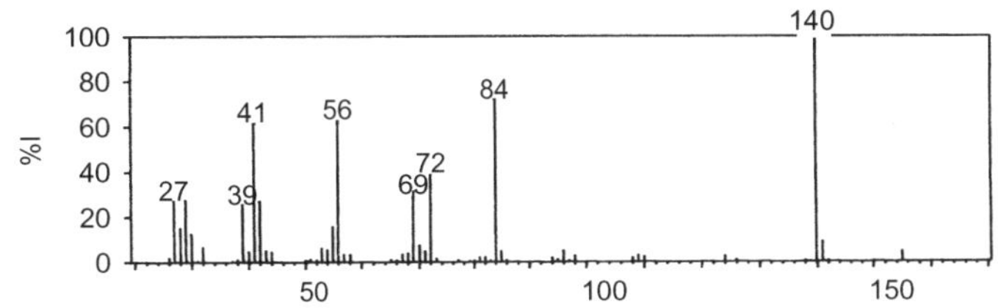

Dose. 7.5 to 80 mg of pempidine tartrate daily.

Penciclovir

Antiviral

Synonyms. PCV; BRL-39123
Proprietary names. Denavir; Famvir; Vectavir.
2-Amino-1,9-dihydro-9-[4-hydroxy-3-(hydroxymethyl)butyl]-6*H*-purin-6-one
$C_{10}H_{15}N_5O_3 = 253.3$
CAS—39809-25-1

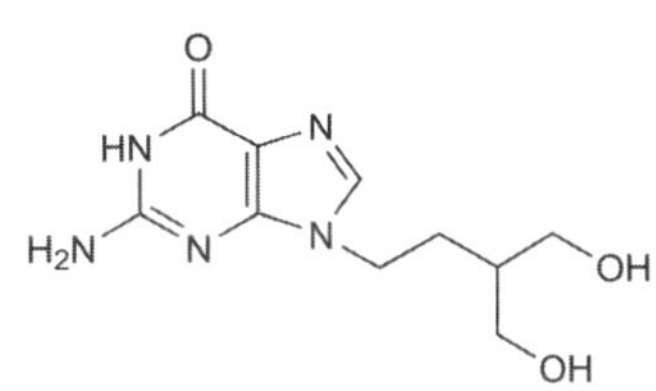

White crystalline solid. M.p. 275° to 277°. Also reported as colourless matted needles. M.p. 272° to 275°. Soluble in water (1.7 mg/mL, 20°, pH 7).

Penciclovir Sodium

Synonym. BRL-39123A
$C_{10}H_{15}N_5O_3Na, H_2O = 294.3$
CAS—97845-62-0
Crystalline solid. Soluble in water.

Partition Coefficient. Log *P* (octanol/water), –1.62.

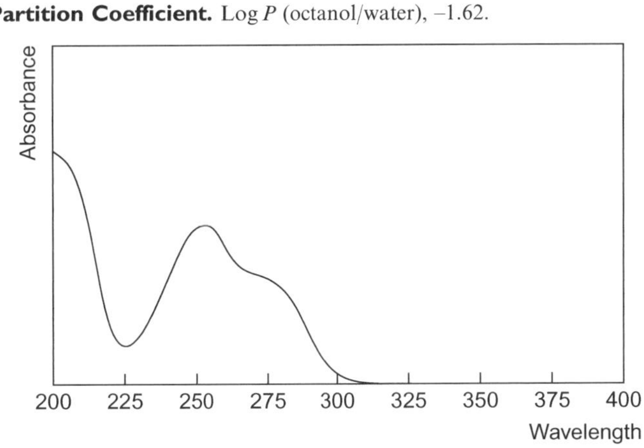

Quantification

High performance liquid chromatography. In plasma and urine: limit of quantification 0.1 mg/L and 50 mg/L, respectively. UV detection—S. E. Fowles and D. M. Pierce, *Analyst*, 1989, *114*, 1373–1375.

Disposition in the Body. The drug is poorly absorbed from the gastrointestinal tract. For systemic use, it is usually administered orally as the prodrug, famciclovir, which is rapidly converted to penciclovir, producing peak plasma concentrations to the dose after 45 min to 1 h. Metabolites include a triphosphate derivative which is active. Minor metabolites include 6-deoxypenciclovir, monoacetylated penciclovir and monoacetylated 6-deoxypenciclovir. It is mainly excreted unchanged in the urine.

Therapeutic concentration

Following the administration of a single 500 mg dose of famciclovir to 9 patients with normal renal function, mean peak plasma penciclovir concentrations were 2.83 mg/L (range 1.30 to 3.82 mg/L) reached in 0.89 h (mean, range 0.5 to 1.5 h). Another 18 patients, split into three groups according to their renal impairment: mild, moderate and severe, were also administered the drug regimen. Mean peak plasma concentrations were 3.26 mg/L, 4.45 mg/L and 5.31 mg/L for the three groups, respectively, and reached in 0.79, 1.38 and 1.13 h (all mean times) [S. C. Boike *et al.*, *Clin. Pharmacol. Ther.*, 1994, *55*, 418–426].

20 healthy males (mean age 36 years old, range 23 to 59 years), fasted from both fluids and solids for ten hours pre-dosing, were administered 4 single oral doses of famciclovir (125, 250, 500 and 750 mg) on 4 separate days and at least one week apart. Penciclovir concentrations were detected 15 to 30 min after oral administration at all four dosages. Mean peak plasma penciclovir concentrations were 0.84 mg/L, 1.59 mg/L, 3.34 mg/L and 5.09 mg/L for the 125, 250, 500 and 750 mg does respectively, reached at 0.51, 0.75, 0.75 and 0.75 h, respectively [M.A. Pue *et al.*, *J. Antimicrob. Chemother.*, 1994, *33*, 119–127].

Following the IV administration of 10, 15 or 20 mg/kg penciclovir over 60 min to 15 healthy male subjects, mean peak plasma concentrations were 12.1, 19.6 and 22.7 mg/L respectively. Peak plasma concentrations coincided with the end of the infusion [S. E. Fowles *et al.*, *Eur. J. Clin. Pharmacol.*, 1992, *43*, 513–516].

Bioavailability. About 77%.

Half-life. In plasma, approximately 2 h.

Volume of distribution. Reported as 111.9 L or 1.5 L/kg (mean values).

Clearance. Reported as 25.5 to 32.0 L/h in young healthy subjects.

Protein binding. Less than 20%.

Dose. Topically as 1% cream every 2 h for 4 days in the treatment of *herpes labialis*. For systemic use, penciclovir is administered orally as the prodrug famciclovir.

Penfluridol

Tranquilliser

Proprietary name. Semap

1-[4,4-Bis(4-fluorophenyl)butyl]-4-[4-chloro-3-(trifluoromethyl)phenyl]-4-piperidinol

$C_{28}H_{27}ClF_5NO = 524.0$

CAS—26864-56-2

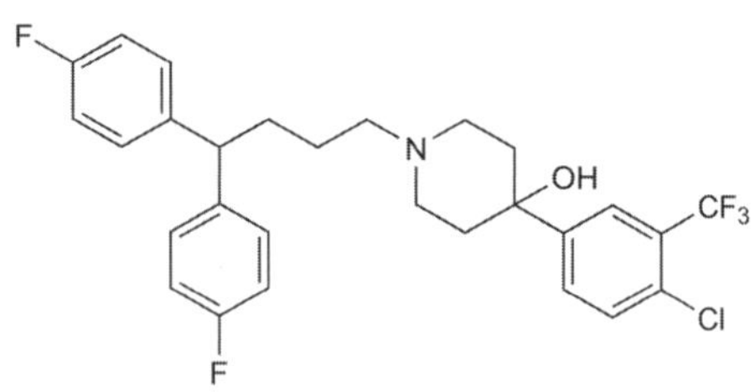

A white crystalline or microcrystalline powder. M.p. 105° to 107°. Practically insoluble in water; very soluble in ethanol, acetone, and chloroform; freely soluble in ether.

Partition Coefficient. Log *P* (octanol/water), 2.7.

Colour Test. Liebermann's Test—brown.

Thin-layer Chromatography. System TA—Rf 76; system TB—Rf 17; system TC—Rf 60; system TE—Rf 84; system TL—Rf 60; system TAE—Rf 72; system TAF—Rf 89. (Dragendorff spray.)

Gas Chromatography. System GA—penfluridol RI 3360; M (*N*-desalkyl-) RI 2210; M (*N*-desalkyl-oxo-)-$2H_2O$ RI 1920; M (desamino-OH-) RI 2120; M (desamino-carboxy-) RI 2230.

High Performance Liquid Chromatography. System HX—RI 659; system HY—RI 656; system HZ—Retention time 43.4 min; system HAA—Retention time 20.2 min.

Ultraviolet Spectrum. Aqueous acid—267 nm ($A_1^1 = 47a$), 273 nm. No alkaline shift.

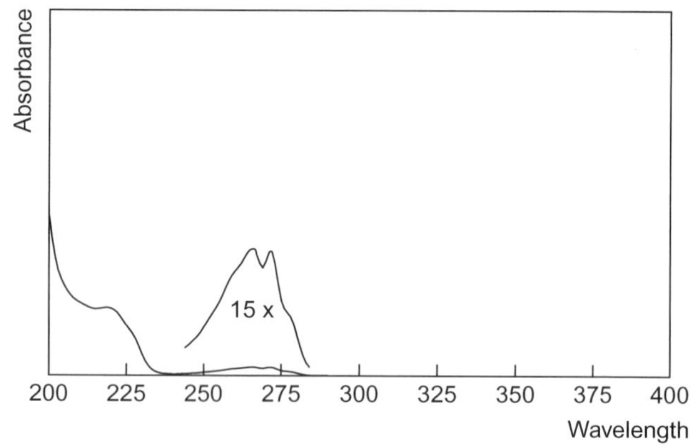

Infra-red Spectrum. Principal peaks at wavenumbers 1500, 1138, 1225, 1315, 1157, 825 (KBr disk).

Mass Spectrum. Principal ions at *m/z* 42, 292, 56, 294, 109, 203, 201, 44.

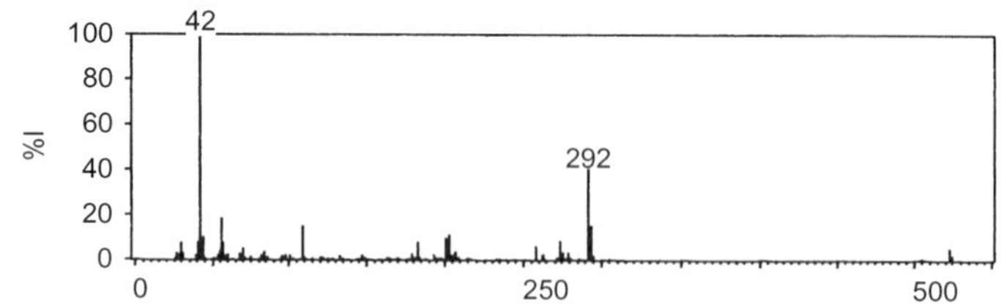

Quantification

Gas chromatography. In plasma: limit of detection 1 to 2 μg/L, ECD—S. F. Cooper *et al.*, *Int. Pharmacopsychiatry*, 1975, *10*, 78–88.

Disposition in the Body. Incompletely absorbed after oral administration. It has a very long duration of action. About 5% of a dose is excreted in the urine in 7 days, mainly as 4,4′-bis(4-fluorophenyl)butyric acid; about 80% of a dose is eliminated in the faeces, mostly as unchanged drug.

Therapeutic concentration.

Following weekly oral administration of 30, 60 and 120 mg for 13 weeks to 7, 7 and 8 subjects, mean steady-state plasma concentrations of about 0.004 to 0.01, 0.006 to 0.012 and 0.008 to 0.025 mg/L were reported. In all subjects maximum concentrations were attained within 12 h of a dose; concentrations declined rapidly between 12 and 24 h followed by a much slower decline during the next 120 h and were still significant (about 0.001 mg/L) 168 h after the dose [S. F. Cooper *et al.*, *Clin. Pharmacol. Ther.*, 1975, *18*, 325–329.]

Dose. Usually 20 to 60 mg weekly, by mouth; doses of up to 120 mg weekly have been given.

Penicillamine

Chelating Agent

Synonyms. (−)-*β*,*β*-Dimethylcysteine; D-3-Mercaptovaline; D-Penicillamine.

Proprietary names. Adalken; Artamin; Atamir; Cuprimine; Cupripen; Depen; Distamine; Kelatin; Mercaptyl; Metalcaptase; D-Penamine; Pendramine; Rheumantin; Sufortan; Sufortanon; Trisorcin; Trolovol.

3,3-Dimethyl-(*s*)-cysteine

$C_5H_{11}NO_2S = 149.2$

CAS—52-67-5

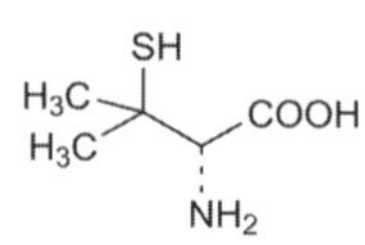

A white, finely crystalline powder. M.p. 202° to 206°.

Soluble 1 in 9 of water and 1 in 530 of ethanol; practically insoluble in chloroform and ether.

Penicillamine Hydrochloride
Proprietary name. Pemine
$C_5H_{11}NO_2S,HCl=185.7$
CAS—2219-30-9
A white, hygroscopic, finely crystalline powder. M.p. about 175°, with decomposition.
Soluble 1 in 1 of water, 1 in 1.5 of ethanol and 1 in 230 of chloroform; practically insoluble in ether.

Dissociation Constant. pK_a 1.8, 7.9, 10.5.

Partition Coefficient. Log *P* (octanol/water), −1.8.

Colour Tests. Mandelin's Test—yellow; Palladium Chloride—yellow.

Thin-layer Chromatography. System TA—Rf 36; system TB—Rf 01; system TC—Rf 03; system TE—Rf 03; system TL—Rf 03; system TAE—Rf 44. (Acidified iodoplatinate solution, positive.)

Infra-red Spectrum. Principal peaks at wavenumbers 1595, 1525, 1615, 1550, 1090, 1055 cm^{-1} (Nujol mull). Two polymorphic forms occur.

Mass Spectrum. Principal ions at *m/z* 75, 41, 57, 70, 43, 59, 56, 47.

Quantification
High performance liquid chromatography. In whole blood, plasma or urine: limit of detection 75 μg/L for plasma and urine, 450 μg/L for whole blood, electrochemical detection—R. F. Bergström *et al.*, *J. Chromatogr.*, 1981, *222*; *Biomed. Appl.*, *11*, 445–452. In serum: limit of detection 130 μg/L, fluorescence detection—E. P. Lankmayr *et al.*, *J. Chromatogr.*, 1981, *222*; *Biomed. Appl.*, *11*, 249–255. In blood: limit of detection 10 μg/L, electrochemical detection—O. H. Drummer *et al.*, *J. Chromatogr.*, 1986, *374*, 251–257. In plasma: D-penicillamine-albumin sulfide, limit of detection 1.2 μmol/L, electrochemical detection—D. A. Joyce and D. N. Wade, *J. Chromatogr.*, 1988, *430*, 319–327. In plasma, erythrocytes or urine: penicillamine, penicillamine disulfide and penicillamine glutathione mixed disulfide, limit of detection 30 μg/L for penicillamine disulfide, electrochemical detection—G. T. Yamashita and D. L. Rabenstein, *J. Chromatogr.*, 1989, *491*, 341–354. In plasma or urine: penicillamine, homocysteine, homocystine and disulfides, electrochemical detection—D. L. Rabenstein and G. T. Yamashita, *Anal. Biochem.*, 1989, *180*, 259–263.

Reviews. For reviews of assay methods see D. R. Lecavalier and J. C. Crawhall, *J. Rheumatol.*, 1981, *Suppl.* 7, 20–27 and N. Kucharczyk and S. Shahinian, *J. Rheumatol.*, 1981, *Suppl.* 7, 28–34.

Disposition in the Body. Readily but incompletely absorbed after oral administration. About 50% of an oral dose is excreted in the urine in 48 h with about 10% as unchanged drug, up to 25% as cysteine-penicillamine disulfide, about 15% as penicillamine disulfide and less than 10% as *S*-methyl-D-penicillamine; about 35% of an oral dose is eliminated in the faeces in 3 days. After intravenous administration, about 80% of the dose is excreted in the urine in 24 h; traces of penicillamine remain in the plasma after 48 h owing to protein binding.

Therapeutic concentration
Following daily oral doses of 500 to 750 mg to 10 subjects, peak plasma concentrations of 1.7 to 5.6 mg/L (mean 3.7) were attained 1.5 to 3 h after a dose [M. Butler *et al.*, *Arthritis Rheum.*, 1982, *25*, 111–116.]

Half-life. Plasma half-life, about 2 to 6 h.

Protein binding. In plasma, up to 90%.

Note. For further details of penicillamine metabolism and kinetics see R. F. Bergström *et al.*, *Clin. Pharmacol. Ther.*, 1981, *30*, 404–413 and J. C. Crawhall *et al.*, *Biopharm. Drug Dispos.*, 1979, *1*, 73–95.

Dose. 0.125 to 4 g daily.

Pentachlorophenol

Preservative

Synonyms. PCP; Penta.
$C_6HCl_5O=266.3$
CAS—87-86-5

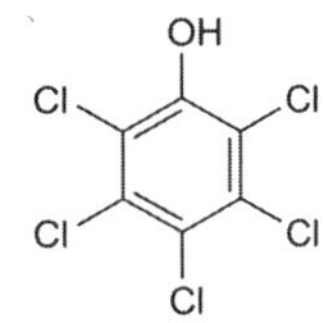

Note. The name PCP has also been used as a synonym for phencyclidine hydrochloride.
White crystals. M.p. 190° to 191°.
Practically insoluble in water; freely soluble in ethanol and ether; soluble in benzene.

Dissociation Constant. pK_a 4.7 (25°).

Partition Coefficient. Log *P* (octanol/water), 5.1.

Colour Test. Fuming Nitric Acid—red/red/brown-violet.

Gas Chromatography. System GA—pentachlorophenol RI 1760, pentachlorophenol-Me RI 1815.

Ultraviolet Spectrum. Aqueous alkali—319 nm ($A_1^1=194b$); ethanol—295 nm ($A_1^1=89b$), 303 nm ($A_1^1=115b$).

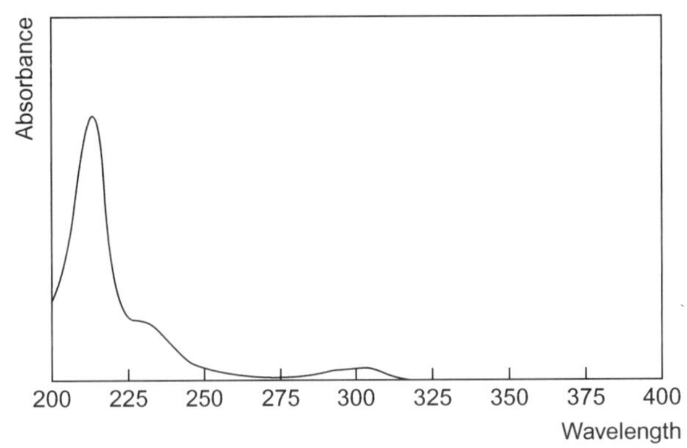

Infra-red Spectrum. Principal peaks at wavenumbers 1307, 774, 1222, 711, 1196, 1553 cm^{-1} (KBr disk).

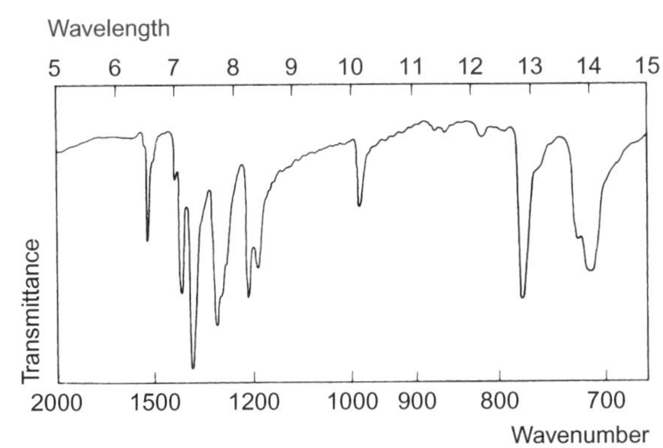

Mass Spectrum. Principal ions at *m/z* 266, 268, 264, 167, 165, 270, 202, 132.

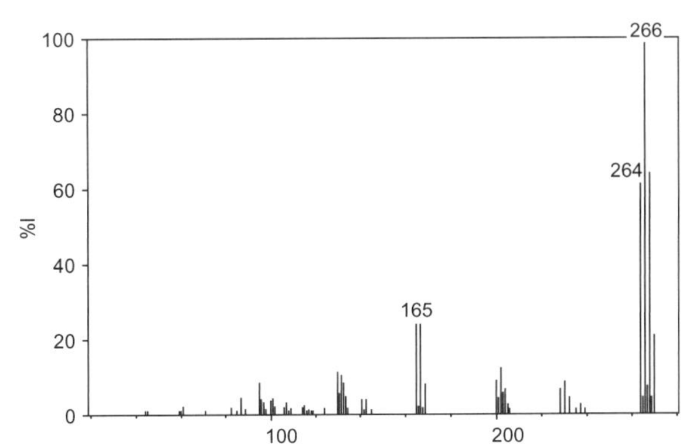

Quantification

Gas chromatography. In serum, whole blood or urine: limit of detection 1 µg/L, ECD—L. L. Needham *et al.*, *J. Anal. Toxicol.*, 1981, *5*, 283–286. In plasma or urine: limit of detection 10 µg/L, ECD—D. L. Rick *et al.*, *J. Anal. Toxicol.*, 1982, *6*, 297–300. In urine: ECD—K. Noren and J. Sjovall, *J. Chromatogr.*, 1987, *414*, 55–63.

Gas chromatography–mass spectrometry. In postmortem tissues: pentachlorophenol and other chlorinated compounds—S. L. Wagner *et al.*, *Arch. Environ. Contam. Toxicol.*, 1991, *21*, 596–606. In urine: pentachlorophenol and other chlorophenols, limit of detection for pentachlorophenol 3.6 µg/L, SIM—H. Kontsas *et al.*, *Analyst*, 1995, *120*, 1745–1749.

High performance liquid chromatography. In urine: limit of detection 30 µg/L, UV detection—K. Pekari and A. Aitio, *J. Chromatogr.*, 1982, *232*; *Biomed. Appl.*, *21*, 129–136.

Disposition in the Body. Readily absorbed after ingestion, inhalation or through intact skin. Pentachlorophenol and its oxidised metabolite, tetrachlorohydroquinone, are excreted in the urine in free and conjugated forms, with about 74% of a dose being excreted unchanged in 7 days. About 4% of a dose is eliminated in the faeces. Urinary concentrations in 130 pest-control operators exposed to pentachlorophenol ranged from 0.003 to 35.7 mg/L (mean 1.8) [A. Bevenue *et al.*, *Bull. Environ. Contam. Toxicol.*, 1967, *2*, 319–332.]

Blood concentration

Plasma concentrations of 0.99 to 9.1 mg/L were reported in 6 occupationally exposed subjects and blood concentrations of 0.34 to 6.0 mg/L were reported in 7 exposed workers [A. Bevenue *et al.*, *J. Chromatogr.*, 1968, *38*, 467–472.]

A sample of 15 women with long-term (5 to 17 years) low exposure to pentachlorophenol contained in wood-preservative had a mean pentachlorophenol serum level of 43.6 µg/L [M. Peper *et al.*, *Am. J. Ind. Med.*, 1999, *35*, 632–641.]

Toxicity. The estimated minimum lethal dose is 1 g and the maximum permissible atmospheric concentration is 0.5 mg/m^3. Blood concentrations greater than 30 mg/L are usually toxic. Numerous fatalities after absorption, inhalation or ingestion have been reported.

In two fatalities, the following postmortem tissue concentrations (mg/L or µg/g) were reported: blood 113, 156; brain 14, 35; kidney –, 123; liver 94, 134; urine –, 520 [M. F. Mason *et al.*, *J. Forensic Sci.*, 1965, *10*, 136–147.]

In one fatality, the following postmortem tissue concentrations were reported: blood 173 mg/L, kidney 116 µg/g, liver 225 µg/g, urine 75 mg/L [M. J. Cretney, *Bull. Int. Assoc. Forensic Toxicol.*, 1976, *12*(3), 10.]

Half-life. Plasma half-life, about 30 h.

Distribution in blood. Plasma:whole blood ratio, 1.8.

Protein binding. In plasma, about 99%.

Pentaerithrityl Tetranitrate *Anti-anginal Vasodilator*

Synonyms. Erynite; Nitropentaerythrol; Nitropenthrite; Pentaerythritol Tetranitrate; Pentanitrol.

Proprietary names. Cardiacap; Dilcoran; Hasethrol; Lentrat; Mycardol; Neo-Corovas; Nirason S; Nitrodex; Nitropenton; Pentafin; Pentalong; Pentanitrine; Pentral 60; Pentrite; Pentritol; Pentryate; Pentylan; Peritrate; Pergitral; Perityl; Prevangor; Quintrate; Subicard; Terpate; Vasodiatol.

2,2-Bis[(nitrooxy)methyl]-1,3-propanediol dinitrate (ester)

$C_5H_8N_4O_{12}$=316.1

CAS—115-77-5 (pentaerithrityl); 78-11-5 (tetranitrate)

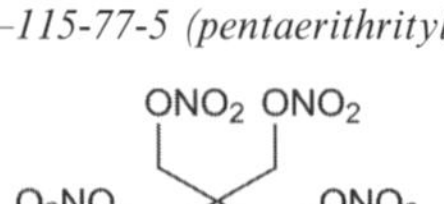

A white crystalline powder. M.p. 140°.

Practically insoluble in water; slightly soluble in ethanol and ether; soluble in acetone.

Note. For medicinal purposes pentaerithrityl tetranitrate is supplied diluted with an inert substance such as lactose, since the undiluted compound may explode upon percussion or on exposure to heat.

Partition Coefficient. Log *P* (octanol/water), 2.4.

Thin-layer Chromatography. System TE—Rf 72; system TAE—Rf 92.

High Performance Liquid Chromatography. System HX—RI 663 (pentaerithrityl tetranitrate); system HAA—Retention time 23.1 min (pentaerithrityl).

Ultraviolet Spectrum. Aqueous acid—255 nm; aqueous alkali—294 nm.

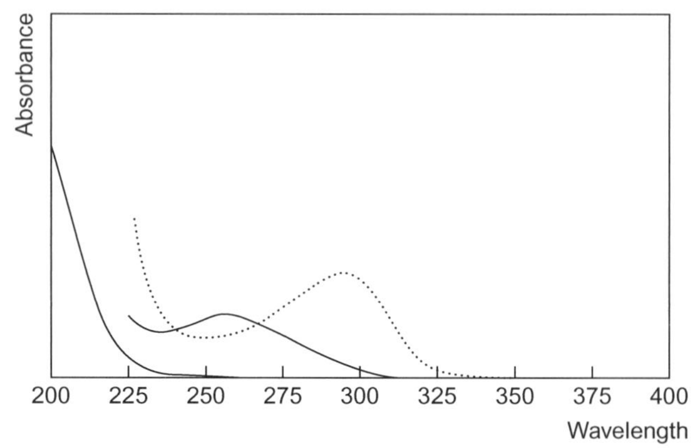

Mass Spectrum. Principal ions at *m/z* 46, 76, 57, 55, 56, 60, 47, 97.

Quantification

Gas chromatography. In blood or urine: pentaerithrityl tetranitrate and de-esterified metabolites, limits of detection 100 ng/L to 2 µg/L in blood, ECD—G. B. Neurath and M. Düünger, *Arzneimittelforschung*, 1977, *27*, 416–419.

Gas chromatography–mass spectrometry. In plasma: pentaerithrityl tetranitrate and its metabolites, limit of detection <50 ng/L—D. Stalleicken *et al.*, *Arzneimittelforschung*, 1997, *47*, 347–352.

High performance liquid chromatography. In plasma: limit of detection 100 pg—W. C. Yu and E. U. Goff, *Anal. Chem.*, 1983, *55*, 29–32.

Disposition in the Body. Incompletely absorbed from the gastrointestinal tract; it may be absorbed through intact skin. The main metabolic reaction is stepwise de-esterification ultimately to pentaerithrityl. The nitrate ester metabolites may be conjugated with glucuronic acid. About 50 to 60% of a dose is excreted in the urine in 48 h, mainly as pentaerithrityl and pentaerithrityl mononitrate, with small amounts of the dinitrate ester. About 30 to 40% of a dose is eliminated in the faeces in 72 h, partly as unchanged drug, with the main metabolite present being pentaerithrityl, together with small quantities of the dinitrate and mononitrate esters.

Half-life. About 7 h.

Protein binding. In plasma, about 85%.

Dose. 30 to 240 mg daily.

Pentamidine *Antiprotozoal*

4,4′-[1,5-Pentanediylbis(oxy)]bisbenzenecarboximidamide

$C_{19}H_{24}N_4O_2$=340.4

CAS—100-33-4

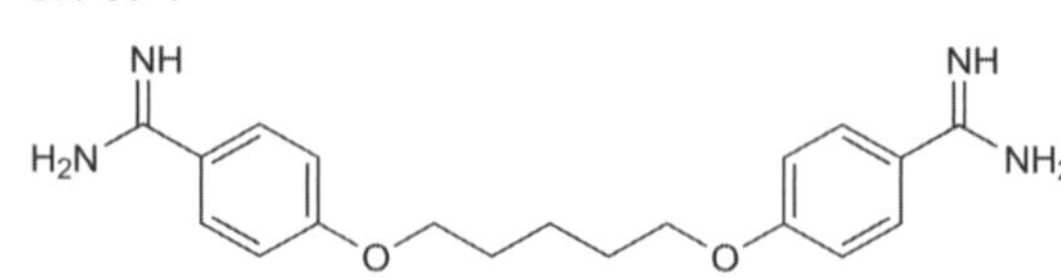

Pentamidine Isetionate

Synonyms. Pentamidine Di-isetionate; Pentamidine Isethionate

Proprietary names. NebuPent; Pentacarinet; Pentam; Pentamina; Pneumopent

$C_{19}H_{24}N_4O_2,2C_2H_6O_4S$=592.7

CAS—140-64-7

White, hygroscopic crystals or powder. M.p. about 180°.

Soluble 1 in 10 of water; slightly soluble in ethanol; insoluble in acetone, chloroform and ether.

Pentamidine Mesilate
Synonyms. Pentamidine Dimethylsulfonate; Pentamidine Mesylate; Pentamidine Methanesulfonate.
Proprietary name. Lomidine
$C_{19}H_{24}N_4O_2,2CH_4O_3S=532.6$
CAS—6823-79-6
A white or very faintly pink granular powder.
Slightly soluble in water and ethanol; practically insoluble in chloroform and ether.

Partition Coefficient. Log *P* (octanol/water), 2.8.

Thin-layer Chromatography. System TA—Rf 01; system TB—Rf 01; system TC—Rf 00; system TL—Rf 00; system TAD—Rf 00; system TAE—Rf 00. (Acidified iodoplatinate solution, positive.)

Gas Chromatography. System GA—RI 3010.

Ultraviolet Spectrum. Aqueous acid—262 nm ($A_1^1=840a$); aqueous alkali—249 nm. (See below.)

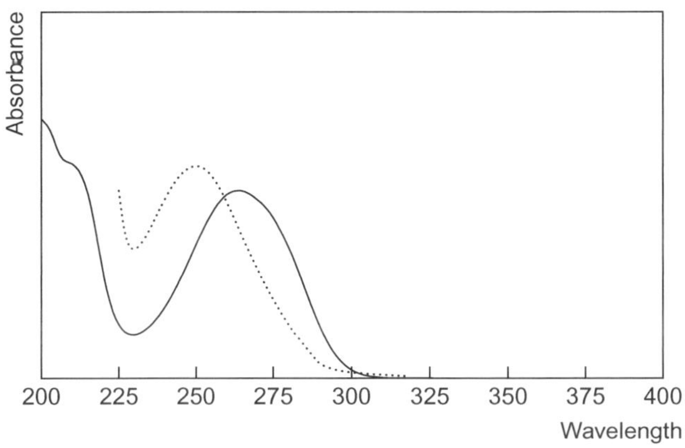

Infra-red Spectrum. Principal peaks at wavenumbers 1188, 1604, 1260, 1028, 1676, 1003 cm^{-1} (pentamidine isetionate, KBr disk). (See below.)

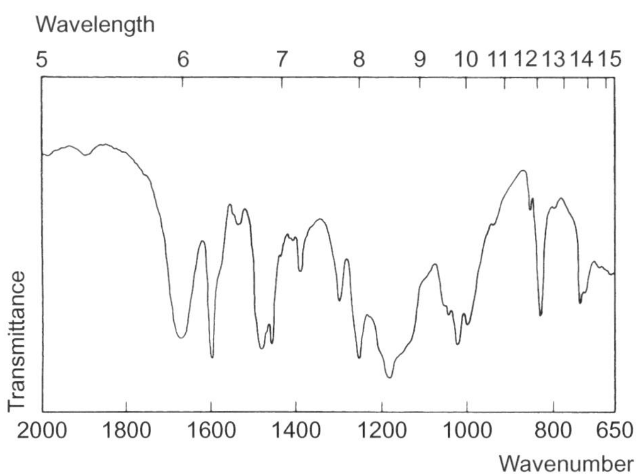

Quantification
High performance liquid chromatography. In plasma: limit of detection 15 nmol/L, UV detection—L. J. Dusci *et al.*, *Ther. Drug Monit.*, 1987, *9*, 422–425. In whole blood, plasma or urine: limits of detection 16 nmol/L (plasma, whole blood) and 27.7 nmol/L (urine), fluorescence detection—O. Ericsson and M. Rais, *Ther. Drug Monit.*, 1990, *12*, 362–365.

Disposition in the Body
Therapeutic concentration
In 6 subjects treated for *Pneumocystis carinii* pneumonia with intravenous pentamidine isetionate 3 mg/kg given once daily as a 2 h intravenous infusion, the plasma concentration at the end of the first infusion was 249 (±80) µg/L; this value was 179 (±185) µg/L in a further 4 patients. In 9 patients undergoing haemodialysis, the mean peak plasma concentration was 275 (±184) µg/L after a 3 mg/kg dose and 227 (±110) µg/L after a 4 mg/kg dose [J. E. Conte, *J. Infect. Dis.*, 1991, *163*, 169–175.]

Dose. Usually the equivalent of 2 to 4 mg/kg of pentamidine daily, by intramuscular injection.

Pentapiperide Metilsulfate
Anticholinergic

Synonyms. Pentapiperide Methylsulfate; Pentapiperium Metilsulfate; Valpipamate Methylsulfate.
Proprietary names. Crilin; Crylène.
Note. Pentapiperide metilsulfate and pentapiperium methylsulfate are identical but pentapiperide differs from pentapiperium in having one less methyl group.
1,1-Dimethyl-4-(3-methyl-2-phenylvaleryloxy)piperidinium methylsulfate
$C_{19}H_{30}NO_2,CH_3SO_4=415.5$
CAS—7009-54-3 (pentapiperide); 26372-86-1 (pentapiperium); 7681-80-3 (pentapiperide metilsulfate or pentapiperium methylsulfate)

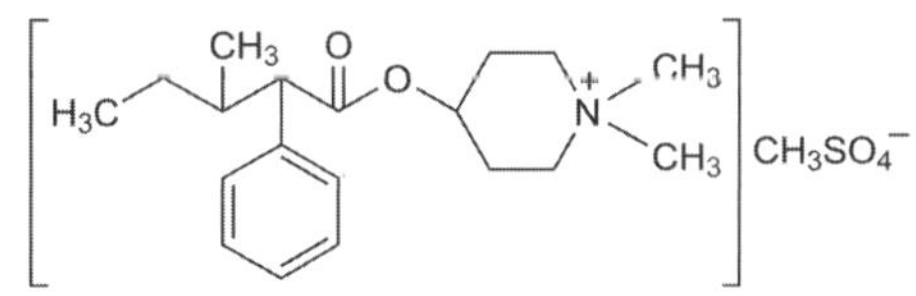

A white crystalline powder. M.p. 140° to 148°.
Freely soluble in water, chloroform and methanol; soluble in ethanol.

Colour Tests. Liebermann's Test—red-orange; Marquis Test—orange.

Thin-layer Chromatography. System TA—Rf 01; system TB—Rf 00; system TC—Rf 01; system TL—Rf 00. (Acidified iodoplatinate solution, positive.)

Gas Chromatography. System GA—not eluted.

Ultraviolet Spectrum. Aqueous acid —253, 258, 265 nm.

Infra-red Spectrum. Principal peaks at wavenumbers 1210, 1730, 1252, 755, 1008, 1162 cm^{-1} (Nujol mull).

Mass Spectrum. Principal ions at *m/z* 96, 97, 98, 91, 136, 31, 29, 55.

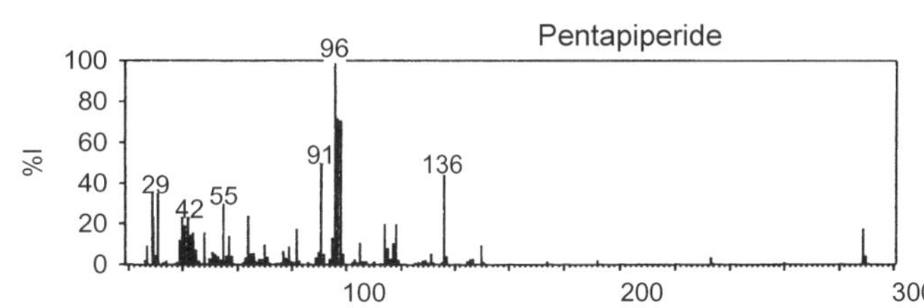

Dose. 20 to 30 mg daily.

Pentazocine
Narcotic Analgesic

Synonyms. IH-7958; NSC-107430; Pentazocinum; Win 20228.
Proprietary names. Fortal; Fortalgesic; Fortral; Fortralin; Ospronim; Pentalgina; Rafazocine; Sosegon; Sosenol; Talwin; Talwin NX. It is an ingredient of Emergent-Ez, Fortagesic and Talacen (includes proprietary names of pentazocine salts).
(2*R*,6*R*,11*R*-*rel*)-1,2,3,4,5,6-Hexahydro-6,11-dimethyl-3-(3-methyl-2-butenyl)-2,6-methano-3-benzazocin-8-ol
$C_{19}H_{27}NO=285.4$
CAS—359-83-1

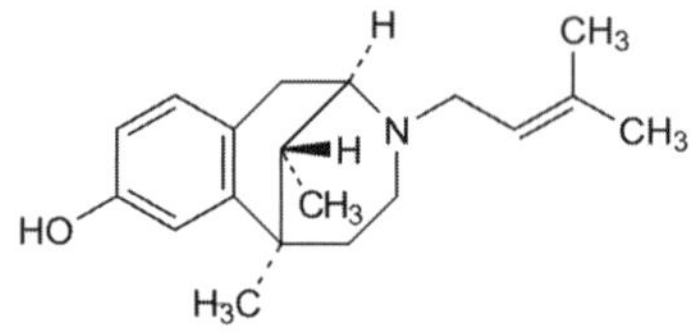

A white or pale tan-coloured powder. M.p. 145.4° to 147.2°.
Practically insoluble in water; soluble 1 in about 15 of ethanol, 1 in 2 of chloroform, and 1 in 33 of ether.

Pentazocine Hydrochloride
$C_{19}H_{27}NO,HCl=321.9$
CAS—2276-52-0; 64024-15-3
A white to pale cream-coloured crystalline powder. There are 2 forms, melting at about 218° and about 254°.
Soluble 1 in 30 of water, 1 in 16 of ethanol, and 1 in 4 of chloroform; practically insoluble in ether.

Pentazocine Lactate
$C_{19}H_{27}NO,C_3H_6O_3=375.5$
CAS—17146-95-1
A white to cream-coloured powder.
Soluble 1 in 25 of water, 1 in 12 of ethanol, 1 in 25 of chloroform, and 1 in 1500 of ether.

Dissociation Constant. pK_a 8.5, 10.0 (20°).

Partition Coefficient. Log *P* (octanol/pH 7.4), 2.0.

Colour Tests. Folin–Ciocalteu Reagent—blue; Mandelin's Test—green; Marquis Test—red→green.

Thin-layer Chromatography. System TA—Rf 61; system TB—Rf 16; system TC—Rf 12; system TE—Rf 70; system TL—Rf 28; system TAE—Rf 34; system TAF—Rf 72; system TAJ—Rf 02; system TAK—Rf 03; system TAL—Rf 57. (Acidified iodoplatinate solution, positive.)

Gas Chromatography. System GA—pentazocine RI 2280, pentazocine-AC RI 2330, pentazocine-PFP RI 2120, pentazocine-TFA RI 2075, pentazocine-TMS RI 2320, M (desalkyl-)-AC_2 RI 2380, M (OH-) RI 2545; system GB—pentazocine RI 2356, M (desalkyl-) RI 2019, M (OH-) RI 2649; system GC—RI 2225; system GF—RI 3030; system GM—RRT 0.870 (relative to iprindole).

High Performance Liquid Chromatography. System HA—*k* 1.8; system HC—*k* 0.67; system HX—RI 372; system HY—RI 288; system HZ—retention time 3.8 min; system HAA—retention time 12.5 min; system HAX—retention time 9.9 min; system HAY—retention time 5.5 min.

Ultraviolet Spectrum. Aqueous acid—278 (A^1_1=69a); aqueous alkali—240 (A^1_1=330a), 300 nm (A^1_1=106a).

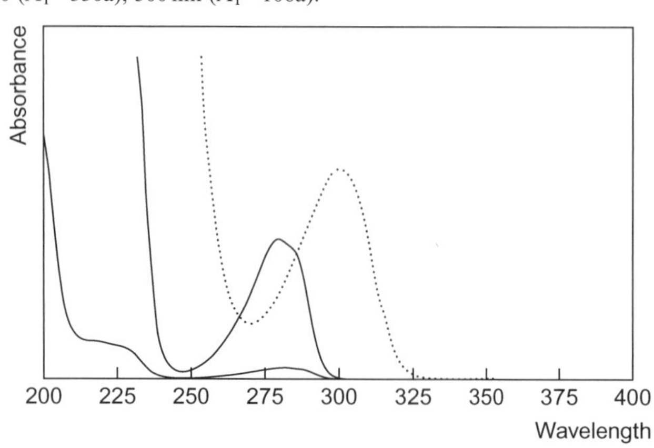

Infra-red Spectrum. Principal peaks at wavenumbers 1238, 1264, 1609, 1214, 854, 1054 cm^{-1} (KBr disk). Polymorphism may occur.

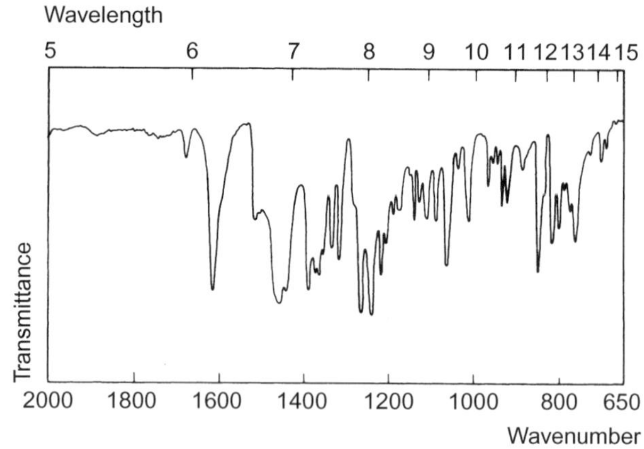

Mass Spectrum. Principal ions at *m/z* 45, 217, 70, 41, 69, 110, 285, 202.

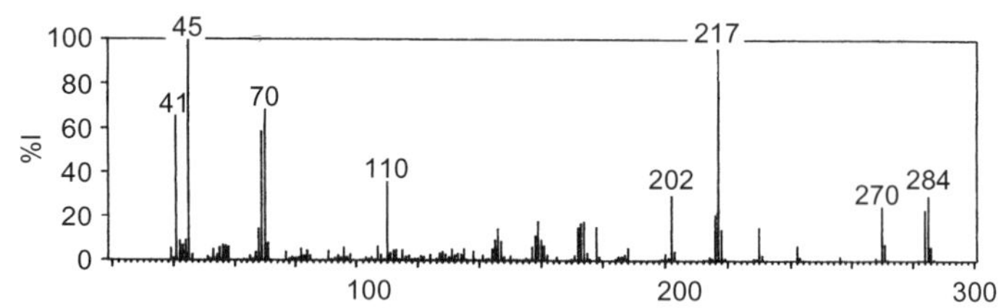

Quantification

Gas chromatography. In blood: pentazocine and tripelennamine, AFID—M. A. Mackell and A. Poklis, *J. Chromatogr.*, 1982, *235*, 445–452.

Gas chromatography–mass spectrometry. In blood: limit of detection 0.5 µg/L—H. Seno *et al., J. Mass Spectrom.*, 2000, *35*, 33–38.

High performance liquid chromatography. In serum: limit of detection 15 µg/L, UV detection (λ=220 nm) —E. Ameyibor and J. T. Stewart, *J. Chromatogr.* 1997, *703 B Biomed. Sci. Appl.*, 273–278. In serum: limit of detection 5 µg/L, fluorescence detection (λ_{ex}=275 nm; λ_{em}=335 nm)—J. W. Kelly *et al., Biomed. Chromatogr.*, 1994, *8*, 255–257. In plasma—G. Misztal and L. Przyborowski, *Pharmazie*, 1991, *46*, 464–465.

Disposition in the Body. Well absorbed after oral, IM, or rectal administration, but undergoes extensive first-pass metabolism after oral administration. Metabolism occurs mainly by extensive oxidation of the methyl groups of the dimethylallyl side-chain to produce the *cis*-hydroxy and the *trans*-carboxylic acid metabolites; the *trans*-hydroxy metabolite appears to be rapidly oxidised to the acid and is not detectable. Glucuronic acid conjugation of unchanged drug and metabolites also occurs; the 3-(3-hydroxy-3-methylbutyl) derivative has also been detected in the urine after overdoses. There is considerable intersubject variation in the rate of metabolism, and smokers appear to metabolise 40% more pentazocine than non-smokers. After IM administration, 65 to 76% of a dose is excreted in the urine in 48 h. After an oral dose, up to 13% is excreted as unchanged drug and 12 to 30% as the conjugate in 24 h, the major proportion being excreted in the first 12 h. Less than 2% of a dose is eliminated in the faeces. Pentazocine crosses the placenta.
In plasma, usually in the range 0.05 to 0.20 mg/L. Blood concentrations may be erratic and, after IM or oral administration, more than one peak may occur.

Therapeutic concentration

6 healthy former drug abusers, aged between 21 and 55 years, were administered 40 or 80 mg IM pentazocine. Mean peak plasma concentrations at 15 min were 102 and 227 µg/L, respectively. [S. Y. Yeh *et al., Clin. Pharmacol. Ther.*, 1986, *39*, 669–676.]

After an IM dose of 45 mg given to 8 subjects, peak plasma concentrations of 0.11 to 0.24 mg/L (mean 0.14) were attained in 1 h. After a single oral dose of 75 mg given to 5 subjects, peak plasma concentrations of 0.11 to 0.30 mg/L (mean 0.16) were attained in 1 to 3 h. [B. A. Berkowitz *et al., Clin. Pharmacol. Ther.*, 1969, *10*, 320–328.]

Toxicity. The estimated minimum lethal dose is 0.3 g, although recovery after ingestion of 1.2 g has been reported. Blood concentrations of 1 mg/L or more may be lethal. Some cases of abuse have been reported resulting in a mild form of addiction. Pentazocine abuse has been reported to be widespread among 'street addicts' in the USA, in combination with tripelennamine ('T's and Blues').

A 26-year-old woman was found dead at home. Postmortem examination revealed the following pentazocine concentrations: stomach contents, 2.15 mg/g; blood, 41 mg/L; liver, 12.1 µg/g. Zopiclone was also found at the following levels: stomach contents, 0.15 mg/g; blood, 1.18 mg/L; liver 5.10 µg/g. [J. Van Bocxlaer *et al.*, *J. Anal. Toxicol.*, 1996, *20*, 52–54.]

In 2 fatalities due to pentazocine ingestion, the following postmortem tissue concentrations were reported: blood 9.2 and 3.3 mg/L, liver 43 and 34 µg/g, and urine - and 4.5 mg/L; ethanol was also detected in blood at concentrations of 200 and 1760 mg/L. Blood and liver pentazocine concentrations in other cases taken from the literature were reported to range from 0.8 to 38 mg/L and 3 to 197 µg/g respectively. [A. Poklis and M. A. Mackell, *Forensic Sci Int.*, 1982, *20*, 89–95.]

In 17 fatalities involving IV abuse of pentazocine and tripelennamine, pentazocine blood concentrations of 0 to 11 mg/L (mean 3) were reported; tripelennamine concentrations ranged from 0 to 3.0 mg/L (mean 0.5). [J. R. Monforte *et al.*, *J. Forensic Sci.*, 1983, *28*, 90–101.]

Bioavailability. About 20%.

Half-life. Plasma half-life, about 4 h.

Volume of distribution. About 5 L/kg.

Clearance. Plasma clearance, about 18 mL/min/kg.

Distribution in blood. Plasma:whole blood ratio, about 0.93.

Protein binding. In plasma, about 60%.

Note. For a review of pentazocine, see G. Goldstein, *Drug Alcohol Depend.*, 1985, *14*, 313–323. For a review of the pharmacokinetics of narcotic agonists–antagonists, see R. E. S. Bullingham *et al.*, *Clin. Pharmacokinet.*, 1983, *8*, 332–343.

Dose. The equivalent of up to 600 mg of pentazocine daily, orally; up to 360 mg daily, given parenterally.

Pentetrazol

Respiratory Stimulant

Synonyms. Corazol; Leptazol; Pentamethazol; 1,5-Pentamethylenetetrazole; Pentazol; Pentylenetetrazol.
Proprietary names. Cardiazol; Cenalene-M; Coranormol; Corazole; Corvasol; Deumacard; Gewazol; Korazol; Metrazol; Phrenazol; Ventrazol.
6,7,8,9-Tetrahydro-5*H*-tetrazolo[1,5-*a*]azepine
$C_6H_{10}N_4$ = 138.2
CAS—54-95-5

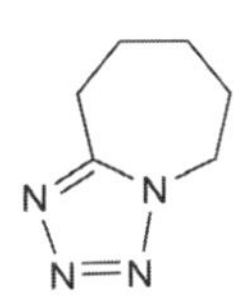

Colourless crystals or white crystalline powder. M.p. 57° to 60°.
Soluble 1 in less than 1 of water, of ethanol, and of chloroform, and 1 in less than 4 of ether.

Partition Coefficient. Log *P* (octanol/water), 0.1.

Thin-layer Chromatography. System TA—Rf 72; system TB—Rf 07; system TC—Rf 64; system TE—Rf 60; system TL—Rf 63; system TAE—Rf 72; system TAF—Rf 74; system TAJ—Rf 70; system TAK—Rf 41; system TAL—Rf 95. (Acidified iodoplatinate solution, positive.)

Gas Chromatography. System GA—RI 1550; system GB—RI 1579; system GC—RI 2021.

High Performance Liquid Chromatography. System HX—RI 290.

Ultraviolet Spectrum. No significant absorption, 230 to 360 nm.

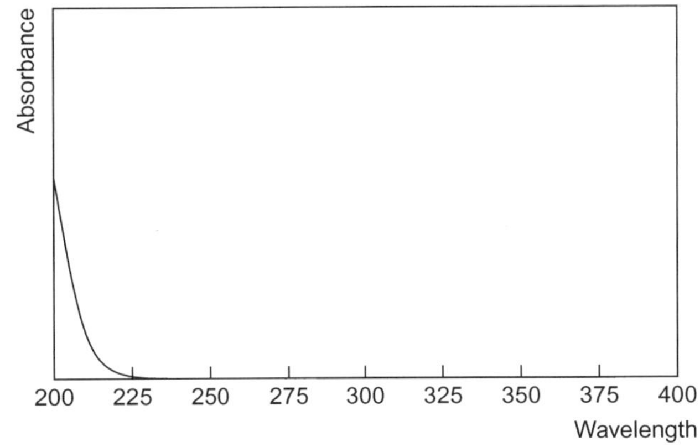

Infra-red Spectrum. Principal peaks at wavenumbers 1535, 1115, 1250, 1000, 900, 800 cm^{-1} (KBr disk).

Mass Spectrum. Principal ions at *m/z* 55, 82, 41, 39, 54, 42, 56, 109.

Quantification
Gas chromatography. In plasma: limit of detection 100 µg/L, AFID—L. D. Bo *et al.*, *J Pharmacol Methods*, 1979, *2*, 29–33. In plasma or urine: limit of detection 500 µg/L, FID—H. W. Jun *et al.*, *J. Pharm. Sci.*, 1975, *64*, 1843–1846.

Disposition in the Body. Readily absorbed after oral or parenteral administration and rapidly metabolised. About 60% of an oral dose is excreted in the urine in 24 h with about 10% as unchanged drug and the remainder as metabolites.

Therapeutic concentration
Following an oral dose of 100 mg to 3 subjects, who were taking the drug regularly, peak plasma concentrations of 1.5 to 3.1 mg/L (mean 2.2) were attained in 1.3 to 5 h [H. W. Jun *et al.*, *J. Pharm. Sci.*, 1975, *64*, 1843–1846.]

Dose. Usually 100 mg parenterally.

Penthienate Methobromide

Anticholinergic

Synonym. Penthienate Bromide
Proprietary name. Monodral
2-[(Cyclopentylhydroxy-2-thienylacetyl)oxy]-*N*,*N*-diethyl-*N*-methylethanaminium bromide
$C_{18}H_{30}BrNO_3S$ = 420.4
CAS—22064-27-3 ($C_{18}H_{30}NO_3S$); 60-44-6 (methobromide)

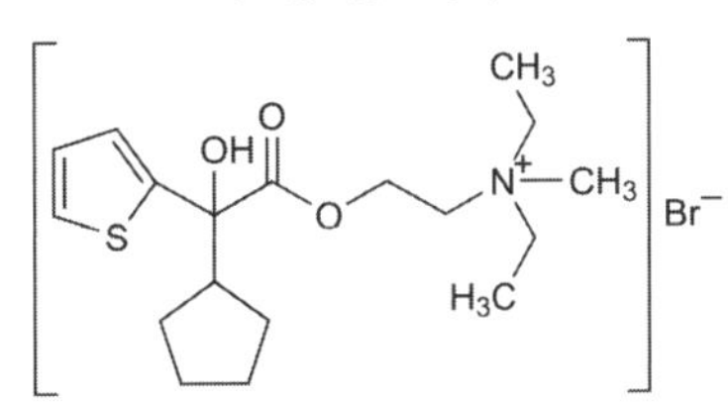

A white crystalline powder. M.p. about 125°.
Soluble 1 in 5 of water; freely soluble in ethanol and chloroform; insoluble in ether.

Partition Coefficient. Log *P* (octanol/water), −0.5.

Colour Tests. The following tests are performed on the nitrate (see p. 128): Liebermann's Test—violet; Mandelin's Test—violet; Marquis Test—violet; Sulfuric Acid—orange.

Thin-layer Chromatography. System TA—Rf 02; system TE—Rf 03; system TAE—Rf 09. (Acidified iodoplatinate solution, positive.)

High Performance Liquid Chromatography. System HA—*k* 3.2.

Ultraviolet Spectrum. Aqueous acid—238 nm (A^1_1 = 188a).

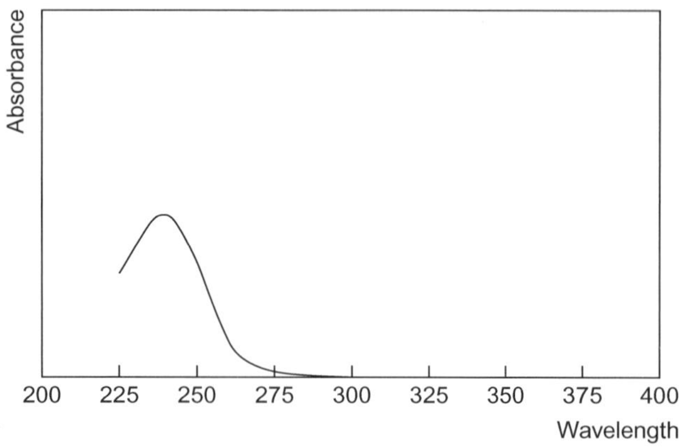

Infra-red Spectrum. Principal peaks at wavenumbers 1739, 1227, 1234, 704, 1064, 1130 cm^{-1} (KBr disk).

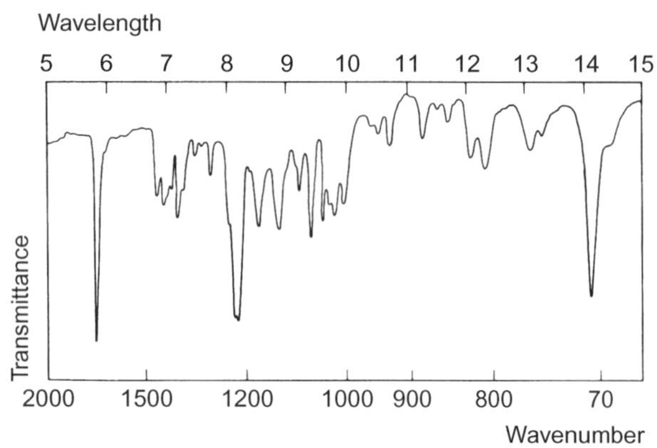

Dose. 7.5 to 40 mg daily.

Pentifylline

Vasodilator

Synonym. 1-Hexyltheobromine
Proprietary name. Cosaldon
1-Hexyl-3,7-dihydro-3,7-dimethyl-1*H*-purine-2,6-dione
$C_{13}H_{20}N_4O_2$=264.3
CAS—1028-33-7

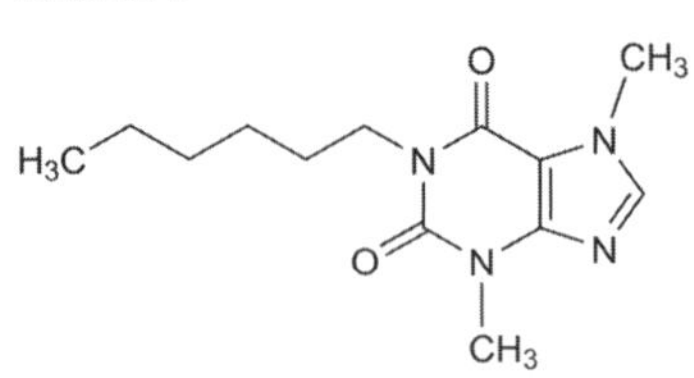

A crystalline solid. M.p. 82° to 83°.
Practically insoluble in water; soluble in ethanol, chloroform and hydrochloric acid.

Partition Coefficient. Log *P* (octanol/water), 2.6.

Colour Test. Amalic Acid Test—pink-orange/violet.

Thin-layer Chromatography. System TA—Rf 55; system TB—Rf 06; system TC—Rf 66; system TE—Rf 66; system TL—Rf 46; system TAE—Rf 72. (Acidified iodoplatinate solution, positive.)

Gas Chromatography. System GA—pentifylline RI 2240, M (OH-)-AC RI 2560, M (OH-) isomer-1 RI 2295, M (OH-) isomer-2 RI 2505, M (di-OH-)-H_2O isomer-1 RI 2250, M (di-OH-)-H_2O isomer-2 RI 2285, M (di-OH-) RI 2700.

Ultraviolet Spectrum. Aqueous acid—275 nm (A^1_1=335b).

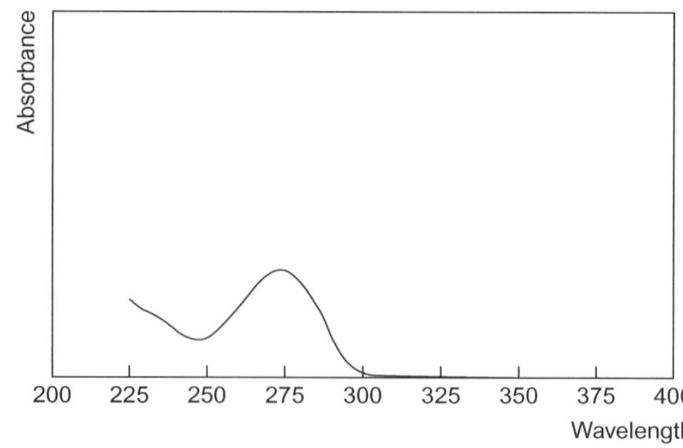

Infra-red Spectrum. Principal peaks at wavenumbers 1652, 1700, 1548, 1220, 760, 750 cm^{-1} (KBr disk).

Mass Spectrum. Principal ions at *m/z* 180, 264, 193, 109, 194, 181, 67, 42.

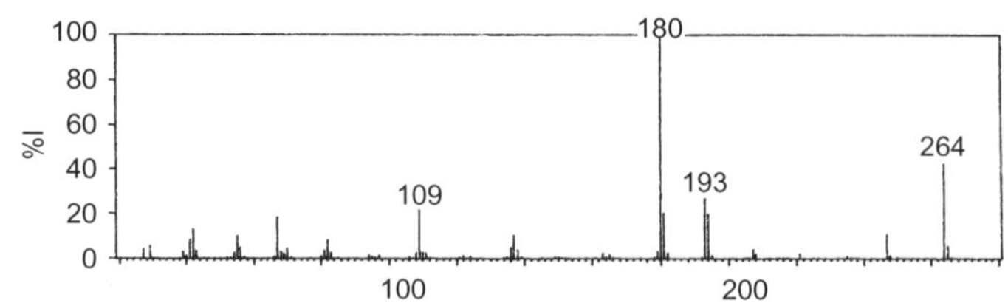

Dose. Pentifylline has been given in doses of up to 800 mg daily.

Pentobarbital

Hypnotic/Barbiturate

Synonyms. Aethaminalum; Mebubarbital; Mebumal; Pentobarbitalum; Pentobarbitone.
Proprietary name. Hypnol
5-Ethyl-5-(1-methylbutyl)-2,4,6(1*H*,3*H*,5*H*)-pyrimidinetrione
$C_{11}H_{18}N_2O_3$=226.3
CAS—76-74-4

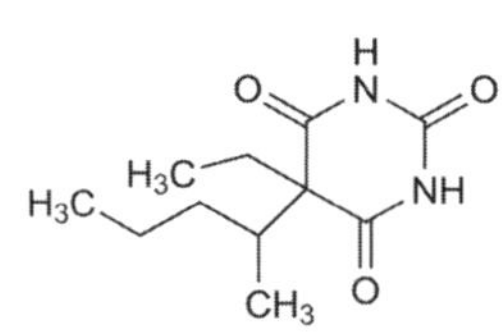

Colourless crystals or a white crystalline powder. M.p. 129° to 130° (from alcohol). A polymorphic form may occur, with an m.p. of about 115°; it gradually reverts to the more stable form on heating at about 110°.
Very slightly soluble in water; soluble 1 in 4.5 of ethanol, 1 in 4 of chloroform, and 1 in 10 of ether; very soluble in acetone and methanol.

Pentobarbital Calcium
Synonym. Pentobarbitone Calcium
Proprietary name. Repocal
$(C_{11}H_{17}N_2O_3)_2Ca$=490.6
CAS—7563-42-0 ($C_{11}H_{18}N_2O_3$,xCa)
A fine white crystalline powder.
Sparingly soluble in water; slightly soluble in ethanol; practically insoluble in ether.

Pentobarbital Sodium
Synonyms. Ethaminal Sodium; Mebumalnatrium; Pentobarbitone Sodium; Soluble Pentobarbitone.
Proprietary names. Nembutal; Nova Rectal; Pentone; Petab. It is an ingredient of Cafatine PB and Cafergot-PB.
$C_{11}H_{17}N_2NaO_3$=248.3
CAS—57-33-0
A white, hygroscopic, crystalline powder or granules. Decomposes at about 127°.

Freely soluble in water and ethanol; practically insoluble in benzene and ether. A solution in water slowly decomposes.

Dissociation Constant. pK_a 8.0 (20°).

Partition Coefficient. Log *P* (octanol/buffer pH 7.4), 1.9.

Colour Tests. Koppanyi–Zwikker Test—violet; Mercurous Nitrate—black; Vanillin Reagent—brown-red/violet.

Thin-layer Chromatography. System TD—Rf 55; system TE—Rf 45; system TF—Rf 66; system TH—Rf 76; system TAD—Rf 59; system TAE—Rf 90. (Mercuric chloride–diphenylcarbazone reagent, positive; mercurous nitrate spray, black; Zwikker's reagent, pink.)

Gas Chromatography. System GA—pentobarbital RI 1735, pentobarbital-Me_2 RI 1630, M (3′-OH-) RI 1955, M (3′-OH-)-Me_2 RI 1820; system GB—pentobarbital RI 1776, M (3′-OH-) RI 2039; system GF—RI 2465; system GAJ—RRT 0.803 (relative to methylphenobarbital).

High Performance Liquid Chromatography. System HG—*k* 10.96; system HH—*k* 8.07; system HX—RI 424; system HY—RI 383; system HZ—retention time 4.1 min; system HAX—retention time 5.9 min; system HAY—retention time 5.6 min.

Ultraviolet Spectrum. Borax buffer 0.05 M (pH 9.2)—239 (A_1^1=438a); 1 M sodium hydroxide (pH 13)—255 nm (A_1^1=327b).

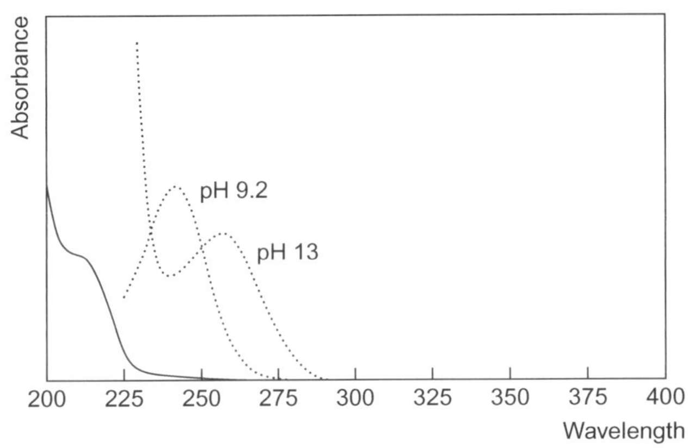

Infra-red Spectrum. Principal peaks at wavenumbers 1685, 1719, 1744, 1315, 1218, 845 cm^{-1} (KBr disk). (See below)

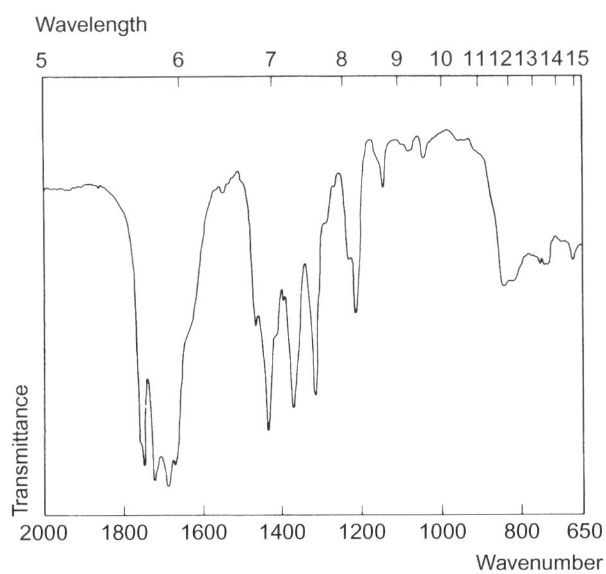

Mass Spectrum. Principal ions at *m/z* 141, 156, 43, 41, 157, 55, 39, 98; 3′-hydroxypentobarbital 45, 156, 141, 69, 41, 43, 157, 55.

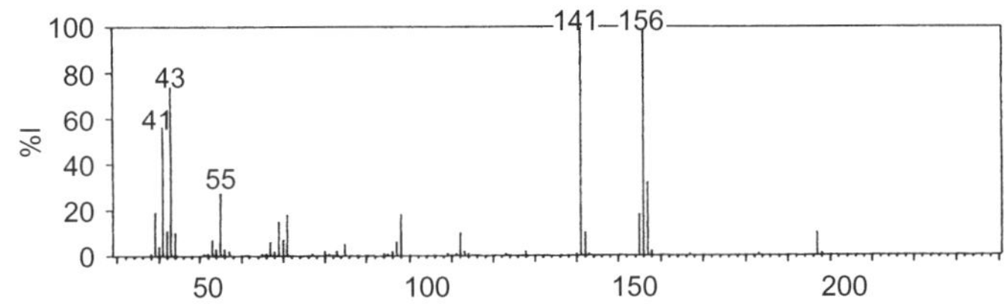

Quantification. See also under Amylobarbital.

Gas chromatography. In serum: limit of detection 80 µg/L, AFID—S.-R. Sun and D. J. Hoffman, *J. Pharm. Sci.*, 1979, *68*, 386–388. In plasma: limit of detection 500 µg/L, FID—A. Hulshoff *et al.*, *Anal. Chim. Acta*, 1979, *105*, 139–146.

Gas chromatography–mass spectrometry. In plasma: pentobarbital and thiopental, limits of detection 5 µg/L and 10 µg/L respectively—J. Martens-Lobenhoffer, *Pharmazie*, 1999, *54*, 597–599.

Disposition in the Body. More than 90% of the sodium salt is absorbed after oral administration. About 80% of a dose is excreted in the urine in 5 days, with about 7% as (+)-3′-hydroxypentobarbital, 30% as the (−)-3′-hydroxy isomer, up to 13% as the *N*-hydroxy metabolite, 7 to 14% as the 3′-oxo metabolite, and about 10 to 15% as the 3′-carboxy derivative. About 1% of a dose is excreted in the urine unchanged.
Pentobarbital is a metabolite of thiopental.

Therapeutic concentration. In plasma, usually in the range 1 to 10 mg/L.

Following a single oral dose of 50 mg to 5 fasting subjects, peak plasma concentrations of 0.62 to 0.88 mg/L (mean 0.73) were attained in 1 h. [R. B. Smith *et al.*, *J. Pharmacokinet. Biopharm.*, 1973, *1*, 5–16.]

After an IV injection of 100 mg to 7 subjects, mean plasma concentrations of 3 mg/L were reported in 6 min. [M. Ehrnebo, *J. Pharm. Sci.*, 1974, *63*, 1114–1118.]

Toxicity. The estimated minimum lethal dose is 1 g. Toxic effects are usually associated with blood concentrations greater than about 8 mg/L and concentrations of 12 mg/L or more may produce coma. Fatalities have been associated with plasma concentrations of 8 to 24 to 73 mg/L.

In 55 fatalities, the following postmortem concentrations were reported: blood 5 to 169 mg/L (mean 30), liver 23 to 550 µg/g (mean 130). [R. C. Baselt and R. H. Cravey, *J. Anal. Toxicol.*, 1977, *1*, 81–103.]

A 51-year-old veterinary official, who committed suicide by self-injecting pentobarbital, had the following postmortem tissue concentrations, 24 h after discovery of the corpse (mg/L or µg/g): peripheral blood 13.5, plasma from peripheral blood 21.7, urine 7.2, gastric contents 18.1 (0.7 mg total), vitreous humour 12.6, brain cortex 33.2, CSF 13.9, bile 67.4, liver 27.5; approximately 1.6 g of pentobarbital was thought to have been administered. [N. Romain *et al.*, *Forensic Sci. Int.*, 2003, *131*, 103–107.]

In 3 fatalities caused by pentobarbital, the following postmortem tissue distribution, mg/L or µg/g, was reported:

	Pentobarbital	3′-Hydroxy metabolite
Blood	51, 10, 25	ND, ND, 4
Bile	152, 148, 59	-, -, 13
Kidney (left)	46, 16, 38	4, 7, 7
Liver	165, 20, 46	5, 8, 9
Urine	7, 5, 62	-, 82, 65

(ND=not detected)

[A. E. Robinson and R. D. McDowall, *J. Pharm. Pharmacol.*, 1979, *31*, 357–365.]

Half-life. Plasma half-life, about 15 to 50 h (mean 27).

Volume of distribution. About 0.7 to 1 L/kg.

Clearance. Plasma clearance, about 0.3 to 0.5 mL/min/kg.

Distribution in blood. Plasma:whole blood ratio, 0.93.

Saliva. Plasma:saliva ratio, about 3.

Protein binding. In plasma, about 60 to 70%.

Note. For a review of the pharmacokinetics of hypnotic drugs, see D. D. Breimer, *Clin. Pharmacokinet.*, 1977, *2*, 93–109.

Dose. 100 mg by mouth or up to 200 mg rectally, as a hypnotic.

Pentolonium Tartrate

Antihypertensive

Synonyms. Pentapyrrolidinium Bitartrate; Pentolinium Tartrate.
Proprietary names. Ansolysen; Pentilium.
1,1′-(1,5-Pentanediyl)bis[1-methylpyrrolidinium] salt with [*R*-(*R**,*R**)]-2,3-dihydroxybutanedioic acid (1:2)
$C_{23}H_{42}N_2O_{12}$=538.6
CAS—144-44-5 (pentolonium); 52-62-0 (tartrate)

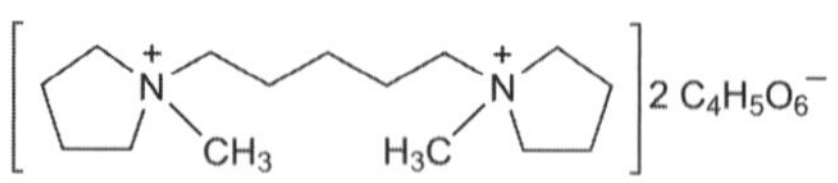

A white powder. M.p. 203°, with decomposition.
Soluble 1 in 0.4 of water and 1 in 810 of ethanol; insoluble in chloroform and ether.

Thin-layer Chromatography. System TA—Rf 00; system TB—Rf 00; system TC—Rf 00; system TE—Rf 00; system TL—Rf 00; system TAE—Rf 00; system TAF—Rf 01. (Acidified iodoplatinate solution, positive.)

High Performance Liquid Chromatography. System HX—RI 48.

Ultraviolet Spectrum. No significant absorption, 230 to 360 nm.

Infra-red Spectrum. Principal peaks at wavenumbers 1299, 1256, 1064, 1208, 1129, 676 cm^{-1} (KBr disk).

Disposition in the Body. Incompletely and irregularly absorbed after oral administration. Excreted in the urine as unchanged drug.

Dose. 2.5 to 25 mg intravenously. Doses of 20 to 900 mg daily have been given by mouth.

Pentostatin

Antineoplastic

Synonyms. CI-825; CL-67310405; NSC-218321; PD-81565; Covidarabine; 2′-Deoxycoformycin; DCF; 2′-dCF.
Proprietary name. Nipent
(8*R*)-3-(2-Deoxy-*β*-D-*erythro*-pentofuranosyl)-3,4,7,8-tetrahydroimidazole[4,5-*d*][1,3]diazepin-8-ol
$C_{11}H_{16}N_4O_4$=268.3
CAS—53910-25-1

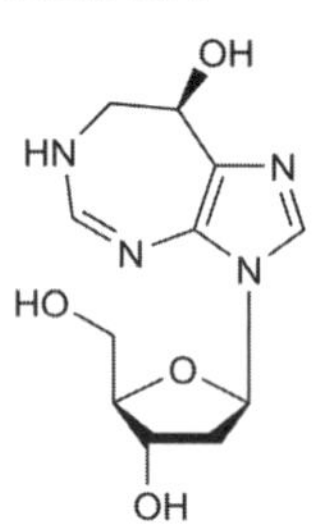

White crystals from methanol/water. M.p. 220° to 225°; also reported as 204° to 209.5° with darkening at >150°.

Dissociation Constant. pK_a 5.2.

Partition Coefficient. Log *P* (octanol/water), −2.54.

Quantification
Enzyme inhibition assay. In plasma: limit of quantification 1 μg/L—A. E. Staubus *et al.*, *Biochem. Pharmacol.*, 1984, *33(10)*, 1633–1637.

Disposition in the Body. Pentostatin penetrates the blood–brain barrier and the concentration in the cerebrospinal fluid reaches 10 to 12% of that observed in plasma within 2 to 4 h after an intravenous administration of a 5 to 30 mg/m^2 (0.25 mg/kg) dose. The drug is metabolised by phosphorylation to mono-, di- and triphosphate derivatives, and is recovered in urine unchanged. 50 to 96% of a single dose is excreted through the kidney in 24 h.

Therapeutic concentration
An intravenous dose of 0.25 to 1 mg/kg (7.5 to 30 mg/m^2) generates peak plasma concentrations of 2 to 6 μmol/L observed at 1 h. No accumulation of the drug occurs with greater than three consecutive doses of 1 mg/kg pentostatin. [P. M. Venner *et al.*, *Cancer Res.*, 1981, *41*, 4508–4511].

Toxicity
In early clinical trials, considerable toxicity was observed with the administration of pentostatin, affecting the kidneys (acute renal failure), central nervous system (depression, seizures and coma) and the immune system with severe and often fatal opportunistic infections. These are frequently associated with the higher doses; 10 to 20 mg/m^2 daily for 3 to 5 consecutive days). [R. N. Brogden and E. M. Sorkin, *Drugs*, 1993, *46*, 652–677].

Half-life. Plasma, 3 to 15 h (measured with sampling for 24 h); may be increased in patients with impaired renal function.

Volume of distribution. 42.4 L (terminal phase); 36.9 L (steady state).

Clearance. Total body plasma, 52.5 to 64 mL/min/m^2 (3.14 to 3.84 L/h/m^2); 27 mL/min/m^2 (1.6 L/h/m^2) in patients with renal impairment.

Protein binding. 1.9 to 4.9% (at therapeutic plasma concentrations).

Note. For a review of the pharmacokinetics of pentostatin, see R. N. Brogden and E. M. Sorkin, *Drugs*, 1993, *46*, 652–677.

Dose. 4 mg/m^2 every 1 to 2 weeks.

Pentoxifylline

Vasodilator

Synonym. Oxpentifylline
Proprietary names. Torental; Trental.
3,7-Dihydro-3,7-dimethyl-1-(5-oxohexyl)-1*H*-purine-2,6-dione
$C_{13}H_{18}N_4O_3$=278.3
CAS—6493-05-6

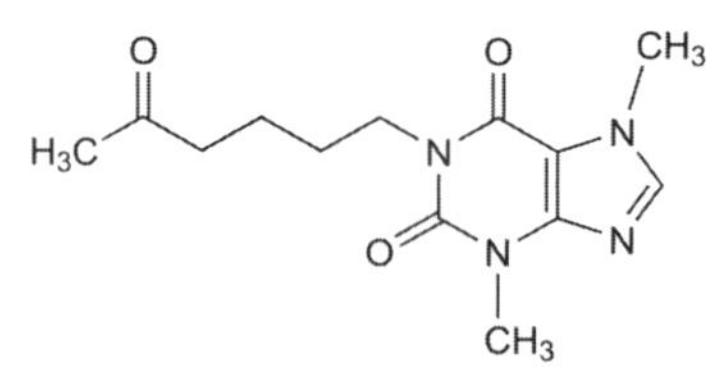

A white crystalline powder. M.p. 102° to 105°.
Soluble in water; sparingly soluble in ethanol; freely soluble in chloroform and methanol; slightly soluble in ether.

Dissociation Constant. pK_a 0.3.

Partition Coefficient. Log *P* (octanol/water), 0.3.

Colour Test. Amalic Acid Test—pink/violet.

Thin-layer Chromatography. System TE—Rf 55; system TAE—Rf 64; system TAJ—Rf 49; system TAK—Rf 12; system TAL—Rf 90.

Gas Chromatography. System GA—RI 2406.

High Performance Liquid Chromatography. System HX—RI 355; system HY—RI 274; system HZ—Retention time, 2.1 min; system HAA—Retention time, 11.5 min; system HAX—Retention time, 5.0 min; system HAY—Retention time, 4.2 min.

Ultraviolet Spectrum. Aqueous acid—274 nm (A_1^1=380a). No alkaline shift.

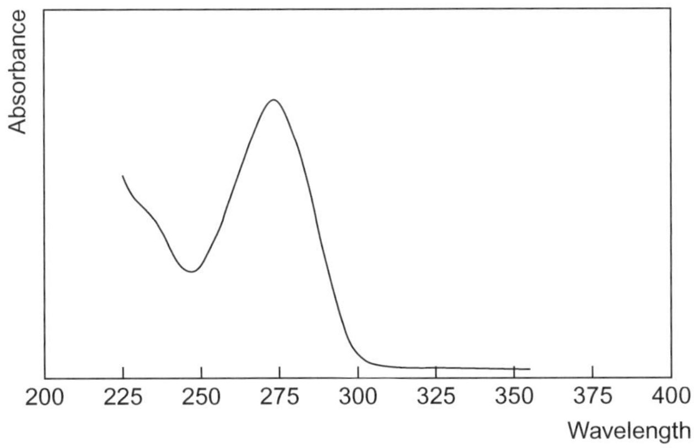

Infra-red Spectrum. Principal peaks at wavenumbers 1660, 1700, 1720, 1550, 762, 752 cm^{-1} (KBr disk).

Quantification

Gas chromatography. In plasma: pentoxifylline and 5-hydroxyhexyl metabolite, limit of detection 3 to 10 μg/L, AFID—T. A. Bryce and J. L. Burrows, *J. Chromatogr.*, 1980, *181*; *Biomed. Appl.*, *7*, 355–361.

Gas chromatography–mass spectrometry. In serum: pentoxifylline and its major metabolite, limits of detection 2 μg/L and 10 μg/L respectively—V. Marko and K. Bauerova, *Biomed. Chromatogr.*, 1991, *5*, 256–261.

High performance liquid chromatography. In plasma: pentoxifylline and 5-hydroxyhexyl metabolite, limit of detection 150 μg/L, UV detection—W. Rieck and D. Platt, *J. Chromatogr.*, 1984, *305*; *Biomed. Appl.*, *30*, 419–427. In plasma or urine: pentoxifylline and its metabolites—W. E. Lambert *et al.*, *Clin. Chem.*, 1989, *35*, 298–301. In plasma: pentoxifylline and its metabolites, limit of detection 25 μg/L, UV detection—A. Mancinelli *et al.*, *J. Chromatogr.*, 1992, *575*, 101–107. In plasma: limit of detection 3 μg/L, UV detection—J. W. Wong *et al.*, *J. Chromatogr. B. Biomed. Sci. Appl.*, 1998, *716*, 387–391.

Disposition in the Body. Readily absorbed after oral administration. It is extensively metabolised and several metabolites have been identified in the urine. About 60% of a dose is excreted in the urine as metabolites in 24 h, mostly in the first 4 h; the major urinary metabolite, 1-(3-carboxypropyl)-3,7-dimethylxanthine (inactive), accounts for about 80% of the material excreted in the urine; less than 1% is excreted as unchanged drug. Other metabolites include 1-(5-hydroxyhexyl)-3,7-dimethylxanthine, which is active and is the major metabolite detected in blood, 1-(5,6-dihydroxyhexyl)-3,7-dimethylxanthine, 1-(4,5-dihydroxyhexyl)-3,7-dimethylxanthine, 1-(4-carboxybutyl)-3,7-dimethylxanthine, 3-methyl-1-(5-oxohexyl)xanthine and 1-(5-hydroxyhexyl)-3-methylxanthine, all of which are inactive.

Therapeutic concentration

Following a single oral dose of 400 mg to 16 fasting subjects, mean peak plasma concentrations of 1.3 mg/L of pentoxifylline and 1.8 mg/L of the 5-hydroxy metabolite were attained in 0.8 and 1.3 h, respectively [R. J. Wills *et al.*, *Drug Dev. Ind. Pharm.*, 1981, *7*, 385–396].

Toxicity

A 54-year-old man died after intentional ingestion of a massive overdose of pentoxifylline (estimated to be 20 to 24 g); plasma concentrations were as high as 32.5 mg/L [J. M. Suárez-Peñaranda *et al.*, *Int. J. Legal Med.*, 1998, *111*, 151–153].

Half-life. Plasma half-life, pentoxifylline, about 1 h, 5-hydroxy metabolite about 1 h; 1-(3-carboxypropyl)-3,7-dimethylxanthine, derived from urinary excretion data, about 1.4 h.

Volume of distribution. About 5 L/kg.

Clearance. Plasma clearance, about 70 mL/min/kg.

Distribution in blood. Plasma : whole blood ratio, about 1.2.

Dose. Usually 300 to 600 mg daily; sustained-release tablets are given in doses of 0.8 to 1.2 g daily.

Perazine

Tranquilliser

Synonyms. Pemazine; P-725.
10-[3-(4-Methyl-1-piperazinyl)propyl]-10*H*-phenothiazine
$C_{20}H_{25}N_3S = 339.5$
CAS—84-97-9

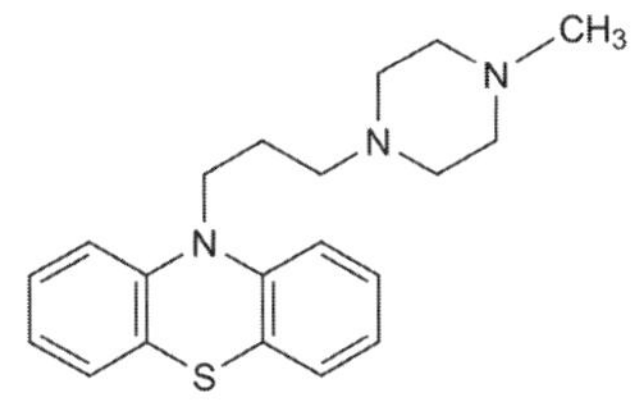

Crystals. M.p. 51° to 53°.

Perazine Dimalonate
Proprietary name. Taxilan
$C_{20}H_{25}N_3S,2C_3H_4O_4 = 547.6$
CAS—14777-25-4
A white crystalline powder. M.p. 114° to 116°.
Soluble 1 in 1 of water, 1 in 33 of ethanol, and 1 in 250 of chloroform.

Dissociation Constant. pK_a 8.0.

Partition Coefficient. Log *P* (octanol/pH 7.4), 2.9.

Colour Tests. Formaldehyde–Sulfuric Acid—red-violet; Forrest Reagent—brown-orange; FPN Reagent—brown-orange; Mandelin's Test—green→violet; Marquis Test—violet; Sulfuric Acid—violet.

Thin-layer Chromatography. System TA—Rf 48; system TB—Rf 25; system TC—Rf 37; system TE—Rf 47; system TL—Rf 03; system TAE—Rf 21; system TAF—Rf 23. (Acidified iodoplatinate solution, positive.)

Gas Chromatography. System GA—perazine RI 2798, M (OH-) RI 3175, M (phenothiazine) RI 2120.

High Performance Liquid Chromatography. System HX—RI 403; system HY—RI 371; system HZ—retention time 6.3 min.

Ultraviolet Spectrum. Aqueous acid—251 (A^1_1=875a), 300 nm.

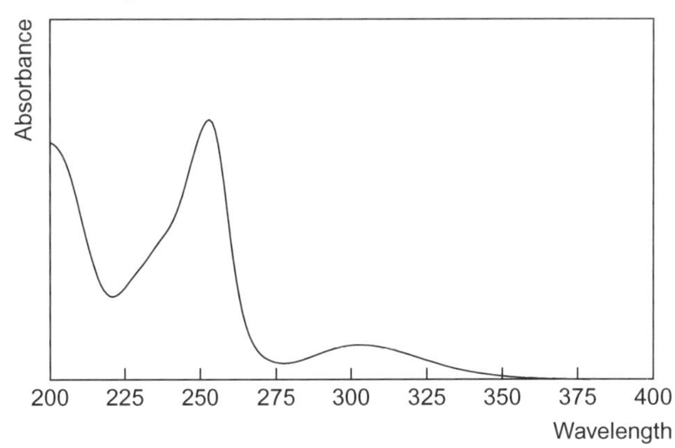

Infra-red Spectrum. Principal peaks at wavenumbers 748, 1279, 1244, 1163, 1143, 1570 cm^{-1} (KBr disk).

Mass Spectrum. Principal ions at *m/z* 113, 339, 44, 70, 141, 43, 60, 340.

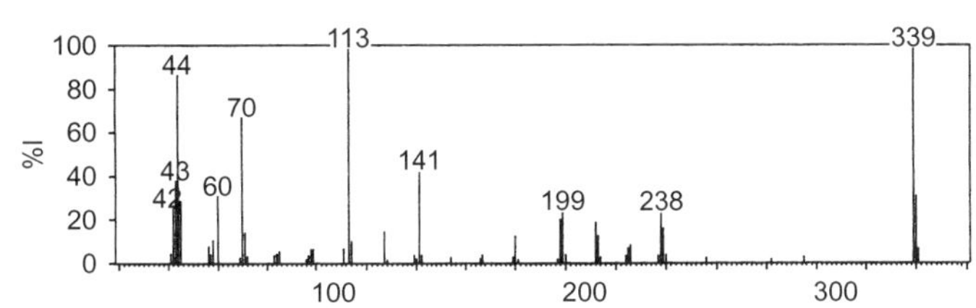

Quantification

Gas chromatography. In serum: limit of detection 20 μg/L, FID—J. Schley *et al.*, *J. Clin. Chem. Clin. Biochem.*, 1978, *16*, 307–311.

High performance liquid chromatography. In serum: perazine as internal standard. UV detection—C. Dilger *et al.*, *Arzneimittelforschung*, 1988, *38*, 1522–1525.

Thin-layer chromatography. In plasma: perazine and desmethylperazine, limit of detection 10 µg/L—M. Kresse *et al.*, *J. Chromatogr.* 1980, *183*(9) *B Biomed. Appl.*, 475–482.

Disposition in the Body. Absorbed after oral administration but undergoes extensive metabolism by demethylation, sulfoxidation, *N*-oxidation and aromatic hydroxylation, followed by conjugation with glucuronic acid. About 15 to 30% of an oral dose is excreted in the urine mainly as conjugated phenolic metabolites.

Therapeutic concentration

Following daily oral doses of 300 to 400 mg given to 14 subjects for at least 4 days, plasma concentrations of 0.02 to 0.34 mg/L (mean 0.11) of perazine and 0.04 to 0.54 mg/L (mean 0.17) of the desmethyl metabolite were reported. [U. Breyer and K. Villumsen, *Eur. J. Clin. Pharmacol.*, 1976, *9*, 457–465.]

Toxicity

A 22-year-old woman who died after ingesting perazine had the following postmortem tissue concentrations: heart blood 9.6 µg/g, muscle 4.1 µg/g, brain 32 µg/g, liver 176 µg/g, kidney 64 µg/g, lungs 83 µg/g. Analytical results led to the assumption that 14 to 30 Taxilan 100-mg tablets had been ingested, probably intentionally. [H. Kaferstein *et al.*, *Arch. Kriminol.*, 2000, *206*, 82–87.]

A 51-year-old woman who committed suicide by ingesting perazine and moclobemide had a blood concentration of 1.27 and 49.9 mg/L, respectively; some metabolites were also detected in the blood. [F. Musshoff *et al.*, *Int. J. Legal Med.*, 1998, *111*, 196–198.]

Protein binding. In plasma, about 94 to 97%.

Dose. Usually the equivalent of 25 to 600 mg of perazine daily; up to 1000 mg daily in resistant cases.

Pergolide

Dopaminergic/Antiparkinsonian

Synonym. LY-141B

(8β)-8-[(Methylthio)methyl]-6-propylergoline

$C_{19}H_{26}N_2S$=314.5

CAS—66104-22-1

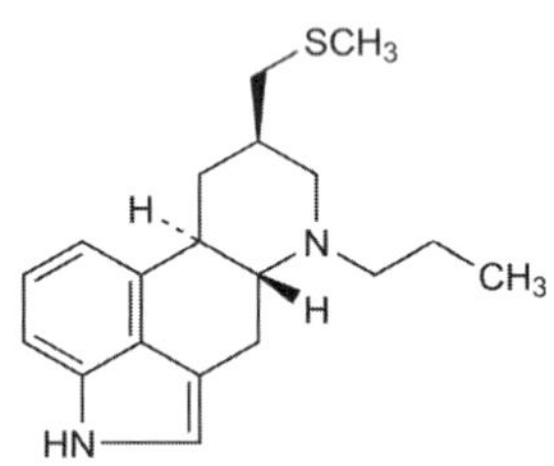

M.p. 206° to 209°.

Pergolide Mesilate

Synonym. LY-127809

Proprietary names. Celance; Nopar; Permax.

$C_{19}H_{26}N_2S,CH_3SO_3H$=410.6

CAS—66104-23-2

A white to off-white crystalline powder. M.p. 225°; also reported as 258° to 260° (decomposition). It is sparingly soluble in dimethylformamide and methanol; slightly soluble in water, 0.01 M hydrochloric acid, chloroform, acetonitrile, dichloromethane and dehydrated ethanol; very slightly soluble in acetone; practically insoluble in 0.1 M sodium hydroxide and 0.1 M hydrochloric acid and ether.

Dissociation Constant. pK_a 7.8.

Partition Coefficient. Log *P* (octanol/water), 4.02 (pergolide); log *P* (chloroform/water, pH 2.19), 6.14; (chloroform/water, pH 4.02), 119.6 (pergolide mesylate).

Colour Test. Neubauer rhode—deep purplish blue.

Thin-layer Chromatography. Plate: silica gel 60 F_{254}. Mobile phase: methanol:$CHCl_3$:acetone:NH_4OH (7:63:27:3). UV detection (λ=254 and 280 nm). Rf 0.70. [A. Rubin *et al.*, *Clin. Pharm. Ther.*, 1981, *30*, 258–265].

High Performance Liquid Chromatography. System HZ—retention time 5.4 min.

Column: ODS Hypersil (100 × 4.6 mm i.d., 5 µm). Mobile phase: methanol, flow rate 0.5 mL/min. UV diode array detection. Retention time(s): 3.6 min. [T. Mills and J. C. Roberson, *Instrumental Data for Drug Analysis*, 1993, CRC Press, Boca Raton, US. 2nd Edn, Vol. 6, pp. 196–197].

Ultraviolet Spectrum. (Pergolide mesylate) Aqueous acid (0.2 M H_2SO_4)—222, 279 nm; (methanol)—280 nm; (dehydrated ethanol)—281 nm; basic—279 nm.

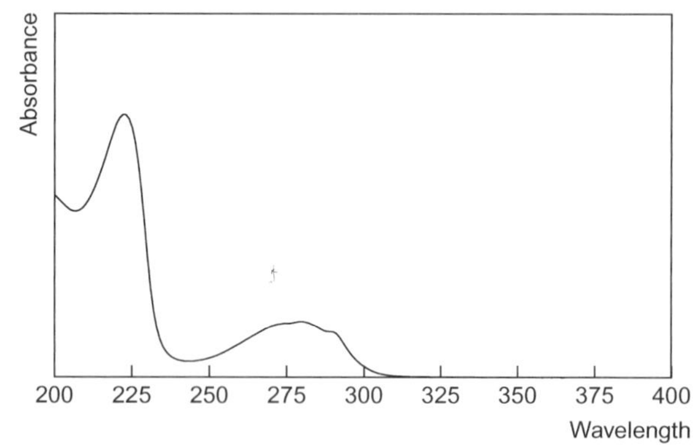

Infra-red Spectrum. Principal peaks at wavenumbers 1456, 1157, 1038 and 775 cm^{-1} (pergolide mesilate) (KBr disk).

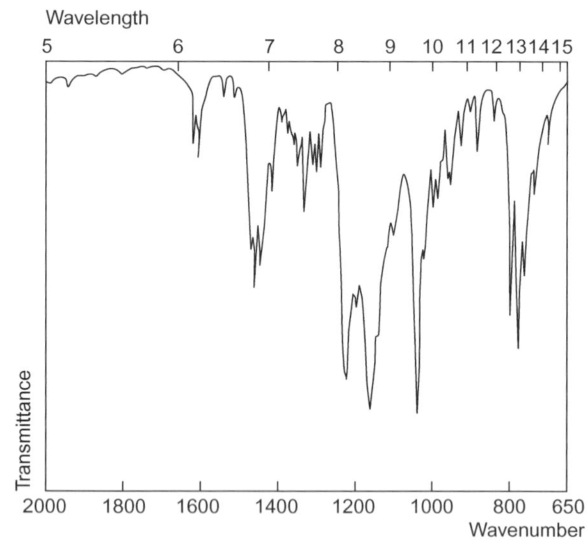

Mass Spectrum. Principal ions at *m/z* 314, 285, 154, 87, 315, 155, 144, 167.

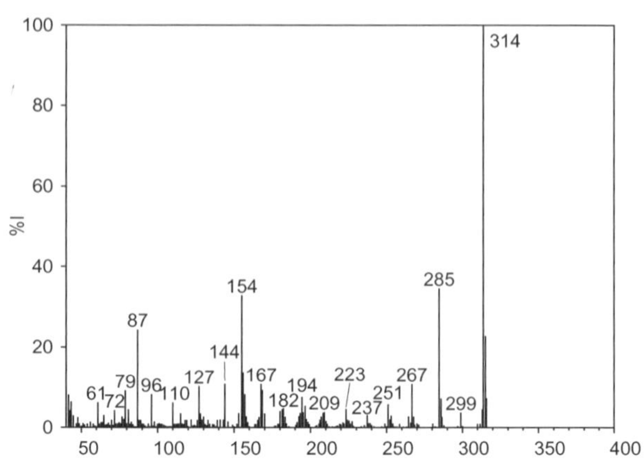

Disposition in the Body. Pergolide is rapidly absorbed after oral administration from the gastro-intestinal tract and appears in plasma 15 to 30 min after dosing. Ten metabolites have been identified including *N*-despropylpergolide, pergolide sulfoxide and pergolide sulfone. It is known that these are not produced by β-glucuronidation or sulfate conjugation. It is excreted mainly as the metabolites in urine (55% of an administered dose), 40% in faeces, 5% in expired carbon dioxide and the remainder is absorbed.

Therapeutic concentration

Three healthy male volunteers, aged 31, 42 and 47 years, were administered a dose equivalent to 0.138 mg pergolide base. Peak plasma concentrations of 1.8 mg/L were reached within 1 to 2 h. The dose was completely cleared within 4 to 5 days. [A. Rubin *et al*., *Clin. Pharm. Ther*., 1981, *30*, 258–265].

Toxicity

Overdoses of 60 mg on one day, 19 mg daily for 3 days, and 14 mg daily for 23 days have occurred. Vomiting, hypotension, agitation, severe hallucinations, severe involuntary movements and tingling sensations were observed. Another patient administered with 7 mg pergolide, instead of 0.7 mg suffered from palpitations and hypotension. [Data as supplied by Eli Lilly and Company Ltd.].

Protein binding. 90%

Dose. The initial dose is 50 µg daily for 2 days. This may be increased over the next 12 days as 100 to 150 µg steps every third day. Further increases of 250 µg every third day until an optimal therapeutic dosage is reached. The usual maintenance dose is 2 to 2.5 mg daily.

Perhexiline

Anti-anginal

2-(2,2-Dicyclohexylethyl)piperidine
$C_{19}H_{35}N$=277.5
CAS—6621-47-2

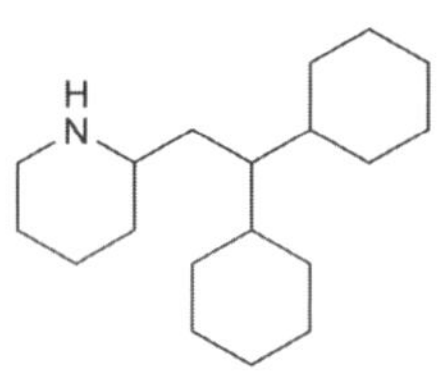

Perhexiline Maleate

Proprietary names. Pexid; Pexsig.
$C_{19}H_{35}N,C_4H_4O_4$=393.6
CAS—6724-53-4
A white crystalline powder. M.p. 188° to 191°.
Slightly soluble in water; soluble in chloroform and methanol.

Partition Coefficient. Log *P* (octanol/water), 7.5.

Thin-layer Chromatography. System TA—Rf 41; system TB—Rf 57; system TC—Rf 08; system TE—Rf 59; system TL—Rf 06; system TAE—Rf 08. (Acidified iodoplatinate solution, strong reaction.)

Gas Chromatography. System GA—Perhexiline, RI 2245; M (OH-), RI 2485; M (diOH-), RI 2660; M (diOH-)–H_2O, RI 2510.

High Performance Liquid Chromatography. System HA—*k* 0.2.

Ultraviolet Spectrum. No significant absorption, 230 to 360 nm.

Infra-red Spectrum. Principal peaks at wavenumbers 1582, 873, 990, 730, 1029, 1081 cm^{-1} (perhexiline maleate, KBr disk).

Mass Spectrum. Principal ions at *m/z* 84, 194, 55, 85, 56, 41, 30, 99.

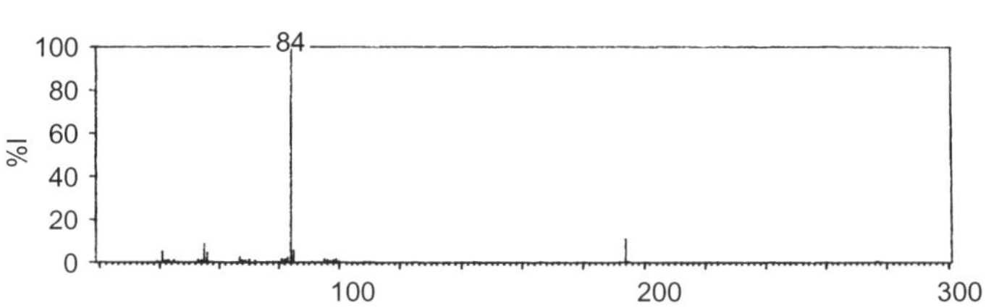

Quantification

Gas chromatography. In plasma: limit of detection 20 µg/L, AFID—N. Grgurinovich, *J. Chromatogr*., 1983, *274*; *B Biomed. Appl*., *25*, 361–365.

High performance liquid chromatography. In plasma: limit of detection 5 µg/L, fluorescence detection—J. D. Horowitz *et al*., *J. Pharm. Sci*., 1981, *70*, 320–322. In plasma, urine, or bile: perhexiline and its monohydroxy metabolites, limits of detection 0.1 mg/L (perhexiline) and 0.025 mg/L (metabolites), ECD—R. G. Cooper *et al*., *J. Chromatogr*., 1986, *381*, 305–314. In plasma: perhexiline and its monohydroxy metabolite, limits of detection 0.03 mg/L and 0.02 mg/L respectively, UV detection—N. Grgurinovich, *J. Chromatogr. B Biomed. Sci. Appl*., 1997, *696*, 75–80.

Disposition in the Body. Incompletely absorbed after oral administration. It is metabolised by hydroxylation to mono- and dihydroxylated derivatives which are slowly excreted in the urine and faeces; very little unchanged drug is excreted in the urine.

Therapeutic concentration

After a single oral dose of 150 mg given to 5 subjects, peak plasma concentrations of 0.02 to 0.12 mg/L (mean 0.07) were attained in about 6 h; following a single oral dose of 300 mg to the same subjects, peak plasma concentrations of 0.14 to 0.44 mg/L (mean 0.27) were reported at 7 h; absorption was considerably delayed in one subject with both doses [J. D. Horowitz *et al*., *J. Pharm. Sci*., 1981, *70*, 320–322].

Following chronic oral doses of 100 to 400 mg daily to 14 subjects, minimum steady-state plasma-perhexiline concentrations of 0.35 to 2.8 mg/L (mean 1.07) were reported; steady-state plasma concentrations of the major monohydroxylated metabolite ranged from 1.25 to 7.4 mg/L (mean 3.8). Steady-state plasma concentrations in 13 subjects who had been receiving similar daily doses but had developed toxic effects were: perhexiline 2.2 to 6.5 mg/L (mean 3.8), monohydroxy metabolite 0.6 to 3.8 mg/L (mean 1.6) [E. Singlas *et al*., *Eur. J. Clin. Pharmacol*., 1978, *14*, 195–201].

Forty subjects receiving perhexiline maleate 400 mg daily for 3 days followed by 200 mg daily thereafter had widely varying plasma perhexiline levels at 72 to 96 h (mean 0.46 mg/L, range 0.11 to 1.77) [S. Stewart *et al*., *Ther. Drug Monit*., 1996, *18*, 635–639].

Half-life. Plasma half-life, about 2 to 6 days; the rate of elimination appears to be decreased in subjects with toxic effects, and may be dose-dependent.

Dose. 100 to 400 mg of perhexiline maleate daily.

Pericyazine

Tranquilliser

Synonyms. Periciazine; Propericiazine; RP-8909; SKF-20716.
Proprietary names. Aolept; Neulactil; Neuleptil.
10-[3-(4-Hydroxy-1-piperidinyl)propyl]-10*H*-phenothiazine-2-carbonitrile
$C_{21}H_{23}N_3OS$=365.5
CAS—2622-26-6

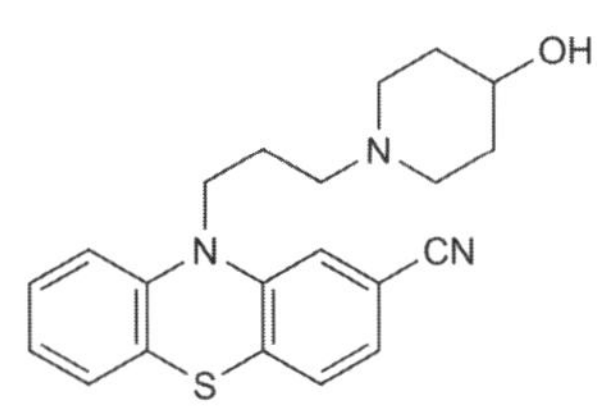

A yellow crystalline powder. M.p. 116° to 117°.
Practically insoluble in water; soluble in ethanol and acetone; freely soluble in chloroform; slightly soluble in ether.

Partition Coefficient. Log *P* (octanol/water), 3.5.

Colour Tests. Formaldehyde–Sulfuric Acid—red; Forrest Reagent—brown-orange; FPN Reagent—orange; Mandelin's Test—red; Marquis Test—red.

Thin-layer Chromatography. System TA—Rf 58; system TB—Rf 04; system TC—Rf 16; system TE—Rf 51; system TL—Rf 18; system TAE—Rf 46; system TAF—Rf 61. (Acidified iodoplatinate solution, positive.)

Gas Chromatography. System GA—pericyazine RI 3260, M (ring) RI 2555; system GB—RI 3486.

High Performance Liquid Chromatography. System HA—*k* 1.3; system HX—RI 410; system HY—RI 356; system HZ—retention time 4.4 min; system HAX—retention time 10.2 min; system HAY—retention time 5.1 min.

Ultraviolet Spectrum. Aqueous acid—232, 268 (A_1^1=761a); aqueous alkali—272 nm.

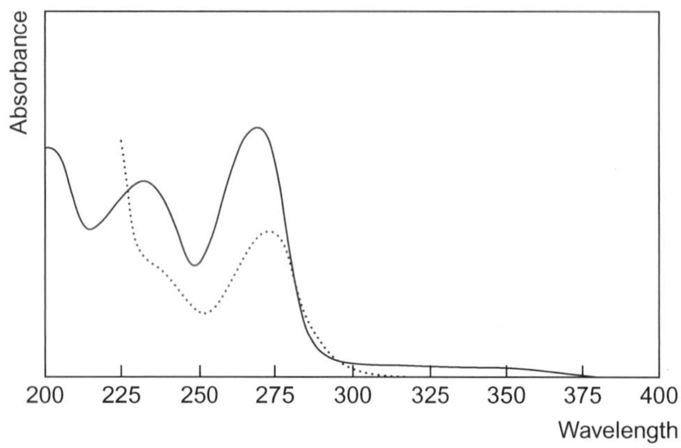

Infra-red Spectrum. Principal peaks at wavenumbers 736, 1066, 811, 746, 1245, 1260 cm^{-1} (KBr disk).

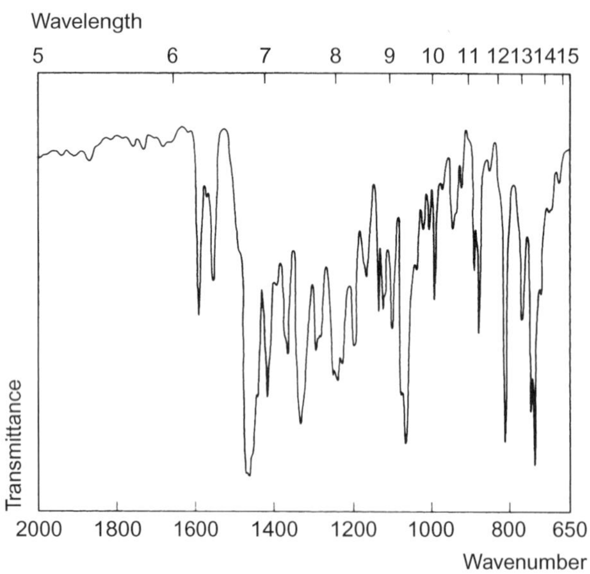

Mass Spectrum. Principal ions at *m*/*z* 114, 44, 142, 365, 42, 223, 115, 205.

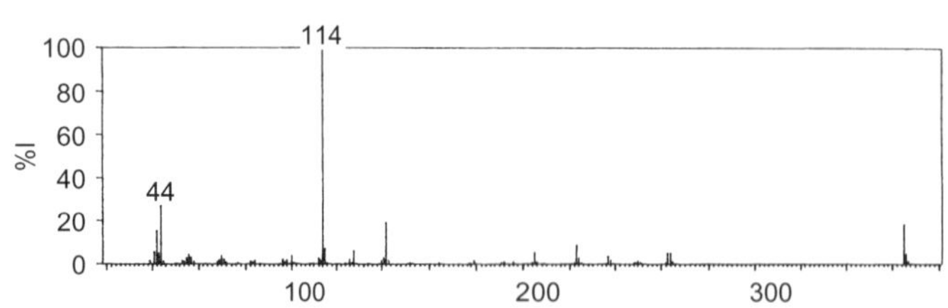

Dose. 15 to 30 mg daily for severe anxiety or behaviour disorders; initially 75 mg daily in psychoses increasing up to 300 mg daily in severe cases.

Perindopril

Antihypertensive

Synonyms. McN-A-2833; S-9490.
(2*S*,3a*S*,7a*S*)-1-[(2*S*)-2-[[(1*S*)-1-(Ethoxycarbonyl)butyl]amino]-1-oxopropyl]octahydro-1*H*-indole-2-carboxylic acid

$C_{19}H_{32}N_2O_5$=368.5
CAS—82834-16-0

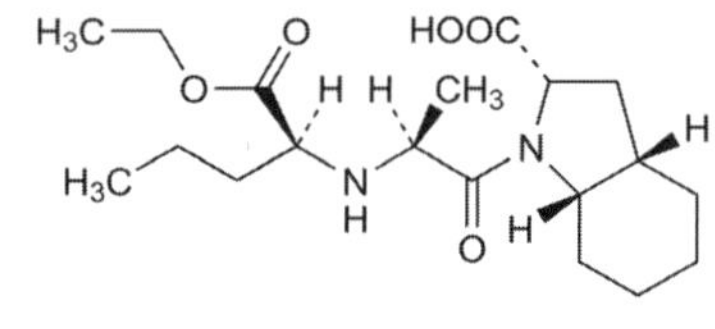

Perindoprilat
Synonym. S-9780
$C_{17}H_{28}N_2O_5$=340.4
CAS—95153-31-4

Perindopril Erbumine (Perindopril *tert-butylamine*)
Synonyms. MCN-A-2833-109; S-9490-3.
Proprietary names. Aceon; Coversum; Coversyl; Procaptan.
$C_{19}H_{32}N_2O_5,C_4H_{11}N$=441.6
CAS—107133-36-8
White crystalline powder. Freely soluble in water, alcohol and chloroform.

Thin-layer Chromatography. System TE—Rf 06 (perindopril), Rf 03 (perindoprilat); system TF—Rf 00 (perindopril), Rf 00 (perindoprilat).

Gas Chromatography. System GP—RI 2450 perindopril-ME; RI 2470 M(perindoprilat)-ME3; RI 2560 M(perindoprilat-H_2O)-ME3.

High Performance Liquid Chromatography. System HX—RI 314 (perindoprilat); system HZ—retention time 1.6 min (perindoprilat); system HAA—retention time 13.7 min.

Mass Spectrum. Principal ions at *m*/*z* 172, 98, 73, 367, 173, 56, 124, 55 (TMS (tetramethylsilane) derivative).

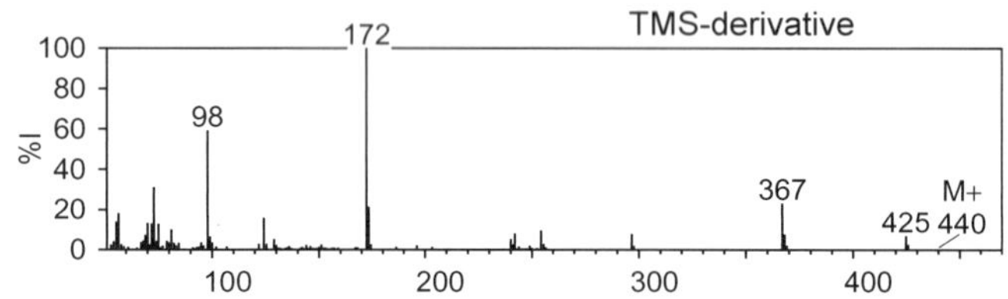

Quantification
Gas chromatography–mass spectrometry. In plasma: limit of detection 2 μg/L—C. Tsaconas *et al.*, *J. Chromatogr.*, 1989, *488*; *Biomed. Appl.*, 237–248.

Disposition in the Body. Perindopril is rapidly and extensively absorbed after oral administration and approx. 30 to 50 % is hydrolysed to the active drug perindoprilat. Other metabolites include perindopril and perindoprilat glucuronides, dehydrated perindopril and the diastereoisomers of dehydrated perindoprilat. Peak plasma concentrations of perindopril are reached within 1 h and of perindoprilat in 3 to 4 h. The metabolism of perindopril to perindoprilat is affected by the presence of food in the gastro-intestinal tract. Around 75% of the dose is excreted in urine as perindopril, perindoprilat and other metabolites, and the remainder in faeces. Only 4 to 12% of the dose is recovered as unchanged drug in urine. Excretion is reduced in those with renal impairment.

Therapeutic concentration
12 healthy males, 19 to 33 years old, were administered a single 4 mg oral dose of perindopril erbumine after 12 h fasting or during breakfast. Peak plasma perindopril concentrations were 64.2 μg/L for those in the fasted state and 52.4 μg/L for those in the fed state. These levels were reached within 0.9 and 1.1 h, respectively. The peak concentrations of the metabolite, pendoprilat were 4.7 and 3.6 μg/L in the fasted and fed individuals, observed 3.6 to 3.9 h after administration. [B. Lecocq *et al.*, *Clin. Pharmacol. Ther.*, 1990, *47*, 397–402].

Bioavailability. Perindopril, 65 to 70%; perindoprilat, 25%.

Half-life. Perindopril: 2.9 h (fasted individuals) and 3.4 h (fed). Perindoprilat: 10.9 h (fasted) and 12.0 h (fed). For perindoprilat, the distribution half-life is also reported as 5 h with an elimination half-life of 25 to 30 h.

Volume of distribution. Perindoprilat, 0.2 L/kg; also reported as 4.3 L/kg.

Clearance. Perindoprilat, 4.9 L/h.

Protein binding. Perindopril, 60%; perindoprilat, <30% (concentration dependent).

Note. For a review of the pharmacokinetics of ACE (angiotensin-converting enzyme) inhibitors, see J. C. Song and C. M. White, *Clin. Pharmacokinet.*, 2002, *41*, 207–224.

Dose. 2 to 4 mg daily with a maximum of 8 mg daily.

Perphenazine

Tranquilliser

Synonyms. Chlorpiprazine; Chlorpiprozine; Perphenazinum.
Proprietary names. Decentan; Fentazin; Peratsin; Perphenan; Phenazine; Trilafon; Trilifan. It is an ingredient of Etrafon, Triavil, and Triptafen.
4-[3-(2-Chloro-10*H*-phenothiazin-10-yl)propyl]-1-piperazineethanol
$C_{21}H_{26}ClN_3OS = 404.0$
CAS—58-39-9

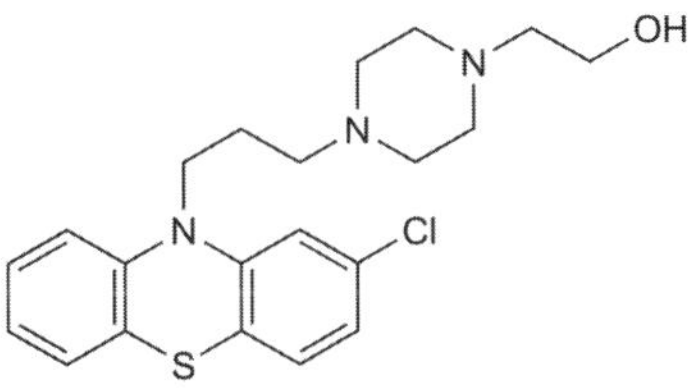

A white or creamy-white powder, sensitive to light. M.p. 94° to 100°. Practically insoluble in water; soluble 1 in 20 of ethanol, 1 in 1 of chloroform, and 1 in 80 of ether.

Dissociation Constant. pK_a 7.8 (24°).

Partition Coefficient. Log *P* (octanol/pH 7.0), 3.1.

Colour Tests. Formaldehyde–Sulfuric Acid—violet; Forrest Reagent—violet-red; FPN Reagent—violet-red; Liebermann's Test—red-brown; Mandelin's Test—violet; Marquis Test—violet.

Thin-layer Chromatography. System TA—Rf 55; system TB—Rf 07; system TC—Rf 29; system TE—Rf 42; system TL—Rf 09; system TAE—Rf 40; system TAF—Rf 40; system TAJ—Rf 00; system TAK—Rf 03; system TAL—Rf 56. (Dragendorff spray, positive; FPN reagent, pink; acidified iodoplatinate solution, positive; Marquis reagent, pink; ninhydrin spray, positive.)

Gas Chromatography. System GA—perphenazine RI 3380, M (ring) RI 2100; system GB—RI 3594.

High Performance Liquid Chromatography. System HA—*k* 1.9; system HX—RI 428; system HY—RI 395; system HZ—retention time 7.2 min; system HAA—retention time 16.0 min; system HAX—retention time 13.1 min; system HAY—retention time 6.3 min; system HAZ—*k* 3.28.

Ultraviolet Spectrum. Aqueous acid—254 (A^1_1 = 805a), 307; aqueous alkali—257 (A^1_1 = 791a), 310 nm.

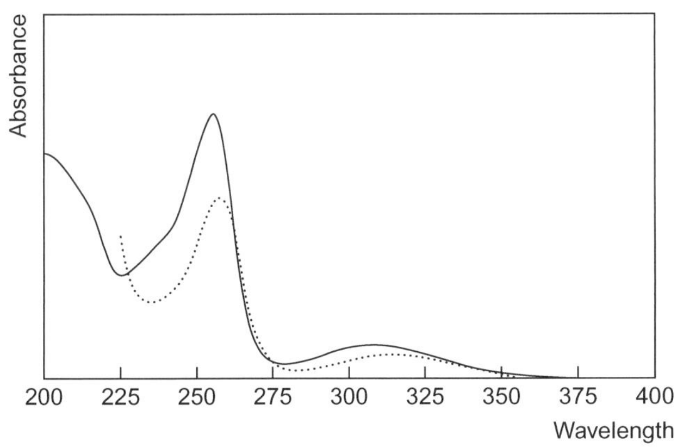

Infra-red Spectrum. Principal peaks at wavenumbers 757, 1294, 917, 1145, 1247, 1155 cm^{-1} (KBr disk).

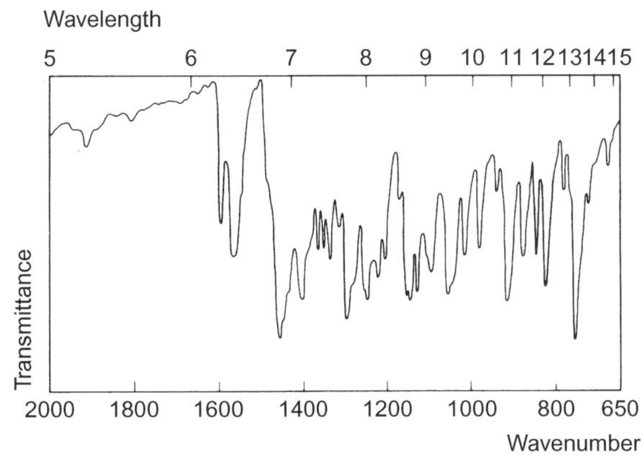

Mass Spectrum. Principal ions at *m*/*z* 246, 143, 403, 70, 404, 42, 248, 113.

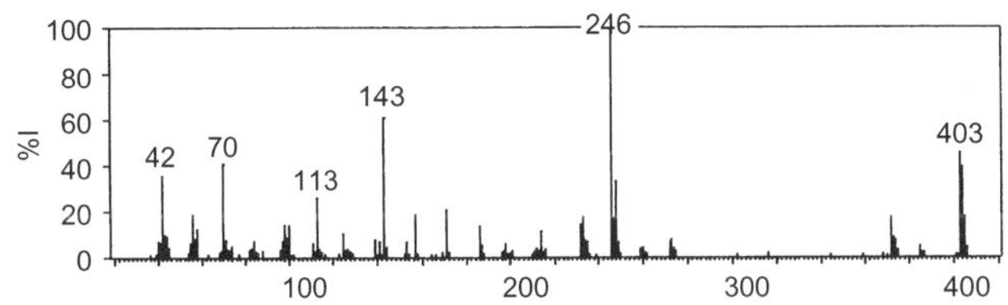

Quantification

Gas chromatography. In plasma: perphenazine and perphenazine sulfoxide, limit of detection 200 ng/L, ECD—N.-E. Larsen and J. Naestoft, *J. Chromatogr.*, 1975, *109*, 259–264.

High performance liquid chromatography. In serum: perphenazine and *N*-deshydroxyethylperphenazine, limit of detection 1 μg/L, UV detection—M. Larsson and A. Forsman, *Ther. Drug Monit.*, 1983, *5*, 225–228. In plasma: perphenazine and its metabolites, limit of quantification for perphenazine 0.5 μg/L, coulometric detection—J. P. Foglia *et al.*, *J. Chromatogr.* 1995, *668 B Biomed. Appl.*, 291–297. In serum: perphenazine and other antipsychotics, limit of quantification 1 nmol/L, UV detection—H. R. Angelo and A. Petersen, *Ther. Drug Monit.*, 2001, *23*, 157–162.

Radioimmunoassay. In plasma: limit of detection 250 ng/L—K. K. Midha *et al.*, *Br. J. Clin. Pharmacol.*, 1981, *11*, 85–88.

Disposition in the Body. Absorbed after oral administration but subject to first-pass metabolism. Small amounts are found in breast milk The main metabolic reactions are oxidation to the sulfoxide, which may have some pharmacological activity, *N*-dealkylation to form the *N*-deshydroxyethyl metabolite, *N*-oxidation, cleavage of the piperazine ring, and phenolic hydroxylation, followed by glucuronide conjugation. After oral administration, about 1 to 2% of the daily dose is excreted in the urine as unchanged drug, with about 13% as the sulfoxide and 30% as perphenazine glucuronide; after chronic administration of perphenazine enantate intramuscularly, excretion of unchanged drug and the sulfoxide is increased to about 6% and 22% of the dose, respectively.

Therapeutic concentration

After daily oral doses of 12 to 48 mg to 16 subjects, steady-state plasma concentrations of 0.3 to 25 μg/L (mean 4) of perphenazine and 0.4 to 18 μg/L (mean 4) of the sulfoxide were reported. [L. B. Hansen and N.-E. Larsen, *Psychopharmacologia*, 1977, *53*, 127–130.]

Toxicity

The following postmortem tissue concentrations were reported in a fatality due to the ingestion of about 1 g of perphenazine: blood 3 mg/L, brain 11 μg/g, liver 149 μg/g; a blood alcohol concentration of 1700 mg/L was also reported. [R. H. Cravey, per R. C. Baselt, *Disposition of Toxic Chemicals and Drugs in Man*, 5th Edn., Davis, California, Biomedical Publications, 2000, pp. 672–674.]

A 34-year-old female whose death was attributed to suicide by means of multiple drug intoxication, was found to have a heart blood concentration of 4.4 mg/L perphenazine and 950 mg/L valproic acid at *post mortem*. [B. Levine *et al.*, *J. Anal. Toxicol.*, 1999, *23*, 127–129.]

Bioavailability. About 60 to 80%

Half-life. Plasma half-life, about 8 to 12 h.

Volume of distribution. 10 to 35 L/kg.

Clearance. Plasma clearance, about 12 to 38 mL/min/kg.

Note. For a study of the pharmacological profile of perphenazine metabolites, see R.A. Sweet *et al.*, *J. Clin. Psychopharmacol.*, 2000, *20*, 181–187.

Dose. Usually 12 to 24 mg daily; up to 64 mg daily has been given.

Pethidine

Narcotic Analgesic

Synonyms. Isonipecaine; Meperidine.
1-Methyl-4-phenyl-4-piperidinecarboxylic acid ethyl ester
$C_{15}H_{21}NO_2$=247.3
CAS—57-42-1

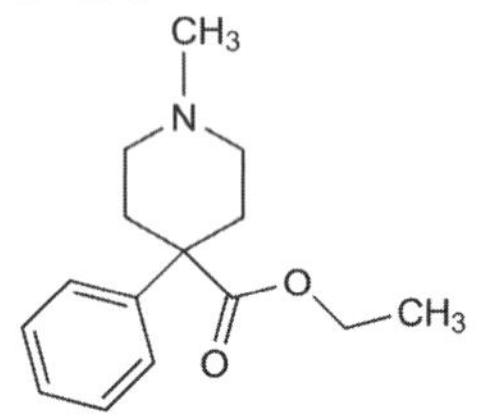

An oily liquid which slowly crystallises.

Pethidine Hydrochloride

Proprietary names. Alodan; Centralgine; Demerol; Dispadol; Dolantine; Dolantin(a); Dolestine; Dolosal; Mefedina; Pethoid. It is an ingredient of Mepergan and Pamergan P100.
$C_{15}H_{21}NO_2$,HCl=283.8
CAS—50-13-5
A white crystalline powder. M.p. 186° to 189°.
Soluble in water, acetone, and ethyl acetate; slightly soluble in alcohol and isopropanol; practically insoluble in ether and benzene.

Dissociation Constant. pK_a 8.7 (20°).

Partition Coefficient. Log *P* (octanol/water), 2.7.

Colour Tests. Liebermann's Test—red-orange; Marquis Test—orange.

Thin-layer Chromatography. System TA—Rf 52; system TB—Rf 37; system TC—Rf 34; system TE—Rf 60; system TL—Rf 11; system TAE—Rf 34; system TAF—Rf 40; system TAJ—Rf 14; system TAK—Rf 06; system TAL—Rf 72. (Dragendorff spray, positive; acidified iodoplatinate solution, positive; Marquis reagent, brown.)

Gas Chromatography. System GA—pethidine RI 1754, M (nor-) RI 1885, M (nor-)-AC RI 2240, M (OH-) RI 2045, M (OH-)-AC RI 2205, M (nor-OH-)-AC_2 RI 2600; system GB—pethidine RI 1809, M (nor-) RI 1842, M (nor-)-AC RI 2256, M (OH-) RI 2145; system GC—RI 2025; system GF—RI 1995; system GM—pethidine RRT 0.319, M (nor-) RRT 0.357 (both relative to iprindole).

High Performance Liquid Chromatography. System HA—pethidine *k* 2.8 (tailing peak), M (nor-) *k* 1.7 (tailing peak), pethidinic acid *k* 2.8 (tailing peak); system HC—pethidine *k* 0.55, M (nor-) *k* 2.04; system HX—RI 345; system HY—RI 281; system HZ—retention time 3.2 min; system HAA—retention time 11.8 min; system HAX—retention time 9.2 min; system HAY—retention time 4.8 min.

Ultraviolet Spectrum. Aqueous acid—251, 257 (A_1^1=8.5a), 263 nm. No alkaline shift.

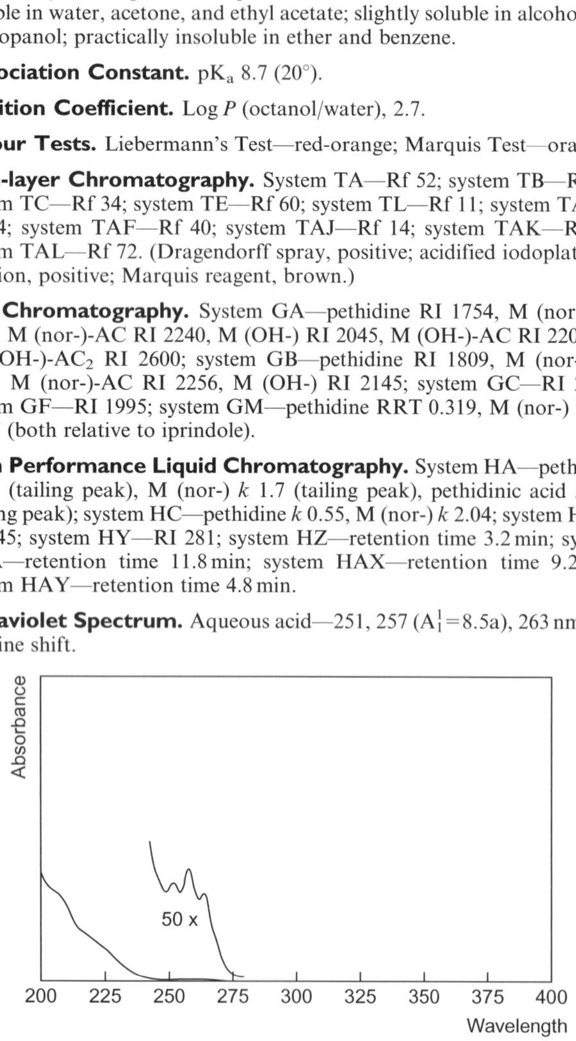

Infra-red Spectrum. Principal peaks at wavenumbers 1708, 1218, 1166, 1148, 688, 730 cm^{-1} (pethidine hydrochloride, KBr disk).

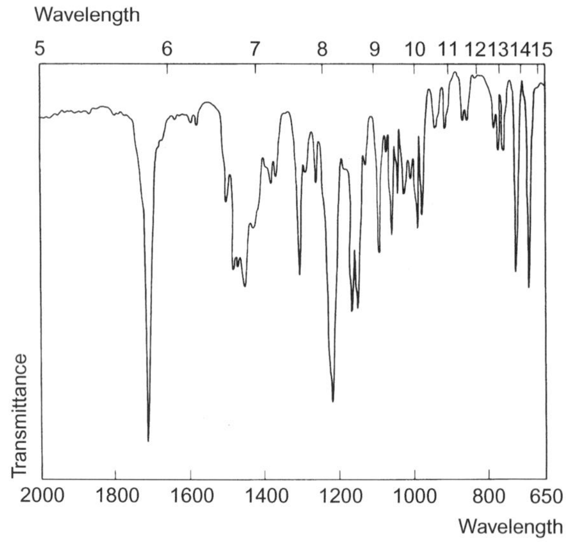

Mass Spectrum. Principal ions at *m/z* 71, 70, 44, 57, 42, 247, 43, 246; norpethidine 57, 233, 42, 56, 158, 43, 160, 103; pethidinic acid 71, 70, 57, 43, 219, 42, 218, 44.

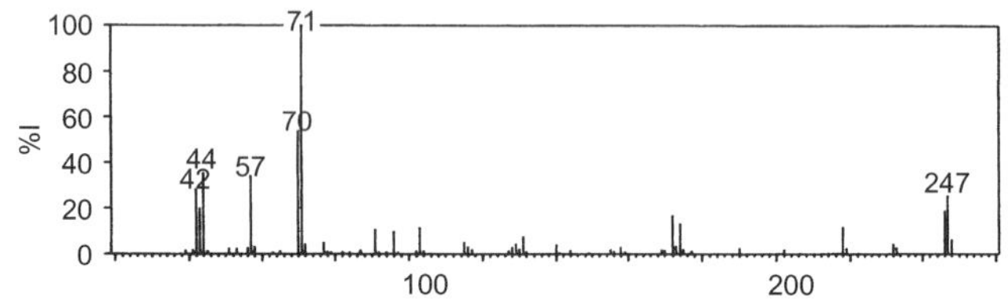

Quantification

Gas chromatography. In blood, plasma, or urine: pethidine and norpethidine, limit of detection 5 µg/L for pethidine and 2.5 µg/L for norpethidine, AFID—P. Jacob *et al.*, *J. Pharm. Sci.*, 1982, *71*, 166–168. In plasma: pethidine and norpethidine, limit of detection 20 µg/L, ECD—P. Hartvig and C. Fagerlund, *J. Chromatogr.* 1983, 274(25) *B Biomed. Appl.*, 355–360. In urine: pethidine and its major metabolites, NPD—K. Chan *et al.*, *J. Chromatogr.*, 1991, *565*, 247–254. In urine: FID—F. Liu *et al.*, *J. Chromatogr.* 1994, *658 B Biomed. Appl.*, 375–379. In urine: limit of detection 1 µg/L. NPD—S. W. Myung *et al.*, *Analyst*, 1999, *124*, 1283–1286.

Gas chromatography–mass spectrometry In plasma or serum: pethidine and norpethidine, limit of detection 170 ng/L for pethidine and 500 ng/L for norpethidine—E. L. Todd *et al.*, *J. Anal. Toxicol.*, 1979, *3*, 256–259. In urine: pethidinic and norpethidinic acids, limit of detection 500 µg/L—C. Lindberg *et al.*, *Acta Pharm Suec.*, 1978, *15*, 327–336. In urine: limit of detection 20 µg/L—H. Y. Hu *et al.*, *Yao Xue Xue Bao*, 1994, *1291*, 116–121. In breast milk—L. Borgatta *et al.*, *J. Clin. Pharmacol.*, 1997, *37*, 186–192. In blood: limit of detection 0.02 µg/L—A. Ishii *et al.*, *J. Chromatogr. B Biomed. Sci. Appl.*, 2001, *758*, 117–121.

Disposition in the Body. Readily absorbed after oral administration and rapidly and extensively distributed throughout the tissues. It undergoes considerable first-pass metabolism. The major metabolites are the *N*-demethylated derivative, norpethidine, and the hydrolysis product, pethidinic acid, and its conjugates. Norpethidine is about half as active an analgesic and about twice as toxic as pethidine; it may accumulate in the plasma on chronic administration, particularly in subjects with renal failure. The excretion of pethidine and its metabolites is dependent on the urinary pH. In normal subjects, about 70% of a dose is excreted in the urine in 24 h, up to 10% as unchanged drug, 10% as norpethidine, 20% as pethidinic acid, 16% as conjugated pethidinic acid, 8% as norpethidinic acid, and 10% as conjugated norpethidinic acid; other metabolites identified in the urine in minor amounts include the *N*-hydroxy and *N*-hydroxyphenyl derivatives and pethidine *N*-oxide. Urinary excretion of pethidine and norpethidine may both be enhanced to about 30% of a dose if the urine is acid; in alkaline urine, less than 5% is excreted as pethidine and norpethidine. In pregnant women and in women taking oral contraceptives, the excretion of unchanged pethidine appears to be increased; less

unchanged drug is eliminated in older subjects and, in subjects with cirrhosis, excretion of pethidine is delayed. Pethidine and norpethidine are distributed in the CSF. Pethidine crosses the placenta and is excreted in breast milk.
Pethidine is a metabolite of phenoperidine.

Therapeutic concentration. In plasma, usually in the range 0.2 to 0.8 mg/L. Higher plasma concentrations are found in elderly subjects.

Following a single oral dose of 50 mg to 6 subjects, a mean peak serum concentration of 0.14 mg/L was attained in 2 h; after an IM injection of 50 mg to the same subjects, a mean peak serum concentration of 0.20 mg/L in 1 h was reported, and a mean serum concentration of 0.52 mg/L was obtained 1 min after an IV injection of 50 mg. [J. E. Stambaugh *et al.*, *J. Clin. Pharmacol.*, 1976, *16*, 245–256.]

Following multiple oral doses of 75 to 100 mg to 4 subjects, plasma concentrations of 0.16 to 0.54 mg/L (mean 0.36) of pethidine and 0.13 to 0.48 mg/L (mean 0.27) of norpethidine were reported 1 to 4 h after a dose. [H. H. Szeto *et al.*, *J. Chromatogr.*, 1976, *125*, 503–510.]

Toxicity. The estimated minimum lethal dose is 1 g. Toxic effects are usually associated with blood concentrations greater than 2 mg/L but fatalities involving pethidine are uncommon.

Bioavailability. About 55%.

Half-life. Plasma half-life, pethidine 3 to 6 h, increased in neonates and in renal impairment; norpethidine about 20 h.

Volume of distribution. About 4.4 L/kg.

Clearance. Plasma clearance, about 17 mL/min/kg, decreased in subjects with liver disease and in the elderly.

Distribution in blood. Plasma:whole blood ratio, about 0.9.

Protein binding. In plasma, about 50 to 60%.

Note. For reviews of the pharmacokinetics of pethidine, see L. E. Mather and P. J. Meffin, *Clin. Pharmacokinet.*, 1978, *3*, 352–368, and D. J. Edwards *et al.*, *Clin. Pharmacokinet.*, 1982, *7*, 421–433; for a general review of pethidine, see K. S. Latta *et al.*, *Am. J. Ther.*, 2002, *9*, 53–68.

Dose. Usually 50 to 150 mg of pethidine hydrochloride, by mouth or 25 to 100 mg by IM injection every 4 h.

Phanquinone

Anti-amoebic/Antibacterial

Synonyms. Phanquone; Ciba 11925
Proprietary name. Entobex
4,7-Phenanthroline-5,6-dione
$C_{12}H_6N_2O_2$=210.2
CAS—84-12-8

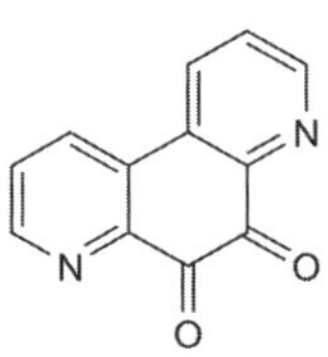

An orange crystalline powder. M.p. 295°, with decomposition.
Slightly soluble in water; practically insoluble in ethanol and chloroform; soluble in dilute mineral acids.

Partition Coefficient. Log *P* (octanol/water), 1.2.

Colour Tests. Marquis Test—yellow; Methanolic Potassium Hydroxide—yellow→brown-violet.

Thin-layer Chromatography. System TA—Rf 49; system TB—Rf 03; system TC—Rf 45; system TE—Rf 54; system TL—Rf 17; system TAE—Rf 86; system TAJ—Rf 11; system TAK—Rf 00; system TAL—Rf 00. (Acidified iodoplatinate solution, positive.)

Ultraviolet Spectrum. Aqueous acid—265 (A^1_1=500a), 272 (A^1_1=500a), 292 nm (A^1_1=480b).

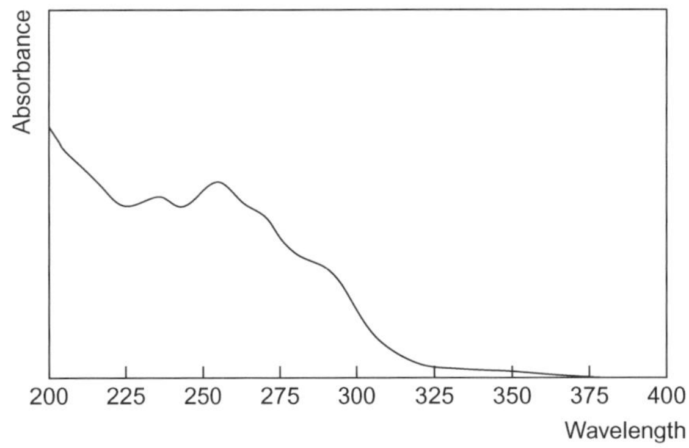

Infra-red Spectrum. Principal peaks at wavenumbers 1700, 1283, 1584, 1275, 1683, 950 cm^{-1} (KBr disk).

Quantification
Gas chromatography. In biological fluids: limit of detection 15 μg/L—P. H. Degen *et al.*, *J. Chromatogr.*, 1976, *118*, 363–370.

Dose. 150 to 300 mg daily.

Phenacaine

Anaesthetic (local)

Synonym. Phenetidylphenacetin
N,N′-Bis(4-ethoxyphenyl)ethanimidamide
$C_{18}H_{22}N_2O_2$=298.4
CAS—101-93-9

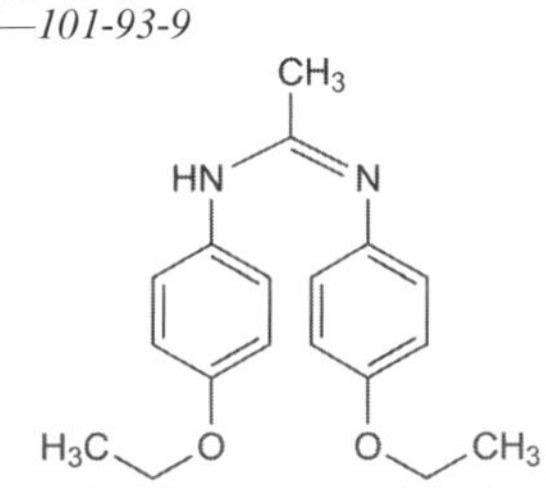

Phenacaine Hydrochloride Monohydrate
Proprietary name. Holocaine
$C_{18}H_{22}N_2O_2$,HCl,H_2O=352.9
CAS—620-99-5 (anhydrous); 6153-19-1 (monohydrate)
White crystals. M.p. 190° to 192°.
Soluble 1 in 50 of water; freely soluble in ethanol and chloroform; insoluble in ether.

Partition Coefficient. Log *P* (octanol/water), 5.6.

Gas Chromatography. System GA—RI 2617.

Infra-red Spectrum. Principal peaks at wavenumbers 1646, 1520, 1256, 1300, 1046, 815 cm^{-1} (KBr disk).

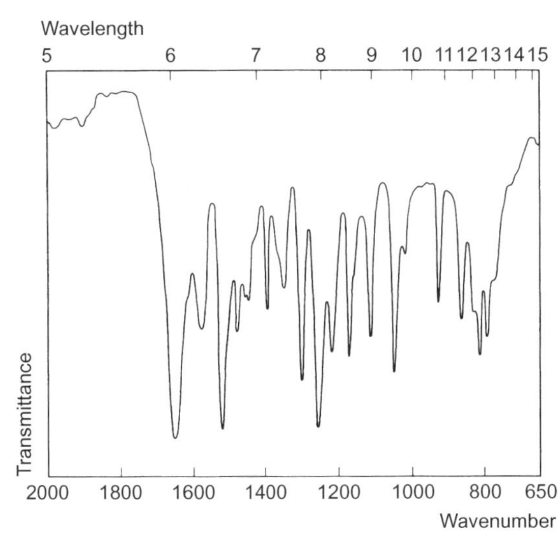

Uses. Phenacaine hydrochloride has been used as a 1% aqueous solution or as a 1 or 2% ointment.

Phenacemide

Anticonvulsant

Synonyms. Carbamidum Phenylaceticum; Phenacetylurea.
Proprietary name. Phenurone
N-(Aminocarbonyl)benzeneacetamide
$C_9H_{10}N_2O_2$=178.2
CAS—63-98-9

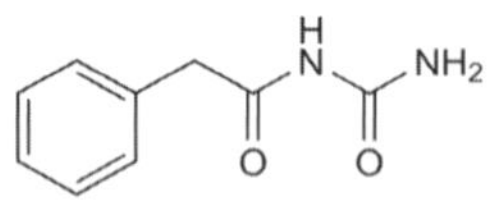

A white crystalline powder. M.p. about 212° to 216°.
Very slightly soluble in water; slightly soluble in acetone, ethanol, chloroform, ether and methanol.

Partition Coefficient. Log *P* (octanol/water), 0.9.

Colour Tests. Liebermann's Test—red-orange; Nessler's Reagent—brown-orange (slow).

Thin-layer Chromatography. System TD—Rf 22; system TE—Rf 65; system TF—Rf 40; system TAD—Rf 50.

Gas Chromatography. System GA—RI 1473.

High Performance Liquid Chromatography. System HX—RI 339; system HY—RI 266.

Ultraviolet Spectrum. Methanol—258 (A^1_1=18a), 265 nm.

Infra-red Spectrum. Principal peaks at wavenumbers 1660, 1090, 716, 1618, 1170, 970 cm^{-1} (KBr disk).

Mass Spectrum. Principal ions at *m/z* 91, 92, 118, 44, 43, 135, 65, 178.

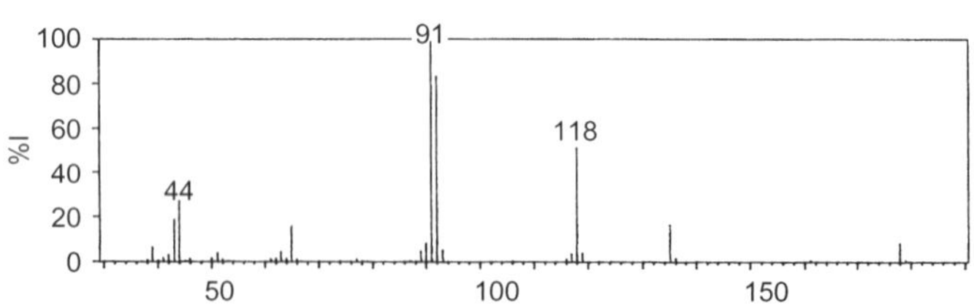

Disposition in the Body. Well absorbed after oral administration. It is extensively metabolised to inactive metabolites, principally by *p*-hydroxylation of the phenyl ring; the metabolites are excreted in the urine.

Toxicity. The estimated minimum lethal dose is 5 g.

Dose. 1.5 to 3 g daily.

Phenacetin

Analgesic

Synonyms. *p*-Acetiphenetidide; Aceto-*p*-phenetidide; Acetophenetidin; Acetylphenetidin; Fenacetina; Paracetophenetidin.
Proprietary names. It is an ingredient of APC tablets and was included in Gripponyl, Hemagene Tailleur, Polypirine and Cratodin Rectal.
N-(4-Ethoxyphenyl)acetamide
$C_{10}H_{13}NO_2$=179.2
CAS—62-44-2

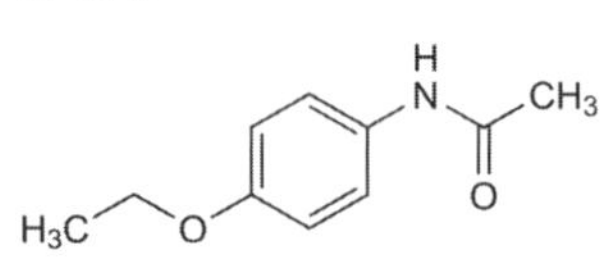

White glistening crystalline scales or fine white crystalline powder. M.p. 134° to 135°.

Soluble 1 in 1300 of water, 1 in 15 of ethanol, 1 in 14 of chloroform, and 1 in 90 of ether.

Dissociation Constant. pK_a 2.2.

Partition Coefficient. Log *P* (octanol/water), 1.6.

Colour Tests. Liebermann's Test—violet.
Boil 0.1 g with 1 mL of hydrochloric acid for 3 min, dilute with 10 mL of water, cool, filter, and add one drop of 0.02 M potassium dichromate to the filtrate—violet→red.

Thin-layer Chromatography. System TD—Rf 38; system TE—Rf 68; system TF—Rf 37; system TAD—Rf 52; system TAE—Rf 83; system TAJ—Rf 58; system TAK—Rf 41; system TAL—Rf 89. (Acidified potassium permanganate solution, positive.) See also under Paracetamol.

Gas Chromatography. System GA—phenacetin RI 1675, M (hydroquinone) RI 1240, M (*p*-phenetidine) RI 1275, paracetamol RI 1687; system GB—RI 1730; system GF—RI 2325.

High Performance Liquid Chromatography. System HD—phenacetin *k* 0.6 ; paracetamol *k* 0.1; system HW—phenacetin *k* 4.4; paracetamol *k* 0.3; system HX—phenacetin RI 377; paracetamol RI 264; system HY—phenacetin RI 335; paracetamol RI 241; system HZ—Retention time, phenacetin 3.0 min; paracetamol 1.9 min.

Ultraviolet Spectrum. Aqueous acid—244 nm (A^1_1=649a). No alkaline shift.

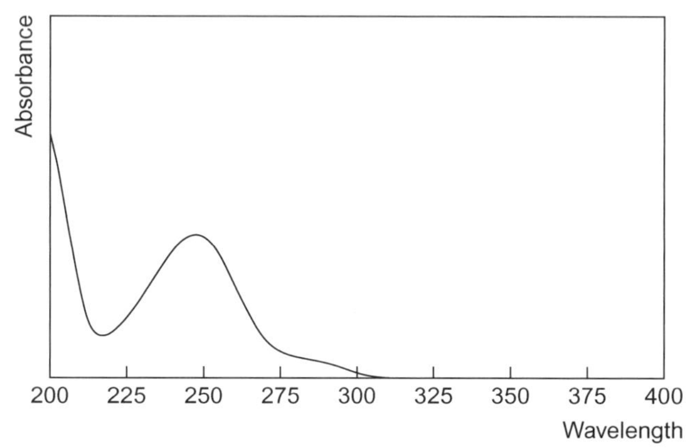

Infra-red Spectrum. Principal peaks at wavenumbers 1244, 1655, 1513, 1555, 1265, 836 cm^{-1} (KBr disk).

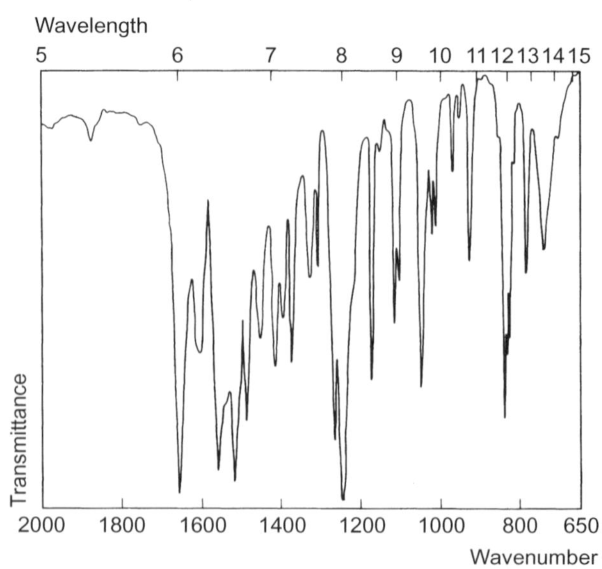

Mass Spectrum. Principal ions at *m/z* 108, 109, 179, 137, 43, 81, 80, 110; paracetamol 109, 151, 43, 80, 108, 81, 53, 52.

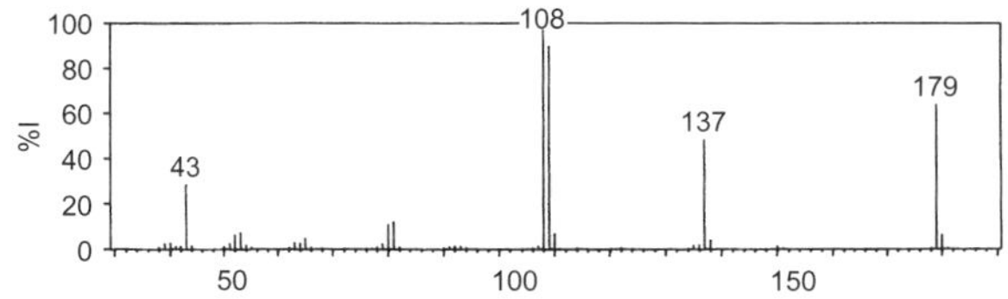

Quantification See also under Paracetamol.

Gas chromatography. In plasma: phenacetin and paracetamol, limit of detection <100 μg/L, FID—M. A. Evans and R. D. Harbison, *J. Pharm. Sci.*, 1977, *66*, 1628–1629.

Gas chromatography–mass spectrometry. In plasma: phenacetin and paracetamol, limit of detection 1 μg/L for phenacetin and 100 μg/L for paracetamol—W. A. Garland *et al.*, *J. Pharm. Sci.*, 1977, *66*, 340–344. In plasma: limit of detection 1 pg—S. Murray and A. R. Boobis, *J. Chromatogr.*, 1991, *568*, 341–350.

High performance liquid chromatography. In plasma: phenacetin and paracetamol, limit of detection 500 μg/L, UV detection—G.R. Gotelli *et al.*, *Clin. Chem.*, 1977, *23*, 957–959.

Disposition in the Body. Readily absorbed after oral administration, but subject to extensive first-pass metabolism. It is metabolised mainly in the liver by *O*-dealkylation to paracetamol and acetaldehyde, followed by conjugation of the paracetamol with sulfate or glucuronic acid (see under Paracetamol); other reactions are deacetylation to phenetidine (*p*-ethoxyaniline), *N*-, 2-, and α-hydroxylation forming mainly 2-hydroxyphenetidine and also 2-hydroxyphenacetin, sulfate conjugation of deacetylated metabolites, and glutathione conjugation to form *S*-(1-acetamido-4-hydroxyphenyl)cysteine and its corresponding mercapturic acid.
2-Hydroxyphenetidine appears to be the nephrotoxic metabolite and is possibly involved in the formation of methaemoglobinaemia. As the dose is increased so the percentage of the dose which is deacetylated is increased, producing proportionately more phenetidine and 2-hydroxyphenetidine; production of these metabolites is also increased by concomitant administration of aspirin, caffeine, and codeine. Phenacetin is not hepatotoxic despite being converted to paracetamol; this is because the enzyme systems which convert paracetamol to its toxic metabolite are also involved in the conversion of phenacetin to paracetamol and the two conversions therefore compete, resulting in reduced paracetamol oxidation. Phenacetin metabolism is stimulated by cigarette smoking. The extent of *O*-dealkylation appears to be genetically determined. About 80 to 90% of a dose is excreted in the urine in 24 h with 50 to 80% of the dose as the sulfate and glucuronide conjugates of paracetamol, 6 to 8% as 2-hydroxyphenetidine sulfate, about 2% as *S*-(1-acetamido-4-hydroxyphenyl)cysteine, about 0.3% as phenetidine and 2-hydroxyphenacetin, 0.2% as unchanged drug, and 2 to 3% as unconjugated paracetamol.

Therapeutic concentration

After a single oral dose of 0.9 g to 9 subjects, peak plasma-phenacetin concentrations of 0.2 to 7.4 mg/L (mean 2.3) were attained in 1 to 2 h, and peak plasma-paracetamol concentrations of 3.1 to 11.9 mg/L (mean 7.9) were attained in 2 to 3.5 h; plasma-phenacetin concentrations were reported to be lower in 9 smokers [E. J. Pantuck *et al.*, *Clin. Pharmacol. Ther.*, 1974, *15*, 9–17].

Toxicity. The estimated minimum lethal dose is 5 g. Prolonged use of phenacetin is associated with analgesic nephropathy; it may also produce haemolytic anaemia and methaemoglobinaemia.

In a fatality involving the intentional overdosage of a preparation containing codeine, aspirin, phenacetin and caffeine, a blood-phenacetin concentration of 136 mg/L was reported; the codeine and salicylate blood concentrations were 5.3 and 265 mg/L respectively [J. A. Wright *et al.*, *Clin Toxicol.*, 1975, *8*, 457–463].

Half-life. Plasma half-life, phenacetin 0.7 to 1.5 h, paracetamol 1.5 to 3 h.

Volume of distribution. About 1 to 2 L/kg.

Clearance. Plasma clearance, about 20 mL/min/kg.

Distribution in blood. Plasma : whole blood ratio, 0.93.

Protein binding. In plasma, about 30%.

Note. For a review of the general properties of phenacetin, see S. P. Clissold, *Drugs*, 1986, *32* (Suppl.4), 46–59.

Dose. Phenacetin has been given as a single dose of 300 to 600 mg; maximum daily dose of 3 g.

Phenaglycodol

Tranquilliser

Proprietary name. Felixyn
2-(4-Chlorophenyl)-3-methylbutane-2,3-diol
$C_{11}H_{15}ClO_2=214.7$
CAS—79-93-6

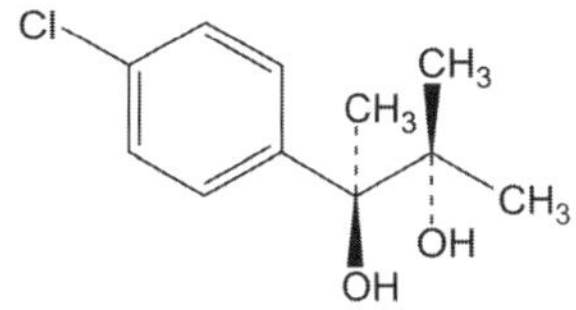

A crystalline solid. M.p. 77° to 78°.
Practically insoluble in water; soluble in ethanol.

Colour Tests. Liebermann's Test—brown; Mandelin's Test—blue.

Thin-layer Chromatography. System TE—Rf 71; system TAE—Rf 84.

Ultraviolet Spectrum. Ethanol—259, 266 (A^1_1=13.5a), 275 nm.

Infra-red Spectrum. Principal peaks at wavenumbers 1095, 1085, 1015, 1180, 807, 830 cm^{-1} (KBr disk).

Mass Spectrum. Principal ions at *m/z* 43, 59, 155, 121, 156, 31, 157, 158.

Quantification

Ultraviolet spectrophotometry. In blood or urine—J. E. Wallace, *J. Pharm. Sci.*, 1968, *57*, 426–429.

Dose. 0.9 to 1.2 g daily.

Phenazocine

Narcotic Analgesic

Synonyms. Phenethylazocine; Phenobenzorphan.
1,2,3,4,5,6-Hexahydro-6,11-dimethyl-3-(2-phenethyl)-2,6-methano-3-benzazocin-8-ol
$C_{22}H_{27}NO=321.5$
CAS—127-35-5

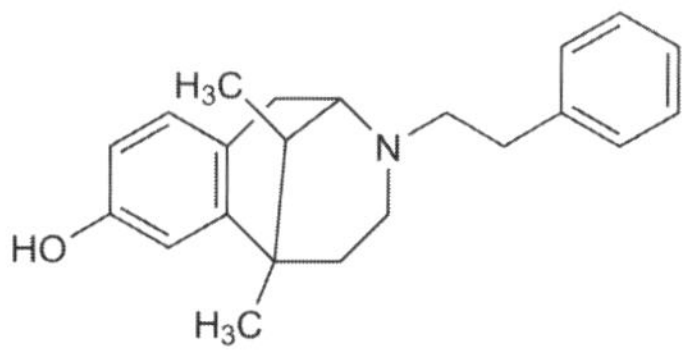

Crystals. M.p. 181° (±-form) and M.p. about 159° (− -form).

Phenazocine Hydrobromide

Proprietary name. Narphen
$C_{22}H_{27}NO,HBr,½H_2O=411.4$
CAS—1239-04-9 (anhydrous)
A white microcrystalline powder, which can exist in 3 polymorphic forms. M.p. about 166° to 170°.
Soluble 1 in 350 of water, 1 in 45 of ethanol and 1 in 140 of chloroform; practically insoluble in ether.

Dissociation Constant. pK_a 8.5.

Partition Coefficient. Log *P* (octanol/water), 5.2.

Colour Test. Marquis Test—brown.

Thin-layer Chromatography. System TA—Rf 68; system TB—Rf 16; system TC—Rf 39; system TE—Rf 74; system TL—Rf 49; system TAE—Rf 50; system TAF—Rf 81; system TAJ—Rf 26; system TAK—Rf 20; system TAL—Rf 90. (Dragendorff spray, positive; acidified iodoplatinate solution, positive; Marquis reagent, brown.)

Gas Chromatography. System GA—RI 2686; system GB—RI 2833.

High Performance Liquid Chromatography. System HA—*k* 1.3; system HC—*k* 0.3; system HX—RI 409; system HY—RI 299.

Ultraviolet Spectrum. Aqueous acid—278 nm (A^1_1=64a); aqueous alkali—238, 298 nm.

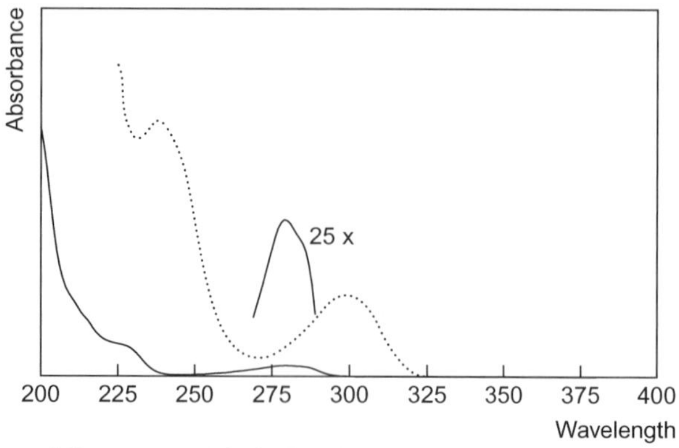

Infra-red Spectrum. Principal peaks at wavenumbers 1224, 1497, 1241, 705, 1613, 758 cm^{-1} (phenazocine hydrobromide, Nujol mull).

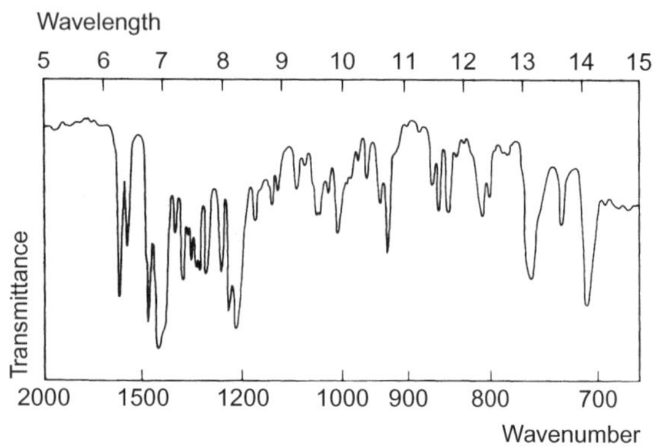

Mass Spectrum. Principal ions at *m/z* 230, 231, 58, 44, 42, 105, 173, 159.

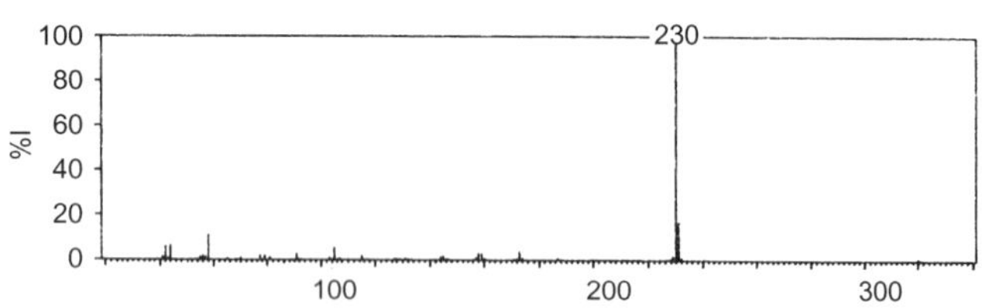

Disposition in the Body. Readily absorbed after oral, sublingual or intramuscular administration; metabolised in the liver.

Toxicity. The estimated minimum lethal dose is 0.2 g. Phenazocine is addictive although tolerance develops more slowly and to a lesser extent than with morphine.

Dose. Usually 5 mg of phenazocine hydrobromide every 4 to 6 h; single doses of 20 mg may be given.

Phenazone

Analgesic

Synonyms. Analgésine; Antipyrin(e); Azophenum; Fenazona; Phenazonum; Phenyldimethylpyrazolone.
Proprietary names. Aequiton-P; Aurone; Erasol; Migrane-Kranit-mono; Oto-Phen; Tropex. It is an ingredient of Allergen; Auralgan, Auralgicin; Auroto, Otocalm, and Tympagesic.
1,2-Dihydro-1,5-dimethyl-2-phenyl-3*H*-pyrazol-3-one
$C_{11}H_{12}N_2O = 188.2$
CAS—60-80-0

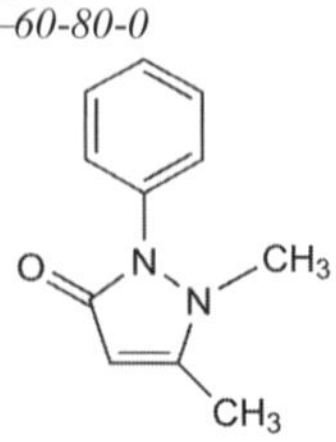

Small, colourless crystals or white crystalline powder. M.p. 111° to 113°. Soluble 1 in less than 1 of water, 1 in 1.3 of ethanol, 1 in 1 of chloroform, and 1 in 43 of ether.

Dissociation Constant. pK_a 1.5 (25°).

Partition Coefficient. Log *P* (octanol/pH 7.4), 0.4.

Colour Tests. *p*-Dimethylaminobenzaldehyde (100°, 5 min) —red/violet; Ferric Chloride—red; Liebermann's Test (100°)—orange; Mandelin's Test—green; Nitrous Acid—green.

Thin-layer Chromatography. System TA—Rf 65; system TB—Rf 04; system TD—Rf 18; system TE—Rf 45; system TF—Rf 14; system TAD—Rf 50; system TAE—Rf 66; system TAF—Rf 66; system TAJ—Rf 51; system TAK—Rf 18; system TAL—Rf 83. (Ferric chloride solution, red-brown; acidified iodoplatinate solution, positive; mercuric chloride–diphenylcarbazone reagent, positive; acidified potassium permanganate solution, positive; Van Urk reagent, pink.)

Gas Chromatography. System GA—phenazone RI 1835, M (4-OH-) RI 1855; system GB—RI 1951; system GF—RI 2445.

High Performance Liquid Chromatography. System HA—*k* 0.2; system HD—*k* 0.1; system HW—*k* 0.95; system HX—RI 333; system HY—RI 299; system HZ—retention time 2.1 min; system HAX—retention time 5.4 min; system HAY—retention time 4.5 min.

Ultraviolet Spectrum. Aqueous acid—230 ($A_1^1 = 590a$); aqueous alkali—242 ($A_1^1 = 494a$), 256 nm.

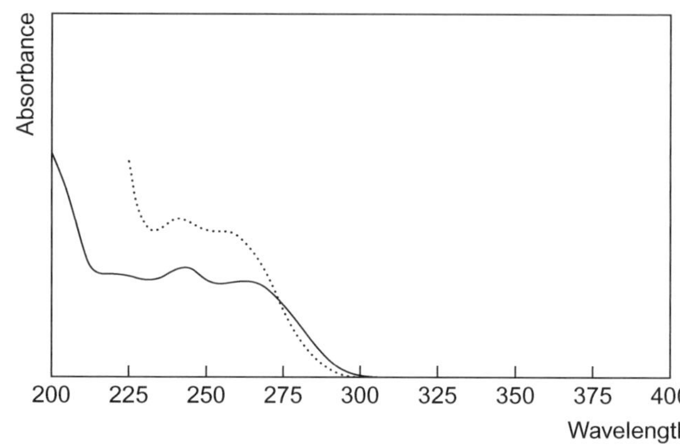

Infra-red Spectrum. Principal peaks at wavenumbers 1660, 770, 1318, 1305, 1590, 1580 cm^{-1} (KBr disk).

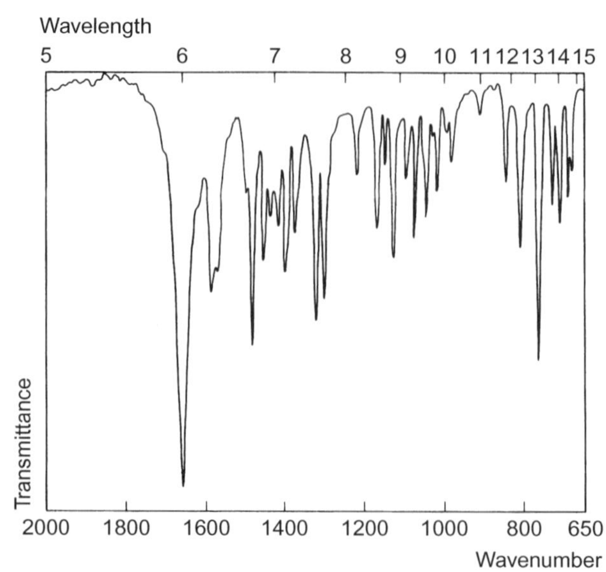

Mass Spectrum. Principal ions at *m/z* 188, 96, 77, 56, 105, 189, 55, 51; norphenazone 174, 77, 91, 105, 132, -, -, -.

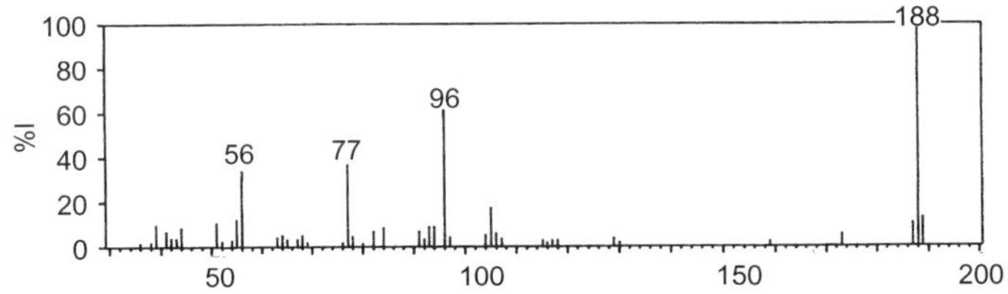

Quantification

Gas chromatography. In plasma: limit of detection 1 mg/L, AFID—D. R. Abernethy *et al.*, *J. Chromatogr.* 1981, *223*(12) *B Biomed. Appl.*, 432–437.

High performance liquid chromatography. In plasma: limit of detection 500 μg/L, UV detection—T. M. Campbell *et al.*, *J. Chromatogr.* 1979, *163*(5) *B Biomed. Appl.*, 236–238. In urine: phenazone, 3-hydroxymethylphenazone, 4-hydroxyphenazone and norphenazone, limit of detection 1 to 2 mg/L, UV detection—M. Eichelbaum *et al.*, *Pharmacology*, 1981, *23*, 192–202. In saliva—J. Gartzke and H. Jager, *J. Pharm. Biomed. Anal.*, 1991, *9*, 977–979. In urine: phenazone metabolites—C. Palette *et al.*, *J. Chromatogr.*, 1991, *563*, 103–113. In urine: phenazone and its metabolites—M. A. Sarkar *et al.*, *Biomed. Chromatogr.*, 1992, *6*, 300–304. In biological fluids: phenazone sulfo- and glucuro-conjugated metabolites—C. Palette *et al.*, *Biomed. Chromatogr.*, 1994, *8*, 77–84. In plasma: phenazone and its major metabolites, UV detection—V. L. Lanchote *et al.*, *Ther. Drug Monit.*, 1997, *19*, 705–710.

High performance liquid chromatography–mass spectrometry. In plasma: limit of detection 0.3 μg/L—S. A. Coolen *et al.*, *J. Chromatogr. B Biomed. Sci. Appl.*, 1999, *732*, 103–113.

Radioimmunoassay. In plasma or saliva: limit of detection 10 μg/L—R. L. Chang *et al.*, *Clin. Pharmacol. Ther.*, 1976, *20*, 219–226.

Disposition in the Body. Rapidly and completely absorbed after oral administration. It is widely distributed in body fluids, with saliva and breast milk levels being about the same as those found in plasma. It is metabolised to 3-hydroxymethylphenazone, 4-hydroxyphenazone, and norphenazone, followed by glucuronic acid conjugation; demethylation also occurs. The rate of biotransformation is variable and appears to be genetically determined. Phenazone and its metabolites are excreted in the urine mainly as glucuronides, although sulfate conjugation has also been reported. About 30 to 40% of a dose is excreted in the urine in 48 h as conjugated 4-hydroxyphenazone, 10 to 40% as the 3-hydroxymethyl derivative, up to about 20% as norphenazone, 3 to 6% as 4,4′-dihydroxyphenazone, 8 to 12% as 4,5-dioxypyrazoline, and less than 5% as unchanged drug; 3-carboxyphenazone has also been identified in the urine. A total of about 95% of a dose is excreted in the urine in 4 days.

Therapeutic concentration

After a single oral dose of 10 mg/kg to 5 subjects, peak plasma concentrations of 10 to 15.5 mg/L (mean 13.4) were attained in 1 h. Concentrations in saliva were similar to those in plasma. [C. J. van Boxtel, *et al.*, *Eur. J. Clin. Pharmacol.*, 1976, *9*, 327–332.]

Toxicity. The estimated minimum lethal dose is 5 g, but fatalities from acute poisoning are rare. Prolonged therapeutic administration may give rise to agranulocytosis.

In a suicide due to ingestion of phenazone, a postmortem blood concentration of 110 mg/L was reported; alcohol was also detected in the blood at a concentration of 260 mg/L. [C. Péclet and M. Rousseau, *Bull. Int. Assoc. Forensic Toxicol.*, 1981, *16(1)*, 32.]

During the course of a clinical trial of the efficacy of oxerutins in venous ulceration, an 87-year-old woman died within 2 h of the IV injection of phenazone 500 mg (administered over 10 min). Postmortem analysis revealed a blood phenazone concentration of 22 mg/L and the cause of death was certified as 'cardiac arrest following injection of antipyrine'. [A. F. Travers, *Clin. Pharmacol. Ther.*, 1991, *49*, 695–696.]

Half-life. Plasma half-life, about 7 to 15 h (mean 10); increased in subjects with renal impairment or hypothyroidism and in the elderly, decreased in subjects with hyperthyroidism; the half-life is also readily influenced by concomitant administration of other drugs.

Volume of distribution. About 0.6 L/kg.

Clearance. Plasma clearance, about 0.7 mL/min/kg.

Distribution in blood. Plasma:whole blood ratio, about 0.93.

Protein binding. In plasma, less than 10%.

Note. For a review of the pharmacokinetics of phenazone, see D. Vital-Durand *et al.*, *Therapie*, 1988, *43*, 263–266.

Dose. Phenazone has been given in doses of 300 to 600 mg; maximum daily dose of 4 g.

Phenazopyridine

Analgesic

3-(Phenylazo)-2,6-pyridinediamine
$C_{11}H_{11}N_5$=213.2
CAS—94-78-0

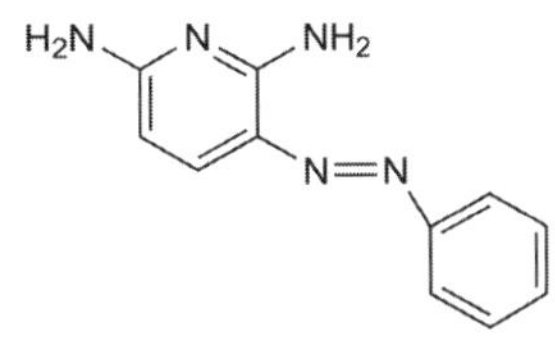

M.p. 139°.

Phenazopyridine Hydrochloride

Proprietary names. Phenazo; Pyridacil; Pyridium. It is an ingredient of Azo Gantanol, Azo Gantrisin, Azo-Mandelamine, Azotrex, and Uromide.
$C_{11}H_{11}N_5$,HCl=249.7
CAS—136-40-3
A light or dark red to dark violet crystalline powder. M.p. about 235°, with decomposition.
Soluble 1 in 300 of cold water, 1 in 20 of boiling water, 1 in about 60 of ethanol, and 1 in about 330 of chloroform; very slightly soluble in ether; soluble in glacial acetic acid. Phenazopyridine hydrochloride readily forms supersaturated aqueous solutions which deposit slowly on storage.

Partition Coefficient. Log *P* (octanol/water), 2.8.

Colour Tests. Mandelin's Test—green; Marquis Test—red.

Thin-layer Chromatography. System TA—Rf 59; system TB—Rf 01; system TC—Rf 50; system TE—Rf 70; system TL—Rf 53; system TAE—Rf 80; system TAJ—Rf 46; system TAK—Rf 56; system TAL—Rf 91. (Acidified potassium permanganate solution, positive.)

Gas Chromatography. System GA—phenazopyridine RI 2245, 4-aminophenol RI 1265, aniline RI 1158; system GB—RI 2370.

High Performance Liquid Chromatography. System HY—RI 314.

Ultraviolet Spectrum. Ethanol—238 (A_1^1=455a), 277 nm. (See below)

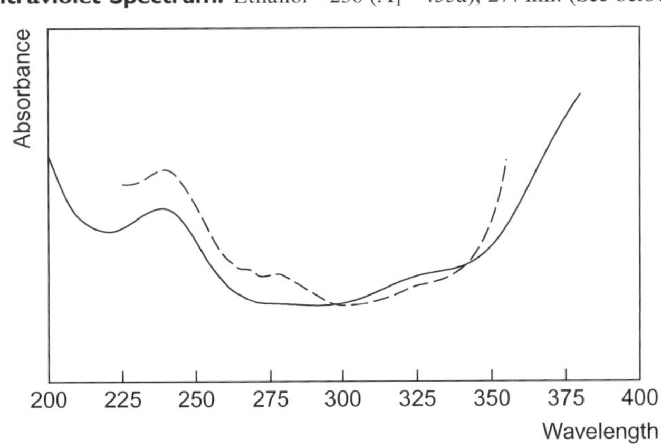

Infra-red Spectrum. Principal peaks at wavenumbers 1585, 1656, 762, 685, 1248, 1493 cm^{-1} (Nujol mull). (See below)

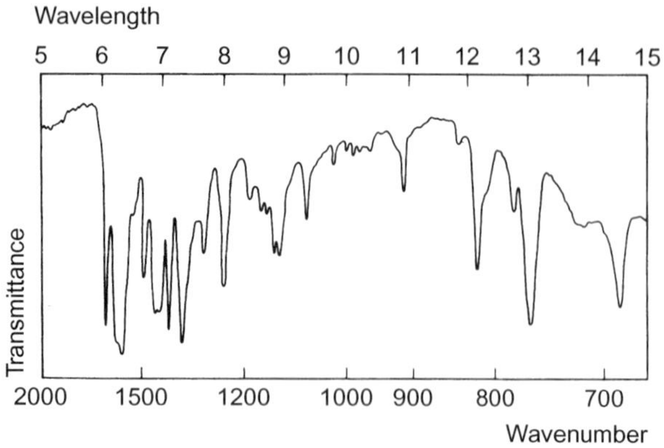

Mass Spectrum. Principal ions at *m/z* 108, 81, 213, 54, 77, 136, 51, 43; 4-aminophenol 109, 80, 53, 81, 108, 52, 54, 110.

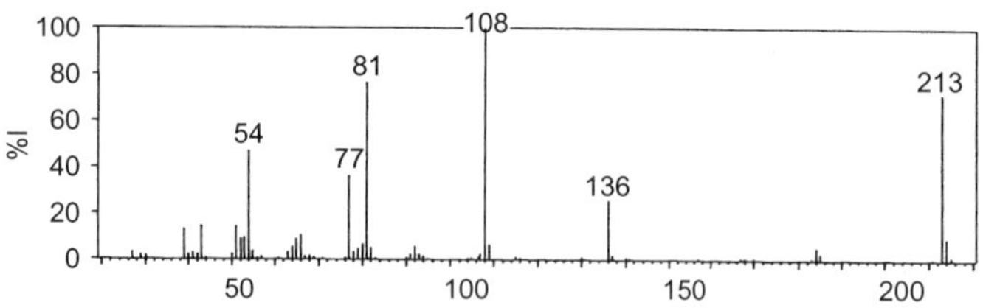

Disposition in the Body. Absorbed after oral administration. Rapidly eliminated by the kidneys, giving an orange-red colour to the urine; about 90% of a dose is excreted in the urine in 24 h, of which 7% is aniline, 20% is *N*-acetyl-4-aminophenol, 25% is 4-aminophenol, and 45% is unchanged drug.

Toxicity. Methaemoglobinaemia and acute renal failure have been reported after overdoses.

Dose. Usually 600 mg of phenazopyridine hydrochloride daily.

Phencyclidine

Hallucinogen

Note. Phencyclidine is also known as Angel Dust, Crystal, Cyclone, Killer Weed, PCP, Peace Pills, and T. For other names applied to illicitly used Phencyclidine and Phencyclidine Hydrochloride, see *Martindale, The complete drug reference*, 33rd Edn, Pharmaceutical Press, London, 2002.

1-(1-Phenylcyclohexyl)piperidine

$C_{17}H_{25}N$=243.4

CAS—77-10-1

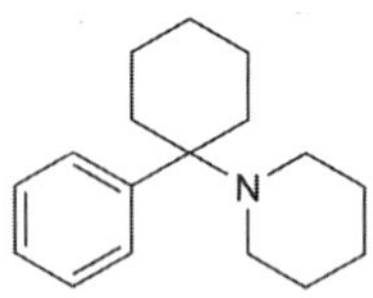

Crystals. M.p. 46° to 46.5°.

Phencyclidine Hydrochloride

Synonyms. CI-395; CN-25253-2; GP-121; NSC-40902; PCP.

$C_{17}H_{25}N,HCl$=279.9

CAS—956-90-1

A white crystalline powder. M.p. 233° to 235° (from 2-propanol).

Soluble 1 in 6 of water, 1 in 7 of ethanol, and 1 in 2 of chloroform; very slightly soluble in ether.

Phencyclidine Hydrobromide

Crystals. M. p. 214° to 218°.

Dissociation Constant. pK_a 8.5.

Partition Coefficient. Log *P* (octanol/water), 4.7.

Colour Test. *p*-Dimethylaminobenzaldehyde (100°, 3 min)—red.

Thin-layer Chromatography. System TA—Rf 59; system TB—Rf 73; system TC—Rf 35; system TE—Rf 84; system TL—Rf 66; system TAE—Rf 23; system TAF—Rf 69; system TAJ—Rf 24; system TAK—Rf 04; system TAL—Rf 48. (Acidified iodoplatinate solution, positive.)

Gas Chromatography. System GA—RI 1900; system GB—RI 1981; system GF—RI 2150.

High Performance Liquid Chromatography. System HA—*k* 2.4 (tailing peak); system HX—RI 375; system HY—RI 285.

Ultraviolet Spectrum. Aqueous acid—252, 258, 263 (A_1^1=13.5a), 270 nm.

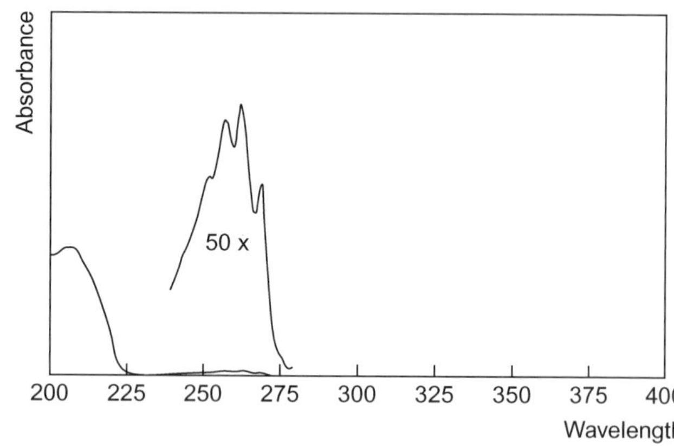

Infra-red Spectrum. Principal peaks at wavenumbers 700, 760, 1298, 1020, 892, 869 cm^{-1} (phencyclidine hydrochloride, KBr disk).

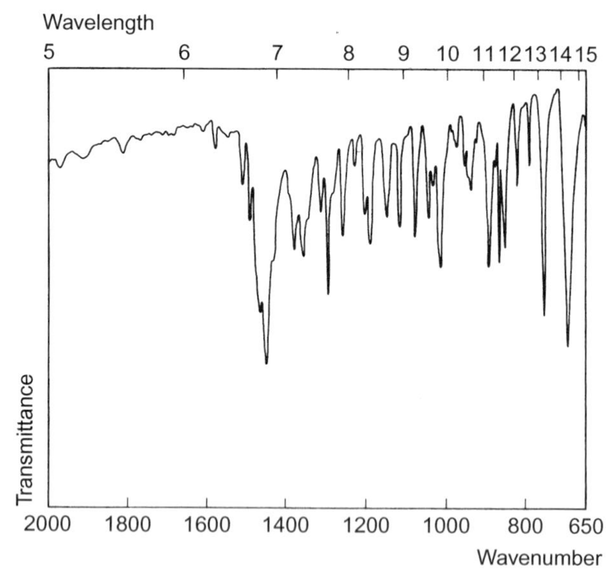

Mass Spectrum. Principal ions at *m/z* 200, 91, 243, 242, 84, 186, 166, 201; 1-(1-phenylcyclohexyl)-4-hydroxypiperidine 91, 216, 77, 259, -, -, -, -; 4-phenyl-4-piperidinocyclohexanol 200, 91, 84, 86, 186, 259, -, -.

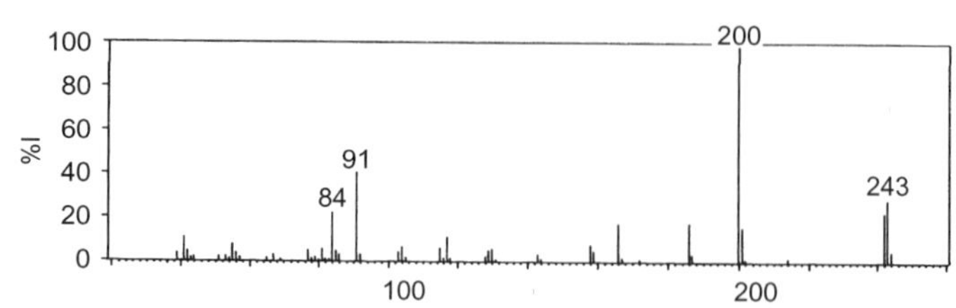

Quantification

Gas chromatography. In CSF, serum, or urine: limit of detection 5 μg/L, AFID—J. N. Miceli *et al.*, *J. Anal. Toxicol.*, 1981, *5*, 29–32. In urine: NPD—C. T. Kandiko *et al.*, *J. Chromatogr.*, 1990, *528*, 208–213. In plasma or urine: limit of detection 0.75 μg/L, surface-ionisation detection—A. Ishii *et al.*, *Int. J. Legal Med.*, 1996, *108*, 244–247. In urine: phencyclidine and amfetamines, limit of detection for phencyclidine 15 μg/L, PDHID—C. Casari and A. R. Andrews, *Forensic Sci. Int.*, 2001, *120*, 165–171. In plasma, serum, saliva, tissues, or urine: limit of detection 5 ng/L, AFID—F. N. Pitts *et al.*, *J. Chromatogr.*, 1980, *193*, 157–159. In plasma: phencyclidine and opioid analgesics, limit of quantification 10 μg/L, nitrogen-selective detection—P. Kintz *et al.*, *Methods Find. Exp. Clin. Pharmacol.*, 1990, *12*, 193–196.

Gas chromatography–mass spectrometry. In urine: phencyclidine and two monohydroxy metabolites, limit of detection for phencyclidine 10 μg/L—E. J. Cone *et al.*, *J. Chromatogr.* 1981, *223*(12) *B Biomed. Appl.*, 331–339. In urine: limit of detection 0.47 μg/L—C. C. Stevenson *et al.*, *J. Anal. Toxicol.*, 1992, *16*, 337–339. In hair: limit of quantification 0.1 ng/mg—M. H. Slawson *et al.*, *J. Anal. Toxicol.*, 1996, *20*, 350–354. In hair: phencyclidine and its metabolites—Y. Nakahara *et al.*, *J. Anal. Toxicol.*, 1997, *21*, 356–362. In urine: phencyclidine and other drugs of abuse, comparisons of SIM, SIS, or full scan mode—S. P. Vorce *et al.*, *J. Anal. Toxicol.*, 2000, *24*, 595–601.

Radioimmunoassay. In serum: limit of detection 500 ng/L—S. M. Owens *et al.*, *Clin. Chem.*, 1982, *28*, 1509–1513.

Note. For a review of the analysis of phencyclidine and its metabolites—see T. N. V. Veselovskaia *et al.*, *Sud. Med. Ekspert*, 1999, *42*, 20–25.

Disposition in the Body. Phencyclidine is a drug of abuse which is self-administered orally, IV, by nasal insufflation, or by smoking impregnated plant material. The main metabolic reaction is hydroxylation and two metabolites have been identified in the urine as glucuronide conjugates: 4-phenyl-4-piperidinocyclohexanol and 1-(1-phenylcyclohexyl)-4-hydroxypiperidine (PCHP). The product of *N*-dealkylation (1-phenylcyclohexylamine) has also been identified in urine, together with an oxidised derivative, 5-(1-phenylcyclohexylamino)valeric acid. About 73% of a dose is excreted in the urine and 5% is eliminated in the faeces in 10 days, of which about 16% of the dose is unchanged and 30% is conjugated hydroxylated metabolites; the rate of excretion of unchanged drug is increased in acidic urine.

Blood concentration

Following an oral dose of 1 mg, given to 5 subjects, a mean peak plasma concentration of 2.7 μg/L was reported at 2.5 h. [C. E. Cook *et al.*, *Clin. Pharmacol. Ther.*, 1982, *31*, 625–634.]

Toxicity. Blood concentrations in the region of 0.1 mg/L produce abnormal behaviour and concentrations of about 0.3 mg/L or more cause severe toxic symptoms which may be followed by death although there is considerable intersubject variation. Many deaths have been due, not to the toxic effects of phencyclidine itself, but to the effects of irrational behaviour caused by the drug. In 53 cases of death reported in the literature as not directly due to phencyclidine, blood concentrations ranged from 0.01 to 2.1 mg/L (mean 0.36); in 22 of these cases urine concentrations ranged from 0.1 to 10.6 mg/L (mean 2.1); alcohol was also present in a number of these cases.

In 9 fatalities directly attributable to phencyclidine overdose, the following postmortem concentrations were reported: blood 0.3 to 12 mg/L (mean 2.4, 8 cases), brain 0.1 to 32 μg/g (mean 7.3, 6 cases), liver 0.9 to 80 μg/g (mean 20, 9 cases), urine 0.4 to 48.6 mg/L (mean 21.7, 5 cases). [R. H. Cravey *et al.*, *J. Anal. Toxicol.*, 1979, *3*, 199–201.]

A 28-year-old man survived a massive overdose of phencyclidine, despite plasma concentrations reaching a maximum of 1.879 mg/L 2 days after admission to hospital (the highest recorded thus far in a survivor). On hospital day 11 (13 days after the ingestion) he passed 2 plastic bags (one of which was ruptured) via his rectum and his cerebrospinal phencyclidine concentration was 0.245 mg/L; the patient made a rapid neurological recovery starting on hospital day 12. [J. E. Jackson, *Ann. Intern. Med.*, 1989, *111*, 613–615.]

In a 29-year-old man who swallowed a plastic bag containing phencyclidine, serum levels were persistently elevated for several weeks, with the patient remaining in a coma for 24 days. On hospital day 20, following nasogastric administration of oral colonic lavage solution on days 11 to 14, a plastic bag (presumed to have contained phencyclidine) was passed via the rectum; the serum phencyclidine levels declined, and the patient recovered neurological function. The following course of serum phencyclidine concentrations was reported: 0.85 mg/L on day 4, 1.01 mg/L on day 7, 1.69 mg/L on day 10, 1.65 mg/L on day 14, 1.16 mg/L on day 16, 0.57 mg/L on day 18, 0.62 mg/L on day 21, and 0.06 mg/L on day 23. [J. D. Young and L. M. Crapo, *Arch. Intern. Med.*, 1992, *152*, 859–860.]

Half-life. Plasma half-life, 7 to 46 h (mean 17), increased up to 4 days in severe poisoning cases.

Volume of distribution. About 6 L/kg.

Distribution in blood. Plasma: whole blood ratio, about 1.0.

Protein binding. In plasma, about 65 to 80%.

Phendimetrazine

Anorectic

3,4-Dimethyl-2-phenylmorpholine
$C_{12}H_{17}NO = 191.3$
CAS—634-03-7

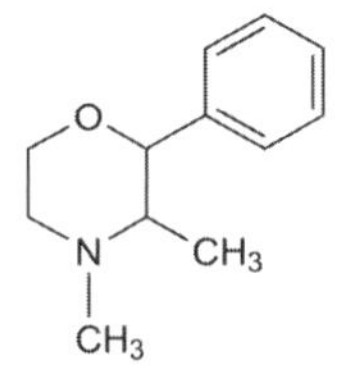

Phendimetrazine Tartrate

Synonyms. Phendimetrazine Acid Tartrate; Phendimetrazine Bitartrate.
Proprietary names. Adipost; Adphen; Anoran; Anorex; Bacarate; Bontril; Dyrexan-OD; Melfiat; Obalan; Obesan-X; Obex-LA; Plegine; Prelu-2; Rexigen Forte; Statobex; Trimstat; Trimtabs; Wehless; Weightrol; X-trozine.
$C_{12}H_{17}NO,C_4H_6O_6 = 341.4$
CAS—50-58-8
A white crystalline powder.
Freely soluble in water; very slightly soluble in ethanol; practically insoluble in acetone, benzene, chloroform and ether.

Dissociation Constant. pK_a 7.6.

Partition Coefficient. Log *P* (octanol/water), 1.7.

Colour Test. Liebermann's Test—red-orange.

Thin-layer Chromatography. System TA—Rf 57 ; system TB—Rf 36; system TC—Rf 51; system TE—Rf 62; system TL—Rf 24; system TAE—Rf 49; system TAF—Rf 41. (Dragendorff spray, positive; acidified iodoplatinate solution, positive; acidified potassium permanganate solution, positive.). See also Phenmetrazine.

Gas Chromatography. System GA—phendimetrazine RI 1334, phenmetrazine RI 1432; system GB—phendimetrazine RI 1504, phenmetrazine RI 1483; system GC—phendimetrazine RI 1735, phenmetrazine RI 1873.

High Performance Liquid Chromatography. System HA—*k* 0.9 phendimetrazine; *k* 1.7 phenmetrazine; system HC—*k* 0.3; system HX—phendimetrazine RI 263; phenmetrazine RI 258; system HY—phendimetrazine RI 218; phenmetrazine RI 241.

Ultraviolet Spectrum. Aqueous acid—251, 257 nm ($A^1_1 = 12.7a$), 261, 267 nm. No alkaline shift.

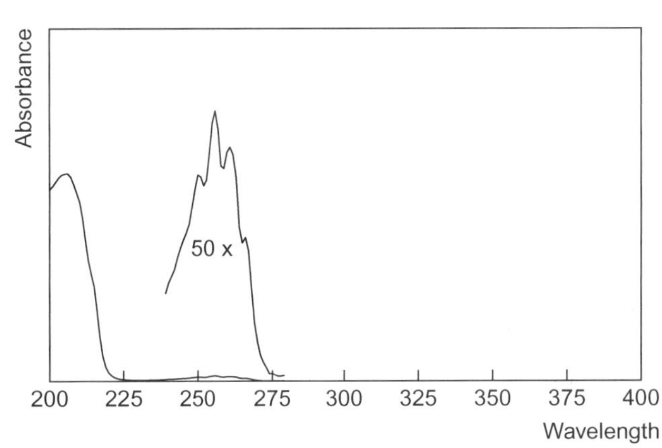

Infra-red Spectrum. Principal peaks at wavenumbers 1120, 1105, 697, 1083, 752, 1630 cm^{-1} (KBr disk).

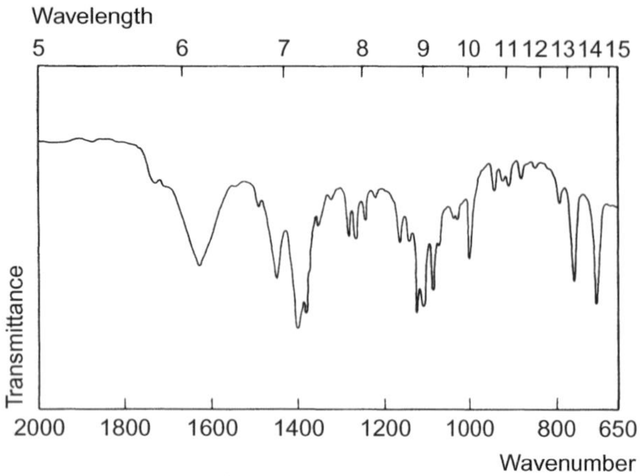

Mass Spectrum. Principal ions at *m/z* 57, 85, 42, 56, 76, 191, 70, 77; phenmetrazine 71, 42, 56, 43, 177, 77, 178, 105.

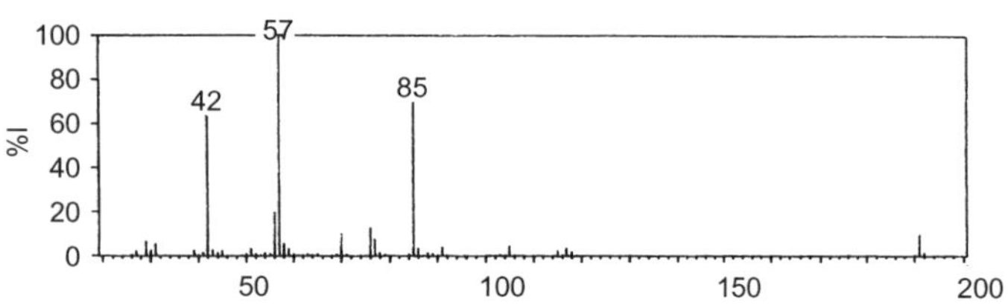

Quantification

Gas chromatography. In plasma, serum or urine: limit of detection 2 μg/L, AFID—G. R. Rudolph *et al.*, *J. Pharm. Sci.*, 1983, *72*, 519–521. In serum or urine: phendimetrazine and phenmetrazine, limit of detection 10 μg/L, AFID—G. Long *et al.*, *Drug Dev. Ind. Pharm.*, 1982, *8*, 203–213. In plasma or urine: phendimetrazine and other CNS stimulants, FID—P. Kintz *et al.*, *Forensic Sci. Int.*, 1989, *40*, 153–159.

Disposition in the Body. Readily absorbed after oral administration. Metabolised by *N*-demethylation to phenmetrazine, which is active, and by *N*-oxidation. About 5 to 30% of a dose is excreted in the urine unchanged in 24 h together with up to 30% as phenmetrazine and 20% as the *N*-oxide.

Therapeutic concentration

Following a single oral dose of 35 mg to 20 subjects, a mean peak plasma concentration of about 0.07 mg/L was attained in about 1 h [G. R. Rudolph *et al.*, *J. Pharm. Sci.*, 1983, *72*, 519–521].

Toxicity

A blood concentration of 300 μg/L was reported in a fatality attributed to phendimetrazine [I. Hood *et al.*, *Clin. Toxicol.*, 1988, *26*, 249–255].

Half-life. Plasma half-life, about 2 to 3 h.

Dose. Usually 70 to 105 mg of phendimetrazine tartrate daily; maximum of 210 mg daily.

Phenelzine

Antidepressant

(2-Phenethyl)hydrazine
$C_8H_{12}N_2=136.2$
CAS—51-71-8

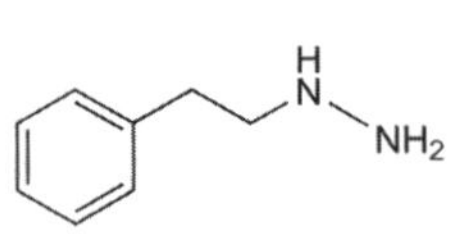

Practically insoluble in water; soluble in chloroform and ether.

Phenelzine Sulfate
Proprietary names. Nardelzine; Nardil.
$C_8H_{12}N_2,H_2SO_4=234.3$
CAS—156-51-4
A white or yellowish-white powder or pearly platelets. M.p. 164° to 168°. Soluble 1 in 7 of water; practically insoluble in ethanol, chloroform, and ether.

Partition Coefficient. Log *P* (octanol/water), 1.0.

Colour Tests. Benedict's Reagent—orange; Liebermann's Test—orange; Mandelin's Test—brown; Nessler's Reagent—black; Palladium Chloride—black.

Thin-layer Chromatography. System TA—Rf 77; system TB—Rf 37; system TC—Rf 12; system TE—Rf 83; system TL—Rf 63; system TAE—Rf 29; system TAF—Rf 82; system TAJ—Rf 74; system TAK—Rf 74; system TAL—Rf 93. (Dragendorff spray, positive; acidified iodoplatinate solution, positive; Marquis reagent, brown; ninhydrin spray, positive.)

Gas Chromatography. System GA—RI 1335; system GB—RI 1278; system GC—RI 1460.

High Performance Liquid Chromatography. System HA—*k* 1.0; system HB—*k* 5.91; system HC—*k* 0.37; system HX—RI 184.

Ultraviolet Spectrum. Aqueous acid—247, 252, 257 nm ($A^1_1=12.9a$), 263 nm.

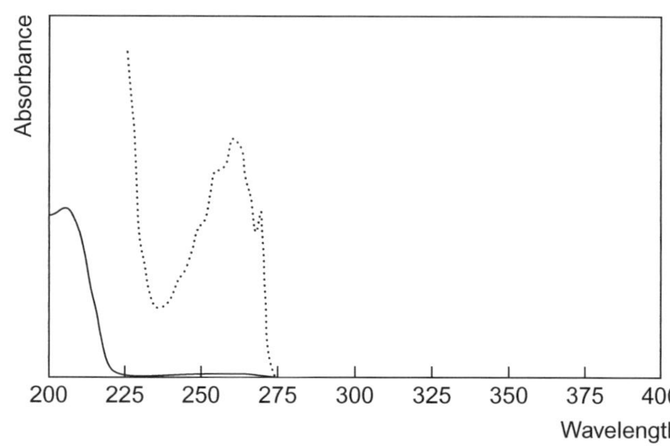

Infra-red Spectrum. Principal peaks at wavenumbers 1016, 1108, 1050, 1080, 940, 699 cm^{-1} (phenelzine sulfate, KBr disk).

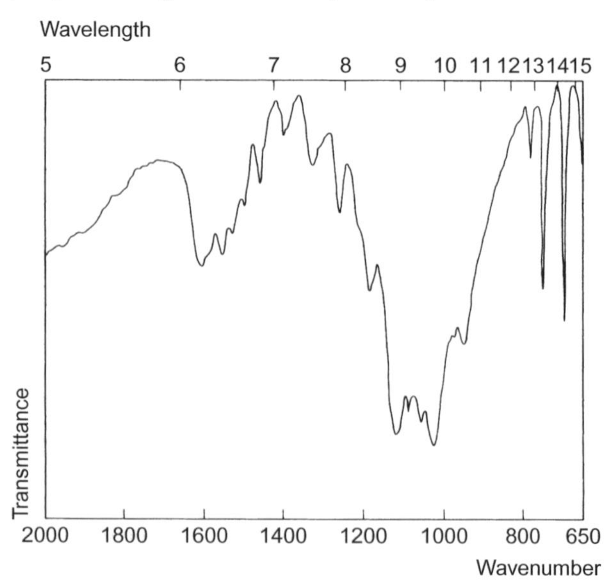

Mass Spectrum. Principal ions at *m/z* 31, 45, 46, 29, 27, 59, 74, 43.

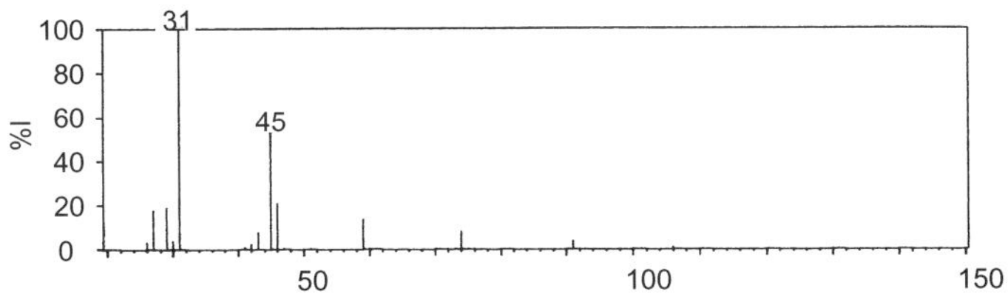

Quantification

Gas chromatography. In plasma: limit of detection 2 µg/mL, AFID—I. J. McGilveray *et al.*, *J. Pharm. Pharmacol.*, 1982, *34*, *Suppl.*, 98P. In urine: limit of detection 50 µg/mL, FID—B. Caddy and A. H. Stead, *Analyst*, 1977, *102*, 42–49. In urine: ECD—T. S. Rao *et al.*, *J. Pharmacol. Methods*, 1987, *17*, 297–304. In plasma and other biological fluids: limit of detection <1 µg/L, nitrogen specific detection—M. Lichtenwalner *et al.*, *J. Anal. Toxicol.*, 1988, *12*, 98–101.

Gas chromatography–mass spectrometry. In plasma: limit of detection 1 to 2 µg/L—S. P. Jindal *et al.*, *J. Chromatogr.* 1980, *221(10) B Biomed. Appl.*, 301–308.

Disposition in the Body. Readily absorbed after oral administration and widely distributed throughout the body. It is believed to be metabolised by acetylation, followed by glutamine conjugation, producing phenylacetylglutamine. Aromatic hydroxylation and conjugation with glucuronic acid may also occur. Less than 5% of a dose is excreted in the urine unchanged.

Therapeutic concentration

Following a single oral dose of 50 mg, given as a solution to 1 subject, a peak plasma concentration of 0.05 mg/L was reported at 0.25 h. [I. J. McGilveray *et al.*, *J. Pharm. Pharmacol.*, 1982, *34*, *Suppl.*, 98P.]

Following a single oral dose of 30 mg to 1 subject, a peak plasma concentration of 2 µg/L was attained in 2 h. In a subject who had been receiving daily oral doses of 30 mg for 6 weeks, a trough steady-state plasma concentration of 0.2 µg/L was reported. [T. B. Cooper *et al.*, *Commun. Pyschopharmacol.*, 1978, *2*, 505–512.]

Toxicity

In a fatality attributed to phenelzine and alcohol, postmortem urine concentrations were: phenelzine 58 mg/L, alcohol 1700 mg/L; in a second non-fatal overdose subject, blood and plasma concentrations of 1.5 and 1.26 mg/L were reported, 12 h after ingestion. [B. Caddy and A. H. Stead, *J. Forensic Sci. Soc.*, 1978, *18*, 207–208.]

Phenelzine was held to be the cause of death in two cases, even though other drugs were present in elevated concentrations. The postmortem blood concentration in case 1 was 3.1 mg/L and a total of 62 g was found in the stomach contents. Postmortem tissue concentrations in case 2 were: blood 0.68 mg/L, urine 4.60 mg/L, and the ante-mortem serum concentration was 0.72 mg/L. [M. R. Lichtenwalner *et al.*, *J. Anal. Toxicol.*, 1995, *19*, 265–266.]

Half-life. Plasma half-life, about 7 h.

Dose. The equivalent of 45 to 60 mg of phenelzine daily.

Phenethylamine

Putrefactive Base

Synonym β-Aminoethylbenzene
Benzeneethanamine
$C_8H_{11}N$=121.2
CAS—64-04-0

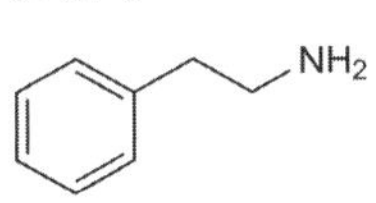

A strongly basic liquid which absorbs carbon dioxide from the air. B.p. 194° to 195°.
Soluble in water; freely soluble in ethanol and ether.

Dissociation Constant. pK_a 10.0 (19°).

Partition Coefficient. Log P (octanol/water), 1.4.

Colour Test. Marquis Test—orange.

Thin-layer Chromatography. System TA—Rf 49; system TB—Rf 28; system TC—Rf 28; system TE—Rf 54; system TL—Rf 39; system TAE—Rf 44; system TAJ—Rf 03; system TAK—Rf 16; system TAL—Rf 50. (Acidified iodoplatinate solution, positive.)

Gas Chromatography. System GA—RI 1111.

High Performance Liquid Chromatography. System HA—*k* 1.2; system HB—*k* 3.6; system HC—*k* 1.3.

Ultraviolet Spectrum. Aqueous acid—242 (A^1_1=15b), 247 (A^1_1=17.2b), 252 (A^1_1=19.8b), 257 (A^1_1=21.3b), 263 nm (A^1_1=16b).

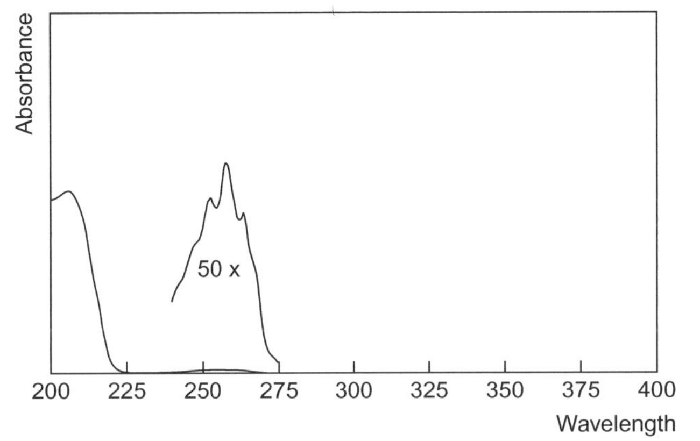

Infra-red Spectrum. Principal peaks at wavenumbers 695, 745, 755, 942, 1146, 1608 cm^{-1} (KBr disk).

Mass Spectrum. Principal ions at *m/z* 30, 91, 65, 92, 51, 39, 121, 103.

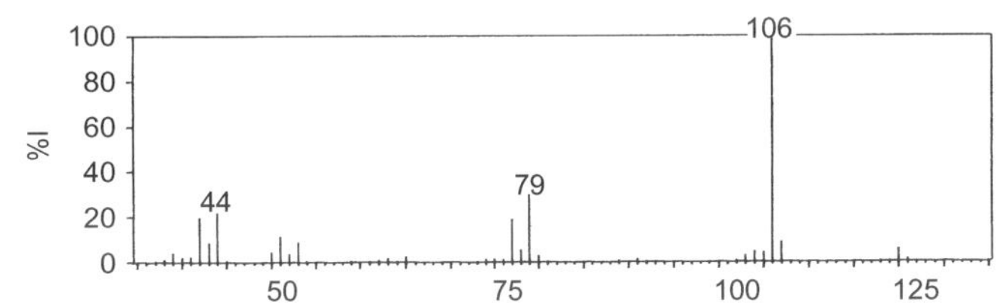

Disposition in the Body. Phenethylamine is the putrefactive base obtained from phenylalanine by decarboxylation.

Pheneticillin

Antibiotic

Synonyms. Penicillin B; Phenethicillin; α-Phenoxyethylpenicillin.
(2*S*,5*R*,6*R*)-3,3-Dimethyl-7-oxo-6-[(1-oxo-2-phenoxypropyl)amino]-4-thia-1-azabicyclo[3.2.0]heptane-2-carboxylic acid
$C_{17}H_{20}N_2O_5S$=364.4
CAS—147-55-7

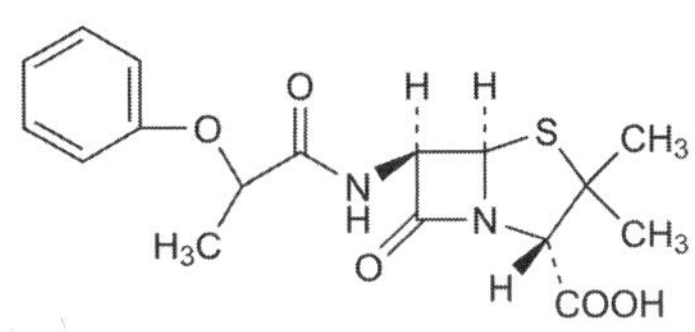

Pheneticillin Potassium

Synonym. Phenethicillin Potassium
Proprietary names. Alfacillin; Brocosil; Broxil; Chemipen; Darcil; Dramcillin-S; Maxipen; Optipen; Peniplus; Penorale; Penova; Pensig; Syncillin; Synthecilline; Synthepen.
$C_{17}H_{19}KN_2O_5S$=402.5
CAS—132-93-4
A white, fine, crystalline powder. M.p. 230° to 232°, with decomposition.
Soluble 1 in 1.5 of water, 1 in 85 of ethanol, and 1 in 800 of dehydrated alcohol; slightly soluble in chloroform; practically insoluble in ether.

Dissociation Constant. pK_a 2.7 (25°).

Partition Coefficient. Log *P* (octanol/water), 2.2.

Ultraviolet Spectrum. Pheneticillin potassium: aqueous acid—271 (A^1_1=44b), 275 nm. No alkaline shift.

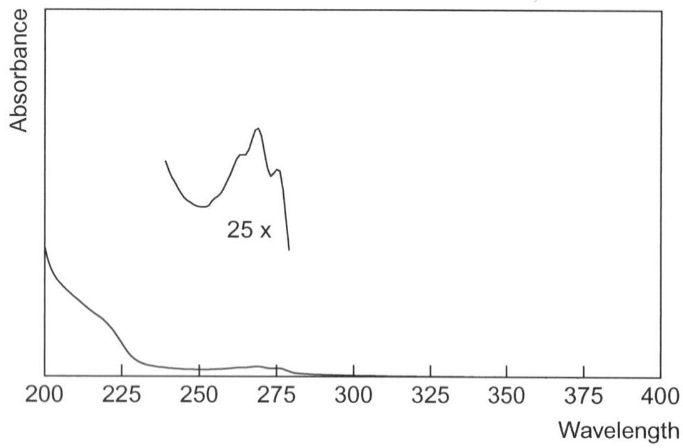

Infra-red Spectrum. Principal peaks at wavenumbers 1610, 1778, 1510, 1238, 1690, 752 cm^{-1} (pheneticillin potassium, KBr disk).

Dose. The equivalent of 1 to 2 g of pheneticillin daily.

Pheneturide

Anticonvulsant

Synonyms. Ethylphenacemide; EPA; PBU.
Proprietary names. Benuride; Laburide.
N-(Aminocarbonyl)-α-ethylbenzeneacetamide
$C_{11}H_{14}N_2O_2$=206.2
CAS—90-49-3

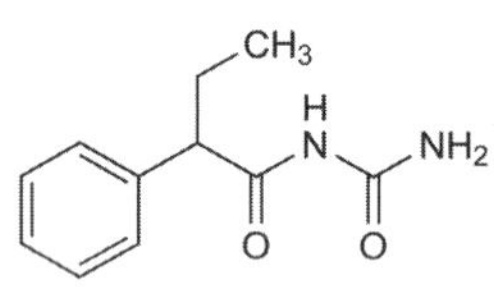

A white crystalline powder.
Practically insoluble in water and ether; slightly soluble in ethanol; very soluble in glacial acetic acid.

Partition Coefficient. Log *P* (octanol/water), 1.6.

Colour Test. Nessler's Reagent—orange-brown (slow).

Thin-layer Chromatography. System TA—Rf 76; system TD—Rf 38; system TE—Rf 71; system TF—Rf 53; system TAD—Rf 59.

Gas Chromatography. System GA—RI 1465.

High Performance Liquid Chromatography. System HE—*k* 6.8.

Ultraviolet Spectrum. Chloroform—259 (A^1_1=18b), 265 nm (A^1_{1s}=11b).

Infra-red Spectrum. Principal peaks at wavenumbers 1672, 1700, 1093, 694, 1176, 1615 cm^{-1} (KBr disk).

Mass Spectrum. Principal ions at *m/z* 91, 146, 44, 119, 206, 41, 78, 77.

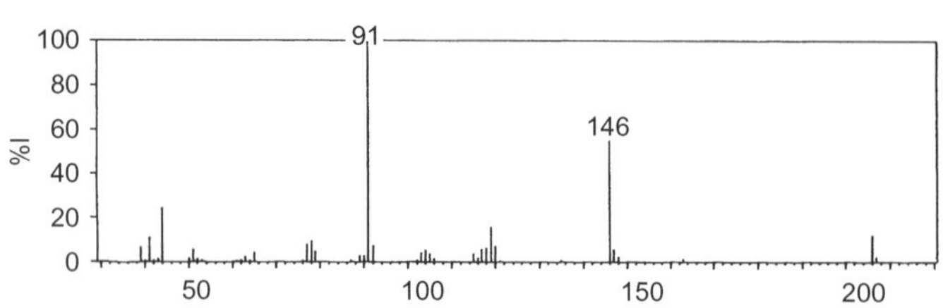

Quantification

High performance liquid chromatography. In plasma or serum: pheneturide and other anticonvulsants, limit of detection 1.4 mg/L, UV detection—J. A. Christofides and D. E. Fry, *Clin. Chem.*, 1980, *26*, 499–501.

Thin-layer chromatography–ultraviolet spectrophotometry. In plasma, serum or urine: limit of detection 500 µg/L in serum—R. L. Galeazzi *et al.*, *J. Pharmacokinet. Biopharm.*, 1979, *7*, 453–462.

Disposition in the Body. Slowly absorbed after oral administration. Pheneturide is thought to be completely metabolised as only traces of unchanged drug have been found in the urine. It may induce its own metabolism.

Toxicity. Pheneturide has been reported to be less likely to cause toxic effects than phenacemide, to which it is chemically related.

Half-life. Plasma half-life, 30 to 90 h (mean 54) after single doses and about 40 h after chronic administration.

Volume of distribution. About 3 L/kg.

Clearance. Plasma clearance, about 0.7 mL/min/kg.

Dose. Pheneturide has been given in doses of 0.6 to 1 g daily.

Phenformin

Antidiabetic

Synonyms. Fenformina; Phenethyldiguanide β-PEBG; PEDG.
N-(2-Phenylethyl)imidodicarbonimidic diamide
$C_{10}H_{15}N_5$=205.3
CAS—114-86-3

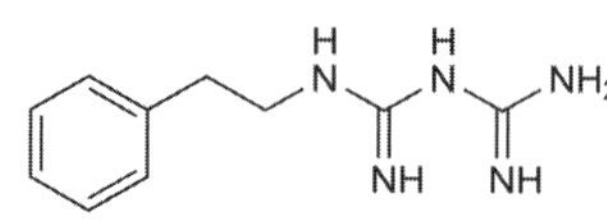

Phenformin Hydrochloride
Proprietary names. Azucaps; Debei; Debein; Debeuna; Debeone; Debinyl; Dibotin; Dipar; Feguanide; Glucopostin; Insoral; Lentobetic; Meltrol; Normoglucina.
$C_{10}H_{15}N_5$,HCl=241.7
CAS—834-28-6
A white crystalline powder. M.p. 175° to 178°.
Soluble 1 in 8 of water and 1 in 15 of ethanol; practically insoluble in chloroform and ether.

Dissociation Constant. pK_a 2.7, 11.8 (32°).

Partition Coefficient. Log *P* (octanol/water), –0.8.

Colour Tests. Mandelin's Test—green; Marquis Test—orange→brown.

Thin-layer Chromatography. System TA—Rf 03; system TB—Rf 00; system TC—Rf 00; system TL—Rf 00; system TAJ—Rf 00; system TAK—Rf 03; system TAL—Rf 29. (Marquis reagent, positive.)

High Performance Liquid Chromatography. System HX—RI 250.

Ultraviolet Spectrum. Aqueous acid—251 (A^1_1=11a), 258 (A^1_1=11a), 264, 267 nm.

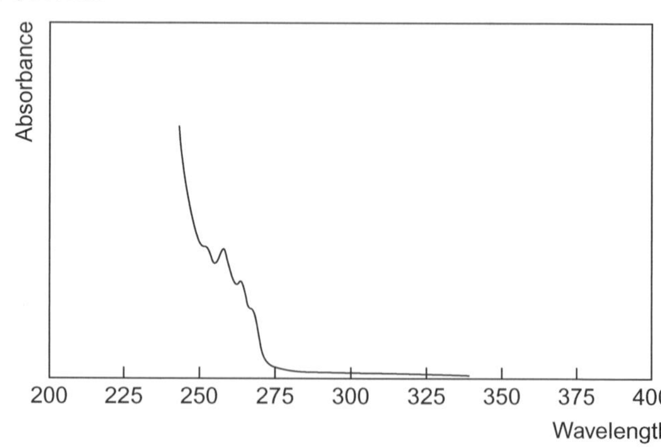

Infra-red Spectrum. Principal peaks at wavenumbers 1568, 1537, 1590, 1625, 1650, 1500 cm^{-1} (phenformin hydrochloride, KBr disk).

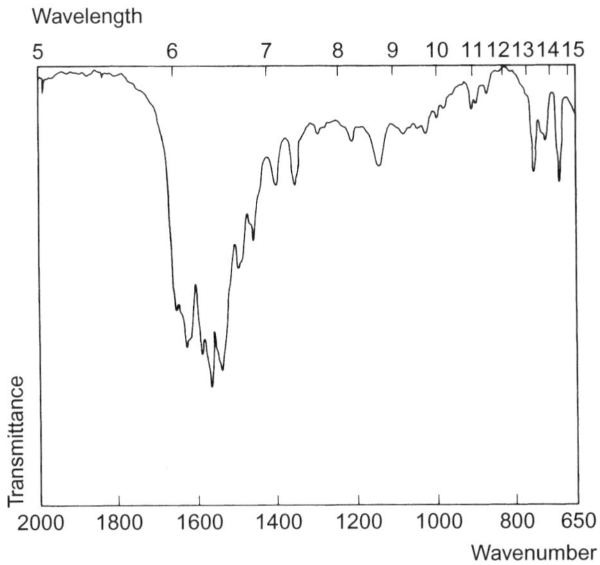

Mass Spectrum. Principal ions at m/z 91, 30, 92, 42, 29, 146, 44, 104 (no peaks above 150).

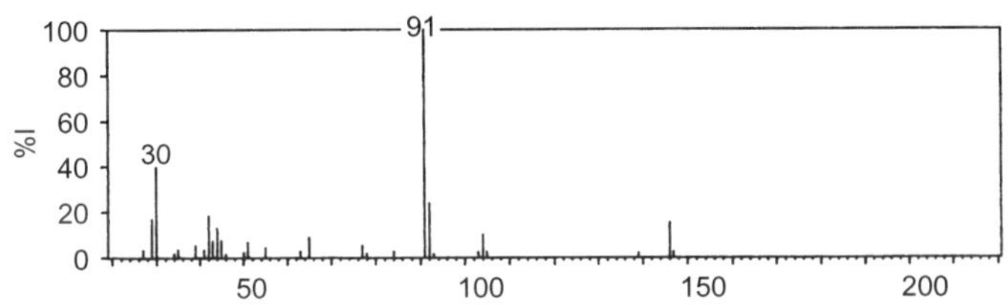

Quantification

Gas chromatography. In plasma or urine: phenformin and other biguanides, limit of detection <1 μg/L in plasma, ECD—S. B. Matin *et al.*, *Anal. Chem.*, 1975, *47*, 545–548.

High performance liquid chromatography. In plasma or urine: limit of detection 10 μg/L in plasma, UV detection—H. M. Hill and J. Chamberlain, *J. Chromatogr.*, 1978, *149*, 349–358. In urine: phenformin and 4-hydroxyphenformin, limit of detection 1 mg/L for phenformin and 500 μg/L for 4-hydroxyphenformin, UV detection—N. S. Oates *et al.*, *J. Pharm. Pharmacol.*, 1980, *32*, 731–732. In serum: phenformin and buformin, fluorimetric detection—Y. Kobayashi *et al.*, *J. Chromatogr.*, 1988, *430*, 65–71.

Disposition in the Body. Well absorbed after oral administration. The major metabolic reaction is aromatic hydroxylation to form 4-hydroxyphenformin which is then conjugated with glucuronic acid. Up to about 50% of a dose is excreted in the urine in 24 h, about two-thirds in the form of unchanged drug and one-third as the hydroxy metabolite.

Therapeutic concentration

Following a single oral dose of 50 mg to 8 subjects, peak plasma concentrations of 0.08 to 0.18 mg/L (mean 0.13) were attained in about 3 h; plasma concentrations were higher in 4 subjects who were poor metabolisers of debrisoquine in comparison with the 4 extensive metabolisers [N. S. Oates *et al.*, *Clin. Pharmacol. Ther.*, 1983, *34*, 827–834].

Following daily oral doses of 50 mg three times a day to 8 subjects, plasma concentrations of 0.10 to 0.24 mg/L (mean 0.18) were reported 2 h after a dose [J. Karam *et al.*, *Diabetes*, 1974, *23*, *Suppl.* 1, 375].

Toxicity

A 44-year-old woman ingested 1.5 g in slow-release capsules and died 30 h later. A postmortem blood concentration of 3 mg/L and liver concentration of 60 μg/g were reported [J. P. Bingle *et al.*, *BMJ*, 1970, *3*, 752].

Half-life. Plasma half-life, 10 to 15 h.

Protein binding. In plasma, about 12 to 20%.

Note. For a review of phenformin-induced lactic acidosis, see S. C. Kwong and J. Brubacher, *J. Emerg. Med.*, 1998, *16*, 881–886.

Dose. 50 to 100 mg of phenformin hydrochloride daily.

Phenglutarimide

Anticholinergic/Antiparkinsonian

3-[2-(Diethylamino)ethyl]-3-phenyl-2,6-piperidinedione
$C_{17}H_{24}N_2O_2 = 288.4$
CAS—1156-05-4

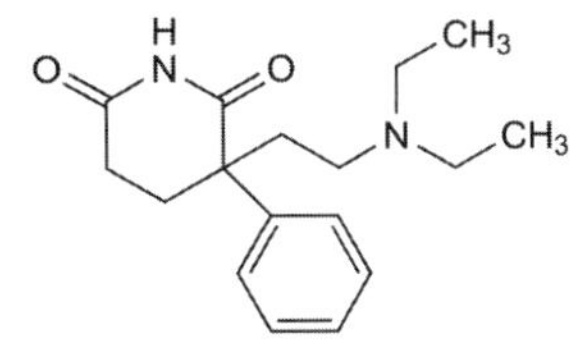

Crystals. M.p. 125° to 127°.

Phenglutarimide Hydrochloride
Proprietary names. Aturbal; Aturbane.
$C_{17}H_{24}N_2O_2,HCl = 324.8$
CAS—1674-96-0
A white crystalline powder. M.p. 168° to 172° and also 176° to 177°, with decomposition.
Soluble 1 in 1 of water and 1 in 1.5 of ethanol; very slightly soluble in ether.

Partition Coefficient. Log *P* (octanol/water), 1.9.

Colour Tests. Koppanyi-Zwikker Test—violet; Liebermann's Test—red-orange.

Thin-layer Chromatography. System TA—Rf 40; system TB—Rf 17; system TC—Rf 08; system TL—Rf 08. (Acidified iodoplatinate solution, positive.)

Gas Chromatography. System GA—Phenglutarimide RI 2235; M (desethyl-) RI 2370.

High Performance Liquid Chromatography. System HA—*k* 2.9.

Ultraviolet Spectrum. Aqueous acid—251, 257 ($A^1_1 = 13.3a$), 263 nm.

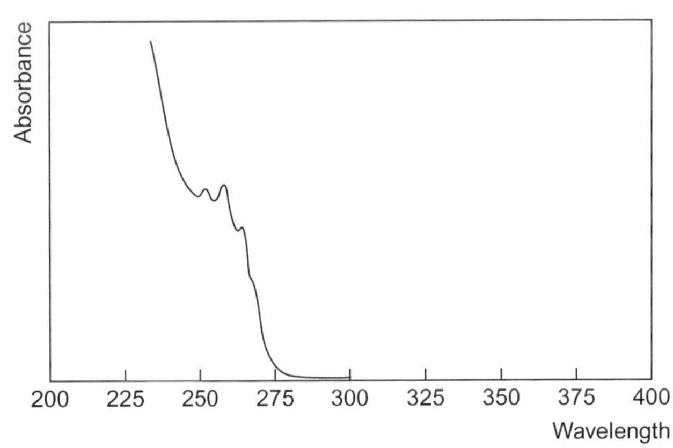

Infra-red Spectrum. Principal peaks at wavenumbers 1698, 1194, 1181, 1250, 700, 1150 cm^{-1} (phenglutarimide hydrochloride, KBr disk).

Mass Spectrum. Principal ions at m/z 86, 30, 216, 87, 58, 100, 99, 56.

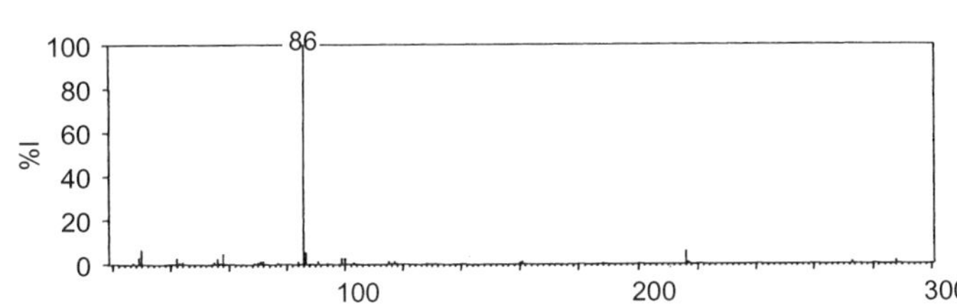

Dose. Phenglutarimide hydrochloride has been given in doses of 10 to 50 mg daily.

Phenindamine

Antihistamine

Synonym. Nu-1504
2,3,4,9-Tetrahydro-2-methyl-9-phenyl-1*H*-indeno[2,1-*c*]pyridine
$C_{19}H_{19}N=261.4$
CAS—82-88-2

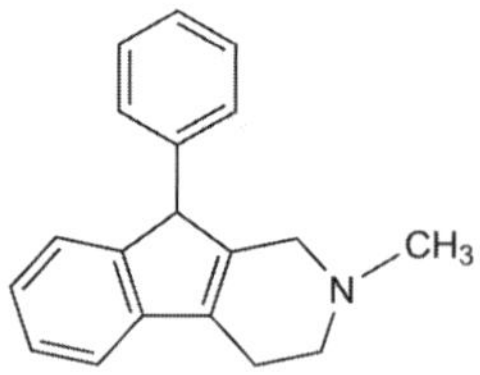

Crystals. M.p. 90° to 91°.

Phenindamine Tartrate
Proprietary names. Nolahist; Thephorin.
$C_{19}H_{19}N,C_4H_6O_6=411.5$
CAS—569-59-5
A white voluminous powder. M.p. 160°; on further heating it solidifies and melts again at about 168°, with decomposition.
Soluble 1 in 70 of water and 1 in 300 of ethanol; practically insoluble in chloroform and ether.

Dissociation Constant. pK_a 8.3 (25°).

Partition Coefficient. Log *P* (octanol/water), 4.2.

Colour Tests. Mandelin's Test—green; Marquis Test—grey-green.

Thin-layer Chromatography. System TA—Rf 63; system TB—Rf 45; system TC—Rf 57; system TE—Rf 68; system TL—Rf 21; system TAD—Rf 41; system TAF—Rf 49; system TAJ—Rf 37; system TAK—Rf 02; system TAL—Rf 82. (Dragendorff spray, positive; acidified iodoplatinate solution, positive; Marquis reagent, grey-brown.)

Gas Chromatography. System GA—Phenindamine RI 2165, M (OH-) RI 2300, M (*N*-oxide) RI 2230, M (nor-) RI 2210, M (nor-OH-) RI 2590; system GB—RI 2245; system GC—RI 2926; system GF—RI 2515.

High Performance Liquid Chromatography. System HA—*k* 2.5; system HX—RI 397.

Ultraviolet Spectrum. Aqueous acid—259 ($A^1_1=347a$); aqueous alkali—263 nm ($A^1_1=385a$).

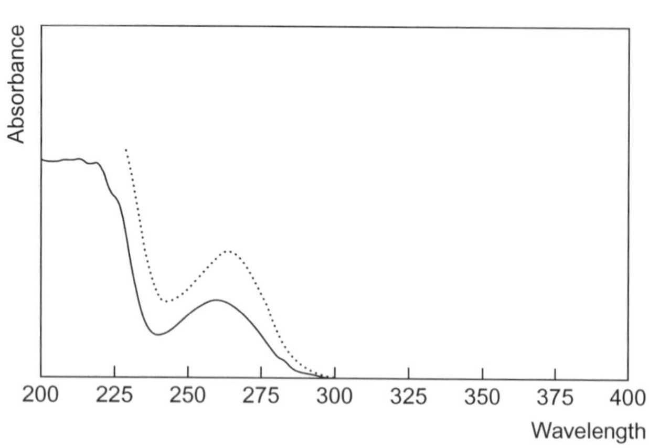

Infra-red Spectrum. Principal peaks at wavenumbers 1751, 1302, 1585, 752, 1072, 693 cm^{-1} (phenindamine tartrate, KBr disk).

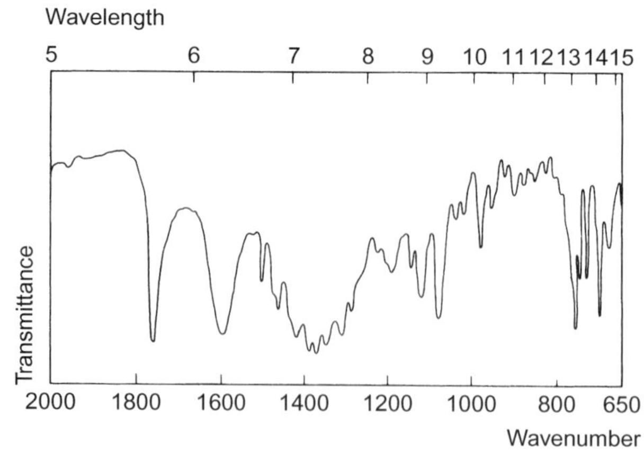

Mass Spectrum. Principal peaks at *m/z* 260, 261, 42, 57, 184, 215, 217, 262.

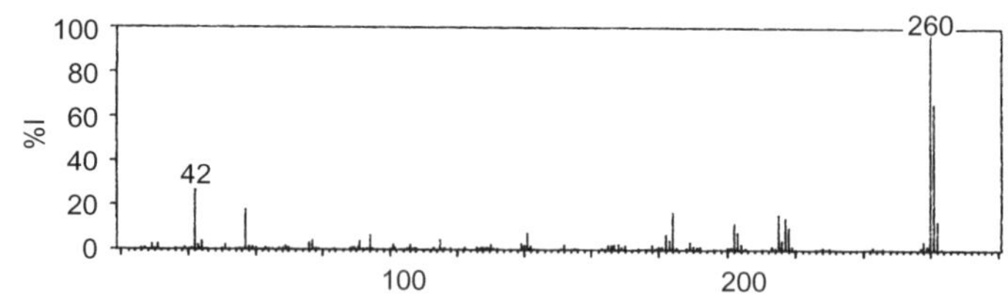

Dose. Up to 150 mg of phenindamine tartrate daily.

Phenindione

Anticoagulant

Synonyms. Phenylindanedione; Phenylinium PID.
Proprietary names. Danilone; Dindevan; Hedulin; Pindione; Fenilin; Rectadione.
2-Phenyl-1*H*-indene-1,3(2*H*)-dione
$C_{15}H_{10}O_2=222.2$
CAS—83-12-5

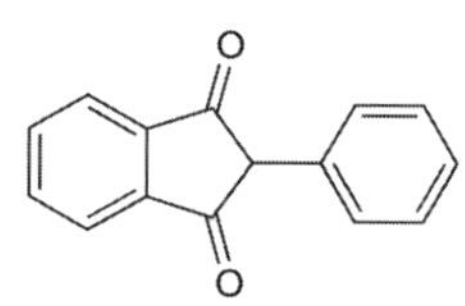

Soft, white or creamy-white or pale yellow crystals or crystalline powder. M.p. 149° to 151°.
Very slightly soluble in water; soluble 1 in about 125 of ethanol, 1 in 6.5 of chloroform, and 1 in 110 of ether; soluble in methanol, benzene, and acetone; forms yellow to red solutions.

Dissociation Constant. pK_a 4.1.

Partition Coefficient. Log *P* (octanol/water), 2.9.

Colour Tests. Methanolic Potassium Hydroxide—red; Sulfuric Acid—violet.

Thin-layer Chromatography. System TD—Rf 65; system TE—Rf 21; system TF—Rf 56; system TAD—Rf 70.

Gas Chromatography. System GA—RI 2055.

High Performance Liquid Chromatography. System HAA—Retention time 18.1 min.

Ultraviolet Spectrum. Aqueous alkali—278 ($A^1_1=1310a$), 330 nm ($A^1_1=400b$).

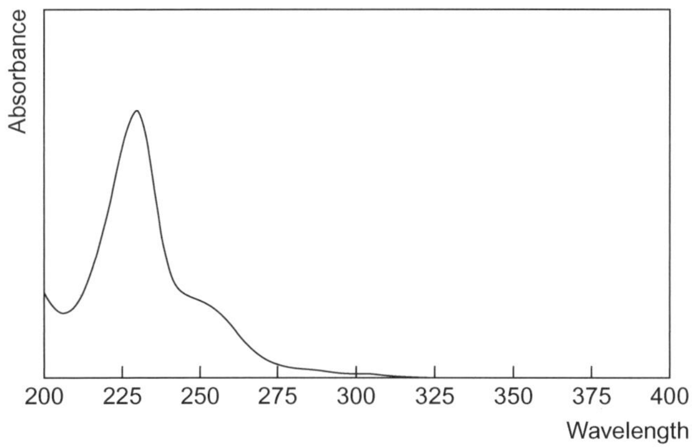

Infra-red Spectrum. Principal peaks at wavenumbers 1700, 700, 766, 1219, 1740, 1280 cm^{-1} (KBr disk).

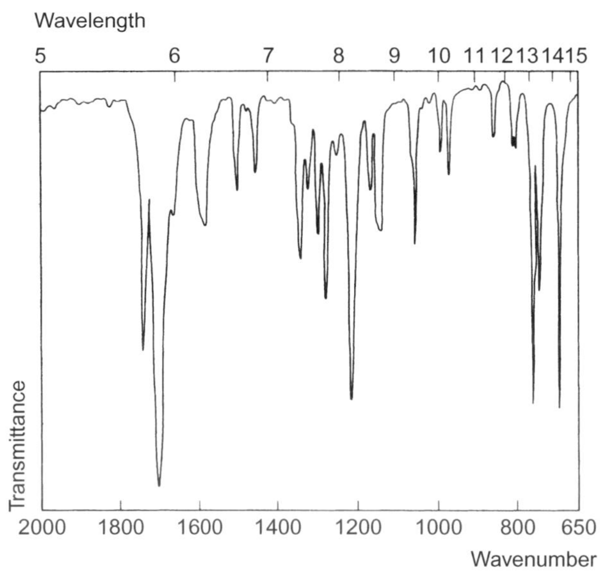

Mass Spectrum. Principal ions at *m/z* 222, 165, 76, 223, 166, 105, 104, 90.

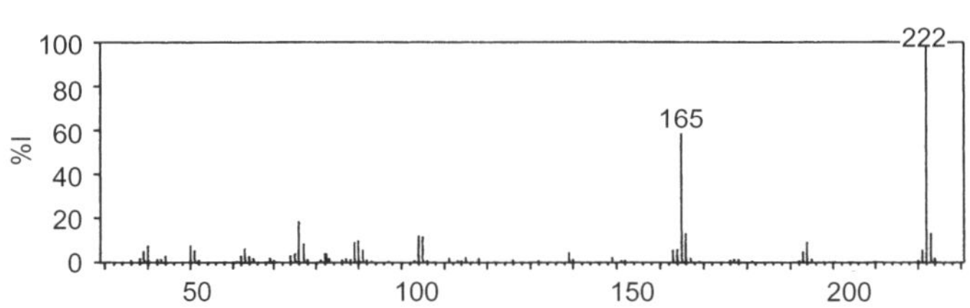

Quantification

Polarography. In serum: limit of detection 4 mg/L—E. Jacobsen and K. H. Klevan, *Analytica Chim. Acta*, 1972, *62*, 405–413.

Disposition in the Body. Well absorbed after oral administration. The urine may be coloured red-orange due to the excretion of a metabolite.

Toxicity. Fatalities have occurred after therapeutic doses.

Half-life. Plasma half-life, about 6 h.

Dose. Maintenance, 25 to 150 mg daily.

Pheniramine

Antihistamine

Synonym. Prophenpyridamine
N,N-Dimethyl-*γ*-phenyl-2-pyridinepropanamine
$C_{16}H_{20}N_2$=240.3
CAS—86-21-5

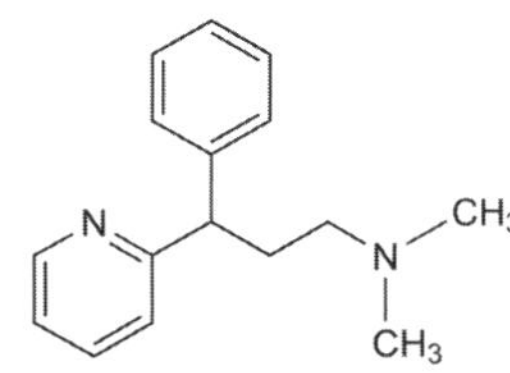

A slightly yellow oily liquid.
Practically insoluble in water; soluble in ethanol, benzene, chloroform, and ether.

Pheniramine Aminosalicylate
$C_{16}H_{20}N_2,C_7H_7NO_3$=393.5
CAS—3269-83-8
Crystals. M.p. 142°, with decomposition.
Soluble 1 in 10 of water; freely soluble in ethanol; sparingly soluble in ethyl acetate, ether, and acetone.

Pheniramine Maleate
Proprietary names. Avil; Daneral; Fenamine; Inhiston.
$C_{16}H_{20}N_2,C_4H_4O_4$=356.4
CAS—132-20-7
A white crystalline powder. M.p. 107° (crystals from amyl alcohol).
Soluble 1 in 0.3 of water, 1 in 2.5 of ethanol, and 1 in 1.5 of chloroform; slightly soluble in ether and benzene.

Dissociation Constant. pK_a 4.2, 9.3 (25°).

Partition Coefficient. Log *P* (octanol/water), 3.2.

Colour Tests. Cyanogen Bromide—orange; Liebermann's Test—red-orange.

Thin-layer Chromatography. System TA—Rf 45; system TB—Rf 35; system TC—Rf 13; system TE—Rf 46; system TL—Rf 03; system TAE—Rf 14; system TAF—Rf 26. (Dragendorff spray, positive; acidified iodoplatinate solution, positive.)

Gas Chromatography. System GA—pheniramine RI 1805, M (nor-) RI 2080; system GB—pheniramine RI 1874, M (nor-) RI 1890; system GF—RI 2100.

High Performance Liquid Chromatography. System HA—*k* 4.1; system HX—RI 283; system HY—RI 206; system HAX—retention time 9.5 min; system HAY—retention time 4.5 min.

Ultraviolet Spectrum. Aqueous acid—261 (A^1_1=305a), 266 (A^1_1=310a); aqueous alkali—258, 263 (A^1_1=206a), 268 nm.

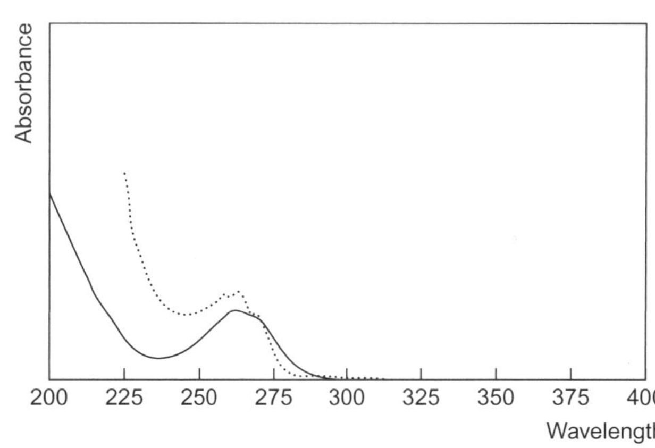

Infra-red Spectrum. Principal peaks at wavenumbers 1584, 690, 860, 870, 990, 1010 cm^{-1} (pheniramine maleate, KBr disk).

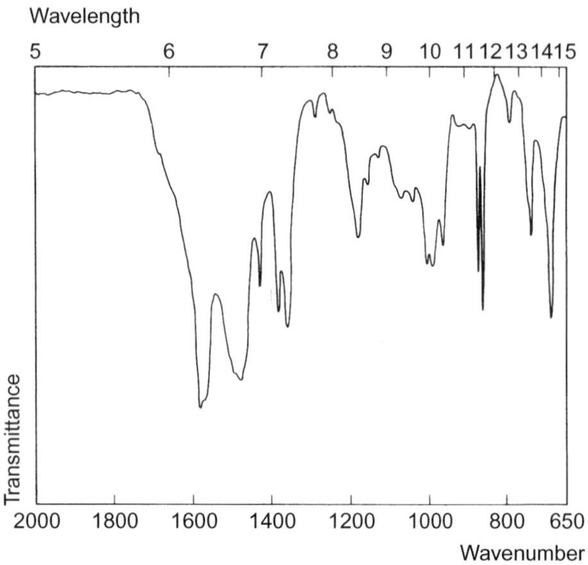

Mass Spectrum. Principal ions at m/z 169, 58, 168, 170, 72, 167, 44, 42 (no peaks above 200).

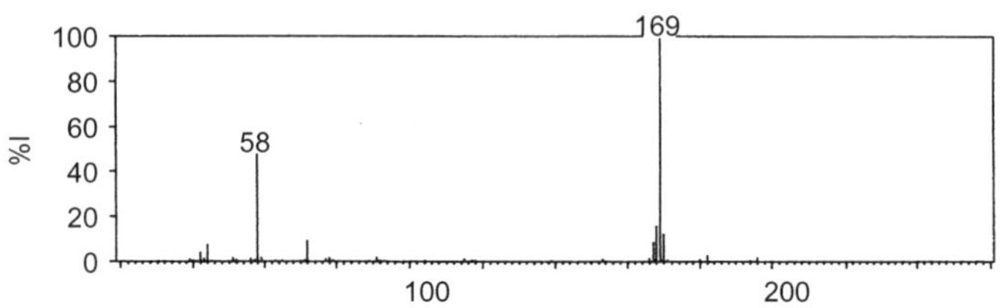

Quantification

Gas chromatography. In blood, urine, or tissues: limit of detection 50 µg/L, AFID—E. A. Querée *et al.*, *J. Anal. Toxicol.*, 1979, *3*, 253–255.

Gas chromatography–mass spectrometry. In serum: pheniramine and loratadine, limit of detection for pheniramine 0.5 µg/L—J. Martens, *J. Chromatogr.* 1995, *673 B. Biomed. Appl.*, 183–188.

Disposition in the Body. Absorbed after oral administration. About 17% of a dose is excreted in the urine as unchanged drug in 24 h, increasing to 23% over a period of 6 days; after chronic oral administration about 24% is excreted daily as monodesmethylpheniramine, and 0.5% as didesmethylpheniramine.

Therapeutic concentration

After a single oral dose of 75 mg to 6 subjects, blood concentrations of 0.01 to 0.19 mg/L (mean 0.11) were reported at 2 h. [E. A. Querée *et al.*, *J. Anal. Toxicol.*, 1979, *3*, 253–255.]

Toxicity. The estimated minimum lethal dose is 25 mg/kg.

In a fatality due to pheniramine overdose, the following postmortem tissue concentrations were reported: blood 1.9 mg/L, brain 5.3 µg/g, kidney 4.0 µg/g, liver 6.6 µg/g, urine 149 mg/L; in a second fatality in which methadone, pentobarbital, phenobarbital, and alcohol had also been ingested, postmortem blood and liver concentrations of 30 mg/L and 115 µg/g, respectively, were reported. [E. A. Querée *et al.*, *J. Anal. Toxicol.*, 1979, *3*, 253–255.]

In a fatality due to the ingestion of 3.75 g of pheniramine, the following postmortem tissue concentrations were reported: blood 10.7 mg/L, bile 109 mg/L, liver 33 µg/g, urine 362 mg/L. [L. F. T. Chan and W. J. Allender, *Bull. Int. Assoc. Forensic Toxicol.*, 1983, *17(2)*, 25–26.]

Note. For a review of the clinical pharmacokinetics of antihistamines, see D. M. Paton and D. R. Webster, *Clin. Pharmacokinet.*, 1985, *10*, 477–497.

Dose. Up to 90 mg of pheniramine maleate daily.

Phenmetrazine

Anorectic

3-Methyl-2-phenylmorpholine
$C_{11}H_{15}NO$=177.2
CAS—134-49-6

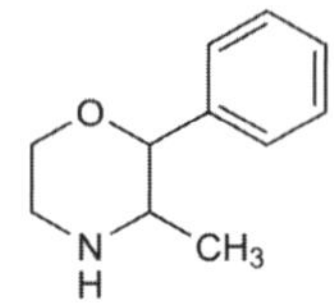

A liquid.

Phenmetrazine Hydrochloride
Synonym. Oxazimédrine
Proprietary name. Preludin
$C_{11}H_{15}NO,HCl$=213.7
CAS—1707-14-8
A white crystalline powder. M.p. 182° (crystals from ethanol and ether). Soluble 1 in 0.4 of water, 1 in 2 of ethanol, and 1 in 2 of chloroform; sparingly soluble in ether.

Phenmetrazine Teoclate
Synonyms. Phenmetrazine 8-Chlorotheophyllinate; Phenmetrazine Theoclate.
$C_{11}H_{15}NO,C_7H_7ClN_4O_2$=391.9
CAS—13931-75-4
A white powder.
Soluble in water and ethanol; slightly soluble in acetone and ether.

Dissociation Constant. pK_a 8.4 (25°).

Partition Coefficient. Log *P* (octanol/water), 1.5.

Colour Test. Liebermann's Test—red-orange.

Thin-layer Chromatography. System TA—Rf 50; system TB—Rf 14; system TC—Rf 27; system TE—Rf 46; system TL—Rf 14; system TAE—Rf 34; system TAF—Rf 45; system TAJ—Rf 20; system TAK—Rf 08; system TAL—Rf 60. (Acidified iodoplatinate solution, positive; acidified potassium permanganate solution, positive.)

Gas Chromatography. System GA—phenmetrazine RI 1432, phenmetrazine-TFA RI 1530, phenmetrazine-TMS RI 1620, phenmetrazine-AC RI 1810, M (OH-) isomer 1 RI 1830, M (OH-) isomer 2 RI 1865, M (OH-methoxy-) RI 1900, M (OH-) isomer 1-AC_2 RI 2150, M (OH-) isomer 2-AC_2 RI 2200, M (OH-methoxy-)-AC_2 RI 2320; system GB—phenmetrazine RI 1483; system GC—RI 1873.

High Performance Liquid Chromatography. System HA—*k* 1.7; system HX—RI 258; system HY—RI 241.

Ultraviolet Spectrum. Aqueous acid—250, 256 (A_1^1=13.3a), 261, 263, 267 nm.

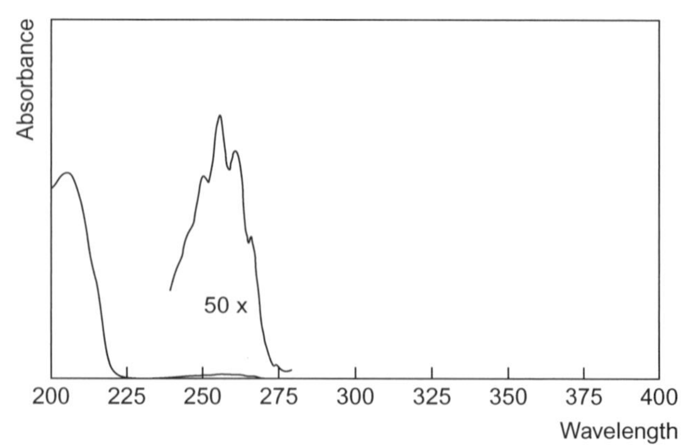

Infra-red Spectrum. Principal peaks at wavenumbers 1083, 757, 695, 965, 990, 1030 cm^{-1} (phenmetrazine hydrochloride, KBr disk).

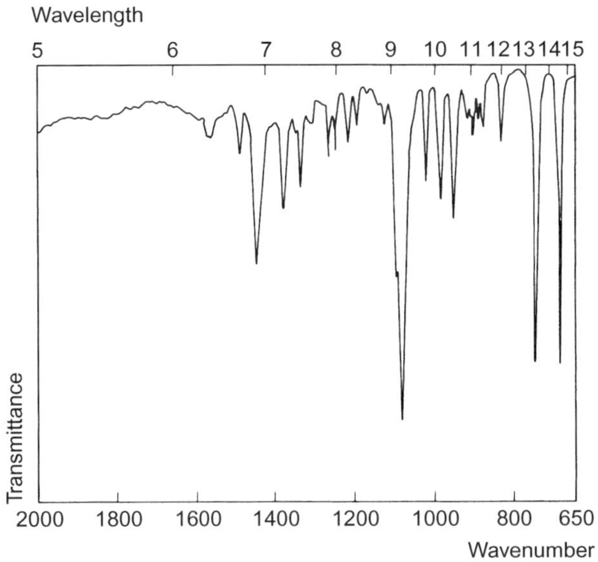

Mass Spectrum. Principal ions at *m/z* 71, 42, 56, 43, 177, 77, 178, 105.

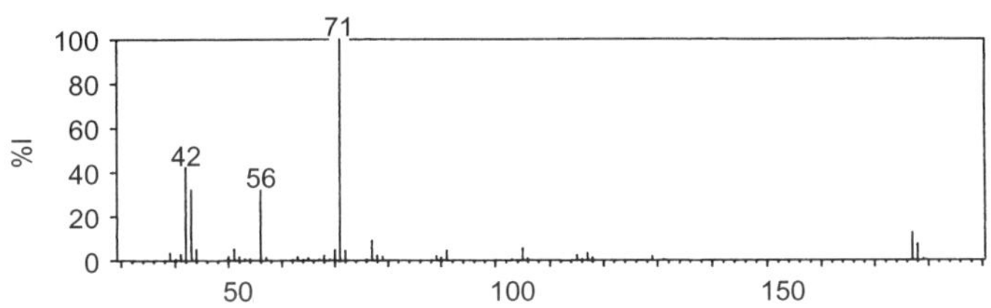

Quantification

Gas chromatography. In serum or urine: phendimetrazine and phenmetrazine, limit of detection 10 µg/L, AFID—G. Long *et al.*, *Drug Dev. Ind. Pharm.*, 1982, *8*, 203–213. In urine: phenmetrazine, phentermine, and amfetamines, NPD—J. Jonsson *et al.*, *J. Forensic Sci.*, 1996, *41*, 148–151.

Gas chromatography–mass spectrometry. In urine: limit of quantification 50 µg/L—R. Kronstrand *et al.*, *J. Anal. Toxicol.*, 1996, *20*, 277–280. In urine: limit of detection 0.2 to 0.5 mg/L—A. Dasgupta and C. E. Mahle, *J. Forensic Sci.*, 1997, *42*, 937–941; A. Dasgupta *et al.*, *J. Forensic Sci.*, 1998, *43*, 630–635; A. Dasgupta *et al.*, *J. Forensic Sci.*, 1998, *43*, 636–640.

Disposition in the Body. Readily absorbed after oral administration. About 70% of a dose is excreted in the urine in 24 h with about 19% as unchanged drug, 19% as the lactam (5-methyl-3-oxo-6-phenylmorpholine), 12% as free 4-hydroxyphenmetrazine, 10% as conjugated 4-hydroxyphenmetrazine, and about 5% as the *N*-oxide.
Phenmetrazine is a metabolite of phendimetrazine.

Therapeutic concentration

After a single oral dose of 75 mg given to 5 subjects, peak plasma concentrations of 0.10 to 0.24 mg/L (mean 0.16) were attained in about 2 h. Following a single oral dose of 75 mg of a slow-release preparation, average peak plasma concentrations of about 0.07 mg/L were reported at 5 h; concentrations remained almost constant over the period 5 to 24 h. [G. P. Quinn *et al.*, *Clin. Pharmacol. Ther.*, 1967, *8*, 369–373.]

Toxicity. Estimated minimum lethal dose for children up to 2 years of age, 200 mg. Large doses and prolonged treatment may lead to severe mental depression and dependence of the amfetamine type.

In a fatality following IV overdosage, the following postmortem distribution was reported: blood 4 mg/L, bile 7 mg/L, liver 5 µg/g, urine 24 mg/L. [G. Norheim, *J. Forensic Sci. Soc.*, 1973, *13*, 287–289.]

The following postmortem tissue concentrations were reported in 12 fatalities: blood 0.1 to 4.9 mg/L (mean 1.1), bile 0.2 to 23 mg/L (mean 5.5), brain 0.1 to 15 µg/g (mean 2.9), kidney 0.1 to 8 µg/g (mean 1.5), liver 0.1 to 20 µg/g (mean 3.1), urine 0.1 to 90 mg/L (mean 21). [L. Gottschalk, per R. C. Baselt, *Disposition of toxic chemicals and drugs in man*, 5th Edn., Davis, California, Biomedical Publications, 2000, pp. 687–688.]

Half-life. Plasma half-life, about 8 h.

Dose. 25 to 75 mg of phenmetrazine hydrochloride daily.

Phenobarbital

Hypnotic/Sedative/Barbiturate

Synonyms. Fenobarbital; Phenemalum; Phenobarbitalum; Phenobarbitone; Phenylethylbarbituric Acid; Phenylethylmalonylurea.
Proprietary names. Aparoxal; Comizial; Edhanol; Fenemal; Fenocriz; Gardenal(e); Kaneuron; Luminal(e); Luminaletas; Luminalette; Luminaletten; Neurobiol; Phenaemal; Phenaemaletten; Solfoton. It is an ingredient of many proprietary preparations—*Martindale, The complete drug reference*, 33rd Edn, Pharmaceutical Press, London, 2002.
5-Ethyl-5-phenyl-2,4,6(1*H*,3*H*,5*H*)-pyrimidinetrione
$C_{12}H_{12}N_2O_3$=232.2
CAS—50-06-6

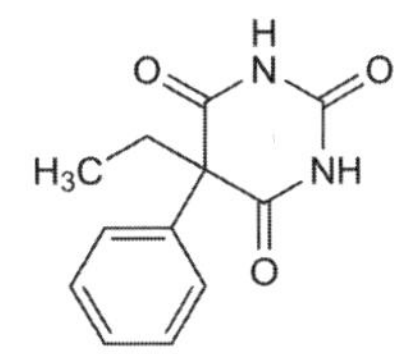

Colourless crystals or a white crystalline powder which may exhibit polymorphism. M.p. 174° to 178°.
Soluble 1 in 1000 of water, 1 in 8 of ethanol, 1 in 40 of chloroform, 1 in 13 of ether, and 1 in about 700 of benzene.

Phenobarbital Sodium

Synonyms. Phenemalnatrium; Phenobarbitone Sodium; Sodium Phenylethylbarbiturate; Soluble Phenobarbitone.
Proprietary names. Garnenal(e); Luminal(e). It is an ingredient of Garoin.
$C_{12}H_{11}N_2NaO_3$=254.2
CAS—57-30-7
A white hygroscopic powder, granules, or flakes. M.p. about 175°.
Soluble 1 in about 1 of water and 1 in about 10 of ethanol; practically insoluble in chloroform and ether.

Dissociation Constant. pK_a 7.4 (25°).

Partition Coefficient. Log *P* (octanol/water), 1.5.

Colour Tests. Koppanyi–Zwikker Test—violet; Liebermann's Test—red-orange; Mercurous Nitrate—black.

Thin-layer Chromatography. System TD—Rf 47; system TE—Rf 28; system TF—Rf 65; system TH—Rf 38; system TAD—Rf 53; system TAE—Rf 85. (Mercuric chloride–diphenylcarbazone reagent, positive; mercurous nitrate spray, black; Zwikker's reagent, pink.)

Gas Chromatography. System GA—phenobarbital RI 1953, M (4-OH-) RI 2295, phenobarbital-Me_2 RI 1855, M (4-OH-)-Me_3 RI 2200; system GB—phenobarbital RI 2031, M (4-OH-) RI 2378; system GE—RRT 0.74 (relative to phenytoin); system GF—RI 2960; system GAJ—RRT 1.150 (relative to methylphenobarbital).

High Performance Liquid Chromatography. System HE—*k* 2.76; system HG—*k* 3.09; system HH—*k* 1.23; system HX—RI 379; system HY—RI 335; system HZ—retention time 3.0 min; system HAA—retention time 14.0 min; system HAK—not detected; system HAM—retention time 2.8 min; system HAX—retention time 5.6 min; system HAY—retention time 4.7 min; system HAZ—phenobarbital *k* 0.39, M (4-OH-) *k* 0.14.

Ultraviolet Spectrum. Borax buffer 0.05 M (pH 9.2) —239 (A_1^1=452a); 1 M sodium hydroxide (pH 13) —254 nm (A_1^1=342b).

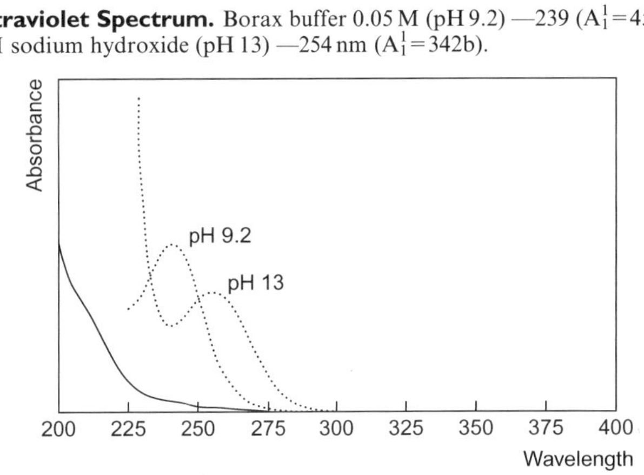

Infra-red Spectrum. Principal peaks at wavenumbers 1712, 1684, 1670, 1770, 1310, 1300 cm^{-1} (KBr disk).

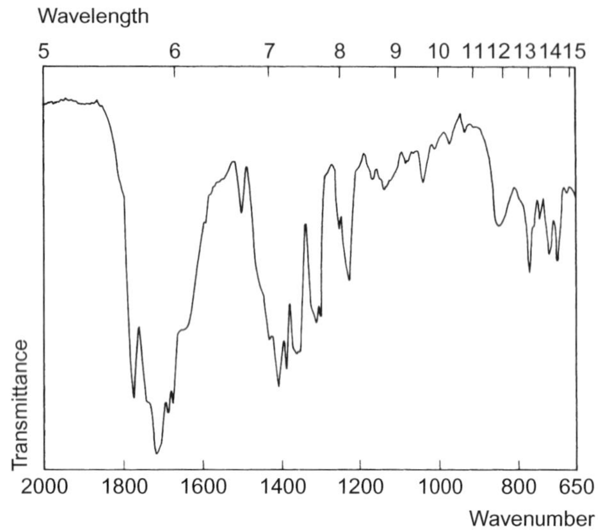

Mass Spectrum. Principal ions at *m/z* 204, 117, 146, 161, 77, 103, 115, 118; 4-hydroxyphenobarbital 219, 248, 148, 220, 120, 218, 133, 64.

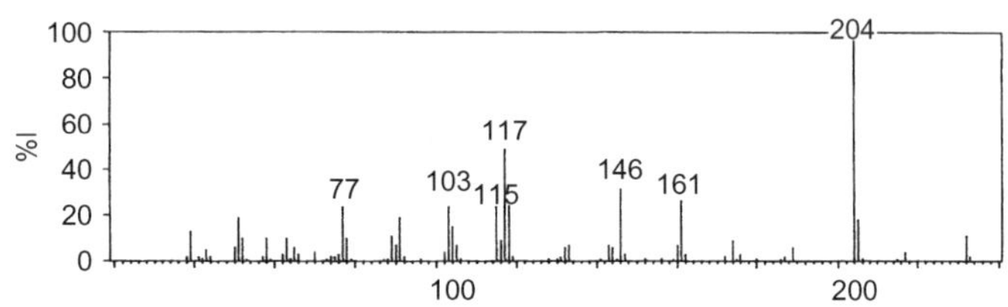

Quantification. See also under Amylobarbital.

Gas chromatography In serum: limit of detection 500 μg/L, FID—A. Di Corcia *et al., J. Chromatogr.* 1982, *229*(18) *B Biomed. Appl.*, 365–372. In serum: phenobarbital and other anticonvulsants, limits of quantification 50 to 200 μg/L, thermionic specific detection—M. E. Queiroz *et al., J. Chromatogr. Sci.*, 2002, *40*, 219–223.

Gas chromatography–mass spectrometry. In plasma or urine: phenobarbital and 4-hydroxyphenobarbital, limit of detection 100 μg/L—I. H. Patel *et al., J. Pharm. Sci.*, 1980, *69*, 1218–1219. In hair—J. P. Goulle *et al., Forensic Sci. Int.*, 1995, *70*, 191–202. In blood or liver: phenobarbital and other anticonvulsants—D. J. Speed *et al., J. Anal. Toxicol.*, 2000, *24*, 685–690. In hair: phenobarbital, phenytoin, and their metabolites—K. Saisho *et al., Biol. Pharm. Bull.*, 2001, *24*, 59–64.

High performance liquid chromatography. In plasma or serum: phenobarbital and other anticonvulsants, limit of detection about 600 μg/L for phenobarbital, UV detection—J. A. Christofides and D. E. Fry, *Clin. Chem.*, 1980, *26*, 499–501. In serum: phenobarbital, phenytoin, and theophylline, comparison with immunoassay—D. Hannak *et al., Wien. Klin. Wochenschr.* 1992, *191, Suppl.*, 27–31. In serum, saliva, or urine: phenobarbital, other anticonvulsants, and their metabolites, photodiode-array detection—H. Liu *et al., J. Chromatogr.*, 1993, *616*, 105–115. In serum: phenobarbital and other anticonvulsants, UV detection—Y. Kouno *et al., J. Chromatogr.*, 1993, *622*, 47–52. In plasma: phenobarbital and other anticonvulsants, UV detection—L. A. Romanyshyn *et al., Ther. Drug Monit.*, 1994, *16*, 90–99. In plasma: phenobarbital and other anticonvulsants, UV detection—K. Johansen *et al., J. Chromatogr.* 1995, *669 B Biomed. Appl.*, 281–288. In biological samples: phenobarbital and other barbiturates—E. Tanaka *et al., Forensic Sci. Int.*, 1997, *85*, 73–82. In urine: phenobarbital and its metabolites, UV detection—S. G. Paibir and W. H. Soine, *J. Chromatogr. B Biomed. Sci. Appl.*, 1997, *691*, 111–117. In serum: phenobarbital and other anticonvulsants, UV detection—Y. Kouno *et al., J. Chromatogr. B Biomed. Sci.Appl.*, 1997, *695*, 349–353. In plasma: phenobarbital and other anticonvulsants—K. M. Matar *et al., Ther. Drug Monit.*, 1999, *21*, 559–566. In serum: phenobarbital and other anticonvulsants, limit of quantification for phenobarbital about 1 μg/L, UV detection—H. Levert *et al., Biomed. Chromatogr.*, 2002, *16*, 19–24.

High performance liquid chromatography–mass spectrometry. In plasma: phenobarbital and other sedatives—H. Kanazawa *et al., J. Chromatogr. A*, 1998, *797*, 227–236.

Polarisation fluoroimmunoassay. In plasma or serum: limit of detection 800 μg/L—A. M. Sidki *et al., Ther. Drug Monit.*, 1982, *4*, 397–403. In serum: phenobarbital and other anticonvulsants—L. S. Steijns *et al., Ther. Drug Monit.*, 2002, *24*, 432–435.

Disposition in the Body. Readily absorbed after oral administration. The major metabolites are *N*-glucopyranosylphenobarbital and 4-hydroxyphenobarbital, together with its glucuronide conjugate. Other metabolites include two dihydrodiol compounds and hydroxymethylphenylbarbituric acid. During chronic dosing, up to about 25% of a dose is excreted in the urine in 24 h as unchanged drug and up to about 17% as total 4-hydroxyphenobarbital, about half of which is the glucuronide conjugate. Urinary excretion of unchanged drug is increased when the urine is alkaline or when the urinary volume is increased; the excretion of conjugated 4-hydroxyphenobarbital is reduced in patients with liver disease. After a single dose, about 80 to 90% is excreted in the urine in 16 days; the *N*-glucoside accounts for about 30% of a single dose. Phenobarbital crosses the placenta and is found in breast milk.
Phenobarbital is a metabolite of methylphenobarbital and primidone.

Therapeutic concentration. In plasma, usually in the range 2 to 30 mg/L. However, there is considerable intersubject variation and there does not appear to be any correlation between plasma concentration and clinical effect. Concentrations in CSF reach about 50% of those in plasma.

Following a single oral dose of 100 mg to 6 subjects, peak serum concentrations of 2.1 to 3.8 mg/L (mean 2.9) were attained in 0.5 to 4 h (mean 1.5). [A. J. Wilensky *et al., Eur. J. Clin. Pharmacol.*, 1982, *23*, 87–92.]

Following daily oral doses of 100 mg to 10 subjects for 15 days, serum concentrations of 10.6 to 22.1 mg/L (mean 17) were reported 12 h after a dose. [P. V. Luoma *et al., Ther. Drug Monit.*, 1982, *4*, 65–68.]

Toxicity. The estimated minimum lethal dose is 1.5 g although recovery has occurred after ingestion of as much as 16 g. Toxic effects have been associated with blood concentrations of 4 to 17 to 90 mg/L and fatalities with concentrations of 4 to 45 to 120 mg/L. However, a degree of tolerance may develop in chronic dosing.

Blood concentrations ranged from 10 to 300 mg/L (mean 86) in 113 fatalities attributed to phenobarbital overdose. [K. D. Parker *et al., Clin Toxicol.*, 1970, *3*, 131–145.]

In 20 fatalities caused by phenobarbital overdose, the following post-mortem concentrations were reported: blood 15 to 540 mg/L (mean 113), brain 0 to 833 μg/g (mean 135), kidney 17 to 867 μg/g (mean 152), liver 24 to 1450 μg/g (mean 236), spleen 0 to 850 μg/g (mean 137). [I. Sunshine and E. Hackett, *J. Forensic Sci.*, 1957, *2*, 149–158.]

Bioavailability. Almost 100%

Half-life. Plasma half-life, about 90 to 100 h in adults, prolonged in neonates and reduced to about 65 to 70 h in children; increased in subjects with liver disease.

Volume of distribution. About 0.5 L/kg.

Clearance. Plasma clearance, about 0.06 mL/min/kg.

Distribution in blood. Plasma:whole blood ratio, 0.93.

Saliva. Plasma:saliva ratio, about 3.

Protein binding. In plasma, about 50%.

Dose. 60 to 180 mg daily.

Phenol

Disinfectant/Anaesthetic (Topical)

Synonyms. Carbolic Acid; Fenol; Oxybenzene; Phenyl Hydrate; Phenylic Acid.
Proprietary names. Chloraseptic; Phenaseptic; Septosol.
Hydroxybenzene
C_6H_5O=94.11
CAS—108-95-2

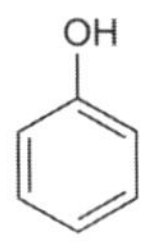

Colourless or faintly pink, deliquescent crystals or crystalline masses, becoming pink on storage. M.p. 40° to 41°; commercial products may contain impurities which raise the m.p. B.p. about 182°.
Soluble 1 in about 15 of water, 6 in 1 of ethanol, 2 in 1 of chloroform, and 5 in 1 of ether; soluble in glycerol.
Caution. Phenol is caustic to the skin.

Dissociation Constant. pK_a 10.0 (25°).

Partition Coefficient. Log *P* (octanol/water), 1.5.

Colour Tests. *p*-Dimethylaminobenzaldehyde—orange/violet; Ferric Chloride—blue; Folin–Ciocalteu Reagent—blue; Liebermann's Test—green; Potassium Dichromate (Method 1)—yellow→brown (2 min).

Gas Chromatography. System GA—RI 981.

High Performance Liquid Chromatography. System HAA—Retention time 13.4 min.

Ultraviolet Spectrum. Aqueous acid—270 (A^1_1=172b); aqueous alkali—287 nm (A^1_1=281a).

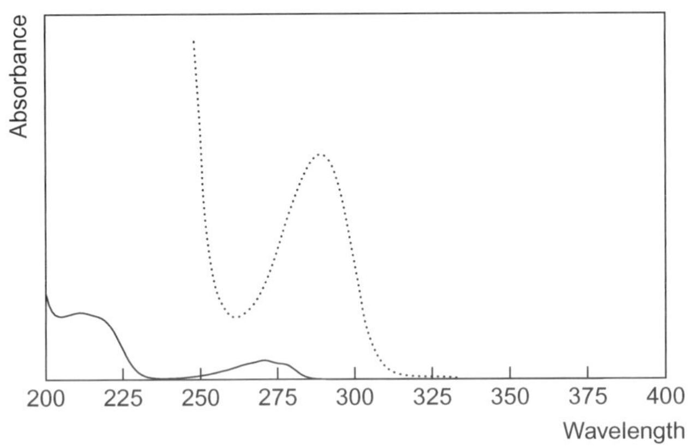

Infra-red Spectrum. Principal peaks at wavenumbers 690, 755, 1235, 1595, 1497, 811 cm^{-1} (Nujol mull).

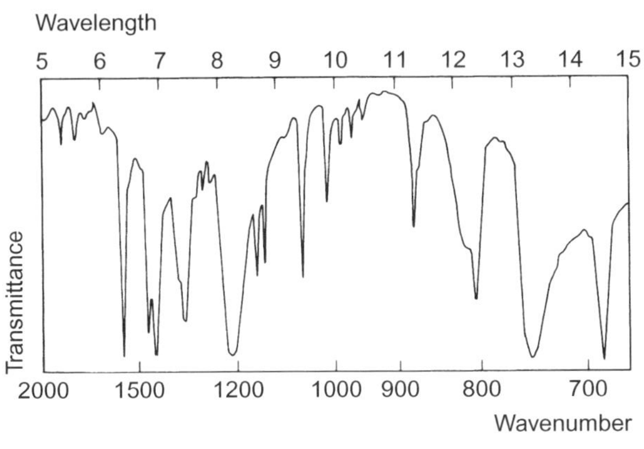

Mass Spectrum. Principal ions at *m/z* 94, 66, 39, 65, 40, 55, 38, 95.

Quantification

Gas chromatography. In urine: FID—D. L. Rick *et al.*, *J. Anal. Toxicol.*, 1982, *6*, 297–300. In urine: FID—M. K. Baldwin *et al.*, *Analyst*, 1981, *106*, 763–767. In urine: limit of detection 1 mg/L—N. Ahmed and K. Hale, *Clin. Chim. Acta*, 1994, *230*, 201–208. In urine, phenol and other phenolic compounds, limit of detection 0.1 to 0.2 mg/L—G. Bieniek, *J. Chromatogr. B Biomed. Appl.*, 1996, *682*, 167–172.

Gas chromatography–mass spectrometry. In plasma—L. M. Harrison *et al.*, *Clin. Chem.*, 1991, *37*, 1739–1742. In serum: limit of detection 1 mg/L—A. P. Hart and A. Dasgupta, *J. Forensic Sci.*, 1997, *42*, 693–696.

High performance liquid chromatography. In urine: limit of detection <500 μg/L, UV detection—C. V. Eadsforth and P. C. Coveney, *Analyst*, 1984, *109*, 175–176. In urine: phenol, hydroquinone, and catechol, fluorimetric detection—B. L. Lee *et al.*, *J. Chromatogr.*, 1993, *619*, 259–266. In urine, limit of detection 10 ppb, fluorescence detection—J. F. Jen and M. Y. Tsai, *J. Chromatogr. B Biomed. Appl.*, 1994, *658*, 87–92. In urine or faeces: phenol and *p*-cresol, UV detection—A. M. Birkett *et al.*, *J. Chromatogr. B Biomed. Appl.*, 1995, *674*, 187–191. In urine: phenol and *p*-cresol, limits of detection 0.17 pmol and 0.25 pmol per injection respectively, fluorescence detection—Y. Tsuruta *et al.*, *Anal. Biochem.*, 1996, *243*, 86–91.

Disposition in the Body. Rapidly absorbed from the gastrointestinal tract and readily penetrates the skin. It is metabolised by conjugation to yield phenyl glucuronide and phenyl sulfate; small amounts are oxidised to catechol and quinol which are also conjugated. Oxidation of these metabolites to quinones may tint the urine green. Acid-labile phenol conjugates are present endogenously in serum at concentrations of about 0.1 mg/L. Phenol is a metabolite of benzene. Endogenous phenol concentrations in urine average about 5 to 10 mg/L.

Toxicity. Phenol denatures and precipitates cellular proteins and thus may cause rapid poisoning. The minimum lethal dose by mouth is about 1 g. Severe and even fatal poisoning may also arise from absorption of phenol from open wounds or through the intact skin. The maximum permissible atmospheric concentration is 5 ppm.

In a fatality due to the deliberate ingestion of a mixture containing phenol, the following postmortem tissue concentrations were reported: blood, phenol 56 mg/L, alcohol 300 mg/L; liver, phenol 74 μg/g. In a second fatality due to accidental percutaneous absorption, postmortem blood concentrations of 27 mg/L of phenol and 300 mg/L of alcohol were reported [E. R. Soares and J. P. Tift, *J. Forensic Sci.*, 1982, *27*, 729–731].

In a fatality resulting from the ingestion of phenol, the following postmortem concentrations were reported: blood 130 mg/L, urine 47 mg/L, bile 187 mg/L, brain 486 μg/g, kidney 331 μg/g, muscle 204 μg/g, liver 228 μg/g, stomach content 668 mg [C. Lo Dico *et al.*, *J. Forensic Sci.*, 1989, *34*, 1013–1015].

In a fatality due to accidental dermal exposure to phenol, the following postmortem concentrations were reported: blood 4.7 mg/L, unhydrolysed liver 3.3 μg/g, hydrolysed liver 7.1 μg/g [J. F. Lewin and W. T. Cleary, *Forensic Sci. Int.*, 1982, *19*, 177–179].

Phenolphthalein

Purgative

Synonyms. Dihydroxyphthalophenone; Fenolftaleina.
Proprietary names. Alophen Pills; Bonomint; Brooklax; Easylax; Euchessina; Laxen Busto; Laxettes; Laxicaps P; Nylax; Purmolax; Regulim; Sure Lax. It is an ingredient of Agarol and Alophen. For a list of other preparations which contain phenolphthalein, see Martindale, The complete drug reference, 33rd Edn., Pharmaceutical Press, London, 2002.
3,3-Bis(4-hydroxyphenyl)-1-(3*H*)-isobenzofuranone
$C_{20}H_{14}O_4$=318.3
CAS—77-09-8

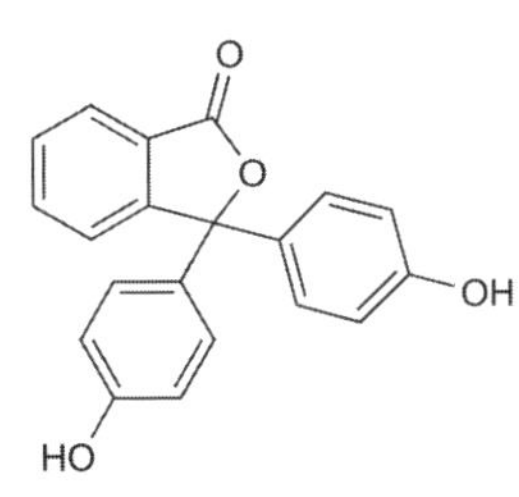

A white or yellowish-white crystalline or amorphous powder. M.p. 258° to 262°.
Practically insoluble in water; soluble 1 in 12 of ethanol, and 1 in about 100 of ether; soluble in dilute solutions of alkali hydroxides.

Dissociation Constant. pK_a 9.7 (25°).

Partition Coefficient. Log *P* (octanol/water), 2.4.

Colour Test. Folin–Ciocalteu Reagent—blue.

Thin-layer Chromatography. System TD—Rf 38; system TE—Rf 53; system TF—Rf 59; system TAD—Rf 39; system TAE—Rf 86. (Acidified potassium permanganate solution, positive.)

High Performance Liquid Chromatography. System HX—RI 436; system HZ—Retention time 4.2 min.

Ultraviolet Spectrum. Methanol—277 nm (A^1_1 = 150a).

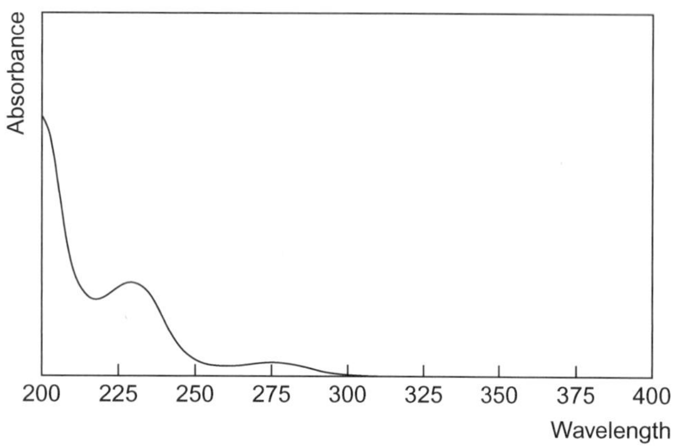

Infra-red Spectrum. Principal peaks at wavenumbers 1740, 1178, 1230, 1265, 1278, 1510 cm^{-1} (KBr disk).

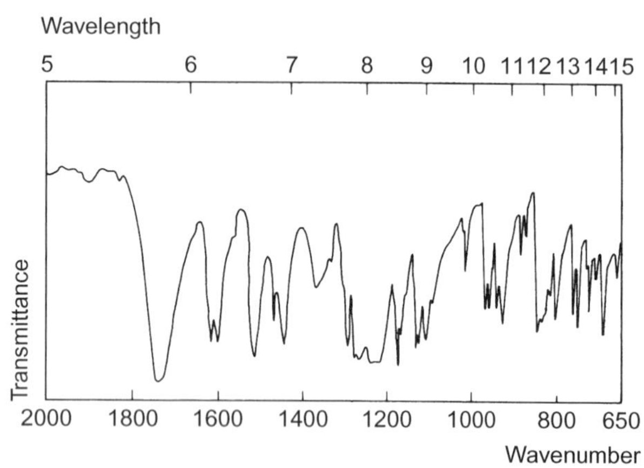

Mass Spectrum. Principal ions at *m/z* 274, 225, 318, 273, 275, 226, 257, 121.

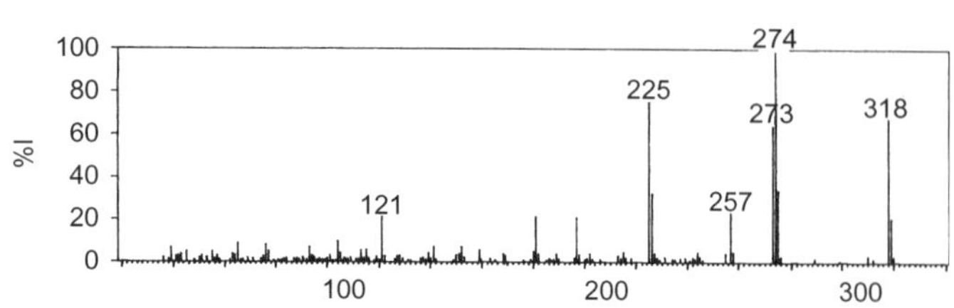

Quantification

Colorimetry. In serum or urine—S. M. Morris and D. W. Powell, *Anal Biochem.*, 1979, *95*, 465–471.

Disposition in the Body. Poorly absorbed after oral administration (up to about 15%), and partly excreted in the bile as the active glucuronide, and in the urine; if the urine is alkaline the excreted compound will impart a red colour. The greater part of the ingested material is eliminated in the faeces in both free and conjugated forms.

Toxicity. Phenolphthalein is usually non-toxic even in relatively large doses, although fatalities have occurred in young children after ingestion of 0.6 to 1.8 g.

A 32-year-old woman (suspected of being a chronic laxative abuser) eventually died due to massive liver necrosis after ingesting an unknown quantity of Nylax tablets containing phenolphthalein. The serum-phenolphthalein concentration on the day after hospital admission was 0.4 μg/L [P. S. Sidhu *et al.*, *Hum. Toxicol.*, 1989, *8*, 381–384].

Dose. 50 to 300 mg.

Phenoperidine

Narcotic Analgesic

1-(3-Hydroxy-3-phenylpropyl)-4-phenyl-4-piperidinecarboxylic acid ethyl ester

$C_{23}H_{29}NO_3$ = 367.5

CAS—562-26-5

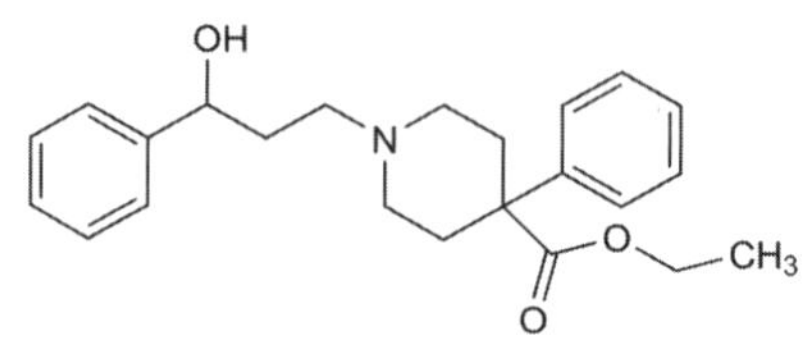

Phenoperidine Hydrochloride

Proprietary names. Lealgin; Operidine; R 1406.

Note. Operidine has been used as a synonym for pethidine hydrochloride in *Jap. Pharmacopeia.*

$C_{23}H_{29}NO_3$,HCl = 403.9

CAS—3627-49-4

A white crystalline powder. M.p. 200° to 202°.

Soluble 1 in 50 of water, 1 in 10 of ethanol (90%), and 1 in 3 of chloroform; practically insoluble in ether.

Partition Coefficient. Log *P* (octanol/water), 4.0.

Colour Test. Marquis Test—red.

Thin-layer Chromatography. System TA—Rf 71; system TB—Rf 26; system TC—Rf 64; system TE—Rf 76; system TL—Rf 58; system TAE—Rf 70; system TAF—Rf 82. (Dragendorff spray, positive; acidified iodoplatinate solution, positive; Marquis reagent, faint red.) See also Pethidine.

Gas Chromatography. System GA—phenoperidine RI 2872, norpethidine RI 1885, pethidine RI 1754; system GB—phenoperidine RI 2983, norpethidine RI 1842, pethidine RI 1809.

High Performance Liquid Chromatography. System HA—phenoperidine *k* 0.8, norpethidine *k* 1.7 (tailing peak), pethidine *k* 2.8 (tailing peak); system HC—phenoperidine *k* 0.10, norpethidine *k* 2.04, pethidine *k* 0.55; system HX—RI 434 (phenoperidine; see also Pethidine).

Infra-red Spectrum. Principal peaks at wavenumbers 1710, 698, 1230, 1136, 1175, 1205 cm^{-1} (phenoperidine hydrochloride, KBr disk).

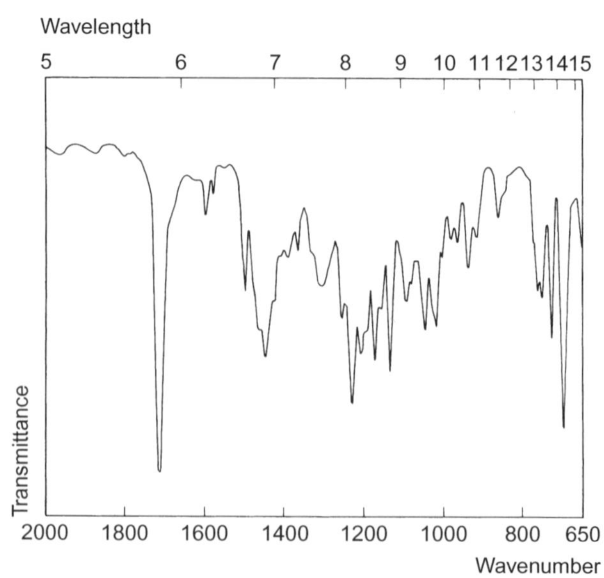

Mass Spectrum. Principal ions at *m/z* 246, 42, 367, 247, 57, 56, 91, 77;

norpethidine 57, 233, 42, 56, 158, 43, 160, 103; pethidine 71, 70, 44, 57, 42, 247, 43, 246.

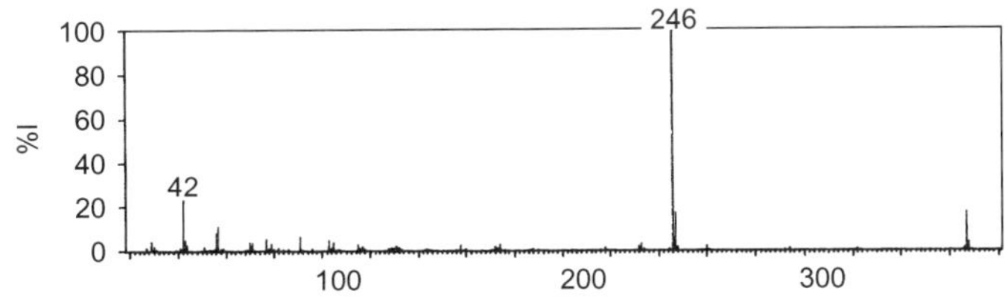

Quantification
Gas chromatography. In plasma: limit of detection 2 µg/L, AFID—K. Chan *et al.*, *J. Chromatogr.* 1981, *223(12) B Biomed. Appl.*, 213–218. In plasma: phenperidine, pethidine and norpethidine, limits of detection about 5 µg/L, selective nitrogen detection—P. Kintz *et al.*, *Forensic Sci. Int.*, 1989, *43*, 267–273. In plasma: phenoperidine and other narcotic analgesics, limit of detection 10 µg/L, selective nitrogen detection—P. Kintz *et al.*, *Methods Find. Exp. Clin. Pharmacol.*, 1990, *12*, 193–196.

Disposition in the Body. Absorbed from the gastro-intestinal tract but there is extensive first-pass metabolism. It is metabolised to pethidine and norpethidine. Up to about 5% of a dose is excreted unchanged in the urine, with about 18% as norpethidine and 2% as pethidine, in 2 to 3 days. The urinary excretion of unchanged phenoperidine is increased to about 7% when the urine is acidified.

Therapeutic concentration
After a single intravenous dose of 2 mg administered to 5 patients during general anaesthesia, a mean plasma concentration of 0.02 mg/L was reported at 2 min. [L. Milne *et al.*, *Br. J. Anaesth.*, 1980, *52*, 537–540.]

Bioavailability. About 30%.

Half-life. Plasma half-life, about 1 h.

Volume of distribution. About 2 L/kg.

Clearance. Plasma clearance, about 20 mL/min/kg.

Protein binding. In plasma, about 80%.

Dose. 0.5 to 1 mg of phenoperidine hydrochloride intravenously. With assisted ventilation, an initial intravenous dose of 2 to 5 mg may be given.

Phenothiazine

Anthelmintic (Veterinary)

Synonyms. Bibenzothiazine; Thiodiphenylamine
Proprietary names. AFI-Tiazin; Antiverm; Fentiazin; Helmetina; Lethelmin; Nemazine; Orimon; Phenegic; Phenoverm; Phenovis; Phenoxur; Reconox; Souframine; Vermitin.
10H-Phenothiazine
$C_{12}H_9NS = 199.3$
CAS—92-84-2

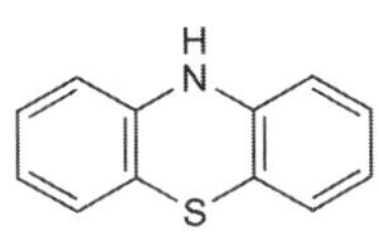

A yellow crystalline powder. It is slowly oxidised in air and darkens on exposure to light acquiring a greenish-brown tint. M.p. about 185°.
Practically insoluble in water and chloroform; freely soluble in benzene; soluble 1 in 60 of ethanol and 1 in 5 of acetone.

Dissociation Constant. pK_a 2.5.

Partition Coefficient. Log *P* (octanol/water), 4.2.

Colour Tests. Ferric Chloride—green; Formaldehyde–Sulfuric Acid—red-violet; Forrest Reagent—orange; FPN Reagent—orange; Liebermann's Test—green; Sulfuric Acid—green.

Thin-layer Chromatography. System TA—Rf 79; system TB—Rf 11; system TC—Rf 79; system TE—Rf 82; system TL—Rf 71; system TAE—Rf 82; system TAF—Tf 89; system TAJ—Rf 90; system TAK—Rf 77; system TAL—Rf 96.

Gas Chromatography. System GA—RI 2120; system GB—RI 2130; system GF—RI 2845.

High Performance Liquid Chromatography. System HA—*k* 0.1; system HX—RI 665; system HY—RI 637; system HAA—Retention time 14.1 min (phenothiazine ring); Retention time 14.3 min (phenothiazine ring 2).

Ultraviolet Spectrum. Ethanol—254 (A^1_1=2160b), 317 nm (A^1_1=266b).

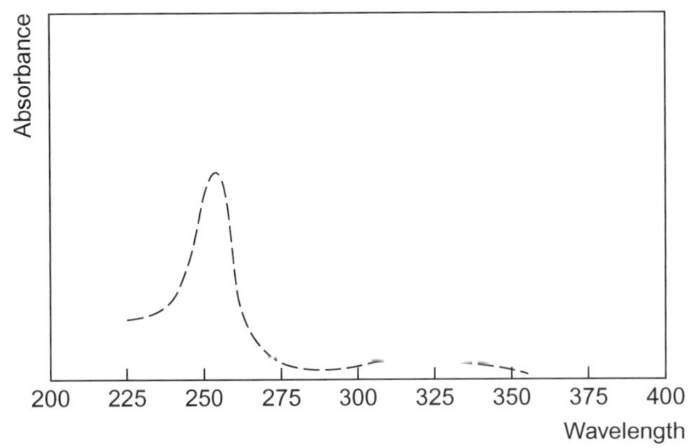

Infra-red Spectrum. Principal peaks at wavenumbers 735, 750, 1310, 710, 1300, 1590 cm^{-1} (KBr disk).

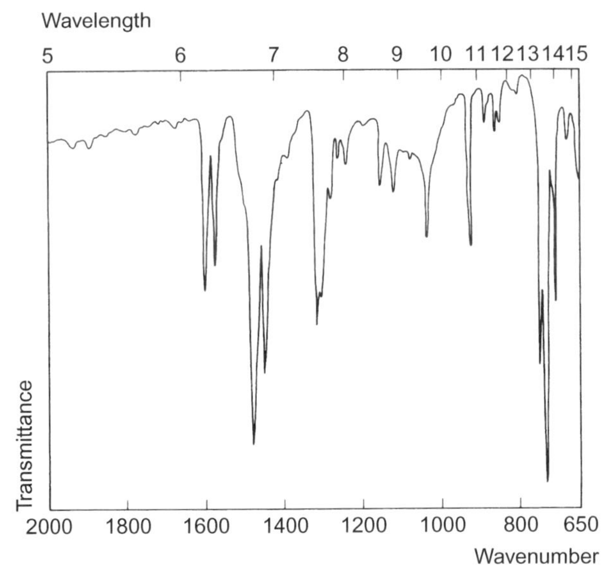

Mass Spectrum. Principal ions at *m/z* 199, 167, 198, 166, 99, 154, 69, 77.

Phenoxybenzamine

Antihypertensive

Synonyms. 688-A; bensylyt.
N-(2-Chloroethyl)-*N*-(1-methyl-2-phenoxyethyl)benzenemethanamine
$C_{18}H_{22}ClNO = 303.8$
CAS—59-96-1

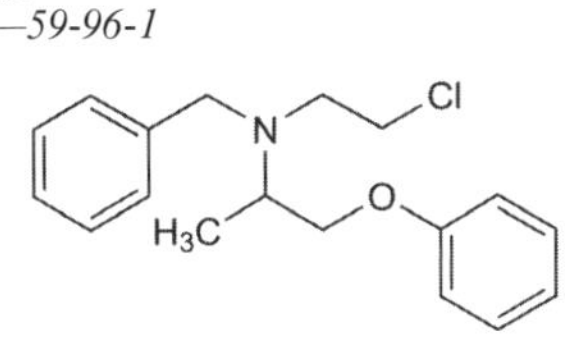

Crystals. M.p. 38° to 40°.
Soluble in benzene.

Phenoxybenzamine Hydrochloride
Proprietary names. Dibenyline; Dibenzyline; Dibenzyran.
$C_{18}H_{22}ClNO,HCl=340.3$
CAS—63-92-3
A white crystalline powder. M.p. 137° to 141°.
Soluble 1 in 25 of water, 1 in 9 of ethanol, and 1 in 9 of chloroform; practically insoluble in ether. Neutral and alkaline solutions are unstable.
Caution. Phenoxybenzamine hydrochloride in powder form should not be allowed to come into contact with eyes or skin, as it may cause irritation.

Partition Coefficient. Log *P* (octanol/water), 4.6.

Colour Tests. Mandelin's Test—green→violet; Marquis Test—violet.

Thin-layer Chromatography. System TA—Rf 73; system TB—Rf 63; system TC—Rf 76; system TE—Rf 87; system TL—Rf 68; system TAE—Rf 84; system TAF—Rf 97; system TAJ—Rf 65; system TAK—Rf 04; system TAL—Rf 51. (Acidified iodoplatinate solution, positive.)

Gas Chromatography. System GA—RI 2235; system GB—RI 2332; system GF—RI 2600.

High Performance Liquid Chromatography. System HA—*k* 0.1; system HX—RI 396.

Ultraviolet Spectrum. Aqueous acid—262, 268 (A^{1}_{1}=48a), 274 nm.

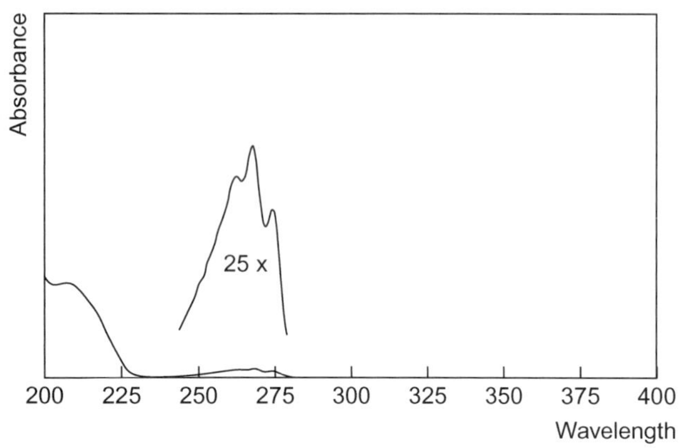

Infra-red Spectrum. Principal peaks at wavenumbers 1240, 750, 698, 1494, 1598, 1586 cm^{-1} (phenoxybenzamine hydrochloride, KBr disk).

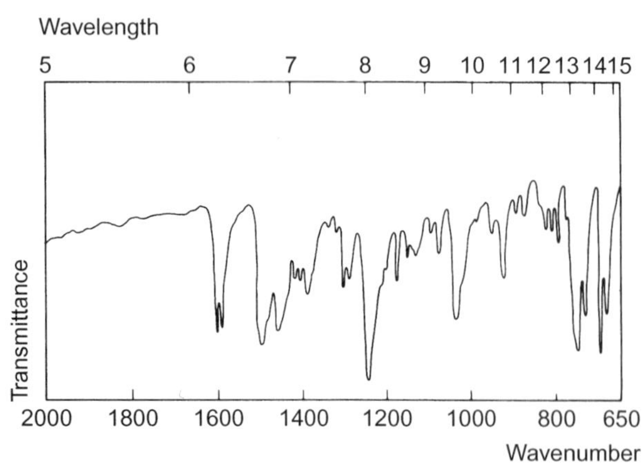

Mass Spectrum. Principal ions at *m/z* 91, 196, 198, 92, 197, 65, 77, 56.

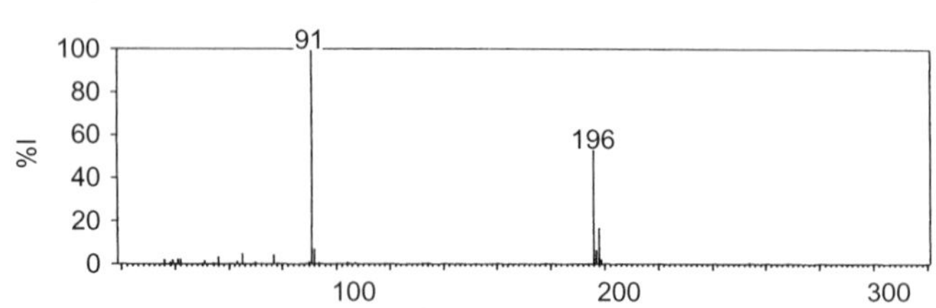

Dose. 10 to 60 mg of phenoxybenzamine hydrochloride daily; up to 200 mg daily has been given.

Phenoxymethylpenicillin *Antibiotic*

Synonyms. Fenoximetilpenicilina; Penicillin V; Phénomycilline.
Proprietary names. Acipen V; Compocillin; Fenospen; Kopen; Meracilina; Ospen; Pen-V; Pen-Vee; Rafapen.
(2*S*,5*R*,6*R*)-3,3-Dimethyl-7-oxo-6-[(phenoxyacetyl)amino]-4-thia-1-azabicyclo[3.2.0]heptane-2-carboxylic acid
$C_{16}H_{18}N_2O_5S=350.4$
CAS—87-08-1

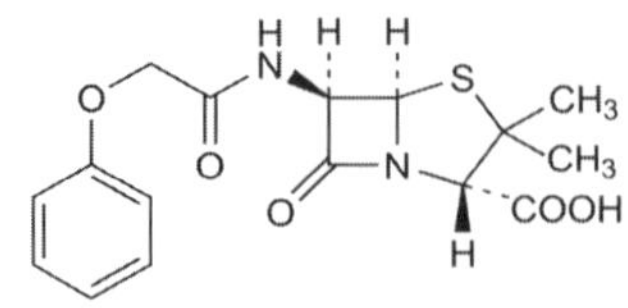

An antimicrobial acid produced by the growth of certain strains of *Penicillium notatum* or related organisms.
A white crystalline powder. M.p. 120° to 128°, with decomposition.
Soluble 1 in 1700 of water, 1 in 7 of ethanol, and 1 in 6 of acetone; soluble in chloroform.

Phenoxymethylpenicillin Calcium
Synonym. Penicillin V Calcium
Proprietary names. Calcipen; Calvepen; Milcopen.
$(C_{16}H_{17}N_2O_5S)_2Ca,2H_2O=774.9$
CAS—147-48-8 (anhydrous); 73368-74-8 (dihydrate)
A white, finely crystalline powder.
Slowly soluble 1 in 20 of water.

Phenoxymethylpenicillin Potassium
Synonyms. Fenoximetilcilina Potássica; Penicillin V Potassium.
Proprietary names. Acipen; Apocillin; Apo-Pen-VK; Apsin VK; Arcasin; Beepen-VK; Betapen-VK; Brunocillin; Calciopen; Cilicaine VK; Cliacil; Colipen VK; Copen; Darocillin; Deltacillin; Distaquaine V-K; Fenoxicillin; InfectoCillin; Isocillin; Ledercillin VK; Len V.K; LPV; Mack Pen; Megacillin(e); Milcopen; Nadopen-V; NovoPen-VK; Oracilin; Oracilline; Ospen; Pen; Penbene; Penhexal VK; Peni-Oral; Penstad; Pen-V; Pen-Vee-K; Pen-Ve-Oral; Pen-Vi-K; PVFK; PVK; Robicillin VK; Rocilin; Tikacillin; V-Cil-K; V-Cillin K; Veekay; Veetids; Vepenicillin.

Note. Megacillin is also used as a proprietary name for benzylpenicillin potassium or benzathine benzylpenicillin and Megacilline for clemizole penicillin. Oracilline, Pen-V and Pen-Vee are also used as proprietary names for benzathine phenoxymethylpenicillin and Arcasin for cisapride.
$C_{16}H_{17}KN_2O_5S=388.5$
CAS—132-98-9
A white crystalline powder.
Soluble 1 in 1.5 of water and 1 in 150 of ethanol; practically insoluble in ether; insoluble in acetone.

Dissociation Constant. pK_a 2.7 (25°).

Partition Coefficient. Log *P* (octanol/water), 2.1.

Ultraviolet Spectrum. Phenoxymethylpenicillin potassium: water—268 (A^{1}_{1}=31b), 275 nm (A^{1}_{1}=25b).

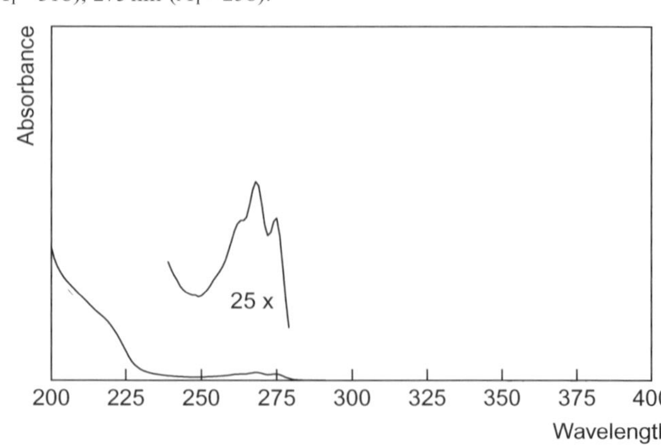

Infra-red Spectrum. Principal peaks at wavenumbers 1754, 1660, 1181, 1202, 1174, 1532 cm^{-1} (KBr disk).

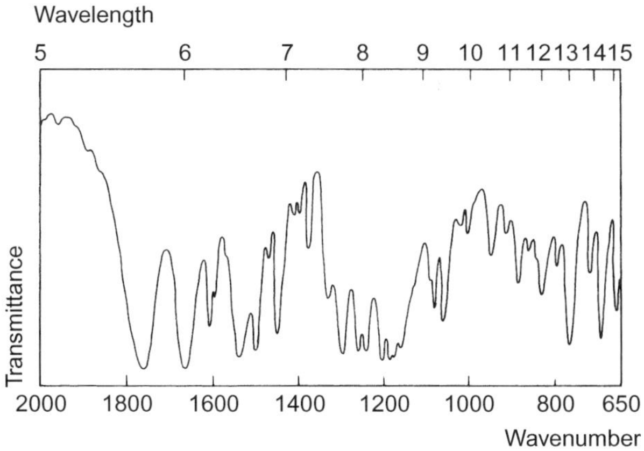

Quantification

High performance liquid chromatography. In serum: limit of detection 30 μg/L—R. L. Lindberg *et al.*, *Antimicrob. Agents Chemother.*, 1984, *26*, 300–302. In serum: phenoxymethylpenicillin and other penicillins, limit of detection <0.5 mg/L, UV detection—E. Mendez-Alvarez *et al.*, *Biomed. Chromatogr.*, 1991, *5*, 78–82. In plasma: limit of detection 0.1 mg/L, UV detection—W. J. Krauwinkel and N. J. Volkers-Kamermans, *J. Chromatogr. B Biomed. Appl.*, 1996, *679*, 129–135.

Disposition in the Body. Rapidly but incompletely absorbed after oral administration; peak plasma concentrations are attained about 2 h after a dose. About 20 to 35% of an oral dose is excreted in the urine unchanged in 24 h and about 34% is excreted as penicilloic acid in the same period.

Half-life. Plasma half-life, about 0.5 h.

Protein binding. In plasma, about 80%.

Dose. 0.5 to 3 g daily.

Phenprobamate

Tranquilliser/Muscle Relaxant (Skeletal)

Synonyms. Proformiphen; MH-532.
Proprietary names. Extacol; Gamaquil; Spantol.
Benzenepropanol carbamate
$C_{10}H_{13}NO_2$ = 179.2
CAS—673-31-4

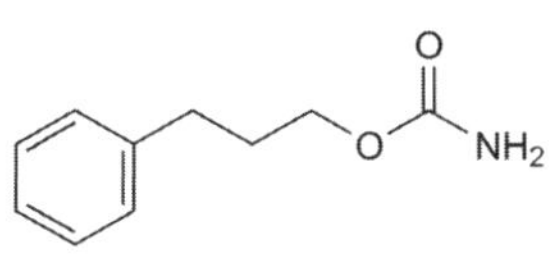

A fine, white, crystalline powder. M.p. 101° to 104°.
Practically insoluble in water; soluble in ethanol and chloroform; slightly soluble in ether.

Partition Coefficient. Log *P* (octanol/water), 2.0.

Colour Test. Marquis Test—red-brown.

Thin-layer Chromatography. System TA—Rf 75; system TD—Rf 47; system TE—Rf 73; system TF—Rf 55; system TAD—Rf 60; system TAE—Rf 82. (Furfuraldehyde reagent, positive.)

Gas Chromatography. System GA—RI 1520.

Ultraviolet Spectrum. Ethanol—254, 259 (A_1^1 = 11.6b), 261 (A_1^1 = 11.6b), 265 nm, 269 nm.

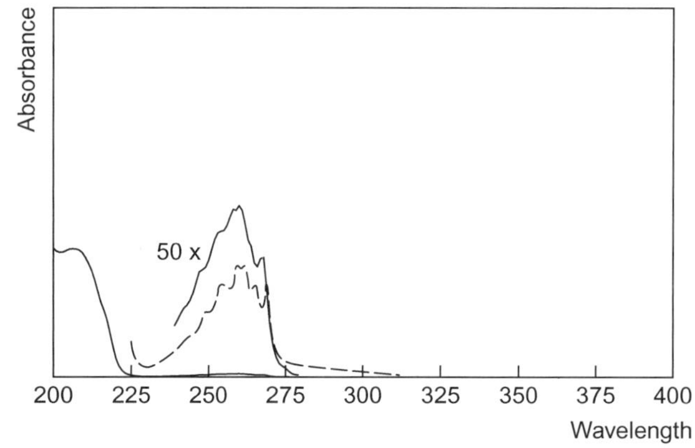

Infra-red Spectrum. Principal peaks at wavenumbers 1690, 1088, 1064, 700, 1605, 1623 cm^{-1} (KBr disk).

Mass Spectrum. Principal ions at *m/z* 118, 117, 91, 92, 119, 65, 77, 103.

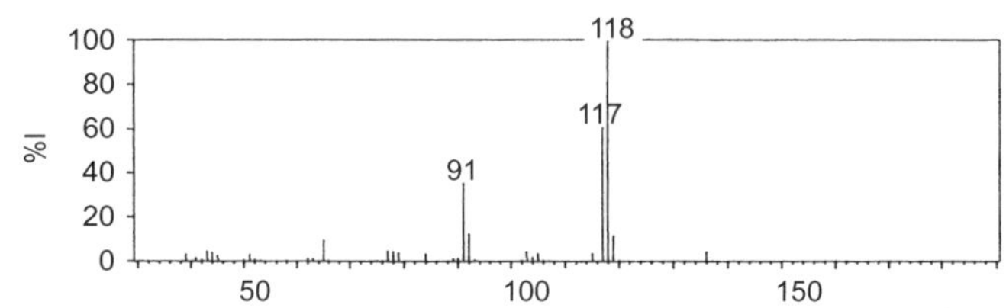

Quantification

Colorimetry and thin-layer chromatography. In blood or urine: phenprobamate and metabolites—F. Schatz and U. Jahn, *Arzneimittelforschung*, 1966, *16*, 866–870.

High performance liquid chromatography. In plasma: UV detection—J. X. Sun *et al.*, *Biopharm. Drug Dispos.*, 1987, *8*, 341–351.

Disposition in the Body. Rapidly absorbed after oral administration and metabolised by oxidative degradation of the side chain and *p*-hydroxylation of the phenyl ring. About 7% of a dose is excreted unchanged in the urine in 48 h and about 76% as metabolites, mostly as hippuric acid and free and conjugated 3-hydroxyphenprobamate. The 3-hydroxy metabolite, which is active, is present in blood at concentrations greater than those of unchanged drug.

Half-life. Plasma half-life, 5 to 8 h.

Dose. 1.2 to 2.4 g daily.

Phenprocoumon

Anticoagulant

Synonym. Phenylpropylhydroxycoumarin
Proprietary names. Falithrom; Liquamar; Marcoumar; Marcumar; marcuphen; Phenpro.
4-Hydroxy-3-(1-phenylpropyl)-2*H*-1-benzopyran-2-one
$C_{18}H_{16}O_3$ = 280.3
CAS—435-97-2

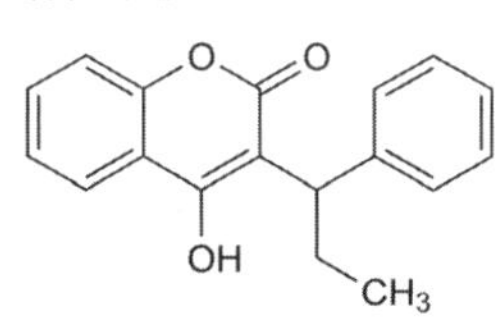

A fine white crystalline powder. M.p. 179° to 180°.
Practically insoluble in water; soluble in chloroform, methanol, and solutions of alkali hydroxides.

Partition Coefficient. Log *P* (octanol/water), 3.6.

Thin-layer Chromatography. System TD—Rf 62; system TE—Rf 19; system TF—Rf 58; system TAD—Rf 61; system TAE—Rf 93.

Gas Chromatography. System GA—phenprocoumon isomer 1-Me RI 2375, isomer 2-Me RI 2395; M (OH-) isomer-1 Me_2 RI 2655, isomer-2 Me_2 RI 2675, isomer 3 Me_2 RI 2705; M (OH-methoxy)-Me_2 RI 2770; M (di-OH-)-Me_3 RI 2770.

High Performance Liquid Chromatography. System HX—RI 616; system HZ—Retention time 12.6 min.

Ultraviolet Spectrum. Aqueous alkali—310 (A_1^1=540b); methanol—285 (A_1^1=394a), 310 nm (A_1^1=440a).

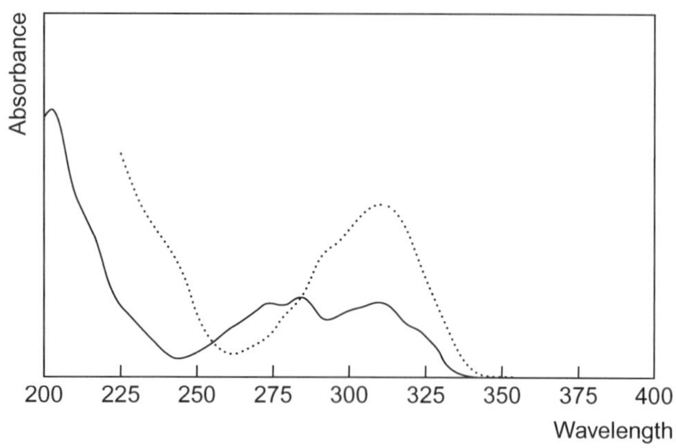

Infra-red Spectrum. Principal peaks at wavenumbers 1656, 759, 696, 1613, 1163, 1113 cm^{-1} (Nujol mull).

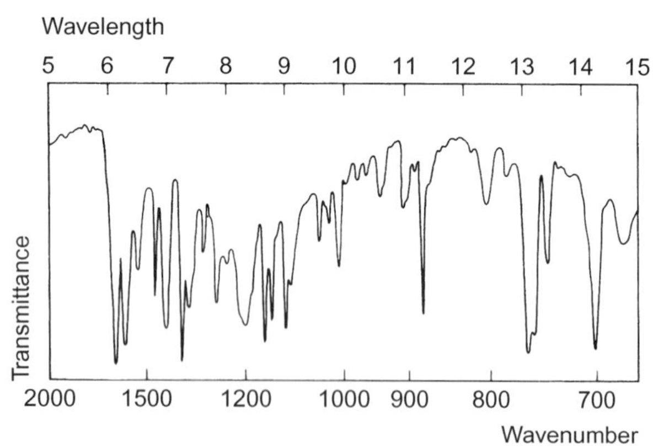

Mass Spectrum. Principal ions at *m/z* 251, 280, 118, 91, 121, 119, 252, 189.

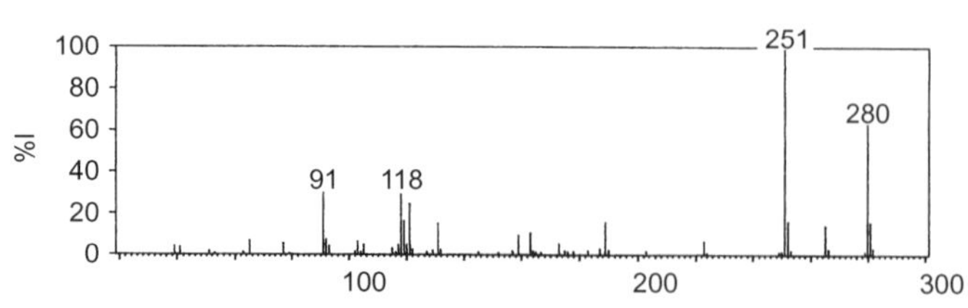

Quantification

Gas chromatography. In plasma: limit of detection 125 μg/L, FID—K. K. Midha *et al.*, *J. Pharm. Sci.*, 1976, 65, 387–391.

High performance liquid chromatography. In plasma or urine: limit of detection 100 μg/L in plasma, UV detection—J. X. De Vries *et al.*, *J. Chromatogr.*, 1982, *231*; *B Biomed. Appl.*, *20*, 83–92. In urine: phenprocoumon and its metabolites—P. M. Edelbroek *et al.*, *J. Chromatogr.*, 1990, *530*, 347–358. In serum—D. Petersen *et al.*, *Haemostasis*, 1993, *23*, 83–90. In plasma, urine, or breast milk: phenprocoumon and its metabolites, UV and fluorescence detection—J. X. de Vries and E. Schmitz-Kummer, *J. Chromatogr. B Biomed. Appl.*, 1994, *655*, 63–71.

High performance liquid chromatography–mass spectrometry. In plasma: phenprocoumon, warfarin, and acenocoumarol, limits of detection 1 μg/L (phenprocoumon and warfarin) and 10 μg/L (acenocoumarol)—M. Kollroser and C. Schober, *Clin. Chem.*, 2002, *48*, 84–91 and 1372.

Thin-layer chromatography–fluorescence densitometry. In plasma: limit of detection 5 μg/L—P. Haefelfinger, *J. Chromatogr.*, 1979, *162*; *B Biomed. Appl.*, *4*, 215–222.

Disposition in the Body. Well absorbed after oral administration. The *S*-enantiomer is stated to be considerably more potent as an anticoagulant than the *R*-form but there appears to be little difference in pharmacokinetic properties. Phenprocoumon is thought to be excreted almost entirely as a glucuronide conjugate with less than 10% of the dose as unchanged drug.

Therapeutic concentration

Following an IV injection of 3 mg to 1 subject, a plasma concentration of 0.8 mg/L was reported at 5 min; in a subject receiving daily doses of 1.6 mg, a steady-state plasma concentration of 1.8 mg/L was reported [P. Haefelfinger, *J. Chromatogr.*, 1979, *162*; *B Biomed. Appl.*, *4*, 215–222].

Half-life. Plasma half-life, 3 to 9 days (mean 5).

Volume of distribution. 0.1 to 0.2 L/kg.

Clearance. Plasma clearance, about 0.01 mL/min/kg.

Protein binding. In plasma, more than 99%.

Note. For a review of the clinical pharmacokinetics of oral anticoagulants see J. G. Kelly and K. O'Malley, *Clin. Pharmacokinet.*, 1979, *4*, 1–15.

Dose. Maintenance, 0.75 to 4.5 mg daily.

Phensuximide

Anticonvulsant

Synonym. Fensuximid
Proprietary names. Lifene; Milontin; Mirontin; Succitimal.
1-Methyl-3-phenyl-2,5-pyrrolidinedione
$C_{11}H_{11}NO_2$=189.2
CAS—86-34-0

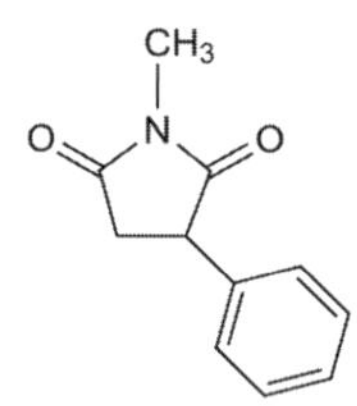

A white crystalline powder. M.p. 71° to 73°.
Soluble 1 in 250 of water, 1 in 20 of ethanol, 1 in 1.5 of chloroform, and 1 in 35 of ether; readily soluble in methanol.

Partition Coefficient. Log *P* (octanol/water), 1.0.

Colour Test. Liebermann's Test—red-orange.

Thin-layer Chromatography. System TA—Rf 75; system TD—Rf 71; system TE—Rf 77; system TF—Rf 59; system TAD—Rf 72; system TAJ—Rf 81; system TAK—Rf 71; system TAL—Rf 96. (Acidified potassium permanganate solution, positive.)

Gas Chromatography. System GA—RI 1634; system GE—Retention time 0.4 relative to phenytoin.

High Performance Liquid Chromatography. System HY—RI 347.

Ultraviolet Spectrum. Ethanol—247 (A_1^1=17.2b), 252 (A_1^1=16.2b), 258 (A_1^1=14.5b), 264 nm (A_1^1=9.6b). (See below)

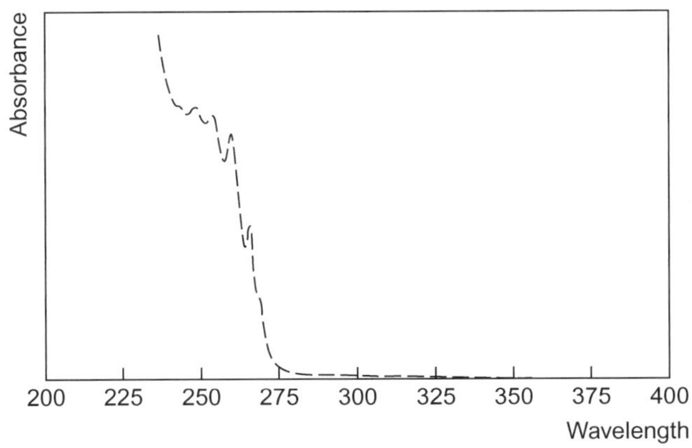

Infra-red Spectrum. Principal peaks at wavenumbers 1686, 1275, 1637, 1111, 695, 751 cm^{-1} (KBr disk). (See below)

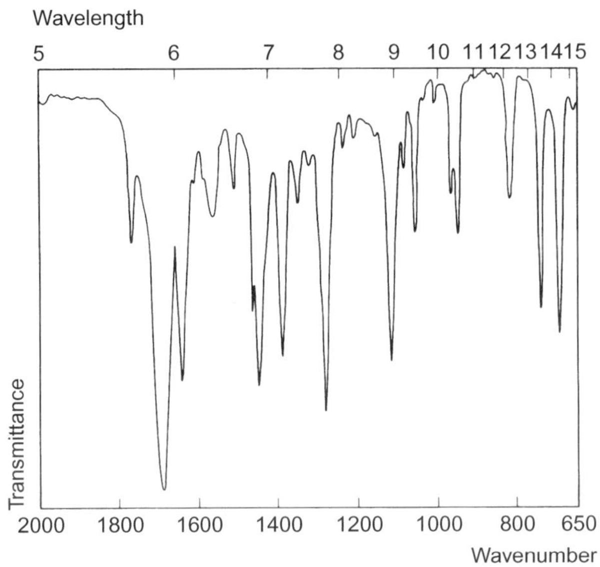

Mass Spectrum. Principal ions at m/z 104, 189, 103, 78, 51, 77, 105, 52.

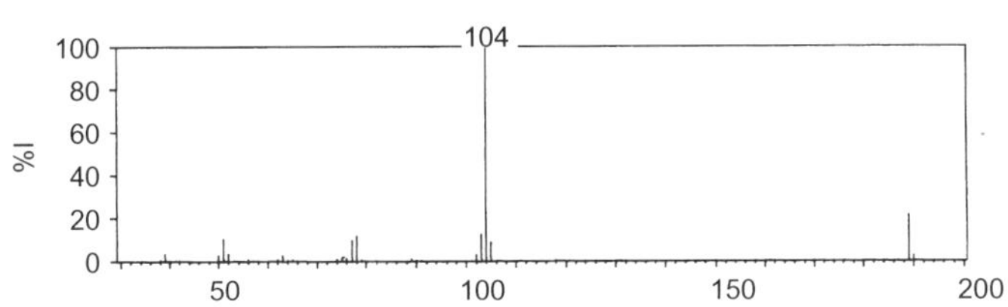

Quantification

Gas chromatography. In serum: phensuximide and other succinimide anticonvulsants, limit of detection 1 to 5 mg/L for phensuximide, FID—J. Bonitati, *Clin. Chem.*, 1976, *22*, 341–345. In plasma or urine: limit of detection 2.5 mg/L, FID—E. van der Kleijn *et al.*, *J. Pharm. Pharmacol.*, 1973, *25*, 324–327.

Disposition in the Body. Readily absorbed after oral administration and rapidly metabolised to the *N*-desmethyl derivative, which is active. About 27% of a dose is excreted in the urine in 48 h, mostly as 4′-hydroxyphensuximide and its conjugate.

Therapeutic concentration

After a single oral dose of 1 g to 12 subjects, peak plasma concentrations of 10.6 to 15.6 mg/L were attained in 0.5 to 1.5 h [A. J. Glazko and W. A. Dill, Other Succinimides: Methuximide and Phensuximide, in *Antiepileptic Drugs*, D. M. Woodbury *et al.* (Eds.), New York, Raven Press, 1972, pp. 455–464].

Following daily oral doses of 3 g to 5 subjects with intractable seizures, steady-state plasma concentrations of 3.9 to 7.9 mg/L (mean 5.7) of phensuximide and 1.5 to 2.1 mg/L (mean 1.7) of *N*-desmethylphensuximide, were reported [R. J. Porter *et al.*, *Neurology*, 1977, *27*, 1006–1011].

Toxicity. The estimated minimum lethal dose is 5 g.

Half-life. Plasma half-life, 4 to 12 h (mean 8).

Protein binding. In plasma, not significantly bound.

Dose. 0.5 to 3 g daily.

Phentermine

Anorectic

Proprietary names. Duromine; Ionamin(e); Mirapront (all as resin complexes).

α,α-Dimethylbenzeneethanamine

$C_{10}H_{15}N = 149.2$

CAS—122-09-8

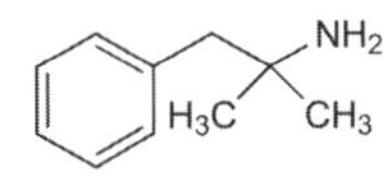

A colourless oily liquid.

Slightly soluble in water; soluble in ethanol, chloroform, and ether.

Note. Phentermine is an isomer of metamfetamine.

Phentermine Hydrochloride

Proprietary names. Adipex-P; Fastin; Panbesy; Pronidin; Umine.

$C_{10}H_{15}N,HCl = 185.7$

CAS—1197-21-3

A white crystalline powder. M.p. 198°.

Very soluble in water, ethanol, and chloroform; practically insoluble in ether.

Dissociation Constant. pK_a 10.1.

Partition Coefficient. Log P (octanol/water), 1.9.

Colour Test. Marquis Test—orange.

Thin-layer Chromatography. System TA—Rf 46; system TB—Rf 26; system TC—Rf 24; system TE—Rf 48; system TL—Rf 12; system TAE—Rf 11; system TAF—Rf 78; system TAJ—Rf 02; system TAK—Rf 05; system TAL—Rf 36. (Acidified iodoplatinate solution, positive.)

Gas Chromatography. System GA—phentermine RI 1155, phentermine-TFA RI 1100, phentermine-PFP RI 1305, phentermine-TMS RI 1195, phentermine-AC RI 1510; system GB—RI 1191; system GC—RI 1450.

High Performance Liquid Chromatography. System HA—k 0.6; system HB—k 19.46; system HC—k 0.86; system HY—RI 245; system HZ—retention time 2.4 min.

Ultraviolet Spectrum. Aqueous acid—247, 251, 257 ($A^1_1 = 13.9$b), 263 nm. No alkaline shift.

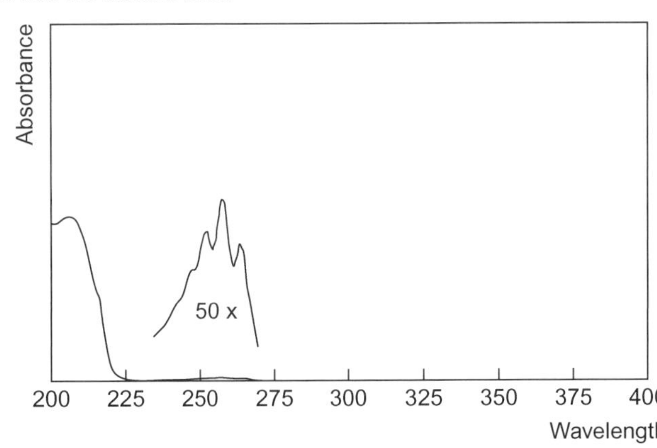

Infra-red Spectrum. Principal peaks at wavenumbers 730, 1285, 705, 1495, 1610, 1510 cm^{-1} (phentermine hydrochloride, KCl disk).

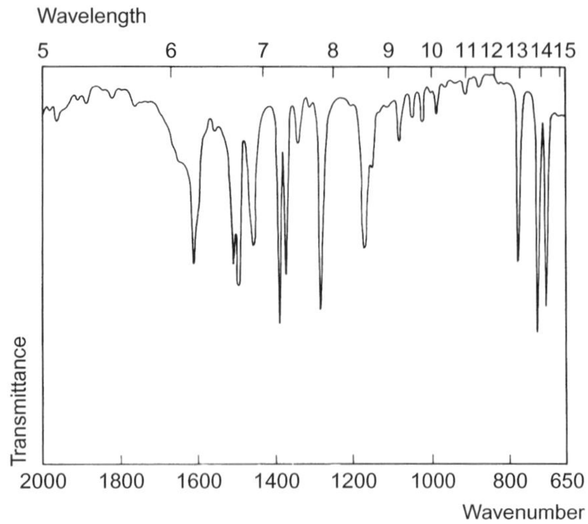

Mass Spectrum. Principal ions at m/z 58, 91, 42, 41, 134, 65, 59, 40.

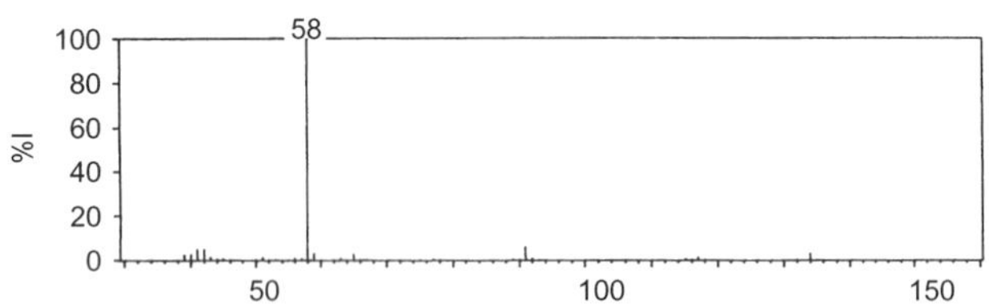

Quantification

Gas chromatography. In blood or urine: amfetamine and phentermine, limit of detection 10 µg/L in blood, FID—J. E. O'Brien *et al.*, *J. Chromatogr. Sci.*, 1972, *10*, 336–341. In urine: phentermine, chlorphentermine, and mephentermine, FID—A. H. Beckett and L. G. Brookes, *J. Pharm. Pharmacol.*, 1971, *23*, 288–294. In urine: phentermine and amfetamines, limit of quantification for phentermine 0.07 mg/L, NPD—J. Jonsson *et al.*, *J. Forensic Sci.*, 1996, *41*, 148–151.

Gas chromatography–mass spectrometry. In urine: phentermine and fenfluramine—R. B. Palmer *et al.*, *Ther. Drug Monit.*, 2000, *22*, 418–422. In urine: phentermine and other amfetamine-related drugs—A. Namera *et al.*, *J. Chromatogr. Sci.*, 2002, *40*, 19–25.

High performance liquid chromatography. In serum or urine: phentermine and other amfetamine-related drugs, limits of detection 0.01 to 0.03 mg/L (UV detection, single wavelength) or 0.05 to 0.1 mg/L (diode-array detection); also MS detection—M. J. Bogusz *et al.*, *J. Anal. Toxicol.*, 1997, *21*, 59–69. In plasma: phentermine and other sympathomimetic amines, limits of detection about 0.3 to 23 pmol, UV detection—A. Kaddoumi *et al.*, *Biomed. Chromatogr.*, 2001, *15*, 379–388. In plasma: phentermine and fenfluramine, fluorescence detection—A. Kaddoumi *et al.*, *J. Chromatogr. B Biomed. Sci. Appl.*, 2001, *763*, 79–90.

High performance liquid chromatography–mass spectrometry. In serum: phentermine and other amfetamine-related drugs, limits of detection 1 to 5 µg/L—M. J. Bogusz *et al.*, *J. Anal. Toxicol.*, 2000, *24*, 77–84.

Disposition in the Body. Readily absorbed after oral administration. About 70 to 80% of a dose is excreted in the urine as unchanged drug in 24 h together with small amounts of the *N*-hydroxy and nitroso metabolites and traces of free and conjugated 4-hydroxyphentermine.
Phentermine is a metabolite of mephentermine.

Therapeutic concentration

The following postmortem tissue concentrations were reported in a subject who had been receiving daily oral doses of 40 mg of a slow-release preparation and who died of natural causes: blood 0.9 mg/L, bile 6.5 mg/L, liver 4 µg/g, urine 50 mg/L. [K. Price, *Bull. Int. Assoc Forensic Toxicol.*, 1974, *10(1)*, 12–13.]

Following single oral doses of 0.375 mg/kg, peak blood concentrations of about 0.1 mg/L were attained in about 4 h. [O. N. Hinsvark *et al.*, *J. Pharmacokinet. Biopharm.*, 1973, *1*, 319–328.]

Toxicity

In a fatality involving the ingestion of phentermine, the following postmortem tissue concentrations were reported: blood 7.6 mg/L, kidney 16 µg/g, liver 14 µg/g, urine 88 mg/L; amylobarbital and ethchlorvynol were also detected in blood at concentrations of 10 mg/L and 12 mg/L, respectively. [B. Levine *et al.*, *J. Forensic Sci.*, 1984, *29*, 1242–1245.]

Half-life. Plasma half-life, about 19 to 24 h.

Volume of distribution. About 3 to 4 L/kg.

Dose. 15 to 30 mg daily as the resin complex; 15 to 37.5 mg daily as the hydrochloride.

Phentolamine

Antihypertensive

Synonym. C-7337
3-[[(4,5-Dihydro-1*H*-imidazol-2-yl)methyl](4-methylphenyl)amino]-phenol
$C_{17}H_{19}N_3O = 281.4$
CAS—50-60-2

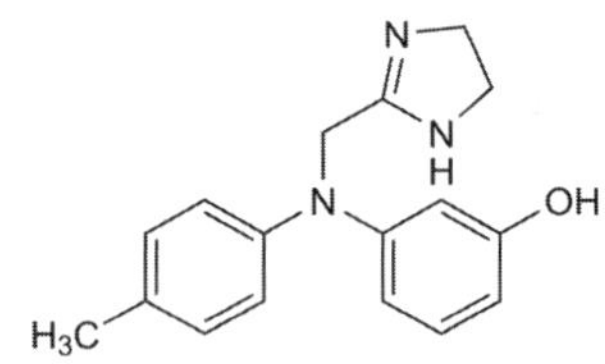

A white crystalline powder. M.p. 174° to 175°.

Phentolamine Hydrochloride

$C_{17}H_{19}N_3O,HCl = 317.8$
CAS—73-05-2
A white or faintly cream-coloured crystalline powder. M.p. 239° to 240°. Soluble 1 in 50 of water and 1 in about 70 of ethanol; very slightly soluble in chloroform and ether; practically insoluble in acetone. Solutions in water foam on shaking.

Phentolamine Mesilate

Synonyms. Phentolamine Mesylate; Phentolamine Methanesulfonate.
Proprietary names. Q-Tech; Regitine; Rogitine; Z-Max.
$C_{17}H_{19}N_3O,CH_3SO_3H = 377.5$
CAS—65-28-1
A white, slightly hygroscopic, crystalline powder. M.p. 177° to 181°. Soluble 1 in 1 of water, 1 in 4 of ethanol, and 1 in 700 of chloroform.

Dissociation Constant. pK_a 7.7.

Partition Coefficient. Log *P* (octanol/water), 3.4.

Colour Tests. Mandelin's Test—blue-green; Marquis Test—yellow.

Thin-layer Chromatography. System TA—Rf 32; system TB—Rf 01; system TC—Rf 03; system TE—Rf 33; system TL—Rf 02; system TAE—Rf 06; system TAJ—Rf 00; system TAK—Rf 01; system TAL—Rf 34. (Acidified iodoplatinate solution, positive.)

Gas Chromatography. System GA—not eluted.

High Performance Liquid Chromatography. System HA—*k* 1.7; system HX—RI 368; system HZ—Retention time 3 min.

Ultraviolet Spectrum. Aqueous acid—278 nm; aqueous alkali—291 nm.

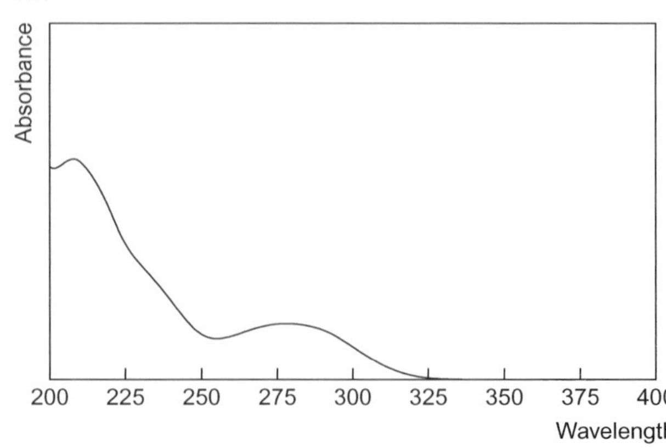

Infra-red Spectrum. Principal peaks at wavenumbers 1195, 1508, 1610, 1580, 1592, 1247 cm^{-1} (KBr disk). (See below)

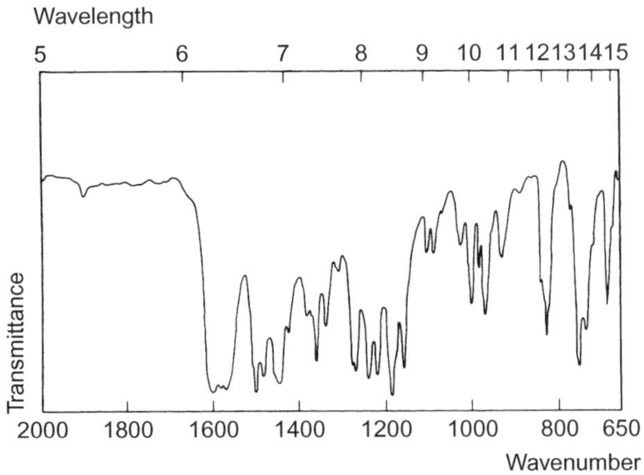

Mass Spectrum. Principal ions at m/z 281, 120, 91, 122, 280, 160, 68, 282.

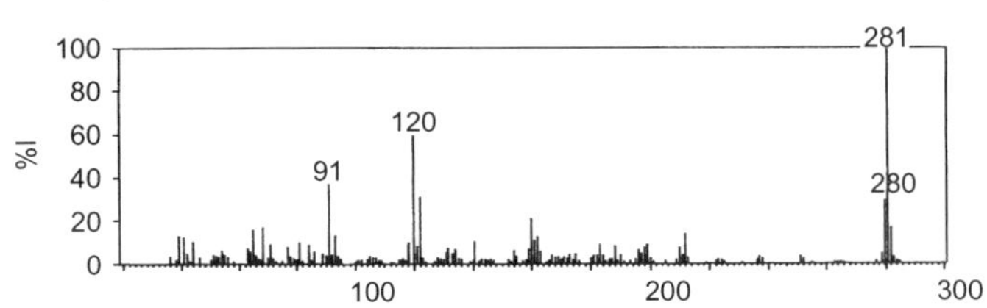

Quantification

Gas chromatography. In plasma or urine: phentolamine and conjugates, limits of detection 5 µg/L (phentolamine in plasma) and 25 µg/L (phentolamine and conjugates in urine), ECD—A. Sioufi *et al.*, *J. Chromatogr.*, 1981, *222*, 429–435.

High performance liquid chromatography. In plasma or urine: phentolamine metabolite, limit of detection 200 µg/L, UV detection—J. Godbillon and G. Carnis, *J. Chromatogr.*, 1981, *222*, 461–466.

Dose. 5 to 10 mg of phentolamine mesilate intravenously. Phentolamine hydrochloride has been given in doses of 200 to 300 mg daily, by mouth.

Phenylbutazone

Analgesic

Synonyms. Butadione; Fenilbutazona.
Proprietary names. Aflamina; Ambene; Basireuma; Bresal; Buta; Butacote; Butadion; Butazolidina; Butazolidin(e); Butazolon; Butazona; Butazone; Butazonil; Carudol; Delbulasa; Demoplas; exrheudon OPT; Feniben; Fezona; Inflazone; Kadol; Peralgin; Rudesol; Tisatin.
4-Butyl-1,2-diphenyl-3,5-pyrazolidinedione
$C_{19}H_{20}N_2O_2$ = 308.4
CAS—50-33-9

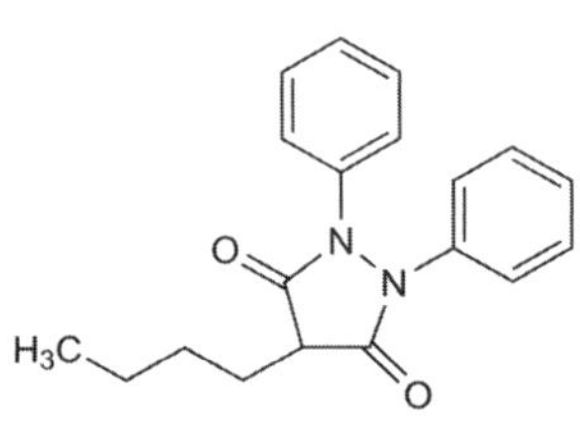

A fine, white, crystalline powder. M.p. 105°.
Practically insoluble in water; soluble 1 in 28 of ethanol, 1 in 1.25 of chloroform, and 1 in 15 of ether; freely soluble in acetone; soluble in alkaline solutions.

Dissociation Constant. pK_a 4.4 (20°).

Partition Coefficient. Log P (octanol/pH 7.4), 0.7; (octanol/water), 3.2.

Colour Tests. Liebermann's Test (100°)—brown; Mandelin's Test—violet.

Thin-layer Chromatography. System TA—Rf 79; system TD—Rf 78; system TE—Rf 65; system TF—Rf 68; system TG—Rf 23; system TAD—Rf 76; system TAE—Rf 87; system TAJ—Rf 90; system TAK—Rf 76; system TAL—Rf 97. (Chromic acid solution, brown; Ludy Tenger reagent, orange; mercurous nitrate spray, positive; acidified potassium permanganate solution, positive.)

Gas Chromatography. System GA—phenylbutazone RI 2367, phenylbutazone-Me RI 2290, oxyphenbutazone not eluted; system GB—RI 2472; system GD—phenylbutazone RRT 2.05 and 1.81, oxyphenbutazone RRT 2.11, both as methyl derivatives relative to n-$C_{16}H_{34}$; system GF—RI 2860; system GL—phenylbutazone-Me RI 2290, M (OH-alkyl)-Me RI 2500.

High Performance Liquid Chromatography. System HD—phenylbutazone k 6.5; oxyphenbutazone k 1.95; system HV—phenylbutazone RRT 0.95; oxyphenbutazone RRT 0.7, both relative to meclofenamic acid; system HX—phenylbutazone RI 672; oxyphenbutazone RI 501; system HY—phenylbutazone RI 643; oxyphenbutazone RI 459; system HZ—phenylbutazone Retention time 19.5 min oxyphenbutazone 6.7 min; system HAA—Retention time 24.1 min.

Ultraviolet Spectrum. Aqueous acid—237 (A^1_1=456a); aqueous alkali—264 nm (A^1_1=660a).

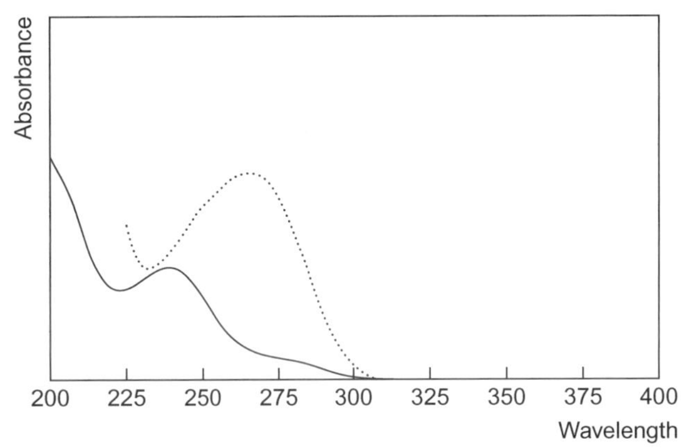

Infra-red Spectrum. Principal peaks at wavenumbers 1714, 1300, 1755, 755, 1492, 1275 cm^{-1} (KBr disk).

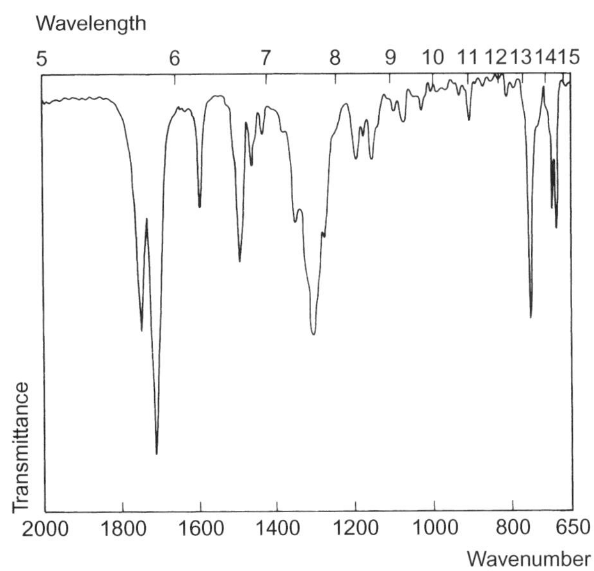

Mass Spectrum. Principal ions at m/z 77, 183, 308, 184, 105, 55, 51, 41; oxyphenbutazone 199, 324, 93, 77, 65, 55, 121, 135.

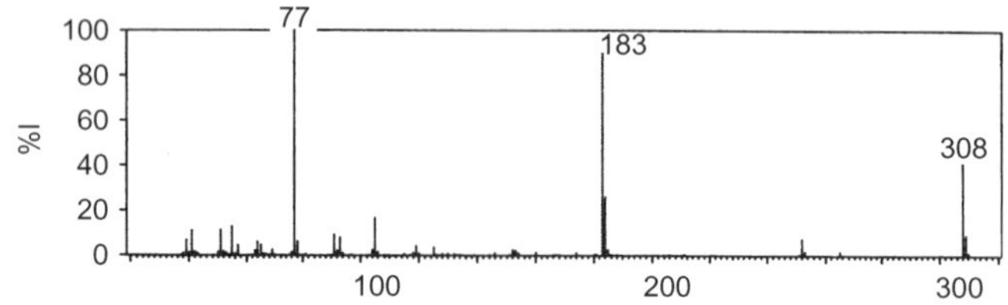

Quantification

Gas chromatography. In blood, plasma, bile, or urine: limit of detection 1 mg/L—R. D. Budd, *J. Chromatogr.*, 1982, *243*, 368–371. In plasma: sensitivity 10 µg/L, ECD—A. Sioufi *et al.*, *J. Pharm. Sci.*, 1978, *67*, 243–245.

High performance liquid chromatography. In plasma or urine: phenylbutazone, oxyphenbutazone and 3′-hydroxyphenylbutazone, limit of detection 50 µg/L, UV detection—T. Marunaka *et al.*, *J. Chromatogr.*, 1980, *183*; *B Biomed. Appl.*, *9*, 331–338. In plasma: phenylbutazone, oxyphenbutazone and 3′-hydroxyphenylbutazone, limit of detection 5.5 mg/L for phenylbutazone, UV detection—L. Aarons and C. Higham, *Clinica Chim. Acta*, 1980, *105*, 377–382. In plasma: phenylbutazone and other NSAIDs, UV detection—S. G. Owen *et al.*, *J. Chromatogr.*, 1987, *416*, 293–302. In plasma: phenylbutazone, oxyphenbutazone and other NSAIDs, limit of detection 0.05 mg/L, UV detection—M. C. Caturla and E. Cusido, *J. Chromatogr.*, 1992, *581*, 101–107. In serum: phenylbutazone and oxyphenbutazone, limits of detection 0.1 mg/L and 1 mg/L respectively, UV detection—B. R. Simmons *et al.*, *J. Pharm. Biomed. Anal.*, 1995, *13*, 59–64.

Disposition in the Body. Readily absorbed after oral or rectal administration and slowly absorbed after IM injection. The major metabolic reactions are *C*-glucuronidation at the 4-position of the pyrazolidine ring and 4-hydroxylation of one of the phenyl rings to form the active metabolite, oxyphenbutazone; 3-hydroxylation of the butyl side-chain to form 3′-hydroxyphenylbutazone, and formation of 4,3′-dihydroxyphenylbutazone also occur. About 61% of a dose is slowly excreted in the urine over a period of about 21 days, together with up to 27% in the faeces. Of the material excreted in the urine, the 4-*C*-glucuronide of phenylbutazone accounts for about 40%, free phenylbutazone and free oxyphenbutazone about 1%, 4,3′-dihydroxyphenylbutazone about 6%, 3′-hydroxyphenylbutazone about 3%, and the remainder consists of the *C*-glucuronide of 3′-hydroxyphenylbutazone (about 12%), oxyphenbutazone *O*-glucuronide and two other metabolites.

Therapeutic concentration. In plasma, usually in the range 50 to 100 mg/L.

Following single oral doses of 100, 300 and 600 mg to 6 subjects, peak plasma concentrations of 12.5 to 17.1 mg/L (mean 14), 30.8 to 46.3 mg/L (mean 38), and 51.2 to 88.1 mg/L (mean 75), respectively, were obtained in 1 to 7 h (mean 3) [A. Sioufi *et al.*, *J. Pharm. Sci.*, 1980, *69*, 1413–1416].

After daily oral doses of 100, 200, and 300 mg to 7 subjects, mean steady-state plasma concentrations of 52, 83, and 95 mg/L respectively were reported; in 3 subjects given 400 mg daily, the mean steady-state concentration was 99 mg/L [M. Orme *et al.*, *Br. J. Clin. Pharmacol.*, 1976, *3*, 185–191].

Following daily oral doses of 200 mg to 1 subject for 7 days, the following plasma concentrations were found: phenylbutazone about 50 mg/L, oxyphenbutazone about 20 mg/L, and 3′-hydroxyphenylbutazone about 12 mg/L [K. K. Midha *et al.*, *J. Pharm. Sci.*, 1974, *63*, 1751–1754].

Toxicity. The estimated minimum lethal dose is 5 g. Toxic effects during treatment are frequent and may occur even when the dose does not exceed 400 mg daily; they are usually associated with plasma concentrations above 100 mg/L. A considerable number of deaths have occurred, especially from blood disorders.

In a fatality due to an accidental overdose by a 5-year-old child, the following postmortem concentrations were reported: blood 400 mg/L, bile 475 mg/L, kidney 250 µg/g, liver 250 µg/g [K. L. Lam and K. Chien, *Bull. Int. Assoc. Forensic Toxicol.*, 1976, *12*(2), 20].

A plasma concentration of 670 mg/L was reported in one subject, one day after ingestion of 8 g. The concentration of phenylbutazone declined rapidly with a half-life of 23 h but concentrations of 3′-hydroxyphenylbutazone were unusually high and exceeded those of unchanged drug after 48 h; the subject recovered after about 3 days [L. F. Prescott *et al.*, *BMJ*, 1980, *281*, 1106–1107].

A racetrack worker ingested at least 17 g of phenylbutazone (intended for equine use) over a 24-h period in an attempt to treat toothache. He had a serum-phenylbutazone concentration of 900 mg/L and a serum-oxyphenbutazone concentration of 60 mg/L approximately 8 h after presentation [T. A. Newton and S. R. Rose, *Ann. Emerg. Med.*, 1991, *20*, 204–207].

Half-life. Plasma half-life, phenylbutazone 2 to 5 days (mean 3), but dose-dependent and increased in subjects with renal failure and in the elderly; oxyphenbutazone about 2 to 3 days, 3′-hydroxyphenylbutazone about 32 h.

Distribution in blood. Plasma : whole blood ratio, 1.8.

Protein binding. In plasma, about 99% at therapeutic concentrations; decreased at higher concentrations when the binding sites become saturated.

Note. For a review of the pharmacokinetics of phenylbutazone see J. Aarbakke, *Clin. Pharmacokinet.*, 1978, *3*, 369–380.

Dose. Initially 300 to 600 mg daily; maintenance, 100 to 400 mg daily.

Phenylephrine

Sympathomimetic

Synonyms. Néosynéphrine; *m*-Synephrine.
Note. Synephrine has been used as a synonym for oxedrine.
Proprietary name. It is an ingredient of Vibrocil.
(αR)-3-Hydroxy-α-[(methylamino)methyl]benzenemethanol
$C_9H_{13}NO_2$=167.2
CAS—59-42-7

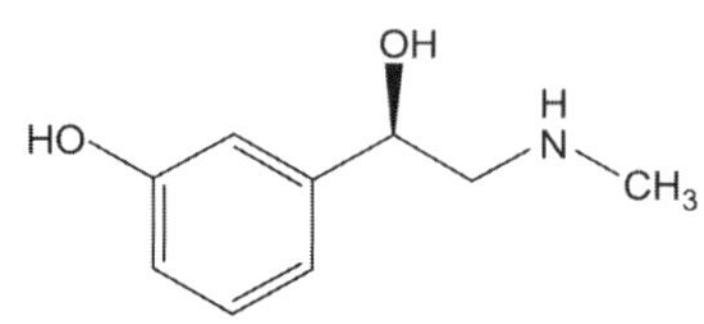

A white or almost white crystalline powder. M.p. about 174°.
Slightly soluble in water and ethanol; sparingly soluble in methanol; soluble in dilute mineral acids and solutions of alkali hydroxides.

Phenylephrine Hydrochloride

Synonyms. Mesatonum; Metaoxedrini Chloridum.
Proprietary names. Ak-Dilate; Ak-Nefrin; Albalon; Analux; Dionephrine; Fenox; Isonefrine; Isopto Frin; Mydfrin; Neofrin; Neo-Mydrial; Neo-Synephrine; Ocu-Phrin; Phenoptic; Prefrin; Rectacaine; Releif; Rhinall; Rico-bid D; Sinex; Visadron; Vistafrin. It is an ingredient of many preparations for the relief of nasal congestion – see *Martindale: The complete drug reference*, 33rd Edn., Pharmaceutical Press, London, 2002 or the latest edition of the *British National Formulary*, BMA and RPSGB, London.
$C_9H_{13}NO_2$,HCl=203.7
CAS—61-76-7
A white crystalline powder. M.p. 140° to 145°. A solution in water is laevorotatory.
Soluble 1 in 2 of water and 1 in 4 of ethanol.

Dissociation Constant. pK_a 8.9 (–OH), 10.1 (–NH–), (20°).

Partition Coefficient. Log *P* (octanol/water), –0.3.

Colour Tests. Mandelin's Test—brown; Marquis Test—red.

Thin-layer Chromatography. System TA—Rf 33; system TB—Rf 01; system TC—Rf 01; system TE—Rf 12; system TL—Rf 00; system TAE—Rf 08; system TAF—Rf 67; system TAJ—Rf 00; system TAK—Rf 00; system TAL—Rf 22. (Acidified potassium permanganate solution, positive.)

Gas Chromatography. System GC—RI 1934.

High Performance Liquid Chromatography. System HA—*k* 1.3; system HC—*k* 1.6; system HX—RI 80; system HY—RI 79.

Ultraviolet Spectrum. Aqueous acid—273 (A^1_1=110a); aqueous alkali—238 (A^1_1=534a), 291 nm (A^1_1=182a). (See below)

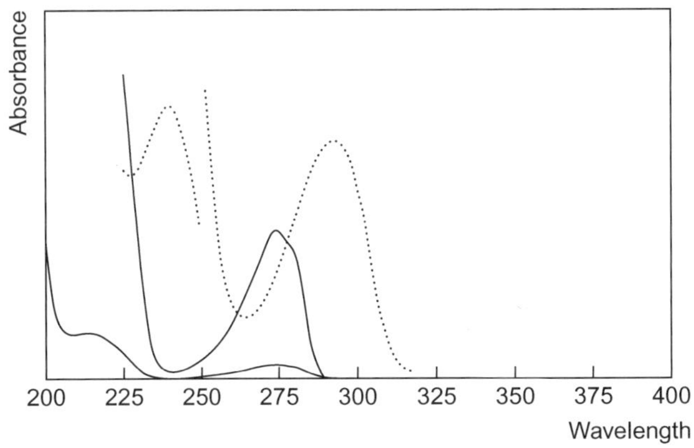

Infra-red Spectrum. Principal peaks at wavenumbers 1594, 1273, 784, 696, 1304, 900 cm^{-1} (phenylephrine hydrochloride, KBr disk). (See below)

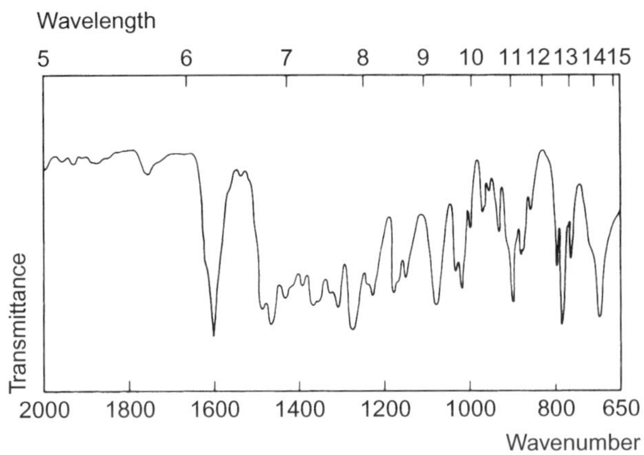

Mass Spectrum. Principal ions at *m/z* 44, 76, 77, 29, 45, 42, 95, 65.

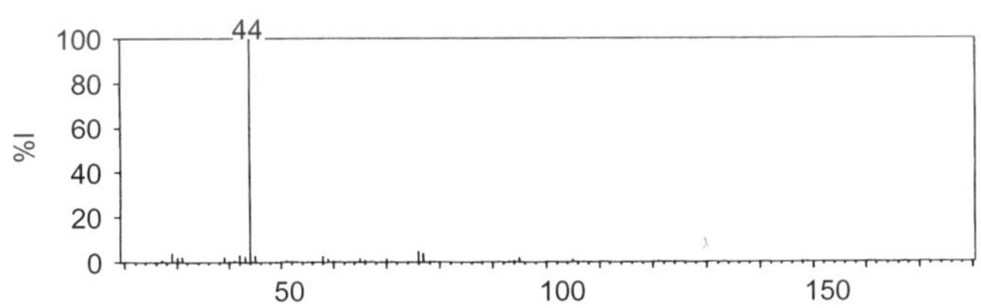

Quantification

Gas chromatography. In plasma: limit of detection 12.5 μg/L, ECD—L. J. Dombrowski *et al.*, *J. Pharm. Sci.*, 1973, *62*, 1761–1763.

Gas chromatography–mass spectrometry. In urine: phenylephrine and four metabolites—K. E. Ibrahim *et al.*, *J. Pharm. Pharmacol.*, 1983, *35*, 144–147.

High performance liquid chromatography. In plasma: limit of detection 0.5 μg/L, fluorescence detection—D. S. Chien and R. D. Schoenwald, *J. Pharm. Sci.*, 1985, *74*, 562–564. In serum: limit of detection 5 μg/L, fluorescence detection—M. Yamaguchi *et al.*, *J. Chromatogr. B Biomed. Appl.*, 1994, *661*, 93–99. In plasma: phenylephrine and its conjugates, limits of detection 2 μg/L for phenylephrine and 25 μg/L for its conjugates, electrochemical detection—K. Gumbhir and W. D. Mason, *J. Pharm. Biomed. Anal.*, 1996, *14*, 623–630. In serum: limit of detection about 0.3 μg/L, coulometric detection—V. Vuma and I. Kanfer, *J. Chromatogr. B Biomed. Appl.*, 1996, *678*, 245–252. In aqueous humour: phenylephrine and tropicamide, UV detection—M. J. Galmier *et al.*, *Biomed. Chromatogr.*, 2000, *14*, 202–204.

Disposition in the Body. Readily absorbed after oral administration, but undergoes extensive first-pass metabolism; bioavailability about 38%. It is metabolised by conjugation with sulfate and glucuronic acid and by oxidative deamination to *m*-hydroxymandelic acid (MHMA) and *m*-hydroxyphenylglycol (MHPG). About 80% of an oral dose is excreted in the urine in 24 h, mainly as sulfate conjugates of phenylephrine and MHPG; about 30% of a dose is excreted as unconjugated MHMA.

Therapeutic concentration

After a single oral dose of 9 mg of ^3H-labelled phenylephrine hydrochloride to 6 subjects, peak plasma concentrations of 0.23 to 0.47 mg/L (mean 0.31) of total phenylephrine and metabolites were attained in 1 to 2 h [C. J. Cavallito *et al.*, *J. Pharm. Sci.*, 1963, *52*, 259–263].

Following a single oral dose of 1 mg to 3 subjects, a mean peak plasma concentration of unconjugated phenylephrine of 0.0009 mg/L was attained in about 1.3 h [J. H. Hengstmann and J. Goronzy, *Eur. J. Clin. Pharmacol.*, 1982, *21*, 335–341].

Toxicity. The estimated minimum lethal dose, for children up to 2 years is 100 mg intranasally and for adults is 1 g.

Half-life. Plasma half-life, about 2 to 3 h.

Volume of distribution. About 5 L/kg.

Clearance. Plasma clearance, about 30 mL/min/kg.

Dose. 30 to 40 mg of phenylephrine hydrochloride daily, by mouth.

Phenylmethylbarbituric Acid

Barbiturate/ Anticonvulsant

Synonym. Heptobarbitalum (distinguish from Heptabarbital).
Proprietary name. Rutonal
5-Methyl-5-phenyl-2,4,6(1*H*,3*H*,5*H*)-pyrimidinetrione
$C_{11}H_{10}N_2O_3$=218.2
CAS—76-94-8

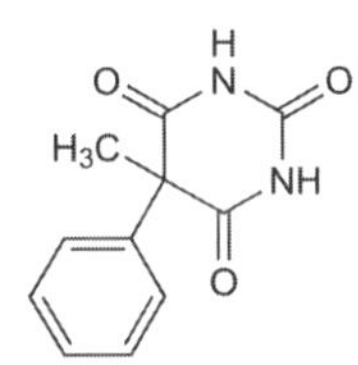

A white crystalline powder. M.p. about 226°.
Practically insoluble in water; soluble 1 in 60 of ethanol; soluble in ether and aqueous solutions of alkalis.

Dissociation Constant. pK_a 7.7 (25°).

Partition Coefficient. Log *P* (octanol/water), 0.9.

Colour Test. Liebermann's Test—red-orange.

Thin-layer Chromatography. System TD—Rf 29; system TE—Rf 24; system TF—Rf 61; system TH—Rf 27. (Mercurous nitrate spray, black; Zwikker's reagent, pink.)

Gas Chromatography. System GA—phenylmethylbarbituric acid RI 1880, phenylmethylbarbituric acid-Me_2 RI 1790; system GAJ—RRT 1.087 (relative to methylphenobarbital).

High Performance Liquid Chromatography. System HG—*k* 1.5; system HH—*k* 0.9.

Ultraviolet Spectrum. Borax buffer 0.05 M (pH 9.2)—238 nm (A^1_1=494b); M sodium hydroxide (pH 13)—253 nm (A^1_1=350b).

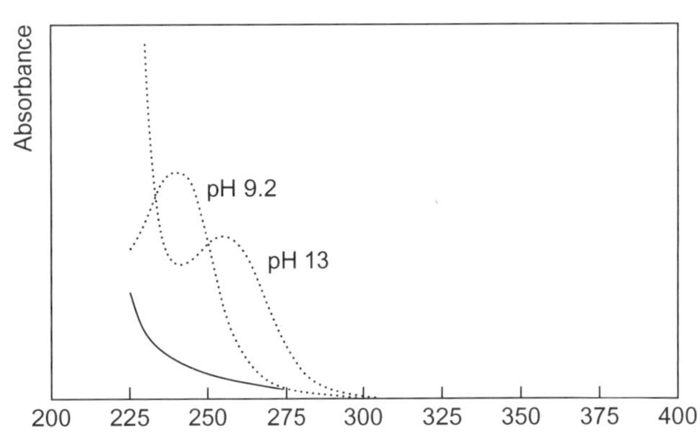

Infra-red Spectrum. Principal peaks at wavenumbers 1702, 1720, 1751, 1240, 802, 716 cm^{-1}.

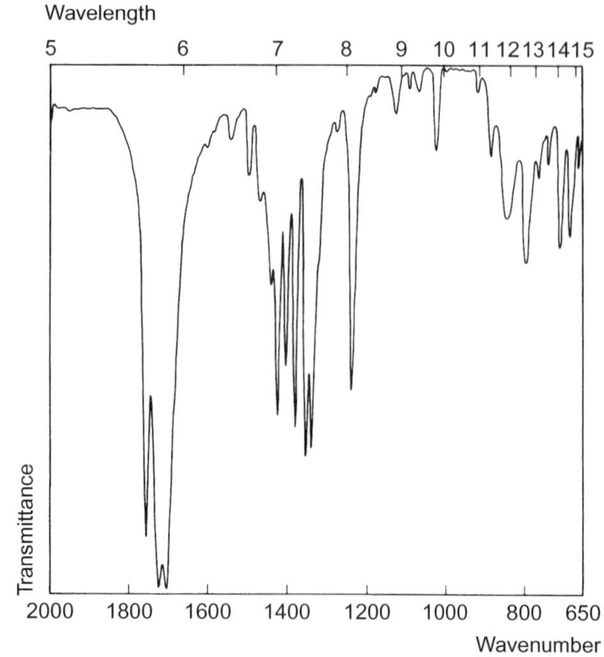

Mass Spectrum. Principal ions at *m/z* 104, 132, 218, 51, 103, 77, 78, 52.

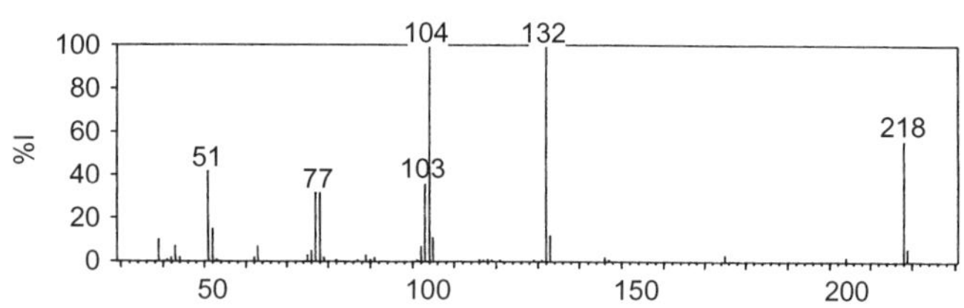

Dose. Phenylmethylbarbituric acid has been given in doses of 400 mg daily.

Phenylpropanolamine *Sympathomimetic*

Synonym. DL-Norephedrine
(αS)-*rel*-α-[(1*R*)-1-Aminoethyl]benzenemethanol
$C_9H_{13}NO = 151.2$
CAS—14838-15-4

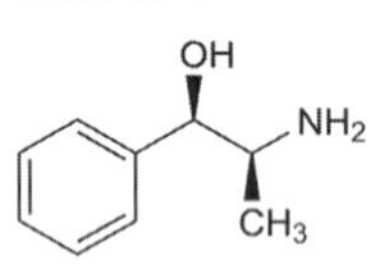

(+)-Form

M.p. about 101°.

Phenylpropanolamine Hydrochloride

Synonym. Mydriatin
Proprietary names. Acutrim; Appedrine; Capton Diet; Centapp; Control; Dexatrim; Fansia; Fasupond; Just One Per Day; Kontexin; Merex; Monydrin; Phenoxine; Phenyldrine; Procol; Propagest; Recatol mono; Restaslim; Rinexin; Slimomin; Spray-U-Thin; Stay Trim; Unitrol. It is an ingredient of many preparations for the relief of cold and cough symptoms – see *Martindale: The complete drug reference*, 33rd Edn., Pharmaceutical Press, London, 2002 or the latest edition of the *British National Formulary*, BMA and RPSGB, London.
$C_9H_{13}NO,HCl = 187.7$
CAS—154-41-6
A white to creamy-white crystalline powder. M.p. 190° to 194°.

Soluble 1 in 1 of water and 1 in about 7 of ethanol; practically insoluble in chloroform and ether.

Dissociation Constant. pK_a 9.4 (20°).

Partition Coefficient. Log *P* (octanol/water), 0.7.

Thin-layer Chromatography. System TA—Rf 44; system TB—Rf 04; system TC—Rf 04; system TAJ—Rf 01; system TAK—Rf 02; system TAL—Rf 29. (Dragendorff spray, positive; FPN reagent, violet; acidified iodoplatinate solution, positive; Marquis reagent, yellow; ninhydrin spray, positive; acidified potassium permanganate solution, positive.)

Gas Chromatography. System GA—RI 1313; system GB—RI 1353; system GC—RI 1383.

High Performance Liquid Chromatography. System HA—*k* 0.9; system HB—*k* 3.9; system HC—*k* 0.7; system HY—RI 201.

Ultraviolet Spectrum. Aqueous acid—251, 257 ($A^1_1 = 11.7a$), 262 nm. No alkaline shift.

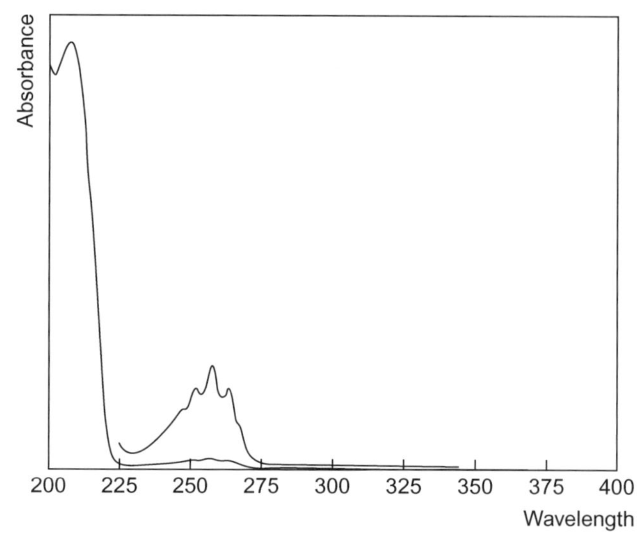

Infra-red Spectrum. Principal peaks at wavenumbers 700, 746, 1030, 1500, 1055, 1590 cm^{-1} (phenylpropanolamine hydrochloride, KBr disk).

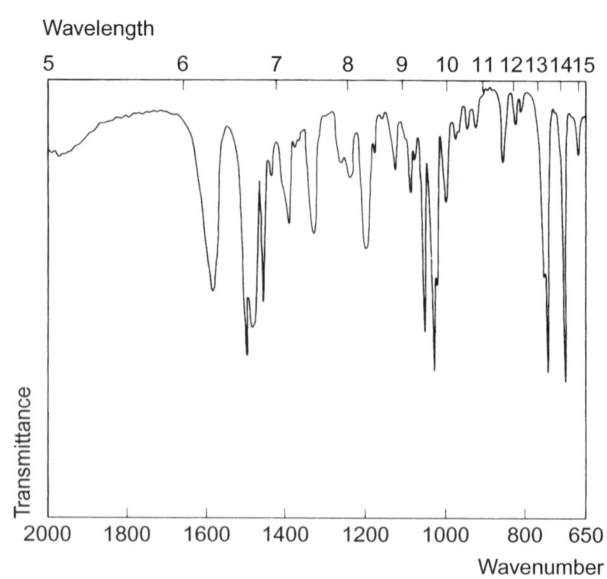

Mass Spectrum. Principal ions at *m/z* 44, 77, 79, 51, 45, 42, 107, 105.

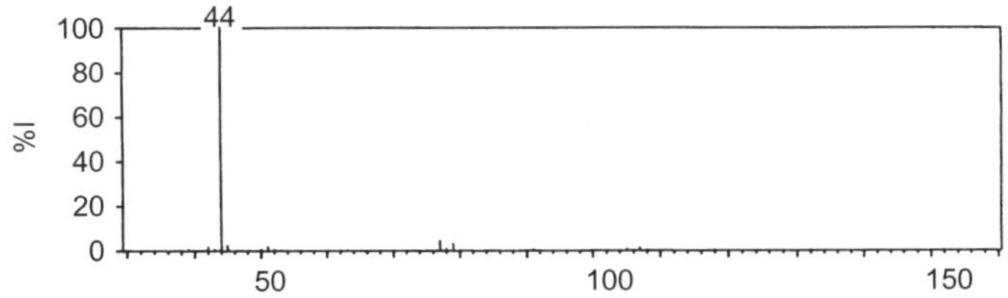

Quantification

Gas chromatography. In plasma: limit of detection 1 µg/L, ECD—N. Crisologo *et al.*, *J. Pharm. Sci.*, 1984, *73*, 1313–1315.

High performance liquid chromatography. In plasma: limit of detection 5 µg/L, fluorescence detection—W. D. Mason and E. N. Amick, *J. Pharm. Sci.*, 1981, *70*, 707–709. In plasma or urine: limits of detection 0.4 µg/L and 8 µg/L respectively, UV detection—K. Yamashita *et al.*, *J. Chromatogr.*, 1990, *527*, 103–114. In plasma: phenylpropanolamine enantiomers, limit of detection <10 µg/L, UV detection—C. S. Stockley *et al.*, *Ther. Drug Monit.*, 1991, *13*, 332–338.

Disposition in the Body. Absorbed after oral administration. More than 90% of a dose is excreted in the urine as unchanged drug in 24 h, together with small amounts of hippuric acid. Phenylpropanolamine is a metabolite of amfetamine, diethylpropion, and ephedrine.

Therapeutic concentration

Following a single oral dose of 25 mg to 12 subjects, a mean peak plasma concentration of about 0.08 mg/L was attained in about 2 h [W. D. Mason and E. N. Amick, *J. Pharm. Sci.*, 1981, *70*, 707–709].

Toxicity

In a fatality due to a phenylpropanolamine overdose, the following postmortem tissue concentrations were reported: blood 48 mg/L, brain 86 µg/g, liver 460 µg/g [R. H. Cravey, per R. C. Baselt, *Disposition of Toxic Chemicals and Drugs in Man*, 5th Edn, Davis, California, Biomedical Publications, 2002, pp. 700–702].

A 9-month-old infant died due to non-intentional overdosage with over-the-counter cough and cold preparations. Postmortem analysis revealed the following phenylpropanolamine levels: heart blood 1.4 mg/L, liver 0.5 mg/kg; elevated blood levels of pseudoephedrine and dextromethorphan were also found [V. L. Gunn *et al.*, *Pediatrics*, 2001, *108*, e52].

Half-life. Plasma half-life, about 4 h.

Dose. 75 to 200 mg of phenylpropanolamine hydrochloride daily.

Phenyltoloxamine

Antihistamine

Synonyms. Phenyltolyloxamine; PRN; C-5581H.
Proprietary name. It is an ingredient of Pholtex.
N,*N*-Dimethyl-2-[2-(phenylmethyl)phenoxy]ethanamine
$C_{17}H_{21}NO=255.4$
CAS—92-12-6

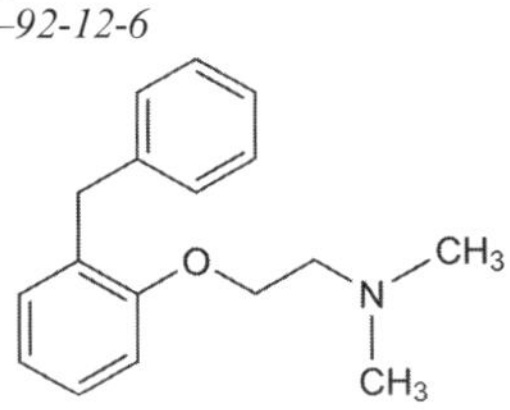

An oily liquid.
Note. Phenyltoloxamine is a structural isomer of diphenhydramine.

Phenyltoloxamine Citrate

Proprietary names. It is an ingredient of Aceta-Gesic, Anabar, Codipront, Comhist LA, Mobigesic, Momentum, Naldecon, Nalex-A, Percogesic, Phenylgesic, Poly-Histine, Sinutab Nightime, and Tetra-Mag.
$C_{17}H_{21}NO,C_6H_8O_7=447.5$
CAS—1176-08-5
Crystals. M.p. 138° to 140°.
Soluble in water.

Dissociation Constant. pK_a 9.1.

Partition Coefficient. Log *P* (octanol/water), 3.8.

Colour Tests. Mandelin's Test—green; Marquis Test—violet.

Thin-layer Chromatography. System TA—Rf 53; system TB—Rf 38; system TC—Rf 48; system TE—Rf 67; system TL—Rf 15; system TAE—Rf 32; system TAJ—Rf 27; system TAK—Rf 15; system TAL—Rf 69. (Acidified iodoplatinate solution, positive.)

Gas Chromatography. System GA—phenyltoloxamine RI 1940; M ((*N*-oxide)-ME_2 NOH) RI 1500; M (nor-) RI 2140; M (O-desalkyl-) RI 1680; M (O-desalkyl-OH-) RI 2220; M (OH-) isomer 1 RI 2280; M (OH-) isomer 2 RI 2300; M (nor-OH-) isomer 1 RI 2320; M (nor-OH-) isomer 2 RI 2340; M (OH-methoxy-) RI 2320; M (desamino-OH-) RI 1830; system GB—phenyltoloxamine RI 2030; M ((*N*-oxide)-ME_2 NOH) RI 1580; M (nor-) RI 2002; M (O-desalkyl-) RI 1724; M (nor-OH-) isomer 1 RI 2398; M (nor-OH-) isomer 2 RI 2402; M (desamino-OH-) RI 1928.

High Performance Liquid Chromatography. System HA—*k* 3.1; system HX—RI 415.

Ultraviolet Spectrum. Aqueous acid—270 (A^1_1=73b), 276 nm.

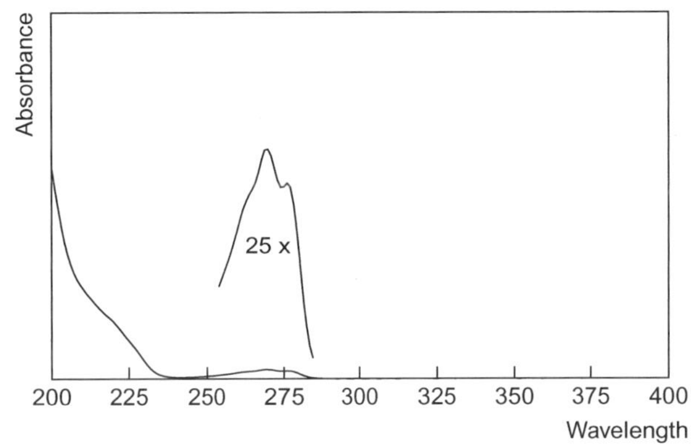

Infra-red Spectrum. Principal peaks at wavenumbers 1245, 1491, 752, 1030, 697, 1111 cm^{-1} (KBr disk).

Mass Spectrum. Principal ions at *m/z* 58, 255, 42, 71, 59, 44, 181, 165.

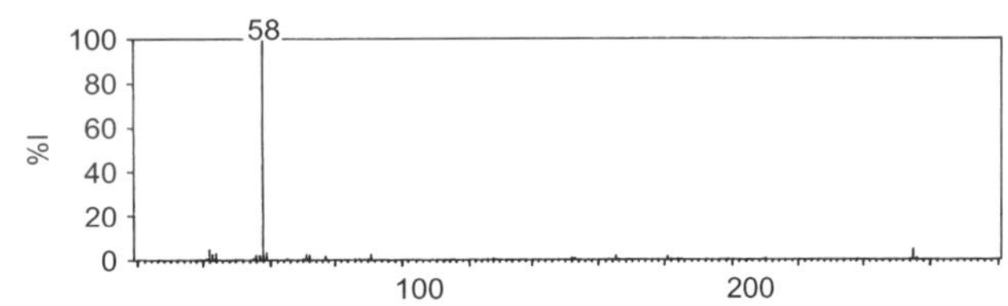

Dose. 75 to 200 mg of phenyltoloxamine citrate daily.

Phenytoin

Anticonvulsant

Synonyms. Diphenylhydantoin; Fenitoína; Phenantoinum; Phenytoinum.
Proprietary names. Aurantin; Dantoin; Di-Hydan; Dilantin; Diphantoine; Diphenylan; Epanutin; Epelin; Epilan-D; Epilantine; Epinat; Hidantal; Hydantin; Neosidantoina; Phenhydan; Pyorédol; Sinergina; Zentropil.
5,5-Diphenyl-2,4-imidazolidinedione
$C_{15}H_{12}N_2O_2=252.3$
CAS—57-41-0

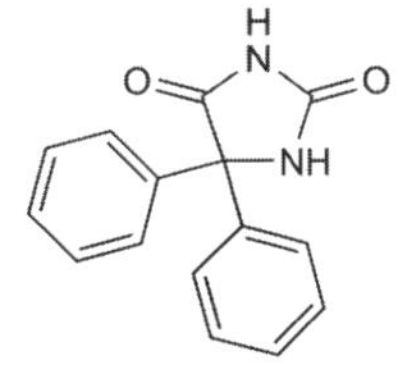

A white crystalline powder. M.p. 295° to 298°.
Practically insoluble in water; soluble 1 in about 60 of ethanol, 1 in 500 of chloroform, 1 in about 30 of acetone, and 1 in 600 of ether; soluble in solutions of alkali hydroxides.

Phenytoin Sodium

Synonyms. Diphenin; Phenytoinum Natricum; Sodium Diphenylhydantoin; Soluble Phenytoin.

Proprietary name. Phenytoin sodium is an ingredient of Garoin.
$C_{15}H_{11}N_2NaO_2$=274.3
CAS—630-93-3
A white, slightly hygroscopic, crystalline powder which on exposure to air absorbs carbon dioxide with the liberation of phenytoin.
Soluble 1 in about 66 of water and 1 in 10.5 of alcohol; practically insoluble in chloroform and ether. In aqueous solution it is partly hydrolysed to the base and turbidity develops.

Dissociation Constant. pK_a 8.3 (25°).

Partition Coefficient. Log *P* (octanol/water), 2.5.

Colour Tests. Koppanyi–Zwikker Test—violet; Liebermann's Test—red-orange; Mercurous Nitrate—black.

Thin-layer Chromatography. System TD—Rf 33; system TE—Rf 41; system TF—Rf 55; system TAD—Rf 53; system TAE—Rf 86; system TAJ—Rf 48; system TAK—Rf 84; system TAL—Rf 96. (Mercuric chloride–diphenylcarbazone reagent, positive; mercurous nitrate spray, black.)

Gas Chromatography. System GA—phenytoin RI 2320, M (OH-) RI 2795, phenytoin-Me RI 2245, M (4-OH-)-Me_2 RI 2720, M (4-OH-methoxy-) RI 2770, M (4-OH-methoxy-)-Me_2 RI 2740. Phenytoin is used as the reference substance in system GE.

High Performance Liquid Chromatography. System HE—*k* 9.71; system HX—RI 431; system HY—RI 381; system HZ—retention time 3.7 min; system HAA—retention time 16.3 min; system HAK—not detected; system HAM—retention time 3.5 min; system HAX—retention time 6.1 min; system HAY—retention time 5.3 min; system HAZ—*k* 0.60.

Ultraviolet Spectrum. Methanol—258 (A^1_1=27a), 264 nm (A^1_1=16a).

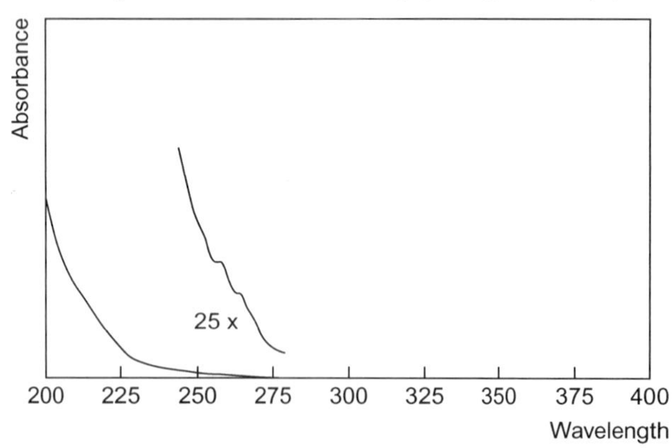

Infra-red Spectrum. Principal peaks at wavenumbers 1720, 1740, 1774, 748, 698, 785 cm^{-1} (KBr disk).

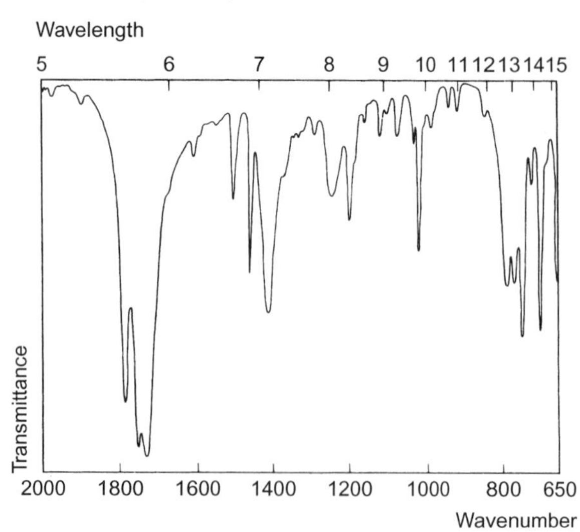

Mass Spectrum. Principal ions at *m/z* 180, 104, 223, 77, 209, 252, 51, 165; 5-(4-hydroxyphenyl)-5-phenylhydantoin 239, 196, 268, 120, 197, 225, 77, 104.

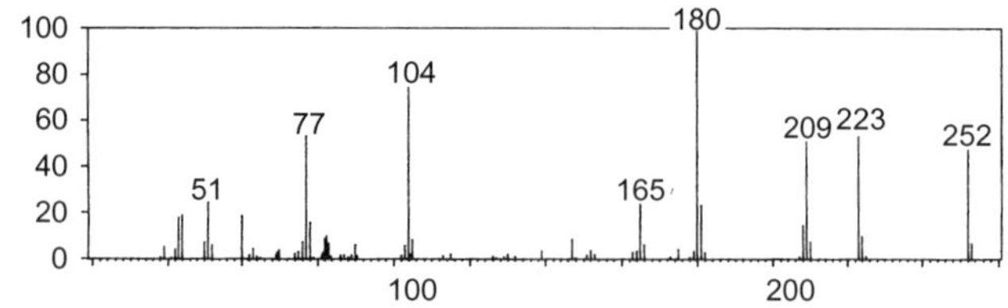

Quantification

Gas chromatography. In plasma: limits of detection 500 to 1000 µg/L, FID—J. Gordos *et al.*, *J. Chromatogr.* 1977, *143*(1) *B Biomed. Appl.*, 171–181. In plasma: limit of detection 200 µg/L, FID—A. Zarghi *et al.*, *Boll. Chim. Farm.*, 1999, *138*, 508–510. In plasma: phenytoin and other anticonvulsants, limits of quantification 50 to 200 µg/L, thermionic detection—M. E. Queiroz *et al.*, *J. Chromatogr. Sci.*, 2002, *40*, 219–223.

Gas chromatography–mass spectrometry. In plasma—M. H. Nelson *et al.*, *J. Pharm. Biomed. Anal.*, 1998, 17, 1311–1323. In blood or liver: phenytoin and other anticonvulsants—D. J. Speed *et al.*, *J. Anal. Toxicol.*, 2000, *24*, 685–690. In hair: phenytoin, other anticonvulsants and their metabolites—K. Saisho *et al.*, *Biol. Pharm. Bull.*, 2001, *24*, 59–64.

High performance liquid chromatography. In serum: phenytoin, phenobarbital, and theophylline, comparison with immunoassay—D. Hannak *et al.*, *Wien. Klin. Wochenschr.*, 1992, *191, Suppl.*, 27–31. In plasma or urine: phenytoin and its major metabolites, UV detection—M. T. Maya *et al.*, *J. Pharm. Biomed. Anal.*, 1992, *10*, 1001–1006. In serum, saliva, or urine: phenytoin and other anticonvulsants, photodiode-array detection—H. Liu *et al.*, *J. Chromatogr.*, 1993, *616*, 105–115. In plasma—A. T. Andresen *et al.*, *J. Chromatogr.*, 1993, *621*, 189–198. In plasma: phenytoin and other anticonvulsants, UV detection—Y. Kouno *et al.*, *J. Chromatogr.*, 1993, *622*, 47–52. In serum: comparison with immunoassay—B. Rambeck *et al.*, *Ther. Drug Monit.*, 1994, *16*, 608–612. In plasma: phenytoin and other anticonvulsants, UV detection—L. A. Romanyshyn *et al.*, *Ther. Drug Monit.*, 1994, *16*, 90–99; K. Johansen *et al.*, *J. Chromatogr.* 1995, *669 B Biomed. Appl.*, 281–288. In serum: phenytoin and other anticonvulsants, UV detection—Y. Kouno *et al.*, *J. Chromatogr.* 1997, *695 B Biomed. Sci. Appl.*, 349–353. In hair: phenytoin and carbamazepine, limit of detection for phenytoin 2 ng/mg, UV detection—Z. Mei and J. Williams, *Ther. Drug Monit.*, 1997, *19*, 92–94. In serum: phenytoin and other anticonvulsants, limits of detection 150 to 350 µg/L, UV detection—G. L. Lensmeyer *et al.*, *Ther. Drug Monit.*, 1997, *19*, 292–300. In plasma: phenytoin and other anticonvulsants, limit of quantification 50 µg/L, UV detection—M. M. Bhatti *et al.*, *J. Pharm. Biomed. Anal.*, 1998, *16*, 1233–1240. In maternal plasma, cord blood, or breast milk: limit of quantification 50 µg/L, UV detection—R. Shimoyama *et al.*, *J. Pharm. Biomed. Anal.*, 1998, *17*, 863–869. In hair: comparison with immunoassay—A. M. Tsatsakis *et al.*, *Boll. Chim. Farm.*, 1998, *137*, 459–466; A. M. Tsatsakis *et al.*, *J. Clin. Psychopharmacol.*, 2000, *20*, 560–573. In serum: comparison with immunoassay—T. W. May *et al.*, *Ther. Drug Monit.*, 1998, *20*, 619–623. In plasma: phenytoin and other anticonvulsants, UV detection—K. M. Matar *et al.*, *Ther. Drug Monit.*, 1999, *21*, 559–566. In serum: phenytoin and other anticonvulsants, limit of quantification for phenytoin about 3 µg/L, UV detection—H. Levert *et al.*, *Biomed. Chromatogr.*, 2002, *16*, 19–24.

Disposition in the Body. Slowly but almost completely absorbed after oral administration; the rate of absorption is variable, being prolonged after large doses, and the bioavailability may vary considerably between different formulations. It is metabolised mainly by P450 isoenzyme CYP2C9 and to a lesser extent by CYP2C19. Metabolism is affected by genetic polymorphism. It undergoes enterohepatic recirculation. About 50 to 70% of a dose may be excreted as free or conjugated 5-(4-hydroxyphenyl)-5-phenylhydantoin (HPPH) in 24 h; the excretion of this metabolite is dose-dependent and decreases as the dose is increased. Phenytoin hydroxylation is capacity-limited, and is therefore readily inhibited by agents which compete for its metabolic pathways. Less than 5% of a dose is excreted as unchanged drug. Minor metabolites include 5-(3-hydroxyphenyl)-5-phenylhydantoin, 3,4-dihydro-3,4-dihydroxyphenytoin, catechol, and 3-*O*-methylcatechol. Up to about 15% of a dose may be eliminated in the faeces. Phenytoin crosses the placenta; low concentrations are found in breast milk

Therapeutic concentration. In plasma, usually in the range 10 to 20 mg/L.

In 332 adults treated for epilepsy with phenytoin for an average of 7.7 months, the average optimized dose was 305.8 (range 100 to 500) mg daily, which produced an average steady-state serum concentration of 62.7 (range

15 to 133) μmol/L. [P. N. Valodia *et al.*, *J. Clin. Pharm. Ther.*, 1999, *24*, 381–385.]

Following daily oral doses of 300 mg, mean steady-state plasma concentrations of 1.3 to 6.6 mg/L (mean 3.6) were reported in 5 subjects with short phenytoin half-lives, in comparison to mean steady-state plasma concentrations of 5.0 to 27.2 mg/L (mean 13.4) in 4 subjects with long phenytoin half-lives; the corresponding concentrations of HPPH were 1.3 to 2.7 mg/L (mean 2.0) and 0.7 to 1.3 mg/L (mean 1.0), respectively. [A. J. Glazko *et al.*, *Ther. Drug Monit.*, 1982, *4*, 281–292.]

A single oral dose of 15 mg/kg phenytoin produced a peak serum concentration of 11.95 mg/L at 7.26 h in 19 healthy subjects. To achieve a target serum concentration of 15 mg/L, an oral loading dose of 18.7 mg/kg was needed in males and 24.8 mg/kg in females; a peak serum concentration of 23.89 mg/L was attained in 9.71 h in males and 21.46 mg/L was attained in 7.71 h in females. [D. Ratanakorn *et al.*, *J. Neurol. Sci.*, 1997, *147*, 89–92.]

Toxicity. The estimated minimum lethal dose is 5 g but few deaths from overdosage have been reported. Side-effects have been associated with plasma concentrations greater than 20 mg/L and severe toxic effects with concentrations greater than 40 mg/L. Fatalities have been associated with blood concentrations greater than 70 mg/L.

A 4½-year-old girl ingested 2 g of phenytoin and 24 h later the blood concentration was found to be 94 mg/L. She died on the third day and postmortem concentrations were: blood 45 mg/L, brain 78 μg/g, kidney 112 μg/g, liver 272 μg/g. [F. A. Laubscher, *JAMA*, 1966, *198*, 1120–1121.]

In 9 patients displaying signs of phenytoin toxicity during the course of therapy, initial serum levels ranged from 34.0 to 57.5 mg/L. In 3 patients levels remained relatively constant for 2 to 5 days before declining steadily; in the remaining patients levels declined almost linearly. In 7 patients, levels declined between 4.6 and 5.9 mg/L per day. [H. C. Chua *et al.*, *Clin. Neurol. Neurosurg.*, 2000, *102*, 6–8.]

A 15-year-old boy survived after ingesting 19.6 g (15 g verifiable; 392 mg/kg) phenytoin sodium in a suicide attempt, despite having a peak serum level of 100.8 mg/L. [L. B. Mellick *et al.*, *Am. J. Emerg. Med.*, 1989, *7*, 61–67.]

Following an apparent suicide attempt by an adult non-epileptic man who ingested an unkown amount of phenytoin, an unusual absorption profile was observed. Twelve hours after the ingestion, the serum phenytoin concentration was 45 mg/L. This steadily increased, reaching a maximum of 114 mg/L 4 days later, fluctuated at about 100 mg/L for a week, and then slowly declined to undetectable levels over the following week. The protracted absorption appeared to result from the presence of a large concretion of phenytoin in the gastro-intestinal tract, slowly disintegrating and dissolving and also to the patient's diminished intestinal motility. [P. Chaikin and J. Adir, *J. Clin. Pharmacol.*, 1987, *27*, 70–73.]

Half-life. Plasma half-life, varies considerably within the approximate range of 7 to 42 h, and is dose-dependent, increasing as the dose increases; at steady-state about 22 h.

Volume of distribution. About 0.5 to 1.2 L/kg.

Distribution in blood. Plasma:whole blood ratio, about 1.6.

Saliva. Plasma:saliva ratio, about 10.

Protein binding. In plasma, about 90%.

Note. For a review of phenytoin disposition and toxicity, see T.I. Edeki and D. A. Brase, *Drug Metab. Rev.*, 1995, *27*, 449–469; for a review of phenytoin dosing methods, see R. D. Pryka *et al.*, *Clin. Pharmacokinet.*, 1991, *20*, 209–217; for a review of the clinical features and management of poisoning due to phenytoin, see J. R. Larsen and L. S. Larsen, *Med. Toxicol. Adverse Drug Exp.*, 1989, *4*, 229–245; for a review of the pharmacokinetics of phenytoin, see A. Richens, *Clin. Pharmacokinet.*, 1979, *4*, 153–169.

Dose. 300 to 600 mg of phenytoin or phenytoin sodium daily.

Pholcodine

Antitussive

Synonyms. Folcodina; Pholcodinum; MEM; Morpholinylethylmorphine.
Proprietary names. Benylin Childrens Dry Coughs; Evaphol; Expulin Dry Cough; Famel Linctus; Galenphol; Hill's Balsam Dry Cough; Pavacol-D; Pholcomed; Tixylix Daytime. It is an ingredient of many proprietary preparations, see *Martindale, The complete drug reference* 33rd Edn, Pharmaceutical Press, London, 2002.
(5α,6α)-7,8-Didehydro-4,5-epoxy-17-methyl-3-[2-(4-morpholinyl)-ethoxy]morphinan-6-ol monohydrate
$C_{23}H_{30}N_2O_4,H_2O$=416.5
CAS—509-67-1 (anhydrous)

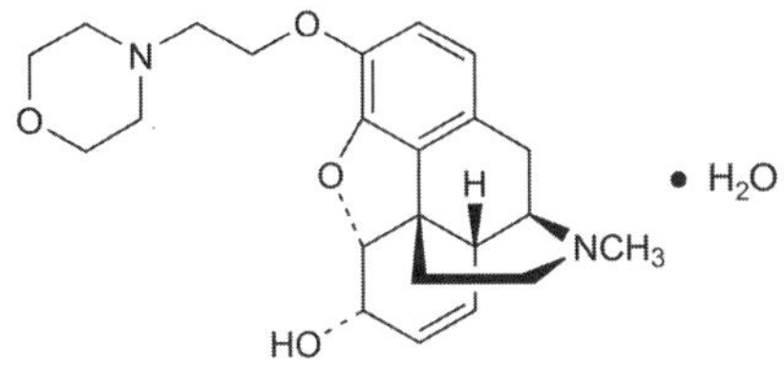

Colourless crystals or a white crystalline powder. M.p. 91°.
Soluble 1 in 50 of water and 1 in 3 of dehydrated alcohol; soluble in benzene and chloroform.

Pholcodine Tartrate

$C_{23}H_{30}N_2O_4,2C_4H_6O_6,3H_2O$ = 752.7
A white crystalline powder.
Soluble 1 in 8 of water; very slightly soluble in ethanol; slightly soluble in chloroform and ether.

Dissociation Constant. pK_a 8.0, 9.3 (37°).

Partition Coefficient. Log *P* (octanol/water), 0.6.

Colour Tests. Liebermann's Test—black; Marquis Test—violet.

Thin-layer Chromatography. System TA—Rf 36; system TB—Rf 03; system TC—Rf 18; system TE—Rf 25; system TL—Rf 02; system TAE—Rf 15. (Dragendorff spray, positive; acidified iodoplatinate solution, positive; Marquis Reagent, violet.)

Gas Chromatography. System GA—phocoldine RI 3070, phocoldine-AC RI 3260, phocoldine-PFP RI 2980, phocoldine-TFA RI 2800, phocoldine-TMS RI 3140; system GB—pholcodine RI 3348, pholcodine-TMS RI 3410.

High Performance Liquid Chromatography. System HA—*k* 6.0 (tailing peak); system HC—*k* 1.63; system HX—RI 65; system HY—RI 92; system HAA—retention time 2.7 min.

Ultraviolet Spectrum. Aqueous acid—283 nm (A_1^1=40a). No alkaline shift.

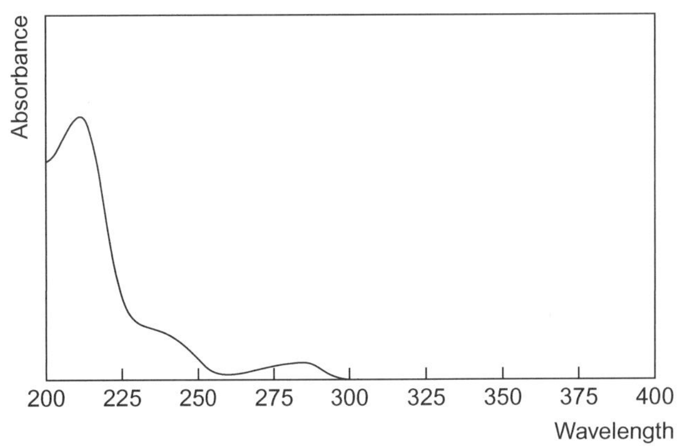

Infra-red Spectrum. Principal peaks at wavenumbers 1118, 969, 1250, 1043, 1500, 1098 cm^{-1} (KBr disk).

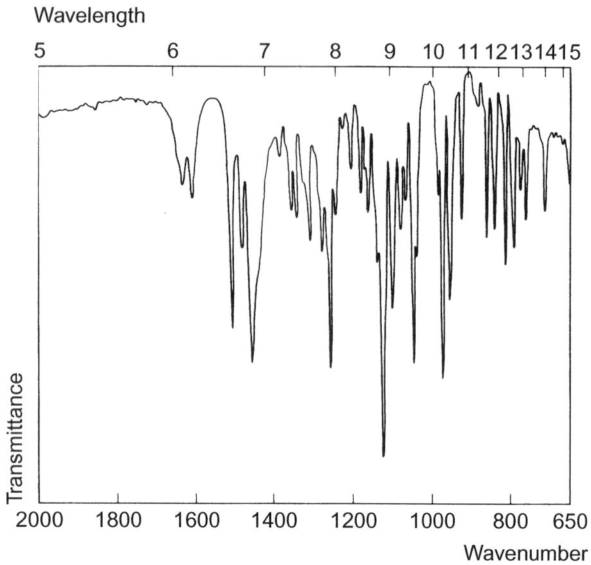

Mass Spectrum. Principal ions at m/z 114, 100, 56, 42, 115, 101, 70, 398.

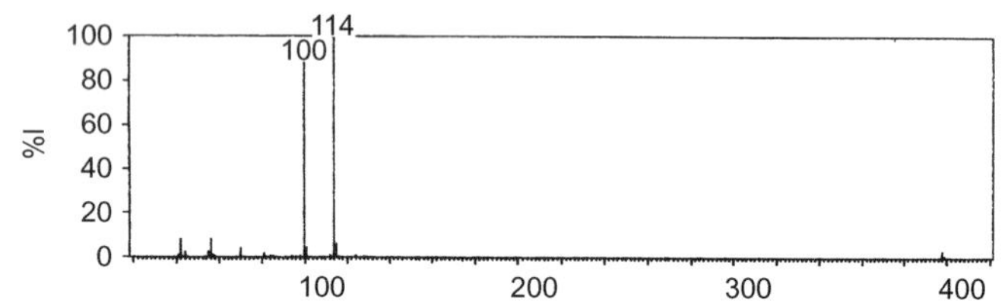

Quantification

Gas chromatography. In urine: pholcodine and its metabolites, nitrogen detection—M. Johansen *et al.*, *J. Chromatogr.*, 1990, 532, 277–284.

Gas chromatography–mass spectrometry. In urine or hair: pholcodine and its metabolites, comparison with immunoassay—H. H. Maurer and C. F. Fritz, *Int. J. Legal Med.*, 1990, *104*, 43–46. In plasma or whole blood: pholcodine and other opioids—M. Krogh *et al.*, *J. Chromatogr.*, 1993, *621*, 41–48. In urine: pholcodine and other opioids—V. Sautou *et al.*, *J. Pharm. Belg.*, 1994, *49*, 383–389.

High performance liquid chromatography. In urine: pholcodine and its metabolites, fluorescence and electrochemical detection—M. Johansen *et al.*, *J. Chromatogr.*, 1992, *573*, 283–288. In plasma or whole blood: fluorescence detection—A. T. Andresen *et al.*, *J. Chromatogr.*, 1992, *582*, 123–130. In urine: pholcodine and other opioids, limits of detection 4 to 20 μg/L, comparison with EMIT—A. S. Low and R. B. Taylor, *J. Chromatogr.* 1995, *663 B Biomed. Appl.*, 225–233.

Disposition in the Body. Pholcodine is partly metabolised to morphine and other metabolites; it also forms a glucuronic acid conjugate. About 29% of an oral dose is excreted in the urine as unchanged pholcodine and a further 15% as the glucuronide; about 0.5 to 1% is excreted in the urine as morphine glucuronide. Other metabolites have been identified as desmorpholinohydroxy-, nordesmorpholinohydroxy-, hydroxy-, oxo-, nor-, and noroxo-pholcodine.

Therapeutic concentration

6 healthy subjects received single oral doses of 20 and 60 mg pholcodine (with 3 weeks between the doses) and subsequently received 20 mg pholcodine orally every 8 h for 10 days. After single doses pholcodine was absorbed rapidly (t_{max}=1.6 h), with the mean peak plasma concentration being 12.8 μg/L after the 20-mg dose and 26.3 μg/L after the 60-mg dose. Multiple dosing did not alter the pharmacokinetics. [Z. R. Chen *et al.*, *Br. J. Clin. Pharmacol.*, 1988, *26*, 445–453.]

Note. For interpretation of GC–MS opiate results in the presence of pholcodine, see C. Meadway *et al.*, *Forensic Sci. Int.*, 2002, *127*, 131–135.

Dose. Usually up to 40 mg daily.

Pholedrine

Sympathomimetic

Synonyms. Isodrine; Sympropaminum.
4-[2-(Methylamino)propyl]phenol
$C_{10}H_{15}NO$=165.2
CAS—370-14-9

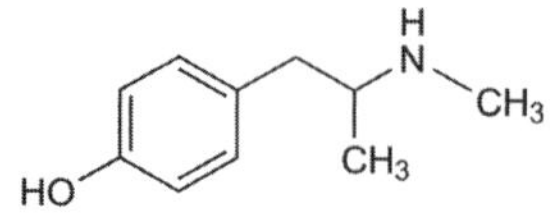

Crystals. M.p. 162° to 163°.
Slightly soluble in water; soluble in ethanol and ether.

Pholedrine Sulfate

Synonym. Pholedrine Sulfate
Proprietary name. Paredrinol; Pulsotyl; Veritol
$(C_{10}H_{15}NO)_2,H_2SO_4$=428.5
CAS—6114-26-7
A white crystalline powder. M.p. about 320° to 323°, with decomposition. Soluble 1 in 20 of water; practically insoluble in ethanol, chloroform, and ether.

Dissociation Constant. pK_a 9.4 (25°).

Partition Coefficient. Log *P* (octanol/water), 1.7.

Colour Test. Marquis Test—grey→green.

Thin-layer Chromatography. System TA—Rf 29; system TB—Rf 03; system TC—Rf 03; system TE—Rf 27; system TL—Rf 03; system TAE—Rf 09. (Acidified potassium permanganate solution, positive.)

Gas Chromatography. System GA—RI 1490.

High Performance Liquid Chromatography. System HX—RI 205.

Ultraviolet Spectrum. Aqueous acid—275 (A^1_1=82a); aqueous alkali—238 (A^1_1=640b), 295 nm (A^1_1=150b).

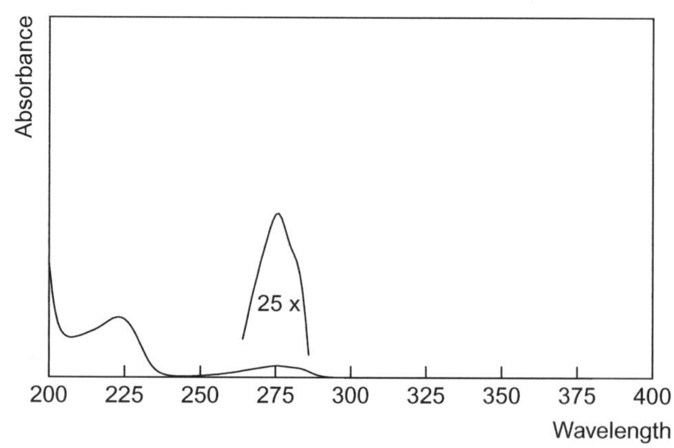

Infra-red Spectrum. Principal peaks at wavenumbers 1258, 1513, 1274, 1590, 1610, 810 cm^{-1} (KBr disk).

Mass Spectrum. Principal ions at m/z 58, 30, 107, 59, 77, 56, 42, 43.

Quantification

High performance liquid chromatography. In serum: amperometric detection—G. P. Peinhardt, *J. Chromatogr. B Biomed. Sci. Appl.*, 1999, *726*, 309–312.

Radioimmunoassay. In plasma—G. Peinhardt, *Pharmazie*, 1997, *52*, 937–939.

Disposition in the Body

Toxicity

In a fatality involving the ingestion of pholedrine, the following postmortem concentrations were reported: blood 15 μg/g, kidney 122 μg/g, liver 73 μg/g [H.-J. Hammer *et al.*, *Dtsch. GesundhWes.*, 1980, *35*, 1352–1354].

Dose. Pholedrine sulfate has been given parenterally in doses of up to 20 mg.

Phthalylsulfacetamide

Antibacterial/Sulfonamide

Synonyms. Ftalicetimida; Phthaloylsulfacetamide; Phthalylsulfacetamide; Sulfanilacetamidum Phthalylatum.
Proprietary names. Enterocid; Enterosulfamid; Enterosulfon; Talecid; Thalacet; Rabalan; Sterathal.
2-[[[4-[(Acetylamino)sulfonyl]phenyl]amino]carbonyl]benzoic acid
$C_{16}H_{14}N_2O_6S=362.4$
CAS—131-69-1

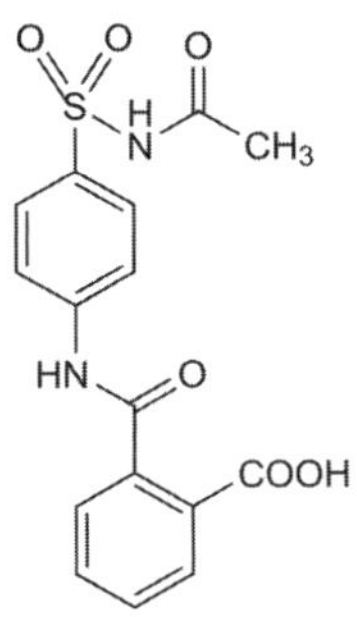

White or creamy-white crystals or crystalline powder. M.p. 196°.
Very slightly soluble in water; slightly soluble in ethanol; soluble in acetone; freely soluble in solutions of alkali hydroxides.

Partition Coefficient. Log *P* (octanol/water), 1.3.

Colour Test. Copper Sulfate (Method 1)—blue.

Thin-layer Chromatography. System TD—Rf 00; system TE—Rf 00; system TF—Rf 00; system TAD—Rf 00.

Gas Chromatography. See sulfacetamide.

Ultraviolet Spectrum. Aqueous acid—268 nm (broad); aqueous alkali—265 nm (broad).

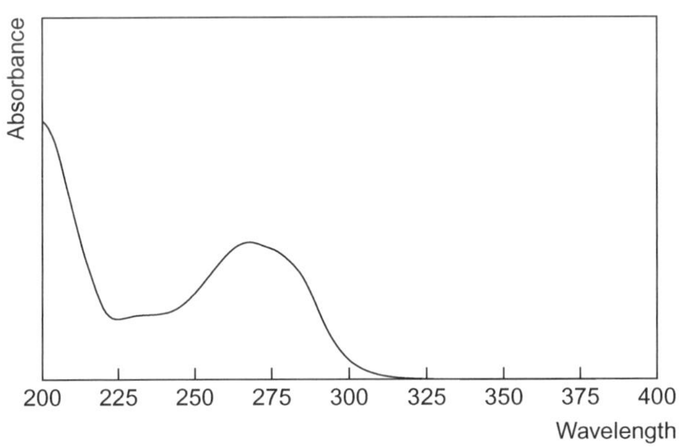

Infra-red Spectrum. Principal peaks at wavenumbers 1170, 1681, 1527, 837, 1302, 1592 cm^{-1}.

Mass Spectrum. Principal ions at *m/z* 109, 76, 104, 92, 239, 65, 108, 43.

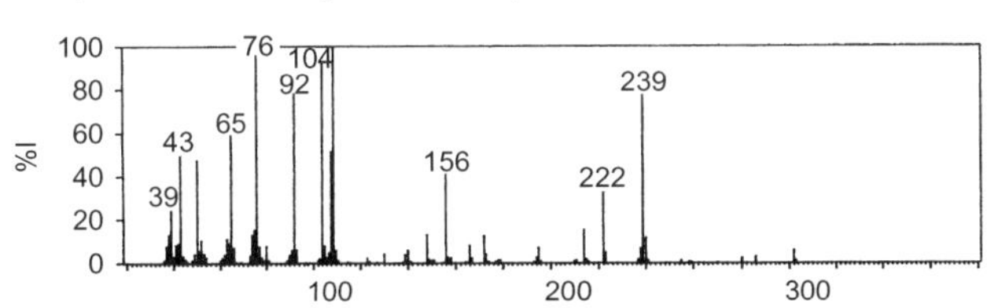

Dose. 6 to 12 g daily.

Phthalylsulfathiazole

Antibacterial/Sulfonamide

Synonyms. Ftalilsulfatiazol; Phthalazolum; Phthalylsulfathiazole; Sulfaphtalylthiazol.
Proprietary names. AFI-Ftalyl; Entexidina; Ftalazol; Intestiazol; Kaotalil; Sulfathalidine; Sulfalyl; Taleudron; Talidine; Thalazole; Ultratiazol.
2-[[[4-[(2-Thiazolylamino)sulfonyl]phenyl]amino]carbonyl]benzoic acid
$C_{17}H_{13}N_3O_5S_2=403.4$
CAS—85-73-4

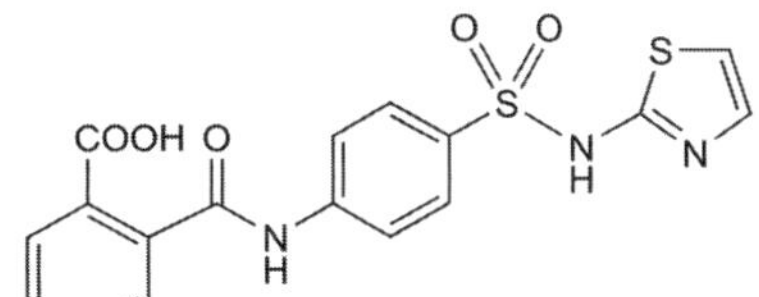

White or yellowish-white crystals, or powder, which darken on prolonged exposure to light. Effervesces at 244° to 250°. M.p. 272° to 277°, with decomposition.
Practically insoluble in water, chloroform, and ether; soluble 1 in 600 of ethanol; freely soluble in dimethylformamide and solutions of alkali hydroxides and carbonates, and in hydrochloric acid.

Partition Coefficient. Log *P* (octanol/water), 0.9.

Colour Test. Copper Sulfate (Method 1)—green.

Thin-layer Chromatography. System TD—Rf 00; system TE—Rf 00; system TF—Rf 00; system TT—Rf 02; system TU—Rf 04; system TV—Rf 04; system TAD—Rf 00; system TAJ—Rf 00; system TAK—Rf 04; system TAL—Rf 42.

Gas Chromatography. See sulfathiazole

High Performance Liquid Chromatography. System HU—*k* 14.0.

Ultraviolet Spectrum. Aqueous acid—282; aqueous alkali—260 ($A^1_1=600a$); methanol—260 ($A^1_1=497a$), 288 nm ($A^1_1=648a$).

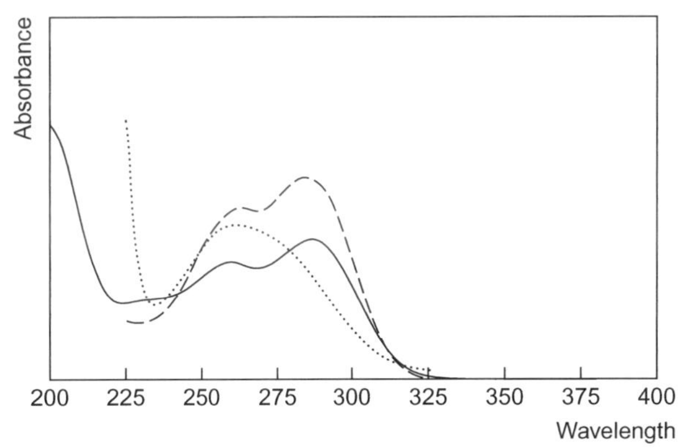

Infra-red Spectrum. Principal peaks at wavenumbers 1532, 1142, 1084, 1710, 1585, 1560 cm^{-1} (KBr disk).

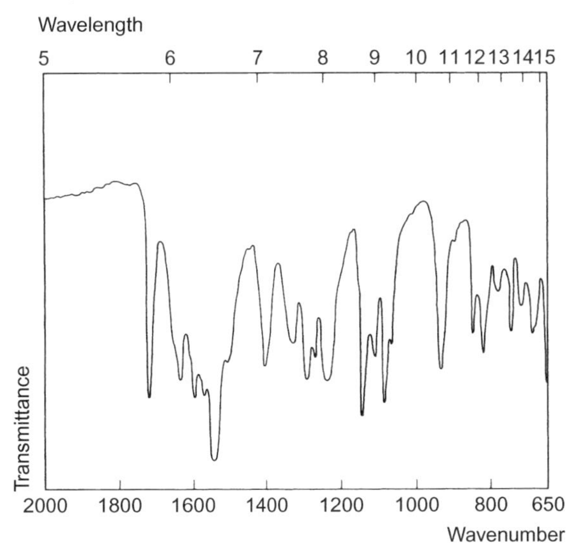

Mass Spectrum. Principal ions at *m/z* 92, 156, 191, 65, 108, 76, 104, 50.

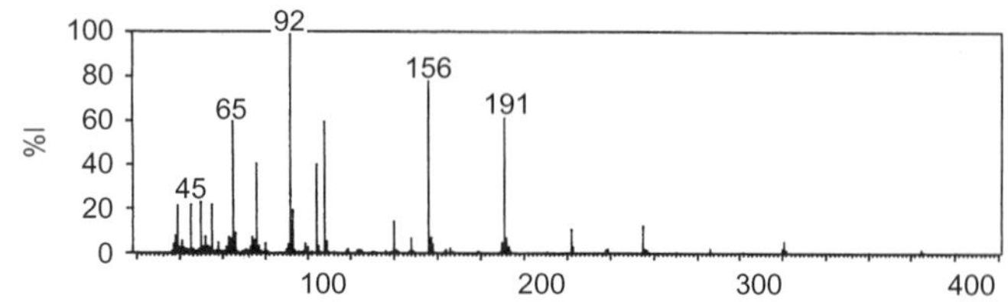

Disposition in the Body. Only about 5% of a dose is absorbed after oral administration and blood concentrations are therefore very low compared to other sulfonamides, usually less than 15 mg/L. It is slowly hydrolysed to sulfathiazole in the gastro-intestinal tract.

Dose. 2 to 12 g daily.

Physostigmine

Anticholinesterase

Synonyms. Eserine; Physostigmina.
(3a*S*-*cis*)-1,2,3,3a,8,8a-Hexahydro-1,3a,8-trimethylpyrrolo[2,3-*b*]-indol-5-ol methylcarbamate ester
$C_{15}H_{21}N_3O_2$=275.3
CAS—57-47-6

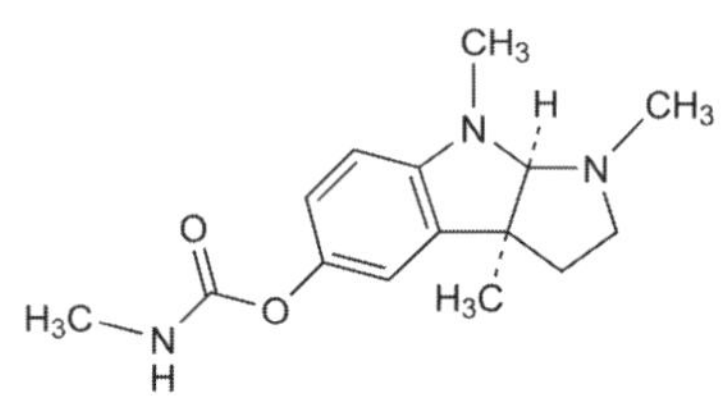

An alkaloid obtained from the calabar bean (ordeal bean; chopnut), the seed of *Physostigma venenosum* (Leguminosae).
Colourless crystals, or a white microcrystalline powder. M.p. 105° to 106°; also unstable, low-melting form, m.p. 86° to 87°.
Soluble 1 in 75 of water, 1 in 10 of ethanol, 1 in 1 of chloroform, and 1 in 30 of ether.
Physostigmine, its salts and their aqueous solutions become red on exposure to heat, light, air, and on contact with traces of metals, owing to the formation of rubreserine; the change is less rapid in acid solution.

Physostigmine Salicylate

Synonym. Eserine Salicylate
Proprietary names. Anticholium; Antilirium.
$C_{15}H_{21}N_3O_2,C_7H_6O_3$=413.5
CAS—57-64-7
Colourless or white crystals or white powder. M.p. 185° to 187°.
Soluble 1 in 75 to 1 in 90 of water, 1 in 16 of ethanol, 1 in 6 of chloroform, and 1 in 250 of ether.

Physostigmine Sulfate

Synonym. Eserine Sulfate
$(C_{15}H_{21}N_3O_2)_2,H_2SO_4$=648.8
CAS—64-47-1
A white deliquescent, microcrystalline powder. M.p. 140°.
Soluble 1 in 4 of water and 1 in 0.4 of ethanol; soluble in chloroform; very slightly soluble in ether.

Dissociation Constant. pK_a 1.8, 7.9 (25°).

Partition Coefficient. Log *P* (octanol/water), 1.6.

Colour Test. Mandelin's Test—yellow-brown.

Thin-layer Chromatography. System TA—Rf 55; system TB—Rf 12; system TC—Rf 36; system TE—Rf 55; system TL—Rf 18; system TAE—Rf 40; system TAF—Rf 38; system TAJ—Rf 18; system TAK—Rf 03; system TAL—Rf 50. (Acidified potassium permanganate solution, positive.)

Gas Chromatography. System GA—RI 1804, 2035, and 2190.

High Performance Liquid Chromatography. System HA—*k* 2.6; system HX—RI 296; system HY—RI 240; system HZ—Retention time 2.2 min.

Ultraviolet Spectrum. Aqueous acid—246 (A_1^1=462a), 302 nm.

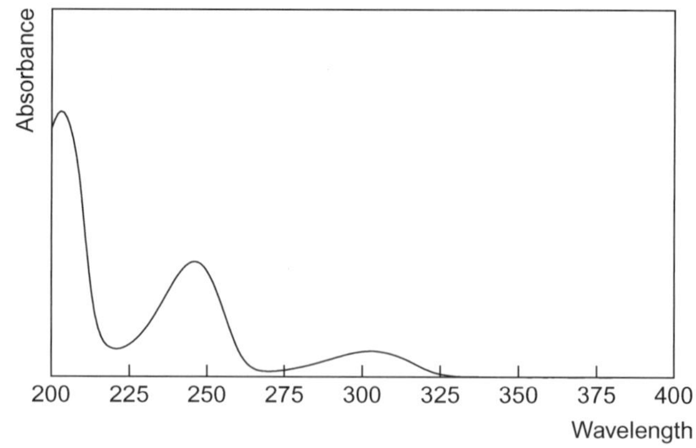

Infra-red Spectrum. Principal peaks at wavenumbers 1724, 1243, 1200, 1495, 1120, 1162 cm^{-1} (KBr disk).

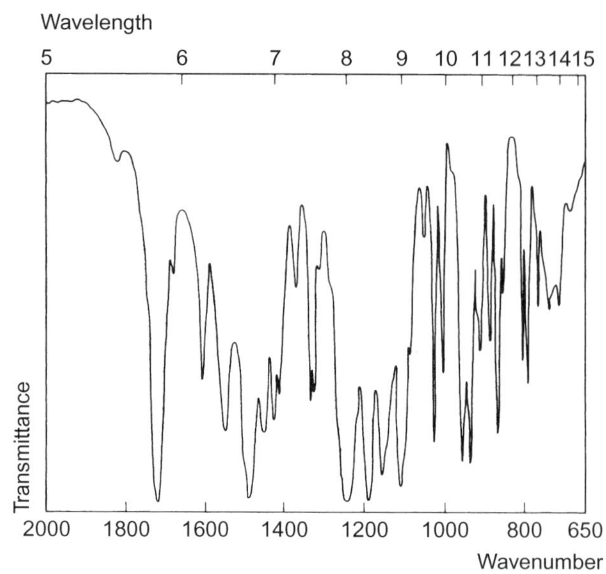

Mass Spectrum. Principal ions at *m/z* 218, 174, 160, 161, 275, 219, 175, 162.

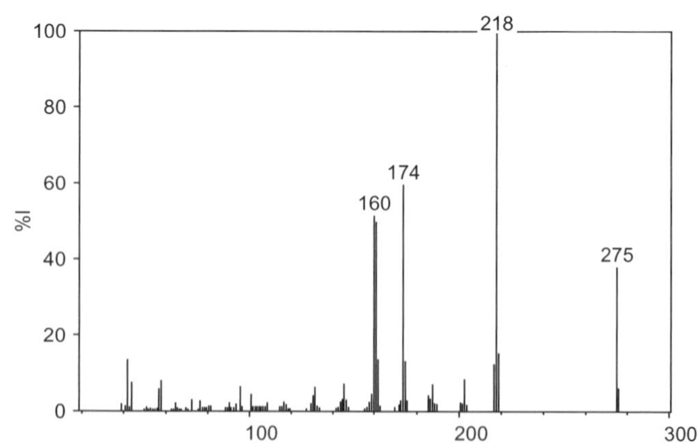

Quantification

High performance liquid chromatography. In plasma: limit of detection 500 ng/L, electrochemical detection—R. Whelpton, *J. Chromatogr.*, 1983, *272*; *B Biomed. Appl.*, *23*, 216–220. In plasma: limits of detection 25 to 50 pg/mol, electrochemical detection—R. Whelpton and T. Moore, *J. Chromatogr.*, 1985, *341*, 361–371. In plasma: limit of detection 100 ng/L, fluorescence detection—N. M. Elsayed *et al.*, *Anal. Biochem.*, 1989, *177*, 207–211. In plasma or cerebrospinal fluid: limit of detection 500 ng/L, electrochemical detection—L. K. Unni *et al.*, *Clin. Chem.*, 1989, *35*,

292–295. In plasma, whole blood, or cerebrospinal fluid, physostigmine and eseroline, electrochemical detection—G. D. Lawrence and N. Yatim, *J. Pharmacol. Methods*, 1990, *24*, 137–143. In serum: physostigmine and eseroline, limits of detection 2 μg/L and 5 μg/L respectively, fluorescence detection—K. D. Quinn and J. T. Stewart, *Biomed. Chromatogr.*, 1991, *5*, 8–13.

Disposition in the Body. Readily absorbed after oral or subcutaneous administration and from mucous membranes. Physostigmine readily penetrates the CNS. It is rapidly hydrolysed by cholinesterases and most of a dose is destroyed in 2 h. Very little is excreted in the urine.

Therapeutic concentration

After a single subcutaneous injection of 1 mg of physostigmine salicylate (equivalent to 0.67 mg base) to one subject, a peak plasma concentration of 0.0036 mg/L was achieved after 15 min [R. Whelpton, *J. Chromatogr.*, 1983, *272*; *B Biomed. Appl.*, *23*, 216–220].

After a single oral dose of 4 mg of physostigmine salicylate to one subject, a peak plasma concentration of about 0.001 mg/L was attained in 0.75 h [M. Gibson *et al.*, *Lancet*, 1985, *1*, 695–696].

Toxicity. Fatalities have occurred following ingestion of 6 mg of physostigmine orally and administration of 1.2 mg intravenously. The ingestion of 6 calabar beans by a child has proved fatal.

Physostigmine Aminoxide

Anticholinesterase

Synonyms. Eseridine; Eserine Aminoxide; Physostigmine *N*-Oxide.
(4a*S*-*cis*)-2,3,4,4a,9,9a-Hexahydro-2,4a,9-trimethyl-1,2-oxazino[6,5-*b*]-indol-6-ol methylcarbamate ester
$C_{15}H_{21}N_3O_3$=291.3
CAS—25573-43-7

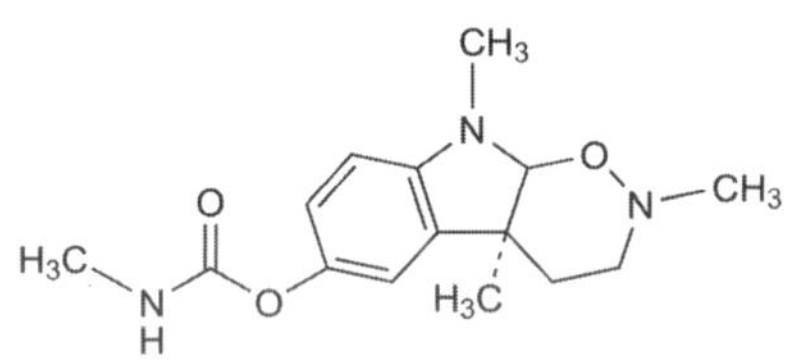

Crystals. M.p. 129°.
Practically insoluble in water; soluble in ethanol, chloroform, benzene, acetone, and ether.

Physostigmine Aminoxide Salicylate

Synonyms. Eseridine Salicylate; Eserine Aminoxide Salicylate; Physostigmine *N*-Oxide Salicylate.
Proprietary name. Génésérine 3
$C_{15}H_{21}N_3O_3,C_7H_6O_3$=429.5
CAS—5995-96-0
Crystals which become red on exposure to heat, light, and air. M.p. 90°.

Partition Coefficient. Log *P* (octanol/water), 2.1.

Thin-layer Chromatography. System TA—Rf 31. (Acidified potassium permanganate solution, positive.)

Ultraviolet Spectrum. Aqueous acid—241 $(A^1_1=411b)$, 300 nm.

Infra-red Spectrum. Principal peaks at wavenumbers 1720, 1250, 1204, 1268, 1495, 1289 cm^{-1} (KBr disk).

Quantification

High performance liquid chromatography–mass spectrometry. In plasma: limit of detection 25 ng/L—A. Pruvost *et al.*, *J. Mass Spectrom.*, 2000, *35*, 625–633.

Dose. Physostigmine aminoxide salicylate has been given in doses of 9 mg daily.

Phytomenadione

Vitamin

Synonyms. Methylphytylnaphthochinonum; Phylloquinone; Phytonadione; Vitamin K_1.

Proprietary names. Aquamephyton; Kanakion; Kanavit; Konakion; Mephyton; Vitamon K.
2-Methyl-3-[(2*E*,7*R*,11*R*)-3,7,11,15-tetramethyl-2-hexadecenyl]-1,4-naphthalenedione
$C_{31}H_{46}O_2$=450.7
CAS—84-80-0

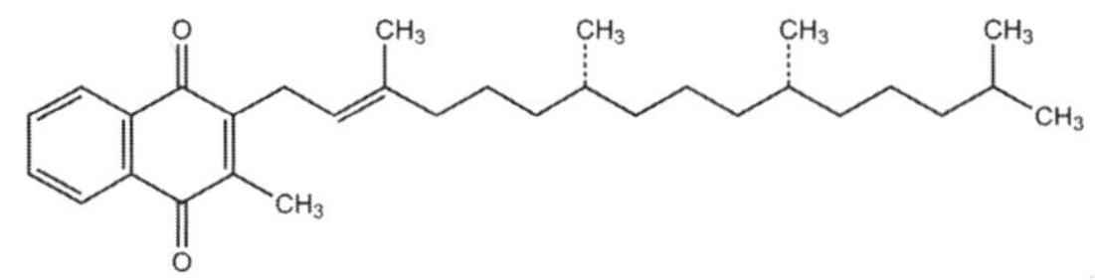

A clear, deep yellow, very viscous oil which is stable in air but decomposes on exposure to light. Sp. gr. about 0.967. Refractive index 1.5255 to 1.5285. Practically insoluble in water; soluble 1 in 70 of ethanol; more soluble in dehydrated alcohol; sparingly soluble in methanol; freely soluble in chloroform and ether.

Partition Coefficient. Log *P* (octanol/water), 11.7.

Colour Test. Methanolic Potassium Hydroxide—green-yellow→violet→brown.

Gas Chromatography. System GA—RI 3287.

Ultraviolet Spectrum. Methanol—244, 249 $(A^1_1=394a)$, 263 $(A^1_1=350b)$, 270 $(A^1_1=349a)$, 331 nm $(A^1_1=68a)$.

Infra-red Spectrum. Principal peaks at wavenumbers 1285, 1650, 714, 1587, 690, 1610 cm^{-1}.

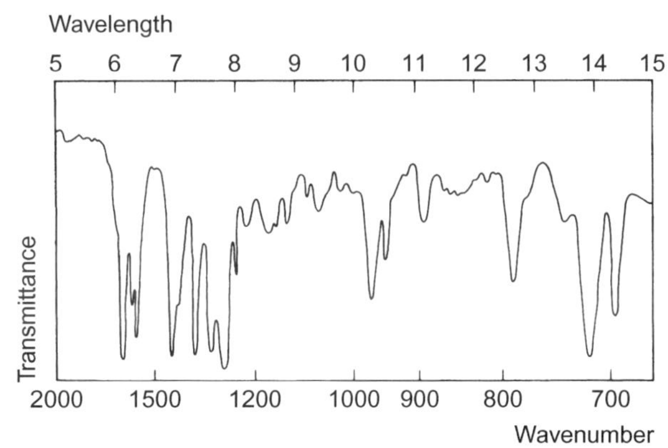

Quantification

High performance liquid chromatography. In plasma: limit of detection 500 pg, UV detection—M. J. Shearer *et al.*, *Lancet*, 1982, *2*, 460–463. In plasma: limit of detection 0.05 μg/L, fluorescence detection—Y. Haroon *et al.*, *Clin Chem.*, 1986, *32*, 1925–1929. In plasma: phytomenadione, its epoxides, and menaquinone-4, limit of detection 30 to 50 ng/L, fluorescence detection—K. Hirauchi *et al.*, *J. Chromatogr.*, 1988, *430*, 21–29. In liver: phytomenadione and menaquinone, fluorescence detection—Y. Usui *et al.*, *J. Chromatogr.*, 1989, *489*, 291–301. In serum: phytomenadione, limit of detection 30 pg/inj., fluorescence detection—B. E. Cham *et al.*, *Clin. Chem.*, 1989, *35*, 2285–2289. In serum: limit of detection about 20 ng/L, fluorescence detection—W. A. MacCrehan and E. Schonberger, *J. Chromatogr. B Biomed. Appl.*, 1995, *670*, 209–217. In plasma: phytomenadione and vitamins A and E, and beta-carotene, limit of detection 0.04 μg/L for phytomenadione, fluorescence detection—E. Jakob and I. Elmadfa, *Int. J. Nutr. Res.*, 1995, *65*, 31–35.

Disposition in the Body. Absorbed from the gastro-intestinal tract in the presence of bile. Rapidly metabolised and excreted as conjugates in the urine, bile and faeces. Endogenous plasma concentrations are usually in the range 0.0001 to 0.0007 mg/L.

Therapeutic concentration

Phytomenadione given in a dose of 10 mg as a mixed micellar preparation to 30 subjects, produced a mean maximum plasma concentration of 67 μg/L (range 16 to 113) after 9.2 h (range 2 to 24) after IM injection [J. R. Soedirman *et al.*, *Br. J. Clin. Pharmacol.*, 1996, *41*, 517–523].

Phytomenadione given by IV injection to 18 neonates at a dose of 0.3 mg/kg, resulted in a mean blood concentration of 191.3 μg/L after 22.9 h; a further blood sample taken after 111.8 h from 10 of the neonates revealed a concentration of 98.7 µg/L [W. Raith *et al.*, *Thromb. Res.*, 2000, *99*, 467–472].

Half-life. Plasma half-life, about 2 h.

Dose. Initially 2.5 to 25 mg by subcutaneous or IM injection, or 5 to 20 mg by mouth.

Picotamide

Anticoagulant/Antithrombotic

Synonyms. G-137.
4-Methoxy-*N*,*N'*-bis(3-pyridinylmethyl)-1,3-benzenedicarboxamide
$C_{21}H_{20}N_4O_3$=376.4
CAS—32828-81-2

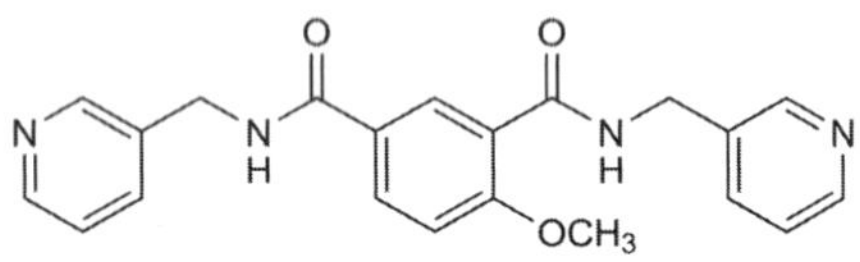

A white or almost white crystalline powder with m.p. 124°. It is slightly soluble in water; soluble in ethanol, methanol and dichloromethane. It dissolves in dilute mineral acids.

Picotamide Monohydrate

Synonym. Picotamidum Monohydricum.
Proprietary name. Plactidil
$C_{21}H_{20}N_4O_3,H_2O$=394.4

Partition Coefficient. Log *P* (octanol/water), 1.53.

Thin-layer Chromatography. Plate: Merck F-254 silica gel plates (0.25 mm thick). Mobile phase: (A) chloroform:methanol (9:1); (B) methanol:concentrated ammonia (100:105); (C) benzene:ethylacetate:acetic acid (2:1:0.1); (D) ethylacetate:ethanol (2:1). UV detection (λ=254 nm). Picotamide monohydrate (A) Rf 0.41; Picotamide (B) Rf 0.60; (C) Rf 0.0; (D) Rf 0.21. [G. Orzalesi *et al.*, *Int. J. Pharm.*, 1989, *52*, 225–229].

High Performance Liquid Chromatography. Column: LiChrosorb RP-Select B C_8 (250 × 4 mm i.d., 5 µm). Mobile phase: acetonitrile:sodium dihydrogen phosphate (50 mM, pH 5.5) (28:72), flow rate 1 mL/min. IS: bamifylline. UV detection (λ=230 nm). Retention time(s): picotamide, 10 min; IS, 7 min. [T. Fossati *et al.*, *J. Chromatogr.*, 1992, *577*, 382–386].

Column: Spherisorb S5 ODS1 (250 × 40 mm, 6 mm i.d.). Mobile phase: methanol:phosphate buffer, pH 7.9 (60:40), flow rate 0.8 mL/min. Retention time(s): 9.35 min. [G. Orzalesi *et al.*, *Int. J. Pharm.*, 1989, *52*, 225–229].

Quantification

Thin-layer chromatography. Limit of detection 0.1 µg—G. Orzalesi *et al.*, *Int. J. Pharm.*, 1989, *52*, 225–229.

High performance liquid chromatography. In blood and urine: limit of quantification is 5 µg/L and 1 µg/L, respectively. UV detection (λ=230 nm)—T. Fossati *et al.*, *J. Chromatogr.*, 1992, *577*, 382–386.

Dose. Initial daily dose, 900 to 1200 mg; maintenance dose of 300 to 600 mg daily.

Picrotoxin

Respiratory Stimulant

Synonym. Cocculin
$C_{30}H_{34}O_{13}$=602.6
CAS—124-87-8
An active principle from the seeds of *Anamirta cocculus* (=*A. paniculata*) (Menispermaceae). The fruits of *A. cocculus* are sometimes known as 'fish berries' or 'Levant berries'.
Colourless, flexible, shining prismatic crystals or white microcrystalline powder. M.p. 203°.
Soluble 1 in 350 of water and 1 in 16 of ethanol; soluble in glacial acetic acid and solutions of acids and alkali hydroxides; slightly soluble in chloroform and ether.

Partition Coefficient. Log *P* (octanol/water), –2.8.

Colour Tests. Dissolve in sulfuric acid—yellow→red-brown (slow). Add 1 drop of fuming nitric acid to the material—blue-green, discharged by excess acid.

Infra-red Spectrum. Principal peaks at wavenumbers 1780, 1755, 1795, 1123, 990, 1162 cm^{-1} (KBr disk).

Mass Spectrum. Principal ions at *m/z* 95, 55, 41, 43, 59, 27, 39, 67.

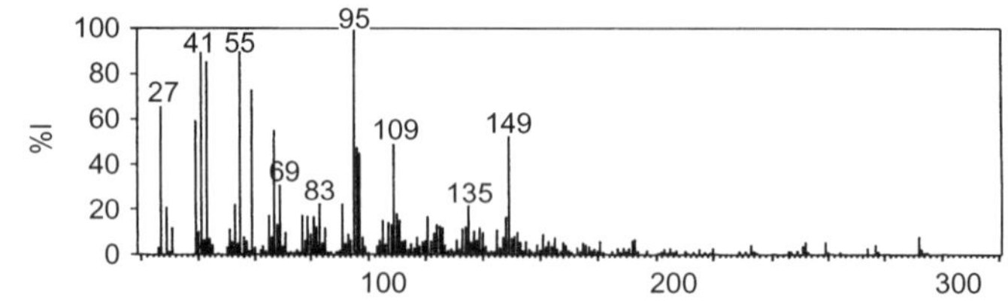

Dose. Picrotoxin was formerly given in doses of 3 to 6 mg intravenously.

Pilocarpine

Parasympathomimetic

Proprietary names. Ocusert Pilo; Pilocarpol; Piloftal; Pilomann-Ol; Piloplex.
(3*S*-*cis*)-3-Ethyldihydro-4-[(1-methyl-1*H*-imidazol-5-yl)methyl]-2(3*H*)-furanone
$C_{11}H_{16}N_2O_2$=208.3
CAS—92-13-7

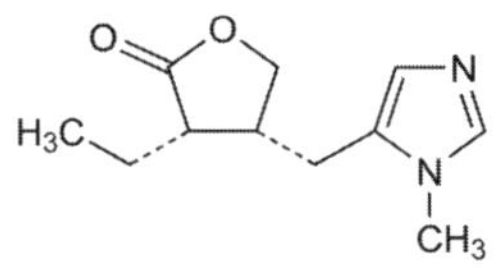

An alkaloid obtained from the leaves of jaborandi, *Pilocarpus microphyllus* (Rutaceae) and other species of *Pilocarpus*.
A viscous, hygroscopic, colourless, oily liquid or crystals. M.p. about 34°. Soluble in water, ethanol, and chloroform; sparingly soluble in ether and benzene.

Pilocarpine Hydrochloride

Proprietary names. Adsorbocarpine; Akarpine; Asthenopin; Borocarpin-S; Isopto Carpine; Diocarpine; Dropilton; Glaucocarpine Liocarpina; Miocarpine; Mi-Pilo; Ocu-Carpine; Pilax; Pilo; Pilocar; Pilocarcil; Pilogel; Pilomann; Pilopt; Piloptic; Pilostat; Pilo-Stulln; Pilotonina; PV Carpine; Salagen; Sno Pilo; Spersacarpin(e); Storzine; Vistacarpin. It is an ingredient of E-Pilo and PE.
$C_{11}H_{16}N_2O_2,HCl$=244.7
CAS—54-71-7
Hygroscopic, colourless crystals or white crystalline powder. M.p. 204° to 205°. Soluble 1 in less than 1 of water, 1 in 3 of ethanol, and 1 in 360 of chloroform; practically insoluble in ether.

Pilocarpine Nitrate

Proprietary names. Chibro-Pilocarpine; Licarpin; Pilagan; Pilo; Pilopos.
$C_{11}H_{16}N_2O_2,HNO_3$=271.3
CAS—148-72-1
Colourless crystals or white crystalline powder. M.p. 173° to 174°, with decomposition.
Soluble 1 in 4 of water and 1 in 75 of ethanol; insoluble in chloroform and ether.

Dissociation Constant. pK_a 1.6, 7.1 (15°).

Partition Coefficient. Log *P* (octanol/water), 0.1.

Thin-layer Chromatography. System TA—Rf 53; system TB—Rf 00; system TC—Rf 32; system TE—Rf 44; system TL—Rf 12; system TAE—Rf 52; system TAF—Rf 45; system TAJ—Rf 22; system TAK—Rf 00; system TAL—Rf 44. (Acidified iodoplatinate solution, positive.)

Gas Chromatography. System GA—RI 2014.

High Performance Liquid Chromatography. System HAA—Retention time 4.6 min; system HY—RI 158.

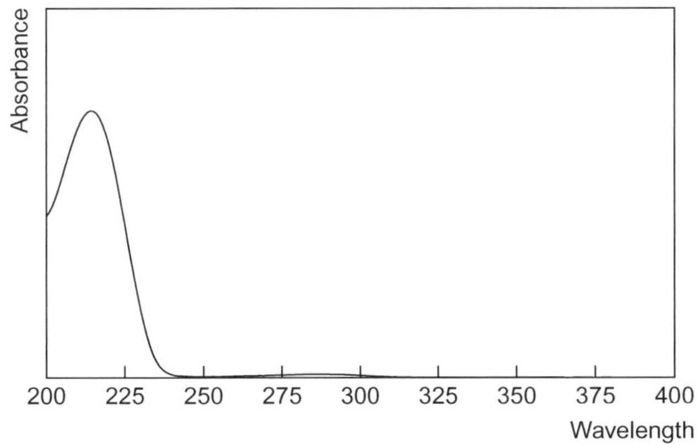

Infra-red Spectrum. Principal peaks at wavenumbers 1752, 1168, 1104, 660, 1505, 1020 cm^{-1} (thin film).

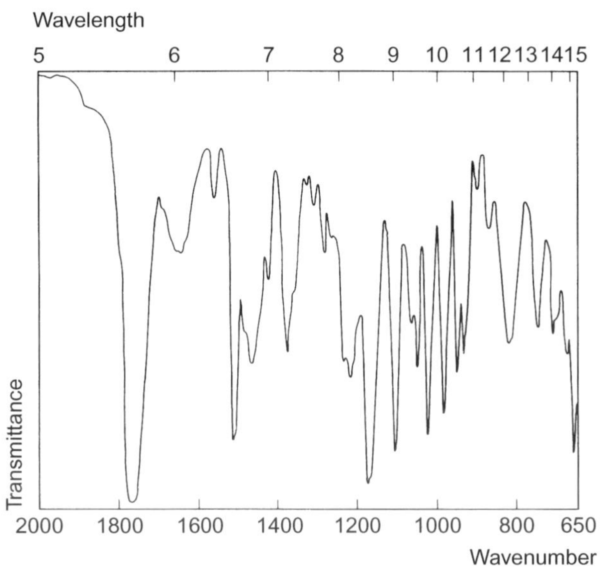

Mass Spectrum. Principal ions at *m/z* 95, 96, 42, 109, 41, 208, 54, 39.

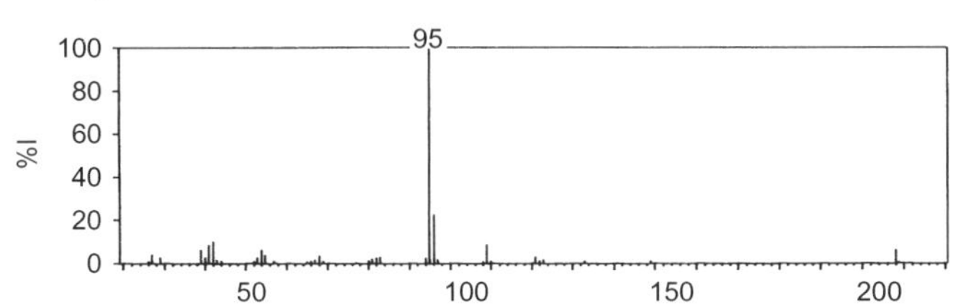

Quantification

Gas chromatography–mass spectrometry. In plasma: pilocarpic acid, limit of detection <1 µg/L—K. L. Birk *et al.*, *J. Chromatogr. B Biomed. Sci Appl.*, 1998, *719*, 93–102.

High performance liquid chromatography. In plasma: limit of detection 10 µg/L—M. L. Weaver *et al.*, *J. Chromatogr.* 1992, *581*, 293–296. In biological fluids: limit of detection 1 µg/L—C. Aromdee *et al.*, *J. Chromatogr. B Biomed. Appl.*, 1996, *677*, 313–318.

High performance liquid chromatography–mass spectrometry. In plasma or urine: pilocarpine, isopilocarpine, pilocarpic acid, and isopilocarpic acid—N. C. van de Merbel *et al.*, *J. Chromatogr. B Biomed. Sci Appl.*, 1998, *708*, 103–112.

Therapeutic concentration

18 subjects receiving a single oral dose (2.5 to 20 mg) of pilocarpine had a mean peak plasma concentration of 20.5 µg/L (range 12.5 to 33.2) at 1.21 h (0.50 to 1.87); the mean peak plasma concentration in 8 patients with renal failure receiving a similar dose was 30.9 µg/L (range 12.7 to 47.0) at 0.61 h (range 0.57 to 0.65) [J. V. St Peter *et al.*, *J. Clin. Pharmacol.*, 2000, *40*, 1470–1475].

8 subjects given 15 mg of a controlled-release pilocarpine formulation every 12 h for 3 doses had a mean peak plasma concentration of 8.2 µg/L approx. 1 h after the first dose and 11.5 µg/L after the third dose; 24 h after the final dose the level had declined to 0.06 µg/L [P. B. Lockhart *et al.*, *Oral Surg. Oral Med. Oral Pathol. Oral Radiol. Endod.*, 1996, *82*, 517–524].

Uses. Pilocarpine hydrochloride is used as a 0.5 to 5% ophthalmic solution and in the treatment of xerostomia/xerophthalmia.

Piminodine

Narcotic Analgesic

4-Phenyl-1-[3-(phenylamino)propyl]-4-piperidinecarboxylic acid ethyl ester

$C_{23}H_{30}N_2O_2$=366.5

CAS—13495-09-5

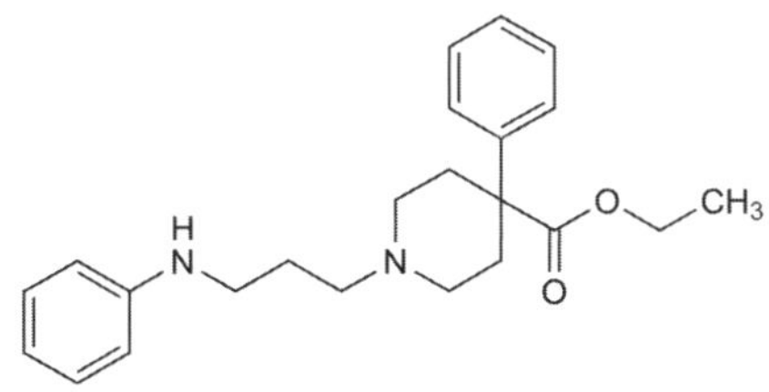

Piminodine Esilate

Synonyms. Piminodine Esylate; Piminodine Ethanesulfonate.

$C_{23}H_{30}N_2O_2,C_2H_6O_3S$=476.6

CAS—7081-52-9

A colourless crystalline powder. M.p. 128° to 135°.

Slightly soluble in water and ether; soluble 1 in 6 of ethanol and 1 in 2 of chloroform.

Partition Coefficient. Log *P* (octanol/water), 4.8.

Colour Test. Marquis Test—orange.

Thin-layer Chromatography. System TA—Rf 67; system TB—Rf 36; system TC—Rf 64; system TE—Rf 88; system TL—Rf 59; system TAE—Rf 63; system TAF—Rf 77; system TAJ—Rf 51; system TAK—Rf 24; system TAL—Rf 90. (Acidified iodoplatinate solution, positive; acidified potassium permanganate solution, positive.)

Gas Chromatography. System GA—RI 2884.

High Performance Liquid Chromatography. System HA—*k* 1.0.

Ultraviolet Spectrum. Aqueous acid—247, 253, 257, 263 nm.

Mass Spectrum. Principal ions at *m/z* 246, 45, 42, 366, 58, 57, 43, 106.

Dose. Piminodine esilate has been given in doses of 25 to 50 mg by mouth and 10 to 20 mg parenterally.

Pimozide

Tranquilliser

Synonym. R-6238

Proprietary names. Antolan; Opiran; Orap; Pizide.

1-[1-[4,4-Bis(4-fluorophenyl)butyl]-4-piperidinyl]-1,3-dihydro-2*H*-benzimidazol-2-one

$C_{28}H_{29}F_2N_3O$=461.6

CAS—2062-78-4

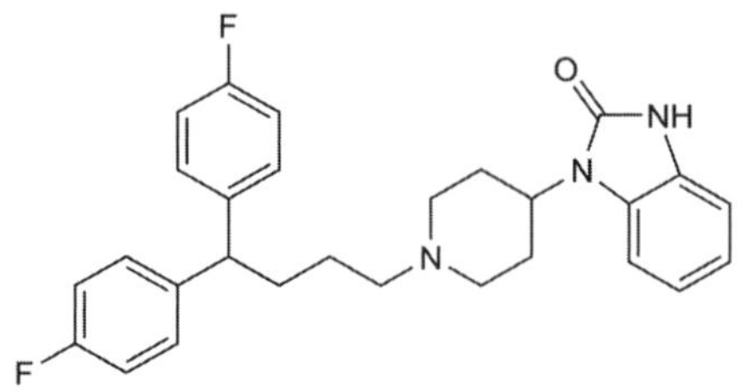

A colourless microcrystalline powder. M.p. 214° to 218°.
Practically insoluble in water; soluble 1 in 1000 of ethanol, ether, and methanol, 1 in 10 of chloroform, and 1 in 100 of acetone.

Dissociation Constant. pK_a 7.3.

Partition Coefficient. Log *P* (octanol/water), 6.3.

Colour Tests. Koppanyi–Zwikker Test—violet; Liebermann's Test—brown; Mandelin's Test—brown; Marquis Test—violet.

Thin-layer Chromatography. System TA—Rf 71; system TB—Rf 03; system TC—Rf 60; system TE—Rf 71; system TL—Rf 40; system TAE—Rf 73; system TAF—Rf 82. (Acidified iodoplatinate solution, positive.)

Gas Chromatography. System GA—pimozide RI 3870, M (*N*-desalkyl-) RI 2415, M (benzimidazolone) RI 1950, M (desamino-OH-) RI 2120, M (desamino-carboxy-) RI 2130; system GB—not eluted.

High Performance Liquid Chromatography. System HA—*k* 0.7; system HX—RI 504; system HZ—Retention time 11.9 min; system HAA—Retention time 17.2 min.

Ultraviolet Spectrum. Acid isopropyl alcohol—273, 280 nm (A^1_1 = 145a).

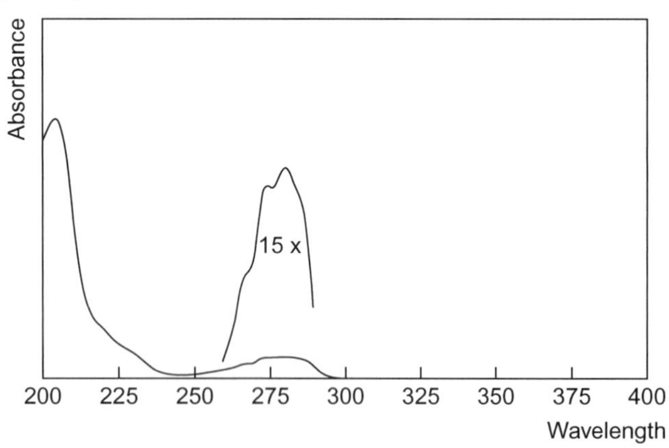

Infra-red Spectrum. Principal peaks at wavenumbers 1695, 1505, 753, 1220, 1230, 825 cm^{-1} (KBr disk).

Mass Spectrum. Principal ions at *m/z* 230, 187, 42, 217, 83, 82, 461, 96.

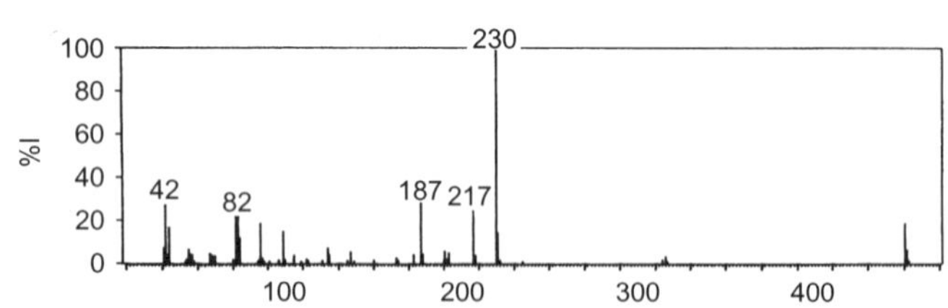

Quantification

Gas chromatography. In plasma: limit of detection 30 µg/L, FID—M. P. Quaglio *et al.*, *Boll. Chim. Farm.*, 1982, *121*, 276–284.

High performance liquid chromatography. In plasma: limit of detection < 5 µg/L, fluorescence detection—Y. Miyao *et al.*, *J. Chromatogr.*, 1983, *275*; *B Biomed. Appl.*, *26*, 443–449. In plasma: limit of detection 1 µg/L, fluorescence detection—T. Kerbusch *et al.*, *J. Chromatogr. B Biomed. Sci. Appl.*, 1997, *694*, 163–168.

Radioimmunoassay. In plasma: limit of detection 50 pg—L. J. M. Michiels *et al.*, *Life Sci.*, 1975, *16*, 937–944.

Disposition in the Body. Readily but slowly absorbed after oral administration. About 40% of a dose is excreted in the urine in 4 days. Two metabolites which have been identified in the urine are 4-bis(4-fluorophenyl)butyric acid and 1-(4-piperidyl)benzimidazolin-2-one. Very little unchanged drug is excreted in the urine. Both unchanged drug and the butyric acid metabolite are eliminated in the faeces.

Therapeutic concentration
Following a single oral dose of 6 mg to 9 subjects, a mean peak plasma concentration of about 0.004 mg/L was attained in 4 to 12 h (mean 8) [R. G. McCreadie *et al.*, *Br. J. Clin. Pharmacol.*, 1979, *7*, 533–534].

Half-life. Plasma half-life, about 2 days.

Note. For a review of pimozide see R. M. Pinder *et al.*, *Drugs*, 1976, *12*, 1–39.

Dose. 2 to 20 mg daily.

Pindolol

Beta-blocker

Synonyms. Prindolol; Prinodolol; LB-46.
Proprietary names. Apo-Pindol; Barbloc; Betapindol; durapindol; Hexapindol; Novo-Pindol; Nu-Pindol; Pinden; Pindocor; Pindol; Pindoptan; Pinloc; Pinsken; Viskeen; Visken; Viskene; Vypen. It is an ingredient of Viskaldix, Viskazide, and Viskenit.
1-(1*H*-Indol-4-yloxy)-3-[(1-methylethyl)amino]-2-propanol
$C_{14}H_{20}N_2O_2$ = 248.3
CAS—13523-86-9

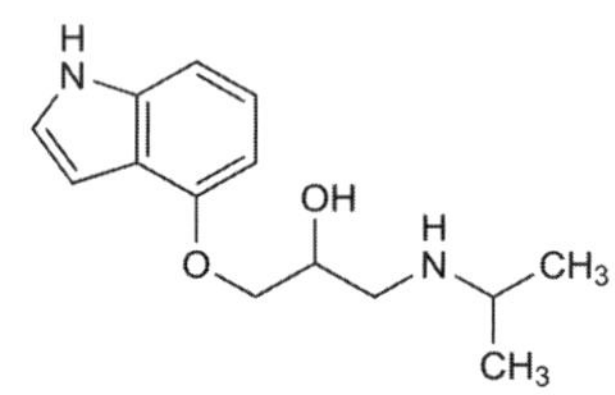

A white or almost white crystalline powder. M.p. 171° to 173°.
Practically insoluble in water; slightly soluble in dehydrated alcohol, methanol, and chloroform; soluble in mineral acids.

Dissociation Constant. pK_a 9.7 (24°).

Partition Coefficient. Log *P* (octanol/pH 7.0), −0.9.

Colour Tests. *p*-Dimethylaminobenzaldehyde—red/violet; Liebermann's Test—blue-green; Mandelin's Test—green; Marquis Test—yellow→brown.

Thin-layer Chromatography. System TA—Rf 49; system TB—Rf 02; system TC—Rf 05; system TE—Rf 43; system TL—Rf 08; system TAE—Rf 18; system TAF—Rf 78; system TAJ—Rf 00; system TAK—Rf 06; system TAL—Rf 56.

Gas Chromatography. System GA—RI 2245; system GB—RI 2335.

High Performance Liquid Chromatography. System HA—*k* 1.2; system HX—RI 300; system HY—RI 253; system HZ—Retention time 2.4 min; system HAA—Retention time 8.6 min.

Ultraviolet Spectrum. Aqueous acid—264 (A^1_1 = 292b), 287; methanol—264 (A^1_1 = 330a), 287 nm (A^1_1 = 182a). No alkaline shift.

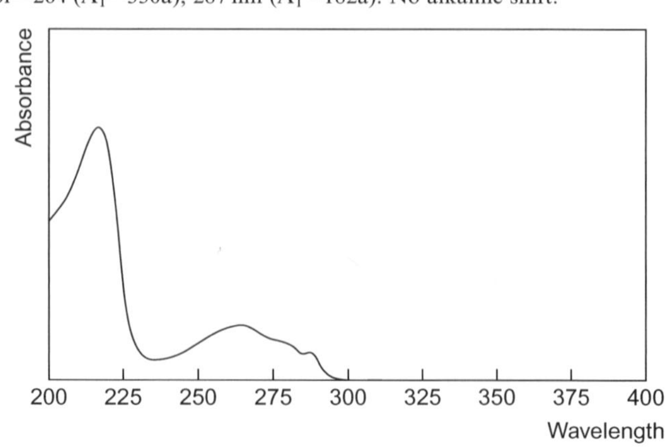

Infra-red Spectrum. Principal peaks at wavenumbers 768, 1096, 1250, 1288, 1053, 890 cm^{-1}.

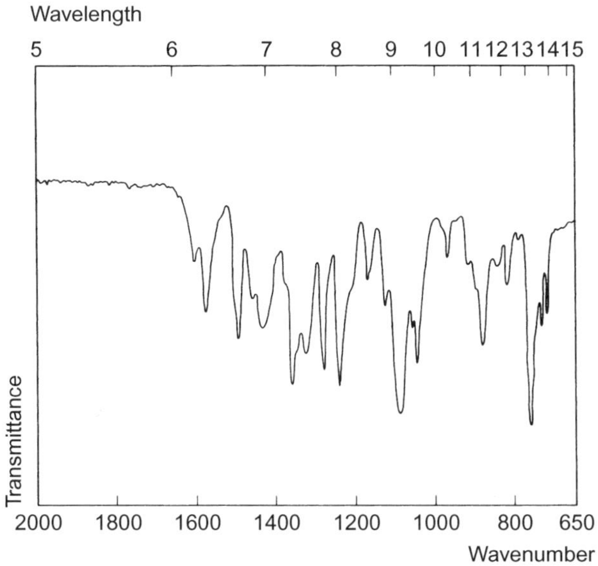

Mass Spectrum. Principal peaks at *m/z* 72, 133, 30, 116, 248, 134, 56, 41.

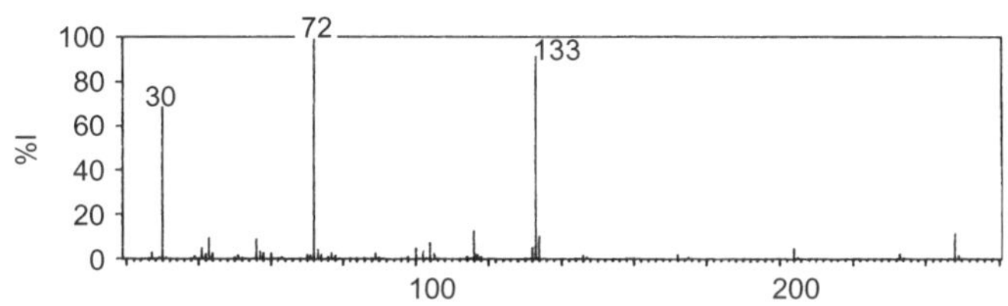

Quantification

Gas chromatography (Capillary column). In plasma: limit of detection 500 ng/L, ECD—M. Guerret, *J. Chromatogr.*, 1980, *221*; *B Biomed. Appl.*, *10*, 387–392.

High performance liquid chromatography. In plasma: limit of detection 2 µg/L, fluorescence detection—M. Bangah *et al.*, *J. Chromatogr.*, 1980, *183*; *B Biomed. Appl.*, *9*, 255–259; H. T. Smith, *J. Chromatogr.*, 1987, *415*, 95–103. In plasma or urine—B. J. Shields *et al.*, *J. Chromatogr.*, 1986, *378*, 163–171. In plasma: pindolol and other beta-blockers, UV or fluorescence detection—G. Musch *et al.*, *J. Pharm. Biomed. Anal.*, 1989, *7*, 483–497. In serum: limit of detection 2 µg/L—D. Chmielowiec *et al.*, *J. Chromatogr. Sci.* 1991, *29*, 37–39. In plasma: limit of detection 15 µg/L, amperometric detection—M. Telting-Diaz *et al.*, *J. Pharm. Biomed. Anal.*, 1991, *9*, 889–893. In serum or urine: pindolol enantiomers, limits of detection 1.2 µg/L (R+) and 4.3 µg/L (R–) in serum and 21 µg/L (R+) and 76 µg/L (R–) in urine, fluorescence detection—H. Zwang *et al.*, *J. Chromatogr. B Biomed. Appl.*, 1995, *668*, 309–313. In plasma or urine: fluorescence detection—J. L. Beal and S. E. Tett, *J. Chromatogr. B Biomed. Sci. Appl.*, 1998, *715*, 409–415.

Disposition in the Body. Well absorbed after oral administration. Metabolised by conjugation with glucuronic acid and sulfate. About 20 to 30% of an oral dose is excreted in the urine in 24 h as unchanged drug.

Therapeutic concentration

After a single oral dose of 5 mg given to 12 subjects, peak plasma concentrations of 0.02 to 0.08 mg/L (mean 0.04) were attained in 0.5 to 3 h [R. Gugler *et al.*, *Eur. J. Clin. Pharmacol.*, 1974, *7*, 17–24].

After daily oral dosing of 6 subjects with 5 mg three times a day, a mean steady-state plasma concentration of 0.015 mg/L was reported [R. Gugler and G. Bodem, *Eur. J. Clin. Pharmacol.*, 1978, *13*, 13–16].

Half-life. Plasma half-life, 2 to 4 h.

Volume of distribution. About 1 to 2 L/kg.

Clearance. Plasma clearance, about 7 mL/min/kg.

Distribution in blood. Plasma:whole blood ratio, 1.5.

Protein binding. In plasma, 40 to 70%.

Note. For a review of the pharmacokinetics of the beta-blocking agents see G. Johnsson and C.-G. Regärdh, *Clin. Pharmacokinet.*, 1976, *1*, 233–263.

Dose. Up to 45 mg daily.

Pipamperone

Tranquilliser

Synonyms. Floropipamide; R-3345.

1′-[4-(4-Fluorophenyl)-4-oxobutyl]-[1,4′-bipiperidine]-4′-carboxamide

$C_{21}H_{30}FN_3O_2$=375.5

CAS—1893-33-0

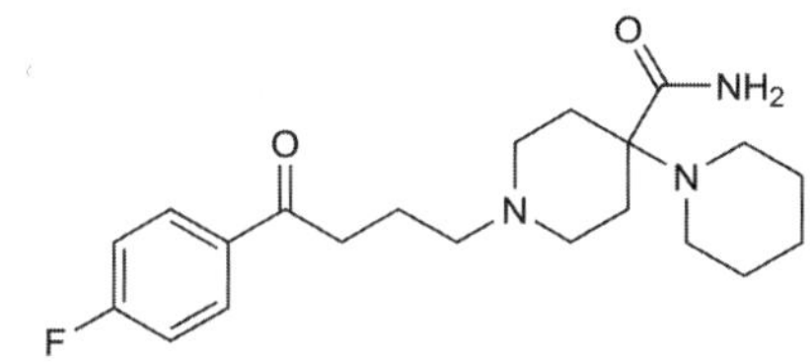

Pipamperone Hydrochloride

Proprietary names. Dipiperon; Piperonil.

$C_{21}H_{30}FN_3O_2$,2HCl=448.4

CAS—2448-68-2

Crystals. M.p. 124.5° to 126.0°.

Partition Coefficient. Log *P* (octanol), 2.4; (octanol/water), 2.0.

Thin-layer Chromatography. System TA—Rf 56; system TB—Rf 01; system TC—Rf 12; system TE—Rf 43; system TL—Rf 08; system TAE—Rf 33; system TAF—Rf 61. (Acidified potassium permanganate solution, positive.)

Gas Chromatography. System GA—pipamperone RI 3040, M (OH-) RI 3250.

High Performance Liquid Chromatography. System HX—RI 299; system HY—RI 241; system HZ—retention time 2.7 min; system HAA—retention time 10.9 min.

Ultraviolet Spectrum. Aqueous acid—248 nm (A^1_1=315a).

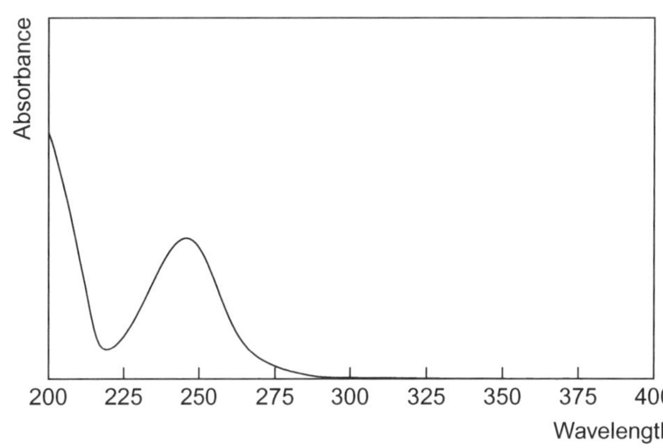

Infra-red Spectrum. Principal peaks at wavenumbers 1660, 1685, 1600, 1239, 1157, 1212 cm^{-1} (KBr disk).

Mass Spectrum. Principal ions at *m/z* 165, 138, 331, 123, 110, 194, 42, 41.

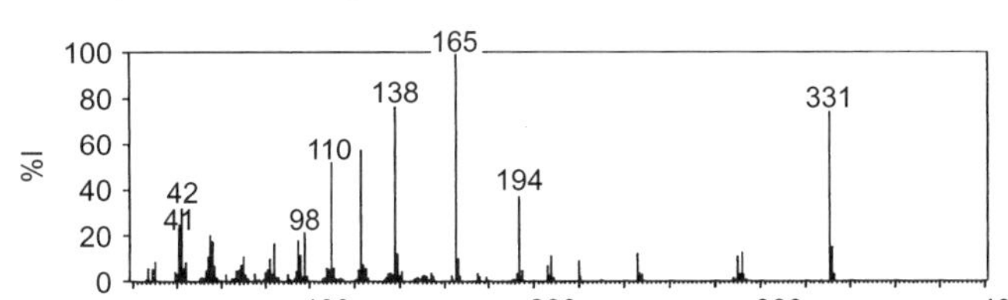

Quantification

Gas chromatography. In whole blood or urine: pipamperone and other butyrophenones, limit of detection about 0.1 nmol/L, SID—H. Seno *et al.*, *Nippon Hoigaku Zasshi*, 1993, *47*, 367–371.

High performance liquid chromatography. In plasma: limit of detection 2 µg/L, UV detection—I. Luhmann *et al.*, *Arzneimittelforschung*, 1992, *42*, 1069–1072.

Disposition in the body

Therapeutic concentration

Pipamperone dihydrochloride (≡120 mg pipamperone), given as either a reference tablet or one of two test tablets, to 24 subjects as a single oral dose, produced mean maximum plasma concentrations of 0.266 mg/L (range 0.161 to 0.455) for the reference product, 0.266 mg/L (range 0.087 to 0.509) for one of the test products and 0.263 mg/L (range 0.123 to 0.502) for the other. The time taken to reach maximum plasma concentrations was 1 h for all preparations. [G. E. Potgieter *et al.*, *Arzneimittelforschung*, 2002, *52*, 430–434.]

Mean plasma concentrations of 0.04403 (±0.01744) mg/L were attained 1.5 h after a single oral dose of 40 mg to 12 subjects. [I. Luhmann *et al.*, *Arzneimittelforschung*, 1992, *42*, 1069–1072.]

Dose. The equivalent of 120 to 360 mg of pipamperone daily.

Pipazetate

Antitussive

Synonyms. Pipazethate; Piperestazine; D-254.

10*H*-Pyrido[3,2-*b*][1,4]benzothiadiazine-10-carboxylic acid 2-(2-piperidinoethoxy)ethyl ester

$C_{21}H_{25}N_3O_3S$=399.5

CAS—2167-85-3

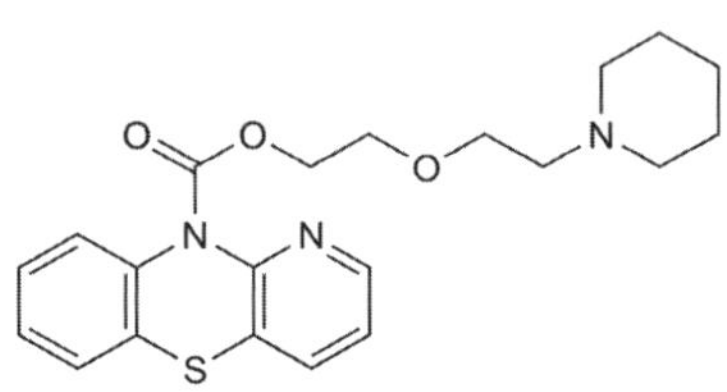

Pipazetate Hydrochloride

Proprietary names. Selvigon; Selvjgon; Transpulmin; Lenopect; Theratuss.

$C_{21}H_{25}N_3O_3S$,HCl=436.0

CAS—6056-11-7

A white crystalline powder. M.p. 160° to 161°.

Very soluble in water; soluble in ethanol and methanol. Practically insoluble in acetone.

Partition Coefficient. Log *P* (octanol/water), 4.9.

Colour Tests. Aromaticity (Method 2—colourless/yellow; Liebermann's Test—brown (→red at 100°).

Thin-layer Chromatography. System TA—Rf 47; system TB—Rf 17; system TC—Rf 13; system TE—Rf 48; system TL—Rf 06; system TAE—Rf 12. (Acidified iodoplatinate solution, positive.)

Gas Chromatography. System GA—RI 2037.

High Performance Liquid Chromatography. System HA—*k* 5.4; system HX—RI 385.

Ultraviolet Spectrum. Aqueous acid—251 nm (A_1^1=210a).

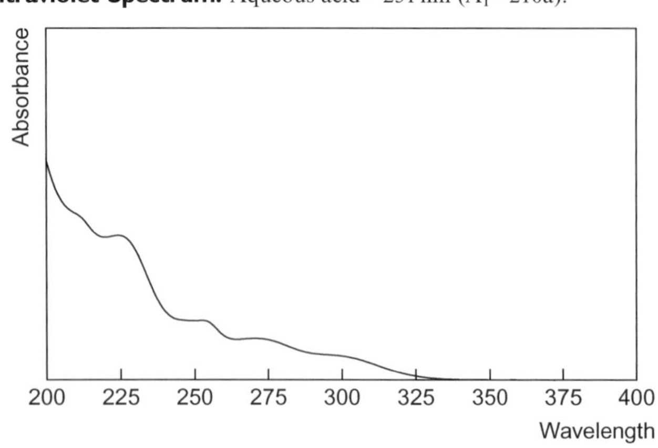

Infra-red Spectrum. Principal peaks at wavenumbers 1717, 1225, 1315, 1300, 1095, 1050 cm^{-1} (KBr disk).

Mass Spectrum. Principal ions at *m/z* 98, 111, 99, 199, 41, 288, 200, 55.

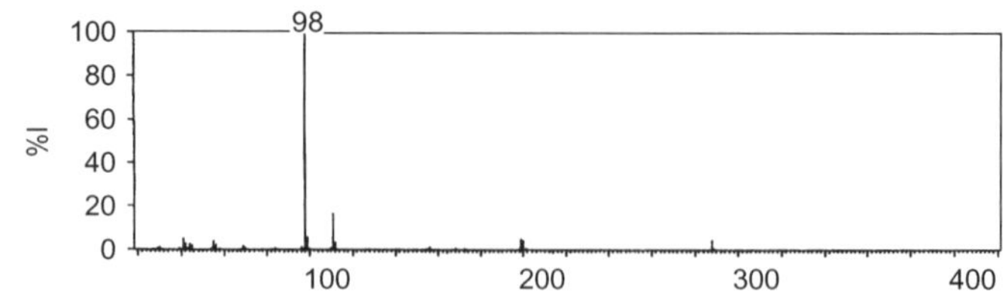

Dose. Pipazetate hydrochloride has been given in doses of 60 to 120 mg daily.

Pipenzolate Bromide

Anticholinergic

Synonyms. Pipenzolate Methobromide; Pipenzolone Bromide; JB-323.

Proprietary names. Expal; Ila-med m; Piptal; Poliptal; Propedil. It is an ingredient of Finprod, Pedriachol, and Piptalin.

1-Ethyl-3-[(hydroxydiphenylacetyl)-oxy]-1-methylpiperidinium bromide

$C_{22}H_{28}BrNO_3$=434.4

CAS—13473-38-6 (pipenzolate); 125-51-9 (bromide)

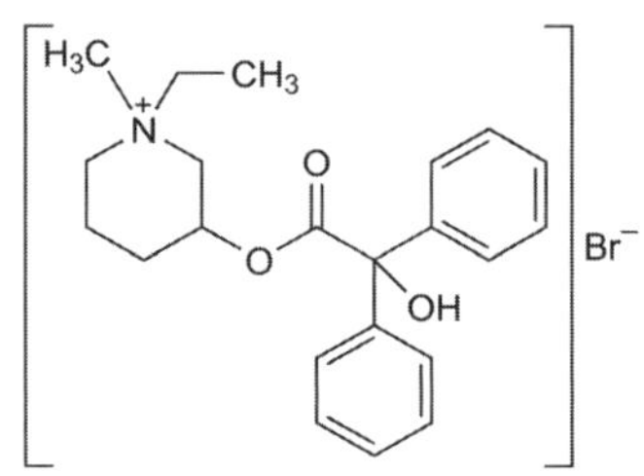

A white crystalline powder. M.p. 179° to 180°.

Freely soluble in water.

Partition Coefficient. Log *P* (octanol/water), –0.3.

Colour Tests. The following tests are performed on pipenzolate nitrate (see Chapter 19): Mandelin's Test—orange→green; Marquis Test—orange→green→blue.

Thin-layer Chromatography. System TA—Rf 04. (Acidified iodoplatinate solution, positive.)

Ultraviolet Spectrum. Aqueous acid—252, 258 nm (A_1^1=11a), 262 nm.

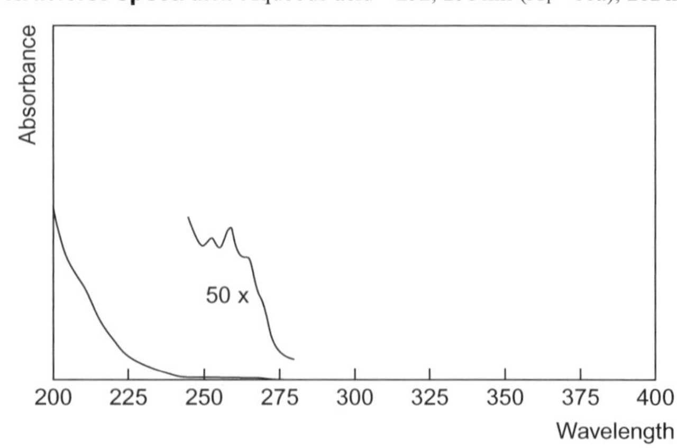

Infra-red Spectrum. Principal peaks at wavenumbers 1726, 698, 1220, 1160, 763, 1055 cm^{-1} (KBr disk).

Mass Spectrum. Principal ions at *m/z* 105, 111, 77, 96, 97, 183, 42, 51.

Dose. Usually 20 to 25 mg daily.

Piperacetazine

Tranquilliser

Synonym. PC-1421
Proprietary name. Quide
1-[10-[3-[4-(2-Hydroxyethyl)-1-piperidinyl]propyl]-10*H*-phenothiazin-2-yl]ethanone
$C_{24}H_{30}N_2O_2S = 410.6$
CAS—3819-00-9

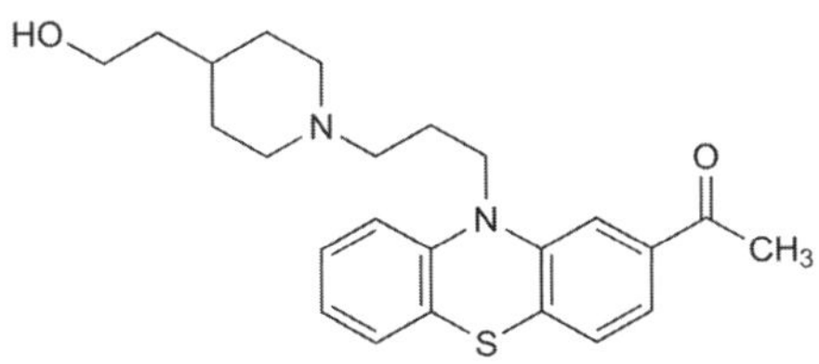

A yellow granular powder. M.p. 100° to 110°.
Practically insoluble in water; soluble 1 in 11 of ethanol, 1 in 1.3 of chloroform, and 1 in 1200 of ether.

Partition Coefficient. Log *P* (octanol/water), 5.1.

Colour Tests. Formaldehyde–Sulfuric Acid—blue-violet; Forrest Reagent—red; FPN Reagent—brown-orange; Mandelin's Test—green→red→violet; Marquis Test—red; Sulfuric Acid—yellow→red.

Thin-layer Chromatography. System TA—Rf 56; system TB—Rf 06; system TC—Rf 19; system TL—Rf 17; system TAJ—Rf 04; system TAK—Rf 00; system TAL—Rf 30. (Acidified iodoplatinate solution, positive.)

Gas Chromatography. System GA—not eluted.

High Performance Liquid Chromatography. System HA—*k* 1.9.

Ultraviolet Spectrum. Aqueous acid—243, 278 nm.

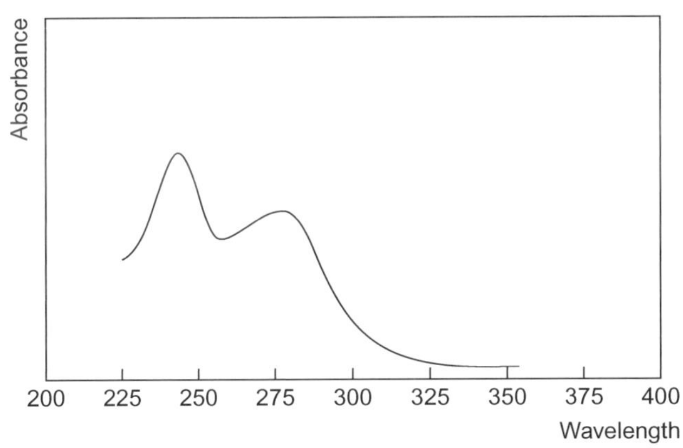

Infra-red Spectrum. Principal peaks at wavenumbers 1675, 1222, 1269, 1592, 748, 1560 cm^{-1} (KBr disk).

Mass Spectrum. Principal ions at *m/z* 142, 170, 44, 410, 42, 143, 43, 41.

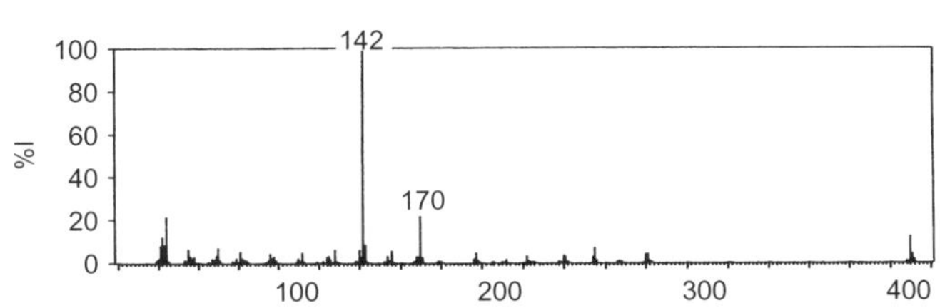

Dose. 20 to 160 mg daily.

Piperazine

Anthelmintic

Proprietary names. Lombrimade; Lu-Peracina; Ortovermin; Oxiurazina; Overpon; Pipemed; Piperazil; Pipercream; Pipermel; Pipertox; Pipervermin; Pirzinol; Trivermon; Verfid; Vermilen; Vermin; Versol.

$C_4H_{10}N_2 = 86.1$
CAS—110-85-0

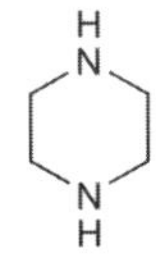

Crystals. M.p. 106°.
Soluble in water and ethanol; practically insoluble in ether.

Piperazine Adipate

Proprietary names. Adelmintex; Antepar; Entacyl; Vermi.
$C_4H_{10}N_2,C_6H_{10}O_4 = 232.3$
CAS—142-88-1
A white crystalline powder. M.p. 256° to 257°.
Soluble 1 in 18 of water; practically insoluble in ethanol, chloroform, and ether.

Piperazine Calcium Edetate

Synonym. Piperazine Calcium Edathamil
$C_4H_{10}N_2,C_{10}H_{14}CaN_2O_8 = 416.4$
CAS—12002-30-1
Freely soluble in water; very slightly soluble in ethanol and chloroform; practically insoluble in ether.

Piperazine Citrate

Synonym. Hydrous Tripiperazine Dicitrate
Proprietary names. Antepar; Citrazine; Citropiperazina; Ectodyne; Helmifar; Pipermed; Piprine; Pripsen Elixir; Tasnon; Veriga; Verimex; Vermex; Worm; Wormex; Wormilex.
$(C_4H_{10}N_2)_3,2C_6H_8O_7,xH_2O = 642.7$ (anhydrous)
CAS—144-29-6 (anhydrous); 41372-10-5 (hydrate)
A fine, white, crystalline or granular powder. M.p. about 190°.
Soluble 1 in 1.5 of water; practically insoluble in ethanol, chloroform, and ether.

Piperazine Hydrate

Synonyms. Diethylenediamine; Hexahydropyrazine; Piperazidine.
Proprietary names. Antelmina; Antepar; Ascarin; Desparasil; Pipralen; Solucamphre; Vermifran; Vermifuge.
$C_4H_{10}N_2,6H_2O = 194.2$
CAS—142-63-2
Colourless, glassy, deliquescent crystals. M.p. about 43°.
Soluble 1 in 3 of water and 1 in 1 of ethanol; very slightly soluble in ether.

Piperazine Phosphate

Proprietary name. It is an ingredient of Pripsen.
$C_4H_{10}N_2,H_3PO_4,H_2O = 202.1$
CAS—14538-56-8 (anhydrous); 18534-18-4 (monohydrate)
A white crystalline powder.
Soluble 1 in about 60 of water; practically insoluble in ethanol, chloroform, and ether; soluble in dilute hydrochloric acid.

Dissociation Constant. pK_a 5.7, 9.8 (20°).

Partition Coefficient. Log *P* (octanol/water), −1.5.

Colour Test. Simon's Test—blue.

Thin-layer Chromatography. System TA—Rf 05; system TB—Rf 01; system TC—Rf 01; system TL—Rf 00; system TAE—Rf 01; system TAF—Rf 04. (Acidified iodoplatinate solution, positive.)

Gas Chromatography. System GA—RI 813.

Ultraviolet Spectrum. No significant absorption, 230 to 360 nm.

Infra-red Spectrum. Principal peaks at wavenumbers 1592, 955, 870, 1080, 1055, 1115 cm^{-1} (piperazine citrate, KBr disk).

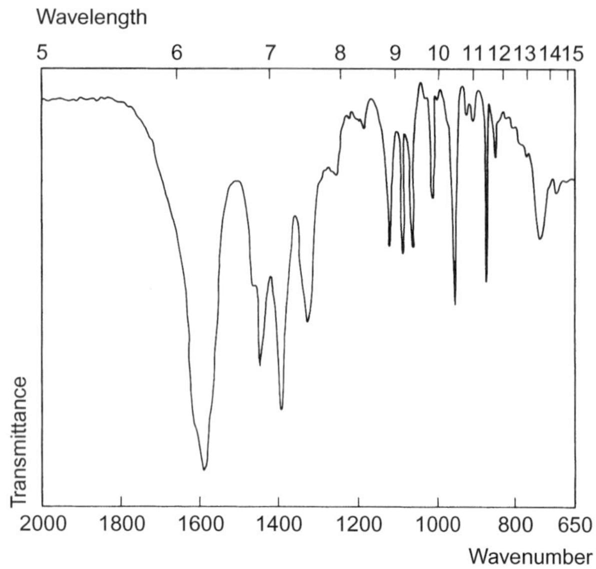

Mass Spectrum. Principal ions at *m/z* 44, 100, 41, 60, 29, 27, 30, 86 (piperazine adipate).

Quantification

Colorimetry. In urine—S. Hanna and A. Tang, *J. Pharm. Sci.*, 1973, *62*, 2024–2025.

Gas chromatography. In urine: limits of detection 20 µg/L and 1 µg/L, nitrogen-selective or mass-selective detection, respectively—G. Skarping *et al.*, *J. Chromatogr.*, 1986, *370*, 245–258.

Disposition in the Body. Readily absorbed after oral administration and excreted in the urine as unchanged drug and metabolites. There is wide variation in the rate of excretion between individuals, 15 to 75% of a dose being excreted in 24 h.

Toxicity. Toxic effects are rare and are usually due to accumulation after large doses. Three children had symptoms of toxicity after doses of 6, 9, and 12 g but they subsequently recovered.

Dose. The equivalent of 4 g of piperazine hydrate as a single dose, or 2 g daily for 7 days.

Piperidolate

Anticholinergic

Synonym. JB-305

α-Phenylbenzeneacetic acid 1-ethyl-3-piperidinyl ester

$C_{21}H_{25}NO_2$ = 323.4

CAS—82-98-4

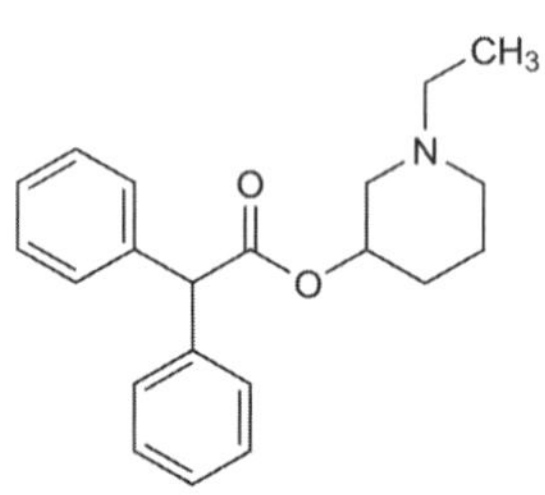

A liquid. B.p. 191° to 192°.

Piperidolate Hydrochloride

Proprietary name. Dactil

$C_{21}H_{25}NO_2,HCl$ = 359.9

CAS—129-77-1

A white or cream-coloured powder. M.p. 195° to 196°.

Soluble 1 in about 18 of water, 1 in about 52 of ethanol, 1 in about 4 of chloroform, and 1 in about 5 of methanol.

Partition Coefficient. Log *P* (octanol/water), 4.7.

Colour Tests. Liebermann's Test—orange-brown; Mandelin's Test—brown; Marquis Test—orange.

Thin-layer Chromatography. System TA—Rf 69; system TB—Rf 55; system TC—Rf 81; system TE—Rf 82; system TL—Rf 55; system TAE—Rf 54; system TAF—Rf 52; system TAJ—Rf 49; system TAK—Rf 11; system TAL—Rf 64. (Dragendorff spray, positive; acidified iodoplatinate solution, positive; Marquis reagent, yellow.)

Gas Chromatography. System GA—RI 2318; system GF—RI 2660.

High Performance Liquid Chromatography. System HA—*k* 1.7; system HX—RI 429.

Ultraviolet Spectrum. Aqueous acid—252, 258 (A_1^1 = 13.4a), 264 nm. No alkaline shift.

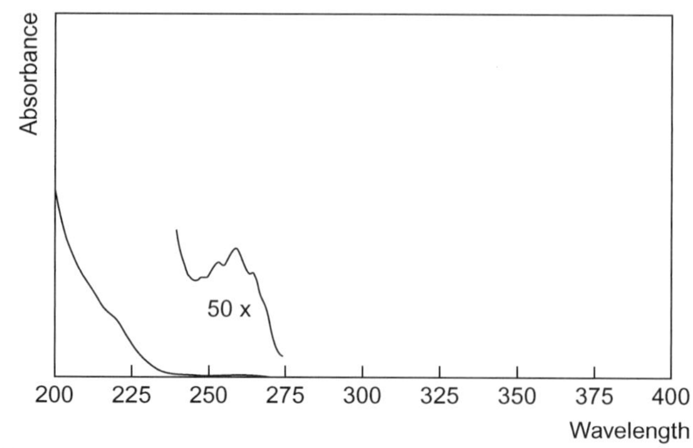

Infra-red Spectrum. Principal peaks at wavenumbers 1192, 1715, 1163, 1101, 700, 1149 cm^{-1} (piperidolate hydrochloride, KBr disk).

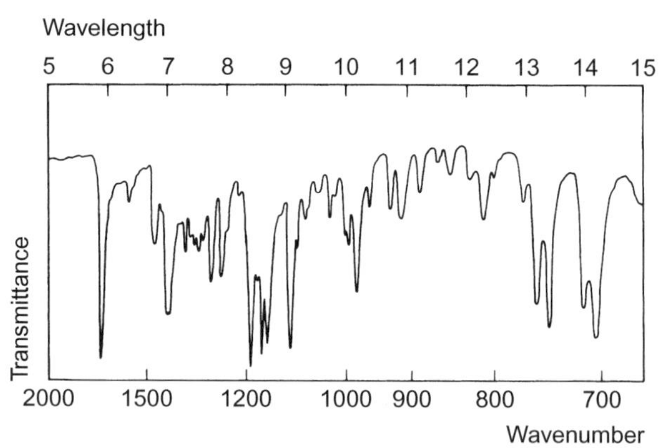

Mass Spectrum. Principal ions at *m/z* 111, 96, 167, 112, 165, 71, 43, 42.

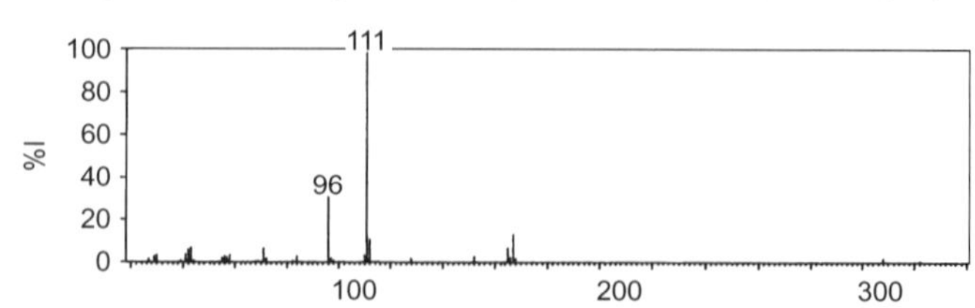

Dose. 200 mg of piperidolate hydrochloride daily.

Piperocaine

Anaesthetic (local)

2-Methyl-1-piperidinepropanol benzoate

$C_{16}H_{23}NO_2$ = 261.4

CAS—136-82-3

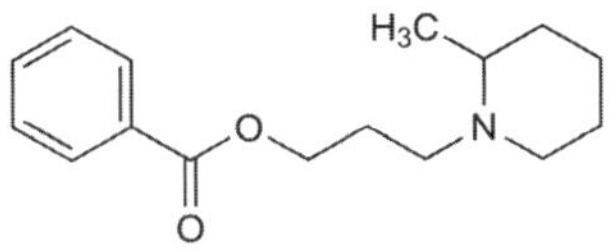

Piperocaine Hydrochloride
Proprietary name. Metycaine Hydrochloride
$C_{16}H_{23}NO_2,HCl=297.8$
CAS—533-28-8
Small white crystals or white crystalline powder. M.p. 167° to 169°.
Soluble 1 in 1.5 of water and 1 in 4.5 of ethanol; soluble in chloroform; practically insoluble in ether.

Partition Coefficient. Log *P* (octanol/water), 3.8.

Thin-layer Chromatography. System TA—Rf 55; system TB—Rf 53; system TC—Rf 37; system TE—Rf 76; system TL—Rf 27; system TAE—Rf 24; system TAF—Rf 56. (Dragendorff spray, positive; Acidified iodoplatinate solution, positive.)

Gas Chromatography. System GA—RI 1980.

High Performance Liquid Chromatography. System HQ—*k* 4.59; system HX—RI 357; system HY—RI 312.

Ultraviolet Spectrum. Aqueous acid—231, 274 nm.

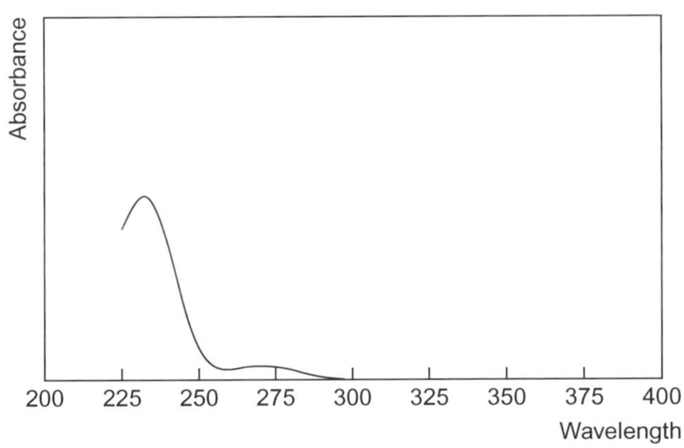

Infra-red Spectrum. Principal peaks at wavenumbers 1278, 1703, 711, 1115, 1310, 1040 cm^{-1} (piperocaine hydrochloride, KBr disk).

Mass Spectrum. Principal ions at *m/z* 112, 246, 105, 77, 55, 41, 44, 247.

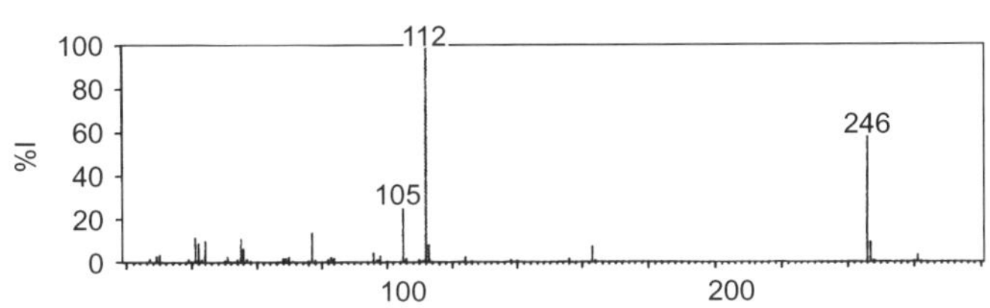

Uses. Piperocaine hydrochloride is used in concentrations of 0.5 to 10%.

Piperonyl Butoxide

Insecticide Synergist

Synonym. ENT 14250
Proprietary names. Butacide; Nusyn-noxfish; Prentox; Pybuthrin; Synpren-fish.
5-[[2-(2-Butoxyethoxy)ethoxy]methyl]-6-propyl-1,3-benzodioxole
$C_{19}H_{30}O_5=338.4$
CAS—51-03-6

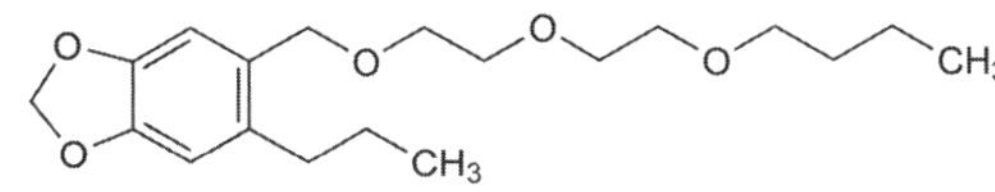

A yellow/ pale brown oily liquid. M.p. <25° and B.p. 180° at 1 mm Hg. Miscible with methanol, ethanol, benzene, freons, geons, other organic solvents, and oils. Very slightly soluble in water (14.3 mg/L at 25°).

Partition Coefficient. Log *P* (octanol/water), 4.75.

Gas Chromatography. System GA—RI 2376.

High Performance Liquid Chromatography. System HAA—retention time 27.6 min.

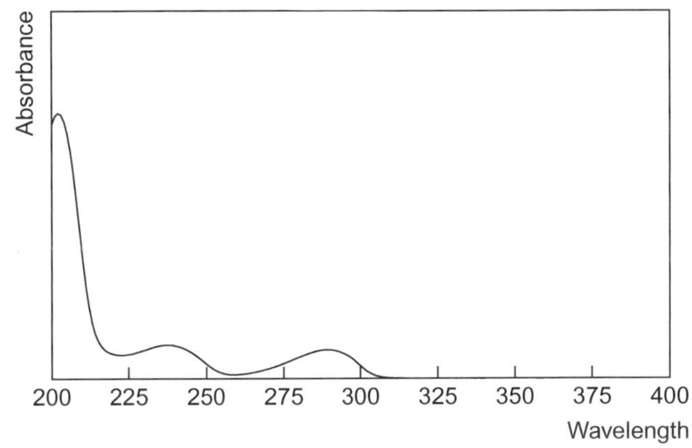

Mass Spectrum. Principal ions at *m/z* 176, 177, 149, 57, 119, 193, 41, 147.

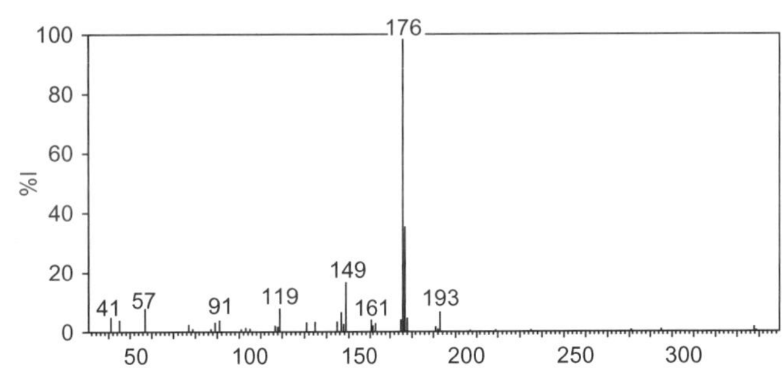

Disposition in the Body. Piperonyl is eliminated as the glucuronide or amino acid derivative.

Toxicity. Gastro-intestinal tract effects and mild CNS depression: coma, convulsions, hepatic, and renal damage. Poison via skin contact; moderately toxic by ingestion and intraperitoneal routes.

Pipobroman

Antineoplastic

Proprietary names. Vercite 25; Vercyte; Amedel.
1,4-Bis-(3-bromo-1-oxopropyl)piperazine
$C_{10}H_{16}Br_2N_2O_2=356.1$
CAS—54-91-1

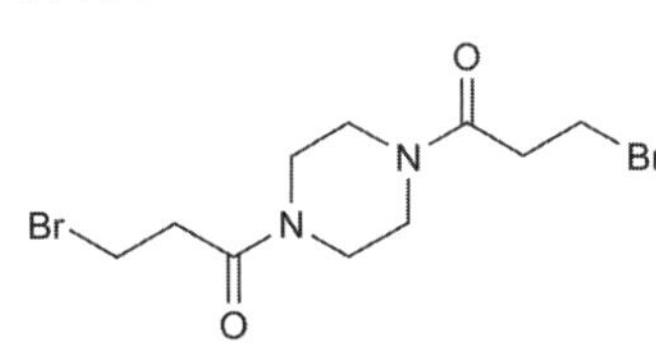

A white crystalline powder. M.p. 106° to 107°.
Soluble 1 in 230 of water, 1 in 35 of ethanol, 1 in 4.8 of chloroform, and 1 in 530 of ether; soluble in acetone.

Partition Coefficient. Log *P* (octanol/water), 0.4.

Colour Test. Add 2 mg to 2 mL of water and heat to dissolve; add 2 mL of hydroxylamine hydrochloride solution and 2 mL of 3 M sodium hydroxide, mix, and allow to stand for 30 min; acidify with dilute hydrochloric acid and add 2 mL of a 9% ferric chloride solution—red–orange.

Thin-layer Chromatography. System TA—Rf 66; system TB—Rf 02; system TC—Rf 58; system TL—Rf 41. (Acidified iodoplatinate solution, positive.)

Gas Chromatography. System GA—RI 1811.

Ultraviolet Spectrum. No significant absorption, 230 to 360 nm.

Infra-red Spectrum. Principal peaks at wavenumbers 1626, 1219, 1003, 1266, 923, 892 cm^{-1} (KBr disk).

Mass Spectrum. Principal ions at *m/z* 85, 56, 69, 55, 27, 44, 42, 109.

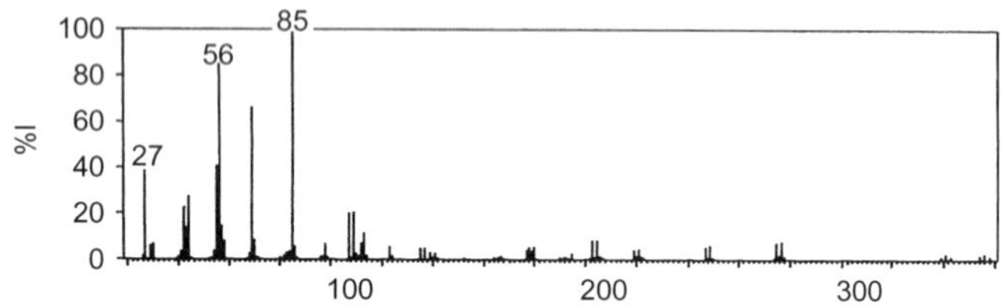

Dose. Initially 1 to 1.5 mg/kg daily, by mouth; maintenance, 7 to 175 mg daily.

Pipotiazine

Tranquilliser

Synonyms. Pipothiazine; RP-19366
Proprietary name. Piportil
10-[3-[4-(2-Hydroxyethyl)-1-piperidinyl]propyl]-*N*,*N*-dimethyl-10*H*-phenothiazine-2-sulfonamide
$C_{24}H_{33}N_3O_3S_2$=475.7
CAS—39860-99-6

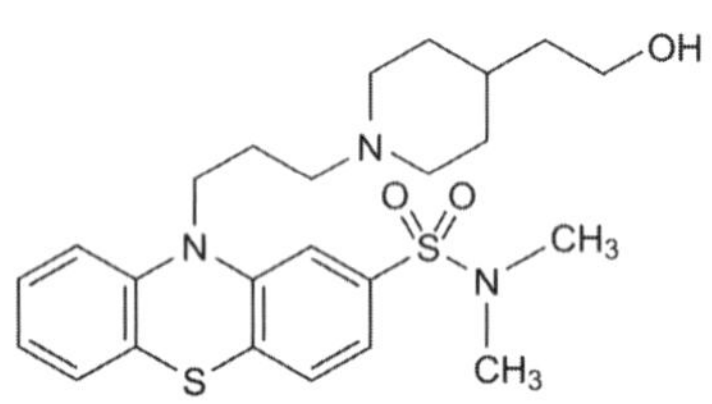

Pipotiazine Palmitate

Synonym. Pipothiazine Palmitate; RP-19552.
Proprietary names. Lonseren; Piportil L4.
$C_{40}H_{63}N_3O_4S_2$=714.1
CAS—37517-26-3
A pale yellow crystalline powder.
Practically insoluble in water; sparingly soluble in ethanol; freely soluble in chloroform and ether.

Pipotiazine Undecylenate

Synonym. RP-19551
Proprietary name. Piportil M2
$C_{35}H_{51}N_3O_4S_2$=641.9

Partition Coefficient. Log *P* (octanol/water), 4.4.

Thin-layer Chromatography. System TA—Rf 66; system TB—Rf 03; system TC—Rf 32; system TE—Rf 53; system TL—Rf 21; system TAE—Rf 40; system TAF—Rf 59.

Gas Chromatography. System GA—RI 2932; system GB—not eluted.

High Performance Liquid Chromatography. System HX—RI 431; system HAA—Retention time 14.7 min.

Ultraviolet Spectrum. Pipotiazine palmitate: ethanol—265 (A^1_1=500b), 315 nm.

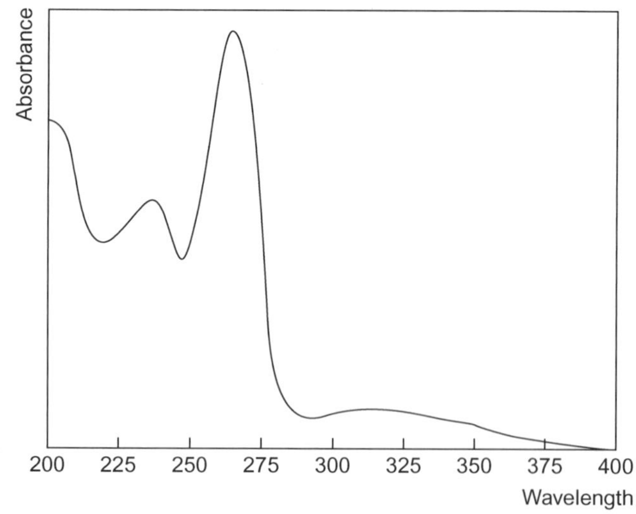

Infra-red Spectrum. Principal peaks at wavenumbers 1165, 1735, 710, 745, 1250, 955 cm^{-1} (pipotiazine palmitate, solution in carbon tetrachloride–carbon disulfide).

Mass Spectrum. Principal ions at *m/z* 142, 44, 140, 42, 198, 170, 41, 96.

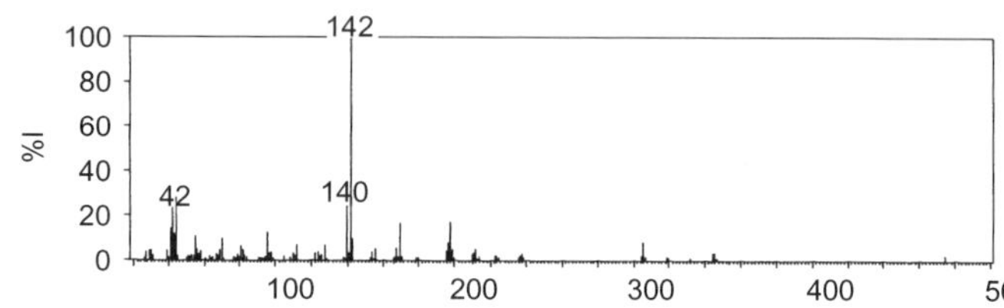

Quantification

Gas chromatography. In plasma: limit of detection 10 µg/L, ECD—S. F. Cooper and Y. D. Lapierre, *J. Chromatogr.*, 1981, *222*; *B Biomed. Appl.*, *11*, 291–296.

High performance liquid chromatography. In plasma or urine: limit of detection 250 ng/L for plasma and 2 µg/L for urine, fluorescence detection—Y. Le Roux *et al.*, *J. Chromatogr.*, 1982, *230*; *B Biomed. Appl.*, *19*, 401–408. In plasma—D. A. Ogden *et al.*, *J. Pharm. Biomed. Anal.*, 1989, *7*, 1273–1280.

Disposition in the Body. Pipotiazine palmitate is very slowly absorbed from the site of IM injections and gradually releases pipotiazine into the body. After oral administration of pipotiazine, about 1% of a dose is excreted in the urine unchanged in 24 h.

Therapeutic concentration

Following monthly IM injections of 25 to 112.5 mg to 5 subjects, plasma concentrations of 0.018 to 0.058 mg/L (mean 0.038) were reported immediately before a dose [S. F. Cooper and Y. D. Lapierre, *J. Chromatogr.*, 1981, *222*; *B Biomed. Appl.*, *11*, 291–296].

Dose. Usually 10 to 20 mg of pipotiazine daily, by mouth. Pipotiazine palmitate is given intramuscularly in doses of 25 to 200 mg, at intervals of about 4 weeks.

Pipoxolan

Antispasmodic

Synonym. BR-18
5,5-Diphenyl-2-[2-(1-piperidinyl)ethyl]-1,3-dioxolan-4-one
$C_{22}H_{25}NO_3$=351.4
CAS—23744-24-3

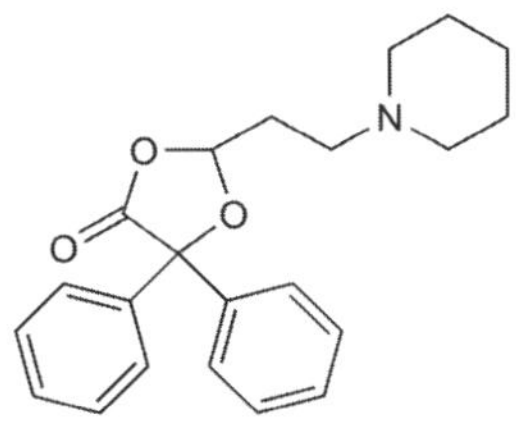

Pipoxolan Hydrochloride
Proprietary name. Rowapraxin
$C_{22}H_{25}NO_3,HCl=387.9$
CAS—18174-58-8
A white crystalline powder. M.p. 207° to 209°.
Soluble in water.

Colour Tests. Liebermann's Test—brown; Mandelin's Test—green→brown; Marquis Test—violet→grey; Sulfuric Acid—red.

Thin-layer Chromatography. System TA—Rf 77; system TB—Rf 53; system TC—Rf 68; system TL—Rf 56. (Acidified iodoplatinate solution, positive.)

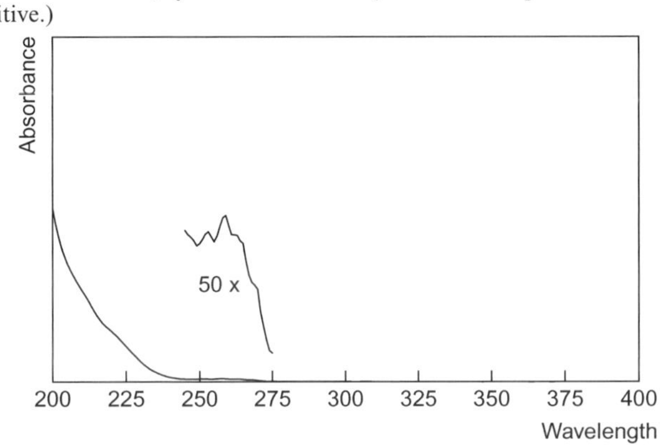

Infra-red Spectrum. Principal peaks at wavenumbers 1786, 1176, 1205, 1111, 1149, 698 cm^{-1} (KBr disk).

Mass Spectrum. Principal ions at *m/z* 98, 194, 166, 157, 55, 42, 165, 99.

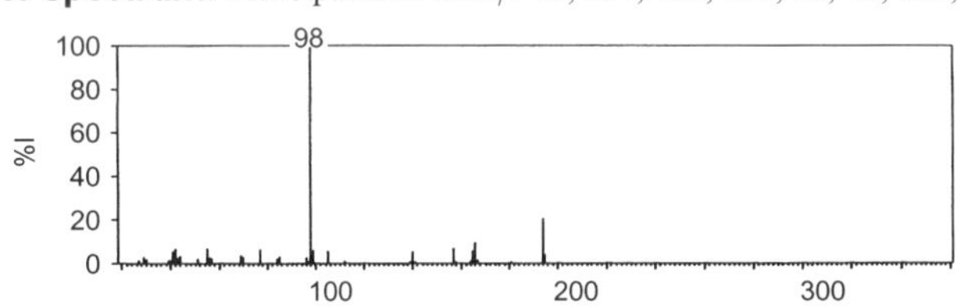

Dose. Pipoxolan hydrochloride has been given in doses of 20 to 90 mg daily.

Pipradrol

Central Stimulant

Synonyms. MRD-108; alpha-pipradrol; pipradol.
α,α-Diphenyl-2-piperidinemethanol
$C_{18}H_{21}NO=267.4$
CAS—467-60-7

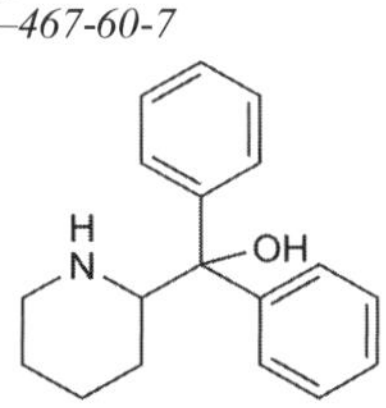

Pipradrol Hydrochloride
Proprietary names. Meratran; Stimolag. It is an ingredient of Alertonic.
$C_{18}H_{21}NO,HCl=303.8$
CAS—71-78-3
Small white crystals or white crystalline powder. M.p. 308° to 309° (crystals from butanone).
Soluble 1 in 60 of hot water, 1 in 35 of ethanol, 1 in 1000 of chloroform, and 1 in 8 of methanol; practically insoluble in ether.

Partition Coefficient. Log *P* (octanol/water), 3.4.

Colour Test. Marquis Test—yellow-orange.

Thin-layer Chromatography. System TA—Rf 54; system TB—Rf 59; system TC—Rf 38; system TE—Rf 81; system TL—Rf 39; system TAE—Rf 19; system TAF—Rf 79. (Dragendorff spray, positive; acidified iodoplatinate solution, positive; Marquis reagent, red-brown; ninhydrin spray, positive.)

Gas Chromatography. System GA—RI 2145; system GB—RI 2242; system GC—RI 2478.

High Performance Liquid Chromatography. System HA—*k* 1.2; system HC—*k* 0.69; system HX—RI 355.

Ultraviolet Spectrum. Aqueous acid—252, 258 nm ($A^1_1=17a$). No alkaline shift. (See below)

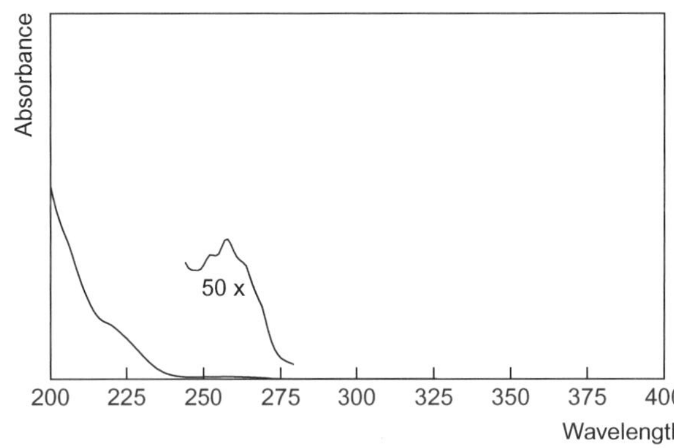

Infra-red Spectrum. Principal peaks at wavenumbers 701, 740, 690, 1585, 1300, 1065 cm^{-1} (pipradrol hydrochloride, KBr disk).

Mass Spectrum. Principal ions at *m/z* 84, 56, 85, 77, 105, 55, 30, 42.

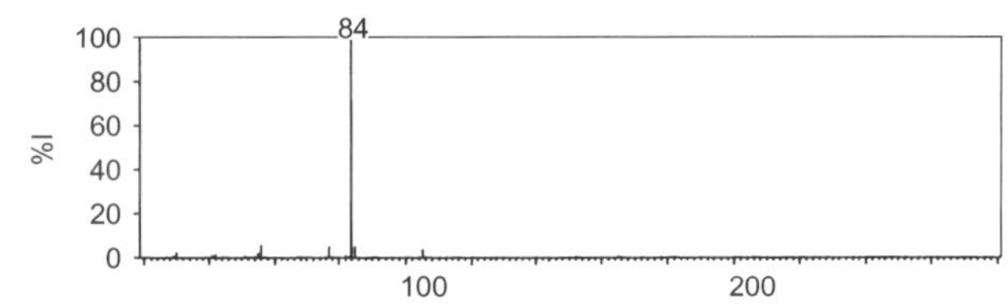

Dose. Pipradrol hydrochloride has been given in doses of 2 to 6 mg daily.

Pirenzepine

Treatment of Gastric Ulcers/Antiulcerative

Synonym. LS-519
5,11-Dihydro-11-[(4-methyl-1-piperazinyl)acetyl]-6*H*-pyrido[2,3-*b*]-[1,4]benzodiazepin-6-one
$C_{19}H_{21}N_5O_2=351.4$
CAS—28797-61-7

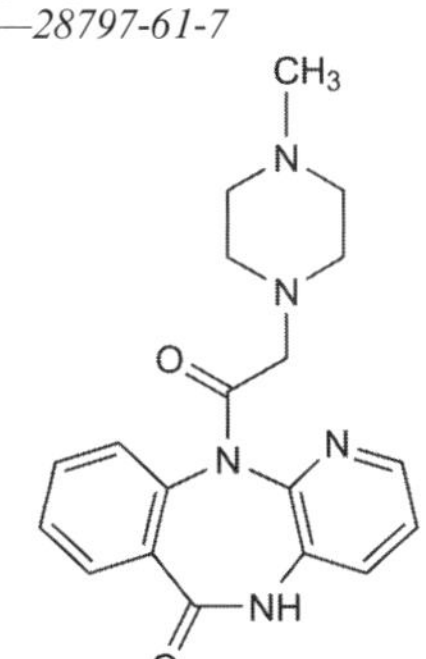

Pirenzepine Hydrochloride
Synonym. LS-519-cl2
Proprietary names. Cevanil; Duogastral; Frazim; Gastricur; Gastrol; Gastropin; Gastropiren; Gastrosed; Gastrozepin(a); Ulcepin; Ulcin; Ulcoprotect; Ulcosafe; Leblon; Maghen; Tabe.

$C_{19}H_{21}N_5O_2,2HCl=424.3$
CAS—29868-97-1
A white crystalline powder. M.p. 248° to 253°, with decomposition.
Freely soluble in water; practically insoluble in ether; very slightly soluble in methanol.

Dissociation Constant. pK_a 2.1, 8.1.

Partition Coefficient. Log *P* (octanol/water), 1.7.

Thin-layer Chromatography. System TB—pirenzepine Rf 00; M (desamide) Rf 04; M (*N*-desmethyl) Rf 00; system TE—pirenzepine Rf 16; M (desamide) Rf 70; M (*N*-desmethyl) Rf 03; system TAE—pirenzepine Rf 18; M (desamide) Rf 81; M (*N*-desmethyl) Rf 04.

High Performance Liquid Chromatography. System HA—*k* 2.7; system HX—pirenzepine RI 293; M (desamide) RI 373; M (*N*-desmethyl) RI 291.

Ultraviolet Spectrum. Aqueous acid—280 (A_1^1=237a); aqueous alkali—297 nm (A_1^1=282b).

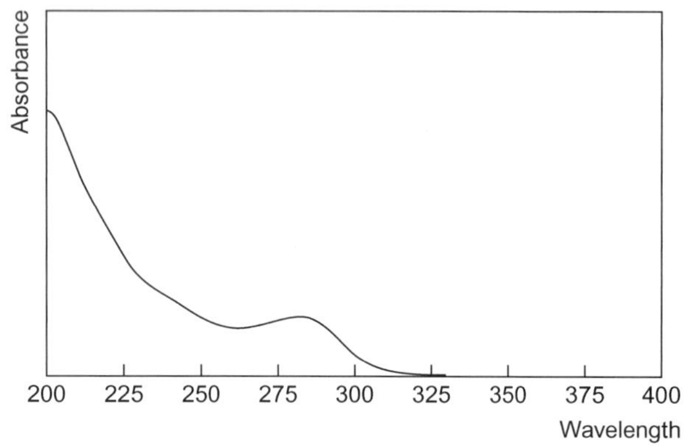

Infra-red Spectrum. Principal peaks at wavenumbers 1665, 1703, 1318, 1300, 1278, 1593 cm^{-1} (pirenzepine hydrochloride, KBr disk).

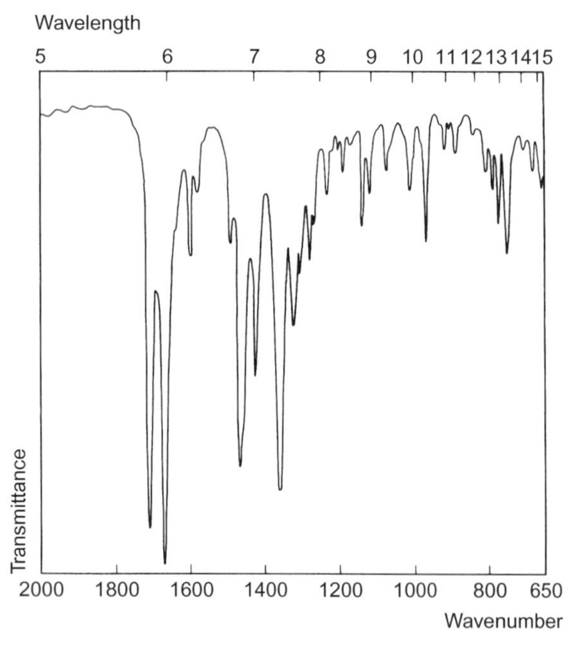

Mass Spectrum. Principal ions at *m/z* 113, 70, 42, 211, 351, 43, 71, 56.

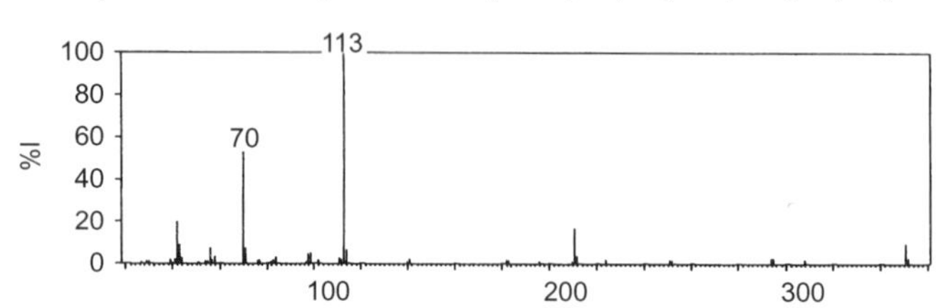

Quantification
High performance liquid chromatography. In plasma: limit of detection 2.5 μg/L—I. Meineke *et al.*, *J Chromatogr.*, 1986, *375*, 369–375.

Radioimmunoassay. In plasma or urine: limits of detection 0.25 μg/L in plasma and 4 μg/L in urine—P. Tanswell *et al.*, *J. Immunol. Methods*, 1986, *93*, 247–258.

Disposition in the Body. Incompletely absorbed after oral administration. Excreted in the urine and faeces largely as unchanged drug with less than 10% of a dose as the desmethyl metabolite.

Therapeutic concentration
Following a single oral dose of 50 mg to 87 subjects, a mean peak plasma concentration of 0.05 mg/L was attained in 2 h [G. Bozler and R. Hammer, *Scand. J. Gastroenterol.*, 1980, *15*, *Suppl.* 66, 27–33].

Bioavailability. About 20 to 30%.

Half-life. Plasma half-life, about 11 h.

Clearance. Plasma clearance, about 3.5 mL/min/kg.

Protein binding. In plasma, about 10%.

Dose. 100 to 150 mg of pirenzepine hydrochloride daily.

Piritramide

Narcotic Analgesic

Synonyms. Pirinitramide; A-65; R-3356.
Proprietary names. Dipidolor; Piridolan.
1′-(3-Cyano-3,3-diphenylpropyl)-[1,4′-bipiperidine]-4′-carboxamide
$C_{27}H_{34}N_4O=430.6$
CAS—302-41-0

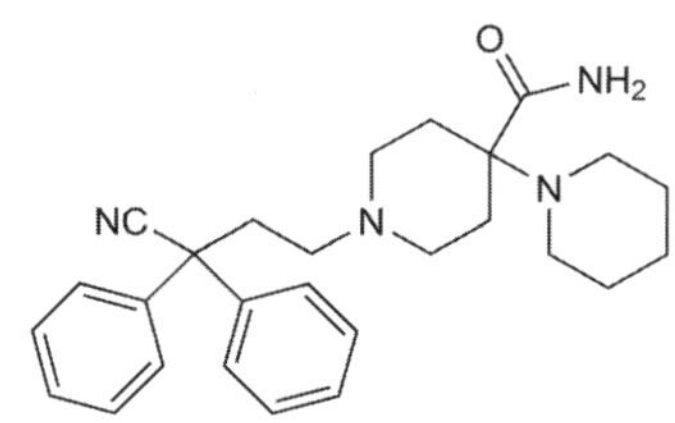

A crystalline powder. M.p. 149° to 150°.
Soluble in dilute acetic acid.

Partition Coefficient. Log *P* (octanol/water), 3.9.

Thin-layer Chromatography. System TA—Rf 70; system TB—Rf 01; system TC—Rf 45; system TE—Rf 61; system TL—Rf 42; system TAE—Rf 73; system TAF—Rf 74. (Dragendorff spray, positive; acidified iodoplatinate solution, positive; Marquis reagent, orange; ninhydrin spray, positive.)

Gas Chromatography. System GA—RI 3560.

High Performance Liquid Chromatography. System HA—*k* 0.6; system HC—*k* 0.1; system HX—RI 377; system HY—RI 343.

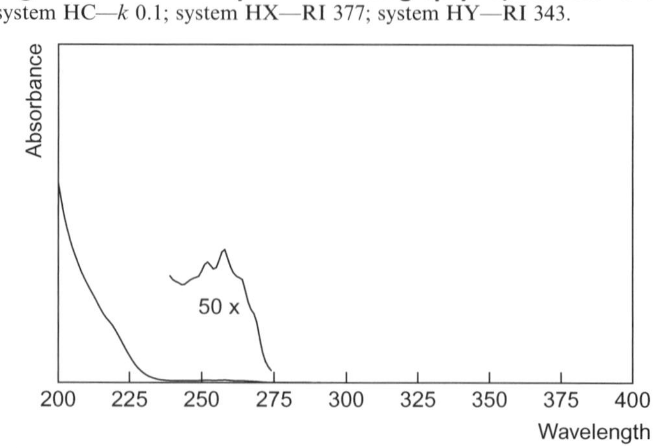

Infra-red Spectrum. Principal peaks at wavenumbers 1669, 701, 757, 1087, 1190, 1592 cm^{-1} (KBr disk).

Mass Spectrum. Principal ions at m/z 386, 138, 387, 84, 110, 42, 301, 263.

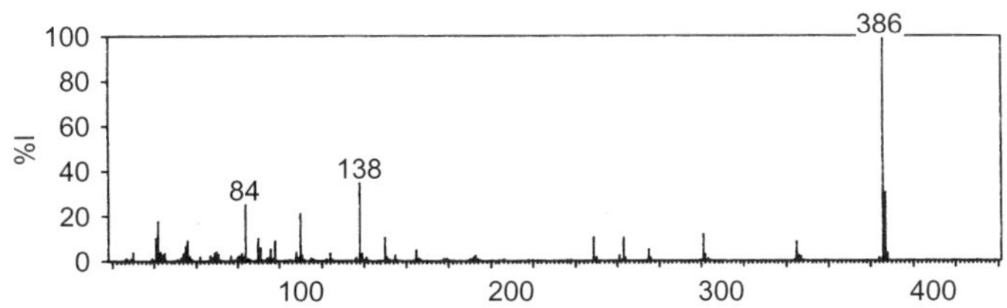

Dose. 20 mg by IM injection.

Piroxicam

Analgesic

Synonym. CP-16171
Proprietary names. Antiflog; Brexidol; Brexin(e); Candyl; Cycladol; Fasax; Felden(e); Fexicam; Flamatrol; Flexase; Flexirox; Geroxicam; Inflaced; Jenapirox; Larapam; Olcam; Pericam; Piro; Pirocam; Piroflam; Piroxil; Piroxistad; Proxalyoc; Zofora; Sasulen; Zunden.
4-Hydroxy-2-methyl-*N*-2-pyridinyl-2*H*-1,2-benzothiazine-3-carboxamide 1,1-dioxide
$C_{15}H_{13}N_3O_4S = 331.3$
CAS—36322-90-4

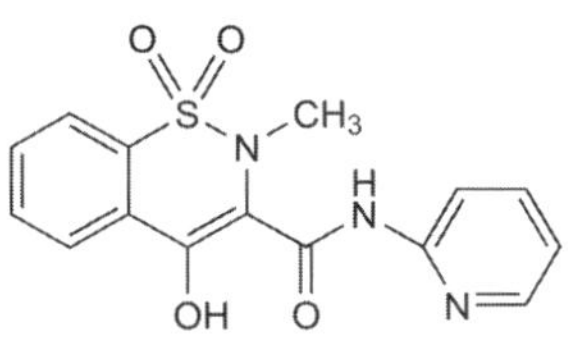

Crystals. M.p. 198° to 200°.
Practically insoluble in water; slightly soluble in dehydrated ethanol and aqueous alkaline solutions.

Dissociation Constant. pK_a 6.3.

Partition Coefficient. Log P (octanol/water), 3.1.

Colour Tests. Koppanyi–Zwikker Test (omit pyrrolidine)—orange; Liebermann's Test—yellow.

Thin-layer Chromatography. System TB—M (5-hydroxy) Rf 00; system TD—piroxicam Rf 51; M (5-hydroxy) Rf 08; system TE—piroxicam Rf 17; M (5-hydroxy) Rf 03; system TF—piroxicam Rf 38; M (5-hydroxy) Rf 18; system TAD—Rf 71; system TAE—piroxicam Rf 88; M (5-hydroxy) Rf 88; system TAJ—Rf 69; system TAK—Rf 45; system TAL—Rf 94.

Gas Chromatography. System GA—RI 1413.

High Performance Liquid Chromatography. System HD—*k* 0.6; system HW—*k* 7.7; system HX—piroxicam RI 431; M (5-hydroxy) RI 446; system HY—RI 382; system HZ—Retention time 4.9 min; system HAA—Retention time 16.6 min.

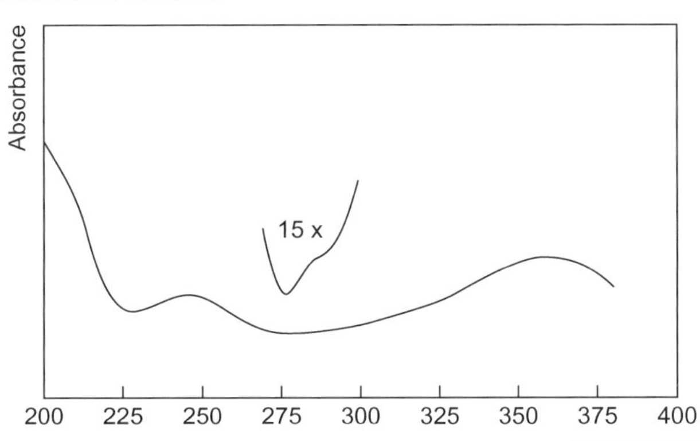

Infra-red Spectrum. Principal peaks at wavenumbers 1524, 1180, 1298, 1147, 1573, 770 cm^{-1}.

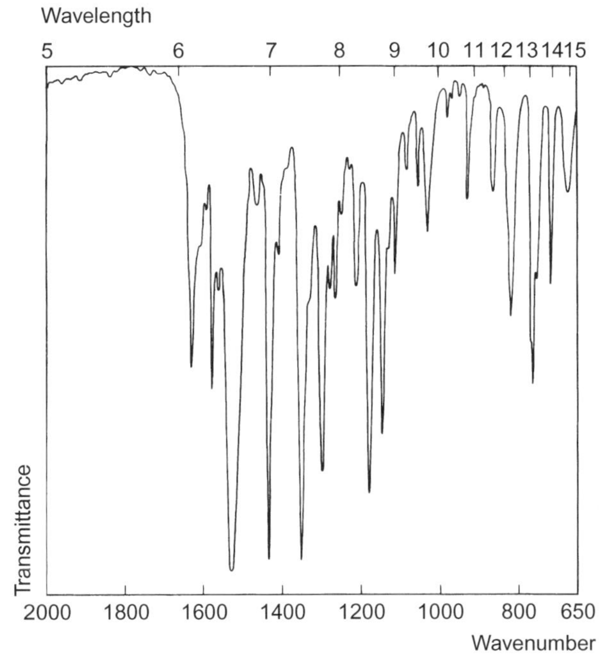

Mass Spectrum. Principal ions at m/z 173, 117, 145, 78, 104, 94, 76, 147.

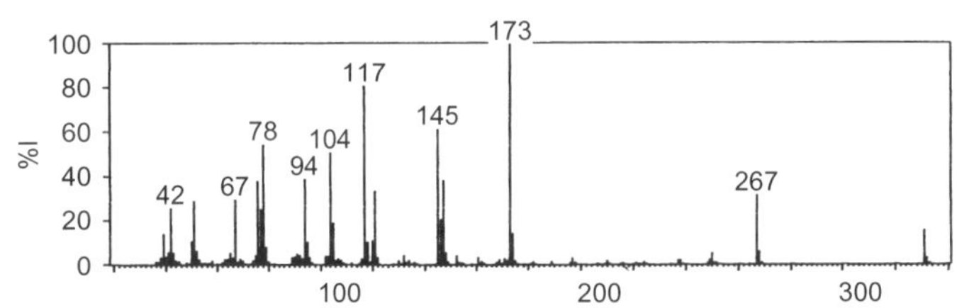

Quantification

High performance liquid chromatography. In serum: limit of detection 500 µg/L, UV detection—A. D. Fraser and J. F. L. Woodbury, *Ther. Drug Monit.*, 1983, *5*, 239–242. In plasma or serum: piroxicam and other NSAIDs, UV detection—P. J. Streete, *J. Chromatogr.*, 1989, *495*, 179–193. In plasma: limit of detection 0.2 mg/L, UV detection—K. Saeed and M. Becher, *J. Chromatogr.*, 1991, *567*, 185–193. In plasma, urine, or bile: piroxicam and its metabolites, limit of detection 50 µg/L, UV detection—P. A. Milligan, *J. Chromatogr.*, 1992, *576*, 121–128. In plasma or urine: piroxicam and 5′-hydroxypiroxicam, limit of detection 50 µg/L, UV detection—A. Avgerinos *et al.*, *J. Chromatogr. B Biomed. Appl.*, 1995, *673*, 142–146. In urine: piroxicam and other NSAIDs, limit of detection 50 µg/L, UV detection—T. Hirai *et al.*, *J. Chromatogr. B Biomed. Sci. Appl.*, 1997, *692*, 375–388. In plasma, subcutaneous tissue, synovial capsule, and synovial fluid, limit of detection in plasma 0.72 µg/L, electrochemical detection—A. D. de Jager *et al.*, *J. Chromatogr. B Biomed. Sci. Appl.*, 1999, *729*, 183–189. In plasma: limit of detection 50 to 100 µg/L, UV detection—M. Yritia *et al.*, *J. Chromatogr. A*, 1999, *846*, 199–205.

Disposition in the Body. Readily absorbed after oral or rectal administration. It is extensively metabolised to inactive metabolites; the major metabolite is produced by hydroxylation of the pyridyl ring and exists free and conjugated with glucuronic acid. About 10% of an oral dose is excreted in the urine as unchanged drug in 8 days.

Therapeutic concentration. Piroxicam accumulates on repeated administration; steady-state plasma concentrations are attained after approximately 7 days. The normal therapeutic level is between 5 and 10 mg/L.

Following oral administration of 40 mg to 20 subjects, peak plasma concentrations of 1.7 to 6.8 mg/L (mean 4.3) were reported; multiple peak concentrations were observed in 16 subjects, suggesting possible enterohepatic circulation. After daily oral administration of 10, 20, and 30 mg to 5 subjects for 14 days, maximum steady-state plasma concentrations of 2.1 to 4.3 (mean 3.2), 3.6 to 6.5 (mean 4.5), and 9.0 to 16.5 (mean 11.7) mg/L were reported [D. C. Hobbs and T. M. Twomey, *J. Clin. Pharmacol.*, 1979, *19*, 270–281].

Administration of 20 mg piroxicam daily for at least 4 weeks to 85 osteoarthritis patients produced mean steady-state free plasma concentrations of 0.057 mg/L when all patients were considered and 0.004 to 0.117 mg/L in newly diagnosed patients (fraction of unbound piroxicam was 0.87%) [O. Hundal and H. E. Rugstad, *Clin. Rheumatol.*, 1993, *12*, 221–230].

Toxicity
After ingesting approximately 1800 mg of piroxicam, a 54-year-old woman had a maximum serum concentration of 241.6 mg/L (measured at about 12 h after the overdosage), which is about 30 times the normal therapeutic level (5 to 10 mg/L) [J. Mosvold *et al.*, *Acta Med. Scand.*, 1984, *216*, 335–336].

Half-life. Plasma half-life, about 30 to 60 h, increased in elderly subjects.

Volume of distribution. About 0.1 L/kg.

Clearance. Plasma clearance, about 0.03 mL/min/kg.

Protein binding. In plasma, about 99%.

Note. For a review of the pharmacokinetics of piroxicam see R. N. Brogden *et al.*, *Drugs*, 1984, *28*, 292–323.

Dose. Usually 20 mg daily; doses of 40 mg daily may be given for 7 days.

Pivampicillin

Antibiotic

Synonym. MK-191.
Proprietary names. Lervipan; Pondocil; Pondocillin; Proampi.
(2*S*,5*R*,6*R*)-6-[[(2*R*)-Aminophenylacetyl]amino]-3,3-dimethyl-7-oxo-4-thia-1-azabicyclo[3.2.0]heptane-2-carboxylic acid (2,2-dimethyl-1-oxopropoxy)methyl ester
$C_{22}H_{29}N_3O_6S = 463.5$
CAS—33817-20-8

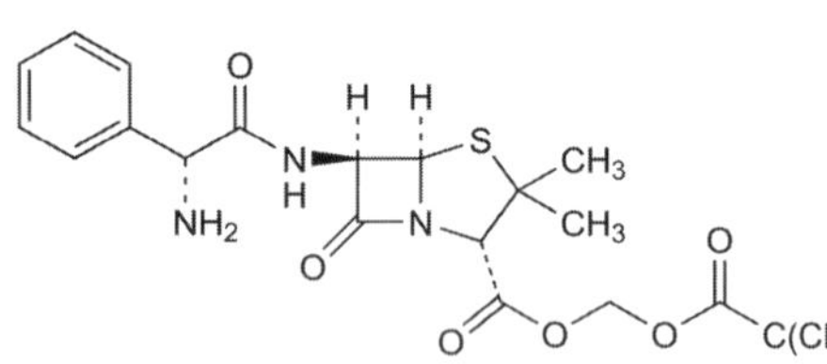

Pivampicillin Hydrochloride

Proprietary name. Pivamiser; Pondocil; Sanguicillin.
$C_{22}H_{29}N_3O_6S,HCl = 500.0$
CAS—26309-95-5
A white, hygroscopic, crystalline powder.
Soluble 1 in 2 of water and 1 in 1.5 of chloroform; very slightly soluble in ether.

Dissociation Constant. pK_a 7.0.

High Performance Liquid Chromatography. System HAA—Retention time 15.8 min.

Ultraviolet Spectrum. Aqueous acid—256, 261, 268 nm; aqueous alkali—257, 311 nm.

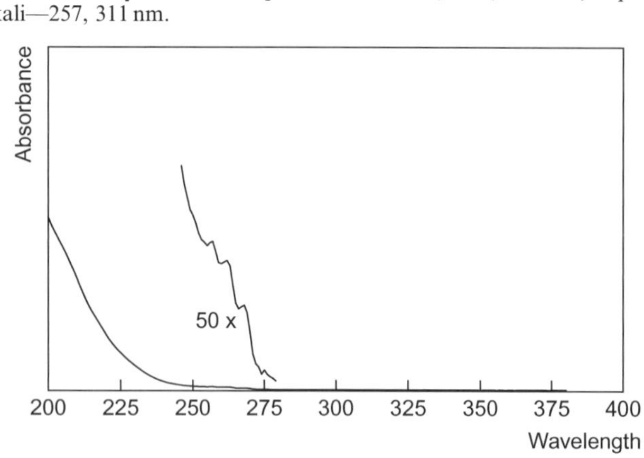

Infra-red Spectrum. Principal peaks at wavenumbers 1760, 1742, 1104, 1683, 972, 1150 cm^{-1} (KBr disk).

Therapeutic concentration
10 cystic fibrosis patients given pivampicillin 50 mg/kg daily alone or combined with pivmecillinam 40 mg/kg daily for 14 days displayed mean peak pivampicillin serum concentrations of 6.0 mg/L and 6.9 mg/L, respectively, 2 h after oral dosing [H. K. Johansen *et al.*, *Curr. Med. Res. Opin.*, 1999, *15*, 300–309].

Dose. 1 to 2 g daily.

Pizotifen

Antimigraine/Antihistamine (sedating)

Synonyms. Pizotyline; BC-105.
4-(9,10-Dihydro-4*H*-benzo[4,5]cyclohepta[1,2-*b*]thien-4-ylidene)-1-methylpiperidine
$C_{19}H_{21}NS = 295.4$
CAS—15574-96-6

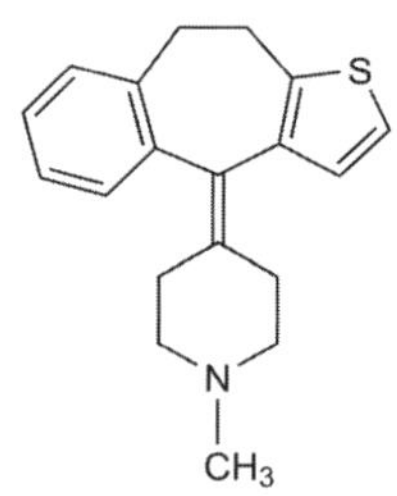

A white to yellow crystalline powder. M.p. 261° to 263°, with decomposition.
Soluble in dilute acetic acid and in chloroform:methanol (1:1).

Pizotifen Malate

Proprietary names. Anorsia; Litec; Mosegor; Pizomed; Sandomigran; Sanmigran; Sanomigran; Zofen.
$C_{19}H_{21}NS,C_4H_6O_5 = 429.5$
CAS—5189-11-7
Crystals. M.p. 185° to 186°, with decomposition.

Dissociation Constant. pK_a 7.0.

Partition Coefficient. Log *P* (octanol/water), 5.2.

Colour Tests. Liebermann's Test—black; Mandelin's Test—violet→green; Marquis Test—orange→red; Sulfuric Acid—orange-yellow→violet.

Thin-layer Chromatography. System TA—Rf 48; system TB—Rf 45; system TE—Rf 64; system TAE—Rf 28. (Acidified iodoplatinate solution, positive.)

Gas Chromatography. System GA—RI 2375.

High Performance Liquid Chromatography. System HA—*k* 3.4; system HX—RI 435; system HZ—Retention time 6.6 min; system HAA—Retention time 15.2 min.

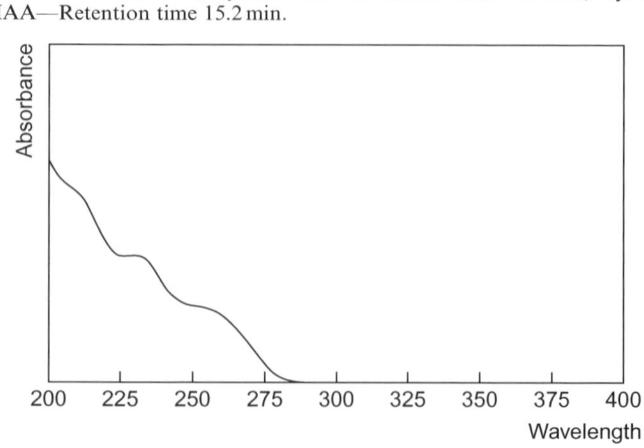

Infra-red Spectrum. Principal peaks at wavenumbers 1577, 756, 1212, 1703, 1124, 1274 cm^{-1} (KBr disk).

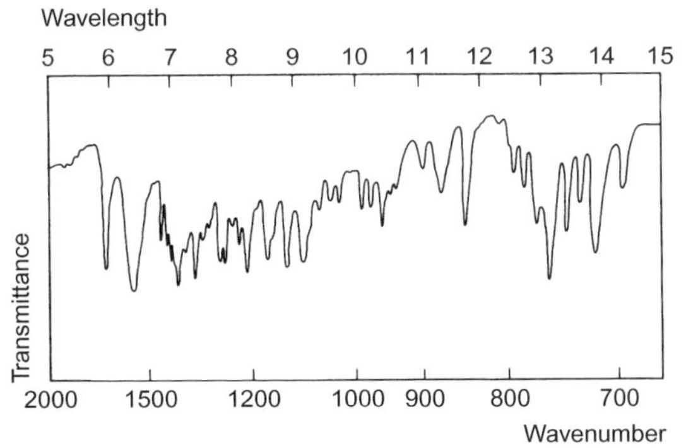

Disposition in the Body. Absorbed after oral administration. Peak blood concentrations of total radioactivity were attained in 5 to 7 h after a single oral dose of 1 mg of ^{3}H-pizotifen. About 62% of a dose is excreted in the urine and 24% is eliminated in the faeces in 120 h, with about 36% of the dose being excreted in the first 24 h.

Half-life. Derived from urinary excretion data (total radioactivity), about 26 h.

Dose. The equivalent of 0.5 to 6 mg of pizotifen daily.

Poldine Metilsulfate

Anticholinergic

Synonyms. Poldine Methosulfate; Poldine Methylsulfate; IS-499; MeN-R-726-47.
Proprietary names. Nactate; Nacton.
2-[[(Hydroxydiphenylacetyl)oxy]methyl]-1,1-dimethylpyrrolidinium methyl sulfate
$C_{21}H_{26}NO_3,CH_3SO_4$=451.5
CAS—596-50-9 (poldine); 545-80-2 (metilsulfate)

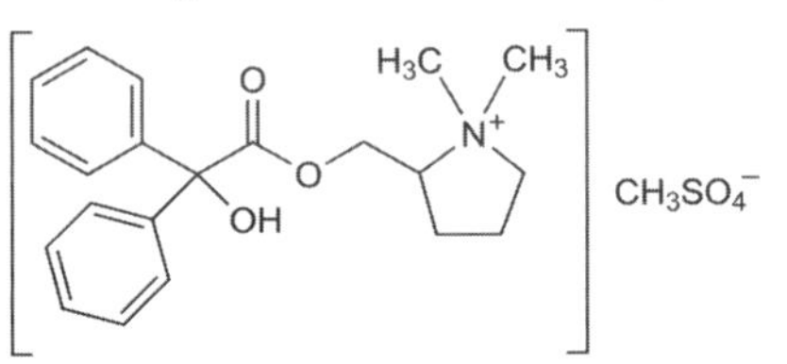

A white to creamy-white crystalline powder. M.p. 154° to 155°.
Soluble 1 in 1 of water, 1 in 20 of ethanol, and 1 in 1000 of chloroform; practically insoluble in ether.

Partition Coefficient. Log *P* (octanol/water), 0.9.

Colour Tests. Mandelin's Test—orange→green→violet; Marquis Test—orange→green→blue.

Thin-layer Chromatography. System TA—Rf 02. (Acidified iodoplatinate solution, positive.)

High Performance Liquid Chromatography. System HA—*k* 3.3 (tailing peak).

Ultraviolet Spectrum. Aqueous acid—252, 258 nm (A^1_1=10.5a). No alkaline shift.

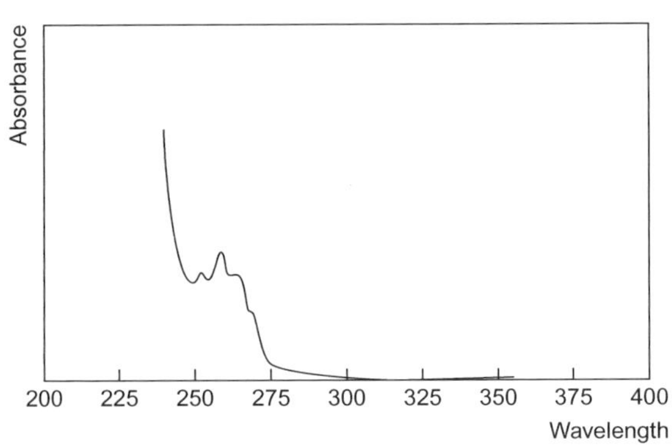

Infra-red Spectrum. Principal peaks at wavenumbers 1222, 701, 1061, 1008, 765, 1751 cm^{-1} (KBr disk).

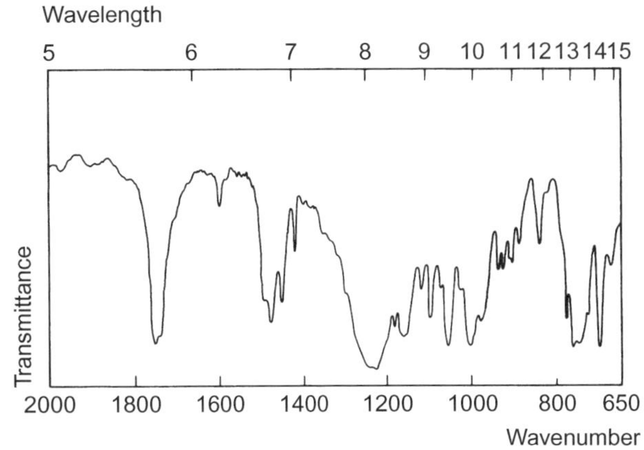

Dose. 8 to 16 mg daily.

Polythiazide

Diuretic

Proprietary names. Drenusil; Nephril; Renese.
6-Chloro-3,4-dihydro-2-methyl-3-[[(2,2,2-trifluoroethyl)thio]methyl]-2*H*-1,2,4-benzothiadiazine-7-sulfonamide 1,1-dioxide
$C_{11}H_{13}ClF_3N_3O_4S_3$=439.9
CAS—346-18-9

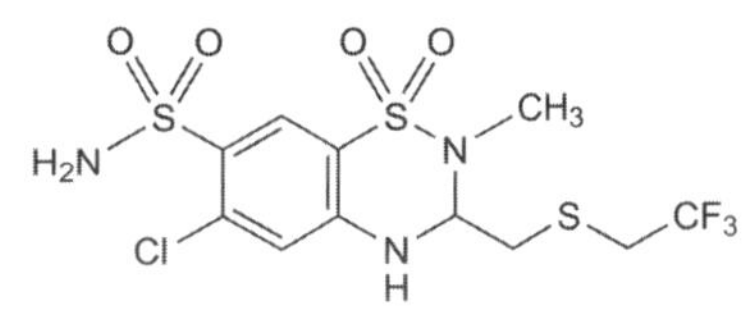

A white crystalline powder. M.p. about 214°, with decomposition.
Practically insoluble in water and chloroform; soluble 1 in 40 of ethanol; soluble in acetone and methanol.

Partition Coefficient. Log *P* (octanol/water), 1.9.

Colour Tests. Koppanyi–Zwikker Test—violet; Liebermann's Test—red-brown; Palladium Chloride—orange; Sulfuric Acid—orange.

Thin-layer Chromatography. System TD—Rf 22; system TE—Rf 63; system TF—Rf 60; system TAD—Rf 32; system TAJ—Rf 35; system TAK—Rf 08; system TAL—Rf 70.

Gas Chromatography. System GA—polythiazide RI 2380; polythiazide-ME3 RI 2985; system GX—polythiazide-ME3 Retention time 11.0 min.

High Performance Liquid Chromatography. System HN—*k* 15.09.

Ultraviolet Spectrum. Methanol—268 (A^1_1=500a), 317 nm.

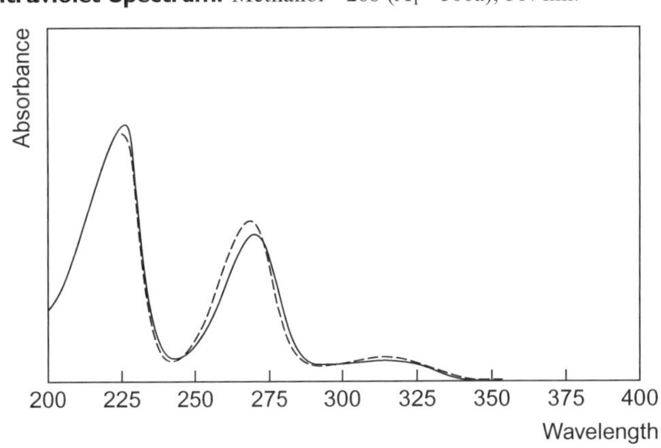

Infra-red Spectrum. Principal peaks at wavenumbers 1162, 1120, 1597, 1071, 1240, 1500 cm^{-1} (KBr disk).

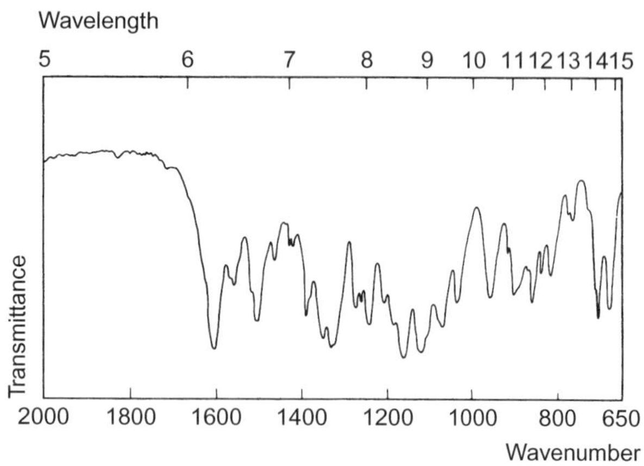

Mass Spectrum. Principal ions at *m/z* 310, 206, 42, 64, 312, 299, 45, 48.

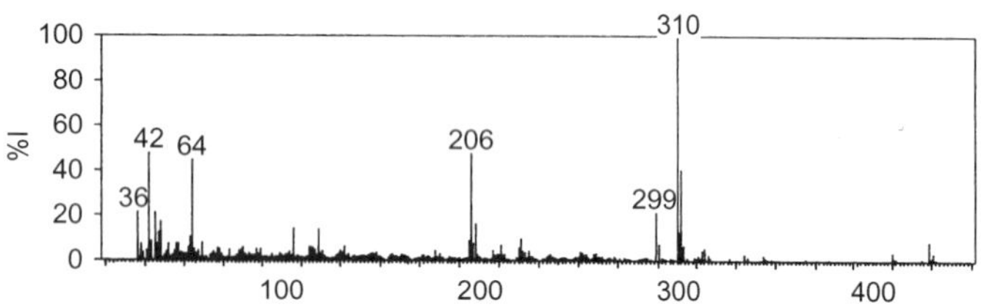

Quantification

Gas chromatography. In plasma: limit of detection 200 ng/L, ECD—D. C. Hobbs and T. M. Twomey, *Clin. Pharmacol. Ther.*, 1978, *23*, 241–246.

High performance liquid chromatography. In plasma: limit of detection 0.5 µg/L, spectrophotometric detection—J. Dokladalova *et al.*, *J. Chromatogr.*, 1981, *224*, 33–41.

Disposition in the Body. Well absorbed after oral administration. About 20% of a single oral dose is excreted in the urine as unchanged drug in 48 h.

Therapeutic concentration

After a single oral dose of 1 mg to 18 subjects, peak plasma concentrations of 0.002 to 0.007 mg/L (mean 0.004) were attained in 5 to 12 h [D. C. Hobbs and T. M. Twomey, *Clin. Pharmacol. Ther.*, 1978, *23*, 241–246].

Half-life. Plasma half-life, about 26 h.

Protein binding. In plasma, about 80 to 85%.

Dose. 1 to 4 mg daily.

Practolol

Beta-blocker

Synonyms. AY-21011; ICI-50172.
Proprietary name. Eraldin; Dalzic.
N-[4-[2-Hydroxy-3-[(1-methylethyl)amino]propoxy]phenyl]acetamide
$C_{14}H_{22}N_2O_3$ = 266.3
CAS—6673-35-4; 23313-50-0 (±)

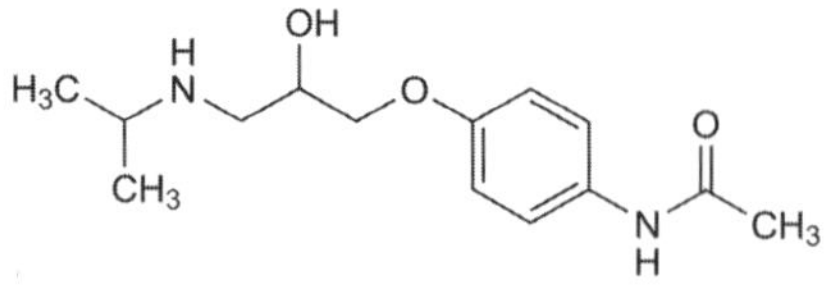

A fine, white powder. M.p. 134° to 136°.
Soluble 1 in 400 of water, 1 in 40 of ethanol, and 1 in 200 of chloroform; very soluble in dilute solutions of acetic acid.

Dissociation Constant. pK_a 9.5 (20°).

Partition Coefficient. Log *P* (octanol/pH 8.0), −1.3.

Colour Test. Liebermann's Test—black.

Thin-layer Chromatography. System TA—Rf 45; system TB—Rf 00; system TC—Rf 01; system TL—Rf 04. (Acidified potassium permanganate solution, positive.)

Gas Chromatography. System GA—not eluted; system GB—RI 2440.

High Performance Liquid Chromatography. System HA—*k* 0.5.

Ultraviolet Spectrum. Aqueous acid—243 (A_1^1=467a); methanol—248 nm (A_1^1=620a). (See below.)

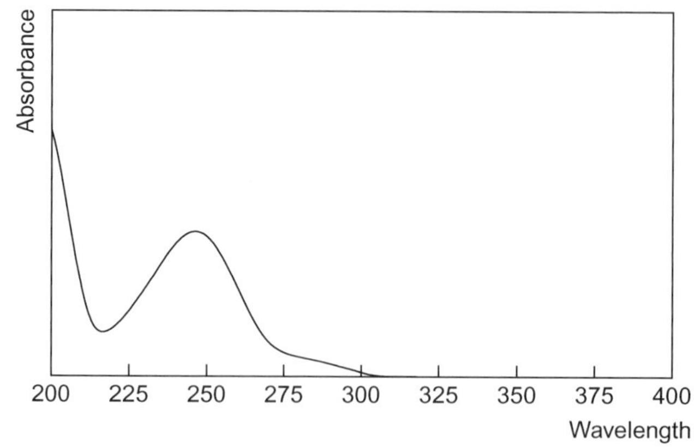

Infra-red Spectrum. Principal peaks at wavenumbers 1642, 1497, 1234, 1515, 822, 1019 cm^{-1} (KBr disk).

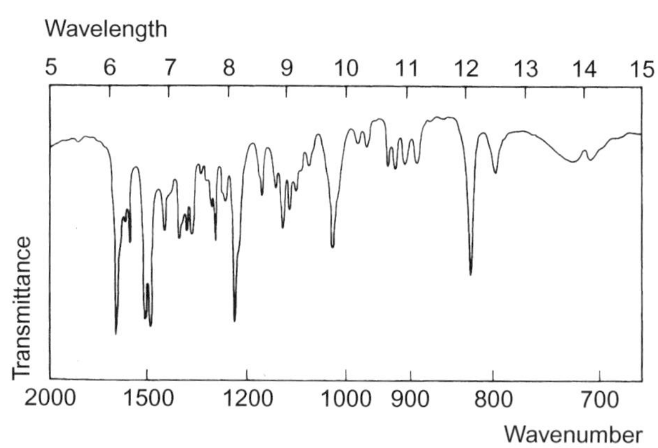

Mass Spectrum. Principal ions at *m/z* 72, 30, 151, 43, 109, 56, 57, 108.

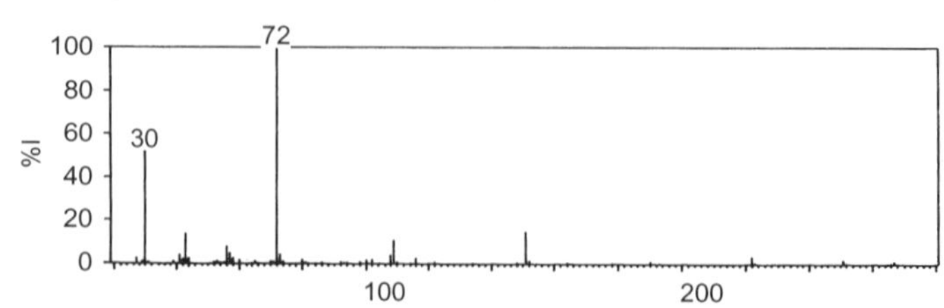

Quantification

Spectrofluorimetry. In blood or urine: limit of detection 200 µg/L—G. Bodem and C. A. Chidsey, *Clin. Chem.*, 1972, *18*, 363–365.

Gas chromatography. In plasma or urine: limit of detection 10 µg/L, ECD—J. P. Desager and C. Harvengt, *J. Pharm. Pharmacol*, 1975, *27*, 52–54.

High performance liquid chromatography. In plasma: limit of detection 30 ng/mL, UV detection—A. C. Mehta and R. T. Calvert, *J. Chromatogr.*, 1983, *276*; *B Biomed. Appl.*, *27*, 208–212. In plasma: practolol and other beta-blockers—G. Musch *et al.*, *J. Pharm. Biomed. Anal.*, 1989, *7*, 483–497.

Disposition in the Body. Completely absorbed after oral administration and almost entirely excreted in the urine as unchanged drug. Up to about 70% of a dose is excreted in the urine in 24 h.

Therapeutic concentration

After a single oral dose of 200 mg to 13 subjects, a mean peak plasma concentration of 1.3 mg/L was attained in 2 h [C. M. Castleden *et al.*, *Br. J. Clin. Pharmacol.*, 1975, *2*, 303–306].

Daily oral doses of 200 mg, 400 mg, and 800 mg to 8 subjects produced mean steady-state serum concentrations of 1.6, 2.9, and 4.5 mg/L, respectively [E. L. Alderman *et al.*, *Clin. Pharmacol. Ther.*, 1973, 14, 175–181].

Toxicity. The use of practolol has been restricted by serious adverse effects, notably the oculomucocutaneous syndrome which is characterised by adverse effects on the skin, eyes and mucous membranes, deafness, systemic lupus erythematosus, and sclerosing peritonitis.

Half-life. Plasma half-life, 10 to 13 h.

Volume of distribution. About 1.6 L/kg.

Clearance. Plasma clearance, about 2 mL/min/kg.

Protein binding. In plasma, less than 10%.

Dose. Practolol has been given in doses of 0.2 to 1.2 g daily.

Prajmalium Bitartrate

Anti-arrhythmic

Synonym. NPAB; GT-1012.
Proprietary names. Neo Aritmina; Neo-Gilurytmal; Neorythmin.
(17*R*,21α)-17,21-Dihydroxy-4-propylajmalinium hydrogen tartrate
$C_{23}H_{33}N_2O_2,C_4H_5O_6=518.6$
CAS—35080-11-6 (prajmalium); 2589-47-1 (bitartrate)

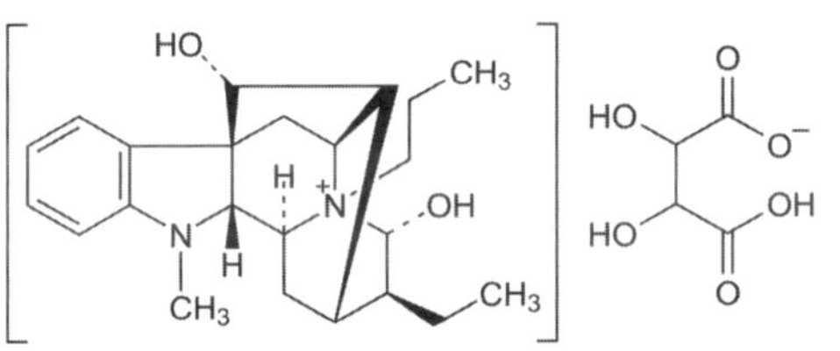

A white to pale yellow powder. M.p. 149° to 152°.
Soluble in water; readily soluble in ethanol, glacial acetic acid, and dilute mineral acids; moderately soluble in chloroform; practically insoluble in ether.

Colour Tests. Liebermann's Test—red; Mandelin's Test—red.

Thin-layer Chromatography. System TA—Rf 59; system TAE—Rf 08. (Acidified potassium permanganate solution, positive.)

Gas Chromatography. System GA—prajmalium RI 2925; M (OH-) Art RI 3130; M (methoxy-) Art RI 2895; M (OH-methoxy-) Art RI 3200.

High Performance Liquid Chromatography. System HA—*k* 2.2 (tailing peak); system HY—RI 340.

Ultraviolet Spectrum. Aqueous acid—246, 290 nm.

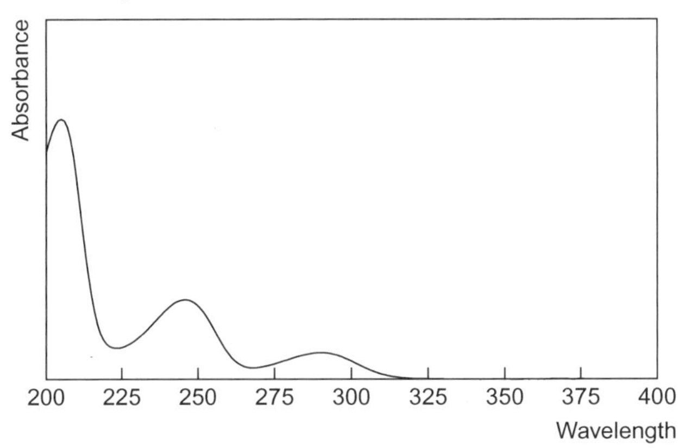

Quantification

Gas chromatography. In plasma: limit of detection 5 µg/L, AFID—M. Thoma *et al.*, *Arzneimittelforschung.*, 1981, *31*, 1020–1021.

High performance liquid chromatography. In plasma: limit of detection about 5 µg/L, fluorescence detection—I. Grundevik and B. A. Persson, *J. Liq. Chromatogr.*, 1982, *5*, 141–150.

Disposition in the Body

Therapeutic concentration

Following oral administration of 20 mg four times a day to 8 subjects, steady-state plasma concentrations of 0.08 to 0.55 mg/L (mean 0.2) were reported [A. T. Trompler *et al.*, *Arzneimittelforschung.*, 1983, *33*, 436–439].

Half-life. Plasma half-life, about 7 h.

Dose. 20 to 40 mg daily.

Pralidoxime Chloride

Cholinesterase Reactivator/Antidote (nerve gas and organophosphate insecticide poisoning)

Synonyms. Chloride Oxime; 2-PAM Chloride; 2-PAMCl; Pyraloxime Chloride; 2-Pyridine Aldoxime Methochloride.
Proprietary name. Protopam Chloride
2-[(Hydroxyimino)methyl]-1-methylpyridinium chloride
$C_7H_9ClN_2O=172.6$
CAS—6735-59-7 (pralidoxime); 51-15-0 (chloride)

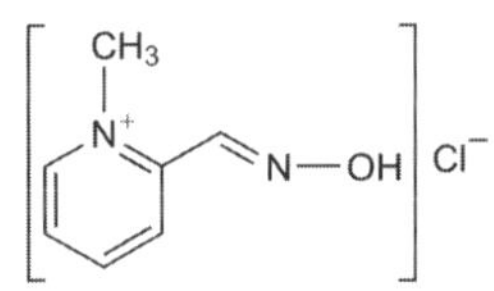

A white or pale yellow crystalline powder. M.p. 235° to 238°, with decomposition.
Soluble 1 in less than 2 of water and 1 in 100 of ethanol.

Pralidoxime Iodide

Synonyms. PAM; P-2-AM; 2-PAM Iodide; 2-PAMI; Pamium; Pyraloxime Iodide; 2-Pyridine Aldoxime Methiodide.
$C_7H_9IN_2O=264.1$
CAS—94-63-3
A yellow, hygroscopic, crystalline powder. M.p. 225° to 226°, with decomposition.
Soluble 1 in 20 of water; practically insoluble in ethanol, chloroform, and ether. Aqueous solutions are unstable.

Pralidoxime Mesilate

Synonyms. 2-PAMM; Pralidoxime Mesylate; Pralidoxime Methanesulfonate; P2S; 2-Pyridine Aldoxime Methyl Mesilate.
$C_8H_{12}N_2O_4S=232.3$
CAS—154-97-2
A colourless or white, hygroscopic, crystalline or granular powder. M.p. 155°.
Soluble 1 in 2 of water and 1 in 12 of ethanol; practically insoluble in chloroform and ether.

Pralidoxime Metilsulfate

Synonym. Pralidoxime Methylsulfate
Proprietary name. Contrathion
$C_8H_{12}N_2O_5S=248.3$
CAS—1200-55-1
A white crystalline powder. M.p. about 111°.
Very soluble in water; slightly soluble in chloroform.

Dissociation Constant. pK_a 8.0 (20°).

Thin-layer Chromatography. System TA—Rf 05; system TB—pralidoxime mesilate Rf 00; system TE—pralidoxime mesilate Rf 00; system TF—pralidoxime mesilate Rf 00; system TAE—pralidoxime mesilate Rf 00. (Acidified iodoplatinate solution, positive.)

High Performance Liquid Chromatography. System HAA—Retention time 2.9 min.

Ultraviolet Spectrum. Aqueous acid—242, 292; aqueous alkali—332, inflexion at 280 nm.

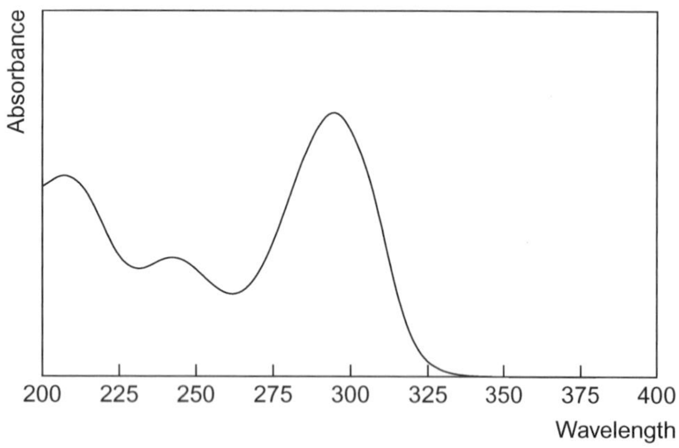

Disposition in the Body. Pralidoxime chloride is slowly absorbed from the gastro-intestinal tract; the mesilate is more readily absorbed. After IV administration as the chloride, about 86% of a dose is excreted in the urine in 24 h, mostly in the first 3 h. After oral administration as the mesilate, about 30% of a dose is excreted in the 24-h urine. 1-Methyl-2-cyanopyridinium ion has been detected in urine as a metabolite.

Half-life. Plasma half-life, about 1 h.

Volume of distribution. About 0.6 L/kg.

Clearance. Plasma clearance, about 7 mL/min/kg.

Protein binding. In plasma, not significantly bound.

Dose. 1 to 2 g of pralidoxime chloride parenterally, repeated if necessary; up to 15 g daily, by mouth.

Pramipexole

Antiparkinsonian/Dopamine D_2-agonist

Synonyms. SUD919Y; U-98528E.
(*S*)-2-Amino-4,5,6,7-tetrahydro-6-(propylamino)benzothiazole
$C_{10}H_{17}N_3S$=211.3
CAS—104632-26-0

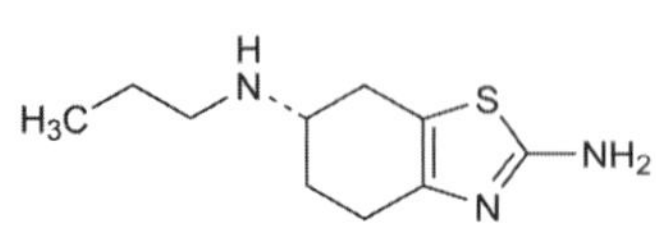

White to off-white crystals.

Pramipexole Dihydrochloride Monohydrate

Synonyms. SND-919-CL-2Y; PNU-98528-E
Proprietary names. Mirapex; Mirapexin; Sifrol.
$C_{10}H_{17}N_3S,2HCl,H_2O$=302.3
CAS—191217-81-9
White to off-white crystals. M.p. 296° to 301°. It is soluble in water (>20%); 8% soluble in methanol; 0.5% soluble in ethanol; practically insoluble in dichloromethane.

Dissociation Constant. pKa_1 5.0; pKa_2 9.6.

Partition Coefficient. Log *P* (octanol/water), 0.87.

High Performance Liquid Chromatography. Column: Zorbax Rx C_8 (250 × 4.6 mm, 5 μm). Mobile phase: 10.2 g potassium dihydrogen phosphate, 10.2 g sodium acetate and 4.5 g heptanesulfonic acid sodium salt in 3 L water, pH adjusted to 3.5 with acetic acid, flow rate 1.2 mL/min. Electrochemical and UV detection (λ=286 nm). Retention time(s): 14.4 min. [Y. Lau *et al.*, *J. Chromatogr.* 1996, *683*; *Biomed. Appl.*, 217–223.

Ultraviolet Spectrum. Aqueous acid (pH 2.38)—216, 264 nm.

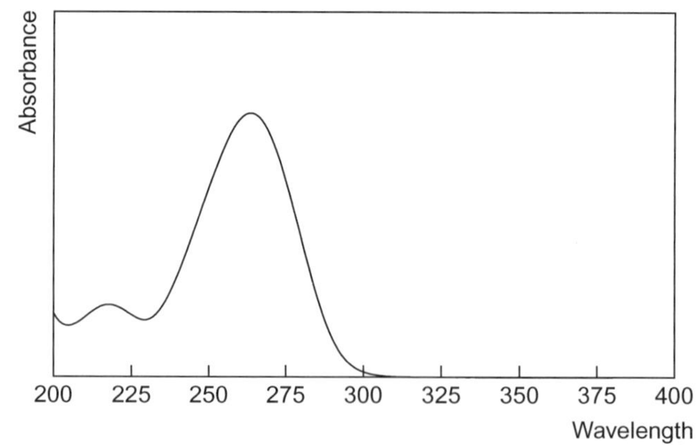

Mass Spectrum. Principal ions at *m/z* 126, 56, 70, 211, 127, 151, 152, 85.

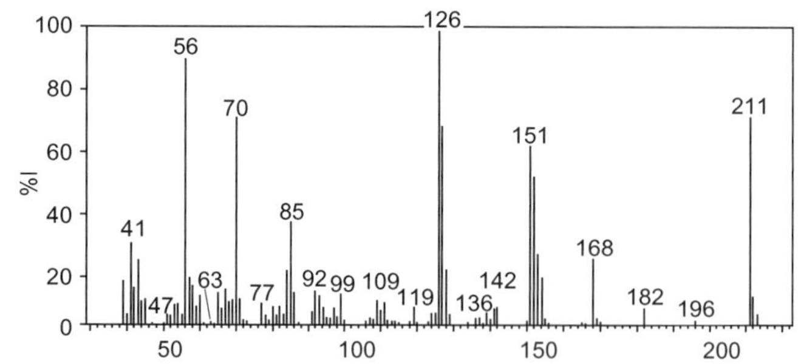

Quantification

High performance liquid chromatography. In plasma and urine: limit of quantification 0.05 and 10 μg/L, respectively—C. E. Wright *et al.*, *J. Clin. Pharmacol.*, 1997, *37*, 520–525. In plasma: limit of quantification 0.05 μg/L, MS–MS detection—Y. Lau *et al.*, *J. Chromatogr.*, 1996, *683*; *Biomed. Appl.*, 209–216. In plasma and urine: 0.05 and 10 μg/L, respectively, electrochemical (plasma) and UV (urine) detection—Y. Lau *et al.*, *J. Chromatogr.*, 1996, *683*; *Biomed. Appl.*, 217–223.

Disposition in the Body. Pramipexole is readily, rapidly and completely absorbed from the gastro-intestinal tract. It is widely and extensively distributed throughout the body. Metabolism is minimal. More than 90% of the dose is excreted unchanged in urine via renal tubular secretion. Steady state is achieved by 2 days. No metabolites have been identified in plasma or urine.

Therapeutic concentration

16 healthy males (aged 19.5 to 52.1 years, mean 28 years) and females (42.6 to 53.7 years, mean age 48.3 years) were administered 0.125, 0.5, 1.0, and 1.5 mg doses of pramipexole dihydrochloride monohydrate every 8 h. The maximum steady state concentrations, when measured, reached 0.39, 1.65, 3.55 and 5.44 μg/L for the males at doses 0.125, 0.5, 1.0 and 1.5 mg. For the females, these concentrations were 0.50, 2.12, 4.63 and 7.17 μg/L, respectively. These concentrations were observed by day 3. [C. E. Wright *et al.*, *J. Clin. Pharmacol.*, 1997, *37*, 520–525].

Toxicity

No clinical experience with massive overdose. One patient with a 10 year history of schizophrenia took 11 mg daily for 2 days (2 to 3 times the recommended amount) and showed no adverse reaction. [*ABPI Medicines Compendium 2002*, Epsom, Surrey: Datapharm Communications.].

Bioavailability. 90%.

Half-life. Men, 11.6 h; women, 14.1 h; also reported as 8 to 12 h.

Volume of distribution. Men, 7.34 L/kg; women, 7.01 L/kg; also reported as 400 L.

Clearance. Total 500 mL/min. Renal clearance is approx. 400 mL/min (3 times higher than the glomerular filtration rate) or 5.5 mL/min/kg. Clearance is about 30% lower in women compared to men, elderly compared to young people and those with Parkinson's disease compared to healthy people. It is about 75% lower for people with renal impairment.

Distribution in blood. The erythrocyte:plasma ratio is 2.

Protein binding. 15%.

Dose. 125 to 500 µg three times daily. Maximum 4.5 mg/day.

Pramocaine

Anaesthetic (local)

Synonyms. Pramoxine; Proxazocain.
4-[3-(4-Butoxyphenoxy)propyl]morpholine
$C_{17}H_{27}NO_3$=293.4
CAS—140-65-8

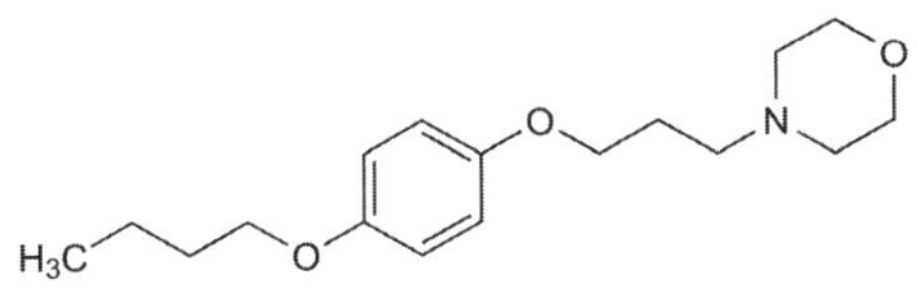

Pramocaine Hydrochloride
Proprietary names. Anti Itch; Balsabit; PramOtic; Prax; Proctofoam-NS; Tronotene; Tronothane.
$C_{17}H_{27}NO_3$,HCl=329.9
CAS—637-58-1
A white crystalline powder. M.p. 181° to 183°.
Freely soluble in water and ethanol; soluble 1 in 35 of chloroform; very slightly soluble in ether.

Partition Coefficient. Log *P* (octanol/water), 3.4.

Colour Test. Marquis Test—yellow→green.

Thin-layer Chromatography. System TA—Rf 70; system TB—Rf 43; system TC—Rf 55; system TE—Rf 73; system TL—Rf 41; system TAE—Rf 62; system TAF—Rf 60; system TAJ—Rf 59; system TAK—Rf 20; system TAL—Rf 90. (Dragendorff spray, positive; Acidified iodoplatinate solution, positive; Marquis reagent, green.)

Gas Chromatography. System GA—RI 2281; system GF—RI 2600.

High Performance Liquid Chromatography. System HA—*k* 0.6; system HR—*k* 2.48; system HX—RI 415; system HZ—Retention time 6.5 min.

Ultraviolet Spectrum. Aqueous acid—286 nm (A_1^1=80c). No alkaline shift.

Infra-red Spectrum. Principal peaks at wavenumbers 1510, 1230, 1118, 1210, 824, 1635 cm^{-1} (KBr disk).

Mass Spectrum. Principal ions at *m/z* 100, 128, 70, 41, 42, 293, 56, 101.

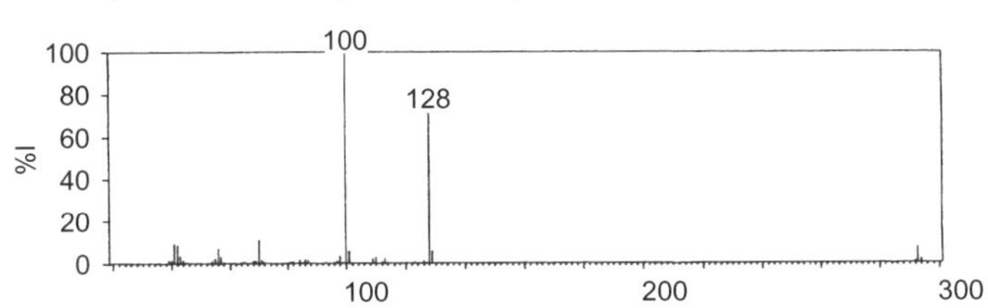

Uses. Pramocaine hydrochloride is used as a 1% cream or jelly.

Pravastatin

HMG CoA Reductase Inhibitor/ Antihyperlipoproteinaemic

($\beta R,\delta R$,1*S*,2*S*,6*S*,8*S*,8a*R*)-1,2,6,7,8,8a-Hexahydro-β,δ,6-trihydroxy-2-methyl-8-[(2*S*)-2-methyl-1-oxobutoxy]-1-naphthaleneheptanoic acid
$C_{23}H_{36}O_7$=425.5
CAS—81093-37-0

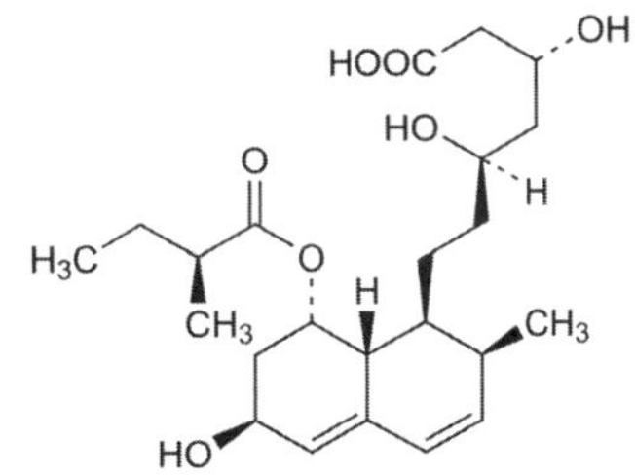

Pravastatin Sodium
Synonyms. CS-514; SQ-31000; Eptastatin Sodium; 3β-Hydroxycompactin Sodium.
Proprietary names. Elisor; Lipostat; Liprevil; Mevalotin; Oliprevin; Pravachol; Pravaselect; Selectin; Selipran; Vasten.
$C_{23}H_{35}O_7Na$=446.5
CAS—81131-70-6
A hygroscopic white to off-white crystalline powder. It is freely soluble in water and methanol; relatively insoluble in chloroform, ether, acetone and acetonitrile.

Pravastatin Lactone
$C_{23}H_{34}O_6$=406.5
Colourless plate-like crystals with m.p. 138° to 142°.

Partition Coefficient. Log *P* (octanol/water), −0.23 (pravastatin sodium).

High Performance Liquid Chromatography. Column: ODS Hypersil (100 × 4.6 mm i.d., 5 µm). Mobile phase: methanol, flow rate 0.5 mL/min. UV diode array detection. Retention time(s): pravastatin sodium, 2.9 min. [T. Mills and J. C. Roberson, *Instrumental Data for Drug Analysis*, 1993, CRC Press, Boca Raton, US. 2nd Edn, Vol. 6, pp. 206–207].

Column: ODS-2 (Inertsil, 150 × 4.6 mm i.d., 5 µm). Mobile phase: acetonitrile:ammonium acetate (0.01 M) (60:40) containing 0.02% glacial acetic acid and 0.06% triethylamine, flow rate, 1 mL/min. MS detection (NIAPCI, *m/z* 423). Retention time(s): 2.1 min; metabolite, 2.5 min. [K. Kawabata *et al.*, *Biomed. Chromatogr.*, 1998, *12*, 271–275].

Column: RP C_{18} endcapped (Purospher, 250 × 4.0 mm i.d., 5 µm) with an RP C_{18} (LiChrospher 100, 4 × 4 mm i.d., 5 µm). Mobile phase: sodium dihydrogen phosphate (20 mM containing 1 mM dodecyl sulfate): acetonitrile (65:35), adjusted to pH 2 with phosphoric acid, flow rate 1 mL/min. Internal standard (IS): triamcinolone acetonide. UV detection (λ=239 nm). Retention time(s): pravastatin, 6.8 min; IS, 11.0 min. [K. Otter *et al.*, *J. Chromatogr. B, Biomed. Sci. Appl.*, 1998, *708*, 235–241].

Ultraviolet Spectrum. (Sodium salt) methanol—230, 237, 245 nm; aqueous acid—238 nm; basic—238 nm. (Lactone) methanol—230, 237, 245 nm.

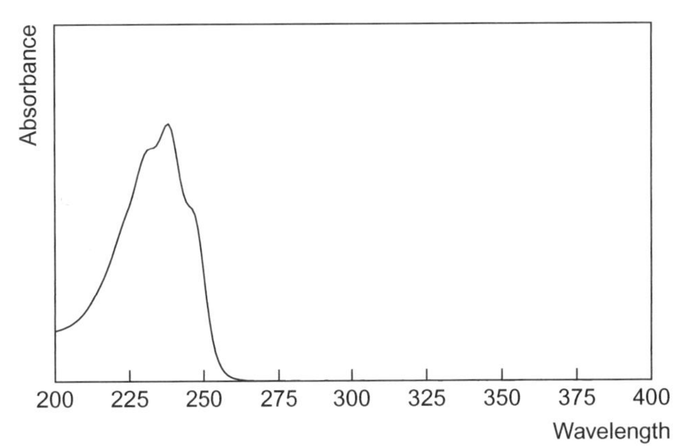

Infra-red Spectrum. (Sodium salt) Principal peaks at wavenumbers 1727, 1579, 1187 cm^{-1} (KBr disk).

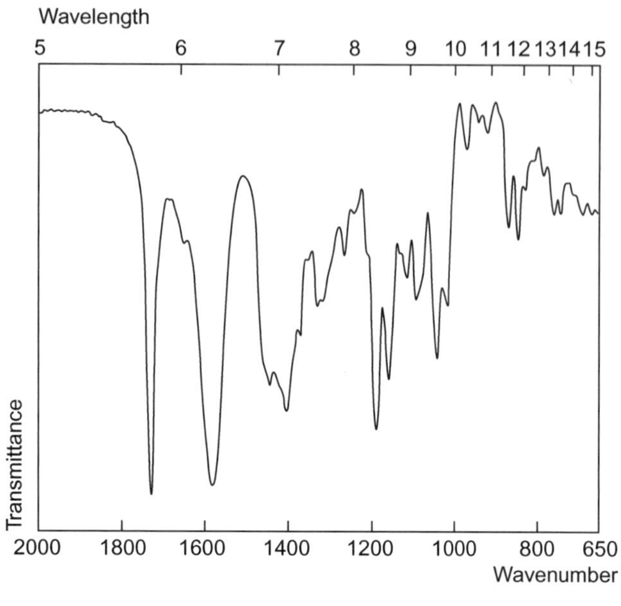

Quantification

Gas chromatography–mass spectrometry. In serum: limit of quantification 0.5 µg/L for pravastatin and its metabolites—H. Y. Pan *et al.*, *J. Clin. Pharmacol.*, 1990, *30*, 1128–1135. In serum and plasma: limit of detection 0.3 µg/L—P. T. Funke *et al.*, *Biomed. Env. Mass Spectrom.*, 1989, *18(10)*, 904–909.

High performance liquid chromatography. In plasma: limit of quantification 2 µg/L. UV detection (λ=239 nm)—K. Otter and C. Mignat, *J. Chromatogr. B, Biomed. Sci. Appl.*, 1998, *708(1-2)*, 235–241. In plasma: limit of quantification is 0.625 µg/L, MS detection—K. Kawabata *et al.*, *Biomed. Chromatogr.*, 1998, *12*, 271–275. In serum: limit of quantification 0.5 µg/L for the drug and analytes. MS–MS detection—D. Mulvana *et al.*, *J. Pharm. Biomed. Anal.*, 2000, *23(5)*, 851–866

Disposition in the Body. Pravastatin is rapidly absorbed after oral administration and peak plasma concentrations are observed 1 to 1.5 h after dosing. Approx. 34% of a dose is absorbed after ingestion. It undergoes extensive hepatic metabolism to a 3-α-hydroxy isomeric compound (SQ-31906; R-416), which has one-tenth to one-fortieth the activity of the parent compound, and a 3-α,5-β,6-β-trihydroxy isomeric metabolite (SQ-31945). Peak plasma concentrations of the metabolite, SQ-31906, are observed between 0.9 and 1.3 h after ingestion of pravastatin. It is excreted mainly in faeces (approx. 70%) via bile and also, urine (20%) with 80% of urine excretion being completed within the first 12 h. The drug and/or its metabolites may accumulate in patients with renal or hepatic insufficiency. A negligible amount of the drug is distributed into breast milk.

Therapeutic concentration

20 healthy male volunteers, 19 to 36 years old (mean 25), fasted overnight and were administered an oral daily dose of 40 mg pravastatin, followed by an additional 1 h fast. The mean peak plasma concentration was 64.1 µg/L observed 1.05 h after ingestion. [H. Y. Pan *et al.*, *J. Clin. Pharmacol.*, 1990, *30*, 1128–1135].

16 healthy males (18 to 40 years old) were administered a 20 mg single dose after an 8 h fast and fasted for another 4 h after ingestion or alternatively, co-administered with 40 mg twice daily propranolol. The peak plasma drug concentrations were 38.4 and 29.1 µg/L, respectively. The peak concentration for the metabolite SQ-31906 was 16.4 µg/L for pravastatin alone and 7.8 µg/L for co-administration with propranolol. Peak concentrations for the metabolite, SQ-31945, were 5.3 and 4.4 µg/L, respectively. All peak concentrations were reached within 1 to 1.4 h. [H. Y. Pan *et al.*, *Br. J. Clin. Pharmacol.*, 1991, *31*, 665–670].

Bioavailability. 17%.

Half-life. 1.3 to 2.6 h (pravastatin); 0.8 to 1.3 h (metabolites).

Volume of distribution. 0.46 L/kg at steady state.

Protein binding. 50%.

Dose. The usual dose is 10 to 40 mg daily.

Prazepam

Tranquilliser

Synonyms. Prazepamum; W-4020.
Proprietary names. Centrax: Demetrin; Lysanxia; Pozapam; Prasepine; Prazene; Reapam; Trepidan.
7-Chloro-1-(cyclopropylmethyl)-1,3-dihydro-5-phenyl-2*H*-1,4-benzodiazepin-2-one
$C_{19}H_{17}ClN_2O$=324.8
CAS—2955-38-6

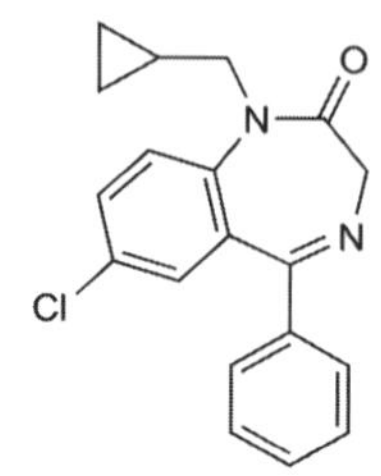

A white crystalline powder. M.p. 145° to 146° (crystals from methanol). Soluble in ethanol, chloroform, and dilute mineral acids.

Dissociation Constant. pK_a 2.7.

Partition Coefficient. Log *P* (octanol/pH 7.4), 3.7.

Colour Test. Formaldehyde–Sulfuric Acid—orange.

Thin-layer Chromatography. System TA—Rf 65; system TB—Rf 36; system TC—Rf 74; system TD—Rf 64; system TE—Rf 81; system TF—Rf 55; system TL—Rf 63; system TAD—Rf 72; system TAE—Rf 84; system TAF—Rf 89; system TAJ—Rf 75; system TAK—Rf 69; system TAL—Rf 94. (Acidified iodoplatinate solution, positive; acidified potassium permanganate solution, positive.)

Gas Chromatography. System GA—prazepam RI 2648, M (3-OH-) RI 2860, nordazepam RI 2490, oxazepam RI 2325; system GB—prazepam RI 2783, nordazepam RI 2625, oxazepam RI 2438; system GC—prazepam RI 3145, oxazepam RI 2803.

High Performance Liquid Chromatography. System HJ—*k* 4.60; system HK—prazepam *k* 2.19; nordazepam *k* 1.99; oxazepam *k* 0.73; system HX—RI 648; system HY—RI 570; system HZ—retention time 17.6 min; system HAA—retention time 23.4 min; system HAX—retention time 10.5 min; system HAY—retention time 12.8 min; system HB—*k* 29.99; system HBI—*k* 4.28.

Ultraviolet Spectrum. Aqueous acid—240 (A_1^1=1760a), 285, 360 nm.

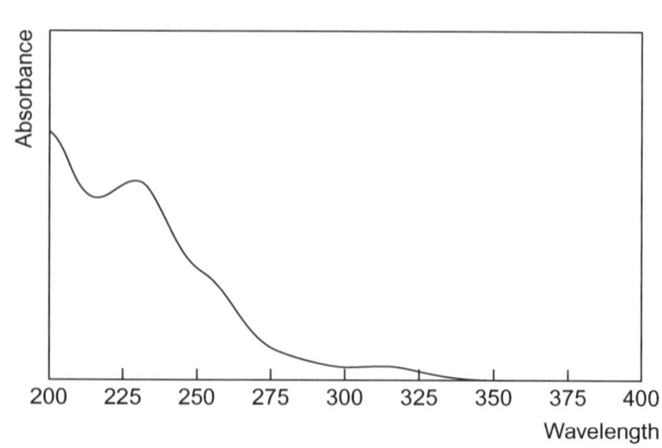

Infra-red Spectrum. Principal peaks at wavenumbers 1667, 1316, 740, 694, 1602, 704 cm^{-1} (KBr disk).

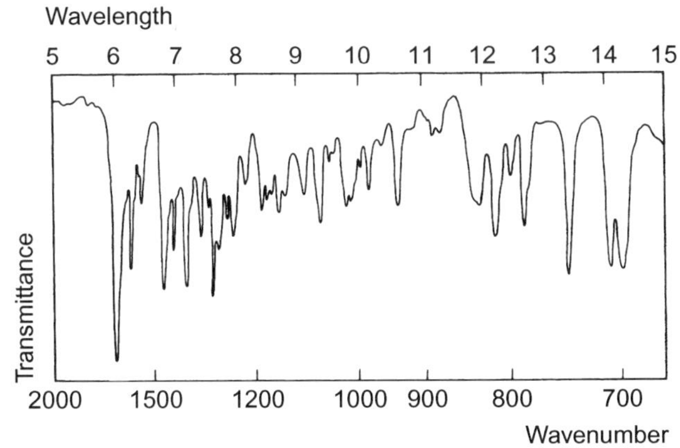

Mass Spectrum. Principal ions at *m*/*z* 91, 269, 324, 55, 296, 295, 323, 297; nordazepam 242, 269, 270, 241, 243, 271, 244, 272; 3-hydroxyprazepam 257, 55, 311, 77, 259, 313, 44, 312; oxazepam 257, 77, 268, 239, 205, 267, 233, 259.

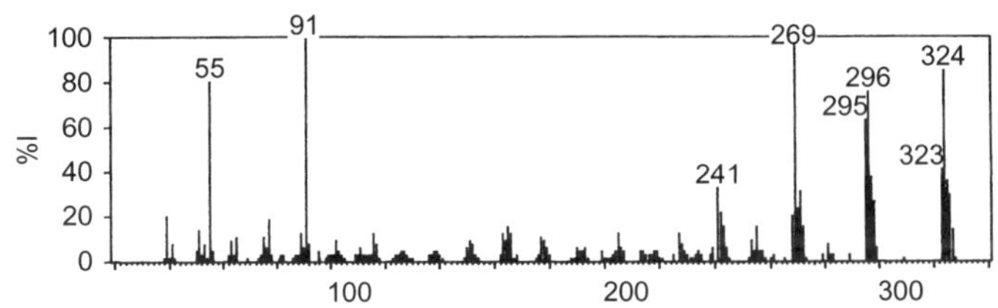

Quantification

Gas chromatography. In serum: prazepam, desmethyldiazepam, 3-hydroxyprazepam, and oxazepam, limit of detection 1 μg/L, ECD—H. Nau *et al.*, *J. Chromatogr.* 1978, *146*(3) *B Biomed. Appl.*, 227–239.

Disposition in the Body. Slowly and variably absorbed after oral administration. Desmethyldiazepam (nordazepam) is the major metabolite found in plasma and accounts for most of the activity. Prazepam is excreted in the urine mainly as glucuronide conjugates of oxazepam and 3-hydroxyprazepam with only trace amounts of desmethyldiazepam or unchanged drug. Up to about 20% of a dose is excreted in the urine in 24 h and about 60% over a period of 7 days; about 7% of a dose is eliminated in the faeces in 48 h. Desmethyldiazepam is found in breast milk after administration of prazepam.

Therapeutic concentration

After a single oral dose of 30 mg to 10 subjects, peak plasma concentrations of 0.19 to 0.40 mg/L (mean 0.3) of desmethyldiazepam were reported in 2 to 8 h; a second peak plasma concentration was reported for each subject. Following oral administration of 20 mg three times a day for 3 days to 5 subjects, plasma concentrations averaged 0.8 mg/L 12 h after the final dose. [R. R. Brodie *et al.*, *Biopharm. Drug Dispos.*, 1981, *2*, 59–68.]

Half-life. Plasma half-life, desmethyldiazepam about 40 to 100 h but there is considerable intersubject variation—see under Nordazepam.

Volume of distribution. Desmethyldiazepam, 0.5 to 2.5 L/kg, increased in elderly subjects.

Clearance. Plasma clearance, desmethyldiazepam about 0.1 to 0.3 mL/min/kg.

Distribution in blood. Plasma:whole blood ratio, desmethyldiazepam about 1.7. Plasma:breast milk ratio, desmethyldiazepam 9.6.

Protein binding. In plasma, desmethyldiazepam about 97%.

Dose. 10 to 60 mg daily.

Prazosin

Antihypertensive

Synonym. Furazosin

1-(4-Amino-6,7-dimethoxy-2-quinazolinyl)-4-(2-furanylcarbonyl)-piperazine

$C_{19}H_{21}N_5O_4$=383.4

CAS—19216-56-9

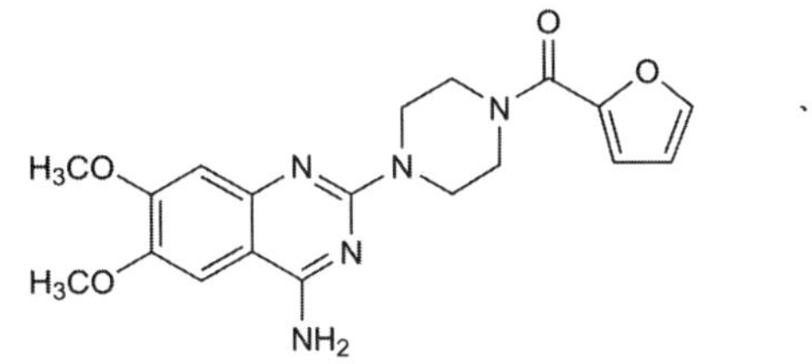

Crystals. M.p. 278° to 280°.

Prazosin Hydrochloride

Synonym. CP-12299-1

Proprietary names. Adversuten; Alphavase; Alpress; Apo-Prazo; Duramipress; Hexapress; Hypovase; Hyprosin; Hypotens; Minipress; Mipraz; Novo-Prazin; Nu-Prazo; Parabowl; Patsolin; Peripress; Prasig; Pratsiol; Prazac; Prazocor; Prazohexal; Pressin.

$C_{19}H_{21}N_5O_4$,HCl=419.9

CAS—19237-84-4

A white to tan-coloured powder. M.p. about 264°, with decomposition.

Very slightly soluble in water; slightly soluble in ethanol and methanol; practically insoluble in acetone and chloroform.

Dissociation Constant. pK_a 6.5.

Colour Test. Liebermann's Test—brown-pink (→red-orange at 100°).

Thin-layer Chromatography. System TA—Rf 60; system TB—Rf 01; system TC—Rf 47; system TE—Rf 59; system TL—Rf 49; system TAE—Rf 68; system TAF—Rf 74; system TAJ—Rf 39; system TAK—Rf 00; system TAL—Rf 54.

Gas Chromatography. System GA—Not eluted.

High Performance Liquid Chromatography. System HA—*k* 0.8; system HX—RI 352; system HZ—Retention time 2.5 min; system HAA—Retention time 10.6 min.

Ultraviolet Spectrum. Aqueous acid—247 (A^1_1=1470b), 331 (A^1_1=281b); aqueous alkali—252 (A^1_1=1642b), 345 nm (A^1_1=150b).

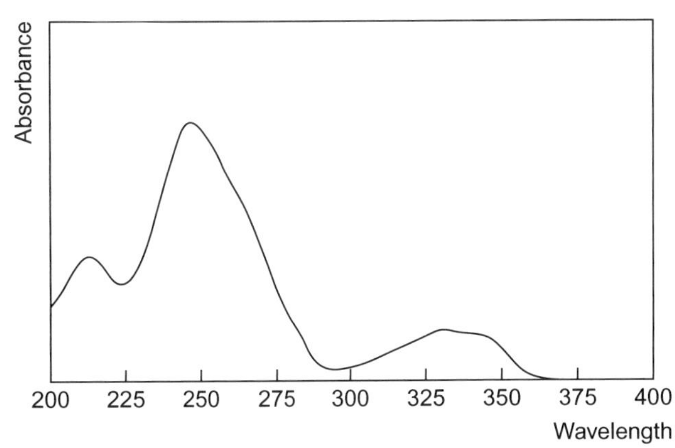

Infra-red Spectrum. Principal peaks at wavenumbers 1603, 1643, 1293, 1125, 1252, 1540 cm^{-1} (prazosin hydrochloride).

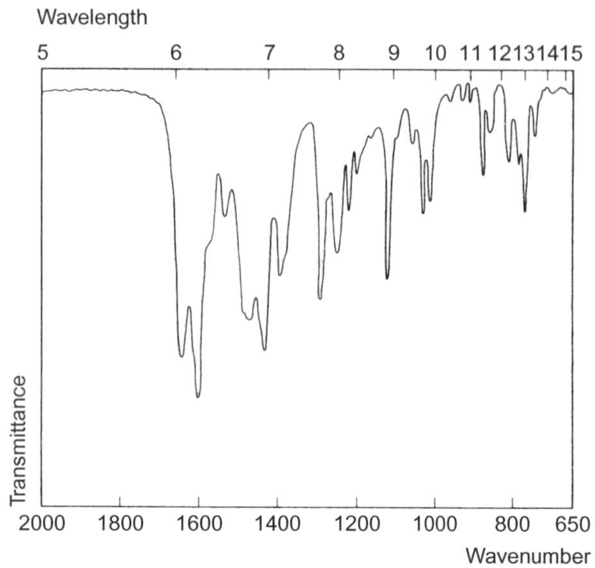

Mass Spectrum. Principal ions at *m/z* 233, 383, 259, 245, 95, 56, 246, 234.

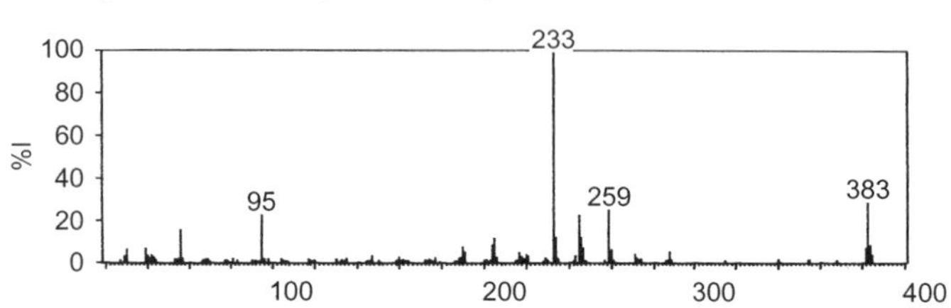

Quantification

High performance liquid chromatography. In plasma, blood or urine: limit of detection 1 µg/L, fluorescence detection—E. T. Lin *et al.*, *J. Chromatogr.*, 1980, *183*; *B Biomed. Appl.*, *9*, 367–371. In plasma: limit of detection 500 mg/L, fluorescence detection—P. A. Reece, *J. Chromatogr.*, 1980, *221*; *B Biomed. Appl.*, *10*, 188–192.

Disposition in the Body. Readily absorbed after oral administration; bioavailability about 60%. Extensively metabolised by 6-*O*- and 7-*O*-demethylation and glucuronic acid conjugation; less than 5% of a dose is excreted in the urine as unchanged drug in 24 h.

Therapeutic concentration

After single oral doses of 0.5 mg and 1.5 mg given to 5 subjects, peak plasma concentrations of 0.001 to 0.005 mg/L (mean 0.003) and 0.004 to 0.009 mg/L (mean 0.006), respectively, were attained in 1 to 3 h [M. K. Dynon *et al.*, *Clin. Pharmacokinet.*, 1980, *5*, 583–590].

Following oral administration of 0.5 mg three times a day to 8 subjects, mean steady-state plasma concentrations of 0.001 to 0.007 mg/L (mean 0.003) were reported; after dosing with 2 mg three times a day in 7 subjects, mean steady-state plasma concentrations were 0.008 to 0.019 mg/L (mean 0.013) [A. Grahnén *et al.*, *Clin. Pharmacol. Ther.*, 1981, *30*, 439–446].

Half-life. Plasma half-life, about 3 h.

Volume of distribution. About 0.6 L/kg.

Clearance. Plasma clearance, about 3 mL/min/kg.

Distribution in blood. Plasma:whole blood ratio, 1.4.

Protein binding. In plasma, about 95%.

Note. For a review of the pharmacokinetics of prazosin see P. Jaillon, *Clin. Pharmacokinet.*, 1980, *5*, 365–376.

Dose. 0.5 to 20 mg of prazosin hydrochloride daily.

Prednisolone

Corticosteroid

Synonyms. 1,2-Dehydrohydrocortisone; Deltahydrocortisone; Δ^1-Hydrocortisone; Hydroretrocortine; Metacortandralone.

Proprietary names. Codelcortone; Cortalone; Decaprednil; Decortin H; Delta-Cortef; Deltacortril; Deltasolone; Flamasone; Hydeltra; Hydrodeltalone; Klismacort; Meticortolone; Paracortol; Precortilon; Precortisyl; Prednelan; Solone; Sterolone.

(11*β*)-11,17,21-Trihydroxypregna-1,4-diene-3,20-dione

$C_{21}H_{28}O_5$=360.4

CAS—50-24-8 (anhydrous); 52438-85-4 (sesquihydrate)

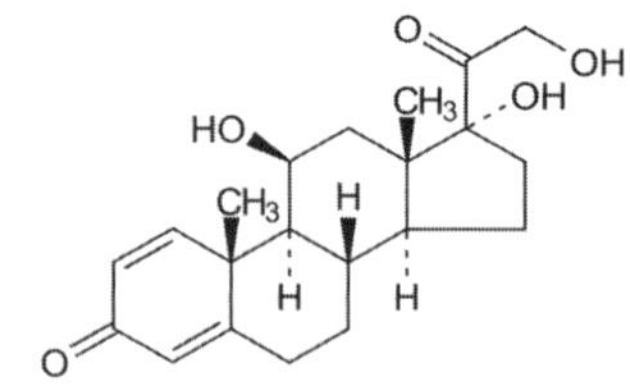

A white hygroscopic crystalline powder. M.p. 240° to 241°, with decomposition.

Soluble 1 in 1300 of water, 1 in 30 of ethanol, 1 in 27 of dehydrated alcohol, 1 in 180 of chloroform and 1 in 50 of acetone; soluble in dioxan and methanol.

Prednisolone Acetate

Synonym. Prednisolone 21-Acetate

Proprietary names. Deltastab; Econopred; Pred Forte; Pred Mild; Ultracortenol.

$C_{23}H_{30}O_6$=402.5

CAS—52-21-1

A white crystalline powder. M.p. 237° to 239°, with decomposition.

Practically insoluble in water; soluble 1 in 120 of ethanol, 1 in 170 of dehydrated alcohol, and 1 in 150 of chloroform; slightly soluble in acetone.

Prednisolone Pivalate

Synonyms. Prednisolone 21-Pivalate; Prednisolone Trimethylacetate.

Proprietary name. Ultracortenol

$C_{26}H_{36}O_6$=444.6

CAS—1107-99-9

A white crystalline powder. M.p. 233° to 236°.

Practically insoluble in water; soluble 1 in 150 of ethanol and 1 in 16 of chloroform.

Prednisolone Sodium Phosphate

Synonym. Prednisolone 21-(Disodium Orthophosphate)

Proprietary names. Codelsol; Hefasolon; Hydeltrasol; Inflamase; Metreton; Prednesol; Predsol; Solucort; Solu-Predalone.

$C_{21}H_{27}Na_2O_8P$=484.4

CAS—125-02-0

A white or slightly yellow hygroscopic powder or granules.

Soluble 1 in 3 or 1 in 4 of water, 1 in 1000 of dehydrated alcohol, and 1 in 13 of methanol; practically insoluble in chloroform.

Prednisolone Steaglate

Synonym. Prednisolone 21-Stearoylglycolate

Proprietary name. Sintisone

$C_{41}H_{64}O_8$=684.9

CAS—5060-55-9

A white powder. M.p. 105° to 107°.

Soluble in ethanol, acetone, and methanol.

Prednisolone Succinate

Synonym. Prednisolone 21-Hydrogen Succinate

Proprietary name. Solu-Dacortin (sodium salt)

$C_{25}H_{32}O_8$=460.5

CAS—2920-86-7; 1715-33-9 (sodium salt)

A fine creamy-white powder with friable lumps. M.p. about 205°, with decomposition.

Very slightly soluble in water; soluble 1 in about 6 of ethanol and 1 in about 250 of ether; soluble in acetone; very slightly soluble in chloroform.

Prednisolone Tebutate

Synonyms. Prednisolone Butylacetate; Prednisolone 21-(3,3-Dimethylbutyrate); Prednisolone Tertiary-butylacetate.

Proprietary names. Codelcortone TBA; Hydeltra-TBA.

$C_{27}H_{38}O_6,H_2O$=476.6

CAS—7681-14-3 (anhydrous)

A white to slightly yellow hygroscopic powder.

Very slightly soluble in water; sparingly soluble in ethanol and methanol; soluble in acetone; freely soluble in chloroform and dioxan.

Partition Coefficient. Log *P* (octanol/water), 1.6.

Colour Tests. Naphthol–Sulfuric Acid—brown/brown; Sulfuric Acid—orange-pink.

Thin-layer Chromatography. Prednisolone: system TB—Rf 00; system TE—Rf 41; system TF—Rf 24; system TP—Rf 20; system TQ—Rf 00; system TR—Rf 02, streaking may occur; system TS—Rf 00; system TAE—Rf 86; system TAJ—Rf 19; system TAK—Rf 03; system TAL—Rf 65; system TAM—Rf 54. (DPST solution.)

Prednisolone pivalate: System TP—Rf 69; system TQ—Rf 04; system TR—Rf 44; system TS—Rf 00. (DPST solution.)

Prednisolone sodium phosphate: System TP—Rf 00; system TQ—Rf 00; system TR—Rf 00; system TS—Rf 00.

High Performance Liquid Chromatography. System HT—*k* 8.4; system HX—RI 401; system HY—RI 361; system HZ—Retention time 2.5 min; system HAA—Retention time 14.1 min.

Ultraviolet Spectrum. Ethanol—240 nm (A^1_1=415a).

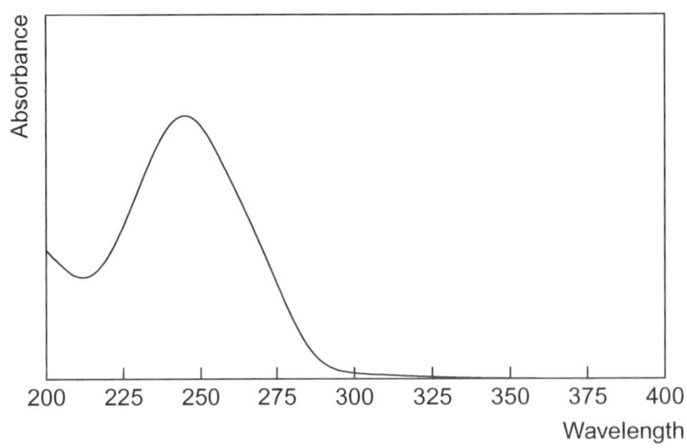

Infra-red Spectrum. Principal peaks at wavenumbers 1654, 1612, 1708, 887, 1112, 1085 cm^{-1} (KBr disk).

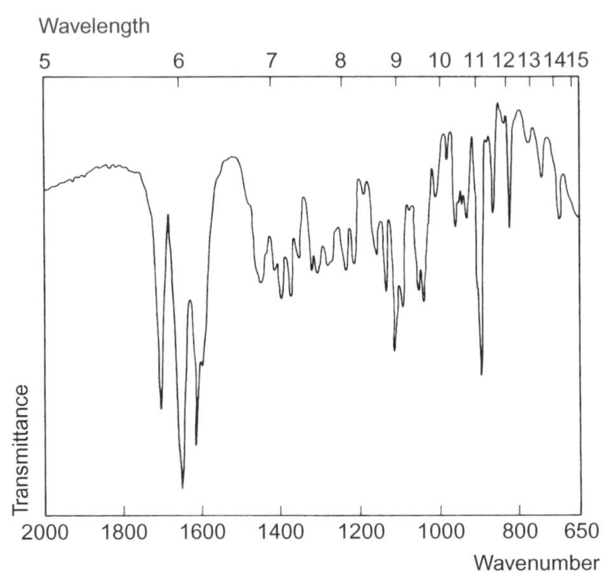

Mass Spectrum. Principal peaks at *m/z* 121, 122, 91, 147, 225, 43, 135, 120.

Quantification

Gas chromatography–mass spectrometry. In plasma: prednisolone and prednisone—S. B. Matin and B. Amos, *J. Pharm. Sci.*, 1978, *67*, 923–926.

High performance liquid chromatography. In plasma: limit of detection 10 µg/L, UV detection—R. Hartley and J. T. Brocklebank, *J. Chromatogr.*, 1982, *232; B Biomed. Appl.*, *21*, 406–412. In plasma, saliva, or urine: prednisolone, prednisone and hydrocortisone, limit of detection 5 µg/L, UV detection—J. Q. Rose and W. J. Jusko, *J. Chromatogr.*, 1979, *162; B Biomed. Appl.*, *4*, 273–280. In plasma, saliva, or urine, prednisolone and other corticosteroids, limits of detection 10 µg/L in plasma and saliva and 25 µg/L in urine—S. M. al-Habet and H. J. Rogers, *J. Pharm. Sci.*, 1989, *78*, 660–666.

Radioimmunoassay. In serum: limit of detection 10 µg/L—A. Olivesi *et al.*, *Clin. Chem.*, 1983, *29*, 1358–1362.

Dose. Usually 5 to 60 mg of prednisolone daily.

Prednisone

Corticosteroid

Synonyms. 1,2-Dehydrocortisone; Deltacortisone; Deltadehydrocortisone; Metacortandracin; NSC-10023.
Proprietary names. Colisone; Contancyl; Dacortin; Deltacortone; Deltason(e); Meprosona-F; Meticorten; Ofisolona; Orasone; Panafcort; Paracort; Predeltin; Predicor; Prednicort; Prednicorten; Prednidib; Prednitone; Promifen; Pulmison; Rectodelt; Sterapred; Trolic; Winpred.
17,21-Dihydroxypregna-1,4-diene-3,11,20-trione
$C_{21}H_{26}O_5$=358.4
CAS—53-03-2

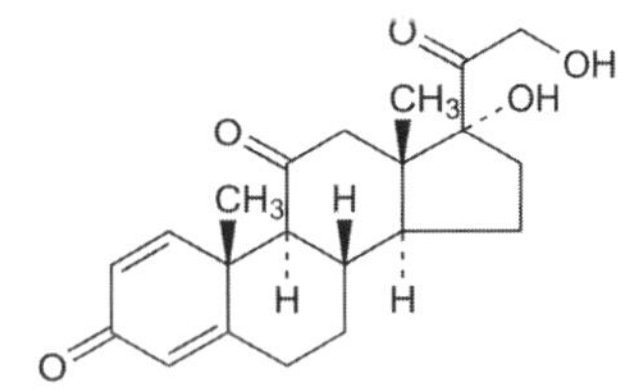

A white crystalline powder. M.p. 233° to 235°, with decomposition.
Practically insoluble in water; soluble 1 in about 150 of ethanol, 1 in 300 of dehydrated alcohol, and 1 in 200 of chloroform; slightly soluble in methanol.

Prednisone Acetate

Synonym. Prednisone 21-Acetate
$C_{23}H_{28}O_6$=400.5
CAS—125-10-0
A white crystalline powder. M.p. 226° to 232°, with decomposition.
Practically insoluble in water; soluble 1 in about 120 of ethanol, 1 in 160 of dehydrated alcohol, and 1 in 6 of chloroform.

Partition Coefficient. Log *P* (octanol/water), 1.5.

Colour Tests. Naphthol–Sulfuric Acid—brown/orange; Sulfuric Acid—yellow (green fluorescence under UV light).

Thin-layer Chromatography. System TB—Rf 00; system TE—Rf 45; system TF—Rf 28; system TP—Rf 41; system TQ—Rf 00; system TR—Rf 10; system TS—Rf 00; system TAE—Rf 84; system TAJ—Rf 33; system TAK—Rf 04; system TAL—Rf 74; system TAM—Rf 60. (DPST solution.)

High Performance Liquid Chromatography. System HT—*k* 3.4; system HX—RI 250; system HY—RI 340; system HZ—Retention time 2.6 min; system HAA—Retention time 14.2 min.

Ultraviolet Spectrum. Ethanol—240 nm (A^1_1=420a).

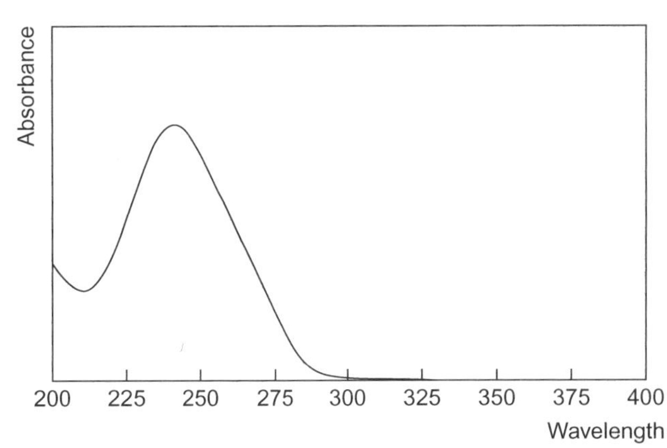

Infra-red Spectrum. Principal peaks at wavenumbers 1668, 1707, 904, 1622, 1610, 1246 cm^{-1} (KBr disk).

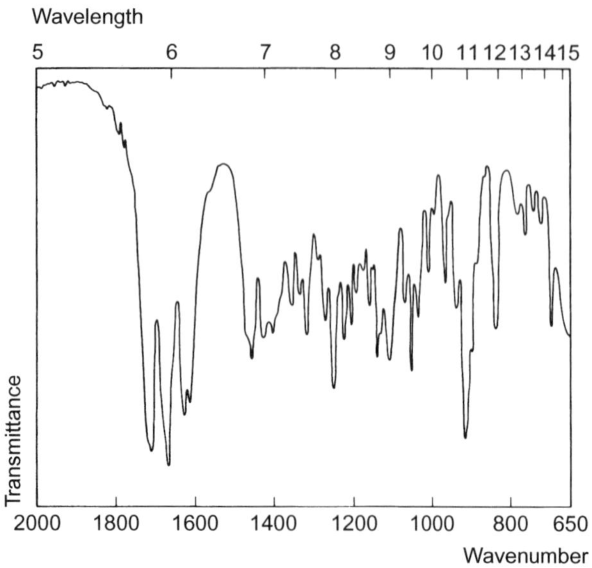

Quantification See under Prednisolone.

Dose. Usually 5 to 60 mg daily.

Prenalterol

Sympathomimetic

4-[(2*S*)-2-Hydroxy-3-[(1-methylethyl)amino]propoxy]phenol
$C_{12}H_{19}NO_3$=225.3
CAS—57526-81-5

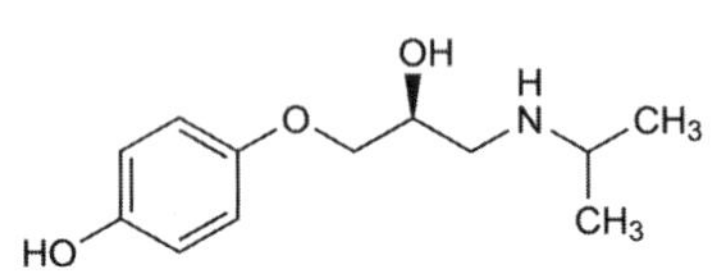

Prenalterol Hydrochloride

Synonym. H-133/22; CGP-7760B; (-)H-80/62.
Proprietary names. Hyprenan; Varbian.
$C_{12}H_{19}NO_3$,HCl=261.7
CAS—61260-05-7
A white crystalline powder. M.p. about 128°.
Freely soluble in water and ethanol; slightly soluble in acetone; very slightly soluble in ether.

Dissociation Constant. pK_a 9.5 (ammonium ion), 10.0 (phenol).

Partition Coefficient. Log *P* (octanol/water), 0.9.

Thin-layer Chromatography. System TA—Rf 47; system TB—Rf 01; system TC—Rf 09; system TD—Rf 02; system TE—Rf 25; system TF—Rf 02. (Dragendorff spray, positive; Ferric chloride solution, violet; Acidified iodoplatinate solution, positive; Marquis reagent, green→black; acidified potassium permanganate solution, positive.)

Gas Chromatography. System GA—RI 1933.

Ultraviolet Spectrum. Aqueous acid—287 (A_1^1=105a); aqueous alkali—235 (A_1^1=444b), 305 nm.

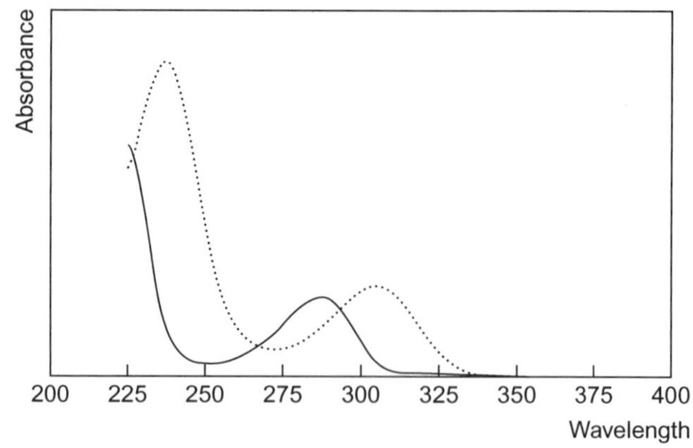

Infra-red Spectrum. Principal peaks at wavenumbers 1518, 1242, 1213, 1099, 840, 772 cm^{-1} (prenalterol hydrochloride, KBr disk).

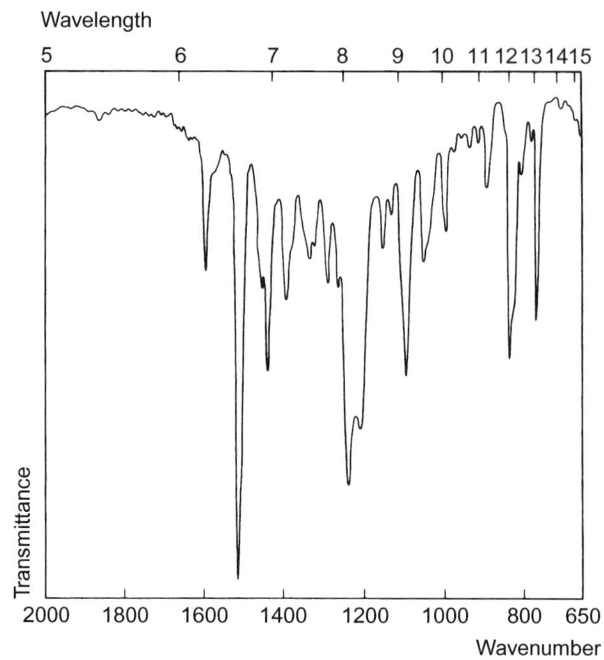

Mass Spectrum. Principal ions at *m*/*z* 72, 30, 56, 43, 27, 41, 39, 110.

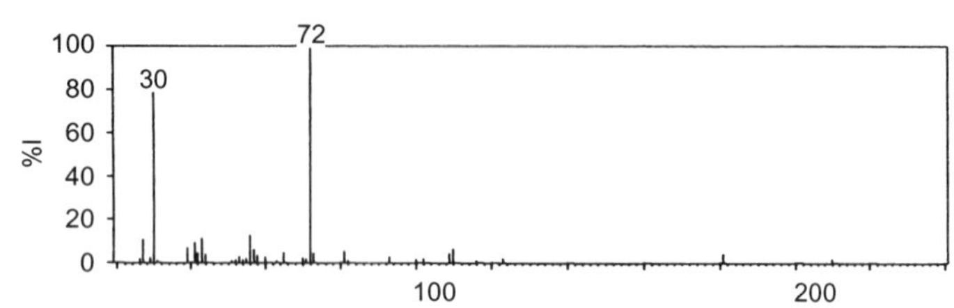

Quantification

Gas chromatography. In plasma or urine: limit of detection 2 µg/L, ECD—P. H. Degen and M. Ervik, *J. Chromatogr.*, 1981, *222*; *B Biomed. Appl.*, *11*, 437–444.

Gas chromatography–mass spectrometry. In plasma or urine: limit of detection 1 µg/L—M. Ervik *et al.*, *J. Chromatogr.*, 1982, *229*; *B Biomed. Appl.*, *18*, 87–94.

High performance liquid chromatography. In plasma: limit of detection 1 µg/L, fluorescence detection—C. J. Oddie *et al.*,*J. Chromatogr.*, 1982, *231*; *B Biomed. Appl.*, *20*, 473–477. In plasma: prenalterol and other beta-blockers, UV and fluorescence detection—G. Musch *et al.*, *J. Pharm. Biomed. Anal.*, 1989, *7*, 483–497.

Disposition in the Body. Rapidly and completely absorbed after oral administration, but subject to extensive first-pass metabolism. The main metabolic reaction is conjugation with sulfate at the phenol position; minor metabolites formed are β-(4-hydroxyphenoxy)lactic acid and prenalterol glucuronide. About 90% of a dose is excreted in the urine in 24 h. After an IV dose, about 60% is excreted unchanged with about 35% as the sulfate; after oral administration, about 15% is excreted unchanged, with about 80% as the sulfate.

Bioavailability. About 25%.

Half-life. Plasma half-life, about 2 h.

Volume of distribution. About 3.5 L/kg.

Clearance. Plasma clearance, about 20 mL/min/kg.

Distribution in blood. Plasma : whole blood ratio, about 0.9.

Protein binding. In plasma, less than 5%.

Dose. 0.5 mg of prenalterol hydrochloride per min by IV infusion, to a total of not more than 20 mg.

Prenylamine

Anti-anginal

Synonym. B-436
Proprietary name. Elecor
N-(1-Methyl-2-phenylethyl)-γ-phenylbenzenepropanamine
$C_{24}H_{27}N$=329.5
CAS—390-64-7

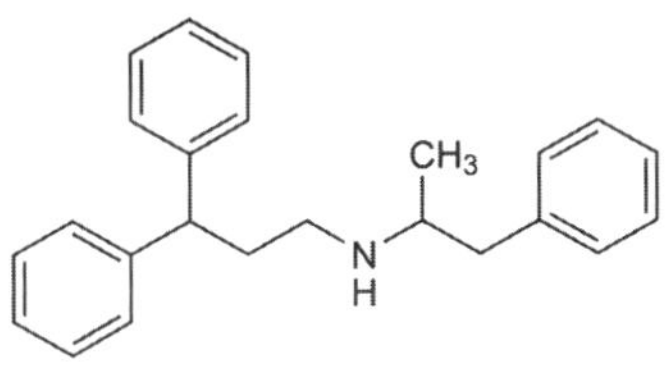

M.p. 36.5° to 37.5°.

Prenylamine Lactate

Proprietary names. Angormin; Bismetin; Carditin-Same; Coredamin; Corontin; Crepasin; Daxauten; Hostaginan; Incoran; Irrorin; Lactamin; Plactamin; Reocorin; Roinin; Seccidin; Sedolatan; Segontin(e); Synadrin.
$C_{24}H_{27}N,C_3H_6O_3$=419.6
CAS—69-43-2
A white crystalline powder. M.p. 140° to 142°.
Soluble 1 in about 200 of water, 1 in 5 of ethanol, and 1 in 2 of chloroform; very soluble in glacial acetic acid.

Partition Coefficient. Log *P* (octanol/water), 6.0.

Colour Tests. Mandelin's Test—green; Marquis Test—red.

Thin-layer Chromatography. System TA—Rf 68; system TB—Rf 55; system TC—Rf 68; system TE—Rf 84; system TL—Rf 56; system TAE—Rf 43; system TAF—Rf 85; system TAJ—Rf 47; system TAK—Rf 63; system TAL—Rf 90. (Acidified iodoplatinate solution, positive.)

Gas Chromatography. System GA—prenylamine RI 2555; M (desamino-OH-)-H_2O RI 1940.

High Performance Liquid Chromatography. System HA—*k* 1.0.

Ultraviolet Spectrum. Methanol—253, 258 (A^1_1=18.8a), 268 nm.

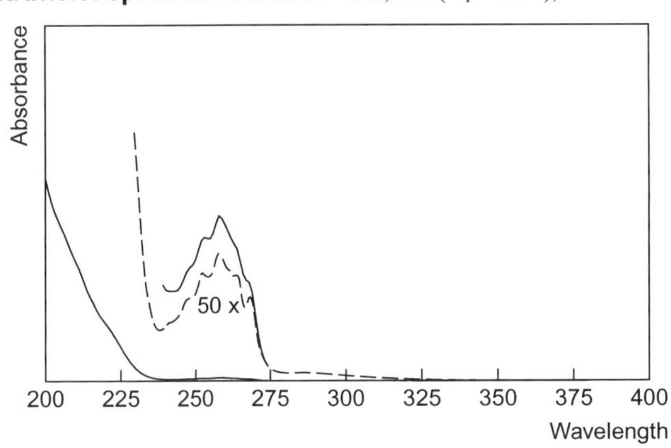

Infra-red Spectrum. Principal peaks at wavenumbers 700, 747, 1136, 1027, 1592, 1075 cm^{-1} (KBr disk).

Mass Spectrum. Principal ions at *m/z* 58, 238, 91, 45, 239, 167, 165, 56.

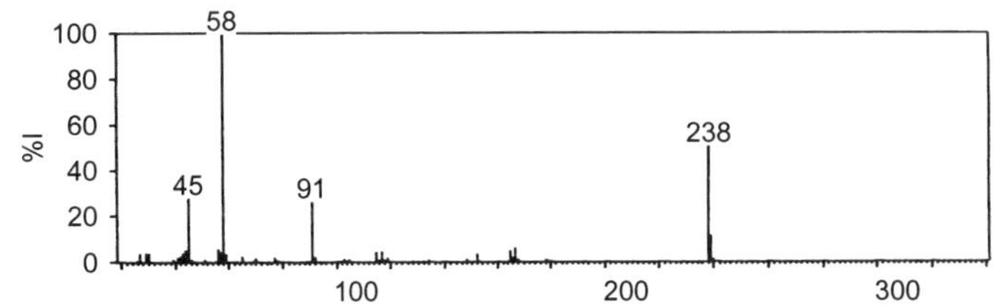

Quantification
Gas chromatography. In serum or urine: prenylamine and metabolites, limits of detection 10 to 50 μg/L, FID—M. Eichelbaum *et al.*, *Arzneimittelforschung*, 1973, *23*, 74–77.

High performance liquid chromatography. In plasma or urine: *R*- and *S*-prenylamine, limits of detection 1 μg/L in plasma and 2 μg/L in urine, fluorimetric detection—Y. Gietl *et al.*, *J. Chromatogr.*, 1988, *426*, 304–314.

Disposition in the Body. Readily absorbed after oral administration but extensively metabolised. Numerous metabolites, including traces of amfetamine, have been detected in the urine; some unchanged drug is eliminated in the faeces.

Half-life. Plasma half-life, about 7 h.

Protein binding. In plasma, about 97%.

Dose. The equivalent of 180 to 300 mg of prenylamine daily.

Prilocaine

Local Anaesthetic

Synonym. Propitocaine
N-(2-Methylphenyl)-2-(propylamino)propanamide
$C_{13}H_{20}N_2O$=220.3
CAS—721-50-6

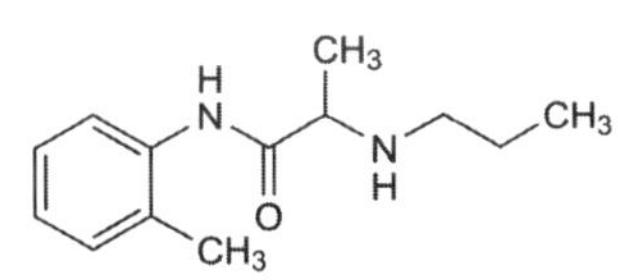

A white crystalline powder. M.p. 37° to 38°.
Freely soluble in ethanol, chloroform, and ether.

Prilocaine Hydrochloride

Synonyms. Astra-1512; L-67.
Proprietary names. Citanest; Citocaina; Xylonest. It is an ingredient of EmLa.
$C_{13}H_{20}N_2O,HCl$=256.8
CAS—1786-81-8
A white crystalline powder. M.p. 167° to 168°(crystals from ethanol and isopropyl ether).
Soluble 1 in 5 of water, 1 in 6 of ethanol, and 1 in 175 of chloroform; practically insoluble in ether.

Dissociation Constant. pK_a 7.9 (25°).

Partition Coefficient. Log *P* (octanol/water), 2.1.

Colour Test. Mandelin's Test—violet.

Thin-layer Chromatography. System TA—Rf 77; system TB—Rf 29; system TC—Rf 64; system TE—Rf 75; system TL—Rf 60; system TAE—Rf 62; system TAF—Rf 79; system TAJ—Rf 50; system TAK—Rf 22; system TAL—Rf 69.

Gas Chromatography. System GA—prilocaine RI 1823, M (OH-) RI 2155, M (OH-desacyl-) RI 1160, prilocaine-AC RI 2060, M (desacyl-)-AC RI 1350; system GQ—Retention time 5.7 min.

High Performance Liquid Chromatography. System HA—*k* 1.0; system HQ—*k* 1.38; system HZ—Retention time 2.7 min.

Ultraviolet Spectrum. Methanol—230 nm (A^1_1=295a).

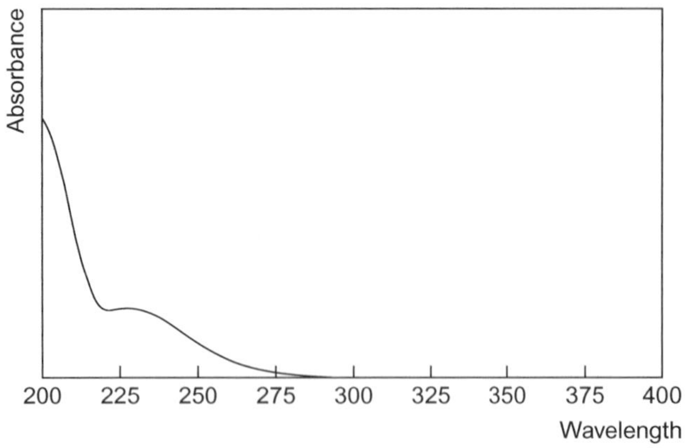

Infra-red Spectrum. Principal peaks at wavenumbers 1695, 1543, 766, 754, 1299, 1258 cm^{-1} (prilocaine hydrochloride, KBr disk).

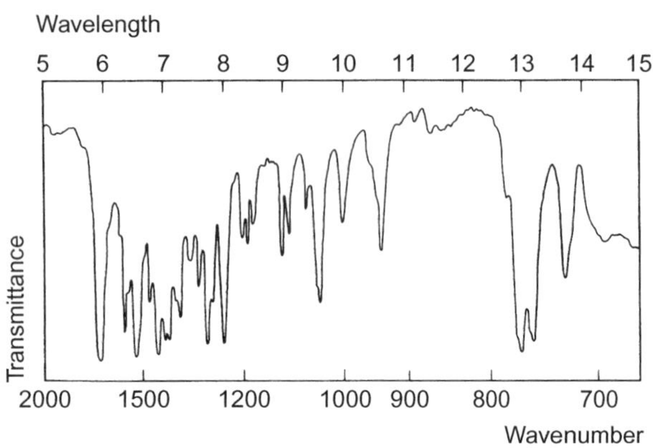

Mass Spectrum. Principal ions at *m/z* 86, 44, 87, 107, 43, 106, 56, 41.

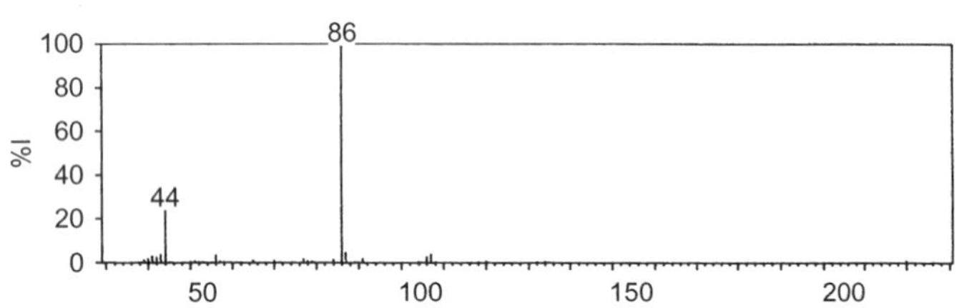

Quantification

Gas chromatography. In biological samples: prilocaine and other local anaesthetics, nitrogen sensitive detection—O. W. Lau *et al.*, *Methods Find. Exp. Clin. Pharmacol.*, 1991, *13*, 475–481.

Gas chromatography–mass spectrometry. In blood: prilocaine and other local anaesthetics—T. Watanabe *et al.*, *J. Chromatogr. B Biomed. Sci. Appl.*, 1998, *709*, 225–232. In plasma and urine: limit of quantification is 100 µg/L and limit of detection is 80 µg/L (SIM, *m/z* 86)—T. Ohshima and T. Takayasu, *J. Chromatogr. B Biomed. Sci. Appl.*, 1999, *726*, 185–194.

High performance liquid chromatogrpahy. In plasma: prilocaine enantiomers—G. T. Tucker *et al.*, *Br. J. Anaesth.*, 1990, *65*, 333–336. In plasma: limit of detection 10 mg/L—B. Bachmann-Mennenga *et al.*, *Arzneimittelforschung*, 1991, *41*, 520–524. In serum: prilocaine enantiomers, limit of quantification 10 µg/L, UV detection—M. Siluveru and J. T. Stewart, *J. Pharm. Biomed. Anal.*, 1996, *15*, 389–392.

Disposition in the Body. Metabolised by hydrolysis and hydroxylation resulting in deacetylated and hydroxylated metabolites which are excreted mainly as conjugates. About 35% of a dose is excreted in the urine as 4-hydroxy-2-methylaniline (*p*-hydroxytoluidine), 3% as 6-hydroxy-2-methylaniline, 1% as 2-methylaniline (*o*-toluidine), and less than 5% as unchanged drug. Prilocaine crosses the placenta and is excreted in breast milk.

Therapeutic concentration. In plasma, usually in the range 1 to 5 mg/L. 4-Hydroxy-2-methylaniline has been detected in plasma at concentrations similar to those of prilocaine.

In 30 patients receiving 40 mL of a 0.5% solution of prilocaine intravenously, the mean peak plasma concentration was 4.4 mg/L reached immediately after release of the tourniquet [M. A. Simon *et al.*, *Reg. Anesth.*, 1997, *22*, 29–34.]

After the epidural administration of 200, 400, and 600 mg to 10 subjects, mean peak plasma concentrations determined within 10 to 20 min were 1.69, 2.67, and 4.47 mg/L, respectively; after the intercostal administration of 20 mL of a 2% solution, the mean peak concentration was 4.5 mg/L [D. B. Scott *et al.*, *Br. J. Anaesth.*, 1972, *44*, 1040–1049].

Toxicity. Toxic effects are usually associated with plasma concentrations greater than 5 mg/L. 4-Hydroxy-2-methylaniline is thought to be responsible for the methaemoglobinaemia which may occur after large doses.

Half-life. Plasma half-life, about 1 to 2 h.

Distribution in blood. Plasma:whole blood ratio, 0.80.

Protein binding. In plasma, about 50%.

Dose. Maximum dose of prilocaine hydrochloride, 400 mg, or 300 mg in solutions with felypressin.

Primaquine

Antimalarial

Synonym. Primachin
N^4-(6-Methoxy-8-quinolinyl)-1,4-pentadiamine
$C_{15}H_{21}N_3O$=259.4
CAS—90-34-6

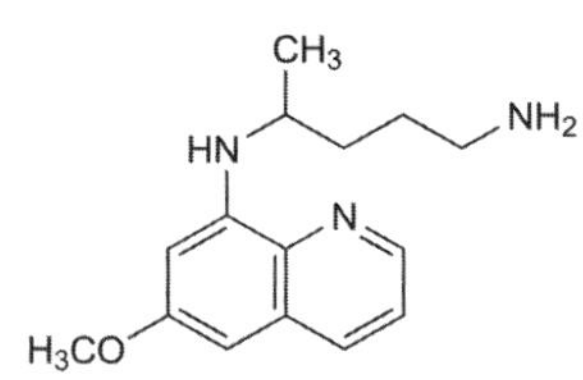

A viscous liquid.
Moderately soluble in water; soluble in ether.

Primaquine Phosphate

Proprietary name. Primacin
$C_{15}H_{21}N_3O,2H_3PO_4$=455.3
CAS—63-45-6
An orange-red crystalline powder. M.p. 197° to 198°.
Soluble 1 in about 15 of water; practically insoluble in ethanol, chloroform, and ether.

Partition Coefficient. Log *P* (octanol/water), 3.2.

Colour Tests. Mandelin's Test—violet→orange; Marquis Test—orange. Dissolve 10 mg in 5 mL of water and add 1 mL of a 5% solution of ceric ammonium sulfate in dilute nitric acid—violet (distinction from chloroquine).

Thin-layer Chromatography. System TA—Rf 19; system TB—Rf 13; system TC—Rf 05; system TL—Rf 15. (Acidified iodoplatinate solution, positive.)

Gas Chromatography. System GA—RI 2314.

High Performance Liquid Chromatography. System HA—*k* 1.4; system HY—RI 276.

Ultraviolet Spectrum. Aqueous acid—265 (A^1_1=579a), 282 (A^1_1=574a), 334 nm.

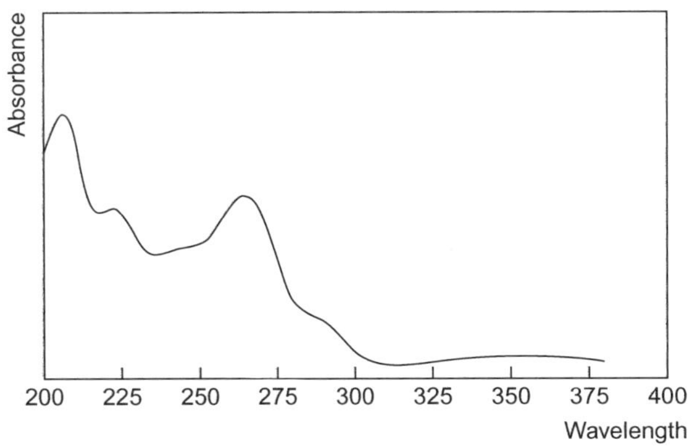

Infra-red Spectrum. Principal peaks at wavenumbers 1611, 1595, 815, 1230, 1572, 1170 cm^{-1} (KBr disk).

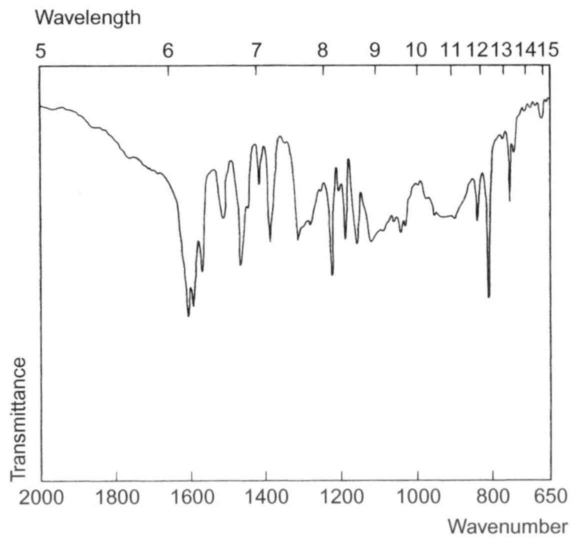

Mass Spectrum. Principal ions at *m/z* 201, 81, 98, 175, 259, 176, 202, 242.

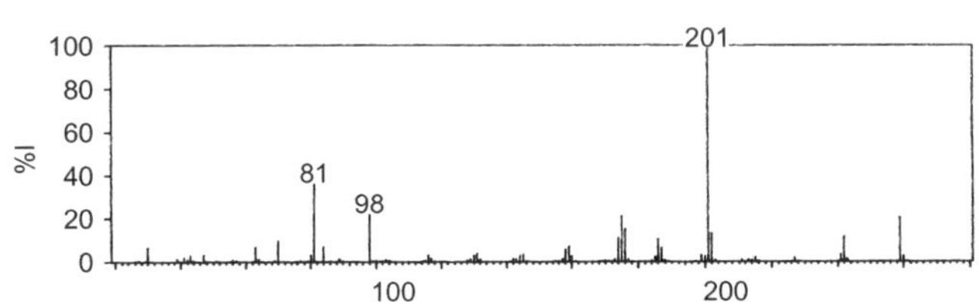

Quantification

Gas chromatography. In blood: limit of detection 10 µg/L, ECD—T. G. Rajagopalan *et al., J. Chromatogr.*, 1981, *224*; *B Biomed. Appl.*, *13*, 265–273.

Gas chromatography–mass spectrometry. In plasma or urine—J. Greaves *et al., Biomed. Mass Spectrom.*, 1979, *6*, 109–112.

High performance liquid chromatography. In plasma: limit of detection 1 µg/L, UV detection—S. A. Ward *et al., J. Chromatogr.*, 1983, *305*; *B Biomed. Appl.*, *30*, 239–243. In plasma or urine: carboxyprimaquine and *N*-acetylprimaquine, limit of detection 75 µg/L and 10 µg/L, respectively, UV detection—G. W. Mihaly *et al., Br. J. Clin. Pharmacol.*, 1984, *17*, 441–446. In plasma: primaquine and carboxyprimaquine, limits of detection 5 µg/L and 20 µg/L respectively, electrochemical detection—R. A. Dean *et al., J. Chromatogr. B Biomed. Appl.*, 1994, *655*, 89–96. In plasma or blood cells: primaquine and carboxyprimaquine, UV detection—V. K. Dua *et al., J. Chromatogr. B Biomed. Appl.*, 1996, *675*, 93–98.

Disposition in the Body. Readily absorbed after oral administration. It is extensively metabolised by oxidation to carboxyprimaquine which is the major plasma metabolite. Other reactions which may occur are demethylation and oxidation to the 5,6-diol, which is then converted to an active quinone, *N*-dealkylation to 8-amino-6-methoxyquinoline, and *N*-acetylation. Less than 5% of a dose is excreted in the urine unchanged in 24 h.

Therapeutic concentration

Following a single oral dose of 45 mg to 5 subjects, peak plasma concentrations of 0.13 to 0.18 mg/L (mean 0.15) were attained in 2 to 3 h; peak plasma concentrations of carboxyprimaquine of 1.1 to 1.8 mg/L (mean 1.4) were attained in 2 to 12 h (mean 7) [G. W. Mihaly *et al., Br. J. Clin. Pharmacol.*, 1984, *17*, 441–446].

Half-life. Plasma half-life, about 4 to 10 h (mean 7).

Volume of distribution. About 3 to 4 L/kg.

Protein binding. In plasma, extensively bound.

Dose. The equivalent of 15 to 45 mg of primaquine daily.

Primidone

Anticonvulsant

Synonyms. Hexamidinum; Primaclone; Primidonum.
Note. The name Hexamidine is applied to a compound with antibacterial and fungistatic properties.
Proprietary names. Cyral; Liskantin; Midone; Mylepsin; Mylepsinum; Mysoline; Prysoline; Resimatil; Sertan.
5-Ethyldihydro-5-phenyl-4,6(1*H*,5*H*)-pyrimidinedione
$C_{12}H_{14}N_2O_2$=218.3
CAS—125-33-7

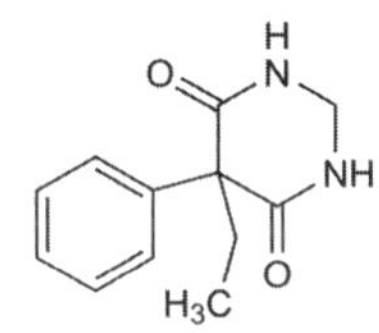

A white crystalline powder. M.p. 281° to 282°.
Soluble 1 in 2000 of water and 1 in 170 of ethanol; practically insoluble in most other organic solvents.

Partition Coefficient. Log *P* (octanol/water), 0.9.

Thin-layer Chromatography. System TA—Rf 88; system TD—Rf 08; system TE—Rf 41; system TF—Rf 23; system TAD—Rf 28; system TAE—Rf 76; system TAJ—Rf 29; system TAK—Rf 60; system TAL—Rf 86. (Mercuric chloride–diphenylcarbazone reagent, positive; mercurous nitrate spray, positive.)

Gas Chromatography. System GA—primidone RI 2250, M (phenobarbital) RI 1953, M (phenylethylmalondiamide (PEMA)) RI 1884, M (diamide) RI 1935, M (acetyl-) RI 2115; system GB—primidone RI 2384, primidone-Me_2 RI 2161, M (PEMA) RI 1996, M (acetyl-) RI 2189; system GE—primidone RRT 0.89, M (phenobarbital) RRT 0.74, and M (PEMA) RRT 0.65 (all relative to phenytoin); system GAJ—primidone RRT 1.674, M (PEMA) RRT 1.074 (both relative to methylphenobarbital).

High Performance Liquid Chromatography. System HE—primidone *k* 1.35, M (phenobarbital) *k* 2.76; system HX—RI 322; system HY—RI 288; system HZ—Retention time 2.1 min; system HAA—Retention time 11.1 min; system HAM—Retention time 2.2 min.

Ultraviolet Spectrum. Methanol—252, 258 (A^1_1=9.7c), 264 nm.

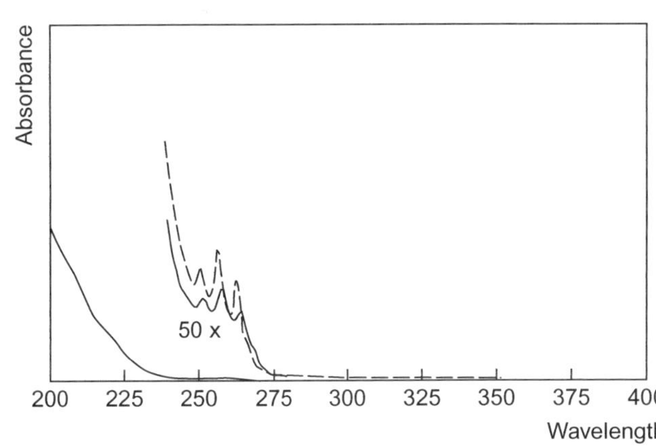

Infra-red Spectrum. Principal peaks at wavenumbers 1662, 1705, 1496, 700, 765, 1120 cm^{-1} (KBr disk).

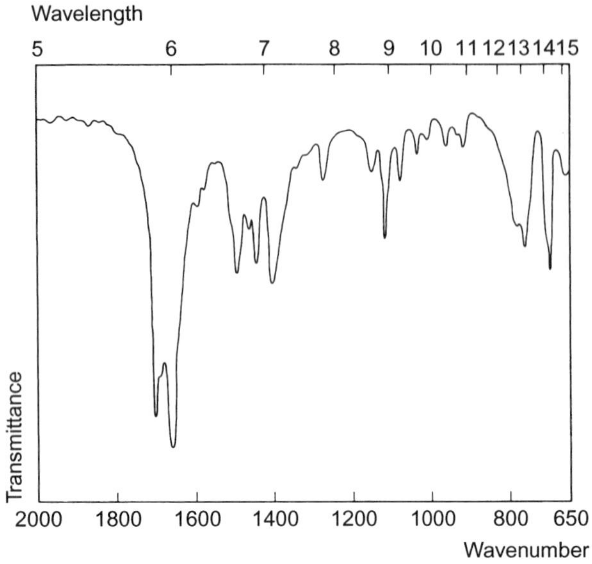

Mass Spectrum. Principal ions at *m/z* 146, 190, 117, 118, 161, 189, 103, 91; phenobarbital 204, 117, 146, 161, 77, 103, 115, 118; phenylethylmalondiamide 163, 148, 91, 103, 117, 120, 44, 77.

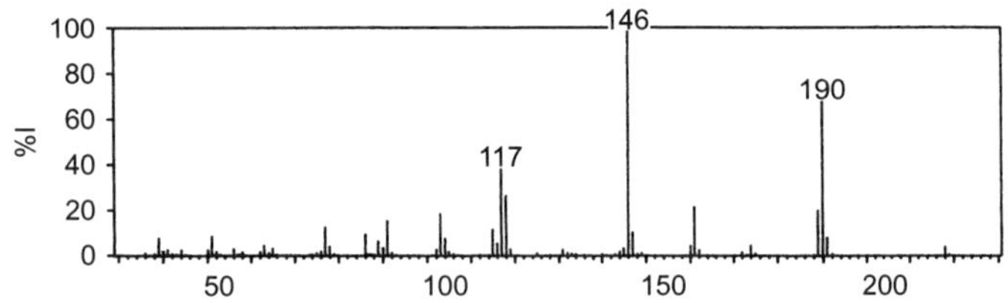

Quantification

Gas chromatography. In plasma: primidone and other anticonvulsants, limits of quantification 0.05 to 0.2 mg/L, thermionic specific detection—M. E. Queiroz *et al.*, *J. Chromatogr. Sci.*, 2002, *40*, 219–223.

Gas chromatography–mass spectrometry. In serum, urine, saliva, breast milk or tissues: primidone, phenobarbital, 4-hydroxyphenobarbital and phenylethylmalondiamide, limits of detection between 1.4 and 3.7 µg/L—H. Nau *et al.*, *J. Chromatogr.*, 1980, *182*; *B Biomed. Appl.*, *8*, 71–79. In whole blood or liver: primidone and other anticonvulsants—D. J. Speed *et al.*, *J. Anal. Toxicol.*, 2000, *24*, 685–690.

High performance liquid chromatography. In plasma or serum: primidone and phenobarbital, limit of detection about 550 µg/L for primidone, UV detection—J. A. Christofides and D. E. Fry, *Clin. Chem.*, 1980, *26*, 499–501. In serum, saliva, or urine: primidone and other anticonvulsants, photodiode-array detection—H. Liu *et al.*, *J. Chromatogr.*, 1993, *616*, 105–115. In plasma: primidone and other anticonvulsants, UV detection—L. A. Romanyshyn *et al.*, *Ther. Drug Monit.*, 1994, *16*, 90–99.

Disposition in the Body. Readily absorbed after oral administration. Rapidly metabolised to phenylethylmalondiamide (PEMA) and more slowly metabolised to phenobarbital; both metabolites are active anticonvulsants. Aromatic hydroxylation to form 4-hydroxyphenobarbital also occurs followed by glucuronic acid conjugation. The formation of phenobarbital is stimulated by phenytoin. During chronic treatment, about 92% of the daily dose is excreted in the urine in 24 h, of which 15 to 65% (mean 42%) is unchanged drug, 16 to 65% (mean 45%) is PEMA, and 1 to 8% (mean 5%) is phenobarbital or its hydroxylated metabolites and conjugates. Primidone is widely distributed in all organs and tissues. It crosses the blood–brain barrier and placental barrier and is excreted in breast milk.

Therapeutic concentration. In plasma, usually in the range 5 to 12 mg/L but there is considerable intersubject variation. At the beginning of treatment there is a delay of several days before phenobarbital appears in the plasma. Concentrations of phenobarbital and PEMA accumulate during chronic treatment, and steady-state plasma-phenobarbital concentrations are often used to monitor therapy.

After daily oral dosing of a number of subjects at various dose levels, steady-state plasma concentrations were as follows: 26 subjects at 250 mg per day, 0 to 13 mg/L (mean 3.2); 26 subjects at 500 mg per day, 1 to 14 mg/L (mean 6.7); 78 subjects at 750 mg per day, 2 to 23 mg/L (mean 8.7); 52 subjects at 1000 mg per day, 3 to 20 mg/L (mean 10.5); 9 subjects at 1250 mg per day, 10 to 19 mg/L (mean 14.7). In 30 subjects given primidone but no barbiturate, the mean primidone concentration was 9.2 mg/L and the mean phenobarbital concentration was 31 mg/L [H. E. Booker *et al.*, *Epilepsia*, 1970, *11*, 395–402].

Following oral doses of 75 to 250 mg three times a day to 7 subjects, the following steady-state serum concentrations were reported: primidone 5.0 to 13.4 mg/L (mean 8.3), phenobarbital 3.3 to 34.6 mg/L (mean 12.6), PEMA 1.4 to 9.9 mg/L (mean 4.6) [J. C. Cloyd *et al.*, *Clin. Pharmacol. Ther.*, 1981, *29*, 402–407].

Toxicity. The estimated minimum lethal dose is 5 g but instances of survival after the ingestion of 25 to 30 g have been reported. Toxic effects are usually associated with plasma concentrations greater than 10 mg/L and concentrations greater than 50 mg/L may be lethal.

In a fatality due to primidone ingestion, postmortem blood concentrations of 65 mg/L of primidone and 3 mg/L of phenobarbital were reported [J. A. Wright per R. C. Baselt, *Disposition of Toxic Chemicals and Drugs in Man*, 5th Edn, Davis, California, Biomedical Publications, 2000, pp. 724–726].

Serum concentrations of 95 mg/L of primidone and 175 mg/L of phenobarbital were reported about 12 h after a non-fatal suicide attempt by a 10-year-old epileptic subject; the corresponding urine concentrations were 1570 and 50 mg/L, respectively [J. C. Cate and R. Tenser, *Clin Toxicol.*, 1975, *8*, 385–389].

Half-life. Plasma half-life, primidone about 10 to 15 h, phenobarbital 50 to 150 h, PEMA 24 to 48 h.

Volume of distribution. In children after oral dosing, about 0.6 L/kg.

Clearance. Plasma clearance, after oral administration, about 0.7 mL/min/kg.

Saliva. Plasma:saliva ratio, about 1.0.

Protein binding. In plasma, less than 20%.

Dose. Initially 125 mg daily, increasing to 0.5 to 1.5 g daily.

Probenecid

Uricosuric

Proprietary names. Bencid; Benemid(e); Benuryl; Probalan; Probecid; Proben; Procid.

4-[(Dipropylamino)sulfonyl]benzoic acid

$C_{13}H_{19}NO_4S$=285.4

CAS—57-66-9

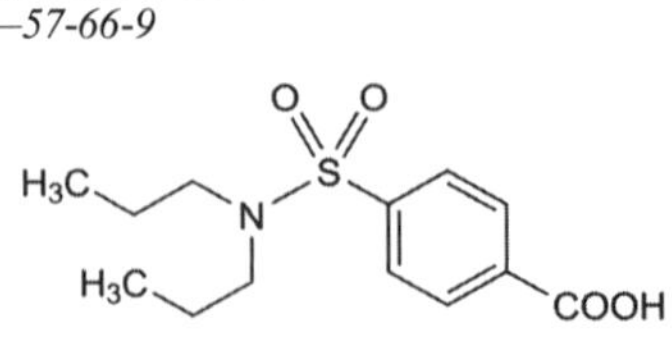

A white crystalline powder. M.p. 194° to 196°.

Practically insoluble in water and dilute acids; soluble 1 in 25 of ethanol and 1 in 12 of acetone; soluble in chloroform and dilute alkalis.

Dissociation Constant. pK_a 3.4 (20°).

Partition Coefficient. Log *P* (octanol/water), 3.2.

Thin-layer Chromatography. System TD—Rf 13; system TE—Rf 05; system TF—Rf 23; system TAD—Rf 24; system TAE—Rf 87; system TAJ—Rf 28; system TAK—Rf 71; system TAL—Rf 90.

Gas Chromatography. System GA—RI 2336.

High Performance Liquid Chromatography. System HX—RI 526; system HY—RI 507; system HZ—Retention time 7.8 min.

Ultraviolet Spectrum. Ethanolic acid—248 nm (A_1^1=332a).

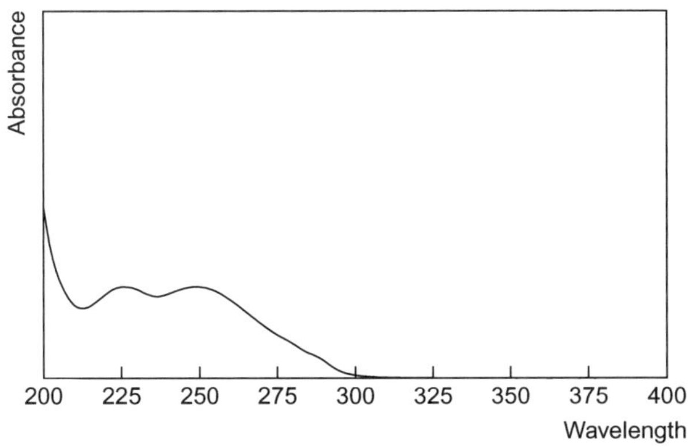

Infra-red Spectrum. Principal peaks at wavenumbers 1683, 1156, 1285, 1307, 1125, 1180 cm^{-1} (KBr disk).

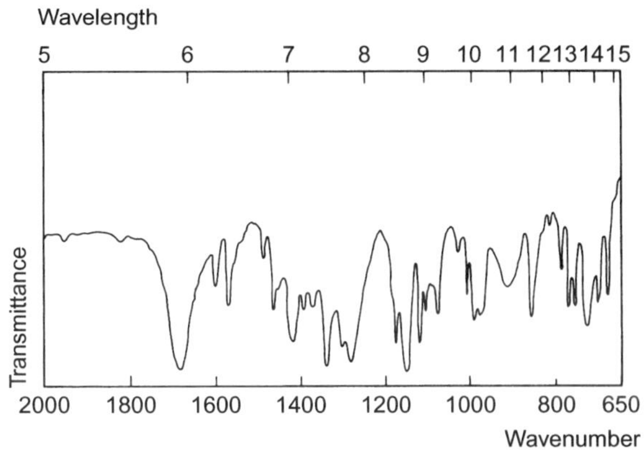

Mass Spectrum. Principal ions at *m/z* 256, 121, 185, 43, 257, 65, 42, 214.

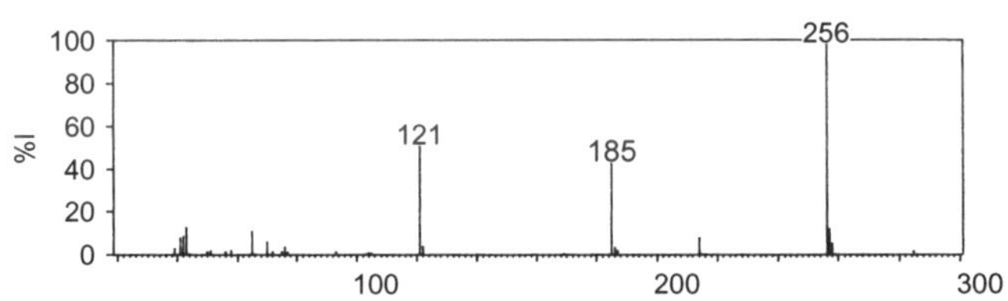

Quantification

Spectrofluorimetry. In plasma—R. F. Cunningham *et al., J. Pharm. Sci.*, 1978, *67*, 434–436.

Gas chromatography. In plasma or cerebrospinal fluid: limit of detection 20 µg/L, ECD—B. E. Roos *et al., Eur. J. Clin. Pharmacol.*, 1980, *17*, 223–226.

High performance liquid chromatography. In plasma or urine: limit of detection 500 µg/L, UV detection—P. Hekman *et al., J. Chromatogr.*, 1980, *182*; *B Biomed. Appl.*, *8*, 252–256. In urine: probenecid and its glucuronide—J. Hansen-Moller and U. Schmit, *J. Pharm. Biomed. Anal.*, 1991, *9*, 65–73. In plasma or urine: probenecid and its metabolites—T. B. Vree *et al., Pharm. Weekbl. (Sci.)*, 1992, *14*, 83–87.

Disposition in the Body. Readily absorbed after oral administration. Metabolised by side-chain oxidation, glucuronic acid conjugation, and *N*-dealkylation. Up to about 90% of a dose is excreted in the urine, the major urinary metabolite, probenecid acyl glucuronide, accounting for up to 50% of a dose; up to 25% of a dose is excreted as hydroxylated and carboxylic acid metabolites, and 5 to 15% as *N*-dealkylated metabolites. About 5 to 10% of a dose is excreted as unchanged drug but this appears to be variable, increasing with increasing urinary pH values and urinary flow.

Therapeutic concentration

Following single oral doses of 0.5, 1.0, and 2.0 g to 5 subjects, mean peak plasma concentrations of 35.3, 69.6, and 149 mg/L were reported at 3 to 4 h [A. Selen *et al., J. Pharm. Sci.*, 1982, *71*, 1238–1242].

After daily oral administration of 0.5 g four times a day to 19 subjects for 4 weeks, a mean plasma concentration of 22.5 mg/L was reported [R. F. Cunningham *et al., Clin. Pharmacokinet.*, 1981, *6*, 135–151].

Toxicity. Probenecid is relatively non-toxic and recovery has occurred after the ingestion of 47 g.

A 36-year-old man died after deliberately ingesting approximately 75 g of probenecid. Postmortem tissue concentrations were highest in serum (710 mg/L) and the liver (550 µg/g); ethanol was also detected in blood (1.3 g/L) [I. M. McIntyre *et al., J. Forensic Sci.*, 1992, *37*, 1190–1193].

Half-life. Plasma half-life, 4 to 17 h (dose-dependent).

Volume of distribution. About 0.1 to 0.2 L/kg.

Protein binding. In plasma, about 90%.

Note. For a review of the clinical pharmacokinetics of probenecid see R. F. Cunningham *et al., Clin. Pharmacokinet.*, 1981, *6*, 135–151.

Dose. 0.5 to 2 g daily.

Procainamide

Anti-arrhythmic

Synonym. Procaine Amide

4-Amino-*N*-(2-diethylaminoethyl)benzamide

$C_{13}H_{21}N_3O$=235.3

CAS—51-06-9

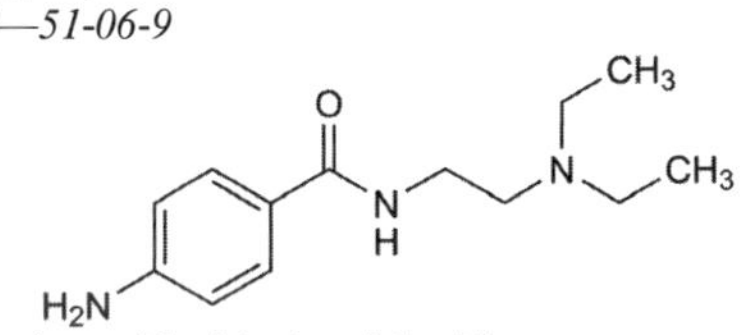

Procainamide Hydrochloride

Synonym. Novocainamidum

Proprietary names. Biocoryl; Novocamid; Procamide; Procan SR; Procanbid; Procapan; Pronestyl.

$C_{13}H_{21}N_3O$,HCl=271.8

CAS—614-39-1

A white to tan-coloured, hygroscopic, crystalline powder. M.p. 165° to 169°. Soluble 1 in 0.25 of water, 1 in 2 of ethanol, and 1 in 140 of chloroform; slightly soluble in acetone; practically insoluble in ether.

Dissociation Constant. pK_a 9.2 (20°).

Partition Coefficient. Log *P* (ethyl acetate/pH 7.4), −1.5; (octanol/water), 0.9.

Colour Tests. Coniferyl Alcohol—orange; Diazotisation—red; Ninhydrin—yellow.

Thin-layer Chromatography. System TA—Rf 49; system TB—Rf 01; system TC—Rf 05; system TE—Rf 39; system TL—Rf 09; system TAE—Rf 17; system TAF—Rf 33. (Acidified iodoplatinate solution, positive.)

Gas Chromatography. System GA—procainamide RI 2255, *N*-acetylprocainamide RI 2550; system GB—procainamide RI 2332, *N*-acetylprocainamide RI 2724; system GF—RI 2965.

High Performance Liquid Chromatography. System HA—procainamide *k* 1.3, *N*-acetylprocainamide *k* 3.0; system HX—RI 208; system HY—RI 160; system HZ—procainamide Retention time 1.9 min; *N*-acetylprocainamide 1.8 min.

Ultraviolet Spectrum. Aqueous alkali—275 nm (A^1_1=693a).

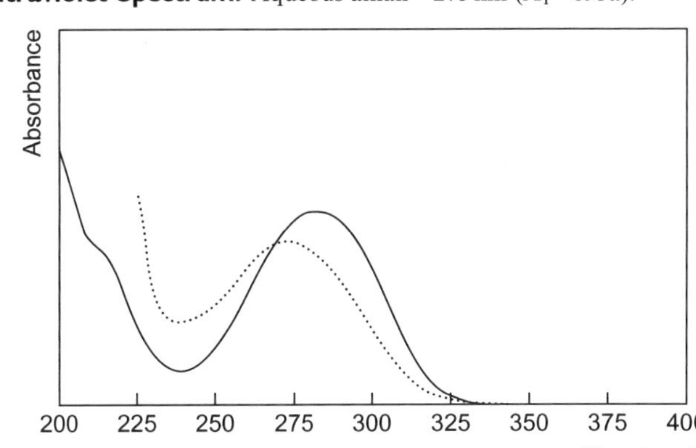

Infra-red Spectrum. Principal peaks at wavenumbers 1600, 1512, 1639, 1297, 1545, 1570 cm^{-1} (procainamide hydrochloride, KBr disk).

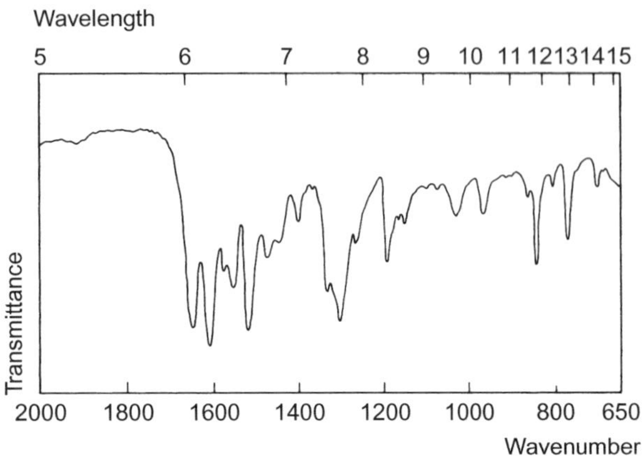

Mass Spectrum. Principal ions at *m/z* 86, 99, 120, 30, 92, 87, 58, 65; *N*-acetylprocainamide 86, 58, 99, 56, 162, 132, 149, 205.

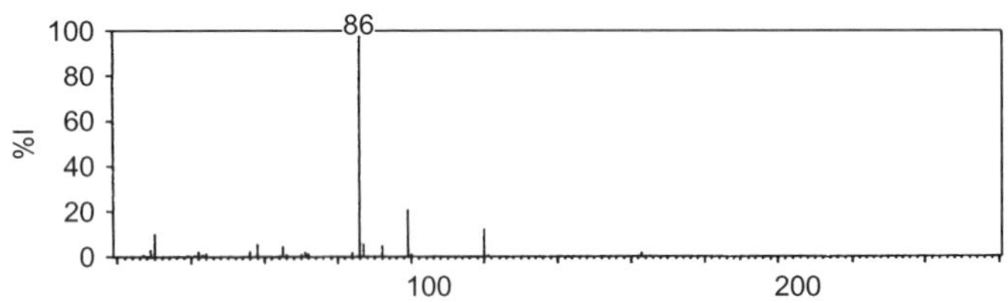

Quantification

Gas chromatography. In serum: limit of detection 100 ng, ECD—T. M. Ludden *et al.*, *J. Pharm. Sci.*, 1978, *67*, 371–373.

High performance liquid chromatography. In plasma: procainamide, *N*-acetylprocainamide, and other anti-arrhythmic agents, limit of detection 500 µg/L, UV detection—R. R. Bridges and T. A. Jennison, *J. Anal. Toxicol.*, 1983, *7*, 65–68. In plasma: procainamide and *N*-acetylprocainamide, limit of detection 1 mg/L, UV detection—K. Carr *et al.*, *J. Chromatogr.*, 1976, *129*, 363–368. In plasma or urine: procainamide and *N*-acetylprocainamide, limit of detection 50 µg/L in plasma, UV detection—C.-M. Lai *et al.*, *J. Pharm. Sci.*, 1980, *69*, 982–984. In plasma: procainamide and *N*-acetylprocainamide, limits of detection 0.1 mg/L and 0.25 mg/L respectively, spectrofluorimetric detection—D. Raphanaud *et al.*, *Ther. Drug Monit.*, 1986, *8*, 365–367. In serum or urine: procainamide and metabolites, limit of detection 50 µg/L, UV detection—J. D. Coyle *et al.*, *J. Pharm. Sci.*, 1987, *76*, 402–405. In plasma: procainamide and other anti-arrhythmics, UV or fluorescence detection—R. Verbesselt *et al.*, *Ther. Drug Monit.*, 1991, *13*, 157–165. In plasma: procainamide and *N*-acetylprocainamide, limit of detection 2 µg/L, UV detection—E. Lessard *et al.*, *J. Chromatogr. Sci.*, 1998, *36*, 49–54.

Disposition in the Body. Readily absorbed after oral administration and widely distributed throughout the body. The major metabolite, *N*-acetylprocainamide (acecainide), has similar pharmacological activity to procainamide; the acetylation of procainamide is subject to genetic polymorphism. Up to about 80% of a dose is excreted in the urine of normal subjects in 24 h, about 50 to 60% as unchanged drug and up to about 30% as *N*-acetylprocainamide (less in slow acetylators). Other metabolites include monodesethylprocainamide and monodesethyl-*N*-acetylprocainamide.

Therapeutic concentration. There is considerable intersubject variation in plasma concentrations. The therapeutic effect has been correlated with plasma concentrations of about 4 to 10 mg/L of procainamide and 5 to 30 mg/L of combined procainamide and *N*-acetylprocainamide. *N*-Acetylprocainamide may accumulate during chronic administration in fast acetylators and in subjects with renal impairment.

After a single oral dose of 1 g to 5 normal subjects, peak plasma concentrations of 3.5 to 5.3 mg/L of procainamide (mean 4.2) were attained in 1 to 2 h; concentrations of *N*-acetylprocainamide reached a peak of 0.6 to 2.1 mg/L (mean 1.6) in 3 to 8 h [E.-G. V. Giardina *et al.*, *Clin. Pharmacol. Ther.*, 1976, *19*, 339–351].

The following steady-state plasma concentrations were reported in 10 subjects receiving maintenance treatment: procainamide, 2.6 to 20.7 mg/L (mean 10.6); *N*-acetylprocainamide, 4.6 to 43.6 mg/L (mean 15.9); monodesethyl-*N*-acetylprocainamide 0.4 to 11.9 mg/L (mean 2.7) [T. I. Ruo *et al.*, *J. Pharmacol. Exp. Ther.*, 1981, *216*, 357–362].

Following IV infusion of 84 to 374 mg/h to 34 subjects, steady-state plasma concentrations of 1.7 to 17 mg/L (mean 6.5) of procainamide and 1.1 to 20 mg/L (mean 5.7) of *N*-acetylprocainamide were reported [J. J. Lima *et al.*, *Am. J. Cardiol.*, 1979, *43*, 98–105].

Subjects received 1, 2 or 4 g of procainamide daily by mouth, given either in four divided doses as a conventional-release capsule or in two divided doses as an extended-release tablet. The peak plasma concentrations of procainamide after twice daily and four times daily administration, respectively, were 2.74 and 2.77 mg/L for all dose levels (at 4.0 and 2.0 h). Corresponding values for *N*-acetylprocainamide were 2.61 and 2.92 mg/L (at 4.4 and 2.6 h) [B. B. Yang *et al.*, *J. Clin. Pharmacol.*, 1996, *36*, 623–633].

Toxicity. Toxic effects are usually associated with plasma-procainamide concentrations of about 12 mg/L or more and fatalities with concentrations greater than 20 mg/L. As little as 200 mg intravenously can be fatal.

In 4 fatalities attributed to procainamide intoxication in subjects receiving therapeutic doses, plasma-procainamide concentrations shortly before death ranged from 17.6 to 25.2 mg/L [J. Koch-Weser and S. W. Klein, *J. Am. Med. Assoc.*, 1971, *215*, 1454–1460].

The following postmortem concentrations were reported in a fatality attributed to procainamide: blood 114 mg/L, liver 283 µg/g, urine 556 mg/L [L. Kopjak and T. A. Jennison, *Bull. Int. Assoc. Forensic Toxicol.*, 1976, *12*(1), 12–13].

A 14-year-old boy had a serum procainamide level of 63 mg/L and an *N*-acetylprocainamide level of 80.4 mg/L approximately 2.5 h after intentionally ingesting about 21 g of procainamide; after 43 h, the levels were 0.3 and 0.6 mg/L for procainamide and *N*-acetylprocainamide, respectively [S. R. White *et al.*, *Pediatr. Emerg. Care*, 2002, *18*, 185–188].

Bioavailability. About 75 to 95%.

Half-life. Plasma half-life: procainamide about 3 h in normal subjects, increased in subjects with renal failure or with heart disease; *N*-acetylprocainamide about 6 to 9 h.

Volume of distribution. About 2 L/kg.

Clearance. Plasma clearance, about 5 to 15 mL/min/kg.

Protein binding. In plasma, about 15%.

Note. For a review of the clinical pharmacokinetics of procainamide see E. Karlsson, *Clin. Pharmacokinet.*, 1978, *3*, 97–107.

Dose. Maintenance, 0.5 to 1 g of procainamide hydrochloride, by mouth, every 4 to 6 h.

Procaine

Local Anaesthetic

Synonym. Ethocaine

2-Diethylaminoethyl 4-aminobenzoate

$C_{13}H_{20}N_2O_2$ = 236.3

CAS—59-46-1

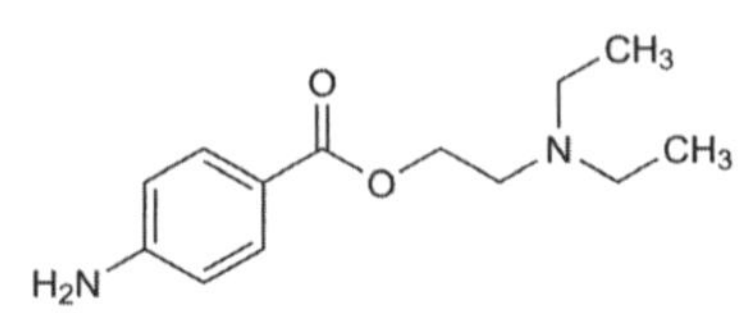

M.p. 61°.

Soluble 1 in 200 of water (when freshly precipitated); soluble in ethanol, benzene, chloroform, and ether.

Procaine Hydrochloride

Synonyms. Allocaine; Novocainum; Procaini Hydrochloridum; Procainii Chloridum; Procainum Chloride; Syncaine.

Proprietary names. Geroaslan H3; Gerovital H3; Lenident; NovanaestNovocain; Procaneural; Syntocaine; Venocaina.
$C_{13}H_{20}N_2O_2$,HCl=272.8
CAS—51-05-8
Colourless crystals or a white crystalline powder. M.p. 153° to 156°.
Soluble 1 in 1 of water, 1 in 30 of ethanol, and 1 in 30 of dehydrated alcohol; slightly soluble in chloroform; practically insoluble in ether.

Dissociation Constant. pK_a 9.0 (20°).

Partition Coefficient. Log *P* (octanol/water), 2.1.

Colour Test. Diazotisation—red-orange.

Thin-layer Chromatography. System TA—Rf 54; system TB—Rf 05; system TC—Rf 31; system TE—Rf 71; system TL—Rf 30; system TAE—Rf 36; system TAF—Rf 42; system TAJ—Rf 06; system TAK—Rf 00; system TAL—Rf 22. (Dragendorff spray, positive; acidified iodoplatinate solution, positive; ninhydrin spray, positive.)

Gas Chromatography. System GA—procaine RI 2010, procaine-AC RI 2350, 4-aminobenzoic acid RI 1547; system GF—RI 2580; system GQ—Retention time 6.8 min.

High Performance Liquid Chromatography. System HA—*k* 1.9; system HQ—*k* 0.00; system HX—RI 264; system HY—RI 225; system HAA—Retention time 5.2 min; system HAX—Retention time 7.3 min; system HAY—Retention time 4.0 min.

Ultraviolet Spectrum. Aqueous acid—294, 222 nm; methanol—296 nm (A^1_1=954a).

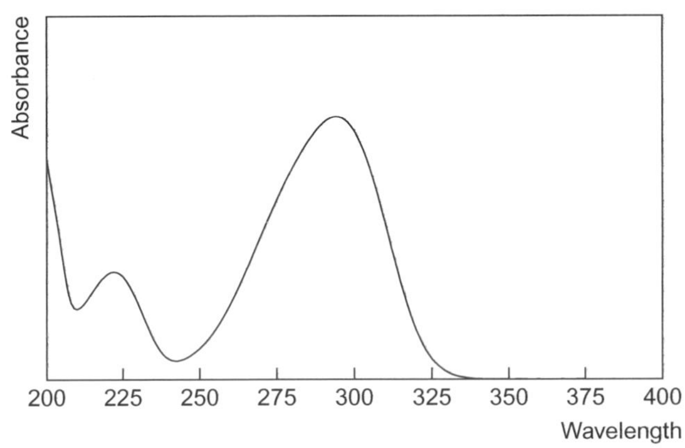

Infra-red Spectrum. Principal peaks at wavenumbers 1690, 1274, 1605, 1174, 1116, 772 cm^{-1} (procaine hydrochloride, KBr disk). (See below)

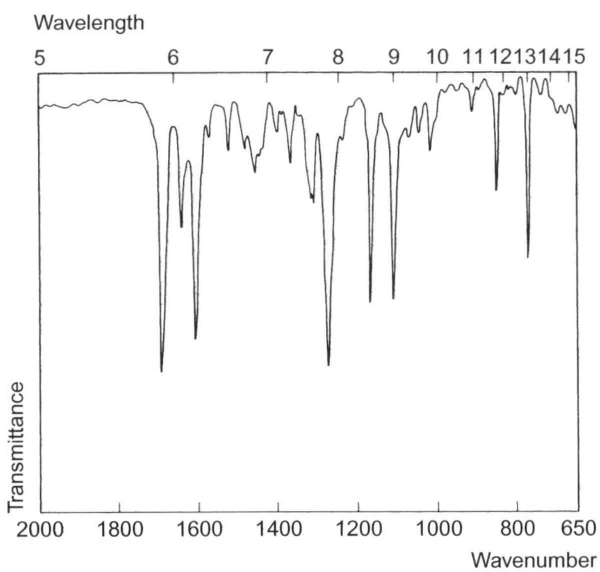

Mass Spectrum. Principal ions at *m/z* 86, 99, 120, 58, 87, 30, 92, 71; 4-aminobenzoic acid 137, 120, 92, 65, 39, 138, 121, 63.

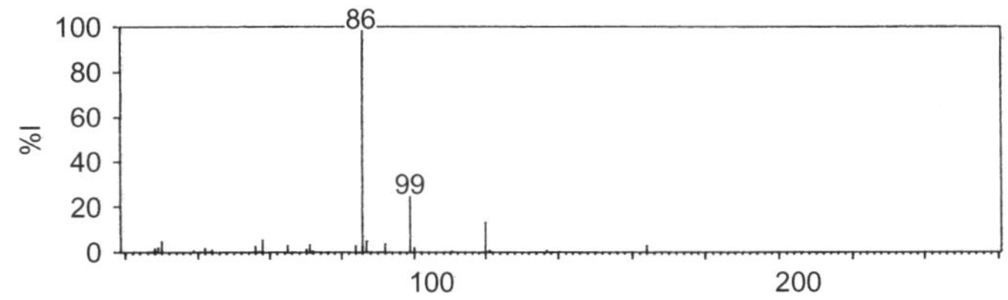

Quantification

Gas Chromatography. In plasma: procaine and chloroprocaine, limit of detection 0.1 mg/L, FID—R. H. Smith *et al.*, *Clin. Chem.*, 1978, *24*, 1599–1601. In plasma: FID—R. L. Green *et al.*, *New Engl. J. Med.*, 1974, *291*, 223–226. In whole blood or CSF: procaine and other local anaesthetics, limits of detection 5 to 10 pg per injection, SID—H. Hattori *et al.*, *J. Chromatogr.*, 1991, *564*, 278–282. In serum: procaine and other local anaesthetics, limits of detection about 60 to 70 pg per injection, NPD—M. Terada *et al.*, *J. Anal. Toxicol.*, 1996, *20*, 318–322.

Gas chromatography–mass spectrometry. In plasma and urine: limit of quantification 100 µg/L and limit of detection 80 µg/L (SIM, *m/z* 86)—T. Ohshima and T. Takayasu, *J. Chromatogr. B Biomed. Sci. Appl.*, 1999, *726(1–2)*, 185–194.

Disposition in the Body. Poorly absorbed from mucous membranes; readily absorbed after parenteral administration and rapidly hydrolysed in the plasma to 4-aminobenzoic acid and diethylaminoethanol. About 80% of the 4-aminobenzoic acid is excreted unchanged or conjugated in the urine, together with about 30% of the diethylaminoethanol, the remainder being metabolised in the liver; about 2% of a dose is excreted in the urine as unchanged drug.

Therapeutic concentration

A mean steady-state plasma concentration of 12.7 mg/L was reported during the continuous IV infusion of 1.0 mg/kg/min to 6 subjects; following continuous IV infusion of 1.5 mg/kg/min to a further 6 subjects, a mean steady-state plasma concentration of 42.7 mg/L was reported [A. B. Seifen *et al.*, *Anesth. Analg. Curr. Res.*, 1979, *58*, 382–386].

Toxicity

Following IV injection to 10 subjects until convulsions were induced (total dose 18 to 55 mg/kg), plasma concentrations of 21 to 86 mg/L (mean 49) of procaine and 0.6 to 80 mg/L (mean 23) of 4-aminobenzoic acid were reported [J. E. Usubiaga *et al.*, *Anesth. Analg. Curr. Res.*, 1966, *45*, 611–620].

Following the accidental IV injection of 4 g to 1 subject, a peak blood concentration of 96 mg/L was reported; the subject recovered [J. A. Wikinski *et al.*, *JAMA.*, 1970, *213*, 621–623].

Half-life. Plasma half-life, about 0.1 h.

Protein binding. Plasma, about 6%.

Dose. Up to 1 g of procaine hydrochloride may be administered by injection with adrenaline.

Procaine Benzylpenicillin

Antibacterial

Synonyms. Benzylpenicillin Novocaine; Penicillin G Procaine; Procaine Penicillin; Procaine Penicillin G.
Proprietary names. Aqucilina; Atracilina; Ayercillin; Cilicaine; Crysticillin AS; Farmaproina; Fradicilina; Jenacillin O; Novocillin; Pfizerpen AS; Probecilin; Procillin; Wycillin. It is an ingredient of Bicillin.

Note. Bicillin is also used as a proprietary name for benzathine benzylpenicillin.
(2S,5*R*,6*R*)-3,3-Dimethyl-7-oxo-6-[(phenylacetyl)amino]-4-thia-1-azabicyclo[3.2.0]heptane-2-carboxylic acid compound with 2-(diethylamino)ethyl 4-aminobenzoate (1:1) monohydrate
$C_{13}H_{20}N_2O_2$,$C_{16}H_{18}N_2O_4S$,H_2O=588.7
CAS—54-35-3 (anhydrous); 6130-64-9 (monohydrate)
A white crystalline powder. M.p. 106° to 110°, with decomposition.
Soluble 1 in 200 of water, 1 in 30 of ethanol, and 1 in 60 of chloroform; very slightly soluble in ether.

Ultraviolet Spectrum. Aqueous acid—278 (A^1_1=53b); aqueous alkali—280 (A^1_1=256b); methanol—295 nm (A^1_1=367b).

Infra-red Spectrum. Principal peaks at wavenumbers 1266, 1600, 1779, 1692, 1176, 1120 cm^{-1} (KBr disk).

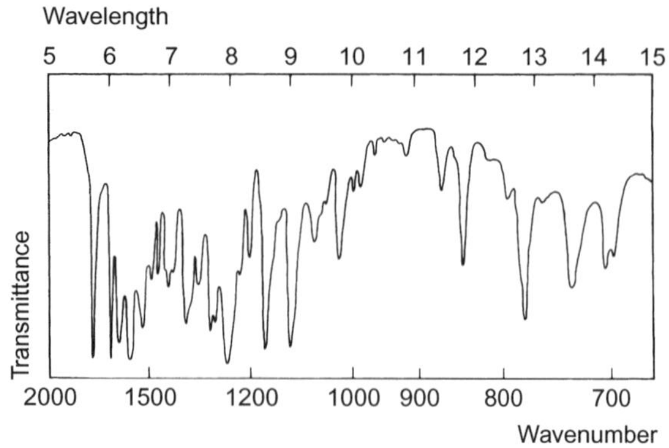

Dose. 300 to 600 mg daily, by deep IM injection.

Procarbazine

Antineoplastic

Synonym. Ibenzmethyzin; MIH; Ro-4-6467.
N-(1-Methylethyl)-4-[(2-methylhydrazino)methyl]benzamide
$C_{12}H_{19}N_3O$=221.3
CAS—671-16-9

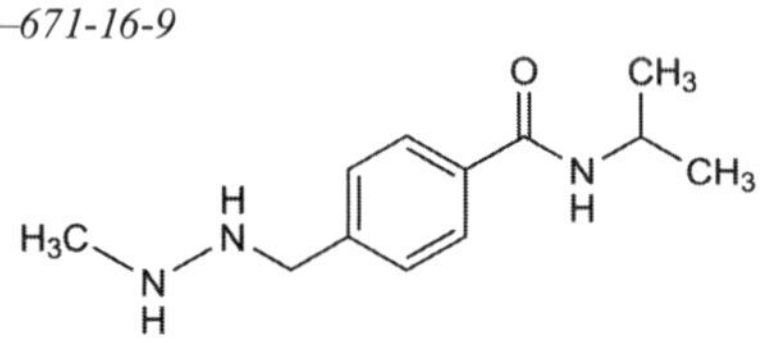

Procarbazine Hydrochloride

Proprietary names. Matulane; Natulan.
$C_{12}H_{19}N_3O,HCl$=257.8
CAS—366-70-1
A white to pale yellow crystalline powder. M.p. 223° to 226°, with decomposition.
Freely soluble in water; sparingly soluble in ethanol; slightly soluble in chloroform; practically insoluble in ether; soluble in methanol. Solutions in water are unstable.

Dissociation Constant. pK$_a$ 6.8.

Partition Coefficient. Log *P* (octanol/water), 0.1.

Colour Tests. Liebermann's Test (100°)—blue (15 s); Nessler's Reagent (room temperature) —black; Palladium Chloride—black.

Thin-layer Chromatography. System TA—Rf 49; system TB—Rf 02; system TC—Rf 10; system TE—Rf 80; system TL—Rf 04; system TAD—Rf 68; system TAE—Rf 88; system TAJ—Rf 34; system TAK—Rf 03; system TAL—Rf 90. (Acidified potassium permanganate solution, positive.)

Gas Chromatography. System GA—RI 1990.

Ultraviolet Spectrum. Aqueous acid—232 nm (A^1_1=570a).

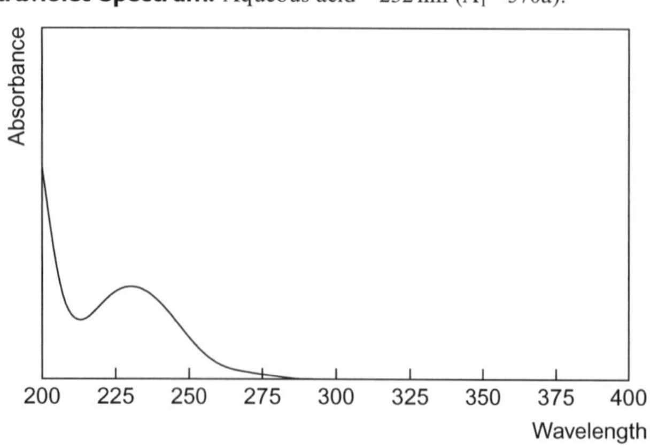

Infra-red Spectrum. Principal peaks at wavenumbers 1632, 1555, 1661, 1301, 861, 1176 cm^{-1} (procarbazine hydrochloride, KBr disk).

Mass Spectrum. Principal ions at *m/z* 177, 118, 45, 135, 90, 91, 221, 119.

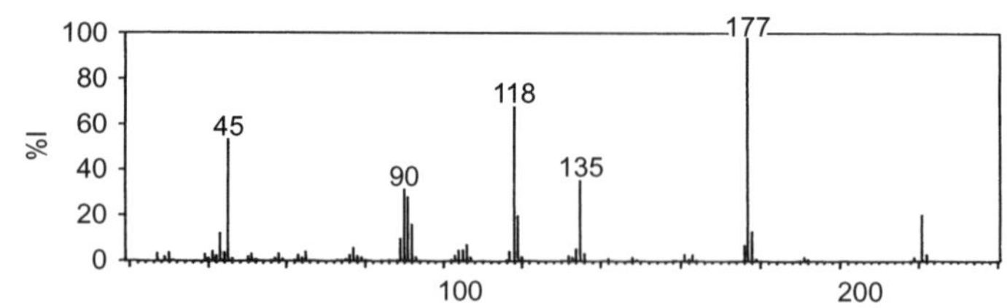

Quantification

Gas chromatography–mass spectrometry. In plasma: procarbazine and metabolites, limit of detection 10 µg/L—R. M. Gorsen *et al.*, *J. Chromatogr.*, 1980, *221*; *B Biomed. Appl.*, *10*, 309–318.

High performance liquid chromatography. In plasma or urine: limit of detection 10 ng, electrochemical detection—R. J. Rucki and S. A. Moros, *J. Chromatogr.*, 1980, *190*, 359–365. In plasma: procarbazine metabolites, UV detection—D. A. Shiba and R. J. Weinkam, *J. Chromatogr.*, 1982, *229*; *B Biomed. Appl.*, *18*, 397–407.

Disposition in the Body. Readily absorbed after oral administration; peak plasma concentrations are attained in 0.5 to 1 h. Rapidly metabolised to active azo derivatives and by oxidation to *N*-isopropylterephthalamic acid. Up to about 75% of a dose is excreted in the urine with about 5% of a dose consisting of unchanged drug.

Dose. Initially the equivalent of 50 mg of procarbazine daily, increasing to 250 or 300 mg daily.

Prochlorperazine

Tranquilliser

Synonyms. Chlormeprazine; Prochlorpemazine; Proclorperazine; SKF-4657; Bayer A 173; RP-6140.
Proprietary names. Compazine; Compro; Stemetil (suppositories).
2-Chloro-10-[3-(4-methyl-1-piperazinyl)propyl]-10*H*-phenothiazine
$C_{20}H_{24}ClN_3S$=373.9
CAS—58-38-8

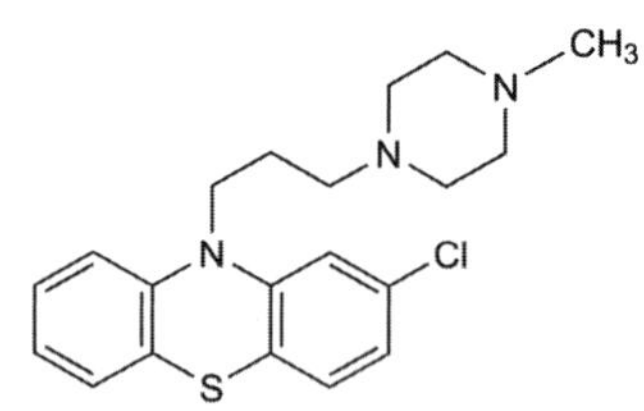

A clear, pale yellow, viscous liquid which is sensitive to light.
Very slightly soluble in water; freely soluble in ethanol, chloroform, and ether.

Prochlorperazine Edisilate

Synonyms. Prochlorperazine Edisylate; Prochlorperazine Ethanedisulfonate.
Proprietary name. Compazine
$C_{20}H_{24}ClN_3S,C_2H_6O_6S_2$=564.1
CAS—1257-78-9
A white to very light yellow crystalline powder.
Soluble 1 in 2 of water and 1 in 1500 of ethanol; practically insoluble in chloroform and ether.

Prochlorperazine Maleate

Synonyms. Prochlorperazine Dihydrogen Maleate; Prochlorperazine Dimaleate.
Proprietary names. Anti-Naus; Buccastem; Compazine; Dhaperazine; Meterazine; Mitil; Proclozine; Proziere; Scripto-Metic; Stemetil (tablets); Stemzine.
$C_{20}H_{24}ClN_3S,2C_4H_4O_4$=606.1
CAS—84-02-6
A white or pale yellow crystalline powder. M.p. 228°.
Practically insoluble in water, ethanol, and ether; slightly soluble in warm chloroform.

Prochlorperazine Mesilate

Synonyms. Prochlorperazine Dimethanesulfonate; Prochlorperazine Mesylate; Prochlorperazine Methanesulfonate.
Proprietary name. Stemetil (injection and syrup); Novamin; Tementil.
$C_{20}H_{24}ClN_3S,2CH_3SO_3H=566.2$
CAS—51888-09-6
A white powder. M.p. about 242°.
Soluble 1 in less than 0.5 of water and 1 in 40 of ethanol; slightly soluble in chloroform; practically insoluble in ether.

Dissociation Constant. pK_a 8.1 (24°).

Partition Coefficient. Log *P* (octanol/water), 4.9.

Colour Tests. Formaldehyde–Sulfuric Acid—red-violet; Forrest Reagent—red; FPN Reagent—red; Mandelin's Test—brown→violet; Marquis Test—violet.

Thin-layer Chromatography. System TA—Rf 49; system TB—Rf 34; system TC—Rf 37; system TE—Rf 55; system TL—Rf 7; system TAE—Rf 26; system TAF—Rf 26; system TAJ—Rf 18; system TAK—Rf 09; system TAL—Rf 74. (Acidified iodoplatinate solution, positive.)

Gas Chromatography. System GA—Prochlorperazine RI 2954; M (*N*-oxide) RI 2100; system GB—Prochlorperazine RI 3129; M (*N*-oxide) RI 2356; M (norsulfoxide) RI 3571; M (sulfoxide) RI 3758.

High Performance Liquid Chromatography. System HA—*k* 3.9; system HX—RI 450; system HY—RI 323; system HZ—Retention time 10.4 min.

Ultraviolet Spectrum. Aqueous acid—254 (A^1_1=875a), 305 nm.

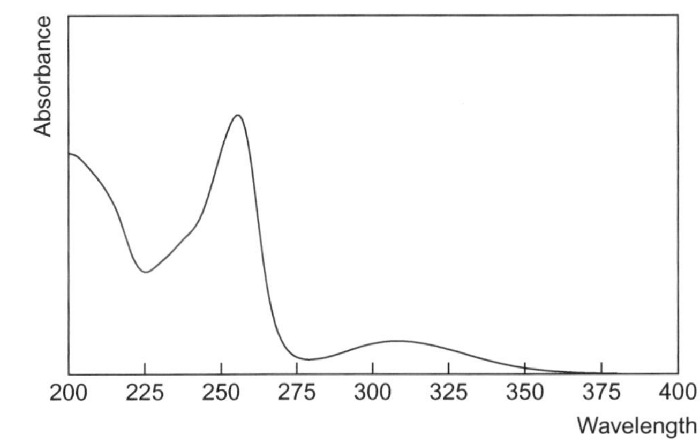

Infra-red Spectrum. Principal peaks at wavenumbers 752, 1280, 1569, 1165, 1242, 1145 cm^{-1} (KBr disk).

Mass Spectrum. Principal ions at *m/z* 113, 70, 373, 141, 43, 72, 42, 127.

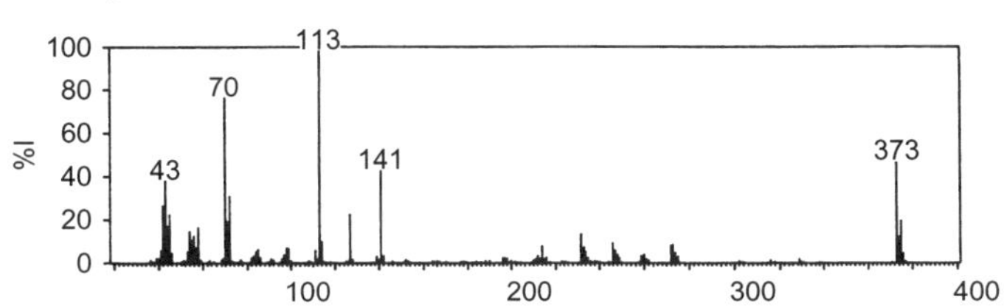

Quantification

High performance liquid chromatography. In plasma: limit of detection about 200 ng/L, electrochemical detection—M. G. Sankey *et al.*, *Br. J. Clin. Pharmacol.*, 1982, *13*, 578–580.

Radioimmunoassay. In plasma: limit of detection 156 ng/L—K. K. Midha *et al.*, *Ther. Drug Monit.*, 1983, *5*, 117–121.

Disposition in the Body. Absorbed after oral administration but extensively metabolised.

Therapeutic concentration
Following a single oral dose of 12.5 mg to 1 subject, a peak plasma concentration of about 0.0008 mg/L was attained in 6 h [M. G. Sankey *et al.*, *Br. J. Clin. Pharmacol.*, 1982, *13*, 578–580].

High prochlorperazine plasma levels of >600 µg/L were sustained for up to 24 h in patients treated with 135 mg/m^2 by IV infusion given over 2 h, as a doxorubicin-efflux blocker [K. S. Sridhar *et al.*, *Cancer Chemother. Pharmacol.*, 1994, *34*, 377–384].

Toxicity
Serum concentrations of 1.2 to 1.6 mg/L were found in 4 cases of non-fatal overdose [S. L. Tompsett, *Acta Pharmacol.Toxicol.*, 1968, *26*, 298–302].

Dose. Usually 15 to 30 mg of prochlorperazine maleate daily, as an anti-emetic; 50 to 100 mg daily for the treatment of psychoses.

Procyclidine

Anticholinergic

α-Cyclohexyl-α-phenyl-1-pyrrolidinepropanol
$C_{19}H_{29}NO=287.4$
CAS—77-37-2

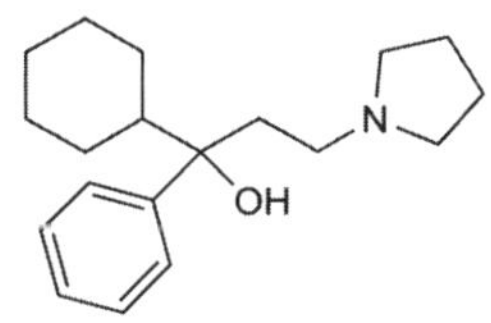

Crystals. M.p. 85.5° to 86.5° (crystals from petroleum ether).

Procyclidine Hydrochloride

Proprietary names. Arpicolin; Kemadren; Kemadrin; Muscinil; Osnervan; Procyclid.
$C_{19}H_{29}NO,HCl=323.9$
CAS—1508-76-5
A white crystalline powder. M.p. 226° to 227° (crystals from ethanol and ethyl acetate), with decomposition.
Soluble 1 in about 40 of water, 1 in 15 of ethanol, and 1 in 6 of chloroform; very slightly soluble in ether.

Partition Coefficient. Log *P* (octanol/water), 4.8.

Colour Tests. Mandelin's Test—black; Marquis Test—violet; Sulfuric Acid—yellow.

Thin-layer Chromatography. System TA—Rf 48; system TB—Rf 62; system TC—Rf 31; system TE—Rf 74; system TL—Rf 23; system TAE—Rf 20; system TAF—Rf 68; system TAJ—Rf 00; system TAK—Rf 00; system TAL—Rf 36. (Dragendorff spray, positive; acidified iodoplatinate solution, positive; Marquis reagent, violet-brown.)

Gas Chromatography. System GA—procyclidine RI 2156, M (oxo-)-H_2O RI 2490; system GB—procyclidine RI 2261, M (OH-isomer-1) RI 2487, M (OH-isomer-2) RI 2517, M (oxo-)-H_2O RI 2669; system GF—RI 2485.

High Performance Liquid Chromatography. System HA—*k* 2.0; system HX—RI 406; system HZ—Retention time 6.2 min; system HAX—not eluted after 20 min; system HAY—Retention time 4.7 min.

Ultraviolet Spectrum. Aqueous acid—251, 257 (A^1_1=6.9a), 263 nm.

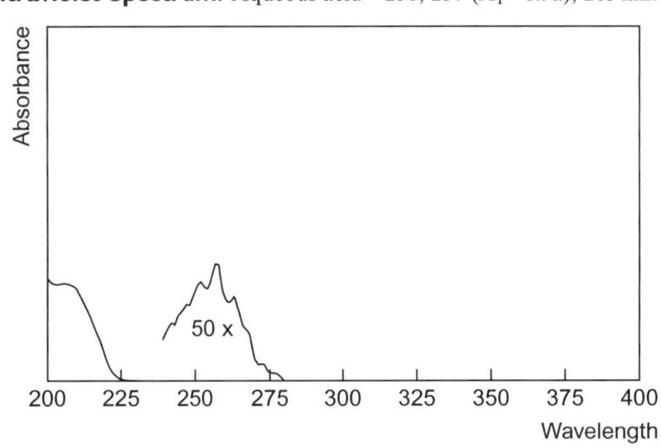

Infra-red Spectrum. Principal peaks at wavenumbers 700, 756, 746, 1128, 1075, 1175 cm^{-1} (procyclidine hydrochloride, KBr disk).

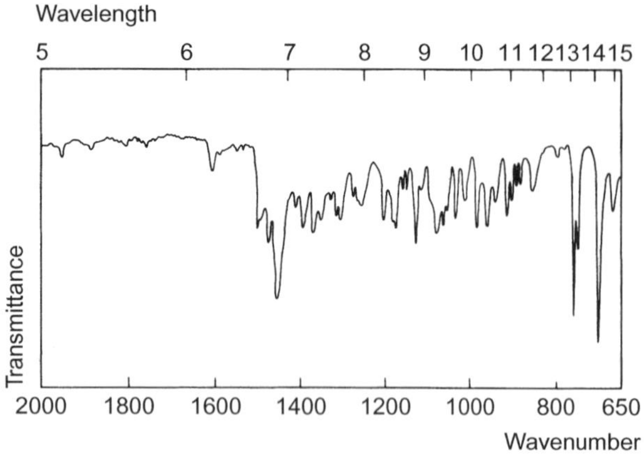

Mass Spectrum. Principal ions at *m/z* 84, 204, 205, 85, 42, 55, 105, 77.

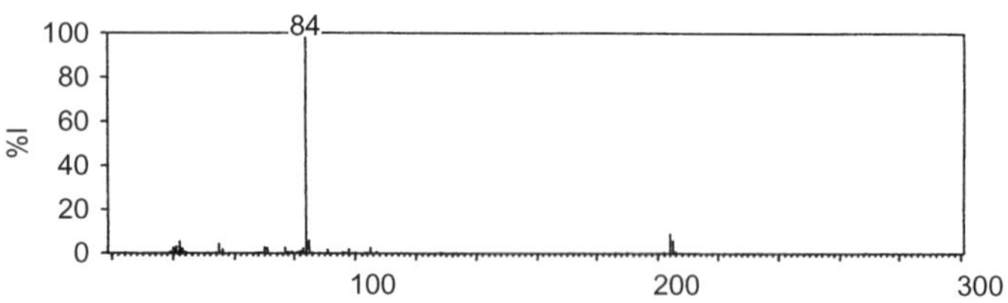

Quantification

Gas Chromatography. In plasma or urine: limit of detection 20 μg/L, AFID—K. Dean *et al.*, *J. Chromatogr.*, 1980, *221*; *B Biomed. Appl.*, *10*, 408–413. In blood: limit of detection 100 μg/L, AFID—A. W. Missen *et al.*, *J. Anal. Toxicol.*, 1978, *2*, 238–240. In biological fluids: procyclidine, cycrimine and trihexyphenidyl, limit of detection 50 to 100 ng/L, flame thermionic detection—J. A. Owen *et al.*, *J. Chromatogr.*, 1989, *494*, 135–142.

Disposition in the Body. Absorbed after oral administration. It rapidly disappears from the tissues. Metabolised by hydroxylation of the benzyl or cyclohexyl rings and then conjugated with glucuronic acid.

Therapeutic concentration

Following a single oral dose of 10 mg to 6 subjects, a mean peak plasma concentration of 0.12 mg/L was reported; in 5 of the subjects the peak concentrations were attained in about 1 h, whereas in the sixth subject the time to peak concentration was 8 h [P. D. Whiteman *et al.*, *Eur. J. Clin. Pharmacol.*, 1985, *28*, 73–78].

In 6 patients undergoing therapy with daily oral doses of 10 to 30 mg, mean steady-state blood concentrations of 0.15 to 0.63 mg/L were reported [A. W. Missen *et al.*, *J. Anal. Toxicol.*, 1978, *2*, 238–240].

Toxicity

In 2 fatalities involving procyclidine, postmortem tissue concentrations were: blood 4 and 4.4 mg/L, liver 15 and 11 μg/g, urine 7 and 1.8 mg/L; in the second case benzatropine and chlorpromazine were also detected [P. G. Ashton, *Bull. Int. Assoc. Forensic Toxicol.*, 1980, *15(2)*, 9–11].

Bioavailability. About 75%.

Half-life. Plasma half-life, 8 to 16 h (mean 12).

Volume of distribution. About 1 L/kg.

Clearance. Plasma clearance, about 1 mL/min/kg.

Dose. 7.5 to 30 mg of procyclidine hydrochloride daily; up to 60 mg daily has been given.

Profadol

Narcotic Analgesic

3-(1-Methyl-3-propylpyrrolidin-3-yl)phenol
$C_{14}H_{21}NO$=219.3
CAS—428-37-5

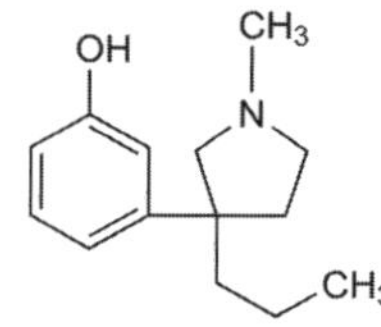

Profadol Hydrochloride
$C_{14}H_{21}NO,HCl$=255.8
CAS—2324-94-9
A white solid. M.p. 145° to 146°.
Soluble in water and chloroform.

Colour Tests. Folin–Ciocalteu Reagent—blue; Liebermann's Test—black; Mandelin's Test—blue-green→green; Marquis Test—orange→red-brown.

Thin-layer Chromatography. System TA—Rf 42; system TB—Rf 08; system TC—Rf 06; system TL—Rf 08. (Acidified iodoplatinate solution, positive.)

Gas Chromatography. System GA—RI 1748.

Ultraviolet Spectrum. Aqueous acid—272 (A^1_1=87b); aqueous alkali—237, 290 nm.

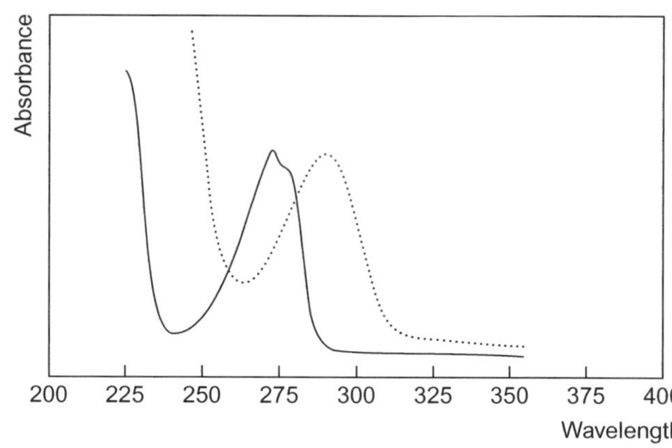

Infra-red Spectrum. Principal peaks at wavenumbers 1575, 1590, 1234, 752, 702, 1267 cm^{-1} (KBr disk).

Mass Spectrum. Principal ions at *m/z* 57, 42, 44, 177, 58, 219, 133, 107.

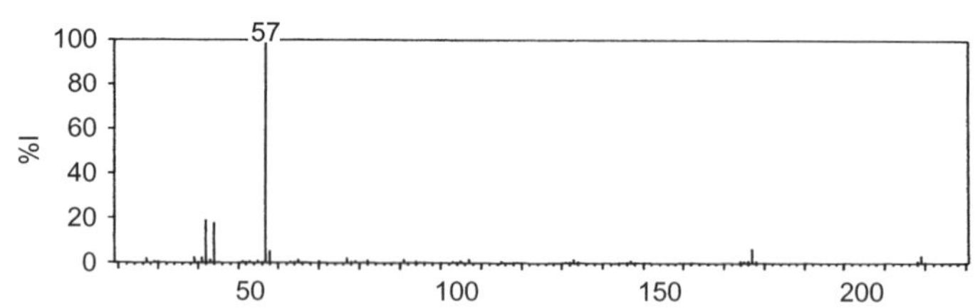

Profenamine

Anticholinergic

Synonyms. Ethopropazine; Isothazine; Phenopropazine.
N,*N*-Diethyl-α-methyl-10*H*-phenothiazine-10-ethanamine
$C_{19}H_{24}N_2S$=312.5
CAS—522-00-9

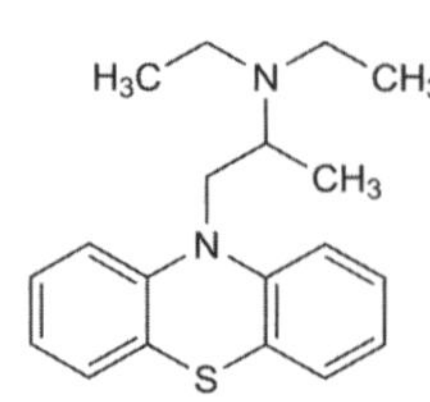

Crystals. M.p. 53° to 55°.

Profenamine Hibenzate
Synonym. Profenamine Hybenzate
$C_{19}H_{24}N_2S,C_{14}H_{10}O_4$=554.7
A white crystalline powder. M.p. about 188°, with decomposition.
Practically insoluble in water; slightly soluble in methanol.

Profenamine Hydrochloride
Synonyms. Profenamini Hydrochloridum; Prophenamini Chloridum.
Proprietary name. Parsitan
$C_{19}H_{24}N_2S,HCl$=348.9
CAS—1094-08-2
A white crystalline powder, which darkens in colour on exposure to light. M.p. 223° to 225°, with some decomposition.
Soluble 1 in 400 of water at 20° and 1 in 20 at 40°, 1 in 35 of ethanol, and 1 in 7 of chloroform; sparingly soluble in acetone; practically insoluble in ether and benzene.

Dissociation Constant. pK_a 9.6 (20°).

Partition Coefficient. Log *P* (octanol/water), 4.8.

Colour Tests. Formaldehyde–Sulfuric Acid—red-violet; Forrest Reagent—pink; FPN Reagent—orange→yellow; Liebermann's Test—red-brown; Mandelin's Test—green→violet; Marquis Test—violet.

Thin-layer Chromatography. System TA—Rf 67; system TB—Rf 64; system TC—Rf 47; system TE—Rf 83; system TL—Rf 66; system TAE—Rf 31; system TAF—Rf 55; system TAJ—Rf 22; system TAK—Rf 10; system TAL—Rf 57. (Dragendorff spray, positive; FPN reagent, pink; acidified iodoplatinate solution, positive; Marquis reagent, orange; ninhydrin spray, positive.)

Gas Chromatography. System GA—profenamine RI 2340, M (bis-desethyl-)-AC RI 2450, M (bis-desethyl-OH-)-AC_2 RI 2900, M (desethyl-)-AC RI 2515, M (desethyl-OH-)-AC_2 RI 2880; system GF—RI 2775.

High Performance Liquid Chromatography. System HA—*k* 2.4; system HX—RI 444; system HY—RI 338; system HAX—retention time 16.6 min; system HAY—retention time 8.3 min.

Ultraviolet Spectrum. Aqueous acid—250 (A_1^1=881a), 299; aqueous alkali—253, 302 nm.

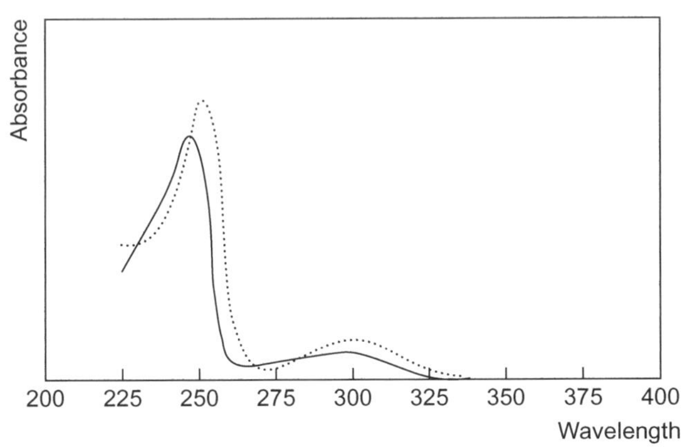

Infra-red Spectrum. Principal peaks at wavenumbers 748, 1248, 1590, 1282, 1568, 1125 cm^{-1} (KBr disk).

Mass Spectrum. Principal ions at *m/z* 100, 101, 44, 72, 198, 180, 42, 29.

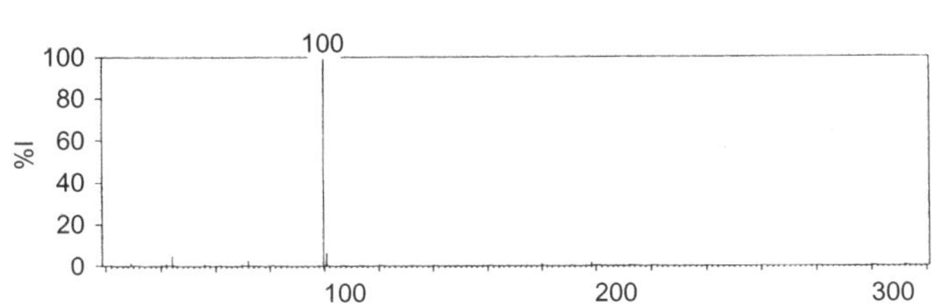

Dose. 50 to 500 mg of profenamine hydrochloride daily.

Proflavine Hemisulfate

Disinfectant/Topical Antiseptic

Synonyms. Neutral Proflavine Sulfate; Proflavine Hemisulfate.
3,6-Acridinediamine sulfate dihydrate
$(C_{13}H_{11}N_3)_2,H_2SO_4,2H_2O$=552.6
CAS—92-62-6 (proflavine); 553-30-0 (sulfate, anhydrous)

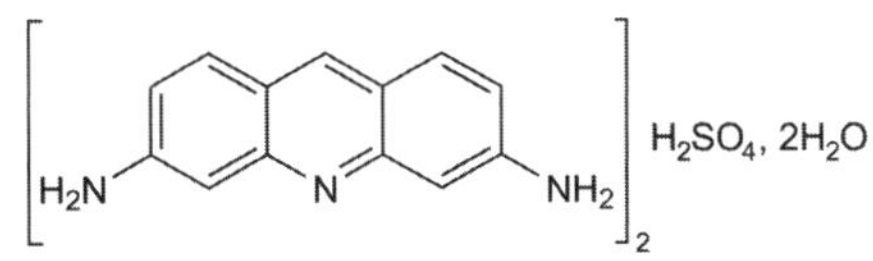

An orange to red, hygroscopic, crystalline powder.
Soluble 1 in 300 of water, 1 in 1 of boiling water, and 1 in 35 of glycerol; very slightly soluble in ethanol; practically insoluble in chloroform and ether. A saturated solution in water is deep orange in colour and gives a green fluorescence when freely diluted.

Dissociation Constant. Proflavine: pK_a 8.1 (20°).

Partition Coefficient. Proflavine: Log *P* (octanol/water), 1.8.

Colour Tests. Mandelin's Test—green; Marquis Test—yellow→orange.

Thin-layer Chromatography. System TA—Rf 16.

Ultraviolet Spectrum. Ethanol—261 nm (A_1^1=1091b).

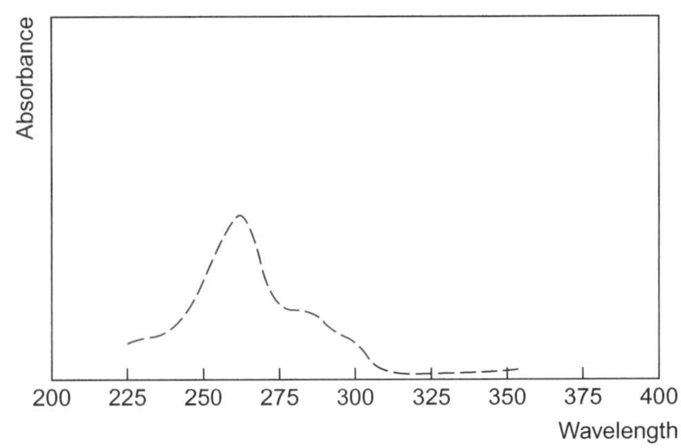

Infra-red Spectrum. Principal peaks at wavenumbers 1605, 1625, 1125, 1160, 1218, 1263 cm^{-1} (KBr disk).

Progesterone

Progestational Steroid

Synonyms. Corpus Luteum Hormone; Luteal Hormone; Luteine; Pregnenedione; Progestin.
Proprietary names. Crinone; Cutifitol; Cyclogest; Esolut; Estima; Evapause; Gesterol; Gestone; Lugesteron; Progeffik; Progenar; Progestan; Progestasert; Progestilin; Progestogel; Progestol; Progestosol; Prolidon; Proluton; Prometrium; Prontogest; Utrogest; Utrogestan.
Pregn-4-ene-3,20-dione
$C_{21}H_{30}O_2$=314.5
CAS—57-83-0

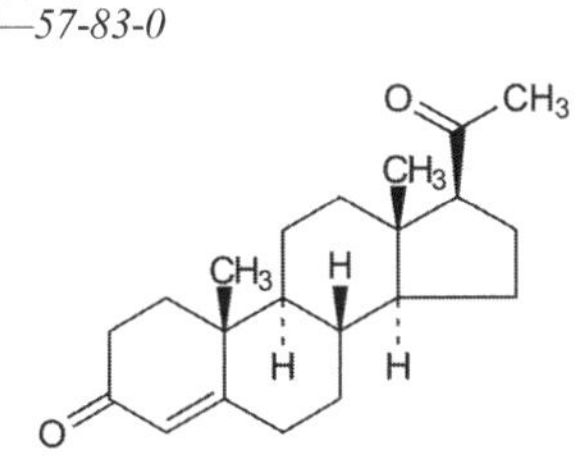

Colourless crystals or a white or slightly yellowish-white crystalline powder. There are two forms, one known as the α-form melts at 127° to 131° and the other, known as β-progesterone, at about 121°.

Practically insoluble in water; soluble 1 in 8 of ethanol, 1 in less than 1 of chloroform, and 1 in 16 of ether.

Partition Coefficient. Log *P* (octanol/water), 3.9.

Colour Tests. Naphthol–Sulfuric Acid—brown/yellow; Sulfuric Acid—yellow (green fluorescence under UV light).

Thin-layer Chromatography. System TB—Rf 36; system TE—Rf 79; system TF—Rf 56; system TP—Rf 81; system TQ—Rf 20; system TR—Rf 99; system TS—Rf 95; system TAE—Rf 83; system TAF—Rf 89; system TAJ—Rf 76; system TAK—Rf 68; system TAL—Rf 95; system TAM—Rf 97.

Gas Chromatography. System GA—RI 2793.

High Performance Liquid Chromatography. System HX—RI 672; system HY—RI 698; system HAA—Retention time 23.8 min.

Ultraviolet Spectrum. Dehydrated alcohol—240 nm (A_1^1=540a).

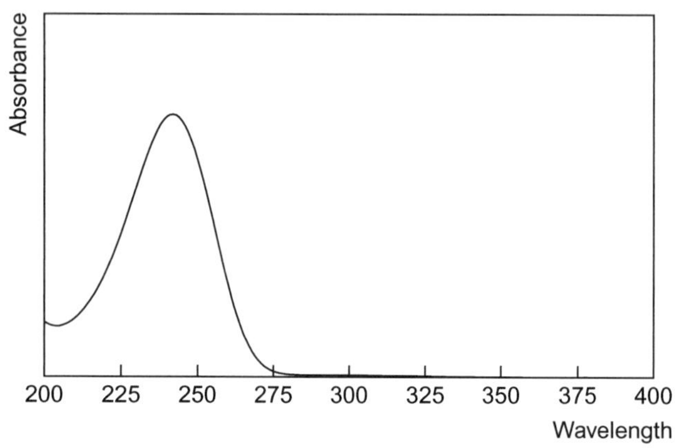

Infra-red Spectrum. Principal peaks at wavenumbers 1662, 1614, 1700, 872, 1209, 1232 cm^{-1} (KBr disk).

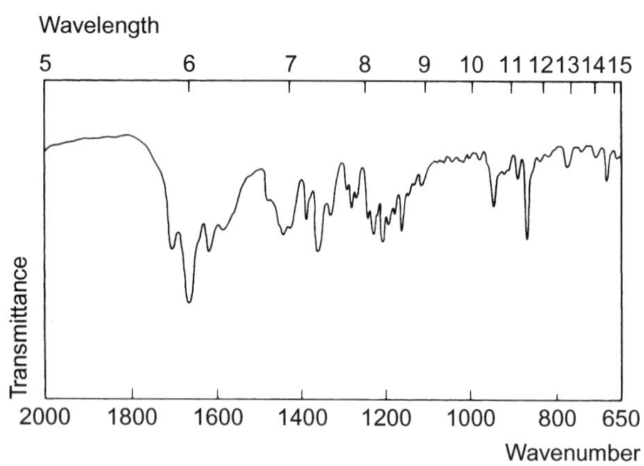

Mass Spectrum. Principal ions at *m/z* 124, 43, 314, 79, 91, 229, 272, 105.

Dose. Up to 50 mg daily by IM injection.

Proguanil

Antimalarial

Synonyms. Chloriguane; Chlorguanide; Chloroguanide; Proguanide.
N-(4-Chlorophenyl)-*N′*-(1-methylethyl)imidodicarbonimidic diamide
$C_{11}H_{16}ClN_5$=253.7
CAS—500-92-5

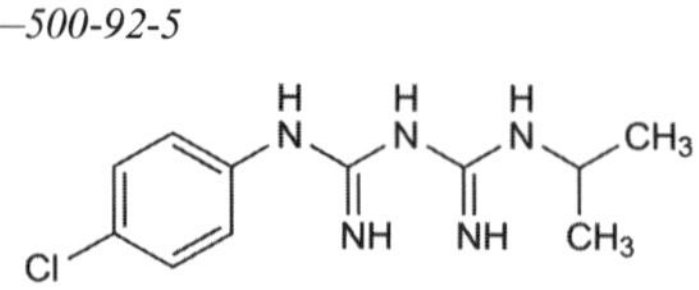

Colourless crystals. M.p. 129°.

Proguanil Hydrochloride

Synonym. Bigumalum; M-4888; RP-3359; SN-12837.
Proprietary names. Paludrine. It is an ingredient of Malarone.
$C_{11}H_{16}ClN_5,HCl$=290.2
CAS—637-32-1
A white crystalline powder. M.p. 243° to 244°.
Soluble 1 in 110 of water and 1 in 40 of ethanol; practically insoluble in chloroform and ether.

Dissociation Constant. pK_a 2.3, 10.4 (22.5°).

Partition Coefficient. Log *P* (octanol/water), 2.5.

Colour Test. To 10 mL of a saturated solution of proguanil hydrochloride add 1 drop of 10% copper sulfate solution and 2.5 mL of dilute ammonia solution and shake well; add 5 mL of toluene and shake again—toluene layer is violet-red.

Thin-layer Chromatography. System TA—Rf 03; system TB—Rf 00; system TC—Rf 01; system TE—Rf 18; system TL—Rf 01; system TAE—Rf 07; system TAF—Rf 79. (Acidified iodoplatinate solution, positive.)

High Performance Liquid Chromatography. System HX—RI 379; system HZ—Retention time 3.8 min; system HAA—Retention time 13.6 min.

Ultraviolet Spectrum. Methanol—259 nm (A_1^1=886b).

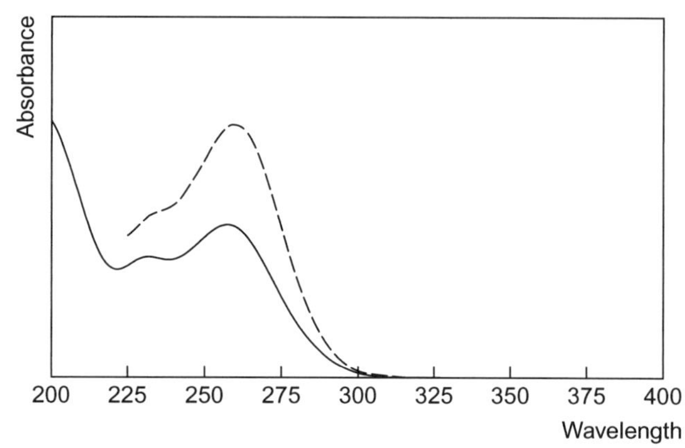

Infra-red Spectrum. Principal peaks at wavenumbers 1534, 1635, 1492, 1575, 1600, 1170 cm^{-1} (proguanil hydrochloride, KBr disk).

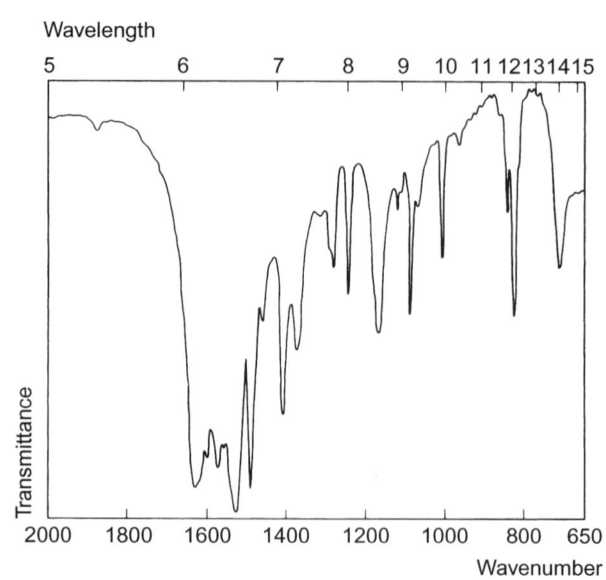

Mass Spectrum. Principal ions at *m/z* 43, 127, 195, 85, 44, 36, 152, 58.

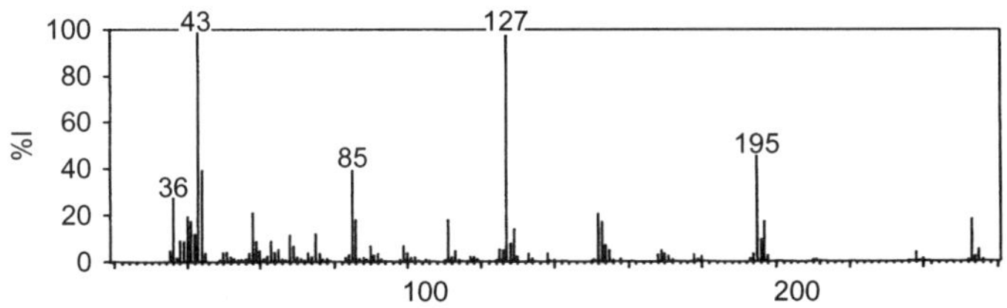

Quantification

High performance liquid chromatography. In serum: proguanil, cycloguanil and 4-chlorophenylbiguanide, limit of detection 60 µg/L, UV detection—R. R. Moody *et al.*, *J. Chromatogr.*, 1980, *182*; *B Biomed. Appl.*, *8*, 359–367. In plasma, erythrocytes, or urine: proguanil, chloroquine and their metabolites, limit of detection for proguanil 9 µg/L, UV detection—J. F. Chaulet *et al.*, *J. Pharm. Biomed. Anal.*, 1994, *12*, 111–117. In plasma or blood (dried on filter paper): proguanil, cycloguanil and 4-chlorophenylbiguanide, limit of detection for proguanil about 12 µg/L—J. A. Kolawole *et al.*, *J. Chromatogr. B Biomed. Appl.*, 1995, *674*, 149–154. In plasma or urine: proguanil, cycloguanil and 4-chlorophenylbiguanide, limits of detection 1 µg/L and 5 µg/L in plasma and urine respectively—M. Kusaka *et al.*, *Am. J. Trop. Med. Hyg.*, 1996, *54*, 189–196. In plasma, blood, or urine: limits of detection 20 nmol/L and 50 nmol/L in plasma and whole blood respectively—Y. Bergqvist *et al.*, *Ther. Drug Monit.*, 1998, *20*, 325–330. In blood (dried on sampling paper): proguanil, cycloguanil, and 4-chlorophenylbiguanide, limit of detection for proguanil 125 nmol/L—Y. Bergqvist *et al.*, *J. Chromatogr. B Biomed. Sci. Appl.*, 1998, *719*, 141–149.

Disposition in the Body. Readily absorbed after oral administration; peak plasma concentrations are attained in about 3 h. About 60% of a dose is excreted in the urine unchanged, together with about 30% as the active metabolite cycloguanil; 4-chlorophenylbiguanide is also a metabolite.

Therapeutic concentration

Six healthy subjects given proguanil 200 mg daily by mouth for 7 days, co-administered with dapsone (10 mg), had peak plasma concentrations of 151 µg/L 3.5 h after the final dose; the peak plasma concentration of cycloguanil was 55.5 µg/L after 6 h [M. D. Edstein *et al.*, *Chemotherapy*, 1990, *36*, 169–176].

Children given proguanil 100–300 mg daily by mouth (mean, 7 mg/kg daily) for 3 days after having received atovaquone (250–750 mg; mean, 17 mg/kg daily) for 3 days, had peak plasma concentrations of 306 µg/L 6 h after the final dose; the peak plasma concentration of cycloguanil was 44.3 µg/L after 6 h [A. Sabchareon *et al.*, *Trans. R. Soc. Trop. Med. Hyg.*, 1998, *92*, 201–208].

Protein binding. In plasma, about 75%.

Dose. 100 to 300 mg of proguanil hydrochloride daily.

Prolintane

Central Stimulant

1-[1-(Phenylmethyl)butyl]pyrrolidine
$C_{15}H_{23}N = 217.4$
CAS—493-92-5

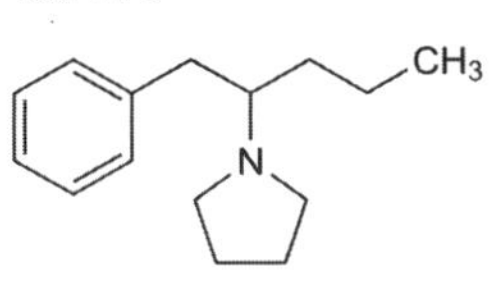

Prolintane Hydrochloride

Proprietary names. Catorid; Catovit N; Promotil. It is an ingredient of Katovit and Villescon.
$C_{15}H_{23}N,HCl = 253.8$
CAS—1211-28-5
A white powder. M.p. about 133° to 134°.
Soluble in water, ethanol and chloroform; practically insoluble in ether.

Partition Coefficient. Log *P* (octanol/water), 4.3.

Colour Tests. Liebermann's Test—red-orange; Mandelin's Test—red; Marquis Test—orange→brown.

Thin-layer Chromatography. System TA—Rf 50; system TB—Rf 67; system TC—Rf 32; system TE—Rf 79; system TL—Rf 25; system TAE—Rf 22. (Dragendorff spray, positive; acidified iodoplatinate solution, positive; Marquis reagent, orange-brown; acidified potassium permanganate solution, positive.)

Gas Chromatography. System GA—prolintane RI 1634; M (oxo-) RI 1895; M (OH-phenyl-) RI 2135, M (OH-phenyl-)-AC RI 2110, M (OH-methoxy-phenyl-)-AC RI 2115; M (oxo-OH-alkyl-) RI 2200, M (oxo-OH-alkyl-)-AC RI 2255; M (oxo-OH-methoxy-phenyl-) RI 2240, M (oxo-OH-methoxy-phenyl-)-AC RI 2360; M (oxo-di-OH-)-AC_2 RI 2485, M (oxo-di-OH-phenyl-) RI 2475, M (oxo-di-OH-phenyl-)-AC_2 RI 2450, M (oxo-OH-phenyl-)-AC RI 2275, M (oxo-di-OH-methoxy-)-AC_2 RI 2560, M (di-OH-phenyl-)-AC_2 RI 2295, M (tri-OH-)-AC_3 RI 2630, system GB—prolintane RI 1660; system GC—prolintane RI 1849.

High Performance Liquid Chromatography. System HA—*k* 2.0; system HC—*k* 1.3; system HX—RI 370.

Ultraviolet Spectrum. Aqueous acid—252, 258 nm ($A^1_1 = 8.6a$), 264 nm.

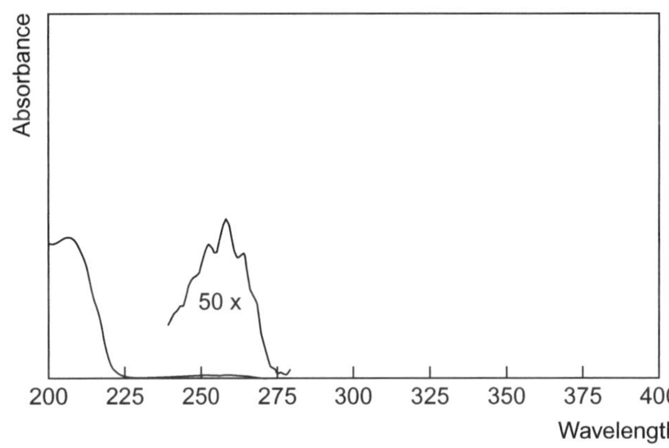

Infra-red Spectrum. Principal peaks at wavenumbers 776, 714, 752, 1501, 1141, 1020 cm^{-1} (prolintane hydrochloride, KBr disk).

Mass Spectrum. Principal ions at *m/z* 126, 127, 174, 91, 70, 69, 55, 42.

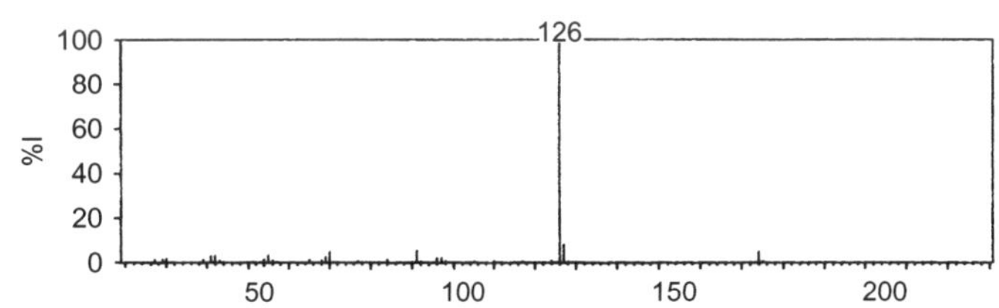

Dose. 20 mg of prolintane hydrochloride daily.

Promazine

Tranquilliser

Synonyms. RP-3276; Wy-1094; A-145.
N,N-Dimethyl-10*H*-phenothiazine-10-propanamine
$C_{17}H_{20}N_2S = 284.4$
CAS—58-40-2

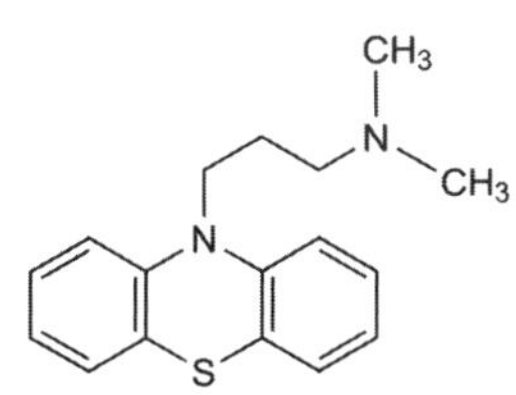

An oily liquid.

Promazine Embonate

Synonym. Promazine Pamoate
Proprietary names. Protactyl (suspension); Sparine (suspension).
$(C_{17}H_{20}N_2S)_2,C_{23}H_{16}O_6 = 957.2$

Promazine Hydrochloride

Synonym. Propazinum

Proprietary names. Liranol; Prazine; Promabec; Promanyl; Promwill; Protactyl (injection and tablets); Sparine (injection and tablets); Talofen.

$C_{17}H_{20}N_2S,HCl=320.9$

CAS—53-60-1

A white or slightly yellow, slightly hygroscopic, crystalline powder. It is affected by air and light and traces of heavy metals. Decomposed solutions may be coloured pink, red, or blue. M.p. 181°, with decomposition.

Soluble 1 in 3 of water, 1 in 2 of ethanol, and 1 in 2 of chloroform; soluble in methanol; practically insoluble in ether and benzene.

Dissociation Constant. pK_a 9.4 (25°).

Partition Coefficient. Log *P* (octanol/pH 7.4), 2.5.

Colour Tests. Formaldehyde–Sulfuric Acid—red; Forrest Reagent—red-brown; FPN Reagent—red-brown; Liebermann's Test—green-brown; Mandelin's Test—green→violet; Marquis Test—violet.

Thin-layer Chromatography. System TA—Rf 44; system TB—Rf 38; system TC—Rf 30; system TE—Rf 62; system TL—Rf 11; system TAE—Rf 18; system TAF—Rf 35; system TAJ—Rf 06; system TAK—Rf 02; system TAL—Rf 41. (Dragendorff spray, positive; FPN reagent, pink; Acidified iodoplatinate solution, positive; Marquis reagent, red; ninhydrin spray, positive.)

Gas Chromatography. System GA—Promazine RI 2315; M (nor-) RI 2405; M (sulfoxide) RI 2705; M (phenothiazine) RI 2120; M (OH-) RI 2685; system GB—promazine RI 2425; M (nor-) RI 2452; M (sulfoxide) RI 2840; M (norsulfoxide) RI 2875; M (phenothiazine) RI 2130; M (OH-) RI 2781; M (nor-OH-) RI 2797; system GF—RI 2745.

High Performance Liquid Chromatography. System HA—*k* 5.9; system HX—RI 407; system HY—RI 326; system HZ—Retention time 5.9 min.

Ultraviolet Spectrum. Aqueous acid—251 ($A_1^1=1055a$), 302; aqueous alkali—254, 306 nm.

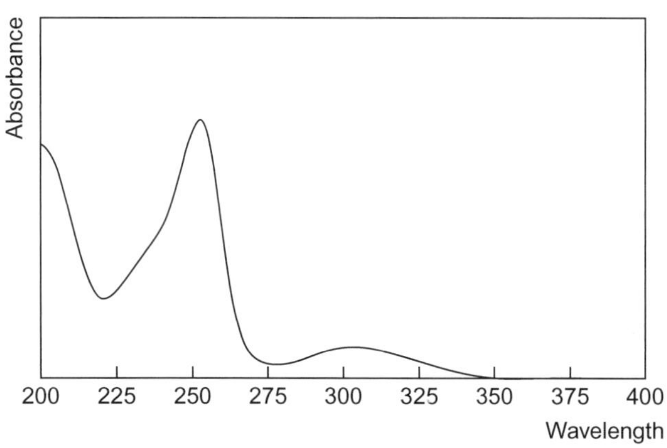

Infra-red Spectrum. Principal peaks at wavenumbers 751, 1250, 1234, 1287, 770, 1162 cm^{-1} (promazine hydrochloride, KBr disk). (See below.)

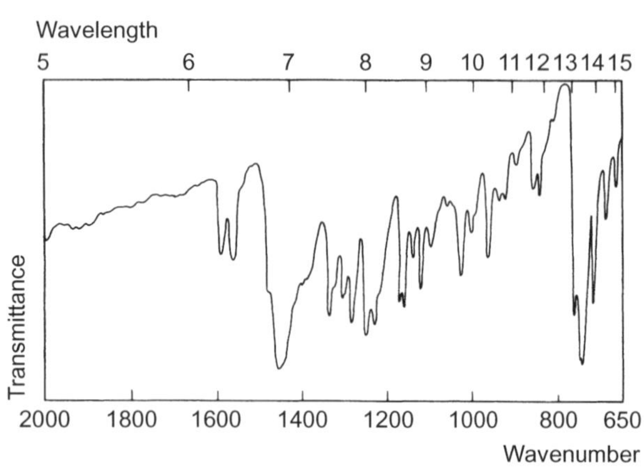

Mass Spectrum. Principal ions at *m/z* 58, 284, 86, 238, 198, 199, 85, 42.

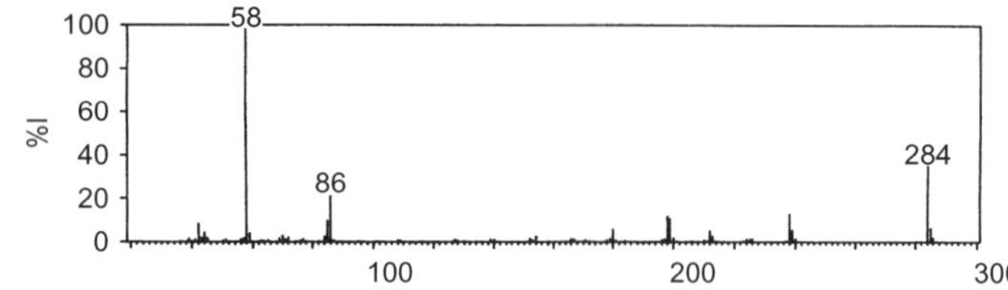

Quantification.

Gas chromatography. In blood or urine: promazine and other phenothiazines, limits of detection 250 to 500 ng/L, SID—H. Hattori *et al.*, *J. Chromatogr.*, 1992, *579*, 247–252.

High performance liquid chromatography. In plasma: electrochemical detection—V. Larsimont *et al.*, *J. Chromatogr. B Biomed. Sci. Appl.*, 1998, *719*, 222–226.

Dose. Usually up to 400 mg of promazine hydrochloride daily; maximum of 1 g daily.

Promethazine

Antihistamine

Proprietary names. Fenergan Creme; Phenergan.

N,*N*,α-Trimethyl-10*H*-phenothiazine-10-ethanamine

$C_{17}H_{20}N_2S=284.4$

CAS—60-87-7

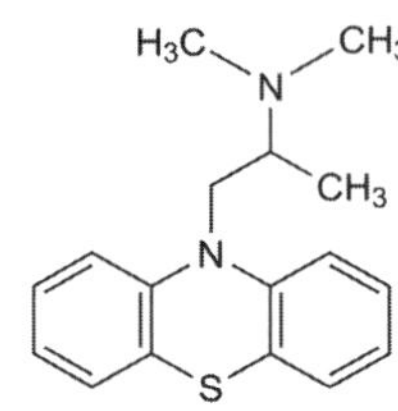

A crystalline solid. M.p. 60°.

Promethazine Hydrochloride

Synonyms. Diprazinum; Proazamine Chloride; Promethazini Hydrochloridum; Promethazinium Chloride.

Proprietary names. Anergan; Atosil; Fenergan; Histantil; Insomn-Eze; Pamergan; Phenergan; Phenhalal; Prothiazine; Q-Mazine; Sominex; Ziz. It is an ingredient of Medised, Mepergan, Night Nurse, Pamergan P100, Phensedyl Plus, and Tixylix Night-Time.

$C_{17}H_{20}N_2S,HCl=320.9$

CAS—58-33-3

A white or faintly yellow, crystalline powder, which is slowly oxidised on prolonged exposure to air, becoming blue in colour. M.p. 230° to 232° (crystals from ethylene dichloride), with some decomposition.

Soluble 1 in 0.6 of water, 1 in 9 of ethanol, and 1 in 2 of chloroform; practically insoluble in acetone, ether, and ethyl acetate.

Promethazine Teoclate

Synonyms. Promethazine Chlorotheophyllinate; Promethazine Theoclate.

Proprietary names. Avomine.

$C_{17}H_{20}N_2S,C_7H_7ClN_4O_2=499.0$

CAS—17693-51-5

A white powder.

Very slightly soluble in water; soluble 1 in 70 of ethanol and 1 in 2.5 of chloroform; practically insoluble in ether.

Dissociation Constant. pK_a 9.1 (25°).

Partition Coefficient. Log *P* (octanol/pH 7.4), 2.9.

Colour Tests. Formaldehyde–Sulfuric Acid—blue–violet; Forrest Reagent—red; FPN Reagent—orange; Mandelin's Test—green→violet; Marquis Test—violet.

Thin-layer Chromatography. System TA—Rf 50; system TB—Rf 36; system TC—Rf 35; system TE—Rf 65; system TL—Rf 17; system TAE—Rf 30; system TAF—Rf 44. (Dragendorff spray, positive; FPN reagent, positive; acidified iodoplatinate solution, positive; Marquis reagent, violet; ninhydrin spray, positive.)

Gas Chromatography. System GA—promethazine RI 2259, M (nor-) RI 2250, M (phenothiazine) RI 2020, M (sulfoxide) RI 2710, M (nor-OH-) RI 2580, M (OH-) RI 2590; system GB—promethazine RI 2383, M (nor-) RI 2333, M (phenothiazine) RI 2120, M (sulfoxide) RI 2797, M (norsulfoxide) RI 2732, M (nor-OH-) RI 2717; system GC—RI 2546; system GF—RI 2675.

High Performance Liquid Chromatography. System HA—*k* 5.0; system HX—RI 409; system HY—RI 324; system HZ—Retention time 5.7 min; system HAA—Retention time 14.5 min; system HAX—Retention time 13.2 min; system HAY—Retention time 6.4 min.

Ultraviolet Spectrum. Aqueous acid—249 (A_1^1=1032a), 298; aqueous alkali—254, 305 nm.

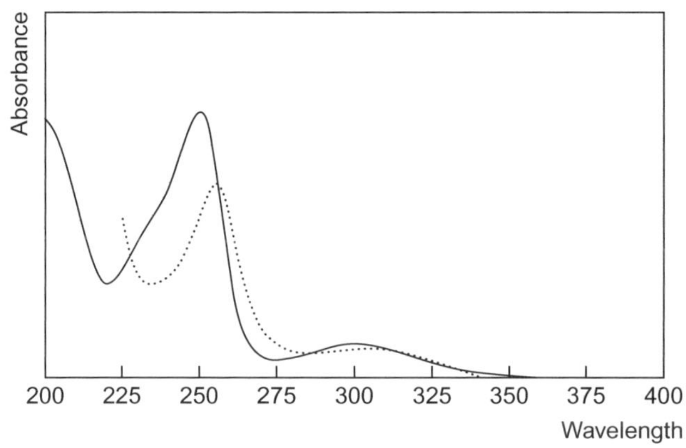

Infra-red Spectrum. Principal peaks at wavenumbers 758, 1229, 733, 1129, 1259, 1287 cm^{-1} (promethazine hydrochloride, KBr disk).

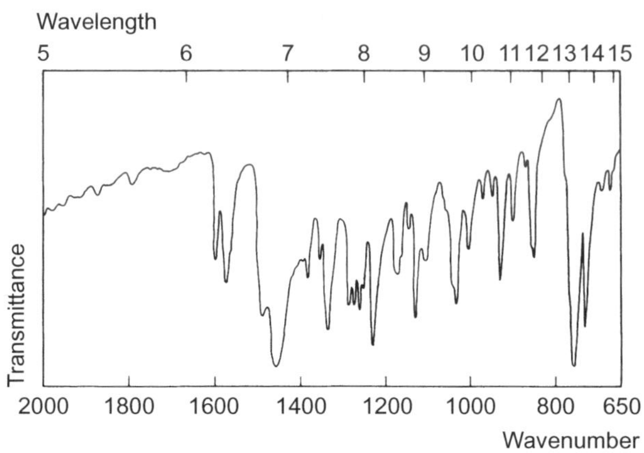

Mass Spectrum. Principal ions at *m/z* 72, 73, 284, 198, 213, 199, 180, 56; *N*-monodesmethylpromethazine (M(nor-)) 58, 213, 198, 180, 214, 57, 212, 270.

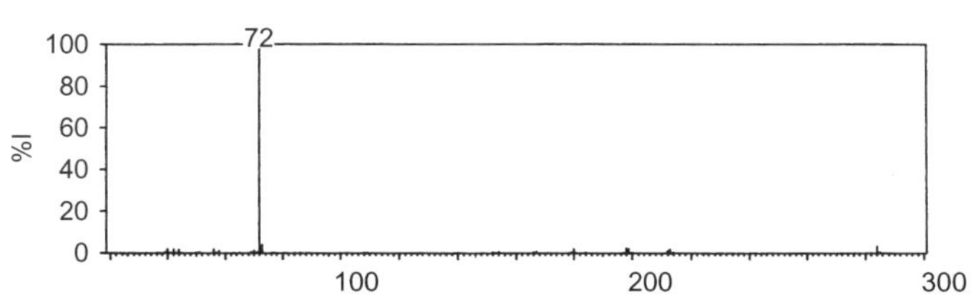

Quantification

High performance liquid chromatography. In blood: promethazine, *N*-monodesmethylpromethazine and promethazine sulfoxide, limit of detection for promethazine 200 ng/L, UV detection—G. Taylor and J. B. Houston, *J. Chromatogr.*, 1982, *230*; *B Biomed. Appl.*, *19*, 194–198. In plasma or serum: limit of detection 200 ng/L, electrochemical detection—J. E. Wallace *et al.*, *Anal. Chem.*, 1981, *53*, 960–962. In postmortem samples: promethazine and metabolites, UV detection—W. J. Allender and A. W. Archer, *J. Forensic Sci.*, 1984, *29*, 515–526. In serum: limit of quantification 0.2 µg/L, electrochemical detection—A. R. Fox and D. A. McLoughlin, *J. Chromatogr.*, 1993, *631*, 255–259. In serum: promethazine and other neuroleptics, limit of detection for promethazine 0.1 µg/L, coulometric electrochemical detection—M. Bagli *et al.*, *J. Chromatogr. B Biomed. Appl.*, 1994, *657*, 141–148. In serum: promethazine enantiomers, limit of detection 2 µg/L, UV detection—J. Liu and J. T. Stewart, *J. Pharm. Biomed. Anal.*, 1997, *16*, 303–309. In plasma: promethazine and its metabolites, limit of detection for promethazine 1 µg/L, UV detection—S. R. Vanapalli *et al.*, *J. Chromatogr. Sci.*, 2001, *39*, 70–72.

Disposition in the Body. Readily absorbed after oral administration but bioavailability is low because of extensive first-pass metabolism. About 2% of a dose is excreted in the urine unchanged. It is excreted slowly via urine and bile. The major urinary metabolite is the sulfoxide; glucuronic acid conjugation also occurs. *N*-Monodesmethylpromethazine has been detected in plasma and urine. Promethazine crosses the blood–brain and placental barriers and it is excreted in breast milk

Therapeutic concentration

Following an oral dose of 25 mg to 10 subjects, a mean peak blood concentration of 0.005 mg/L was attained in 2 h; saliva concentrations averaged 0.008 mg/L consistently from 1 to 6 h after administration. After an intramuscular dose of 25 mg to the same subjects, mean peak concentrations of 0.022 mg/L at 4 h and 0.003 mg/L at 2 h were reported for blood and saliva, respectively [G. J. DiGregorio and E. Ruch, *J. Pharm. Sci.*, 1980, *69*, 1457–1459].

Following single oral doses of 25 mg to 7 subjects, peak blood concentrations of 0.002 to 0.018 mg/L were attained in 1.5 to 3 h [G. Taylor *et al.*, *Br. J. Clin. Pharmacol.*, 1983, *15*, 287–293].

Toxicity. The estimated minimum lethal dose is 200 mg/kg.

In 2 fatalities involving the ingestion of promethazine, the following postmortem tissue concentrations were reported (mg/L or µg/g):

	Promethazine	Promethazine sulfoxide	*N*-Monodesmethyl-promethazine
Blood	5.2, 2.4	3.1, 0.8	0.8, 1.2
Bile	82.6, 11.6	23.5, 27.0	14.5, 3.0
Liver	30.6, 23.2	8.4, 5.4	6.3, 16.2
Urine	6.0, 14.0	26.0, 42.0	1.0, 3.0

Other drugs were detected in both cases [W. J. Allender and A. W. Archer, *J. Forensic Sci.*, 1984, *29*, 515–526].

Half-life. Plasma half-life, 10 to 15 h.

Volume of distribution. About 13 L/kg.

Clearance. Plasma clearance, about 16 mL/min/kg.

Distribution in blood. Plasma:whole blood ratio, 1.5.

Protein binding. In plasma, about 75 to 93%.

Dose. 20 to 100 mg of promethazine hydrochloride daily.

Prometryne

Herbicide

Synonym. Prometryn
Proprietary names. Caparol; Gesagard.
N,*N'*-Bis(1-methylethyl)-6-methylthio-1,3,5-triazine-2,4-diamine
$C_{10}H_{19}N_5S$=241.4
CAS—*7287-19-6*

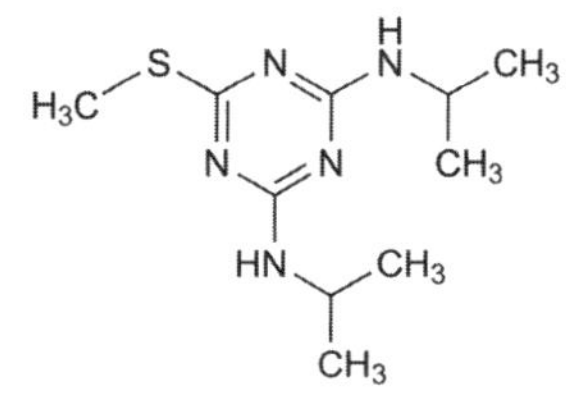

A white crystalline solid. M.p. 118° to 120°.
Practically insoluble in water; readily soluble in organic solvents.

Dissociation Constant. pK_a 4.1.

Partition Coefficient. Log *P* (octanol/water), 3.5.

Thin-layer Chromatography. System TA—Rf 76; system TX—Rf 32; system TY—Rf 31. (Dragendorff spray, positive.)

Gas Chromatography. System GA—RI 1930.

High Performance Liquid Chromatography. System HAA—Retention time 21.9 min.

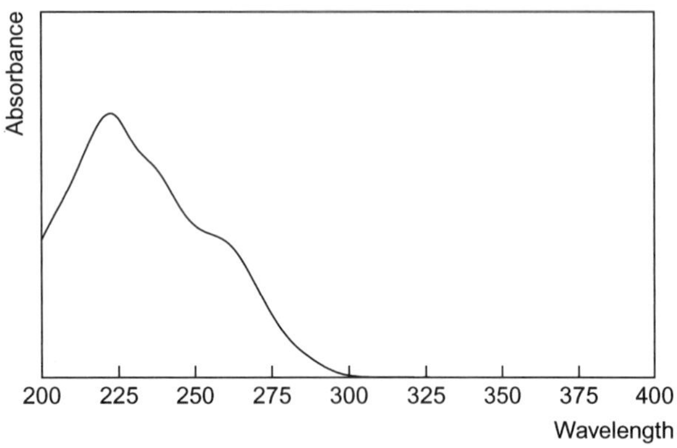

Infra-red Spectrum. Principal peaks at wavenumbers 1510, 1592, 1171, 1299, 809, 1217 cm^{-1} (KBr disk).

Propamidine

Antibacterial/Antifungal

4,4′-[1,3-Propanediylbis(oxy)]bisbenzenecarboximidamide
$C_{17}H_{20}N_4O_2$=312.4
CAS—104-32-5

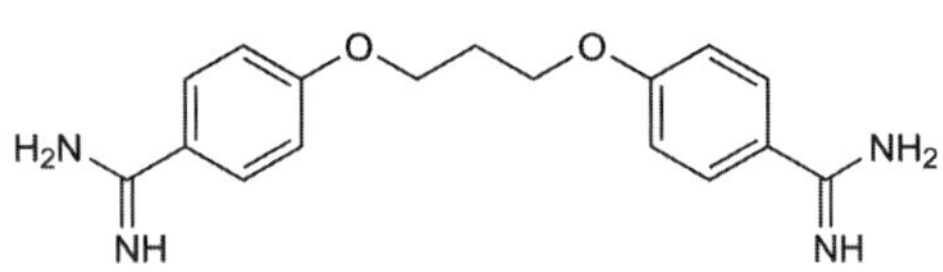

Propamidine Isetionate
Synonym. Propamidine Isethionate
Proprietary name. Brolene
$C_{17}H_{20}N_4O_2,2C_2H_6O_4S$=564.6
CAS—140-63-6
A white, granular, hygroscopic powder. M.p. 235°.
Soluble 1 in 5 of water and 1 in 33 of ethanol; practically insoluble in organic solvents.

Partition Coefficient. Log *P* (octanol/water), 1.8.

Thin-layer Chromatography. System TA—Rf 01; system TB—Rf 01; system TC—Rf 01; system TL—Rf 01. (Acidified iodoplatinate solution, positive.)

Ultraviolet Spectrum. Ethanol—267 nm (A^1_1=1224b).

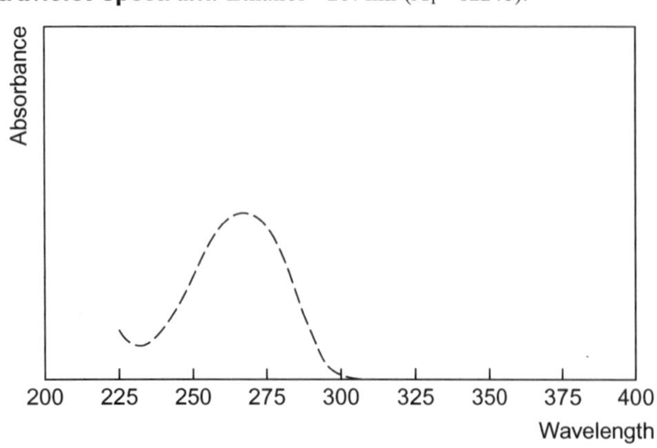

Infra-red Spectrum. Principal peaks at wavenumbers 1200, 1219, 1613, 1048, 1280, 1495 cm^{-1} (propamidine isetionate, KBr disk).

Mass Spectrum. Principal ions at *m/z* 41, 132, 102, 160, 96, 29, 27, 44.

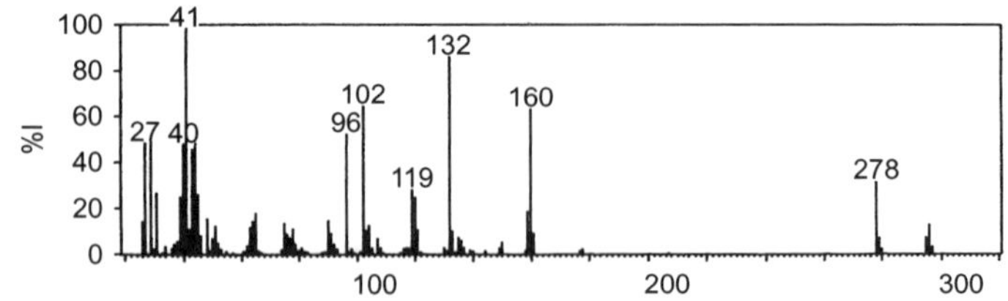

Uses. Propamidine isetionate is used in concentrations of 0.1 to 0.15%.

Propanidid

Anaesthetic (General)

Proprietary names. Epontol; Inductol; Panitol; Sombrevin.
4-[2-(Diethylamino)-2-oxoethoxyl]-3-methoxybenzeneacetic acid propyl ester
$C_{18}H_{27}NO_5$=337.4
CAS—1421-14-3

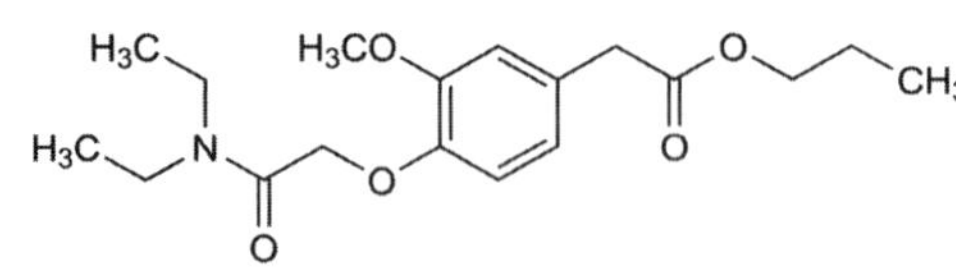

A pale greenish-yellow, hygroscopic, viscous liquid. B.p. 210° to 212°. Very slightly soluble in water; miscible with ethanol, chloroform, and ether.

Partition Coefficient. Log *P* (octanol/water), 2.4.

Colour Tests. Aromaticity (Method 2)—yellow/orange; Liebermann's Test—black.

Thin-layer Chromatography. System TA—Rf 66; system TB—Rf 20; system TC—Rf 70; system TE—Rf 72; system TL—Rf 55; system TAE—Rf 80. (Dragendorff spray, positive.)

Gas Chromatography. System GA—RI 2433.

Ultraviolet Spectrum. Ethanol—280 nm (A^1_1=82a).

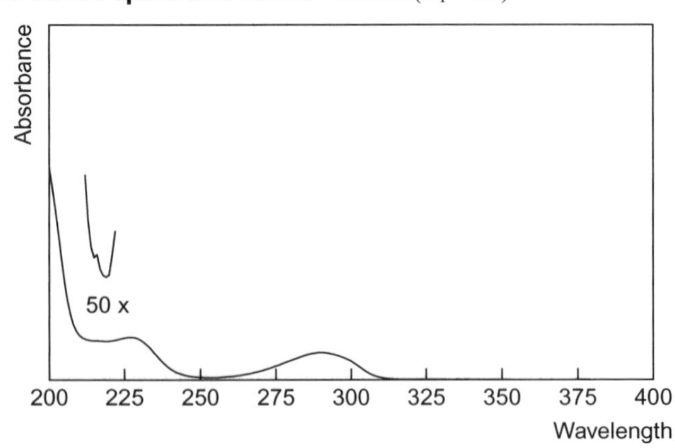

Infra-red Spectrum. Principal peaks at wavenumbers 1258, 1508, 1637, 1142, 1724, 1220 cm^{-1} (thin film).

Mass Spectrum. Principal ions at *m/z* 114, 72, 43, 100, 29, 44, 337, 86.

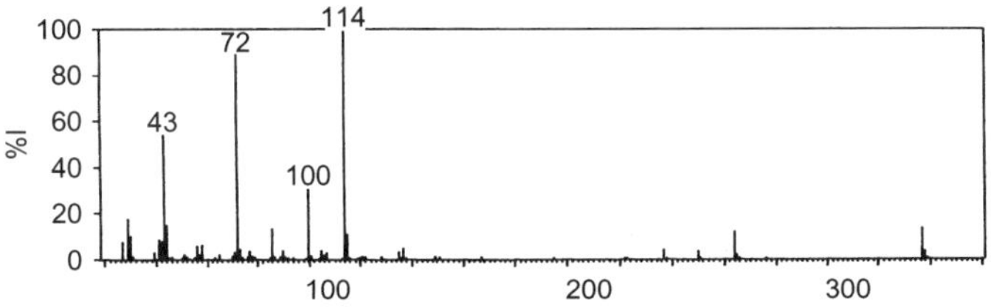

Disposition in the Body. Rapidly metabolised by hydrolysis and demethylation to inactive metabolites which are excreted in the urine. About 90% of a dose is excreted in the urine in 2 h and up to 6% is eliminated in the faeces.

Therapeutic concentration

Following IV administration of 7 mg/kg to 10 subjects, a mean serum concentration of about 14 mg/L was reported at 1 min [A. Doenicke *et al.*, *Br. J. Anaesth.*, 1968, *40*, 415–428].

Half-life. Plasma half-life, about 0.2 h.

Protein binding. In plasma, about 75%.

Dose. Usually 5 to 10 mg/kg intravenously.

Propanil

Herbicide, Nematocide

Synonyms. Bay 30130; Cekupropanil; DCPA; DPA; FW-734; S10145.
Proprietary names. Arrosol; ChemRice; Dropaven; Erban; Herbax; Propanex; Riselect; Rogue; Stam; Stampede; Strel; Surcopur; Surpur; Vertac.
N-(3,4-Dichlorophenyl)propanamide
$C_9H_9Cl_2NO = 218.1$
CAS—709-98-8

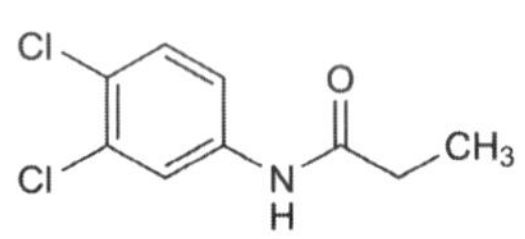

A white crystalline solid with M.p. 91° to 93° (the technical state is brownish in colour). It is soluble in water (19.73 mg/L at 25°), toluene, isopropanol and xylene, and very soluble in benzene (70 g/L at 25°), ethanol (1100 g/L at 25°), acetone (1700 g/L at 25°), cyclohexane (350 g/L at 20°) and methyl ethyl ketone (250 g/L at 20°).

Partition Coefficient. Log *P* (octanol/water), 3.07.

Gas Chromatography. System GK—RRT 0.94 (relative to caffeine).

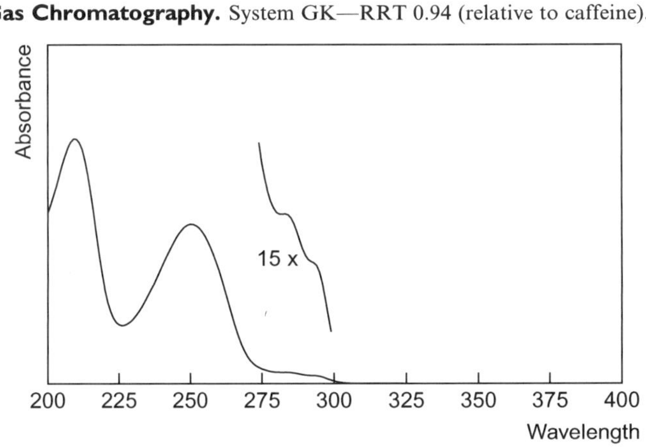

Infra-red Spectrum. Principal peaks at wavenumbers 1729, 1282, 1590, 1136 cm^{-1}.

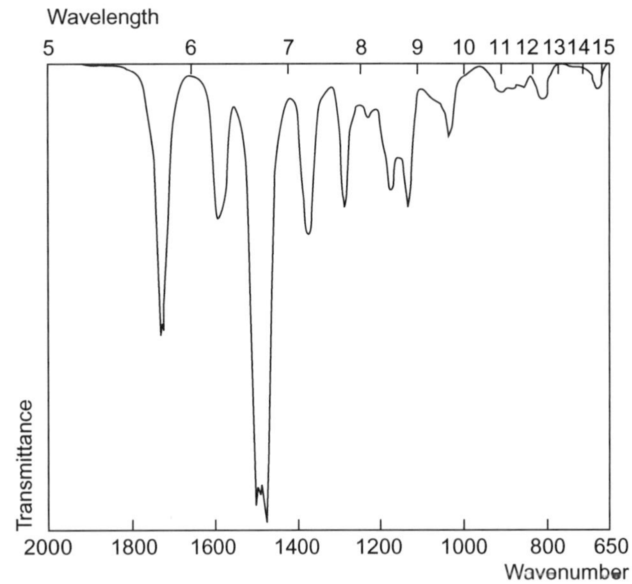

Mass Spectrum. Principal ions at *m/z* 161, 57, 163, 217, 219, 63, 165, 90.

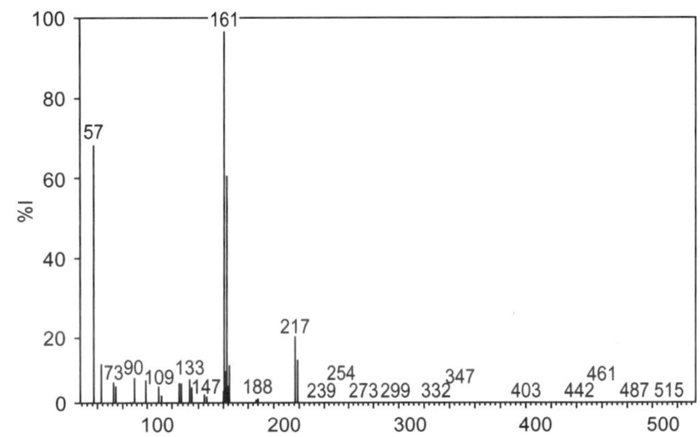

Disposition in the Body. Propanil is absorbed into the bloodstream after ingestion and metabolised in the liver to aniline derivatives: 3,4-dichloroaniline and *N*-hydroxy-3,4-dichloroaniline. Metabolism is responsible for the formation of methaemoglobin. Propanil is lipid/fat soluble. It is recovered in faeces and urine.

Propanol

Solvent

Synonyms. Normal Propyl Alcohol; Primary Propyl Alcohol; Propyl Alcohol.
Proprietary name. Satinazid
Propan-1-ol
$C_3H_7OH = 60.1.$
CAS—71-23-8

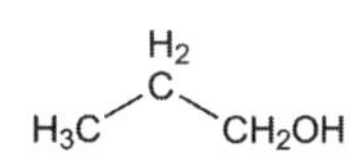

A clear, colourless, flammable liquid. Wt per mL about 0.804 g. B.p. about 96°.
Miscible with water, ethanol, chloroform, and ether.

Dissociation Constant. pK_a 16.1.

Partition Coefficient. Log *P* (octanol/water), 0.3.

Colour Test. Potassium Dichromate (Method 2)—green.

Gas Chromatography. System GA—RI 571; system GI—Retention time 5.5 min.

Mass Spectrum. Principal ions at *m/z* 31, 59, 42, 60, 27, 29, 45, 41.

Propantheline Bromide

Anticholinergic

Proprietary names. Bropantil; Ercoril; Ercotina; Pantheline; Pro-Banthine; Propantel; Propanthel.
N-Methyl-*N*-(1-methylethyl)-*N*-[2-[(9*H*-xanthen-9-ylcarbonyl)oxy] ethyl]-2-propanaminium bromide
$C_{23}H_{30}BrNO_3$=448.4
CAS—298-50-0 (propantheline); 50-34-0 (bromide)

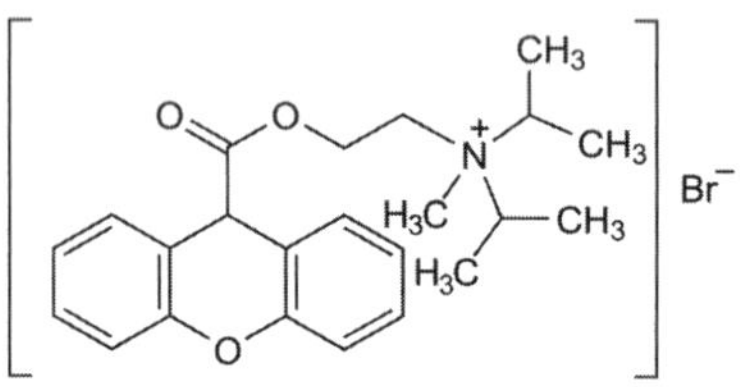

A white or yellowish-white powder. M.p. 159° to 160°.
Very soluble in water, ethanol, and chloroform; practically insoluble in ether and benzene.

Note. The dust is irritant to mucous membranes.

Partition Coefficient. Log *P* (octanol/water), 2.5.

Colour Tests. The following tests are performed on the nitrate: Mandelin's Test—orange; Marquis Test—orange.

Thin-layer Chromatography. System TA—propantheline bromide Rf 04; system TB—propantheline bromide Rf 00; system TC—propantheline bromide Rf 04; system TE—propantheline bromide Rf 04; xanthanoic acid Rf 05; system TF—xanthanoic acid Rf 08; system TL—Rf 00; system TAE—propantheline bromide Rf 03; xanthanoic acid Rf 87; system TAF—propantheline bromide Rf 31; system TAJ—Rf 00; system TAK—Rf 00; system TAL—Rf 20. (Acidified iodoplatinate solution, positive.)

Gas Chromatography. System GA—Not eluted.

High Performance Liquid Chromatography. System HA—k 4.4; system HX—RI 454 (propantheline bromide); RI 499 (xanthanoic acid).

Ultraviolet Spectrum. Aqueous acid—243 (A_1^1=103a), 281 nm; aqueous alkali—249, 282 nm.

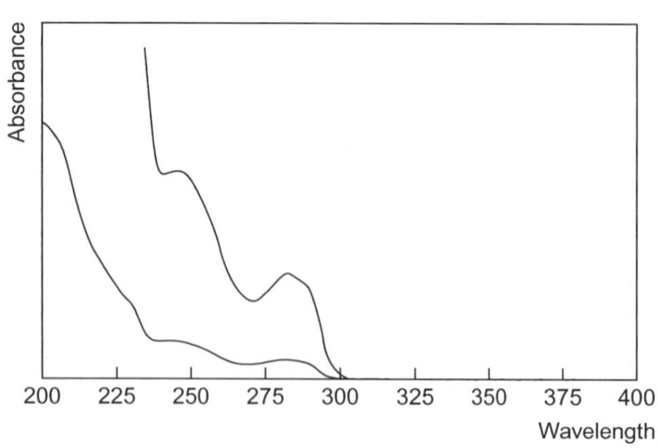

Infra-red Spectrum. Principal peaks at wavenumbers 1255, 761, 1208, 1733, 745, 1158 cm^{-1} (KBr disk).

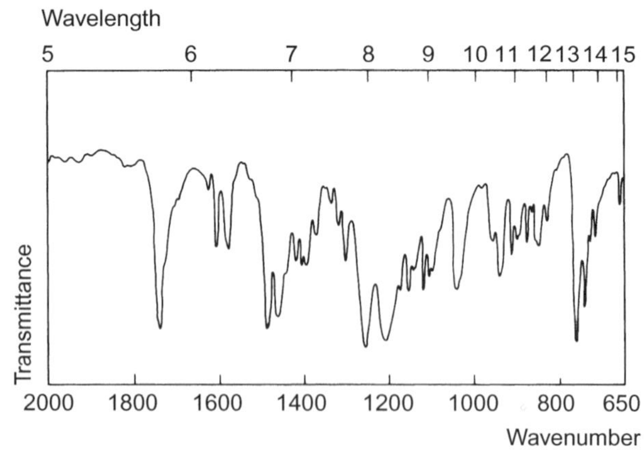

Mass Spectrum. Principal ions at *m/z* 86, 181, 43, 44, 41, 114, 42, 152 (propantheline).

Quantification

Gas chromatography–mass spectrometry. In plasma or urine: limit of detection 5 µg/L and 10 µg/L respectively—G. C. Ford *et al.*, *Biomed. Mass Spectrom.*, 1977, *4*, 94–97.

Mass spectrometry. In urine: propantheline bromide and other quaternary ammonium compounds, limits of detection 20 to 150 µg/L—M. Nisikawa *et al.*, *Forensic Sci. Int.*, 1991, *51*, 131–138.

High performance liquid chromatography. In serum: limit of detection 2 µg/L, UV detection—D. K. Moses *et al.*, *Br. J. Clin. Pharmacol.*, 1983, *16*, 758–759.

Disposition in the Body. Poorly absorbed after oral administration due to decomposition in the small intestine. It undergoes extensive metabolism mainly by hydrolysis and glucuronide conjugation; aromatic hydroxylation also occurs. About 50 to 65% of an oral dose is excreted in the urine in 24 h with less than 10% as unchanged drug. The major urinary metabolite is xanthanoic acid glucuronide conjugate; other metabolites include free xanthanoic acid, hydroxyxanthanoic acid, propantheline, and hydroxypropantheline.

Therapeutic concentration. Following single oral doses of 30 mg and 60 mg to 6 subjects, peak plasma concentrations of 0.0 to 0.038 mg/L (mean 0.024) and 0.033 to 0.162 mg/L (mean 0.06), respectively, were attained in about 0.5 to 1 h [C. W. Vose *et al.*, *Eur. J. Drug Metab. Pharmacokinet.*, 1980, *5*, 29–34].

Half-life. Plasma half-life, 1 to 3 h.

Clearance. Plasma clearance, about 20 mL/min/kg.

Dose. Usually 75 mg daily; maximum of 120 mg daily.

Propazine

Herbicide

Synonyms. G-30028; Geigy 30028.
Proprietary names. Gesamil; Milocep; Milogard; Milo-Pro; Plantulin; Primatol P; Propazin; Propinex; Prozinex.
6-Chloro-*N*,*N*′-bis(1-methylethyl)-1,3,5-triazine-2,4-diamine
$C_9H_{16}ClN_5$=229.7
CAS—139-40-2

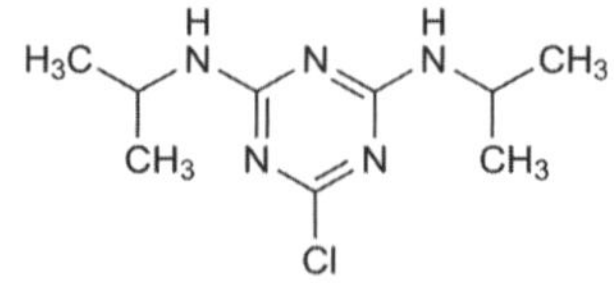

A colourless crystalline solid. M.p. 213°. It is practically insoluble in water (5 mg/L at 20°, 8.6 mg/L at 22°). It is slightly soluble in benzene (6.2 g/kg at 20°), diethyl ether (5.0 g/kg at 20°), carbon tetrachloride (2.5 g/kg at 20°) and toluene (6.2 g/kg at 20°).

Dissociation Constant. pK_a 1.7 (21°).

Partition Coefficient. Log *P* (octanol/water), 2.93.

Gas Chromatography. System GA—RI 1738.

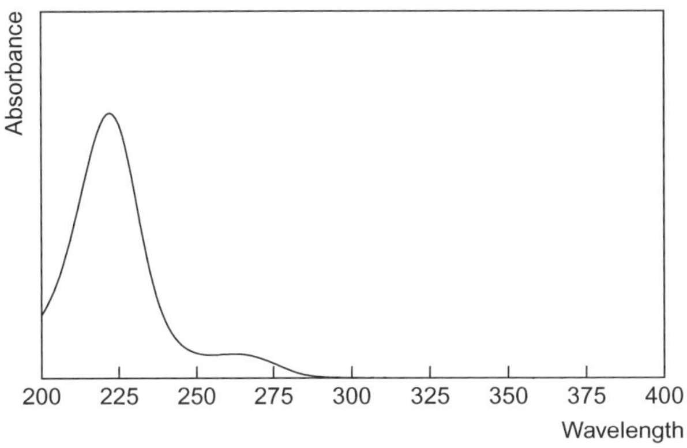

Infra-red Spectrum. Principal peaks at wavenumbers 1571, 1496, 1173, 1323 cm^{-1}.

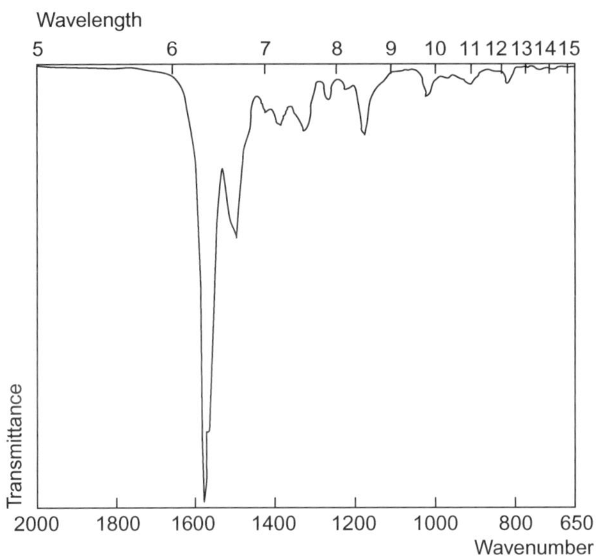

Mass Spectrum. Principal ions at *m/z* 58, 214, 229, 43, 172, 187, 216, 69.

Disposition in the Body. Propazine is readily absorbed into the bloodstream after ingestion and metabolised in the body. It is excreted in both urine (approx. 65%) and faeces (25%).

Toxicity. Slightly toxic by ingestion.

Propicillin

Antibacterial

Synonym. α-Phenoxypropylpenicillin
(2*S*,5*R*,6*R*)-3,3-Dimethyl-7-oxo-6-[(1-oxo-2-phenoxybutyl)amino]-4-thia-1-azabicyclo[3.2.0]heptane-2-carboxylic acid
$C_{18}H_{22}N_2O_5S$=378.4
CAS—551-27-9

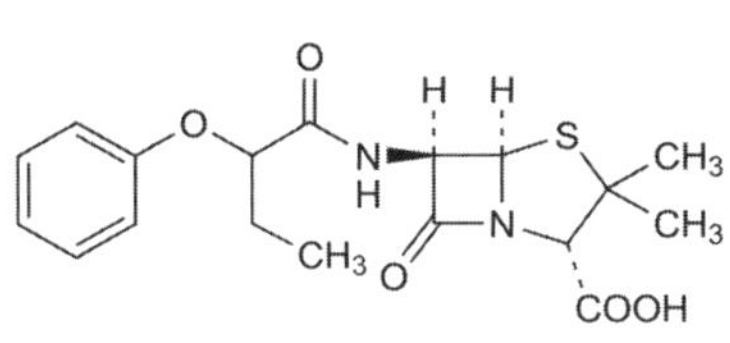

Propicillin Potassium

Synonym. Potassium α-Phenoxypropylpenicillin; BRL-284; PA-248.
Proprietary names. Baycillin; Oricillin; Propibay; Ultrapen.
$C_{18}H_{21}KN_2O_5S$=416.5
CAS—1245-44-9
A white, hygroscopic, finely crystalline powder. M.p. 195° to 197°, with decomposition.
Soluble 1 in about 1 of water, 1 in about 25 of ethanol, and 1 in 65 of dehydrated alcohol; practically insoluble in chloroform and ether.

Dissociation Constant. pK_a 2.7 (25°).

Partition Coefficient. Log *P* (octanol/water), 2.6.

Ultraviolet Spectrum. Propicillin potassium: water—269 (A^1_1=27b), 276 nm (A^1_1=21.5b).

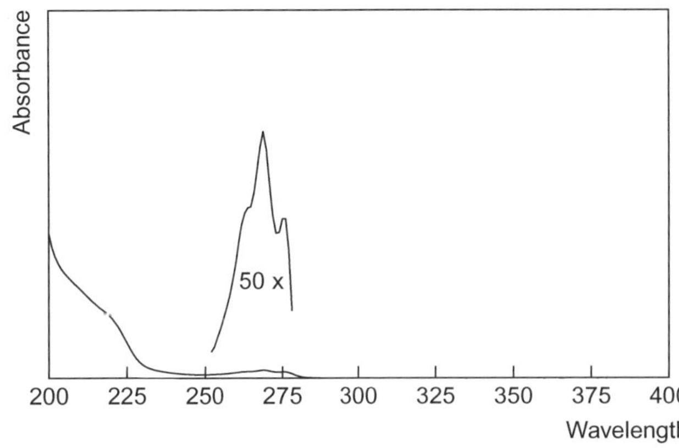

Infra-red Spectrum. Principal peaks at wavenumbers 1600, 1757, 1669, 1224, 1314, 750 cm^{-1} (propicillin potassium, KBr disk).

Dose. The equivalent of 0.5 to 1.5 g of propicillin daily.

Propiomazine

Antihistamine/Sedative

Synonym. Wy-1359
1-[10-[2-(Dimethylamino)propyl]-10*H*-phenothiazin-2-yl]-1-propanone
$C_{20}H_{24}N_2OS$=340.5
CAS—362-29-8

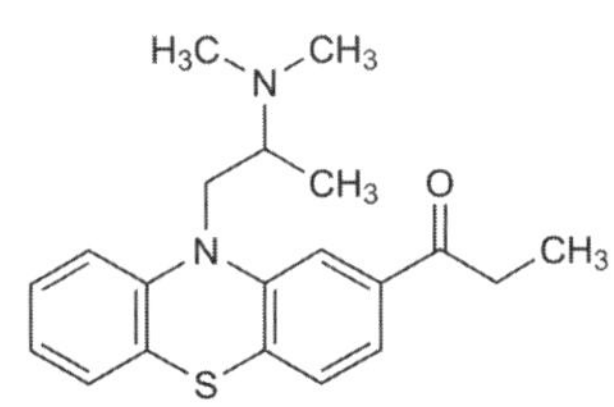

Propiomazine Hydrochloride

Proprietary name. Largon
$C_{20}H_{24}N_2OS,HCl$=376.9
CAS—1240-15-9
A yellow powder.
Soluble 1 in less than 1 of water, 1 in 6 of ethanol, and 1 in 2 of chloroform; practically insoluble in ether and benzene.

Propiomazine Maleate

Synonym. Propiomazine Hydrogen Maleate
Proprietary name. Propavan
$C_{20}H_{24}N_2OS,C_4H_4O_4$=456.6
CAS—3568-23-8
A yellow microcrystalline powder. M.p. 160° to 161° (from propan-2-ol).
Soluble 1 in 500 of water, 1 in 60 of ethanol, and 1 in 140 of dehydrated alcohol.

Dissociation Constant. pK_a 6.6.

Partition Coefficient. Log *P* (octanol/water), 4.8.

Colour Tests. Formaldehyde–Sulfuric Acid—blue–violet; Forrest Reagent—red; FPN Reagent—pink–orange→red→fades; Liebermann's Test—violet; Mandelin's Test—violet; Marquis Test—red–violet.

Thin-layer Chromatography. System TA—Rf 55; system TB—Rf 34; system TC—Rf 42; system TE—Rf 68; system TL—Rf 26; system TAE—

Rf 30; system TAF—Rf 52; system TAJ—Rf 34; system TAK—Rf 16; system TAL—Rf 81. (Location under UV light, pink fluorescence; Dragendorff spray, positive; FPN reagent, yellow; acidified iodoplatinate solution, positive; Marquis reagent, red.)

Gas Chromatography. System GA—RI 2738; system GF—RI 3225.

High Performance Liquid Chromatography. System HA—*k* 2.1; system HX—RI 440; system HY—RI 359; system HAX—Retention time 14.1 min; system HAY—Retention time 7.1 min.

Ultraviolet Spectrum. Aqueous acid—241 (A_1^1=749a), 273, 360; aqueous alkali—243, 283 nm.

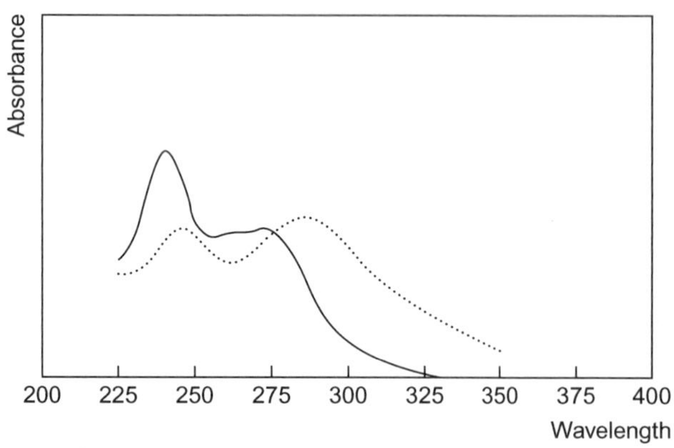

Infra-red Spectrum. Principal peaks at wavenumbers 754, 1653, 1221, 1186, 1575, 1316 cm^{-1} (propiomazine hydrochloride, KBr disk). (See below)

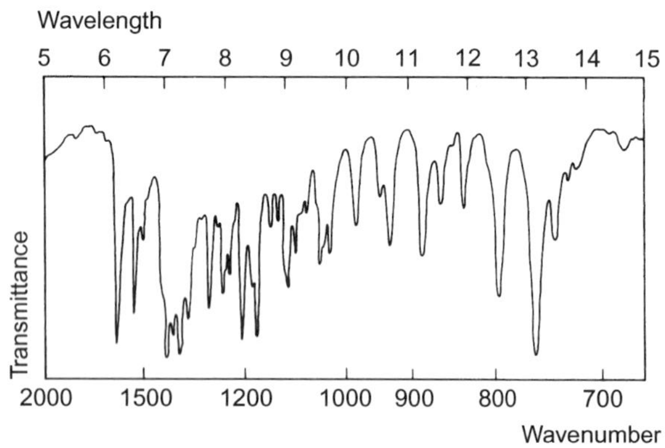

Mass Spectrum. Principal ions at *m*/*z* 72, 73, 340, 269, 197, 71, 70, 56.

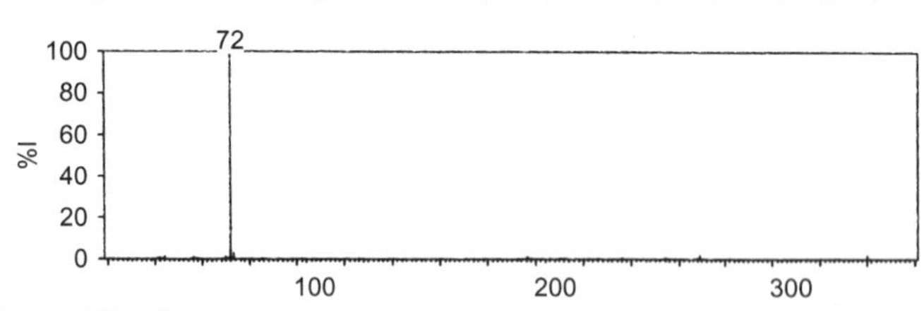

Quantification

Gas chromatography. In plasma: propiomazine and *N*-monodesmethylpropiomazine, limit of detection 10 to 20 µg/L, AFID—P. Hartvig *et al.*, *J. Chromatogr.*, 1980, *183*; *B Biomed. Appl.*, *9*, 229–233.

Disposition in the Body. Slowly absorbed after oral administration. Metabolised by *N*-demethylation.

Therapeutic concentration

After a single oral dose of 50 mg to one subject, a peak serum concentration of about 0.05 mg/L was attained in 2 to 3 h. In several subjects, low concentrations (<0.01 mg/L) of *N*-monodesmethylpropiomazine were also observed [P. Hartvig *et al.*, *Curr. Ther. Res.*, 1981, *29*, 351–362].

Bioavailability. About 33%.

Half-life. Plasma half-life, 2 to 15 h (mean 9).

Volume of distribution. About 2 to 3 L/kg.

Clearance. Plasma clearance, 3 to 10 mL/min/kg (mean 5).

Dose. The equivalent of 25 to 50 mg of propiomazine daily, by mouth.

Propofol

Anaesthetic

Synonyms. ICI-35868; Disoprofol.
Proprietary names. Ansiven; Diprivan; Disoprivan; Rapinovet.
2,6-Bis(1-methylethyl)phenol
$C_{12}H_{18}O$=178.3
CAS—2078-54-8

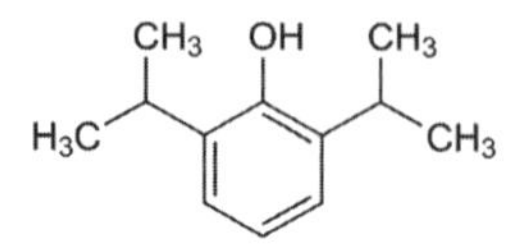

M.p. 19°. It is very slightly soluble in water.

Dissociation Constant. pK_a 11.1.

Partition Coefficient. Log *P* (octanol/water), 3.79.

High Performance Liquid Chromatography. System HZ—retention time 35.0 min; system HAX—retention time 10.1 min; system HAY—retention time 15.2 min.

Ultraviolet Spectrum. Aqueous acid—271 nm; basic—240, 291 nm.

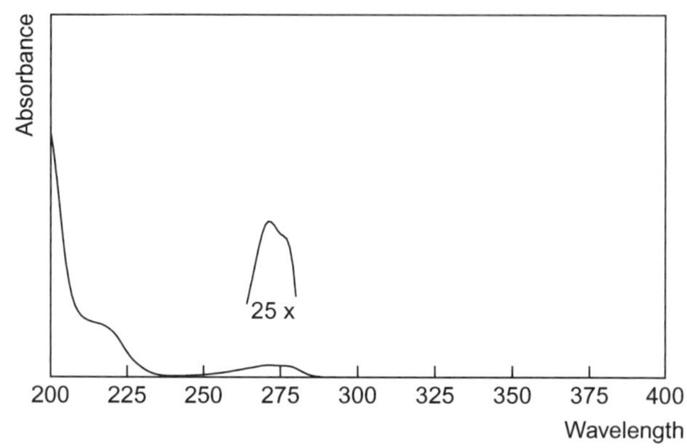

Infra-red Spectrum. Principal peaks at wavenumbers 1461, 1202, 748 cm^{-1} (KBr disk).

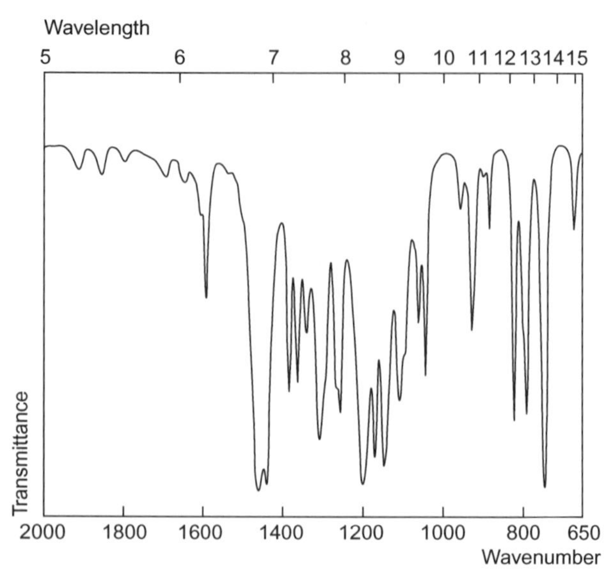

Mass Spectrum. Principal ions at *m*/*z* 163, 178, 91, 117, 41, 164, 77, 121 (propofol); *m*/*z* 235, 73, 250, 207, 161, 115, 128, 177 (TMS (tetramethylsilane) derivative).

Quantification

Gas chromatography–mass spectrometry. In plasma: limit of detection 0.02 µg/L—P. L. Stetson *et al.*, *J. Chromatogr.*, 1993, *620*; *Biomed. Appl.*, 260–267.

High performance liquid chromatography. In serum: limit of detection 0.1 mg/L. UV detection (λ=270 nm)—I. Pavan *et al.*, *J. Chromatogr. Sci.*, 1992, *30(5)*, 164–166. In serum: limit of detection 0.08 mg/L. Coulometric detection—R. A. Uebel *et al.*, *J. Chromatogr.*, 1990, *526*, 293–295. In blood: limit of detection 0.02 mg/L. Electrochemical detection—G. Mazzi and M. Schinella, *J. Chromatogr.*, 1990, *528*, 537–541.

Disposition in the Body. Propofol is rapidly absorbed and distributed from circulation into the tissues. Extensive tissue distribution occurs. It has a two-phase distribution, with the second phase being the slower phase when significant hepatic metabolism (conjugation) takes place before excretion via urine. Inactive conjugates of propofol are formed and its corresponding quinol. Also detected in urine is the unchanged drug, propofol glucuronide, 1-glucuronide, 4-glucuronide and the 4-sulfate conjugates of 2,6-diisopropyl 1,4-quinol. Approx. 2% of a dose is excreted in faeces. Propofol crosses the placental barrier and is also excreted in breast milk. It is extensively distributed and rapidly cleared from the body.

Therapeutic concentration. Sedation can be maintained at serum concentrations of 0.001 to 0.004 mg/L.

7 male patients, 38 to 67 years old, admitted for oral or neck surgery, were administered a dose between 403 and 1800 mg to reach a state of anaesthesia. Doses were administered at a maintenance infusion rate of 3.5 and 6.1 mg/kg lean body mass/h and after 15 min of infusion, blood concentrations were relatively stable ranging between 1.5 and 2.5 mg/L. [D. J. Morgan *et al.*, *Br. J. Clin. Pharmacol.*, 1990, *30*, 144–148].

Toxicity. The toxic blood concentration is 0.22 mg/L, as noted from abuse.

A 29-year-old female committed suicide by IV injection of 400 mg propofol. Postmortem concentrations were 0.22 mg/L in femoral blood and 1.4 mg/kg in liver. [O. H. Drummer, *J. Forensic Sci.*, 1992, *37*, 1186–1189].

Half-life. 2 to 4 min (first phase); 30 to 60 min (second phase); 3 to 12 h (terminal half-life).

Volume of distribution. Steady state, 171 to 349 L; elimination, 209 to 1008 L. Also reported as 2 to 12 L/kg and 60 L/kg.

Clearance. Total, 94 to 139 L/h.

Protein binding. >95% (haemoglobin, erythrocytes and other serum proteins); hypoalbuminaemia may increase free fraction.

Dose. Adults: Induction of anaesthesia: 1.5 to 2.5 mg/kg. Maintenance of anaesthesia: 25 to 50 mg repeated according to response, or 4 to 12 mg/kg/h. Children >3 years: 9 to 15 mg/kg/h. Sedation: 0.3 to 4.5 mg/kg/h.

Propoxycaine

Anaesthetic (local)

4-Amino-2-propoxybenzoic acid 2-diethylaminoethyl ester
$C_{16}H_{26}N_2O_3$=294.4
CAS—86-43-1

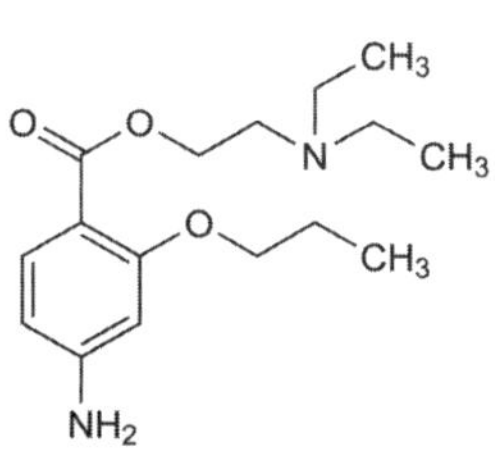

Propoxycaine Hydrochloride

Proprietary names. It is an ingredient of Ravocaine and Novocain.
$C_{16}H_{26}N_2O_3$,HCl=330.9
CAS—550-83-4
A white crystalline powder which discolours on prolonged exposure to light and air. M.p. 148° to 150°.
Soluble 1 in 2 of water, 1 in 10 of ethanol, and 1 in 80 of ether; practically insoluble in acetone and chloroform.

Dissociation Constant. pK_a 8.6.

Partition Coefficient. Log *P* (octanol/water), 1.5.

Colour Tests. Coniferyl Alcohol—orange; Diazotisation—red; Mandelin's Test—brown.

Thin-layer Chromatography. System TA—Rf 58; system TB—Rf 03; system TC—Rf 33; system TL—Rf 28; system TAJ—Rf 11; system TAK—Rf 00; system TAL—Rf 45. (Acidified iodoplatinate solution, positive.)

Gas Chromatography. System GA—RI 2335.

High Performance Liquid Chromatography. System HQ—*k* 1.1.

Ultraviolet Spectrum. Aqueous acid—235 (A^1_1=270b), 298 nm.

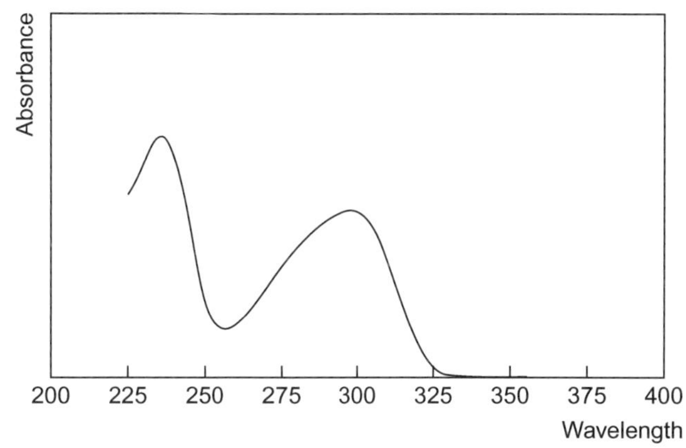

Infra-red Spectrum. Principal peaks at wavenumbers 1605, 1278, 1246, 1670, 1210, 1700 cm^{-1} (KBr disk).

Mass Spectrum. Principal ions at *m/z* 86, 99, 136, 30, 58, 178, 87, 71.

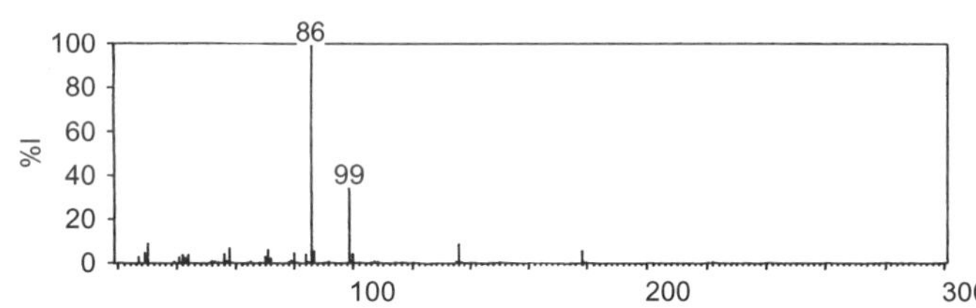

Uses. Propoxycaine hydrochloride has been used as a 0.5% solution.

Propranolol

Beta-adrenoceptor Blocking Agent

1-[(1-Methylethyl)amino]-3-(1-naphthalenyloxy)-2-propanol
$C_{16}H_{21}NO_2$=259.3
CAS—525-66-6; 13013-17-7 (±)

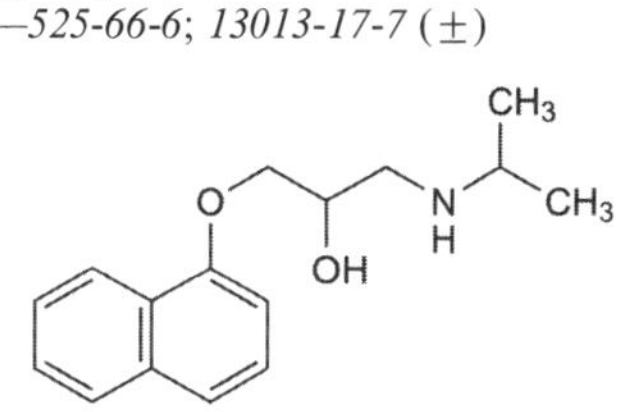

Crystals. M.p. 96° (from cyclohexane).

Propranolol Hydrochloride

Synonyms. AY-64043; ICI-45520; NSC-91523; Propranololi Hydrochloridum.
Proprietary names. Adrexan; Angilol; Apsolol; Avlocardyl; Bedranol; Berkolol; Betachron; Beta-Prograne; Betadur CR; Cardinol; Dociton; Efektolol; Elbrol; Half Beta-Prograne; Half Betadur; Half Inderal; Indobloc; Hemipralon; Inderal; Lopranol LA; Obsidan; Probeta LA; Propabloc; Propanix; Prophylux; Proprnur; Syprol; Tiperal. It is an ingredient of Inderetic, Inderex, and Inderide.
$C_{16}H_{21}NO_2$,HCl=295.8
CAS—318-98-9; 3506-09-0 (±)
A white powder. M.p. 163° to 164° (crystals from *n*-propanol).

Soluble 1 in 20 of water and ethanol; slightly soluble in chloroform; practically insoluble in ether, benzene, and ethyl acetate.

Dissociation Constant. pK_a 9.5 (24°).

Partition Coefficient. Log *P* (octanol/pH 7.4), 1.2.

Colour Tests. Mandelin's Test—green; Marquis Test—green.

Thin-layer Chromatography. System TA—Rf 50; system TB—Rf 06; system TC—Rf 10; system TE—Rf 49; system TL—Rf 07; system TAE—Rf 21; system TAF—Rf 79; system TAJ—Rf 00; system TAK—Rf 05; system TAL—Rf 49. (Acidified iodoplatinate solution, positive.)

Gas Chromatography. System GA—propranolol RI 2147, M (1-naphthol-) RI 1505, M (desamino-OH-) RI 2065; system GB—propranolol RI 2234, M (4-OH-) RI 2546, M (1-naphthol-) RI 1534.

High Performance Liquid Chromatography. System HA—propranolol *k* 1.3, 4-hydroxypropranolol *k* 1.1; system HX—RI 377; system HY—RI 299; system HZ—Retention time 3.7 min; system HAA—Retention time 13.1 min; system HAM—not detected; system HAV—*k* 2.3; system HAX—Retention time 9.2 min; system HAY—Retention time 4.9 min.

Ultraviolet Spectrum. Aqueous acid—288 (A^1_1=222 a), 305, 319; methanol—290 (A^1_1=240 a), 306 (A^1_1=143 a), 319 nm (A^1_1=86 a). No alkaline shift.

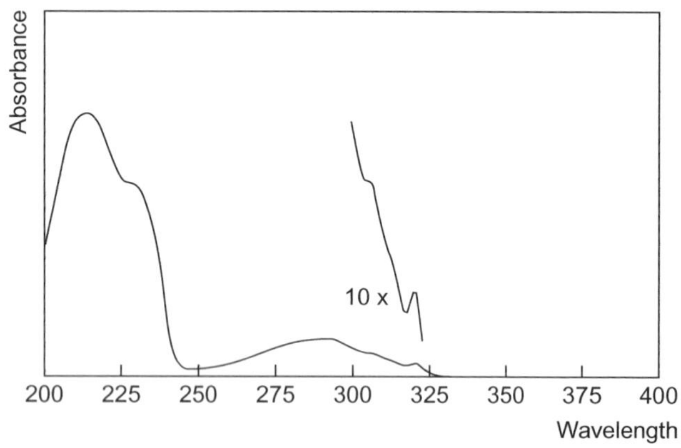

Infra-red Spectrum. Principal peaks at wavenumbers 1103, 1270, 772, 1580, 795, 1240 cm^{-1} (propranolol hydrochloride, KBr disk).

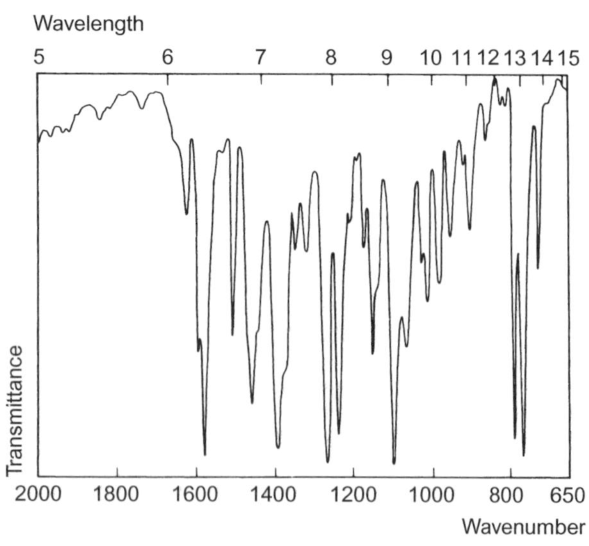

Mass Spectrum. Principal ions at *m/z* 72, 56, 30, 43, 98, 115, 144, 41; 4-hydroxypropranolol 72, 30, 116, 56, 43, 160, 41, 158.

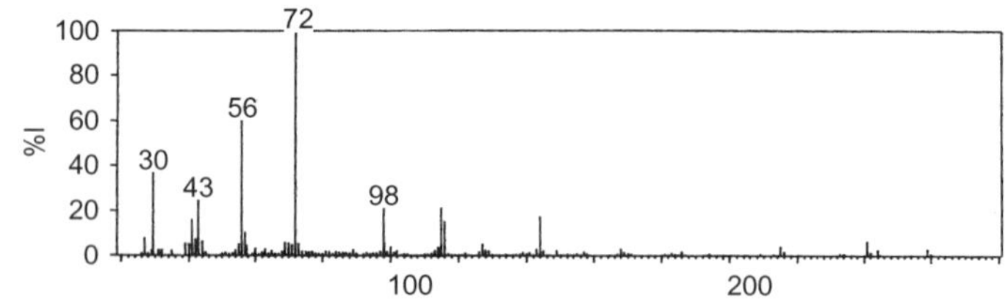

Quantification

Gas chromatography. In plasma: limit of detection <1 μg/L, ECD—R. E. Kates and C. L. Jones, *J. Pharm. Sci.*, 1977, *66*, 1490–1492. In plasma: propranolol and metoprolol, FID—M. P. Quaglio *et al.*, *Farmaco*, 1992, *47 (5 Suppl.)*, 799–809.

Gas chromatography–mass spectrometry. In plasma: propranolol and metoprolol in presence of butyrophenones, limit of detection 10 μg/L (or 50 μg/L with FID)—M. P. Quaglio *et al.*, *J. Pharm. Sci.*, 1993, *82*, 87–90. In urine: *N*-desisopropylpropranolol—A. Noda *et al.*, *Biol. Pharm. Bull.*, 1995, *18*, 1454–1455. In urine: propranolol and other beta-blockers, limit of detection for propranolol 40 μg/L—K. Hartonen and M. L. Riekkola, *J. Chromatogr. B Biomed. Appl.*, 1996, *676*, 45–52. In postmortem blood or urine: propranolol and other beta-blockers—S. B. Stenhouse *et al.*, *J. Chromatogr. B Biomed. Appl.*, 1996, *685*, 67–80.

High performance liquid chromatography. In plasma or urine: propranolol enantiomers, limits of quantification 1 to 2 μg/L—H. Spahn-Langguth *et al.*, *J. Anal. Toxicol.*, 1991, *15*, 209–213. In urine: propranolol and 4-hydroxypropranolol, fluorescence detection—V. L. Herring and J. A. Johnson, *J. Chromatogr.*, 1993, *612*, 215–221. In plasma or urine: propranolol enantiomers and conjugates, limit of detection about 1 μg/L, fluorescence detection—C. Pham-Huy *et al.*, *J. Pharm. Biomed. Anal.*, 1994, *12*, 1189–1198. In plasma or urine: propranolol enantiomers, limit of detection about 1.5 μg/L, fluorescence detection—C. Pham-Huy *et al.*, *J. Chromatogr. B Biomed. Appl.*, 1995, *665*, 125–132. In plasma or serum: fluorescence detection—G. S. Rekhi *et al.*, *J. Pharm. Biomed. Anal.*, 1995, *13*, 1499–1505. In serum: propranolol enantiomers, limit of detection 4 μg/L—D. O. Rumiantsev and T. V. Ivanova, *J. Chromatogr. B Biomed. Appl.*, *1995*, *674*, 301–305. In plasma: propranolol enantiomers and 4-hydroxypropranolol, fluorescence detection—S. T. Wu *et al.*, *J. Chromatogr. B Biomed. Sci. Appl.*, 1997, *692*, 133–140.

High performance liquid chromatography–mass spectrometry. In serum or urine: propranolol and other beta-blockers and their metabolites, limits of detection 0.1 to 1.2 μg/L—H. Kataoka *et al.*, *Anal. Chem.*, 1999, *71*, 4237–4244. In blood or plasma: propranolol and other beta-blockers—C. Mislanova and M. Hutta, *J. Chromatogr. B Biomed. Sci. Appl.*, 2001, *765*, 167–177.

Radioimmunoassay. In plasma: limit of detection 600 ng/L—G. P. Mould *et al.*, *Biopharm Drug Disp.*, 1981, *2*, 49–57.

Review. For a review of HPLC methods for propranolol and other beta-blockers—G. Egginger *et al.*, *Biomed. Chromatogr.*, 1993, *7*, 277–295.

Disposition in the Body. Rapidly and almost completely absorbed after oral administration, but undergoes extensive first-pass metabolism with considerable intersubject variation. It is very soluble in lipids. It is rapidly distributed throughout the body with highest levels being found in the lungs, liver, kidney, brain and heart. It crosses the placenta; it is excreted in breast milk. Metabolic reactions include ring hydroxylation, *N*-demethylation, oxidative deamination, and conjugation. In 48 h, about 10% of a dose is excreted in the urine as propranolol glucuronide and less than 4% as unchanged drug. Metabolites found in the urine, in free and conjugated forms, include naphthoxylactic acid (14 to 22% of the dose in 48 h) and the active metabolite, 4-hydroxypropranolol and its glucuronide (5 to 8% of the dose); propranolol glycol, *N*-desisopropylpropranolol, and naphthoxyacetic acid each account for less than 2% of the dose and 4-hydroxypropranolol sulfate accounts for about 18% of the dose. After IV doses, a greater proportion of naphthoxylactic acid (up to 40% of the dose) is excreted in the urine and 4-hydroxypropranolol is not found in the urine. Less than 5% of a dose is eliminated in the faeces.

Therapeutic concentration. In plasma, usually in the range 0.05 to 1 mg/L. However, there is considerable intersubject variation and a correlation between plasma concentration and therapeutic effect has not been established.

After a single oral dose of 80 mg administered to 6 subjects, the following mean peak concentrations of drug and metabolites were found in the plasma after 2 h: propranolol 0.05 mg/L, naphthoxylactic acid 0.53 mg/L, 4-hydroxypropranolol 0.009 mg/L, naphthoxyacetic acid 0.024 mg/L, propranolol glycol 0.005 mg/L [D. W. Schneck *et al.*, *Clin. Pharmacol. Ther.*, 1980, *27*, 744–755].

Following oral administration of 160 mg twice a day to 12 subjects, mean steady-state plasma concentrations of 0.38 mg/L of propranolol and 0.03 mg/L of 4-hydroxypropranolol were reported [B. G. Charles *et al.*, *J. Pharm. Pharmacol.*, 1982, *34*, 403–404].

Administration of a single 40-mg dose of propranolol hydrochloride, either sublingually or orally, to 14 severely hypertensive patients, produced mean peak plasma concentrations of 0.147 and 0.041 mg/L, respectively, at 34 and 52 min [A. P. Mansur *et al.*, *Braz. J. Med. Biol. Res.*, 1998, *31*, 691–696].

Toxicity. Toxic effects have been associated with plasma concentrations greater than 2 mg/L and fatalities with concentrations greater than 4 mg/L.

In a case of suicide attributed to propranolol overdose, the following concentrations were found: blood 14 mg/L, brain 67 µg/g, liver 171 µg/g, urine 0.9 mg/L; alcohol was also present [J. Kristinsson and T. Johannesson, *Acta Pharmacol. Toxicol.*, 1977, *41*, 190–192].

In a fatality due to the ingestion of 9.6 g of propranolol, in which death occurred 8 h after ingestion, the following postmortem tissue concentrations were reported: blood 20 mg/L, brain 6 µg/g, kidney 26 µg/g, liver 10 µg/g, lung 69 µg/g [J. W. Jones *et al.*, *J. Forensic Sci.*, 1982, *27*, 213–216].

In postmortem examination performed 5 days after a 60-year-old man was found dead near an empty box of Inderal, the following propranolol concentrations were reported: blood 7 mg/L, urine 0.28 mg/L, gastric contents 2000 mg/L; death was attributed to cardiocirculatory failure resulting from the suicidal ingestion of a massive dose of Inderal [N. Fucci and C. Offidani, *Am. J. Forensic Med. Pathol.*, 2000, *21*, 56–58].

Bioavailability. 10 to 50% (mean 30).

Half-life. Plasma half-life, 3 to 6 h (dose-dependent elimination has been reported).

Volume of distribution. About 4 L/kg.

Clearance. Plasma clearance, about 10 to 20 mL/min/kg.

Distribution in blood. Plasma : whole blood ratio, about 1.3.

Protein binding. In plasma, about 90%.

Note. For a review of the pharmacokinetics of long-acting propranolol, see G. S. Nace and A. J. Wood, *Clin. Pharmacokinet.*, 1987, *13*, 51–64; see also P. A. Routledge and D. G. Shand, *Clin. Pharmacokinet.*, 1979, *4*, 73–90; and B. M. Silber *et al.*, *J. Pharm. Sci.*, 1983, *72*, 725–732.

Dose. 30 to 400 mg of propranolol hydrochloride daily.

Propyl Hydroxybenzoate

Preservative

Synonyms. Propagin; Propyl Parahydroxybenzoate; Propylis Oxybenzoas; Propylparaben.
Proprietary names. Nipasol M; Propyl Parasept; Solbrol P. It is an ingredient of Nipasept and Nipastat.
4-Hydroxybenzoic acid propyl ester
$C_{10}H_{12}O_3$=180.2
CAS—94-13-3

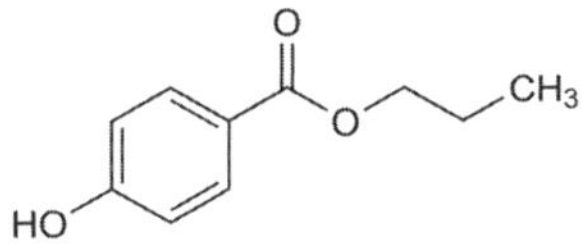

Colourless crystals or a white crystalline powder. M.p. 96° to 97°.
Soluble 1 in 2500 of cold water, 1 in 400 of boiling water, 1 in 1.5 of ethanol, 1 in 4 of chloroform, and 1 in 3 of ether.

Sodium Propyl Hydroxybenzoate

Synonyms. Sodium Propylparaben; Soluble Propyl Hydroxybenzoate.
Proprietary name. Nipasol M Sodium
$C_{10}H_{11}NaO_3$=202.2
CAS—35285-69-9
A white, hygroscopic, crystalline powder.
Soluble 1 in 1 of water, 1 in 50 of ethanol, and 1 in 2 of ethanol (50%).

Dissociation Constant. pK_a 8.4 (22°).

Partition Coefficient. Log *P* (octanol/water), 3.0.

Thin-layer Chromatography. System TE—Rf 53; system TF—Rf 67; system TAD—Rf 56; system TAE—Rf 90.

Gas Chromatography. System GA—RI 1567.

High Performance Liquid Chromatography. System HX—473; system HY—RI 458; system HAA—Retention time 18.3 min.

Ultraviolet Spectrum. Aqueous acid—255 (A^1_1=877b); aqueous alkali—296 nm (A^1_1=1324b).

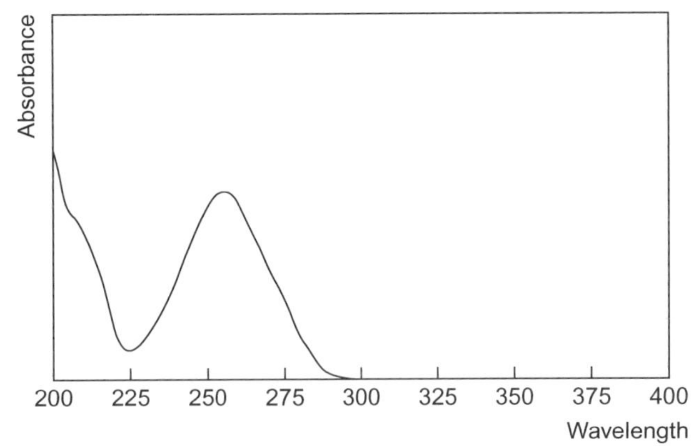

Infra-red Spectrum. Principal peaks at wavenumbers 1276, 1165, 1220, 1317, 1665, 1600 cm^{-1} (KBr disk).

Propylhexedrine

Sympathomimetic/Anorectic

Synonyms. Hexahydrodesoxyephedrine; Propylhexed.
Proprietary names. Benzedrex; Colloidine.
N,α-Dimethylcyclohexaneethanamine
$C_{10}H_{21}N$=155.3
CAS—101-40-6; 3595-11-7 (±)

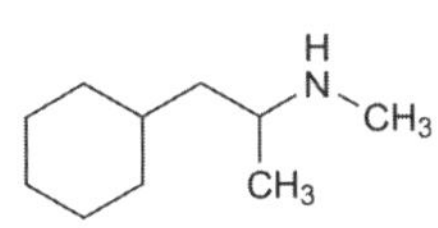

A clear colourless liquid which slowly volatilises at room temperature and absorbs carbon dioxide from the air. Mass per mL 0.853 to 0.861 g. B.p. about 204°.
Very slightly soluble in water; miscible with ethanol, chloroform, and ether.

Propylhexedrine Hydrochloride

Proprietary name. Eventin(e)
$C_{10}H_{21}N,HCl$=191.7
CAS—1007-33-6; 6192-95-6 (±)
A crystalline solid. M.p. 127° to 128°, with decomposition.
Soluble in water, ethanol, and chloroform; slightly soluble in ether.

Dissociation Constant. pK_a 10.7 (25°).

Partition Coefficient. Log *P* (octanol/water), 3.5.

Thin-layer Chromatography. System TA—Rf 26; system TB—Rf 34; system TE—Rf 34; system TAE—Rf 14; system TAJ—Rf 00; system TAK—Rf 24; system TAL—Rf 65. (Acidified iodoplatinate solution, positive.)

Gas Chromatography. System GA—propylhexedrine RI 1175, propylhexedrine-TFA RI 1385, propylhexedrine-PFP RI 1385, propylhexedrine-AC RI 1570, M (OH-) RI 1475, M (OH-)-AC_2 RI 1915; system GB—RI 1192; system GC—RI 1500.

Ultraviolet Spectrum. No significant absorption, 230 to 360 nm.

Infra-red Spectrum. Principal peaks at wavenumbers 1058, 1015, 885, 913, 1153, 966 cm^{-1} (propylhexedrine hydrochloride, Nujol mull).

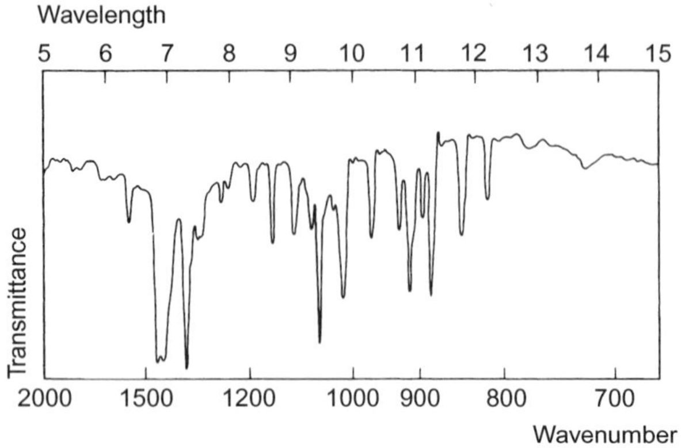

Mass Spectrum. Principal ions at *m/z* 58, 140, 67, 72, 83, 81, 155, 156.

Quantification

High performance liquid chromatography. In serum or urine: propylhexedrine and other sympathomimetics and amfetamines, limits of detection 0.01 to 0.03 mg/L (UV detection single wavelength) and 0.05 to 0.1 mg/L (diode-array detection), (also MS)—M. J. Bogusz *et al.*, *J. Anal. Toxicol.*, 1997, *21*, 59–69.

High performance liquid chromatography–mass spectrometry. In serum: propylhexedrine and other sympathomimetics and amfetamines, limits of detection 1 to 5 µg/L—M. J. Bogusz *et al.*, *J. Anal. Toxicol.*, 2000, *24*, 77–84.

Disposition in the Body. Norpropylhexedrine, cyclohexylacetoxime, and *cis/trans*-4-hydroxypropylhexedrine have been identified as urinary metabolites.

Toxicity. The estimated minimum lethal dose for children up to 2 years of age is 200 mg.

In a fatality attributed to propylhexedrine ingestion, the following postmortem tissue concentrations were reported: blood 35 mg/L, bile 20 mg/L, brain 24 µg/g, kidney 30 µg/g, liver 36 µg/g, lung 50 µg/g, urine 60 mg/L [L. Riddick and R. Reisch, *J. Forensic Sci.*, 1981, *26*, 834–839].

The following postmortem tissue concentrations were reported in 2 fatalities involving IV abuse: blood 1.8 and 2.7 mg/L, kidney 1.5 and 9.5 µg/g, liver 2.8 and 11.8 µg/g, urine 12.6 mg/L (first case) [W. Q. Sturner *et al.*, *J. Forensic Sci.*, 1974, *19*, 572–574].

In a fatality attributed to acute IV propylhexedrine abuse, postmortem tissue concentrations were: blood 2 mg/L, bile 9.4 mg/L, kidney 4.0 µg/g, liver 7.4 µg/g, urine 69.5 mg/L [V. J. M. DiMaio and J. C. Garriott, *J. Forensic Sci.*, 1977, *22*, 152–158].

Note. For a review of propylhexedrine, see D. R. Wesson, *Drug Alcohol Depend.*, 1986, *17*, 273–278.

Dose. Usually 75 to 100 mg of propylhexedrine hydrochloride daily.

Propyliodone

Diagnostic Aid (Radiopaque Medium)

Synonym. Propiodone
Proprietary name. Dionosil
3,5-Diiodo-4-oxo-1(4*H*)-pyridineacetic acid propyl ester
$C_{10}H_{11}I_2NO_3$=447.0
CAS—587-61-1

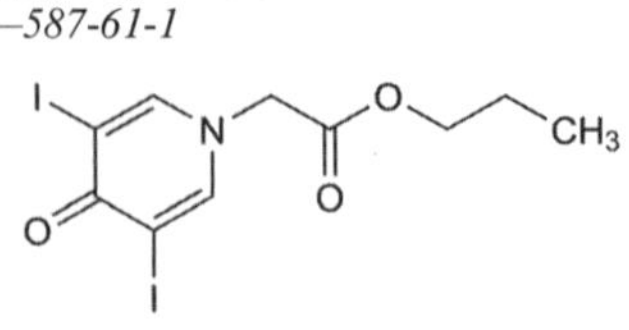

A white crystalline powder. M.p. 186° to 187°.
Practically insoluble in water; soluble 1 in 500 of ethanol and 1 in 150 of chloroform; soluble in acetone and ether.

Partition Coefficient. Log *P* (octanol/water), 2.1.

Colour Test. Iodine Test—positive.

Thin-layer Chromatography. System TA—Rf 81. (Acidified iodoplatinate solution, positive.)

Gas Chromatography. System GA—not eluted.

Ultraviolet Spectrum. Dehydrated alcohol—239 (A_1^1=320a), 281 nm (A_1^1=260a).

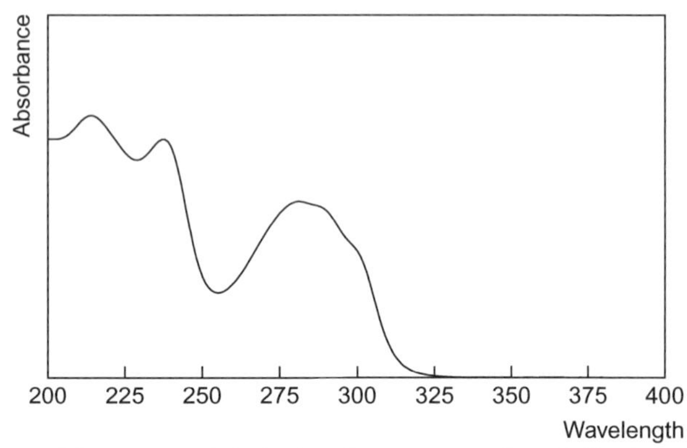

Infra-red Spectrum. Principal peaks at wavenumbers 1730, 1200, 1567, 1608, 751, 1227 cm^{-1} (KBr disk).

Uses. Administered as a 50% aqueous suspension or as a 60% oily suspension.

Propylthiouracil

Antihyperthyroid

Proprietary names. Propacil; Propycil; Propylthiocil; Propyl-Thyracil; Prothiucil; Thyreostat II; Tiotil.
2,3-Dihydro-6-propyl-2-thioxo-4(1*H*)pyrimidinone
$C_7H_{10}N_2OS$=170.2
CAS—51-52-5

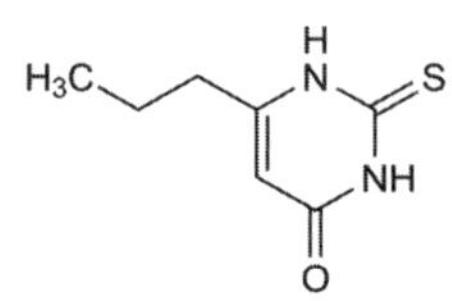

White or pale cream-coloured crystals or crystalline powder. M.p. 219° to 221°.
Soluble 1 in about 900 of water, 1 in about 60 of ethanol, and 1 in 60 of acetone; slightly soluble in chloroform and ether; soluble in solutions of alkali hydroxides.

Dissociation Constant. pK_a 8.3 (20°).

Partition Coefficient. Log *P* (octanol/water), 1.0.

Ultraviolet Spectrum. Aqueous acid—275 (A_1^1=987b); aqueous alkali—260 nm (A_1^1=703a).

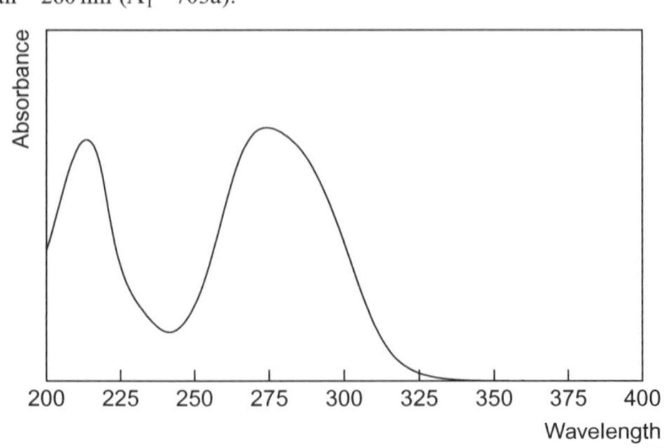

Infra-red Spectrum. Principal peaks at wavenumbers 1658, 1563, 1193, 1625, 1166, 1241 cm^{-1} (KBr disk).

Quantification

High performance liquid chromatography. In blood: limit of detection 300 µg/L, UV detection—C. Kim, *J. Chromatogr.*, 1983, *272*; *B Biomed. Appl.*, *23*, 376–379. In plasma: limit of detection 40 µg/L—G. R. Cannell *et al.*, *J. Chromatogr.*, 1991, *564*, 310–314.

Radioimmunoassay. In serum: limit of detection 2.5 ng—D. S. Cooper *et al.*, *J. Clin. Endocr. Metab.*, 1981, *52*, 204–213.

Disposition in the Body. Rapidly and almost completely absorbed after oral administration; concentrated in the thyroid. Metabolised by conjugation with glucuronic acid and sulfate. Less than 10% of a dose is excreted in the urine as unchanged drug.

Therapeutic concentration

Following a single oral dose of 400 mg to 17 subjects, serum concentrations of 1.6 to 7.5 mg/L (mean 4.2) were reported at 1 h [J. P. Kampmann and J. E. M. Hansen, *Br. J. Clin. Pharmacol.*, 1981, *12*, 681–686].

A single oral administration of 300 mg to 7 subjects produced peak plasma concentrations of 3.50 mg/L about 2 h after a conventional-release tablet and 0.50–1.25 mg/L about 3 h after sustained-release tablets [L. Kabanda et al., *J. Pharm. Pharmacol.*, 1996, *48*, 1023–1026].

Half-life. Plasma half-life, about 1 to 2 h, increased in renal failure.

Volume of distribution. About 0.4 L/kg.

Clearance. Plasma clearance, about 4 mL/min/kg.

Protein binding. In plasma, about 80%.

Note. For a review of the pharmacokinetics of antithyroid drugs, see J. P. Kampmann and J. E. M. Hansen, *Clin. Pharmacokinet.*, 1981, *6*, 401–428.

Dose. Initially 200 to 600 mg daily; maintenance, 50 to 200 mg daily.

Propyphenazone *Analgesic*

Synonyms. Isopropylantipyrine; Isopropylphenazone; Propifenazona.
Proprietary names. Cibalgina; Demex; Dim-Antos; Eufibron; Isoprochin P; Pireuma.
1,2-Dihydro-1,5-dimethyl-4-(1-methylethyl)-2-phenyl-3*H*-pyrazol-3-one
$C_{14}H_{18}N_2O$=230.3
CAS—479-92-5

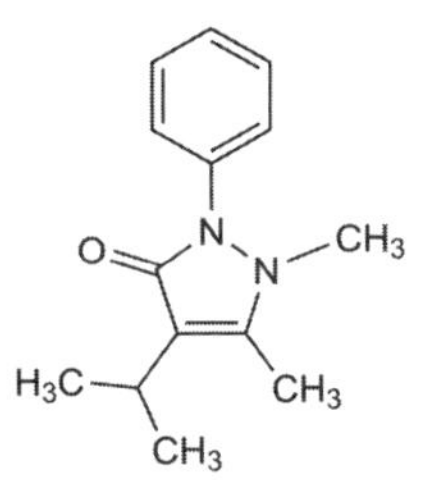

White crystals or white crystalline powder. M.p. 103°.
Soluble 1 in 400 of water; freely soluble in ethanol and chloroform; soluble in ether.

Partition Coefficient. Log *P* (octanol/water), 1.9.

Colour Tests. Ferric Chloride—orange; Liebermann's Test (100°)—blue (red with water).

Thin-layer Chromatography. System TA—Rf 71; system TB—Rf 32; system TD—Rf 61; system TE—Rf 74; system TF—Rf 49; system TAD—Rf 65; system TAE—Rf 81. (Acidified potassium permanganate solution, positive.)

Gas Chromatography. System GA—RI 1920; system GB—RI 2030; system GF—RI 2310.

High Performance Liquid Chromatography. System HD—*k* 1.3; system HW—*k* 11.0; system HX—RI 441; system HY—RI 370; system HZ—Retention time 4.7 min.

Ultraviolet Spectrum. Aqueous acid—240 (A_1^1=400a); aqueous alkali—245 (A_1^1=385b), 265 nm.

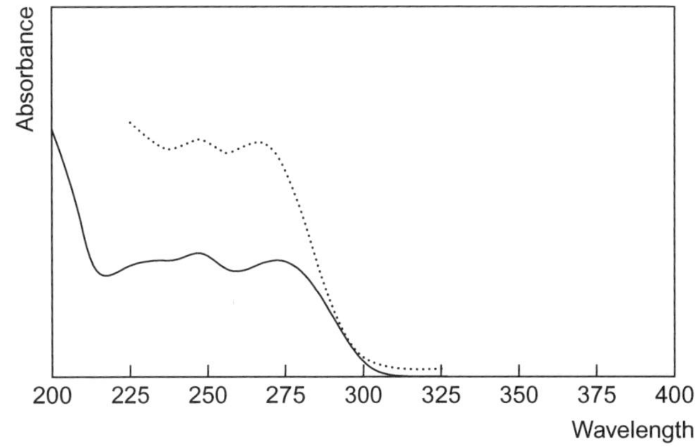

Infra-red Spectrum. Principal peaks at wavenumbers 1650, 1618, 1131, 1590, 1500, 750 cm^{-1} (KBr disk).

Mass Spectrum. Principal ions at *m/z* 215, 230, 56, 77, 216, 96, 41, 39.

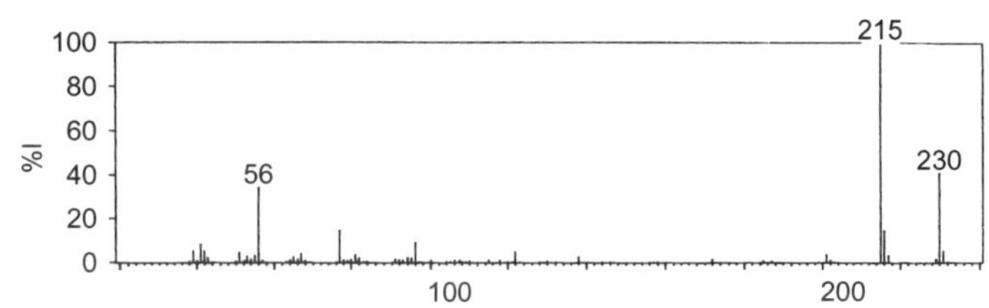

Quantification

High performance liquid chromatography. In plasma: limit of detection 100 µg/L, UV detection—M. C. Rouan *et al.*, *J. Chromatogr.*, 1992, *577*, 387–90.

Dose. Propyphenazone has been given in doses of 0.3 to 1.5 g daily.

Prothipendyl *Tranquilliser*

Synonym. Phrenotropin
N,N-Dimethyl-10*H*-pyrido[3,2-*b*][1,4]benzothiazine-10-propanamine
$C_{16}H_{19}N_3S$=285.4
CAS—303-69-5

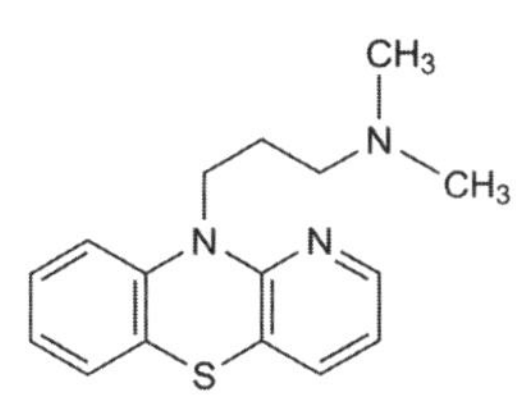

Prothipendyl Hydrochloride

Synonym. D-206
Proprietary name. Dominal; Tolnate.
$C_{16}H_{19}N_3S,HCl,H_2O$=339.9
CAS—1225-65-6 (anhydrous)
A crystalline powder. M.p. 108° to 112°.
Freely soluble in water and methanol; practically insoluble in ether.

Dissociation Constant. pK_a 2.3 (25°).

Partition Coefficient. Log *P* (octanol/water), 4.0.

Colour Test. Marquis Test—orange.

Thin-layer Chromatography. System TA—Rf 47; system TAE—Rf 15; system TAF—Rf 29; system TL—Rf 09; system TB—Rf 43; system TC—Rf 23; system TE—Rf 59. (Dragendorff spray, positive; FPN reagent, yellow; Acidified iodoplatinate solution, positive; Marquis reagent, orange.)

Gas Chromatography. System GA—Prothipendyl RI 2345; M (OH-) RI 2720; M (OH-ring) RI 2800; M (ring) RI 2045; M (sulfoxide) RI 2750; system GF—RI 2800.

High Performance Liquid Chromatography. System HA—*k* 4.4; system HX—RI 388.

Ultraviolet Spectrum. Aqueous acid—242 (A_1^1=928a); aqueous alkali—250 (A_1^1=909a), 320 nm (A_1^1=163b).

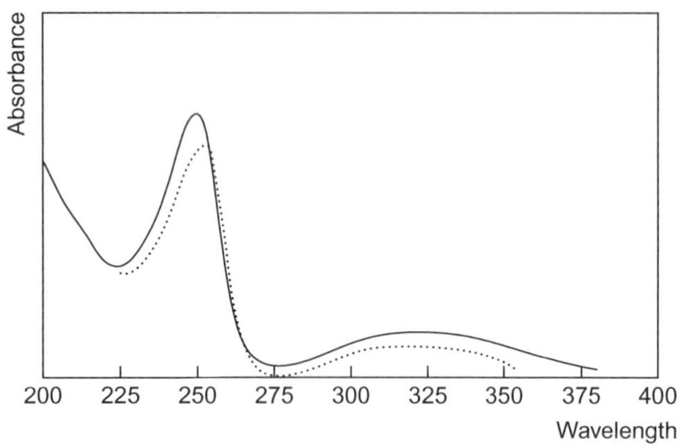

Infra-red Spectrum. Principal peaks at wavenumbers 757, 1295, 780, 1592, 1162, 1110 cm^{-1} (prothipendyl hydrochloride, KBr disk).

Mass Spectrum. Principal ions at *m/z* 58, 285, 214, 200, 86, 227, 85, 213.

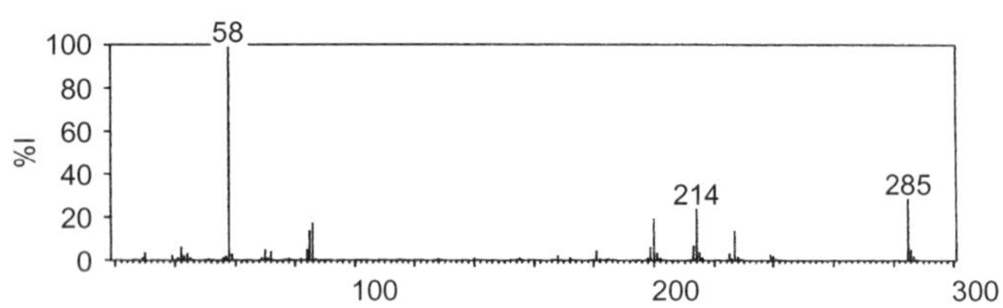

Quantification

High performance liquid chromatography. In plasma: prothipendyl and zolpidem, UV detection—G. Debailleul *et al.*, *J. Anal. Toxicol.*, 1991, *15*, 35–37.

Toxicity

In 2 cases of fatal poisoning with prothipendyl, the highest concentrations were found in the liver (1.2 to 1.8 mg/g) and kidney (0.6 mg/g) and far exceeded those found in the blood (which in one of the cases was 200 times over the therapeutic range). It was suggested that more than 4 g of prothipendyl is fatal [M. Wu *et al.*, *Arch. Kriminol.*, 1994, *193*, 158–162].

Dose. The equivalent of up to 960 mg of prothipendyl daily.

Protionamide

Tuberculostatic

Synonym. Prothionamide

Proprietary names. Ektebin; Peteha; Trevintix.

2-Propyl-4-pyridinecarbothioamide

$C_9H_{12}N_2S$=180.3

CAS—14222-60-7

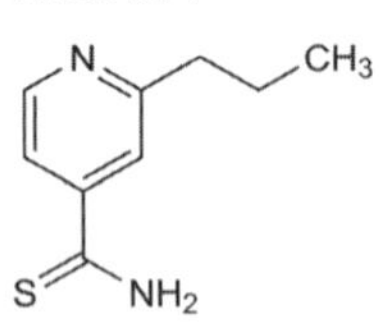

Yellow crystals or crystalline powder. M.p. 142°.

Practically insoluble in water; soluble 1 in 30 of ethanol, 1 in 200 of chloroform, 1 in 300 of ether, and 1 in 16 of methanol; soluble in acetone.

Partition Coefficient. Log *P* (octanol/water), 2.0.

Colour Tests. Nessler's Reagent—brown-orange; Palladium Chloride—brown.

Thin-layer Chromatography. System TA—Rf 66; system TAE—Rf 77; system TL—Rf 57; system TB—Rf 01; system TC—Rf 38. (Acidified iodoplatinate solution, positive.)

Gas Chromatography. System GA—RI 1816.

Ultraviolet Spectrum. Ethanol—291 nm (A_1^1=390b).

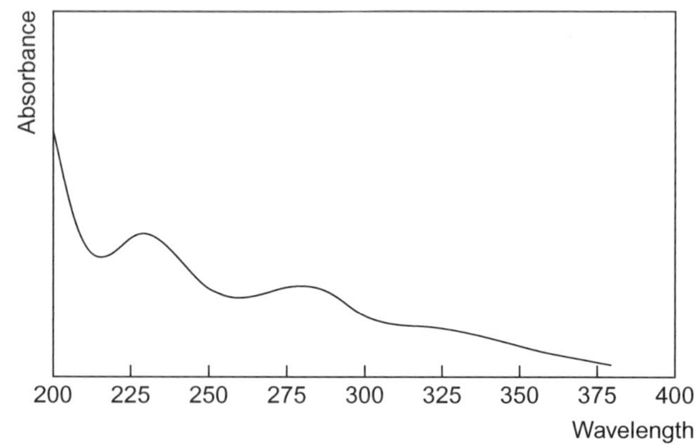

Infra-red Spectrum. Principal peaks at wavenumbers 828, 1590, 1284, 902, 1148, 710 cm^{-1} (KBr disk).

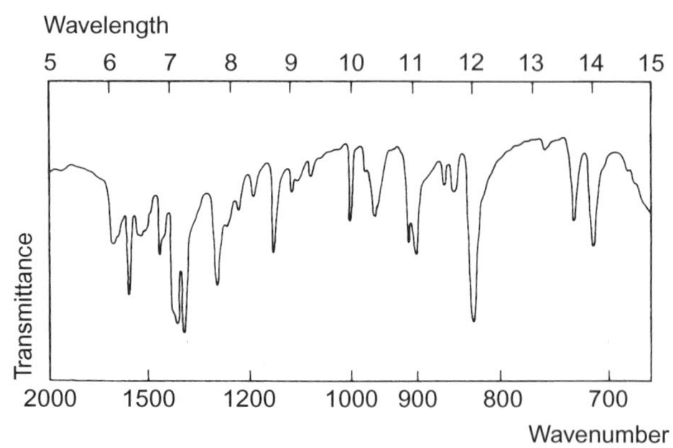

Mass Spectrum. Principal ions at *m/z* 152, 119, 165, 163, 180, 60, 179, 153.

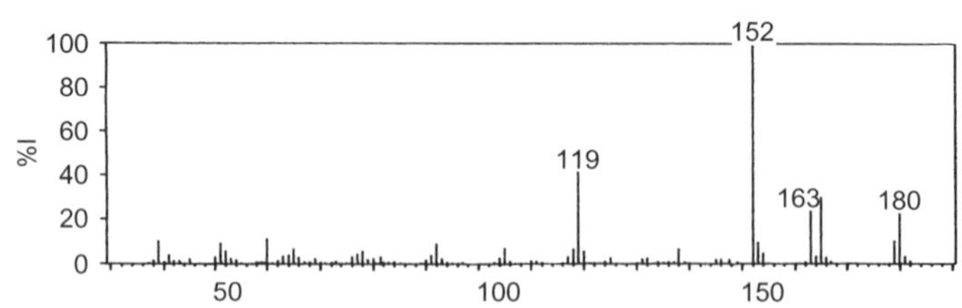

Quantification

High performance liquid chromatography. In plasma, serum or urine: limit of detection 10 µg/L, UV detection—P. J. Jenner and G. A. Ellard, *J. Chromatogr.*, 1981, *225*; *B Biomed. Appl.*, 14, 245–251. In serum: limit of detection 27 µg/L, UV detection—H. Bartels and R. Bartels, *J. Chromatogr. B Biomed. Sci. Appl.*, 1998, *707*, 338–341.

Disposition in the Body. Readily absorbed after oral administration. Metabolised to the sulfoxide and excreted in the urine mainly as metabolites.

Therapeutic concentration

Following a single oral dose of 500 mg to 10 subjects, mean peak plasma concentrations of 3 mg/L of unchanged drug and 2.7 mg/L of the sulfoxide were attained in 1 h [J. Pütter, *Arzneimittelforschung.*, 1972, *22*, 1027–1031].

Dose. Usually 0.5 to 1 g daily.

Protokylol

Bronchodilator

Synonym. Protochylol
4-[2-[[2-(1,3-Benzodioxol-5-yl)-1-methylethyl]amino]-1-hydroxyethyl]-1,2-benzenediol
$C_{18}H_{21}NO_5$=331.4
CAS—136-70-9

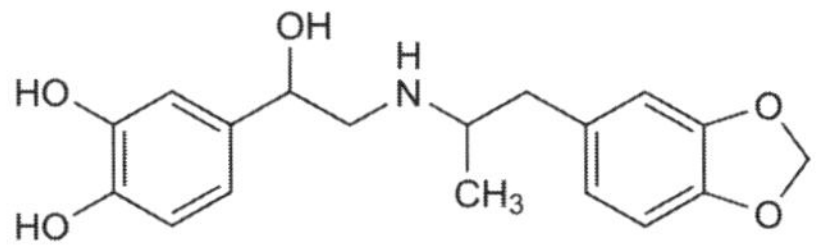

Protokylol Hydrochloride
Synonym. JB-251
Proprietary names. Caytime; Ventaire.
$C_{18}H_{21}NO_5$,HCl=367.8
CAS—136-69-6
A white crystalline powder. M.p. 126° to 127°.
Soluble in water.

Partition Coefficient. Log *P* (octanol/water), 1.8.

Colour Tests. Ammoniacal silver nitrate—red-grey/brown; Ferric chloride—green; Folin–Ciocalteu reagent—blue; Liebermann's test—black; Mandelin's test—yellow→brown; Marquis test—grey-green; Methanolic potassium hydroxide—orange→yellow; Nessler's reagent—black; Potassium dichromate—brown→red-brown (on warming).

Thin-layer Chromatography. System TA—Rf 65; system TB—Rf 01; system TC—Rf 03; system TL—Rf 06; system TAJ—Rf 00; system TAK—Rf 02; system TAL—Rf 48. (Acidified potassium permanganate solution, positive.)

Gas Chromatography. System GA—RI 1487.

High Performance Liquid Chromatography. System HA—*k* 3.1 (tailing peak).

Ultraviolet Spectrum. Aqueous acid—281 nm (A_1^1=168b).

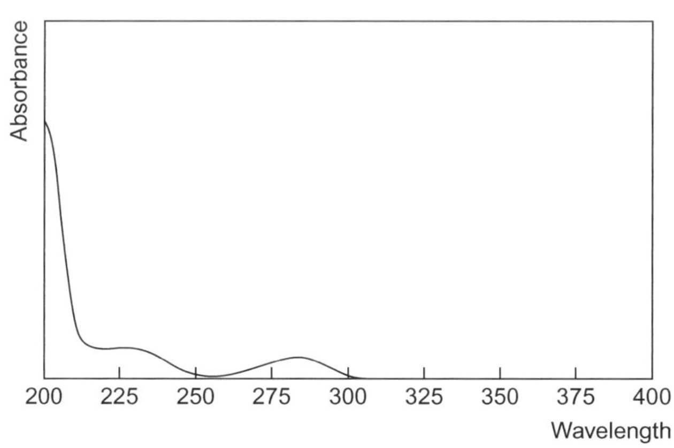

Infra-red Spectrum. Principal peaks at wavenumbers 1492, 1250, 1271, 1227, 1036, 1128 cm^{-1}(KBr disk).

Mass Spectrum. Principal ions at *m/z* 178, 44, 163, 135, 77, 196, 176, 179.

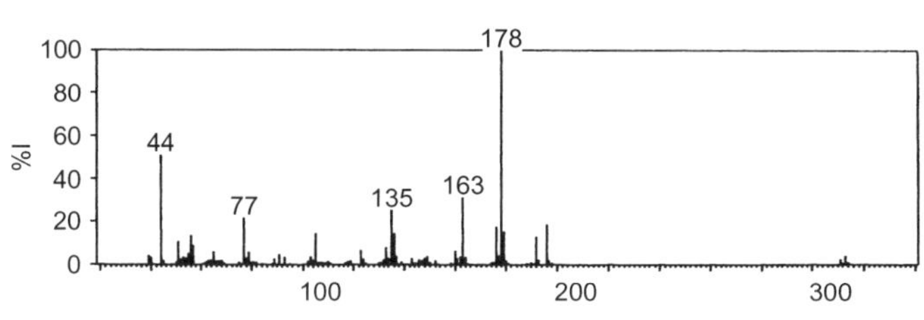

Dose. Protokylol hydrochloride has been given in doses of 8 to 16 mg daily.

Protoveratrine A

Antihypertensive

Proprietary name. Protalba
[3β(*S*),4α,6α,7α,15α(*R*),16β]-4,9-Epoxycevane-3,4,6,7,14,15,16,20-octol 6,7-diacetate
$C_{41}H_{63}NO_{14}$=793.9
CAS—143-57-7

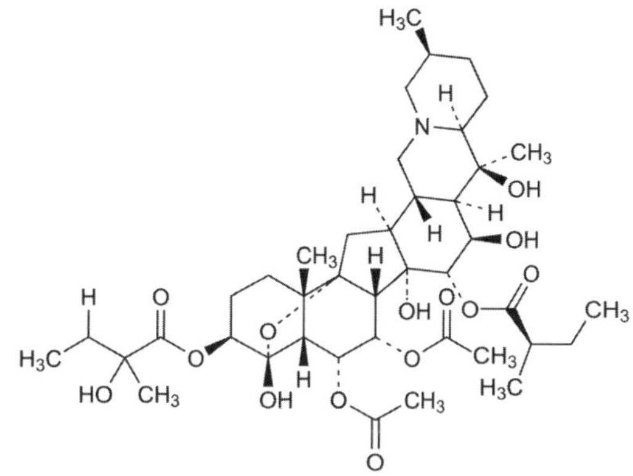

An alkaloid obtained from the roots and rhizomes of white veratrum, *Veratrum album* (Liliaceae).
White crystals. M.p. 267° to 269°, with decomposition.
Practically insoluble in water; soluble in hot ethanol and in chloroform.

Protoveratrine B

Synonyms. Neoprotoveratrine; Veratetrine.
[3β(2*R*,3*R*),4α,6α,7α,15α(*R*),16β]-4,9-Epoxycevane-3,4,6,7,14,15,16,20-octol 6,7-diacetate
$C_{41}H_{63}NO_{15}$=809.9
CAS—124-97-0

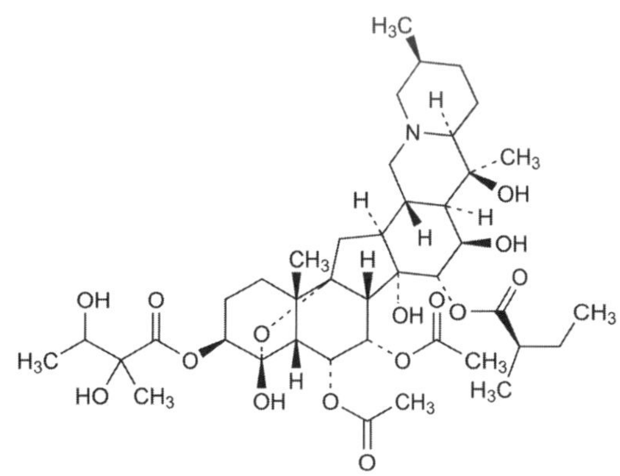

An alkaloid obtained from the roots and rhizomes of white veratrum, *Veratrum album* (Liliaceae).
White crystals. M.p. 268° to 270°, with decomposition.
Practically insoluble in water; soluble in hot ethanol and in chloroform.

Protoveratrines A and B
Proprietary names. Provell; Tensatrin.
CAS—8053-18-7
A white crystalline powder with a strong sternutatory action. M.p. 256° to 262°, with decomposition.
Practically insoluble in water; soluble in chloroform; very slightly soluble in ether. It is rapidly decomposed in alkaline and alcoholic solutions.

Thin-layer Chromatography. Protoveratrine A: System TA—Rf 72. Protoveratrine B: System TA—Rf 70. (Acidified iodoplatinate solution, positive; acidified potassium permanganate solution, positive.)

Gas Chromatography. System GA—protoveratrines A and B, RI 2465.

Infra-red Spectrum. Principal peaks at wavenumbers 1742, 1200, 1182, 1240, 1150, 1055 cm^{-1} protoveratrines A and B, KCl disk).

Dose. Protoveratrines A and B have been given in a dose of 1.6 to 6 mg daily.

Protriptyline

Antidepressant

Synonym. Amimetilina
N-Methyl-5*H*-dibenzo[*a*,*d*]cycloheptene-5-propanamine
$C_{19}H_{21}N$=263.4
CAS—438-60-8

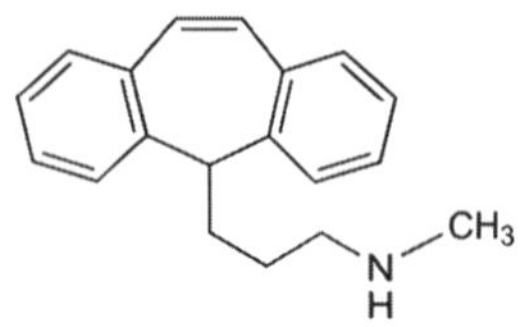

Protriptyline Hydrochloride

Synonym. MK-240
Proprietary names. Concordin(e); Triptil; Vivactil.

Note. The name Vivactil has also been applied to a vitamin/amino acid preparation.
$C_{19}H_{21}N,HCl$=299.8
CAS—1225-55-4
A white to yellowish powder. M.p. about 169° to 171°.
Soluble 1 in 2 of water, 1 in 3.5 of ethanol and 1 in 2.5 of chloroform; practically insoluble in ether.

Dissociation Constant. pK_a 8.2 (protriptyline HCl).

Partition Coefficient. Log *P* (octanol/water), 4.9.

Colour Tests. Mandelin's test—violet→brown; Marquis test—green; Sulfuric acid—green.

Thin-layer Chromatography. System TA—Rf 19; system TB—Rf 18; system TC—Rf 07; system TE—Rf 38; system TL—Rf 02; system TAE—Rf 06; system TAF—Rf 69; system TAJ—Rf 04; system TAK—Rf 28; system TAL—Rf 76. (Acidified iodoplatinate solution, positive.)

Gas Chromatography. System GA—RI 2253; system GB—protriptyline RI 2329; M (nor-) RI 2343; system GF—RI 2590; system GM—RRT 0.878 (relative to iprindole).

High Performance Liquid Chromatography. System HA—*k* 2.1; system HF—*k* 3.6; system HX—RI 418; system HY—RI 362.

Ultraviolet Spectrum. Methanolic acid—292 nm (A^1_1=530a). No alkaline shift.

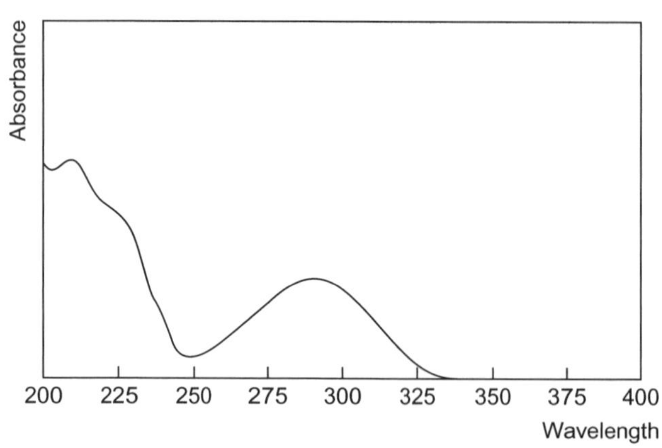

Infra-red Spectrum. Principal peaks at wavenumbers 792, 750, 768, 1490, 730, 1595 cm^{-1} (protriptyline hydrochloride, KBr disk).

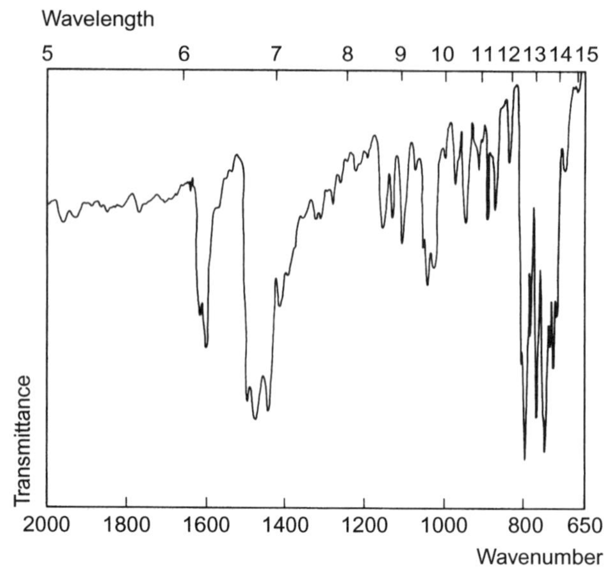

Mass Spectrum. Principal ions at *m/z* 70, 44, 191, 192, 188, 59, 165, 71; 10,11-dihydro-10,11-dihydroxyprotriptyline 44, 70, 179, 178, 207, 280, 250, 236; 10-hydroxyprotriptyline 70, 44, 207, 178, 279, 249, -, -.

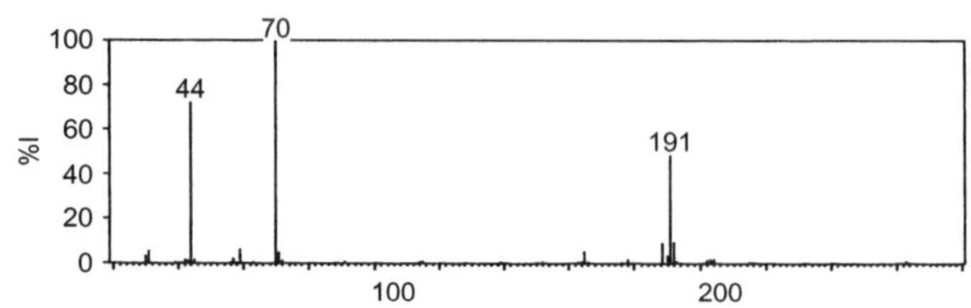

Quantification

Gas chromatography. In serum: protriptyline and other tricyclic antidepressants, limit of detection 10 to 20 µg/L, AFID—J. Kristinsson, *Acta Pharmacol. Toxicol.*, 1981, *49*, 390–398. In serum: protripyline and other antidepressants and metabolites, limit of detection 25 µg/L, nitrogen-selective detection—N. Rifai *et al.*, *Ther. Drug Monit.*, 1988, *10*, 194–196.

Gas chromatography–mass spectrometry In plasma: protriptyline and other tricyclic antidepressants, limit of detection 10 µg/L—J. T. Biggs *et al.*, *J. Pharm. Sci.*, 1976, *65*, 261–268.

High performance liquid chromatography. In plasma: limit of detection 60 µg/L, UV detection—L. P. Hackett and L. J. Dusci, *Clin Toxicol.*, 1979, *15*, 55–61.

Disposition in the Body. Protriptyline is slowly but well absorbed after oral administration. It is metabolised by oxidation to form the 10-hydroxy and 10,11-dihydro-10,11-dihydroxy derivatives and 5,10-dihydro-10-formylanthracen-5-ylpropylamine; glucuronic acid conjugation also occurs. About 50% of a dose is excreted in the urine in 16 days with only small amounts of unchanged drug; about 2% of a dose is eliminated in the faeces.

Therapeutic concentration. In plasma, usually in the range 0.07 to 0.25 mg/L.

After a single oral dose of 30 mg to 8 subjects, peak plasma concentrations of 0.010 to 0.022 (mean 0.014) mg/L were attained in 6 to 12 h. [V. E. Ziegler *et al.*, *Clin. Pharmacol. Ther.*, 1978, *23*, 580–584].

Following daily oral doses of 40 mg to 30 subjects, steady-state plasma concentrations of 0.11 to 0.38 (mean 0.22) mg/L were reported. [J. P. Moody *et al.*, *Eur. J. Clin. Pharmacol.*, 1977, *11*, 51–56].

Toxicity. Toxic effects are associated with plasma concentrations greater than 0.5 mg/L; concentrations above 1 mg/L may be lethal.

Bioavailability. About 75 to 90% (10 to 25% first-pass metabolism).

Half-life. Plasma half-life, during chronic dosing, about 3 to 8 (mean 4) days.

Volume of distribution. About 22 L/kg.

Clearance. Plasma clearance, 2 to 5 mL/min/kg.

Protein binding. In plasma, about 92%.

Note. For a review of tricyclic antidepressants, see G. Molnar and R. N. Gupta, *Biopharm. Drug Disp.*, 1980, *1*, 283–305.

Dose. 15 to 60 mg of protriptyline hydrochloride daily.

Proxymetacaine

Local Anaesthetic

Synonym. Proparacaine
3-Amino-4-propoxybenzoic acid 2-(diethylamino)ethyl ester
$C_{16}H_{26}N_2O_3$=294.4
CAS—499-67-2

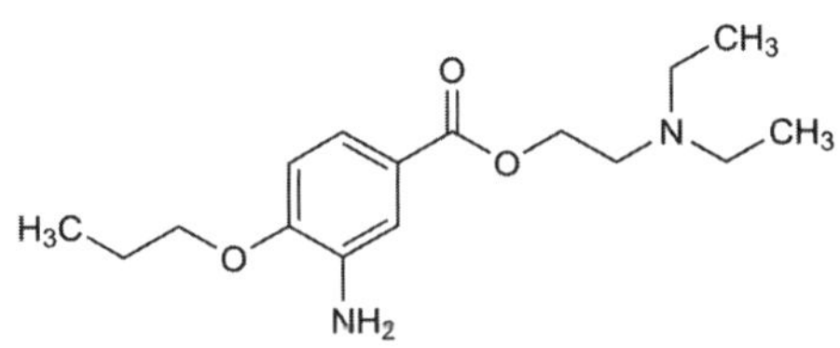

Proxymetacaine Hydrochloride

Proprietary names. Ak-Taine; Alcaine; Anestalcon; Diocaine; Kéracaine; Ocu-Caine; Ophthaine; Ophthetic; Parcaine; Visonest.
$C_{16}H_{26}N_2O_3$,HCl=330.9
CAS—5875-06-9
A white or faintly buff-coloured crystalline powder. It discolours on heating or exposure to air and solutions exposed to air become yellow and then dark brown. M.p. 182° to 183°.
Soluble 1 in 30 of water and 1 in 50 of ethanol; practically insoluble in ether; soluble in chloroform and methanol.

Partition Coefficient. Log *P* (octanol/water), 3.2.

Colour Tests. Coniferyl alcohol—orange; Diazotisation—red; Ninhydrin—yellow.

Thin-layer Chromatography. System TA—Rf 62; system TB—Rf 26; system TC—Rf 41; system TL—Rf 35. (Acidified iodoplatinate solution, positive; Van Urk reagent, yellow.)

Gas Chromatography. System GA—RI 2323.

High Performance Liquid Chromatography. System HA—*k* 2.1; system HQ—*k* 1.38; system HY—RI 269.

Ultraviolet Spectrum. Water—231 nm, 268 nm (A_1^1=326b), 310 nm (A_1^1=182a).

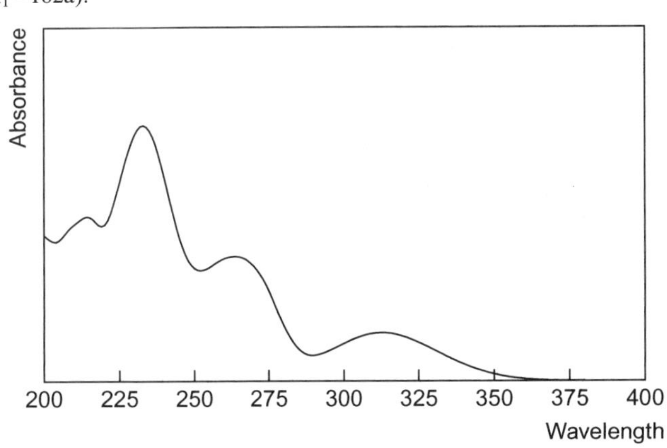

Infra-red Spectrum. Principal peaks at wavenumbers 1213, 1708, 1305, 1104, 1590, 1520 cm^{-1} (proxymetacaine hydrochloride, KCl disk).

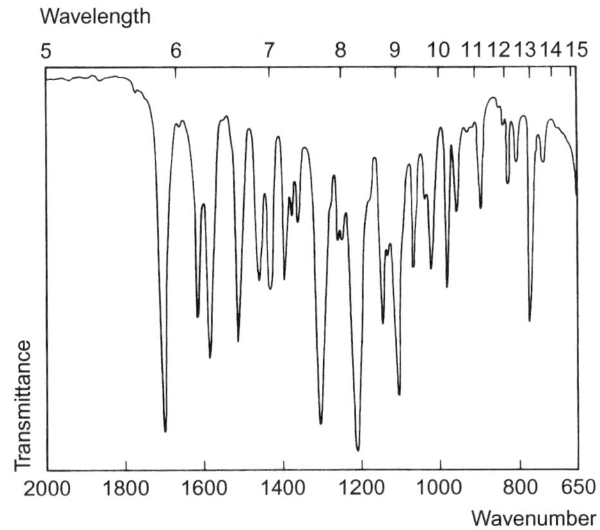

Mass Spectrum. Principal ions at *m/z* 86, 99, 30, 87, 58, 71, 136, 100.

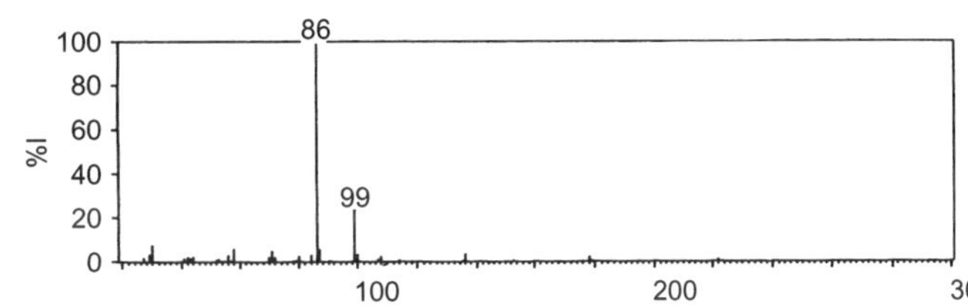

Use. Proxymetacaine hydrochloride is used as a 0.5% ophthalmic solution.

Proxyphylline

Xanthine Bronchodilator

Proprietary names. Brontyl; Neofyllin; Pantafillina; Purofilina; Spantin; Spasmolysin; Thean; Theon.
3,7-Dihydro-7-(2-hydroxypropyl)-1,3-dimethyl-1*H*-purine-2,6-dione
$C_{10}H_{14}N_4O_3$=238.2
CAS-603-00-9

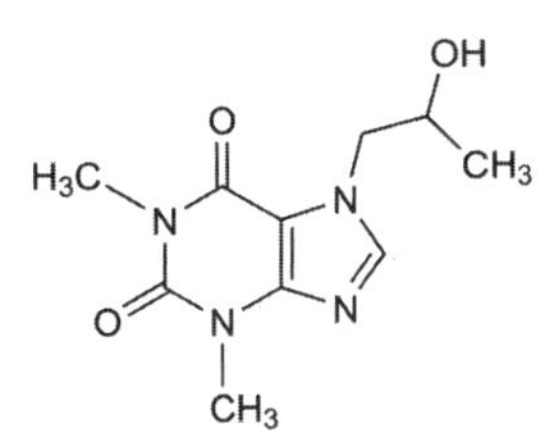

A white crystalline powder. M.p. 135° to 136°.
Soluble 1 in 1 of water, 1 in 12 of ethanol, 1 in 6 of chloroform and 1 in 500 of ether.

Partition Coefficient. Log *P* (octanol/water), −0.8.

Colour Test. Amalic acid test—yellow/violet.

Thin-layer Chromatography. System TA—Rf 58; system TB—Rf 02; system TC—Rf 33; system TE—Rf 49; system TL—Rf 29; system TAE—Rf 71. (Acidified potassium permanganate solution, positive.)

Gas Chromatography. System GA—RI 2103.

High Performance Liquid Chromatography. System HA—*k* 0.1; system HX—RI 293.

Ultraviolet Spectrum. Aqueous acid—273 nm (A_1^1=372a). No alkaline shift.

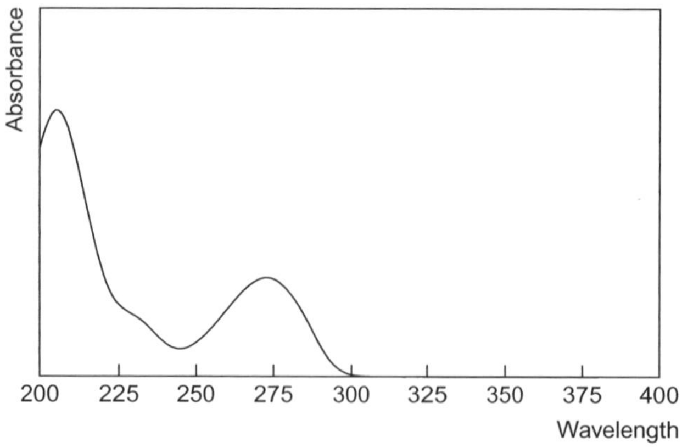

Infra-red Spectrum. Principal peaks at wavenumbers 1656, 1690, 750, 1538, 763, 1282 cm^{-1} (KBr disk).

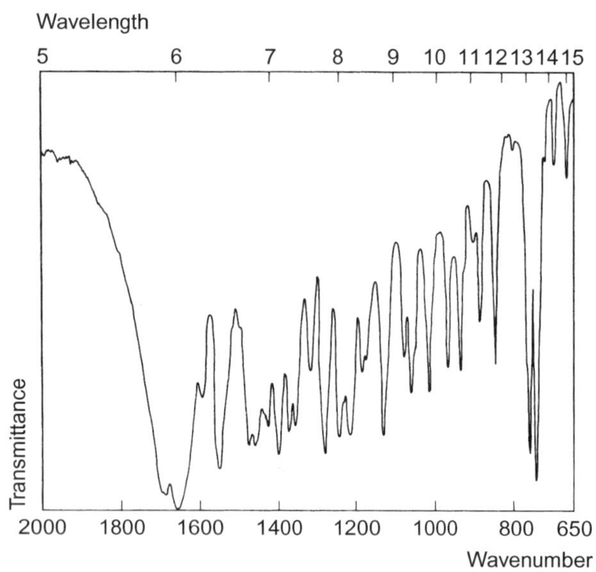

Mass Spectrum. Principal ions at *m/z* 194, 180, 109, 193, 238, 95, 137, 81.

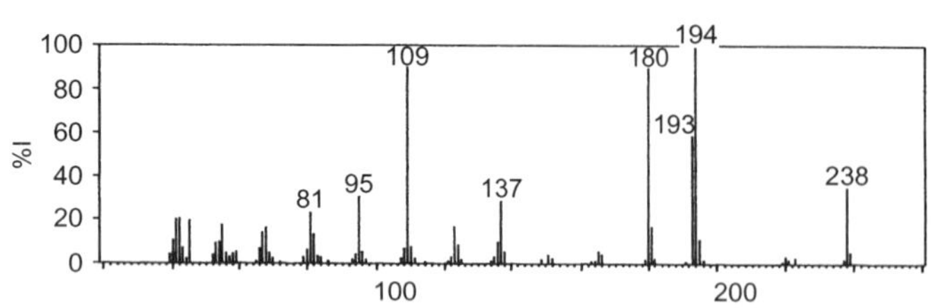

Quantification

Gas chromatography. In plasma: limit of detection 100 µg/L, ECD—A. Arbin *et al.*, *Acta Pharm. Suec.*, 1976, *13*, 235–240.

High performance liquid chromatography. In serum: limit of detection 12 µg/L, UV detection—K. Selvig and K. S. Bjerve, *Scand. J. Clin. Lab. Invest.*, 1977, *37*, 373–378. In plasma: (*R*)- and (*S*)-proxyphylline, limit of detection 0.2 mg/L—M. Ruud-Christensen *et al.*, *J. Chromatogr.*, 1989, *491*, 355–366.

Disposition in the Body. Proxyphylline is rapidly and completely absorbed after oral administration. More than 95% of a dose is excreted in the urine in 96 h with about 30% as unchanged drug, 58% as 1-methyl-7-(2-hydroxypropyl)xanthine, 10% as proxyphylline glucuronide, and 2% as 1-methyl-7-(2-hydroxypropyl)uric acid.

Therapeutic concentration
After a single oral dose of 400 mg given to 5 subjects, plasma concentrations of 7 to 13 (mean 10) mg/L were attained in 1 h. Oral dosing of 5 subjects with 400 mg three times a day for 5 days, produced peak plasma concentrations of 12 to 25 (mean 18) mg/L on the 5th day. [C. Graffner *et al.*, *Acta Pharm. Suec.*, 1973, *10*, 425–434].

Half-life. Plasma half-life, 8 to 12 (mean 9) h.

Volume of distribution. About 0.6 L/kg.

Clearance. Plasma clearance, about 0.8 mL/min/kg.

Dose. Usually 900 mg daily.

Pseudoephedrine *Sympathomimetic*

Synonyms. *d*-ψ-Ephedrine; *d*-Isoephedrine.
(α*S*)-α-[(1*S*)-1-(Methylamino)ethyl]benzenemethanol
$C_{10}H_{15}NO=165.2$
CAS—90-82-4

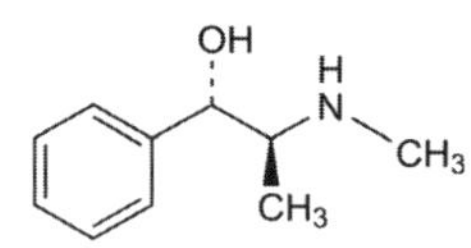

An alkaloid obtained from *Ephedra* spp. It is a stereoisomer of ephedrine.
M.p. 118.0° to 118.7° (crystals from ether).
Sparingly soluble in water; freely soluble in ethanol and ether.

Pseudoephedrine Hydrochloride

Proprietary names. Afrin; Allermed; Bronalin Decongestant; Cenafed; Contac; Decofed; DeFed; Dimetapp Decongestant; Dorcol Children's Decongestant; Drixoral Non-Drowsy; Efidac; Galpseud; Genaphed; Halofed; Seudotabs; Silfedrine; Sinustop Pro; Sudafed; Triaminic Decongestant. It is an ingredient of many proprietary preparations—see *Martindale, The complete drug reference*, 33rd Edn, London, Pharmaceutical Press, 2002.
$C_{10}H_{15}NO,HCl=201.7$
CAS—345-78-8
White crystals or powder. M.p. 182.5° to 183.5°. A solution in water is dextrorotatory.
Soluble 1 in 1.6 of water, 1 in 4 of ethanol, and 1 in 60 of chloroform; very slightly soluble in ether.

Pseudoephedrine Sulfate

Synonym. Sch-4855
Proprietary names. Drixora; Afrinol.
$(C_{10}H_{15}NO)_2,H_2SO_4=428.5$
CAS—7460-12-0
A white crystalline powder. M.p. 174° to 179°. A solution in water is dextrorotatory.
Soluble in water.

Dissociation Constant. pK_a 9.8.

Partition Coefficient. Log *P* (octanol/water), 0.9.

Thin-layer Chromatography. System TA—Rf 33; system TB—Rf 54; system TC—Rf 04; system TE—Rf 17; system TL—Rf 63; system TAE—Rf 09; system TAJ—Rf 00; system TAK—Rf 01; system TAL—Rf 30. (Acidified potassium permanganate solution, positive.)

Gas Chromatography. System GA—RI 1365; system GB—RI 1410; system GC—RI 1543.

High Performance Liquid Chromatography. System HA—pseudoephedrine *k* 1.2, norpseudoephedrine *k* 1.0; system HB—*k* 5.90; system HC—*k* 1.77; system HX—RI 237; system HY—RI 230.

Ultraviolet Spectrum. Aqueous acid—251, 257 ($A_1^1=11.9a$), 263 nm. No alkaline shift.

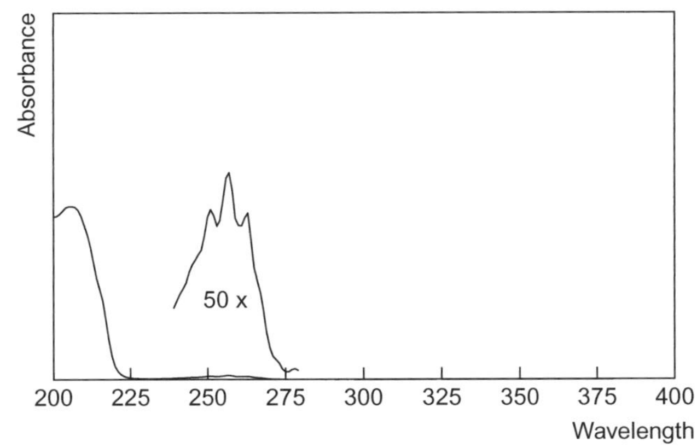

Infra-red Spectrum. Principal peaks at wavenumbers 704, 1036, 764, 1005, 1210, 1595 cm^{-1} (pseudoephedrine hydrochloride, KBr disk).

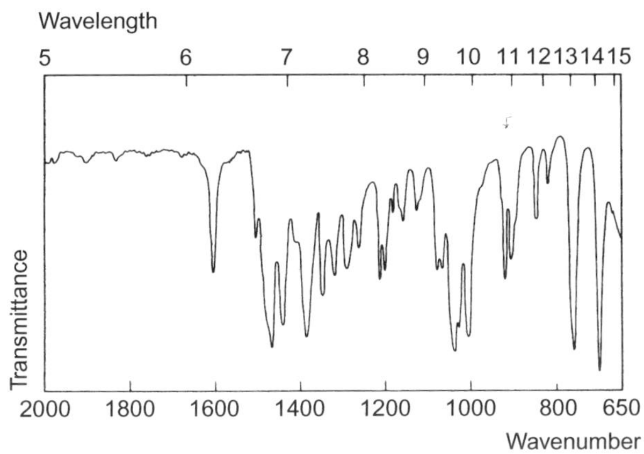

Mass Spectrum. Principal ions at *m/z* 58, 77, 59, 56, 51, 42, 105, 91.

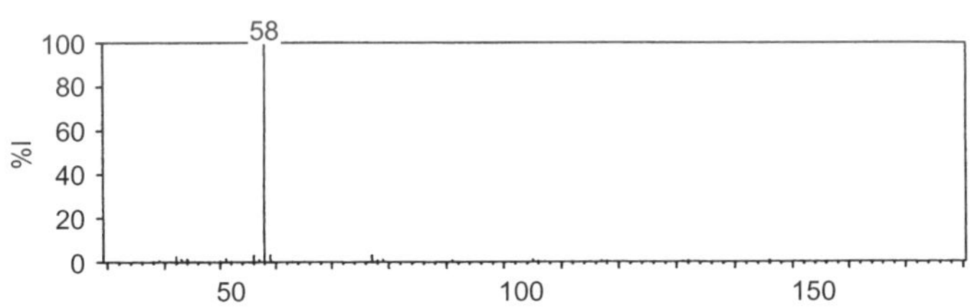

Quantification

Gas chromatography. In plasma or urine: pseudoephedrine and norpseudoephedrine, limit of detection 20 µg/L for pseudoephedrine in plasma, ECD—L. Y. Lo *et al.*, *J. Chromatogr.*, 1981, *222*; *B Biomed. Appl.*, *11*, 297–302. In serum: limit of detection 20 µg/L, ECD—S.-R. Sun and M. J. Leveque, *J. Pharm. Sci.*, 1979, *68*, 1567–1568. In urine: pseudoephedrine and other ephedrines, nitrogen–phosphorus detection—P. Van Eenoo *et al.*, *J. Chromatogr. B Biomed. Sci. Appl.*, 2001, *760*, 255–261.

High performance liquid chromatography. In urine: pseudoephedrine and other ephedrines, UV detection—C. Imaz *et al.*, *J. Chromatogr.*, 1993, *631*, 201–205. In urine: pseudoephedrine and other ephedrines, limit of quantification 0.5 mg/L, UV detection—P. J. van der Merwe *et al.*, *J. Chromatogr. B Biomed. Appl.*, 1994, *661*, 357–361. In plasma: pseudoephedrine and ephedrine, limit of quantification 1 µg/L, fluorescence detection—G. Shao *et al.*, *Yao Xue Xue Bao*, 1995, *30*, 384–389. In plasma: limit of detection 12 µg/L—P. Guo *et al.*, *Biomed. Chromatogr.*, 1999, 13, 61–64. In plasma: limit of quantification 5.8 µg/L, spectrophotometric detection—J. Macek *et al.*, *J. Chromatogr. B Anal. Technol. Biomed. Life Sci.*, 2002, *766*, 289–294.

Radioimmunoassay. In plasma: limit of detection 0.2 to 2.5 µg/L depending on the method—J. W. A. Findlay *et al.*, *J. Pharm. Sci.*, 1981, *70*, 624–631.

Disposition in the Body. Rapidly and completely absorbed after oral administration. Up to about 90% of a dose is excreted unchanged in the urine in 24 h with less than 1% as norpseudoephedrine (cathine) (pH-dependent).

Therapeutic concentration

After a single oral dose of 180 mg to 3 subjects, peak plasma concentrations of 0.72 to 0.81 mg/L were attained in 2 to 3 h [R. G. Kuntzman *et al.*, *Clin. Pharmacol. Ther.*, 1971, *12*, 62–67].

Following oral administration of 60 mg 4 times a day to 17 subjects, maximum steady-state plasma concentrations of 0.41 to 0.79 mg/L (mean 0.55) were reported about 1.5 h after a dose [J. G. Perkins *et al.*, *Curr. Ther. Res.*, 1980, *28*, 650–668].

Toxicity. Toxic effects have occurred after single doses of 60 mg.

The following postmortem tissue concentrations were reported in a fatality involving pseudoephedrine: blood 19 mg/L, brain 22 µg/g, liver 33 µg/g, urine 105 mg/L [Registry of Human Toxicology, American Academy of Forensic Sciences, 1978].

Half-life. Plasma half-life, 5 to 8 h but may be increased when the urine is alkaline and decreased when it is acid.

Volume of distribution. About 3 L/kg.

Dose. Usually 180 to 240 mg of pseudoephedrine hydrochloride daily.

Pseudomorphine

Synonyms. 2,2′-Bimorphine; Oxydimorphine
(5′α,6′α)-7,7′,8,8′-Tetradehydro-4,5:4′,5′-diepoxy-17,17′-dimethyl-[2,2′-bimorphinan]-3,3′,6,6′-tetrol
$C_{34}H_{36}N_2O_6,3H_2O = 622.7$
CAS—125-24-6 (anhydrous); 6472-73-7 (trihydrate)
White crystals (trihydrate). Becomes anhydrous at 150°; m.p. 327°, with decomposition.
Practically insoluble in water, ethanol, and ether; soluble in dilute hydrochloric acid, dilute acetic acid, and pyridine (pseudomorphine trihydrate).

Colour Test. Marquis Test—green.

Thin-layer Chromatography. System TA—Rf 46; system TB—Rf 00; system TC—Rf 00; system TL—Rf 00; system TAJ—Rf 00; system TAK—Rf 00; system TAL—Rf 02. (Acidified iodoplatinate solution, positive.)

Gas Chromatography. System GA—RI 2770.

Ultraviolet Spectrum. Aqueous acid—231 nm ($A_1^1 = 308$b).

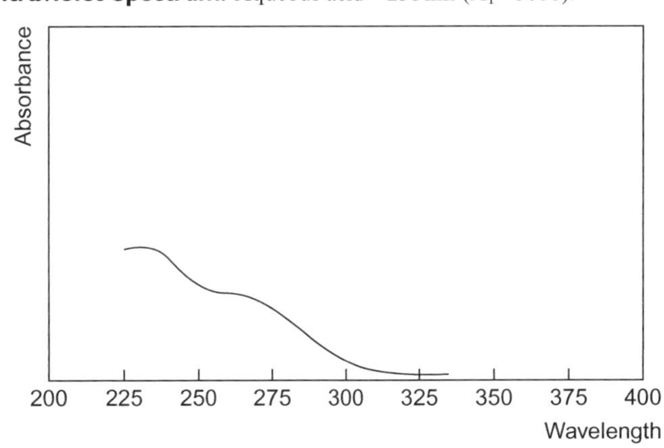

Infra-red Spectrum. Principal peaks at wavenumbers 1118, 1098, 1069, 1044, 1195, 1210 cm^{-1} (KBr disk).

Mass Spectrum. Principal ions at *m/z* 30, 44, 42, 568, 31, 58, 27, 81.

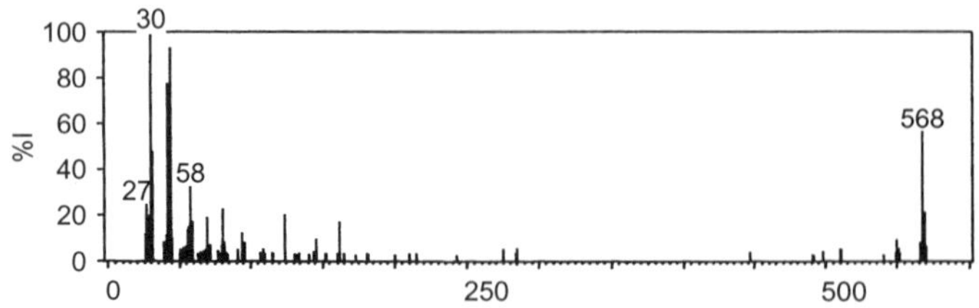

Note. Pseudomorphine may be found as an oxidation product of morphine in decomposed viscera.

Psilocin

Hallucinogen

Synonym. 4-Hydroxy-*N*,*N*-dimethyltryptamine
3-[2-(Dimethylamino)ethyl]-1*H*-indol-4-ol
$C_{12}H_{16}N_2O$=204.3
CAS—520-53-6

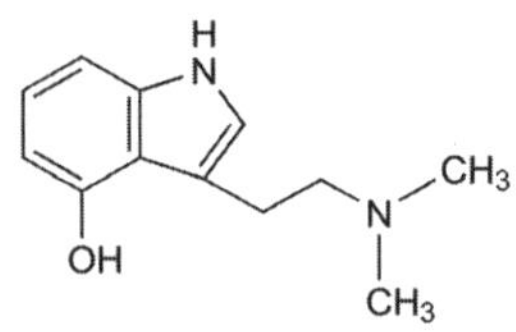

An indole alkaloid obtained from the Mexican mushroom (Teonanácatl) *Psilocybe mexicana* (Agaricaceae).
White crystals. M.p. 173° to 176°.
Soluble in ethanol and dilute acetic acid; very slightly soluble in water. Unstable in solution, especially alkaline solution.

Partition Coefficient. Log *P* (octanol/water), 1.5.

Colour Test. Marquis Test—green-brown.

Thin-layer Chromatography. System TA—psilocin Rf 39; system TB—psilocin Rf 05, psilocin-ethyl Rf 09; system TC—psilocin Rf 09, psilocin-ethyl Rf 15; system TE—psilocin Rf 47, psilocin-ethyl Rf 65; system TL—psilocin Rf 09, psilocin-ethyl Rf 25; system TAE—psilocin Rf 14, psilocin-ethyl Rf 15; system TAF—psilocin Rf 48, psilocin-ethyl Rf 67. (Van Urk reagent, faint blue.)

Gas Chromatography. System GA—psilocin RI 1985; psilocin-AC RI 2270; psilocin-AC_2 RI 2340; system GB—psilocin RI 2080.

High Performance Liquid Chromatography. System HA—*k* 3.1 (tailing peak); system HX—RI 240; system HY—RI 226.

Ultraviolet Spectrum. Aqueous acid—266, 283, 292 nm; aqueous alkali—270, 293 nm.

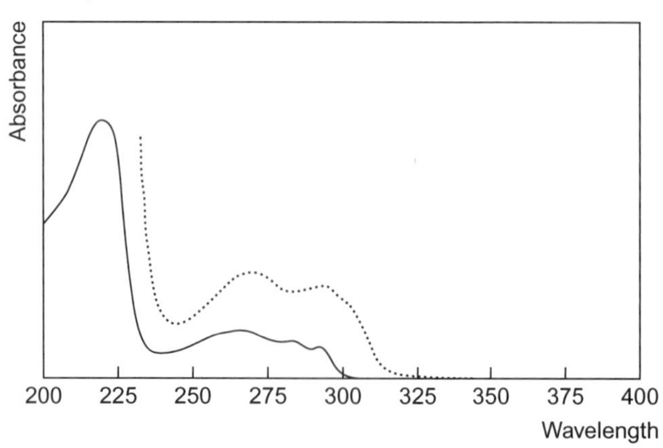

Infra-red Spectrum. Principal peaks at wavenumbers 836, 1261, 1236, 1042, 1061, 733 cm^{-1}.

Mass Spectrum. Principal ions at *m/z* 58, 204, 59, 42, 30, 146, 77, 44.

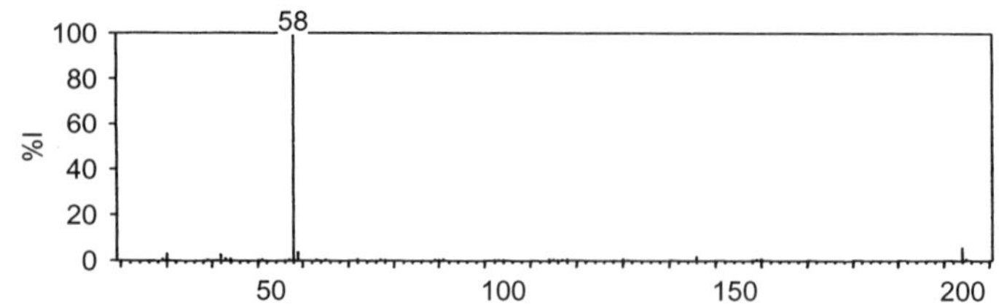

Quantification
Gas chromatography–mass spectrometry. In plasma or urine—G. Sticht and H. Kaferstein, *Forensic Sci. Int.*, 2000, *113*, 403–407. In urine: limit of detection 10 µg/L—A. F. Greishaber *et al.*, *J. Forensic Sci.*, 2001, *46*, 627–630.

High performance liquid chromatography. In plasma: psilocin and 4-hydroxyindole-3-acetic acid, ECD—F. Hasler *et al.*, *Pharm. Acta Helv.*, 1997, *72*, 175–184. In plasma: limit of detection 10 µg/L, ECD—H. Lindenblatt *et al.*, *J. Chromatogr. B. Biomed. Sci. Appl.*, 1998, *709*, 255–263.

Disposition in the Body. Absorbed from the gastro-intestinal tract. It is a metabolite of psilocybine. An oral dose of several milligrams may produce hallucinations and related effects.

Psilocybine

Hallucinogen

Synonyms. 4-Phosphoryloxy-*N*,*N*-dimethyltryptamine; CY-39; Psilocybin.
3-[2-(Dimethylamino)ethyl]-1*H*-indol-4-ol dihydrogen phosphate ester
$C_{12}H_{17}N_2O_4P$=284.3
CAS—520-52-5

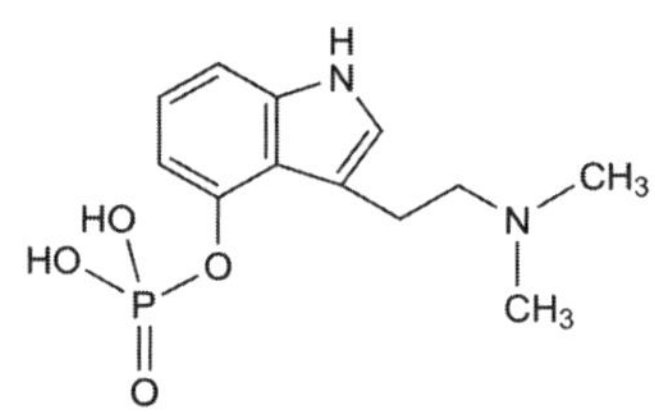

The main indole alkaloid present in the sacred Mexican mushroom (Teonanácatl), *Psilocybe mexicana* (Agaricaceae). In the UK, psilocybine is present in the indigenous mushroom *Psilocybe semilanceata* (magic mushroom; liberty cap). Psilocybine is also present in the mushrooms *Stropharia cubensis* and *Conocybe* spp.
White crystals. M.p. 185° to 195°(crystals from boiling methanol), with decomposition.
Soluble in 20 parts boiling water, in 120 parts boiling methanol and dilute acetic acid; practically insoluble in chloroform and benzene.

Partition Coefficient. Log *P* (octanol/water), 1.00.

Colour Test. Marquis Test—orange.

Thin-layer Chromatography. System TA—Rf 05; system TB—Rf 00; system TE—Rf 00; system TL—Rf 00; system TAE—Rf 80; system TAF—Rf 01. (Van Urk reagent, grey-violet.)

Gas Chromatography. System GA—RI 2046; system GAM—Retention time 6.9 min.

High Performance Liquid Chromatography. System HY—RI 185; system HBF—*k* 3.20.

Ultraviolet Spectrum. Aqueous acid—268; aqueous alkali—269, 282, 292 nm.

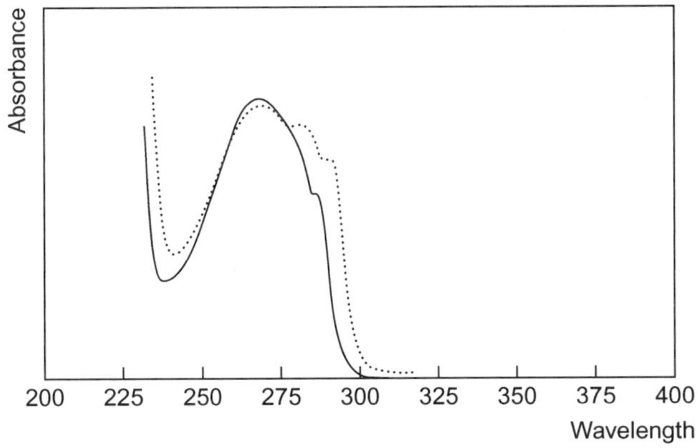

Infra-red Spectrum. Principal peaks at wavenumbers 1105, 1045, 1062, 1183, 1160, 932 cm^{-1} (KBr disk).

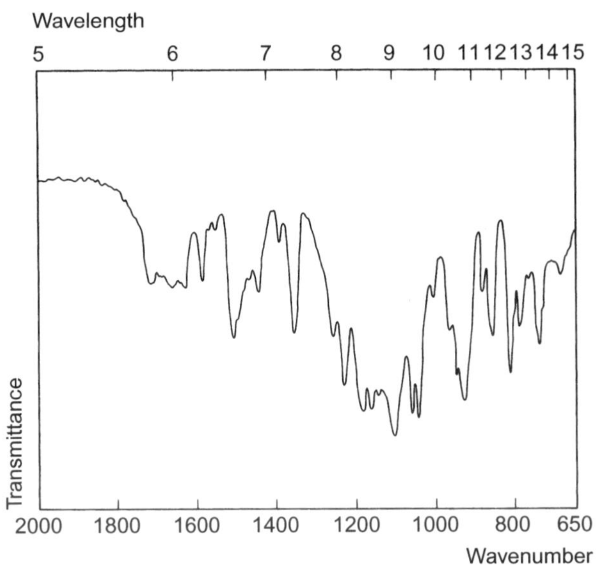

Mass Spectrum. Principal ions at *m/z* 58, 42, 30, 51, 204, 146, 77, 44.

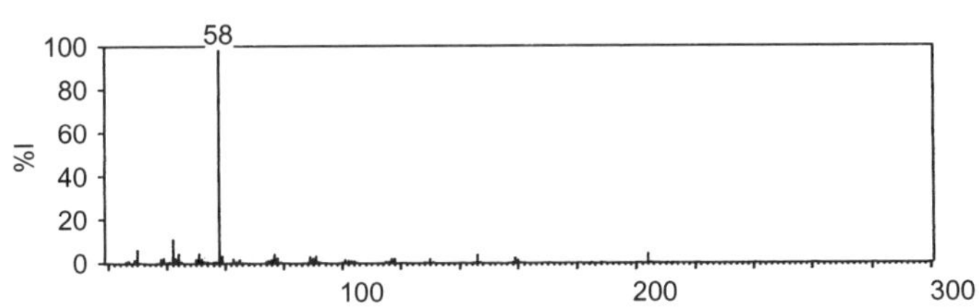

Quantification

Gas chromatography–mass spectrometry. In blood or urine: psilocybine and psilocin—G. Sticht and H. Kaferstein, *Forensic Sci. Int.*, 2000, *113*, 403–407. In urine: limit of quantification 10 μg/L—A. F. Grieshaber *et al.*, *J. Forensic Sci.*, 2001, *46*, 627–630.

High performance liquid chromatography. In plasma: psilocin and 4-hydroxyindole-3-acetic acid, electrochemical detection—F. Hasler *et al.*, *Pharm. Acta Helv.*, 1997, *72*, 175–184. In plasma: limit of quantification 10 μg/L psilocin, ECD—H. Lindenblatt *et al.*, *J. Chromatogr. B Biomed. Sci. Appl.*, 1998, *709*, 255–263.

Disposition in the Body. Absorbed from the gastro-intestinal tract; hallucinogenic effects usually occur within 30 min of ingestion with a duration of effect of about 6 h. It is rapidly dephosphorylated to psilocin which appears to be the psychoactive compound.

Blood concentration

6 healthy volunteers were administered a single 10 to 20 mg (mean, 0.22 mg/kg body weight) oral dose and 1 mg IV dose of psilocybine. After the oral dose, the mean peak plasma psilocin concentration was 8.2 μg/L at 105 min and the peak 4-hydroxyindole-3-acetic acid concentration was 150 μg/L at 113 min. After the IV dose, the mean psilocin concentration was 12.9 μg/L 1.9 min after administration [F. Hasler *et al.*, *Pharm. Acta Helv.*, 1997, *72*, 175–184].

Toxicity

In one case where 2 young males ingested 4 to 5 g of 'magic mushrooms', the majority of psilocybine was metabolised to psilocin and excreted as the glucuronide. Psilocin was detected in serum at a concentration of 0.018 mg/L (free psilocin) and 0.052 mg/L (total). The concentration of free psilocin in urine was 0.23 mg/L with a total amount of 1.76 mg/L. It was noted that, 5 to 6 h after ingestion, they showed unstable and sluggish walking, inarticulate speech, enlarged pupils, dazed consciousness, depression and retarded behaviour [G. Sticht and H. Kaferstein, *Forensic Sci. Int.*, 2000, *113*, 403–407].

Note. For a study of the renal excretion profiles of psilocin in man following oral administration of psilocybine, see F. Hasler *et al.*, *J. Pharm. Biomed. Anal.*, 2002, *30*, 331.

Pumactant

Pulmonary Surfactant

Synonym. ALEC

Dipalmitoylphosphatidylcholine and egg phosphatidylglycerol in a 7:3 (w/w) ratio

Fine crystalline powder.

Note. For a study of pumactant for treatment of respiratory distress syndrome in neonates, see S. B. Ainsworth *et al.*, *Lancet*, 2000, *355*, 1387–1392; for a review of natural versus synthetic surfactants in neonatal respiratory distress syndrome, see H. L. Halliday, *Drugs*, 1996, *51*, 226–237.

Putrescine

Putrefactive Base

Synonym. Tetramethylenediamine

1,4-Butanediamine

$NH_2[CH_2]_4NH_2=88.2$

CAS—110-60-1

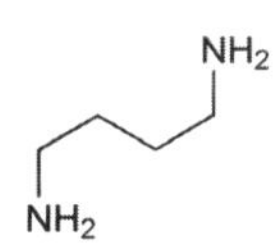

Crystals with a strong odour. M.p. 23° to 24°. B.p. 158° to 160°.

Very soluble in water.

Dissociation Constant. pK_a 10.8 (20°).

Partition Coefficient. Log *P* (octanol/water), −0.7.

Colour Test. Ninhydrin—violet.

Thin-layer Chromatography. System TA—Rf 09. (Acidified iodoplatinate solution, positive.)

Gas Chromatography. System GA—RI 930.

Infra-red Spectrum. Principal peaks at wavenumbers 1118, 874, 1288, 923, 1026, 1036 cm^{-1} (KBr disk).

Quantification

Gas chromatography. In urine: putrescine and other polyamines and their metabolites, nitrogen–phosphorus detection—F. A. Muskiet *et al.*, *Clin. Chem.*, 1984, *30*, 687–695. In serum: putrescine and cadaverine, limit of detection 0.5 to 0.6 ng/injection, FID—M. Y. Khuhawar *et al.*, *J. Chromatogr. B, Biomed. Sci. Appl.*, 1999, *723*, 17–24.

High performance liquid chromatography. In cancer cell homogenates: putrescine and other natural polyamines and monoacetyl conjugates: limits of detection 30 to 130 fmol for putrescine, fluorescence detection—T. Weiss *et al.*, *Anal. Biochem.*, 1997, *247*, 294–304. In urine: putrescine and other polyamines, limits of detection 2 to 10 μg/L—C. Molins-Legua *et al.*, *Analyst*, 1999, *124*, 477–482.

Pyrantel

Anthelmintic

Synonym. Pirantel
(*E*)-1,4,5,6-Tetrahydro-1-methyl-2-[2-(2-thienyl)ethenyl]pyrimidine
$C_{11}H_{14}N_2S$=206.3
CAS—15686-83-6

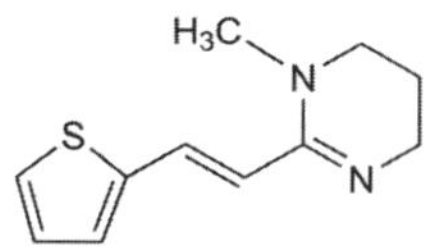

Crystals. M.p. 178° to 179°.

Pyrantel Embonate

Synonyms. Pyrantel Pamoate; CP-10423-16.
Proprietary names. Anthel; Antiminth; Ascarical; Banminth (vet.); Bantel; Canex (vet.); Combantrin; Early Bird; Helmex; Helmintox; Lombriareu; Nemex (vet.); Pin-Rid; Pin-X; Pirantrim; Pyral; Pyrantrin; Pyrapam; Reese's Pinworm; Strongid (vet.); Trilombrin.
$C_{11}H_{14}N_2S,C_{23}H_{16}O_6$=594.7
CAS—22204-24-6
A yellow to tan-coloured crystalline powder.
Practically insoluble in water, ethanol and methanol; soluble in dimethyl sulfoxide.

Pyrantel Tartrate

Synonym. CP-10423-18
$C_{11}H_{14}N_2S,C_4H_6O_6$=356.4
CAS—33401-94-4
A white to pale greenish-yellow, crystalline powder. M.p. 148° to 150°.
Soluble 1 in 5 of water and 1 in 9 of methanol; slightly soluble in chloroform; practically insoluble in ether.

Dissociation Constant. pK_a 11.0 (20°).

Partition Coefficient. Log *P* (octanol/water), 3.1.

Colour Tests. Liebermann's test—black; Mandelin's test—violet; Marquis test—blue-violet; Sulfuric acid—orange→violet.

Thin-layer Chromatography. System TA—Rf 06. (Acidified iodoplatinate solution, positive.)

Gas Chromatography. System GA—not eluted.

High Performance Liquid Chromatography. System HX—RI 299.

Ultraviolet Spectrum. Methanolic acid—315 nm (A_1^1=920a).

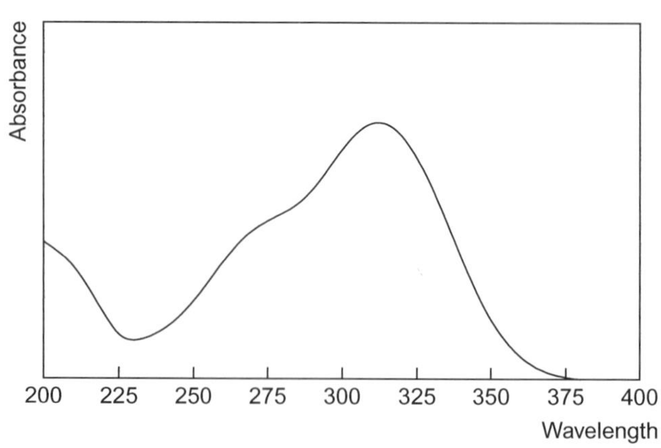

Infra-red Spectrum. Principal peaks at wavenumbers 1640, 1605, 1305, 1208, 1132, 1065 cm^{-1} (pyrantel tartrate, KBr disk).

Mass Spectrum. Principal ions at *m/z* 205, 42, 135, 173, 206, 123, 145, 45.

Dose. The equivalent of 10 to 20 mg/kg of pyrantel, as a single dose.

Pyrazinamide

Tuberculostatic

Synonym. Pyrazinoic Acid Amide; D-50.
Proprietary names. Braccopiral; Pirafoid; Piraldina; Piraside; Pirazer; Pirilene; Pramide; Premox; Pyrafat; Pyratab; PZA; Rozide; Tebezide; Tebrazid; Tisamid; Zinamide.
Pyrazinecarboxamide
$C_5H_5N_3O$=123.1
CAS—98-96-4

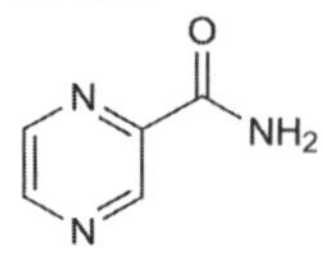

A white crystalline powder. M.p. 189° to 191°; begins to sublime at 60°. Soluble 1 in about 60 of water and 1 in 175 of dehydrated ethanol, 1 in 135 of chloroform, 1 in 1000 of ether and 1 in 72 of methanol.

Dissociation Constant. pK_a 0.5.

Partition Coefficient. Log *P* (octanol/water), −0.6.

Colour Test. Nessler's reagent—brown-orange.

Thin-layer Chromatography. System TA—Rf 63; system TB—Rf 03; system TC—Rf 42; system TE—Rf 54; system TL—Rf 46; system TAD—Rf 44; system TAE—Rf 71; system TAF—Rf 70.

Gas Chromatography. System GA—RI 1250.

High Performance Liquid Chromatography. System HAA—Retention time(s) 3.8 min.

Ultraviolet Spectrum. Aqueous acid—269 nm (A_1^1=659a), 312 nm. No alkaline shift. (See below)

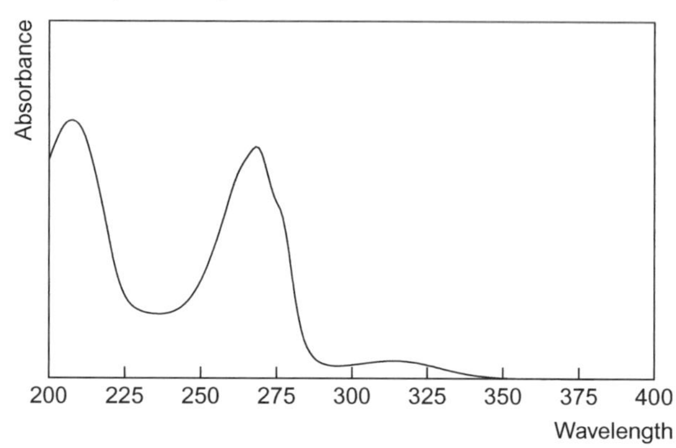

Infra-red Spectrum. Principal peaks at wavenumbers 1685, 1020, 1600, 1584, 1050, 1165 cm^{-1} (KBr disk).

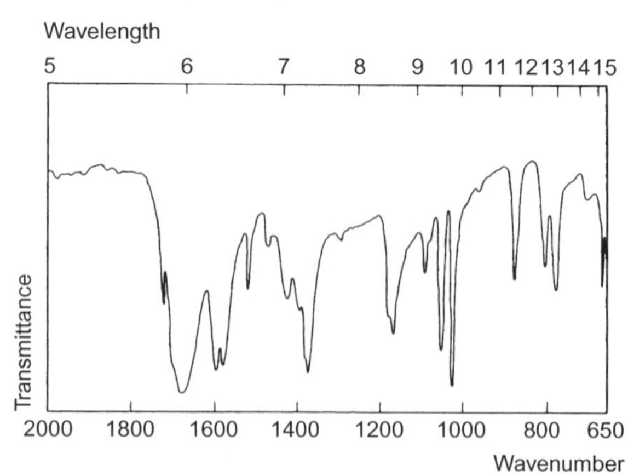

Quantification

Gas chromatography–mass spectrometry. In serum or urine: pyrazinamide, pyrazine-2-carboxylic acid and 5-hydroxypyrazine-2-carboxylic acid, limit of detection 10 μg/L for pyrazinamide—J. Roboz *et al.*, *J. Chromatogr.*, 1978, *147*, 337–347.

High performance liquid chromatography. In plasma: limit of detection 0.2 mg/0.2 mL—S. N. Revankar *et al.*, *J. Postgrad. Med.*, 1994, *40*, 7–9. In plasma: pyrazinamide and its metabolites—H. J. Kraemer *et al.*, *J. Chromatogr. B, Biomed. Sci. Appl.*, 1998, *706*, 319–328. In plasma, bronchoalveolar lavage, or alveolar cells: UV detection—J. E. Conte *et al.*, *J. Chromatogr. Sci.*, 2000, *38*, 33–37. In plasma: pyrazinamide, rifampicin and isoniazid, UV detection—A. Walubo *et al.*, *J. Chromatogr. B, Biomed. Appl.*, 1994, *658*, 391–396. In plasma: pyrazinamide, rifampicin and isoniazid—P. J. Smith *et al.*, *Int. J. Tuberc. Lung Dis.*, 1999, *3 (Suppl. 3)*, S325–S328 and S351–S352. In serum: pyrazinamide and other antituberculosis drugs, limit of detection about 90 µg/L—M. C. Gennaro *et al.*, *J. Chromatogr. B, Biomed. Sci. Appl.*, 2001, *754*, 477–486. In blood: pyrazinamide, isoniazid and rifampicin, limits of detection 0.11, 0.2 and 13 ng/5 µL, respectively, UV detection—M. Y. Khuhawar and F. M. Rind, *J. Chromatogr. B, Analyt. Technol. Biomed. Life Sci.*, 2002, *766*, 357–363.

Disposition in the Body. Pyrazinamide is well absorbed after oral administration. It is metabolised by hydrolysis to pyrazine-2-carboxylic acid and subsequent hydroxylation to 5-hydroxypyrazine-2-carboxylic acid. In 24 h, about 30 to 40% of a dose is excreted in the urine as pyrazine-2-carboxylic acid and less than 4% as unchanged drug; the 5-hydroxy metabolite is also excreted in the urine.

Therapeutic concentration

After an oral dose of 3 g to one subject, a peak serum concentration of 134 mg/L was attained in 1 h; the serum concentration of pyrazine-2-carboxylic acid was 20 to 30 mg/L after the first hour and the concentration of 5-hydroxypyrazine-2-carboxylic acid ranged between 3 and 8 mg/L over a period of 12 h. [J. Roboz *et al.*, *J. Chromatogr.*, 1978, *147*, 337–347].

Half-life. Plasma half-life, 4 to 10 h.

Protein binding. About 50%.

Dose. 20 to 35 mg/kg to a maximum of 3 g daily.

Pyrazophos

Fungicide

Synonyms. HOE 2873; W11099.
Proprietary names. Afugan; Curamil; Missile; Pokon Mildew Spray; Siafos.
2-[(Diethoxyphosphinothioyl)oxy]-5-methylpyrazolo[1,5-*a*]pyrimidine-6-carboxylic acid ethyl ester
$C_{14}H_{20}N_3O_5PS = 373.4$
CAS—13457-18-6

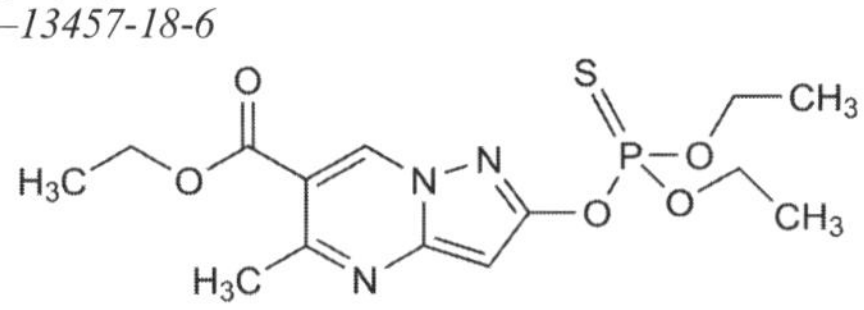

A yellow oil. M.p. 38° to 40°. It is soluble in water (4.2 mg/L at 20°), acetone (1212 g/L at 25°), toluene (>980 g/L at 25°), ethyl acetate (898 g/L at 25°), ethanol (95 g/L at 25°) and hexane (11 g/L at 25°); readily soluble in most organic solvents.

Partition Coefficient. Log *P* (octanol/water), 3.80.

Thin-Layer Chromatography. System TX—Rf 32; system TY—Rf 47.

Gas Chromatography. System GA—RI 2590.

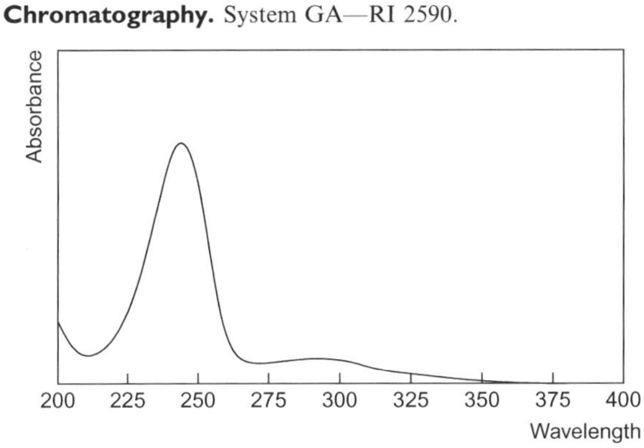

Mass Spectrum. Principal ions at *m/z* 221, 232, 97, 237, 373, 65, 265, 193.

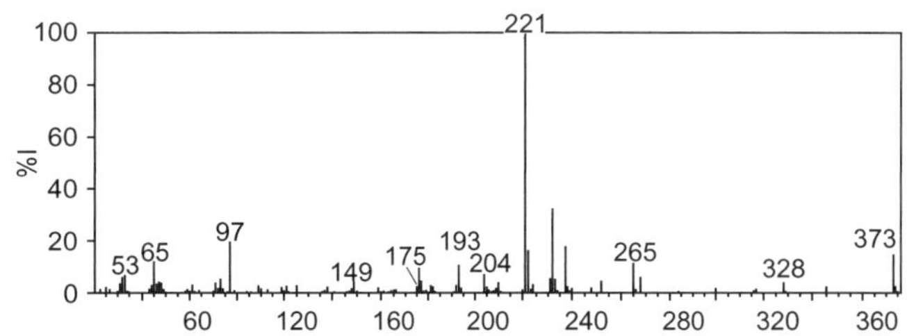

Toxicity. The allowed daily intake is 0.004 mg/kg bodyweight.

Pyrethrum

Insecticide, Scabicide

Synonyms. Pyrethrum Flower; Chrysantheme Insecticide; Insektenbluten; Pyrethriflos.
Proprietary names. Allethrin; Anerin; Buhach; Chrysanthenum Cinerariaefolium; Cypermethrin; Dalmatian Insect Powder; Decamethrin; Firmotox; Flucythrinate; Moskill; Ofirmotox; Parexan; Persian Insect Powder; Piretro; Prothrin; Resmethrin.
$C_{(20-22)}H_{(28,30)}O_{(3,5)} = 316–374$
CAS—8000-33-47

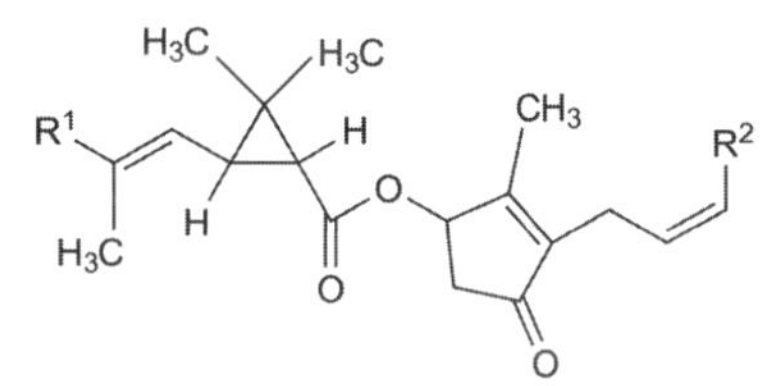

	R1	R2
Pyrethrin-I	CH_3	$CH{=}CH_2$
Pyrethrin-II	$COOCH_3$	$CH{=}CH_2$
Cinerin-I	CH_3	CH_3
Cinerin-II	$COOCH_3$	CH_3

Pyrethrum extract is a mixture of three naturally occurring esters of chrysanthemic acid (Pyrethrins I: pyrethrin 1, cinerin 1 and jasmolin 1) and three esters of pyrethric acid (Pyrethrins II: pyrethrin 2, cinerin 2 and jasmolin 2) with the molecular weight varying between 316 and 374. It is a pale yellow to brown viscous liquid or oil. It is practically insoluble in water but soluble in liquid paraffin and most organic solvents including alcohol, kerosene, nitromethane, petroleum ether, carbon tetrachloride and ethylene dichloride.

Pyrethrin I

Synonyms. Chrysanthemummonocarboxylic Acid Pyrethrolone Ester; Pyrethronyl (+)-*trans*-chrysanthemate.
$C_{21}H_{28}O_3 = 328.5$
CAS—121-21-1
A viscous liquid with solubility as for the pyrethrum extract.

Pyrethrin II

Synonyms. Pyrethrine; Pyrethronyl (+)-pyrethrate.
$C_{22}H_{28}O_5 = 372.5$
CAS—121-29-9
A viscous liquid with solubility as for the pyrethrum extract.

Gas Chromatography. System GK— Pyrethrin I RRT 1.27, pyrethrin II RRT 1.59 (both relative to caffeine).

Ultraviolet Spectrum. Ethanol—225 nm (Pyrethrin I) and 229 nm (Pyrethrin II).

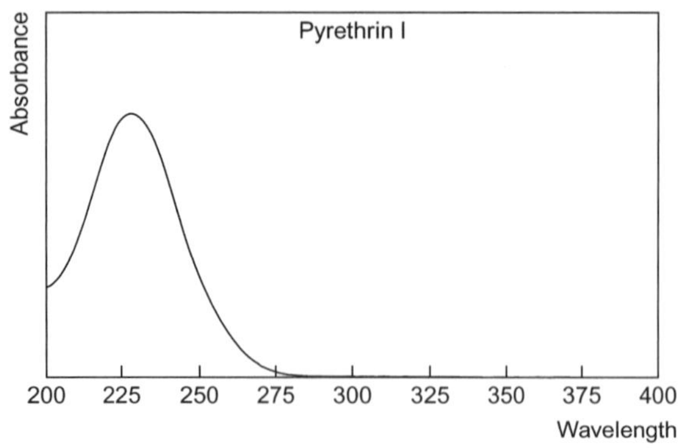

Disposition in the Body. Pyrethrum is absorbed through the stomach, intestines and the skin quite slowly and more quickly through the lungs during respiration. It is metabolised to chrysanthemumic acid and alcohol which can be further metabolised to aldehyde and acid or conjugated with glucuronide. It is excreted in urine and faeces. The metabolites are less toxic than the parent compound. Pyrethrins I and II are excreted unchanged in faeces and the other pyrethrum components undergo rapid destruction and detoxification in the liver and gastro-intestinal tract.

Toxicity. The lowest lethal oral dose for children is 750 mg/kg bodyweight and for adults, 1000 mg/kg. The allowed daily intake is 0.04 mg/kg bodyweight.

Pyridostigmine Bromide

Anticholinesterase

Proprietary names. Mestinon; Regonol.
3-[[(Dimethylamino)carbonyl]oxy]-1-methylpyridinium bromide
$C_9H_{13}BrN_2O_2$=261.1
CAS—155-97-5 (pyridostigmine); 101-26-8 (bromide)

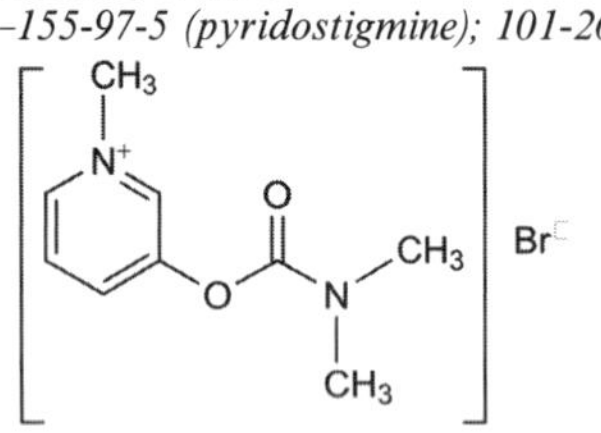

A white, deliquescent, crystalline powder. M.p. 152° to 154°.
Soluble 1 in less than 1 of water, 1 in less than 1 of ethanol and 1 in 1 of chloroform; practically insoluble in ether, acetone and benzene.

Partition Coefficient. Log *P* (octanol/water), −3.7.

Thin-layer Chromatography. System TA—Rf 04; system TB—Rf 00; system TE—Rf 00; system TF—Rf 00; system TAE—Rf 00. (Acidified iodoplatinate solution, positive.)

Gas Chromatography. System GA—RI 1515.

High Performance Liquid Chromatography. System HA—*k* 6.3 (tailing peak); system HX—RI 65; system HZ—Retention time(s) 1.8 min; system HAA—Retention time(s) 3.2 min.

Ultraviolet Spectrum. Aqueous acid—270 nm (A^1_1=186a).

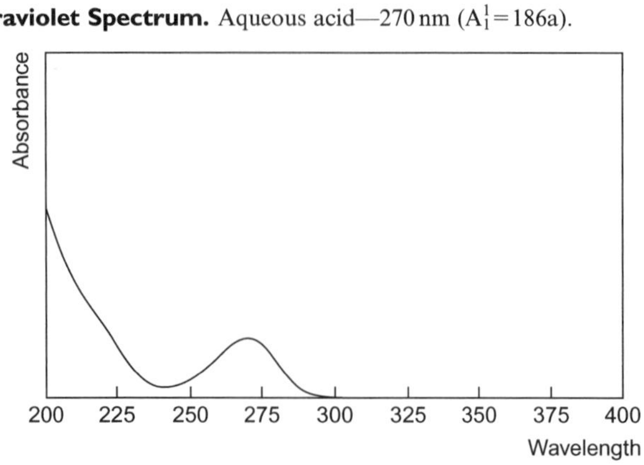

Infra-red Spectrum. Principal peaks at wavenumbers 1728, 1156, 1249, 1500, 1630, 1010 cm^{-1} (KBr disk).

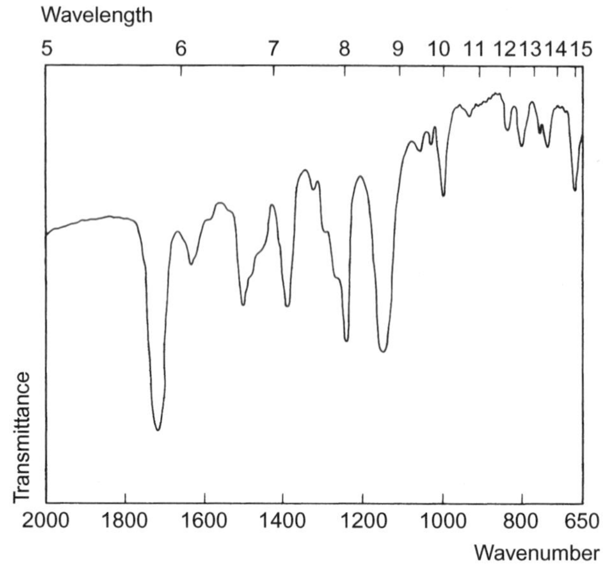

Mass Spectrum. Principal ions at *m*/*z* 72, 39, 42, 38, 94, 56, 51, 81.

Quantification

Gas chromatography. In plasma: limit of detection 5 µg/L, AFID—K. Chan *et al.*, *J. Chromatogr.*, 1976, *120*, 349–358.

Gas chromatography–mass spectrometry. In plasma: limit of detection 50 µg/L—S. M. Aquilonius *et al.*, *Eur. J. Clin. Pharmacol.*, 1980, *18*, 423–428.

High performance liquid chromatography. In blood or urine: limit of detection 40 µg/L—R. I. Ellin *et al.*, *J. Chromatogr.*, 1982, *228*; *Biomed. Appl.*, *17*, 235–244.

High performance liquid chromatography–mass spectrometry. In plasma: limit of detection 1 µg/L—S. L. Malcolm *et al.*, *J. Pharm. Biomed. Anal.*, 1990, *8*, 771–776.

Disposition in the Body. Pyridostigmine bromide is poorly and irregularly absorbed after oral administration and may undergo significant first-pass metabolism. Up to about 16% of an oral dose is excreted in the urine unchanged, together with small amounts of 3-hydroxy-*N*-methylpyridinium. After intravenous administration, up to about 90% is excreted in the urine unchanged.

Therapeutic concentration. In plasma, usually in the range 0.05 to 0.1 mg/L.

After a single oral dose of 120 mg to 5 subjects, peak plasma concentrations of about 0.04 to 0.07 mg/L were attained in 1 to 2 h. [S. M. Aquilonius *et al.*, *Eur. J. Clin. Pharmacol.*, 1980, *18*, 423–428].

Following daily oral doses of 60 to 660 mg to 6 subjects, maximum steady-state plasma concentrations of 0.04 to 0.08 mg/L were reported. [T. N. Calvey and K. Chan, *Clin. Pharmacol. Ther.*, 1977, *21*, 187–193].

Half-life. Plasma half-life, 0.3 to 2 h, increased in subjects with renal disease.

Volume of distribution. About 1 L/kg.

Clearance. Plasma clearance, about 8 to 16 mL/min/kg.

Dose. Usually 0.3 to 1.2 g daily.

Pyridoxine

Vitamin

Synonyms. Adermine; Pyridoxol; Vitamin B_6.
5-Hydroxy-6-methyl-3,4-pyridinedimethanol
$C_8H_{11}NO_3$=169.2
CAS—65-23-6

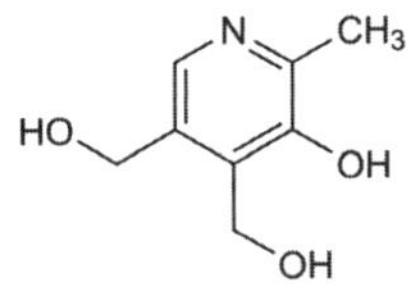

Pyridoxine Hydrochloride

Proprietary names. Aminoxin; Anacrodyne; Bécilan; Bedoxine; Beesix; Benadon; Bonasanit; Carthamex; Comploment; Conductasa; Dermo 6; Heksavit; Hexobion; Lactosec; Memosprint; Metadoxil; Pyroxin; Surfoxide; Vicotrat; Vita-B6; Xanturenasi.

$C_8H_{11}NO_3,HCl=205.6$

CAS—58-56-0

A white crystalline powder or crystals. M.p. 205° to 212°, with decomposition. Soluble 1 in 5 of water and 1 in about 90 of ethanol; practically insoluble in chloroform and ether; sparingly soluble in acetone.

Dissociation Constant. pK_a 5.0 (–N=), 9.0 (–OH), (25°).

Partition Coefficient. Log P (octanol/water), −0.8 (pyridoxine).

Colour Test. Mandelin's test–blue→grey-green.

Thin-layer Chromatography. System TA—Rf 59; system TB—Rf 00; system TC—Rf 08; system TE—Rf 15; system TL—Rf 05; system TAE—Rf 75; system TAF—Rf 67. (Acidified potassium permanganate solution, positive.)

High Performance Liquid Chromatography. System HAA—Retention time(s) 2.9 min; system HX—RI 65.

Ultraviolet Spectrum. Aqueous acid—290 .nm ($A_1^1=523a$); phosphate buffer (pH 6.88)—254 nm ($A_1^1=219a$), 324 nm ($A_1^1=426a$).

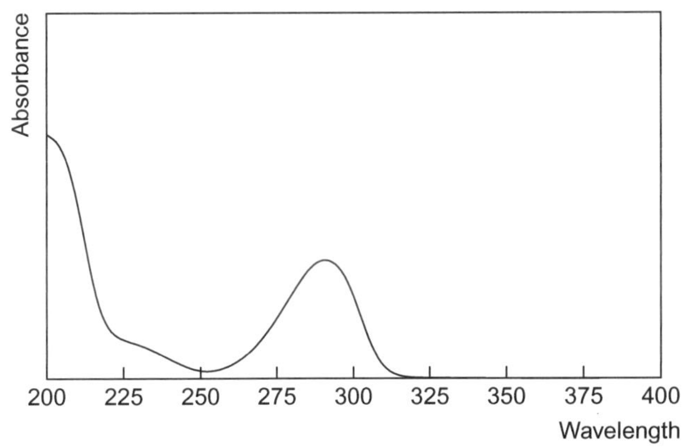

Infra-red Spectrum. Principal peaks at wavenumbers 1277, 1212, 1015, 1540, 870, 1086 cm^{-1} (pyridoxine hydrochloride, KBr disk).

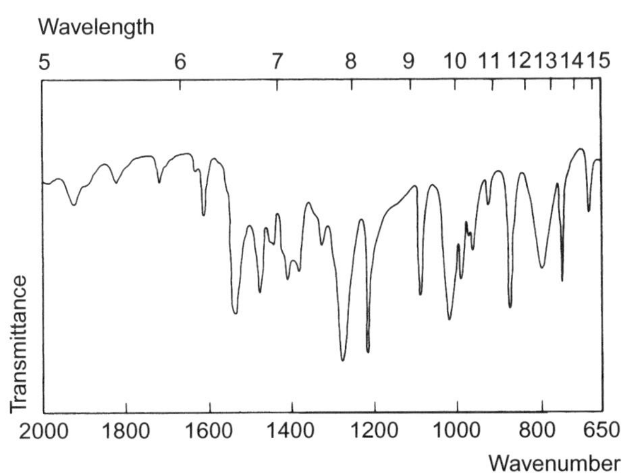

Mass Spectrum. Principal ions at *m/z* 151, 94, 122, 106, 51, 53, 149, 150.

Quantification

High performance liquid chromatography. In plasma or urine: pyridoxine, pyridoxal and 4-pyridoxic acid, limit of detection 300 µg/L for plasma, 500 µg/L for urine, UV detection—W. J. O'Reilly *et al.*, *J. Chromatogr.*, 1980, *183*; *Biomed. Appl.*, *9*, 492–498. In plasma: pyridoxal 5′-phosphate, fluorescence detection—N. Hirose *et al.*, *J. Nutr. Sci. Vitaminol. (Tokyo)*, 1990, *36*, 521–529. In plasma: pyridoxal 5′-phosphate, limit of detection 50 fmol, fluorescence detection—S. Kurioka *et al.*, *Biomed. Chromatogr.*, 1993, *7*, 162–165. In plasma: pyridoxal, limit of detection 2 µg/L, fluorescence detection—H. Mascher, *J. Pharm. Sci.*, 1993, *82*, 972–974. In plasma: pyridoxal and pyridoxal 5′-phosphate, fluorescence detection—M. Kimura *et al.*, *J. Chromatogr. A*, 1996, *722*, 296–301. In plasma: pyridoxine, pyridoxal 5′-phosphate, pyidoxal, pyridoxamine and pyridoxamine 5′-phosphate, fluorescence detection—M. R. Bisp *et al.*, *Anal. Biochem.*, 2002, *305*, 82–89.

Disposition in the Body. Pyridoxine is absorbed from the gastrointestinal tract and converted to the active form, pyridoxal phosphate. It is excreted in the urine, mainly as 4-pyridoxic acid.

Protein binding. In plasma, pyridoxine not significantly bound, pyridoxal phosphate almost completely bound.

Dose. 20 to 200 mg of pyridoxine hydrochloride daily.

Pyrimethamine

Antimalarial

Proprietary names. Daraprim; Erbaprelina; Malocide. It is an ingredient of Fansidar, Maloprim, Madomine; Supacox (vet.), Vivaxine and Whitsyn S (vet.).

5-(4-Chlorophenyl)-6-ethyl-2,4-pyrimidinediamine

$C_{12}H_{13}ClN_4=248.7$

CAS—58-14-0

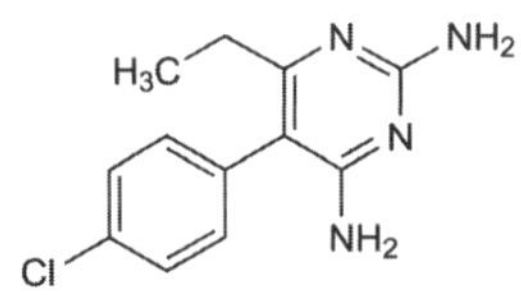

A white crystalline powder. M.p. 233°to 234°(capillary); m.p. 240° to 242° (copper block).

Practically insoluble in water; soluble 1 in 200 of ethanol and 1 in 125 of chloroform; slightly soluble in acetone; soluble in warm dilute mineral acids.

Dissociation Constant. pK_a 7.3 (20°).

Partition Coefficient. Log *P* (octanol/water), 2.7.

Thin-layer Chromatography. System TA—Rf 61; system TB—Rf 02; system TC—Rf 31; system TE—Rf 58; system TL—Rf 21; system TAE—Rf 66. (Acidified iodoplatinate solution, positive.)

Gas Chromatography. System GA—RI 2138.

High Performance Liquid Chromatography. System HA—*k* 1.0; system HY—RI 289; system HAA—Retention time(s) 12.5 min.

Ultraviolet Spectrum. Aqueous acid—272 nm ($A_1^1=320a$); aqueous alkali—286 nm ($A_1^1=381b$).

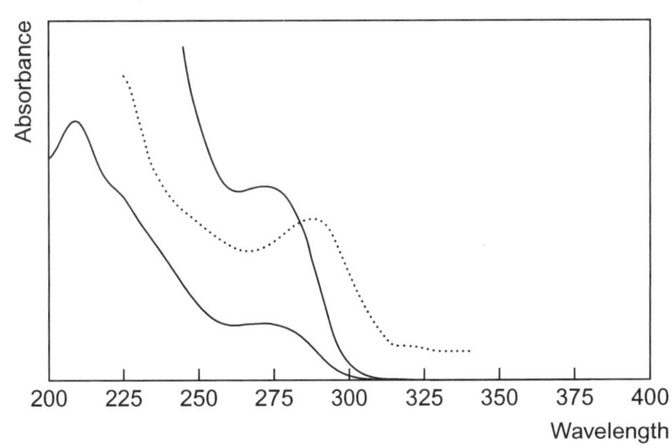

Infra-red Spectrum. Principal peaks at wavenumbers 1628, 1575, 1640, 1075, 835, 805 cm^{-1} (KBr disk).

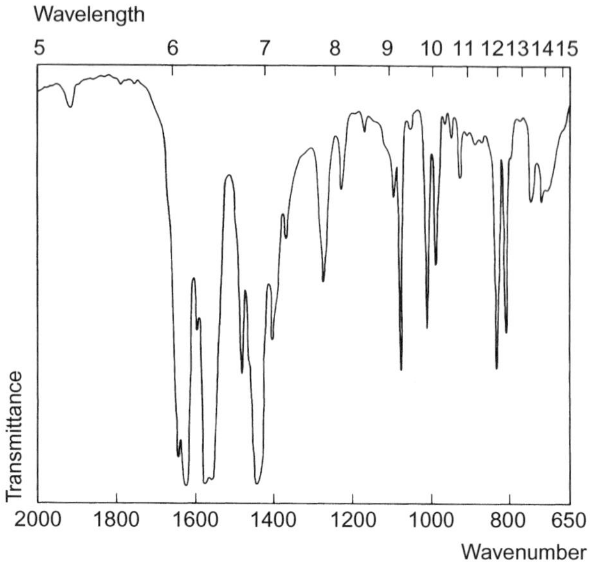

Mass Spectrum. Principal ions at *m/z* 247, 248, 249, 250, 219, 212, 106, 221.

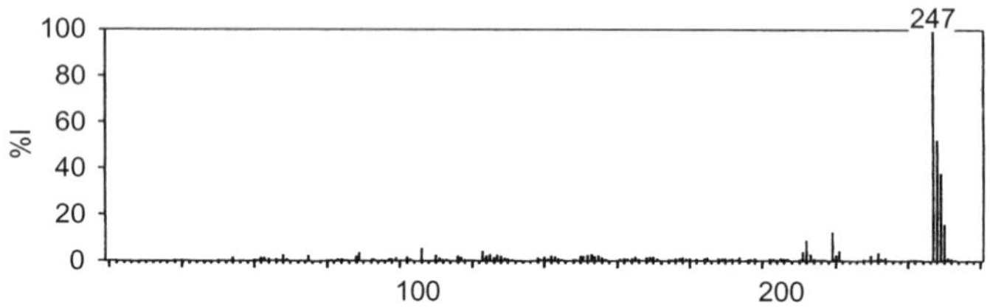

Quantification

Gas chromatography. In plasma or urine: limit of detection 5 μg/L, ECD—C. Midskov, *J. Chromatogr.*, 1984, *306*; *Biomed. Appl.*, *31*, 388–393.

High performance liquid chromatography. In plasma: limit of detection 10 μg/L, fluorescence detection—U. Timm and E. Weidekamm, *J. Chromatogr.*, 1982, *230*; *Biomed. Appl.*, *19*, 107–114. In plasma: limit of detection 1 μg/L—A. Le Liboux *et al.*, *Eur. J. Drug Metab. Pharmacokinet.*, 1991, *Spec. 3*, 284–290. In plasma: enzyme inhibition analysis—W. L. Roberts *et al.*, *Am. J. Clin. Pathol.*, 1995, *104*, 82–88. In plasma: limit of detection, 3 μg/L, UV detection—K. Na-Bangchang *et al.*, *J. Chromatogr. B*, *Biomed. Sci. Appl.*, 1997, *689*, 433–437. In plasma: pyrimethamine and mefloquine, limit of detection 10 μg/L, UV detection—A. Guenzi *et al.*, *J. Chromatogr.*, 1989, *494*, 219–230. In plasma: pyrimethamine, sulfadoxine and mefloquine, UV detection—Y. Bergqvist *et al.*, *J. Chromatogr.*, 1991, *571*, 169–177. In plasma: pyrimethamine and other antimalarials, limit of detection for pyrimethamine 15 μg/L, UV detection—J. Eljaschewitsch *et al.*, *Ther. Drug Monit.*, 1996, *18*, 592–597. In plasma: pyrimethamine and sulfadoxine, limit of detection for pyrimethamine 10 μg/L, UV detection—H. Astier *et al.*, *J. Chromatogr. B*, *Biomed. Sci. Appl.*, 1997, *698*, 217–223. In blood (dried on filter paper): limit of detection 1 to 10 mg/L—M. D. Green *et al.*, *J. Chromatogr. B*, *Analyt. Technol. Biomed. Life Sci.*, 2002, *767*, 159–162.

Disposition in the Body. Pyrimethamine is well absorbed after oral administration, and very slowly excreted in the urine, about 20% of a dose being excreted in 7 days.

Therapeutic concentration

A single oral dose of 50 mg given to 5 subjects produced a peak plasma concentration of 0.21 to 0.43 (mean 0.34) mg/L in 2 to 4 h, followed by a slow decline over several days. [L. Donno *et al.*, *Curr. Ther. Res.*, 1980, *27*, 346–355].

6 subjects given 8 weekly doses of 12.5 mg pyrimethamine plus 100 mg dapsone, had a pyrimethamine peak plasma concentrations of 116.2 μg/L 3.7 h after the last dose. [M. D. Edstein *et al.*, *Br. J. Clin. Pharmacol.*, 1990, *30*, 259–265].

In 3 severely ill patients with advanced AIDS (acquired immunodeficiency syndrome), maximum plasma pyrimethamine concentrations were 254, 34 and 610 μg/L after receiving maintenance doses of 0.5, 1.4 and 1.6 mg/kg, respectively, for cerebral toxoplasmosis (lower end of therapeutic range: 750 mg/L). [P. Winstanley *et al.*, *J. Antimicrob. Chemother.*, 1995, *36*, 435–439].

Toxicity. Children have died following ingestion of 0.4 to 1 g.

Accidental prolonged overdosage with pyrimethamine (30 mg daily instead of the usual dose of 3 mg daily, for 10 days) in a 7-week-old infant treated for toxoplasmosis produced initial plasma concentrations of 6.22 mg/L. Plasma levels were still within the normal therapeutic range 7 days after stopping therapy. [A. Tracqui *et al.*, *J. Anal. Toxicol.*, 1993, *17*, 248–250].

Half-life. Plasma half-life, about 4 days.

Dose. Up to 75 mg daily.

Pyritidium Bromide

Trypanocide (Veterinary)

Synonym. Pyrithidium Bromide
3-Amino-8-(2-amino-1,6-dimethylpyrimidinium-4-ylamino)-6-(4-aminophenyl)-5-methylphenanthridinium dibromide
$C_{26}H_{27}Br_2N_7 = 597.4$
CAS—3616-05-5 (pyritidium); 14222-46-9 (bromide)

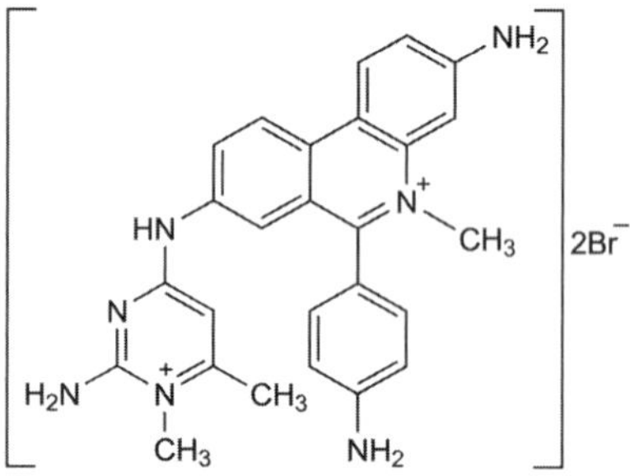

A brick-red to reddish-purple, hygroscopic powder.
Soluble 1 in 40 of water and 1 in 1900 of ethanol.

Thin-layer Chromatography. System TA—Rf 01. (Location under ultraviolet light, yellow fluorescence; Acidified iodoplatinate solution, positive.)

Ultraviolet Spectrum. Aqueous acid—256 nm (A_1^1=425a), 313 nm (A_1^1=813a).

Infra-red Spectrum. Principal peaks at wavenumbers 1615, 1642, 1515, 1250, 1562, 1298 cm^{-1} (KBr disk).

Pyrrobutamine

Antihistamine

Proprietary name. Pyronil
1-[4-(4-Chlorophenyl)-3-phenyl-2-butenyl]pyrrolidine
$C_{20}H_{22}ClN = 311.9$
CAS—91-82-7

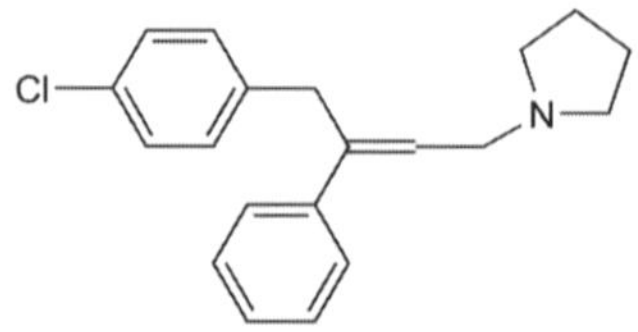

An oily liquid. On standing gives crystals. M.p. 48° to 49°.

Pyrrobutamine Phosphate
Proprietary name. It is an ingredient of Co-Pyronil
$C_{20}H_{22}ClN,2H_3PO_4 = 507.8$
CAS—135-31-9
A white crystalline powder. M.p. 129° to 130°.
Soluble in water; soluble 1 in 20 of ethanol; practically insoluble in chloroform and ether.

Dissociation Constant. Pyrrobutamine pK_a 8.8 (25°); Pyrrobutamine phosphate pK_a 8.8, 5.2.

Partition Coefficient. Log *P* (octanol/water), 6.3.

Colour Tests. Liebermann's test—brown; Mandelin's test—violet; Marquis test—grey-violet.

Thin-layer Chromatography. System TA—Rf 54; system TB—Rf 54; system TC—Rf 37; system TE—Rf 71; system TL—Rf 18; system TAE—Rf 25; system TAF—Rf 66; system TAJ—Rf 24; system TAK—Rf 25; system TAL—Rf 86. (Dragendorff spray, positive; Acidified iodoplatinate solution, positive; Marquis reagent, grey.)

Gas Chromatography. System GA—pyrrobutamine RI 2419; M (oxo-) RI 2920; system GF—RI 2815.

High Performance Liquid Chromatography. System HA—*k* 2.8; system HX—RI 477.

Infra-red Spectrum. Principal peaks at wavenumbers 995, 1018, 1087, 772, 1492, 820 cm^{-1} (pyrrobutamine phosphate, KBr disk).

Mass Spectrum. Principal ions at *m/z* 205, 240, 91, 84, 125, 242, 206, 186.

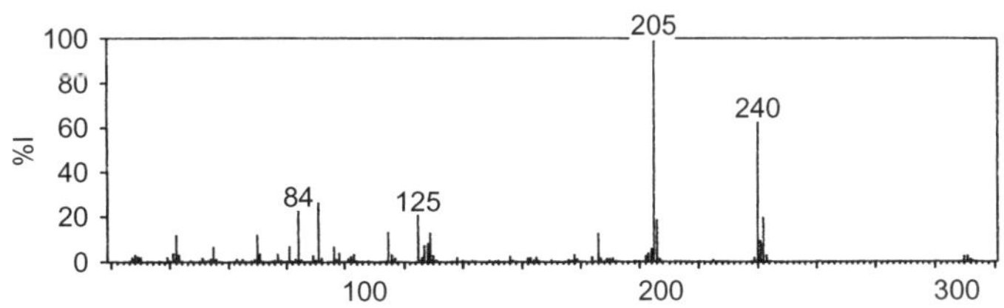

Dose. 30 to 90 mg of pyrrobutamine phosphate daily.

Pyrvinium Embonate

Anthelmintic

Synonyms. Pyrvinium Pamoate; Viprynium Embonate; Viprynium Pamoate.
Proprietary names. Molevac; Pamovin; Pamoxan; Povan; Povanyl; Pyrcon; Pyr-Pam; Pyrvin; Vanquin.
6-(Dimethylamino)-2-[2-(2,5-dimethyl-1-phenyl-1*H*-pyrrol-3-yl)-ethenyl]-1-methylquinolinium salt with 4,4′-methylenebis[3-hydroxy-2-naphthalenecarboxylic acid] (2:1)
$C_{52}H_{56}N_6,C_{23}H_{14}O_6$=1151.4
CAS—3546-41-6

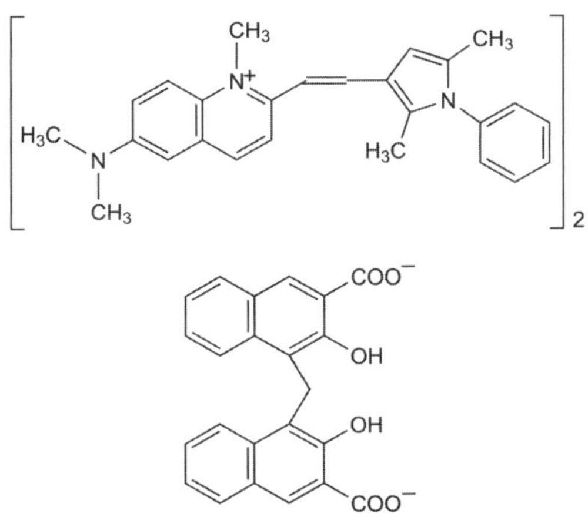

A bright orange or orange-red to almost black, crystalline powder. M.p. 210° to 215° (softens at 190°).
Practically insoluble in water and ether; very slightly soluble in ethanol; slightly soluble in chloroform and methoxyethanol; freely soluble in glacial acetic acid.

Pyrvinium Chloride
Synonyms. Viprynium Chloride; SN-4395.
$C_{26}H_{27}N_3$,HCl=418.0
CAS—548-84-5
Deep-red powder. M.p. 249° to 251° with decomposition.
Sparingly soluble in water.

Colour Tests. Mandelin's Test—yellow; Marquis Test—yellow

Thin-layer Chromatography. System TA—Rf 67. (Acidified potassium permanganate solution, weak reaction.)

Ultraviolet Spectrum. 2-Methoxyethanol—239, 358 nm (A_1^1=380b).

Infra-red Spectrum. Principal peaks at wavenumbers 1592, 1618, 1294, 1188, 1500, 1513 cm^{-1} (KBr disk).

Dose. The equivalent of 5 mg/kg of pyrvinium as a single dose.

Quazepam

Sedative/Hypnotic

Synonym. Sch-16134
Proprietary names. Doral; Dormalin; Dorme; Oniria; Prosedar; Quazium; Quiedorm; Selepam.
7-Chloro-5-(2-flurophenyl)-1,3-dihydro-1-(2,2,2-trifluroethyl)-2*H*-1,4-benzodiazepine-2-thione
$C_{17}H_{11}ClF_4N_2S$=386.8
CAS—36735-22-5

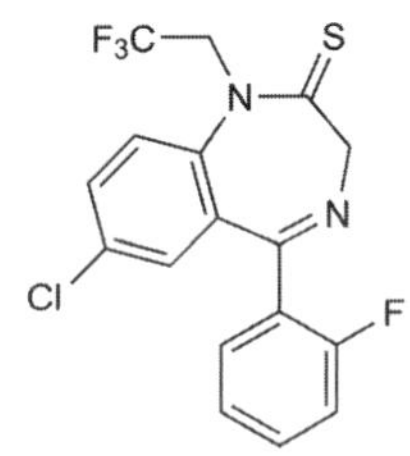

An off-white to yellowish powder with m.p. 137.5° to139°. It is insoluble in water; soluble in alcohol.

Partition Coefficient. Log *P* (octanol/water), 4.03.

Thin-layer Chromatography. System TA—Rf 74 quazepam, Rf 79 quazepam-CFTB, Rf 78 M(2-oxo), Rf 71 M(3-hydroxy-2-oxo), Rf 67 M(3-hydroxy-*N*-dealkyl-2-oxo), Rf 75 M(*N*-dealkyl-2-oxo); system TB—Rf 27 quazepam, Rf 44 quazepam-CFTB, Rf 16 M(2-oxo), Rf 2 M(3-hydroxy-2-oxo), Rf 0 M(3-hydroxy-*N*-dealkyl-2-oxo), Rf 2 M(*N*-dealkyl-2-oxo); system TC—Rf 75 quazepam, Rf 77 quazepam-CFTB, Rf 89 M(2-oxo), Rf 55 M(3-hydroxy-2-oxo), Rf 30 M(3-hydroxy-*N*-dealkyl-2-oxo), Rf 56 M(*N*-dealkyl-2-oxo); system TD—Rf 78 quazepam, Rf 74 quazepam-CFTB, Rf 59 M(2-oxo), Rf 42 M(3-hydroxy-2-oxo), Rf 15 M(3-hydroxy-*N*-dealkyl-2-oxo), Rf 34 M(*N*-dealkyl-2-oxo); system TE—Rf 83 quazepam, Rf 85 quazepam-CFTB, Rf 80 M(2-oxo), Rf 69 M(3-hydroxy-2-oxo), Rf 49 M(3-hydroxy-*N*-dealkyl-2-oxo), Rf 72 M(*N*-dealkyl-2-oxo); system TF—Rf 71 quazepam, Rf 73 quazepam-CFTB, Rf 57 M(2-oxo), Rf 52 M(3-hydroxy-2-oxo), Rf 28 M(3-hydroxy-*N*-dealkyl-2-oxo), Rf 45 M(*N*-dealkyl-2-oxo); system TL—Rf 76 quazepam, Rf 73 quazepam-CFTB, Rf 71 M(2-oxo), Rf 59 M(3-hydroxy-2-oxo), Rf 38 M(3-hydroxy-*N*-dealkyl-2-oxo), Rf 58 M(*N*-dealkyl-2-oxo); system TAD—Rf 78 quazepam, Rf 80 quazepam-CFTB, Rf 70 M(2-oxo), Rf 58 M(3-hydroxy-2-oxo), Rf 35 M(3-hydroxy-*N*-dealkyl-2-oxo), Rf 60 M(*N*-dealkyl-2-oxo); system TAE—Rf 87 quazepam, Rf 77 quazepam-CFTB, Rf 87 M(2-oxo), Rf 88 M(3-hydroxy-2-oxo), Rf 88 M(3-hydroxy-*N*-dealkyl-2-oxo), Rf 88 M(*N*-dealkyl-2-oxo); system TAF—Rf 96 quazepam, Rf 93 quazepam-CFTB, Rf 90 M(2-oxo), Rf 90 M(3-hydroxy-2-oxo), Rf 89 M(3-hydroxy-*N*-dealkyl-2-oxo), Rf 88 M(*N*-dealkyl-2-oxo).

Gas Chromatography. System GA—RI 2440, RI 2255 M (2-oxo-); system GB—RI 2576.

High Performance Liquid Chromatography. System HY—RI 766; system HZ—retention time 37.5 min; system HAX—retention time 11.9 min; system HAY—retention time 17.7 min.

Column: C_{18} (Nova-Pak, 75 × 3.9 mm i.d.). Mobile phase: methanol: phosphate buffer (2 mM, pH 7.2) (60:40), flow rate 1 mL/min. Internal standard (IS): diazepam. UV detection (λ=265 nm). Retention time(s): quazepam, 17.6 min; IS, 8.1 min. [S. Gupta *et al.*, *Pharm. Res.*, 1988, *5*, 365–368].

Column: (analytical) Si-10 porous silica (300 × 4 mm, 10 µm), (guard) Porasil A (5 cm). Mobile phase: ethanol. Flow rate 0.5 mL/min. UV detection. Retention time(s): 2.7 min. [T. Mills and J. C. Roberson, *Instrumental Data for Drug Analysis*, 1993, CRC Press, Boca Raton, US. 2nd Edn,].

Ultraviolet Spectrum. Aqueous acid—283 nm; basic—281 nm.

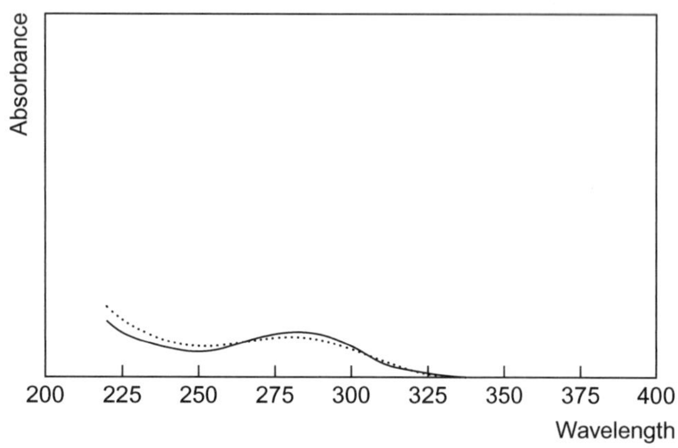

Infra-red Spectrum. Principal peaks at wavenumbers 1141, 1405 and 1253 cm^{-1} (KBr disk).

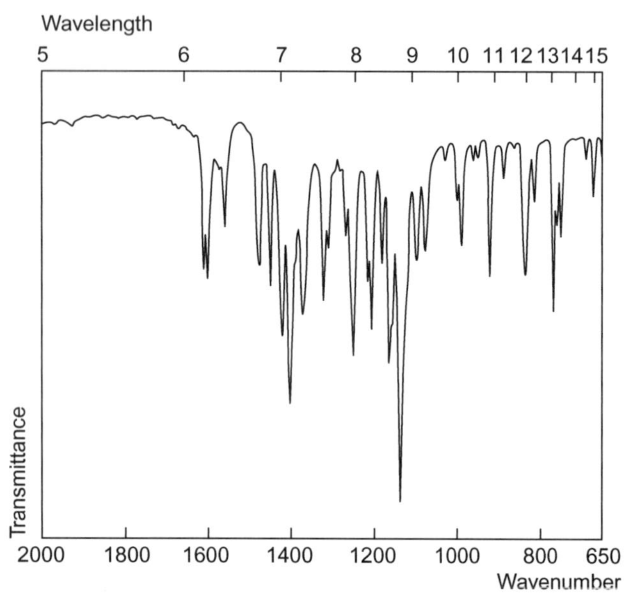

Mass Spectrum. Principal ions at *m/z* 386, 359, 323, 388, 245, 303, 342, 361.

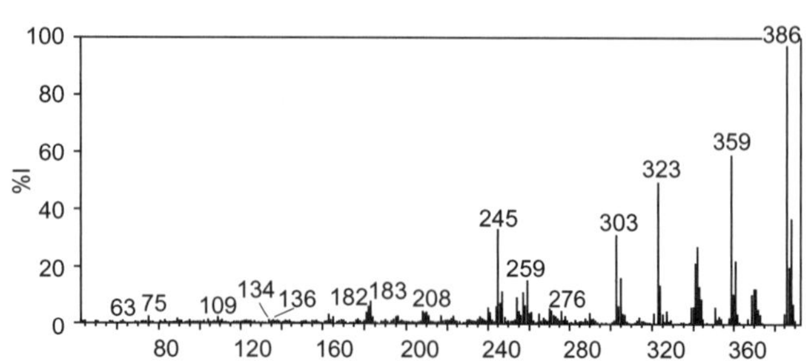

Quantification

Gas chromatography. In plasma: limit of quantification 0.75 µg/L. ECD—J. Hilbert *et al.*, *J. Pharm. Sci.*, 1984, *73(4)*, 516–519.

High performance liquid chromatography. In blood: limit of quantification 2 µg/L. UV detection (λ=265 nm)—S. Gupta and E. Ellinwood, *Pharm. Res.*, 1988, *5(6)*, 365–368.

Enzyme immunoassay. In serum: EMIT-tox serum benzodiazepines assay, concentration 30 µg/L—W. Huang and D. Moody, *J. Anal. Toxicol.*, 1995, *19*, 333–342.

Disposition in the Body. Quazepam is readily and rapidly absorbed from the gastro-intestinal tract after oral administration. It is distributed widely throughout the body into most body tissues and fluids and metabolised extensively in the liver. The principal active metabolites are 2-oxo-quazepam (half-life 40 h), *O,N*-desalkyl-2-oxoquazepam (half-life, 69 h) and 3-hydroxy-2-oxoquazepam glucuronide. It is excreted in urine (31%) and faeces (23%), mainly as the conjugated metabolites. Only trace amounts of the unchanged drug are present in urine. Elimination is prolonged in the elderly. Steady state is achieved by day 7 and maintained for up to 14 days due to slow elimination. Quazepam and its metabolites readily cross the blood–brain barrier.

Therapeutic concentration. The serum therapeutic concentration range is 10 to 150 µg/L.

> 6 healthy males were administered 25 mg quazepam in solution. Peak plasma concentrations of the unchanged drug were 148 µg/L and observed at 1.5 h post-dosing. [N. Zampaglione *et al.*, *Drug Metab. Dispos.*, 1985, *13(1)*, 25–29].

Toxicity. Quazepam has the same toxic potential as the benzodiazepines.

Bioavailability. Approx. 80%.

Half-life. 39 h.

Volume of distribution. At bedtime, 5 L/kg and in the morning, 8.6 L/kg.

Clearance. The total body clearance is 890 mL/min.

Protein binding. Greater than 95%.

Note. Active metabolites accumulate with chronic use.

Dose. An oral dose of 15 mg is administered at bedtime which may be reduced to 7.5 mg in the elderly and debilitated.

Quetiapine

Antipsychotic

2-[2-(4-Dibenzo[*b,f*][1,4]thiazepin-11-yl-1-piperazinyl)ethoxy]ethanol
$C_{21}H_{25}N_3O_2S$=383.5
CAS—111974-69-7

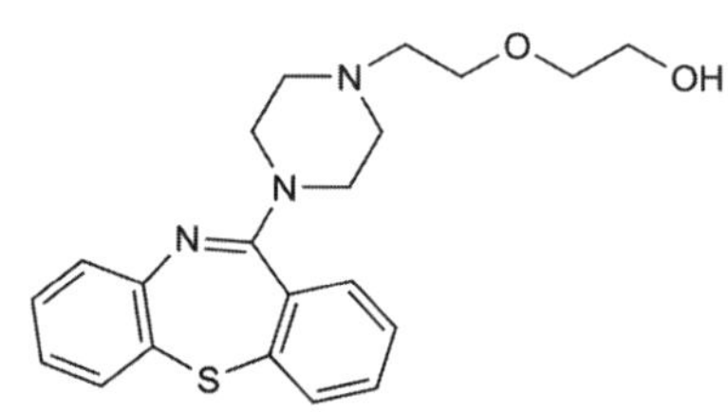

A white to off-white crystalline powder. It is moderately soluble in water.

Quetiapine Hemifumarate
Synonym. ICI-204636
Proprietary name. Seroquel
$(C_{21}H_{25}N_3O_2S)_2C_4H_4O_4$=883.1
CAS–111974-72-2
Crystals from ethanol. M.p. 172° to 173°.

Dissociation Constant. pK_{a_1} 3.3; pK_{a_2} 6.8.

Gas Chromatography. System GB—RI 3400.

Column: cross-linked methylsilicone (30 m × 0.25 mm i.d., 0.1 µm film thickness). Column temperature: 190° for 1.6 min to 295° at 30°/min, held for 8.9 min. Injector temperature: 290°. Carrier gas: helium, flow rate 0.75 mL/min. MS detection (EI, SIM at *m/z* 322 and 340). Retention time(s): TMS (trimethylsilane) derivatives: quetiapine, 10.1 min; 7-hydroxyquetiapine, 13.0 min. [R. H. Pullen *et al.*, *J. Chromatogr.*, 1992, *573*, 49–57].

High Performance Liquid Chromatography. Column: stablebond phenyl (SB-Ph) (Zorbax, 150 × 2.1 mm i.d., 5 µm). Mobile phase: phosphate buffer (20 mM, pH 7.4 with 30 mM potassium chloride): methanol:acetonitrile (40:50:10), flow rate 0.25 mL/min. UV detection (λ=225 nm). Retention time(s): 7.8 min. [P. Davis *et al.*, *J. Pharm. Biomed. Anal.*, 1999, *20*, 271–282].

Column: (analytical) ODS (Hypersil, 250 × 4.6 mm i.d., 5 µm); (guard) C_8 (Newguard, 15 × 3.2 mm i.d., 7 µm). Mobile phase: acetonitrile: methanol:potassium phosphate (5 mM, pH 7.0) (2:1:2), flow rate 1 mL/min. UV detection (λ=250 nm). Retention time(s): quetiapine, 9.7 min; 7-hydroxyquetiapine, 4.0 min. [R. H. Pullen *et al.*, *J. Chromatogr.*, 1992, *573*, 49–57].

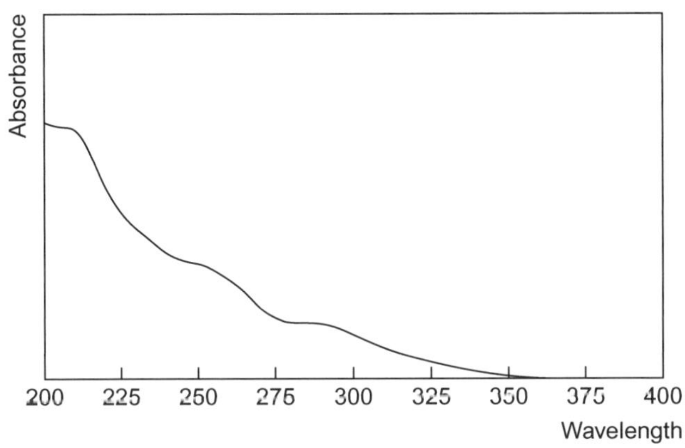

Infra-red Spectrum. Principal peaks at wavenumbers 1600, 1575, 1410, 765 cm^{-1}.

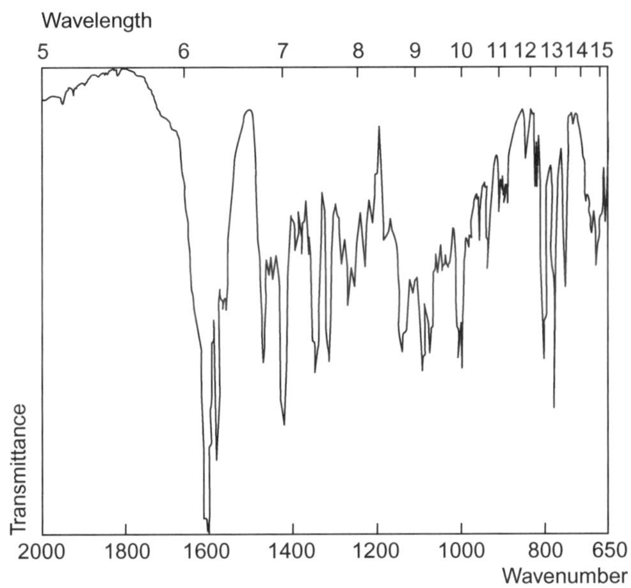

Mass Spectrum. Principal ions at *m/z* 210, 144, 239, 45, 321, 209, 95, 211.

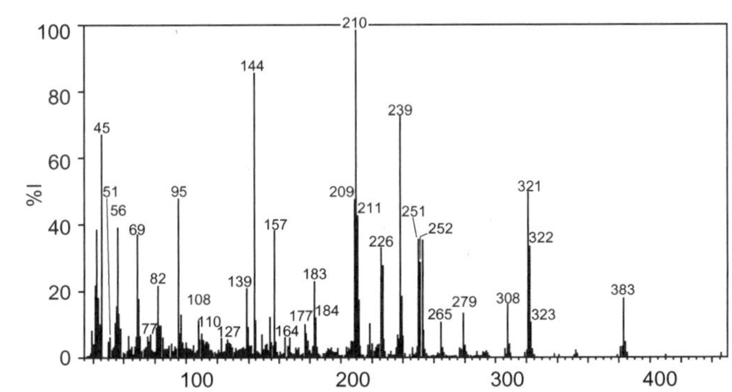

Quantification

High performance liquid chromatography. In plasma: limit of quantification 2.5 µg/L. UV detection (λ=225 nm)—P. Davis *et al.*, *J. Pharm. Biomed. Anal.*, 1999, *20*, 271–282.

Disposition in the Body. Quetiapine is well and rapidly absorbed following oral administration. It is widely distributed throughout the body and extensively metabolised in the liver by sulfoxidation, carboxylic acid formation on the ethoxyethanol side-chain and 7-hydroxylation. At least 20 metabolites have been detected but only 7-hydroxyquetiapine has significant pharmacological activity. CYP3A4 is the main isoenzyme responsible for cytochrome P450-mediated metabolism. Elimination is mainly by hepatic metabolism. The drug is excreted as its inactive metabolite: 73% in urine and 20% in faeces. 1% of an administrated dose is excreted unchanged. Peak plasma concentrations are observed within 1.5 to 2 h after administration. Steady state is achieved within 2 days of the dose. Linear pharmacokinetics are observed.

Therapeutic concentration. The effective dose is 200 to 750 mg daily. The therapeutic concentration is 0.4 mg/L.

12 hospitalised patients with schizophrenia were administered increasing doses of quetiapine over 21 days. A 75 mg oral dose produced a peak serum concentration of 0.278 mg/L on the last day of treatment. [L. F. Fabre *et al.*, *Clin Ther.*, 1995, *17(3)*, 366–378].

Toxicity. The lethal concentration is 7 mg/L.

A physically healthy 40-year-old woman with extensive psychiatric history was being treated with 100 mg quetiapine fumarate twice daily as well as clonazepam, chloral hydrate and valproic acid. After being discharged from hospital (after treatment for another overdose) she overdosed on 3000 mg quetiapine fumarate. Upon admission at hospital, she was drowsy, confused, suffered from hypotension, tachycardia and was mildly obtunded; other symptoms were also present. She was treated with activated charcoal and after 90 min was more obtunded and could not continue with this treatment. The serum quetiapine concentration was 1.824 mg/L. She became progressively worse but improved after systolic blood pressure support and saline solution. 8 h after overdosing, serum concentration was 0.963 mg/L; 22 h, 0.180 mg/L; 42 h, 0.015 mg/L and 48 h, 0.005 mg/L. The drug was still detectable after 7 days. Tachycardia persisted until 42 h after overdosing. [P. T. Pollak and K. Zbuk, *Clin. Pharmacol. Ther.*, 2000, *68(1)*, 92–97].

A 40-year-old male was found decomposed in a hotel room. Postmortem examination revealed the following quetiapine concentrations: 49 mg/L in heart blood, 112 mg/kg in liver, 7.6 mg total gastric content, 4.0 mg/kg in spleen. Other substances detected in the heart blood were: alprazolam (2.6 mg/L), fluoxetine (2.1 mg/L), norfluoxetine (2.1 mg/L), prochlorperazine (0.83 mg/L) and ethanol (0.41 g%). [D. T. Anderson and K. L. Fritz, *J. Anal. Toxicol.*, 2000, *24*, 300–304].

A young woman who overdosed with 10 000 mg quetiapine was initially treated with gastric lavage and activated charcoal within 75 min of overdosing. Serum drug concentrations reached 12.7 mg/L. Her level of consciousness decreased 180 min after ingestion requiring intubation for 240 min. Alertness was regained at 16 h but her persistent tachycardia was not resolved until 42 h after ingestion. A full recovery was made. [T. J. Harman *et al.*, *J. Toxicol. Clin. Toxicol.*, 1998, *36*, 599–602].

Bioavailability. 100% bioavailability of tablets relative to solution. Absolute bioavailability 9%.

Half-life. 6 to 7 h; also reported as 2.7 to 9.3 h.

Volume of distribution. 10 L/kg.

Protein binding. 83%.

Dose. 25 mg twice daily on day 1; 50 mg twice daily on day 2; 100 mg twice daily on day 3; 150 mg twice daily on day 4; then increased as necessary. The usual dose is 300 to 450 mg daily in two divided dose with a maximum of 750 mg. In the elderly the initial dose is 25 mg.

Quinagolide

Prolactin Inhibitor/Dopaminergic

(3*R*,4a*R*,10a*S*)-*rel*-*N*,*N*-Diethyl-*N′*-(1,2,3,4,4a,5,10,10a-octahydro-6-hydroxy-1-propylbenzo[*g*]quinolin-3-yl)sulfamide
$C_{20}H_{33}N_3O_3S$=395.6
CAS—87056-78-8

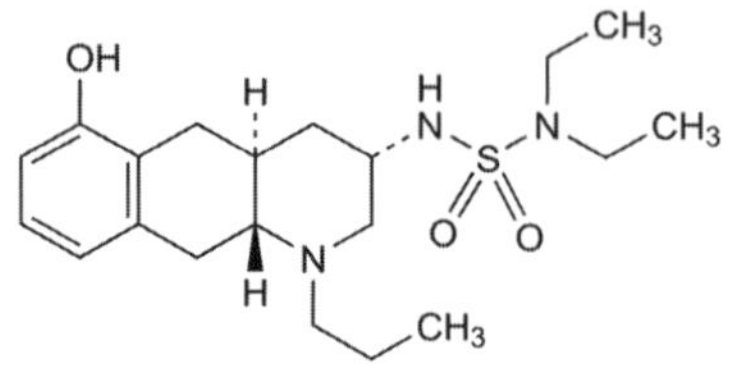

A beige powder with m.p. 122.5° to 124°.

Quinagolide Hydrochloride

Proprietary name. Norprolac
$C_{20}H_{33}N_3O_3S,HCl$=432.0
CAS—94424-50-7
Crystals with m.p. 234° to 236°.

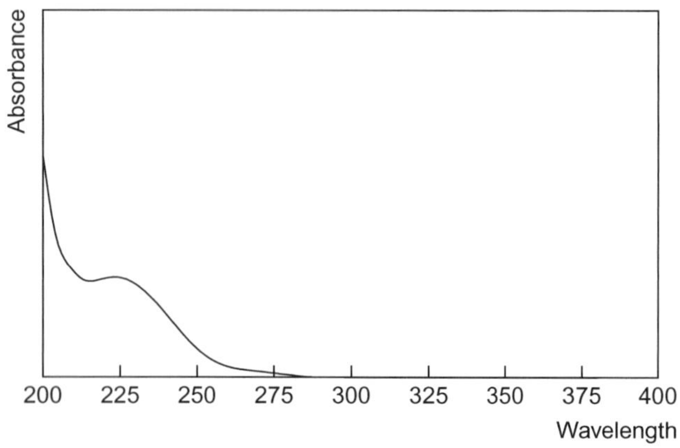

Disposition in the Body. Quinagolide is rapidly and well absorbed from the gastro-intestinal tract. There is extensive first-pass metabolism to the *N*-desethyl analogue which is biologically active and the *N,N*-didesethyl analogue. 95% of the drug is excreted as its metabolites with approximately equal amounts of a dose appearing in urine and in faeces. Excretion occurs in urine as sulfate or glucuronide conjugates of quinagolide and its metabolites and in faeces as the unconjugated forms.

Bioavailability. 100% after oral administration.

Half-life. 11.5 h after a single dose and 17 h at steady state.

Volume of distribution. Approx. 100 L after single a oral dose.

Protein binding. About 90%.

Dose. 25 to 150 µg daily. Maximum 300 µg.

Quinapril

Antihypertensive

Proprietary names. (Quinapril with Hydrochlorothiazide) Accuretic; Acequide; Koretic.
(3*S*)-2-[(2*S*)-2-[[(1*S*)-1-(Ethoxycarbonyl)-3-phenylpropyl]amino]-1-oxopropyl]-1,2,3,4-tetrahydro-3-isoquinolinecarboxylic acid
$C_{25}H_{30}N_2O_5$=438.5
CAS—85441-61-8

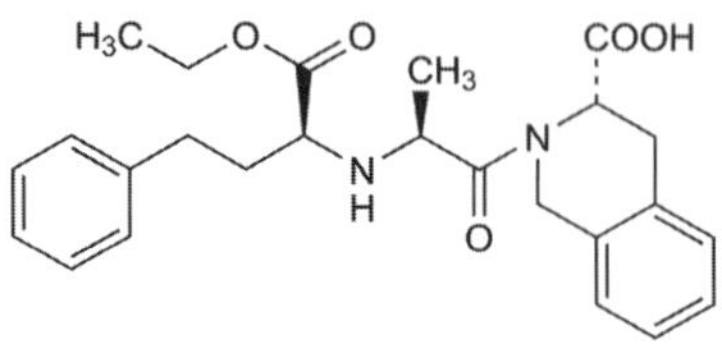

Quinaprilat (Diacid of quinapril)

Synonym. CI-928
$C_{23}H_{26}N_2O_5$=410.5
CAS—82768-85-2
Hydrate crystals from methanol–ethyl ether. M.p. 166° to 168°.

Quinapril Hydrochloride

Synonyms. CI-906; PD-109452-2.
Proprietary names. Accupril; Accuprin; Accupro; Acequin; Acuitel; Korec; Quinazil.
$C_{25}H_{30}N_2O_5,HCl$=475.0
CAS—82586-55-8
Crystals from ethyl acetate–toluene. M.p. 120° to 130°. Also reported as white crystalline solid (from acetonitrile) with m.p. 119° to 121.5°.

Partition Coefficient. Log *P* (octanol/water), 3.72.

Gas Chromatography. System GP—RI 3110 quinapril-ME; RI 3080 M (quinaprilate)-ME3; RI 3310 M (quinaprilate-H_2O)-ME3.

Column: fused-silica capillary (DB-1, 10 m × 0.32 mm i.d., 0.25 µm film thickness). Column temperature: 150°, held 0.1 min, to 300° at 25°/min, held 1.5 min. Injector temperature: 70° to 300° at 10°/min, held for 5 min. Carrier gas: helium. MS detection (NICI, SIM at *m/z* 302 for quinapril and 288 for quinaprilat). Retention time(s): quinapril, 6.20 min; quinaprilat, 6.15 min. [W. Hammes *et al., J. Chromatogr.*, 1995, *670*; *Biomed. Appl.*, 81–89].

High Performance Liquid Chromatography. System HZ—retention time 5.4 min; system HAA—retention time 16.8 min.

Column: C_{18} (µBondapak, 300 × 3.9 mm i.d., 10 µm). Column temperature: 30°. Mobile phase: 1-propanol:acetonitrile:phosphoric acid (0.01 M) (20:15:78), flow rate 1.0 mL/min. UV detection (λ=206 nm). Retention time(s): quinapril, 7.6 min; quinaprilat, 5.7 min. [J. A. Prieto *et al., J. Chromatogr. Sci.*, 2001, *39(4)*, 153–159].

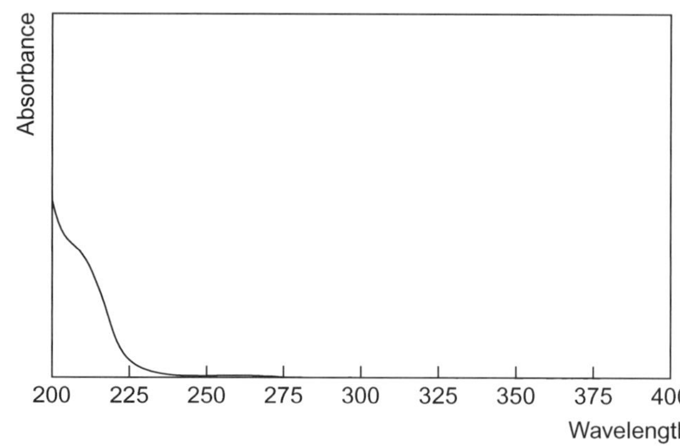

Mass Spectrum. Principal ions at *m/z* 316, 270, 91, 130, 117, 104, 132, 231.

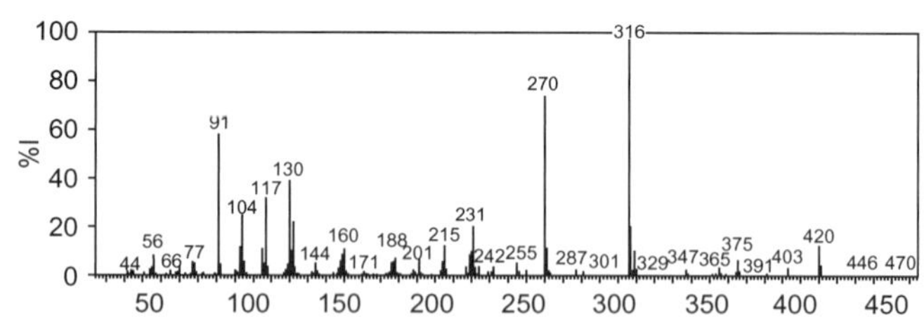

Quantification

Gas chromatography. In plasma and urine: limit of detection 10 and 50 µg/L, respectively, ECD—J. J. Ferry *et al., J. Chromatogr.*, 1987, *421*; *Biomed. Appl.*, 187–191.

Gas chromatography–mass spectrometry. In plasma and urine: limit of quantification for quinapril and quinaprilat 0.05 µg/L in plasma and 0.5 µg/L in urine—N. Goto *et al., J. Chromatogr.*, 1992, *578(2)*, 195–201. In plasma and urine: limit of quantification for dioxopiperazine metabolites of quinapril 0.2 and 1.0 µg/L in plasma and urine, respectively; limit of detection 0.1 and 0.5 µg/L, respectively—N. Goto *et al., J. Chromatogr.*, 1992, *578(2)*, 203–206.

High performance liquid chromatography. In urine: limit of detection 60 µg/L for quinapril and 50 µg/L for quinaprilat; limit of quantification 190 and 160 µg/L, respectively. UV detection (λ=206 nm)—J. A. Prieto *et al., J. Chromatogr. Sci.*, 2001, *39(4)*, 153–159.

Disposition in the Body. Approx. 60% of a dose is absorbed after oral administration and is metabolised mainly in the liver to quinaprilat and inactive metabolites. Peak plasma concentrations of the active metabolite are reached within 2 h of administration. Up to 60% of the dose is excreted in urine as the unchanged drug, quinaprilat and inactive metabolites. The remainder is excreted in faeces. Elimination of quinaprilat is reduced in elderly patients (>65 years).

Therapeutic concentration

12 patients with terminal renal failure were involved in the study, 6 of whom were on maintenance haemodialysis (at 4 h, three times a week), mean age 58.5 years (range 25 to 71 years) and 6 on continuous peritoneal dialysis (CAPD) treatment (4 exchanges daily), mean 50.2 years old (range 32 to 68 years). Patients were administered a single oral dose of 2.5 mg quinapril. Peak plasma concentrations for those undergoing haemodialysis were 83.5 (range 45.8 to 103.2) μg/L observed at 4 h and for those being treated by CAPD, 64.3 (47.1 to 83.8) μg/L at 4.7 (4 to 8) h. [K. Wolter and E. Fritschka, *Eur. J. Clin. Pharmacol.*, 1993, *44 (Suppl 1)*, S53–S56].

22 normotensive subjects, aged 18 to 75 years, were divided into three groups according to their creatinine clearance rates and treated with 20 mg quinapril hydrochloride on day 1 and on days 4 to 10. The dose was administered after an 8 h fast which was continued for another 4 h after dosing. Group 1: creatinine clearance, >60 mL/min (6 subjects); group 2: 30 to 59 mL/min (6 subjects); group 3: <29 mL/min (10 subjects). For the single dose, peak plasma quinapril concentrations reached 153, 136 and 161 μg/L for groups 1, 2 and 3, respectively. These were observed at 0.75, 0.8 and 1.29 h, respectively. The peak quinaprilat concentrations were 607, 663 and 885 μg/L at 1.88, 2.25 and 3.57 h, respectively, for groups 1, 2 and 3. For the multiple dosing, peak drug concentrations for groups 1, 2 and 3, were 149, 115 and 211 μg/L observed at 0.75, 1.0 and 1.07 h, respectively. The metabolite concentrations were 578, 686 and 1330 μg/L at 1.75, 2.33 and 2.43 μg/L for the three groups, respectively. These concentrations were measured on day 10. [C. E. Halstenson *et al.*, *J. Clin. Pharmacol.*, 1992, *32*, 344–350].

Bioavailability. Quinapril, 60%.

Half-life. Quinapril, approx. 1 h; quinaprilat, 3 h (increased in those with creatinine clearance ⩽40 mL/min).

Volume of distribution. 0.31 L/kg (range 0.18 to 0.52 L/kg) for patients undergoing haemodialysis; 0.3 (0.26 to 0.4) L/kg for those undergoing continuous peritoneal dialysis treatment.

Clearance. Quinapril, 111 L/h; quinaprilat 13 L/h.

Protein binding. 97% (quinapril and its metabolites).

Dose. Hypertension: An initial dose of 10 mg once daily is administered. In the elderly, those with renal impairment and those taking diuretics: 2.5 mg. The usual maintenance dose is 20 to 40 mg daily. Heart failure: initially 2.5 mg daily followed by a maintenance dose of 10 to 20 mg.

Quinethazone

Diuretic

Synonym. Chinethazonum; CL-36010.
Proprietary names. Aquamox; Hydromox.
7-Chloro-2-ethyl-1,2,3,4-tetrahydro-4-oxo-6-quinazolinesulfonamide
$C_{10}H_{12}ClN_3O_3S = 289.7$
CAS—73-49-4

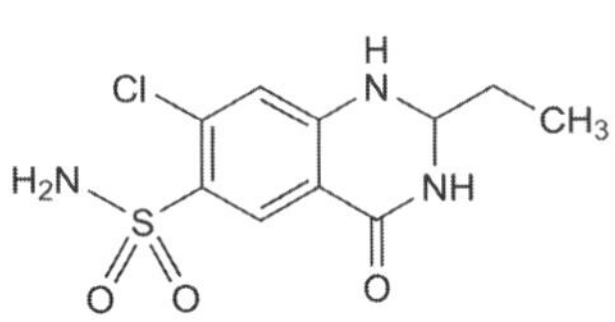

A white to yellowish-white, crystalline powder. M.p. 250° to 252°.
Very slightly soluble in water; slightly soluble in ethanol; freely soluble in solutions of alkali hydroxides and carbonates.

Dissociation Constant. pK_a 9.3, 10.7.

Partition Coefficient. Log *P* (octanol/water), 0.2.

Colour Test. Koppanyi–Zwikker test—violet.

Thin-layer Chromatography. System TA—Rf 75; system TAD—Rf 15; system TD—Rf 04; system TE—Rf 40; system TF—Rf 21; system TAJ—Rf 11; system TAK—Rf 06; system TAL—Rf 56. (Location under ultraviolet light, blue fluorescence; Acidified iodoplatinate solution, positive.)

Gas Chromatography. System GA—not eluted.

High Performance Liquid Chromatography. System HN—*k* 0.67.

Ultraviolet Spectrum. Ethanol—234 nm ($A^1_1 = 1532a$), 278 nm, 345 nm.

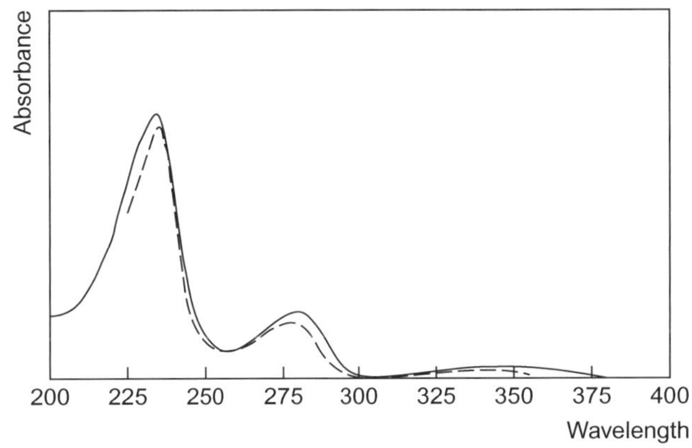

Infra-red Spectrum. Principal peaks at wavenumbers 1600, 1650, 1160, 960, 1510, 1040 cm^{-1} (KBr disk).

Mass Spectrum. Principal ions at *m/z* 260, 262, 180, 287, 261, 145, 286, 124.

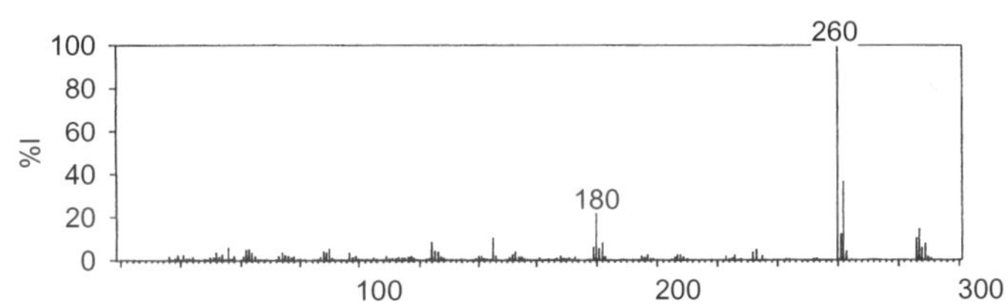

Quantification

High performance liquid chromatography. In urine: quinethazone and other diuretics, average limit of detection 1 mg/L, UV detection—S. F. Cooper *et al.*, *J. Chromatogr.*, 1989, *489*, 65–88.

Dose. 50 to 200 mg daily.

Quinidine

Anti-arrhythmic

Synonyms. Chinidinum; Quinidina.
(9*S*)-6′-Methoxycinchonan-9-ol
$C_{20}H_{24}N_2O_2,2H_2O = 360.5$
CAS—56-54-2 (anhydrous); 63717-04-4 (dihydrate)

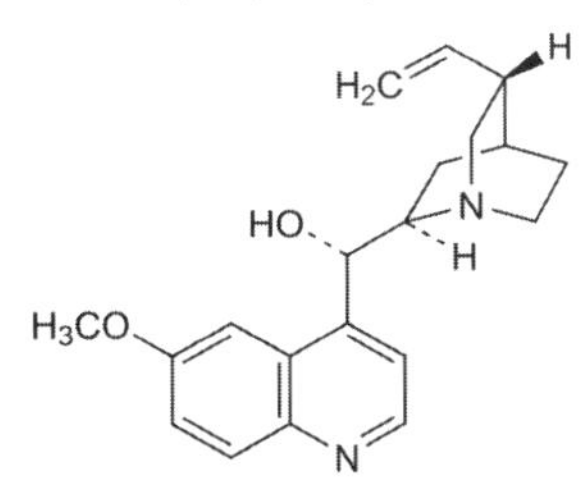

A dextrorotatory stereoisomer of quinine, obtained from the bark of species of *Cinchona* (Rubiaceae). Commercial samples may contain 20 to 30% of hydroquinidine.
A white amorphous powder or acicular crystals. M.p. 174° to 175° (anhydrous).

The anhydrous alkaloid is soluble 1 in about 2000 of cold water, 1 in 800 of boiling water, 1 in 36 of alcohol, 1 in 1.6 of chloroform, and 1 in 56 of ether; very soluble in methanol; practically insoluble in petroleum ether.

Quinidine Bisulfate
Proprietary names. Biquin; Biquinate; Kiditard; Kinidin(e); Kiniduron; Quini; Quiniduran; Quinidurule.
$C_{20}H_{24}N_2O_2,H_2SO_4,4H_2O$=494.6
CAS—747-45-5 (anhydrous); 6151-39-9 (tetrahydrate)
Colourless crystals.
Soluble 1 in 8 of water and 1 in 3 of ethanol; practically insoluble in ether.

Quinidine Gluconate
Proprietary names. Quinaglute; Quinate.
$C_{20}H_{24}N_2O_2,C_6H_{12}O_7$=520.6
CAS—7054-25-3
A white powder. M.p. 175.0° to 176.5°.
Soluble 1 in 9 of water and 1 in 60 of alcohol.

Quinidine Polygalacturonate
Proprietary names. Cardioquin(e); Galactoquin.
$C_{20}H_{24}N_2O_2,(C_6H_{10}O_7)_x,xH_2O$
CAS—27555-34-6 (anhydrous); 65484-56-2 (hydrate)
An amorphous powder. M.p. 180°, with decomposition.
The anhydrous product is sparingly soluble in water; insoluble in ethanol, chloroform, ether, acetone, dioxane, and methanol.

Quinidine Sulfate
Synonyms. Chinidini Sulfas; Chinidin sulfate; Chinidinum Sulfuricum; Quinidini Sulfas.
Proprietary names. Kinidin; Quinicardina; Quinicardine; Quinidex; Quinora; Systodin.
$(C_{20}H_{24}N_2O_2)_2,H_2SO_4,2H_2O$=783.0
CAS—50-54-4 (anhydrous); 6591-63-5 (dihydrate)
White acicular crystals or fine white powder, darkening on exposure to light. M.p. about 207°, with decomposition.
Soluble 1 in about 90 of water (1 in 15 boiling water), 1 in 10 of ethanol, 1 in 3 of methanol, and 1 in 12 of chloroform; insoluble in ether and benzene.

Dissociation Constant. pK_a 4.2, 8.8 (20°).

Partition Coefficient. Log *P* (octanol/water), 3.4.

Colour Tests. Sulfuric Acid—yellow (fluoresces under UV light); Thalleioquin Test—green.

Thin-layer Chromatography. System TA—Rf 51; system TB—Rf 04; system TC—Rf 12; system TE—Rf 49; system TL—Rf 06; system TAE—Rf 30; system TAF—Rf 63; system TAJ—Rf 00; system TAK—Rf 02; system TAL—Rf 68. (Location under UV light, blue fluorescence; Dragendorff spray, positive; acidified iodoplatinate solution, positive.)

Gas Chromatography. System GA—quinidine RI 2790, M (*N*-oxide) RI 2950; system GB—quinidine RI 2979, M (*N*-oxide) RI 3086.

High Performance Liquid Chromatography. System HA—*k* 2.1; system HX—RI 322; system HY—RI 245; system HZ—Retention time 2.6 min; system HAA—Retention time 11.0 min; system HAX—Retention time 8.7 min; system HAY—Retention time 4.6 min.

Ultraviolet Spectrum. Aqueous acid—250 (A_1^1=959a), 317, 345; aqueous alkali—280, 330 nm.

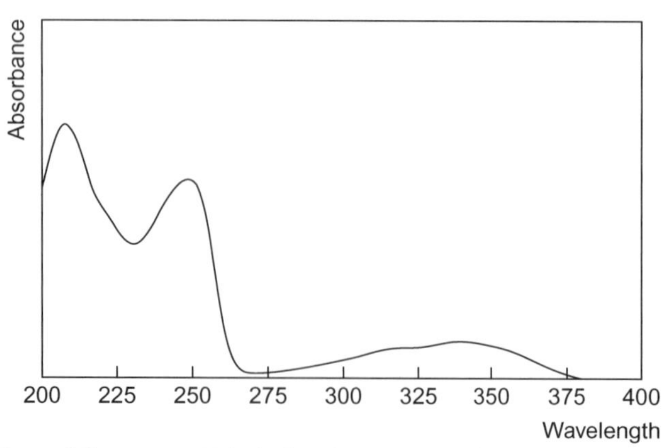

Infra-red Spectrum. Principal peaks at wavenumbers 1258, 1514, 1619, 1040, 860, 820 cm^{-1} (KBr disk).

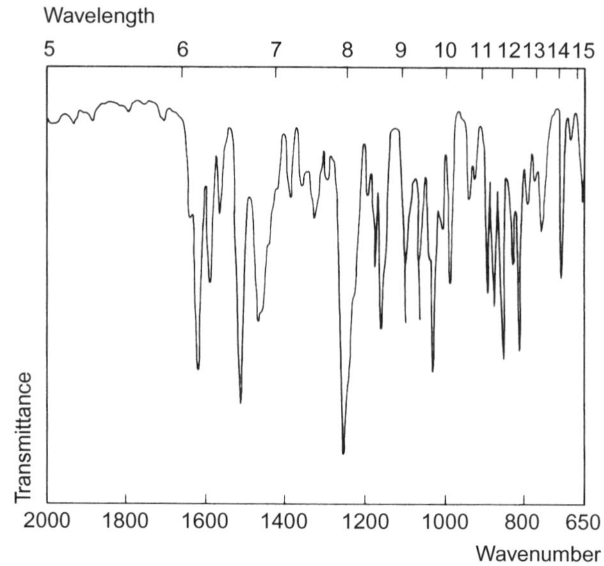

Mass Spectrum. Principal ions at *m/z* 136, 81, 322, 188, 55, 42, 41, 172.

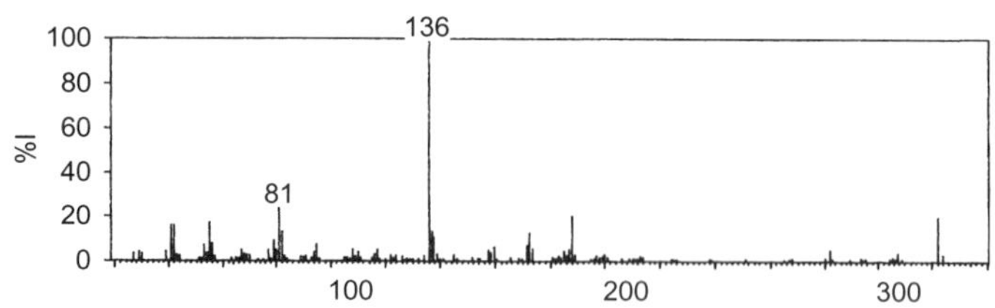

Quantification
Gas chromatography. In serum: quinidine and other anti-arrhythmic agents, AFID—K. M. Kessler *et al.*, *Clin. Chem.*, 1982, *28*, 1187–1190.

High performance liquid chromatography. In plasma: quinidine and other anti-arrhythmic agents, limit of detection 500 μg/L, UV detection—R. R. Bridges and T. A. Jennison, *J. Anal. Toxicol.*, 1983, *7*, 65–68. In plasma: quinidine, hydroquinidine, and 2 quinidine metabolites, limit of detection 50 μg/L for quinidine, fluorescence detection—L. K. Pershing *et al.*, *J. Anal. Toxicol.*, 1982, *6*, 153–156. In plasma or urine: quinidine, hydroquinidine and quinidine metabolites, limit of detection 10 μg/L for quinidine, fluorescence and UV detection—T. W. Guentert *et al.*, *J. Chromat.*, 1980, *183*; *B Biomed. Appl.*, *9*, 514–518. In plasma: quinidine and quinine, fluorescence detection—M. D. Edstein *et al.*, *Ther. Drug Monit.*, 1990, *12*, 493–500. In serum: quinidine and metabolites, limit of detection 0.1 mg/L, UV detection—G. L. Hoyer *et al.*, *J. Chromatogr.*, 1991, *572*, 159–169. In plasma—E. Brandsteterova *et al.*, *J. Chromatogr. A.*, 1994, *665*, 101–104. In plasma or urine: quinidine and its metabolites, limit of quantification 3.6 μg/L, fluorescence detection—F. Nielsen *et al.*, *J. Chromatogr. B Biomed. Appl.*, 1994, *660*, 103–110. In plasma: quinidine and diltiazem, limit of quantification for quinidine 4 μg/L, UV and fluorescence detection—G. Carignan *et al.*, *J. Chromatogr. B Biomed. Appl.*, 1995, *672*, 261–269.

Disposition in the Body. Rapidly absorbed after oral administration and undergoes first-pass metabolism in the liver. Extensively metabolised, mainly by the cytochrome P450 isoenzyme CYP3A4. The major metabolites, 3-hydroxyquinidine and quinidin-2′-one appear to be pharmacologically active. Hydroquinidine which may occur in quinidine as an impurity, at concentrations of up to about 30%, has similar pharmacological activity to quinidine. About 10 to 30% of a dose is excreted in the urine as unchanged drug in 48 h and the remainder is mostly excreted in the urine as metabolites; *O*-desmethylquinidine accounts for about 2% of a dose; quinidine-10,11-dihydrodiol and an *N*-oxide metabolite have been detected in plasma and urine. The proportion of unchanged drug is dependent on the urinary pH, being decreased if the urine is alkaline.
Quinidine crosses the placenta and is excreted in breast milk.

Therapeutic concentration. In plasma, usually in the range 2 to 6 mg/L; there is, however, considerable intersubject variation. Concentrations appear to be higher in subjects with congestive heart failure.

After single oral doses of 4.5 mg/kg of quinidine sulfate to 10 subjects, peak plasma concentrations of 0.9 to 1.8 mg/L (mean 1.2) were attained in about 50 min [T. W. Guentert *et al.*, *J. Pharmacokinet. Biopharm.*, 1979, *7*, 315–330].

Following daily oral doses of 8 to 19 mg/kg (mean 12) to 5 subjects, steady-state serum concentrations of 0.5 to 2.5 mg/L (mean 1.8) of quinidine, 0.38 to 0.94 mg/L (mean 0.55) of 3-hydroxyquinidine, and 0.02 to 0.12 mg/L (mean 0.07) of quinidin-2′-one, were reported; following daily oral doses of 8.6 to 13.3 mg/kg (mean 10.7) to 8 subjects with mild renal dysfunction, steady-state serum-quinidine concentrations ranged from 1.4 to 3.6 mg/L (mean 2.3) [D. E. Drayer *et al.*, *Clin. Pharmacol. Ther.*, 1978, *24*, 31–39].

Toxicity. Plasma concentrations greater than 6 mg/L are progressively associated with toxicity, and concentrations of about 15 mg/L may cause toxic reactions in about 50% of patients; concentrations in excess of about 30 mg/L may be lethal.

The following postmortem tissue concentrations were reported in one fatality: blood 75 mg/L, brain 11 µg/g, kidney 89 µg/g, liver 145 µg/g, spleen 136 µg/g, urine 52 mg/L; 3-hydroxyquinidine, and lactone conjugates of quinidine and 3-hydroxyquinidine were also detected [J. G. Leferink *et al.*, *J. Anal. Toxicol.*, 1977, *1*, 62–65].

In a fatality involving the ingestion of about 5 g of a sustained-release preparation by a 2-year-old child, the following postmortem tissue concentrations were reported: blood 45 mg/L, kidney 180 µg/g, liver 220 µg/g; death occurred 28 h after ingestion [A. J. McBay and R. F. Turk, *Bull. Int. Assoc. Forensic Toxicol.*, 1972, *8(4)*, 2–3].

Bioavailability. About 70 to 80% but there is considerable intersubject variation.

Half-life. Plasma half-life, about 4 to 12 h (mean 7).

Volume of distribution. About 2 to 3 L/kg, decreased in subjects with congestive heart failure.

Clearance. Plasma clearance, about 5 mL/min/kg.

Distribution in blood. Plasma : whole blood ratio, about 1.0.

Protein binding. In plasma, quinidine about 75 to 95%, 3-hydroxyquinidine about 60%, and quinidin-2′-one about 55%.

Note. For a review of the pharmacokinetic interactions of antimalarial agents, see P. T. Giao and P. J. de Vries, *Clin. Pharmacokinet.*, 2001, *40*, 343–373. For a general review of quinidine, see A.A. Grace and A. J. Camm, *N. Engl. J. Med.*, 1998, *338*, 35–45. For a review of the pharmacokinetics of quinine and quinidine in malaria, see N. J. White, *Acta Leiden.*, 1987, *55*, 65–76. For a review of the pharmacokinetics of quinidine see H.R.Ochs *et al.*, *Clin. Pharmacokinet.*, 1980, *5*, 150–168.

Dose. Usually 0.6 to 1.6 g of quinidine sulfate daily.

Quinine

Antimalarial

Synonyms. Chinina; Chininum; Quinina.
Proprietary name. It is an ingredient of Nicobrevin.
(8α,9*R*)-6′-Methoxycinchonan-9-ol trihydrate
$C_{20}H_{24}N_2O_2,3H_2O = 378.5$
CAS—130-95-0 (anhydrous)

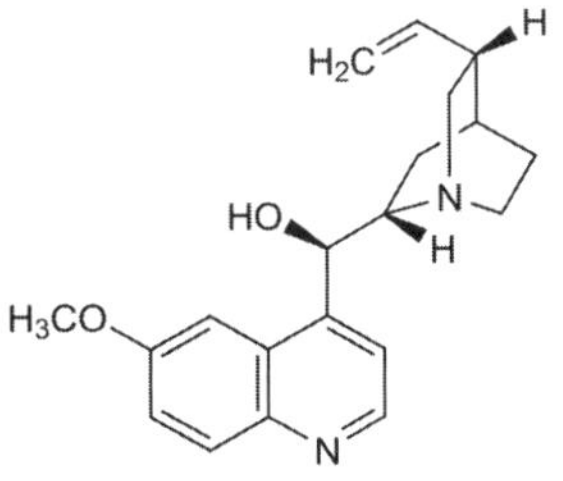

The chief alkaloid of various species of *Cinchona* (Rubiaceae). It is a laevorotatory stereoisomer of quinidine.
A white, slightly efflorescent, flaky, granular or microcrystalline powder. M.p. 57° (trihydrate).
The anhydrous form is soluble 1 in 1900 of water, 1 in 760 of boiling water, 1 in 0.8 of alcohol, 1 in 80 of benzene, 1 in 1.2 of chloroform, 1 in 250 of dry ether, and 1 in 20 of glycerol; almost insoluble in petroleum ether.

Quinine Bisulfate

Synonyms. Chininum Bisulfuricum; Neutral Quinine Sulfate; Quinine Acid Sulfate; Quinine Bisulphate; Quinini Bisulfas.
Proprietary names. Biquin; Biquinate; Myoquin; Quinbisul.
$C_{20}H_{24}N_2O_2,H_2SO_4,7H_2O = 548.6$
CAS—549-56-4 (anhydrous); 6183-68-2 (heptahydrate)
Colourless crystals or white crystalline powder. It effloresces in dry air and becomes yellow when exposed to light.
Soluble 1 in 8 of water, 1 in 50 of ethanol, and 1 in 625 of chloroform.

Quinine Dihydrobromide

Synonyms. Neutral Quinine Hydrobromide; Quinine Acid Hydrobromide.
$C_{20}H_{24}N_2O_2,2HBr,3H_2O = 540.3$
Yellowish or white crystals or powder.
Soluble 1 in 7 of water; soluble in ethanol; practically insoluble in ether.

Quinine Dihydrochloride

Synonyms. Chinini Dihydrochloridum; Neutral Quinine Hydrochloride; Quinine Acid Hydrochloride; Quinini Dihydrochloridum.
$C_{20}H_{24}N_2O_2,2HCl = 397.3$
CAS—60-93-5
A white powder.
Soluble 1 in about 0.6 of water, 1 in about 12 of ethanol, and 1 in 7 of chloroform; very slightly soluble in ether.

Quinine Ethyl Carbonate

Synonyms. Euquinina; Euquinine; Quinine Etabonate.
$C_{23}H_{28}N_2O_4 = 396.5$
CAS—83-75-0
White masses of silky crystals which darken on exposure to light. M.p. 91° to 95°.
Very slightly soluble in water; soluble 1 in 2 of ethanol, 1 in 1 of chloroform, and 1 in 10 of ether.

Quinine Hydrobromide

Synonyms. Basic Quinine Hydrobromide; Chinini Bromidum; Quinine Monohydrobromide.
$C_{20}H_{24}N_2O_2,HBr,2H_2O = 441.4$
CAS—549-49-5 (anhydrous)
White, silky, efflorescent crystals which darken on exposure to light.
Soluble 1 in about 55 of water, 1 in 0.7 of ethanol, and 1 in 1 of chloroform, the solution in chloroform being turbid due to separation of water.

Quinine Hydrochloride

Synonyms. Basic Quinine Hydrochloride; Chinini Hydrochloridum; Chinini Chloridum; Chininium Chloratum; Chininum Hydrochloricum; Quinine Monohydrochloride.
Proprietary names. Kinin; Surquina.
$C_{20}H_{24}N_2O_2,HCl,2H_2O = 396.9$
CAS—130-89-2 (anhydrous); 6119-47-7 (dihydrate)
Colourless, fine, silky, acicular crystals which effloresce in dry air and gradually become yellowish on exposure to light.
Soluble 1 in 16 of water (1 in 0.5 of boiling water), 1 in 1 of ethanol, 1 in 7 of glycerol, 1 in about 350 of ether, and 1 in about 1 of chloroform to give a turbid solution.

Quinine Salicylate

$C_{20}H_{24}N_2O_2,C_7H_6O_3,H_2O = 480.6$
CAS—750-90-3 (anhydrous)
White silky crystals or a crystalline powder; it becomes pink on storage.
Very slightly soluble in water; soluble 1 in 24 of ethanol and 1 in 25 of chloroform.

Quinine Sulfate

Synonyms. Basic Quinine Sulphate; Chinini Sulfas; Chininum Sulfuricum; Quinine Sulphate.
Proprietary names. Q200; Q300; Quinate; Quinoc; Quinoctal; Quinora; Quinsul.
$(C_{20}H_{24}N_2O_2)_2,H_2SO_4,2H_2O = 783.0$
CAS—804-63-7 (anhydrous); 6119-70-6 (dihydrate)
Colourless acicular crystals or a white crystalline powder, becoming brown on exposure to light.
Soluble 1 in about 810 of water (1 in 32 of boiling water) and 1 in 120 of ethanol; slightly soluble in chloroform and ether; readily soluble in a 2:1 mixture of chloroform and dehydrated alcohol.

Dissociation Constant. pK_a 4.1, 8.5 (20°).

Partition Coefficient. Log *P* (octanol/water), 3.4.

Colour Tests. Sulfuric Acid—yellow (fluoresces under UV light); Thalleioquin Test—green.

Thin-layer Chromatography. System TA—Rf 51; system TB—Rf 02; system TC—Rf 11; system TE—Rf 45; system TL—Rf 04; system TAE—Rf 26; system TAF—Rf 65. (Location under UV light, blue fluorescence; Dragendorff spray, positive; acidified iodoplatinate solution, positive.)

Gas Chromatography. System GA—quinine RI 2800, quinine-AC RI 2760, M (OH-)-AC_2 RI 3195, M (*N*-oxide)-AC RI 2945, M (di-OH-dihydro-)-AC_3 RI 3360.

High Performance Liquid Chromatography. System HA—*k* 2.4; system HS—*k* 2.02; system HX—RI 327; system HY—RI 246; system HZ—Retention time 2.6 min; system HAA—Retention time 11.3 min; system HAX—Retention time 8.3 min; system HAY—Retention time 4.5 min.

Ultraviolet Spectrum. Aqueous acid—250 (A_1^1=959a), 317, 346; aqueous alkali—280, 330 nm.

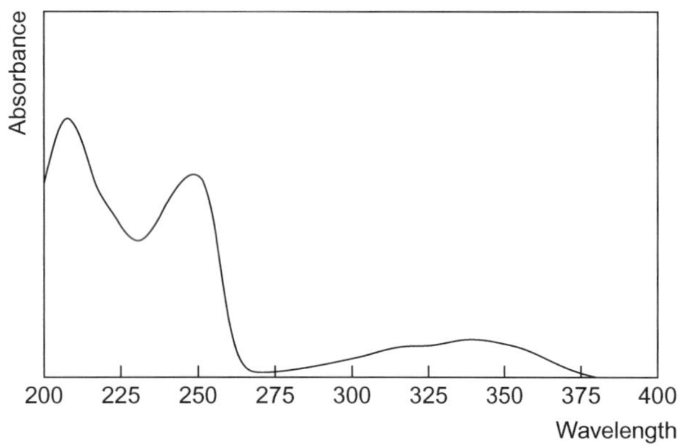

Infra-red Spectrum. Principal peaks at wavenumbers 1235, 1215, 1510, 1619, 1030, 1105 cm^{-1} (KBr disk).

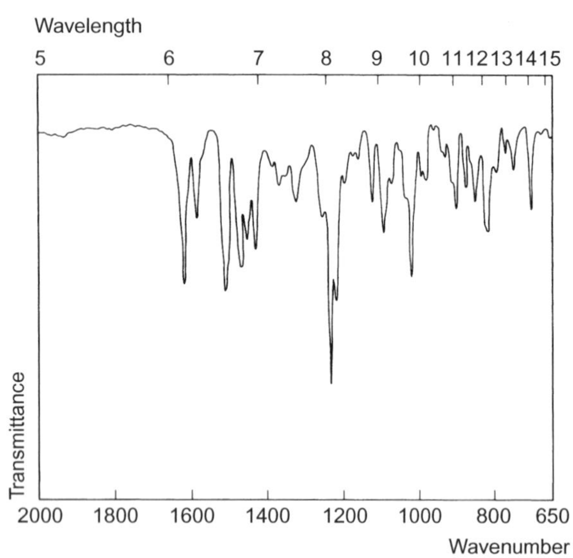

Mass Spectrum. Principal ions at *m/z* 136, 137, 81, 42, 41, 189, 55, 117.

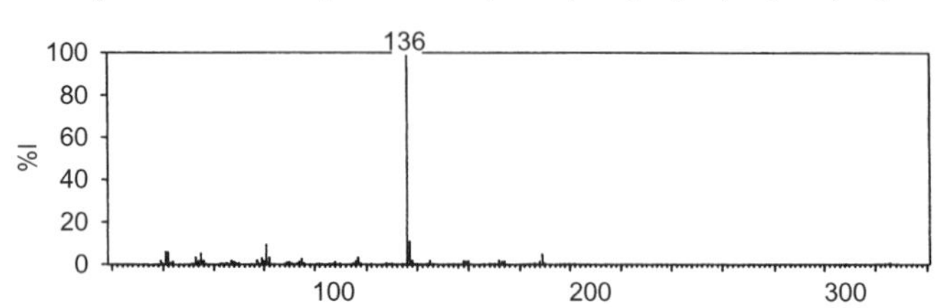

Quantification

Spectrofluorimetry. In plasma or urine—A. P. Hall *et al.*, *Clin. Pharmacol. Ther.*, 1973, *14*, 580–585.

Gas chromatography–mass spectrometry. In urine: limit of detection 50 pg—R. L. Furner *et al.*, *J. Anal. Toxicol.*, 1981, *5*, 275–278.

High performance liquid chromatography. In serum: UV detection, comparison with spectrofluorometric method—J. H. Galloway *et al.*, *J. Anal. Toxicol.*, 1990, *14*, 345–347. In plasma: quinine and quinidine, fluorescence detection—M. D. Edstein *et al.*, *Ther. Drug Monit.*, 1990, *12*, 493–500. In blood (on filter paper)—E. K. Mberu *et al.*, *J. Chromatogr.*, 1991, *570*, 180–184. In plasma, erythrocytes, or urine: quinine and chloroquine, limit of detection for quinine about 23 μg/L, fluorescence detection—J. F. Chaulet *et al.*, *J. Chromatogr.*, 1993, *613*, 303–310. In serum, plasma, red blood cells or whole blood (on filter paper): fluorescence detection—V. K. Dua *et al.*, *J. Chromatogr.*, 1993, *614*, 87–93. In plasma, saliva, or urine: limit of detection 10 μg/L, UV detection—C. P. Babalola *et al.*, *J. Chromatogr.*, 1993, *616*, 151–154. In whole blood, plasma or urine (and dried on filter paper): limit of detection 2 nmol/L in plasma and 50 nmol/L in whole blood, dried samples and urine, fluorescence detection—O. Ericsson *et al.*, *Ther. Drug Monit.*, 1993, *15*, 334–337. In serum or whole blood (or dried on filter paper): quinine and chloroquine and related compounds, limit of quantification for quinine 50 μg/L, fluorescence detection—K. Croes *et al.*, *J. Anal. Toxicol.*, 1994, *18*, 255–260. In plasma or urine: 3-hydroxyquinine, limit of quantification in plasma 4.5 nmol/L, fluorescence detection—R. A. Mirghani *et al.*, *J. Chromatogr. B Biomed. Sci. Appl.*, 1998, *708*, 209–216. In plasma or whole blood (on filter paper): limit of quantification 0.1 mg/L, UV and fluorescence detection—J. A. Kolawole and A. Mustapha, *Biopharm. Drug Dispos.*, 2000, 21, 345–352. In plasma or urine: quinine and its metabolites, limits of quantification 0.024 to 0.081 μmol/L, fluorescence detection—R. A. Mirghani *et al.*, *J. Chromatogr. B Biomed. Sci. Appl.*, 2001, *754*, 57–64.

Disposition in the Body. Readily absorbed after oral administration but more slowly absorbed after IM or subcutaneous doses. Hydroquinine may occur in quinine as an impurity at concentrations up to about 10%. Metabolised by oxidation to hydroxylated metabolites, mainly the 2-hydroxyquinoline and 6-hydroxyquinoline derivatives, 3-hydroxyquinine, and the corresponding dihydro compounds; quinine-10,11-epoxide and quinine-10,11-dihydrodiol have also been detected in urine. Up to about 20% of a single dose is excreted in the urine in 24 h with less than 5% as unchanged drug. Less than 5% of a dose is eliminated in the faeces. The urinary excretion of quinine is increased when the urine is acid; quinine is excreted to some extent in the bile and saliva. Quinine crosses the placenta and is excreted in breast milk.

Therapeutic concentration. In plasma, usually in the range 3 to 7 mg/L. Malarial infection inhibits hepatic metabolism and thus plasma concentrations resulting from a given dose will vary according to the severity of the infection.

Single oral doses of 300 mg quinine bisulfate administered to 8 healthy subjects and to 8 patients with chronic renal failure on haemodialysis, resulted in mean maximum plasma concentrations of 2.60 mg/L in healthy subjects and 4.56 mg/L in dialysis patients; the time to reach peak concentrations was similar in both groups (1.6 vs 1.9 h) [L. Roy *et al.*, *Br. J. Clin. Pharmacol.*, 2002, *54*, 604–609].

Following a single oral dose of quinine sulfate 600 mg to 4 healthy subjects, a mean maximum concentration of 2.88 mg/L was attained in the plasma at 2.75 h and 0.90 mg/L in the saliva at 4.25 h [C. P. Babalola *et al.*, *Ther. Drug Monit.*, 1996, *18*, 30–33].

Oral doses of 540 mg, given 8-hourly for 3 days to 11 subjects, resulted in a mean peak plasma concentration of 4 mg/L after 72 h [A. P. Hall *et al.*, *Clin. Pharmacol. Ther.*, 1973, *14*, 580–585].

Toxicity. The estimated minimum lethal dose is 8 g. Blood concentrations greater than about 10 mg/L may cause toxic effects and can be lethal.

Fatal quinine poisoning occurred in three young females, and the following postmortem concentrations (mg/L or μg/g) were reported: blood -, 11, -; kidney 300, 96, 410; liver 1500, 39, 150; spleen 600, 87, -; urine -, -, 860 [G. W. Walker, personal communication, 1964].

In a fatality involving the ingestion of 32.5 g of quinine sulfate, postmortem brain and liver concentrations of 292 and 3000 μg/g, respectively, were reported [S. Andrtauskas *et al.*, *Bull. Int. Assoc. Forensic Toxicol.*, 1974, *10(3)*, 7–8].

Half-life. Plasma half-life, 4 to 15 h (mean 9); it appears to be increased during malarial infection.

Volume of distribution. About 2 L/kg; reduced in malaria infection.

Distribution in blood. Plasma : whole blood ratio, about 0.93 in normal subjects. In malarial subjects, the plasma concentration rises but this does not seem to be accompanied by a rise in the amount taken up by erythrocytes; under these conditions there may be twice as much in the plasma as in the erythrocytes.

Protein binding. In plasma, 70% in healthy subjects increasing to 90% or higher in malaria infection.

Note. For a review of the pharmacokinetics of quinine, chloroquine and amodiaquine, see S. Krishna and N. J. White, *Clin. Pharmacokinet.*, 1996, *30*, 263–299. For a review of the pharmacokinetics of quinine and quinidine in malaria, see N. J. White, *Acta Leiden*, 1987, *55*, 65–76; for a review of the pharmacokinetic interactions of antimalarial agents, see P. T. Giao and P. J. de Vries, *Clin. Pharmacokinet.*, 2001, *40*, 343–373. For a toxicity study of quinine when given with doxycycline and mefloquine, see J. Karbwang *et al.*, *Southeast Asian J. Trop. Med. Public Health*, 1994, *25*, 397–400.

Dose. 1.8 g of quinine sulfate or other salt, by mouth daily, for 7 days for treatment of falciparum malaria. For nocturnal leg cramps 200 mg to 300 mg of sulfate or bisulfate at night.

Quinisocaine

Local Anaesthetic

Synonyms. Chinisocaine; Dimethisoquin.
2-[(3-Butyl-1-isoquinolinyl)oxy]-*N*,*N*-dimethylethanamine
$C_{17}H_{24}N_2O = 272.4$
CAS—86-80-6

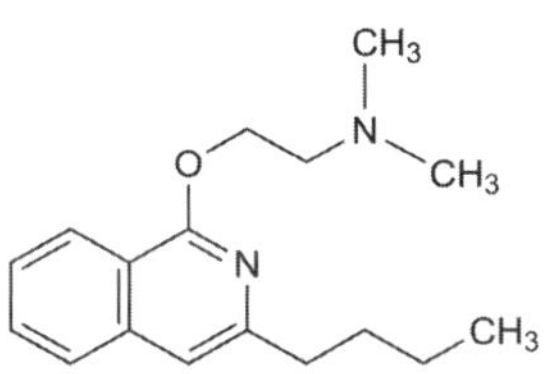

A liquid. B.p. 155° to 157°.

Quinisocaine Hydrochloride

Proprietary names. Haenal; Isochinol; Pruralgan; Pruralgin; Quotane.
$C_{17}H_{24}N_2O,HCl = 308.9$
CAS—2773-92-4
A white crystalline powder. M.p. 144° to 148°.
Soluble 1 in 8 of water, 1 in 3 of ethanol, and 1 in 2 of chloroform; practically insoluble in ether.

Partition Coefficient. Log *P* (octanol/water), 4.4.

Thin-layer Chromatography. System TA—Rf 61; system TB—Rf 55; system TC—Rf 46; system TL—Rf 28; system TAJ—Rf 25; system TAK—Rf 13; system TAL—Rf 66. (Acidified iodoplatinate solution, positive.)

Gas Chromatography. System GA—RI 2030.

High Performance Liquid Chromatography. System HA—*k* 2.2; system HR—*k* 11.24.

Ultraviolet Spectrum. Aqueous acid—261, 269 nm ($A_1^1 = 159a$), 331 nm.

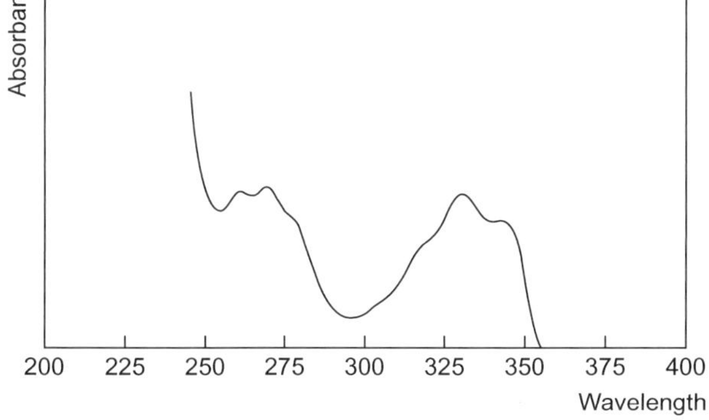

Infra-red Spectrum. Principal peaks at wavenumbers 1576, 1631, 1499, 1155, 1115, 751 cm^{-1} (KBr disk).

Mass Spectrum. Principal ions at *m/z* 71, 58, 72, 43, 159, 56, 42, 201.

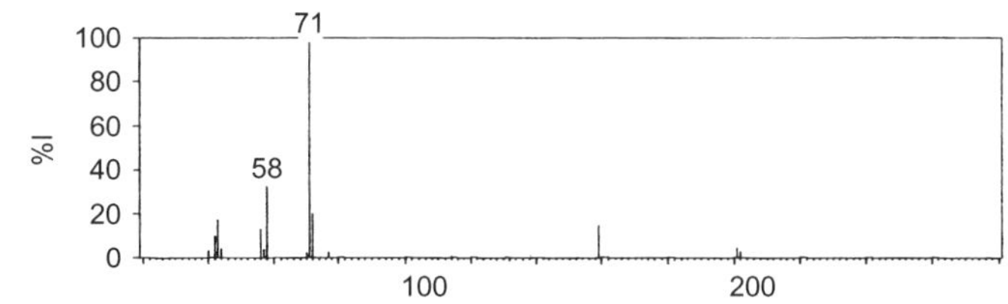

Use. Quinisocaine hydrochloride is used in a concentration of 0.5%.

Quinuronium Sulfate

Antiprotozoal (Veterinary)

Synonym. SN-5870
Proprietary names. Acaprin; Atral; Babesan; Baburan; Pirevan; Pyroplasmin; Zothelone.
6,6′-Ureylenebis[1,1′-dimethylquinolinium]sulfate
$C_{23}H_{26}N_4O_9S_2 = 566.6$
CAS—135-14-8

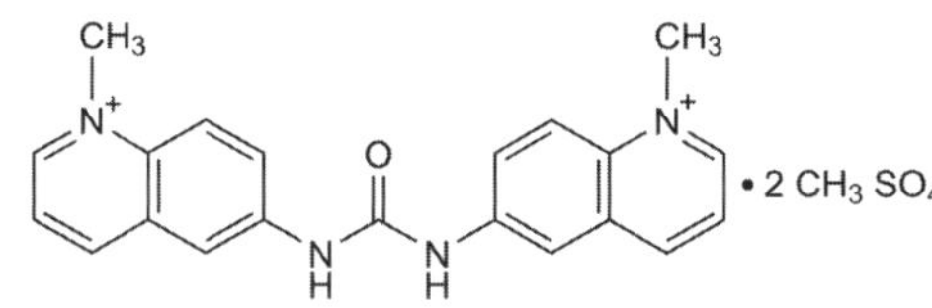

A creamy-white to yellow, crystalline powder. M.p. 237°, with decomposition.
Very soluble in water; very slightly soluble in organic solvents. On heating, aqueous solutions darken and some decomposition may occur.

Colour Test. Aromaticity (Method 2)—yellow/orange.

Thin-layer Chromatography. System TA—Rf 00. (Acidified iodoplatinate solution, positive.)

Ultraviolet Spectrum. Aqueous acid—274 nm ($A_1^1 = 1527a$), 323 nm, 359 nm.

Infra-red Spectrum. Principal peaks at wavenumbers 1210, 1248, 1276, 1572, 1025, 1525 cm^{-1} (KBr disk).

Rabeprazole

Proton Pump Inhibitor

Synonyms. LY-307640; Pariprazole.
2-[[[4-(3-Methoxypropoxy)-3-methyl-2-pyridinyl]methyl]sulfinyl]-1*H*-benzimidazole
$C_{18}H_{21}N_3O_3S = 359.4$
CAS—117976-89-3

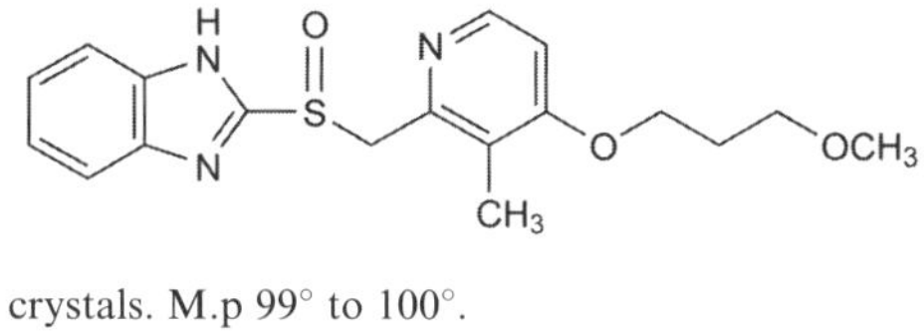

White crystals. M.p 99° to 100°.

Rabeprazole Sodium

Synonyms. E-3810; SHKA.
Proprietary names. AcipHex; Pariet.
$C_{18}H_{20}N_3NaO_3S = 381.4$
CAS— 117976-90-6
A white to slightly yellowish white crystalline solid. M.p 140° to 141°. It is very soluble in water and methanol; freely soluble in ethanol, chloroform and ethyl acetate; insoluble in ether and *n*-hexane.

High Performance Liquid Chromatography. Column: C_8 (Inertsil, 150 × 4.6 mm i.d., 5 μm). Column temperature: 40°. Mobile phase: acetonitrile:phosphate buffer (0.1 M, pH 7.0) (28:72), flow rate 1.4 mL/min. UV detection (λ=288 nm). Retention time(s): rabeprazole sodium, 6.5 min;

demethylated metabolite, 2.8 min; demethylated thioether metabolite, 6.0 min; sulfone metabolite, 8.0 min; thioether metabolite, 19.7 min. [H. Nakai *et al.*, *J. Chromatogr.*, 1994, *660*; *Biomed. Appl.*, 211–220].

Ultraviolet Spectrum. Aqueous base (0.01 M NaOH)—292 nm.

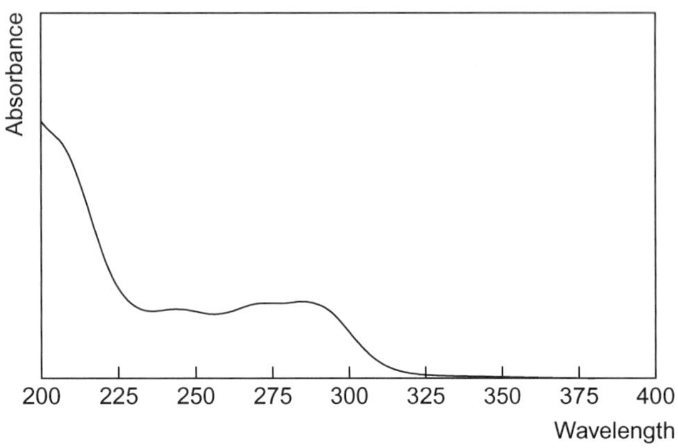

Infra-red Spectrum. Principal peaks at wavenumbers 1584, 1298, 1462, 1081 cm^{-1}.

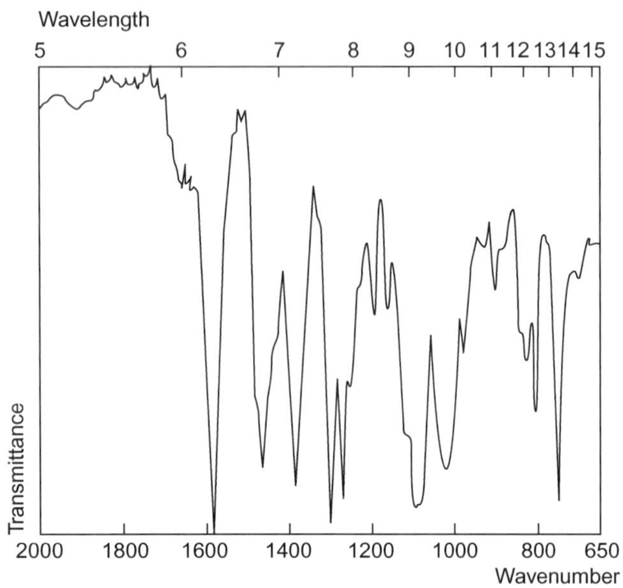

Quantification

High performance liquid chromatography. In plasma: limit of quantification 0.03 mg/L. UV detection (λ=290 nm)—N. Mano *et al.*, *J. Pharm. Sci.*, 1996, *85*, 903–907. In plasma: limit of quantification 5 μg/L for the drug and 20 μg/L for the metabolites. UV detection (λ=288 nm)—H. Nakai *et al.*, *J. Chromatogr.*, 1994, *660*; *Biomed. Appl.*, 211–220.

Disposition in the Body. Rabeprazole is well absorbed (at least 30%) and can be detected in the plasma within 1 h. Food delays absorption. It is extensively and rapidly metabolised; this is regulated by the CYP2C19 isoenzyme in the liver and to some extent by CYP3A4. The primary metabolite is the rabeprazole thioether. Other metabolites are sulfone E3810, desmethyl E3810, desmethylated thioether E3810 and thioether carboxylic acid E3810. 90% of the administered drug is excreted in urine with 30% as the thioether carboxylic acid metabolite and its glucuronide. No unchanged rabeprazole has been recovered in urine or faeces. Renal excretion accounts for 30 to 35%. There is no accumulation following multiple dosing.

Therapeutic concentration. A maximum plasma concentration of 0.406 mg/L can be achieved with a single 20 mg dose of rabeprazole. A maximum concentration of 0.418 mg/L is reached after 40 mg for 7 days. Time to reach maximum plasma concentration is about 3.1 h. [A. Prakash and D. Faulds, *Drugs*, 1998, *55(2)*, 261–267].

6 healthy volunteers were administered with doses between 10 and 80 mg rabeprazole sodium. The maximum plasma concentration reached for the 20 mg dose was 0.406 mg/L, observed after 3.5 h. The 80 mg dose produced concentrations of approx. 1.4 mg/L at 4 h; 40 mg dose approx. 0.9 mg/L at 3.5 h; and the 10 mg dose, approx. 0.15 mg/L at 4.5 h. [H. Nakai *et al.*, *J. Chromatogr.*, 1994, *660*; *Biomed. Appl.*, 211–220].

Bioavailability. 52%.

Half-life. 1 to 2 h

Clearance. 35.3 L/h; 4.37 to 8.40 mL/min/kg.

Protein binding. 96.3%.

Dose. 20 mg daily.

Racemorphan

Narcotic Analgesic

Synonym. Methorphinan

17-Methylmorphinan-3-ol

$C_{17}H_{23}NO$=257.4

CAS—297-90-5

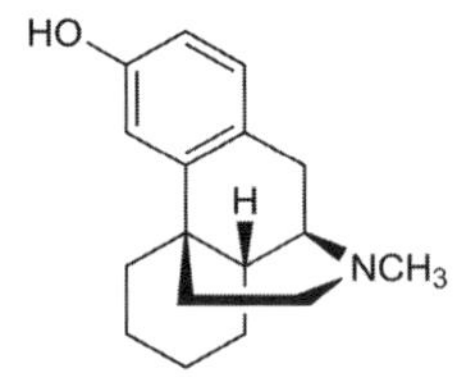

A white powder. M.p. 251° to 253°.

Soluble in dilute acetic acid.

Thin-layer Chromatography. System TA—Rf 34; system TB—Rf 14; system TC—Rf 09; system TL—Rf 02. (Dragendorff spray, positive; acidified iodoplatinate solution, positive.)

Gas Chromatography. System GA—racemorphan RI 2138; M (nor-) RI 2193; system GB—racemorphan RI 2237; M (nor-) RI 2244; M (OH-) RI 2420.

Ultraviolet Spectrum. Aqueous acid—279 (A_1^1=79a); aqueous alkali—240 (A_1^1=339a), 299 nm (A_1^1=119a).

Infra-red Spectrum. Principal peaks at wavenumbers 1242, 1280, 1580, 1495, 1505, 760 cm^{-1} (KBr disk).

Mass Spectrum. Principal ions at *m/z* 257, 59, 150, 256, 31, 157, 42, 200.

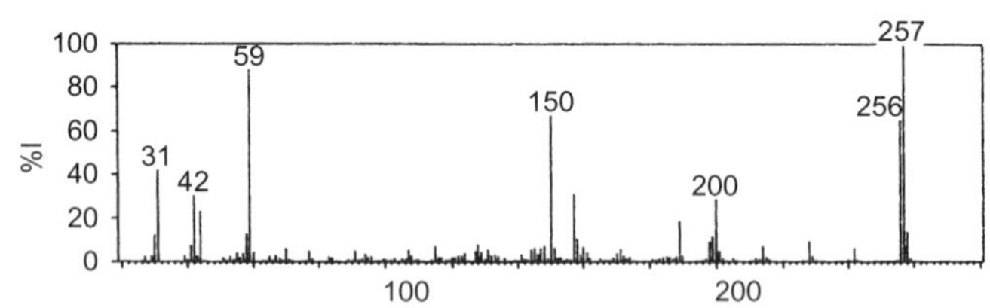

Racephedrine

Sympathomimetic

Synonyms. *dl*-Ephedrine; Racemic Ephedrine.

Proprietary name. It is an ingredient of Riddofan.

[α-(Methylamino)ethyl]benzenemethanol

$C_{10}H_{15}NO$=165.2

CAS—90-81-3

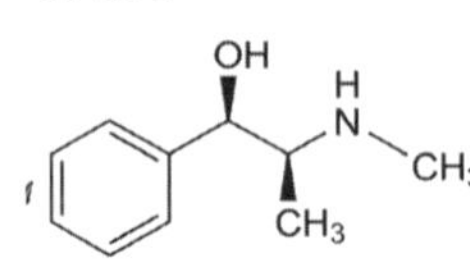

Crystals. M.p. 75°.

Soluble in water, ethanol, chloroform and ether.

Racephedrine Hydrochloride
Proprietary names. Efetonina; Ephetonin.
$C_{10}H_{15}NO,HCl=201.7$
CAS—134-71-4
Fine, white, crystals or powder. M.p. 189°.
Soluble 1 in about 4 of water and 1 in about 4 of ethanol; practically insoluble in ether.

Partition Coefficient. Log *P* (octanol/water), 0.7.

For analytical data see under Ephedrine.

Dose. 50 to 200 mg of racephedrine hydrochloride daily.

Rafoxanide

Anthelmintic (Veterinary)

Synonym. MK-990
Proprietary names. Flukanide; Flukex; Ranide; Ridafluke.
N-[3-Chloro-4-(4-chlorophenoxy)phenyl]-2-hydroxy-3,5-diiodobenzamide
$C_{19}H_{11}Cl_2I_2NO_3=626.0$
CAS—22662-39-1

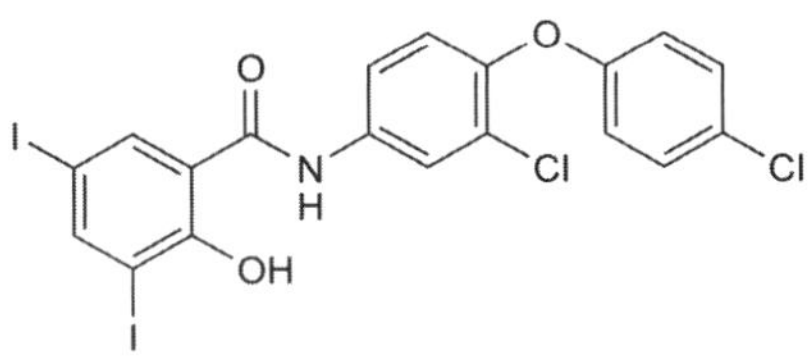

A greyish-white to brown powder. M.p. 168° to 170°.
Practically insoluble in water; soluble 1 in 25 of acetone, 1 in 40 of chloroform, 1 in 35 of ethyl acetate, and 1 in 200 of methanol.

Partition Coefficient. Log *P* (octanol/water), 8.1.

Colour Test. Iodine test—positive.

Thin-layer Chromatography. System TA—Rf 89. (Acidified potassium permanganate solution, positive.)

Gas Chromatography. System GA—not eluted.

Ultraviolet Spectrum. Methanolic acid—280 nm (A_1^1=243b), 335 nm (A_1^1=149a).

Infra-red Spectrum. Principal peaks at wavenumbers 1215, 1562, 1592, 1257, 1087, 1275 cm^{-1} (KBr disk).

Raltitrexed

Antineoplastic

Synonyms. ICI-D-1694; ZD-1694.
Proprietary name. Tomudex
N-[[5-[[(1,4-Dihydro-2-methyl-4-oxo-6-quinazolinyl)methyl]-methylamino]-2-thienyl]carbonyl]-L-glutamic acid
$C_{21}H_{22}N_4O_6S=458.5$
CAS—112887-68-0

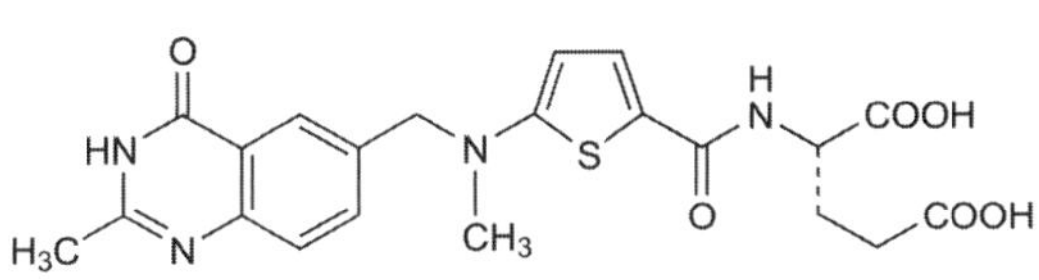

Pale yellow powder. Soluble in water.

Raltitrexed Monohydrate
Crystals with m.p. 180° to 184°.

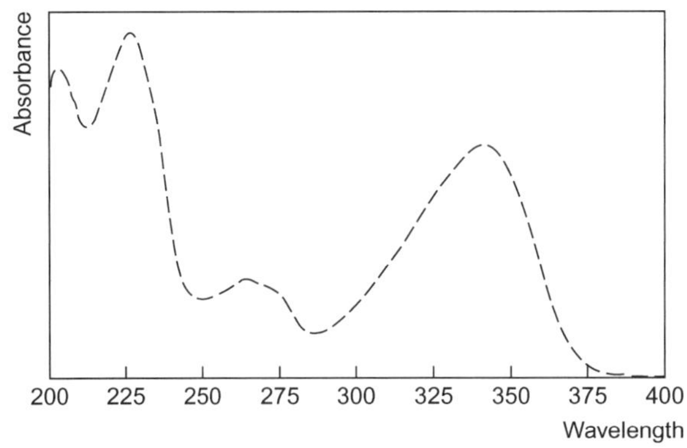

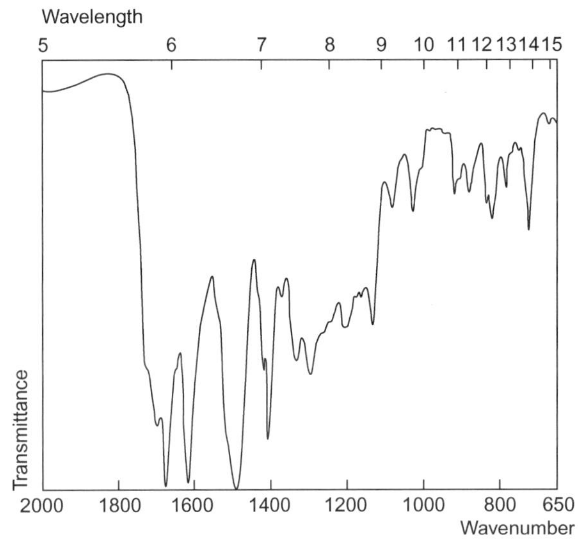

Disposition in the Body. Following intravenous administration of raltitrexed, triphasic pharmacokinetics are displayed. There is a rapid decline from peak plasma concentration followed by a slow terminal elimination phase. The maximum plasma concentration is reached within 15 min. The drug is actively transported into cells and metabolised to active polyglutamate forms. The reminder of the dose is excreted unchanged with approx. 50% of the dose appearing in urine and 15% in faeces. No accumulation occurs of the drug after multiple dosing.

Therapeutic concentration
The peak plasma concentration after a 3 mg/m^2 dose was 833 µg/L. The mean observed peak plasma concentration in cancer patients was 700.6 µg/L. [P. Beale *et al.*, *Cancer Chemother. Pharmacol.*, 1998, *42*, 71–76].

Toxicity
Increasing the dosage above 3 mg/m^2, increases the incidence of life threatening or fatal toxicity. [*ABPI Data Sheets*].

Bioavailability. Following intraperitoneal administration, it is fully bioavailable. Following oral administration, 10 to 20%.

Half-life. 8 days (257 h).

Volume of distribution. Steady state, 548 L.

Clearance. Following a 3 mg/m^2 dose clearance is 51.6 mL/min and the renal clearance is 25.1 mL/min. It is reduced in those with renal impairment by 25%.

Protein binding. 93%.

Dose. 3 mg/m^2 intravenously every 3 weeks.

Ramipril

Antihypertensive

Synonyms. HOE-498; Ramiprilum.
Proprietary names. Acovil; Altace; Cardace; Delix; Pramace; Quark; Ramace; Triatec; Tritace; Unipril; Vespril. It is also an ingredient of Arelix; Composto; Delix Plus; and Triapin.

(2*S*,3a*S*,6a*S*)-1-[(2*S*)-2-[[(1*S*)-1-(Ethoxycarbonyl)-3-phenylpropyl] amino]-1-oxopropyl]octahydrocyclopenta[*b*]pyrrole-2-carboxylic acid
$C_{23}H_{32}N_2O_5$=416.5
CAS—87333-19-5

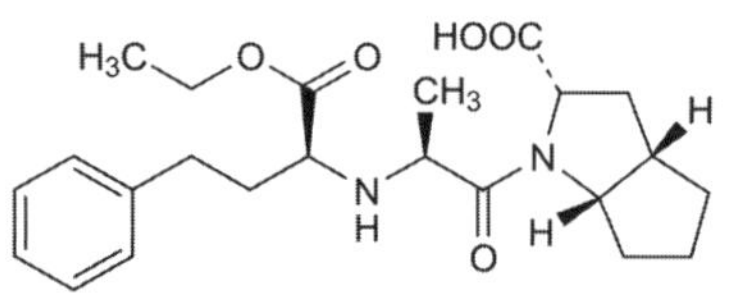

Needle-shaped crystals (from ether), m.p. 109°. It is soluble in methyl alcohol; sparingly soluble in water.

Ramiprilat
CAS—87269-97-4

Partition Coefficient. Log *P* (octanol/water), 3.32 for ramipril; 0.22 for ramiprilat.

Gas Chromatography. System GP—RI 2880 ramipril-ME; RI 2865 M (ramiprilat)-ME3; RI 2925 M (ramiprilate-H_2O)-ME3.

High Performance Liquid Chromatography. System HAA—retention time 15.7 min; system HZ—retention time 4.2 min.

Column: LC-8 (Supelcosil, 150 × 4.6 mm i.d., 5 µm). Mobile phase: acetonitrile:sodium perchlorate solution (0.1 M), pH 2.5, flow rate 1.5 mL/min. IS: clobazam. UV detection (λ=210 nm). Retention time(s): ramipril, 5.1 min; IS, 3.4 min. [F. Belal *et al.*, *J. Pharm. Biomed. Anal.*, 2001, *24*, 335–342].

Ultraviolet Spectrum. Aqueous acid (0.2 M H_2SO_4)—252, 258 nm; basic—252, 258, 267 nm.

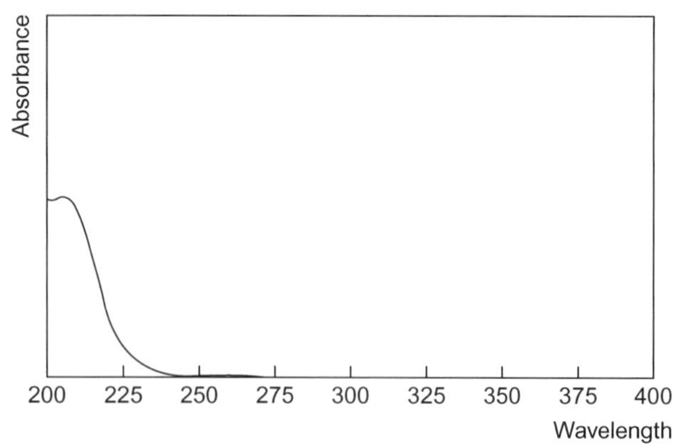

Infra-red Spectrum. Principal peaks at wavenumbers 1743, 1652, 1187, 756 cm^{-1} (KBr pellet).

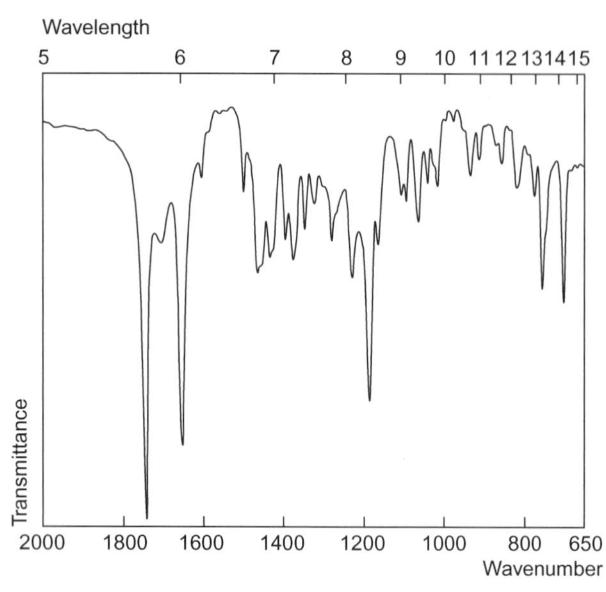

Mass Spectrum. Principal ions at *m/z* 294, 248, 91, 110, 117, 209, 160, 297.

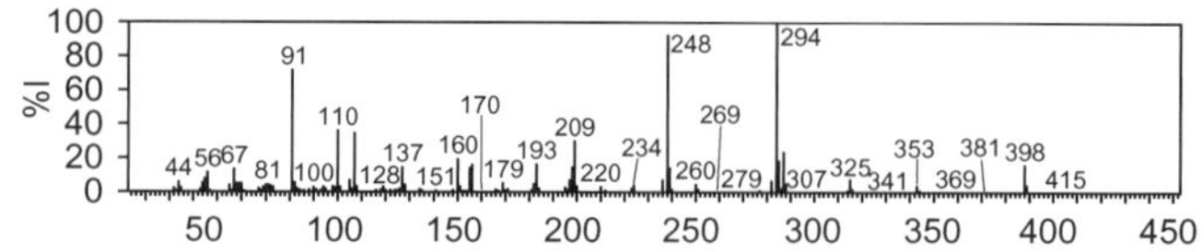

Disposition in the Body. Ramipril is rapidly absorbed after oral administration, with 54 to 65% of the dose absorbed. Absorption is not affected by the presence of food. It is metabolised in the liver to the active drug ramiprilat, a dicarboxylic acid, by hydrolysis, as well as ramipril glucuronide, ramiprilat glucuronide and diketopiperazine derivatives. Peak plasma concentrations of the parent drug are reached within 0.25 and 1 h and for the metabolite, ramiprilat, 2 to 4 h. The drug is excreted mainly in urine (60%) and faeces (40%) with little unchanged drug detected. The drug is rapidly cleared from the blood and distributed to all body tissues especially to the liver, kidneys and lungs where high concentrations are found. The drug can still be detected in serum up to 24 h after dosing.

Therapeutic concentration

12 healthy male volunteers were administered 2.5 mg ramipril orally, intravenously and ramiprilat 2.5 mg intravenously on three separate occasions, after an overnight fast. The peak plasma ramipril concentration after the oral ramipril dose was 6.2 µg/L and 2.7 µg/L for the metabolite, ramiprilat. These were observed at 48 and 151 min, respectively. The peak drug concentration was 261 µg/L after the intravenous dose and 14 µg/L for the metabolite at 5.3 and 158 min, respectively. For the ramiprilat dose, the peak concentration was 301 µg/L at 6.9 min. [J. M. T. van Griensven *et al.*, *Eur. J. Clin. Pharmacol.*, 1995, *47*, 513–518].

Bioavailability. Ramipril, 28%; ramiprilat 44%.

Half-life. Ramipril, 1 to 2 h; ramiprilat, 9 to 18 h.

Volume of distribution. Ramipril, 90 L.

Clearance. Ramiprilat clearance reduced in renal impairment.

Protein binding. Ramipril, 73%; ramiprilat, 56%.

Dose. 1.25 to 5 mg daily with a maximum of 10 mg daily.

Ranitidine

Histamine H_2-Receptor Antagonist

N-[2-[[[-5-[(Dimethylamino)methyl]-2-furanyl]methyl]thio]ethyl]-*N*′-methyl-2-nitro-1,1-ethenediamine
$C_{13}H_{22}N_4O_3S$=314.4
CAS—66357-35-5

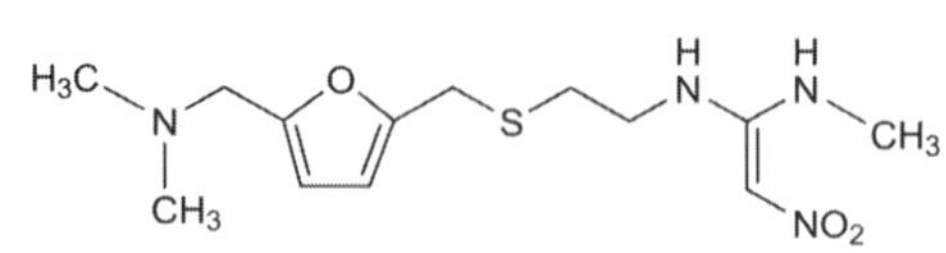

A solid. M.p. 69° to 70°.

Ranitidine Hydrochloride
Synonyms. AH-19065; Ranitidini Hydrochloridum.
Proprietary names. Ausran; Azantac; Azuranit; Digestosan; Gertac; Ranaps; Rani; Ranic; Ranihexal; Raniplex; Raniprotect; Ranitic; Ranopine; Ranoxyl; Rantec; Sostril; Ulcidine; Ulcirex; Ulsal; Xanomel; Zaedoc; Zandin(e); Zantac; Zantic; Zidac.
$C_{13}H_{22}N_4O_3S,HCl$=350.9
CAS—66357-59-3
A yellowish-grey powder. M.p. 133° to 134°.
Freely soluble in water and acetic acid; soluble in methanol; sparingly soluble in ethanol; practically insoluble in chloroform.

Ranitidine Bismuth Citrate
Synonyms. GR-122311X; (Ranitidine Bismutrex)
Proprietary names. Pylorid; Tritec.
Compound with bismuth (3+)citrate (1:1)
$C_{13}H_{22}N_4O_3S.C_6H_5BiO_7$=712.5
CAS—128345-62-0

Dissociation Constant. pK_a 2.3, 8.2.

Partition Coefficient. Log *P* (octanol/water), 0.3.

Thin-layer Chromatography. System TA—Rf 50; system TE—Rf 30; system TAJ—Rf 02; system TAK—Rf 00; system TAL—Rf 10.

Gas Chromatography. System GA—RI 2087.

High Performance Liquid Chromatography. System HA—*k* 2.3; system HAA—Retention time 3.7 min; system HAX—Retention time 5.9 min; system HAY—3.3 min; system HY—RI 175; system HZ—Retention time 1.8 min.

Column: (analytical) C_{18} (μBondapak, 250 × 4.6 mm i.d., 10 μm); (guard) C_{18} (μBondapak, 6 × 5.0 mm i.d., 10 μm). Mobile phase: disodium hydrogen phosphate (21 mM):TEA:acetonitrile, pH 3.5 (1000:60:150), flow rate 1.3 mL/min. Retention time: 6.7 min. [A. Ahmadiani and H. Amini, *J. Chromatogr. Biomed. Sci. Appl.*, 2001, *751*, 291–296].

Ultraviolet Spectrum. Water—313 nm (A^1_1=499a).

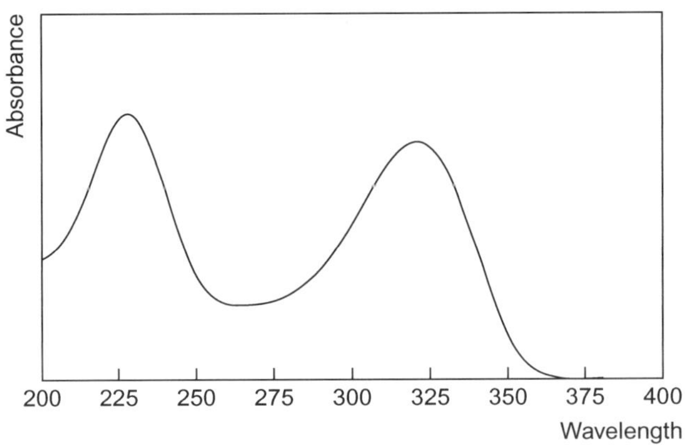

Infra-red Spectrum. Principal peaks at wavenumbers 1220, 1620, 1192, 1570, 1590, 1260 cm^{-1} (ranitidine hydrochloride, KBr disk).

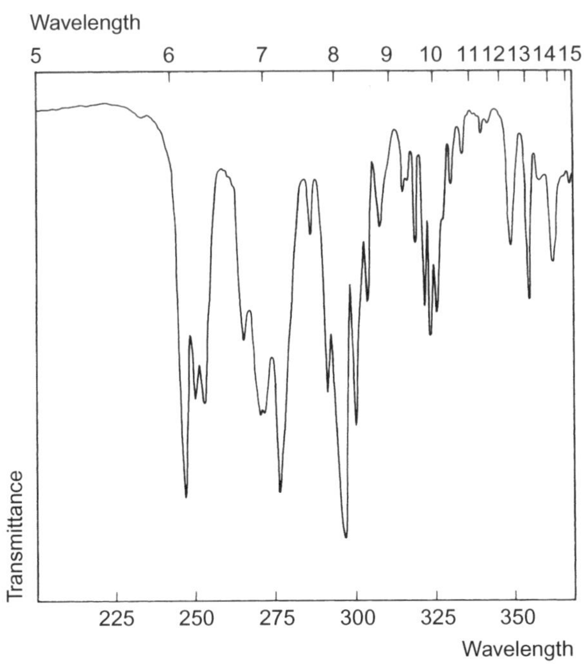

Quantification

High performance liquid chromatography. In plasma or urine: limit of detection 5 μg/L for ranitidine, 15 μg/L for desmethylranitidine, UV detection—G. W. Mihaly *et al.*, *J. Pharm. Sci.*, 1980, *69*, 1155–1157. In urine: ranitidine and metabolites, UV detection—P. F. Carey *et al.*, *J. Chromatogr.*, 1981, *225*; *B Biomed Appl.*, *14*, 161–168. In plasma or serum: limit of quantification 10 μg/L—T. L. Lloyd *et al.*, *Biomed. Chromatogr.*, 1992, *6*, 311–316. In plasma: limit of detection 10 μg/L, UV detection—D. Farthing *et al.*, *J. Chromatogr. B Biomed. Sci. Appl.*, 1997, *688*, 350–353. In serum: limit of detection 2 μg/L, UV detection—C. Lopez-Calull *et al.*, *J. Chromatogr. B Biomed. Sci. Appl.*, 1997, *693*, 228–232. In plasma or urine: ranitidine and its *N*-oxide and *S*-oxide metabolites, limit of detection for ranitidine 32 μg/L, fluorescence detection—P. Vinas *et al.*, *J. Chromatogr. B Biomed. Sci. Appl.*, 1997, *693*, 443–449. In plasma: limit of detection 1 μg/L—C. F. Wong *et al.*, *J. Chromatogr. B Biomed. Sci. Appl.*, 1998, *718*, 205–210. In plasma: limit of detection 5 μg/L, UV detection—A. Ahmadiani and H. Amini, *J. Chromatogr. B Biomed. Sci. Appl.*, 2001, *751*, 291–296. In plasma: limit of detection 2 μg/L, UV detection—L. G. Hare *et al.*, *J. Pharm. Pharmacol.*, 2001, *53*, 1265–1272.

Radioimmunoassay. In biological fluids: limit of detection 2 μg/L—W. N. Jenner *et al.*, *Life Sci.*, 1981, *28*, 1323–1329.

Disposition in the Body. Readily absorbed after oral administration. It is metabolised by *N*-oxidation, *S*-oxidation, and demethylation, its major metabolite being ranitidine *N*-oxide, but is excreted mainly as unchanged drug. After oral administration, about 30% is excreted unchanged in the urine in 24 h (dose-dependent), together with small amounts of the metabolites; after an intravenous dose, about 70 to 80% is excreted unchanged in the urine in 24 h, mainly by active tubular secretion. Ranitidine crosses the placenta and is excreted in breast milk.

The pharmacokinetics of the ranitidine component of ranitidine bismuth citrate is dose-proportional and similar to that observed after administration of ranitidine alone. Ranitidine bismuth citrate is rapidly absorbed and dissociates into ranitidine and bismuth compounds after oral administration. About 0.5% of the bismuth dose is absorbed and accumulates in plasma after repeated dosing (peak plasma concentration around 19 μg/L) and is eliminated via urine. Bismuth absorption is increased more than proportionally with the dose at 1600 mg. Low levels of bismuth can be detected in plasma and urine up to 5 months after the last dose. Because of the risk of bismuth accumulation, ranitidine bismuth citrate is not suitable for those with renal impairment or for long-term maintenance therapy.

Therapeutic concentration

Following single oral administration of an over-the-counter 75-mg preparation of ranitidine to 19 children with heartburn, a median peak plasma concentration of 0.477 mg/L was attained in 2.5 h [S. R. Orenstein *et al.*, *Aliment. Pharmacol. Ther.*, 2002, *16*, 899–907].

A study of IV ranitidine administration to 23 critically ill children revealed that a mean bolus dose of 1.37 mg/kg rapidly reduced gastric acidity, producing a peak plasma concentration of 0.373 mg/L at 2.3 h. Subsequent administration of ranitidine as a continuous IV infusion to 18 of the same subjects showed that a dose of 0.17 mg/kg/h and steady-state concentration of 0.287 mg/L was associated with gastric pH control. It was determined that a loading dose of 0.45 mg/kg followed by a continuous infusion of 0.15 mg/kg/h would be necessary to achieve a steady-state concentration of 0.287 mg/L [R. A. Lugo *et al.*, *Crit. Care Med.*, 2001, *29*, 759–764].

A total of 60 healthy males, aged between 19 and 40 years, were administered with either a 200, 400, 800 or 1600 mg dose of ranitidine bismuth citrate (equal number of volunteers for each dose), after an overnight fast and followed by a further 4 h after ingestion. The peak plasma ranitidine concentrations were 182, 480, 956 and 1983 μg/L for the doses, respectively, and these were observed between 1 and 5 h. The peak bismuth concentrations were 2.89, 2.85, 3.31 and 11.6 μg/L for the 200, 400, 800 and 1600 mg dose, respectively, and were reached 0.25 to 1.0 h after ingestion [K. M. Koch, *Br. J. Clin. Pharmacol.*, 1996, *42*, 201–205].

Bioavailability. About 50% but there is considerable intersubject variability.

Half-life. Plasma half-life, about 2 to 3 h, increased in elderly subjects, and in renal impairment.

Volume of distribution. 1 to 2 L/kg.

Clearance. Plasma clearance, about 10 mL/min/kg.

Protein binding. In plasma, about 15%.

Note. For a review of ranitidine bismuth citrate in the treatment of *Helicobacter pylori* infection and duodenal ulcer, see T. G. Vondracek, *Ann. Pharmacother.*, 1998, *32*, 672–679; for a general review of ranitidine, see S. M. Grant *et al.*, *Drugs*, 1989, 37, 801–870; for a review of the drug interaction potential of ranitidine, see U. Klotz and H. K. Kroemer, *Pharmacol.Ther.*, 1991, *50*, 233–244.

Dose. The equivalent of 150 to 600 mg of ranitidine daily. Ranitidine bismuth citrate is used in a 7 day triple therapy regimen: 400 mg twice daily or 14 day dual therapy with clarithromycin, amoxicillin and/or metronidazole. It is not used in those with moderate to severe renal impairment.

Rapacuronium Bromide

Anaesthetic

Synonym. Org-9487
Proprietary name. Raplon
1-[(2β,3α,5α,16β,17β)-3-(Acetyloxy)-17-(1-oxopropoxy)-2-(1-piperidinyl)androstan-16-yl]-1-(2-propenyl)piperidinium bromide
$C_{37}H_{61}N_2O_4,Br = 677.8$
CAS—156137-99-4

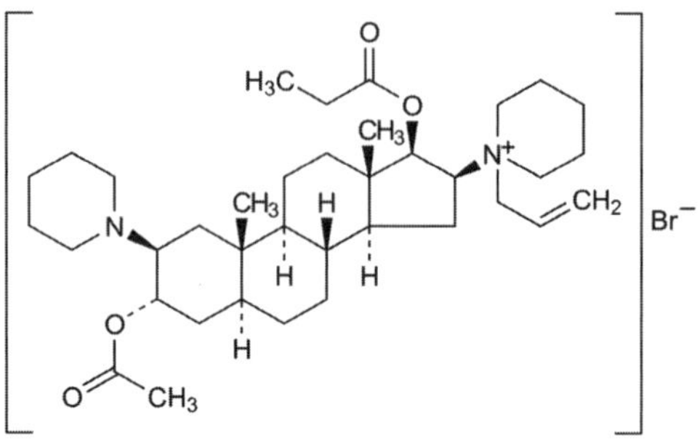

Disposition in the Body. Rapacuronium rapidly enters the neuromuscular junction (its effect compartment) and is subsequently rapidly cleared from the plasma. After intramuscular injection, peak plasma concentrations are observed at 4 and 5 min in infants and children, respectively. After 30 min, less than 25% of a dose has been absorbed. It is metabolised by spontaneous hydrolysis and/or hepatic metabolism. The major metabolite is 3-desacetylrapacuronium and represents 10% of the drug plasma concentration. Rapacuronium is excreted by the hepatic and renal pathways; 22% of the drug and metabolite in urine over a 24 h period.

Therapeutic concentration

10 patients undergoing elective surgery, aged 18 to 57 years (mean 28 years) were treated with fentanyl and propofol to induce anaesthesia. They were then treated with rapacuronium as an intravenous bolus dose of 1.5 mg/kg, followed by an infusion of 3.4 mg/kg/h for 45 min, to maintain a neuromuscular block of 83%, and in the final 15 min, 2.5 mg/kg/h. 10 min after the beginning of the infusion, peak plasma concentrations were 5979 μg/L for the drug and 340 μg/L for its metabolite; 60 min afterwards the concentrations were 5029 and 650 μg/L for the drug and metabolite, respectively. However, 240 min after the infusion period had finished, the plasma concentrations were 89 and 205 μg/L, respectively. [L. Van den Broek *et al.*, *Br. J. Anaesth.*, 1994, *73*, 331–335].

Toxicity. Rapacuronium is associated with bronchospasm which may lead to death.

Bioavailability. Intramuscular bioavailability, 56%.

Half-life. Approx. 90 min (range 72 to 184 min).

Volume of distribution. Total apparent, 221 (124 to 285) mL/kg (healthy individuals); 331 (284 to 488) mL/kg (patients with cirrhosis); steady state, 0.193 to 0.457 L/kg; lower in those with chronic renal failure compared to those with normal function and in men compared with women.

Clearance. Plasma, 4.77 mL/min/kg (infants and children); 5.3 mL/min/kg (healthy adults); 6.9 mL/min/kg (patients with cirrhosis).

Dose. The recommended dose is 1.5 to 2.5 mg/kg as a rapid intravenous bolus after anaesthetic induction.

Reboxetine

Antidepressant

(2*R*)-*rel*-2-[(*R*)-(2-Ethoxyphenoxy)phenylmethyl]morpholine
$C_{19}H_{23}NO_3 = 313.4$
CAS—71620-89-8; 98769-81-4

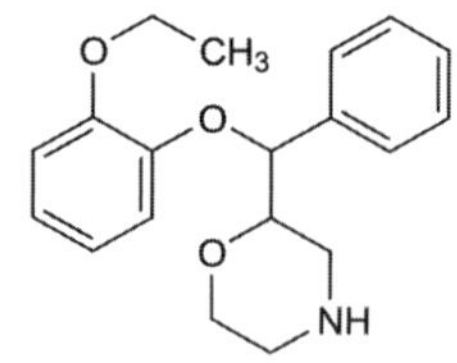

M.p. 170° to 171°.

Reboxetine Methanesulfonate (Mesilate)
Synonyms. FCE-20124; PNU-155950E.
Proprietary names. Edronax; Prolift; Vestra.
$C_{19}H_{23}NO_3,CH_3SO_3H = 409.5$
CAS—98769-82-5
M.p. 145° to 146°.

High Performance Liquid Chromatography. Column: phenyl (Zorbax, 150 × 3.0 mm i.d.). Column temperature: 30°. Mobile phase: acetonitrile:phosphate buffer (10 mM, pH 4.9) (27:73), flow rate 0.5 mL/min. UV detection (λ = 210 nm). Retention time(s): 13.0 min. [D. Ohman *et al.*, *Ther. Drug Monit.*, 2001, *23*, 27–34].

Ultraviolet Spectrum. Aqueous acid—274 nm.

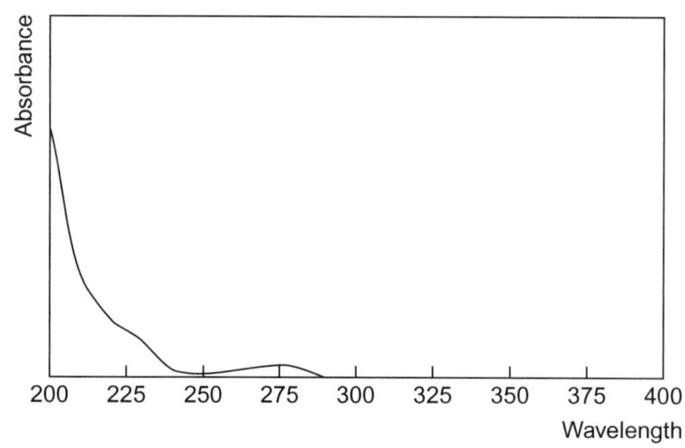

Mass Spectrum. Principal peaks at *m/z* 175, 56, 176, 91, 104, 86, 174, 85.

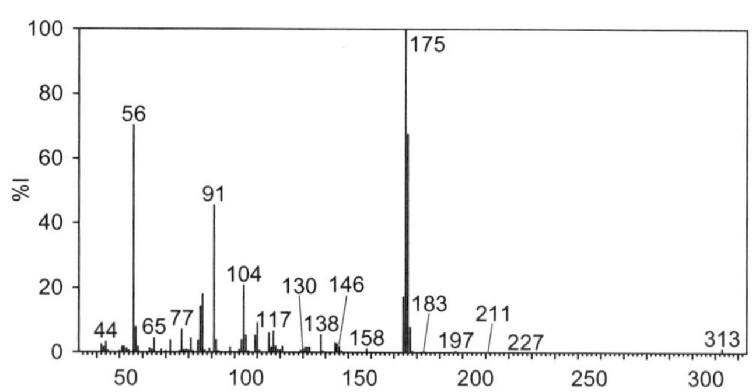

Quantification

High performance liquid chromatography. In blood: limit of quantification is 1 μg/L. Fluorescence detection ($\lambda_{ex} = 260$ nm, $\lambda_{em} = 315$ nm)—E. Frigerio *et al.*, *J. Chromatogr. A*, 1994, *660*, 351–358. In blood and urine: limit of quantification 10 μg/L, UV detection (λ = 210 nm)—D. M. F. Edwards *et al.*, *Biopharm. Drug. Dispos.*, 1995, *16*, 443–460. In plasma: limit of quantification 1.1 μg/L for each enantiomer. Fluorescence detection ($\lambda_{ex} = 260$ nm, $\lambda_{em} = 315$ nm)—T. Denolle *et al.*, *Clin. Pharmacol. Ther.*, 1999, *66(3)*, 282–287. In plasma: limit of quantification 10 μg/L. UV detection (λ = 210 nm)—F. Coulomb *et al.*, *J. Clin. Pharmacol.*, 2000, *40*, 482–487.

Disposition in the Body. Reboxetine is rapidly and well absorbed from the gastro-intestinal tract and peak plasma levels occur in about 2 h. The presence of food decreases the peak concentration reached and lengthens the time to reach this. The drug is metabolised by dealkylation, hydroxylation and oxidation followed by glucuronide or sulfate conjugation. Traces of hydroxyl-, desethyl- and 3-morpholine metabolites have been identified in plasma as well as glucuronide and sulfate conjugates of these. Elimination is mainly renal via urine (78%) with 10% excreted as the unchanged drug. Linear pharmacokinetics are displayed. Multiple dosing and gender do not affect the pharmacokinetics. Steady state concentrations are reached within 4 days.

Therapeutic concentration

9 healthy males, 19 to 29 years (mean 23 years) were administered a single oral dose of 4 mg reboxetine and 2 mg *R,R*-enantiomer, after an overnight fast. The peak plasma concentration was 109 μg/L observed at 1.9 h for the parent drug, 77 μg/L at 1.8 h for the *R,R*-enantiomer and 35 μg/L for the *S,S*-enantiomer 2.3 h after reboxetine administration. The peak concentration of *R,R*-enantiomer observed after its administration was 75 μg/L at 1.4 h. [T. Denolle *et al., Clin. Pharmacol. Ther.*, 1999, *66(3)*, 282–287].

6 patients with mild renal dysfunction (mean age 54 years; creatinine clearance 60 to 80 mL/min), 6 with moderate dysfunction (mean 45 years; creatinine clearance 30 to 50 mL/min), 6 with severe dysfunction (mean 55 years; creatinine clearance 10 to 20 mL/min) and healthy volunteers, were administered a 4 mg dose after an overnight fast and continued fasting 4 h after dosing. Peak plasma concentrations were 151, 176, 203 and 111 μg/L for the four groups of individuals, observed at 1.83, 1.08, 1.58 and 2.4 h, respectively. [F. Coulomb *et al., J. Clin. Pharmacol.*, 2000, *40*, 482–487].

Bioavailability. 60%.

Half-life. 13 to 15 h.

Volume of distribution. 32 L; steady state, 0.39 L/kg (*R,R*)-(−)-reboxetine; 0.92 L/kg (*S,S*)-(+)-reboxetine.

Clearance. Plasma, 2.21 L/h.

Protein binding. Approx. 97% primarily to α_1-acid glycoprotein. 92% in the elderly.

Dose. A usual dose of 8 mg daily. Maximum 12 mg.

Remifentanil

Narcotic Analgesic

Synonyms. GI-87084; remifentanyl.

4-(Methoxycarbonyl)-4-[(1-oxopropyl)phenylamino]-1-piperidinepropanoic acid methyl ester

$C_{20}H_{28}N_2O_5$=376.5

CAS—132875-61-7

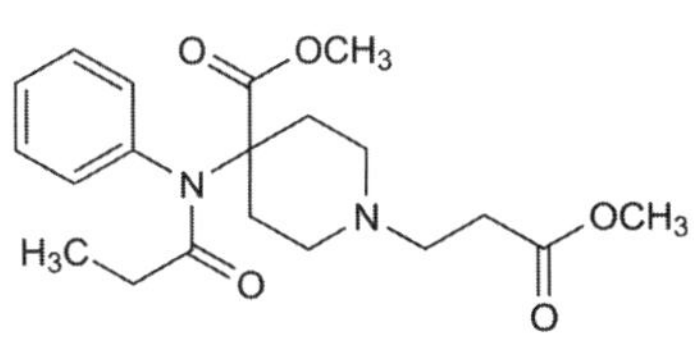

A white to off-white lyophilised powder.

Remifentanil Hydrochloride

Synonym. GI-87084B

Proprietary name. Ultiva

$C_{20}H_{28}N_2O_5$,HCl=412.9

Dissociation Constant. pK_a 7.1.

High Performance Liquid Chromatography. Column: (analytical) Cyano SB-CN (Zorbax, 250 × 4.6 mm i.d., 5 μm) (guard) cyano (15 × 3.2 mm i.d.). Column temperature: 30°. Mobile phase: acetonitrite:methanol:water:phosphate buffer (0.03 M, pH 3.0) (14:28:52:6), flow rate 1.5 mL/min. UV detection (λ=210 nm). Retention time: remifentanil, 8.5 min; carboxylic acid metabolite, 4.5 min. [K. Selinger *et al. J. Pharm. Biomed. Anal.*, 1994, *42(2)*, 243–248.]

Column: RP C_8 column (150 × 4.6 mm i.d., 5 μm). Mobile phase: acetonitrile:sodium hydrogen phosphate buffer (0.05 M, pH 3.5) (27:73) with 300 μl/L TEA, flow rate 1.5 mL/min. UV detection (λ=210 nm). Retention time: 6 min. [S. Haidar *et al. J. Pharm. Biomed. Anal.*, 1996, *14*, 1727–1732.]

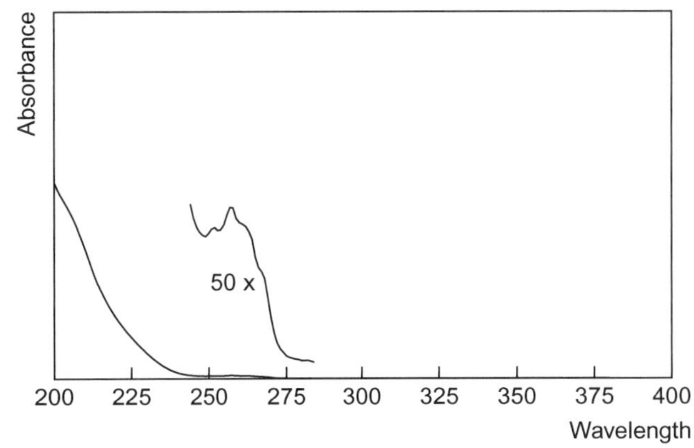

Mass Spectrum. Principal ions at *m/z* 168, 227, 55, 212, 303, 140, 93, 42.

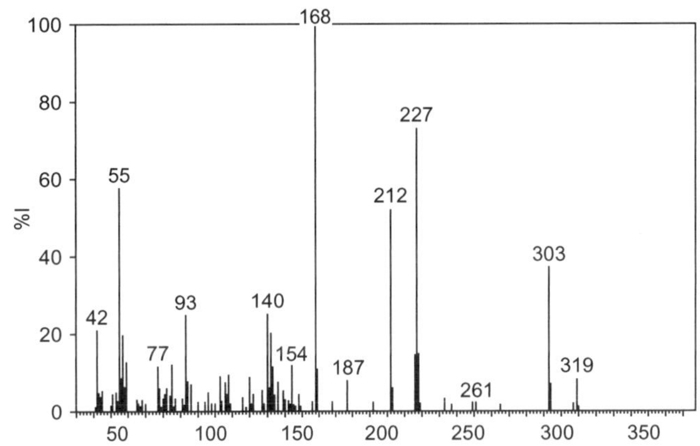

Quantification

Gas chromatography–mass spectrometry. In blood: limit of quantification 0.1 μg/L—C. Grosse *et al., J. Pharm. Biomed. Anal.*, 1994, *12(2)*, 195–203.

High performance liquid chromatography. In blood: limit of quantification 1 μg/L, UV detection (λ=210 nm)—K. Selinger *et al., J. Pharm. Biomed. Anal.*, 1994, *12(2)*, 243–248. In blood: limit of quantification 0.1 μg/L, MS–MS detection—J. Bender *et al., J. Pharm. Biomed. Anal.*, 1999, *21*, 559–567.

Disposition in the Body. Parenteral administration results in rapid onset and there is short duration of action. Remifentanil is metabolised by non-specific plasma and tissue esterases that hydrolyse the drug prior to its secretion by the kidneys to an inactive carboxylic acid metabolite (with a half-life of 90 min). There is rapid distribution throughout the body and elimination is independent of duration of the drug. 95% of a dose is excreted in urine as the metabolite. Linear and dose-independent pharmacokinetics are seen while the pharmacokinetics are gender independent. Age and lean body mass alter pharmacokinetics. Pharmacokinetics are not changed in renal or hepatic impairment.

Therapeutic concentration. 1 to 40 μg/L after an infusion rate of 0.04 to 2 μg/kg bodyweight per min. Steady state is achieved within 5 to 10 min with a volume of 350 mL/kg.

Half-life. 6 to 16 min (independent of dose).

Volume of distribution. 0.39 L/kg; steady-state volume of distribution, 24 to 40 L; children (2 to 12 years old), steady-state, 0.21 L/kg.

Clearance. 40 mL/min/kg (reduced by 25% in the elderly); total clearance, 2.5 to 3.8 L/min; systemic clearance, 2.8 L/min.

Protein binding. About 70%.

Note. For a review of remifentanil, see T. D. Egan, *Clin. Pharmacokinet.*, 1995, *29*, 80–94.

Dose. 0.5 to 1 μg/kg/min. Initial dose reduced in the elderly by 50%.

Remoxipride

Antipsychotic

Synonyms. BRN4323708; A-33547; FLA-731.
Proprietary names. Psyloc; Roxiam.
3-Bromo-*N*-[[(2*S*)-1-ethyl-2-pyrrolidinyl]methyl]-2,6-dimethoxybenzamide
$C_{16}H_{23}BrN_2O_3$=371.3
CAS—80125-14-0

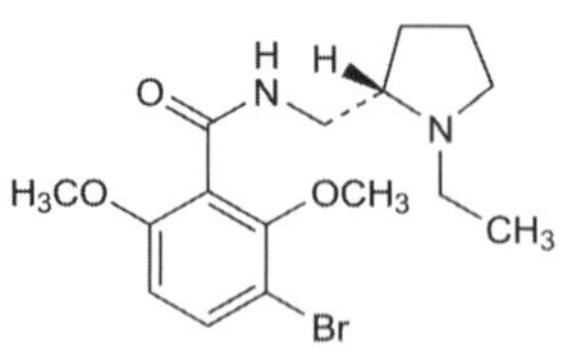

Remoxipride Hydrochloride
3-Bromo-*N*-[[(2*S*)-1-ethyl-2-pyrrolidinyl]methyl]-2,6-dimethoxybenzamide hydrochloride monohydrate
$C_{16}H_{23}BrN_2O_3,HCl,H_2O$=425.8
CAS—73220-03-8 (anhydrous remoxipride hydrochloride); 117591-79-4 (remoxipride hydrochloride monohydrate)
A white to off-white crystalline solid with m.p. 173°. It is soluble in water, ethanol, dichloromethane and acetone.

Dissociation Constant. pK_a 8.9.

Partition Coefficient. Log *P* (octanol/water), 2.10.

Thin-layer Chromatography. System TB—Rf 14 remoxipride, Rf 00 M(FLA-838), Rf 00 M(NCM-001), Rf 00 M(NCM-009); system TE—Rf 54 remoxipride, Rf 23 M(FLA-838), Rf 41 M(NCM-001), Rf 27 M(NCM-009); system TAE—Rf 26 remoxipride, Rf 08 M(FLA-838), Rf 82 M(NCM-001), Rf 82 M(NCM-009).

Plate: Merck 254. Mobile phase: Acetone:toluene:ethanol:concentrated ammonia (150:150:20:2). Detection: Dragendorff's reagent. Rf 0.4. [M. Segerberg-Konttinen *et al.*, *J. Forensic Sci.*, 1989, *34(2)*, 500–503].

Gas Chromatography. System GB—RI 2588.

High Performance Liquid Chromatography. System HX—RI 334 remoxipride, RI 316 M(FLA-838), RI 364 M(NCM-001), RI 341 M(NCM-009); system HZ—3.0 min; system HAX—retention time 8.8 min; system HAY—retention time 4.6 min.

Column: 120-3 C_{18} (Nucleosil, 100 × 4.6 mm i.d., 3 μm). Mobile phase: in plasma, acetonitrile:phosphate buffer (pH 2) (30:70), containing 0.4 mM *N*,*N*-dimethyloctylamine and 0.5 mM decylsulfate; in urine, acetonitrile:phosphate buffer (pH 2) (25:75) containing 0.2 mM *N*,*N*-dimethyloctylamine, flow rate 1.3 mL/min. IS: 3-bromo-*N*-[(1-propyl-2-pyrrolidinyl)methyl]-2,6-dimethoxybenzamide. UV detection (λ=206 nm). Retention time(s): in urine, remoxipride, 2.2 min; IS, 3.6 min; in plasma, remoxipride 3 min; IS 5.3 min. [L. Nilsson. *J. Chromatogr.*, 1990, *526*, 139–150].

Column: C_{18} (Analytichem, 50 × 4.6 mm i.d., 3 μm). Column temperature: 40°. Mobile phase: in plasma, aqueous buffer (0.2 M sodium perchlorate, 0.1 M phosphoric acid, pH 1.7):acetonitrile (25:75); in urine, (69:31), 1.3 mL/min flow rate. UV detection (λ=214 nm). Retention time(s): 2.8 min (plasma); 1.8 min (urine). [R. H.-Y. Chiou *et al.*, *J. Chromatogr.*, 1992, *581*, 300–305].

Ultraviolet Spectrum. Aqueous solution (neutral)—286 nm; Ethanol—287 nm; aqueous acid (0.1 M hydrochloric acid)—286 nm.

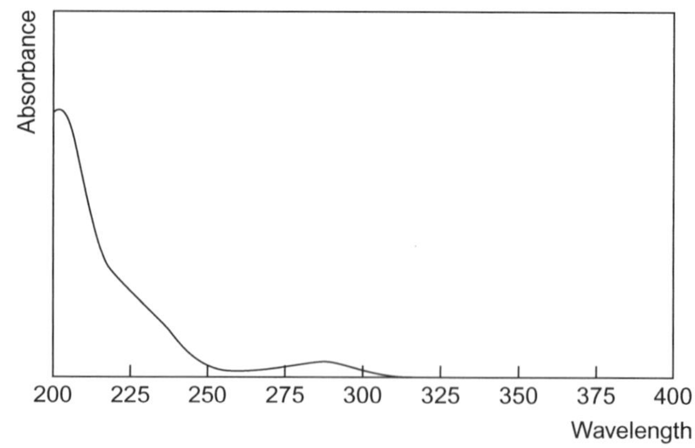

Mass Spectrum. Principal peaks at *m/z* 98, 99, 70, 228, 230, 243, 245, 185.

Quantification
High performance liquid chromatography. In blood: limit of detection <2.5 μg/L. Electrochemical detection—M. Aravagiri *et al.*, *J. Pharm. Sci.*, 1993, *82*, 447–449. In blood and urine: limit of quantification 0.002 μg/L. UV detection (λ=206 nm)—L. Nilsson, *J. Chromatogr.*, 1990, *526*, 139–150. In plasma and urine: limit of quantification 12.5 and 50 μg/L, respectively. UV detection (λ=214 nm)—R. H.-Y. Chiou *et al.*, *J. Chromatogr.*, 1992, *581*, 300–305.

Disposition in the Body. Remoxipride is almost completely absorbed following oral administration in healthy subjects, mainly in the small intestine although some absorption does take place in the large intestine. Distribution is rapid. Peak plasma levels are reached within 1 to 2 h of oral administration. The drug is metabolised to lactam, hydroxy-substituted lactam, *N*-de-ethylated lactam and *N*-de-ethylated hydroxy-substituted lactam metabolites. Most of the oral dose is excreted in urine, 10 to 40% unchanged and the remainder as metabolites. Elimination may be impaired in the elderly and individuals with severe renal dysfunction. Steady state was achieved within 2 days of initial treatment. Pharmacokinetics are not altered by alcohol, warfarin or diazepam.

Therapeutic concentration. The recommended therapeutic level should not exceed 7 to 8 mg/L.

Doses of 70 to 140 mg are safe, but above 140 mg side effects become apparent. A single dose of 75 mg results in a therapeutic plasma level of 1 mg/L after 1 h. [From *TIAFT Bulletin Case Notes*, October 1997, Vol. 27, No. 3].

6 healthy volunteers were administered 100 mg remoxipride hydrochloride monohydrate and plasma concentrations reached 3.8 μmol/L. The concentrations for the lactam, hydroxy-substituted lactam, *N*-de-ethylated lactam and *N*-de-ethylated hydroxy-substituted lactam metabolites were 1.5, 0.5, 0.3 and 0.2 μmol/L, respectively. [M. Widman *et al.*, *Eur. J. Clin. Pharmacol.*, 1990, *183(5)*, Abst P. th.245].

Toxicity
A 23-year-old woman was found dead at her home and was known to be receiving psychiatric treatment. At the scene at empty bottle of triazolam and three empty bottles of remoxipride were found. Remoxipride was detected at concentrations of 230 mg/L, 220 mg/L and 490 mg/kg in blood, urine and liver, respectively. No triazolam was detected and ethanol was found at a concentration of 0.048 g/100 L in urine. Death was attributed to remoxipride poisoning. [M. Segerberg-Konttinen *et al.*, *J. Forensic Sci.*, 1989, *34(2)*, 500–503].

Bioavailability. Greater than 90%.

Half-life. 4 to 7 h. Longer in elderly patients and those with renal dysfunction.

Volume of distribution. 0.5 to 0.7 L/kg.

Clearance. Plasma, 120 mL/min.

Protein binding. 80% bound to plasma protein.

Dose. By mouth, intramuscular or intravenously, starting dose of 300 mg in 2 divided doses and adjusted to control symptoms. Initial dose may be halved for elderly patients. The majority of patients are administered 300 to 450 mg daily.

Repaglinide

Antidiabetic

Synonyms. AG-EE-338 ZW; AG-EE-623 ZW; AG-EE-6232W.
Proprietary Names. Novonorm; Prandin.
2-Ethoxy-4-[2-[[(1*S*)-3-methyl-1-[2-(1-piperidinyl)phenyl]butyl]amino]-2-oxoethyl]benzoic acid
$C_{27}H_{36}N_2O_4$=452.6
CAS—135062-02-1

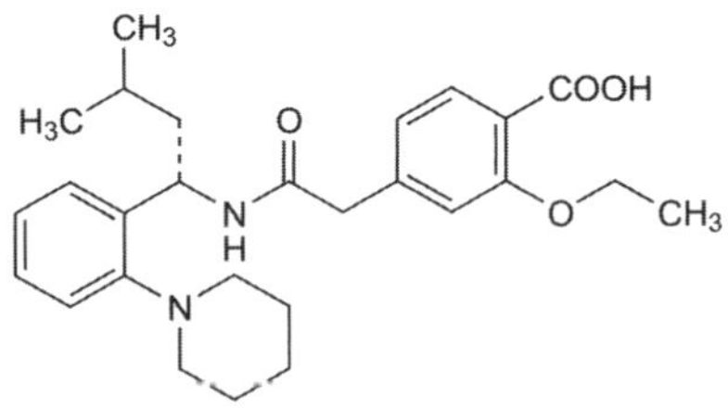

A white, odourless, crystalline powder. M.p. 126° to 128°.

High Performance Liquid Chromatography. Columns: (analytical) 100 RP_{18} (LiChrospher, 125 × 4 mm i.d., 5 µm); (guard) ODS (Hypersil, 17 × 4.6 mm i.d., 5 µm); (precolumn) Perisorb RP_2 (17 × 2.9 mm i.d., 30 to 40 µm). Mobile phase: (A) methanol:acetonitrile:dioxane (68:24:8); (B) potassium dihydrogenphosphate (21 mM) with lithium perchlorate (0.5 g/L), pH 2.7. (A:B) (76:24), flow rate 1 mL/min. Electrochemical detection. Retention time(s): 8.8 to 9.1 min. [A. Greischel *et al.*, *J. Chromatogr.*, 1991, *568(1)*; *Biomed. Appl.*, 246–252].

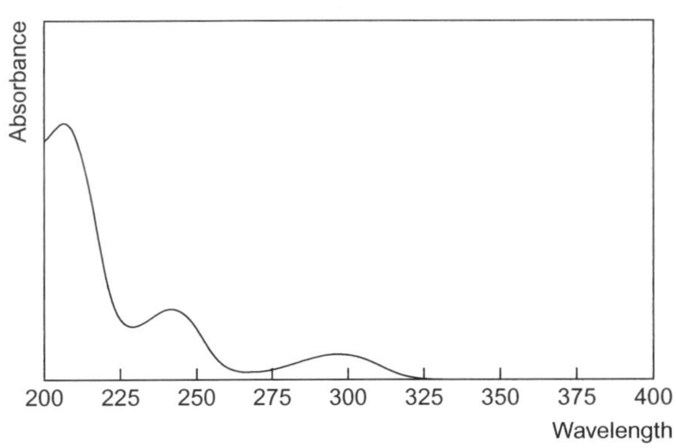

Infra-red Spectrum. Principal peaks at wavenumbers 1688, 1636, 1215, 1588, 1150, 1607 cm^{-1}.

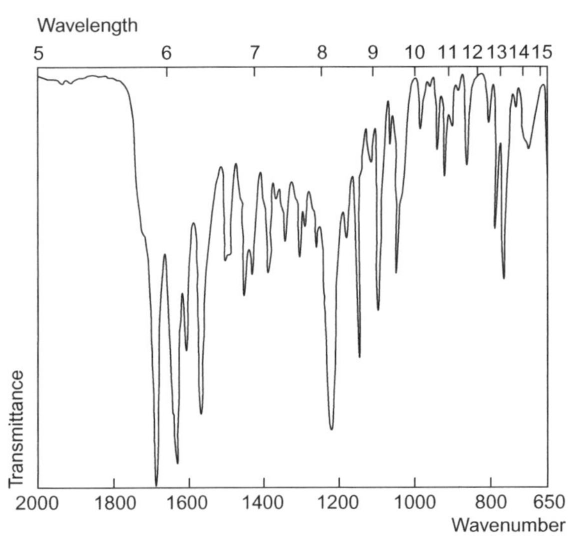

Mass Spectrum. Principal ions at *m/z* 409, 172, 452, 186, 245, 228, 130, 396.

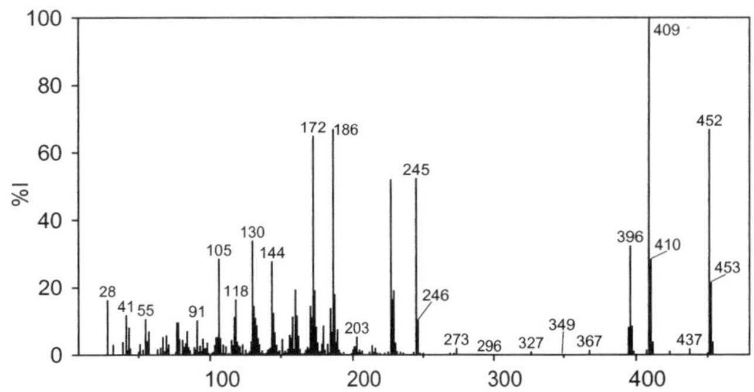

Quantification

High performance liquid chromatography. In plasma: limit of detection 5 µg/L, electrochemical detection—A. Greischel *et al.*, *J. Chromatogr.*, 1991, *568(1)*; *Biomed. Appl.*, 246–252.

Enzyme immunoassay. In serum: limit of quantification 1.88 µg/L, limit of detection 0.35 µg/L—V. Hatorp *et al.*, *J. Clin. Pharmacol.*, 2000, *40(2)*, 142–152.

Disposition in the Body. Repaglinide is rapidly and almost completely absorbed after oral administration and peak concentrations are observed in approx. 1 h. The presence of food does not affect the absorption or pharmacokinetics of repaglinide. Plasma levels decrease rapidly once the peak concentration has been reached. It undergoes almost complete hepatic metabolism involving cytochrome P450 CYP3A4. Major metabolites include the oxidised dicarboxylic acid, aromatic amine and the acyl glucuronide, none of which are active with clinically relevant hypoglycaemic activity. The drug is eliminated rapidly, usually within 4 to 6 h, and excreted primarily via bile as both the parent compound and its metabolites. Less than 8% of an administered dose is excreted in urine, mainly as the metabolites, and less than 1% of the dose is detected in faeces as the unchanged drug.

Therapeutic concentration

12 male volunteers aged between 37 and 62 years (mean age 52.9 years) with moderate to severe chronic liver damage, and 12 healthy males, 42 to 62 years old (mean age 53.2 years) participated in this study. All subjects were fasted overnight and administered 4 mg repaglinide. An additional fast of 1 h after dosing was required. The peak plasma concentration for the patients was 105.4 µg/L at 0.8 h and for the healthy individuals, 46.7 µg/L at 0.8 h. [V. Hatorp *et al.*, *J. Clin. Pharmacol.*, 2000, *40(2)*, 142–152].

12 healthy volunteers; young adults aged 18 to 40 years (mean 33 years) and elderly individuals (mean 67 years) participated in this study. On day 1, after a 10 h fast, subjects were administered 2 mg repaglinide and continued fasting until noon that day. On days 2 to 8: 2 mg repaglinide 15 min before each of the 3 meals was administered and on day 9: a single 2 mg dose was administered. The mean peak plasma concentrations for the young adults were 47.9 µg/L (range 18.0 to 127.0 µg/L) on day 1 and 58.5 (range 26.0 to 212.0) µg/L on day 9. These concentrations were observed at 0.8 (0.5 to 2.5) h and 0.6 (0.5 to 0.8) h, respectively. For the elderly adults, the peak concentrations on day 1 were 47.5 (range 20.0 to 115.0) µg/L at 0.7 (0.5 to 1.3) h and on day 9, 52.8 (range 21.0 to 109.0) µg/L at 0.8 (0.3 to 1.5) h. [V. Hatorp *et al.*, *Clin. Ther.*, 1999, *21(4)*, 702–710].

Bioavailability. Approx. 63%; also reported as 56%.

Half-life. 1 h.

Clearance. Plasma, 143 mL/min.

Volume of distribution. 20 to 30 L.

Protein binding. >98%.

Dose. The initial dose is 0.5 to 2.0 mg administered 30 min before meals. 1.0 mg or above is administered to patients who have had previous hypoglycaemic treatment. The dose is adjusted every 1 to 2 weeks up to 4.0 mg. A total daily dose of 16.0 mg should not be exceeded.

Reproterol

Bronchodilator

Synonym. D-1959
Proprietary name. Allergospasmin
7-[3-[[2-(3,5-Dihydroxyphenyl)-2-hydroxyethyl]amino]propyl]-3,7-dihydro-1,3-dimethyl-1*H*-purine-2,6-dione
$C_{18}H_{23}N_5O_5$=389.4
CAS—*54063-54-6*

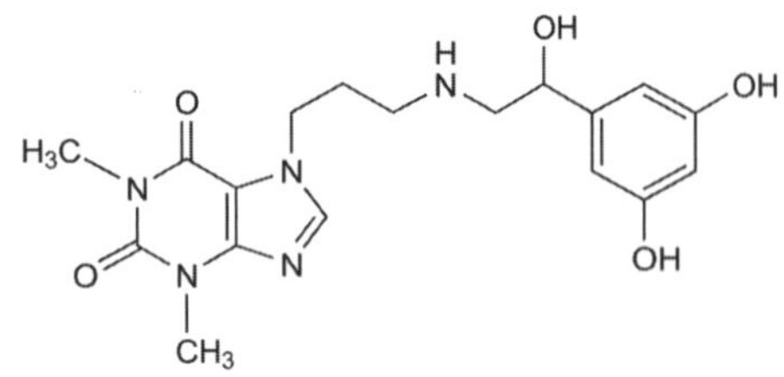

Reproterol Hydrochloride

Synonym. W-2946M
Proprietary names. Aarane; Asmaterolo; Bronchodil; Bronchospasmin.
$C_{18}H_{23}N_5O_5$,HCl=425.9
CAS- 13055-82-8
Crystals. M.p. 249° to 250°.

Partition Coefficient. Log *P* (octanol/water), −0.39.

Gas Chromatography. Column: HP Ultra-1 (OV1, 16.8 m × 0.22 mm i.d., film thickness 0.11 µm). Column temperature: 140° with 20°/min to 320°, held 3 min. Carrier gas: helium, split flow 11 mL/min. MS detection (EI, SIM *m/z* at 527, 369, 368, 356, 262, 250). Retention time(s): 9.5 min (TMS (trimethylsilane) derivative). [M. K. Henze *et al.*, *J. Chromatogr. B, Biomed. Sci. Appl.*, 2001, *751(1)*, 93–105].

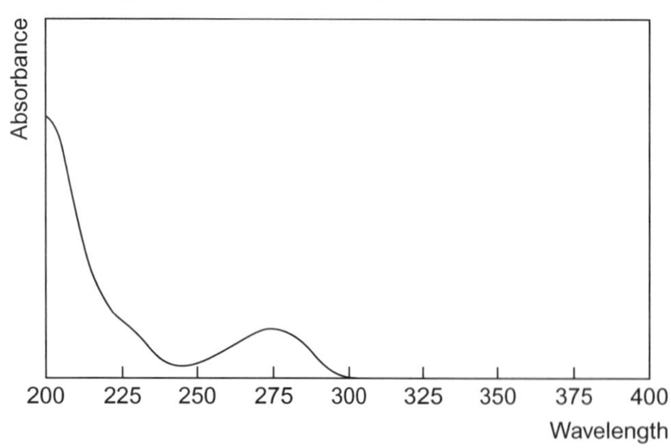

Mass Spectrum. Principal ions at *m/z* 527, 368, 526, 73, 396, 528, 306, 369 (C,N-methylene-reproterol tris-TMS)

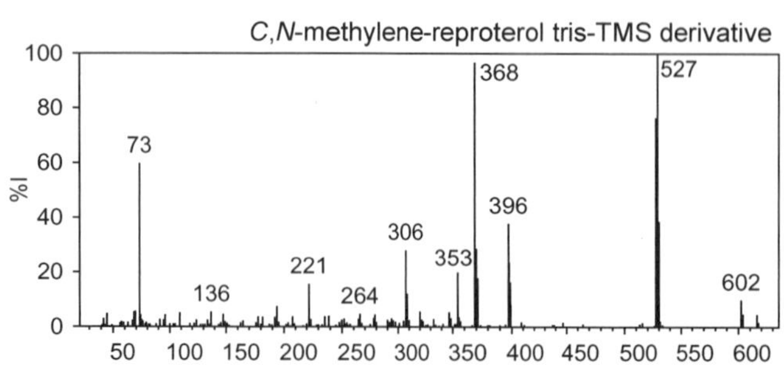

Quantification

Gas chromatography–mass spectrometry. In urine: limit of detection 10 µg/L—M. K. Henze *et al.*, *J. Chromatogr. B, Biomed. Sci. Appl.*, 2001, *751(1)*, 93–105.

High performance liquid chromatography–mass spectrometry. In plasma: limit of quantification 0.4 µg/L—N. Knebel and M. Winkler, *J. Chromatogr. B, Biomed. Sci. Appl.*, 1997, *702*, 119–129.

Disposition in the Body. Reproterol is rapidly and well absorbed after oral, intravenous and aerosol administration. Intravenously: the drug is rapidly distributed and very low plasma levels are observed. Elimination is predominantly renal. By aerosol: it is quickly absorbed and is present at very low concentrations in plasma; peak concentrations are reached in 10 min. Orally: reproterol is rapidly and well absorbed with peak plasma concentrations at 1 to 3 h. Elimination is mainly renal but some biotransformation does take place. The drug is metabolised mainly in the liver and also in the small intestine. Up to 80% is excreted in urine unchanged. There is substantial extracellular distribution of the administered dose. Pharmacokinetics are linear.

Therapeutic concentration

3 healthy volunteers, aged 20 years, were orally administered 20 or 40 mg reproterol hydrochloride or 270 or 540 µg reproterol intravenously over 10 to 15 min or were administered with 1 mg as two separate aerosol puffs, after an overnight fast. Peak plasma concentrations were observed shortly after administration of an oral dose. Plasma concentrations were 3.1 and 6.0 µg/L at 90 to 120 min for the 20 mg dose and 9.9 and 18.5 µg/L for the 2 individuals at 90 to 180 min for 40 mg. For the intravenous dose, the maximum concentrations were 8.4 µg/L for the 270 µg dose and 17.9 and 21.2 µg/L for the 2 individuals receiving the 540 µg dose. Peak plasma concentrations of 0.6 µg/L were observed with the inhaled dose (after the second puff) after 6 to 30 min. [R. J. Hageman *et al.*, *Biopharm. Drug Dispos.*, 1988, *9(3)*, 301–314].

Bioavailability. 50%, after oral administration.

Protein binding. Negligible.

Dose. Adults: 0.5 to 1 mg aerosol inhalation 3 times a day. 10 to 20 mg orally 3 times a day. Single or repeated dose of 90 µg ampoule intravenously. Child: 500 µg.

Rescinnamine

Antihypertensive

Synonym. Reserpinine
Proprietary names. Anaprel; Apoterin S; Cartric, Cinnaloid; Moderil.
(3β,16β,17α,18β,20α)-11,17-Dimethoxy-18-[[1-oxo-3-(3,4,5-trimethoxyphenyl)-2-propenyl]oxy]-3,20-yohimban-16-carboxylic acid methyl ester
$C_{35}H_{42}N_2O_9$=634.7
CAS—24815-24-5

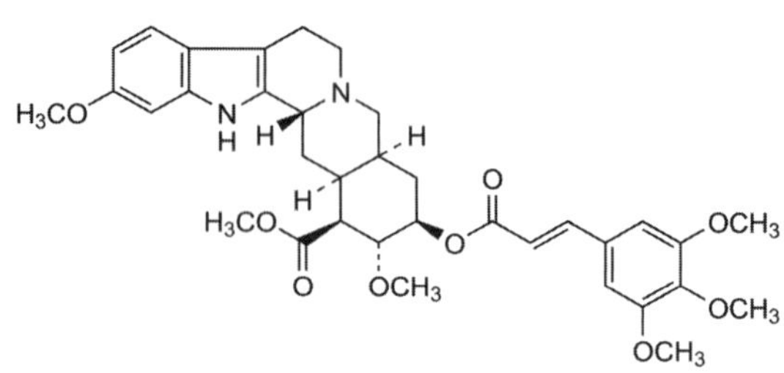

An alkaloid obtained from the roots of certain species of *Rauwolfia* (Apocynaceae), mainly *R. serpentina* and *R. vomitoria* or by synthesis.
A white or pale buff to cream-coloured, crystalline powder. It slowly darkens on exposure to light but more rapidly when in solution. M.p. 238° to 239°.
Practically insoluble in water; soluble in methanol, ethanol, benzene, acetic acid and chloroform.

Partition Coefficient. Log *P* (octanol/water), 3.8.

Colour Tests. Mandelin's test—brown; Marquis test—grey-green.

Thin-layer Chromatography. System TA—Rf 73; system TB—Rf 01; system TC—Rf 75; system TE—Rf 81; system TL—Rf 64; system TAE—Rf 77; system TAF—Rf 79. (Acidified potassium permanganate solution, positive.)

Gas Chromatography. System GA—RI 2180.

High Performance Liquid Chromatography. System HA—*k* 0.6; system HX—RI 496; system HY—RI 407.

Ultraviolet Spectrum. Aqueous acid—299 nm; aqueous alkali—306 nm.

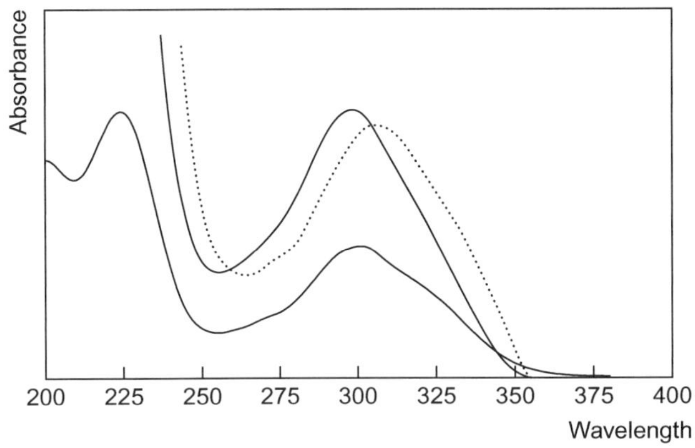

Infra-red Spectrum. Principal peaks at wavenumbers 1266, 1147, 1124, 1165, 1233, 1715 cm^{-1} (KBr disk).

Mass Spectrum. Principal ions at *m/z* 221, 199, 200, 186, 395, 251, 77, 214.

Dose. 0.25 to 1 mg daily.

Reserpine

Antihypertensive

Proprietary names. Crystoserpine; Eskaserp; Ortoserpina; Rau-Sed; Rauserpin; Reserpoid; Rivasin; Sandril; Sedaraupin; Serfin; Serfinato; Serpalan; Serpasil. It is an ingredient of Diupres, Hydropres, Metatensin, Naquival, Regroton, Renese-R, Salutensin and Tri-Hydroserpine.

(3β,16β,17α,18β,20α)-11,17-Dimethoxy-18-[(3,4,5-trimethoxybenzoyl)-oxy]yohimban-16-carboxylic acid methyl ester

$C_{33}H_{40}N_2O_9$=608.7

CAS—50-55-5

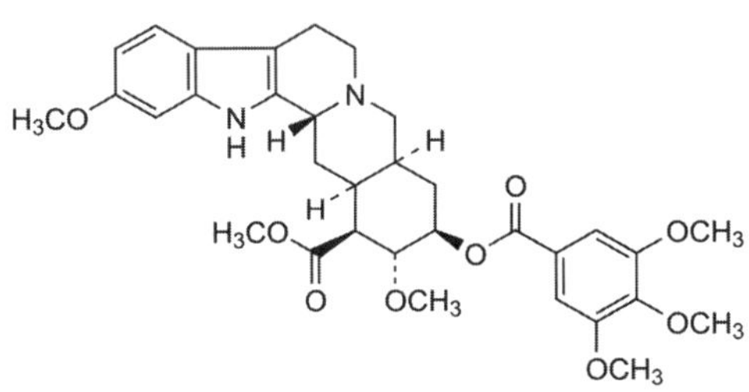

An alkaloid obtained from the roots of certain species of *Rauwolfia* (Apocynaceae), mainly *R. serpentina* and *R. vomitoria* or by synthesis.

Fine, white or pale buff to slightly yellow-coloured crystals or crystalline powder. It darkens slowly on exposure to light, but more rapidly when in solution. M.p. about 264° to 265°, with decomposition.

Practically insoluble in water and ether; soluble 1 in 2000 of ethanol and 1 in 6 of chloroform; freely soluble in glacial acetic acid; slightly soluble in acetone and methanol.

Dissociation Constant. pK_a 6.6 (25°).

Partition Coefficient. Log *P* (octanol/water), 3.3.

Colour Tests. Mandelin's test—green; Marquis test—grey-green→brown.

Thin-layer Chromatography. System TA—Rf 69; system TB—Rf 02; system TC—Rf 74; system TE—Rf 77; system TL—Rf 63; system TAE—Rf 76; system TAF—Rf 80; system TAJ—Rf 56; system TAK—Rf 06; system TAL—Rf 92. (Acidified potassium permanganate solution, positive.)

Gas Chromatography. System GA—not eluted; M (trimethoxybenzoic acid) RI 1780; M (trimethoxyhippuric acid) RI 2085; M (trimethoxybenzoic acid)-ME RI 1740; (trimethoxyhippuric acid)-ME RI 2350.

High Performance Liquid Chromatography. System HX—RI 467; system HY—RI 351; system HAA—Retention time(s) 16.4 min.

Ultraviolet Spectrum. Ethanol—267 nm (A^1_1=272a), 295 nm.

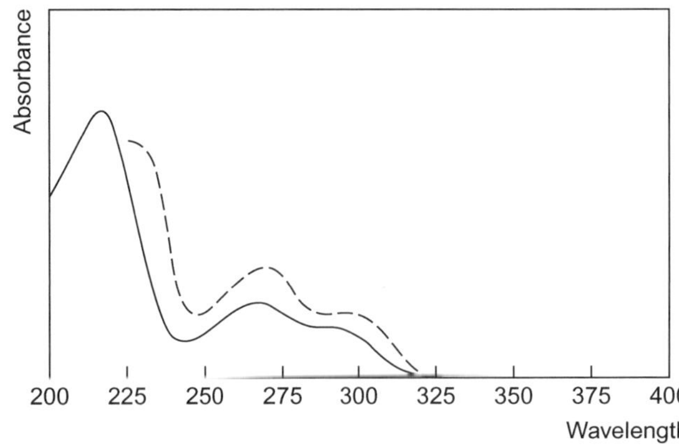

Infra-red Spectrum. Principal peaks at wavenumbers 1220, 1120, 1700, 1240, 1720, 1265 cm^{-1} (KBr disk).

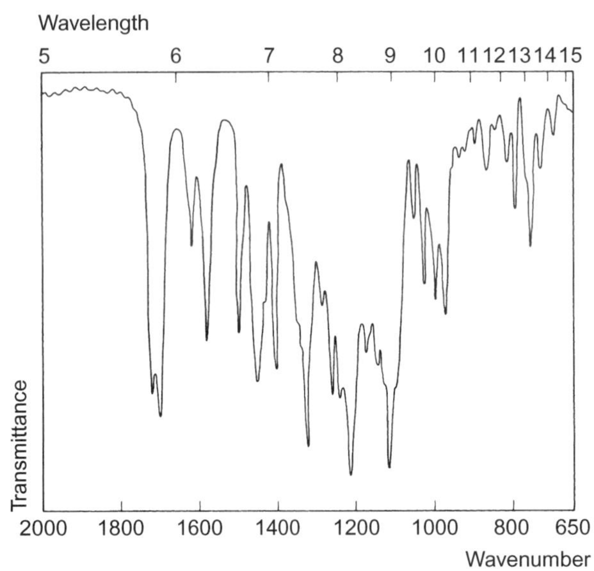

Mass Spectrum. Principal ions at *m/z* 608, 606, 195, 609, 395, 397, 212, 396.

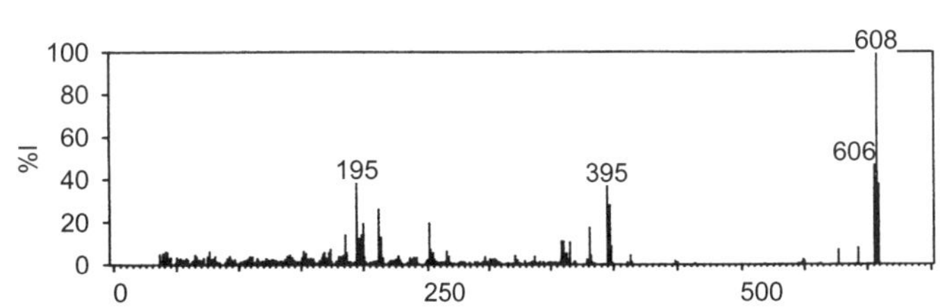

Quantification

High performance liquid chromatography. In plasma: limit of detection 300 ng/L, fluorescence detection—R. F. Suckow *et al.*, *J. Liq. Chromatogr.*, 1983, *6*, 1111–1122.

Thin-layer chromatography. In plasma: limit of detection 50 ng/L—S. L. Tripp *et al.*, *Life Sci.*, 1975, *16*, 1167–1177.

Disposition in the Body. Reserpine is readily but somewhat erratically absorbed after oral administration. It is rapidly and extensively metabolised by hydrolysis and *O*-demethylation; the major metabolites are trimethoxybenzoic acid and methyl reserpate, together with reserpic acid, syringomethyl reserpate and syringic acid; metabolites may be conjugated with glucuronic acid or sulfate. About 6% of an oral dose is excreted in the urine in 24 h and about 8% in the first 4 days, mainly as trimethoxybenzoic acid; less than 3% of a dose is excreted in the urine unchanged. About 60% of the dose is eliminated in the faeces in 4 days, mainly as unchanged drug.

Therapeutic concentration

After a single oral dose of 1 mg to 2 subjects, peak plasma concentrations of 0.0004 to 0.0006 mg/L were attained in 2 to 3 h. [S. L. Tripp *et al.*, *Life Sci.*, 1975, *16*, 1167–1177.].

Toxicity. High dosage may occasionally cause a Parkinsonian-like syndrome and severe depression; several cases of accidental poisoning have been reported in children but fatalities are unlikely.

Half-life. Plasma half-life, extremely variable and may be up to 11 days.

Distribution in blood. Plasma : whole blood ratio, 1.1.

Protein binding. In plasma, about 40%.

Dose. Usually 250 to 500 µg daily, for hypertension. Doses of 0.1 to 1 mg or more daily have been given as a sedative.

Resorcinol

Dermatological

Synonyms. *m*-Dihydroxybenzene; Dioxybenzolum; Resorcin.
Proprietary names. Astriderm; Castel. It is an ingredient of Acnomel and Eskamel.
1,3-Benzenediol
$C_6H_6O_2$=110.1
CAS—108-46-3

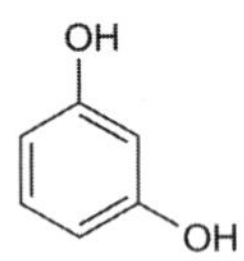

Colourless or slightly pinkish-grey, acicular crystals or crystalline powder. It becomes red on exposure to air and light. M.p. 109° to 111°; it sublimes on further heating.
Soluble 1 in less than 1 of water and 1 in 1 of ethanol; slightly soluble in chloroform; freely soluble in ether and glycerol.

Resorcinol Monoacetate

Synonyms. 3-Acetoxyphenol; Resorcin Acetate.
Proprietary name. Euresol
$C_8H_8O_3$=152.1
CAS—102-29-4
A pale yellow or amber viscous liquid. Relative density 1.203 to 1.207. B.p. about 283°, with decomposition.
Sparingly soluble in water; soluble in ethanol and most organic solvents.

Dissociation Constant. pK_a 9.5, 10.1 (20°).

Partition Coefficient. Log *P* (octanol/water), 0.8.

Colour Test. Liebermann's test—violet.

Thin-layer Chromatography. System TAE—Rf 86; system TAF—Rf 91; system TB—Rf 00; system TE—Rf 50; system TAJ—Rf 34; system TAK—Rf 20; system TAL—Rf 68.

Gas Chromatography. System GA—RI 1258.

High Performance Liquid Chromatography. System HX—RI 243; system HY—RI 211; system HAA—Retention time(s) 8.0 min.

Ultraviolet Spectrum. Aqueous acid—273 nm (A^1_1=172a); aqueous alkali—290 nm (A^1_1=315a).

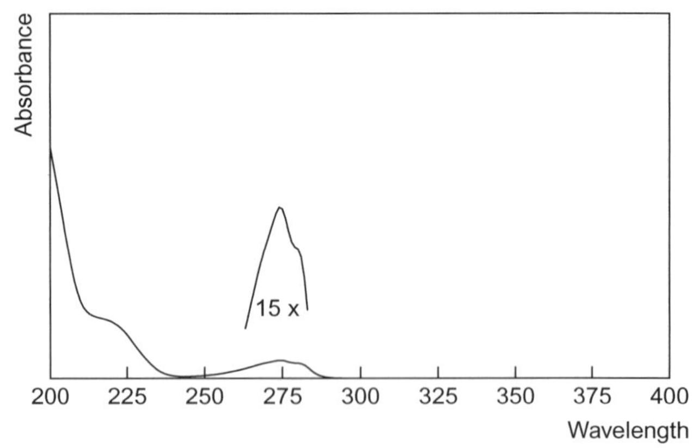

Infra-red Spectrum. Principal peaks at wavenumbers 1149, 1603, 774, 962, 1164, 1289 cm^{-1} (KBr disk).

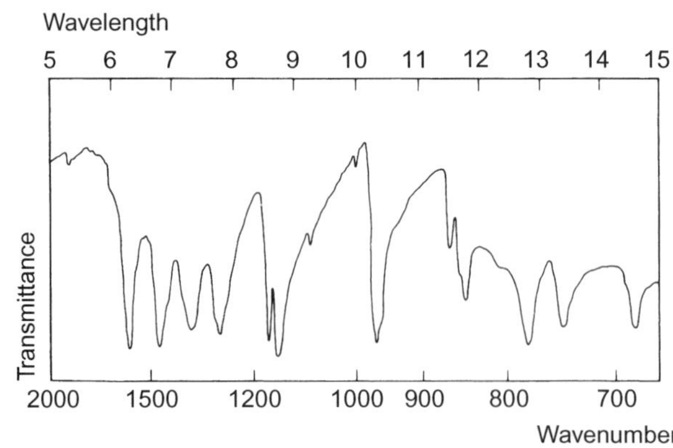

Mass Spectrum. Principal ions at *m/z* 110, 82, 39, 81, 53, 69, 55, 111.

Quantification

High performance liquid chromatography. In plasma or urine: limit of detection 500 µg/L, UV detection—D. Yeung *et al.*, *J. Chromatogr.*, 1981, *224*; *Biomed Appl.*, *13*, 513–518.

Disposition in the Body. Resorcinol may be absorbed through the skin or from ulcerated surfaces.

Toxicity. The estimated minimum lethal dose is 2 g and the maximum permissible atmospheric concentration is 10 ppm. The systemic effects of resorcinol are similar to those of phenol but convulsions may be more frequent.

Use. Topically in concentrations of 2 to 5%.

Reteplase

Thrombolytic/Acute Myocardial Infarction

Synonyms. BM-06.022; r-PA.
Proprietary names. Rapilysin; Retavase.
173-L-Serine-174-L-tyrosine-175-L-glutamine-173-527-plasminogen activator
$C_{1736}H_{2653}N_{499}O_{522}S_{22}$=39571.1
CAS—133652-38-7

Disposition in the Body. Elimination is both hepatic and renal. Hepatic clearance appears to be less than that of renal clearance. The drug is also cleared from circulation by α_2-antiplasmin, C_1 inactivator and α_1-antitrypsin, however the extent by these factors is unknown.

Half-life. 170 to 173 min.

Volume of distribution. 6 L in healthy individuals.

Clearance. The total plasma clearance is 17.4 to 22.3 L/h. In individuals with acute myocardial infarction, 7.3 L/h.

Note. For a review of reteplase, see S. Noble and D. McTavish, *Drugs*, 1996, *52*, 589–605.

Dose. 10 Units over 2 min by intravenous administration followed by another 10 Units after 30 min. 10 Units = 1.16 g.

Riboflavin

Vitamin

Synonyms. Lactoflavin; Riboflavine; Vitamin B_2; Vitamin G.
Proprietary names. Beflavin(e); Berivine; Boflavin; Flavaxin; Hibon; Ribon.
7,8-Dimethyl-10-(D-*ribo*-2,3,4,5-tetrahydroxypentyl)isoalloxazine
$C_{17}H_{20}N_4O_6 = 376.4$
CAS—83-88-5

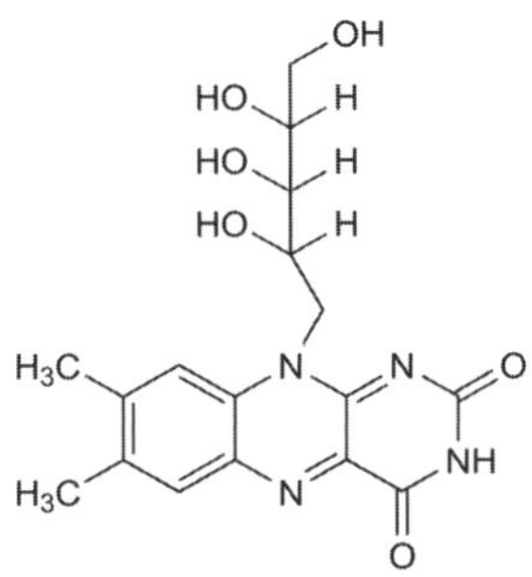

A yellow or orange-yellow, crystalline powder. M.p. 278° to 282°, with decomposition (darkens at about 240°). Solutions deteriorate on exposure to light.
Soluble 1 in 3000 to 1 in 20 000 of water, the variation in solubility being due to the variation in the internal crystalline structure; practically insoluble in ethanol, acetone, chloroform and ether; very soluble in dilute solutions of alkali hydroxides.

Dissociation Constant. pK_a 1.9, 10.2 (20°).

Partition Coefficient. Log *P* (octanol/water), −1.5.

Colour Test. Dissolve 1 mg in 100 mL of water—the solution is green-yellow when viewed by transmitted light and shows an intense yellow-green fluorescence which disappears on adding mineral acids, alkalis and reducing agents such as sodium dithionite.

Ultraviolet Spectrum. Aqueous acid—267 nm ($A^1_1 = 820a$); aqueous alkali—270 nm, 356 nm.

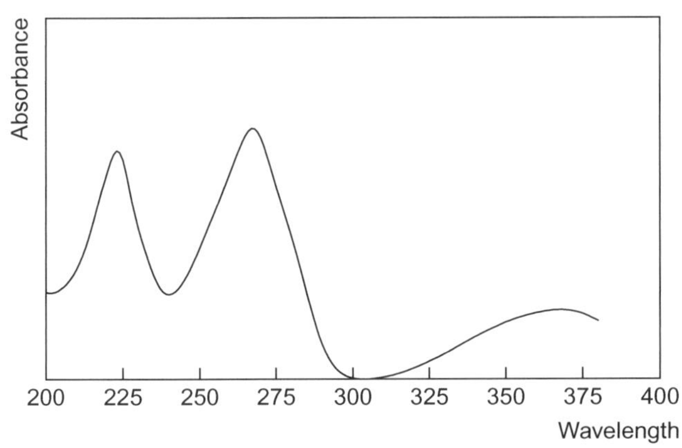

Infra-red Spectrum. Principal peaks at wavenumbers 1544, 1575, 1641, 1715, 1235, 1070 cm^{-1} (KBr disk).

Quantification

High performance liquid chromatography. In urine: limit of detection 50 µg/L, fluorescence detection—M. D. Smith, *J. Chromatogr.*, 1980, *182*; *Biomed Appl.*, *8*, 285–291. In plasma or urine: riboflavin, riboflavin 5′-phosphate and flavin adenine dinucleotide, fluorimetric detection—A. Lopez-Anaya and M. Mayersohn, *J. Chromatogr.*, 1987, *423*, 105–113. In whole blood or serum: riboflavin, thiamine and pyridoxine, UV and fluorescence detection—B. Botticher and D. Botticher, *Int. J. Vitam. Nutr. Res.*, 1987, *57*, 273–278. In plasma: riboflavin and flavocoenzymes, limits of detection < 3 nmol/L (riboflavin) and 9 nmol/L (flavocoenzymes), fluorescence detection—J. Zempleni, *Ann. Nutr. Metab.*, 1995, *39*, 224–226. In plasma: riboflavin and riboflavin cofactors—C. D. Capo-chichi *et al.*, *J. Chromatogr. B Biomed. Sci. Appl.*, 2000, *739*, 219–224.

Disposition in the Body. Riboflavin is readily absorbed after oral administration. It is widely distributed throughout the body but little is stored, and amounts in excess of the body's requirements are excreted in the urine. It is metabolised by phosphorylation to flavine mononucleotide (FMN) and then to flavine adenine dinucleotide (FAD). The recommended daily intake is up to 500 µg/kg. Endogenous plasma concentrations are usually less than 0.1 µg/mL.

Half-life. Plasma half-life, about 1 h.

Protein binding. In plasma, about 60%.

Note. For a review of the chemical and biological actions of riboflavin, see V. Massey, *Biochem. Soc. Trans.*, 2000, *28*, 283–296.

Dose. 2 to 10 mg daily.

Rifabutin

Antimycobacterial/Rifamycin Antibiotic

Synonyms. Ansamicin; Ansamycin; LM-427; Rifabutine.
Proprietary names. Alfacid; Ansatipine; Mycobutin.
(9*S*,12*E*,14*S*,15*R*,16*S*,17*R*,18*R*,19*R*,20*S*,21*S*,22*E*,24*Z*)-6,16,18,20-Tetrahydroxy-1′-isobutyl-14-methoxy-7,9,15,17,19,21,25-heptamethyl-spiro[9,4-(epoxypentadeca-[1,11,13]trienimino)-2*H*-furo-[2′,3′:7-,8]naphth[1,2-d]imidazole-2,4′-piperidine]-5,10,26-(3*H*,9*H*)-trione-16-acetate
$C_{46}H_{62}N_4O_{11} = 847.0$
CAS—72559-06-9

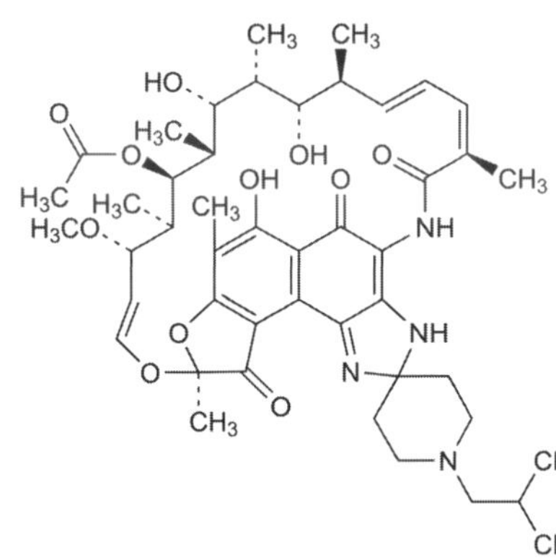

A violet/red crystalline powder. It is highly soluble in chloroform; soluble in methanol; sparingly soluble in ethanol; minimal solubility in water.

Partition Coefficient. Log *P* (*n*-octanol/water), 3.2.

High Performance Liquid Chromatography. System HAA—RT 17.6 min.

Column: RP C_8 (Symmetry Shield, 250 × 4.6 mm i.d., 5 µm). Mobile phase: acetonitrile:potassium dihydrogen phosphate buffer (0.05 M, pH 4.10) (48.7:51.3), flow rate 1 mL/min. Internal standard (IS): medazepam. UV detection (λ = 275 nm). RT: rifabutin, 4.5 min; IS, 6.4 min [G. Gatti *et al.*, *J. Chromatogr. B Biomed. Sci. Appl.*, 1999, *728*, 233–239].

Column: (analytical) ODS (Ultrasphere, 250 × 4.6 mm i.d., 5 µm); (guard) RP-18 (Newguard, 15 × 3.2 mm i.d.). Mobile phase: acetonitrile:monobasic potassium phosphate (0.05 M, pH 4.2):TEA (38:61.5:0.5), flow rate 1 mL/min. IS: medazepam. UV detection (λ = 275 nm). Retention times: rifabutin, 22 min; 25-deacetylrifabutin, 9 min; IS, 19 min [R. C. Lewis *et al.*, *Pharm. Res.*, 1991, *8(11)*, 1434–1440].

Ultraviolet Spectrum. Aqueous acid—208, 237, 277, 326 nm.

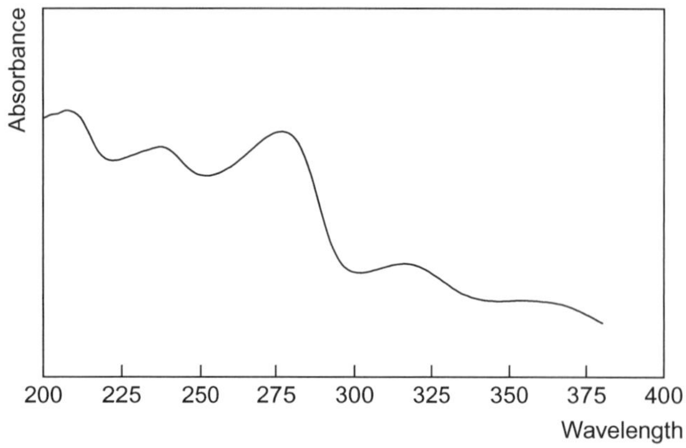

Quantification

High performance liquid chromatography. In plasma: limit of quantification 5 μg/L. UV detection (λ=275 nm)—G. Gatti *et al.*, *J. Chromatogr. B Biomed. Sci. Appl.*, 1999, *728*, 233–239. In plasma: limit of quantification 30 μg/L. UV detection (λ=275 nm)—M. H. Skinner *et al.*, *Antimicrob. Agents Chemother.*, 1989, *33*, 1237–1241. In plasma: limit of quantification is 5 μg/L for rifabutin and 2.5 μg/L for the metabolite, 25-deacetylrifabutin, and in urine, 100 μg/L for both. UV detection (λ=275 nm)—R. C. Lewis *et al.*, *Pharm. Res.*, 1991, *8(11)*, 1434–1440.

Disposition in the Body. The absorption of rifabutin from the gastro-intestinal tract is poor but rapid with peak concentrations (0.4 to 0.7 mg/L) observed at 2 to 4 h. Absorption is delayed by co-administration with food but the extent is not affected. Rifabutin undergoes extensive tissue distribution especially with lung tissues (concentrations can be 5 to 10 times higher than those detected in plasma over 24 h). This drug induces hepatic enzymes and is thought to induce its own metabolism. It appears to have more than 20 metabolites, out of which 25-deacetylrifabutin (25-*o*-deacetyl-rifabutin-*N*-oxide) has antibacterial activity similar to the parent drug. Following administration, rifabutin and its main metabolite, 25-deacetylrifabutin, are excreted in urine and faeces (30%). 31-Hydroxy-rifabutin (another predominant metabolite), 32-hydroxy-rifabutin and 32-hydroxydeactyl-rifabutin have also been identified in urine.

Therapeutic concentration. The trough serum therapeutic concentration is 50 μg/L and peak, 150 μg/L.

15 healthy male volunteers with a mean age of 24.7 years (19 to 39 years old) were either administered with 150 mg rifabutin solution in a fasted state, 150 mg capsule in a fasted state or 150 mg capsule after breakfast. The peak plasma concentrations for the fasted and fed volunteers were 156.2 and 187.9 μg/L, respectively for rifabutin, and 23.3 and 27.2 μg/L for the metabolite, 25-deacetylrifabutin. These concentrations were observed 5.4 and 3 h after administration, respectively. The peak concentration detected for the solution was higher than that observed for the capsule formulation; 237.5 μg/L compared with 187.9 μg/L for the drug and 34.5 versus 27.2 μg/L for the metabolite. These were observed at 2.5 and 3 h [P. K. Narang *et al.*, *Clin. Pharmacol. Ther.*, 1992, *52*, 335–341].

Toxicity

Dose-limiting toxicity was observed in 9 out of 10 patients (with AIDS-related complex) administered with doses greater than 1050 mg over 4 to 66 weeks. A reversible syndrome of arthritis was observed [F. P. Siegal *et al.*, *AIDS*, 1990, *4*, 433–441].

Bioavailability. 20%.

Half-life. Mean, 45 h (range, 16 to 69 h).

Volume of distribution. 8 to 9 L/kg (in HIV-infected patients).

Clearance. Systemic, healthy volunteers: mean, 0.69 L/h/kg (range, 0.46 to 1.34 L/h/kg).

Protein binding. 70 to 90%.

Dose. Dose varies between 150 and 600 mg daily depending on symptoms and use, but the recommended dose is 300 mg once daily.

Rifampicin

Tuberculostatic

Synonyms. Rifaldazine; Rifampin; Rifamycin AMP.
Proprietary names. Eremfat; Fampin; Ramfin; Rifa; Rifadin(e); Rifagen; Rifaldin; Rifapiam; Rifasynt; Rifcin; Rifex; Rifocina; Rifoldin(e); Rimactan(e); Rimapen; Rofact. It is an ingredient of Rifater, Rifinah and Rimactazid.
3-[[(4-Methyl-1-piperazinyl)imino]methyl]rifamycin
$C_{43}H_{58}N_4O_{12}$=822.9
CAS—13292-46-1

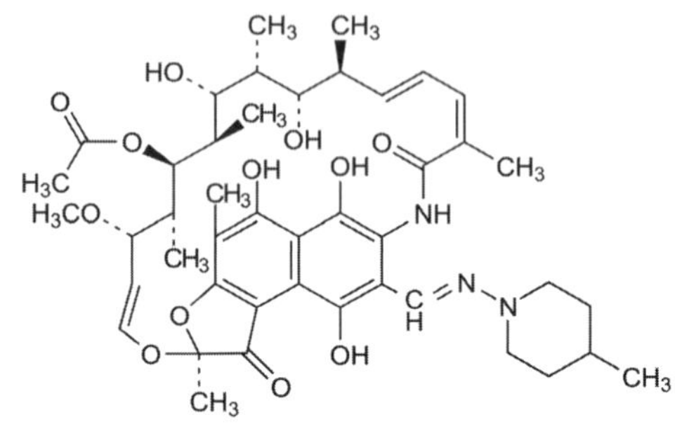

A brick-red to reddish-brown, crystalline powder. M.p. 183° to 188°, with decomposition.
Slightly soluble in water, ethanol, acetone and ether; freely soluble in chloroform; soluble in ethyl acetate and methanol.

Dissociation Constant. pK_a 1.7, 7.9.

Partition Coefficient. Log *P* (octanol/water), 4.2.

Colour Test. Mandelin's test—orange-brown.

Thin-layer Chromatography. System TA—Rf 79; system TAE—Rf 83. (Visible red-brown spot; Acidified potassium permanganate solution, positive.)

High Performance Liquid Chromatography. System HAA—Retention time(s) 16.2 min; system HY—RI 417.

Ultraviolet Spectrum. Aqueous acid—231 nm (A_1^1=320a), 263 nm, 336 nm (A_1^1=250a).

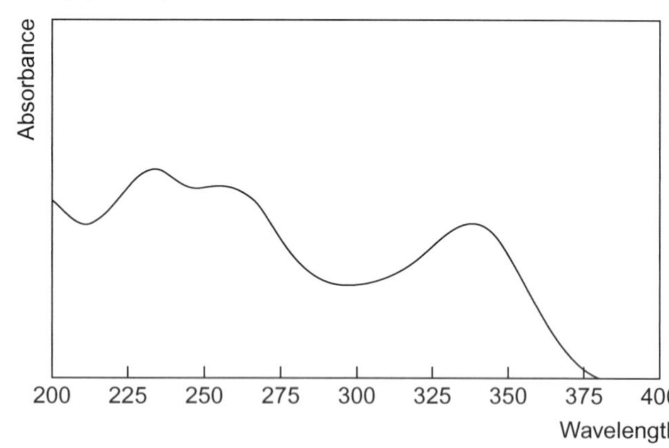

Infra-red Spectrum. Principal peaks at wavenumbers 1250, 1567, 976, 1098, 1064, 1650 cm^{-1} (KBr disk).

Mass Spectrum. Principal ions at *m/z* 43, 45, 60, 58, 95, 99, 398, 206.

Quantification

High performance liquid chromatography. In plasma, urine or saliva: rifampicin and metabolites, limit of detection 100 μg/L, UV detection—J. B. Lecaillon *et al.*, *J. Chromatogr.*, 1978, *145*; *B Biomed Appl.*, *2*, 319–324. In serum: rifampicin and desacetylrifampicin, limits of detection 17 and 10 μg/L, respectively—M. Guillaumont *et al.*, *J. Chromatogr.*, 1982, *232*; *B Biomed Appl.*, *21*, 369–376. In plasma, bronchoalveolar lavage fluid, or alveolar cells: limits of detection 0.5, 0.015 and 0.03 mg/L, respectively—J. E. Conte *et al.*, *J. Chromatogr. Sci.*, 2000, *38*, 72–76.

Disposition in the Body. Rifampicin is readily absorbed after oral administration; peak plasma concentrations are attained in about 2 h after a single dose. It is widely distributed in the tissues and fluids, and undergoes enterohepatic circulation. It is metabolised to desacetylrifampicin, which is active and is excreted in the urine and bile.

Therapeutic concentration

14 subjects ingested single doses of 600 mg rifampicin, under fasting conditions and after a high-fat meal and with an aluminium–magnesium antacid. The fasting mean peak plasma concentration was 10.54 mg/L at 2.42 h; this was unaltered by the antacid (10.89 mg/L at 2.36 h) but was reduced and delayed by the high-fat meal (7.27 mg/L at 4.43 h). [C. A. Peloquin *et al.*, *Chest*, 1999, *115*, 12–18].

Half-life. Plasma half-life, about 2 to 6 h (dose-dependent), decreased during chronic dosing; prolonged in subjects with liver disease.

Volume of distribution. About 1 L/kg.

Protein binding. In plasma, about 80%.

Note. For a review of the pharmacokinetics of rifampicin, see G. Acocella, *Clin. Pharmacokinet.*, 1978, *3*, 108–127.

Dose. Usually 600 mg daily.

Rifamycin SV

Antibacterial

Synonyms. Rifamicine SV; Rifomycin SV.
5,6,9,17,19,21-Hexahydroxy-23-methoxy-2,4,12,16,18,20,22-heptamethyl-2,7-(epoxypentadeca[1,11,13]trienimino)-naphtho[2,1-*b*]furan-1,11(2*H*)dione 21-acetate
$C_{37}H_{47}NO_{12}$=697.8
CAS—6998-60-3
Rifamycin SV is a semi-synthetic antibiotic derived from rifamycin B, a substance produced during growth of certain strains of *Streptomyces mediterranei*.
Dark yellow crystals. M.p. 300° (decomposes at 140°).
Practically insoluble in water; very soluble in ethanol, methanol, acetone and ethyl acetate; soluble in chloroform and ether.

Rifamycin Sodium

Synonyms. Rifamycin SV Sodium; Rifamastene.
Proprietary names. Otofa; Rifocin(e); Rifocina; Rifocyna.
$C_{37}H_{46}NNaO_{12}$=719.8
CAS—15105-92-7; 14897-39-3

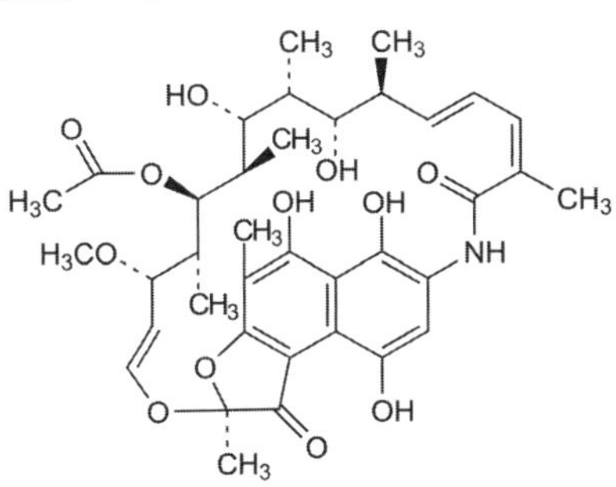

A brick-red, fine or slightly granular powder.
Soluble in water and chloroform; freely soluble in dehydrated alcohol and methanol; practically insoluble in ether.

Partition Coefficient. Log *P* (octanol/water), 5.0.

Colour Test. Mandelin's test—yellow-brown.

Thin-layer Chromatography. System TA—Rf 84. (Visible orange spot.)

High Performance Liquid Chromatography. System HAA—Retention time(s) 20.9 min.

Ultraviolet Spectrum. Ethanol—315 nm (A_1^1=420b).

Dose. 0.5 to 1 g of rifamycin sodium daily, by intramuscular injection.

Riluzole

Glutamate Antagonist/Neuroprotective

Synonyms. PK-26124; RP-54274.
Proprietary name. Rilutek
6-(Trifluoromethoxy)-2-benzothiazolamine
$C_8H_5F_3N_2OS$=234.2
CAS—1744-22-5

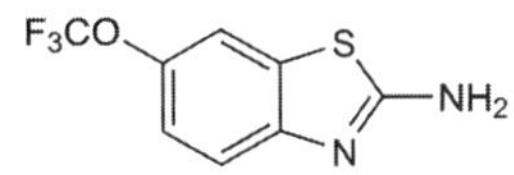

A white to slightly yellow crystalline powder with m.p. 119°. It is very slightly soluble in water and 0.1 M sodium hydroxide; very soluble in dimethylformamide and methanol; sparingly soluble in 0.1 M hydrochloric acid.

High Performance Liquid Chromatography. Column: (analytical) C_{18} (μBondapak, 300 × 4.6 mm i.d.); (guard) C_{18} (μBondapak, 39 × 4.6 mm i.d.). Mobile phase: acetonitrile:methanol:acetic acid:dipotassium hydrogen phosphate (10:55:1:35), flow rate 1 mL/min. Internal standard (IS): riluzole *N*-methyl derivative. UV detection (λ=265 nm). Retention time: riluzole, 9.2 min; IS, 12.4 min [A. Le Liboux *et al.*, *J. Clin. Pharmacol.*, 1997, *37*, 820–827].

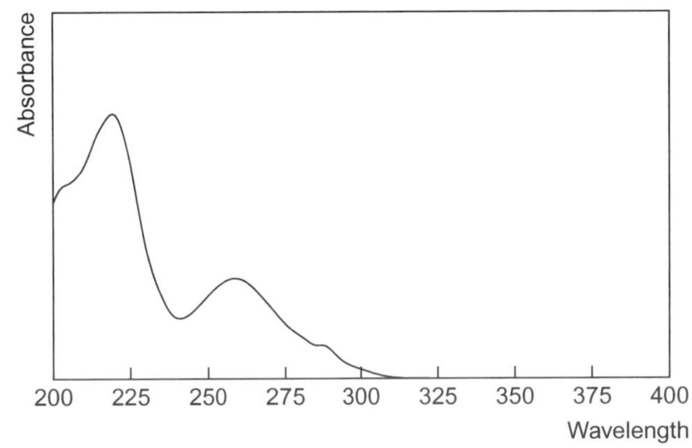

Quantification

High performance liquid chromatography. In blood and urine: limit of detection 5 μg/L and 10 μg/L, respectively. UV detection (λ=265 nm)—A. Le Liboux *et al.*, *J. Clin. Pharmacol.*, 1997, *37*, 820–827. In plasma: limit of quantification 0.5 μg/L. MS–MS detection—A. Le Liboux *et al.*, *J. Clin. Pharmacol.*, 1999, *39*, 480–486.

Disposition in the Body. At least 90% of an administered dose is absorbed 1 to 1.5 h after an oral dose. Absorption is rapid from the gastro-intestinal tract following oral administration and metabolism occurs via hepatic hydroxylation and glucuronidation with several inactive metabolites. The rate and the extent of absorption may be reduced when a high-fat meal is taken with the dose. The drug is widely and extensively distributed throughout the body. The main metabolites are three phenolic derivatives, one ureido derivative and unchanged riluzole. Excretion is mainly renal via urine and predominately as glucuronides. 2% of a dose is excreted unchanged in urine and a small amount in faeces. Decreased renal function will result in higher plasma concentrations. The drug displays linear pharmacokinetics, which are dose independent. Steady state is achieved in less than 5 days. The unchanged drug is the main component in plasma. There is no change in pharmacokinetics in the elderly or those with renal impairment.

Therapeutic concentration

16 healthy, young, white males (18 to 40 years) were administered with a single dose of 100 mg riluzole with or without a high-fat meal. The peak plasma concentrations were decreased when the drug was administered with food; 216 μg/L compared with 387 μg/L for those in the fasting state. These concentrations were observed at 2 h and 0.8 h, respectively.

16 males were administered with a single intravenous dose of 50 mg and two single oral doses of 100 mg riluzole. The peak concentration for the oral dose was 318 μg/L at 1.1 h and 584 μg/L for the intravenous dose at 0.5 h.

24 males were administered with four incremental doses of 25, 75, 150 and 250 mg (group 1); 50, 100, 200 and 300 mg (group 2). The peak plasma concentrations observed were 91, 247, 557 and 889 µg/L at 1.0, 0.9, 1.1, 1.3 h (group 1) and 214, 428, 1117 and 1611 µg/L at 1.4, 1.4, 1.5 and 1.3 h, respectively for group 2.

In the final part of this study, 12 males were administered with single oral doses of 25, 50 and 100 mg riluzole and then multiple dosing twice daily for 10 days. For the single doses, the peak concentrations were 52, 180 and 282 µg/L at 1.1, 0.9 and 1.6 h for the 25, 50 and 100 mg doses. The multiple doses produced peak concentrations of 77, 173 and 357 µg/L at 0.8, 0.8 and 1.3 h, respectively [A. Le Liboux *et al.*, *J. Clin. Pharmacol.*, 1997, *37(9)*, 820–827].

Bioavailability. 60%.

Half-life. 9 to 15 h.

Volume of distribution. 245 L (3.4 L/kg).

Clearance. This can vary between individuals because CYP 1A2 has considerable inter-individual variability. Cigarette smoking and reduced hepatic function may reduce or delay clearance. Japanese patients clear riluzole 50% less efficiently than Caucasians. Possible genetic and environmental factors might be involved.

Protein binding. 97% (mainly to albumin and lipoproteins).

Dose. 100 mg daily.

Rimantadine

Antiviral

Synonym. α-Methyl-1-adamantanemethylamine
α-Methyltricyclo[3.3.1.1^{3,7}]decane-1-methenamine
$C_{12}H_{21}N$=179.3
CAS—13392-28-4

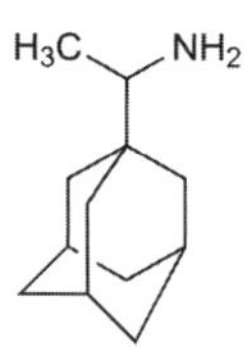

Rimantadine Hydrochloride

Synonym. EXP-126
Proprietary names. Flumadine; Meradan(e); Roflual.
$C_{12}H_{21}N,HCl$=215.8
CAS—1501-84-4
A white crystalline powder. M.p. 373° to 375° (sealed tube).
Soluble 1 in 17 of water, 1 in 20 of ethanol and 1 in 6 of chloroform.

Colour Test. Ninhydrin—pink-violet.

Thin-layer Chromatography. System TA—Rf 37; system TL—Rf 35; system TB—Rf 50; system TC—Rf 11. (Acidified iodoplatinate solution, strong reaction.)

Gas Chromatography. System GA—RI 1388.

Infra-red Spectrum. Principal peaks at wavenumbers 1538, 1600, 1266, 1277, 1160, 1117 cm^{-1} (KBr disk).

Mass Spectrum. Principal ions at *m/z* 44, 43, 79, 93, 41, 135, 91, 81.

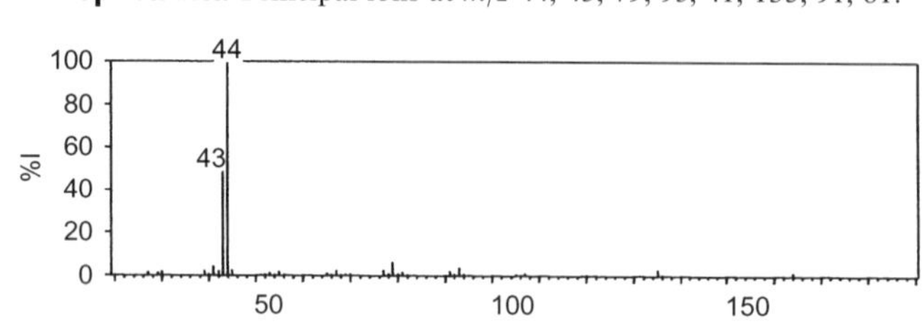

Note. For a review of the clinical use of rimantadine, see S. M. Wintermeyer and M. C. Nahata, *Ann. Pharmacother.*, 1995, *29*, 299–310.

Dose. 300 to 400 mg of rimantadine hydrochloride daily.

Rimiterol

Bronchodilator

4-(Hydroxy-2-piperidinylmethyl)-1,2-benzenediol
$C_{12}H_{17}NO_3$=223.3
CAS—32953-89-2

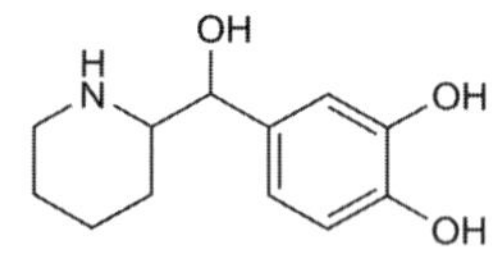

Crystals. M.p. 203° to 204°.

Rimiterol Hydrobromide

Synonyms. R-798; WG-253.
Proprietary name. Pulmadil
$C_{12}H_{17}NO_3,HBr$=304.2
CAS—31842-61-2
A white or pale grey, crystalline powder. M.p. about 220°, with decomposition. Soluble 1 in 10 of water and 1 in 20 of methanol.

Dissociation Constant. pK$_a$ 8.7, 10.3 (25°).

Partition Coefficient. Log *P* (octanol/water), 0.6.

Colour Tests. Ammoniacal silver nitrate—red/brown; Ferric chloride—green; Liebermann's test—black; Marquis test—brown→black; Methanolic potassium hydroxide—orange-pink; Nessler's reagent—black; Palladium chloride—orange; Potassium dichromate—green→brown; Sulfuric acid—yellow.

Thin-layer Chromatography. System TB—Rf 00; system TE—Rf 06; system TAE—Rf 07.

High Performance Liquid Chromatography. System HX—RI 150.

Ultraviolet Spectrum. Aqueous acid—280 nm (A^1_1=131a).

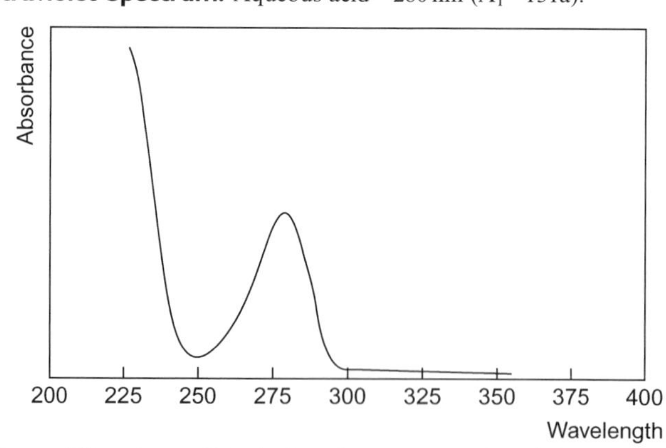

Infra-red Spectrum. Principal peaks at wavenumbers 1020, 1230, 1290, 1210, 1530, 1605 cm^{-1} (rimiterol hydrobromide, KCl disk).

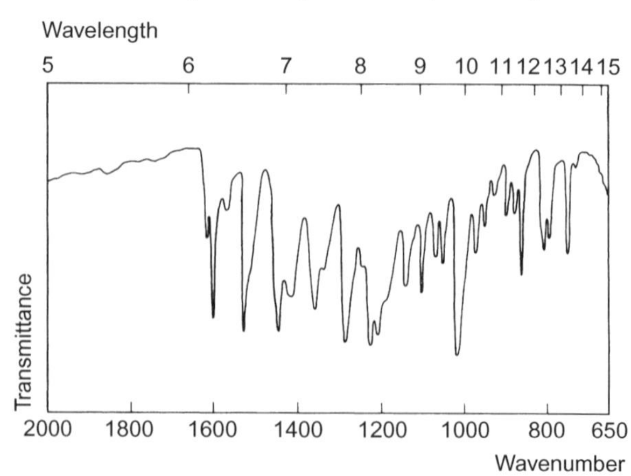

Disposition in the Body. Rimiterol is rapidly absorbed from the lungs, but most of an inhaled dose is swallowed; it is readily absorbed from the gastro-intestinal tract. It is subject not only to extensive first-pass metabolism by sulfate and glucuronide conjugation, but also to metabolism by catechol-*O*-methyltransferase (COMT) forming 3-*O*-methylrimiterol. It also appears to be metabolised by COMT in the lungs. After intrabronchial administration, about 70% of a dose is excreted in the urine in 24 h, mainly as free and conjugated 3-*O*-methylrimiterol, together with some free and conjugated rimiterol. A proportion of a dose is excreted in the bile. After oral or aerosol administration, less than 50% of a dose is excreted in the urine, mainly as conjugates of rimiterol.

Half-life. Plasma half-life, about 3 min after intravenous administration.

Dose. 200 to 600 µg of rimiterol hydrobromide, by aerosol inhalation; maximum of 8 doses daily.

Risperidone

Antipsychotic

Synonym. R-64766

Proprietary names. Belivon; Risperdal; Rispolin.

3-[2-[4-(6-Fluoro-1,2-benzisoxazol-3-yl)-1-piperidinyl]ethyl]-6,7,8,9-tetrahydro-2-methyl-4*H*-pyrido[1,2-*a*]pyrimidin-4-one

$C_{23}H_{27}FN_4O_2$=410.5

CAS—106266-06-2

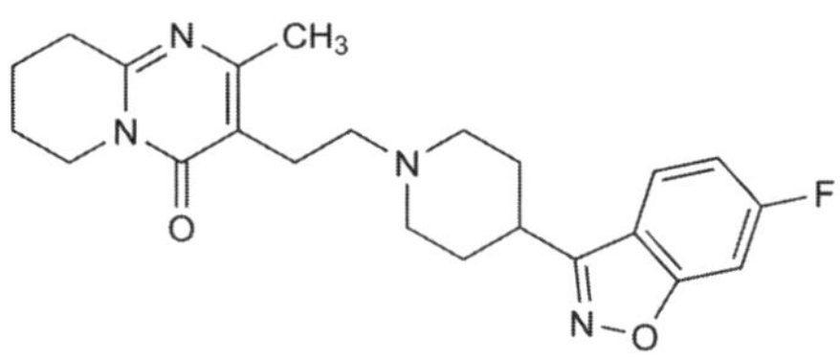

White or almost white powder. M. p. 170°. Practically insoluble in water; sparingly soluble in alcohol; freely soluble in dichloromethane and dilute acid solutions.

Partition Coefficient. Log *P* (octanol/water), 3.49.

High Performance Liquid Chromatography. System HZ—Retention time 3.1 min (risperidone), Retention time 2.8 min (9-hydroxy-risperidone); system HAX—Retention time 9.1 min; system HAY—Retention time 4.6 min.

Column: cyano (Ultrasphere, 250 × 4.6 mm i.d., 5 µm). Column temperature: 40°. Mobile phase: ammonium acetate buffer (0.04 M, pH 6.8):methanol:acetonitrile (10:8:82), flow rate 1.5 mL/min. Internal standard (IS): remoxipride. Electrochemical detection. Retention times: risperidone, 14 min; IS, 17 min [M. Aravagiri *et al.*, *J. Pharm. Sci.*, 1993, *82(5)*, 447–449].

Ultraviolet Spectrum. Aqueous acid—237, 275 nm; ethanol—237, 279, 285 nm.

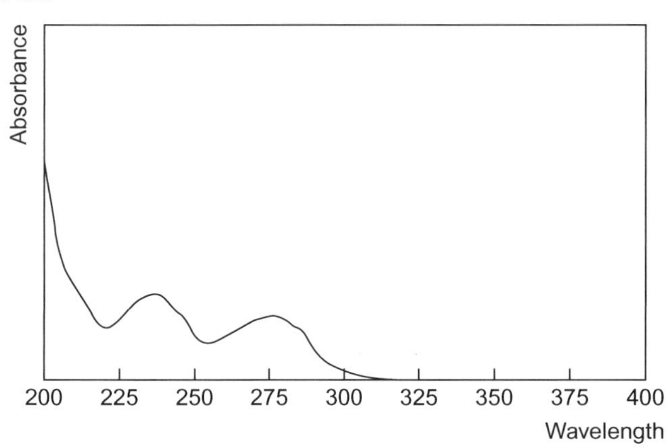

Mass Spectrum. Principal ions at *m*/*z* 220, 191, 204, 178, 192, 221, 233, 410.

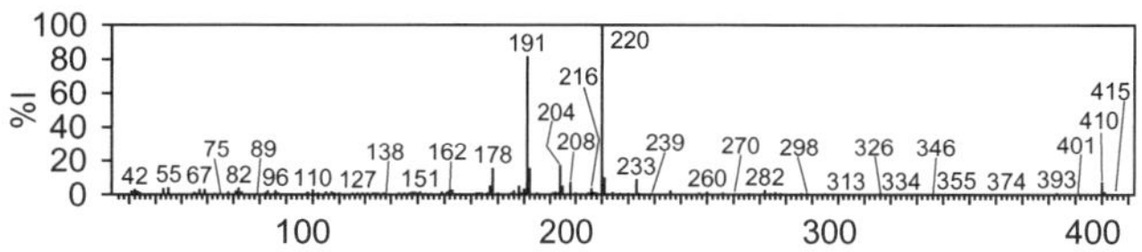

Quantification

High performance liquid chromatography. In plasma: limit of detection 1 to 2 µg/L. Electrochemical detection—J. P. Le Moing *et al.*, *J. Chromatogr.*, 1993, *614*, 333–339. In plasma and urine: limit of quantification 2 µg/L for risperidone and 9-hydroxyrisperidone. UV detection (λ=280 nm)—R. Woestenborghs *et al.*, *J. Chromatogr.*, 1992, *583*, 223–230. In plasma: limit of quantification 0.1 µg/L. Electrochemical detection— M. Aravagiri *et al.*, *J. Pharm. Sci.*, 1993, *82(5)*, 447–449.

Bioassay. Limit of detection 0.1 to 0.2 µg/L.—E. Reid and I. D. Wilson, *Methodological Surveys in Biochemistry and Analysis*, Royal Society of Chemistry, 1990, *20*, 241–246. Published by Plenum Press.

Disposition in the Body. Risperidone is well absorbed after oral administration with peak plasma concentrations reached within 1 to 2 h. It undergoes metabolism by hydroxylation and oxidative *N*-dealkylation to 9-hydroxyrisperidone which is active. Other metabolites include 7-hydroxyrisperidone (an acid derivative of the drug and metabolite), as well as glucuronides. The hydroxylation process is mediated by the cytochrome P450 isoenzyme CYP2D6 which is subject to genetic polymorphism, but the effect of this on the pharmacokinetics of risperidone and 9-hydroxyrisperidone is not thought to be clinically significant as the absolute bioavailability of the active (antipsychotic) components remains unaffected. The drug and metabolites are extensively distributed within the body. Excretion is via urine (70%), mainly as the metabolite, and faeces (15%) over 7 days following a dose.

Therapeutic concentration. The serum therapeutic concentration range is between 10 and 90 µg/L and the total sum of parent drug and its metabolite, hydroxyrisperidone, 10 to 100 µg/L.

12 healthy males (mean age, 24 years; range, 19 to 41 years) were treated, on three separate occasions, with 1 mg risperidone as an intravenous infusion (over a 30 min period), as an intramuscular injection or orally. At least 2 weeks were allowed between treatments. The individuals were fasted overnight for at least 10 h and for an additional 2 h after dosing. After the oral dose, the peak plasma drug concentrations were 7.90 µg/L for the extensive metabolisers (9 subjects); 4.97 µg/L for the intermediate metaboliser, and 20.8 and 12.1 µg/L for the poor metabolisers (2 subjects). These concentrations were observed at 0.8, 3.0, 1.0 and 1.5 h, respectively. After the intramuscular injection, peak concentrations were 13.9, 7.54, and 28.1 and 18.4 µg/L for the extensive, intermediate and poor metabolisers, respectively observed at 0.35, 0.13, and 0.5 and 0.13 h. Peak concentrations for the metabolite, 9-hydroxyrisperidone, were 6.5, 1.61, and 0.85 and 1.05 µg/L for the extensive, intermediate and poor metabolisers observed at 3.2, 8.0, and 48 and 24 h, respectively, after the oral dose. For the intramuscular dose, the peak metabolite concentrations were 5.0, 1.3, and 1.8 and 0.86 µg/L at 6.9, 5.0, and 8.0 and 16.0 h, respectively for the different metabolisers [M. L. Huang *et al.*, *Clin. Pharmacol. Ther.*, 1993, *54*, 257–268].

Toxicity

A 45-year-old male was found dead with several empty bottles of risperidone by his side. Postmortem examination revealed the following risperidone concentrations: blood, 1.8 mg/L; urine, 14.4 mg/L and gastric contents, 34.6 mg/L. The 9-hydroxyrisperidone metabolite was not detected in the blood or gastric contents, however, the urine concentration was found to be 17.8 mg/L [A. C. Springfield and E. Bodiford, *J. Anal. Toxicol.*, 1996, *20*, 202–203].

Bioavailability. 66% (extensive metabolisers), 82% (slow metabolisers).

Half-life. Approximately, 19 h (active fraction). Also reported as extensive metabolisers: risperidone $t_{1/2\beta}$ 2.8 h, 9-hydroxyrisperidone $t_{1/2\beta}$ 20.5 h. Poor metabolisers: risperidone 16 h. Both groups, total active moiety 24 h. Increases in the elderly and those with moderate to severe renal impairment.

Volume of distribution. 1.1 L/kg (extensive metabolisers); 2.1 L/kg (intermediate); 0.7 L/kg (poor).

Clearance. Total plasma, 394 mL/min (extensive metabolisers); 192 (intermediate); 54 mL/min (poor metabolisers).

Protein binding. Risperidone, 88 to 90%; 9-hydroxyrisperidone, 77%

Dose. Day 1: 2 mg; day 2: 4 mg. The usual dose ranges between 4 and 6 mg daily with a maximum of 16 g. In the elderly and those with hepatic or renal impairment: 500 μg twice daily increased in 500 μg steps to 1 to 2 mg daily.

Ritodrine

Sympathomimetic

(αS)-*rel*-4-Hydroxy-α-[(1*R*)-1-[[2-(4-hydroxyphenyl)ethyl]amino]-ethyl]benzenemethanol
$C_{17}H_{21}NO_3$=287.4
CAS—26652-09-5

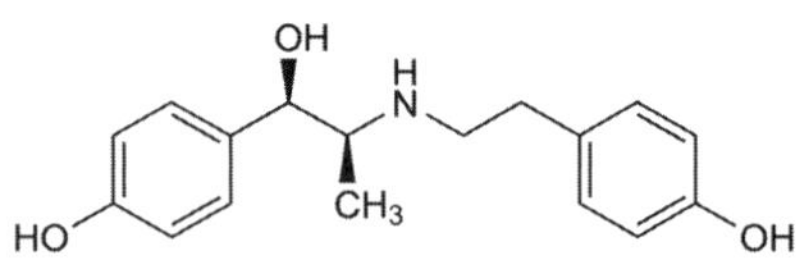

M.p. 88° to 90°.

Ritodrine Hydrochloride

Synonym. DU-21220
Proprietary names. Miodrina; Miolene; Prempar; Pre-Par; Utemerin; Utopar; Yutopar.
$C_{17}H_{21}NO_3$,HCl=323.8
CAS—23239-51-2
A white crystalline powder. M.p. 193° to 195°, with decomposition.
Soluble in chloroform and dilute acetic acid.

Colour Tests. Folin–Ciocalteu reagent—blue; Liebermann's test–black; Mandelin's test—green; Marquis test—yellow-brown.

Thin-layer Chromatography. System TA—Rf 73. (Acidified iodoplatinate solution, positive.)

Gas Chromatography. System GA—not eluted.

Ultraviolet Spectrum. Aqueous acid—274 nm (A^1_1=98a).

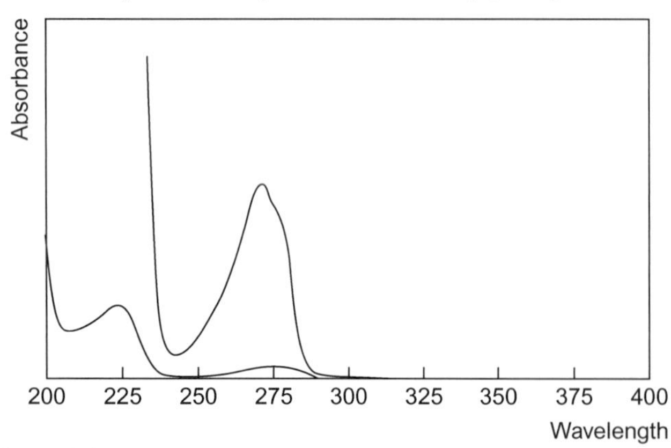

Infra-red Spectrum. Principal peaks at wavenumbers 1510, 1209, 1256, 1610, 833, 1170 cm^{-1} (KBr disk).

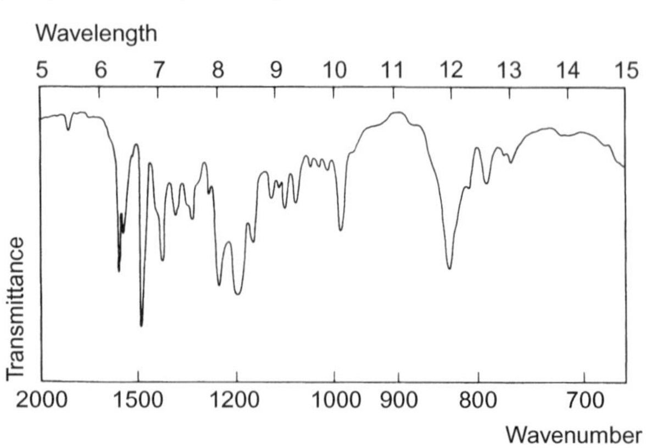

Mass Spectrum. Principal ions at *m/z* 121, 164, 77, 57, 56, 165, 162, 122.

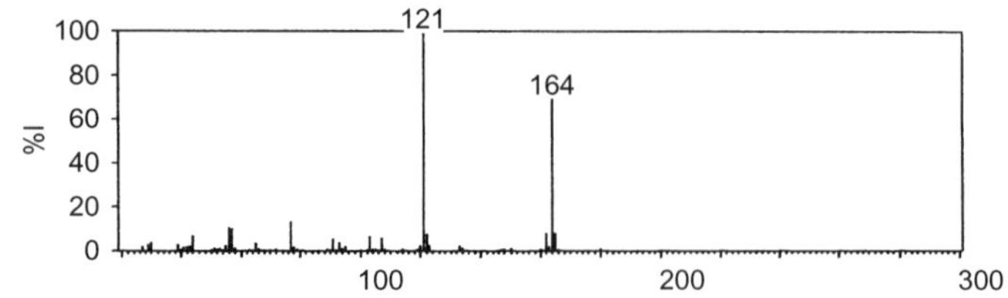

Quantification

High performance liquid chromatography. In serum: limit of detection 2 μg/L, electrochemical detection—L. S. Lin *et al.*, *J. Pharm. Sci.*, 1984, *73*, 131–133.

Radioimmunoassay. In plasma or serum: limit of detection 300 ng/L—R. Gandar *et al.*, *Eur. J. Clin. Pharmacol.*, 1980, *17*, 117–122.

Disposition in the Body. Ritodrine is readily absorbed after oral administration but subject to considerable first-pass metabolism. About 70 to 90% of an oral dose is excreted in the urine in 24 h, mainly as sulfate and glucuronide conjugates with about 5% of the dose as unchanged drug.

Therapeutic concentration

Following oral and intramuscular administration of 10 mg to 4 subjects, mean peak serum concentrations of 0.01 and 0.02 mg/L were attained in 20 to 40 min and 10 min, respectively. [R. Gandar *et al.*, *Eur. J. Clin. Pharmacol.*, 1980, *17*, 117–122].

Intravenous ritodrine hydrochloride, administered at a dose of 50 μg/min and increased by 50 μg/min every 30 min, if necessary, to a maximum of 350 μg/min, produced average plasma ritodrine levels of 27.8 to 113.3 μg/L in patients undergoing tocolytic therapy, whereas levels fell to 9.8 to 13.8 μg/L upon switching to oral therapy at a dose of 60 to 120 mg per 24 h. [E. Schiff *et al.*, *Am. J. Obstet. Gynecol.*, 1993, *169*, 1059–1064].

Bioavailability. About 30%.

Half-life. Plasma half-life, about 1 to 2 h; a longer elimination half-life of about 15 to 20 h has also been reported.

Protein binding. In plasma, about 32%.

Note. For a review of ritodrine, see B. W. Finklestein, *Drug Intell. Clin. Pharm.*, 1981, *15*, 425–433.

Dose. 50 to 350 μg/min of ritodrine hydrochloride by intravenous infusion; up to 120 mg daily, by mouth.

Ritonavir

Protease Inhibitor/Antiviral

Synonyms. A-84538, Abbott-84538, ABJ-538.
Proprietary name. Norvir
[5*S*,8*S*,10*S*,11*S*)]-10-Hydroxy-2-methyl-5-(1-methylethyl)-1-[2-(1-methylethyl)-4-thiazolyl]-3,6-dioxo-8,11-bis(phenylmethyl)-2,4,7,12-tetraazatridecan-13-oic acid 5-thiazolylmethyl ester
$C_{37}H_{48}N_6O_5S_2$=721.0
CAS—155213-67-5

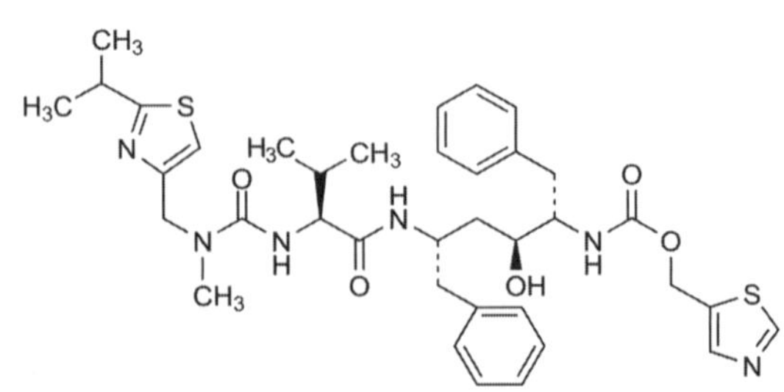

White to light-tan powder. Practically insoluble in water, freely soluble in methanol and ethanol; soluble in isopropanol.

High Performance Liquid Chromatography. System HAC—k 7.1; HAE—Retention time 22.2 min.

Column: ODS-AQ (50 × 4.0 mm i.d., 3 μm). Mobile phase: acetonitrile:methanol:0.1% trifluoroacetic acid (with 0.01 M tetramethylammonium perchlorate) (40:5:55), flow rate 1 mL/min. UV detection (λ=205 nm). Retention time: 8 min [K. C. Marsh *et al.*, *J. Chromatogr. B Biomed. Sci. Appl.*, 1997, *704*, 307–313].

Ultraviolet Spectrum. Aqueous acid—238 nm. No alkaline shift.

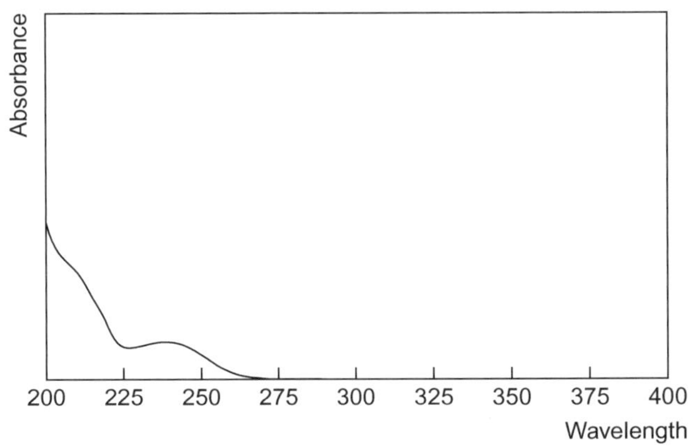

Infrared Spectrum. Principal peaks at wavenumber 3355, 3328, 2964, 1714, 1618, 1522, 1235 cm^{-1}.

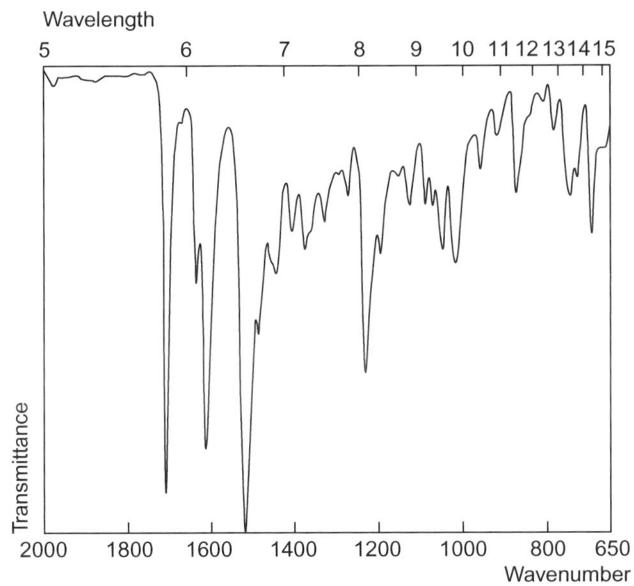

Quantification

High performance liquid chromatography. In serum: limit of detection 0.51 mg/L. UV detection (λ=250 nm)—V. A. Simon *et al.*, *J. Chromatogr. A*, 2001, *913(1–2)*, 447–453. In plasma: limit of quantification 0.05 mg/L—G. Aymard *et al.*, *J. Chromatogr. B Biomed. Sci. Appl.*, 2000, *744*, 227–240. In plasma: limit of quantification 0.1 mg/L. UV detection (λ=260 nm)—V. Proust *et al.*, *J. Chromatogr. B Biomed. Sci. Appl.*, 2000, *742*, 453–458. In plasma: lower limit of quantification 0.012 mg/L. UV detection λ=205 nm)—K. C. Marsh *et al.*, *J. Chromatogr. B Biomed. Sci. Appl.*, 1997, *704*, 307–313.

Disposition in Body. Approximately 60 to 80% of a dose is absorbed. Ritonavir is extensively metabolised in the liver by oxidation principally by cytochrome P450 CYP3A and CYP2D6, to three major metabolites; desthiazolyl carbamate, an isopropylthiazolyl oxidative product and a des-isopropylthiazolyl product. It induces its own metabolism. Ritonavir is excreted mainly in faeces (86%) with a minor amount in urine (11% over a 148 h period). The plasma concentration is generally higher during the first few days of administration. Linear pharmacokinetics have been observed after multiple dosing and steady state is achieved after administration for 2 weeks.

Therapeutic concentration

12 HIV-positive male patients, aged 40 to 49 years, were fasted overnight and co-administered ritonavir as three dosing regimens. Group 1: 800 mg indinavir twice daily and 100 mg ritonavir twice daily. Group 2: 1200 mg indinavir twice daily and 100 mg ritonavir twice daily. The peak plasma ritonavir concentration for group 1 was 1.4 mg/L (range, 0.7 to 2.1 mg/L) and group 2, 1.9 mg/L. These levels were observed at 2.8 (1.5 to 6.9) and 1.5 to 5.0 h, respectively [R. P. van Heeswijk *et al.*, *AIDS*, 1999, *13(14)*, F95–F99].

18 males confirmed as asymptomatic HIV positive but otherwise healthy, mean age 37.4 years (range, 28 to 49 years), were administered 300 mg ritonavir every 6 h for 4 days. The peak plasma concentration was 12.31 mg/L at 3.8 h, and the minimum concentration was 4.93 mg/L after multiple dosing [A. Cato III *et al.*, *Antimicrob. Agents Chemother.*, 1998, *42(7)*, 1788–1793].

64 HIV positive males, mean 29 years old (range, 21 to 45 years) with no AIDS defining illness other than non-visceral Kaposi's sarcoma, were involved in the study. They were divided into equal groups and received ritonavir in the following doses. Group 1: 200 mg every 12 h; group 2: 300 mg/12 h; group 3: 400 mg/12 h; group 4: 500 mg/12 h. Peak plasma concentrations on day 1 were 2.0, 4.4, 9.0 and 9.6 g/L at 4.3, 3.9, 3.6 and 3.9 h, respectively, for the four groups. On day 16, the peak concentrations were 4.5, 6.5, 11.7 and 14.2 g/L for groups 1, 2, 3 and 4, respectively, at 3.8, 4.6, 4.3 and 4.3 h. The minimum concentrations on day 16 were 0.6, 0.7, 1.1 and 2.3 g/L, respectively [A. Hsu *et al.*, *Antimicrob. Agents Chemother.*, 1997, *41(5)*, 898–905].

Half-life. 3 to 5 h.

Volume of distribution. 20 to 40 L (after single 600 mg dose). Also reported as 0.41 L/kg.

Clearance. Apparent oral, 40 L/h (100 mg dose); 5 L/h (600 mg); clearance increases in children.

Protein binding. 98 to 99%.

Dose. An oral dose of 1.2 g daily in two divided doses.

Rituximab

Immunosuppressant

Synonyms. IDEC-102; IDEC-C2B8.
Proprietary names. MabThera; Rituxan.
IgG_1 kappa immunoglobulin (145 kDa)
CAS—174722-31-7

Quantification

Enzyme immunoassay. In serum: limit of quantification is 6.6 mg/L, limit of detection 2.0 mg/L—I. Iacona *et al.*, *Ther. Drug Monit.*, 2000, *22(3)*, 295–301.

Disposition in the Body. Serum concentrations of rituximab are proportional to the dose administered. The drug can be detected in serum for a long period of time after the completion of treatment, on average 3 to 6 months, and accumulation of the drug occurs.

Therapeutic concentration

Patients were administered with either a 125, 250 or 375 mg/m^2 body surface dose of rituximab once weekly for 4 weeks. The serum antibody concentration increased with increasing dose. For the 375 mg/m^2 dose, peak serum concentrations were 238.7 mg/L after the first infusion and 480.7 mg/L after the fourth infusion [Roche Products Limited product information, 1999].

7 patients with follicular non-Hodgkin's lymphoma were administered 375 mg/m^2 rituximab infusion once weekly, after chemotherapy, for 4 weeks. Maximum serum concentrations were 349.1 mg/L after the first infusion; 332.0 mg/L after the second; 447.5 mg/L after the third infusion and 660.0 mg/L after the fourth. These concentrations were observed by the end of the infusion [I. Iacona *et al.*, *Ther. Drug Monit.*, 2000, *22(3)*, 295–301].

14 patients with relapsed indolent lymphoma were administered 375 mg/m^2 rituximab once weekly for 4 weeks. After the first infusion, the maximum serum concentration was 206 mg/L at the end and following the fourth infusion, the maximum was 465 mg/L [N. L. Berinstein *et al.*, *Ann. Oncol.*, 1998, *9*, 995–1001].

Toxicity. Rituximab is associated with cytokine-release syndrome including fevers and rigors, usually within 2 h of beginning the treatment. Tumour lysis syndrome, respiratory failure and cardiac arrhythmias (both serious and life-threatening) and even death may occur.

Half-life. The serum half-life is proportional to the dose administered. A mean serum half-life is 60 (range, 11 to 105) h after a 10 mg/m^2 intravenous infusion and 174 (26 to 442) h after 250 mg/m^2.

Clearance. Plasma, 0.046 L/h (after an 375 mg/m^2 body surface dose, first infusion); 0.015 L/h (after fourth infusion).

Dose. The recommended dose is 375 mg/m^2 body surface once weekly as an intravenous dose for 4 doses. The first infusion is given at a rate of 50 mg/h which is increased in steps of 50 mg/h every 30 min to a maximum of 400 mg/h.

Rivastigmine

Acetyl-cholinesterase Inhibitor/Nootropic

Ethylmethylcarbamic acid 3-[(1*S*)-1-(dimethylamino)ethyl]phenyl ester
$C_{14}H_{22}N_2O_2$=250.3
CAS—123441-03-2

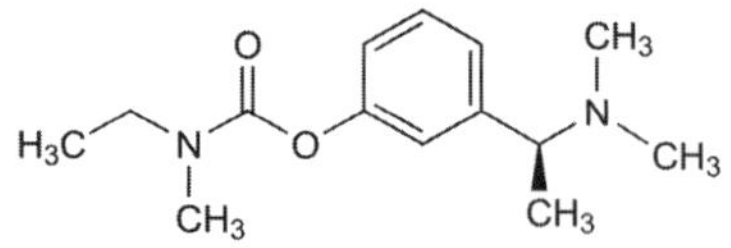

Rivastigmine Hydrogen Tartrate

Synonyms. ENA-713; SDZ-ENA-713; SDZ-212-713.
Proprietary names. Exelon; Prometax.
$C_{14}H_{22}N_2O_2$, $C_4H_6O_6$=400.4
CAS—129101-54-8
M. p. 123° to 125°. White to off-white fine crystalline powder. Very soluble in water, soluble in ethanol and acetonitrile, slightly soluble in *n*-octanol and very slightly soluble in ethyl acetate.

Partition Coefficient. Log *P* (octanol/buffer pH 7.0), 3.0.

Gas Chromatography. Column: wide bore fused silica coated with cross bonded 50% phenyl/5% methyl silicone. Carrier gas: helium, flow rate 5 mL/min. MS detection: Retention time: 3.2 min [K. Habucky *et al.*, *Biopharm. Drug. Dispos.*, 1998, *19*, 285–290].

High Performance Liquid Chromatography. System HZ—RT 2.3 min.

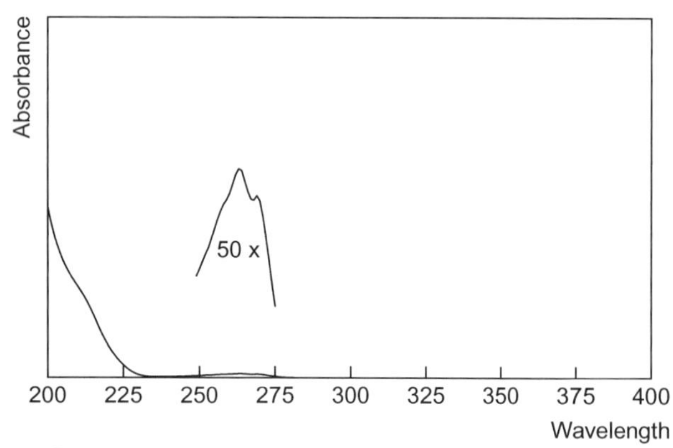

Quantification

Gas chromatography–mass spectrometry. In blood: limit of quantification 0.25 μg/L—F. Tse and R. Laplanche, *Pharm. Res.*, 1998, *15*, 1614–1620.

Disposition in the Body. Rivastigmine is rapidly and completely absorbed from the gastro-intestinal tract after administration. Peak plasma concentrations are reached in about 1 h. Administration with food delays absorption by 1.5 h and reduces the maximum plasma concentration. The drug is rapidly and extensively metabolised by cholinesterase-mediated hydrolysis to a weakly active decarbamylated metabolite. Rivastigmine undergoes a significant first-pass effect and it is widely distributed throughout the body. 90% of the dose is excreted in urine within 24 h and <1% appears in faeces. Metabolism and excretion of rivastigmine and its metabolite may be altered by renal impairment. The drug has a prolonged duration of action. There is no accumulation of the parent drug or its metabolite.

Toxicity. Most accidental overdoses resulted in no clinical signs or symptoms. After ingestion of a 46 mg dose full recovery was made within 24 h following conservative management. Nausea, vomiting and diarrhoea may occur.

Bioavailability. Approximately 36% following a 3 mg dose which may increase when taken with food.

Half-life. Approx. 1 h.

Volume of distribution. Apparent, 1.8 to 2.7 L/kg.

Clearance. Plasma, 130 L/h (0.2 mg intravenous dose); 70 mL/h (2.7 mg).

Distribution in blood. Blood: plasma ratio is 0.8 to 0.9 with 40 to 50% of the drug associated with red blood cells; independent of concentration.

Protein binding. 40%.

Dose. The initial dose is 1.5 mg twice daily which is increased to 3 mg twice daily over a two week interval; 4.5 mg twice daily to a maximum 6 mg twice daily. The effective dose is 3 to 6 mg daily.

Rizatriptan

Selective Serotonin 5-HT1 agonist/Antimigraine

N,N-Dimethyl-5-(1*H*-1,2,4-triazol-1-ylmethyl)-1*H*-indole-3-ethanamine
$C_{15}H_{19}N_5$=269.4
CAS—144034-80-0

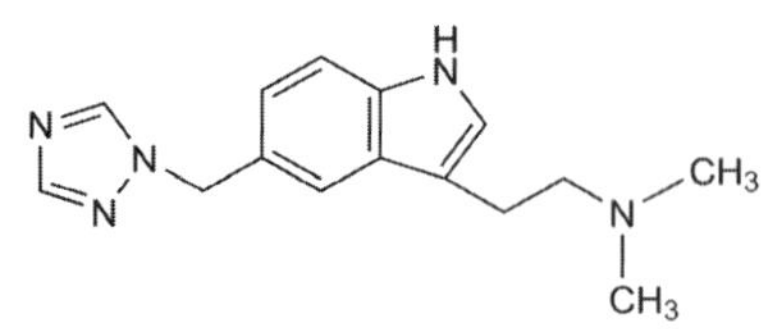

A white to off white crystalline solid. M. p. 120° to 121°. It is soluble in water (42 g/L at 25°) as the free base.

Rizatriptan Benzoate

Synonyms. MK-0462; MK-462.
Proprietary name. Maxalt
$C_{15}H_{19}N_5$, C_6H_5COOH=391.5
CAS—145202-66-0
A white to off white crystalline solid. M. p. 178° to 180°.

High Performance Liquid Chromatography. Column: (analytical) silica (Alltech, 150 × 2.1 mm i.d., 5 μm); (guard) C_8 (Optiguard, 1 mm).

Mobile phase: ammonium acetate (20 mM, pH 4 with glacial acetic acid, then to pH 2.7 with formic acid):methanol:acetonitrile (80:10:10), flow rate 300 μL/min. MS–MS detection (ESI, SIM *m/z* at 270→201). Retention time: 3.48 min [K. Vishwanathan *et al.*, *Rapid Commun. Mass Spectrom.*, 2000, *14(3)*, 168–172].

Column: SB-phenyl (Zorbax, 250 × 4.6 mm i.d., 5 μm). Mobile phase: (A)-acetonitrile:0.1% trifluroacetic acid in water (16:84); (B)-acetonitrile:0.1% phosphoric acid in water (12:88), flow rate 1.5 mL/min. UV detection (λ=280 nm). Retention times: rizatriptan, (A)-6.3 min; (B)-6.7 min [V. Antonucci *et al.*, *J. Liq. Chromatogr. Rel. Technol.*, 1998, *21*, 1649–1670].

Ultraviolet Spectrum. Aqueous acid—225, 282 nm.

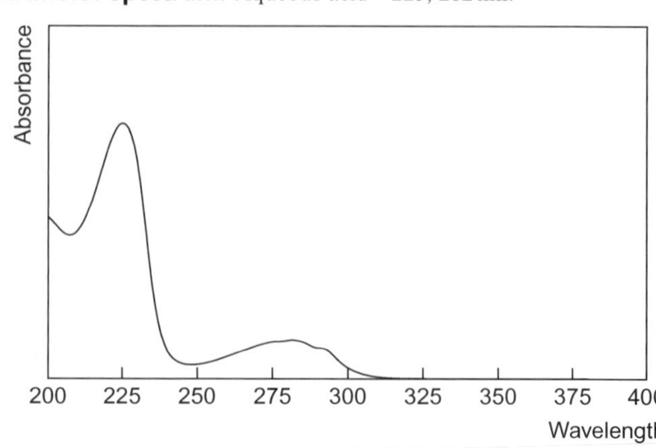

Mass Spectrum. Principal ions at *m/z* 58, 143, 115, 42, 156, 211, 128, 269.

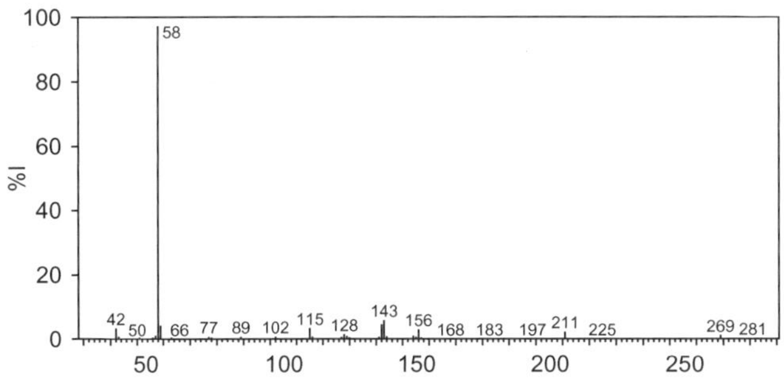

Quantification

High performance liquid chromatography–mass spectrometry. In serum: limit of detection 0.1 μg/L. MS–MS detection—K. Vishwanathan *et al.*, *Rapid Commun. Mass Spectrom.*, 2000, *14(3)*, 168–172. In plasma and urine: limit of quantification 0.5 μg/L and 1 μg/L, respectively. MS–MS detection—Y.Lee *et al. Br. J. Clin. Pharmacol.*, 1999, *47*, 373–378. In plasma: limit of quantification 0.5 μg/L. MS detection—D.A. McLoughlin *et al., J. Chromatogr. A.*, 1996, *726*, 115–124.

Disposition in the Body. Rizatriptan is rapidly and completely absorbed after an oral dose. Peak plasma concentrations are reached after 1 to 1.5 h or 1.6 to 2.5 (disintegrating tablets) h depending on formulation. Food may delay time to peak plasma concentration by up to 1 h. It is metabolised primarily by monoamine oxidase type A to the inactive indole acetic acid derivative. The active *N*-monodesmethyl-rizatriptan metabolite is formed to a small degree. Other minor non-active metabolites include *N*-oxide, 6-hydroxy compound and the sulfate conjugate of the 6-hydroxy metabolite. 80% of a dose is excreted in urine with approximately 14% as the unchanged drug, 51% as the indole acetic acid metabolite and 1% as *N*-monodesmethyl-rizatriptan. This indicates substantial first-pass metabolism. 10% is excreted in the faeces. No accumulation occurs. The drug is rapidly cleared from the plasma. Renal impairment did not effect pharmacokinetics. Hepatic impairment increased plasma concentrations by 30%.

Therapeutic concentration

6 healthy males were administered with 60 mg rizatriptan. The mean peak plasma concentration was 19.8 μg/L which was observed at 1.4 h [K. P. Vyas *et al.*, *Drug Metab. Dispos.*, 2000, *28(1)*, 89–95].

24 healthy male and female individuals, aged between 19 and 49 years (mean, 32.9 years) were administered with a single dose of 10 mg rizatriptan followed, 48 h later, by a second 10 mg dose every 2 h for three doses on 4 consecutive days. The mean peak plasma rizatriptan concentration reached on day 1 was 19.6 μg/L at 0.9 h; day 3, 35.7 μg/L at 5.0 h and on day 6, 37.0 μg/L at 4.8 h. For the metabolite, *N*-monodesmethyl-rizatriptan, peak concentrations were 2.2, 3.4 and 3.8 g/L at 1.5, 5.3 and 5.0 h, respectively, on days 1, 3 and 6 [M. R. Goldberg *et al.*, *J. Clin. Pharmacol.*, 2000, *40(1)*, 74–83].

Bioavailability. 40 to 45%.

Half-life. 2 to 3 h.

Volume of distribution. 140 L in males and 110 L in females.

Clearance. 1000 to 1500 mL/min (males); 900 to 1100 mL/min (females). About 20 to 30% of this is renal clearance.

Protein binding. 14%.

Dose. 10 mg.

Rocuronium

Neuromuscular Blocker/ Muscle Relaxant

1-[(2β,3α,5α,16β,17β)-17-(Acetyloxy)-3-hydroxy-2-(4-morpholinyl)-androstan-16-yl]-1-(2-propenyl)pyrrolidinium
$[C_{32}H_{53}N_2O_4]^+$ = 529.8
CAS—143558-00-3

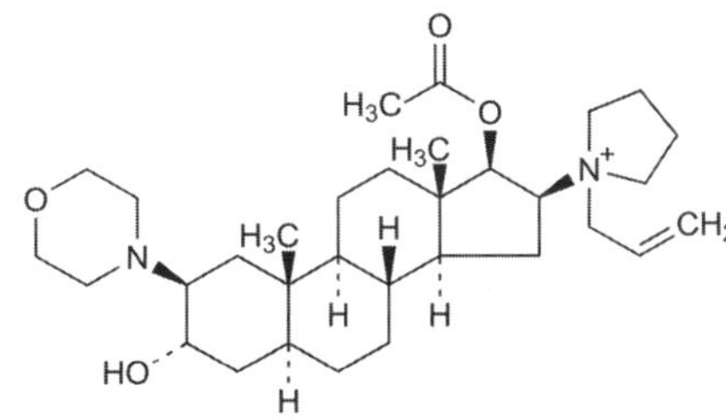

Rocuronium Bromide
Synonym. Org-9426
Proprietary names. Esmeron; Zemuron.
$C_{32}H_{53}BrN_2O_4$ = 609.7
CAS—119302-91-9
Crystals. M.p. 161° to 169°.

Partition Coefficient. Log *P* (octanol/water), 0.5.

Thin-layer Chromatography. Silica gel plates (20 × 20 cm). Mobile phase: solution of 2% sodium iodide in 2-propanol. Detected with iodoplatinate reagent. Rf 31.8 [U. W. Kleef *et al.*, *J. Chromatogr.*, 1993, *621*, 65–76].

Quantification

High performance liquid chromatography. In plasma, urine, bile, stoma fluid and tissue homogenates: limit of quantification 10, 25, 100, 20 and 100 μg/L, respectively, and limit of detection 3, 4, 4 and 5 μg/L, for plasma, urine, bile and tissue respectively. Fluorescence detection (λ_{ex} = 385 nm; λ_{em} = 452 nm)—U. W. Kleef *et al.*, *J. Chromatogr.*, 1993, *621*, 65–76.

Disposition in the Body. Rocuronium has two distribution phases following intravenous administration. The initial phase has a half-life of 1 to 2 min and the slower phase a half-life of 14 to 18 min. It undergoes metabolism and the metabolite 17-desacetylrocuronium has weak neuromuscular blocking activity. Up to 30% of the dose is excreted in urine with the majority being excreted in bile.

Therapeutic concentration

9 patients with renal failure with a mean age of 51 years (range, 22 to 61 years) requiring regular haemodialysis and 9 subjects with normal renal function, mean 46 years old (range, 27 to 64 years), undergoing elective dental or ophthalmic surgery were involved in this study. After anaesthesia was induced with nitrous oxide, fentanyl and isoflurane, a 0.6 mg/kg single bolus dose of rocuronium was administered. The plasma concentration during clinical relaxation was 1.229 (range, 0.843 to 1.657) mg/L for those with renal failure and 0.891 (0.430 to 1.560) mg/L for those with normal renal function. The duration of clinical relaxation was 55 min for the patients with renal failure and 42 min for those without [R. A. Cooper *et al.*, *Br. J. Anaesth.*, 1993, *71*, 222–226].

Half-life. 1.4 to 1.6 h may be increased by hepatic impairment.

Volume of distribution. Steady state, 0.28 L/kg (0.6 mg/kg dose); 0.27 L (1.0 mg/kg dose).

Clearance. 0.17 L/kg/h (0.6 mg/kg dose); 0.24 L/kg/h (1.0 mg/kg dose); 0.32 L/kg/h (individuals with hepatic dysfunction after a 0.6 mg/kg dose).

Protein binding. 30%.

Dose. Intravenous injection: 600 μg/kg with a maintenance dose of 150 μg/kg. IV infusion: 300 to 600 μg/kg/h.

Rofecoxib

Anti-inflammatory/Cyclo-oxygenase inhibitor

Synonym. MK-0966
Proprietary name. Vioxx
4-[4-(Methylsulfonyl)phenyl]-3-phenyl-2(5*H*)-furanone
$C_{17}H_{14}O_4S$ = 314.4
CAS—162011-90-7

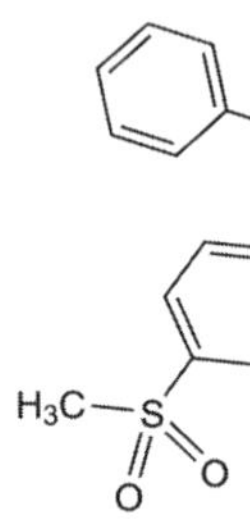

White to off-white yellow powder. Insoluble in water, sparingly soluble in acetone, slightly soluble in methanol and isopropyl acetate, very slightly soluble in ethanol and practically insoluble in octanol.

Gas Chromatography. System GB—RI 3119.

High Performance Liquid Chromatography. Column: C_{18} (100 x 4.6 mm i.d., 5 μm). Mobile phase: water:acetonitrile:acetic acid: triethylamine (770:230:1:0.3), flow rate 1 mL/min. Internal standard: ketoprofen. UV detection (λ=272 nm). Retention time(s): rofecoxib 13 min, I.S. 24 min (F. Jamali and S. Sattari, *J. Pharm. Pharm. Sci.*, 2000, *3*, 312–317).

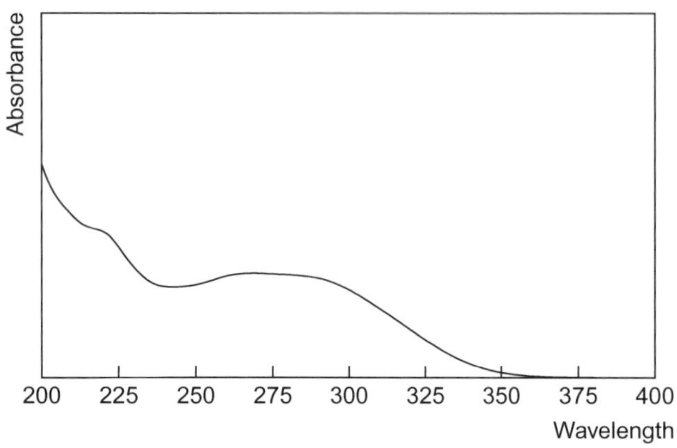

Quantification

High performance liquid chromatography. In plasma: limit of quantification 0.5 μg/L. Fluorescence detection—E. Woolf *et al.*, *J. Chromatogr. B Biomed. Sci. Appl.*, 1999, *730*, 221–227. In plasma: limit of quantification 10 μg/L, UV detection (λ=272 nm)—F. Jamali and S. Sattari, *J. Pharm. Pharm. Sci.*, 2000, *3*, 312–317. In serum: limit of quantification 20 μg/L—M. K. Aravind *et al.*, *J. Chromatogr. Sci.*, 2002, *40*, 26–28.

High performance liquid chromatography–mass spectrometry. In plasma: limit of quantification 0.1 μg/L. MS–MS detection—C. M. Chavez-Eng *et al.*, *J. Chromatogr. B Biomed. Sci. Appl.*, 2002, *767*, 117–129.

Disposition in the Body. Rofecoxib is well absorbed from the gastro-intestinal tract after oral administration. Peak plasma concentration are reached in approximately 2 h. It is extensively metabolised in the liver, mainly by reduction to *cis*- and *trans*-dihydrorofecoxib, accounting for 56% of a dose recovered in urine and an additional 8.8% as the 5-hydroxy glucuronide metabolite. None of the metabolites demonstrates measurable activity as cyclo-oxygenase inhibitors. Excretion is mainly via the urine (72%) with only 14% of a dose appearing in the faeces.

Bioavailability. Approximately 93%.

Half-life. Steady state, 17 h.

Volume of distribution. Approximately 91 to 100 L (1.55 L/kg).

Clearance. About 120 mL/min.

Protein binding. About 85%.

Toxicity. Administration of single doses of up to 1000 mg rofecoxib have not resulted in significant toxicity.

Dose. In osteoarthritis, 12.5 mg once daily to a maximum of 25 mg. Patients with mild hepatic impairment should not exceed 12.5 mg daily. An initial dose of 50 mg once daily is permitted for the short-term treatment of acute symptomatic pain.

Rolitetracycline

Antibacterial

Synonyms. PMT; Pyrrolidinomethyltetracycline.
Proprietary names. Reverin; Syntetrin; Tetraverin; Transcycline.
[4*S*-(4α,4aα,5aα,6β,12aα)]-4-(Dimethylamino)-1,4,4a,5,5a,6,11,12a-octa-hydro-3,6,10,12,12a-pentahydroxy-6-methyl-1,11-dioxo-*N*-(1-pyrro-lidinylmethyl)-2-naphthacenecarboxamide
$C_{27}H_{33}N_3O_8$=527.6
CAS—751-97-3

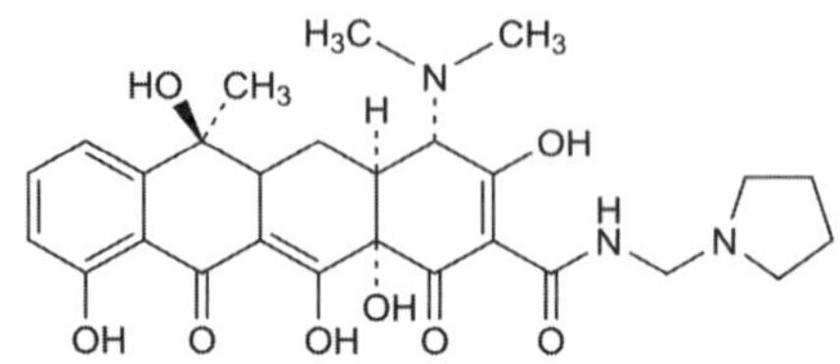

A light yellow crystalline powder. M.p. 162° to 165°, with decomposition. Soluble 1 in 1.1 of water and 1 in 200 of ethanol; soluble in acetone; very slightly soluble in ether; soluble in dilute acids and alkalis.

Rolitetracycline Nitrate

$C_{27}H_{33}N_3O_8$,HNO_3,1½H_2O=617.6
CAS—20685-78-3 (anhydrous); 26657-13-6 (sesquihydrate)
A yellow crystalline powder.
Soluble 1 in 40 of water.

Dissociation Constant. pK_a 7.4.

Partition Coefficient. Log *P* (octanol/water), −0.7.

Colour Tests. Benedict's reagent—red; Formaldehyde–Sulfuric acid—green-yellow (→yellow-brown); Mandelin's test—violet→red→orange; Marquis test—orange; Sulfuric acid—violet.

Thin-layer Chromatography. System TA—Rf 05, streaking; system TAE—Rf 00. (Location under ultraviolet light, orange fluorescence; acidified potassium permanganate solution, positive.)

Ultraviolet Spectrum. Aqueous acid—272 nm (A^1_1=325a), 357 nm; aqueous alkali—248 nm (A^1_1=261b), 268 nm (A^1_1=266b).

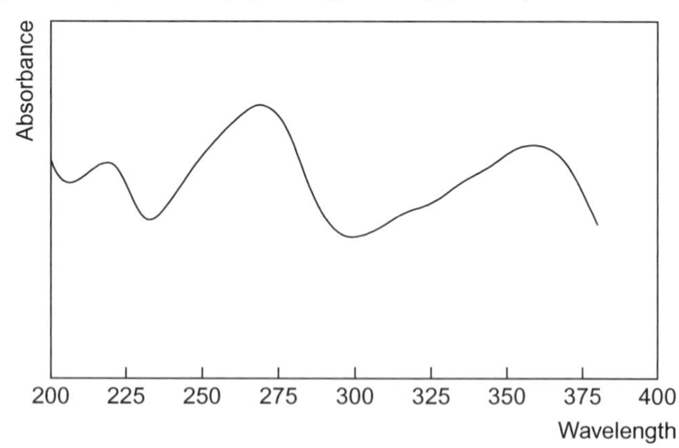

Dose. Up to 700 mg daily, given parenterally.

Ropinirole

Dopamine D_2-agonist/ Antiparkinsonian

Synonym. SKF-101468
4-[2-(Dipropylamino)ethyl]-1,3-dihydro-2*H*-indol-2-one
$C_{16}H_{24}N_2O$=260.4
CAS—91374-21-9

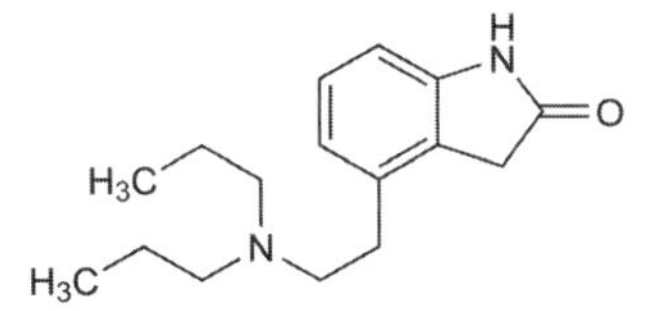

Ropinirole Hydrochloride
Synonym. SKF-101468A
Proprietary name. Requip
$C_{16}H_{25}ClN_2O$=296.8
CAS—91374-20-8
A white to greenish-yellow crystalline powder with m.p. 243° to 250°. It is soluble in water (133 g/L).

Partition Coefficient. Log *P* (octanol/water), 2.70.

High Performance Liquid Chromatography. Column: LC-ABZ (Supelcosil, 150 × 4.6 mm i.d., 5 μm). Column temperature: 40°. Mobile phase: (A)-acetonitrile; (B)-ammonium acetate (0.1 M, pH 4). Elution program: (A:B) (0:100) to (15:85) in 10 min to (100:0) in 12 min, held 15 min, flow rate 1 mL/min. UV detection (λ=250 nm). Retention time: 15 min [J. C. Bloomer *et al.*, *Drug Metab. Dispos.*, 1997, *25*, 840–844].

Column: RP C_{18} (Ultrasphere, 250 × 4.6 mm i.d., 5 μm). Mobile phase: acetonitrile:ammonium formate buffer (0.07 M, pH 3.8, containing 0.3% EDTA and 0.005% sodium octyl sulfate) (25:75), flow rate 1 mL/min. UV detection (λ=250 nm). RT: 9.4 min [J. Swagzdis and B. Mico, *J. Pharm. Sci.*, 1986, *75(1)*, 90–91].

Ultraviolet Spectrum. Aqueous acid—205, 248 nm.

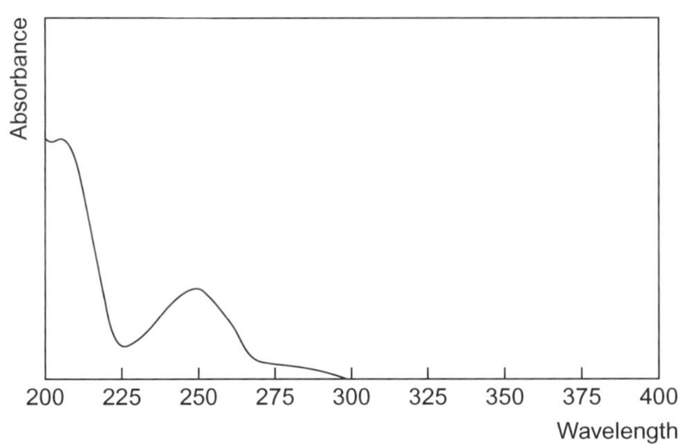

Mass Spectrum. Principal ions at *m/z* 114, 115, 160, 72, 43, 86, 229, 42.

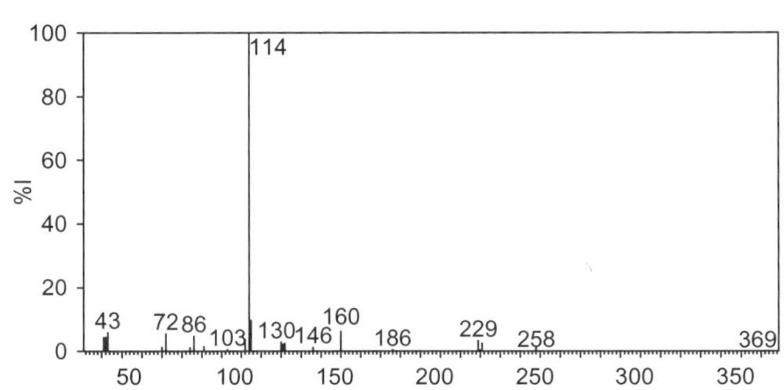

Quantification
High performance liquid chromatography. In plasma: limit of detection 5 μg/L, limit of quantification 10 μg/L. UV detection (λ=250 nm)—J. Swagzdis and B. Mico, *J. Pharm. Sci.*, 1986, *75*, 90–91.

Disposition in the Body. Ropinirole is rapidly and completely absorbed from the gastro-intestinal tract after oral administration and is widely distributed throughout the body. The rate, but not the extent, of absorption may be reduced if taken with food. Extensive metabolism in the liver occurs primarily by oxidative metabolism via cytochrome P450 isoenzyme CYP1A2 and excreted in urine as metabolites. The major metabolic pathways are *N*-despropylation and hydroxylation to form the inactive *N*-despropyl and hydroxy metabolites. *N*-despropyl ropinirole is the predominant metabolite in urine (40%) followed by the carboxylic acid metabolite (10%) and the glucuronide of the hydroxy metabolite (10%). 88% of dose is recovered in urine with less than 10% as the unchanged drug. There is wide inter-individual variability with its pharmacokinetics. Steady state is achieved within 2 days. The drug displays linear pharmacokinetics over dosing range 1 to 8 mg twice daily. Accumulation from multiple dosing is predictive from single dosing.

Therapeutic concentration
Mean maximum plasma concentrations of 1.16 μg/L after a 1 mg dose and 5.11 μg/L after 5 mg have been observed. These concentrations are reached within 1.5 h after oral administration [B. Boothman and E. Spokes, *Lancet*, 1990, *336*, 814].

Toxicity
10 patients ingested more than 24 mg daily and there were no significant effects. The largest overdose in pre-marketing clinical trials was 435 mg taken over a 7 day period (62.1 mg daily) [SmithKline Beecham Information].

Bioavailability. Absolute approximately, 50 to 55%. Relative bioavailability from tablet to an oral solution is 85%.

Half-life. 6 h.

Volume of distribution. 7.5 to 8 L/kg.

Clearance. 47 L/h.

Distribution in blood. Blood:plasma ratio is 1:1.

Protein binding. 10 to 40%.

Dose. 3 to 9 mg daily.

Ropivacaine

Local Anaesthetic

Synonyms. AL-281; LEA-103.
(2*S*)-*N*-(2,6-Dimethylphenyl)-1-propyl-2-piperidinecarboxamide
$C_{17}H_{26}NO_2$=274.4
CAS—84057-95-4

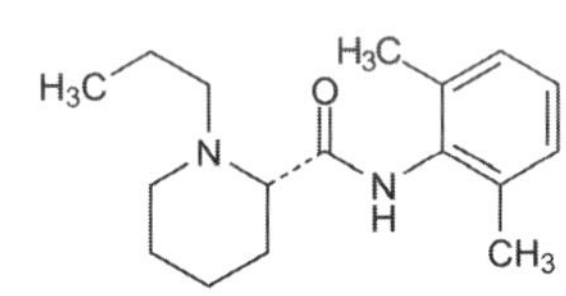

A white crystalline powder with m.p. 144° to 146°.

Ropivacaine Hydrocloride
$C_{17}H_{26}N_2O$, HCl=310.9
CAS—98717-15-8
Crystals with m.p. 260° to 262°.

Ropivacaine Hydrocloride Monohydrate
Proprietary name. Naropin
$C_{17}H_{26}N_2O$, HCl, H_2O=328.9
CAS— 132112-35-7
A white crystalline powder with m.p. 269.5° to 270.6°. It is soluble in water (53.8 g/L).

Dissociation Constant. pK_a 8.16.

Partition Coefficient. Log *P* (octanol/buffer), 2.9.

Gas Chromatography. Column: fused silica (12 m × 0.2 mm i.d., film thickness 0.33 μm). Column temperature: 150° to 230° at 40°/min. Carrier gas: helium. MS detection: (PICI, SIM at *m/z* 275). Retention time: 4.02 min [B. Emanuelsson *et al.*, *Eur. J. Pharm. Sci.*, 1997, *5*, 171–177].

High Performance Liquid Chromatography. Column: Lichrospher RP-SelectB-C_8 (125 × 4.0 mm i.d., 5 μm). Column temperature: 30°. Mobile phase: acetonitrile:potassium dihydrogen phosphate (pH 2.1, 0.01 M) (20:80), flow rate 1 mL/min. Internal standard (IS): mepivacaine. UV detection (λ=205 nm). *k* value: ropivacaine, 11.3; IS, 15.9 [S. Reif *et al.*, *J. Chromatogr. B Biomed. Sci. Appl.*, 1998, *719*, 239–244].

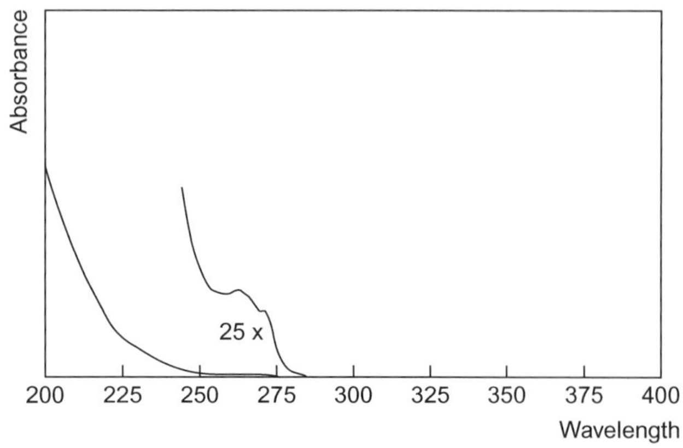

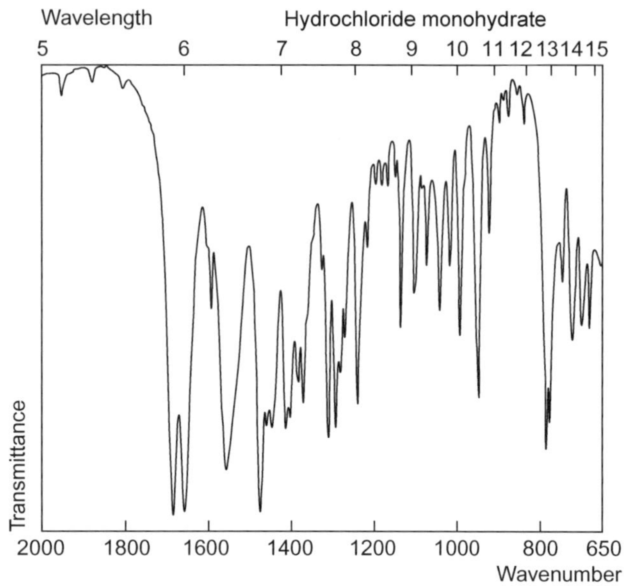

Mass Spectrum. Principal ions at *m/z* 126, 127, 84, 56.

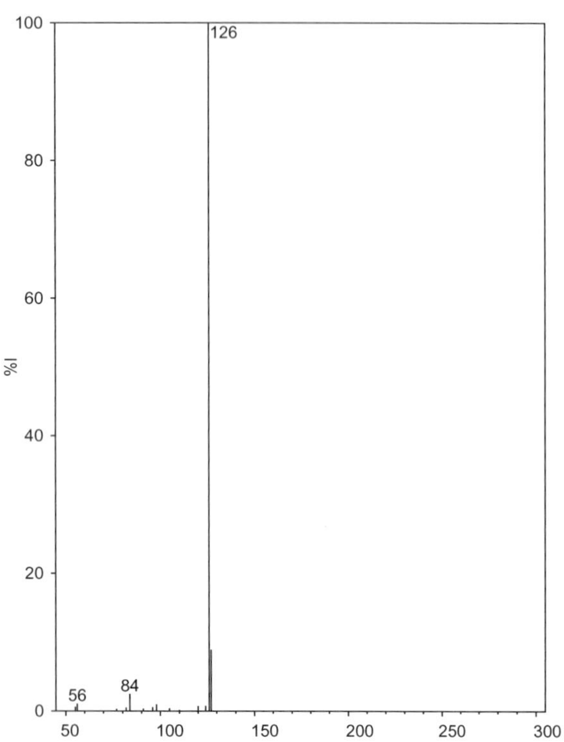

Quantification

Gas chromatography–mass spectrometry. In plasma: limit of quantification is 3 μg/L—B. Emanuelsson *et al.*, *Eur. J. Pharm. Sci.*, 1997, *5*, 171–177. In plasma: limit of detection 10 g/L—C-J. Erichsen *et al.*, *Anaesthesiology*, 1996, *84*, 834.

High performance liquid chromatography. In plasma: limit of detection 0.9 μg/L. UV detection (λ=205 m)—S. Reif *et al.*, *J. Chromatogr. B Biomed. Sci. Appl.*, 1998, *719*, 239–244.

Disposition in the Body. Ropivacaine is readily absorbed and extensively metabolised in the liver, predominately by aromatic hydroxylation, which is mediated by cytochrome P450 isoenzyme CYP1A. The metabolites are mainly excreted in urine with 86% of the dose excreted after intravenous administration. 1% of the dose is excreted as the unchanged drug. The major metabolites are 3-hydroxyropivacaine, 37% of which is excreted in urine mainly in the conjugated form, and 4-hydroxyropivacaine, the *N*-dealkylated metabolite and 4-hydroxy-dealkylated metabolite. The drug displays linear pharmacokinetics and has a long duration of action and has been shown to cross the placenta.

Therapeutic concentration. Plasma concentrations are dependent on the dose, route of administration and the vascularity of injection site. The mean maximum tolerated and free arterial plasma concentration is 4.3 and 0.6 mg/L.

An 80 mg intravenous dose resulted in a mean peak plasma concentration of 1.9 ±0.3 mg/L, and an infusion of 50 mg over a 15 min period produced mean plasma concentrations of 1.5 mg/L [Markham and Faulds, *Drugs*, 1996, *52(3)*, 429–449].

Toxicity. Ropivacaine is associated with central nervous system toxicity in particular symptoms resembling those caused by seizure activity in the temporal lobe (psychomotor epilepsy). Including spasms of facial muscles, behavioural manifestations and motor movements. Accidental intravenous injection results in immediate toxic effects. Acute systemic toxicity. The toxic plasma concentration is >4 mg/L.

A 45-year-old woman with rheumatoid arthritis was treated with ropivacaine for regional anaesthesia prior to surgery on her right wrist. A total of 40 mL ropivacaine (7.5 g/L) was slowly injected in doses of 5 mL 1 to 2 min apart (the total dose was 6 mg/kg). 3 min after the injection had been completed, the patient experienced oral numbness and twitching in her throat. Her speech became irrational, her arterial blood pressure increased, she experienced sinus tachycardia and her heart beat increased. She finally lost consciousness but regained after subsequent treatment. The total plasma concentration of ropivacaine was 6.0 mg/L 40 min after injection; 5.4 mg/L after 60 min; 4.6 mg/L after 80 min and 4.0 mg/L after 98 min.

6 weeks later, a second attempt at the surgery was planned. A total dose of 30 mL ropivacaine (7.5 g/L) was administered, total dose 4.5 mg/kg followed by 10 mL lidocaine–adrenaline (20 g/L). Her heart rate increased over the first 10 min and after 25 min, she experienced a strange feeling in her tongue and speech disorders due to loss of muscle control relating to the central nervous system. She did not respond when spoken to and experienced involuntary spasms around the head and neck. The total plasma concentrations of ropivacaine were 4.0 mg/L 25 min after injection; 2.5 mg/L after 37 min and 2.0 mg/L after 56 min [T. I. Ala-Kokko *et al.*, *Acta Anaesthesiol. Scand.*, 2000, *44*, 623–626].

A 13-year-old male patient with chronic pain due to bladder spasm was given an epidural IV infusion of ropivacaine hydrochloride (2 mL at a concentration of 10 mg/mL) over 15 s. Facial numbness was experienced immediately and within 1 min, classical grand mal seizure. Convulsions lasted for 2 min and he returned to a normal state of consciousness within the next 15 min. The blood ropivacaine concentration, 30 to 40 min after the convulsion, was 1.4 mg/L and at the time of the seizure this would have been considerably higher, possibly a concentration of 6 to 30 mg/L [A. N. Plowman *et al.*, *Anaesth. Intensive Care*, 1998, *26*, 204–206].

Half-life. 1.8 h.

Volume of distribution. Steady state, 41 to 59 L.

Clearance. Total plasma clearance, 387 ±107 mL/min; unbound plasma clearance, 7.2 ±1.6 L/min.

Protein binding. 94% (α_1-acid glycoprotein).

Dose. Maximum single dose is 200 mg.

Rotenone

Pesticide

[2*R*-(2α,6*a*α,12*a*α)]-1,2,12,12a-Tetrahydro-8,9-dimethoxy-2-(1-methylethenyl)[1]benzopyrano[3,4-*b*]furo[2,3-*h*][1]benzopyran-6(6a*H*)-one
$C_{23}H_{22}O_6$=394.4
CAS—83-79-4

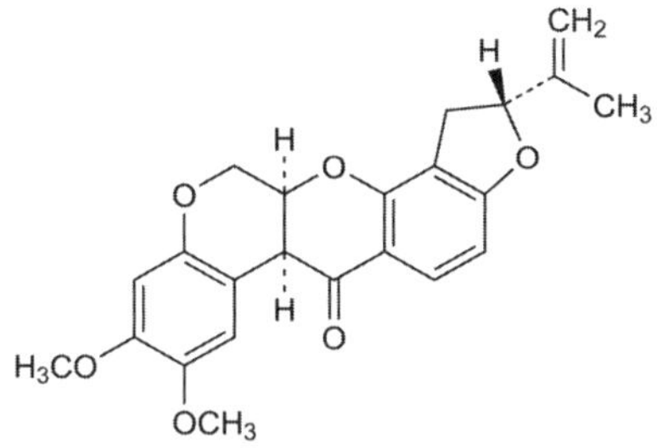

Rotenone is the principal active insecticidal constituent of derris, the dried rhizome and roots of *Derris elliptica*, *D. malaccensis* (Leguminosae) and other species of *Derris* (also known as tuba root or akertuba), and of lonchocarpus, the dried root of *Lonchocarpus utilis*, *L. urucu* and other species of *Lonchocarpus* (Leguminosae).
Colourless to brownish crystals, or a white to brownish-white crystalline powder; it decomposes on exposure to light and air. M.p. 165° to 166°. A dimorphic form melts at 185° to 186°.
Practically insoluble in water; soluble 1 in 300 of ethanol, 1 in 12 of acetone, 1 in 3 of chloroform and 1 in 200 of ether.
Caution. Inhalation may cause severe pulmonary irritation. Symptoms of overexposure are irritation of eyes, skin and respiratory system, numbness of mucous membranes, nausea, vomiting, abdominal pain, muscle tremors, incontinence, clonic convulsions and stupor.

Partition Coefficient. Log *P* (octanol/water), 4.1.

Colour Tests. Antimony Pentachloride—brown; Liebermann's Test—black; Sulfuric Acid—orange.

Gas Chromatography. System GA—RI 3195.

Ultraviolet Spectrum. Aqueous acid—235 nm (A^1_1=480b), 292 nm (A^1_1=550b).

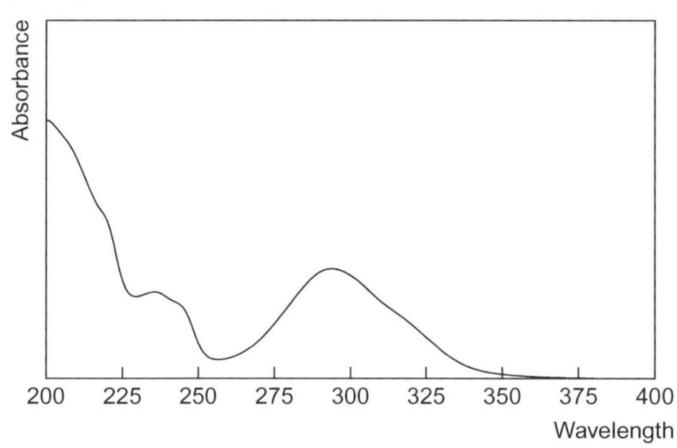

Roxithromycin

Antibacterial

Synonyms. Roxithromycinum; RU-965; RU-28965.
Proprietary names. Assoral; Biaxin; Biaxsig; Cirumyan; Claramid; Forilin; Macrosil; Overal; Rossitrol; Rotesan; Rotramin; Rulid; Surlid.
Erythromycin 9-[*O*-[(2-methoxyethoxy)methyl]oxime]
$C_{41}H_{76}N_2O_{15}$=837.0
CAS—80214-83-1

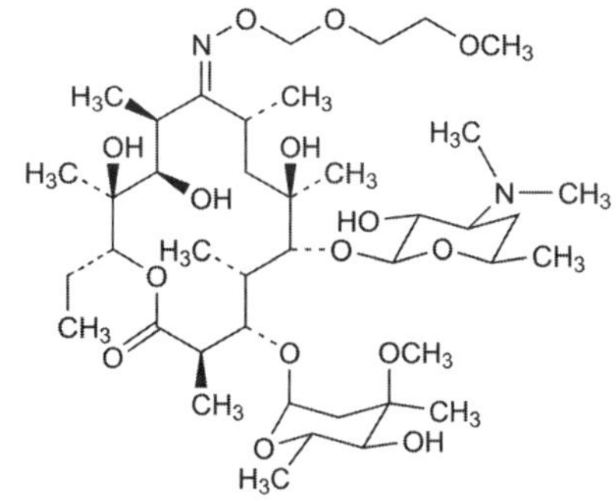

A white crystalline powder which exhibits polymorphism. It is very slightly soluble in water; freely soluble in alcohol, acetone and dichloromethane; slightly soluble in dilute hydrochloric acid.

Partition Coefficient. Log *P* (octanol/water), 2.75.

High Performance Liquid Chromatography. System HAA—Retention time 15.8 min; system HBA—Retention time 17.1 min; system HBB—Retention time 16.3 min.

Column: (analytical) C_{18} (Nucleosil 100-3, 150 × 4.6 mm i.d., 3 µm); (guard) C_{18} (Nucleosil 120-5, 10 × 4.0 mm i.d., 5 µm). Column temperature: 60°. Mobile phase: methanol:potassium dihydrogen phosphate buffer (15 mM, pH 6.0 with potassium hydroxide) (70:30), flow rate 1.2 mL/min. Internal standard (IS): clarithromycin. UV detection (λ=220 nm). Retention times: roxithromycin, 8.5 min; IS, 10.2 min. [J. Macek *et al.*, *J. Chromatogr. B Biomed. Sci. Appl.*, 1999, *723*, 233–238].

Column: ODS (Kromasil, 200 × 4.6 mm i.d., 5 µm). Mobile phase: acetonitrile:methanol:aqueous buffer (3 mM EDTA and 60 mM sodium dihydrogen phosphate, pH 7.0 with sodium hydroxide) (39:11:49), flow rate 1.0 mL/min. Electrochemical detection. Retention times: roxithromycin, 31.5 min; descladinosine derivative, 13.4 min; erythromycin-oxime, 14.5 min; *N*-demethylated derivative, 19.8 min; *O*-demethylated derivative, 14.1 min; *N,O*-di-demethylated derivative, 10.2 min; *N*-mono-demethylated derivative of the erythromycin-oxime metabolite, 10.7 min; *N*-di-demethylated derivative of the erythromycin-oxime metabolite, 9.96 min [D. Zhong *et al.*, *Drug Metab. Dispos.*, 2000, *28(5)*, 552–559].

Quantification

High performance liquid chromatography. In plasma: limit of quantification 0.5 mg/L. UV detection (λ=220 nm)—J. Macek *et al.*, *J. Chromatogr. B Biomed. Sci. Appl.*, 1999, *723(1–2)*, 233–238. In plasma: limit of quantification 0.1 mg/L—C. Taninaka *et al.*, *J. Chromatogr. B. Biomed. Sci. Appl.*, 2000, *738*, 405–411. In bile, urine and plasma: limit of detection 0.01 mg/L. Electrochemical detection—D. Zhong *et al.*, *Drug Metab. Dispos.*, 2000, *28(5)*, 552–559.

Disposition in the Body. Roxithromycin is well absorbed but this is reduced when taken with food. It is widely distributed in tissue and body fluids. A small amount is metabolised in the liver by isomerisation, *O*-demethylation, *N*-demethylation, hydrolysis and dealkylation. Secondary metabolism may also occur involving these pathways. Metabolites include a descladinosine derivative of the drug, an erythromycin-oxime, *N*-, *O*-, and *N,O*-di-demethylated derivatives of the drug and *N*-mono- and *N*-di-demethylated derivatives of the erythromycin-oxime metabolite. The majority of the dose is excreted in faeces as the unchanged drug and as its metabolites. Approximately 7 to 12% is excreted in urine and 15% via the lungs. It crosses the placenta and is distributed in breast milk. Steady state is achieved by day 4.

Therapeutic concentration

18 paediatric patients suffering from a respiratory tract infection were administered with a 2.5 mg/kg oral dose of roxithromycin. The patients were divided into three groups; group 1: patients aged < 18 months; 2: aged < 5 years; 3: aged < 13 years. The maximum plasma concentration on day 6 was observed at 1 to 2 h post-administration and was measured at 10.1, 8.7 and 8.8 mg/L, respectively, for the three groups [F. M. Demotes-Mainard *et al.*, *J. Clin. Pharmacol.*, 1989, *29(8)*, 752–756].

12 healthy men with a mean age of 20.8 years (range, 18 to 28 years) were administered with 150 mg roxithromycin after an overnight fast and continued fasting for 4 h post-dosing. 150 mg 12-hourly was also administered in a multiple dosing study for 5 days. The peak plasma concentration after the single dose was 5.69 (1.59 to 9.57) mg/L observed at 2.19 (0.5 to 8.0) h. The peak concentration for the multiple dosing was 6.76

(2.32 to 9.35) mg/L at 2.4 (0.5 to 6.17) h [D. J. Birket *et al.*, *Ther. Drug Monit.*, 1990, *12(1)*, 65–71].

Bioavailability. 50%.

Half-life. 8 to 13 h (prolonged in patients with hepatic and renal impairment); 20 to 21 h in children aged < 18 months to 13 years.

Protein binding. 96% (mainly α_1-acid glycoprotein). Binding is saturable and only 86% is bound at peak concentrations.

Note. For a review of roxithromycin antibacterial activity, pharmacokinetic properties and clinical efficacy, see R. A. Young *et al.*, *Drugs*, 1989, *37*, 8–41.

Dose. 150 mg twice daily.

Saccharin

Sweetener

Synonyms. Benzoic Acid Sulphimide; Benzoic Sulfimide; Benzosulphimide; Garantose; Gluside; Sacarina; Saccarina; Zaharina.
1,2-Benzisothiazol-3(2*H*)-one 1,1-dioxide
$C_7H_5NO_3S$ = 183.2
CAS—81-07-2

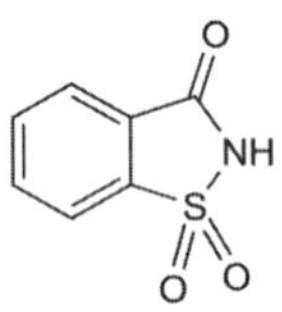

White crystals or crystalline powder. M.p. 228° to 230°.
Soluble 1 in 290 of water, 1 in 31 of ethanol and 1 in 12 of acetone; slightly soluble in chloroform and ether; readily soluble in dilute ammonia solution and in solutions of alkali hydroxides and, with the evolution of carbon dioxide, in solutions of alkali bicarbonates and carbonates.

Saccharin Calcium

Synonym. Calcium Benzosulphimide
$C_{14}H_8CaN_2O_6S_2,3\frac{1}{2}H_2O$ = 467.5
CAS—6485-34-3 (anhydrous); 6381-91-5 (hydrate)
White crystals or crystalline powder.
Soluble 1 in about 2.5 of water and 1 in about 5 of ethanol.

Saccharin Sodium

Synonyms. Saccharoidum Natricum; Sodium Benzosulphimide; Soluble Gluside; Soluble Saccharin.
$C_7H_4NNaO_3S,2H_2O$ = 241.2
CAS—128-44-9 (anhydrous); 6155-57-3 (dihydrate)
White efflorescent crystals or a white crystalline powder.
Soluble 1 in 1.5 of water and 1 in 50 of ethanol; practically insoluble in chloroform and ether.

Dissociation Constant. pK_a 1.6 (20°); 1.3 (25°).

Partition Coefficient. Log *P* (octanol/water), 0.9.

Colour Tests. Koppanyi–Zwikker test—violet; Mercurous nitrate—black.

Thin-layer Chromatography. System TD—Rf 01; system TE—Rf 07; system TF—Rf 01; system TAD—Rf 04; system TAE—Rf 87; system TAJ—Rf 00; system TAK—Rf 19; system TAL—Rf 25.

Gas Chromatography. System GA—RI 1819.

High Performance Liquid Chromatography. System HX—RI 291; system HY—RI 234; system HAA—Retention time(s) 5.9 min.

Ultraviolet Spectrum. Aqueous alkali—235 nm (A^1_1=351b), 268 nm (A^1_1=82a).

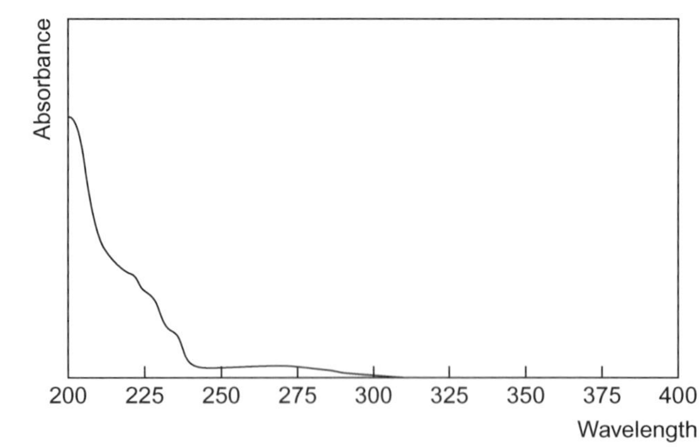

Infra-red Spectrum. Principal peaks at wavenumbers 1260, 1154, 1646, 750, 678, 1120 cm^{-1} (saccharin sodium, KBr disk).

Mass Spectrum. Principal ions at *m/z* 183, 76, 90, 50, 91, 120, 106, 92.

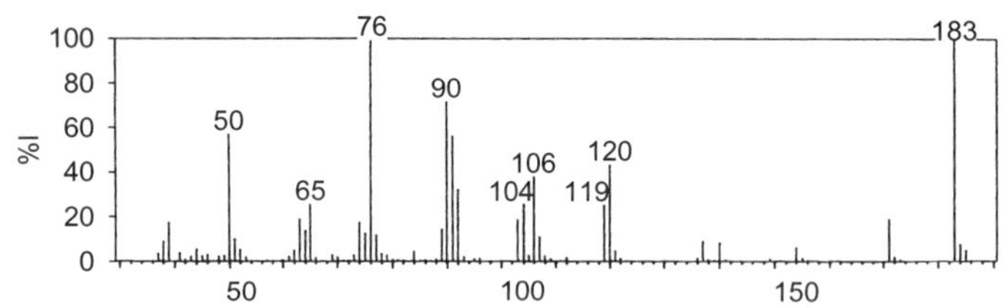

Quantification

Gas chromatography. In urine: limit of detection 10 µg/L, ECD—P. Hartvig *et al.*, *J. Chromatogr.*, 1978, *151*, 232–236.

Gas chromatography–mass spectrometry. In plasma or urine: limit of detection 50 µg/L—C. Pantarotto *et al.*, *J. Pharm. Sci.*, 1981, *70*, 871–874.

High performance liquid chromatography. In urine: saccharin sodium, limit of detection 10 ppm, UV detection—C. L. Holder and M. C. Bowman, *Toxicol. Lett.*, 1980, *5*, 27–38.

Disposition in the Body. Saccharin is rapidly absorbed after oral administration; peak plasma concentrations are attained in 0.5 to 1 h. About 60% of a dose is excreted in the urine unchanged in 6 h and 80% in 24 h.

Half-life. Plasma half-life, about 5 to 9 h in regular saccharin users.

Salbutamol

Sympathomimetic/Bronchodilator

Synonyms. Albuterol; AH-3365; Salbutamolum; Sch-13949W.
Proprietary names Accuneb; Aerolin; Airet; Airomir; Asmasal; Asmaven; Buventol; Kentamol; Libetist; Maxivent; Proventil; Rimasal; Salamol; Salapin; Salbulin; Ventmax; Ventodisks; Ventolin(e); Volmax. It is an ingredient of Aerocrom, Combivent, DuoNeb, and Ventide. (Includes proprietary names of Salbutamol and Salbutamol Sulfate.)
α^1-[[(1,1-Dimethylethyl)amino]methyl]-4-hydroxy-1,3-benzenedimethanol
$C_{13}H_{21}NO_3$ = 239.3
CAS—18559-94-9

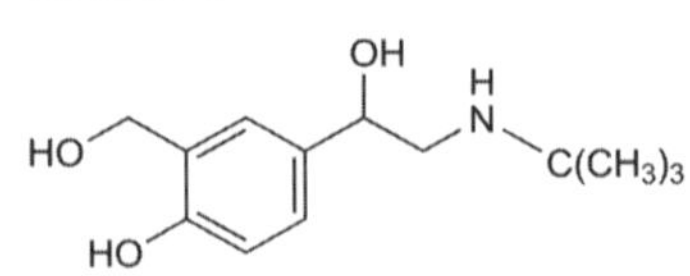

A white crystalline powder. M.p. 151° also reported as 157° to 158°.
Soluble 1 in 70 of water and 1 in 25 of ethanol; slightly soluble in ether.

Salbutamol Sulfate

Synonyms. Albuterol Sulfate; Salbutamol Hemisulfate; Salbutamol Sulphate.
$(C_{13}H_2NO_3)_2,H_2SO_4$ = 576.7

CAS—51022-70-9
A white powder.
Soluble 1 in 4 of water; slightly soluble in ethanol, chloroform, and ether.

Dissociation Constant. pK_a 9.3, 10.3.

Partition Coefficient. Log *P* (octanol/water), 0.6.

Colour Tests. Liebermann's Test—black; Mandelin's Test—blue rim→brown rim; Marquis Test—yellow; Sulfuric Acid—yellow.

Thin-layer Chromatography. System TA—Rf 46; system TB—Rf 01; system TC—Rf 01; system TE—Rf 20; system TF—Rf 00; system TL—Rf 04; system TAE—Rf 16; system TAF—Rf 74. (Acidified potassium permanganate solution, positive.)

Gas Chromatography. System GA—salbutamol-AC_2 RI 2230, salbutamol-AC_3 RI 2250, salbutamol-H_2O RI 1850.

High Performance Liquid Chromatography. System HA—*k* 1.0; system HX—RI 220; system HY—RI 238.

Ultraviolet Spectrum. Aqueous acid—276 (A^1_1=71a); aqueous alkali—245 (A^1_1=510a), 295 nm (A^1_1=133a).

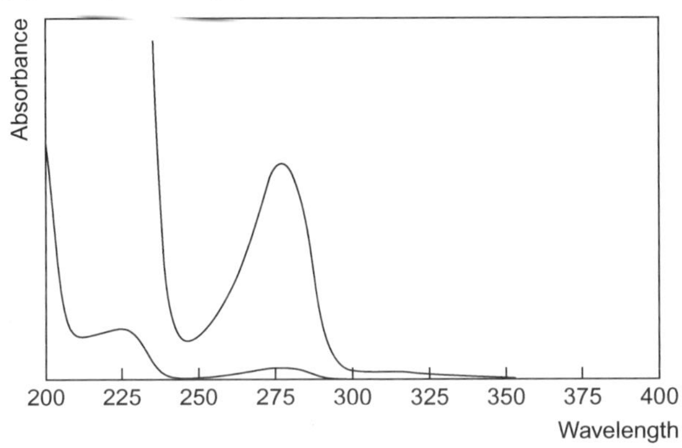

Infra-red Spectrum. Principal peaks at wavenumbers 1075, 1038, 1263, 1228, 1213, 822 cm^{-1} (KBr disk).

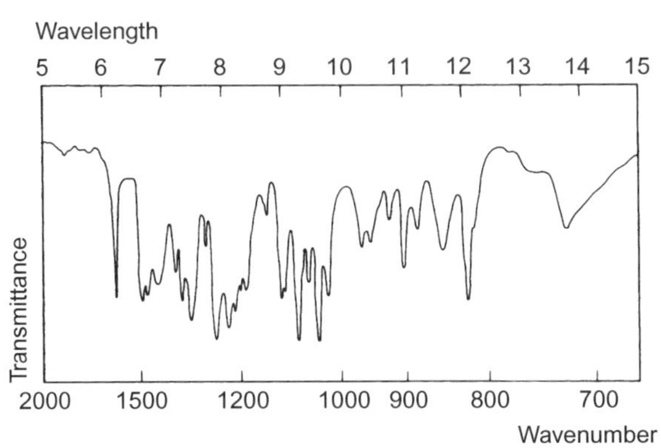

Mass Spectrum. Principal ions at *m/z* 30, 86, 57, 41, 77, 135, 29, 206.

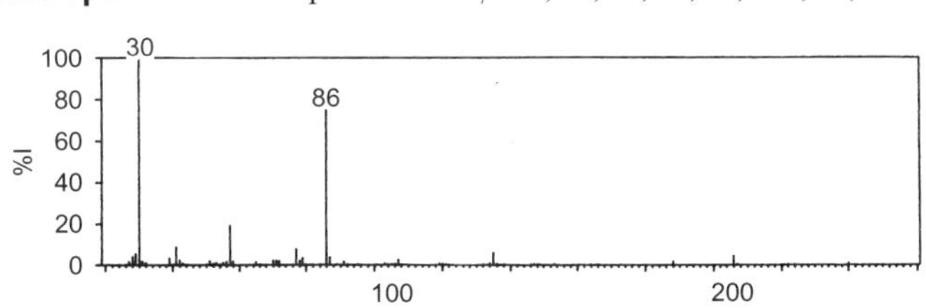

Quantification

Gas chromatography-mass spectrometry. In serum: limit of detection 1 µg/L—J. G. Leferink *et al., J. Chromatogr.*, 1982, *229*; *B Biomed. Appl.*, *18*, 217–221. In postmortem blood: salbutamol and other *β*-agonists, limit of quantification 1 µg/L—F. J. Couper and O. H. Drummer, *J. Chromatogr. B Biomed. Appl.*, 1996, *685*, 265–272. In plasma: limit of quantification 50 ng/L—T. W. Logsdon *et al., J. Chromatogr. B Biomed. Sci. Appl.*, 1997, *692*, 472–477. In postmortem blood or urine: salbutamol and other *β*-agonists, SIM—S. B. Black and R. C. Hansson, *J. Anal. Toxicol.*, 1999, *23*, 113–118. In serum: limit of detection 2 µg/L—M. I. Saleh *et al., Analyst*, 2000, *125*, 1569–1572.

High performance liquid chromatography. In plasma: limit of detection 500 ng/L, electrochemical detection—B. Oosterhuis and C. J. van Boxtel, *J. Chromatogr.*, 1982, *232*; *B Biomed. Appl.*, *21*, 327–334. In plasma: limit of detection 0.5 µg/L, amperometric detection—L. Tamisier-Karolak *et al., Ther. Drug Monit.*, 1992, *14*, 243–248. In serum: salbutamol enantiomers, limit of detection 1 µg/L, fluorescence detection—L. He and J. T. Stewart, *Biomed. Chromatogr.*, 1992, *6*, 291–294. In plasma: salbutamol and terbutaline, limit of detection for salbutamol 1 µg/L, fluorescence detection—P. T. McCarthy *et al., Biomed. Chromatogr.*, 1993, *7*, 25–28. In plasma: salbutamol and terbutaline, limit of detection for salbutamol 1 µg/L, electrochemical detection—K. A. Sagar *et al., Biomed. Chromatogr.*, 1993, *7*, 29–33. In plasma or urine: salbutamol enantiomers, limit of detection 250 ng/L, fluorescence detection—D. W. Boulton and J. P. Fawcett, *J. Chromatogr. B Biomed. Appl.*, 1995, *672*, 103–109. In plasma: salbutamol enantiomers, limit of detection 125 ng/L, fluorescence detection—K. M. Fried *et al., Chirality*, 1998, *10*, 484–491. In urine: salbutamol enantiomers, limit of detection 20 µg/L, electrochemical detection—K. H. Kim and T. K. Kim, *Arch. Pharm. Res.*, 1998, 21, 217–222. In urine: salbutamol enantiomers, fluorescence detection—R. Berges *et al., J. Chromatogr. B Biomed. Sci. Appl.*, 1999, *723*, 173–184.

High performance liquid chromatography–mass spectrometry. In plasma: limit of quantification 0.2 µg/L—K. Schmeer *et al., J. Chromatogr. A.*, 1997, *777*, 67–72.

Disposition in the Body. Rapidly absorbed after oral administration and after inhalation. It is not metabolised in the lung. About 10 to 20% of an inhaled dose reaches the lower airways; the remainder is retained in the delivery system or deposited on the oropharynx and swallowed. Orally administered salbutamol, or the swallowed portion of an inhaled dose, undergoes first-pass metabolism in the liver and possibly in the gut wall to the phenolic sulfate. About 60 to 90% of a dose is excreted in the urine in 24 h, of which approximately 50% is unchanged salbutamol and 50% is the 4′-*O*-sulfate of salbutamol. Up to about 12% is eliminated in the faeces.

Therapeutic concentration

Following oral or rectal administration of racemic salbutamol solution (dose 0.1 mg/kg) to 5 healthy subjects, a peak serum concentration of 0.0179 mg/L was attained in 0.67 h after rectal administration compared with a concentration of 0.017 mg/L in 1.5 h after oral administration [N. Kurosawa *et al., J. Clin. Pharm. Ther.*, 1993, *18*, 103–108].

In 11 asthmatic patients attending hospital with acute asthma who had been receiving salbutamol as part of their maintenance therapy (5 mg nebulised salbutamol), the plasma salbutamol concentration before treatment was <0.003 to 0.0346 mg/L (median <0.003); one hour after dosing, the concentration was <0.003 to 0.056 mg/L (median 0.0074) [L. D. Lewis *et al., Aust N. Z. J. Med.*, 1990, *20*, 204–207].

Toxicity. Hypokalaemia has been reported after overdosage; recovery has occurred after the ingestion of up to 240 mg.

In a study of 17 patients admitted to emergency departments who had recently ingested an overdose of salbutamol, the mean dose ingested was 89 mg, which resulted in plasma concentrations of 0.018 to 0.449 mg/L (median 0.166) [L. D. Lewis *et al., Hum. Exp. Toxicol.*, 1993, *12*, 397–401].

Bioavailability. After oral administration, about 50%.

Half-life. Plasma half-life, 4 to 6 h.

Protein binding. In plasma, about 10%.

Note. For a review of salbutamol clinical efficacy in the 1980s, see A. H. Price and S. P. Clissold, *Drugs*, 1989, *38*, 77–122. For a review of the pharmacokinetics of levosalbutamol, see D. W. Boulton and J. P. Fawcett, *Clin. Pharmacokinet.*, 2001, *40*, 23–40.

Dose. Usually the equivalent of 6 to 16 mg of salbutamol daily by mouth.

Salicylamide

Analgesic

Proprietary names. Isosal. It is an ingredient of Anabar, Lobac, Intralgin, Saleto, and Trim-Elim.
2-Hydroxybenzamide
$C_7H_7NO_2$=137.1

CAS—65-45-2

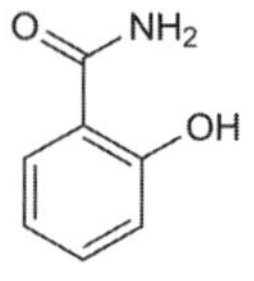

A white crystalline powder. M.p. 140°.
Soluble 1 in 500 of water, 1 in 15 of ethanol, 1 in 100 of chloroform, and 1 in 35 of ether; soluble in solutions of alkalis.

Dissociation Constant. pK_a 8.2 (37°).

Partition Coefficient. Log P (octanol/water), 1.3.

Colour Tests. Ferric Chloride—blue-violet (after hydrolysis); McNally's Test—orange; Nessler's Reagent—brown-orange (weak).

Thin-layer Chromatography. System TB—Rf 00; system TD—Rf 38; system TE—Rf 50; system TF—Rf 55; system TAD—Rf 43; system TAE—Rf 83; system TAF—Rf 84. (Location under UV light, violet fluorescence; ferric chloride solution, violet; acidified potassium permanganate solution, positive.)

Gas Chromatography. System GA—salicylamide RI 1414, salicylamide-AC RI 1660, M (OH-)-AC_2 RI 1860; system GB—RI 1489.

High Performance Liquid Chromatography. System HD—*k* 0.4; system HW—*k* 2.5; system HX—RI 327; system HY—RI 289.

Ultraviolet Spectrum. Aqueous acid—235 (A^1_1=572a), 298; aqueous alkali—241 (A^1_1=547a), 328 nm.

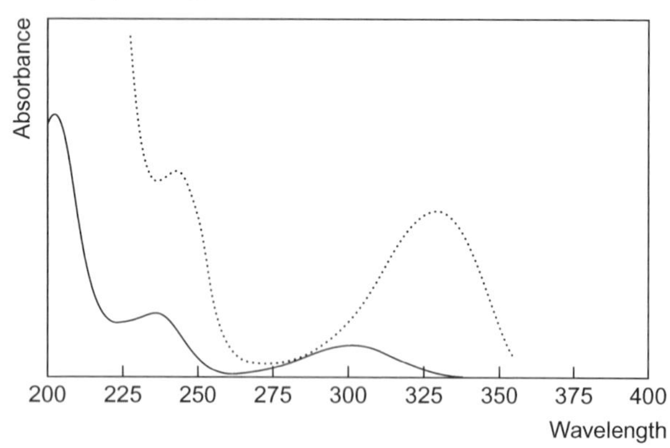

Infra-red Spectrum. Principal peaks at wavenumbers 1250, 752, 758, 1670, 1626, 1587 cm^{-1} (Nujol mull).

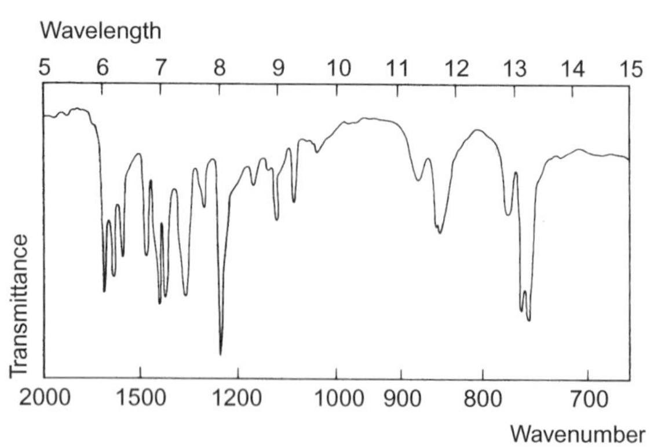

Mass Spectrum. Principal ions at *m/z* 120, 92, 137, 65, 121, 39, 64, 53.

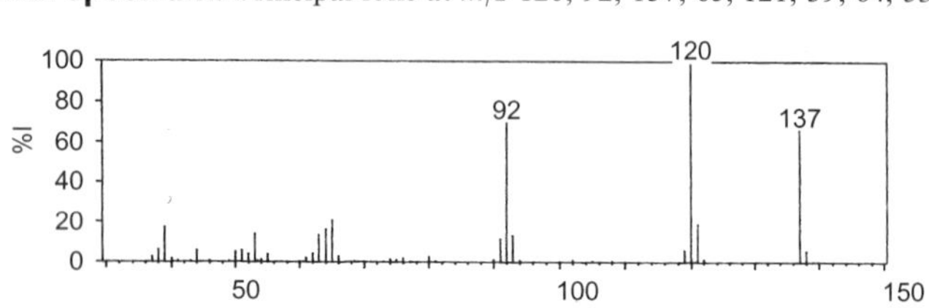

Quantification

Spectrofluorimetry. In blood, serum or urine: limit of detection 100 µg/L—S. A. Varesh *et al.*, *J. Pharm. Sci.*, 1971, *60*, 1092–1095.

Gas chromatography. In plasma, saliva or urine: limit of detection 1 mg/L in plasma and saliva, 5 mg/L in urine, AFID—A. G. de Boer *et al.*, *J. Chromatogr.*, 1979, *162*; *B Biomed. Appl.*, *4*, 457–460.

High performance liquid chromatography. In plasma: limit of detection 500 pg, fluorescence detection—S. R. Gautam *et al.*, *Anal. Lett.* (Part B), 1981, *14*, 577–582. In serum, saliva or urine: salicylamide and metabolites, limit of detection 1 to 2 mg/L, UV detection—M. E. Morris and G. Levy, *J. Pharm,. Sci.*, 1983, *72*, 612–617.

Disposition in the Body. Readily absorbed after oral administration but undergoes significant first-pass metabolism; widely distributed throughout the body. It is rapidly excreted in the urine mainly as the sulfate and glucuronide conjugates together with small amounts of gentisamide glucuronide and traces of gentisamide and gentisamide sulfate; only traces are excreted unchanged.

Therapeutic concentration

After a single oral dose of 1.3 g given to 5 subjects, mean peak plasma concentrations of about 2 mg/L of free salicylamide and about 18 mg/L of total (free + conjugated) salicylamide were attained in 0.3 and 2 h respectively; following similar doses of a solution of sodium salicylamide, peak plasma concentrations were higher and were attained more rapidly [L. Fleckenstein *et al.*, *Clin. Pharmacol. Ther.*, 1976, *19*, 451–458].

Following a single oral dose of 1.5 g of sodium salicylamide given as an aqueous solution to 5 subjects, peak plasma concentrations of 21.8 to 44.6 mg/L (mean 31) of salicylamide were attained in 5 to 10 min [A. G. de Boer *et al.*, *Biopharm. Drug Dispos.*, 1983, *4*, 321–330].

Half-life. Derived from urinary excretion data, about 1 h.

Dose. Salicylamide is given in doses of about 1 to 2.5 g daily, usually with other analgesics.

Salicylic Acid

Dermatological Agent/Analgesic

Synonyms. Acido Ortóxibenzoico; Acidum Salicylicum; Salizylsäure.
Proprietary names. It is an ingredient of many proprietary preparations—see Martindale, *The complete drug reference*, 33rd Edn, London, Pharmaceutical Press, 2002.
2-Hydroxybenzoic acid
$C_7H_6O_3$=138.1
CAS—69-72-7

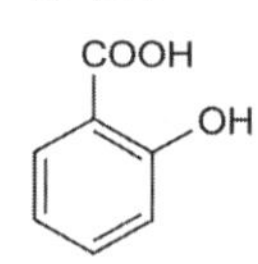

Colourless, feathery crystals or a white crystalline powder. M.p. 159°.
Soluble 1 in about 550 of water, 1 in about 4 of ethanol, 1 in 45 of chloroform, and 1 in 3 of ether.

Choline Salicylate
Synonym. (2-Hydroxyethyl)trimethylammonium Salicylate
Proprietary names. Arthropan; Audax; Teejel. It is an ingredient of Bonjela.
$C_{12}H_{19}NO_4$=241.3
CAS—2016-36-6
A white, crystalline, very hygroscopic powder. M.p. 49.5° to 50.0°.
Very freely soluble in water; soluble in ethanol and acetone; practically insoluble in ether, petroleum ether, benzene, and oils.

Sodium Salicylate
Synonym. Sodium 2-Hydroxybenzoate
Proprietary names. Dodds; Jackson's Febrifuge. It is an ingredient of Cystex, Doans Backache Pills, and TCP Cream.
$C_7H_5NaO_3$=160.1
CAS—54-21-7
Colourless crystals, crystalline flakes, or white or faintly pink powder. M.p. 440°.
Soluble 1 in 1 of water and 1 in 11 of ethanol; practically insoluble in chloroform and ether. Concentrated aqueous solutions are liable to deposit crystals of the hexahydrate on standing.

Dissociation Constant. pK_a 3.0, 13.4 (25°).

Partition Coefficient. Log *P* (octanol/water), 2.3.

Colour Tests. Ferric Chloride—blue-violet; Folin–Ciocalteu Reagent—blue; McNally's Test—red.

Thin-layer Chromatography. System TD—Salicylic acid Rf 07, salicyluric acid Rf 00; system TE—salicylic acid Rf 10, salicyluric acid Rf 00; system TF—salicylic acid Rf 01, salicyluric acid Rf 00; system TAD—Rf 24; system TAE—Rf 86; system TAJ—Rf 12; system TAK—Rf 71; system TAL—Rf 70. (Location under UV light, violet fluorescence; ferric chloride solution, violet; acidified potassium permanganate solution, positive.)

Gas Chromatography. System GA—Salicylic acid RI 1307, salicylic acid-Me RI 1200, salicylic acid-Me_2 RI 1195, M (glycine conjugate) RI 1825, M (glycine conjugate)-Me RI 1810, M (glycine conjugate)-Me_2 RI 1845; system GB—salicylic acid RI 1340, salicylic acid-Me RI 1228; system GL—salicylic acid-Me_2 RI 1210, M (5-OH-)-Me_3 RI 1530.

High Performance Liquid Chromatography. System HD—salicylic acid *k* 0.7, choline salicylate *k* 0.7; system HW—salicylic acid *k* 4.6, choline salicylate *k* 4.8; system HX—RI 350; system HY—RI 355; system HAA—Retention time 12.1 min; system HAX—Retention time 5.2 min; system HAY—Retention time 4.4 min.

Ultraviolet Spectrum. Aqueous acid—236 (A^1_1=647a), 303; aqueous alkali—298 (A^1_1=259a). Choline salicylate: methanol—298 nm (A^1_1=170b). (See below)

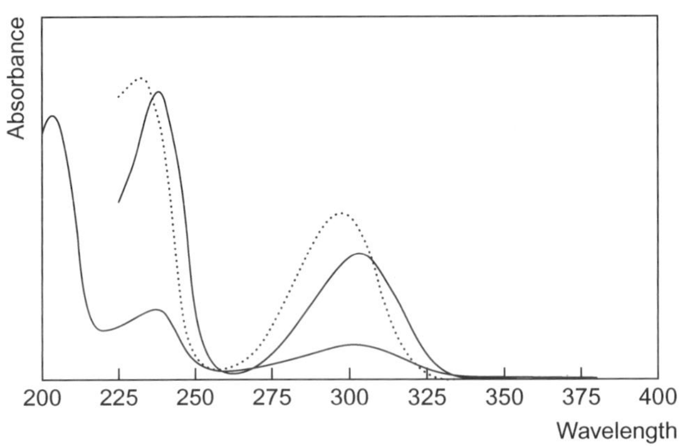

Infra-red Spectrum. Principal peaks at wavenumbers 758, 1657, 1288, 1210, 1250, 1150 (salicylic acid, KBr disk); 1587, 1724, 1176, 1515, 699, 1041 cm^{-1} (choline salicylate).

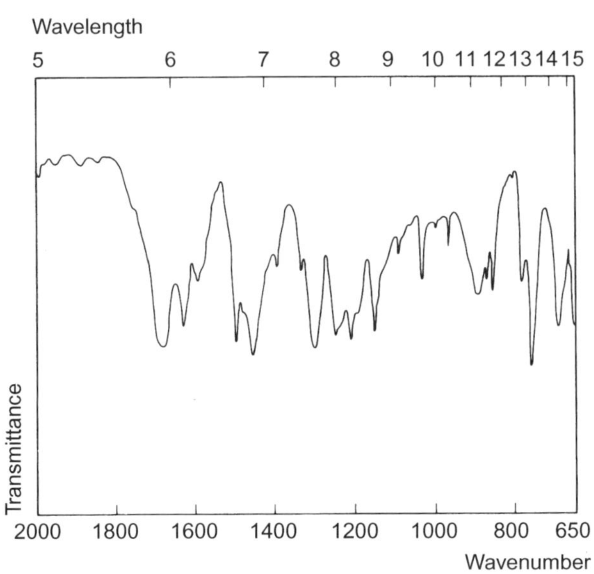

Mass Spectrum. Principal ions at *m/z* 120, 92, 138, 64, 39, 63, 121, 65; salicyluric acid 121, 120, 69, 92, 195, 39, 93, 45.

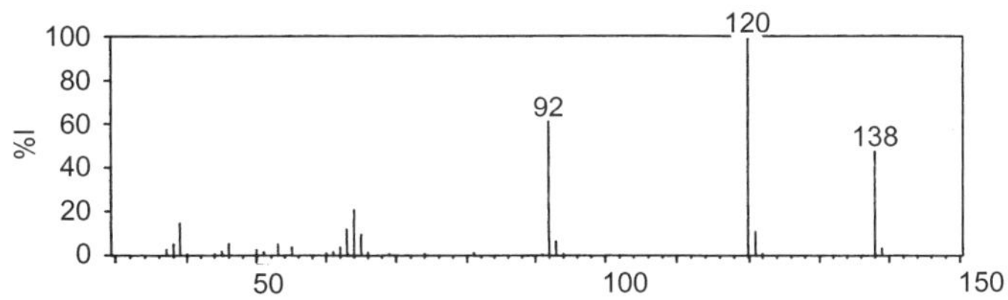

Quantification. See under Aspirin.

Disposition in the Body. Rapidly absorbed and distributed throughout the body. Metabolised by conjugation with glucuronic acid and glycine to give salicyluric acid, salicyl *O*-glucuronide, and salicyl ester glucuronide; hydroxylation to gentisic acid, gentisuric acid, and dihydroxy and trihydroxy derivatives also occurs. Excreted in the urine as unchanged drug and metabolites.
Salicylic acid is the major metabolite of aspirin, methyl salicylate, and salsalate.

Therapeutic concentration

Following daily oral doses of 9 mg/kg of sodium salicylate to 20 female and 20 male subjects, mean peak plasma concentrations of 57 and 58 mg/L were attained in 0.9 and 0.5 h respectively [S. L. Miaskiewicz *et al.*, *Clin. Pharmacol. Ther.*, 1982, *31*, 30–37].

After daily oral doses of choline salicylate, equivalent to 3.8 g of aspirin, a mean steady-state serum concentration of 166 mg/L was reported [P. D. Hansten and W. L. Hayton, *J. Clin. Pharmacol.*, 1980, *20*, 326–331].

Toxicity. The estimated minimum lethal dose is 15 g. Plasma concentrations greater than 300 mg/L are likely to produce toxic effects and concentrations greater than 500 mg/L are associated with moderate to severe intoxication.

In 80 subjects who had ingested an overdose of salicylate either in the form of aspirin tablets (n=42) or as topical medicaments containing methyl salicylate or wintergreen oil (n=38), the plasma salicylate concentrations on admission to hospital were generally higher in the subjects who had ingested aspirin tablets, although the 2 highest readings (4.3 and 3.5 nmol/L) belonged to subjects who had taken topical medicaments [T. Y. Chan, *Postgrad. Med. J.*, 1996, *72*, 109–112].

A blood salicylic acid concentration of 6.04 mmol/L was reported in a patient with psoriasis 19 h after he had applied 40% salicylic acid ointment to approximately 41% of his body surface; following haemodialysis, the patient was discharged after 14 days [J. Pec *et al.*, *Cutis*, 1992, *50*, 307–309].

Half-life. Plasma half-life, dose-dependent (2 to 4 h after salicylate doses of less than 3 g, increasing to about 19 h after large doses).

Volume of distribution. About 0.1 to 0.2 L/kg (dose-dependent).

Protein binding. In plasma, about 50 to 90% (dose-dependent, about 90% bound at concentrations below 100 mg/L, decreasing to 50% at concentrations above 400 mg/L).

Note. For a review of the pharmacokinetics of salicylates see C. J. Needs and P. M. Brooks, *Clin. Pharmacokinet.*, 1985, *10*, 164–177; for a review of drug interactions involving aspirin and salicylic acid, see J. O. Miners, *Clin. Pharmacokinet.*, 1989, *17*, 327–344; for a brief review of ototoxicity associated with salicylates, see J. A. Brien, *Drug Saf.*, 1993, *9*, 143–148.

Use. Salicylic acid is applied topically in concentrations usually ranging from 1 to about 6% as a keratolytic; up to 60% is used as a caustic in preparations for the removal of warts. Sodium salicylate is given by mouth in doses of up to 5.4 g daily.

Salinazid

Tuberculostatic

Synonyms. *o*-Hydroxybenzal Isonicotinylhydrazone; INSH; SAH; Salizid.
Proprietary names. Acozid; Nupa-Sal.
[(2-Hydroxyphenyl)methylene]hydrazide 4-pyridinecarboxylic acid
$C_{13}H_{11}N_3O_2$=241.2
CAS—495-84-1

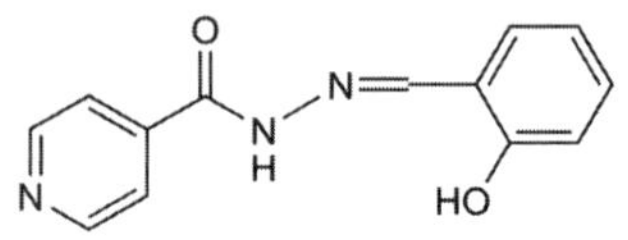

A pale cream-coloured powder. M.p. 232° to 233°; also reported as m.p. 251°.
Very slightly soluble in water; soluble in dilute acids and alkalis.

Partition Coefficient. Log *P* (octanol/water), 1.8.

Colour Tests. Aromaticity (Method 2)—yellow/orange; Ferric chloride—yellow-brown; Folin–Ciocalteu reagent—blue; Liebermann's test—orange; Mandelin's test—brown; Marquis test—yellow; Nessler's reagent (100°)—black; Sulfuric acid—yellow.

Thin-layer Chromatography. System TA—Rf 84; system TL—Rf 25; system TB—Rf 01; system TC—Rf 20. (Acidified iodoplatinate solution, positive.)

Ultraviolet Spectrum. Aqueous acid—257 nm (A_1^1=697a), 327 nm (broad); aqueous alkali—264 nm.

Infra-red Spectrum. Principal peaks at wavenumbers 1290, 1680, 1565, 1270, 687, 772 cm^{-1} (KBr disk).

Mass Spectrum. Principal ions at *m/z* 106, 123, 78, 51, 119, 79, 77, 107.

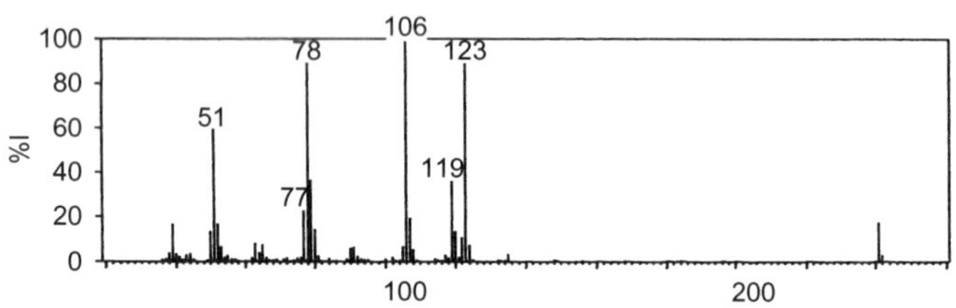

Dose. Salinazid was formerly given in doses of 0.2 to 3 g daily.

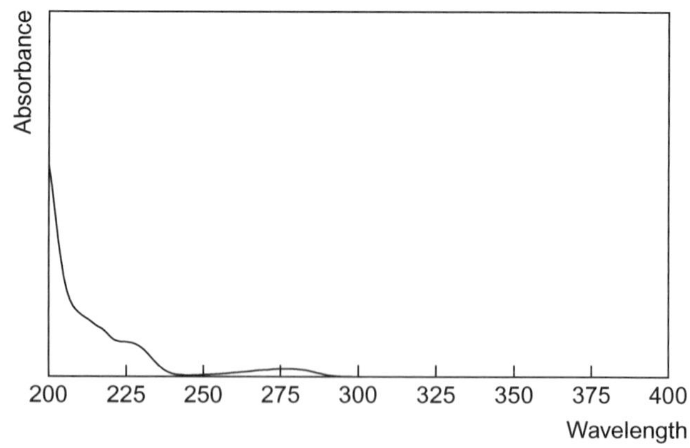

Quantification

High performance liquid chromatography. In plasma: limit of detection 10 µg/L. Fluorescence detection (λ_{ex}=310 nm; λ_{em}=410 nm)—A. S. Chilton *et al.*, *J. Pharm. Biomed. Anal.*, 1995, *13(2)*, 165–169.

Disposition in the Body. Salmeterol is extensively metabolised by P450 cytochrome CYP3A4 by aliphatic oxidation to α-hydroxy-salmeterol, which is primarily excreted in faeces (57%) and also urine (23%). Less than 5% of the unchanged drug is detected in urine. After taking salmeterol xinafoate, xinafoic acid is detected in the systemic circulation and steady state concentrations are approximately, 100 µg/L. This is 1000-fold less than the steady state concentration observed in toxicity studies. Very low plasma concentrations have been observed at therapeutic doses (<200 ng/L) after an inhaled dose.

Therapeutic concentration

Healthy individuals administered with single oral doses of 50 µg and 400 µg salmeterol produced peak plasma concentrations of 0.1 to 0.2 µg/L and 1 to 2 µg/L, respectively within 5 to 15 min. After a 1 mg dose, peak concentrations were approximately 0.6 µg/L at 45 min.

Repeated dosing of 50 µg twice daily to 6 patients with asthma, resulted in levels of 0.15 µg/L and dosing was continued for 10 months, a second peak could be observed between 0.07 and 0.2 µg/L 45 to 90 min after administration [Glaxo Wellcome data on file, 1996].

Toxicity. Associated with cardiovascular and other non-pulmonary effects including headaches, tremors and palpitations.

Half-life. 5.5 h for salmeterol; 15 days (healthy individuals); 30 days (patients with renal impairment) for xinafoic acid.

Volume of distribution. Steady state, 7.26 L.

Clearance. Plasma, 18.6 mL/h (healthy); 10.8 mL/h (renal impairment).

Protein binding. 94 to 98%.

Note. For a review of salmeterol, see J. C. Adkins and D. McTavish, *Drugs*, 1997, *54*, 331–354.

Dose. 50 to 100 µg twice daily (by inhalation).

Salmeterol

Beta₂-adrenoceptor Receptor Agonist/Bronchodilator

Synonym. GR-33343X
4-Hydroxy-α[1]-[[[6-(4-phenylbutoxy)hexyl]amino]methyl]-1,3-benzenedimethanol
$C_{25}H_{37}NO_4$=415.6
CAS—89365-50-4

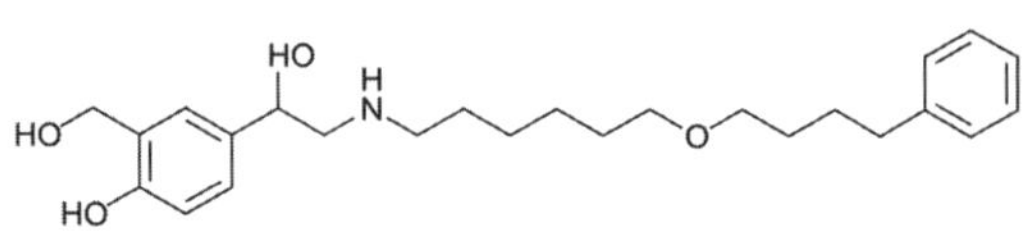

M.p. 75.5° to 76.5°.

Salmeterol Xinafoate

Synonym. GR-33343G
Proprietary names. Arial; Aeromax; Beglan; Betamican; Dilamax; Inaspir; Salmetedur; Seretide; Serevent.
$C_{25}H_{37}NO_4$, $C_{11}H_8O_3$=603.7
CAS—94749-08-3
White to off-white powder. M.p. 137° to 138°. It is freely soluble in methanol; sparingly soluble in water; slightly soluble in ethanol, chloroform and isopropanol.

High Performance Liquid Chromatography. Column: (analytical) Spherisorb ODS II cartridge (100 × 4.6 mm i.d., 5 µm); (guard) ODS II (10 × 4.6 mm i.d.). Mobile phase: phosphate buffer (0.05 M, pH 5):methanol (6:4), flow rate 1 mL/min. Fluorescence detection (λ_{ex}=310 nm; λ_{em}=410 nm). Retention time: salmeterol xinafoate, 4.4 min [A. S. Chilton *et al.*, *J. Pharm. Biomed. Anal.*, 1995, *13(2)*, 165–169].

Salol

Analgesic/Antipyretic/Anti-inflammatory

Synonym. Phenyl Salicylate
Proprietary name. Aussie Tan Sunstick
2-Hydroxybenzoic acid phenyl ester
$C_{13}H_{10}O_3$=214.2
CAS—118-55-8

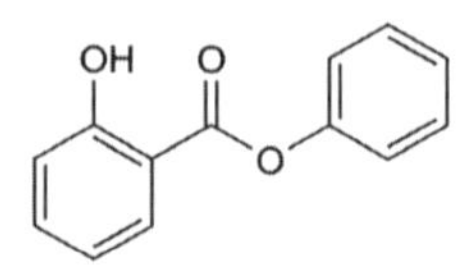

Colourless acicular crystals, or white crystalline powder. M.p. 41° to 43°. Soluble 1 in about 7000 of water, 1 in 6 of ethanol and 1 in 0.3 of chloroform and of ether.

Partition Coefficient. Log *P* (octanol/water), 3.8.

Gas Chromatography. System GA—RI 1685.

High Performance Liquid Chromatography. System HD—*k* 15.6.

Ultraviolet Spectrum. Ethanol—242 nm (A^1_1=664a), 310 nm (A^1_1=248a).

Use. Topically in concentrations of 5 to 10%.

Salsalate

Analgesic

Synonyms. Salicyl Salicylate; Salicylosalicylic Acid; Salicylsalicylic Acid; Salysal; Sasapyrine; NSC-49171.
Proprietary names. Amigesic; Argesic-SA; Artha-G; Disalcid; Marthritic; Mono-Gesic; Salflex; Salsitab; Umbradol.
2-Hydroxybenzoic acid 2-carboxyphenyl ester
$C_{14}H_{10}O_5$=258.2
CAS—552-94-3

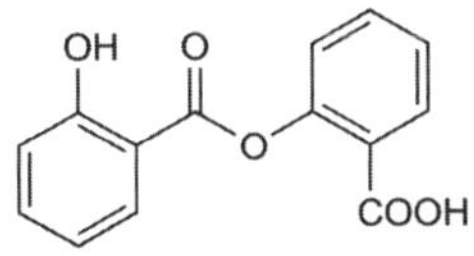

Colourless crystals or white crystalline powder. M.p. about 147° to 149°. Practically insoluble in water but gradually hydrolysed to 2 molecules of salicylic acid; soluble in ethanol and ether; sparingly soluble in benzene.

Dissociation Constant. pK_a 3.5, 9.8 (25°).

Partition Coefficient. Log *P* (octanol/water), 3.4.

Thin-layer Chromatography. System TG—Rf 23. (Chromic acid solution, brown.)

Gas Chromatography. System GD—RRT of methyl derivative 0.4 and 0.6 relative to n-$C_{16}H_{34}$.

High Performance Liquid Chromatography. System HD—*k* 3.6; system HV—RRT 0.69 relative to meclofenamic acid.

Ultraviolet Spectrum. Aqueous acid—204, 235, 310 nm; aqueous alkali—341 nm.

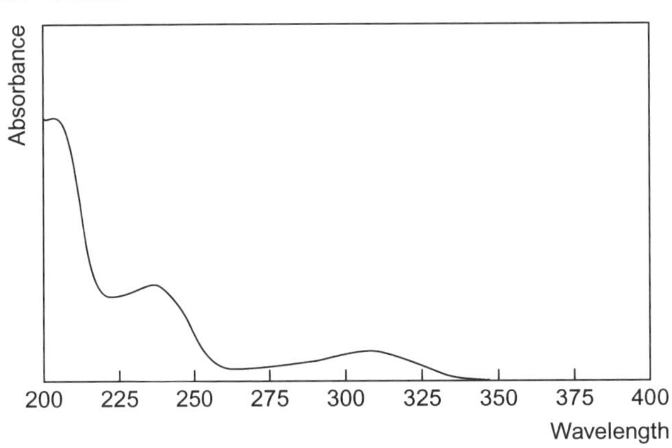

Infra-red Spectrum. Principal peaks at wavenumbers 1690, 1205, 1170, 1310, 1620, 1270 cm^{-1} (KBr disk).

Quantification.
High performance liquid chromatography. In plasma or urine: limit of detection 1 mg/L for salsalate and salicylic acid, UV detection—L. I. Harrison *et al.*, *J. Pharm. Sci.*, 1980, *69*, 1268–1271.

Disposition in the Body. Salsalate is rapidly absorbed after oral administration and extensively hydrolysed to salicylic acid. Less than 1% of a dose is excreted in the urine as unchanged salsalate in 24 h, and the remainder is excreted in the urine by the normal metabolic route for salicylic acid.

Therapeutic concentration
Following a single oral dose of 1 g of salsalate to 12 subjects, a mean peak plasma concentration of 21 mg/L of salsalate was attained in 1.5 h and peak plasma-salicylic acid concentrations of 38 to 77 mg/L (mean 54) were reported at 2 to 4 h. [L. I. Harrison *et al.*, *J. Clin. Pharmacol.*, 1981, *21*, 401–404].

Half-life. Plasma half-life, about 1 h.

Dose. Up to 4 g daily.

Santonin

Anthelmintic

Synonyms. Santolactone; α-Santonin.
[3*S*-(3α,3aα,5aβ,9bβ)]-3a5,5a,9b-Tetrahydro-3,5a,9-trimethylnaphtho-[1,2-*b*]furan-2,8(3*H*,4*H*)-dione
$C_{15}H_{18}O_3$=246.3
CAS—481-06-1

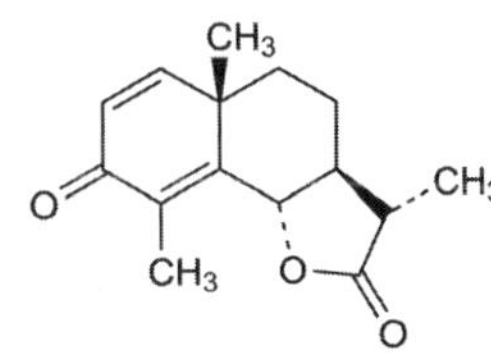

A crystalline lactone obtained from the dried unexpanded flowerheads of *Artemesia cina* (santonica, wormwood) and other species of *Artemesia* (Compositae).
Colourless crystals, or white crystalline powder, becoming yellow on exposure to light. M.p. about 173°.
Practically insoluble in water; soluble 1 in 50 of ethanol, 1 in about 4 of chloroform and 1 in 125 of ether.

Partition Coefficient. Log *P* (octanol/water), 1.8.

Thin-layer Chromatography. System TD—Rf 64; system TE—Rf 75; system TF—Rf 50; system TAD—Rf 69; system TAF—Rf 79. (Acidified iodoplatinate solution, positive; Acidified potassium permanganate solution, positive.)

Gas Chromatography. System GA—RI 2174.

Ultraviolet Spectrum. Methanol—239 nm (A^1_1=493a).

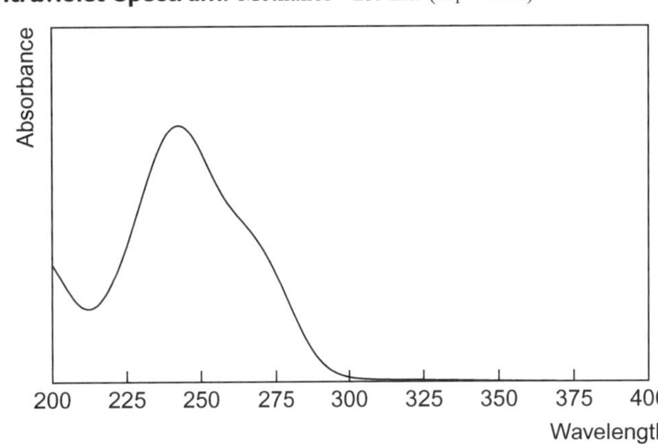

Mass Spectrum. Principal ions at *m/z* 41, 173, 91, 135, 77, 55, 44, 69.

Dose. Santonin was formerly given in doses of 60 to 200 mg daily for 3 days.

Saquinavir

Antiviral

(2*S*)-N^1-[(1*S*,2*R*)-3-[(3*S*,4a*S*,8a*S*)-3-[[(1,1-Dimethylethyl)amino] carbonyl]octahydro-2(1*H*)-isoquinolinyl]-2-hydroxy-1-(phenylmethyl)propyl]-2-[(2-quinolinylcarbonyl)amino]butanediamide
$C_{38}H_{50}N_6O_5$ = 670.8

CAS—127779-20-8

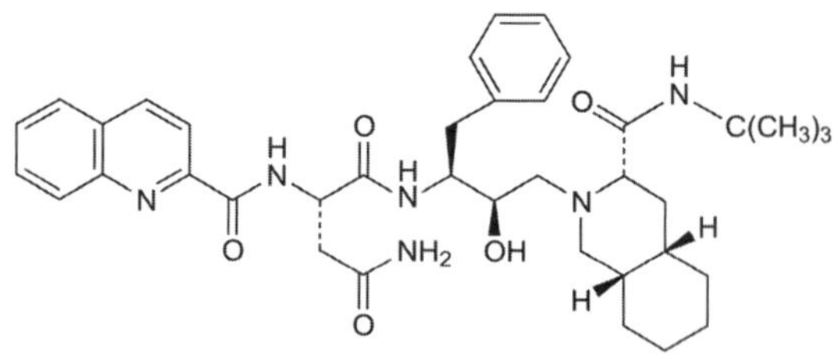

A white crystalline solid. Solubility: 0.22 g/100mL water.

Saquinavir Mesilate
Synonyms. Ro-31-8959/003; Ro-31-8959.
Proprietary names. Invirase; Fortovase.
$C_{38}H_{50}N_6O_5.CH_3SO_3H = 767.0$
CAS—149845-06-7

High Performance Liquid Chromatography. System HAC—k 9.5; HAE—Retention time, 22.2 min.

Ultraviolet Spectrum. Aqueous acid—204, 238, 292 nm. (saquinavir mesilate).

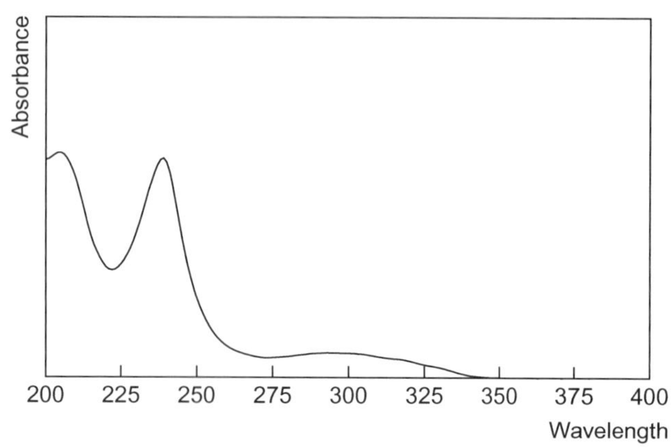

Infra-red Spectrum. Principal peaks at wavenumber 1670, 1658, 1198, 1173 cm^{-1} (saquinavir mesilate).

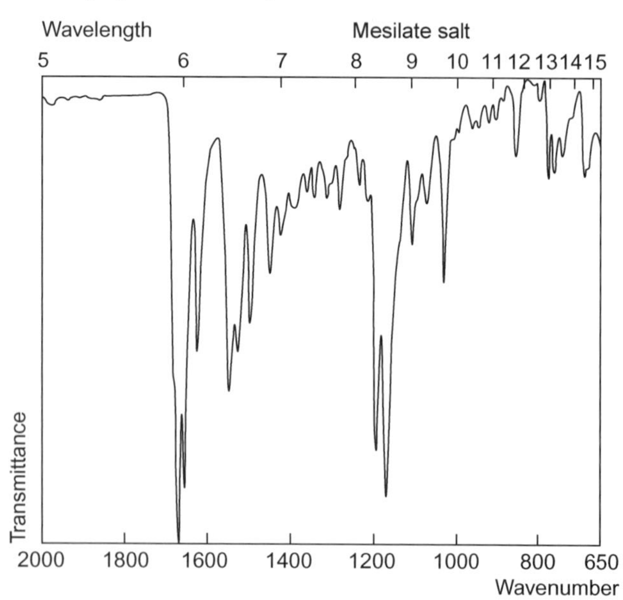

Mass Spectrum. Principal ions at *m/z* 129, 172, 128, 102, 101, 130, 76, 77 (saquinavir mesilate).

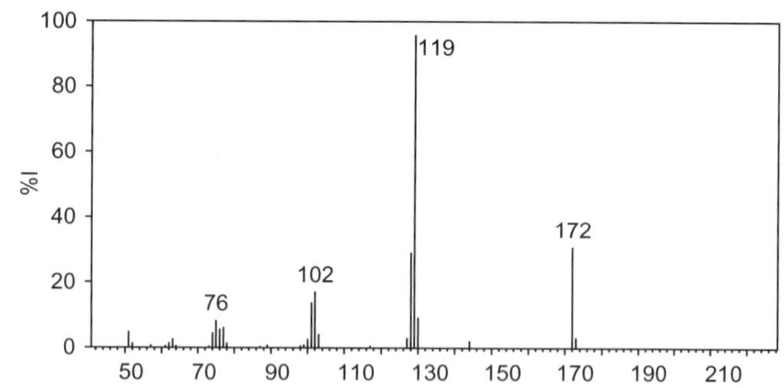

Quantification
High performance liquid chromatography. In plasma: limit of detection 1 μg/L. UV detection (λ = 240 nm)—H. R. Ha *et al., J. Chromatogr. B. Biomed. Sci. Appl.*, 1997, *694*, 427–433. In plasma: limit of quantification 5 μg/L. UV detection (λ = 241 nm)—G. Aymard *et al., J. Chromatogr. B. Biomed. Sci. Appl.*, 2000, *744*, 227–240. In plasma: limit of quantification 100 μg/L—V. Proust *et al., J. Chromatogr. B. Biomed. Sci. Appl.*, 2000, *742*, 453–458. In serum: limit of detection 100 μg/L, UV detection (λ = 250 nm)—V. A. Simon *et al., J. Chromatogr. A*, 2001, *913(1–2)*, 447–453.

Disposition in the Body. Saquinavir is absorbed but to a limited extent (30%) following oral administration and undergoes extensive first-pass metabolism in the liver. Peak plasma concentrations are observed approximately 0.77 h after administration of a suspension formulation and 3 to 4 h after capsules. It is extensively distributed into tissues but CNS concentrations are minimal. Metabolism is rapid by the cytochrome P450 system (CYP3A4) and a number of inactive monohydroxylated and dihydroxylated metabolites are formed. The drug is excreted mainly in faeces (88%) with only 1% in urine.

Therapeutic concentration

8 starved volunteers were administered with 600 mg saquinavir mesilate. Mean peak plasma concentrations of 20 μg/L were reached in less than an hour with a second peak of approximately, 0.4 μg/L after 5 h (after lunch) [H. R. Ha *et al., J. Chromatogr. B Biomed. Sci. Appl.*, 1997, *694*, 427–433].

100 HIV-infected patients with $CD4^+$ cell counts between 50 and 301 cells/mm^3, mean age 41.5 years, were administered with 600 mg saquinavir three times a day plus 200 mg zidvudine three times a day for 24 weeks. The mean weekly peak saquinavir concentration was 70.8 μg/L after 3.11 h [G. F. Vanhove *et al., Antimicrob. Agents Chemother.*, 1997, *41(11)*, 2428–2432].

Bioavailability. The oral bioavailability of saquinavir is low and is affected by the presence of food. In healthy volunteers receiving a single 600 mg dose after a heavy breakfast the bioavailability was found to be around 4%.

Half-life. 13.2 h.

Volume of distribution. 700 L following an intravenous dose of 12 mg.

Clearance. 1.14 L/h/kg. Plasma, 98.8 L/h.

Protein binding. Approx. 98% (independent of concentration over range 15 to 700 ng/mL).

Dose. 1800 mg daily as 600 mg three times a day.

Secbutabarbital

Sedative/Barbiturate

Synonyms. Butabarbital; Butabarbitone (distinguish from Butobarbital, Butobarbitone); Secbutobarbital; Secbutobarbitone.
5-Ethyl-5-(1-methylpropyl)-2,4,6(1*H*,3*H*,5*H*)-pyrimidinetrione
$C_{10}H_{16}N_2O_3 = 212.2$
CAS—125-40-6

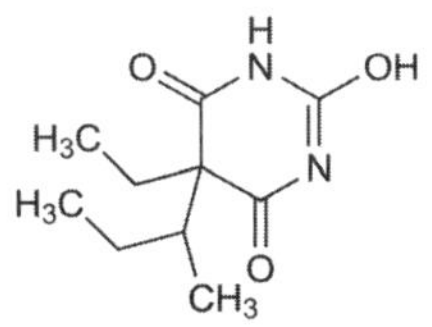

A fine, white, microcrystalline powder. M.p. 165° to 168°.
Soluble 1 in 1400 of water, 1 in 12 of ethanol, 1 in 30 of chloroform, and 1 in 30 of ether; soluble in aqueous solutions of alkali hydroxides and carbonates.

Secbutabarbital Sodium
Synonyms. Butabarbital Sodium; Butabarbitone Sodium; Secumalnatrium; Secbutobarbital Sodium; Secbutobarbitone Sodium; Sodium Butabarbital.
Proprietary names. Asturidon; Busotran; Butabon; Butak; Buta-Kay; Butalan; Butanotic; Butased; Butatran; Butazem; Butex; Butisol; Butrate; Butte; Carrbutabarb; Loubarb; Neravan; Prelital; Sarisol. It is an ingredient of Butibel.
$C_{10}H_{15}N_2NaO_3$=234.2
CAS—143-81-7
A white powder.
Soluble 1 in 2 of water and 1 in 7 of ethanol; very slightly soluble in chloroform; practically insoluble in ether.

Dissociation Constant. pK_a 8.0 (20°).

Partition Coefficient. Log *P* (octanol/water), 1.6.

Colour Tests. Koppanyi–Zwikker Test—violet; Mercurous Nitrate—black; Vanillin Reagent—orange/violet.

Thin-layer Chromatography. System TD—Rf 50; system TE—Rf 48; system TF—Rf 64; system TH—Rf 69; system TAD—Rf 57; system TAE—Rf 88. (Mercurous nitrate spray, black.)

Gas Chromatography. System GA—secbutabarbital RI 1655, secbutabarbital-Me_2 RI 1565, 2′-hydroxysecbutabarbital RI 1926.

High Performance Liquid Chromatography. System HG—*k* 4.9; system HH—*k* 3.3; system HX—RI 377; system HY—RI 331.

Ultraviolet Spectrum. Borax buffer 0.05 M (pH 9.2)—239 (A^1_1=428a); M sodium hydroxide (pH 13) —254 nm (A^1_1=354b).

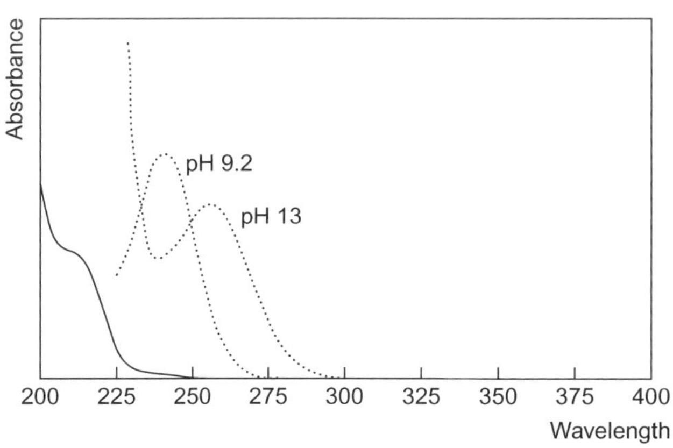

Infra-red Spectrum. Principal peaks at wavenumbers 1675, 1760, 1317, 1303, 1230, 853 cm^{-1} (KBr disk).

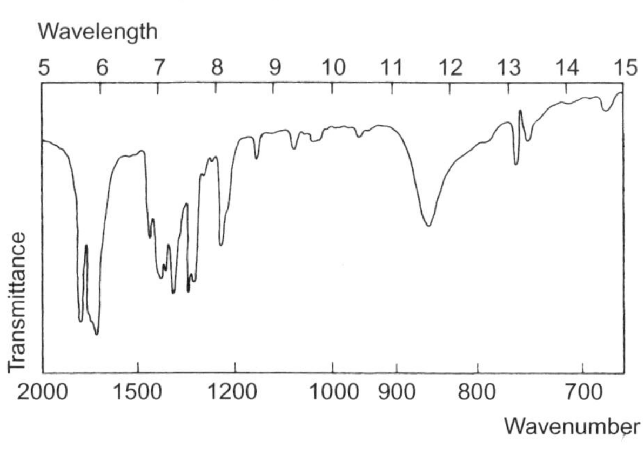

Mass Spectrum. Principal ions at *m/z* 141, 156, 41, 57, 39, 98, 157, 47.

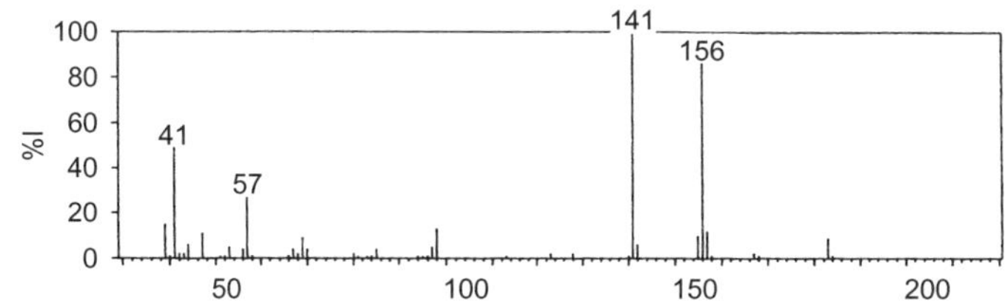

Quantification. See also under Amylobarbital.

Gas chromatography–mass spectrometry. In urine: secbutabarbital and other barbiturates—R. Pocci *et al.*, *J. Anal. Toxicol.*, 1992, *16*, 45–47.

Disposition in the Body. Well absorbed after oral administration. Rapidly metabolised by ω- and (ω-1)-oxidation of the methylpropyl side-chain. About 40 to 60% of a dose is slowly excreted in the urine, 5 to 9% as unchanged drug, 30% as 5-(2-carboxy-1-methylethyl)-5-ethylbarbituric acid, 3% as 2′-hydroxysecbutabarbital, and 1% as 2′-oxosecbutabarbital; greater amounts of unchanged drug may be excreted after excessive doses.

Toxicity. The estimated minimum lethal dose is 2 g. Blood concentrations greater than about 10 mg/L are likely to cause toxic reactions, and concentrations greater than 30 mg/L may be fatal.

Following oral administration of 600 mg, given in 3 doses over a period of 3 h to 5 subjects, peak blood concentrations of 7.6 to 16.9 mg/L (mean 12.3) were reported, 0.5 h after the third dose. Tests 2 h after the first dose indicated depression of the central nervous system in all subjects [K. D. Parker *et al.*, *Clin Toxicol.*, 1970, *3*, 131–145].

In 4 fatalities attributed to secbutabarbital overdose, blood concentrations of 30 to 88 mg/L (mean 58) and liver concentrations of 51 to 250 μg/g (mean 112) were reported [R. C. Baselt and R. H. Cravey, *J. Anal. Toxicol.*, 1977, *1*, 81–102].

Half-life. Plasma half-life, 34 to 42 h.

Protein binding. In plasma, about 26%.

Dose. Usually 45 to 120 mg daily.

Secobarbital

Barbiturate

Synonyms. Meballymal; Quinalbarbitone; Secobarbitalum; Secobarbitone.
5-(1-Methylbutyl)-5-(2-propenyl)-2,4,6(1*H*,3*H*,5*H*)-pyrimidinetrione
$C_{12}H_{18}N_2O_3$=238.3
CAS—76-73-3

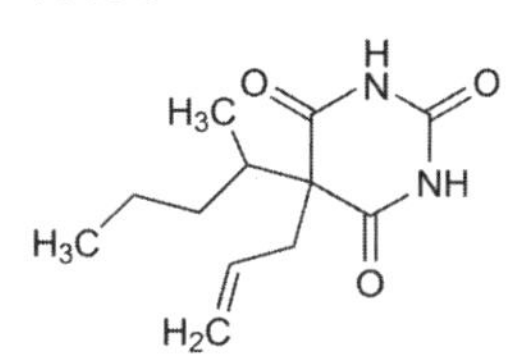

A white amorphous or crystalline powder. M.p. 100°.
Very slightly soluble in water; freely soluble in ethanol and ether; soluble in chloroform.

Secobarbital Sodium
Synonyms. Meballymalnatrium; Quinalbarbitone Sodium; Secobarbitalum Natricum; Secobarbitone Sodium.
Proprietary names. Seconal. It is an ingredient of Somolose (vet.) and Tuinal.
$C_{12}H_{17}N_2NaO_3$=260.3
CAS—309-43-3
A white hygroscopic powder.
Soluble 1 in 3 of water and 1 in 5 of ethanol; practically insoluble in chloroform and ether.

Dissociation Constant. pK_a 7.9 (20°).

Partition Coefficient. Log *P* (octanol/water), 2.0.

Colour Tests. Koppanyi–Zwikker Test—violet; Mercurous Nitrate—black; Vanillin Reagent—brown-red/violet.

Thin-layer Chromatography. System TD—Rf 55; system TE—Rf 45; system TF—Rf 68; system TH—Rf 78; system TAD—Rf 62; system TAE—Rf 88. (Mercuric chloride–diphenylcarbazone reagent, positive; mercurous nitrate spray, black; acidified potassium permanganate solution, yellow-brown; Zwikker's reagent, pink.).

Gas Chromatography. System GA—secobarbital RI 1786, M (3′-OH-) RI 1865, M (desallyl-) RI 1665, secobarbital-Me_2 RI 1690; system GB—secobarbital RI 1827, M (3′-OH-) RI 2029; system GF—RI 2510; system GAJ—secobarbital RRT 0.865, M (3′-OH-) RRT 1.206 (both relative to methylphenobarbital).

High Performance Liquid Chromatography. System HG—*k* 16.28; system HH—*k* 11.47; system HX—RI 437; system HY—RI 407; system HZ—Retention time 4.7 min; system HAA—Retention time 17.4 min; system HAX—Retention time 6.2 min; system HAY—Retention time 5.9 min.

Ultraviolet Spectrum. Borax buffer 0.05 M (pH 9.2) —239 (A_1^1=393a); 1 M sodium hydroxide (pH 13)—254 nm (A_1^1=330b).

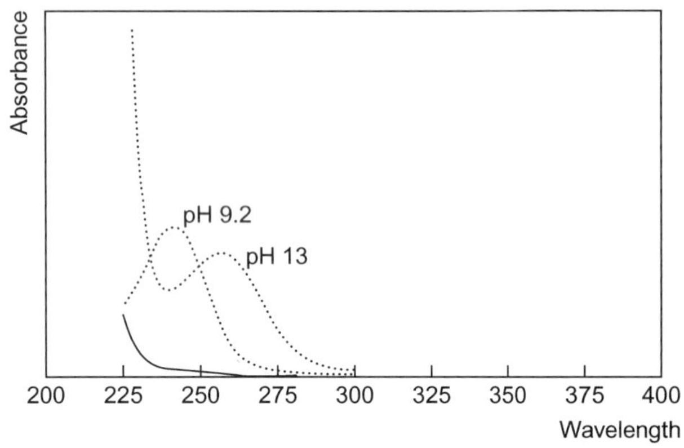

Infra-red Spectrum. Principal peaks at wavenumbers 1559, 1648, 1690, 1298, 1270, 925 cm^{-1} (secobarbital sodium, KBr disk).

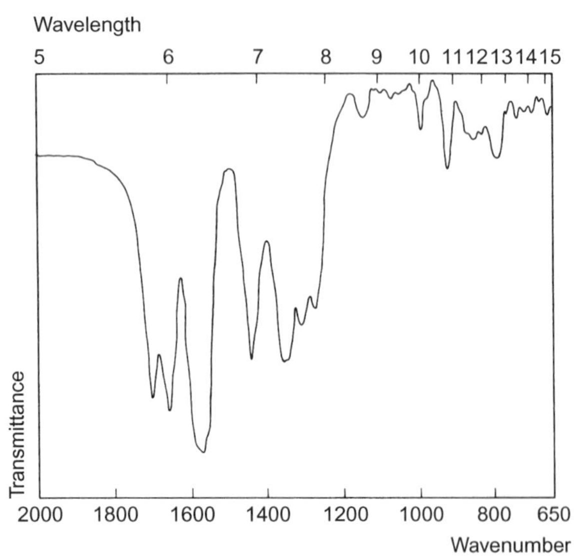

Mass Spectrum. Principal ions at *m/z* 167, 168, 41, 43, 97, 124, 39, 55; 5-(2,3-dihydroxypropyl)secobarbital 171, 43, 143, 41, 128, 55, 141, 159; 3′-hydroxysecobarbital 41, 45, 43, 168, 39, 70, 69, 167; 3′-ketosecobarbital 43, 69, 168, 41, 85, 167, 86, 169.

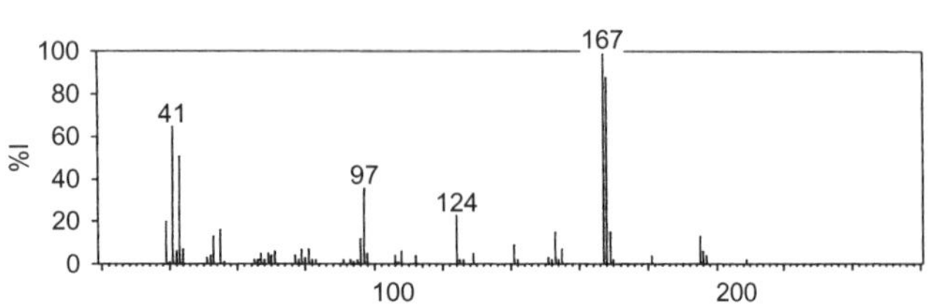

Quantification. See also under Amylobarbital.

Gas chromatography. In plasma or urine: limit of detection 200 μg/L in plasma, FID—J. L. Valentine *et al.*, *Anal. Lett.* (Part B), 1982, *15*, 343–361.

High performance liquid chromatography. In serum: limit of detection 20 μg/L, UV detection—H. L. Levine *et al.*, *J. Pharm. Sci.*, 1982, *71*, 1281–1283.

Disposition in the Body. About 90% of a dose is absorbed after oral administration. The major metabolic reactions are hydroxylation of both side-chains at the C_5-position with further oxidation of the ω-position on the butyl side-chain. Less than 5% of an oral dose is excreted unchanged in the urine. Two diastereoisomeric forms of the following metabolites have been found in the urine, each metabolite accounting for about 4% of the dose in 24 h: 5-allyl-5-(3-hydroxy-1-methylbutyl)barbituric acid (3′-hydroxysecobarbital), 5-allyl-5-(3-carboxy-l-methylpropyl)barbituric acid, and 5-(2,3-dihydroxy-propyl)secobarbital; an additional metabolite, 5-allyl-5-(1-methyl-3-oxobutyl)barbituric acid (3′-ketosecobarbital), accounts for about 3% of the dose in 96 h. A total of about 45% of the dose is excreted in the urine over a period of 108 h.

Therapeutic concentration. In plasma, usually in the range 2 to 10 mg/L.

After an oral dose of 3.3 mg/kg to 6 subjects, peak blood concentrations of 2.0 to 2.2 mg/L (mean 2.1) were attained in about 3 h [J. M. Clifford *et al.*, *Clin. Pharmacol. Ther.*, 1974, *16*, 376–389].

Toxicity. The estimated minimum lethal dose is 2 g. Toxic effects are usually associated with blood concentrations greater than about 8 mg/L. In 276 reported fatalities attributed to secobarbital, blood concentrations ranged from 4 to 132 mg/L (mean 30).

The following postmortem tissue distribution was reported in 5 fatalities: blood 35 to 123 mg/L (mean 66), brain 109 μg/g (1 case), kidney 67 to 270 μg/g (mean 152, 3 cases), liver 25 to 605 μg/g (mean 271, 4 cases), spleen 42 μg/g (1 case), urine 12 to 182 mg/L (mean 72, 3 cases) [C. J. Rehling, Poison Residues in Human Tissues, in *Progress in Chemical Toxicology*, Vol. 3, A. Stolman (Ed.), New York, Academic Press Inc., 1967, p. 371].

The following postmortem tissue concentrations (mg/L or μg/g) were reported in 3 fatalities due to secobarbital:

	Secobarbital 3′	Hydroxysecobarbital
Blood	12, 9, 13	0, –, 2
Bile	–, 42, 79	–, –, 0
Left kidney	37, 25, 25	3, –, 17
Right kidney	69, 24, 28	4, –, 16
Liver	77, 51, 44	4, –, 25
Urine	6, 3, 32	0, –, 33

[A. E. Robinson and R. D. McDowall, *J. Pharm. Pharmacol.*, 1979, *31*, 357–365].

Following a fatality involving the suicidal ingestion of secobarbital, nitrazepam, and codeine, the respective blood concentrations were reported as 11.48, 1.72, and 0.036 mg/L [A. Tracqui *et al.*, *Am. J. Forensic Med. Pathol.*, 1989, *10*, 130–133].

Half-life. Plasma half-life, 19 to 34 h (mean 28).

Volume of distribution. About 1.5 L/kg.

Clearance. Plasma clearance, about 0.8 mL/min/kg.

Saliva. Plasma : saliva ratio, about 3.3.

Protein binding. In plasma, about 70%.

Dose. 100 mg daily as secobarbital sodium.

Selegiline

Antiparkinsonian

Synonyms. Synonyms used in the literature are confusing and include (−)-Deprenil; L-Deprenil; Deprenyl; (−)-Deprenyl; L-Deprenyl; L-Deprenaline and E-250. It is the (−)-isomer which is active.

(αR)-*N*,α-Dimethyl-*N*-2-propynylbenzeneethanamine

$C_{13}H_{17}N$=187.3

CAS—14611-51-9

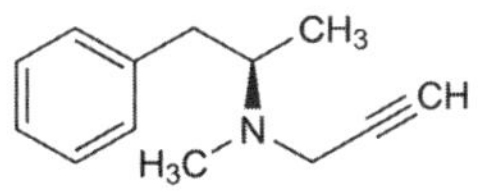

An oil.

Selegiline Hydrochloride

Proprietary names. Amboneural; Amindan; Antiparkin; Atapryl; Carbex; Centrapryl; Cognitiv; Deprilan; Egibren; Eldepryl; Elepril; Jumex; Jumexil; MAOtil; Movergan; Niar; Regepar; Selegam; Selgene; Seline; Selpar; Stilline; Tremorex; Vivapryl; Zelapar.

$C_{13}H_{17}N,HCl = 223.7$

CAS—14611-52-0

A white crystalline solid. M.p. 141° to 142°.

Thin-layer Chromatography. System TA—Rf 74; system TB—Rf 57; system TC—Rf 69. (Dragendorff spray, positive; acidified iodoplatinate solution, positive; Marquis reagent, orange.)

Gas Chromatography. System GA—selegiline RI 1450, M (OH-) RI 1580, M (OH-)-AC RI 1860; M (nor-) RI 1350, M (nor-)-AC RI 1735, M (nor-OH-) RI 1550, M (nor-OH-)-AC_2 RI 2030, amfetamine RI 1125, metamfetamine RI 1175, system GB—selegiline RI 1453, amfetamine RI 1150, metamfetamine RI 1200.

High Performance Liquid Chromatography. System HAA—Retention time 10.7 min.

Ultraviolet Spectrum. Aqueous acid—252, 258 nm ($A_1^1 = 9.1b$), 264 nm; aqueous alkali—259, 269 nm.

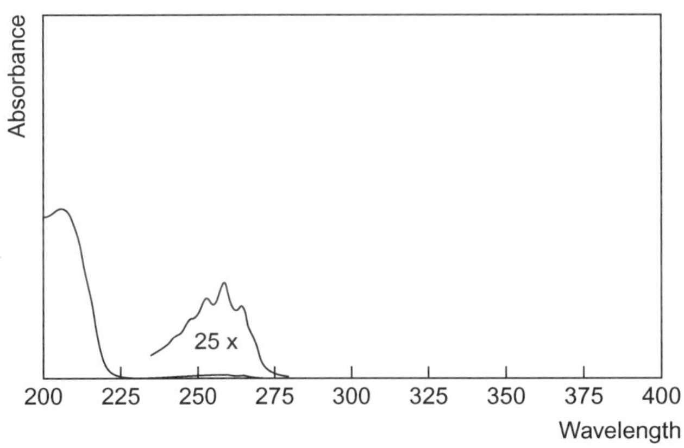

Infra-red Spectrum. Principal peaks at wavenumbers 704, 765, 740, 1492, 1092, 981 cm^{-1} (selegiline hydrochloride, KBr disk).

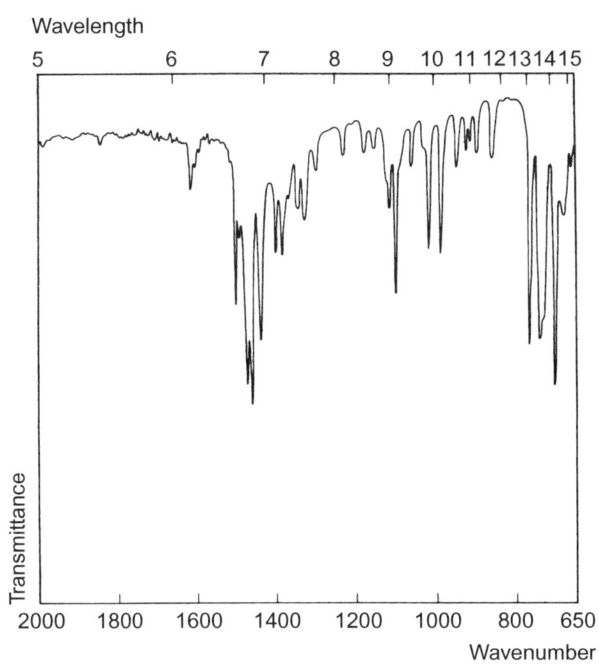

Mass Spectrum. Principal ions at *m/z* 96, 56, 42, 91, 97, 39, 65, 58; amfetamine 44, 91, 40, 42, 65, 45, 39, 43; metamfetamine 58, 91, 59, 134, 65, 56, 42, 57.

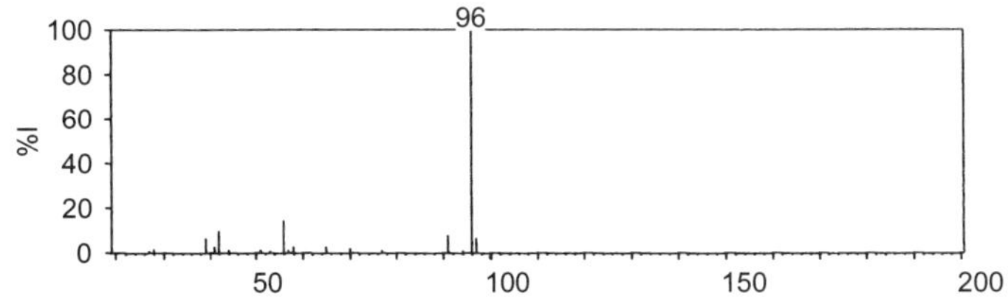

Quantification. See also under amfetamine and metamfetamine.

Gas chromatography. In plasma or urine: (−)-metamfetamine, (−)-amfetamine and norselegiline (or (+)-metamfetamine and (+) -amfetamine associated with metamfetamine abuse)—M. Hasegawa *et al.*, *Forensic Sci. Int.*, 1999, *101*, 95–106.

Gas chromatography–mass spectrometry. In hair; selegiline, desmethylselegiline, metamfetamine and amfetamine, SIM—R. Kikura and Y. Nakahara, *Biol. Pharm. Bull.*, 1995, *18*, 267–272.

High performance liquid chromatography. In plasma: norselegiline, amfetamine and metamfetamine, limit of detection 0.5 µg/L, fluorescence detection—R. La Croix *et al.*, *J. Chromatogr.*, 1994, *656*, *Biomed. Appl.*, 251–258R. La Croix *et al.*, *J. Chromatogr.*, 1996, *681*, *Biomed. Appl.*, 185–190. In urine: enantiomers of metamfetamine and amfetamine, limit of detection 2.8 to 8.8 fmol/5 mL, fluorescence detection—O. al-Dirbashi *et al.*, *Analyst*, 1998, *123*, 2333–2337.

High performance liquid chromatography–mass spectrometry. In urine: selegiline-*N*-oxide, metamfetamine, amfetamine and desmethylselegiline, limit of detection 0.1 to 0.5 µg/L, ESI–MS detection—M. Katagi *et al.*, *J. Chromatogr. B. Biomed. Sci. Appl.*, 2001, *759*, 125–133.

Disposition in the Body. Rapidly absorbed after oral administration and distributed to the tissues. Selegiline is almost completely metabolised to form metamfetamine and amfetamine. About 50% of a dose is excreted in the urine in 24 h and 75% in 72 h; excreted mainly as metamfetamine with lesser amounts of amfetamine. The excretion of metabolites is increased in acid urine. About 15% of a dose is eliminated in the faeces in 72 h.

Half-life. Derived from urinary excretion data (total radioactivity), about 39 h.

Note. For a review of the pharmacology of selegeline see M. Gerlach *et al.*, *Neurology*, 1996, *47* (Suppl. 3), S137–S145.

Dose. 5 to 10 mg of selegiline hydrochloride daily.

Serotonin

Synonyms. Enteramine; 5-HT; 5-Hydroxytryptamine; Thrombocytin; Thrombotonin.

3-(2-Aminoethyl)-1*H*-indol-5-ol

$C_{10}H_{12}N_2O = 176.2$

CAS—50-67-9

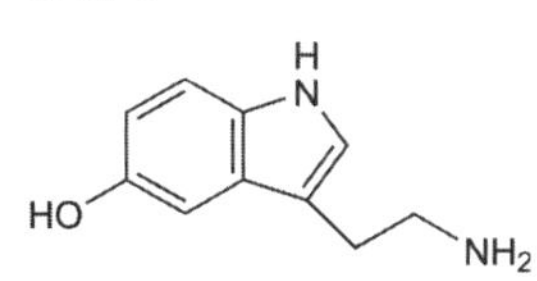

Serotonin Hydrochloride

White crystals. M.p. about 167°.

Soluble in water.

Dissociation Constant. pK_a 9.1, 9.8.

Partition Coefficient. Log *P* (octanol/water), 0.2.

Colour Test. Marquis test—brown (slow).

Thin-layer Chromatography. System TA—Rf 25. (Acidified potassium permanganate solution, positive.)

Ultraviolet Spectrum. Aqueous acid—276 nm; aqueous alkali—274, 323 nm.

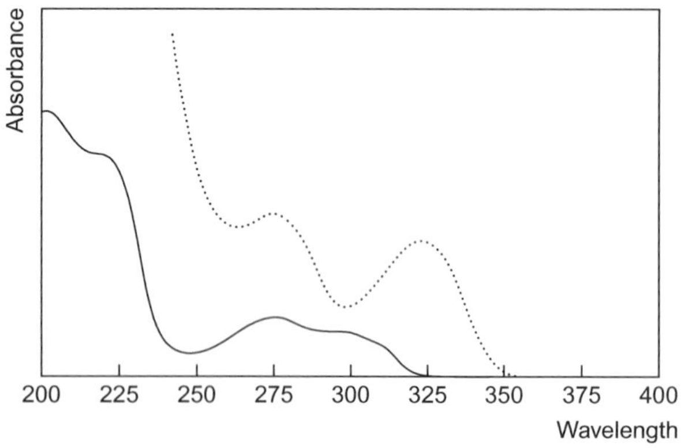

Infra-red Spectrum. Principal peaks at wavenumbers 1195, 1225, 1582, 1627, 720, 1105 cm^{-1} (serotonin oxalate, KBr disk).

Quantification

Gas chromatography–mass spectrometry. In plasma: SIM—S. Baba *et al.*, *J. Chromatogr.*, 1984, *307*, 1–9.

High performance liquid chromatography. In urine: serotonin, catecholamines and their metabolites, fluorescence detection—T. J. Panholzer *et al.*, *Clin. Chem.*, 1999, *45*, 262–268. In urine: serotonin and 5-hydroxyindoleacetic acid, limit of quantification for serotonin, 2.4 nM, fluorescence detection—M. Kai *et al.*, *J. Chromatogr. B Biomed. Sci. Appl.*, 1998, *720*, 25–31.

Disposition in the Body. Serotonin is widely distributed in the body, arising from the hydroxylation and subsequent decarboxylation of tryptophan. It is metabolised chiefly by oxidative deamination to 5-hydroxyindol-3-ylacetic acid; *N*-methylation of the side chain may also occur.

Sertindole

Antipsychotic

Synonym. LU-23-174
Proprietary name. Serdolect
1-[2-[4-[5-Chloro-1-(4-fluorophenyl)-1*H*-indol-3-yl]-1-piperidinyl]ethyl]-2-imidazolidinone
$C_{24}H_{26}ClFN_4O = 440.9$
CAS—106516-24-9

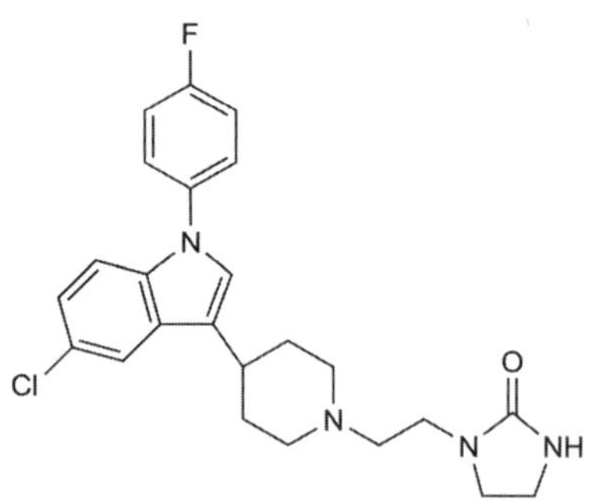

A white to off-white, fine powder with m.p. 166°. It is soluble in 0.1 M acetic acid; practically insoluble in water; sparingly soluble in ethanol 96%; freely soluble in dichloromethane.

Dissociation Constant. pK_a 8.9.

Partition Coefficient. Log *P* (octanol/buffer pH 7.4), 3.9.

High Performance Liquid Chromatography. System HZ—Retention time 9.8 min.

Column: (analytical) C_{18} (Spherisorb, 250 × 4.6 mm i.d., 5 µm); (guard) (Partisil, 20 × 2 mm i.d.). Mobile phase: hexane:isopropyl alcohol: methanol:tetrahydrofuran:28% ammonium hydroxide (73.6:15:9.6:1.3:0.5), flow rate 1 mL/min. Fluorescence detection (λ_{ex} = 260 nm; λ_{em} 340 nm). Retention time: 12.1 min [T. B. Tzeng *et al.*, *J. Chromatogr. B Biomed. Appl.*, 1994, *661*, 299–306].

Ultraviolet Spectrum. Methanol—227, 258, 302; ethanol—226, 259, 302 nm.

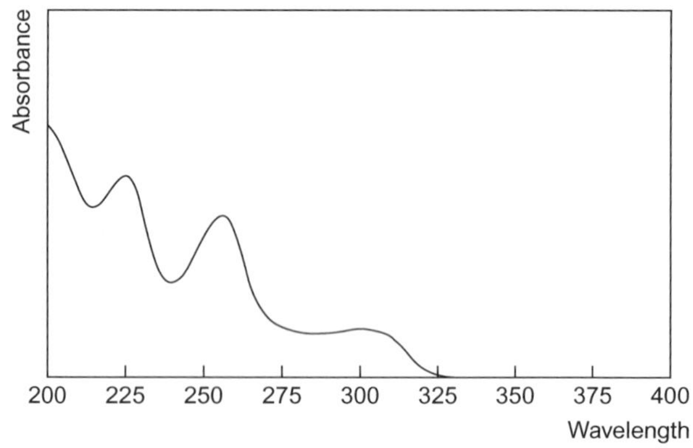

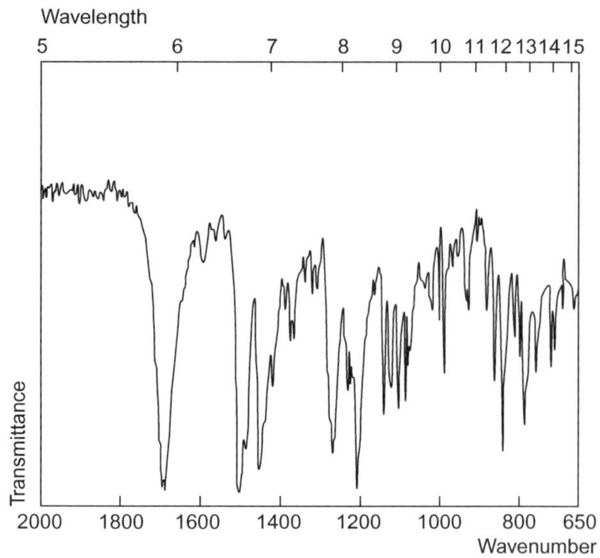

Mass Spectrum. Principal ions at *m/z* 341, 44, 343, 342, 440, 70, 18, 344.

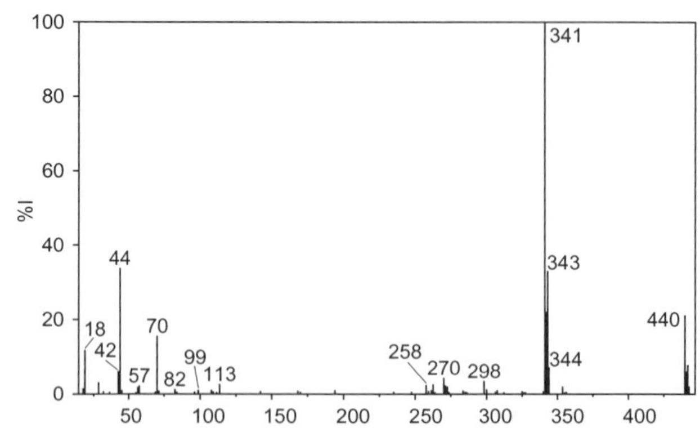

Quantification

High performance liquid chromatography. In plasma: limit of detection 0.01 µg/L, limit of quantification 0.025 µg/L. Fluorescence detection (λ_{ex} = 260 nm; λ_{em} 340 nm)—T-B. Tzeng *et al.*, *J. Chromatogr. B Biomed. Appl.*, 1994, *661*, 299–306.

Disposition in the Body. Sertindole is absorbed slowly after oral administration with peak plasma concentrations being reached after about 10 h. It is extensively metabolised in the liver by the cytochrome P450 isoenzymes CYP2D6 and CYP3A. Poor metabolisers (deficient in isoenzyme CYP2D6) may have plasma concentrations of sertindole which are 2 to 3 times greater. Two metabolites have been identified: dehydrosertindole and norsertindole which appear to be inactive. Excretion is slow and mainly via faeces with a small amount in urine. It readily crosses the placenta.

Therapeutic concentration

12 young, healthy males (mean age, 29 years), 12 elderly males (mean, 71 years), 11 young females (mean, 22 years) and 12 elderly females (mean, 73 years) participated in this study. Each received 4 mg sertindole daily for 3 consecutive days, 8 mg daily for 3 consecutive days and 12 mg daily for 10 consecutive days. After the 4 mg single dose, peak plasma concentrations for sertindole were 1.41 μg/L for the young males and the elderly males, 2.34 μg/L for the young females and 1.83 μg/L for the elderly females. These were observed at 9.7, 10.2, 10.2 and 11.8 h, respectively. Peak dehydro-sertindole concentrations were 0.78 and 0.90 μg/L for the young and elderly males, respectively, and 0.89 and 0.97 μg/L for the young and elderly females. These concentrations were seen at 23.0, 23.3, 22.2 and 21.7 h for the four groups, respectively. After 12 mg sertindole daily for 10 days, the peak concentrations were 53.13, 43.91, 63.74 and 57.6 μg/L for the young males, elderly males, young females and elderly females, respectively, at 7.5, 9.3, 8.9 and 10.3 h, respectively. Peak concentrations for the metabolite, dehydro-sertindole were 38.34, 34.06, 43.29 and 51.58 μg/L for the four groups of volunteers at 8.5, 9.6, 6.0 and 7.3 h, respectively [S. L. Wong *et al.*, *Clin. Pharmacol. Ther.*, 1997, *62(2)*, 157–164].

7 healthy males, aged 18 to 37 years, were administered with 4 mg sertindole daily for 2 days and then the dose was increased 4 mg every 3 days until 20 mg daily was reached. The peak serum concentration for the 20 mg dose was 69.8 μg/L on day 11, observed at 8.9 h. 6 alternative healthy males were administered with 4 mg daily for 7 days followed by 8 mg daily for an additional 7 days. After a 4 mg dose (day 1), the peak concentration was 2.3 μg/L at 9.3 h and 9.6 μg/L at 10.0 h (day 7). For the 8 mg dose on day 14, peak concentration was 28.7 μg/L at 9.3 h [S. L. Wong and G. R. Granneman, *J. Pharm. Sci.*, 1998, *87(12)*, 1629–1631].

Toxicity. Cardiac arrhythmia, sudden cardiac death.

Half-life. 3 days.

Volume of distribution. 1887 to 2447 L (single doses of 4 and 8 mg); 809 L (multiple dosing 20 mg).

Clearance. Plasma, 22 to 31 L/h (single doses of 4 and 8 mg); 9.8 L/h (multiple dosing of 20 mg).

Protein binding. 99.5%.

Dose. An initial dose of 4 mg daily which may be increased by 4 mg every 4 to 5 days. The usual maintenance dose is 12 to 20 mg daily with a maximum of 24 mg.

Sertraline

Antidepressant

Synonym. CP-51974

(1*S*,4*S*)-4-(3,4-Dichlorophenyl)-1,2,3,4-tetrahydro-*N*-methyl-1-naphthalenamine

$C_{17}H_{17}Cl_2N = 306.2$

CAS—79617-96-2

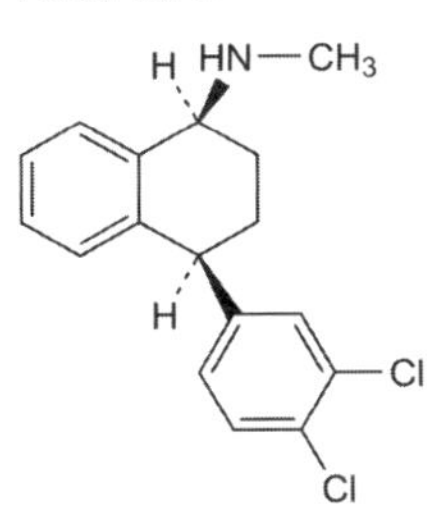

Sertraline Hydrochloride

Synonym. CP-51974-01

Proprietary names. Altruline; Aremis; Besitran; Gladem; Lustral; Sealdin; Serad; Tatig; Zoloft.

(1*S*,4*S*)-4-(3,4-Dichlorophenyl)-1,2,3,4-tetrahydro-*N*-methyl-1-naphthalenamine hydrochloride

$C_{17}H_{17}Cl_2N,HCl = 342.7$

CAS—79559-97-0

A white to off-white crystalline powder (irritant). M. p. onset of change 160° to 180°, partial melt 218°, total melt 243° to 245°. Solubility: water 3.8 mg/mL (pH 5.3)-pH dependent. It is soluble in chloroform:methanol (1:1), methanolic 0.1 M hydrochloric acid, dimethyl sulfoxide, ethanol and *N*,*N*-dimethylformamide; practically insoluble in aqueous 0.1 M hydrochloric acid, aqueous 0.1 M sodium hydroxide, isopropyl alcohol, acetone, ethyl acetate and acetonitrile.

Dissociation Constant. pK_a 9.48 ± 0.04 (water); 8.5 (ethanol:water (1:1)); 8.6 (methanol:water (40:60)).

Partition Coefficient. Log *P* (octanol/water), 5.29.

Thin-layer Chromatography. System TB—Rf 46; system TE—Rf 72; system TAE—Rf 25.

Gas Chromatography. System GB—RI 2481; RI 2468 sertraline M (nor-); RI 2496 sertraline M (ketone); system GM—RRT 1.166; RRT 1.218 sertraline M (nor-) (relative to iprindole).

Column: methyl silicone (HP1, 0.2 mm i.d., 0.33 μm film thickness). Column temperature: 250°. Carrier gas: helium, 0.9 mL/min flow rate. MS detection. RI: 2401 [T. Mills and J. C. Roberson, *Instrumental Data for Drug Analysis*, CRC Press, *2nd Edn.*, *6*, 222–223].

Column: 3% Silar 10C on Gas Chrom Q 80-100 mesh (0.8 m × 0.2 mm i.d.), glass column. Column temperature: 255°. Injector temperature: 200°. Carrier gas: helium, 40 mL/min flow rate. MS detection (EI, SIM at *m/z*:274). Retention time: 3.9 min [H. G. Fouda *et al.*, *J. Chromatogr. B Biomed.. Appl.*, 1987, *417*, 197–202].

High Performance Liquid Chromatography. System HAX—Retention time 14.5 min; system HAY—Retention time 7.7 min; system HX—RI 460; system HZ—Retention time 8.2 min (sertraline); Retention time 7.0 min (desmethylsertraline).

Ultraviolet Spectrum. Aqueous acid (0.01 M hydrochloric acid/methanol or methanol only)—265, 273, 281 nm (no alkaline shift).

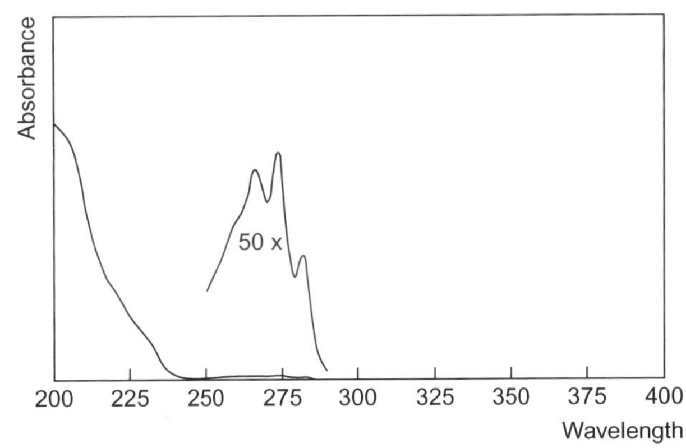

Infra-red Spectrum. Principal peaks at wavenumber 1470, 1135, 825, 800, 790, 760 cm^{-1} (KBr disk).

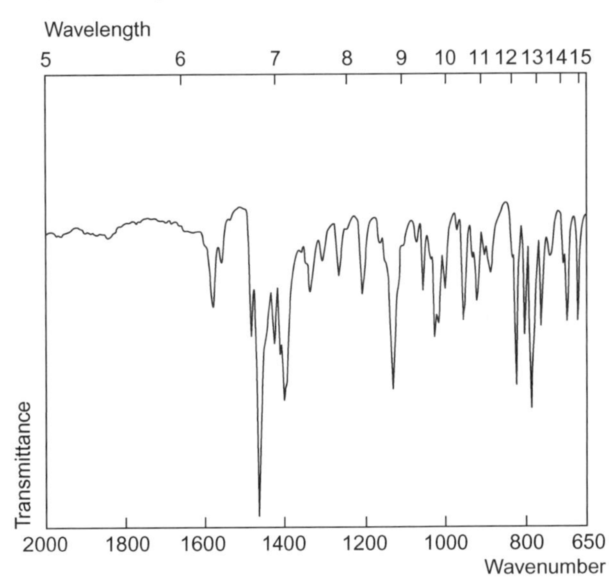

Mass Spectrum. Principal ions at *m/z* 274, 276, 159, 103, 262, 275, 278, 132.

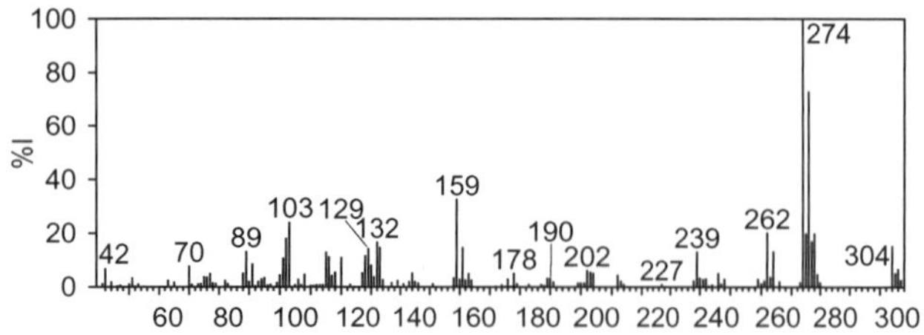

Quantification

Gas chromatography. In plasma: limit of detection 1 µg/L—L. M. Tremaine and E. A. Joerg, *J. Chromatogr.*, 1989, *496*, 59–67.

High performance liquid chromatography. In plasma: limit of detection 5 µg/L. UV detection (λ = 210 nm)—J. H. Kristensen *et al.*, *Br. J. Clin. Pharmacol.*, 1998, *45*, 453–457.

High performance liquid chromatography, gas chromatography and mass spectrometry. In serum: limit of detection, 10 µg/L—D. Rogowsky *et al.*, *J. Chromatogr. B Biomed. Appl.*, 1994, *655*, 138–141.

Disposition in the Body. Sertraline is absorbed slowly after oral administration with peak plasma concentrations being reached within 4.5 to 8.4 h. Steady state levels are achieved after one week of daily dosing. It is widely distributed throughout the body. Sertraline and its metabolite *N*-desmethylsertraline (inactive in *in vivo* models of depression) are extensively metabolised (sertraline: *N*-demethylation, oxidative deamination and subsequent reduction, hydroxylation and glucuronide conjugation; *N*-desmethylsertraline: oxidative deamination and subsequent reduction, hydroxylation and glucuronide conjugation) and excreted in urine and faeces. 40 to 45% of an administered dose is excreted in urine over 9 days with less than 0.2% as the unchanged drug. It is distributed in breast milk.

Therapeutic concentration. The serum therapeutic range is 50 to 250 µg/L.

44 healthy volunteers, aged between 18 and 45 years, and >65 years (male and female) were administered with a single 50 mg daily dose of sertraline. The initial dose was titrated to 200 mg over 30 days which is the maximum dose. On day 30, peak sertraline plasma concentrations were determined as 118 µg/L for the young males and 166 µg/L for the young females. Concentrations were reached in 6.9 and 6.7 h, respectively. Peak plasma concentrations of the metabolite, *N*-demethylsertraline, were 156 µg/L in 9.1 h and 244 µg/L in 5.9 h for the males and females, respectively. For the older patients, peak plasma concentrations of the drug were 135 µg/L and 147 µg/L for the males and females, respectively and were reached in 7.8 and 6.4 h, respectively. For the metabolite, 237 µg/L and 274 µg/L in 13.8 and 8.2 h, respectively [R. A. Ronfeld *et al.*, *Clin. Pharmacokinet.*, 1997, *32(suppl.1)*, 22–30].

10 patients, aged 35 to 69 years, with stable chronic hepatic insufficiency due to cirrhosis (mild to severe) and 10 equally matched healthy individuals were administered with a single 100 mg sertraline base dose after an overnight fast. For patients, mean peak plasma concentrations for the drug were 35.2 (range, 20.0 to 40.8) µg/L, observed at 4 (2 to 6) h and for the metabolite, *N*-demethylsertraline, 7.9 (5.5 to 9.7) µg/L at 168 (96 to 216) h. For the healthy volunteers, mean peak drug concentrations were 20.6 (12.6 to 27.5) µg/L at 6 (4 to 6) h and 11.2 (10.6 to 13.0) µg/L for the metabolite at 6 (6 to 10) h [J. L. Demolis *et al.*, *Br. J. Clin. Pharmacol.*, 1996, *42*, 394–397].

Toxicity

A 51-year-old white woman was admitted into hospital after ingesting 8000 mg of sertraline. She had been treated 3 days before for acute alcohol intoxication. Symptoms included somnolence, nausea, tachycardia, anxiety and dilated pupils. On admission, serum concentrations were 2930 µg/L and 1679 µg/L for sertraline and desmethylsertraline, respectively. Other drugs detected included norpropoxyphene (268 µg/L) and nortriptylene (26 µg/L). No ethanol was found. On day 4, sertraline and desmethyl sertraline serum concentrations were 453 µg/L and 1132 µg/L, respectively. The drug concentration went down further to 305 µg/L on day 5 and the patient was discharged on day 6 after receiving supportive measures [D. H. Brendel *et al.*, *Ann. Emerg. Med.*, 2000, *36*, 524–526].

Half-life. Sertraline, approximately 26 h (mean for young and elderly 22 to 36 h); *N*-desmethylsertraline, 62 to 104 h; prolonged in hepatic impairment.

Volume of distribution. 20 L/kg.

Protein binding. Approx. 98%.

Dose. 50 to 200 mg daily.

Setiptiline

Antidepressant

Proprietary name. Tecipul
2,3,4,9-Tetrahydro-2-methyl-1*H*-dibenzo[3,4:6,7]cyclohepta-[1,2-c]pyridine
$C_{19}H_{19}N = 261.4$
CAS—57262-94-9

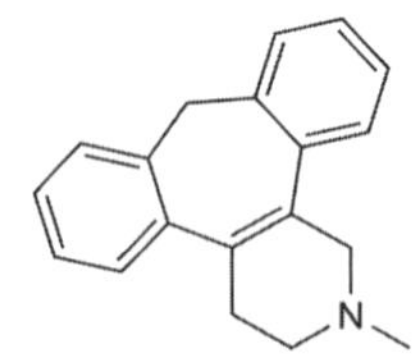

Gas Chromatography. Column: SPB-1 fused-silica (Supelco, 30 m × 0.32 mm i.d., 0.25 µm film thickness). Column temperature: 100° for 5 min, to 280° at 20°/min. Carrier gas: helium, flow rate 0.8 mL/min. Internal standard (IS): imipramine. MS detection (SIM at *m/z* 202, 217, 261 for setiptiline; 243 for IS). Retention times: setiptiline, 14.1 min; IS, 13.7 min [A. Namera *et al.*, *J. Anal. Toxicol.*, 1998, *22(5)*, 396–400].

Mass Spectrum. Principal ions at *m/z* 83, 70, 261, 202, 217, 203, 82, 215.

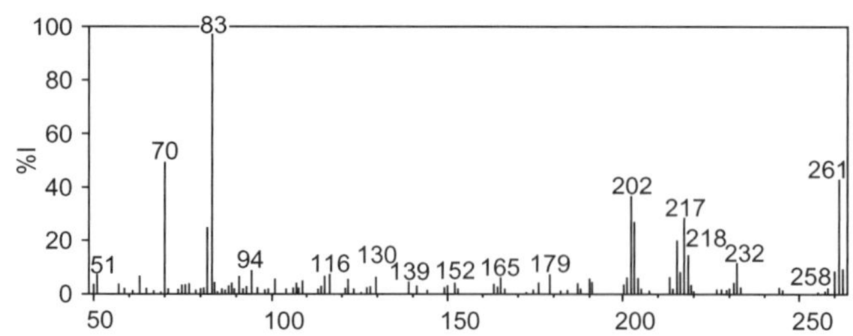

Quantification

Gas chromatography–mass spectrometry. In blood: limit of detection 0.005 µg/g—A. Namera *et al.*, *J. Anal. Toxicol.*, 1998, *22(5)*,396–400.

Disposition in the Body. Setiptiline is metabolised via glucuronide conjugation, demethylation and hydroxylation in the liver. About 10.7% of a dose is excreted in urine as the glucuronide conjugate and approx. 9% as the other metabolites, in 48 h, resulting from aromatisation and hydroxylation following demethylation.

Therapeutic concentration

45 outpatients, aged between 22 and 86 years (male's mean, 48.8 years; female's mean, 59.3 years), being treated for depression were administered with setiptiline at doses and frequency determined by the attending doctors according to symptoms and illness. The mean dose administered to the female volunteers was 0.08 mg/kg daily (range, 0.04 to 0.16 mg/kg) and to the male volunteers, 0.07 mg/kg daily (0.04 to 0.12 mg/kg). The mean plasma concentration observed was 3.54 (0.05 to 7.12) µg/L for the females and 2.24 (0.08 to 6.40) µg/L for the males. In terms of age, the mean plasma concentrations for mean ages of 23.8, 33.4, 44.0, 54.8, 65.6, 74.8 and 83.1 years were 1.92, 2.00, 3.06, 2.17, 2.61, 3.32 and 5.63 µg/L, respectively. The daily doses for these ages were 0.051, 0.057, 0.079, 0.062, 0.094, 0.086 and 0.064 mg/kg, respectively [M. Kamimura *et al.*, *Prog. Neuropsychopharmacol. Biol. Psychiatry*, 1994, *18*, 1015–1026].

Toxicity

Heart blood samples were taken from a subject whose death was suspected to be caused by acute setiptiline poisoning. A concentration of setiptiline of 1.77 µg/g was determined in blood taken from the left hand side of the heart and 0.78 µg/g from the right. [A. Namera *et al.*, *J. Anal. Toxicol.*, 1998, *22(5)*, 396–400].

Half-life. 11 h.

Sevoflurane

Anaesthetic

Synonyms. BAX-3084; MR-654.
Proprietary names. Sevofrane; Sevorane; Ultane.
1,1,1,3,3,3-Hexafluoro-2-(fluoromethoxy)propane

$C_4H_3F_7O = 200.1$
CAS—28523-86-6

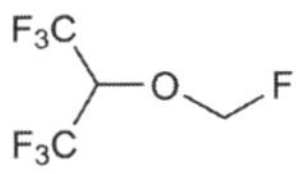

A clear, colourless, volatile liquid with a non-pungent light odour. It is non-flammable with m.p. less than 25°. B.p 58.5°. It is slightly soluble in water and miscible with ethanol, ether, chloroform and petroleum benzene.

Partition Coefficient. Log *P* (octanol/water), 1.75.

Gas Chromatography. System GR—Retention time, 2.8 min.

Column: PoraPLOT Q (25 m × 0.32 mm i.d., 10 µm film thickness). Column temperature: 30° for 2 min, increase by 15°/min to 250° and held for 5 min. Carrier gas: helium, flow rate 3.8 mL/min. Detection: flame ionisation/FT–IR. IS: diethyl ketone. Retention time: (relative to IS) 0.758 [I. Ojanpera *et al.*, *J. Anal. Toxicol.*, 1998, *22*, 290–295].

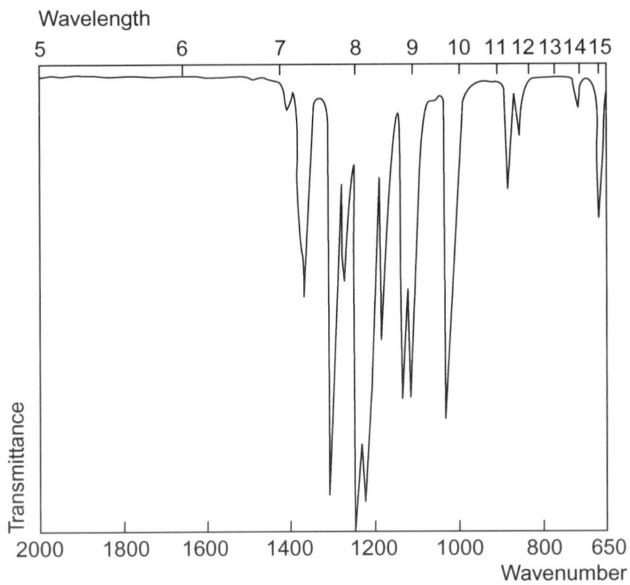

Mass Spectrum. Principal ions at *m/z* 33, 131, 69, 79, 181, 51, 151, 101.

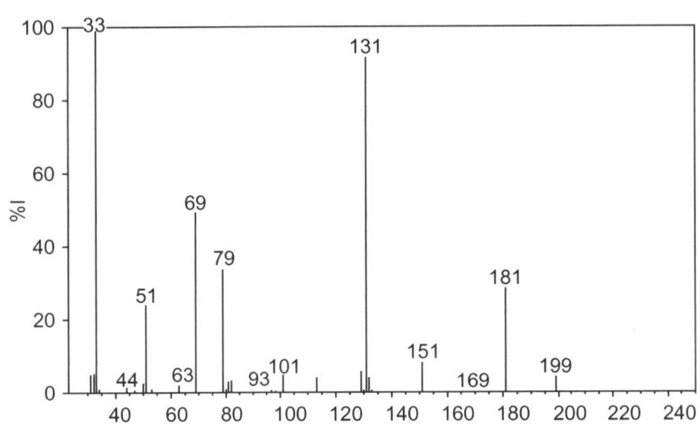

Quantification

Gas chromatography–FT–IR. In blood: limit of detection 0.01 mg/L, FT–IR detection—I. Ojanpera *et al.*, *J. Anal. Toxicol.*, 1998, *22*, 290–295.

Gas chromatography–mass spectrometry. In blood: limit of detection 0.2 mg/L, pulse-heating method—K. Saito *et al.*, *J. Anal. Toxicol.*, 1995, *19*, 115–119.

Disposition in the Body. Sevoflurane is readily absorbed via the pulmonary capillary system. Up to 5% is metabolised by the hepatic cytochrome P450-2E1 isoenzyme to hexafluroisopropanol (HFIP) with the release of inorganic fluoride and carbon dioxide. HFIP is rapidly conjugated with glucuronic acid and eliminated in the urine. No other metabolic pathway has been identified suggesting that only 5% of the dose is metabolised. Approximately 3.5% of an administered dose appears in urine as the fluoride. Low solubility facilitates rapid uptake and elimination via the lungs. The blood/gas coefficient is low (0.60). Changes in the clinical effects rapidly follow changes in the inspired concentration. The rapid and extensive pulmonary elimination minimises the amount available for metabolism. Alveolar equilibration is rapid (85% within 30 min). Between 95 and 98% of the amount taken up is eliminated through the lungs. Distribution partition coefficients at 37° water/gas 0.36 and oil/gas 47.2.

Toxicity. Toxic effects are related to the metabolism.

Half-life. Sevoflurane, 9.5 min; HFIP glucuronide, 55 h.

Clearance. Mean pulmonary elimination clearance, 3.58 L/min; total body clearance, 3.6 L/min.

Dose. Administered by inhalation using a calibrated vaporiser. In adults, inspired concentrations of up to 5% sevoflurane usually produce surgical anaesthesia in less than 2 min. In children, inspired concentrations of up to 7% sevoflurane usually produce surgical anaesthesia in less than 2 min. Surgical levels may be sustained with concentrations of 0.5 to 3% sevoflurane with or without nitrous oxide. Less in the elderly.

Sildenafil

Vasodilator

Synonym. UK-92480-10
1-[[3-(4,7-Dihydro-1-methyl-7-oxo-3-propyl-1*H*-pyrazolo[4,3-*d*]-pyrimidin-5-yl)-4-ethoxyphenyl]sulfonyl]-4-methylpiperazine
$C_{22}H_{30}N_6O_4S = 474.6$
CAS—139755-83-2

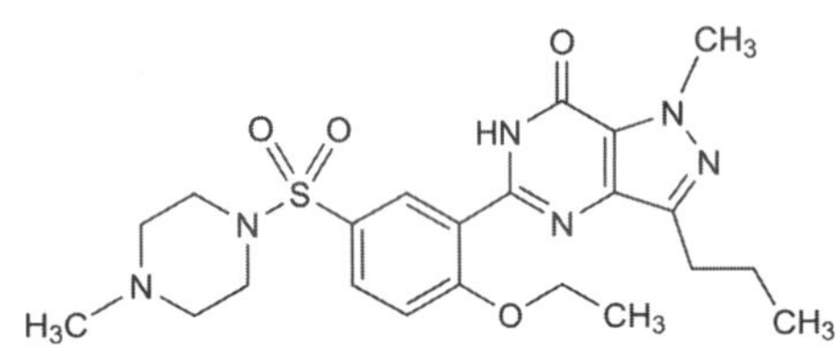

Crystals. M. p. 187° to 189°.

Sildenafil Citrate
Proprietary name. Viagra
$C_{22}H_{30}N_6O_4S,C_6H_8O_7 = 666.7$
CAS—171599-83-0
A white to off-white crystalline powder.

Dissociation Constant. pK_a 8.7.

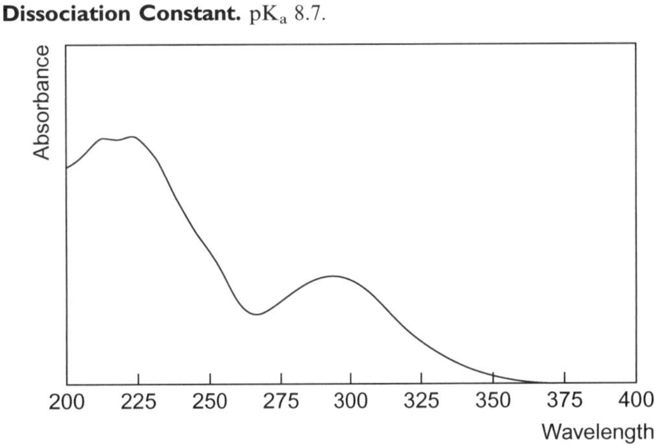

Infrared Spectrum. Principal peaks at wavenumber 760, 1695, 1169, 946 cm^{-1}

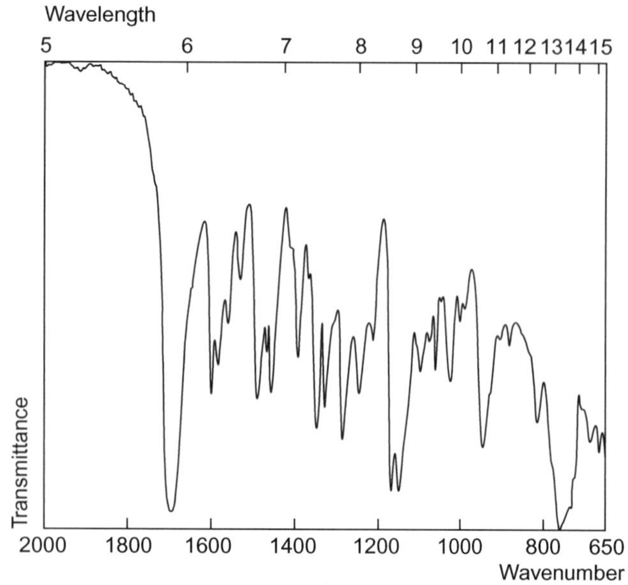

Mass Spectrum. Principal ions at *m/z* 99, 404, 56, 100, 405, 70, 312, 381.

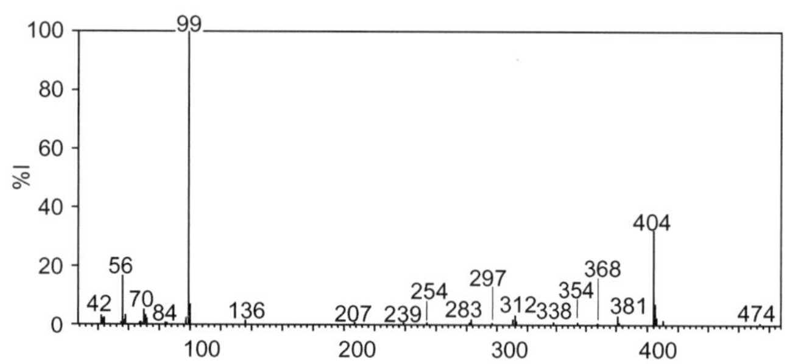

High Performance Liquid Chromatography. Column: RP C_4 (Kromasil, 150 × 4.6 mm i.d., 5 μm). Column temperature: 40°. Mobile phase: acetonitrile:potassium dihydrogen phosphate (0.5 M, with diethylamine hydrochloride (10 mM)) (32:68), flow rate 0.7 mL/min. UV detection (λ = 230 nm). Retention time: 10.3 min [M. Lee and D. I. Min, *Ther. Drug Monit.*, 2001, *23*, 21–26].

Column: C_{18} (μBondapak, 300 × 3.9 mm i.d., 10 μm). Mobile phase: ammonium acetate (0.2 M, pH 7.0):acetonitrile (1:1), flow rate 1 mL/min. UV detection (λ = 240 nm). Retention time: 9.0 min [N. Daraghmeh *et al.*, *J. Pharm. Biomed. Anal.*, 2001, *25*, 483–492].

Quantification

Gas chromatography. In hair: limit of quantification 0.1 ng/g. MS detection—K. Saisho *et al.*, *Biol. Pharm. Bull.*, 2001, *24*, 1384–1388.

High performance liquid chromatography. In plasma: sildenafil and *N*-desmethylsildenafil, limit of quantification 1 μg/L. UV detection (λ = 230 nm)—J. D. H. Cooper *et al.*, *J. Chromatogr. B Biomed. Sci. Appl.*, 1997, *701*, 87–95.

Disposition in the Body. Sildenafil is rapidly absorbed after oral administration. Peak plasma concentrations occur within about 30 to 120 min. Rate of absorption is reduced when taken with food. It is widely distributed into tissues and metabolised in the liver primarily by CYP3A4; some is also metabolised by CYP2C9. The major metabolite formed, *N*-desmethylsildenafil (UK-103,320) has some activity and makes up 30 to 40% of the total plasma drug concentration after a single dosing regimen. Sidenafil is excreted predominantly as metabolites in faeces (about 80% of administered dose) and to a lesser extent in urine (about 13% of administered dose with <2% as the parent drug). Clearance may be reduced in the elderly and in patients with severe renal or hepatic impairment.

Therapeutic concentration

4 groups of healthy males, approximately 14 per group, aged between 18 and 45 years, were administered with a single oral dose of 100 mg sildenafil. The mean peak drug concentrations were 0.296, 0.302, 0.321 and 0.325 mg/L observed at 2.1, 3.1, 2.0 and 2.3 h, respectively. Peak concentrations for the metabolite, UK-103,320, were 0.116, 0.118, 0.132 and 0.160 mg/L at 2.5, 3.5, 2.0 and 2.5 h [G. J. Muirhead *et al.*, *Br. J. Clin. Pharmacol.*, 2000, *50(2)*, 99–107].

Toxicity

Since 6 million prescriptions have been dispensed, the US Food and Drug Administration have reported 130 deaths in males taking sildenafil. The cause of death was unknown for 48 of these cases, 41 were caused by known or suspected myocardial function, 27 suffered from cardiac arrest, 6 with other cardiac symptoms and 3 with coronary artery disease. All were a known risk factor or contraindication to use of drug, for example, co-administration with another drug or substance. [US Food & Drug Administration report, Rockville, MD, USA, 1998].

A 43-year-old man, treated for cardiovascular disease and erectile dysfunction with sildenafil citrate (Viagra), was found dead in a hotel room. Several tablets of verapamil, trimetazidine, yohimbine and bromazepam were found at the scene as well as a box of Viagra with two 25 mg tablets missing. Postmortem examination revealed sildenafil concentrations of 105, 246, 1206 and 754 μg/L in blood, urine, bile and gastric content, respectively. Hair concentration was 177 ng/g. The desmethyl metabolite was measured as 143 μg/L in urine. Blood levels of verapamil and trimetazidine were found to be 659 and 2133 μg/L respectively. Trinitrine and yohimbine were not detected [V. Dumestre-Toulet *et al.*, *Forensic. Sci. Int.*, 2002, *126*, 71–76].

A 42-year-old female ingested 20 tablets of Viagra (100 mg per tablet) in a suicide attempt. Upon admission, she was oriented but nervous and complained of general weakness, palpitations, headache, dizziness and abdominal fullness. She underwent a gastro-intestinal decontamination procedure, recovered and was discharged 12 h later [D. Z. Hung and D. Y. Yang, *J. Toxicol. Clin. Toxicol.*, 2001, *39*, 423–424].

Bioavailability. 40%.

Half-life. Plasma half-life, sildenafil, 3 to 5 h; *N*-desmethylsildenafil, 4 h.

Clearance. Plasma clearance, 41 L/h.

Volume of distribution. Approx. 105 L.

Protein binding. In plasma, 96% (both sildenafil and *N*-desmethylsildenafil).

Note. For a review of sildenafil see H. D. Langtry and A. Markham, *Drugs*, 1999, *57*, 967–989.

Dose. Usually the equivalent of 50 mg of sildenafil.

Simazine

Herbicide

Proprietary names. Gesatop; Princep; Simadex. It is an ingredient of Pathclear.

6-Chloro-*N*,*N*′-diethyl-1,3-5-triazine-2,4-diamine

$C_7H_{12}ClN_5$=201.7

CAS—122-34-9

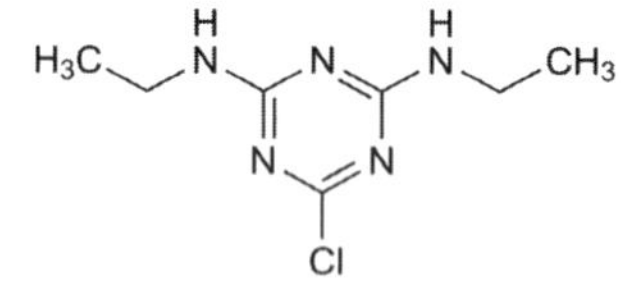

A white crystalline powder. M.p. 226° to 227°.

Practically insoluble in water; very slightly soluble in chloroform and ether.

Dissociation Constant. pK_a 1.6 (20°).

Partition Coefficient. Log *P* (octanol/water), 2.2.

Thin-layer Chromatography. System TA—Rf 73; system TX—Rf 22; system TY—Rf 18.

Gas Chromatography. System GA—RI 1690; system GK—RRT 0.8 (relative to caffeine).

High Performance Liquid Chromatography. System HAA—Retention time 15.7 min.

Ultraviolet Spectrum. Ethanol—262 nm (A_1^1=162b). (See below.)

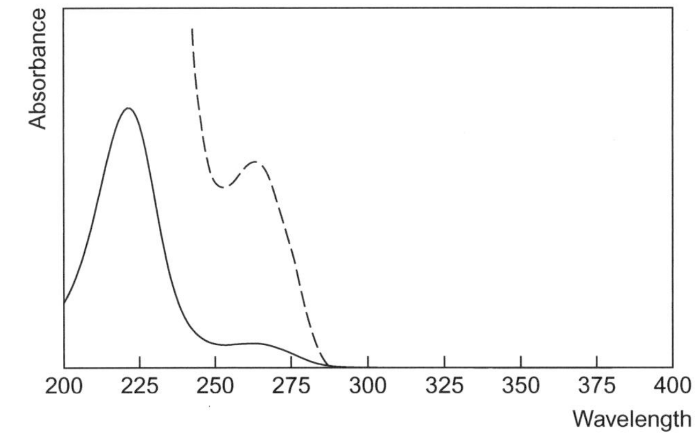

Infra-red Spectrum. Principal peaks at wavenumbers 1553, 1621, 1289, 797, 1103, 1129 cm^{-1} (KBr disk).

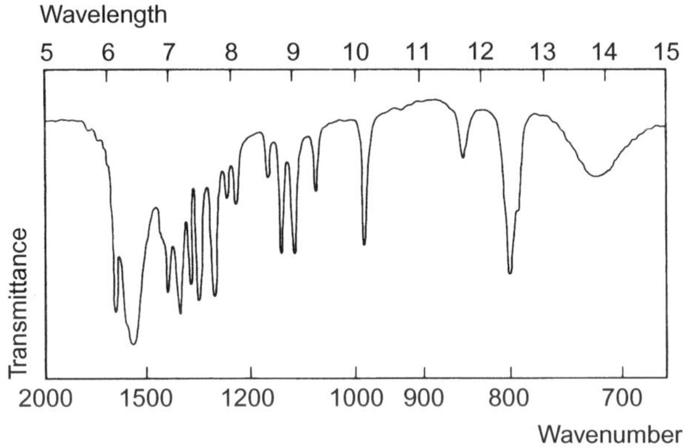

Mass Spectrum. Principal ions at *m/z* 201, 44, 186, 68, 173, 96, 158, 203.

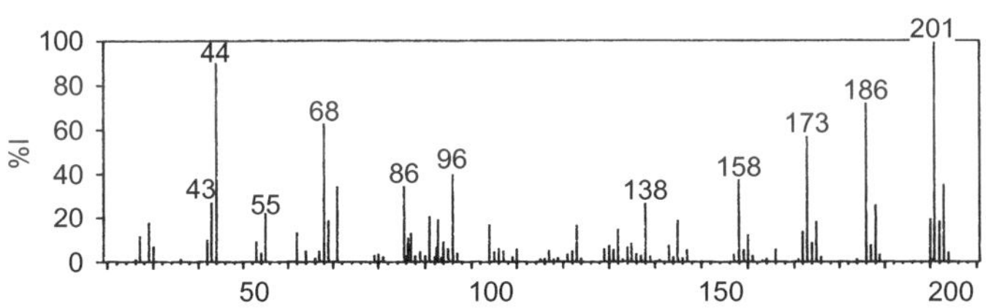

Simvastatin

HMG-CoA reductase inhibitor/ Antihyperlipidaemic

Synonyms. L-644128-000U; MK-733; Synvinolin; Velastatin.
Proprietary names. Denan; Lipex; Liponorm; Lipovas; Lodalès; Simovil; Sinvacor; Sivastin; Zocor; Zocord.
2,2-Dimethylbutanoic acid (1*S*,3*R*,7*S*,8*S*,8a*R*)-1,2,3,7,8,8a-hexahydro-3,7-dimethyl-8-[2-[(2*R*,4*R*)-tetrahydro-4-hydroxy-6-oxo-2*H*-pyran-2-yl]ethyl]-1-naphthalenyl ester
$C_{25}H_{38}O_5 = 418.6$
CAS—*79902-63-9*

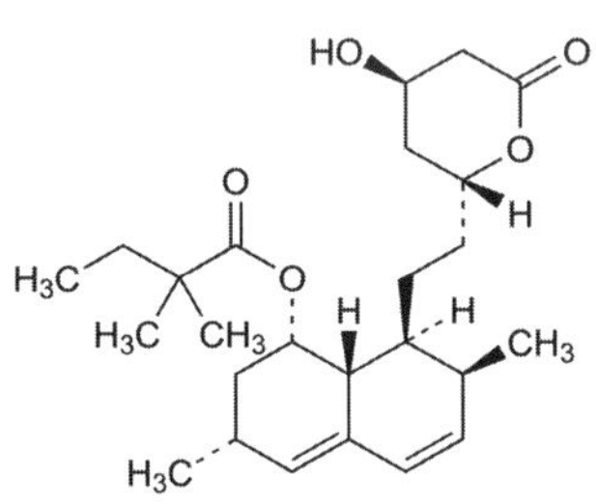

A white crystalline powder. M. p. 135° to 138°. It is insoluble in water (0.03 g/L), *n*-hexane (0.15 g/L) and hydrochloric acid (0.1 M) (0.06 g/L); soluble in chloroform (610 g/L), dimethyl sulfoxide (540 g/L), methanol (200 g/L), ethanol (160 g/L), polyethylene glycol (70 g/L), sodium hydroxide (0.1 M) (70 g/L) and propylene glycol (30 g/L).

Partition Coefficient. Log *P* (octanol/water), 4.68.

Thin-layer Chromatography. System TE—Rf 68; system TF—Rf 44.

Gas Chromatography. Column: methyl silicone (HP1, 0.2 mm i.d., 0.33 μm film thickness). Column temperature: 280°. Carrier gas: helium, flow rate 0.9 mL/min. MS detection. RI: 3158. [T. Mills and J. C. Roberson, *Instrumental Data for Drug Analysis*, CRC Press, *2nd Edn.*, *6*, 224–225].

High Performance Liquid Chromatography. System HX—RI 814.

Column: ODS (Hypersil, 100 × 4.6 mm i.d., 5 μm). Mobile phase: methanol, flow rate 0.5 mL/min. UV diode array detection. Retention time: 3.4 min [T. Mills and J. C. Roberson, *Instrumental Data for Drug Analysis*, CRC Press, *2nd Edn.*, *6*, 224–225].

Column: (analytical) ODS (Hypersil, 250 × 4.6 mm i.d., 5 μm); (guard) Pelliguard precolumn (20 mm). Mobile phase: sodium dihydrogen phosphate (25 mM, pH 4.5):acetonitrile (35:65), flow rate 1.5 mL/min. UV detection (λ = 238 nm). Retention times: simvastatin, 7.2 min; simvastatin β,δ-dihydroxyacid, 3.6 min [G. Carlucci *et al.*, *J. Pharm. Biomed. Anal.*, 1992, *10*, 693–697].

Ultraviolet Spectrum. Acetonitrile—231, 238, 247 nm; basic—229, 237, 246 nm.

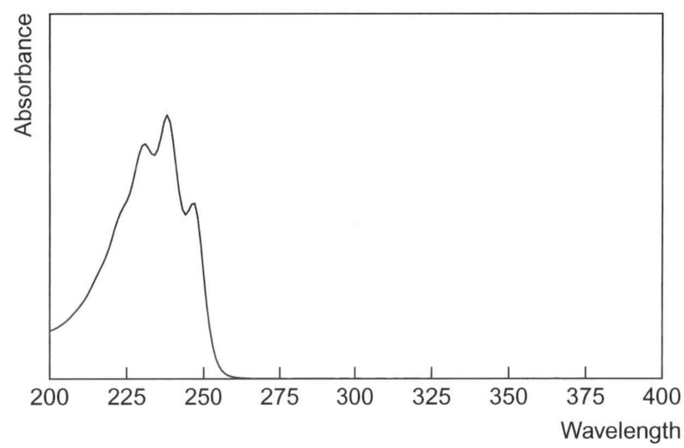

Infra-red Spectrum. Principal peaks at wavenumber 1718, 1459, 1389, 1267 cm^{-1}.

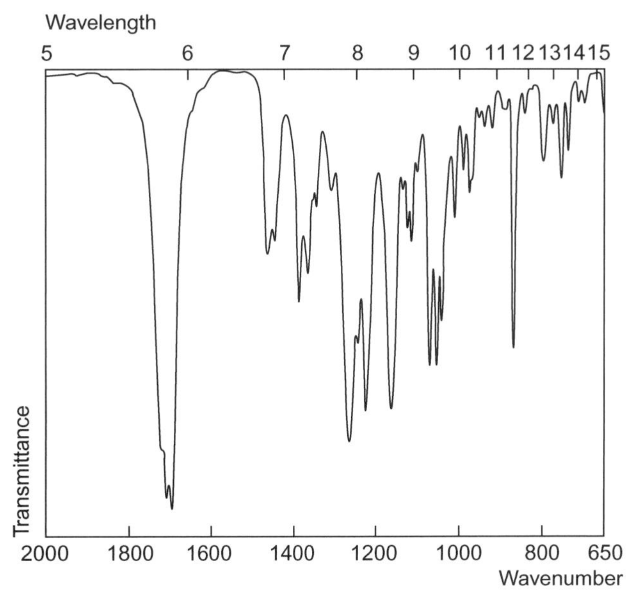

Mass Spectrum. Principal ions at *m/z* 159, 157, 43, 198, 71, 172, 143, 105.

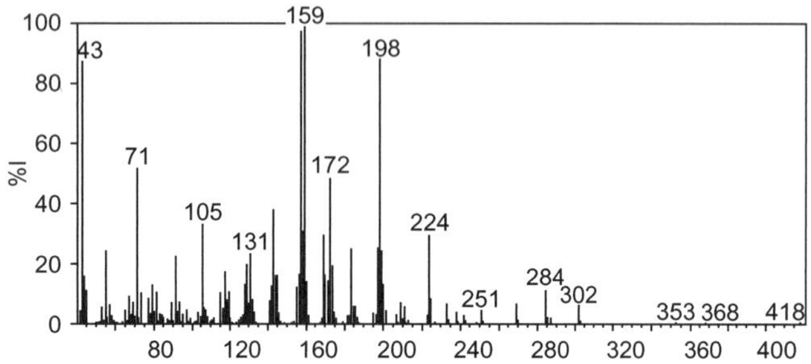

Quantification.

Gas chromatography–mass spectrometry. In plasma: limit of detection 0.1 μg/L—A. Scoppola et al., *J. Lipid Res.*, 1991, *32*(6), 1057–1060. In plasma: limit of quantification 0.1 μg/L—T. Takano *et al.*, *Biomed. Env. Mass Spectrom.*, 1990, *19(9)*, 577.

High performance liquid chromatography. In plasma: limit of quantification 0.1 μg/L. Fluorescence detection (λ_{ex} = 360 nm, λ_{em} = 430 nm)—H. Ochiai *et al.*, *J. Chromatogr. B Biomed. Sci. Appl.*, 1997, *694*, 211–217.

Disposition in the Body. Simvastatin is a pharmacologically inactive pro-drug which is rapidly metabolised mainly to simvastatin β-hydroxy acid analogue (with maximum concentrations being reached within 1.3 to 2.4 h after dosing) which is an inhibitor of HMC-CoA reductase. Other metabolites include 3-hydroxy-, 3-hydroxy-3-methyl-, and 3-oxomethylene derivatives and analogues of 6-hydroxymethyl- and 6-carboxylic acid of which the chiral centre at position 6 has been inverted (these are the biliary metabolites). The drug and its metabolites are excreted in urine (13%) and faeces (60%) which includes both the unabsorbed drug and drug excreted in bile.

Therapeutic concentration

12 healthy males, aged between 22 and 29 years, were administered with a single 40 mg dose of simvastatin. The peak plasma concentration of the active inhibitors was 10.3 μg (equivalent)/L and total inhibitors 34.5 μg (equivalent)/L, reached in 2.5 and 2.3 h, respectively [P. J. Pentikeinen *et al.*, *J. Clin. Pharmacol.*, 1992, *32*, 136–140].

Bioavailability. β-hydroxyacid, 5%.

Half-life. Simvastatin, 2 h; β-hydroxyacid, 1.9 h.

Protein binding. Simvastatin, 98% and β-hydroxyacid, 94%.

Note. For a review of simvastatin, see G. L. Plosker and D. McTavish, *Drugs*, 1995, *50*, 334–363.

Dose. The usual daily dose is 10 to 80 mg.

Sirolimus

Immunosuppressant

Synonyms. AY-22989; AY-022989; NSC 226080; Rapamycin; RPM; SILA 9268A; WY-090217.

Proprietary name. Rapamune

(3*S*,6*R*,7*E*,9*R*,10*R*,12*R*,14*S*,15*E*,17*E*,19*E*,21*S*,23*S*,26*R*,27*R*,34a*S*)-9,10,12,13,14,21,22,23,24,25,26,27,32,33,34,34a-Hexadecahydro-9,27-dihydroxy-3-((1*R*)-2-((1*S*,3*R*,4*R*)-4-hydroxy-3-methoxycyclohexyl)-1-methylethyl)-10,21-dimethoxy-6,8,12,14,20,26-hexamethyl-23,27-epoxy-3*H*-pyrido[2,1-c][1,4]oxaazacyclohentriacontine-1,5,11,28,29-(4*H*,6*H*,31*H*)-pentone

$C_{51}H_{79}NO_{13}$ = 914.2

CAS—53123-88-9

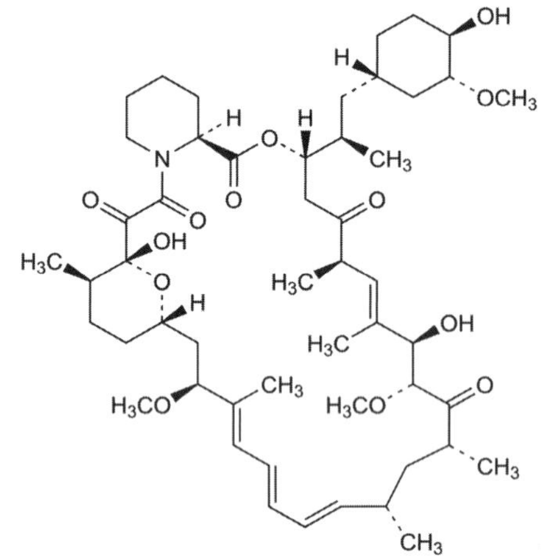

Colourless crystalline solid. M. p. 183° to 185°. Insoluble in water; soluble in ether, chloroform, acetone, methanol and dimethylformamide; very sparingly soluble in hexane and petroleum ether.

High Performance Liquid Chromatography. Column: BDS C_{18} (Hypersil, 100 × 3.0 mm i.d., 3 μm). Column temperature: 70°. Mobile phase: acetonitrile:methanol:water (38:34:28), flow rate 0.3 mL/min. UV detection (λ = 278 nm). Retention time: 8.4 min [J. O. Svensson *et al.*, *Ther. Drug Monit.*, 1997, *19(1)*, 112–116].

Column: C_{18} (Novapak, 150 × 2.1 mm i.d., 4 μm). Column temperature: 50°. Mobile phase: methanol:ammonium acetate buffer (50 mM, pH 5.1) (80:20), flow rate 0.2 mL/min. Internal standard: 32-*O*-desmethoxysirolimus. MS detection (ESI, SIM at *m/z* 931.8→864.6 for sirolimus; 901.8→834.4 for IS). Retention times: sirolimus, 7.8 min; IS, 8.4 min [P. J. Taylor and A. G. Johnson, *J. Chromatogr. B. Biomed. Sci. Appl.*, 1998, *718(2)*, 251–257].

Ultraviolet Spectrum. Aqueous acid—267, 277, 288 nm.

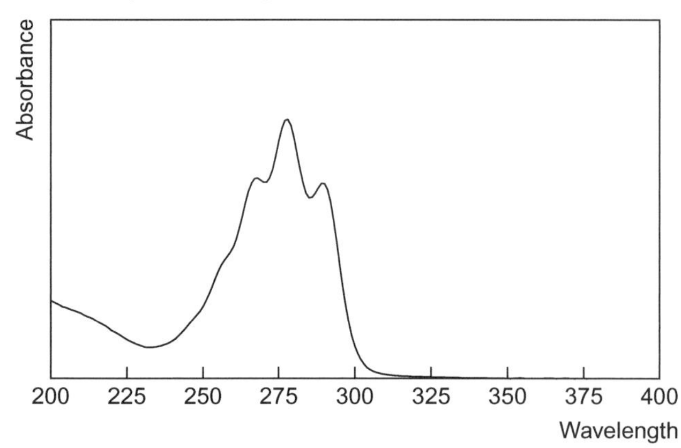

Quantification

High performance liquid chromatography. In blood: limit of quantification 0.25 μg/L, MS detection—P. J. Taylor *et al.*, *Ther. Drug Monit.*, 2000, *22(5)*, 608–612. In whole blood: limit of detection 2.5 μg/L. UV detection (λ = 278 nm)—S. Maleki *et al.*, *Clin. Ther.*, 2000, *22 (Suppl. B)*, B25–B37. In whole blood: limit of quantification 6.5 μg/L. UV detection (λ = 278 nm)—D. W. Holt *et al.*, *Clin. Ther.*, 2000, *22 (Suppl. B)*, B38–B48. In blood: limit of quantification is 0.2 μg/L, tandem MS detection—P. J. Taylor and A. G. Johnson, *J. Chromatogr. B. Biomed. Sci. Appl.*, 1998, *718(2)*, 251–257. In whole blood: limit of detection is 0.4 μg/L. UV detection (λ = 278 nm)—J. O. Svensson *et al.*, *Ther. Drug Monit.*, 1997, *19(1)*, 112–116.

Immunoassay. In whole blood: limit of detection is 1.0 μg/L—K. Jones *et al.*, *Clin. Ther.*, 2000, *22 (Suppl. B)*, B49–B61.

Disposition in the Body. Sirolimus is rapidly but incompletely absorbed (within 1 h); it is more slowly absorbed with a high-fat meal compared with those in the fasting state. Peak concentrations are reduced and the times taken to reach these levels are increased. Peak whole blood concentrations increase proportionally with the dose administered. Sirolimus is extensively distributed to a variety of tissues and organs. It is a substrate for both cytochrome P4503A4 and *p*-glycoprotein. It is metabolised in both the intestine and liver by *O*-demethylation and hydroxylation to 7 known metabolites including hydroxyl, demethyl and hydroxydemethyl derivatives. It is excreted mainly in faeces (90%) and a small amount in urine (2%).

Therapeutic concentration

30 patients treated with a stable renal transplant were administered 0.5, 1.0, 1.5, 2.5, 3.0, 3.5, 4.0, 5.0 and 6.5 mg/m^2 every 12 h for 13 days and a single dose on day 14. Each participant was treated with cyclosporin for at least 3 months beforehand and steady state therapeutic blood concentrations had been achieved. The steady state concentrations were 10.1, 20.4, 22.0, 40.5, 44.9, 112.0, 93.6, 110.0 and 210.0 µg/L for the doses, respectively. These concentrations were observed at 1.1, 0.8, 0.9, 2.7, 0.8, 1.3, 3.0, 1.0 and 0.7 h, respectively [J. J. Zimmerman and B. D. Kahan, *J. Clin. Pharmacol.*, 1997, *37*, 405–415].

16 patients, aged 24 to 63 years, who had received a renal transplant at least 6 months before inclusion in the study and diagnosed as clinically stable for at least 3 months before treatment participated in the study. After an overnight fast, all were administered either 3, 5, 10 or 15 mg/m^2 as an oral solution (5 mg/mL). Mean peak plasma concentrations were 1.00, 0.83, 2.93 and 3.23 µg/L for the 4 doses observed at 1.3, 3.7, 3.0, 2.3 h, respectively. The peak whole blood concentrations were 78.0, 46.3, 119.7 and 190.7 µg/L for the 3, 5, 10 and 15 mg/m^2 doses at 0.83, 2.67, 1.17 and 1.67 h, respectively [C. Brattstrom *et al.*, *Ther. Drug Monit.*, 1997, *19(4)*, 397–406].

Toxicity

Sirolimus toxicity is associated with thrombocytopenia, leucopenia, anaemia and hyperlipidaemia and whole blood concentrations of >15 µg/L increase this risk. Concentrations of <6 µg/L are associated with acute rejection [H. U. Meier-Kriesche and B. Kaplan, *Clin. Ther.*, 2000, *22 (Suppl. B)*, B93–B100].

Bioavailability. Approx. 15%.

Half-life. Mean, 57 h (range, 44 to 87 h).

Volume of distribution. Steady state, mean, 23 L/kg (healthy); 11.2 L/kg (patients treated by renal transplant).

Clearance. Mean, 278 mL/h/kg (healthy); 199.5 mL/h/kg (patients with renal transplant).

Distribution in blood. Whole blood: plasma concentration ratio is 49.1.

Protein binding. 92%, mainly to albumin.

Dose. 2 mg daily.

Sodium Cromoglicate

Anti-allergic

Synonyms. Cromolyn Sodium; Disodium Cromoglicate; Sodium Cromoglycate; FPL-670; DSCG.

Proprietary names. Acromax; Allercrom; Brol-eze; Clariteyes; Colimune; Cromabak; Cromogen; Cromo(l); Cromolyn; Flenid; Frenal; Gastrocrom; Glinor; Hay-Crom; Intal; Lecrolyn; Lomudal; Lomusol; Nalcrom; Nasalcrom; Opticrom; Rynacrom; Vividrin.

Disodium-5,5′-[(2-Hydroxy-1,3-propanediyl)bis(oxy)]bis[4-oxo-4*H*-1-benzopyran-2-carboxylate]

$C_{23}H_{14}Na_2O_{11}$ = 512.3

CAS—16110-51-3 (cromoglycic acid); 15826-37-6 (disodium salt)

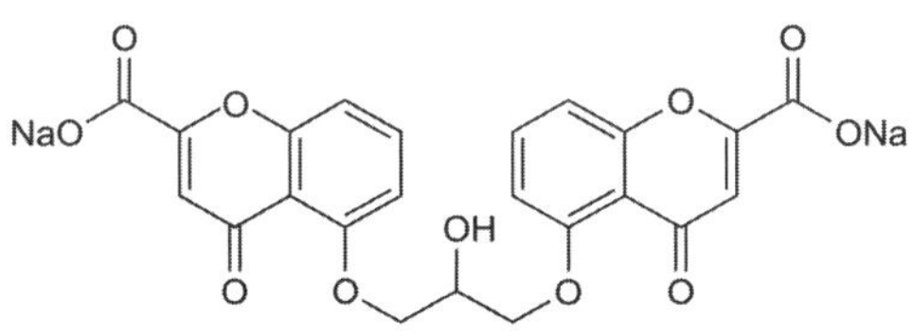

A white, hygroscopic, crystalline powder. M.p. 241° to 242°, with decomposition (cromoglycic acid).

Soluble 1 in 20 of water; practically insoluble in ethanol, ether and chloroform.

Dissociation Constant. Cromoglycic acid: pK_a 2.5 (20°).

Partition Coefficient. Cromoglycic acid: Log *P* (octanol/water), 1.9.

Colour Tests. Copper sulfate (Method 2)—blue (1 to 2 min); Mandelin's test—red; Marquis test—yellow; Methanolic potassium hydroxide—yellow; Sulfuric acid—yellow.

Thin-layer Chromatography. Cromoglycic acid: System TAD—Rf 00; system TD—Rf 00; system TE—Rf 00; system TF—Rf 00.

Ultraviolet Spectrum. Phosphate buffer (pH 7.4)—238 nm (A_1^1 = 600b), 326 nm (A_1^1 = 164a).

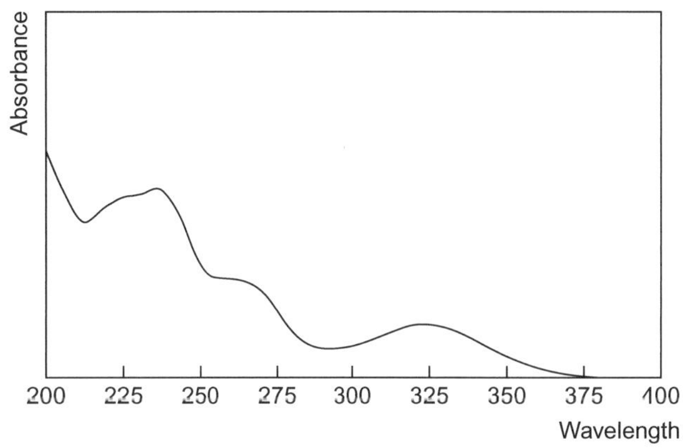

Infra-red Spectrum. Principal peaks at wavenumbers 1635, 1305, 1264, 805, 1069, 1047 cm^{-1} (KBr disk).

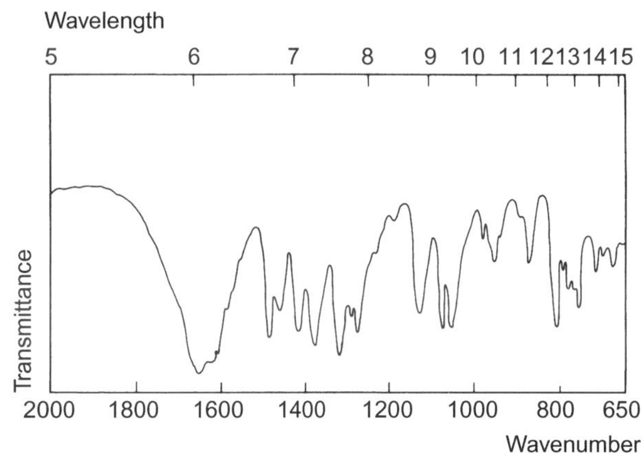

Mass Spectrum. Principal ions at *m/z* 44, 206, 162, 108, 51, 207, 201, 178 (cromoglycic acid).

Quantification

Spectrofluorimetry. In plasma: limit of detection 100 µg/L—G. F. Moss *et al.*, *Toxicol. Appl. Pharmacol.*, 1971, *20*, 147–156.

High performance liquid chromatography. In urine: limit of detection 50 µg/L, UV detection—J. J. Gardner, *J. Chromatogr.*, 1984, *305*; *Biomed. Appl.*, *30*, 228–232. In urine: limit of detection 250 µg/L, UV detection—O. A. Aswania *et al.*, *J. Chromatogr. B*, *Biomed. Sci. Appl.*, 1997, *690*, 373–378. In urine: fluorescence detection—K. Mawatari *et al.*, *Analyst*, 1997, *122*, 715–717.

High performance liquid chromatography–mass spectrometry. In plasma: limit of detection 0.1 µg/L—M. L. Ozou *et al.*, *J. Chromatogr. B*, *Biomed. Sci. Appl.*, 2001, *765*, 179–185.

Polarography. In urine: limit of detection 500 µg/L—A. G. Fogg and N. Fayad, *Anal. Chim. Acta*, 1978, *102*, 205–210.

Disposition in the Body. Sodium cromoglicate is poorly absorbed after oral or subcutaneous administration. After inhalation most of a dose is swallowed with less than 10% reaching the lungs, from where it is rapidly absorbed; the amount absorbed after inhalation is dependent on particle size, smaller particles being absorbed better than large ones. It does not appear to be metabolised. Up to about 3% of an inhaled dose is excreted unchanged in the urine in 24 h and up to about 87% is eliminated unchanged in the faeces in 3 days. After oral administration less than 1% is excreted in the urine, and after an intravenous dose about 50% is excreted in the urine and 50% is eliminated in the faeces.

Therapeutic concentration

Following inhalation of a ^{14}C-labelled 20-mg dose by 12 asthmatic subjects, peak plasma concentrations of 0.006 to 0.012 mg/L (mean 0.009) were attained in 15 min. [S. R. Walker *et al.*, *J. Pharm. Pharmacol.*, 1972, *24*, 525–531].

After inhalation of a single 60 mg dose by 3 subjects, peak plasma concentrations of about 0.2 to 0.3 mg/L were reported in 10 to 15 min. [G. F. Moss *et al.*, *Toxicol. Appl. Pharmacol.*, 1971, *20*, 147–156].

Half-life. Plasma half-life, about 1 to 1.5 h.

Clearance. Plasma clearance, about 8 mL/min/kg.

Protein binding. In plasma, about 60 to 70%.

Dose. 20 mg inhaled as a dry powder 4 times daily; 800 mg daily, by mouth.

Solanidine

Alkaloid

Synonym. Solatubine
(3*β*)-Solanid-5-en-ol
$C_{27}H_{43}NO$=397.6
CAS—80-78-4

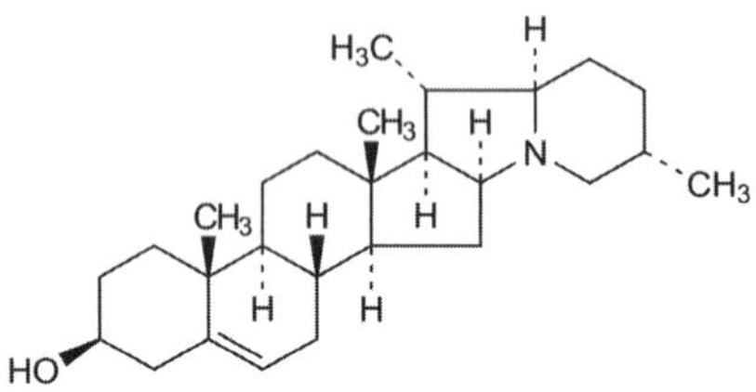

An alkaloid present in various species of *Solanum* (Solanaceae). It is the aglycone of solanine.
A white crystalline powder. M.p. 218° to 219°, with decomposition.
Practically insoluble in water and ether; slightly soluble in ethanol; freely soluble in chloroform; soluble in dilute acids.

Partition Coefficient. Log *P* (octanol/water), 7.3.

Colour Tests. Mandelin's test—orange→violet→blue; Marquis test—violet.

Thin-layer Chromatography. System TA—Rf 68.

Quantification

High performance liquid chromatography. In serum: solanidine and glycoalkaloids, limit of detection 0.3 µg/L, UV detection—K. E. Hellenas *et al.*, *J. Chromatogr.*, 1992, *573*, 69–78.

Radioimmunoassay. In plasma: limit of detection 200 ng/L—J. A. Matthew *et al.*, *Food Chem. Toxicol.*, 1983, *21*, 637–640.

Solanine

Alkaloid

Synonym. Solatunine
$C_{45}H_{73}NO_{15}$=868.1
CAS—20562-02-1

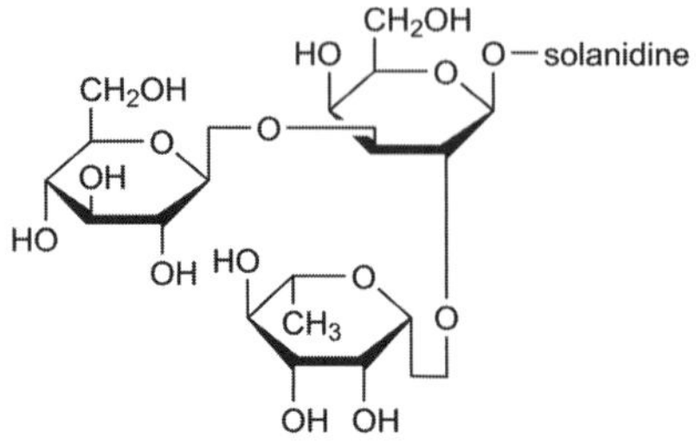

A glycoalkaloid present in various species of *Solanum*, particularly *S. tuberosum* (Solanaceae).
A white crystalline powder which decomposes at about 285°.
Practically insoluble in water, chloroform and ether; soluble in hot ethanol, dilute acids and amyl alcohol.

Dissociation Constant. pK_a 6.65 (15°).

Partition Coefficient. Log *P* (octanol/water), 2.0.

Colour Tests. Mandelin's test—orange→violet→blue; Marquis test—yellow→violet.

Thin-layer Chromatography. System TA—Rf 52. (Marquis reagent, positive.)

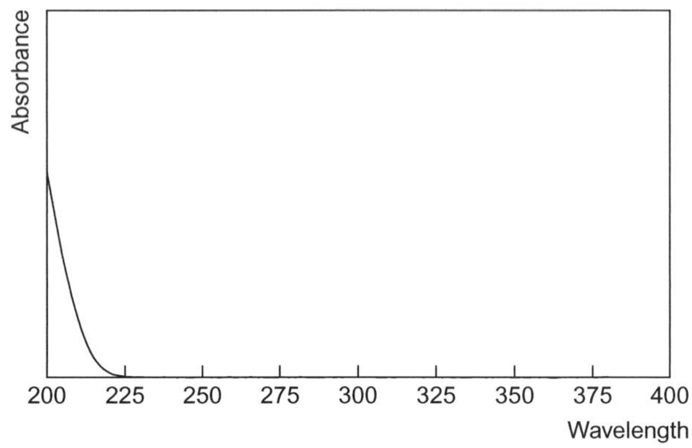

Quantification. See under Solanidine.

Somatropin

Growth Stimulant

Synonyms. CB-311; hGH; Human growth hormone; LY-137998; Somatotropin.
Proprietary names. Asellacrin; Crescormon; Genotropin; Grorm; Humatrope; Nanormon; Norditropin; Nutropin; Saizen; Umatrope; Zomacton.
Adenohypophyseal growth hormone
$C_{990}H_{1529}N_{263}O_{299}S_7$=22124.1
CAS—12629-01-5
A white or almost white powder.

High Performance Liquid Chromatography. Column: G3000SW (TSK, 300 × 21.5 mm). Mobile phase: sodium borate (20 mM) with EDTA (1.44 mM), pH 7.3 with hydrochloric acid, flow rate 0.5 mL/min. UV detection (λ = 280 nm). Retention times: dimer, 13.3 min; monomer, 14.5 min [J. P. Chang *et al.*, *J. Chromatogr. A*, 1996, *736*, 97–104].

Column: Vydac 218TP104. Mobile phase: A-acetonitrile:trifluoroacetic acid (0.1%):water (10.5:70:19.5); B-acetonitrile:trifluoroacetic acid (0.1%):water 21:70:9. Gradient elution: (A:B) (100:0) to (0:100) in 30 min, flow rate 1 mL/min. UV detection (λ = 214 nm). Retention times: monomer, 22.5 min; dimer, 25.0 min [J. P. Chang *et al.*, *J. Chromatogr. A*, 1996, *736*, 97–104].

Disposition in the Body. Somatropin is well absorbed after subcutaneous or intramuscular injection. It is metabolised in the liver and the kidney and excreted in bile and a little in urine. Maximum plasma concentrations are reached within 2 to 6 h.

Therapeutic concentration

Adult male volunteers administered with 100 µg/kg somatropin reached peak serum concentrations of approximately 55 µg/L after infusion/injection. [Data as supplied by Eli Lilly & Company Ltd.]

Toxicity. Acromegaly reported. Results in premature death.

Bioavailability. 60 to 80%.

Half-life. After intravenous administration: 20 to 30 min; after intramuscular or subcutaneous administration: 3 to 5 h due to prolonged release from the injection site.

Volume of distribution. At steady state, 50 mL/kg body weight.

Clearance After intravenous administration, 116 to 174 mL/h/kg.

Protein binding. 20%.

Dose. In paediatric patients: recommended dose is 25 to 35 µg/kg bodyweight daily by subcutaneous or intramuscular injection. In adults: 6 µg/kg bodyweight daily as subcutaneous injection. This can be increased to 12 μg/kg daily as required. Patients with Turner's Syndrome and paediatric patients with chronic renal insufficiency: 45 to 50 μg/kg daily by subcutaneous administration.

Sorbic Acid

Preservative

Proprietary name. Sorbistat
(2*E*,4*E*)-2,4-Hexadienoic acid
$C_6H_8O_2$=112.1
CAS—110-44-1; 22500-92-1

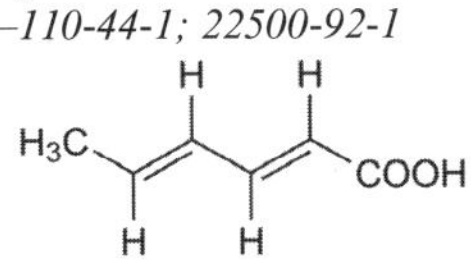

A white or creamy-white crystalline powder. M.p. about 134°.
Soluble 1 in 1000 of water, 1 in 10 of ethanol, 1 in 15 of chloroform, 1 in 30 of ether, 1 in 8 of methanol and 1 in 19 of propylene glycol.
Caution. Sorbic acid is irritant to the eyes and possibly also to the skin.

Potassium Sorbate

Proprietary name. Sorbistat-K
$C_6H_7KO_2$=150.2
CAS—590-00-1; 24634-61-5
White or creamy-white crystals or powder. M.p. about 270°, with decomposition.
Soluble 1 in 4.5 of water and 1 in 35 of ethanol; very slightly soluble in acetone, chloroform and ether; soluble in propylene glycol.

Dissociation Constant. pK_a 4.8.

Partition Coefficient. Log *P* (octanol/water), 1.3.

Ultraviolet Spectrum. Aqueous acid—264 nm (A_1^1=2343a); aqueous alkali—254 nm (A_1^1=2211b).

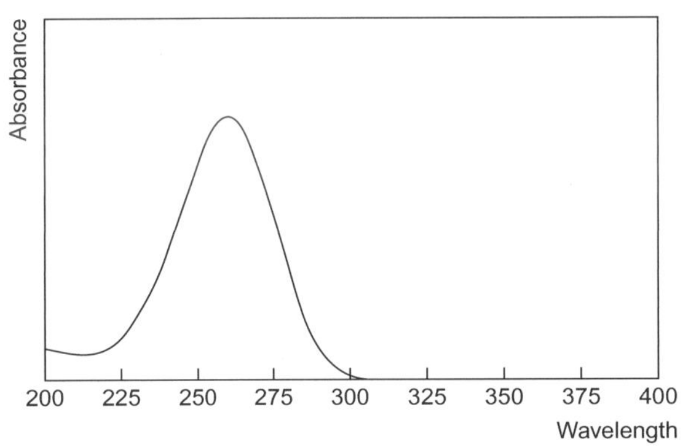

Infra-red Spectrum. Principal peaks at wavenumbers 1550, 1005, 1616, 1602, 1647, 882 cm^{-1} (potassium sorbate, KBr disk).

Quantification
Gas chromatography–mass spectrometry. In urine: limit of detection 0.7 μg/L—T. Renner *et al.*, *J. Chromatogr.*, 1999, *847*, 127–133.

Use. In concentrations of 0.1 to 0.2%.

Sotalol

Antihypertensive/Anti-arrhythmic/Antianginal

N-[4-[1-Hydroxy-2-[(1-methylethyl)amino]ethyl]phenyl]-methanesulfonamide
$C_{12}H_{20}N_2O_3S$=272.4
CAS—3930-20-9

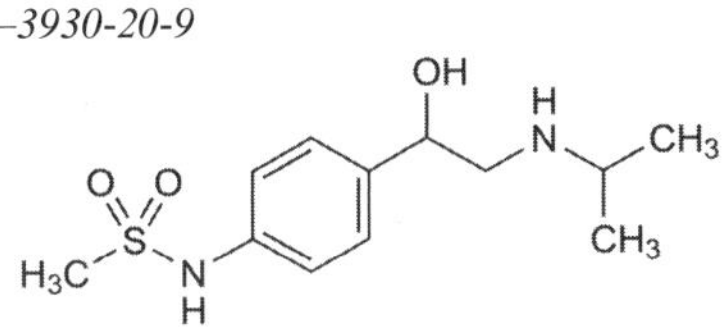

Crystals. M.p.about 207°.

Sotalol Hydrochloride

Proprietary names. Beta-Cardone; Cardol; CorSotalol; Darob; Dutacor; Favorex; Gilucor; Rentibloc; Rylosol; Rytmobeta; Sotab; Sotabet; Sotacor; Sotahexal; Sotalex; Sotalin; Sotamed; Sotamol; Sotaper; Sotapor; Sotaryt; Sotastad; Tachytalol.
$C_{12}H_{20}N_2O_3S,HCl$=308.8
CAS—959-24-0
An off-white to pale cream crystalline powder. M.p. 206° to 207°, with decomposition.
Freely soluble in water; sparingly soluble in chloroform.

Dissociation Constant. pK_a 8.2, 9.8.

Partition Coefficient. Log *P* (octanol/water), 0.2.

Colour Tests. Liebermann's test (100°)—brown; Mercurous nitrate—black.

Thin-layer Chromatography. System TA—Rf 53; system TAE—Rf 19; system TL—Rf 05; system TB—Rf 01; system TC—Rf 03; system TE—Rf 30.

Gas Chromatography. System GA—RI 2413; system GB—RI 2520.

High Performance Liquid Chromatography. System HA—*k* 1.2; system HAA—Retention time(s) 3.8 min; system HX—RI 226; system HZ—Retention time(s) 2.0 min.

Ultraviolet Spectrum. Aqueous acid—269 nm (A_1^1=16a); aqueous alkali—249 nm (A_1^1=552b).

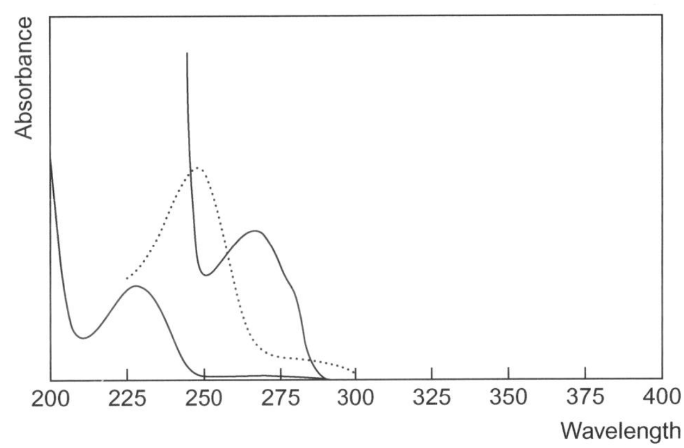

Infra-red Spectrum. Principal peaks at wavenumbers 1160, 992, 785, 1512, 1230, 1585 cm^{-1} (sotalol hydrochloride, KBr disk).

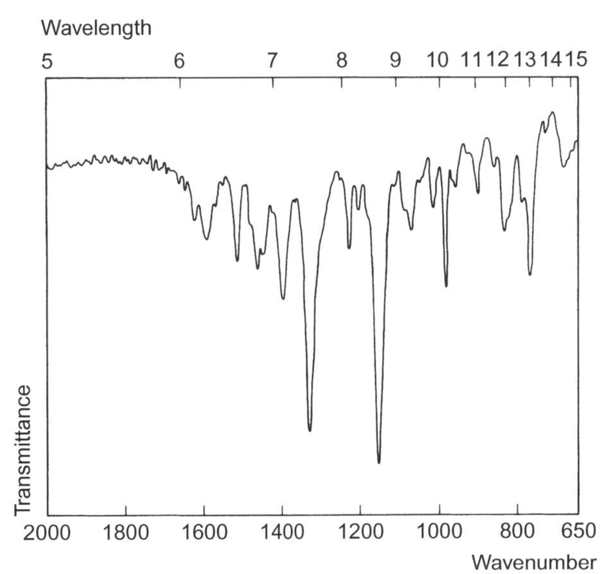

Mass Spectrum. Principal ions at *m*/*z* 72, 30, 43, 122, 73, 41, 106, 121.

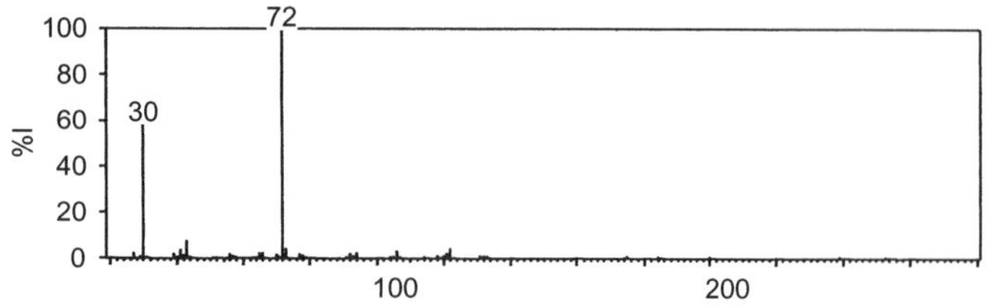

Quantification

High performance liquid chromatography. In plasma: limit of detection 20 μg/L, fluorescence detection—M. A. Lefebvre *et al.*, *J. Pharm. Sci.*, 1980, *69*, 1216–1217. In plasma or urine: sotalol enantiomers, limit of detection 12.5 μg/L, fluorescence detection—C. Fiset *et al.*, *J. Chromatogr.*, 1993, *612*, 231–237; L. C. da Cunha *et al.*, *Boll. Chim. Farm.*, 2001, *140*, 448–454. In plasma or urine: sotalol enantiomers, limits of detection 22 μg/L and 220 μg/L respectively, UV detection—T. Shimizu *et al.*, *J. Chromatogr.*, 1995, *674*; *B Biomed. Appl.*, 77–83. In plasma: sotalol enantiomers, fluorescence detection—W. D. Hooper and P. V. Baker, *J. Chromatogr.*, 1995, *672*; *Biomed. Appl.*, 89–96. In plasma: limit of detection 90 μg/L, fluorescence detection—S. Laer *et al.*, *J. Chromatogr.*, 2001, *753*; *B Biomed. Appl.*, 421–425. In plasma: racemic sotalol, limit of detection 20 μg/L, fluorescence detection—S. R. Papini *et al.*, *Braz. J. Med. Biol. Res.*, 2000, *33*, 199–204. In cardiac tissue, blood or plasma: limit of detection in tissue 0.27 μg/g, UV detection—S. Laer *et al.*, *J. Chromatogr.*, 1996, *681*; *B Biomed. Appl.*, 291–298.

Disposition in the Body. Sotalol is almost completely absorbed after oral administration. It is excreted almost entirely in the urine as unchanged drug, 50 to 80% of a dose being excreted in 24 h. Less than 10% is eliminated in the faeces.

Therapeutic concentration

A single oral dose of 160 mg given to 8 subjects produced peak plasma concentrations of 1.1 to 1.4 mg/L in about 3 h. [M. Anttila *et al.*, *Acta Pharmacol.Toxicol.*, 1976, *39*, 118–128].

Following daily oral doses of 400 mg for 5 days to 5 subjects, a mean plasma concentration of 6 mg/L was reported 3 h after the last dose. [D. G. McDevitt and R. G. Shanks, *Br. J. Clin. Pharmacol.*, 1977, *4*, 153–156].

Toxicity

A man ingested about 3 g of sotalol and subsequently died; the following postmortem concentrations were reported: blood 40 mg/L, brain 0.59 μg/g, heart 42.7 μg/g, kidney 116 μg/g, liver 88 μg/g, lung 59.7 μg/g, urine 416 mg/L. [M. Montagna and A. Groppi, *Arch. Toxicol.*, 1980, *43*, 221–226].

Postmortem tissue concentrations in a woman who ingested 14.4 g of sotalol (and 50 mg triazolam) were: plasma 40 mg/L, brain 11.5 μg/g, heart 104.4 μg/g, lung 242.2 μg/g, liver 102.6 μg/g, kidney 103.2 μg/g, muscle 352.2 μg/g, bile 37.1 mg/L; the plasma sotalol concentration at admission had been 65 mg/L. [D. Perrot *et al.*, *J. Toxicol. Clin. Toxicol.*, 1988, *26*, 389–396].

A 37-year-old man who took 11.2 g of sotalol in a suicide attempt had serum concentrations of 20.6 mg/L after 3 h and 1.8 mg/L after 59 h. [C. G. Gustavsson *et al.*, *Ann. Pharmacother.*, 1997, *31*, 856–859].

Bioavailability. About 90%.

Half-life. Plasma half-life, 10 to 17 h, increased in renal insufficiency and in elderly subjects.

Volume of distribution. About 1 to 2 L/kg.

Clearance. Plasma clearance, about 1 to 2 mL/min/kg.

Protein binding. In plasma, not significantly bound.

Dose. Usually 120 to 600 mg of sotalol hydrochloride daily.

Sparteine

Treatment of Cardiac Insufficiency

Synonyms. Lupinidine; (−)-Sparteine; *l*-Sparteine.
[7*S*-(7α,7aα,14α,14aβ)]-Dodecahydro-7,14-methano-2*H*,6*H*-dipyrido-[1,2-a:1′,2′-e][1,5]diazocine
$C_{15}H_{26}N_2$=234.4
CAS—90-39-1

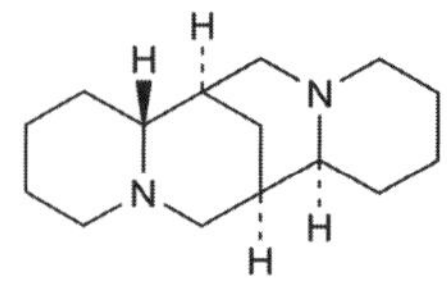

A dibasic alkaloid obtained from scoparium, the dried tops of broom, *Sarothamnus scoparius* (= *Cytisus scoparius*) (Leguminosae).
A viscous oily liquid.
Soluble 1 in 325 of water; very soluble in ethanol, chloroform and ether.

Sparteine Sulfate

Synonyms. Sparteine Sulphate; Sparteinum Sulfuricum; Sulfato de Esparteina.
Proprietary names. Depasan; Tocosamine.
$C_{15}H_{26}N_2,H_2SO_4,5H_2O$=422.5
CAS—299-39-8 (anhydrous); 6160-12-9 (pentahydrate)
Colourless crystals or white crystalline granules or powder which decompose at 136°.
Soluble 1 in about 1 of water and 1 in 3 of ethanol; practically insoluble in chloroform and ether.

Partition Coefficient. Log *P* (octanol/water), 2.7.

Thin-layer Chromatography. System TA—Rf 05; system TAE—Rf 04; system TAF—Rf 10; system TL—Rf 05; system TB—Rf 67; system TC—Rf 03; system TE—Rf 40; system TAJ—Rf 00; system TAK—Rf 00; system TAL—Rf 27. (Acidified iodoplatinate solution, positive.)

Gas Chromatography. System GA—RI 1801.

Ultraviolet Spectrum. No significant absorption, 230 to 360 nm.

Infra-red Spectrum. Principal peaks at wavenumbers 1118, 1070, 1045, 980, 962, 1015 cm^{-1} (sparteine sulfate, KBr disk).

Mass Spectrum. Principal ions at *m/z* 98, 137, 97, 136, 41, 193, 84, 110.

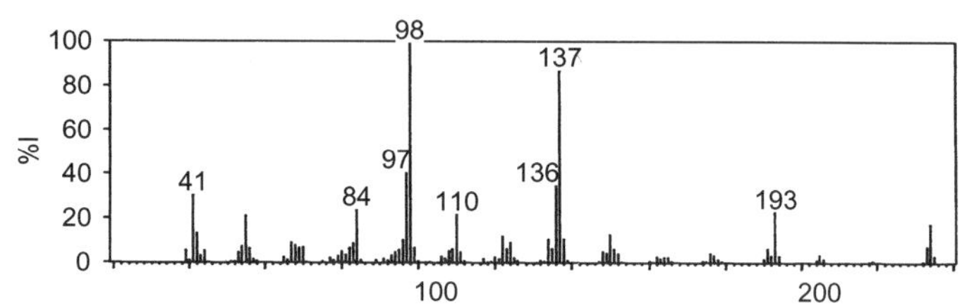

Quantification

Gas chromatography. In urine: sparteine and metabolites, limit of detection 50 μg/L, FID—M. Eichelbaum *et al.*, *Eur. J. Clin. Pharmacol.*, 1979, *16*, 183–187. In plasma: sparteine and metabolites, limit of detection 30 μg/L, FID—M. Eichelbaum *et al.*, *Eur. J. Clin. Pharmacol.*, 1979, *16*, 189–194. In urine: sparteine metabolites—T. Inaba *et al.*, *Br. J. Clin. Pharmacol.*, 1986, *21*, 473–480. In biological fluids: NPD—P. Kintz *et al.*, *Methods Find. Exp. Clin. Pharmacol.*, 1989, *11*, 115–118.

High performance liquid chromatography. In urine: sparteine and dehydro metabolites, electrochemical detection—J. Moncrieff, *J. Chromatogr.*, 1990, *529*, 194–200.

Disposition in the Body. Sparteine is metabolised by N-oxidation followed by rearrangement to 2- and 5-dehydrosparteine. About 5% of the population are non-metabolisers (greater than 90% of a dose excreted in the urine unchanged in 24 h). In metabolisers, about 55% of a dose is excreted in the urine in 24 h, about 30% of the dose as unchanged drug, 7% as 5-dehydrosparteine and 18% as 2-dehydrosparteine.

Half-life. Plasma half-life, about 3 h in metabolisers and 7 h in non-metabolisers.

Dose. Sparteine sulfate has been given intramuscularly in a dose of 150 mg.

Spiramycin

Antibiotic

Synonyms. Espiramicina; Spiramycinum; RP-5337.
Proprietary names. Dicorvin; Provamicina; Rovamycin(e); Rovamicina; Selectomycin.

A mixture of basic antimicrobial substances produced by the growth of *Streptomyces ambofaciens* and consisting of Spiramycin I, $C_{43}H_{74}N_2O_{14}$=843.1 (about 63%), Spiramycin II, $C_{45}H_{76}N_2O_{15}$=885.1 (about 24%) and Spiramycin III, $C_{46}H_{78}N_2O_{15}$=899.1 (about 13%).

Note. The stated molecular formulae for the spiramycins may vary.
CAS—8025-81-8

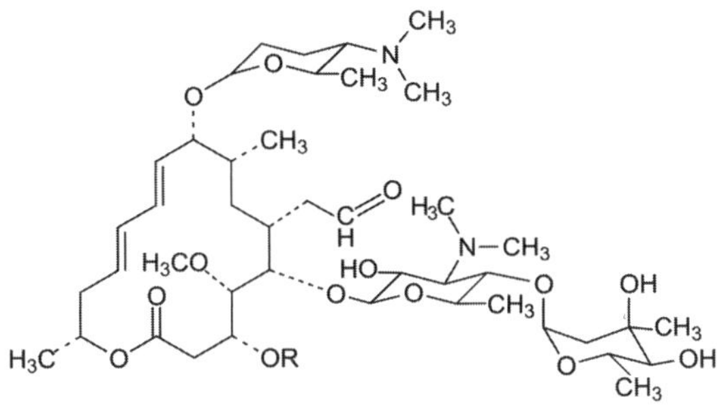

Spiramycin I R = H
Spiramycin II R = $COCH_3$
Spiramycin III R = $COCH_2CH_3$

A white or slightly yellowish amorphous powder.
Soluble 1 in 50 of water; very soluble in ethanol, methanol, acetone and chloroform.

Dissociation Constant. pK_a 8.0.

Colour Tests. Mandelin's test—orange-brown; Marquis test—orange.

Thin-layer Chromatography. System TA—Rf 42; system TAE—Rf 46. (Acidified potassium permanganate solution, positive.)

Ultraviolet Spectrum. Aqueous acid—233 nm (A_1^1=160b). No alkaline shift.

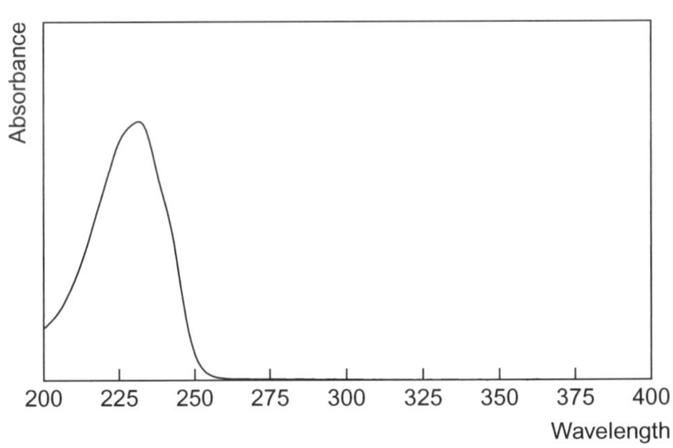

Infra-red Spectrum. Principal peaks at wavenumbers 1052, 1163, 1122, 994, 1016, 1730 cm^{-1} (KBr disk).

Quantification
High performance liquid chromatography. In plasma—J. Dow *et al., J. Chromatogr.*, 1985, *344*, 275–283. In plasma or vitreous: limit of detection 200 µg/L, UV detection—D. Carlhant *et al., Biomed. Chromatogr.*, 1989, *3*, 1–4.

Dose. 2 to 4 g daily.

Spirapril

Antihypertensive

(8*S*)-7-[(2*S*)-2-[[(1*S*)-1-(Ethoxycarbonyl)-3-phenylpropyl]amino]-1-oxopropyl]-1,4-dithia-7-azaspiro[4.4]nonane-8-carboxylic acid
$C_{22}H_{30}N_2O_5S_2$=466.6
CAS—83647-97-6

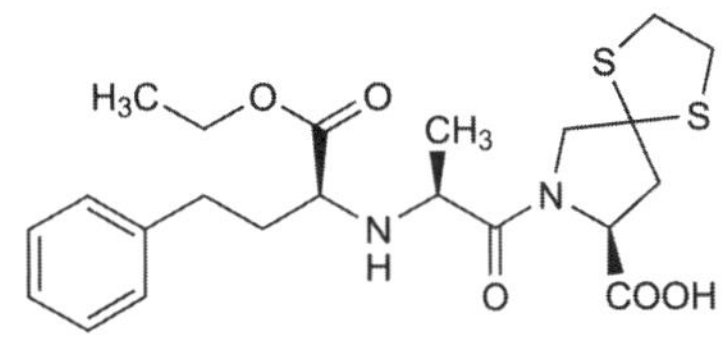

White foam (hemihydrate).

Spiraprilat
Synonyms. Spiraprilic acid; Sch-33861.
$C_{20}H_{26}N_2O_5S_2$=438.6
CAS—83602-05-5
White foam (hemihydrate), M.p. 163° to 165°.

Spirapril Hydrochloride
Synonyms. Sch-33844; TI-211-950.
Proprietary names. Cardiopril; Quadropril; Renormax, Renpress, Sandopril; Setrilan.
$C_{22}H_{30}N_2O_5S_2$.HCl=503.1
CAS—94841-17-5
A white solid, M.p. 192° to 194° (dec).

Partition Coefficient. Log *P* (octanol/water), 3.89.

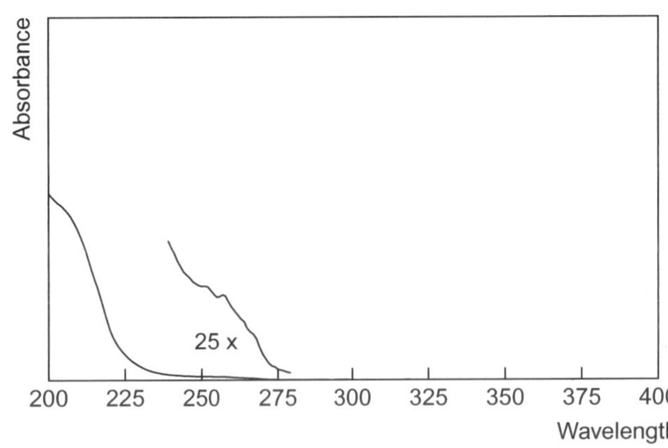

Disposition in the Body. After oral administration, spirapril is rapidly absorbed with peak plasma concentrations observed at 0.65 to 1.1 h. Elimination is mainly via conversion to the active metabolite spiraprilat (approximately 42%) and a small amount (3%) is eliminated unchanged in urine. The metabolite is observed at peak concentrations at 1.8 to 3 h. Sprilaprilat is excreted via both the renal (12.5%) and hepatobiliary routes; spiraprilat is not detected in plasma or urine.

Therapeutic concentration
18 patients with liver cirrhosis (mean age of 46 years old) or chronic, non-cirrhotic disease (41 years old) and 16 healthy male and female volunteers (mean age 29 years) were administered with a 25 mg dose after an overnight fast. The peak plasma concentrations for spirapril were 0.430 mg/L for the healthy individuals, 0.415 mg/L for those with liver cirrhosis and 0.289 mg/L for patients with non-cirrhotic disease. These were observed at 0.9, 1.1 and 0.8 h, respectively. Peak concentrations of the metabolite, spiraprilat, were 0.345 mg/L for the healthy volunteers, 0.203 mg/L for patients with liver cirrhosis and 0.257 mg/L for those with non-cirrhotic liver disease. These concentrations were reached at 2.0, 2.2 and 1.9 h, respectively [S. Krähenbühl *et al., Eur. J. Clin. Pharmacol.*, 1993, *45*, 247–253].

Bioavailability. After oral administration in healthy volunteers: spirapril, the mean bioavailability is 50% (range, 28 to 69%).

Half-life. Spirapril (oral administration in healthy volunteers) 0.9 to 1.6 h; spiraprilat (biphasic disposition) approximately 1 to 2 h and 30 to 40 h.

Volume of distribution. 57.5 L (healthy individuals); 48.5 L (patients with liver cirrhosis); 83.3 L (non-cirrhotic liver disease).

Clearance. Spirapril (total plasma clearance in healthy volunteers) 50 to 55 L/h; value of 117.8 L/h (renal 3.3 L/h; non-renal 114.5 L/h) has also been reported; spiraprilat 24 L/h.

Dose. The recommended dose is 6 mg daily.

Spironolactone

Diuretic

Synonyms. Espironolactona; Spirolactone.
Proprietary names. Aldactone; Aldopur; Altone; Deverol; Hexalacton; Laractone; Osiren; Spiractin; Spiretic; Spirix; Spiro(x); Spiroctan; Spirobene; Spirolone; Spironex; Spirospare; Spirotone. It is an ingredient of Aldactide, Aldactazide and Lasilactone.

Note. The name Aldactone is also used in some countries as a proprietary name for canrenoate potassium.
(7α,17α)-7-(Acetylthio)-17-hydroxy-3-oxopregn-4-ene-21-carboxylic acid γ-lactone
$C_{24}H_{32}O_4S = 416.6$
CAS—52-01-7

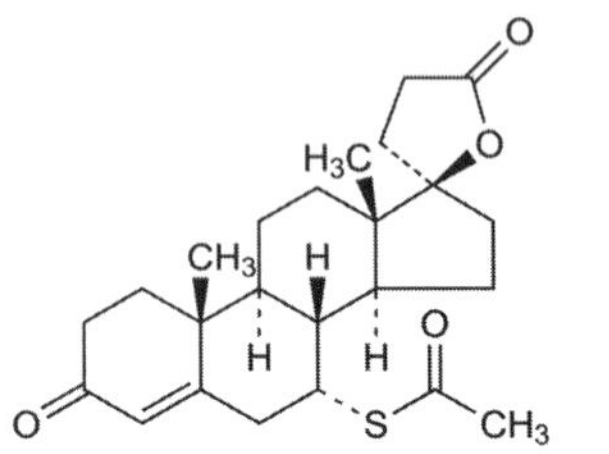

A white to light tan powder. M.p. 134° to 135°.
Practically insoluble in water; soluble 1 in 80 of ethanol, 1 in 3 of chloroform and 1 in 100 of ether; slightly soluble in methanol and fixed oils.

Partition Coefficient. Log *P* (octanol/water), 2.8.

Colour Tests. Palladium chloride—brown; Sulfuric acid—orange→yellow-green (yellow-green fluorescence under ultraviolet light).

Thin-layer Chromatography. System TD—Rf 66; system TE—Rf 78; system TF—Rf 51; system TAD—Rf 75; system TAE—Rf 84; system TAJ—Rf 73; system TAK—Rf 64; system TAL—Rf 96.

Gas Chromatography. System GA—spironolactone RI 3280; M (canrenone) RI 3250; M (canrenoic acid) RI 3100; M (canrenoic acid)-ME RI 3130.

High Performance Liquid Chromatography. System HX—RI 592; system HY—RI 539; system HZ—Retention time(s) 9.5 min; system HAA—Retention time(s) 20.7 min.

Ultraviolet Spectrum. Aqueous acid—242 nm ($A^1_1 = 464a$); aqueous alkali—247 nm ($A^1_1 = 405a$).

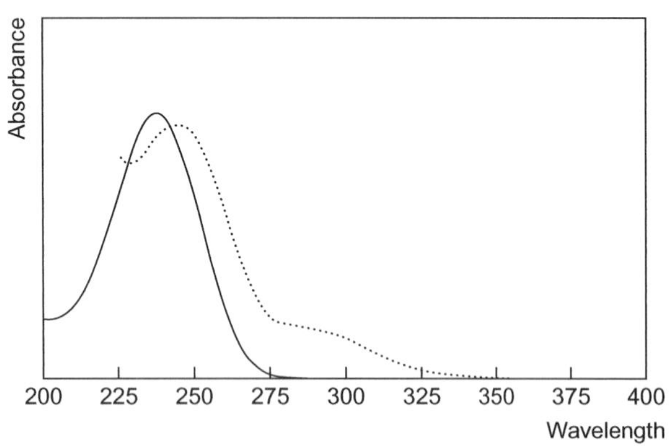

Infra-red Spectrum. Principal peaks at wavenumbers 1773, 1676, 1170, 1127, 1115, 1185 cm^{-1} (KBr disk).

Mass Spectrum. Principal ions at *m/z* 341, 43, 340, 374, 267, 107, 55, 342.

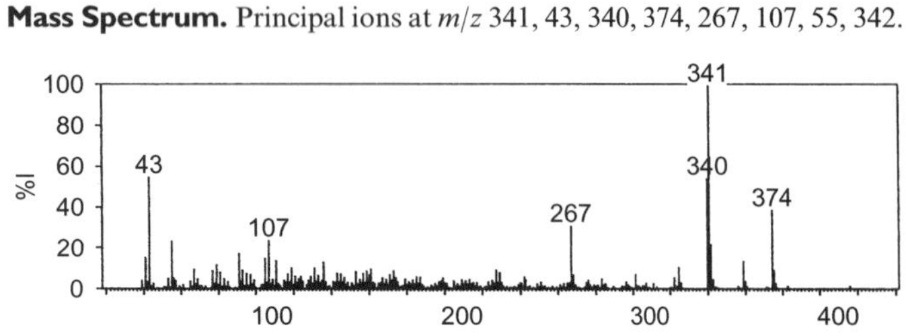

Quantification

Gas chromatography. In urine: canrenone, limit of detection 20 ng, FID—T. Fehér *et al.*, *J. Chromatogr.*, 1976, *123*, 460–462.

High performance liquid chromatography. In serum: canrenone, limit of detection 5 μg/L, UV detection—E. Besenfelder and R. Endele, *J. High Resolut. Chromatogr., Chromatogr. Commun.*, 1981, *4*, 419–421. In serum or urine: canrenone, limit of detection 5 μg/L in serum, UV detection—G. B. Neurath and D. Ambrosius, *J. Chromatogr.*, 1979, *163*; *B Biomed. Appl.*, *5*, 230–235. In serum: spironolactone and metabolites, UV detection—J. W. Overdiek *et al.*, *J. Chromatogr.*, 1985, *341*, 279–285. In plasma or urine: spironolactone and major metabolites—F. Varin *et al.*, *J. Chromatogr.*, 1992, *574*, 57–64. In urine: spironolactone and canrenone, limit of detection 20 μg/L—R. Herraez-Hernandez *et al.*, *J. Chromatogr.*, 1994, *658*; *B Biomed. Appl.*, 303–310. In plasma: spironolactone and major metabolites, UV detection—A. Jankowski *et al.*, *J. Pharm. Biomed. Anal.*, 1996, *14*, 1359–1365.

Note. Plasma-canrenone concentrations are apparently overestimated when determined by spectrofluorimetry in comparison to HPLC methods [U. Abshagen *et al.*, *Eur. J. Clin. Pharmacol.*, 1979, *16*, 255–262].

Disposition in the Body. Spironolactone is rapidly but incompletely absorbed after oral administration; it is subject to extensive first-pass metabolism and enterohepatic circulation. The metabolism of spironolactone is very complex and there are a large number of metabolites; the initial step appears to be the formation of a thiol intermediate which is subsequently hydrolysed to canrenone, and which may also be methylated to thiomethylspironolactone. The transformation is rapid and spironolactone cannot be measured in the plasma. Canrenone, which is an active metabolite, is in enzymatic equilibrium with canrenoic acid, which may be conjugated with glucuronic acid; canrenone may also be hydroxylated to 15α-hydroxycanrenone. Other active sulfur-containing metabolites are thought to be formed from hydroxylation and sulfoxidation of thiomethylspironolactone. About 25 to 55% of a dose is excreted in the urine in 6 days and up to 40% may be eliminated in the faeces. About 11% of a dose is excreted in the urine as canrenone, canrenoic acid and its glucuronide conjugate, and about 6% as the 6β-hydroxysulfoxide metabolite; the 6β-hydroxysulfone derivative has also been detected in the urine.

Therapeutic concentration

Following a single oral dose of 100 mg to 20 subjects, a mean peak serum-canrenone concentration of 0.13 mg/L was attained in 2.5 to 3 h; after daily oral doses of 100 mg to 20 subjects, the mean maximum steady-state serum concentration was reported to be 0.20 mg/L. [U. Abshagen *et al.*, *Eur. J. Clin. Pharmacol.*, 1979, *16*, 255–262].

Half-life. Plasma half-life, canrenone 13 to 24 (mean 18) h.

Distribution in blood. Plasma : whole blood ratio, canrenone 1.85.

Protein binding. In plasma, canrenone, about 98%.

Note. For a review of spironolactone, see A. Karim, *Drug Metab. Rev.*, 1978, *8*, 151–188.

Dose. 100 to 400 mg daily.

Stanozolol

Anabolic Steroid

Synonyms. Androstanazole; Methylstanazole; Stanazolol.
Proprietary names. Stromba; Strombaject; Winstrol.
(5α,17β)-17-Methyl-2′*H*-androst-2-enol[3,2-*c*]pyrazol-17-ol
$C_{21}H_{32}N_2O = 328.5$
CAS—10418-03-8

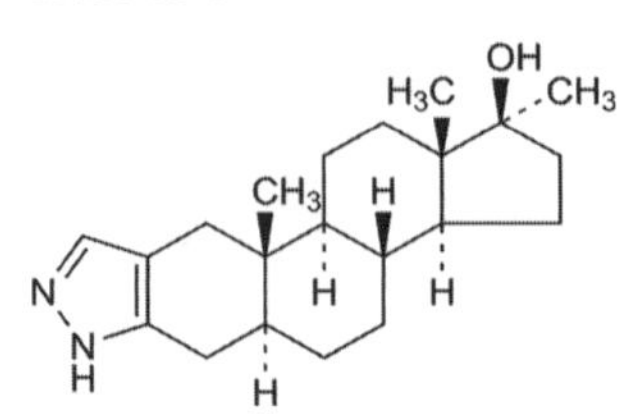

A white crystalline powder. It exists as needles, M.p. 155°, or prisms, M.p. about 235°.

Practically insoluble in water; soluble 1 in about 40 of ethanol, 1 in about 75 of chloroform and 1 in 370 of ether; slightly soluble in acetone and ethyl acetate; soluble in dimethylformamide.

Colour Tests. Mandelin's Test—brown; Marquis Test—orange-yellow.

Thin-layer Chromatography. System TA—Rf 78; system TAJ—Rf 43; system TAK—Rf 56; system TAL—Rf 91; system TAM—Rf 78. (Acidified iodoplatinate solution, positive.)

Gas Chromatography. System GA—stanozolol RI 3085, stanozolol-TMS_2 RI 3025, stanozolol-AC RI 2120; system GAI—stanozolol RRT 1.310, 3′-hydroxystanozolol RRT 1.380, 4β-hydroxystanozolol RRT 1.393 (all relative to 17α-methyl-5α-androstan-3β,17β-diol); system GAR—stanozolol Retention time 15.4 min.

High Performance Liquid Chromatography. System HX—RI 693.

Ultraviolet Spectrum. Methanolic acid—230 nm (A^{1}_{1} = 200b).

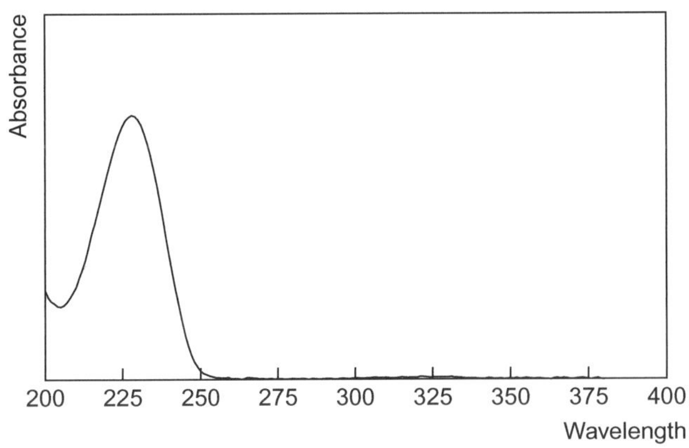

Infra-red Spectrum. Principal peaks at wavenumbers 1096, 950, 1068, 982, 1175, 1125 cm^{-1} (KCl disk).

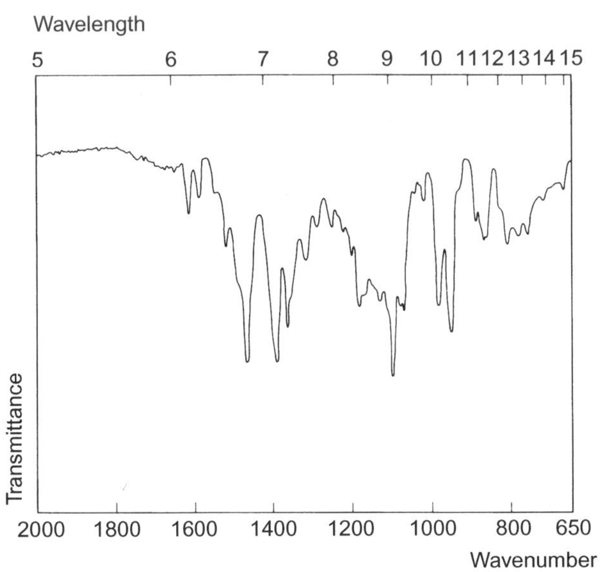

Quantification

Gas chromatography–mass spectrometry. In urine: limit of detection 2 µg/L—O. Lantto *et al.*, *J. Steroid Biochem.*, 1981, *14*, 721–727. In urine: stanozolol and 3′-hydroxystanozolol, limit of detection about 1 µg/L—H. Y. Choo *et al.*, *J. Anal. Toxicol.*, 1990, *14*, 109–112. In hair: limit of detection 2 ng/g—V. Cirimele *et al.*, *J. Chromatogr. B. Biomed. Sci. Appl.*, 2000, *740*, 265–271.

Dose. 5 to 10 mg daily.

Stavudine

Nucleoside Reverse Transcriptase Inhibitor/Antiviral

Synonyms. D4T, BMY-27857.
Proprietary names. Zerit; Zeritavir.
2′,3′-Didehydro-3′-deoxy-thymidine
$C_{10}H_{12}N_2O_4$ = 224.2
CAS—3056-17-5

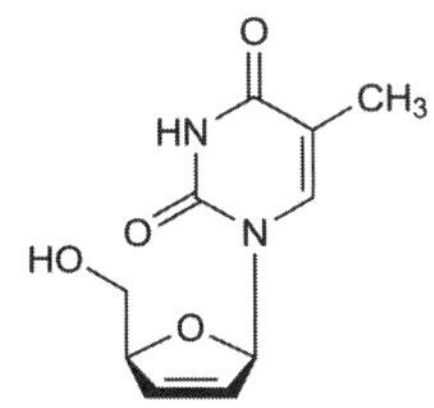

Crystals from ethanol/ether. M.p. 174°. Also reported as a colourless, granular solid from ethanol/benzene, m.p. 165° to 166°. Soluble in water and in propylene glycol.

Partition Coefficient. Log *P* (octanol/water), −0.72 (also quoted as 0.14).

High Performance Liquid Chromatography. System HAD—*k* 3.8.

Column: ODS (Apex, 250 × 4.6 mm i.d., 5 µm). Mobile phase: ammonium phosphate (10 mM): acetonitrile (9:1) (with 7.2 mM TEA, pH 2.5 with 85% phosphoric acid), flow rate 0.8 mL/min. UV detection (λ = 266 nm). Retention time: 7 to 7.5 min [J. S. Janiszewski *et al.*, *J. Chromatogr.*, 1992, *577(1)*, 151–156].

Ultraviolet Spectrum. Aqueous acid—266 nm.

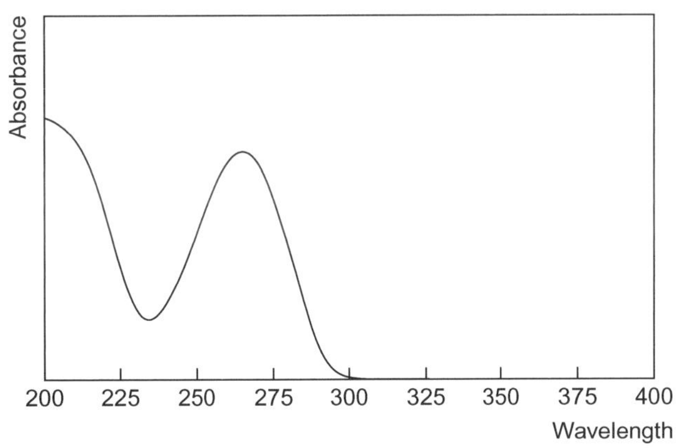

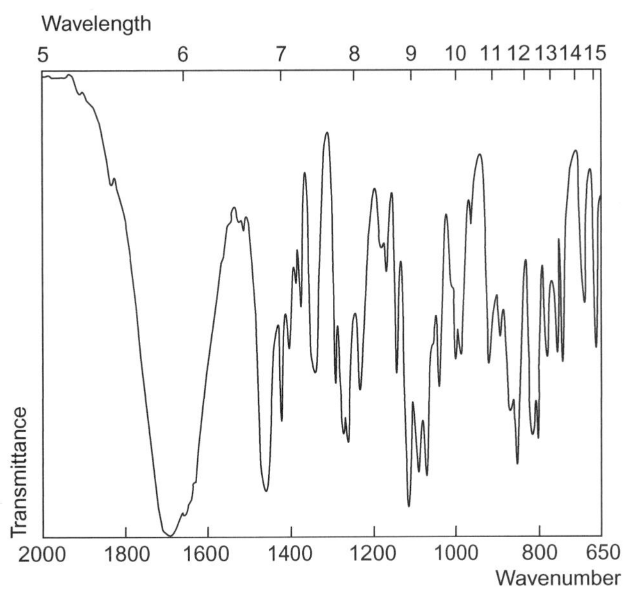

Quantification

High performance liquid chromatography. In plasma and urine: limit of quantification 0.025 mg/L and 0.5 mg/L in urine. UV detection (λ = 266 nm)—J. S. Janiszewski *et al.*, *J. Chromatogr.*, 1992, *577(1)*, 151–156. In plasma: limit of quantification 0.01 mg/L. UV detection (λ = 260 nm)—G. Aymard *et al.*, *J. Chromatogr. B Biomed. Sci. Appl.*, 2000, *744*, 227–240. In serum: limit of detection 0.04 mg/L. UV detection (λ = 250 nm)—V. A. Simon *et al.*, *J. Chromatogr. A*, 2001, *913(1–2)*, 447–453.

Disposition in the Body. Stavudine is rapidly absorbed after oral administration and is metabolised intracellularly to an active form; stavudine triphosphate. Absorption is delayed but not reduced in the presence of food. Around 40% of the dose is excreted via urine 6 to 24 h after administration with approximately half as the unchanged drug. Stavudine crosses the blood–brain barrier and the CSF: plasma ratio is 0.4 after about 4 h. It also distributes into total body water and crosses the placenta.

Therapeutic concentration

Male and female patients with hepatic impairment (creatinine clearance, >50 mL/min), at least 18 years of age, and healthy individuals were administered with a 40 mg oral dose of stavudine after an 8 h fast. The mean peak concentrations were 0.856 and 1.215 mg/L, respectively, and were reached at about 0.6 h [H. J. Schaad *et al.*, *Antimicrob. Agents Chemother.*, 1997, *41*, 2793–2796].

22 patients with a HIV infection (8 people with AIDS and 14 with the AIDS-related complex), aged between 22 and 59 years (mean, 35 years old) were split into 4 groups for different treatment. Group 1: 2 mg/kg daily (0.67 mg/kg three times daily). Group 2: 4 mg/kg daily (1.33 mg/kg three times daily). Group 3: 8 mg/kg (2.67 mg/kg three times daily). Group 4: 12 mg/kg (4 mg/kg three times daily). The mean peak plasma concentrations observed for the groups were 1.19, 1.56, 3.49 and 4.15 mg/L, respectively, all measured within 2 h of administration [M.N. Dudley *et al.*, *J.Infect. Dis.*, 1992, *166*, 480–485].

Bioavailability. 86% (adults); 61 to 78% (children).

Half-life. Elimination, 1.0 to 1.5 h (single dose); intracellular stavudine triphosphate, 3.5 h (measured *in vitro*); 0.82 to 1.24 h (children).

Volume of distribution. 0.88 to 1.06 L/kg (also reported as 58 ± 21 L); 16.8 to 19 L/m^2 (children).

Clearance. Oral, 0.46 to 0.6 L/h/kg (also reported as 35.5 L/h); children, 212 to 256 mL/min/m^2 (also reported as 333 mL/min/m^2).

Protein binding. Negligible.

Dose. Patients >60 kg: recommended dose is 40 mg every 12 h. Patients <60 kg: 30 mg every 12 h. Children >3 years and <30 kg: 1 mg/kg bodyweight every 12 h. Dose may be reduced in those with renal impairment.

Stilbazium Iodide

Anthelmintic

1-Ethyl-2,6-bis[4-(pyrrolidin-1-yl)styryl]pyridinium iodide

$C_{31}H_{36}IN_3$ = 577.6

CAS—3784-99-4

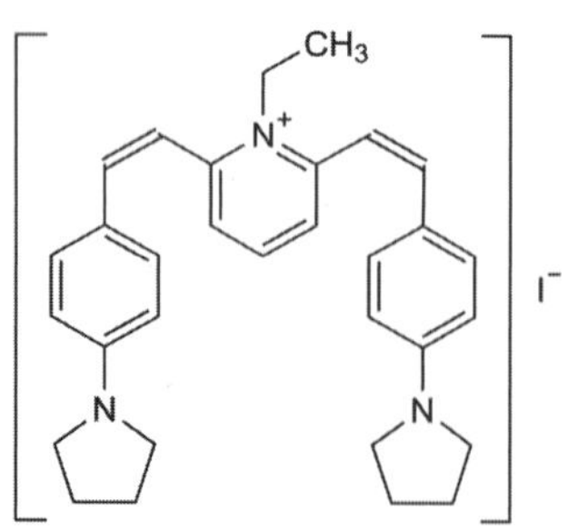

M.p. about 282°.

Soluble in ethanol and dilute acetic acid.

Thin-layer Chromatography. System TA—Rf 10. (Acidified iodoplatinate solution, positive.)

Ultraviolet Spectrum. Aqueous acid—264 nm (A^1_1 = 274b), 355 nm (A^1_1 = 310b).

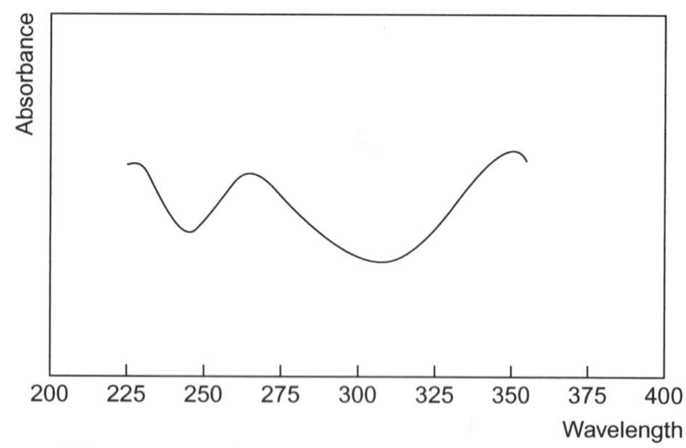

Infra-red Spectrum. Principal peaks at wavenumbers 1175, 1538, 1582, 1510, 1307, 1274 cm^{-1} (KBr disk).

Dose. Stilbazium iodide has been given in doses of 10 mg/kg once or twice daily for up to 3 days.

Streptomycin

Antibacterial

Synonym. Estreptomicina

O-2-Deoxy-2-(methylamino)-α-L-glucopyranosyl-(1→2)-*O*-5-deoxy-3-*C*-formyl-α-L-lyxofuranosyl-(1→4)-*N*,*N*′-bis(aminoiminomethyl)-D-streptamine

$C_{21}H_{39}N_7O_{12}$ = 581.6

CAS—57-92-1

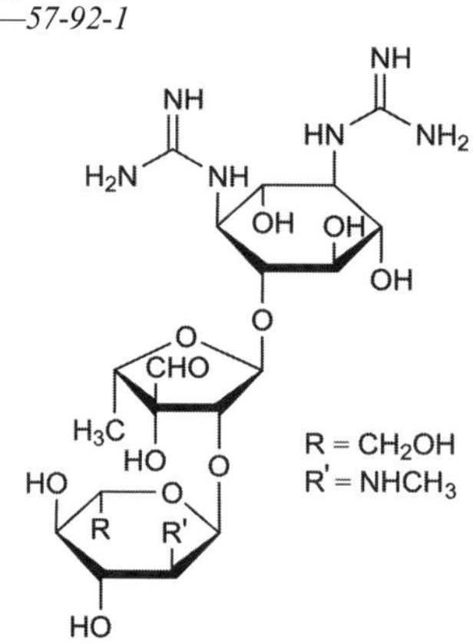

An antimicrobial organic base produced by the growth of certain strains of *Streptomyces griseus*, or by any other means.

Caution. Streptomycin may cause severe dermatitis in sensitised persons.

Streptomycin Sulfate

Synonyms. Streptomycin Sesquisulfate; Streptomycin Sulfate.

Proprietary names. Agristrep (vet.); Novostrep; Solustrep; Strepto; Streptobrettin; Streptocol; Sulfestrep; Vetstrep (vet.).

$(C_{21}H_{39}N_7O_{12})_2,3H_2SO_4$ = 1457.4

CAS—3810-74-0

A white hygroscopic powder.

Very soluble in water; practically insoluble in ethanol, chloroform and ether.

Partition Coefficient. Log *P* (octanol/water), –7.5.

Colour Tests. Benedict's reagent—orange-brown.

Boil a small quantity of streptomycin sulfate with 1 M sodium hydroxide, add a slight excess of hydrochloric acid and a few drops of ferric chloride solution—violet.

Thin-layer Chromatography. System TA—Rf 00; system TAE—Rf 00. (Acidified potassium permanganate solution, positive.)

Quantification

High performance liquid chromatography. In serum: UV detection—N. Kurosawa *et al.*, *J. Chromatogr.*, 1985, *343*, 379–385. In serum: limit of detection 1 mg/L, fluorescence detection—H. Kubo *et al.*, *Anal. Biochem.*, 1987, *162*, 219–223.

Disposition in the Body. Streptomycin is poorly and irregularly absorbed from the gastro-intestinal tract. It is rapidly absorbed after IM administration and widely distributed throughout the body. About 30 to 90% of a parenteral dose is excreted unchanged in the urine in 24 h.

Half-life. Plasma half-life, about 2 to 4 h, increased in neonates, in elderly subjects, and in renal impairment.

Distribution in blood. Plasma:whole blood ratio, about 1.9.

Protein binding. In plasma, about 20 to 30%.

Dose. The equivalent of 0.5 to 1 g of streptomycin daily, by IM injection.

Strophanthin-K

Cardiac Glycoside

Synonyms. Estrofantina; Kombé Strophanthin; K-Strophanthin; Strophanthoside-K.
Proprietary names. Kombetin; Laevostrophan.
A mixture of glycosides from strophanthus, the dried ripe seeds of *Strophanthus kombe* (Apocynaceae), adjusted by admixture with a suitable diluent such as lactose so as to possess 40% of the activity of anhydrous ouabain.

Note. Do not confuse with K-strophanthin-α which is Cymarin.
CAS—11005-63-3
A white or yellowish-white powder containing microscopic crystals.
Soluble in water and ethanol; practically insoluble in chloroform and ether.

Colour Tests. Antimony pentachloride—orange→red.
Dissolve in a cold mixture of sulfuric acid and water (4:1)—green, immediately (distinction from ouabain).

Thin-layer Chromatography. System TB—Rf 00; system TE—Rf 00; system TAE—Rf 81.

High Performance Liquid Chromatography. System HX—RI 356.

Infra-red Spectrum. Principal peaks at wavenumbers 1071, 1035, 1733, 1140, 1165, 1640 cm^{-1} (KBr disk).

Dose. Strophanthin-K has been given intravenously in doses of 125 to 500 μg daily.

Strychnine

Alkaloid

Synonym. Estricnina
Strychnidin-10-one
$C_{21}H_{22}N_2O_2$=334.4
CAS—57-24-9

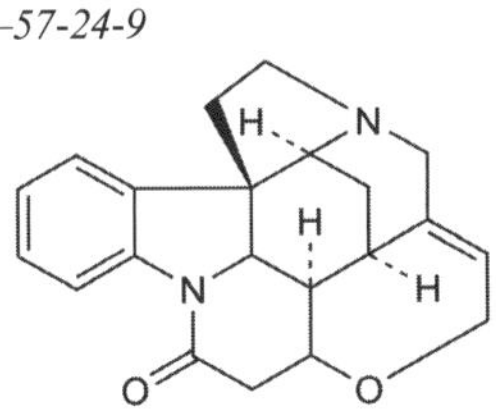

An alkaloid obtained from *nux vomica* and the seeds of other species of *Strychnos*.
Translucent colourless crystals or white crystalline powder. M.p. 275° to 285°(crystals from chloroform-ether).
Very slightly soluble in water and ether; soluble 1 in 182 of ethanol, 1 in 250 of methanol, 1 in 150 of benzene, 1 in 83 of pyridine, and 1 in 6.5 of chloroform.

Strychnine Hydrochloride

$C_{21}H_{22}N_2O_2$,HCl,$2H_2O$=406.9
CAS—1421-86-9 (anhydrous); 6101-04-8 (dihydrate)
Colourless crystals or white crystalline powder.
Soluble 1 in about 40 of water and 1 in about 80 of ethanol; practically insoluble in ether.

Strychnine Nitrate

Proprietary names. It is an ingredient of Dysurgal, Neuroftal, and Tesso-palmed Forte cum Yohimbine.
$C_{21}H_{22}N_2O_2$,HNO_3=397.4
CAS—66-32-0
Colourless glistening crystals.
Soluble 1 in 42 of water (1 in 10 of boiling water), 1 in 150 of ethanol, 1 in 50 of glycerol, and 1 in 105 of chloroform; practically insoluble in ether.

Strychnine Sulfate

Synonym. Strychnine Sulphate
Proprietary name. It is an ingredient of Hemo-Cyto-Serum.
$(C_{21}H_{22}N_2O_2)_2$,H_2SO_4,$5H_2O$=857.0
CAS—60-41-3 (anhydrous); 60491-10-3 (pentahydrate)
Colourless crystals or white crystalline powder. It is efflorescent in dry air. Melts when anhydrous at about 200°, with decomposition.
Soluble 1 in 35 of water (1 in 7 of boiling water), 1 in 81 of ethanol, 1 in 220 of chloroform, 1 in 6 of glycerol; practically insoluble in ether.

Dissociation Constant. pK_a 2.3, 8.0 (25°).

Partition Coefficient. Log *P* (octanol/water), 1.9.

Colour Test. Mandelin's Test—violet.

Thin-layer Chromatography. System TA—Rf 26; system TB—Rf 08; system TC—Rf 19; system TE—Rf 32; system TL—Rf 02; system TAE—Rf 8; system TAF—Rf 11; system TAJ—Rf 04; system TAK—Rf 02; system TAL—Rf 44. (Dragendorff spray, positive; acidified iodoplatinate solution, positive.)

Gas Chromatography. System GA—RI 3116.

High Performance Liquid Chromatography. System HA—*k* 13.0 (tailing peak); system HS—*k* 2.43; system HX—RI 302; system HY—RI 257, system HZ—Retention time 2.2 min; system HAA—Retention time 9.2 min; system HAX—Retention time 7.5 min; system HAY—Retention time 3.9 min.

Ultraviolet Spectrum. Aqueous acid—254 (A_1^1=373a); aqueous alkali—255, 278 nm.

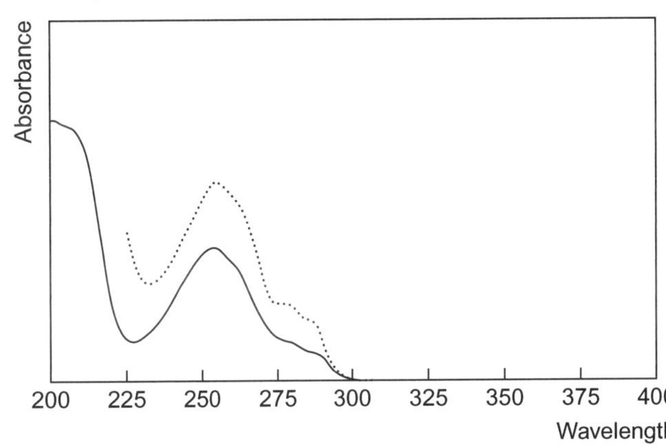

Infra-red Spectrum. Principal peaks at wavenumbers 1664, 764, 1050, 1110, 1282, 775 cm^{-1} (KBr disk).

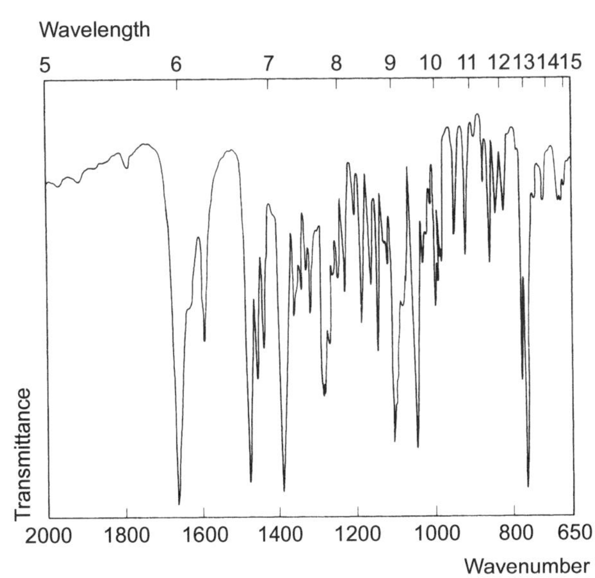

Mass Spectrum. Principal ions at *m/z* 334, 335, 162, 120, 107, 144, 143, 130.

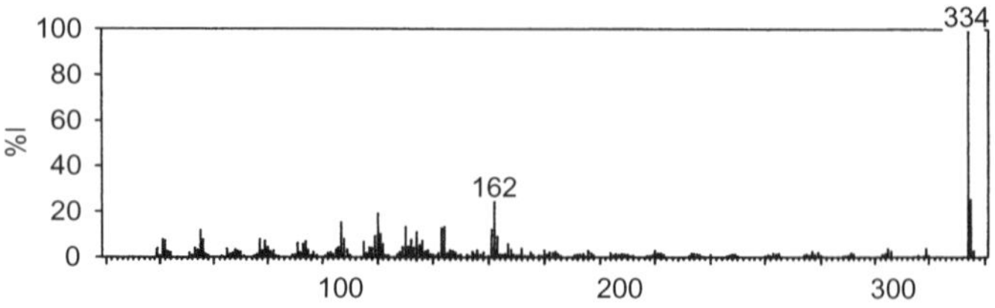

Quantification

Gas chromatography–mass spectrometry. In biological samples: limit of quantification 0.1 mg/L (or µg/g)—E. P. Marques *et al.*, *Forensic Sci. Int.*, 2000, *110(2)*, 145–152.

High performance liquid chromatography. In plasma or urine: limit of detection 625 µg/L, UV detection—L. Alliot *et al.*, *J. Chromatogr.*, 1982, *232*; *B Biomed. Appl.*, *21*, 440–442. In postmortem tissue:—M. Cingolani *et al.*, *J. Anal. Toxicol.*, 1999, *23*, 219–221.

Disposition in the Body. Readily absorbed after oral or parenteral administration and rapidly oxidised. It is taken up to some extent by the red blood cells. About 20% of a dose is excreted unchanged in the urine.

Toxicity. The minimum lethal dose is about 15 to 30 mg for children and 50 to 100 mg for adults, although with adequate treatment recovery may occur after the ingestion of 250 mg or more.

A 42-year-old man survived after ingesting an unknown quantity of strychnine powder despite his serum level being 4.73 mg/L at 1.5 h. After respiratory arrest, the patient underwent intensive supportive management and his serum concentration fell to 0.38 mg/L at 74 h post-ingestion (and to zero at 100 h) [D. Wood *et al.*, *Crit. Care*, 2002, *6*, 456–459].

In a fatal strychnine poisoning case, strychnine concentrations in blood were 1.82 mg/L (subclavian blood); 3.32 mg/L (inferior vena cava); in urine, 3.35 mg/L; bile, 11.4 mg/L; liver, 98.6 µg/g; lung, 12.3 µg/g; spleen, 11.8 µg/g; brain, 2.42 µg/g; skeletal muscle, 2.32 µg/g [T. G. Rosano *et al.*, *J. Anal. Toxicol.*, 2000, *24(7)*, 642–647].

A 50-year-old woman was admitted to hospital with classic signs of strychnine poisoning, including marked pain in the muscles of her lower limbs, dermal sensitivity and stiffness of the jaw. A strychnine concentration of 0.196 mg/L was detected in her plasma and 6.85 mg/L in her urine. She did not die from this amount [R. Greene and R. Meatherall, *J. Anal. Toxicol.*, 2001, *25(5)*, 344–347].

The following postmortem tissue concentrations were reported in a case of acute strychnine poisoning: bile 2.40 mg/L, stomach contents 14.2 mg, liver 6.68 µg/g, kidney 2.68 µg/g. After preservation of the tissues in formaldehyde solution for 8 weeks, the concentrations were: liver 1.59 µg/g, formaldehyde from liver 1.80 mg/L, kidney 0.98 µg/g, formaldehyde from kidney 1.11 mg/L [M. Cingolani *et al.*, *J. Anal. Toxicol.*, 1999, *23*, 219–221].

Note. For a review of strychnine poisoning, see B. A. Smith, *J. Emerg. Med.*, 1990, *8*, 321–325 and B. A. Smith, *J. Emerg. Med.*, 1990, *9*, 555; for a review of the toxicokinetics of acute strychnine poisoning, see W. Palatnick *et al.*, *J. Toxicol. Clin. Toxicol.*, 1997, *35*, 617–620.

Dose. Strychnine has been given, as a bitter and analeptic, in doses of 2 to 8 mg, usually as its salts.

Styramate

Muscle Relaxant

Proprietary name. Sinaxar
β-Hydroxyphenethyl carbamate
$C_9H_{11}NO_3$=181.2
CAS—94-35-9

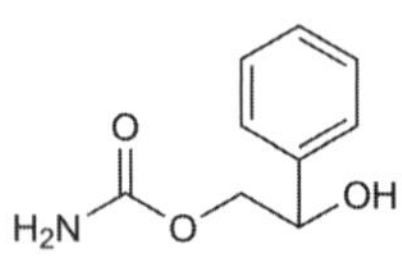

A crystalline powder. M.p. 110° to 111°.
Sparingly soluble in water; soluble in ethanol, chloroform and ether.

Partition Coefficient. Log *P* (octanol/water), 0.2.

Thin-layer Chromatography. System TA—Rf 62; system TB—Rf 01; system TC—Rf 20; system TD—Rf 13; system TE—Rf 53; system TF—Rf 39; system TL—Rf 53; system TAD—Rf 30. (Furfuraldehyde reagent, positive; Van Urk reagent, positive.)

Gas Chromatography. System GA—RI 1667.

Ultraviolet Spectrum. Aqueous acid—251, 257 (A^1_1=11b), 263 nm.

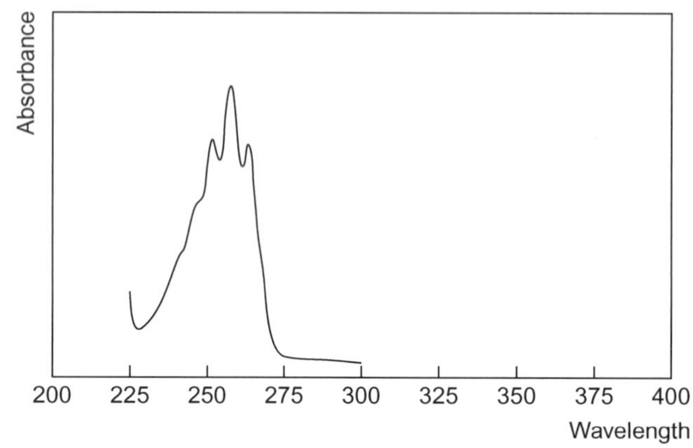

Infra-red Spectrum. Principal peaks at wavenumbers 1660, 1059, 1630, 750, 699, 1115 cm^{-1} (KBr disk).

Mass Spectrum. Principal ions at *m/z* 107, 120, 79, 75, 77, 44, 91, 45.

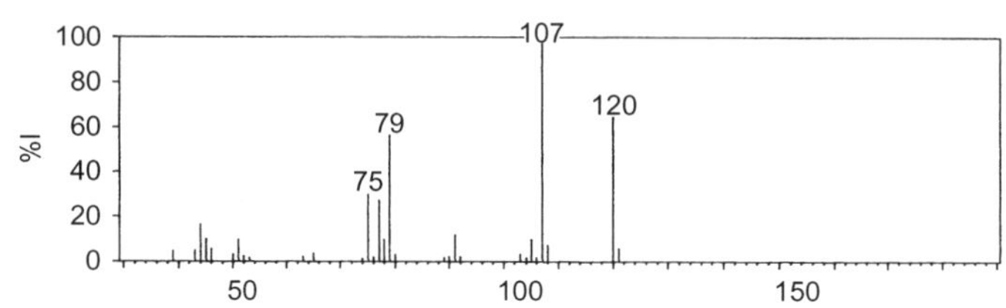

Dose. Usually 0.8 to 1.6 g daily.

Succinimide

Antiurolithic

Synonyms. Butanimide; 3,4-Dihydropyrrolidine; 3,4-Dihydropyrrole-2,5-dione; Dihydro-3-pyrroline-2,5-dione; 2,5-Diketopyrrolidine; 2,5-Dioxopyrrolidine; Lubrizol 6406; Succinic acid imide; Succinic imide; Succinimide-Sauba.
Proprietary name. Orotric
2,5-Pyrrolidinedione
$C_4H_5NO_2$=99.1
CAS—123-56-8

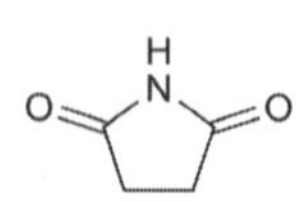

A white to off-white crystalline nitrogenous powder. M.p. 122° to 124°. B.p. 287° to 289°.
It is very soluble in water, slightly soluble in alcohol, and insoluble in ether and chloroform.

Dissociation Constant. pK_a 9.5.

Partition Coefficient. Log *P* (octanol/water), −0.85.

High Performance Liquid Chromatography. System HZ—retention time 2.4 min (dimethyl-methyl-succinimide).

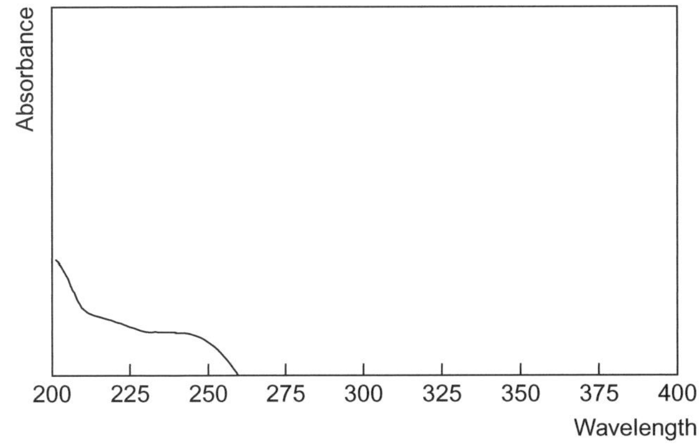

Infra-red Spectrum. Principal peaks at wavenumber 1777, 1145, 648, 896 cm^{-1}.

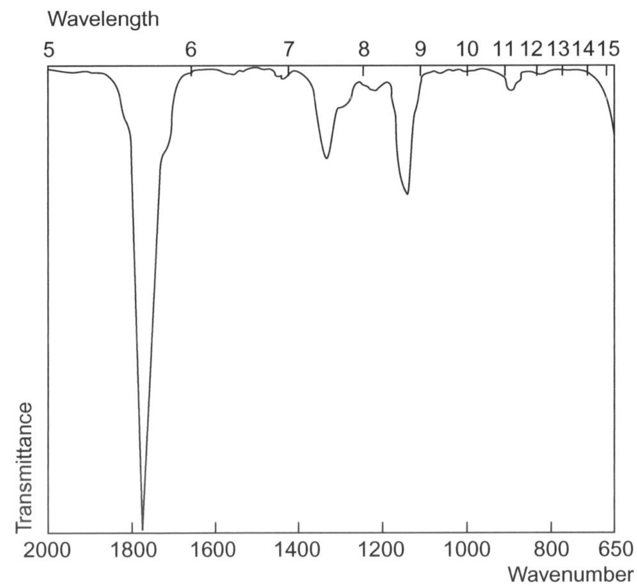

Mass Spectrum. Principal ions at *m/z* 28, 99, 56, 27, 26, 55, 42, 100.

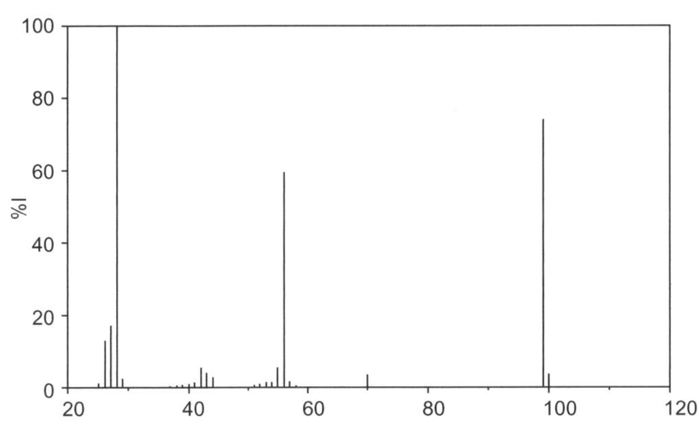

Dose. The usual oral dose is 3 g 3 times a day.

Succinylsulfathiazole

Antibacterial/Sulfonamide

Synonyms. Succinilsolfatiazolo; Succinylsulfathiazole; Sulfasuccithiazole.
Proprietary name. Sulfasuxidine
4-Oxo-4-[[4-[(2-thiazolylamino)sulfonyl]phenyl]amino]butanoic acid monohydrate

$C_{13}H_{13}N_3O_5S_2,H_2O$=373.4
CAS—116-43-8 (anhydrous)

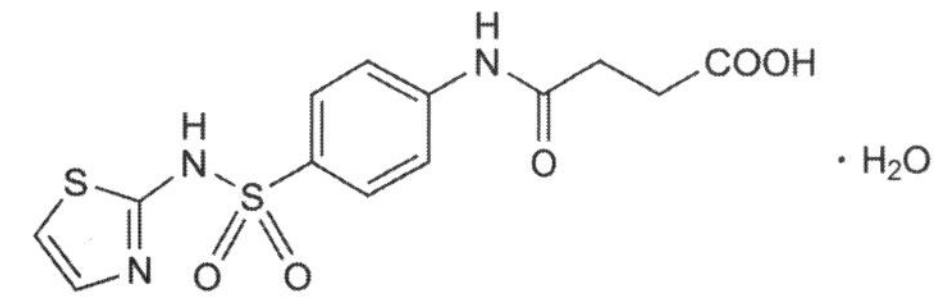

White or yellowish-white crystals or powder which darken on exposure to light. M.p. 184° to 186°; also reported as m.p.192° to 195°.
Soluble 1 in about 4800 of water, 1 in 200 of ethanol, and 1 in 150 of acetone; practically insoluble in chloroform and ether; soluble in aqueous solutions of alkali hydroxides and carbonates.

Dissociation Constant. pK_a 4.5.

Partition Coefficient. Log *P* (octanol/water), 1.2.

Colour Tests. Copper Sulfate (Method 1)—green (→violet); Koppanyi–Zwikker Test—red-violet; Mercurous Nitrate—black.

Thin-layer Chromatography. System TD—Rf 00; system TE—Rf 00; system TF—Rf 00; system TT—Rf 02; system TU—Rf 01; system TV—Rf 01; system TAD—Rf 02.

Gas Chromatography. See sulfathiazole.

High Performance Liquid Chromatography. System HU—*k* 16.8.

Ultraviolet Spectrum. Aqueous acid—258 (A^1_1=570a), 281; aqueous alkali—257 nm (A^1_1=651a).

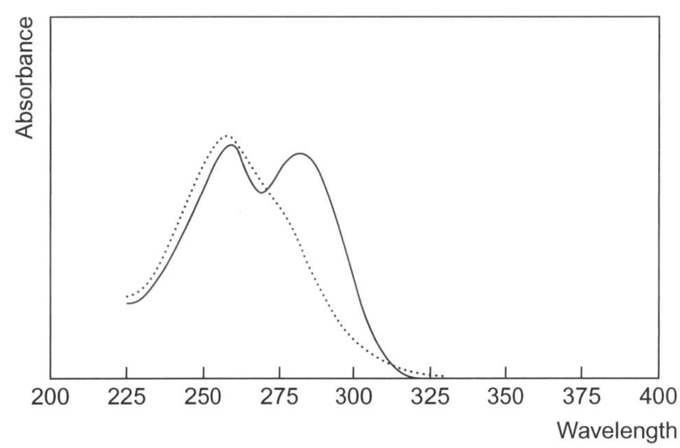

Infra-red Spectrum. Principal peaks at wavenumbers 1143, 1585, 1091, 840, 1529, 1667 cm^{-1} (Nujol mull).

Mass Spectrum. Principal ions at *m/z* 92, 156, 65, 191, 108, 55, 45, 174.

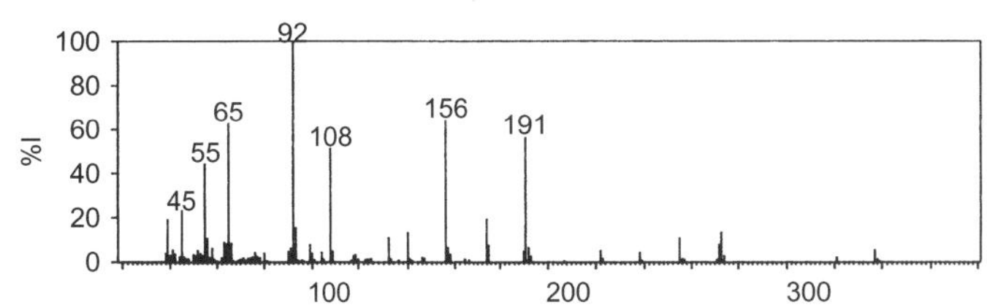

Disposition in the Body. Only about 5% of a dose is absorbed after oral administration and blood concentrations are therefore very low compared to other sulfonamides, usually less than 40 mg/L. It is slowly hydrolysed to sulfathiazole in the gastro-intestinal tract. Considerable amounts of sulfathiazole are eliminated in the faeces.

Dose. Usually 10 to 20 g daily.

Sulfacarbamide

Sulfonamide

Synonyms. Sulfanilcarbamide; Sulfaurea; Sulphacarbamide; Sulphanilylurea; Sulphaurea; Urosulphanum.

Proprietary names. Euvernil; Uractyl; Uramid; Urenil; Urosulfan.
4-Amino-*N*-(aminocarbonyl)benzenesulfonamide monohydrate
$C_7H_9N_3O_3S,H_2O=233.2$
CAS—547-44-4 (anhydrous); 6101-35-5 (monohydrate)

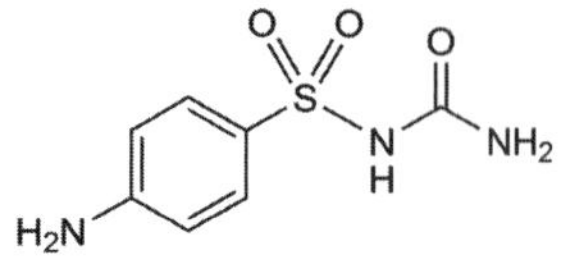

A white crystalline powder. M.p. 125° to 127°.
Soluble 1 in 430 of water; slightly soluble in ethanol; practically insoluble in chloroform and ether; soluble in acetone, dilute mineral acids, and solutions of alkali hydroxides.

Partition Coefficient. Log *P* (octanol/water), –1.0.

Colour Tests. Copper Sulfate (Method 1)—blue; Koppanyi–Zwikker Test—violet; Palladium Chloride—black.

Thin-layer Chromatography. System TA—Rf 76; system TB—Rf 00; system TC—Rf 01; system TL—Rf 08; system TAD—Rf 14; system TAE—Rf 81.

Ultraviolet Spectrum. Aqueous acid—266 (A^1_1=188b), 272; aqueous alkali—255 nm. (See below.)

Infra-red Spectrum. Principal peaks at wavenumbers 1694, 1149, 1587, 1086, 1612, 684 cm^{-1}.

Disposition in the Body. Readily absorbed after oral administration. It is rapidly excreted in the urine, most of a single dose being eliminated in 12 h. About 10 to 15% of the material in the urine is the inactive N^4-acetyl metabolite and the remainder is unchanged drug.

Half-life. Plasma half-life, about 2.5 h.

Dose. 3 g daily.

Sulfacetamide

Antibacterial/Sulfonamide

Synonym. Acetosulfaminum.
Proprietary names. Sulfanil; Vista-Cetamide. It is an ingredient of Sultrin.
N-[(4-Aminophenyl)sulfonyl]acetamide
$C_8H_{10}N_2O_3S=214.2$
CAS—144-80-9

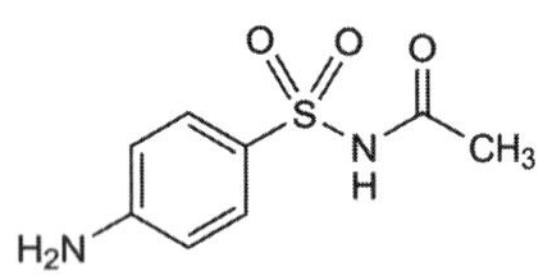

A white or yellowish-white crystalline powder. M.p. 182° to 184°.
Soluble 1 in 150 of water, 1 in 15 of ethanol, and 1 in 7 of acetone; very slightly soluble in chloroform; slightly soluble in ether; soluble in mineral acids and alkali hydroxides.

Sulfacetamide Sodium

Synonyms. Soluble Sulfacetamide; Sulfacylum Natrium; Sulfacetamide Sodium.
Proprietary names. Acetopt; Ak-Sulf; Albucid; Antebor; Beocid Puroptal; Bleph-10; Cetamide; Cetazin; Diosulf; Optamid(e); Optisol; Optosulfex; Prontamid; Sebizon; Sodium Sulamyd; Sulf-10; Sulfac; Sulfex; Ultra; Vanocin. It is an ingredient of Ocusol.
$C_8H_9N_2NaO_3S,H_2O=254.2$
CAS—127-56-0 (anhydrous); 6209-17-2 (monohydrate)
White or yellowish-white crystals or crystalline powder. It slowly darkens on exposure to light; on exposure to moist air it absorbs carbon dioxide and becomes less soluble.
Soluble 1 in 1.5 of water; slightly soluble in ethanol; sparingly soluble in acetone; practically insoluble in chloroform and ether.

Dissociation Constant. pK_a 1.8, 5.4.

Partition Coefficient. Log *P* (octanol/water), –1.0.

Colour Tests. Coniferyl Alcohol—orange; Copper Sulfate (Method 1)—blue; Koppanyi–Zwikker Test—blue-violet.

Thin-layer Chromatography. System TA—Rf 70; system TD—Rf 17; system TE—Rf 04; system TF—Rf 42; system TT—Rf 53; system TU—Rf 37; system TV—Rf 04; system TAD—Rf 28; system TAE—Rf 87. (Mercuric chloride–diphenylcarbazone reagent, blue; acidified potassium permanganate solution, positive; Van Urk reagent, yellow.)

Gas Chromatography. System GA—RI 2132; System GJ—RRT of methyl derivative 0.16 (relative to griseofulvin).

High Performance Liquid Chromatography. System HU—*k* 7.7; system HY—RI 241.

Ultraviolet Spectrum. Aqueous acid—271 (A^1_1=260a); aqueous alkali—256 nm (A^1_1=750a).

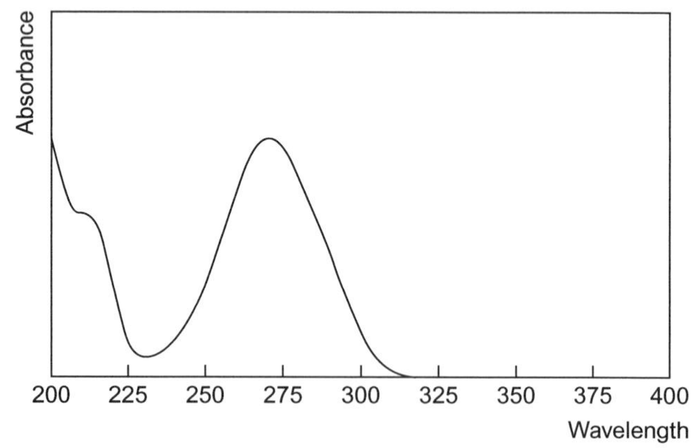

Infra-red Spectrum. Principal peaks at wavenumbers 1145, 1264, 1552, 1090, 825, 1600 cm^{-1} (sulfacetamide sodium, KBr disk).

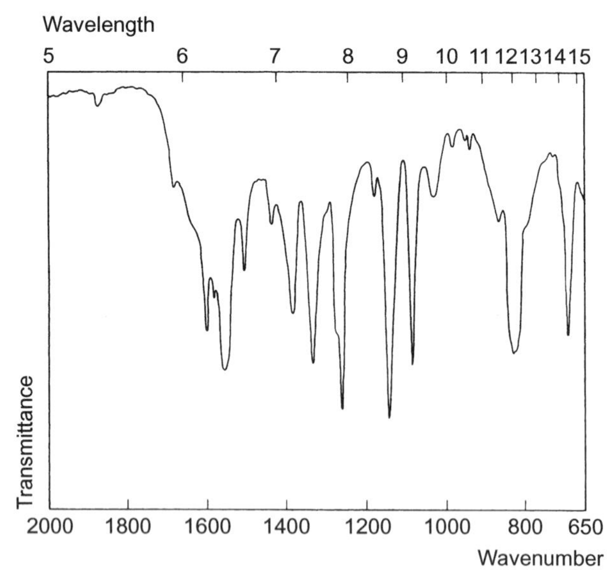

Mass Spectrum. Principal ions at *m/z* 172, 92, 156, 65, 108, 39, 44, 41.

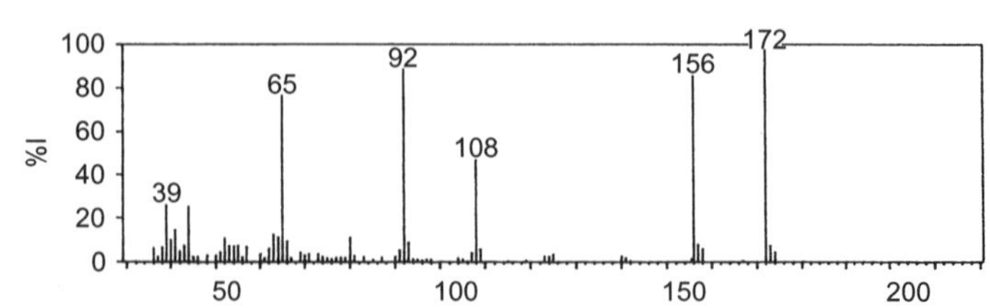

Quantification

High performance liquid chromatography. The methods referred to under sulfamethoxazole may be used.

Disposition in the Body. After oral administration sulfacetamide is readily absorbed and rapidly excreted in the urine, mainly as unchanged drug. However, it is usually only used topically in the treatment of eye infections; absorption into the blood may occur after application to the eye if the conjunctiva is inflamed.

Half-life. Plasma half-life, 7 to 14 h.

Protein binding. In plasma, 15 to 18%.

Use. Sulfacetamide sodium is used as a 10 to 30% ophthalmic solution.

Sulfachlorpyridazine

Antibacterial/Sulfonamide

Synonym. Sulphachlorpyridazine; Ba-10370.
Proprietary names. Cosulid; Cosumix; Nefrosul; Sonilyn.
4-Amino-*N*-(6-chloro-3-pyridazinyl)benzenesulfonamide
$C_{10}H_9ClN_4O_2S$=284.7
CAS—80-32-0

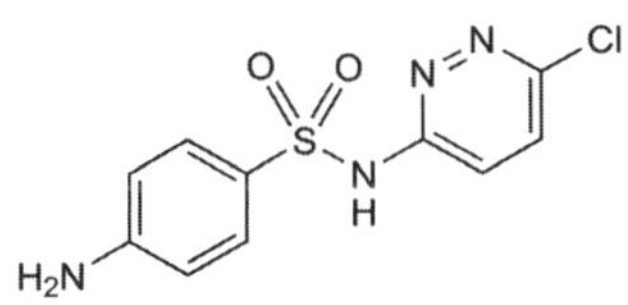

A yellowish crystalline powder.
Soluble in bicarbonate solutions.

Sulfachlorpyridazine Sodium

Proprietary names. Prinzone; Vetisulid.
$C_{10}H_8ClN_4O_2S,Na$=306.7
CAS—23282-55-5

Partition Coefficient. Log *P* (octanol/water), 0.3.

Colour Tests. Coniferyl Alcohol—orange; Copper Sulfate (Method 1)—green; Koppanyi–Zwikker Test—pink; Mercurous Nitrate—black; Nitrous Acid—yellow.

Thin-layer Chromatography. System TA—Rf 70; system TAJ—Rf 41; system TAK—Rf 23; system TAL—Rf 80. (Van Urk reagent, positive.)

High Performance Liquid Chromatography. System HU—*k* 3.3.

Ultraviolet Spectrum. Aqueous acid—256; aqueous alkali—257 nm.

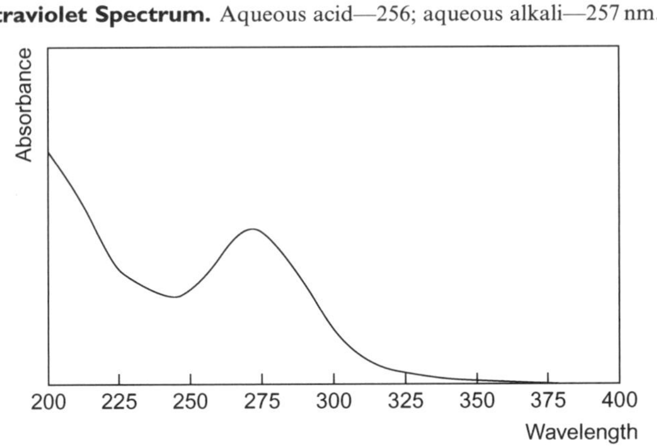

Infra-red Spectrum. Principal peaks at wavenumbers 1124, 1220, 1087, 1208, 963, 1618 cm^{-1} (KBr disk).

Disposition in the Body. Readily absorbed after oral administration and rapidly excreted in the urine.

Therapeutic concentration
After a single oral dose of 500 mg to 10 subjects, peak plasma concentrations of 39.7 to 85.5 mg/L (mean 59.6) were attained in about 1 h [E. L. Marino *et al.*, *Int. J. Clin. Pharmacol. Ther. Toxicol.*, 1980, *18*, 10–14].

Half-life. Plasma half-life, about 3 to 4 h.

Volume of distribution. About 0.1 L/kg.

Clearance. Plasma clearance, about 0.5 mL/min/kg.

Protein binding. In plasma, about 94 to 99%.

Dose. Sulfachlorpyridazine has been given in an initial dose of 4 g, followed by 2 to 4 g daily.

Sulfadiazine

Antibacterial/Sulfonamide

Synonyms. Solfadiazina; Solfapirimidina; Sulfadiazine.
Proprietary names. Adiazine; Balin; Diazyl; Labdiazina; Sulfolex. It is an ingredient of Geatrim-Boli, Norodine, Scorprin, Synutrim, Tribrissen, Triglobe, and Vesuprim.
4-Amino-*N*-2-pyrimidinylbenzenesulfonamide
$C_{10}H_{10}N_4O_2S$=250.3
CAS—68-35-9

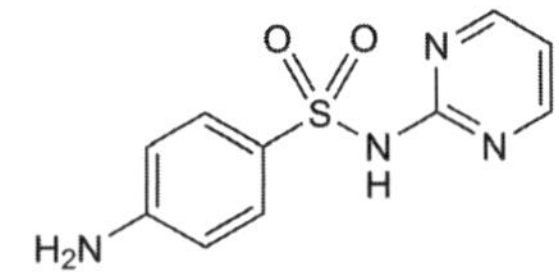

White, yellowish-white, or pinkish-white crystals or powder, slowly darkening on exposure to light. M.p. about 255°, with decomposition.
Practically insoluble in water, chloroform, and ether; very slightly soluble in ethanol; soluble 1 in 300 of acetone; soluble in dilute mineral acids and in solutions of alkali hydroxides and carbonates.

Sulfadiazine Sodium

Synonyms. Soluble Sulfadiazine; Sulfadiazine Sodium.
$C_{10}H_9N_4NaO_2S$=272.3
CAS—547-32-0
A white or yellowish-white powder. It slowly darkens on exposure to light; on exposure to moist air it absorbs carbon dioxide with the liberation of sulfadiazine and becomes incompletely soluble in water.
Soluble 1 in 2 of water; slightly soluble in ethanol; practically insoluble in chloroform and ether.

Dissociation Constant. pK_a 6.5 (25°).

Partition Coefficient. Log *P* (octanol/pH 7.5), –1.3.

Colour Tests. Coniferyl Alcohol—orange; Copper Sulfate (Method 1)—violet-brown; Koppanyi–Zwikker Test—violet-pink; Mercurous Nitrate—black.

Thin-layer Chromatography. System TA—Rf 64; system TD—Rf 22; system TE—Rf 04; system TF—Rf 39; system TT—Rf 24; system TU—Rf 22; system TV—Rf 03; system TAD—Rf 38; system TAE—Rf 81; system TAJ—Rf 40; system TAK—Rf 11; system TAL—Rf 70.

Gas Chromatography. System GA—sulfadiazine RI 2502; sulfadiazine-Me RI 2625; M (acetyl-)-Me_2 RI 3710; System GJ—sulfadiazine-Me RRT 0.66, N^4-acetylsulfadiazine-Me RRT 1.69 (both relative to griseofulvin).

High Performance Liquid Chromatography. System HU—*k* 8.7; system HY—RI 234; system HAA—Retention time 8.4 min.

Ultraviolet Spectrum. Aqueous acid—242 (A_1^1=587a); aqueous alkali—240 (A_1^1=867a), 254 nm (A_1^1=868a).

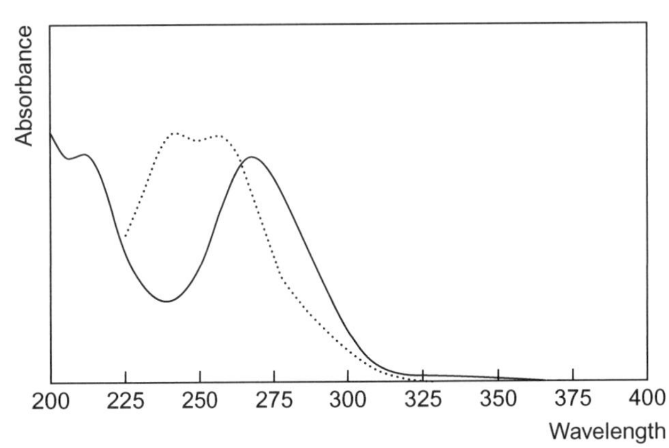

Infra-red Spectrum. Principal peaks at wavenumbers 1580, 1159, 1494, 682, 940, 797 cm^{-1} (KBr disk).

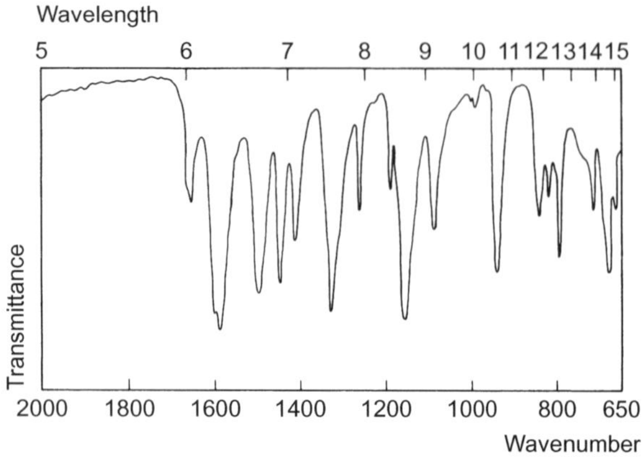

Mass Spectrum. Principal ions at *m/z* 186, 185, 92, 65, 108, 39, 93, 187.

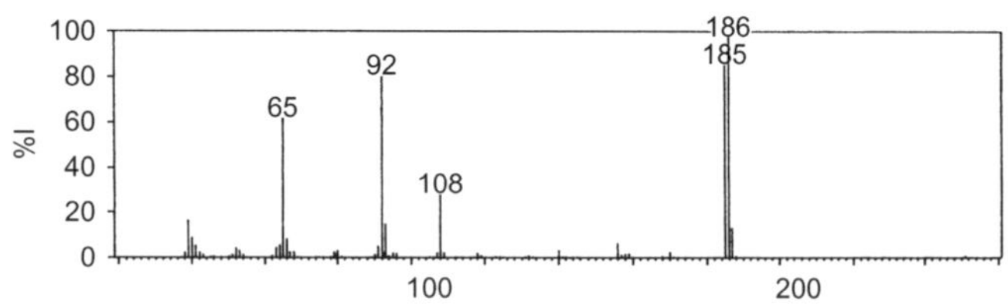

Quantification

Gas chromatography. In plasma or urine: sulfadiazine and acetyl derivative, limit of detection 1 ng, ECD—A. Bye and G. Land, *J. Chromatogr.*, 1977, *139*, 181–185.

High performance liquid chromatography. In plasma or urine: limit of detection 400 μg/L for sulfadiazine in plasma, 5 and 7 mg/L for sulfadiazine and the acetyl derivative, respectively, in urine, UV detection—D. Westerlund and A. Wijkström, *J. Pharm. Sci.*, 1982, *71*, 1142–1145. In serum or urine: UV detection—V. Springolo and G. Coppi, *J. Pharm. Biomed. Anal.*, 1989, *7*, 57–65; H. N. Alkaysi *et al.*, *Biomed. Chromatogr.*, 1991, *5*, 265–268. In plasma or urine: —R. Metz *et al.*, *J. Chromatogr.*, 1996, *729*, 243–249. In urine: sulfadiazine and other sulfonamides, limit of detection 0.1 to 0.3 mg/L—E. F. Simo-Alfonso *et al.*, *J. Chromatogr. B Biomed. Appl.*, 1995, *670*, 183–187.

Disposition in the Body. Readily absorbed after oral administration. It is acetylated in the body and up to 15% of the sulfadiazine in the blood is in the form of the inactive N^4-acetyl derivative. About 50% of a dose is excreted in the urine in 24 h; up to about 40% of the excreted material is the acetyl derivative and up to about 50% is unchanged drug. Excretion is influenced by the pH of the urine, the rate being increased when the urine is alkaline.

Therapeutic concentration

After a single oral dose of 820 mg to 5 subjects, peak serum concentrations of sulfadiazine plus metabolites of 19 to 40 mg/L (mean 33) were attained in 4 h [T. Bergan *et al.*, *Clin. Pharmacol. Ther.*, 1977, *22*, 211–224].

Half-life. Plasma half-life, 6 to 17 h.

Volume of distribution. About 0.3 L/kg.

Clearance. Plasma clearance, about 0.3 mL/min/kg.

Distribution in blood. Plasma : whole blood ratio, 0.93.

Protein binding. In plasma, about 50%.

Dose. An initial dose of 2 to 4 g, followed by 1 g every 4 to 6 h.

Sulfadimethoxine

Antibacterial/Sulfonamide

Synonym. Solfadimetossina.
Proprietary names. Agribon; Albon; Arnosulfan; Diasulfa; Madribon; Maxulvet; Neostreptal; Sudine; Suldixine; Sulfabon; Sulxin; Symbio; Ultrasulfon.

4-Amino-*N*-(2,6-dimethoxy-4-pyrimidinyl)benzenesulfonamide
$C_{12}H_{14}N_4O_4S = 310.3$
CAS—122-11-2

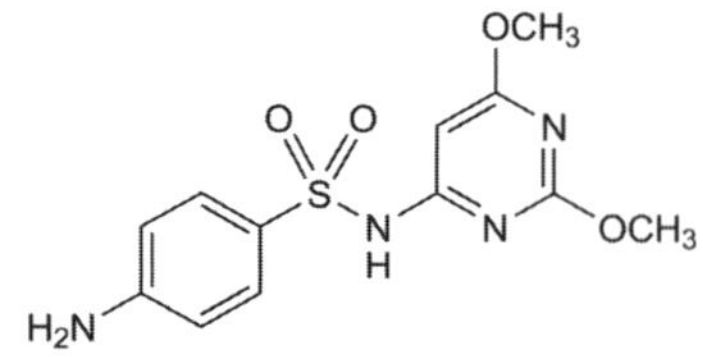

A white or creamy-white crystalline powder. M.p. 201° to 204°.
Very slightly soluble in water; soluble 1 in 200 of ethanol, 1 in 800 of chloroform, and 1 in 2000 of ether; soluble in dilute mineral acids and in solutions of alkali hydroxides and carbonates.

Dissociation Constant. pK_a 5.9 (25°).

Partition Coefficient. Log *P* (octanol/water), 1.6.

Colour Tests. Coniferyl Alcohol—orange; Copper Sulfate (Method 1)—green; Koppanyi–Zwikker Test—violet-pink; Mercurous Nitrate—black.

Thin-layer Chromatography. System TA—Rf 65; system TD—Rf 31; system TE—Rf 10; system TF—Rf 51; system TT—Rf 85; system TU—Rf 52; system TV—Rf 34; system TAD—Rf 48; system TAE—Rf 86; system TAJ—Rf 53; system TAK—Rf 28; system TAL—Rf 98.

Gas Chromatography. System GA—sulfadimethoxine-TMS RI 3060.

High Performance Liquid Chromatography. System HY—RI 352; system HAA—Retention time 14.7 min.

Ultraviolet Spectrum. Aqueous acid—275 (A^1_1=449a); aqueous alkali—269 nm (A^1_1=845a).

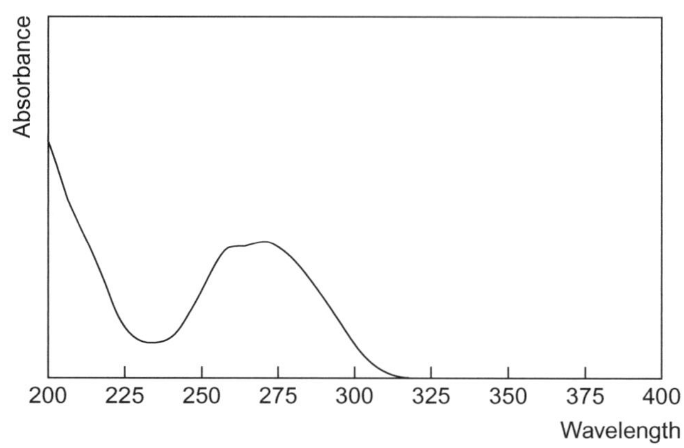

Infra-red Spectrum. Principal peaks at wavenumbers 1590, 1147, 1090, 1314, 685, 1066 cm^{-1} (KBr disk).

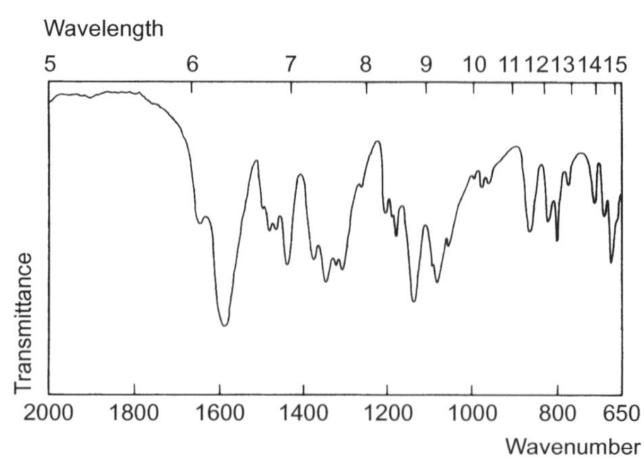

Mass Spectrum. Principal ions at *m/z* 246, 92, 65, 245, 108, 247, 39, 260.

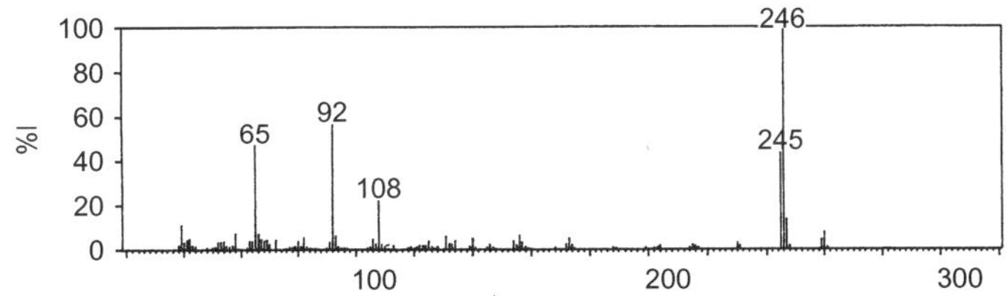

Quantification. In plasma or urine: sulfadimethoxine and its N^1-glucuronide, N^4-acetyl, and N^4-acetyl-N^1-glucuronide metabolites—T. B. Vree *et al.*, *J. Chromatogr.*, 1990, *526*, 119–128.

Disposition in the Body. Sulfadimethoxine is a long-acting sulfonamide which is readily absorbed after oral administration. After a single dose, peak blood concentrations are attained in about 4 to 6 h. It is acetylated in the body and about 10% of the sulfadimethoxine in the blood is present as the inactive N^4-acetyl derivative, and about 5% as the N^1-glucuronide. About 50% of a dose is excreted in the urine in 48 h, about 20% of the excreted material being the acetyl derivative, about 5% unchanged drug, and 60 to 80% the N^1-glucuronide. Both unchanged drug and the N^1-glucuronide are excreted in the bile.

Therapeutic concentration. In plasma, usually in the range 50 to 100 mg/L.

Following an oral dose of 2 g, peak blood concentrations of 120 to 180 mg/L were attained [H. Seneca, *J. Am. Med. Assoc.*, 1966, *198*, 975–980].

Half-life. Plasma half-life, 20 to 40 h.

Volume of distribution. About 0.1 to 0.2 L/kg.

Protein binding. In plasma, 90 to 99%.

Dose. An initial dose of 1 or 2 g, followed by 0.5 to 1 g daily.

Sulfadimidine

Antibacterial/Sulfonamide

Synonyms. Solfametazina; Sulfadimerazine; Sulfadimezinum; Sulfamethazine; Sulfadimethylpyrimidine; Sulfamethazine.
Note. Sulfadimethylpyrimidine has been used as a synonym for sulfasomidine. Care should be taken to avoid confusion between the two compounds, which are isomeric.
Proprietary names. Diazil; Dimidin-R; Neazina; S-Dimidine Sulfadine; Sulmet. It is an ingredient of Trisulfaminic and Sulfatril.
4-Amino-*N*-(4,6-dimethyl-2-pyrimidinyl)benzenesulfonamide
$C_{12}H_{14}N_4O_2S = 278.3$
CAS—57-68-1

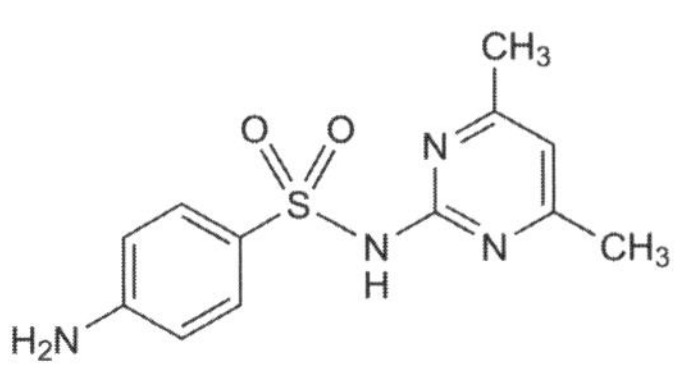

White or yellowish-white crystals or powder which darken and decompose on exposure to light. M.p. 176°; also reported as 178° to 179°, 198° to199°, and 205° to 207°.
Very slightly soluble in water; soluble 1 in 120 of ethanol, 1 in 30 of acetone, 1 in 600 of chloroform, and 1 in 2500 of ether; soluble in dilute mineral acids and in aqueous solutions of alkali hydroxides and carbonates.

Sulfadimidine Sodium

Synonyms. Soluble Sulfadimethylpyrimidine; Soluble Sulfadimidine; Soluble Sulfamethazine; Sulfadimidine Sodium.
Proprietary names. Intradine; Sulfoxine 33; Vesadin.
$C_{12}H_{13}N_4NaO_2S = 300.3$
CAS—1981-58-4
White or creamy-white hygroscopic crystals or powder. It slowly discolours and decomposes on exposure to light; on exposure to air it absorbs carbon dioxide and becomes less soluble in water.
Soluble 1 in 2.5 of water and 1 in 60 of ethanol.

Dissociation Constant. pK_a 7.4 (25°).

Partition Coefficient. Log *P* (octanol/water), 0.9.

Colour Tests. Coniferyl Alcohol—orange; Copper Sulfate (Method 1)—green→brown; Koppanyi–Zwikker Test—violet-pink; Mercurous Nitrate—black; Nitrous Acid—yellow.

Thin-layer Chromatography. System TA—Rf 62; system TD—Rf 23; system TE—Rf 13; system TF—Rf 45; system TT—Rf 50; system TU—Rf 27; system TV—Rf 62; system TAD—Rf 44; system TAE—Rf 79; system TAJ—Rf 43; system TAK—Rf 17; system TAL—Rf 95. (Mercuric chloride–diphenylcarbazone reagent, blue; acidified potassium permanganate solution, positive; Van Urk reagent, yellow.)

Gas Chromatography. System GA—RI 2613; System GJ—RRT of methyl derivative 0.71 (relative to griseofulvin).

High Performance Liquid Chromatography. System HU—*k* 7.1; system HX—RI 333; system HY—RI 257.

Ultraviolet Spectrum. Aqueous acid—243 ($A_1^1 = 541a$), 301; aqueous alkali—242 ($A_1^1 = 760a$), 258 nm ($A_1^1 = 783a$).

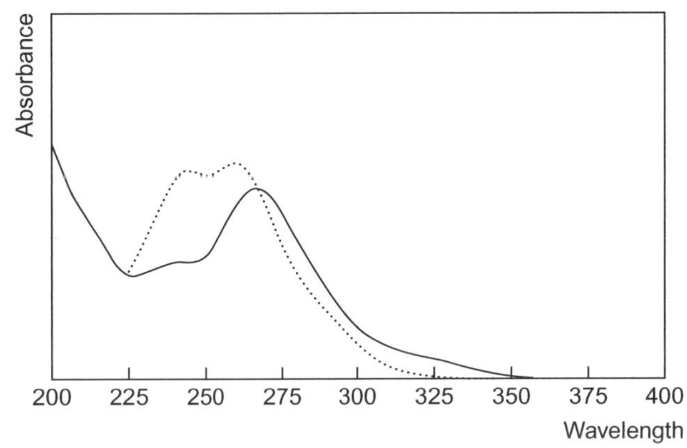

Infra-red Spectrum. Principal peaks at wavenumbers 1145, 1595, 1304, 1635, 682, 1090 cm^{-1} (KCl disk).

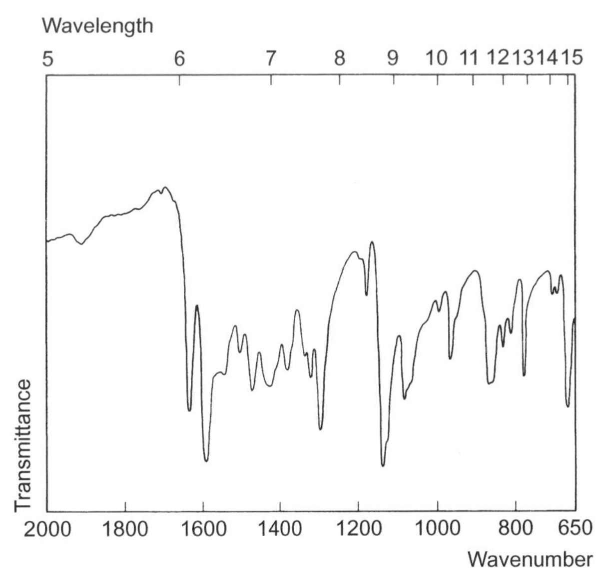

Mass Spectrum. Principal ions at *m/z* 214, 213, 92, 65, 215, 108, 39, 42.

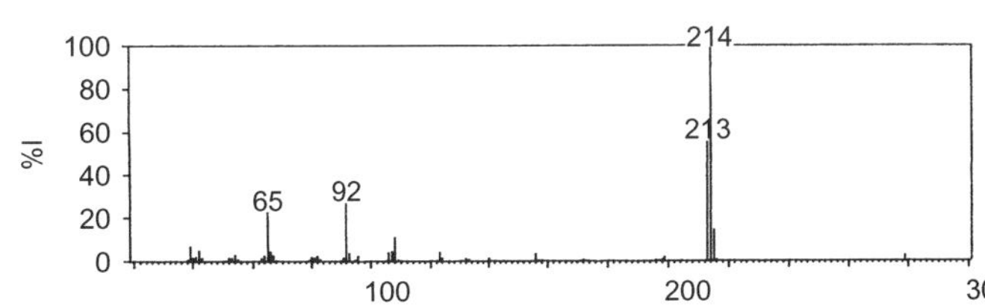

Quantification

High performance liquid chromatography. In plasma or blood: sulfadimidine and acetyl metabolite, limit of detection 6 mg/L, UV detection—R. Whelpton *et al.*, *Clin. Chem.*, 1981, 27, 1911–1914.

Disposition in the Body. Readily absorbed after oral administration. It is acetylated in the body, the degree of acetylation being dependent on the acetylator status of the subject. In rapid acetylators, 60 to 90% of the sulfadimidine in the blood is present as the N^4-acetyl derivative whereas, in slow acetylators, the proportion is only about 16 to 37%. About 50% of a dose is excreted in the urine in 48 h. Of the excreted material, up to about 15% is unchanged drug and up to about 95% may be the acetyl derivative.

Therapeutic concentration. In plasma, free sulfadimidine, usually in the range 50 to 100 mg/L.

Following a single oral dose of 1.5 g to 8 slow acetylators, plasma-sulfadimidine concentrations of 64.0 to 88.4 mg/L (mean 80.7) were attained in 3 to 4 h; after a similar dose to 8 rapid acetylators, peak plasma concentrations ranged from 38.8 to 64.1 mg/L (mean 45.7) at 3 h [U. M. Woolhouse and L. C. Atu-Taylor, *Clin. Pharmacol. Ther.*, 1982, *31*, 377–383].

Half-life. Derived from urinary excretion data, 1 to 5 h for rapid acetylators and 3 to 11 h (mean 6) for slow acetylators.

Volume of distribution. About 0.6 L/kg.

Protein binding. In plasma, 60 to 90%.

Dose. An initial dose of up to 3 g, followed by 0.5 to 1.5 g every 6 h.

Sulfadoxine

Antibacterial/Sulfonamide

Synonyms. Sulformethoxine; Sulforthomidine; Sulfadoxine; Sulformethoxine; Sulforthodimethoxine.
Proprietary names. Fanasil; Fanzil. It is an ingredient of Bimotrim (vet.), Borgal (vet.), Fansidar, and Trivetrin (vet.).
4-Amino-*N*-(5,6-dimethoxy-4-pyrimidinyl)benzenesulfonamide
$C_{12}H_{14}N_4O_4S = 310.3$
CAS—2447-57-6

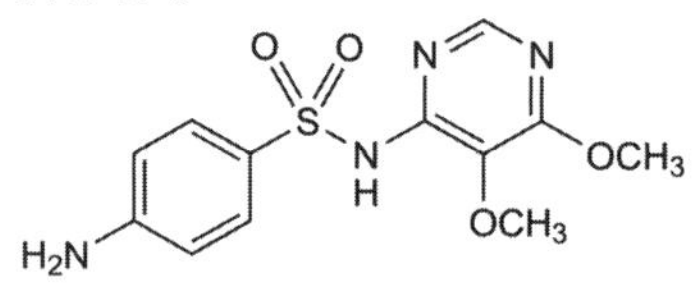

A white or creamy-white crystalline powder. M.p. 190° to 194°.
Very slightly soluble in water; slightly soluble in ethanol and in methanol; practically insoluble in ether; soluble in solutions of alkali hydroxides and mineral acids.

Partition Coefficient. Log *P* (octanol/water), 0.7.

Colour Tests. Coniferyl Alcohol—orange; Copper Sulfate (Method 1)—green; Mercurous Nitrate—black; Nitrous Acid—yellow.

Thin-layer Chromatography. System TA—Rf 67; system TB—Rf 63; system TD—Rf 37; system TE—Rf 79; system TF—Rf 51; system TAD—Rf 55; system TAE—Rf 78; system TAJ—Rf 53; system TAK—Rf 28; system TAL—Rf 90.

High Performance Liquid Chromatography. System HU—*k* 4.4; system HX—RI 364; system HAA—Retention time 13.3 min.

Ultraviolet Spectrum. Aqueous acid—264; aqueous alkali—272 nm ($A^1_1 = 762a$).

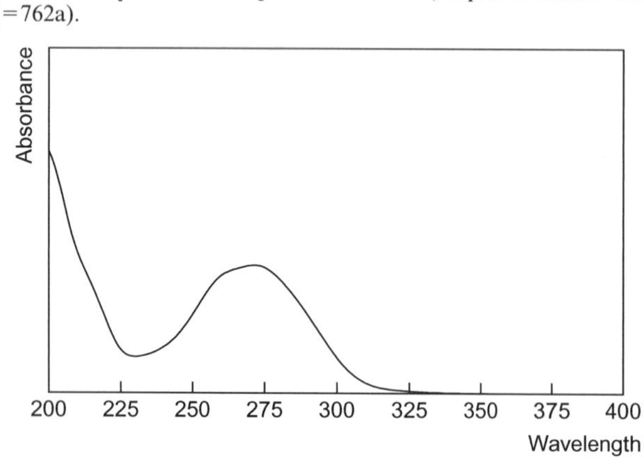

Infra-red Spectrum. Principal peaks at wavenumbers 1583, 1161, 1596, 1315, 1091, 1305 cm^{-1} (KBr disk).

Quantification
High performance liquid chromatography. In plasma, red blood cells or whole blood: sulfadoxine and other sulfonamides, limit of detection 50 μg/L, UV detection—V. K. Dua *et al.*, *J. Pharm. Biomed. Anal.*, 1994, *12*, 1317–1323. In plasma: sulfadoxine and other antimalarials, limit of detection 25 μg/L for sulfadoxine, UV detection—J. Eljaschewitsch *et al.*, *Ther. Drug Monit.*, 1996, *18*, 592–597. In plasma: sulfadoxine and pyrimethamine, limits of detection 22 mg/L (sulfadoxine) and 10 μg/L (pyrimethamine), UV detection—H. Astier *et al.*, *J. Chromatogr. B Biomed. Sci. Appl.*, 1997, *698*, 217–223. In blood: sulfadoxine and pyrimethamine—M. D. Green *et al.*, *J. Chromatogr. B Analyt. Technol. Biomed. Life Sci.*, 2002, *767*, 159–162.
The methods referred to under sulfamethoxazole may also be used.

Disposition in the Body. Sulfadoxine is a long-acting sulfonamide which is readily absorbed after oral administration. The main metabolic reaction is N^4-acetylation together with glucuronidation. High concentrations of sulfadoxine are attained in the blood in about 4 h with about 5% as the acetyl derivative and 2% as the glucuronide. It is excreted very slowly in the urine, about 8% of a dose being excreted in 24 h and 30% in 7 days. The excreted material consists of 30 to 60% acetyl derivative and 30 to 60% unchanged sulfadoxine of which up to 40% may be conjugated with glucuronic acid and up to 10% with sulfate.

Therapeutic concentration

Blood concentrations of 130 to 200 mg/L were attained by 31 patients receiving 1.5 to 2 g weekly [V. Haegi, *Schweiz. Med. Wochenschr.*, 1966, *96*, 1308, per *Int. Pharm. Abstr.*, 1967, *4*, 93].

Half-life. Plasma half-life, about 4 to 8 days.

Protein binding. In plasma, about 90%.

Dose Initially 2 g, followed by 1 to 1.5 g weekly.

Sulfaethidole

Antibacterial/Sulfonamide

Synonyms. Aethazolum; Ethazol; SETD; Sulfaethidole; Sulfaethylthiadiazole.
Proprietary name. Sul-Spantab
4-Amino-*N*-(5-ethyl-1,3,4-thiadiazol-2-yl)benzenesulfonamide
$C_{10}H_{12}N_4O_2S_2 = 284.4$
CAS—94-19-9

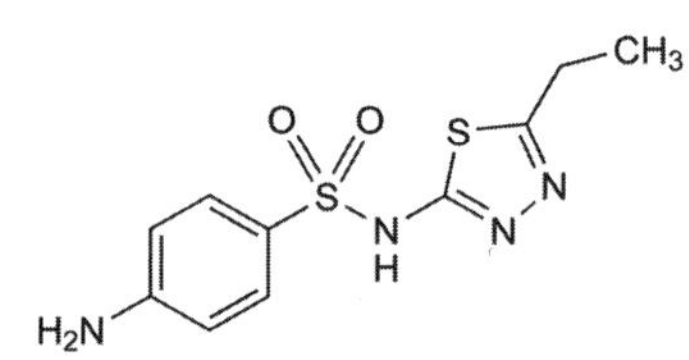

A white or yellowish-white crystalline powder. M.p. about 186°.
Very slightly soluble in water; soluble 1 in 30 of ethanol, 1 in 40 of methanol, 1 in 10 of acetone, 1 in 2800 of chloroform, and 1 in 1350 of ether; freely soluble in solutions of alkali hydroxides.

Dissociation Constant. pK_a 5.6.

Partition Coefficient. Log *P* (octanol/water), 1.0.

Colour Tests. Coniferyl Alcohol—orange; Copper Sulfate (Method 1)—green; Koppanyi–Zwikker Test—violet; Mercurous Nitrate—black; Nitrous Acid—yellow.

Thin-layer Chromatography. System TA—Rf 67; system TD—Rf 14; system TE—Rf 08; system TF—Rf 35; system TAD—Rf 34.

Gas Chromatography. System GA—sulfaethidole RI 2620; sulfaethidole-Me RI 3060; sulfaethidole-ME$_2$ RI 2840; M (acetyl-) RI 2490; M (acetyl-)-Me$_2$ RI 3410.

High Performance Liquid Chromatography. System HY—RI 314.

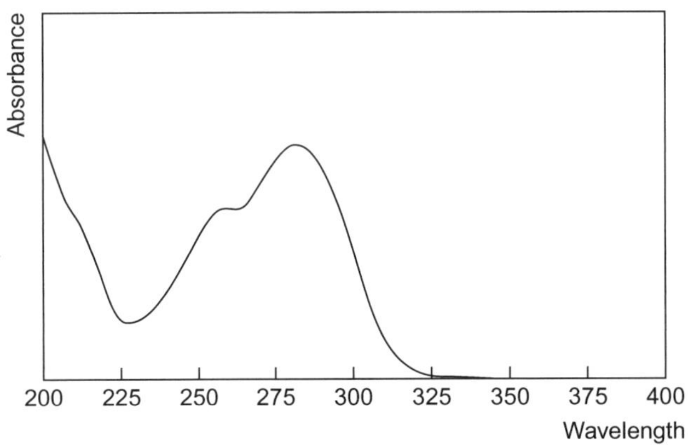

Infra-red Spectrum. Principal peaks at wavenumbers 1086, 1298, 1538, 1149, 689, 917 cm^{-1}.

Mass Spectrum. Principal ions at *m/z* 92, 284, 156, 108, 65, 106, 93, 220.

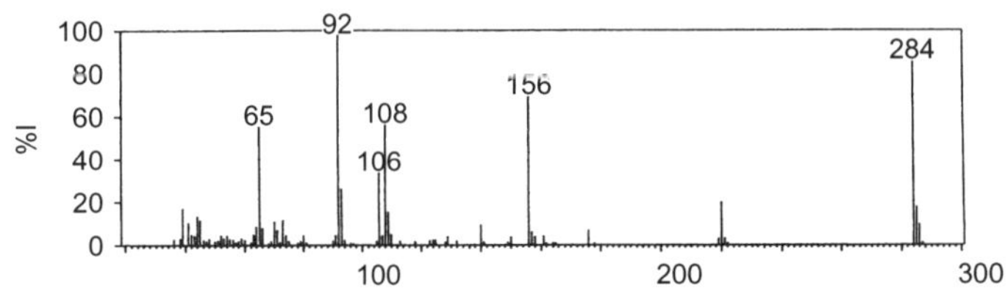

Quantification

High performance liquid chromatography. The methods referred to under sulfamethoxazole may be used.

Disposition in the Body. Readily absorbed after oral administration and only slightly acetylated in the body. More than 75% of a dose is excreted in the urine in 48 h as unchanged drug.

Therapeutic concentration

Following oral administration of 3.9 g to 6 subjects, peak blood concentrations of 138 to 275 mg/L (mean 227) were attained in about 2 h [A. E. Nicholson *et al.*, *J. Am. Pharm. Assoc.*, 1960, *49*, 40–44].

Half-life. Plasma half-life, about 10 to 12 h.

Volume of distribution. About 0.1 L/kg.

Protein binding. In plasma, 96 to 99%.

Dose. Sulfaethidole has been given in sustained-release form in a dose of up to 3.9 g.

Sulfafurazole

Antibacterial/Sulfonamide

Synonym. Sulfafuraz; Sulfafurazolum; Sulfisoxazole; Sulfafurazole.
Proprietary names. Gantrisin (tablets); Koro-Sulf; Novo-Soxazole; Sosol; Soxisol; Soxomide; Sulfalar; Sulfazin; Sulfizax; Sulfoxol.
4-Amino-*N*-(3,4-dimethyl-5-isoxazolyl)benzenesulfonamide
$C_{11}H_{13}N_3O_3S = 267.3$
CAS—127-69-5

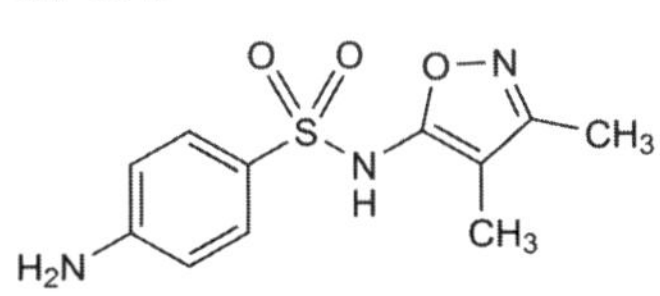

A white or yellowish-white crystalline powder. M.p. 191° to 194°.
Soluble 1 in 7700 of water, 1 in 50 of ethanol, 1 in 1000 of chloroform, and 1 in 800 of ether; freely soluble in acetone; soluble in methanol.

Acetyl Sulfafurazole

Synonym. Sulfisoxazole Acetyl.
Proprietary names. Gantrisin (suspension and syrup). It is an ingredient of Pediazole.

Note. Acetyl sulfafurazole [*N*-[(4-aminophenyl)sulfonyl]-*N*-(3,4-dimethyl-5-isoxazolyl)acetamide] should be distinguished from the N^4-acetyl derivative formed from sulfafurazole by acetylation in the body.
$C_{13}H_{15}N_3O_4S = 309.3$
CAS—80-74-0
A white to slightly yellow crystalline powder. M.p. 193° to 194°.
Practically insoluble in water; soluble 1 in about 180 of ethanol, 1 in 35 of chloroform, 1 in about 1100 of ether, and 1 in about 200 of methanol.

Sulfafurazole Diethanolamine

Synonyms. Sulfisoxazole Diolamine; Sulfafurazole Diolamine.
Proprietary name. Gantrisin (injection)
$C_{11}H_{13}N_3O_3S, C_4H_{11}NO_2 = 372.4$
CAS—4299-60-9
A white, fine, crystalline powder. M.p. 119° to 124°.
Soluble 1 in 2 of water, 1 in 16 of ethanol, 1 in 1000 of chloroform, and 1 in 4 of methanol; practically insoluble in ether.

Dissociation Constant. pK_a 5.0 (20°).

Partition Coefficient. Log *P* (octanol/pH 7.5), –0.9.

Colour Tests. Coniferyl Alcohol—orange; Copper Sulfate (Method 1)—brown; Koppanyi–Zwikker Test—blue-violet; Mercurous Nitrate—black; Nitrous Acid—orange.

Thin-layer Chromatography. System TA—Rf 65; system TD—Rf 25; system TE—Rf 06; system TF—Rf 52; system TT—Rf 74; system TU—Rf 48; system TV—Rf 04; system TAD—Rf 33; system TAE—Rf 81; system TAJ—Rf 39; system TAK—Rf 11; system TAL—Rf 70. (Mercuric chloride–diphenylcarbazone reagent, blue; acidified potassium permanganate solution, positive; Van Urk reagent, yellow.)

Gas Chromatography. System GA—RI 1212; system GJ—RRT of methyl derivative 0.42 (relative to griseofulvin).

High Performance Liquid Chromatography. System HU—*k* 6.0; system HY—RI 333.

Ultraviolet Spectrum. Aqueous acid—265; aqueous alkali—253 nm ($A_1^1 = 783a$).

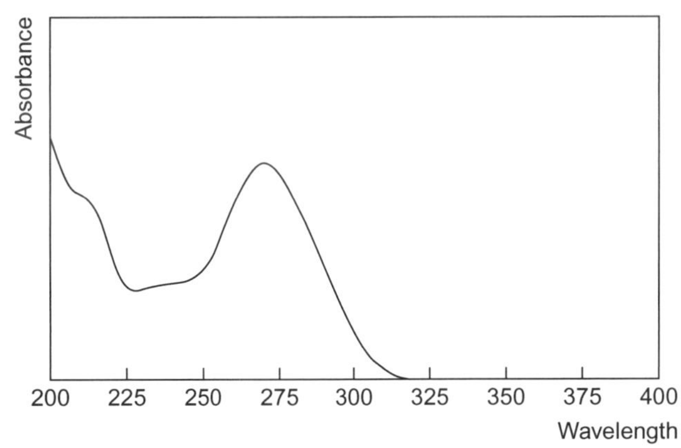

Infra-red Spectrum. Principal peaks at wavenumbers 1166, 1633, 1598, 1092, 1647, 690 cm^{-1} (KBr disk).

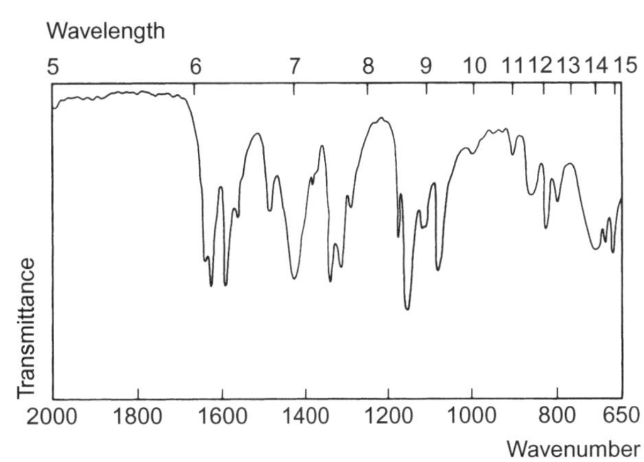

Mass Spectrum. Principal ions at *m/z* 156, 92, 108, 65, 140, 43, 157, 42.

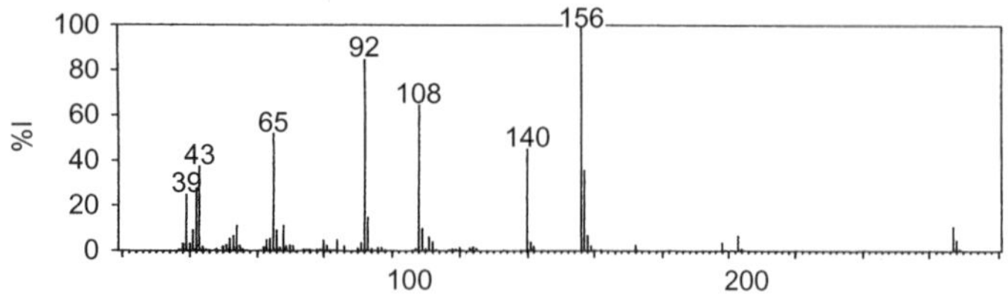

Quantification

High performance liquid chromatography. In plasma or urine: sulfafurazole and acetylsulfafurazole, limit of detection 50 µg/L, UV detection—D. Jung and S. Øie, *Clin. Chem.*, 1980, *26*, 51–54. In plasma: sulfafurazole and other sulfonamides, electrochemical detection—J. Klimes and M. Mokry, *Pharmazie*, 1997, *52*, 448–450.

Disposition in the Body. Rapidly absorbed after oral administration. It is acetylated in the body, about 30% of the sulfafurazole in the blood being in the form of the inactive N^4-acetyl derivative. It is rapidly excreted in the urine, almost the entire dose being excreted within 48 h, with up to about 60% as unchanged drug and up to about 30% as the acetyl derivative. Excretion is influenced by the pH of the urine, the rate being increased when the urine is alkaline.

Therapeutic concentration

After a single oral dose of 2 g to 7 subjects, peak plasma concentrations of sulfafurazole of 127 to 210 mg/L (mean 169) were attained in 1 to 4 h [S. A. Kaplan *et al.*, *J. Pharm. Sci.*, 1972, *61*, 773–778].

Half-life. Plasma half-life, 4 to 7 h.

Volume of distribution. About 0.1 to 0.2 L/kg.

Clearance. Plasma clearance, about 0.3 mL/min/kg.

Protein binding. In plasma, 85 to 95%.

Dose. An initial dose of 2 to 4 g, followed by 1 to 2 g every 4 to 6 h.

Sulfaguanidine

Antibacterial/Sulfonamide

Synonyms. Solfaguanidina; Sulfamidinum; Sulfanilylguanidine; Sulginum.

Proprietary names. Diacta; Enteropathyl; Ganidan; Guanicil; Resulfon; Shigatox.

4-Amino-*N*-(aminoiminomethyl)benzenesulfonamide

$C_7H_{10}N_4O_2S$=214.3

CAS—57-67-0

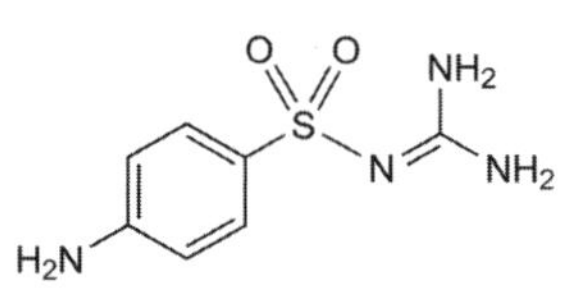

Sulfaguanidine Monohydrate

$C_7H_{10}N_4O_2S,H_2O$=232.3

CAS—6190-55-2

White crystals or powder, slowly darkening on exposure to light. M.p. 190° to 193°.

Soluble 1 in 1000 of water and 1 in 250 of ethanol; slightly soluble in acetone; practically insoluble in ether; readily soluble in dilute mineral acids.

Partition Coefficient. Log *P* (octanol/water), −1.2.

Colour Tests. Coniferyl Alcohol—orange; Copper Sulfate (Method 1)—blue; Koppanyi–Zwikker Test—violet (transient).

Thin-layer Chromatography. System TA—Rf 65; system TD—Rf 01; system TE—Rf 25; system TF—Rf 06; system TT—Rf 21; system TU—Rf 90; system TV—Rf 48; system TAD—Rf 07; system TAE—Rf 75.

Gas Chromatography. System GA—not eluted.

High Performance Liquid Chromatography. System HY—RI 92; system HAA—Retention time 3.8 min.

Ultraviolet Spectrum. Aqueous acid—264 (A^1_1=115a), 271 (A^1_1=107c); aqueous alkali—259 nm (A^1_1=758a).

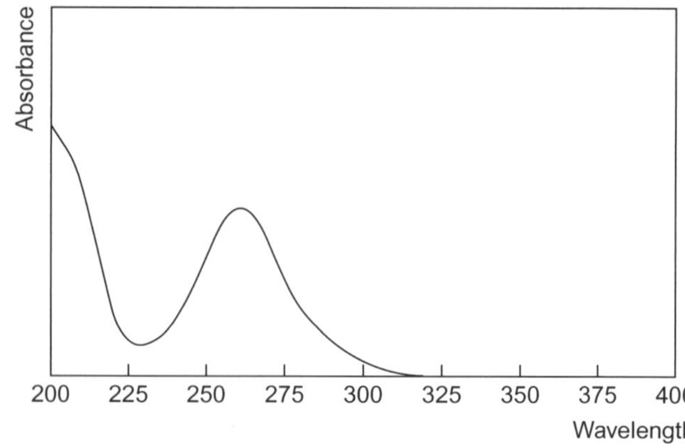

Infra-red Spectrum. Principal peaks at wavenumbers 1620, 1129, 1230, 1537, 1075, 1176 cm^{-1} (KBr disk).

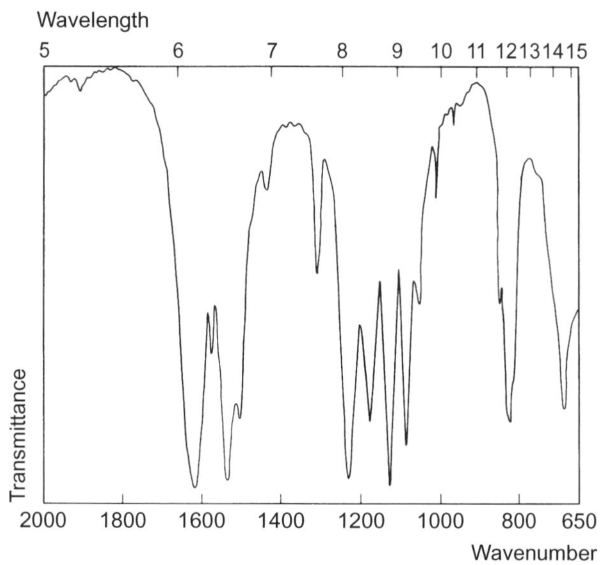

Mass Spectrum. Principal ions at *m/z* 92, 65, 108, 214, 156, 39, 109, 43.

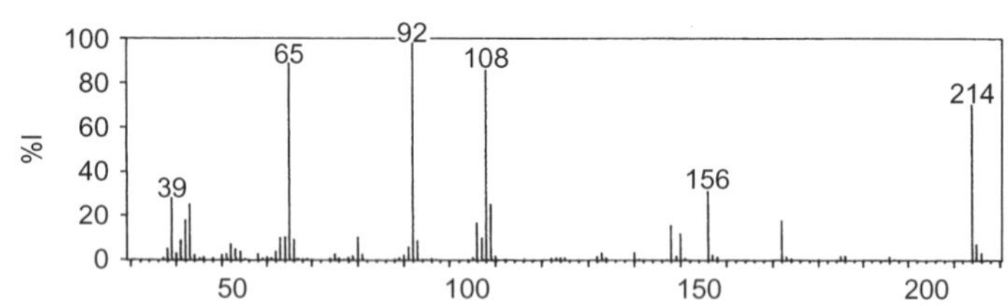

Quantification

High performance liquid chromatography. In plasma: limit of detection 10 µg/L, UV detection—R. L. Suber and G. T. Edds, *J. Liq. Chromatogr.*, 1980, *3*, 257–268. In urine: sulfaguanidine and other sulfonamides, limit of detection 0.1 to 0.3 mg/L—E. F. Simo-Alfonso *et al.*, *J. Chromatogr. B Biomed. Appl.*, 1995, *670*, 183–187.

Disposition in the Body. Absorption is variable after oral administration. It is rapidly excreted in the urine, about 30% of the excreted material being in the form of the inactive N^4-acetyl derivative. Large amounts are also eliminated in the faeces.

Therapeutic concentration. In plasma, usually in the range 15 to 40 mg/L.

Protein binding. In plasma, about 8%.

Dose. Sulfaguanidine has been given in doses of 9 g daily for 3 days.

Sulfamerazine

Antibacterial/Sulfonamide

Synonyms. Solfamerazina; Sulfamethyldiazine; Sulfamethylpyrimidine; Sulfamerazine.
Proprietary names. It is an ingredient of Berlocombin, Sulfatril, and Trisulfaminic.
4-Amino-*N*-(4-methyl-2-pyrimidinyl)benzenesulfonamide
$C_{11}H_{12}N_4O_2S$=264.3
CAS—127-79-7

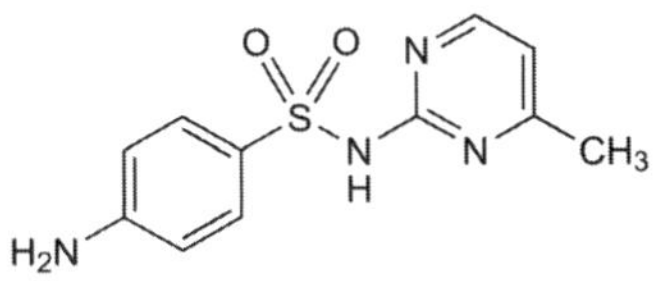

A white or faintly yellowish-white crystalline powder which slowly darkens on exposure to light. M.p. 234° to 238°, with decomposition.
Soluble 1 in 6250 of water, 1 in 550 of ethanol, and 1 in 60 of acetone; very slightly soluble in ether and chloroform; soluble in dilute mineral acids and in solutions of alkali hydroxides and carbonates.

Sulfamerazine Sodium

Synonyms. Soluble Sulfamerazine; Sulfamerazine Sodium.
$C_{11}H_{11}N_4NaO_2S$=286.3
CAS—127-58-2
A white or yellowish-white powder. It slowly darkens on exposure to light; on exposure to moist air it absorbs carbon dioxide and becomes less soluble in water.
Soluble 1 in 3.6 of water; slightly soluble in ethanol; insoluble in chloroform and ether.

Dissociation Constant. pK_a 7.1 (20°).

Partition Coefficient. Log *P* (octanol/pH 7.5), –0.1.

Colour Tests. Coniferyl Alcohol—orange; Copper Sulfate (Method 1)—green→brown; Koppanyi–Zwikker Test—pink; Mercurous Nitrate—black.

Thin-layer Chromatography. System TA—Rf 65; system TD—Rf 23; system TE—Rf 08; system TF—Rf 41; system TT—Rf 33; system TU—Rf 18; system TV—Rf 07; system TAD—Rf 42; system TAE—Rf 80.

Gas Chromatography. System GA—sulfamerazine RI 2566; sulfamerazine-Me RI 2625; System GJ—sulfamerazine-Me RRT 0.69 (relative to griseofulvin).

High Performance Liquid Chromatography. System HU—*k* 8.1; system HY—RI 247.

Ultraviolet Spectrum. Aqueous acid—242 (A_1^1=596a), 304; aqueous alkali—242 (A_1^1=820b), 255 nm (A_1^1=828b).

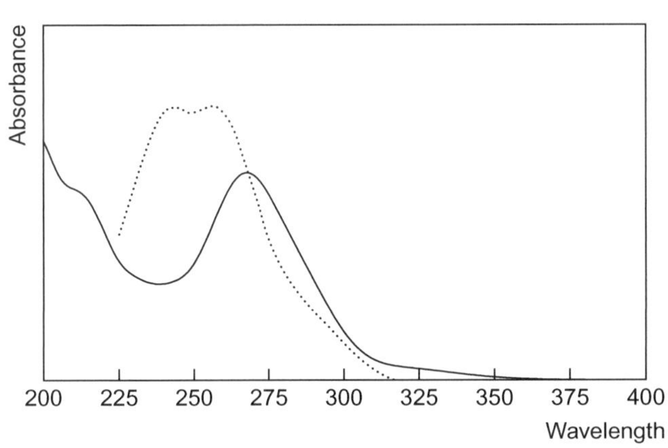

Infra-red Spectrum. Principal peaks at wavenumbers 1149, 1590, 1560, 1316, 1088, 1618 cm^{-1} (KBr disk).

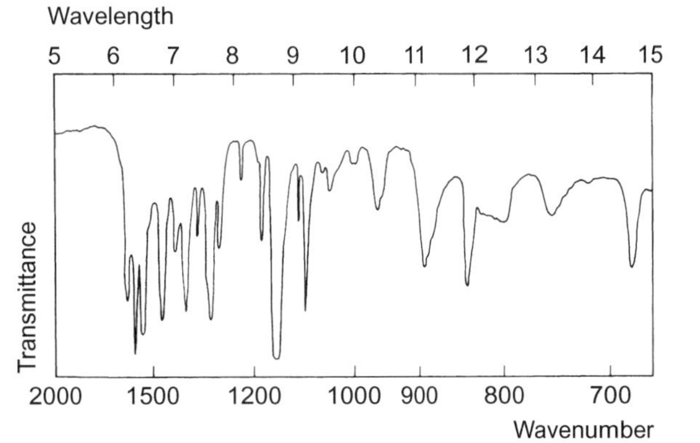

Mass Spectrum. Principal ions at *m/z* 199, 200, 92, 65, 108, 39, 66, 201.

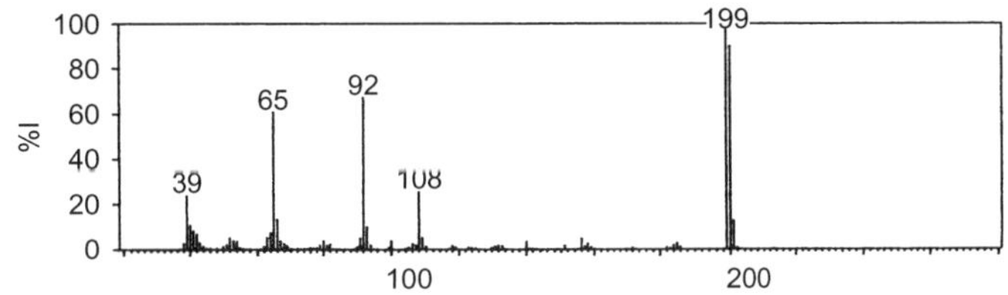

Quantification

High performance liquid chromatography. In plasma or urine: sulfamerazine and acetylsulfamerazine, limit of detection 300 µg/L, UV detection—T. B. Vree *et al.*, *Biopharm. Drug Disp.*, 1983, *4*, 271–291.

Disposition in the Body. Rapidly absorbed after oral administration. It penetrates into the CSF to produce concentrations about one-half of those in blood. Metabolised by N^4-acetylation, the extent of which is genetically determined; in slow acetylators about 15% of the sulfamerazine in the blood is in the form of the acetyl derivative compared with 35% in rapid acetylators. About 60% of a dose is excreted in the urine in 48 h; approximately half of the excreted material is in the form of the acetyl derivative.

Toxicity. Serious toxic effects, sometimes fatal, have occurred in young children, after therapeutic doses.

Half-life. Plasma half-life, 9 to 14 h in rapid acetylators and about 24 h in slow acetylators.

Volume of distribution. About 0.4 L/kg.

Protein binding. In plasma, about 80 to 90%.

Dose. 4 g daily.

Sulfamethizole

Antibacterial/Sulfonamide

Synonym. Sulfamethylthiadiazole.
Proprietary names. Famet; Luco-Oph; Lucosil; Methazol; Renisul; Rufol; Salimol; Sulfapyelon; Thidicur; Thiosulfil; Urolex; Urolucosil.
4-Amino-*N*-(5-methyl-1,3,4-thiadiazol-2-yl)benzenesulfonamide
$C_9H_{10}N_4O_2S_2$=270.3
CAS—144-82-1

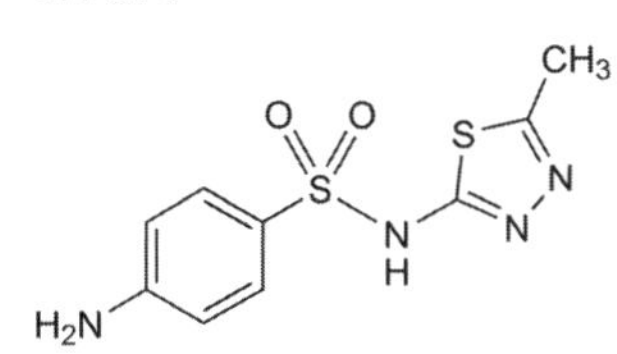

Colourless crystals or white or creamy-white crystalline powder. M.p. 208°.
Soluble 1 in 2000 of water, 1 in 30 of ethanol, 1 in 40 methanol, 1 in 10 to 1 in 13 of acetone, 1 in 1370 of ether, and 1 in 2800 of chloroform; soluble in solutions of alkali hydroxides and in dilute mineral acids.

Dissociation Constant. pK_a 5.5 (25°).

Partition Coefficient. Log *P* (octanol/pH 7.5), –1.1; (octanol/water), 0.5.

Colour Tests. Coniferyl Alcohol—orange; Copper Sulfate (Method 1)—green; Koppanyi–Zwikker Test—red-violet; Mercurous Nitrate—black; Nitrous Acid—yellow.

Thin-layer Chromatography. System TA—Rf 65; system TD—Rf 12; system TE—Rf 04; system TF—Rf 23; system TT—Rf 46; system TU—Rf 36; system TV—Rf 02; system TAD—Rf 27; system TAE—Rf 83; system TAJ—Rf 34; system TAK—Rf 14; system TAL—Rf 75. (Mercuric chloride–diphenylcarbazone reagent, blue; acidified potassium permanganate solution, positive; Van Urk reagent, yellow.)

Gas Chromatography. System GA—Sulfamethizole-Me RI 2660; System GJ—RRT of methyl derivative 0.98 (relative to griseofulvin).

High Performance Liquid Chromatography. System HZ—Retention time 2.3 min.

Ultraviolet Spectrum. Aqueous acid—268 (A^1_1=542a); aqueous alkali—260 nm.

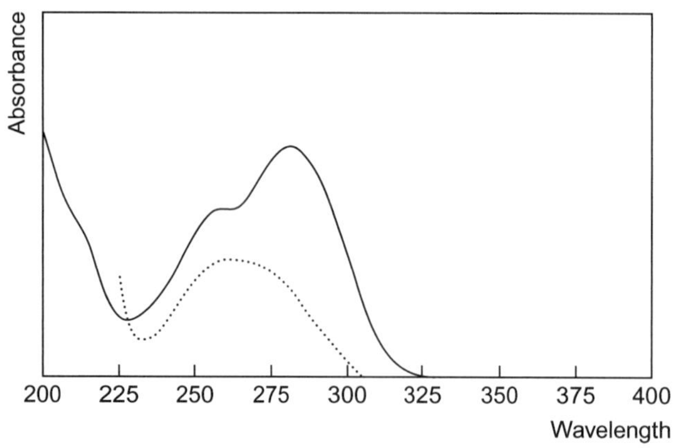

Infra-red Spectrum. Principal peaks at wavenumbers 1549, 1134, 699, 1084, 1152, 1600 cm^{-1} (KBr disk). (See below)

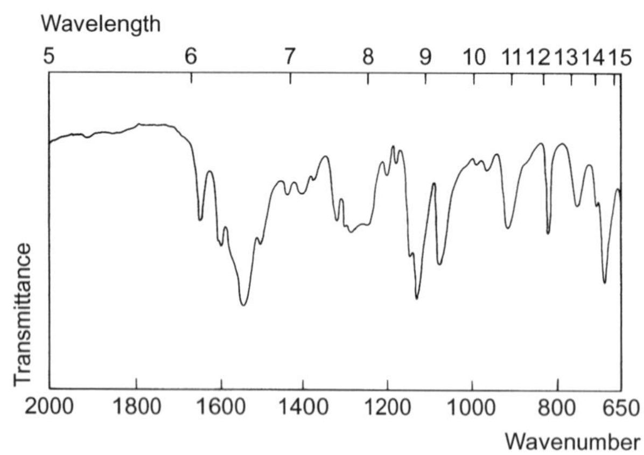

Mass Spectrum. Principal ions at *m/z* 92, 270, 65, 156, 108, 106, 93, 59.

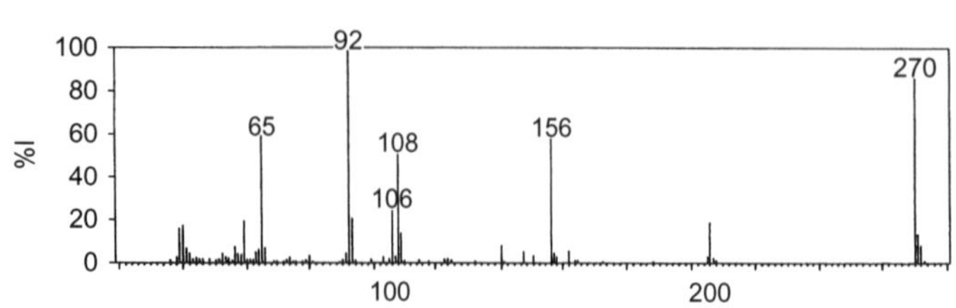

Quantification

High performance liquid chromatography. In urine: sulfamethizole and other sulfonamides, limit of detection 0.1 to 0.3 mg/L—E. F. Simo-Alfonso *et al.*, *J. Chromatogr. B Biomed. Appl.*, 1995, *670*, 183–187.

The methods referred to under sulfamethoxazole may also be used.

Disposition in the Body. Readily absorbed after oral administration and only slightly acetylated in the body. It is rapidly excreted in the urine, up to 90% of a dose being excreted within 24 h, mainly as unchanged drug.

Therapeutic concentration

Following oral administration of 0.5 g of sulfamethizole to 5 subjects, a mean peak blood concentration of 20 mg/L was attained in about 2 h [G. L. Mattock and I. J. McGilveray, *J.Pharm. Sci.*, 1972, *61*, 746–749].

Half-life. Plasma half-life, 1 to 2 h.

Volume of distribution. About 0.3 L/kg.

Clearance. Blood clearance, about 3 mL/min/kg.

Protein binding. In plasma, about 90%.

Dose. 1 to 4 g daily.

Sulfamethoxazole

Sulfonamide

Synonyms. Ro-4-2130; Sulfamethoxazole; Sulfisomezole.
Proprietary names. Gantanol; Urobak. It is an ingredient of many proprietary preparations—see Martindale, *The complete drug reference*, 33rd Edn., Pharmaceutical Press, London, 2002.
4-Amino-*N*-(5-methyl-3-isoxazolyl)benzenesulfonamide
$C_{10}H_{11}N_3O_3S$=253.3
CAS—723-46-6

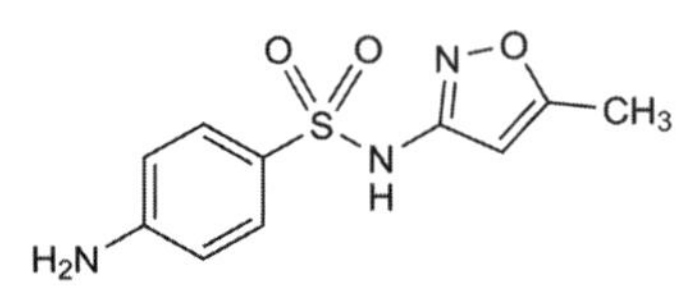

A white or yellowish-white crystalline powder. M.p. 167° (crystals from dilute ethanol).
Very slightly soluble in water; soluble 1 in 50 of ethanol and 1 in 3 of acetone; practically insoluble in chloroform and ether; soluble in solutions of alkali hydroxides.

Dissociation Constant. pK_a 5.6 (25°).

Partition Coefficient. Log *P* (octanol/water), 0.9.

Colour Tests. Coniferyl Alcohol—orange; Copper Sulfate (Method 1)—green; Koppanyi–Zwikker Test—blue-violet; Mercurous Nitrate—black; Nitrous Acid—yellow

Thin-layer Chromatography. System TA—Rf 65; system TD—Rf 26; system TE—Rf 05; system TF—Rf 54; system TT—Rf 88; system TU—Rf 33; system TV—Rf 02; system TAD—Rf 41; system TAE—Rf 79; system TAJ—Rf 45; system TAK—Rf 26; system TAL—Rf 81. (Mercuric chloride–diphenylcarbazone reagent, blue; acidified potassium permanganate solution, positive; Van Urk reagent, yellow.)

Gas Chromatography. System GA—sulfamethoxazole-Me RI 2500, sulfamethoxazole-Me_2 RI 2460, M (N^4-acetyl-)-Me RI 3255; system GJ—sulfamethoxazole-Me RRT 0.40, M (N^4-acetyl-)-Me RRT 0.91 (both relative to griseofulvin).

High Performance Liquid Chromatography. system HU—sulfamethoxazole *k* 4.8, (N^4-acetyl-) *k* 4.9; system HY—RI 320; system HZ—Retention time, 2.9 min; system HAA—Retention time, 13.4 min; system HAM—Retention time 2.7 min.

Ultraviolet Spectrum. Aqueous acid—265 nm (A^1_1=175a); aqueous alkali—256 nm (A^1_1=673a).

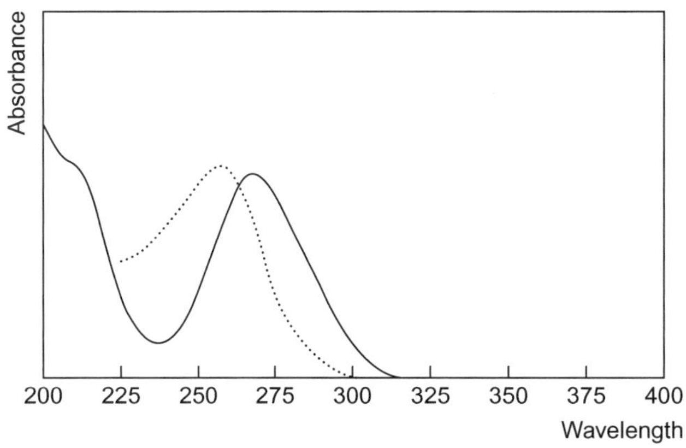

Infra-red Spectrum. Principal peaks at wavenumbers 1145, 1160, 1599, 1621, 685, 1306 cm^{-1} (KBr disk).

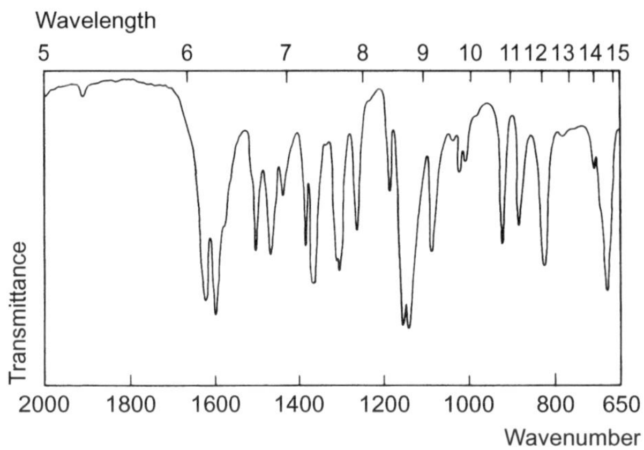

Mass Spectrum. Principal ions at *m/z* 156, 92, 108, 65, 140, 253, 157, 43.

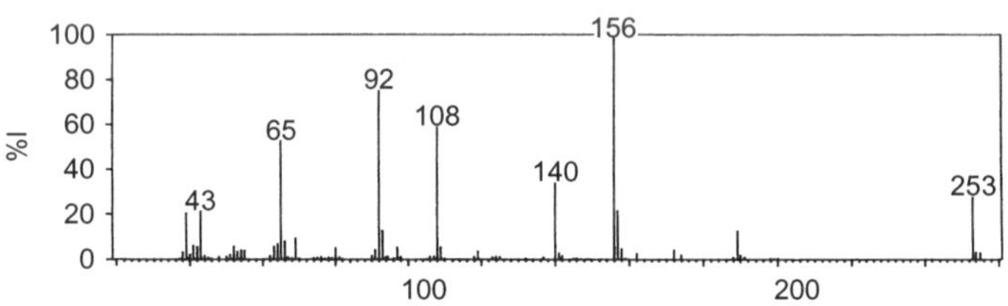

Quantification

High performance liquid chromatography. In serum or urine: limit of detection 0.5 mg/L, UV detection—T. B. Vree *et al.*, *J. Chromatogr.*, 1978, *146*; *Biomed. Appl.*, *3*, 103–112. In plasma or urine: sulfamethoxazole and its metabolites, limit of quantification for sulfamethoxazole 0.1 mg/L, UV detection—T. B. Vree *et al.*, *J. Chromatogr.*, 1994, *658*, *Biomed. Appl.*, 327–340. In blood: sulfamethoxazole and trimethoprim, limits of quantification 1 mg/L and 0.1 mg/L, respectively—A. M. Ronn *et al.*, *Ther. Drug Monit.*, 1999, *21*, 609–614.

Disposition in the Body. Readily absorbed after oral administration and widely distributed; it is found in saliva, sweat, bile, CSF, peritoneal, ocular and synovial fluids; it is found in pleural and other effusions. It crosses the placenta and is excreted in breast milk. It is metabolised mainly by acetylation with the formation of the N^1-acetyl and N^4-acetyl derivatives; about 15% of the sulfamethoxazole in the blood is present as acetylated metabolites. Excreted in the urine mostly as the N^4-acetyl derivative and unchanged sulfamethoxazole together with some glucuronide conjugates. Urinary excretion is variable and is dependent on the pH of the urine, the proportion of unchanged drug excreted being increased when the urine is alkaline. Up to about 25% of the dose is excreted unchanged when the urine is acid, rising to 40% or more in alkaline urine. The amount of the N^4-acetyl derivative excreted may be 30 to 70% of the dose. Sulfamethoxazole is oxidised to form a hydroxylamine which may be involved in adverse reactions to sulfonamides.

Sulfamethoxazole is frequently administered together with trimethoprim but this does not affect its metabolism.

Therapeutic concentration

7 healthy males (aged 22 to 32 years; mean 28.2) were administered with a mean trimethoprim dose of 20.2 (range 19.3 to 20.9) mg/kg daily and 101.1 (96.3 to 104.7) mg/kg daily sulfamethoxazole for 3 days, as even doses administered every 6 h. Volunteers were fasted for 1 h before dosing and 2 h after administration. The mean peak serum concentrations observed were 13.6 (range 10.6 to 16.1) mg/L trimethoprim, 372 (277 to 469) mg/L sulfamethoxale and 50.1 (39.5 to 70.3) mg/L acetylsulfamethoxale. These concentrations were observed at 1.9 (0.3 to 2.7), 2.6 (0.7 to 3.5) and 2.8 (0.3 to 6.0) h, respectively [R. C. Stevens *et al.*, *Antimicrob. Agents Chemother.*, 1991, *35*, 1884–1890].

Administration of a single oral dose of sulfamethoxazole and trimethoprim (800 mg and 160 mg, respectively) and metronidazole (2 g) to 24 patients, 1.5 to 10.5 h before colorectal surgery, produced sulfamethoxazole serum concentrations of 15 to 65 mg/L (median 35) at the start of the operation and 13 to 70 mg/L (median 33) at the end. Corresponding concentrations of trimethoprim were 0.7 to 2.6 mg/L (median 1.4) and 1.0 to 2.8 mg/L (median 1.3) at the start and end of surgery, respectively [Y. Raab *et al.*, *Eur. J. Surg.*, 2001, *167*, 46–49].

Toxicity. Plasma concentrations greater than 400 mg/L may be associated with toxic effects.

Half-life. Plasma half-life, 9 to 12 h.

Volume of distribution. About 0.25 L/kg.

Clearance. Plasma clearance, about 0.3 mL/min/kg.

Distribution in blood. Plasma : whole blood ratio, about 1.35.

Saliva. Plasma : saliva ratio, about 14.

Protein binding. In plasma, 50 to 70%.

Note. For a review of the clinical pharmacokinetics of sulfonamides and their N^4-acetyl derivatives, see C. A. Hekster and T. B. Vree, *Antibiot. Chemother.*, 1982, *31*, 22–118; for a review of the clinical pharmacokinetics of sulfamethoxazole and trimethoprim, see R. B. Patel and P. G. Welling, *Clin. Pharmacokinet.*, 1980, *5*, 405–423.

Dose. Usually 2 g initially, followed by 1 g twice daily; maximum of 3 g daily.

Sulfamethoxypyridazine

Antibacterial/Sulfonamide

Synonyms. CL-13494; RP-7522

Proprietary names. Dibasul; Exasul; Kynex; Lederkyn; Midicel; Midikel; Sulfalex; Sulfdurazin; Sultirene.

4-Amino-*N*-(6-methoxy-3-pyridazinyl)benzenesulfonamide

$C_{11}H_{12}N_4O_3S = 280.3$

CAS—80-35-3

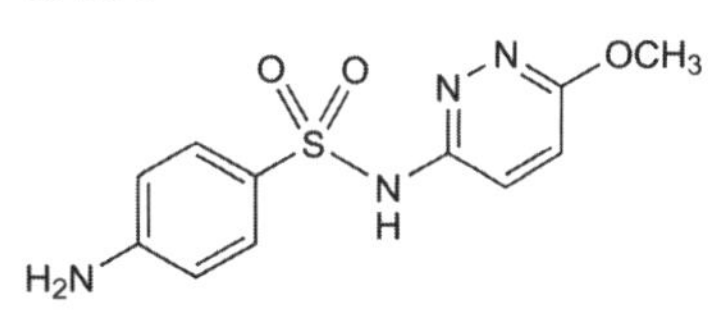

A white or yellowish-white crystalline powder which slowly darkens on exposure to light. M.p. 182° to 183°.

Very slightly soluble in water; soluble 1 in 200 of ethanol, 1 in 50 of acetone, and 1 in 400 of chloroform; slightly soluble in methanol; practically insoluble in ether; freely soluble in dilute mineral acids and solutions of alkali hydroxides.

Sulfamethoxypyridazine Sodium

Proprietary names. Davosin, Sulfoxine LA.

$C_{11}H_{11}N_4O_3S\ Na = 302.3$

CAS—2577-32-4

Acetyl Sulfamethoxypyridazine

Note. Acetyl sulfamethoxypyridazine [*N*-(6-methoxypyridazin-3-yl)-*N*-sulfanilylacetamide] should be distinguished from the N^4-acetyl derivative formed from sulfamethoxypyridazine by acetylation in the body.

$C_{13}H_{14}N_4O_4S = 322.3$
CAS—3568-43-2
Crystals. M.p. 186° to 187°, with decomposition.
Very soluble in water.

Dissociation Constant. pK_a 7.2 (20°).

Partition Coefficient. Log *P* (octanol/water), 0.3.

Colour Tests. Coniferyl Alcohol—orange; Copper Sulfate (Method 1)—green-brown; Koppanyi–Zwikker Test—red-violet; Mercurous Nitrate—black; Nitrous Acid—yellow.

Thin-layer Chromatography. System TA—Rf 65; system TD—Rf 19; system TE—Rf 09; system TF—Rf 39; system TT—Rf 53; system TU—Rf 26; system TV—Rf 50; system TAD—Rf 43; system TAE—Rf 83; system TAJ—Rf 46; system TAK—Rf 20; system TAL—Rf 84.

Gas Chromatography. System GJ—RRT of methyl derivative 0.93 (relative to griseofulvin).

High Performance Liquid Chromatography. System HAA—Retention time 11.2 min; system HU—*k* 7.5; system HX—RI 335.

Ultraviolet Spectrum. Aqueous acid—316 (A^1_1 = 163b); aqueous alkali—250 nm (A^1_1 = 712a).

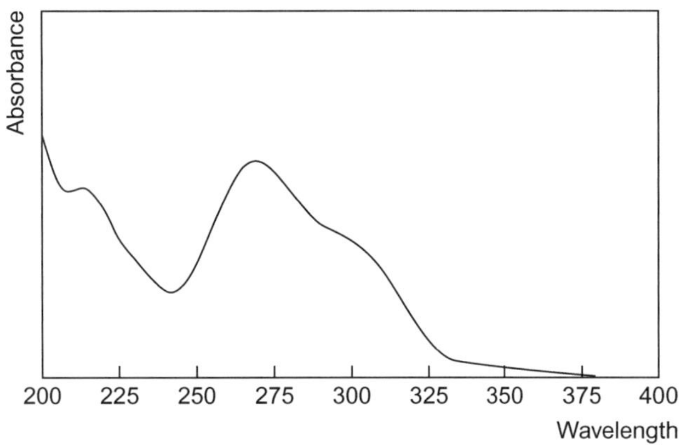

Infra-red Spectrum. Principal peaks at wavenumbers 1159, 1599, 1130, 1305, 1630, 1088 cm^{-1} (KBr disk).

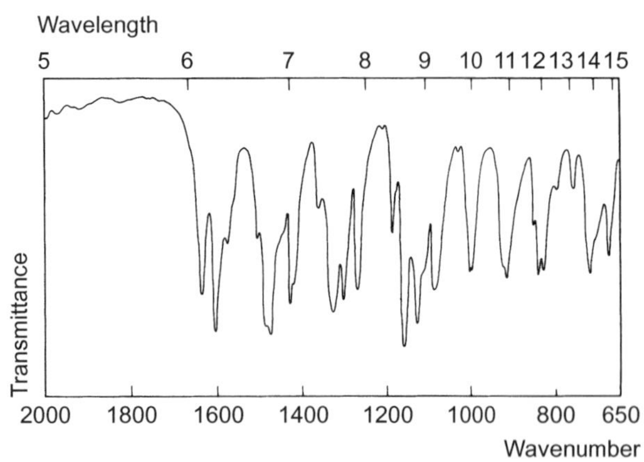

Mass Spectrum. Principal ions at *m/z* 215, 92, 216, 65, 108, 53, 69, 39.

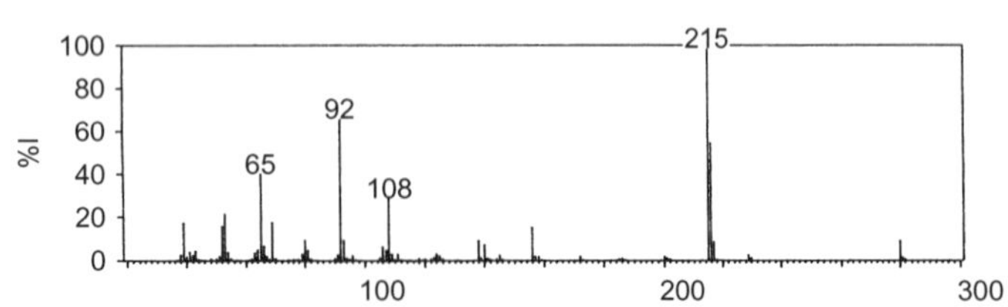

Quantification

High performance liquid chromatography. The methods referred to under sulfamethoxazole may be used.

Disposition in the Body. Sulfamethoxypyridazine is a long-acting sulfonamide which is readily absorbed after oral administration and may be detected in blood for up to 7 days after discontinuation of treatment. It is acetylated in the body and 10 to 15% of the sulfamethoxypyridazine in the blood is present as the inactive N^4-acetyl derivative. About 45% of a dose is excreted in the urine in 48 h, with 40 to 70% of the excreted material as the acetyl derivative, about 20% as unchanged drug, and about 13% as glucuronide conjugates. Excretion is influenced by the pH of the urine, the rate being increased when the urine is alkaline.

Therapeutic concentration

Blood concentrations of 110 to 180 mg/L were attained in 5 h following an oral dose of 4 g [H. Seneca, *J. Am. Med. Assoc.*, 1966, *198*, 975–980].

Half-life. Plasma half-life, 1 to 3 days.

Volume of distribution. About 0.2 L/kg.

Distribution in blood. Small amounts are taken up by the erythrocytes.

Protein binding. In plasma, 80 to 90%.

Dose. An initial dose of 1 to 2 g, followed by 500 mg daily.

Sulfametopyrazine

Antibacterial/Sulfonamide

Synonyms. Solfametopirazina; Solfametossipirazina; Sulfalene; Sulfamethoxypyrazine; Sulfapyrazin Methoxyne; Sulfalene.
Proprietary names. Dalysep; Kelfizina; Kelfizine W; Longum; Policydal; Vetkelfizina.
4-Amino-*N*-(3-methoxypyrazinyl)benzenesulfonamide
$C_{11}H_{12}N_4O_3S = 280.3$
CAS—152-47-6

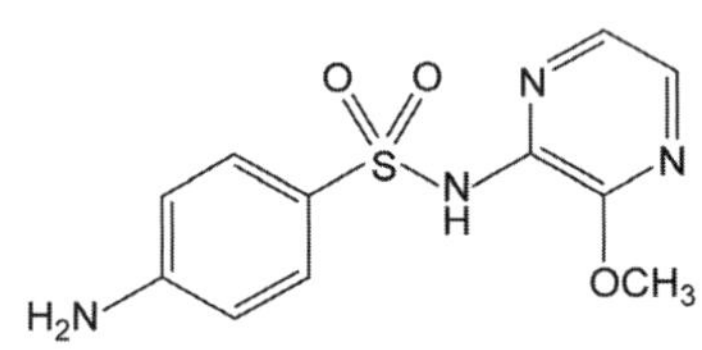

A white or yellowish-white crystalline powder. M.p. 176°.
Practically insoluble in water; slightly soluble in ethanol and chloroform; freely soluble in acetone and in dilute mineral acids and solutions of alkali hydroxides.

Dissociation Constant. pK_a 7.0.

Partition Coefficient. Log *P* (octanol/water), 0.7.

Colour Tests. Coniferyl Alcohol—orange; Copper Sulfate (Method 1)—green; Mercurous Nitrate—black; Nitrous Acid—yellow.

Thin-layer Chromatography. System TA—Rf 67; system TD—Rf 40; system TE—Rf 08; system TF—Rf 50; system TAD—Rf 54. (Van Urk reagent, positive.)

Gas Chromatography. System GJ—sulfametopyrazine-Me RRT 0.69 (relative to griseofulvin).

High Performance Liquid Chromatography. System HX—RI 353.

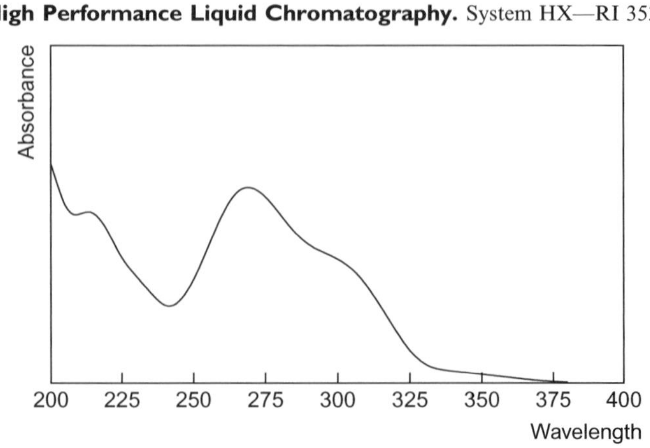

Infra-red Spectrum. Principal peaks at wavenumbers 1145, 1315, 1162, 1601, 1642, 1085 cm^{-1} (KBr disk).

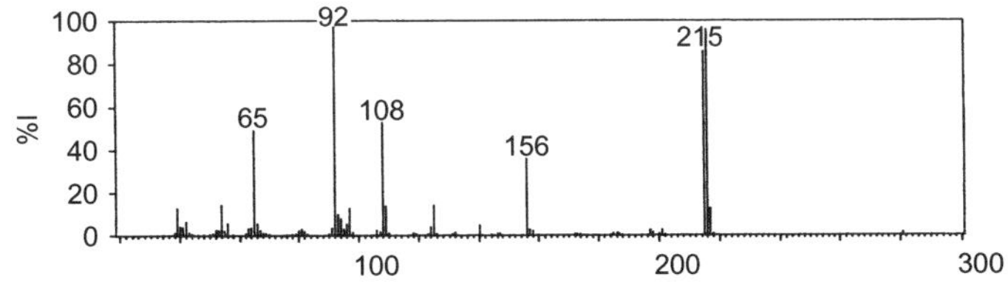

Quantification

High performance liquid chromatography. In plasma, red blood cells and whole blood: limit of detection 50 µg/L, UV detection—V. K. Dua *et al.*, *J. Chromatogr.*, 1991, *563*, 333–340; V. K. Dua *et al.*, *J. Chromatogr. B Biomed. Sci. Appl.*, 1998, *714*, 390–394.

Disposition in the Body. Sulfametopyrazine is a long-acting sulfonamide and is readily absorbed after oral administration. It is acetylated in the body, 5 to 10% of the sulfametopyrazine in the blood being in the form of the N^4-acetyl derivative which is inactive. It is slowly excreted in the urine, about 70% of the excreted material being the acetyl derivative and about 14 to 20% being unchanged drug.

Therapeutic concentration

After a single oral dose of 500 mg to 3 subjects, peak plasma concentrations of 25 to 33 mg/L (mean 29) were attained in 2 to 4 h [R. L. Herting *et al.*, *Antimicrob. Agents Chemother.*, 1964, 554–561].

Maximum steady-state plasma concentrations of 51 to 69 mg/L (mean 58) were reported on the seventh day after 6 subjects had received an initial dose of 600 mg followed by 200 mg daily [D. S. Reeves *et al.*, *J. Antimicrob. Chemother.*, 1980, *6*, 647–656].

Half-life. Plasma half-life, 2 to 4 days.

Volume of distribution. About 0.2 to 0.3 L/kg.

Protein binding. In plasma, 65 to 80%.

Dose. 2 g once a week.

Sulfametoxydiazine

Antibacterial/Sulfonamide

Synonyms. Sulfameter; Sulfametin; Sulfametorinum; Sulfamethoxydiazine; Sulfamethoxydin.

Proprietary names. Bayrena; Durenat; Kinecid; Kirocid; Sulla; Ultrax.

4-Amino-*N*-(5-methoxy-2-pyrimidinyl)benzenesulfonamide

$C_{11}H_{12}N_4O_3S$ = 280.3

CAS—651-06-9

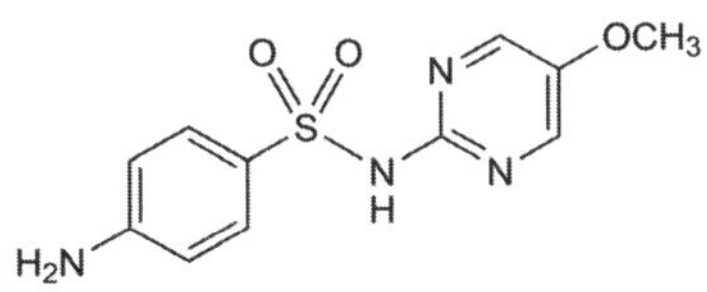

A white or yellowish-white crystalline powder. M.p. 214° to 216°.

Very sparingly soluble in water, ethanol, and ether; sparingly soluble in acetone; freely soluble in aqueous solutions of alkali hydroxides and carbonates.

Dissociation Constant. pK_a 7.0.

Partition Coefficient. Log *P* (octanol/water), 0.4.

Colour Tests. Coniferyl Alcohol—orange; Copper Sulfate (Method 1)—violet-brown; Koppanyi–Zwikker Test—pink; Mercurous Nitrate—black; Nitrous Acid—yellow.

Thin-layer Chromatography. System TA—Rf 60; system TD—Rf 24; system TE—Rf 12; system TF—Rf 43; system TT—Rf 55; system TU—Rf 17; system TV—Rf 15; system TAD—Rf 47; system TAE—Rf 82.

Gas Chromatography. System GA—sulfamethoxydiazine-Me_3 RI 2925; M (acetyl-)-Me RI 3620; System GJ—RRT of methyl derivative 1.38 (relative to griseofulvin).

High Performance Liquid Chromatography. System HU—*k* 8.2.

Ultraviolet Spectrum. Aqueous alkali—245 nm (A^1_1 = 920a).

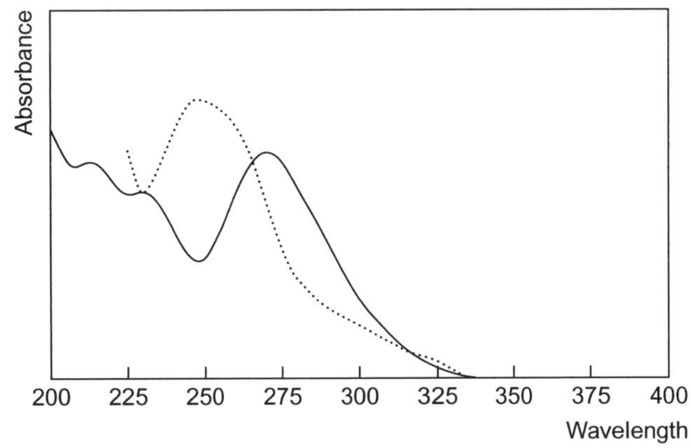

Infra-red Spectrum. Principal peaks at wavenumbers 1153, 1597, 1140, 1284, 1090, 925 cm^{-1} (KBr disk).

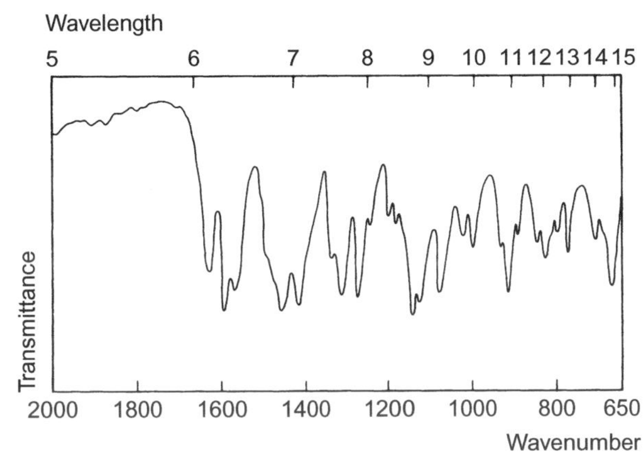

Mass Spectrum. Principal ions at *m/z* 216, 215, 92, 65, 108, 54, 125, 39.

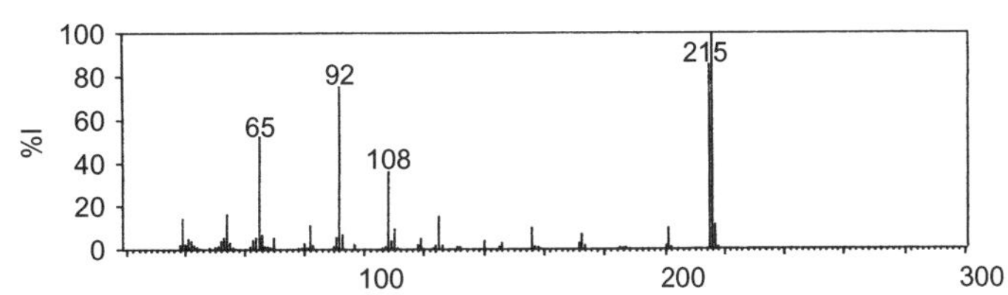

Quantification

High performance liquid chromatography. In plasma: sulfametoxydiazine and other sulfonamides, electrochemical detection—J. Klimes and M. Mokry, *Pharmazie*, 1997, *52*, 448–450.

Disposition in the Body. Sulfametoxydiazine is a long-acting sulfonamide which is readily absorbed after oral administration. It is acetylated in the body, about 10% being present in the blood as the inactive N^4-acetyl derivative. It is excreted slowly in the urine, 20 to 40% of a dose being excreted in 24 h and about 70% in 3 days. About 50% of the excreted material is unchanged drug, about 25% is the acetyl derivative, and about 20% is a glucuronide conjugate.

Therapeutic concentration

After a single oral dose of 1 g to 4 subjects, peak serum concentrations of 62 to 90 mg/L (mean 80) were attained in about 6 to 8 h; following a single oral dose of 2 g to a further 4 subjects, peak serum concentrations of 113 to 148 mg/L (mean 134) were reported at 6 to 8 h; mean peak serum concentrations of 86 mg/L and 166 mg/L respectively were reported following daily oral doses of 0.5 and 1 g for 3 days [W. H. Chew *et al.*, *Clin. Pharmacol. Ther.*, 1965, *6*, 307–315].

Half-life. Plasma half-life, 29 to 59 h (mean 37).

Volume of distribution. About 0.3 L/kg.

Protein binding. In plasma, about 80%.

Dose. An initial dose of 1 or 1.5 g, followed by 500 mg daily.

Sulfamoxole

Antibacterial/Sulfonamide

Synonyms. SDMO; Sulphadimethyloxazole; Sulphamoxole.
Proprietary names. Justamil; Sulfmidil; Sulfuno; Tardamide. It is an ingredient of Co-Fram and Supristol.
4-Amino-*N*-(4,5-dimethyl-2-oxazolyl)benzenesulfonamide
$C_{11}H_{13}N_3O_3S$=267.3
CAS-729-99-7

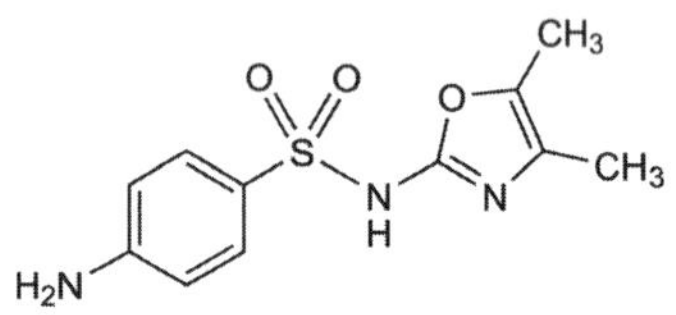

A white crystalline powder. M.p. about 193°.
Slightly soluble in water.

Dissociation Constant. pK_a 7.4.

Partition Coefficient. Log *P* (chloroform/pH 7.4), −0.3; (octanol/water), 1.0.

Colour Tests. Coniferyl Alcohol—orange; Copper Sulfate (Method 1)—green-brown; Mercurous Nitrate—black; Nitrous Acid—yellow.

Thin-layer Chromatography. System TA—Rf 67. (Van Urk reagent, positive.)

Gas Chromatography. System GA—not eluted; system GJ—RRT of methyl derivative 0.40 (relative to griseofulvin).

High Performance Liquid Chromatography. System HU—*k* 12.6.

Ultraviolet Spectrum. Aqueous acid—249 nm (A_1^1=375b); aqueous alkali—250 nm (A_1^1=685b).

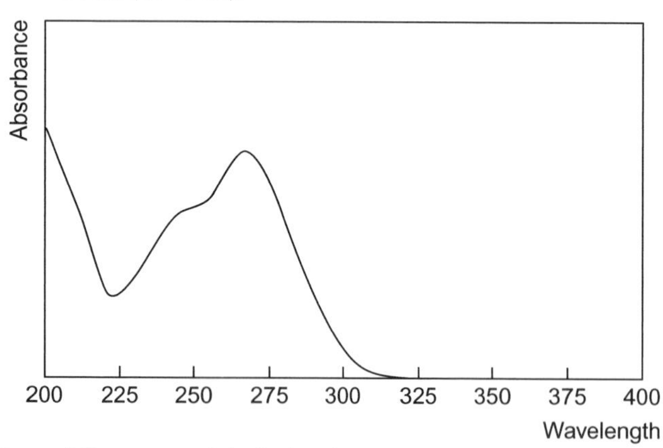

Infra-red Spectrum. Principal peaks at wavenumbers 1605, 1626, 1127, 1145, 1276, 1094 cm^{-1} (KBr disk).

Quantification

High performance liquid chromatography. In plasma: sulfamoxole and other sulfonamides, electrochemical detection—J. Klimes and M. Mokry, *Pharmazie*, 1997, *52*, 448–450.

Disposition in the Body. Rapidly absorbed after oral administration. About 65 to 71% of a dose is excreted in the urine, mainly as unchanged drug, the N^4-acetyl conjugate, and sulfanilamide.

Therapeutic concentration

Following single oral doses of 1, 2 and 4 g to 4 subjects, peak serum concentrations of 73.5 to 94.8 (mean 88), 138 to 182 (mean 157), and 215 to 290 mg/L (mean 241), respectively, were attained in about 2 h [C. G. vom Bruck *et al.*, *Arzneimittelforschung*, 1960, *10*, 621–626].

Following oral administration of 400 mg twice a day to 10 subjects (in combination with trimethoprim 80 mg), a mean maximum steady-state plasma concentration of 75 mg/L and a mean trough concentration of 42 mg/L were reported [I. D. Watson *et al.*, *Br. J. Clin. Pharmacol.*, 1982, *14*, 437–443].

Half-life. Plasma half-life, 4 to 11 h.

Volume of distribution. About 0.1 L/kg.

Distribution in blood. Plasma : whole blood ratio, about 1.8.

Protein binding. In plasma, about 25%.

Dose. 2 g daily for 1 or 2 days, followed by 1 g daily.

Sulfanilamide

Antibacterial/Sulfonamide

Synonyms. Solfammide; Streptocidum; Sulfaminum; 1162-F.
Proprietary names. Astreptine; AVC; Azol; Prontosil album; Prontylin; Streptozide.
4-Aminobenzenesulfonamide
$C_6H_8N_2O_2S$=172.2
CAS-63-74-1

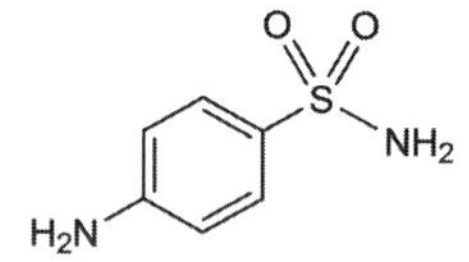

A white crystalline powder. On heating the dry powder it becomes violet-blue and eventually aniline and ammonia are produced. M.p. about 165°. Soluble 1 in 170 of water, 1 in 37 of ethanol and 1 in 5 of acetone; practically insoluble in chloroform and ether; soluble in hydrochloric acid and solutions of alkali hydroxides.

Dissociation Constant. pK_a 10.6 (20°).

Partition Coefficient. Log *P* (octanol/water), −0.6.

Colour Tests. Coniferyl Alcohol—orange; Copper Sulfate (Method 1)—blue; Koppanyi–Zwikker Test—blue-violet; Mercurous Nitrate—black.

Thin-layer Chromatography. System TA—Rf 67; system TD—Rf 13; system TE—Rf 51; system TF—Rf 46; system TT—Rf 61; system TU—Rf 96; system TV—Rf 66; system TAD—Rf 22; system TAE—Rf 83; system TAJ—Rf 22; system TAK—Rf 05; system TAL—Rf 50. (Mercuric chloride–diphenylcarbazone reagent, blue; acidified potassium permanganate solution, positive; Van Urk reagent, yellow.)

Gas Chromatography. System GA—sulfanilamide RI 2185; sulfanilamide-Me RI 2135; sulfanilamide-Me_4 RI 2095; M (acetyl-) RI 2690; M (acetyl-)-Me RI 2600.

High Performance Liquid Chromatography. System HU—sulfanilamide *k* 8.9, N^4-acetylsulfanilamide *k* 9.6; system HY—RI 86.

Ultraviolet Spectrum. Aqueous acid—262 nm (A_1^1=106a), 269 nm (A_1^1=85a); aqueous alkali—250 nm (A_1^1=932b).

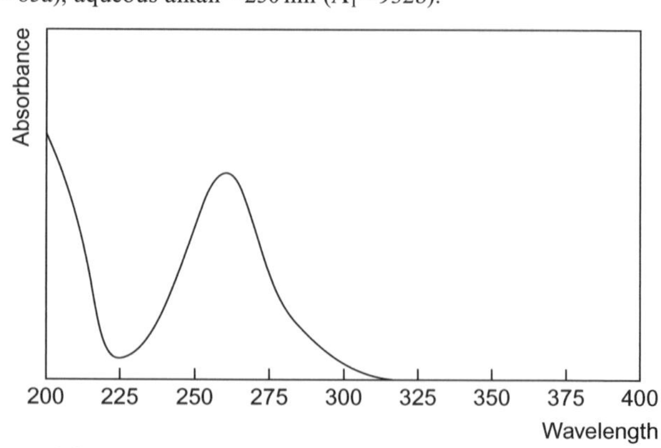

Infra-red Spectrum. Principal peaks at wavenumbers 1149, 1603, 1316, 1637, 1099, 1294 cm^{-1} (KBr disk).

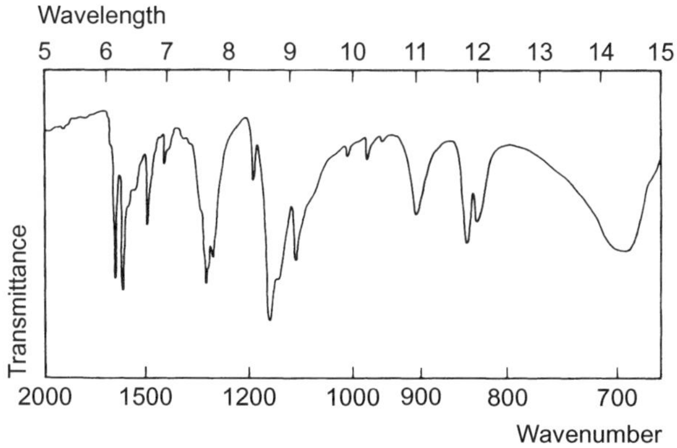

Mass Spectrum. Principal ions at m/z 172, 92, 156, 65, 108, 173, 39, 174.

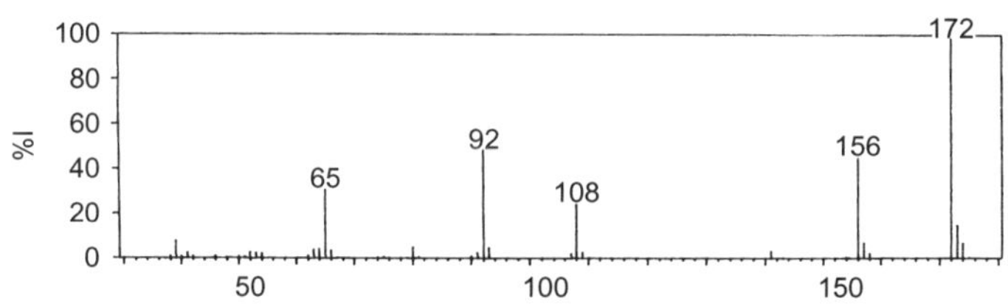

Dose. Sulfanilamide has been given in an initial dose of 3 g, followed by 1 to 1.5 g every 4 h.

Sulfaphenazole

Antibacterial/Sulfonamide

Synonyms. Sulphaphenazole; Sulphaphenylpyrazol.
Proprietary names. Isarol V; Orisul; Orisulf.
4-Amino-*N*-(1-phenyl-1*H*-pyrazol-5-yl)benzenesulfonamide
$C_{15}H_{14}N_4O_2S$=314.4
CAS–526-08-9

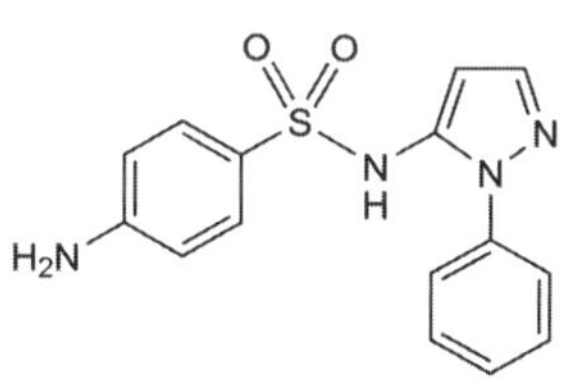

A white crystalline powder. When heated, the powder becomes brown; when further heated, it produces yellow fumes and an odour of sulfur dioxide. M.p. 179° to 183°.
Very slightly soluble in water, ethanol, chloroform and ether; soluble in acetone, mineral acids and solutions of alkali hydroxides.

Dissociation Constant. pK_a 6.5.

Partition Coefficient. Log *P* (octanol/water), 1.5.

Colour Tests. Coniferyl Alcohol—orange; Copper Sulfate (Method 1)—blue; Koppanyi–Zwikker Test—blue-violet; Mercurous Nitrate—black; Nitrous Acid—yellow.

Thin-layer Chromatography. System TA—Rf 69; system TD—Rf 29; system TE—Rf 09; system TF—Rf 51; system TT—Rf 89; system TU—Rf 70; system TV—Rf 13; system TAD—Rf 43; system TAE—Rf 89.

Gas Chromatography. System GJ—RRT of methyl derivative 1.71 (relative to griseofulvin).

Ultraviolet Spectrum. Aqueous alkali—249 nm (A^1_1=700b).

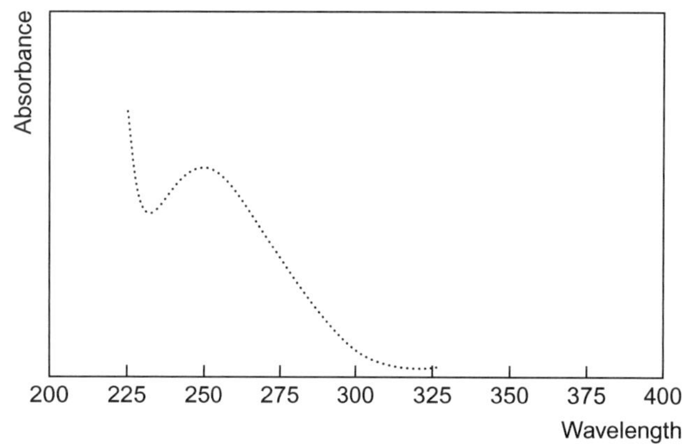

Infra-red Spectrum. Principal peaks at wavenumbers 1148, 1507, 1313, 1592, 675, 1630 cm^{-1} (KBr disk).

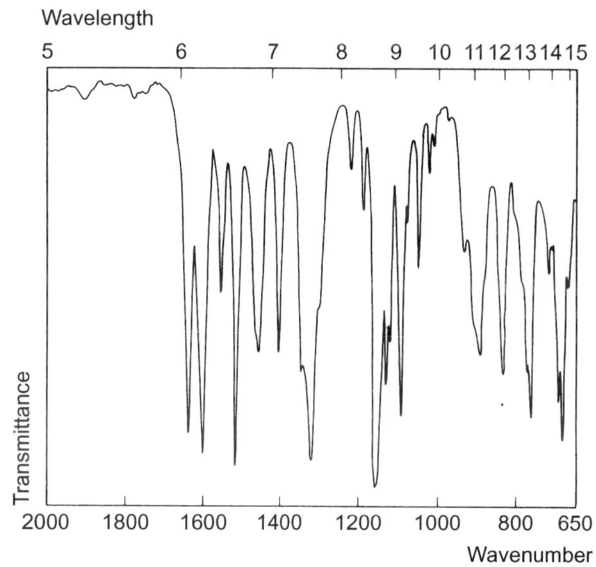

Mass Spectrum. Principal ions at m/z 156, 158, 92, 77, 157, 314, 108, 65.

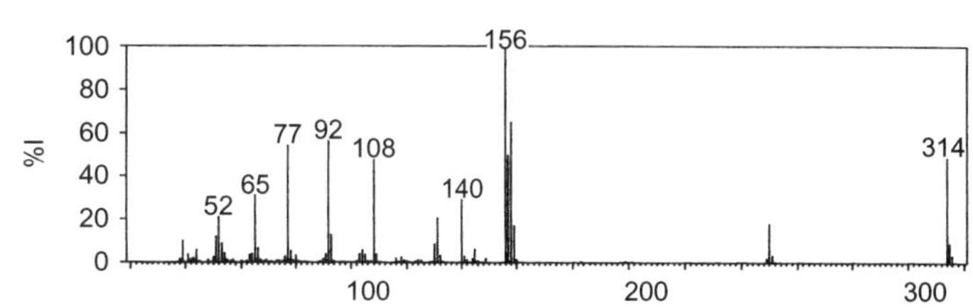

Quantification

High performance liquid chromatography. In urine: sulfaphenazole–N^2-glucuronide—T. B. Vree *et al.*, *Pharm. Weekbl. (Sci.)*, 1990,*12*, 243–246. The methods referred to under sulfamethoxazole may also be used.

Disposition in the Body. Readily absorbed after oral administration. It is acetylated in the body and slowly excreted in the urine, about 70 to 80% of a dose being excreted in 72 h, 30% as the acetyl derivative.

Half-life. Plasma half-life, 8 to 12 h.

Protein binding. In plasma, about 90 to 99%.

Dose. 2 to 3 g daily for 2 days, followed by 1 g daily.

Sulfapyridine

Antibacterial/Sulfonamide

Synonym. Sulphapyridine
Proprietary names. Coccoclase; Dagenan; Eubasin; M & B 693; Pyriamid; Septipulmon. It is an ingredient of Trinamide (vet.).
4-Amino-*N*-2-pyridinylbenzenesulfonamide
$C_{11}H_{11}N_3O_2S=249.3$
CAS—144-83-2

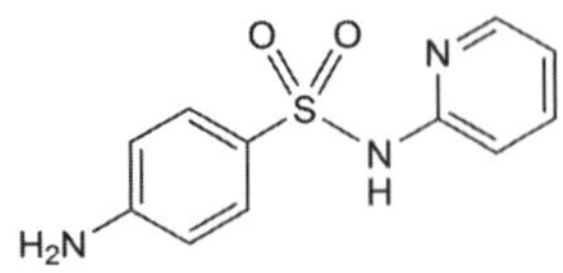

A white or yellowish-white crystalline powder or granules. It slowly darkens on exposure to light. M.p. 190° to 192°.
Soluble 1 in 3500 of water, 1 in about 440 of ethanol and 1 in 65 of acetone; practically insoluble in chloroform and ether; soluble in dilute mineral acids and aqueous solutions of alkali hydroxides.

Sulfapyridine Sodium Monohydrate

Synonym. Soluble Sulfapyridine
Proprietary names. Izopiridina; Soludagenan.
$C_{11}H_{10}N_3NaO_2S,H_2O=289.3$
CAS—127-57-1 (anhydrous); 6101-41-3 (monohydrate)
A white or yellowish-white crystalline powder. On exposure to air, it slowly absorbs carbon dioxide with the liberation of sulfapyridine and becomes incompletely soluble in water.
Soluble 1 in 1.5 of water and 1 in 10 of ethanol.

Dissociation Constant. pK_a 8.4 (25°).

Partition Coefficient. Log *P* (octanol/water), 0.4.

Colour Tests. Coniferyl Alcohol—orange; Copper Sulfate (Method 1)—green→brown-green; Koppanyi–Zwikker Test—pink; Mercurous Nitrate—black; Nitrous Acid—yellow.

Thin-layer Chromatography. System TA—Rf 67; system TD—Rf 16; system TE—Rf 24; system TF—Rf 42; system TT—Rf 47; system TU—Rf 43; system TV—Rf 73; system TAD—Rf 34; system TAJ—Rf 50; system TAK—Rf 19; system TAL—Rf 85.

Gas Chromatography. System GA—RI 2600; System GJ—RRT of methyl derivative 0.47 (relative to griseofulvin).

High Performance Liquid Chromatography. System HU—*k* 3.8; system HX—RI 312; system HY—RI 242; system HZ—Retention time 2.2 min (sulfapyridine); Retention time 1.9 min (N^4-acetylsulfapyridine).

Ultraviolet Spectrum. Aqueous acid—240 nm ($A_1^1=392a$); aqueous alkali—247 nm.

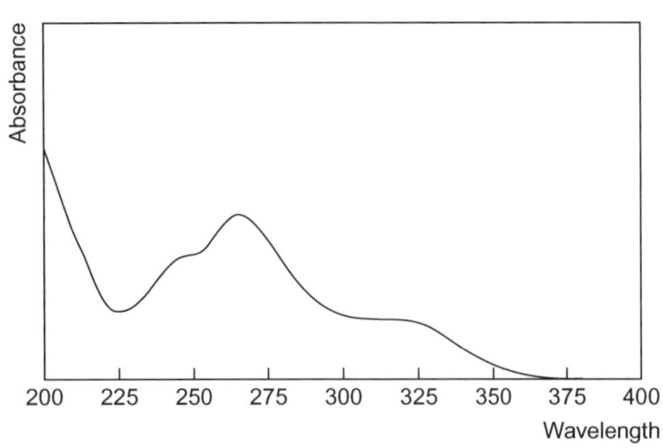

Infra-red Spectrum. Principal peaks at wavenumbers 1585, 1264, 1127, 1078, 1639, 950 cm^{-1} (KBr disk).

Mass Spectrum. Principal ions at *m/z* 184, 92, 185, 65, 39, 108, 66, 186.

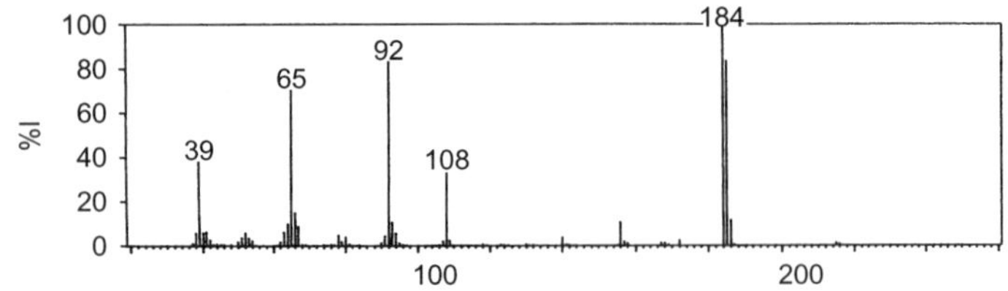

Quantification. See also under Sulfasalazine.

Colorimetry. In serum, saliva or plasma: limit of detection 1.5 mg/L for sulfapyridine or the acetyl metabolite—T. R. Bates and H. J. Pieniaszek, *Anal. Lett. (Part B)*, 1978, *11*, 709–720.

High performance liquid chromatography. In plasma: sulfapyridine and metabolites, limit of detection 1 mg/L, UV detection—C. Fischer and U. Klotz, *J. Chromatogr.*, 1978, *146*; *Biomed. Appl.*, *3*, 157–162. In plasma, saliva or urine: comparison with GC, limits of detection 50 ng for HPLC (fluorescence detection), 10 ng for GC (ECD)—M. E. Sharp *et al.*, *Can. J. Pharm. Sci.*, 1980, *15*, 35–38.

Disposition in the Body. Irregularly absorbed after oral administration. It is acetylated in the body, about 30 to 70% of the sulfapyridine in the blood being present as the inactive N^4-acetyl derivative; the extent of acetylation is genetically determined. The rate of excretion appears to be irregular but about 25% of a dose may be excreted in the urine as the acetyl derivative and about 20% as unchanged drug in 60 h. Other metabolites include the 5-hydroxy derivative and its glucuronide conjugate. Sulfapyridine is a metabolite of sulfasalazine.

Therapeutic concentration
After an oral dose of 2.5 g given to 5 subjects, peak serum concentrations of sulfapyridine plus metabolites of about 35 to 60 mg/L were attained in 3 to 5 h [H. Schröder and D. E. S. Campbell, *Clin. Pharmacol. Ther.*, 1972, *13*, 539–551].

Toxicity. Toxic effects are associated with plasma concentrations greater than 50 mg/L.

Half-life. Plasma half-life, about 6 h in rapid acetylators, increased in slow acetylators to about 13 h.

Volume of distribution. About 0.4 L/kg.

Saliva. Plasma : saliva ratio, about 1.8.

Protein binding. In plasma, about 40 to 60%.

Dose. Initially 3 or 4 g daily, followed by 0.5 to 1 g daily.

Sulfaquinoxaline

Coccidiostat (Veterinary)

Synonyms. Solfabenzpyrazine; Sulfabenzpyrazine; Sulfaquinoxaline.
Proprietary names. Sulfa-Q; Sul-Q-Nox. It is an ingredient of Tribrissen (SQX).
4-Amino-*N*-2-quinoxalinylbenzenesulfonamide
$C_{14}H_{12}N_4O_2S=300.3$
CAS—59-40-5

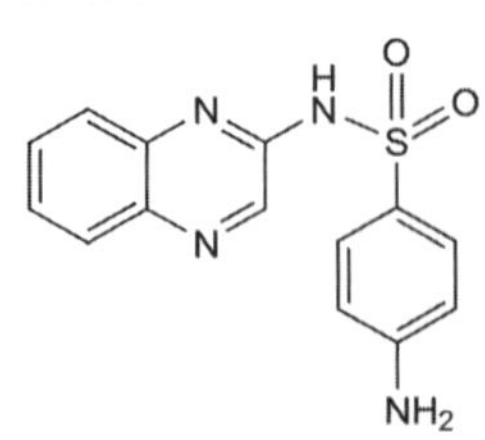

A yellow powder. M.p. 247° to 248°, with decomposition.
Practically insoluble in water and ether; very slightly soluble in ethanol and chloroform; soluble in dilute solutions of mineral acids and in solutions of alkalis.

Sulfaquinoxaline Sodium

Proprietary name. Aviochina.
$C_{14}H_{11}N_4O_2S, Na=322.3$
Very soluble in water.

Dissociation Constant. pK_a 5.5 (20°).

Partition Coefficient. Log *P* (octanol/water), 1.7.

Colour Test. Copper Sulfate (Method 1)—green.

Thin-layer Chromatography. System TA—Rf 71.

High Performance Liquid Chromatography. System HU—*k* 4.8.

Ultraviolet Spectrum. Aqueous acid—248 (A^1_1=648b), 263 (A^1_1=540b), 348 (A^1_1=263b); aqueous alkali—252 (A^1_1=1085a), 357 nm (A^1_1=265b).

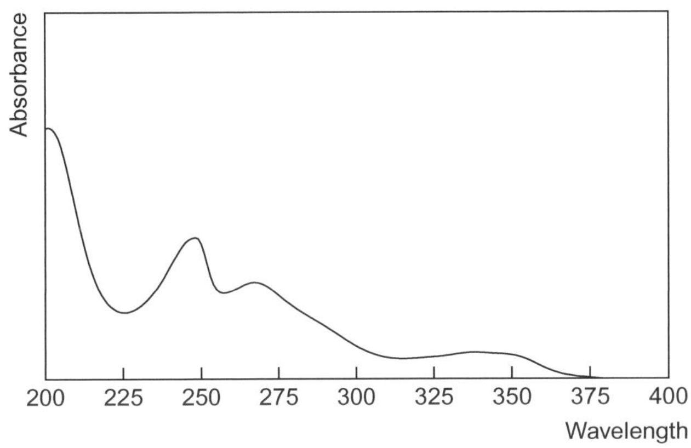

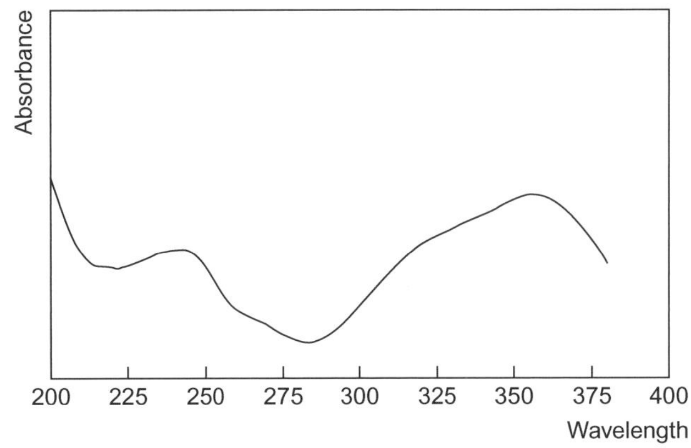

Infra-red Spectrum. Principal peaks at wavenumbers 1078, 1123, 772, 1634, 1175, 1672 cm^{-1} (Nujol mull).

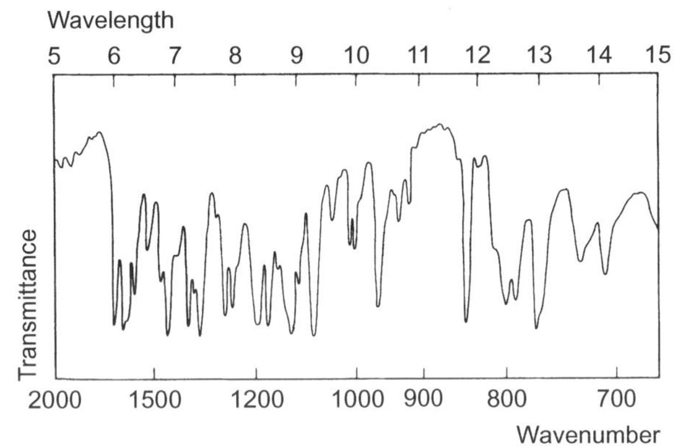

Sulfasalazine

Anti-inflammatory/Antibacterial/Sulfonamide

Synonyms. Salazosulfapyridine; Salicylazosulphapyridine; Sulphasalazine.
Proprietary names. Aculfin; Azulfidine; Azulfin; Colo-Pleon; Pleon RA; Pyralin; Salazine; Salazopirina; Salazopyrin(e); Salazopyrina; Saridine; SAS; Sulazine; Ucine.
2-Hydroxy-5-[[4-[(2-pyridinylamino)sulfonyl]phenyl]azo]benzoic acid
$C_{18}H_{14}N_4O_5S$=398.4
CAS—599-79-1

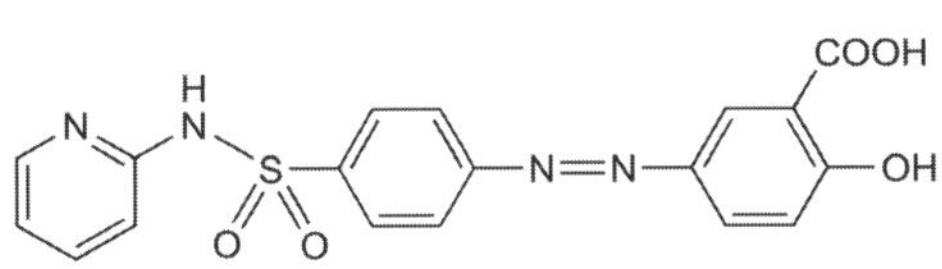

A fine bright yellow to brownish-yellow powder. M.p. about 240° to 245°, with decomposition.
Practically insoluble in water, chloroform and ether; soluble 1 in 2900 of ethanol and 1 in 1500 of methanol; soluble in aqueous solutions of alkali hydroxides.

Dissociation Constant. pK_a 0.6, 2.4, 9.7, 11.8.

Partition Coefficient. Log *P* (octanol/water), 3.8.

Colour Tests. Copper Sulfate (Method 1)—orange-brown; Palladium Chloride—black.

Thin-layer Chromatography. System TA—Rf 66; system TD—Rf 00; system TE—Rf 00; system TF—Rf 00; system TAD—Rf 02; system TAE—Rf 85; system TAJ—Rf 00; system TAK—Rf 30; system TAL—Rf 39. (Visible orange spot.)

High Performance Liquid Chromatography. System HX—RI 433; system HZ—Retention time 1.9 min.

Mass Spectrum. Principal ions at *m/z* 169, 92, 289, 65, 290, 39, 333, 184.

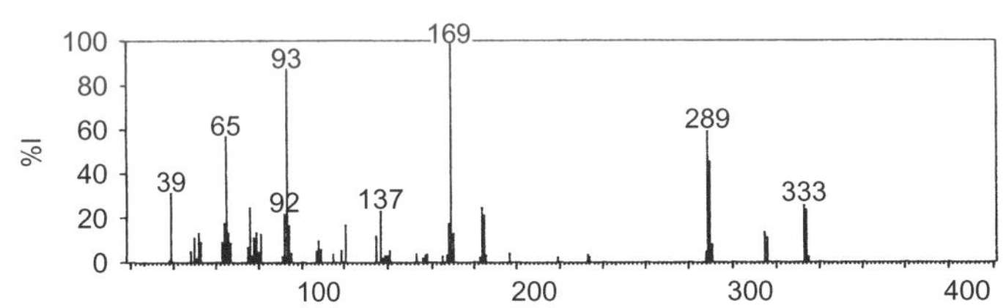

Quantification

High performance liquid chromatography. In plasma: sulfapyridine, acetylsulfapyridine, 5-aminosalicylic acid and 5-acetamidosalicylic acid, limit of detection 500 μg/L, UV and fluorescence detection—P. N. Shaw *et al., J. Chromatogr.*, 1983, *274*; *Biomed. Appl.*, *25*, 393–397. In plasma or urine: 5-aminosalicylic acid and 5-acetamidosalicylic acid, limit of detection 20 μg/L, fluorescence detection—C. Fischer *et al., J. Chromatogr.*, 1981, *225*; *Biomed. Appl.*, *14*, 498–503. In bile: 5-aminosalicylic acid and 5-acetamidosalicylic acid, fluorescence detection—C. Fischer *et al., Br. J. Clin. Pharmacol.*, 1983, *15*, 273–274. In plasma, urine or faeces: sulfasalazine metabolites and conjugates, limit of detection 1 mg/L or less, UV, fluorescence or electrochemical detection—S. H. Hansen, *J. Chromatogr.*, 1989, *491*, 175–185. In serum: sulfasalazine, sulfapyridine and *N*-acetylsulfapyridine, limit of detection 0.1 to 0.25 mg/L, UV detection—C. J. Bugge *et al., J. Pharm. Sci.*, 1990, *79*, 1095–1098.

Disposition in the Body. Partially and irregularly absorbed after oral administration. The absorbed material is not metabolised but is excreted unchanged in the urine and accounts for up to about 10% of the dose. The greater part of the dose passes unchanged into the colon where it is metabolised by bacteria to sulfapyridine and 5-aminosalicylic acid, which is thought to be the active moiety. The sulfapyridine so formed is absorbed, and metabolised by N^4-acetylation, ring hydroxylation and glucuronidation. The degree of acetylation is dependent on the acetylator status of the subject. About 60% of the dose is excreted in the urine as free and acetylated sulfapyridine and their glucuronides, and about 25% of the dose is eliminated as sulfapyridine in the faeces. The 5-aminosalicylic acid is partially absorbed and metabolised by *N*-acetylation; about 30% is excreted in the urine as unchanged drug and 5-acetamidosalicylic acid, and most of the remainder is eliminated unchanged in the faeces.

Therapeutic concentration

Following a single oral dose of 2 g to 8 subjects, peak plasma concentrations of 7 to 32 mg/L (mean 17) of sulfasalazine were attained in about 3 h; peak plasma concentrations of sulfapyridine averaged about 20 mg/L [E. M. Ryde and J. J. Lima, *Curr. Ther. Res.*, 1981, *29*, 728–737].

Following daily oral doses of 3 g to 6 subjects, minimum steady-state plasma concentrations of 0.04 to 0.34 mg/L of 5-aminosalicylic acid and 0.2 to 1.4 mg/L of 5-acetamidosalicylic acid were reported [C. Fischer *et al.*, *J. Chromatogr.*, 1981, *225*; *Biomed. Appl.*, *14*, 498–503].

After daily oral doses of 4 g to 9 subjects, steady-state serum concentrations of 37 to 92 mg/L (median 50) for total sulfapyridine and its metabolites, 4.7 to 45 mg/L (median 12) for sulfasalazine, and less than 2 mg/L for 5-aminosalicylic acid metabolites were reported on the 5th day [H. Schröder and D. E. S. Campbell, *Clin. Pharmacol. Ther.*, 1972, *13*, 539–551].

Toxicity. Toxic effects are associated with plasma concentrations of sulfapyridine greater than 50 mg/L.

The serum salicylate concentration in a 26-year-old man who had taken 50 g of sulfasalazine at some point in the previous 12 h was 128 mg/L [R. J. Dunn, *J. Toxicol. Clin. Toxicol.*, 1998, *36*, 239–242].

Half-life. Plasma half-life, sulfasalazine, 6 to 17 h (mean 10).

Note. For a review of the pharmacokinetics of sulfasalazine see K. M. Das and R. Dubin, *Clin. Pharmacokinet.*, 1976, *1*, 406–425.

Dose. Initially 4 to 8 g daily; maintenance, 1.5 to 2 g daily.

Sulfathiazole

Antibacterial/Sulfonamide

Synonyms. Norsulfazole; Solfatiazolol; Sulfanilamidothiazolum; Sulfathiazolum; Sulfonazolum; Sulphathiazole.
Proprietary names. Cibazol: Stopex; Sulfagine; Sulfamul; Sulfavitina; Sulzol; Thiazamide. It is an ingredient of Sultrin and Triple Sulfa.
4-Amino-*N*-2-thiazolylbenzenesulfonamide
$C_9H_9N_3O_2S_2$=255.3
CAS—72-14-0

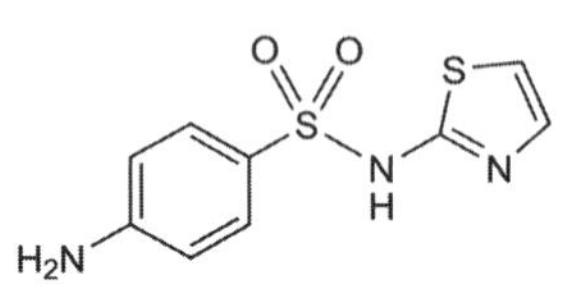

A white crystalline powder which slowly darkens on exposure to light. M.p. about 202°.
Soluble 1 in 2500 of water and 1 in 120 of ethanol; practically insoluble in chloroform and ether; soluble in acetone, dilute mineral acids and solutions of alkali hydroxides and carbonates.

Sulfathiazole Sodium

Synonym. Soluble Sulfathiazole
$C_9H_8N_3NaO_2S_2,5H_2O$=367.4
CAS—144-74-1 (anhydrous); 6791-71-5 (pentahydrate)
A white or yellowish-white microcrystalline powder. It slowly darkens on exposure to light; on exposure to moist air it absorbs carbon dioxide and becomes incompletely soluble in water.
Soluble 1 in 3 of water and 1 in 20 of ethanol.

Dissociation Constant. pK_a 7.1 (25°).

Partition Coefficient. Log *P* (octanol/pH 7.5), −0.4.

Colour Tests. Coniferyl Alcohol—orange; Copper Sulfate (Method 1)—violet-brown; Koppanyi–Zwikker Test—red-violet; Mercurous Nitrate—black; Nitrous Acid—yellow.

Thin-layer Chromatography. System TA—Rf 66; system TD—Rf 09; system TE—Rf 08; system TF—Rf 20; system TT—Rf 53; system TU—Rf 40; system TV—Rf 05; system TAD—Rf 27; system TAE—Rf 79. (Mercuric chloride–diphenylcarbazone reagent, blue; acidified potassium permanganate solution, positive; Van Urk reagent, yellow.)

Gas Chromatography. System GA—not eluted; system GJ—RRT of methyl derivative 0.49 (relative to griseofulvin).

High Performance Liquid Chromatography. System HU—*k* 13.4; system HX—RI 310; system HAA—Retention time 9.0 min.

Ultraviolet Spectrum. Aqueous acid—280 nm (A_1^1=498a); aqueous alkali—256 nm (A_1^1=716b).

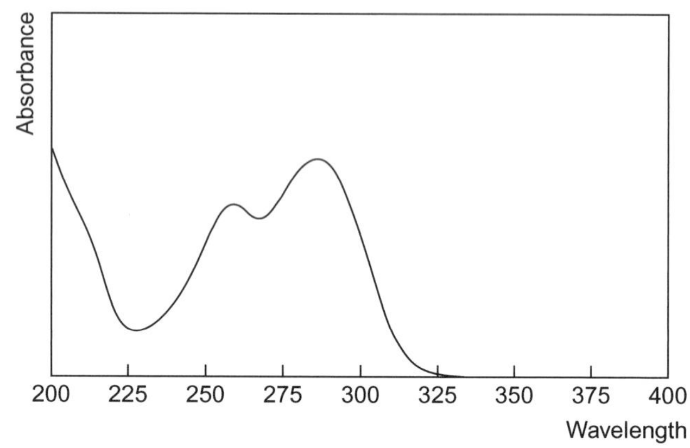

Infra-red Spectrum. Principal peaks at wavenumbers 1130, 1527, 929, 1274, 1082, 1592 cm^{-1} (Nujol mull).

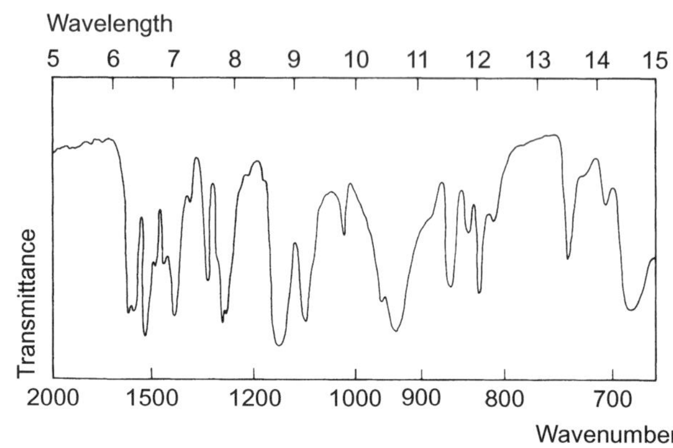

Mass Spectrum. Principal ions at *m/z* 92, 156, 65, 108, 191, 45, 39, 55.

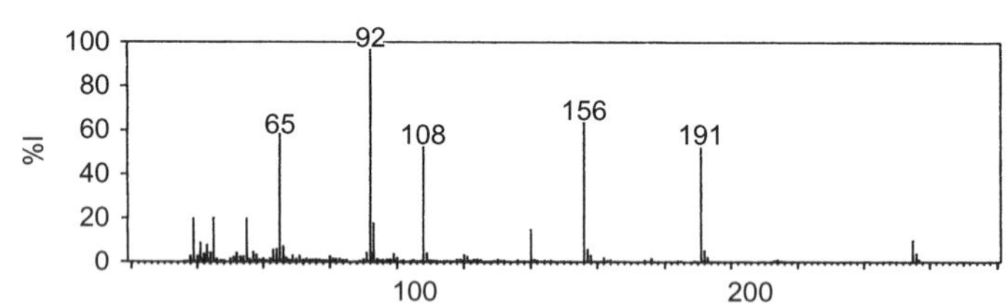

Quantification

High performance liquid chromatography. In plasma or urine: limit of detection 250 μg/L in plasma, 2.5 mg/L in urine, UV detection—A. Sioufi *et al.*, *J. Chromatogr.*, 1980, *221*; *Biomed. Appl.*, *10*, 419–424. In urine: sulfathiazole and other sulfonamides, limit of detection 0.1 to 0.3 mg/L—E. F. Simo-Alfonso *et al.*, *J. Chromatogr.*, 1995, *670*, *Biomed. Appl.*, 183–187.

Disposition in the Body. Readily absorbed after oral administration and acetylated in the body, about 20% of the sulfathiazole in the blood is in the form of the inactive N^4-acetyl derivative. It is rapidly excreted in the urine, about 60 to 90% of a dose being excreted in 24 h; about 20% of the excreted material is the acetyl derivative. Sulfathiazole is a metabolite of phthalylsulfathiazole and succinylsulfathiazole.

Half-life. Plasma half-life, about 4 h.

Protein binding. In plasma, 55 to 80%.

Dose. An initial dose of 2 to 3 g, followed by 1 g every 4 to 6 h.

Sulfinpyrazone

Uricosuric/Antithrombotic

Synonyms. Sulphinpyrazone; Sulfoxyphenylpyrazolidine.
Proprietary names. Anturan(e); Enturen; Sulfinona.
1,2-Diphenyl-4-[2-(phenylsulfinyl)ethyl)-3,5-pyrazolidinedione
$C_{23}H_{20}N_2O_3S = 404.5$
CAS—57-96-5

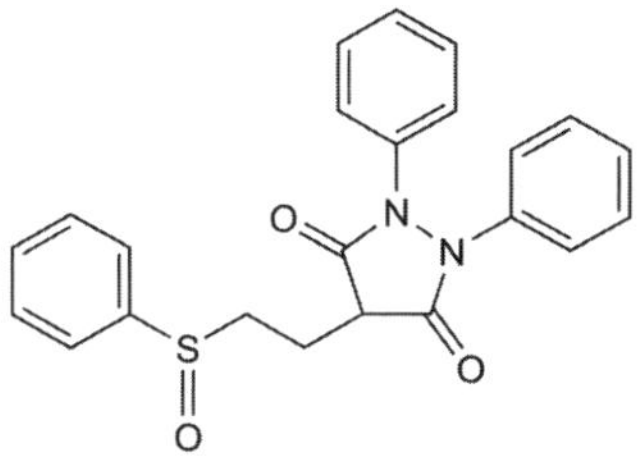

A white powder. M.p. 136° to 137°.
Practically insoluble in water; soluble 1 in 40 of ethanol, 1 in about 10 of acetone, 1 in 2 of chloroform and 1 in 750 of ether.

Dissociation Constant pK_a 2.8 (22°).

Partition Coefficient. Log *P* (octanol/water), 2.3.

Colour Tests. Copper sulfate (method 1)—blue; Koppanyi–Zwikker test—violet (transient); Liebermann's test—orange; Nitrous acid—yellow.

Thin-layer Chromatography. System TAD—Rf 30; system TD—Rf 04; system TE—Rf 16; system TF—Rf 04.

Gas Chromatography. System GA—RI 2253.

High Performance Liquid Chromatography. System HY—RI 474; system HZ—Retention time(s) 4.7 min.

Ultraviolet Spectrum. Aqueous acid—237 (A^1_1=436a); aqueous alkali—260 nm (A^1_1=559a).

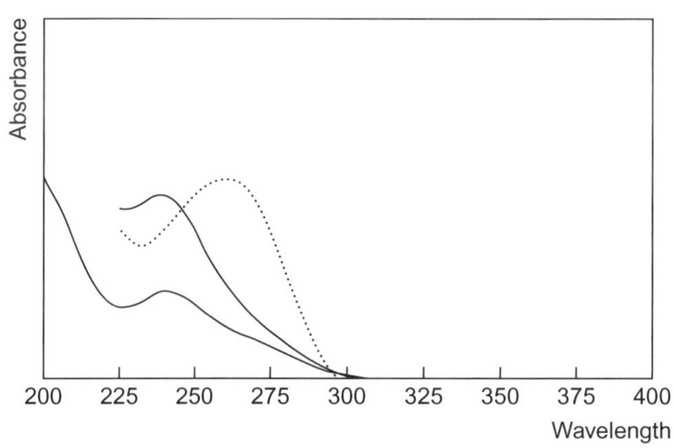

Infra-red Spectrum. Principal peaks at wavenumbers 1716, 1305, 750, 688, 1750, 1595 cm^{-1} (KBr disk).

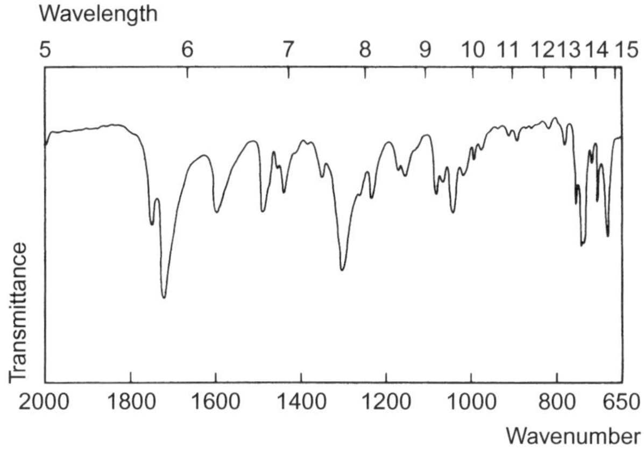

Mass Spectrum. Principal ions at *m/z* 77, 278, 105, 78, 51, 279, 252, 130.

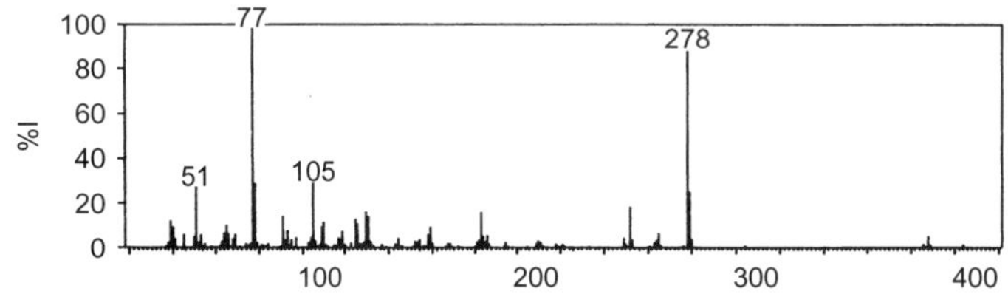

Quantification

Gas chromatography. In plasma or urine: sulfinpyrazone and its *p*-hydroxy and sulfone metabolites, limit of detection for sulfinpyrazone 100 μg/L using AFID or 10 μg/L using ECD—P. Jakobsen and A. K. Pedersen, *J. Chromatogr.*, 1979, *163*; *B Biomed. Appl.*, *5*, 259–269.

Gas chromatography–mass spectrometry. In plasma or urine: sulfide and *p*-hydroxysulfide metabolites, limit of detection 5 μg/L for sulfide and 30 μg/L for *p*-hydroxysulfide—P. Jakobsen and A. K. Pedersen, *J. Pharm. Pharmacol.*, 1981, *33*, 89–92.

High performance liquid chromatography. In plasma or urine: sulfinpyrazone and its *p*-hydroxy and sulfone metabolites, limit of detection 50 μg/L for sulfinpyrazone, UV detection—T. D. Bjornsson *et al.*, *J. Chromatogr.*, 1980, *181*; *B Biomed. Appl.*, *7*, 417–425. In plasma: sulfinpyrazone and metabolites, limit of detection 30 μg/L, UV detection—B.-S. Kuo *et al.*, *Arzneimittelforschung*, 1984, *34*, 548–550. In plasma or urine: sulfinpyrazone and its *p*-hydroxy, sulfone, sulfide and *p*-hydroxysulfide metabolites, limits of detection 10 μg/L (sulfinpyrazone and sulfide metabolite) and 50 μg/L (other metabolites)—E. G. Lentjes *et al.*, *Pharm. Weekbl. (Sci.)*, 1985, *7*, 252–259.

Disposition in the Body. Sulfinpyrazone is readily absorbed after oral administration. It is metabolised by reduction to the sulfide which is active and is the predominant circulating metabolite, reaching a concentration about 25% of that of sulfinpyrazone. It is also oxidised to the sulfone (active) and there are several hydroxy metabolites. All metabolites are excreted in the urine as the *C*-glucuronides, only a small proportion being excreted in *O*-glucuronidated or unconjugated form. Up to 50% of a dose is excreted in the urine as unchanged drug or its glucuronide. About 80% of a single dose is recovered within the first 24 h and more than 95% within 4 days (85% from urine and 10% from faeces).

Therapeutic concentration

Following single oral doses of 200 mg to 6 subjects, peak plasma concentrations of 6.0 to 17.0 (mean 13) mg/L of sulfinpyrazone were attained in 1 to 4 h; peak plasma concentrations of the metabolites attained in about 4, 4, and 11 h, respectively, were: sulfone 0.2 to 1.1 mg/L, *p*-hydroxysulfinpyrazone 0.1 to 0.48 mg/L, sulfide 0.6 to 8.9 mg/L. [C. Mahony *et al.*, *Clin. Pharmacol. Ther.*, 1983, *33*, 491–497].

Following oral administration of 200 mg four times a day to 6 subjects, mean maximum steady-state plasma concentrations were: sulfinpyrazone 20.7 mg/L about 2 h after a dose, sulfide 13.9 mg/L about 7 h after a dose, sulfone 3.4 mg/L 2 h after a dose. [B. Rosenkranz *et al.*, *Eur. J. Clin. Pharmacol.*, 1983, *24*, 231–235].

Daily oral doses of 600 to 800 mg to 8 people with diabetes, treated for 2.5 years or more, produced sulfinpyrazone plasma concentrations of 2.5 to 13.2 (mean 7) mg/L before the first morning dose of 200 mg and 9.1 to 23.2 (mean 16) mg/L 2 h later. The corresponding sulfide plasma concentrations were 1.0 to 6.0 (mean 2.8) μg/mL and 1.5 to 8.6 (mean 4.3) μg/mL [A. K. Pedersen *et al.*, *Br. J. Clin. Pharmacol.*, 1981, *11*, 597–603].

Half-life. Plasma half-life, about 3 to 5 h, sulfide metabolite about 14 to 21 h.

Volume of distribution. About 0.06 L/kg.

Clearance. Plasma clearance, about 0.3 mL/min/kg.

Distribution in blood. Plasma:whole blood ratio, 1.8.

Protein binding. In plasma, about 98%.

Note. For a review of the pharmacokinetics of sulfinpyrazone, see A. Kirstein-Pedersen *et al.*, *Clin. Pharmacokinet.*, 1982, *7*, 42–56.

Dose. 100 to 800 mg daily.

Sulfisomidine

Antibacterial/Sulfonamide

Synonyms. Sulfa-isodimérazine; Sulfaisodimidine; Sulfasomidine; Sulphasomidine.
Note. Sulfadimethylpyrimidine has been used as a synonym for sulfisomidine and is sometimes used as a synonym for sulfadimidine. Care should be taken to avoid confusion between the two compounds, which are isomeric.
Proprietary names. Aristamid; Domain; Elcosine; Elkosil; Elkosin(e).
4-Amino-*N*-(2,6-dimethyl-4-pyrimidinyl)benzenesulfonamide
$C_{12}H_{14}N_4O_2S$=278.3
CAS—515-64-0

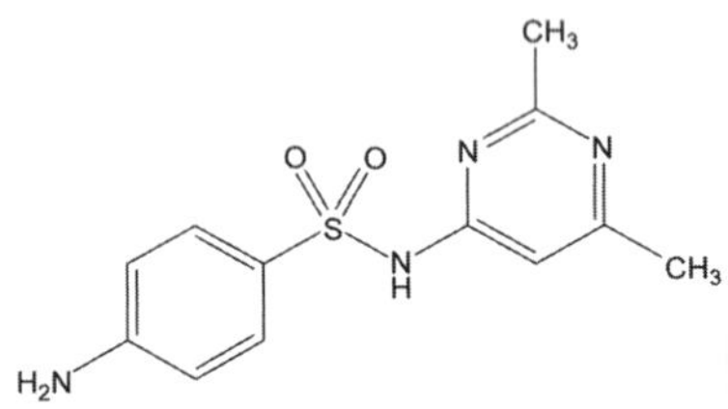

A white or creamy-white finely crystalline powder which slowly darkens on exposure to light. M.p. 243°.
Very slightly soluble in water, chloroform and ether; slightly soluble in ethanol and acetone; readily soluble in dilute mineral acids and solutions of alkali hydroxides.

Dissociation Constant. pK_a 7.5 (27°).

Partition Coefficient. Log *P* (octanol/water), −0.3.

Colour Tests. Coniferyl Alcohol—orange; Copper Sulfate (Method 1)—green; Koppanyi–Zwikker Test—blue-violet (transient); Mercurous Nitrate—black; Nitrous Acid—yellow.

Thin-layer Chromatography. System TA—Rf 64; system TAD—Rf 27; system TAE—Rf 80; system TD—Rf 05; system TE—Rf 05; system TF—Rf 16; system TT—Rf 11; system TU—Rf 49; system TV—Rf 20.

Gas Chromatography. System GJ—RRT of methyl derivative 0.50 (relative to griseofulvin).

High Performance Liquid Chromatography. System HX—RI 290.

Ultraviolet Spectrum. Aqueous acid—262 nm; aqueous alkali—262 nm (A_1^1=764b); methanol—272 nm (A_1^1=745a).

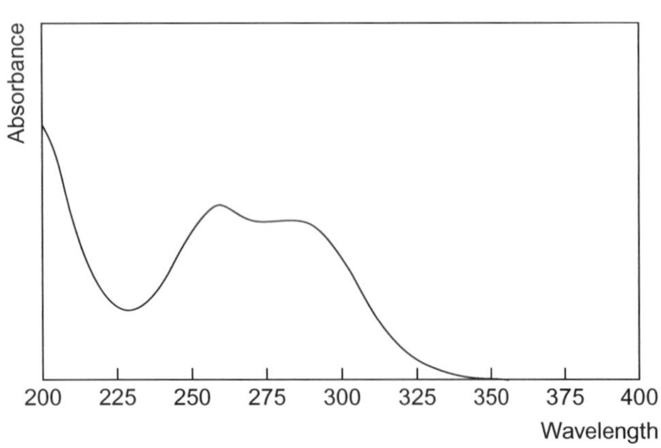

Infra-red Spectrum. Principal peaks at wavenumbers 1125, 1260, 1138, 1595, 1650, 1070 cm^{-1} (KBr disk).

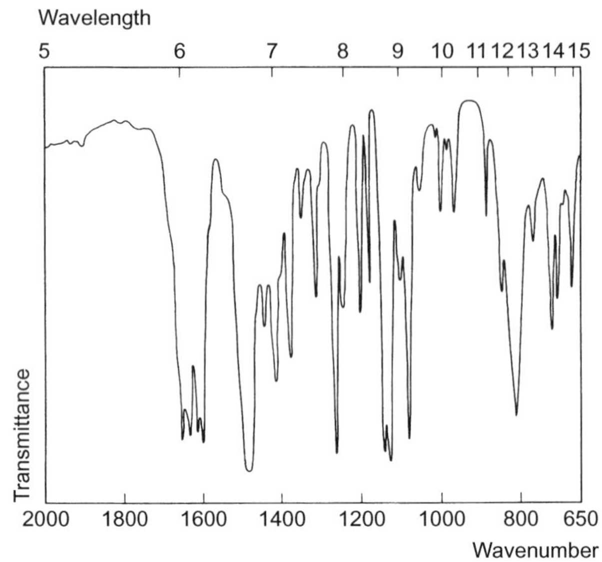

Mass Spectrum. Principal ions at *m/z* 214, 92, 65, 213, 108, 42, 215, 39.

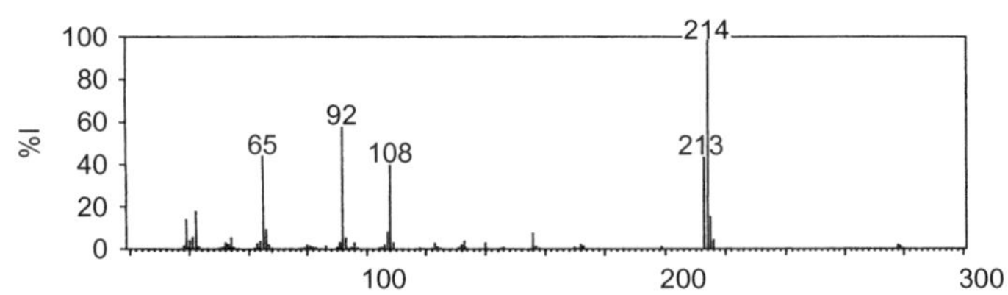

Quantification

High performance liquid chromatography. The methods referred to under sulfamethoxazole may be used.

Disposition in the Body. Absorbed after oral administration. It is acetylated in the body to only a small extent, about 10 to 25% of the material in the blood being in the form of the inactive N^4-acetyl derivative. It is rapidly excreted in the urine, about 87% of the dose being excreted within 48 h as unchanged drug together with about 6% as the acetyl derivative.

Half-life. Plasma half-life, 6 to 8 h.

Protein binding. In plasma, 40 to 90% (dose-dependent).

Dose. Sulfisomidine has been given in an initial dose of 2 to 4 g, followed by 6 g daily.

Sulfiram

Parasiticide

Synonym. Monosulfiram
Proprietary names. Kutkasin; Tetmosol; Tiosol; Thiosan.
Tetraethylthiodicarbonic diamide
$C_{10}H_{20}N_2S_3$=264.5
CAS—95-05-6

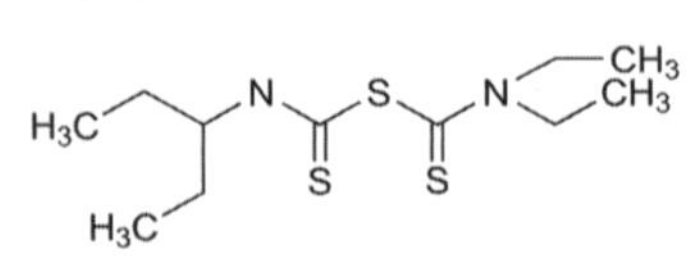

A yellow or yellowish-brown, soft crystalline powder. M.p. 28.5° to 32°.
Practically insoluble in water; soluble 1 in 3 of ethanol; freely soluble in chloroform, ether, and most other organic solvents.

Partition Coefficient. Log *P* (octanol/water), 2.7.

Colour Test. Sodium Nitroprusside (Method 3)—violet.

Thin-layer Chromatography. System TA—Rf 75. (Acidified iodoplatinate solution, positive.)

Ultraviolet Spectrum. Methanol—281 nm (A_1^1=650a).

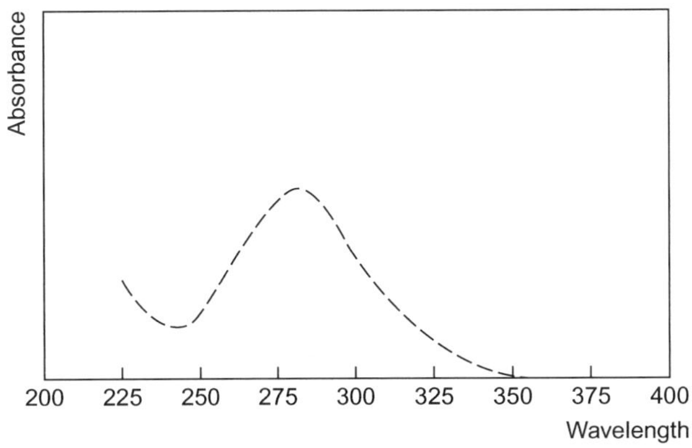

Infra-red Spectrum. Principal peaks at wavenumbers 1270, 1490, 1198, 1142, 968, 915 cm^{-1} (KBr disk).

Use. As a 25% alcoholic solution, diluted with 2 or 3 parts of water immediately before use.

Sulforidazine

Tranquilliser

Synonym. Sulphoridazine
Proprietary names. Imagotan; Inofal.
10-[2-(1-Methyl-2-piperidinyl)ethyl]-2-(methylsulfonyl)-10*H*-phenothiazine
$C_{21}H_{26}N_2O_2S_2$=402.6
CAS—14759-06-9

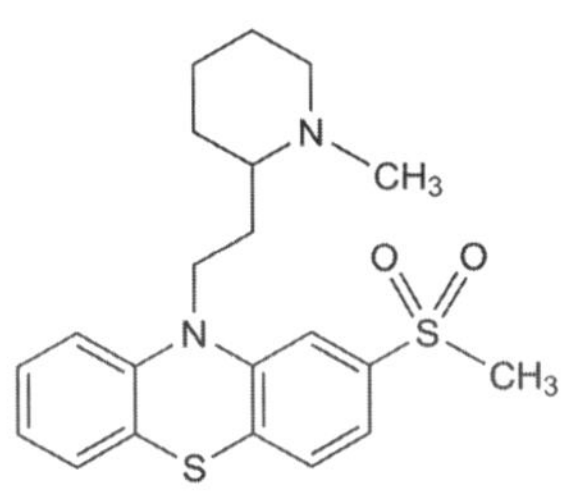

Crystals. M.p. 121° to 123°.

Partition Coefficient. Log *P* (octanol/water), 4.5.

Thin-layer Chromatography. System TE—Rf 54; system TF—Rf 00.

Gas Chromatography. System GA—sulforidazine RI 3415; M (ring) RI 3180; system GB—RI 3690.

High Performance Liquid Chromatography. System HX—RI 421; system HZ—Retention time(s) 4.8 min.

Ultraviolet Spectrum. Aqueous acid—265 (A^1_1=700b), 311 (A^1_1=75b); aqueous alkali—266 nm (A^1_1=659b).

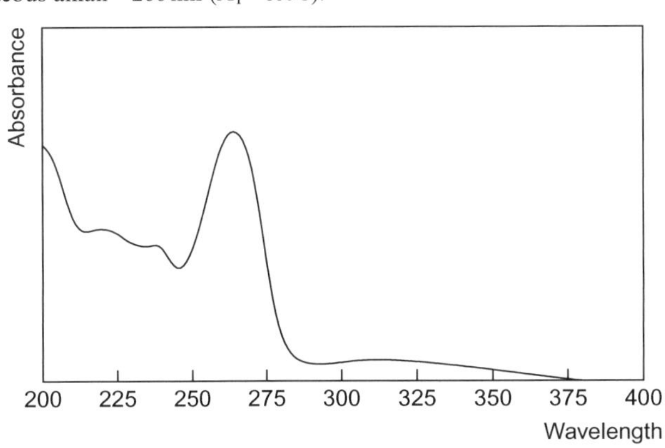

Quantification

Radioimmunoassay. In plasma: limit of detection 40 pg—B. S. Chakraborty *et al.*, *Ther. Drug Monit.*, 1988, *10*, 205–214.

See also under Thioridazine.

Disposition in the Body. Sulforidazine is an active metabolite of mesoridazine and thioridazine.

Dose. Sulforidazine has been given in doses of 150 to 300 mg daily.

Sulindac

Analgesic

Synonym. MK-231
Proprietary Names. Aclin; Apo-Sulin; Artribid; Arthrocine; Cenlidac; Citireuma; Clinoril; Copal; Daclin; Kenalin; Lyndak; Novo-Sundac; Saldac; Sulartrene; Sulene; Sulindal; Sulreuma.
(1*Z*)-5-Fluoro-2-methyl-1-[[4-(methylsulfinyl)phenyl]methylene]-1*H*-indene-3-acetic acid
$C_{20}H_{17}FO_3S$=356.4
CAS—38194-50-2

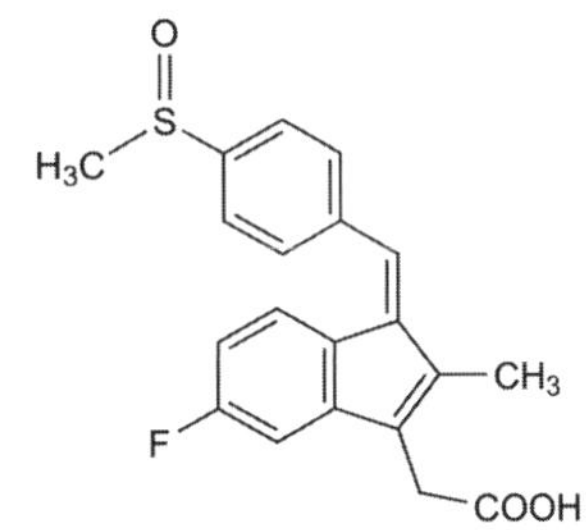

A yellow crystalline powder. M.p. about 182° to 185°.
Practically insoluble in water; slightly soluble in ethanol, acetone, chloroform and methanol.

Dissociation Constant. pK_a 4.7.

Partition Coefficient. Log *P* (octanol/water), 3.4.

Colour Tests. Liebermann's test—brown; Mandelin's test—orange; Marquis test—green (slow); Sulfuric acid—brown.

Thin-layer Chromatography. System TD—Rf 14; system TE—Rf 04; system TF—Rf 10; system TG—Rf 13; system TAD—Rf 34; system TAE—Rf 87; system TAJ—Rf 39; system TAK—Rf 40; system TAL—Rf 92. (Chromic acid solution, white; Ludy Tenger reagent, orange-brown.)

Gas Chromatography. System GA—sulindac RI 2890; M (sulfide) RI 2896; sulindac-ME RI 3220; system GD—RRT of methyl derivative 0.49 relative to *n*-$C_{16}H_{34}$.

High Performance Liquid Chromatography. System HD—*k* 1.25; system HV—RRT 0.78 relative to meclofenamic acid; system HX—RI 488; system HY—RI 462; system HZ—Retention time(s) 3.9 min (sulindac); Retention time(s) 7.2 min (sulindac sulfoxide); system HAA—Retention time(s) 16.6 min.

Ultraviolet Spectrum. Methanolic acid—284 (A^1_1=420a), 327 (A^1_1=373a); aqueous alkali—280 (A^1_1=442b), 327 nm (A^1_1=364b).

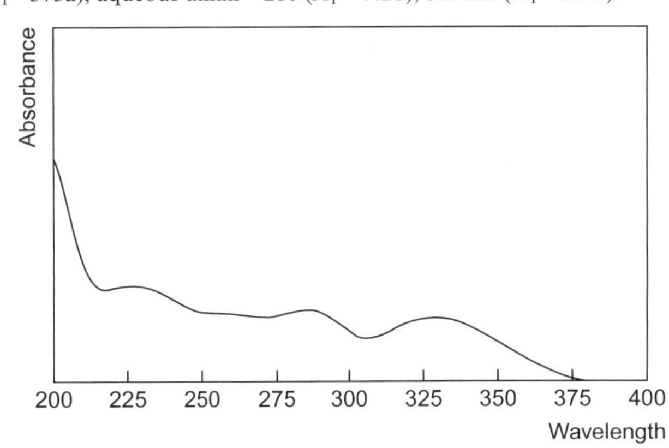

Infra-red Spectrum. Principal peaks at wavenumbers 1704, 1006, 1018, 1160, 1270, 1603 cm^{-1} (KBr disk).

Mass Spectrum. Principal ions at *m/z* 341, 233, 356, 246, 247, 248, 234, 281.

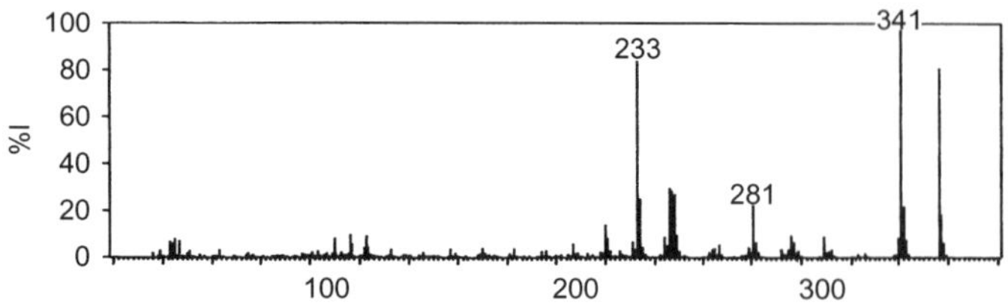

Quantification

High performance liquid chromatography. In plasma or urine: sulindac and its sulfide and sulfone metabolites, limit of detection 100 µg/L in plasma, UV detection—B. N. Swanson and V. K. Boppana, *J. Chromatogr.*, 1981, *225*; *B Biomed. Appl.*, *14*, 123–130. In plasma, urine, bile, or gastric fluid: sulindac and its sulfide and sulfone metabolites, limit of detection 250 µg/L, UV detection—D. G. Musson *et al.*, *J. Pharm. Sci.*, 1984, *73*, 1270–1273. In plasma or urine: sulindac and its sulfide and sulfone metabolites, limit of detection 0.1 mg/L, UV detection—J. Stubbs *et al.*, *J. Chromatogr.*, 1987, *413*, 171–180. In serum: sulindac and its sulfide and sulfone metabolites, limit of detection 10 µg/L, fluorescence detection—M. Siluveru and J. T. Stewart, *J. Chromatogr.* 1995, *673*; *B. Biomed. Appl.*, 91–96.

Disposition in the Body. Sulindac is readily absorbed after oral administration. It is metabolised by oxidation to the sulfone and by reduction to the sulfide which is thought to be responsible for most of the pharmacological activity. A total of about 36% of a dose is excreted in the urine in 24 h and about 75% in 4 days. In 4 days, about 30% of a dose is excreted as the sulfone and its conjugate, and 20% as unchanged drug and its conjugate; no significant amount of the sulfide or its conjugate is found in the urine. Sulindac and its metabolites are excreted in the bile and undergo extensive enterohepatic circulation. Up to about 25% of a dose is eliminated in the faeces in 4 days, with less than 2% as unchanged drug.

Therapeutic concentration

A single dose of 200 mg to 14 subjects produced a mean peak plasma concentration of about 4 mg/L after 1 h; mean peak plasma concentrations for the sulfide and sulfone were about 3 and about 2 mg/L, respectively, after 2 h. [D. F. Duggan *et al.*, *Clin. Pharmacol. Ther.*, 1977, *21*, 326–335].

Following daily oral doses of 200 mg, twice a day to 12 subjects, mean maximum steady-state plasma concentrations were: sulindac 5.0 mg/L, sulfide 6.9 mg/L, sulfone 2.6 mg/L; a diurnal variation in plasma concentrations was reported with lower concentrations being attained after the evening dose. After oral administration of 400 mg once daily to 12 subjects, maximum steady-state plasma concentrations were: sulindac 8.7 mg/L, sulfide 8.8 mg/L, sulfone 3.9 mg/L. [B. N. Swanson *et al.*, *Clin. Pharmacol. Ther.*, 1982, *32*, 397–403].

In 6 patients with end-stage renal failure a single 300-mg oral dose of sulindac produced a mean maximum plasma concentration of 6.26 mg/L and 0.87 mg/L of sulindac and sulindac sulfide, respectively, at 1.6 h and 2.6 h, compared with 11.4 mg/L and 7.68 mg/L at 1.67 h and 7.68 h in normal subjects. [W. R. Ravis *et al.*, *J. Clin. Pharmacol.*, 1993, *33*, 527–534].

Toxicity

Postmortem concentrations of sulindac in a 4-year-old child who accidentally overdosed with disopyramide and sulindac were: blood 12.2 mg/L, liver 12.4 µg/g, bile 1.251 g/L, and urine 29.8 mg/L. [P. Singer and A. Mozayani, *J. Anal. Toxicol.*, 1995, *19*, 529–530].

Half-life. Plasma half-life, sulindac about 7 h, sulfide metabolite about 16 to 18 h.

Protein binding. In plasma, sulindac, sulfone, and sulfide, about 95%.

Note. For a review of the pharmacokinetics of sulindac, see R. N. Brogden *et al.*, *Drugs*, 1978, *16*, 97–114.

Dose. 200 to 400 mg daily.

Sulpiride

Tranquilliser

Proprietary names. Abilit; Aiglonyl; Arminol; Championyl; Depex; Desisulpid; Dobren; Dogmatil; Dolmatil; Eglonyl; Equilid; Espiride; Guastil; Intrasil; Levobren; Levopraid; Lisopride; Meresa; Neogama; Omperan; Sernevin; Sulp; Sulpitil; Sulpivert; Sulpor; Sulpril; Synedil.

5-(Aminosulfonyl)-*N*-[(1-ethyl-2-pyrrolidinyl)methyl]-2-methoxybenzamide

$C_{15}H_{23}N_3O_4S = 341.4$

CAS—15676-16-1

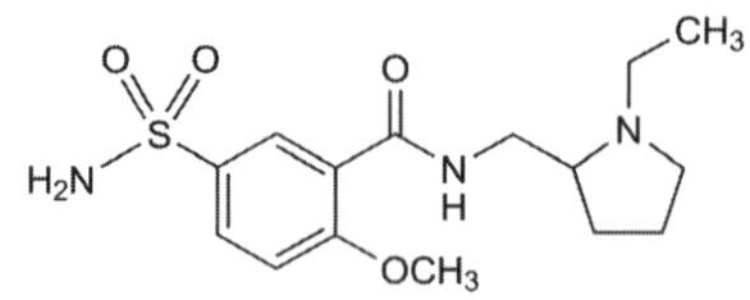

A white to almost white crystalline powder. M.p. 178° to 180°.

Soluble 1 in about 2200 of water, 1 in 100 of ethanol, 1 in about 220 of chloroform, 1 in about 2600 of ether and 1 in 50 of methanol; practically insoluble in benzene. Dissolves in dilute solutions of mineral acids and alkali hydroxides.

Dissociation Constant. pK_a 8.9; 10.19.

Partition Coefficient. Log *P* (octanol/water), 0.57.

Thin-layer Chromatography. System TA—Rf 38; system TB—Rf 00; system TE—Rf 34; system TAE—Rf 17.

Plate: Silica gel F_{254} (20 × 10 cm, 0.2 mm layer). Mobile phase: methylene chloride:methanol:ammonia solution (25%; 18:2.8:0.4). Developed with ninhydrin solution and UV. Rf (× 100), 84.8 [D. Agbaba *et al.*, *J. AOAC Int.*, 1999, *82*, 825–829].

Gas Chromatography. System GA—sulpiride RI 3102, sulpiride-Me RI 3125, sulpiride-Me_2 RI 2995, art (-SO_2NH) RI 2295; system GB—not eluted.

High Performance Liquid Chromatography. System HX—RI 259; system HY—RI 235; system HZ—Retention time, 2.0 min; system HAA—Retention time, 3.9 min; system HAZ—*k* 0.02.

Column: Spherisorb ODS-II-5 (250 × 4.6 mm i.d., 5 µm). Mobile phase: acetonitrile:phosphate buffer (0.01 M monopotassium phosphate adjusted to pH 3.0 with phosphoric acid) (50:50), flow rate 1.0 mL/min. Fluorescence detection (excitation, 300 nm; emission, 365 nm). Retention time: 7.7 min. [H. Tokunaga *et al.*, *J. Chromatogr. B Biomed. Sci. Appl.*, 1997, *691*, 203–207].

Ultraviolet Spectrum. Aqueous acid—292 nm (A_1^1 = 70a). No alkaline shift.

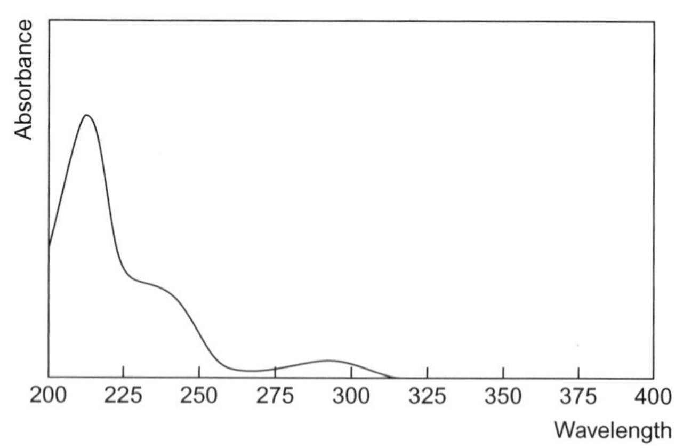

Mass Spectrum. Principal ions at *m/z* 98, 70, 214, 111, 134, 341, 199, 326.

Quantification

High performance liquid chromatography. In plasma: limit of detection 1 µg/L, fluorescence detection (λ_{ex} = 300 nm; λ_{em} = 365 nm)—H. Tokunaga *et al.*, *J. Chromatogr. B. Biomed. Sci. Appl.*, 1997, *691*, 203–207. In plasma: limit of quantification 5 µg/L, UV detection (λ = 240 nm) and 10 µg/L (MS, full scan or SIM, *m/z* 339)—N. Jitsufuchi *et al.*, *J. Chromatogr. B. Biomed. Sci. Appl.*, 1997, *690*, 153–159. In plasma: limit of detection 10 µg/L, fluorescence detection (λ_{ex} = 300 nm; λ_{em} = 365 nm)—P. Nicolas *et al.*, *J. Chromatogr.*, 1986, *381(2)*, 393–400. In plasma: limit of quantification

20 µg/L, fluorescence detection—M. C. Huang *et al.*, *J. Chromatogr. B. Biomed. Sci. Appl.*, 2001, *763*, 157–163.

Disposition in the Body. Slowly and incompletely absorbed after oral administration. It is rapidly distributed to tissues; passage across the blood–brain barrier, however, is not significant. Sulpiride is not metabolised to a significant extent. About 70% of an intravenous dose is excreted as unchanged drug in the urine in 36 h; up to about 20% of an oral dose is excreted in the urine as unchanged drug. A high percentage of the drug is recovered in faeces. Sulpiride has been detected in breast milk.

Therapeutic concentration. The therapeutic serum concentration is 0.04 to 0.6 mg/L.

After a single oral dose of 200 mg given to 10 subjects, peak plasma concentrations of 0.18 to 0.32 mg/L (mean 0.24) were attained in 3 to 4 h [F. R. Sugnaux *et al.*, *Eur. J. Drug Metab. Pharmacokinet.*, 1983, *8*, 189–200].

Following oral administration of 50 mg, three times a day to 14 subjects, steady-state plasma concentrations of 0.03 to 0.6 mg/L (mean 0.18) were reported, 4 to 7 h after the final dose [J. K. Salminen *et al.*, *Curr. Ther. Res.*, 1980, *27*, 109–115].

Toxicity

A 38-year-old woman with a lengthy history of mental illness was found dead at her home. Empty containers of sulpiride medication were found in her bedroom along with a variety of other pharmaceutical drugs, including cyamemazine, clorazepate and maprotiline. The postmortem blood sulpiride concentration was 38 mg/L; and the other drugs were detected in minute amounts [P. P. Rop *et al.*, *J. Anal. Toxicol.*, 1999, *23*, 294–296].

A 55-year-old woman poisoned herself with sulpiride and was admitted to the intensive care unit with cardiovascular shock. The woman died 10 h after admission to hospital despite medical treatment. The postmortem blood sulpiride concentration was 38.7 mg/L; in urine the concentration was 803.2 mg/L and in the gastric contents, 155.6 mg/L. The blood drug concentration was approx. 60 times the therapeutic level; the cause of death was determined as sulpiride intoxication [P. Kintz *et al.*, *TIAFT Bulletin Case Notes*, 1994, *24*, http://www.tiaft.org/].

Bioavailability. About 30%.

Half-life. Plasma half-life, after intravenous administration 4 to 13 h; after oral administration variously reported as 6 to 15 h (mean 10) and 13 to 41 h (mean 25).

Volume of distribution. About 2 to 3 L/kg.

Clearance. Plasma clearance, about 6 mL/min/kg.

Protein binding. <40%.

Dose. Adults: 200 to 400 mg twice daily; maximum 1200 mg twice daily orally; intramuscularly, 200 to 800 mg daily. Children >14 years old: 3 to 5 mg/kg body weight daily.

Sultiame

Anticonvulsant

Synonym. Sulthiame
Proprietary name. Ospolot
4-(Tetrahydro-2*H*-1,2-thiazin-2-yl)benzenesulfonamide- *S,S*-dioxide
$C_{10}H_{14}N_2O_4S_2$=290.4
CAS—61-56-3

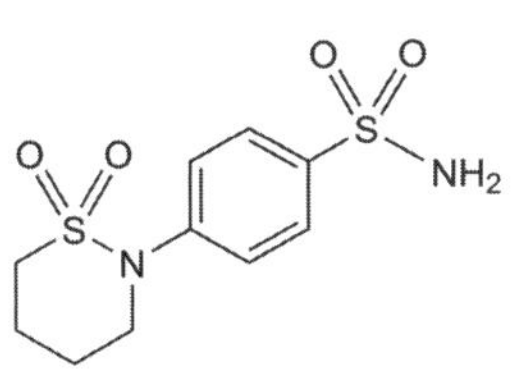

A white crystalline powder. M.p. 180° to 182°.
Soluble 1 in 2000 of water, 1 in 350 of ethanol, 1 in 700 of chloroform and 1 in 500 of ether; readily soluble in alkaline solutions.

Dissociation Constant. pK_a 10.0.

Partition Coefficient. Log *P* (octanol/water), 1.0.

Colour Tests. Copper Sulfate (Method 1)—blue; Koppanyi–Zwikker Test—violet-blue.

Thin-layer Chromatography. System TD—Rf 23; system TE—Rf 57; system TF—Rf 43; system TAD—Rf 42; system TAE—Rf 81.

Gas Chromatography. System GA—Sultiame RI 3000, sultiame-Me RI 2880, sultiame-Me_2 RI 2815.

High Performance Liquid Chromatography. System HE—*k* 1.57; system HX—RI 344; system HY—RI 275.

Ultraviolet Spectrum. Methanol—246 nm (A^1_1=390a).

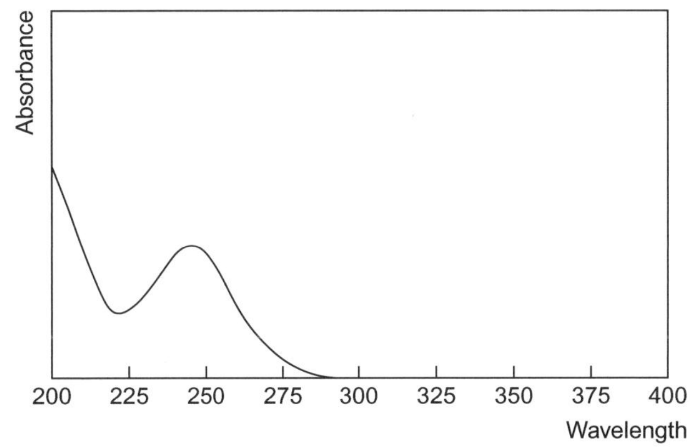

Infra-red Spectrum. Principal peaks at wavenumbers 1138, 1158, 1172, 1293, 889, 1192 cm^{-1} (KBr disk). (See below)

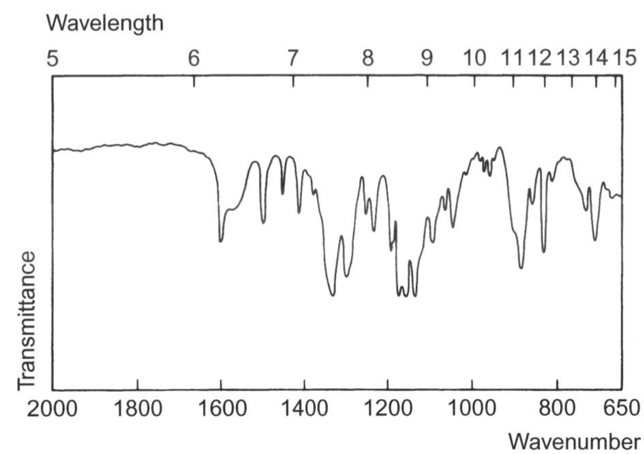

Mass Spectrum. Principal ions at *m/z* 290, 184, 185, 104, 77, 168, 291, 198.

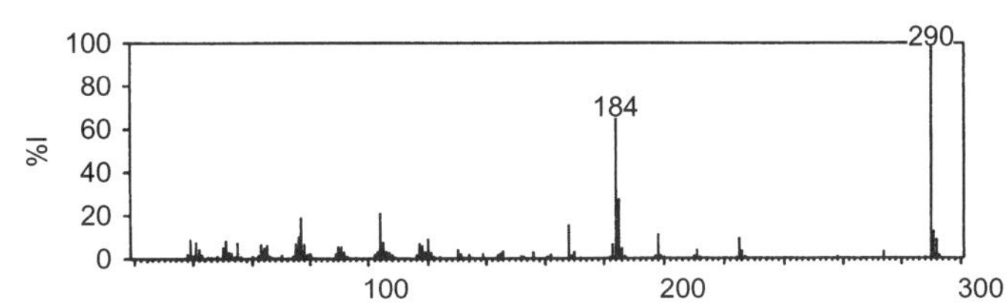

Quantification

High performance liquid chromatography. In plasma: UV detection—D. J. Berry *et al.*, *J. Chromatogr.*, 1979, *171*, 363–370. In plasma: limit of detection 150 µg/L, UV detection—T. Sadanaga *et al.*, *Chem. Pharm. Bull. (Tokyo)*, 1981, *29*, 872–874. In serum—U. H. Juergens, *J. Chromatogr.*, 1991, *553*, 7–13.

Disposition in the Body. Readily but variably absorbed after oral administration. During long-term therapy 17 to 70% (mean 32) of the daily dose is excreted in 24 h, of which about 60% is unchanged drug and the remainder is an inactive metabolite. Up to 15% of a dose may be eliminated in the faeces.

Therapeutic concentration

Following daily oral doses of 3 to 14.5 mg/kg to 36 subjects, serum concentrations ranged from 0.5 to 12.5 mg/L; peak concentrations were attained 1 to 5 h after a dose [O. V. Olesen, *Acta Pharmacol. Toxicol.*, 1968, *26*, 22–28].

Toxicity. Recovery has occurred after the ingestion of 4 to 5 g. Blood concentrations of 12 to 26 mg/L have been reported in fatalities.

Dose. 200 to 600 mg daily.

Suprofen

Analgesic

Synonym. Sutoprofen

Proprietary names. Masterfen; Profenol; Srendam; Sulprotin; Supranol; Suprocil; Suprol; Topalgic.

α-Methyl-4-(2-thienylcarbonyl)benzeneacetic acid

$C_{14}H_{12}O_3S$=260.3

CAS—40828-46-4

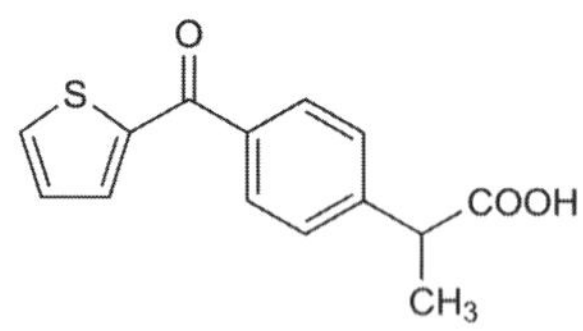

A white to slightly yellowish powder. M.p. 124°.

Sparingly soluble in water; soluble 1 in 5 of ethanol, 1 to 3 of acetone, 1 in about 4 of chloroform and 1 in about 20 of ether.

Dissociation Constant. pK_a 3.9.

Partition Coefficient. Log *P* (octanol/water), 2.8.

Thin-layer Chromatography. System TAJ—Rf 37; system TAK—Rf 62; system TAL—Rf 87.

High Performance Liquid Chromatography. System HY—RI 95.

Ultraviolet Spectrum. Isopropyl alcohol—265 (A^1_1=550b), 291 nm (A^1_1=550b).

Infra-red Spectrum. Principal peaks at wavenumbers 1590, 1220, 1722, 1050, 1308, 743 cm^{-1}(KBr disk).

Quantification

High performance liquid chromatography. In plasma: limit of detection 100 μg/L, UV detection—K. B. Alton and J. E. Patrick, *J. Pharm. Sci.*, 1978, *67*, 985–987. In plasma or urine: limit of detection less than 0.05 mg/L—H. Muller *et al.*, *Arzneimittelforschung*, 1982, *32*, 257–260.

Disposition in the Body. Suprofen is rapidly and well absorbed after oral administration. About 72% of a dose is excreted in the urine in 6 h, mainly as dihydrosuprofen glucuronide.

Therapeutic concentration

After a single oral dose of 200 mg to 6 subjects, peak plasma concentrations of 4.5 to 28.9 (mean 17.5) mg/L were attained in 0.25 to 2 h. [H. W. Zulliger and A. Fassolt, *Arzneimittelforschung*, 1983, *33*, 1322–1326].

Half-life. Plasma half-life, about 2 h.

Protein binding. In plasma, about 99.5%.

Dose. 600 to 800 mg daily.

Suxamethonium Chloride

Muscle Relaxant

Synonyms. Choline Chloride Succinate; Succicurarium Chloride; Succinylcholine Chloride.

Proprietary names. Anectine; Celocurin; Curacit; Ectinex; Ethicholine; Lysthenon; Midarine; Mioflex; Myotenlis; Pantolax; Quelicin; Scoline; Succicuran; Succinolin; Succinyl; Sucostrin; Sukolin; Uxicolin.

2,2′-[(1,4-Dioxo-1,4-butanediyl)bis(oxy)]bis[*N*,*N*,*N*-trimethylethanaminium] dichloride dihydrate

$C_{14}H_{30}Cl_2N_2O_4,2H_2O$=397.3

CAS—306-40-1 (suxamethonium); 71-27-2 (chloride, anhydrous); 6101-15-1 (chloride, dihydrate)

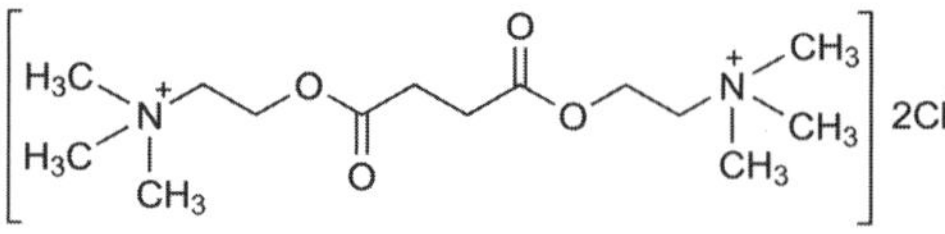

A white, hygroscopic, crystalline powder. M.p. about 156° to 163°; anhydrous form m.p. about 190°.

Soluble 1 in 1 of water and 1 in 350 of ethanol; practically insoluble in chloroform and ether; soluble in methanol.

Suxamethonium Bromide

Synonyms. Choline Bromide Succinate; Succinylcholine Bromide.

Proprietary name. Brevidil M

$C_{14}H_{30}Br_2N_2O_4,2H_2O$=486.2

CAS—55-94-7

A white or creamy-white powder. M.p. about 225°.

Soluble 1 in 0.3 of water and 1 in 5 of ethanol; practically insoluble in chloroform and ether.

Suxamethonium Iodide

Synonyms. Dithylinum; Succinylcholine Iodide.

Proprietary name. Célocurine

$C_{14}H_{30}I_2N_2O_4$=544.2

CAS—541-19-5

A white, slightly hygroscopic, crystalline powder. M.p. about 243° to 245°.

Freely soluble in water; very slightly soluble in ethanol; practically insoluble in ether.

Partition Coefficient. Log *P* (octanol/water), –7.9.

Thin-layer Chromatography. System TA—Rf 01; system TAE—Rf 00; system TAF—Rf 00; system TL—Rf 00; system TB—Rf 00; system TC—Rf 00; system TE—Rf 00; system TN—Rf 35; system TO—Rf 10. (Acidified iodoplatinate solution, positive.)

Gas Chromatography. System GA—not eluted.

Ultraviolet Spectrum. No significant absorption, 230 to 360 nm.

Infra-red Spectrum. Principal peaks at wavenumbers 1724, 1148, 1308, 961, 952, 1612 cm^{-1} (KBr disk).

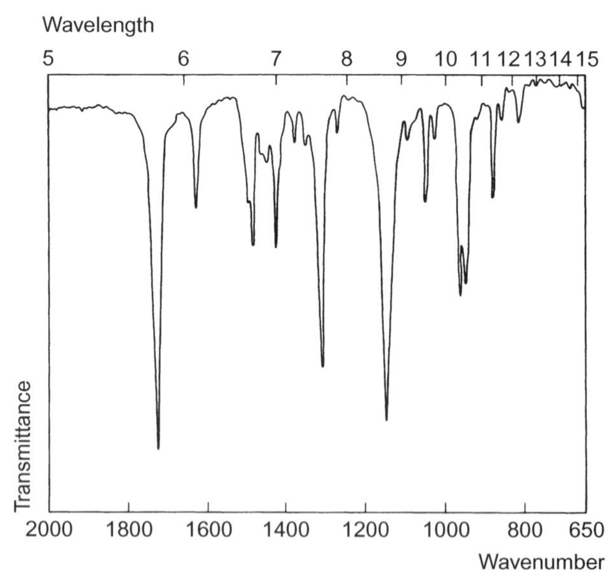

Quantification

Mass spectrometry. In plasma—J. J. Roy *et al.*, *Anal. Biochem.*, 2001, *290*, 238–244.

High performance liquid chromatography. In plasma: limit of detection 100 μg/L, fluorescence detection—A. J. Lagerwerf *et al.*, *J. Chromatogr.*, 1991, *570*, 390–395. In plasma: limit of detection 250 μg/L, electrochemical detection—H. Gao *et al.*, *J. Chromatogr. B. Biomed. Sci. Appl.*, 1998, *718*, 129–134. In plasma: limit of detection 156 nmol, electrochemical detection—N. I. Pitts *et al.*, *Br. J. Anaesth.*, 2000, *85*, 592–598.

Disposition in the Body. Suxamethonium chloride is slowly and incompletely absorbed after oral administration; it is absorbed after IM administration but generally given by the IV route. It is rapidly distributed into the extracellular fluids throughout the body. Suxamethonium is rapidly hydrolysed in plasma and body tissues to succinylmonocholine (weak activity) and choline. Succinylmonocholine is then slowly hydrolysed to succinic acid and choline. Less than 3% of a dose is excreted unchanged in the urine.

Toxicity

A 33-year-old anaesthesiologist, who committed suicide by injecting suxamethonium and thiobarbital, had a postmortem blood suxamethonium concentration of 14.3 mg/L 3 h after administration. [G. Somogyi *et al.*, *Forensic Sci. Int.*, 1989, *43*, 257–266].

Half-life. Plasma half-life, about 3 min.

Dose. Usually 20 to 100 mg of suxamethonium chloride, intravenously.

Suxethonium Bromide

Muscle Relaxant

Proprietary name. Brevidil E

2,2′-Succinyldioxybis(diethyldimethylammonium) dibromide

$C_{16}H_{34}Br_2N_2O_4$=478.3

CAS—111-00-2

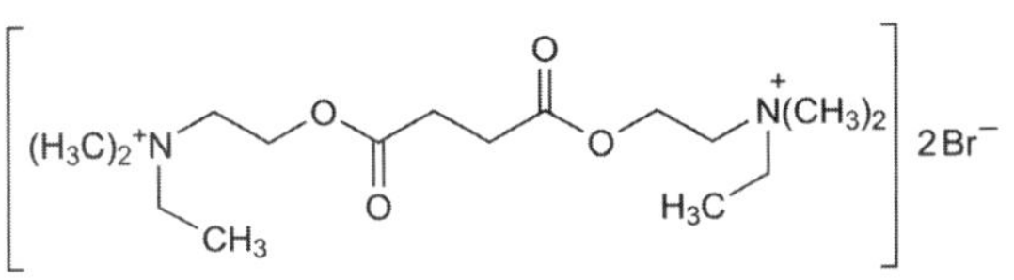

A slightly hygroscopic, white or slightly cream, crystalline powder. M.p. 158°.

Readily soluble in water, yielding weakly acidic solutions.

Partition Coefficient. Log *P* (octanol/water) −7.0.

Thin-layer Chromatography. System TA—Rf 01; system TN—Rf 40; system TO—Rf 23. (Acidified iodoplatinate solution, positive.)

Ultraviolet Spectrum. No significant absorption, 230 to 360 nm.

Infra-red Spectrum. Principal peaks at wavenumbers 1740, 1163, 1638, 1270, 962, 1012 cm^{-1} (KBr disk).

Disposition in the Body. After intravenous administration it is rapidly hydrolysed in plasma and body tissues to succinic acid and choline.

Dose. 1.5 to 1.9 mg/kg intravenously.

Syrosingopine

Antihypertensive

Synonym. Methyl Carbethoxysyringoyl Reserpate

Proprietary names. Isotense; Londomin; Raunova; Serinamin; Singoserp; Siringina.

18-[[4-[(Ethoxycarbonyl)oxy]-3,5-dimethoxybenzoyl]oxy]-11,17-dimethoxyyohimban-16-carboxylic acid methyl ester

$C_{35}H_{42}N_2O_{11}$=666.7

CAS—84-36-6

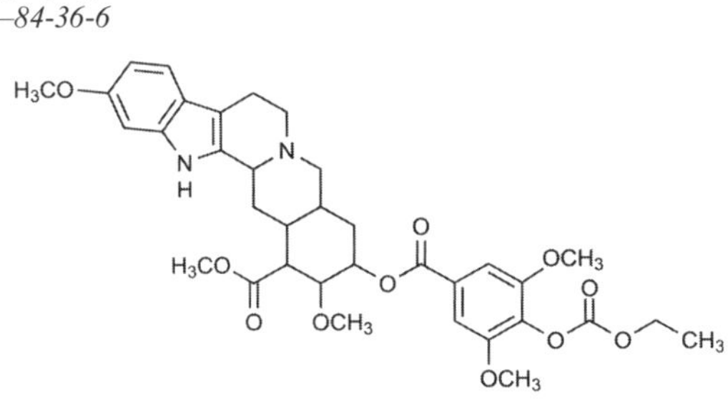

A white or slightly yellowish crystalline powder. M.p. 175° to 179°.

Practically insoluble in water; freely soluble in chloroform and acetic acid; slightly soluble in ether.

Colour Tests. Mandelin's Test—green-brown; Marquis Test—brown.

Thin-layer Chromatography. System TA—Rf 78. (Acidified potassium permanganate solution, positive.)

Ultraviolet Spectrum. Ethanol—258 nm (A^1_1=242a), 298 nm.

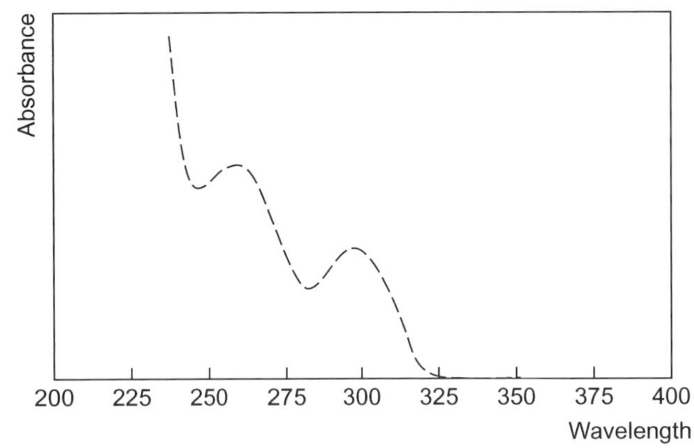

Infra-red Spectrum. Principal peaks at wavenumbers 1209, 1130, 1247, 1180, 1770, 1727 cm^{-1} (KBr disk).

Mass Spectrum. Principal ions at *m/z* 181, 395, 198, 251, 397, 396, 199, 666.

Dose. 0.5 to 3 mg daily.

Tacrine

Anticholinesterase/Central Stimulant

Synonym. Tetrahydroaminoacridine

1,2,3,4-Tetrahydro-9-acridinamine

$C_{13}H_{14}N_2$=198.3

CAS—321-64-2

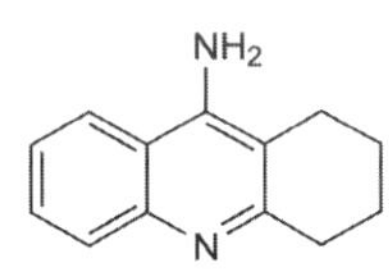

M.p. 183° to 184°.

Tacrine Hydrochloride

Synonyms. CI-970; Tetrahydroaminoacridine Hydrochloride; THA.

Proprietary names. Cognex; Tacrinal.

$C_{13}H_{14}N_2$,HCl=234.7

CAS—1684-40-8

A pale yellow crystalline powder. M.p. 283° to 284°.

Soluble in water.

Dissociation Constant. pK_a 9.95 (20°).

Partition Coefficient. Log *P* (octanol/water), 2.71.

Thin-layer Chromatography. System TA—Rf 43; system TB—Rf 05; system TC—Rf 04; system TL—Rf 10. (Acidified iodoplatinate solution, positive.)

Gas Chromatography. System GA—RI 2165.

High Performance Liquid Chromatography. System HA—*k* 1.6.

Column: LiChrospher RP-select B (250 × 4 mm i.d., 5 μm). Mobile phase: acetate buffer (0.2 M, pH 4): acetonitrile (87:13), flow rate 1.25 mL/min (0 to 16 min) and 2.5 mL/min (16 to 40 min). Fluorescence detection (λ_{ex} = 330 nm; λ_{em} = 365 nm). Retention time: 29 to 30 min [L. L. Hansen *et al.*, *J. Chromatogr. B Biomed. Sci. Appl.*, 1998, *712*, 183-191].

Ultraviolet Spectrum. Aqueous acid—240 nm (A^1_1=2032a), 323, 336 nm; aqueous alkali—237, 317 nm.

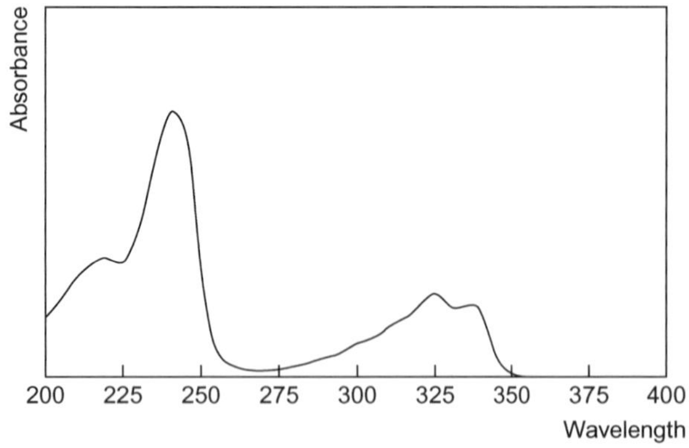

Infra-red Spectrum. Principal peaks at wavenumbers 1650, 1590, 765, 1496, 774, 1176 cm^{-1} (KBr disk).

Mass Spectrum. Principal ions at *m/z* 198, 197, 170, 199, 182, 169, 77, 183.

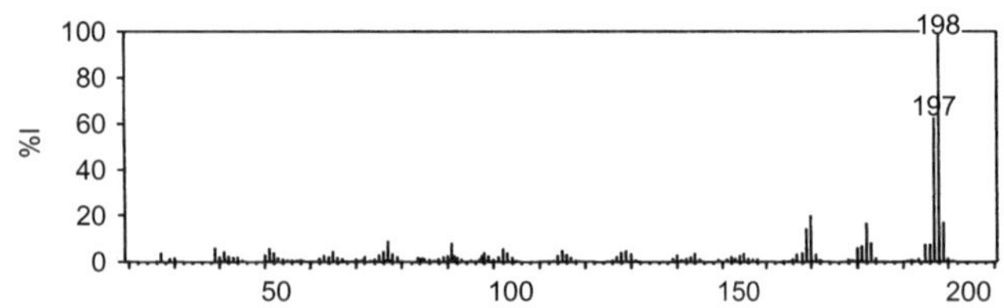

Quantification

High performance liquid chromatography. In plasma: tacrine and its metabolites, limit of quantification for tacrine 0.5 µg/L, fluorescence detection—D. B. Haughey *et al.*, *J. Pharm. Sci.*, 1994, *83*, 1582–1585; G. Aymard *et al.*, *Ther. Drug Monit.*, 1998, *20*, 422–429. In plasma and urine: limit of detection 0.5 nmol/L and limit of quantification 2.5 nmol/L for 2-hydroxytacrine and 4-hydroxytacrine, 2.0 nmol/L and 10.0 nmol/L for 1-hydroxytacrine and tacrine in plasma. In urine, the limit of detection is 60 nmol/L for 2-hydroxytacrine and 4-hydroxytacrine, 30 nmol/L for 1-hydroxytacrine and 80 nmol/L for tacrine; limit of quantification 120 nmol/L for all analytes in urine, fluorescence detection (λ_{ex} = 330 nm; λ_{em} = 365 nm)—L. L. Hansen *et al.*, *J. Chromatogr. B Biomed. Sci. Appl.*, 1998, *712(1-2)*, 183–191. In plasma—D. F. Chollet *et al.*, *Ther. Drug Monit.*, 2000, *22*, 225–229.

Disposition in the Body. Tacrine is rapidly absorbed from the gastro-intestinal tract after oral administration, but there is large inter-individual variation in oral bioavailability and the extent of absorption decreases when administered with food. It is metabolised in the liver by the cytochrome P450 enzymes, principally CYP1A2 to several metabolites, the main one being 1-hydroxytacrine, velnacrine. Little unchanged drug is excreted in urine.

Therapeutic concentration

7 patients received tacrine 40 to 140 mg daily for Alzheimer's disease, as part of a 6-week clinical trial. At the end of this period, patients had a mean concentration of 8.01 ± 7.07 µg/L in the plasma and 5.21 ± 6.00 µg/L in the cerebrospinal fluid 30 min after the morning dose (10 to 40 mg, given in the fasting state) [D. R. Grothe *et al.*, *J. Clin. Psychopharmacol.*, 1998, *18*, 78–81].

5 patients with Alzheimer's disease who had the disease for 2 to 12 years, aged between 57 and 72 years were administered with 40 to 160 mg tacrine daily, during a 12 to 31 month treatment period. The mean steady-state plasma concentrations were 1.3, 5.5, 11.9 and 30.0 µg/L for the 40, 80, 120 and 160 mg doses, respectively. After the morning 80 mg dose, the mean maximum plasma concentration was 8.7 µg/L observed at 1.3 h. The mean plasma concentration was 2.6 to 5.6 µg/L [M. Johansson *et al.*, *Dementia*, 1996, *7(2)*, 111–117].

24 healthy, mature volunteers (aged 50 to 76 years; mean 64 years) were administered with a single 40 mg dose of tacrine after an 8 h overnight fast; 1 h before a standard breakfast; 15 min after the start of breakfast (i.e. during breakfast); and 2 h after a standard breakfast was finished. There was a 1 week washout period in between doses. The mean maximum plasma concentration was 15.8 µg/L for the fasting individuals (i.e. after the overnight fast and before breakfast), 17.9 µg/L 1 h before breakfast, 9.9 µg/L when tacrine was administered during breakfast and 11.6 µg/L when the dose was administered 2 h after breakfast. These concentrations were observed at 1.9, 1.7, 3.6 and 2.8 h, respectively [D. F. Welty *et al.*, *J. Clin. Pharmacol.*, 1994, *34(10)*, 985–988].

Toxicity. A serum concentration greater than 20 µg/L is associated with a high risk of adverse reaction.

A 75-year-old woman with Alzheimer's disease was treated with 40 mg tacrine daily for 14 months. She was admitted to hospital with jaundice and was very confused. Her liver span measured 13 cm. She had excessive levels of bilirubicin in the blood and decreased transaminase levels. Drug-induced hepatotoxicity was suspected. All medications were stopped but transaminase levels decreased further and she had urosepsis and acute renal failure. She died 3 weeks after admission to hospital. Postmortem examination showed massive hepatic necrosis which was believed to have been caused by tacrine and possibly the production of toxic metabolites in the liver [W. G. Blackard *et al.*, *J. Clin. Gastroenterol.*, 1998, *26(1)*, 57–59].

Bioavailability. About 17% with a large inter-individual variation.

Half-life. 1.5 to 2 h.

Protein binding. Approximately 55%.

Note. For a review of the clinical pharmacokinetics of tacrine, see S. Madden *et al.*, *Clin. Pharmacokinet.*, 1995, *28*, 449–457; for a review of the pharmacokinetics of cholinesterase inhibitors, see M. W. Jann *et al.*, *Clin. Pharmacokinet.*, 2002, *41*, 719–739.

Dose. Up to 160 mg daily by mouth.

Tacrolimus

Immunosuppressant

Synonyms. FK506; FR-900506.

Proprietary names. Prograf; Protopic.

(3*S*,4*R*,5*S*,8*R*,9*E*,12*S*,14*S*,15*R*,16*S*,18*R*,19*R*,26a*S*)-5,6,8,11,12,13,14,15,16,17,18,19,24,25,26,26a-Hexadecahydro-5,19-dihydroxy-3-[(1*E*)-2-[(1*R*,3*R*,4*R*)-4-hydroxy-3-methoxycyclohexyl]-1-methylethenyl]-14,16-dimethoxy-4,10,12,18-tetramethyl-8-(2-propenyl)-15,19-epoxy-3*H*-pyrido[2,1-c][1,4]oxaazacyclotricosine-1,7,20,21(4*H*,23*H*)-tetrone

$C_{44}H_{69}NO_{12}$ = 804.0

CAS—104987-11-3

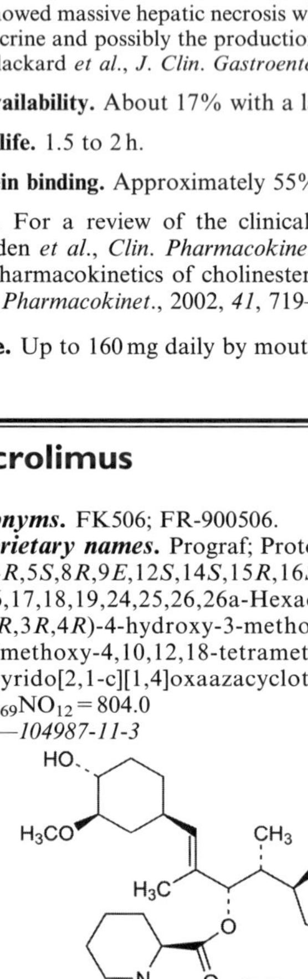

Tacrolimus Monohydrate

$C_{44}H_{69}NO_{12}$, H_2O = 822.0

CAS—109581-93-3

A white crystalline powder with m.p. 127° to 129°. It is practically insoluble in water; soluble in methanol, ethanol, acetone, ethyl acetate, trichloromethane and diethylether; sparingly soluble in hexane and petroleum ether.

High Performance Liquid Chromatography. Column: ODS (Hypersil, 100 × 2.1 mm i.d., 5 µm). Mobile phase: methanol:ammonium acetate (5 mM, pH 9.0 ammonium hydroxide) (99:1), flow rate 0.3 mL/min. MS detection (SIM *m/z* 802.5→168.2). Retention time: 0.97 min [A. Alak *et al.*, *J. Pharm. Biomed. Anal.*, 1997, *16*, 7–13].

Column: RP C_{18} (Spherical, 150 × 3.9 mm i.d., 5 µm). Mobile phase: methanol:water (90:10), flow rate 0.4 mL/min. MS detection (NCI, SIM at *m/z* 803.7). Retention time: 5.2 min [A. Gonschior *et al.*, *Ther. Drug. Monit.*, 1995, *17*, 504–510].

Column: C_{18} (Novapak, 150 × 2.1 mm i.d., 4 µm). Column temperature: 50°. Mobile phase: methanol:ammonium acetate buffer (40 mmol, pH 5.1)

(76:24), flow rate 0.2 mL/min. MS detection (ESI, SIM at *m/z* 821.5→768.5). Retention time: 7.3 min (ammoniated adduct) [P. J. Taylor *et al.*, *Ther. Drug Monit.*, 2000, *22*, 608–612].

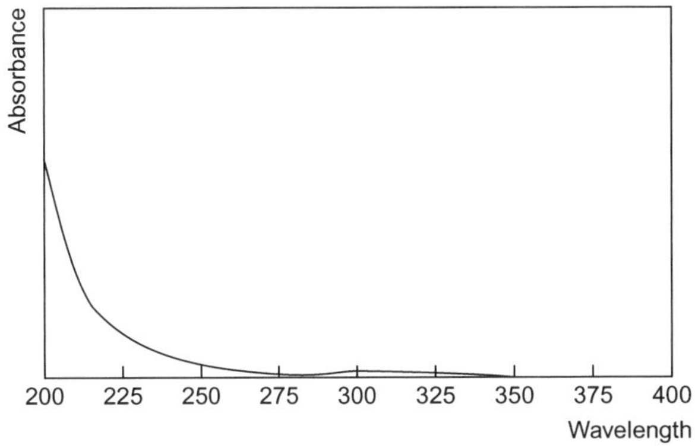

Quantification

High performance liquid chromatography–mass spectrometry. In blood: limit of quantification 0.25 µg/L. MS detection—P. J. Taylor *et al.*, *Ther. Drug Monit.*, 2000, *22(5)*, 608–612. In blood: limit of detection 0.10 µg/L. MS detection—A. Alak *et al.*, *J. Pharm. Biomed. Anal.*, 1997, *16*, 7–13. In blood: limit of quantification 0.025 µg/L. MS detection—H. Hill *et al.*, *Pharm. Res.*, 1997, *14*, S261. In blood and urine: limit of quantification 200 µg/L. MS detection—A. Gonschior *et al.*, *Ther. Drug. Monit.*, 1995, *17*, 504–510.

Immunoassay. In serum: limit of detection 0.1 µg/L—M.C. Friob *et al.*, *Transplant. Proc.*, 1991, *23*(6), 2750–2752.

Disposition in the Body. Absorption of tacrolimus after oral administration is erratic and generally poor. It undergoes extensive tissue distribution and metabolism is hepatic with greater than 99% of the drug being metabolised. At least 15 metabolites have been detected and are produced mainly by demethylation and hydroxylation, via the hepatic cytochrome P450 enzyme (CYP3A), and some metabolism may occur in the gastrointestinal tract. Several hydroxylated and demethylated metabolites have been identified, including 13-*O*-desmethyl tacrolimus and 15-*O*-desmethyl tacrolimus. It is widely and extensively distributed throughout the tissues of the body after intravenous administration. Elimination is primarily via bile (>90% of an absorbed dose is excreted in bile as metabolites. Less than 1% of the dose is excreted in urine as the unchanged drug. A peak plasma concentration of 0.4 to 5.6 µg/L is reached after a single oral dose of 0.15 mg/kg and 10 to 24 µg/L after intravenous infusion of 0.5 mg/kg over 2 h. Hepatic impairment causes increased plasma concentration, prolonged half-life and reduced clearance. Renal impairment causes no change in the pharmacokinetics.

Therapeutic concentration The reference range is 0.5 to 2 µg/L and the therapeutic peak is 0.2 to 6 µg/L. In blood, the therapeutic reference concentration at its trough is 3 to 15 µg/L and its peak, 10 to 25 µg/L.

10 African American (mean age, 32.2 years), 12 white (mean age, 44.6 years) and 12 Latin-American (mean age, 35.7 years) healthy patients were administered with a single, oral dose of 5 mg tacrolimus after an overnight fast. The mean maximum drug concentrations after the oral dose were 20.8, 37.8 and 33.0 µg/L for the three ethnic groups observed at 1.6, 1.3 and 1.3 h, respectively. For the intravenous dose, the mean concentrations were 28.3, 26.4 and 27.4 µg/L detected at the end of the infusion. The metabolite, 13-*O*-desmethyl tacrolimus, was observed at concentrations of 2.0, 4.8 and 3.6 µg/L for the ethnic groups at 1.3, 1.5 and 1.6 h, respectively following oral administration [L. M. Mancinelli *et al.*, *Clin. Pharmacol. Ther.*, 2001, *69(1)*, 24–31].

Toxicity The toxic blood reference concentration is 12 to 15 µg/L.

A 54-year-old male patient waiting for a liver transplant was co-administered with mibefradil for the treatment of hypertension. He subsequently developed dizziness, fatigue and shoulder muscle ache as well as reversible renal impairment. Tacrolimus levels were observed at 54 µg/L (originally in the therapeutic range, 5 to 8 µg/L). Treatment with mibefradil was stopped and tacrolimus levels decreased to normal and all symptoms and clinical changes were reversed. It was decided that these toxic effects were due to interaction between the two drugs. [K. W. Ocran *et al.*, *Z. Gastroenterol.*, 1999, *37(10)*, 1025].

Bioavailability. Oral: 5 to 67% (mean, 30%).

Half-life. 43 h in healthy volunteers and 12 to 16 h in transplant patients.

Volume of distribution. Plasma, 5 to 65 L/kg; blood: 0.5 to 1.4 L/kg (1300 L).

Clearance. Plasma, 0.6 to 5.4 (mean, 1.8) L/h/kg; blood: 0.03 to 0.09 (mean, 0.06) L/h/kg; also reported as 2.43 L/kg.

Distribution in blood. Tacrolimus is primarily associated with red blood cells and the blood:plasma ratio is between 4 and 39.

Protein binding. 77 to 99%. Predominately to the non-lipoprotein fractions containing albumin and α_1-acid glycoprotein.

Dose. Intravenous administration: 0.1 mg/kg/day. Oral: 0.3 mg/kg/day.

Talbutal

Sedative/Barbiturate

Proprietary name. Lotusate
5-(1-Methylpropyl)-5-(2-propenyl)-2,4,6(1*H*,3*H*,5*H*)-pyrimidinetrione
$C_{11}H_{16}N_2O_3$ = 224.3
CAS—115-44-6

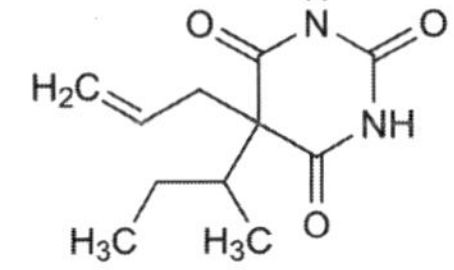

A white crystalline powder. It occurs in 2 polymorphic forms with M.p. about 108° and 110°.
Soluble 1 in 500 of water, 1 in 1 of ethanol, 1 in 2 of chloroform and 1 in 40 of ether.

Dissociation Constant. pK_a 7.9 (20°).

Partition Coefficient. Log *P* (octanol/pH 7.4), 1.3; (octanol/water), 1.5.

Colour Tests. Koppanyi–Zwikker Test—violet; Mercurous Nitrate—black; Vanillin Reagent—brown-orange/violet.

Thin-layer Chromatography. System TD—Rf 53; system TE—Rf 46; system TF—Rf 67; system TH—Rf 71; system TAD—Rf 60; system TAE—Rf 92.

Gas Chromatography. System GA—talbutal RI 1703, talbutal-Me_2 RI 1600.

High Performance Liquid Chromatography. System HG—*k* 7.2; system HH—*k* 4.7; system HX—RI 403; system HY—RI 370.

Ultraviolet Spectrum. Borax buffer 0.05 M (pH 9.2)—239 nm (A_1^1=415a); 1 M sodium hydroxide (pH 13)—255 nm (A_1^1=313b).

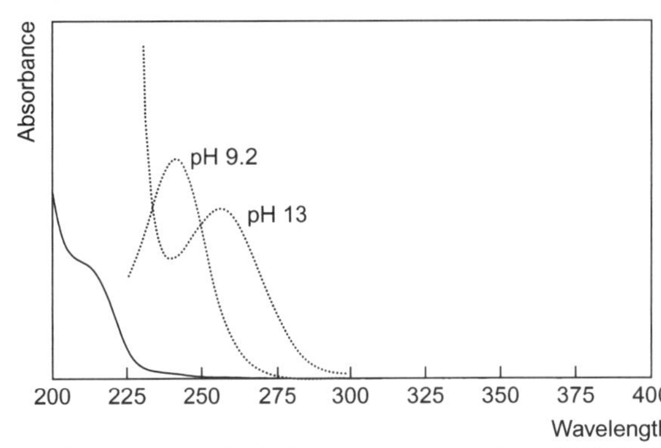

Infra-red Spectrum. Principal peaks at wavenumbers 1703, 1728, 1752, 1315, 1211, 829 cm^{-1} (KBr disk).

Mass Spectrum. Principal ions at *m/z* 167, 168, 41, 97, 124, 39, 57, 53.

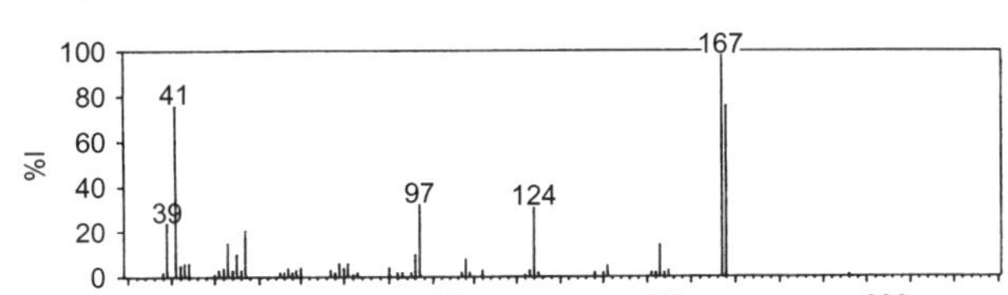

Disposition in the Body
Toxicity. The estimated minimum lethal dose is 2 g.

In one fatality involving talbutal, a blood concentration of 13 mg/L and a liver concentration of 305 μg/g was reported [R. C. Baselt and R. H. Cravey, *J. Anal. Toxicol.*, 1977, *1*, 81–102].

Dose. 60 to 150 mg daily.

Tamsulosin

Alpha$_1$-adrenoreceptor Blocker

5-[(2*R*)-2-[[2-(2-Ethoxyphenoxy)ethyl]amino]propyl]-2-methoxybenzenesulfonamide
$C_{20}H_{28}N_2O_5S = 408.5$
CAS—106133-20-4

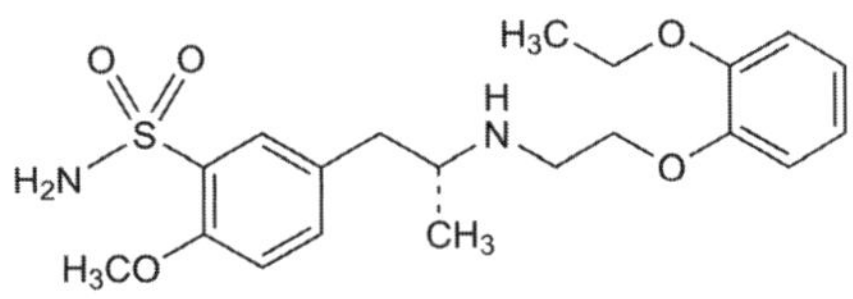

M.p. 254° to 256°.

Tamsulosin Hydrochloride

Synonyms. LY-253351; R-(-)-YM-12617; YM-617; YM-12617-1.
Proprietary names. Alna; Flomax; Harnal; Omiz; Omnic; Pradif.
$C_{20}H_{28}N_2O_5S, HCl = 445.0$
CAS—106463-17-6
White crystals. M.p. 228° to 230°. It is sparingly soluble in water and methanol; slightly soluble in glacial acetic acid and ethanol; practically insoluble in ether.

Dissociation Constant. pK_a 8.4 (secondary amine), 10.2 (sulfonamide).

Partition Coefficient. Log *P* (octanol/pH 6.9), 0.51.

High Performance Liquid Chromatography. Column: C_{18} (Nucleosil, 150 × 4.0 mm i.d., 5 μm). Mobile phase: A- potassium dihydrogen phosphate (100 mM, pH 4.5), B- acetonitrile:potassium dihydrogen phosphate (100 mM, pH 4.9) (20:80). Elution program: (A:B) (100:0) for 5 min, to (0:100) over 60 min, held for 60 min, flow rate 1 mL/min. UV detection (λ = 275 nm). Retention time: 80 min [Y. Soeishi *et al.*, *Xenobiotica*, 1996, *26*, 355–365].

Ultraviolet Spectrum. Aqueous acid—225 nm, 280 nm.

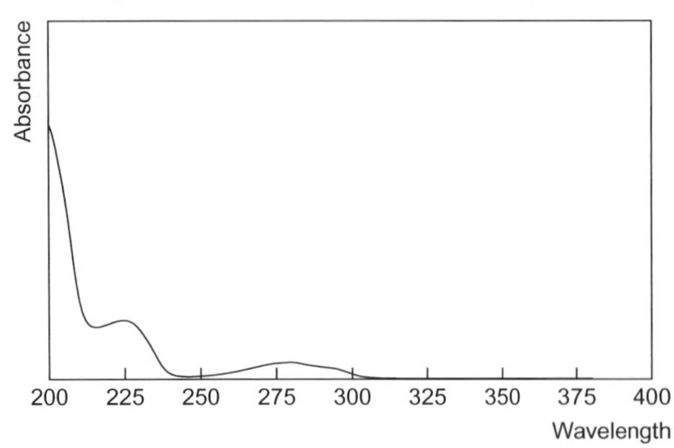

Infra-red Spectrum. Principal peaks at wavenumber 1500, 1340, 1255, 1165 cm^{-1}.

Mass Spectrum. Principal ions at *m/z* 409, 271, 257, 228, 208, 70.

Quantification
High performance liquid chromatography. In blood: limit of quantification 0.5 μg/L. Fluorescence detection (λ_{ex} = 352 nm; λ_{em} = 500 nm)—H. Matsushima *et al.*, *Drug Metab. Dispos.*, 1998, *26*, 240–245. In plasma dialysate, plasma and urine: lower limit of quantification is 0.01 μg/L. MS detection—H. Matsushima *et al.*, *J. Chromatogr. B. Biomed. Sci. Appl.*, 1997, *695(2)*, 317–327.

Disposition in the Body. Tamsulosin is absorbed from the gastrointestinal tract; 90% following oral administration. The extent and rate of absorption is reduced in the presence of food. It is distributed into extracellular fluid in the body. The drug is metabolised slowly in the liver by hepatic metabolism while first-pass metabolism is negligible. It is mainly metabolised by the cytochrome P_{450} CYP3A enzyme and less than 10% of the dose is excreted in urine unchanged. The metabolites of tamsulosin hydrochloride undergo extensive conjugation to glucuronide or sulfate prior to renal excretion. It is excreted mainly in urine as metabolites and some unchanged drug. There are linear kinetics following single and multiple doses. Steady state concentrations have been observed by the fifth day. Tamsulosin is highly bound to α_1-acid glycoprotein. There appears to be no or little possibility of binding interactions between tamsulosin and other drugs in clinically concomitant use, despite its strong binding to α_1-acid glycoprotein [H. Matsushima *et al.*, *Eur. J. Clin. Pharmacol.*, 1999, *55*, 437–443]. In patients with renal impairment, the pharmacokinetics of tamsulosin are affected by the change in protein binding that is associated with alteration of plasma α_1-acid glycoprotein concentration, but are not largely affected by the decrease in the renal excretion. Although total tamsulosin levels increased as plasma protein binding increased, unbound tamsulosin levels (which are directly associated with the pharmacological effects) remained unchanged in these patients [K. Koiso *et al.*, *J. Clin. Pharmacol.*, 1996, *36*, 1029–1038], indicating that no dose modification is required in symptomatic BPH patients with renal impairment [M. Wolzt *et al.*, *Eur. J. Clin. Pharmacol.*, 1998, *54*, 367–73]. There are no data available on the hepatically impaired.

Therapeutic concentration
Young, healthy, male volunteers were administered with 0.4 mg tamsulosin (as modified release tablets) and the median peak plasma concentration was 16 μg/L. This was reached after 5 h and decreased to 2 μg/L at around 23.5 h [K. Taguchi *et al.*, *Br. J. Clin. Pharmacol.*, 1998, *45(1)*, 49–55].

4 healthy males were administered with a single oral dose of 0.2 mg tamsulosin. The mean peak plasma concentration of the unchanged drug was 13.0 μg/L observed with the hour [Y. Soeishi *et al.*, *Xenobiotica*, 1996, *26(6)*, 637–645].

Bioavailability. 100%.

Half-life. 5 to 7 h. Prolonged in the elderly. Due to absorption rate-controlled pharmacokinetics, the apparent half-life is approximately 9 to 13 h in healthy individuals and 14 to 15 h in the target population.

Volume of distribution. Steady state after intravenous administration, 16 L or 0.2 L/kg.

Clearance. 2.88 L/h or 48 mL/min.

Distribution in blood. Blood:plasma ratio is 0.53.

Protein binding. 94 to 99%, primarily to α_1-acid glycoprotein.

Dose. 0.4 to 0.8 mg daily.

Tandospirone

Anxiolytic/Antidepressant

(3aα,4β,7β,7aα)-Hexahydro-2-[4-[4-(2-pyrimidinyl)-1-piperazinyl]-butyl]-4,7-methano-1*H*-isoindole-1,3(2*H*)-dione
$C_{21}H_{29}N_5O_2 = 383.5$
CAS—87760-53-0

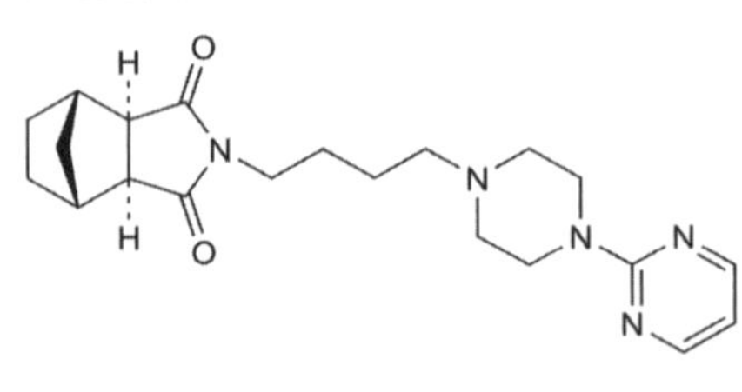

Crystals. M.p. 112° to 113.5°.

Tandospirone Citrate

Synonyms. Metanopirone Citrate; SM-3997.
Proprietary name. Sediel
$C_{21}H_{29}N_5O_2, C_6H_8O_7 = 575.6$
CAS—112457-95-1
Crystals. M.p. 169.5° to 170°.

Tandospirone Hydrochloride

$C_{21}H_{29}N_5O_2, HCl = 420.0$
Crystals from isopropanol. M. p. 227° to 229°.

Disposition in the Body. Tandospirone is metabolised to 1-(2-pyrimidinyl)-piperazine (1-PP). Maximum plasma concentrations after oral administration are reached in 0.5 to 2 h and are 3- to 8-fold higher for the metabolites than the parent drug. Approximately 70% of the administered drug is excreted in urine, with only 0.1% of the dose excreted as the unchanged drug. Dose-dependent pharmacokinetics do not seem to occur.

Therapeutic concentration. The maximum plasma concentration after a 30 mg dose is 3 μg/L.

Half-life. Parent drug, 2 to 3 h; metabolite, 3 to 5 h.

Protein binding. Parent drug, 30.4%; metabolite, 1-PP, 87.5%.

Note. For a review of tandospirone, see L. B. Barradell and A. Fitton, *CNS Drugs*, 1996, *5*, 147–153.

Dose. 30 or 60 mg daily.

Teicoplanin

Antibacterial

Synonyms. A-8327; DL-507-IT; L-12507; MDL-507; Teichomycin A_2.
Proprietary names. Targocid; Targosid; Teicomid.
CAS—61036-62-2 (teichoplanin); 61036-64-4 (teichoplanin A_2)

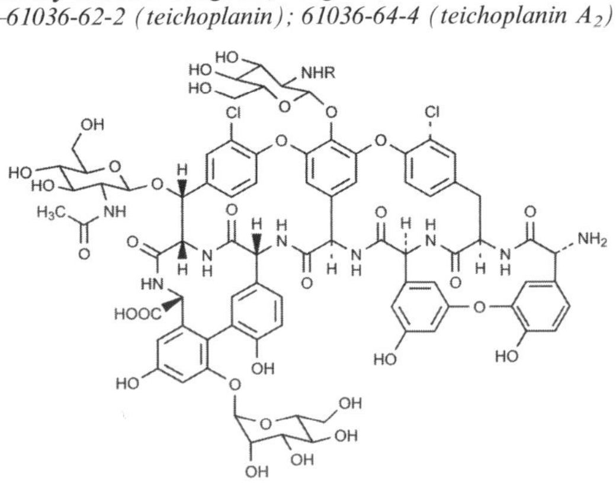

	R
Teicoplanin A_2-1	(*Z*)-4-decenoic acid
A_2-2	8-methylnonanoic acid
A_2-3	*n*-decanoic acid
A_2-4	8-methyldecanoic acid
A_2-5	9-methyldecanoic acid

A glycopeptide antibiotic obtained from cultures of *Actinoplanes teichomyceticus*. An amorphous powder. M.p. 260°. It is soluble in aqueous solutions at pH 7, in propylene glycol, dimethylformamide and dimethylsulfoxide; partially soluble in methanol and ethanol; insoluble in carbon tetrachloride, acetone, butanol, ethylether and in diluted mineral acids.

High Performance Liquid Chromatography. Column: RP C_{18} (150 × 4.6 mm i.d., 5 μm). Mobile phase: (A)-acetonitrile:sodium dihydrogen phosphate (15.4 mM) (5:95); (B)-acetonitrile:sodium dihydrogen phosphate (75:25), flow rate 1 mL/min. Elution program: (A:B) (90:10) for 5 min; to (70:30) in 10 min, held 20 min; to initial conditions over 12 min. UV detection (λ = 214 nm). Retention times: component A_3, 13.7 min; A_2-1, 18.7 min; A_2-2, 20.0 min; A_2-3, 21.0 min; A_2-4, 25.0 min; A_2-5, 26.3 min [F. Jehl *et al.*, *J. Antimicrob. Chemother.*, 1988, *21*, *Suppl.* A, 53–59].

Column: RP C_{18} (150 × 3.9 mm i.d., 5 μm). Mobile phase: aqueous tetrabutylammonium phosphate solution (0.01 M, pH 7.5):methanol:*n*-butanol (10:10:1), flow rate 1.3 mL/min. Fluorescence detection (λ_{ex} = 390 nm; λ_{em} = 490). Retention times: A_2-1, 10.2 min; A_2-2, 13.7 min; A_2-3, 15.7 min; A_2-3a, 17.9 min; A_2-4, 23.2 min; A_2-5, 25.4 min [B. Joos and R. Lüthy, *Antimicrob. Agents Chemother.*, 1987, *31*, 1222–1224].

Ultraviolet Spectrum. Aqueous acid (0.1 M hydrochloric acid)—278 nm; aqueous alkali (0.1 M sodium hydroxide)—297 nm.

Quantification

High performance liquid chromatography. In serum: limit of detection 0.5 mg/L. Fluorescence detection (λ_{ex} = 390 nm; λ_{em} = 490 nm)—B. Joos and R. Lüthy, *Antimicrob. Agents Chemother.*, 1987, *31*, 1222–1224. In serum: limit of detection 5 mg/L. UV detection (λ = 210 nm)—J. Levy, *et al.*, *J. Antimicrob. Chemother.*, 1987, *19*, 533–539. In plasma or urine: limit of detection 0.1 mg/L. UV detection (λ = 240 nm)—E. Riva *et al.*, *J. Chromatogr.*, 1987, *421*; *B Biomed. Appl.*, *65*, 99–110. In blood or urine: limit of detection 0.5 mg/L. UV detection (λ = 214 nm)—F. Jehl *et al.*, *J. Antimicrob. Chemother.*, 1988, *21*, *Suppl.* A, 53–59. In plasma: limit of detection 0.2 mg/L. UV detection (λ = 240 nm)—A. Georgopoulos *et al.*, *J. Chromatogr.*, 1989, *494*; *B Biomed. Appl.*, *86*, 340–346. In plasma: limit of detection 0.05 mg/L. UV detection (λ = 210 nm)—R. B. Taylor *et al.*, *J. Chromatogr.*, 1991, *563*; *B Biomed. Appl.*, *101*, 451–457. In plasma: limit of quantification 0.09 mg/L, limit of detection 0.03 mg/L—M. Cociglio *et al.*, *J. Chromatogr. B Biomed. Sci. Appl.*, 1998, *705*, 79–85.

Review. For a comparison of methods for the determination of teicoplanin see W. M. Awni *et al.*, *Ther. Drug Monit.*, 1991, *13*, 511–517.

Disposition in the Body. Teicoplanin is a mixture of several components and the pharmacokinetics of individual components vary slightly depending on their lipophilicity. The drug is poorly absorbed after oral administration and therefore administered by the parenteral route. It is well absorbed after intramuscular injection with a bioavailability of 90% and it rapidly penetrates tissues including skin, fat, and bone. Highest concentrations are observed in the kidneys, trachea, lungs, and adrenals. Penetration into CSF is poor. It is taken up into white blood cells. No metabolites have been identified and it is excreted almost entirely by glomerular filtration in the urine as unchanged drug. Approx. 80% in urine and a minor amount in faeces. It is not removed by haemodialysis.

Therapeutic concentration. The trough serum therapeutic concentration range is 10 to 40 mg/L.

Teicoplanin was administered to 6 healthy males, aged 22 to 23 years old, as a single intramuscular dose of 3 mg/kg, an intravenous dose of 3 mg/kg or 6 mg/kg after an overnight fast and continued fasting for 2 h after dosing. The mean peak plasma concentrations were 7.12, 53.48 and 111.81 mg/L at 2.02 h and by the end of the infusion, respectively [L. Verbist *et al.*, *Antimicrob. Agents Chemother.*, 1984, *26*, 881–886].

Toxicity. The toxic serum concentration is 200 mg/L.

Several overdoses of 100 mg/kg daily administered to a 4-year-old and an 8-year-old neutropenic paediatric patient by mistake, resulted in high plasma concentrations up to 300 mg/L but no symptoms or laboratory abnormalities were observed. [Data on file from manufacturer.]

Bioavailability. 90%.

Half-life. Plasma half-life, 30 to over 160 h in normal subjects (depending on the sampling time), increased in renal impairment; an effective half-life of about 60 h has been suggested in calculating dosage regimens.

Volume of distribution. 0.9 to 1.6 L/kg.

Clearance. Plasma clearance, 0.18 mL/min/kg.

Protein binding. In plasma, 90 to 95%.

Note. For reviews of teicoplanin see A. P. Wilson, *Clin. Pharmacokinet.*, 2000, *39*, 167–183 and R. N. Brogden and D. H. Peters, *Drugs*, 1994, *47*, 823–854.

Dose. Initially 400 mg intravenously followed by 200 mg intravenously or intramuscularly on each subsequent day of treatment.

Telmisartan

Angiotensin II Receptor Antagonist

Synonyms. BIBR-277-SE; BIBR-277.
Proprietary names. Micardis; Pritor.
4′-[(1,4′-Dimethyl-2′-propyl[2,6′-bi-1*H*-benzimidazol]-1′-yl)methyl]-[1,1′-biphenyl]-2-carboxylic acid
$C_{33}H_{30}N_4O_2$ = 514.6
CAS—144701-48-4

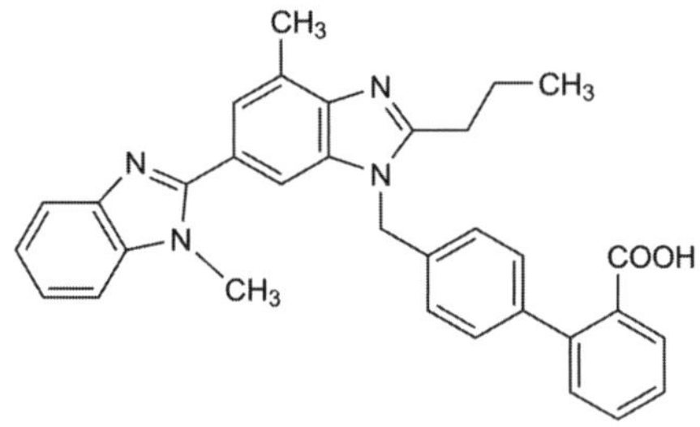

A white to off-white, odourless crystalline powder. M. p. 261° to 263°. It is practically insoluble in water; sparingly soluble in strong acid; soluble in strong base.

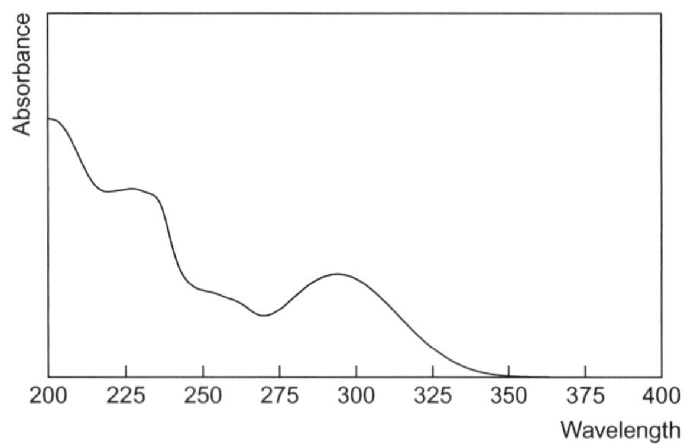

Quantification

High performance liquid chromatography. In plasma: limit of quantification 1 µg/L. Fluorescence detection (λ_{ex} = 300 nm; λ_{em} = 385 nm)—J. Stangier *et al.*, *J. Clin. Pharmacol.*, 2000, *40*, 1312–1322. In plasma and dialysate samples: limit of quantification is 0.5 µg/L. Fluorescence detection (λ_{ex} = 305 nm; λ_{em} = 365 nm)—J. Stangier *et al.*, *J. Clin. Pharmacol.*, 2000, *40*, 1365–1372.

Disposition in the Body. After oral administration, telmisartan is rapidly absorbed and the peak concentration is achieved within 0.5 to 1 h. Most of a dose is eliminated unchanged in faeces via biliary excretion (>97%) with minute amounts detected in urine. Telmisartan is metabolised to form its acylglucuronide (pharmacologically inactive) and this is the only metabolite that has been detected in human plasma and urine. The glucuronide makes up approximately 11% of the plasma concentration of the drug.

Therapeutic concentration

13 healthy males (mean age, 51.2 years; range, 33 to 62 years) and 13 patients with hepatic impairment (mean, 53.5 years; range, 44 to 60 years) were fasted overnight and then administered 20 mg telmisartan. After a 14 day 'wash-out' period, another dose of 120 mg was given to the individuals. After the 20 mg dose, mean peak plasma concentrations of 105 (range, 10.5 to 265) µg/L were observed for the patients and 16.2 (range, 7.8 to 267) µg/L for the healthy individuals. These were detected in a time range between 0.5 and 4.0 h. After the 120 mg, the mean peak concentration for the patients was 1520 (514 to 3280) µg/L and 475 (167 to 760) µg/L for the healthy individuals. These concentrations were observed at a time range between 0.5 and 2.0 h [J. Stangier *et al.*, *J. Clin. Pharmacol.*, 2000, *40*, 1355–1364].

6 patients with severe renal insufficiency and undergoing regular maintenance dialysis, aged 37 years (range, 21 to 46 years) and 12 healthy males (mean age, 51.2 years; range, 33 to 62 years) were fasted overnight and then administered with a 120 mg dose telmisartan. The healthy individuals reached a mean peak plasma concentration of 438 µg/L after 1 h. The patients receiving the dose between dialysis periods reached concentrations of 100 µg/L at 1 h and for those receiving telmisartan during dialysis, the peak concentration was 169 µg/L at 0.5 h [J. Stangier *et al.*, *J. Clin. Pharmacol.*, 2000, *40*, 1365–1372].

Bioavailability. Administration with food slightly reduces the bioavailability and this is also dose dependent. With a 40 mg dose the absolute bioavailability is 42% and with a 160 mg dose, 58%.

Half-life. 24 h.

Volume of distribution. 500 L.

Clearance. Plasma clearance, >800 mL/min.

Protein binding. >99.5% bound to, mostly, albumin and α_1-acid glycoprotein.

Dose. The usual daily dose is 40 mg.

Temazepam

Hypnotic

Synonyms. ER-115; 3-Hydroxydiazepam; K-3917; *N*-Methyloxazepam; Oxydiazepam; Ro-5-5345; Temazepamum; Wy-3917.
Proprietary names. Euhypnos; Euipnos; Gelthix; Levanxene; Levanxol; Maeva; Nocturne; Normison; Nortem; Perdorm; Planum; Remestan; Restoril; Somapam; Temaze; Temtabs; Tenox.
7-Chloro-1,3-dihydro-3-hydroxy-1-methyl-5-phenyl-2*H*-1,4-benzodiazepin-2-one
$C_{16}H_{13}ClN_2O_2$=300.7
CAS—846-50-4

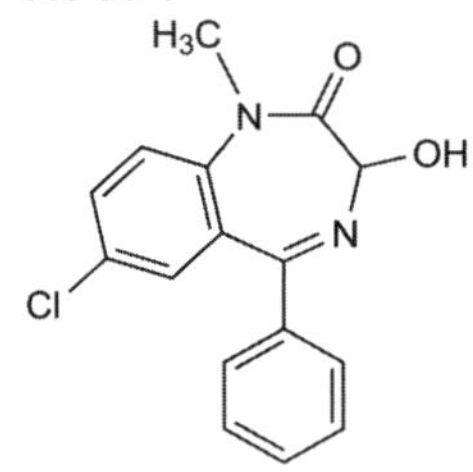

A white to almost white crystalline powder. M.p. 156° to 159°.
Very slightly soluble in water; soluble 1 in 10 of ethanol and 1 in 10 of chloroform; freely soluble in dichloromethane.

Dissociation Constant. pK_a 1.6.

Partition Coefficient. Log *P* (octanol/water), 2.19.

Colour Test. Formaldehyde–Sulfuric Acid—orange.

Thin-layer Chromatography. System TA—Rf 53; system TB—Rf 08; system TC—Rf 59; system TD—Rf 51; system TE—Rf 62; system TF—Rf 47; system TL—Rf 53; system TAD—Rf 65; system TAE—Rf 82; system TAF—Rf 82; system TAJ—Rf 65; system TAK—Rf 54; system TAL—Rf 92. (Dragendorff spray, positive; acidified iodoplatinate solution, positive; acidified potassium permanganate solution, positive.)

Gas Chromatography. System GA—temazepam RI 2595, temazepam-AC RI 2730, temazepam-Me RI 2600, M (OH-) RI 2670, M (OH-)-AC RI 2790, oxazepam RI 2325; system GB—temazepam RI 2727, temazepam-TMS RI 2713, oxazepam RI 2438; system GG—temazepam RI 3125, oxazepam RI 2803.

High Performance Liquid Chromatography. System HI—temazepam *k* 5.68, oxazepam *k* 4.62; system HK—temazepam *k* 0.60, oxazepam *k* 0.73; system HX—RI 472; system HY—RI 438; system HZ—Retention time, 5.5 min; system HAA—Retention time, 18.6 min; system HAX—Retention time 8.9 min; system HAY—Retention time 6.7 min; system HAZ—*k* 1.43; system HBH—*k* 6.80; system HBI—*k* 1.49.

Ultraviolet Spectrum. Aqueous acid—237 nm (A^1_1=980b), 284 nm (A^1_1=283b), 358 nm (A^1_1=68b); aqueous alkali—231, 313 nm; methanol—230 nm (A^1_1=1090a), 314 nm(A^1_1=76b).

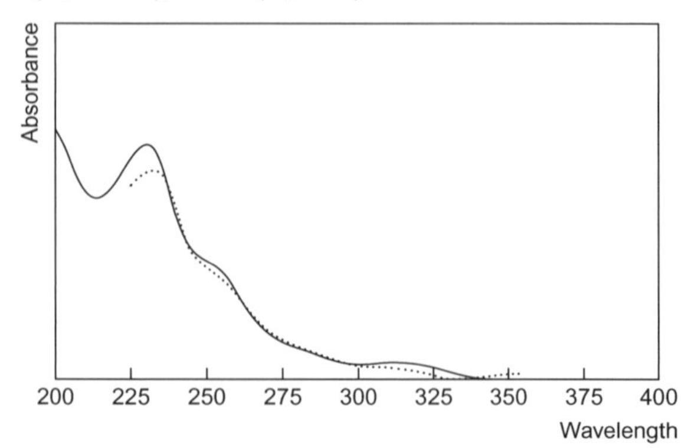

Infra-red Spectrum. Principal peaks at wavenumbers 1687, 1670, 1112, 1603, 705, 1150 cm^{-1} (KBr disk).

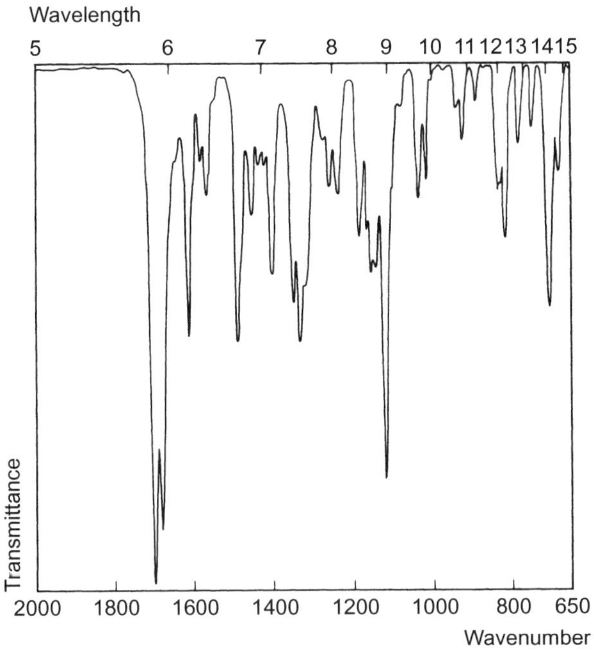

Mass Spectrum. Principal ions at *m/z* 271, 273, 300, 272, 256, 77, 255, 257; oxazepam 257, 77, 268, 239, 205, 267, 233, 259.

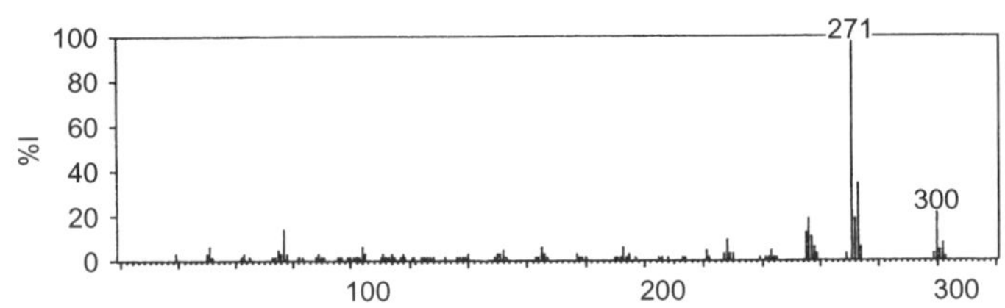

Quantification

Gas chromatography. In plasma: limit of detection 5 μg/L, ECD—M. Divoll and D. J. Greenblatt, *J. Chromatogr.*, 1981, *222*; *Biomed. Appl.*, *11*, 125–128. In biological fluids: limit of detection 0.13 ng/injection—T. V. Beischlag and T. Inaba, *J. Anal. Toxicol.*, 1992, *16(4)*, 236–239.

Gas chromatography–mass spectrometry. In urine: temazepam and other benzodiazepines, limit of quantification < 10 μg/L—P. H. Dickson *et al.*, *J. Anal. Toxicol.*, 1992, *16*, 67–71. In urine: temazepam and other benzodiazepine metabolites—R. E. West and D. P. Ritz, *J. Anal. Toxicol.*, 1993, *17*, 114–116; R. L. Fitzgerald *et al.*, *J. Anal. Toxicol.*, 1993, *17*, 342–347.

High performance liquid chromatography. In plasma and urine: limit of quantification and detection 10 μg/L, UV detection ($\lambda = 232$ nm)—R. M. Azzam *et al.*, *J. Chromatogr. B Biomed. Sci. Appl.*, 1998, *708*, 304–309. In urine: limit of detection 2 μg/L—K. Chiba *et al.*, *J. Chromatogr.*, 1995, *668*, *Biomed. Appl.*, 77–84. In plasma and urine: limit of detection is 15.5 μg/L and limit of quantification, 46.5 μg/L, UV detection ($\lambda = 230$ nm)—G. W. Kunsman *et al.*, *J. Chromatogr.*, 1991, *568*, 427–436. In plasma or urine: temazepam and other benzodiazepine glucuronides, limits of detection 5 to 10 μg/L—C. Franzelius and K. Besserer, *J. Chromatogr.*, 1993, *613*, 162–167. In whole blood—K. S. Scott and J. S. Oliver, *J. Anal. Toxicol.*, 1997, *21*, 297–300. In serum: temazepam and other benzodiazepines, photodiode-array detection—B. Ahrens *et al.*, *Arzneimittelforschung*, 2000, *50*, 1057–1062. In urine: temazepam and other benzodiazepines, limit of detection for temazepam 333 μg/L, UV detection—W. M. Mullett and J. Pawliszyn, *Anal. Chem.*, 2002, *74*, 1081–1087. In serum: temazepam and other benzodiazepines, limit of detection for temazepam 29 μg/L—W. M. Mullett *et al.*, *J. Chromatogr. A.*, 2002, *963*, 325–334.

High performance liquid chromatography–mass spectrometry. In serum and urine: limit of detection 0.02 to 2.0 μg/L—H. Yuan *et al.*, *J. Anal. Toxicol.*, 2000, *24(8)*, 718–725.

Disposition in the Body. Rapidly absorbed after oral administration. The exact rate of absorption is determined by the formulation of the drug administered. Metabolised principally by glucuronic acid conjugation; demethylation to oxazepam occurs to a small extent and it is also found as a conjugate. About 80% of a dose is excreted in the urine, mostly as the inactive glucuronide conjugates; less than 2% of a dose is excreted as unchanged drug. About 12% of a dose is eliminated in the faeces. Small amounts of the demethylated derivative, oxazepam, and its conjugated form have also been detected. Temazepam can be found in breast milk and cerebrospinal fluid.

Temazepam is a metabolite of several benzodiazepines, including diazepam, ketazolam and medazepam.

Therapeutic concentration. The therapeutic serum concentration is 0.3 to 0.9 mg/L.

10 healthy male volunteers (21 to 52 years old) were rectally administered, after an overnight fast, 10 mg temazepam as a polyethylene glycol-based suppository, a liquid-filled capsule and a micro-enema. The same dose was also administered orally as a liquid-filled capsule. A 1 week washout period was allowed between doses. The mean peak serum concentrations of temazepam were 0.202, 0.182 and 0.205 mg/L for the suppository, capsule (administered rectally) and micro-enema, respectively. These were observed at 1.48, 4.08 and 0.49 h, respectively. For the capsule administered orally, the mean peak serum concentration was 0.326 mg/L at 0.8 h [L. M. Hanff and W. J. Rutten, *Pharm. World Sci.*, 1996, *18(3)*, 114–119].

24 healthy, male and female volunteers (aged 18 to 43 years; mean 29 years) were administered a single oral 20 mg dose of temazepam as a soft-gelatin capsule and a liquid-filled capsule. Administration was after a 10 h fast which continued for 4 h after dosing and a 1 week washout period was allowed between doses. The peak plasma concentration observed for the first type of formulation was 0.617 mg/L, observed at approx. 40 min (median value). For the liquid-filled capsule, however, the peak plasma concentration was 0.708 mg/L at 30 min [J. Drake *et al.*, *J. Clin. Pharm. Ther.*, 1991, *16(5)*, 345–351].

13 male patients were administered 20 mg of temazepam orally 1 to 2 h before undergoing spinal anaesthesia for a urological procedure. The total plasma temazepam concentrations just before insertion of the anaesthetic were 0.116 to 0.534 mg/L (mean 0.309 mg/L). The mean concentration in the cerebrospinal fluid was 5.2% of that in the plasma [N. R. Badcock *et al.*, *Eur. J. Clin. Pharmacol.*, 1990, *38*, 153–155].

Toxicity. Toxic effects may be produced by serum concentrations greater than 1.0 mg/L.

Half-life. Plasma half-life, about 8 to 15 h; there is considerable inter-subject variation, and sex differences have been reported.

Volume of distribution. About 1 L/kg.

Clearance. Plasma clearance, about 1 to 2 mL/min/kg.

Distribution in blood. Plasma : whole blood ratio, 1.9.

Protein binding. In plasma, about 96%.

Note. For a review of the pharmacokinetics of temazepam, see R. C. Heel *et al.*, *Drugs*, 1981, *21*, 321–340; for a review of temazepam and new trends in its clinical application, see F. Fraschini and B. Stankov, *Pharmacol. Res.*, 1993, *27*, 97–113; for a review of alcohol and benzodiazepines in fatal poisonings see A. Koski *et al.*, *Alcohol Clin. Exp. Res.*, 2002, *26*, 956–959.

Dose. For insomnia, 10 to 20 mg at night; exceptional circumstances, 30 to 40 mg; premedication usually 20 to 40 mg.

Temozolomide

Antineoplastic

Synonyms. BRN-5547136; CCRG-81045; MB 39831; Methazolastone; NSC-632856.

Proprietary name. Temodal

3,4-Dihydro-3-methyl-4-oxoimidazo[5,1-*d*]-1,2,3,5-tetrazine-8-carboxamide

$C_6H_6N_6O_2 = 194.2$

CAS—85622-93-1

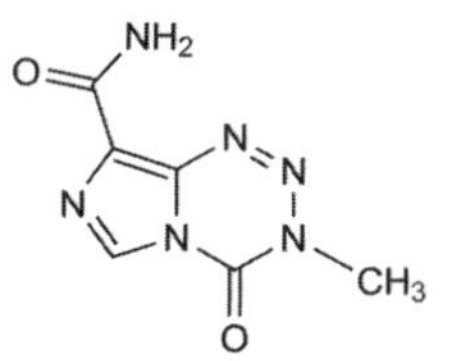

A white to light tan/pink powder, M. p. 212°.

High Performance Liquid Chromatography. Column: ODS (Ultrasphere, 150 × 4.6 mm i.d., 5 μm). Mobile phase: aqueous acetic acid (0.1%):acetonitrile (90:10), flow rate 1.0 mL/min. Internal standard (IS): ethazolastone. UV detection (λ = 316 nm). Retention times: temozolomide, 2.7 min; IS, 5.0 min [H. Kim *et al.*, *J. Pharm. Biomed. Anal.*, 2001, *24*, 461–468].

Column: SCD-100 (Synchropak, 150 × 4.6 mm i.d., 5 μm). Mobile phase: ammonium acetate (0.02 M):acetonitrile (92:8), flow rate 1.1 mL/min. IS: hydrochlorothiazide. UV detection (λ = 316 nm). Retention times: MTIC, 4.5 min; IS, 6.5 min [H. K. Kim *et al.*, *J. Chromatogr. B Biomed. Sci. Appl.*, 1997, *703(1-2)*, 225–233].

Column: (analytical) RP HP ODS (Hypersil, 100 × 4.6 mm i.d., 5 μm); (guard) HP ODS (Hypersil, 20 × 4.0 mm i.d., 5 μm). Mobile phase: methanol:acetic acid (0.5%) (10:90), flow rate 1.0 mL/min. UV detection (λ = 330 nm). IS: ethazolastone. Retention times: 3.2 min; IS, 7.4 min [F. Shen *et al.*, *J. Chromatogr. B Biomed.. Appl.*, 1995, *667*, 291–300].

Ultraviolet Spectrum. Ethanol—327 nm.

Quantification

High performance liquid chromatography. In plasma: limit of quantification 0.1 mg/L, UV detection (λ = 316 nm)—H. Kim *et al.*, *J. Pharm. Biomed. Anal.*, 2001, *24(3)*, 461–468. In plasma: limit of quantification 0.01 mg/L, UV detection (λ = 316 nm)—H. K. Kim *et al.*, *J. Chromatogr. B Biomed. Sci. Appl.*, 1997, *703(1–2)*, 225–233. In plasma and urine: limit of quantification 0.2 mg/L and 2.0 mg/L, respectively—F. Shen *et al.*, *J. Chromatogr. B Biomed.. Appl.*, 1995, *667*, 291–300.

Disposition in the Body. Temozolomide is rapidly and completely absorbed after oral administration, with peak plasma concentrations observed within 0.5 to 1.5 h after administration. Food reduces the rate and the extent of absorption. Peak concentrations are reduced by approximately 32%, and the time to reach these concentrations is extended to over 2 h after a high-fat breakfast. Temozolomide undergoes spontaneous non-enzymatic hydrolysis to its active metabolite 5-(3-methyltriazen-1-yl)imidazole-4-carboxamide (MTIC), the hydrolysis of which is faster in alkaline pH compared with neutral pH. MTIC is further hydrolysed to 5-amino-imidazole-4-carboxamide (AIC). Temozolomide is also metabolised to the temozolomide acid metabolite. The drug is largely eliminated by the kidneys, about 5 to 10% as the unchanged drug. The majority of the dose is recovered in urine, and a small amount in the faeces. Temozolomide is detected mainly as AIC, the unchanged drug, the temozolomide acid metabolite and other unidentified polar metabolites.

Therapeutic concentration

24 patients with solid malignancies untreatable with conventional therapy, aged 32 to 78 years, were fasted 8 h prior to treatment and for an additional 2 h after dosing. All were administered a single oral dose of 100, 150 or 200 mg/m^2 daily for 5 consecutive days. On day 1, the mean peak plasma concentration was 5.4 mg/L for the 100 mg/m^2 dose, 7.7 mg/L for the 150 mg/m^2 dose and 11.0 mg/L for the 200 mg/m^2 dose. These concentrations were observed at 1.0, 0.85 and 0.89 h, respectively. On day 5 the concentrations were 6.4, 9.9 and 16.0 mg/L for the three doses at 1.0, 0.64 and 0.53 h, respectively [L. A. Hammond *et al.*, *J. Clin. Oncol.*, 1999, *17(8)*, 2604–2613].

15 patients with a short life expectancy of approximately 12 weeks, and with histologically confirmed malignancies untreatable by standard therapy, aged 25 to 71 years (mean, 50 years) participated in the study. All were fasted overnight (and for 2 h after dosing) and administered 100, 150, 200 or 250 mg/m^2 daily for 5 days. On day 1, the peak plasma concentration was 7.0 mg/L for the 100 mg/m^2 dose; 5.84 mg/L for the 150 mg/m^2 dose; 13.9 mg/L for 200 mg/m^2 and 13.7 mg/L for 250 mg/m^2. These concentrations were observed at 0.5, 0.94, 0.94 and 1.0 h, respectively. On day 5, the concentrations were 6.92, 5.71, 13.0 and 12.2 mg/L for the 4 doses at 0.39, 1.17, 1.25 and 1.33 h, respectively.

15 patients were also administered 200 mg/m^2 daily for 5 days, either in the fasting state (overnight fast and an additional 4 h after dosing), or in the fed state (ate a high-fat breakfast 1 h before dosing). This was repeated every 4 weeks. The peak plasma concentration for those who were administered temozolomide whilst fasting was 9.55 mg/L at 1.07 h, and for those who were allowed food 6.51 mg/L at 2.25 h [M. Brada *et al.*, *Br. J. Cancer*, 1999, *81(6)*, 1022–1030].

Advanced cancer patients were administered an oral dose of 250 mg/m^2 temozolomide daily for 5 consecutive days. On day 1, the peak plasma concentration was 13.7 mg/L observed at 1 h. On day 5, the peak concentration was 12.2 mg/L at 1.33 h. The drug could be quantified in plasma between 0.25 and 12.0 h after dosing [H. Kim *et al.*, *J. Pharm. Biomed. Anal.*, 2001, *24(3)*, 461–468].

Toxicity. Haematologic toxicity is dose-limiting with values of 1 g/m^2 and 1.25 g/m^2 being associated. Myelosuppression and thrombocytopenia are also dose-limiting.

Bioavailability. 100%.

Half-life. 1.8 h (temozolomide); 2.5 min (MTIC).

Volume of distribution. Apparent, 0.4 L/kg; 17 L/m^2.

Clearance. Systemic clearance, mean, 115 mL/min/m^2 after a single dose and 102 mL/min/m^2 after 5 days multiple dosing.

Protein binding. 15%.

Dose. Orally, 150 to 200 mg/m^2 body surface daily for 5 days, repeated every 28 days.

Tenoxicam

Analgesic

Synonym. Ro-12-0068

Proprietary names. Alganex; Artriunic; Dolmen; Liman; Mobiflex; Reutenox; Rexalgan; Tilatil; Tilcotil.

4-Hydroxy-2-methyl-*N*-(2-pyridyl)-2*H*-thieno[2,3-*e*][1,2]thiazine-3-carboxamide1,1-dioxide

$C_{13}H_{11}N_3O_4S_2 = 337.38$

CAS—59804-37-4

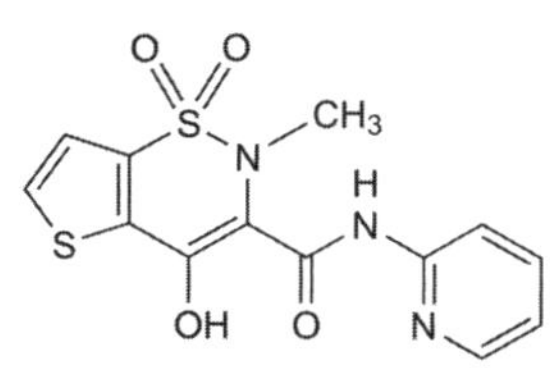

A yellow, polymorphic, crystalline powder. M. p. 205° to 213°. It is practically insoluble in water; very slightly soluble in alcohol; sparingly soluble in dichloromethane; it dissolves in solutions of acids and alkalis.

Dissociation Constant. pK_a 5.3; 1.1.

Partition Coefficient. Log *P* (octanol/water), 2.40; log *P* (octanol/pH 7.4 buffer), 0.3.

Thin-layer Chromatography. System TE—Rf 14; system TF—Rf 06; system TAE—Rf 87.

Gas Chromatography. System GA—RI 2690 (tenoxicam-ME2)

High Performance Liquid Chromatography. System HX—RI 366; system HAA—Retention time 12.7 min.

Column: RP C_{18} (Nucleosil, 250 × 4.6 mm, 5 μm). Mobile phase: sodium dihydrogen orthophosphate (10 mM), sodium lauryl sulfate (1 mM) and acetonitrile:water (pH 2.8) (35:65), flow rate 1.5 mL/min. UV detection (λ = 355 nm). Internal standard (IS) : ketorolac. Retention times: tenoxicam, 4.6 min; IS, 10.3 min [J. L. Mason and G. J. Hobbs, *J. Chromatogr. B Biomed. Appl.*, 1995, *665*, 410–415].

Column: 100 RP-18 (Lichrospher, 125 × 4 mm i.d., 5 μm). Mobile phase: phosphate buffer (0.1 M, pH 7.4):methanol (3:2), flow rate 1.1 mL/min. UV detection (λ = 335 nm). IS: prioxicam. Retention times: tenoxicam, 3.4 min; IS, 4.5 min [M. I. Múnera-Jaramillo and S. Botero-Garcés, *J. Chromatogr.*, 1993, *616*; *B Biomed. Appl.*, *127*, 349–352].

Ultraviolet Spectrum. Aqueous acid—263, 377 nm; basic—263, 289 nm.

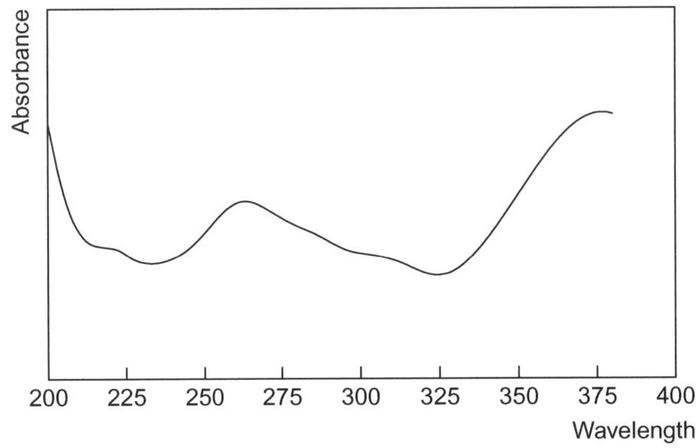

Infra-red Spectrum. Principal peaks at wavenumber 1607, 1325, 1423 cm^{-1} (KBr disk).

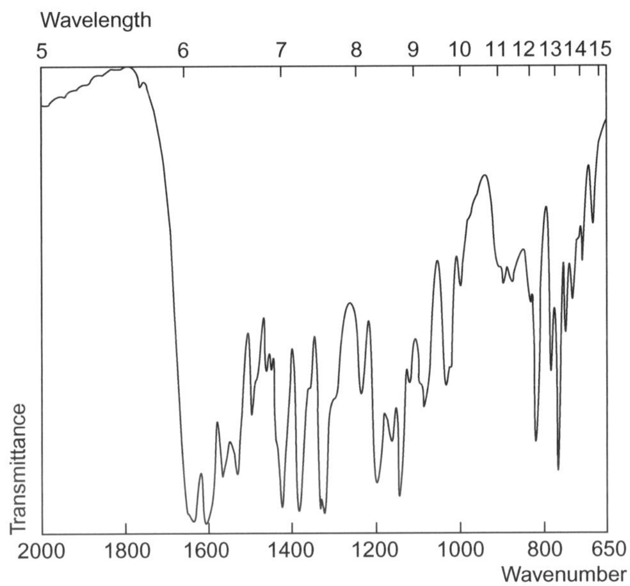

Mass Spectrum. Principal ions at *m/z* 78, 350, 135, 176, 77, 97, 123, 110. (tenoxicam-ME2).

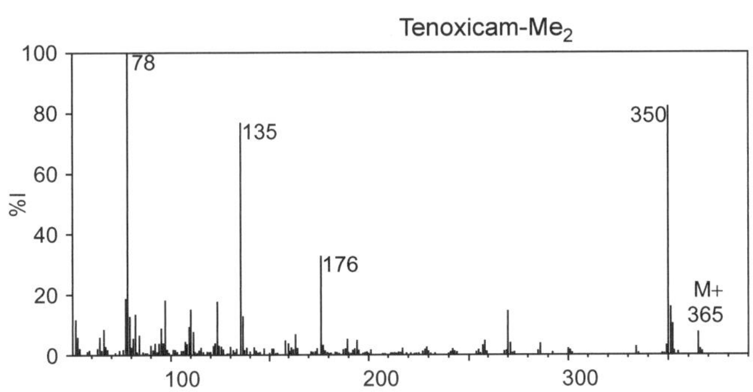

Quantification

High performance liquid chromatography. In plasma: limit of detection 0.2 mg/L, UV detection (λ = 361 nm)—J. S. Dixon *et al.*, *J. Chromatogr.*, 1984, *310*; *B Biomed. Appl.*, *35*, 455–459. In urine: tenoxicam and hydroxy-metabolites, limit of detection 0.05 mg/L, UV detection (λ = 371 nm)—D. Dell *et al.*, *J. Chromatogr.*, 1984, *317*, 483–492. In plasma: limit of detection 0.02 mg/L, UV detection (λ = 371 nm)—P. Heizmann *et al.*, *J. Chromatogr.*, 1986, *374*; *B Biomed. Appl.*, *47*, 95–102. In plasma: limit of detection 0.05 mg/L, UV detection (λ = 361 nm)—M. E. Pickup *et al.*, *J. Chromatogr.*, 1981, *225*; *B Biomed. Appl.*, *14*, 493–497. In plasma: limit of detection 0.005 mg/L, UV detection (λ = 355 nm)—M. I. Múnera-Jaramillo and S. Botero-Garcés, *J. Chromatogr.*, 1993, *616*; *B Biomed. Appl.*, *127*, 349–352. In plasma: limit of detection 0.04 mg/L, UV detection (λ = 355 nm)—J. L. Mason and G. J. Hobbs, *J. Chromatogr. B Biomed. Appl.*, 1995, *665*, 410–415.

Disposition in the Body. Tenoxicam is rapidly and completely absorbed after oral administration. Peak plasma concentrations occur within about 2 h in fasting subjects, but may be delayed up to 6 h after food, although the extent of absorption is not affected. It is over 98.5% protein bound and penetrates sinovial fluid. Tenoxicam is completely metabolised to its inactive metabolites, and about two-thirds of the administered dose is excreted in urine, primarily as the active 5-hydroxypyridyl metabolite. The remainder is excreted in bile as glucuronide conjugates (glucuronidated 6-*O*-metabolite and glucuronide metabolites of the hydroxy-metabolite). 0.4% of the drug is excreted unchanged in urine. Steady state concentrations are achieved within 10 to 15 days. The drug is not known to accumulate.

Therapeutic concentration

After oral administration of 20 mg to 12 healthy subjects, aged between 21 and 52 years, in the fasting state and then following food, mean peak plasma concentrations of 3.0 mg/L and 2.4 mg/L, respectively, were obtained at 1.8 and 5.8 h (R. O. Day *et al.*, *Br. J. Clin. Pharmacol.*, 1987, *24*, 323–328).

6 healthy male volunteers with a mean age of 25.5 years (between 20 and 31 years) were administered with 20 mg tenoxicam after an overnight fast. The mean maximum concentration was 7.66 μmol/L after 1.3 h [C. Benveniste *et al.*, *Eur. J. Clin. Pharmacol.*, 1990, *38*, 547–549].

Half-life. Plasma half-life, 60 to 70 h.

Volume of distribution. 10 to 12 L.

Clearance. Plasma, 0.09 to 0.14 L/h.

Protein binding. In plasma, over 98.5%.

Note. For reviews of tenoxicam see J. P. Gonzalez and P. A. Todd, *Drugs*, 1987, *34*, 289–310 and P. A. Todd and S. P. Clissold, *Drugs*, 1991, *41*, 625–646.
For a review of the pharmacokinetics of tenoxicam see O. G. Nilsen, *Clin. Pharmacokinet.*, 1994, *26*, 16–43.

Dose. Usually 20 mg daily.

Terazosin

Alpha$_1$-adrenoceptor Blocker

Proprietary names. Abbott-45975; Deflox; Flotrin; Heitrin; Hytrin; Hytrinex; Itrin; Magnurol; Sinalfa; Teraprost; Urodie; Uroflow; Vasocard; Vicard.

1-(4-Amino-6,7-dimethoxy-2-quinazolinyl)-4-[(tetrahydro-2-furanyl)-carbonyl]-piperazine

$C_{19}H_{25}N_5O_4$ = 387.4

CAS—63590-64-7

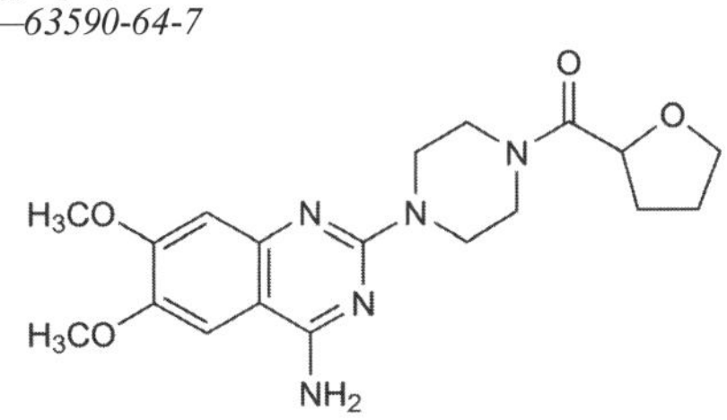

A white, fine crystalline powder with no discernible odour. M. p. 272° to 274°. It is soluble in water (29.7 g/L), methanol (33.7 g/L), ethanol (4.1 g/L), 0.1 M aqueous hydrochloric acid (3.8 g/L), chloroform (1.2 g/L) and acetone (0.01 g/L); freely soluble in isotonic saline; practically insoluble in hexane.

Terazosin Hydrochloride

$C_{19}H_{25}N_5O_4$,HCl = 423.9

CAS—63074-08-8

Hygroscopic crystals with M. p. 278° to 279°. It is soluble in water (761.2 g/L).

Terazosin Hydrochloride Dihydrate

$C_{19}H_{25}N_5O_4$,HCl,$2H_2O$ = 459.9

CAS—70024-40-7

M. p. 271° to 274°. It is soluble in water (24.2 g/L).

Dissociation Constant. pK_a 7.1 (0.1 M sodium hydroxide).

Partition Coefficient. Log *P* (octanol/water), 1.47.

Thin-layer Chromatography. Plate: silica Gel 60 F_{254}. Mobile phase: chloroform:toluene:methanol (9:1:6). Fluorescence detection (λ_{ex} = 257 nm; λ_{em} = 345 nm). Rf 0.60 [Z. L. Chang and J. F. Bauer, *Anal. Profiles Drug Subs. Excip.*, 1991, *20*, 693–727].

High Performance Liquid Chromatography. System HZ—Retention time 2.2 min.

Column: KR100-5-C_{18} (metaphase, 150 × 4 mm i.d., 5 µm); (guard) RP-$_{18}$ (Perisorb, 30 to 40 µm pellicular). Mobile phase: disodium hydrogen phosphate (0.01 M):acetonitrile:tetrahydrofuran (76:22:2) (pH 6.5), flow rate 1 mL/min. Internal standard (IS): prazosin. Fluorescence detection (λ_{ex} = 250 nm; λ_{em} = 370 nm)). Retention times: terazosin, 4.1 min; IS, 8.24 min [P. Y. Cheah *et al.*, *J. Chromatogr. B Biomed. Sci. Appl.*, 2000, *745(2)*, 439–443].

Column: AD (Chiralpak, 100 × 2.1 mm i.d., 10 µm). Mobile phase: hexane:2-propanol containing 0.05% diethylamine (65:35), flow rate 0.15 mL/min. IS: prazosin. Detection: MS–MS (terazosin, *m/z* →388.2; IS, *m/z* →384.2). Retention times: terazosin, 4.8 min; IS, 4.92 min [A. Zavitsanos *et al.*, *J. Chromatogr. A*, 1998, *794*, 46–56].

Column: ODS (250 × 4.6 mm i.d., 5 µm). Mobile phase: methanol: acetonitrile:disodiumhydrogen orthophosphate (0.04 M) (22:22:56), flow rate 1.2 mL/min. IS: prazosin. Fluorescence detection (λ_{ex} = 250 nm; λ_{em} = 370 nm). Retention times: terazosin 3.8 min; IS, 4.9 min [E. Sekhar *et al.*, *J. Chromatogr. B Biomed. Sci. Appl.*, 1998, *710*, 137–142].

Ultraviolet Spectrum. Aqueous solution (water)—212 (A_1^1 = 65.7), 245 (A_1^1 = 127.5), 330 nm (A_1^1 = 24.0); aqueous acid—246, 212, 331 nm; basic—250, 273 nm.

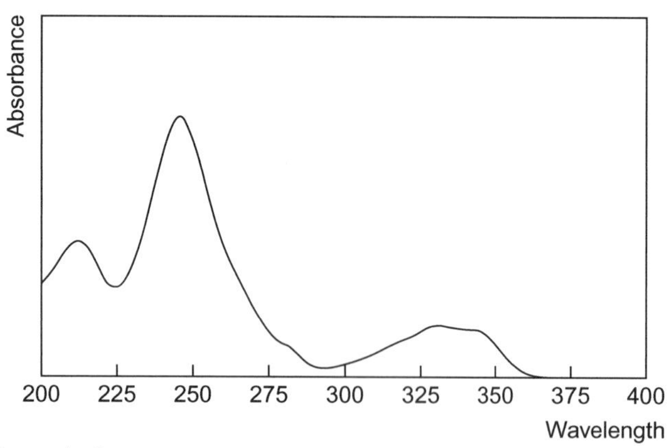

Infra-red Spectrum. Principal peaks at wavenumber 1594, 1437, 1247 cm^{-1} (KBr disk).

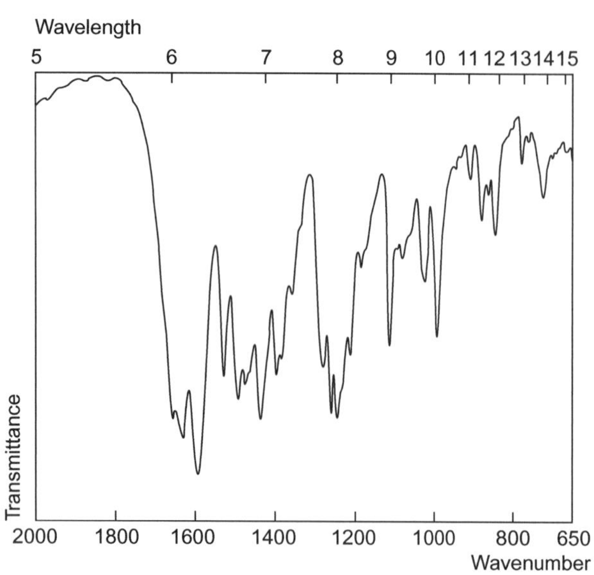

Mass Spectrum. Principal ions at *m/z* 233, 71, 316, 245, 43, 387, 234, 205, 259.

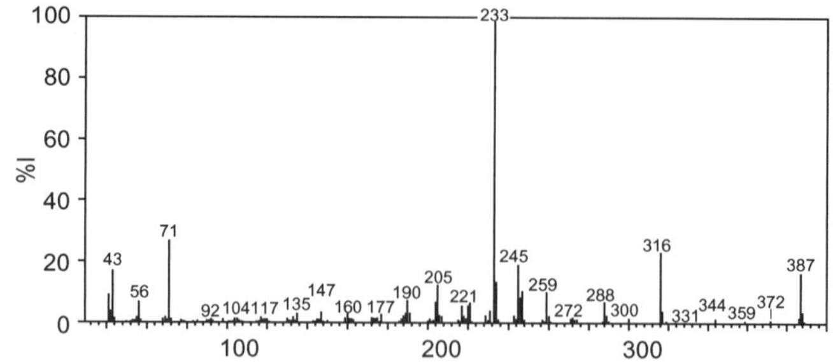

Quantification

High performance liquid chromatography. In plasma: limit of quantification 0.25 µg/L—P. Y. Cheah *et al.*, *J. Chromatogr. B Biomed. Sci. Appl.*, 2000, *745(2)*, 439–443. In blood: limit of quantification 0.0625 µg/L—A. Zavitsanos *et al.*, *J. Chromatogr. A*, 1998, *794*, 46–56. In blood: limit of detection 1 µg/L—E. Sekhar *et al.*, *J. Chromatogr. B Biomed. Sci. Appl.*, 1998, *710*, 137–142.

Disposition in the Body. The onset of action occurs after approximately 15 min and the duration is about 24 h. Terazosin is rapidly and almost completely absorbed from the gastro-intestinal tract after oral administration, and is extensively metabolised in the liver to yield piperazine and three other inactive metabolites. Absorption is not affected by the presence of food. The major route of elimination is via the biliary tract, and the drug is excreted in faeces (60%) and urine (40%). 10% is excreted as the parent drug and the remainder as its metabolites. Renal impairment shows no significant effect on pharmacokinetics. The drug displays linear kinetics after oral and IV doses.

Therapeutic concentration

Young, healthy, male volunteers were administered with 5 mg terazosin and the median peak plasma concentration was 91 µg/L. This was reached after 1 h and decreased to 11 µg/L at around 23.5 h [K. Taguchi *et al.*, *Br. J. Clin. Pharmacol.*, 1998, *45(1)*, 49–55].

Bioavailability. 90 to 94%.

Half-life. 8 to 13 h; increased in the elderly.

Volume of distribution. 15 to 30 L.

Clearance. Plasma, 76.3 to 86.6 mL/min (after an 0.5 to 2.0 mg IV dose); decreased in patients with hypertension, 53 to 57 mL/min.

Protein binding. 90 to 95%.

Dose. The usual dose is 1 to 3 mg daily but up to 20 mg daily may be administered.

Terbutaline

Sympathomimetic

5-[2-[(1,1-Dimethylethyl)amino]-1-hydroxyethyl]-1,3-benzenediol
$C_{12}H_{19}NO_3$=225.3
CAS—23031-25-6

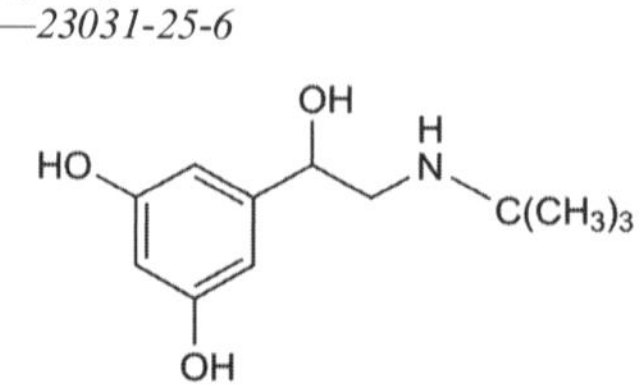

Crystals. M.p. 119° to 122°.

Terbutaline Sulfate

Proprietary names. Aerodur; Arubendol; Asmaline; Asthmoprotect; Ataline; Brethaire; Brethine; Bricalin; Bricanyl; Butaliret; Butalitab; Butylin; Contimit; Dhatalin; Monovent; Taziken; Tedipulmo; Terbasmin; Terbul(in); Terbuturmant; Tolbin; Vacanyl.
$(C_{12}H_{19}NO_3)_2,H_2SO_4$=548.6
CAS—23031-32-5
A white to greyish-white crystalline powder. M.p. 246° to 248°.

Soluble 1 in 4 of water; slightly soluble in ethanol and methanol; practically insoluble in chloroform and ether.

Dissociation Constant. pK_a 8.7, 10.0, 11.0 (20°).

Colour Tests. *p*-Dimethylaminobenzaldehyde—orange/violet; Folin–Ciocalteu reagent—blue; Liebermann's test—black; Mandelin's test—grey-green; Marquis test—yellow; Potassium dichromate (Method 1)—brown (slow).

Thin-layer Chromatography. System TA—Rf 47; system TB—Rf 01; system TC—Rf 01; system TE—Rf 21; system TL—Rf 05; system TAE—Rf 18; system TAF—Rf 77; system TAJ—Rf 00; system TAK—Rf 00; system TAL—Rf 29. (Acidified potassium permanganate solution, strong reaction.)

High Performance Liquid Chromatography. System HA—*k* 0.9; system HAA—Retention time(s) 3.7 min; system HX—RI 225.

Ultraviolet Spectrum. Aqueous acid—276 (A^1_1=85a); aqueous alkali—297 nm (A^1_1=150b).

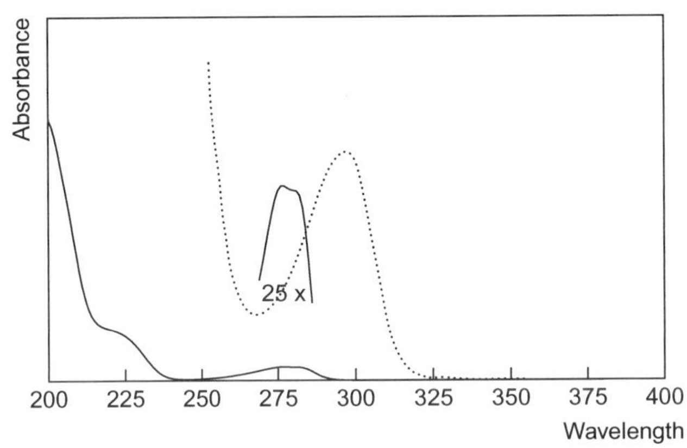

Infra-red Spectrum. Principal peaks at wavenumbers 1210, 1231, 1155, 1069, 1610, 1042 cm^{-1} (terbutaline sulfate, KBr disk).

Mass Spectrum. Principal ions at *m/z* 30, 86, 57, 41, 29, 39, 192, 42.

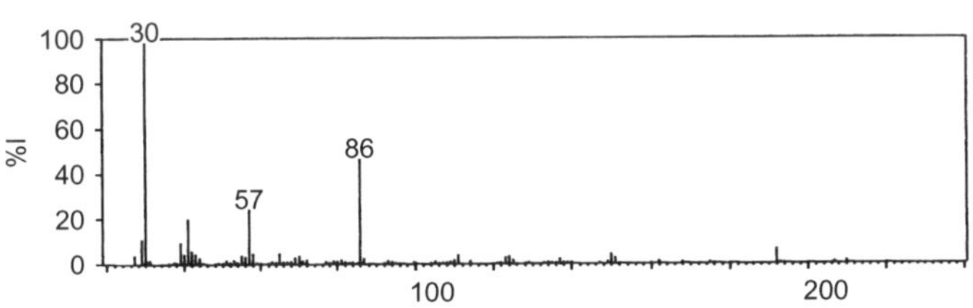

Quantification

Gas chromatography–mass spectrometry. In plasma: unconjugated terbutaline, limit of detection 100 ng/L—S.-E. Jacobsson *et al.*, *Biomed. Mass Spectrom.*, 1980, *7*, 265–268. In plasma or urine: unconjugated and total terbutaline, limit of detection 300 ng/L—R. A. Clare *et al.*, *Biomed. Mass Spectrom.*,1979, *6*, 31–37. In postmortem tissues: unconjugated terbutaline, limit of detection 1.5 ng/g—J. G. Leferink *et al.*, *J. Anal. Toxicol.*, 1978, *2*, 86–88. In postmortem blood or urine: terbutaline and other beta-agonists, SIM—S.B. Black and R.C. Hansson, *J. Anal. Toxicol.*, 1999, *23*, 113–118.

High performance liquid chromatography. In plasma: limit of detection about 1 μg/L, electrochemical detection—S. Bergquist and L.-E. Edholm, *J. Liq. Chromatogr.*, 1983, *6*, 559–574. In plasma: limit of detection 0.8 to 1 μg/L, electrochemical detection—K.A. Sagar *et al.*, *J. Chromatogr.*, 1992, *577*, 109–116; K.A. Sagar *et al.*, *Biomed. Chromatogr.*, 1993, *7*, 29–33; V.L. Herring and J.A. Johnson, *J. Chromatogr. B. Biomed. Appl.*, 2000, *741*, 307–312. In plasma: limit of detection 2.5 μg/L, fluorescence detection—P.T. McCarthy *et al.*, *Biomed. Chromatogr.*, 1993, *7*, 25–28. In plasma: terbutaline enantiomers, limit of detection 1 μg/L, fluorescence detection—K.H. Kim *et al.*, *Arch. Pharm. Res.*, 2000, *23*, 441–445. In urine: terbutaline enantiomers, limit of detection 0.3 μg/L, fluorescence detection—K.H. Kim *et al.*, *J. Chromatogr. B. Biomed. Sci. Appl.*, 2001, *751*, 69–77.

Disposition in the Body. Terbutaline is incompletely absorbed after oral administration. Extensive first-pass metabolism occurs in the liver and gut wall to produce the sulfate conjugate (the main metabolite) but some glucuronic acid conjugation also occurs. Less than 15% of an oral dose is present as free drug in the plasma. It is excreted in the urine as unchanged drug and the inactive conjugates, the concentration of each being dependent upon the route of administration. After oral administration, up to about 50% of a dose is excreted in the urine, predominantly as the sulfate conjugate, with up to 10% as unchanged drug. Up to about 60% of a dose is eliminated in the faeces, mainly in unchanged form. After IV or subcutaneous administration, more than 80% of a dose is excreted in the urine, with up to about 60% as unchanged drug and only about 2 to 3% is eliminated in the faeces.

Therapeutic concentration

After single oral doses of 5 mg to 8 subjects, peak serum concentrations of 0.002 to 0.005 (mean 0.003) mg/L were attained in 2 to 4 h. In 3 subjects there were 2 peaks; the first occurred in 1 to 2 h and the second in 3 to 4 h. After single subcutaneous doses of 0.5 mg to the same subjects, peak serum concentrations of 0.005 to 0.011 (mean 0.007) mg/L were attained in 0.2 to 0.6 h. [J. G. Leferink *et al.*, *Arzneimittelforschung*, 1982, *32*, 159–164].

Toxicity

A female subject took several tablets of terbutaline during a severe night attack of asthma and died the next morning. The following postmortem tissue concentrations were reported: serum 0.014 mg/L, heart 0.036 μg/g, kidney 0.054 μg/g, liver 0.055 μg/g, lung 0.026 μg/g, muscle 0.063 μg/g [J. G. Leferink *et al.*, *J. Anal. Toxicol.*, 1978, *2*, 86–88].

Approximately 6 h after taking 500 mg of terbutaline, a 22-year-old woman presented with a plasma concentration of 0.2 mg/L, about 50 times the normal therapeutic concentration, which fell to therapeutic levels within 36 h. [A. Heath and B.-Å. Hultén, *Hum. Exp. Toxicol.*, 1987, *6*, 525–526].

Half-life. Plasma half-life, about 3 to 4 h.

Volume of distribution. About 1 L/kg.

Clearance. Plasma clearance, about 4 mL/min/kg.

Protein binding. In plasma, about 15 to 25%.

Dose. 10 to 15 mg of terbutaline sulfate daily.

Terbutryne

Herbicide

Synonym. Terbutryn

Proprietary names. Clarosan; Prebane. It is an ingredient of Opogard.

2-*tert*-Butylamino-4-ethylamino-6-methylthio-1,3,5-triazine

$C_{10}H_{19}N_5S$=241.4

CAS—886-50-0

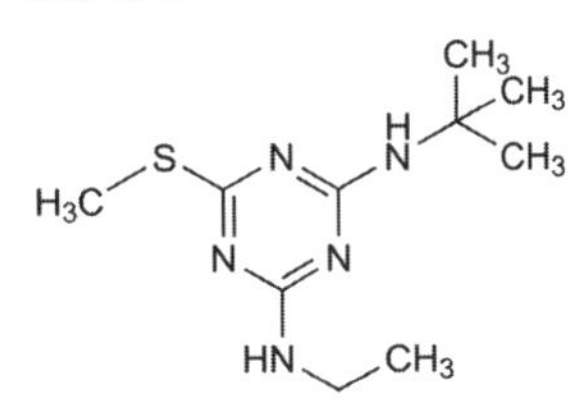

A white crystalline powder. M.p. 104°.

Practically insoluble in water; readily soluble in chloroform, ether and methanol.

Dissociation Constant. pK_a 4.3.

Partition Coefficient. Log *P* (octanol/water), 3.7.

Thin-layer Chromatography. System TA—Rf 77; system TX—Rf 32; system TY—Rf 32; system TAB—Rf 07; system TAC—Rf 12. (Dragendorff spray, positive.)

Gas Chromatography. System GA—RI 1940; system GK—RRT 0.99 (relative to caffeine).

High Performance Liquid Chromatography. System HY—RI 442; system HAO—*k* 12.09; system HAP—*k* 1.68.

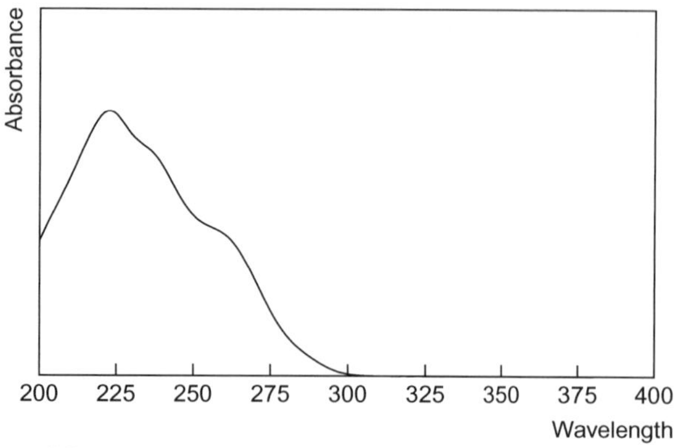

Infra-red Spectrum. Principal peaks at wavenumbers 1520, 1587, 1215, 806, 1266, 1133 cm^{-1} (KBr disk).

Terbutylazine

Herbicide

Synonyms. Diethylterbutylazine; GS-13529; Terbuthylazine.
Proprietary names. Gardoprim; Primatol M; Sorgoprim.
6-Chloro-*N*-(1,1-dimethylethyl)-*N'*-ethyl-1,3,5-triazine-2,4-diamine
$C_9H_{16}ClN_5$=229.7
CAS—5915-41-3

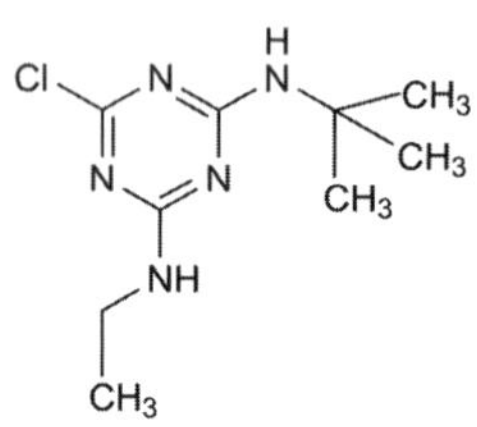

A colourless powder/white solid. M.p. 177° to 179°. It is soluble in water (8.5 mg/L at 20°), dimethylformamide (100 g/L at 20°), ethyl acetate (40 g/L at 20°), isopropanol (10 g/L at 20°), tetralin (10 g/L at 20°), xylene (10 g/L at 20°) and octanol (14.3 g/L at 20°).

Dissociation Constant. pK_a 2.0.

Partition Coefficient. Log *P* (octanol/water), 3.21.

Gas Chromatography. System GA—RI 1805.

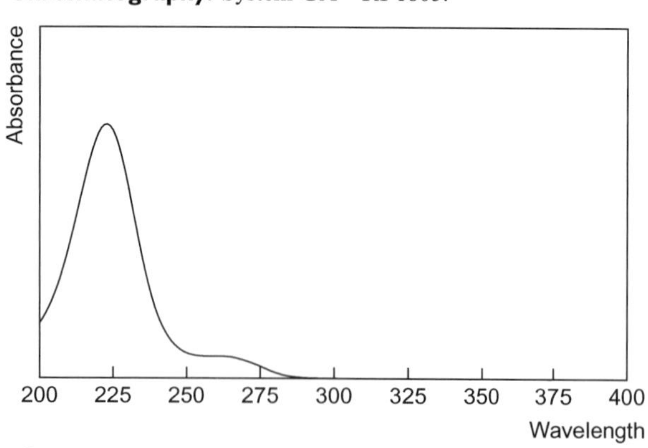

Mass Spectrometry. Principal ions at *m/z* 214, 173, 216, 229, 132, 68, 138, 175.

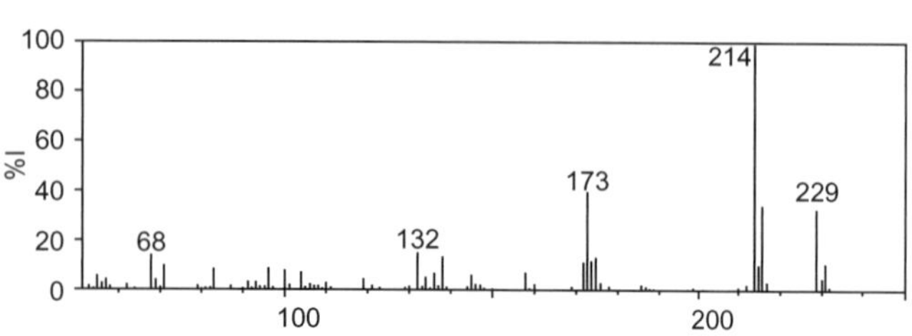

Disposition in the Body. Terbutylazine is excreted in urine and faeces, approximately 85% of a dose within the first 24 h.

Tertatolol

Beta-blocker/Antihypertensive

1-[(3,4-Dihydro-2*H*-1-benzothiopyran-8-yl)oxy]-3-[(1,1-dimethylethyl)-amino]-2-propanol
$C_{16}H_{25}NO_2S$=295.4
CAS—34784-64-0

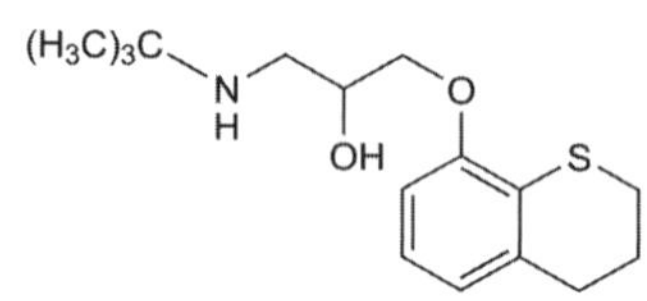

M. p. 180° to 183°

Tertatolol Hydrochloride
Proprietary names. Artex; Artexal; Prenalex.
$C_{16}H_{25}NO_2S,HCl$=331.9
CAS—33580-30-2
White crystals. M.p. 180° to 183°. It is freely soluble in aqueous solution and alcohol, and has high lipid solubility.

Dissociation Constant. pK_a 9.8.

Partition Coefficient. Log *P* (octanol/water), 2.5 (pH 7, 24°).

Thin-layer Chromatography. System TB—Rf 13; system TE—Rf 43; system TF—Rf 1; system TAE—Rf 17.

Gas Chromatography. System GA—RI 2310.

Column: 3% SE-30 on 100-120 mesh Chromosorb W AW DMCS (glass, 2.1 m x 2 mm i.d.). Column temperature: oven, 260°. Carrier gas: helium, flow rate 20 mL/min. MS detection (SIM at *m/z* 368 for tertatolol; 456 for IS). IS: 4-hydroxytertalolol. Retention times: tertatolol, 2.13 min; IS, 2.92 min [C. Efthymiopoulos *et al.*, *J. Chromatogr.*, 1987, *421*, 360–366].

High Performance Liquid Chromatography. System HX—RI 381.

Column: XLODS (Ultrasphere, 70 × 4.6 mm i.d., 3 μm). Mobile phase: acetonitrile:water (40:60), flow rate 2 mL/min. IS: (–)-alprenolol. Fluorescence detection (λ_{ex}=220 nm; λ_{em}=320 nm) Retention times: (–)-tertatolol, 15 min; (+)-tertatolol, 17 min; IS, 12.5 min [T. Lave *et al.*, *J. Chromatogr.*, 1991, *572*, 203–210].

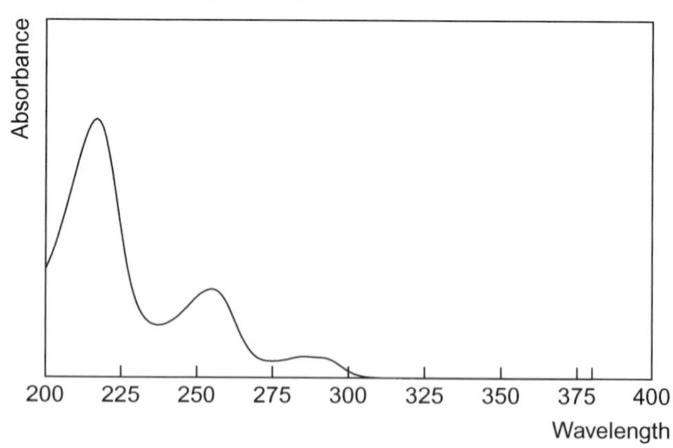

Mass Spectrum. Principal ions at *m/z* 86, 166, 251, 280, 57, 151, 70, 165.

Quantification
Gas chromatography–mass spectrometry. In urine: limit of detection 1 μg/L—C. Efthymiopoulos *et al.*, *J. Chromatogr.*, 1987, *421*, 360–366.

High performance liquid chromatography. In blood and urine: limit of quantification 6 μg/L—T. Lave *et al.*, *J. Chromatogr.*, 1991, *572*, 203–210.

Disposition in the Body. Tertatolol is rapidly and almost completely absorbed, and peak plasma levels are reached within 1 to 2 h after administration. First-pass hepatic metabolism is low and there is limited extravascular distribution. There are linear pharmacokinetics in the dose range of 1 to 10 mg. The three main metabolic routes are sulfoxidation, hydroxylation and conjugation. Inactive metabolites make up 70% of urine excretion. 4-OH-tertatolol is the active metabolite and makes up less than 10% of urine. Repeated dose results in no change in the pharmacokinetics and there is no change in pharmacokinetics in the elderly or renal impaired. Steady state is achieved from first administration without accumulation.

Therapeutic concentration

22 hypertensive patients (12 men and 10 women) with a mean age of 52.6 years and chronic renal failure were used in the study. The patients were orally administered 5 mg tertatolol daily for 4 weeks. The mean peak concentration of the drug was 160 µg/L observed at 1.2 h [M. Rainfray *et al.*, *Am. J. Hypertens.*, 1989, *2*, 266S–277S].

10 patients, with cirrhosis and oesophageal varices, were administered with 2.5 mg tertatolol orally and 1.25 mg intravenously. The mean peak plasma concentration was 70 µg/L at 0.75 h [P. Cales *et al.*, *J. Hepatol.*, 1993, *19(1)*, 43–50].

Toxicity. High therapeutic safety index. LD_{50} is high. 3800 to 13 000 higher than human clinical dose.

Bioavailability. 60% after oral administration.

Half-life. 3 h.

Volume of distribution. 30 to 40 L (0.7 L/kg); increased to 50 L in patients with cirrhosis.

Clearance. Plasma clearance, 130 mL/min; decreased to 49 mL/min in patients with cirrhosis. Systemic clearance, 0.1 L/h.

Protein binding. 95% to mainly α_1-glycoprotein; 85% in patients with cirrhosis.

Dose. 5 mg daily.

Testosterone

Androgen

Proprietary names. Androderm; Androgel; Andropatch; Atmos; Histerone; Hydrotest; Malogen Aqueous; Oreton; Tesamone; Testandro; Testoderm; Testopel; Testotop; Testozzard.
17β-Hydroxyandrost-4-en-3-one
$C_{19}H_{28}O_2$=288.4
CAS—58-22-0

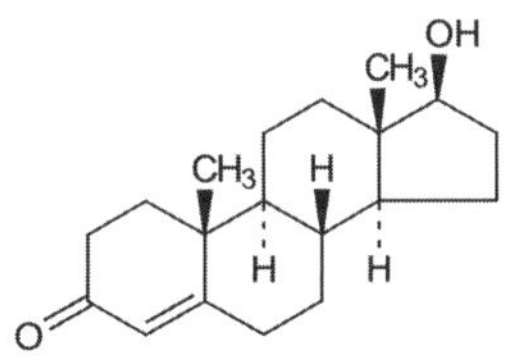

White or creamy-white crystals or crystalline powder. M.p. 152° to 157°.
Practically insoluble in water; soluble 1 in 6 of dehydrated alcohol, 1 in 2 of chloroform and 1 in 100 of ether.

Testosterone Cipionate

Synonyms. Testosterone Cyclopentylpropionate; Testosterone Cypionate.
Proprietary names. Andronate; depAndro; Depotesteron; Duratest; Pertestis; Testex; Testiormina; Virilon.
$C_{27}H_{40}O_3$=412.6
CAS—58-20-8
A white or creamy-white crystalline powder. M.p. 101° to 102°.
Insoluble in water; freely soluble in ethanol, chloroform and ether.

Testosterone Enantate

Synonyms. Testosterone Enanthate; Testosterone Heptanoate; Testosterone Oenanthate.
Proprietary names. Andro; Andropository; Androtardyl; Delatestryl; Durathate Everone; Malogen LA; Malogex; Primoteston-Depot; Testate; Testo-Enant; Testone LA; Testostroval-PA; Testoviron-Depot.
$C_{26}H_{40}O_3$=400.6
CAS—315-37-7
A white or creamy-white crystalline powder. M.p. 36° to 38°.
Practically insoluble in water; soluble 1 in 0.3 of ethanol, chloroform and ether.

Testosterone Isocaproate

Synonym. Testosterone Isohexanoate
Proprietary names. It is an ingredient of Durateston, Estandron P, Mixogen, Sostanon and Sustanon.
$C_{25}H_{38}O_3$=386.6
CAS—15262-86-9
White to creamy-white crystals or crystalline powder. M.p. about 80°.
Practically insoluble in water; very soluble in ethanol and chloroform.

Testosterone Phenylpropionate

Proprietary names. It is an ingredient of Durateston, Estandron P, Mixogen, Sostanon and Sustanon.
$C_{28}H_{36}O_3$=420.6
CAS—1255-49-8
A white crystalline powder. M.p. 114° to 117°.
Practically insoluble in water; soluble 1 in 40 of ethanol.

Testosterone Propionate

Proprietary names. Malogen in Oil; Testoviron; Tesurene; Virormone. It is an ingredient of Durateston, Estandron P, Mixogen, Sostenon and Sustanon.
$C_{22}H_{32}O_3$=344.5
CAS—57-85-2
Colourless or yellowish-white crystals or a white or creamy-white crystalline powder. M.p. 118° to 122°.
Practically insoluble in water; soluble 1 in 6 of ethanol and 1 in 4 of acetone; very soluble in chloroform; freely soluble in ether and in methanol.

Testosterone Undecylate

Synonym. Testosterone Undecanoate
Proprietary names. Andriol; Androxon; Panteston(e); Restandol; Undestor.
$C_{29}H_{48}O_3$=444.7
CAS—5949-44-0

Partiton Coefficient. Log *P* (octanol/water), 3.3.

Colour Tests. Naphthol–Sulfuric Acid—yellow/green, brown dichroism; Sulfuric Acid—no initial colour (green fluorescence under ultraviolet light).

Thin-layer Chromatography. Testosterone: system TB—Rf 14; system TE—Rf 70; system TF—Rf 45; system TP—Rf 60; system TQ—Rf 07; system TR—Rf 90; system TS—Rf 63; system TAE—Rf 85; system TAF—Rf 88; system TAJ—Rf 59; system TAK—Rf 63; system TAL—Rf 92; system TAM—Rf 92. Testosterone phenylpropionate: system TP—Rf 86; system TQ—Rf 28; system TR—Rf 99; system TS—Rf 98. Testosterone propionate: system TP—Rf 78; system TQ—Rf 12; system TR—Rf 99; system TS—Rf 98.

Gas Chromatography. System GA—testosterone RI 2620, testosterone-AC RI 2750, testosterone enol-TMS_2 RI 2690, testosterone propionate RI 2815, testosterone dipropionate RI 3350; system GAG—methyltestosterone RRT 1.05, testosterone acetate RRT 1.21, testosterone propionate RRT 1.43, testosterone isobutyrate RRT 1.54, testosterone cipionate RRT 2.19, testosterone enantate RRT 1.92, testosterone undecylate RRT 2.56, testosterone isocaproate RRT 1.77, testosterone decanoate RRT 2.36 (all relative to testosterone); system GAI—RRT 0.970 (relative to 17α-methyl-5α-androstan-3β,17β-diol); system GAR—testosterone Retention time 12.9 min, methyltestosterone 13.1 min, testosterone acetate 13.5 min, testosterone propionate 14.2 min, testosterone isocaproate 15.9 min, testosterone enantate 16.7 min, testosterone benzoate 18.0 min, testosterone cipionate 18.7 min, testosterone decanoate 19.8 min, testosterone phenylpropionate 20.2 min.

High Performance Liquid Chromatography. System HX—RI 534; system HY—testosterone RI 508, testosterone acetate RI 894; testosterone propionate RI 1003; system HAR—methyltestosterone RRT 1.17, testosterone acetate RRT 1.76, testosterone propionate RRT 2.01, testosterone isobutyrate RRT 2.17, testosterone cipionate. RRT 2.63, testosterone enantate RRT 2.60, testosterone undecanoate RRT 3.18 (all relative to testosterone); system HATa—testosterone propionate RRT 1.31, testosterone phenylpropionate RRT 1.48, testosterone isocaproate RRT 1.62, testosterone enantate RRT 1.80, testosterone cipionate RRT 2.05, testosterone undecenoate RRT 2.53, testosterone decanoate RRT 2.78, testosterone undecylate RRT 3.27 (all relative to testosterone); system HATb—methyltestosterone RRT 1.27, testosterone acetate RRT 2.59, testosterone propionate RRT 4.06 (all relative to testosterone).

Ultraviolet Spectrum. Dehydrated alcohol—240 nm (A^1_1=560a).

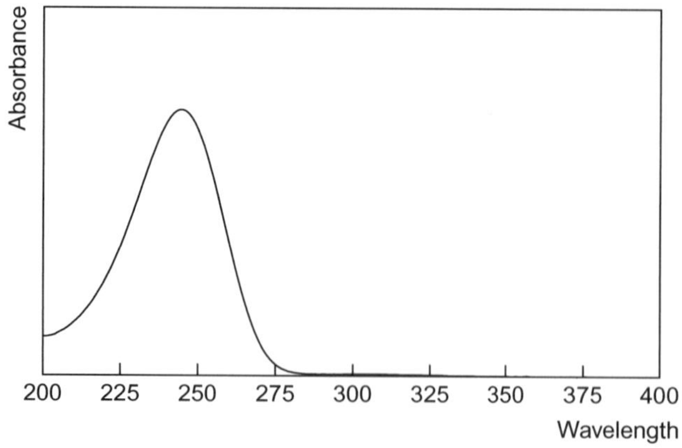

Infra-red Spectrum. Principal peaks at wavenumbers 1660, 871, 1615, 1057, 1236, 1066 cm^{-1} (KBr disk).

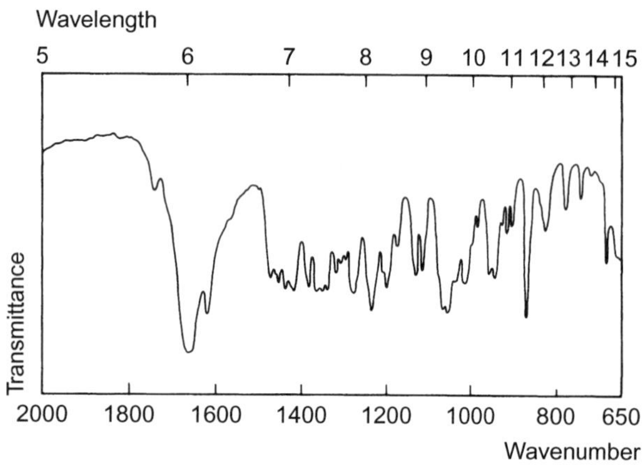

Quantification

Gas chromatography–mass spectrometry. In urine: testosterone and metabolites—M. Becchi *et al.*, *Rapid Commun. Mass Spectrom.*, 1994, *8*, 304–308.

High performance liquid chromatography. In semen: testosterone and other sex hormones—R. Hampl *et al.*, *J. Steroid Biochem. Mol. Biol.*, 2003, *84*, 307–316. In urine: limit of quantification for testosterone 20 μg/L and 30 μg/L for epitestosterone, UV detection (λ=240 nm)—R. Navajas *et al.*, *J. Chromatogr.*, 1995, *673*; *Biomed. Appl.*, 159–164. In serum: testosterone and other sex hormones, limit of detection 250 nmol/L to 7.5 μg/L—Y. Suzuki *et al.*, *J. Chromatogr.*, 1988, *426*, 33-40.

Radioimmunoassay. In hair—M. J. Wheeler *et al.*, *J. Endocrinol.*, 1998, *159*, R5–R8 In plasma or other biological fluids: limit of detection 8 pg—C. S. Corker and D. W. Davidson, *J. Steriod Biochem.*, 1978, *9*, 373–374.

Enzyme immunoassay. In plasma or saliva: limit of detection 4 pg—A. Turkes *et al.*, *Steroids*, 1979, *33*, 347–359.

Note. For a review of methods in urinary testosterone analysis, see E. Venturelli *et al.*, *J. Chromatogr.*, 1995, *671*; *Biomed. Appl.*, 363–380.

Disposition in the Body. Testosterone is the androgenic hormone formed in the testes. In man, it is metabolised to 5α-androstane-3α,17β-diol, androsterone, etiocholanolone and 5α-androstene-3,17-dione. In the horse, the major metabolites are 5α-androstane-3β,17α-diol, which is excreted in the urine as the glucuronide conjugate, and the 17β-epimer which is excreted in the urine as the sulfate conjugate.

Therapeutic concentration

Administration of weekly injections of 25, 50, 125, 300 or 600 mg testosterone enantate to eugonadal males who had received a long-acting gonadotropin-releasing hormone agonist to suppress endogenous testosterone secretion resulted in mean peak concentrations of 25.3, 30.6, 54.2, 134.5 and 237.0 ng/L, respectively [S. Bhasin *et al.*, *Am. J. Physiol. Endocrinol. Metab.* 2001, *281*, E1172–E1181].

In 45 hypogonadal males receiving long-term treatment with 200 mg testosterone enantate or cipionate intramuscularly every 2 weeks, the mean blood testosterone concentration was 31.09 ± 2.00 ng/L (mean bioavailable testosterone was 4.25 ± 0.29 ng/L) [R.R. Hajjar *et al.*, *J. Clin. Endocrinol. Metab.*, 1997, *82*, 3793–3796].

Dose. 10 to 30 mg daily, sublingually; 200 to 600 mg by implantation.

Tetrabenazine

Tranquilliser

Synonym. TBZ
Proprietary names. Nitoman; Xenazine.
1,3,4,6,7,11b-Hexahydro-9,10-dimethoxy-3-(2-methylpropyl)-2*H*-benzo[*a*]quinolizin-2-one
$C_{19}H_{27}NO_3$=317.4
CAS—58-46-8

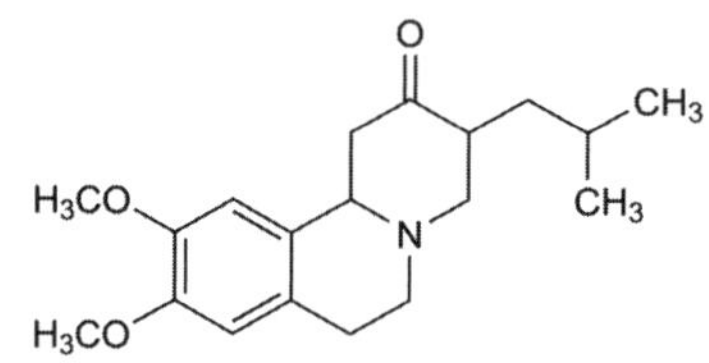

A white crystalline powder. M.p. 125° to 128°.
Soluble in hot water, ethanol and chloroform.

Partition Coefficient. Log *P* (octanol/water) 2.7.

Colour Tests. Liebermann's Test—black; Mandelin's Test—brown; Marquis Test—yellow.

Thin-layer Chromatography. System TA—Rf 69; system TB—Rf 41; system TC—Rf 78; system TE—Rf 79; system TL—Rf 67; system TAE—Rf 80; system TAJ—Rf 83; system TAK—Rf 33; system TAL—Rf 97. (Acidified iodoplatinate solution, positive.)

Gas Chromatography. System GA—tetrabenazine RI 2490; M (*O*-desmethyl-OH-) RI 2500; system GB—tetrabenazine RI 2579; M (*O*-desmethyl-OH-) RI 2638.

High Performance Liquid Chromatography. System HZ—Retention time 4.4 min.

Ultraviolet Spectrum. Aqueous acid—282 nm (A_1^1=108a). No alkaline shift.

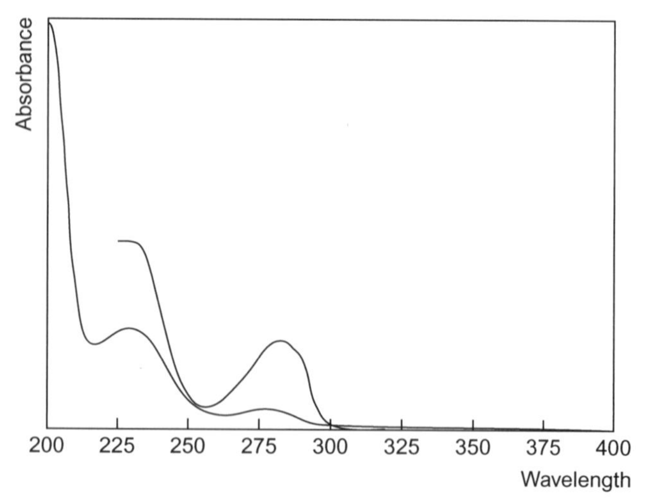

Infra-red Spectrum. Principal peaks at wavenumbers 1694, 1260, 1520, 1155, 1140, 1222 cm^{-1} (KBr disk).

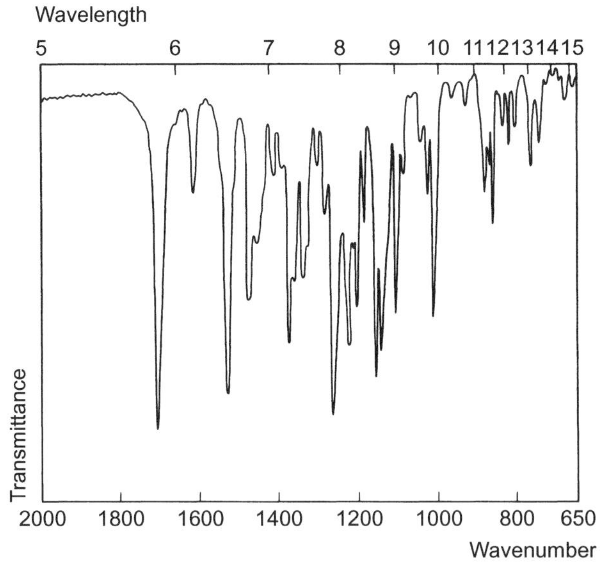

Mass Spectrum. Principal ions at m/z 191, 261, 274, 260, 316, 192, 190, 176.

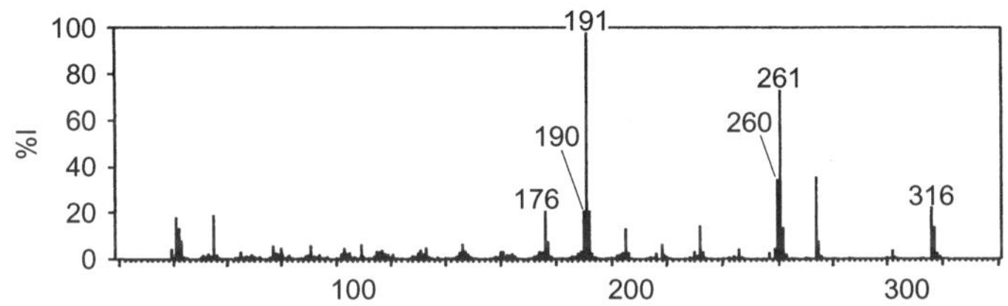

Quantification

High performance liquid chromatography. In plasma: tetrabenazine and 2-hydroxy metabolite, limits of detection 100 to 500 ng/L and 1 to 2 μg/L, respectively, fluorescence detection—M. S. Roberts *et al.*, *J. Chromatogr.*, 1981, *226*; *Biomed. Appl.*, *15*, 175–182; R. Mehvar *et al.*, *J. Pharm. Sci.*, 1986, *75*, 1006–1009.

Disposition in the Body. Absorbed after oral administration. It is extensively metabolised and excreted in the urine as free and conjugated metabolites; nine metabolites have been identified in the urine. 2-Hydroxytetrabenazine is an active metabolite.

Therapeutic concentration

Following a single oral dose of 50 mg to 1 subject, peak plasma concentrations of about 0.015 mg/L of tetrabenazine and 0.085 mg/L of the 2-hydroxy metabolite were attained in 1 and 2 h, respectively [M. S. Roberts *et al.*, *J. Chromatogr.*, 1981, *226*; *Biomed Appl.*, *15*, 175–182].

Dose. 75 to 200 mg daily.

Tetracaine

Local Anaesthetic

Synonym. Amethocaine

Proprietary names. Ametop; Anestesico; Pontocaine. It is an ingredient of Stypto-Caine.

4-(Butylamino)benzoic acid 2-(dimethylamino)ethyl ester

$C_{15}H_{24}N_2O_2$=264.4

CAS—94-24-6

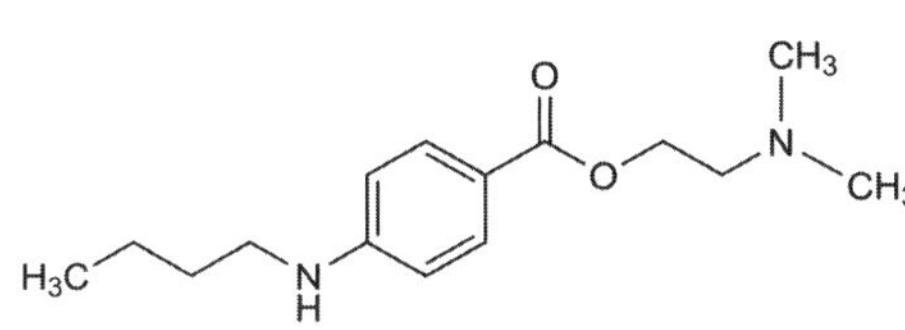

A white or light yellow, waxy solid. M.p. 41° to 46°.

Very slightly soluble in water; soluble 1 in 5 of ethanol, 1 in 2 of chloroform, and 1 in 2 of ether.

Tetracaine Hydrochloride

Synonyms. Butethanol; Dicainum.

Proprietary names. Ametop; Anestesico; Anethaine; Cepacol Viractin; Covostet; Hemonet; Pontocaine. It is an ingredient of Anestesiol; Anevrase; Cetacaine; Dynexan; Eludril (spray); Herviros; Hexomedine; Neocones; Osmogenol.

$C_{15}H_{24}N_2O_2$,HCl=300.8

CAS—136-47-0

A white, hygroscopic, crystalline powder. It melts at about 148° or may occur in either of two polymorphic modifications which melt at about 134° and 139°. Mixtures of the forms may melt within the range 134° to 147°.

Soluble 1 in 7.5 of water, 1 in 40 of ethanol, and 1 in 30 of chloroform; practically insoluble in acetone, benzene, and ether.

Dissociation Constant. pK_a 8.2.

Partition Coefficient. Log *P* (octanol/water), 3.5.

Colour Tests. Aromaticity (Method 2)—yellow/red; Liebermann's Test (100°)—blue.

Thin-layer Chromatography. System TA—Rf 57; system TB—Rf 15; system TC—Rf 32; system TE—Rf 64; system TL—Rf 16; system TAE—Rf 43; system TAF—Rf 39; system TAJ—Rf 12; system TAK—Rf 00; system TAL—Rf 25. (Dragendorff spray, positive; acidified iodoplatinate solution, positive.)

Gas Chromatography. System GA—tetracaine RI 2220, 4-aminobenzoic acid RI 1547; system GF—RI 2715; system GQ—retention time 8.0 min.

Column: HP-1 100% dimethylpolysiloxane (12 m × 0.2 mm i.d., 0.33 μm film thickness). Column temperature: 100° held for 2 min, ramp to 300° at 20°/min, held for 1 min. Injector temperature: 280°. Carrier gas: helium, flow rate 1 mL/min. Detection: MS (SIM). Retention time 8.7 min. [K. Kudo *et al.*, *Forensic Sci. Int.*, 2001, *116*, 9–14.]

Column: methylsilicone fused-silica wide-bore DB-1 (15 m × 0.53 mm i.d., 1.0 μm film thickness). Column temperature: 60° to 220° at 8°/min. Injector temperature: 250°. Carrier gas: helium, 15 mL/min. Detection: nitrogen-phosphorus. [M. Terada *et al.*, *J. Anal. Toxicol.*, 1996, *20(5)*, 318–322.]

High Performance Liquid Chromatography. System HA—*k* 2.0; system HQ—*k* 16.25; system HR—*k* 1.33; system HX—RI 389; system HY—RI 321; system HZ—retention time 4.4 min; system HAX—retention time 10.8 min; system HAY—retention time 5.4 min.

Column: C_{18} (μBondapak, 300 × 4 mm i.d., 10 μm). Mobile phase: water: acetonitrile:methanol (60:20:20) containing 0.06% sulfuric acid, 0.5% sodium sulfate, 0.02% sodium heptane sulfonate, pH 2.6. Flow rate, 2 mL/min. UV detection (λ=305 nm). Retention time 6.0 min. [G. N. Menon and B.J. Norris, *J. Pharm. Sci.*, 1981, *70(5)*, 569–570.]

Ultraviolet Spectrum. Aqueous acid—229 (A_1^1=561a), 281, 312 aqueous alkali—227, 303 nm.

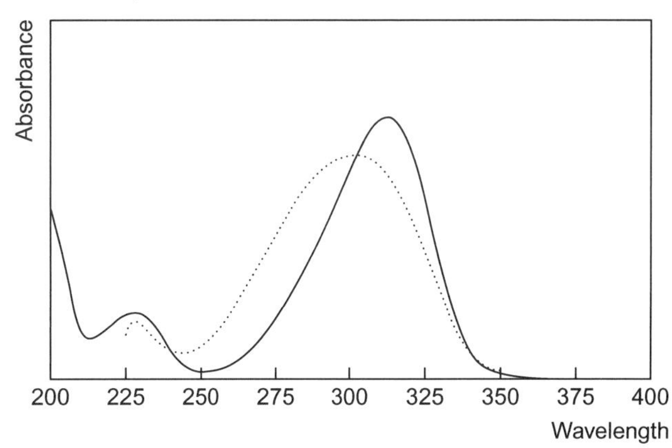

Infra-red Spectrum. Principal peaks at wavenumbers 1600, 1286, 1174, 1688, 1126, 1532 cm^{-1} (tetracaine hydrochloride, KBr disk).

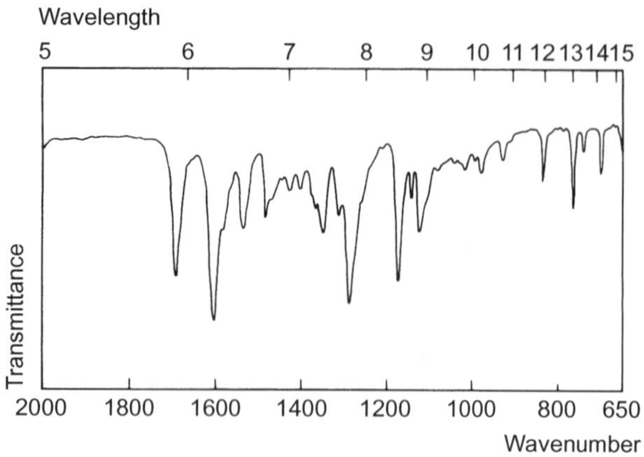

Mass Spectrum. Principal ions at *m/z* 58, 71, 150, 176, 72, 193, 105, 59 (no peaks above 200); 4-aminobenzoic acid 137, 120, 92, 65, 39, 138, 121, 63.

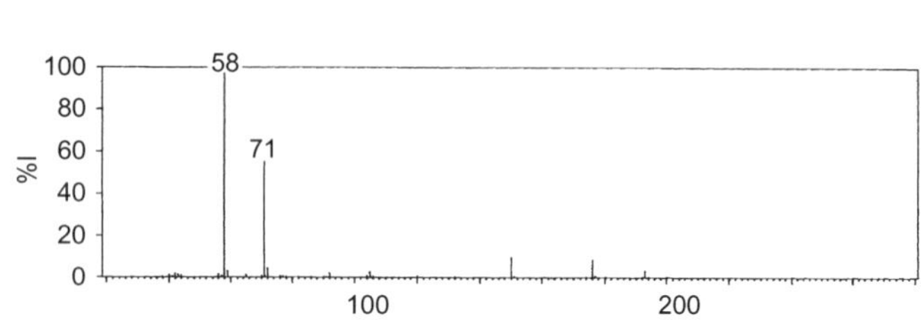

Quantification

High performance liquid chromatography. Limit of detection: tetracaine, 0.4 g/L; *p-n*-butylaminobenzoic acid, 0.003 g/L—G. N. Menon and B.J. Norris, *J. Pharm. Sci.*, 1981, *70(5)*, 569–570. In plasma: tetracaine and *p-n*-butylaminobenzoic acid—B. Mazumdar *et al.*, *Br. J. Anaesth.*, 1991, *67*, 432–436. In plasma: tetracaine, *p*-butylaminobenzoic acid, and mepivacaine, limit of detection for tetracaine and *p*-butylaminobenzoic acid 50 μg/L, multiwavelength detection—R. Murtaza *et al.*, *J. Pharmacol. Toxicol. Methods*, 2001, *46*, 131–136.

Gas chromatography. In biological samples: tetracaine and other local anaesthetics, nitrogen sensitive detection—O. W. Lau *et al.*, *Methods Find. Exp. Clin. Pharmacol.*, 1991, *13*, 475–481. In serum: tetracaine and other local anaesthetics, limit of quantification, 24 μg/L, NPD—M. Terada *et al.*, *J. Anal. Toxicol.*, 1996, *20*, 318–322.

Gas chromatography–mass spectrometry. In plasma and urine: limit of quantification 100 μg/L and limit of detection 80 μg/L (SIM, *m/z* 58)—T. Ohshima and T. Takayasu, *J. Chromatogr. B Biomed. Sci. Appl.*, 1999, *726(1–2)*, 185–194. In whole blood and tissues: tetracaine and 4-butylaminobenzoic acid, limits of detection 10 ng/g and 0.6 ng/g respectively—Y. Hino *et al.*, *J. Anal. Toxicol.*, 2000, *24*, 165–169. In blood: tetracaine and its metabolites—K. Kudo *et al.*, *Forensic Sci. Int.*, 2001, *116*, 9–14.

Disposition in the Body. Tetracaine is rapidly hydrolysed in the blood to 4-aminobenzoic acid by plasma pseudocholinesterase; it is completely metabolised within 1 h of injection. It can rarely be isolated from blood even within a few minutes of administration. Metabolites are excreted mainly by kidneys. The maximum amount that may be safely administered by injection is probably 50 mg.

Therapeutic concentration

Following intraspinal administation of 8 to 14 mg of tetracaine to 10 patients, no trace of tetracaine was revealed in the blood, but mean concentrations of the metabolite, 4-aminobenzoic acid, at 1, 2, and 6 h after injection were 126.5, 97.9, and 43.3 μg/L respectively. [K. Kudo *et al.*, *Forensic Sci. Int.*, 2001, *116*, 9–14.]

Dose. 5 to 20 mg of tetracaine hydrochloride (0.5% solution) is injected for spinal anaesthesia; 0.5 to 2% solutions have been used for surface anaesthesia.

Tetrachloroethane

Solvent

Synonym. Acetylene Tetrachloride
1,1,2,2-Tetrachloroethane
$C_2H_2Cl_4$=167.8
CAS—79-34-5

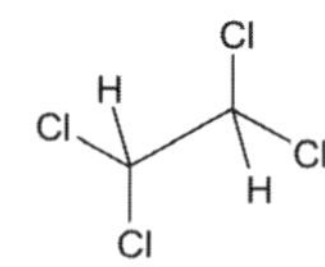

A clear, colourless, heavy, non-flammable, mobile liquid. Wt per mL 1.590 to 1.595 g. M.p. -44°. B.p. 146°. Refractive index, at 25°, 1.4918.
Soluble 1 in 350 of water; miscible with ethanol, chloroform and ether.

Partition Coefficient. Log *P* (octanol/water), 2.4.

Gas Chromatography. System GA—RI 910; system GI—Retention time(s) 24.9 min.

Disposition in the Body. Tetrachloroethane is absorbed from the gastro-intestinal tract, lungs, and through the skin.

Toxicity. Tetrachloroethane is probably the most toxic of the chlorinated hydrocarbons. The estimated lethal dose is 3 mL.

Tetrachloroethylene

Anthelmintic/Solvent

Synonyms. Ethylene Tetrachloride; Perchloroethylene; Tetrachloroethene.
Proprietary names. Ankilostin; Didakene; Nema; Perclene; Tetracap; Tetropil.
C_2Cl_4=165.8
CAS—127-18-4

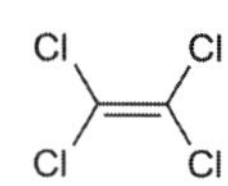

A colourless, heavy, non-flammable, mobile liquid. Wt per mL 1.620 to 1.626 g. M.p.– 22°. B.p. 121°.
Tetrachloroethylene (*B.P.*) contains thymol 0.01% as a preservative.
Practically insoluble in water; soluble in ethanol; miscible with chloroform and ether.

Partition Coefficient. Log *P* (octanol/water), 3.4.

Colour Test. Tetrachloroethylene may be distinguished from carbon tetrachloride and chloroform by the following test: to 5 mL in a stoppered cylinder add 5 mL of bromine solution and shake vigorously at intervals of 15 min for 1 h—bromine colour fades and there is a white turbidity in the lower layer.

Gas Chromatography. System GA—RI 789; system GI—Retention time(s) 24.3 min.

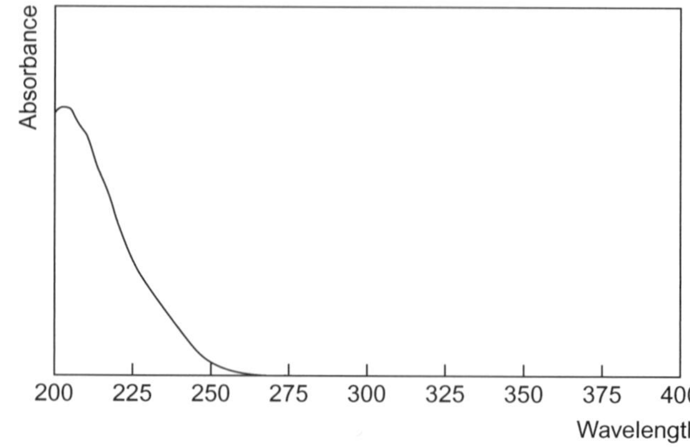

Mass Spectrum. Principal ions at m/z 166, 164, 129, 131, 168, 94, 133, 96.

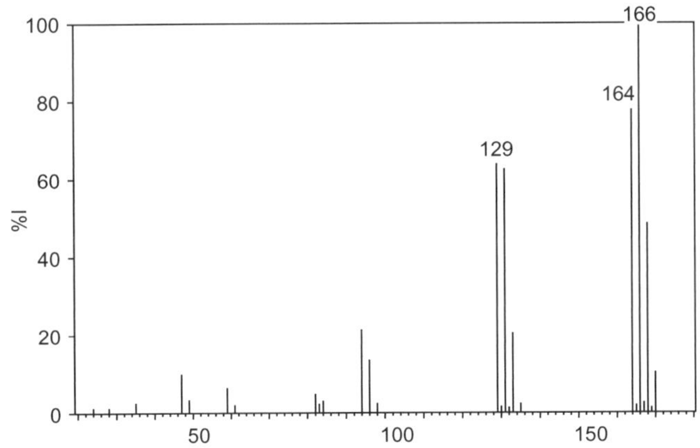

Quantification

Gas chromatography. In blood or tissues: ECD—B. Levine *et al., J. Forens. Sci.*, 1981, *26*, 206–209. In urine: tetrachloroethylene and other solvents, FID—S. Ghittori *et al., G. Ital. Med. Lav.*, 1987, *9*, 21–24.

Gas chromatography–mass spectrometry. In blood or tissues—T. Lukaszewski, *Clin. Toxicol.*, 1979, *15*, 411–415.

Disposition in the Body. Tetrachloroethylene is slightly absorbed from the gastro-intestinal tract and through the skin; it is well absorbed from the lungs. It has an affinity for lipid-rich tissues from which it is slowly released. About 25% of an inhaled dose is excreted unchanged in expired air in 40 h and this is thought to be the major route of excretion; small amounts are eliminated through the skin. Less than about 3% of a dose is metabolised and excreted in the urine, partly as trichloroacetic acid, in 3 days.

Toxicity. The maximum permissible atmospheric concentration is 100 ppm. Exposure to air concentrations of more than 1000 ppm may cause unconsciousness within a short time.

A 53-year-old man was found dead after exposure to tetrachloroethylene vapour. The following postmortem concentrations were reported: blood 4.5 mg/L, brain 69 μg/g, kidney 71 μg/g, liver 240 μg/g, and lung 30 μg/g. [B. Levine *et al., J. Forensic Sci.*, 1981, *26*, 206–209].

In a case of fatal exposure to tetrachloroethylene vapour, a 33-year-old man had the following postmortem concentrations: blood 44 mg/L, brain 360 μg/g, and lung 3 μg/g. [T. Lukaszewski, *Clin. Toxicol.*, 1979, *15*, 411–415].

Postmortem tissue concentrations in a 2-year-old child accidentally fatally exposed to tetrachloroethylene vapour were as follows: blood 66 mg/L, urine 0.3 mg/L (also expressed as 1.7 mg/L of trichloroethanol and 0.9 mg/L of trichloroacetic acid, to which trichloroethylene is metabolised), brain 79.9 μg/g, lungs 46 μg/g. [Y. Gaillard *et al., Forensic Sci. Int.*, 1995, *76*, 161–168].

Half-life. About 72 h.

Dose. Usually 0.1 mL/kg, to a maximum of 5 mL, as a single dose.

Tetracycline

Antibiotic

Proprietary names. Tetracycline and Tetracycline Hydrochloride are ingredients of many proprietary preparations—see Martindale, *The Complete Drug Reference*, 33rd Edn, London, Pharmaceutical Press, 2002.

A hydrated form of [4*S*-(4α,4aα,5aα,6β,12aα)]-4-(dimethylamino)-1,4,4a,5,5a,6,11,12a-octahydro-3,6,10,12,12a-pentahydroxy-6-methyl-1,11-dioxo-2-naphthacenecarboxamide

$C_{22}H_{24}N_2O_8$=444.4

CAS—60-54-8 (anhydrous); 6416-04-2 (trihydrate)

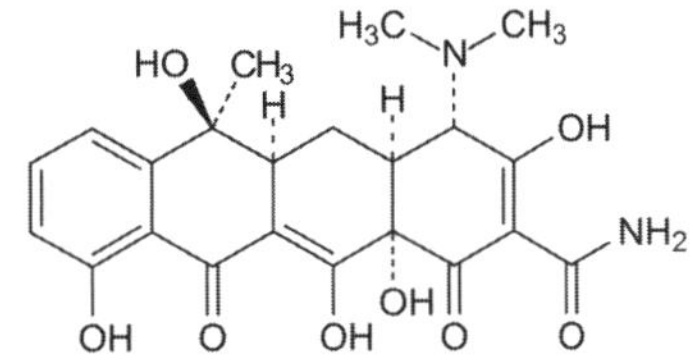

A yellow, crystalline, amphoteric powder which darkens in moist air on exposure to strong sunlight.

Soluble 1 in 2500 of water and 1 in 50 of ethanol; practically insoluble in chloroform and ether; freely soluble in dilute acids and, with decomposition, in solutions of alkali hydroxides.

Tetracycline Hydrochloride

$C_{22}H_{24}N_2O_8$,HCl=480.9

CAS—64-75-5

A yellow, hygroscopic, crystalline, amphoteric powder which darkens in moist air on exposure to strong sunlight. M.p. about 214°, with decomposition.

Soluble 1 in 10 of water and 1 in 100 of ethanol; practically insoluble in chloroform and ether; soluble in methanol and in aqueous solutions of alkali hydroxides and carbonates. Solutions in water become turbid on standing owing to hydrolysis and precipitation of tetracycline.

Dissociation Constant. pK_a 3.3, 7.7, 9.7 (25°).

Partition Coefficient. Log *P* (octanol/pH 7.4) 1.4.

Colour Tests. Benedict's Reagent—red; Formaldehyde–Sulfuric Acid—green-yellow→yellow-brown; Liebermann's Test—black; Mandelin's Test—violet→red→orange; Marquis Test—orange; Sulfuric Acid—violet.

Thin-layer Chromatography. System TA—Rf 05, streaking; system TB—Rf 00; system TAE—Rf 88. (Location under ultraviolet light, orange fluorescence; acidified potassium permanganate solution, positive.)

Gas Chromatography. System GA—RI 1950.

High Performance Liquid Chromatography. System HX—RI 314; system HY—RI 265; system HAA—Retention time 9.9 min.

Ultraviolet Spectrum. Aqueous acid—270 nm (A_1^1=417a), 356 nm.

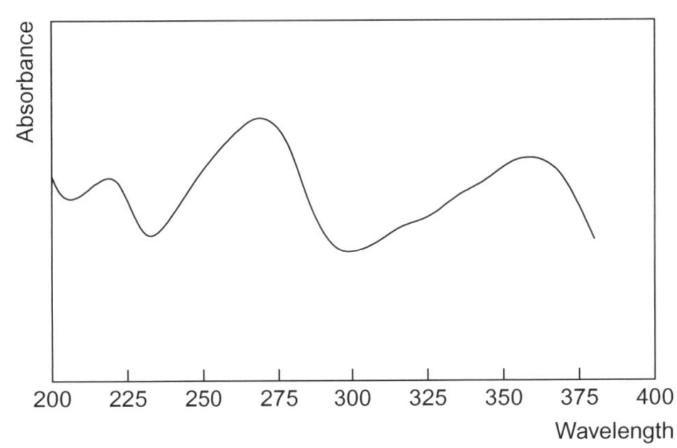

Infra-red Spectrum. Principal peaks at wavenumbers 1612, 1580, 1660, 1226, 1248, 1530 cm^{-1} (tetracycline hydrochloride, KCl disk) (see below).

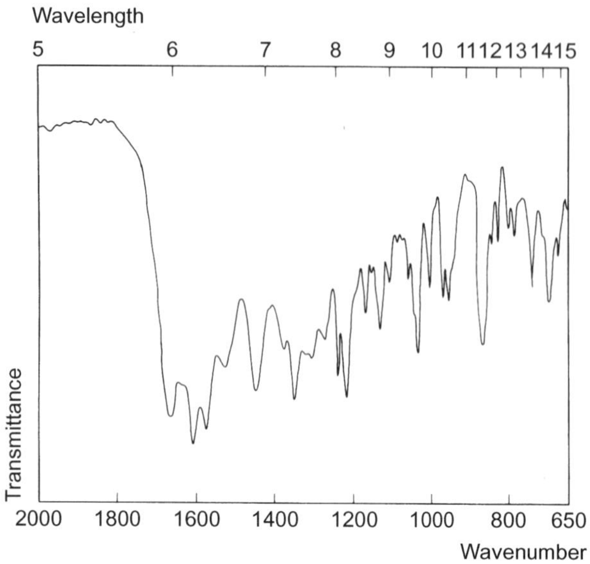

Quantification

High performance liquid chromatography. In plasma or urine: limit of detection 100 µg/L, UV detection—J. Hermansson, *J. Chromatogr.*, 1982, *232*; *Biomed. Appl.*, *21*, 385–393.

Radioimmunoassay. In plasma or urine: limit of detection about 20 µg/L—B. A. Faraj and F. M. Ali, *J. Pharmacol. Exp. Ther.*, 1981, *217*, 10–14.

Disposition in the Body. Irregularly and incompletely absorbed after oral administration; widely distributed throughout the body. Up to about 60% of an intravenous dose and 20 to 50% of an oral dose is excreted in the urine unchanged in 48 h. Excreted in the bile and undergoes some enterohepatic circulation.

Therapeutic concentration. In plasma, usually in the range 1 to 5 mg/L.

6 patients with symptomatic pleural effusions and 1 patient with recurrent pneumothorax were administered 150 mg lidocaine, immediately followed by 20 mg/kg tetracycline instilled in the pleural space through a chest tube. Mean peak plasma concentrations for lidocaine and tetracaine were 1.3 mg/L and 3.6 mg/L, respectively, and these were reached after 86 and 96 min, respectively [S. A. Wooten *et al.*, *Chest*, 1988, *94*, 960–963].

Half-life. Plasma half-life, about 9 h.

Volume of distribution. About 1.3 L/kg.

Clearance. Plasma clearance, about 2 mL/min/kg.

Distribution in blood. Plasma:whole blood ratio, about 0.97.

Protein binding. In plasma, 25 to 65%.

Dose. 1 to 2 g daily.

Tetramisole

Anthelmintic (Veterinary)

2,3,5,6-Tetrahydro-6-phenylimidazo[2,1-*b*]thiazole
$C_{11}H_{12}N_2S$=204.3
CAS—5036-02-2

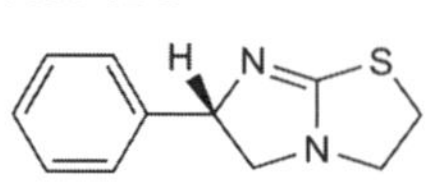

Crystals. M.p. 87° to 89°.
Practically insoluble in water; soluble in chloroform.

Tetramisole Hydrochloride

Proprietary names. Ascarotrat; Ascaverm; Cofasol; Tetramizotil.
$C_{11}H_{12}N_2S$,HCl=240.8
CAS—5086-74-8
A white to pale cream-coloured crystalline powder. M.p. 264° to 265°.

Soluble 1 in 5 of water, 1 in 50 of ethanol, 1 in 3000 of chloroform and 1 in 10 of methanol; very slightly soluble in ether.
For analytical data see also under Levamisole.

Thin-layer Chromatography. System TA—Rf 69; system TB—Rf 18; system TC—Rf 54; system TE—Rf 66; system TL—Rf 46; system TAE—Rf 51; system TAF—Rf 53; system TAJ—Rf 09; system TAK—Rf 00; system TAL—Rf 06.

High Performance Liquid Chromatography. System HX—RI 261; system HY—RI 222; system HAA—retention time 7.0 min.

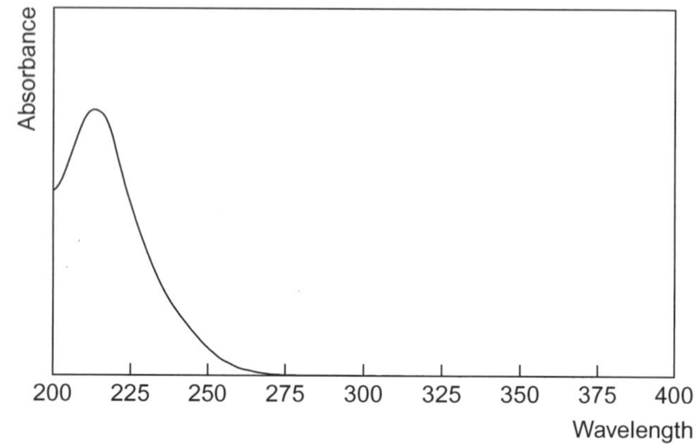

Note. For a review of the pharmacokinetics of anthelmintic drugs, see G. Edwards and A. M. Breckenridge, *Clin. Pharmacokinet.*, 1988, *15*, 67–93.

Dose. 2.5 to 5 mg/kg of tetramisole hydrochloride as a single dose.

Tetrazepam

Muscle Relaxant/Tranquilliser

Proprietary names. Megavix; Miolastan; Mobiforton; Musapam; Musaril; Muskelat; Myolastan; Myospasmal; Panos; Rilex; Tepam; Tethexal; Tetra-saar; Tetramdura; Tetrazep.
7-Chloro-5-(1-cyclohexen-1-yl)-1,3-dihydro-1-methyl-2*H*-1,4-benzodiazepin-2-one
$C_{16}H_{17}ClN_2O$=288.8
CAS—10379-14-3

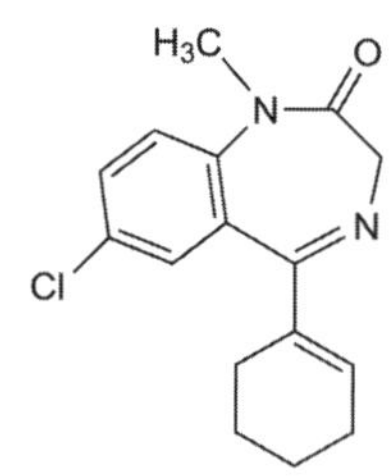

Yellow-brown crystals. M.p. 144°.

Partition Coefficient. Log *P* (octanol/water), 3.2.

Colour Test. Formaldehyde–sulfuric acid—orange.

Thin-layer Chromatography. System TA—tetrazepam Rf 78; M (nor-) Rf 77; system TAD—tetrazepam Rf 67; M (nor-) Rf 56; system TAE—tetrazepam Rf 84; M (nor-) Rf 85; system TAF—tetrazepam Rf 89; M (nor-) Rf 92; system TL—tetrazepam Rf 66; M (nor-) Rf 60; system TB—tetrazepam Rf 32; M (nor-) Rf 5; system TC—tetrazepam Rf 69; M (nor-) Rf 58; system TD—tetrazepam Rf 57; M (nor-) Rf 35; system TE—tetrazepam Rf 79; M (nor-) Rf 73; system TF—tetrazepam Rf 49; M (nor-) Rf 45.

Gas Chromatography. System GA—tetrazepam RI 2430; M (nor-) RI 2530; M (OH-) isomer 1 RI 2570; M (OH-) isomer 2 RI 2580; M (oxo-) RI 2430. (Tetrazepam does not form a TMS derivative.)

High Performance Liquid Chromatography. System HX—RI 511; system HY—RI 483; system HAA—Retention time(s) 22.4 min.

Ultraviolet Spectrum. Aqueous acid—239 (A^1_1=940b), 284, 345; aqueous alkali—305 nm (A^1_1=84b).

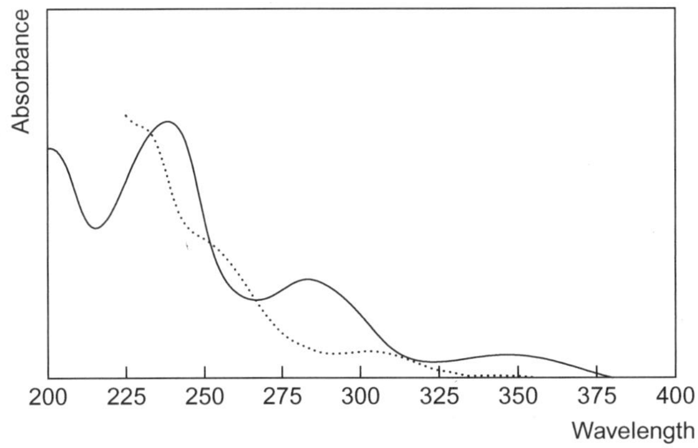

Infra-red Spectrum. Principal peaks at wavenumbers 1678, 1602, 825, 1132, 1310, 800 cm^{-1} (KBr disk).

Mass Spectrum. Principal ions at *m/z* 253, 288, 287, 289, 225, 259, 254, 41.

Quantification

High performance liquid chromatography. In serum: limit of detection 100 ng/L for tetrazepam and 500 ng/L for desmethyltetrazepam, UV detection—M. G. Baumgärtner *et al.*, *Arzneimittelforschung*, 1984, *34*, 724–729.

Disposition in the Body. Tetrazepam is rapidly absorbed after oral administration. It is extensively metabolised by *N*-demethylation and hydroxylation. Urinary metabolites include 3-hydroxytetrazepam, 3-hydroxydesmethyltetrazepam, 3′-hydroxytetrazepam and 3′-hydroxydesmethyltetrazepam.

Therapeutic concentration

Following a single oral dose of 50 mg to 12 subjects, peak serum concentrations of 0.49 to 0.63 (mean 0.57) mg/L of tetrazepam and 0.005 to 0.008 mg/L of desmethyltetrazepam were attained in about 2 h and 4 h, respectively. [M. G. Baumgärtner *et al.*, *Arzneimittelforschung*, 1984, *34*, 724–729].

Half-life. Plasma half-life, 10 to 25 (mean 15) h.

Dose. 25 to 150 mg daily.

Tetryzoline

Sympathomimetic

Synonym. Tetrahydrozoline

4,5-Dihydro-2-(1,2,3,4-tetrahydro-1-naphthalenyl)-1*H*-imidazole

$C_{13}H_{16}N_2$=200.3

CAS—84-22-0

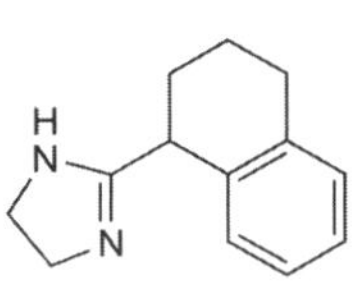

A white crystalline powder.

Soluble in water and chloroform.

Tetryzoline Hydrochloride

Proprietary names. Azoline; Caltheon; Constrilia; Demetil; Diabenyl T; Edolzine; Exrhinin; Mallazine; Octilia; Ophtalmin N; Optazine Fresh; Optizoline; Rhinopront; Stilla; Tetrasine; Tetrilin; Tyzine; Vasopos N; Visine; Vispring; V-Zoline; Yxin.

$C_{13}H_{16}N_2$,HCl=236.7

CAS—522-48-5

A white crystalline powder. M.p. about 256° to 257°, with decomposition. Soluble 1 in 3.5 of water and 1 in 7.5 of ethanol; very slightly soluble in chloroform; practically insoluble in ether.

Partition Coefficient. Log *P* (octanol/water) 3.7.

Colour Tests. Aromaticity (Method 2)—colourless/yellow; Liebermann's Test—brown-orange.

Thin-layer Chromatography. System TA—Rf 13; system TB—Rf 07; system TC—Rf 02; system TE—Rf 26; system TL—Rf 02; system TAE—Rf 05; system TAF—Rf 60. (Acidified iodoplatinate solution, positive.)

Gas Chromatography. System GA—RI 1833.

Ultraviolet Spectrum. Aqueous acid—265 nm (A^1_1=21a), 272 nm. No alkaline shift.

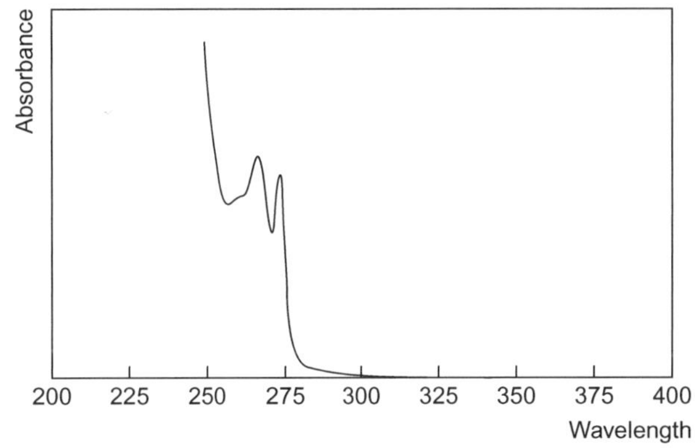

Infra-red Spectrum. Principal peaks at wavenumbers 1600, 742, 1293, 1250, 763, 1500 cm^{-1} (tetryzoline hydrochloride, KBr disk).

Mass Spectrum. Principal ions at *m/z* 200, 185, 199, 171, 44, 84, 71, 131.

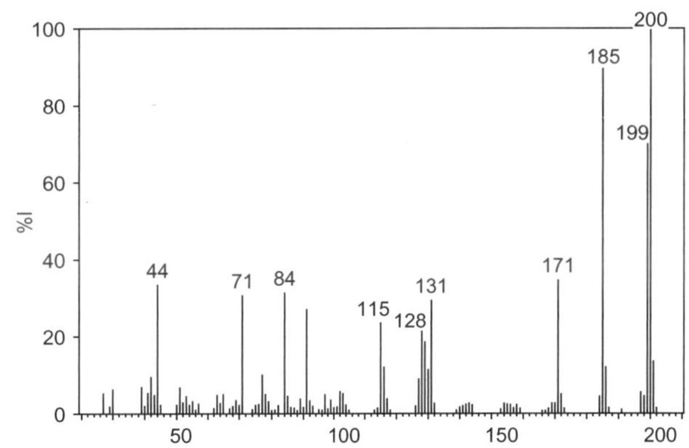

Use. Tetryzoline hydrochloride is used as a 0.1% nasal solution.

Thalidomide

Hypnotic/Immunosuppressant

Proprietary name. Thalomid

2-(2,6-Dioxo-3-piperidinyl)-1*H*-isoindole-1,3(2*H*)-dione

$C_{13}H_{10}N_2O_4$=258.2

CAS—50-35-1

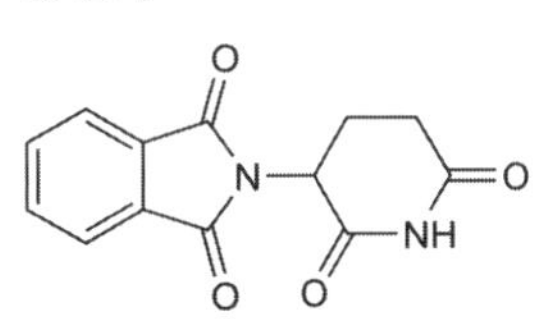

A white crystalline powder. M.p. 269° to 271°.

Sparingly soluble in water, methanol, ethanol and acetone; practically insoluble in chloroform, ether and benzene; very soluble in dimethylformamide, dioxan and pyridine.

Partition Coefficient. Log *P* (octanol/water), 0.3.

Ultraviolet Spectrum. Aqueous acid—240 (A^1_1=385b), 300 nm (A^1_1=94b).

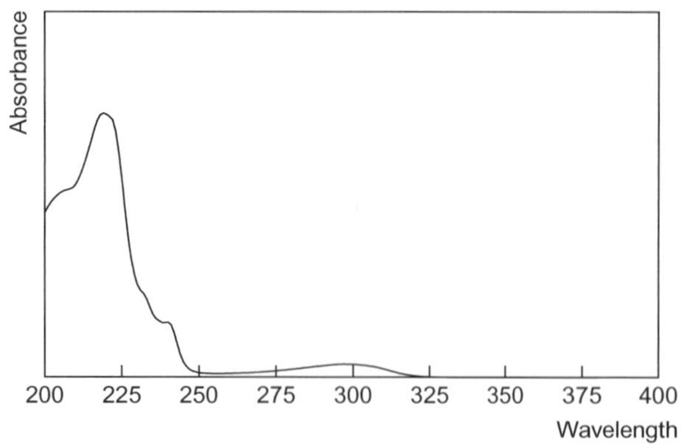

Infra-red Spectrum. Principal peaks at wavenumbers 1681, 727, 1205, 1250, 1316, 1110 cm^{-1} (Nujol mull).

Mass Spectrum. Principal ions at *m*/*z* 76, 173, 104, 111, 148, 50, 169, 130.

Quantification

High performance liquid chromatography. In serum: thalidomide and metabolites—M. J. Czejka and H.P. Koch, *J. Chromatogr.*, 1987, *413*, 181–187. In plasma: limit of detection 200 µg/L—B. J. Boughton *et al.*, *Ann. Clin. Biochem.*, 1995, *32*, 79–83. In serum: limit of detection 222 µg/L to 21 mg/L, UV detection —J. S. Torano *et al.*, *J. Chromatogr. B. Biomed. Sci. Appl.*, 1999, *734*, 203–210.

Ultraviolet spectrophotometry. In blood, plasma or urine—J. N. Green and B. C. Benson, *J. Pharm. Pharmacol.*, 1961, *13*, 117T–121T.

Disposition in the Body. Thalidomide is absorbed from the gastrointestinal tract and hydrolysed in the body, forming mainly 2-(*o*-carboxybenzamido)glutarimide, although many other hydrolysis products are also detectable.

Toxicity. Thalidomide has a low acute toxicity; in 2 cases of reported overdose there was no evidence of respiratory or cardiac depression. Thalidomide has teratogenic effects when administered to women early in pregnancy.

Dose. 50 to 400 mg daily, in the treatment of lepra reactions.

Thebacon

Narcotic Analgesic

Synonyms. Acethydrocodone; Acetyldihydrocodeinone; Dihydrocodeinone Enol Acetate.

(5α)-6,7-Didehydro-4,5-epoxy-3-methoxy-17-methylmorphinan-6-ol acetate

$C_{20}H_{23}NO_4$=341.4

CAS—466-90-0

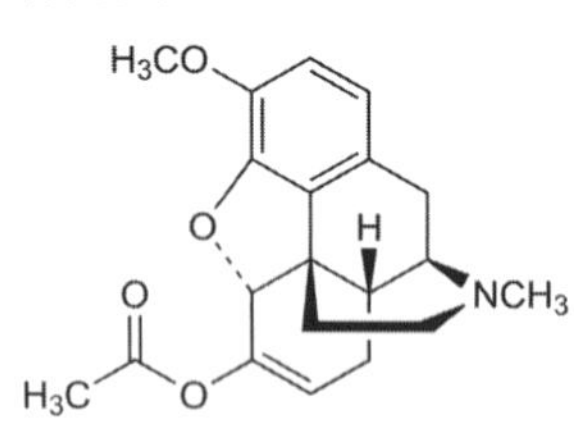

A white powder. M.p. 154°.

Practically insoluble in water; soluble in ethanol, chloroform and ether.

Thebacon Hydrochloride

Proprietary name. Acedicon

$C_{20}H_{23}NO_4$,HCl=377.9

CAS—20236-82-2

White crystals. M.p. 132° to 135°, with decomposition.

Soluble in water.

Partition Coefficient. Log *P* (octanol/water), 2.4.

Colour Test. Marquis Test—yellow→violet.

Thin-layer Chromatography. System TA—Rf 45; system TB—Rf 20; system TC—Rf 34; system TE—Rf 49; system TL—Rf 11; system TAE—Rf 24; system TAF—Rf 25. (Acidified iodoplatinate solution, positive.)

Gas Chromatography. System GA—RI 2533; system GB—RI 2559. Also metabolised to dihydrocodeine.

High Performance Liquid Chromatography. System HA—*k* 3.7 (tailing peak); system HC—*k* 0.85; system HX—RI 333.

Ultraviolet Spectrum. Aqueous acid—281 nm (A_1^1=41b).

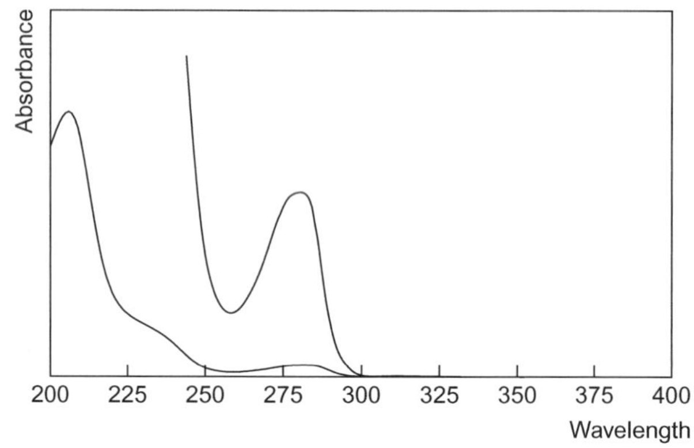

Infra-red Spectrum. Principal peaks at wavenumbers 1208, 1138, 1744, 1500, 905, 1194 cm^{-1} (KBr disk).

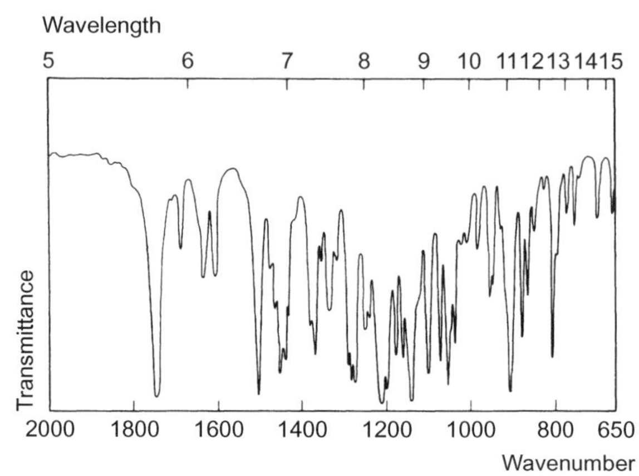

Mass Spectrum. Principal ions at *m*/*z* 341, 298, 43, 44, 55, 284, 242.

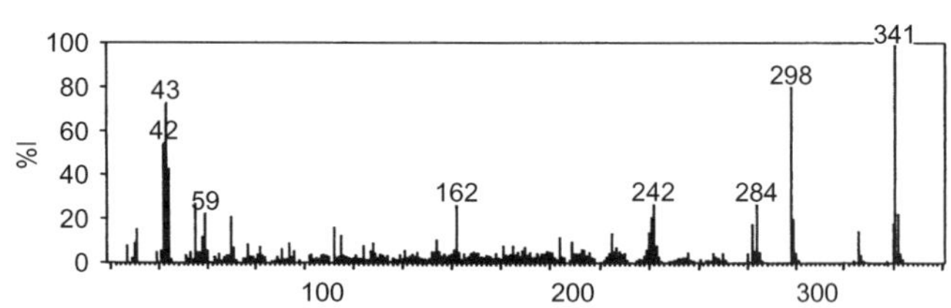

Dose. Usually 10 mg of thebacon hydrochloride daily.

Thebaine

Alkaloid

Synonym. Paramorphine

(5α)-6,7,8,14-Tetradehydro-4,5-epoxy-3,6 dimethoxy-17-methylmorphinan

$C_{19}H_{21}NO_3$=311.4

CAS—115-37-7

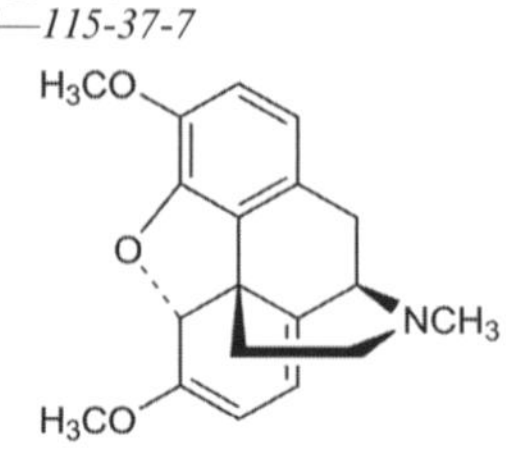

An alkaloid present in opium.

A white powder. M.p. 193°.

Soluble 1 in 1460 of water, 1 in about 15 of hot ethanol, 1 in 13 of chloroform, 1 in 200 of ether and 1 in 25 of benzene.

Dissociation Constant. pK_a 6.1 (15°); 8.2 (20°).

Partition Coefficient. Log *P* (octanol/buffer pH 7.5), 0.3; (octanol/water), 2.0.

Colour Tests. Mandelin's test—orange→brown; Marquis test—red→orange.

Thin-layer Chromatography. System TA—Rf 45; system TB—Rf 24; system TC—Rf 37; system TE—Rf 45; system TL—Rf 05; system TAE—Rf 23; system TAF—Rf 32; system TAJ—Rf 22; system TAK—Rf 11; system TAL—Rf 76. (Dragendorff spray, positive; FPN reagent, faint brown; Acidified iodoplatinate solution, positive; Marquis reagent, yellow.)

Gas Chromatography. System GA—RI 2517.

High Performance Liquid Chromatography. System HA—*k* 4.6 (tailing peak); system HC—*k* 0.9; system HS—*k* 0.8; system HX—RI 340; system HY—RI 276.

Ultraviolet Spectrum. Aqueous acid—284 nm (A^1_1=253a). No alkaline shift.

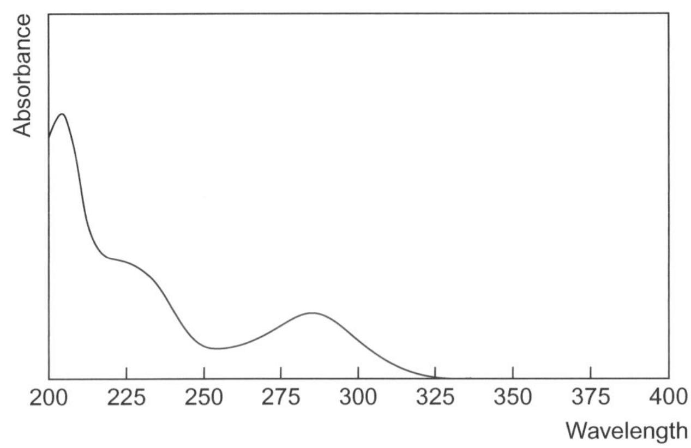

Infra-red Spectrum Principal peaks at wavenumbers 1234, 1605, 1144, 1270, 1030, 910 cm^{-1} (KBr disk).

Mass Spectrum. Principal ions at *m/z* 311, 255, 42, 44, 296, 310, 312, 174.

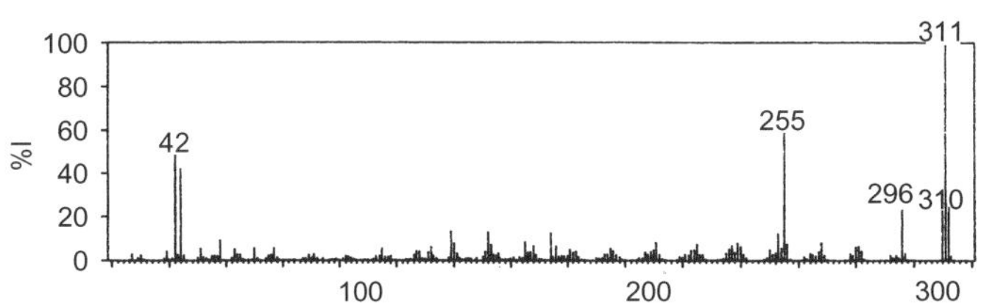

Quantification

Gas chromatography–mass spectrometry. In urine: limit of detection 2 to 81 µg/L—G. Cassella *et al.*, *J. Anal. Toxicol.*, 1997, *21*, 376–383. In hair: thebaine and drugs of abuse—G. Achilli *et al.*, *J. Chromatogr.*, 1996, *729*, 273–277.

Thenalidine

Antihistamine

Synonyms. Thenaldine; Thenophenopiperidine; Thenopiperidine.

1-Methyl-*N*-phenyl-*N*-(2-thienylmethyl)-4-piperidinamine

$C_{17}H_{22}N_2S$=286.4

CAS—86-12-4

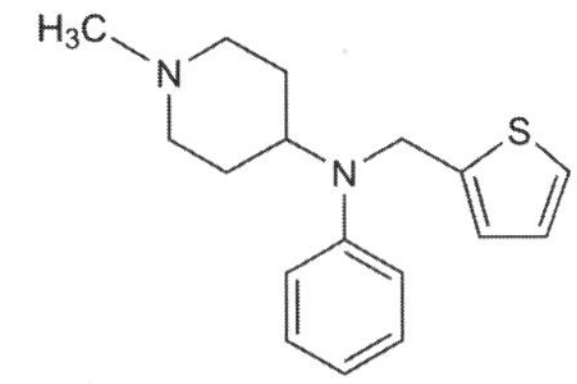

M.p. 95° to 97°.

Practically insoluble in water; soluble in chloroform.

Thenalidine Tartrate

$C_{17}H_{22}N_2S,C_4H_6O_6$=436.5

CAS—16509-35-6

A white crystalline powder. M.p. 170° to 172°.

Soluble in water.

Partition Coefficient. Log *P* (octanol/water), 3.9.

Colour Tests. Mandelin's test—orange→brown; Marquis test—grey-violet.

Thin-layer Chromatography. System TA—Rf 50; system TB—Rf 38; system TC—Rf 44; system TE—Rf 52; system TL—Rf 12; system TAE—Rf 20. (Acidified iodoplatinate solution, positive.)

Gas Chromatography. System GA—RI 2318.

High Performance Liquid Chromatography. System HA—*k* 3.5.

Ultraviolet Spectrum. Aqueous acid—234 nm (A^1_1=280b).

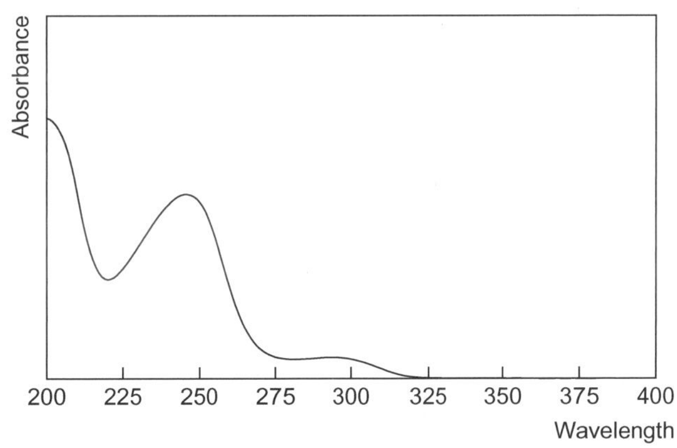

Infra-red Spectrum. Principal peaks at wavenumbers 1505, 748, 1600, 693, 1279, 755 cm^{-1} (KBr disk).

Mass Spectrum. Principal ions at *m/z* 97, 70, 99, 43, 98, 44, 42, 188.

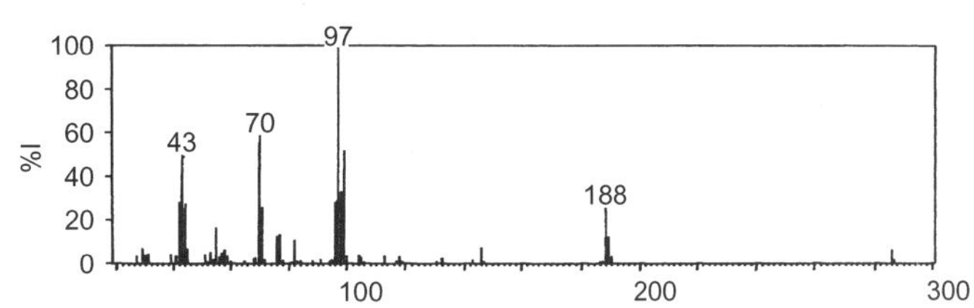

Dose. Thenalidine tartrate has been given in doses of 100 to 150 mg daily.

Thenium Closilate

Anthelmintic (Veterinary)

Synonym. Thenium Closylate; 611CSS.

N,N-Dimethyl-*N*-(2-phenoxyethyl)-2-thiophenemethanaminium salt with 4-chlorobenzenesulfonic acid (1:1)

$C_{21}H_{24}ClNO_4S_2$=454.0

CAS—16776-64-0 (thenium); 4304-40-9 (closilate)

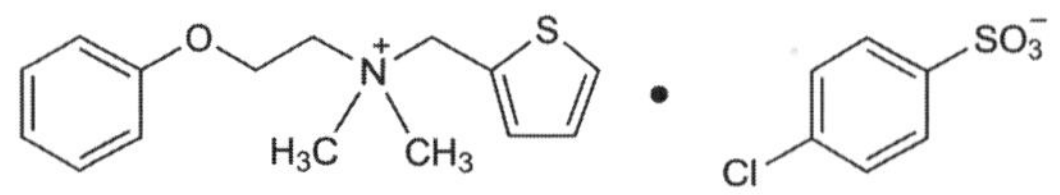

A white crystalline powder. M.p. 159° to 160°.
Soluble 1 in 200 of water, 1 in 25 of ethanol and 1 in 35 of chloroform.

Colour Tests. Mandelin's test—green; Marquis test—violet.

Thin-layer Chromatography. System TA—Rf 02. (Acidified iodoplatinate solution, positive.)

Ultraviolet Spectrum. Aqueous acid—268 (A^1_1=45b), 275 nm (A^1_1=36b).

Infra-red Spectrum. Principal peaks at wavenumbers 1210, 1174, 1042, 1135, 760, 1010 cm^{-1} (KBr disk).

Thenyldiamine

Antihistamine

N,*N*-Dimethyl-*N*′-2-pyridinyl-*N*′-(3-thienylmethyl)-1,2-ethanediamine
$C_{14}H_{19}N_3S$=261.4
CAS—91-79-2

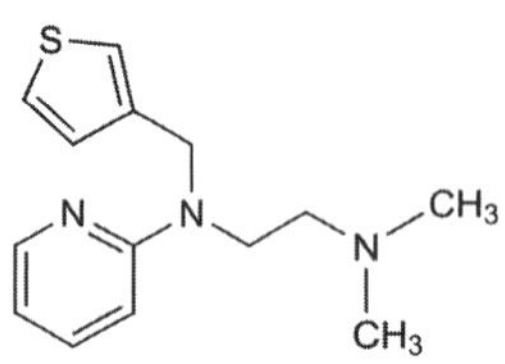

A liquid.
Practically insoluble in water; soluble in chloroform.

Thenyldiamine Hydrochloride

Proprietary names. It is an ingredient of Asafen, NTR and Sinefricol.
$C_{14}H_{19}N_3S,HCl$=297.8
CAS—958-93-0
A white crystalline powder. M.p. about 170°.
Soluble 1 in 5 of water, 1 in 5 of ethanol and 1 in 5 of chloroform; practically insoluble in ether.

Dissociation Constant. pK_a 3.9, 8.9 (25°).

Partition Coefficient. Log *P* (octanol/water), 2.6.

Colour Tests. Mandelin's test—green; Marquis test—black→violet.

Thin-layer Chromatography. System TA—Rf 53; system TAE—Rf 21; system TAF—Rf 36; system TL—Rf 12; system TB—Rf 42; system TC—Rf 25; system TE—Rf 65. (Dragendorff spray, positive; Acidified iodoplatinate solution, positive; Marquis reagent, violet.)

Gas Chromatography. System GA—RI 1999; system GB—RI 2034; system GC—RI 2300; system GF—RI 2340.

High Performance Liquid Chromatography. System HA—*k* 4.0; system HX—RI 317.

Ultraviolet Spectrum. Aqueous acid—239 (A^1_1=703a), 315; aqueous alkali—246, 310 nm.

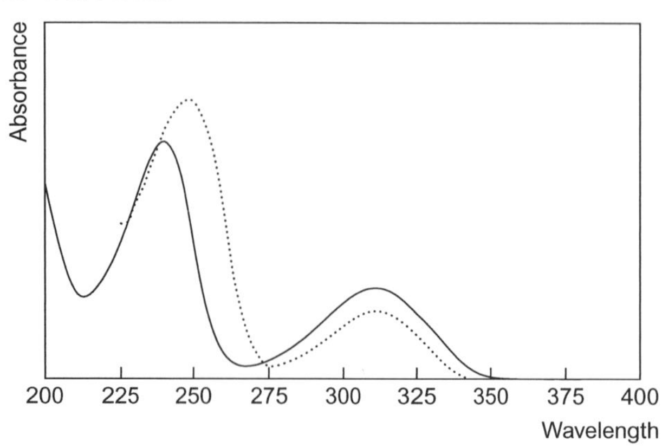

Infra-red Spectrum. Principal peaks at wavenumbers 1597, 766, 1242, 976, 1159, 1311 cm^{-1}.

Mass Spectrum. Principal ions at *m/z* 58, 97, 72, 71, 203, 191, 190, 42.

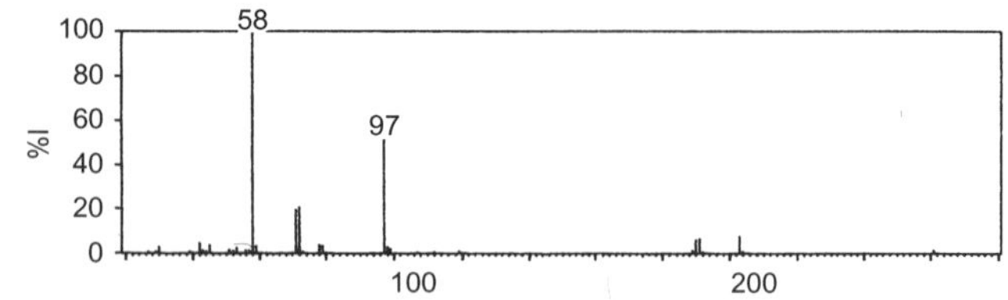

Dose. Thenyldiamine hydrochloride has been given in doses of up to 90 mg daily.

Theobromine

Xanthine Derivative

Synonyms. 3,7-Dimethylxanthine; Santheose; Theobrominum.
Proprietary names. It is an ingredient of Asthma-Hilfe, Propyre T and Urodonal.
3,7-Dihydro-3,7-dimethyl-(1*H*)-purine-2,6-dione
$C_7H_8N_4O_2$=180.2
CAS—83-67-0

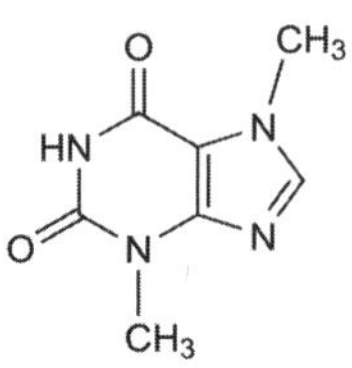

An alkaloid contained in the seeds of *Theobroma cacao* (Sterculiaceae).
A white microcrystalline powder which sublimes at 290° to 295°.
Soluble 1 in 2000 of water, 1 in 2220 of 95% ethanol and 1 in 6000 of chloroform; almost insoluble in benzene, carbon tetrachloride and ether; freely soluble in dilute mineral acids and aqueous solutions of alkali hydroxides.

Dissociation Constant. pK_a <1, 10.0 (25°).

Partition Coefficient. Log *P* (octanol/water), −0.8.

Colour Test. Amalic Acid Test—yellow/violet.

Thin-layer Chromatography. System TA—Rf 53; system TB—Rf 01; system TC—Rf 31; system TE—Rf 34; system TF—Rf 4; system TG—Rf 47; system TL—Rf 21; system TAE—Rf 59; system TAF—Rf 54; system TAJ—Rf 32; system TAK—Rf 08; system TAL—Rf 65. (Ludy Tenger reagent, orange.)

Gas Chromatography. System GA—RI 1807; system GB—RI 1920.

High Performance Liquid Chromatography. System HA—*k* 0.1; system HX—RI 262; system HY—RI 201; system HZ—Retention time, 1.6 min; system HAA–Retention time, 3.8 min.

Ultraviolet Spectrum. Aqueous acid—272 nm (A^1_1=563a); aqueous alkali—274 nm.

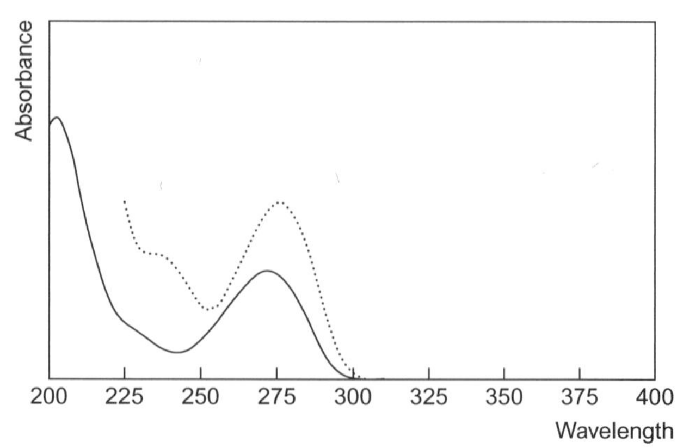

Infra-red Spectrum. Principal peaks at wavenumbers 1690, 1665, 1221, 1550, 1595, 680 cm^{-1} (KBr disk).

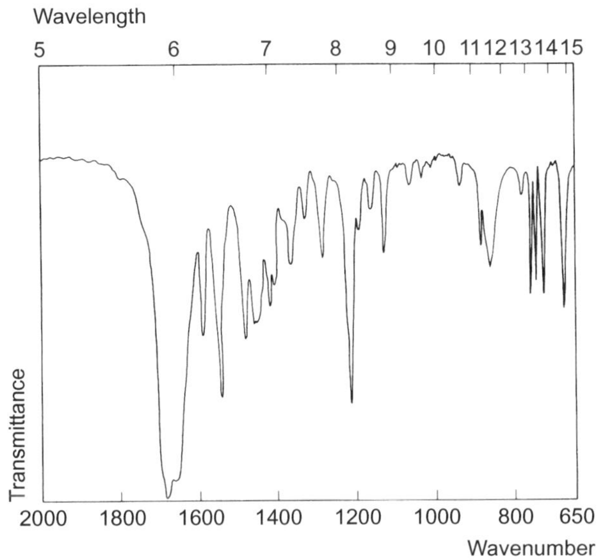

Mass Spectrum. Principal ions at *m/z* 180, 55, 67, 109, 82, 42, 137, 70; 3-methylxanthine 166, 68, 95, 41, 53, 123, –, –; 7-methylxanthine 166, 68, 123, 53, 42, 41, 95, –.

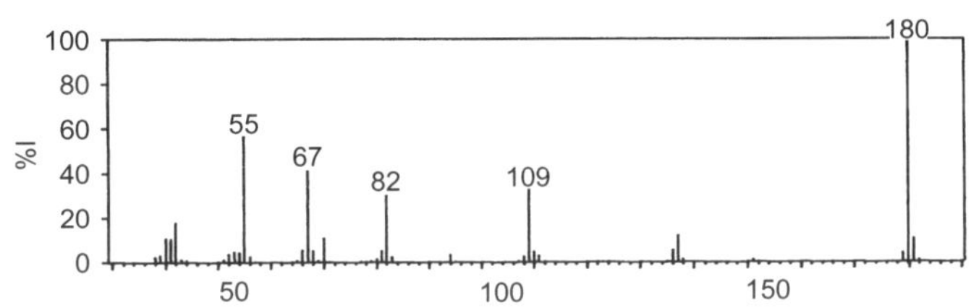

Disposition in the Body. Well absorbed after oral administration. It is metabolised by demethylation, mainly to 7-methylxanthine, together with some 3-methylxanthine. The 7-methylxanthine is further oxidised to 7-methyluric acid. About 90% of a dose is excreted in the urine in 48 h, of which about 40% is 7-methylxanthine, 20% is 3-methylxanthine, 11% is 7-methyluric acid and 15% is unchanged drug. An additional metabolite, 6-amino-5-(*N*-methylformylamino)-1-methyluracil, accounts for about 7% of a dose.
Theobromine is a metabolite of caffeine.

Half-life. Plasma half-life, 5 to 11 h (mean 8) after a single dose, increased on chronic administration.

Volume of distribution. About 0.5 to 1 L/kg.

Clearance. Plasma clearance, about 0.8 mL/min/kg.

Saliva. Plasma : saliva ratio, about 1.0.

Dose. 300 to 600 mg.

Theophylline

Xanthine Bronchodilator

Synonyms. Anhydrous Theophylline, 1,3-Dimethylxanthine; Teofilina; Theophyllinum.
Proprietary names Accurbron; Aerolate; Aquaphyllin; Asmalix; Elixomin; Elixophyllin; Lasma; Nuelin (tablets); Quibron-T; Respbid; Slo-Bid; Slo-Phyllin; Sustaire; Theo-24; Theobid; Theochron; Theoclear; Theo-Dur; Theolair; Theospan; Theovent; Theo-X; T-Phyl; Uni-Dur; Uniphyl; Uniphyllin Continus (includes proprietary names of the hydrate). It is an ingredient of Elixophyllin-GG, Elixophyllin-KI, Franol, Franol Plus, Franolyn Expectorant, Franyl, Glyceryl-T, Hydrophed, Marax, Quadrinal, Quibron, Slo-Phyllin GG, Tedrigen, Theodrine and Theomax DF.
3,7-Dihydro-1,3-dimethyl-1*H*-purine-2,6-dione
$C_7H_8N_4O_2$=180.2
CAS—58-55-9

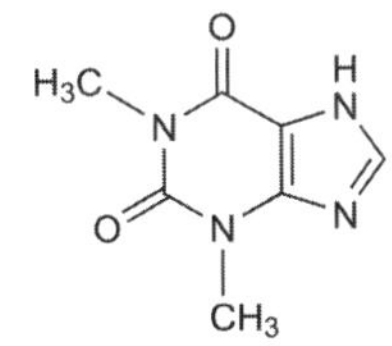

A white crystalline powder. M.p. 270° to 274°.
Soluble 1 in 120 of water, 1 in 80 of ethanol and 1 in 110 of chloroform; sparingly soluble in ether; soluble in dilute acids, ammonia and alkali hydroxide solutions.

Aminophylline

Synonyms. Euphyllinum; Metaphyllin; Theophyllaminum; Theophylline and Ethylenediamine; Theophylline Ethylenediamine Compound.
Proprietary names. Aminocont; Aminomal; Amnivent; Clonofilin; Elixophyllin; Escophylline; Euphyllin(a); Filotempo; Mundiphyllin; Norphyllin SR; Phyllocontin; Phyllotemp; Tefamin; Teofylamin; Truphylline. It is an ingredient of Emergent-Ez, Mudrane, Mudrane GG and Mudrane GG-2.
A stable mixture containing 78 to 84% of anhydrous theophylline and 13 to 14% of ethylenediamine with a variable quantity of water.
Its composition approximately corresponds to the formula
$(C_7H_8N_4O_2)_2,C_2H_4(NH_2)_2,2H_2O$=456.5
CAS—317-34-0 (anhydrous)
White or slightly yellowish granules or powder.
Soluble 1 in 5 of water at 25°, but the addition of ethylenediamine or ammonia solution may be necessary to give complete solution. Practically insoluble in ethanol and ether.

Choline Theophyllinate

Synonyms. Oxtriphylline; Theophylline Cholinate.
Proprietary names. Brondecon Elixir; Choledyl; Euspirax; Rouphylline; Sabidal; Teovent.
$C_{12}H_{21}N_5O_3$=283.3
CAS—4499-40-5
A white crystalline powder. M.p. 185° to 192°.
Soluble 1 in less than 1 of water and 1 in 10 of ethanol; very slightly soluble in chloroform and ether.

Theophylline Hydrate

Synonym. Theophylline Monohydrate
$C_7H_8N_4O_2,H_2O$=198.2
CAS—5967-84-0
A white crystalline powder. M.p. about 272°, after drying.
Soluble 1 in 120 of water and 1 in 80 of ethanol; very slightly soluble in ether; soluble in solutions of alkali hydroxides.

Theophylline Monoethanolamine

Synonym. Theophylline Olamine
An equimolecular compound of anhydrous theophylline and monoethanolamine.
$C_7H_8N_4O_2,C_2H_7NO$=241.2
CAS—573-41-1
A white crystalline powder.
Soluble 1 in 20 of water.

Theophylline Sodium Glycinate

Synonym. Theophylline Sodium Aminoacetate
Proprietary name. Nuelin (liquid).
An equilibrium mixture of theophylline sodium ($C_7H_7N_4NaO_2$=202.1) and glycine ($C_2H_5NO_2$=75.07) in approximately equimolecular proportions, buffered with an additional mole of glycine.
CAS—8000-10-0
A white crystalline powder. Darkens at 180°.
Soluble 1 in 6 of water; very slightly soluble in ethanol; practically insoluble in chloroform.

Dissociation Constant. pK_a 8.6 (25°).

Partition Coefficient. Log *P* (octanol/water), 0.0.

Colour Tests. Amalic Acid Test—yellow/violet; Folin–Ciocalteu Reagent—blue.

Thin-layer Chromatography. System TA—Rf 75; system TB—Rf 01; system TC—Rf 30; system TE—Rf 11; system TF—Rf 9; system TG—Rf 33; system TL—Rf 11; system TAE—Rf 74; system TAF—Rf 66; system TAJ—Rf 40; system TAK—Rf 21; system TAL—Rf 78. (Ludy Tenger reagent, orange.)

Plate: silica gel 60 F_{254} (0.25 mm layer thickness). Mobile phase: chloroform:methanol (9:1). Visualised with UV detection (λ = 254 nm). Rf 0.54 [P. V. Devarajan *et al.*, *J. Chromatogr. B Biomed. Sci. Appl.*, 1999, *736*, 289–293].

Gas Chromatography. System GA—RI 2005; system GF—RI 2745.

High Performance Liquid Chromatography. System HA—*k* 0.1; system HX—RI 276; system HY—RI 249; system HZ—Retention time, 1.7 min; system HAA—Retention time, 4.9 min; system HAM—Retention time 1.8 min; system HAX—Retention time 4.5 min; system HAY—Retention time 3.5 min.

Column: RP Ultrasphere-ODS (150 × 4.6 mm i.d., 5 μm); (pre-column), RP-2 (Lichrosorb, 400 × 2.5 mm i.d., 10 μm). Mobile phase: sodium acetate (10 mM):acetonitrile:tetrahydrofuran (96.9:3.0:0.1) containing tetrabutylammonium hydrogensulfate (5 mM), pH 4.7, flow rate 1.5 mL/min. UV detection (280 nm). *k* value: 4.31 (Retention time, 8.5 min) [H. Tajerzadeh and S. Dadashzadeh, *J. Pharm. Biomed. Anal.*, 1995, *13*, 1507–1512].

Column: RP ODS-2 (150 × 4.6 mm i.d., 5 μm). Mobile phase: acetonitrile:tetrahydrofuran:concentrated acetic acid:distilled water (20:20:5:955), flow rate 1 mL/min. UV detection (λ = 273 nm). Retention time: 5.0 min [E. Schreiber-Deturmeny and B. Bruguerolle, *J. Chromatogr.*, 1996, *677*; *Biomed. Appl.*, 305–312].

Ultraviolet Spectrum. Aqueous acid—270 nm (A_{1}^{1} = 536a); aqueous alkali—275 nm (A_{1}^{1} = 650a).

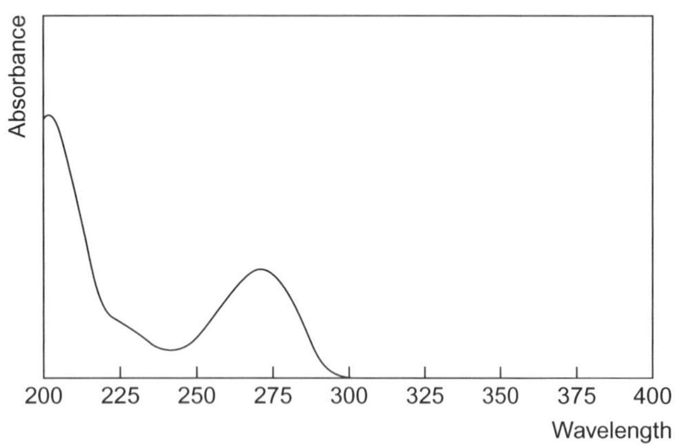

Infra-red Spectrum. Principal peaks at wavenumbers 1670, 1717, 1567, 745, 980, 1190 cm^{-1} (KBr disk). (See below)

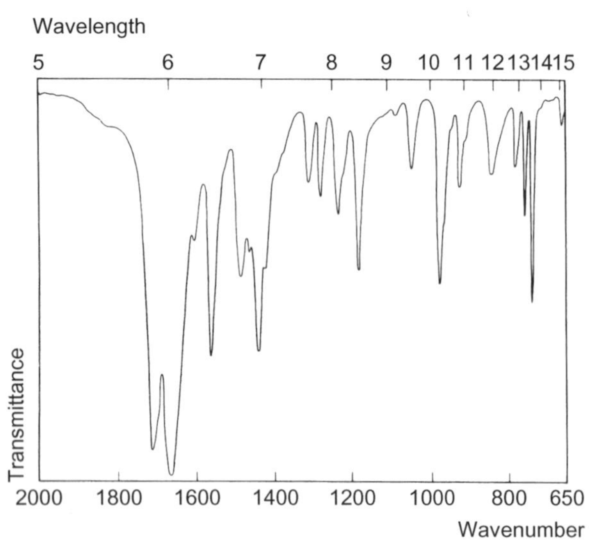

Mass Spectrum. Principal ions at *m/z* 180, 95, 68, 41, 53, 181, 96, 40; 3-methylxanthine 166, 68, 95, 41, 53, 123, –, –.

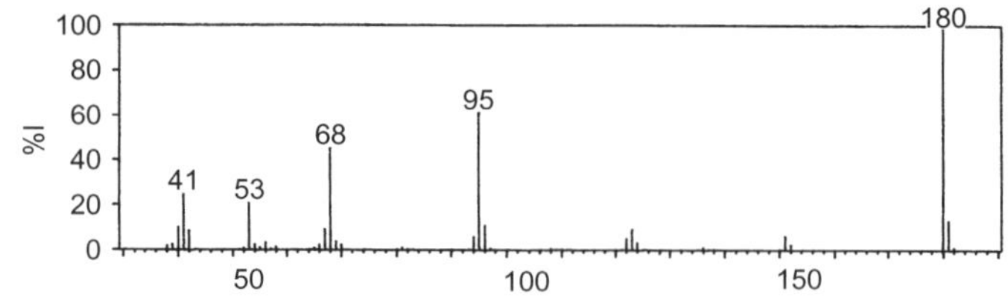

Quantification

Gas chromatography. In serum: limit of detection 2.5 mg/L, FID—H. A. Schwertner, *Clin. Chem.*, 1979, *25*, 212–214.

High performance liquid chromatography. In plasma and urine: limit of quantification 0.5 μg/L, UV detection (λ = 280 nm)—M. Kamberi *et al.*, *Ther. Drug Monit.*, 1999, *21*, 335–340. In serum: limit of detection is 0.2 μg/L, UV detection (λ = 273 nm)—T. Umemura *et al.*, *Analyst*, 1998, *123*, 1767–1770. In plasma: limit of detection 0.1 μg/L, UV detection (λ = 273 nm)—E. Schreiber-Deturmeny and B. Bruguerolle, *J. Chromatogr.*, 1996, *677*; *Biomed. Appl.*, 305–312. In plasma and urine: limit of detection is 0.1 to 0.2 μg/L in plasma and 1 to 2 μg/L in urine for its metabolites, UV detection (λ = 273 nm)—B. B. Rasmussen and K. Brosen, *J. Chromatogr.*, 1996, *676*; *Biomed. Appl.*, 169–174. In urine: limit of detection 1 μg/L for theophylline and 0.5 μg/L for its metabolites, UV detection (λ = 280 nm)—H. Tajerzadeh and S. Dadashzadeh, *J. Pharm. Biomed. Anal.*, 1995, *13(12)*, 1507–1512.

High performance liquid chromatography–mass spectrometry. In blood spots: limit of quantification 0.012 mg/L, (SIM, *m/z* 179)—D. G. Watson *et al.*, *J. Pharm. Pharmacol.*, 2001, *53*, 413–416.

Chemiluminescent immunoassay. In serum and plasma: limit of quantification 0.2 mg/L—D. P. Malliaros *et al.*, *Ther. Drug Monit.*, 1997, *19(2)*, 224–229.

Thin-layer chromatography. In plasma: limit of detection, 20 ng—P. V. Devarajan *et al.*, *J. Chromatogr. B Biomed. Sci. Appl.*, 1999, *736(1-2)*, 289–293.

Disposition in the Body. Readily absorbed after oral administration of aminophylline; less rapidly absorbed when given as theophylline; irregularly absorbed after rectal administration. The presence of food or antacids does not affect absorption. Rapidly and widely distributed throughout the tissues; unbound theophylline distributes into body water but poorly into body fat. It also passes freely across the placenta, into breast milk and into cerebrospinal fluid. Metabolised by *N*-demethylation to form 3-methylxanthine (which is active but less potent than theophylline), 1,3-dimethyluric acid and 1-methyluric acid (by further hydroxylation of 1-methylxanthine). Approximately 90% of a dose is metabolised in adults and children > 1 year old; 6% to caffeine by *N*-methylation. In adults, about 13% of a dose is excreted in the urine in 24 h as unchanged drug, with about 15% as 3-methylxanthine, 35 to 50% as 1,3-dimethyluric acid and about 20% as 1-methyluric acid. In premature neonates, most of a dose is excreted as unchanged drug with up to 10% as caffeine.
Theophylline is a metabolite of caffeine.

Therapeutic concentration. There is considerable inter-subject variation in serum-theophylline concentrations; therapeutic effect has been correlated with concentrations of 10 to 15 mg/L. 3-Methylxanthine accumulates in the serum to concentrations of about 25% of those of theophylline. Diurnal variations in plasma concentrations have been reported with higher concentrations in the morning. Steady-state concentrations are reached within 30 to 65 h (mean 40) and levels reach 60% of the mean peak therapeutic concentration.

18 healthy males, aged 20 to 30 years, were administered either a 1000 mg once daily dose in the evening (equivalent to 13 mg/kg) or two 500 mg doses in the morning and evening. Each dose was administered 30 min after a standard meal. The mean peak plasma concentration for the once daily dose was 15.2 (range 11.9 to 19.4) mg/L on days 5/6 and 15.0 (11.6 to 19.3) mg/L on days 8/9. For the twice daily dosing, the peak concentration was 11.8 (9.0 to 15.3) mg/L and 12.1 (9.0 to 16.2) mg/L, respectively [J. Gotz *et al.*, *Int. J. Clin. Pharmacol. Ther.*, 1994, *32(4)*, 168–173].

12 healthy, young, non-smoking males, aged 23 to 30 years, were administered a single oral dose of 200 mg theophylline in solution diluted with either water or grapefruit juice, after an overnight fast. The mean peak plasma concentration was 6.2 (range 4.7 to 9.6) mg/L for the dose

administered with the water and 5.6 (4.2 to 7.8) mg/L with grapefruit, observed at 0.25 to 2.0 h and 0.5 to 1.5 h, respectively [U. Fuhr *et al.*, *Int. J. Clin. Pharmacol. Ther.*, 1995, *33(6)*, 311–314].

12 debilitated elderly patients were administered theophylline either orally (dose 360 mg daily) or via a nasogastric tube (320 mg daily, by means of emptying capsule contents and mixing with 10 mL of water; dose not significantly different from that given orally). Trough and peak levels in the nasogastric-tube group were 0.5 to 10.7 mg/L (mean 3.7) and 1.3 to 13.3 mg/L (mean 6.5), respectively, with the time to reach peak concentration being 6.5 h. Trough and peak levels in the orally administered group were 0 to 15.61 mg/L (mean 8.63) and 4.3 to 16.2 mg/L (mean 10.5), respectively, with a time to peak concentration of 5.5 h [M. Berkovitch *et al.*, *Ther. Drug Monit.*, 2002, *24*, 594–597].

Toxicity. The estimated minimum lethal dose after intravenous administration is 0.1 g; fatalities have occurred after oral doses of 8.4 mg/kg in a child and after 25 to 100 mg/kg of aminophylline given as a suppository. Recovery has been reported after ingestion of choline theophyllinate equivalent to 12.8 g of theophylline. Toxic effects are usually associated with plasma concentrations greater than 30 mg/L and fatalities with concentrations above 50 mg/L; premature neonates appear to be relatively resistant to theophylline poisoning. Premature neonates, patients with hepatic cirrhosis, the elderly and women during the third trimester of pregnancy may show toxic signs at serum concentrations in the therapeutic range, 10 to 20 mg/L (owing to an increase in unbound pharmacologically active drug.

In a 44-year-old female who was found dead next to an empty container of theophylline capsules (maximum possible dose ingested was 100 × 350 mg), toxicological analysis revealed a serum theophylline concentration of 127 mg/L and a concentration of 154 mg/L in the fluid gathered from cutaneous blisters on regions exposed to pressure [M. Tsokos and J. P. Sperhake, *Am. J. Forensic Med. Pathol.*, 2002, *23*, 292–294].

A 17-year-old male was found dead the following morning after complaining of a headache the night before which he treated with 1 to 2 Panadol (500 mg paracetamol). Postmortem toxicological analysis showed a serum theophylline concentration of 145 mg/L; liver, 91 μg/g; urine, 182 mg/L; vitreous humour, 48 mg/L and a total of 320 mg and 3 part tablets were detected in the stomach contents. All tissue/fluid theophylline concentrations were at a fatal level [J. E. Ryall, *TIAFT Bulletin Case Notes*, 1997, *27(1)*, http://www.tiaft.org/].

Of 249 patients classed as having theophylline intoxication (defined as a peak serum concentration of 30 mg/L; 167 μmol/L), 119 had acute intoxication without having previously received theophylline therapy. These patients had a mean peak serum theophylline concentration of 67.4 mg/L (158.4 mg/L in 4 who died). In 38 patients who had acute intoxication while receiving theophylline therapy, the mean peak serum concentration was 381 μmol/L. In 92 patients who had intoxication caused by chronic overmedication, the mean peak serum level was 279 μmol/L [M. Shannon, *Ann. Intern. Med.*, 1993, *119*, 1161–1167].

Half-life. Plasma half-life, 3 to 13 h in normal subjects (mean 7) but decreased in smokers and in children, and increased in premature neonates and in certain disease states such as hepatic disease, heart failure, and chronic obstructive pulmonary disease. The half-life may also be affected by the amount of dietary methylxanthines ingested.

Volume of distribution. About 0.5 L/kg; increases in premature neonates, patients with hepatic cirrhosis, the elderly and in women during the third trimester of pregnancy.

Clearance. Plasma clearance, about 0.5 to 2 mL/min/kg in normal subjects; decreases by approximately 30% in the elderly and 50% in patients with hepatic impairment and congestive heart failure.

Distribution in blood. Plasma : whole blood ratio, 1.2.

Saliva. Plasma : saliva ratio, about 2, but there is considerable inter-subject variation.

Protein binding. In plasma, about 40% (temperature and pH-dependent); decreased in neonates and in subjects with hepatic cirrhosis.

Note. For reviews of the clinical pharmacokinetics of theophylline see R. I. Ogilvie, *Clin. Pharmacokinet.*, 1978, *3*, 267–293 and T. J. Haley, *Drug Metab. Rev.*, 1983, *14*, 295–335; for a review of theophylline intoxication see C. A. Stegeman and J. G. Jordans, *Neth. J. Med.*, 1991, *39*, 115–125.

Dose. 0.18 to 1 g daily.

Thialbarbital

Anaesthetic/Barbiturate

Synonym. Thialbarbitone

5-(2-Cyclohexen-1-yl)dihydro-5-(2-propenyl)-2-thioxo-4,6(1*H*,5*H*)-pyrimidinedione

$C_{13}H_{16}N_2O_2S = 264.3$

CAS—467-36-7

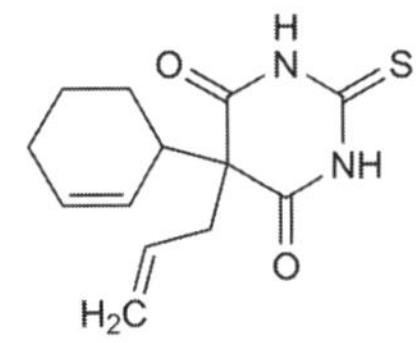

Crystals. M.p. 148° to 150°.

Sparingly soluble in water; readily soluble in most organic solvents.

Thialbarbital Sodium

Synonyms. Natrium Cyclohexenylallylthiobarbituricum; Thiohexallymalnatrium.

$C_{13}H_{15}N_2NaO_2S = 286.3$

CAS-3546-29-0

A pale yellow hygroscopic powder. M.p. 130° to 132°.

Very soluble in water and ethanol; slightly soluble in chloroform; practically insoluble in ether.

Partition Coefficient. Log *P* (octanol/water), 3.4.

Colour Tests. Palladium Chloride—orange-yellow; Vanillin Reagent—brown-orange/violet (transient).

Thin-layer Chromatography. System TD—Rf 77; system TE—Rf 43; system TF—Rf 72; system TH—Rf 75; system TAD—Rf 69. (Mercurous nitrate spray, black; acidified potassium permanganate solution, yellow-brown; Zwikker's reagent, green.)

Gas Chromatography. System GA—RI 2116.

High Performance Liquid Chromatography. System HX—RI 480.

Ultraviolet Spectrum. Borax buffer 0.05 M (pH 9.2)—256, 307 nm ($A_1^1 = 1236b$); M sodium hydroxide (pH 13)—306 nm ($A_1^1 = 1271b$).

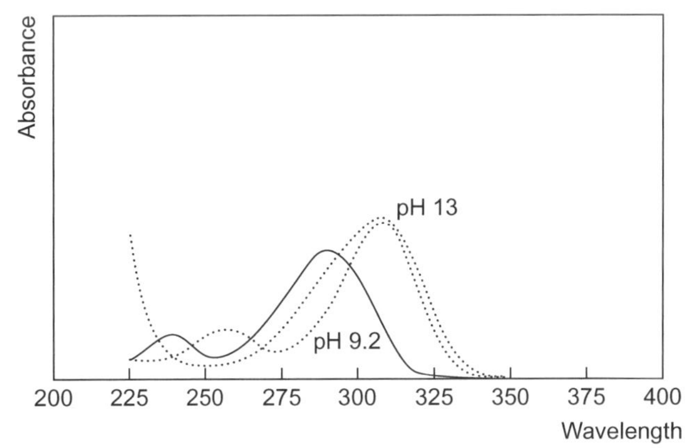

Infra-red Spectrum. Principal peaks at wavenumbers 1685, 1610, 1300, 1130, 1270, 1000 cm^{-1} (thialbarbital sodium, KBr disk).

Mass Spectrum. Principal ions at *m/z* 81, 223, 79, 41, 80, 157, 185, 77.

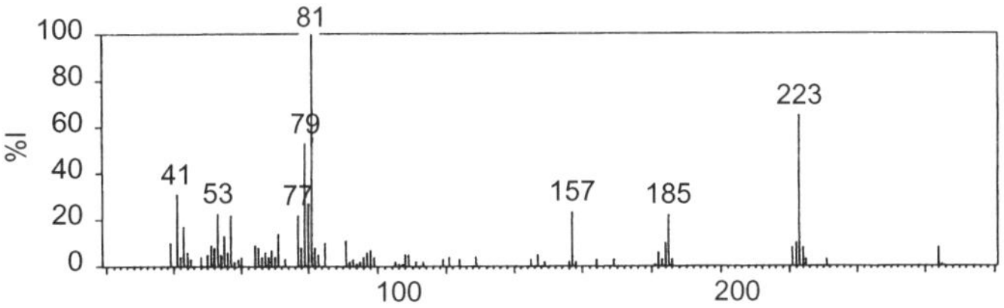

Dose. Thialbarbital sodium has been given in doses of 0.2 to 1 g intravenously.

Thiamazole

Antithyroid Agent

Synonyms. Mercazolylum; Methimazole; Tiamazol.
Proprietary names. Favistan; Mercaptizol; Metibasol; Strumazol; Tapazol(e); Thacapzol; Thycapzol; Thyrozol; Tirodril.
1,3-Dihydro-1-methyl-2*H*-imidazole-2-thione
$C_4H_6N_2S = 114.2$
CAS—60-56-0

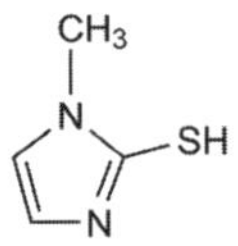

A white to pale buff, crystalline powder. M.p. 144° to 147°.
Soluble 1 in 5 of water, 1 in 5 of ethanol, and 1 in about 5 of chloroform; freely soluble in acetone; sparingly soluble in ether, petroleum ether, and benzene.

Partition Coefficient. Log *P* (octanol/water), −0.3.

Colour Test. Palladium Chloride—orange.

Thin-layer Chromatography. System TA—Rf 62; system TB—Rf 01; system TC—Rf 52; system TE—Rf 41; system TL—Rf 59; system TAE—Rf 80. (Acidified iodoplatinate solution, positive.)

Gas Chromatography. System GA—RI 1550.

Ultraviolet Spectrum. Aqueous acid—252 nm ($A^1_1 = 1505a$).

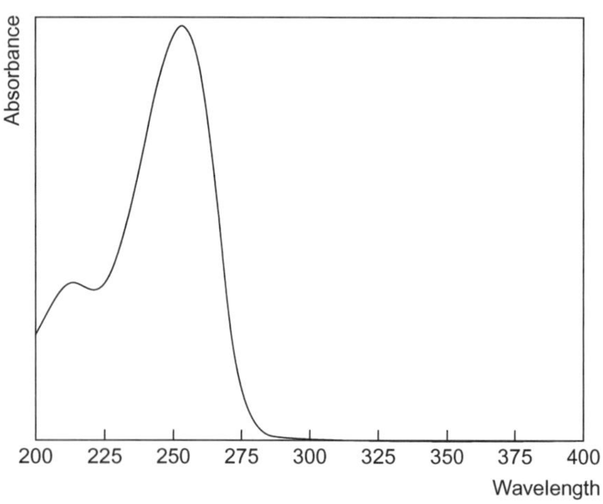

Infra-red Spectrum. Principal peaks at wavenumbers 1570, 1271, 740, 1250, 765, 675 $^{-1}$ (KBr disk).

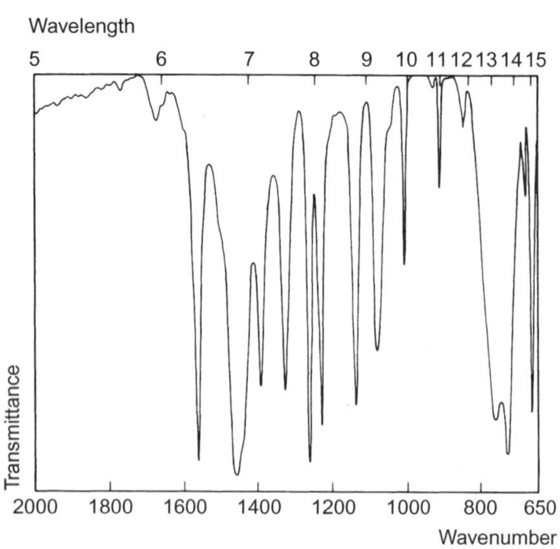

Mass Spectrum. Principal ions at *m/z* 114, 42, 72, 113, 69, 81, 54, 115.

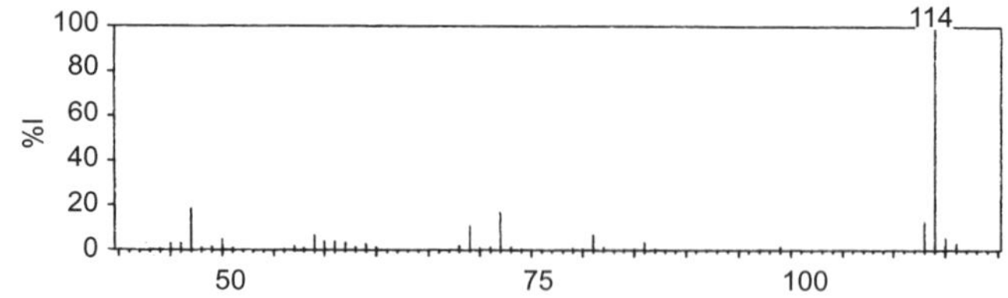

Quantification. See under Carbimazole.

Disposition in the Body. Absorbed after oral administration and widely distributed throughout the body. About 10% of a dose is excreted in the urine as unchanged drug. 3-Methyl-2-thiohydantoin has been identified in plasma and urine as a minor metabolite.
Thiamazole is the active metabolite of carbimazole.

Therapeutic concentration

Following a single oral dose of 60 mg given to 11 subjects, peak serum concentrations of 0.5 to 2.5 mg/L (mean 1.3) were attained in about 1 to 3 h [A. Melander *et al.*, *Eur. J. Clin. Pharmacol.*, 1980, *17*, 295–299.]

Half-life. Plasma half-life, about 3 to 5 h.

Volume of distribution. About 0.5 L/kg.

Protein binding. In plasma, not significantly bound.

Note. For a review of the pharmacokinetics of antithyroid agents see J. P. Kampmann and J. M. Hansen, *Clin. Pharmacokinet.*, 1981, *6*, 401–428.

Dose. Initially, 15 to 60 mg daily; maintenance, 5 to 15 mg daily.

Thiambutosine

Antileprotic

Synonym. DPT
Proprietary name. Ciba-1906
1-(4-Butoxyphenyl)-3-(4-dimethylaminophenyl)thiourea
$C_{19}H_{25}N_3OS = 343.5$
CAS—500-89-0

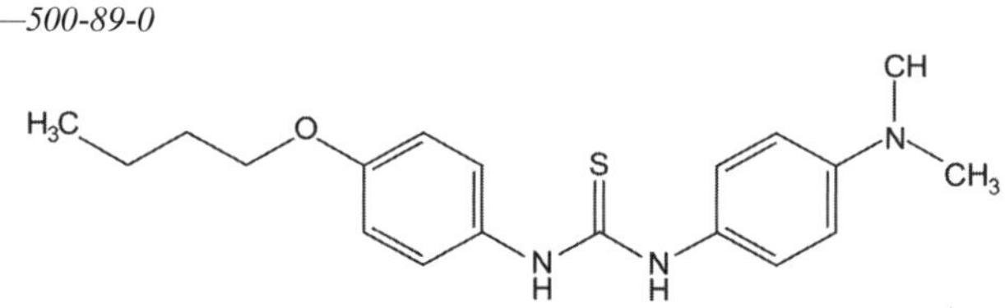

A white or creamy-white crystalline powder. M.p. 123° to 127°.
Practically insoluble in water; soluble 1 in 1.5 of chloroform and 1 in 300 of ether; soluble in acetone.

Thin-layer Chromatography. System TA—Rf 76; system TL—Rf 69; system TB—Rf 6; system TC—Rf 77.

Gas Chromatography. System GA—RI 1715.

Ultraviolet Spectrum. Ethanol—270 nm ($A^1_1 = 720a$).

Infra-red Spectrum. Principal peaks at wavenumbers 1234, 720, 1307, 1499, 813, 1093 cm^{-1}.

Mass Spectrum. Principal ions at *m/z* 151, 109, 136, 178, 177, 29, 207, 135.

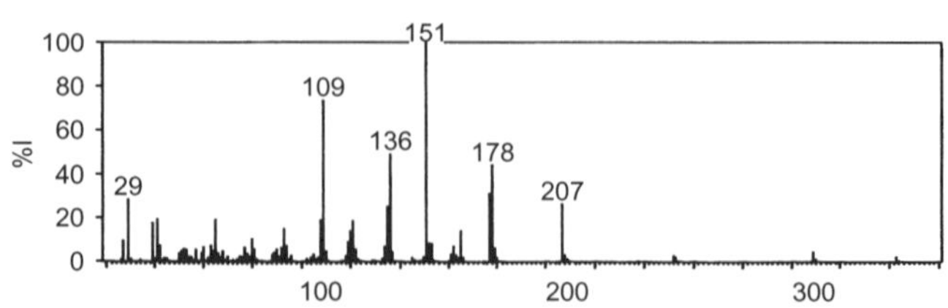

Disposition in the Body. Thiambutosine is poorly absorbed after oral administration; aqueous suspensions are slowly and possibly incompletely absorbed after IM injection. About 10% of a dose is metabolised to water-soluble compounds and rapidly excreted in the urine; about 75% of a dose is eliminated unchanged in the faeces.

Dose. 1 to 3 g daily.

Thiamine

Vitamin

Synonyms. Aneurine; Vitamin B_1.
3-[(4-Amino-2-methyl-5-pyrimidinyl)methyl]-5-(2-hydroxyethyl)-4-methylthiazolium chloride
$C_{12}H_{17}ClN_4OS=300.8$
CAS—59-43-8

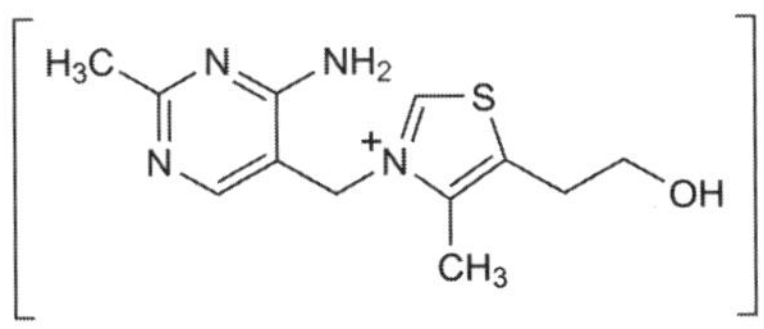

Thiamine Hydrochloride

Synonym. Aneurine Chloride Hydrochloride
Proprietary names. Benerva; Beneuran; Betabion; Betamin(e); Beta-Sol; Betaxin; Bevitine; Bevitol; Bewon; Neuramin; Vita-B1. It is an ingredient of Labiton and Quiet Life.
$C_{12}H_{17}ClN_4OS,HCl=337.3$
CAS—67-03-8
Colourless crystals or white crystalline powder. M.p. 248°, with decomposition.
Soluble 1 in about 1 of water, 1 in 100 of 95% ethanol and 1 in 18 of glycerol; practically insoluble in dehydrated alcohol, benzene, hexane, chloroform and ether; soluble in methanol.

Thiamine Mononitrate

Synonyms. Aneurine Mononitrate; Thiamine Nitrate; Vitamin B_1 Mononitrate.
Proprietary name. B_1-Vicotrat
$C_{12}H_{17}N_5O_4S=327.4$
CAS—532-43-4
White crystals or crystalline powder. M.p. 196° to 200°, with decomposition.
Soluble 1 in 44 of water; slightly soluble in ethanol and chloroform.

Dissociation Constant. pK_a 4.8 (20°).

Partition Coefficient. Log *P* (octanol/water), −3.9.

Colour Test. Dissolve about 5 mg of thiamine hydrochloride in a mixture of 1 mL of lead acetate solution and 1 mL of 10% sodium hydroxide solution—yellow; after heating on a steam-bath—brown; on standing—a black precipitate of lead sulfide.

Thin-layer Chromatography. Thiamine hydrochloride: system TA—Rf 01; system TB—Rf 00; system TC—Rf 00; system TE—Rf 01; system TL—Rf 00; system TAE—Rf 02; system TAF—Rf 18. (Acidified iodoplatinate solution, positive.)

Gas Chromatography. System GA—not eluted.

High Performance Liquid Chromatography. System HA—*k* 2.0; system HX—RI 09 (hydrochloride); system HY—RI 21 (hydrochloride).

Ultraviolet Spectrum. Aqueous acid—246 nm ($A_1^1=450a$); aqueous alkali—232 nm ($A_1^1=566b$), 336 nm.

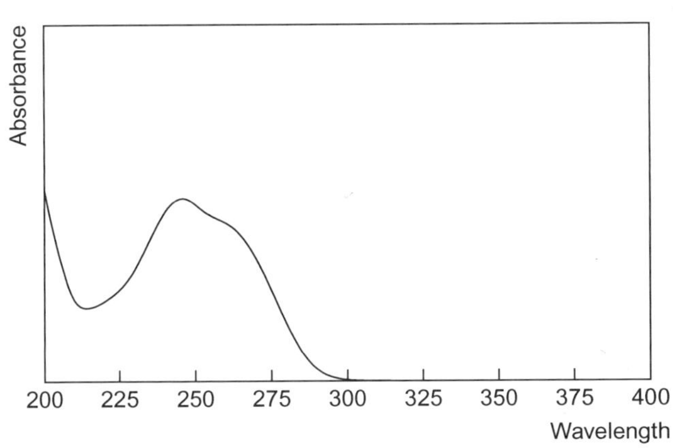

Infra-red Spectrum. Principal peaks at wavenumbers 1660, 1618, 1048, 1237, 1595, 1228 cm^{-1} (thiamine hydrochloride, KBr disk).

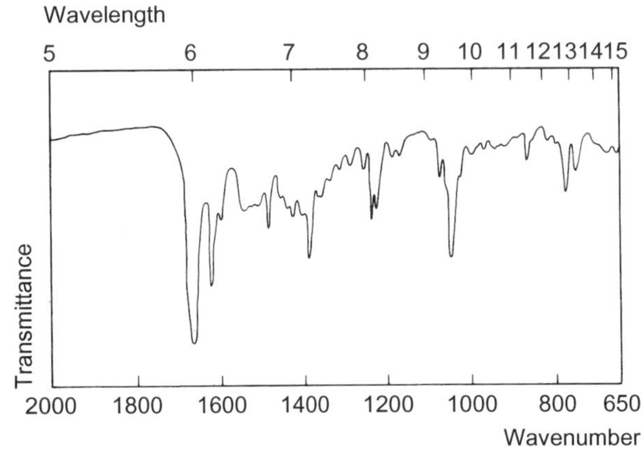

Quantification

High performance liquid chromatography. In plasma: limit of detection 150 ng/L, fluorescence detection—W. Weber and H. Kewitz, *Eur. J. Clin. Pharmacol.*, 1985, *28*, 213–219.

Disposition in the Body. Well absorbed from the gastro-intestinal tract and widely distributed throughout the body. It is converted in the body to thiamine pyrophosphate. Thiamine is not stored to any appreciable extent in the body and amounts in excess of the body's requirements are excreted in the urine unchanged or as metabolites. About 1 mg of thiamine is metabolised in the body daily.

Blood concentration. Endogenous blood concentrations are about 0.010 to 0.015 mg/L and concentrations of thiamine pyrophosphate in erythrocytes are usually 0.03 to 0.11 mg/L.

Endogenous plasma concentrations in 91 subjects ranged from 0.002 to 0.013 mg/L (median 0.004) [W. Weber and H. Kewitz, *Eur. J. Clin. Pharmacol.*, 1985, *28*, 213–219].

Note. For a general review of thiamine see H. Inui and Y. Nakano, *Nippon Rinsho*, 1999, *57*, 2187–2192.

Dose. 10 to 100 mg daily.

Thiamylal

Barbiturate

Dihydro-5-(1-methylbutyl)-5-(2-propenyl)-2-thioxo-4,6(1*H*,5*H*)-pyrimidinedione
$C_{12}H_{18}N_2O_2S=254.3$
CAS—77-27-0

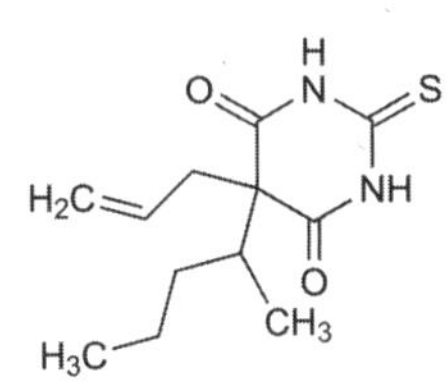

Crystals. M.p. 132° to 133°.

Sodium Thiamylal

Proprietary name. Surital
$C_{12}H_{17}N_2NaO_2S=276.3$
CAS—337-47-3
Thiamylal sodium for injection is a mixture of sodium thiamylal with anhydrous sodium carbonate. It is a pale yellow hygroscopic powder.
Soluble in water.

Dissociation Constant. pK_a 7.5.

Partition Coefficient. Log *P* (octanol/water), 3.23.

Thin-layer Chromatography. System TE—Rf 55; system TF—Rf 75.

Gas Chromatography. System GA—RI 1899.

Column: glass coil packed with 3% poly-A-103 on Gas Chrom Q (80–100 mesh) (0.5 m × 2.6 mm i.d.). Column and injector temperatures: 255° and 270°, respectively. Carrier gas: helium, flow rate 40 mL/min. IS: thiopental. MS detection (EI, SIM at *m/z* 184 for thiamylal and 172 for IS). Retention time(s): thiamylal, 1.2 min; IS, 1.1 min [K. Kudo *et al.*, *Forensic Sci. Int.*, 1988, *37(3)*, 193–200).

High Performance Liquid Chromatography. System HX—RI 516; system HY—RI 476.

Column: Chiral-AGP (100 × 4.0 mm i.d.); guard, Chiral-AGP (10 × 3.0 mm). Mobile phase: 20 mM potassium dihydrogen phosphate containing 3% 2-propanol, pH 4.7, flow rate 0.9 mL/min. UV detection (λ = 288 nm). Retention time(s): *R*-(+)-thiamylal, 10.0 min; *S*-(−)-thiamylal, 11.7 min [M. Sueyasu *et al.*, *J. Chromatogr.*, 1995, *665(1)*; *Biomed. Appl.*, 133–137].

Ultraviolet Spectrum. Aqueous acid—238, 287 nm; aqueous alkali—305 nm.

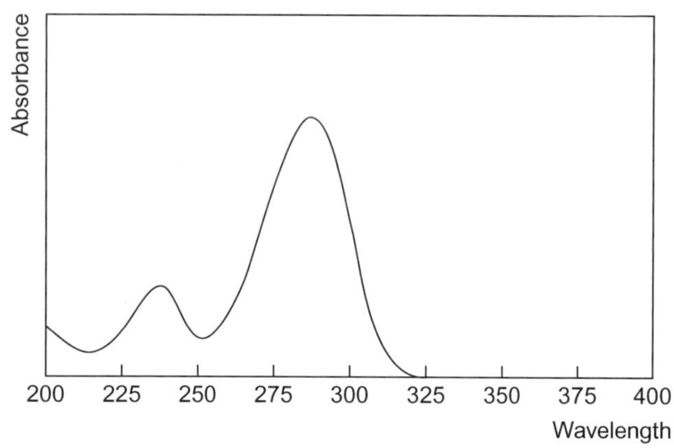

Infra-red Spectrum. Principal peaks at wavenumbers 1668, 1541, 1731, 1170, 1318, 1291 cm^{-1} (KBr disk).

Mass Spectrum. Principal ions at *m/z* 43, 41, 184, 168, 167, 97, 55, 53.

Quantification

Gas chromatography–mass spectrometry. In biological samples: limit of detection is 0.01 μg/g—K. Kudo *et al.*, *Forensic Sci. Int.*, 1988, *37*, 193–200.

High performance liquid chromatography. In serum: limit of quantification 0.05 mg/L, UV detection (λ = 288 nm)—M. Sueyasu *et al.*, *J. Chromatogr.*, 1995, *665(1)*; *Biomed. Appl.*, 133–137.

Disposition in the Body

Therapeutic concentration

6 patients with liver dysfunction, aged 0.3 to 72 years, were intravenously administered with a total dose of 15.1 to 307.4 mg/kg (concentration of 25 or 50 g/L; infusion rate 0.45 to 4.0 mg/kg/h, over a period of 4.7 to 108.3 h). The unbound *R*-(+)-thiamylal serum concentration was 0.57 to 3.11 mg/L and the total concentration was 2.94 to 18.51 mg/L. The unbound *S*-(−)-thiamylal concentration was 0.78 to 3.74 mg/L and total 5.28 to 33.35 mg/L. All concentrations were observed after 10 min following administration [M. Sueyasu *et al.*, *Int. J. Clin. Pharmacol. Ther.*, 1997, *35(3)*, 128–132].

Toxicity

A fatal intoxication of intravenous thiamylal administration is reported. After toxicological analysis, thiamylal was detected in blood at a concentration of 129 mg/L; in liver 366 μg/g and in brain 116 μg/g. It was not detected in urine, gastric contents or bile [T. L. Stockham *et al.*, *J. Anal. Toxicol.*, 1991, *15(3)*, 155–156].

A 28-year-old student was found dead at his hotel room, hanging by his neck, and was intravenously connected to a bottle of thiamylal sodium. Thiamylal was detected at a concentration of 29 mg/L in blood, 1.4 mg/L in urine, 16 mg/L in bile and was present in liver at 135 μg/g, in kidney 25 μg/g and was present in his stomach contents at 0.4 mg. Alcohol and other drugs were not detected in the blood [A. G. Costantino *et al.*, *J. Forensic Sci.*, 1990, *35(1)*, 89–96].

Dose. Initially 3 to 6 mL of a 2.5% solution of sodium thiamylal intravenously.

Thiazinamium Metilsulfate

Antihistamine

Synonyms. Methylpromethazinium Methylsulfuricum; Thiazinamium Methylsulfate; RP-3554.

Proprietary name. Multergan

N,N,N-α-Tetramethyl-10*H*-phenothiazine-10-ethanaminium methyl sulfate

$C_{19}H_{26}N_2O_4S_2$=410.6

CAS—2338-21-8 (thiazinamium); 58-34-4 (metilsulfate)

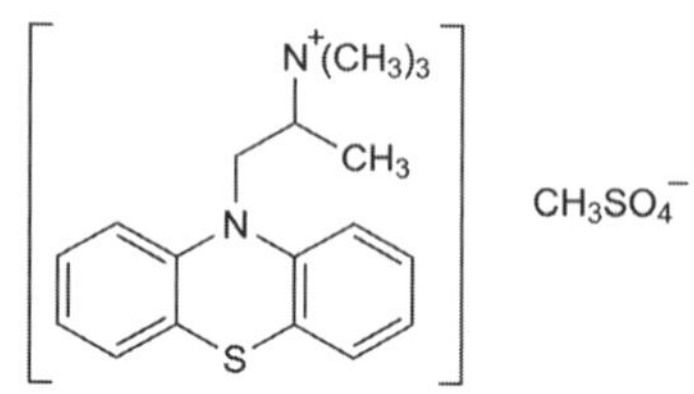

A white crystalline powder which discolours on exposure to light. M.p. 206° to 210°, with decomposition.

Soluble 1 in 10 of water; very soluble in ethanol; practically insoluble in ether.

Partition Coefficient. Log *P* (octanol/water), 2.7.

Colour Tests. Formaldehyde–Sulfuric acid—brown-violet; Forrest reagent—red; FPN reagent—red; Liebermann's test—red.

Thin-layer Chromatography. System TA—Rf 02; system TAE—thiazinamium metilsulfate Rf 01; M (sulfoxide) Rf 00; system TAF—Rf 25; system TL—Rf 00; system TB—thiazinamium metilsulfate Rf 00; M (sulfoxide) Rf 00; system TC—Rf 00; system TE—thiazinamium metilsulfate Rf 00; M (sulfoxide) Rf 00; system TF—M (sulfoxide) Rf 00. (Acidified iodoplatinate solution, positive.)

Gas Chromatography. System GA—RI 2339; system GB—RI 2383 (both for thiazinamium methylsulfate Art (promethazine)).

High Performance Liquid Chromatography. System HX—RI 326 (M-sulfoxide); system HZ—Retention time(s) 6.4 min.

Ultraviolet Spectrum. Aqueous acid—251 (A_1^1=450b), 299 nm.

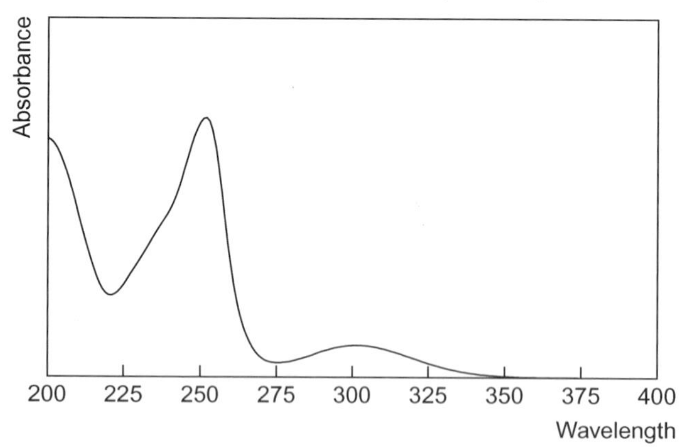

Infra-red Spectrum. Principal peaks at wavenumbers 1224, 1010, 1059, 764, 743, 1036 cm^{-1}.

Quantification

Gas chromatography. In plasma or urine: limit of detection 20 μg/L, AFID—J. H. G. Jonkman *et al.*, *J. Pharm. Pharmacol.*, 1975, *27*, 849–854.

Disposition in the Body. Thiazinamium metilsulfate is incompletely absorbed after oral administration and undergoes considerable first-pass metabolism to thiazinamium sulfoxide; it is well absorbed after IM administration. About 40% of a parenteral dose is excreted in the urine unchanged in 8 hours, together with 9% of the dose as the sulfoxide.

Therapeutic concentration

Following single oral doses equivalent to 300 mg and 900 mg of thiazinamium to 10 subjects, peak plasma concentrations of 0.03 to 0.13 (mean 0.07) mg/L and 0.06 to 0.36 (mean 0.17) mg/L were attained in about

2.4 h and 5 h, respectively [J. H. G. Jonkman *et al.*, *Clin. Pharmacol. Ther.*, 1977, *21*, 457–463].

Dose. 0.6 to 1.2 g daily.

Thiethylperazine

Anti-emetic

2-(Ethylthio)-10-[3-(4-methyl-1-piperazinyl)propyl]phenothiazine
$C_{22}H_{29}N_3S_2=399.6$
CAS—1420-55-9

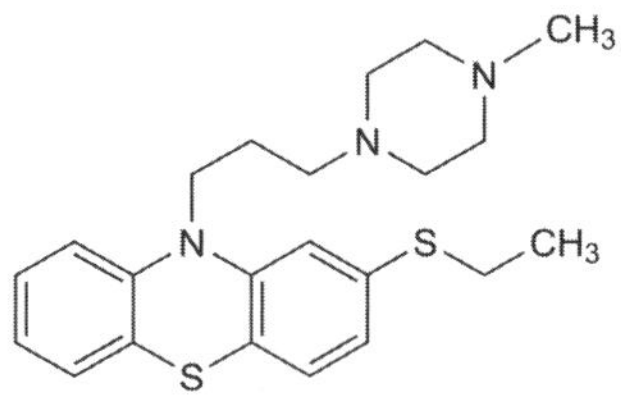

Crystals. M.p. 62° to 64°.
Practically insoluble in water.

Thiethylperazine Malate
Proprietary name. Torecan (injection)
$C_{22}H_{29}N_3S_2,2C_4H_6O_5=667.8$
CAS—52239-63-1
A white to faintly yellow crystalline powder. M.p. 139°.
Soluble 1 in 40 of water, 1 in 90 of ethanol, 1 in 525 of chloroform and 1 in 3400 of ether.

Thiethylperazine Maleate
Proprietary name. Torecan (suppositories and tablets)
$C_{22}H_{29}N_3S_2,2C_4H_4O_4=631.8$
CAS—1179-69-7
A yellowish granular powder. M.p. about 188° to 190°, with decomposition.
Soluble 1 in 1700 of water and 1 in 530 of ethanol; practically insoluble in chloroform and ether.

Partition Coefficient Log *P* (octanol/water), 5.4.

Colour Tests. Formaldehyde–Sulfuric acid—green; Forrest reagent—blue; FPN reagent—blue; Mandelin's test—violet; Marquis test—red→green.

Thin-layer Chromatography. System TA—Rf 51; system TB—Rf 30; system TC—Rf 41; system TE—thiethylperazine Rf 52; M Rf 30; system TL—Rf 08; system TAE—thiethylperazine Rf 27; M Rf 13; system TAJ—Rf 22; system TAK—Rf 11; system TAL—Rf 83. (Acidified iodoplatinate solution, positive.)

Gas Chromatography. System GA—RI 3247.

High Performance Liquid Chromatography. System HA—*k* 3.8; system HX—RI 487; system HZ—Retention time(s) 16.3 min.

Ultraviolet Spectrum. Aqueous acid—255 ($A_1^1=857b$), 309 nm ($A_1^1=98b$).

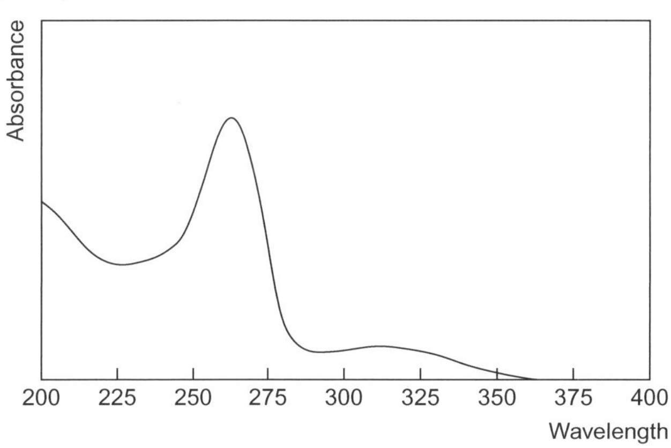

Infra-red Spectrum. Principal peaks at wavenumbers 1563, 864, 1613, 1212, 1105, 1067 cm^{-1} (KBr disk).

Mass Spectrum. Principal ions at *m*/*z* 70, 113, 141, 399, 43, 26, 72, 42.

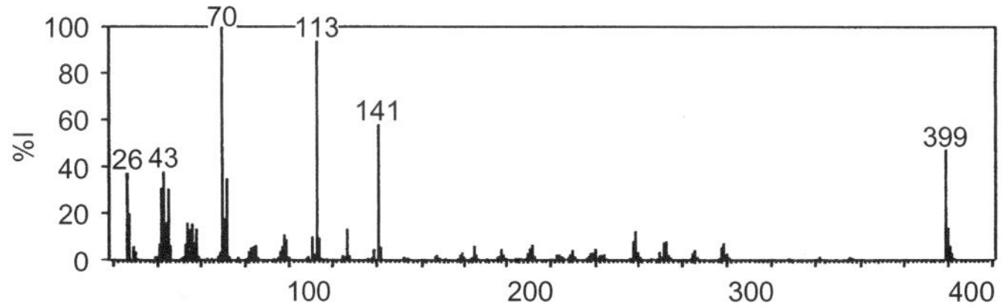

Quantification
Gas chromatography. In blood or urine: thiethylperazine and other phenothiazines, limit of detection 250 to 500 ng/L, SID—H. Hattori *et al.*, *J. Chromatogr.*, 1992, *579*, 247–252.

High performance liquid chromatography–mass spectrometry. In blood: limit of detection 0.5 μg/L—H. Seno *et al.*, *Rapid Comm. Mass Spectrom.*, 1999, *13*, 2394–2398.

Dose. Usually 20 to 30 mg of thiethylperazine maleate daily.

Thioacetazone

Antibacterial/Tuberculostatic

Synonyms. Amithiozone; Tebezonum; Thiacetazone; TbI-698.
Proprietary Names. Conteben; Livazore; Neustab; Panrone; Seroden.
N-[4-[[(Aminothioxomethyl)hydrazono]methyl]phenyl]acetamide
$C_{10}H_{12}N_4OS=236.3$
CAS—104-06-3

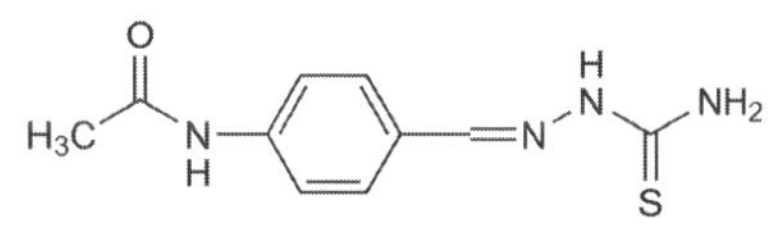

Pale yellow crystals or crystalline powder. M.p. 225° to 230°, with decompostion.
Insoluble in water, acetone, benzene and chloroform; soluble 1 in 500 of ethanol and 1 in 100 of propylene glycol; practically insoluble in ether.

Partition Coefficient. Log *P* (octanol/water), 1.1.

Colour Tests. Nessler's reagent (100°)—black; Palladium chloride—orange.

Thin-layer Chromatography System TA—Rf 78. (Acidified iodoplatinate solution, positive.)

Gas Chromatography. System GA—RI 2038.

Ultraviolet Spectrum. Ethanol—328 nm ($A_1^1=1870a$).

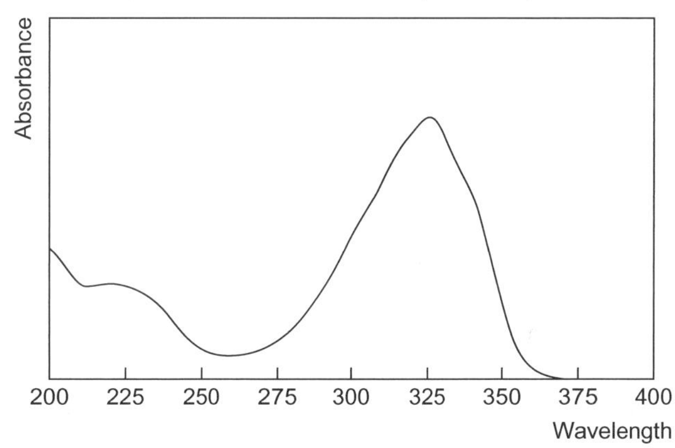

Infra-red Spectrum. Principal peaks at wavenumbers 1515, 1603, 1580, 1661, 1250, 1305 cm^{-1} (KBr disk).

Quantification
High performance liquid chromatography. In plasma or urine: limit of detection 3 μg/L, UV detection—P. J. Jenner, *J. Chromatogr.*, 1983, *276*;

Biomed. Appl., *27*, 463–470; P. J. Jenner *et al.*, *Lepr. Rev.*, 1984, *55*, 121–128.

Disposition in the Body. Thioacetazone is slowly absorbed after oral administration. Most of a dose is metabolised and excreted in the urine; about 20% of a dose is excreted in the urine unchanged.

Therapeutic concentration

Following a single oral dose of 4 mg/kg to 10 subjects, peak serum concentrations of 1.3 to 4.0 (mean 3.1) mg/L were attained in about 5 h [P. K. Sen *et al.*, *J. Indian Med. Assoc.*, 1973, *61*, 306–308].

Half-life. About 8 to 12 h.

Dose. Up to 150 mg daily.

Thiopental

Barbiturate

Synonyms. Penthiobarbital; Thiomebumal; Thiopentone.

5-Ethyldihydro-5-(1-methylbutyl)-2-thio-4,6(1*H*,3*H*,5*H*)-pyrimidinedione

$C_{11}H_{18}N_2O_2S = 242.3$

CAS—76-75-5

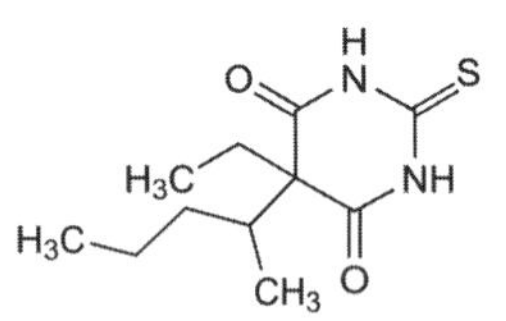

Thiopental Sodium

Synonyms. Penthiobarbital Sodique; Soluble Thiopentone; Thiomebumalnatrium cum Natrii Carbonate; Thiopental Sodium and Sodium Carbonate; Thiopentalum Natricum; Thiopentobarbitalum Solubile; Thiopentone Sodium.

Proprietary names. Farmotal; Intraval Sodium; Nesdonal; Pentothal; Trapanal.

$C_{11}H_{17}N_2NaO_2S = 264.3$

CAS—71-73-8

A white to yellowish-white to pale green, hygroscopic powder. It usually contains anhydrous sodium carbonate in the proportion of 6 parts to each 100 parts of thiopental sodium.

Soluble 1 in 1.5 of water; partly soluble in ethanol; insoluble in ether, benzene and petroleum ether.

Dissociation Constant. pK_a 7.6 (20°).

Partition Coefficient. Log *P* (octanol/water), 2.85.

Colour Tests. Koppanyi–Zwikker Test—violet; Palladium Chloride—orange; Vanillin Reagent—brown-red/violet.

Thin-layer Chromatography. System TD—Rf 77; system TE—Rf 49; system TF—Rf 74; system TH—Rf 80; system TAD—Rf 68. Thiopental sodium: system TAJ—Rf 73; system TAK—Rf 71; system TAL—Rf 92. (Mercuric chloride–diphenylcarbazone reagent, positive; mercurous nitrate spray, black; acidified potassium permanganate solution, yellow-brown; Zwikker's reagent, green.)

Gas Chromatography. System GA—thiopental RI 1857, thiopental-Me_2 RI 1825, pentobarbital RI 1735; system GB—thiopental RI 1923, M (OH-) RI 2134; system GF—RI 2600; system GAJ—RRT 0.948 (relative to methylphenobarbital).

High Performance Liquid Chromatography. System HX—RI 485; system HY—RI 433; system HZ—Retention time, 6.9 min; system HAA—Retention time, 19.2 min.

Column: ODS C_{18} (150 × 4.6 mm i.d., 4 μm). Mobile phase: water:methanol:acetonitrile (50:40:10), adjusted to pH 2.70 with phosphoric acid, flow rate 1.5 mL/min. UV detection (λ = 290 nm). IS: tolylbarb. Retention time(s): thiopental, 9.5 min; thiopental isomer, 8.4 min; IS, 5.4 min [G. Coppa *et al.*, *Clin. Chim. Acta*, 2001, *305*, 41–45].

Column: C_8 (Whatman PatriSphere, 110 × 4.6 mm i.d.. Mobile phase: 50% acetonitrile:phosphate buffer (120 mM, pH 6.2) UV detection (270 nm). Retention time 4.3 min [R. W. Schmid and C. Wolf, *J. Pharm. Biomed. Anal.*, 1989, *7(12)*, 1749–1755].

Column: Chiral AGP (100 × 4.0 mm i.d.); guard, (10 × 3.0 mm i.d.). Mobile phase: 20 mM phosphate buffer:2-propanol:methanol (93.5:5.0:1.5), pH 5.0, flow rate 0.9 mL/min. UV detection. *k* value (Retention time(s)): (*R*)-(+)-thiopental, 2.7 (4.8 min); (*S*)-(−)-thiopental, 3.7 (6.2 min) [D. J. Jones *et al.*, *J. Chromatogr.*, 1996, *67(1)*; *Biomed. Appl.*, 174–179].

Ultraviolet Spectrum. Borax buffer 0.05 M (pH 9.2)—255, 304 nm (A_1^1 = 1138b); 1 M sodium hydroxide (pH 13)—303 nm (A_1^1 = 1170b).

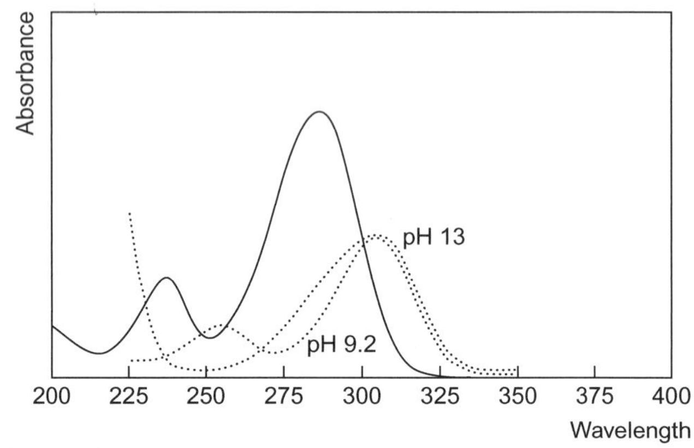

Infra-red Spectrum. Principal peaks at wavenumbers 1670, 1540, 1300, 1170, 1735, 1220 cm^{-1} (KBr disk).

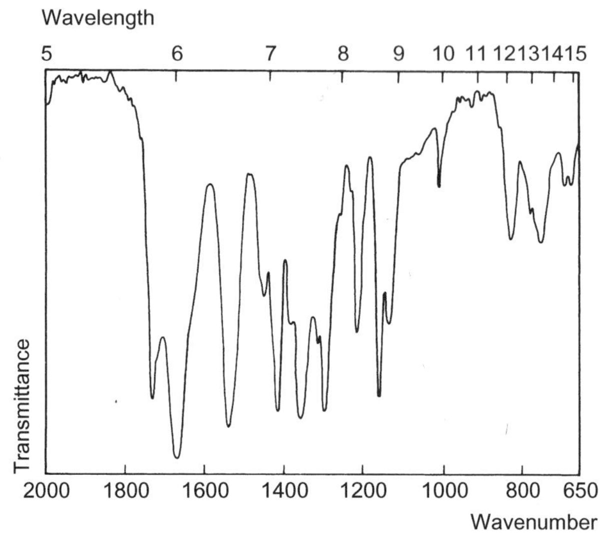

Mass Spectrum. Principal ions at *m*/*z* 172, 157, 173, 43, 41, 55, 69, 71.

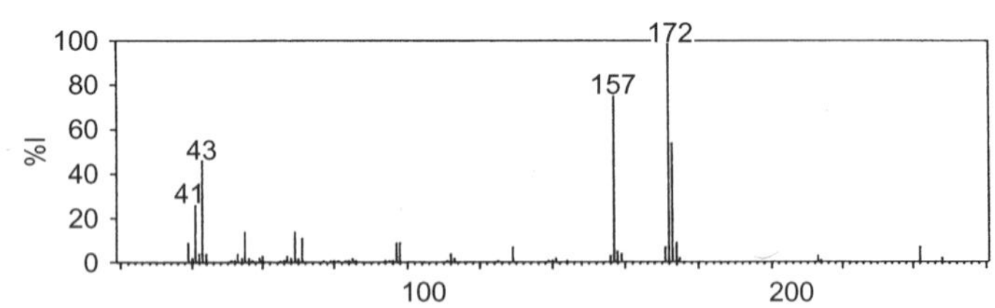

Quantification. See also under Amylobarbital.

Gas chromatography. In plasma: limit of detection 0.025 mg/L, AFID—D. Jung *et al.*, *Clin. Chem.*, 1981, *27*, 113–115.

High performance liquid chromatography. In plasma: limit of detection 0.2 mg/L, UV detection—C. Salvadori *et al.*, *Ther. Drug Monit.*, 1981, *3*, 171–176. In blood or tissues: limit of detection 1 mg/L, UV detection—B. Levine *et al.*, *J. Anal. Toxicol.*, 1983, *7*, 207–208. In plasma: limit of quantification 0.01 mg/L, UV detection (λ = 280 nm)—D. J. Jones *et al.*, *J. Chromatogr.*, 1996, *675*; *Biomed. Appl.*, 174–179. In blood: limit of detection 0.2 mg/L, UV detection (λ = 270 nm)—R. W. Schmid and C. Wolf, *J. Pharm. Biomed. Anal.*, 1989, *7*, 1749–1755. In serum: limit of detection 0.1 mg/L, UV detection ($\lambda = 280$ nm)—P. Altmayer *et al.*, *Methods Find Exp. Clin. Pharmacol.*, 1987, *9(12)*, 817–822.

Disposition in the Body. About 10% of a dose is concentrated in the brain within 1 min of an intravenous injection and it is then rapidly distributed throughout the body, eventually accumulating in body fat; about 50% of a dose accumulates in this way after 30 to 90 min. The very short action of thiopental is due to the brief α-phase half-life and the redistribution of the drug from the brain to other fatty tissues. Metabolic reactions include ω-hydroxylation, further oxidation and, to a lesser extent, desulfuration to pentobarbital. Metabolism occurs almost exclusively in the liver and mostly inactive metabolites are produced. Less than 1% of a dose is excreted in the urine as unchanged drug. 5-(3-Carboxy-1-methylpropyl)-5-ethyl-2-thiobarbituric acid has been reported to be a urinary metabolite. Repeated or continuous administration of thiopental may result in accumulation of the drug in fatty tissues which may result in extended anaesthesia and possibly respiratory and/or cardiovascular depression. Thiopental readily diffuses across the placenta and has been detected in breast milk.

Therapeutic concentration

Plasma concentrations of 4.2 to 134 mg/L (mean 28) were reported in 22 patients after intravenous injections [K. E. Becker, *Anesthesiology*, 1976, *45*, 656–660].

After multiple intravenous doses of 250 (5 subjects) or 500 mg (2 subjects) every 2 h for up to 7 days to neurosurgical patients, the steady-state trough plasma concentrations were 4.8 to 30 mg/L (mean 16.0) and the peak concentrations were 8.35 to 45 mg/L (mean 25.4) [H. Russo *et al.*, *Eur. J. Clin. Pharmacol.*, 1995, *49*, 127–137].

Toxicity. The estimated minimum lethal dose is 1 g. Numerous fatalities have occurred owing to accidental or intentional overdosage, and blood concentrations from 6 to 392 mg/L have been reported in fatalities.

The following postmortem tissue distribution was reported in one suicide case: blood 6 mg/L, brain 24 µg/g, heart 22 µg/g, kidney 31 µg/g, and liver 63 µg/g [A. M. Bruce *et al.*, *Forensic Sci.*, 1977, *9*, 205–207].

In a fatality caused by intravenous self-administration of thiopental, the following postmortem tissue concentrations were reported: blood 285 mg/L, brain 414 µg/g, kidney 195 µg/g, liver 440 µg/g [E. Reed and J. R. Monforte, *Bull. Int. Assoc. Forensic Toxicol.*, 1973, *9 (3&4)*, 12].

The blood concentration of an individual who died following intravenous administration of a clinical dose was 0.6 mg/L. The brain concentration was 11.9 mg/kg and thiopental was also detected in the thymus at a concentration of 7.66 µg/g [T. Yasuda *et al.*, *Int. J. Legal Med.*, 1993, *105(4)*, 239–241].

Half-life. Plasma half-life, 4 to 20 h (mean 9), increased after high doses (25 mg/min), up to 60 h.

Volume of distribution. 0.5 to 4 L/kg.

Clearance. Plasma clearance, 1 to 4 mL/min/kg.

Distribution in blood. Plasma : whole blood ratio, 1.0.

Protein binding. In plasma, about 75 to 90%.

Dose. Premedicated adults, 100 to 150 mg of thiopental sodium intravenously over 10 to 15 s (25 g/L solution), repeated if necessary, or up to 4 mg/kg. Children, 2 to 7 mg/kg.

Thiopropazate

Tranquilliser

4-[3-(2-Chlorophenothiazin-10-yl)propyl]-1-piperazineethanol acetate
$C_{23}H_{28}ClN_3O_2S = 446.0$
CAS—84-06-0

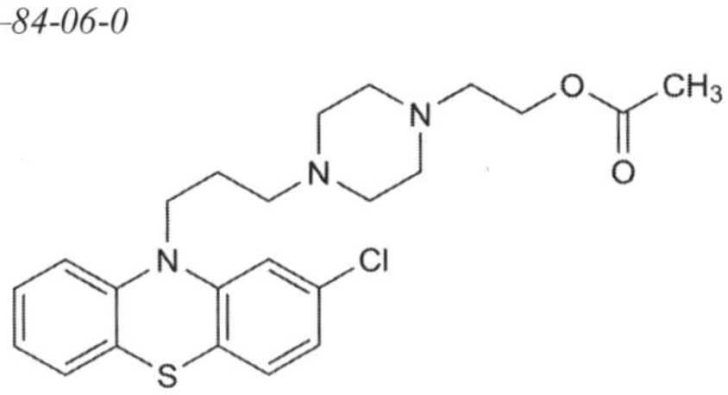

Practically insoluble in water; soluble in chloroform and ether.

Thiopropazate Hydrochloride

Proprietary names. Dartal; Dartalan.
$C_{23}H_{28}ClN_3O_2S,2HCl = 518.9$
CAS—146-28-1

A white or pale yellow crystalline powder. M.p. 223° to 229°, with decomposition.

Soluble 1 in 4 of water, 1 in 130 of ethanol and 1 in 65 of chloroform; practically insoluble in ether.

Caution. Thiopropazate hydrochloride may cause severe dermatitis in sensitised persons.

Dissociation Constant. pK_a 7.3 (24°).

Partition Coefficient. Log *P* (octanol/water), 4.8.

Colour Tests. Formaldehyde–Sulfuric acid—red-violet; Forrest reagent—red; FPN reagent—red; Liebermann's test—green-brown; Mandelin's test—violet; Marquis test—violet.

Thin-layer Chromatography. System TA—Rf 61; system TB—Rf 35; system TC—Rf 53; system TE—thiopropazate Rf 74; M Rf 46; system TL—Rf 42; system TAE—thiopropazate Rf 62; M Rf 48; system TAF—Rf 59; system TAJ—Rf 52; system TAK—Rf 36; system TAL—Rf 91. (Dragendorff spray, positive; FPN reagent, pink; Acidified iodoplatinate solution, positive; Marquis reagent, red; Ninhydrin spray, positive.)

Gas Chromatography. System GA—RI 3467 (metabolised to perphenazine, see monograph for data).

High Performance Liquid Chromatography. System HA—*k* 1.0; system HX—RI 483.

Ultraviolet Spectrum. Aqueous acid—255 (A^1_1=733a), 305; aqueous alkali—257 nm.

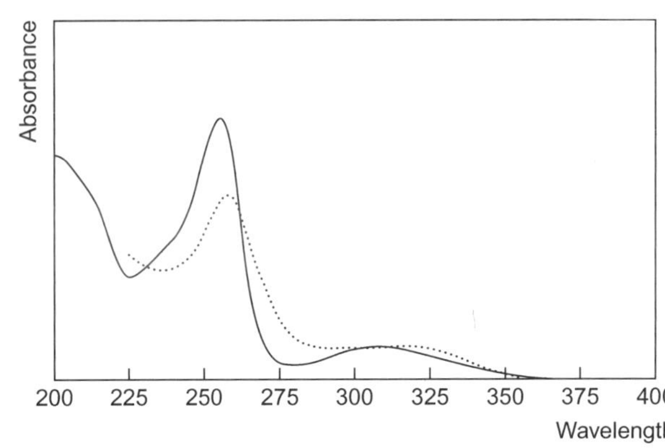

Infra-red Spectrum. Principal peaks at wavenumbers 1222, 1728, 746, 1265, 1250, 1200 cm^{-1} (thiopropazate hydrochloride, KBr disk).

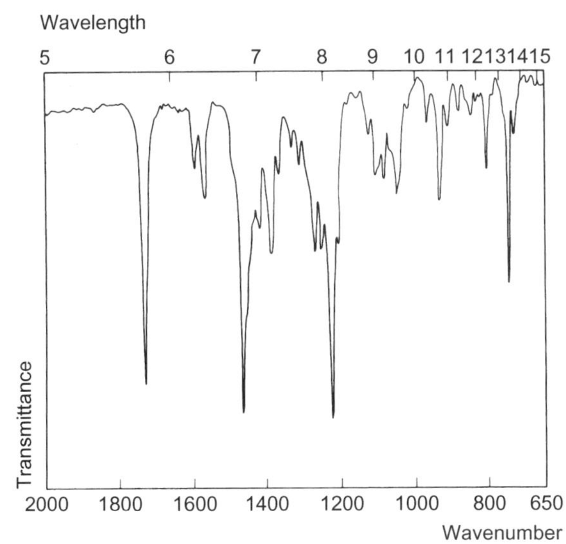

Mass Spectrum. Principal ions at *m/z* 42, 43, 70, 246, 185, 55, 56, 445.

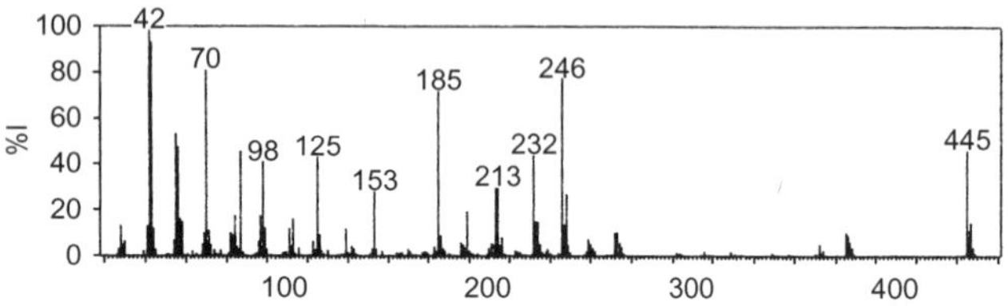

Dose. Initially 15 to 30 mg of thiopropazate hydrochloride daily; maximum of 100 mg daily.

Thioproperazine

Tranquilliser

Synonyms. RP-7843; SKF-5883.
N,*N*-Dimethyl-10-[3-(4-methyl-1-piperazinyl)propyl]phenothiazine-2-sulfonamide
$C_{22}H_{30}N_4O_2S_2$=446.6
CAS—316-81-4

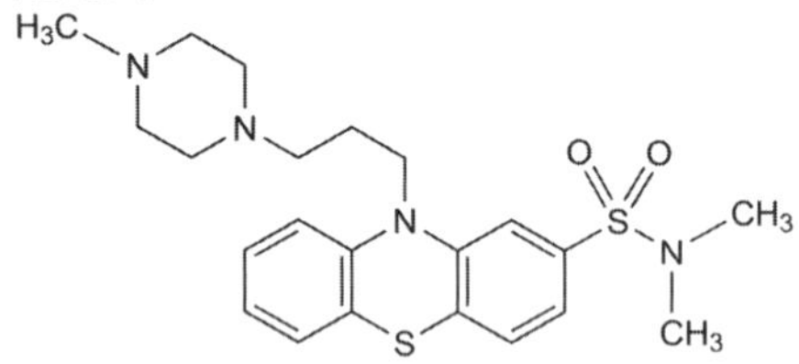

Crystals. M.p. 140°.
Practically insoluble in water.

Thioproperazine Mesilate
Synonyms. Thioproperazine Dimethanesulfonate; Thioproperazine Mesylate; Thioproperazine Methanesulfonate.
Proprietary name. Majeptil; Vontil
$C_{22}H_{30}N_4O_2S_2,2CH_4O_3S$=638.8
CAS—2347-80-0
A fine, white or pale cream powder, which becomes coloured on exposure to light. M.p. about 227°.
Soluble in water; slightly soluble in ethanol.

Partition Coefficient Log *P* (octanol/water), 2.9.

Colour Tests. Formaldehyde–Sulfuric acid—pink; Forrest reagent—red; FPN reagent—orange; Mandelin's test—brown→green→violet; Marquis test—red.

Thin-layer Chromatography. System TA—Rf 46; system TB—Rf 07; system TC—Rf 34; system TE—thioproperazine Rf 43; M Rf 26; system TL—Rf 06; system TAE—thioproperazine Rf 22; M Rf 13; system TAF—Rf 22. (Acidified iodoplatinate solution, positive.)

Gas Chromatography. System GA—thioproperazine RI 3552; M (ring) RI 3200.

High Performance Liquid Chromatography. System HA—*k* 4.1; system HX—RI 427; system HY—RI 305; system HZ—Retention time(s) 15.4 min; system HAA—Retention time(s) 15.2 min.

Ultraviolet Spectrum. Aqueous acid—234, 263 (A^1_1=668a), 312 nm. No alkaline shift.

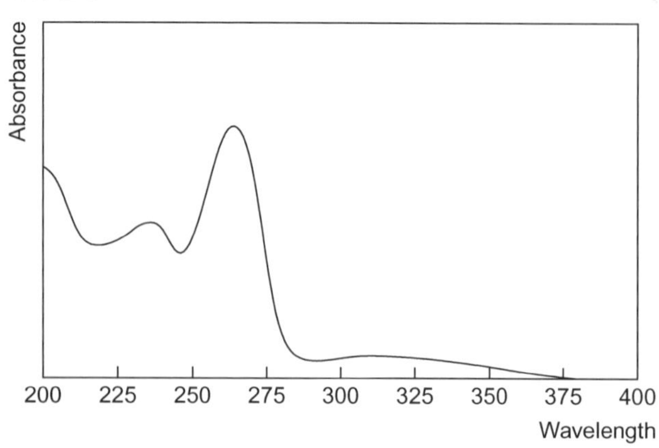

Infra-red Spectrum. Principal peaks at wavenumbers 1156, 1042, 1212, 720, 960, 762 cm^{-1} (thioproperazine mesilate, Nujol mull).

Mass Spectrum. Principal ions at *m/z* 79, 96, 31, 113, 81, 70, 127, 78.

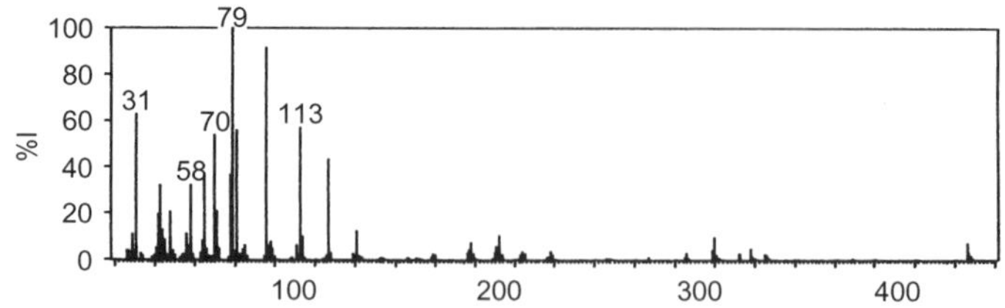

Quantification
Gas chromatography. In blood or urine: limit of detection 250–500 ng/L, SID—H Hattori *et al.*, *J. Chromatogr.*, 1992, *579*, 247–252.

Dose. Usually 15 to 30 mg of thioproperazine mesilate daily; up to 90 mg daily has been given.

Thioridazine

Tranquilliser

Proprietary names. Mellaril-S; Melleretten; Melleril; Rideril.
10-[2-(1-Methyl-2-piperidinyl)ethyl]-2-(methylthio)-10*H*-phenothiazine
$C_{21}H_{26}N_2S_2$=370.6
CAS—50-52-2

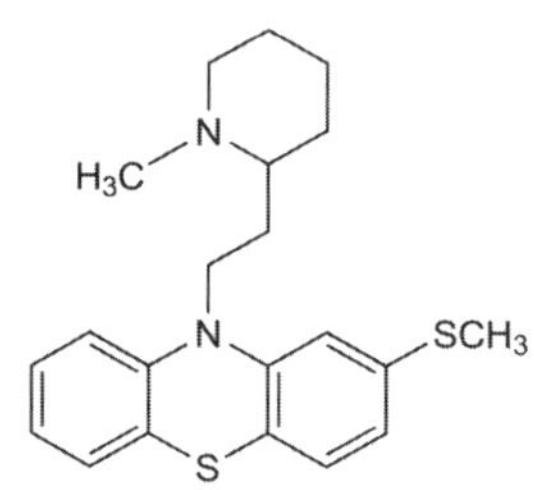

A white or slightly yellow crystalline powder which darkens on exposure to light. M.p. 72° to 74°.
Practically insoluble in water; soluble 1 in 6 of ethanol, 1 in 0.8 of chloroform and 1 in 3 of ether; freely soluble in dehydrated alcohol.

Thioridazine Hydrochloride
Proprietary names. Aldazine; Mallorol; Mellaril; Melleretten (tablets); Melleril (tablets); Melzine; Novoridazine; Orsanil; Thioril; Thiozine.
$C_{21}H_{26}N_2S_2,HCl$=407.0
CAS—130-61-0
A white or slightly yellow crystalline powder. M.p. 158° to 160° (from acetone). Soluble 1 in 9 of water, 1 in 10 of ethanol and 1 in 1.5 of chloroform; freely soluble in methanol; practically insoluble in ether.

Dissociation Constant. pK_a 9.5 (24°).

Partition Coefficient. Log *P* (octanol/water), 5.90.

Colour Tests. Formaldehyde–Sulfuric Acid—blue; Forrest Reagent—blue; FPN Reagent—blue; Mandelin's Test—blue→violet; Marquis Test—violet-red→blue-green.

Thin-layer Chromatography. System TA—Rf 48; system TB—Rf 42; system TC—Rf 30; system TE—Rf 67; system TL—Rf 13; system TAE—Rf 20; system TAF—Rf 55; system TAJ—Rf 09; system TAK—Rf 02; system TAL—Rf 51. (Dragendorff spray, positive; Marquis reagent, grey-violet.)

Gas Chromatography. System GA—thioridazine RI 3115, mesoridazine RI 3380, M (oxo-) RI 3500, M (ring sulfone) RI 3420, M (side chain sulfone) RI 3800; system GB—thioridazine RI 3292, M (nor-) RI 3275, mesoridazine RI 3629, M (ring) RI 2639, M (ring sulfone) RI 3626; system GW—Retention time 31.1 min.

High Performance Liquid Chromatography. System HA—thioridazine *k* 5.2, mesoridazine *k* 5.0; system HX—RI 490; system HY—RI 427; system HZ—Retention time 13.5 min; system HAA—Retention time

17.2 min; system HAM—not detected; system HAX—not eluted; system HAY—Retention time 9.8 min; system HAZ—*k* 3.88.

Ultraviolet Spectrum. Aqueous acid—262 nm (A_1^1=987a), 310 nm; (0.1 M hydrochloric acid)—230, 263 nm; aqueous alkali—275 nm; (0.1 M sodium hydroxide)—313 nm.

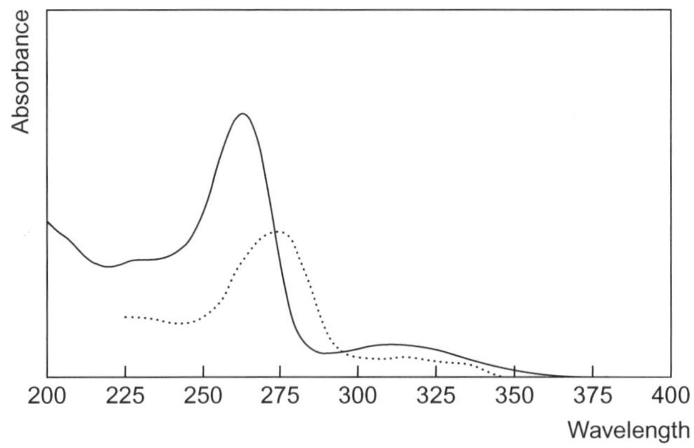

Infra-red Spectrum. Principal peaks at wavenumbers 754, 1248, 796, 1234, 1281, 1211 cm^{-1} (thioridazine hydrochloride, KBr disk).

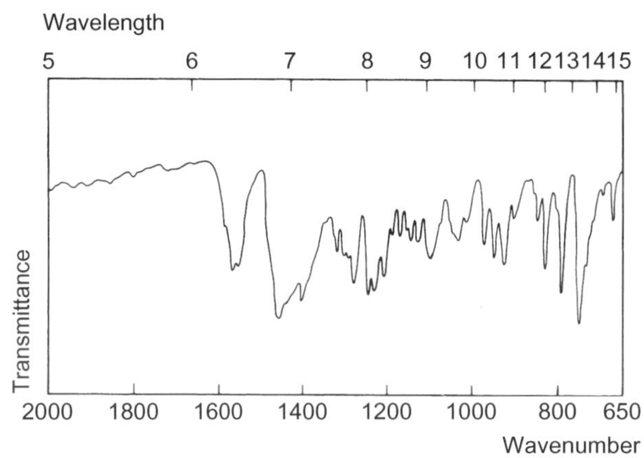

Mass Spectrum. Principal ions at *m/z* 98, 370, 126, 99, 40, 70, 371, 258; mesoridazine 98, 70, 99, 42, 386, 126, 55, 41.

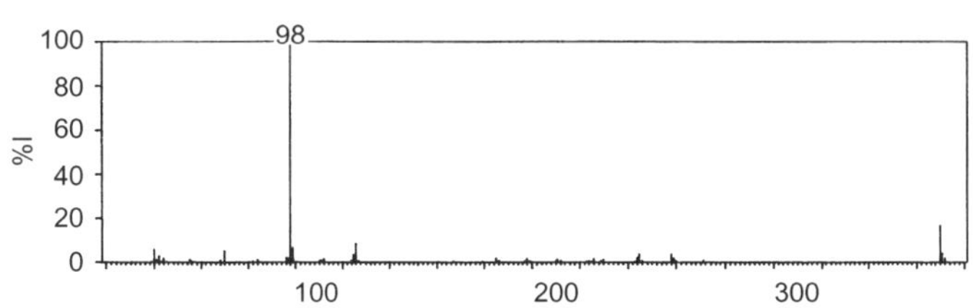

Quantification

Gas chromatography. In plasma: limit of detection 5 to 200 µg/L, depending on the extraction procedure, NPD—H. Tokunaga *et al.*, *Nippon Hoigaku Zasshi*, 1996, *50(3)*, 196–202.

High performance liquid chromatography. In plasma: limit of quantification 15 µg/L for thioridazine and 5 µg/L for the metabolites—C. B. Eap *et al.*, *J. Chromatogr.*, 1995, *669*; *Biomed. Appl.*, 271–279. In serum: lower limit of quantification 50 µg/L; limit of detection, 12.5 µg/L, UV detection (λ = 263 nm)—S. A. Jortani and A. Poklis, *J. Anal. Toxicol.*, 1993, *17(6)*, 374–377. In biological tissues/fluids: limit of quantification 0.05 mg/L, UV detection (λ = 263 nm)—S. A. Jortani *et al.*, *Forensic Sci. Int.*, 1994, *64(2–3)*, 165–170.

Disposition in the Body. Readily absorbed after oral administration. It is metabolised mainly by sulfoxidation to give the side-chain sulfoxide (mesoridazine), the side-chain sulfone (sulforidazine), both of which are active and the ring sulfoxide and sulfone; *N*-demethylation also occurs. Other metabolites are produced by combinations of these metabolic reactions. It is metabolised in the liver, secreted in the bile and excreted mainly in the faeces. Less than about 10% of a dose is excreted in the urine, with less than 1% as unchanged drug; mesoridazine and sulforidazine are also excreted in the urine in amounts slightly greater than unchanged drug.

Therapeutic concentration. Plasma concentrations of drug and metabolites show considerable inter-subject variation. Concentrations appear to be independent of dose and tend to decrease during chronic treatment. The therapeutic serum concentration is 0.2 to 1.0 mg/L (thioridazine); 0.3 mg/L (mesoridazine).

After a single oral dose of 100 mg administered to 5 subjects, the following peak serum concentrations were found: thioridazine 0.05 to 0.50 mg/L (mean 0.24) in 1 to 4 h, mesoridazine 0.10 to 0.51 mg/L (mean 0.32) in 2 to 6 h, sulforidazine 0.02 to 0.11 mg/L (mean 0.07) in 5 to 8 h, ring sulfoxide 0.07 to 0.38 mg/L (mean 0.18) in 4 to 8 h [R. Axelsson and E. Martensson, *Curr. Ther. Res.*, 1977, *21*, 561–586].

Following daily oral doses of 100 to 800 mg (mean 382) to 17 subjects, serum concentrations, determined 12 h after a dose, were: thioridazine 0.4 to 2.0 mg/L (mean 0.9), mesoridazine 0.2 to 1.6 mg/L (mean 0.8), sulforidazine 0 to 0.6 mg/L (mean 0.2), ring sulfoxide 0.06 to 4.0 mg/L (mean 1.5) [R. Axelsson *et al.*, *Eur. J.Clin. Pharmacol.*, 1982, *23*, 359–363].

Toxicity. The estimated minimum lethal dose is 1 g. Blood concentrations greater than about 2 mg/L may produce toxic effects and can be lethal; and with sulforidazine, a total concentration of 3 mg/L drug and metabolite is toxic.

A 68-year-old male with known severe depressive illness self-administered a high dose of thioridazine; approx. 80 tablets (each 200 mg slow release). He was admitted to hospital 4 h after ingestion and gastric lavage was able to remove 25 tablets. On arrival at hospital, he was drowsy and progressively lost consciousness over the next 6 h, resulting in coma and failing respiratory. Over a period of 9 days, the central nervous, cardiovascular and gastro-intestinal systems showed thioridazine toxicity. At high toxic levels of the drug, 6.06 to 6.48 mg/L, life-threatening malignant ventricular arrhythmias occurred as well as bradycardia. The thioridazine concentration was 3.34 mg/L when the patient slipped into a coma. The patient recovered following the appropriate treatment; 10 days after ingestion, he was transferred from the intensive care unit [W. Schmidt and K. Lang, *Crit. Care Med.*, 1997, *25(11)*, 1925–1930].

In 2 fatalities attributed to thioridazine overdose, the following post-mortem concentrations were reported, mg/L or µg/g:

	Blood	Liver*
Thioridazine	8.85, 2.43	138, 50
Mesoridazine	26.8, 0.29	–
Sulforidazine	0.87, 0	–

*Total thioridazine plus metabolites determined by a non-specific fluorimetric assay.

The determination of two stereoisomeric ring sulfoxides is also discussed [A. Poklis *et al.*, *J. Anal. Toxicol.*, 1982, *6*, 250–252].

Half-life. Plasma half-life, 10 to 36 h.

Distribution in blood. Plasma : whole blood ratio, 0.79.

Protein binding. In plasma, thioridazine greater than 99.5%; mesoridazine and sulforidazine, about 99%.

Dose. 50 to 300 mg of thioridazine hydrochloride daily; maximum of 600 mg daily.

Thiotepa

Antineoplastic

Synonyms. TESPA; Thiophosphamide; Triethylenethiophosphoramide; TSPA.

Proprietary names. Ledertepa; Tespamin; Thioplex; Tifosyl.

1,1′,1″-Phosphinothioylidynetrisaziridine

$C_6H_{12}N_3PS$ = 189.2

CAS—52-24-4

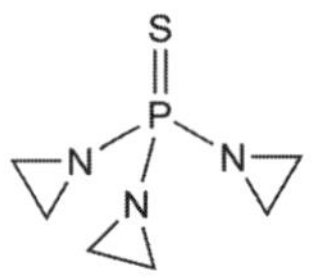

Fine white crystalline flakes. M.p. 51.5°.
Soluble 1 in 13 of water, 1 in about 8 of ethanol, 1 in 2 of chloroform and 1 in about 4 of ether.

Caution. Thiotepa is irritant; avoid contact with skin and mucous membranes.

Partition Coefficient. Log *P* (octanol/water), 0.5.

Thin-layer Chromatography. System TAE—Rf 75.

Gas Chromatography. System GA—RI 1504.

Ultraviolet Spectrum. No significant absorption, 230 to 360 nm.

Infra-red Spectrum. Principal peaks at wavenumbers 932, 1255, 729, 718, 669, 815 cm^{-1} (solution in carbon disulfide).

Quantification

Gas chromatography. In plasma or urine: thiotepa and metabolites, selective nitrogen/phosphorus detection—M. J. van Maanen *et al.*, *Int. J. Pharm.*, 2000, *200*, 187–194.

High performance liquid chromatography. In plasma—P.W. Tinsley *et al.*, *J. Chromatogr.*, 1989, *495*, 18–23.

Dose. Up to 60 mg in single or divided doses by injection or by instillation.

Thonzylamine

Antihistamine

Synonym. Histylamine
N-[(4-Methoxyphenyl)methyl]-*N′*,*N′*-dimethyl-*N*-2-pyrimidinyl-1,2-ethanediamine
$C_{16}H_{22}N_4O$=286.4
CAS—91-85-0

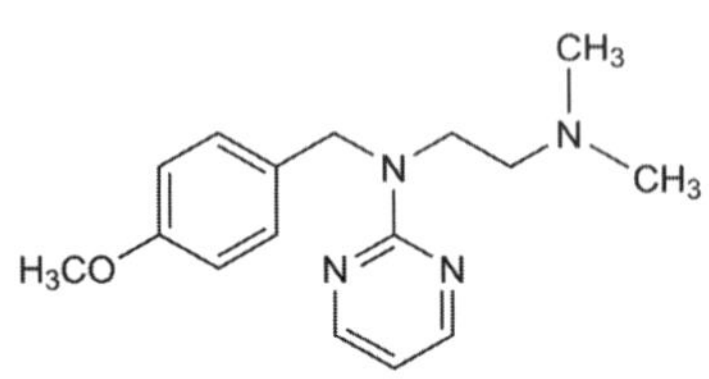

An oily liquid.
Practically insoluble in water; soluble in chloroform.

Thonzylamine Hydrochloride

Proprietary name. Tonamil
$C_{16}H_{22}N_4O,HCl$=322.8
CAS—63-56-9
A white crystalline powder. M.p. 173° to 176°.
Soluble 1 in 1 of water, 1 in 6 of ethanol and 1 in 4 of chloroform; practically insoluble in ether.

Dissociation Constant. pK_a 2.1, 8.8 (25°).

Colour Test. Mandelin's test—red-violet.

Thin-layer Chromatography. System TA—Rf 55; system TB—Rf 38; system TC—Rf 28; system TE—Rf 65; system TL—Rf 14; system TAE—Rf 22; system TAF—Rf 31. (Dragendorff spray, positive; Acidified iodoplatinate solution, positive.)

Gas Chromatography. System GA—RI 2203; system GC—RI 2576.

High Performance Liquid Chromatography. System HA—*k* 3.2.

Ultraviolet Spectrum. Aqueous acid—236 (A^1_1=857a), 274, 316 nm.

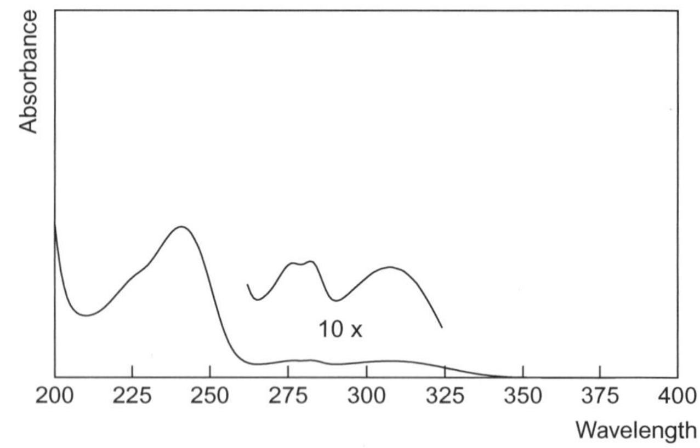

Infra-red Spectrum. Principal peaks at wavenumbers 1515, 1593, 1550, 1250, 1613, 1175 cm^{-1} (KBr disk).

Mass Spectrum. Principal ions at *m*/*z* 58, 121, 72, 71, 216, 215, 122, 78.

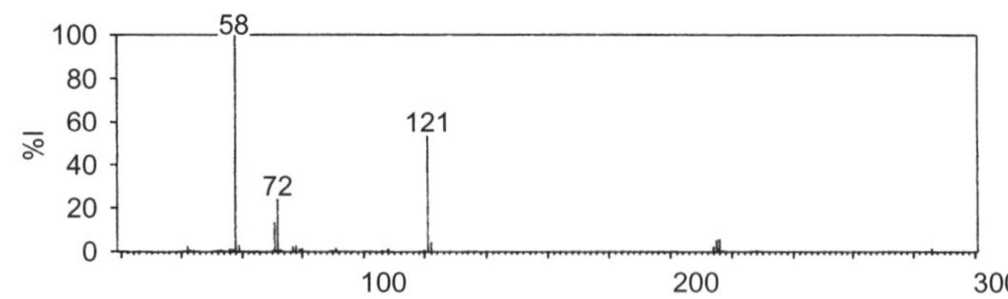

Dose. Usually 50 to 100 mg of thonzylamine hydrochloride daily.

Thymol

Antiseptic

Synonyms. Acido Timico; Isopropylmetacresol; Timol.
Proprietary names. Flavinol; Intrasol; Medophyll.
5-Methyl-2-(1-methylethyl)phenol
$C_{10}H_{14}O$=150.2
CAS—89-83-8

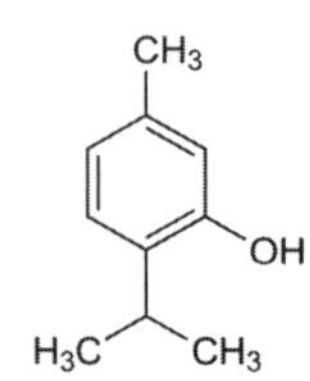

Colourless crystals or white crystalline powder. M.p. 51.5°; when melted it remains liquid at a considerably lower temperature.
Soluble 1 in 1000 of water, 1 in 1 of ethanol, 1 in 0.6 of chloroform, 1 in 1.5 of ether and 1 in 1.7 of olive oil.

Dissociation Constant. pK_a 10.6 (20°).

Partition Coefficient. Log *P* (octanol/water), 3.3.

Colour Test. Liebermann's test—black.

Thin-layer Chromatography. System TD—Rf 73; system TE—Rf 81; system TF—Rf 68; system TAD—Rf 65; system TAF—Rf 92.

Gas Chromatography. System GA—RI 1260.

High Performance Liquid Chromatography. System HY—RI 544.

Ultraviolet Spectrum. Aqueous acid—272 (A^1_1=137b); aqueous alkali—292 nm (A^1_1=257b).

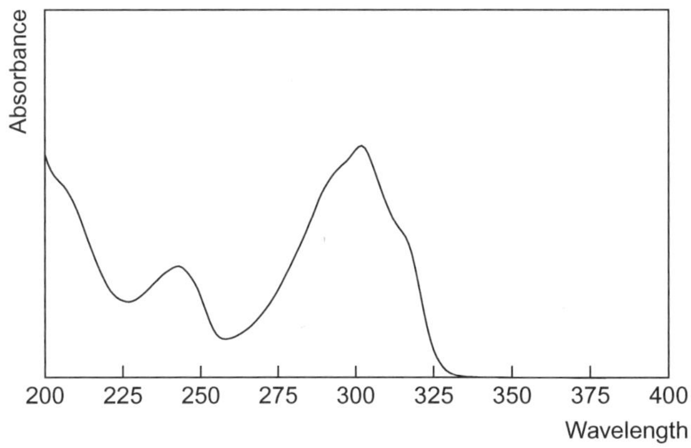

Infra-red Spectrum. Principal peaks at wavenumbers 817, 1248, 1290, 1095, 1160, 952 cm^{-1}.

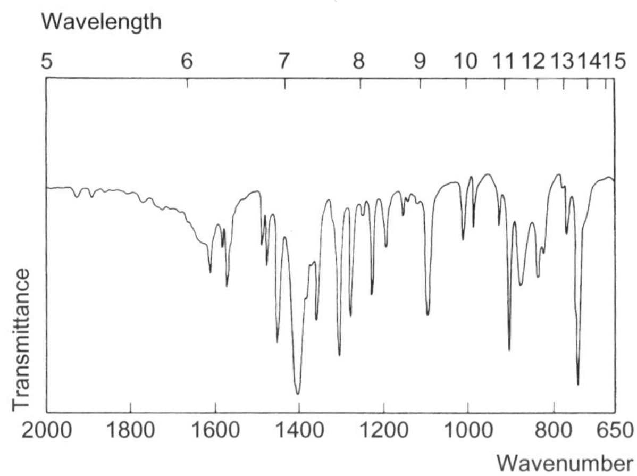

Mass Spectrum. Principal ions at m/z 135, 150, 91, 107, 117, -, -, -.

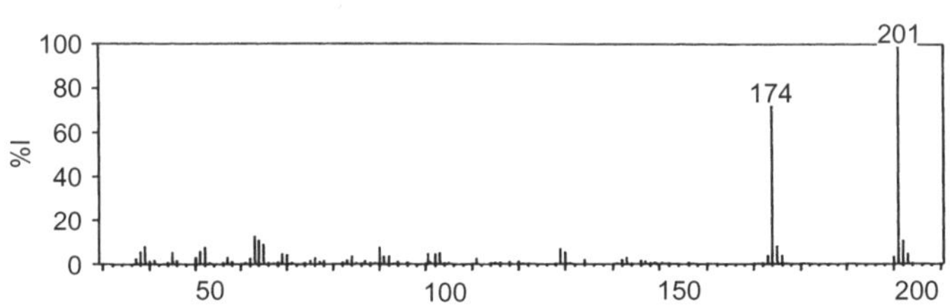

Quantification

Gas chromatography. In plasma or urine: thymol metabolites, FID—C. Kohlert *et al.*, *J. Clin. Pharmacol.*, 2002, *42*, 731–737.

Tiabendazole

Anthelmintic

Synonym. Thiabendazole; TBZ.
Proprietary names. Eprofil; Equizole (vet.); Foldan; Folderm; Mintezol; Storite; Tecto; Thiaben; Thiprazole (vet.); Tiabiose; Triasox; Tutiverm.
2-(4-Thiazolyl)-1*H*-benzimidazole
$C_{10}H_7N_3S$=201.3
CAS—148-79-8

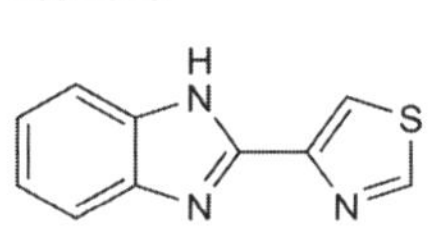

A white or cream-coloured powder. M.p. 300° to 305°.
Practically insoluble in water; soluble 1 in 150 of ethanol, 1 in 300 of chloroform and 1 in 2000 of ether; soluble in dilute mineral acids.

Dissociation Constant. pK_a 4.6 (25°).

Partition Coefficient. Log *P* (octanol/water), 2.5.

Thin-layer Chromatography. System TA—Rf 67; system TB—Rf 07; system TC—Rf 54; system TL—Rf 53; system TAE—Rf 75; system TAJ—Rf 46; system TAK—Rf 02; system TAL—Rf 59. (Acidified iodoplatinate solution, positive.)

Gas Chromatography. System GA—RI 2040; system GK—RRT 1.18 relative to caffeine.

High Performance Liquid Chromatography. System HY—RI 234.

Ultraviolet Spectrum. Aqueous acid—243, 302 nm (A_1^1=1230a).

Infra-red Spectrum. Principal peaks at wavenumbers 740, 1306, 902, 1095, 1279, 1231 cm^{-1} (KBr disk).

Mass Spectrum. Principal ions at m/z 201, 174, 63, 202, 64, 65, 175, 90.

Quantification

High performance liquid chromatography. In serum: tiabendazole and 5-hydroxythiabendazole, limit of detection 100 µg/L and 400 µg/L, respectively, fluorescence detection—M. T. Watts *et al.*, *J. Chromatogr.*, 1982, *230*; *B Biomed. Appl.*, *19*, 79–86.

Disposition in the Body. Tiabendazole is readily absorbed after oral administration; peak plasma concentrations are attained in 1 to 2 h. It is metabolised to the 5-hydroxy derivative and excreted in the urine as conjugates. About 90% of a dose is excreted in the urine in 48 h and 5% is eliminated in the faeces. Less than 1% of a dose is excreted in the urine unchanged.

Half-life. Plasma half-life, about 1 h.

Dose. Usually 25 mg/kg twice daily, to a maximum daily dose of 3 g.

Tiagabine

Anticonvulsant/Antidiabetic

Synonyms. Abbot-70569; ABT-569; NNC-05-0328; NO-05-0328; TGB.
Proprietary name. Gabitril
(3*R*)-1-[4,4,-Bis(3-methyl-2-thienyl)-3-butenyl]-3-piperidinecarboxylic acid
$C_{20}H_{25}NO_2S_2$=375.6
CAS—115103-54-3

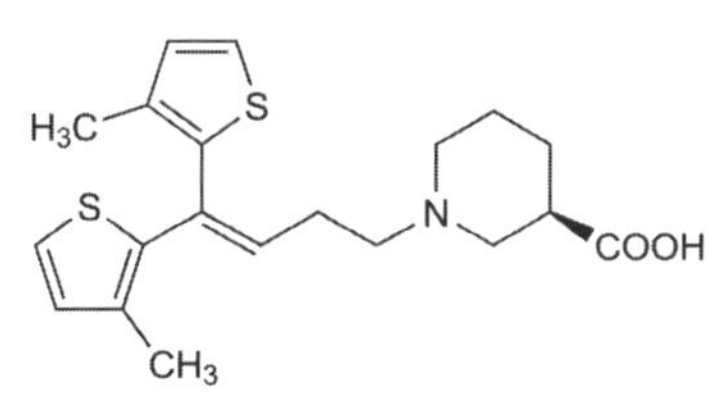

Tiagabine Hydrochloride
Proprietary name. Gabitril
$C_{20}H_{25}NO_2S_2$,HCl=412.0
CAS—145821-59-6
A white to off-white odourless crystalline powder. M.p. 192°. It is sparingly soluble in water; practically insoluble in hexane and heptane; soluble in aqueous base.

Dissociation Constant. pK_a 3.3, 9.4 (tiagabine hydrochloride).

Gas Chromatography. Column: cross-linked 5% phenyl methyl siloxane (HP-5MS, 30 m × 0.25 mm i.d., film thickness 0.25 µm). Column temperature: 100° increased at 20°/min to 300°. Carrier gas: helium. MS detection (EI, SIM mode, m/z: 156) IS: monomethyl analogue of tiagabin. Retention time(s): tiagabin, 11.9 min; IS, 11.5 min [D Chollet *et al. J. Pharm. Biomed. Anal.*, 1999, *21*, 641–646].

High Performance Liquid Chromatography. Column: OD (Chiracel, 250 × 4.6 mm i.d.). Mobile phase: ethanol:hexane:isopropanol: trifluoroacetic acid (6:80:14:0.5). UV detection (λ=290 nm). Retention time(s): (*S*-(+)-tiagabine), 10.1 min; (*R*-(−)-tiagabine) 14.2 min [A. Rustum and V. Estrad, *J. Chromatogr. B Biomed. Sci. Appl.*, 1998, *705*, 111–117].

Column: l-phenylglycine (250 × 4.6 mm i.d., 5 µm). Mobile phase: ammonium acetate (0.1 M, pH 3.7):acetonitrile (69:31), flow rate 1.5 mL/min. UV detection (λ=230 nm). Retention time(s): *S*-(+)-tiagabine, 13.0 min; *R*-(−)-tiagabine, 15.7 min [A. M. Rustum *et al.*, *J. Pharm. Biomed. Anal.*, 1998, *17*, 1439–1447].

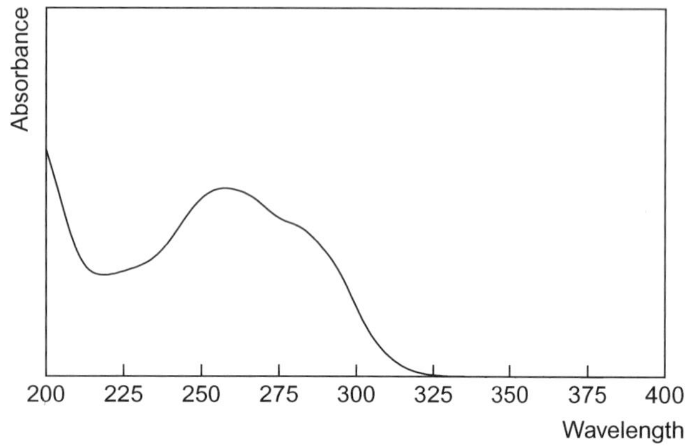

Mass Spectrum. Principal ions at *m/z* 156, 157, 113, 111, 358, 96, 97, 81 (Tiagabine-Me).

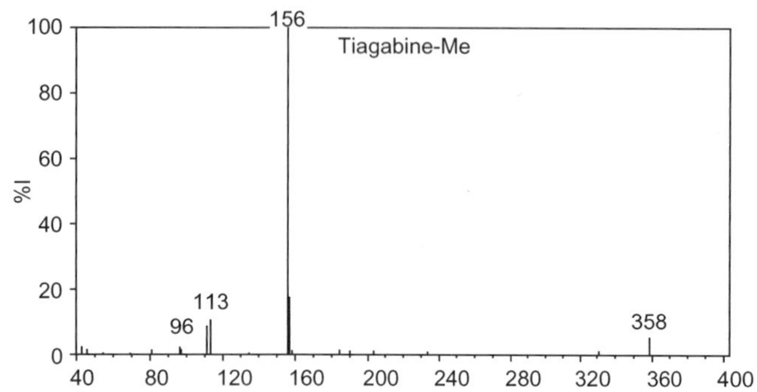

Quantification

Gas chromatography–mass spectrometry. In serum: limit of quantification 5 µg/L and limit of detection 0.4 µg/L—D. Chollet *et al.*, *J. Pharm. Biomed. Anal.*, 1999, *21*, 641–646.

High performance liquid chromatography. In plasma: limit of quantification 2 µg/L—L. Gustavson and S. Chu, *J. Chromatogr.*, 1992, *574*; *Biomed. Appl.*, 313–318.

Disposition in the Body. Tiagabine is readily and virtually completely absorbed after oral administration, within one hour of administration. Food prolongs absorption, however this reduces the rate, but not the extent. Absorption and elimination pharmacokinetics are linear within the therapeutic dosage range. The drug is widely distributed throughout the body. It is extensively metabolised in the liver and excreted as the metabolite in faeces (64%) or to a lesser extent in urine (25%). Only 2% is eliminated as the unchanged drug. Hepatic metabolism occurs via cytochrome P450 enzymes CYP3A subfamily and no active metabolites have been identified. Two metabolic pathways have been identified: thiophene ring oxidation leading to the formation of 5-oxo-tiagabine and glucuronidation. There is no drug accumulation after multiple doses and no change in pharmacokinetics in patients with renal impairment.

Therapeutic concentration

25 patients, aged 19 to 64 years (mean 44 years) with varying degrees of renal function-group (1): healthy volunteers; (2): mild renal impairment (creatinine clearance, 40 to 80 mL/min); (3): moderate (20 to 39 mL/min); (4): severe (5 to 19 mL/min); (5): patients requiring haemodialysis, were involved in the study. Groups 1 to 4 were orally administered with 4 mg doses of tiagabine hydrochloride as a single dose on day 1, multiple doses every 12 h for days 2 to 4 and a single dose on day 5. Group 5 was administered with a single 4 mg dose 2 h after haemodialysis. The mean total tiagabine plasma concentrations, after single doses, were 68.64, 108.09, 82.18, 80.50 and 51.65 µg/L for the five groups observed at 0.60, 0.50, 0.60, 0.63 and 1.20 h, respectively. For the multiple doses, the peak concentrations were 89.64, 125.25, 104.51 and 80.50 µg/L for groups 1 to 4 at 0.80, 0.44, 0.55 and 0.75 h, respectively [A. Cato *et al.*, *Epilepsia*, 1998, *39(1)*, 43–47].

4 patients with mild hepatic impairment, 2 with moderate hepatic impairment and 6 normal, healthy subjects were administered twice daily with oral tiagabine hydrochloride for 5.5 days. The healthy individuals produced peak plasma concentrations of 117 µg/L, the patients with mild hepatic impairment, 172 µg/L and moderate hepatic impairment, 172 µg/L. Minimum concentrations were 13, 27 and 28 µg/L for the three groups, respectively [A. H. Lau *et al.*, *Epilepsia*, 1997, *38(4)*, 445–451].

Toxicity

Reports of overdose are few and all episodes have recovered within 24 h. There is a broad therapeutic index. Median lethal doses are at least 50-fold higher than the maximum recommended doses (56 mg/day) [N. M. Graves *et al.*, *Ann. Pharmacother.*, 1998, *32(11)*, 1239–1243].

Bioavailability. 90 to 95%.

Half-life. 7 to 9 h. May be reduced to 2 to 3 h by the concomitant administration of liver enzyme inducing drugs.

Volume of distribution. 1 to 1.3 L/kg.

Clearance. Mean systemic plasma clearance is 109 mL/min.

Protein binding. About 96% mainly to serum albumin and α-1 acid glycoprotein over the concentration range 10 to 10 000 µg/L.

Note. For a review of the pharmacokinetics of tiagabine see J. C. Adkins and S. Noble, *Drugs*, 1998, *55*, 437–460.

Dose. The usual dose is 30 to 45 mg daily.

Tianeptine

Antidepressant

Proprietary name. Stablon

7-[(3-Chloro-6,11-dihydro-6-methyldibenzo[*c,f*][1,2]thiazepin-11-yl)-amino]heptanoic acid *S,S*-dioxide

$C_{21}H_{25}ClN_2O_4S$=436.5

CAS—66981-73-5

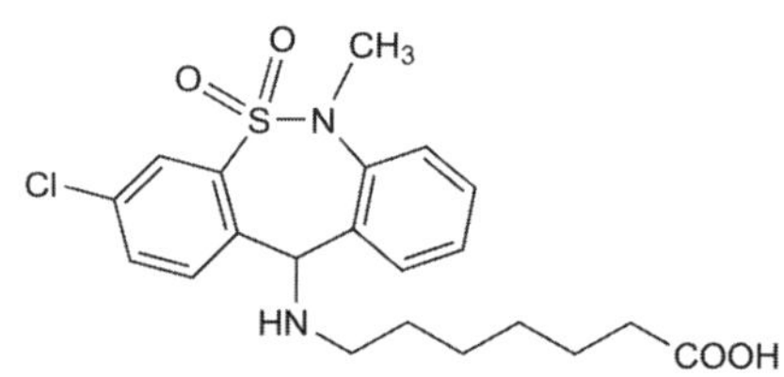

Tianeptine Sodium

$C_{21}H_{25}ClN_2NaO_4S$=459.9

M. p. 180°.

High Performance Liquid Chromatography. System HAA—Retention time 14.9 min.

Column: C_{18} (Nucleosil, 150 × 4.6 mm i.d., 5 µm). Mobile phase: acetonitrile:sodium heptane sulfonate buffer (1.5 g/L, pH 3) (40:60), flow rate 1.3 mL/min. Internal standard (IS): pentanoic acid. UV detection (diode array at λ=220 nm). Retention times: tianeptine, 9.5 min; IS, 6.2 min [J.-M. Gaulier *et al.*, *J. Chromatogr. B Biomed. Sci. Appl.*, 2000, *748*, 407–414].

Column: C_{18} (Nova-Pack, 300 × 3.9 mm i.d., 4 µm). Mobile phase: methanol:THF:potassium dihydrogen phosphate (10 mM, 0.68 g/L) (pH 2.6) (65:5:30), flow rate 0.8 mL/min. UV detection (λ=210 nm). Retention time: 5.40 min [A. Tracqui *et al.*, *J. Forensic Sci.*, 1995, *40*, 254–262].

Column: ODS (microbore Hypersil, 100 × 2.1 mm i.d.). Mobile phase: (A) phosphate buffer (20 mmol/L, containing triethylamine at 500 µL/L): (B) acetronitrile. Elution programme: (A:B) initial conditions (85:15), to (60:40) at 10 min, to (25:75) in 3.5 min, to (20:80) in 2.5 min, flow rate 0.4 mL/min. IS: prazepam. UV detection (λ=230 nm). Retention times: tianeptine, 9.0 min; IS, 13.7 min [A. Turcant *et al.*, *Clin. Chem.*, 1991, 37/7, 1210–1215].

Quantification

High performance liquid chromatography. In plasma: limit of quantification 5 µg/L for tianeptine and its metabolite MC_5, UV detection (λ=220 nm) —

J. M. Gaulier *et al.*, *J. Chromatogr. B Biomed. Sci. Appl.*, 2000, *748(2)*, 407–414. In blood: limit of detection <120 µg/L—A. Tracqui *et al.*, *J. Forensic Sci.*, 1995, *40*, 254–262. In blood and urine: limit of detection 10 µg/L—G. Nicot *et al.*, *J. Chromatogr.*, 1986, *381*, 115–126.

Disposition in the Body. The drug is completely absorbed, although food delays absorption. It is completely metabolised by the liver and is not subject to first-pass metabolism. Metabolism occurs mainly by extrarenal routes. Beta-oxidation is the major metabolic pathway, and the principal metabolites in plasma and urine are propanoic acid (MC_3, inactive metabolite) and pentanoic acid (MC_5, active metabolite). Pharmacokinetics is linear to the dosage. Less than 3% of the dose is excreted unchanged in urine. MC_5 half-life is 7.2 h. It is eliminated partly unchanged by the kidney, and undergoes biotransformation. Plasma concentrations reach steady state in one month and are maintained at month three.

Therapeutic concentration

12 elderly patients, aged between 72 and 81 years, were administered with a single oral dose of 12.5 mg tianeptine twice daily for 18 days. The maximum plasma concentration of tianeptine was 353 µg/L after 1.81 h and for its metabolite MC_5, 81 µg/L after 2.96 h for the single dose [F. Demotes-Mainard *et al.*, *J. Clin. Pharmacol.*, 1991, *31(2)*, 174–178].

12 healthy volunteers were administered with a single oral dose of 12.5 mg tianeptine, following either an overnight fast or after a standard breakfast. Peak plasma concentrations reached 322 µg/L in the fasted individuals after 1.29 h and those who had their dose administered after a meal, peak concentrations were lowered to 241.5 µg/L at approx. 1.79 h [A. Dresse *et al.*, *J. Clin. Pharmacol.*, 1988, *28(12)*, 1115–1119].

Bioavailability. Approx. 99% and in the elderly, 85%.

Half-life. 2.5 h; increased in patients with renal failure; prolonged in patients suffering from depression (6.3 h).

Volume of distribution. 0.5 to 0.8 L/kg; elderly, 0.41 L/kg.

Clearance. Total plasma clearance, 14.5 L/h; 40% lower in the elderly.

Protein binding. 95%.

Dose. Oral administration: 12.5 mg three times daily which may be reduced to a maximum of 25 mg daily in the elderly and patients with renal impairment.

Tiaprofenic Acid

Analgesic

Synonyms. FC-3001; RU-15060.
Proprietary names. Anafen; Artiflam; Artroreuma; Fengam; Flamirex; Gasam; Lindotab; Suralgan; Surdolin; Surgam; Surgamic; Surgamyl; Tiaprofen; Tiaprorex.
5-Benzoyl-α-methyl-2-thiopheneacetic acid
$C_{14}H_{12}O_3S=260.3$
CAS—33005-95-7

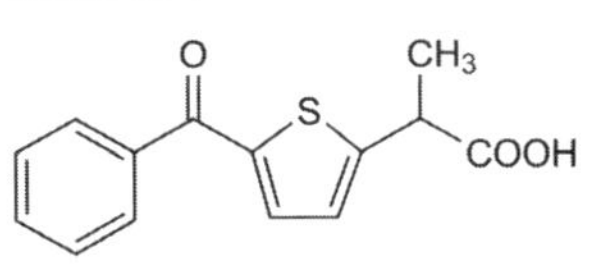

A white microcrystalline powder. M.p. 96°.
Slightly soluble in water; soluble in ethanol, chloroform and ether.

Dissociation Constant. pK_a 3.0.

Partition Coefficient. Log *P* (octanol/water), 2.8.

Thin-layer Chromatography. System TE—Rf 04; system TF—Rf 05; system TAE—Rf 86; system TAJ—Rf 30; system TAK—Rf 80; system TAL—Rf 98.

Gas Chromatography. System GA—tiaprofenic acid RI 1976; tiaprofenic acid-ME2 RI 2180.

High Performance Liquid Chromatography. System HAA—Retention time(s) 17.6 min; system HX—RI 484; system HY—RI 452; system HZ—Retention time(s) 5.8 min.

Ultraviolet Spectrum. Ethanolic acid—260 (A^1_1=370a), 305 nm (A^1_1=575a).

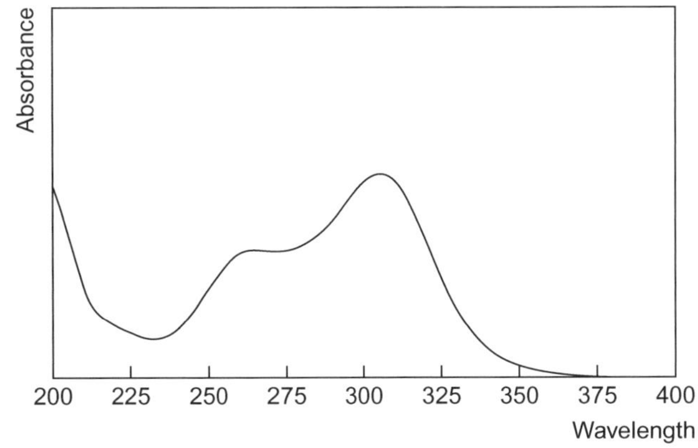

Infra-red Spectrum. Principal peaks at wavenumbers 1727, 718, 1593, 1198, 1605, 1572 cm^{-1} (Nujol mull).

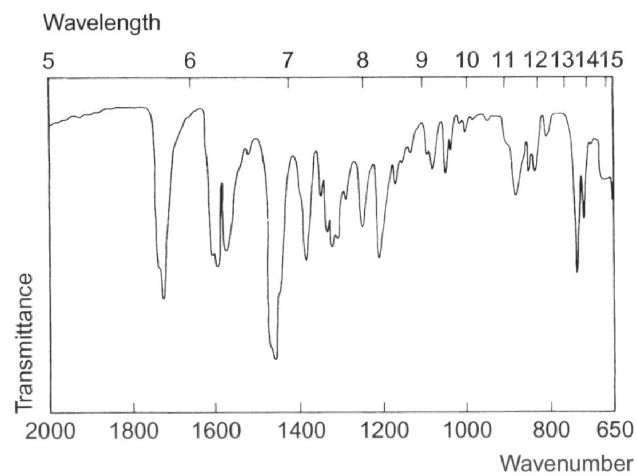

Quantification

Gas chromatography–mass spectrometry. In urine: tiaprofenic acid and other NSAIDs, limits of detection 10 to 50 µg/L—H. H. Maurer *et al.*, *J. Anal. Toxicol.*, 2001, *25*, 237–244.

High performance liquid chromatography. In plasma: limit of detection 500 µg/L, UV detection—G. T. Ward *et al.*, *J. Liq. Chromatogr.*, 1982, *5*, 165–174. In plasma: tiaprofenic acid enantiomers, limit of detection 25 µg/L, UV detection—G. Geisslinger *et al.*, *J. Chromatogr. B, Biomed. Appl.*, 1996, *675*, 77–81; M. Vakily and F. Jamali, *J. Pharm. Sci.*, 1996, *85*, 638–642.

Disposition in the Body. Tiaprofenic acid is rapidly and almost completely absorbed after oral administration. It is metabolised by reduction to 2-(5-α-hydroxybenzyl-2-thienyl)propionic acid, oxidation to 2-(5-*p*-hydroxybenzoyl-2-thienyl)propionic acid, and conjugation with glucuronic acid. About 60% of an oral dose is excreted in the urine in 24 h, about 55% as tiaprofenic acid (excreted mainly as an acylglucuronide conjugate), and about 5% as the two metabolites, excreted partly as acylglucuronides.

Therapeutic concentration

Following daily oral administration of 300 mg twice a day to 6 subjects, maximum steady-state serum concentrations of 18.6 to 73.3 (mean 48) mg/L were reported 0.5 to 1.5 h after a dose. [T. J. Daymond and R. Herbert, *Br. J. Clin. Pharmacol.*, 1983, *15*, 157P–158P].

Half-life. Plasma half-life, 1 to 2 h.

Clearance. Plasma clearance, about 1.4 mL/min/kg.

Protein binding. In plasma, about 98%.

Note. For a review of tiaprofenic acid, see E. N. Sorkin and R. N. Brogden, *Drugs*, 1985, *29*, 208–235 and N. M. Davies, *Clin. Pharmacokinet.*, 1996, *31*, 331–347.

Dose. 600 mg daily.

Ticlopidine

Antithrombotic

5-[(2-Chlorophenyl)-methyl]-4,5,6,7-tetrahydrothieno[3,2-*c*]pyridine
$C_{14}H_{14}ClNS$=263.8
CAS—55142-85-3

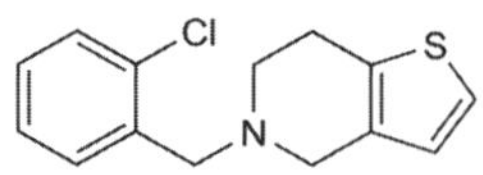

Ticlopidine Hydrochloride

Proprietary names. Anagregal; Antigreg; Aplaket; Clox; Fluilast; Klodin; Opteron; Parsilid; Thrombodine; Thrombopat; Ticlid; Ticlodone; Ticloproge; Ticlosan; Tiklid; Tiklyd.
$C_{14}H_{14}ClNS,HCl$=300.2
CAS—53885-35-1
A white or almost white crystalline powder. It is sparingly soluble in water and in dehydrated alcohol; very slightly soluble in ethyl acetate; practically insoluble in ether.

Dissociation Constant. pK_a 7.6.

Gas Chromatography. Column: methyl silicone (HP1, 0.2 mm i.d., 0.33 µm film thickness). Column temperature: 250°. Carrier gas: helium, flow rate 0.9 mL/min. MS detection. RI: 2167 [T. Mills and J. C. Roberson, *Instrumental Data for Drug Analysis*, CRC Press, *2nd Edn.*, *5*, 392–393].

Column: 3% OV1 on Gas Chrom Q, 80 to 100 mesh (glass, 1.8 m × 3 mm i.d.). Column temperature: 252°. Carrier gas: helium, flow rate 30 mL/min. Internal standard (IS): *S*-(2,4-dichlorophenyl)-4,5,6,7-tetrahydrothieno[3,2-*c*]pyridine. MS detection (SIM at *m/z* 110). Retention times: ticlodipine, 70 s; IS, 100 s [J. B. Knudsen *et al.*, *Xenobiotica*, 1992, *22(5)*, 579–589].

High Performance Liquid Chromatography. System HAA—Retention time 13.8 min.

Column: LC-8-DB (Supelcosil, 150 × 4.6 mm i.d., 5 µm); (guard) LC-8-DB (Supelguard, 20 × 4.6 mm i.d., 5 µm). Mobile phase: acetonitrile:methanol:potassium dihydrogen phosphate (0.05 M, pH 3, containing 0.2% triethylamine) (20:25:55), flow rate 1 mL/min. UV detection (λ=235 nm). Retention time: 7.6 min [L. Dal Bo *et al.*, *J. Chromatogr. B Biomed. Appl.*, 1995, *665*, 404–409].

Column: ODS (Hypersil, 100 × 4.5 mm i.d., 5 µm). Mobile phase: methanol:water:concentrated ammonia solution (80:20:1), flow rate 1 mL/min. IS: *S*-(2,4-dichlorophenyl)-4,5,6,7-tetrahydrothieno[3,2-*c*]pyridine. UV detection (λ=210 nm). Retention times: ticlodipine, 5.5 min; IS, 10 min [J. B. Knudsen *et al.*, *Xenobiotica*, 1992, *22(5)*, 579–589].

Column: ODS (Hypersil, 100 × 4.6 mm i.d., 5 µm). Mobile phase: methanol:dihydrogen potassium phosphate buffer (0.01 M, pH 3.5) (90:10), flow rate 1 mL/min. UV detection. Retention time: 2.5 min [T. Mills and J. C. Roberson, *Instrumental Data for Drug Analysis*, CRC Press, *2nd Edn.*, *5*, 392–393].

Ultraviolet Spectrum. Aqueous acid—214, 231, 268, 275 nm.

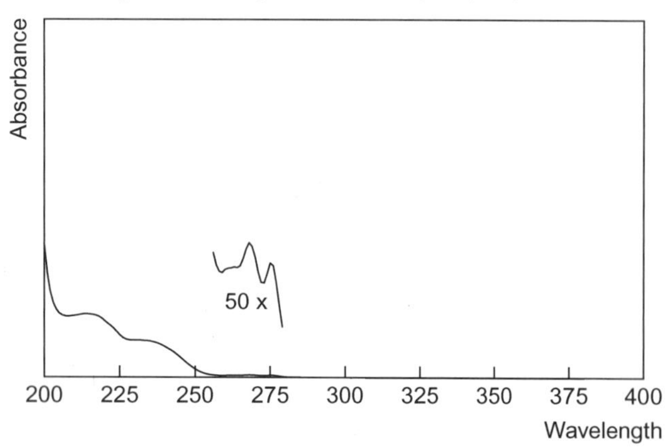

Infra-red Spectrum. Principal peaks at wavenumber 1457, 971, 717 cm^{-1} (KBr disk).

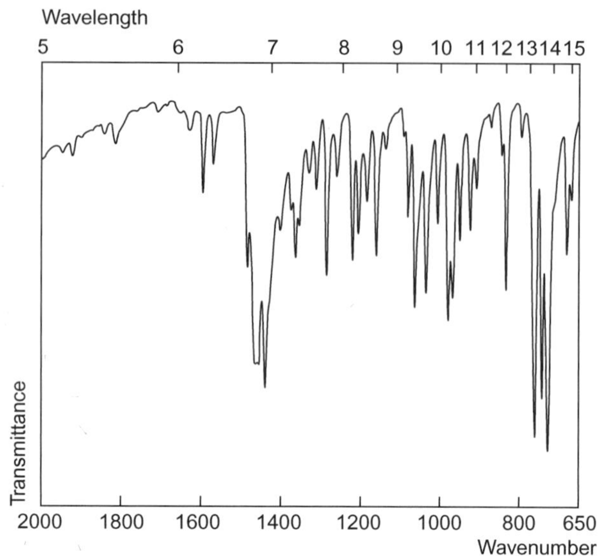

Mass Spectrum. Principal ions at *m/z* 110, 263, 125, 262, 265, 264, 111, 89.

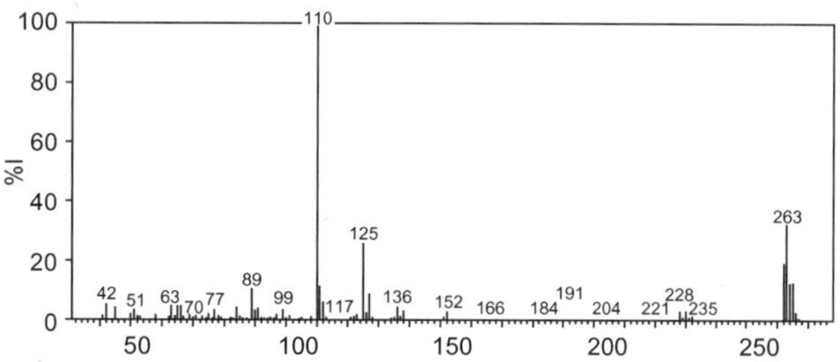

Quantification

Gas chromatography. In plasma: limit of detection 0.01 mg/L, NPD—J. Shah *et al.*, *Br. J. Clin. Pharmacol.*, 1991, *32*, 761–764. In plasma: limit of detection 0.002 mg/L, NPD—J. P. Desager *et al.*, *Int. J. Clin. Pharm. Res.*, 1990, *10(4)*, 247–250.

Gas chromatography–mass spectrometry. In plasma: limit of detection 5 g/L—J. B. Knudsen *et al.*, *Xenobiotica*, 1992, *22(5)*, 579–589.

High performance liquid chromatography. In plasma: limit of detection 0.005 mg/L, UV detection (λ=235 nm)—L. Dal Bo *et al.*, *J. Chromatogr. B Biomed. Appl.*, 1995, *665*, 404–409. In plasma: limit of quantification is 0.01 mg/L and detection 0.005 mg/L, UV detection (λ=215 nm)—K. Róna *et al.*, *J. Chromatogr. B Biomed. Sci. Appl.*, 1997, *693*, 393–398.

Disposition in the Body. Ticlopidine is rapidly and almost completely absorbed (80 to 90%) after oral administration. The bioavailability is improved when the drug is administered with food, especially a high-fat meal, and the rate and extent of absorption is slightly improved. Peak plasma concentrations occur after about 2 h. Pharmacokinetics are non-linear with clearance decreasing markedly on repeated dosing. The drug is rapidly and extensively metabolised in the liver by *N*-dealkylation and oxidation with a number of highly polar urinary and biliary metabolites, which have not been identified. Further metabolism and conjugation may also occur. Approximately 60% of an administered dose is excreted in urine as metabolites, and 25% is eliminated in faeces. Less than 1% of the drug appears in urine unchanged. Accumulation of the drug may occur with repeated dosing.

Therapeutic concentration

Administration of a single oral dose of 250 mg to 12 young subjects (mean 28.6 years) and 13 elderly subjects (mean 69.5 years) after a light breakfast, resulted in mean peak plasma concentrations of 0.41 and 0.70 mg/L, respectively at 2 h. Administration of 250 mg twice a day for 21 days, resulted in mean peak plasma concentrations of 0.89 mg/L in the young group and 1.42 mg/L in the elderly group after 1 and 2 h, respectively (J. Shah *et al.*, *Br. J. Clin. Pharmacol.*, 1991, *32*, 761–764).

12 healthy male volunteers with a mean age of 32 years were fasted from midnight the evening before and administered with a single dose of 250 mg in a fasted state, 30 min after a high-fat breakfast, or immediately after

ingestion of an antacid. The peak concentrations were 0.573 mg/L for the fasted individuals, 0.695 mg/L for the fed individuals and 0.375 mg/L for those who also took antacid. These concentrations were observed 1.917, 1.708 and 2.000 h after administration [J. Shah *et al.*, *J. Clin. Pharmacol.*, 1990, *30*, 733–736].

Half-life. Plasma half-life, 7.9 h (in young volunteers) and 12.7 h (elderly) after a single dose; 91 h (young) and 98 h (elderly) after repeated dosing.

Protein binding. In plasma, 98%.

Note. For reviews of ticlopidine see E. Saltiel and A. Ward, *Drugs*, 1987, *34*, 222–262 and D. McTavish *et al.*, *Drugs*, 1990, *40*, 238–259.
For a review of the pharmacokinetics of ticlopidine, see J.-P. Desager, *Clin. Pharmacokinet.*, 1994, *26*, 347–355.

Dose. 250 mg of the hydrochloride twice daily.

Tienilic Acid

Diuretic

Synonyms. Thienylic Acid; Ticrynafen; ANP-3624; CE-3624; SKF-62698.
Proprietary names. Diflurex; Selacryn.
[2,3-Dichloro-4-(2-thienylcarbonyl)phenoxy]acetic acid
$C_{13}H_8Cl_2O_4S$=331.2
CAS—40180-04-9

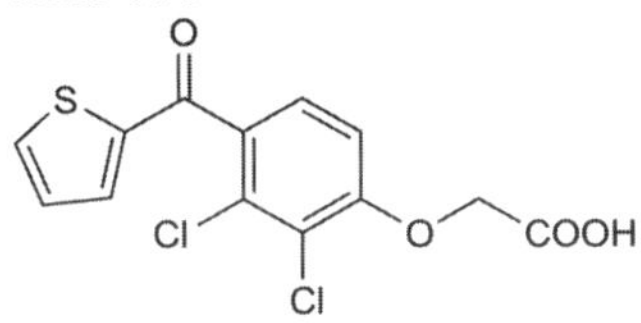

A white crystalline powder. M.p. 148° to 149°; also reported as 157°. Very slightly soluble in water; soluble 1 in 14 of ethanol, 1 in about 5 of acetone, 1 in 77 of chloroform and 1 in about 6 of methanol.

Dissociation Constant. pK_a 2.7 (25°).

Partition Coefficient. Log *P* (octanol/water), 3.6.

Ultraviolet Spectrum. Ethanol—267 (A^1_1=343a), 296 nm (A^1_1=384a).

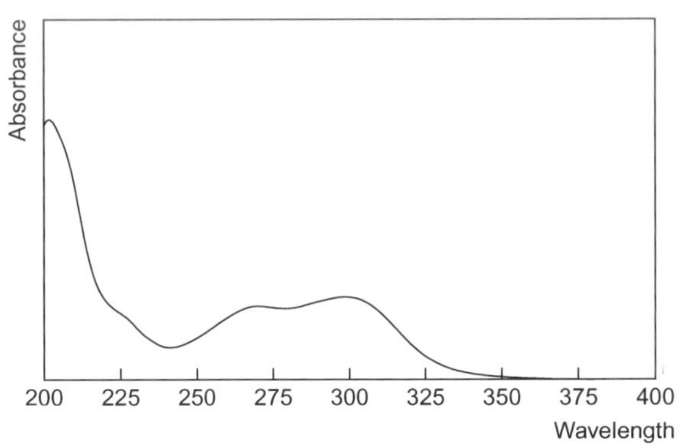

Infra-red Spectrum. Principal peaks at wavenumbers 1185, 1620, 1075, 1762, 1580, 1290 cm^{-1} (KBr disk).

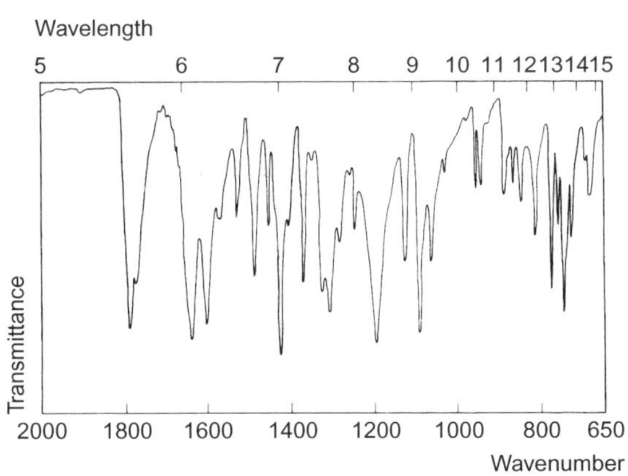

Quantification

Gas chromatography. In plasma, serum or urine: tienilic acid and metabolites, limit of detection 10 µg/L, ECD—B. Hwang *et al.*, *J. Pharm. Sci.*, 1978, *67*, 1095–1098.

High performance liquid chromatography. In plasma or urine: tienilic acid and monohydroxy metabolite, limit of detection 200 µg/L, UV detection—A. L. M. Kerremans *et al.*, *Eur. J. Clin. Pharmacol.*, 1982, *22*, 515–521. In urine: tienilic acid and 5-hydroxy-tienilic acid—D. Mansuy *et al.*, *Biochem. Pharmacol.*, 1984, *33*, 1429–1435.

Disposition in the Body. Tienilic acid is absorbed after oral administration. It is metabolised by hydroxylation and oxidation. About 40% of a dose is excreted in the urine in 24 h; about 20% of the dose is excreted in the urine as unchanged drug, up to 10% as [2,3-dichloro-4-(α-hydroxy-2-thenyl)phenoxy]acetic acid, about 15% as a dihydroxylated metabolite, and 1 to 2% as (2,3-dichloro-4-carboxyphenoxy)acetic acid.

Therapeutic concentration

After a single oral dose of 250 mg to 8 subjects, mean peak plasma concentrations of 11 mg/L of tienilic acid, 0.7 mg/L of the monohydroxylated metabolite, and 0.07 mg/L of the *p*-carboxy metabolite were attained in 3 to 4 h. [B. Hwang *et al.*, *J. Pharm. Sci.*, 1978, *67*, 1095–1098].

Following a single oral dose of 250 mg to 8 subjects, peak plasma concentrations of 7.7 to 27.4 (mean 16) mg/L of tienilic acid were attained in 1 to 2 h. [A. L. M. Kerremans *et al.*, *Eur. J. Clin. Pharmacol.*, 1982, *22*, 515–521].

Half-life. Plasma half-life, 1.5 to 4 h.

Distribution in blood. Plasma:whole blood ratio, about 1.6.

Protein binding. In plasma, about 99%.

Dose. Tienilic acid has been given in doses of 0.25 to 1 g daily.

Tigloidine

Anticholinergic

Synonym. Tiglylpseudotropeine
2-Methyl-2-butenoic acid [1α,3α(*E*),5α]-8-methyl-8-azabicyclo[3.2.1]oct-3-yl ester
$C_{13}H_{21}NO_2$=223.3
CAS—495-83-0

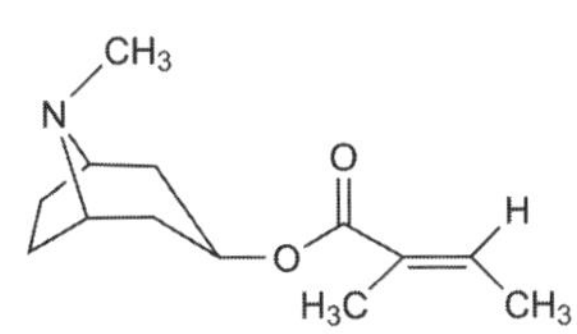

Tigloidine was first isolated from *Duboisia myoporoides* (*Solanaceae*) but is now synthesised.
A thin syrupy liquid.

Tigloidine Hydrobromide

Proprietary name. Tiglyssin
$C_{13}H_{21}NO_2$,HBr=304.2
CAS—22846-83-9
A white crystalline solid. M.p. 234° to 235°.
Soluble in water and chloroform.

Thin-layer Chromatography. System TA—Rf 42; system TL—Rf 07; system TB—Rf 39; system TC—Rf 21. (Acidified iodoplatinate solution, positive.)

Gas Chromatography. System GA—RI 1687.

High Performance Liquid Chromatography. System HA—*k* 3.6 (tailing peak).

Infra-red Spectrum. Principal peaks at wavenumbers 1700, 1266, 1136, 1036, 1156, 1073 cm^{-1} (thin film).

Mass Spectrum. Principal ions at *m*/*z* 124, 82, 83, 94, 55, 42, 67, 96.

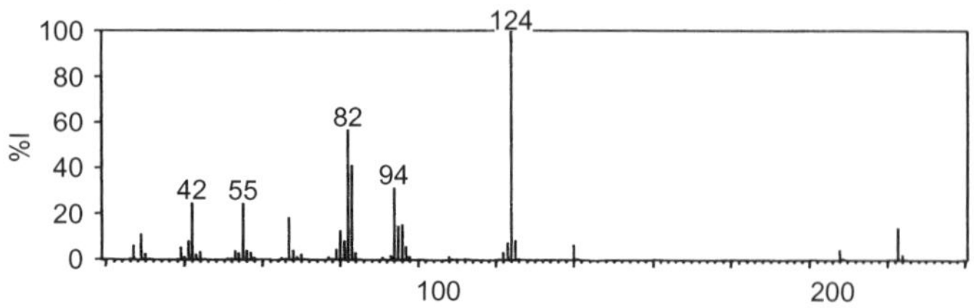

Dose. 1 to 2 g of tigloidine hydrobromide daily.

Tilidate

Narcotic Analgesic

Synonym. Tilidine
(1*R*,2*S*)-*rel*-2-(Dimethylamino)-1-phenyl-3-cyclohexene-1-carboxylic acid ethyl ester
$C_{17}H_{23}NO_2$=273.4
CAS—20380-58-9

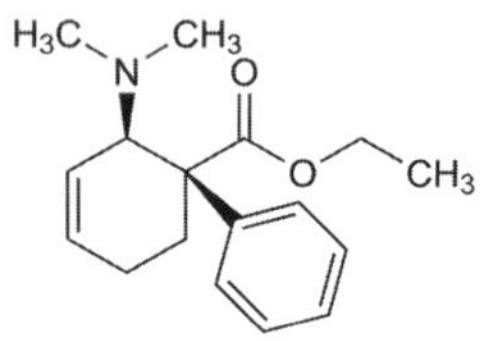

Tilidate Hydrochloride
Proprietary names. Findol N; Tili; Tilicomp; Tilidalor; Tilidin; Tiligetic; Tilimerck; Tilitrate; Tilnalox; Valoron; Valtran
$C_{17}H_{23}NO_2$,HCl,½H_2O=318.8
CAS—27107-79-5 (anhydrous)
A white crystalline powder. M.p. 125°.
Soluble in water.

Partition Coefficient. Log *P* (octanol/water), 3.7.

Thin-layer Chromatography. System TE—Rf 84; system TAE—Rf 61; system TAJ—Rf 47; system TAK—Rf 03; system TAL—Rf 38.

Gas Chromatography. System GA—tilidate RI 1838, bisnortilidate RI 1827, nortilidate RI 1830.

High Performance Liquid Chromatography. System HY—RI 290.

Ultraviolet Spectrum. Aqueous acid—251 nm (A^1_1=6.2b), 257 nm (A^1_1=7.6b), 262 nm (A^1_1=6.1b).

Infra-red Spectrum. Principal peaks at wavenumbers 1714, 1238, 1182, 1263, 1167, 703 cm^{-1} (tilidate hydrochloride). (See below)

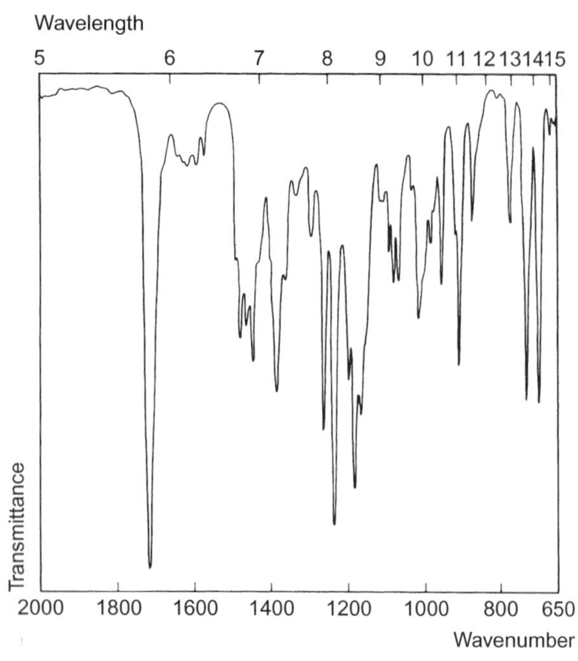

Mass Spectrum. Principal ions at *m/z* 103, 77, 82, 29, 97, 42, 51, 104; bisnortilidate 69, 68, 70, 77, 103, 56, 54, 51; nortilidate 83, 68, 82, 72, 84, 77, 103, 115.

Quantification
Gas chromatography. In plasma or urine: tilidate, nortilidate and bisnortilidate, limit of detection 1 μg/L, AFID—H. Hengy *et al., J. Pharm. Sci.*, 1978, *67*, 1765–1768.

Disposition in the Body. Rapidly and almost completely absorbed after oral administration. It is rapidly metabolised by *N*-demethylation to form nortilidate and bisnortilidate; these metabolites may then be conjugated with glucuronic acid. About 80% of an oral dose is excreted in the urine in 24 h, with less than 0.1% of a dose as unchanged drug, about 1.5% as nortilidate, 2.5% as bisnortilidate and the rest as unknown metabolites. Up to 10% may be eliminated in the faeces.

Therapeutic concentration
Following a single oral dose of 50 mg to 1 subject, peak plasma concentrations of 0.127 g/L of (+)-nortilidate and 0.121 g/L of (−)-nortilidate were attained in about 2 h [H. Hengy *et al., Clin. Chem.*, 1978, *24*, 692–697].

Toxicity
In a fatal intoxication involving the ingestion of an unknown quantity of tilidate by a 29-year-old man, the postmortem tissue concentrations were as follows (nortilidate and bisnortilidate given, respectively, in brackets): blood 1.74 (4.41 and 0.15) mg/L, lung 5.75 (21.70 and 2.12) μg/g, liver 9.40 (13.70 and 3.51 μg/g, bile 2.88 (6.54 and 0.90) mg/L, kidney 2.78 (12.30 and 1.01) μg/g, urine 0.94 (6.75 (6.75 and 4.10) mg/L [J. Cordonnier *et al., J. Anal. Toxicol.*, 1987, *11*, 105–109].

A 28-year-old woman had a serum tilidate concentration of 38.1 mg/L 3 h after ingesting 100 mL of a preparation containing 6.94 g of tilidate (and about 0.56 g of naloxone) in a suicide attempt; the concentration of nortilidate was 18.8 mg/L [R. Regenthal *et al., Hum. Exp. Toxicol.*, 1998, *17*, 593–597].

Dose. The equivalent of up to 400 mg of the anhydrous hydrochloride daily.

Tilmicosin

Antibacterial (Veterinary)

Synonyms. EL-870; LY-177370.
Proprietary names. Micotil; Pulk motil.
4^A-*O*-De(2,6-dideoxy-3-*C*-methyl-α-L-*ribo*-hexopyranosyl)-20-deoxo-20-(3,5-dimethyl-1-piperidinyl)tylosin
$C_{46}H_{80}N_2O_{13}$=869.2
CAS—108050-54-0

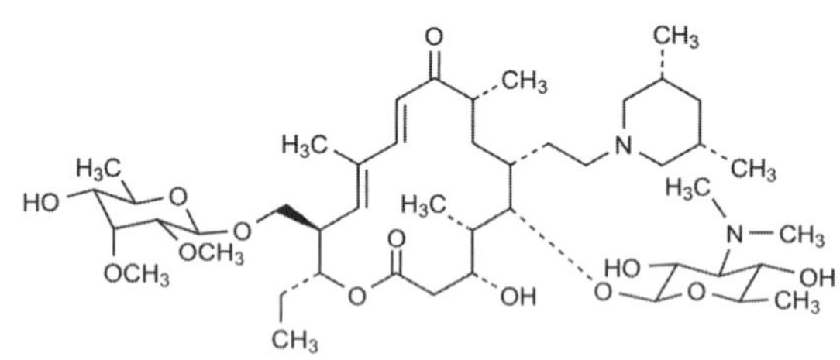

cis-form

Tilmicosin contains not less than 85% $C_{46}H_{80}N_2O_{13}$, calculated on an anhydrous basis. The content of Tilmicosin *cis*-isomers is between 82% and 88%, and the content of Tilmicosin *trans*-isomers is between 12% and 18%.

Dissociation Constant. pK_a (25°) 8.18.

Partition Coefficient. Log *P* (octanol/water), 3.80.

High Performance Liquid Chromatography. Column: RP18 (Lichrospher, 125 × 4 mm i.d., 5 μm). Mobile phase: acetonitrile:methanol:trifluroacetic acid (0.1%) in water (20:20:60 to 25:55:20 in 10 min), flow rate 0.5 mL/min. Detection: MS–MS (NCI: isotopic M$^-$, *m/z* → 869; M$^-$, *m/z* → 868; isotopic, *m/z* → 678). Retention time: 5.7 min [B. Delepine *et al., J. AOAC Int.*, 1996, *79*, 397–404].

Ultraviolet Spectrum. Aqueous solution—283 nm.

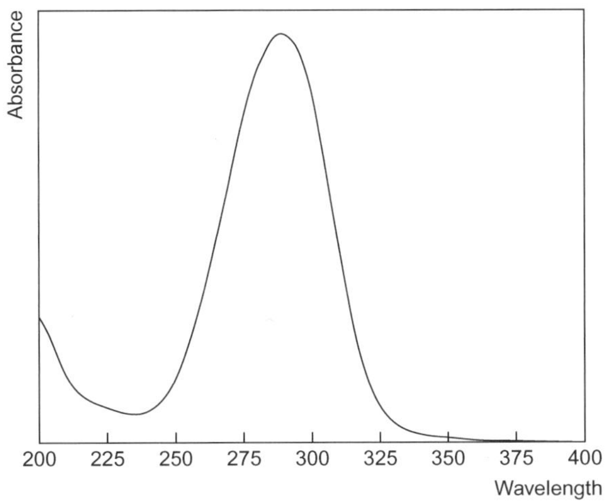

Infra-red Spectrum. Principal peaks at wavenumber 1592, 1167, 1141, 1081, 1058 cm^{-1} (acetate).

Quantification

High performance liquid chromatography. In serum: limit of detection 0.05 mg/L—J. W. Moran *et al.*, *J. AOAC Int.*, 1997, *80(6)*, 1183–1189.

Toxicity. May be fatal in humans.

There are 36 cases of accidental exposure where less than 1 mL was given. All medical outcomes were benign [M. McGuigan, *Vet. Hum. Toxicol.*, 1994, *36*, 306–308].

Tiludronic Acid

Bone resorption inhibitor

Synonyms. ACPMD; Cl-TMBP; ME-3737; SR-41319; Tiludronate.
Proprietary name. Skelid
[[(4-Chlorophenyl)thio]methylene]bisphosphonic acid
$C_7H_9ClO_6P_2S = 318.6$
CAS—89987-06-4

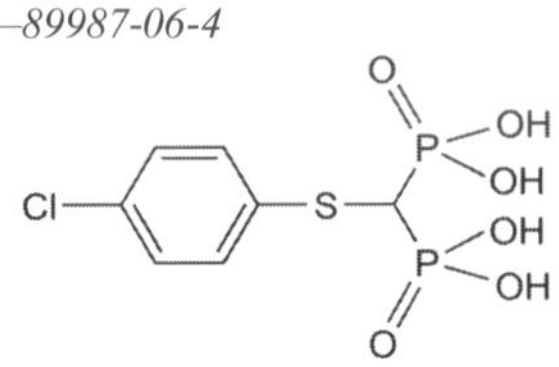

Disodium Tiludronate

Synonyms. Disodium dihydrogen; SR-41319B; Tiludronate disodium.
Proprietary name Skelid
$C_7H_7ClNa_2O_6P_2S = 362.6$
CAS—149845-07-8 (anhydrous); *155453-10-4* (hemihydrate)
M.p. 253°.

High Performance Liquid Chromatography. Column: PRP-1 (Hamilton, 5 µm, 150 × 4.1 mm i.d.). Mobile phase: tetrabutyl ammonium phosphate (0.005 M)-sodium hydrogen phosphate (0.05 M):acetonitrile, (pH 11.8) (87:13), flow rate 1.0 mL/min. UV detection (λ = 280 nm). Retention time: 2.5 min [J-P. Fels *et al.*, *J. Chromatogr. B. Biomed. Appl.*, 1988, *430*, 73–79].

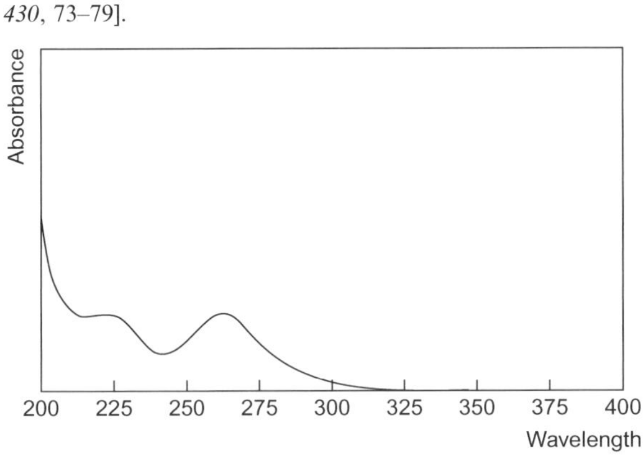

Quantification

High performance liquid chromatography. In plasma and urine: limit of quantification 0.05 mg/L and 0.2 mg/L, respectively—J-P. Fels *et al.*, *J. Chromatogr. B. Biomed. Appl.*, 1988, *430*, 73–79.

Disposition in the Body. The drug is rapidly absorbed following oral administration and is absorbed as the free acid. Absorption is decreased by food, especially by products containing calcium or other polyvalent cations. Approximately half of the absorbed portion is bound to bone, and is only very slowly excreted. The remainder is excreted unchanged in urine. After an intravenous dose, approximately 50% of a dose is excreted in urine over 13 days. Peak plasma concentrations are reached within 1 to 2 h but are below the limit of detection within 24 h. Steady state is achieved within 9 to 12 days. Concentration of the drug in the bone continues to increase for around 30 days.

Therapeutic concentration

12 healthy individuals were administered with 400 mg tiludronate 1 h after an antacid containing aluminium and magnesium hydroxide was administered. Peak plasma concentrations were 3.35, 1.59 and 2.90 mg/L for the three dosing regimens observed at 1.7, 1.3 and 1.9 h, respectively [L. N. Sansom *et al.*, *Bone*, 1995, *17(5)*, 479S–483S].

Bioavailability. Approx. 6% in the fasting state. Reduced by 90% when administered within 2 h of food.

Half-life. 40 to 150 h.

Volume of distribution. 30 to 60 L.

Clearance. Plasma, 1.3 L/h.

Distribution in blood. Binding to red blood cells is less than 5% of the total concentration.

Protein binding. 90%, mainly to albumin.

Dose. 400 mg daily for 3 months.

Timolol

Beta-blocker

(2*S*)-1-[(1,1-Dimethylethyl)amino]-3-[[4-(4-morpholinyl)-1,2,5-thiadiazol-3-yl]oxy]-2-propanol
$C_{13}H_{24}N_4O_3S = 316.4$
CAS—26839-75-8

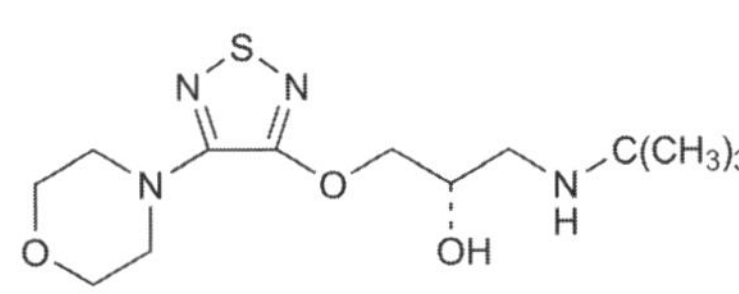

Timolol Maleate

Synonym. MK-950
Proprietary names. Aquanil; Betim(ol); Blocadren; Cusimolol; Dispatim; Glau-opt; Glaucol; Nyogel; Nyolol; Oftamolol; Oftan; Optimol; Timabak; Timacor; Timoftal; Timoptic; Timoptol; Timosil. It is an ingredient of Cosopt, Moducren and Prestim.
$C_{13}H_{24}N_4O_3S,C_4H_4O_4 = 432.5$
CAS—26921-17-5
A white crystalline powder. M.p. 201.5° to 202.5°.
Soluble in water, ethanol and methanol; sparingly soluble in chloroform; practically insoluble in ether.

Partition Coefficient. Log *P* (octanol/water), 1.8.

Colour Test. Liebermann's test (100°)—violet.

Thin-layer Chromatography. System TA—Rf 52; system TAE—Rf 20; system TAF—Rf 75; system TL—Rf 09; system TB—Rf 06; system TC—Rf 11; system TE—Rf 50.

Gas Chromatography. System GA—timolol RI 2266; timolol-Art RI 2275; system GB—timolol RI 2373; timolol-Art RI 2380.

High Performance Liquid Chromatography. System HA—*k* 1.2; system HAA—Retention time(s) 10.3 min; system HX—RI 317; system HY—RI 250; system HZ—Retention time(s) 2.1 min.

Ultraviolet Spectrum. Aqueous acid—295 nm (A_1^1=279a). No alkaline shift.

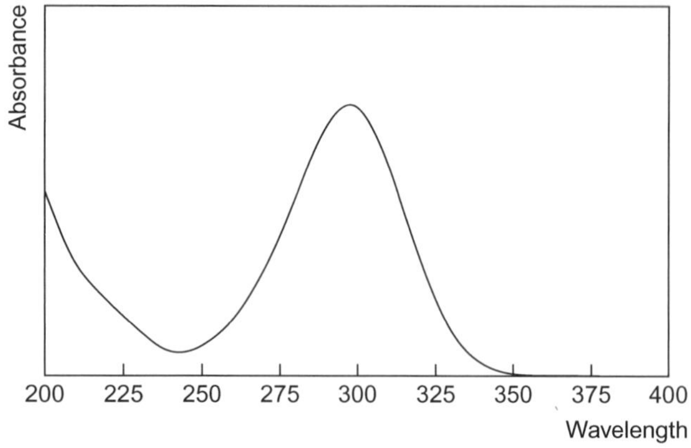

Infra-red Spectrum. Principal peaks at wavenumbers 1497, 1527, 1120, 1230, 1590, 1620 cm^{-1} (timolol maleate, KBr disk).

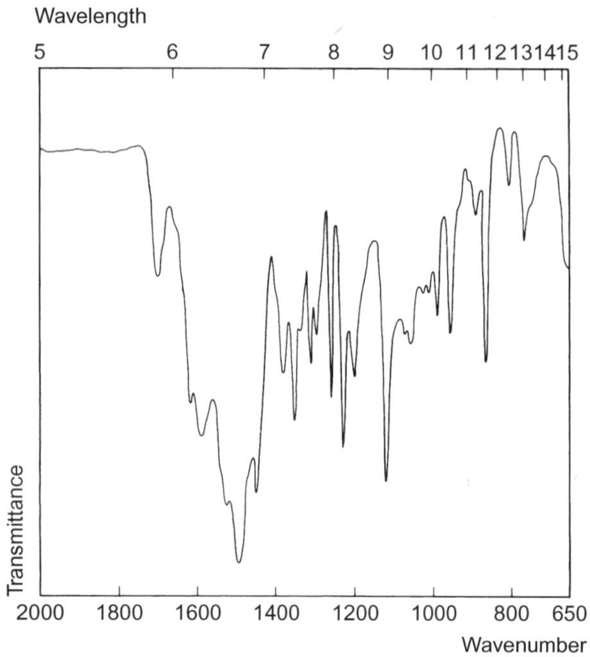

Mass Spectrum. Principal ions at *m/z* 30, 86, 57, 129, 74, 56, 41, 114.

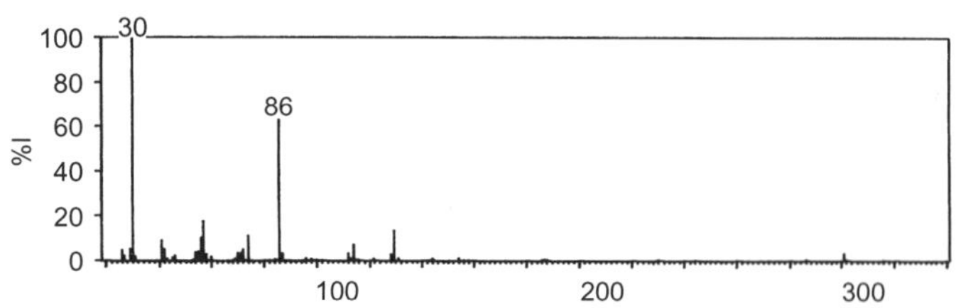

Quantification

Gas chromatography. In plasma or urine: limit of detection 2 µg/L and 20 µg/L, respectively, ECD—D. J. Tocco *et al.*, *J. Pharm. Sci.*, 1975, *64*, 1879–1881.

Gas chromatography–mass spectrometry. In plasma or urine: limit of detection 5 µg/L—J. B. Fourtillan *et al.*, *J. Pharm. Sci.*, 1981, *70*, 573–575. In hair: timolol and other beta-blockers, limit of detection 2 to 10 ng/g—P.Kintz *et al.*, *J. Forens. Sci.*, 2000, *45*, 170–174.

High performance liquid chromatography. In plasma or urine: limit of detection 40 µg/L, UV detection—M. A. Lefebvre *et al.*, *J. Liq. Chromatogr.*, 1981, *4*, 483–500. In plasma or urine: timolol and other beta-blockers, limit of detection 4 to 27 µg/L—A. Tracqui *et al.*, *Forens. Sci. Int.*, 1988, 38, 37–41; A. Tracqui *et al.*, *Acta Med. Leg. Soc. (Liege)*, 1989, *39*, 397–400. In plasma or breast milk: ECD—M. R. Gregg and D. B. Jack, *J. Chromatogr.*, 1984, *305*, 244–249. In urine: timolol and other beta-blockers, limit of detection 15 ppb to 500 ppb, amperometric detection—M. I. Maguregui *et al.*, *J. Chromatogr.*, 1995, *674*; *B. Biomed. Appl.*, 85–91.

High performance liquid chromatography–gas chromatography. In serum or urine: timolol and other beta-blockers, limit of detection 18 to 44 µg/L—T. Hyotylainen *et al.*, *J. Chromatogr. Sci.*, 1997, *35*, 280–286.

High performance liquid chromatography–mass spectrometry. In plasma: limit of detection 0.5 µg/L—T. V. Olah *et al.*, *J. Pharm. Biomed. Anal.*, 1993, *11*, 157–163.

Electrophoresis. In urine: limit of detection 190 µg/L, UV detection—M. I. Maguregui *et al.*, *J. Chromatogr.*, 2002, *949*, 91–97.

Disposition in the Body. Timolol is almost completely absorbed after oral administration. It is metabolised mainly by oxidation and hydrolytic cleavage of the morpholine ring. About 70% of a dose is excreted in the urine in 24 h, with about 20% of the dose as unchanged drug.

Therapeutic concentration

After a single oral dose of 20 mg to 5 subjects, peak plasma concentrations of 0.05 to 0.11 (mean 0.08) mg/L were attained in 0.5 to 3 h. [J. B. Fourtillan *et al.*, *Eur. J. Clin. Pharmacol.*, 1981, *19*, 193–196].

Following daily oral administration of 15 mg three times a day to 8 subjects, maximum steady-state plasma concentrations of 0.04 to 0.23 (mean 0.11) mg/L were reported. [B. N. Singh *et al.*, *Clin. Pharmacol. Ther.*, 1980, *28*, 159–166].

One, two, or three patches, each releasing 97.5 mg timolol, were applied at weekly intervals to subjects' inner arm for 48 h and produced mean plasma timolol concentrations of 5, 11 and 14 µg/L, respectively. A study of suppression of exercise heart rate and plasma timolol concentrations showed the 50% inhibitory concentration of timolol to be 2 to 4 µg/L. [J. B. McCrea *et al.*, *Pharmacotherapy*, 1990, *10*, 289–293].

Bioavailability. 50 to 75%.

Half-life. Plasma half-life, about 2 to 6 h.

Volume of distribution. 1 to 3 L/kg.

Clearance. Plasma clearance, about 5 to 10 mL/min/kg.

Dose. 10 to 60 mg of timolol maleate daily.

Tinidazole

Antiprotozoal

Synonym. CP-12574

Proprietary names. Amebysol; Ametricid; Amplium; Asiazole-TN; Dyzole; Estovyn-T; Fa-Cyl; Fasigin; Fasigyn(e); Funida; Ginosutin; Idazole; Pletil; Protocide; Simplotan; Sorquetan; Sporinex; Tini; Tonid; Trichonas; Tricolam; Trimonase; Trinizol; Triseptil.

1-[2-(Ethylsulfonyl)ethyl]-2-methyl-5-nitro-1*H*-imidazole

$C_8H_{13}N_3O_4S$=247.3

CAS—19387-91-8

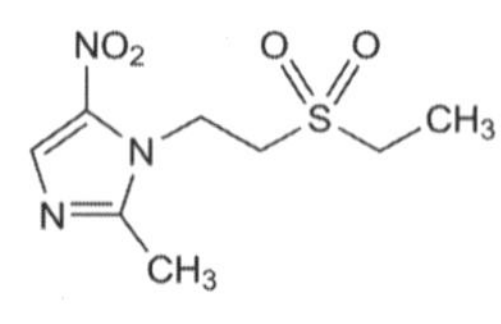

Colourless crystals. M.p. 127° to 128°.

Practically insoluble in water; soluble in acetone; sparingly soluble in methanol.

Partition Coefficient. Log *P* (octanol/water), –0.4.

Gas Chromatography. System GA—RI 2024.

High Performance Liquid Chromatography. System HAA—Retention time(s) 10.6 min.

Ultraviolet Spectrum. Aqueous acid—277 (A_1^1=245b); methanol—230 (A_1^1=148b), 311 nm (A_1^1=354b).

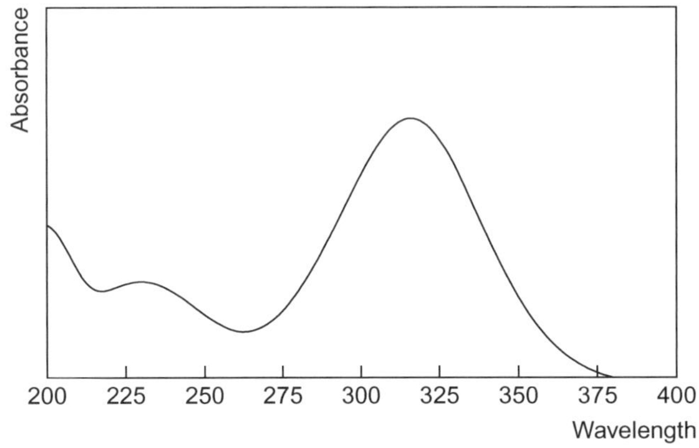

Quantification

Gas chromatography. In plasma or tissues: limit of detection 100 µg/L and 50 ng/g, respectively, AFID—H. Laufen *et al*, *J. Chromatogr.*, 1979, *163*; *B Biomed. Appl.*, *5*, 217–220.

High performance liquid chromatography. In serum or urine: limit of detection 300 µg/L and 600 µg/L, respectively, UV detection—I. Nilsson-Ehle *et al.*, *Antimicrob. Agents Chemother.*, 1981, *19*, 754–760. In serum: limit of detection 50 µg/L, UV/vis detection—K. Rajnarayana *et al.*, *Pharmazie*, 2002, *57*, 535–537.

Disposition in the Body. Tinidazole is well absorbed after oral administration. It is excreted in the bile. About 25% of a dose is excreted in the urine unchanged in 72 h together with small amounts of 2-hydroxymethyl-tinidazole and its glucuronide.

Therapeutic concentration

Following a single oral dose of 2 g to 3 subjects, peak serum concentrations of 35.7, 35.7 and 46.3 mg/L were attained in 2 to 3 h; serum concentrations of 0.19, 0.24 and 0.46 mg/L of the hydroxymethyl metabolite were reported, 6 h after the dose. [R. A. Robson *et al.*, *Clin. Pharmacokinet.*, 1984, *9*, 88–94].

A single oral dose of 2 g in 10 subjects produced serum tinidazole concentrations of 3.2 to 46.5 mg/L (concentrations in gingival crevicular fluid were similar); 24 h after the dose, the mean serum tinidazole concentration was 13 ± 3 mg/L. [V. Liew, *J. Dent. Res.*, 1991, *70*, 910–912].

Bioavailability. Greater than 90%.

Half-life. Plasma half-life, about 12 to 17 h.

Volume of distribution. About 0.7 L/kg.

Clearance. Plasma clearance, about 0.6 mL/min/kg.

Protein binding. In plasma, about 12%.

Note. For a review of tinidazole, see A. A. Carmine *et al.*, *Drugs*, 1982, *24*, 85–117.

Dose. Usually 2 g initially, by mouth, followed by 1 g daily.

Tiocarlide

Tuberculostatic

Synonym. Thiocarlide; DATC
Proprietary names. Disocarban; Datamil; Isoxyl
N,N'-[4-(3-Methylbutoxy)phenyl]thiourea
$C_{23}H_{32}N_2O_2S$ = 400.6
CAS—910-86-1

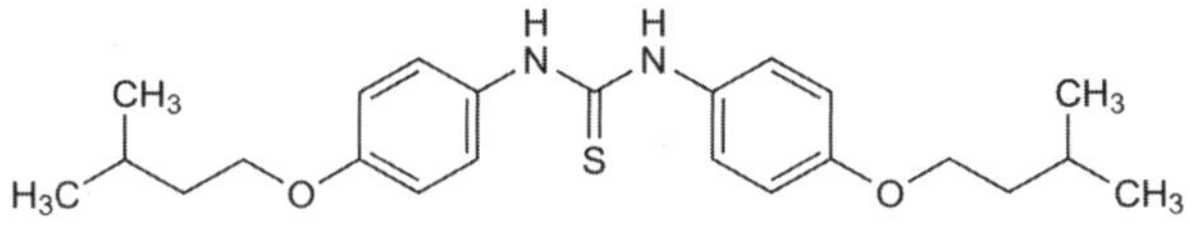

A white crystalline powder. M.p. 134° to 145°.
Practically insoluble in water; soluble in ethanol and chloroform.

Partition Coefficient. Log *P* (octanol/water), 7.2.

Colour Tests. Liebermann's test—green; Mandelin's test—green→yellow.

Thin-layer Chromatography. System TA—Rf 80; system TB—Rf 07; system TC—Rf 78; system TL—Rf 72. (Acidified iodoplatinate solution, positive.)

Gas Chromatography. System GA—RI 2005.

Infra-red Spectrum. Principal peaks at wavenumbers 1228, 1499, 1534, 823, 1163, 1285 cm^{-1} (KBr disk).

Mass Spectrum. Principal ions at *m/z* 109, 151, 43, 41, 221, 179, 29, 108.

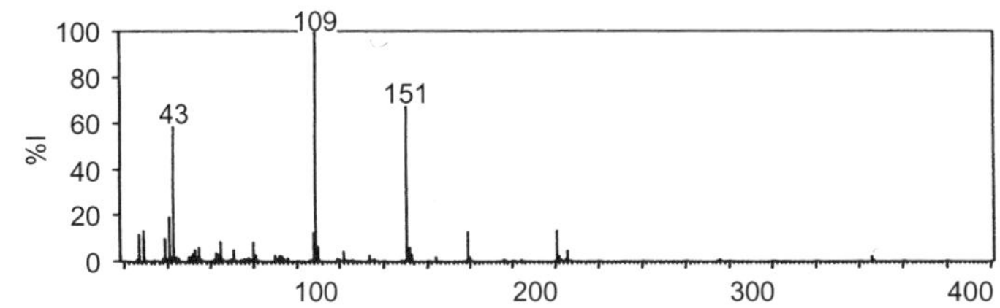

Dose. 6 g daily.

Tioguanine

Antineoplastic

Synonyms. 6-TG; Thioguanine.
Proprietary name. Lanvis
2-Amino-1,7-dihydro-6*H*-purine-6-thione
$C_5H_5N_5S$ = 167.2
CAS—154-42-7 (anhydrous); 5580-03-0 (hemihydrate)

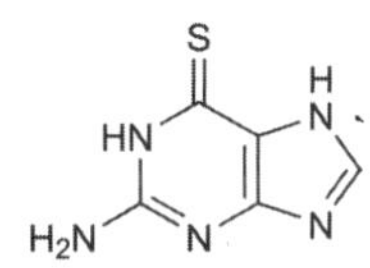

A pale yellow crystalline powder. M.p. >360°.
Practically insoluble in water, ethanol and chloroform; freely soluble in dilute solutions of alkali hydroxides.

Partition Coefficient. Log *P* (octanol/water), –0.1.

Ultraviolet Spectrum. Aqueous acid—258 (A^1_1 = 490b), 348 (A^1_1 = 1240a); aqueous alkali—320 nm (A^1_1 = 1015b).

Infra-red Spectrum. Principal peaks at wavenumbers 1625, 1668, 1257, 1539, 1231, 971 cm^{-1} (KBr disk).

Quantification

Spectrofluorimetry. In plasma: limit of detection 5 µg/L—T. Dooley and J. L. Maddocks, *Br. J. Clin. Pharmacol.*, 1980, *9*, 77–82.

High performance liquid chromatography. In plasma or urine: limit of detection 200 µg/L, UV detection—H. Breithaupt and G. Goebel, *J. Chromatogr. Sci.*, 1981, *19*, 496–499. In plasma: tioguanine and metabolites, limit of detection about 130 µg/L, UV detection—P. A. Andrews *et al.*, *J. Chromatogr.*, 1982, 227; *Biomed. Appl.*, *16*, 83–91. In plasma, urine or cerebrospinal fluid—J. L. Rudy *et al.*, *Ann. Clin. Biochem.*, 1988, *25*, 504–509.

Disposition in the Body. Tioguanine is incompletely and variably absorbed after oral administration. It is rapidly activated by intracellular conversion to thioguanylic acid. It is inactivated by methylation to aminomethylthiopurine and by deamination to thioxanthine. About 40% of an oral dose is excreted in the urine as metabolites in 24 h; only traces of tioguanine have been detected.

Dose. Initially 2 to 2.5 mg/kg daily.

Tiotixene

Tranquilliser

Synonym. Thiothixene
Proprietary names. Navane (capsules and tablets); Orbinamon.
N,N-Dimethyl-9-[3-(4-methyl-1-piperazinyl)propylidene]thioxanthene-2-sulfonamide
$C_{23}H_{29}N_3O_2S_2$ = 443.6

CAS—5591-45-7; 3313-26-6 (Z)

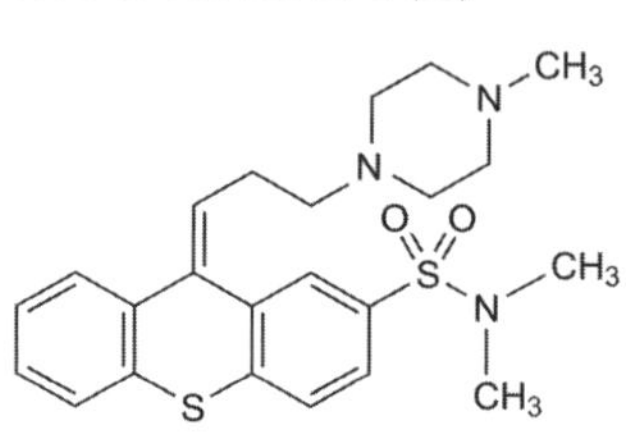

cis-form

A white to tan-coloured crystalline powder. M.p. 147° to 149°.
Practically insoluble in water; soluble 1 in 110 of dehydrated alcohol, 1 in 2 of chloroform and 1 in 120 of ether; slightly soluble in acetone and in methanol.

Tiotixene Hydrochloride

Proprietary names. Navane (oral concentrate); Thixit.
$C_{23}H_{29}N_3O_2S_2,2HCl,2H_2O=552.6$
CAS—58513-59-0 (anhydrous); 49746-04-5 (anhydrous, Z); 22189-31-7 (dihydrate); 49746-09-0 (dihydrate, Z)
A white crystalline powder.
Soluble 1 in 8 of water, 1 in 270 of dehydrated alcohol and 1 in 280 of chloroform; practically insoluble in acetone, in ether and in benzene.

Partition Coefficient. Log *P* (octanol/water), 3.8.

Colour Tests. Formaldehyde–Sulfuric acid—red; Liebermann's test—red; Mandelin's test—red; Marquis test—red; Sulfuric acid—orange.

Thin-layer Chromatography. System TA—Rf 49; system TAE—tiotixene Rf 26; M Rf 12; system TAF—Rf 24; system TL—Rf 07; system TB—Rf 10; system TC—Rf 40; system TE—tiotixene Rf 44; M Rf 36; system TAJ—Rf 19; system TAK—Rf 05; system TAL—Rf 71. (Acidified iodoplatinate solution, positive.)

Gas Chromatography. System GA—RI 3060.

High Performance Liquid Chromatography. System HA—*k* 3.8; system HX—RI 442; system HY—RI 374; system HZ—Retention time(s) 6.8 min.

Ultraviolet Spectrum. Aqueous acid—308 nm ($A_1^1=191a$).

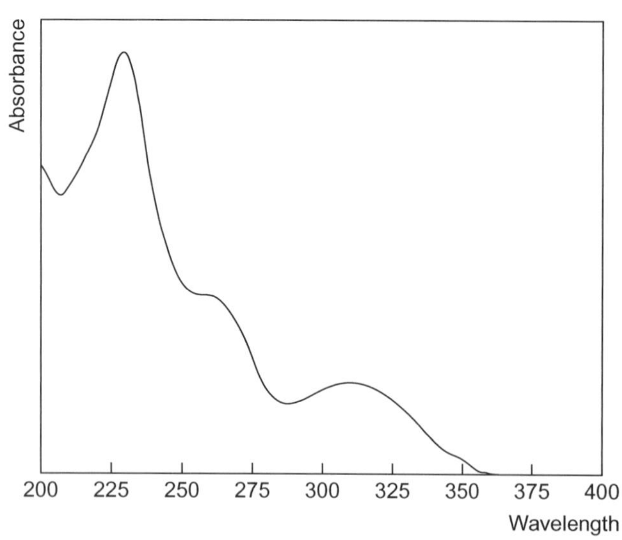

Infra-red Spectrum. Principal peaks at wavenumbers 1156, 719, 765, 1176, 957, 747 cm^{-1} (KBr disk).

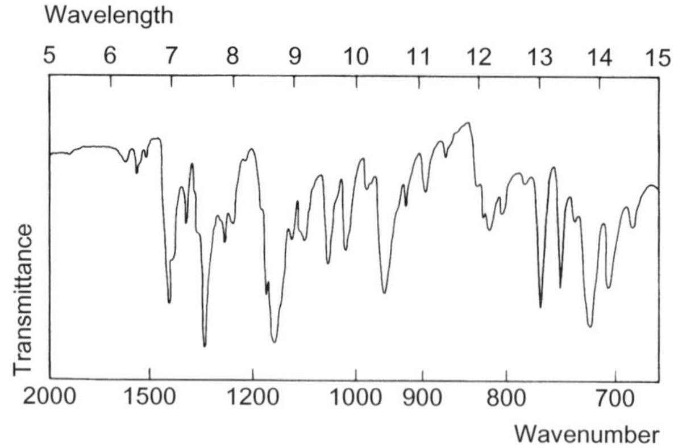

Mass Spectrum. Principal ions at *m/z* 113, 70, 114, 42, 221, 222, 56, 43.

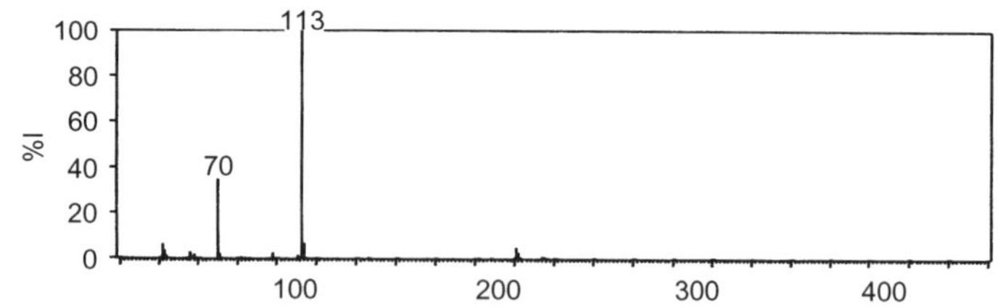

Quantification

Gas chromatography–mass spectrometry. In plasma: limit of detection <1 µg/L—D. C. Hobbs *et al., Clin. Pharmacol. Ther.*, 1974, *16*, 473–478.

High performance liquid chromatography. In plasma: *cis*- and *trans*-tiotixene, UV detection—S. C. Bogema *et al., J. Chromatogr.*, 1982, *233*; *Biomed. Appl.*, *22*, 257–267. In serum: limit of detection 0.05 µg/L, UV detection—C. Dilger *et al., Arzneimittelforschung*, 1988, *38*, 1522–1525. In plasma: *cis*-tiotixene, limit of detection 200 ng/L, coulometric detection—M. Hariharan *et al., Ther. Drug Monit.*, 1991, *13*, 79–85.

Disposition in the Body. Tiotixene is rapidly absorbed after oral administration. The *N*-desmethyl derivative accounts for about 10% of the plasma concentration; other unidentified metabolites may accumulate on chronic administration.

Therapeutic concentration

Following chronic oral administration of 15 to 60 mg daily in divided doses to 15 subjects, plasma concentrations, determined 2 to 2½ h after the last daily dose, were in the range 0.010 to 0.023 (mean 0.016) mg/L. [D. C. Hobbs *et al., Clin. Pharmacol. Ther.*, 1974, *16*, 473–478].

A study in 42 schizophrenic patients showed that a median plasma concentration of 12 to 15 µg/L might be expected with a daily dose of 60 mg of tiotixene. [L. E. Hollister *et al., Int. Clin. Psychopharmacol.*, 1987, *2*, 77–82].

Toxicity

In a fatality involving the ingestion of 250 mg of tiotixene and an unknown quantity of doxepin, a postmortem blood concentration of 0.13 mg/L of tiotixene was reported. [R. C. Baselt, *Disposition of Toxic Drugs and Chemicals in Man*, 5th Edn, Davis, California, Biomedical Publications, 2000, pp. 830–831].

A blood concentration of 0.53 mg/L was detected in acute overdosage with tiotixene before it declined to 0.047 mg/L in 12 h. [M. Kemal and R. H. Imami, *J. Anal. Toxicol.*, 1985, *9*, 94–95].

Half-life. Plasma half-life, about 34 h.

Dose. Usually 10 to 30 mg daily; up to 60 mg daily may be given.

Tirofiban

Antithrombotic

N-(Butylsulfonyl)-*O*-[4-(4-piperidinyl)butyl]-L-tyrosine
$C_{22}H_{36}N_2O_5S=440.6$
CAS—144494-65-5

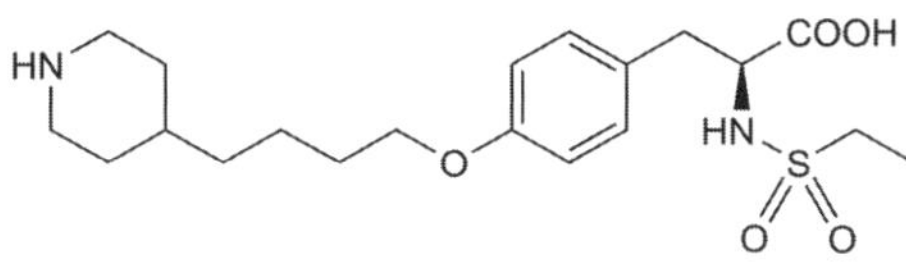

A white solid, m.p. 223° to 225°.

Tirofiban Hydrochloride Monohydrate
Synonyms. L-700462; MK-0383; MK-383.
Proprietary name. Aggrastat
$C_{22}H_{36}N_2O_5S,HCl,H_2O = 495.1$
CAS—142373-60-2 (anhydrous); *150915-40-5* (monohydrate)
A white to off-white, non-hygroscopic, free-flowing powder, m.p. 131° to 132°. It is very slightly soluble in water.

High Performance Liquid Chromatography. Column: RX-C_{18} (Zorbax, 250 × 4.6 mm i.d., 5 µm). Mobile phase: acetonitrile:ammonium acetate (1 mM) (pH 6.0) (41.5 : 58.5), flow rate 1 mL/min. Internal standard (IS): L-702,128. Detection: MS–MS (Aggrastat, *m/z* 535 → 415; IS, *m/z* 555 → 141). Retention times: Tirofiban, 5.2 min; IS, 5.1 min [J. D. Ellis *et al.*, *J. Pharm. Biomed. Anal.*, 1997, *15(5)*, 561–569].

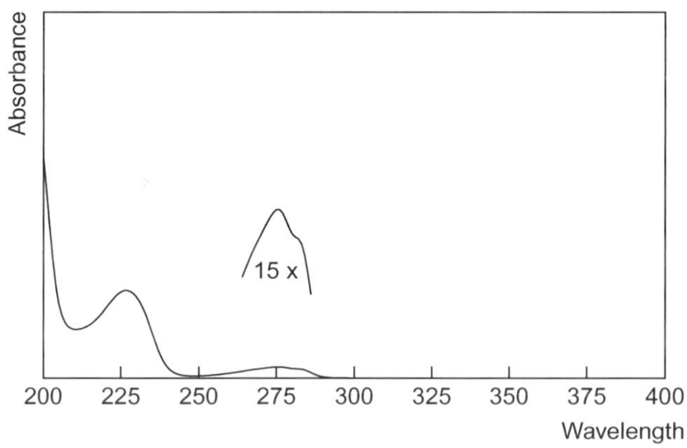

Quantification
High performance liquid chromatography–mass spectrometry. In plasma: limit of quantification is 0.4 µg/L, tandem MS detection—J. D. Ellis *et al.*, *J. Pharm. Biomed. Anal.*, 1997, *15(5)*, 561–569.

Disposition in the Body. Tirofiban is mainly cleared from plasma by renal excretion. Approximately 65% of a dose is recovered in urine and 25% in faeces mainly as the unchanged drug. Metabolism is limited.

Therapeutic concentration

18 healthy males were administered 0.05, 0.10, 0.15, 0.25 and 0.40 µg/kg/min doses of tirofiban hydrochloride as a 1 h infusion. A separate group of 20 healthy males were administered 0.10, 0.15 and 0.20 µg/kg/min doses as a 4 h infusion. The peak plasma concentrations after the 1 h infusion were 5.4, 10.9, 12.0, 30.1 and 47.8 µg/L for the 5 doses and after the 4 h infusion, 20.7, 42.2 and 42.6 µg/L for the 0.10, 0.15 and 0.20 µg/kg/min doses, respectively. As part of the study, the volunteers were administered 0.15 µg/kg/min tirofiban hydrochloride as a 4 h infusion with 325 mg aspirin administered the day before treatment and approximately 1 h before the tirofiban dose. The peak concentration of tirofiban was 29.3 µg/L [J. S. Barrett *et al.*, *Clin. Pharmacol. Ther.*, 1994, *56*, 377–388].

Toxicity. Overdosing may result in bleeding, primarily minor mucocutaneous bleeding and minor bleeding at the sites of cardiac catheterisation. Tirofiban has also been associated with a higher incidence of thrombocytopenia.

Half-life. 1.2 to 2.0 h.

Volume of distribution. Steady state, 22 to 42 L.

Clearance. Plasma, 213 to 329 mL/min; 152 to 267 mL/min in patients with coronary artery disease. This value is decreased further in elderly patients, and is reduced in patients with severe renal insufficiency (creatinine clearance, < 30 mL/min) by approximately 50%.

Protein binding. Not highly plasma protein bound.

Dose. IV infusion, 0.4 µg/kg/min initially for 30 min followed by 0.1 µg/kg/min for at least 48 h (continued during and for 12 to 24 h after percutaneous coronary invention). Maximum duration is 108 h.

Tizanidine

Muscle Relaxant/Alpha$_2$ Adrenergic Agonist

Synonyms. AN-021; DS-103-282; DS-103-282-ch.
Proprietary names. Sirdalud; Temelin; Zanaflex.
5-Chloro-*N*-(4,5-dihydro-1*H*-imidazol-2-yl)-2,1,3-benzothiadiazol-4-amine
$C_9H_8ClN_5S = 253.7$
CAS—51322-75-9

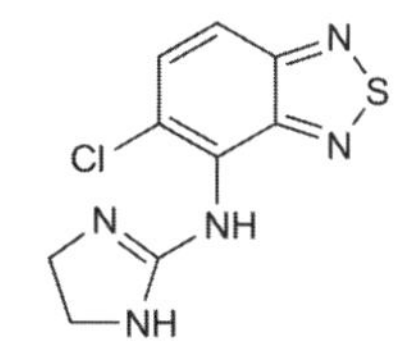

A white to off-white fine crystalline odourless powder with M. p. 221° to 223°. It is slightly soluble in water and methanol.

Tizanidine Hydrochloride
$C_9H_9Cl_2N_5S,HCl = 290.2$
CAS—64461-82-1
A white to off-white fine crystalline odourless powder. It is slightly soluble in water and methanol. Its solubility in water decreases as the pH increases.

Thin-layer Chromatography. System TB—Rf 04; system TE—Rf 56; system TAE—Rf 51.

High Performance Liquid Chromatography. System HX—RI 247; system HZ—Retention time 2.3 min.

Ultraviolet Spectrum. Aqueous acid—227, 313, 319 nm.

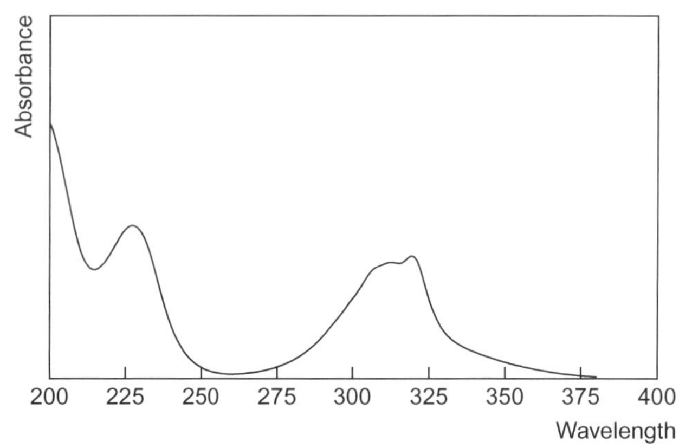

Mass Spectrum. Principal ions at *m/z* 253, 218, 196, 255, 42, 198, 43, 44.

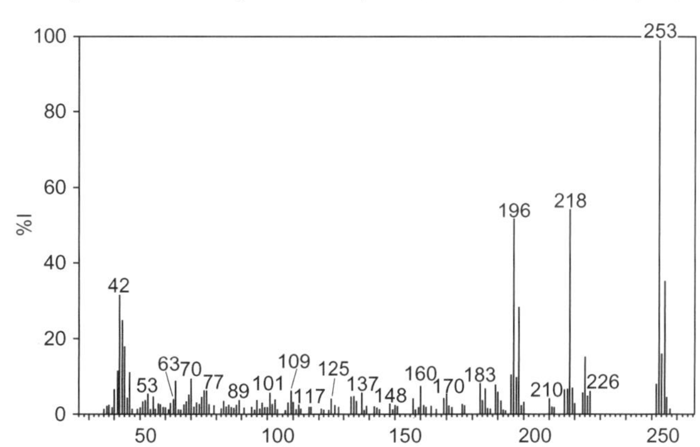

Disposition in the Body. Tizanidine is rapidly absorbed from the gastro-intestinal tract with 53 to 66% of the dose being absorbed. Peak plasma concentrations are reached within 1 to 2 h after oral administration. The drug is widely distributed throughout the body and undergoes rapid and extensive first-pass metabolism in the liver (approximately 95% of a dose). Metabolism is via oxidation of the imidazoline moiety, the aromatic system and the sulfur atom. Approximately 70% of the dose is excreted in urine as the inactive metabolite, and 20% is excreted in faeces. Renal excretion of the parent compound is approximately 53% after a single 5 mg dose. Tizanidine has a short duration of action. Food has no influence on its pharmacokinetics. The drug displays linear pharmacokinetics within the dose 1 to 20 mg.

Therapeutic concentration

15 healthy males, aged between 19 and 27 years (mean, 23.5 years), were administered with 4 mg twice daily for seven consecutive doses. The volunteers fasted for 10 h before the first dose and for 2 h after each subsequent dose. The mean peak plasma concentration was 2.51 μg/L observed at 0.9 h [M. Kent Shellenberger *et al.*, *Drug Metab. Dispos.*, 1999, *27(2)*, 201–204].

Toxicity. Low order of acute toxicity.

A 46-year-old male with multiple sclerosis fell into coma very shortly after ingesting one hundred 4 mg tablets of tizanidine. Respiratory depression occurred but the patient recovered [*Physicians Desk Reference*, 56th Edn., Thomson Healthcare, Montvale, NJ, 2001].

Bioavailability. 34 to 40%.

Half-life. 2.1 to 4.2 h.

Volume of distribution. Steady state, 2.4 L/kg.

Clearance. Reduced by 50% in the elderly, renal impairment and women taking oral contraceptives.

Protein binding. 30%.

Dose. The usual initial dose is 2 mg which may be increased in steps of 2 mg daily over 3 to 4 days, depending on response. The maximum is 36 mg daily and the usual is 24 mg.

Tobramycin

Antibiotic

Synonym. Nebramycin Factor 6
Proprietary names. AkTob; Brulamycin; Defy; Distobram; Gernebcin; Mytobrin; Nebcin(a); Nebcine; Obracin; Tobi; Tobra(l); Tobra-cell; Tobracil; Tobradistin; Tobralex; Tobramaxin; Tobramina; Tobrasix; Tobrex; Tobridavi; Tomycin(e); Trazil.
O-3-Amino-3-deoxy-α-D-glucopyranosyl-(1→6)-*O*-[2,6-diamino-2,3,6-trideoxy-α-D-*ribo*-hexopyranosyl-(1→4)]-2-deoxy-D-streptamine
$C_{18}H_{37}N_5O_9$=467.5
CAS—32986-56-4; 49842-07-1 (sulfate: xH_2SO_4); 79645-27-5 (sulfate: 5H_2SO_4)

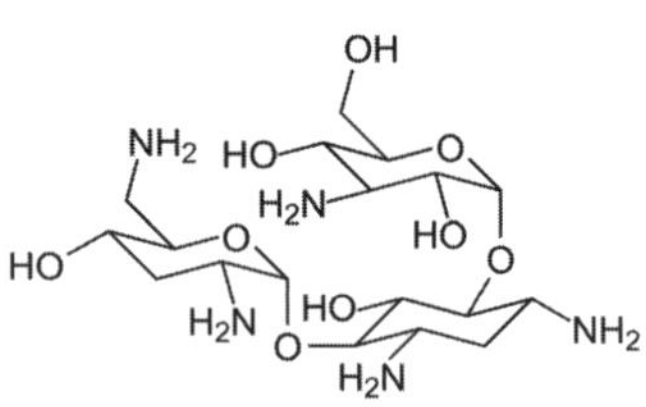

A white hygroscopic powder. A solution in water is dextro-rotatory.
Soluble 1 in 1.5 of water and 1 in 2000 of ethanol; practically insoluble in chloroform and ether.

Dissociation Constant. pK_a 6.7, 8.3, 9.9.

Partition Coefficient. Log *P* (octanol/water), –5.8.

Thin-layer Chromatography. System TAE—Rf 00.

High Performance Liquid Chromatography. System HAA—Retention time(s) 13.4 min.

Ultraviolet Spectrum. No significant absorption, 230 to 360 nm.

Infra-red Spectrum. Principal peaks at wavenumbers 1040, 1590, 845, 770, 660, 1260 cm^{-1} (KBr disk).

Quantification See also under Amikacin.

High performance liquid chromatography. In serum or urine: limit of detection 200 μg/L, fluorescence detection—D. B. Haughey *et al.*, *Antimicrob. Agents Chemother.*, 1980, *17*, 649–653. In serum: limit of detection 500 μg/L, UV detection—D. M. Barends *et al.*, *J Chromatogr.*, 1981, *225*, 417–426. In serum: tobramycin and other aminoglycosides—L. Essers, *J. Chromatogr.*, 1984, *305*, 345–352.

Disposition in the Body. Tobramycin is poorly absorbed after oral administration, but rapidly absorbed after IM injection. Up to 90% of a dose is excreted unchanged in the urine in 24 h, most being excreted within the first 6 h. It accumulates in the tissues and may be detected in serum and urine for several days after cessation of treatment.

Therapeutic concentration. During treatment, the serum concentration should be in the range 4 to 10 mg/L and should be monitored regularly, especially in patients who have renal insufficiency. During multiple dosing the trough concentration immediately preceding a dose should not exceed 2 mg/L.

After an IV infusion of 100 mg administered over 1 h to 4 subjects, peak serum concentrations of 4.1 to 5.1 (mean 4.6) mg/L were achieved at the end of the infusion. After a single IM injection of 100 mg administered to 3 subjects, a mean peak serum concentration of 5.16 mg/L was achieved after 0.3 to 0.75 h. [C. Regamey *et al.*, *Clin. Pharmacol. Ther.*, 1973, *14*, 396–403].

Cystic fibrosis patients inhaling 300 mg tobramycin twice daily as an aerosol, in 28-day on/off treatment cycles, had a mean serum concentration of 0.95 mg/L 1 hour after the dose. The mean peak sputum concentration of tobramycin was 1.237 mg/g. [D. E. Geller *et al.*, *Chest*, 2002, *122*, 219–226].

Toxicity. Toxic effects may be produced at serum concentrations of 12 mg/L or more or, during chronic treatment, if the trough serum concentration exceeds 2 mg/L.

Half-life. Plasma half-life, about 2 to 3 h, increased in renal failure; a long terminal elimination phase of about 6 days has also been reported.

Volume of distribution. About 0.3 L/kg.

Clearance. Plasma clearance, about 1.5 mL/min/kg.

Protein binding. In plasma, up to 10%.

Dose. Usually the equivalent of 3 to 5 mg/kg of tobramycin daily, given parenterally.

Tocainide

Anti-arrhythmic

2-Amino-*N*-(2,6-dimethylphenyl)propanamide
$C_{11}H_{16}N_2O$=192.3
CAS—41708-72-9

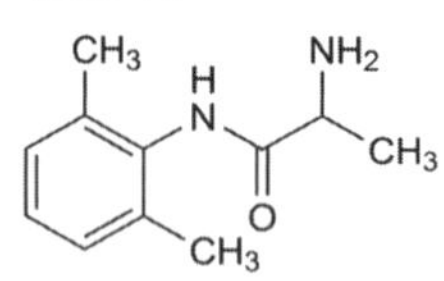

A white waxy solid. M.p. 53° to 55°.
Sparingly soluble in water; freely soluble in organic solvents.

Tocainide Hydrochloride

Proprietary names. Tonocard; Xylotocan.
$C_{11}H_{16}N_2O$,HCl=228.7
CAS—71395-14-7 ((±)-Form); *CAS—53984-74-0* (R-(–)-Form); *CAS—53984-76-2* (S-(–)-Form)
A white crystalline powder. M.p. about 245°, with decomposition.
Freely soluble in water and ethanol; practically insoluble in chloroform and ether.

Dissociation Constant. pK_a 7.8.

Partition Coefficient. Log *P* (octanol/water), 0.8.

Thin-layer Chromatography. System TA—Rf 60; system TB—Rf 02; system TC—Rf 23; system TE—Rf 44; system TAE—Rf 42; system TAF—Rf 74.

Gas Chromatography. System GA—RI 1714; system GB—RI 1769.

High Performance Liquid Chromatography. System HA—*k* 1.2; system HX—RI 247; system HY—RI 208; system HZ—Retention time(s) 2.1 min.

Ultraviolet Spectrum. Aqueous acid—262 (A_1^1=22a), 270 nm (A_1^1=18b).

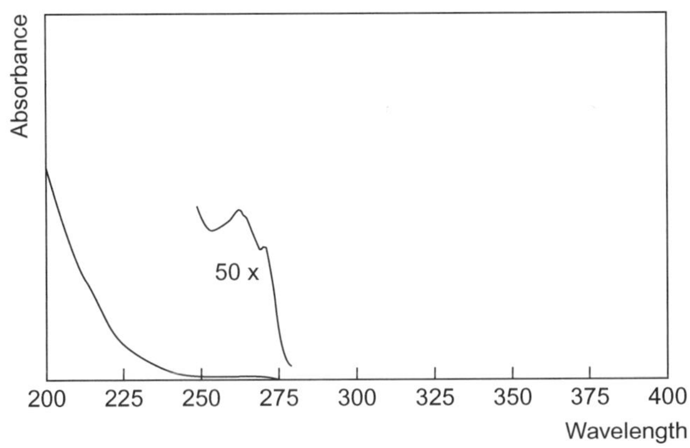

Infra-red Spectrum. Principal peaks at wavenumbers 1675, 1540, 765, 1128, 772, 1240 cm^{-1} (tocainide hydrochloride, KBr disk).

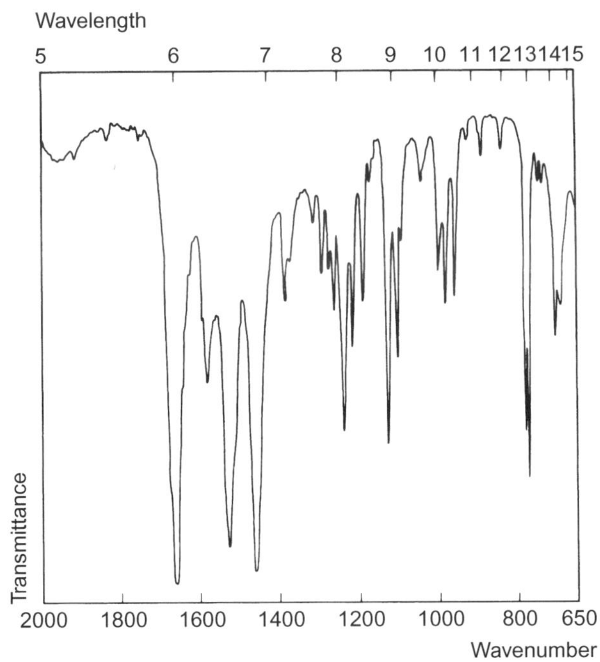

Mass Spectrum. Principal ions at *m/z* 44, 121, 77, 120, 42, 106, 91, 39.

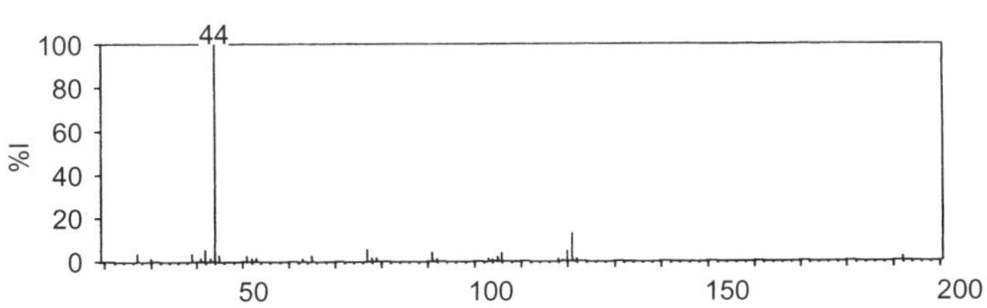

Quantification

Gas chromatography. In plasma or urine: limit of detection 2 pg, ECD—G. K. Pillai *et al.*, *J. Chromatogr.*, 1982, *229*; *B Biomed. Appl.*, *18*, 103–109. In plasma or serum: limit of detection 200 µg/L, FID—S. D. Gettings *et al.*, *J. Chromatogr.*, 1981, *225*; *B Biomed. Appl.*, *14*, 469–475.

High performance liquid chromatography. In plasma: limit of detection 100 µg/L, fluorescence detection—A. J. Sedman and J. Gal, *J. Chromatogr.*, 1982, *232*; *B Biomed. Appl.*, *21*, 315–326. In serum or plasma: tocainide and other anti-arrhythmics—T. Annesley *et al.*, *Res. Commun. Chem. Path. Pharmacol.*, 1986, *51*, 173–181; E. vasBinder and T. Annesley, *Biomed. Chromatogr.*, 1991, *5*, 19–22. In serum: tocainide and other anti-arrhythmics and metabolites, limit of detection 100 to 200 µg/L—H. F. Proelss and T. B. Townsend, *Clin. Chem.*, 1986, *32*, 1311–1317. In plasma: tocainide and other anti-arrhythmics, fluorescence or UV detection—R. Verbesselt *et al.*, *Ther. Drug Monit.*, 1991, *13*, 157–165. In plasma: limit of detection 250 µg/L, fluorescence detection—R. A. Carr *et al.*, *J. Chromatogr.*, 1991, *566*, 155–162.

Disposition in the Body. Tocainide is almost completely absorbed after oral administration. About 20 to 50% of a dose is excreted in the urine as unchanged drug in 24 h, and about 20 to 30% as a glucuronide conjugate, which is thought to be tocainide carbamoyl *O*-β-D-glucuronide (TOCG); an additional metabolite, lactoxylidide has also been detected in urine.

Therapeutic concentration. In plasma, usually in the range 4 to 12 mg/L.

Following a single oral dose of 400 mg to 3 subjects, peak plasma concentrations of 1.6 to 1.8 mg/L were attained in 0.5 to 2 h. After oral administration of 400 mg three times a day to 4 subjects, steady-state plasma concentrations of 4.9 to 7.1 (mean 5.9) mg/L were reported. [C. Graffner *et al.*, *Clin. Pharmacol. Ther.*, 1980, *27*, 64–71].

Toxicity

A 26-year-old woman who committed suicide by ingesting a large amount of tocainide was found to have a serum concentration of 68 mg/L. [K. Sperry *et al.*, *J. Forensic Sci.*, 1987, *32*, 1440–1446].

Half-life. Plasma half-life, 8 to 25 (mean 14) h.

Volume of distribution. About 1 to 3 L/kg.

Clearance. Plasma clearance, about 2 to 3 mL/min/kg.

Protein binding. In plasma, variously reported as 10 to 50%.

Note. For a review of tocainide, see B. Holmes *et al.*, *Drugs*, 1983, *26*, 93–123.

Dose. 1.2 to 2.4 g of tocainide hydrochloride daily, by mouth.

Tofenacin

Antidepressant

Synonyms. *N*-Demethylorphenadrine; Desmethylorphenadrine.
N-Methyl-2-[(2-methylphenyl)phenylmethoxy]ethanamine
$C_{17}H_{21}NO$=255.4
CAS—15301-93-6

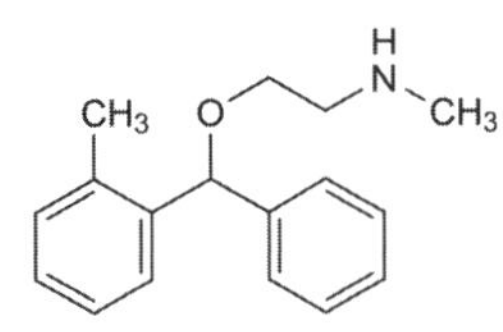

A liquid.

Tofenacin Hydrochloride

Synonym. BS-7331
Proprietary names. Elamol; Tofacine.
$C_{17}H_{21}NO,HCl$=291.8
CAS—10488-36-5
A white to off-white crystalline powder. M.p. 147° to 148°.
Soluble 1 in about 3 of water, 1 in 8 of ethanol and 1 in 3 of chloroform; slightly soluble in acetone; practically insoluble in ether.

Partition Coefficient. Log *P* (octanol/water), 3.4.

Colour Tests. Liebermann's test—red-orange; Mandelin's test—yellow; Marquis test—yellow; Sulfuric acid—orange.

Thin-layer Chromatography. System TA—Rf 45; system TB—Rf 26; system TC—Rf 21; system TE—Rf 48; system TL—Rf 7; system TAE—Rf 14. (Acidified potassium permanganate solution, positive.)

Gas Chromatography. System GA—RI 1920; system GB—RI 2013; system GM—RRT 0.420 (relative to iprindole).

High Performance Liquid Chromatography. System HA—*k* 1.7; system HZ—Retention time(s) 5.3 min.

Ultraviolet Spectrum. Ethanol—259, 265, 272 nm.

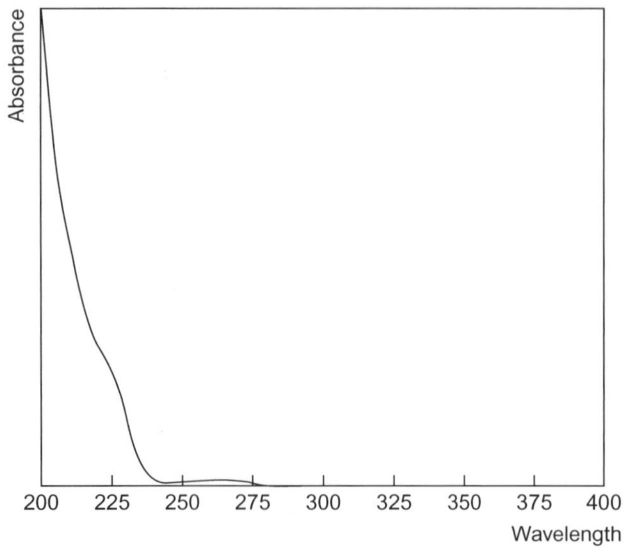

Infra-red Spectrum. Principal peaks at wavenumbers 1102, 704, 757, 1117, 1042, 917 cm^{-1} (tofenacin hydrochloride, KBr disk).

Mass Spectrum. Principal ions at *m/z* 44, 59, 165, 166, 181, 179, 178, 43.

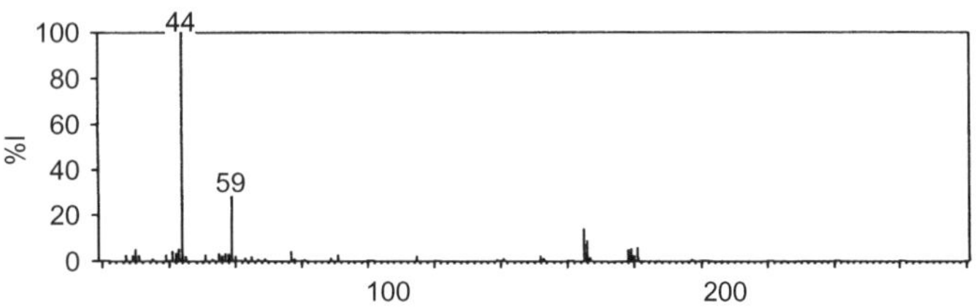

Quantification. See under Orphenadrine.

Disposition in the Body. Tofenacin is a metabolite of orphenadrine.

Dose. Up to 240 mg of tofenacin hydrochloride daily.

Tolazamide

Antidiabetic

Proprietary names. Diabewas; Norglycin; Tolanase; Tolinase.

N-[[(Hexahydro-1*H*-azepin-1-yl)amino]carbonyl]-4-methylbenzenesulfonamide

$C_{14}H_{21}N_3O_3S$=311.4

CAS—1156-19-0

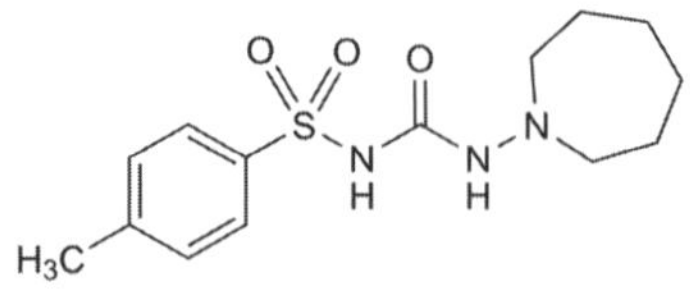

A white crystalline powder. M.p. 170° to 173°.

Very slightly soluble in water; slightly soluble in ethanol; soluble in acetone; freely soluble in chloroform.

Dissociation Constant. pK_a 3.5 (25°), 5.7 (37.5°)

Partition Coefficient. Log *P* (octanol/water), 2.7.

Thin-layer Chromatography. System TAD—Rf 66; system TAE—Rf 86; system TB—Rf 00; system TD—Rf 52; system TE—Rf 07; system TF—Rf 50; system TAJ—Rf 65; system TAK—Rf 71; system TAL—Rf 95. (Acidified potassium permanganate solution, positive.)

Gas Chromatography. System GA—RI 1651.

High Performance Liquid Chromatography. System HX—RI 452; system HY—RI 445; system HZ—Retention time(s) 6.8 min.

Ultraviolet Spectrum. Methanol—257, 263 (A^1_1=21a), 268, 275 nm.

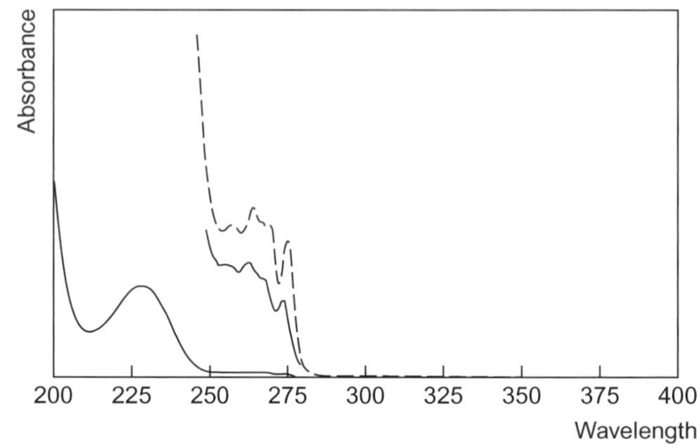

Infra-red Spectrum. Principal peaks at wavenumbers 1694, 1176, 884, 819, 675, 1086 cm^{-1} (KBr disk). Polymorphism may occur.

Mass Spectrum. Principal ions at *m/z* 91, 155, 114, 65, 197, 42, 41, 85.

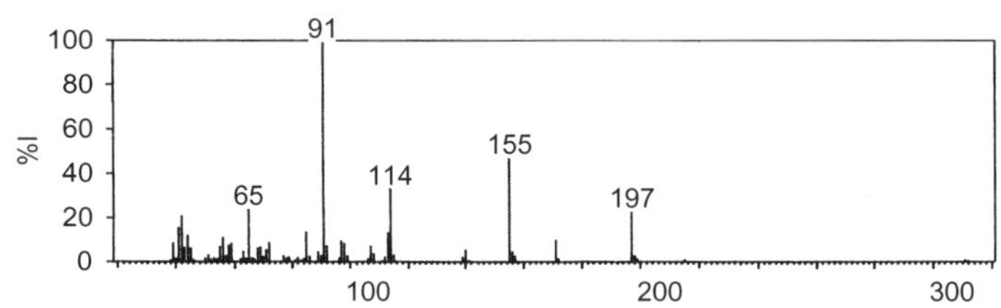

Quantification

High performance liquid chromatography. In serum: limit of detection 1 mg/L, UV detection—P. G. Welling *et al.*, *J. Pharm. Sci.*, 1982, *71*, 1259–1263.

Micellar electrokinetic chromatography. In urine: tolazamide and other hypoglycaemic drugs, limit of detection 50 µg/L—M. Nunez *et al.*, *Anal. Chem.*, 1995, *67*, 3668–3675.

Disposition in the Body. Tolazamide is slowly absorbed after oral administration. About 85% of a dose is excreted in the urine in 5 days, mostly in the first 24 h. Of the urinary material, about 17% is the *p*-carboxy derivative, 25% is 4-hydroxytolazamide, 10% is *p*-hydroxymethyltolazamide, 26% is *p*-toluenesulfonamide, and 7% is unchanged drug.

Therapeutic concentration

Following a single oral dose of 500 mg to 20 subjects, a mean peak serum concentration of 27.8 mg/L was attained in 3 h. [P. G. Welling *et al.*, *J. Pharm. Sci.*, 1982, *71*, 1259–1263].

Half-life. Plasma half-life, about 5 h.

Protein binding. In plasma, about 94%.

Note. For a review of the pharmacokinetics of sulfonylurea hypoglycaemic drugs, see J. E. Jackson and R. Bressler, *Drugs*, 1981, *22*, 211–245.

Dose. 0.1 to 1 g daily.

Tolazoline

Vasodilator

Synonym. Benzazoline

4,5-Dihydro-2-(phenylmethyl)-1*H*-imidazole

$C_{10}H_{12}N_2$=160.2

CAS—59-98-3

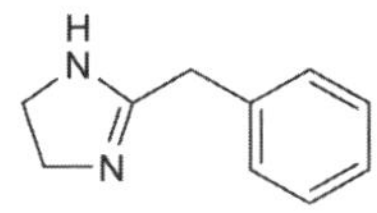

Soluble in water and chloroform.

Tolazoline Hydrochloride

Proprietary names. Priscol; Priscoline; Vaso-Dilatan.
$C_{10}H_{12}N_2,HCl = 196.7$
CAS—59-97-2
A white or creamy-white crystalline powder. M.p. 174°.
Soluble 1 in 0.5 of water, 1 in 2 of ethanol and 1 in 3 of chloroform; practically insoluble in ether.

Dissociation Constant. pK_a 10.6 (20°).

Partition Coefficient. Log *P* (octanol/water), 2.7.

Colour Tests. Aromaticity (Method 2)—colourless/orange; Liebermann's test—orange.

Thin-layer Chromatography. System TA—Rf 13; system TB—Rf 02; system TC—Rf 02; system TE—Rf 25; system TL—Rf 02; system TAE—Rf 03; system TAF—Rf 55. (Acidified iodoplatinate solution, positive.)

Gas Chromatography. System GA—RI 1598.

High Performance Liquid Chromatography. System HA—*k* 2.1; system HX—RI 225; system HY—RI 179.

Ultraviolet Spectrum. Aqueous acid—257 ($A_1^1 = 14.7a$), 263 nm.

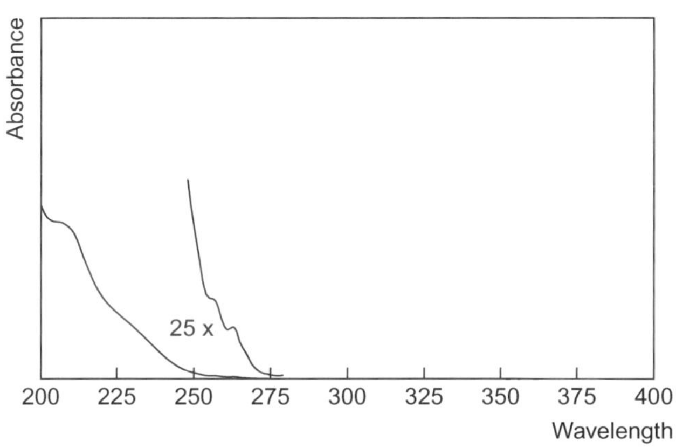

Infra-red Spectrum. Principal peaks at wavenumbers 1608, 1296, 721, 1580, 690, 775 cm^{-1} (KBr disk).

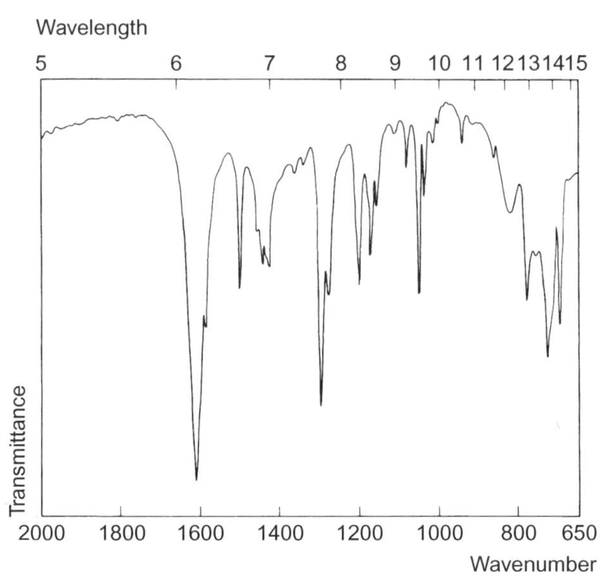

Mass Spectrum. Principal ions at *m/z* 91, 159, 160, 131, 65, 92, 81, 39.

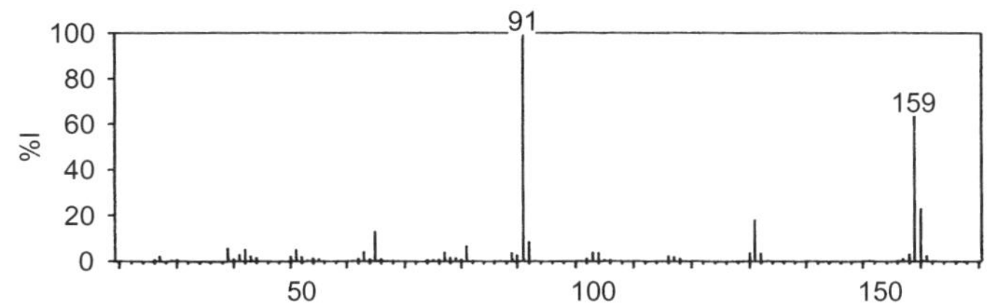

Quantification

High performance liquid chromatography. In plasma: limit of detection 200 µg/L, UV detection—V. Rovei *et al.*, *J. Chromatogr.*, 1982, *231*; *B Biomed. Appl.*, *20*, 210–215. In serum or urine: limit of detection 100 µg/L, UV detection—M. J. Cwik *et al.*, *J. Chromatogr.*, 1985, *338*, 123–130. In serum: limit of detection 50 to 250 µg/L, UV detection—L. M. Todesco *et al.*, *Ther. Drug Monit.*, 1987, *9*, 78–84.

Capillary isotachophoresis. In serum or urine: limit of detection 40 mg/L and 3 mg/L, respectively—A. Hercegova *et al.*, *Acta Pol. Pharm.*, 1998, *55*, 167–171.

Disposition in the Body. Tolazoline is well absorbed after oral or parenteral administration. It is excreted in the urine, about 90% of an oral dose being eliminated unchanged in 12 h.

Therapeutic concentration

After a bolus intravenous injection of 2 mg/kg followed by continuous IV infusion to provide a maintenance dose of 2 mg/kg to 1 neonate, plasma concentrations attained a steady-state of 7 to 8 mg/L and declined with a half-life of 5 h at the end of the infusion. [V. Rovei *et al.*, *J. Chromatogr.*, 1982, *231; B Biomed. Appl.*, *20*, 210–215].

Toxicity

A 54-year-old woman found comatose after ingesting 2.5 g of tolazoline hydrochloride died about 3 h later. Postmortem concentrations were: femoral blood 130 mg/L, liver 102 µg/g. [L. K. Turner, personal communication, 1964].

Dose. 12.5 to 200 mg of tolazoline hydrochloride daily.

Tolbutamide

Antidiabetic

Synonyms. Butamidum; Tolglybutamide.
Proprietary names. Arcosal; Artosin; Diabetil; Diatelan; Diatol; Diaval; Dolipol; Flusan; Glyconon; Ifumelus; Ipoglusan; Mobenol; Novobutamide; Orabet; Orinase; Orsinon; Rastinon (tablets); Tol-Tab.
N-[(Butylamino)carbonyl]-4-methylbenzenesulfonamide
$C_{12}H_{18}N_2O_3S = 270.3$
CAS—64-77-7

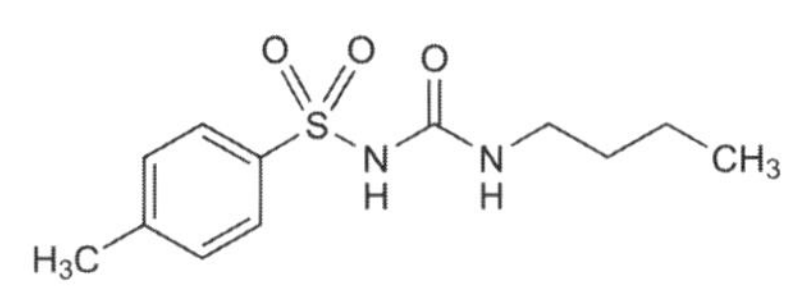

A white crystalline powder. M.p. about 129°.
Practically insoluble in water; soluble 1 in 10 of ethanol and 1 in 3 of acetone; soluble in chloroform; slightly soluble in ether.

Tolbutamide Sodium

Proprietary names. Orinase Diagnostic; Rastinon (injection).
$C_{12}H_{17}N_2NaO_3S = 292.3$
CAS—473-41-6
A white crystalline powder. M.p. 130° to 133°.
Freely soluble in water; soluble in ethanol and chloroform; very slightly soluble in ether.

Dissociation Constant. pK_a 5.3 (20°).

Partition Coefficient. Log *P* (octanol/water), 2.3.

Colour Tests. Koppanyi–Zwikker test—violet; Mercurous nitrate—black.

Thin-layer Chromatography. System TA—Rf 76; system TD—Rf 51; system TE—Rf 12; system TF—Rf 55; system TT—Rf 98; system TU—Rf 35; system TV—Rf 04; system TAD—Rf 62; system TAE—Rf 88; system

TAF—Rf 88; system TAJ—Rf 69; system TAK—Rf 74; system TAL—Rf 93.

Gas Chromatography. System GA—RI 1683.

High Performance Liquid Chromatography. System HX—RI 477; system HY—RI 424; system HZ—Retention time(s) 5.9 min.

Ultraviolet Spectrum. Methanol—257, 263 (A^1_1=22a), 268, 275 nm.

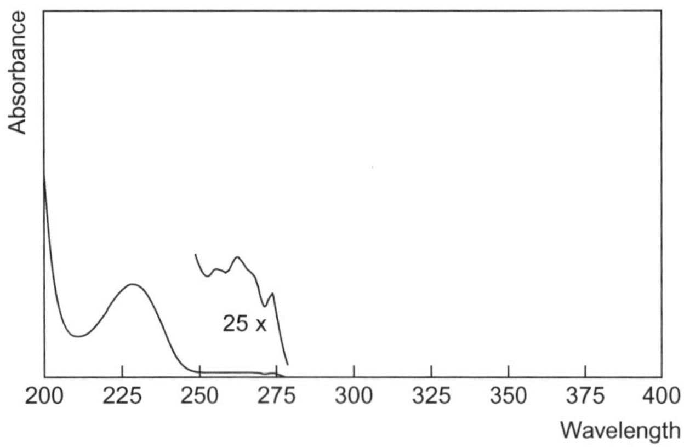

Infra-red Spectrum. Principal peaks at wavenumbers 1658, 1157, 1552, 668, 1090, 905 cm^{-1} (KBr disk). Polymorphism may occur.

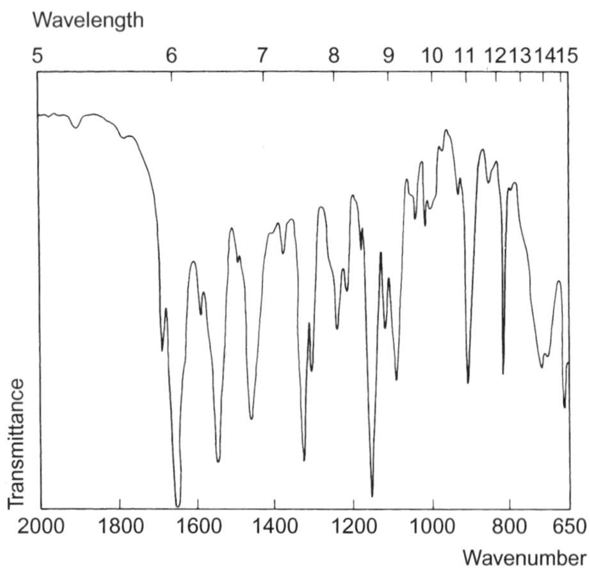

Mass Spectrum. Principal ions at *m/z* 91, 30, 155, 108, 65, 197, 39, 107.

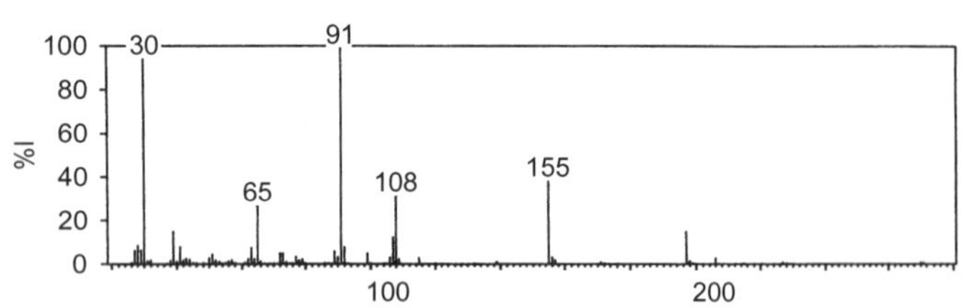

Quantification. See also under Chlorpropamide.

Gas chromatography. In plasma or urine: tolbutamide and two metabolites, limit of detection 1 mg/L, ECD—S. B. Matin and M. Rowland, *Anal. Lett. (Part B)*, 1973, *6*, 865–876.

High performance liquid chromatography. In plasma: tolbutamide and carboxytolbutamide, limit of detection 2 mg/L for tolbutamide and 100 μg/L for the carboxy metabolite, UV detection—G. Raghow and M. C. Meyer, *J. Pharm. Sci.*, 1981, *70*, 1166–1168. In plasma: limit of detection 200 μg/L, UV detection—H. M. Hill and J. Chamberlain, *J. Chromatogr.*, 1978, *149*, 349–358. In plasma or urine: tolbutamide and metabolites, photodiode-array detection—K. Csillag *et al.*, *J. Chromatogr.*, 1989, *490*, 353–363. In plasma or urine: tolbutamide and metabolites, limit of detection 0.1 to 1.5 μM in plasma and 0.5 to 2 μM in urine, UV detection—L. L. Hansen and K. Brosen, *Ther. Drug Monit.*, 1999, *21*, 664–671.

Mass spectrometry. In serum: tolbutamide and other sulfonylureas, limits of detection and quantification 2 and 10 μg/L, respectively—F. Magni *et al.*, *Anal. Biochem.*, 2000, *282*, 136–141.

Disposition in the Body. Tolbutamide is readily absorbed after oral administration. About 85% of an oral dose is excreted in the urine in 48 h, of which about two-thirds is the 4-carboxy metabolite and about one-third is the 4-hydroxymethyl metabolite; less than 5% is excreted as unchanged drug. About 9% of a dose is eliminated in the faeces in 48 h.

Therapeutic concentration

Following a single oral dose of 500 mg to 1 subject, a peak plasma-tolbutamide concentration of 49 mg/L was attained in about 4 h and a peak plasma concentration of the 4-carboxy metabolite of about 2.2 mg/L was attained in 6 h. [G. Raghow and M. C. Meyer, *J. Pharm. Sci.*, 1981, *70*, 1166–1168].

In 20 patients treated for non-insulin-dependent diabetes mellitus with tolbutamide (average daily dose 2 g), the plasma concentration was 19.8 (range 4.3 to 58.2) mg/L before their morning dose and a maximum of 92.2 (39.8 to 154.7) mg/L 85 (35 to 370) min after the dose. [R. E. Ferner *et al.*, *Eur. J. Clin. Pharmacol.*, 1991, *40*, 163–168].

Toxicity. Several fatalities from hypoglycaemia have been reported.

The following postmortem tissue distribution was reported in one suicide after the ingestion of 50 g: blood 640 mg/L, kidney 1073 μg/g, liver 930 μg/g, urine 3510 mg/L. [O. Pribilla, *Arch. Toxicol.*, 1968, *23*, 153–159].

Half-life. Plasma half-life, usually in the range 4 to 12 (mean 7) h but may vary up to 70 h during concomitant administration of other drugs such as sulfonamides, phenylbutazone, or dicoumarol.

Volume of distribution. 0.1 to 0.2 L/kg.

Clearance. Plasma clearance, about 0.3 mL/min/kg.

Protein binding. In plasma, about 95% at concentrations up to 100 μg/mL, decreasing to about 90% at plasma concentrations of 200 μg/mL.

Note. For a review of sulfonylurea hypoglycaemic drugs, see J. E. Jackson and R. Bressler, *Drugs*, 1981, *22*, 211–245.

Dose. 0.25 to 3 g daily.

Tolfenamic Acid

Analgesic

Proprietary names. Bifenac; Clotam; Clotan; Flocur; Migea; Rociclyn.
2-[(3-Chloro-2-methylphenyl)amino]benzoic acid
$C_{14}H_{12}ClNO_2$=261.7
CAS—13710-19-5

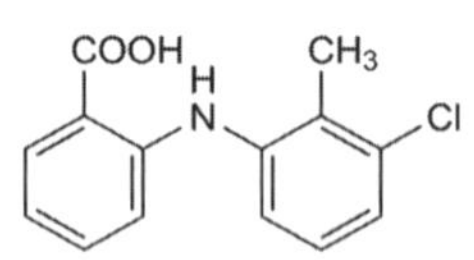

A white crystalline powder. M.p. about 207°.
Practically insoluble in water; soluble 1 in 70 of ethanol, 1 in 140 of chloroform, 1 in 15 of dimethylformamide and 1 in 45 of ether.

Partition Coefficient. Log *P* (octanol/water) 5.2.

Thin-layer Chromatography. System TE—Rf 14; system TF—Rf 31.

Gas Chromatography. System GL—Tolfenamic acid-ME RI 2255.

High Performance Liquid Chromatography. System HX—RI 690; system HZ—Retention time 37.9 min.

Ultraviolet Spectrum. Dehydrated alcohol—294, 330 nm.

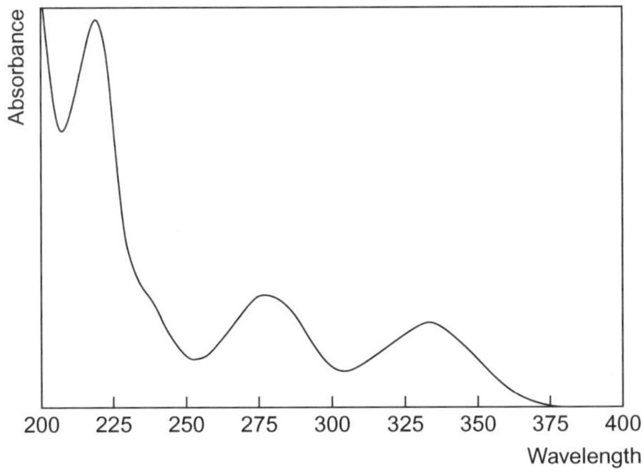

Infra-red Spectrum. Principal peaks at wavenumbers 1670, 1270, 1590, 755, 1500, 1575 cm^{-1} (KBr disk).

Quantification

High performance liquid chromatography. In plasma or urine: limit of detection 20 µg/L, UV detection—P. J. Pentikäinen *et al.*, *Eur. J. Clin. Pharmacol.*, 1981, *19*, 359–365. In urine, tolfenamic acid and other anthranilic acid derivatives, limit of detection, about 2 ng, UV detection—E. Mikami *et al.*, *J. Chromatogr. B. Biomed. Sci. Appl.*, 2000, *744*, 81–89.

Disposition in the Body. Readily absorbed after oral administration. It is metabolised by hydroxylation to *N*-[(2-hydroxymethyl-3-chlorophenyl)amino]benzoic acid and *N*-[(2-methyl-3-chloro-4-hydroxyphenyl)-amino]benzoic acid, which are the major metabolites. About 50% of an oral dose is excreted in the urine in 48 h mainly as glucuronide conjugates of the two hydroxylated metabolites. Less than 10% of a dose is excreted in the urine as unchanged drug or its glucuronide conjugate. Tolfenamic acid and its metabolites are excreted in the bile.

Therapeutic concentration

Following single oral doses of 100 and 200 mg to 6 subjects, mean peak plasma concentrations of 2.0 and 3.0 mg/L were attained in 1.3 and 1.5 h respectively [P. J. Pentikäinen *et al.*, *Eur. J. Clin. Pharmacol.*, 1981, *19*, 359–365].

Bioavailability. About 60%.

Half-life. Plasma half-life, about 2.5 h.

Volume of distribution. About 0.5 L/kg.

Clearance. Plasma clearance about 2.5 mL/min/kg.

Protein binding. In plasma, more than 99.5%.

Dose. Tolfenamic acid has been given in doses of 300 to 600 mg daily.

Tolmetin

Analgesic

1-Methyl-5-(4-methylbenzoyl)-1*H*-pyrrole-2-acetic acid
$C_{15}H_{15}NO_3$ = 257.3
CAS—26171-23-3

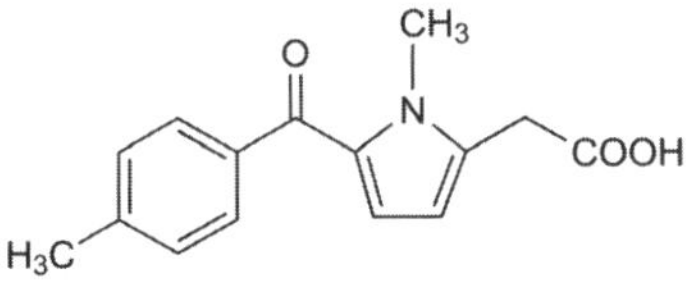

Crystals. M.p. 155° to 157°, with decomposition.

Tolmetin Sodium

Proprietary names. Artrocaptin; Tolectin.
$C_{15}H_{14}NNaO_3,2H_2O$ = 315.3
CAS—35711-34-3 (anhydrous); *64490-92-2* (dihydrate)

Dissociation Constant. pK_a 3.5.

Partition Coefficient. Log *P* (octanol/water) 2.8.

Colour Tests. Formaldehyde–Sulfuric Acid—brown-red; Liebermann's Test (100°)—red.

Thin-layer Chromatography. System TD—Rf 13; system TE—Rf 5; system TF—Rf 20; system TG—Rf 10; system TAD—Rf 30; system TAE—Rf 85; system TAJ—Rf 20; system TAK—Rf 59; system TAL—Rf 83. (Ludy Tenger reagent, black.)

Gas Chromatography. System GA—RI 1890; tolmetin-ME RI 2247; System GD—Relative retention times of methyl derivative 1.77 and 1.36, relative to *n*-$C_{16}H_{34}$; system GL—tolmetin-ME RI 2235; M (COOH-)-ME_2 RI 2600.

High Performance Liquid Chromatography. System HD—*k* 2.05; system HV—Relative retention times 0.60 and 0.99 relative to meclofenamic acid; system HX—RI 470; system HY—RI 434; system HZ—Retention time 5.4 min.

Ultraviolet Spectrum. Aqueous acid—262 nm (A^1_1=345b), 315 nm (A^1_1=735b); aqueous alkali—260 nm (A^1_1=333b), 323 nm (A^1_1=762b).

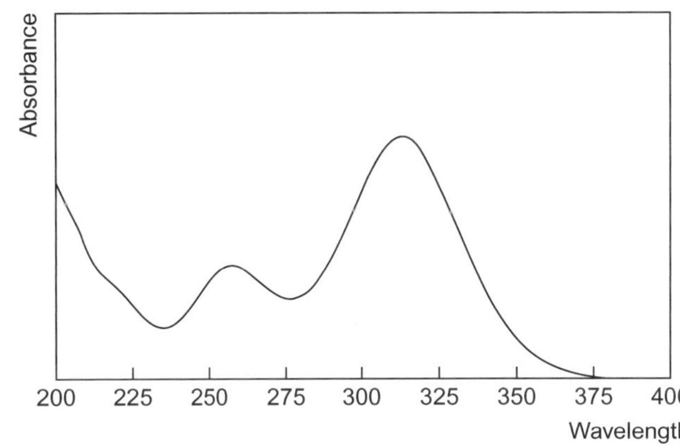

Mass Spectrum. Principal ions at *m*/*z* 212, 213, 122, 198, 44, 53, 91, 65.

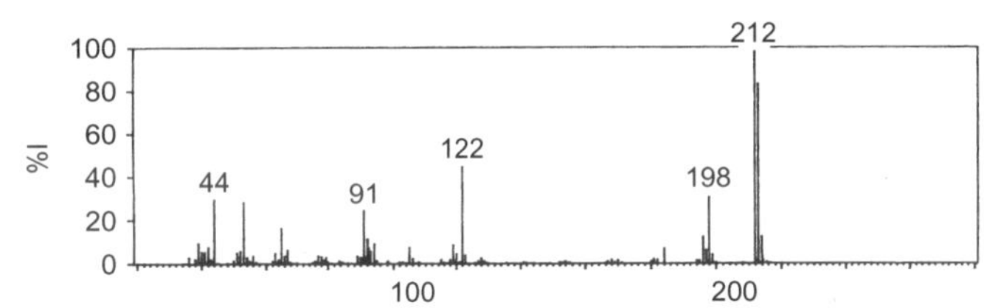

Quantification

Gas chromatography. In plasma: limit of detection 100 µg/L, ECD—K.-T. Ng, *J. Chromatogr.*, 1978, *166*, 527–535.

High performance liquid chromatography. In plasma or urine: limit of detection for tolmetin and the dicarboxylated metabolite, 40 µg/L in plasma, UV detection—R. K. Desiraju *et al.*, *J. Chromatogr.*, 1982, *232*; *Biomed. Appl.*, *21*, 119–128. In plasma or urine, tolmetin, tolmetin glucuronide and isomeric conjugates, range of detection 0.05 to 50 mg/L in plasma and 0.025 to 50 mg/L in urine, UV detection—M. L. Hyneck *et al.*, *J Chromatogr.*, 1987, *420*, 349–56.

Disposition in the Body. Rapidly and almost completely absorbed after oral administration. Metabolised mainly by oxidation to inactive metabolites. More than 90% of a dose is excreted in the urine in 24 h, mostly in the first 8 h. The urinary material consists mostly of free and conjugated (glucuronide) 5-(4-carboxybenzoyl)-1-methylpyrrol-2-ylacetic acid and conjugated (glucuronide) tolmetin; up to 15% is excreted in the urine as unchanged drug.

Therapeutic concentration

After a single oral dose of 300 mg to 5 subjects, a mean peak plasma concentration of 29.3 mg/L of tolmetin was attained in 0.25 to 1 h; plasma concentrations of the dicarboxylated metabolite reached a peak of about 5 mg/L in 1.5 to 3 h [M. L. Selley *et al.*, *Clin. Pharmacol. Ther.*, 1975, *17*, 599–605].

Following oral administration of 400 mg four times a day to 5 subjects for 7 days, maximum steady-state plasma concentrations of 8.3 to 78.9 mg/L (mean 45) of tolmetin and 4.1 to 13.6 mg/L (mean 10) of the dicarboxylated metabolite were reported about 0.75 and 1.75 h after a dose, respectively [S. H. Dromgoole *et al.*, *Clin. Pharmacol. Ther.*, 1982, *32*, 371–377].

Toxicity. Toxic effects are associated with plasma concentrations greater than about 60 µg/mL.

Half-life. Plasma half-life, about 6 h.

Clearance. Plasma clearance, about 1 to 2 mL/min/kg.

Distribution in blood. Plasma:whole blood ratio, 1.8.

Protein binding. In plasma, tolmetin more than 99% but displaced by salicylic acid; dicarboxylated metabolite about 70%.

Note. For a review of the pharmacokinetics of tolmetin see R. N. Brogden *et al.*, *Drugs*, 1978, *15*, 429–450.

Dose. The equivalent of 0.6 to 1.8 g of tolmetin daily.

Tolnaftate

Antifungal

Proprietary names. Absorbine Antifungal; Aftate; Blis-To-Sol; Curatin; Devorfungi; Excelsior; Micoisdin; Mycil; Pitrex; Podactin; Quinsana Plus; Sorgoa; Sorgoran; Sporiline; Tinactin; Tinatox; Tineafax; Tinaderm(e); Tinasol; Tolnaderm; Tonoftal; Trinaderm.
Methyl(3-methylphenyl)-carbamothioic acid *O*-2-naphthalenyl ester
$C_{19}H_{17}NOS = 307.4$
CAS—2398-96-1

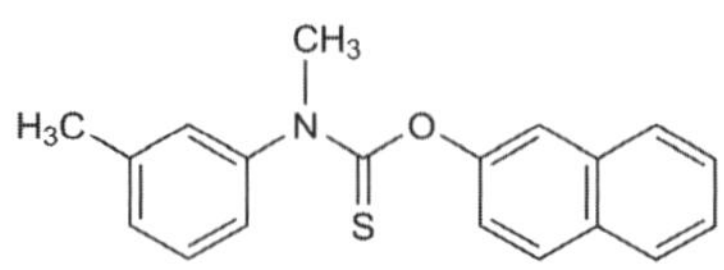

A white to creamy-white powder. M.p. about 111°.
Practically insoluble in water; sparingly soluble in ethanol and methanol; soluble 1 in 8 of acetone, 1 in 2.5 of chloroform and 1 in 55 of ether.

Partition Coefficient. Log *P* (octanol/water) 5.8.

Colour Tests. Mandelin's Test—brown; Marquis Test—blue-green.

Thin-layer Chromatography. System TAJ—Rf 96; system TAK—Rf 83; system TAL—Rf 97.

High Performance Liquid Chromatography. System HY—RI 867.

Ultraviolet Spectrum. Methanol—257 nm ($A_1^1 = 708a$).

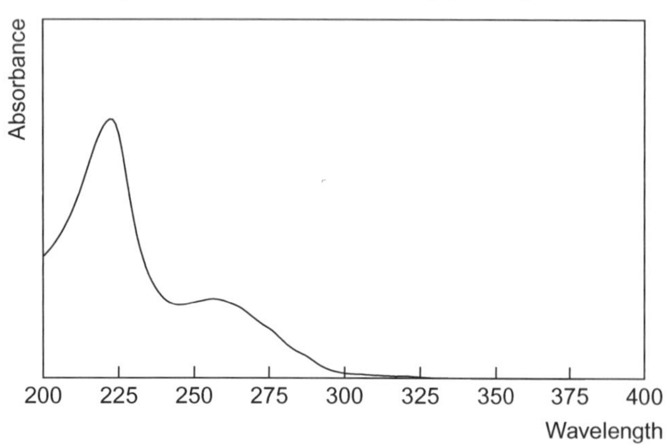

Infra-red Spectrum. Principal peaks at wavenumbers 1211, 1170, 1156, 754, 1234, 810 cm^{-1} (KBr disk).

Use. Topically as a 1% solution, powder or cream.

Toloxatone

Antidepressant

Proprietary name. Humoryl
5-(Hydroxymethyl)-3-(3-methylphenyl)-2-oxazolidinone
$C_{11}H_{13}NO_3 = 207.2$
CAS—29218-27-2

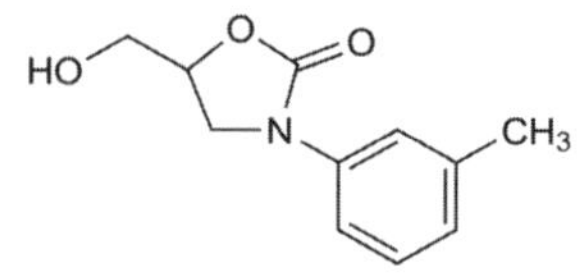

A white to off-white crystalline powder with M. p. 76°. It is slightly soluble in water (4.5 g/L), 0.1 M hydrochloric acid and 0.1 M sodium hydroxide solution.

Partition Coefficient. Log *P* (octanol/water), 1.88.

Thin-layer Chromatography. Plate: silica gel coated plates (Kieselgel 60). Mobile phase: chloroform:diethyl ether:methanol:ammonia (25%) (85:15:20:0.5). Detection: colour reaction with nitrous gas. Rf 0.68. Limit of detection, 0.005 mg/L [M. Strolin Benedetti *et al.*, *Arzneimittelforschung.*, 1982, *32*, 276–279].

Gas Chromatography. Column: 3% OV-101 Supelcoport 80-100 mesh (2000 × 2 mm i.d.), silanised glass. Column temperature: 200°. Carrier gas: helium, flow rate 35 mL/min. Detection: nitrogen-phosphorus. Retention time: (TMS derivative) 2.5 min [S. Vajta *et al.*, *J. Chromatogr.*, 1983, *274*, 139–148].

High Performance Liquid Chromatography. System HAA—RT 14.1 min.

Column: Nova-Pack C_{18} (300 × 3.9 mm, 4 μm). Mobile phase: methanol:THF:potassium dihydrogen phosphate (10 mM, pH 2.6) (65:5:30), flow rate 0.8 mL/min. UV detection (λ=238 nm). Retention time: 3.4 min [A. Tracqui *et al.*, *J. Forensic Sci.*, 1995, *40*, 254–262].

Ultraviolet Spectrum. Aqueous acid—204, 238, 271, 279 nm.

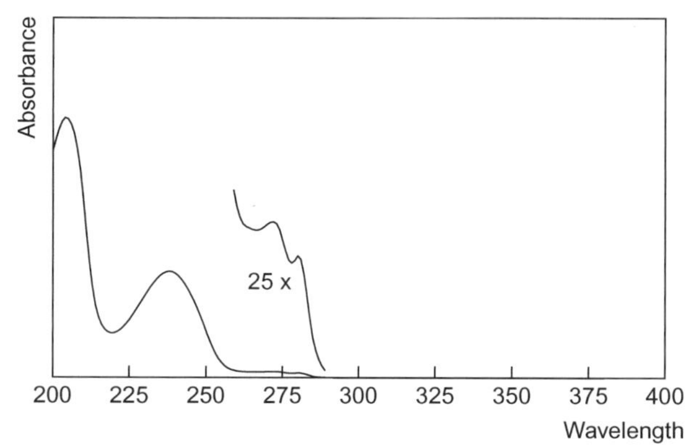

Quantification

High performance liquid chromatography. In blood: limit of detection <0.12 mg/L— A. Tracqui *et al.*, *J. Forensic Sci.*, 1995, *40*, 254–262.

Disposition in the Body. Toloxatone is rapidly absorbed from the gastro-intestinal tract after oral administration. It is rapidly and extensively metabolised and no unchanged drug is found in urine. The major metabolite is 3-(3-carboxyphenyl)-5-hydroxymethyl-2-oxozalidinone produced by methyl-oxidation of the drug. The drug is eliminated extensively in urine (80%), mostly as its metabolites.

Therapeutic concentration

5 healthy adult volunteers, aged between 23 and 42 years, were administered with a single oral dose of 1 mg/kg 1 h after a standard breakfast. 3 weeks later, the volunteers received a 1 mg/kg intravenous infusion of toloxatone. The mean peak toloxatone concentration for the oral dose was 0.474 (range, 0.384 to 0.640) mg/L at 0.83 h (0.53 to 1.00 h). The drug concentration after the intravenous dose was 0.623 to 0.840 mg/L observed at the end of the 30 min infusion [M. Strolin Benedetti *et al.*, *Arzneimittelforschung.*, 1982, *32*, 276–279].

Toxicity

The minimum toxic dose reported in cases of toloxatone poisoning is 2 g. The first symptoms, including drowsiness and mild adrenergic effects, are observed after an hour. In cases of massive overdose, coma and jerks have occurred. In cases where toloxatone was co-administered with tricyclic antidepressants, two patients died and symptoms included muscular rigidity, hyperthermia and cardiovascular collapse [P. Azoyan *et al.*, *Therapie.*, 1990, *45(2)*, 139–144 (French)].

Bioavailability 50 to 62%.

Half-life. 0.88 to 2.46 h.

Volume of distribution. 1.09 to 1.64 L/kg.

Clearance. Plasma, 0.462 to 0.860 L/h/kg.

Protein binding. 49 to 53% (mainly to albumin).

Dose. Orally, 200 mg three times a day.

Tolpropamine

Antihistamine

N,*N*,4-Trimethyl-γ-phenylbenzenepropanamine
$C_{18}H_{23}N$=253.4
CAS—5632-44-0

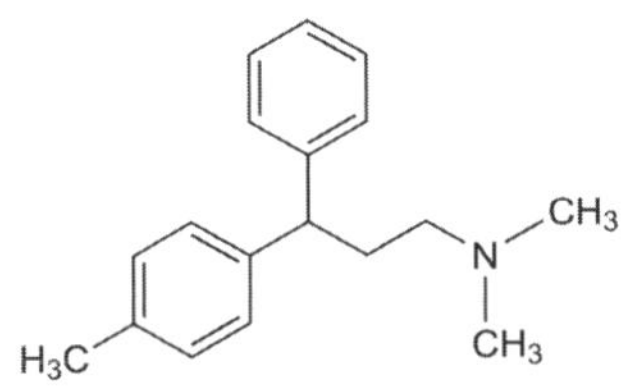

Practically insoluble in water; soluble in chloroform.

Tolpropamine Hydrochloride

Proprietary name. Pragman
$C_{18}H_{23}N,HCl$=289.8
CAS—3339-11-5
A white crystalline powder. M.p. 182° to 184°.
Soluble in water and ethanol; practically insoluble in chloroform and ether.

Partition Coefficient. Log *P* (octanol/water) 4.4.

Colour Tests. Mandelin's Test—brown; Marquis Test—red.

Thin-layer Chromatography. System TA—Rf 51; system TB—Rf 52; system TC—Rf 32; system TE—Rf 68; system TL—Rf 15; system TAE—Rf 26. (Acidified iodoplatinate solution, positive.)

Gas Chromatography. System GA—tolpropamine RI 1900; M (OH-) RI 2150; M (nor-) RI 2100; M (nor-OH-) RI 2200; M (*N*-oxide) RI 1750.

High Performance Liquid Chromatography. System HA—*k* 2.9.

Ultraviolet Spectrum. Aqueous acid—260 nm (A^1_1=25a), 265 nm (A^1_1=25a), 273 nm.

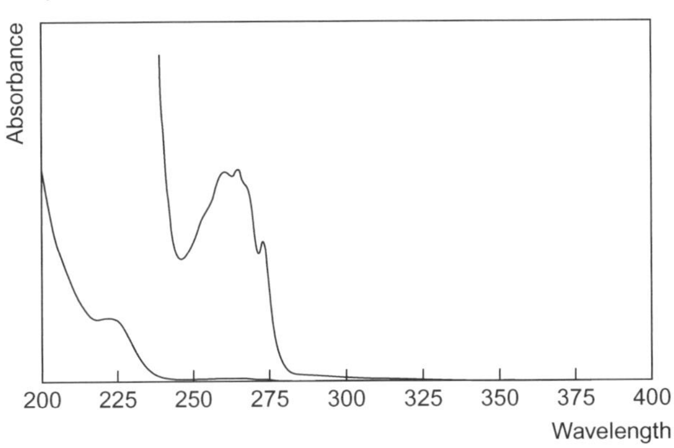

Infra-red Spectrum. Principal peaks at wavenumbers 727, 776, 700, 802, 1515, 970 cm^{-1} (tolpropamine hydrochloride, KBr disk).

Use. Topically in a concentration of 1% of the hydrochloride.

Tolrestat

Antidiabetic

Synonym. AY-27773
Proprietary names. Alredase; Lorestat.
N-[[6-Methoxy-5-(trifluoromethyl)-1-naphthalenyl]thioxomethyl]-*N*-methylglycine
$C_{16}H_{14}F_3NO_3S$=357.3
CAS—82964-04-3

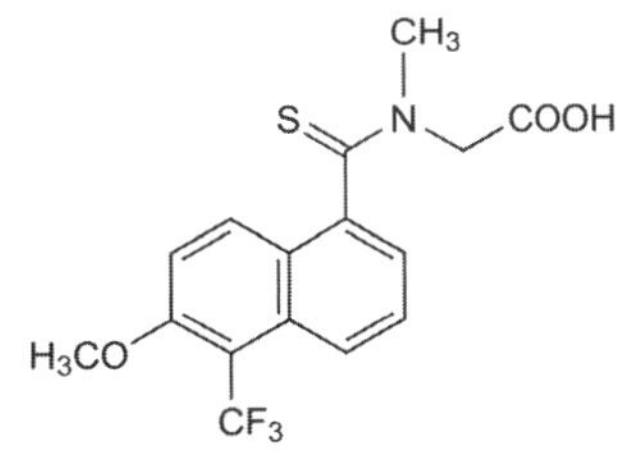

M. p. 164° to 165°.

High Performance Liquid Chromatography. Column: ODS (Hypersil, 250 × 4.6 mm i.d., 5 μm). Mobile phase: acetonitrile:phosphate buffer (100 mM, pH 6.0) (30:70), flow rate 1.1 mL/min. UV detection (λ=240 nm). Retention time: 6.4 min [D. Hicks and M. Kraml. *Ther. Drug Monit.*, 1984, *6*, 328–333].

Mass Spectrum. Principal ions at *m/z* 357, 269, 226, 356, 207, 312, 279, 324.

Quantification
High performance liquid chromatography. In serum and tissue: limit of detection 25 μg/L (2 mL serum), 200 μg/L (1 mL serum), 50 ng/g (tissue). UV detection (λ=226 nm)—D. Hicks and M. Kraml, *Ther. Drug Monit.*, 1984, *6*, 328–333.

Disposition in the Body. Tolrestat is well absorbed within 2 h and rapidly distributed throughout the body. Elimination is renal (63 to 68%) and faecal (25 to 27%) mainly as the unchanged drug, along with conjugated tolrestat and sulfo-tolrestat as minor metabolites. No accumulation was observed after multiple dosing. The majority of the dose (approximately 95%) is excreted within 7 days of administration.

Therapeutic concentration
20 healthy, young females (mean age 25 years) and males (mean age 31 years), were administered with a single 200 mg dose of tolrestat after an overnight fast, and were fasted for an additional 4 h after dosing. Multiple dosing of 200 mg every 12 h for 5 days was administered. 25 healthy, elderly males, mean age 74 years, and females, 73 years, were also included in the study. Mean peak plasma concentrations were 27 (19 to 34), 21 (12 to 30) mg/L, observed at mean times 1.2 (0.6 to 1.8), 1.3 (0.5 to 2.1) h, for the females and males respectively [R. Fruncillo *et al.*, *Clin. Pharmacol. Ther.*, 1996, *59(6)*, 603–612].

Bioavailability. Linearly proportional to dose over 25 to 800 mg.

Half-life. 10 to 13 h.

Volume of distribution. 0.27 to 0.41 L/kg.

Clearance. Oral clearance, 18 to 30 mL/h/kg.

Protein binding. 99%.

Dose. 200 mg.

Tolterodine

Antimuscarinic

Proprietary names. Detrol; Difluorasone Topical.
2-[(1*R*)-3-[Bis(1-methylethyl)amino]-1-phenylpropyl]-4-methylphenol
$C_{22}H_{31}NO$=325.5
CAS—124937-51-5

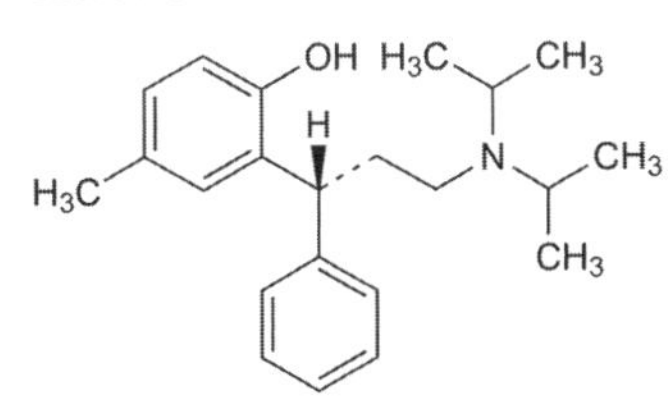

Tolterodine Tartrate

Proprietary names. Detrol; Detrusitol.
$C_{22}H_{31}NO,C_4H_6O_6$=475.6
A white crystalline powder. It is soluble in water (12 g/L at room temperature); soluble in methanol; slightly soluble in ethanol; practically insoluble in toluene.

Dissociation Constant. pK_a 9.9.

Gas Chromatography. Column: fused silica capillary with 5% phenyl methyl silicon (25 m × 0.2 mm i.d., 0.33 µm film thickness). Column temperature: initially, 120° for 0.5 min, increased by 35°/min to 300° maintained for 5 to 10 min. Carrier gas: helium. Internal standard (IS): [$^2H_5$] tolterodine. MS detection (EI, SIM at *m/z* 382 for tolterodine and 387 for IS). Retention times: tolterodine, (plasma) 7.45 min, (urine) 8.25 min; IS, (plasma) 7.41 min, (urine) 8.22 min [L. Palmer *et al.*, *J. Pharm. Biomed. Anal.*, 1997, *16*, 155–165].

High Performance Liquid Chromatography. Column: (analytical) PKB 100 (Supelco 150 × 4.5 mm i.d.); (guard) PKB 100 (Supelco 20 × 4.5 mm i.d.). Mobile phase: A: methanol; B: ammonium acetate (20 mM, pH 4.5); (A:B); (10:90) to (20:80) in 5 min, to (45:55) in 30 min, to (100:0) in 5 min, maintain for 10 min, flow rate 1 mL/min. UV detection (λ=280 nm). RT: 29 min [S. Andersson *et al.*, *Drug Metab. Dispos.*, 1998, *26*, 528–535].

Mass Spectrum. Principal ions at *m/z* 114, 382, 73, 397, 116, 30, 72, 135 (TMS derivative).

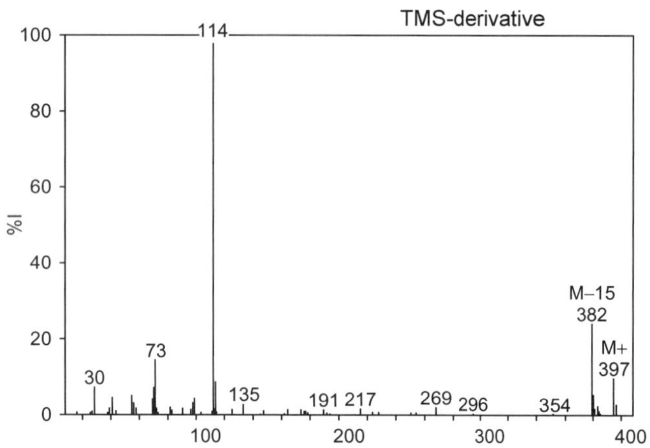

Quantification

Gas chromatography–mass spectrometry. In plasma, serum and urine: limit of quantification 0.5 µg/L—L. Palmer *et al.*, *J. Pharm. Biomed. Anal.*, 1997, *16*, 155–165.

Disposition in the Body. Tolterodine is rapidly absorbed, and levels increase when co-administered with food. Peak plasma concentrations are reached within 1 to 3 h following an oral dose. Metabolism is mainly by the cytochrome P450 isoenzyme, CYP2D6 to the active 5-hydroxymethyl derivative. In a minority of people with no functional gene of CYP2D6, it is metabolised by CYP3A4 to the inactive *N*-dealkylated derivative. Tolterodine is excreted primarily in urine (77%) with approx. 17% appearing in faeces. Less than 1% of a dose is excreted as the unchanged drug, and 4% as its metabolites. The half-life is prolonged in poor metabolisers and results in a 7-fold increase in the concentration of tolterodine. Steady state concentrations are achieved within 2 days. Pharmacokinetics are effected by hepatic impairment.

Therapeutic concentration

19 healthy male and female volunteers with a mean age of 33 years (range, 18 to 55 years), were classified as being either a poor metaboliser of tolterodine (i.e. no functional gene of CYP2D6) or extensive metabolisers. They were then administered with 4 mg once daily of extended release formulation of tolterodine or 2 mg instant release twice daily, for 6 days. A washout period of 7 days was allowed between the doses. The peak plasma tolterodine concentrations for the extended release dose were 6.1 (1.1 to 59.0) nmol/L at 4 (2 to 6) h for the extensive metabolisers and 35 (28 to 130) nmol/L at 4 (3 to 6) h for the poor metabolisers. After the instant release formulation, concentrations observed for the extensive metabolisers were 12.0 (1.2 to 57.0) nmol/L after the morning dose and 9.2 (1.5 to 50.0) nmol/L after the evening dose. For the poor metabolisers, 51 (40 to 143) nmol/L in the morning and 45 (34 to 99) nmol/L in the evening. After the morning dose, peak concentrations were observed at approx. 1 h, and in the evening, between 1.5 and 1.8 h (and up to 3 h). These steady state concentrations were observed on day 6 [B. Olsson and J. Szamosi, *Clin. Pharmacokinet.*, 2001, *40(3)*, 227–235].

Toxicity. The highest dose of tolterodine L-tartrate given to human volunteers is 12.8 mg as a single dose. The most severe adverse effects were accommodation disturbances and micturition difficulties. Overdose can potentially result in severe central anticholinergic effects.

Bioavailability. 17% in extensive metabolisers; 65% in poor metabolisers.

Half-life. 2 to 3 h in extensive metabolisers; 10 h in poor metabolisers.

Volume of distribution. Mean, 113 L.

Clearance. In extensive metabolisers: systemic clearance is 30 L/h, apparent oral clearance is approximately 8900 following a single 4 mg dose of the drug, and 6919 mL/min following multiple oral doses of the drug, respectively. Poor metabolisers (deficient of CYP2D6) show reduced clearance of 283 mL/min, and apparent oral clearance of 183 mL/min. Clearance of oral tolterodine, approx. 18 mL/min/kg in individuals with liver cirrhosis or 95 mL/min/kg in healthy individuals.

Distribution in blood. Neither tolterodine nor the metabolite distributes significantly to erythrocytes. Blood:serum ratio 0.6 (tolterodine); 0.8 (5-hydroxy metabolite).

Protein binding. 96.3% (tolterodine) 64% (5-hydroxymethyl metabolite), primarily to orosomucoids and α_1-acid glycoprotein.

Dose. 2 mg twice daily.

Toluene

Solvent

Synonyms. Methylbenzene; Phenylmethane; Toluol(e).

$C_6H_5{\cdot}CH_3=92.1$

CAS—108-88-3

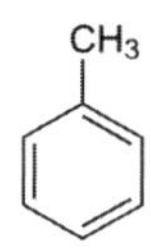

A colourless, mobile, highly flammable liquid which burns with a smoky flame. Wt per mL about 0.87 g. B.p. about 111°.

Practically insoluble in water; miscible with ethanol, chloroform, ether, acetone and glacial acetic acid.

Partition Coefficient. Log *P* (octanol/water) 2.7.

Gas Chromatography. System GA—RI 756; system GI—Retention time 24.8 min.

High Performance Liquid Chromatography. System HAA—Retention time 21.9 min.

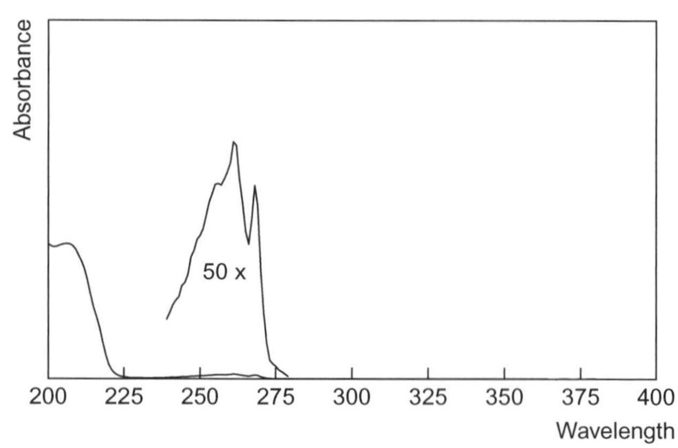

Mass Spectrum. Principal ions at *m/z* 91, 92, 65, 39, 63, 93, 51, 89.

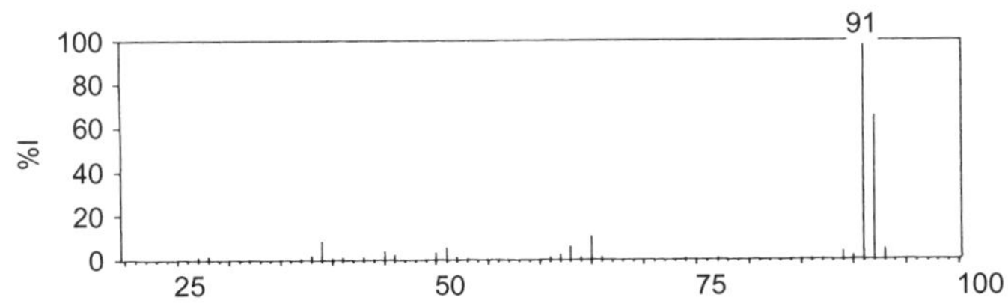

Quantification

Gas chromatography. In blood or breath: limit of detection 1 mg/L, FID—J. C. Garriott *et al.*, *Clin. Toxicol.*, 1981, *18*, 471–479. In blood or urine: toluene and other volatile compounds, limit of detection 0.5 to 5 µg/0.5 L, using headspace analysis—X. P. Lee *et al.*, *Int. J. Legal Med.*, 1995, *107*, 310–313; X. P. Lee *et al.*, *Analyst*, 1998, *123*, 147–150; K. Watanabe-Suzuki *et al.*, *Anal. Bioanal. Chem.*, 2002, *373*, 75–80.

Gas chromatography and gas chromatography–mass spectrometry. In blood or tissues: toluene and other volatile compounds, using headspace analysis—J. A. Bellanca *et al.*, *J. Anal. Toxicol.*, 1982, *6*, 238–240. In blood or urine: toluene, using H-SPME (solid phase micro-extraction)—N. Y. Kim and S. W. Park, *J. Forensic Sci.*, 2000, *45*, 702–770.

High performance liquid chromatography. In urine: hippuric acid and *o*-cresol, limit of detections hippuric acid 50 mg/L and *o*-cresol 5 µg/L, fluorescence and UV detection—S. H. Hansen and M. Døssing, *J. Chromatogr.*, 1982, *229*; *Biomed. Appl.*, *18*, 141–148.

Disposition in the Body. Toluene is absorbed from the gastro-intestinal tract, through the skin and mucous membranes, and from the lungs. It has an affinity for lipid-rich tissues from which it is slowly released. About 80% of an inhaled dose is oxidised to benzoic acid which is conjugated with glycine to give hippuric acid and excreted in the urine. Conjugation with glucuronic acid also occurs when large amounts of toluene are absorbed. About 20% of the dose is excreted unchanged in expired air with less than 0.1% in the urine.

Blood concentration

Exposure to a concentration of 100 ppm of toluene produced a mean venous-blood concentration of about 0.39 mg/L in 6 healthy subjects at rest and about 1.16 mg/L in 6 subjects during light exercise, after 20 to 30 min. Exposure to 200 ppm for the same time produced a mean blood concentration of about 0.55 mg/L in 4 subjects at rest [I. Astrand *et al.*, *Scand. J. Work Environ. Health*, 1972, *9*, 119–130].

Toxicity. Toluene has about the same acute toxicity as benzene but is a less serious industrial hazard. The maximum permissible atmospheric concentration of toluene is 100 ppm. Exposure to air concentrations of 10 000 to 30 000 ppm may cause unconsciousness within a few minutes. A blood concentration of more than 10 µg/mL may be lethal although higher concentrations have been found in habitual abusers.

7 children aged from 9 to 13 years, with an acute encephalopathy caused by toluene intoxication from glue-sniffing were found to have blood-toluene concentrations of 0.8 to 7.7 µg/g (mean 2.3) [M. D. King *et al.*, *BMJ*, 1981, *283*, 663–665].

A boy of 13 years found dead after sniffing glue had the following postmortem concentrations of toluene in body tissues: blood 11 mg/L, brain 44 µg/g, kidney 39 µg/g, liver 47 µg/g [W. D. Collom and C. L. Winek, *Clin. Toxicol.*, 1970, *3*, 125–130].

The following postmortem tissue concentrations of toluene were reported in a 16-year-old boy found dead with a plastic bag over his head: blood 20.6 mg/L, brain 297 µg/g, liver 89 µg/g; acetone was also detected in blood at a concentration of 3 mg/L [S. C. Paterson and R. Sarvesvaran, *Med. Sci. Law*, 1983, *23*, 64–66].

Half-life. Blood half-life about 7.5 h.

Topiramate

Antiepileptic

Synonyms. McN-4853; RWJ-17021-000.
Proprietary names. Topamax; Topimax.
2,3:4,5-Bis-*O*-(1-methylethylidene)-*β*-D-fructopyranose sulfamate
$C_{12}H_{21}NO_8S$ = 339.4
CAS—97240-79-4

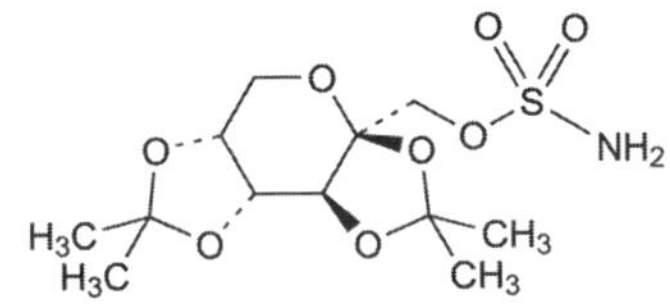

A white crystalline powder. It is freely soluble in acetone, in alcohol, in chloroform and in dimethyl sulfoxide.

Gas Chromatography. System GB—RI 2253.

Column: DB-1 methylsilicone (30 m × 0.25 mm, 0.25 µm film thickness). Column temperature: 230°. Carrier gas: hydrogen, flow rate 31 mL/min. Detection: flame ionisation. Retention time: 3.2 min. [B. E. Gidal and G. L. Lensmeyer, *Ther. Drug. Monit.*, 1999, *21*, 567–576].

Column: DB-5 fused silica capillary (25 m × 0.32 mm i.d., 0.25 µm film thickness). Column temperature: 165° to 205° at 9°/min. Carrier gas: helium, flow rate 3 mL/min. Detection: flame ionisation. Retention time 5 min [M. L. Holland *et al.*, *J. Chromatogr.*, 1988, *433*; *Biomed. Appl.*, *77*, 276–281].

Quantification

Gas chromatography. In plasma: limit of detection 0.1 mg/L, FID—M. L. Holland *et al.*, *J. Chromatogr.*, 1988, *433*; *Biomed. Appl.*, *77*, 276–281.

Disposition in the Body. Topiramate is rapidly and well absorbed after oral administration. The rate of absorption is delayed with the presence of food but the extent is not affected. Peak plasma concentrations are attained after about 2 h. It displays linear pharmacokinetics. Topiramate undergoes rapid distribution and there is significant binding to red blood cells. It is not extensively metabolised (about 20%); up to 50% of a dose may undergo metabolism in patients taking other enzyme-inducing anti-epileptics, for example, phenytoin. The presence of these antiepileptics may also reduce the plasma concentration of topiramate, increase the clearance of the drug and decrease its half-life. Metabolic pathways include, hydroxylation, hydrolysis and glucuronidation and in total six metabolites have been identified. The drug is eliminated mainly in urine as the unchanged drug (a total of 55 to 66% of the dose) and its metabolites (35%). There is some renal tubular reabsorption. It is removed by haemodialysis.

Therapeutic concentration

Healthy volunteers were administered with 100, 200, 400, 800 and 1200 mg topiramate and peak concentrations of 1.7, 3.7, 7.7, 18.4 and 28.7 mg/L were observed, respectively. These concentrations were seen 1.8 to 4.3 h after administration of the drug [D. E. Easterling *et al.*, *Epilepsia*, 1988, *29*, 662].

Group 1: 7 renally impaired patients with creatinine clearance <30 mL/min. Group 2: 7 renally impaired patients with creatinine clearance between 30 and 69 mL/min. Groups 3 and 4: 7 individuals with normal renal function, creatinine clearance ⩾70 mL/min. Each group was administered with a single, oral dose of 100 mg topiramate and peak concentrations were 2.1, 2.2, 1.9 and 1.6 mg/L, respectively for the four groups [L. G. Gisclon *et al.*, *Pharm. Res.*, 1993, *10 (Suppl. 10)*, S397].

Bioavailability. 80 to 95%.

Half-life. Plasma, 20 to 30 h.

Volume of distribution. 0.6 to 0.8 L/kg. In women it is approximately half of that in men although this difference is not considered clinically significant.

Clearance. Plasma, 1.2 to 2.4 L/h; decreased in patients with renal or hepatic impairment.

Distribution in blood. Topiramate significantly binds red blood cells and the major proportion of the circulating drug is bound to erythrocytes. Saturation of the binding sites occurs rapidly with higher drug concentrations and hence, the blood:plasma ratio decreases with increasing drug concentration.

Protein binding. In plasma, 13 to 17%.

Note. For reviews of topiramate see H. D. Langtry *et al.*, *Drugs*, 1997, *54*, 752–773 and R. C. Sachdeo, *Clin. Pharmacokinet.*, 1998, *34*, 335–346; for reviews of the pharmacokinetics of topiramate see M. Bialer, *Clin. Pharmacokinet.*, 1993, *24*, 441–452 and E. Perucca and M. Bialer, *Clin. Pharmacokinet.*, 1996, *31*, 29–46.

Dose. Usually 200 to 400 mg daily.

Topotecan

Antineoplastic

Synonyms. Hycamptamine; SKF-104864A; SKFS-104864-A.
Proprietary name. Hycamtin
(4*S*)-10-[(Dimethylamino)methyl]-4-ethyl-4,9-dihydroxy-1*H*-pyrano-[3′,4′:6,7]indolizino[1,2-*b*]quinoline-3,14(4*H*,12*H*)-dione
$C_{23}H_{23}N_3O_5$=421.5
CAS—123948-87-8

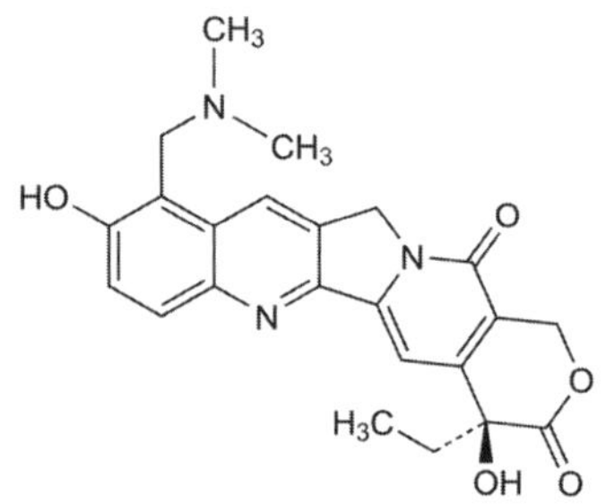

It is soluble in water, methanol and dimethylformamide; insoluble in ethanol.

Topotecan Hydrochloride
Synonym. NSC-609669
Proprietary name. Hycamtin
$C_{23}H_{23}N_3O_5$,HCl=457.9
CAS—*119413-54-6*
A light yellow to greenish powder with m.p. 213° to 218°. It is soluble in water up to 1 g/L.

Dissociation Constant. pK_a 10.5.

Partition Coefficient. Log *P* (octanol/water), -0.88.

High Performance Liquid Chromatography. Column: RP-18 (Lichrosorb, 125 × 4 mm i.d., 5 μm). Mobile phase: methanol:water:sodium dioctylsulfosuccinate (DOSS, 0.25 M):phosphate buffer:triethylamine (1.0 M), (pH 6.0), (567:375:35:20:3), flow rate 1.0 mL/min. Fluorescence detection (λ_{ex}=381 nm; λ_{em}=527 nm). Retention time: 5.52 min [J. Beijen *et al.*, *J. Pharm. Biomed. Anal.*, 1990, *8*, 789–794].

Column: BDS C_{18} (Hypersil, 100 × 3 mm i.d., 3 m). Mobile phase: potassium hydrogen phosphate (10 mM, pH 6.0) containing methanol (25%) and ethylamine (0.2%), flow rate 0.70 mL/min. Fluorescence detection (λ_{ex}=381 nm, λ_{em}=525 nm). Retention times: topotecan (closed ring form), 6.5 min; (open ring form), 2.5 min [W. J. Loos *et al.*, *J. Chromatogr. B Biomed. Appl.*, 1996, *678*, 309–315].

Ultraviolet Spectrum. Aqueous acid—223, 267, 295, 316 nm.

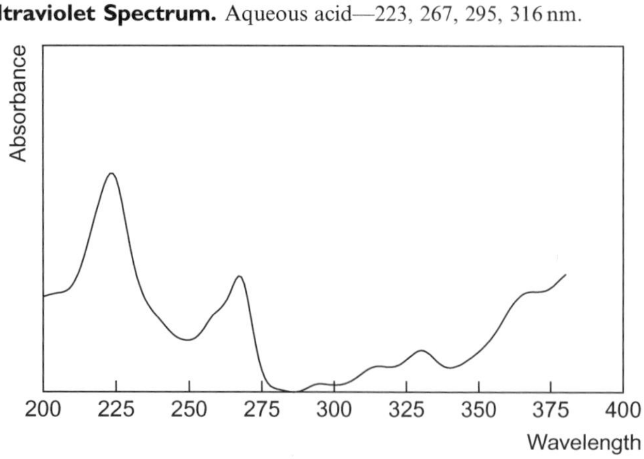

Mass Spectrum. Principal ions at *m/z* 44, 45, 42, 58, 43, 59, 41, 57.

Quantification
High performance liquid chromatography. In plasma: limit of quantification 1.0 μg/L, limit of detection 0.2 μg/L, fluorescence detection (λ_{ex}=381 nm; λ_{em}=527 nm)—J. Beijen *et al.*, *J. Pharm. Biomed. Anal.*, 1990, *8*, 789–794. In plasma: limit of quantification 0.05 μg/L. Fluorescence detection (λ_{ex}=361 nm, λ_{em}=527 nm)—H. Rosing *et al.*, *J. Chromatogr. B Biomed. Appl.*, 1995, *668*, 107–115. In plasma: limit of quantification 0.10 μg/L. Fluorescence detection (λ_{ex}=381 nm, λ_{em}=525 nm)—Loos *et al.*, *J. Chromatogr. B Biomed. Appl.*, 1996, *678*, 309–315.

Disposition in the Body. Topotecan is rapidly absorbed following oral administration. It is widely and rapidly distributed throughout the body following IV administration. Topotecan undergoes reversible hydrolysis of the lactone ring to the inactive hydroxy acid form, and only small amounts are demethylated in the liver. A significant proportion (30%) of a dose is excreted in urine via the kidneys. Peak maximum concentrations are reached within 45 min. The concentration of the drug in cerebrospinal fluid is 29% of the plasma concentration. Topotecan exhibits substantial inter-individual pharmacokinetics.

Therapeutic concentration
The lactone mean peak plasma concentrations following a 30 min infusion ranged from 9 to 35 μg/L after dosages. Following 21 days of continuous infusion of dose 0.4 to 0.6 mg/m^2 per day, steady state plasma lactone and total concentrations were 2.3 to 5.5 μg/L and 6.7 to 8.9 μg/L, respectively. Following oral administration peak plasma lactone concentrations were 5.9 and 48 μg/L after 1.5 and 14 mg/m^2 [Herben *et al.*, *Clin. Pharmacokinet.*, 1996, *31(2)*, 85–102].

Toxicity. One patient on a single dose regimen of 17.5 mg/m^2 was given on day one of a 21-day cycle a single dose of 35 mg/m^2. They experienced severe neutropenia 14 days later but recovered without incident.

Bioavailability. Oral, 20 to 55%.

Half-life. 2 to 3 h.

Volume of distribution. Initial, 17 to 22 L/m^2. At steady state, 75 to 91 L/m^2.

Clearance. Approx. 24%. Clearance is higher in males than females. It decreases to about 67% of the normal value in patients with mild renal impairment; to about 34% of the normal value in those with moderate renal impairment; and about 67% of the norm in patients with hepatic impairment.

Protein binding. Approx. 35%.

Dose. 1.5 mg/m^2.

Torasemide

Diuretic

Synonyms. AC-4464; BM-02015; JDL-464; Torsemide.
Proprietary names. Demadex; Dilutol; Isodiur; Sutril; Torem, Torrem; Unat.
N-[[(1-Methylethyl)amino]carbonyl]-4-[(3-methylphenyl)amino]-3-pyridinesulfonamide
$C_{15}H_{20}N_4O_3S$=348.4
CAS—56211-40-6

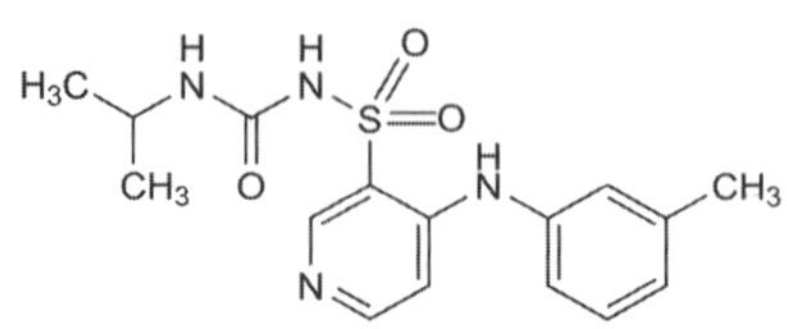

M.p. 163° to 164°.

Torasemide Sodium
CAS—72810-59-4

Dissociation Constant. pK_a 6.44, 7.1.

Gas Chromatography. Column: DB-1701 capillary (30 m × 0.25 mm i.d., 0.25 μm film thickness). Column temperature: 40°, held 1 min, then 20°/min to 300°. Carrier gas: helium. MS detection (EI, MID at *m/z* 197 and 305). Retention time: 18.24 min [M. B. Barroso *et al.*, *J. Chromatogr. B Biomed. Sci. Appl.*, 1997, *690(1–2)*, 105–113].

High Performance Liquid Chromatography. Column: Nucleosil C_{18} (250 × 4.6 mm i.d., 5 μm). Mobile phase: A: acetonitrile; B: potassium dihydrogen phosphate (100 mM, pH 4.5). Elution programme: (A:B) initial conditions; (14:86) for 8 min, (30:70) for 3.5 min, (21:79) for 8.5 min, (40:60) for 2 min, (21:79) for 10 min, (14:86) for 6 min, flow rate 1.3 mL/min. UV detection (λ=290 nm). Retention time: 18.2 min [C. March *et al.*, *J. Pharm. Sci.*, 1990, *79*, 453–457].

Column: ODS (Ultrasphere, 75 × 4.6 mm i.d., 3 μm). Mobile phase: A: acetonitrile; B: ammonium acetate (100 mM, pH 3). Elution programme: (A:B): (10:90) to (15:85) in 2 min, to (55:45) in 3 min, to (60:40) in 3 min, held for 1 min, decreased to (10:90) in 1 min, held for 2 min, flow rate 1 mL/min. UV detection (λ=270, 290 nm). Retention time: 5.2 min [R. Ventura *et al.*, *J. Chromatogr. A.*, 1993, *655*, 233–242].

Column: C_{18} (Nucleosil 10, 250 × 4.6 mm i.d.). Mobile phase: A: acetonitrile; B: sodium dihydrogen phosphate (0.0 1M pH 3.0). Elution programme: (A:B) initial conditions (78:22) to (60:40) in 5 min, (40:60) in 5 min, (25:75) in 5 min, (78:22) in 20 min. Retention time: 10 min [E. Besenfelder, *J. Pharm. Biomed. Anal.*, 1987, *5(3)*, 259–266].

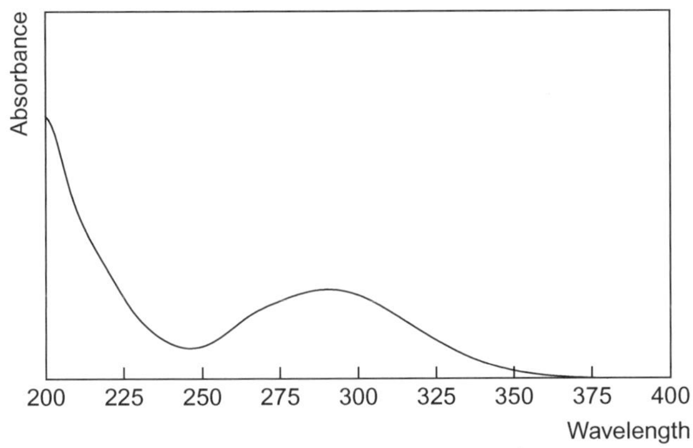

Mass Spectrum. Principal ions at *m/z* 181, 263, 246, 182, 198, 154, 91, 65.

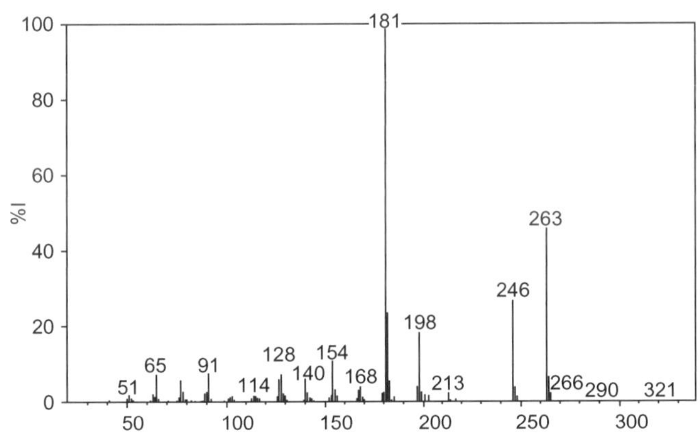

Quantification

Gas chromatography–mass spectrometry. In urine: limit of quantification is 0.5 ng (1 μL injection)—M. B. Barroso *et al.*, *J. Chromatogr. B Biomed. Sci. Appl.*, 1997, *690(1–2)*, 105–113.

High performance liquid chromatography. In plasma and urine: limit of quantification 0.01 mg/L and 0.02 mg/L, respectively, UV detection (λ=290 nm)—C. March *et al.*, *J. Pharm. Sci.*, 1990, *79*, 453–457. In plasma: limit of detection 0.04 mg/L—E. Besenfelder, *J. Pharm. Biomed. Anal.*, 1987, *5(3)*, 259–266. In plasma and urine: limit of detection 0.02 mg/L and 0.05 mg/L, respectively, UV detection (λ=290 nm)—J. Broekhuysen *et al.*, *Eur. J. Clin. Pharmacol.*, 1986, *31*, *Suppl.*, 29–34.

Disposition in the Body. Torasemide is almost completely absorbed rapidly from the gastro-intestinal tract with little first-pass metabolism. Food does not alter the absorption and is unaffected by renal or hepatic dysfunction. Peak serum concentrations are achieved within 1 h of oral administration. It is cleared from circulation by both hepatic metabolism and excretion into urine (≈20% of total clearance). Very little drug enters urine via glomerular filtration. Most renal clearance occurs via active secretion of the drug by the proximal tubules into tubular urine. Three metabolites are formed M1, M3 and M5 by stepwise oxidation, hydroxylation or ring hydroxylation. The total amount of torasemide and metabolites recovered in urine is 83%; 25% torasemide, 11% M1, 3% M3 (both active) and 44% M5 (inactive). Kinetics are linear with dosage.

Therapeutic concentration

15 patients with moderate chronic renal insufficiency (creatinine clearance, 30 to 60 mL/min), mean age of 63.3 years, and 16 patients with severe insufficiency (creatinine clearance, <30 mL/min), mean age 52.8 years, were administered with 20, 50 and 100 mg oral doses of torasemide, and 50, 100 and 200 mg doses, respectively. The mean peak drug concentrations were 2.95, 6.68 and 11.1 mg/L for the 20, 50 and 100 mg doses received by the patients with moderate impairment. These concentrations were observed at 0.94, 1.03 and 1.36 h, respectively. The mean drug concentration for the 50, 100 and 200 mg doses administered to the patients with severe impairment were 6.11, 11.3 and 18.5 mg/L at 1.18, 1.05 and 1.56 h, respectively [T. W. B. Gehr *et al.*, *Clin. Pharmacol. Ther.*, 1994, *56*, 31–38].

12 patients with ascites caused by cirrhosis, aged between 38 and 66 years, with a creatinine clearance 63 to 127 mL/min, were administered with an oral dose of 10 mg or intravenously over a 30-min period. The patients fasted overnight and for 4 h after dosing. The peak plasma concentrations were 1.7 mg/L for the intravenous dose observed at 0.52 h and 1.45 mg/L at 0.71 h for the oral dose. For healthy individuals receiving the same oral dose, the peak concentration was 1.27 mg/L at 0.86 h [S. Schwartz *et al.*, *Clin. Pharmacol. Ther.*, 1993, *54(1)*, 90–97].

16 patients with congestive heart failure (New York Heart Association class II or III), aged between 39 and 81 years, were administered with 10 mg orally or intravenously (over a 30-min infusion). The peak concentration with the intravenous dose was 2.9 mg/L after 0.6 h and 1.5 mg/L at 1.1 h for the orally administered dose [D. L. Vargo *et al.*, *Clin. Pharmacol. Ther.*, 1995, *57(6)*, 601–609].

Bioavailability. 80 to 90%; 76% (elderly).

Half-life 2.2 to 3.5 h.

Volume of distribution. 11 to 16.5 L or 0.09 to 0.31 L/kg; this value may increase by approximately double in individuals with hepatic cirrhosis.

Clearance. Following a 10 mg dose, total clearance is 0.72 ±0.23 mL/s; renal clearance 0.11 ±0.04 mL/s. After a 20 mg oral dose, total clearance is 3.4 L/h; renal clearance 0.43 L/h. After an IV dose, total clearance is 2.2 to 2.6 L/h and renal clearance 0.38 to 0.53 L/h. Systemic clearance is 41 mL/min. Renal clearance is reduced in individuals with renal impairment.

Protein binding. Greater than 99%.

Dose. Oedema: usual dose is 5 mg, increased to 20 mg once daily if necessary, maximum 40 mg. Hypertension: 2.5 mg daily, increased to 5 mg if necessary.

Toremifene

Anti-oestrogen/Antineoplastic

Proprietary name. Fareston

2-[4-[(1*Z*)-4-Chloro-1,2-diphenyl-1-butenyl]phenoxy]-*N*,*N*-dimethyl-ethanamine

$C_{26}H_{28}ClNO$=406.0

CAS—*89778-26-7*

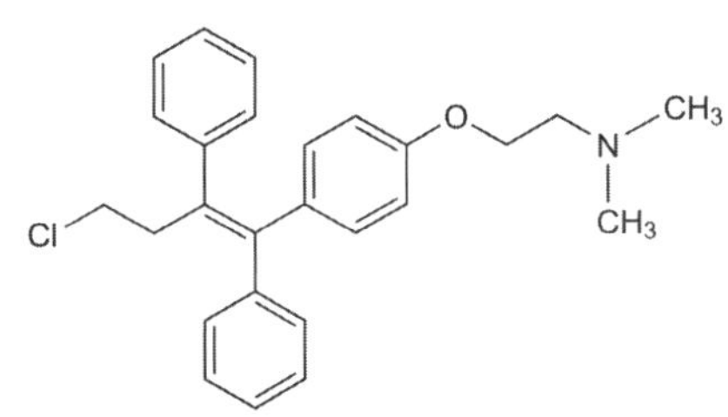

M.p. 108° to 110°.

Toremifene Citrate

Proprietary name. Fareston

$C_{26}H_{28}ClNO,C_6H_8O_7$=598.1

CAS—89778-27-8

M.p. 160° to 162°.

Dissociation Constant. pK_a 8.0.

High Performance Liquid Chromatography. Column: C_{18} (Nova-Pak, 250 × 4 mm i.d., 5 µm). Mobile phase: acetonitrile:ammonium acetate (100 mM):triethylamine (pH 6) (46:54:0.05), flow rate 1 mL/min. UV detection (λ=220 nm). Retention time: 25 min [F. Berthou and Y Dréano, *J. Chromatogr.*, 1993, *616*, 117–127].

Column: CN (Zorbax, 250 × 4.6 mm i.d., 5 µm). Mobile phase: ammonium acetate (0.1 M, pH 8) in 70% methanol, flow rate 1.2 mL/min. MS detection (API, SIM at toremifene, *m/z* 392; *N*-desmethyltoremifene, *m/z* 406; 4-hydroxytoremifene, *m/z* 408). Retention times: toremifene, 19.5 min; *N*-desmethyltoremifene, 16.0 min; 4-hydroxytoremifene, 13.7 min [N. Watanabe *et al.*, *J. Chromatogr.*, 1989, *497*; B *Biomed. Appl.*, *89*, 169–180].

Ultraviolet Spectrum. Aqueous acid—236 nm.

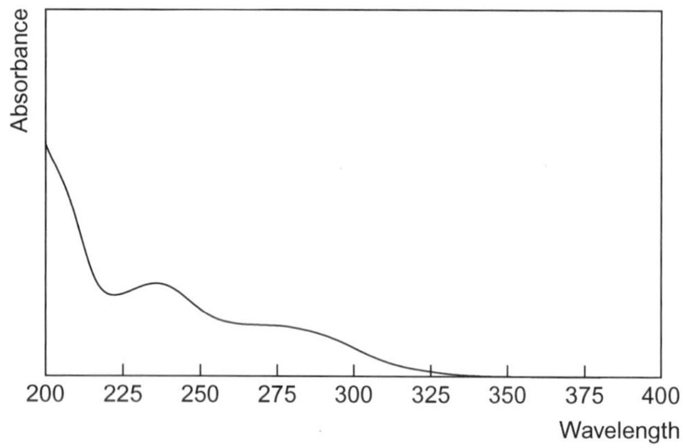

Mass Spectrum. Principal ions at *m/z* 58, 72, 59, 405.

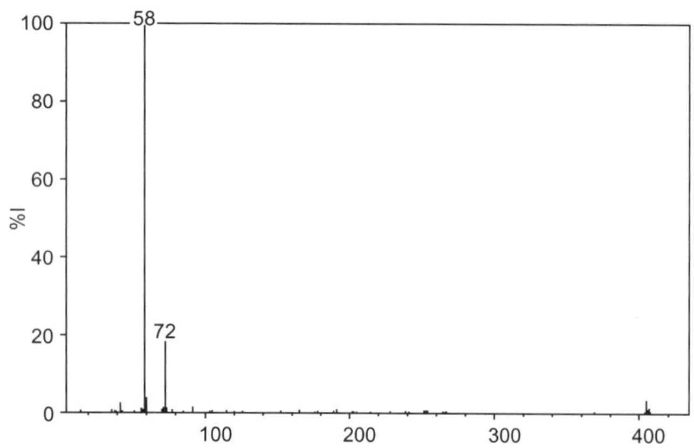

Quantification

High performance liquid chromatography. In plasma or urine: toremifene and metabolites, limit of detection is about 0.2 mg/L in plasma, UV detection (λ=277 nm)—L. K. Webster *et al.*, *J. Chromatogr.*, 1991, *565*; B *Biomed. Appl.*, *103*, 482–487.

High performance liquid chromatography–mass spectrometry. In urine: metabolites—N. Watanabe *et al.*, *J. Chromatogr.*, 1989, *497*; B *Biomed. Appl.*, *89*, 169–180.

Disposition in the Body. Toremifene is well absorbed after oral administration and absorption is not influenced by food. Peak plasma concentrations are attained within 3 h. This drug shows linear pharmacokinetics. Toremifene is extensively metabolised primarily by CYP3A4. It is metabolised by *N*-demethylation, *p*-hydroxylation and side chain oxidation to *N*-desmethyltoremifene, which also has anti-oestrogenic properties but only weak *in vitro* antitumour activity. Other metabolites include deaminohydroxy-toremifene, 4-hydroxy-toremifene and di-desmethyl-toremifene. It also undergoes entero-hepatic circulation. The drug is eliminated as metabolites mainly in faeces (70%). About 10% is excreted in urine during a 1-week period as metabolites. Toremifene accumulates during repeated dosing.

Therapeutic concentration

4 groups of subjects, aged between 32 and 75 years, were administered with a single oral dose of 120 mg after an overnight fast and fasting was continued for 3 h after dosing. Group 1 comprised 10 normal, healthy subjects; group 2 comprised 10 patients with impaired liver function (alcohol related); group 3 comprised 10 patients with drug-activated liver dysfunction; and group 4 comprised 10 subjects with impaired renal function (stable, chronic renal impairment). Mean peak plasma drug concentrations were 0.414, 0.523, 0.384 and 0.498 mg/L for the four groups, respectively. These concentrations were observed after 2 h (range 0.5 to 8 h). Peak concentrations for the metabolite, *N*-desmethyltoremifene, were 0.130, 0.142, 0.196 and 0.136 µg/L for groups 1, 2, 3 and 4 observed at approx. 72, 7, 16 and 24 h, respectively (M. Anttila *et al.*, *Clin. Pharmacol. Ther.*, 1995, *57*, 628–635).

Half-life. Plasma half-life, toremifene, 5 days; *N*-desmethyltoremifene, 6 days.

Protein binding. In plasma, more than 99.5%, mainly to albumin.

Note. For a review of toremifene see L. R. Wiseman and K. L. Goa, *Drugs*, 1997, *54*, 141–160.

Dose. The equivalent of 60 mg of toremifene daily.

Tosylchloramide Sodium

Disinfectant

Synonyms. Chloramidum; Chloramine; Chloramine T; Cloramina; Mianin; Natrium Sulfaminochloratum.
Proprietary names. Hydroclonazone; Klortee.
Note. The name Chloramin is applied to a preparation of chlorphenamine maleate.
Sodium *N*-chloro-4-methylbenzenesulfonamide trihydrate
$C_7H_7ClNNaO_2S,3H_2O$=281.7
CAS—127-65-1 (anhydrous)

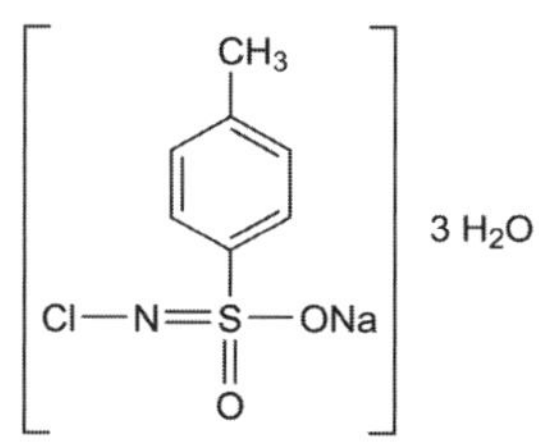

A white or slightly yellow crystalline powder. It effloresces in air, losing chlorine, becoming yellow in colour and less soluble in water.
Soluble 1 in 7 of water and 1 in 2 of boiling water; soluble 1 in 12 of ethanol, with slow decomposition; practically insoluble in benzene, chloroform, and ether.

Thin-layer Chromatography. System TAJ—Rf 40; system TAK—Rf 18; system TAL—Rf 68.

Ultraviolet Spectrum. No significant absorption, 230 to 360 nm.

Infra-red Spectrum. Principal peaks at wavenumbers 1165, 1316, 1105, 825, 710, 920 cm^{-1} (KCl disk).

Use. As a 2% solution for wound irrigation.

Tramadol

Narcotic Analgesic

(1*R*,2*R*)-*rel*-2-[(Dimethylamino)methyl]-1-(3-methoxyphenyl)cyclohexanol
$C_{16}H_{25}NO_2$=263.4
CAS—27203-92-5

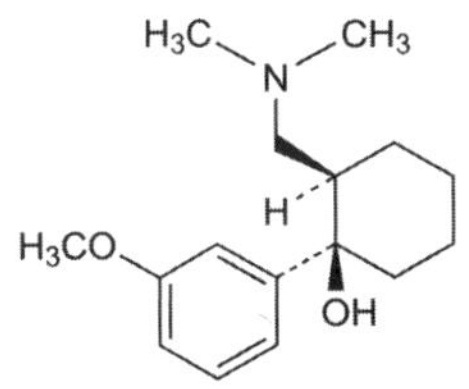

Tramadol Hydrochloride

Synonyms. CG-315; CG-315E; U-26225A.
Proprietary names. Dromadol; Tramake; Tramal; Ultram; Zamadol; Zydol.
$C_{16}H_{25}NO_2$,HCl=299.8
CAS—22204-88-2
A white, bitter, odourless crystalline powder. M.p. 180° to 181°.
Readily soluble in water and ethanol.

Dissociation Constant. pK_a 8.3, 9.41.

Partition Coefficient. Log *P* (octanol/water), 3.01.

Thin-layer Chromatography. System TE—Rf 78; system TAE—Rf 30.

Gas Chromatography. System GA—tramadol RI 1943, M (nor-)-AC RI 2295, M (*O*-desmethyl-) RI 1995, M (*O*-desmethyl-)-AC RI 1998, M (*N,O*-didesmethyl-)-AC_2 RI 2464, M (OH-) RI 2200; system GB—tramadol RI 2021, M (nor-) RI 2049, M (*O*-desmethyl-) RI 2093, M (*N,O*-didesmethyl-) RI 2122, M (OH-) RI 2252.

Column: capillary (RTX 10024, 30 m × 0.32 mm i.d., 0.25 μm film thickness). Column temperature: 100°; increased to 250° at 10°/min; held 8 min. Carrier gas: nitrogen, 1 mL/min flow rate. Detection: Flame ionisation. *k* value (Retention time): 13.41 (11.53 min). [S.-T. Ho *et al.*, *J. Chromatogr. B Biomed. Sci. Appl.*, 1999, *736*, 89–96].

Column: HP-5-MS capillary (30 m × 0.25 mm i.d., 0.25 μm). Column temperature: 140°; increased to 260° at 24°/min; held 4 min. Carrier gas: helium, flow rate 1 mL/min. MS detection, SIM (*m*/*z* 263, 179). Retention time: 6.03 min [M. Merslavic and L. Zupancic-Kralj, *J. Chromatogr. B Biomed. Sci. Appl.*, 1997, *693*, 222–227].

High Performance Liquid Chromatography. System HX—RI 328; system HY—RI 267; system HZ—Retention time, 2.9 min.

Column: RP-18 (LiChrosorb, 250 × 4.6 mm i.d., 5 μm); guard, RP-18 (Supelcosil, 4 × 4 mm i.d., 5 μm). Mobile phase: 70% phosphate buffer (0.01 M, pH 5.9): 30% acetonitrile with 0.1% triethylamine, flow rate 0.75 mL/min. UV detection (λ = 218 nm). *k* value (Retention time): 2.09 (11.4 min) [S. H. Gan and R. Ismail, *J. Chromatogr. B Biomed. Sci. Appl.*, 2001, *759*, 325–335].

Column: ODP-50 (Asahipack, 125 × 4.0 mm i.d., 5 μm). Mobile phase: 0.01 M borate buffer (pH 9):methanol (40:60), flow rate 0.7 mL/min. ECD. Retention time: 10.5 min [M. Valle *et al.*, *J. Chromatogr. B Biomed. Sci. Appl.*, 1999, *724(1)*, 83–89].

Column (1): analytical, Separon SGX C_{18} (150 × 3.3 mm i.d., 5 μm), compact glass cartridge; guard, (30 × 3.3 mm i.d.). Mobile phase: 4 g hexanesulfonic acid sodium salt monohydrate dissolved in 400 mL 0.02 M phosphoric acid (1.28 mL 85% phosphoric acid in 1000 mL water), and mixed with 600 mL acetonitrile, flow rate 0.9 mL/min. UV detection (λ = 275 nm) and fluorescence detection (λ_{ex} = 202 nm; λ_{em} = 296 nm). Retention time: 4.34 min.

Column (2): LiChrospher 100 RP-18 (250 × 4 mm, 5 μm); precolumn, (4 × 4 mm i.d.). Mobile phase: 4 g hexanesulfonic acid sodium salt monohydrate in 600 mL phosphoric acid and 400 mL acetonitrile. Retention time: 4.4 min [M. Nobilis *et al.*, *J. Chromatogr.*, 1996, *681*; *Biomed. Appl.*, 177–183].

Ultraviolet Spectrum. Aqueous acid—272 nm (A_1^1=70a), shoulder at 279 nm. No alkaline shift.

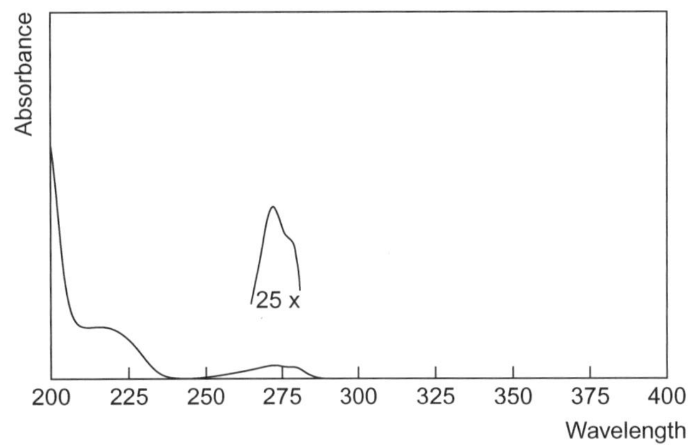

Infra-red Spectrum. Principal peaks at wavenumbers 1284, 1601, 1042, 1238, 1575, 702 cm^{-1} (tramadol hydrochloride, KBr disk).

Quantification

Gas chromatography. In serum: limit of detection 3 μg/L, NSD—R. Becker and W. Lintz, *J. Chromatogr.*, 1986, *377*, 213–220. In plasma: limit of detection 8 μg/L, FID—S.-T. Ho *et al.*, *J. Chromatogr. B Biomed. Sci. Appl.*, 1999, *736*, 89–96.

Gas chromatography–mass spectrometry. In plasma: limit of detection 1 μg/L, SIM (*m*/*z* 263, 179)—M. Merslavic and L. Zupancic-Kralj, *J. Chromatogr. B Biomed. Sci. Appl.*, 1997, *693(1)*, 222–227. In serum: 4 μg/L, SIM—W. Lintz and H. Uragg, *J. Chromatogr.*, 1985, *341(1)*, 65–79.

High performance liquid chromatography. In plasma: limit of quantification 50 μg/L, UV detection (λ = 218 nm)—S. H. Gan and R. Ismail, *J. Chromatogr. B Biomed. Sci. Appl.*, 2001, *759(2)*, 325–335. In plasma: limit of detection 8 μg/L, FID—S. T. Ho *et al.*, *J. Chromatogr. B Biomed. Sci. Appl.*, 1999, *736(1-2)*, 89–96. In plasma: limit of quantification < 15 μg/L tramadol and < 10 μg/L *O*-desmethyltramadol, ECD—M. Valle *et al.*, *J. Chromatogr. B Biomed. Sci. Appl.*, 1999, *724*, 83–89. In plasma: limit of detection 9 μg/L, UV detection (λ = 225 nm)—G. C. Yeh *et al.*, *J. Chromatogr. B Biomed. Sci. Appl.*, 1999, *723*, 247–253. In liver: limit of detection 500 μg/L tramadol, 200 μg/L *O*-desmethyltramadol and mono-*N*-desmethyltramadol, fluorescence detection (λ_{ex} = 280 nm; λ_{em} = 310 nm)—W. D. Paar *et al.*, *J. Chromatogr.*, 1996, *686*; *Biomed. Appl.*, 221–227. In plasma: limit of quantification is 17 μg/L, UV detection (λ = 275 nm) and fluorescence detection (λ_{ex} = 202 nm; λ_{em} = 296 nm)—M. Nobilis *et al.*, *J. Chromatogr.*, 1996, *681*; *Biomed. Appl.*, 177–183.

Disposition in the Body. Tramadol is rapidly and almost completely absorbed after oral or parenteral administration. The presence of food does not significantly affect the rate or extent of absorption. As the drug is administered as the racemate, both the (−) and (+) drug and metabolites are detected in circulation. Peak serum concentrations are achieved in about 2 h. Tramadol is extensively metabolised. The main metabolic reactions are *N*- and *O*-demethylation and conjugation with glucuronic acid and sulfate. The major metabolites formed are *O*-monodesmethyltramadol, *N,O*-didesmethyltramadol and their conjugates, and *N*-monodesmethyltramadol. *O*-Monodesmethyltramadol is an active metabolite and has a greater analgesic activity than the parent drug. The extent of metabolism is reduced in patients with hepatic impairment. About 90% of an oral dose is excreted in the urine in 3 days, about 30% of the dose as unchanged drug and the rest as metabolites. The remainder of the dose is eliminated in the faeces. The rate and extent of excretion is reduced in patients with renal impairment. The drug is widely distributed throughout the body and crosses the placenta; it has also been detected in breast milk. Steady-state concentrations of both the drug and main metabolite are achieved within 2 days of multiple dosing.

Therapeutic concentration. The therapeutic tramadol blood concentration is 100 to 800 μg/L.

12 male and female healthy subjects (mean age 30.1 years; range 21 to 41 years) were fasted overnight for 12 h and orally administered with a single 50 mg dose of tramadol hydrochloride (as drops without ethanol) in the morning and as an intravenous 30 min infusion, with a 1 week washout period between doses. The mean peak serum concentration was 136 μg/L observed at a median of 1.1 h (minimum 0.74 h and maximum 1.5 h). After

the intravenous dose, a maximum concentration of 286.8 µg/L at 0.52 h was observed [W. Lintz *et al.*, *Arzneimittelforschung*, 2000, *50(2)*, 99–108].

12 healthy males received a single 50 mg dose of tramadol hydrochloride either as an intramuscular injection or as a 30 min intravenous infusion, after an overnight fast (with a 1 week washout period between doses). After intramuscular injection, a mean peak serum tramadol concentration of 0.166 mg/L was reached after 0.75 h and after intravenous infusion, a peak of 0.293 mg/L was reached at 0.5 h [W. Lintz *et al.*, *Int. J. Clin. Pharmacol. Ther.*, 1999, *37*, 175–183].

92 patients who were recovering from major gynaecological surgery were intravenously administered with a maximum dose of 200 mg (+)-tramadol, (−)-tramadol or racemic tramadol and 20 mg doses of each were also administered, as requested, for 24 h. Drug and metabolite serum concentrations were measured before each additional dose. The mean tramadol concentration was 470 µg/L for (+)-drug, 590 µg/L for the racemate and 771 µg/L for the (−)-drug. The mean *O*-desmethyltramadol concentration was 57, 84 and 96 µg/L for the three drug types, respectively [S. Grond *et al.*, *Br. J. Clin. Pharmacol.*, 1999, *48(2)*, 254–257].

10 healthy, female subjects (aged 38 to 57 years; mean 48.7 years) were rectally administered with 100 mg tramadol hydrochloride (as a suppository and as an intravenous injection; washout period 1 week between doses) after a 12 h overnight fast. The mean maximum serum concentration was 294 µg/L observed at 3.3 h (range 2 to 6 h) for the suppository dose. After the intravenous dose, a concentration of 603.1 µg/L was observed at 0.25 h [W. Lintz *et al.*, *Arzneimittelforschung*, 1998, *48(9)*, 889–899].

Toxicity. The toxic tramadol blood concentration is 1.0 mg/L; lethal, 2.0 mg/L.

A 26-year-old male nurse returned home from work after a night shift and went to bed to sleep. Later that evening he was found dead face down on his bed. A bottle of tramadol was found in his pocket. The peripheral blood tramadol concentration was 9.6 mg/L, which is approximately 30 times the observed therapeutic concentration range (0.1 to 0.3 mg/L). The heart blood concentration was 13.1 mg/L; urine, 46.0 mg/L; bile, 46.1 mg/L; liver, 6.2 µg/g and kidney, 3.1 µg/g. There was also a trace of the drug detected in the gastric contents. No other drugs or alcohol were detected [F. Musshoff and B. Madea, *Forensic Sci. Int.*, 2001, *116(2-3)*, 197–199].

A 30-year-old woman was found dead at her home after ingestion of unknown amounts of alprazolam, tramadol and alcohol (empty packages of each found at the scene). She had a history of depression. Toxicological analysis showed concentrations of tramadol in her peripheral blood at 38.3 mg/L (approx 100 times the therapeutic concentration). Alprazolam was found at a concentration of 0.21 mg/L and alcohol at 1.29 mg/g. Tramadol was also detected at concentrations of 44.0 mg/L, 27.6 µg/g and 130 mg total in the bile, liver and gastric contents, respectively, and alprazolam at 0.27 mg/L, 0.23 µg/g and 2.73 mg, respectively [K. Michaud *et al.*, *Forensic Sci. Int.*, 1999, *105(3)*, 185–189].

In a fatal overdose case involving tramadol, the tramadol concentration in various tissues and fluids was: blood, 20 mg/L; liver, 68.9 µg/g; kidney, 37.5 µg/g and urine, 110.2 mg/L. In all body tissues and blood, the drug concentration was greater than the metabolites *N*-desmethyl and *O*-desmethyltramadol, and *O*-desmethyltramadol was always greater in concentration than the *N*-desmethyl metabolite [K. A. Moore *et al.*, *Am. J. Forensic Med. Pathol.*, 1999, *20(1)*, 98–100].

Analysis of 12 blood samples from tramadol-related death and 4 from non-fatal tramadol intoxications revealed concentrations ranging from 0.03 to 22.59 mg/L for tramadol, 0.02 to 1.84 mg/L for *O*-desmethyltramadol and 0.01 to 2.08 mg/L for *N*-desmethyltramadol. 3 of the fatalities were attributable to morphine and 1 to doxapin; 6 were multiple drug overdoses [K. E. Goeringer *et al.*, *J. Anal. Toxicol.*, 1997, *21*, 529–537].

Bioavailability. About 75%.

Half-life. Plasma half-life, tramadol about 6 h (increases to 7 h with multiple dosing), *O*-monodesmethyltramadol, about 9 h.

Volume of distribution. About 3 L/kg; slightly higher in females compared with males (2.9 L/kg versus 2.6 L/kg).

Clearance. Plasma clearance, about 6 mL/min/kg; slightly higher in males compared with females (6.4 mL/min/kg versus 5.7 mL/min/kg).

Protein binding. In plasma, 20%.

Dose. Tramadol hydrochloride is given in doses of 50 to 100 mg; orally, not more often than every 4 h (no more than 400 mg daily required); intramuscular injection or intravenous injection/infusion, 50 to 100 mg every 4 to 6 h (for post-operative pain, 100 mg initially followed by 50 mg every 10 to 20 min; total maximum, 250 mg in first hour, then as before).

Tramazoline

Sympathomimetic

4,5-Dihydro-*N*-(5,6,7,8-tetrahydro-1-naphthalenyl)-1*H*-imidazol-2-amine
$C_{13}H_{17}N_3$=215.3
CAS—1082-57-1

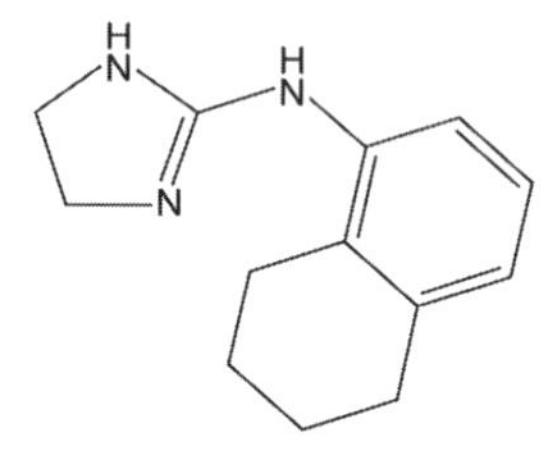

Crystals. M.p. 142° to 143°.

Tramazoline Hydrochloride

Proprietary names. Biciron; Bisolnasal; Ellatun; Rhinospray; Rinogutt Spray-Fher; Spray-Tish. It is an ingredient of Dexa-Rhinaspray.
$C_{13}H_{17}N_3$,HCl=251.8
CAS—3715-90-0
A white crystalline solid. M.p. 171°.
Soluble 1 in 6 of water.

Partition Coefficient. Log *P* (chloroform/pH 7.4) 0.8; (octanol/water) 2.5.

Colour Tests. Mandelin's Test—brown; Marquis Test—red-violet.

Thin-layer Chromatography. System TA—Rf 06; system TAE—Rf 04; system TL—Rf 02; system TB—Rf 04; system TC—Rf 02; system TE—Rf 30. (Acidified potassium permanganate solution, positive.)

Gas Chromatography. System GA—RI 2440.

High Performance Liquid Chromatography. System HA—*k* 1.8; system HX—RI 341.

Ultraviolet Spectrum. Aqueous acid—267, 275 nm.

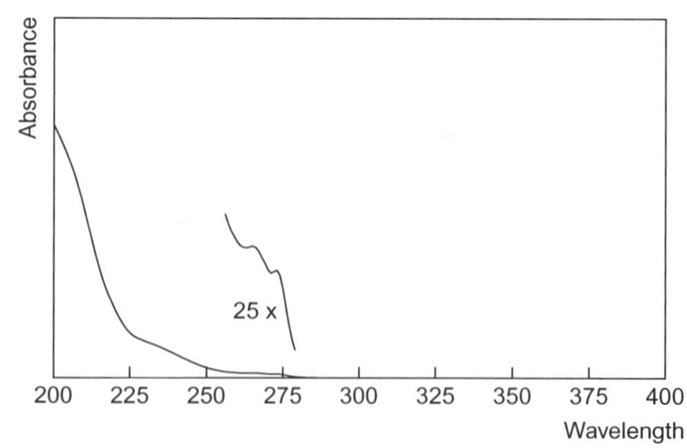

Infra-red Spectrum. Principal peaks at wavenumbers 1667, 1626, 1590, 1302, 797, 1289 cm^{-1} (tramazoline hydrochloride, KBr disk).

Mass Spectrum. Principal ions at *m/z* 215, 214, 44, 185, 200, 216, 157, 186.

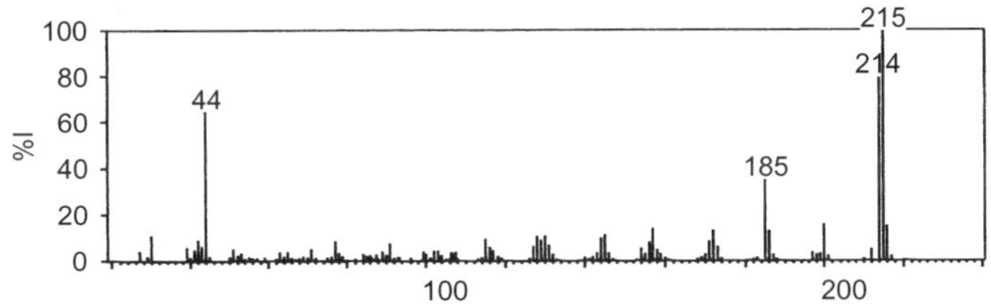

Trandolapril

Antihypertensive

Synonyms. RU-44570; RU-44403.
Proprietary names. Gopten; Mavik; Odrik; Zeddan.
(2*S*,3a*R*,7a*S*)-1-[(2*S*)-2-[[1*S*)-1-(Ethoxycarbonyl)-3-phenylpropyl]-amino]-1-oxopropyl]octahydro-1*H*-indole-2-carboxylic acid
$C_{24}H_{34}N_2O_5$=430.5
CAS—87679-37-6

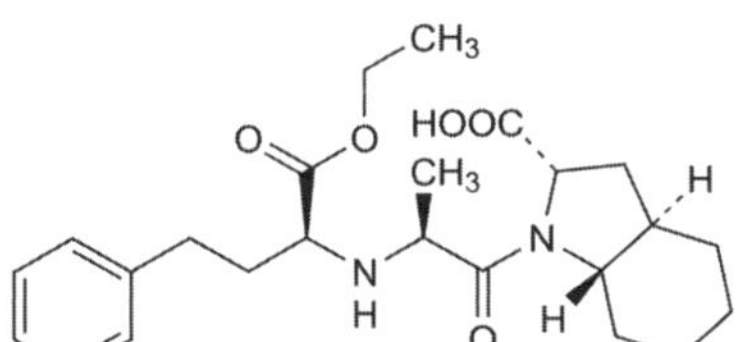

Gas Chromatography. System GP—trandolapril-ME RI 2970; M perindoprilate-ME3 RI 3005; M perindoprilate-H_2O-ME3 RI 3070.

High Performance Liquid Chromatography. System HAA—RT 17.0 min; system HZ—trandolapril retention time 6.1 min; trandolaprilat retention time 2.1 min.

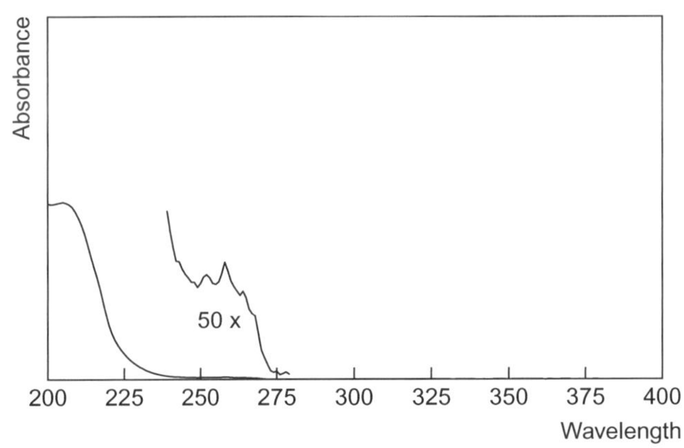

Mass Spectrum. Principal ions at *m/z* 262, 308, 91, 124, 117, 223, 179, 160.

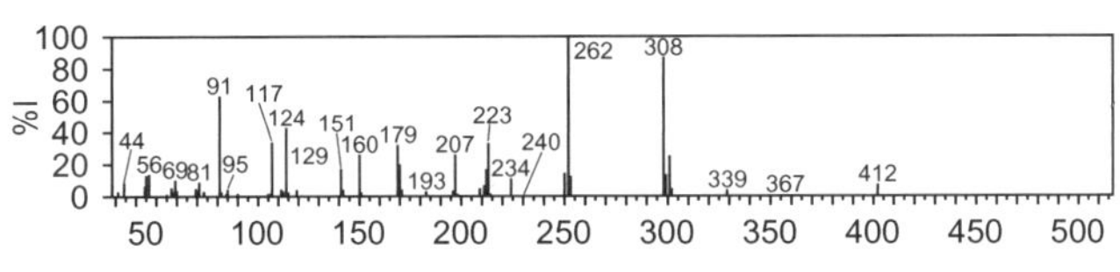

Quantification
Gas chromatography–mass spectrometry. In urine: limit of detection 10 µg/L—H. H. Maurer *et al.*, *Ther. Drug. Monit.*, 1998, *20*, 706–713.

Disposition in the Body. Trandolapril is very rapidly absorbed after oral administration and is not affected by food. It is a pro-drug of its metabolite, diacid trandolaprilat, which is a specific angiotensin-converting enzyme (ACE) inhibitor. The effective half-life for accumulation of trandolaprilat is 16 to 24 h following multiple dosing. Trandolapril is metabolised in the liver to trandolaprilat and some inactive metabolites. Peak plasma concentrations of trandolapril following an oral dose are achieved within 30 to 60 min. Peak plasma concentrations of trandolaprilat range from 4 to 6 h. Approximately 33% of an oral dose is excreted in urine, mainly as trandolaprilat, and the remainder is excreted in faeces. Excretion is virtually complete (99.2%) after 7 days, except in patients with impaired renal function where excretion is decreased. Steady state concentrations are reached in about 4 days. Trandolaprilat is eliminated in urine in the unchanged form and accounts for 10 to 15% of the dose of trandolapril administered. Modest accumulation of trandolapril occurs during multiple dosing.

Therapeutic concentration
10 patients with a mean age of 44.1 years, and 14 patients with a mean age 69.3 years, all with mild to moderate hypertension, were administered 2 mg trandolapril for 10 consecutive days. Steady state plasma concentrations were reached after 4 days and absorption is rapid, in less than 1 h. The steady state concentration was 7.49 µg/L for the young individuals and 8.35 µg/L in the elderly [P. Arner *et al.*, *J. Cardiovasc. Pharmacol.*, 1994, *23 (Suppl.4)*, S44–S49].

Bioavailability. Trandolapril approx. 9.5%; trandolaprilat, 40 to 60%.

Half-life. Trandopril, 1.3 h (healthy individuals and patients with mild to moderate hypertension); trandolaprilat, steady state, 16 to 24 h.

Protein binding. Trandolapril, >80%, not saturable over 0.1 to 1.0 µg/L; trandolaprilat, 65% at 1000 µg/L to 94% at 0.1 µg/L; will bind to saturation with a strong affinity in serum.

Dose. The usual dose is 1 to 2 mg, maximum 4 mg.

Tranylcypromine

Antidepressant

Synonyms. Tranilcipromina; Transamine.
(1*R*,2*S*)-*rel*-2-Phenylcyclopropanamine
$C_9H_{11}N$=133.2
CAS—155-09-9

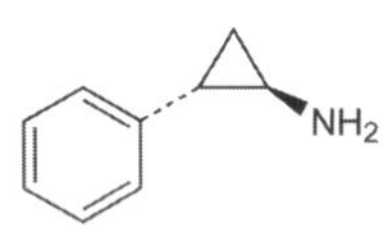

A liquid.

Tranylcypromine Sulfate
Proprietary names. Jatrosom N; Parnate; Tylciprine. It is an ingredient of Parmodalin, Parstelin and Stelapar.
$(C_9H_{11}N)_2,H_2SO_4$=364.5
CAS—13492-01-8
A white crystalline powder.
Soluble 1 in 20 to 1 in 25 of water and 1 in 2000 of ether; very slightly soluble in ethanol; practically insoluble in chloroform.

Dissociation Constant. pK_a 8.2.

Partition Coefficient. Log *P* (octanol/chloroform), 0.6; (octanol/water), 1.6.

Colour Tests. Liebermann's Test—red-orange; Mandelin's Test—green→violet; Marquis Test—red→brown.

Thin-layer Chromatography. System TA—Rf 54; system TB—Rf 39; system TC—Rf 33; system TE—Rf 58; system TL—Rf 48; system TAE—Rf 41; system TAF—Rf 67; system TAJ—Rf 19; system TAK—Rf 17; system TAL—Rf 52. (Dragendorff spray, positive; FPN reagent, yellow; acidified iodoplatinate solution, positive; Marquis reagent, orange-brown; ninhydrin spray, positive.)

Gas Chromatography. System GA—RI 1220; system GB—RI 1252; system GC—RI 1759; system GF—RI 1455.

High Performance Liquid Chromatography. System HA—*k* 1.0; system HC—*k* 0.26; system HX—RI 230; system HY—RI 196; system HZ—Retention time 2.0 min.

Ultraviolet Spectrum. Aqueous acid—258, 264 nm (A^1_1=22a), 271 nm; aqueous alkali—260, 266, 273 nm.

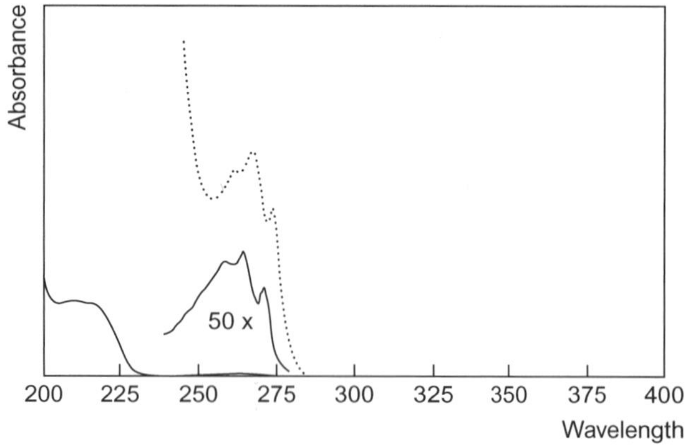

Infra-red Spectrum. Principal peaks at wavenumbers 1023, 1112, 695, 963, 1153, 743 cm^{-1} (tranylcypromine sulfate, Nujol mull).

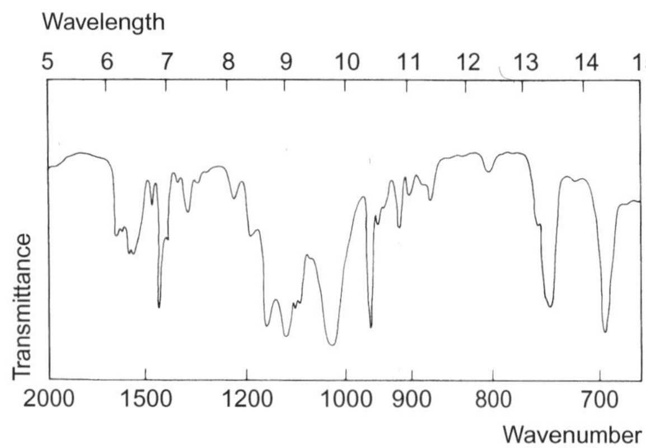

Mass Spectrum. Principal ions at *m/z* 133, 132, 56, 115, 30, 117, 91, 77.

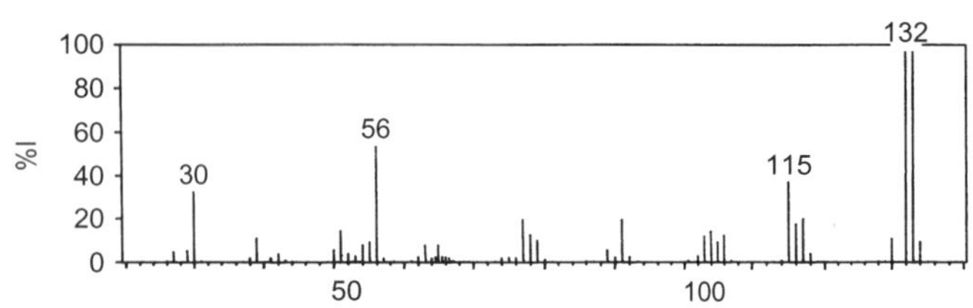

Quantification

Gas chromatography. In serum or urine: limit of detection 1 µg/L, ECD—R. C. Baselt *et al.*, *J. Anal. Toxicol.*, 1977, *1*, 215–217. In plasma or urine: limit of detection 2.5 µg/L, AFID—E. Bailey and E. J. Barron, *J. Chromatogr.*, 1980, *183*; *Biomed. Appl.*, *9*, 25–31.

Disposition in the Body. Readily absorbed after oral administration and extensively metabolised. Less than 2% of a dose is excreted as unchanged drug in the urine in 24 h; this increases to about 8% if the urine is maintained at an acid pH.

Therapeutic concentration

A single oral dose of 30 mg administered to 2 subjects produced a peak serum concentration of about 0.04 mg/L in 1 h. During chronic treatment of 42 patients with 10 to 30 mg daily, serum concentrations of 0.005 to 0.01 mg/L were found when measured 12 h after the last dose [R. C. Baselt *et al.*, *J. Anal. Toxicol.*, 1977, *1*, 215–217].

Toxicity. Several cases of addiction to tranylcypromine have been reported.

The following postmortem tissue concentrations were reported in a fatality involving the ingestion of 300 mg of tranylcypromine: blood 3.7 mg/L, brain 1.0 µg/g, liver 7.3 µg/g, urine 25 mg/L; several other drugs were detected [R. C. Baselt *et al.*, *J. Anal. Toxicol.*, 1977, *1*, 168–170].

A man who ingested 400 mg tranylcypromine with suicidal intent had a blood tranylcypromine concentration of 0.51 mg/L approx. 3 h later; another man, who was found dead 48 h after taking an unknown quantity of tranylcypromine, had the following tranylcypromine tissue concentrations: blood 0.7 mg/L, liver 1.9 mg/g, urine 238.0 mg/L [S. Iwersen and A. Schmoldt, *J. Anal. Toxicol.*, 1996, *20*, 301–304].

A 41-year-old man survived after ingesting 4 g of tranylcypromine in a suicide attempt. Approx. 8 h after ingestion of the overdose, the tranylcypromine concentration in the blood was 19.88 mg/L and decreased to 1.14 mg/L on day 2, 0.028 mg/L on day 3, 0.006 mg/L on day 4 and 0.001 mg/L on day 8 [J. M. Pennings *et al.*, *J. Clin. Psychopharmacol.*, 1997, *17*, 430–432].

Half-life. Plasma half-life, about 2 h.

Dose. The equivalent of 10 to 30 mg of tranylcypromine daily.

Trazodone

Antidepressant

2-[3-[4-(3-Chlorophenyl)-1-piperazinyl]propyl]-1,2,4-triazolo[4,3-*a*]-pyridin-3(2*H*)-one

$C_{19}H_{22}ClN_5O = 371.9$

CAS—19794-93-5

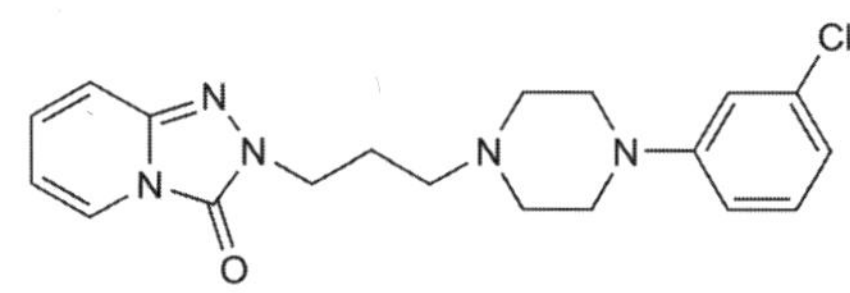

Crystals. M.p. 86° to 87°. Also reported as 96°.

Soluble 1 in 50 of ethanol and methanol; freely soluble in acetone and benzene; slightly soluble in ether.

Trazodone Hydrochloride

Proprietary names. Azona; Deprax; Depyrel; Desirel; Desyrel; Molipaxin; Sideril; Thombran; Trazodil; Trazolan; Trazone; Trazorel; Triticum; Trittico.

$C_{19}H_{22}ClN_5O,HCl = 408.3$

CAS—25332-39-2

White crystals. M.p. 223°.

Sparingly soluble in water, ethanol and methanol; soluble in chloroform; practically insoluble in common organic solvents.

Partition Coefficient. Log *P* (octanol/water), 3.2.

Colour Tests. Liebermann's Test—violet (transient); Mandelin's Test—grey→violet.

Thin-layer Chromatography. System TA—Rf 63; system TB—Rf 10; system TC—Rf 58; system TE—Rf 66; system TL—Rf 37; system TAE—Rf 64; system TAF—Rf 61; system TAJ—Rf 55; system TAK—Rf 00; system TAL—Rf 66. (Location under ultraviolet light, violet fluorescence; Dragendorff spray, positive; acidified iodoplatinate solution, positive.)

Gas Chromatography. System GA—trazodone RI 3330; M (OH-acetyl-) RI 3380; system GB—trazodone RI 3562; M (mCPP) RI 1806; M (OH-acetyl-) RI 3640; M (desalkylacetyl-) RI 2261; system GM—trazodone, not eluted.

High Performance Liquid Chromatography. System HA—*k* 0.6; system HX—RI 378; system HY—RI 305; system HZ—Retention time 3.3 min; system HAA—Retention time 12.7 min.

Ultraviolet Spectrum. Aqueous acid—246 nm (A_1^1 = 314a), 274, 310 nm. No alkaline shift.

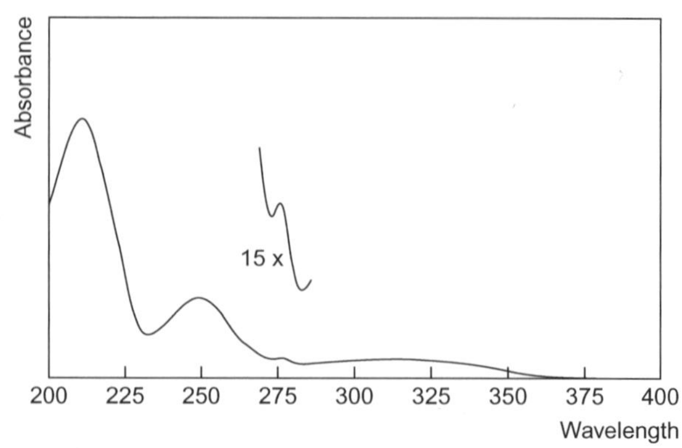

Infra-red Spectrum. Principal peaks at wavenumbers 1705, 1595, 943, 1640, 742, 1272 cm^{-1} (trazodone hydrochloride, KBr disk). (See below)

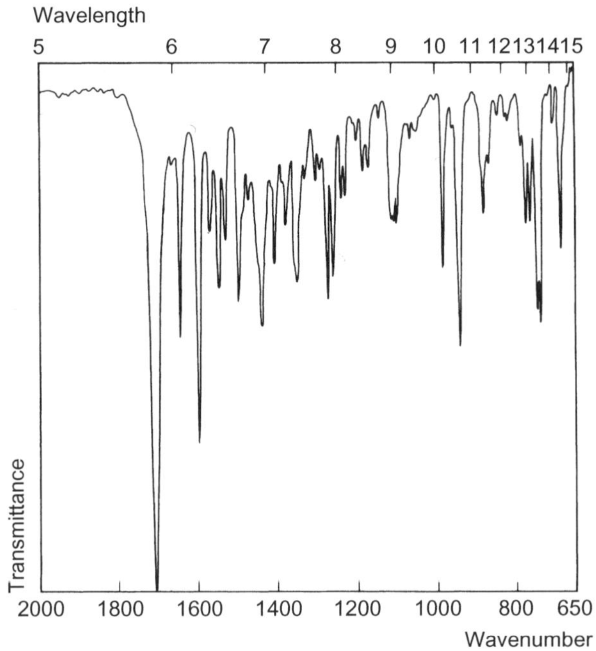

Mass Spectrum. Principal ions at *m/z* 205, 70, 231, 78, 135, 136, 42, 166.

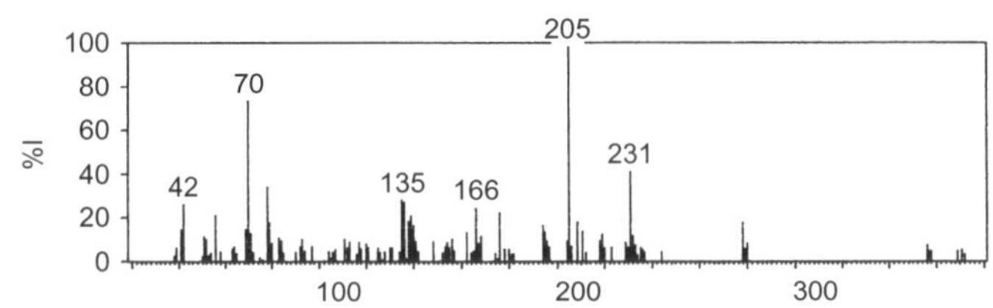

Quantification

Gas chromatography. In plasma or brain: trazodone and 1-(3-chlorophenyl)piperazine, detection limits 50 µg/L and 10 µg/L, respectively, AFID—S. Caccia *et al., J. Chromatogr.*, 1981, *210*, 311–318.

High performance liquid chromatography. In plasma: limit of detection 20 µg/L, UV detection—S. I. Ankier *et al., Br. J. Clin. Pharmacol.*, 1981, *11*, 505–509. In biological fluids—R. Caldwell and R. J. Flanagan, *J Chromatogr.*, 1985, *345*, 187–91.

Disposition in the Body. Rapidly and almost completely absorbed after oral administration. It is extensively metabolised by hydroxylation and oxidation. About 75% of a dose is excreted in the urine as metabolites and 15% is eliminated in the faeces, in 72 h. Less than 1% of a dose is excreted in the urine as unchanged drug. The major urinary metabolites are a propionic acid derivative (3-oxo-1,2,4-triazolo[4,3-*a*]pyridine-2-propionic acid), *p*-hydroxytrazodone, and a dihydrodiol derivative and its glucuronide and sulfate conjugates, which account for about 35%, 20% and 15% of the urinary material respectively; an *N*-oxide has also been identified. In plasma, the major metabolite is 1-(3-chlorophenyl)piperazine (active), but this accounts for less than 1% of a dose in the urine.

Therapeutic concentration

After an oral dose of 50 mg to 13 subjects, peak plasma concentrations of 0.49 to 2.3 mg/L (mean 1.1) were attained in 0.5 to 2.5 h [S. I. Ankier *et al., Br. J. Clin. Pharmacol.*, 1981, *11*, 505–509].

Following a single oral dose of 150 mg to 4 subjects, mean peak plasma concentrations of 2.05 mg/L of trazodone and 0.01 mg/L of 1-(3-chlorophenyl)piperazine were reported at about 2 h and 2 to 4 h, respectively [S. Caccia *et al., J. Pharm. Pharmacol.*, 1982, *34*, 605–606].

Following oral administration of 25 mg three times a day to 10 subjects, steady-state serum concentrations averaged 0.7 mg/L on the 12th day [B. Catanese *et al., Boll. Chim. Farm.*, 1978, *117*, 424–427].

Toxicity

In a fatality in which a woman was found drowned in a bath following the ingestion of about 2 to 4 g of trazodone, the following postmortem concentrations were reported: blood 15 mg/L, bile 45 mg/L, liver 57 µg/g, urine 2.5 mg/L [D. Demorest, *J. Anal. Toxicol.*, 1983, *7*, 63].

Postmortem tissue concentrations of trazodone in 2 women, aged 53 and 48, were reported, respectively, as follows: blood 14.4 and 15.5 mg/L, brain 48.6 and 20.9 µg/g, liver 73.7 and 82.4 µg/g, lung 12.9 to 13.3 and 35.3 to 40.1 µg/g, fat 18.5 and 16.5 µg/g, kidneys 34.7 and 39.6 µg/g, heart 30.9 and 28.9 µg/g [A. Martin and D. J. Pounder, *Forensic Sci. Int.* 1992, *56*, 201–207].

Trazodone was the primary cause of death in 3 subjects (2 suicides and 1 probable suicide), all of whom had blood concentrations greater than 9 mg/L (9.06, 24.32 and 32.91 mg/L) [K. E. Goeringer *et al., J. Forensic Sci.*, 2000, *45*, 850–856].

Half-life. Plasma half-life, about 4 to 7 h.

Protein binding. In plasma, about 90%.

Note. For a review of the pharmacokinetics of trazodone see R. N. Brogden *et al., Drugs*, 1981, *21*, 401–429.

Dose. 100 to 300 mg of trazodone hydrochloride daily; maximum of 600 mg daily.

Trenbolone

Anabolic Steroid

Synonyms. Trienbolone; Trienolone; β-TBOH; RU-1697.
Proprietary names. Parabolan; Regumate.
(17β)-17-Hydroxyestra-4,9,11-trien-3-one
$C_{18}H_{22}O_2$=270.4
CAS—10161-33-8

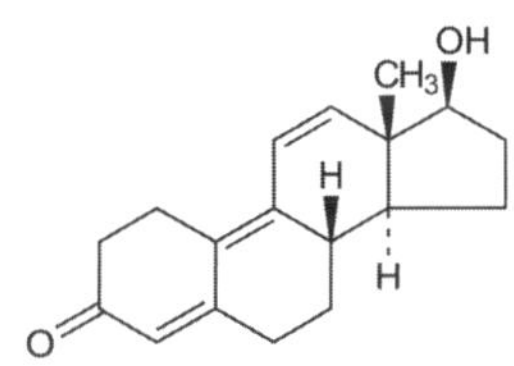

Crystals. M.p. 183° to 186°.

Trenbolone Acetate

Proprietary names. Finajet; Finaplix.
$C_{20}H_{24}O_3$=312.4
CAS—10161-34-9
Crystals. M.p. 96° to 97°.

Trenbolone Hexahydrobenzylcarbonate

Proprietary names. Hexabolan; Parabolan.
$C_{26}H_{34}O_4$=410.5
CAS—23454-33-3

Gas Chromatography. System GAI—urinary metabolite: 17α-trenbolone RRT 0.943 (relative to 17α-methyl-5α-androstan-3β,17β-diol).

Column: methyl silicone (HP1, 0.2 mm i.d., 0.33 µm film thickness). Column temperature: 280°. Carrier gas: helium, flow rate 0.9 mL/min. MS detection. Retention index: trenbolone acetate, 2811 [T. Mills and J. C. Roberson, *Instrumental Data for Drug Analysis*, CRC Press, 2nd Edn., Vol 5, Boca Raton, 1993, 402-403].

High Performance Liquid Chromatography. System HATa—trenbolone hexahydrobenzylcarbonate RRT 1.65 (relative to testosterone); system HATb—trenbolone acetate RRT 1.71 (relative to testosterone).

Column: ODS (Zorbax, 250 × 4 mm i.d., 5 µm). Mobile phase: (A)-methanol:water (10:90); (B)-acetonitrile. Elution programme; A:B (85:15) to (63:37) over 10 min, held for 10 min, to (0:100) over 5 min, flow rate 1 mL/min. UV detection (λ=340 nm). Retention time(s): 17β-trenbolone, 33 min; 17α-trenbolone, 35 min [B. Spranger *et al. J. Chromatogr.*, 1991, *564*, 485–492].

Ultraviolet Spectrum. Alcohol—237, 340 (A=between 92.0 and 97.6) nm; ethanol—338 nm.

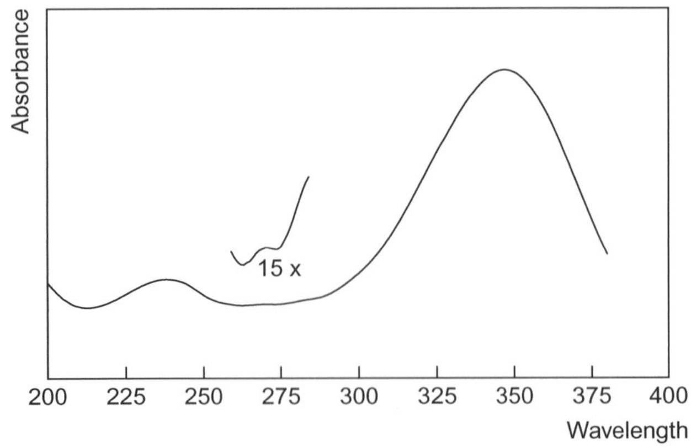

Infra-red Spectrum. Principal peaks at wavenumbers 1636, 1568, 1225, 1100 cm^{-1}; for acetate, principal peaks at wavenumbers 1652, 1739, 1244, 1023 cm^{-1}.

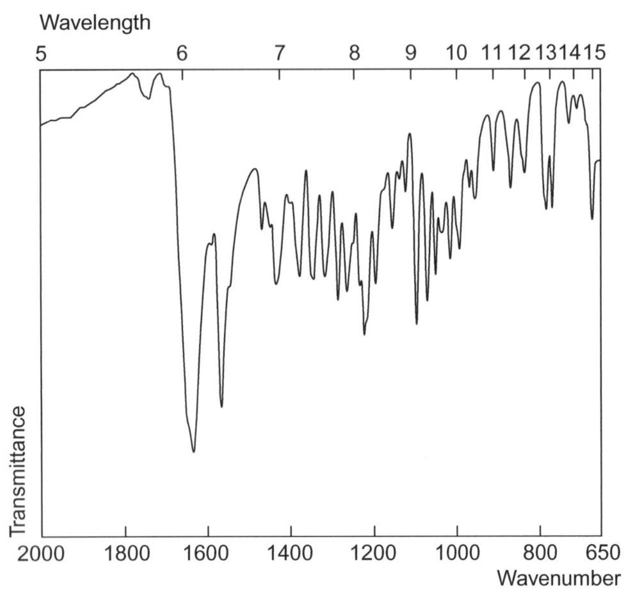

Mass Spectrum. Principal ions at *m/z* 270, 198, 252, 226, 141, 115; 155, 128; for acetate *m/z* 252, 312, 253, 237, 141, 198, 213, 270.

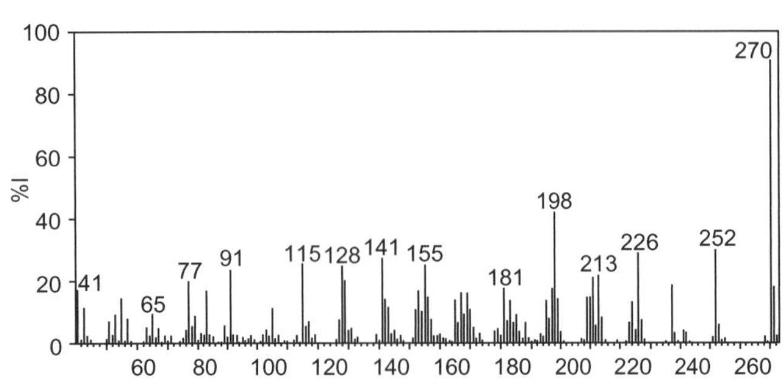

Quantification

High performance liquid chromatography. In faeces and bile: limit of detection 0.5 ng/g and 0.5 μg/L, respectively—S. Hewitt *et al., J. Chromatogr.*, 1993, *639*, 185–191.

Disposition in the Body. After administration, trenbolone undergoes metabolism to epitrenbolone and hydroxytrenbolone, possibly the main metabolites. These metabolites, mainly as the glucuronide form, have been identified in urine, along with a little trenbolone and estra-4,9,11-trien-3,17-dione and other polar metabolites in the unconjugated and sulfate forms.

Triamcinolone

Corticosteroid

Synonyms. 9α-Fluoro-16α-hydroxyprednisolone; Fluoxiprednisolonum.
Proprietary names. Aristocort; Atolone; Berlicort; Delphicort; Ipercortis; Kenacort; Ledercort; Sterocort; Triam-Oral; Triamsicort; Volon.
(11β,16α)-9-Fluoro-11,16,17,21-tetrahydroxypregna-1,4-diene-3,20-dione
$C_{21}H_{27}FO_6$=394.4
CAS—124-94-7

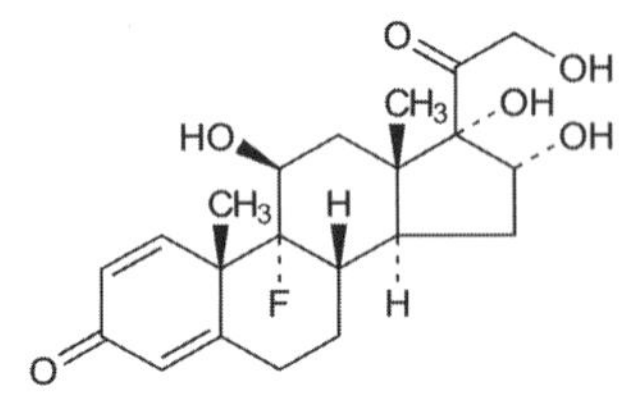

A white, slightly hygroscopic, crystalline powder. M.p. about 269° to 271°. Soluble 1 in 500 of water and 1 in 240 of ethanol; slightly soluble in methanol; very slightly soluble in chloroform and ether.

Triamcinolone Acetonide

Proprietary names. Adcortyl; Aftab; Aftach; Albicort; Aristocort; Arutrin; Azmacort; Berlicort; Delphi(cort); Denkacort; Dermacort; Extracort; Facort; Generlog; Kanolone; Kela; Kemzid; Kenacort; Kenalog; Kenalone; Ledercort; Nasacor(t); Omcilon; Oracort; Orcilone; Sta-Cort A; Steronase; Triaderm; Triam; Triamonide; Tri-Anemul; Triderm; Trigon; Trilog; Trimacort; Volon A; Volonimat; Zamacort.
$C_{24}H_{31}FO_6$=434.5
CAS—76-25-5
A white or cream-coloured crystalline powder. M.p. about 292° to 294°.
Very slightly soluble in water; soluble 1 in 150 of ethanol, 1 in 11 of acetone and 1 in 40 of chloroform; sparingly soluble in dehydrated alcohol and methanol.

Triamcinolone Diacetate

Proprietary names. Aristocort; Articulose LA; Delphicort;; Delphimix; Kenacort; Ledercort; Proctosteroid; Tracilon; Triamolone; Trilone; Tristoject.
$C_{25}H_{31}FO_8$=478.5
CAS—67-78-7
A fine, white, crystalline powder.
Practically insoluble in water; soluble 1 in 13 of ethanol, 1 in 80 of chloroform and 1 in 40 of methanol; slightly soluble in ether.

Triamcinolone Hexacetonide

Synonym. Triamcinolone Acetonide 21-(3,3-Dimethylbutyrate)
Proprietary names. Aristospan; Hexatrione; Lederlon; Lederspan.
$C_{30}H_{41}FO_7$=532.6
CAS—5611-51-8
A white to cream-coloured powder. M.p. 295° to 296°, with decomposition. Practically insoluble in water; soluble in chloroform; slightly soluble in methanol.

Partition Coefficient. Log *P* (octanol/water), 1.2.

Colour Tests. Naphthol–Sulfuric Acid—green, yellow dichroism/yellow; Sulfuric Acid—orange.

Thin-layer Chromatography. Triamcinolone: System TA—Rf 79; system TE—Rf 27; system TP—Rf 09; system TQ—Rf 00; system TR—Rf 00; system TS—Rf 00; system TAJ—Rf 14; system TAK—Rf 06; system TAL—Rf 65; system TAM—Rf 33. (DPST solution.) Triamcinolone acetonide: System TP—Rf 32; system TQ—Rf 00; system TR—Rf 20; system TS—Rf 06. (DPST solution.)

Gas Chromatography. System GA—RI 2970 and 3107.

High Performance Liquid Chromatography. Triamcinolone: System HX—RI 438; system HY—RI 312. Triamcinolone acetonide: System HT—*k* 2.5.

Ultraviolet Spectrum. Methanol—238 nm (A^1_1=390a).

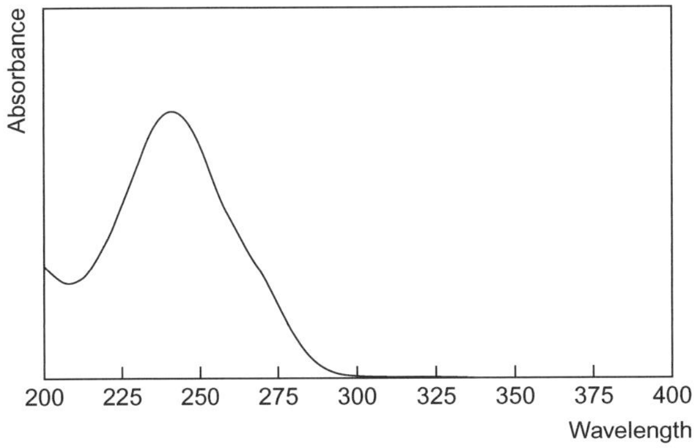

Infra-red Spectrum. Principal peaks at wavenumbers 1663, 1057, 1618, 1609, 902, 1080 cm^{-1} (triamcinolone acetonide, KBr disk).

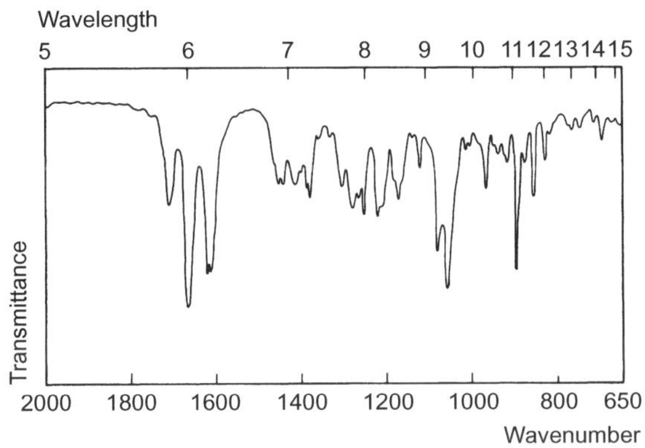

Quantification

Gas chromatography–mass spectrometry. In bronchoalveolar lavage: limit of detection triamcinolone acetonide 6.0 ng/L—W. C. Hubbard *et al.*, *Anal. Biochem.* 2001, *290*, 18–25.

High performance liquid chromatography. In blood or urine: limit of detection 200 pg, UV detection—Z. Saito *et al.*, *Nippon Naibunpi Gakki Zasshi*, 1979, *55*, 1296–1306. In plasma: limit of detection triamcinolone acetonide 0.6 μg/L, UV detection—S.A. Doppenschmitt *et al.*, *J. Chromatogr. B. Biomed. Appl.*, 1996, *682*, 79–88.

High performance liquid chromatography–mass spectrometry. In hair: limit of detection 0.03 to 0.17 μg/g—V. Cirimele *et al.*, *Forensic Sci. Int.*, 2000, *107*, 381–388.

Radioimmunoassay. In plasma: limit of detection <12.5 μg/L—J. C. K. Loo and N. Jordan, *Res. Commun. Chem. Pathol. Pharmacol.*, 1979, *23*, 493–504.

Note. For a review of the pharmacokinetics of intranasal corticosteroids, see S. J. Szefler, *J. Allergy Clin. Immunol.*, 2001, *108*, S26–S31.

Dose. 4 to 48 mg daily.

Triamterene

Diuretic

Synonyms. NSC-77625; SKF-8542; Triamterenum; Triantereno.
Proprietary names. Dyrenium; Dytac; Jatropur. It is an ingredient of Dyazide, Dytenzide, Dytide, Frusene, Kalspare, Maxzide, Triamaxco and Triamco.
6-Phenyl-2,4,7-pteridinetriamine
$C_{12}H_{11}N_7$=253.3
CAS—396-01-0

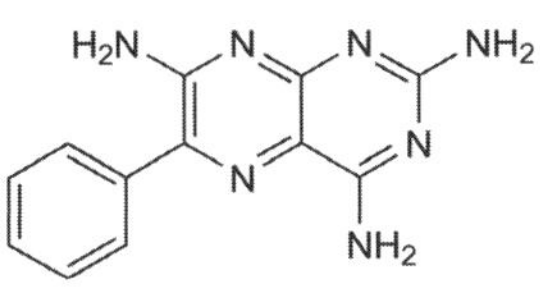

A yellow crystalline powder. Acidified solutions give a blue fluorescence. M.p. 316°.

Soluble 1 in 1000 of water, 1 in 3000 of ethanol, 1 in 4000 of chloroform and 1 in 30 of formic acid; soluble in dilute ammonia, dilute aqueous ammonium hydroxide and dimethylformamide; very slightly soluble in acetic acid and dilute mineral acids; practically insoluble in ether and dilute solutions of alkali hydroxides.

Dissociation Constant. pK_a 6.2.

Partition Coefficient. Log *P* (octanol/water), 0.98.

Colour Tests. Liebermann's Test—red-orange; Marquis Test—yellow.

Thin-layer Chromatography. System TA—Rf 51; system TB—Rf 01; system TC—Rf 08; system TE—Rf 30; system TL-Rf 04; system TAD—Rf 13; system TAE—Rf 50; system TAF—Rf 65; system TAJ—Rf 04; system TAK—Rf 00; system TAL—Rf 40. (Location under ultraviolet light, blue fluorescence.)

Gas Chromatography. System GA—triamterene RI 2010, triamterene-Me_6 RI 2875; system GX—triamterene-Me_6 Retention time 9.2 min.

High Performance Liquid Chromatography. System HX—RI 298; system HY—RI 263; system HZ—Retention time, 2.3 min; system HAA—Retention time, 8.7 min; system HAX—Retention time 6.7 min; system HAY—Retention time 3.9 min.

Ultraviolet Spectrum. Aqueous acid—250 nm (A^1_1=634b), 360 nm (A^1_1=840a); (0.1 M hydrochloric acid)—228 nm (A^1_1=1618), 360 nm (A^1_1=840); aqueous alkali (0.1 M sodium hydroxide)—232 nm (A^1_1=1633), 270 nm (A^1_1=555a), 370 nm (A^1_1=741); methanol—233 nm (A^1_1=1570a), 267 nm (A^1_1=580a).

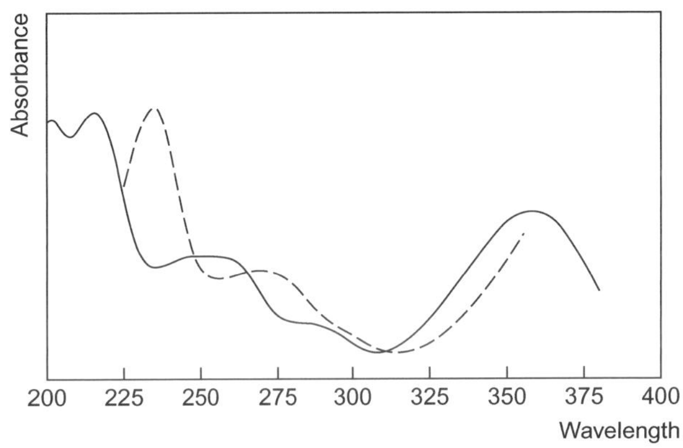

Infra-red Spectrum. Principal peaks at wavenumbers 1574, 1610, 1584, 1536, 761, 822 cm^{-1} (KBr disk). (See below)

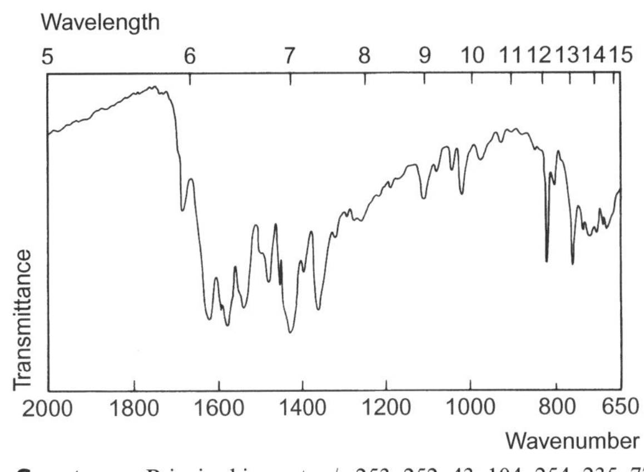

Mass Spectrum. Principal ions at *m/z* 253, 252, 43, 104, 254, 235, 77, 89.

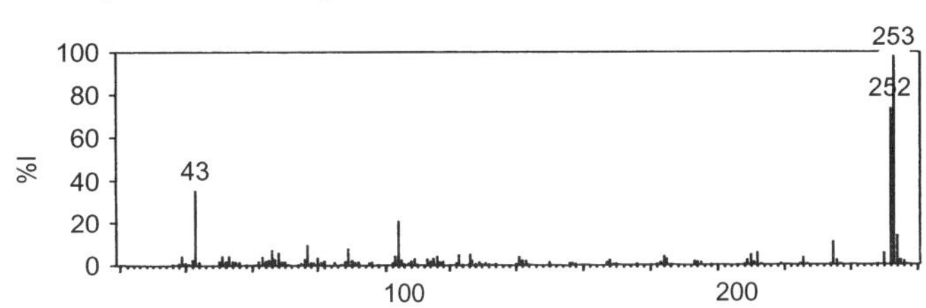

Quantification

High performance liquid chromatography. In plasma: triamterene and *p*-hydroxytriamterene, limit of detection 20 µg/L, UV detection—G. J. Yakatan and J. E. Cruz, *J. Pharm. Sci.*, 1981, *70*, 949–951. In plasma, whole blood or urine: triamterene and *p*-hydroxytriamterene sulfate, limit of detection, for blood, 1 µg/L and 2 µg/L, respectively, for urine, 40 µg/L and 100 µg/L, respectively, fluorescence detection—F. Sörgel *et al.*, *J. Pharm. Sci.*, 1984, *73*, 831–833.

Disposition in the Body. Rapidly but incompletely absorbed after oral administration and extensively metabolised. After oral administration, about 30 to 70% of a dose is excreted in the urine, mainly as the sulfate conjugate of *p*-hydroxytriamterene, with about 5 to 10% of a dose as unchanged drug; variable amounts are excreted in the bile. *p*-Hydroxytriamterene sulfate is an active metabolite. Triamterene crosses the placenta and it may be detected in breast milk.

Therapeutic concentration

After single oral doses of 150 to 300 mg to 7 subjects, peak plasma-triamterene concentrations of 0.03 to 0.15 mg/L (mean about 0.1) were attained in 1 to 2 h; peak plasma concentrations of *p*-hydroxytriamterene sulfate averaged about 1 mg/L at 2 to 4 h; both unchanged drug and the metabolite exhibited a second peak concentration several hours later, possibly due to enterohepatic circulation [U. Gundert-Remy *et al.*, *Eur. J. Clin. Pharmacol.*, 1979, *16*, 39–44].

Following a single oral dose of 100 mg to 6 subjects, peak plasma concentrations of 0.06 to 0.18 mg/L (mean 0.13) of triamterene and 1.3 to 3.2 mg/L (mean 1.8) of *p*-hydroxytriamterene sulfate were attained in about 1 to 2 h [J. Hasegawa *et al.*, *J. Pharmacokinet. Biopharm.*, 1982, *10*, 507–523].

Triamterene, 200 mg daily for 10 days, administered to 7 healthy subjects, produced an average plasma concentration during the dosage interval of 0.045 mg/L triamterene and 0.967 mg/L of hydroxytriamterene sulfate in healthy subjects; in 6 patients with cirrhosis and ascites, the respective levels were 0.586 and 0.747 mg/L (a 13-fold increase compared with healthy subjects) [M. T. Dao and J. P. Villeneuve, *Clin. Invest. Med.*, 1988, *11*, 6–9].

Toxicity. The toxic low oral dose for a woman is 42 mg/kg body weight at 3 weekly intervals. It is moderately toxic by subcutaneous administration. May be poisonous by ingestion and intraperitoneal routes.

Bioavailability. 30 to 70%.

Half-life. Plasma half-life, triamterene about 2 to 4 h, *p*-hydroxytriamterene sulfate, about 3 h; half-life derived from urinary excretion data, 6 to 12 h.

Distribution in blood. Plasma : whole blood ratio, triamterene 0.97, *p*-hydroxytriamterene sulfate, 1.7.

Protein binding. In plasma, triamterene about 45 to 70%, *p*-hydroxytriamterene sulfate about 90%.

Dose. 150 to 250 mg daily; reduced to alternate days after 1 week.

Triazolam

Hypnotic

Synonyms. Clorazolam; U-33030.
Proprietary names. Apo-Triazo; Halcion; Hypam; Rilamir; Somese; Songar; Trilam; Trycam.
8-Chloro-6-(2-chlorophenyl)-1-methyl-4*H*-[1,2,4]-triazolo[4,3-*a*]-[1,4]-benzodiazepine
$C_{17}H_{12}Cl_2N_4$=343.2
CAS—28911-01-5

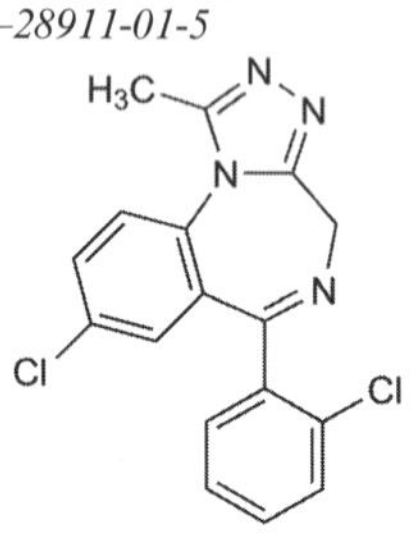

A white or pale yellow crystalline powder. M.p. 233° to 235°.
Practically insoluble in water and ether; soluble 1 in 1000 of alcohol; 1 in 25 chloroform; 1 in 600 0.1 M hydrochloric acid.

Partition Coefficient. Log *P* (octanol/water), 2.42.

Thin-layer Chromatography. System TA—Rf 60; system TB—Rf 01; system TC—Rf 40; system TD—Rf 05; system TE—Rf 44; system TF—Rf 02; system TL—Rf 16; system TAD—Rf 41; system TAE—Rf 68; system TAF—Rf 65.

Gas Chromatography. System GA—triazolam RI 3080, M (α-OH-) RI 3000; system GB—triazolam RI 3219, M (α-OH-) not eluted, M (α-OH-)-TMS RI 3308.

Column: fused silica (15 m × 0.25 mm i.d., 0.25 µm film thickness). Column temperature: 200° for 1 min, to 235° at 35°/min, to 265° at 5°/min, held for 1 min. Carrier gas: helium with auxiliary gas of 5% argon in methane, flow rates 0.6 and 30 mL/min, respectively. IS: flunitrazepam. Detection: electron capture. Retention time: triazolam, 8.66 min; IS, 4.7 min [T. Edeki *et al.*, *J. Chromatogr.*, 1992, *577(1)*, 190–194].

High Performance Liquid Chromatography. System HI—*k* 4.38; system HK—*k* 1.83; system HX—RI 476; system HY—RI 390; system HZ–Retention time, 4.2 min; system HAA—Retention time, 17.4 min; system HAF—Retention time 13.7 min; system HAL—Retention time 6.6 min; system HAM—not detected; system HAX—Retention time 6.4 min; system HAY—Retention time 6.7 min; system HAZ—*k* 1.07; system HBH—*k* 5.18; system HBI—*k* 1.13.

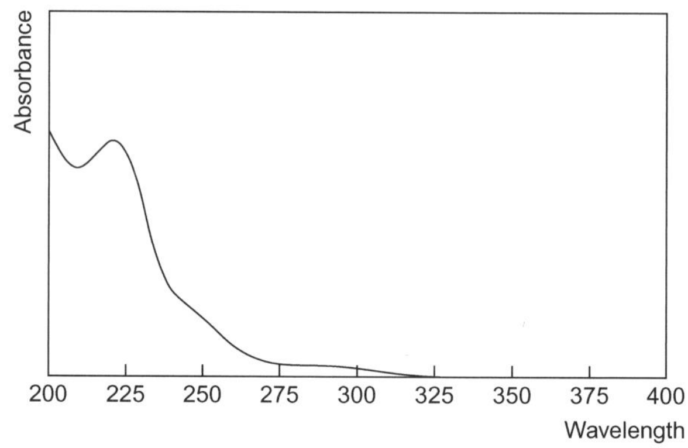

Infra-red Spectrum. Principal peaks at wavenumbers 761, 842, 1618, 1003, 1310, 827 cm^{-1} (KBr disk).

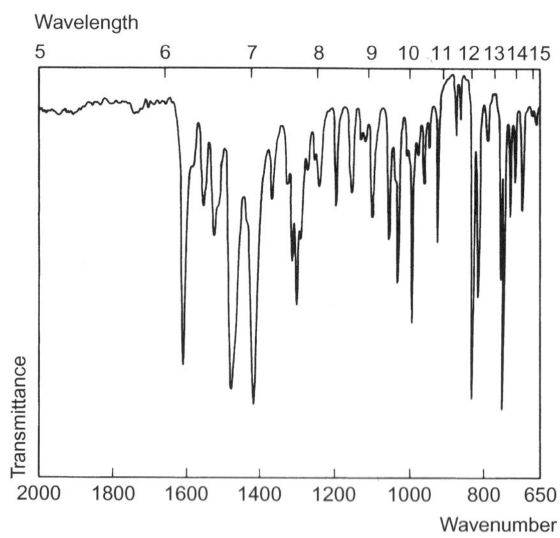

Mass Spectrum. Principal ions at *m/z* 313, 238, 342, 315, 75, 344, 239, 137.

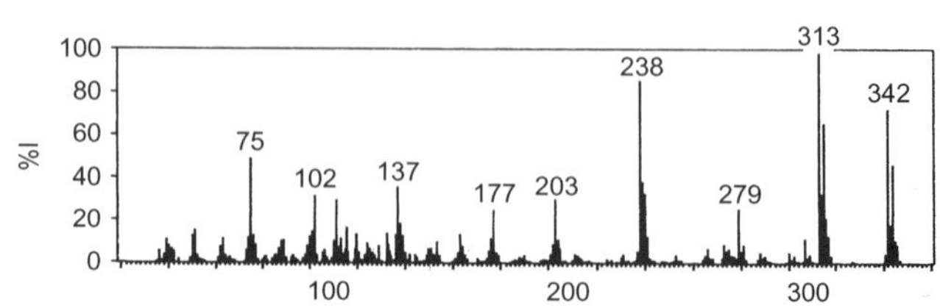

Quantification

Gas chromatography. In plasma: limit of detection 0.25 µg/L, ECD—D. J. Greenblatt *et al.*, *J. Chromatogr.*, 1981, *225*; *Biomed. Appl.*, *14*, 202–207. In plasma or urine: limit of detection 0.5 µg/L, ECD—P. Coassolo *et al.*, *J. Chromatogr.*, 1983, *274*; *Biomed. Appl.*, *25*, 161–170. In serum: limit of detection 0.5 µg/L, ECD—R. Nishioka, *J. Chromatogr.*, 1996, *681*; *Biomed. Appl.*, 401–404. In plasma: limit of detection 0.02 6 µg/L—T. Edeki *et al.*, *J. Chromatogr.*, 1992, *577*, 190–194. In tissue: limit of detection is 0.5 ng/g, NPD—K. Kudo *et al.*, *Int. J. Legal Med.*, 1991, *104(2)*, 67–69.

Gas chromatography–mass spectrometry. Limit of quantification is 2.5 to 5 µg/L (full scan) and 0.1 to 0.5 µg/L (SIMm/z 313)—D. Borrey *et al.*, *J. Chromatogr. A*, 2001, *910*, 105–118. In muscle: limit of detection is 0.5 ng/g—H. Inoue *et al.*, *J. Chromatogr. B Biomed. Sci. Appl.*, 1997, *701(1)*, 47–52.

High performance liquid chromatography. In serum: limit of detection 0.001 µg, UV detection—W. J. Adams *et al.*, *Anal. Lett.* (Part B), 1980, *13*, 149–161. In urine: limit of detection 5 µg/L, UV detection (λ = 220 nm)—T. Inoue and S. Suzuki, *J. Chromatogr.*, 1987, *422*, 197–204. In urine: limit of detection 10 µg/L, UV detection (λ = 220 nm)—M. T. Kinirons *et al.*, *Br. J. Clin. Pharmacol.*, 1996, *41(1)*, 69–72.

Disposition in the Body. Rapidly and almost completely absorbed after oral administration. It is metabolised mainly by hydroxylation. The major metabolite, 1-hydroxymethyltriazolam, has a hypnotic potency approximately equivalent to that of triazolam. Other metabolites include 4-hydroxytriazolam, 1-hydroxymethyl-4-hydroxytriazolam and three dichlorotriazolylbenzophenone derivatives. About 80% of a dose is excreted in the urine in 48 h mainly as the unconjugated metabolite (only a small amount as the unchanged drug) and about 7% is eliminated in the faeces in 72 h.

Therapeutic concentration

Following oral administration of 0.88 mg of ^{14}C-labelled triazolam to 6 subjects, peak plasma concentrations of 6 to 17 µg/L (mean 9) of triazolam were attained in 0.75 to 3 h; peak plasma concentrations of the glucuronide conjugates of the 1-hydroxymethyl and 4-hydroxy metabolites of 3 to 10 µg/L (mean 6) and 2 to 9 µg/L (mean 6) were attained in 0.75 to 2.5 h and 1.5 to 5 h, respectively [F. S. Eberts *et al.*, *Clin. Pharmacol. Ther.*, 1981, *29*, 81–93].

9 healthy children, 6 to 9 years old, were orally administered with 0.025 mg/kg triazolam before dental treatment; the total dose administered ranged from 0.5 to 0.9 mg (median dose 0.75 mg). The mean peak plasma concentration was 8.5 (range 4.7 to 13.7) µg/L, which was reached in 74 min (45 to 128 min) [H. W. Karl *et al.*, *J. Clin. Psychopharmacol.*, 1997, *17(3)*, 169–172].

Peak plasma triazolam concentrations of 4.9 ± 2.0 µg/L (mean ± s.d.) were attained in 75 min in 9 healthy children given 0.25 or 0.375 mg of sublingual triazolam before dental treatment [C. M. Tweedy *et al.*, *J. Clin. Psychopharmacol.*, 2001, *21*, 268–272].

6 male volunteers were administered with 0.125, 0.250 and 0.375 mg triazolam. The mean peak plasma concentrations observed were 2.2, 4.3 and 5.0 µg/L for the three doses and the times to reach these concentrations were 0.7, 0.6 and 0.8 h, respectively [T. Edeki *et al.*, *J. Chromatogr.*, 1992, *577(1)*, 190–194].

Toxicity. Manifestations of overdosage including somnolence, confusion, impaired co-ordination, slurred speech and even coma, may occur with doses of 2 mg (four times the recommended therapeutic dose). Seizures, respiratory depression and even death have also been reported.

A 77-year-old woman who was found dead in her bathtub (her head was above the water line and an empty bottle of triazolam was discovered in the bin), was revealed to have a heart-blood triazolam concentration of 120 µg/L; the cause of death was ruled to be triazolam intoxication and the manner of death was suicide [B. Levine *et al.*, *J. Anal. Toxicol.*, 2002, *26*, 52–54].

The lowest triazolam blood concentration that has been associated with death is 7 µg/L in whole blood. Ethanol at a concentration of 2300 mg/L was also detected in the blood of this individual [K. Uemura and S. Komura, *Am. J. Forensic Med. Pathol.*, 1995, *16(1)*, 66–68].

Of 6 fatal poisonings by triazolam alone or in combination with ethanol, in the 1 case where only triazolam was detected, the blood concentration was 110 µg/L. Because of putrefaction, blood was not available for analysis in the other case involving only triazolam. In the 4 cases also involving ethanol (blood concentration 1100 to 2020 mg/L), the triazolam concentration was 40 to 220 µg/L [A. Steentoft and K. Worm, *J. Forensic Sci. Soc.*, 1993, *33*, 45–48].

A 38-year-old drug addict who was being treated with methadone was found dead at home. At the scene were syringes containing a liquid later identified to be blood with traces of triazolam and a number of bottles containing Halcion (triazolam). Toxicological analysis of blood, bile, urine and stomach contents showed concentrations of triazolam (blood: 15 µg/L; urine: traces); morphine (blood: 0.12 mg/L; bile: total of 0.0037 mg: urine: traces) and codeine (blood: 0.30 µg/L; urine: traces). The blood drug concentrations were also found to be at therapeutic concentrations only. The cause of death was determined as being due to combined adverse effects of triazolam and morphine. This is the first case where triazolam was injected rather that taken orally [Kammie Hon *et al.*, *TIAFT Bulletin Case Notes* (http://www.tiaft.org/, 1988, *20(1)*].

Half-life. Plasma half-life, triazolam 1.5 to 3 h, 1-hydroxymethyltriazolam about 4 h.

Volume of distribution. About 1 to 2 L/kg, also quoted as 65 L (mean).

Clearance. Plasma clearance, about 10 mL/min/kg, also quoted as 300 mL/min (mean).

Protein binding. In plasma, about 89%.

Note. For a review of the pharmacokinetics of triazolam see C. J. Klett, *J. Clin. Psychiatry*, 1992, *53*, S61–S67; P.D. Garzone and P.D. Kroboth, *Clin. Pharmacokinet.*, 1989, *16*, 337–364; G. E. Pakes *et al.*, *Drugs*, 1981, *22*, 81–110.

Dose. 125 to 250 µg, as a hypnotic.

Triazophos

Acaricide, Insecticide

Synonyms. HOE 2960; HOE 2960 OJ; Triazofos.
Proprietary name. Hostathion
Phosphorothioic acid *O*,*O*-diethyl-*O*-(1-phenyl-1*H*-1,2,4-triazol-3-yl)-ester
$C_{12}H_{16}N_3O_3PS = 313.3$
CAS—24017-47-8

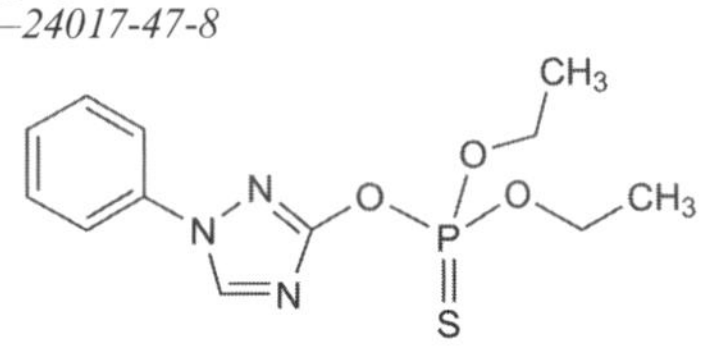

A yellowish to light brown oil. M.p. 2° to 5° (technical); 0.5° (pure). It is soluble in water (39 mg/L at 20°), *n*-hexane (0.7 g/100 mL at 25°), toluene (30 g/100 mL at 25°), ethyl acetate (30 g/100 mL at 25°), acetone (30 g/100 mL at 25°) and ethanol (30 g/100 mL at 25°).

Partition Coefficient. Log *P* (octanol/water), 3.34.

Thin-layer Chromatography. System TX—Rf 21; system TY—Rf 38.

Gas Chromatography. System GA—RI 2258.

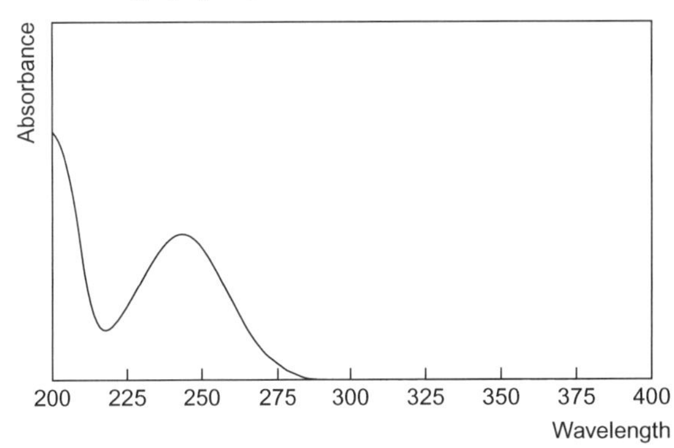

Mass Spectrum. Principal ions at *m/z* 161, 162, 172, 257, 285, 77, 208, 177.

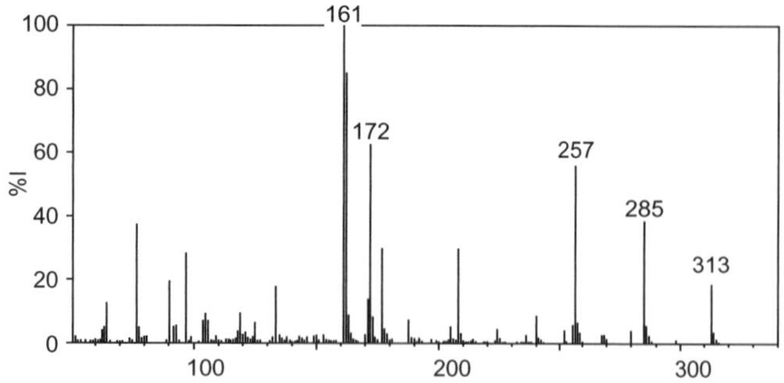

Disposition in the Body. Triazophos is absorbed through the skin, respiratory tract and the gastro-intestinal tract. It acts on the central nervous system.

Toxicity. The allowed daily intake is 0.001 mg/kg bodyweight and the highest dose to show no toxic effect is 0.0125 mg/kg.

Tributyl Phosphate

Plasticiser

Synonyms. BP; Tributhylphosphate; Tributoxyphosphine Oxide.
Proprietary names. Celluphos 4; Disflammol TB.
Tributyl phosphate
$C_{12}H_{27}O_4P = 266.3$
CAS—126-73-8

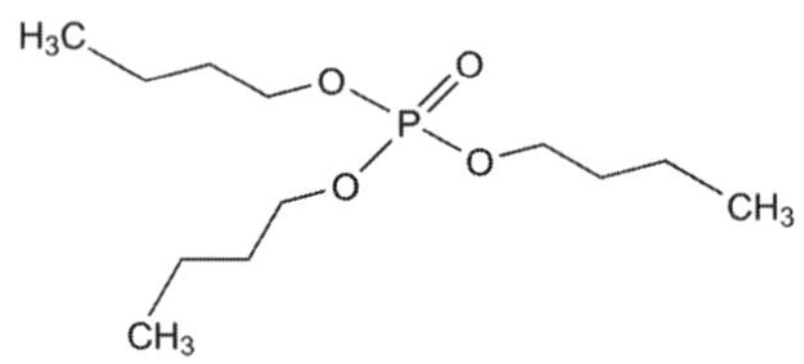

A colourless to pale yellow liquid with M.p. −79° to −80° and B.p. 289°. It is slightly soluble in water (<1 mg/L at 20.5°); soluble in DMSO, 95% ethanol and acetone (⩾100 g/L at 20.5°), ether and benzene.

Partition Coefficient. Log *P* (octanol/water), 4.00.

Gas Chromatography. System GA—RI 1690.

Infra-red Spectrum. Principal peaks at wavenumbers 1031, 1293, 907 cm^{-1}.

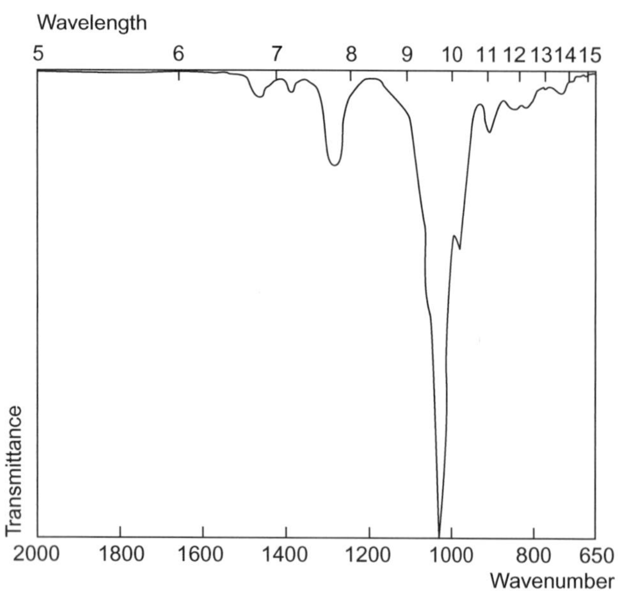

Mass Spectrum. Principal ions at *m/z* 99, 156, 41, 29, 57, 211, 125, 137.

Disposition in the Body. Tributyl phosphate is absorbed through skin and after ingestion. During metabolism, oxidation and dealkylation occur to produce dibutylhydrogen phosphate, butyldihydrogen phosphate and butyl-bis(3-hydroxybutyl)phosphate. Excretion occurs mainly within the first 48 h in urine mostly but also in faeces and via exhalation.

Toxicity. Tributyl phosphate is highly toxic via intravenous and intraperitoneal routes and moderately toxic via oral administration.

Trichlorfon

Insecticide, Anthelmintic

Synonyms. BayerL13/59; Chlorofos; DEP; DETF; Dipherex; Foschlor; Metrifonate; Metrifonatum; Metriphonate; TCF; Trichlorofon; Trichlorphon.
Proprietary names. Anthon; Bilarcil; Bovinox; Briten; Chlorofos; Chlorophos; Ciclosom; Combot; Dipterex; Ditrifon; Dylox; Dyrex; Leivasom; Neguvon; Proxol; Trinex; Vermicide Masoten Promem.
O,*O*-Dimethyl-2,2,2-trichloro-1-hydroxyethylphosphonate
$C_4H_8Cl_3O_4P = 257.4$
CAS—52-68-6

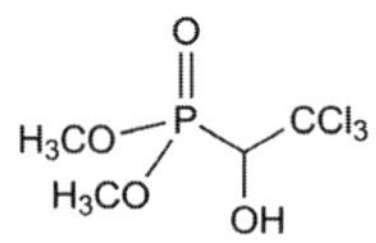

A white crystalline powder. M.p. between 75° and 84°. It is very soluble in water (15.4 g/100 mL at 20°); soluble in dichloromethane, 2-propanol, diethyl ether (17 g/100 mL at 20°), alcohol, acetone, chloroform (75 g/100 mL at 20°), benzene (15.2 g/100 mL at 20°) and toluene; very slightly soluble in *n*-hexane (0.08 g/100 mL at 20°) and pentane.

Partition Coefficient. Log *P* (octanol/water), 0.52.

Thin-layer Chromatography. System TE—Rf 61; system TX—Rf 07; system TY—Rf 02; system TZ—Rf 15; system TAA—Rf 05; system TAB—Rf 02; system TAC—Rf 01; system TAE—Rf 90.

Gas Chromatography. System GA—trichlorfon RI 1438; trichlorfon-Me RI 1395; system GK—RRT 0.27 (relative to caffeine).

High Performance Liquid Chromatography. System HY—RI 738.

Infra-red Spectrum. Principal peaks at wavenumbers 1109, 1154, 854, 978, 1323 cm^{-1}.

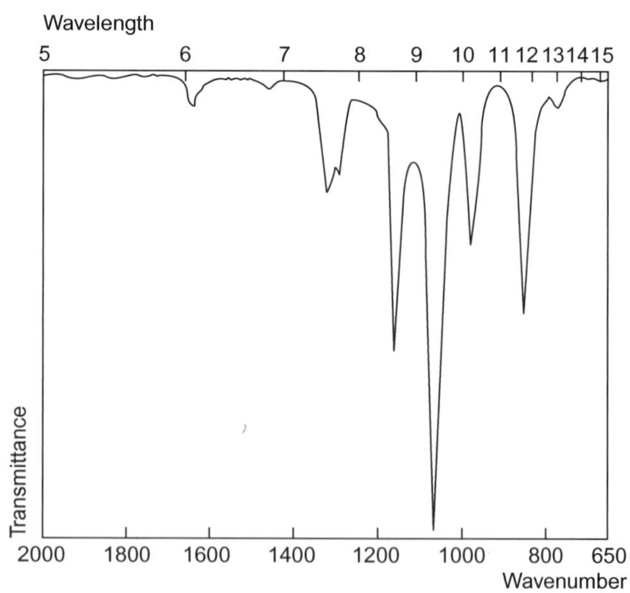

Mass Spectrum. Principal ions at *m/z* 109, 79, 110, 145, 139, 47, 15, 112.

Quantification

Gas chromatography. In blood and urine: limit of quantification trichlorfon 0.01 mg/L, ECD—R. Heinig *et al.*, *J. Chromatogr. Biomed. Sci. Appl.*, 2000, *741(2)*, 257–269. In serum: limit of detection 2.5 µg/L, FTD—K. Ameno *et al.*, *J. Anal. Toxicol.*, 1989, *13*, 150–151.

Gas chromatography–mass spectrometry. In serum: limit of detection of the metabolite, dimethylphosphate (DMP) 0.06 mg/L—F. A. Tarbah *et al.*, *TIAFT Poster Session 4*, 1998. In blood and urine: limit of quantification of the metabolite dichlorvos (DDVP) 0.001 mg/L—R. Heinig *et al.*, *J. Chromatogr. Biomed. Sci. Appl.*, 2000, *741(2)*, 257–269.

High performance liquid chromatography. In plasma: limit of quantification for trichlorfos and the metabolite DDVP 1 mg/L and 0.04 mg/L, respectively—L. K. Unni *et al.*, *J. Chromatogr.*, 1992, *573(1)*, 99–103.

Disposition in the Body. Trichlorfon is rapidly absorbed after oral administration and some of the dose is converted to dichlorvos (DDVP) which is the active moiety. Another metabolite observed is dimethylphosphate (DMP) as well as dimethylphosphoric acid, phosphoric acid, desmethyldichlorvos and monomethylphosphoric acid. It is excreted via the kidneys mainly as glucuronides. Approximately 70% of a dose is recovered in urine and also a small amount in faeces. Trichlorfon is readily absorbed through the skin and absorption, distribution and excretion are quick. It is distributed to the main organs with the highest concentrations observed in the liver, kidney and lungs.

Blood concentration

6 healthy male volunteers were administered with a single oral dose of 7.5 mg/kg trichlorfon. Trichlorfon was quickly absorbed and peak plasma concentrations were observed 0.7 to 1 h after administration at levels of 50.5 µmol/L. DDVP concentrations were approx. 1% of that for trichlorfon. [Y. A. Abdi and T. Villen, *Pharmacol. Toxicol.*, 1991, *68(2)*, 137–139.]

Toxicity. Moderately toxic by ingestion and dermal absorption. The allowed daily intake is 0.01 mg/kg.

A 76-year-old man committed suicide by ingesting 50 mL of Dipterex and died after 8 h. An autopsy revealed that his trichlorfon blood concentration was 215 µg/g and his gastric lavage liquid sample contained 15 mg/g of the pesticide. These samples were taken 1 h after admission [M. Yashiki *et al.*, *Nippon Hoigaku Zasshi*, 1988, *42*, 94–98].

A 70-year-old woman died from acute trichlorfon poisoning after ingesting 50% emulsifiable concentrate. Postmortem toxicology showed a blood concentration of 310 µg/g, liver 487 µg/g, brain 465 µg/g, kidney 416 µg/g, urine 2240 µg/g and a total of 7.2 g in her stomach contents [M. Yashiki *et al.*, *Nippon Hoigaku Zasshi*, 1982, *36*, 426–430].

Half-life. The mean half-life is 2.07 h for healthy volunteers.

Clearance. The mean clearance, for healthy males, is 0.34 L/h/kg.

Dose. (As an anthelmintic agent), 7.5 to 10 mg/kg bodyweight every two weeks for three doses.

Trichlormethiazide

Diuretic

Synonym. Hydrotrichlorothiazide
Proprietary names. Diurese; Metahydrin; Naqua. It is an ingredient of Esmalorid, Metatensin and Rulun.
6-Chloro-3-(dichloromethyl)-3,4-dihydro-2*H*-1,2,4-benzothiadiazine-7-sulfonamide 1,1-dioxide
$C_8H_8Cl_3N_3O_4S_2$=380.7
CAS—133-67-5

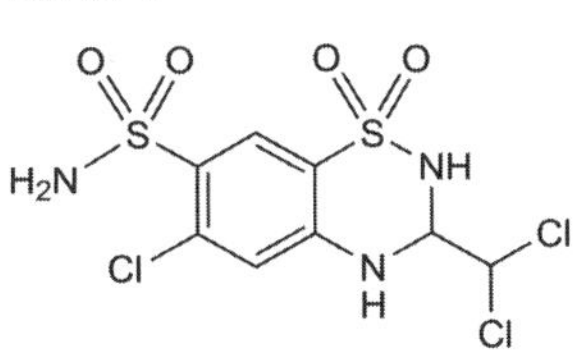

A white crystalline powder. M.p. about 270°, with decomposition.
Very slightly soluble in water, chloroform, and ether; soluble 1 in 48 of ethanol, 1 in 17 of methanol, 1 in about 9 of dioxan, and 1 in about 4 of dimethylformamide; freely soluble in acetone.

Dissociation Constant. pK_a 8.6.

Partition Coefficient. Log *P* (octanol/water) 0.6.

Colour Test. Sulfuric Acid—yellow.

Thin-layer Chromatography. System TA—Rf 80; system TD—Rf 15; system TE—Rf 14; system TF—Rf 60; system TAD—Rf 23; system TAE—Rf 88; system TAJ—Rf 24; system TAK—Rf 05; system TAL—Rf 61. (Acidified potassium permanganate solution, positive.)

Gas Chromatography. System GA—RI 2810; system GX—Retention time 10.7 min (Both for trichlormethiazide-ME_4).

High Performance Liquid Chromatography. System HN—*k* 3.10; system HY—RI 341; system HAA—Retention time 14.9 min.

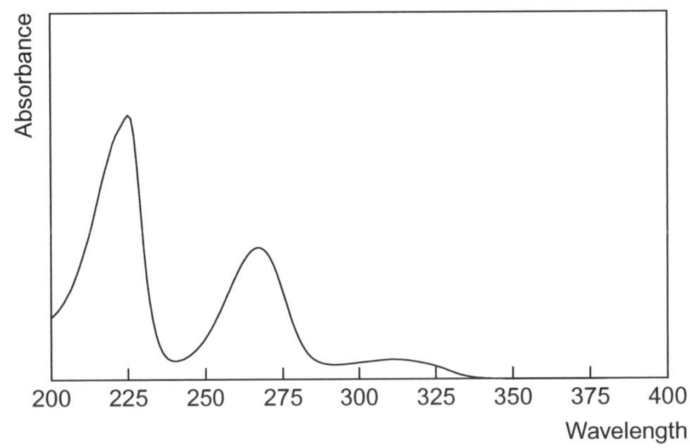

Infra-red Spectrum. Principal peaks at wavenumbers 1158, 1177, 1597, 772, 1073, 1509 cm^{-1} (KBr disk).

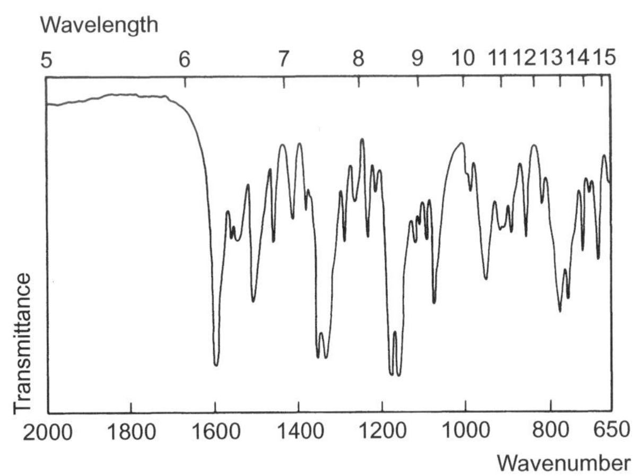

Mass Spectrum. Principal ions at *m/z* 296, 298, 279, 205, 36, 64, 117, 62.

Quantification

High performance liquid chromatography. In plasma or urine: limit of detection 10 µg/L for plasma, UV detection—M. C. Meyer and P. T. R. Hwang, *J. Chromatogr.*, 1981, *223*; *Biomed. Appl.*, *12*, 466–472.

Disposition in the Body. Readily absorbed after oral administration. About 70% of a dose is excreted in the urine unchanged in 48 h, mostly in the first 8 h.

Therapeutic concentration

Following a single oral dose of 4 mg to 7 subjects, peak plasma concentrations of 0.027 to 0.067 mg/L (mean 0.04) were attained in 1 to 3.5 h (mean 2) [I. S. Sketris *et al.*, *Eur. J. Clin. Pharmacol.*, 1981, *20*, 453–457].

Half-life. Plasma half-life, about 1 to 4 h (mean 2), increased in renal impairment.

Dose. Usually 2 to 4 mg daily; initial doses of 4 to 8 mg daily may be given.

Trichloroethane

Solvent

Synonyms. Chlorothene; Methylchloroform; α-Trichloroethane.
Proprietary name. Zoff
1,1,1-Trichloroethane
CCl_3CH_3=133.4
CAS—71-55-6

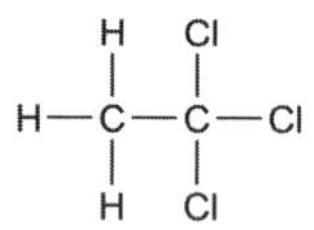

A colourless non-flammable liquid. M.p. −32.5°. B.p. 74°.
Practically insoluble in water; miscible with ethanol, methanol, acetone, benzene, ether and chloroform.

Partition Coefficient. Log *P* (octanol/water) 2.5.

Colour Test. Fujiwara Test—red.

Gas Chromatography. System GA—RI 634; system GI—Retention time 8.2 min.

Mass Spectrum. Principal ions at *m/z* 97, 99, 61, 117, 119, 63, 101, 62.

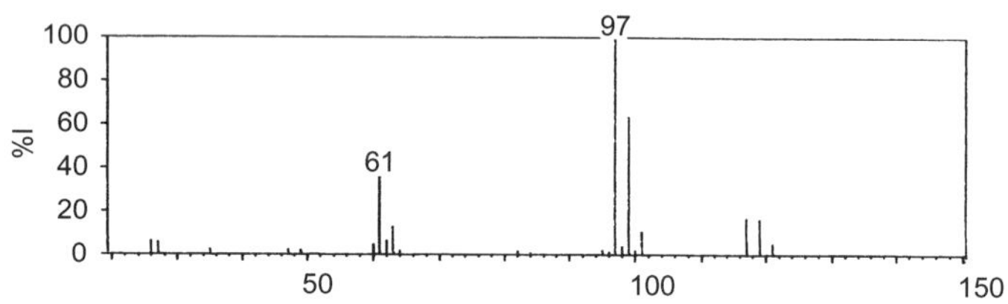

Quantification

Gas chromatography. In blood, bile or tissues: using headspace analysis and FID—Y. H. Caplan *et al.*, *Clin. Toxicol.*, 1976, *9*, 69–74. In urine: using FID—S. Ghittori *et al.*, *G. Ital. Med. Lav.*, 1987, *9*, 21–24.

Gas chromatography–mass spectrometry. In breath: sensitivity in ppb range—K.W. Thomas *et al.*, *J. Anal. Toxicol.*, 1991, *15*, 54–59.

Disposition in the Body. Rapidly absorbed from the gastro-intestinal tract and the lungs; poorly absorbed through the skin. It is metabolised by oxidation and conjugation; only a small proportion of an absorbed dose is excreted in the urine as trichloroethanol glucuronide (urochloralic acid) and trichloroacetic acid. About 60 to 80% of a dose is excreted unchanged in expired air in one week.

Toxicity. The estimated minimum lethal dose by ingestion or inhalation is 5 mL and the maximum permissible atmospheric concentration is 350 ppm. Exposure to air concentrations of more than 5000 ppm may cause unconsciousness within a short time. Fatalities have been associated with blood concentrations greater than 15 mg/L.

The following postmortem tissue concentrations were reported in a fatality involving the accidental inhalation of trichloroethane: blood 18 mg/L, brain 80 μg/g, liver 80 μg/g, lungs 31 μg/g, urine 0.9 mg/L [A. Franc, *Bull. Int. Assoc. Forensic Toxicol.*, 1983, *17*(2), 22–25].

A postmortem blood tetrachloroethane concentration of 1.7 mg/L was found following fatal cerebral oedema in a 15-year-old boy who had been sniffing typewriter correction fluid [D. F. D'Costa and N. P. R. Gunasekera, *J. R. Soc. Med.*, 1990, *83*, 533–534].

There was a broad correlation between blood tetrachloroethane concentration and severity of poisoning in 48 patients referred to a poisons unit (plus data from 18 other deaths); concentrations ranged from 0.1 to 60 mg/L [T. J. Meredith *et al.*, *Hum. Toxicol.*, 1989, *8*, 277–286].

Half-life. Blood half-life, about 10 to 12 h.

Trichloroethanol

Hypnotic

Synonym. 2,2,2-Trichloroethyl Alcohol
2,2,2-Trichloroethanol
CCl_3CH_2OH=149.4
CAS—115-20-8

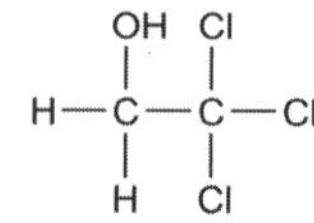

A hygroscopic liquid or crystals. M.p. 18°. B.p. 151° to 153°.
Soluble 1 in about 12 of water; miscible with ethanol and ether.

Dissociation Constant. pK_a 12.2 (25°).

Partition Coefficient. Log *P* (octanol/water) 1.4.

Colour Test. Fujiwara Test—yellow.

Gas Chromatography. System GA—RI 857; system GI—Retention time 25.5 min.

Mass Spectrum. Principal ions at *m/z* 31, 49, 77, 113, 115, 82, 51, 117.

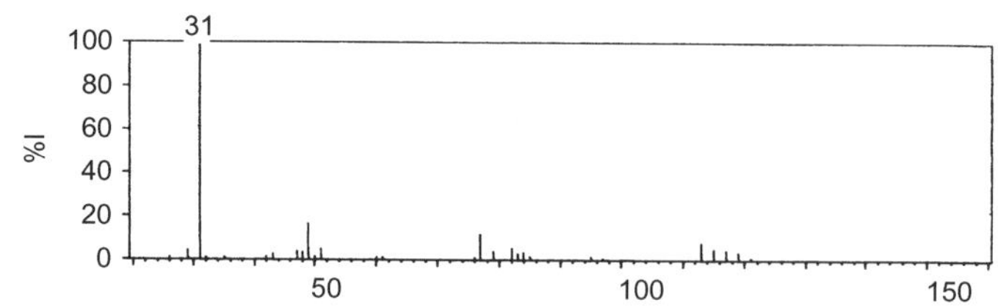

Quantification. See under Cloral Hydrate.

Disposition in the Body. Trichloroethanol is a metabolite of cloral hydrate, trichloroethane, trichloroethylene and triclofos; it has hypnotic activity. It is further metabolised by conjugation with glucuronic acid to form urochloralic acid and by oxidation to trichloroacetic acid.

Toxicity. See under Cloral Hydrate.

Half-life. Plasma half-life, about 8 h.

Volume of distribution. About 0.6 L/kg.

Distribution in blood. Plasma:whole blood ratio, about 0.9.

Protein binding. In plasma, about 35%.

Trichloroethylene

General Anaesthetic/Solvent

Synonyms. Trichlorethylene; Trichloroethene.
Proprietary name. Trilene.
$CHCl{:}CCl_2$=131.4
CAS—79-01-6

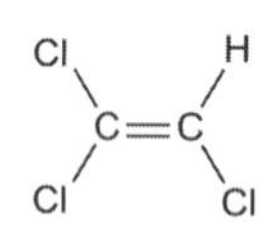

A clear, colourless or pale blue, mobile, non-flammable liquid. It decomposes in light in the presence of moisture with the formation of hydrochloric acid. Relative density 1.464 to 1.470. B.p. 87°.
Trichloroethylene (*B.P.*) contains thymol 0.01% w/w as a preservative and may contain not more than 0.001% w/w of a suitable blue colouring matter to distinguish it from chloroform.
Practically insoluble in water; miscible with dehydrated alcohol, chloroform and ether.

Partition Coefficient. Log *P* (octanol/water) 2.4.

Colour Test. Fujiwara Test—red.

Gas Chromatography. System GA—RI 710; system GI—Retention time 14.8 min.

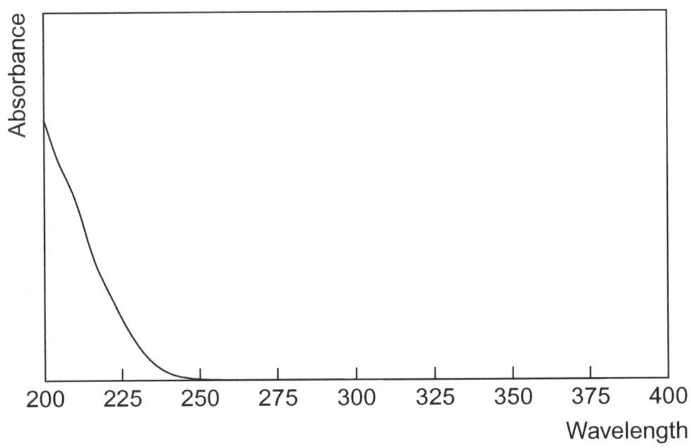

Mass Spectrum. Principal ions at *m/z* 95, 130, 132, 60, 97, 35, 134, 47; trichloroacetic acid 44, 83, 85, 36, 28, –, –, –.

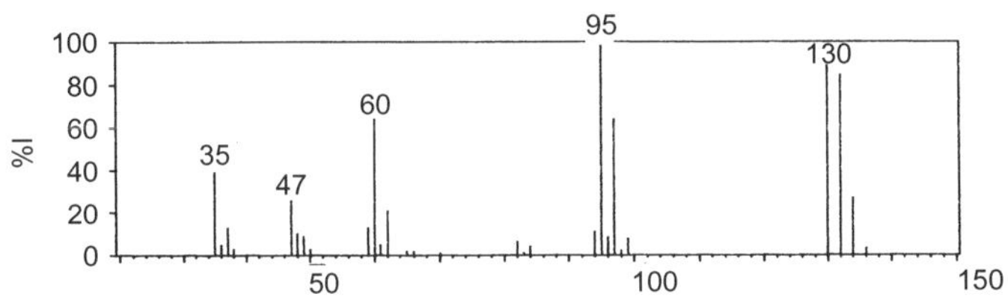

Quantification

Gas chromatography. In blood: using headspace analysis, FID—F. N. Prior, *Anaesthesia*, 1972, *27*, 379–389. In blood or urine: trichloroethanol and trichloroacetic acid, using headspace analysis, limit of detection 500 µg/L for trichloroethanol, ECD—D. D. Breimer *et al.*, *J. Chromatogr.*, 1974, *88*, 55–63. In urine: trichloroethanol and trichloroacetic acid, using headspace analysis, limit of detection 5 µg/L for trichloroethanol—A. Ohara *et al.*, *Sangyo Igaku*, 1991, *33*, 94–103.

Gas chromatography–mass spectrometry. In urine: trichloroethylene, using headspace analysis—M. Imbriani *et al.*, *Ind. Health*, 2001, *39*, 225–230.

High performance liquid chromatography. In urine: trichloroacetic acid, limit of detection 0.5 µg—M. Ogata and Y. Yamazaki, *Acta Med. Okayama*, 1979, *33*, 479–81.

Disposition in the Body. Rapidly absorbed from the lungs; about 50 to 65% of an inhaled dose is retained. Absorbed from the gastro-intestinal tract and through the skin. It is highly soluble in lipid-rich tissues, from which it is slowly released. Cloral hydrate is a transient metabolite which is further metabolised by reduction to trichloroethanol and oxidation to trichloroacetic acid. Trichloroethanol is mainly excreted as its glucuronide conjugate (urochloralic acid). Monochloroacetic acid is a minor metabolite. About 45% of an absorbed dose is excreted as urochloralic acid and about 30% as trichloroacetic acid in the urine in 3 weeks; small amounts are eliminated in the faeces. About 16% is excreted unchanged in expired air.

Therapeutic concentration. In blood, for anaesthesia, usually in the range 26 to 82 mg/L.

During anaesthesia, exposure to an induction level of 1% of trichloroethylene for 30 min to 20 patients, produced blood concentrations of 34 to 90 mg/L (mean 65) [F. N. Prior, *Anaesthesia*, 1972, *27*, 379–389].

Toxicity. The estimated minimum lethal dose by ingestion or inhalation is 5 mL and the maximum permissible atmospheric concentration is 100 ppm.

A man of 56 years was found dead after exposure to trichloroethylene fumes. The following postmortem concentrations of trichloroethylene were reported: blood about 90 mg/L, brain about 270 µg/g, lung about 40 µg/g [A. Alha *et al.*, *Bull. Int. Assoc. Forensic Toxicol.*, 1974, *10*(1), 14–15].

In 19 cases of fatal trichloroethylene poisoning, the following postmortem concentrations were reported: blood 1 to 41 mg/mL (mean 14, 15 cases), brain 4 to 74 µg/g (mean 31, 5 cases), kidney 4 to 140 µg/g (mean 30, 8 cases), liver 1 to 250 µg/g (mean 64, 9 cases), lung 1 to 15 µg/g (mean 7, 6 cases), urine a trace to 91 mg/L (mean 35, 5 cases) [R. Bonnichen and A. C. Maehly, *J. Forensic Sci.*, 1966, *11*, 414–427].

A 17-year-old male ingested about 70 mL of trichloroethylene in a suicide attempt. The highest blood concentration of trichloroethylene (4.05 mg/L) was reached at 13 h after ingestion [T. Brüning *et al.*, *Toxicol. Sci.* 1998, *41*, 157–165].

Half-life. About 30 to 38 h.

Dose. To produce light anaesthesia, 0.5 to 2% of the vapour by inhalation.

Trichlorofluoromethane

Aerosol Propellent/Refrigerant

Synonyms. Fluorocarbon 11; Fluorotrichloromethane; Propellent 11; Refrigerant 11; Trichloromonofluoromethane.
Proprietary name. It was formerly an ingredient of PR Spray.
$CCl_3F = 137.4$
CAS—75-69-4

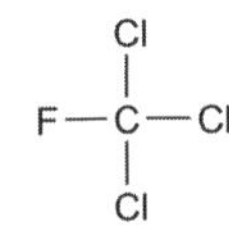

A clear, colourless, non-flammable volatile liquid. B.p. about 24°.
In the liquid state it is practically immiscible with water but miscible with dehydrated alcohol, ether and other organic solvents.

Partition Coefficient. Log *P* (octanol/water) 2.5.

Gas Chromatography. System GA—RI 484; system GI—Retention time 3.0 min.

Mass Spectrum. Principal ions at *m/z* 101, 103, 105, 66, 47, 35, 31, 82.

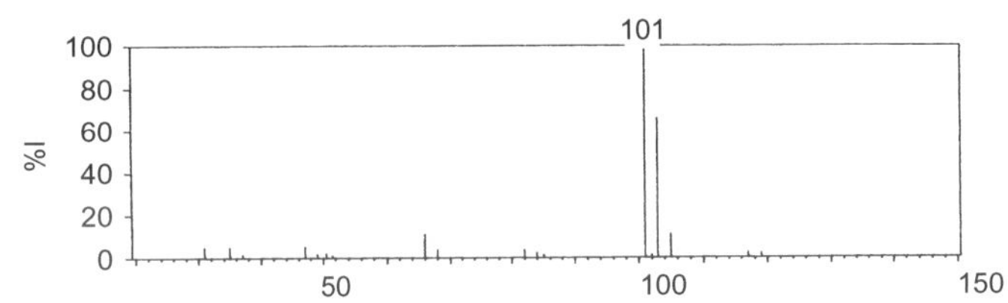

Toxicity

A 33-year-old man, working in an expanded polyurethane factory where trichlorofluoromethane was used as a foaming agent, was found dead on the floor in a 4 m² room. Postmortem examination revealed the following concentrations: blood, 62.8 mg/L; brain 108.9 mg/kg; lung, 149.1 mg/kg; liver 74.1 mg/kg and less than 0.1 mg/L in urine [A. Groppi *et al.*, *J. Forensic Sci.*, 1994, *39*, 871–876].

Trichlorophenoxyacetic Acid

Herbicide

Synonym. 2,4,5-T
Proprietary names. Boots Nettle Killer; Marks Brushwood Killer; Phortox; Silvapron T; Trioxone 50. It is an ingredient of Econal, Nettle Ban, Spontox and Stancide BWK 75.
(2,4,5-Trichlorophenoxy)acetic acid
$C_8H_5Cl_3O_3 = 255.5$
CAS—93-76-5; 35915-18-5

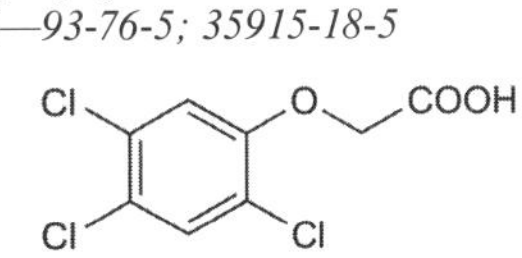

A white crystalline solid. M.p. 153°.
Very slightly soluble in water; soluble in ethanol, acetone and ether.

Dissociation Constant. pK_a 2.8 (25°).

Partition Coefficient. Log *P* (octanol/water), 3.3.

Colour Test. Liebermann's Test—pink(→brown).

Thin-layer Chromatography. System TAB—Rf 04; system TAC—Rf 02.

Gas Chromatography. System GA—2,4,5-T RI 1850, 2,4,5-T-methyl ester RI 1750, 2,4,5-T-isobutyl ester RI 2280, 2,4,5-T-isopropyl ester RI 1825, 2,4,5-T-isooctil ester RI 2320, M (trichlorophenol) RI 1440; system GK—2,4,5-T-methyl ester RRT 0.80; 2,4,5-T-isooctil ester 1.24 and 1.31 (both relative to caffeine).

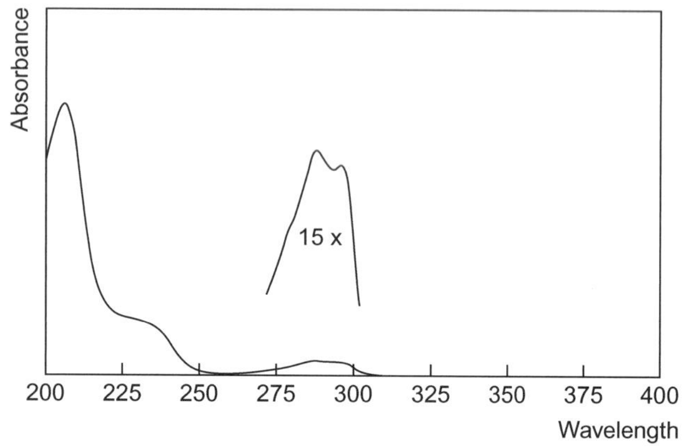

Mass Spectrum. Principal ions at m/z 233, 45, 42, 59, 179, 146, 109, 235 (methyl ester); 43, 57, 41, 55, 71, 69, 56, 70 (isooctil ester).

Triclocarban

Disinfectant/Antiseptic

Synonyms. TCC; 3,4,4′-Trichlorocarbanilide.
Proprietary names. Citrosil Sapone; Cuticura; Cutisan; Derso TCC; Nobacter; Solubacter; Valderma.
N-(4-Chlorophenyl)-*N*′-(3,4-dichlorophenyl)urea
$C_{13}H_9Cl_3N_2O$=315.6
CAS—101-20-2

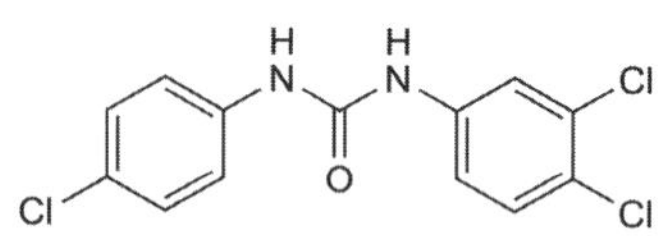

Fine white plates. M.p. 255° to 256°.
Practically insoluble in water; soluble 1 in 25 of acetone and 1 in 100 of propylene glycol.

Partition Coefficient. Log *P* (octanol/water), 4.9.

Thin-layer Chromatography. System TD—Rf 60; system TE—Rf 75; system TF—Rf 59; system TAD—Rf 63.

Ultraviolet Spectrum. Ethanol—265 nm (A^1_1=1391 b).

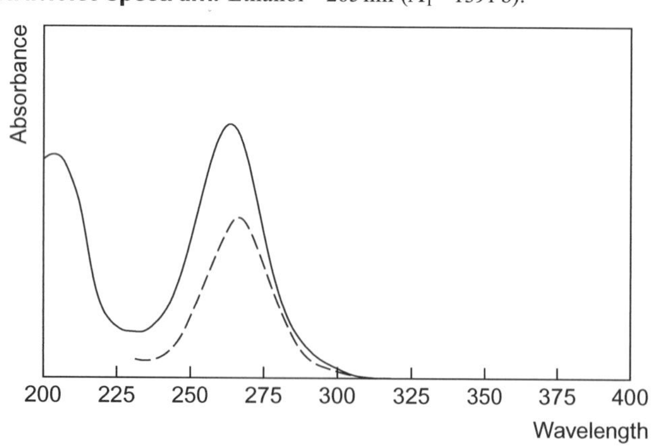

Infra-red Spectrum. Principal peaks at wavenumbers 1634, 1587, 1550, 820, 1089, 1232 cm^{-1}(KBr disk).

Mass Spectrum. Principal ions at m/z 127, 161, 163, 153, 129, 187, 90, 189.

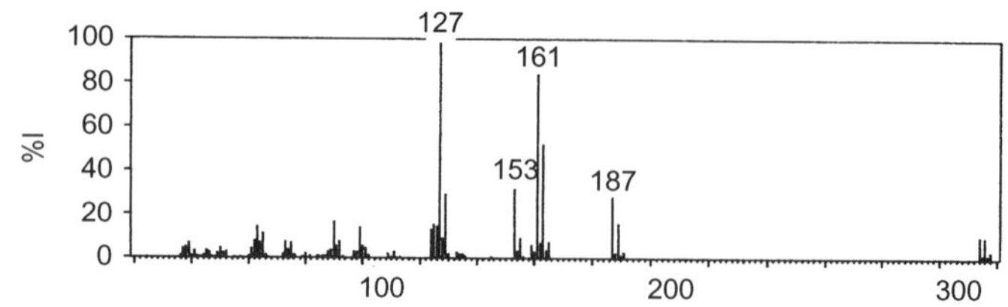

Quantification

Gas chromatography. In blood: limit of detection 12.5 ng/mL, ECD—D. R. Hoar and M. H. Bowen, *J. Pharm. Sci.*, 1977, *66*, 725–726.

Gas chromatography–mass spectrometry. In plasma or urine: limit of detection for 2′-hydroxy sulfate metabolite in plasma, 1.5 ng/mL and for *N*-glucuronide in urine, 3 ng/mL—L.D. Gruenke *et al.*, *J. Anal. Toxicol.*, 1997, *11*, 75–80.

Use. In concentrations of 1 to 2%.

Triclofos Sodium

Sedative/Hypnotic

Proprietary names. Triclonam; Tricloryl; Triclos.
Sodium 2,2,2-trichloroethanol hydrogen phosphate
$C_2H_3Cl_3NaO_4P$=251.4
CAS—306-52-5 (triclofos); *7246-20-0* (sodium salt)

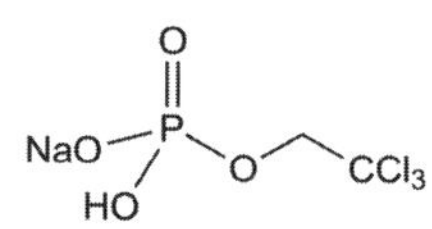

A white hygroscopic powder.
Soluble 1 in 2 of water and 1 in 250 of ethanol; practically insoluble in ether.

Partition Coefficient. Log *P* (octanol/water), 1.1.

Colour Test. Phosphorus Test—yellow precipitate.

Gas Chromatography. System GB—RI 1952.

Infra-red Spectrum. Principal peaks at wavenumbers 1107, 1227, 926, 1124, 709, 876 cm^{-1}(triclofos sodium, Nujol mull).

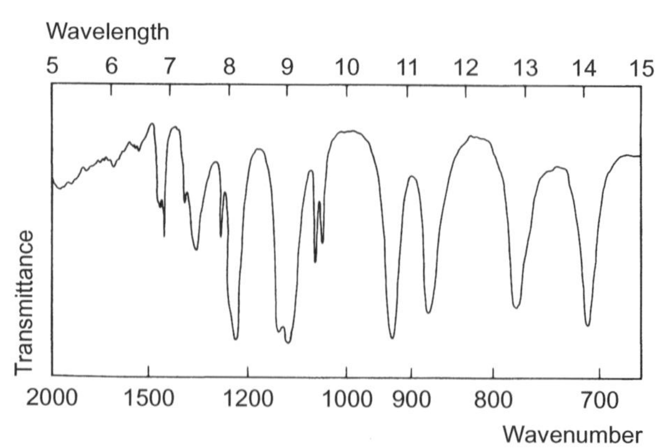

Mass Spectrum. Principal ions at m/z 31, 49, 77, 29, 113, 51, 48, 115, no peaks above 120 (triclofos); trichloroacetic acid 44, 83, 85, 36, 28, -, -, -; trichloroethanol 31, 49, 77, 113, 115, 82, 51, 117.

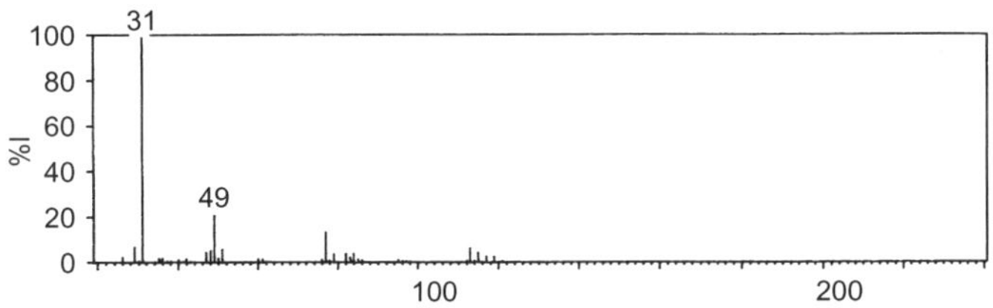

Quantification Determination of trichloroethanol – see under Cloral Hydrate.

Disposition in the Body. Rapidly hydrolysed in the stomach to trichloroethanol which is readily absorbed. Trichloroethanol, the active metabolite, is conjugated with glucuronic acid to give urochloralic acid, and oxidised to trichloroacetic acid. About 12% of a dose is excreted in the urine in 24 h as metabolites.

Therapeutic concentration. In plasma, trichloroethanol, usually in the range 1.5 to 15 mg/L.

After an oral dose of 22 mg/kg given to 7 subjects, peak plasma concentrations of trichloroethanol and urochloralic acid of about 8 mg/L and 2 mg/L, respectively, were reported; no unchanged triclofos was detectable in plasma [E. M. Sellers *et al.*, *Clin. Pharmacol. Ther.*, 1973, *14*, 147].

Toxicity. Plasma concentrations greater than 40 mg/L of trichloroethanol are likely to produce toxic effects, and concentrations greater than 100 mg/L may be fatal.

The following postmortem tissue concentrations of trichloroethanol were reported in a fatality due to triclofos ingestion: blood 335 μg/mL, bile 696 mg/L, brain 326 μg/g, kidney 928 μg/g, liver 690 μg/g, urine 195 mg/L; other drugs were also detected [D. J. Doedens and J. A. Benz, *Bull. Int. Assn. Forens Toxicol.*, 1976, *12*(2), 10–11].

Half-life. Plasma half-life, trichloroethanol about 8 h, urochloralic acid about 7 h, trichloroacetic acid about 4 days.

Volume of distribution. Trichloroethanol, about 0.6 L/kg.

Distribution in blood. Plasma: whole blood ratio, trichloroethanol about 0.9.

Protein binding. In plasma, trichloroethanol about 35% and trichloroacetic acid about 94%.

Dose. 1 to 2 g, as a hypnotic.

Triclosan

Disinfectant

Synonym. Cloxifenol
Proprietary names. Acneclear; Adasept; Aquasept; Bioband; Dermax; Dermo-Steril; Fisohex; Gamophen; Geroderm; Irgasan DP300; Novaderm; Procoutol; Proderm; Sapoderm; Septisol; Solyptol; Ster-Zac; Stri-Dex; Tersaseptic; Zalclense.
5-Chloro-2-(2,4-dichlorophenoxy)phenol
$C_{12}H_7Cl_3O_2$ = 289.5
CAS—3380-34-5

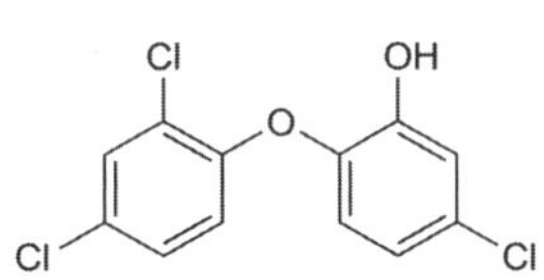

A white crystalline powder or soft agglomerates. M.p. 54° to 57°.
Practically insoluble in water; very soluble in most organic solvents.

Dissociation Constant. pK_a 7.9.

Partition Coefficient. Log *P* (octanol/water), 4.8.

Ultraviolet Spectrum. Ethanol—283 nm (A^1_1 = 179 b); alkaline ethanol—295 nm.

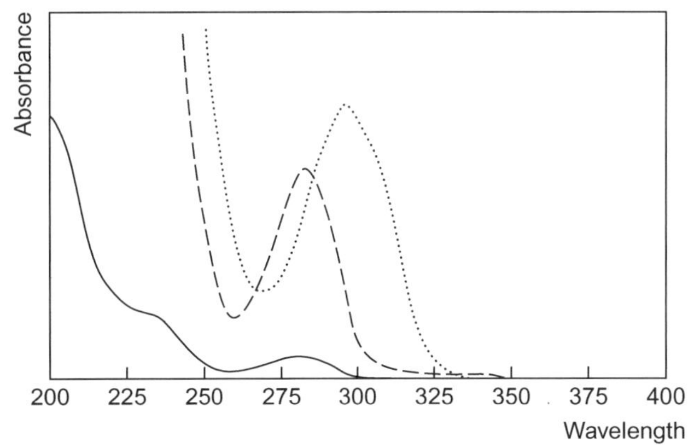

Mass Spectrum. Principal ions at *m/z* 288, 290, 218, 146, 114, 63, 51, 148.

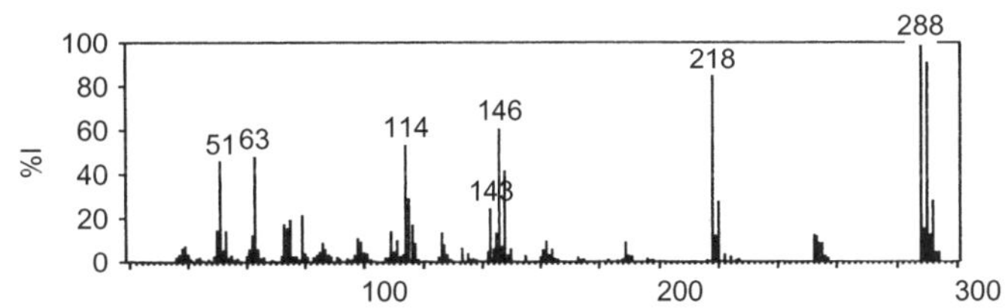

Quantification
Gas chromatography. In plasma or urine: limit of detection 2 μg/L, ECD—A. Sioufi *et al.*, *J. Pharm. Sci.*, 1977, *66*, 1166–1168.

Disposition in the Body.
Therapeutic concentration
In a single dose study, subjects brushed one time with 1.25 g dentifrice containing 0.3% triclosan (3.75 mg) and ingested all of the dentifrice. Blood samples were collected at multiple time points from pre-dose to 72 h post-dose. In a multiple dose study, the same subjects brushed 3 times daily as in the single dose study. After 12 days of 3 times daily toothbrushing and ingestion of the dental slurry, the mean triclosan plasma concentration was 352 μg/L in the steady state period. There was no significant difference between results obtained in the single dose study, suggesting a complete elimination of daily triclosan dose and no increase in the triclosan level during repeated brushing/ingestion. [D. M. Bagley and Y. J. Lin, *Am. J. Dent.*, 2000, *13*, 148–152].

Use. In concentrations of 0.05 to 2%.

Tricyclamol Chloride

Anticholinergic

1-(3-Cyclohexyl-3-hydroxy-3-phenylpropyl)-1-methylpyrrolidinium chloride
$C_{20}H_{32}ClNO$ = 337.9
CAS—3818-88-0

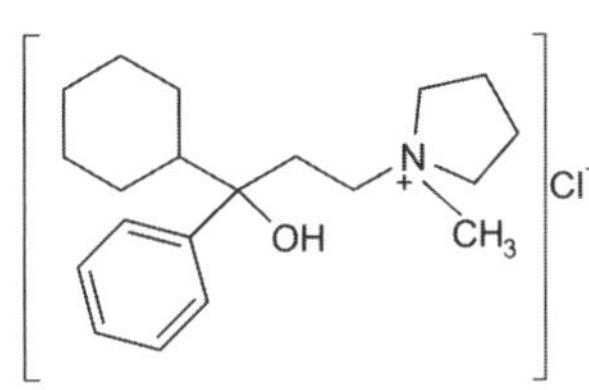

A white crystalline powder. M.p. 165° to 168°.
Soluble 1 in 3 of water, 1 in 3 of ethanol, and 1 in 25 of chloroform; practically insoluble in ether.

Colour Tests. Mandelin's Test—grey-violet; Marquis Test—violet.

Thin-layer Chromatography. System TA—Rf 06. (Acidified iodoplatinate solution, positive.)

Ultraviolet Spectrum. Aqueous acid—251, 257 (A^1_1 = 5.7 a), 263 nm. No alkaline shift.

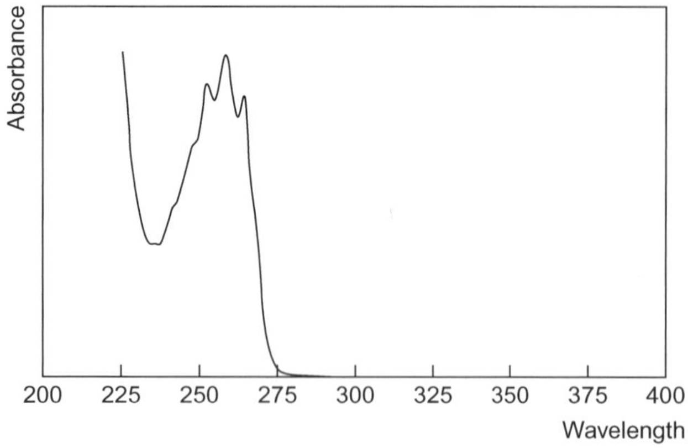

Infra-red Spectrum. Principal peaks at wavenumbers 705, 920, 1115, 772, 1045, 1061 cm^{-1}(KBr disk).

Dose. Tricyclamol chloride has been given in doses of 50 to 100 mg.

Tridihexethyl Chloride

Anticholinergic

Proprietary names. Pathilon. It is an ingredient of Milpath.
γ-Cyclohexyl-*N*,*N*,*N*-triethyl-γ-hydroxybenzenepropanaminium chloride
$C_{21}H_{36}ClNO$=354.0
CAS—60-49-1 (tridihexethyl); *4310-35-4* (chloride)

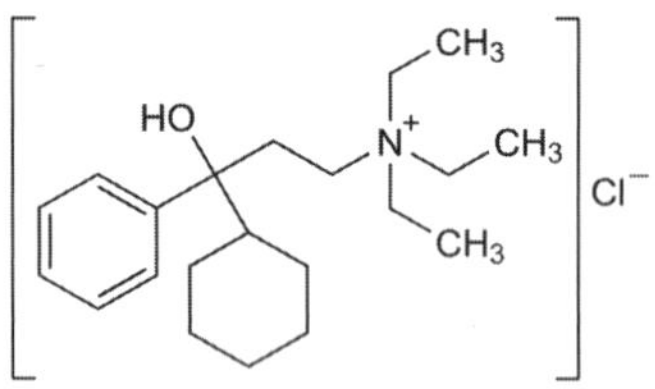

A white crystalline powder. M.p. 196° to 202°.
Soluble 1 in 3 of water, 1 in 3 of ethanol, and 1 in 2 of chloroform; practically insoluble in ether.

Colour Tests. Mandelin's Test—violet; Marquis Test—brown-violet.

Thin-layer Chromatography. System TA—Rf 07. (Acidified iodoplatinate solution, positive.)

Ultraviolet Spectrum. Aqueous acid—251, 257, 263 nm. No alkaline shift.

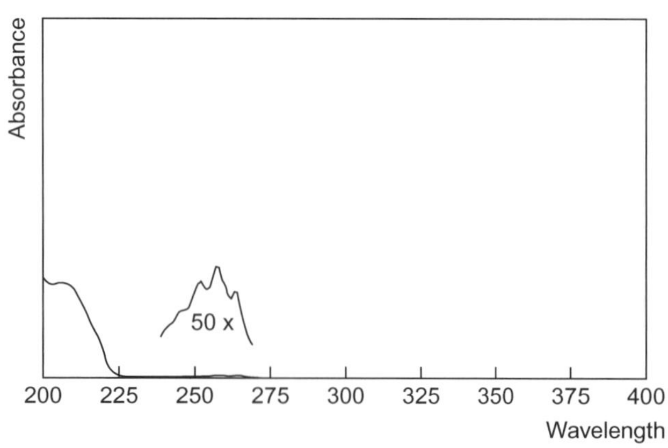

Infra-red Spectrum. Principal peaks at wavenumbers 717, 1492, 710, 769, 1162, 729 cm^{-1} (KBr disk).

Mass Spectrum. Principal ions at *m/z* 86, 58, 88, 105, 206, 87, 55, 77.

Dose. 75 to 300 mg daily.

Trientine

Copper Chelator

Synonym. Triethylenetetramine; Trien; TETA; TECZA.
N,*N'*-Bis-(2-aminoethyl)-1,2-ethanediamine
$C_6H_{18}N_4$=146.2
CAS—112-24-3

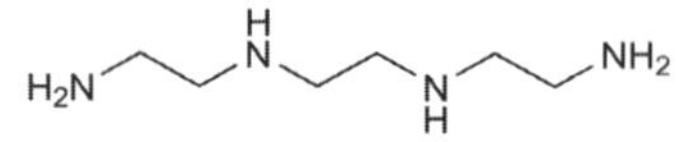

An oily liquid with M. p. of 12° and b. p. of 266° to 267°. It is soluble in water and alcohol, and is corrosive.

Trientine Dihydrochloride

Synonyms. MK-0681; TECZA; TETA; Trien hydrochloride; Trientine hydrochloride; Triethylenetetramine dihydrochloride.
Proprietary name. Syprine
$C_6H_{18}N_4$,2HCl=219.2
CAS—38260-01-4
A white to pale yellow crystalline powder. M.p. 115° to 118°. It is freely soluble in water; soluble in methyl alcohol; slightly soluble in alcohol; practically insoluble in chloroform and ether.

Dissociation Constant. pK_a 9.92 (20°).

Partition Coefficient. Log *P* (octanol/water), −2.65.

High Performance Liquid Chromatography. Column: Nucleosil 5-CN (250 × 4.6 mm i.d., 5 μm). Mobile phase: acetonitrile:ammonium chloride (140 mM) (containing sodium benzene sulfonate (48 mM), and acetic acid (9.2 mM), pH 6) (27:73), flow rate 0.5 mL/min. Fluorescence detection (λ_{ex}=380 nm, λ_{em}=485 nm). RT: 9.5 min [K Miyazaki *et al.*, *Chem. Pharm. Bull.*, 1990, *38*, 1035–1038].

Quantification

High performance liquid chromatography. In blood: limit of detection 100 μg/L. Fluorescence detection (λ_{ex}=380 nm, λ_{em}=485 nm)—K. Miyazaki *et al.*, *Chem. Pharm. Bull.*, 1990, *38*, 1035–1038.

Disposition in the Body. Trientine is rapidly absorbed after oral administration. High concentrations of the metabolites are detected in the blood at the early stages following administration. It is widely distributed throughout the body. Urine and faeces are the major routes of elimination, with a large amount of metabolites being detected in urine. 1-*N*-acetyltriethylene tetramine (acetyltrien) has been identified in urine. This metabolite has chelating activity which is significantly lower than trientine. Both drug and metabolite are capable of combining with copper, iron and zinc. After oral administration, approx. 1.6% of an administered dose is detected in urine unchanged, and 8% as acetyltrien. The majority of the drug is excreted within the first 6 h, and the metabolite excreted over 26 h.

Bioavailability. 90 to 95%.

Dose. Adults: (US guidelines) the usual initial dose is 750 to 1250 mg daily which may be increased to a maximum of 2 g daily; (UK guidelines) 1.2 to 2.4 g daily is recommended. Children: the usual initial dose is 500 to 750 mg which may be increased to a maximum of 1.5 g daily if necessary.

Trifluomeprazine

Tranquilliser (Veterinary)

Synonym. Triflutrimeprazine
N,*N*,*β*-Trimethyl-2-(trifluoromethyl)-10*H*-phenothiazine-10-propanamine
$C_{19}H_{21}F_3N_2S$=366.4
CAS—2622-37-9

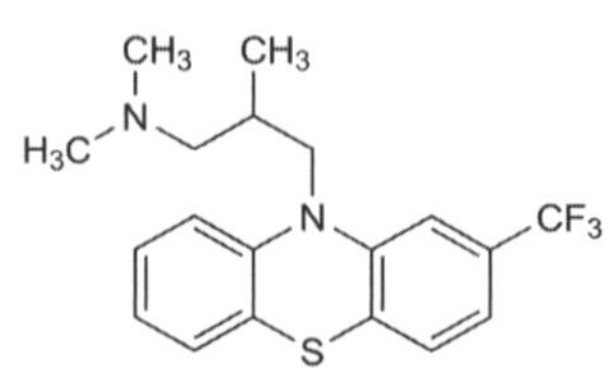

Trifluomeprazine Maleate

Proprietary name. Nortran
$C_{19}H_{21}F_3N_2S,C_4H_4O_4$=482.5
A white crystalline powder. M.p. about 178°.

Very slightly soluble in water; soluble 1 in 25 of ethanol and 1 in 25 of chloroform; practically insoluble in ether.

Colour Tests. Mandelin's Test—green→red-violet; Marquis Test—red-violet; Sulfuric Acid—red-violet.

Thin-layer Chromatography. System TA—Rf 65; system TB—Rf 60; system TC—Rf 58; system TL—Rf 52. (Acidified iodoplatinate solution, positive.)

Gas Chromatography. System GA—RI 2250.

Ultraviolet Spectrum. Aqueous acid—255 (A_1^1=803 a), 305 nm, less well-defined.

Mass Spectrum. Principal ions at *m/z* 58, 366, 59, 100, 266, 248, 84, 44.

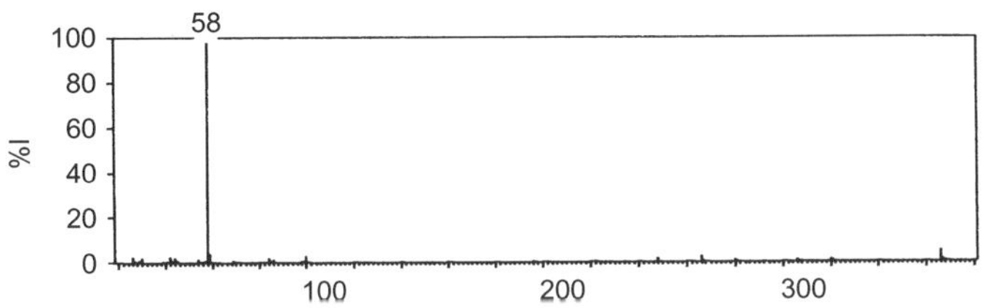

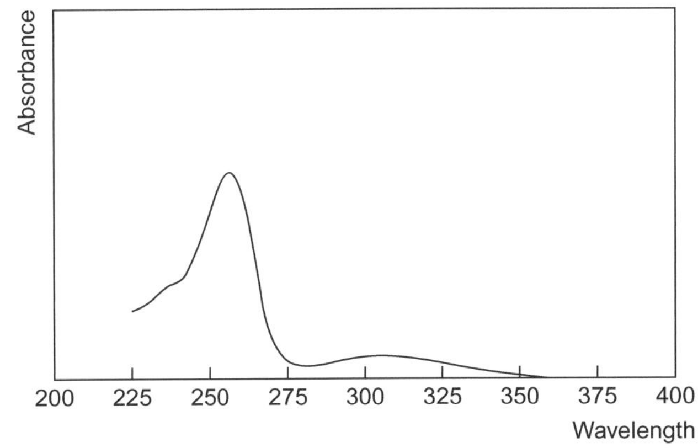

Trifluoperazine

Antipsychotic

10-[3-(4-Methyl-1-piperazinyl)propyl]-2-(trifluoromethyl)-10*H*-phenothiazine
$C_{21}H_{24}F_3N_3S$=407.5
CAS—117-89-5

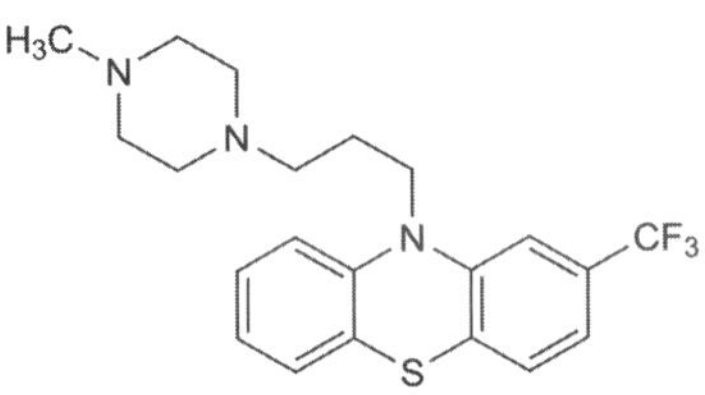

Trifluoperazine Hydrochloride

Synonym. Triphthazinum
Proprietary names. Eskazine; Flupazine; Jatroneural; Modalina; Novoflurazine; Stelazine; Terfluzine; Triplex. It is an ingredient of Parstelin, and Stelabid.
$C_{21}H_{24}F_3N_3S,2HCl$=480.4
CAS—440-17-5
A white to pale yellow, hygroscopic, crystalline powder. M.p. 242° to 243°. Soluble 1 in 2 of water, 1 in 11 of ethanol, and 1 in 100 of chloroform; practically insoluble in ether.

Dissociation Constant. pK_a 8.1 (24°).

Partition Coefficient. Log *P* (octanol/water), 5.0.

Colour Tests. Formaldehyde-Sulfuric Acid—pink; Forrest Reagent—orange; FPN Reagent—orange; Liebermann's Test—red; Mandelin's Test—red-brown; Marquis Test—red-violet.

Thin-layer Chromatography. System TA—Rf 53; system TB—Rf 33; system TC—Rf 30; system TE—Rf 55; system TL—Rf 08; system TAE—Rf 30; system TAF—Rf 29. (Dragendorff spray, positive; FPN reagent, pink; Acidified iodoplatinate solution, positive; Marquis reagent, pink.)

Gas Chromatography. System GA—RI 2683 trifluoperazine; RI 2190 M (ring); RI 2990 M (sulfoxide); system GB—RI 2798 trifluoperazine; RI 3145 M (sulfoxide); RI 3191 M (norsulfoxide); system GF—RI 3050.

High Performance Liquid Chromatography. System HA—*k* 3.0; system HX—RI 480; system HY—RI 344; system HZ—Retention time 13.2 min; system HAA—Retention time 17.7 min.

Ultraviolet Spectrum. Aqueous acid—256 (A_1^1=743 a), 305 nm; aqueous alkali—258, 308 nm.

Infra-red Spectrum. Principal peaks at wavenumbers 1114, 1316, 1145, 1081, 755, 1255 cm^{-1} (trifluoperazine hydrochloride, KBr disk).

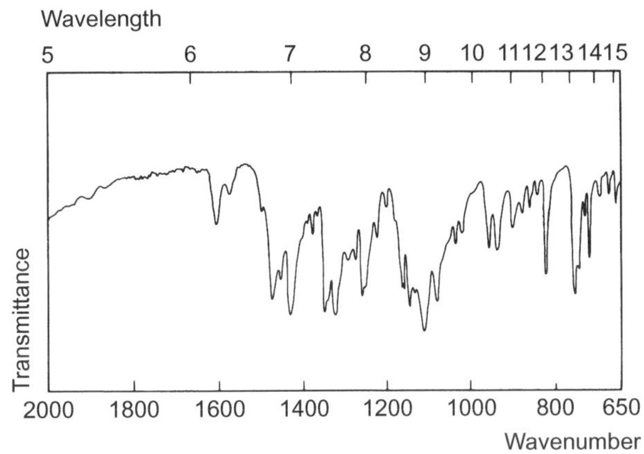

Mass Spectrum. Principal ions at *m/z* 113, 70, 407, 43, 141, 42, 127, 71.

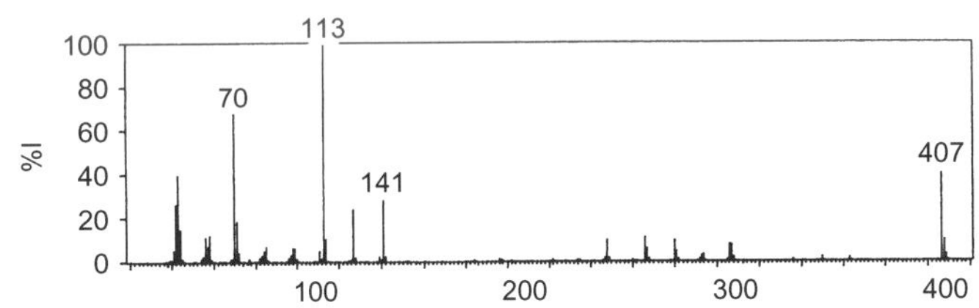

Quantification

Gas chromatography. In plasma: limit of detection 0.2 µg/L, AFID—J. I. Javaid *et al.*, *J. Pharm. Sci.*, 1982, *71*, 63–66.

Radioimmunoassay. In plasma: limit of detection 0.25 µg/L—K. K. Midha *et al.*, *Br. J. Clin. Pharmacol.*, 1981, *12*, 189–193.

Disposition in the Body. Absorbed after oral administration. About 1% of a daily dose is excreted in the 24-h urine as unchanged drug and up to 6% of a dose as the sulfoxide. Metabolism to 7-hydroxytrifluoperazine and desmethyltrifluoperazine has been reported.

Therapeutic concentration

Following a single oral dose of 5 mg to 5 healthy subjects, peak plasma concentrations of 0.5 to 3.1 µg/L (mean, 1.4 µg/L) were reached between 2.3 and 3.2 h [K. K. Midha *et al.*, *Br. J. Clin. Pharmacol.*, 1983, *15*, 380–382]

Following a single oral dose of 20 mg to 4 subjects, peak plasma concentrations of 1 to 4 µg/L (mean 2) were attained in 3 to 6 h [T. J. Gillespie and I. Sipes, *J. Chromatogr.*, 1981, *223*; B *Biomed. Appl.*, *12*, 95–102].

Following daily oral doses of 80 mg to 1 subject, a peak plasma concentration of 0.028 mg/L was reported 8 h after a dose [S. H. Curry *et al.*, *Lancet*, 1981, *1*, 395–396].

Toxicity

Postmortem blood and liver concentrations of 0.06 mg/L and 0.31 mg/kg respectively were reported in a woman who died of suspected trifluoperazine overdose while receiving daily oral doses of 40 mg [E. Street, per R. C. Baselt, *Disposition of Toxic Drugs and Chemicals in Man*, 5th Edn, Davis, California, Biomedical Publications, 2000, 860–861].

The following postmortem concentrations were reported in a fatality attributed to trifluoperazine ingestion: blood 0.4 mg/L, kidney 83 mg/kg, liver 198 mg/kg; 7-hydroxytrifluoperazine, kidney 61 mg/kg, liver 161 mg/kg; desmethyltrifluoperazine, kidney 89 mg/kg, liver 205 mg/kg [I. Quai *et al.*, *J. Anal. Toxicol.*, 1985, *9*, 43–44].

Half-life. Plasma half-life, 7 to 18 h (mean 12).

Dose. For psychoses, the equivalent of 10 to 20 mg of trifluoperazine daily; more than 40 mg daily has been given.

Trifluperidol

Antipsychotic

Synonym. Flumoperone

1-(4-Fluorophenyl)-4-[4-hydroxy-4-[3-(trifluoromethyl)phenyl]-1-piperidinyl]-1-butanone

$C_{22}H_{23}F_4NO_2$=409.4

CAS—749-13-3

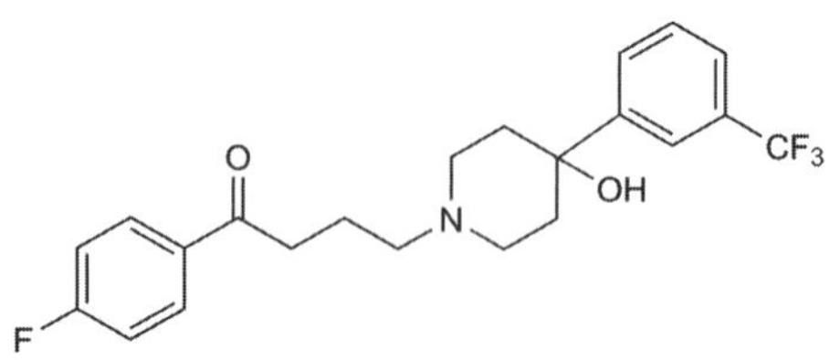

A white crystalline powder. M.p. 93° to 95°.

Trifluperidol Hydrochloride

Proprietary names. Psicoperidol; Triperidol.

$C_{22}H_{23}F_4NO_2$,HCl=445.9

CAS—2062-77-3

A white, amorphous or crystalline, flocculent powder which is stable in air but darkens slowly on exposure to light. M.p. about 201°.

Slightly soluble in water and chloroform; soluble in ethanol; practically insoluble in ether; freely soluble in methanol.

Partition Coefficient. Log *P* (octanol/water), 4.5.

Thin-layer Chromatography. System TA—Rf 73; system TB—Rf 13; system TD—Rf 02; system TE—Rf 77; system TF—Rf 05; system TAD—Rf 26; system TAE—Rf 55; system TAF—Rf 76. (Acidified iodoplatinate solution, positive.)

Gas Chromatography. System GA—RI 2675; RI 1570 M (*N*-desalkyl-oxo) – $2H_2O$; RI 1970 M (*N*-desalkyl-).

High Performance Liquid Chromatography. System HA—*k* 1.2; system HX—RI 459; system HY—RI 306; system HAA—Retention time 21.6 min.

Ultraviolet Spectrum. Aqueous acid—248 nm (A^1_1=308 a).

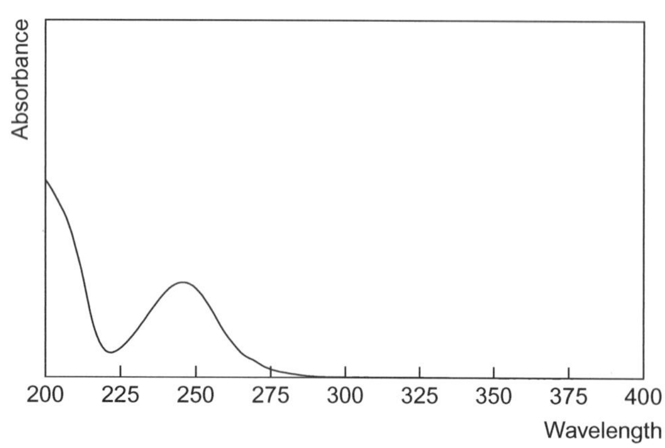

Infra-red Spectrum. Principal peaks at wavenumbers 1317, 1150, 1665, 1170, 1110, 1595 cm^{-1} (trifluperidol hydrochloride, KBr disk).

Mass Spectrum. Principal ions at *m/z* 42, 271, 258, 123, 56, 83, 240, 95.

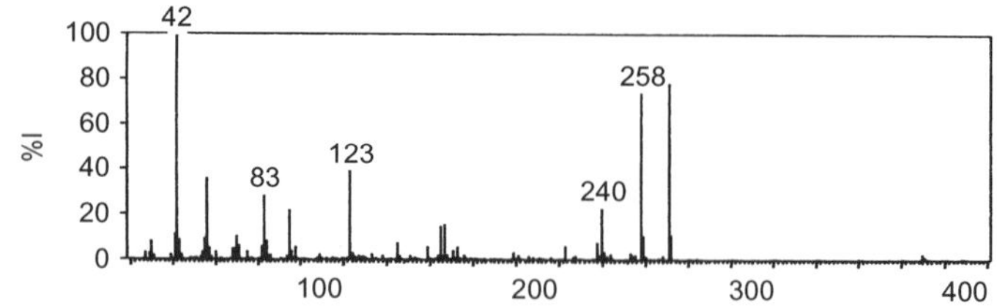

Quantification

Gas chromatography. In plasma or tissues: ECD—F. Marcucci *et al.*, *J. Chromatogr.*, 1971, *59*, 174–177.

High performance liquid chromatography. In plasma—L. Przyborowski and G. Misztal, *Pharmazie*, 1991, *46*, 813–814.

Dose. Initially the equivalent of 500 µg of trifluperidol daily, increased to a maximum dose of 8 mg daily.

Triflupromazine

Tranquilliser

Synonym. Fluopromazine

N,*N*-Dimethyl-2-(trifluoromethyl)-10*H*-phenothiazine-10-propanamine

$C_{18}H_{19}F_3N_2S$=352.4

CAS—146-54-3

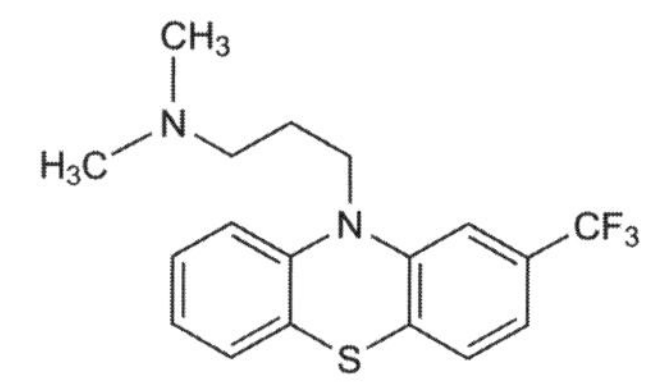

A pale amber viscous oily liquid, which forms into large irregular crystals during prolonged storage.

Practically insoluble in water.

Triflupromazine Hydrochloride

Proprietary names. Psyquil; Siquil; Vesprin.

$C_{18}H_{19}F_3N_2S$,HCl=388.9

CAS—1098-60-8

A white to pale tan crystalline powder. M.p. 170° to 178°.

Soluble 1 in less than 1 of water and of ethanol, and 1 in 1.7 of chloroform; soluble in acetone; practically insoluble in ether.

Dissociation Constant. pK_a 9.2 (24°).

Partition Coefficient. Log *P* (octanol/water), 5.5.

Colour Tests. Formaldehyde–Sulfuric Acid—red; Forrest Reagent—orange; FPN Reagent—orange; Mandelin's Test—red-brown; Marquis Test—red-violet.

Thin-layer Chromatography. System TA—Rf 54; system TB—Rf 47; system TC—Rf 35; system TE—Rf 75; system TL—Rf 22; system TAE—Rf 32; system TAF—Rf 49. (Acidified iodoplatinate solution, positive.)

Gas Chromatography. System GA—triflupromazine RI 2230, M (ring) RI 2190; system GB—triflupromazine RI 2318; system GF—triflupromazine RI 2550; system GW—triflupromazine Retention time 19.3 min.

High Performance Liquid Chromatography. System HA—*k* 2.7; system HX—RI 484; system HY—RI 454; system HZ—Retention time, 12.3 min; system HAX—Retention time 17.3 min; system HAY—Retention time 8.9 min.

Ultraviolet Spectrum. Aqueous acid—256 nm (A^1_1=874a), 305 nm.

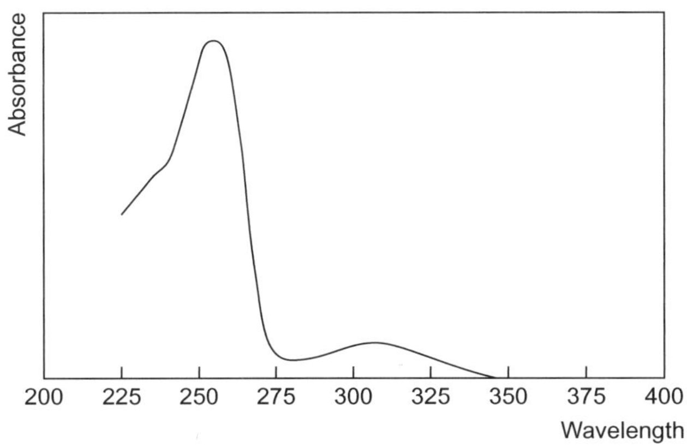

Infra-red Spectrum. Principal peaks at wavenumbers 1117, 1316, 1159, 1237, 1075, 1030 cm^{-1} (KBr disk).

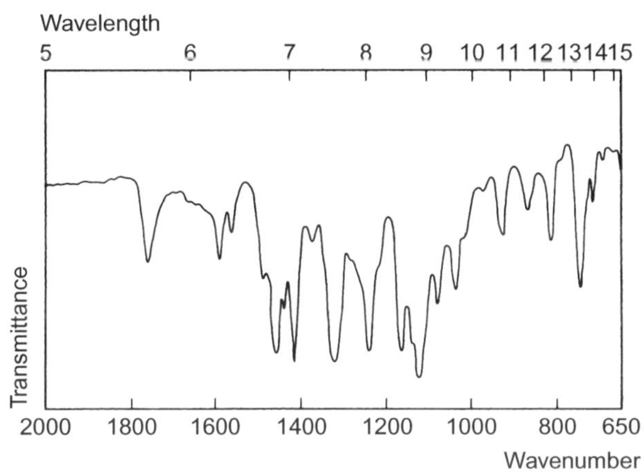

Mass Spectrum. Principal ions at *m/z* 58, 352, 86, 353, 85, 306, 42, 266.

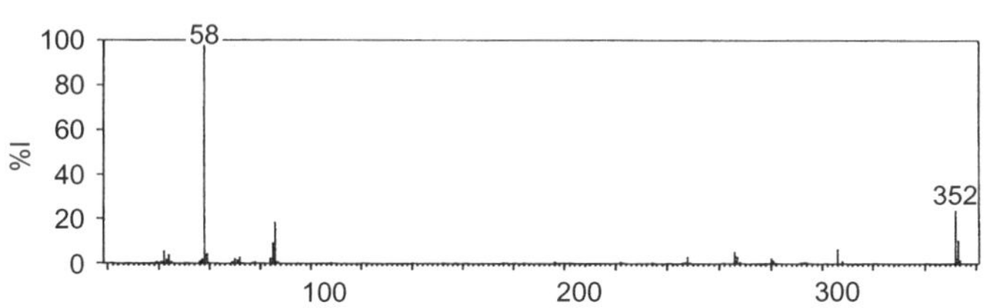

Quantification.

Gas chromatography–mass spectrometry. In urine—H. H. Maurer and K. Pfleger, *Arch. Toxicol.*, 1988, *62*, 185–191.

High performance liquid chromatography. In plasma: triflupromazine as internal standard—T. L. Schwinghammer *et al.*, *Biopharm. Drug Dispos.*, 1984, *5*, 185–194.

Dose. 20 to 150 mg of triflupromazine hydrochloride daily.

Trihexyphenidyl

Anticholinergic

Synonym. Benzhexol

α-Cyclohexyl-α-phenyl-1-piperidinepropanol

$C_{20}H_{31}NO$=301.5

CAS—144-11-6

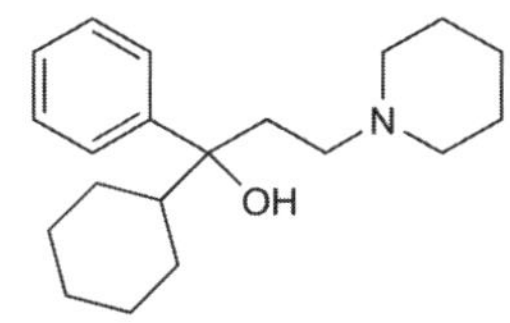

M.p. 114.3° to 115.0°.

Trihexyphenidyl Hydrochloride

Synonyms. Cyclodolum; Trihexyphenidylium Chloride.

Proprietary names. Aparkane; Apo-Trihex; Artandyl; Artane; Broflex; Cyclodol; Hipokinon; Kexidil; Novohexidyl; Pacitane; Paralest; Pargitan; Parkinane; Parkopan; Partane; Peragit; Pipanol; Sedrena; Tremin, Trihexy; Triphedinon; Triphedinyl; Tsiklodol; Trixyl. It is an ingredient of Largatrex and Spasman.

$C_{20}H_{31}NO,HCl$=337.9

CAS—52-49-3

A white or creamy-white crystalline powder. M.p. about 258.5°, with decomposition.

Soluble 1 in 100 of water, 1 in 6 of alcohol, and 1 in 5 chloroform. More soluble in methanol, very slightly soluble in ether and benzene.

Partition Coefficient. Log *P* (octanol/water), 5.27.

Colour Tests. Mandelin's Test—grey-green; Marquis Test—grey-violet.

Thin-layer Chromatography. System TA—Rf 68; system TB—Rf 66; system TC—Rf 61; system TE—Rf 83; system TL—Rf 59; system TAE—Rf 43; system TAF—Rf 75; system TAJ—Rf 38; system TAK—Rf 22; system TAL—Rf 80. (Acidified iodoplatinate solution, positive.)

Gas Chromatography. System GA—trihexyphenidyl RI 2245, M (OH-) RI 2500; system GB—trihexyphenidyl RI 2354, M (OH-) RI 2618.

Column: BP1 methyl silicone (12.5 m × 0.22 mm i.d., 0.12 μm film thickness). Column temperature: 90° for 45 s to 270° at 25°/min, held for 3 min. Injector temperature: 250°. Carrier gas: helium, flow rate 1 mL/min. MS detection. Retention time 8.05 min. [M. Desage *et al.*, *J. Chromatogr.*, 1991, *571 (1–2)*, 250–256.]

High Performance Liquid Chromatography. System HA—*k* 1.8; system HX—RI 429; system HY—RI 381; system HZ—retention time 7.6 min; system HAA—retention time 15.3 min.

Ultraviolet Spectrum. Aqueous acid—252 (A_1^1=6c), 258 (A_1^1=7c), 264 nm (A_1^1=6c).

Infra-red Spectrum. Principal peaks at wavenumbers 702, 756, 973, 1206, 1196, 935 cm^{-1} (trihexyphenidyl hydrochloride, KBr disk).

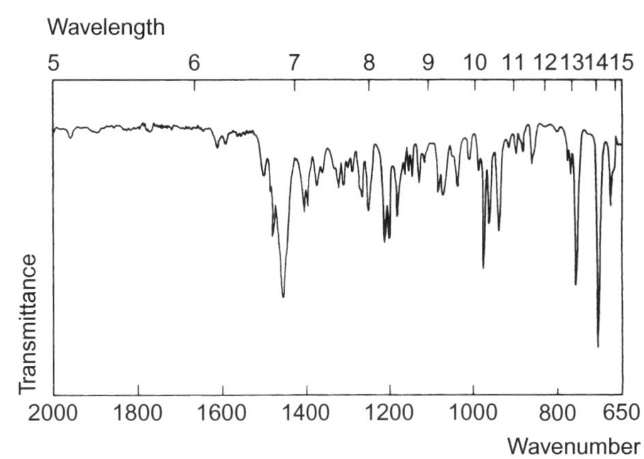

Mass Spectrum. Principal ions at *m/z* 98, 105, 55, 41, 99, 77, 218, 84.

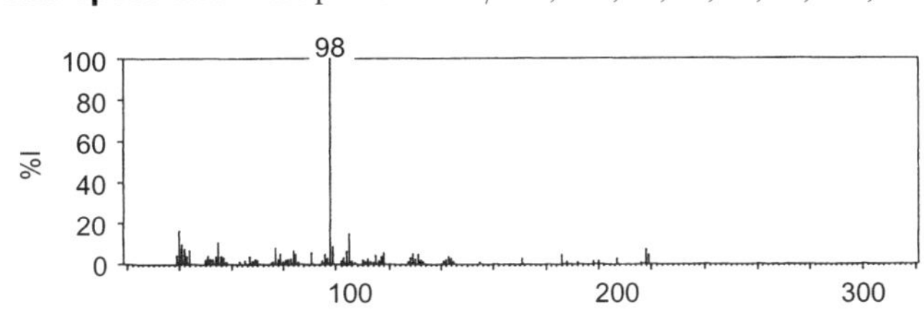

Quantification

Capillary electrophoresis. In serum: limit of detection, 0.17 mg/L—G. Vargas *et al.*, *J. Capillary Electrophor.*, 1998, *5*, 153–158.

Gas chromatography. In biological fluids: trihexyphenidyl, and procyclidine, limit of detection 50 to 100 ng/L—J. A. Owen *et al.*, *J. Chromatogr.*, 1989, *494*, 135–142. In plasma or urine: trihexyphenidyl and its hydroxylated metabolite, limits of detection 2 µg/L and 1 µg/L respectively, NPD—P. Kintz *et al.*, *J. Anal. Toxicol.*, 1989, *13*, 47–49.

Gas chromatography–mass spectrometry. In plasma: limit of detection 1 µg/L, limit of quantification 5 µg/L—M. Desage *et al., J. Chromatogr.*, 1991, *571*, 250–256.

Radioimmunoassay. In plasma: limit of quantification 40 ng/L—H. He *et al., J. Pharm. Sci.*, 1995, *84*, 561–567.

Disposition in the Body. Absorbed after oral administration; disappears rapidly from the tissues.

Toxicity. In some patients, doses of more than 12 mg daily may produce severe mental disturbance and excitement.

The following postmortem concentrations were observed in a 48-year-old schizophrenic male: femoral artery blood 0.12 mg/L, liver 0.5 µg/g, gastric contents 0.4 mg trihexyphenidyl. Other drugs were not detected. It is suggested that for fatalities to occur following trihexyphenidyl intoxication, secondary contributory factors, which probably further alter the patient's conscious state, are necessary. [J. A. Gall *et al., Forensic Sci. Int.*, 1995, *71(1)*, 9–14.]

The following postmortem concentrations were observed in a 16-year-old youth who experienced hallucinations and was found dead in a nearby lake 2 days after the ingestion of 20 mg of trihexyphenidyl: blood 0.03 mg/L, urine 0.38 mg/L. [L. Kopjak and T. A. Jennison, *Bull. Int. Assoc. Forensic Toxicol.*, 1976, *12(1)*, 8.]

Dose. 1 mg of trihexyphenidyl hydrochloride daily, increased gradually; usual maintenance dose 5 to 15 mg in 3 to 4 divided doses.

Trilostane

Adrenocortical Suppressant

Proprietary name. Modrenal

(4α,5α,17β)-4,5-Epoxy-3,17-dihydroxyandrost-2-ene-2-carbonitrile

$C_{20}H_{27}NO_3$=329.4

CAS—13647-35-3

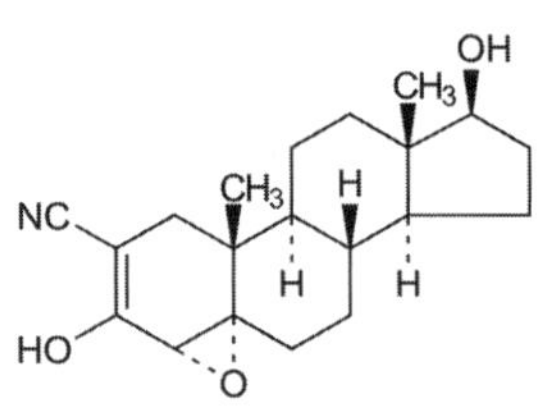

Tan crystals. M.p. 258° to 270°, with some decomposition.

Practically insoluble in water, chloroform and ether; slightly soluble in a mixture of equal parts of chloroform and methanol.

Partition Coefficient. Log *P* (octanol/water) 2.0.

Thin-layer Chromatography. System TA—Rf 88; system TB—Rf 0; system TC—Rf 18; system TD—Rf 30; system TE—Rf 7; system TF—Rf 45. (Marquis reagent, red; mercuric chloride–diphenylcarbazone, violet, fades to pink; acidified potassium permanganate solution, positive.)

Gas Chromatography. System GA—RI 3075, decomposition occurs.

Ultraviolet Spectrum. Aqueous alkali—281 nm; ethanol—253 nm (A^{1}_{1}=234b).

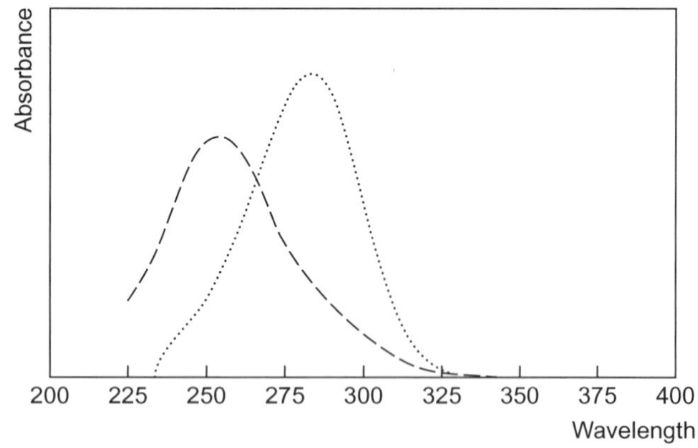

Infra-red Spectrum. Principal peaks at wavenumbers 1665, 1060, 1050, 1320, 1205, 1180 cm^{-1} (KBr disk).

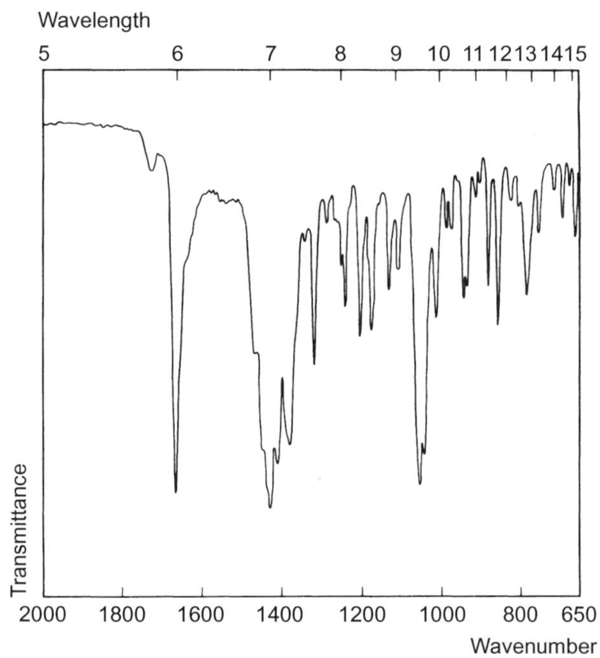

Mass Spectrum. Principal ions at *m/z* 41, 147, 79, 93, 55, 105, 67, 91.

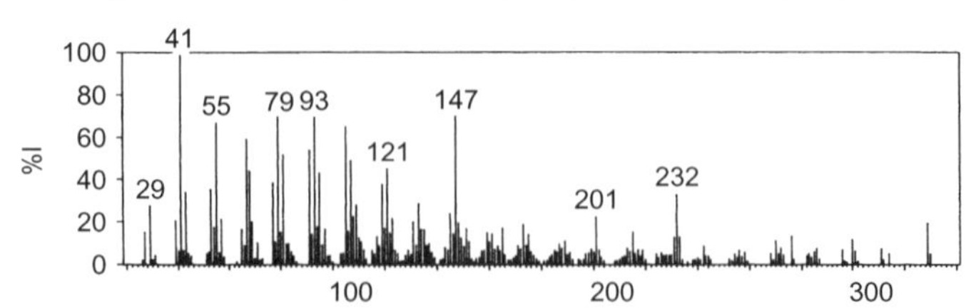

Quantification

High performance liquid chromatography. In plasma: trilostane and ketotrilostane—P. Powles *et al., J. Chromatogr.*, 1984, *311*, 434–442; R.R. Brown *et al., J. Chromatogr.*, 1995, *339*, 440–444.

Dose. 120 to 480 mg daily.

Trimeperidine

Narcotic Analgesic

Synonym. Promedol

1,2,5-Trimethyl-4-phenyl-4-piperidinol propanoate

$C_{17}H_{25}NO_2$=275.4

CAS—64-39-1

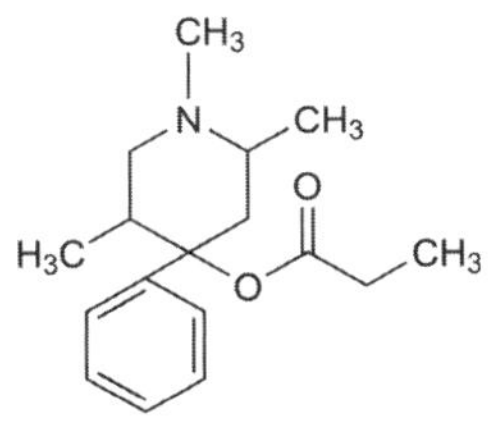

Soluble 1 in about 27 of water.

Trimeperidine Hydrochloride

$C_{17}H_{25}NO_2,HCl=311.9$

CAS—125-80-4

A white crystalline powder.

Freely soluble in water and chloroform; soluble in ethanol; practically insoluble in ether.

Partition Coefficient. Log *P* (octanol/water), 3.1.

Colour Test. Marquis Test—red-violet.

Thin-layer Chromatography. System TA—Rf 58; system TB—Rf 41; system TC—Rf 41; system TL—Rf 17. (Dragendorff spray, positive; acidified iodoplatinate solution, positive; Marquis reagent, red-violet.)

Gas Chromatography. System GA—RI 1808; system GB—RI 1895.

High Performance Liquid Chromatography. System HA—*k* 2.1.

Ultraviolet Spectrum. Aqueous acid—251, 257 nm ($A^1_1=7.6b$), 263 nm. No alkaline shift.

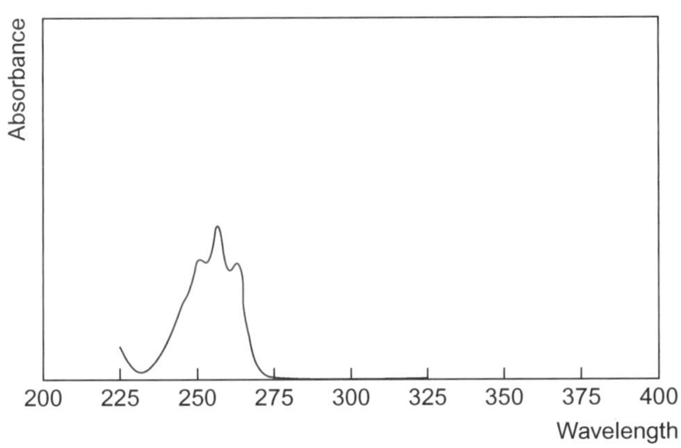

Infra-red Spectrum. Principal peaks at wavenumbers 1738, 1181, 1141, 1162, 1195, 1077 cm^{-1} (KBr disk).

Mass Spectrum. Principal ions at *m/z* 186, 42, 201, 56, 57, 187, 202, 71.

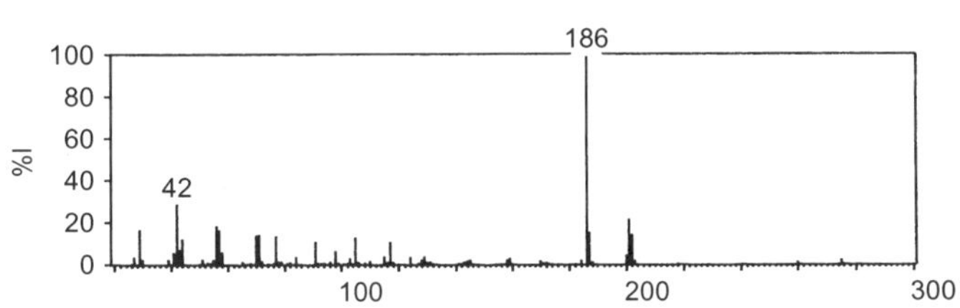

Dose. Trimeperidine hydrochloride has been given in doses of up to 200 mg daily.

Trimetaphan Camsilate

Antihypertensive

Synonyms. Méthioplégium; Trimetaphan Camphorsulfonate; Trimethaphan Camsylate.

Proprietary name. Arfonad

Decahydro-2-oxo-1,3-bis(phenylmethyl)thieno[1′,2′:1,2]thieno-[3,4-*d*]imidazol-5-ium salt with (1*S*)-7,7-dimethyl-2-oxobicyclo[2,2,1]heptane-1-methanesulfonic acid (1:1)

$C_{22}H_{25}N_2OS,C_{10}H_{15}O_4S=596.8$

CAS—7187-66-8 (trimetaphan); 68-91-7 (camsilate)

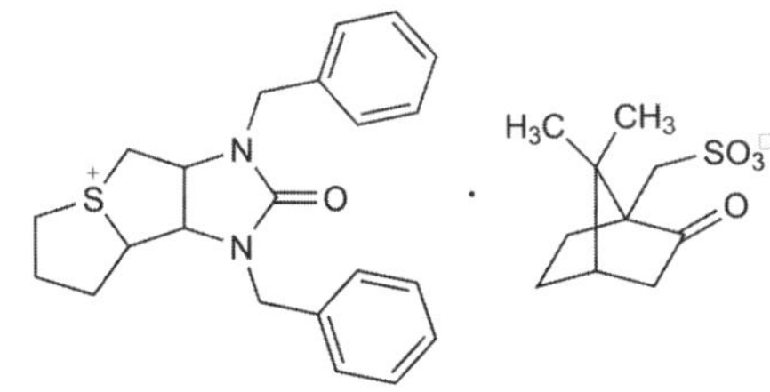

Colourless crystals or white crystalline powder. M.p. about 245°, with decomposition.

Soluble 1 in less than 5 of water and 1 in 2 of ethanol; freely soluble in chloroform; slightly soluble in acetone and ether.

Partition Coefficient. Log *P* (octanol/water) 6.9.

Colour Tests. Aromaticity (Method 2)—colourless/yellow; Liebermann's Test—orange.

Thin-layer Chromatography. System TA—Rf 02; system TB—Rf 00; system TE—Rf 00; system TF—Rf 00; system TAE—Rf 00; system TAJ—Rf 00; system TAK—Rf 01; system TAL—Rf 20. (Acidified iodoplatinate solution, positive.)

High Performance Liquid Chromatography. System HX—RI 386.

Ultraviolet Spectrum. Aqueous acid—252 nm ($A^1_1=8.2a$), 258 nm ($A^1_1=8.3a$), 264 nm. No alkaline shift.

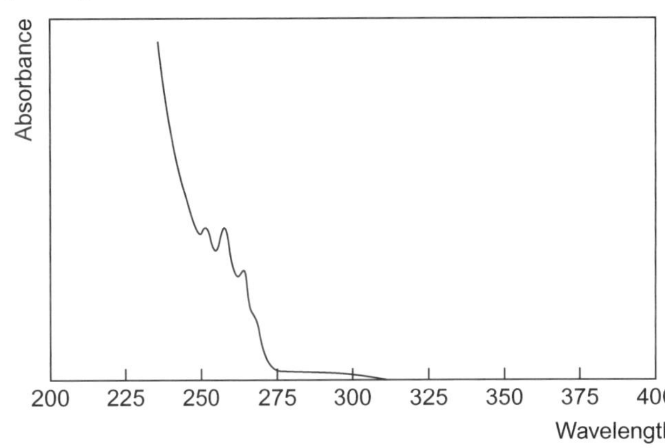

Infra-red Spectrum. Principal peaks at wavenumbers 1701, 1220, 1184, 1735, 1052, 1672 cm^{-1} (KBr disk).

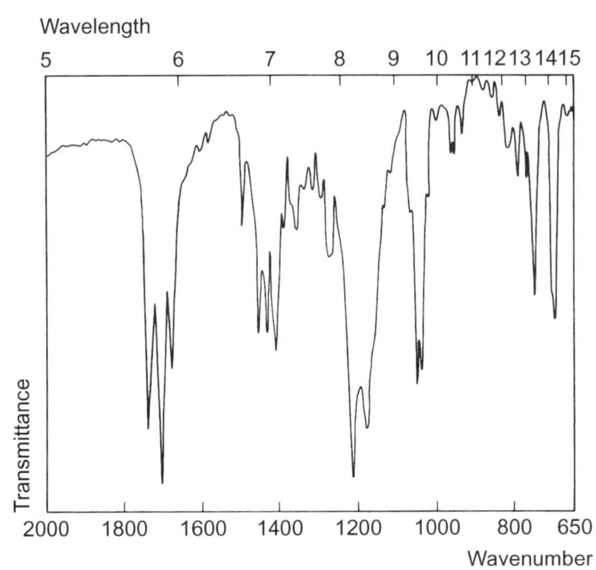

Mass Spectrum. Principal ions at *m/z* 91, 65, 187, 92, 277, 259, 90, 273.

Dose. Initially 3 to 4 mg/min by intravenous infusion.

Trimetazidine

Anti-anginal Vasodilator

Synonym. Trimetazine
1-[(2,3,4-Trimethoxyphenyl)methyl]piperazine
$C_{14}H_{22}N_2O_3 = 266.3$
CAS—5011-34-7

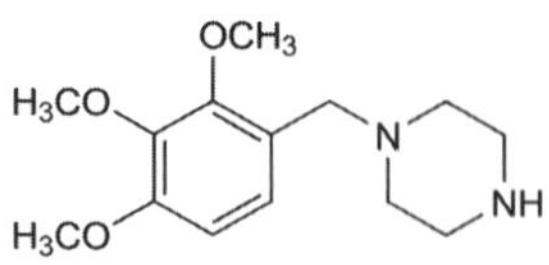

Trimetazidine Hydrochloride

Proprietary names. Cardiazidine; Centrophene; Idaptan; Oxygirex; Vastarel; Vastinol.
$C_{14}H_{22}N_2O_3,2HCl = 339.3$
CAS—13171-25-0
A white crystalline powder. M.p. 225° to 228°.
Freely soluble in water; sparingly soluble in ethanol.

Partition Coefficient. Log *P* (octanol/water), 0.6.

Colour Tests. Mandelin's Test—violet; Marquis Test—yellow (fades).

Thin-layer Chromatography. System TA—Rf 22; system TB—Rf 05; system TC—Rf 04; system TL—Rf 01. (Acidified iodoplatinate solution, positive.)

High Performance Liquid Chromatography. System HA—k 3.0 (tailing peak); system HAA—RT 6.1 min.

Ultraviolet Spectrum. Aqueous acid—231 (A_1^1 = 424 a), 269 nm.

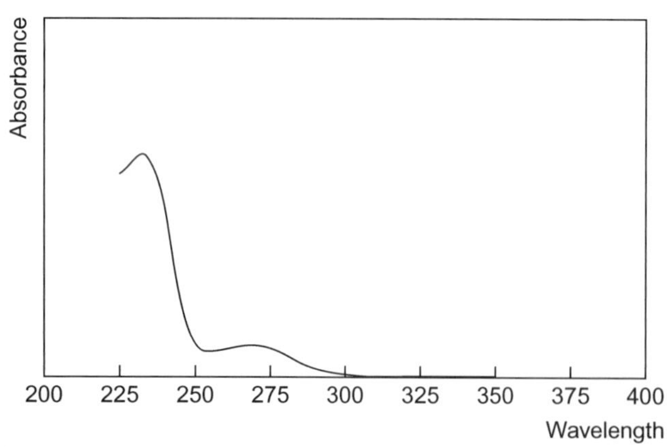

Infra-red Spectrum. Principal peaks at wavenumbers 1093, 1494, 1280, 1011, 1042, 1600 cm^{-1} (KBr disk).

Mass Spectrum. Principal ions at *m/z* 181, 85, 56, 166, 266, 182, 179, 91.

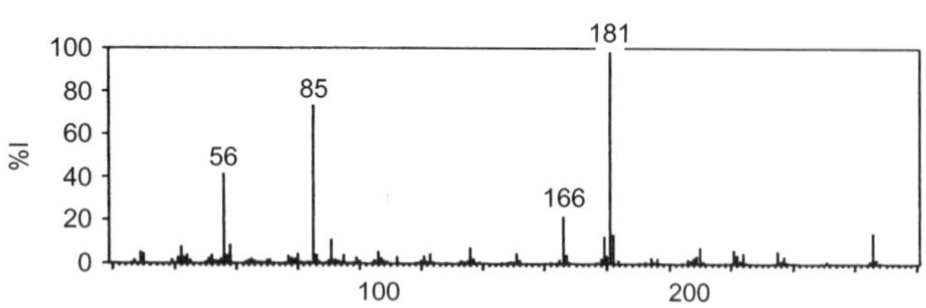

Quantification

Gas chromatography–mass spectrometry. In biological fluids—L. Fay *et al.*, *J. Chromatogr.*, 1989, *490*, 198–205.

High performance liquid chromatography. In plasma: fluorescence detection—S. Courte and N. Bromet, *J Chromatogr.*, 1981, *224*, 162–167.

Dose. Trimetazidine hydrochloride has been given in doses of 40 to 60 mg daily.

Trimethadione

Anticonvulsant

Synonyms. Trimetadiona; Trimethadionum; Trimethinum; Troxidone.
Proprietary names. Absentol; Epidione; Petidon; Ptimal; Tridione.
3,5,5-Trimethyl-2,4-oxazolidinedione
$C_6H_9NO_3 = 143.1$
CAS—127-48-0

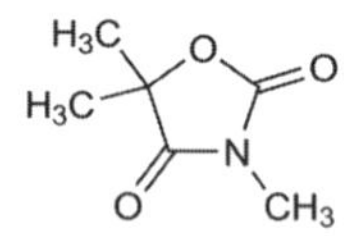

Colourless or white granular crystals. M.p. 46°.
Soluble 1 in 20 of water; freely soluble in ethanol, chloroform, benzene and ether.

Partition Coefficient. Log *P* (octanol/water), 0.6.

Thin-layer Chromatography. System TE—Rf 00; system TF—Rf 00; system TAE—Rf 00.

Gas Chromatography. System GA—trimethadione RI 1090, M (nor-) RI 1060; system GE—RRT 0.04 (relative to phenytoin).

High Performance Liquid Chromatography. System HX—RI 286.

Infra-red Spectrum. Principal peaks at wavenumbers 1730, 1802, 1098, 1200, 770, 1295 cm^{-1} (KBr disk).

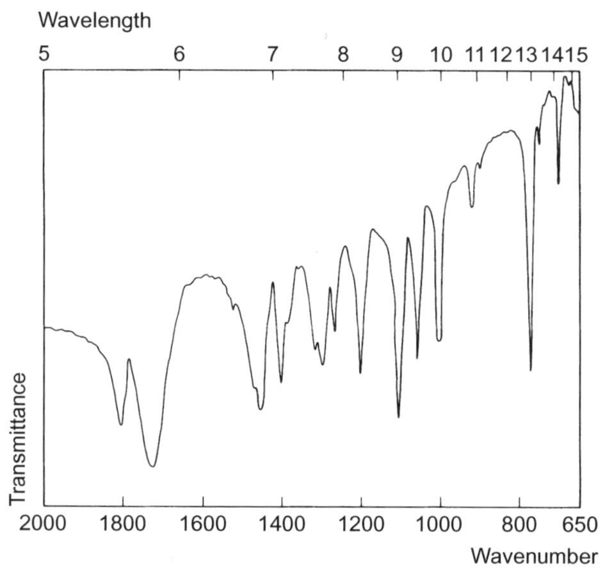

Mass Spectrum. Principal ions at *m/z* 43, 58, 143, 42, 41, 40, 39, 128.

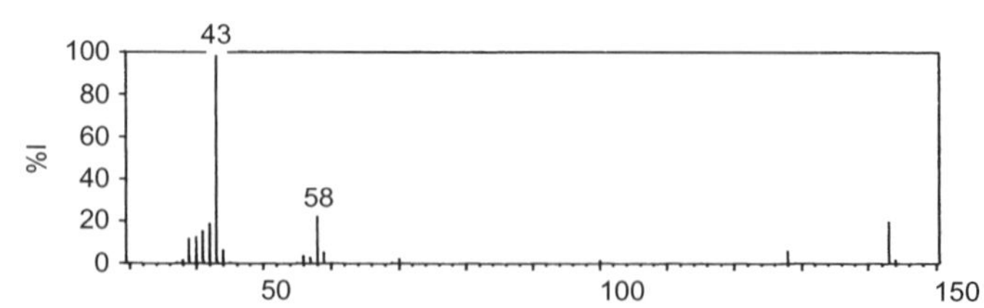

Quantification

Gas chromatography. In plasma: trimethadione and dimethadione, FID—D. L. Bius *et al.*, *Ther. Drug Monit.*, 1979, *1*, 495–505. In serum: trimethadione and dimethadione, limits of detection 10 µg/L and 50 µg/L, respectively—E. Tanaka and S. Misawa, *J. Chromatogr.*, 1992, *584*, 267–269.

Disposition in the Body. Readily absorbed after oral administration and extensively metabolised in the liver to the active metabolite, dimethadione, which is thought to be primarily responsible for the pharmacological activity. It is very slowly excreted in the urine over a period of several days, almost entirely in the form of dimethadione; the excretion of dimethadione is increased in alkaline urine.

Therapeutic concentration. Dimethadione attains plasma concentrations about 20 times greater than those of trimethadione and accumulates on chronic administration; there is considerable intersubject variation in plasma concentrations.

Steady-state plasma concentrations of 19 to 41 mg/L (mean 25) of trimethadione and 350 to 1033 mg/L (mean 550) of dimethadione were reported in 5 subjects during chronic treatment with trimethadione [D. L. Bius *et al.*, *Ther. Drug Monit.*, 1979, *1*, 495–505.]

Toxicity. The estimated minimum lethal dose is 5 g. Toxic effects may be associated with plasma-dimethadione concentrations greater than 1000 mg/L.

Half-life. Plasma half-life, trimethadione about 16 h; dimethadione, half-life derived from urinary excretion data, 6 to 13 days.

Protein binding. In plasma, not significantly bound.

Dose. Initially 900 mg daily, increasing to 1.8 g daily.

Trimethobenzamide

Antihistamine

N-[(2-Dimethylaminoethoxy)benzyl]-3,4,5-trimethoxybenzamide
$C_{21}H_{28}N_2O_5 = 388.5$
CAS—138-56-7

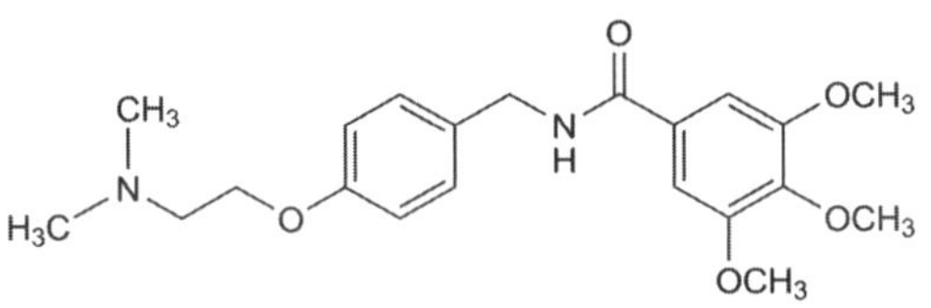

Trimethobenzamide Hydrochloride

Proprietary names. Tebamide; T-Gen; Ticon; Tigan; Trimazide.
$C_{21}H_{28}N_2O_5,HCl = 424.9$
CAS—554-92-7
A white crystalline powder. M.p. 188° to 190°.
Soluble 1 in 2 of water, 1 in about 60 of ethanol, 1 in 67 of chloroform, and 1 in 720 of ether.

Dissociation Constant. pK_a 8.8.

Partition Coefficient. Log *P* (octanol/water), 2.3.

Colour Tests. Liebermann's Test—black; Mandelin's Test—violet-brown.

Thin-layer Chromatography. System TA—Rf 42; system TB—Rf 02; system TE—Rf 47; system TAE—Rf 24. (Acidified iodoplatinate solution, positive.)

Gas Chromatography. System GA—RI 3281.

High Performance Liquid Chromatography. System HA—k 4.7; system HX—RI 347.

Ultraviolet Spectrum. Aqueous acid—258 (A^1_1 = 312 b). No alkaline shift.

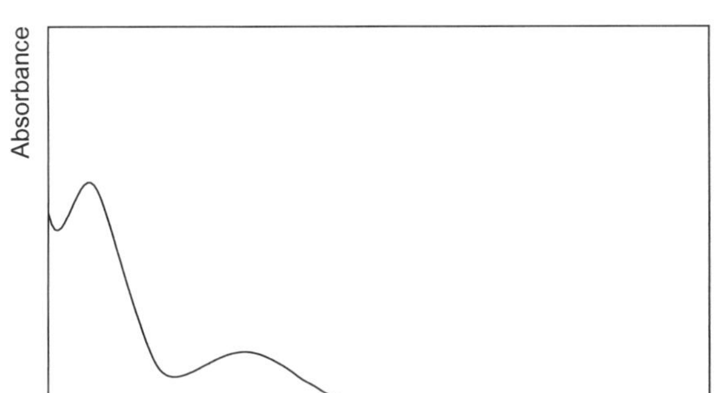

Infra-red Spectrum. Principal peaks at wavenumbers 1123, 1230, 1575, 1505, 1616, 990 cm^{-1} (KBr disk).

Mass Spectrum. Principal ions at *m/z* 58, 195, 59, 72, 388, 89, 315, 42.

Quantification

Gas chromatography–mass spectrometry. In saliva: limit of detection <100 µg/L—T. A. Robert *et al.*, *J. Chromatogr.*, 1981, *224*; *B Biomed. Appl.*, *13*, 116–121.

High performance liquid chromatography. In serum: UV detection—T. A. Robert *et al.*, *J. Clin. Pharmacol.*, 1982, *22*, 53–58.

Disposition in the Body

Therapeutic concentration

Following a single oral dose of 250 mg to 4 subjects, peak blood concentrations of 1.3 to 2.4 µg/mL (mean 1.7) were attained in 1.5 h [R. C. Baselt and R. H. Cravey, *J. Anal. Toxicol.*, 1977, *1*, 81–103].

Toxicity

In a fatality involving the ingestion of trimethobenzamide, postmortem blood and bile concentrations of 184 mg/L and 1150 mg/L, respectively, were reported; a postmortem blood-alcohol concentration of 1100 mg/L was also reported [J. C. Harrill, *Bull. Int. Assn. Forens. Toxicol.*, 1976, *12*(2), 29–30].

Dose. 0.75 to 1 g daily.

Trimethoprim

Antimicrobial

Synonyms. BW-56-72; NSC-106568; Trimethoprimum; Trimethoxyprim.
Proprietary names. Ipral; Monotrim; Primsol; Proloprim; Tiempe; Trimogal; Trimopan; Trimpex; Uretrim; Wellcoprim. It is an ingredient of Bactrim, Borgal (vet.), Chemotrim, Cotrim, Fectrim, Laratrim, Polytrim, Septra, Septrin, SMZ-TMP, Sulfatrimand Trivetrin (vet.).
5-[(3,4,5-Trimethoxyphenyl)methyl]-2,4-pyrimidinediamine
$C_{14}H_{18}N_4O_3 = 290.3$
CAS—738-70-5

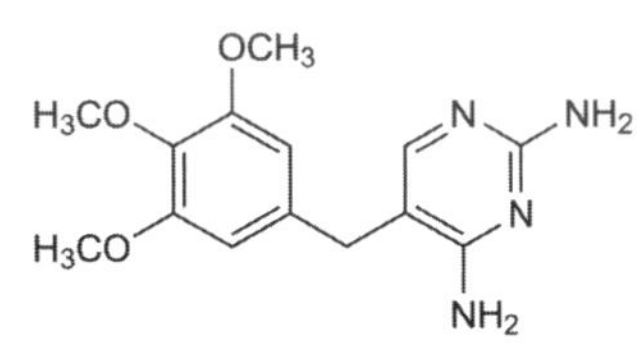

White or yellowish-white crystals or crystalline powder. M.p. 199° to 203°. Soluble 1 in 2500 of water, 1 in 300 of ethanol, 1 in 55 of chloroform and 1 in 80 of methanol; practically insoluble in ether.

Dissociation Constant. pK_a 7.2; 6.6.

Partition Coefficient. Log *P* (octanol/water), 0.91.

Colour Tests. Aromaticity (Method 2)—yellow/red; Mandelin's Test—yellow-brown; Marquis Test—orange.
Cold nitric acid gives a red colour which fades to yellow on heating.

Thin-layer Chromatography. System TA—Rf 55; system TB—Rf 00; system TC—Rf 22; system TE—Rf 45; system TL—Rf 12; system TAD—Rf 20; system TAE—Rf 45; system TAF—Rf 59; system TAJ—Rf 14; system TAK—Rf 08; system TAL—Rf 66. (Acidified iodoplatinate solution, positive.)

Gas Chromatography. System GA—trimethoprim RI 2558, trimethoprim-AC_2 RI 3000.

High Performance Liquid Chromatography. System HA—*k* 1.2; system HX—RI 299; system HY—RI 254; system HZ—Retention time, 2.1 min; system HAA—Retention time, 8.3 min; system HAX—Retention time 6.7 min; system HAY—Retention time 3.7 min.

Ultraviolet Spectrum. Aqueous acid—271 nm (A^1_1=218a); aqueous alkali—287 nm (A^1_1=250a).

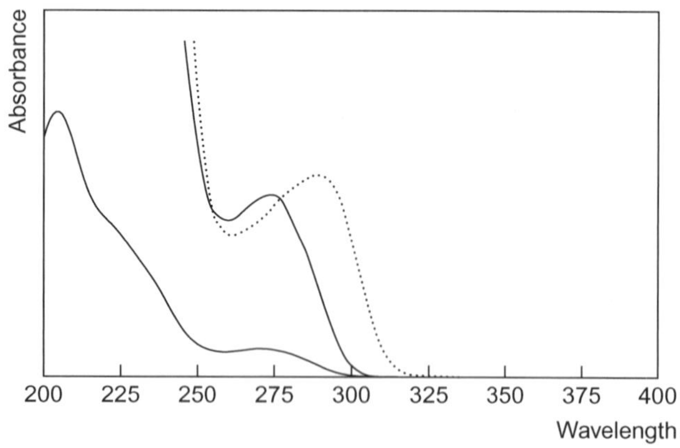

Infra-red Spectrum. Principal peaks at wavenumbers 1126, 1630, 1596, 1235, 1650, 1565 cm^{-1} (KBr disk).

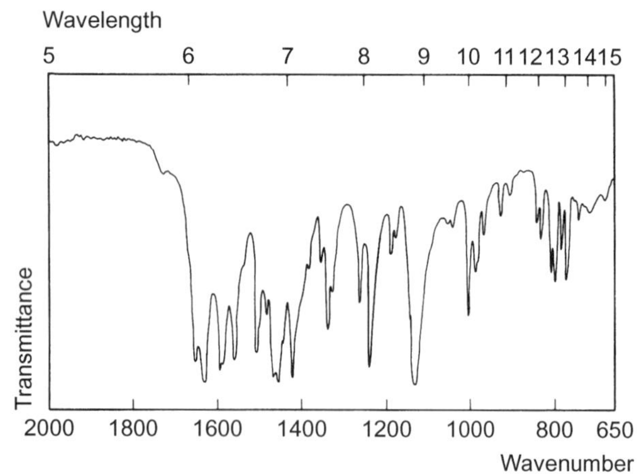

Mass Spectrum. Principal ions at *m/z* 290, 259, 275, 291, 243, 123, 200, 43.

Quantification

Gas chromatography. In plasma or urine: limit of detection 0.1 mg/L, AFID—G. Land *et al.*, *J. Chromatogr.*, 1978, *146*; *Biomed. Appl.*, *3*, 143–147.

High performance liquid chromatography. In serum or urine: limit of detection 0.01 mg/L, electrochemical detection—L. Nordholm and L. Dalgaard, *J. Chromatogr.*, 1982, *233*; *Biomed. Appl.*, *22*, 427–431. In serum or urine: limit of detection 0.1 mg/L, UV detection—R. Gochin *et al.*, *J. Chromatogr.*, 1981, *223*; *Biomed. Appl.*, *12*, 139–145.

High performance liquid chromatography–mass spectrometry. In tissues: limit of detection is 4 μg/kg, (SIM: *m/z* 291)—A. Cannavan *et al.*, *Analyst*, 1997, *122(11)*, 1379–1381.

Disposition in the Body. Readily and rapidly absorbed after oral administration. Trimethoprim is widely distributed around the body to tissues and fluids including kidneys, liver, lung and bronchial secretions, saliva, aqueous humour and vaginal secretions. Metabolic reactions include oxidation of the methylene group to a hydroxymethyl group, *N*-oxidation, *O*-demethylation, hydroxylation and conjugation with glucuronic acid or sulfate. 10 to 20% of a dose is metabolised. Metabolites are excreted in the urine as conjugates but the greater part of the dose is excreted as unchanged drug. Urinary excretion is pH-dependent and is increased in acid urine. About 40 to 75% of a dose is excreted in 24 h, up to 60% being in the form of unchanged drug, with about 4% each as the 3′-hydroxymethyl and 4′-hydroxymethyl metabolites, and 2% as the N^1-oxide. Less than 4% is eliminated in the faeces. It readily crosses the placenta and has been detected in breast milk.

Therapeutic concentration. The serum therapeutic concentration ranges from 1.5 to 2.5 mg/L.

Following oral administration of 300 mg once daily to 6 subjects, maximum steady-state plasma concentrations of 3.1 to 9.5 mg/L (mean 6.0) were attained in 1 to 4 h (mean 2) [B. Odlind *et al.*, *Eur. J. Clin. Pharmacol.*, 1984, *26*, 393–397].

For further references to trimethoprim when administered with sulfamethoxazole, see under Sulfamethoxazole.

Toxicity. Toxic effects have been associated with plasma concentrations greater than 20 mg/L. Bone marrow depression may result owing to the administration of high doses of trimethoprim or use for extended periods of time.

A 28-year-old man ingested 8 g of trimethoprim and 14 h later the plasma concentration was 19.6 mg/L. It was estimated that the actual amount of trimethoprim absorbed was about 3 g. The patient subsequently recovered [K. Hoppu *et al.*, *Lancet*, 1980, *1*, 778].

Half-life. Plasma half-life, 8 to 17 h (mean 11).

Volume of distribution. About 1.4 L/kg.

Clearance. Plasma clearance, about 2 mL/min/kg.

Distribution in blood. Plasma:whole blood ratio, about 0.78.

Saliva. Plasma:saliva ratio, about 1.3.

Protein binding. In plasma, 40 to 70%.

Note. For a review of the clinical pharmacokinetics of sulfamethoxazole and trimethoprim see R. B. Patel and P. G. Welling, *Clin. Pharmacokinet.*, 1980, *5*, 405–423.

Dose. Doses of 1.5 g daily for 3 days have been given for malaria. For acute infection (oral): adults, 100 to 200 mg twice daily or a 100 to 300 mg single dose; children, 6 to 8 mg/kg daily; (6 to 12 years old) 100 mg twice daily; (6 month to 5 years old) 50 mg twice daily; (6 weeks to 5 months) 25 mg twice daily. (Intravenous): 200 mg every 12 h (adults); 6 to 9 mg/kg daily (children).

Trimethoxyamfetamine

Hallucinogen

Synonym. Trimethoxyamphetamine

α-Methyl-3,4,5-trimethoxyphenethylamine

$C_{12}H_{19}NO_3 = 225.3$

CAS—1082-88-8

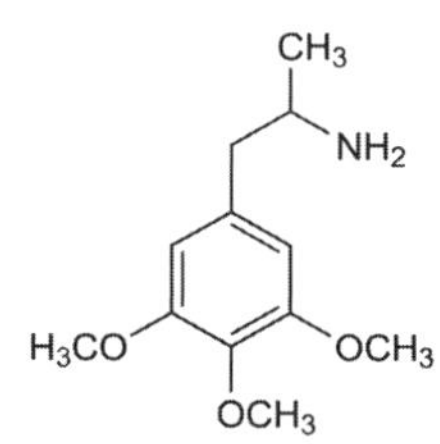

Trimethoxyamfetamine is the α-methyl homologue of mescaline.

An oil.

Practically insoluble in water; soluble in chloroform.

Trimethoxyamfetamine chloride

The hydrochloride is soluble in water; m.p. 219° to 220°.

Partition Coefficient. Log *P* (octanol/water), 1.2.

Colour Test. Marquis Test—orange.

Thin-layer Chromatography. System TA—Rf 33 (2,4,6-TMA); system TB—Rf 06 (2,4,6-TMA); system TC—Rf 11 (2,4,6-TMA); system TE—Rf 29 (2,4,6-TMA); system TL—Rf 12 (2,4,6-TMA); system TAE—Rf 07 (2,4,6-TMA); system TAF—Rf 70 (2,4,6-TMA). (Acidified iodoplatinate solution, positive.)

Gas Chromatography. System GA—RI 1748.

High Performance Liquid Chromatography. System HC—k 1.48; system HX—RI 290 (2,4,6-TMA); system HY—RI 232 (3,4,5-TMA); 298 (2,4,6-TMA).

Ultraviolet Spectrum. Aqueous acid—269 (A_1^1 = 26 b). No alkaline shift.

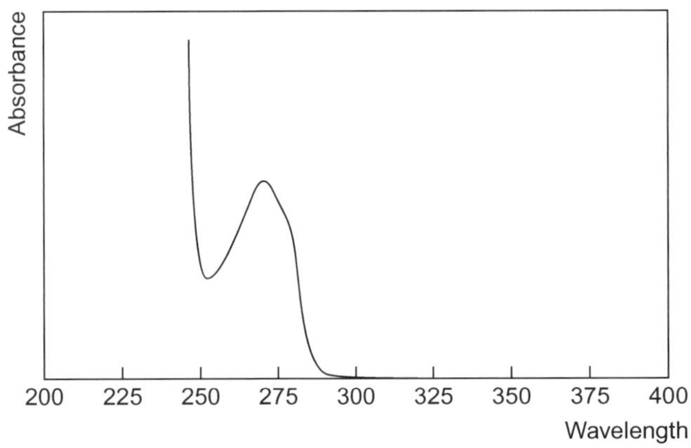

Infra-red Spectrum. Principal peaks at wavenumbers 1130, 1595, 1510, 1240, 1000, 1151 cm^{-1} (KBr disk).

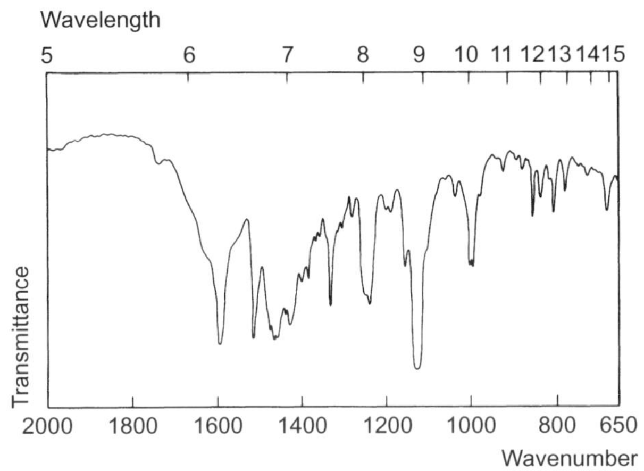

Mass Spectrum. Principal ions at *m/z* 43, 182, 167, 225, 181, 183, 151, 142.

Trimetozine

Tranquilliser

Synonyms. Trimethoxazine; Trimolide.
Proprietary names. Opalene; Trioxazine
4-(3,4,5-Trimethoxybenzoyl)morpholine
$C_{14}H_{19}NO_5$ = 281.3
CAS—635-41-6

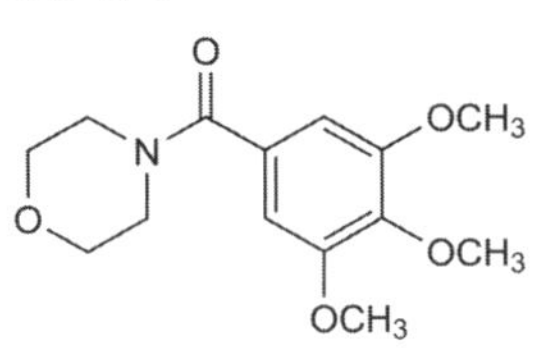

A white crystalline powder. M.p. about 120° to 122°.
Slightly soluble in water and ethanol; freely soluble in chloroform and methanol.

Partition Coefficient. Log *P* (octanol/water) −0.2.

Colour Tests. Liebermann's Test—black; Marquis Test—red-brown.

Thin-layer Chromatography. System TA—Rf 61; system TAE—Rf 80; system TL—Rf 52; system TB—Rf 11; system TC—Rf 72; system TE—Rf 68. (Acidified iodoplatinate solution, positive.)

Gas Chromatography. System GA—RI 2253.

Ultraviolet Spectrum. Methanol—245 nm (A_1^1 = 259b).

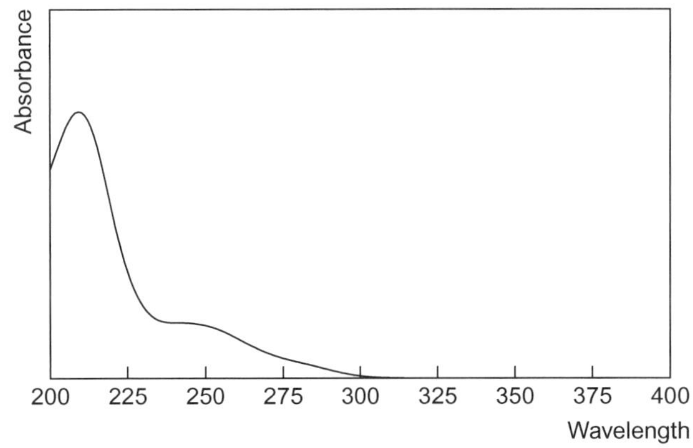

Infra-red Spectrum. Principal peaks at wavenumbers 1131, 1642, 1229, 1110, 1592, 1001 cm^{-1} (KBr disk).

Mass Spectrum. Principal ions at *m/z* 195, 281, 196, 152, 280, 81, 77, 66.

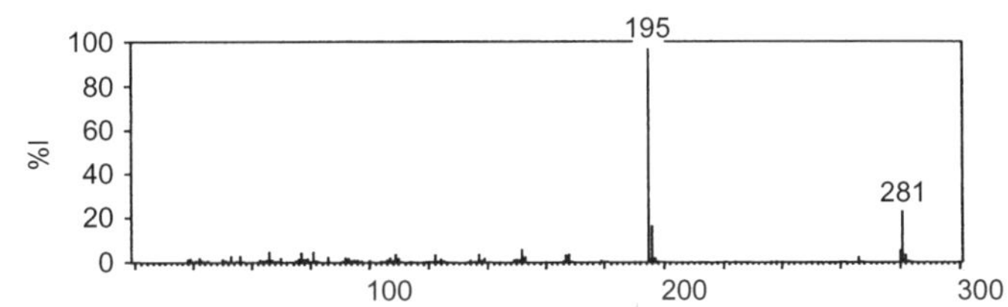

Dose. Usually 0.6 to 1.8 g daily; maximum of 3 g daily.

Trimetrexate

Antineoplastic

Synonyms CI-898; JB-11; NSC-249008.
5-methyl-6-[[(3,4,5-trimethoxyphenyl)amino]methyl]-2,4-quinazoline-diamine
$C_{19}H_{23}N_5O_3$ = 369.4
CAS—52128-35-5

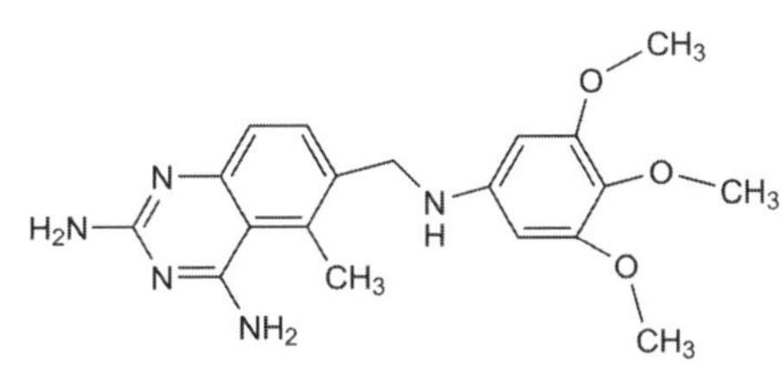

M. p. 215° to 217°. It is practically insoluble in water (<0.1 g/L).

Trimetrexate D-Glucuronate

Synonyms. NSC-352122; 2,4-Diamino-5-methyl-6-[(3,4,5-triethoxyanilino)methyl] quinazoline mono-D-glucuronate; Trimetrexate D-glucuronate; D-Glucuronic acid compound with 5-methyl-6-{[(3,4,5-trimethoxyphenyl)amino]methyl.
Proprietary names. NeuTrexin; Oncotrex.
$C_{25}H_{33}N_5O_{10}$ = 563.6
CAS—82952-64-5
A pale greenish to yellow powder or cake. It is soluble in water (>50 g/L).

Dissociation Constant. pK_a (50% methanol/water), 8.0.

Partition Coefficient. Log *P* (octanol/water), 1.63; 2.55.

Gas Chromatography Column: fused silica (5 m × 0.32 mm i.d.), cross-linked methyl silicone liquid (0.17 mm film thickness). Column temperature: 200° (0.1 min hold) at 15°/min to 300°. Carrier gas: helium, 1.0 mL/min. MS detection: electron ionisation, SIM. Reference compound: 2,4-diamino-5-methyl-6-[(4-chloroanilino)-methyl] quinazoline. Retention time: 3.7 min [P. L. Stetson and W. D. Ensminger *et al.*, *J. Chromatogr., B Biomed. Appl.*, 1986, *383*, 69–76].

High Performance Liquid Chromatography. Column: TMS (Zorbax, 250 × 4.6 mm i.d., 5 µm). Mobile phase: acetonitrile:$(NH_4)H_2PO_4$ (50 mM) containing 0.8% triethylamine and 0.2% phosphoric acid (pH 4.5), flow rate 1.2 mL/min. Internal standard (IS): *N*-6-(phenylmethyl)-2,4,6-quinazolinetriamine. UV detection (λ = 241 nm). Retention times: trimetrexate, 9.4 min; IS, 12.0 min [W. Bullen *et al.*, *J. Chromatogr.*, 1990, *526*, 266–272].

Column: ODS C_{18} (Hypersil 100 × 4.6 mm i.d., 5 µm). Mobile phase: (gradient elution) (A)-acetonitrile; (B)-buffer—0.16% triethylamine containing 0.08% orthophosphoric acid (85%), pH 4.2. (A:B) initial conditions (9:91) to (35:65), re-equilibrated at initial conditions for 5 min, flow rate 1.5 mL/min. IS: trimethoprin. UV detection (λ = 241 nm). RT: trimetrexate 11.0 min; IS, 5.8 min [P. Tinsley and F. LaCreta, *J. Chromatogr.*, 1990, *529*, 468–472].

Column: ODS (Spherisorb, 100 × 4.6 mm i.d., 5 µm). Mobile phase: acetonitrile:triethylamine (0.08%) (15:85 to 40:60 over 10 min), flow rate 1.5 mL/min. UV detection (λ = 241 nm). Retention time: 7.6 min [G. Hudes *et al.*, *Cancer Chemother. Pharmacol.*, 1989, *24*, 117–122].

Mass Spectrum. Principal ions at *m/z* 331, 332, 73, 201, 315, 333, 513, 217 (bis TMS derivative).

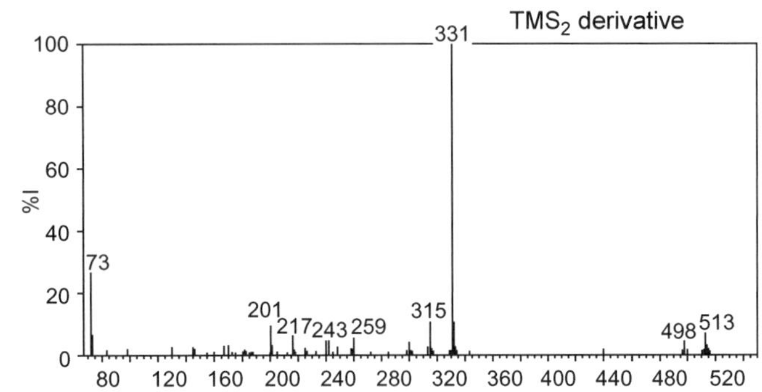

Quantification

Gas chromatography–mass spectrometry. In plasma: limit of detection 0.005 µg/L—P. L. Stetson and W. D. Ensminger, *J. Chromatogr.*, *B Biomed. Appl.*, 1986, *383(1)*, 69–76.

High performance liquid chromatography. In blood: limit of quantification 2.4 µg/L, UV detection (λ = 241 nm)—W. Bullen *et al.*, *J. Chromatogr.*, 1990, *526*, 266–272. In urine: limit of quantification 100 µg/L, UV detection (λ = 241 nm)—P. Tinsley and F. La Creta, *J. Chromatogr.*, 1990, *529*, 468–472. In blood and urine: limit of quantification 100 µg/L, UV detection (λ = 241 nm)—G. Hudes *et al.*, *Cancer Chemother. Pharmacol.*, 1989, *24*, 117–122. In blood, faeces and urine: limit of quantification is 0.02 µg/L, 0.05 µg/L and 0.05 µg/L, respectively, UV detection (λ = 254 nm)—J. Lin *et al.*, *Cancer Res.*, 1987, *47*, 609–619.

Disposition in the Body. Metabolism has not been characterised in humans for trimetrexate. However, pre-clinical data suggest that the major metabolic pathway is oxidative *O*-demethylation, followed by conjugation to either its glucuronide or the sulfate. *N*-demethylation and oxidation are related minor pathways. Preliminary findings in humans indicate the presence of a glucuronide conjugate with DHFR inhibition and a demethylated metabolite in urine. Trimetrexate is extensively metabolised by the liver and eliminated by hepatic metabolism via cytochrome P450 system. At least two metabolites are active and two are conjugated with glucuronic acid. Hepatic degradation may account for the low and variable oral absorption. About 50% of dose is excreted in urine with 10 to 30% as the unchanged drug, and 0.1 to 8% in faeces.

Therapeutic concentration

A paediatric patient with AIDS and PCP was administered with a 30 mg/m² dose trimetrexate daily for 21 days. A peak plasma concentration of 8 mg/L was reached [M. J. Smit *et al.*, *Pediatr. Infect. Dis. J.*, 1990, *9*, 212–214 (discussion 215)].

49 adult patients with AIDS and PCP (in combination with calcium folinate) were administered with 30 mg/m² trimetrexate for 21 days and peak plasma concentrations of 4.4 mg/L were observed by the end of infusion [C. J. Allegra *et al.*, *N. Engl. J. Med.*, 1987, *317*, 978–985].

6 adult patients with AIDS and PCP (in combination with calcium folinate) were administered with 30 mg/m² daily for 21 days and peak plasma concentrations of 3.1 mg/L were detected. A dose of 60 mg/m² daily for 3 days, produced peak concentrations of 1.2 mg/L [P. Rogers *et al.*, *Antimicrob. Agents Chemother.*, 1988, *32*, 324–326].

Toxicity. Administration without concurrent leucovorin can cause lethal complications.

Bioavailability. Mean oral bioavailability, 44% (range, 19 to 67%).

Half-life. 11 to 16.4 h.

Volume of distribution. Plasma, 0.17 L/kg; steady state, 0.62 L/kg (20 L/m²); steady state in AIDS patients, 11 to 20 L/m²; in cancer patients, 12 to 42 L/m².

Clearance. Plasma clearance, 53 mL/min.

Protein binding. >97%.

Dose. 45 mg/m²/day.

Trimipramine

Antidepressant

Synonyms. IL-6001; 7162-R; Trimeprimine; Trimeproprimine.
Proprietary name. Tydamine
10,11-Dihydro-*N*,*N*,*β*-trimethyl-5*H*-dibenz[*b*,*f*]azepine-5-propanamine
$C_{20}H_{26}N_2$=294.4
CAS—739-71-9

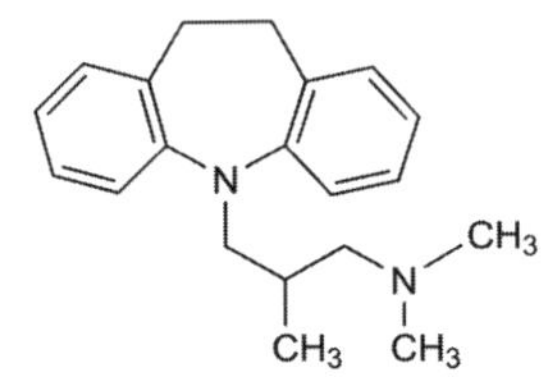

A pale yellowish-white waxy solid. M.p 45°.
Practically insoluble in water; readily soluble in ethanol.

Trimipramine Maleate

Synonym. Trimipramine Hydrogen Maleate
Proprietary names. Apo-Trimip; Herphonal; Novo-Tripramine; Rhotrimine; Stangyl; Surmontil; Tripress.
$C_{20}H_{26}N_2,C_4H_4O_4$=410.5
CAS—521-78-8
A white to almost white crystalline powder. M.p. 142°.
Slightly soluble in water and ethanol; soluble in chloroform; practically insoluble in ether.

Partition Coefficient. Log *P* (octanol/water), 5.43.

Colour Tests. Forrest Reagent—blue; FPN Reagent—blue; Mandelin's Test (add water)—blue.

Thin-layer Chromatography. System TA—Rf 59; system TB—Rf 62; system TC—Rf 54; system TE—Rf 80; system TL—Rf 37; system TAE—Rf 36; system TAF—Rf 56. (Acidified iodoplatinate solution, positive.)

Gas Chromatography. System GA—trimipramine RI 2215, M (OH-) RI 2575, M (OH-methoxy-) RI 2590, M (nor-ring) RI 1930; system GB—trimipramine RI 2302, M (nor-) RI 2335, M (OH-) RI 2631, M (nor-OH-) RI 2662, M (OH-methoxy-) RI 2715, M (nor-ring) RI 2107; system GF—RI 2505; system GS—Retention time: 16.3 min.

Column: OV-1 fused silica (25 m × 0.32 mm i.d., 0.2 µm film thickness). Column and injector temperatures: 195° and 280°, respectively. Carrier gas: helium, flow rate 2.5 mL/min. Detection: nitrogen–phosphorous. ISs: clomipramine and maprotiline. Retention time(s): trimipramine, 5.9 min; desmethyltrimipramine, 6.9 min; 2-hydroxytrimipramine, 16.0 min; 2-hydroxydesmethyltrimipramine, 18.0 min; clomipramine, 12.0 min; maprotiline, 8.5 min [N. Jourdil *et al.*, *J. Chromatogr.*, 1993, *613*, 59–65].

High Performance Liquid Chromatography. System HA—trimipramine *k* 2.7, M (nor-) *k* 1.8; system HF—*k* 6.17; system HX—RI 454; system HY—RI 345; system HZ—Retention time, 8.3 min; system HAA—Retention time, 15.9 min; system HAX—Retention time 15.5 min; system HAY—Retention time, 7.7 min.

Column: Chiralcel OD-R (250 × 4.6 mm i.d., 10 µm); guard, RP C_8 (15 × 1.0 mm i.d.). Mobile phase: 0.3 M aqueous sodium perchlorate:acetonitrile (58:42), flow rate 0.5 mL/min. UV detection (λ = 210 nm). k values (Retention time(s)): *R*-trimipramine, 2.41 (19.6 min); *S*-trimipramine, 2.87 (22.3 min) [J. Liu and J. T. Stewart, *J. Chromatogr. B Biomed. Sci. Appl.*, 1997, *700(1-2)*, 175–182].

Ultraviolet Spectrum. Aqueous acid—250 nm (A_1^1 = 300a).

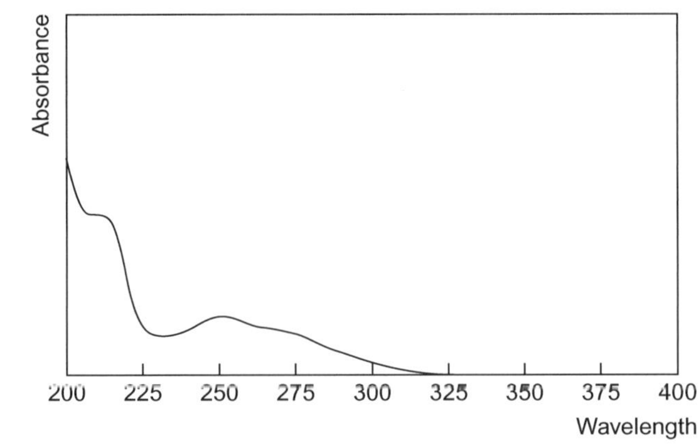

Infra-red Spectrum. Principal peaks at wavenumbers 1490, 762, 1240, 1230, 741, 749 (KBr disk).

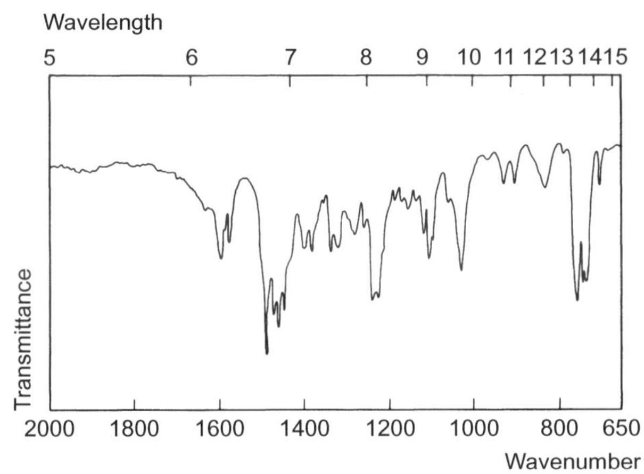

Mass Spectrum. Principal ions at *m/z* 58, 249, 208, 99, 193, 234, 84, 248.

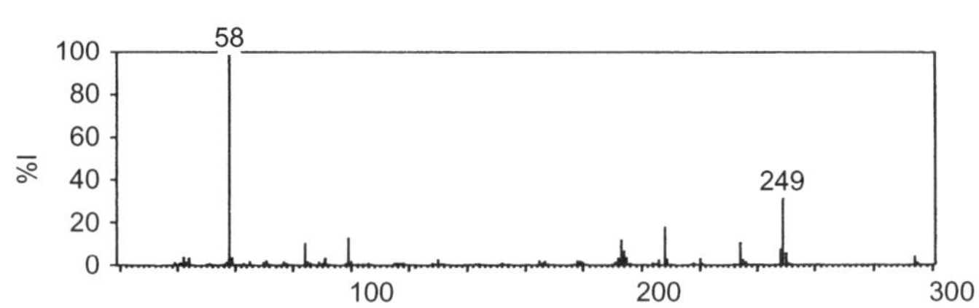

Quantification

Gas chromatography. In plasma: limit of quantification 125 µg/L, NPD—S. Ulrich and J. Martens, *J. Chromatogr. B Biomed. Sci. Appl.*, 1997, *696*, 217–234. In whole blood: limit of detection 32 to 50 µg/L, FID—X. P. Lee *et al.*, *J. Chromatogr. Sci.*, 1997, *35*, 302–308. In plasma and red blood cells: limit of detection 3 µg/L for trimipramine and 4 µg/L for desmethyltrimipramine and hydroxytrimipramine, NSD—N. Jourdil *et al.*, *J. Chromatogr.*, 1993, *613(1)*, 59–65.

Gas chromatography–mass spectrometry. In plasma: limit of quantification is 4 µg/L for trimipramine and 2 µg/L for desmethyltrimipramine, SIM (*m/z* 249)—C. B. Eap *et al.*, *J. Chromatogr.*, 1994, *652(1)*, 97–103.

High performance liquid chromatography. In serum: limit of quantification 15 µg/L and limit of detection 10 µg/L, UV detection (λ = 210 nm)—J. Liu and J. T. Stewart, *J. Chromatogr. B Biomed. Sci. Appl.*, 1997, *700(1-2)*, 175–182. In plasma: limit of detection is 5 µg/L—T. Visser *et al.*, *J. Chromatogr.*, 1984, *309(1)*, 81–93.

Disposition in the Body. Readily absorbed after oral administration but undergoes considerable first-pass metabolism to the active metabolite, *N*-monodesmethyltrimipramine. Didesmethyltrimipramine, 2-hydroxytrimipramine and 2-hydroxydesmethyltrimipramine have also been detected as metabolites. Excreted in the urine mainly as metabolites.

Therapeutic concentration

A single oral dose of 50 mg administered to 9 subjects, resulted in peak plasma concentrations of 15 to 51 µg/L (mean 28) in 1 to 6 h [D. R. Abernethy *et al.*, *Clin. Pharmacol. Ther.*, 1984, *35*, 348–353].

Following daily oral doses of 75 or 150 mg to 29 subjects, the following steady-state plasma concentrations were reported: trimipramine 10 to 240 µg/L (mean 90), *N*-monodesmethyltrimipramine 3 to 380 µg/L (mean 70), 2-hydroxytrimipramine 3 to 40 µg/L (mean 16), and 2-hydroxy-*N*-monodesmethyltrimipramine 3 to 50 µg/L (mean 17) [R. F. Suckow and T. B. Cooper, *J. Pharm. Sci.*, 1984, *73*, 1745–1748].

10 patients receiving 75 mg of trimipramine daily had a mean steady-state plasma concentration of 53.8 µg/L trimipramine and 26.3 µg/L desmethyl trimipramine, whereas 10 others receiving 150 mg daily had a mean concentration of 122.5 µg/L trimipramine and 133.8 µg/L desmethyltrimipramine, representing a markedly disproportionate increase [M. N. Musa, *J. Clin. Pharmacol.*, 1989, *29*, 746–747].

Toxicity. Toxic effects have been associated with plasma concentrations greater than 1 mg/L; serum concentrations greater than 0.5 mg/L. A lethal serum concentration of 8.7 mg/L has been noted.

In a fatality involving the ingestion of up to 6 g of trimipramine, the following postmortem tissue concentrations were reported: blood 9.5 mg/L, brain 27 mg/kg, kidney 42 mg/kg, liver 224 mg/kg, spleen 31 mg/kg [J. J. Rousseau and M. Rousiseau, *Bull. Int. Assoc. Forensic Toxicol.*, 1970, *7(3)*, 5–6].

In a fatality involving the ingestion of trimipramine and clomipramine, postmortem concentrations were: blood, trimipramine 11.6 mg/L, clomipramine 2.1 mg/L; liver, trimipramine 544 mg/kg, clomipramine 56 mg/kg [R. S. Hucker, *Bull. Int. Assoc. Forensic Toxicol.*, 1983, *17(2)*, 20–22].

Investigation into the death of a 53-year-old woman concluded that she had taken an acute (suicidal) overdose of trimipramine and citalopram. Postmortem toxicological examination revealed the following tissue concentrations (in mg/L or mg/kg; TM = trimipramine; DTM = desmethyltrimipramine; CP = citalopram; DCP = desmethylcitalopram):

	TM	DTM	CP	DCP
Heart blood	11.81	4.07	4.82	2.30
Femoral blood	2.33	1.13	4.81	2.45
Liver	38.35	12.06	11.89	5.89
Kidney	30.57	–	13.34	–
Urine	8.46	–	13.00	–
Brain	10.39	–	1.98	–
Bile	–	–	3.31	–

Zolpidem was also detected (0.07 mg/L in heart blood, 1.12 mg/L in femoral blood, 0.19 mg/kg in kidney) [F. Musshoff *et al.*, *Forensic Sci. Int.*, 1999, *106*, 125–131].

Bioavailability. About 40% with wide inter-subject variation.

Half-life. Plasma half-life, 16 to 40 h (mean 24).

Volume of distribution. About 20 to 50 L/kg (mean 30).

Clearance. Plasma clearance, 10 to 25 mL/min/kg (mean 16).

Distribution in blood. Plasma:whole blood ratio, 1.2.

Protein binding. In plasma, about 94%.

Dose. Initially, 50 to 75 mg trimipramine daily; increased as necessary to 150 to 300 mg. In the elderly, 10 to 25 mg is administered initially and increased as necessary. (In the USA, initially 50 mg is administered and a maximum of 100 mg to the elderly).

Trioxysalen

Pigmenting Agent

Synonyms. 4,5′,8-Trimethylpsoralen; Trioxsalen.
Proprietary names. Puvadin; Tripsor; Trisoralen.
2,5,9-Trimethyl-7*H*-furo[3,2-*g*][1]benzopyran-7-one
$C_{14}H_{12}O_3$=228.2
CAS—3902-71-4

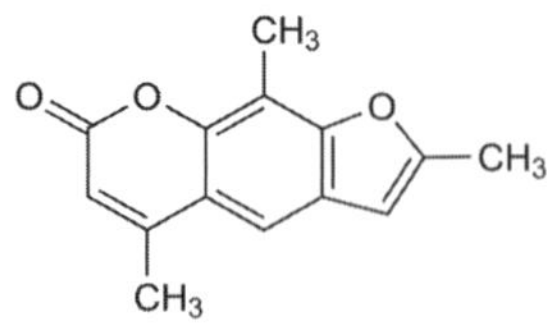

A white or greyish crystalline solid. M.p. about 230°.
Practically insoluble in water; soluble 1 in 1150 of ethanol, 1 in 84 of chloroform and 1 in 43 of methylene chloride.

Partition Coefficient. Log *P* (octanol/water), 3.7.

Gas Chromatography. System GA—RI 2155.

Ultraviolet Spectrum. Methanol—248 nm (A^1_1=981b), 296 nm (A^1_1=428b), 338 nm (A^1_1=276b).

Infra-red Spectrum. Principal peaks at wavenumbers 1710, 1600, 1110, 880, 930, 1620 cm^{-1} (Nujol mull).

Mass Spectrum. Principal ions at *m/z* 228, 200, 199, 128, 229, 185, 115, 201.

Quantification
Gas chromatography–mass spectrometry. In blood or skin—A. M. Ros *et al.*, *Photodermatology*, 1988, *5*, 121–125.

High performance liquid chromatography. In blood, ophthalmic fluid or skin: limit of detection 2 µg/L, UV detection—S. G. Chakrabarti *et al.*, *J. Invest. Dermatol.*, 1982, *79*, 374–377.

Dose. 5 to 10 mg daily.

Tripelennamine

Antihistamine

N,*N*-Dimethyl-*N*′-(phenylmethyl)-*N*′-2-pyridinyl-1,2-ethanediamine
$C_{16}H_{21}N_3$=255.4
CAS—91-81-6

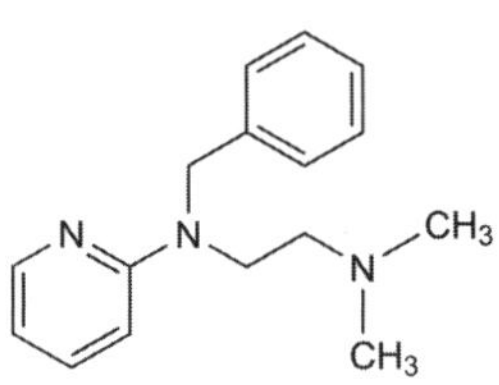

An oily yellow liquid.
Miscible with water.

Tripelennamine Citrate
Proprietary name. PBZ (elixir)
$C_{16}H_{21}N_3,C_6H_8O_7$=447.5
CAS—6138-56-3
A white crystalline powder. M.p. 106° to 110°.
Freely soluble in water and ethanol; practically insoluble in benzene and chloroform; very slightly soluble in ether.

Tripelennamine Hydrochloride
Proprietary names. Azaron; Etono; Fenistil; PBZ (tablets); Pyribenzamine; Vaginex.
$C_{16}H_{21}N_3$,HCl=291.8
CAS—154-69-8
A white crystalline powder which slowly darkens on exposure to light. M.p. 192° to 193°.
Soluble 1 in about 0.8 of water, 1 in 6 of ethanol, 1 in 6 of chloroform and 1 in about 350 of acetone; practically insoluble in ether and benzene.

Dissociation Constant. pK_a 3.9, 9.0 (25°).

Partition Coefficient. Log *P* (octanol/water), 2.7.

Colour Tests. Cyanogen Bromide—yellow; Liebermann's Test—orange→brown; Mandelin's Test—yellow-brown; Marquis Test—red-brown.

Thin-layer Chromatography. System TA—Rf 55; system TB—Rf 44; system TC—Rf 27; system TE—Rf 68; system TL—Rf 15; system TAE—Rf 22; system TAF—Rf 34; system TAJ—Rf 02; system TAK—Rf 00; system TAL—Rf 18. (Dragendorff spray, positive; acidified iodoplatinate solution, positive; Marquis reagent, brown.)

Gas Chromatography. System GA—tripelennamine RI 1976; M (OH-) RI 2400, M (OH-)-AC RI 2390, M (benzylpyridylamine) RI 1650; M (nor-) RI 2420, M (nor-)-AC RI 2420, M (nor-OH-)-AC_2 RI 2860.

High Performance Liquid Chromatography. System HA—*k* 3.6; system HX—RI 336; system HY—RI 265.

Ultraviolet Spectrum. Aqueous acid—239 nm (A^1_1=562a), 314 nm; aqueous alkali—249, 312 nm.

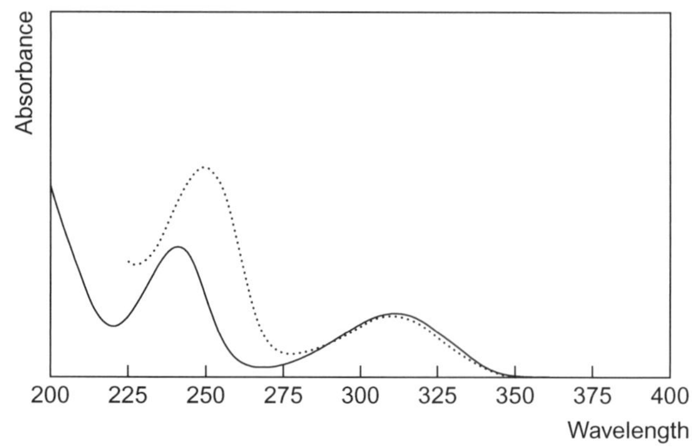

Infra-red Spectrum. Principal peaks at wavenumbers 1496, 1592, 770, 1250, 955, 735 cm^{-1} (tripelennamine hydrochloride, KBr disk).

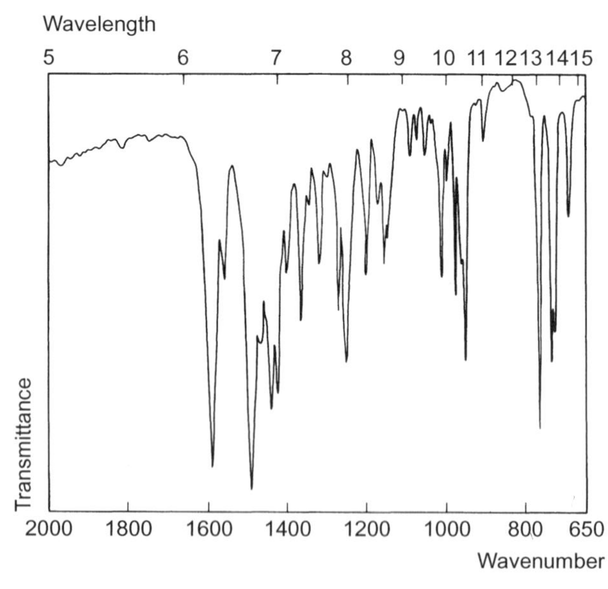

Mass Spectrum. Principal ions at *m/z* 58, 91, 72, 71, 197, 185, 184, 92.

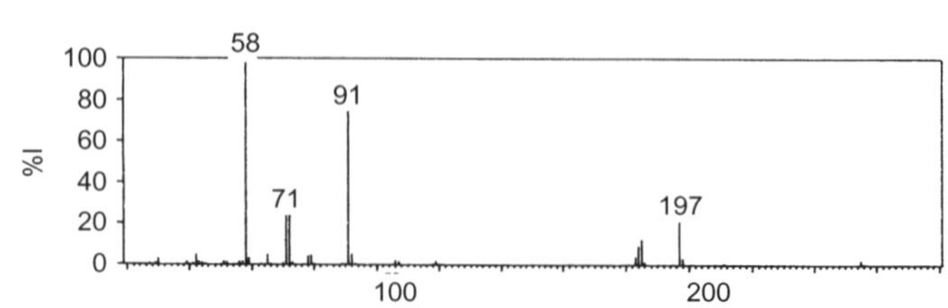

Quantification

Gas chromatography. In postmortem tissues: FID—J. R. Monforte *et al.*, *J. Forensic Sci.*, 1983, *28*, 90–101.

Disposition in the Body. Rapidly absorbed after oral administration. Metabolised by ring hydroxylation and demethylation followed by conjugation with glucuronic acid. It is excreted in the urine, mainly as metabolites, and in the bile, and appears to undergo enterohepatic circulation. The major urinary metabolites are tripelennamine-*N*-glucuronide, conjugated hydroxytripelennamine and the conjugated hydroxydesmethyl metabolite; the *N*-oxide is a minor metabolite.

Therapeutic concentration

After a single oral dose of 100 mg, a peak plasma concentration of 0.06 mg/L was reported to have been attained in 2 to 3 h [M. Bayley *et al.*, *J. Forensic Sci.*, 1975, *20*, 539–543.]

Toxicity

Fatal intracranial haemorrhage occurred in a 30-year-old man following intravenous abuse of pentazocine and tripelennamine (approx. 125 mg of each was injected over the 6 h before admission) together with oral phenylpropanolamine (a 75 mg extended-release preparation was taken 20 h before onset of neurological symptoms); gastric aspirate from admission contained pentazocine 8.2 mg/L and tripelennamine 2.0 mg/L [C. Jackson *et al.*, *J. Emerg. Med.*, 1985, *3*, 127–132.]

In one fatality arising from the ingestion of about 1 g, in which death occurred about 7 h after ingestion, the following postmortem tissue distribution was reported: blood 10 mg/L, brain 43 µg/g, kidney 35 µg/g, liver 83 µg/g, urine 287 mg/L [M. Bayley *et al.*, *J.Forensic Sci.*, 1975, *20*, 539–543].

In 17 fatalities involving the intravenous abuse of tripelennamine and pentazocine, tripelennamine blood concentrations of 0 to 3.0 mg/L (mean 0.5) were reported; kidney concentrations of 0.4 to 2.0 µg/g (mean 1.1) were reported in 4 subjects and liver concentrations of 1.0 to 6.5 µg/g (mean 3.1) in 5 subjects; pentazocine blood concentrations ranged from 0 to 11 mg/L (mean 3) [J. R. Monforte *et al.*, *J. Forensic Sci.*, 1983, *28*, 90–101.]

Dose. 25 to 50 mg of tripelennamine hydrochloride every 4 to 6 h; up to 600 mg daily has been given.

Triphenyltetrazolium Chloride

Diagnostic Agent

Synonyms. Red Tetrazolium; RT; TPTZ; TTC.
Proprietary name. VitaStain
2,3,5-Triphenyl-2*H*-tetrazolium chloride
$C_{19}H_{15}ClN_4$=334.8
CAS—298-96-4

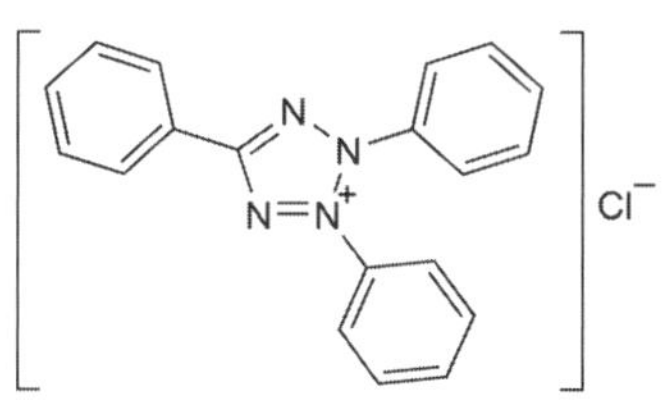

A white crystalline powder which turns yellow on exposure to light. M.p. 243°, with decomposition.
Soluble in water, ethanol and acetone; insoluble in ether.

Partition Coefficient. Log *P* (octanol/water), −2.4.

Colour Tests. Liebermann's Test—red-orange; Mandelin's Test—blue (slow).

Thin-layer Chromatography. System TA—Rf 61. (Acidified iodoplatinate solution, positive.)

Ultraviolet Spectrum. Aqueous acid—246 nm (A_1^1=680b).

Infra-red Spectrum. Principal peaks at wavenumbers 691, 769, 1529, 720, 1164, 998 cm^{-1} (KBr disk).

Triprolidine

Antihistamine

2-[(1E)-1-(4-Methylphenyl)-3-(1-pyrrolidinyl)-1-propenyl]pyridine
$C_{19}H_{22}N_2$=278.4
CAS—486-12-4

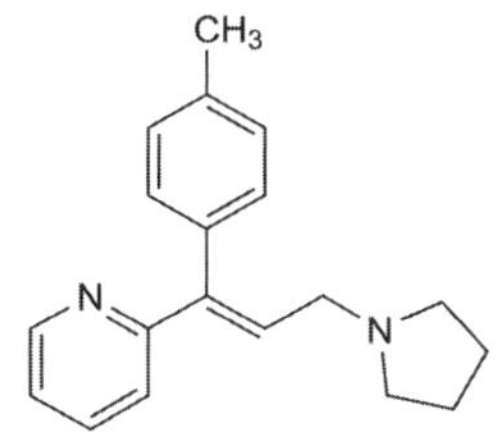

Crystals. M.p. 59° to 61°.

Triprolidine Hydrochloride

Proprietary names. Actidil; Actidilon; Myidyl; Pro-Actidil. It is an ingredient of Actifed.
$C_{19}H_{22}N_2,HCl,H_2O$=332.9
CAS—550-70-9 (anhydrous); 6138-79-0 (monohydrate)
A white crystalline powder. M.p. 116° to 118°.
Soluble 1 in about 2 of water, 1 in about 1.5 of ethanol, 1 in less than 1 of chloroform and 1 in 2000 of ether.

Dissociation Constant. pK_a 6.5.

Partition Coefficient. Log *P* (octanol/water), 3.9.

Colour Tests. Cyanogen Bromide—orange-pink (after 1 to 2 min); Liebermann's Test—orange.

Thin-layer Chromatography. System TA—Rf 51; system TB—Rf 11; system TC—Rf 20; system TE—Rf 55; system TL—RF 06; system TAE—Rf 19; system TAF—Rf 30; system TAJ—Rf 95; system TAK—Rf 03; system TAL—Rf 69. (Dragendorff spray, positive; Acidified iodoplatinate solution, positive.)

Gas Chromatography. System GA—RI 2253; system GB—RI 2340; system GC—RI 2954; system GF—RI 2600.

High Performance Liquid Chromatography. System HA—*k* 3.2; system HX—RI 388; system HY—RI 270; system HAA—Retention time 13.1 min.

Ultraviolet Spectrum. Aqueous acid—290 nm (A_1^1=347a). (See below.)

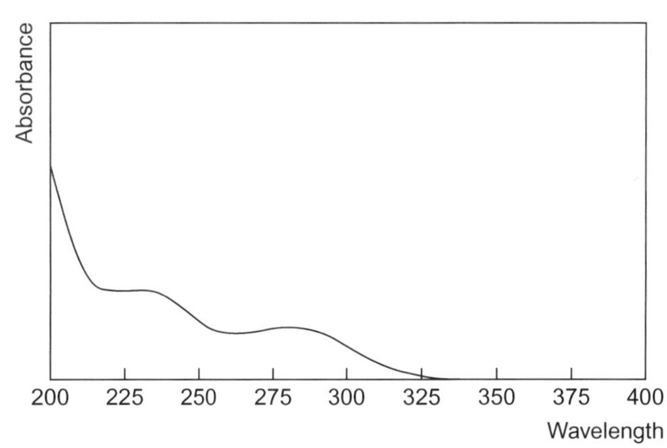

Infra-red Spectrum. Principal peaks at wavenumbers 775, 1580, 825, 990, 1509, 1146 cm^{-1} (triprolidine hydrochloride, KBr disk). (See below.)

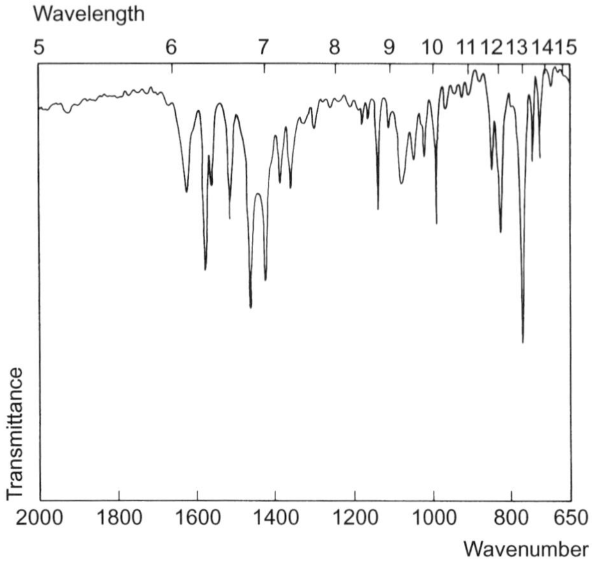

Mass Spectrum. Principal ions at *m/z* 208, 209, 278, 207, 193, 200, 194, 84.

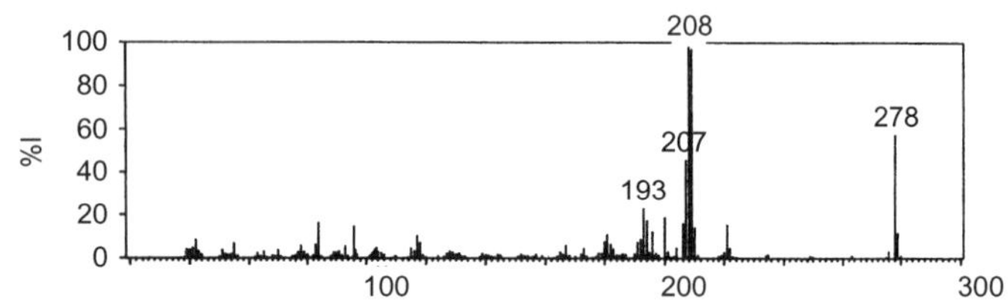

Quantification

High performance liquid chromatography–mass spectrometry. In biological samples: triprolidine and its metabolite hydroxymethyltriprolidine, limit of detection 10 μg—E. B. Hansen *et al.*, *J. Anal. Toxicol.*, 1989, *13*, 185–187.

Thin-layer chromatography–densitometry. In plasma: limit of detection 800 ng/L—R. L. DeAngelis *et al.*, *J. Pharm. Sci.*, 1977, *66*, 841–843.

Disposition in the Body. Irregularly absorbed after oral administration.

Therapeutic concentration

Following oral administration of 15 mL of a syrup containing 3.75 mg of triprolidine hydrochloride to 16 subjects, peak plasma concentrations of 0.004 to 0.017 mg/L (mean 0.009) were attained in about 2 h [R. L. DeAngelis *et al.*, *J. Pharm. Sci.*, 1977, *66*, 841–843.]

Following oral administration of 2.5 mg of triprolidine hydrochloride and 60 mg of pseudoephedrine hydrochloride four times a day to 17 subjects for 5 days, peak plasma-triprolidine concentrations of 0.004 to 0.044 mg/L (mean 0.013) were reported about 1.6 h after a dose [J. G. Perkins *et al.*, *Curr. Ther. Res.*, 1980, *28*, 650–668.]

In 6 subjects receiving single oral doses of triprolidine hydrochloride (2.5 mg), peak plasma concentrations of 0.0027 to 0.0085 mg/L (mean 0.0056) were achieved at 0.8 to 3.2 h (mean 2.0). After wearing transdermal patches releasing triprolidine (base) 5 or 10 mg for 24 h, the same subjects had peak plasma concentrations of 0.001 to 0.003 mg/L (mean 0.002) at 6.1 to 17.9 h (mean 12.0) and 0.0022 to 0.0062 mg/L (mean 0.0042) at 4.4 to 24.2 h (mean 14.3), respectively [M. V. Miles *et al.*, *J. Clin. Pharmacol.*, 1990, *30*, 572–575.]

Half-life. Plasma half-life, 1.5 to 20 h (mean 5).

Dose. Usually 7.5 to 15 mg of triprolidine hydrochloride daily.

Troglitazone

Antidiabetic

Synonyms. CL-991; CS-045; GR-92132X; Romglizone.
Proprietary names. Noscal; Rezulin; Romozin.
5-[[4-[(3,4-Dihydro-6-hydroxy-2,5,7,8-tetramethyl-2H-1-benzopyran-2-yl)-methoxy]phenyl]methyl]-2,4-thiazolidineodione
$C_{24}H_{27}NO_5S = 441.5$

CAS—97322-87-7

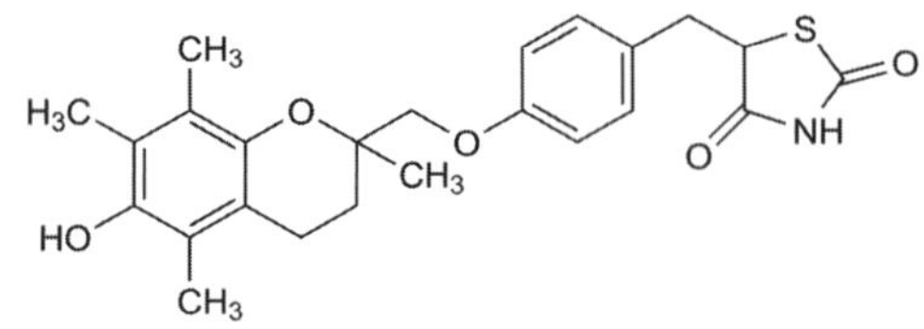

A white to yellowish crystalline compound with a characteristic odour. M.p. 184° to 186°. It is practically insoluble in water; soluble in *N,N*-dimethylformamide and acetone; sparingly soluble in ethyl acetate; slightly soluble in acetonitrile, anhydrous ethanol and ether.

High Performance Liquid Chromatography. Column: ODS (300 × 6.0 mm i.d., 5 μm). Mobile phase: acetonitrile:water:phosphoric acid (60:40:0.08), flow rate 1.2 mL/min. UV detection (λ=230 nm). Retention time: 23.2 min [C. Loi *et al.*, *J. Clin. Pharmacol.*, 1997, *37*, 1114–1120].

Ultraviolet Spectrum. acetonitrile—225 nm.

Quantification

Gas chromatography. In plasma: limit of quantification is 40 nmol/L—M. Bjork and K. Pettersson, *J. Chromatogr.*, 1990, *533*; *Biomed. Appl.*, 229–234.

High performance liquid chromatography. In blood: limit of quantification 0.1 mg/L—C. Loi *et al.*, *J. Clin. Pharmacol.*, 1997, *37*, 1114–1120. In tablets: limit of detection is 0.05 mg/L. UV detection (λ=225 nm)—J. Lambropoulos and A. B. Bergholdt, *J. Pharm. Biomed. Anal.*, 2000, *24(2)*, 251–258.

Disposition in the Body. Troglitazone is rapidly absorbed and widely distributed into body tissues following oral administration. Absorption is increased in the presence of food, and peak plasma concentrations are reached generally 1 to 3 h after administration. It is extensively metabolised in the liver primarily by conjugation, and is excreted largely in the faeces as its metabolites. A few metabolites are also excreted in urine (3%). Steady state concentrations are achieved between 2 and 6 weeks. Three metabolites have been identified, a sulfate conjugate, a quinone conjugate and a glucuronide conjugate. The sulfate conjugate is the most abundant (7 to 10 times that of the parent drug). 85% of the drug is recovered in faeces and 3.1 % in urine. Pharmacokinetics are linear over clinical dosage range of 200 to 600 mg. No accumulation of the drug or its metabolites has been noted.

Therapeutic concentration

12 healthy volunteers and 12 patients with type 2 diabetes were administered 400 mg troglitazone once a day for 15 days. Steady state plasma concentrations were reached by day 5 and peaked at 1.42 mg/L for the healthy individuals and 1.54 mg/L for those with diabetes. These concentrations were observed at 2.63 and 3.25 h, respectively [C. M. Loi *et al.*, *J. Clin. Pharmacol.*, 1997, *37(12)*, 1114–1120].

Toxicity

A 44-year-old woman with a history of type 1 diabetes began treatment with 200 mg troglitazone daily for 4 weeks and then the dose was increased to 400 mg daily. On admission she was icteric, her liver was tender and enlarged with subacute hepatic necrosis, fibrosis and cholestasis. Troglitazone treatment was stopped and after 3 months the patient gradually improved.

A 65-year-old woman with a history of type 2 diabetes was admitted with a 3-week history of nausea, anorexia, pruritus and jaundice. She was currently being treated with 400 mg daily troglitazone (had been for 6 weeks). Histologic tests showed chronic hepatitis (severe activity), hepatocyte necrosis and fibrosis. 3 months after treatment was discontinued, the patient showed improvement [N. Gitlin *et al.*, *Ann. Intern. Med.*, 1998, *129(1)*, 36–38].

Bioavailability. 53%.

Half-life. 10 to 39 h.

Volume of distribution. Steady state 2.5 L/kg.

Clearance. Systemic plasma clearance, 172 mL/min.

Distribution in blood. Distribution into red blood cells is low.

Protein binding. ⩾ 99% at concentrations of 0.5 to 3 mg/L. Primarily to albumin.

Dose. 200 mg.

Troleandomycin

Antibiotic

Synonym. Triacetyloleandomycin
Proprietary names. TAO; Triocetin.
The triacetyl ester of oleandomycin.
$C_{41}H_{67}NO_{15}$=814.0
CAS—2751-09-9
A white crystalline powder. M.p. 176° with decomposition.
Slightly soluble in water and ether; soluble 1 in 10 of ethanol and 1 in 1 of chloroform.

Dissociation Constant. pK_a 6.6.

Partition Coefficient. Log *P* (octanol/water), 2.5.

Colour Tests. Mandelin's Test—violet (slow); Marquis Test—yellow-brown.

Thin-layer Chromatography. System TA—Rf 65. (Acidified iodoplatinate solution, positive.)

Infra-red Spectrum. Principal peaks at wavenumbers 1744, 1239, 1735, 1053, 1004, 1123 cm^{-1} (KBr disk).

Dose. The equivalent of 1 to 2 g of oleandomycin daily.

Trometamol

Treatment of Acidosis

Synonyms. THAM; Trihydroxymethylaminomethane; TRIS; Tris(hydroxymethyl)aminomethane; Tromethamine.
Proprietary names. Addex-THAM; Pleomix-Alpha; Tham: Thamacet; Thamesol; Thioctacid; Tris; TromLipon.
2-Amino-2-hydroxymethyl-1,3-propanediol
$C_4H_{11}NO_3$=121.1
CAS—77-86-1

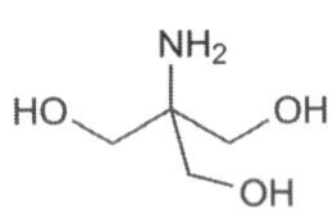

A white crystalline powder. M.p. 171° to 172°.
Soluble 1 in 1.8 of water, 1 in 45 of ethanol and 1 in 38 of methanol; practically insoluble in chloroform; slightly soluble in acetone and ether.

Dissociation Constant. pK_a 8.3 (20°).

Partition Coefficient. Log *P* (octanol/water), −1.6.

Thin-layer Chromatography. System TA—Rf 57. (Ninhydrin spray, positive.)

Gas Chromatography. System GA—RI 1645.

Infra-red Spectrum. Principal peaks at wavenumbers 1031, 1018, 1076, 975, 1582, 1279 cm^{-1} (KBr disk).

Quantification

Gas chromatography. In plasma: limit of detection 5 µg/L, FID—A. Hulshoff and H. B. Kostenbauder, *J. Chromatogr.*, 1978, *145*; *Biomed. Appl.*, *2*, 155–159.

High performance liquid chromatography. In plasma: limit of detection about 0.28 mg/L, UV detection—K. Gumbhir and W. D. Mason, *J. Chromatogr.*, 1992, *583*, 99–104. In plasma or urine: fluorescence detection—M. J. Morris and J. Y. Hieh, *J. Chromatogr.*, 1993, *622*, 87–92.

Thin-layer chromatography. In serum: limit of detection 20 µg—G. Andermann and C. Andermann, *J. High Resolut. Chromatogr. Chromatogr. Commun.*, 1980, *3*, 36–37.

Disposition in the Body. About 75% of a dose is excreted in the urine as unchanged drug in 8 h and the remainder is excreted over a period of 3 days. Trometamol may accumulate in the body if large doses are given frequently.

Therapeutic concentration
Following an intravenous injection of 109 mg to an infant, a plasma concentration of 430 mg/L was reported at 0.5 h, declining to 86 mg/L at 4.5 h [A. Hulshoff and H. B. Kostenbauder, *J. Chromatogr.*, 1978, *145*; *Biomed. Appl.*, *2*, 155–159.]

Dose. Up to 500 mg/kg by intravenous infusion.

Tropicamide

Anticholinergic

Synonym. Bistropamide
Proprietary names. Diotrope; Mydral; Mydramide; Mydriacil; Mydriacyl; Mydrian; Mydriaticum; Mydrum; Myriacyl; Ocu-Tropic; Opticyl; Tropicacyl; Tropicil Top; Tropicol; Tropimil; Visumidriatic.
N-Ethyl-α-(hydroxymethyl)-*N*-(4-pyridinylmethyl)benzeneacetamide
$C_{17}H_{20}N_2O_2$=284.4
CAS—1508-75-4

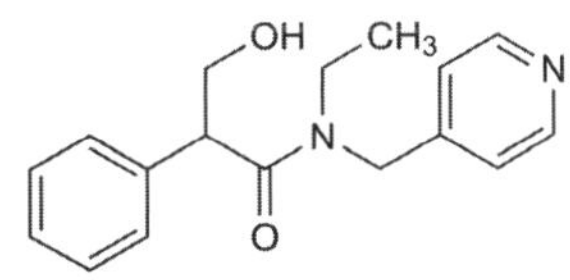

A white crystalline powder. M.p. 96° to 97°.
Soluble 1 in 160 of water, 1 in 3.5 of ethanol, and 1 in 2 of chloroform.

Dissociation Constant. pK_a 5.2.

Partition Coefficient. Log *P* (octanol/water), 1.2.

Colour Tests. Cyanogen Bromide—violet-pink; Liebermann's Test—yellow.

Thin-layer Chromatography. System TA—Rf 65; system TE—Rf 51; system TF—Rf 03; system TAA—Rf 00. (Acidified iodoplatinate solution, positive.)

Gas Chromatography. System GA—tropicamide RI 2335, tropicamide-CH_2O RI 2230, tropicamide-H_2O RI 2250, tropicamide-AC RI 2410; system GB—tropicamide RI 2442.

High Performance Liquid Chromatography. System HX—RI 311.

Ultraviolet Spectrum. Aqueous acid—254 nm (A_1^1=180a); aqueous alkali—256 nm.

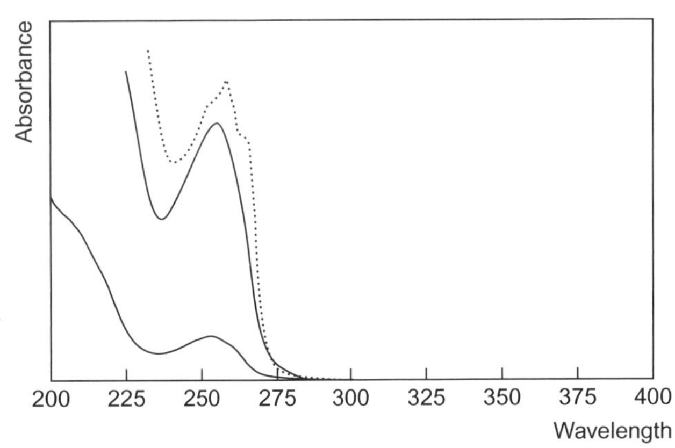

Infra-red Spectrum. Principal peaks at wavenumbers 1627, 1601, 709, 1266, 761, 1070 cm^{-1} (KBr disk).

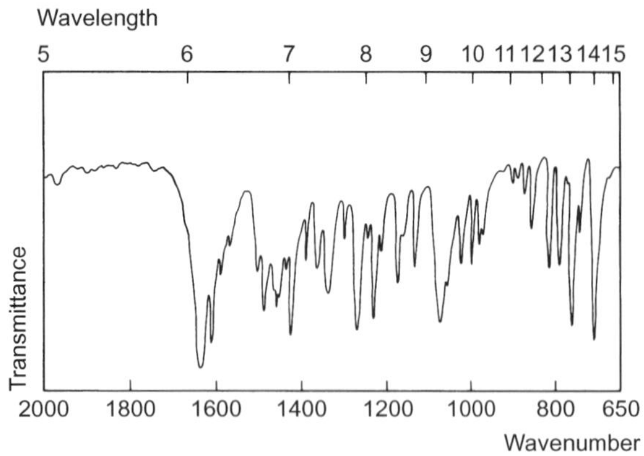

Mass Spectrum. Principal ions at *m/z* 92, 91, 65, 103, 93, 39, 163, 77.

Quantification

High performance liquid chromatography. In aqueous humour: tropicamide and phenylephrine, UV detection—M. J. Galmier *et al.*, *Biomed. Chromatogr.*, 2000, *14*, 202–204.

Use. As a 0.5 to 1% ophthalmic solution.

Tropisetron

Anti-emetic/5-HT$_3$-receptor Antagonist

Synonym. ICS-205-930

1*H*-Indole-3-carboxylic acid (3-*endo*)-8-methyl-azabicyclo[3.2.1]oct-3-yl ester

$C_{17}H_{20}N_2O_2$=284.4

CAS—89565-68-4

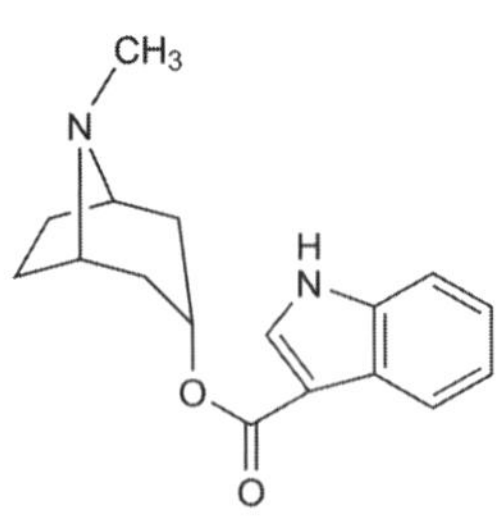

M.p. 201° to 202°.

Tropisetron Hydrochloride

Proprietary names. Navaban; Navoban.

$C_{17}H_{21}ClN_2O_2$=320.8

CAS—105826-92-4

M.p 283° to 285°.

High Performance Liquid Chromatography. Column: Lichrosorb RP18 (250 × 7 mm i.d., 7 µm). Mobile phase: acetonitrile:water and 0.3% triethylamine (5:95 to 15:85 over 30 min, to 20:80 over 10 min, to 90:10 over 20 min). UV detection (λ=283 nm). Retention time: 60 min [V. Fischer *et al.*, *Drug Metab. Dispos.*, 1992, *20(4)*, 603–607].

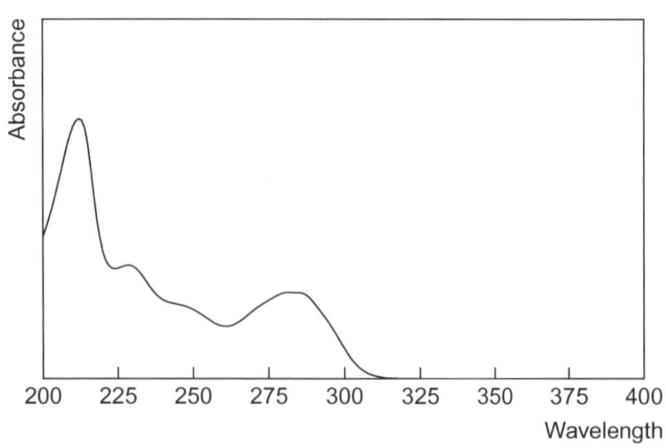

Mass Spectrum. Principal ions at *m/z* 124, 82, 94, 83, 140, 144, 67, 284.

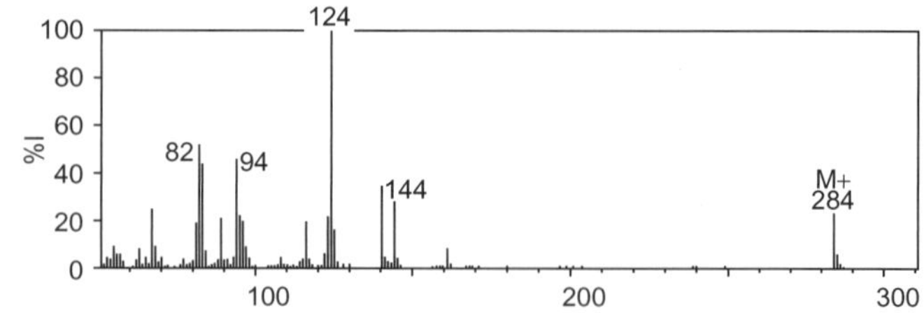

Quantification

High performance liquid chromatography. In plasma: limit of quantification is 0.3 µg/L, UV detection (λ=283 nm)—V. Fischer *et al.*, *Drug Metab. Dispos.*, 1992, *20(4)*, 603–607.

Disposition in the Body. Tropisetron is rapidly and extensively absorbed from the gastro-intestinal tract in approx. 20 min. Peak plasma concentrations are reached in about 3 h. Metabolism is saturable, which results in non-linear pharmacokinetics. It occurs by hydroxylation at the 5, 6 or 7 position of the indole ring, followed by a conjugation reaction to form the glucuronide or sulfate. These metabolites are excreted in urine or bile with a urine:bile ratio of 5:1. Metabolism is linked to a genetically determined sparteine/debrisoquin polymorphism. 8% of the Caucasian population are thought to be poor metabolisers, but there is no change in metabolism in cases of renal impairment or in the elderly. Tropisetron is not accumulative.

Therapeutic concentration. In serum, the trough therapeutic concentration is 20 to 30 mg/L and the peak serum concentrations are 50 to 100 mg/L.

Following an oral dose of 20 or 100 mg, the mean and peak plasma concentrations are 24.7 and 173 µg/L which occurred after 1.3 and 1.1 h [C. Lee *et al.*, *Drugs*, 1993, *46*, 925–943].

12 healthy males were administered 20 or 100 mg single, oral doses and the maximum concentrations observed were 0.087 and 0.608 µg/L, respectively [V. Fischer *et al.*, *Drug Metab. Dispos.*, 1992, *20(4)*, 603–607].

Toxicity. At very high doses of 100 mg for 5 days, visual hallucinations may occur.

Bioavailability. ⩾ 95%. Absolute bioavailability depends on the dose.

Half-life. 7.3 h (intravenous), 8.6 h (oral) in extensive metabolisers; 30.3 h (intravenous) and 41.9 h (oral) in poor metabolisers.

Volume of distribution. 400 to 600 L.

Clearance. In extensive metabolisers, the total clearance is 1 L/min, renal clearance is 10%. In poor metabolisers, total clearance is 0.1 to 0.2 L/min and the renal clearance is unchanged.

Protein binding. 59 to 71%, mainly to α_1 glycoprotein.

Dose. 2 to 5 mg intravenously; 5 mg orally.

Tryptamine

Putrefactive Base

1*H*-Indole-3-ethanamine

$C_{10}H_{12}N_2$=160.2

CAS—61-54-1

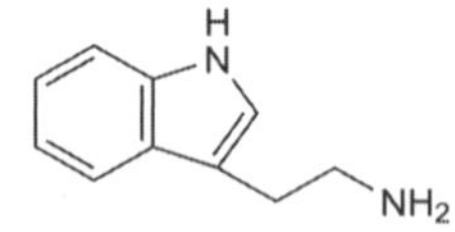

A white crystalline powder. M.p. 118°.

Practically insoluble in water, chloroform, benzene and ether; soluble in ethanol and acetone.

Tryptamine Hydrochloride

$C_{10}H_{12}N_2$,HCl=196.7

CAS—343-94-2

A white crystalline powder. M.p. 248°.

Soluble in water.

Partition Coefficient. Log *P* (octanol/water), 1.6.

Colour Tests. *p*-Dimethylaminobenzaldehyde—red/violet; Formaldehyde–Sulfuric Acid—brown; Marquis Test—orange.

Thin-layer Chromatography. System TA—Rf 23; system TB—Rf 01; system TC—Rf 02; system TE—Rf 26; system TL—Rf 11; system TAE—Rf 06; system TAJ—Rf 00; system TAK—Rf 05; system TAL—Rf 36. (Acidified iodoplatinate solution, positive.)

Gas Chromatography. System GA—Tryptamine RI 1725, tryptamine-AC RI 2390, tryptamine-AC_2 RI 2440.

High Performance Liquid Chromatography. System HA—*k* 1.2; system HY—RI 190.

Ultraviolet Spectrum. Aqueous acid—278 nm (A^1_1=353a), 287 nm.

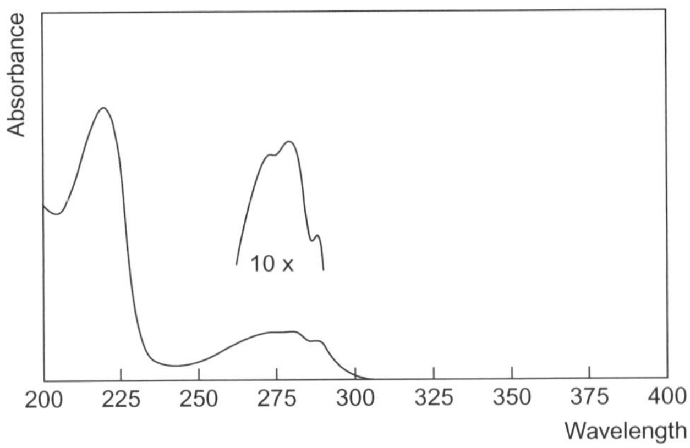

Infra-red Spectrum. Principal peaks at wavenumbers 742, 1585, 1233, 1035, 909, 1494 cm^{-1} (KBr disk).

Mass Spectrum. Principal ions at *m/z* 130, 131, 30, 160, 77, 103, 132, 102.

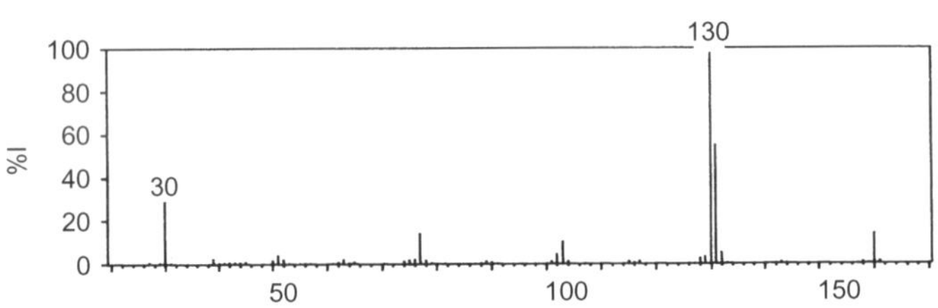

Quantification. See under Tryptophan.

Tryptophan

Amino Acid

Synonyms. L-Trp; L-Tryptophan; Tryptophanum.
Proprietary names. Ardeytropin; Kalma; Optimax; Pacitron; Trofan; Tryptan.
(*S*)-α-Amino-1*H*-indole-3-propanoic acid
$C_{11}H_{12}N_2O_2$=204.2
CAS—73-22-3

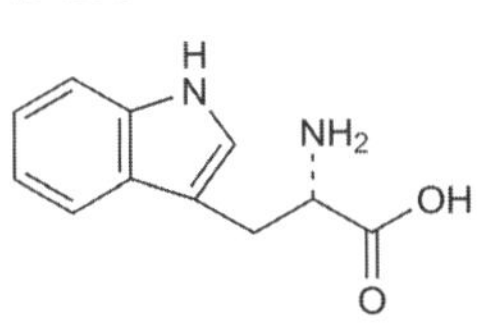

White to slightly yellowish-white crystals or crystalline powder.
Soluble 1 in about 100 of water; very slightly soluble in ethanol; soluble in hot ethanol; insoluble in chloroform; practically insoluble in ether; soluble in solutions of dilute mineral acids and alkali hydroxides.

Gas Chromatography. System GA—tryptophan-Me-AC RI 2150, trytophan-Me_2-AC RI 2170; M (OH-skatole) RI 1370, M (indole acetic acid)-Me RI 1900, M (indole formic acid)-Me RI 1940; M (tryptamine) RI 1725.

Ultraviolet Spectrum. Aqueous acid—278 nm (A^1_1=290b), 286 nm (A^1_1=234b); aqueous alkali—280, 288 nm.

Quantification
High performance liquid chromatography. In urine: tryptamine, fluorescence detection—H. Tsuchiya *et al.*, *Clin. Chem.*, 1989, *35*, 43–47. In serum: limit of detection about 0.6 μmol/L, UV detection—A. Tang *et al.*, *Hunan Yi Ke Da Xue Xue Bao*, 1998, *23*, 605–607, 610. In serum: tryptophan and other amino acids, limit of quantification 5 μM—Y. V. Tcherkas *et al.*, *J. Chromatogr. A.*, 2001, *913*, 303–308.

High performance liquid chromatography–mass spectrometry. In plasma or dried blood: tryptophan and other amino acids—B. Casetta *et al.*, *Clin. Chem. Lab. Med.*, 2000, *38*, 391–401.

Review. In biological tissues or fluids: tryptophan and its metabolites—I. Molnar-Perl, *Adv. Exp. Med. Biol.*, 1999, *467*, 801–816.

Dose. 3 to 6 g daily.

Tuaminoheptane

Sympathomimetic

2-Heptanamine
$C_7H_{17}N$=115.2
CAS—123-82-0

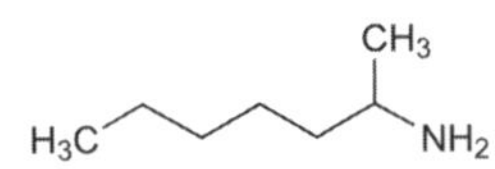

A colourless or pale yellow volatile liquid. B.p.142° to 144°.
It absorbs carbon dioxide on exposure to air, forming a white precipitate of tuaminoheptane carbonate. Sp. gr. 0.760 to 0.763.
Slightly soluble in water; freely soluble in ethanol, ether, chloroform and benzene.

Tuaminoheptane Sulfate

Proprietary names. Tuamine Sulfate. It is an ingredient of R(h)inofluimucil.
$(C_7H_{17}N)_2,H_2SO_4$=328.5
CAS—6411-75-2
A white powder.
Freely soluble in water; soluble in ethanol; sparingly soluble in ether.

Dissociation Constant. pK_a 10.6.

Partition Coefficient. Log *P* (octanol/water), 2.4.

Thin-layer Chromatography. System TA—Rf 33; system TB—Rf 01; system TC—Rf 07; system TL—Rf 24. (Acidified iodoplatinate solution, positive.)

Gas Chromatography. System GA—RI 888; system GC—RI 1287.

Ultraviolet Spectrum. No significant absorption, 230 to 360 nm.

Mass Spectrum. Principal ions at *m/z* 44, 30, 42, 41, 29, 27, 100, 55.

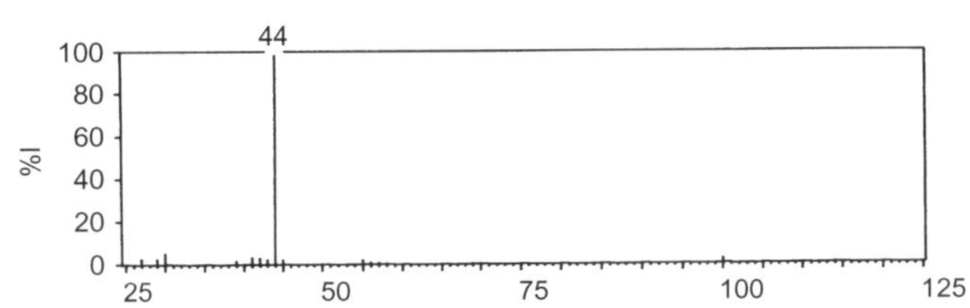

Use. As a 1% solution of the sulfate for nasal drops or spray.

Tubocurarine Chloride

Muscle Relaxant

Synonyms. D-Tubocurarine Chloride; Dextrotubocurarine Chloride.
Proprietary names. Curarina Miro; Curarine; Jexin; Tubarine.
7′,12′-Dihydroxy-6,6′-dimethoxy-2,2′,2′-trimethyltubocuraranium dichloride pentahydrate
$C_{37}H_{42}Cl_2N_2O_6,5H_2O$=771.7
CAS—57-95-4 (tubocurarine); 57-94-3 (chloride, anhydrous); 6989-98-6 (chloride, pentahydrate)

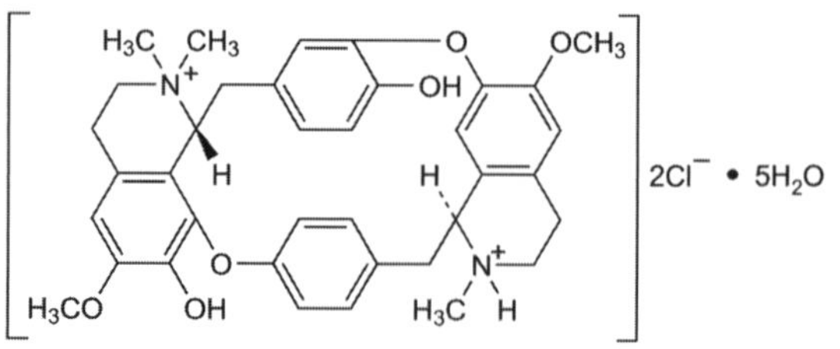

The chloride of an alkaloid, (+)-tubocurarine. It may be obtained from extracts of the stems of *Chondodendron tomentosum* (Menispermaceae).
A white or slightly yellowish-white or greyish-white crystalline powder. M.p. about 270°, with decomposition.
Soluble 1 in 20 of water; soluble in ethanol and methanol; insoluble in chloroform, benzene, acetone and ether.

Dissociation Constant. pK_a 8.0, 9.2 (22°).

Colour Tests. Aromaticity (Method 2)—yellow/brown; Folin–Ciocalteu Reagent—blue; Liebermann's Test—black; Mandelin's Test—brown; Millon's Reagent (hot)—red. Cold nitric acid gives a black colour.

Thin-layer Chromatography. System TA—Rf 00; system TB—Rf 00; system TC—Rf 00; system TE—Rf 00; system TL—Rf 00; system TN—Rf 85; system TO—Rf 40; system TAE—Rf 00; system TAF—Rf 11. (Acidified iodoplatinate solution, positive.)

Gas Chromatography. System GA—RI 2495.

High Performance Liquid Chromatography. System HX—RI 321; system HY—RI 257.

Ultraviolet Spectrum. Water—280 nm (A_1^1=119a).

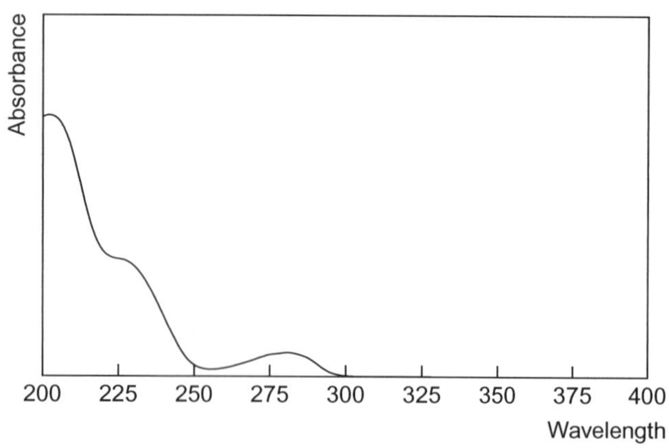

Infra-red Spectrum. Principal peaks at wavenumbers 1516, 1228, 1120, 1280, 1265, 1165 cm^{-1} (KBr disk).

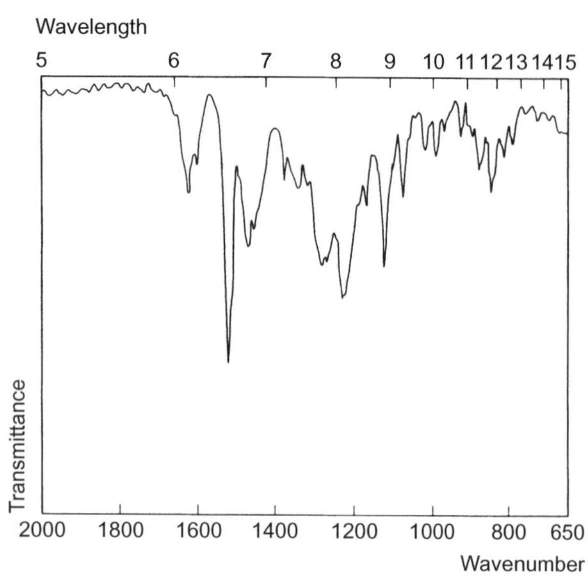

Mass Spectrum. Principal ions at *m/z* 298, 594, 58, 593, 299, 609, 595, 564.

Quantification

Ultraviolet spectrophotometry. In postmortem tissues—H. M. Stevens and R. H. Fox, *J. Forensic Sci. Soc.*, 1971, *11*, 177–182.

High performance liquid chromatography. In plasma: limit of detection 25 µg/L, UV detection—A. Meulemans *et al.*, *J. Chromatogr.*, 1981, *226*; *Biomed. Appl.*, *15*, 255–258.

Radioimmunoassay. In serum or urine: limit of detection 5 µg/L—P. E. Horowitz and S. Spector, *J. Pharmacol. Exp. Ther.*, 1973, *185*, 94–100.

Disposition in the Body. After intravenous administration it is widely distributed throughout the tissues and is concentrated at the neuromuscular junctions; slowly and irregularly absorbed following intramuscular injection. About 45% of a dose is excreted in the urine unchanged in 24 h.

Therapeutic concentration. In plasma, usually in the range 0.7 to 1 mg/L.

After an intravenous bolus of 540 µg/kg followed by constant intravenous infusion of 2.9 µg/kg/min to 9 subjects, a mean steady-state plasma concentration of 1.1 mg/L was attained in about 1 h [M. I. Ramzan *et al.*, *Br. J. Anaesth.*, 1980, *52*, 893–899.]

Toxicity.

In a fatality caused by tubocurarine, a postmortem liver concentration of about 0.8 µg/g was reported [H. M. Stevens and R. H. Fox, *J. Forensic Sci. Soc.*, 1971, *11*, 177–182.]

Half-life. Plasma half-life, about 2 to 4 h.

Volume of distribution. About 0.3 to 0.6 L/kg.

Clearance. Plasma clearance, about 2 mL/min/kg.

Distribution in blood. Plasma:whole blood ratio, 1.9.

Protein binding. In plasma, 33 to 50%.

Note. For a review of the pharmacokinetics of neuromuscular blocking agents see M. I. Ramzan *et al.*, *Clin. Pharmacokinet.*, 1981, *6*, 25–60.

Dose. Initially 10 to 15 mg intravenously, with additional doses of 5 mg.

Tybamate

Tranquilliser

Proprietary names. Nospan; Solacen; Tybatran.
Butylcarbamic acid 2-[[(aminocarbonyl)oxy]methyl]-2-methylpentyl ester
$C_{13}H_{26}N_2O_4$=274.4
CAS—4268-36-4

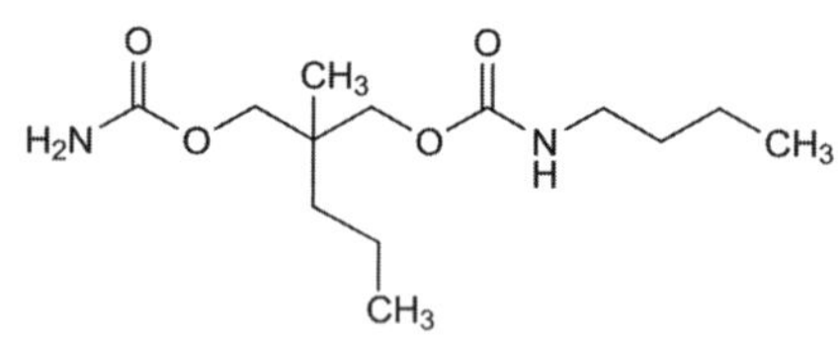

A white crystalline powder or clear viscous liquid which may congeal to a solid form on standing. M.p. of the powder 49° to 51°.
Very slightly soluble in water; very soluble in ethanol and acetone; freely soluble in ether.

Partition Coefficient. Log *P* (octanol/water), 2.9.

Thin-layer Chromatography. System TA—Rf 77; system TD—Rf 35; system TE—Rf 65; system TF—Rf 68. (Furfuraldehyde reagent, positive.)

Gas Chromatography. System GA—RI 1725; system GF—RI 2130.

Ultraviolet Spectrum. No significant absorption, 230 to 360 nm.

Infra-red Spectrum. Principal peaks at wavenumbers 1695, 1250, 1065, 1538, 1600, 1140 cm^{-1} (KBr disk).

Mass Spectrum. Principal ions at *m/z* 55, 72, 97, 41, 56, 158, 118, 57.

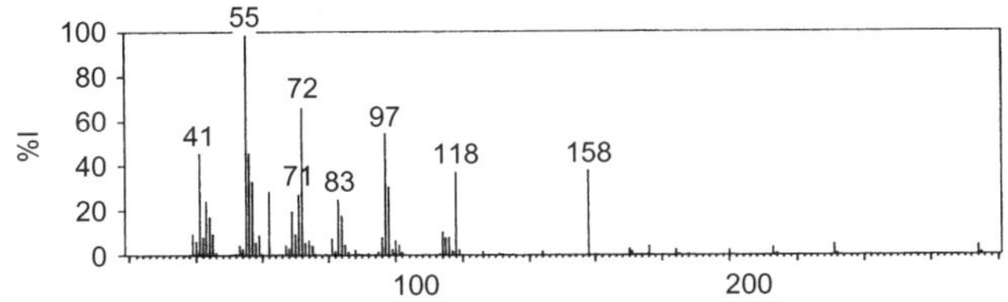

Disposition in the Body. Readily absorbed after oral administration. Metabolised in the liver and excreted in the urine, mainly as hydroxylated compounds. Meprobamate can appear as a minor metabolite.

Half-life. Plasma half-life, about 3 h.

Dose. Usually 0.75 to 2 g daily; maximum of 3 g daily.

Tylosin

Antibiotic (Veterinary)

Proprietary names Bilosin; Norotyl; Tylacre; Tylamix; Tylan; Tyluvet (includes proprietary names of Tylosin salts). Tylosin Tartrate is an ingredient of Tylan Soluble, Tylo and Tylomix. Tylosin phosphate is an ingredient of Tylan G and Tylasul-G.
$C_{46}H_{77}NO_{17}$=916.1
CAS—1401-69-0

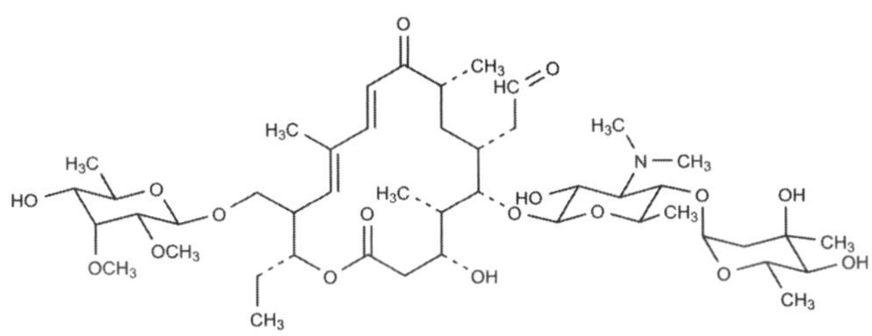

An antimicrobial substance with a macrolide structure, produced by a strain of *Streptomyces fradiae*.
An almost white to buff-coloured powder. M.p. 128° to 132°.
Slightly soluble in water; soluble in lower alcohols, esters, ketones, chlorinated hydrocarbons, benzene and ether.

Tylosin Tartrate
CAS—1405-54-5
A white to buff-coloured hygroscopic powder. M.p. 140° to 146°.
Soluble 1 in 10 of water; slightly soluble in ethanol; very slightly soluble in chloroform; practically insoluble in ether.

Dissociation Constant. pK_a 7.73 (25°).

Partition Coefficient. Log *P* (octanol/water), 1.6.

Colour Tests. Mandelin's Test—yellow→yellow—brown; Marquis Test—yellow-brown; Sulfuric Acid—yellow-brown (slow).

Thin-layer Chromatography. System TA—Rf 72. (Acidified iodoplatinate solution, positive.)

Ultraviolet Spectrum. Aqueous acid—290 nm (A_1^1=225b).

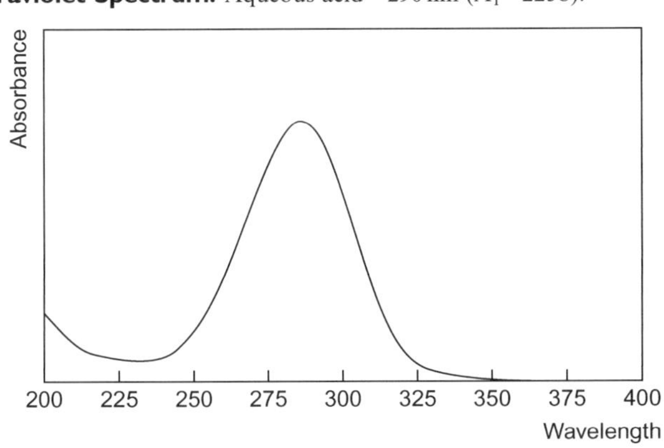

Infra-red Spectrum. Principal peaks at wavenumbers 1075, 1052, 1162, 1111, 1010, 1587 cm^{-1}.

Tyramine

Diagnostic Agent/Sympathomimetic

Synonyms. *p*-Tyramine; Tyrosamine.
4-(2-Aminoethyl)phenol
$C_8H_{11}NO$=137.2
CAS—51-67-2

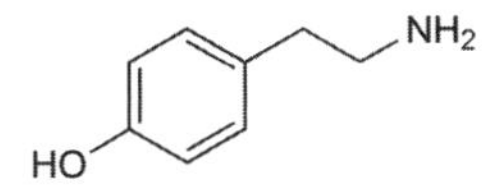

Colourless crystals. M.p. 164° to 165°.
Soluble 1 in 95 of water and 1 in 10 of boiling ethanol; sparingly soluble in benzene and xylene.

Tyramine Hydrochloride
Proprietary name. Mydrial
$C_8H_{11}NO,HCl$=173.6
CAS—60-19-5
Crystals. M.p. 269°.
Soluble in water.

Dissociation Constant. pK_a 9.5 (phenol), 10.8 (-NH_2).

Partition Coefficient. Log *P* (octanol/water), 0.9.

Colour Tests. *p*-Dimethylaminobenzaldehyde—orange/violet; Marquis Test—brown→green.

Thin-layer Chromatography. System TA—Rf 31. (Acidified potassium permanganate solution, positive.)

Gas Chromatography. System GA—tyramine RI 1745; tyramine-AC_2 RI 1950.

High Pressure Liquid Chromatography. System HA—*k* 1.2; system HB—*k* 0.81; system HC—*k* 1.47; system HY—RI 77.

Ultraviolet Spectrum. Aqueous acid—274 nm (A_1^1=110a); aqueous alkali—294 nm (A_1^1=182b).

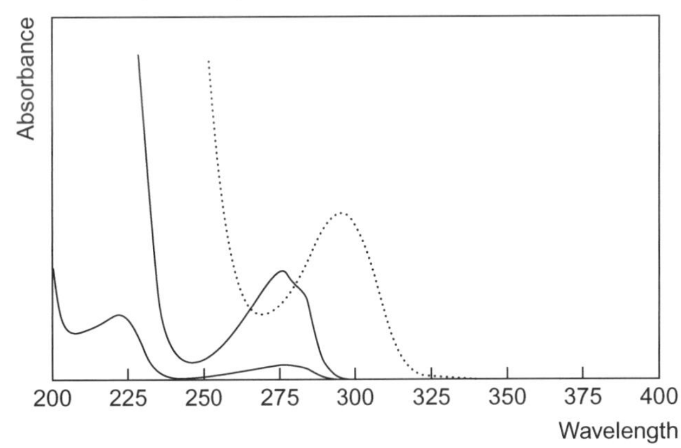

Infra-red Spectrum. Principal peaks at wavenumbers 1266, 1518, 1595, 822, 1495, 1612 cm^{-1} (KBr disk).

Mass Spectrum. Principal ions at *m/z* 30, 108, 107, 77, 39, 51, 137, 27.

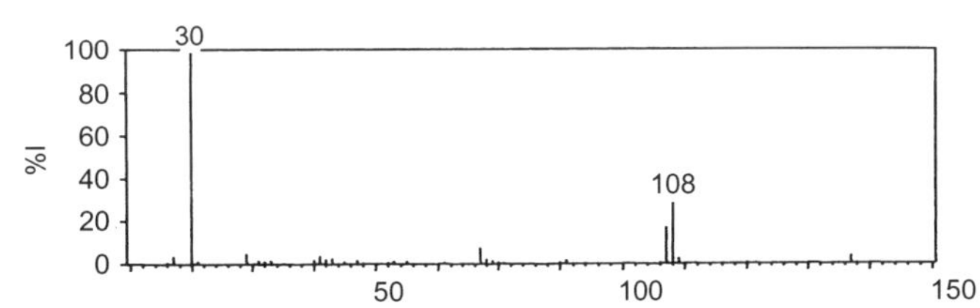

Quantification
Gas chromatography. In urine: limit of detection 25 ng, ECD—R. T. Coutts *et al., Res. Commun. Chem. Pathol. Pharmacol.*, 1980, *28*, 177–184.

Dose. Tyramine hydrochloride has been given by mouth in doses of up to 250 mg daily in the investigation of migraine.

Urea

Diuretic

Synonyms. Carbamide; Ureia; Ureum.
Proprietary names. Aquacare; Aquadrate; Balisa; Basodexan; Calmurid; Calmuril; Carmol; Dermaflex; Elacutan; Fenuril; Gormel; Karbasal; Lanaphilic; Monilen; Nubral; Nutraplus; Ti-U-Lac; Ultra-Mide; Ureacin; Ureaphil; Urecare; Urecrem; Urederm; Uree; Uremol; Urisec.
Carbonyldiamide
$CH_4N_2O=60.1$
CAS—57-13-6

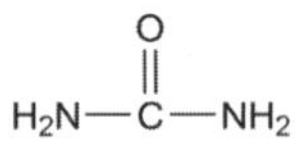

Colourless, slightly hygroscopic, prismatic crystals or pellets, or white crystalline powder. M.p. 133°; decomposes on further heating.
Soluble 1 in about 1 of water, 1 in 6 of methanol, 1 in 10 of ethanol, 1 in 1 of boiling ethanol and 1 in 2 of glycerol; practically insoluble in chloroform and ether.

Dissociation Constant. pK_a 0.1 (21°).

Partition Coefficient. Log *P* (octanol/water), −2.1.

Colour Test. Nessler's Reagent—brown-orange.

Thin-layer Chromatography. System TA—Rf 55; system TE—Rf 15; system TAJ—Rf 05; system TAK—Rf 15; system TAL—Rf 30.

Gas Chromatography. System GA—not eluted.

Mass Spectrum. Principal ions at *m/z* 60, 44, 28, –, –, –, –, –.

Disposition in the Body. Rapidly absorbed after oral administration. Excreted in the urine as unchanged drug and also metabolised to ammonium salts in the colon. Endogenous urinary excretion is in the range 10 to 35 g in 24 h; urea is not usually found in the faeces.

Therapeutic concentration. Endogenous concentrations in blood are about 300 mg/L in adults and lower in infants.

After intravenous infusion of 0.6 to 1.2 g/kg of a solution containing 30% urea and 10% invert sugar to 7 subjects over a period of 0.5 to 2 h, plasma concentrations at the end of the infusion were reported to range from 1160 to 3400 mg/L (mean 2430) [P. R. Yarnell *et al.*, *Clin. Pharmacol. Ther.*, 1972, *13*, 558–562.]

Half-life. Biological half-life, about 1 h.

Dose. 40 to 80 g by intravenous infusion, not exceeding 1.5 g/kg daily.

Urethane

Antineoplastic

Synonyms. Ethyl carbamate; Ethylurethane; Urethan.
Carbamic acid ethyl ester
$C_3H_7NO_2=89.1$
CAS—51-79-6

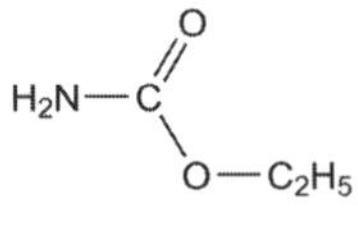

Colourless crystals or white granular powder. M.p. 48° to 50°. B.p. 182° to 184°.
Soluble 1 in 0.5 of water, 1 in 0.8 of ethanol, 1 in 0.9 of chloroform, 1 in 1.5 of ether, 1 in 2.5 of glycerol and 1 in 32 of olive oil.

Partition Coefficient. Log *P* (octanol/water), −0.2.

Gas Chromatography. System GA—RI 838.

Infra-red Spectrum. Principal peaks at wavenumbers 1713, 1075, 1610, 805, 1010 cm^{-1} (KBr disk).

Dose. Formerly given in doses of 3 g daily; maximum of 6 g daily.

Valaciclovir

Antiviral

Synonyms. Valacyclovir; 256U87.
L-Valine 2-[(2-amino-1,6-dihydro-6-oxo-9*H*-purin-9-yl)methoxy]ethyl ester
$C_{13}H_{20}N_6O_4=324.3$
CAS—124832-26-4

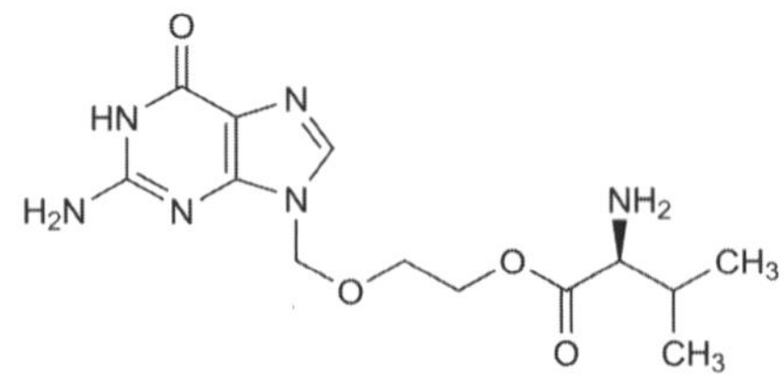

Valaciclovir Hydrochloride

Proprietary names. Valtrex; Zelitrex.
$C_{13}H_{21}ClN_6O_4=360.8$
CAS—124832-27-5
A white to off-white crystalline powder. It is soluble in water (174 g/L at 25°).

Dissociation Constant. pK_a 1.90, 7.47, 9.43.

High Performance Liquid Chromatography. Column: (analytical) RP-8 (SymmetryShield, 250 × 4.6 mm i.d., 5 μm); (guard) RP-8 (20 × 3.9 mm). Mobile phase: acetonitrile:monoammonium phosphate buffer (0.025 M, pH 4.0), flow rate 1.0 mL/min. UV detection (λ=254 nm). Retention time: 9.7 min [C. Pham-Huy *et al.*, *J. Chromatogr. B Biomed. Sci. Appl.*, 1999, *732*, 47–53].

Ultraviolet Spectrum. Aqueous solution—252.8 nm.

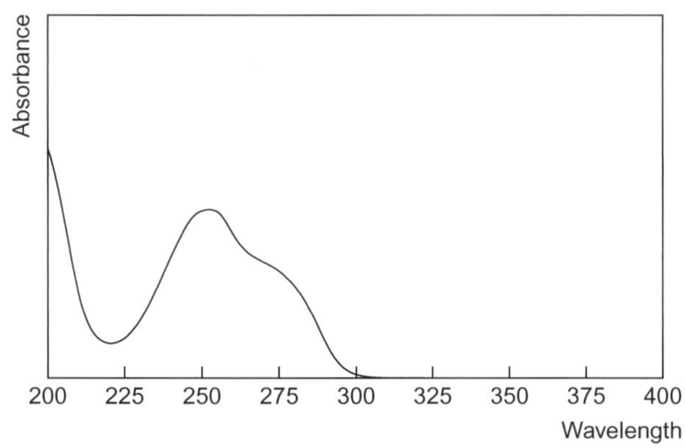

Quantification

High performance liquid chromatography. In plasma: limit of detection 0.625 mg/L—J. M. Poirier *et al.*, *Ther. Drug Monit.*, 1999, *21(1)*, 129–133. In tissue: limit of quantification 0.001 mg/L—P.J. Sinko *et al.*, *Biopharm. Drug. Dispos.*, 1998, *19*, 209–217. In serum: limit of detection is 0.07 mg/L and lower limit of quantification 0.25 mg/L, UV detection (λ=254 nm)—C. Pham-Huy *et al.*, *J. Chromatogr. B Biomed. Sci. Appl.*, 1999, *732*, 47–53.

Disposition in the Body. Valaciclovir is absorbed easily and rapidly from the gastro-intestinal tract after oral administration. Absorption is unaffected by administration with food. Valaciclovir is rapidly converted to aciclovir (99% of a dose) and valine by first-pass intestinal and/or hepatic metabolism, mediated by valaciclovir hydrolase. Plasma concentrations of valaciclovir are undetectable after 3 h and plasma aciclovir concentrations can be detected as early as 15 min. Elimination is renal as aciclovir, and the metabolites 9-carboxymethoxymethylguanine (CMMG) and 8-hydroxy-aciclovir (8-OHACV). Less than 1% of the administered dose of valaciclovir is recovered unchanged in urine over a 24 h period. Peak plasma valaciclovir concentrations are generally less than 0.5 mg/L at all doses. Hepatic impairment does not affect pharmacokinetics. No accumulation of aciclovir occurs after administration of valaciclovir at the recommended dosage regimens in healthy individuals.

Therapeutic concentration

39 elderly normotensive or hypertensive volunteers with a mean age of 72 years were administered the following dose regimen: 500 or 1000 mg valaciclovir twice on day 1; 500 or 1000 mg three times a day for days 2 to 7; and either doses once on day 8 (a total of 21 doses). Peak alaciclovir

concentrations for the normotensive patients receiving 500 mg valaciclovir were 4.14 mg/L on day 1 and 4.30 mg/L on day 8 (steady state) observed at 1.41 and 1.22 h, respectively. For the 1000 mg dose, however, peak concentrations were 5.66 mg/L at 1.67 h on day 1 and 5.98 mg/L at 2.06 h at steady state. For the hypertensive patients, also receiving thiazide diuretics, peak concentrations with the 500 mg dose were 3.56 mg/L on day 1 observed after 1.22 h and 3.89 mg/L in the steady state at 1.47 h [L. H. Wang *et al.*, *Antimicrob. Agents Chemother*., 1996, *40(1)*, 80–85].

20 pregnant women (at 36 weeks' gestation) with a history of reoccurring genital herpes simplex virus infections (with positive herpes simplex virus 2 serological results) were administered 500 mg valaciclovir twice daily for 2 weeks. Peak aciclovir plasma concentrations were 3.14 mg/L after the initial dose and 3.03 mg/L at steady state (after 2 weeks dosing) [D. F. Kimberlin *et al.*, *Am. J. Obstet. Gynecol*., 1998, *179(4)*, 846–851].

Bioavailability. Approx. 54%.

Half-life. 3 h as aciclovir which may be increased to 14 h in patients with end stage renal disease.

Volume of distribution. Has not been calculated, as the drug has not been administered intravenously and the elimination rate constant has not been accurately measured. Aciclovir is 50 L in a typical adult.

Clearance. Aciclovir, 679 mL/min/1.73 m^2 in healthy individuals and 86 mL/min/1.73 m^2 in dialysis patients. The mean renal clearance is 15.3 L/h after a single 1000 mg dose of valaciclovir.

Protein binding. 13.5 to 17.9%.

Dose. 1 g oral dose.

Valethamate Bromide

Anticholinergic

Proprietary name. Epidosin

N,*N*-Diethyl-*N*-methyl-2-[(3-methyl-1-oxo-2-phenylpentyl)oxy]-ethanaminium bromide

$C_{19}H_{32}BrNO_2$ = 386.4

CAS—16376-74-2 (valethamate); 90-22-2 (bromide)

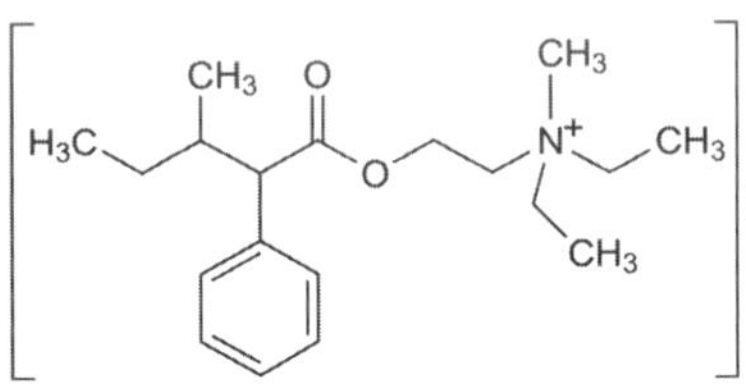

A white crystalline powder. M.p. 100° to 101°.

Freely soluble in water; very soluble in ethanol; practically insoluble in ether.

Partition Coefficient. Log *P* (octanol/water), 1.1.

Thin-layer Chromatography. System TA—Rf 02. (Acidified iodoplatinate solution, positive.)

Ultraviolet Spectrum. Aqueous acid—253, 259 nm (A^1_1 = 5.4b), 265 nm.

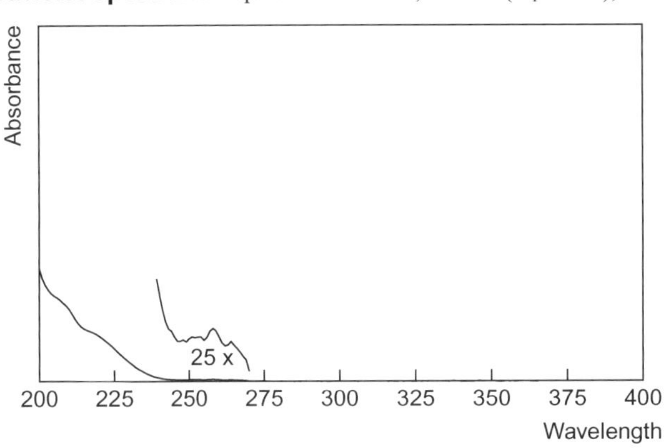

Infra-red Spectrum. Principal peaks at wavenumbers 1730, 1230, 695, 726, 1163, 1265 cm^{-1} (KBr disk).

Dose. 30 to 80 mg daily.

Valproic Acid

Anticonvulsant

Proprietary names. Convulex (capsules); Cryoval; Depakene (capsules); Deproic; Ergenyl; Mylproin; Proteval; Provetal; Valcaps; Valken; Valporal; Valprosid.

2-Propylpentanoic acid

$C_8H_{16}O_2$ = 144.2

CAS—99-66-1

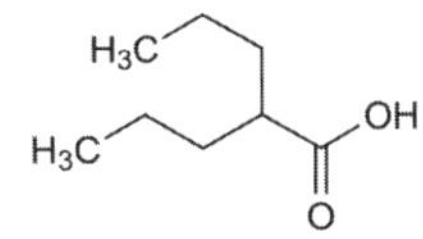

A colourless liquid.

Very slightly soluble in water.

Sodium Valproate

Proprietary names. Absenor; Convulex (solution and tablets); Delepsine; Depacon; Depakene (syrup); Depakin(e); Deplexil; Deproic; Encorate; Epilim; Ergenyl; Leptilan; Leptilanil; Orfiril; Orlept; Selenica; Valpakine; Valparin; Valporal; Valpro; Valprosid.

$C_8H_{15}NaO_2$ = 166.2

CAS—1069-66-5

A white, crystalline, deliquescent powder.

Soluble 1 in 0.4 of water; soluble 1 in 5 of ethanol; practically insoluble in common organic solvents.

Dissociation Constant. pK_a 4.6.

Partition Coefficient. Log *P* (octanol/water), 2.8.

Colour Test. Ferric Chloride—orange.

Thin-layer Chromatography. system TD—Rf 00; system TE—Rf 00; system TF—Rf 52; systemTAD—Rf 00.

Gas Chromatography. system GA—RI 1064; system GB—RI 1098; system GE—RRT 0.09 (relative to phenytoin); system GAJ—RRT 0.350 (relative to methylphenobarbital).

High Performance Liquid Chromatography. System HZ—Retention time 8.0 min.

Infra-red Spectrum. Principal peaks at wavenumbers 1708, 1213, 1250, 1278, 946, 1107 cm^{-1} (thin film).

Mass Spectrum. Principal ions at *m/z* 73, 102, 41, 57, 43, 27, 55, 29.

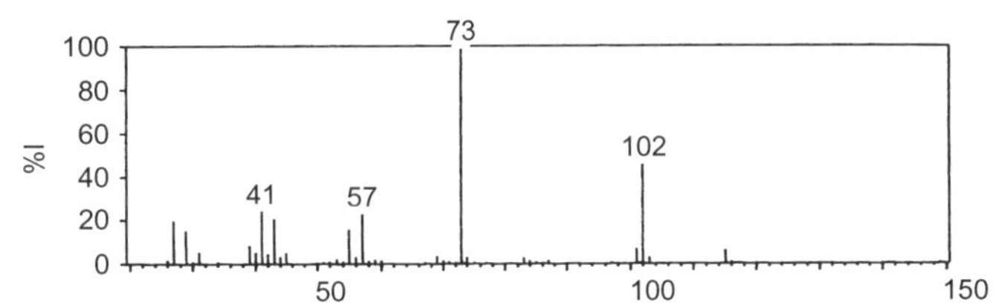

Quantification

Gas chromatography. In plasma: limit of detection 1 to 2 mg/L, FID—R. Riva *et al.*, *J. Pharm. Sci*., 1982, *71*, 110–111. In plasma or serum: limit of detection 1 mg/L—W. Lin and A. R. Kelly, *Ther. Drug Monit*., 1985, *7*, 336–343. In plasma or brain: valproic acid and *E*-delta 2-valproic acid, limits of detection 0.1 µg/g in brain tissue and 0.2 mg/L in plasma, FID—R. L. Semmes and D. D. Shen, *J. Chromatogr*., 1988, *432*, 185–197. In plasma: valproic acid and valpromide, limit of detection 2 mg/L, FID—M. Pokrajac *et al.*, *Pharm. Acta Helv*., 1992, *67*, 237-240. In plasma: limit of detection 1 mg/L, FID—M. Krogh *et al.*, *J. Chromatogr*., 1995, *673*, *Biomed. Appl*, 299–305. In plasma or brain: with or without HPLC clean-up, ECD—R. L. Dills and D. D. Shen, *J. Chromatogr. B. Biomed. Sci. Appl*., 1997, *690*, 139–152.

Gas chromatography–mass spectrometry. In serum, urine or breast-milk: valproic acid and several metabolites, limits of detection between 2.8 and 18 µg/L in serum—H. Nau *et al.*, *J. Chromatogr*., 1981, *226*; *Biomed. Appl*.,

15, 69–78. In serum or saliva: limit of detection 2 μg/L—K. Kassahun *et al.*, *Biomed. Environ. Mass Spectrom.*, 1989, *18*, 918–926.

High performance liquid chromatography. In serum: limit of detection 9 mg/L, UV detection—J. P. Moody and S. M. Allan, *Clin. Chim. Acta*, 1983, *127*, 263–269. In plasma: valproic acid and other antiepileptic drugs—K. Kushida and T. Ishizaki, *J. Chromatogr.*, 1985, *338*, 131–139. In plasma: comparison with immunological assay—F. A. van der Horst *et al.*, *J. Chromatogr.*, 1988, *456*, 191–199; H. Lui *et al.*, *Ther Drug Monit.*, 1992, *14*, 513–521. In serum: sodium valproate, fluorescence detection—E. Bousquet *et al.*, *Pharmazie*, 1991, *46*, 257–258. In serum: photodiode-array and fluorescence detection—H. Liu *et al.*, *J. Chromatogr.*, 1992, *576*, 163–169. In serum: limit of detection 0.1 mg/L, fluorescence detection—S. Hara *et al.*, *Biol. Pharm. Bull.*, 1999, *22*, 975–977.

Disposition in the Body. Well absorbed after oral administration. Metabolised mainly by oxidation to a number of metabolites, including 3-oxovalproic acid, 2-propylglutaric acid, 3-hydroxyvalproic acid, 4-hydroxyvalproic acid, 5-hydroxyvalproic acid and valpro-1,4-lactone. About 20% of a dose is excreted in the urine as the glucuronide of valproic acid in 72 h; most of the remainder is excreted as glucuronides of metabolites, less than 5% of a dose being excreted as unchanged drug.

Therapeutic concentration. In plasma, usually in the range 40 to 100 mg/L, but there is no clear correlation with therapeutic effect.

Following a single oral dose of 500 mg to 6 subjects, peak plasma concentrations of 36 to 73 mg/L (mean 58) were attained in 1 to 5 h (mean 3) [C. A. May and W. R. Garnett, *Clin. Pharm.*, 1983, *2*, 143–147].

Daily oral doses in the range 1 to 3.75 g were administered to 20 patients; at the end of 10 weeks, minimum serum concentrations were 30 to 135 mg/L (mean 82) and maximum concentrations were 70 to 190 mg/L (mean 109). About 75% of the patients had serum concentrations within 55 to 100 mg/L [J. Bruni *et al.*, *Clin. Pharmacol. Ther.*, 1978, *24*, 324–332.]

Rapid intravenous infusion of valproic acid to 21 subjects (dose range 21 to 28 mg/kg (mean 24.2)) at a rate of 3 or 6 mg/kg/min produced peak serum concentrations of 105 to 204.1 mg/L (mean 132.6) 20 min after the end of infusion; in 2 subjects the serum valproic acid levels were 64 and 74 mg/L 30 to 40 min post infusion [V Venkataraman and J. W. Wheless, *Epilepsy Res.*, 1999, *35*, 147–153.]

Toxicity. Plasma concentrations greater than 200 mg/L are associated with toxic effects but valproic acid is relatively non-toxic after overdose and recovery after the ingestion of up to 75 g has been reported. Hepatotoxicity has been reported during therapeutic administration.

A 43-year-old female recovered following haemodialysis after becoming comatose owing to ingesting a large amount of valproic acid; her serum valproic acid concentration on admission to hospital was 1380 mg/L [L. Z. Johnson *et al.*, *Am. J. Kidney Dis.*, 1999, *33*, 786–789.]

A 25-year-old female became comatose after ingesting an unknown quantity of valproic acid (concentrations increased to >1200 mg/L); she was successfully treated with haemodialysis [S. L. Kane *et al.*, *Ann. Pharmacother.*, 2000, *34*, 1146–1151.]

A multicentre case-series study of valproic acid intoxication revealed that of 335 reports, 186 had serum levels of >100 mg/L. Peak serum valproic acid concentrations were 110 to 1840 mg/L (mean 378.3) at 1 to 18 h (mean 7.4). A peak concentration of >850 mg/L was more likely to be associated with coma, respiratory depression, aspiration or metabolic acidosis [H. S. Spiller *et al.*, *J. Toxicol. Clin. Toxicol.*, 2000, *38*, 755–760.]

Bioavailability. Almost 100%.

Half-life. Plasma half-life, about 6 to 20 h, reduced when administered in combination with other anticonvulsants.

Volume of distribution. About 0.1 to 0.2 L/kg.

Clearance. Plasma clearance, about 0.1 to 0.3 mL/min/kg.

Distribution in blood. Plasma:whole blood ratio, about 1.8.

Protein binding. In plasma, about 90% (concentration-dependent; decreased at plasma concentration >100 mg/L).

Note. For a review of the clinical pharmacokinetics of valproic acid, see R. Gugler and G. E. von Unruh, *Clin. Pharmacokinet.*, 1980, *5*, 67–83; for a review of its toxicity, see M. D. Sztajukrycer, *J. Toxicol. Clin. Toxicol.*, 2002, *40*, 789–801; and for a review of its pharmacological and therapeutic properties, see E. Perucca, *CNS Drugs*, 2002, *16*, 695–714.

Dose. Initially 600 mg of sodium valproate daily, increasing to 2.6 g daily.

Valsartan

Angiotension II Receptor Antagonist

Synonym. CGP-48933
Proprietary names. Diovan; Tareg.
N-[*p*-(*o*-1*H*-Tetrazol-5-ylphenyl)benzyl]-*N*-valeryl-L-valine
$C_{24}H_{29}N_5O_3$=435.5
CAS—137862-53-4

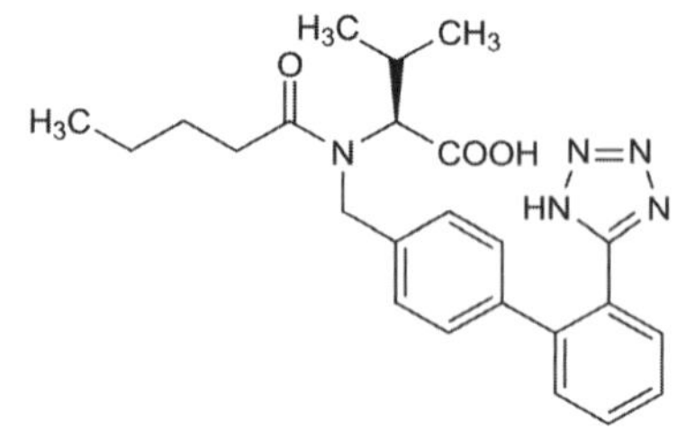

A white to practically white fine powder. M.p. 116° to 117°. It is soluble in ethanol and methanol; slightly soluble in water.

Gas Chromatography. System GP—RI 3420 valsartan-ME$_2$.

High Performance Liquid Chromatography. Column: ODS Hypersil C_{18} (150 × 4.6 mm i.d., 5 μm). Mobile phase: phosphate buffer (pH 2.8):acetonitrile (50:50), flow rate 1.3 mL/min. Fluorescence detection (λ_{ex}=265 nm; λ_{em}=378 nm). Retention time: 5 min [A. Sioufi *et al.*, *J. Liq. Chromatogr.*, 1994, *17(10)*, 2179–2186].

Column: Chiral AGP (ChromTech) silica bonded α_1-acid glycoprotein (100 × 4 mm i.d., 5 μm). Mobile phase: phosphate buffer (pH 7.0, containing 2% 2-propanol), flow rate 0.8 mL/min. UV detection (λ=227 nm). Retention times: 10 min; CGP 49309, 6 min [E. Francotte *et al.*, *J. Chromatogr. B*, 1996, *686*, 77–83].

Ultraviolet Spectrum. Aqueous acid—203, 248 nm.

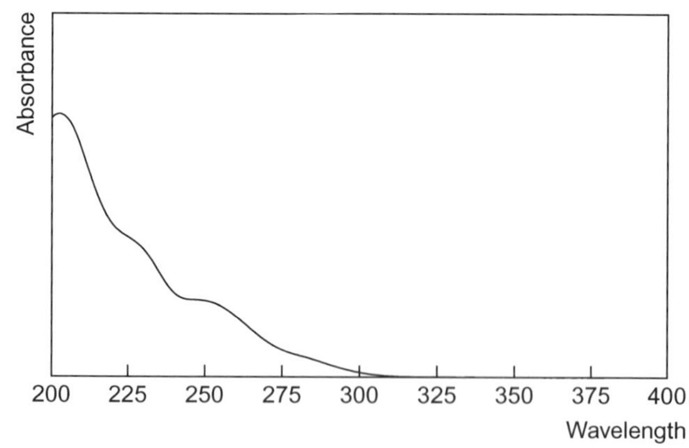

Mass Spectrum. Principal ions at *m/z* 264, 378, 192, 250, 320, 58, 165, 251 (valsartan-ME$_2$).

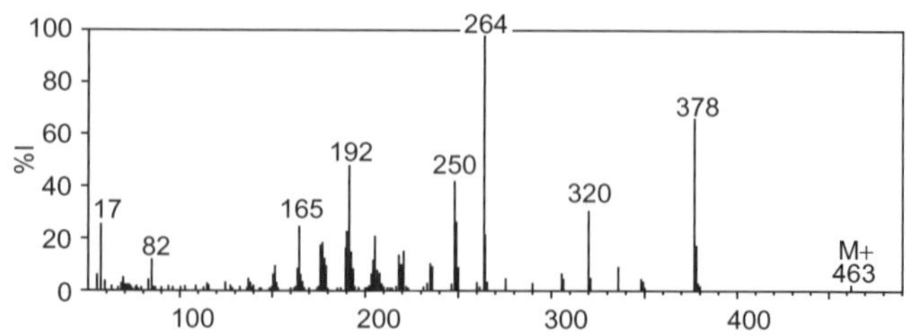

Quantification

Gas chromatography–mass spectrometry. In urine: limit of detection 10 μg/L—H. H. Maurer *et al.*, *Ther. Drug. Monit.*, 1998, *20*, 706–713.

High performance liquid chromatography. In plasma, urine and bile: limit of quantification 5 μg/L (plasma) and 10 μg/L (urine and bile), fluorometric detection—L. Brookman *et al.*, *Clin. Pharmcol. Ther.*, 1997, *62 (3)*, 272–278. In plasma, urine and bile: limit of quantification 5 μg/L in plasma and 10 μg/L in urine and bile, fluorescence detection (λ_{ex}=265 nm; λ_{em}=378 nm)—A. Sioufi *et al.*, *J. Liq. Chromatogr.*, 1994, *17*, 2179–2186.

Disposition in the Body. Valsartan is rapidly absorbed following oral administration. It is quickly eliminated from the body and no significant metabolism takes place. A pharmacologically inactive metabolite, valeryl-4-hydroxyvalsartan, is formed by oxidative biotransformation, accounting for 9% of the dose, and can be detected in plasma after 2 h. Following an oral dose, 86% is excreted in faeces, mainly as the unchanged drug and 13% in urine, 10% as the unchanged drug. After intravenous administration, 30% of a dose is detected unchanged in urine. The bulk of the drug is excreted within 4 days; and 99% of a dose is excreted in 7 days. The drug displays linear pharmacokinetics. Little accumulation occurs following multiple dosing.

Therapeutic concentration

A peak plasma concentration of 1.64 mg/L occurs in 2 h following a single 80 mg dose and 3.46 mg/L following 200 mg [A. Markham and K. L. Goa, *Drugs*, 1997, *54*, 299–311].

12 patients, 6 with mild impairment of liver function and 6 with moderate impairment, and 12 healthy individuals were orally administered a single dose of 160 mg valsartan. The patients with mild impairment produced mean peak concentrations of 5.91 (range 4.06 to 7.16) mg/L at 3.5 h; those with moderate impairment, 3.91 (2.44 to 6.5) mg/L at 4.0 h and the healthy individuals produced peak concentrations of 3.30 (1.27 to 5.12) mg/L at 2.5 h [L. J. Brookman *et al.*, *Clin. Pharmacol. Ther.*, 1997, *62(3)*, 272–278].

Bioavailability. 23%.

Half-life. Mean 7.5 h (range 5 to 9 h).

Volume of distribution. Steady state, 16.9 L.

Clearance. Plasma, 2.2 L/h.

Protein binding. 94 to 97% mainly to albumin.

Dose. Usually 80 to 160 mg and a maximum of 320 mg.

Vancomycin

Antibiotic

An amphoteric glycopeptide antimicrobial substance produced by the growth of certain strains of *Streptomyces orientalis*.

$C_{66}H_{75}Cl_2N_9O_{24}$=1449.3

CAS—1404-90-6

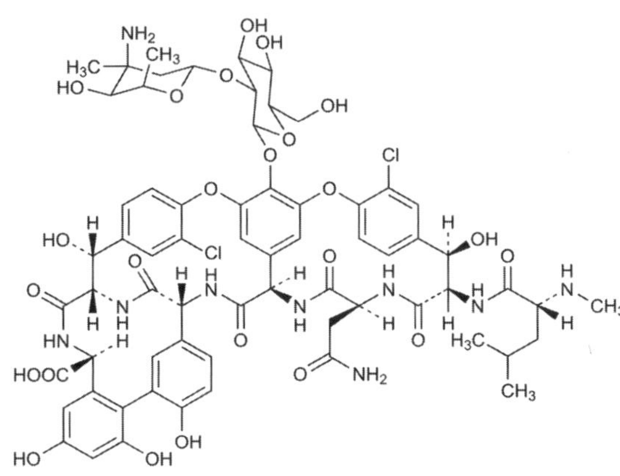

Vancomycin Hydrochloride

Proprietary names. Balcoran; Diatracin; Edicin; Glipep; Lyphocin; Orivan; Vancocin(e); Vancocina; Vancoled; Vancoscand; Vancox

$C_{66}H_{75}Cl_2N_9O_{24}$,HCl=1485.7

CAS—1404-93-9

A light brown powder.

Soluble 1 in 10 of water; moderately soluble in dilute methanol; insoluble in higher alcohols, acetone, and ether.

Colour Test. Marquis Test—yellow.

Thin-layer Chromatography. System TA—Rf 22. (Acidified potassium permanganate solution, positive.)

Ultraviolet Spectrum. Vancomycin hydrochloride: aqueous acid—281 nm (A_1^1=34b).

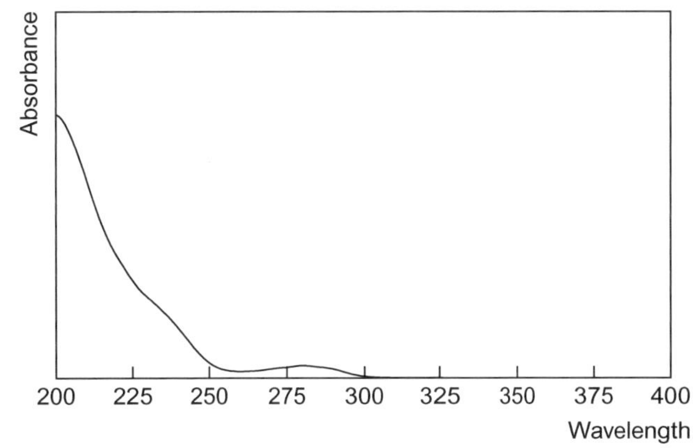

Quantification

High performance liquid chromatography. In serum: limit of detection 2 mg/L, UV detection—R. J. Hoagland *et al.*, *J. Anal. Toxicol.*, 1984, *8*, 75–77. In serum, cerebrospinal fluid or peritoneal fluid: limit of detection 100 μg/L—F. Jehl *et al.*, *Antimicrob. Agents Chemother.*, 1985, *27*, 503–507. In plasma, bone atrial appendage tissue, or pericardial fluid: limit of detection in fluids 3 mg/L and in bone 0.75 μg/g, UV detection—S. V. Greene *et al.*, *J. Chromatogr.*, 1987, *417*, 121–128. In serum: vancomycin and its crystalline degradation product CDP-1 (comparison with EMIT and fluorescence polarisation immunoassay (FPIA))—M. W. Hu *et al.*, *Ther. Drug Monit.*, 1990, *12*, 562–569. In serum: (comparison with EMIT)—F. Demotes-Mainard *et al.*, *Ther. Drug Monit.*, 1994, *16*, 293–297. In plasma—J. Luska and A. Marusic, *J. Chromatogr.*, 1995, *667*, *Biomed. Appl.*, 277–281. In plasma or serum: UV detection—L. Li *et al.*, *Ther. Drug Monit.*, 1995, *17*, 366–370. In serum: vancomycin and CDP-1, UV detection—D. W. Backes *et al.*, *J. Pharm. Biomed. Anal.*, 1998, *16*, 1281–1287. In plasma and tissues: UV detection (comparison with FPIA)—D. Farin *et al.*, *J. Pharm. Biomed. Anal.*, 1998, *18*, 367–372. In serum: limit of detection 0.5 mg/L, UV detection (comparison with FPIA)—I. Furuta *et al.*, *Clin. Chim. Acta*, 2000, *301*, 31–39. In plasma: electrochemical detection (comparison with EMIT)—P. Favetta *et al.*, *J. Chromatogr. B Biomed. Sci. Appl.*, 2001, *751*, 377–382.

Fluorescence polarisation immunoassay (FPIA) In serum: limit of detection <2 mg/L—M. Adamczyk *et al.*, *Ther. Drug Monit.*, 1998, *20*, 191–201. In serum: (comparison with HPLC and EMIT)—P. F. Smith *et al.*, *Ther. Drug Monit.*, 1998, *20*, 231–235.

Radioimmunoassay. In serum or urine: limit of detection 40 ng/L—K.-L. L. Fong *et al.*, *Antimicrob. Agents Chemother.*, 1981, *19*, 139–143.

Disposition in the Body. Not absorbed from the gastro-intestinal tract. About 90% of an intravenous dose is excreted in the urine with about 50% of the dose being excreted in 4 h.

Therapeutic concentration. In plasma, usually in the range 10 to 40 mg/L.

In 101 infants who received vancomycin 15 mg/kg by intravenous infusion over 60 min, every 12 or 18 h, trough serum concentrations of 0.6 to 23.4 mg/L (median 7.1) and peak serum concentrations of 9.0 to 47.2 mg/L (median 25.5) were attained. Target trough concentrations of 1 to 10 mg/L were achieved by 46.5% and 1 to 12 mg/L by 55.4%; peak concentrations of 20 to 40 mg/L were found in 83.2% and 15 to 60 mg/L in 99.0% [W. H. Tan *et al.*, *Arch. Dis. Child. Fetal Neonatal Ed.*, 2002, *87*, F214–F216.]

Half-life. Plasma half-life, about 4 to 10 h.

Volume of distribution. About 0.4 to 1 L/kg.

Clearance. Plasma clearance, about 1 mL/min/kg.

Protein binding. In plasma, about 55%.

Note. For a review of vancomycin see B. A. Cunha and A. M. Ristuccia, *Clin. Pharmacol.*, 1983, *2*, 417–424.

Dose. The equivalent of up to 2 g of vancomycin daily, by mouth or by intravenous infusion.

Vanillin

Flavouring Agent

Synonyms. Vainillina; Vanillic Aldehyde; Vanillinum.
4-Hydroxy-3-methoxybenzaldehyde
$C_8H_8O_3=152.1$
CAS—121-33-5

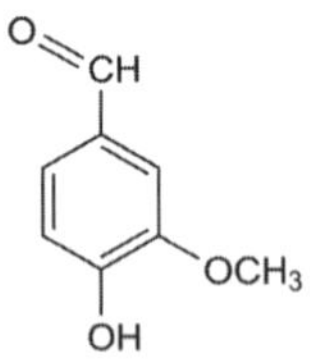

White or slightly yellow crystalline needles or powder. M.p. 81° to 83°. Soluble 1 in 100 of water; freely soluble in ethanol, chloroform and ether; soluble in glycerol and hot water.

Dissociation Constant. pK_a 7.4 (20°).

Partition Coefficient. Log *P* (octanol/water), 1.2.

Gas Chromatography. System GA—RI 1630; system GB—RI 1632; system GN—Retention time 86.5 min.

High Performance Liquid Chromatography. System HAA—Retention time 11.7 min.

Ultraviolet Spectrum. Aqueous acid—230, 278 nm (A^1_1=685b), 309 nm; aqueous alkali—248, 348 nm (A^1_1=1640b).

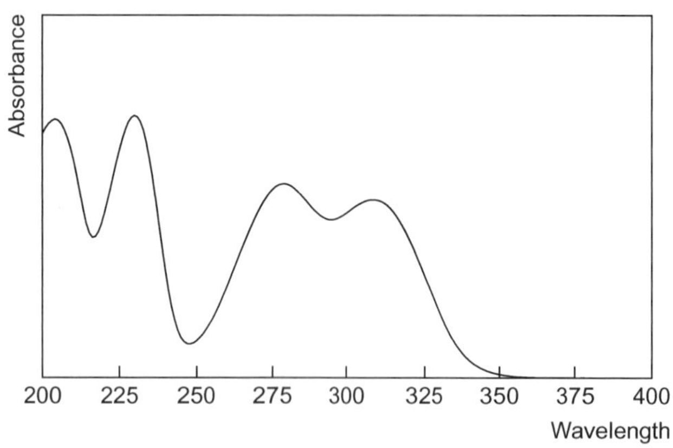

Infra-red Spectrum. Principal peaks at wavenumbers 1660, 1153, 1267, 735, 1590, 1300 cm^{-1} (KCl disk).

Mass Spectrum. Principal ions at *m/z* 152, 151, 81, 109, 51, –, –, –.

Quantification

High performance liquid chromatography. In plasma, red blood cells or urine: vanillin and vanillic acid, limit of detection 1 mg/L, UV detection—D. Farthing *et al.*, *J. Chromatogr. B Biomed. Sci. Appl.*, 1999, *726*, 303–307.

Venlafaxine

Antidepressant

Synonym. Venlafexine
1-[2-(Dimethylamino)-1-(4-methoxyphenyl)ethyl]cyclohexanol
$C_{17}H_{27}NO_2=277.4$
CAS—93413-69-5

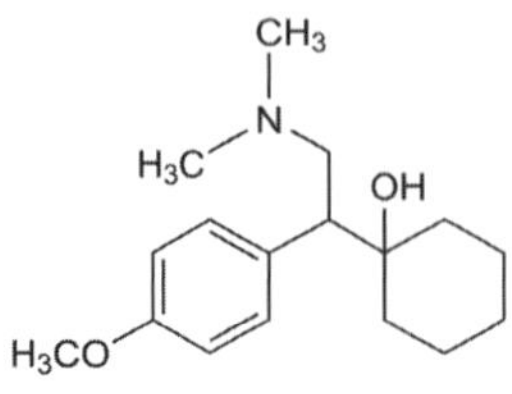

(−) and (+) forms: crystals from ethyl acetate. M.p. 102° to 104°.

Venlafaxine Hydrochloride

Synonym. Wy-45030

Proprietary names. Dobupal; Efexor; Effexor; Trevilor; Trewilor; Vandral.
$C_{17}H_{27}NO_2,HCl=313.9$
CAS—99300-78-4

A white to off-white crystalline solid with M.p. 215° to 217°. It is soluble in water at 572 g/L.
(−) and (+) forms: crystals from methanol/ether. M.p. 240°.

Partition Coefficient. Log *P* (octanol/water), 0.43.

Gas Chromatography. System GB—venlafaxine RI 2163; M (*N*-desmethyl-) RI 2196; M (*O*-desmethyl-) RI 2230; M (*N,O*-didesmethyl) RI 2264; M (nor OH-) RI 2450; M (*O*-desmethyl OH-) isomer 1 RI 2373; M (*O*-desmethyl OH-) isomer 2 RI 2408; system GM—venlafaxine RRT 0.544; M (*N*-desmethyl-) RRT 0.570; M (*O*-desmethyl-) RRT 0.625; M (*N,O*-didesmethyl) RRT 0.687 (all relative to iprindole).

High Performance Liquid Chromatography. System HZ—venlafaxine retention time 3.1 min; *O*-desmethylvenlafaxine retention time 2.2 min.

Column: C_{18} ODS/CN (Spherisorb, 250 × 4.6 mm i.d., 5 μm). Mobile phase: potassium phosphate buffer (0.05 M, pH 4.8):methanol (30:70), flow rate 1 mL/min. Detection: coulometric detection. Retention times: venlafaxine, 8.8 min; *O*-desmethylvenlafaxine, 5.4 min [E. M. Clement *et al.*, *J. Chromatogr. B Biomed. Sci. Appl.*, 1998, *705*, 303–308].

Ultraviolet Spectrum. Aqueous acid—225, 273, 280 nm; (0.025 M sulfuric acid)—226.5, 274.5 nm; basic—274, 280 nm.

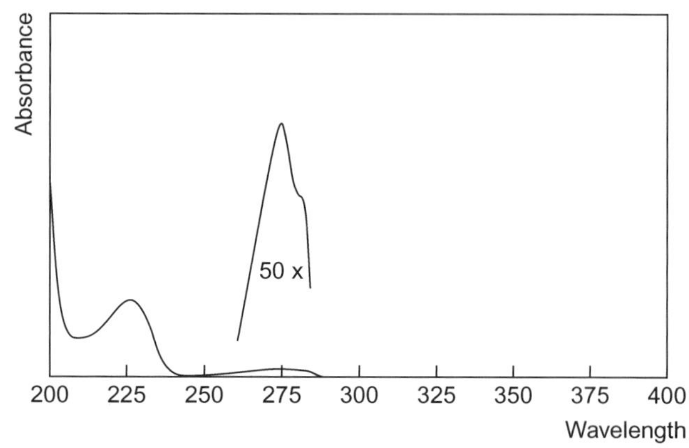

Infra-red Spectrum. (Venlafaxine hydrochloride) Principal peaks at wavenumbers 1513, 1243, 1179 cm^{-1} (KBr disk).

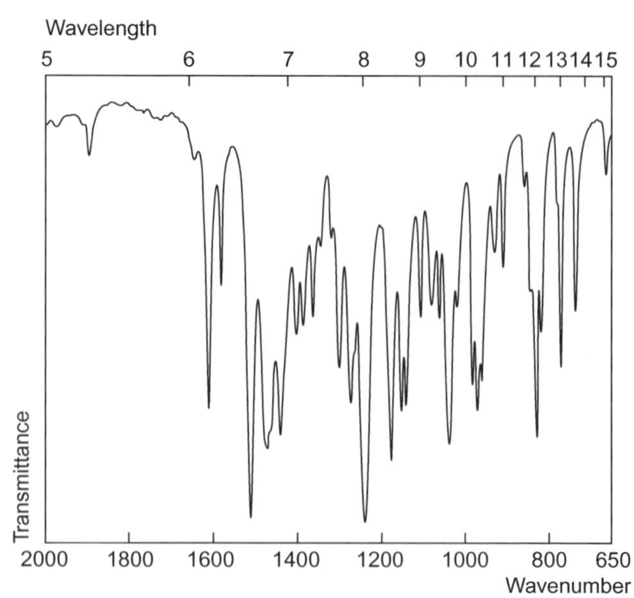

Mass Spectrum. Principal ions at *m/z* 58, 134, 91, 119, 179, 121, 42, 55.

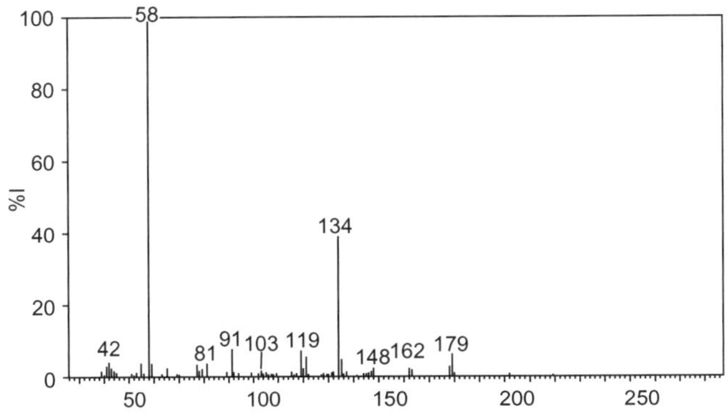

Quantification

Gas chromatography–mass spectrometry. In urine: limit of detection < 100 µg/L—J. Bickeboeller-Friedrich and H. H. Maurer, *Ther. Drug Monit.*, 2001, *23*, 61–70.

High performance liquid chromatography. In plasma or urine: venlafaxine and *O*-desmethylvenlafaxine, limit of detection 10 µg/L in plasma and 100 µg/L in urine, UV detection—D. R. Hicks *et al.*, *Ther. Drug Monit.*, 1994, *16*, 100–107. In plasma: venlafaxine and *O*-desmethylvenlafaxine, limit of detection 2 µg/L, electrochemical detection—E. M. Clement *et al.*, *J. Chromatogr. B Biomed. Sci. Appl.*, 1998, *705*, 303–308.

Disposition in the Body. Venlafaxine is well absorbed after oral administration and undergoes extensive first-pass metabolism in the liver, mainly to the active metabolite *O*-desmethylvenlafaxine. Two less active minor metabolites are also produced; *N*-desmethylvenlafaxine and *N,O*-didesmethylvenlafaxine. It is excreted predominantly in urine, mainly in the form of its metabolites (either free or conjugated); 1 to 10% as the unchanged drug, 30% *O*-desmethylvenlafaxine, 6 to 19% *N,O*-didesmethylvenlafaxine and 1% *N*-desmethylvenlafaxine. Approx. 2% is excreted in faeces.

Therapeutic concentration The serum therapeutic range is 250 to 750 µg/L for the total drug and metabolites.

18 healthy male volunteers (mean age of 27 years) were administered single oral doses of 25, 75 or 150 mg on day 1, and the same dose every 8 h on days 2 to 4. A single dose was then administered on day 5. The mean peak concentrations from day 1 were 37, 102 and 163 µg/L for the three doses at 2.4, 2.1 and 2.1 h, respectively. The mean peak plasma *O*-desmethylvenlafaxine concentrations were 61, 168 and 325 µg/L for the three doses at 4.0 (1.5 to 7.8), 4.4 (1.2 to 6.7) and 4.6 (3.1 to 5.9) h, respectively [K. J. Klamerus *et al.*, *J. Clin. Pharmacol.*, 1992, *32*, 716–724].

Toxicity. Toxic effects may be produced by blood concentrations greater than 1.0 mg/L.

Two venlafaxine-related deaths were reported. Blood concentrations in case 1 were 7.27 mg/L venlafaxine, and 5.03 mg/L *O*-desmethylvenlafaxine. Blood concentrations in case 2 were 89.67 mg/L venlafaxine, and 3.44 mg/L *O*-desmethylvenlafaxine [C. Long *et al.*, *J. Anal. Toxicol.*, 1997, *21*, 166–169].

Half-life. Plasma half-life, venlafaxine 4 h; *O*-desmethylvenlafaxine 10 h.

Volume of distribution. Venlafaxine 6.8 L/kg; *O*-desmethylvenlafaxine 5.7 L/kg.

Clearance. Plasma clearance, venlafaxine 1.2 to 1.7 L/h/kg; *O*-desmethylvenlafaxine 0.4 L/h/kg.

Protein binding. In plasma, venlafaxine and *O*-desmethylvenlafaxine, 30%.

Note. For a review of venlafaxine see S. M. Holliday and P. Benfield, *Drugs*, 1995, *49*, 280–294.

Dose. The usual dose is 75 mg venlafaxine daily with a maximum of 375 mg. The dose is reduced by 50% in those with moderate hepatic impairment and 25% with mild to moderate renal impairment.

Verapamil

Anti-arrhythmic

Synonyms. CP-16533-1; D-365; Iproveratril.
α-[3-[[2-(3,4-Dimethoxyphenyl)ethyl]methylamino]propyl]-3,4-dimethoxy-α-(1-methylethyl)benzeneacetonitrile
$C_{27}H_{38}N_2O_4$=454.6
CAS—52-53-9

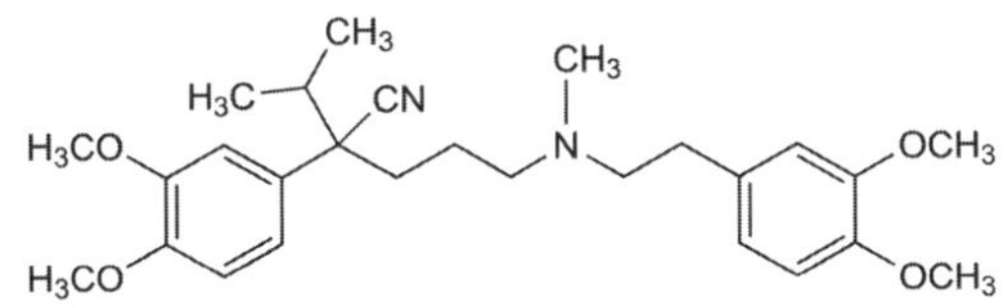

A pale yellow viscous oil.
Practically insoluble in water; freely soluble in the lower alcohols, acetone, ethyl acetate and chloroform; soluble in benzene and ether.

Verapamil Hydrochloride

Proprietary names. Angimon; Berkatens; Calan; Cordilox; Covera; Half Securon; Isoptin(e); Securon; Univer; Verapress; Verelan; Vertab; Zolvera.
$C_{27}H_{38}N_2O_4$,HCl=491.1
CAS—152-11-4
A white crystalline powder. M.p. 138.5° to 140.5°, with decomposition.
Soluble 1 in 20 of water, 1 in 25 of ethanol and 1 in 1.5 of chloroform; practically insoluble in ether.

Dissociation Constant. pK_a 8.9.

Partition Coefficient. Log *P* (octanol/water), 3.8.

Colour Tests. Liebermann's Test—black; Marquis Test—yellow-green→grey.

Thin-layer Chromatography. System TA—Rf 59; system TB—Rf 23; system TC—Rf 70; system TE—Rf 73; system TL—Rf 42; system TAE—Rf 43; system TAF—Rf 61. (Acidified iodoplatinate solution, positive.)

Gas Chromatography. System GA—verapamil RI 3150, M (nor-) RI 3180, M (*N*-desalkyl-) RI 2100, M (*N*-desalkyl-acetyl-) RI 2460, M (*N*-didesalkyl-acetyl-) RI 2545; system GB—verapamil RI 3305, M (nor-) RI 3371, M (*N*-desalkyl-) RI 2193, M (*O*-desmethyl-didesalkyl-) RI 2169, M (*O*-desmethyl-desalkyl-) RI 2246, M (didesalkyl-) RI 2300, M (*N*-desalkyl-acetyl-) RI 2546, M (*N*-didesalkyl-acetyl-) RI 2579.

Column: fused-silica capillary cross-linked with 5% phenylmethyl silicone (SE-54) (25 m × 0.2 mm i.d., 0.3 µm film thickness). Column temperature: 100°; increased to 310° at 20°/min, held 10 min. Carrier gas: helium, flow rate 0.9 mL/min. Internal standard: zipeprol. NPD. Retention time: 17.5 min [H. S. Shin *et al.*, *J. Chromatogr.*, 1996, *677(2)*; *Biomed. Appl.*, 369–373].

High Performance Liquid Chromatography. System HA—verapamil *k* 2.6, M (nor-) *k* 1.7; system HX—RI 447; system HY—RI 386; system HZ—verapamil Retention time, 7.0 min, M (nor-) Retention time, 6.6 min; system HAA—Retention time, 15.4 min; system HAV—*k* 8.2; system HAX—Retention time 13.3 min; system HAY—Retention time 7.0 min.

Column: NovaPak C_{18} RP (150 × 3.9 mm i.d., 4 µm). Mobile phase: methanol:0.04 M ammonium acetate:acetonitrile:triethylamine (2:2:1:0.04), pH adjusted to 7.1 with 0.1 M acetic acid, flow rate 1.2 mL/min. UV detection (λ=210 nm). Retention time: verapamil, 4.9 min; norverapamil, 3.6 min [M. A. Garcia *et al.*, *J. Chromatogr. B Biomed. Sci. Appl.*, 1997, *693(2)*, 377–382].

Column: (analytical) Chiral-AGP (150 × 4 mm i.d.); (guard) Chiral-AGP (10 × 3 mm i.d.). Mobile phase: phosphate buffer (pH 6.65, 0.01 M):acetonitrile (91:9), flow rate 0.9 mL/min. Fluorescence detection (λ_{ex} = 227 nm; λ_{em} = 308 nm). Resolution: 3.3 [G. Stagni and W. R. Gillespie, *J. Chromatogr.*, 1995, *667(2)*; *Biomed. Appl.*, 349–354].

Ultraviolet Spectrum. Aqueous acid—278 nm (A_1^1=127a).

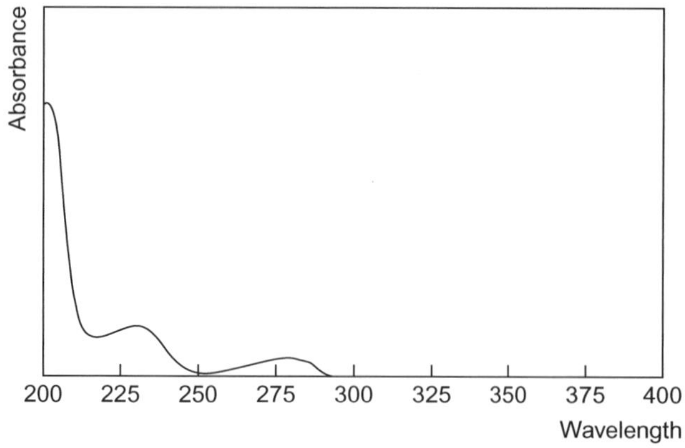

Infra-red Spectrum. Principal peaks at wavenumbers 1510, 1253, 1026, 1232, 1149, 1587 (thin film).

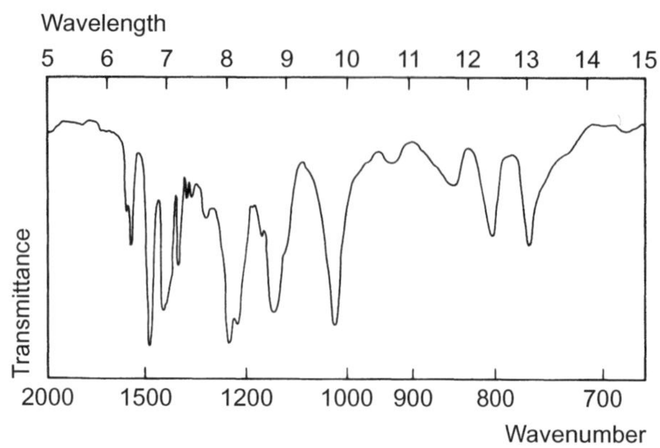

Mass Spectrum. Principal ions at *m/z* 303, 58, 43, 304, 151, 44, 42, 57.

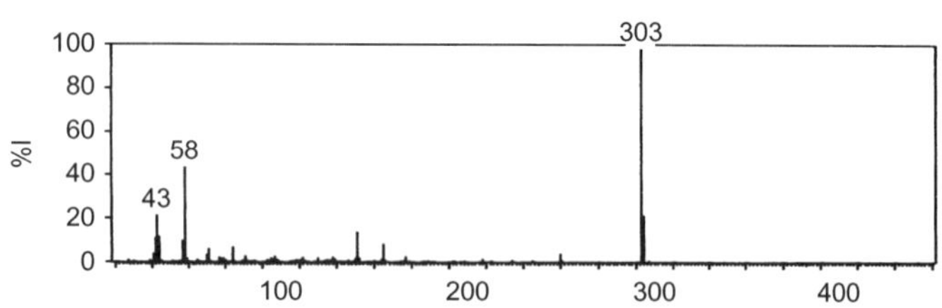

Quantification

Gas chromatography. In plasma: limit of detection 2 μg/L, NPD—H. S. Shin *et al.*, *J. Chromatogr.*, 1996, *677(2)*; *Biomed. Appl.*, 369–373.

High performance liquid chromatography. In plasma and urine: limit of detection is 10 μg/L, fluorescence detection (λ_{ex} = 280 nm; λ_{em} = 315 nm)—P. C. Ho *et al.*, *Eur. J. Clin. Pharmacol.*, 2000, *56(9-10)*, 693–698. In serum: limit of quantification 3 μg/L for verapamil and 5 μg/L for norverapamil, fluorescence detection—E. Brandsteterova and I. W. Wainer, *J. Chromatogr. B Biomed. Sci. Appl.*, 1999, *732*, 395–404. In urine: limit of quantification 3 μg/L, fluorescence detection (λ_{ex} = 230 nm; λ_{em} = 312 nm)—E. B. Asafu-Adjaye and G. K. Shiu, *J. Chromatogr. B Biomed. Sci. Appl.*, 1998, *707(1-2)*, 161–167. In biological samples: limit of detection 5 μg/L for verapamil and 3 μg/L norverapamil, UV detection, (λ = 210 nm)—M. A. Garcia *et al.*, *J. Chromatogr. B Biomed. Sci. Appl.*, 1997, *693(2)*, 377–382. In plasma: limit of detection 1.3 μg/L verapamil and 1.4 μg/L norverapamil; limit of quantification 4.3 and 4.8 μg/L, respectively, fluorescence detection (λ_{ex} = 275 nm; λ_{em} = 310 nm)—A. Ceccato *et al.*, *J. Chromatogr. A*, 1996, *750(1-2)*, 351–360. In plasma: limit of quantification is 3 μg/L for verapamil and 2 μg/L for norverapamil, fluorescence detection (λ_{ex} = 227 nm; λ_{em} = 308 nm)—G. Stagni and W. R. Gillespie, *J. Chromatogr.*, 1995, *667(2)*; *Biomed. Appl.*, 349–354.

Disposition in the Body. Almost completely absorbed after oral administration but undergoes extensive first-pass metabolism. The main metabolic reactions are *N*-dealkylation (*N*-demethylation gives norverapamil which is thought to be active) and *O*-demethylation of the resulting compounds. About 70% of a dose is excreted in the urine in 5 days with about 50% in the first 24 h; less than 5% is excreted as unchanged drug. The urinary metabolites consist mainly of *N*-dealkylated compounds together with about 10% of the dose as norverapamil or its *O*-demethylated derivative; conjugated *O*-demethylated products account for about 17% of the urinary material. About 16% of a dose is eliminated in the faeces.

Therapeutic concentration

12 healthy subjects, aged 20 to 38 years, were administered a single dose of verapamil 20 mg either as a buccal formulation or orally as a tablet, with a 7-day gap between doses. A mean peak verapamil plasma concentration of 51.28 μg/L was attained at 1.5 h after buccal administration and 31.67 μg/L at 1 h after oral administration. The equivalent concentrations of norverapamil were 5.03 μg/L at 6 h after buccal administration and 27.35 μg/L at 1 h after oral administration [W. Sawicki and S. Janicki, *Int. J. Pharm.*, 2002, *238*, 181–189].

30 young and 30 elderly healthy subjects were administered verapamil 180 mg via a controlled-release gastro-intestinal therapeutic system (approximately half of each age group were males and half were females). Mean steady-state plasma concentrations were reported as follows: *R*-verapamil, 155.0 μg/L in elderly and 108.6 μg/L in young subjects (in 10.0 h); *S*-verapamil, 40.9 μg/L in elderly and 24.2 μg/L in young subjects (in 10.2 and 10.0 h, respectively); *R*-norverapamil, 150.3 μg/L in elderly and 121.3 μg/L in young patients (in 11.2 and 10.9 h, respectively); *S*-norverapamil, 56.9 μg/L in elderly and 43.2 μg/L in young patients (in 11.0 h) [S. K. Gupta *et al.*, *Br. J. Clin. Pharmacol.*, 1995, *40*, 325–331].

12 healthy men (aged 19 to 37 years) received a single 240 mg oral dose of racemic verapamil as either an immediate-release formulation (in the fasting state) or as a sustained-release. A peak plasma verapamil concentration of 327 μg/L was attained at 1.71 h with the immediate-release preparation and 73 μg/L at 10.8 h after the sustained-release preparation. Measurement of the total (*R*)-verapamil and (*S*)-verapamil levels in the plasma revealed the *R*/*S* ratio (at C_{max} and at several other times) to be lower with the immediate-release preparation for both verapamil (4.52 versus 5.83%) and norverapamil (2.48 versus 3.04%) [A. Karim and A. Piergies, *Clin. Pharmacol. Ther.*, 1995, *58*, 174–184].

9 healthy, male volunteers (mean age 26 years; range 19 to 40 years) were administered 120 mg verapamil twice daily for 3 days before the actual study day. Grapefruit juice or orange juice (control), 200 mL, was also taken twice daily for 5 days beforehand. On the study day, a single oral dose of 120 mg verapamil was administered with either orange or grapefruit juice, after an overnight fast. The steady-state maximum plasma concentration of (*S*)-verapamil was 41 μg/L for the dose taken with grapefruit juice compared with orange juice which was 26 μg/L. For (*R*)-verapamil, the maximum concentration was 132 μg/L with grapefruit juice and 94 μg/L with orange juice. These concentrations were observed at 4.6, 3.9, 4.3 and 4.0 h, respectively. The peak (*S*)-norverapamil concentrations were 33 and 29 μg/L at 5.8 and 5.1 h for grapefruit and orange, respectively. For (*R*)-norverapamil, these concentrations were 84 and 75 μg/L at 5.2 and 4.0 h, respectively [P. C. Ho *et al.*, *Eur. J. Clin. Pharmacol.*, 2000, *56(9-10)*, 693–698].

Toxicity

A 30-year-old woman being treated with verapamil for supraventricular tachycardia, ingested the equivalent of 2.4 g verapamil with an unknown quantity of alcohol. On admission to hospital she was unconscious, her blood pressure could not be recorded and she was hypotensive and bradycardic. Toxicological analysis showed that her blood verapamil concentration was 5.18 mg/L. She deteriorated rapidly but was stabilised with plasmapheresis (this reduced the verapamil blood concentration by approximately 40%). After 4 h of treatment, she developed acute lung, liver and renal failure. She died 38 h after admission to hospital owing to multi-organ failure [U. Kuhlmann *et al.*, *Artif. Cells Blood Substit. Immobil. Biotechnol.*, 2000, *28(5)*, 429–440].

A 45-year-old woman overdosed on 4 g ordinary-release verapamil tablets. 1 to 2 h after ingestion, she was admitted to hospital; she was unconscious, hypotensive and had a low heart beat. The maximum plasma verapamil concentration observed was 2.7 mg/L 2 to 3 h after the overdose.

A 22-year-old male ingested 3.2 mg verapamil with an unknown quantity of alcohol. 2 h after the overdose, he was admitted to hospital with complete heart block and a low blood pressure. The maximum plasma concentration detected was 2.2 mg/L 2 to 3 h after ingestion.

In both the above cases these concentrations were 10- to 20-fold higher than the expected therapeutic range [K. T. Kivisto *et al.*, *Hum. Exp. Toxicol.*, 1997, *16(1)*, 35–37].

A man was found dead in his home and in the room were an empty container of verapamil and a partly emptied bottle of vodka. Verapamil was found in his blood at a concentration of 402 mg/L; in his stomach at 49.3 μg/g and in his liver at 42.1 μg/g. The blood alcohol concentration was 1100 mg/L [E. J. Janowska and E. M. Chudzikiewicz, *Vet. Hum. Toxicol.*, 1996, *38(3)*, 210–211].

Bioavailability. About 20%.

Half-life. Plasma half-life, verapamil about 2 to 7 h, increased during long term oral dosing and in subjects with liver disease; norverapamil about 5 to 13 h.

Volume of distribution. About 2 to 6 L/kg.

Clearance. Plasma clearance, about 10 to 20 mL/min/kg.

Distribution in blood. Plasma : whole blood ratio, about 1.2.

Protein binding. In plasma, about 90%.

Note. For a general review of verapamil, see D. McTavish and E. M. Sorkin, *Drugs*, 1989, *38*, 19–76.

Dose. 120 to 480 mg of verapamil hydrochloride daily.

Veratrine

Topical Counterirritant

A mixture of alkaloids from sabadilla, the dried ripe seeds of *Schoenocaulon officinale* (Liliaceae).
Note. Veratrine should be distinguished from protoveratrines obtained from veratrum.
CAS—8051-02-3 (mixture)
A white or greyish-white powder. M.p. 145° to 155°.
Soluble 1 in 1800 of water; soluble 1 in 2.8 of ethanol, 1 in 0.7 of chloroform, 1 in 4.2 of ether and 1 in 80 of olive oil; freely soluble in benzene and amyl alcohol; slightly soluble in glycerol.
Caution. Veratrine has a violent irritant action on mucous membranes, even in minute doses, and must be handled with great care.

Partition Coefficient. Log *P* (octanol/water), 4.0.

Colour Tests. Liebermann's Test—brown; Mandelin's Test—yellow→orange→violet-brown; Marquis Test—orange; Sulfuric Acid—yellow→violet.

Thin-layer Chromatography. System TA—Rf 59; system TB—Rf 04; system TC—Rf 35; ;system TE—Rf 71; system TL—Rf 17; system TAE—Rf 17.

High Performance Liquid Chromatography. System HAA—Retention time 13.6 min.

Ultraviolet Spectrum. Aqueous acid—262 nm (A_1^1=67b), 292 nm.

Infra-red Spectrum. Principal peaks at wavenumbers 1270, 1085, 1111, 1136, 1234, 1035 cm^{-1} (KBr disk).

Vigabatrin

Anti-epileptic

Synonyms. Gamma-vinyl-GABA; γ-vinyl-GABA; GVG; MDL-71754; RMI-71754.
Proprietary names. Sabril; Sabrilex.
4-Amino-5-hexenoic acid
$C_6H_{11}NO_2$=129.2
CAS—60643-86-9

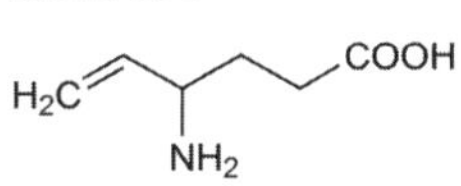

A white to almost white powder. M.p. 209°. It is very soluble in water.

Dissociation Constant. pK_a 4.02, 9.72.

Gas Chromatography. System GB—not eluted; system GAJ—not eluted.

Column: megabore Chirasil-Val non-packed (20 m × 0.53 mm i.d., 0.125 μm film thickness). Column temperature: initially 80°, held 1 min; 20°/min to 129°, held 2 min; 1°/min to 135°, held 20 min; 20°/min to 200°, held 10 min. Carrier gas: helium, flow rate 2.0 mL/min. IS: *S*-γ-ethynyl-GABA. Detection: thermionic specific. Retention time(s): (*R*)-(—)-vigabatrin, 21.5 min; (*S*)-(+)-vigabatrin, 22.2 min; IS 23.2 min [T. M. Schramm *et al.*, *J. Chromatogr.*, 1993, *616*; *Biomed. Appl.*, *127*, 39–44].

High Performance Liquid Chromatography. Column: RP (Spherisorb 3ODS2, 150 × 4.6 mm i.d.). Mobile phase: (A)-acetonitrile; (B)-55 mM sodium acetate (pH 7.6), flow rate 1.0 mL/min. Elution programme: (A:B): initial condition (5:95) to (17.5:82.5) in 20 min, to (35:65) in 1 min, held for 3 min; back to (5:95) in 1 min, held for 2 min. IS: l-homoargenine. Fluorescence detection (λ_{ex}=330; λ_{em}=450). Retention time(s): (*R*)-(—)-vigabatrin, 14.2 min; (*S*)-(+)-vigabatrin, 16.4 min; IS, 13.1 min [T. A. C. Vermeij and P. M. Edelbroek, *J. Chromatogr. B Biomed. Sci. Appl.*, 1998, *716*, 233–238].

Mass Spectrum. Principal ions at *m/z* 56, 84, 111, 69, 82, 54, 67, 45.

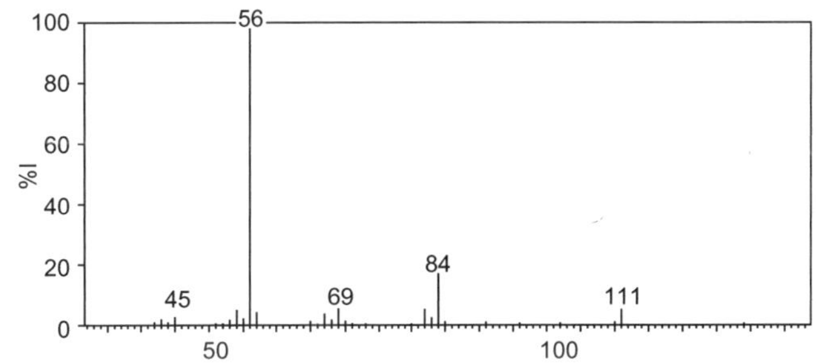

Quantification

Gas chromatography. In plasma: enantiomers, limit of detection (*R*)-(—) 1 mg/L, (*S*)-(+) 0.5 mg/L, thermionic detection—T. M. Schramm *et al.*, *J. Chromatogr.*, 1993, *616*; *Biomed. Appl.*, *127*, 39–44.

Gas chromatography–mass spectrometry. In plasma: enantiomers—K. D. Haegele *et al.*, *J. Chromatogr.*, 1983, *274*; *Biomed. Appl.*, *25*, 103–110.

High performance liquid chromatography. In plasma or urine: limit of detection 0.2 mg/L, fluorescence detection (λ_{ex}=340 nm; λ_{em}=440 nm)—J. Grove *et al.*, *J. Chromatogr.*, 1984, *306*; *Biomed. Appl.*, *31*, 383–387. In plasma or urine: limit of detection 0.5 mg/L in plasma and 10 mg/L in urine, fluorescence detection (λ_{ex}=345 nm; λ_{em}=418 nm)—J. A. Smithers *et al.*, *J. Chromatogr.*, 1985, *341*; *Biomed. Appl.*, *42*, 232–238. In plasma: limit of detection 0.54 mg/L, fluorescence detection (λ_{ex}=370 nm; λ_{em}=418 nm)—L. M. Tsanaclis *et al.*, *Ther. Drug Monit.*, 1991, *13*, 251–253. In serum: enantiomers, limit of detection 0.20 mg/L (*R*)-(—) and 0.14 mg/L (*S*)-(+), fluorescence detection (λ_{ex}=330 nm; λ_{em}=450 nm)—T. A. C. Vermeij and P. M. Edelbroek, *J. Chromatogr. B Biomed. Sci. Appl.*, 1998, *716*, 233–238.

Disposition in the Body. Vigabatrin is rapidly and completely absorbed after oral administration, and food does not alter the extent of absorption. The inactive (*R*)-(—)-enantiomer is reported to be present at much higher plasma concentrations than the active (*S*)-(+)-enantiomer. It is widely distributed and readily crosses the blood–brain barrier. CSF concentrations are about 10 to 15% of those in plasma. Most of a dose is excreted in urine as the unchanged drug as little or no metabolism occurs. 50% is excreted as the (*S*)-(+)-enantiomer and 65% as (*R*)-(—)-enatiomer. There does not appear to be any correlation between plasma concentrations and efficacy or toxicity. Haemodialysis reduces plasma concentrations by about 40 to 60%.

Therapeutic concentration. Plasma concentrations show considerable inter-patient variation.

8 healthy, male subjects aged between 18 and 40 years, were fasted overnight and orally administered with 1 g vigabatrin on an empty stomach, or 1 h after breakfast. The individuals were fasted for a further 4 h after dosing. Mean peak plasma concentrations were 30.5 mg/L and 25.3 mg/L for the fasted and fed individuals at 1.1 and 1.6 h, respectively [M. Frisk-Holmberg *et al.*, *Br. J. Clin. Pharmacol.*, 1989, *27*, 23S–25S].

12 individuals (group 1: 6 with a mean age of 12.1 months; group 2: 6 with a mean age of 8.7 years) suffering from refractory epilepsy, were

administered with a single oral dose of 50 mg/kg (not exceeding 1.5 g in the older children). 24 h after the single treatment multiple dosing at 50 mg/kg twice daily was continued. The mean peak concentration after the single dose was 13.8 mg/L (*S*)-(+)-vigabatrin and 20.6 mg/L (*R*)-(−)-vigabatrin at 2.85 and 2.35 h, respectively for those in group 1. The peak concentrations for group 2 were 19.4 and 34.7 mg/L for the (*S*)-(+)- and (*R*)-(−)-enantiomers, respectively, observed at 1.36 and 1.28 h. The mean concentrations for the multiple dosing were 13.6 (1.2 to 29.2) and 20.7 (0.6 to 37.5) mg/L for the (S)-(+)- and R(−)-enantiomers, respectively 1 h after dosing for group 1. In group 2 these concentrations were 11.8 (5.0 to 24.0) and 21.0 (3.5 to 55.1) mg/L for the two enantiomers, respectively [E. Ray *et al.*, *Br. J. Clin. Pharmacol.*, 1990, *30*, 253–257].

Half-life. Plasma half-life, 5 to 8 h.

Volume of distribution. 0.8 L/kg.

Clearance. Plasma, 1.7 mL/min/kg (0.1 L/h/kg).

Protein binding. In plasma, not bound.

Note. For a review of vigabatrin see S. M. Grant and R. C. Heel, *Drugs*, 1991, *41*, 889–926; for reviews of the pharmacokinetics of vigabatrin see E. Rey *et al.*, *Clin. Pharmacokinet.*, 1992, *23*, 267–278, M. Bialer, *Clin. Pharmacokinet.*, 1993, *24*, 441–452 and R. D. C. Elwes and C. D. Binnie, *Clin. Pharmacokinet.*, 1996, *30*, 403–415.

Dose. The usual dose is 3 g daily; increased in increments of 0.5 to 1 g daily up to a maximum of 4 mg daily or 50 mg/kg.

Viloxazine

Antidepressant

2-[(2-Ethoxyphenoxy)methyl]morpholine
$C_{13}H_{19}NO_3$=237.3
CAS—46817-91-8

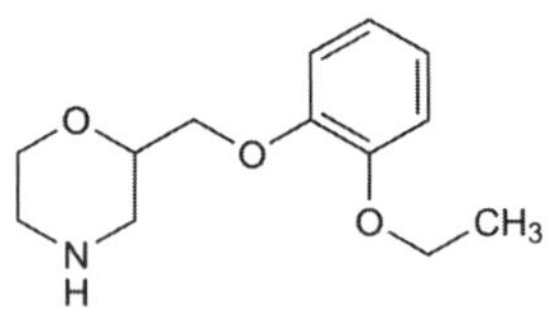

Viloxazine Hydrochloride

Proprietary names. Vicilan; Vivalan; Vivarint.
$C_{13}H_{19}NO_3$,HCl=273.8
CAS—35604-67-2
M.p. 185° to 186°.

Dissociation Constant. pK_a 8.1.

Partition Coefficient. Log *P* (octanol/water), 1.8.

Colour Tests. Liebermann's Test—black; Mandelin's Test—blue-green; Marquis Test—violet.

Thin-layer Chromatography. System TA—Rf 42; system TB—Rf 06; system TC—Rf 23; system TE—Rf 36; system TL—Rf 06; system TAE—Rf 25.

Gas Chromatography. System GA—viloxazine RI 1855, viloxazine-AC RI 2220; M (OH-)-AC_2 RI 2590, M (*O*-desethyl-)-AC_2 RI 2360, M (di-oxo-) RI 2325; system GB—viloxazine RI 1923.

High Performance Liquid Chromatography. System HF—*k* 2.7; system HX—RI 325; system HY—RI 273; system HAA—Retention time 11.0 min.

Ultraviolet Spectrum. Aqueous acid—273 nm (A^1_1=92b). No alkaline shift.

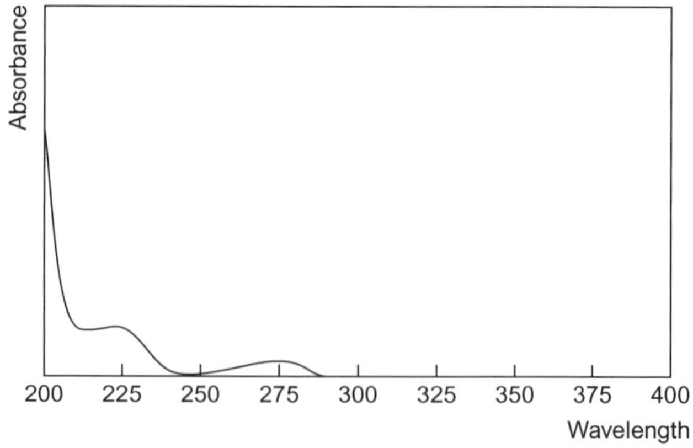

Infra-red Spectrum. Principal peaks at wavenumbers 1217, 1121, 1252, 739, 1511, 1031 cm^{-1} (viloxazine hydrochloride, KBr disk).

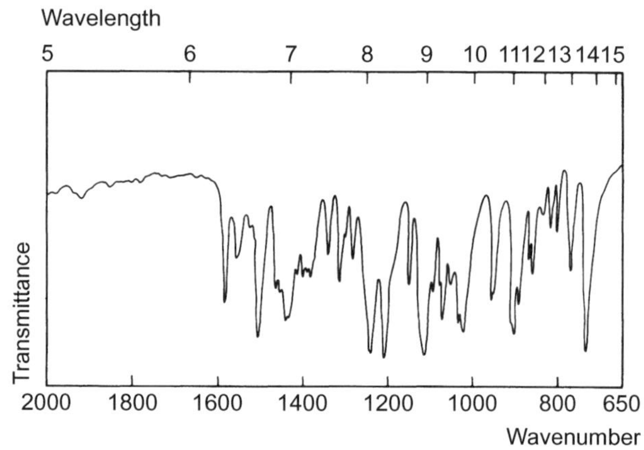

Mass Spectrum. Principal ions at *m/z* 56, 100, 138, 110, 57, 237, 70, 41.

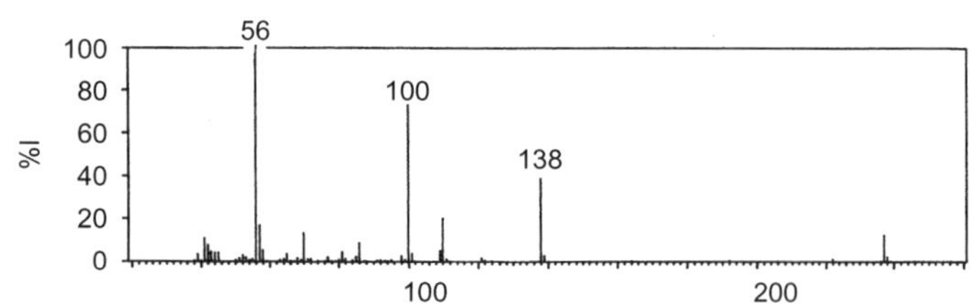

Quantification

Gas chromatography. In plasma: limit of detection 200 µg/L, FID—T. R. Norman *et al.*, *Br. J. Clin. Pharmacol.*, 1979, *8*, 169–171. In blood: viloxazine and other antidepressants, limits of detection 21 µg/L to 100 µg/L, nitrogen–phosphorus detection—M. A. Martinez *et al.*, *J. Anal. Toxicol.*, 2002, *26*, 296–302.

Gas chromatography–mass spectrometry. In serum: viloxazine and other antidepressants, limit of detection <500 µg/L—E. Lacassie *et al.*, *Acta Clin. Belg.*, 1999, *Suppl*, *1*, 20–24.

High performance liquid chromatography. In plasma or urine: limits of detection 25 µg/L and 1 mg/L, respectively, fluorescence detection—R. Gillilan and W. D. Mason, *J. Pharm. Sci.*, 1981, *70*, 220–221.

Disposition in the Body. Rapidly and completely absorbed after oral administration and crosses the blood–brain barrier. It is extensively metabolised by hydroxylation. About 90% of an oral dose is excreted in the urine in 24 h, of which 12 to 15% is unchanged drug, 3% is the free 4- and 5-hydroxy metabolites, and more than 40% is the glucuronide conjugate of 5-hydroxyviloxazine; about 16% is excreted as the glucuronide of a hydroxylated 5-oxo metabolite.

Therapeutic concentration.

Following single oral doses of 100 mg to 10 subjects, peak plasma concentrations of 1.11 to 2.93 mg/L (mean 1.7) were attained in about 1.5 h [B. Vandel *et al.*, *Eur. J. Drug Metab. Pharmacokinet.*, 1982, *7*, 65–68.]

Following oral doses of 400 mg daily in divided doses to 13 subjects, a mean steady-state blood concentration of about 1.3 mg/L was reported [P. F. C. Bayliss and D. E. Case, *Br. J. Clin. Pharmacol.*, 1975, *2*, 209–214.]

In 11 subjects receiving 300 mg viloxazine, peak blood concentrations of 3.6 mg/L were achieved in 86 min; when the same dose was given as a sustained-release preparation, peak concentrations of 1.92 mg/L were achieved in 215 min. 12 h after administration, plasma levels were 0.54 to 1.60 mg/L and 0.66 to 2.12 mg/L with the conventional and sustained-release dosage forms, respectively [M. F. Kergueris *et al.*, *Neuropsychobiology*, 1989, *20*, 136–140.]

Toxicity. A number of attempted suicides have been reported but recovery has occurred after the ingestion of up to 6.5 g of viloxazine together with other drugs.

The following postmortem tissue concentrations were reported in a fatality attributed to viloxazine: blood 45 mg/L, liver 185 μg/g, urine 640 mg/L; death occurred about 8 to 12 h after ingestion [M. Bailey, *Bull. Int. Assoc. Forensic Toxicol.*, 1976, *12*(3), 22.]

Half-life. Plasma half-life, 2 to 5 h.

Volume of distribution. About 0.5 to 1.5 L/kg.

Protein binding. In plasma, about 85 to 90%.

Note. For a review of viloxazine see R. M. Pinder *et al.*, *Drugs*, 1977, *13*, 401–421.

Dose. The equivalent of 100 to 400 mg of viloxazine daily.

Vinbarbital

Sedative/Barbiturate

Synonyms. Butenemal; Vinbarbitone.
5-Ethyl-5-(1-methyl-1-butenyl)-2,4,6(1*H*,3*H*,5*H*)-pyrimidinetrione
$C_{11}H_{16}N_2O_3$=224.3
CAS—125-42-8

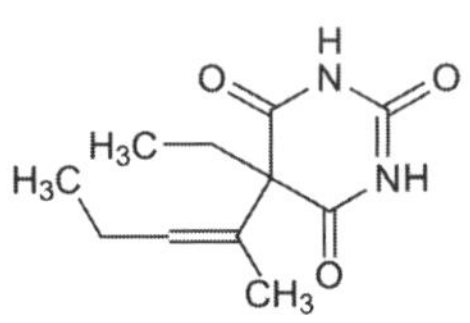

A white powder. M.p. 160° to 163°.
Very slightly soluble in water; soluble in ethanol; sparingly soluble in ether.

Dissociation Constant. pK_a 7.5 (20°).

Colour Tests. Koppanyi–Zwikker Test—violet; Mercurous Nitrate—black; Vanillin Reagent—violet-brown/colourless.

Thin-layer Chromatography. System TD—Rf 50; system TE—Rf 34; system TF—Rf 65; system TH—Rf 56; system TAD—Rf 57; system TAE—Rf 89; system TAJ—Rf 56; system TAK—Rf 62; system TAL—Rf 91. (Mercurous nitrate spray, black; Acidified potassium permanganate solution, yellow-brown; Zwikker's reagent, pink.)

Gas Chromatography. System GA—vinbarbital RI 1753, vinbarbital-Me_2 RI 1670, M (5-(1-ethylpropyl)-5-hydroxybarbituric acid) RI 1790, M (5-(1-ethylpropyl)barbituric acid) RI 1660, M (5-(3-hydroxy-1-methylbutyl)-5-vinylbarbituric acid) RI 1930, M (OH-) RI 2070, M (OH-)-H_2O RI 2020; system GF—RI 2495.

High Performance Liquid Chromatography. System HG—*k* 4.83; system HH—*k* 2.32; system HX—RI 379; system HY—RI 363.

Ultraviolet Spectrum. Borax buffer 0.05 M (pH 9.2)—238 nm (A_1^1=452a); M sodium hydroxide (pH 13)—254 nm (A_1^1=374b).

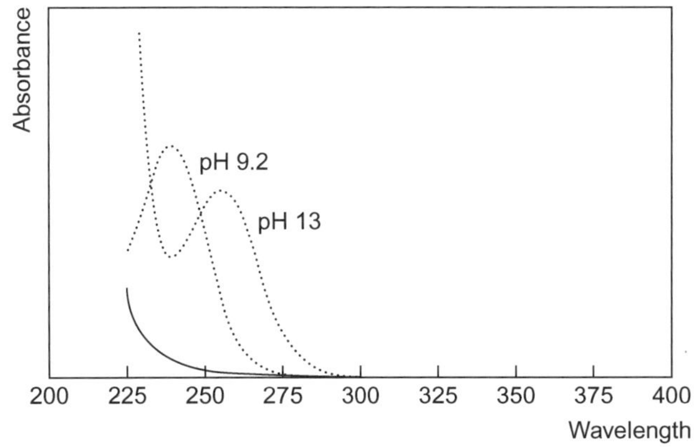

Infra-red Spectrum. Principal peaks at wavenumbers 1675, 1760, 1725, 1234, 1282, 1298 cm^{-1} (KBr disk).

Mass Spectrum. Principal ions at *m/z* 195, 41, 141, 69, 39, 152, 135, 196.

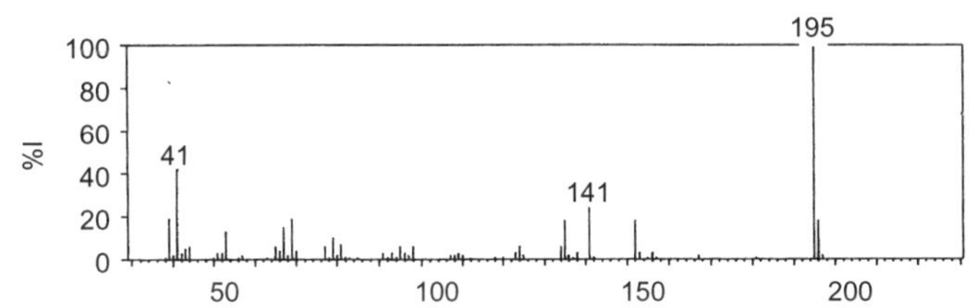

Quantification. See under Amylobarbital.

Dose. 100 to 200 mg daily.

Vinblastine

Antineoplastic

Synonyms. Vinblastini; Vincaleucoblastine; Vincaleukoblastine; VLB.
$C_{46}H_{58}N_4O_9$=811.0
CAS—865-21-4

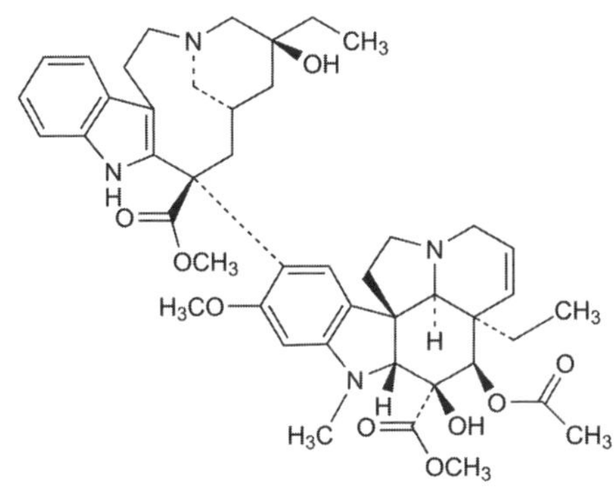

An alkaloid extracted from periwinkle, *Vinca rosea* (*Catharanthus roseus*) (Apocynaceae).
Crystals. M.p. 211° to 216°.
Practically insoluble in water; soluble in ethanol, acetone and chloroform.

Vinblastine Sulfate

Proprietary names. Blastovin; Cellblastin; Lemblastin; Solblastin; Velban; Velbe.
$C_{46}H_{58}N_4O_9,H_2SO_4$=909.1
CAS—143-67-9
A white to slightly yellow, very hygroscopic, amorphous or crystalline powder. M.p. 284° to 285°.
Soluble 1 in 10 of water and 1 in 50 of chloroform; very slightly soluble in ethanol; practically insoluble in ether.

Dissociation Constant. pK_a 5.4, 7.4.

Partition Coefficient. Log *P* (octanol/water), 3.7.

Colour Test. Marquis Test—red

Thin-layer Chromatography. System TA—Rf 60; system TB—Rf 01; system TC—Rf 60; system TE—Rf 57; system TL—RF 29; system TAE—Rf 46.

High Performance Liquid Chromatography. System HY—RI 355; system HAA—Retention time 8.4 min.

Ultraviolet Spectrum. Aqueous acid—268 nm (A_1^1 = 176b).

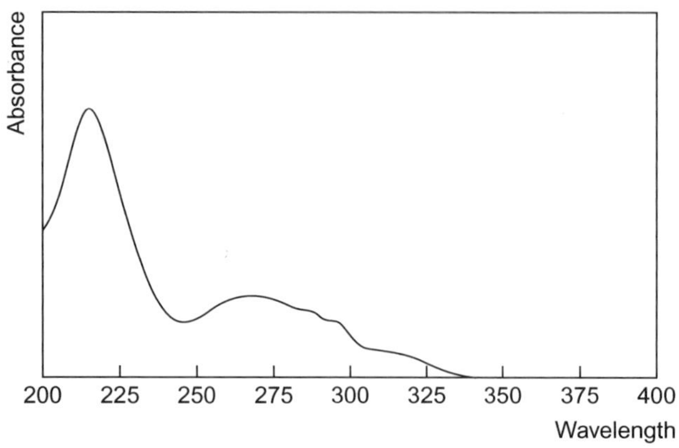

Infra-red Spectrum. Principal peaks at wavenumbers 1227, 1136, 1111, 1724, 1176, 1613 cm^{-1} (vinblastine sulfate, KBr disk).

Quantification

High performance liquid chromatography. In plasma or urine: vinblastine, vincristine and vindesine—M. de Smet *et al.*, *J. Chromatogr.*, 1985, *345*, 309–321. In plasma or urine: vinblastine, desacetylvinblastine, vincristine and vindesine, limit of detection 100 pg, electrochemical detection—D. E. Vendrig *et al.*, *J. Chromatogr.*, 1988, *424*, 83–94. In plasma or urine: vinblastine and metabolites, limit of detection 1 μg/L for vinblastine, fluorescence detection—O. van Tellingen *et al.*, *J. Chromatogr.*, 1991, *553*, 47–53.

Radioimmunoassay. In plasma: vinblastine and vincristine, limit of detection 2.1 μg/L and 3.8 μg/L, respectively—J. D. Teale *et al.*, *Br. J. Clin. Pharmacol.*, 1977, *4*, 169–172.

Disposition in the Body. Poorly absorbed after oral administration. After intravenous administration, it is metabolised to desacetylvinblastine which is active. About 14% of a radioactively labelled dose is excreted in the urine in 72 h and 10% is eliminated in the faeces in the same period.

Therapeutic concentration

After a bolus intravenous dose of 3 mg/m^2 given before or after cisplatin (100 mg/m^2) to 16 subjects, plasma vinblastine concentrations at 10 h were 3.2 to 6.3 μg/L (mean 4.8) and 2.7 to 7.1 μg/L (mean 4.9), respectively. Neutropenia was less severe in patients with plasma vinblastine levels less than 2.75 μg/L at 10 h [M. Links *et al.*, *Cancer Invest.*, 1999, *17*, 479–485.]

Toxicity

A vinblastine overdose in an 18-month-old child, who received 1.5 mg/kg instead of 0.15 mg/kg, was succesfully treated with steroids and citrovorum factor [V. Conter *et al.*, *Pediatr. Hematol. Oncol.*, 1991, *8*, 165–169.]

Half-life. Plasma half-life (total radioactivity), about 20 h.

Protein binding. In plasma, about 99%.

Dose. Initially 100 μg/kg of vinblastine sulfate weekly, by intravenous injection.

Vincristine

Antineoplastic

Synonym. Leurocristine
22-Oxovincaleukoblastine
$C_{46}H_{56}N_4O_{10}$ = 825.0
CAS—57-22-7

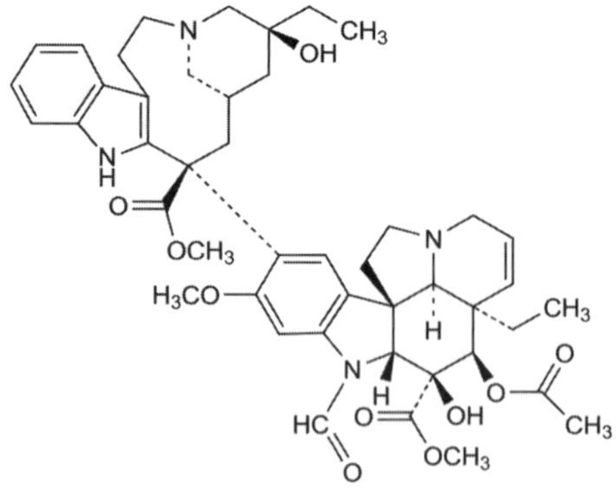

An alkaloid obtained from *Vinca rosea* (*Catharanthus roseus*) (Apocynaceae).
Crystals. M.p. 218° to 220°.

Vincristine Sulfate

Proprietary names. Cellcristin; Citomid RU; Farmistin; Faulcris; Filcrin; Oncovin; Pericristine; Vincasar; Vincrin; Vincrisul; Vintec.
$C_{46}H_{56}N_4O_{10},H_2SO_4$ = 923.0
CAS—2068-78-2
A white to slightly yellow, very hygroscopic, amorphous or crystalline powder.
M.p. about 277°.
Soluble 1 in 2 of water and 1 in 30 of chloroform; slightly soluble in ethanol; practically insoluble in ether; soluble in methanol.

Dissociation Constant. pK_a 5.0, 7.4.

Partition Coefficient. Log *P* (octanol/water), 2.8.

High Performance Liquid Chromatography. System HAA—Retention time 13.8 min.

Ultraviolet Spectrum. Aqueous acid—256 nm (A_1^1 = 181b), 297 nm (A_1^1 = 179b).

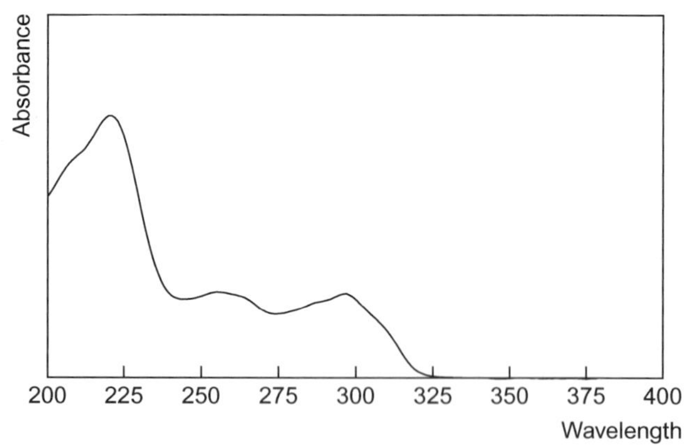

Infra-red Spectrum. Principal peaks at wavenumbers 1230, 1745, 1170, 1685, 1030, 1130 cm^{-1} (vincristine sulfate, KBr disk).

Quantification. See also under Vinblastine.

High performance liquid chromatography. In serum: limit of detection 0.3 μg/L, electrochemical detection—H. Bloemhof *et al.*, *J. Chromatogr.*, 1991, *572*, 171–179. In plasma: limit of detection < 28 μg/L, UV detection—L. Embree *et al.*, *J. Pharm. Biomed. Anal.*, 1997, *16*, 675–687. In plasma: electrochemical detection—P. Koopmans *et al.*, *Ther. Drug Monit.*, 2001, *23*, 406–409.

Disposition in the Body. Poorly absorbed after oral administration. After intravenous injection it disappears rapidly from the blood and is excreted mainly in the bile. About 12% of a dose is excreted in the urine in 72 h and 70% is eliminated in the faeces in the same period.

Toxicity.

A vincristine overdose (7.5 mg/m^2) was accidentally administered to 3 children, 2 of whom survived and 1 of whom died. The children were treated with double-volume exchange transfusions. In the 2 children who survived, the vincristine plasma levels were, respectively: pre-exchange 39.5 and 14.4 μg/L, post-exchange 16.7 and 4.1 μg/L, 8th day 2.6 and 2.9 μg/L;

in the child who died the levels were: pre-exchange 26.0 μg/L, post-exchange 24.0 μg/L, 8th day 5.6 μg/L [H. V. Kosmidis *et al.*, *Pediatr. Hematol. Oncol.*, 1991, *8*, 171–178.]

Half-life. Plasma half-life, about 3 h; a terminal elimination half-life of about 23 h has also been reported.

Dose. Initially 25 to 75 μg/kg of vincristine sulfate weekly, by intravenous injection.

Vindesine

Antineoplastic

Synonyms. Desacetyl Vinblastine Amide; VDS.
3-(Aminocarbonyl)-O^4-deacetyl-3-de(methoxycarbonyl)-vincaleukoblastine
$C_{43}H_{55}N_5O_7$=753.9
CAS—53643-48-4

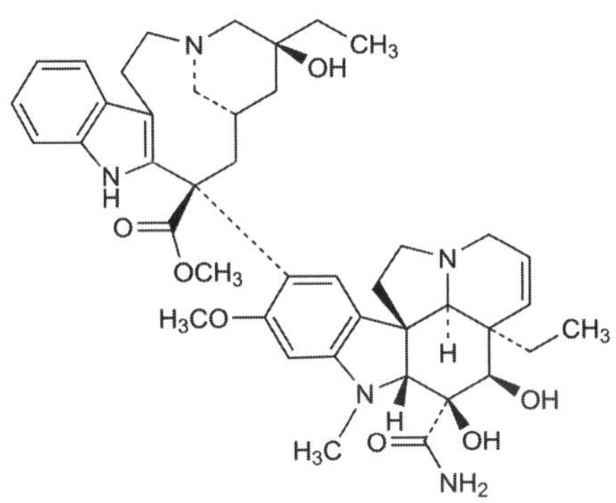

Crystals. M.p. 230° to 232°.

Vindesine Sulfate
Proprietary names. Eldisin(e); Enison; Gesidine.
$C_{43}H_{55}N_5O_7,H_2SO_4$=852.0
CAS—59917-39-4
An amorphous solid.
Freely soluble in water.

Dissociation Constant. pK_a (DMF 66%) 5.4, 7.4; (water) 6.0, 7.7.

Partition Coefficient. Log *P* (octanol/water), 4.4.

Ultraviolet Spectrum. Methanol—270 nm (A_1^1=235b).

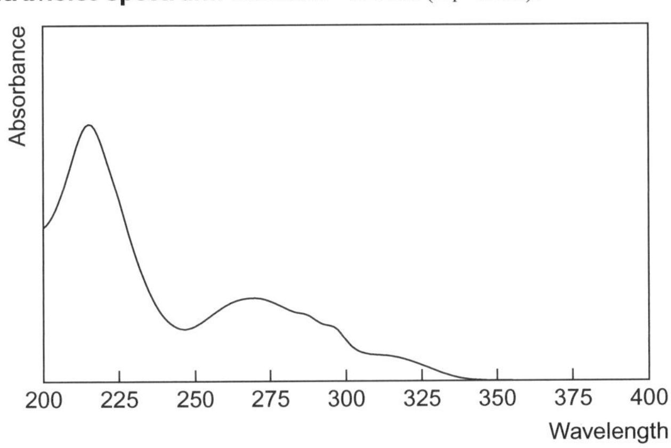

Infra-red Spectrum. Principal peaks at wavenumbers 1120, 1230, 1680, 1175, 1610, 1038 cm^{-1} (vindesine sulfate, KBr disk).

Quantification. See also under Vinblastine.

Radioimmunoassay. In plasma: limit of detection 50 ng/L—R. Rahmani *et al.*, *Clin. Chim. Acta*, 1983, *129*, 57–69.

Disposition in the Body. Poorly absorbed after oral administration. After intravenous injection, about 13% of a dose is excreted in the urine in 24 h.

Therapeutic concentration
15 subjects received therapy with vindesine either by intravenous bolus injection at doses ranging from 0.7 to 1.2 mg/m^2 or by 5 day infusions (total dose 5 mg/m^2) in combination with cisplatin (20 mg/m^2 daily) and bleomycin (6 mg/m^2 daily) for 5 days. Steady-state vindesine concentrations of 4 to 15 μg/L were reached after about 30 h of infusion administration [R. Rahmani *et al*, *Cancer Treat. Rep.*, 1985, *69*, 839–844].

Half-life. Plasma half-life, about 24 h.

Dose. Initially 3 mg/m^2 of vindesine sulfate weekly, by intravenous injection.

Vinorelbine

Antineoplastic

Synonyms. nor-5′-Anhydrovinblastine; NVBKW-2307.
Proprietary name. Navelbine
3′,4′-Didehydro-4′-deoxy-*C*′-norvincaleukoblastine
$C_{45}H_{54}N_4O_8$=779.0
CAS—71486-22-1

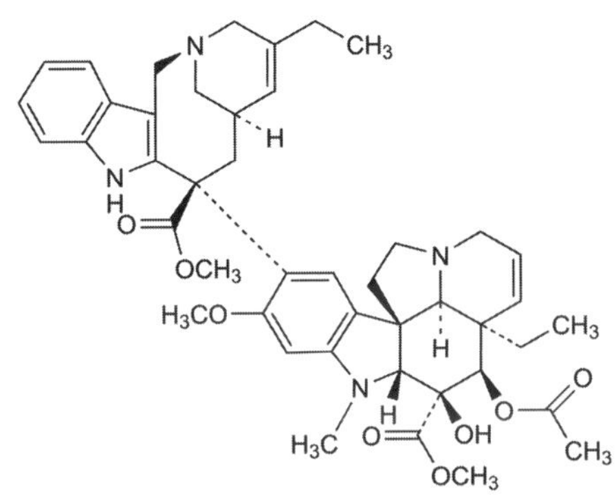

Vinorelbine Tartrate
Synonym. Vinorelbine Ditartrate
Proprietary names. Biovelbin; Eunades; Navelbine.
$C_{45}H_{54}N_4O_8,2C_4H_6O_6$=1079.1
CAS—125317-39-7
A yellow to white amorphous powder. It is soluble in water and in alcohol.

Dissociation Constant. pK_a 5.4.

Partition Coefficient. Log *P* (octanol/buffer, pH 7.2), 16.

High Performance Liquid Chromatography. Column: cyano (Spherisorb, 250 × 4.6 mm i.d., 5 μm). Mobile phase: acetonitrile:ammonium acetate (80 mM, pH 2.5) (50:50), flow rate 1 mL/min. IS: vinoblastine sulfate. Fluorescence detection (λ_{ex}=280 nm; λ_{em}=360 nm). Retention times: vinorelbine, 5.4 min; IS, 4.5 min [A. Gauvin *et al.*, *J Chromatogr. B Biomed. Sci. Appl.*, 2000, *748 (2)*, 389–399].

Column: C_{18} (Novapak, 300 × 3.9 mm i.d.); (guard) C_{18} (Novapak, 300 × 3.9 mm i.d.). Mobile phase: acetonitrile:phosphate buffer (pH 2.7) (60:40), flow rate 0.9 mL/min. Fluorescence detection (λ_{ex}=280 nm; λ_{em}=360 nm). Retention time: 13 min [I. Robieux *et al.*, *J. Chromatogr.*, 1996, *675*, *Biomed. Appl.*, 183–187].

Ultraviolet Spectrum. Ethanol—215, 268, 282, 293, 310 nm.

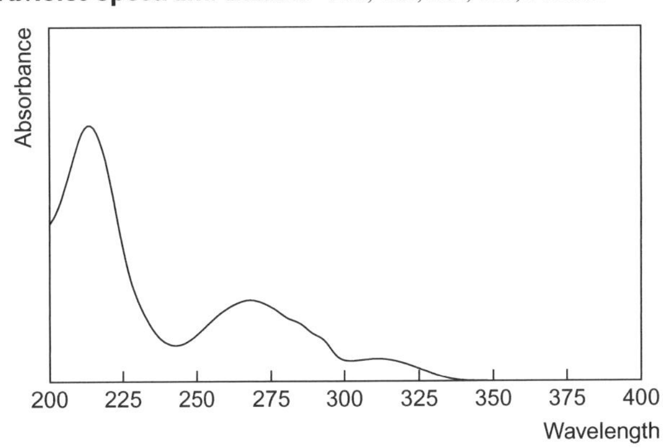

Quantification

High performance liquid chromatography. In serum or urine: vinorelbine and desacetylvinorelbine, limit of detection is 2.5 μg/L in serum and 5.0 μg/L in urine, UV detection (λ=268 nm)—F. Jehl *et al.*, *J. Chromatogr.*, 1990, *525*; *Biomed. Appl.*, *90*, 225–233. In plasma or urine: limit of detection is about 1 μg/L in plasma and 20 μg/L in urine, ECD—G. Nicot *et al.*, *J. Chromatogr.*, 1990, *528*; *Biomed. Appl.*, *93*, 258–266. In plasma or urine: limit of detection is 1.5 μg/L in plasma and 15 μg/L in urine, fluorescence detection (λ_{ex}=270 nm; λ_{em}=320 nm)—O. van Tellingen *et al.*, *J. Chromatogr.*, 1992, *573*; *Biomed. Appl.*, *111*, 328–332. In plasma: limit of detection 2 μg/L, fluorescence detection (λ_{ex}=280 nm; λ_{em}=360 nm)—I. Robieux *et al.*, *J. Chromatogr.*, 1996, *675*, *Biomed. Appl.*, 183–187.

Disposition in the Body. Vinorelbine is rapidly absorbed and peak plasma concentrations increase with dose between 0.9 and 2.0 h after administration. The drug shows triphasic pharmacokinetics after intravenous administration. It is widely distributed and highly bound to platelets (78%) and lymphocytes. Vinorelbine is metabolised in the liver to desacetylvinorelbine which has antineoplastic activity. It is excreted primarily in faeces via bile, and to a lesser extent it is also excreted in urine as the unchanged drug and as metabolites. Recovery of the drug is incomplete which suggests that it may be retained in tissue.

Therapeutic concentration

8 male patients with lung cancer (stage III or IV), aged between 51 and 74 years, were intravenously administered a weekly dose of 30 mg/m^2 over 15 min. A mean peak plasma concentration of 780 μg/L (range 260 to 1230 μg/L) was observed [P. Marquet *et al.*, *Eur. J. Clin. Pharmacol.*, 1992, *42*, 545–547].

5 patients, with a mean age of 56.7 years, with advanced breast cancer were treated with 30 mg/m^2 vinorelbine intravenously over a 20 min infusion. Mean peak plasma concentrations of 179 μg/L were observed at 0.5 h and plasma concentrations remained above 2 μg/L for 48 h or longer after administration [I. Robieux *et al.*, *J. Chromatogr.*, 1996, *675*, *Biomed. Appl.*, 183–187].

Toxicity

In a study carried out in 8 male patients with lung cancer, 2 patients died resulting from haematological toxicity, namely anaemia. Other toxicological effects observed were leucopenia and neurological toxicity [P. Marquet *et al.*, *Eur. J. Clin. Pharmacol.*, 1992, *42*, 545–547].

Half-life. Plasma half-life, 28 to 44 h.

Volume of distribution. 25 to 100 L/kg; steady state mean 47.6 L/kg (range 13.8 to 156).

Clearance. Plasma clearance, 16 to 21 mL/min/kg (mean 1.28 L/h/kg (range 0.58 to 2.61).

Distribution in blood. Vinorelbine, 84% bound to red blood cells, mainly platelets.

Protein binding. In plasma, 14%.

Note. For a review of the pharmacokinetics of vinorelbine see D. Levêque and F. Jehl, *Clin. Pharmacokinet.*, 1996, *31*, 184–197.

Dose. Initially the equivalent of 25 to 30 mg per m^2 of vinorelbine intravenously weekly.

Vinylbital

Hypnotic/Barbiturate

Synonyms. Butyvinal; Vinylbitone; Vinymalum.
Proprietary names. Optanox; Speda.
5-Ethenyl-5-(1-methylbutyl)-2,4,6-(1*H*,3*H*,5*H*)-pyrimidinetrione
$C_{11}H_{16}N_2O_3$=224.3
CAS—2430-49-1

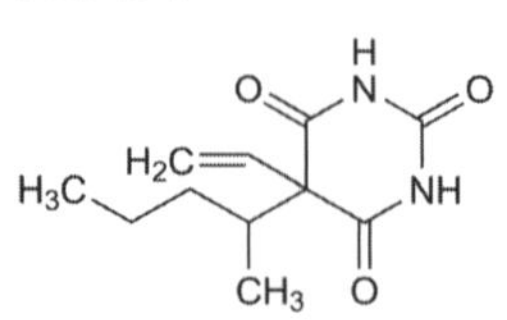

Crystals. M.p. 90° to 92°.

Partition Coefficient. Log *P* (octanol/water), 1.9.

Thin-layer Chromatography. System TD—Rf 38; system TE—Rf 39; system TF—Rf 64; system TAD—Rf 66; system TAE—Rf 89.

Gas Chromatography. System GA—vinylbital RI 1729, vinylbital-Me$_2$ RI 1655, M (OH-)-H_2O RI 1995, M (desvinyl-) RI 1665; system GAJ—vinylbital RRT 0.798 (relative to methylphenobarbital).

High Performance Liquid Chromatography. System HX—RI 424; system HZ—Retention time 4.1 min; system HAA—Retention time 16.6. min.

Ultraviolet Spectrum. Aqueous alkali—247 nm (A^1_1=298b).

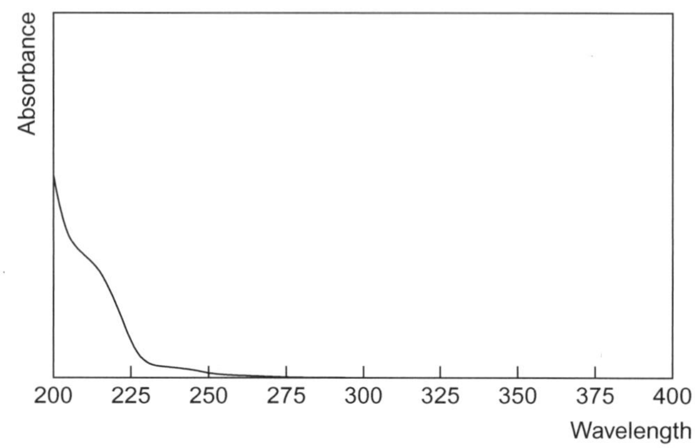

Infra-red Spectrum. Principal peaks at wavenumbers 1692, 1730, 1750, 1318, 1220, 1630 cm^{-1}.

Quantification. See also under Amylobarbital.

Gas chromatography. In plasma: limit of detection <125 μg/L, AFID—D. D. Breimer and A. G. de Boer, *Arzneimittelforschung*, 1976, *26*, 448–454.

Disposition in the Body. Readily absorbed after oral administration. Metabolites which have been identified in urine are 3′-hydroxyvinylbital and the corresponding desvinyl derivative, 5-(3-hydroxy-1-methylbutyl)barbituric acid. Less than 5% of a dose is excreted in the urine unchanged in 72 h.

Therapeutic concentration

Following a single oral dose of 150 mg to 6 subjects, peak plasma concentrations of 2.2 to 3.9 mg/L were attained in 1 to 2 h [D. D. Breimer and A. G. de Boer, *Arzneimittelforschung*, 1976, *26*, 448–454].

Half-life. Plasma half-life, 18 to 34 h (mean 24).

Volume of distribution. About 0.7 L/kg.

Dose. 100 to 200 mg, as a hypnotic.

Voglibose

Antidiabetic/Alpha-glucosidase Inhibitor

Synonym. AO-128.
Proprietary name. Basen
3,4-Dideoxy-4-[[2-hydroxy-1-(hydroxymethyl)ethyl]amino]-2-*C*-(hydroxymethyl)-D-epi-inositol
$C_{10}H_{21}NO_7$=267.3
CAS—83480-29-9

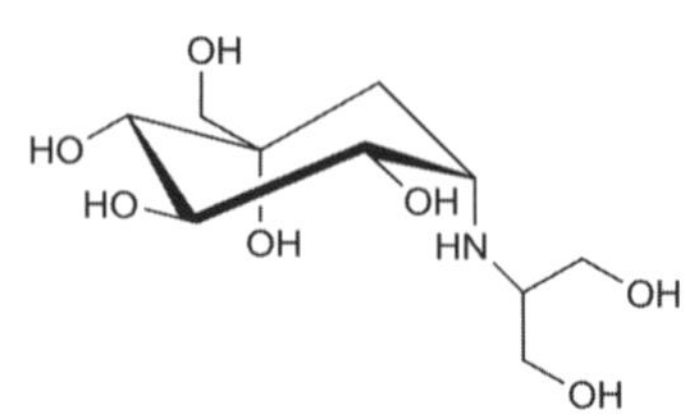

Colourless crystals, M.p. 162° to 163°

Disposition in the Body. Voglibose is slowly and poorly absorbed, and is rapidly excreted. Little metabolism occurs and no metabolites have as yet been identified. Within 48 h of oral administration, it is almost totally excreted in the faeces (93%) as the unchanged drug with a small amount in urine (4%). Maximum concentrations are reached in tissues up to 1 h after oral administration. Penetration of the blood–brain barrier and erythrocyte membrane is low.

Toxicity. Voglibose competitively and reversibly inhibits the alpha-glucosidase enzymes; glucoamylase, sucrase, maltase and isomaltase, found in the small intestine, and this delays hydrolysis of complex carbohydrates. It is unlikely to produce hypoglycaemia in overdose, but abdominal discomfort and diarrhoea may occur.

Bioavailability. Less than 6%.

Volume of distribution. Low tissue affinity.

Protein binding. Less than 15%.

Dose. 200 to 300 μg orally 3 times a day.

Warfarin

Anticoagulant/Rodenticide

Proprietary names. Biotrol; Dethmor; Sorexa (all rodenticides).
4-Hydroxy-3-(3-oxo-1-phenylbutyl)-2*H*-1-benzopyran-2-one
$C_{19}H_{16}O_4$=308.3
CAS—81-81-2

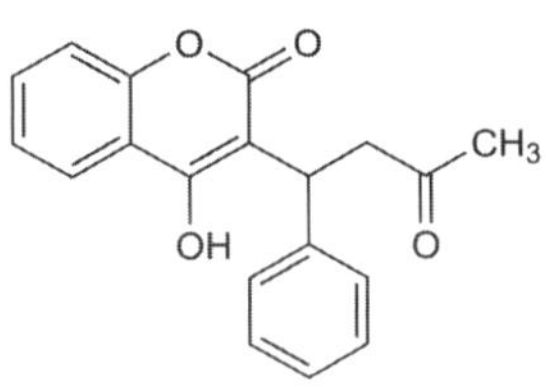

Colourless crystals. M.p. of the purified compound 159° to 160°; of the technical grade 157°.
Practically insoluble in water, benzene and cyclohexane; moderately soluble in alcohols; freely soluble in alkaline aqueous solutions; soluble in acetone and dioxane.

Warfarin Potassium

Proprietary name Athrombin-K
$C_{19}H_{15}KO_4$=346.4
CAS—2610-86-8
A white crystalline powder which discolours on exposure to light.
Soluble 1 in 1.5 of water and 1 in 1.9 of ethanol; very slightly soluble in chloroform and ether.

Warfarin Sodium

Proprietary names. Aldocumar; Coumadin(e); Marevan; Panwarfin; Varfine; Waran; Warfilone.
$C_{19}H_{15}NaO_4$=330.3
CAS—129-06-6
A white amorphous or crystalline powder which discolours on exposure to light.
Soluble 1 in less than 1 of water and ethanol; very slightly soluble in chloroform and ether.

Dissociation Constant. pK_a 5.0 (20°).

Partition Coefficient. Log *P* (octanol/pH 8.0), 0.0; (octanol/water), 2.60.

Colour Test. Liebermann's Test—red-orange.

Thin-layer Chromatography. System TD—Rf 64; system TE—Rf 18; system TF—Rf 62; system TX—Rf 12; system TY—Rf 11; system TAD—Rf 64. (Acidified potassium permanganate solution, positive.)

Gas Chromatography. System GA—warfarin RI 1432, warfarin-Me RI 2580, M (OH-) isomer-1-Me_2 RI 2810, M (OH-) isomer-2-Me_2 RI 2830, M (OH-) isomer 3-Me_2 RI 2870.

High Performance Liquid Chromatography. System HX—RI 546; system HY—RI 514; system HZ—Retention time, 9.4 min; system HAX—Retention time 8.0 min; system HAY—Retention time 8.3 min.

Column: (analytical) *β*-cyclodextrin (Astec, 250 × 4.6 mm i.d., 5 μm); (guard) *β*-cyclodextrin (50 × 4.6 mm, 5 μm). Mobile phase: acetonitrile:glacial acetic acid:triethylamine (1000:3:2.5), flow rate 1.0 mL/min. UV detection (λ = 320 nm). Retention time(s): (*S*)-warfarin, 6.9 min; (*R*)-warfarin, 7.7 min [P. R. Ring and J. M. Bostick, *J. Pharm. Biomed. Anal.*, 2000, *22*, 573–581].

Column: Chiralcel OD (250 × 4.6 mm i.d., 10 μm); Chiralcel OD guard (50 × 4.6 mm i.d.). Mobile phase: isopropanol:acetic acid:hexane (18:0.5:81.5), flow rate 1.0 mL/min. Fluorescence detection (λ_{ex} = 320 nm; λ_{em} = 415 nm). Resolution factor: warfarin, 5.6; 7-hydroxywarfarin, 4.5 [H. Takahashi *et al.*, *J. Chromatogr. Biomed. Sci. Appl.*, 1997, *701(1)*, 71–80].

Ultraviolet Spectrum. Aqueous acid—270, 280, 303 nm; aqueous alkali—293, 308 nm (A_1^1=462a).

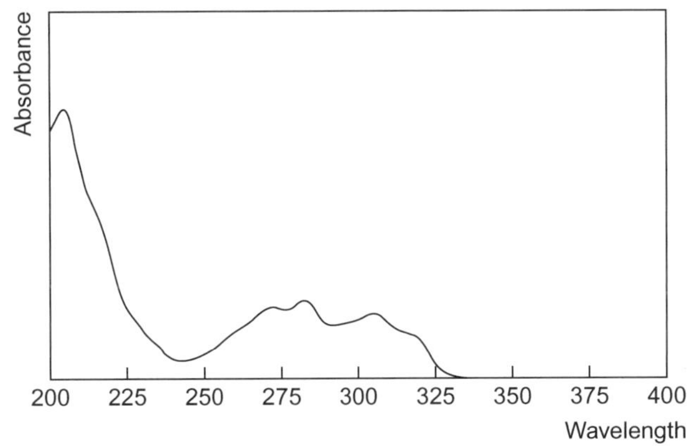

Infra-red Spectrum. Principal peaks at wavenumbers 1517, 1599, 1640, 750, 1700, 692 cm^{-1} (warfarin sodium, KBr disk).

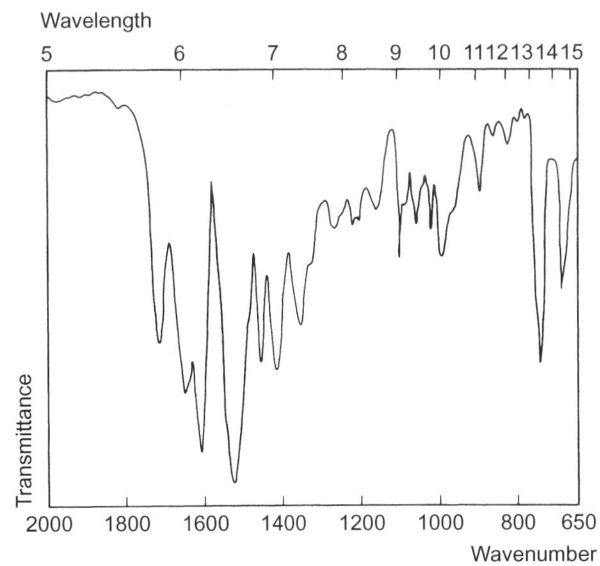

Mass Spectrum. Principal ions at *m/z* 265, 308, 121, 43, 266, 187, 213, 251.

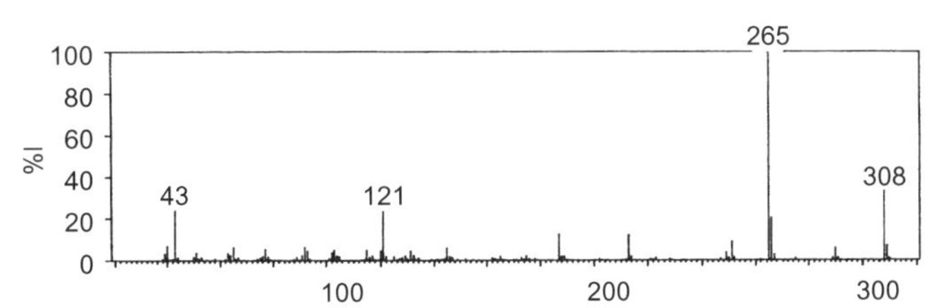

Quantification

Gas chromatography. In plasma: limit of detection 0.3 mg/L, FID—S. Hanna *et al.*, *J. Pharm. Sci.*, 1978, *67*, 84–86.

High performance liquid chromatography. In plasma: limit of quantification 12.5 μg/L—P. R. Ring and J. M. Bostick, *J. Pharm. Biomed. Anal.*, 2000, *22*, 573–581. In plasma and urine: limit of detection 20 μg/L for (*R*)-warfarin, 40 μg/L for (*S*)-warfarin, 2.5 μg/L for (R)-7-hydroxywarfarin and 4.5 μg/L for (*S*)-7-hydroxywarfarin, UV or fluorescence detection (λ_{ex} = 320 nm; λ_{em} = 415 nm)—H. Takahashi *et al., J. Chromatogr. B Biomed. Sci. Appl.*, 1997, *701(1)*, 71–80. In serum: limit of quantification 3 μg/L for fluorescence detection and 20 μg/L for UV detection—E. A. Kuijpers *et al., J. Anal. Toxicol.*, 1995, *19*, 557–562. In plasma: limit of detection 8.05 μg/L for (*S*)-warfarin and 6.21 μg/L for (*R*)-warfarin, fluorescence detection—W. M. Cai *et al., Ther. Drug Monit.*, 1994, *16(5)*, 509–512. In plasma: limit of quantification 12.5 μg/L, UV detection—W. Naidong and J. W. Lee, *J. Pharm. Biomed. Anal.*, 1993, *11(9)*, 785–792.

Disposition in the Body. Warfarin is readily and almost completely absorbed after oral administration with peak concentrations observed within the first 4 h. The (*R*)-enantiomer of warfarin is metabolised mainly by reduction to (*RS*)-3′-hydroxywarfarin although 6-hydroxylation also occurs. The (*S*)-enantiomer is metabolised mainly by 6- and 7-hydroxylation with smaller amounts of the (*SS*)-3′-hydroxy metabolite; the reduced metabolites are less active than warfarin; the 6- and 7-hydroxy metabolites are inactive. Other metabolites include warfarin sodium alcohols, including dehydrowarfarin sodium and two diastereoisomer alcohols, which have minimum activity. Less than 1% of a dose is excreted in the urine as unchanged drug. About 16 to 43% of a single dose is excreted in the urine as free or conjugated metabolites in 6 days. Excretion also occurs, to a lesser extent, through bile.

Therapeutic concentration. In plasma, usually in the range 1 to 3 mg/L but there are considerable inter-subject variations in sensitivity to warfarin and measurement of the plasma concentration is generally of little value since the pharmacological effect can be easily measured.

Following a single oral dose of 50 mg to 8 subjects, peak plasma concentrations of 5.2 to 10.9 mg/L (mean 7.2) were attained in 0.3 to 3 h (mean 1.5) [A. Welle-Watne *et al., Medd. Nor. Farm. Selsk.*, 1980, *42*, 103–113].

In 6 subjects receiving daily oral doses of 5 to 11 mg, steady-state plasma concentrations of 1.2 to 2.6 mg/L were attained [M. L'E. Orme *et al., BMJ*, 1977, *1*, 1564–1565].

6 male ischaemic stroke patients, aged between 61 and 69 years, participating in a warfarin–aspirin recurrent stroke study were administered 4 to 6 mg warfarin daily for at least 1 week. The mean (*S*)-warfarin plasma concentration observed was 0.47 (0.16 to 0.66) mg/L and for (R)-warfarin, 0.69 (0.42 to 0.97) mg/L [W. M. Cai *et al., Ther. Drug Monit.*, 1994, *16(5)*, 509–512].

Toxicity. Toxic effects are associated with plasma concentrations greater than 10 mg/L. The maximum permissible atmospheric concentration is 0.1 mg/m^3.

In a patient who took an overdose of warfarin (2000 mg by mouth plus 25 × 10^4 U administered subcutaneously), a plasma concentration of 111 mg/L was reported on the day of admission (the day after the overdose). Concentrations fell steadily in an approximate first-order fashion to 0.2 mg/L 10 days after the overdose [L. P. Hackett *et al., Med. J. Aust.*, 1985, *142*, 642–643].

Half-life. Plasma half-life, 15 to 85 h (mean, 42), decreased in subjects with renal disease. The half-life of the *R*-enantiomer (mean about 45 h; range 37 to 89 h) appears to be longer than that of the *S*-enantiomer (mean about 30 h; range 21 to 43 h).

Volume of distribution. 0.05 to 0.25 L/kg (mean 0.15).

Clearance. Plasma clearance, 0.02 to 0.08 mL/min/kg (mean 0.04).

Distribution in blood. Plasma : whole blood ratio, about 1.8.

Protein binding. In plasma, 97 to 99%, reduced in renal impairment.

Note. For a review of warfarin metabolism and mode of action, see B. K. Park, *Biochem. Pharmacol.*, 1988, *37*, 19–27.

Dose. Maintenance, 3 to 12 mg of warfarin sodium daily.

Xamoterol

Cardiotonic/ Beta-adrenocepter Partial Agonist

N-[2-[[2-Hydroxy-3-(4-hydroxyphenoxy)propyl]amino]ethyl]-4-morpholinecarboxamide
$C_{16}H_{25}N_3O_5$ = 339.4
CAS—81801-12-9

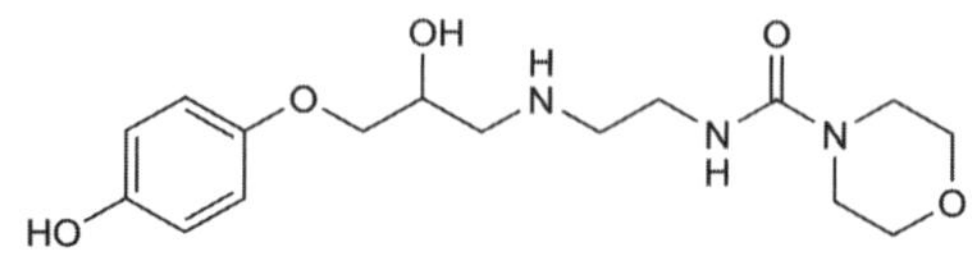

Crystals. M.p. 168° to 169°.

Xamoterol Hemifumarate

Synonym. ICI-118587
Proprietary names. Corwil; Corwin; Xamtol.
$(C_{16}H_{25}N_3O_5)_2$, $C_4H_4O_4$ = 794.8
CAS—90730-93-1

Partition Coefficient. Log *P* (octanol/water), −1.11.

Thin-layer Chromatography. System TB—Rf 00; system TE—Rf 15; system TF—Rf 00; system TAE—Rf 18.
Plate: silica gel (Merck 60 F_{254}). Mobile phase: toluene:ethanol:ethyl acetate:ammonium hydroxide (6:4:2:1). Rf value: 0.10 (sulfate conjugate) [T. R. Marten *et al., Drug Metab. Dispos.*, 1984, *12(5)*, 652–670].

High Performance Liquid Chromatography. System HX—RI 239.

Column: Hypersil-ODS (150 × 4.1 mm i.d., 5 μm). Mobile phase: methanol:tetrahydrofuran (THF):perchloric acid (30 mM) (8.0:0.6:91.4), flow rate 1.5 mL/min. Retention time: 8 min. Electrochemical detection [P.C. Davis, *J. Chromatogr.*, 1987, *417*, 233–235].

Column: Lichrospher 60 RP Select B (125 × 4 mm i.d., 5 μm). Mobile phase: acetonitrile:ammonium acetate (20 mM) (55:45), flow rate 2 mL/min. IS: prenalterol. Fluorescence detection (λ_{ex} = 190 nm; λ_{em} = 320 to 400 nm). Retention times: xamoterol, 6.9 min; IS, 5.8 min [C. J. Oddie *et al., J. Chromatogr.*, 1984, *308*, 370–375].

Ultraviolet Spectrum. Aqueous acid—280 nm (xamoterol); 270 nm (sulfate metabolite); 275 nm (glucuronide metabolite); aqueous alkali—300 nm (xamoterol).

Quantification

High performance liquid chromatography. In blood: limit of detection 0.002 mg/L—P.C. Davis, *J. Chromatogr.*, 1987, *417*, 233–235. In blood and urine: limit of detection 0.001 mg/L and 0.01 mg/L, respectively, fluorescence detection (λ_{ex} = 190 nm; λ_{em} = 320 to 400 nm)—C. J Oddie *et al., J. Chromatogr.*, 1984, *308*, 370–375.

Disposition in the Body. The drug is poorly absorbed from the gastro-intestinal tract. A small amount is metabolised to inactive sulfate conjugates. Glucuronide metabolites have also been identified. Xamoterol is excreted mainly in urine as the unchanged drug and its metabolite(s). Most of the absorbed drug is eliminated within 24 h. Maximum plasma concentrations are reached within 1 to 2 h, although in the elderly the plasma concentrations are increased.

Therapeutic concentration

The mean maximal plasma concentration after a 200 mg oral dose is 0.189 mg/L in young healthy individuals, and 0.134 mg/L in the elderly. In individuals with ischaemic heart disease, the mean maximum plasma concentrations were 0.128, 0.264 and 0.403 mg/L after 200, 400 and 600 mg doses, respectively [R. Furlong and R. Brogden, *Drugs*, 1988, *36(4)*, 455–474].

6 patients with liver disease (mostly alcohol induced), aged between 29 and 69 years (mean 56.5 years) and 6 healthy individuals (34 to 68 years; mean 56 years) were administered 0.2 mg/kg xamoterol intravenously over 5 min followed by a single oral dose of 200 mg. The peak plasma concentrations after the intravenous dose were 0.715 mg/L for the patients and 0.691 mg/L for the healthy individuals. For the oral dose, peak concentrations were 0.149 and 0.138 mg/L, respectively [D. P. Nicholls *et al, Br. J. Clin. Pharmacol.*, 1989, *28*, 718–721].

Bioavailability. 5%.

Half-life. 16 h.

Volume of distribution. 1.12 L/kg.

Clearance. Total plasma clearance, 0.18 to 0.3 L/h/kg.

Protein binding. 3%.

Dose. 200 to 400 mg daily.

Xantinol Nicotinate

Vasodilator

Synonym. Xanthinol Nicotinate; Xantinol Niacinate
Proprietary names. Complamin; Frigol; Vedrin.
3-Pyridinecarboxylic acid compound with 3,7-dihydro-7-[2-hydroxy-3-[(2-hydroxyethyl)methylamino]propyl]-1,3-dimethyl-1*H*-purine-2,6-dione (1:1)
$C_{13}H_{21}N_5O_4,C_6H_5NO_2$=434.5
CAS—2530-97-4 (xantinol); 437-74-1 (nicotinate)

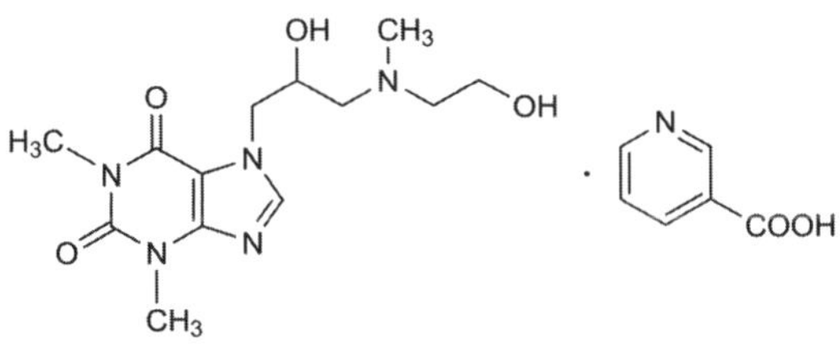

Colourless crystals. M.p. 180°.
Freely soluble in water.

Partition Coefficient. Log *P* (octanol/water), −1.8.

Colour Tests. Amalic Acid Test—orange/violet; Cyanogen Bromide—orange

Thin-layer Chromatography. System TA—Rf 41; system TE—Rf 21; system TF—Rf 00; system TAE—Rf 26. (Acidified potassium permanganate solution, positive.)

Gas Chromatography. System GA—xantinol-AC_2 RI 2870.

High Performance Liquid Chromatography. System HX—RI 215.

Ultraviolet Spectrum. Aqueous acid—267 nm (A^1_1=300a). Xantinol: aqueous acid—273 nm (A^1_1=270b).

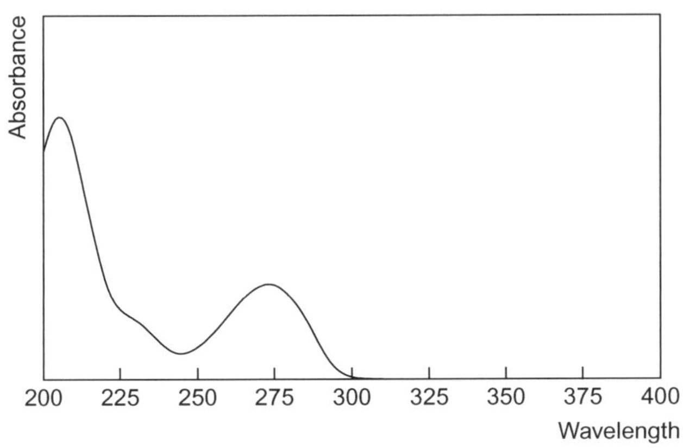

Infra-red Spectrum. Principal peaks at wavenumbers 1658, 1695, 1548, 763, 750, 1029 cm^{-1} (xantinol, KBr disk).

Dose. 450 to 900 mg daily.

Xipamide

Diuretic

Proprietary names. Aquaphor; Aquaphoril; Chronexan; Demiax; Diurexan; Lumitens.
4-Chloro-5-sulfamoyl-2′,6′-salicyloxylidide
$C_{15}H_{15}ClN_2O_4S$=354.8
CAS—14293-44-8

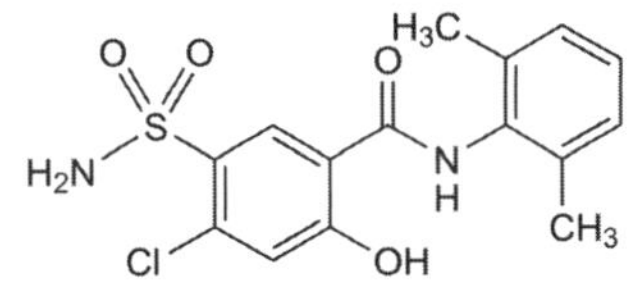

A white crystalline substance. M.p. about 260°, with decomposition. Practically insoluble in water; soluble in ethanol; very soluble in acetone; slightly soluble in chloroform and ether.

Dissociation Constant. pK_a 4.8 (phenol), 10.0 (sulfonamide).

Partition Coefficient. Log *P* (octanol/water), 2.2.

Colour Tests. Koppanyi–Zwikker Test—violet; Liebermann's Test—orange; Mandelin's Test—blue; Mercurous Nitrate—black

Thin-layer Chromatography. System TB—Rf 00; system TD—Rf 38; system TE—Rf 13; system TF—Rf 64; system TAD—Rf 36; system TAE—Rf 93.

Gas Chromatography. System GA—xipamide-Me_2 RI 3350, xipamide-Me_4 RI 2780, M (OH-)-Me_4 RI 3000, xipamide isomer-1 Me_3 RI 2800, xipamide isomer-2 Me_3 RI 3320, art (-SO_2NH) RI 2385, art (-SO_2NH)-Me RI 2480, art (-SO_2NH)-Me_2 RI 2115.

High Performance Liquid Chromatography. System HX—RI 488; system HAA—Retention time 18.8 min.

Ultraviolet Spectrum. Aqueous acid—296 nm (A^1_1=92b); aqueous alkali—330 nm (A^1_1=160b).

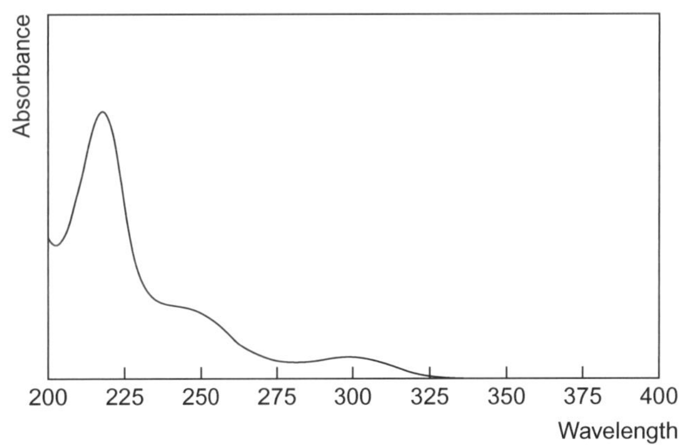

Infra-red Spectrum. Principal peaks at wavenumbers 1163, 1635, 1578, 1560, 975, 1525 cm^{-1} (KBr disk). (See below.)

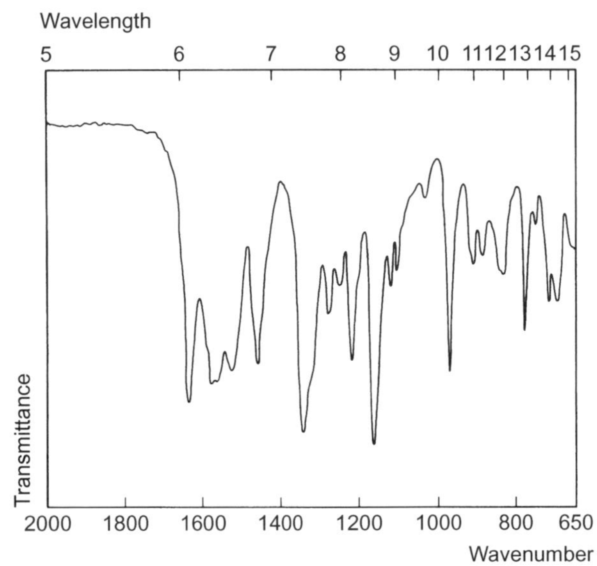

Mass Spectrum. Principal ions at m/z 121, 120, 354, 122, 43, 234, 106, 64.

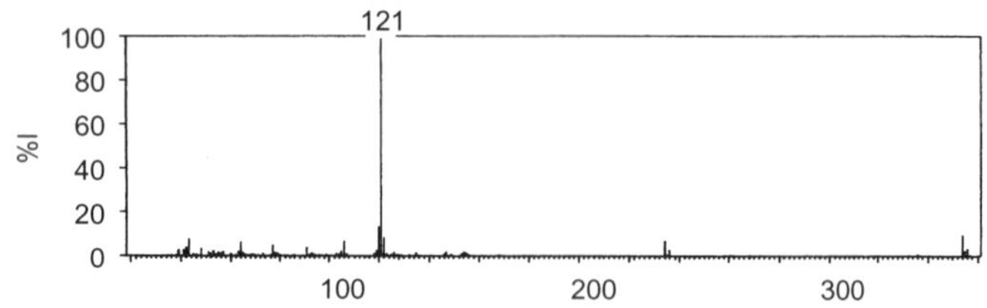

Quantification

High performance liquid chromatography. In urine: UV detection—W. Diembeck *et al.*, *Arzneimittelforschung*, 1982, *32*, 1482–1485. In urine: UV detection—A. Rosado-Maria *et al.*, *J. Chromatogr. B. Biomed. Sci. Appl.*, 2000, *748*, 415–424.

Thin-layer chromatography–spectrofluorimetry. In plasma or urine: limit of detection <10 µg/L in plasma—M. Sobel and E. Mutschler, *J. Chromatogr.*, 1980, *183 Biomed. Appl.*, *9*, 124–130.

Disposition in the Body. Completely and fairly rapidly absorbed after oral administration. About 88% of a dose is excreted in the urine in 48 h with about 50% as unchanged drug and 30% as xipamide-*O*-glucuronide; free amine metabolites have also been detected. In normal subjects, only traces are excreted in the bile, but biliary excretion may be extensive in renal failure.

Half-life. Plasma half-life, about 5 to 8 h.

Protein binding. In plasma, about 99%.

Dose. Usually 20 to 40 mg daily; doses of 80 mg daily have been given.

Xylazine

Sedative/Analgesic (Veterinary)

N-(2,6-Dimethylphenyl)-5,6-dihydro-4*H*-1,3-thiazin-2-amine
$C_{12}H_{16}N_2S$=220.3
CAS—7361-61-7

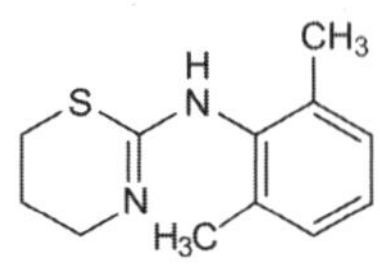

Colourless crystals. M.p. 140° to 142°; also reported as 136° to 139°.
Practically insoluble in water and alkalis; soluble in dilute acids, benzene, acetone and chloroform; sparingly soluble in petroleum ether.

Xylazine Hydrochloride

Synonym. Bay-Va-1470.
Proprietary names. Narcoxyl; Rompun; Xylapan; Xylasol.
$C_{12}H_{16}N_2S,HCl$=256.8
CAS—23076-35-9
A white powder. M.p. 164° to 167°.
Readily soluble in water, ethanol and methanol; very slightly soluble in chloroform and ether.

Partition Coefficient. Log *P* (octanol/water), 4.52.

Colour Tests. Liebermann's Test—red; Mandelin's Test—blue.

Thin-layer Chromatography. System TA—Rf 60; system TE—Rf 78; system TAJ—Rf 08; system TAK—Rf 06; system TAL—Rf 70. (Acidified iodoplatinate solution, positive.)

Gas Chromatography. System GV—Retention time, 11.6 min.

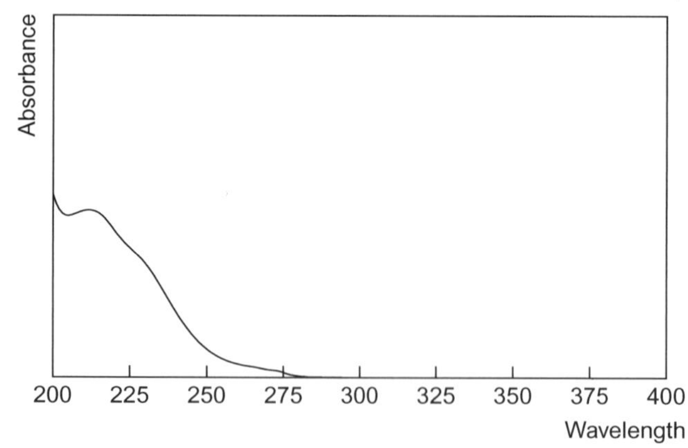

Infra-red Spectrum. Principal peaks at wavenumbers 1613, 1585, 1164, 1314, 1085, 1099 cm^{-1} (KBr disk).

Mass Spectrum. Principal ions at m/z 205, 77, 41, 39, 220, 130, 145, 131.

Quantification

Gas chromatography–mass spectrometry. In urine: limit of detection 0.02 mg/L (m/z 187, 177, 220, 205)—M. L. Olmos-Carmona and M. Hernandez-Carrazquilla, *J. Chromatogr. Biomed. Sci. Appl.*, 1999, *734*, 113–120.

High performance liquid chromatography. In plasma: limit of detection 5 µg/L; limit of quantification 25 µg/L, UV detection (λ=220 nm)—U. Hoffmann *et al.*, *J. Anal. Toxicol.*, 2001, *25(4)*, 245–249.

Disposition in Body. Xylazine is metabolised in the liver to approximately 20 metabolites. A major metabolite is 2,6-dimethylaniline. Both the unchanged drug and metabolites have been detected in urine.

Toxicity

In a suicide by hanging, xylazine was the sole drug detected in tissues; the concentrations were as follows: heart blood 2.3 mg/L, peripheral (subclavian) blood 2.9 mg/L, bile 6.3 mg/L, urine 0.01 mg/L, liver 6.1 µg/g, kidney 7.8 µg/g [K. A. Moore *et al.*, *J. Anal. Toxicol.*, 2003, 27, 110–112].

A 27-year-old farmer attempted to commit suicide by intramuscularly injecting himself with 1.5 g xylazine (approx. 75 mL of a 2% xylazine solution). As a result he became comatose, he had no light/pain response, he was hypotensive, bradycardic and mildly glycaemic, and suffered from respiratory depression. He was admitted to hospital 2 h after ingestion and was treated in the intensive care unit with artificial respiration and intravenous fluid therapy. The highest concentration of xylazine in plasma was 4.6 mg/L, gastric fluid 446 mg/L and urine 194 mg/L. The level of drug decreased over 12 h and he regained consciousness after 20 h. He was discharged from hospital 4 days after admission [U. Hoffmann *et al.*, *J. Anal. Toxicol.*, 2001, *25(4)*, 245–249].

The 16-year-old son of a horse breeder developed signs consistent with α-adrenergic agonist toxicity 2 h after an overdose of xylazine (the xylazine solution had been dried on a CD case, scraped up into a bag and then snorted). The patient recovered after appropriate supportive measures. A sample of blood taken approx. 2 h after inhalation contained 0.54 mg/L xylazine [A. J. Capraro *et al.*, *Pediatr. Emerg. Care*, 2001, 17, 447–448].

A 59-year-old woman who was a known former alcoholic was found dead at her home. Various empty containers of a number of drugs were found in her bedroom. After toxicological analysis, xylazine was found in her urine at a concentration of 30 mg/L; in her blood at 16 mg/L and a large amount in her stomach contents. Traces of lorazepam could also be detected and ethanol was found in her blood at 0.78 mg/g [Th. A. Briellmann *et al.*, *TIAFT Bulletin Case Notes*, 1994, *24(1)*].

Xylene

Solvent

Synonym. Xylol(e)
Proprietary names. Cerulisina; Cerulyse; Novo-Cerusol.
A mixture of *o*-, *m*- and *p*-dimethylbenzene in which the *m*-isomer predominates.
C_8H_{10}=106.2

CAS—1330-20-7; 108-38-3 (m-xylene); 95-47-6 (o-xylene); 106-42-3 (p-xylene)

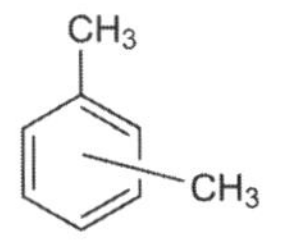

A colourless, flammable liquid. Mass per mL about 0.86 g. B.p. 137° to 140°.
Practically insoluble in water; miscible with absolute ethanol, ether and other organic solvents.

Partition Coefficient. Log *P* (octanol/water), 3.2.

Gas Chromatography. System GA—*o*-xylene RI 884, *m*-xylene RI 863, *p*-xylene RI 860; system GI—*o*-xylene Retention time 34.5 min, *m*-xylene Retention time 33.2 min, *p*-xylene Retention time 34.2 min.

High Performance Liquid Chromatography. System HAA—retention time 24.0 min.

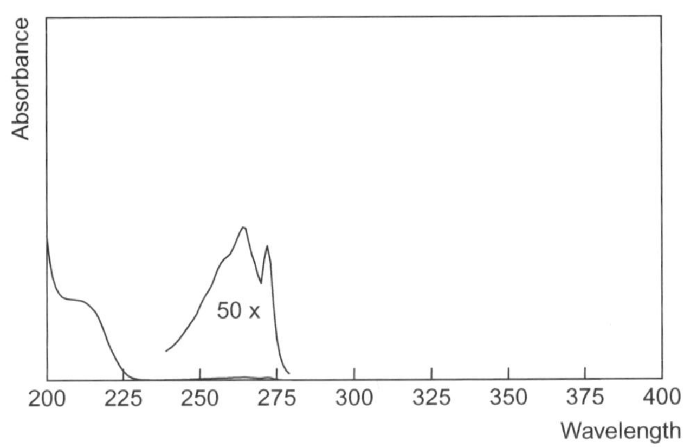

Mass Spectrum. Principal ions at *m/z* 91, 106, 105, 77, 51, 39, 29, 92 (*m*-xylene).

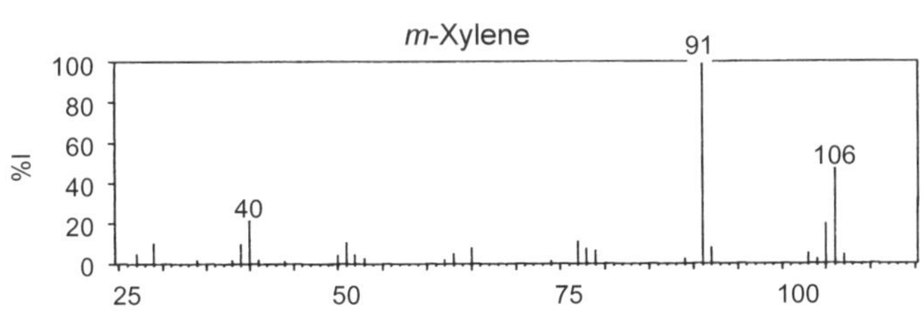

Quantification

Gas chromatography. In urine: *m*- and *p*-methylhippuric acids, limit of detection 1.0 mg/L, AFID—M. Morin *et al.*, *J. Chromatogr.*, 1981, *210*, 346–349. In urine: xylenol isomers and other phenolics, limits of detection 0.1 to 0.2 mg/L—G. Bieniek, *J. Chromatogr.*, 1996, *682 Biomed. Appl.*, 167–172. In blood and postmortem tissue: xylene isomers and other volatile organic compounds, ion-trap detection—J. Schuberth, *J. Chromatogr. Sci.*, 1996, *34*, 314–319. In blood: musk xylene (a synthetic musk), ECD—J. Angerer and H. U. Kafferlein, *J. Chromatogr. B. Biomed. Sci. Appl.*, 1997, *693*, 71–78. In urine: xylene and other volatile compounds, limits of detection 26 to 67 ng/L, PID, ECD, FID—H. J. Schroers *et al.*, *Analyst*, 1998, *123*, 715–720. In blood: *o*-, *m*- and *p*-xylenes, limit of detection about 20 µg/L—H. Hattori *et al.*, *J. Chromatogr. B. Biomed. Sci. Appl.*, 1998, *718*, 285–289. In body fluids: xylene isomers and other volatile organic compounds—K. Watanabe-Suzuki *et al.*, *Anal. Bioanal. Chem.*, 2002, *373*, 75–80.

Gas chromatography and gas chromatography–mass spectrometry. In blood or tissues: xylenes and other volatile compounds, using headspace analysis—J. A. Bellanca *et al.*, *J. Anal. Toxicol.*, 1982, *6*, 238–240. In urine: xylenes, benzene, toluene and ethylbenzene, using headspace analysis, limits of detection 12 to 34 ng/L—S. Fustioni *et al.*, *J. Chromatogr. B. Biomed. Sci. Appl.*, 1999, *723*, 105–115.

High performance liquid chromatography. In urine: *o*-, *m*- and *p*-xylene metabolites—M. Ogata and T. Taguchi, *Int. Arch. Occup. Environ. Health*, 1987, *59*, 263–272; M. Ogata and T. Taguchi, *Int. Arch. Occup. Environ. Health*, 1988, *61*, 131–140; A. Astier, *J. Chromatogr.*, 1992, *573*, 318–322. In urine: xylene isomers and metabolites and other organic solvents—D. H. Moon *et al.*, *J. Chromatogr. B. Biomed. Sci. Appl.*, 1997, *694*, 367–374. In urine: *o*-, *m*- and *p*-methylhippuric acids and other aromatic hydrocarbon metabolites—C. Burrini, *Med. Lav.*, 1998, *89*, 404–411.

Disposition in the Body. The three isomers of xylene are absorbed from the gastro-intestinal tract, through the skin and from the lungs. The main metabolic reactions are oxidation of a methyl group to give the corresponding *o*-, *m*- or *p*-toluic acid and conjugation with glycine to *o*-, *m*- or *p*-methylhippuric acid; about 70% of the absorbed material is excreted as these conjugates in the urine in 18 h. Hydroxylation of the xylenes to the corresponding xylenols also occurs and these may be excreted in the urine as conjugates. About 5% of a dose is excreted unchanged in expired air and less than 0.01% in the urine.

Blood concentration

Exposure to a concentration of 100 ppm of *m*-xylene, for 6 h, produced a mean peak blood-xylene concentration of about 1.0 mg/L in 4 subjects at rest; when the concentration was increased to 200 ppm for 3 h, the mean peak blood concentration was about 2.1 mg/L [K. Savolainen *et al.*, *Int. Arch. Occup. Environ. Health*, 1979, *44*, 201–211].

In a paint factory, average ambient-air concentrations of xylene were 5 to 58 ppm (average 29) during production and 3 to 21 ppm (average 8) during spraying; the blood concentrations of xylenes in 10 production workers were 63 to 715 µg/L (average 380) and 49 to 308 µg/L (average 130) in 10 spray workers [A. Kramer *et al.*, *Int. Arch. Occup. Environ. Health*, 1999, *72*, 52–55].

Toxicity. Xylene has about the same acute toxicity as benzene or toluene. The maximum permissible atmospheric concentration is 100 ppm. Exposure to air concentrations of 10 000 ppm has been reported to cause unconsciousness or death.

2 men, aged 51 and 55 years, died in two separate incidents after ingestion of petrol which contained xylenes. The following postmortem concentrations of xylene in body tissues were reported: blood 20 and 3.0 mg/L, and liver 1.0 µg/g for both subjects. A woman of 55, found dead, had the following postmortem concentrations of xylene in body tissues: blood 40 mg/L, liver 1.0 µg/g [R. Bonnichen *et al.*, *J. Forensic Sci.*, 1966, *11*, 186–204].

A 27-year-old man committed suicide by ingesting a large quantity of xylene. A high level was detected in his blood (0.11 g/L), gastric contents (8.8 g/L), and duodenal contents (33 g/L) [S. Abu Al Ragheb *et al.*, *Am. J. Forensic Med. Pathol.*, 1986, *7*, 327–329].

A 20-year-old man who attempted suicide by intravenously injecting 8 mL of xylene (0.1 mL/kg) developed acute pulmonary failure after 10 min and eventually recovered following haemoperfusion and haemodialysis [P. Sevcik *et al.*, *Intensive Care Med.*, 1992, *18*, 377–378].

Half-life. Blood half-life, about 20 to 30 h.

Xylometazoline

Sympathomimetic

2-[[4-(1,1-Dimethylethyl)-2,6-dimethylphenyl]methyl]-4,5-dihydro-1-*H*-imidazole
$C_{16}H_{24}N_2$=244.4
CAS—526-36-3

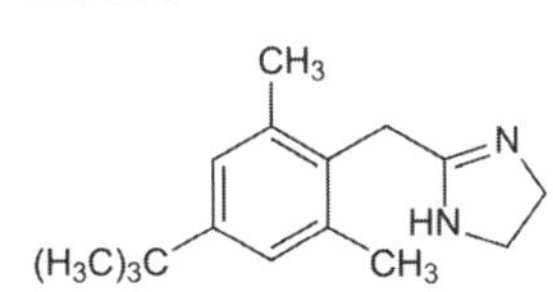

M.p. 131° to 133°.

Xylometazoline Hydrochloride

Proprietary names. Amidrin; Balkis; Dorenasin; Gelonasal; Nasolin; Olynth; Otalgicin; Otradrops; Otraspray; Otrivin(e); Otrivina; Otrix; Passagen; Rhinidine; Rinosedin; Xylo; Xylolin; Xyloma; Xylovit; Zymelin.
$C_{16}H_{24}N_2$,HCl=280.8

CAS—1218-35-5
A white crystalline powder. M.p. above 300°, with decomposition.
Soluble 1 in 33 of water; soluble in ethanol and methanol; practically insoluble in ether or benzene.

Partition Coefficient. Log *P* (chloroform/water), 5.4.

Colour Tests. Mandelin's Test—red; Marquis Test—orange.

Thin-layer Chromatography. System TA—Rf 13; system TB—Rf 07; system TC—Rf 05; system TE—Rf 30; system TL—Rf 03; system TAE—Rf 05; system TAF—64. (Acidified iodoplatinate solution, positive.)

Gas Chromatography. System GA—xylometazoline RI 2020, xylometazoline-AC RI 2260.

High Performance Liquid Chromatography. System HA—*k* 1.6; system HX—RI 413.

Ultraviolet Spectrum. Aqueous acid—265 nm (A_1^1=11.5a).

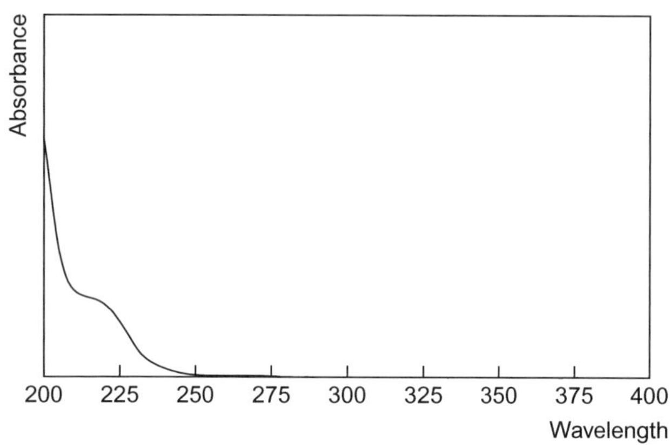

Infra-red Spectrum. Principal peaks at wavenumbers 1602, 1253, 1298, 871, 1237, 800 cm^{-1} (xylometazoline hydrochloride, KBr disk).

Mass Spectrum. Principal ions at *m/z* 244, 229, 44, 173, 40, 230, 243, 245.

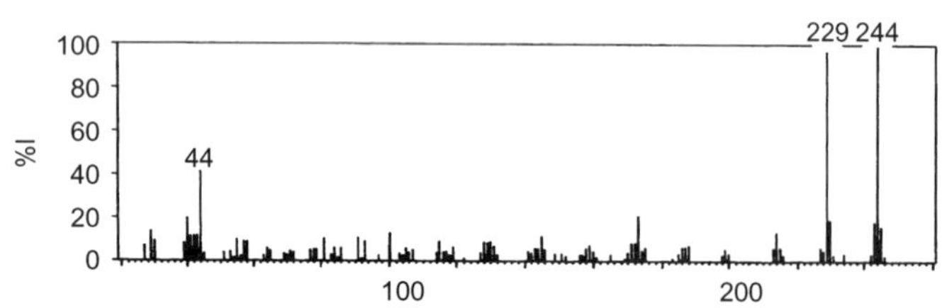

Quantification
Gas chromatography. In plasma or urine: ECD—A. Sioufi *et al.*, *J. Chromatogr.*, 1989, *487*, 81–89.

Disposition in the Body
Toxicity
The following postmortem concentrations were reported in a 23-year-old man who died after the intravenous self-administration of xylometazoline: blood 0.14 mg/L, liver blood 0.37 mg/L [P. Vanezis and P. A. Toseland, *Med., Sci. Law*, 1980, *20*, 35–36].

Use. In concentrations of 0.05 to 0.1% of the hydrochloride, as nasal drops or spray.

Yohimbine

Alkaloid

Synonyms. Aphrodine; Corynine; Québrachine.
(16α, 17α)-17-Hydroxyyohimban-16-carboxylic acid methyl ester
$C_{21}H_{26}N_2O_3$=354.4
CAS—146-48-5

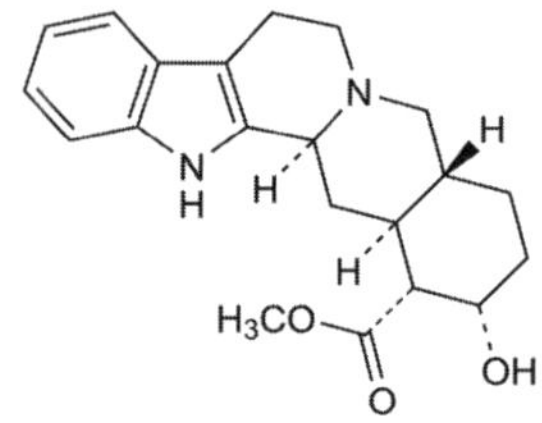

The principal alkaloid of the bark of the yohimbe tree, *Pausinystalia yohimbe* (= *Corynanthe yohimbi*) (Rubiaceae).
Crystals. M.p. about 234°.
Sparingly soluble in water; soluble in ethanol and chloroform; moderately soluble in ether.

Yohimbine Hydrochloride
Proprietary names. Antagonil; Dayto Himbin; Erex; Pluriviron mono; Prowess Plain; Urobine; Yobine; Yocon; Yocoral; Yohimex; Yohydrol; Yomax; Yovital; Zumba.
$C_{21}H_{26}N_2O_3$,HCl=390.9
CAS—65-19-0
A white crystalline powder. M.p. about 302°, with decomposition.
Soluble 1 in 100 of water; soluble 1 in 400 of ethanol; more soluble in hot water and ethanol.

Partition Coefficient. Log *P* (octanol/water), 2.7.

Colour Tests. Liebermann's Test—blue; Mandelin's Test—blue→green.

Thin-layer Chromatography. System TA—Rf 63; system TB—Rf 06; system TC—Rf 38; system TE—Rf 64; system TL—Rf 52; system TAE—Rf 66; system TAF—RF 70. (Dragendorff spray, positive; acidified iodoplatinate solution, positive; Marquis reagent, grey.)

Gas Chromatography. System GA—yohimbine RI 3155, yohimbine-AC RI 3190.

High Performance Liquid Chromatography. System HX—RI 348; system HY—RI 279; system HZ—Retention time 2.6 min; system HAA—Retention time 11.5 min.

Ultraviolet Spectrum. Aqueous acid—271 nm (A_1^1=211a), 277 nm (A_1^1=207a), 287 nm; aqueous alkali—280 nm.

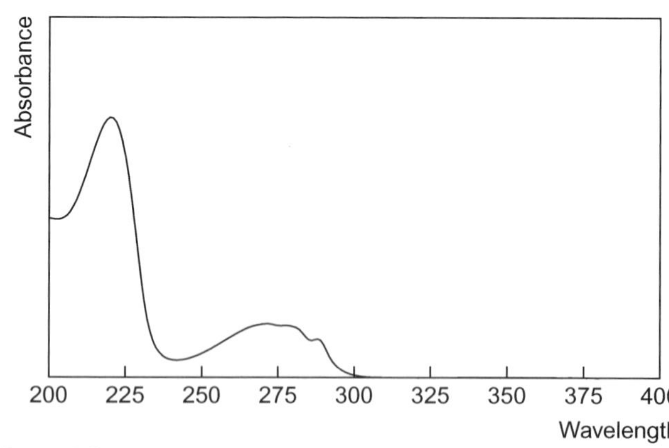

Infra-red Spectrum. Principal peaks at wavenumbers 1705, 741, 1197, 1160, 1290, 1135 cm^{-1} (yohimbine hydrochloride, KBr disk).

Mass Spectrum. Principal ions at *m/z* 353, 354, 169, 170, 355, 156, 184, 144.

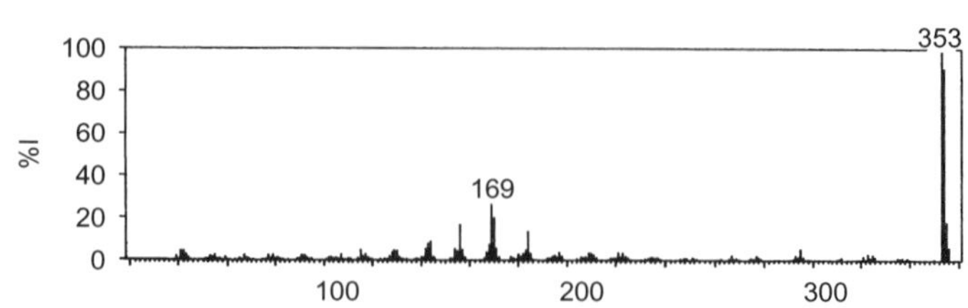

Quantification
High performance liquid chromatography. In plasma: limit of detection 10 μg/L, electrochemical detection—M. R. Goldberg *et al.*, *J. Liq. Chromatogr.*, 1984, *7*, 1003–1012. In blood: limit of detection 50 ng/L,

fluorescence detection—J. A. Owen *et al.*, *J. Chromatogr.*, 1985, *342*, 333–340. In plasma: yohimbine and its main metabolite 11-hydroxyyohimbine, limit of detection 1 μg/L, fluorescence detection—R. Le Verge *et al.*, *J. Chromatogr.*, 1992, *574*, 283–292.

Therapeutic concentration

In 13 subjects receiving an intravenous bolus dose of 0.25 or 0.5 mg/kg yohimbine, peak plasma concentrations of 150 to 1140 μg/L were achieved [T. Hedner *et al.*, *Eur. J. Clin. Pharmacol.*, 1992, *43*, 651–656].

Toxicity

A 38-year-old man experienced atrial fibrillation and memory loss after ingesting 350 mg of yohimbine [S. Varkey, *BMJ.*, 1992, *304*, 548].

A 62-year-old male who ingested 200 mg yohimbine experienced only mild adverse effects (tachycardia, hypertension, anxiety) [K. Friesen *et al.*, *J. Emerg. Med.*, 1993, *11*, 287–288].

Dose. Yohimbine hydrochloride has been given in doses of up to 30 mg daily.

Zafirlukast

Leukotriene D_4 Antagonist/ Anti-asthmatic

Synonyms. ICI-204219; MK-571.
Proprietary name. Accolate
[3-[[2-Methoxy-4-[[[(2-methylphenyl)sulfonyl]amino]carbonyl]phenyl]-methyl]-1-methyl-1*H*-indol-5-yl]carbamic acid cyclopentyl ester
$C_{31}H_{33}N_3O_6S$=575.7
CAS—107753-78-6

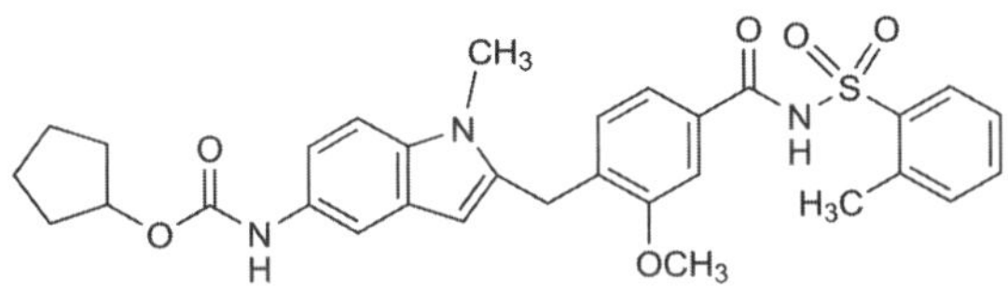

A white to pale yellow powder. M.p. 138° to 140°. It is practically insoluble in water; slightly soluble in methanol; freely soluble in tetrahydrofuran (THF), dimethylsulfoxide and acetone.

High Performance Liquid Chromatography. Column: C_{18} (Vydac reversed-phase, 250 × 4.6 mm, i.d., 10 μm). Column temperature: 24°. Mobile phase: acetonitrile:water (80:20), flow rate 1 mL/min. IS: flavone. UV detection (λ=245 nm). Retention times: zafirlukast 3.22 min; IS, 3.78 min [R. Ficarra *et al.*, *J. Pharm. Biomed. Anal.* 2000, *23*, 169–174].

Column: (analytical) (Zorbax CN, 150 × 4.6 mm i.d., 5 μm); (guard) Zorbax CN (12.5 × 4.0 mm, 5 μm). Mobile phase: THF:hexane:glacial acetic acid (90%) (30:70:0.1). Fluorescence detection (λ_{ex}=250 nm; λ_{em}=452 nm). Retention time: 9 to 10 min [K. Bui *et al.*, *J. Chromatogr. B Biomed. Sci. Appl.*, 1997, *696*, 131–136].

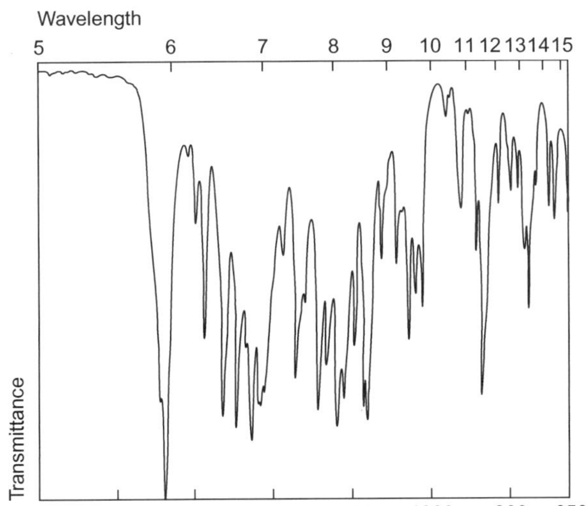

Mass Spectrum. Principal ions at *m/z* 463, 91, 575, 159, 185, 489, 309, 92.

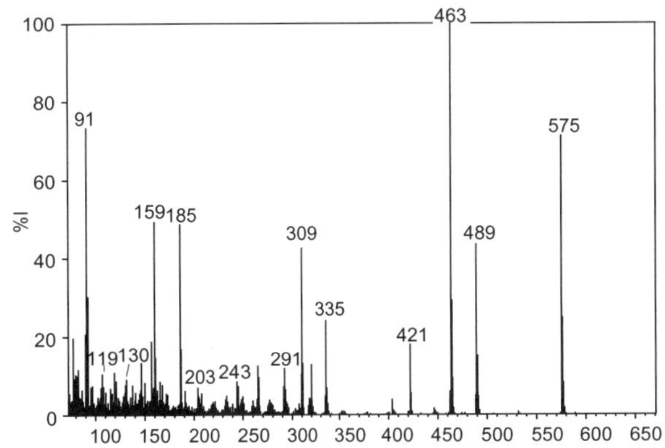

Quantification

High performance liquid chromatography. In blood: limit of quantification 0.75 μg/L, florescence detection (λ_{ex}=250 nm; λ_{em}=452 nm)—K. Bui *et al.*, *J. Chromatogr. B Biomed. Sci Appl.*, 1997, *696*, 131–136.

Disposition in the Body. Zafirlukast is absorbed from the gastrointestinal tract, 1 to 2 h after oral administration. Food decreases the rate and the extent of absorption. It is distributed to tissue, although there is minimal distribution across the blood–brain barrier. The drug is extensively metabolised in the liver by hepatic cytochrome P450; CYO2C9 and CYP3A4. It is excreted primarily in faeces as the unchanged drug and its metabolite. 10% of the dose is excreted in urine following oral administration. The metabolites are at least 90 times less potent than zafirlukast. The onset of action is 1 to 2 h and peak plasma concentrations are reached within 3 h of dosing. Peak serum levels after 20 mg and 40 mg oral dose are about 150 μg/L and 250 μg/L, respectively. The steady state plasma concentration is proportional to the dose and is achieved within 3 days. Pharmacokinetics are not changed in individuals with renal impairment but are with increased age and hepatic impairment.

Therapeutic concentration

5 healthy male volunteers (mean age 25.5 years) were administered 40 mg zafirlukast orally in solution, directly into the colon via an oro-enteric tube. Peak concentrations of 697 μg/L and 194 μg/L were reached for the oral and direct administration, respectively. Median times to reach these concentrations were 2.0 (1.1 to 3.0) and 1.35 (0.5 to 10.0) h, respectively [J. D. Fischer *et al.*, *Pharm. Res.*, 2000, *17(2)*, 154–159].

Half-life. 10 h.

Clearance. Apparent oral clearance, 11.4 L/h; decreased by 50 to 60% in the elderly and those with cirrhosis.

Protein binding. 99%; predominately to albumin.

Dose. 20 mg twice daily.

Zalcitabine

Antiviral

Synonyms. DDC; ddC; ddCyd; Dideoxycytidine; NSC-606170; Ro-24-2027; Ro-24-2027/000.
Proprietary name. Hivid
2′,3′-Dideoxycytidine
$C_9H_{13}N_3O_3$=211.2
CAS—7481-89-2

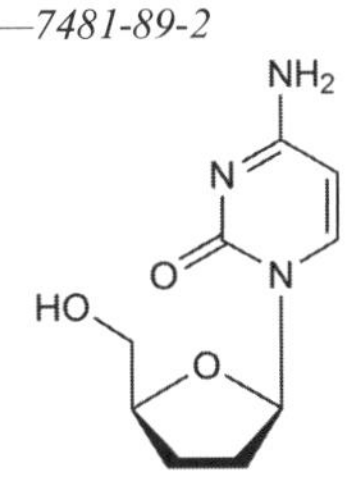

A white to off-white crystalline powder with M.p. 215° to 217°. It is soluble in water and methyl alcohol; sparingly soluble in alcohol in acetonitrile, chloroform and dichloromethane; slightly soluble in cyclohexane.

Partition Coefficient. Log *P* (octanol/water), −1.30.

High Performance Liquid Chromatography. Column: Ultrasphere ODS (250 × 4.6 mm i.d., 5 μm). Mobile phase: methanol:ammonium acetate (50 mM) (10:90), flow rate 1 mL/min. MS detection (SIM at *m/z* 212). Retention time: zalcitabine, 8.9 min [H. Jajoo *et al.*, *J. Chromatogr.*, 1992, *577*, 299–304].

Column: phenyl Hypersil (NC-04, 250 × 4 mm, i.d., 5 μm). Mobile phase:methanol (1.4 g/L):sodium acetate (pH 6.55), flow rate 1 mL/min. Retention time: 10 min [N. Frijus-Plessen *et al.*, *J. Chromatogr.*, 1990, *534*, 101–107].

Column: RSP (cyclobond I, 250 × 4.6 mm, i.d., 5 μm). Mobile phase: aqueous triethylamine (0.25%), flow rate 0.25 mL/min. IS: 2*S-cis*, 2*R-trans* and 2*S-trans* stereoisomers. Retention time: 27.1 min. UV detection (λ=270 nm). Retention times: zalcitabine, 27.1 min; 2*S-cis*, 24.9 min; 2*S-trans*, 29.4 min; 2*R-trans*, 32.2 min [S. Scypinski and A. Ross, *J. Pharm. Biomed. Anal.*, 1994, *12(10)*, 1271–1276].

Ultraviolet Spectrum. Aqueous acid (0.1 M hydrochloric acid)—212, 280 nm; aqueous alkali (0.1 M sodium hydroxide)—270 nm.

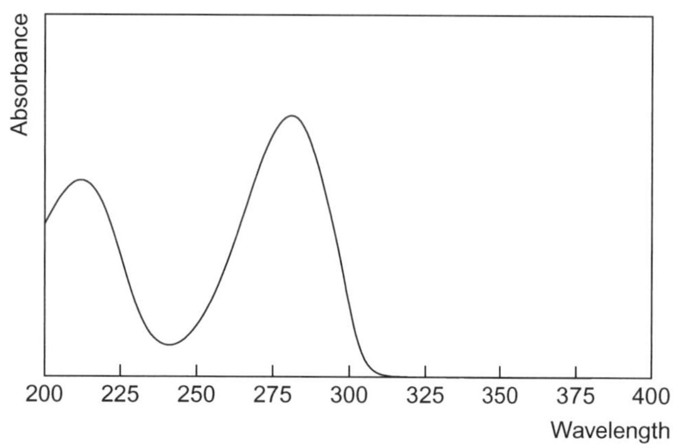

Infra-red Spectrum. Principal peaks at wavenumbers 1646, 1490, 1064 cm^{-1}.

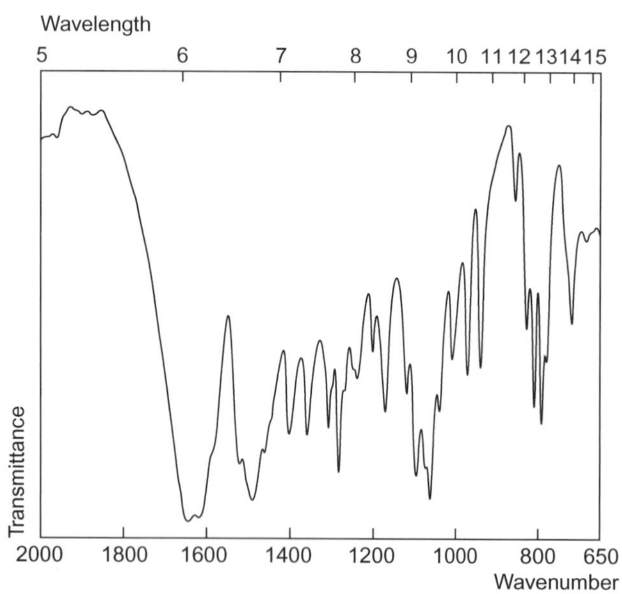

Quantification

Gas chromatography–mass spectrometry. In plasma: limit of quantification 2 μg/L—F.R. Rubio *et al.*, *Biomed. Environ. Mass Spectrom.*, 1988, *17*, 399–404.

High performance liquid chromatography. In serum: limit of detection 440 μg/L, UV detection (λ=250 nm)—V. A. Simon *et al.*, *J. Chromatogr. A*, 2001, *913(1-2)*, 447–453. In plasma and urine: limits of quantification are 0.2 and 5 μg/L, respectively, MS detection—M. Bazunga *et al.*, *J. Clin. Pharmacol.*, 1998, *38(1)*, 28–33. In blood: limit of quantification 0.25 μg/L—H. Jajoo *et al.*, *J. Chromatogr.*, 1992, *577*, 299–304. In blood, cell suspensions and perfusate: limit of detection 50 μg/L—N. Frijus-Plessen *et al.*, *J. Chromatogr.*, 1990, *534*, 101–107.

Disposition in the Body. Zalcitabine is well absorbed from the gastro-intestinal tract. Absorption shows interindividual variation and the rate of absorption is decreased by administration with food. Peak plasma concentrations in the fasting state are achieved in about 1 to 2 h. The cerebrospinal fluid concentration of the drug is 9 to 37% of those in plasma. The drug is phosphorylated intracellularly to an active antiviral triphosphate for HIV-reverse transcriptase. The metabolites have been identified primarily as dideoxyuridine (ddU). The drug does not appear to undergo any substantial hepatic metabolism. Renal excretion is the primary route of elimination (75% excreted in urine after an IV dose, 60 to 70% after an oral dose). Approx. 10% of an orally administered dose appears in faeces, comprised primarily of unchanged drug and ddU. Accumulation is negligible.

Therapeutic concentration

Five individuals were fasted overnight and administered 0.75 mg zalcitabine orally, followed by a further 2 h fasting. Peak plasma concentrations reached 17.27, 16.95 and 12.50 μg/L at 1.3, 1.58 and 1.22 h, respectively [M. Bazunga *et al.*, *J. Clin. Pharmacol.*, 1998, *38(1)*, 28–33].

100 HIV-infected patients with CD4$^+$ cell counts between 50 and 301 cells/mm^3, mean age 31.4 years, were administered 0.75 mg zalcitabine three times a day plus 200 mg zidvudine three times a day for 24 weeks. The mean peak zalcitabine concentration was 5.31 μg/L after 1.75 h [G. F. Vanhove *et al.*, *Antimicrob. Agents Chemother.*, 1997, *41(11)*, 2428–2432].

Toxicity. Use of zalcitabine has been associated with significant clinical adverse reactions, some of which are potentially fatal. However, there have been no reports of acute overdose associated with high zalcitabine doses (over 1.5 mg/kg).

Bioavailability. Adults: greater than 80%. Children: 29 to 100%. Reduced by 14% with food.

Half-life. Adults: 1 to 3 h; children: 0.8 h. Prolonged in patients with renal impairment, up to 8.5 h (with creatinine clearance < 55 mL/min).

Volume of distribution. Adults: 0.54 L/kg; children: 9.3 L/m^3.

Clearance. Adults: total mean clearance, 285 mL/min (range 165 to 447); mean plasma clearance, 227 mL/min/m^2. Children: mean plasma clearance, 149 mL/min/m^2.

Protein binding. < 4%.

Dose. 0.75 mg. Dose may be reduced in patients with renal and hepatic impairment.

Zanamivir

Antiviral

Synonyms. GG-167; GR-121167X.
Proprietary name. Relenza
5-(Acetylamino)-4-[(aminoiminomethyl)amino]-2,6-anhydro-3,4,5-tri-deoxy-D-*glycero*-D-*galacto*-non-2-enonic acid
$C_{12}H_{20}N_4O_7$=332.31
CAS—139110-80-8

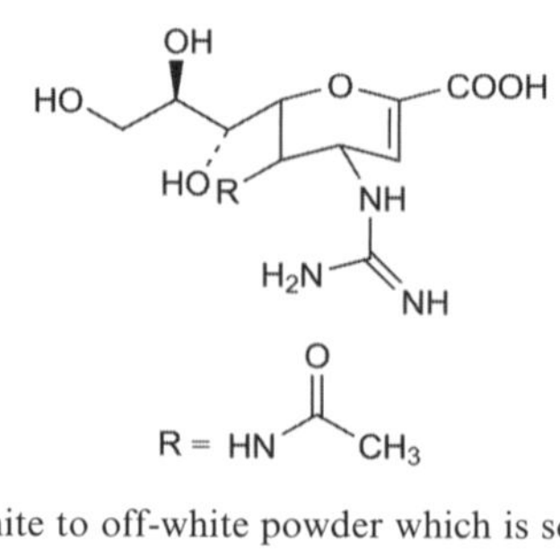

A white to off-white powder which is soluble in water (18 g/L at 20°).

High Performance Liquid Chromatography. Column: (Nucleosil-Diol, 250 × 4.6 mm, 7 μm). Mobile phase: phosphate (20 mM, pH 2.5):acetonitrile (18:82), flow rate 2.0 mL/min. UV detection (λ=238 nm).

Retention time 17 min [D. M. Morris *et al.*, *J. Pharm. Biomed. Anal.*, 1995, *14*, 191–201].

Column: ODS (Hypersil, 100 × 4.6 mm i.d.). Mobile phase: acetonitrile:Tris-HCl buffer (pH 8.5, 0.05 M) (20:80), flow rate 1 mL/min. Fluorescent detection (λ_{ex}=325 nm; λ_{em}=442 nm). Retention time: not specified [R. J. Stubbs and A. J. Harker., *J. Chromatogr.*, 670, 1995, *Biomed. Appl.* 279–285].

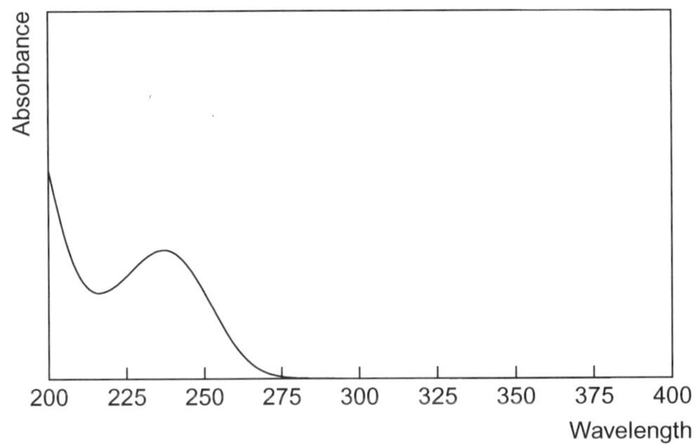

Mass Spectrum. Principal ions at *m/z* 60, 167, 121, 197, 180, 151, 214, 274.

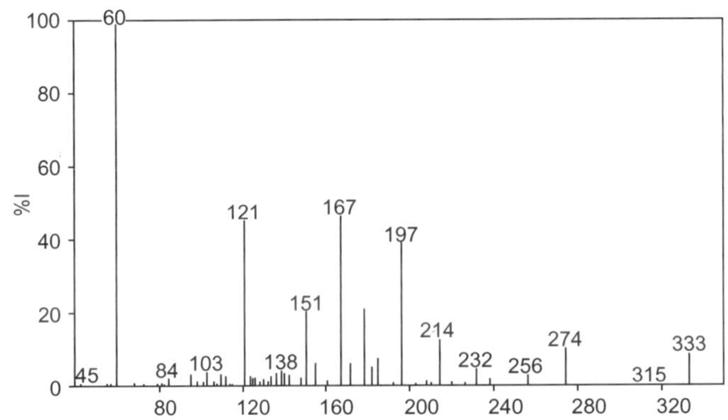

Quantification

High performance liquid chromatography. In serum: limit of detection is 10 µg/L, MS–MS detection (*m/z* 333 to 60)—G. D. Allen *et al.*, *J. Chromatogr. B Biomed. Sci. Appl.*, 1999, *732*, 383–393. In serum: limit of quantification 10 µg/L, fluorescence detection (λ_{ex}=325 nm; λ_{em}=442 nm)—R. J. Stubbs and A. J. Harker, *J. Chromatogr.*, 1995, *670*, *Biomed. Appl.*, 279–285. In urine: limit of quantification 300 µg/L, UV detection (λ=238 nm)—D. M. Morris *et al.*, *J. Pharm. Biomed. Anal.*, 1995, *14*, 191–201.

Disposition in the Body. Zanamivir is not well absorbed. Systemic absorption is between 10 and 20% after an inhaled dose. It does not undergo extensive metabolism or biotransformation, and no metabolites have been detected in humans. The unchanged drug is excreted in urine with 90% of a dose being detected within 24 h. Unabsorbed drug has been detected in faeces.

Therapeutic concentration

92 healthy male volunteers and 12 females, aged 18 to 45 years, were administered with the following: 16 mg zanamivir, single doses, intravenously over a period of 20 to 30 min; 600 mg intravenously as a single dose and repeated doses; 500 mg, single oral dose; and 16 mg administered daily for five days as separate studies. The single 16 mg intravenous dose generated mean maximum plasma concentrations of 1.28 (range 1.14 to 1.47) mg/L at 0.32 h. For the single 600 mg dose concentrations reached 32.76 mg/L at 0.5 h. Steady state concentrations were observed with the repeated dosing, and the maximum concentration was 39.71 mg/L at 0.5 h on day 5. After the single intranasal dose, the maximum serum concentration was 0.042 (0.020 to 0.054) mg/L observed within 1.8 (0.75 to 3.0) h. For the repeated dosing, concentration was 0.086 (0.039 to 0.107) mg/L at 0.5 to 3.0 h. The steady state concentration was 0.071 mg/L. For the oral dose, the maximum concentration was 0.057 to 0.500 mg/L observed at 4 (0.75 to 8.0) h [L. M. R. Cass *et al.*, *Clin. Pharmacokinet.*, 1999, *36*, *Suppl. 1*, 1–11].

Bioavailability. 1 to 5% after oral administration.

Half-life. Serum half-life, 2.5 to 5.1 h.

Volume of distribution. 16 L; decreases in patients with renal impairment (13.4 L in those with severe impairment; 15.1 L for mild–moderate impairment).

Clearance. Total serum clearance, 6.07 to 7.22 (mean 6.67) L/h; decreases in patients with renal impairment.

Protein binding. Less than 10%.

Dose. 10 mg daily.

Zidovudine

Antiviral

Synonyms. Azidodeoxythymidine; Azidothymidine; AZT; BW-A509U; BW-509U; Compound-S; Zidovudinum.
Proprietary names. Combivir; Novo-AZT; Retrovir.
3′-Azido-3′-deoxythymidine
$C_{10}H_{13}N_5O_4$=267.2
CAS—30516-87-1

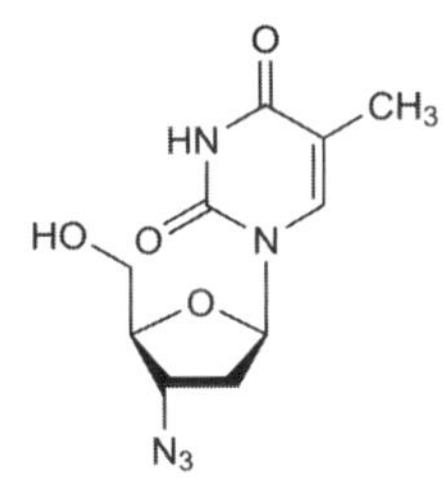

A white to yellowish or brownish odourless crystalline powder with M.p. 124°. It is sparingly soluble in water, freely soluble in alcohol, and soluble in dehydrated alcohol.

Dissociation Constant. pK_a 9.68; 3′-azido-3′-deoxy-5′-β′D-glucopyranuronosyl (GZDV), 3.5.

Partition Coefficient. Log *P* (octanol/water), 0.05.

Gas Chromatography. Column: 3% OV-1 Chromosorb WHP 80/100 mesh (4 inch × ¼ inch). Column temperature: 280°. Carrier gas: nitrogen, flow rate 32 mL/min. Detection: flame ionisation. Retention index: 2307 [T. Mills and J. C. Roberson, *Instrumental Data for Drug Analysis*, CRC Press, Boca Raton, USA, 1993, 2nd Edn, Vol. 5, pp. 42–43].

High Performance Liquid Chromatography. System HAD—*k* 6.6.

Column: RPC_{18} (Novapak, 300 × 3 mm, i.d., 4 µm); (guard) C_{18} (Bondapak, 20 × 2 mm, i.d., 40 µm end-capped). Mobile phase: methanol: tetrahydrofuran:potassium phosphate (0.025 M, pH 3.1) (3.7:2.8:93.5), flow rate 1.0 mL/min. UV detection (λ=270 nm). Retention times: zidovudine, 16.8 min; metabolite GZDV, 11.7 min [I. Schrive and J. C. Plasse, *J. Chromatogr.*, 1994, *657*, *Biomed. Appl.*, 233–237.]

Column: Ultrasphere ODS (75 × 4.6 mm, 3 µm). Mobile phase: phosphoric acid (pH 6.55):MeCN (95:5 to 70:30 over 7 min, to 20:80 over 1.5 min, return to initial ratio over 1 min), flow rate 1 mL/min. IS: G-AZT. UV detection (λ=266). Retention times: zidovudine, 3.6 min; IS, 5.0 min [T. Nadal *et al.*, *J. Chromatogr. A*, 1996, *721*, 127–137].

Column: Novapak phenyl (150 × 3.9 mm i.d., 4 µm). Mobile phase: isopropanol:20 mM, pH 5 sodium citrate (2.5:97.5), flow rate 1 mL/min. UV detection (λ=250 nm). Retention time: 22.4 min [M. Rosell-Rovira *et al.*, *J. Chromatogr.*, 1996, *675*, *Biomed. Appl.*, 89–92].

Ultraviolet Spectrum. Aqueous acid—207, 266 nm: basic—266 nm.

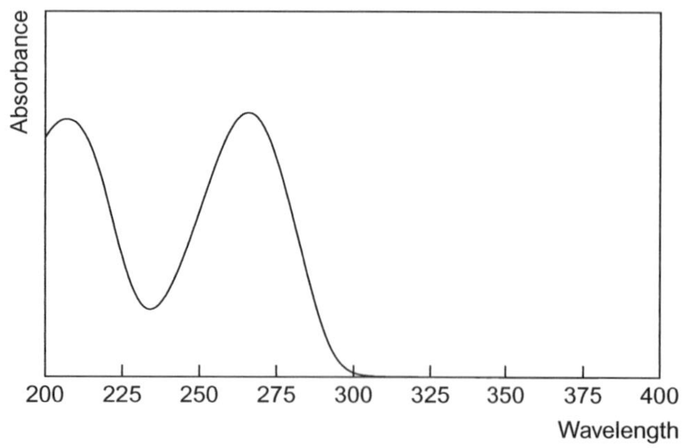

Infra-red Spectrum. Principal peaks at wavenumbers 2077, 1675, 1084 cm^{-1} (KBr disk).

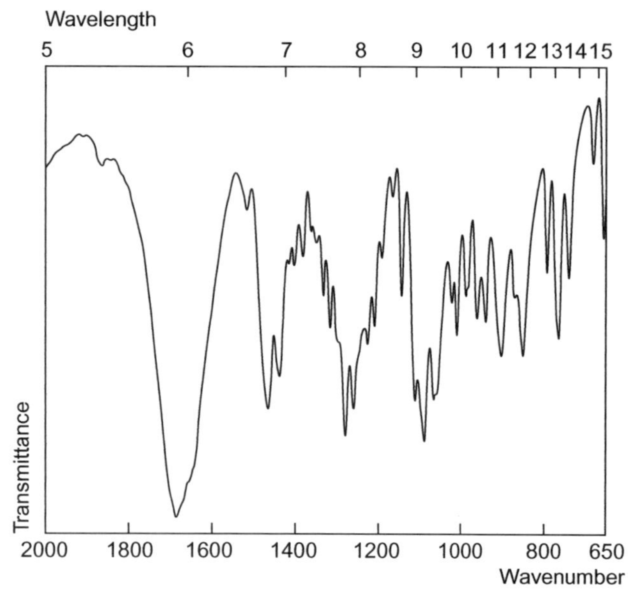

Mass Spectrum. Principal ions at *m/z* 142, 126, 127, 80, 54, 42, 55, 69.

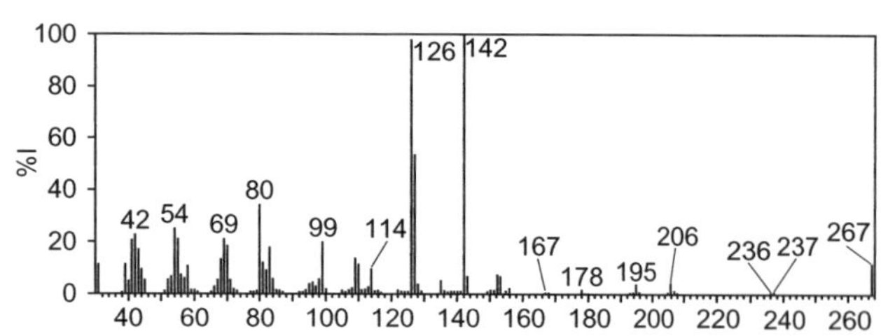

Quantification

High performance liquid chromatography. In serum: limit of detection 30 μg/L, UV detection (λ=250 nm)—V. A. Simon *et al.*, *J. Chromatogr. A*, 2001, *913(1-2)*, 447–453. In serum: limit of detection 2.5 μg/L, MS–MS detection—K. B. Kenney *et al.*, *J. Pharm. Biomed. Anal.*, 2000, *22(6)*, 967–983. In plasma: limit of detection 10 μg/L—G. Aymard *et al.*, *J. Chromatogr. B Biomed. Sci. Appl.*, 2000, *744*, 227–240. In blood: limit of detection 7 μg/L, limit of quantification 22 μg/L, UV detection (diode array at λ=266 nm)—T. Nadal *et al.*, *J. Chromatogr. A*, 1996, *721*, 127–137. In serum: limit of detection 0.05 mg/L—P. Nebinger and M. Koel, *J. Pharm. Biomed. Anal.*, 1994, *12(1)*, 141–143. In plasma and urine: limit of quantification 20 μg/L for zidovudine and 10 μg/L for the 5′-glucuronyl form, GZDV—I. Schrive and J. C. Plasse, *J. Chromatogr.*, 1994, *657(1)*, *Biomed. Appl.*, 233–237.

Disposition in the Body. Zidovudine is rapidly absorbed from the gastro-intestinal tract (66 to 70%), although absorption is delayed if the drug is administered with food. It undergoes extensive first-pass metabolism in the liver where approx. 40% of the oral dose is lost. Metabolism of zidovudine by the kidney is minimal but rapid metabolism occurs intracellularly in the liver to GZDV. Two other hepatic metabolites have been identified, 3′-amino-3′-deoxythymidine (AMT), and its 5′-*O*-glucuronide derivative GAMT. 5′-glucuronide is the major metabolite in plasma and urine accounting for 50 to 80% of an administered dose. Metabolism of zidovudine to AMT occurs in the liver and gastro-intestinal microsomes. Zidovudine is highly lipophilic and is widely distributed. It concentrates in the semen where it may exhibit delayed clearance compared to serum. It is excreted in urine as the unchanged drug and its metabolite (63 to 95%), via both glomerular filtration and tubular secretion. After an oral dose, 72 to 74% is excreted as the metabolite and 14 to 18% as unchanged drug. After IV administration, 45 to 60% is excreted as metabolite and 18 to 29% as the unchanged drug. There is no evidence that zidovudine accumulates in plasma or tissues. There is significant penetration into CNS, with a CNS: plasma ratio of about 0.5.

Therapeutic concentration. The trough serum therapeutic concentration range is 0.1 to 0.3 mg/L and peak, 1.0 to 1.5 mg/L.

13 HIV-positive asymptomatic adults with an average age of 33.1 years were administered 300 mg zidovudine after an 8 h fast. These individuals did not have CD4 cell counts ⩽ 200 cells/mm^3. The mean peak zidovudine concentration was 1.64 mg/L at 0.52 h and the peak GZDV concentration 9.41 mg/L at 0.71 h [L. H. Wang *et al.*, *Antimicrob. Agents Chemother.*, 1999, *43(7)*, 1708–1715].

11 HIV-positive, asymptomatic men (average age 37.4 years, and with CD4 cell counts ⩾ 300 cells/mm^3) were administered 200 mg zidovudine every 8 h for 4 days. Mean peak zidovudine concentrations were 0.714, 0.594 and 0.394 mg/L for three separate dosing regimens (with washout periods of approx. 9 days), observed at 0.9, 0.9 and 1.8 h, respectively. Peak GZDV concentrations were 4.655, 3.346 and 2.508 mg/L at 1.0, 1.2 and 1.7 h, respectively for the three dose intervals [A. Cato III *et al.*, *Antimicrob. Agents Chemother.*, 1998, *42(7)*, 1788–1793].

100 HIV-infected patients with CD4 cell counts between 50 and 301 cells/mm^3, mean age 31.4 years, were administered 0.75 mg zalcitabine three times a day, plus 200 mg zidvudine three times a day for 24 weeks. The mean weekly peak zidovudine concentration was 347 μg/L after 1.29 h [G. F. Vanhove *et al.*, *Antimicrob. Agents Chemother.*, 1997, *41(11)*, 2428–2432].

Toxicity. The serum toxic concentration range is 0.5 to 3 mg/L.

A 34-year-old man with AIDS took a hundred 200 mg tablets of zidovudine with temazepam, after 6 h he experienced symptoms of drowsiness. The blood levels of zidovudine were 185 μmol/L and 5′-gluconuride, 114 μmol/L [M. Hargreaves *et al.*, *Lancet*, 1988, *2/8609*, 509].

A 20-year-old man took an entire month's supply of zidovudine 2 h before presentation. His blood pressure was 90/40 mmHg, and he had tachycardia of 140 bpm. Serum levels 2 h after the overdose were 339.43 μmol/L (zidovudine) and 565.51 μmol/L (G-AZT); after 12 h, 0.33 μmol/L (zidovudine) and 0.88 μmol/L (G-AZT); after 24 h, < 0.05 μmol/L (zidovudine) and < 0.13 μmol/L (G-AZT) [C. Valentine *et al.*, *AIDS*, 1993, *7 (3)*, 436–437].

A 26-year-old male with AIDS ingested 110 to 220 mg/kg zidovudine and unknown amounts of phenobarbital and triazolam. 8 h after ingestion, the man experienced headache and nausea, although the vital signs were normal. 7.75 h after administration, serum levels were 23.82 mg/L (zidovudine) and 89.39 mg/L (G-AZT); after 8.75 h, serum levels were 9.18 mg/L (zidovudine) and 64.29 mg/L (G-AZT); after 9.75 h, serum levels were 9.18 mg/L (zidovudine) and 26.60 mg/L (G-AZT); after 16 h, serum levels were 0.12 mg/L (zidovudine) and 0.47 mg/L (G-AZT) [J. Speat *et al.*, *Ann. Intern. Med.*, 1988, *109 (1)*, 76–77].

Bioavailability. 60 to 70%. This value is erratic in HIV-positive individuals.

Half-life. Zidovudine, 0.9 to 1 h; AMT, 2.7 h; GZDV, 1.6 h.

Volume of distribution. Adults (at steady state): 1.4 to 1.6 L/kg, apparent 3.0 L/kg. Children (at steady state): 22 to 64 L/m^2.

Clearance. Adults: total body clearance, 22 to 27 mL/min/kg; plasma clearance, 1.3 L/h/kg. Children: mean total body clearance, 30.9 mL/min/kg. Reduced clearance in hepatic and renal impairment.

Protein binding. 34 to 38% (predominately to albumin); 20% plasma.

Dose. Adults: oral dose, 500 to 1200 mg daily; intravenous dose, 1 to 2 mg/kg/dose. Children: oral dose, maximum 200 mg; intravenous dose, 100 mg/m^2/dose.

Zimeldine

Antidepressant

Note. Zimeldine was previously known as zimelidine.
(*Z*)-3-(4-Bromophenyl)-*N*,*N*-dimethyl-3-(3-pyridinyl)-2-propen-1-amine
$C_{16}H_{17}BrN_2$=317.2
CAS—56775-88-3

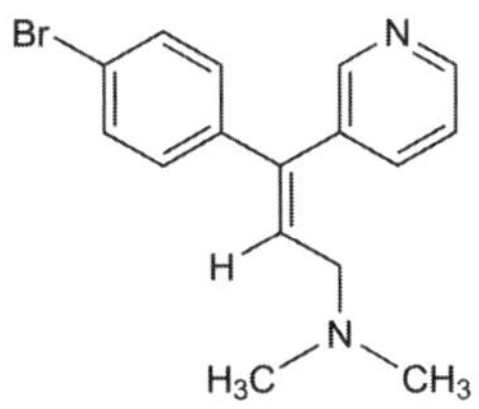

A white crystalline solid.

Zimeldine Hydrochloride

Proprietary names. Normud; Zelmid.
$C_{16}H_{17}BrN_2$,2HCl,H_2O=408.2
CAS—60525 15 7 (anhydrous); 61129-30-4 (monohydrate)
A white to yellowish-white crystalline substance. M.p. 193°.
Soluble 1 in less than 1 of water and 1 in 1000 of ethanol; practically insoluble in chloroform and ether.

Dissociation Constant. pK_a 3.8, 8.6.

Partition Coefficient. Log *P* (octanol/water), 3.18.

Colour Tests. Cyanogen Bromide (30 s)—red; Liebermann's Test—brown

Thin-layer Chromatography. System TA—Rf 47; system TB—Rf 27; system TC—Rf 25; system TE—Rf 48; system TAE—Rf 20. (Location under ultraviolet light, violet fluorescence; Dragendorff spray, positive.)

Gas Chromatography. System GA—zimeldine RI 2270, M (nor-) RI 2223; system GM—zimeldine RRT 0.820, M (nor-) RRT 0.941 (both relative to iprindole).

High Performance Liquid Chromatography. System HA—zimeldine *k* 3.2 (tailing peak), M (nor-) *k* 2.9 (tailing peak); system HF—*k* 0.67; system HY—RI 270.

Ultraviolet Spectrum. Aqueous acid—250 nm (A^1_1 = 630a); aqueous alkali—258 nm.

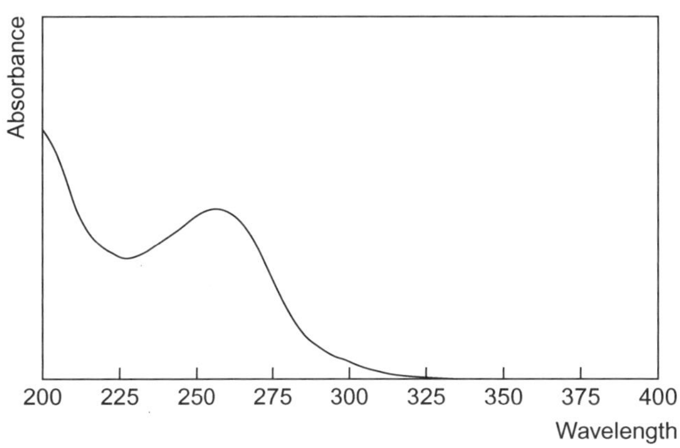

Infra-red Spectrum. Principal peaks at wavenumbers 815, 1492, 699, 953, 1075, 840 cm^{-1} (KBr disk).

Mass Spectrum. Principal ions at *m/z* 58, 70, 318, 316, 317, 193, 319, 161.

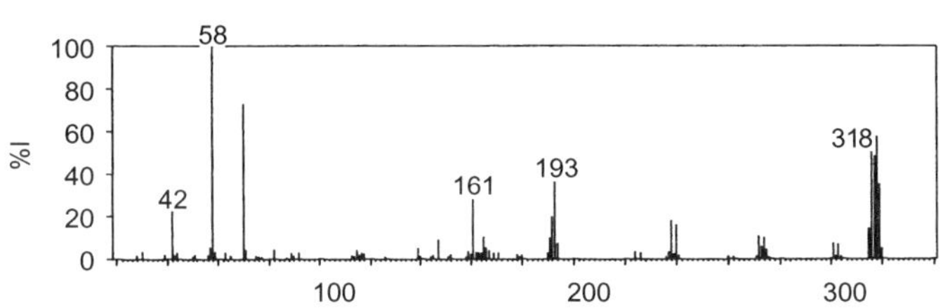

Quantification

Gas chromatography. In plasma: zimeldine and norzimeldine, limit of detection 5 µg/L, ECD—G. Caillé *et al.*, *Clin. Pharmacokinet.*, 1983, *8*, 530–540.

High performance liquid chromatography. In plasma: zimeldine and norzimeldine, limits of detection 1.5 µg/L and 0.7 µg/L, respectively, UV detection—D. Westerlund and E. Erixson, *J. Chromatogr.*, 1979, *185*, 593–603. In plasma: limit of detection 5 µg/L—T. Visser *et al.*, *J. Chromatogr.*, 1984, *309(1)*, 81–93.

Disposition in the Body. Readily absorbed after oral administration and rapidly demethylated by first-pass metabolism to norzimeldine which is active. Other metabolites include zimeldine *N'*-oxide and 3-(4-bromophenyl)-3-(3-pyridyl)acrylic acid; very little unchanged drug is excreted in the urine.

Therapeutic concentration

Following a single oral dose of 100 mg to 10 subjects, peak plasma-zimeldine concentrations of 0.048 to 0.164 mg/L (mean 0.10) were attained in 2 to 3 h and peak plasma-norzimeldine concentrations of 0.012 to 0.092 mg/L (mean 0.04) were attained in 1.5 to 8 h [G. Caillé *et al.*, *Clin. Pharmacokinet.*, 1983, *8*, 530–540].

Following oral doses averaging 225 mg daily, given twice a day to 8 subjects, steady state plasma concentrations of 0.029 to 0.102 mg/L (mean 0.07) of zimeldine and 0.145 to 0.554 mg/L (mean 0.25) of norzimeldine were reported. The corresponding steady-state concentrations in cerebrospinal fluid were 0.003 to 0.007 (mean 0.006) and 0.027 to 0.072 (mean 0.043) for zimeldine and norzimeldine, respectively [H. M. Calil *et al.*, *Clin. Pharmacol. Ther.*, 1982, *31*, 522–527].

Toxicity. Zimeldine has been withdrawn from use because of potentially severe neurological side-effects. Recovery within 48 h of ingestion of 3 g of zimeldine together with half a bottle of vodka has been reported.

The following postmortem tissue distribution was reported in a female subject who had been receiving 300 mg of zimeldine daily and had been found drowned: blood, zimeldine 0.3 mg/L, norzimeldine 0.9 mg/L; bile, zimeldine 5.0 mg/L, norzimeldine 15 mg/L; liver, zimeldine 4.0 µg/g, norzimeldine 16 µg/g [R. Geyer, *Bull. Int. Assoc. Forensic Toxicol.*, 1981, *16(2)*, 30–31].

A 30-year-old woman who was undergoing psychiatric treatment died owing to a self-inflicted gunshot wound. However, zimeldine concentrations exceeded the normal therapeutic levels (ranging from 0.02 to 0.25 mg/L). It was known that she was being treated with 100 mg twice daily and other drugs. The postmortem blood zimeldine concentration was 0.71 mg/L and norzimeldine, 2.2 mg/L. Zimeldine was also detected at a concentration of 24 µg/g in liver, 1.5 mg/L in urine, 0.77 µg/g in brain tissue and in bile, a total of 3.8 mg/L. Norzimeldine was detected at concentrations of 8.2 mg/kg, 11 mg/L, 3.7 mg/kg and 16 mg/L, respectively [D. J. Semple, *J. Anal. Toxicol.*, 1984, *8*, 285–287].

Bioavailability. 20 to 50%.

Half-life. Plasma half-life, zimeldine about 4 to 9 h, norzimeldine about 15 to 25 h.

Volume of distribution. Zimeldine, about 4 L/kg, norzimeldine, about 9 L/kg.

Clearance. Plasma clearance, zimeldine about 7 to 11 mL/min/kg, norzimeldine about 8 mL/min/kg.

Protein binding. In plasma, zimeldine about 90%, norzimeldine about 80%.

Note. For a review of the pharmacokinetics of zimeldine see R. C. Heel *et al.*, *Drugs*, 1982, *24*, 169–206.

Dose. Zimeldine hydrochloride has been given in doses of 100 to 300 mg daily.

Ziprasidone

Antipsychotic

Synonym. CP-88059
Proprietary names. Geoden; Zeldox.
5-[2-[4-(1,2-Benzisothiazol-3-yl)-1-piperazinyl]ethyl]-6-chloro-1,3-dihydro-2*H*-indol-2-one
$C_{21}H_{21}ClN_4OS$=412.9
CAS—146939-27-7

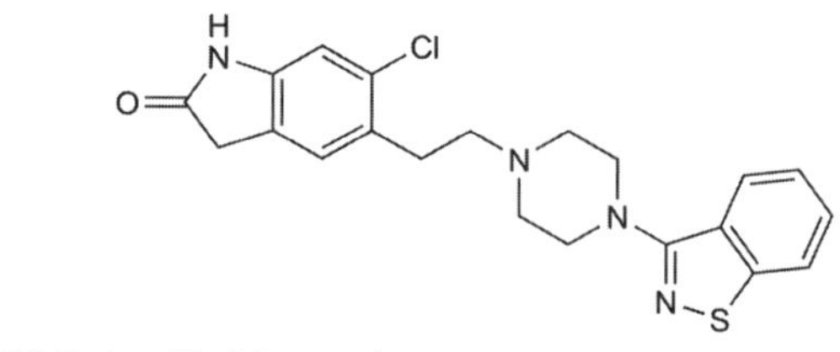

White to off-white powder.

Ziprasidone Hydrochloride Monohydrate
Synonym. CP-88059-1
$C_{21}H_{21}ClN_4OS,HCl,H_2O=467.4$
CAS—138982-67-9

High Performance Liquid Chromatography. Column: LC-18 DB (Supelco, 250 × 2.1 mm i.d.). Mobile phase: water:acetonitrile: trifluoroacetic acid:triethylamine (600:300:0.45:0.72), flow rate 0.27 mL/min. UV detection (λ=215 nm). Retention times: 9.22 to 9.74 min [S. Janiszewski *et al.*, *J. Chromatogr.*, 1995, *668*, *Biomed. Appl.*, 133–139].

Quantification
High performance liquid chromatography. In serum: limit of quantification 0.5 µg/L to 50 µg/L—S. Janiszewski *et al.*, *J. Chromatogr.*, 1995, *668*, *Biomed. Appl.*, 133–139.

Disposition in the Body. Ziprasidone is rapidly absorbed and extensively metabolised by N-dealkylation, oxidation, reductive cleavage, hydration and N-dearylation. Twelve metabolites have been identified in urine and serum; the major ones in urine being oxindole acetic acid and its glucuronide conjugate, benzisothiazole-3-yl-piperazine (BITP), BITP-sulfoxide, BITP-sulfone and its lactam, ziprasidone sulfoxide, and sulfone (the major metabolites in serum). Other metabolites include *S*-methyldihydroziprasidone, *S*-methyldihydroziprasidone sulfoxide and 6-chloro-5-(2-piperazin-1-yl-ethyl)-1,3-dihydro-indol-2-one. After 10 days of treatment with ziprasidone, approx. 20% of an administered dose is excreted in urine, with only a small proportion as the unchanged drug. In patients with mild to moderate impairment of liver function, the serum concentrations were 30% higher than in normal patients. No significant differences in the pharmacokinetics of ziprasidone have been observed in patients with impaired renal function.

Therapeutic concentration

4 healthy male volunteers were fasted overnight and administered a 20 mg suspension of ziprasidone after a standard breakfast, for 11 days. The mean peak plasma concentration was 45.4 µg/L (range 28.8 to 62.0 µg/L) for the four subjects which was observed at approx. 3.5 h (2 to 6 h) [C. Prakash *et al.*, *Drug Metab. Dispos.*, 1997, *25(7)*, 863–872].

39 healthy males, 18 to 45 years old, were administered fixed doses of 10, 40, 40 escalated to 80, and 40 escalated to 120 mg daily. For all doses, a dose of 20 mg was administered on day 1 and a 48 h washout period allowed. On subsequent days dose was administered twice daily and escalated to 80 mg or 120 mg on days 7 and 10, respectively. The peak plasma concentrations on day 1 were 12.2, 26.6, 60.0 and 34.3 µg/L for the four dosing regimens observed at 5.0, 4.8, 3.8 and 4.0 h, respectively. On day 18, the peak plasma concentrations were 14.8, 44.6, 118.6 and 139.4 µg/L for the 10, 40, 80 and 120 mg doses respectively observed at 5.2, 3.8, 3.7 and 4.7 h [J. J. Miceli *et al.*, *Br. J. Clin. Pharmacol.*, 2000, *49 (suppl.1)*, 5S–13S].

Bioavailability. Oral, 59%.

Half-life. 4 h, although the half-life is increased by about 2 h in patients with mild to moderately impaired liver function.

Zolmitriptan

5HT₁ Agonist/Antimigraine

Synonym. 311C90
Proprietary name. Zomig
(4*S*)-4-[[3-[2-(Dimethylamino)ethyl]-1*H*-indol-5-yl]methyl]-2-oxazolidinone
$C_{16}H_{21}N_3O_2=287.4$
CAS—139264-17-8

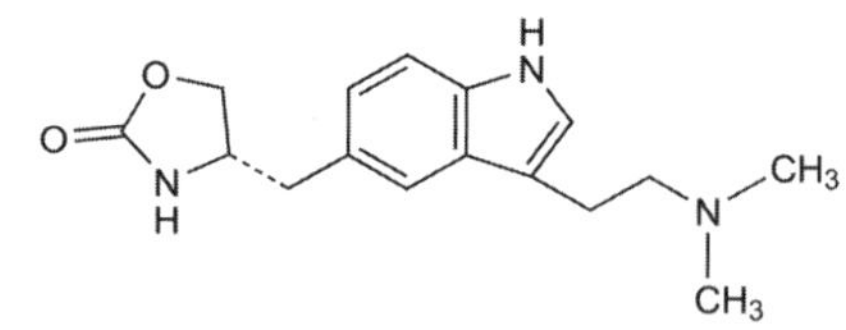

A white to almost white crystalline powder with M.p. 139° to 141°. It is readily soluble in water.

Dissociation Constant. pK_a 9.6.

High Performance Liquid Chromatography. System HZ—retention time 1.8 min.

Column: (analytical) silica (Alltech, 150 × 2.1 mm i.d., 5 µm); (guard) C_8 (Optiguard, 1 mm). Mobile phase: ammonium acetate (20 mM), pH 4 with glacial acetic acid; formic acid:methanol:acetonitrile (80:10:10) (pH 2.7). Detection: MS–MS. Retention time: 2.95 min [K. Vishwanathan *et al.*, *Rapid Commun. Mass Spectrom.*, 2000, *14(3)*, 168–172].

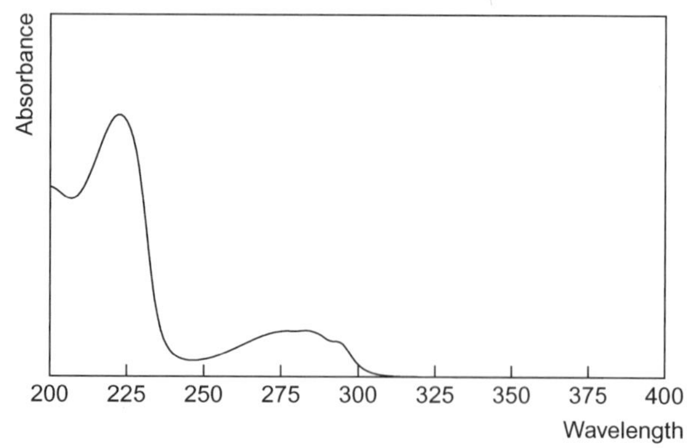

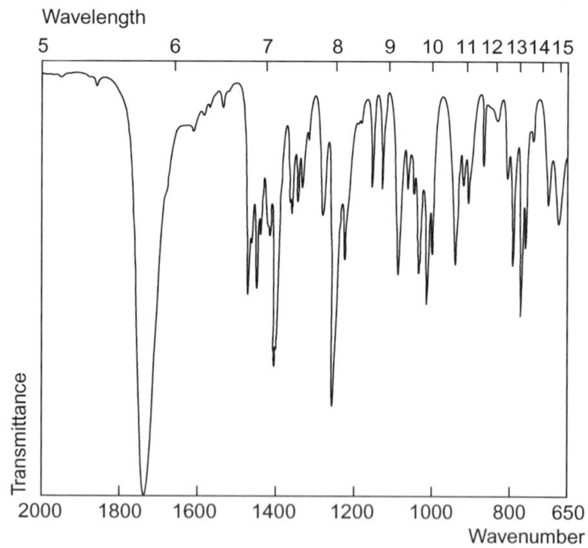

Mass Spectrum. Principal ions at *m/z* 182, 288, 167, 156, 165, 243, 183, 157.

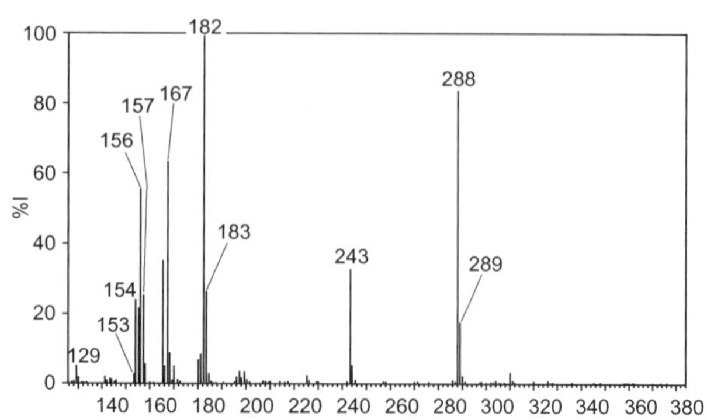

Quantification

High performance liquid chromatography. In serum: limit of detection 0.1 μg/L, electrospray tandem MS detection—K. Vishwanathan *et al.*, *Rapid Commun. Mass Spectrom.*, 2000, *14(3)*, 168–172. In plasma: limit of detection 0.1 μg/L. MS–MS detection—E. J. Seaber *et al.*, *Br. J. Clin. Pharmacol.*, 1998, *46(5)*, 433–439. In plasma and urine: limit of detection 2 μg/L and 100 μg/L, respectively. UV detection (λ=230 nm)—E. Seaber *et al.*, *Br. J. Clin. Pharmacol.*, 1997, *43(6)*, 579–587.

Disposition in the Body. Zolmitriptan is absorbed after oral administration, which is unaffected by food. There is extensive hepatic metabolism, principally to the indole acetic acid, and also the *N*-oxide and *N*-desmethyl analogues. The *N*-desmethyl metabolite is more active than the parent compound in animal studies. Metabolism is primarily mediated by CYP1A2, and monoamine oxidase is responsible for further metabolism of the *N*-desmethyl metabolite. At least 60% of the dose is excreted in urine, mainly as the indole acetic acid. Approx. 30% is excreted in faeces, mainly as the unchanged drug. There is no evidence of accumulation on multiple dosing.

Therapeutic concentration

24 normal individuals, 12 aged between 18 and 39 years, and 12 aged from 65 to 76 years old, were fasted overnight and administered zolmitriptan (5, 10 and 15 mg doses). The peak plasma drug concentrations for the young individuals were 9.1, 18.9 and 23.3 μg/L for the three respective doses. The group aged from 65 to 76 years showed peak zolmitriptan concentrations of 9.9, 18.6 and 22.7 μg/L for the respective doses [R. W. Peck *et al.*, *Clin. Pharmacol. Ther.*, 1998, *63(3)*, 342–353].

20 healthy individuals (average age of 23 years) were administered a single oral dose of 2.5 mg and the equivalent intravenous dosage. Peak drug concentrations were observed within the hour and were sustained for 6 h at levels of 3.3 μg/L (for men), and 3.8 μg/L (for women). For the intravenous doses, the females and males produced peak concentrations of 5.8 and 10.6 μg/L, respectively, when administered 2.5 mg [E. J. Seaber *et al.*, *Br. J. Clin. Pharmacol.*, 1998, *46(5)*, 433–439].

Toxicity. Doses of 50 mg result in sedation. Other side effects include transient increase in blood pressure, myalgia, and muscle weakness.

Bioavailability. 40 to 50%.

Half-life. 2.5 to 3 h, prolonged in patients with hepatic impairment.

Volume of distribution. About 7.0 L/kg.

Clearance. Total plasma clearance, about 31.5 mL/min/kg.

Protein binding. 25%.

Dose. The usual dose is 2.5 mg with a maximum dose of 15 mg in 24 h.

Zolpidem

Hypnotic

Synonym. SL-80.0750

N,*N*-6-Trimethyl-2-(4-methylphenyl)imidazo[1,2-*a*]pyridine-3-acetamide

$C_{19}H_{21}N_3O$=307.4

CAS—82626-48-0

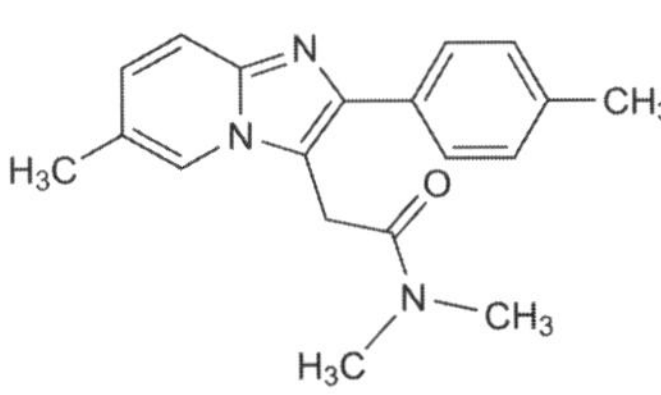

M.p.196°. Insoluble in water.

Zolpidem Tartrate

Synonyms. SL-80.0750-23N; Zolpidem Hemitartrate.

Proprietary names. Ambien; Bikalm; Cedrol; Dalparan; Ivadal; Niotal; Stilnoct; Stilnox.

$(C_{19}H_{21}N_3O)_2,C_4H_6O_6$=764.9

CAS—99294-93-6

A white or almost white hygroscopic crystalline powder. M.p. 193°to 197°. It is slightly soluble in water (23 g/L at 20°); practically insoluble in dichloromethane; sparingly soluble in methanol.

Dissociation Constant. pK_a 6.2.

Partition Coefficient. Log *P* (octanol/water) 3.85.

Gas Chromatography. System GB—RI 2941.

Column: OV-1 fused-silica (25 m × 0.32 mm i.d., 0.2 μm film thickness). Column temperature: 235°. Carrier gas: helium, flow rate 1.3 mL/min. Internal standard: clonazepam. Detection: nitrogen–phosphorus. Retention times: zolpidem, 10.0 min; IS, 10.72 min [F. Stanke *et al.*, *J. Chromatogr.*, 1996, *675*, *Biomed. Appl.*, 43–51].

Column: 5% phenyl methyl silicone fused-silica capillary (Ultra 2, 25 m × 0.32 mm i.d., film thickness 0.52 μm), (guard) deactivated fused-silica tubing (5 m × 0.53 mm i.d.). Column temperature: 210° to 285° at 2.5°/min. Carrier gas: helium, flow rate 2.1 mL/min. IS: prazepam. Detection: electron-capture/nitrogen–phosphorus. Retention times: zolpidem, 1.2 min; IS, 1.0 min [Y. Gaillard *et al.*, *J. Chromatogr.*, 1993, *622*, *Biomed. Appl.*, 197–208].

High Performance Liquid Chromatography. System HY—RI 291; system HZ—retention time 3.2 min; system HAA—retention time 11.9 min.

Column: C_{18} (μBondapak, 300 × 3.9 mm i.d.). Mobile phase: acetonitrile:potassium dihydrogen phosphate (50 nM) (50:50), flow rate 1.5 mL/min. IS: propylzolpidem. Fluorescence detection (λ_{em}=254 nm; λ_{em}=390 nm). Retention times: zolpidem, 3.1 min; IS, 4.7 min [D. J. Greenblatt *et al.*, *J Anal Toxicol.*, 1997, 21, 388–392].

Column: 100-3 C_{18} (Nucleosil, 150 × 4.6 mm i.d.); (guard) 120-5 C_{18} (Nucleosil, 10 × 4 mm i.d.). Column temperature: 35°. Mobile phase: methanol:potassium dihydrogen phosphate (30 mM, pH 6.8):triethylamine (30:69:1), flow rate 0.7 mL/min. Fluorescence detection (λ_{ex}=244 nm; λ_{em}=388 nm). Retention time: 4.7 min [P. Ptácek *et al.*, *J. Chromatogr. B Biomed. Sci. Appl.*, 1997, *694*, 409–413].

Column: C_{18} (Novapak, 300 × 3.9 mm i.d., 4 μm). Column temperature: 30°. Mobile phase: methanol:tetrahydrofuran:phosphate (pH 2.6) (65:5:30), flow rate 0.8 mL/min. UV detection (diode array at λ=210 nm). Retention time: 4.7 min [A. Tracqui *et al.*, *J. Chromatogr.*, 1993, *616*; *Biomed. Appl.*, *127*, 95–103].

Ultraviolet Spectrum. Aqueous acid (pH 2.6)—207 nm; methanol—243, 314 nm; (0.1 M hydrochloric acid)—236, 294 nm; (0.2 M H_2SO_4)—207, 237, 295 nm; (0.025 M sulfuric acid)—238, 294.5 nm; (0.1 M $HCOONH_4$, pH 3)—238, 296 nm; aqueous alkali (0.1 M sodium hydroxide)—242, 311 nm.

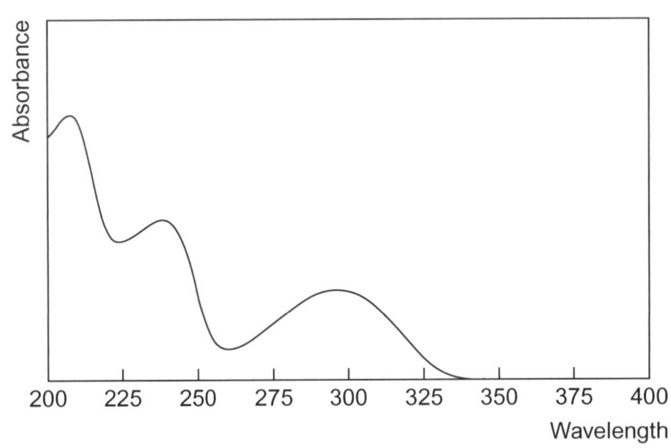

Infra-red Spectrum. (Zolpidem tartrate) Principal peaks at wavenumbers 1637, 1402, 1511, 1136 cm^{-1} (KBr disk).

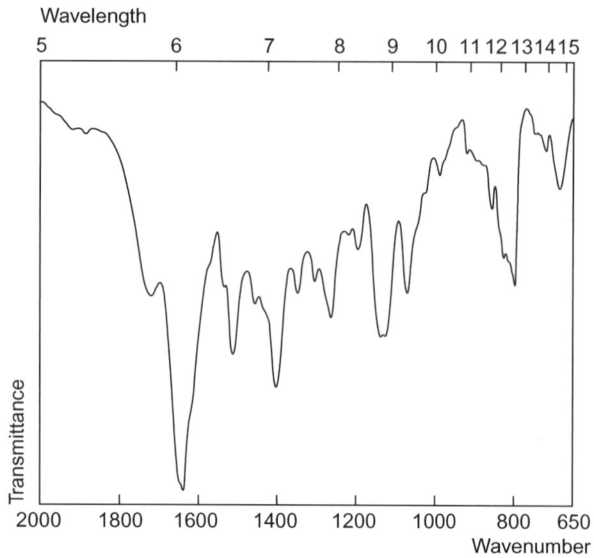

Mass Spectrum. Principal ions at *m/z* 235, 236, 307, 219, 92, 65, 43, 220.

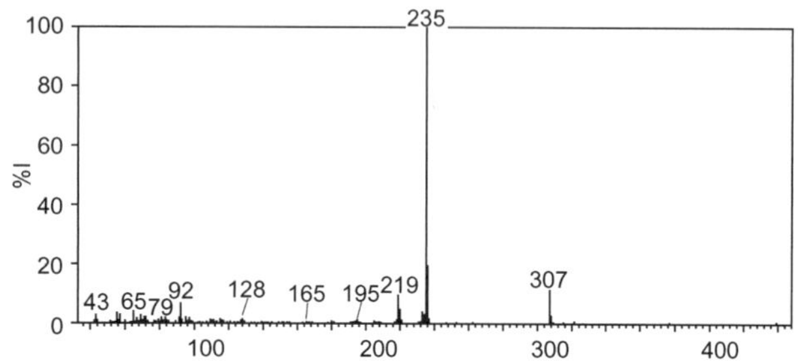

Quantification

Gas chromatography. In plasma: limit of detection 10 µg/L, ECD and AFID—Y. Gaillard *et al.*, *J. Chromatogr.*, 1993, *622*; *Biomed. Appl.*, *133*, 197–208. In plasma: limit of detection 1 µg/L, AFID—F. Stanke *et al.*, *J. Chromatogr.*, 1996, *675*; *Biomed. Appl.*, 43–51.

Gas chromatography–mass spectrometry. In urine: limit of detection < 100 µg/L—J. Bickeboeller-Friedrich and H. H. Maurer, *Ther. Drug Monit.*, 2001, *23*, 61–70.

High performance liquid chromatography. In blood or plasma: limit of detection 1 µg/L in blood and plasma. Fluorescence detection (λ_{ex}=254 nm; λ_{em}=390 nm)—P. Guinebault *et al.*, *J. Chromatogr.*, 1986, *383*; *Biomed. Appl.*, *56*, 206–211. In plasma or urine: zolpidem and metabolites, limit of detection 0.2 µg/L in plasma and 1.0 µg/L in urine, respectively. Fluorescence detection (λ_{ex}=254 nm; λ_{em}=390 nm)—V. Ascalone *et al.*, *J. Chromatogr.*, 1992, *581*; *Biomed. Appl.*, *119*, 237–250. In plasma: limit of detection about 24 µg/L. UV detection (diode array at λ=210 nm)—A. Tracqui *et al.*, *J. Chromatogr.*, 1993, *616*; *Biomed. Appl.*, *127*, 95–103. In plasma: limit of detection 1.5 µg/L. Fluorescence detection (λ_{ex}=244 nm; λ_{em}=388 nm)—P. Ptácek *et al.*, *J. Chromatogr. B Biomed. Sci. Appl.*, 1997, *694*, 409–413.

Disposition in the Body. Absorbed after oral administration; bioavailability about 70%. Peak plasma concentrations are attained within 0.5 and 3 h. The drug displays linear pharmacokinetics within the therapeutic dose range, and undergoes first-pass metabolism by the liver. Metabolic pathways include oxidation and hydroxylation. The inactive metabolites are excreted in urine (56%) and faeces (37%), with less than 1% excreted as the unchanged drug. It is distributed into breast milk and crosses the placenta. It is not removed by dialysis.

Therapeutic concentration. The therapeutic concentration range in serum is 80 to 150 µg/L.

12 males aged between 23 and 36 years, mean 28 years old, were orally administered 10 mg zolpidem. The peak concentration observed at 2.6 h was 76 µg/L [M. Colle *et al.*, *Horm. Res.*, 1991, *35*, 30–34].

18 male volunteers (average age 26) were administered single oral and IV doses of zolpidem. The 12 males who received 20 mg orally showed a mean peak concentration of 55 µg/L at 1.0 h. The remaining males were administered 5 mg intravenously, and the concentration was 244 µg/L at 1.1 h [A. Patat *et al.*, *Psychopharmacology (Berl.)*, 1994, *114*, 138–146].

Toxicity. The serum toxic concentration is 500 µg/L.

Bioavailability. About 70%.

Half-life. Plasma half-life, 1.7 to 2.5 h in normal subjects; increased to about 10 h in patients with cirrhosis.

Volume of distribution. 0.54 to 0.68 L/kg.

Clearance. Plasma clearance, 0.26 L/h/kg.

Protein binding. In plasma, 92%.

Dose. The usual dose is 10 mg, which may be increased to 15 or 20 mg if necessary. In the elderly, the dose is reduced to 5 mg.

Zomepirac

Analgesic

5-(4-Chlorobenzoyl)-1,4-dimethyl-1*H*-pyrrole-2-acetic acid
$C_{15}H_{14}ClNO_3$=291.7
CAS—33369-31-2

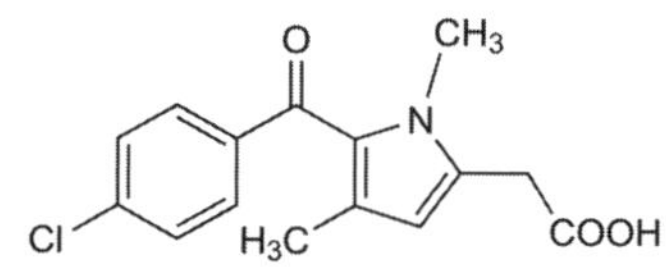

White crystals. M.p. 178° to 179°, with decomposition.

Zomepirac Sodium

Proprietary names. Zomax; Zomaxin; Zopirac.
$C_{15}H_{13}ClNNaO_3,2H_2O$=349.7
CAS—64092-48-4 (anhydrous); 64092-49-5 (dihydrate)
A pale yellow crystalline powder. M.p. 295° to 296°.

Partition Coefficient. Log *P* (octanol/water), 3.21.

Colour Tests. Formaldehyde–Sulfuric Acid—red; Liebermann's Test (100°)—orange; Marquis Test—yellow (→ orange at 100°); Sulfuric Acid—yellow.

Thin-layer Chromatography. System TD—Rf 12; system TE—Rf 04; system TF—Rf 12; system TAE—Rf 88; system TAJ—Rf 19; system TAK—Rf 65; system TAL—Rf 88. (Marquis reagent, yellow → green, slow; mercuric chloride–diphenylcarbazone reagent, blue, pink after heating; acidified potassium permanganate solution, positive; Van Urk reagent, positive, red after heating.)

Gas Chromatography. System GA—zomepirac-ME RI 2343; M (-CO_2) RI 2025.

High Performance Liquid Chromatography. System HD—k 3.7; system HY—RI 495.

Ultraviolet Spectrum. Aqueous acid 262 nm (A_1^1=418b), 324 nm (A_1^1 = 492b); aqueous alkali 261 nm, 330 nm (A_1^1=525a).

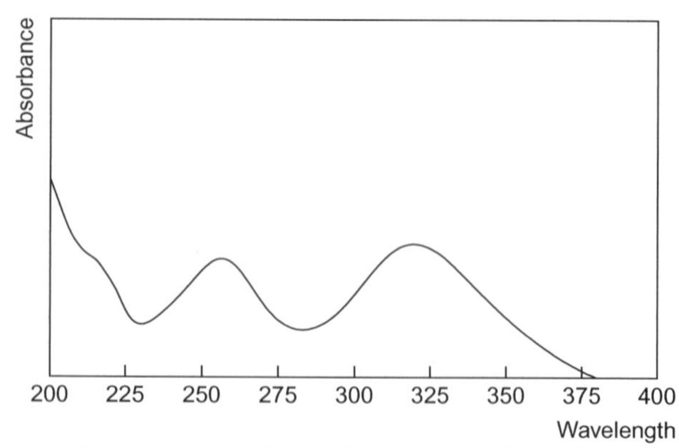

Infra-red Spectrum. Principal peaks at wavenumbers 1587, 1560, 760, 1275, 958, 1493 cm^{-1}(zomepirac sodium, KBr disk).

Mass Spectrum. Principal ions at *m/z* 246, 291, 248, 290, 247, 139, 111, 292.

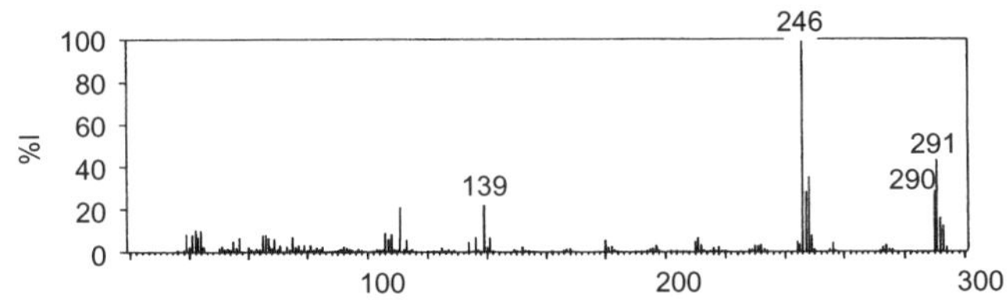

Quantification

Gas chromatography. In plasma: limit of detection 5 µg/L, ECD—K.-T. Ng and J. J. Kalbron, *J. Chromatogr.*, 1983, *276*; *Biomed. Appl.*, *27*, 311–318.

High performance liquid chromatography. In serum or plasma: limit of detection 50 µg/L, UV detection—C. L. Welch *et al.*, *Clin. Chem.*, 1982, *28*, 481–484. In urine: zomepirac and zomepirac glucuronide, limit of detection about 100 µg/L, UV detection—P. Pietta and A. Calatroni, *J. Chromatogr.*, 1983, *275*; *Biomed. Appl.*, *26*, 217–222.

Disposition in the Body. Rapidly and completely absorbed after oral administration. About 90% of a dose is excreted in the urine in 48 h with about 5 to 20% as unchanged drug and about 60 to 80% as a glucuronide conjugate; about 5% of the dose is excreted as a hydroxylated metabolite; 4-chlorobenzoic acid has been reported to be a minor metabolite. Less than 2% of a dose is eliminated in the faeces.

Therapeutic concentration

After a single oral dose of 100 mg to 21 subjects, peak plasma concentrations averaged 4.7 mg/L at about 1 h; following oral administration of 100 mg four times a day to 10 subjects, steady-state plasma concentrations of about 3 to 4 mg/L were reported [R. K. Nayak *et al.*, *Clin. Pharmacol. Ther.*, 1980, *27*, 395–401].

Following a single oral dose of 200 mg to 5 subjects, peak plasma concentrations of 4.5 to 11.3 mg/L (mean 9) were attained in about 1 h; mean peak plasma concentrations of zomepirac glucuronide and hydroxyzomepirac of 3.9 mg/L and 0.2 mg/L, respectively, were attained in 0.5 to 3 h [P. J. O'Neill *et al.*, *J. Clin. Pharmacol.*, 1982, *22*, 470–476].

Toxicity. Zomepirac has been withdrawn from use because of reports of allergic anaphylactoid reactions. In a fatality caused by the ingestion of 9 g of zomepirac sodium, a postmortem blood concentration of 152 mg/L and an ante-mortem blood concentration, obtained 9 h prior to death, of 286 mg/L were reported [R. C. Backer *et al.*, *J. Anal. Toxicol.*, 1983, *7*, 223–224].

Half-life. Plasma half-life, about 4 to 10 h.

Distribution in blood. Plasma: whole blood ratio, 1.9.

Protein binding. In plasma, 98 to 99%.

Note. For a review of zomepirac see P. A. Morley *et al.*, *Drugs*, 1982, *23*, 250–275; for a review on the acute toxicity of zomepirac see D. W. Joubert, *Drug Intell. Clin. Pharm.*, 1982, *16*, 328–330.

Dose. Zomepirac sodium has been given in doses equivalent to 400 to 600 mg of zomepirac daily.

Zonisamide

Anticonvulsant

Synonyms. AD-810; CI-912; PD-110843.
Proprietary names. Excegran; Zonegran.
1,2-Benzisoxazole-3-methanesulfonamide
$C_8H_8N_2O_3S = 212.2$
CAS—68291-97-4

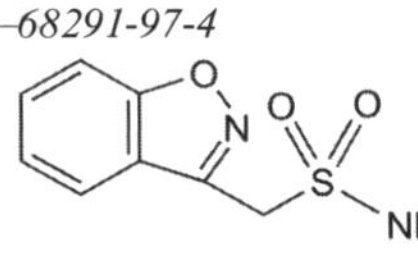

White needles. M.p. 160° to 163°; also reported as 162° to 166°.
Sparingly soluble in water, chloroform, hexane; soluble in methanol, ethanol, ethyl acetate and acetic acid.

Dissociation Constant. pK_a 10.2.

Quantification

High performance liquid chromatography. In serum: limit of detection 0.1 mg/L, UV detection (λ=246 nm)—K. Furuno *et al.*, *J. Chromatogr.*, 1994, *656*; *Biomed. Appl.*, 456–459. In breast milk and plasma: limit of quantification 0.05 mg/L, UV detection (λ=240 nm)—R. Shimoyama *et al.*, *Biomed. Chromatogr.*, 1999, *13*, 370–372.

Disposition in the Body. Zonisamide is rapidly and almost completely absorbed from the gastro-intestinal tract following oral administration. Peak plasma concentrations are achieved within 2 to 6 h of oral administration, however, steady-state concentrations are not achieved for up to 2 weeks owing to the drug's long half-life. It is metabolised via acetylation to *N*-acetylzonisamide and reduction mediated by cytochrome P450 CYP3A4 to 2-sulfamoylacetylphenol (SMAP), further glucuronide conjugation also occurs. Excretion is mainly in the urine, 35% as unchanged drug, 15% as *N*-acetylzonisamide and 50% as the glucuronide of SAMP.

Therapeutic concentration

After single dose oral administration of 200 mg and 800 mg zonisamide to healthy volunteers, peak plasma concentrations were 2.3 mg/L and 12.5 mg/L, respectively, and were reached within 2.4 to 3.6 h [D. H. Peters and E. M. Sorkin, *Drugs*, 1993, *45*, 760–787]

In a study investigating the steady-state pharmacokinetics of zonisamide, 24 healthy volunteers were administered with the following drug regimen: 100 mg/day for a week, followed by 200 mg/day for another week and finishing on 400 mg/day until day 35. The volunteers were split into two groups: group A (*n*=11) receiving their dose divided every 12 h after the first week and group B (*n*=8) receiving their entire dose in the morning. Peak plasma concentrations were 30.3 mg/L and 23.8 mg/L for group A and group B, respectively, reached after 2.1 and 1.8 h, respectively. Steady-state concentrations were 28.3 mg/L for group A and 23.8 mg/L for group B and were reached in an average of 15 days from the last dose adjustment [G. M. Kochak *et al.*, *J. Clin. Pharmacol.*, 1998, *38*, 166–171].

Toxicity. Adverse events, most notably drowsiness, loss of appetite, gastro-intestinal problems and CNS toxicity have been noted with plasma zonisamide concentrations exceeding 30 mg/L.

Bioavailability. Oral, 100%.

Half-life. In plasma, approx. 63 h.

Volume of distribution. Apparent, 1.45 L/kg.

Clearance. Plasma, 0.30 to 0.35 mL/min/kg.

Distribution in Blood. Plasma:red blood cells 1:8.

Protein binding. About 40%.

Note. For a review of zonisamide and its pharmacodynamic and pharmacokinetic properties, and therapeutic potential in epilepsy see D. H. Peters and E. M. Sorkin, *Drugs*, 1993, *45*, 760–787.

Dose. Initially, 100 mg once daily orally, increased to 200 mg daily on one or several doses. Doses of up to 600 mg daily have been administered.

Zopiclone

Hypnotic

Synonym. RP-27267.
Proprietary names. Amoban; Amovane; Datolan; Imovane; Limovan; Rhovane; Siaten; Sopivan; Ximovan; Zileze; Zimovane.
4-Methyl-1-piperazine-carboxylic acid 6-(5-chloro-2-pyridinyl)-6,7-dihydro-7-oxo-5*H*-pyrrolo[3,4-*b*]pyrazin-5-yl ester
$C_{17}H_{17}ClN_6O_3 = 388.8$
CAS—43200-80-2

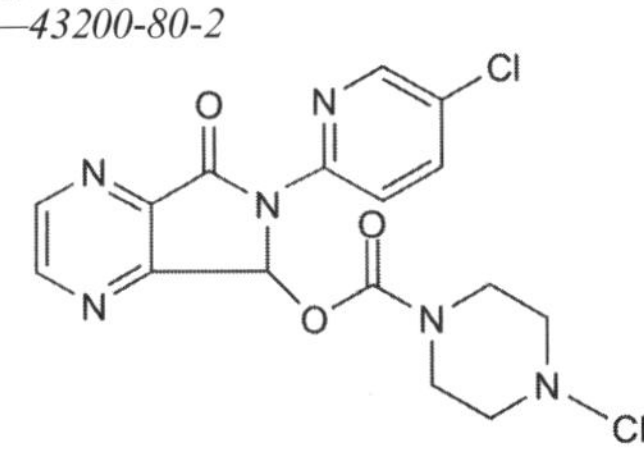

A white or slightly yellow powder. M.p. 178°. It is practically insoluble in water and in alcohol; sparingly soluble in acetone; freely soluble in dichloromethane; dissolves in dilute mineral acids.

Thin-layer Chromatography. System TB—Rf 04; system TE—Rf 47; system TF—Rf 00; system TAE—Rf 42.

Plate: silica gel 60 F_{254} (10 × 10 cm). Mobile phase 1: cyclohexane:toluene:diethylamine (75:15:10); mobile phase 2: chloroform:methanol (90:10); mobile phase 3: chloroform:acetone (80:20).

Dragendorff's reagent. UV detection (λ=366 nm). Rf 21 (mobile phase1); Rf 71 (mobile phase 2); Rf 60 (mobile phase 3) [K. Otsubo *et al.*, *J. Chromatogr.*, 1995, *669*, *Biomed. Appl.*, 408–412].

Gas Chromatography. System GB—zopiclone RI 3263; art (aminochloropyridine) RI 1261.

Column: OV-1 fused-silica (25 m × 0.32 mm i.d., 0.2 µm film thickness). Column temperature: 235°. Carrier gas: helium, flow rate 1.3 mL/min. Detection: nitrogen–phosphorus. Retention time: 19.6 min [F. Stanke *et al.*, *J. Chromatogr.*, 1996, *675*, *Biomed. Appl.*, 43–51].

High Performance Liquid Chromatography. System HX—RI 331; system HY—RI 269; system HZ—retention time 2.3 min; system HAX—retention time 7.5 min; system HAY—retention time 3.8 min.

Column: C_8 (Symmetry, 150 × 3.9 mm i.d., 5 µm). Mobile phase: ammonium acetate (0.05 M):acetonitrile (70:30), flow rate 1.7 mL/min. IS: zopiclone chloride. Fluorescence detection (λ_{ex}=300 nm; λ_{em}=470 nm). Retention time: not specified [J. G. Bramness *et al.*, *J Forensic Sci.*, 2001, *46* (5), 1247–1249].

Column: Chiralcel OD-H chiral (250 × 4.6 mm i.d., 5 µm). Mobile phase: ethanol:hexane (60:40), flow rate 0.6 mL/min. IS: chlordiazepoxide. Fluorescence detection (λ_{ex}=300 nm; λ_{em} = 470 nm). Retention times: (−)-zopiclone, 19 min; (+)-zopiclone, 28 min; IS, 9.5 min [R. T. Foster *et al.*, *J. Chromatogr.*, 1994, *658*, *Biomed. Appl.*, 161–166].

Column: C_{18} (Novapak, 300 × 3.9 mm, i.d., 4 µm). Mobile phase: methanol:tetrahydrofuran:phosphate (pH 2.6) (65:5:30), flow rate 0.8 mL/min. UV detection (diode array at λ=210 nm). *k* value: 0.56. Retention time: 4.1 min [A. Tracqui *et al.*, *J. Chromatogr.*, 1993, *616*; *Biomed. Appl.*, *127*, 95–103].

Ultraviolet Spectrum. Aqueous acid (0.2 M H_2SO_4)—304, 216 nm; (0.1 M hydrochloric acid)—303 nm; (0.1 M $HCOONH_4$, pH 3)—306, 214 nm; aqueous alkali (0.1 M sodium hydroxide)—237, 277 nm.

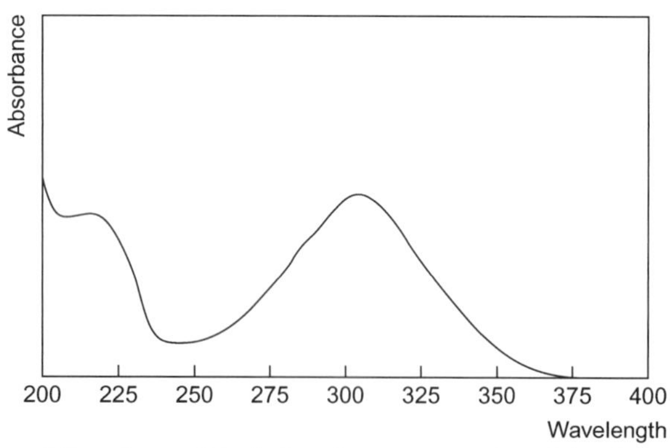

Infra-red Spectrum. Principal peaks at wavenumbers 1715, 1372, 1463, 1087 cm^{-1}.

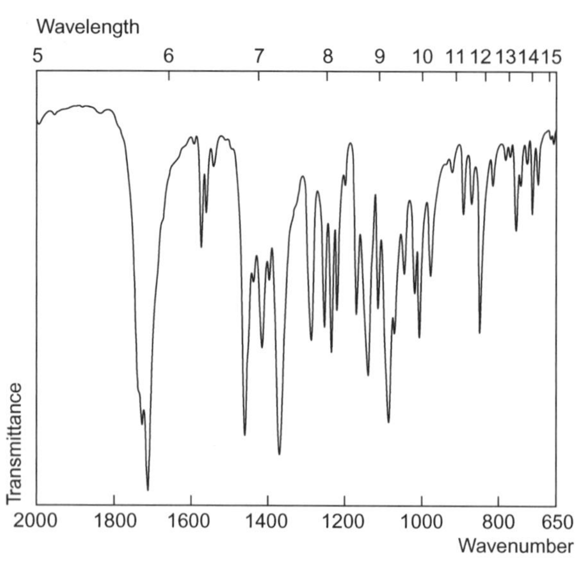

Mass Spectrum. Principal ions at *m*/*z* 143, 245, 112, 99, 56, 139, 217, 247.

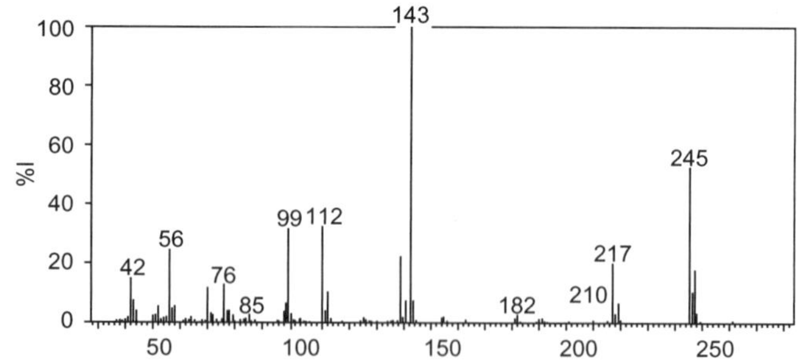

Quantification

Thin-layer chromatography. In serum: limit of detection 100 µg/L. UV detection (λ=366 nm)—K. Otsubo *et al.*, *J. Chromatogr.*, 1995, *669*, *Biomed. Appl.*, 408–412.

Gas chromatography. In plasma: limit of detection 5 µg/L, AFID—S. Kennel *et al.*, *J. Chromatogr.*, 1990, *527*; *Biomed. Appl.*, *92*, 169–173. In plasma: limit of detection 2 µg/L, ECD—Y. Gaillard *et al.*, *J. Chromatogr.*, 1993, *619*; *Biomed. Appl.*, *130*, 310–314. In plasma: limit of detection 2 µg/L. AFID—F. Stanke *et al.*, *J. Chromatogr.*, 1996, *675*, *Biomed. Appl.*, 43–51.

Gas chromatography–mass spectrometry. In urine: limit of detection < 100 µg/L—J. Bickeboeller-Friedrich and H. H. Maurer, *Ther. Drug Monit.*, 2001, *23*, 61–70.

High performance liquid chromatography. In plasma: limit of detection 5 µg/L. UV detection (λ=305 nm)—M. J. Royer-Morrot *et al.*, *J. Chromatogr.*, 1992, *581*; *Biomed. Appl.*, *119*, 297–299. In plasma or urine: limit of detection 5 µg/L for zopiclone; 10 µg/L for metabolites. Fluorescence detection (λ_{ex}=300 nm; λ_{em}=470 nm)—A. Le Liboux *et al.*, *J. Chromatogr.*, 1987, *417*; *Biomed. Appl.*, *61*, 151–158. In plasma: limit of detection 5 µg/L for enantiomers. Fluorescence detection (λ_{ex}=300 nm; λ_{em}=470 nm)—C. Fernandez *et al.*, *J. Chromatogr.*, 1991, *572*; *Biomed. Appl.*, *110*, 195–202. In plasma: limit of detection 5 µg/L. UV detection (λ=305 nm)—M. J. Royer-Morrot *et al.*, *J. Chromatogr.*, 1992, *581*; *Biomed. Appl.*, *119*, 297–299. In whole blood: limit of detection 4 µg/L. UV detection (λ=305 nm)—P. J. Boniface *et al.*, *J. Chromatogr.*, 1992, *584*; *Biomed. Appl.*, *122*, 199–206. In plasma: limit of detection about 25 µg/L. UV detection (diode array at λ=210 nm)—A. Tracqui *et al.*, *J. Chromatogr.*, 1993, *616*; *Biomed. Appl.*, *127*, 95–103.

Disposition in the Body. Zopiclone is rapidly absorbed after oral administration, and is also widely distributed into breast milk. It is extensively metabolised in the liver by demethylation, oxidation and decarboxylation. The 2 major metabolites excreted in urine are zopiclone *N*-oxide, and *N*-demethylzopiclone (inactive). About 50% of a dose is converted by decarboxylation to inactive metabolites, some of which are partly eliminated via the lungs as carbon dioxide. Only 5% of a dose is excreted unchanged in urine and about 16% appears in faeces, the remaining dose being excreted as metabolites.

Therapeutic concentration. The serum therapeutic concentration range is 0.01 to 0.05 mg/L.

12 male Caucasians, 19 to 36 years old, were administered a single oral dose of 15 mg zopiclone after an overnight fast. After 93.8 min, the total drug concentration was 0.131 mg/L (0.087 mg/L as the (+)-enantiomer and 0.044 mg/L as the (−)-enantiomer), observed at 98.8 and 88.8 min, respectively [C. Fernandez *et al.*, *Drug Metab. Dispos.*, 1993, *21(6)*, 1125].

12 healthy, lactating women between 2 and 6 days post-partum, aged 20 to 45 years, were orally administered 7.5 mg zopiclone. The mean peak plasma concentration was 0.08 mg/L at 1.6 h, and the mean milk concentration was 0.034 mg/L at 2.4 h [I. Matheson *et al.*, *Br. J. Clin. Pharmacol.*, 1990, *30*, 267–271].

Toxicity. Toxic symptoms may occur at levels above 0.15 mg/L.

The following postmortem tissue concentrations were reported in a 29-year-old female who committed suicide: portal venous blood, 3.0 mg/L; spleen, 5.8 mg/kg; brainstem, 2.8 mg/kg; myocardium, 1.6 mg/kg; kidney, 1.7 mg/kg; liver, 4.9 mg/kg [D. J. Pounder and J. I. Davies, *Forensic Sci. Int.*, 1994, *65(3)*, 177–183].

A 25-year-old male had ingested 300 mg of zopliclone in a suicide attempt. The maximum plasma concentration was measured as 1.6 mg/L at 4.5 h post-ingestion [M. J. Royer-Morrot *et al.*, *J. Chromatogr.*, 1992, *581*; *Biomed. Appl.*, *119*, 297–299].

The postmortem blood concentrations of 2 individuals who had taken 30 7.5 mg tablets, and up to 100 7.5 mg tablets were 0.62 mg/L and 1.70 mg/L, respectively [P. J. Boniface *et al.*, *J. Chromatogr.*, 1992, *584*; *Biomed. Appl.*, *122*, 199–206].

Half-life. Plasma half-life of zopiclone is 3.5 to 6.5 h, zopiclone *N*-oxide is 3.5 to 6.0 h, *N*-desmethylzopiclone is 7 to 11 h.

Volume of distribution. Approx. 1.3 to 1.6 L/kg.

Clearance. Plasma clearance, 13.9 L/h, also reported as 17.3 L/h (7.5 mg dose).

Protein binding. In plasma, 45 to 80%.
For reviews of zopiclone see K. L. Goa and R. C. Heel, *Drugs*, 1986, *32*, 48–65 and S. Noble *et al.*, *Drugs*, 1998, *55*, 277–302. For a review of the pharmacokinetics of zopiclone see C. Fernandez *et al.*, *Clin. Pharmacokinet.*, 1995, *29*, 431–441.

Dose. The usual dose is 7.5 mg at night, increased to 15 mg if necessary. Initially 3.75 mg may be given to the elderly and those with hepatic/renal impairment and increased if necessary.

Zotepine

Antipsychotic

Proprietary names. Lodopin; Nipolept; Zoleptil.
2-[(8-Chlorodibenzo[*b*,*f*]-thiepin-10-yl)oxy]-*N*,*N*-dimethylethanamine
$C_{18}H_{18}ClNOS = 331.9$
CAS—26615-21-4

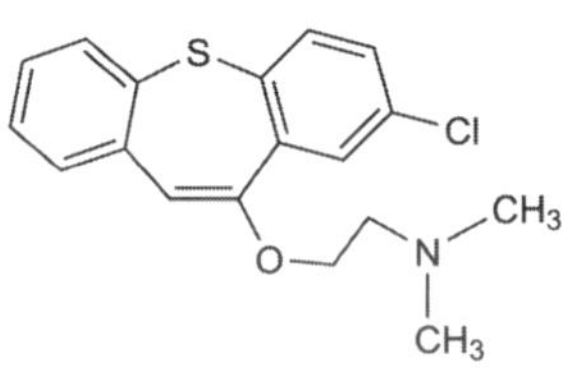

Gas Chromatography. System GA—RI 2660.

Column: HP-5 cross-linked 5% methyl silicone (30 m). Column temperature: 50° held for 1 min, to 300° at 40°/min. IS: clothiapine. MS detection (EI, SIM at *m/z*: 231 for zotepine, and *m/z*: 244 for IS). Retention times: zotepine 8.9 min; IS, 8.4 min [O. Tanaka *et al.*, *Ther. Drug Monit.*, 1996, *18*, 294–296].

High Performance Liquid Chromatography. Column: C_{18} (Novapak, 150 × 3.9 mm i.d., 4 µm). Mobile phase acetonitrile:phosphate (0.067 M, pH 7.95) (45:55), flow rate 1.0 mL/min. IS: Diazepam. UV detection (λ = 304 nm). Retention times: zotepine, 2.6 min; IS, 4.7 min [B. Paw. *et al.*, *J. Pharm. Biomed. Anal.*, 2000, *23(5)*: 819–23].

Ultraviolet Spectrum. Methanol—215, 264, 297 nm.

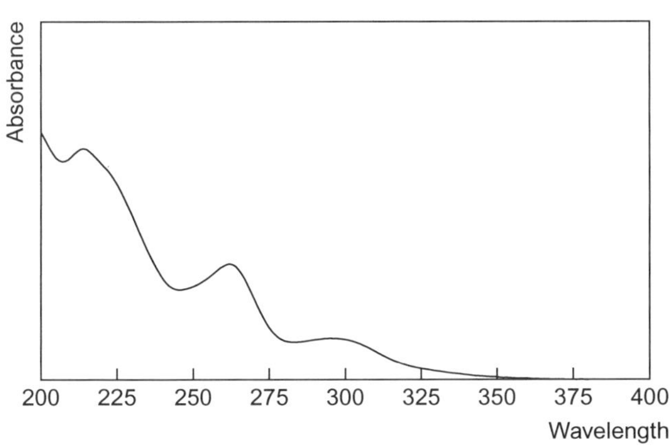

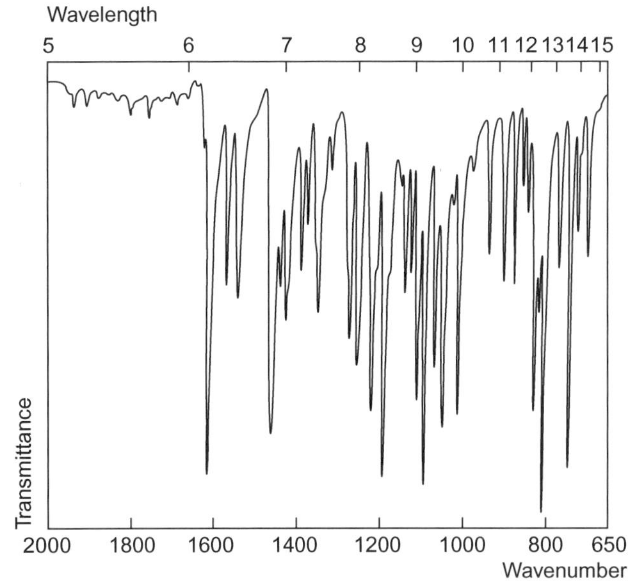

Mass Spectrum. Principal ions at *m/z* 208, 199, 221, 163, 231, 147, 207, 195.

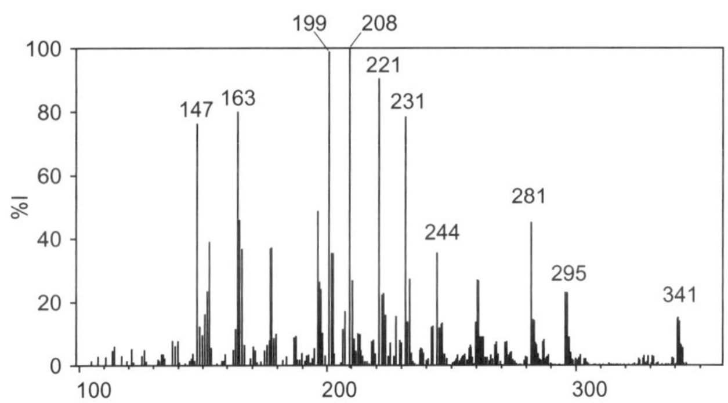

Quantification

Gas chromatography–mass spectrometry. In urine: limit of detection < 100 µg/L—J. Bickeboeller-Friedrich and H. H. Maurer, *Ther. Drug Monit.*, 2001, *23*, 61–70. In plasma: limit of detection 1 µg/L—O. Tanaka *et al.*, *Ther. Drug Monit.*, 1996, *18*, 294–296.

Disposition in the Body. Absorbed after oral administration. Peak plasma concentrations are attained within 2 to 3 h. The drug undergoes extensive first-pass metabolism to the equipotent metabolite norzotepine, and inactive metabolites (hydroxylated, demethylated and *S*-oxide derivatives). CYP1A2 and CYP3A4 are the major cytochrome P450 isozymes involved. It is excreted mainly in urine and faeces as metabolites (ratio 4:6), and is distributed into breast milk.

Therapeutic concentration

2 healthy individuals were administered a single oral dose of 50 mg zotepine. The maximum plasma concentrations observed at 6 and 3 h were 31.7 and 31.0 µg/L, respectively. A second peak was also observed 10 to 12 h after administration [O. Tanaka *et al.*, *Ther. Drug Monit.*, 1996, *18*, 294–296].

Half-life. Plasma half-life, about 15 to 16 h.

Volume of distribution. 1851 to 2856 L.

Clearance. Oral clearance, 81 to 1323 L/h.

Protein binding. In plasma, about 97%.

Dose. Up to 300 mg daily.

Zuclopenthixol

Neuroleptic/Antipsychotic

Synonyms. *Z*-Clopenthixol; *cis*-Clopenthixol; α-Clopenthixol; Lu 0-108.
Proprietary names. Ciatyl; Cisordinol; Clopixol.
(*Z*)-4[3-(2-Chloro-9*H*-thioxan-9-ylidene)propyl]-1-piperazine ethanol
$C_{22}H_{25}ClN_2OS$=401.0
CAS—53772-83-1

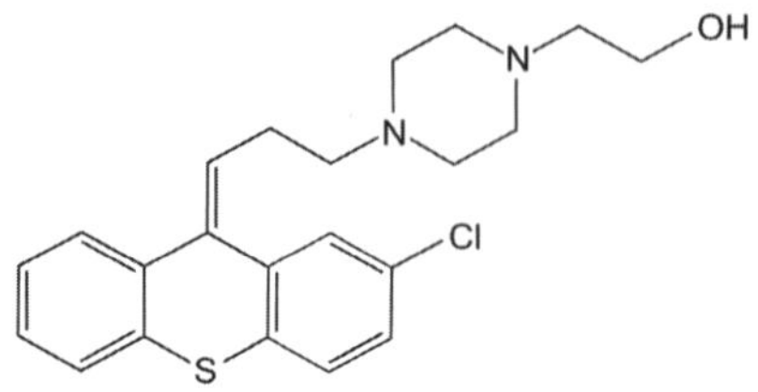

An off-white, granular powder (base). It is very slightly soluble in water; sparingly soluble in diethyl ether; soluble in chloroform; readily soluble in methanol and ethanol (96%).

Zuclopenthixol Acetate

Proprietary name. Viscoleo
$C_{22}H_{25}ClN_2OS,C_2H_2O$=443.0
CAS—85721-05-7
A yellowish, viscous oil. It is very slightly soluble in water; very soluble in alcohol, dichloromethane and ether.

Zuclopenthixol Decanoate

$C_{32}H_{43}ClN_2O_2S$=555.2
CAS—64053-00-5
A yellowish, viscous oil. It is very slightly soluble in water; very soluble in alcohol, dichloromethane and ether.

Zuclopenthixol Hydrochloride

Synonym. Zuclopenthixol Dihydrochloride
Proprietary name. Clopixol
$C_{22}H_{25}ClN_2OS$, 2HCl=473.9
CAS—633-59-0
An off-white granular powder. It is very soluble in water; sparingly soluble in alcohol; slightly soluble in chloroform; very slightly soluble in ether. 1% solution has a pH of 2.0 to 3.0.

Dissociation Constant. pK_a 7.6, 3.3.

Partition Coefficient. Log *P* (octanol/buffer pH 7.4), 3.9; Log *P* (octanol, water (pH 5.0)), 2.22.

Thin-layer Chromatography. System TA—Rf 56; system TB—Rf 7; system TC—Rf 32; system TE—Rf 44; system TL—Rf 11; system TAE—Rf 45.

High Performance Liquid Chromatography. System HZ—retention time 8.0 min; system HAA—retention time 16.3 min.

Column: RP C_{18} (Novapak, 150 × 2 mm i.d., 4 μm). Mobile phase: methanol:ammonium acetate (2 mM, pH 3) (90:10), flow rate 0.2 mL/min. MS detection (ESI, FS (electrospray ionisation, full scan) mode). Retention time: 15 min [A. Tracqui *et al.*, *J. Anal. Toxicol.*, 1997, *21*, 314–318].

Column: C_{18} (Novapak, 300 × 3.9 mm i.d., 4 μm). Mobile phase: methanol:tetrahydrofuran (THF):potassium dihydrogen phosphate (10 mM, pH 2.6) (65:5:30), flow rate 0.8 mL/min. UV detection (λ=228 nm). Retention time: 9 min [A. Tracqui *et al.*, *J. Anal. Toxicol.*, 1997, *21*, 314–318].

Column: S5 CN (Spherisorb, 120 × 4.6 mm i.d.). Mobile phase: acetonitrile:potassium phosphate (200 mM, pH 6.5): water (36:5:59), containing dodecyl-*N*,*N*,*N*-trimethylammonium bromide (6 mM), flow rate 1 mL/min. Fluorescence detection (λ_{ex}=260 nm; λ_{em}=435 nm). Retention time: 9 min [B. Hansen *et al.*, *J. Chromatogr.*, 1994, *658*, *Biomed. Appl.*, 319–325].

Ultraviolet Spectrum. Water—dihydrochloride: 208, 230, 268, 325 nm; Ethanol—acetate: 208, 231, 268, 326 nm; decanoate: 208, 230, 272, 325 nm.

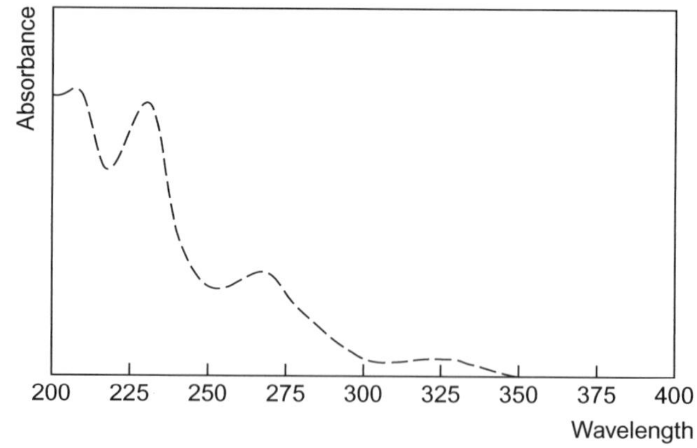

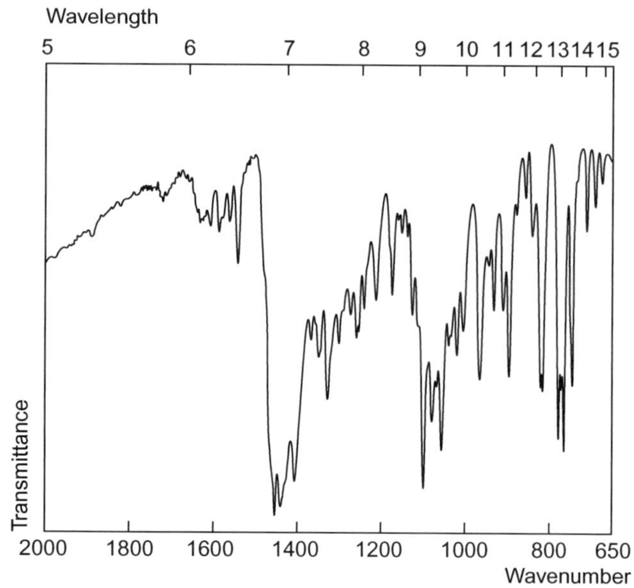

Mass Spectrum. Principal ions at *m/z* 143, 36, 70, 144, 38, 100, 42, 56 (dihydrochloride); 185, 36, 186, 98, 87, 43, 70, 221 (acetate); 297, 298, 36, 98, 125, 143, 70, 43 (decanoate).

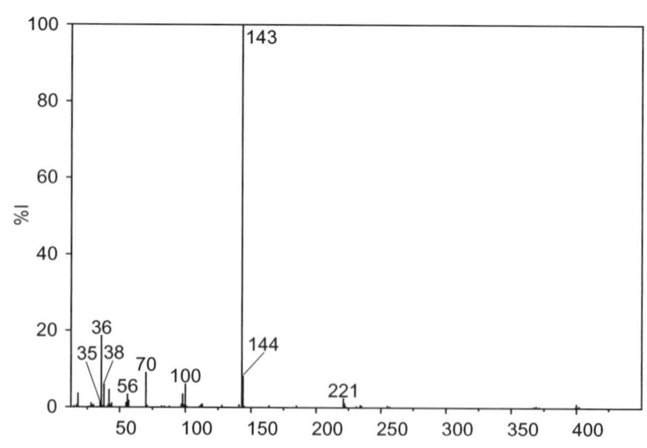

Quantification

High performance liquid chromatography. In blood and urine: limit of detection 0.05 μg/L—B. Hansen *et al.*, *J. Chromatogr.*, 1994, *658*, *Biomed. Appl.*, 319–325. In blood, gastric contents, tissue, urine and vitreous humour: limit of detection 7 μg/L, UV detection (λ=228 nm)—A. Tracqui *et al.*, *J. Anal. Toxicol.*, 1997, *21*, 314–318. In blood: limit of detection 0.5 μg/L—T. Aaes-Jorgensen, *J. Chromatogr.*, 1980, *183*, 239–245.

Disposition in the Body. Following intramuscular injections, the acetate and decanoate esters of zuclopenthixol are hydrolysed to release zuclopenthixol. The acetate has a quick onset after injection, with a duration of action of 2 to 3 h, which is shorter than for the decanoate. The drug is rapidly absorbed from the gastro-intestinal tract. First-pass metabolism occurs in the gut wall, and the drug is also extensively metabolised in the liver. Metabolism occurs by sulfoxidation, side chain N-dealkylation and glucuronic acid conjugation. One known metabolite of zuclopenthixol is *trans*-(*E*)-clopenthixol. The drug is widely distributed in the body with higher concentrations in the liver, lung, intestine and kidney. It is excreted mainly in faeces, but also in urine, in the form of numerous metabolites. There is evidence of enterohepatic recycling and wide inter-subject variation in plasma concentration. The drug also displays linear kinetics.

Therapeutic concentration

19 acutely disturbed Asian patients aged between 18 and 67 years, the majority of whom were suffering from schizophrenia, acute psychosis or mania, were administered 50 mg zuclopenthixol acetate (Viscoleo) by intramuscular injection. The mean serum drug concentrations were taken at 24, 48 and 72 h after administration, and were 19.9 (range 8 to 41.5), 31.5 (12.8 to 52) and 17.8 (8 to 28.8) μg/L, respectively. *trans*-(*E*)-Clopenthixol concentrations ranged between negligible and 39.5 μg/L [C. H. Tan *et al.*, *Ther. Drug Monit.*, 1993, *15(2)*, 108–112].

Toxicity

Postmortem samples were obtained from a 16-year-old Caucasian female who died 40 h after ingesting an undetermined number of clopixol 10 tablets (10 mg each). The following postmortem tissue concentrations were reported: blood 391 μg/L, urine 957 μg/L, gastric contents 105.4 μg/g, liver 0.75 μg/g, kidney 1.413 μg/g, lung 5.21 μg/g, brain 0.12 μg/g [A. Tracqui *et al.*, *J. Anal. Toxicol.* 1997, *21*, 314–318].

Half-life. Zuclopenthixol: mean 20 h (range 12 to 29 h). Zuclopenthixol hydrochloride: 1 day.

Volume of distribution. 15 to 20 L/kg.

Clearance. Systemic clearance, 0.9 L/min.

Protein binding. 98%.

Dose. Zuclopenthixol acetate: 50 to 150 mg (1 to 3 mL). Zuclopenthixol decanoate: 200 to 500 mg every 1 to 4 weeks, with a maximum of 600 mg weekly. Zuclopenthixol hydrochloride: doses between 4 and 150 mg daily have been administered but the usual dose is 20 to 50 mg.

Part Three

Indexes of Analytical Data

CAS Numbers

CAS no.	Compound
50-00-0	Formaldehyde Solution
50-02-2	Dexamethasone
50-03-3	Hydrocortisone Acetate
50-04-4	Cortisone Acetate
50-06-6	Phenobarbital
50-09-9	Hexobarbital Sodium
50-10-2	Oxyphenonium Bromide
50-11-3	Metharbital
50-12-4	Mephenytoin
50-13-5	Pethidine
50-14-6	Ergocalciferol
50-18-0	Cyclophosphamide
50-19-1	Hydroxyphenamate
50-24-8	Prednisolone
50-27-1	Estriol
50-28-2	Estradiol
50-29-3	Clofenotane
50-33-9	Phenylbutazone
50-34-0	Propantheline Bromide
50-35-1	Thalidomide
50-36-2	Cocaine
50-37-3	Lysergide
50-41-9	Clomifene Citrate
50-42-0	Adiphenine Hydrochloride
50-44-2	Mercaptopurine (anhydrous)
50-47-5	Desipramine
50-48-6	Amitriptyline
50-49-7	Imipramine
50-50-0	Estradiol Benzoate
50-52-2	Thioridazine
50-53-3	Chlorpromazine
50-54-4	Quinidine Sulfate (anhydrous)
50-55-5	Reserpine
50-58-8	Phendimetrazine Tartrate
50-59-9	Cefaloridine
50-60-2	Phentolamine
50-62-4	Hexobendine Hydrochloride
50-63-5	Chloroquine Phosphate
50-65-7	Niclosamide
50-67-9	Serotonin
50-76-0	Dactinomycin
50-78-2	Aspirin
50-81-7	Ascorbic Acid
50-98-6	Ephedrine Hydrochloride
51-03-6	Piperonyl Butoxide
51-05-8	Procaine Hydrochloride
51-06-9	Procainamide
51-12-7	Nialamide
51-15-0	Pralidoxime Chloride
51-21-8	Fluorouracil
51-30-9	Isoprenaline Hydrochloride
51-34-3	Hyoscine
51-40-1	Noradrenaline Acid Tartrate (anhydrous)
51-41-2	Noradrenaline
51-42-3	Adrenaline Acid Tartrate
51-43-4	Adrenaline
51-45-6	Histamine
51-48-9	Levothyroxine
51-52-5	Propylthiouracil
51-55-8	Atropine
51-56-9	Homatropine Hydrobromide
51-57-0	Metamfetamine Hydrochloride
51-60-5	Neostigmine Methylsulfate
51-61-6	Dopamine
51-63-8	Dexamfetamine Sulfate
51-64-9	Dexamfetamine
51-67-2	Tyramine
51-68-3	Meclofenoxate
51-71-8	Phenelzine
51-74-1	Histamine Acid Phosphate
51-79-6	Urethane
51-83-2	Carbachol
51-98-9	Norethisterone Acetate
52-01-7	Spironolactone
52-21-1	Prednisolone Acetate
52-24-4	Thiotepa
52-26-6	Morphine Hydrochloride
52-28-8	Codeine Phosphate (anhydrous)
52-31-3	Cyclobarbital
52-39-1	Aldosterone
52-43-7	Allobarbital
52-49-3	Trihexyphenidyl Hydrochloride
52-53-9	Verapamil
52-62-0	Pentolonium Tartrate
52-67-5	Penicillamine
52-68-6	Trichlorfon
52-76-6	Lynestrenol
52-78-8	Norethandrolone
52-86-8	Haloperidol
52-88-0	Atropine Methonitrate
53-03-2	Prednisone
53-06-5	Cortisone
53-16-7	Estrone
53-21-4	Cocaine Hydrochloride
53-33-8	Paramethasone
53-36-1	Methylprednisolone Acetate
53-39-4	Oxandrolone
53-41-8	Androsterone
53-43-0	Dehydroepiandrosterone
53-46-3	Methanthelinium Bromide
53-60-1	Promazine Hydrochloride
53-86-1	Indometacin
54-03-5	Hexobendine
54-04-6	Mescaline
54-05-7	Chloroquine
54-11-5	Nicotine
54-21-7	Sodium Salicylate
54-31-9	Furosemide
54-32-0	Moxisylyte
54-35-3	Procaine Benzylpenicillin
54-36-4	Metyrapone
54-42-2	Idoxuridine
54-49-9	Metaraminol
54-71-7	Pilocarpine Hydrochloride
54-85-3	Isoniazid
54-87-5	Nitrofurantoin Sodium
54-91-1	Pipobroman
54-92-2	Iproniazid
54-95-5	Pentetrazol
55-03-8	Levothyroxine Sodium
55-06-1	Liothyronine Sodium
55-31-2	Adrenaline Hydrochloride
55-38-9	Fenthion
55-48-1	Atropine Sulfate (anhydrous)
55-56-1	Chlorhexidine
55-63-0	Glyceryl Trinitrate
55-65-2	Guanethidine
55-73-2	Bethanidine
55-92-5	Methacholine
55-94-7	Suxamethonium Bromide
55-97-0	Hexamethonium Bromide
55-98-1	Busulfan
56-04-2	Methylthiouracil
56-23-5	Carbon Tetrachloride
56-25-7	Cantharidin
56-29-1	Hexobarbital
56-38-2	Parathion
56-47-3	Desoxycortone Acetate
56-53-1	Diethylstilbestrol
56-54-2	Quinidine
56-65-5	Adenosine Triphosphate
56-72-4	Coumaphos
56-75-7	Chloramphenicol
56-92-8	Histamine Hydrochloride
56-94-0	Demecarium Bromide
56-95-1	Chlorhexidine Acetate
57-12-5	Cyanide
57-13-6	Urea
57-15-8	Chlorobutanol (anhydrous)
57-22-7	Vincristine
57-24-9	Strychnine
57-27-2	Morphine
57-29-4	Nalorphine Hydrochloride
57-30-7	Phenobarbital Sodium
57-33-0	Pentobarbital Sodium
57-37-4	Benactyzine Hydrochloride
57-41-0	Phenytoin
57-42-1	Pethidine
57-43-2	Amobarbital
57-44-3	Barbital
57-47-6	Physostigmine
57-53-4	Meprobamate
57-62-5	Chlortetracycline
57-63-6	Ethinylestradiol
57-64-7	Physostigmine Salicylate
57-66-9	Probenecid
57-67-0	Sulfaguanidine
57-68-1	Sulfadimidine
57-74-9	Chlordane
57-83-0	Progesterone
57-85-2	Testosterone Propionate
57-88-5	Cholesterol
57-92-1	Streptomycin
57-94-3	Tubocurarine Chloride (anhydrous)
57-95-4	Tubocurarine
57-96-5	Sulfinpyrazone
58-00-4	Apomorphine
58-08-2	Caffeine
58-14-0	Pyrimethamine
58-15-1	Aminophenazone
58-18-4	Methyltestosterone
58-19-5	Drostanolone
58-20-8	Testosterone Cipionate
58-22-0	Testosterone
58-25-3	Chlordiazepoxide
58-27-5	Menadione
58-28-6	Desipramine Hydrochloride

CAS no.	*Compound*
58-32-2	Dipyridamole
58-33-3	Promethazine Hydrochloride
58-34-4	Thiazinamium Metilsulfate
58-37-7	Aminopromazine
58-38-8	Prochlorperazine
58-39-9	Perphenazine
58-40-2	Promazine
58-46-8	Tetrabenazine
58-54-8	Etacrynic Acid
58-55-9	Theophylline
58-56-0	Pyridoxine Hydrochloride
58-61-7	Adenosine
58-71-9	Cefalothin Sodium
58-73-1	Diphenhydramine
58-74-2	Papaverine
58-89-9	Lindane
58-93-5	Hydrochlorothiazide
58-94-6	Chlorothiazide
59-01-8	Kanamycin
59-05-2	Methotrexate
59-26-7	Nikethamide
59-30-3	Folic Acid
59-32-5	Chloropyramine
59-33-6	Mepyramine Maleate
59-40-5	Sulfaquinoxaline
59-41-6	Bretylium
59-42-7	Phenylephrine
59-43-8	Thiamine
59-46-1	Procaine
59-47-2	Mephenesin
59-50-7	Chlorocresol
59-52-9	Dimercaprol
59-63-2	Isocarboxazid
59-66-5	Acetazolamide
59-67-6	Nicotinic Acid
59-87-0	Nitrofurazone
59-92-7	Levodopa
59-96-1	Phenoxybenzamine
59-97-2	Tolazoline Hydrochloride
59-98-3	Tolazoline
59-99-4	Neostigmine
60-13-9	Amfetamine Sulfate
60-19-5	Tyramine Hydrochloride
60-26-4	Hexamethonium Bromide
60-29-7	Ether
60-31-1	Acetylcholine Chloride
60-32-2	Aminocaproic Acid
60-40-2	Mecamylamine
60-41-3	Strychnine Sulfate (anhydrous)
60-44-6	Penthienate Methobromide
60-49-1	Tridihexethyl Chloride
60-51-5	Dimethoate
60-54-8	Tetracycline (anhydrous)
60-56-0	Thiamazole
60-57-1	Dieldrin
60-79-7	Ergometrine
60-80-0	Phenazone
60-87-7	Promethazine
60-89-9	Pecazine
60-91-3	Diethazine
60-93-5	Quinine Dihydrochloride
60-99-1	Levomepromazine
61-00-7	Acepromazine
61-12-1	Cinchocaine Hydrochloride
61-16-5	Methoxamine Hydrochloride
61-25-6	Papaverine
61-32-5	Meticillin
61-33-6	Benzylpenicillin
61-49-4	*N*-Methyltryptamine
61-50-7	Dimethyltryptamine
61-51-8	Diethyltryptamine
61-54-1	Tryptamine
61-56-3	Sultiame
61-57-4	Niridazole
61-68-7	Mefenamic Acid
61-72-3	Cloxacillin
61-75-6	Bretylium Tosilate
61-76-7	Phenylephrine Hydrochloride
61-78-9	Aminohippuric Acid
61-82-5	Aminotriazole
62-31-7	Dopamine Hydrochloride
62-44-2	Phenacetin
62-49-7	Choline
62-51-1	Methacholine Chloride
62-53-3	Aniline
62-67-9	Nalorphine
62-73-7	Dichlorvos
62-74-8	Sodium Fluoroacetate
62-90-8	Nandrolone Phenylpropionate
62-97-5	Diphemanil Metilsulfate
63-05-8	Androstenedione
63-12-7	Benzquinamide
63-25-2	Carbaryl
63-45-6	Primaquine Phosphate
63-56-9	Thonzylamine Hydrochloride
63-74-1	Sulfanilamide
63-75-2	Arecoline
63-89-8	Colfosceril Palmitate
63-92-3	Phenoxybenzamine Hydrochloride
63-98-9	Phenacemide
64-04-0	Phenethylamine
64-17-5	Ethanol
64-18-6	Formic Acid
64-19-7	Acetic Acid Glacial
64-31-3	Morphine Sulfate
64-39-1	Trimeperidine
64-43-7	Amobarbital Sodium
64-47-1	Physostigmine Sulfate
64-55-1	Mebutamate
64-65-3	Bemegride
64-72-2	Chlortetracycline Hydrochloride
64-73-3	Demeclocycline Hydrochloride
64-75-5	Tetracycline
64-77-7	Tolbutamide
64-85-7	Desoxycortone
64-86-8	Colchicine
64-95-9	Adiphenine
65-19-0	Yohimbine Hydrochloride
65-23-6	Pyridoxine
65-28-1	Phentolamine Mesilate
65-29-2	Gallamine Triethiodide
65-45-2	Salicylamide
65-49-6	Aminosalicylic Acid
65-64-5	Mebanazine
65-85-0	Benzoic Acid
66-23-9	Acetylcholine Bromide
66-32-0	Strychnine Nitrate
66-76-2	Dicoumarol
66-86-4	Neomycin (neomycin C)
67-03-8	Thiamine Hydrochloride
67-04-9	Oxedrine Tartrate (±)
67-20-9	Nitrofurantoin (anhydrous)
67-45-8	Furazolidone
67-48-1	Choline Chloride
67-52-7	Barbituric Acid
67-56-1	Methanol
67-63-0	Isopropyl Alcohol
67-64-1	Acetone
67-66-3	Chloroform
67-68-5	Dimethyl Sulfoxide
67-73-2	Fluocinolone Acetonide
67-78-7	Triamcinolone Diacetate
67-92-5	Dicycloverine Hydrochloride
67-96-9	Dihydrotachysterol
67-97-0	Colecalciferol
68-19-9	Cyanocobalamin
68-22-4	Norethisterone
68-23-5	Noretynodrel
68-35-9	Sulfadiazine
68-41-7	Cycloserine
68-88-2	Hydroxyzine
68-89-3	Dipyrone
68-90-6	Benziodarone
68-91-7	Trimetaphan Camsilate
68-96-2	Hydroxyprogesterone
69-05-6	Mepacrine Hydrochloride (anhydrous)
69-09-0	Chlorpromazine Hydrochloride
69-22-7	Caffeine Citrate
69-23-8	Fluphenazine
69-43-2	Prenylamine Lactate
69-44-3	Amodiaquine Hydrochloride
69-52-3	Ampicillin Sodium
69-53-4	Ampicillin
69-57-8	Benzylpenicillin Sodium
69-65-8	Mannitol
69-72-7	Salicylic Acid
69-74-9	Cytarabine Hydrochloride
69-81-8	Carbazochrome
70-30-4	Hexachlorophene
70-51-9	Desferrioxamine
71-23-8	Propanol
71-27-2	Suxamethonium Chloride
71-43-2	Benzene
71-55-6	Trichloroethane
71-58-9	Medroxyprogesterone Acetate
71-63-6	Digitoxin
71-68-1	Hydromorphone Hydrochloride
71-73-8	Thiopental Sodium
71-78-3	Pipradrol Hydrochloride
71-81-8	Isopropamide Iodide (iodide)
71-82-9	Levallorphan Tartrate
72-14-0	Sulfathiazole
72-20-8	Endrin
72-33-3	Mestranol
72-43-5	Methoxychlor
72-44-6	Methaqualone
72-63-9	Methandienone
72-69-5	Nortriptyline
72-80-0	Chlorquinaldol
73-05-2	Phentolamine Hydrochloride
73-22-3	Tryptophan
73-48-3	Bendroflumethiazide
73-49-4	Quinethazone
73-78-9	Lidocaine Hydrochloride
74-55-5	Ethambutol
74-83-9	Methyl Bromide
75-07-0	Acetaldehyde
75-09-2	Methylene Chloride
75-69-4	Trichlorofluoromethane
75-71-8	Dichlorodifluoromethane
76-14-2	Cryofluorane
76-22-2	Camphor
76-25-5	Triamcinolone Acetonide
76-38-0	Methoxyflurane
76-40-4	Butylchloral Hydrate
76-41-5	Oxymorphone
76-42-6	Oxycodone
76-43-7	Fluoxymesterone
76-44-8	Heptachlor
76-57-3	Codeine (anhydrous)
76-58-4	Ethylmorphine
76-68-6	Cyclopentobarbital
76-73-3	Secobarbital
76-74-4	Pentobarbital
76-75-5	Thiopental
76-90-4	Mepenzolate Bromide
76-94-8	Phenylmethylbarbituric Acid
76-99-3	Methadone
77-02-1	Aprobarbital
77-07-6	Levorphanol

CAS no.	Compound
77-09-8	Phenolphthalein
77-10-1	Phencyclidine
77-15-6	Ethoheptazine
77-19-0	Dicycloverine
77-20-3	Alphaprodine
77-21-4	Glutethimide
77-22-5	Caramiphen
77-23-6	Carbetapentane
77-26-9	Butalbital
77-27-0	Thiamylal
77-28-1	Butobarbital
77-30-5	Hexethal
77-36-1	Chlortalidone
77-37-2	Procyclidine
77-38-3	Chlorphenoxamine
77-39-4	Cycrimine
77-41-8	Mesuximide
77-51-0	Isoaminile
77-65-6	Carbromal
77-66-7	Acecarbromal
77-67-8	Ethosuximide
77-75-8	Methylpentynol
77-86-1	Trometamol
77-91-8	Choline Dihydrogen Citrate
78-11-5	Pentaerithrityl Tetranitrate
78-28-4	Emylcamate
78-44-4	Carisoprodol
78-93-3	Methyl Ethyl Ketone
79-01-6	Trichloroethylene
79-34-5	Tetrachloroethane
79-55-0	Pempidine
79-57-2	Oxytetracycline Dihydrate (anhydrous)
79-64-1	Dimethisterone (anhydrous)
79-93-6	Phenaglycodol
80-08-0	Dapsone
80-13-7	Halazone
80-32-0	Sulfachlorpyridazine
80-35-3	Sulfamethoxypyridazine
80-49-9	Homatropine Methylbromide
80-50-2	Octatropine Methylbromide
80-74-0	Acetyl Sulfafurazole
80-77-3	Chlormezanone
80-78-4	Solanidine
81-07-2	Saccharin
81-13-0	Dexpanthenol
81-81-2	Warfarin
82-54-2	Cotarnine
82-58-6	Lysergic Acid
82-66-6	Diphenadione
82-88-2	Phenindamine
82-92-8	Cyclizine
82-93-9	Chlorcyclizine
82-95-1	Buclizine
82-98-4	Piperidolate
83-12-5	Phenindione
83-43-2	Methylprednisolone
83-67-0	Theobromine
83-73-8	Diiodohydroxyquinoline
83-74-9	Ibogaine
83-75-0	Quinine Ethyl Carbonate
83-79-4	Rotenone
83-88-5	Riboflavin
83-89-6	Mepacrine
83-98-7	Orphenadrine
84-02-6	Prochlorperazine Maleate
84-06-0	Thiopropazate
84-12-8	Phanquinone
84-16-2	Hexestrol
84-17-3	Dienestrol
84-22-0	Tetryzoline
84-36-6	Syrosingopine
84-66-2	Diethyl Phthalate
84-74-2	Dibutyl Phthalate
84-80-0	Phytomenadione
84-96-8	Alimemazine
84-97-9	Perazine
85-00-7	Diquat Dibromide
85-73-4	Phthalylsulfathiazole
85-79-0	Cinchocaine
86-12-4	Thenalidine
86-13-5	Benzatropine
86-14-6	Diethylthiambutene
86-21-5	Pheniramine
86-22-6	Brompheniramine
86-34-0	Phensuximide
86-35-1	Ethotoin
86-42-0	Amodiaquine
86-43-1	Propoxycaine
86-50-0	Azinphos-methyl
86-54-4	Hydralazine
86-80-6	Quinisocaine
87-00-3	Homatropine
87-08-1	Phenoxymethylpenicillin
87-33-2	Isosorbide Dinitrate
87-67-2	Choline Bitartrate
87-86-5	Pentachlorophenol
88-04-0	Chloroxylenol
89-78-1	Menthol
89-83-8	Thymol
90-22-2	Valethamate Bromide
90-34-6	Primaquine
90-39-1	Sparteine
90-45-9	Aminoacridine
90-49-3	Pheneturide
90-64-2	Mandelic Acid
90-69-7	Lobeline
90-81-3	Racephedrine
90-82-4	Pseudoephedrine
90-84-6	Diethylpropion
90-89-1	Diethylcarbamazine
91-20-3	Naphthalene
91-33-8	Benzthiazide
91-75-8	Antazoline
91-79-2	Thenyldiamine
91-80-5	Methapyrilene
91-81-6	Tripelennamine
91-82-7	Pyrrobutamine
91-84-9	Mepyramine
91-85-0	Thonzylamine
92-12-6	Phenyltoloxamine
92-13-7	Pilocarpine
92-52-4	Diphenyl
92-62-6	Proflavine Hemisulfate
92-84-2	Phenothiazine
93-14-1	Guaifenesin
93-30-1	Methoxyphenamine
93-60-7	Methyl Nicotinate
93-76-5	Trichlorophenoxyacetic Acid
94-07-5	Oxedrine
94-09-7	Benzocaine
94-10-0	Etoxazene
94-13-3	Propyl Hydroxybenzoate
94-16-6	Sodium Aminohippurate
94-19-9	Sulfaethidole
94-20-2	Chlorpropamide
94-24-6	Tetracaine
94-25-7	Butyl Aminobenzoate
94-35-9	Styramate
94-44-0	Benzyl Nicotinate
94-63-3	Pralidoxime Iodide
94-74-6	Methylchlorophenoxyacetic Acid
94-75-7	Dichlorophenoxyacetic Acid
94-78-0	Phenazopyridine
95-05-6	Sulfiram
95-25-0	Chlorzoxazone
95-27-2	Diamthazole
95-47-6	*o*-Xylene
95-48-7	Cresol
95-51-2	2-Chloroaniline
95-81-8	Chloromethylaniline
96-48-0	Gamma-butyrolactone
96-88-8	Mepivacaine
97-23-4	Dichlorophen
97-24-5	Fenticlor
97-31-4	Normetadrenaline
97-44-9	Acetarsone
97-53-0	Eugenol
97-77-8	Disulfiram
98-92-0	Nicotinamide
98-95-3	Nitrobenzene
98-96-4	Pyrazinamide
99-43-4	Oxybuprocaine
99-66-1	Valproic Acid
99-76-3	Methyl Hydroxybenzoate
100-33-4	Pentamidine
100-51-6	Benzyl Alcohol
100-52-7	Benzaldehyde
100-55-0	Nicotinyl Alcohol
100-91-4	Eucatropine
100-92-5	Mephentermine
100-97-0	Methenamine
101-08-6	Diperodon
101-20-2	Triclocarban
101-26-8	Pyridostigmine Bromide
101-31-5	Hyoscyamine
101-40-6	Propylhexedrine
101-93-9	Phenacaine
102-29-4	Resorcinol Monoacetate
102-45-4	Cyclopentamine
103-84-4	Acetanilide
103-86-6	Hydroxyamfetamine
103-90-2	Paracetamol
104-06-3	Thioacetazone
104-29-0	Chlorphenesin
104-31-4	Benzonatate
104-32-5	Propamidine
105-20-4	Ametazole
106-42-3	*p*-Xylene
106-44-5	Cresol
106-46-7	Paradichlorobenzene
106-47-8	4-Chloroaniline
106-48-9	Parachlorophenol
106-50-3	Paraphenylenediamine
107-15-3	Ethylenediamine Hydrate (anhydrous)
107-21-1	Ethylene Glycol
107-43-7	Betaine
108-38-3	*m*-Xylene
108-39-4	Cresol
108-42-9	3-Chloroaniline
108-46-3	Resorcinol
108-88-3	Toluene
108-95-2	Phenol
110-44-1	Sorbic Acid
110-46-3	Amyl Nitrite
110-60-1	Putrescine
110-85-0	Piperazine
111-00-2	Suxethonium Bromide
112-24-3	Trientine
113-07-5	Doxapram Hydrochloride
113-15-5	Ergotamine
113-18-8	Ethchlorvynol
113-42-8	Methylergometrine
113-45-1	Methylphenidate
113-52-0	Imipramine Hydrochloride
113-53-1	Dosulepin
113-59-7	Chlorprothixene
113-69-9	Benzquinamide Hydrochloride
113-92-8	Chlorphenamine maleate
113-98-4	Benzylpenicillin Potassium
114-07-8	Erythromycin A

CAS no.	*Compound*
114-49-8	Hyoscine Hydrobromide (anhydrous)
114-80-7	Neostigmine Bromide
114-85-2	Bethanidine Sulfate
114-86-3	Phenformin
114-90-9	Obidoxime Chloride
115-20-8	Trichloroethanol
115-29-7	Endosulfan
115-33-3	Oxyphenisatine Acetate
115-37-7	Thebaine
115-38-8	Methylphenobarbital
115-44-6	Talbutal
115-46-8	Azacyclonol
115-51-5	Ambutonium Bromide
115-63-9	Hexocyclium Metilsulfate
115-67-3	Paramethadione
115-77-5	Pentaerithrityl
115-79-7	Ambenonium Chloride
116-06-3	Aldicarb
116-38-1	Edrophonium Chloride
116-43-8	Succinylsulfathiazole
117-10-2	Dantron
117-37-3	Anisindione
117-74-8	Berberine
117-89-5	Trifluoperazine
118-08-1	Hydrastine
118-10-5	Cinchonine
118-23-0	Bromazine
118-42-3	Hydroxychloroquine
118-55-8	Salol
119-04-0	Neomycin B
119-36-8	Methyl Salicylate
120-47-8	Ethyl Hydroxybenzoate
120-51-4	Benzyl Benzoate
120-97-8	Diclofenamide
121-21-1	Pyrethrin I
121-25-5	Amprolium Hydrochloride
121-29-9	Pyrethrin II
121-33-5	Vanillin
121-54-0	Benzethonium Chloride
121-59-5	Carbarsone
121-75-5	Malathion
122-09-8	Phentermine
122-11-2	Sulfadimethoxine
122-14-5	Fenitrothion
122-18-9	Cetalkonium Chloride
122-34-9	Simazine
123-03-5	Cetylpyridinium Chloride
123-30-8	4-Aminophenol
123-31-9	Hydroquinone
123-51-3	Amyl Alcohol (3-methyl-1-butanol)
123-56-8	Succinimide
123-63-7	Paraldehyde
123-82-0	Tuaminoheptane
123-92-2	Amyl Acetate (iso)
124-87-8	Picrotoxin
124-90-3	Oxycodone Hydrochloride
124-94-7	Triamcinolone
124-97-0	Protoveratrine B
125-02-0	Prednisolone Sodium Phosphate
125-04-2	Hydrocortisone Sodium Succinate
125-10-0	Prednisone Acetate
125-13-3	Oxyphenisatine
125-24-6	Pseudomorphine
125-28-0	Dihydrocodeine
125-29-1	Hydrocodone
125-30-4	Ethylmorphine Hydrochloride (anhydrous)
125-33-7	Primidone
125-40-6	Secbutabarbital
125-42-8	Vinbarbital
125-51-9	Pipenzolate Bromide
125-52-0	Oxyphencyclimine Hydrochloride
125-53-1	Oxyphencyclimine
125-56-4	Methadone Hydrochloride
125-64-4	Methyprylon
125-69-9	Dextromethorphan Hydrobromide
125-71-3	Dextromethorphan
125-72-4	Levorphanol Tartrate
125-73-5	Dextrorphan
125-80-4	Trimeperidine Hydrochloride
125-84-8	Aminoglutethimide
125-85-9	Caramiphen Hydrochloride
125-86-0	Caramiphen Edisilate
125-88-2	Aprobarbital Sodium
126-02-3	Cycrimine Hydrochloride
126-07-8	Griseofulvin
126-12-5	Anileridine Hydrochloride
126-27-2	Oxetacaine
126-52-3	Ethinamate
126-73-8	Tributyl Phosphate
126-75-0	Demeton-*S*
127-07-1	Hydroxycarbamide
127-18-4	Tetrachloroethylene
127-31-1	Fludrocortisone
127-33-3	Demeclocycline
127-35-5	Phenazocine
127-48-0	Trimethadione
127-56-0	Sulfacetamide Sodium
127-57-1	Sulfapyridine Sodium Monohydrate (anhydrous)
127-58-2	Sulfamerazine Sodium
127-65-1	Tosylchloramide Sodium
127-69-5	Sulfafurazole
127-79-7	Sulfamerazine
128-37-0	Butylated Hydroxytoluene
128-44-9	Saccharin Sodium
128-46-1	Dihydrostreptomycin
128-49-4	Docusate Calcium
128-62-1	Noscapine
129-03-3	Cyproheptadine
129-06-6	Warfarin Sodium
129-20-4	Oxyphenbutazone (anhydrous)
129-49-7	Methysergide Maleate
129-50-0	Ergometrine Tartrate
129-51-1	Ergometrine Maleate
129-74-8	Buclizine Hydrochloride
129-77-1	Piperidolate Hydrochloride
130-26-7	Clioquinol
130-37-0	Menadione Sodium Bisulfite (anhydrous)
130-61-0	Thioridazine Hydrochloride
130-80-3	Diethylstilbestrol Dipropionate
130-83-6	Azapetine Phosphate
130-89-2	Quinine Hydrochloride (anhydrous)
130-95-0	Quinine (anhydrous)
131-01-1	Deserpidine
131-11-3	Dimethyl Phthalate
131-28-2	Narceine (anhydrous)
131-69-1	Phthalylsulfacetamide
132-17-2	Benzatropine Mesilate
132-18-3	Diphenylpyraline Hydrochloride
132-19-4	Diethylthiambutene Hydrochloride
132-20-7	Pheniramine Maleate
132-21-8	Dexbrompheniramine
132-22-9	Chlorphenamine
132-60-5	Cinchophen
132-69-4	Benzydamine Hydrochloride
132-73-0	Chloroquine Sulfate
132-92-3	Meticillin Sodium
132-93-4	Pheneticillin Potassium
132-98-9	Phenoxymethylpenicillin Potassium
133-09-5	Potassium Aminosalicylate
133-10-8	Sodium Aminosalicylate (anhydrous)
133-11-9	Phenyl Aminosalicylate
133-15-3	Calcium Aminosalicylate
133-16-4	Chloroprocaine
133-67-5	Trichlormethiazide
134-03-2	Sodium Ascorbate
134-31-6	Hydroxyquinoline Sulfate
134-36-1	Erythromycin Propionate
134-49-6	Phenmetrazine
134-50-9	Aminoacridine Hydrochloride
134-62-3	Diethyltoluamide
134-63-4	Lobeline Hydrochloride
134-64-5	Lobeline Sulfate
134-71-4	Racephedrine Hydrochloride
134-72-5	Ephedrine Sulfate
134-80-5	Diethylpropion Hydrochloride
134-95-2	Calcium Mandelate
135-07-9	Methyclothiazide
135-09-1	Hydroflumethiazide
135-14-8	Quinuronium Sulfate
135-19-3	Betanaphthol
135-23-9	Methapyrilene Hydrochloride
135-31-9	Pyrrobutamine Phosphate
136-40-3	Phenazopyridine Hydrochloride
136-47-0	Tetracaine Hydrochloride
136-69-6	Protokylol Hydrochloride
136-70-9	Protokylol
136-77-6	Hexylresorcinol
136-82-3	Piperocaine
136-96-9	Diamthazole Hydrochloride
137-32-6	Amyl Alcohol (2-methyl-1-butanol)
137-58-6	Lidocaine
137-88-2	Amprolium Hydrochloride
138-14-7	Desferrioxamine Mesilate
138-37-4	Mafenide Hydrochloride
138-39-6	Mafenide
138-56-7	Trimethobenzamide
138-84-1	Potassium Aminobenzoate
138-92-1	Ametazole Hydrochloride
139-10-6	Amfetamine Phosphate
139-40-2	Propazine
139-62-8	Cyclomethycaine
139-91-3	Furaltadone
140-36-3	Hydroxyamfetamine Hydrobromide (±)
140-40-9	Aminitrozole
140-63-6	Propamidine Isetionate
140-64-7	Pentamidine Isetionate
140-65-8	Pramocaine
141-43-5	Monoethanolamine
141-78-6	Ethyl Acetate
141-94-6	Hexetidine
142-63-2	Piperazine Hydrate
142-88-1	Piperazine Adipate
143-57-7	Protoveratrine A
143-67-9	Vinblastine Sulfate
143-71-5	Hydrocodone Tartrate
143-76-0	Cyclobarbital Calcium
143-81-7	Secbutabarbital Sodium
144-00-3	Hexethal Sodium
144-02-5	Barbital Sodium
144-11-6	Trihexyphenidyl
144-14-9	Anileridine
144-29-6	Piperazine Citrate
144-44-5	Pentolonium
144-49-0	Fluoroacetic Acid
144-62-7	Oxalic Acid (anhydrous)
144-74-1	Sulfathiazole Sodium (anhydrous)

CAS no.	*Compound*
144-80-9	Sulfacetamide
144-82-1	Sulfamethizole
144-83-2	Sulfapyridine
146-22-5	Nitrazepam
146-28-1	Thiopropazate Hydrochloride
146-36-1	Azapetine
146-48-5	Yohimbine
146-54-3	Triflupromazine
146-56-5	Fluphenazine Hydrochloride
147-20-6	Diphenylpyraline
147-24-0	Diphenhydramine Hydrochloride
147-27-3	Dimoxyline
147-48-8	Phenoxymethylpenicillin Calcium
147-55-7	Pheneticillin
147-94-4	Cytarabine
148-01-6	Dinitolmide
148-18-5	Ditiocarb Sodium
148-24-3	Hydroxyquinoline
148-64-1	Chloropyrilene Citrate
148-65-2	Chloropyrilene
148-72-1	Pilocarpine Nitrate
148-79-8	Tiabendazole
148-82-3	Melphalan
149-15-5	Butacaine Sulfate
149-16-6	Butacaine
149-64-4	Hyoscine Butylbromide
150-13-0	Aminobenzoic Acid
150-59-4	Alverine
151-06-4	Chlorphentermine Hydrochloride
151-67-7	Halothane
151-73-5	Betamethasone Sodium Phosphate
151-83-7	Methohexital
152-02-3	Levallorphan
152-11-4	Verapamil Hydrochloride
152-47-6	Sulfametopyrazine
152-62-5	Dydrogesterone
152-72-7	Acenocoumarol
152-97-6	Fluocortolone
153-00-4	Metenolone
153-61-7	Cefalothin
153-76-4	Gallamine Triethiodide
153-87-7	Oxypertine
154-21-2	Lincomycin
154-41-6	Phenylpropanolamine Hydrochloride
154-42-7	Tioguanine
154-68-7	Antazoline Phosphate
154-69-8	Tripelennamine Hydrochloride
154-93-8	Carmustine
154-97-2	Pralidoxime Mesilate
155-09-9	Tranylcypromine
155-41-9	Hyoscine Methobromide
155-97-5	Pyridostigmine Bromide
156-08-1	Benzfetamine
156-34-3	Levamfetamine
156-51-4	Phenelzine Sulfate
156-74-1	Decamethonium Bromide
244-63-3	Norharman
297-76-7	Etynodiol Diacetate
297-88-1	Methadone
297-90-5	Racemorphan
298-04-4	Disulfoton
298-46-4	Carbamazepine
298-50-0	Propantheline Bromide
298-57-7	Cinnarizine
298-59-9	Methylphenidate Hydrochloride
298-81-7	Methoxsalen
298-96-4	Triphenyltetrazolium Chloride
299-26-3	α-Methyltryptamine
299-39-8	Sparteine Sulfate
299-42-3	Anhydrous Ephedrine
299-95-6	Isoprenaline Sulfate
300-08-3	Arecoline Hydrobromide
300-62-9	Amfetamine
302-17-0	Cloral Hydrate
302-22-7	Chlormadinone Acetate
302-27-2	Aconitine
302-31-8	Morphine Tartrate
302-40-9	Benactyzine
302-41-0	Piritramide
302-66-9	Methylpentynol Carbamate
303-25-3	Cyclizine Hydrochloride
303-40-2	Fluocortolone Hexanoate
303-42-4	Metenolone Enantate
303-49-1	Clomipramine
303-53-7	Cyclobenzaprine
303-69-5	Prothipendyl
304-20-1	Hydralazine Hydrochloride
304-21-2	Harmaline
304-84-7	Etamivan
305-03-3	Chlorambucil
305-33-9	Iproniazid Phosphate
306-03-6	Hyoscyamine Hydrobromide
306-07-0	Pargyline Hydrochloride
306-21-8	Hydroxyamfetamine Hydrobromide
306-40-1	Suxamethonium Chloride
306-52-5	Triclofos Sodium
309-00-2	Aldrin
309-29-5	Doxapram
309-36-4	Methohexital Sodium
309-43-3	Secobarbital Sodium
312-48-1	Edrophonium
313-06-4	Estradiol Cipionate
314-19-2	Apomorphine Hydrochloride (anhydrous)
314-35-2	Etamiphylline
315-22-0	Monocrotaline
315-30-0	Allopurinol
315-37-7	Testosterone Enantate
315-72-0	Opipramol
315-80-0	Dibenzepin Hydrochloride
316-05-2	Mepacrine Mesilate (anhydrous)
316-42-7	Emetine Hydrochloride (anhydrous)
316-81-4	Thioproperazine
317-34-0	Aminophylline (anhydrous)
318-23-0	Imolamine
318-98-9	Propranolol Hydrochloride
319-84-6	Benzene Hexachloride (α)
319-85-7	Benzene Hexachloride (β)
319-86-8	Benzene Hexachloride (δ)
321-55-1	Haloxon
321-64-2	Tacrine
322-35-0	Benserazide
326-43-2	Fenyramidol Hydrochloride
329-56-6	Noradrenaline Hydrochloride
330-54-1	Diuron
330-55-2	Linuron
333-31-3	Methacholine Bromide
333-41-5	Dimpylate
337-03-1	Flugestone
337-47-3	Sodium Thiamylal
339-43-5	Carbutamide
340-56-7	Methaqualone Hydrochloride
340-57-8	Mecloqualone
341-69-5	Orphenadrine Hydrochloride
341-70-8	Diethazine Hydrochloride
343-94-2	Tryptamine Hydrochloride
345-78-8	Pseudoephedrine Hydrochloride
346-18-9	Polythiazide
356-12-7	Fluocinonide
357-07-3	Oxymorphone Hydrochloride
357-08-4	Naloxone Hydrochloride (anhydrous)
357-56-2	Dextromoramide
357-57-3	Brucine
357-70-0	Galantamine
359-83-1	Pentazocine
360-70-3	Nandrolone Decanoate
361-37-5	Methysergide
362-29-8	Propiomazine
364-62-5	Metoclopramide
364-98-7	Diazoxide
365-26-4	Hydroxyephedrine
366-70-1	Procarbazine Hydrochloride
370-14-9	Pholedrine
372-66-7	Heptaminol
378-44-9	Betamethasone
379-79-3	Ergotamine Tartrate
389-08-2	Nalidixic Acid
390-28-3	Methoxamine
390-64-7	Prenylamine
395-28-8	Isoxsuprine
396-01-0	Triamterene
404-82-0	Fenfluramine Hydrochloride
426-13-1	Fluorometholone
428-37-5	Profadol
432-60-0	Allylestrenol
434-03-7	Ethisterone
434-05-9	Metenolone Acetate
434-07-1	Oxymetholone
434-22-0	Nandrolone
435-97-2	Phenprocoumon
437-38-7	Fentanyl
437-74-1	Xantinol Nicotinate
438-41-5	Chlordiazepoxide Hydrochloride
438-60-8	Protriptyline
439-14-5	Diazepam
440-17-5	Trifluoperazine Hydrochloride
442-16-0	Ethacridine
442-51-3	Harmine
442-52-4	Clemizole
443-48-1	Metronidazole
446-86-6	Azathioprine
447-41-6	Buphenine
452-35-7	Ethoxzolamide
456-59-7	Cyclandelate
458-24-2	Fenfluramine
458-88-8	Coniine
461-78-9	Chlorphentermine
462-94-2	Cadaverine
464-49-3	Camphor (+)
465-65-6	Naloxone
466-90-0	Thebacon
466-97-7	Normorphine
466-99-9	Hydromorphone
467-14-1	Neopine
467-15-2	Norcodeine
467-36-7	Thialbarbital
467-60-7	Pipradrol
467-83-4	Dipipanone
467-85-6	Normethadone
468-61-1	Oxeladin
469-21-6	Doxylamine
469-62-5	Dextropropoxyphene
469-79-4	Ketobemidone
470-82-6	Cineole
471-53-4	Enoxolone
473-41-6	Tolbutamide Sodium
476-32-4	Chelidonine
477-93-0	Dimethoxanate
478-94-4	Lysergamide
479-18-5	Diprophylline
479-92-5	Propyphenazone
480-30-8	Dichloralphenazone
481-06-1	Santonin
481-37-8	Ecgonine
482-15-5	Isothipendyl

CAS no.	*Compound*
483-17-0	Cephaëline
483-18-1	Emetine
483-63-6	Crotamiton
484-23-1	Dihydralazine
485-35-8	Cytisine
485-71-2	Cinchonidine
486-12-4	Triprolidine
486-16-8	Carbinoxamine
486-17-9	Captodiame
486-67-9	Mersalyl Acid
486-84-0	Harman
487-93-4	Bufotenine
490-55-1	Amiphenazole
492-18-2	Mersalyl Sodium
492-39-7	Cathine
493-75-4	Bialamicol
493-80-1	Histapyrrodine
493-92-5	Prolintane
495-70-5	Meprylcaine
495-83-0	Tigloidine
495-84-1	Salinazid
495-99-8	Hydroxystilbamidine
496-00-4	Dibrompropamidine
496-67-3	Bromisoval
499-67-2	Proxymetacaine
500-89-0	Thiambutosine
500-92-5	Proguanil
501-68-8	Beclamide
502-59-0	Octamylamine
502-85-2	Sodium Gamma-hydroxybutyrate
503-01-5	Isometheptene
508-99-6	Hydrocortisone Cipionate
509-15-9	Gelsemine
509-60-4	Dihydromorphine
509-67-1	Pholcodine
509-86-4	Heptabarb
511-13-7	Clofedanol Hydrochloride
512-15-2	Cyclopentolate
513-10-0	Ecothiopate Iodide
514-36-3	Fludrocortisone Acetate
514-65-8	Biperiden
515-64-0	Sulfisomidine
516-21-2	Cycloguanil
517-18-0	Methallenestril
518-63-8	Dimethoxanate Hydrochloride
519-09-5	Benzoylecgonine
519-37-9	Etofylline
519-88-0	Ambucetamide
520-52-5	Psilocybine
520-53-6	Psilocin
520-85-4	Medroxyprogesterone
521-10-8	Methandriol
521-12-0	Drostanolone Propionate
521-17-5	Androstenediol
521-18-6	Androstanolone
521-35-7	Cannabinol
521-74-4	Broxyquinoline
521-78-8	Trimipramine Maleate
522-00-9	Profenamine
522-40-7	Diethylstilbestrol Diphosphate
522-48-5	Tetryzoline Hydrochloride
522-51-0	Dequalinium Chloride
522-66-7	Hydroquinine
523-87-5	Dimenhydrinate
524-61-8	Cinchonidine Sulfate (anhydrous)
524-81-2	Mebhydrolin
525-66-6	Propranolol
526-08-9	Sulfaphenazole
526-36-3	Xylometazoline
528-92-7	Apronal
530-08-5	Isoetarine
530-31-4	Ammonium Mandelate
530-43-8	Chloramphenicol Palmitate
530-78-9	Flufenamic Acid
532-03-6	Methocarbamol
532-32-1	Sodium Benzoate
532-43-4	Thiamine Mononitrate
532-76-3	Hexylcaine Hydrochloride
532-77-4	Hexylcaine
533-06-2	Mephenesin Carbamate
533-22-2	Hydroxystilbamidine Isetionate
533-28-8	Piperocaine Hydrochloride
533-45-9	Clomethiazole
534-52-1	Dinitro-orthocresol
534-87-2	Etilefrine Hydrochloride
536-24-3	Ethylnoradrenaline
536-33-4	Ethionamide
536-43-6	Dyclonine Hydrochloride
536-71-0	Diminazene
536-93-6	Eucatropine Hydrochloride
537-12-2	Diperodon Hydrochloride
537-21-3	Chlorproguanil
537-46-2	Metamfetamine
537-61-1	Cyclomethycaine
538-71-6	Domiphen Bromide
539-15-1	Hordenine
539-21-9	Ambazone
541-19-5	Suxamethonium Iodide
541-22-0	Decamethonium Bromide
543-15-7	Heptaminol Hydrochloride
545-80-2	Poldine Metilsulfate
545-93-7	Ibomal
546-06-5	Conessine
546-48-5	Pempidine Tartrate
547-32-0	Sulfadiazine Sodium
547-44-4	Sulfacarbamide
548-00-5	Ethyl Biscoumacetate
548-73-2	Droperidol
548-84-5	Pyrvinium Chloride
549-18-8	Amitriptyline Hydrochloride
549-49-5	Quinine Hydrobromide (anhydrous)
549-56-4	Quinine Bisulfate (anhydrous)
550-70-9	Triprolidine Hydrochloride (anhydrous)
550-83-4	Propoxycaine Hydrochloride
550-99-2	Naphazoline Hydrochloride
551-27-9	Propicillin
551-48-4	Guanoclor Sulfate
551-74-6	Mannomustine
551-92-8	Dimetridazole
552-79-4	Methylephedrine
552-94-3	Salsalate
553-30-0	Proflavine Hemisulfate
553-69-5	Fenyramidol
554-13-2	Lithium Carbonate
554-57-4	Methazolamide
554-92-7	Trimethobenzamide Hydrochloride
555-30-6	Methyldopa
555-57-7	Pargyline
561-27-3	Diamorphine
561-48-8	Norpipanone
561-78-4	Alphaprodine Hydrochloride
561-83-1	Nealbarbital
561-86-4	Brallobarbital
562-09-4	Chlorphenoxamine Hydrochloride
562-10-7	Doxylamine Succinate
562-26-5	Phenoperidine
564-25-0	Doxycycline
566-48-3	Formestane
569-57-3	Chlorotrianisene
569-59-5	Phenindamine Tartrate
569-65-3	Meclozine
573-20-6	Acetomenaphthone
573-41-1	Theophylline Monoethanolamine
575-74-6	Buclosamide
577-11-7	Docusate Sodium
577-48-0	Butyl Aminobenzoate Picrate
579-38-4	Diloxanide
579-56-6	Isoxsuprine Hydrochloride
581-88-4	Debrisoquine Sulfate
586-06-1	Orciprenaline
586-60-7	Dyclonine
587-23-5	Methenamine Mandelate
587-61-1	Propyliodone
590-00-1	Potassium Sorbate
590-46-5	Betaine Hydrochloride
590-63-6	Bethanechol Chloride
591-81-1	Gamma-hydroxybutyric Acid
595-33-5	Megestrol Acetate
596-15-6	Morphine Acetate
596-50-9	Poldine Metilsulfate
596-51-0	Glycopyrronium Bromide
599-79-1	Sulfasalazine
603-00-9	Proxyphylline
603-50-9	Bisacodyl
604-51-3	Deptropine
604-75-1	Oxazepam
607-91-0	Myristicin
609-78-9	Cycloguanil Embonate
611-72-3	Mandelic Acid (±)
611-75-6	Bromhexine Hydrochloride
614-18-6	Ethyl Nicotinate
614-39-1	Procainamide Hydrochloride
614-87-9	Dibrompropamidine Isetionate
616-91-1	Acetylcysteine
620-61-1	Hyoscyamine Sulfate (anhydrous)
620-99-5	Phenacaine Hydrochloride Monohydrate
622-64-0	Hordenine Sulfate (anhydrous)
628-63-7	Amyl Acetate
630-56-8	Hydroxyprogesterone Caproate
630-60-4	Ouabain (anhydrous)
630-86-4	Benzylmorphine Hydrochloride
630-93-3	Phenytoin Sodium
633-47-6	Cropropamide
633-59-0	Clopenthixol Hydrochloride
	Zuclopenthixol Hydrochloride
633-65-8	Berberine Hydrochloride
633-66-9	Berberine Sulfate
634-03-7	Phendimetrazine
635-41-6	Trimetozine
636-54-4	Clopamide
637-07-0	Clofibrate
637-32-1	Proguanil Hydrochloride
637-49-0	Coniine Hydrobromide
637-58-1	Pramocaine Hydrochloride
638-94-8	Desonide
640-19-7	Fluoroacetamide
642-72-8	Benzydamine
642-78-4	Cloxacillin Sodium
643-22-1	Erythromycin Stearate
644-62-2	Meclofenamic Acid
645-05-6	Altretamine
645-43-2	Guanethidine Monosulfate
651-06-9	Sulfametoxydiazine
651-48-9	Dehydroepiandrosterone Sulfate
653-03-2	Butaperazine
655-35-6	Carbocromen Hydrochloride
657-24-9	Metformin
665-66-7	Amantadine Hydrochloride
671-16-9	Procarbazine
671-88-5	Disulfamide
673-31-4	Phenprobamate
674-38-4	Bethanechol
692-13-7	Buformin
695-53-4	Dimethadione

CAS no.	Compound
709-55-7	Etilefrine
709-98-8	Propanil
721-50-6	Prilocaine
723-46-6	Sulfamethoxazole
729-99-7	Sulfamoxole
738-70-5	Trimethoprim
739-71-9	Trimipramine
742-20-1	Cyclopenthiazide
745-65-3	Alprostadil
747-36-4	Hydroxychloroquine Sulfate
747-45-5	Quinidine Bisulfate (anhydrous)
749-13-3	Trifluperidol
750-90-3	Quinine Salicylate (anhydrous)
751-94-0	Sodium Fusidate
751-97-3	Rolitetracycline
768-94-5	Amantadine
791-35-5	Clofedanol
804-10-4	Carbocromen
804-63-7	Quinine Sulfate (anhydrous)
808-48-0	Desoxycortone Pivalate
826-39-1	Mecamylamine Hydrochloride
831-61-8	Ethyl Gallate
834-12-8	Ametryne
834-28-6	Phenformin Hydrochloride
835-31-4	Naphazoline
841-06-5	Methoprotryne
846-48-0	Boldenone
846-49-1	Lorazepam
846-50-4	Temazepam
847-84-7	Normethadone Hydrochloride
848-53-3	Homochlorcyclizine
848-75-9	Lormetazepam
849-55-8	Buphenine Hydrochloride
855-19-6	Clostebol Acetate
856-87-1	Dipipanone Hydrochloride
859-18-7	Lincomycin Hydrochloride
865-04-3	Methoserpidine
865-21-4	Vinblastine
870-62-2	Hexamethonium Iodide
886-50-0	Terbutryne
886-74-8	Chlorphenesin Carbamate
894-71-3	Nortriptyline Hydrochloride
897-15-4	Dosulepin Hydrochloride
904-04-1	Captodiame Hydrochloride
908-54-3	Diminazene Aceturate
909-39-7	Opipramol Hydrochloride
910-86-1	Tiocarlide
911-45-5	Clomifene
912-60-7	Noscapine Hydrochloride
914-00-1	Methacycline
915-30-0	Diphenoxylate
919-16-4	Lithium Citrate
919-86-8	Demeton-*S*-methyl
926-93-2	Metallibure
938-73-8	Etenzamide
942-31-4	Amiphenazole Hydrochloride
942-51-8	Hydroxyephedrine Hydrochloride
952-54-5	Morinamide
956-03-6	Meprylcaine Hydrochloride
956-90-1	Phencyclidine Hydrochloride
958-93-0	Thenyldiamine Hydrochloride
959-24-0	Sotalol Hydrochloride
959-98-8	Endosulfan (α)
963-39-3	Demoxepam
964-52-3	Moxisylyte Hydrochloride
965-90-2	Ethylestrenol
968-81-0	Acetohexamide
969-33-5	Cyproheptadine Hydrochloride
972-02-1	Difenidol
979-32-8	Estradiol Valerate
980-71-2	Brompheniramine Maleate
982-24-1	Clopenthixol
982-57-0	Chloramphenicol Sodium Succinate
987-24-6	Betamethasone Acetate
990-73-8	Fentanyl Citrate
991-42-4	Norbormide
992-21-2	Lymecycline
1007-33-6	Propylhexedrine Hydrochloride
1010-95-3	5-Methyltryptamine Hydrochloride
1014-69-3	Desmetryne
1028-33-7	Pentifylline
1041-90-3	Nalorphine Hydrobromide
1050-48-2	Benzilonium Bromide
1055-55-6	Bunamidine Hydrochloride
1063-55-4	Butaperazine Maleate
1069-66-5	Sodium Valproate
1070-11-7	Ethambutol Hydrochloride
1071-83-6	Glyphosate
1082-57-1	Tramazoline
1082-88-8	Trimethoxyamfetamine
1088-11-5	Nordazepam
1093-58-9	Clostebol
1094-08-2	Profenamine Hydrochloride
1095-90-5	Methadone Hydrochloride
1098-60-8	Triflupromazine Hydrochloride
1099-87-2	Dehydroepiandrosterone Sodium Sulfate
1104-22-9	Meclozine Hydrochloride
1107-99-9	Prednisolone Pivalate
1111-39-3	Acetyldigitoxin
1113-02-6	Omethoate
1115-70-4	Metformin Hydrochloride
1131-64-2	Debrisoquine
1134-47-0	Baclofen
1143-38-0	Dithranol
1156-05-4	Phenglutarimide
1156-19-0	Tolazamide
1163-36-6	Clemizole Hydrochloride
1164-38-1	Lachesine Chloride
1165-48-6	Dimefline
1166-52-5	Dodecyl Gallate
1172-18-5	Flurazepam Hydrochloride
1176-08-5	Phenyltoloxamine Citrate
1177-87-3	Dexamethasone Acetate
1179-69-7	Thiethylperazine Maleate
1181-54-0	Clomocycline
1190-53-0	Buformin Hydrochloride
1197-21-3	Phentermine Hydrochloride
1200-55-1	Pralidoxime Metilsulfate
1209-98-9	Fencamfamin
1211-28-5	Prolintane Hydrochloride
1212-72-2	Mephentermine Sulfate (anhydrous)
1213-06-5	Etebenecid
1218-35-5	Xylometazoline Hydrochloride
1225-55-4	Protriptyline Hydrochloride
1225-60-1	Isothipendyl Hydrochloride
1225-65-6	Prothipendyl Hydrochloride
1229-29-4	Doxepin Hydrochloride
1229-35-2	Methdilazine Hydrochloride
1229-69-2	Bamipine Hydrochloride
1231-93-2	Etynodiol
1235-82-1	Biperiden Hydrochloride
1239-04-9	Phenazocine Hydrobromide (anhydrous)
1239-45-8	Homidium Bromide
1240-15-9	Propiomazine Hydrochloride
1245-44-9	Propicillin Potassium
1253-28-7	Gestonorone Caproate
1255-49-8	Testosterone Phenylpropionate
1257-78-9	Prochlorperazine Edisilate
1264-62-6	Erythromycin Ethylsuccinate
1300-94-3	Amylmetacresol
1319-77-3	Cresol
1320-42-9	Aminonitrothiazole
1327-53-3	Arsenic Trioxide
1330-20-7	Xylene
1397-89-3	Amphotericin B
1400-61-9	Nystatin
1401-69-0	Tylosin
1403-66-3	Gentamicin
1404-04-2	Neomycin
1404-90-6	Vancomycin
1404-93-9	Vancomycin Hydrochloride
1405-10-3	Neomycin Sulfate
1405-37-4	Capreomycin Sulfate
1405-41-0	Gentamicin Sulfate
1405-54-5	Tylosin Tartrate
1405-87-4	Bacitracin
1405-89-6	Bacitracin Zinc
1406-04-8	Neomycin Undecylenate
1415-73-2	Aloin
1420-53-7	Codeine Sulfate (anhydrous)
1420-55-9	Thiethylperazine
1421-14-3	Propanidid
1421-28-9	Dihydromorphine Hydrochloride
1421-68-7	Amidefrine Mesilate
1421-86-9	Strychnine Hydrochloride
1422-07-7	Codeine Hydrochloride (anhydrous)
1424-00-6	Mesterolone
1424-27-7	Acetazolamide Sodium
1435-55-8	Hydroquinidine
1473-73-0	Morinamide Hydrochloride
1476-98-8	Hydroquinidine Hydrochloride
1477-40-3	Levacetylmethadol
1480-19-9	Fluanisone
1490-04-6	Menthol
1491-59-4	Oxymetazoline
1501-84-4	Rimantadine Hydrochloride
1502-95-0	Diamorphine Hydrochloride (hydrate)
1508-75-4	Tropicamide
1508-76-5	Procyclidine Hydrochloride
1518-86-1	Hydroxyamfetamine (±)
1524-88-5	Fludroxycortide
1553-34-0	Metixene Hydrochloride (anhydrous)
1597-82-6	Paramethasone Acetate
1620-21-9	Chlorcyclizine Hydrochloride
1622-61-3	Clonazepam
1622-62-4	Flunitrazepam
1639-60-7	Dextropropoxyphene Hydrochloride
1641-17-4	Mexenone
1641-74-3	Nicametate Citrate
1642-54-2	Diethylcarbamazine Citrate
1649-18-9	Azaperone
1668-19-5	Doxepin
1674-96-0	Phenglutarimide Hydrochloride
1684-40-8	Tacrine Hydrochloride
1689-89-0	Nitroxinil
1707-14-8	Phenmetrazine
1715-33-9	Prednisolone Succinate
1722-62-9	Mepivacaine Hydrochloride
1744-22-5	Riluzole
1746-81-2	Monolinuron
1764-85-8	Epithiazide
1786-81-8	Prilocaine Hydrochloride
1798-50-1	Azacyclonol Hydrochloride
1808-12-4	Bromazine Hydrochloride
1812-30-2	Bromazepam
1821-47-2	5-Methyltryptamine
1824-58-4	Ethiazide
1837-57-6	Ethacridine Lactate
1841-19-6	Fluspirilene
1847-24-1	Flucloxacillin Sodium (anhydrous)

CAS no.	*Compound*
1861-21-8	Enallylpropymal
1867-58-9	Clomethiazole Edisilate
1867-66-9	Ketamine Hydrochloride
1892-80-4	Fenetylline Hydrochloride
1893-33-0	Pipamperone
1910-42-5	Paraquat Dichloride
1912-24-9	Atrazine
1918-00-9	Dicamba
1944-12-3	Fenoterol Hydrobromide
1951-25-3	Amiodarone
1953-04-4	Galantamine Hydrobromide
1961-77-9	Chlormadinone
1972-08-3	Δ^9-Tetrahydrocannabinol
1977-10-2	Loxapine
1981-58-4	Sulfadimidine Sodium
1982-37-2	Methdilazine
2002-29-1	Flumetasone Pivalate
2016-36-6	Choline Salicylate
2016-63-9	Bamifylline
2016-88-8	Amiloride Hydrochloride
2022-85-7	Flucytosine
2030-63-9	Clofazimine
2058-46-0	Oxytetracycline Hydrochloride
2058-52-8	Clotiapine
2061-86-1	Methandriol Diacetate
2062-77-3	Trifluperidol Hydrochloride
2062-78-4	Pimozide
2062-84-2	Benperidol
2066-89-9	Isoniazid Aminosalicylate
2068-78-2	Vincristine Sulfate
2078-54-8	Propofol
2081-65-4	Butanilicaine Phosphate
2086-83-1	Berberine
2099-26-5	Androstenediol Diacetate
2127-01-7	Clorexolone
2139-47-1	Nifenazone
2152-34-3	Pemoline
2152-44-5	Betamethasone Valerate
2153-98-2	Cathine Hydrochloride
2165-19-7	Guanoxan
2167-85-3	Pipazetate
2169-75-7	Deptropine Citrate
2180-92-9	Bupivacaine
2192-20-3	Hydroxyzine Hydrochloride
2203-97-6	Hydrocortisone Hydrogen Succinate
2216-51-5	Menthol (−)
2218-68-0	Cloral Betaine
2219-30-9	Penicillamine Hydrochloride
2228-39-9	Dehydroemetine Hydrochloride
2240-14-4	Fencamfamin Hydrochloride
2259-96-3	Cyclothiazide
2265-64-7	Dexamethasone Isonicotinate
2272-11-9	Monoethanolamine Oleate
2276-52-0	Pentazocine
2277-92-1	Oxyclozanide
2297-30-5	Androstenediol Dipropionate
2313-87-3	Etoxazene Hydrochloride
2315-02-8	Oxymetazoline Hydrochloride
2324-94-9	Profadol Hydrochloride
2338-21-8	Thiazinamium
2338-37-6	Levopropoxyphene
2347-80-0	Thioproperazine Mesilate
2375-03-3	Methylprednisolone Sodium Succinate
2391-03-9	Dexbrompheniramine Maleate
2392-39-4	Dexamethasone Sodium Phosphate
2398-96-1	Tolnaftate
2413-38-9	Flupentixol Hydrochloride
2430-49-1	Vinylbital
2438-32-6	Dexchlorphenamine Maleate
2438-72-4	Bufexamac
2447-57-6	Sulfadoxine
2448-68-2	Pipamperone Hydrochloride
2470-73-7	Dixyrazine
2507-91-7	Gloxazone
2508-72-7	Antazoline Hydrochloride
2508-79-4	Methyldopate Hydrochloride
2529-45-5	Flugestone Acetate
2530-97-4	Xantinol
2544-09-4	Methyldopate
2576-92-3	Isoetarine Hydrochloride
2577-32-4	Sulfamethoxypyridazine Sodium
2589-47-1	Prajmalium Bitartrate
2609-46-3	Amiloride
2610-86-8	Warfarin Potassium
2622-26-6	Pericyazine
2622-30-2	Carfenazine
2622-37-9	Trifluomeprazine
2624-43-3	Cyclofenil
2642-71-9	Azinphos-ethyl
2709-56-0	Flupentixol
2740-04-7	Dimefline Hydrochloride
2746-81-8	Fluphenazine Enantate
2751-09-9	Troleandomycin
2751-68-0	Acetophenazine
2753-45-9	Mebeverine Hydrochloride
2764-72-9	Diquat
2773-92-4	Quinisocaine Hydrochloride
2784-73-8	6-Monoacetylmorphine
2870-71-5	Atropine Methobromide
2898-12-6	Medazepam
2920-86-7	Prednisolone Succinate
2921-57-5	Methylprednisolone Hemisuccinate
2921-88-2	Chlorpyrifos
2922-44-3	Dextromoramide Tartrate
2955-38-6	Prazepam
2971-90-6	Clopidol
2975-34-0	Carfenazine Maleate
2975-36-2	Pecazine Hydrochloride
3056-17-5	Stavudine
3093-35-4	Halcinonide
3099-52-3	Nicametate
3131-32-6	Antazoline Mesilate
3146-66-5	Idobutal
3198-07-0	Ethylnoradrenaline Hydrochloride
3200-06-4	Naftidrofuryl Oxalate
3215-70-1	Hexoprenaline
3254-89-5	Difenidol Hydrochloride
3269-83-8	Pheniramine Aminosalicylate
3313-26-6	Tiotixene
3321-80-0	Methylpiperidyl Benzilate
3329-14-4	Fenpiprane Hydrochloride
3339-11-5	Tolpropamine Hydrochloride
3354-67-4	Amidefrine
3362-45-6	Noxiptiline
3380-34-5	Triclosan
3416-26-0	Lidoflazine
3459-06-1	Cyclopentamine Hydrochloride
3459-20-9	Glymidine Sodium
3459-96-9	Amicarbalide
3485-62-9	Clidinium Bromide
3505-38-2	Carbinoxamine Maleate
3506-09-0	Propranolol Hydrochloride
3521-62-8	Erythromycin Estolate
3540-95-2	Fenpiprane
3545-67-3	Chloroquine Hydrochloride
3546-29-0	Thialbarbital Sodium
3546-41-6	Pyrvinium Embonate
3562-63-8	Megestrol
3562-84-3	Benzbromarone
3568-23-8	Propiomazine Maleate
3568-43-2	Acetyl Sulfamethoxypyridazine
3570-46-5	Ethomoxane
3571-53-7	Estradiol Undecylate
3572-43-8	Bromhexine
3572-80-3	Cyclazocine
3576-64-5	Clefamide
3593-85-9	Methandriol Dipropionate
3595-11-7	Propylhexedrine (±)
3598-37-6	Acepromazine Maleate
3614-30-0	Emepronium Bromide
3614-69-5	Dimetindene Maleate
3615-24-5	Isopropylaminophenazone
3616-05-5	Pyritidium Bromide
3624-96-2	Bialamicol Hydrochloride
3625-06-7	Mebeverine
3627-49-4	Phenoperidine Hydrochloride
3639-12-1	Butetamate Citrate
3671-72-5	Amicarbalide Isetionate
3684-46-6	Broxaldine
3685-84-5	Meclofenoxate Hydrochloride
3688-62-8	Aminopromazine Fumarate
3693-39-8	Fluclorolone Acetonide
3697-42-5	Chlorhexidine Hydrochloride
3703-79-5	Bamethan
3706-26-1	Methoxyamfetamine Hydrochloride
3715-90-0	Tramazoline Hydrochloride
3717-88-2	Flavoxate Hydrochloride
3734-33-6	Denatonium Benzoate
3736-08-1	Fenetylline
3736-81-0	Diloxanide Furoate
3737-09-5	Disopyramide
3748-77-4	Bunamidine
3751-730-9	Acebutolol
3784-99-4	Stilbazium Iodide
3785-21-5	Butanilicaine
3810-74-0	Streptomycin Sulfate
3810-80-8	Diphenoxylate Hydrochloride
3811-25-4	Clorprenaline
3818-50-6	Bephenium Hydroxynaphthoate
3818-88-0	Tricyclamol Chloride
3819-00-9	Piperacetazine
3820-67-5	Glafenine
3847-29-8	Erythromycin Lactobionate
3858-89-7	Chloroprocaine Hydrochloride
3902-71-4	Trioxysalen
3922-90-5	Oleandomycin
3930-20-9	Sotalol
3947-65-7	Neomycin A
3963-95-9	Methacycline Hydrochloride
3964-81-6	Azatadine
3978-86-7	Azatadine Maleate
4008-48-4	Nitroxoline
4028-98-2	Dequalinium Acetate
4044-65-9	Bitoscanate
4075-96-1	Dimethylamfetamine
4185-80-2	Levomepromazine Hydrochloride
4205-90-7	Clonidine
4205-91-8	Clonidine Hydrochloride
4255-23-6	Aletamine
4255-24-7	Aletamine Hydrochloride
4268-36-4	Tybamate
4268-37-5	Anileridine Phosphate
4291-63-8	Cladribine
4299-60-9	Sulfafurazole Diethanolamine
4304-40-9	Thenium Closilate
4310-35-4	Tridihexethyl Chloride
4323-43-7	Hexoprenaline Hydrochloride
4330-99-8	Alimemazine Tartrate
4360-12-7	Ajmaline
4378-36-3	Fenbutrazate
4394-00-7	Niflumic Acid
4419-39-0	Beclometasone
4438-22-6	Atropine Oxide
4498-32-2	Dibenzepin
4499-40-5	Choline Theophyllinate

CAS no.	*Compound*
4574-60-1	Atropine Oxide Hydrochloride
4682-36-4	Orphenadrine Citrate
4685-14-7	Paraquat
4697-36-3	Carbenicillin
4759-48-2	Isotretinoin
4764-17-4	Methylenedioxyamfetamine
4800-94-6	Carbenicillin Sodium
4825-53-0	Hexestrol Dipropionate
4845-99-2	Brucine Sulfate (anhydrous)
4884-68-8	Hydrastinine Hydrochloride
4901-03-5	Narceine Hydrochloride
4914-30-1	Dehydroemetine
4936-47-4	Nifuratel
4945-47-5	Bamipine
4969-02-2	Metixene
4985-15-3	Noxiptiline Hydrochloride
5001-32-1	Guanoclor
5001-33-2	Metadrenaline
5002-47-1	Fluphenazine Decanoate
5003-48-5	Benorilate
5011-34-7	Trimetazidine
5026-62-0	Sodium Methyl Hydroxybenzoate
5036-02-2	Tetramisole
5060-55-9	Prednisolone Steaglate
5086-74-8	Tetramisole Hydrochloride
5103-74-2	Chlordane
5104-49-4	Flurbiprofen
5111-12-6	Dihydroergotamine
5144-52-5	Naphazoline Nitrate
5152-30-7	Metocurine Iodide
5189-11-7	Pizotifen Malate
5250-39-5	Flucloxacillin
5355-16-8	Diaveridine
5355-48-6	β-Acetyldigoxin
5370-01-4	Mexiletine Hydrochloride
5377-20-8	Metomidate
5411-22-3	Benzfetamine Hydrochloride
5490-27-7	Dihydrostreptomycin Sulfate
5511-98-8	α-Acetyldigoxin
5534-09-8	Beclometasone Dipropionate
5560-59-8	Alverine Citrate
5560-72-5	Iprindole
5579-84-0	Betahistine Hydrochloride
5580-03-0	Tioguanine
5585-73-9	Butriptyline Hydrochloride
5588-10-3	Methoxyphenamine Hydrochloride
5588-20-5	Clodantoin
5588-22-7	Clorprenaline Hydrochloride (monohydrate)
5588-33-0	Mesoridazine
5591-29-7	Etafedrine Hydrochloride
5591-45-7	Tiotixene
5593-20-4	Betamethasone Dipropionate
5598-13-0	Chlorpyrifos-methyl
5611-51-8	Triamcinolone Hexacetonide
5632-44-0	Tolpropamine
5634-34-4	Bufylline
5635-50-7	Hexestrol
5636-83-9	Dimetindene
5638-76-6	Betahistine
5650-44-2	Methcathinone
5667-46-9	Dimoxyline Phosphate
5697-56-3	Carbenoxolone
5714-00-1	Acetophenazine Dimaleate
5714-04-5	Guanoxan Sulfate
5714-73-8	Methenamine Hippurate
5714-90-9	Levopropoxyphene Napsilate
5716-20-1	Bamethan Sulfate
5743-12-4	Caffeine Hydrate
5786-21-0	Clozapine
5796-31-6	Ecgonine Hydrochloride
5807-87-4	Diphenylpyraline Hydrobromide
5818-17-7	Methanthelinium
5836-29-3	Coumatetralyl
5853-29-2	Cephaëline Hydrochloride
5870-29-1	Cyclopentolate Hydrochloride
5874-97-5	Orciprenaline Sulfate
5875-06-9	Proxymetacaine Hydrochloride
5892-31-9	Chlortetracycline Calcium
5892-48-8	Acetarsone Sodium
5897-19-8	Cyclizine Lactate
5907-38-0	Dipyrone
5908-99-6	Atropine Sulfate (monohydrate)
5913-76-8	Codeine Phosphate (sesquihydrate)
5913-82-6	Conessine Hydrobromide
5915-41-3	Terbutylazine
5934-55-4	Ibogaine Hydrochloride
5936-28-7	Hydrastine Hydrochloride
5949-11-1	Cinchonine Hydrochloride (anhydrous)
5949-44-0	Testosterone Undecylate
5956-60-5	Berberine Hydrochloride
5957-75-5	Δ^8-Tetrahydrocannabinol
5964-56-7	Octamylamine Hydrochloride
5965-13-9	Dihydrocodeine Tartrate
5965-49-1	Ketobemidone Hydrochloride
5967-84-0	Theophylline Hydrate
5974-11-8	Morphine Acetate
5985-38-6	Levorphanol Tartrate
5987-82-6	Oxybuprocaine Hydrochloride
5989-77-5	Dihydroergotamine Tartrate
5991-71-9	Clorazepate Monopotassium
5995-96-0	Physostigmine Aminoxide Salicylate
6000-74-4	Hydrocortisone Sodium Phosphate
6001-64-5	Chlorobutanol (hemihydrate)
6004-24-6	Cetylpyridinium Chloride
6004-98-4	Hexocyclium Metilsulfate
6009-81-0	Morphine
6011-12-7	Ambazone
6018-19-5	Sodium Aminosalicylate
6032-59-3	Morphine Tartrate
6033-41-6	Norpipanone Hydrochloride
6033-42-7	Norpipanone Hydrobromide
6038-78-4	Ethomoxane Hydrochloride
6054-98-4	Olsalazine Sodium
6055-06-7	Morphine Hydrochloride
6055-19-2	Cyclophosphamide
6056-11-7	Pipazetate Hydrochloride
6059-47-8	Codeine (monohydrate)
6080-58-6	Lithium Citrate
6101-04-8	Strychnine Hydrochloride
6101-15-1	Suxamethonium Chloride
6101-35-5	Sulfacarbamide
6101-41-3	Sulfapyridine Sodium Monohydrate
6106-46-3	Hyoscine Methonitrate
6108-05-0	Lidocaine Hydrochloride
6108-10-7	Benzene Hexachloride (ε)
6112-76-1	Mercaptopurine (monohydrate)
6113-17-3	Histapyrrodine Hydrochloride
6114-26-7	Pholedrine Sulfate
6119-47-7	Quinine Hydrochloride (dihydrate)
6119-70-6	Quinine Sulfate (dihydrate)
6130-64-9	Procaine Benzylpenicillin
6138-47-2	Liothyronine Hydrochloride
6138-56-3	Tripelennamine Citrate
6138-79-0	Triprolidine Hydrochloride (monohydrate)
6147-37-1	Menadione Sodium Bisulfite (trihydrate)
6151-30-0	Mepacrine Hydrochloride (dihydrate)
6151-39-9	Quinidine Bisulfate (tetrahydrate)
6153-19-1	Phenacaine Hydrochloride Monohydrate
6153-33-9	Mebhydrolin Napadisilate
6153-56-6	Oxalic Acid (dihydrate)
6153-64-6	Oxytetracycline Dihydrate (dihydrate)
6155-57-3	Saccharin Sodium
6160-12-9	Sparteine Sulfate
6164-87-0	Nicotinyl Tartrate
6168-76-9	Crotetamide
6168-86-1	Isometheptene Hydrochloride
6170-42-9	Chloropyramine Hydrochloride
6183-68-2	Quinine Bisulfate (heptahydrate)
6190-39-2	Dihydroergotamine Mesilate
6190-55-2	Sulfaguanidine Monohydrate
6190-60-9	Mephentermine Sulfate (dihydrate)
6192-95-6	Propylhexedrine Hydrochloride (±)
6202-17-1	Hordenine Sulfate (dihydrate)
6202-23-9	Cyclobenzaprine Hydrochloride
6209-17-2	Sulfacetamide Sodium
6211-15-0	Morphine Sulfate
6292-91-7	Methylenedioxyamfetamine Hydrochloride
6381-91-5	Saccharin Calcium
6385-02-0	Meclofenamate Sodium
6398-98-7	Amodiaquine Hydrochloride
6411-75-2	Tuaminoheptane Sulfate
6416-04-2	Tetracycline (trihydrate)
6452-71-7	Oxprenolol
6452-73-9	Oxprenolol Hydrochloride
6469-93-8	Chlorprothixene Hydrochloride
6472-73-7	Pseudomorphine
6474-85-7	Fenbutrazate Hydrochloride
6485-34-3	Saccharin Calcium
6493-05-6	Pentoxifylline
6500-81-8	Etacrynate Sodium
6506-37-2	Nimorazole
6509-18-8	Aconitine Nitrate
6533-68-2	Hyoscine Hydrobromide (trihydrate)
6536-18-1	Morazone
6556-11-2	Inositol Nicotinate
6591-63-5	Quinidine Sulfate (dihydrate)
6592-85-4	Hydrastinine
6621-47-2	Perhexiline
6673-35-4	Practolol
6700-34-1	Dextromethorphan Hydrobromide
6700-39-6	Isoprenaline Sulfate
6700-56-7	Ethoheptazine Citrate
6703-27-1	Acetylcodeine
6707-58-0	Dequalinium
6724-53-4	Perhexiline Maleate
6735-59-7	Pralidoxime Chloride
6736-03-4	Ecothiopate Iodide (ecothiopate)
6740-88-1	Ketamine
6746-59-4	Ethylmorphine Hydrochloride (dihydrate)
6780-13-8	Ethylenediamine Hydrate (monohydrate)
6791-71-5	Sulfathiazole Sodium (pentahydrate)
6823-79-6	Pentamidine Mesilate
6835-16-1	Hyoscyamine Sulfate (dihydrate)
6854-40-6	Codeine Sulfate (trihydrate)
6888-11-5	Diphenhydramine Di(acefyllinate)
6893-02-3	Liothyronine
6923-22-4	Monocrotophos

CAS no.	*Compound*
6933-90-0	Clorprenaline Hydrochloride (anhydrous)
6989-98-6	Tubocurarine Chloride Pentahydrate
6990-06-3	Fusidic Acid
6998-60-3	Rifamycin SV
7009-54-3	Pentapiperide
7020-55-5	Clidinium
7054-25-3	Quinidine Gluconate
7060-74-4	Oleandomycin Phosphate
7081-38-1	Oxyphenbutazone (monohydrate)
7081-40-5	Metixene Hydrochloride (monohydrate)
7081-44-9	Cloxacillin Sodium
7081-52-9	Piminodine Esilate
7081-53-0	Doxapram Hydrochloride
7083-71-8	Emetine Hydrochloride (hydrate)
7085-44-1	Chlorothiazide Sodium
7085-45-2	Biperiden Lactate
7104-38-3	Levomepromazine Maleate
7177-48-2	Ampicillin Trihydrate
7179-49-9	Lincomycin Hydrochloride
7181-73-9	Bephenium
7187-66-8	Trimetaphan
7195-27-9	Mefruside
7232-21-5	Metoclopramide Hydrochloride
7246-14-2	Meticillin Sodium
7246-20-0	Triclofos Sodium
7247-57-6	Heteronium Bromide
7261-97-4	Dantrolene
7279-75-6	Isoetarine Mesilate
7287-19-6	Prometryne
7327-87-9	Dihydralazine Sulfate
7331-52-4	(S)-3-Hydroxy-gamma-butyrolactone
7361-61-7	Xylazine
7389-45-9	Butaperazine Phosphate
7416-34-4	Molindone
7421-40-1	Carbenoxolone Sodium
7455-39-2	Dimetotiazine Mesilate
7456-24-8	Dimetotiazine
7460-12-0	Pseudoephedrine Sulfate
7481-89-2	Zalcitabine
7491-09-0	Docusate Potassium
7492-31-1	Isometheptene Mucate
7492-32-2	Isopropamide
7527-91-5	Aminoacridine Hexylresorcinate
7528-00-9	Dexamfetamine Phosphate
7554-65-6	Fomepizole
7563-42-0	Pentobarbital Calcium
7599-79-3	Clomifene Citrate (E)
7601-55-0	Metocurine Iodide
7619-53-6	Clomifene Citrate (Z)
7648-98-8	Ambenonium Chloride
7681-14-3	Prednisolone Tebutate
7681-78-9	Mebezonium Iodide
7681-79-0	Etafedrine
7681-80-3	Pentapiperide Metilsulfate
7681-93-8	Natamycin
7683-36-5	Obidoxime
7683-59-2	Isoprenaline
7716-59-8	Etisazole Hydrochloride
7716-60-1	Etisazole
7773-52-6	Cetylpyridinium Chloride
7786-34-7	Mevinphos
8000-10-0	Theophylline Sodium Glycinate
8000-33-47	Pyrethrum
8001-54-5	Benzalkonium Chloride
8006-25-5	Ergotoxine
8008-45-5	Nutmeg Oil
8015-51-8	Cropropamide combination with Crotetamide
8015-61-0	Aloin
8017-89-8	Amyl Nitrite
8025-81-8	Spiramycin
8044-71-1	Cetrimide
8047-28-7	Ergotoxine Esilate
8051-02-3	Veratrine (mixture)
8053-18-7	Protoveratrines A and B
8063-14-7	Cannabis
8063-24-9	Acriflavinium Chloride
8067-24-1	Co-dergocrine Mesilate
8067-69-4	Halquinol
9002-61-3	Chorionic Gonadotropin
9002-91-9	Metaldehyde
9004-10-8	Insulin
9014-67-9	Aloxiprin
9015-68-3	Asparaginase
9041-08-1	Enoxaparin Sodium
9041-93-4	Bleomycin Sulfate
10018-19-6	Cotarnine Chloride
10041-19-7	Docusate Sodium
10075-24-8	Imipramine Embonate
10085-81-1	Benzoctamine Hydrochloride
10118-90-8	Minocycline
10161-33-8	Trenbolone
10161-34-9	Trenbolone Acetate
10238-21-8	Glibenclamide
10246-75-0	Hydroxyzine Embonate
10262-69-8	Maprotiline
10265-92-6	Methamidophos
10347-81-6	Maprotiline Hydrochloride
10379-14-3	Tetrazepam
10418-03-8	Stanozolol
10488-36-5	Tofenacin Hydrochloride
10592-13-9	Doxycycline Hydrochloride
10596-23-3	Clodronic Acid
11003-38-6	Capreomycin
11005-63-3	Strophanthin-K
11018-89-6	Ouabain (octahydrate)
11032-41-0	Co-dergocrine Mesilate
11056-06-7	Bleomycin
11061-68-0	Insulin (human)
12001-72-8	Mafenide Propionate
12002-30-1	Piperazine Calcium Edetate
12629-01-5	Somatropin
12650-69-0	Mupirocin
12789-03-6	Chlordane
13009-99-9	Mafenide Acetate
13013-17-7	Propranolol
13029-44-2	Dienestrol (*E,E*)
13051-01-9	Carbazochrome Salicylate
13055-82-8	Reproterol Hydrochloride
13103-34-9	Boldenone Undecylenate
13115-40-7	Dimetotiazine Mesilate
13171-25-0	Trimetazidine Hydrochloride
13292-46-1	Rifampicin
13392-18-2	Fenoterol
13392-28-4	Rimantadine
13422-51-0	Hydroxocobalamin
13457-18-6	Pyrazophos
13473-38-6	Pipenzolate Bromide
13492-01-8	Tranylcypromine Sulfate
13494-90-1	Gallium Nitrate (anhydrous)
13495-09-5	Piminodine
13501-04-7	Bunamidine Hydroxynaphthoate
13523-86-9	Pindolol
13539-59-8	Azapropazone (anhydrous)
13609-67-1	Hydrocortisone Butyrate
13614-98-7	Minocycline Hydrochloride
13647-35-3	Trilostane
13655-52-2	Alprenolol
13669-70-0	Nefopam
13678-97-2	Alprenolol Hydrochloride
13707-88-5	Alprenolol Hydrochloride
13710-19-5	Tolfenamic Acid
13764-49-3	Etorphine Hydrochloride
13838-16-9	Enflurane
13900-14-6	Domiphen Bromide
13912-80-6	Butoxyethyl Nicotinate
13930-31-9	Oxetacaine Hydrochloride
13931-75-4	Phenmetrazine
13956-29-1	Cannabidiol
13997-19-8	Methyl Benzoquate
14007-49-9	Ambutonium Bromide
14007-53-5	Fenpipramide Hydrochloride (anhydrous)
14007-64-8	Butetamate
14008-44-7	Metopimazine
14028-44-5	Amoxapine
14046-64-1	Benserazide Hydrochloride
14107-37-0	Alfadolone
14116-06-4	Methylthioamfetamine
14214-84-7	Oxyphenonium
14222-46-9	Pyritidium Bromide
14222-60-7	Protionamide
14252-80-3	Bupivacaine Hydrochloride
14255-87-9	Parbendazole
14293-44-8	Xipamide
14297-87-1	Benzylmorphine
14357-78-9	Diprenorphine
14362-31-3	Chlorcyclizine Hydrochloride
14399-14-5	Chloramphenicol Cinnamate
14437-41-3	Clioxanide
14484-47-0	Deflazacort
14521-96-1	Etorphine
14538-56-8	Piperazine Phosphate
14611-51-9	Selegiline
14611-52-0	Selegiline Hydrochloride
14648-14-7	Norcodeine Hydrochloride (anhydrous)
14663-23-1	Dantrolene Sodium
14759-06-9	Sulforidazine
14769-73-4	Levamisole
14777-25-4	Perazine Dimalonate
14779-78-3	Padimate
14838-15-4	Phenylpropanolamine
14897-39-3	Rifamycin Sodium
14919-77-8	Benserazide Hydrochloride
14976-57-9	Clemastine Fumarate
15105-92-7	Rifamycin Sodium
15180-03-7	Alcuronium Chloride
15251-48-6	Oxytetracycline Calcium
15262-86-9	Testosterone Isocaproate
15301-48-1	Bezitramide
15301-69-6	Flavoxate
15301-93-6	Tofenacin
15307-79-6	Diclofenac
15307-86-5	Diclofenac
15351-13-0	Nicofuranose
15356-70-4	Menthol (±)
15500-66-0	Pancuronium Bromide
15537-76-5	Chlorproguanil Hydrochloride
15574-96-6	Pizotifen
15585-70-3	Bibenzonium Bromide
15588-95-1	DOM
15589-00-1	DOM Hydrochloride
15599-39-0	Noxytiolin
15622-65-8	Molindone Hydrochloride
15663-27-1	Cisplatin
15676-16-1	Sulpiride
15686-51-8	Clemastine
15686-61-0	Fenproporex
15686-71-2	Cefalexin
15686-83-6	Pyrantel
15687-14-6	Embutramide
15687-27-1	Ibuprofen
15687-33-9	Metindizate
15687-40-8	Octafonium Chloride (anhydrous)
15690-57-0	Clomifene

CAS no.	*Compound*
15722-48-2	Olsalazine
15823-89-9	Imolamine Hydrochloride
15826-37-6	Sodium Cromoglicate
15867-21-7	Alphaprodine (±)
15876-67-2	Distigmine Bromide
15879-93-3	Alphachloralose
15972-60-8	Alachlor
16051-77-7	Isosorbide Mononitrate
16110-51-3	Sodium Cromoglicate
16203-97-7	Dithranol Triacetate
16210-52-9	Cotarnine Chloride
16320-04-0	Gestrinone
16376-74-2	Valethamate
16509-35-6	Thenalidine Tartrate
16589-24-5	Oxedrine Tartrate
16590-41-3	Naltrexone
16595-80-5	Levamisole Hydrochloride
16676-29-2	Naltrexone Hydrochloride
16776-64-0	Thenium Closilate
16808-86-9	Diprenorphine Hydrochloride
16915-70-1	Nifursol
17086-03-2	Amitriptyline Embonate
17086-28-1	Doxycycline
17086-29-2	Levomepromazine Maleate
17140-78-2	Dextropropoxyphene Napsilate
17140-81-7	Nitrofurantoin (monohydrate)
17146-95-1	Pentazocine
17230-88-5	Danazol
17243-39-9	Benzoctamine
17321-77-6	Clomipramine Hydrochloride
17560-51-9	Metolazone
17575-22-3	Lanatoside C
17598-65-1	Deslanoside
17617-23-1	Flurazepam
17692-31-8	Dropropizine
17693-51-5	Promethazine Teoclate
17737-65-4	Clonixin
17780-72-2	Clorgiline
17780-75-5	Clorgiline Hydrochloride
18010-40-7	Bupivacaine Hydrochloride
18174-58-8	Pipoxolan Hydrochloride
18305-29-8	Fenproporex (hydrochloride)
18323-44-9	Clindamycin
18470-94-5	Nandrolone Cyclohexane-carboxylate
18472-51-0	Chlorhexidine Gluconate
18507-89-6	Decoquinate
18534-18-4	Piperazine Phosphate
18559-94-9	Salbutamol
18652-93-2	Methohexital
18833-13-1	Acefylline Piperazine
19216-56-9	Prazosin
19237-84-4	Prazosin Hydrochloride
19326-29-5	Etamiphylline Camsilate
19387-91-8	Tinidazole
19774-82-4	Amiodarone Hydrochloride
19794-93-5	Trazodone
20236-82-2	Thebacon Hydrochloride
20380-58-9	Tilidate
20432-64-8	Iprindole Hydrochloride
20537-88-6	Amifostine
20562-02-1	Solanine
20574-50-9	Morantel
20594-83-6	Nalbuphine
20684-06-4	Bamifylline Hydrochloride
20685-78-3	Rolitetracycline Nitrate
20830-75-5	Digoxin
20830-81-3	Daunorubicin
21187-98-4	Gliclazide
21245-01-2	Padimate
21245-02-3	Padimate O
21462-39-5	Clindamycin Hydrochloride (anhydrous)
21498-08-8	Lofexidine Hydrochloride
21535-47-7	Mianserin Hydrochloride
21679-14-1	Fludarabine
21829-25-4	Nifedipine
21898-19-1	Clenbuterol Hydrochloride
22059-60-5	Disopyramide
22064-27-3	Penthienate Methobromide
22071-15-4	Ketoprofen
22131-35-7	Butalamine
22131-79-9	Alclofenac
22161-81-5	Dexketoprofen
22189-31-7	Tiotixene Hydrochloride
22204-24-6	Pyrantel Embonate
22204-53-1	Naproxen
22204-88-2	Tramadol Hydrochloride
22212-52-8	Chlordane
22224-92-6	Fenamiphos
22232-54-8	Carbimazole
22232-71-9	Mazindol
22260-51-1	Bromocriptine Mesilate
22298-29-9	Betamethasone Benzoate
22316-47-8	Clobazam
22487-42-9	Benaprizine
22494-42-4	Diflunisal
22500-92-1	Sorbic Acid
22560-50-5	Disodium Clodronate
22662-39-1	Rafoxanide
22664-55-7	Metipranolol
22832-87-7	Miconazole Nitrate
22846-83-9	Tigloidine Hydrobromide
22881-35-2	Famprofazone
22916-47-8	Miconazole
22972-97-0	Oxprenolol Hydrochloride
22972-98-1	Oxprenolol
23031-25-6	Terbutaline
23031-32-5	Terbutaline Sulfate
23047-25-8	Lofepramine
23067-13-2	Erythromycin Gluceptate
23076-35-9	Xylazine Hydrochloride
23093-74-5	Bunitrolol Hydrochloride
23142-01-0	Carbetapentane Citrate
23214-92-8	Doxorubicin
23214-96-2	Alcuronium Chloride
23239-32-9	Methoxyamfetamine
23239-51-2	Ritodrine Hydrochloride
23277-43-2	Nalbuphine Hydrochloride
23282-55-5	Sulfachlorpyridazine Sodium
23313-50-0	Practolol
23325-78-2	Cefalexin
23327-57-3	Nefopam Hydrochloride
23454-33-3	Trenbolone Hexahydrobenzyl-carbonate
23541-50-6	Daunorubicin Hydrochloride
23593-75-1	Clotrimazole
23597-82-2	Hexyl Nicotinate
23651-95-8	Droxidopa
23744-24-3	Pipoxolan
23779-99-9	Floctafenine
23846-70-0	Alprenolol
23887-31-2	Clorazepic Acid
23930-19-0	Alfaxalone
23930-37-2	Alfadolone Acetate
23978-85-0	Δ^9-Tetrahydrocannabinolic Acid
23983-43-9	Dehydroepiandrosterone Enantate
24017-47-8	Triazophos
24169-02-6	Econazole Nitrate
24204-13-5	Dihydrocodeine Phosphate
24219-97-4	Mianserin
24280-93-1	Mycophenolic Acid
24359-81-7	Antazoline Sulfate (anhydrous)
24390-14-5	Doxycycline Hydrochloride
24526-64-5	Nomifensine
24584-09-6	Dexrazoxane
24634-61-5	Potassium Sorbate
24668-75-5	Dexamethasone Tebutate
24729-96-2	Clindamycin Phosphate
24815-24-5	Rescinnamine
24868-20-0	Dantrolene Sodium
25013-16-5	Butylated Hydroxyanisole
25122-41-2	Clobetasol
25122-46-7	Clobetasol Propionate
25122-57-0	Clobetasone Butyrate
25316-40-9	Doxorubicin Hydrochloride
25332-20-1	Dimetridazole Hydrochloride
25332-39-2	Trazodone Hydrochloride
25333-77-1	Acetorphine
25333-78-2	Acetorphine Hydrochloride
25334-00-3	Bemegride Sodium
25389-94-0	Kanamycin Sulfate
25416-65-3	Levothyroxine Sodium
25451-15-4	Felbamate
25507-04-4	Clindamycin Palmitate Hydrochloride
25523-97-1	Dexchlorphenamine
25567-68-4	Chloronitrotoluene
25573-43-7	Physostigmine Aminoxide
25614-03-3	Bromocriptine
25967-29-7	Flutoprazepam
25968-91-6	Hydrocodone Hydrochloride
25990-43-6	Mepenzolate
26097-80-3	Cambendazole
26155-31-7	Morantel Tartrate
26159-34-2	Naproxen Sodium
26171-23-3	Tolmetin
26309-95-5	Pivampicillin Hydrochloride
26372-86-1	Pentapiperide
26570-10-5	Dextropropoxyphene Napsilate
26615-21-4	Zotepine
26652-09-5	Ritodrine
26657-13-6	Rolitetracycline Nitrate
26786-32-3	Lofepramine Hydrochloride
26787-78-0	Amoxicillin
26807-65-8	Indapamide
26839-75-8	Timolol
26844-12-2	Indoramin
26864-56-2	Penfluridol
26921-17-5	Timolol Maleate
26944-48-9	Glibornuride
27060-91-9	Flutazolam
27107-79-5	Tilidate Hydrochloride (anhydrous)
27134-26-5	Chloroaniline
27203-92-5	Tramadol
27220-47-9	Econazole
27223-35-4	Ketazolam
27262-47-1	Levobupivacaine
27262-48-2	Levobupivacaine Hydrochloride
27555-34-6	Quinidine Polygalacturonate (anhydrous)
27833-64-3	Loxapine Succinate
27848-84-6	Nicergoline
27892-33-7	Emepronium
27912-14-7	Levobunolol Hydrochloride
27917-82-4	Nitroxinil Eglumine Salt
28159-98-0	Irgarol
28319-77-9	Choline Alfoscerate
28395-03-1	Bumetanide
28416-66-2	Isoaminile Citrate
28523-86-6	Sevoflurane
28721-07-5	Oxcarbazepine
28797-61-7	Pirenzepine
28860-95-9	Carbidopa
28911-01-5	Triazolam
28981-97-7	Alprazolam
29094-61-9	Glipizide
29122-68-7	Atenolol
29205-06-9	Fluocortolone Pivalate
29216-28-2	Mequitazine

CAS no.	*Compound*
29218-27-2	Toloxatone
29560-58-5	Moracizine Hydrochloride
29868-97-1	Pirenzepine Hydrochloride
29883-15-6	Amygdalin
30272-08-3	Amineptine Hydrochloride
30516-87-1	Zidovudine
30544-47-9	Etofenamate
30652-11-0	Deferiprone
30685-43-9	Metildigoxin
30748-29-9	Feprazone
30909-51-4	Flupentixol Decanoate
31036-80-3	Lofexidine
31329-57-4	Naftidrofuryl Oxalate
31377-23-8	Amantadine Sulfate
31431-39-7	Mebendazole
31677-93-7	Bupropion Hydrochloride
31828-50-9	Cefradine (dihydrate)
31828-71-4	Mexiletine
31842-01-0	Indoprofen
31842-61-2	Rimiterol Hydrobromide
31868-18-5	Mexazolam
31879-05-7	Fenoprofen
31883-05-3	Moracizine
31884-77-2	Meclozine Hydrochloride
32266-10-7	Hexoprenaline Sulfate
32672-69-8	Mesoridazine
32702-55-9	Benaprizine Hydrochloride
32780-64-6	Labetalol Hydrochloride
32795-44-1	Acecainide
32795-47-4	Nomifensine Maleate
32808-09-6	Papaverine
32828-81-2	Picotamide
32865-01-3	Brompheniramine Maleate (±)
32953-89-2	Rimiterol
32986-56-4	Tobramycin
33005-95-7	Tiaprofenic Acid
33032-12-1	Methapyrilene Fumarate
33069-62-4	Paclitaxel
33124-53-7	Indoramin Hydrochloride
33125-97-2	Etomidate
33213-65-9	Endosulfan (β)
33237-74-0	Aprindine Hydrochloride
33286-22-5	Diltiazem Hydrochloride
33342-05-1	Gliquidone
33369-31-2	Zomepirac
33386-08-2	Buspirone Hydrochloride
33401-94-4	Pyrantel Tartrate
33402-03-8	Metaraminol Tartrate
33419-42-0	Etoposide
33580-30-2	Tertatolol Hydrochloride
33817-20-8	Pivampicillin
34118-92-8	Acecainide Hydrochloride
34123-59-6	Isoproturon
34154-59-1	Meptazinol Hydrochloride (±)
34156-56-4	Foscarnet Sodium (hexahydrate)
34195-34-1	Hydrocodone Tartrate
34214-51-2	Flucloxacillin Sodium (monohydrate)
34262-84-5	Mesocarb
34366-67-1	Hydrocodone Phosphate
34368-04-2	Dobutamine
34381-68-5	Acebutolol Hydrochloride
34552-83-5	Loperamide Hydrochloride
34580-13-7	Ketotifen
34580-14-8	Ketotifen Fumarate
34597-40-5	Fenoprofen Calcium (anhydrous)
34642-77-8	Amoxicillin Sodium
34645-84-6	Fenclofenac
34784-64-0	Tertatolol
34911-55-2	Bupropion
34915-68-9	Bunitrolol
35080-11-6	Prajmalium
35285-68-8	Sodium Ethyl Hydroxybenzoate
35285-69-9	Sodium Propyl Hydroxybenzoate
35604-67-2	Viloxazine Hydrochloride
35711-34-3	Tolmetin Sodium
35915-18-5	Trichlorophenoxyacetic Acid
35941-65-2	Butriptyline
35944-74-2	Metomidate Hydrochloride
36104-80-0	Camazepam
36105-20-1	Flurazepam Monohydrochloride
36141-82-9	Diamfenetide
36167-63-2	Halofantrine Hydrochloride
36322-90-4	Piroxicam
36330-85-5	Fenbufen
36393-56-3	Cathine
36418-22-1	6-Monoacetylmorphine Hydrochloride
36505-84-7	Buspirone
36637-18-0	Etidocaine
36637-19-1	Etidocaine Hydrochloride
36653-54-0	Fazadinium
36688-78-5	Clindamycin Palmitate
36735-22-5	Quazepam
36894-69-6	Labetalol
37091-65-9	Azlocillin Sodium
37091-66-0	Azlocillin
37148-27-9	Clenbuterol
37350-58-6	Metoprolol
37517-26-3	Pipotiazine Palmitate
37517-28-5	Amikacin
37612-13-8	Encainide
37640-71-4	Aprindine
37661-08-8	Bacampicillin Hydrochloride
38194-50-2	Sulindac
38260-01-4	Trientine Dihydrochloride
38304-91-5	Minoxidil
38455-90-2	Methylephedrine Hydrochloride
38641-94-0	Glyphosate Isopropylammonium
38677-85-9	Flunixin
38821-49-7	Carbidopa
38821-53-3	Cefradine (anhydrous)
39562-70-4	Nitrendipine
39809-25-1	Penciclovir
39831-55-5	Amikacin Sulfate
39860-99-6	Pipotiazine
40054-69-1	Etizolam
40180-04-9	Tienilic Acid
40542-65-2	Gestrinone
40828-46-4	Suprofen
41294-56-8	Alfacalcidol
41340-25-4	Etodolac
41342-53-4	Erythromycin Ethylsuccinate
41354-29-4	Cyproheptadine Hydrochloride
41354-30-7	Dimethisterone (monohydrate)
41372-08-1	Methyldopa
41372-10-5	Piperazine Citrate
41372-20-7	Apomorphine Hydrochloride (hemihydrate)
41444-62-6	Codeine Phosphate (hemihydrate)
41510-23-0	Biriperone
41587-36-4	Chloronitroaniline
41708-72-9	Tocainide
41859-67-0	Bezafibrate
42200-33-9	Nadolol
42399-41-7	Diltiazem
42408-82-2	Butorphanol
42461-84-7	Flunixin Meglumine
42542-10-9	Methylenedioxymethamfetamine
42864-78-8	Bevantolol Hydrochloride
42882-96-2	Chlorphenamine
42924-53-8	Nabumetone
43033-72-3	Levacetylmethadol Hydrochloride
43200-80-2	Zopiclone
43210-67-9	Fenbendazole
43229-80-7	Formoterol Fumarate Dihydrate
46817-91-8	Viloxazine
47141-42-4	Levobunolol
48141-64-6	Etafedrine
49564-56-9	Fazadinium Bromide
49656-78-2	Methcathinone Hydrochloride
49745-95-1	Dobutamine Hydrochloride
49746-04-5	Tiotixene Hydrochloride
49746-09-0	Tiotixene Hydrochloride
49842-07-1	Tobramycin
50321-35-2	Morazone Hydrochloride
50906-05-3	Ephedrine
50972-17-3	Bacampicillin
50978-10-4	Cyclomethycaine Sulfate
51022-70-9	Salbutamol Sulfate
51022-71-0	Nabilone
51218-45-2	Metolachlor
51264-14-3	Amsacrine
51322-75-9	Tizanidine
51460-26-5	Carbazochrome Sodium Sulfonate
51481-60-8	Naloxone Hydrochloride (dihydrate)
51481-61-9	Cimetidine
51552-99-9	Diperodon
51781-06-7	Carteolol
51781-21-6	Carteolol Hydrochloride
51888-09-6	Prochlorperazine Mesilate
52022-31-8	Ambenonium Chloride
52128-35-5	Trimetrexate
52214-84-3	Ciprofibrate
52225-20-4	Alpha Tocoferil Acetate
52239-63-1	Thiethylperazine Malate
52432-72-1	Oxeladin Citrate
52438-85-4	Prednisolone
52479-85-3	Exifone
52485-79-7	Buprenorphine
52712-76-2	Bunazosin Hydrochloride
52918-63-5	Deltamethrin
53043-14-4	Amylmetacresol
53123-88-9	Sirolimus
53152-21-9	Buprenorphine Hydrochloride
53164-05-9	Acemetacin
53179-11-6	Loperamide
53496-15-4	Amyl Acetate (*sec*)
53597-27-6	Fendosal
53643-48-4	Vindesine
53746-45-5	Fenoprofen Calcium (dihydrate)
53772-83-1	Zuclopenthixol
53885-35-1	Ticlopidine Hydrochloride
53910-25-1	Pentostatin
53984-74-0	Tocainide Hydrochloride
53984-76-2	Tocainide Hydrochloride
53994-73-3	Cefaclor
54063-32-0	Clobetasone
54063-35-3	Dofamium Chloride
54063-54-6	Reproterol
54143-55-4	Flecainide
54143-56-5	Flecainide Acetate
54143-57-6	Metoclopramide Hydrochloride
54340-58-8	Meptazinol
54350-48-0	Etretinate
54739-18-3	Fluvoxamine
54910-89-3	Fluoxetine
54965-21-8	Albendazole
55079-83-9	Acitretin
55096-26-9	Nalmefene
55142-85-3	Ticlopidine
55294-15-0	Muzolimine
55557-30-7	Levopropoxyphene Napsilate
55812-90-3	Dexamethasone Acetate
56180-94-0	Acarbose
56211-40-6	Torasemide
56390-09-1	Epirubicin Hydrochloride
56392-17-7	Metoprolol Tartrate

CAS no.	Compound
56420-45-2	Epirubicin
56775-88-3	Zimeldine
56974-46-0	Butalamine Hydrochloride
56980-93-9	Celiprolol
56995-20-1	Flupirtine
57041-67-5	Desflurane
57109-90-7	Clorazepate Dipotassium
57262-94-9	Setiptiline
57432-61-8	Methylergometrine Maleate
57470-78-7	Celiprolol Hydrochloride
57524-89-7	Hydrocortisone Valerate
57526-81-5	Prenalterol
57574-09-1	Amineptine
57576-44-0	Aclarubicin
57801-81-7	Brotizolam
57852-57-0	Idarubicin Hydrochloride
57982-77-1	Buserelin
57982-78-2	Budipine
58186-27-9	Idebenone
58207-19-5	Clindamycin Hydrochloride (monohydrate)
58513-59-0	Tiotixene Hydrochloride
58579-51-4	Anagrelide Hydrochloride
58786-99-5	Butorphanol Tartrate
58895-64-0	Nalmefene Hydrochloride
58934-46-6	Lorcainide Hydrochloride
58957-92-9	Idarubicin
59122-46-2	Misoprostol
59170-23-9	Bevantolol
59263-76-2	Meptazinol Hydrochloride
59277-89-3	Aciclovir
59302-14-6	Furaltadone (±)
59333-67-4	Fluoxetine Hydrochloride
59467-70-8	Midazolam
59467-94-6	Midazolam Maleate
59467-96-8	Midazolam Hydrochloride
59729-31-6	Lorcainide
59729-32-7	Citalopram Hydrobromide
59729-33-8	Citalopram
59804-37-4	Tenoxicam
59865-13-3	Ciclosporin
59866-76-1	Bibenzonium
59917-39-4	Vindesine Sulfate
60142-96-3	Gabapentin
60491-10-3	Strychnine Sulfate (pentahydrate)
60525-15-7	Zimeldine Hydrochloride (anhydrous)
60583-39-3	Brucine Sulfate (heptahydrate)
60643-86-9	Vigabatrin
60929-23-9	Indeloxazine
60991-48-2	Ajmaline Monoethanolate
61036-62-2	Teicoplanin
61036-64-4	Teicoplanin
61129-30-4	Zimeldine Hydrochloride (monohydrate)
61197-73-7	Loprazolam
61260-05-7	Prenalterol Hydrochloride
61336-70-7	Amoxicillin Trihydrate
61337-67-5	Mirtazapine
61718-82-9	Fluvoxamine Maleate
61802-93-5	Metaclazepam Hydrochloride
61825-94-3	Oxaliplatin
61869-08-7	Paroxetine
62571-86-2	Captopril
62658-63-3	Bopindolol
63074-08-8	Terazosin Hydrochloride
63547-13-7	Adrafinil
63585-09-1	Foscarnet Sodium
63590-64-7	Terazosin
63659-18-7	Betaxolol
63659-19-8	Betaxolol Hydrochloride
63661-61-0	Budipine Hydrochloride
63675-72-9	Nisoldipine
63717-04-4	Quinidine
64024-15-3	Pentazocine
64053-00-5	Zuclopenthixol Decanoate
64057-70-1	Methylenedioxymethamfetamine
64092-48-4	Zomepirac Sodium (anhydrous)
64092-49-5	Zomepirac Sodium (dihydrate)
64228-79-1	Atracurium
64228-81-5	Atracurium Besilate
64461-82-1	Tizanidine Hydrochloride
64490-92-2	Tolmetin Sodium
65043-22-3	Indeloxazine Hydrochloride
65141-46-0	Nicorandil
65271-80-9	Mitozantrone
65277-42-1	Ketoconazole
65484-56-2	Quinidine Polygalacturonate (hydrate)
66051-63-6	Halofantrine (±)
66085-59-4	Nimodipine
66104-22-1	Pergolide
66104-23-2	Pergolide Mesilate
66357-35-5	Ranitidine
66357-59-3	Ranitidine Hydrochloride
66376-36-1	Alendronic Acid
66722-44-9	Bisoprolol
66722-45-0	Bisoprolol Fumarate (hemifumerate)
66778-36-7	Encainide
66794-74-9	Encainide Hydrochloride
66981-73-5	Tianeptine
67037-37-0	Eflornithine
67227-56-9	Fenoldopam
67227-57-0	Fenoldopam Mesilate
67434-14-4	Benoxaprofen
68206-94-0	Cloricromen
68278-23-9	Eflornithine Hydrochloride
68291-97-4	Zonisamide
68359-37-5	Cyfluthrin
68475-42-3	Anagrelide
68630-75-1	Buserelin Acetate
68693-11-8	Modafinil
68797-31-9	Econazole Nitrate
68844-77-9	Astemizole
69049-06-5	Alfentanil Hydrochloride
69049-73-6	Nedocromil
69049-74-7	Nedocromil Sodium
69525-81-1	Morantel Citrate
69655-05-6	Didanosine
69657-51-8	Aciclovir Sodium
69756-53-2	Halofantrine
69815-49-2	Noradrenaline Acid Tartrate (monohydrate)
70024-40-7	Terazosin Hydrochloride Dihydrate
70111-54-5	Loprazolam Mesilate (anhydrous)
70356-03-5	Cefaclor
70393-85-0	Glyphosate Sesquisodium Salt
70476-82-3	Mitozantrone Hydrochloride
70879-28-6	Alfentanil Hydrochloride
70918-01-3	Doxazosin Hydrochloride
70958-86-0	Amosulalol Monohydrochloride
71125-38-7	Meloxicam
71195-58-9	Alfentanil
71320-77-9	Moclobemide
71395-14-7	Tocainide Hydrochloride
71486-22-1	Vinorelbine
71620-89-8	Reboxetine
71675-85-9	Amisulpride
71963-77-4	Artemether
72150-17-5	Eptazocine Hydrobromide
72432-10-1	Aniracetam
72509-76-3	Felodipine
72522-13-5	Eptazocine
72558-82-8	Ceftazidime
72559-06-9	Rifabutin
72810-59-4	Torasemide Sodium
72956-09-3	Carvedilol
73220-03-8	Remoxipride Hydrochloride (anhydrous)
73368-74-8	Phenoxymethylpenicillin Calcium
73384-59-5	Ceftriaxone
73573-87-2	Formoterol
73590-58-6	Omeprazole
73963-72-1	Cilostazol
74011-58-8	Enoxaparin
74103-06-3	Ketorolac
74103-07-4	Ketorolac Trometamol
74197-85-8	Doxazosin
74341-78-9	Methylenedioxyethylamfetamine Hydrochloride
74536-44-0	Metadoxine
74578-69-1	Ceftriaxone Sodium
74697-28-2	Cloricromen Hydrochloride
75272-39-8	Nemonapride
75330-75-5	Lovastatin
75438-57-2	Moxonidine
75438-58-3	Moxonidine Hydrochloride
75507-68-5	Flupirtine Maleate
75607-67-9	Fludarabine Phosphate
75695-93-1	Isradipine
75706-12-6	Leflunomide
75847-73-3	Enalapril
75975-70-1	Cefradine (monohydrate)
76095-16-4	Enalapril Maleate
76420-72-9	Enalaprilat
76547-98-3	Lisinopril
76824-35-6	Famotidine
76932-56-4	Nafarelin
76963-41-2	Nizatidine
77337-73-6	Acamprosate Calcium
77337-76-9	Acamprosate
77472-70-9	Carphedon
77671-31-9	Enoximone
77883-43-3	Doxazosin Mesilate
78110-38-0	Aztreonam
78246-49-8	Paroxetine Hydrochloride Hemihydrate
78415-72-2	Milrinone
78439-06-2	Ceftazidime Pentahydrate
78755-81-4	Flumazenil
79350-37-1	Cefixime
79449-98-2	Cabastine
79516-68-0	Levocabastine
79517-01-4	Octreotide Acetate
79547-78-7	Levocabastine Hydrochloride
79559-97-0	Sertraline Hydrochloride
79617-96-2	Sertraline
79645-27-5	Tobramycin
79794-75-5	Loratadine
79902-63-9	Simvastatin
79983-71-4	Hexaconazole
80012-43-7	Epinastine
80125-14-0	Remoxipride
80214-83-1	Roxithromycin
80474-14-2	Fluticasone Propionate
80573-04-2	Balsalazide
80755-51-7	Bunazosin
81093-37-0	Pravastatin
81098-60-4	Cisapride
81103-11-9	Clarithromycin
81131-70-6	Pravastatin Sodium
81161-17-3	Esmolol Hydrochloride
81403-68-1	Alfuzosin Hydrochloride
81403-80-7	Alfuzosin
81409-90-7	Cabergoline
81591-81-3	Glyphosate Trimesium
81732-46-9	Bambuterol Hydrochloride

CAS no.	*Compound*
81732-65-2	Bambuterol
81801-12-9	Xamoterol
82410-32-0	Ganciclovir
82419-36-1	Ofloxacin
82586-52-5	Moexipril Hydrochloride
82586-55-8	Quinapril Hydrochloride
82586-57-0	Moexipril Diacid Hydrochloride
82626-48-0	Zolpidem
82752-99-6	Nefazodone Hydrochloride
82768-85-2	Quinaprilat
82801-81-8	Methylenedioxyethylamfetamine
82834-16-0	Perindopril
82857-38-3	Bopindolol Malonate
82952-64-5	Trimetrexate D-Glucuronate
82964-04-3	Tolrestat
83150-76-9	Octreotide
83348-52-1	Doxacurium Chloride
83366-66-9	Nefazodone
83380-47-6	Ofloxacin
83480-29-9	Voglibose
83602-05-5	Spiraprilat
83647-97-6	Spirapril
83799-24-0	Fexofenadine
83881-51-0	Cetirizine
83881-52-1	Cetirizine Dihydrochloride
83905-01-5	Azithromycin
83915-83-7	Lisinopril Dihydrate
84031-17-4	Metaclazepam
84057-84-1	Lamotrigine
84057-94-3	Esmolol
84057-95-4	Ropivacaine
84371-65-3	Mifepristone
84625-61-6	Itraconazole
84680-54-6	Enalaprilat
85320-68-9	Amosulalol
85329-89-1	Cabergoline Diphosphate
85441-61-8	Quinapril
85622-93-1	Temozolomide
85721-05-7	Zuclopenthixol Acetate
85721-33-1	Ciprofloxacin
86189-69-7	Felodipine
86197-47-9	Dopexamine
86220-42-0	Nafarelin Acetate Hydrate
86386-73-4	Fluconazole
86393-32-0	Ciprofloxacin Hydrochloride (monohydrate)
86483-48-9	Ciprofloxacin Hydrochloride (anhydrous)
86484-91-5	Dopexamine Dihydrochloride
86541-74-4	Benazepril Hydrochloride
86541-75-5	Benazepril
87056-78-8	Quinagolide
87269-97-4	Ramiprilat
87333-19-5	Ramipril
87679-37-6	Trandolapril
87760-53-0	Tandospirone
87848-99-5	Acrivastine
87913-26-6	Bromantane
88150-42-9	Amlodipine
88150-47-4	Amlodipine Maleate
88495-63-0	Artesunate
88889-14-9	Fosinopril Sodium
89365-50-4	Salmeterol
89371-37-9	Imidapril
89371-44-8	Imidaprilat
89396-94-1	Imidapril Monohydrochloride
89419-40-9	Clospipramine
89565-68-4	Tropisetron
89778-26-7	Toremifene
89778-27-8	Toremifene Citrate
89796-99-6	Aceclofenac
89987-06-4	Tiludronic Acid
90357-06-5	Bicalutamide
90729-43-4	Ebastine
90730-93-1	Xamoterol Hemifumarate
91374-20-8	Ropinirole
91374-21-9	Ropinirole
92077-78-6	Cilazapril
92134-98-0	Fosphenytoin Sodium
92623-85-3	Milnacipran
93390-81-9	Fosphenytoin
93413-69-5	Venlafaxine
93479-97-1	Glimepiride
93633-92-2	Amosulalol Monohydrochloride
93664-94-9	Nemonapride
93957-54-1	Fluvastatin
93957-55-2	Fluvastatin Sodium
94188-84-8	Clopidogrel
94424-50-7	Quinagolide Hydrochloride
94749-08-3	Salmeterol Xinafoate
94841-17-5	Spirapril Hydrochloride
95058-81-4	Gemcitabine
95153-31-4	Perindoprilat
95233-18-4	Atovaquone
95510-70-6	Omeprazole Sodium
96020-91-6	Eflornithine Hydrochloride Monohydrate
96829-58-2	Orlistat
96946-42-8	Cisatracurium Besilate
97240-79-4	Topiramate
97322-87-7	Troglitazone
97682-44-5	Irinotecan
97845-62-0	Penciclovir Sodium
97867-33-9	Ciprofloxacin Lactate
98043-60-8	Clospipramine Dihydrochloride
98048-97-6	Fosinopril
98319-26-7	Finasteride
98717-15-8	Ropivacaine Hydrocloride
98769-81-4	Reboxetine
98769-82-5	Reboxetine Mesilate
99200-09-6	Nebivolol
99283-10-0	Molgramostim
99294-93-6	Zolpidem Tartrate
99300-78-4	Venlafaxine Hydrochloride
99495-87-1	Flecainide (±)
99614-01-4	Ondansetron Hydrochloride (Dihydrate)
99614-02-5	Ondansetron
100286-90-6	Irinotecan Hydrochloride
100286-97-3	Milrinone Lactate
100986-85-4	Levofloxacin
101152-94-7	Milnacipran Hydrochloride
101626-68-0	Nedocromil Calcium
102625-70-7	Pantoprazole
102767-28-2	Levetiracetam
103577-45-3	Lansoprazole
103745-39-7	Fasudil
103775-10-6	Moexipril
103890-78-4	Lacidipine
104227-87-4	Famciclovir
104344-23-2	Bisoprolol Fumarate (hemifumerate)
104376-79-6	Ceftriaxone Sodium
104632-26-0	Pramipexole
104987-11-3	Tacrolimus
105628-07-7	Fasudil Hydrochloride
105826-92-4	Tropisetron Hydrochloride
105827-78-9	Imidacloprid
105857-23-6	Alteplase
106133-20-4	Tamsulosin
106266-06-2	Risperidone
106463-17-6	Tamsulosin Hydrochloride
106516-24-9	Sertindole
106819-53-8	Doxacurium Chloride
106861-44-3	Mivacurium Chloride
107007-99-8	Granisetron Hydrochloride
107133-36-8	Perindopril Erbumine
107753-78-6	Zafirlukast
107868-30-4	Exemestane
107910-75-8	Ganciclovir Sodium
108050-54-0	Tilmicosin
108612-45-9	Mizolastine
108736-35-2	Lanreotide
108929-04-0	Epinastine Hydrochloride
109581-93-3	Tacrolimus Monohydrate
109889-09-0	Granisetron
110429-35-1	Paroxetine Hydrochloride (Hemihydrate)
110942-02-4	Aldesleukin
111470-99-6	Amlodipine Besilate
111974-69-7	Quetiapine
111974-72-2	Quetiapine Hemifumarate
112457-95-1	Tandospirone Citrate
112809-51-5	Letrozole
112887-68-0	Raltitrexed
113665-84-2	Clopidogrel
113775-47-6	Dexmedetomidine
113852-37-2	Cidofovir
114798-26-4	Losartan
114977-28-5	Docetaxel
115007-34-6	Mycophenolate Mofetil
115103-54-3	Tiagabine
115256-11-6	Dofetilide
115956-12-2	Dolasetron
115956-13-3	Dolasetron Methanesulfonate
116644-53-2	Mibefradil
116666-63-8	Mibefradil Dihydrochloride
117591-79-4	Remoxipride Hydrochloride (monohydrate)
117772-70-0	Azithromycin
117976-89-3	Rabeprazole
117976-90-6	Rabeprazole Sodium
119302-91-9	Rocuronium Bromide
119413-54-6	Topotecan Hydrochloride
120011-70-3	Donepezil Hydrochloride
120014-06-4	Donepezil
120202-66-6	Clopidogrel Bisulfate
120511-73-1	Anastrozole
120608-46-0	Duteplase
121268-17-5	Alendronate Sodium
121679-13-8	Naratriptan
121679-19-4	Naratriptan Hydrochloride
122111-03-9	Gemcitabine Hydrochloride
122647-31-8	Ibutilide
122647-32-9	Ibutilide Fumarate
123441-03-2	Rivastigmine
123948-87-8	Topotecan
124750-99-8	Losartan Potassium
124832-26-4	Valaciclovir
124832-27-5	Valaciclovir Hydrochloride
124937-51-5	Tolterodine
125317-39-7	Vinorelbine Tartrate
127779-20-8	Saquinavir
127984-74-1	Lanreotide Acetate
128345-62-0	Ranitidine Bismuth Citrate
128794-94-5	Mycophenolate Mofetil
129101-54-8	Rivastigmine Hydrogen Tartrate
129618-40-2	Nevirapine
130929-57-6	Entacapone
132112-35-7	Ropivacaine Hydrocloride (Monohydrate)
132539-06-1	Olanzapine
132875-61-7	Remifentanil
133652-38-7	Reteplase
134523-00-5	Atorvastatin
134523-03-8	Atorvastatin Calcium
134678-17-4	Lamivudine
135062-02-1	Repaglinide
135886-70-3	Gallium Nitrate (nonahydrate)
136426-54-5	Fluquinconazole
136470-78-5	Abacavir

CAS no.	*Compound*
136572-09-3	Irinotecan Hydrochloride (Trihydrate)
136817-59-9	Delavirdine
137862-53-4	Valsartan
138068-37-8	Lepirudin
138199-71-0	Levofloxacin Hemihydrate
138261-41-3	Imidacloprid
138402-11-6	Irbesartan
138452-21-8	Fexofenadine Hydrochloride
138982-67-9	Ziprasidone Hydrochloride (Monohydrate)
139110-80-8	Zanamivir
139264-17-8	Zolmitriptan
139481-59-7	Candesartan
139755-83-2	Sildenafil
141505-33-1	Levosimendan
142373-60-2	Tirofiban Hydrochloride (Monohydrate)
143201-11-0	Cerivastatin Sodium
143388-64-1	Naratriptan Hydrochloride
143558-00-3	Rocuronium
144034-80-0	Rizatriptan
144494-65-5	Tirofiban
144701-48-4	Telmisartan
145040-37-5	Candesartan Cilexetil
145202-66-0	Rizatriptan Benzoate
145599-86-6	Cerivastatin
145821-59-6	Tiagabine Hydrochloride
146939-27-7	Ziprasidone
147221-93-0	Delavirdine monomethane-sulfonate
148408-66-6	Docetaxel trihydrate
149845-06-7	Saquinavir Mesilate
149845-07-8	Disodium Tiludronate
150378-17-9	Indinavir
150399-21-6	Balsalazide Disodium
150915-40-5	Tirofiban Hydrochloride (Monohydrate)
151767-02-1	Montelukast Sodium
154323-57-6	Almotriptan
154361-50-9	Capecitabine
154598-52-4	Efavirenz
155213-67-5	Ritonavir
155453-10-4	Disodium Tiludronate
156137-99-4	Rapacuronium Bromide
156604-79-4	Dexketoprofen trometamol
157810-81-6	Indinavir Sulfate
158966-92-8	Montelukast
159989-64-7	Nelfinavir
159989-65-8	Nelfinavir
161814-49-9	Amprenavir
162011-90-7	Rofecoxib
164579-32-2	Pantoprazole Sodium (Sesquihydrate)
168146-84-7	Abacavir Succinate
169590-42-5	Celecoxib
171599-83-0	Sildenafil Citrate
174722-31-7	Rituximab
181183-52-8	Almotriptan Maleate
183325-78-2	Calfactant
191217-81-9	Pramipexole Dihydrochloride (Monohydrate)

Molecular Formulae

As_2O_3
Arsenic Trioxide
CCl_2F_2
Dichlorodifluoromethane
CCl_3F
Trichlorofluoromethane
CCl_4
Carbon Tetrachloride
$CHCl_3$
Chloroform
CH_2Cl_2
Methylene Chloride
$CH_2Cl_2Na_2O_6P_2$
Disodium Clodronate
CH_2O
Formaldehyde
CH_2O_2
Formic Acid
CH_3Br
Methyl Bromide
$CH_3Br.20H_2O$
Methyl Bromide Hydrate
$CH_4Cl_2O_6P_2$
Clodronic Acid
CH_4N_2O
Urea
$CH_4N_2O_2$
Hydroxycarbamide
CH_4O
Methanol
CN
Cyanide
CNa_3O_5P
Foscarnet Sodium
$C_2Cl_2F_4$
Cryofluorane
C_2Cl_4
Tetrachloroethylene
$C_2HBrClF_3$
Halothane
C_2HCl_3
Trichloroethylene
$C_2H_2Cl_4$
Tetrachloroethane
$C_2H_2FNaO_2$
Sodium Fluoroacetate
$C_2H_2O_4$
Oxalic Acid
$C_2H_3Cl_3$
Trichloroethane
$C_2H_3Cl_3NaO_4P$
Triclofos Sodium
$C_2H_3Cl_3O$
Trichloroethanol
$C_2H_3Cl_3O_2$
Cloral Hydrate
$C_2H_3FO_2$
Fluoroacetic Acid
C_2H_4FNO
Fluoroacetamide
$C_2H_4N_4$
Aminotriazole
C_2H_4O
Acetaldehyde
$C_2H_4O_2$
Acetic Acid Glacial
C_2H_5OH
Ethanol
C_2H_6OS
Dimethyl Sulfoxide
$C_2H_6O_2$
Ethylene Glycol
C_2H_7NO
Monoethanolamine
$C_2H_7NO,C_{18}H_{34}O_2$
Monoethanolamine Oleate
$C_2H_8NO_2PS$
Methamidophos
$C_2H_8N_2,H_2O$
Ethylenediamine Hydrate
$C_3H_2ClF_5O$
Enflurane
$C_3H_2F_6O$
Desflurane
$C_3H_3N_3O_2S$
Aminonitrothiazole
$C_3H_4Cl_2F_2O$
Methoxyflurane
$C_3H_5NNaO_5P$
Glyphosate Sesquisodium Salt
$C_3H_5N_3O_9$
Glyceryl Trinitrate
$C_3H_6N_2O_2$
Cycloserine
C_3H_6O
Acetone
$C_3H_7NO_2$
Urethane
C_3H_7OH
Propanol
$C_3H_8NO_5P$
Glyphosate
$C_3H_8N_2OS$
Noxytiolin
C_3H_8O
Isopropyl Alcohol
$C_3H_8OS_2$
Dimercaprol
$C_4H_3FN_2O_2$
Fluorouracil
$C_4H_3F_7O$
Sevoflurane
$C_4H_4FN_3O$
Flucytosine
$C_4H_4N_2O_3$
Barbituric Acid
$C_4H_5NO_2$
Succinimide
$C_4H_5N_4NaO_3S_2$
Acetazolamide Sodium
$C_4H_6N_2$
Fomepizole
$C_4H_6N_2S$
Thiamazole
$C_4H_6N_4O_3S_2$
Acetazolamide
$C_4H_6O_2$
Gamma-butyrolactone
$C_4H_6O_3$
(*S*)-3-Hydroxy-gamma-butyrolactone
$C_4H_7Cl_2O_4P$
Dichlorvos
$C_4H_7Cl_3O$
Chlorobutanol
$C_4H_7Cl_3O_2$
Butylchloral Hydrate
$C_4H_8Cl_3O_4P$
Trichlorfon
$C_4H_8NaO_3$
Sodium Gamma-hydroxybutyrate
C_4H_8O
Methyl Ethyl Ketone
$C_4H_8O_2$
Ethyl Acetate
$C_4H_8O_3$
Gamma-hydroxybutyric Acid
$C_4H_{10}N_2$
Piperazine
$C_4H_{10}N_2,6H_2O$
Piperazine Hydrate
$C_4H_{10}N_2,C_6H_{10}O_4$
Piperazine Adipate
$C_4H_{10}N_2,C_{10}H_{14}CaN_2O_8$
Piperazine Calcium Edetate
$C_4H_{10}N_2,H_3PO_4,H_2O$
Piperazine Phosphate
$(C_4H_{10}N_2)_3,2C_6H_8O_7,xH_2O$
Piperazine Citrate
$C_4H_{11}NO_3$
Trometamol
$C_4H_{11}N_5$
Metformin
$C_4H_{11}N_5,HCl$
Metformin Hydrochloride
$C_4H_{12}NNaO_7P_2,3H_2O$
Alendronate Sodium
$C_4H_{12}N_2$
Putrescine
$C_4H_{13}NO_7P_2$
Alendronic Acid
$C_5H_4N_4O$
Allopurinol
$C_5H_4N_4S,H_2O$
Mercaptopurine
$C_5H_5N_3O$
Pyrazinamide
$C_5H_5N_3O_3S$
Aminitrozole
$C_5H_5N_5S$
Tioguanine
$C_5H_6N_2OS$
Methylthiouracil
$C_5H_7NO_3$
Dimethadione
$C_5H_7N_3O_2$
Dimetridazole
$C_5H_7N_3O_2,HCl$
Dimetridazole Hydrochloride
$C_5H_8N_4O_3S_2$
Methazolamide
$C_5H_8N_4O_{12}$
Pentaerithrityl Tetranitrate

$C_5H_9Cl_2N_3O_2$
Carmustine
$C_5H_9NO_3S$
Acetylcysteine
$C_5H_9N_3$
Ametazole
Histamine
$C_5H_9N_3,2HCl$
Ametazole Hydrochloride
Histamine Hydrochloride
$C_5H_9N_3,2H_3PO_4$
Histamine Acid Phosphate
$C_5H_{10}NNaS_2$
Ditiocarb Sodium Trihydrate
$C_5H_{10}NNaS_2,3H_2O$
Ditiocarb Sodium
$C_5H_{10}NS_2$
Ditiocarb
$C_5H_{11}NO_2$
Betaine
Amyl Nitrite
$C_5H_{11}NO_2,HCl$
Betaine Hydrochloride
$C_5H_{11}NO_2S$
Penicillamine
$C_5H_{11}NO_2S,HCl$
Penicillamine Hydrochloride
$C_5H_{12}NO_3PS_2$
Dimethoate
$C_5H_{12}NO_4PS$
Omethoate
$C_5H_{12}O$
Amyl Alcohol
$C_5H_{14}ClNO$
Choline Chloride
$[C_5H_{14}NO]^+$
Choline
$C_5H_{14}N_2$
Cadaverine
$C_5H_{15}NO_2$
Choline Hydroxide
$C_5H_{15}N_2O_3PS$
Amifostine
C_6HCl_5O
Pentachlorophenol
$C_6H_4Cl_2$
Paradichlorobenzene
C_6H_5CHO
Benzaldehyde
$C_6H_5ClN_2O_2$
Chloronitroaniline
C_6H_5ClO
Parachlorophenol
$C_6H_5Li_3O_7,4H_2O$
Lithium Citrate
$C_6H_5NH_2$
Aniline
$C_6H_5NO_2$
Nicotinic Acid
Nitrobenzene
C_6H_5O
Phenol
C_6H_6
Benzene
C_6H_6ClN
2-Chloroaniline
3-Chloroaniline
4-Chloroaniline
Chloroaniline
$C_6H_6Cl_2N_2O_4S_2$
Diclofenamide
$C_6H_6Cl_6$
Lindane
Benzene Hexachloride
$C_6H_6N_2O$
Nicotinamide
$C_6H_6N_4O_3S$
Niridazole
$C_6H_6N_4O_4$
Nitrofurazone
$C_6H_6N_6O_2$
Temozolomide
$C_6H_6O_2$
Hydroquinone
Resorcinol
$C_6H_7KO_2$
Potassium Sorbate
C_6H_7NO
4-Aminophenol
Nicotinyl Alcohol
$C_6H_7NO,C_4H_6O_6$
Nicotinyl Tartrate
$C_6H_7N_3O$
Isoniazid
$C_6H_7N_3O,C_7H_7NO_3$
Isoniazid Aminosalicylate
$C_6H_7NaO_6$
Sodium Ascorbate
C_6H_8ClNS
Clomethiazole
$C_6H_8ClN_7O$
Amiloride
$C_6H_8ClN_7O,HCl,2H_2O$
Amiloride Hydrochloride
$C_6H_8N_2$
Paraphenylenediamine
$C_6H_8N_2O_2S$
Sulfanilamide
$C_6H_8N_2O_8$
Isosorbide Dinitrate
$C_6H_8O_2$
Sorbic Acid
$C_6H_8O_6$
Ascorbic Acid
$C_6H_9NO_3$
Trimethadione
$C_6H_9NO_6$
Isosorbide Mononitrate
$C_6H_9N_3O_3$
Metronidazole
$C_6H_{10}N_4$
Pentetrazol
$C_6H_{10}O$
Methylpentynol
$C_6H_{11}BrN_2O_2$
Bromisoval
$C_6H_{11}NO_2$
Vigabatrin
$C_6H_{12}F_2N_2O_2$
Eflornithine
$C_6H_{12}N_3PS$
Thiotepa
$C_6H_{12}N_4$
Methenamine
$C_6H_{12}N_4,C_8H_8O_3$
Methenamine Mandelate
$C_6H_{12}N_4,C_9H_9NO_3$
Methenamine Hippurate
$C_6H_{13}ClF_2N_2O_2$
Eflornithine Hydrochloride
$C_6H_{13}NO_2$
Aminocaproic Acid
$C_6H_{14}O_6$
Mannitol
$C_6H_{14}O_6S_2$
Busulfan
$C_6H_{15}ClF_2N_2O_3$
Eflornithine Hydrochloride Monohydrate
$C_6H_{15}ClN_2O_2$
Carbachol
$C_6H_{15}N_5$
Buformin
$C_6H_{15}N_5,HCl$
Buformin Hydrochloride
$C_6H_{15}O_3PS_2$
Demeton-S-methyl
$C_6H_{17}N_2O_5P$
Glyphosate Isopropylammonium
$C_6H_{18}N_4$
Trientine
$C_6H_{18}N_4,2HCl$
Trientine Dihydrochloride
$C_7H_3IN_2O_3$
Nitroxinil
$C_7H_3IN_2O_3,C_8H_{19}NO_5$
Nitroxinil Eglumine
$C_7H_4ClNO_2$
Chlorzoxazone
$C_7H_4NNaO_3S,2H_2O$
Saccharin Sodium
$C_7H_5ClN_3NaO_4S_2$
Chlorothiazide Sodium
$C_7H_5Cl_2NO_4S$
Halazone
$C_7H_5NO_3S$
Saccharin
$C_7H_5NaO_3$
Sodium Salicylate
$C_7H_5O_2Na$
Sodium Benzoate
$C_7H_6ClNO_2$
Chloronitrotoluene
$C_7H_6ClN_3O_4S_2$
Chlorothiazide
$C_7H_6KNO_2$
Potassium Aminobenzoate
$C_7H_6KNO_3$
Potassium Aminosalicylate
$C_7H_6NNaO_3,2H_2O$
Sodium Aminosalicylate
$C_7H_6N_2O_5$
Dinitro-orthocresol
$C_7H_6O_2$
Benzoic Acid
$C_7H_6O_3$
Salicylic Acid
$C_7H_7ClNNaO_2S,3H_2O$
Tosylchloramide Sodium
$C_7H_7ClNa_2O_6P_2S$
Disodium Tiludronate
C_7H_7ClO
Chlorocresol
$C_7H_7Cl_2NO$
Clopidol
$C_7H_7Cl_3NO_3PS$
Chlorpyrifos-methyl
$C_7H_7NO_2$
Aminobenzoic Acid
Methyl Nicotinate
Salicylamide
$C_7H_7NO_3$
Aminosalicylic Acid
$C_7H_7N_4NaO_2$
Theophylline Sodium Glycinate
C_7H_8
Toluene
C_7H_8ClN
Chloromethylaniline
$C_7H_8ClN_3O_4S_2$
Hydrochlorothiazide
$C_7H_8N_4O_2$
Theobromine
Theophylline

$C_8H_{19}O_2PS_3$
Disulfoton
$C_8H_{19}O_3PS_2$
Demeton-S
$C_8H_{20}NO_6P$
Choline Alfoscerate
$C_9H_5Br_2NO$
Broxyquinoline
C_9H_5ClINO
Clioquinol
$C_9H_5I_2NO$
Diiodohydroxyquinoline
$C_9H_6Cl_6O_3S$
Endosulfan
$C_9H_6N_2O_3$
Nitroxoline
$C_9H_7Cl_2N_5$
Lamotrigine
C_9H_7NO
Hydroxyquinoline
$C_9H_7N_7O_2S$
Azathioprine
$C_9H_8ClN_5S$
Tizanidine
$C_9H_8N_2O_2$
Pemoline
$C_9H_8N_3NaO_2S_2,5H_2O$
Sulfathiazole Sodium
$C_9H_8O_4$
Aspirin
$C_9H_9ClO_3$
Methylchlorophenoxyacetic Acid
$C_9H_9Cl_2NO$
Propanil
$C_9H_9Cl_2NO_2$
Diloxanide
$C_9H_9Cl_2N_3$
Clonidine
$C_9H_9Cl_2N_3,HCl$
Clonidine Hydrochloride
$C_9H_9Cl_2N_5S,HCl$
Tizanidine Hydrochloride
$C_9H_9N_2NaO_3$
Sodium Aminohippurate
$C_9H_9N_3O_2S_2$
Sulfathiazole
$C_9H_9N_3S$
Amiphenazole
$C_9H_9N_3S,HCl$
Amiphenazole Hydrochloride
$C_9H_9NaO_3$
Sodium Ethyl Hydroxybenzoate
$C_9H_{10}ClN_5O_2$
Imidacloprid
$C_9H_{10}Cl_2N_2O$
Diuron
$C_9H_{10}Cl_2N_2O_2$
Linuron
$C_9H_{10}N_2O_3$
Aminohippuric Acid
$C_9H_{10}N_2O_3S_2$
Ethoxzolamide
$C_9H_{10}N_2S$
Etisazole
$C_9H_{10}N_2S,HCl$
Etisazole Hydrochloride
$C_9H_{10}N_4O_2S_2$
Sulfamethizole
$C_9H_{10}O_3$
Ethyl Hydroxybenzoate
$C_9H_{10}O_5$
Ethyl Gallate
$C_9H_{11}ClN_2O_2$
Monolinuron
$C_9H_{11}ClO_3$
Chlorphenesin
$C_9H_{11}Cl_2N_3O_4S_2$
Methyclothiazide
$C_9H_{11}Cl_3NO_3PS$
Chlorpyrifos
$C_9H_{11}F_2N_3O_4$
Gemcitabine
$C_9H_{11}F_2N_3O_4,HCl$
Gemcitabine Hydrochloride
$C_9H_{11}IN_2O_5$
Idoxuridine
$C_9H_{11}N$
Tranylcypromine
$C_9H_{11}NO_2$
Benzocaine
Etenzamide
$C_9H_{11}NO_3$
Styramate
$C_9H_{11}NO_4$
Levodopa
$C_9H_{11}NO_5$
Droxidopa
$C_9H_{12}ClN_3O_4S_2$
Ethiazide
$C_9H_{12}ClN_5O$
Moxonidine
$C_9H_{12}ClN_5O.xHCl$
Moxonidine Hydrochloride
$C_9H_{12}Cl_2N_4O$
Guanoclor
$C_9H_{12}NO_5PS$
Fenitrothion
Dexamfetamine Phosphate
$C_9H_{12}N_2S$
Protionamide
$C_9H_{12}N_4O_3$
Etofylline
$C_9H_{12}N_5NaO_4$
Ganciclovir Sodium
$C_9H_{13}BrN_2O_2$
Pyridostigmine Bromide
$C_9H_{13}N$
Amfetamine
Dexamfetamine
Levamfetamine
$C_9H_{13}NO$
Cathine
Hydroxyamfetamine
Phenylpropanolamine
$C_9H_{13}NO_2$
Metaraminol
Oxedrine
Ethinamate
Phenylephrine
$C_9H_{13}NO_2,C_4H_6O_6$
Metaraminol Tartrate
$C_9H_{13}NO_2,HCl$
Phenylephrine Hydrochloride
$C_9H_{13}NO_3$
Normetadrenaline
Adrenaline
$C_9H_{13}NO_3,C_4H_6O_6$
Adrenaline Acid Tartrate
$C_9H_{13}NO_3,HCl$
Adrenaline Hydrochloride
$C_9H_{13}NO,HBr$
Hydroxyamfetamine Hydrobromide
$C_9H_{13}NO,HCl$
Cathine Hydrochloride
Phenylpropanolamine Hydrochloride
$C_9H_{13}N_3O$
Iproniazid
$C_9H_{13}N_3O_3$
Zalcitabine
$C_9H_{13}N_3O_5$
Cytarabine
$C_9H_{13}N_3O_5,HCl$
Cytarabine Hydrochloride
$C_9H_{13}N_3O,H_3PO_4$
Iproniazid Phosphate
$C_9H_{13}N_5O_4$
Ganciclovir
$C_9H_{13}N,H_3PO_4$
Amfetamine Phosphate
$C_9H_{14}N_2O_3$
Metharbital
$C_9H_{14}N_4O_3$
Nimorazole
$C_9H_{15}BrN_2O_3$
Acecarbromal
$C_9H_{15}NO_3$
Ecgonine
$C_9H_{15}NO_3,HCl$
Ecgonine Hydrochloride
$C_9H_{15}NO_3S$
Captopril
$C_9H_{15}N_5O$
Minoxidil
$C_9H_{16}ClN_5$
Propazine
Terbutylazine
$C_9H_{16}N_2O_2$
Apronal
$C_9H_{17}NO_2$
Gabapentin
$C_9H_{17}N_5S$
Ametryne
$C_9H_{18}N_2O_4$
Meprobamate
$C_9H_{18}N_6$
Altretamine
$C_9H_{19}N$
Cyclopentamine
Isometheptene
$C_9H_{19}NO_4$
Dexpanthenol
$C_9H_{19}NO_7$
Choline Bitartrate
$C_9H_{19}N,HCl$
Cyclopentamine Hydrochloride
Isometheptene Hydrochloride
$C_9H_{23}INO_3PS$
Ecothiopate Iodide
$C_{10}H_5Cl_7$
Heptachlor
$C_{10}H_6Cl_8$
Chlordane
$C_{10}H_7Cl_2NO$
Chlorquinaldol
$C_{10}H_7Cl_2N_3O$
Anagrelide
$C_{10}H_7N_3S$
Tiabendazole
$C_{10}H_8$
Naphthalene
$C_{10}H_8ClN_4O_2S,Na$
Sulfachlorpyridazine Sodium
$C_{10}H_8Cl_3N_3O$
Anagrelide Hydrochloride
$C_{10}H_8O$
Betanaphthol
$C_{10}H_9ClN_4O_2S$
Sulfachlorpyridazine
$C_{10}H_9N_4NaO_2S$
Sulfadiazine Sodium
$C_{10}H_{10}N_4OS$
Metisazone
$C_{10}H_{10}N_4O_2S$
Sulfadiazine

$C_{10}H_{10}O_4$
Dimethyl Phthalate
$C_{10}H_{11}BrN_2O_3$
Brallobarbital
$C_{10}H_{11}ClF_3N_3O_4S_3$
Epithiazide
$C_{10}H_{11}I_2NO_3$
Propyliodone
$C_{10}H_{11}N_3O_3S$
Sulfamethoxazole
$C_{10}H_{11}N_3O_5S$
Nifuratel
$C_{10}H_{11}N_4NaO_5S$
Carbazochrome Sodium Sulfonate
$C_{10}H_{11}NaO_3$
Sodium Propyl Hydroxybenzoate
$C_{10}H_{12}ClNO$
Beclamide
$C_{10}H_{12}ClNO_2$
Baclofen
$C_{10}H_{12}ClNO_4$
Chlorphenesin Carbamate
$C_{10}H_{12}ClN_3O_3S$
Quinethazone
$C_{10}H_{12}ClN_5O_3$
Cladribine
$C_{10}H_{12}FN_5O_4$
Fludarabine
$C_{10}H_{12}N_2$
Tolazoline
Tryptamine
$C_{10}H_{12}N_2,HCl$
Tolazoline Hydrochloride
Tryptamine Hydrochloride
$C_{10}H_{12}N_2O$
Serotonin
$C_{10}H_{12}N_2O_3$
Allobarbital
$C_{10}H_{12}N_2O_4$
Stavudine
$C_{10}H_{12}N_3O_3PS_2$
Azinphos-methyl
$C_{10}H_{12}N_4OS$
Thioacetazone
$C_{10}H_{12}N_4O_2S_2$
Sulfaethidole
$C_{10}H_{12}N_4O_3$
Carbazochrome
Didanosine
$C_{10}H_{12}O_2$
Eugenol
$C_{10}H_{12}O_3$
Propyl Hydroxybenzoate
$C_{10}H_{12}O_4$
Cantharidin
$C_{10}H_{13}BrN_2O_3$
Ibomal
$C_{10}H_{13}ClN_2O_3S$
Chlorpropamide
$C_{10}H_{13}FN_5O_7P$
Fludarabine Phosphate
$C_{10}H_{13}N$
Debrisoquine
$C_{10}H_{13}NO$
Methcathinone
$C_{10}H_{13}NO_2$
Methylenedioxyamfetamine
Phenacetin
Phenprobamate
$C_{10}H_{13}NO_2$, HCl
Methylenedioxyamfetamine Hydrochloride
$C_{10}H_{13}NO_4,1\frac{1}{2}H_2O$
Methyldopa
$C_{10}H_{13}NO$, HCl
Methcathinone Hydrochloride
$C_{10}H_{13}N_2NaO_3$
Aprobarbital Sodium
$C_{10}H_{13}N_3O_2$
Guanoxan
$C_{10}H_{13}N_5O_4$
Adenosine
Zidovudine
$C_{10}H_{14}ClN$
Chlorphentermine
$C_{10}H_{14}ClN,HCl$
Chlorphentermine Hydrochloride
$C_{10}H_{14}NO_5PS$
Parathion
$C_{10}H_{14}N_2$
Nicotine
$C_{10}H_{14}N_2O$
Nikethamide
$C_{10}H_{14}N_2O_3$
Aprobarbital
$C_{10}H_{14}N_2O_4,H_2O$
Carbidopa
$C_{10}H_{14}N_2O_4S_2$
Sultiame
$C_{10}H_{14}N_4O_2$
Morinamide
$C_{10}H_{14}N_4O_2,HCl$
Morinamide Hydrochloride
$C_{10}H_{14}N_4O_3$
Proxyphylline
$C_{10}H_{14}N_4O_4$
Diprophylline
$C_{10}H_{14}O$
Thymol
$C_{10}H_{14}O_3$
Mephenesin
$C_{10}H_{14}O_4$
Guaifenesin
$C_{10}H_{15}N$
Metamfetamine
Phentermine
$C_{10}H_{15}NO$
Anhydrous Ephedrine
Hordenine
Methoxyamfetamine
Pholedrine
Pseudoephedrine
Racephedrine
$C_{10}H_{15}NO_2$
Etilefrine
Hydroxyephedrine
$C_{10}H_{15}NO_2,HCl$
Etilefrine Hydrochloride
Hydroxyephedrine Hydrochloride
$C_{10}H_{15}NO_3$
Ethylnoradrenaline
Metadrenaline
$C_{10}H_{15}NO_3,HCl$
Ethylnoradrenaline Hydrochloride
$C_{10}H_{15}NO,\frac{1}{2}H_2O$
Ephedrine
$C_{10}H_{15}NO,HCl$
Ephedrine Hydrochloride
Methoxyamfetamine Hydrochloride
Pseudoephedrine Hydrochloride
Racephedrine Hydrochloride
$C_{10}H_{15}NS$
Methylthioamfetamine
$C_{10}H_{15}N_2NaO_3$
Secbutabarbital Sodium
$C_{10}H_{15}N_3$
Bethanidine
$C_{10}H_{15}N_3O_5$
Benserazide
$C_{10}H_{15}N_3O_5,HCl$
Benserazide Hydrochloride
$C_{10}H_{15}N_5$
Phenformin
$C_{10}H_{15}N_5,HCl$
Phenformin Hydrochloride
$C_{10}H_{15}N_5O_3$
Penciclovir
$C_{10}H_{15}N_5O_3Na, H_2O$
Penciclovir Sodium
$C_{10}H_{15}N,HCl$
Metamfetamine Hydrochloride
Phentermine Hydrochloride
$C_{10}H_{15}O_3PS_2$
Fenthion
$C_{10}H_{16}Br_2N_2O_2$
Pipobroman
$C_{10}H_{16}ClNO$
Edrophonium Chloride
$C_{10}H_{16}N_2O_3$
Butobarbital
$C_{10}H_{16}N_2O_3S$
Amidefrine
$C_{10}H_{16}N_2O_3S,CH_3SO_3H$
Amidefrine Mesilate
Secbutabarbital
$C_{10}H_{16}N_5O_{13}P_3$
Adenosine Triphosphate
$C_{10}H_{16}N_6S$
Cimetidine
$C_{10}H_{16}O$
Camphor
$C_{10}H_{17}N$
Amantadine
$C_{10}H_{17}NO_2$
Methyprylon
$C_{10}H_{17}N_3S$
Pramipexole
$C_{10}H_{17}N_3S,2HCl,H_2O$
Pramipexole Dihydrochloride Monohydrate
$C_{10}H_{17}N,\frac{1}{2}H_2SO_4$
Amantadine Sulfate
$C_{10}H_{17}N,HCl$
Amantadine Hydrochloride
$C_{10}H_{18}O$
Cineole
$C_{10}H_{19}N_5S$
Prometryne
Terbutryne
$C_{10}H_{19}O_6PS_2$
Malathion
$C_{10}H_{20}N_2O_4$
Mebutamate
$C_{10}H_{20}N_2S_3$
Sulfiram
$C_{10}H_{20}N_2S_4$
Disulfiram
$C_{10}H_{20}O$
Menthol
$C_{10}H_{21}N$
Pempidine
Propylhexedrine
$C_{10}H_{21}NO_7$
Voglibose
$C_{10}H_{21}N_3O$
Diethylcarbamazine
$C_{10}H_{21}N_3O,C_6H_8O_7$
Diethylcarbamazine Citrate
$C_{10}H_{21}N,C_4H_6O_6$
Pempidine Tartrate
$C_{10}H_{21}N,HCl$
Propylhexedrine Hydrochloride
$C_{10}H_{22}Cl_2N_2O_4,2HCl$
Mannomustine
$C_{10}H_{22}N_4$
Guanethidine

$C_{10}H_{22}N_4,H_2SO_4$
Guanethidine Monosulfate
$C_{10}H_{24}N_2O_2$
Ethambutol
$C_{10}H_{24}N_2O_2,2HCl$
Ethambutol Hydrochloride
$C_{11}H_8N_2$
Norharman
$C_{11}H_8O_2$
Menadione
$C_{11}H_8O_2NaHSO_3,3H_2O$
Menadione Sodium Bisulfite
$C_{11}H_{10}N_2O_3$
Phenylmethylbarbituric Acid
$C_{11}H_{10}N_3NaO_2S,H_2O$
Sulfapyridine Sodium Monohydrate
$C_{11}H_{11}C1O_3$
Alclofenac
$C_{11}H_{11}Cl_2N_3O$
Muzolimine
$C_{11}H_{11}NO_2$
Phensuximide
$C_{11}H_{11}NO_2,HCl$
Hydrastinine Hydrochloride
$C_{11}H_{11}N_3O_2S$
Sulfapyridine
$C_{11}H_{11}N_4NaO_2S$
Sulfamerazine Sodium
$C_{11}H_{11}N_4O_3S$ Na
Sulfamethoxypyridazine Sodium
$C_{11}H_{11}N_5$
Phenazopyridine
$C_{11}H_{11}N_5,HCl$
Phenazopyridine Hydrochloride
$C_{11}H_{12}ClNO_3S$
Chlormezanone
Tetramisole Hydrochloride
$C_{11}H_{12}Cl_2N_2O$
Lofexidine
$C_{11}H_{12}Cl_2N_2O_5$
Chloramphenicol
$C_{11}H_{12}Cl_2N_2O,HCl$
Lofexidine Hydrochloride
$C_{11}H_{12}N_2O$
Phenazone
$C_{11}H_{12}N_2O_2$
Ethotoin
Tryptophan
$C_{11}H_{12}N_2S$
Levamisole
Tetramisole
$C_{11}H_{12}N_2S,HCl$
Levamisole Hydrochloride
$C_{11}H_{12}N_4O_2S$
Sulfamerazine
$C_{11}H_{12}N_4O_3S$
Sulfamethoxypyridazine
Sulfametopyrazine
Sulfametoxydiazine
$C_{11}H_{12}O_3$
Myristicin
$C_{11}H_{13}ClF_3N_3O_4S_3$
Polythiazide
$C_{11}H_{13}N$
Pargyline
$C_{11}H_{13}NO_3$
Hydrastinine
Toloxatone
$C_{11}H_{13}N_3O_3S$
Sulfafurazole
Sulfamoxole
$C_{11}H_{13}N_3O_3S,C_4H_{11}NO_2$
Sulfafurazole Diethanolamine
$C_{11}H_{13}N,HCl$
Pargyline Hydrochloride
$C_{11}H_{14}ClNO_2$
Buclosamide
$C_{11}H_{14}ClN_5$
Cycloguanil
$C_{11}H_{14}N_2$
5-Methyltryptamine
N-Methyltryptamine
α-Methyltryptamine
$C_{11}H_{14}N_2,HCl$
5-Methyltryptamine Hydrochloride
$C_{11}H_{14}N_2O$
Cytisine
$C_{11}H_{14}N_2O_2$
Pheneturide
$C_{11}H_{14}N_2S$
Pyrantel
$C_{11}H_{14}N_2S,C_4H_6O_6$
Pyrantel Tartrate
$C_{11}H_{14}N_2S,C_{23}H_{16}O_6$
Pyrantel Embonate
$C_{11}H_{15}ClO_2$
Phenaglycodol
$C_{11}H_{15}Cl_2N_5$
Chlorproguanil
$C_{11}H_{15}Cl_2N_5,HCl$
Chlorproguanil Hydrochloride
$C_{11}H_{15}N$
Aletamine
$C_{11}H_{15}NO$
Phenmetrazine
$C_{11}H_{15}NO_2$
Butyl Aminobenzoate
Methylenedioxymethamfetamine
$C_{11}H_{15}NO_2,HCl$
Methylenedioxymethamfetamine Hydrochloride
$C_{11}H_{15}NO_3$
Hydroxyphenamate
$C_{11}H_{15}NO_4$
Mephenesin Carbamate
$C_{11}H_{15}NO_4S$
Etebenecid
$C_{11}H_{15}NO_5$
Methocarbamol
$C_{11}H_{15}NO,C_7H_7ClN_4O_2$
Phenmetrazine Teoclate
$C_{11}H_{15}NO,HCl$
Phenmetrazine Hydrochloride
$C_{11}H_{15}N,HCl$
Aletamine Hydrochloride
$C_{11}H_{16}ClNO$
Clorprenaline
$C_{11}H_{16}ClNO,HCl,H_2O$
Clorprenaline Hydrochloride
$C_{11}H_{16}ClN_5$
Proguanil
$C_{11}H_{16}ClN_5,HCl$
Proguanil Hydrochloride
$C_{11}H_{16}N_2O$
Tocainide
$C_{11}H_{16}N_2O_2$
Pilocarpine
$C_{11}H_{16}N_2O_2,HCl$
Pilocarpine Hydrochloride
$C_{11}H_{16}N_2O_2,HNO_3$
Pilocarpine Nitrate
$C_{11}H_{16}N_2O_3$
Butalbital
Enallylpropymal
Idobutal
Talbutal
Vinbarbital
Vinylbital
$C_{11}H_{16}N_2O,HCl$
Tocainide Hydrochloride
$C_{11}H_{16}N_4O_4$
Dexrazoxane
Pentostatin
$C_{11}H_{16}O_2$
Butylated Hydroxyanisole
$C_{11}H_{17}BrN,C_7H_7O_3S$
Bretylium Tosilate
$C_{11}H_{17}Cl_3N_2O_2S$
Clodantoin
$C_{11}H_{17}N$
Dimethylamfetamine
Mephentermine
$C_{11}H_{17}NO$
Methoxymetamfetamine
Methoxyphenamine
Methylephedrine
Mexiletine
$C_{11}H_{17}NO_3$
Isoprenaline
Mescaline
Methoxamine
Orciprenaline
$C_{11}H_{17}NO_3,HCl$
Isoprenaline Hydrochloride
Methoxamine Hydrochloride
Mescaline Hydrochloride
$C_{11}H_{17}NO_3, H_2SO_4$
Mescaline Acid Sulfate
$C_{11}H_{17}NO,HCl$
Methoxyphenamine Hydrochloride
Methylephedrine Hydrochloride
Mexiletine Hydrochloride
$C_{11}H_{17}N_2NaO_2S$
Thiopental Sodium
$C_{11}H_{17}N_2NaO_3$
Amobarbital Sodium
Pentobarbital Sodium
$C_{11}H_{17}N_3O_3S$
Carbutamide
$C_{11}H_{18}N_2O_2S$
Thiopental
$C_{11}H_{18}N_2O_3$
Amobarbital
Pentobarbital
$C_{11}H_{19}N_5O_3$
Bufylline
$C_{11}H_{19}N_5S$
Irgarol
$C_{11}H_{21}N$
Mecamylamine
$C_{11}H_{21}NO_8$
Choline Dihydrogen Citrate
$C_{11}H_{21}N_5OS$
Methoprotryne
$C_{11}H_{21}N,HCl$
Mecamylamine Hydrochloride
$C_{12}H_6N_2O_2$
Phanquinone
$C_{12}H_7Cl_3O_2$
Triclosan
$C_{12}H_7N_5O_9$
Nifursol
$C_{12}H_8Cl_2O_2S$
Fenticlor
$C_{12}H_8Cl_6$
Aldrin
$C_{12}H_8Cl_6O$
Dieldrin
Endrin
$C_{12}H_8O_4$
Methoxsalen
$C_{12}H_9F_3N_2O_2$
Leflunomide
$C_{12}H_9NS$
Phenothiazine

$C_{13}H_{10}N_2$
Aminoacridine
$C_{13}H_{10}N_2,C_{12}H_{18}O_2$
Aminoacridine Hexylresorcinate
$C_{13}H_{10}N_2,HCl,H_2O$
Aminoacridine Hydrochloride
$C_{13}H_{10}N_2O_4$
Thalidomide
$C_{13}H_{10}O_3$
Salol
$C_{13}H_{10}O_7$
Exifone
$C_{13}H_{11}ClN_2O_2$
Clonixin
$C_{13}H_{11}Cl_2NaO_4$
Etacrynate Sodium
$C_{13}H_{11}NO_2$
Benzyl Nicotinate
$C_{13}H_{11}NO_3$
Phenyl Aminosalicylate
$C_{13}H_{11}N_3,2HCl$
Acriflavinium Chloride
$C_{13}H_{11}N_3O_2$
Salinazid
$C_{13}H_{11}N_3O_4S_2$
Tenoxicam
$C_{13}H_{12}Cl_2O_4$
Etacrynic Acid
$C_{13}H_{12}F_2N_6O$
Fluconazole
$C_{13}H_{12}N_2O$
Harmine
$C_{13}H_{13}N_3O_5S_2,H_2O$
Succinylsulfathiazole
$C_{13}H_{14}Cl_2O_3$
Ciprofibrate
$C_{13}H_{14}N_2$
Tacrine
$C_{13}H_{14}N_2,HCl$
Tacrine Hydrochloride
$C_{13}H_{14}N_2O$
Fenyramidol
Harmaline
$C_{13}H_{14}N_2O_2$
Metomidate
$C_{13}H_{14}N_2O_2,HCl$
Metomidate Hydrochloride
$C_{13}H_{14}N_2O_3$
Methylphenobarbital
$C_{13}H_{14}N_2O,HCl$
Fenyramidol Hydrochloride
$C_{13}H_{14}N_3NaO_4S$
Glymidine Sodium
$C_{13}H_{14}N_4O_4S$
Acetyl Sulfamethoxypyridazine
$C_{13}H_{15}Cl_2NO$
Clorgiline
$C_{13}H_{15}Cl_2NO,HCl$
Clorgiline Hydrochloride
$C_{13}H_{15}NO_2$
Glutethimide
$C_{13}H_{15}N_2NaO_2S$
Thialbarbital Sodium
$C_{13}H_{15}N_3O_4S$
Acetyl Sulfafurazole
$C_{13}H_{15}N_5Na_2O_8S_2$
Aztreonam Disodium
$C_{13}H_{16}ClNO$
Ketamine
$C_{13}H_{16}ClNO,HCl$
Ketamine Hydrochloride
$C_{13}H_{16}HgNNaO_6$
Mersalyl Sodium
$C_{13}H_{16}N_2$
Dexmedetomidine
Tetryzoline
$C_{13}H_{16}N_2,HCl$
Tetryzoline Hydrochloride
$C_{13}H_{16}N_2O_2$
Aminoglutethimide
$C_{13}H_{16}N_2O_2S$
Thialbarbital
$C_{13}H_{16}N_3NaO_4S,H_2O$
Dipyrone
$C_{13}H_{16}N_4O_2$
Diaveridine
$C_{13}H_{16}N_4O_6$
Furaltadone
$C_{13}H_{17}ClN_2O_2$
Moclobemide
$C_{13}H_{17}ClN_2O_2,HCl$
Moclobemide Hydrochloride
$C_{13}H_{17}HgNO_6$
Mersalyl Acid
$C_{13}H_{17}N$
Selegiline
$C_{13}H_{17}NO$
Crotamiton
$C_{13}H_{17}N_3$
Tramazoline
$C_{13}H_{17}N_3,HCl$
Tramazoline Hydrochloride
$C_{13}H_{17}N_3O$
Aminophenazone
$C_{13}H_{17}N_3O_2$
Parbendazole
$C_{13}H_{17}N_5O_8S_2$
Aztreonam
$C_{13}H_{17}N,HCl$
Selegiline Hydrochloride
$C_{13}H_{18}ClNO$
Bupropion
$C_{13}H_{18}ClN_3O_4S_2$
Cyclopenthiazide
$C_{13}H_{18}Cl_2N_2O_2$
Melphalan
$C_{13}H_{18}N_2O_3$
Heptabarb
$C_{13}H_{18}N_2O_6$
Metadoxine
$C_{13}H_{18}N_4O_3$
Pentoxifylline
$C_{13}H_{18}O_2$
Ibuprofen
$C_{13}H_{19}ClN_2O$
Butanilicaine
$C_{13}H_{19}ClN_2O_2$
Chloroprocaine
$C_{13}H_{19}ClN_2O_2,HCl$
Chloroprocaine Hydrochloride
$C_{13}H_{19}ClN_2O_5S_2$
Mefruside
$C_{13}H_{19}ClN_2O,H_3PO_4$
Butanilicaine Phosphate
$C_{13}H_{19}Cl_2NO$
Bupropion Hydrochloride
$C_{13}H_{19}NO$
Diethylpropion
$C_{13}H_{19}NO_3$
Viloxazine
$C_{13}H_{19}NO_3,HCl$
Viloxazine Hydrochloride
$C_{13}H_{19}NO_4$
N-Acetylmescaline
$C_{13}H_{19}NO_4S$
Probenecid
$C_{13}H_{19}NO,HCl$
Diethylpropion Hydrochloride
$C_{13}H_{20}N_2O$
Prilocaine
$C_{13}H_{20}N_2O_2$
Dropropizine
Procaine
$C_{13}H_{20}N_2O_2,C_{16}H_{18}N_2O_4S,H_2O$
Procaine Benzylpenicillin
$C_{13}H_{20}N_2O_2,HCl$
Procaine Hydrochloride
$C_{13}H_{20}N_2O,HCl$
Prilocaine Hydrochloride
$C_{13}H_{20}N_4O_2$
Pentifylline
$C_{13}H_{20}N_6O_4$
Valaciclovir
$C_{13}H_{21}ClN_6O_4$
Valaciclovir Hydrochloride
$C_{13}H_{21}NO_2$
Tigloidine
$C_{13}H_{21}NO_2,HBr$
Tigloidine Hydrobromide
$C_{13}H_{21}NO_3$
Isoetarine
Salbutamol
$C_{13}H_{21}NO_3,CH_4O_3S$
Isoetarine Mesilate
$C_{13}H_{21}NO_3,HCl$
Isoetarine Hydrochloride
$C_{13}H_{21}N_3O$
Procainamide
$C_{13}H_{21}N_3O,HCl$
Procainamide Hydrochloride
$C_{13}H_{21}N_5O_2$
Etamiphylline
$C_{13}H_{21}N_5O_4,C_6H_5NO_2$
Xantinol Nicotinate
$C_{13}H_{22}NO_3PS$
Fenamiphos
$C_{13}H_{22}N_2O_6S$
Neostigmine Methylsulfate
$C_{13}H_{22}N_4O_3S$
Ranitidine
$C_{13}H_{22}N_4O_3S,HCl$
Ranitidine Hydrochloride
$C_{13}H_{22}N_4O_3S.C_6H_5BiO_7$
Ranitidine Bismuth Citrate
$C_{13}H_{24}N_2O_2$
Cropropamide
$C_{13}H_{24}N_4O_3S$
Timolol
$C_{13}H_{24}N_4O_3S,C_4H_4O_4$
Timolol Maleate
$C_{13}H_{26}N_2O_4$
Tybamate
$C_{13}H_{29}N$
Octamylamine
$C_{13}H_{29}N,HCl$
Octamylamine Hydrochloride
$C_{14}H_8CaN_2O_6S_2,3\frac{1}{2}H_2O$
Saccharin Calcium
$C_{14}H_8N_2Na_2O_6$
Olsalazine Sodium
$C_{14}H_8O_4$
Dantron
$C_{14}H_9ClF_3NO_2$
Efavirenz
$C_{14}H_9Cl_5$
Clofenotane
$C_{14}H_9N_4NaO_5,3\frac{1}{2}H_2O$
Dantrolene Sodium
$C_{14}H_{10}BrN_3O$
Bromazepam
$C_{14}H_{10}Cl_2NNaO_2$
Diclofenac
Meclofenamate Sodium

$C_{15}H_{13}NO_3$
Ketorolac
$C_{15}H_{13}N_3O_2S$
Fenbendazole
$C_{15}H_{13}N_3O_4S$
Piroxicam
$C_{15}H_{14}ClNO_3$
Zomepirac
$C_{15}H_{14}ClN_3O_4S_3$
Benzthiazide
$C_{15}H_{14}ClN_3O_4S,H_2O$
Cefaclor
$C_{15}H_{14}FN_3O_3$
Flumazenil
$C_{15}H_{14}F_3N_3O_4S_2$
Bendroflumethiazide
$C_{15}H_{14}NNaO_3,2H_2O$
Tolmetin Sodium
$C_{15}H_{14}N_4O$
Nevirapine
$C_{15}H_{14}N_4O_2S$
Sulfaphenazole
$C_{15}H_{14}O_3$
Fenoprofen
Mexenone
$C_{15}H_{14}O_4$
Acetomenaphthone
$C_{15}H_{15}ClN_2O_4S$
Xipamide
$C_{15}H_{15}Cl_2N_2NaO_8$
Chloramphenicol Sodium Succinate
$C_{15}H_{15}NO_2$
Mefenamic Acid
$C_{15}H_{15}NO_2S$
Modafinil
$C_{15}H_{15}NO_3$
Tolmetin
$C_{15}H_{15}NO_3S$
Adrafinil
$C_{15}H_{15}N_3O$
Ethacridine
$C_{15}H_{15}N_3O,C_3H_6O_3$
Ethacridine Lactate
$C_{15}H_{16}N_6O$
Amicarbalide
$C_{15}H_{16}O_2$
Nabumetone
$C_{15}H_{17}FN_4O_2$
Flupirtine
$C_{15}H_{17}FN_4O_2.C_4H_4O_4$
Flupirtine Maleate
$C_{15}H_{17}FN_4O_2.HCl$
Flupirtine Hydrochloride
$C_{15}H_{17}N$
Benethamine
$C_{15}H_{18}Cl_6N_2O_5$
Dichloralphenazone
$C_{15}H_{18}O_3$
Santonin
$C_{15}H_{19}N_5$
Rizatriptan
$C_{15}H_{19}N_5, C_7H_6O_2$
Rizatriptan Benzoate
$C_{15}H_{20}N_2O_4S$
Acetohexamide
$C_{15}H_{20}N_4O_3S$
Torasemide
$C_{15}H_{21}F_3N_2O_2$
Fluvoxamine
$C_{15}H_{21}F_3N_2O_2,C_4H_4O_4$
Fluvoxamine Maleate
$C_{15}H_{21}N$
Fencamfamin
$C_{15}H_{21}NO$
Eptazocine
$C_{15}H_{21}NO_2$
Ketobemidone
Pethidine
$C_{15}H_{21}NO_2,HCl$
Ketobemidone Hydrochloride
Pethidine
$C_{15}H_{21}N_3O$
Primaquine
$C_{15}H_{21}N_3O_2$
Physostigmine
$C_{15}H_{21}N_3O_2,C_7H_6O_3$
Physostigmine Salicylate
$C_{15}H_{21}N_3O_3$
Physostigmine Aminoxide
$C_{15}H_{21}N_3O_3,C_7H_6O_3$
Physostigmine Aminoxide Salicylate
$C_{15}H_{21}N_3O_3S$
Gliclazide
$C_{15}H_{21}N_3O,2H_3PO_4$
Primaquine Phosphate
$C_{15}H_{21}N,HCl$
Fencamfamin Hydrochloride
$C_{15}H_{22}BrNO$
Eptazocine Hydrobromide
$C_{15}H_{22}ClNO_2$
Metolachlor
$C_{15}H_{22}FN_3O_6$
Capecitabine
$C_{15}H_{22}N_2O$
Mepivacaine
Milnacipran
$C_{15}H_{22}N_2O,HCl$
Mepivacaine Hydrochloride
Milnacipran Hydrochloride
$C_{15}H_{23}N$
Prolintane
$C_{15}H_{23}NO$
Meptazinol
$C_{15}H_{23}NO_2$
Alprenolol
$C_{15}H_{23}NO_2,HCl$
Alprenolol Hydrochloride
$C_{15}H_{23}NO_3$
Ethomoxane
Oxprenolol
$C_{15}H_{23}NO_3,HCl$
Ethomoxane Hydrochloride
Oxprenolol Hydrochloride
$C_{15}H_{23}NO,HCl$
Meptazinol Hydrochloride
$C_{15}H_{23}N_3OS$
Diamthazole
$C_{15}H_{23}N_3OS,2HCl$
Diamthazole Hydrochloride
$C_{15}H_{23}N_3O_2$
Acecainide
$C_{15}H_{23}N_3O_2,HCl$
Acecainide Hydrochloride
$C_{15}H_{23}N_3O_4S$
Sulpiride
$C_{15}H_{23}N,HCl$
Prolintane Hydrochloride
$C_{15}H_{24}N_2O_2$
Tetracaine
$C_{15}H_{24}N_2O_2,HCl$
Tetracaine Hydrochloride
$C_{15}H_{24}O$
Butylated Hydroxytoluene
$C_{15}H_{25}NO_3$
Metoprolol
$C_{15}H_{26}N_2$
Sparteine
$C_{15}H_{26}N_2,H_2SO_4,5H_2O$
Sparteine Sulfate
$C_{16}H_8Cl_2FN_5O$
Fluquinconazole
$C_{16}H_{10}ClKN_2O_3$
Clorazepate Monopotassium
$C_{16}H_{10}ClKN_2O_3,KOH$
Clorazepate Dipotassium
$C_{16}H_{11}ClN_2O_3$
Clorazepic Acid
$C_{16}H_{11}NO_2$
Cinchophen
$C_{16}H_{12}ClNO_3$
Benoxaprofen
$C_{16}H_{12}Cl_2N_2O_2$
Lormetazepam
$C_{16}H_{12}FN_3O_3$
Flunitrazepam
$C_{16}H_{12}O_3$
Anisindione
$C_{16}H_{13}ClN_2O$
Diazepam
Mazindol
$C_{16}H_{13}ClN_2O_2$
Clobazam
Temazepam
$C_{16}H_{13}Cl_2NO_4$
Aceclofenac
$C_{16}H_{13}N_2Na_2O_6P$
Fosphenytoin Sodium
$C_{16}H_{13}N_3O_3$
Mebendazole
$C_{16}H_{13}N_5Na_2O_7S$
Cefixime Disodium Salt
$C_{16}H_{14}ClN_3O$
Chlordiazepoxide
$C_{16}H_{14}ClN_3O,HCl$
Chlordiazepoxide Hydrochloride
$C_{16}H_{14}F_2N_3NaO_4S.{}^3/_2H_2O$
Pantoprazole Sodium Sesquihydrate
$C_{16}H_{14}F_3NO_3S$
Tolrestat
$C_{16}H_{14}F_3N_3O_2S$
Lansoprazole
$C_{16}H_{14}N_2O$
Methaqualone
$C_{16}H_{14}N_2O_6S$
Phthalylsulfacetamide
$C_{16}H_{14}N_2O,HCl$
Methaqualone Hydrochloride
$C_{16}H_{14}O_3$
Dexketoprofen
Fenbufen
Ketoprofen
$C_{16}H_{15}ClN_2$
Medazepam
$C_{16}H_{15}Cl_3O_2$
Methoxychlor
$C_{16}H_{15}F_2N_3O_4S$
Pantoprazole
$C_{16}H_{15}N_2NaO_6S_2$
Cefalothin Sodium
$C_{16}H_{15}N_2O_6P$
Fosphenytoin
$C_{16}H_{15}N_3$
Epinastine
$C_{16}H_{15}N_3, HBr$
Epinastine Hydrobromide
$C_{16}H_{15}N_5O_7S_2$
Cefixime
$C_{16}H_{16}ClNO_2S$
Clopidogrel
$C_{16}H_{16}ClNO_2S, H_2SO_4$
Clopidogrel Bisulfate
$C_{16}H_{16}ClNO_3$
Fenoldopam

$C_{17}H_{15}NO_5$
Benorilate
$C_{17}H_{15}N_3O_6$
Balsalazide
$C_{17}H_{16}ClN_3O$
Amoxapine
$C_{17}H_{16}Cl_2N_2O_5$
Clefamide
$C_{17}H_{16}N_2Na_2O_6S$
Carbenicillin Sodium
$C_{17}H_{16}N_4O_2$
Nifenazone
$C_{17}H_{17}ClN_6O_3$
Zopiclone
$C_{17}H_{17}ClO_6$
Griseofulvin
$C_{17}H_{17}Cl_2N$
Sertraline
$C_{17}H_{17}Cl_2N,HCl$
Sertraline Hydrochloride
$C_{17}H_{17}N$
Azapetine
$C_{17}H_{17}NO_2$
Apomorphine
$C_{17}H_{17}NO_2,HCl,\frac{1}{2}H_2O$
Apomorphine Hydrochloride
$C_{17}H_{17}N_3Na_2O_8$
Balsalazide Disodium
$C_{17}H_{17}N,H_3PO_4$
Azapetine Phosphate
$C_{17}H_{18}Br_2N_4O_2$
Dibrompropamidine
$C_{17}H_{18}Br_2N_4O_2,2C_2H_6O_4S$
Dibrompropamidine Isetionate
$C_{17}H_{18}FN_3O_3$
Ciprofloxacin
$C_{17}H_{18}FN_3O_3,C_3H_6O_3$
Ciprofloxacin Lactate
$C_{17}H_{18}FN_3O_3,HCl,H_2O$
Ciprofloxacin Hydrochloride
$C_{17}H_{18}F_3NO$
Fluoxetine
$C_{17}H_{18}F_3NO,C_2H_4$
Fluoxetine Oxalate
$C_{17}H_{18}F_3NO,HCl$
Fluoxetine Hydrochloride
$C_{17}H_{18}N_2O_6$
Nifedipine
$C_{17}H_{18}N_2O_6S$
Carbenicillin
$C_{17}H_{18}N_3O_3S,Na$
Omeprazole Sodium
$C_{17}H_{19}ClN_2S$
Chlorpromazine
$C_{17}H_{19}ClN_2S,HCl$
Chlorpromazine Hydrochloride
$C_{17}H_{19}KN_2O_5S$
Pheneticillin Potassium
$C_{17}H_{19}NO$
Nefopam
$C_{17}H_{19}NO_3$
Hydromorphone
Norcodeine
$C_{17}H_{19}NO_3,C_2H_4O_2,3H_2O$
Morphine Acetate
$C_{17}H_{19}NO_3,HCl$
Hydromorphone Hydrochloride
$C_{17}H_{19}NO_3,HCl,3H_2O$
Morphine Hydrochloride
Norcodeine Hydrochloride
$C_{17}H_{19}NO_3,H_2O$
Morphine
$C_{17}H_{19}NO_4$
Oxymorphone
$C_{17}H_{19}NO_4,HCl$
Oxymorphone Hydrochloride
$C_{17}H_{19}NO,HCl$
Nefopam Hydrochloride
$C_{17}H_{19}N_2NaO_6S,H_2O$
Meticillin Sodium
$C_{17}H_{19}N_3$
Antazoline
Mirtazapine
$C_{17}H_{19}N_3,CH_3SO_3H$
Antazoline Mesilate
$C_{17}H_{19}N_3,HCl$
Antazoline Hydrochloride
$C_{17}H_{19}N_3,H_3PO_4$
Antazoline Phosphate
$C_{17}H_{19}N_3O$
Phentolamine
$C_{17}H_{19}N_3O_3S$
Omeprazole
$C_{17}H_{19}N_3O,CH_3SO_3H$
Phentolamine Mesilate
$C_{17}H_{19}N_3O,HCl$
Phentolamine Hydrochloride
$C_{17}H_{19}N_5$
Anastrozole
$C_{17}H_{20}BrNO$
Bromazine
$C_{17}H_{20}BrNO,HCl$
Bromazine Hydrochloride
$C_{17}H_{20}ClNO$
Clofedanol
$C_{17}H_{20}ClNO_6S$
Fenoldopam Methanesulfonate
$C_{17}H_{20}ClNO,HCl$
Clofedanol Hydrochloride
$C_{17}H_{20}F_6N_2O_3$
Flecainide
$C_{17}H_{20}F_6N_2O_3,C_2H_4O_2$
Flecainide Acetate
$C_{17}H_{20}N_2O_2$
Tropicamide
Tropisetron
$C_{17}H_{20}N_2O_5S$
Bumetanide
Pheneticillin
$C_{17}H_{20}N_2O_6S$
Meticillin
$C_{17}H_{20}N_2S$
Promazine
Promethazine
$C_{17}H_{20}N_2S,C_7H_7ClN_4O_2$
Promethazine Teoclate
$C_{17}H_{20}N_2S,HCl$
Promazine Hydrochloride
Promethazine Hydrochloride
$C_{17}H_{20}N_4O_2$
Propamidine
$C_{17}H_{20}N_4O_2,2C_2H_6O_4S$
Propamidine Isetionate
$C_{17}H_{20}N_4O_6$
Riboflavin
$C_{17}H_{20}O_6$
Mycophenolic Acid
$C_{17}H_{21}ClN_2O_2$
Tropisetron Hydrochloride
$C_{17}H_{21}N$
Benzfetamine
$C_{17}H_{21}NO$
Diphenhydramine
Phenyltoloxamine
Tofenacin
$C_{17}H_{21}NO_3$
Dihydromorphine
Etodolac
Galantamine
Ritodrine
N-Benzoylmescaline
$C_{17}H_{21}NO_3$, HBr
Galantamine Hydrobromide
$C_{17}H_{21}NO_3,HCl$
Dihydromorphine Hydrochloride
Ritodrine Hydrochloride
Galantamine Hydrochloride
$C_{17}H_{21}NO_4$
Cocaine
Fenoterol
Hyoscine
$C_{17}H_{21}NO_4,HBr$
Fenoterol Hydrobromide
$C_{17}H_{21}NO_4,HBr,3H_2O$
Hyoscine Hydrobromide
$C_{17}H_{21}NO_4,HCl$
Cocaine Hydrochloride
$C_{17}H_{21}NO,2C_9H_{10}N_4O_4$
Diphenhydramine Di(acefyllinate)
$C_{17}H_{21}NO,C_6H_8O_7$
Phenyltoloxamine Citrate
$C_{17}H_{21}NO,C_7H_7ClN_4O_2$
Dimenhydrinate
$C_{17}H_{21}NO,HCl$
Diphenhydramine Hydrochloride
Tofenacin Hydrochloride
$C_{17}H_{21}N,HCl$
Benzfetamine Hydrochloride
$C_{17}H_{22}N_2O$
Doxylamine
$C_{17}H_{22}N_2O,C_4H_6O_4$
Doxylamine Succinate
$C_{17}H_{22}N_2S$
Thenalidine
$C_{17}H_{22}N_2S,C_4H_6O_6$
Thenalidine Tartrate
$C_{17}H_{23}NO$
Dextrorphan
Levorphanol
Racemorphan
$C_{17}H_{23}NO_2$
Tilidate
$C_{17}H_{23}NO_2,HCl,\frac{1}{2}H_2O$
Tilidate Hydrochloride
$C_{17}H_{23}NO_3$
Atropine
Hyoscyamine
$C_{17}H_{23}NO_3,HBr$
Hyoscyamine Hydrobromide
$C_{17}H_{23}NO_4$
Atropine Oxide
$C_{17}H_{23}NO_4,HCl$
Atropine Oxide Hydrochloride
$C_{17}H_{23}NO,C_4H_6O_6,2H_2O$
Levorphanol Tartrate
$C_{17}H_{23}N_3O$
Mepyramine
$C_{17}H_{23}N_3O,C_4H_4O_4$
Mepyramine Maleate
$C_{17}H_{24}N_2O$
Quinisocaine
$C_{17}H_{24}N_2O_2$
Phenglutarimide
$C_{17}H_{24}N_2O_2,HCl$
Phenglutarimide Hydrochloride
$C_{17}H_{24}N_2O,HCl$
Quinisocaine Hydrochloride
$C_{17}H_{24}O_3$
Cyclandelate
$C_{17}H_{25}N$
Phencyclidine
$C_{17}H_{25}NO_2$
Trimeperidine

Isoxsuprine
$C_{18}H_{23}NO_3,C_4H_6O_6$
Dihydrocodeine Tartrate
$C_{18}H_{23}NO_3,HCl$
Dobutamine Hydrochloride
Isoxsuprine Hydrochloride
$C_{18}H_{23}NO_3,H_3PO_4$
Dihydrocodeine Phosphate
$C_{18}H_{23}NO,C_6H_8O_7$
Orphenadrine Citrate
$C_{18}H_{23}NO,HCl$
Orphenadrine Hydrochloride
$C_{18}H_{23}N_3O_6$
Imidaprilat
$C_{18}H_{23}N_5O_2$
Fenetylline
$C_{18}H_{23}N_5O_2,HCl$
Fenetylline Hydrochloride
$C_{18}H_{23}N_5O_5$
Reproterol
$C_{18}H_{23}N_5O_5,HCl$
Reproterol Hydrochloride
$C_{18}H_{23}N,HCl$
Tolpropamine Hydrochloride
$C_{18}H_{24}BrNO_4$
Hyoscine Methobromide
$C_{18}H_{24}N_2O_5,2H_2O$
Enalaprilat
$C_{18}H_{24}N_2O_5S$
Amosulalol
$C_{18}H_{24}N_2O_7$
Hyoscine Methonitrate
$C_{18}H_{24}N_4O$
Granisetron
$C_{18}H_{24}N_4O.HCl$
Granisetron Hydrochloride
$C_{18}H_{24}N_6O_5$
Abacavir Succinate
$C_{18}H_{24}O_2$
Estradiol
$C_{18}H_{24}O_3$
Estriol
$C_{18}H_{25}ClN_2O_5S$
Amosulalol Monohydrochloride
$C_{18}H_{25}NO$
Cyclazocine
Dextromethorphan
$C_{18}H_{25}NO,HBr,H_2O$
Dextromethorphan Hydrobromide
$C_{18}H_{26}BrNO_3$
Atropine Methobromide
$C_{18}H_{26}ClN_3$
Chloroquine
$C_{18}H_{26}ClN_3,2HCl$
Chloroquine Hydrochloride
$C_{18}H_{26}ClN_3,2H_3PO_4$
Chloroquine Phosphate
$C_{18}H_{26}ClN_3,H_2SO_4,H_2O$
Chloroquine Sulfate
$C_{18}H_{26}ClN_3O$
Hydroxychloroquine
$C_{18}H_{26}ClN_3O,H_2SO_4$
Hydroxychloroquine Sulfate
$C_{18}H_{26}N_2O_4S$
Glibornuride
$C_{18}H_{26}N_2O_6$
Atropine Methonitrate
$C_{18}H_{26}O_2$
Nandrolone
$C_{18}H_{27}NO_2$
Dyclonine
Caramiphen
$C_{18}H_{27}NO_2,\frac{1}{2}C_2H_6O_6S_2$
Caramiphen Edisilate
$C_{18}H_{27}NO_2,HCl$
Caramiphen Hydrochloride
Dyclonine Hydrochloride
$C_{18}H_{27}NO_5$
Propanidid
$C_{18}H_{28}N_2O$
Bupivacaine
Levobupivacaine
$C_{18}H_{28}N_2O_4$
Acebutolol
$C_{18}H_{28}N_2O_4,HCl$
Acebutolol Hydrochloride
$C_{18}H_{28}N_2O,HCl$
Levobupivacaine Hydrochloride
$C_{18}H_{28}N_2O,HCl,H_2O$
Bupivacaine Hydrochloride
$C_{18}H_{28}N_4O$
Butalamine
$C_{18}H_{28}N_4O,HCl$
Butalamine Hydrochloride
$C_{18}H_{29}NO_3$
Betaxolol
$C_{18}H_{29}NO_3,HCl$
Betaxolol Hydrochloride
$C_{18}H_{29}N_3O_5$
Bambuterol Hydrochloride
Bambuterol
$C_{18}H_{30}BrNO_3S$
Penthienate Methobromide
$C_{18}H_{30}N_2O_2$
Butacaine
$C_{18}H_{31}NO_4$
Bisoprolol
$C_{18}H_{33}ClN_2O_5S$
Clindamycin
$C_{18}H_{33}ClN_2O_5S,HCl,H_2O$
Clindamycin Hydrochloride
$C_{18}H_{34}ClN_2O_8PS$
Clindamycin Phosphate
$C_{18}H_{34}N_2O_6S$
Lincomycin
$C_{18}H_{34}N_2O_6S,HCl,H_2O$
Lincomycin Hydrochloride
$C_{18}H_{36}N_4O_{11}$
Kanamycin
$C_{18}H_{36}N_4O_{11},1.7H_2SO_4$
Kanamycin Acid Sulfate
$C_{18}H_{36}N_4O_{11},H_2SO_4$
Kanamycin Sulfate
$C_{18}H_{37}N_5O_9$
Tobramycin
$C_{19}H_{11}Cl_2I_2NO_3$
Rafoxanide
$C_{19}H_{12}O_6$
Dicoumarol
$C_{19}H_{15}CaNO_7$
Nedocromil Calcium
$C_{19}H_{15}ClN_4$
Triphenyltetrazolium Chloride
$C_{19}H_{15}KO_4$
Warfarin Potassium
$C_{19}H_{15}NO_6$
Acenocoumarol
$C_{19}H_{15}NO_7$
Nedocromil
$C_{19}H_{15}NO_7,Na_2$
Nedocromil Sodium
$C_{19}H_{15}NaO_4$
Warfarin Sodium
$C_{19}H_{16}ClFN_2O$
Flutoprazepam
$C_{19}H_{16}ClFN_3NaO_5S,H_2O$
Flucloxacillin Sodium
$C_{19}H_{16}ClNO_4$
Indometacin
$C_{19}H_{16}O_3$
Coumatetralyl
$C_{19}H_{16}O_4$
Warfarin
$C_{19}H_{17}ClFN_3O_5S$
Flucloxacillin
$C_{19}H_{17}ClN_2O$
Prazepam
$C_{19}H_{17}ClN_2O_4$
Glafenine
$C_{19}H_{17}ClN_3NaO_5S,H_2O$
Cloxacillin Sodium
$C_{19}H_{17}NOS$
Tolnaftate
$C_{19}H_{17}N_3O_4S_2$
Cefaloridine
$C_{19}H_{18}ClFN_2O_3$
Flutazolam
$C_{19}H_{18}ClN_3O_3$
Camazepam
$C_{19}H_{18}ClN_3O_5S$
Cloxacillin
$C_{19}H_{19}N$
Phenindamine
Setiptiline
$C_{19}H_{19}NOS$
Ketotifen
$C_{19}H_{19}NOS,C_4H_4O_4$
Ketotifen Fumarate
$C_{19}H_{19}N_7O_6$
Folic Acid
$C_{19}H_{19}N,C_4H_6O_6$
Phenindamine Tartrate
$C_{19}H_{20}ClNO_4$
Bezafibrate
$C_{19}H_{20}ClN_3$
Clemizole
$C_{19}H_{20}ClN_3,HCl$
Clemizole Hydrochloride
$C_{19}H_{20}FNO_3$
Paroxetine
$C_{19}H_{20}FNO_3,HCl,\frac{1}{2}H_2O$
Paroxetine Hydrochloride Hemihydrate
$C_{19}H_{20}N_2$
Mebhydrolin
$C_{19}H_{20}N_2O_2$
Phenylbutazone
$C_{19}H_{20}N_2O_3$
Dolasetron
$C_{19}H_{20}N_2O_3,CH_3SO_3H$
Dolasetron Methanesulfonate
$C_{19}H_{20}N_2O_3,H_2O$
Oxyphenbutazone
$C_{19}H_{21}F_3N_2S$
Trifluomeprazine
$C_{19}H_{21}F_3N_2S,C_4H_4O_4$
Trifluomeprazine Maleate
$C_{19}H_{21}N$
Nortriptyline
Protriptyline
$C_{19}H_{21}NO$
Doxepin
$C_{19}H_{21}NO_3$
Nalorphine
Thebaine
$C_{19}H_{21}NO_3,HBr$
Nalorphine Hydrobromide
$C_{19}H_{21}NO_3,HCl$
Nalorphine Hydrochloride
$C_{19}H_{21}NO_4$
Naloxone
6-Monoacetylmorphine
$C_{19}H_{21}NO_4,HCl$
6-Monoacetylmorphine Hydrochloride
Naloxone Hydrochloride

$C_{19}H_{35}NO_2,HCl$
Dicycloverine Hydrochloride
$C_{19}H_{35}N,C_4H_4O_4$
Perhexiline Maleate
$C_{19}H_{40}I_2N_2$
Mebezonium Iodide
$C_{20}H_{14}O_4$
Phenolphthalein
$C_{20}H_{15}NO_3$
Oxyphenisatine
$C_{20}H_{16}O_6$
Dithranol Triacetate
$C_{20}H_{17}ClN_2O_3$
Ketazolam
$C_{20}H_{17}FO_3S$
Sulindac
$C_{20}H_{17}F_3N_2O_4$
Floctafenine
$C_{20}H_{18}ClNO_4,2H_2O$
Berberine Hydrochloride
$C_{20}H_{18}Cl_2N_2O_6$
Chloramphenicol Cinnamate
$[C_{20}H_{18}NO_4]^+$
Berberine
$C_{20}H_{18}NO_4,HSO_4$
Berberine Sulfate
$C_{20}H_{19}NO_5$
Chelidonine
$C_{20}H_{20}N_2O_2$
Feprazone
$C_{20}H_{21}FN_2O$
Citalopram
$C_{20}H_{21}FN_2O,HBr$
Citalopram Hydrobromide
$C_{20}H_{21}N$
Cyclobenzaprine
$C_{20}H_{21}NO_3$
Dimefline
$C_{20}H_{21}NO_3,HCl$
Dimefline Hydrochloride
$C_{20}H_{21}NO_4$
Papaverine
$(C_{20}H_{21}NO_4)_2,H_2SO_4,5H_2O$
Papaverine Sulfate Pentahydrate
$C_{20}H_{21}NO_4,HCl$
Papaverine Hydrochloride
$C_{20}H_{21}N,HCl$
Cyclobenzaprine Hydrochloride
$C_{20}H_{22}ClN$
Pyrrobutamine
$C_{20}H_{22}ClN_3O$
Amodiaquine
$C_{20}H_{22}ClN_3O,2HCl,2H_2O$
Amodiaquine Hydrochloride
$C_{20}H_{22}ClN,2H_3PO_4$
Pyrrobutamine Phosphate
$C_{20}H_{22}N_2$
Azatadine
$C_{20}H_{22}N_2,2C_4H_4O_4$
Azatadine Maleate
$C_{20}H_{22}N_2O_2$
Gelsemine
$C_{20}H_{22}N_2S$
Mequitazine
$C_{20}H_{22}N_5NaO_6S$
Azlocillin Sodium
$C_{20}H_{22}N_8O_5$
Methotrexate
$C_{20}H_{23}N$
Amitriptyline
Maprotiline
$C_{20}H_{23}NO_3$
Methylpiperidyl Benzilate
$C_{20}H_{23}NO_4$
Naltrexone
Thebacon
Acetylcodeine
$C_{20}H_{23}NO_4,HCl$
Naltrexone Hydrochloride
Thebacon Hydrochloride
$C_{20}H_{23}NS$
Metixene
$C_{20}H_{23}NS,HCl$
Metixene Hydrochloride
$C_{20}H_{23}N_5O_6S$
Azlocillin
$C_{20}H_{23}N,HCl$
Amitriptyline Hydrochloride
Maprotiline Hydrochloride
$C_{20}H_{24}ClN_3S$
Prochlorperazine
$C_{20}H_{24}ClN_3S,2CH_3SO_3H$
Prochlorperazine Mesilate
$C_{20}H_{24}ClN_3S,2C_4H_4O_4$
Prochlorperazine Maleate
$C_{20}H_{24}ClN_3S,C_2H_6O_6S_2$
Prochlorperazine Edisilate
$C_{20}H_{24}N_2$
Dimetindene
$C_{20}H_{24}N_2,C_4H_4O_4$
Dimetindene Maleate
$C_{20}H_{24}N_2OS$
Propiomazine
$C_{20}H_{24}N_2OS,C_4H_4O_4$
Propiomazine Maleate
$C_{20}H_{24}N_2OS,HCl$
Propiomazine Hydrochloride
$C_{20}H_{24}N_2O_2,2HBr,3H_2O$
Quinine Dihydrobromide
$C_{20}H_{24}N_2O_2,2HCl$
Quinine Dihydrochloride
$C_{20}H_{24}N_2O_2,2H_2O$
Quinidine
$C_{20}H_{24}N_2O_2,3H_2O$
Quinine
$C_{20}H_{24}N_2O_2,C_6H_{12}O_7$
Quinidine Gluconate
$C_{20}H_{24}N_2O_2,C_7H_6O_3,H_2O$
Quinine Salicylate
$C_{20}H_{24}N_2O_2,HBr,2H_2O$
Quinine Hydrobromide
$C_{20}H_{24}N_2O_2,HCl,2H_2O$
Quinine Hydrochloride
$C_{20}H_{24}N_2O_2,H_2SO_4,4H_2O$
Quinidine Bisulfate
$C_{20}H_{24}N_2O_2,H_2SO_4,7H_2O$
Quinine Bisulfate
$C_{20}H_{24}N_2O_5$
Diamfenetide
$C_{20}H_{24}N_2O_6$
Nisoldipine
$C_{20}H_{24}N,CH_3SO_4$
Diphemanil Metilsulfate
$C_{20}H_{24}O_2$
Ethinylestradiol
Exemestane
$C_{20}H_{24}O_3$
Trenbolone Acetate
$C_{20}H_{25}ClNO_5,HCl$
Cloricromen Hydrochloride
$C_{20}H_{25}ClN_2O_5$
Amlodipine
$C_{20}H_{25}ClN_2O_5,C_4H_4O_4$
Amlodipine Maleate
$C_{20}H_{25}ClN_2O_5,C_6H_5SO_3H$
Amlodipine Besilate
$C_{20}H_{25}N$
Fenpiprane
$C_{20}H_{25}NO$
Normethadone
$C_{20}H_{25}NO_2$
Adiphenine
$C_{20}H_{25}NO_2,HCl$
Adiphenine Hydrochloride
$C_{20}H_{25}NO_2S_2$
Tiagabine
$C_{20}H_{25}NO_2S_2,HCl$
Tiagabine Hydrochloride
$C_{20}H_{25}NO_3$
Benactyzine
$C_{20}H_{25}NO_3,HCl$
Benactyzine Hydrochloride
$C_{20}H_{25}NO,HCl$
Normethadone Hydrochloride
$C_{20}H_{25}N_3O$
Lysergide
$C_{20}H_{25}N_3O_2$
Methylergometrine
$C_{20}H_{25}N_3O_2,C_4H_4O_4$
Methylergometrine Maleate
$C_{20}H_{25}N_3S$
Perazine
$C_{20}H_{25}N_3S,2C_3H_4O_4$
Perazine Dimalonate
$C_{20}H_{25}N,HCl$
Fenpiprane Hydrochloride
$C_{20}H_{26}ClNO_3$
Lachesine Chloride
$C_{20}H_{26}ClNO_5$
Cloricromen
$C_{20}H_{26}N_2$
Trimipramine
$C_{20}H_{26}N_2,C_4H_4O_4$
Trimipramine Maleate
$C_{20}H_{26}N_2O$
Ibogaine
$C_{20}H_{26}N_2O_2$
Hydroquinidine
Hydroquinine
Ajmaline
$C_{20}H_{26}N_2O_2,2HCl,2H_2O$
Ajmaline Hydrochloride
$C_{20}H_{26}N_2O_2,C_2H_6O$
Ajmaline Monoethanolate
$C_{20}H_{26}N_2O_2,HCl$
Hydroquinidine Hydrochloride
$C_{20}H_{26}N_2O_5S_2$
Spiraprilat
$C_{20}H_{26}N_2O,HCl$
Ibogaine Hydrochloride
$C_{20}H_{26}O_2$
Norethisterone
Noretynodrel
$C_{20}H_{27}BrN_2O$
Ambutonium Bromide
$C_{20}H_{27}N$
Alverine
$C_{20}H_{27}NO_3$
Trilostane
$C_{20}H_{27}NO_4$
Bevantolol
$C_{20}H_{27}NO_5$
Carbocromen
$C_{20}H_{27}NO_5,HCl$
Carbocromen Hydrochloride
$C_{20}H_{27}NO_{11}$
Amygdalin
$C_{20}H_{27}N_3O_6$
Imidapril
$C_{20}H_{27}N_3O_6.HCl$
Imidapril Monohydrochloride
$C_{20}H_{27}N_5O_3$
Bamifylline
$C_{20}H_{27}N_5O_3,HCl$
Bamifylline Hydrochloride

$C_{21}H_{27}N_3O_2$
Methysergide
$C_{21}H_{27}N_3O_2,C_4H_4O_4$
Methysergide Maleate
$C_{21}H_{27}N_3O_7S$
Bacampicillin
$C_{21}H_{27}N_3O_7S,HCl$
Bacampicillin Hydrochloride
$C_{21}H_{27}N_5O_4S$
Glipizide
$C_{21}H_{27}N,HCl$
Butriptyline Hydrochloride
$C_{21}H_{27}Na_2O_8P$
Prednisolone Sodium Phosphate
$C_{21}H_{28}ClN$
Budipine Hydrochloride
$C_{21}H_{28}N_2O_5$
Trimethobenzamide
$C_{21}H_{28}N_2O_5,HCl$
Trimethobenzamide Hydrochloride
$C_{21}H_{28}O_2$
Dydrogesterone
Ethisterone
$C_{21}H_{28}O_3$
Boldenone Acetate
Pyrethrin I
$C_{21}H_{28}O_5$
Aldosterone
Cortisone
Prednisolone
$C_{21}H_{29}ClO_3$
Clostebol Acetate
$C_{21}H_{29}FO_4$
Flugestone
$C_{21}H_{29}FO_5$
Fludrocortisone
$C_{21}H_{29}NO$
Biperiden
$C_{21}H_{29}NO_2$
Butorphanol
$C_{21}H_{29}NO_2,C_4H_6O_6$
Butorphanol Tartrate
$C_{21}H_{29}NO,C_3H_6O_3$
Biperiden Lactate
$C_{21}H_{29}NO,HCl$
Biperiden Hydrochloride
$C_{21}H_{29}NS_2$
Captodiame
$C_{21}H_{29}NS_2,HCl$
Captodiame Hydrochloride
$C_{21}H_{29}N_3O$
Disopyramide
$C_{21}H_{29}N_3O,H_3PO_4$
Disopyramide Phosphate
$C_{21}H_{29}N_5O_2$
Tandospirone
$C_{21}H_{29}N_5O_2, C_6H_8O_7$
Tandospirone Citrate
$C_{21}H_{29}N_5O_2,HCl$
Tandospirone Citrate
$C_{21}H_{29}Na_2O_8P$
Hydrocortisone Sodium Phosphate
$C_{21}H_{30}BrNO_4$
Hyoscine Butylbromide
$C_{21}H_{30}FN_3O_2$
Pipamperone
$C_{21}H_{30}FN_3O_2,2HCl$
Pipamperone Hydrochloride
$C_{21}H_{30}O_2$
Cannabidiol
Δ^8-Tetrahydrocannabinol
Δ^9-Tetrahydrocannabinol
Progesterone
$C_{21}H_{30}O_3$
Desoxycortone
Hydroxyprogesterone
Nandrolone Propionate
$C_{21}H_{31}N_3O_3,2H_2O$
Lisinopril Dihydrate
$C_{21}H_{31}N_3O_5$
Lisinopril
$C_{21}H_{31}N_5O_2$
Buspirone
$C_{21}H_{31}N_5O_2,HCl$
Buspirone Hydrochloride
$C_{21}H_{32}N_2O$
Stanozolol
$C_{21}H_{32}N_6O_3$
Alfentanil
$C_{21}H_{32}N_6O_3,HCl,H_2O$
Alfentanil Hydrochloride
$C_{21}H_{32}O$
Allylestrenol
$C_{21}H_{32}O_3$
Alfaxalone
Oxymetholone
$C_{21}H_{32}O_4$
Alfadolone
$C_{21}H_{34}BrNO_3$
Oxyphenonium Bromide
$C_{21}H_{36}ClNO$
Tridihexethyl Chloride
$C_{21}H_{38}ClN,H_2O$
Cetylpyridinium Chloride
$C_{21}H_{39}N_7O_{12}$
Streptomycin
$C_{21}H_{41}N_7O_{12}$
Dihydrostreptomycin
$C_{21}H_{45}N_3$
Hexetidine
$C_{22}H_{16}O_8$
Ethyl Biscoumacetate
$C_{22}H_{17}ClN_2$
Clotrimazole
$C_{22}H_{18}Cl_2FNO_3$
Cyfluthrin
$C_{22}H_{19}Br_2NO_3$
Deltamethrin
$C_{22}H_{19}NO_4$
Bisacodyl
$C_{22}H_{19}O_3Cl$
Atovaquone
$C_{22}H_{22}ClKN_6O$
Losartan Potassium
$C_{22}H_{22}FN_3O_2$
Droperidol
$C_{22}H_{22}N_2O_8$
Methacycline
$C_{22}H_{22}N_2O_8,HCl$
Methacycline Hydrochloride
$C_{22}H_{22}N_6O_7S_2$
Ceftazidime
$C_{22}H_{22}N_6O_7S_2,5H_2O$
Ceftazidime Pentahydrate
$C_{22}H_{23}ClN_2O_2$
Loratadine
$C_{22}H_{23}ClN_2O_8$
Chlortetracycline
$C_{22}H_{23}ClN_2O_8,HCl$
Chlortetracycline Hydrochloride
$C_{22}H_{23}ClN_6O$
Losartan
$C_{22}H_{23}F_4NO_2$
Trifluperidol
$C_{22}H_{23}F_4NO_2,HCl$
Trifluperidol Hydrochloride
$C_{22}H_{23}NO_4$
Methyl Benzoquate
$C_{22}H_{23}NO_7$
Noscapine
$C_{22}H_{23}NO_7,HCl,H_2O$
Noscapine Hydrochloride
$C_{22}H_{24}FN_3O_2$
Benperidol
$C_{22}H_{24}N_2O_2$
Acrivastine
$C_{22}H_{24}N_2O_8$
Tetracycline
$C_{22}H_{24}N_2O_8,HCl$
Tetracycline
$C_{22}H_{24}N_2O_8,HCl,\frac{1}{2}C_2H_5OH,\frac{1}{2}H_2O$
Doxycycline Hydrochloride
$C_{22}H_{24}N_2O_8,H_2O$
Doxycycline
$C_{22}H_{24}N_2O_9,2H_2O$
Oxytetracycline Dihydrate
$C_{22}H_{24}N_2O_9,HCl$
Oxytetracycline Hydrochloride
$C_{22}H_{25}ClN_2OS$
Clopenthixol
Zuclopenthixol
$C_{22}H_{25}ClN_2OS,2HCl$
Clopenthixol Hydrochloride
Zuclopenthixol Hydrochloride
$C_{22}H_{25}ClN_2OS,C_2H_2O$
Zuclopenthixol Acetate
$C_{22}H_{25}F_2NO_4$
Nebivolol
$C_{22}H_{25}NO_3$
Pipoxolan
$C_{22}H_{25}NO_3,HCl$
Pipoxolan Hydrochloride
$C_{22}H_{25}NO_4$
Dimoxyline
$C_{22}H_{25}NO_4,H_3PO_4$
Dimoxyline Phosphate
$C_{22}H_{25}NO_6$
Colchicine
$C_{22}H_{25}N_2OS,C_{10}H_{15}O_4S$
Trimetaphan Camsilate
$C_{22}H_{25}N_3O$
Indoramin
$C_{22}H_{25}N_3O_4S$
Moracizine
$C_{22}H_{25}N_3O_4S,HCl$
Moracizine Hydrochloride
$C_{22}H_{25}N_3O,HCl$
Indoramin Hydrochloride
$C_{22}H_{26}BrNO_3$
Clidinium Bromide
$C_{22}H_{26}ClF_2NO_4$
Nebivolol Hydrochloride
$C_{22}H_{26}F_3N_3OS$
Fluphenazine
$C_{22}H_{26}F_3N_3OS,2HCl$
Fluphenazine Hydrochloride
$C_{22}H_{26}N_2O_4S$
Diltiazem
$C_{22}H_{26}N_2O_4S,HCl$
Diltiazem Hydrochloride
$C_{22}H_{27}ClN_2O$
Lorcainide
$C_{22}H_{27}ClN_2O,HCl$
Lorcainide Hydrochloride
$C_{22}H_{27}NO$
Phenazocine
$C_{22}H_{27}NO_2$
Danazol
Amineptine
Lobeline
$C_{22}H_{27}NO_2,HCl$
Lobeline Hydrochloride
$C_{22}H_{27}NO,HBr,\frac{1}{2}H_2O$
Phenazocine Hydrobromide

$C_{23}H_{29}NO,HBr$
Norpipanone Hydrobromide
$C_{23}H_{29}NO,HCl$
Norpipanone Hydrochloride
$C_{23}H_{29}N_3O$
Opipramol
$C_{23}H_{29}N_3O_2$
Oxypertine
$C_{23}H_{29}N_3O_2S$
Acetophenazine
$C_{23}H_{29}N_3O_2S_2$
Tiotixene
$C_{23}H_{29}N_3O_2S_2,2HCl,2H_2O$
Tiotixene Hydrochloride
$C_{23}H_{29}N_3O_2S,2C_4H_4O_4$
Acetophenazine Dimaleate
$C_{23}H_{29}N_3O,2HCl$
Opipramol Hydrochloride
$C_{23}H_{30}BrNO_3$
Propantheline Bromide
$C_{23}H_{30}ClN_3O$
Mepacrine
$C_{23}H_{30}ClN_3O,2CH_3SO_3H,H_2O$
Mepacrine Mesilate
$C_{23}H_{30}ClN_3O,2HCl,2H_2O$
Mepacrine Hydrochloride
$C_{23}H_{30}N_2O_2$
Piminodine
$C_{23}H_{30}N_2O_2,C_2H_6O_3S$
Piminodine Esilate
$C_{23}H_{30}N_2O_4,2C_4H_6O_6,3H_2O$
Pholcodine Tartrate
$C_{23}H_{30}N_2O_4,H_2O$
Pholcodine
$C_{23}H_{30}O_3$
Etretinate
$C_{23}H_{30}O_6$
Cortisone Acetate
Prednisolone Acetate
$C_{23}H_{31}FO_5$
Flugestone Acetate
$C_{23}H_{31}FO_6$
Fludrocortisone Acetate
$C_{23}H_{31}NO_2$
Levacetylmethadol
$C_{23}H_{31}NO_2,HCl$
Levacetylmethadol Hydrochloride
$C_{23}H_{31}NO_7$
Mycophenolate Mofetil
$C_{23}H_{32}N_2O_2S$
Tiocarlide
$C_{23}H_{32}N_2O_5$
Ramipril
$C_{23}H_{32}O_2,H_2O$
Dimethisterone
$C_{23}H_{32}O_3$
Estradiol Valerate
$C_{23}H_{32}O_4$
Desoxycortone Acetate
$C_{23}H_{32}O_6$
Hydrocortisone Acetate
$C_{23}H_{33}IN_2O$
Isopropamide Iodide
$C_{23}H_{33}N_2O_2,C_4H_5O_6$
Prajmalium Bitartrate
$C_{23}H_{34}NO_5P$
Fosinopril Diacid
$C_{23}H_{34}O_4$
Androstenediol Diacetate
$C_{23}H_{34}O_5$
Alfadolone Acetate
$C_{23}H_{34}O_6$
Pravastatin Lactone
$C_{23}H_{35}O_7Na$
Pravastatin Sodium
$C_{23}H_{36}N_2O_2$
Finasteride
$C_{23}H_{36}O_3$
Drostanolone Propionate
$C_{23}H_{36}O_7$
Pravastatin
$C_{23}H_{37}N_5O_6S$
Etamiphylline Camsilate
$C_{23}H_{42}N_2O_{12}$
Pentolonium Tartrate
$C_{23}H_{46}N_6O_{13}$
Neomycin
$C_{24}H_{19}NO_5$
Oxyphenisatine Acetate
$C_{24}H_{20}N_6O_3$
Candesartan
$C_{24}H_{25}FN_6O$
Mizolastine
$C_{24}H_{25}FNNaO_4$
Fluvastatin Sodium
$C_{24}H_{25}NO_3$
Benzylmorphine
$C_{24}H_{25}NO_3,HCl$
Benzylmorphine Hydrochloride
$C_{24}H_{25}NO_4$
Flavoxate
$C_{24}H_{25}NO_4,HCl$
Flavoxate Hydrochloride
$C_{24}H_{26}BrN_3O_3$
Nicergoline
$C_{24}H_{26}ClFN_4O$
Sertindole
$C_{24}H_{26}FN_3O$
Biriperone
$C_{24}H_{26}FNO_4$
Fluvastatin
$C_{24}H_{26}N_2O_4$
Carvedilol
$C_{24}H_{27}N$
Prenylamine
$C_{24}H_{27}NO_5S$
Troglitazone
$C_{24}H_{27}N,C_3H_6O_3$
Prenylamine Lactate
$C_{24}H_{28}N_2O_5$
Benazepril
$C_{24}H_{28}N_2O_5,HCl$
Benazepril Hydrochloride
$C_{24}H_{28}O_4$
Diethylstilbestrol Dipropionate
$C_{24}H_{29}Cl_2FO_5$
Fluclorolone Acetonide
$C_{24}H_{29}NO_3$
Donepezil
$C_{24}H_{29}NO_3,HCl$
Donepezil Hydrochloride
$C_{24}H_{29}N_5O_3$
Valsartan
$C_{24}H_{30}F_2O_6$
Fluocinolone Acetonide
$C_{24}H_{30}N_2O_2$
Doxapram
$C_{24}H_{30}N_2O_2,HCl,H_2O$
Doxapram Hydrochloride
$C_{24}H_{30}N_2O_2S$
Piperacetazine
$C_{24}H_{30}O_4$
Hexestrol Dipropionate
$C_{24}H_{31}FO_6$
Triamcinolone Acetonide
Betamethasone Acetate
Dexamethasone Acetate
Paramethasone Acetate
$C_{24}H_{31}NO$
Dipipanone
$C_{24}H_{31}NO,HCl,H_2O$
Dipipanone Hydrochloride
$C_{24}H_{31}N_3O$
Famprofazone
$C_{24}H_{31}N_3OS$
Butaperazine
$C_{24}H_{31}N_3OS,2C_4H_4O_4$
Butaperazine Maleate
$C_{24}H_{31}N_3OS,2H_3PO_4$
Butaperazine Phosphate
$C_{24}H_{31}N_3O_2S$
Carfenazine
$C_{24}H_{31}N_3O_2S,2C_4H_4O_4$
Carfenazine Maleate
$C_{24}H_{32}ClFO_5$
Halcinonide
$C_{24}H_{32}O_4$
Etynodiol Diacetate
Megestrol Acetate
$C_{24}H_{32}O_4S$
Spironolactone
$C_{24}H_{32}O_6$
Desonide
Methylprednisolone Acetate
$C_{24}H_{33}FO_6$
Fludroxycortide
$C_{24}H_{33}NO_3,C_2H_2O_4$
Naftidrofuryl Oxalate
$C_{24}H_{33}N_3O_2S$
Dixyrazine
$C_{24}H_{33}N_3O_3S_2$
Pipotiazine
$C_{24}H_{34}N_2O_5$
Trandolapril
$C_{24}H_{34}N_4O_5S$
Glimepiride
$C_{24}H_{34}O_4$
Medroxyprogesterone Acetate
$C_{24}H_{35}NO_5$
Decoquinate
$C_{24}H_{36}O_3$
Nabilone
$C_{24}H_{36}O_4$
Methandriol Diacetate
$C_{24}H_{36}O_5$
Lovastatin
$C_{24}H_{40}N_2$
Conessine
$C_{24}H_{40}N_2,2HBr$
Conessine Hydrobromide
$C_{24}H_{40}N_8O_4$
Dipyridamole
$C_{25}H_{19}NO_3$
Fendosal
$C_{25}H_{27}ClN_2$
Meclozine
$C_{25}H_{27}ClN_2,2HCl,H_2O$
Meclozine Hydrochloride
$C_{25}H_{28}N_6O$
Irbesartan
$C_{25}H_{28}O_3$
Estradiol Benzoate
$C_{25}H_{29}I_2NO_3$
Amiodarone
$C_{25}H_{29}I_2NO_3,HCl$
Amiodarone Hydrochloride
$C_{25}H_{30}N_2O_5$
Quinapril
$C_{25}H_{30}N_2O_5,HCl$
Quinapril Hydrochloride
$C_{25}H_{31}FO_8$
Triamcinolone Diacetate
$C_{25}H_{31}F_3O_5S$
Fluticasone Propionate

$C_{25}H_{31}NO_3$
Metindizate
$C_{25}H_{31}NO_3,HCl$
Metindizate Hydrochloride
$C_{25}H_{31}NO_6$
Deflazacort
$C_{25}H_{32}ClFO_5$
Clobetasol Propionate
$C_{25}H_{32}ClN_5O_2$
Nefazodone
$C_{25}H_{32}ClN_5O_2,HCl$
Nefazodone Hydrochloride
$C_{25}H_{32}N_2O_2$
Dextromoramide
$C_{25}H_{32}N_2O_2,C_4H_6O_6$
Dextromoramide Tartrate
$C_{25}H_{32}O_8$
Prednisolone Succinate
$C_{25}H_{33}NO_4$
Etorphine
$C_{25}H_{33}NO_4,HCl$
Etorphine Hydrochloride
$C_{25}H_{33}N_5O_{10}$
Trimetrexate d-Glucuronate
$C_{25}H_{34}O_8$
Hydrocortisone Hydrogen Succinate
$C_{25}H_{35}NO_5$
Mebeverine
$C_{25}H_{35}NO_5,HCl$
Mebeverine Hydrochloride
$C_{25}H_{35}N_3O_6S$
Amprenavir
$C_{25}H_{35}NaO_8$
Hydrocortisone Sodium Succinate
$C_{25}H_{36}O_3$
Nandrolone Cyclohexanecarboxylate
$C_{25}H_{36}O_6$
Hydrocortisone Butyrate
$C_{25}H_{37}NO_4$
Salmeterol
$C_{25}H_{37}NO_4, C_{11}H_8O_3$
Salmeterol Xinafoate
$C_{25}H_{38}N_2O$
Bunamidine
$C_{25}H_{38}N_2O,HCl$
Bunamidine Hydrochloride
$C_{25}H_{38}O_3$
Testosterone Isocaproate
$C_{25}H_{38}O_4$
Androstenediol Dipropionate
$C_{25}H_{38}O_5$
Simvastatin
$C_{25}H_{43}NO_{18}$
Acarbose
$C_{25}H_{44}ClN_3O_2$
Dofamium Chloride
$C_{25}H_{44}N_{14}O_7$
Capreomycin IB
$C_{25}H_{44}N_{14}O_8$
Capreomycin IA
$C_{25}H_{46}ClN$
Cetalkonium Chloride
$C_{25}H_{48}N_6O_8$
Desferrioxamine
$C_{25}H_{48}N_6O_8,CH_3SO_3H$
Desferrioxamine Mesilate
$C_{26}H_{27}Br_2N_7$
Pyritidium Bromide
$C_{26}H_{27}ClN_2O$
Lofepramine
$C_{26}H_{27}ClN_2O,HCl$
Lofepramine Hydrochloride
$C_{26}H_{27}NO_9$
Idarubicin
$C_{26}H_{27}NO_9.HCl$
Idarubicin Hydrochloride
$C_{26}H_{27}N_3,HCl$
Pyrvinium Chloride
$C_{26}H_{28}ClNO$
Clomifene
Toremifene
$C_{26}H_{28}ClNO,C_6H_8O_7$
Clomifene Citrate
Toremifene Citrate
$C_{26}H_{28}Cl_2N_4O_4$
Ketoconazole
$C_{26}H_{28}N_2$
Cinnarizine
$C_{26}H_{29}FN_2O_2$
Levocabastine
$C_{26}H_{29}FN_2O_2,HCl$
Levocabastine Hydrochloride
$C_{26}H_{30}Cl_2F_3NO$
Halofantrine
$C_{26}H_{30}Cl_2F_3NO,HCl$
Halofantrine Hydrochloride
$C_{26}H_{30}O_5$
Boldenone Benzoate
$C_{26}H_{32}ClFO_5$
Clobetasone Butyrate
$C_{26}H_{32}F_2O_7$
Fluocinonide
$C_{26}H_{32}N_2O_7$
Bopindolol Malonate
$C_{26}H_{33}FNNaO_5$
Cerivastatin Sodium
$C_{26}H_{33}NO_6$
Lacidipine
$C_{26}H_{33}NaO_8$
Methylprednisolone Sodium Succinate
$C_{26}H_{34}FNO_5$
Cerivastatin
$C_{26}H_{34}O_4$
Trenbolone Hexahydrobenzylcarbonate
$C_{26}H_{34}O_8$
Methylprednisolone Hemisuccinate
$C_{26}H_{35}NO_4$
Diprenorphine
$C_{26}H_{35}NO_4,HCl$
Diprenorphine Hydrochloride
$C_{26}H_{36}O_3$
Estradiol Cipionate
$C_{26}H_{36}O_6$
Prednisolone Pivalate
$C_{26}H_{37}N_5O_2$
Cabergoline
$C_{26}H_{37}N_5O_2,2H_3PO_4$
Cabergoline Diphosphate
$C_{26}H_{38}O_4$
Desoxycortone Pivalate
Gestonorone Caproate
$C_{26}H_{38}O_6$
Hydrocortisone Valerate
$C_{26}H_{40}O_3$
Dehydroepiandrosterone Enantate
Testosterone Enantate
$C_{26}H_{40}O_4$
Methandriol Dipropionate
$C_{26}H_{44}O_9$
Mupirocin
$C_{27}H_{22}Cl_2N_4$
Clofazimine
$C_{27}H_{29}NO_{10}$
Daunorubicin
$C_{27}H_{29}NO_{10},C_6H_8O_7$
Daunorubicin Lactate
$C_{27}H_{29}NO_{10},HCl$
Daunorubicin Hydrochloride
$C_{27}H_{29}NO_{11}$
Epirubicin
Doxorubicin
$C_{27}H_{29}NO_{11},HCl$
Doxorubicin Hydrochloride
Epirubicin Hydrochloride
$C_{27}H_{30}N_2O_7,HCl$
Moexipril Diacid Hydrochloride
$C_{27}H_{32}N_2O_7$
Bopindolol Maleate
$C_{27}H_{33}N_3O_6S$
Gliquidone
$C_{27}H_{33}N_3O_8$
Rolitetracycline
$C_{27}H_{33}N_3O_8,HNO_3,1\frac{1}{2}H_2O$
Rolitetracycline Nitrate
$C_{27}H_{34}N_2O_7$
Moexipril
$C_{27}H_{34}N_2O_7,HCl$
Moexipril Hydrochloride
$C_{27}H_{34}N_4O$
Piritramide
$C_{27}H_{34}O_3$
Nandrolone Phenylpropionate
$C_{27}H_{35}NO_5$
Acetorphine
$C_{27}H_{35}NO_5,HCl$
Acetorphine Hydrochloride
$C_{27}H_{36}F_2O_6$
Flumetasone Pivalate
$C_{27}H_{36}N_2O_4$
Repaglinide
$C_{27}H_{37}FO_5$
Fluocortolone Pivalate
$C_{27}H_{37}FO_6$
Betamethasone Valerate
$C_{27}H_{38}N_2O_4$
Verapamil
$C_{27}H_{38}N_2O_4,HCl$
Verapamil Hydrochloride
$C_{27}H_{38}O_6,H_2O$
Prednisolone Tebutate
$C_{27}H_{40}O_3$
Testosterone Cipionate
$C_{27}H_{40}O_4$
Hydroxyprogesterone Caproate
$C_{27}H_{42}ClNO_2$
Benzethonium Chloride
$C_{27}H_{42}ClNO,H_2O$
Octafonium Chloride
$C_{27}H_{42}Cl_2N_2O_6$
Chloramphenicol Palmitate
$C_{27}H_{42}O_3$
Metenolone Enantate
$C_{27}H_{43}NO$
Solanidine
$C_{27}H_{44}O$
Colecalciferol
$C_{27}H_{44}O_2$
Alfacalcidol
$C_{27}H_{46}O$
Cholesterol
$C_{28}H_{24}Br_2N_6$
Fazadinium Bromide
$C_{28}H_{27}ClF_5NO$
Penfluridol
$C_{28}H_{29}F_2N_3O$
Pimozide
$C_{28}H_{29}NO_4$
Bephenium Hydroxynaphthoate
$C_{28}H_{31}FN_4O$
Astemizole
$C_{28}H_{32}FNO_6$
Dexamethasone Isonicotinate

$C_{28}H_{33}ClN_2$
Buclizine
$C_{28}H_{33}ClN_2,2HCl$
Buclizine Hydrochloride
$C_{28}H_{34}N_2O_3$
Denatonium Benzoate
$C_{28}H_{35}ClN_4O$
Clospipramine
$C_{28}H_{35}ClN_4O.2HCl$
Clospipramine Dihydrochloride
$C_{28}H_{36}O_3$
Testosterone Phenylpropionate
$C_{28}H_{37}ClO_7$
Beclometasone Dipropionate
$C_{28}H_{37}FO_7$
Betamethasone Dipropionate
$C_{28}H_{38}N_2O_4$
Cephaëline
$C_{28}H_{38}N_2O_4,2HCl$
Cephaëline Hydrochloride
$C_{28}H_{39}FO_5$
Fluocortolone Hexanoate
$C_{28}H_{39}FO_6$
Dexamethasone Tebutate
$C_{28}H_{40}N_2O_2$
Bialamicol
$C_{28}H_{40}N_2O_2,2HCl$
Bialamicol Hydrochloride
$C_{28}H_{41}N_3O_3$
Oxetacaine
$C_{28}H_{42}Cl_4N_4O_2$
Ambenonium Chloride
$C_{28}H_{44}O$
Ergocalciferol
$C_{28}H_{44}O_3$
Nandrolone Decanoate
$C_{28}H_{46}O$
Dihydrotachysterol
$C_{29}H_{31}F_2N_3O$
Fluspirilene
$C_{29}H_{32}O_{13}$
Etoposide
$C_{29}H_{33}ClN_2O_2$
Loperamide
$C_{29}H_{33}ClN_2O_2,HCl$
Loperamide Hydrochloride
$C_{29}H_{33}FO_6$
Betamethasone Benzoate
$C_{29}H_{33}O_{16}P$
Etoposide Phosphate
$C_{29}H_{35}NO_2$
Mifepristone
$C_{29}H_{38}FN_3O_3$
Mibefradil
$C_{29}H_{38}FN_3O_3,2HCl$
Mibefradil Dihydrochloride
$C_{29}H_{38}F_3N_3O_2S$
Fluphenazine Enantate
$C_{29}H_{38}N_2O_4$
Dehydroemetine
$C_{29}H_{38}N_2O_4,2HCl$
Dehydroemetine Hydrochloride
$C_{29}H_{38}N_4O_{10}$
Lymecycline
$C_{29}H_{39}Cl_2F_3NO_7P$
Halofantrine β-Glycerophosphate
$C_{29}H_{40}N_2O_4$
Emetine
$C_{29}H_{40}N_2O_4,2HCl,7H_2O$
Emetine Hydrochloride
$C_{29}H_{41}NO_4$
Buprenorphine
$C_{29}H_{41}NO_4,HCl$
Buprenorphine Hydrochloride
$C_{29}H_{42}O_6$
Hydrocortisone Cipionate
$C_{29}H_{44}O_3$
Estradiol Undecylate
$C_{29}H_{44}O_{12},8H_2O$
Ouabain
$C_{29}H_{48}O_3$
Testosterone Undecylate
$C_{29}H_{53}NO_5$
Orlistat
$C_{30}H_{24}N_4O_{10}$
Nicofuranose
$C_{30}H_{32}N_2O_2$
Diphenoxylate
$C_{30}H_{32}N_2O_2,HCl$
Diphenoxylate Hydrochloride
$C_{30}H_{34}O_{13}$
Picrotoxin
$C_{30}H_{35}F_2N_3O$
Lidoflazine
$C_{30}H_{40}Cl_2N_4$
Dequalinium Chloride
$C_{30}H_{41}FO_7$
Triamcinolone Hexacetonide
$C_{30}H_{44}N_2O_{10}$
Hexobendine
$C_{30}H_{44}N_2O_{10},2HCl$
Hexobendine Hydrochloride
$C_{30}H_{44}O_3$
Boldenone Undecylenate
$C_{30}H_{45}NNaO_7P$
Fosinopril Sodium
$C_{30}H_{46}NO_7P$
Fosinopril
$C_{30}H_{46}O_4$
Enoxolone
$C_{30}H_{60}I_3N_3O_3$
Gallamine Triethiodide
$C_{31}H_{32}N_4O_2$
Bezitramide
$C_{31}H_{33}N_3O_6S$
Zafirlukast
$C_{31}H_{36}IN_3$
Stilbazium Iodide
$C_{31}H_{39}N_5O_5$
Ergotoxine
$C_{31}H_{39}N_5O_5,CH_3SO_3H$
Ergotoxine Esilate
$C_{31}H_{41}N_5O_5,CH_4O_3S$
Co-dergocrine Mesilate
$C_{31}H_{46}O_2$
Phytomenadione
$C_{31}H_{47}NaO_6$
Sodium Fusidate
$C_{31}H_{48}O_6,½H_2O$
Fusidic Acid
$C_{31}H_{52}O_3$
Alpha Tocoferil Acetate
$C_{32}H_{38}N_2O_8$
Deserpidine
$C_{32}H_{39}NO_2$
Ebastine
$C_{32}H_{39}NO_4$
Fexofenadine
$C_{32}H_{39}NO_4, HCl$
Fexofenadine Hydrochloride
$C_{32}H_{39}NO_6, C_4H_4O_4$
Ebastine Fumarate
$C_{32}H_{40}BrN_5O_5$
Bromocriptine
$C_{32}H_{40}BrN_5O_5,CH_4O_3S$
Bromocriptine Mesilate
$C_{32}H_{43}ClN_2O_2S$
Clopenthixol Decanoate
Zuclopenthixol Decanoate
$C_{32}H_{43}N_5O_5,CH_3SO_3H$
Co-dergocrine Mesilate
$C_{32}H_{44}F_3N_3O_2S$
Fluphenazine Decanoate
$C_{32}H_{45}N_3O_4S$
Nelfinavir
$C_{32}H_{45}N_3O_4S,CH_3SO_3H$
Nelfinavir Mesilate
$C_{32}H_{52}Br_2N_4O_4$
Demecarium Bromide
$C_{32}H_{53}BrN_2O_4$
Rocuronium Bromide
$[C_{32}H_{53}N_2O_4]^+$
Rocuronium
$C_{33}H_{25}N_3O_3$
Norbormide
$C_{33}H_{30}N_4O_2$
Telmisartan
$C_{33}H_{33}FN_2O_4$
Atorvastatin Lactone
$C_{33}H_{34}FN_2NaO_5$
Atorvastatin Sodium
$C_{33}H_{34}N_6O_6$
Candesartan Cilexetil
$C_{33}H_{35}FN_2O_5$
Atorvastatin
$C_{33}H_{35}N_5O_5$
Ergotamine
$C_{33}H_{37}N_5O_5$
Dihydroergotamine
$C_{33}H_{37}N_5O_5,CH_3SO_3H$
Dihydroergotamine Mesilate
$C_{33}H_{38}N_4O_6$
Irinotecan
$C_{33}H_{38}N_4O_6,HCl$
Irinotecan Hydrochloride
$C_{33}H_{38}N_4O_6, HCl,3H_2O$
Irinotecan Hydrochloride Trihydrate
$C_{33}H_{40}N_2O_9$
Reserpine
Methoserpidine
$C_{33}H_{43}F_3N_2O_2S$
Flupentixol Decanoate
$C_{33}H_{47}NO_{13}$
Natamycin
$C_{34}H_{36}N_2O_6,3H_2O$
Pseudomorphine
$C_{34}H_{46}N_4O_4$
Dequalinium Acetate
$C_{34}H_{47}NO_{11}$
Aconitine
$C_{34}H_{47}NO_{11},HNO_3$
Aconitine Nitrate
$C_{34}H_{48}Na_2O_7$
Carbenoxolone Sodium
$C_{34}H_{50}O_7$
Carbenoxolone
$C_{34}H_{63}ClN_2O_6S,HCl$
Clindamycin Palmitate Hydrochloride
$C_{35}H_{35}ClNNaO_3S$
Montelukast Sodium
$C_{35}H_{36}ClNO_3S$
Montelukast
$C_{35}H_{38}Cl_2N_8O_4$
Itraconazole
$C_{35}H_{41}N_5O_5,CH_3SO_3H$
Co-dergocrine Mesilate
$C_{35}H_{42}N_2O_9$
Rescinnamine
$C_{35}H_{42}N_2O_{11}$
Syrosingopine
$C_{35}H_{51}N_3O_4S_2$
Pipotiazine Palmitate
$C_{35}H_{60}Br_2N_2O_4$
Pancuronium Bromide

Therapeutic Classes

5-α-Reductase inhibitor

Finasteride

Acaricide

Aldicarb
Azinphos-ethyl
Benzyl Benzoate
Chlorpyrifos
Crotamiton
Fenthion
Methamidophos
Monocrotophos
Omethoate
Triazophos

Aerosol propellent

Cryofluorane
Dichlorodifluoromethane
Trichlorofluoromethane

Alkaloid

Aconitine
Benzoylecgonine
Berberine
Chelidonine
Coniine
Cytisine
Ecgonine
Harman
Hydrastine
Hydrastinine
Hydroquinine
Ibogaine
Monocrotaline
Narceine
Neopine
Solanidine
Solanine
Strychnine
Thebaine
Yohimbine

Alpha$_1$-adrenoceptor blocker

Alfuzosin
Tamsulosin
Terazosin

Anabolic steroid

Androstanolone
Androstenedione
Boldenone
Clostebol
Drostanolone Propionate
Ethylestrenol
Gestrinone
Metenolone
Methandienone
Methandriol
Nandrolone
Norandrostenediol
Norandrostenedione
Norethandrolone
Oxandrolone
Oxymetholone
Stanozolol
Trenbolone

Anaesthetic

Gamma-hydroxybutyric Acid
Levobupivacaine
Methohexital
Propofol
Rapacuronium Bromide
Sevoflurane
Thialbarbital

Analgesic

Acetanilide
Alclofenac
Aletamine
Aloxiprin
Aminophenazone
Aspirin
Azapropazone
Benorilate
Benoxaprofen
Benzydamine
Bufexamac
Cinchophen
Clonixin
Dexmedetomidine
Diclofenac
Diflunisal
Dipyrone
Eptazocine
Etenzamide
Etofenamate
Etoxazene
Famprofazone
Fenbufen
Fenclofenac
Fendosal
Fenoprofen
Fenyramidol
Feprazone
Floctafenine
Flufenamic Acid
Flunixin
Flupirtine
Flurbiprofen
Glafenine
Ibuprofen
Indometacin
Indoprofen
Ketoprofen
Ketorolac
Meclofenamic Acid
Mefenamic Acid
Methyl Salicylate
Morazone
Naproxen
Nefopam
Nifenazone
Niflumic Acid
Oxyphenbutazone
Paracetamol
Phenacetin
Phenazone
Phenazopyridine
Phenylbutazone
Piroxicam
Propyphenazone
Salicylamide
Salicylic Acid
Salol
Salsalate
Sulindac
Suprofen
Tenoxicam
Tiaprofenic Acid
Tolfenamic Acid
Tolmetin
Zomepirac

Analgesic (veterinary)

Isopropylaminophenazone
Xylazine

Anaplasmodastat (veterinary)

Gloxazone

Androgen

Androsterone
Danazol
Fluoxymesterone
Mesterolone
Methyltestosterone
Oxandrolone
Testosterone

Angiotensin II receptor antagonist

Candesartan
Irbesartan
Losartan
Telmisartan
Valsartan

Anionic surfactant

Docusate Sodium

Anorectic

Benzfetamine
Cathine
Chlorphentermine
Diethylpropion
Fenbutrazate
Fenfluramine
Fenproporex
Mazindol
Phendimetrazine
Phenmetrazine
Phentermine

Anthelmintic

Bephenium Hydroxynaphthoate
Bitoscanate
Cambendazole
Dichlorophen
Fenbendazole
Hexylresorcinol
Levamisole
Mebendazole
Naphthalene
Niclosamide
Niridazole
Piperazine
Pyrantel
Pyrvinium Embonate
Santonin
Stilbazium Iodide
Tetrachloroethylene
Tiabendazole
Trichlorfon

Anthelmintic (veterinary)

Albendazole
Bunamidine
Clioxanide
Diamfenetide
Haloxon
Morantel
Nitroxinil
Oxyclozanide
Parbendazole
Phenothiazine
Rafoxanide
Tetramisole
Thenium Closilate

Anti-allergic

Ketotifen
Sodium Cromoglicate

Anti-amoebic

Bialamicol
Carbarsone
Clefamide
Clioquinol
Conessine
Diiodohydroxyquinoline
Diloxanide
Emetine
Phanquinone

Anti-anginal

Lidoflazine
Nicorandil
Perhexiline
Prenylamine
Sotalol

Anti-anginal vasodilator

Amyl Nitrite
Carbocromen
Dipyridamole
Glyceryl Trinitrate
Hexobendine
Imolamine
Isosorbide Dinitrate
Isosorbide Mononitrate
Nifedipine
Pentaerithrityl Tetranitrate
Trimetazidine

Anti-arrhythmic

Acecainide
Adenosine
Ajmaline
Amiodarone
Aprindine
Bretylium Tosilate
Disopyramide
Dofetilide
Encainide
Flecainide
Hydroquinidine
Ibutilide
Lidocaine
Lorcainide
Mexiletine
Moracizine
Prajmalium Bitartrate
Procainamide
Quinidine
Sotalol
Tocainide
Verapamil

Anti-asthmatic

Formoterol
Nedocromil
Zafirlukast

Anti-emetic

Benzquinamide
Cyclizine
Difenidol
Dolasetron
Granisetron
Metoclopramide
Metopimazine
Nabilone
Ondansetron
Thiethylperazine
Tropisetron

Anti-epileptic

Lamotrigine
Levetiracetam
Topiramate
Vigabatrin

Anti-inflammatory

Aceclofenac
Acemetacin
Celecoxib
Deflazacort
Dexketoprofen
Etodolac
Fluticasone Propionate
Ketorolac
Meloxicam
Nabumetone
Olsalazine
Rofecoxib
Salol

Anti-migraine

Almotriptan

Anti-oestrogen

Toremifene

Anti-platelet

Clopidogrel

Anti-psychotic

Clospipramine

Anti-ulcer

Balsalazide

Anti-obesity agent

Orlistat

Antibacterial

Amikacin
Amoxicillin
Azithromycin
Azlocillin
Aztreonam
Bacampicillin
Bacitracin
Capreomycin
Cefaclor
Cefixime
Ceftazidime
Ceftriaxone
Chlorquinaldol
Chlortetracycline
Ciprofloxacin
Clarithromycin
Clomocycline
Demeclocycline
Dequalinium Chloride
Dibrompropamidine
Diminazene
Hydroxyquinoline
Levofloxacin
Lymecycline
Mafenide
Metronidazole
Minocycline
Nitrofurazone
Noxytiolin
Ofloxacin
Oxytetracycline Dihydrate
Phanquinone
Procaine Benzylpenicillin
Propamidine
Propicillin
Rifabutin
Rifamycin SV
Rolitetracycline
Roxithromycin
Streptomycin
Succinylsulfathiazole
Sulfacetamide
Sulfadimethoxine
Sulfaguanidine
Sulfametoxydiazine
Teicoplanin
Thioacetazone

Antibacterial (urinary)

Mandelic Acid
Methenamine
Nalidixic Acid
Nitrofurantoin
Nitroxoline

Antibacterial (veterinary)

Furaltadone
Tilmicosin

Antibacterial (topical)

Mupirocin

Antibiotic

Ampicillin
Benzylpenicillin
Carbenicillin
Cefalexin
Cefaloridine
Cefalothin
Cefradine
Chloramphenicol
Clindamycin
Cloxacillin
Cycloserine
Dihydrostreptomycin
Doxycycline
Erythromycin
Flucloxacillin
Fusidic Acid
Gentamicin
Kanamycin
Lincomycin
Meloxicam
Methacycline
Meticillin
Neomycin
Ofloxacin
Oleandomycin
Pheneticillin
Phenoxymethylpenicillin
Pivampicillin
Rifabutin
Spiramycin
Tetracycline
Tobramycin
Troleandomycin
Vancomycin

Antibiotic (veterinary)

Tylosin

Anticholinergic

Adiphenine
Ambutonium Bromide
Atropine
Atropine Methobromide
Atropine Methonitrate
Atropine Oxide
Benaprizine
Benzatropine
Benzilonium Bromide
Biperiden
Caramiphen
Chlorphenoxamine
Clidinium Bromide
Cyclopentolate
Cycrimine
Dicycloverine
Diethazine
Diphemanil Metilsulfate
Emepronium Bromide
Eucatropine
Glycopyrronium Bromide
Heteronium Bromide
Hexocyclium Metilsulfate
Homatropine
Homatropine Methylbromide
Hyoscine
Hyoscine Butylbromide
Hyoscine Methobromide
Hyoscine Methonitrate
Hyoscyamine
Isopropamide Iodide
Lachesine Chloride
Mepenzolate Bromide
Methanthelinium Bromide
Metixene
Octatropine Methylbromide
Orphenadrine
Oxyphencyclimine
Oxyphenonium Bromide
Pentapiperide Metilsulfate
Penthienate Methobromide
Phenglutarimide
Pipenzolate Bromide
Piperidolate
Poldine Metilsulfate
Procyclidine
Profenamine
Propantheline Bromide
Tigloidine
Tricyclamol Chloride
Tridihexethyl Chloride
Trihexyphenidyl
Tropicamide
Valethamate Bromide

Anticholinesterase

Ambenonium Chloride
Demecarium Bromide
Distigmine Bromide
Ecothiopate Iodide
Edrophonium Chloride
Neostigmine Bromide
Physostigmine
Physostigmine Aminoxide
Pyridostigmine Bromide
Tacrine

Anticoagulant

Acenocoumarol
Anisindione
Dicoumarol
Diphenadione
Enoxaparin
Ethyl Biscoumacetate
Lepirudin
Phenindione
Phenprocoumon
Picotamide
Warfarin

Anticonvulsant

Beclamide
Carbamazepine
Clonazepam
Dimethadione
Ethosuximide
Ethotoin

Antidepressant

Antidiabetic

Antidiarrhoeal

Antidote (barbiturate poisoning)

Antidote (organophosphate insecticide poisoning)

Antidote (nerve gas and organophosphate insecticide poisoning)

Antifilarial

Antifreeze

Antifungal

Antifungal (veterinary)

Antihistamine

Promethazine
Propiomazine
Pyrrobutamine
Thenalidine
Thenyldiamine
Thiazinamium Metilsulfate
Thonzylamine
Tolpropamine
Trimethobenzamide
Tripelennamine
Triprolidine

Antihypercalcaemic

Gallium Nitrate

Antihyperlipidaemic

Simvastatin

Antihyperlipoproteinaemic

Fluvastatin
Lovastatin
Pravastatin

Antihypertensive

Amosulalol
Benazepril
Benzthiazide
Bethanidine
Bopindolol
Bretylium Tosilate
Bunazosin
Captopril
Clonidine
Clopamide
Debrisoquine
Deserpidine
Dihydralazine
Diltiazem
Doxazosin
Enalapril
Felodipine
Fenoldopam
Fosinopril
Guanethidine
Guanoclor
Guanoxan
Hexamethonium Bromide
Hydralazine
Imidapril
Indoramin
Labetalol
Lisinopril
Lofexidine
Mecamylamine
Methoserpidine
Methyldopa
Methyldopate
Minoxidil
Moexipril
Moxonidine
Pargyline
Pempidine
Pentolonium Tartrate
Perindopril
Phenoxybenzamine
Phentolamine
Prazosin
Protoveratrine A
Quinapril
Ramipril
Rescinnamine
Reserpine
Sotalol
Spirapril
Syrosingopine
Tertatolol
Trandolapril
Trimetaphan Camsilate

Antileprotic

Clofazimine
Dapsone
Thiambutosine

Antimalarial

Amodiaquine
Artemether
Artesunate
Chloroquine
Chlorproguanil
Cinchonidine
Cinchonine
Cycloguanil
Halofantrine
Hydroxychloroquine
Mepacrine
Primaquine
Proguanil
Pyrimethamine
Quinine

Antimicrobial

Furazolidone
Halquinol
Hexetidine
Nifuratel
Trimethoprim

Antimigraine

Naratriptan
Pizotifen
Rizatriptan
Zolmitriptan

Antimuscarinic

Tolterodine

Antineoplastic

Aclarubicin
Aldesleukin
Altretamine
Aminoglutethimide
Amsacrine
Anastrozole
Arsenic Trioxide
Asparaginase
Bicalutamide
Bleomycin
Buserelin
Busulfan
Capecitabine
Carmustine
Chlorambucil
Cisplatin
Cladribine
Cyclophosphamide
Cytarabine
Dactinomycin
Daunorubicin
Docetaxel
Doxorubicin
Eflornithine
Epirubicin
Etoposide
Exemestane
Fludarabine
Fluorouracil
Gemcitabine
Hydroxycarbamide
Idarubicin
Irinotecan
Lanreotide
Letrozole
Mannomustine
Melphalan
Mercaptopurine
Methotrexate
Mitozantrone
Molgramostim
Oxaliplatin
Paclitaxel
Pentostatin
Pipobroman
Procarbazine
Raltitrexed
Temozolomide
Thiotepa
Tioguanine
Topotecan
Toremifene
Trimetrexate
Urethane
Vinblastine
Vincristine
Vindesine
Vinorelbine

Antineoplastic (hormonal)

Diethylstilbestrol

Antineoplastic aromatase inhibitor

Formestane

Antineutropenic

Molgramostim

Antiparkinsonian

Amantadine
Benserazide

Bromocriptine
Budipine
Droxidopa
Entacapone
Galantamine
Levodopa
Pergolide
Phenglutarimide
Pramipexole
Quinagolide
Ropinirole
Selegiline

Antiprogestogenic steroid

Mifepristone

Antiprotozoal

Acetarsone
Aminitrozole
Atovaquone
Broxaldine
Broxyquinoline
Dehydroemetine
Diminazene
Eflornithine
Hydroxystilbamidine
Mepacrine
Metronidazole
Nifuratel
Nimorazole
Pentamidine
Tinidazole

Antiprotozoal (veterinary)

Amicarbalide
Aminonitrothiazole
Dimetridazole
Nifursol
Quinuronium Sulfate

Antipruritic

Crotamiton

Antipsychotic

Acetophenazine
Amisulpride
Benperidol
Biriperone
Carfenazine
Clozapine
Droperidol
Nemonapride
Olanzapine
Quetiapine
Remoxipride
Risperidone
Sertindole
Trifluoperazine
Trifluperidol
Ziprasidone
Zotepine
Zuclopenthixol

Antipyretic

Salol

Antirheumatic

Leflunomide

Antiseptic

Acriflavinium Chloride
Aminoacridine
Amylmetacresol
Benzalkonium Chloride
Benzethonium Chloride
Naphthalene
Thymol
Triclocarban

Antispasmodic

Alverine
Ambucetamide
Benactyzine
Butetamate
Dimoxyline
Flavoxate
Hexocyclium Metilsulfate
Mebeverine
Octamylamine
Papaverine
Pipoxolan

Antispasmodic (veterinary)

Aminopromazine
Fenpipramide
Fenpiprane
Metindizate

Antithrombotic

Alteplase
Anagrelide
Cilostazol
Cloricromen
Dipyridamole
Picotamide
Sulfinpyrazone
Ticlopidine
Tirofiban

Antithyroid agent

Carbimazole
Methylthiouracil
Propylthiouracil
Thiamazole

Antituberculous

Aminosalicylic Acid

Antituberculous agent

Ethambutol
Ethionamide

Antitussive

Benzonatate
Benzylmorphine
Bibenzonium Bromide
Caramiphen
Carbetapentane
Clofedanol
Dextromethorphan
Dextrorphan
Dimethoxanate
Dropropizine
Hydrocodone
Isoaminile
Levopropoxyphene
Noscapine
Oxeladin
Pholcodine
Pipazetate

Antiulcerative

Famotidine
Nizatidine
Pirenzepine

Antiurolithic

Succinimide

Antiviral

Abacavir
Aciclovir
Amantadine
Amprenavir
Cidofovir
Delavirdine
Didanosine
Efavirenz
Famciclovir
Foscarnet Sodium
Ganciclovir
Idoxuridine
Indinavir
Lamivudine
Metisazone
Penciclovir
Rimantadine
Ritonavir
Saquinavir
Stavudine
Valaciclovir
Zalcitabine
Zanamivir
Zidovudine

Antiviral (HIV)

Nelfinavir
Nevirapine

Antoparkinsonian

Apomorphine

Antoxidant

Butylated Hydroxyanisole
Butylated Hydroxytoluene
Dodecyl Gallate
Ethyl Gallate
Hydroquinone

Anxiolytic

Alprazolam
Buspirone
Dexmedetomidine
Etizolam
Flutazolam
Flutoprazepam
Metaclazepam
Mexazolam
Tandospirone

Aromatase inhibitor

Exemestane

Azasteroid

Finasteride

Bacteriostat

Ambazone

Barbiturate

Allobarbital
Amobarbital
Aprobarbital
Barbital
Brallobarbital
Butalbital
Butobarbital
Cyclobarbital
Cyclopentobarbital
Enallylpropymal
Heptabarb
Hexethal
Hexobarbital
Ibomal
Idobutal
Metharbital
Methohexital
Methylphenobarbital
Nealbarbital
Pentobarbital
Phenobarbital
Phenylmethylbarbituric Acid
Secbutabarbital
Secobarbital
Talbutal
Thialbarbital
Thiamylal
Thiopental
Vinbarbital
Vinylbital

Benzodiazepine antagonist

Flumazenil

Beta-adrenergic agonist

Bambuterol
Clenbuterol
Dopexamine
Salmeterol

Beta-blocker

Atenolol
Acebutolol
Alprenolol
Betaxolol
Bevantolol
Bisoprolol
Bunitrolol
Carteolol
Carvedilol
Celiprolol
Esmolol
Levobunolol
Metipranolol
Metoprolol
Nadolol
Nebivolol
Oxprenolol
Pindolol
Practolol
Propranolol
Tertatolol
Timolol
Xamoterol

Biological response modifier

Aldesleukin

Bone modulator

Alendronic Acid

Bone resorption inhibitor

Tiludronic Acid

Bronchodilator

Bambuterol
Bamifylline
Butetamate
Protokylol
Reproterol
Rimiterol
Salbutamol
Salmeterol

Calcium antagonist

Amlodipine
Isradipine
Lacidipine
Mibefradil
Nimodipine
Nisoldipine
Nitrendipine

Calcium regulator

Clodronic Acid

Carbonic anhydrase inhibitor

Acetazolamide
Diclofenamide
Ethoxzolamide
Methazolamide

Cardiac glycoside

Acetyldigitoxin
Deslanoside
Digitoxin
Digoxin
Lanatoside C
Metildigoxin
Ouabain
Strophanthin-K

Cardiac stimulant

Heptaminol

Cardioprotective

Dexrazoxane

Cardiotonic

Levosimendan
Milrinone
Ouabain
Xamoterol

Cationic disinfectant

Benzalkonium Chloride
Benzethonium Chloride
Cetalkonium Chloride
Cetrimide
Cetylpyridinium Chloride
Chlorhexidine
Dofamium Chloride
Domiphen Bromide
Octafonium Chloride

Central depressant

Ethanol
Gamma-butyrolactone
Gelsemine

Central stimulant

Amfetamine
Amineptine
Bemegride
Bromantane
Brucine
Carphedon
Dexamfetamine
Dimethylamfetamine
Fencamfamin
Levamfetamine
Meclofenoxate

Ergot derivative

Ergotoxine

Essential oil

Cineole
Eugenol

Estrogen

Estradiol
Ethinylestradiol
Hexestrol
Methallenestril

Expectorant

Cephaëline
Guaifenesin

Flavouring agent

Benzaldehyde
Ethyl Acetate
Vanillin

Fungicide

Hexaconazole
Pyrazophos

Fungistatic

Diphenyl

Gastric and pancreatic lipase inhibitor

Orlistat

General anaesthetic

Alfadolone
Alfaxalone
Chloroform
Desflurane
Enflurane
Ether
Etomidate
Halothane
Ketamine
Methoxyflurane
Trichloroethylene

Glutamate antagonist

Riluzole

Gonad stimulating hormone

Chorionic Gonadotropin

Gonadorelin analogue

Buserelin
Nafarelin

Gout suppressant

Colchicine

Growth stimulant

Somatropin

HMG CoA reductase inhibitor

Atorvastatin
Lovastatin
Pravastatin
Simvastatin

Haemopoietic vitamin

Cyanocobalamin
Hydroxocobalamin

Haemostatic

Aminocaproic Acid
Carbazochrome
Cotarnine

Hallucinogen

5-Methyltryptamine
Bufotenine
DOM
Diethyltryptamine
Dimethyltryptamine
Harmaline
Harmine
Lysergamide
Lysergic Acid
Lysergide
Mescaline
Methoxyamfetamine
Methylenedioxyamfetamine
Methylenedioxyethylamfetamine
Methylenedioxymethamfetamine
Methylpiperidyl Benzilate
Myristicin
N-Methyltryptamine
Phencyclidine
Psilocin
Psilocybine
Trimethoxyamfetamine
α-Methyltryptamine

Herbicide

Alachlor
Ametryne
Aminotriazole
Atrazine
Desmetryne
Dicamba
Dichlorophenoxyacetic Acid
Dinitro-orthocresol
Diquat
Diuron
Glyphosate
Isoproturon
Linuron
Methoprotryne
Methylchlorophenoxyacetic Acid
Metolachlor
Monolinuron
Paraquat
Prometryne
Propanil
Propazine
Simazine
Terbutryne
Terbutylazine
Trichlorophenoxyacetic Acid

Histamine H_2-receptor antagonist

Cimetidine
Famotidine
Nizatidine
Ranitidine

Hypnotic

Acecarbromal
Apronal
Bromisoval
Brotizolam
Butobarbital
Butylchloral Hydrate
Carbromal
Clomethiazole
Cloral Betaine
Cloral Hydrate
Cyclobarbital
Dichloralphenazone
Ethchlorvynol
Ethinamate
Flunitrazepam
Flurazepam
Glutethimide
Ibomal
Idobutal
Loprazolam
Lormetazepam
Mecloqualone
Methaqualone
Methylpentynol
Methyprylon
Midazolam
Nitrazepam
Paraldehyde
Pentobarbital
Phenobarbital
Quazepam
Temazepam
Thalidomide
Triazolam
Trichloroethanol
Triclofos Sodium
Vinylbital
Zolpidem
Zopiclone

Hypothalamus and pituitary suppressant

Metallibure

Immunomodulator

Aldesleukin
Ditiocarb

Immunosuppressant

Azathioprine
Ciclosporin
Mycophenolate Mofetil
Rituximab
Sirolimus
Tacrolimus
Thalidomide

Induction of ovulation

Clomifene
Cyclofenil

Inotrope

Enoximone

Insect repellent

Dibutyl Phthalate
Diethyltoluamide
Dimethyl Phthalate

Insect fumigant

Methyl Bromide

Insecticide

Aldicarb
Aldrin
Azinphos-ethyl
Carbaryl
Chloroaniline
Chloromethylaniline
Chloronitroaniline
Chlorpyrifos
Coumaphos
Cyfluthrin
Deltamethrin
Dichlorvos
Dieldrin
Dinitro-orthocresol
Disulfoton
Endrin
Fenitrothion
Fenthion
Fluquinconazole
Heptachlor
Imidacloprid
Irgarol
Methamidophos
Monocrotophos
Nicotine
Omethoate
Paradichlorobenzene
Pyrethrum
Triazophos
Trichlorfon

Insecticide synergist

Piperonyl Butoxide

Iron chelator

Deferiprone

Leukotriene D_4 antagonist

Zafirlukast

Lipid regulator

Bezafibrate
Cerivastatin
Ciprofibrate
Clofibrate

Local anaesthetic

Benzocaine
Benzyl Alcohol
Bupivacaine
Butacaine
Butanilicaine
Butyl Aminobenzoate
Chloroprocaine
Cinchocaine
Cocaine
Cyclomethycaine
Diperodon
Dyclonine
Etidocaine
Hexylcaine
Lidocaine
Mepivacaine
Meprylcaine
Oxetacaine
Oxybuprocaine
Phenacaine
Piperocaine
Pramocaine
Prilocaine
Procaine
Propoxycaine
Proxymetacaine
Quinisocaine
Ropivacaine
Tetracaine

Lung surfactant

Calfactant
Colfosceril Palmitate
Pumactant

Migraine prophylactic

Methysergide

Molluscicide

Metaldehyde

Mucolytic

Acetylcysteine

Mucolytic expectorant

Bromhexine

Muscle relaxant

Alcuronium Chloride
Baclofen
Carisoprodol
Chlorphenesin Carbamate
Chlorzoxazone
Cyclobenzaprine
Dantrolene
Decamethonium Bromide
Doxacurium Chloride
Emylcamate
Fazadinium Bromide
Fenyramidol
Gallamine Triethiodide
Mebezonium Iodide
Mephenesin
Methocarbamol
Metocurine Iodide
Mivacurium Chloride
Pancuronium Bromide
Rocuronium
Styramate
Suxamethonium Chloride
Suxethonium Bromide
Tetrazepam
Tizanidine
Tubocurarine Chloride

Muscle relaxant (skeletal)

Phenprobamate

Narcotic analgesic

Alfentanil
Alphaprodine
Anileridine
Benzylmorphine
Bezitramide
Buprenorphine
Butorphanol
Codeine
Dextromoramide
Dextropropoxyphene
Diamorphine
Dihydrocodeine
Dihydromorphine
Dipipanone
Embutramide
Ethoheptazine
Ethylmorphine
Fentanyl
Hydrocodone
Hydromorphone
Ketobemidone
Levacetylmethadol
Levorphanol
Meptazinol
Methadone
Morphine
Nalbuphine
Norcodeine
Normethadone

Normorphine
Norpipanone
Oxycodone
Oxymorphone
Pentazocine
Pethidine
Phenazocine
Phenoperidine
Piminodine
Piritramide
Profadol
Racemorphan
Remifentanil
Thebacon
Tilidate
Tramadol
Trimeperidine

Narcotic analgesic (veterinary)

Acetorphine
Etorphine

Narcotic antagonist

Amiphenazole
Cyclazocine
Levallorphan
Nalmefene
Nalorphine
Naloxone
Naltrexone

Narcotic antidiarrhoeal

Diphenoxylate

Nematicide

Aldicarb
Coumaphos
Fenamiphos
Propanil

Neuroleptic

Zuclopenthixol

Neuromuscular blocker

Rocuronium

Neuroprotective

Riluzole

Nitrovasodilator

Nicorandil

Nootropic

Aniracetam
Choline Alfoscerate
Donepezil
Exifone
Idebenone
Indeloxazine
Rivastigmine

Oestrogen

Chlorotrianisene
Dienestrol
Estriol
Estrone
Mestranol

Paracetamol antidote

Acetylcysteine

Parasiticide

Betanaphthol
Sulfiram

Parasympathomimetic

Acetylcholine Chloride
Bethanechol Chloride
Carbachol
Methacholine Chloride
Pilocarpine

Pesticide

Azinphos-methyl
Benzene Hexachloride
Chlordane
Chloronitrotoluene
Clofenotane
Demeton-*S*
Dimethoate
Dimpylate
Endosulfan
Lindane
Malathion
Methoxychlor
Mevinphos
Parathion
Rotenone

Pharmaceutical adjuvant

Benethamine
Ethylenediamine Hydrate

Pigmenting agent

Methoxsalen
Trioxysalen

Plasticiser

Diethyl Phthalate
Tributyl Phosphate

Potassium-channel activator

Nicorandil

Preservative

Benzoic Acid
Chlorobutanol
Ethyl Hydroxybenzoate
Methyl Hydroxybenzoate
Pentachlorophenol
Propyl Hydroxybenzoate
Sorbic Acid

Progestational steroid

Chlormadinone Acetate
Dimethisterone
Dydrogesterone
Ethisterone
Etynodiol Diacetate
Gestonorone Caproate
Hydroxyprogesterone
Lynestrenol
Medroxyprogesterone Acetate
Megestrol Acetate
Norethisterone
Noretynodrel
Progesterone

Progestational steroid (veterinary)

Flugestone

Progestogen

Allylestrenol

Prolactin inhibitor

Quinagolide

Prostaglandin

Alprostadil

Prostaglandin analogue

Misoprostol

Proton pump inhibitor

Lansoprazole
Misoprostol
Omeprazole
Pantoprazole
Rabeprazole

Psychomimetic

Cannabis

Pulmonary surfactant

Calfactant
Pumactant

Purgative

Aloin
Arecoline

Thyroid agent

Levothyroxine
Liothyronine

Topical vasodilator

Butoxyethyl Nicotinate
Ethyl Nicotinate
Hexyl Nicotinate
Methyl Nicotinate

Tranquilliser

Acepromazine
Acetophenazine
Azacyclonol
Benzoctamine
Bromazepam
Butaperazine
Camazepam
Captodiame
Carfenazine
Chlordiazepoxide
Chlormezanone
Chlorpromazine
Chlorprothixene
Clobazam
Clopenthixol
Clorazepic Acid
Clotiapine
Demoxepam
Diazepam
Dixyrazine
Droperidol
Emylcamate
Ethomoxane
Fluanisone
Flupentixol
Fluphenazine
Fluspirilene
Haloperidol
Hydroxyphenamate
Hydroxyzine
Ketazolam
Levomepromazine
Lithium Carbonate
Lorazepam
Loxapine
Mebutamate
Medazepam
Meprobamate
Mesoridazine
Molindone
Nordazepam
Oxazepam
Oxypertine
Pecazine
Penfluridol
Perazine
Pericyazine
Perphenazine
Phenaglycodol
Phenprobamate
Pimozide
Pipamperone
Piperacetazine
Pipotiazine
Prazepam
Prochlorperazine
Promazine
Prothipendyl
Sulforidazine
Sulpiride
Tetrabenazine
Tetrazepam
Thiopropazate
Thioproperazine
Thioridazine
Tiotixene
Triflupromazine
Trimetozine
Tybamate

Tranquilliser (veterinary)

Azaperone
Trifluomeprazine

Trypanocide (veterinary)

Homidium Bromide
Pyritidium Bromide

Tuberculostatic

Cycloserine
Isoniazid
Morinamide
Protionamide
Pyrazinamide
Rifampicin
Salinazid
Thioacetazone
Tiocarlide

Uricosuric

Benzbromarone
Benziodarone
Etebenecid
Probenecid
Sulfinpyrazone

Uterine stimulant

Methylergometrine

Vasodilator

Alprostadil
Azapetine
Bamethan
Benziodarone
Betahistine
Buphenine
Butalamine
Co-dergocrine Mesilate
Cyclandelate
Enoximone
Fasudil
Heptaminol
Inositol Nicotinate
Isoxsuprine
Moxisylyte
Naftidrofuryl Oxalate
Nicametate
Nicergoline
Nicofuranose
Nicotinic Acid
Nicotinyl Alcohol
Pentifylline
Pentoxifylline
Sildenafil
Tolazoline
Xantinol Nicotinate

Vasodilator (coronary)

Cloricromen

Vesicant

Cantharidin

Vitamin

Alfacalcidol
Ascorbic Acid
Colecalciferol
Ergocalciferol
Folic Acid
Nicotinamide
Nicotinic Acid
Phytomenadione
Pyridoxine
Riboflavin
Thiamine

Vitamin B activity

Dexpanthenol

Vitamin D activity

Dihydrotachysterol

Vitamin E activity

Alpha Tocoferil Acetate

Vitamin K activity

Acetomenaphthone

Vitamin K analogue

Menadione

Xanthine bronchodilator

Acefylline Piperazine
Bufylline
Diprophylline
Etamiphylline
Etofylline
Proxyphylline
Theophylline

Xanthine stimulant

Caffeine
Fenetylline

Molecular Weights

Mol. Wt.	*Compound*
26.0	Cyanide
30.0	Formaldehyde
32.0	Methanol
44.1	Acetaldehyde
46.0	Formic Acid
46.07	Ethanol
58.08	Acetone
60.10	Isopropyl Alcohol
60.1	Acetic Acid Glacial
	Propanol
	Urea
61.1	Monoethanolamine
62.1	Ethylene Glycol
72.1	Methyl Ethyl Ketone
73.9	Lithium Carbonate
74.1	Ether
76.1	Hydroxycarbamide
77.1	Fluoroacetamide
78.0	Fluoroacetic Acid
78.1	Dimethyl Sulfoxide
	Ethylenediamine Hydrate
78.1	Benzene
82.1	Fomepizole
84.1	Aminotriazole
84.9	Methylene Chloride
86.1	Gamma-butyrolactone
	Piperazine
88.1	Ethyl Acetate
88.2	Amyl Alcohol
88.2	Putrescine
89.1	Urethane
90.0	Oxalic Acid
92.1	Toluene
93.1	Aniline
94.1	Phenol
94.9	Methyl Bromide
98.1	Methylpentynol
99.1	Succinimide
100.0	Sodium Fluoroacetate
102.0	(*S*)-3-Hydroxy-gamma-butyrolactone
102.1	Cycloserine
102.2	Cadaverine
104.1	Gamma-hydroxybutyric Acid
104.2	Choline
106.1	Benzaldehyde
106.2	Xylene
108·1	Cresol
	Benzyl Alcohol
	Paraphenylenediamine
109.1	4-Aminophenol
	Nicotinyl Alcohol
110.1	Hydroquinone
	Resorcinol
111.1	Ametazole
	Histamine
112.1	Sorbic Acid
114.2	Thiamazole
115.2	Tuaminoheptane
117.1	Amyl Nitrite
117.2	Betaine
119.4	Chloroform
120.2	Noxytiolin

Mol. Wt.	*Compound*
120.9	Dichlorodifluoromethane
121.1	Trometamol
121.2	Choline Hydroxide
	Phenethylamine
122.1	Benzoic Acid
	Nicotinamide
123.1	Nicotinic Acid
	Nitrobenzene
	Pyrazinamide
124.2	Dimercaprol
127.1	Sodium Gamma-hydroxybutyrate
127.2	Coniine
127.6	2-Chloroaniline
	3-Chloroaniline
	4-Chloroaniline
	Chloroaniline
128.1	Barbituric Acid
128.2	Naphthalene
128.6	Parachlorophenol
129.1	Dimethadione
	Flucytosine
129.2	Metformin
	Vigabatrin
130.1	Fluorouracil
130.2	Amyl Acetate
131.2	Aminocaproic Acid
131.4	Trichloroethylene
132.2	Paraldehyde
133.2	Tranylcypromine
133.4	Trichloroethane
135.2	Acetanilide
	Amfetamine
	Dexamfetamine
	Levamfetamine
136.1	Allopurinol
136.2	Betahistine
	Mebanazine
	Phenelzine
137.1	Aminobenzoic Acid
	Isoniazid
	Methyl Nicotinate
	Salicylamide
137.2	Tyramine
137.4	Trichlorofluoromethane
138.1	Salicylic Acid
138.2	Pentetrazol
139.2	Deferiprone
139.6	Choline Chloride
141.1	Dimetridazole
	Methamidophos
141.2	Ethosuximide
	Methylpentynol Carbamate
141.3	Cyclopentamine
	Isometheptene
142.2	Methylthiouracil
142.6	Chlorocresol
143.1	Trimethadione
144.1	Sodium Benzoate
144.2	Betanaphthol
	Valproic Acid
144.6	Ethchlorvynol
145.1	Aminonitrothiazole
145.2	Emylcamate

Mol. Wt.	*Compound*
	Heptaminol
	Hydroxyquinoline
146.2	Trientine
147.0	Paradichlorobenzene
148.3	Ditiocarb
149.2	Metamfetamine
	Penicillamine
	Phentermine
149.4	Trichloroethanol
150.2	Potassium Sorbate
151.2	Cathine
	Ethyl Nicotinate
	Hydroxyamfetamine
	Paracetamol
	Phenylpropanolamine
151.3	Amantadine
152.1	Mandelic Acid
	Methyl Hydroxybenzoate
	Methyl Salicylate
	Resorcinol Monoacetate
	Vanillin
152.2	Camphor
153.1	Aminosalicylic Acid
153.2	Dopamine
153.6	Betaine Hydrochloride
153.8	Carbon Tetrachloride
154.2	Diphenyl
154.3	Cineole
155.2	Arecoline
	Bemegride
155.3	Pempidine
	Propylhexedrine
156.3	Menthol
156.6	Chloroxylenol
157.2	Buformin
	Paramethadione
159.2	Pargyline
160.1	Sodium Salicylate
160.2	Hydralazine
	Tolazoline
	Tryptamine
161.2	Aletamine
161.7	Clomethiazole
162.2	Nicotine
163.2	Acetylcysteine
	Methcathinone
163.3	Dimethylamfetamine
	Mephentermine
164.2	Eugenol
165.0	Methoxyflurane
165.2	Anhydrous Ephedrine
	Benzocaine
	Etenzamide
	Hordenine
	Pholedrine
	Pseudoephedrine
	Racephedrine
165.4	Cloral Hydrate
165.6	Metformin Hydrochloride
165.8	Tetrachloroethylene
166.2	Ethionamide
	Ethyl Hydroxybenzoate
	Sodium Valproate

Mol. Wt.	*Compound*
167.2	Ethinamate
	Metaraminol
	Phenylephrine
	Tioguanine
167.3	Mecamylamine
167.8	Tetrachloroethane
168.0	Desflurane
168.2	Norharman
169.1	Glyphosate
169.2	Ammonium Mandelate
	Noradrenaline
	Pyridoxine
169.6	Chlorzoxazone
170.2	Levetiracetam
	Mercaptopurine
	Propylthiouracil
170.9	Cryofluorane
171.2	Gabapentin
	Metronidazole
171.3	Ditiocarb Sodium
171.6	Chloronitrotoluene
172.2	Menadione
	Sulfanilamide
172.6	Chloronitroaniline
	Pralidoxime Chloride
173.6	Tyramine Hydrochloride
174.1	Sodium Methyl Hydroxybenzoate
174.2	Ephedrine
	5-Methyltryptamine
	N-Methyltryptamine
	α-Methyltryptamine
175.2	Debrisoquine
	Potassium Aminobenzoate
176.1	Ascorbic Acid
176.2	Serotonin
177.2	Bethanidine
	Phenmetrazine
177.5	Chlorobutanol
177.6	Dimetridazole Hydrochloride
177.7	Cyclopentamine Hydrochloride
	Isometheptene Hydrochloride
178.2	Nikethamide
178.3	Amylmetacresol
	Etisazole
	Propofol
179.2	Iproniazid
	Methylenedioxyamfetamine
	Phenacetin
	Phenprobamate
179.3	Methoxymetamfetamine
	Methoxyphenamine
	Methylephedrine
	Mexiletine
	Rimantadine
180.2	Aspirin
	Butylated Hydroxyanisole
	Propyl Hydroxybenzoate
	Theobromine
	Theophylline
180.3	Protionamide
181.2	Etilefrine
	Hydroxyephedrine
	Styramate
181.3	Methylthioamfetamine
181.7	Acetylcholine Chloride
	Heptaminol Hydrochloride
182.2	Eflornithine
	Harman
	Mannitol
	Mephenesin
182.6	Carbachol
183.2	Adrenaline
	Methyprylon
	Normetadrenaline
	Saccharin
183.7	Chlorphentermine
184.1	Histamine Hydrochloride
184.2	Apronal
	Barbital
	Diquat
184.5	Enflurane
185.2	Ecgonine
185.7	Metamfetamine Hydrochloride
	Penicillamine Hydrochloride
	Phentermine Hydrochloride
186.2	Carbimazole
	Mafenide
186.3	Paraquat
187.2	Aminitrozole
187.3	Selegiline
187.7	Amantadine Hydrochloride
	Cathine Hydrochloride
	Phenylpropanolamine Hydrochloride
188.2	Phenazone
	Sodium Ethyl Hydroxybenzoate
188.3	Dimethyltryptamine
	Fenproporex
189.2	Phensuximide
	Thiotepa
189.6	Dopamine Hydrochloride
190.2	Cytisine
	Dihydralazine
	Nitroxoline
190.3	Aldicarb
191.1	Isosorbide Mononitrate
191.2	Potassium Aminosalicylate
191.3	Amiphenazole
	Diethyltoluamide
	Phendimetrazine
191.7	Propylhexedrine Hydrochloride
192.0	Clopidol
	Foscarnet Sodium
192.2	Myristicin
192.3	Bitoscanate
	Tocainide
193.2	Butyl Aminobenzoate
	Methylenedioxymethamfetamine
193.3	Etafedrine
193.5	Butylchloral Hydrate
193.7	Buformin Hydrochloride
194.2	Aminoacridine
	Aminohippuric Acid
	Caffeine
	Dimethyl Phthalate
	Piperazine Hydrate
	Temozolomide
194.3	Hexylresorcinol
195.7	Methacholine Chloride
	Pargyline Hydrochloride
196.2	Cantharidin
196.6	Hydralazine Hydrochloride
196.7	Bethanechol Chloride
	Tolazoline Hydrochloride
	Tryptamine Hydrochloride
197.2	Ethylnoradrenaline
	Levodopa
	Metadrenaline
197.7	Aletamine Hydrochloride
	Beclamide
197.8	Arsenic Trioxide
198.1	Dinitro-orthocresol
	Nitrofurazone
	Sodium Ascorbate
198.2	Ethyl Gallate
	Guaifenesin
	Metharbital
	Theophylline Hydrate
198.3	Guanethidine
	Tacrine
199.3	Diethylcarbamazine
	Phenothiazine
199.4	Octamylamine
199.7	Methcathinone Hydrochloride
200.1	Sevoflurane
200.3	Amantadine Sulfate
	Dexmedetomidine
	Tetryzoline
200.6	Methylchlorophenoxyacetic Acid
201.2	Carbaryl
201.3	Tiabendazole
201.7	Edrophonium Chloride
	Ephedrine Hydrochloride
	Methoxyamfetamine Hydrochloride
	Pseudoephedrine Hydrochloride
	Racephedrine Hydrochloride
	Simazine
202.1	Piperazine Phosphate
	Theophylline Sodium Glycinate
202.2	Sodium Propyl Hydroxybenzoate
202.6	Chlorphenesin
203.2	Mesuximide
203.3	Crotamiton
203.7	Phenylephrine Hydrochloride
203.8	Mecamylamine Hydrochloride
204.2	Ethotoin
	Tryptophan
204.3	Bufotenine
	Ethambutol
	Levamisole
	Psilocin
	Tetramisole
205.3	Dexpanthenol
	Diethylpropion
205.6	Noradrenaline Hydrochloride
	Pyridoxine Hydrochloride
206.2	Barbital Sodium
	Pheneturide
206.3	Ibuprofen
	Isoproturon
	Pyrantel
207.2	Guanoxan
	Hydrastinine
	Toloxatone
207.3	Hexyl Nicotinate
	Methylenedioxyethylamfetamine
208.1	Coniine Hydrobromide
208.2	Allobarbital
208.3	Pilocarpine
209.1	Betahistine Hydrochloride
209.2	Hydroxyphenamate
209.3	Bamethan
	DOM
	Minoxidil
210.2	Aprobarbital
	Phanquinone
210.3	Altretamine
	Naphazoline
210.7	5-Methyltryptamine Hydrochloride
211.1	Sodium Aminosalicylate
211.2	Milrinone
	Nicorandil
	Zalcitabine
211.3	Benethamine
	Isoprenaline
	Mescaline
	Methoxamine
	Orciprenaline
	Pramipexole
212.2	Benzyl Benzoate
	Caffeine Hydrate
	Secbutabarbital

Mol. Wt.	*Compound*
	Zonisamide
212.3	Butobarbital
	Harmine
213.2	Benzyl Nicotinate
	Droxidopa
	Omethoate
	Phenazopyridine
213.3	Desmetryne
213.7	Baclofen
	Clorprenaline
	Phenmetrazine
214.0	Carmustine
214.2	Amifostine
	Niridazole
	Salol
	Sulfacetamide
214.3	Fenyramidol
	Harmaline
	Sulfaguanidine
214.6	Monolinuron
214.7	Etisazole Hydrochloride
	Phenaglycodol
215.3	Fencamfamin
	Tramazoline
215.7	Atrazine
	Methoxyphenamine Hydrochloride
	Methylenedioxyamfetamine Hydrochloride
	Methylephedrine Hydrochloride
	Mexiletine Hydrochloride
215.8	Rimantadine Hydrochloride
216.2	Methoxsalen
	Sodium Aminohippurate
216.3	Diethyltryptamine
217.3	Captopril
	Glutethimide
217.4	Prolintane
217.7	Etilefrine Hydrochloride
	Hydroxyephedrine Hydrochloride
218.1	Propanil
218.3	Carphedon
	Mephenytoin
	Meprobamate
	Metallibure
	Primidone
218.7	Eflornithine Hydrochloride
219.2	Aniracetam
	Trientine Dihydrochloride
219.3	Profadol
219.7	Adrenaline Hydrochloride
220.1	Chlorphentermine Hydrochloride
220.3	Morantel
	Prilocaine
	Xylazine
220.4	Butylated Hydroxytoluene
221.0	Dicamba
	Dichlorophenoxyacetic Acid
	Dichlorvos
221.3	Procarbazine
221.7	Ecgonine Hydrochloride
222.2	Diethyl Phthalate
	Morinamide
	Phenindione
222.3	Acetazolamide
	Nicametate
222.7	Mafenide Hydrochloride
223.1	Bromisoval
223.2	Monocrotophos
223.3	Bufexamac
	Butoxyethyl Nicotinate
	Etamivan
	Rimiterol
	Tigloidine
223.7	Selegiline Hydrochloride
224.1	Mevinphos
224.2	Etofylline
	Stavudine
224.3	Butalbital
	Enallylpropymal
	Idobutal
	Talbutal
	Vinbarbital
	Vinylbital
225.2	Aciclovir
	Dinitolmide
	Furazolidone
	Mephenesin Carbamate
225.3	Ditiocarb Sodium
	N-Methylmescaline
	Prenalterol
	Terbutaline
	Trimethoxyamfetamine
225.7	Hydrastinine Hydrochloride
226.1	Acetylcholine Bromide
226.2	Dithranol
	Nimorazole
226.3	Amobarbital
	Crotetamide
	Metyrapone
	Pentobarbital
226.7	Alclofenac
227.1	Glyceryl Trinitrate
227.3	Ametryne
227.7	Amiphenazole Hydrochloride
	Buclosamide
228.1	Chlorquinaldol
228.2	Glyphosate Isopropylammonium
	Trioxysalen
228.3	Nabumetone
228.7	Tocainide Hydrochloride
229.2	Phenyl Aminosalicylate
229.3	Dimethoate
	Lamivudine
229.6	Amiloride
229.7	Propazine
	Terbutylazine
229.75	Methylenedioxymethamfetamine
229.8	Etafedrine Hydrochloride
230.1	Clonidine
230.3	Demeton-*S*-methyl
	Metomidate
	Naproxen
	Propyphenazone
230.7	Diazoxide
231.3	Aminophenazone
	Eptazocine
	Fenfluramine
	Indeloxazine
	Isocarboxazid
232.1	Hydroxyamfetamine Hydrobromide
232.2	Aprobarbital Sodium
	Nalidixic Acid
	Phenobarbital
232.3	Aminoglutethimide
	Mebutamate
	Piperazine Adipate
	Pralidoxime Mesilate
	Sulfaguanidine Monohydrate
233.1	Diuron
233.2	Amfetamine Phosphate
	Dexamfetamine Phosphate
	Sulfacarbamide
233.3	Methylphenidate
233.4	Meptazinol
233.7	Ethylnoradrenaline Hydrochloride
234.1	Diloxanide
234.2	Riluzole
	Secbutabarbital Sodium
234.3	Cyclopentobarbital
	Lidocaine
	Metisazone
	Phenelzine Sulfate
234.4	Sparteine
234.7	Tacrine Hydrochloride
235.0	Glyphosate Sesquisodium Salt
235.3	Azapetine
	Meprylcaine
	Padimate
	Procainamide
235.8	Octamylamine Hydrochloride
236.1	Arecoline Hydrobromide
	Isosorbide Dinitrate
236.2	Carbazochrome
	Didanosine
236.3	Carbamazepine
	Cyclobarbital
	Dropropizine
	Hexobarbital
	Methazolamide
	Procaine
	Thioacetazone
236.6	Eflornithine Hydrochloride Monohydrate
236.7	Tetryzoline Hydrochloride
237.1	Carbromal
237.3	Cotarnine
	Viloxazine
237.7	Ketamine
238.2	Felbamate
	Methyldopa
	Nitrofurantoin
	Proxyphylline
238.3	Nealbarbital
	Nomifensine
	Secobarbital
239.3	Isoetarine
	Methyldopate
	Salbutamol
239.4	Benzfetamine
239.7	Bupropion
240.1	Methacholine Bromide
240.2	Dantron
240.3	Cropropamide
	Hexethal
	Pheniramine
240.8	Levamisole Hydrochloride
	Tetramisole Hydrochloride
241.2	Methocarbamol
	Saccharin Sodium
	Salinazid
	Theophylline Monoethanolamine
241.3	Choline Salicylate
	Mefenamic Acid
241.4	Prometryne
	Terbutryne
241.7	Moxonidine
	Phenformin Hydrochloride
241.8	Diethylpropion Hydrochloride
242.3	Fenoprofen
	Mexenone
	Thiopental
242.7	Clofibrate
243.2	Cytarabine
243.4	Phencyclidine
243.8	Methylenedioxyethylamfetamine Hydrochloride
244.2	Acetazolamide Sodium
	Carbidopa
244.3	Amidefrine
	Etomidate
	Flurbiprofen
244.4	Isoaminile

Mol. Wt.	*Compound*
	Xylometazoline
244.7	Pilocarpine Hydrochloride
244.9	Clodronic Acid
245.2	Glyphosate Trimesium
245.3	Isopropylaminophenazone
245.7	Chlorphenesin Carbamate
	DOM Hydrochloride
246.3	Busulfan
	Mafenide Acetate
	Methylphenobarbital
	Santonin
246.4	Mepivacaine
	Milnacipran
246.7	Naphazoline Hydrochloride
247.2	Aciclovir Sodium
247.3	Ketobemidone
	Parbendazole
	Pethidine
	Tinidazole
247.7	Isoprenaline Hydrochloride
	Methoxamine Hydrochloride
248.3	Amobarbital Sodium
	Bunitrolol
	Dapsone
	Enoximone
	Pentobarbital Sodium
	Pindolol
	Pralidoxime Metilsulfate
248.7	Aminoacridine Hydrochloride
	Pyrimethamine
249.1	Alendronic Acid
	Linuron
249.3	Cinchophen
	Epinastine
	Sulfapyridine
249.4	Alprenolol
	Benzoctamine
249.7	Phenazopyridine Hydrochloride
250.2	Diflunisal
250.3	Heptabarb
	Methaqualone
	Rivastigmine
	Sulfadiazine
250.7	Fenyramidol Hydrochloride
251.4	Triclofos Sodium
251.7	Cycloguanil
251.8	Fencamfamin Hydrochloride
	Tramazoline Hydrochloride
252.2	Naproxen Sodium
252.3	Anisindione
	Oxcarbazepine
	Phenytoin
252.4	Cimetidine
253.3	Choline Bitartrate
	Ethacridine
	N-Acetylmescaline
	Nefopam
	Penciclovir
	Sulfamethoxazole
	Triamterene
253.4	Irgarol
	Tolpropamine
253.7	Proguanil
	Tizanidine
253.8	Prolintane Hydrochloride
254.2	Diprophylline
	Phenobarbital Sodium
	Sulfacetamide Sodium
254.3	Dexketoprofen
	Fenbufen
	Ketoprofen
	Thiamylal
254.8	Butanilicaine
255.2	Ganciclovir
255.3	Ambazone
	Ketorolac
	Sulfathiazole
255.4	Diphenhydramine
	Phenyltoloxamine
	Tofenacin
	Tripelennamine
255.5	Trichlorophenoxyacetic Acid
255.7	Gallium Nitrate
	Imidacloprid
255.8	Profadol Hydrochloride
256.1	Anagrelide
	Lamotrigine
256.3	Etoxazene
256.8	Prilocaine Hydrochloride
	Xylazine Hydrochloride
257.2	Benserazide
	Choline Alfoscerate
	Paraquat Dichloride
257.3	Etebenecid
	Tolmetin
257.4	Dextrorphan
	Levorphanol
	Racemorphan
	Trichlorfon
257.7	Meclofenoxate
257.8	Procarbazine Hydrochloride
258.2	Salsalate
	Thalidomide
258.3	Acetomenaphthone
	Demeton-*S*
	Ethoxzolamide
	Hexobarbital Sodium
258.7	Morinamide Hydrochloride
259.1	Lofexidine
259.2	Nicotinyl Tartrate
259.3	Propranolol
259.4	Primaquine
260.1	Carbarsone
	Nitrofurantoin Sodium
260.3	Carisoprodol
	Diaveridine
	Imolamine
	Mafenide Propionate
	Secobarbital Sodium
	Suprofen
	Tiaprofenic Acid
260.4	Oxymetazoline
	Ropinirole
261.1	Pyridostigmine Bromide
261.4	Alphaprodine
	Ethoheptazine
	Hexylcaine
	Methapyrilene
	Phenindamine
	Piperocaine
	Setiptiline
	Thenyldiamine
261.7	Prenalterol Hydrochloride
	Tolfenamic Acid
262.3	Hexethal Sodium
	Methohexital
262.7	Clonixin
263.1	Guanoclor
263.2	Gemcitabine
263.4	Butetamate
	Nortriptyline
	Protriptyline
	Tramadol
263.8	Ticlopidine
264.1	Pralidoxime Iodide
264.3	Pentifylline
	Sulfamerazine
	Thialbarbital
	Thiopental Sodium
264.4	Mianserin
	Tetracaine
264.5	Sulfiram
265.3	Albendazole
265.4	Antazoline
	Ethomoxane
	Mirtazapine
	Oxprenolol
266.3	Atenolol
	Dienestrol
	Nevirapine
	Pentachlorophenol
	Practolol
	Tributyl Phosphate
	Trimetazidine
266.4	Cyclizine
	Desipramine
266.6	Clonidine Hydrochloride
266.7	Metomidate Hydrochloride
267.2	Adenosine
	Zidovudine
267.3	Apomorphine
	Lysergamide
	Sulfafurazole
	Sulfamoxole
	Voglibose
267.4	Azacyclonol
	Metoprolol
	Pipradrol
267.7	Fenfluramine Hydrochloride
267.8	Indeloxazine Hydrochloride
268.2	Clorprenaline Hydrochloride
268.3	Dexrazoxane
	Lysergic Acid
	Pentostatin
268.4	Diethylstilbestrol
268.7	Moclobemide
269.1	Dichlorophen
269.3	Bufylline
269.4	Orphenadrine
	Rizatriptan
269.8	Alachlor
	Meptazinol Hydrochloride
	Methylphenidate Hydrochloride
270.1	Halazone
270.2	Leflunomide
270.3	Sulfamethizole
	Tolbutamide
270.4	Doxylamine
	Estrone
	Hexestrol
	Trenbolone
270.7	Mecloqualone
	Nordazepam
270.8	Chloroprocaine
	Medazepam
271.3	Carbutamide
	Normorphine
	Pilocarpine Nitrate
271.4	Cyclazocine
	Dextromethorphan
	Methoprotryne
271.8	Meprylcaine Hydrochloride
	Procainamide Hydrochloride
272.1	Muzolimine
272.2	Clorgiline
272.3	Sulfadiazine Sodium
272.4	Estradiol
	Quinisocaine
	Sotalol
272.8	Procaine Hydrochloride
273.3	Naphazoline Nitrate
273.4	Modafinil

Mol. Wt.	*Compound*
	Tilidate
273.7	Chlormezanone
273.8	Viloxazine Hydrochloride
274.2	Ketamine Hydrochloride
274.3	Phenytoin Sodium
274.4	Disulfoton
	Nandrolone
	Ropivacaine
	Tybamate
274.8	Chlorphenamine
	Dexchlorphenamine
275.1	Acetarsone
275.3	Homatropine
	Physostigmine
275.4	Cyclobenzaprine
	Trimeperidine
275.7	Methyldopate Hydrochloride
275.8	Benzfetamine Hydrochloride
	Isoetarine Hydrochloride
276.2	Bupropion Hydrochloride
276.3	Sodium Thiamylal
276.4	Cyclandelate
	Etidocaine
	Gloxazone
	Mebhydrolin
	Molindone
276.7	Chlorpropamide
277.2	Clenbuterol
	Ethambutol Hydrochloride
	Fenitrothion
	Ganciclovir Sodium
	Iproniazid Phosphate
277.3	Azathioprine
277.4	Acecainide
	Amitriptyline
	Maprotiline
	Padimate O
	Venlafaxine
277.5	Perhexiline
278.2	Exifone
278.3	Dibutyl Phthalate
	Fenthion
	Pentoxifylline
	Sulfadimidine
	Sulfisomidine
278.4	Triprolidine
279.1	Acecarbromal
	Cyclophosphamide
279.2	Cidofovir
279.3	Etamiphylline
279.4	Doxepin
	Fenpiprane
	Moxisylyte
279.7	Cytarabine Hydrochloride
279.9	Phencyclidine Hydrochloride
280.3	Hydroxystilbamidine
	Levosimendan
	Phenprocoumon
	Sulfamethoxypyridazine
	Sulfametopyrazine
	Sulfametoxydiazine
280.4	Bamipine
	Histapyrrodine
	Imipramine
280.8	Xylometazoline Hydrochloride
281.2	Flufenamic Acid
281.3	Diminazene
	Indoprofen
	Nitrazepam
	Trimetozine
281.4	Alverine
	Diphenylpyraline
	Phentolamine
281.7	Tosylchloramide Sodium

Mol. Wt.	*Compound*
282.0	Lithium Citrate
282.2	Acriflavinium Chloride
	Niflumic Acid
282.6	Cloral Betaine
282.8	Mepivacaine Hydrochloride
	Milnacipran Hydrochloride
283.3	Choline Theophyllinate
283.4	Levallorphan
283.8	Ketobemidone Hydrochloride
	Metolachlor
	Pethidine
284.3	Methohexital Sodium
	Psilocybine
284.4	Iprindole
	Lynestrenol
	Promazine
	Promethazine
	Sulfaethidole
	Tropicamide
	Tropisetron
284.7	Diazepam
	Disulfamide
	Mazindol
	Sulfachlorpyridazine
284.8	Bunitrolol Hydrochloride
285.2	Fludarabine
285.3	Hydromorphone
	Letrozole
	Nifuratel
	Norcodeine
285.4	Isothipendyl
	Mepyramine
	Pentazocine
	Probenecid
	Prothipendyl
285.7	Cladribine
285.8	Alprenolol Hydrochloride
	Benzoctamine Hydrochloride
	Epinastine Hydrochloride
286.3	Abacavir
	Sulfamerazine Sodium
	Thialbarbital Sodium
286.4	Androstenedione
	Boldenone
	Methallenestril
	Thenalidine
	Thonzylamine
286.7	Demoxepam
	Oxazepam
286.8	Methaqualone Hydrochloride
287.1	Brallobarbital
287.2	Fenticlor
287.4	Cycrimine
	Cyproheptadine
	Dihydromorphine
	Etodolac
	Galantamine
	N-Benzoylmescaline
	Procyclidine
	Ritodrine
	Zolmitriptan
288.2	Chlorproguanil
288.3	Dihydralazine Sulfate
288.4	Bupivacaine
	Dehydroepiandrosterone
	Estriol
	Levobupivacaine
	Phenglutarimide
	Testosterone
288.5	Ethylestrenol
288.8	Lidocaine Hydrochloride
	Tetrazepam
288.9	Disodium Clodronate
289.1	Ibomal

Mol. Wt.	*Compound*
289.2	Ciprofibrate
289.3	Benzoylecgonine
	Sulfapyridine Sodium Monohydrate
289.4	Adrafinil
	Atropine
	Caramiphen
	Dyclonine
	Hyoscyamine
289.5	Triclosan
289.7	Quinethazone
289.8	Chloropyramine
	Clofedanol
	Nefopam Hydrochloride
	Tolpropamine Hydrochloride
290.0	Nitroxinil
290.2	Proguanil Hydrochloride
	Tizanidine Hydrochloride
290.3	Isoniazid Aminosalicylate
	Trimethoprim
290.4	Androstanolone
	Androstenediol
	Androsterone
	Azatadine
	Sultiame
290.8	Benzene Hexachloride
	Carbinoxamine
	Lindane
291.3	Parathion
	Physostigmine Aminoxide
291.4	Cyclopentolate
	Eucatropine
	Fasudil
	Levobunolol
291.5	Diethylthiambutene
291.7	Cotarnine Chloride
	Zomepirac
291.8	Diphenhydramine Hydrochloride
	Tofenacin Hydrochloride
	Tripelennamine Hydrochloride
292.3	Coumatetralyl
	Methenamine Mandelate
	Tolbutamide Sodium
292.4	Ambucetamide
	Carteolol
	Dimetindene
292.5	Anagrelide Hydrochloride
292.8	Etoxazene Hydrochloride
293.4	Anastrozole
	Budipine
	Diamthazole
	Embutramide
	Ondansetron
	Pramocaine
293.5	Butriptyline
293.7	Benserazide Hydrochloride
294.2	Meclofenoxate Hydrochloride
294.3	Penciclovir Sodium
294.4	Cinchonidine
	Cinchonine
	Noxiptiline
	Propoxycaine
	Proxymetacaine
	Trimipramine
295.3	Choline Dihydrogen Citrate
	Mebendazole
295.4	Dibenzepin
	Dosulepin
	Esmolol
	Normethadone
	Pizotifen
	Tertatolol
295.6	Lofexidine Hydrochloride
295.7	Chlorothiazide
295.8	Chloropyrilene

Mol. Wt.	Compound
	Propranolol Hydrochloride
296.2	Acriflavinium Chloride
	Diclofenac
	Flunixin
	Meclofenamic Acid
296.3	Amicarbalide
296.4	Ethinylestradiol
	Exemestane
	Guanethidine Monosulfate
	Methdilazine
296.5	Disulfiram
296.8	Imolamine Hydrochloride
	Oxymetazoline Hydrochloride
	Ropinirole
297.1	Fenclofenac
297.7	Hydrochlorothiazide
297.8	Alphaprodine Hydrochloride
	Hexylcaine Hydrochloride
	Methapyrilene Hydrochloride
	Piperocaine Hydrochloride
	Thenyldiamine Hydrochloride
298.3	Metadoxine
	Nialamide
298.4	Alimemazine
	Artemether
	Diethazine
	Norethisterone
	Noretynodrel
	Phenacaine
299.3	Fenbendazole
299.4	Buphenine
	Hydrocodone
	Neopine
299.7	Gemcitabine Hydrochloride
299.8	Chlordiazepoxide
	Metoclopramide
	Nortriptyline Hydrochloride
	Protriptyline Hydrochloride
	Tramadol Hydrochloride
300.1	Cisplatin
300.2	Ticlopidine Hydrochloride
300.3	Sulfadimidine Sodium
	Sulfaquinoxaline
300.4	Isotretinoin
	Methandienone
300.5	Allylestrenol
300.7	Temazepam
300.8	Chlorcyclizine
	Clobazam
	Mianserin Hydrochloride
	Tetracaine Hydrochloride
	Thiamine
301.3	Milrinone Lactate
	Oxymorphone
301.4	Dihydrocodeine
	Dobutamine
	Isoxsuprine
301.5	Trihexyphenidyl
301.7	Benoxaprofen
301.8	Antazoline Hydrochloride
	Ethomoxane Hydrochloride
	Oxprenolol Hydrochloride
302.1	Amiloride Hydrochloride
302.2	Olsalazine
302.3	Pramipexole Dihydrochloride Monohydrate
	Sulfamethoxypyridazine Sodium
302.4	Cambendazole
	Formestane
302.5	Metenolone
	Methyltestosterone
	Norethandrolone
302.8	Cyclizine Hydrochloride
	Desipramine Hydrochloride
303.0	Broxyquinoline
303.1	Etacrynic Acid
303.2	Neostigmine Bromide
303.3	Flumazenil
303.4	Cocaine
	Fenamiphos
	Fenoterol
	Hyoscine
	Morphine
303.8	Azacyclonol Hydrochloride
	Chlorphenoxamine
	Phenoxybenzamine
	Pipradrol Hydrochloride
304.2	Chlorambucil
	Rimiterol Hydrobromide
	Tigloidine Hydrobromide
304.3	Flupirtine
304.4	Dimpylate
304.5	Mesterolone
	Methandriol
305.2	Diclofenamide
	Melphalan
	Moclobemide Hydrochloride
305.3	Entacapone
305.4	Atropine Oxide
	Pempidine Tartrate
305.5	Clioquinol
305.8	Fenoldopam
	Orphenadrine Hydrochloride
306.2	Bromantane
	Sertraline
306.3	Fluconazole
306.4	Butacaine
	Oxandrolone
306.7	Sulfachlorpyridazine Sodium
307.1	Histamine Acid Phosphate
307.2	Chloroprocaine Hydrochloride
307.4	Benzatropine
	Betaxolol
	Tolnaftate
	Zolpidem
308.3	Nifenazone
	Warfarin
308.4	Gestrinone
	Oxybuprocaine
	Phenylbutazone
308.6	Clorgiline Hydrochloride
308.8	Alprazolam
	Sotalol Hydrochloride
308.9	Quinisocaine Hydrochloride
309.3	Acetyl Sulfafurazole
	Fluoxetine
309.4	Benzydamine
	Difenidol
	Ketotifen
	Mescaline Acid Sulfate
	Methadone
	Metipranolol
	Nadolol
309.5	Alphachloralose
	Dicycloverine
	Metixene
310.3	Sulfadimethoxine
	Sulfadoxine
310.4	Cannabinol
	Ibogaine
	Mestranol
310.5	Pecazine
310.9	Ropivacaine Hydrocloride
311.4	Adiphenine
	Nalorphine
	Thebaine
	Tolazamide
311.5	Biperiden
311.9	Cyclobenzaprine Hydrochloride
	Pyrrobutamine
	Trimeperidine Hydrochloride
312.2	Eptazocine Hydrobromide
312.4	Ethisterone
	Granisetron
	Olanzapine
	Propamidine
	Trenbolone Acetate
312.5	Dydrogesterone
	Profenamine
312.8	Apomorphine Hydrochloride
	Molindone Hydrochloride
312.9	Etidocaine Hydrochloride
313.3	Benorilate
	Flunitrazepam
	Triazophos
313.4	Ethylmorphine
	Reboxetine
313.8	Acecainide Hydrochloride
	Amoxapine
313.9	Amitriptyline Hydrochloride
	Maprotiline Hydrochloride
	Venlafaxine Hydrochloride
314.2	Hexaconazole
314.3	Dantrolene
314.4	Ranitidine
	Rofecoxib
	Sulfaphenazole
314.5	Cannabidiol
	Δ^8-Tetrahydrocannabinol
	Δ^9-Tetrahydrocannabinol
	Pergolide
	Progesterone
314.7	Clorazepic Acid
314.9	Clomipramine
	Homochlorcyclizine
315.2	Amprolium Hydrochloride
315.3	Tolmetin Sodium
315.4	Oxycodone
315.6	Triclocarban
315.7	Clonazepam
	Efavirenz
315.8	Doxepin Hydrochloride
	Moxisylyte Hydrochloride
315.9	Chlorprothixene
	Fenpiprane Hydrochloride
316–374	Pyrethrum
316.1	Pentaerithrityl Tetranitrate
316.2	Bromazepam
316.4	Butalamine
	Timolol
316.9	Bamipine Hydrochloride
	Histapyrrodine Hydrochloride
	Imipramine Hydrochloride
317.2	Zimeldine
317.3	Azinphos-methyl
	Metaraminol Tartrate
	Oxyphenisatine
317.4	Codeine
	Tetrabenazine
317.7	Chlorothiazide Sodium
317.8	Phentolamine Hydrochloride
317.9	Diphenylpyraline Hydrochloride
318.1	Diclofenac
	Meclofenamate Sodium
318.3	Fluvoxamine
	Phenolphthalein
318.6	Tiludronic Acid
318.8	Tilidate Hydrochloride
318.9	Chlorpromazine
319.2	Brompheniramine
	Dexbrompheniramine
319.4	Methenamine Hippurate

Mol. Wt.	*Compound*
319.9	Chloroquine
320.3	Mycophenolic Acid
320.4	Feprazone
320.8	Tropisetron Hydrochloride
320.9	Iprindole Hydrochloride
	Promazine Hydrochloride
	Promethazine Hydrochloride
321.2	Lorazepam
321.3	Famciclovir
321.5	Phenazocine
321.8	Clopidogrel
	Hydromorphone Hydrochloride
321.9	Isothipendyl Hydrochloride
	Pentazocine
322.3	Acetyl Sulfamethoxypyridazine
	Carbazochrome Sodium Sulfonate
	Sulfaquinoxaline Sodium
322.4	Gelsemine
	Mesocarb
322.5	Aprindine
	Chlorpyrifos-methyl
	Mequitazine
322.8	Thonzylamine Hydrochloride
322.9	Clostebol
323.1	Chloramphenicol
323.4	Dimefline
	Gliclazide
	Lysergide
	Piperidolate
323.8	Dihydromorphine Hydrochloride
	Galantamine Hydrochloride
	Ritodrine Hydrochloride
323.9	Cycrimine Hydrochloride
	Procyclidine Hydrochloride
324.3	Furaltadone
	Valaciclovir
324.4	Acetohexamide
	Citalopram
	Dolasetron
324.6	Chlorproguanil Hydrochloride
324.8	Phenglutarimide Hydrochloride
	Prazepam
324.9	Levobupivacaine Hydrochloride
325.1	Alendronate Sodium
	Etacrynate Sodium
325.4	Ergometrine
	Methylpiperidyl Benzilate
	Monocrotaline
325.5	Bisoprolol
	Tolterodine
325.8	Clemizole
	Ethiazide
	Midazolam
325.9	Caramiphen Hydrochloride
	Dyclonine Hydrochloride
326.3	Clofedanol Hydrochloride
326.4	Acitretin
	Ajmaline
	Hydroquinidine
	Hydroquinine
326.5	Acepromazine
326.8	Clozapine
327.1	Niclosamide
327.4	6-Monoacetylmorphine
	Azaperone
	Benactyzine
	Naloxone
	Thiamine Mononitrate
327.5	Aminopromazine
	Butorphanol
327.8	Fasudil Hydrochloride
	Loxapine
327.9	Cyclopentolate Hydrochloride
	Diethylthiambutene Hydrochloride
	Eucatropine Hydrochloride
	Levobunolol Hydrochloride
328.2	Diloxanide Furoate
328.4	Labetalol
328.5	Boldenone Acetate
	Levomepromazine
	Pyrethrin I
	Stanozolol
	Tuaminoheptane Sulfate
328.8	Carteolol Hydrochloride
	Clorexolone
328.9	Ropivacaine Hydrocloride Monohydrate
329.4	Paroxetine
	Trilostane
329.5	Prenylamine
329.9	Budipine Hydrochloride
	Butriptyline Hydrochloride
	Pramocaine Hydrochloride
330.2	Epinastine Hydrobromide
330.3	Menadione Sodium Bisulfite
	Warfarin Sodium
330.4	Malathion
330.5	Desoxycortone
	Hydroxyprogesterone
	Nandrolone Propionate
330.7	Furosemide
330.9	Noxiptiline Hydrochloride
	Propoxycaine Hydrochloride
	Proxymetacaine Hydrochloride
331.2	Tienilic Acid
331.3	Glymidine Sodium
	Hydroflumethiazide
	Piroxicam
331.4	Ciprofloxacin
	Protokylol
331.5	Nizatidine
331.8	Dibenzepin Hydrochloride
	Esmolol Hydrochloride
331.9	Dosulepin Hydrochloride
	Normethadone Hydrochloride
	Tertatolol Hydrochloride
	Zotepine
332.3	Zanamivir
332.5	Alfaxalone
	Oxymetholone
332.9	Methdilazine Hydrochloride
	Triprolidine Hydrochloride
333.3	Adrenaline Acid Tartrate
	Azapetine Phosphate
333.5	Carbetapentane
	Deptropine
334.3	Bromazine
334.4	Benzylpenicillin
	Neostigmine Methylsulfate
	Strychnine
334.8	Triphenyltetrazolium Chloride
334.9	Diethazine Hydrochloride
335.2	Lormetazepam
335.4	Isoetarine Mesilate
	Naratriptan
335.5	Almotriptan
	Norpipanone
	Oxeladin
335.8	Codeine Hydrochloride
335.9	Buphenine Hydrochloride
	Hydroxychloroquine
336.2	Chlordiazepoxide Hydrochloride
336.3	Dicoumarol
336.4	Acebutolol
	Azapropazone
	Berberine
	Fluoxymesterone
336.5	Fentanyl
337.3	Chlorcyclizine Hydrochloride
	Noradrenaline Acid Tartrate
	Thiamine Hydrochloride
337.3	Tenoxicam
337.4	Propanidid
337.5	Amineptine
	Danazol
	Famotidine
	Lobeline
337.8	Dobutamine Hydrochloride
	Isoxsuprine Hydrochloride
	Oxymorphone Hydrochloride
337.9	Tricyclamol Chloride
	Trihexyphenidyl Hydrochloride
338.4	Dodecyl Gallate
	Idebenone
	Piperonyl Butoxide
338.8	Chlortalidone
339.3	Trimetazidine Hydrochloride
339.4	Methylergometrine
	Nalmefene
	Papaverine
	Topiramate
	Xamoterol
339.5	Dextropropoxyphene
	Disopyramide
	Levopropoxyphene
	Perazine
339.6	Hexetidine
339.8	Cocaine Hydrochloride
339.9	Prothipendyl Hydrochloride
340.3	Chlorphenoxamine Hydrochloride
	Phenoxybenzamine Hydrochloride
340.4	Amidefrine Mesilate
	Diphenadione
	Pentamidine
	Perindoprilat
340.5	Norethisterone Acetate
	Propiomazine
340.8	Flupirtine Hydrochloride
341.4	Acetylcodeine
	Benaprizine
	Fenetylline
	Naltrexone
	Phendimetrazine Tartrate
	Sulpiride
	Thebacon
341.8	Atropine Oxide Hydrochloride
342.4	Calcium Mandelate
	Oxyphenbutazone
342.7	Sertraline Hydrochloride
342.8	Flutoprazepam
342.9	Bupivacaine Hydrochloride
	Etizolam
343.2	Triazolam
343.4	Ethacridine Lactate
343.5	Cinchocaine
	Monoethanolamine Oleate
	Thiambutosine
343.9	Betaxolol Hydrochloride
	Clemastine
	Clotiapine
344.0	Diquat Dibromide
344.4	Formoterol
344.5	Metenolone Acetate
	Oxyphencyclimine
	Testosterone Propionate
344.8	Clotrimazole
345.4	Azinphos-ethyl
	Bevantolol
	Omeprazole
345.7	Methoxychlor
345.8	Fluoxetine Hydrochloride
345.9	Benzydamine Hydrochloride

Mol. Wt.	*Compound*
	Clopamide
	Difenidol Hydrochloride
	Methadone Hydrochloride
	Metixene Hydrochloride
346.0	Dicycloverine Hydrochloride
346.3	Nifedipine
346.4	Warfarin Potassium
346.9	Ibogaine Hydrochloride
347.5	Indoramin
347.7	Clodantoin
347.8	Nalorphine Hydrochloride
347.9	Adiphenine Hydrochloride
	Biperiden Hydrochloride
348.4	Acrivastine
	Torasemide
348.5	Alfadolone
348.9	Granisetron Hydrochloride
	Profenamine Hydrochloride
349.4	Ampicillin
	Cefradine
349.5	Dipipanone
349.7	Zomepirac Sodium
350.4	Phenoxymethylpenicillin
350.6	Chlorpyrifos
350.9	Cyproheptadine Hydrochloride
	Ranitidine Hydrochloride
351.3	Clomipramine Hydrochloride
351.4	Dipyrone
	Meloxicam
	Pipoxolan
	Pirenzepine
352.3	Dithranol Triacetate
352.4	Chlorprothixene Hydrochloride
	Triflupromazine
352.5	Anileridine
	Encainide
352.8	Butanilicaine Phosphate
	Clorazepate Monopotassium
	Griseofulvin
352.9	Butalamine Hydrochloride
	Phenacaine Hydrochloride Monohydrate
353.3	Acenocoumarol
353.4	Chelidonine
353.5	Levacetylmethadol
	Methysergide
354.0	Tridihexethyl Chloride
354.1	Idoxuridine
354.2	Aceclofenac
354.3	Metoclopramide Hydrochloride
354.4	Nomifensine Maleate
	Yohimbine
354.5	Alprostadil
	Clofenotane
	Etretinate
354.8	Xipamide
356.1	Pipobroman
356.3	Homatropine Hydrobromide
356.4	Benzylpenicillin Sodium
	Fluanisone
	Pheniramine Maleate
	Pyrantel Tartrate
	Sulindac
356.5	Cyclizine Lactate
	Dopexamine
	Estradiol Valerate
356.6	Conessine
357.3	Balsalazide
	Tolrestat
357.4	Nalbuphine
357.8	Indometacin
358.0	Cetylpyridinium Chloride
358.4	Prednisone
358.5	Δ^9-Tetrahydrocannabinolic Acid
	Dimethisterone
	Dimethoxanate
359.0	Aprindine Hydrochloride
359.2	Obidoxime Chloride
359.4	Capecitabine
	Rabeprazole
359.5	Cyclomethycaine
359.6	Captodiame
359.9	Dimefline Hydrochloride
	Piperidolate Hydrochloride
360.2	Methyclothiazide
360.4	Aldosterone
	Cortisone
	Nitrendipine
	Prednisolone
360.5	Drostanolone Propionate
	Quinidine
360.8	Valaciclovir Hydrochloride
361.4	Bisacodyl
	Carbocromen
	Levofloxacin
	Ofloxacin
361.5	Antazoline Mesilate
361.8	Bezafibrate
362.2	Hexamethonium Bromide
	Midazolam Hydrochloride
362.3	Clemizole Hydrochloride
	Diphenylpyraline Hydrobromide
	Fosphenytoin
	Octatropine Methylbromide
362.4	Emepronium Bromide
	Phthalylsulfacetamide
362.6	Disodium Tiludronate
362.8	Coumaphos
362.9	Hydroquinidine Hydrochloride
363.2	Mexazolam
363.4	Antazoline Phosphate
363.5	Opipramol
363.8	6-Monoacetylmorphine Hydrochloride
	Naloxone Hydrochloride
363.9	Benactyzine Hydrochloride
	Lachesine Chloride
364.2	Olsalazine Sodium
364.3	Bibenzonium Bromide
	Laxapine Hydrochloride
364.4	Bumetanide
	Cyclofenil
	Pheneticillin
364.5	Flugestone
	Tranylcypromine Sulfate
364.9	Aldrin
	Clostebol Acetate
	Labetalol Hydrochloride
	Levomepromazine Hydrochloride
	Pecazine Hydrochloride
365.2	Fludarabine Phosphate
	Nifursol
365.4	Amoxicillin
	Cefalexin
	Methyl Benzoquate
365.5	Pericyazine
365.8	Indapamide
	Metolazone
365.9	Ondansetron Hydrochloride Dihydrate
366.4	Atropine Methonitrate
	Diamthazole Hydrochloride
	Trifluomeprazine
366.5	Glibornuride
	Piminodine
366.8	Atovaquone
366.9	Cinchonine Hydrochloride
367.4	Dimoxyline
	Omeprazole Sodium
	Sulfathiazole Sodium
367.5	Bambuterol
	Fenbutrazate
	Phenoperidine
367.8	Protokylol Hydrochloride
368.3	Galantamine Hydrobromide
368.5	Amfetamine Sulfate
	Cinnarizine
	Dehydroepiandrosterone Sulfate
	Dexamfetamine Sulfate
	Perindopril
368.8	Ketazolam
369.3	Etofenamate
369.4	Diamorphine
	Lansoprazole
	Trimetrexate
369.5	Amisulpride
	Cilostazol
370.3	Dextromethorphan Hydrobromide
	Homatropine Methylbromide
	Hyoscyamine Hydrobromide
370.4	Levofloxacin Hemihydrate
	Morantel Tartrate
370.6	Thioridazine
370.7	Bromazine Hydrochloride
370.9	Lorcainide
371.3	Nedocromil
	Remoxipride
371.4	Ampicillin Sodium
	Isradipine
371.8	Camazepam
371.9	Naratriptan Hydrochloride
	Norpipanone Hydrochloride
	Trazodone
372.4	Diamfenetide
	Sulfafurazole Diethanolamine
372.5	Ajmaline Monoethanolate
	Benzylpenicillin Potassium
	Desoxycortone Acetate
	Nabilone
	Pyrethrin II
372.6	Finasteride
372.8	Glafenine
372.9	Acebutolol Hydrochloride
373.3	Heptachlor
373.4	Pyrazophos
	Succinylsulfathiazole
373.5	Bunazosin
373.9	Amineptine Hydrochloride
	Lobeline Hydrochloride
	Prochlorperazine
374.5	Androstenediol Diacetate
	Methylprednisolone
374.8	Paroxetine Hydrochloride Hemihydrate
374.9	Hydroxyzine
375.3	Crystal hydrate
375.4	Dexketoprofen trometamol
375.5	Benzylmorphine
	Pentazocine
	Pipamperone
375.6	Tiagabine
375.8	Morphine Hydrochloride
	Norcodeine Hydrochloride
375.9	Dextropropoxyphene Hydrochloride
	Haloperidol
	Nalmefene Hydrochloride
	Papaverine
376.1	Bromhexine
376.2	Fluquinconazole
376.4	Ketorolac Trometamol
	Picotamide

Mol. Wt.	*Compound*
	Riboflavin
376.5	Enalapril
	Estradiol Benzoate
	Fluocortolone
	Fluorometholone
	Remifentanil
376.8	Flutazolam
376.9	Fenpipramide Hydrochloride
	Propiomazine Hydrochloride
377.4	Imidaprilat
377.5	Famprofazone
	Morazone
	Phentolamine Mesilate
377.9	Benaprizine Hydrochloride
	Fenetylline Hydrochloride
	Naltrexone Hydrochloride
	Thebacon Hydrochloride
378.1	Mannomustine
378.4	Carbenicillin
	Propicillin
378.5	Doxapram
	Quinine
379.4	Droperidol
379.5	Celiprolol
	Donepezil
	Oxypertine
379.9	Cinchocaine Hydrochloride
	Cyclopenthiazide
380.3	Neopine Hydrobromide
380.4	Hyoscine Methonitrate
	Meticillin
380.5	Amosulalol
	Bopindolol
	Diethylstilbestrol Dipropionate
	Fludrocortisone
380.7	Trichlormethiazide
380.9	Chlorotrianisene
	Dieldrin
	Endrin
	Hydrocodone Hydrochloride
	Oxyphencyclimine Hydrochloride
381.4	Benperidol
	Celecoxib
	Fendosal
	Rabeprazole Sodium
381.5	Biriperone
381.7	Econazole
381.9	Bevantolol Hydrochloride
382.5	Hexestrol Dipropionate
	Misoprostol
382.6	Bunamidine
382.9	Loratadine
	Mefruside
383.2	Ecothiopate Iodide
383.4	Hydrastine
	Pantoprazole
	Prazosin
383.5	Quetiapine
	Tandospirone
383.9	Indoramin Hydrochloride
384.3	Atropine Methobromide
	Felodipine
	Fenoterol Hydrobromide
384.4	Artesunate
	Enalaprilat
384.5	Caramiphen Edisilate
	Etynodiol Diacetate
	Megestrol Acetate
384.6	Colecalciferol
	Ibutilide
	Nandrolone Cyclohexane-carboxylate
385.5	Bamifylline
	Buspirone
385.8	Cefaclor
	Ciprofloxacin Hydrochloride
385.9	Ethylmorphine Hydrochloride
386.3	Caffeine Citrate
386.4	Valethamate Bromide
386.5	Medroxyprogesterone Acetate
386.6	Mesoridazine
	Testosterone Isocaproate
386.7	Cholesterol
	Fenoldopam Hydrobromide
386.8	Quazepam
387.2	Acetarsone Sodium
387.4	Amoxicillin Sodium
	Terazosin
387.9	Flurazepam
	Nemonapride
	Pipoxolan Hydrochloride
388.4	Hydroxyquinoline Sulfate
	Nisoldipine
388.5	Aminoacridine Hexylresorcinate
	Doxylamine Succinate
	Methandriol Diacetate
	Phenoxymethylpenicillin Potassium
	Trimethobenzamide
388.8	Zopiclone
388.9	Cetirizine
	Encainide Hydrochloride
	Triflupromazine Hydrochloride
389.4	Reproterol
389.5	Alfuzosin
389.9	Cyclothiazide
390.0	Levacetylmethadol Hydrochloride
390.5	Alfadolone Acetate
	Dehydroepiandrosterone sodium sulfate
390.7	Metoclopramide Dihydrochloride
390.9	Chlorphenamine maleate
	Dexchlorphenamine Maleate
	Yohimbine Hydrochloride
391.0	Meclozine
391.4	Ambutonium Bromide
	Diethylcarbamazine Citrate
391.5	Flavoxate
	Rizatriptan Benzoate
391.6	Dimetotiazine
391.9	Phenmetrazine
392.3	Nalorphine Hydrobromide
392.5	Dexamethasone
	Dextromoramide
	Paramethasone
392.8	Chloroquine Hydrochloride
393.5	Amsacrine
	Metindizate
	Pheniramine Aminosalicylate
393.6	Perhexiline Maleate
393.7	Brotizolam
	Metaclazepam
393.9	Nalbuphine Hydrochloride
394.3	Homidium Bromide
394.4	Picotamide Monohydrate
	Rotenone
	Triamcinolone
394.5	Brucine
394.9	Dimethoxanate Hydrochloride
395.6	Quinagolide
395.9	Cloricromen
396.1	Captodiame Hydrochloride
	Cetalkonium Chloride
396.4	Cefalothin
396.5	Quinine Ethyl Carbonate
396.6	Estradiol Cipionate
396.7	Ergocalciferol
396.9	Quinine Hydrochloride
397.0	Diiodohydroxyquinoline
397.3	Oxaliplatin
	Quinine Dihydrochloride
	Suxamethonium Chloride
397.4	Fluoxetine Oxalate
	Strychnine Nitrate
397.6	Solanidine
397.9	Carbocromen Hydrochloride
398.3	Glycopyrronium Bromide
	Hyoscine Methobromide
398.4	Calcium Aminosalicylate
	Sulfasalazine
398.7	Dihydrotachysterol
399.2	Clefamide
399.3	Dantrolene Sodium
399.4	Colchicine
	Dihydrocodeine Phosphate
	Morphine Acetate
399.5	Pipazetate
399.6	Thiethylperazine
400.0	Mepacrine
400.4	Rivastigmine Hydrogen Tartrate
400.5	Acamprosate Calcium
	Prednisone Acetate
400.6	Alfacalcidol
	Dehydroepiandrosterone Enantate
	Testosterone Enantate
	Tiocarlide
401.0	Clopenthixol
	Zuclopenthixol
401.4	Oxyphenisatine Acetate
401.5	Biperiden Lactate
	Mepyramine Maleate
	Oxyclozanide
401.9	Fenoldopam Mesilate
402.5	Cortisone Acetate
	Pheneticillin Potassium
	Prednisolone Acetate
402.6	Androstenediol Dipropionate
	Sulforidazine
403.4	Ampicillin Trihydrate
	Phthalylsulfathiazole
403.5	Benzatropine Mesilate
403.9	Bambuterol Hydrochloride
	Fenbutrazate Hydrochloride
	Phenoperidine Hydrochloride
404.0	Dipipanone Hydrochloride
	Perphenazine
404.4	Abacavir Succinate
404.5	Benzquinamide
	Hydrocortisone Acetate
	Lovastatin
	Sulfinpyrazone
404.9	Chlormadinone Acetate
405.3	Citalopram Hydrobromide
405.4	Imidapril
	Nebivolol
405.5	Lisinopril
405.9	Oxycodone Hydrochloride
406.0	Clomifene
	Toremifene
406.2	Fosphenytoin Sodium
406.4	Artesunate Sodium
	Codeine Phosphate
	Floctafenine
406.5	Carvedilol
	Flugestone Acetate
	Lincomycin
	Pravastatin Lactone
406.6	Nandrolone Phenylpropionate
406.9	Carbinoxamine Maleate
	Endosulfan
	Hexachlorophene
	Strychnine Hydrochloride
407.0	Thioridazine Hydrochloride

Mol. Wt.	*Compound*
407.4	Lorcainide Hydrochloride
407.5	Trifluoperazine
407.8	Berberine Hydrochloride
408.2	Zimeldine Hydrochloride
408.3	Trazodone Hydrochloride
408.4	Ethyl Biscoumacetate
408.5	Dimetindene Maleate
	Tamsulosin
408.9	Amlodipine
	Beclometasone
	Clorazepate Dipotassium
409.4	Trifluperidol
409.5	Reboxetine Mesilate
409.6	Butaperazine
409.8	Chlordane
409.9	Bunazosin Hydrochloride
410.5	Quinaprilat
	Risperidone
	Trenbolone Hexahydrobenzylcarbonate
	Trimipramine Maleate
410.6	Pergolide Mesilate
	Piperacetazine
	Thiazinamium Metilsulfate
411.4	Phenazocine Hydrobromide
411.5	Etorphine
	Fluvastatin
	Nedocromil Calcium
	Phenindamine Tartrate
411.6	Acetophenazine
411.9	Benzylmorphine Hydrochloride
412.0	Tiagabine Hydrochloride
412.3	Heteronium Bromide
412.6	Bromhexine Hydrochloride
	Testosterone Cipionate
412.9	Remifentanil Hydrochloride
	Ziprasidone
413.4	Noscapine
413.5	Physostigmine Salicylate
413.9	Morazone Hydrochloride
414.3	Flecainide
414.4	Bretylium Tosilate
414.5	Diltiazem
	Domiphen Bromide
414.6	Desoxycortone Pivalate
	Gestonorone Caproate
	Metenolone Enantate
415.3	Nedocromil Sodium
415.4	Norpipanone Hydrobromide
415.5	Cefaloridine
	Diperodon
	Pentapiperide Metilsulfate
415.6	Haloxon
	Salmeterol
415.8	Acemetacin
416.0	Celiprolol Hydrochloride
	Donepezil Hydrochloride
416.1	Miconazole
416.5	Alfentanil
	Cyclizine Tartrate
	Desonide
	Methylprednisolone Acetate
	Pholcodine
	Propicillin Potassium
	Ramipril
416.6	Methandriol Dipropionate
	Spironolactone
416.9	Amosulalol Monohydrochloride
417.5	Decoquinate
418.0	Pyrvinium Chloride
418.3	Decamethonium Bromide
418.4	Aloin
	Cefalothin Sodium
	Nimodipine

Mol. Wt.	*Compound*
418.6	Simvastatin
419.0	Bunamidine Hydrochloride
	Lofepramine
419.4	Amoxicillin Trihydrate
419.6	Prenylamine Lactate
419.9	Clopidogrel Bisulfate
	Hydrastine Hydrochloride
	Prazosin Hydrochloride
420.0	Tandospirone Citrate
420.3	Mepenzolate Bromide
	Methanthelinium Bromide
420.4	Flupirtine Maleate
	Meticillin Sodium
	Penthienate Methobromide
420.5	Dolasetron Methanesulfonate
	Hexoprenaline
	Levocabastine
420.6	Testosterone Phenylpropionate
421.1	Broxaldine
421.4	Bendroflumethiazide
	Ciprofloxacin Lactate
421.5	Topotecan
421.9	Bamifylline Hydrochloride
422.0	Buspirone Hydrochloride
422.4	Carbenicillin Sodium
422.5	Boldenone Benzoate
	Fludrocortisone Acetate
	Sparteine Sulfate
422.9	Losartan
423.9	Diamorphine Hydrochloride
	Terazosin Hydrochloride
424.1	Benzbromarone
424.3	Flurazepam Monohydrochloride
	Pirenzepine Hydrochloride
424.5	Benazepril
424.9	Trimethobenzamide Hydrochloride
425.0	Clindamycin
425.4	Anileridine Hydrochloride
425.5	Ketotifen Fumarate
	Pravastatin
425.6	Diprenorphine
425.8	Epithiazide
	Remoxipride Hydrochloride
425.9	Alfuzosin Hydrochloride
	Reproterol Hydrochloride
426.6	Dehydroepiandrosterone Sodium Sulfate Dihydrate
427.5	Moracizine
427.6	Dixyrazine
427.9	Flavoxate Hydrochloride
428.3	Diethylstilbestrol Diphosphate
428.4	Oxyphenonium Bromide
428.5	Irbesartan
	Pholedrine Sulfate
	Pseudoephedrine Sulfate
428.6	Ephedrine Sulfate
	Hexocyclium Metilsulfate
	Hydroxyprogesterone Caproate
428.7	Nandrolone Decanoate
429.4	Dopexamine Dihydrochloride
429.5	Physostigmine Aminoxide Salicylate
	Pizotifen Malate
429.6	Mebeverine
	Mifepristone
430.0	Chlorprothixene Mesilate
	Metindizate Hydrochloride
430.2	Metaclazepam Hydrochloride
430.4	Bicalutamide
430.5	Morantel Citrate
	Trandolapril
430.6	Piritramide
431.9	Benzthiazide
432.0	Quinagolide Hydrochloride
432.3	Cloricromen Hydrochloride

Mol. Wt.	*Compound*
432.4	Clidinium Bromide
	Nicametate Citrate
432.5	Mizolastine
	Pantoprazole Sodium Sesquihydrate
	Timolol Maleate
432.6	Hydrocortisone Butyrate
433.0	Buclizine
	Doxapram Hydrochloride
433.4	Berberine Sulfate
433.5	Fluvastatin Sodium
	Levallorphan Tartrate
	Mycophenolate Mofetil
433.9	Diperodon Hydrochloride
434.0	Hydroxychloroquine Sulfate
434.3	Cyfluthrin
434.4	Benzilonium Bromide
	Fluvoxamine Maleate
	Pipenzolate Bromide
434.5	Betamethasone Acetate
	Dexamethasone Acetate
	Flupentixol
	Paramethasone Acetate
	Triamcinolone Acetonide
	Xantinol Nicotinate
435.3	Brompheniramine Maleate
	Dexbrompheniramine Maleate
435.4	Ajmaline Hydrochloride
	Aztreonam
435.5	Cilazapril
	Fosinopril Diacid
	Valsartan
435.9	Cloxacillin
436.0	Chloroquine Sulfate
	Pipazetate Hydrochloride
436.4	Opipramol Hydrochloride
436.5	Fludroxycortide
	Isoaminile Citrate
	Thenalidine Tartrate
	Tianeptine
436.6	Bialamicol
437.3	Balsalazide Disodium
437.5	Fluphenazine
438.3	Hyoscine Hydrobromide
438.5	Quinapril
438.6	Spiraprilat
439.9	Polythiazide
440.4	Hyoscine Butylbromide
440.5	Candesartan
440.6	Tirofiban
440.7	Estradiol Undecylate
440.9	Sertindole
441.0	Benzquinamide Hydrochloride
441.4	Folic Acid
	Quinine Hydrobromide
441.5	Deflazacort
	Ergometrine Maleate
	Lisinopril Dihydrate
	Troglitazone
441.6	Dofetilide
	Perindopril Erbumine
441.9	Imidapril Monohydrochloride
	Midazolam Maleate
	Nebivolol Hydrochloride
442.4	Methacycline
442.5	Acepromazine Maleate
443.0	Zuclopenthixol Acetate
443.5	Bephenium Hydroxynaphthoate
	Levorphanol Tartrate
443.6	Tiotixene
444.4	Tetracycline
444.5	Levomepromazine Maleate
	Mitozantrone
444.6	Docusate Sodium
	Prednisolone Pivalate

Mol. Wt.	*Compound*
444.7	Econazole Nitrate
	Testosterone Undecylate
445.0	Tamsulosin Hydrochloride
445.2	Chloramphenicol Sodium Succinate
445.5	Glipizide
	Narceine
445.6	Metopimazine
445.9	Loxapine Succinate
	Trifluperidol Hydrochloride
446.0	Thiopropazate
446.4	Hydrocodone Phosphate
446.5	Pravastatin Sodium
446.6	Denatonium Benzoate
	Hydrocortisone Valerate
	Thioproperazine
447.0	Propyliodone
447.5	Phenyltoloxamine Citrate
	Tripelennamine Citrate
447.8	Hydroxyzine Hydrochloride
448.0	Etorphine Hydrochloride
448.1	Benzethonium Chloride
448.4	Pipamperone Hydrochloride
	Propantheline Bromide
448.5	Debrisoquine Sulfate
450.1	Octafonium Chloride
450.5	Anileridine Phosphate
450.7	Phytomenadione
451.0	Diltiazem Hydrochloride
451.5	Dihydrocodeine Tartrate
	Doxazosin
	Poldine Metilsulfate
451.6	Cabergoline
452.5	Fluocinolone Acetonide
452.6	Bethanidine Sulfate
	Diphenoxylate
452.7	Boldenone Undecylenate
453.3	Chloramphenicol Cinnamate
453.5	Cefixime
	Ethoheptazine Citrate
453.6	Acetorphine
453.9	Flucloxacillin
454.0	Thenium Closilate
454.1	Dofamium Chloride
454.4	Methotrexate
454.6	Verapamil
455.0	Halcinonide
455.3	Primaquine Phosphate
455.4	Lofepramine Hydrochloride
455.5	Butetamate Citrate
	Lacidipine
	Methylergometrine Maleate
456.2	Hexamethonium Iodide
456.5	Aminophylline
456.6	Delavirdine
	Propiomazine Maleate
457.0	Levocabastine Hydrochloride
457.4	Amygdalin
457.5	Minocycline
457.6	Cyclomethycaine Sulfate
457.9	Topotecan Hydrochloride
458.5	Raltitrexed
458.6	Astemizole
459.6	Cerivastatin
459.9	Terazosin Hydrochloride Dihydrate
	Tianeptine Sodium
460.0	Clemastine Fumarate
460.5	Prednisolone Succinate
460.6	Fluocortolone Pivalate
	Mephentermine Sulfate
460.7	Docusate Potassium
460.8	Flurazepam Hydrochloride
461.0	Benazepril Hydrochloride
	Lincomycin Hydrochloride
	Losartan Potassium
461.5	Azlocillin
	Orphenadrine Citrate
461.6	Pimozide
461.8	Cetirizine Dihydrochloride
462.0	Diprenorphine Hydrochloride
462.5	Doxycycline
	Hydrocortisone Hydrogen Succinate
463.5	Pivampicillin
464.0	Moracizine Hydrochloride
464.6	Hordenine Sulfate
464.8	Amodiaquine Hydrochloride
464.9	Demeclocycline
	Loprazolam
465.4	Cefixime Disodium
	Dimoxyline Phosphate
465.5	Bacampicillin
466.0	Cisapride
	Mebeverine Hydrochloride
466.5	Brucine tetrahydrate
466.6	Cephaëline
	Spirapril
467.0	Clobetasol Propionate
467.4	Ziprasidone Hydrochloride Monohydrate
467.5	Saccharin Calcium
	Tobramycin
467.6	Buprenorphine
	Oxetacaine
467.9	Noscapine Hydrochloride
469.5	Methysergide Maleate
469.6	Almotriptan Maleate
469.7	Ebastine
470.0	Dimenhydrinate
	Nefazodone
470.2	Dibrompropamidine
470.7	Enoxolone
472.8	Alpha Tocoferil Acetate
473.4	Clofazimine
473.6	Alverine Citrate
	Naftidrofuryl Oxalate
473.9	Clopenthixol Hydrochloride
	Zuclopenthixol Hydrochloride
474.4	Flecainide Acetate
474.5	Methylprednisolone Hemisuccinate
474.6	Fluocortolone Hexanoate
	Sildenafil
475.0	Quinapril Hydrochloride
475.6	Fluspirilene
	Tolterodine Tartrate
475.7	Pipotiazine
475.9	Cloxacillin Sodium
476.6	Betamethasone Valerate
	Piminodine Esilate
	Prednisolone Tebutate
477.0	Loperamide
477.6	Butorphanol Tartrate
478.3	Suxethonium Bromide
478.5	Triamcinolone Diacetate
478.6	Dehydroemetine
478.9	Chlortetracycline
	Methacycline Hydrochloride
479.0	Clobetasone Butyrate
479.1	Clospipramine
	Miconazole Nitrate
479.4	Aztreonam Disodium
479.5	Clindamycin Hydrochloride
480.4	Isopropamide Iodide
	Trifluoperazine Hydrochloride
480.6	Emetine
	Quinine Salicylate
480.9	Tetracycline
481.5	Cerivastatin Sodium
481.9	Meclozine Hydrochloride
	Narceine Hydrochloride
482.5	Trifluomeprazine Maleate
483.5	Azlocillin Sodium
483.9	Mersalyl Acid
484.0	Cisapride Monohydrate
484.4	Nicergoline
	Prednisolone Sodium Phosphate
484.5	Bopindolol Malonate
	Hydrocortisone Sodium Succinate
	Kanamycin
	Oxedrine Tartrate
486.2	Suxamethonium Bromide
486.4	Hydrocortisone Sodium Phosphate
486.6	Hydrocortisone Cipionate
487.4	Fluclorolone Acetonide
487.7	Dimetotiazine Mesilate
488.0	Chloropyrilene Citrate
	Doxazosin Hydrochloride
489.1	Diphenoxylate Hydrochloride
490.0	Acetorphine Hydrochloride
490.6	Dexamethasone Tebutate
	Glimepiride
	Pentobarbital Calcium
491.1	Verapamil Hydrochloride
491.5	Flunixin Meglumine
491.6	Lidoflazine
492.5	Enalapril Maleate
492.6	Bezitramide
492.7	Isometheptene Mucate
493.4	Hexoprenaline Hydrochloride
493.9	Flucloxacillin Sodium
	Minocycline Hydrochloride
494.0	Glibenclamide
494.5	Fluocinonide
	Hydrocodone Tartrate
494.6	Flumetasone Pivalate
	Quinidine Bisulfate
495.1	Tirofiban Hydrochloride Monohydrate
495.6	Mibefradil
495.7	Orlistat
496.5	Methylprednisolone Sodium Succinate
	Oxytetracycline Dihydrate
496.6	Betamethasone Benzoate
	Bopindolol Maleate
496.9	Oxytetracycline Hydrochloride
497.5	Idarubicin
497.6	Dexamethasone Isonicotinate
498.6	Moexipril
499.0	Promethazine Teoclate
499.3	Nitroxinil Eglumine Salt
500.0	Pivampicillin Hydrochloride
500.4	Halofantrine
500.6	Fluticasone Propionate
	Mupirocin
501.3	Demeclocycline Hydrochloride
501.7	Fexofenadine
502.0	Bacampicillin Hydrochloride
503.1	Spirapril Hydrochloride
504.1	Buprenorphine Hydrochloride
504.6	Betamethasone Dipropionate
	Dipyridamole
505.0	Clindamycin Phosphate
505.2	Deltamethrin
505.5	Chlorhexidine
505.6	Amprenavir
505.9	Mersalyl Sodium
506.0	Buclizine Hydrochloride
506.5	Nefazodone Hydrochloride
507.2	Adenosine Triphosphate
507.4	Flupentixol Hydrochloride
507.5	Cefixime Trihydrate
507.8	Pyrrobutamine Phosphate

Mol. Wt.	Compound
508.9	Clomocycline
	Mepacrine Hydrochloride
509.6	Bialamicol Hydrochloride
510.4	Fluphenazine Hydrochloride
510.6	Cyclobarbital Calcium
511.6	Etamiphylline Camsilate
	Norbormide
512.3	Sodium Cromoglicate
512.5	Guanoxan Sulfate
512.9	Doxycycline Hydrochloride
513.5	Clomethiazole Edisilate
	Loperamide Hydrochloride
514.6	Telmisartan
515.3	Chlortetracycline Hydrochloride
515.9	Chloroquine Phosphate
516.4	Betamethasone Sodium Phosphate
	Dexamethasone Sodium Phosphate
516.7	Bamethan Sulfate
517.4	Mitozantrone Hydrochloride
518.1	Benziodarone
518.4	Conessine Hydrobromide
518.6	Hexoprenaline Sulfate
	Prajmalium Bitartrate
518.9	Thiopropazate Hydrochloride
519.0	Dichloralphenazone
520.6	Orciprenaline Sulfate
	Quinidine Gluconate
521.0	Beclometasone Dipropionate
522.6	Azatadine Maleate
524.0	Penfluridol
525.0	Amlodipine Maleate
525.6	Carbetapentane Citrate
	Deptropine Citrate
525.7	Fusidic Acid
527.5	Daunorubicin
527.6	Dequalinium Chloride
	Gliquidone
	Oxeladin Citrate
	Rolitetracycline
528.6	Fentanyl Citrate
529.8	Rocuronium
530.9	Clomocycline Sodium
531.0	Moexipril Diacid Hydrochloride
531.4	Ketoconazole
532.6	Hydroxystilbamidine Isetionate
	Pentamidine Mesilate
	Triamcinolone Hexacetonide
534.0	Idarubicin Hydrochloride
535.0	Moexipril Hydrochloride
536.9	Halofantrine Hydrochloride
538.1	Fexofenadine Hydrochloride
538.6	Pentolonium Tartrate
538.7	Sodium Fusidate
539.5	Cephaëline Hydrochloride
540.3	Quinine Dihydrobromide
540.6	Atorvastatin Lactone
540.7	Mescaline Sulfate Dihydrate
541.5	Clioxanide
542.6	Dextromoramide Tartrate
543.5	Doxorubicin
	Epirubicin
544.2	Suxamethonium Iodide
544.7	Mesoridazine
546.6	Ceftazidime
547.6	Doxazosin Mesilate
	Perazine Dimalonate
548.6	Amicarbalide Isetionate
	Quinine Bisulfate
	Terbutaline Sulfate
549.7	Fluphenazine Enantate
550.3	Mebezonium Iodide
551.6	Dehydroemetine Hydrochloride
552.0	Clospipramine Dihydrochloride
552.6	Proflavine Hemisulfate
	Tiotixene Hydrochloride
552.7	Delavirdine monomethanesulfonate
554.6	Ceftriaxone
554.7	Profenamine Hibenzate
555.2	Clopenthixol Decanoate
	Zuclopenthixol Decanoate
556.6	Isoprenaline Sulfate
558.6	Fenoprofen Calcium
558.7	Atorvastatin
560.7	Desferrioxamine
561.5	Chloramphenicol Palmitate
561.7	Ergotoxine
562.5	Acefylline Piperazine
563.6	Trimetrexate D-Glucuronate
563.7	Fosinopril
564.0	Daunorubicin Hydrochloride
564.1	Prochlorperazine Edisilate
564.6	Propamidine Isetionate
565.7	Dextropropoxyphene Napsilate
	Levopropoxyphene Napsilate
566.2	Prochlorperazine Mesilate
566.6	Quinuronium Sulfate
567.1	Amlodipine Besilate
567.8	Nelfinavir
568.6	Mibefradil Dihydrochloride
570.8	Carbenoxolone
574.8	Dequalinium Acetate
575.6	Tandospirone Citrate
575.7	Zafirlukast
576.3	Distigmine Bromide
576.7	Salbutamol Sulfate
577.6	Stilbazium Iodide
578.4	Chlorhexidine Hydrochloride
578.7	Deserpidine
579.0	Loprazolam Mesilate
580.0	Doxorubicin Hydrochloride
	Epirubicin Hydrochloride
580.6	Atorvastatin Sodium
581.6	Streptomycin
581.7	Ergotamine
582.6	Kanamycin Sulfate
583.6	Dihydrostreptomycin
583.7	Dihydroergotamine
585.6	Amikacin
	Fosinopril Sodium
585.7	Ebastine Fumarate
586.2	Montelukast
586.7	Irinotecan
587.6	Diminazene Aceturate
588.6	Etoposide
588.7	Procaine Benzylpenicillin
588.8	Flupentixol Decanoate
591.8	Fluphenazine Decanoate
592.7	Hexobendine
	Pentamidine Isetionate
594.7	Pyrantel Embonate
596.8	Trimetaphan Camsilate
597.4	Pyritidium Bromide
598.1	Clomifene Citrate
	Toremifene Citrate
600.5	Nicofuranose
602.6	Lymecycline
	Picrotoxin
603	Lymecycline
603.7	Benzonatate
	Salmeterol Xinafoate
604.3	Fazadinium Bromide
605.6	Butaperazine Phosphate
606.1	Prochlorperazine Maleate
608.2	Montelukast Sodium
608.5	Ambenonium Chloride
608.7	Methoserpidine
	Reserpine
609.7	Rocuronium Bromide
610.2	Mepacrine Mesilate
610.7	Candesartan Cilexetil
613.8	Indinavir
614.6	Neomycin
614.7	Carbenoxolone Sodium
615.6	Butyl Aminobenzoate Picrate
617.6	Rolitetracycline Nitrate
622.7	Pseudomorphine
623.2	Irinotecan Hydrochloride
624.3	Guanoclor Sulfate
625.6	Chlorhexidine Acetate
626.0	Rafoxanide
631.8	Thiethylperazine Maleate
634.7	Rescinnamine
636.7	Ceftazidime Pentahydrate
638.8	Thioproperazine Mesilate
641.7	Butaperazine Maleate
641.9	Pipotiazine Palmitate
642.7	Piperazine Citrate
643.7	Acetophenazine Dimaleate
645.3	Amiodarone
645.6	Acarbose
645.7	Aconitine
647.6	Cabergoline Diphosphate
648.8	Physostigmine Sulfate
651.0	Liothyronine
651.2	Kanamycin Acid Sulfate
652.7	Capreomycin
654.6	Bromocriptine
656.8	Desferrioxamine Mesilate
657.7	Carfenazine Maleate
661.6	Ceftriaxone Sodium
663.9	Nelfinavir
664.8	Antazoline Sulfate
665.6	Hexobendine Hydrochloride
665.7	Natamycin
666.7	Syrosingopine
667.8	Thiethylperazine Malate
668.6	Etoposide Phosphate
668.7	Capreomycin
670.8	Abacavir Sulfate
	Saquinavir
671.8	Ergotoxine Esilate
672.5	Halofantrine β-Glycerophosphate
673.0	Liothyronine Sodium
673.8	Co-dergocrine Mesilate
677.2	Irinotecan Hydrochloride Trihydrate
677.8	Rapacuronium Bromide
679.7	Emetine Hydrochloride
679.8	Dihydroergotamine Mesilate
681.8	Amiodarone Hydrochloride
684.8	Metoprolol Tartrate
684.9	Prednisolone Steaglate
687.4	Liothyronine Hydrochloride
687.9	Oleandomycin
694.8	Atropine Sulfate
697.8	Rifamycin SV
699.9	Clindamycin Palmitate Hydrochloride
705.6	Itraconazole
708.8	Aconitine Nitrate
711.0	Butacaine Sulfate
711.9	Indinavir Sulfate
712.5	Ranitidine Bismuth Citrate
712.9	Hyoscyamine Sulfate
714.1	Pipotiazine Palmitate
716.6	Demecarium Bromide
719.6	Daunorubicin Lactate
719.8	Rifamycin Sodium
721.0	Ritonavir
722.4	Dibrompropamidine Isetionate
728.8	Ouabain
731.8	Diphenhydramine Di(acefyllinate)

Mol. Wt.	*Compound*
732.7	Pancuronium Bromide
733.9	Erythromycin
734.0	Colfosceril Palmitate
747.0	Alimemazine Tartrate
748.0	Clarithromycin
749.0	Azithromycin
750.7	Bromocriptine Mesilate
750.9	Codeine Sulfate
752.7	Pholcodine Tartrate
753.9	Vindesine
758.8	Morphine Sulfate
763.3	Hydroxyzine Embonate
764.9	Digitoxin
	Zolpidem Tartrate
767.0	Bisoprolol Fumarate (hemifumerate)
	Saquinavir Mesilate
771.7	Tubocurarine Chloride
773.0	Lobeline Sulfate
774.8	Morphine Tartrate
774.9	Phenoxymethylpenicillin Calcium
776.9	Levothyroxine
779.0	Vinorelbine
780.9	Digoxin
781.8	Amikacin Sulfate
783.0	Quinidine Sulfate
	Quinine Sulfate
785.9	Oleandomycin Phosphate
790.0	Erythromycin Propionate
793.9	Protoveratrine A
794.8	Xamoterol Hemifumarate
795.0	Metildigoxin
798.9	Levothyroxine Sodium
800.9	Ergometrine Tartrate
804.0	Tacrolimus
804.9	Formoterol Fumarate Dihydrate
807.0	Acetyldigitoxin
807.9	Docetaxel
809.9	Protoveratrine A
810.7	Inositol Nicotinate
811.0	Vinblastine
811.8	Aclarubicin
813.0	Cinchonidine Sulfate
814.0	Troleandomycin
822.0	Tacrolimus Monohydrate
822.9	Rifampicin
823.0	α-Acetyldigoxin
825.0	Vincristine
827.9	Alcuronium Chloride
837.0	Roxithromycin
841.1	Mebhydrolin Napadisilate
843.1	Spiramycin
847.0	Rifabutin
848.3	Aclarubicin Hydrochloride
852.0	Vindesine Sulfate
853.9	Paclitaxel
857.0	Strychnine Sulfate
861.9	Docetaxel trihydrate
862.1	Erythromycin Ethylsuccinate
866.9	Papaverine
868.1	Solanine
869.2	Tilmicosin
871.0	Methapyrilene Fumarate
883.1	Quetiapine Hemifumarate
883.2	Docusate Calcium
885.1	Spiramycin
885.2	Ibutilide Fumarate
891.5	Gallamine Triethiodide
891.8	Cycloguanil Embonate
897.8	Chlorhexidine Gluconate Solution
899.1	Spiramycin
906.6	Metocurine Iodide
909.1	Vinblastine Sulfate
914.2	Sirolimus
916.1	Tylosin
923.0	Vincristine Sulfate
924.1	Amphotericin B
926.1	Nystatin
929.2	Atracurium
	Cisatracurium
943.1	Deslanoside
943.2	Amitriptyline Embonate
949.2	Imipramine Embonate
957.2	Promazine Embonate
958.9	Oxytetracycline Calcium
960.1	Erythromycin Gluceptate
985.1	Lanatoside C
1013	Brucine Sulfate
1018.4	Erythromycin Stearate
1019.3	Octreotide
1026.0	Chlorpromazine Embonate
1056.4	Erythromycin Estolate
1079.1	Vinorelbine Tartrate
1092	Erythromycin Lactobionate
1096.3	Lanreotide
1100.2	Mivacurium Chloride
1106.1	Doxacurium Chloride
1151.4	Pyrvinium Embonate
1202.6	Ciclosporin
1209.4	Atorvastatin Calcium
1239.4	Buserelin
1243.5	Atracurium Besilate
	Cisatracurium Besilate
1255.5	Dactinomycin
1299.5	Buserelin Acetate
1313.4	Ergotamine Tartrate
1317.4	Dihydroergotamine Tartrate
1322.5	Nafarelin
1346.4	Hydroxocobalamin
1355.4	Cyanocobalamin
1382.6	Nafarelin Monoacetate
1415.6	Bleomycin
1449.3	Vancomycin
1457.4	Streptomycin Sulfate
1461.4	Dihydrostreptomycin Sulfate
1485.7	Vancomycin Hydrochloride
4000–6000	Enoxaparin
6979.4	Lepirudin
14798.0	Molgramostim
15330.7	Aldesleukin
22124.1	Somatropin
37 000	Chorionic Gonadotropin
39 571.1	Reteplase
59 007.6	Alteplase
64 529.1	Duteplase
136 000	Asparaginase

Melting Points

d = with decomposition

°C	Compound
0.5	Triazophos
2	Chloroquine Phosphate
	Pentazocine
2–5	Triazophos
2.9	Malathion
3.4	Fenitrothion
3.5	Cryofluorane
6	Parathion
7.5	Fenthion
8–9	Ethyl Nicotinate
9	Cadaverine
10	Ethylenediamine Hydrate
10–13	Paraldehyde
12	Trientine
15	Acetic Acid Glacial
15.5–18.5	Fomepizole
18	Trichloroethanol
19	Propofol
22	Tetrachloroethylene
23–24	Putrescine
23–25	Nikethamide
24	Amylmetacresol
25	Sevoflurane
25–30	Monocrotophos
>25	Foscarnet Sodium
	Piperonyl Butoxide
<25	Dichlorvos
27–28	Menthol
28.5–32	Sulfiram
29.5	Chloromethylaniline
30–32	Fluphenazine Decanoate
31d	Carmustine
32–35	Nandrolone Decanoate
33	Fluoroacetic Acid
34	Pilocarpine
35–36	Mescaline
36–38	Testosterone Enantate
36.5–37.5	Prenylamine
37–38	Prilocaine
38–40	Phenoxybenzamine
	Pyrazophos
38.1	Anhydrous Ephedrine
39	Methyl Nicotinate
40	Ephedrine
40–41	Alachlor
	Phenol
40–43	Orlistat
41–42	Chlorpyrifos
41–42.5	Fenpiprane
41–43	Menthol
41–45	Cyclophosphamide
41–46	Tetracaine
	Salol
43	Parachlorophenol
	Piperazine Hydrate
44.6–46.8	Dimethyltryptamine
45	Trimipramine
45d	Metoclopramide Dihydrochloride
45–46	Butanilicaine
45.5–46.5	Chlorpyrifos-methyl
46	Trimethadione
46–46.5	Phencyclidine
46–50	Idebenone
46–52	Ethosuximide
47–49	Diethylcarbamazine
48–49	Pyrrobutamine
48–50	Esmolol
	Urethane
48–55	Butylated Hydroxyanisole
49	Fenamiphos
49–51	Tybamate
49.5–50.0	Choline Salicylate
50–53	Metyrapone
50–56	Mesuximide
50–58	Cloral Hydrate
51	Benactyzine
51–53	Perazine
51.5	Thiotepa
	Thymol
52–52.5	Dimethoate
52–53	Idebenone
53	Azinphos-ethyl
53–54	Paradichlorobenzene
53–55	Profenamine
	Tocainide
53–56	Methylpentynol Carbamate
54	Methamidophos
54–55	Monocrotophos
54–57	Triclosan
55–56.5	Hydroxyphenamate
55–57	Dosulepin
55.0–56.5	Cyclandelate
55.5	Chlorocresol
56–57	Enallylpropymal
56–58	Emylcamate
56–60	Chlorpromazine
57	Quinine
57–59	Alprenolol
	Butyl Aminobenzoate
57–60	Pentetrazol
58–60	Cetalkonium Chloride
59	Hyoscine
59–61	Triprolidine
60	Cyfluthrin
	Promethazine
60–61.5	Levamisole
60–65	Halofantrine β-Glycerophosphate
60.5–61.0	DOM
61	Procaine
62–64	Thiethylperazine
62–68	Hexylresorcinol
63–64	Isoaminile Citrate
64	Cinchocaine
64–67	Dichloralphenazone
66	Chlorambucil
66–67	Cannabidiol
67	Etomidate
67.5–68.5	Fluanisone
68	Alimemazine
68–69	Isometheptene Hydrochloride
	Lidocaine
68–70	Methoprotryne
69–70	Ranitidine
69–71	Diphenyl
70	Butylated Hydroxytoluene
	Disulfiram
	Embutramide
	Isosorbide Dinitrate
	Levacetylmethadol
70–71	Mephenesin
70–72	Betaxolol
70–100	Endosulfan
71	Chloronitrotoluene
71–73	Phensuximide
72–74	Thioridazine
72.5	4-Chloroaniline
73–74	Azinphos-methyl
73–75	Azaperone
	Budipine
74	Emetine
74–75	Methylphenidate
74–77	Methyprylon
75	Etamiphylline
	Racephedrine
75–76	Dextropropoxyphene
	Levopropoxyphene
75–77	Hexobendine
75–80	Oxprenolol
75–84	Trichlorfon
	Ibuprofen
75.5–76.5	Salmeterol
76	Hydroxyquinoline
	Toloxatone
76–77	Cannabinol
	Dimethadione
76–78	Ethylestrenol
77–78	Cathine
	Lidocaine Hydrochloride
	Mupirocin
	Phenaglycodol
77–79	Chlorphenesin
	Mebutamate
77–82	Flurazepam
77–83	Cetylpyridinium Chloride
78	Butylchloral Hydrate
	Chlorobutanol
	Etisazole
	Methadone
78–82	Guaifenesin
80	Allylestrenol
	Anileridine
	Isopropylaminophenazone
	Testosterone Isocaproate
80–80.5	Bamifylline
80–83	Monolinuron
80–85	Lysergide
80.2	Naphthalene
81–82	Anastrozole
81–83	Vanillin
82–83	Pentifylline
82–85	Fenyramidol
83–84	Fentanyl
	Histamine
	Nefazodone
84	Colecalciferol
84–86	Ametryne

°C	Compound
	Desmetryne
85–86	Esmolol Hydrochloride
85–89	Glutethimide
85–90	Atracurium Besilate
85.5–86.5	Procyclidine
86	Dinitro-orthocresol
86–87	Trazodone
86–88	Artemether
86–92	Benzoylecgonine
86.8	Econazole
87–88	Methdilazine
87–89	Diethyltryptamine Hydrochloride
	Tetramisole
87–91	Etidocaine
87–92	Chloroquine
87–95	Chloramphenicol Palmitate
87.5–88.8	Ethambutol
88–90	Metaclazepam
	Noxytiolin
	Ritodrine
88–92	Benzocaine
88–93	Haloxon
89	Anileridine
	Methoxychlor
89–91	Hydroxychloroquine
	Isosorbide Mononitrate
90	Chlorphenesin Carbamate
	Ethotoin
	Physostigmine Aminoxide Salicylate
90–91	Oxeladin Citrate
90–92	Vinylbital
	Clobetasone Butyrate
90–96	Cycrimine
90–98d	Cinchocaine Hydrochloride
	Phenindamine
90–100	Aldicarb
91	Alclofenac
	Buclosamide
	Pholcodine
91–93	Propanil
91–94	Beclamide
91–95	Quinine Ethyl Carbonate
92–93	Carisoprodol
	Ketamine
	Nicorandil
92–94	Maprotiline
92–96	Methohexital
92–97	Dexketoprofen
93	Carbetapentane Citrate
	Mephenesin Carbamate
93–94	Linuron
	Mycophenolate Mofetil
93–95	Trifluperidol
93–96	Halofantrine Hydrochloride
	Ketoprofen
94	Methocarbamol
	N-Acetylmescaline
94–99	Etamivan
94–100	Perphenazine
94–102	Ditiocarb Sodium
95	Coumaphos
	Disopyramide
	Ditiocarb Sodium
	Mebhydrolin
95–96	Heptachlor
	Heptachlor
	Nandrolone Phenylpropionate
95–97	Cilazapril
	Medazepam
	Thenalidine
95–140	Erythromycin Gluceptate
96	Oxyphenbutazone
	Propranolol
	Tiaprofenic Acid
96–97	Propyl Hydroxybenzoate
	Trenbolone Acetate
	Tropicamide
96–97.5	Dodecyl Gallate
96–98	Ethinamate
	Metadoxine
97	Chlorobutanol
97–98	Chlorprothixene
97–99	Bretylium Tosilate
98	Cocaine
98–101	Deltamethrin
98–108	α-Methyltryptamine
99–100	Homatropine
	Rabeprazole
99–102	Mexenone
100	Bisoprolol Fumarate (hemifumerate)
	Orciprenaline
	Secobarbital
100–101	Mepyramine Maleate
	Opipramol
	Valethamate Bromide
100–103	Alverine Citrate
	Butacaine Sulfate
100–104	Doxylamine Succinate
100–110	Piperacetazine
101	Biperiden
	Phenylpropanolamine
101–102	Oxalic Acid
	Testosterone Cipionate
101–104	Phenprobamate
102	Dimethisterone
102–103	Clorgiline Hydrochloride
102–104	Famciclovir
	Venlafaxine
102–104d	Noradrenaline Acid Tartrate
102–105	Pentoxifylline
102–107	Dimenhydrinate
102–108	Gentamicin
102.5–103.5	Isoxsuprine
103	Propyphenazone
103–104	Difenidol
103–107	Dexketoprofen trometamol
103–113	Dexbrompheniramine Maleate
104	Aldrin
	Aldrin
	Diethylstilbestrol Dipropionate
	Oxetacaine
	Terbutryne
104–105	Etretinate
104–106	Meprobamate
104–110	Acetylcysteine
105	Phenylbutazone
105–106	Physostigmine
105–107	Flecainide
	Menadione
	Penfluridol
	Prednisolone Steaglate
105–108	Isocarboxazid
105–109	Metipranolol
105–110	Fenoprofen Calcium
	Methenamine Hippurate
105.0–107.5	Choline Dihydrogen Citrate
105.5–107.5	Cyclizine
106	Captopril
	Lofepramine
	Piperazine
106–107	Pipobroman
106–109	Hyoscyamine
106–110	Tripelennamine Citrate
106–110d	Procaine Benzylpenicillin
107	Pheniramine Maleate
107–109	Aminophenazone
	Oxprenolol Hydrochloride
107–110	Butetamate Citrate
107.5–108	Bupivacaine
108	Disulfoton
	Naftidrofuryl Oxalate
	Talbutal
108–109	Dropropizine
108–110	Endosulfan
	Toremifene
108–111	Alprenolol Hydrochloride
108–112	Prothipendyl Hydrochloride
109	Acecarbromal
	Clofenotane
	Ramipril
109–110	Butyl Aminobenzoate Picrate
	Loxapine
109–111	Resorcinol
109–113	Dextromethorphan
109.8	Cisapride Monohydrate
110	Alprostadil
	Flurbiprofen
	Gallium Nitrate
	Nimorazole
110–111	Styramate
110–112	Celiprolol
110–115	Cetirizine
111	Hexaconazole
	Pralidoxime Metilsulfate
	Tolnaftate
111–112	Buphenine
111–113	Phenazone
111–115	Clomifene
112	Nandrolone
112–113	Dihydrocodeine
	Domiphen Bromide
	Indeloxazine Hydrochloride
112–113.5	Tandospirone
112–115	Acetomenaphthone
	Adiphenine Hydrochloride
112–116	Chloropyrilene Citrate
112.5	Lindane
113	Chlorquinaldol
	Cyproheptadine
	Dihydrotachysterol
	Iproniazid
113–115	Acetanilide
	Azithromycin
	Cyclopentamine Hydrochloride
	Dexchlorphenamine Maleate
	Levorphanol Tartrate
	Levorphanol Tartrate
113–117	Betaxolol Hydrochloride
113–119	Ergocalciferol
114–115	Carvedilol
114–116	Chloroxylenol
	Ciprofibrate
	Dicamba
	Diloxanide Furoate
	Mirtazapine
	Perazine Dimalonate
114–117	Testosterone Phenylpropionate
114–118	Atropine
	Busulfan
114.3–115.0	Trihexyphenidyl
115	Bamipine
115–116	Androstenediol Dipropionate
	Caramiphen Edisilate
	Cephaëline
	Flupirtine
115–118	Trientine Dihydrochloride
116	Ethyl Hydroxybenzoate
	Hydrastine Hydrochloride
116–117	Dibenzepin
	Pericyazine

°C	Compound
	Valsartan
116–118	Triprolidine Hydrochloride
116–119	Carbromal
116–122	Clotiapine
116.2–118.2	Chlormezanone
116.5–118	Clomifene Citrate
117	Hydrastinine
	Levetiracetam
117–118	Hordenine
117–119	Carbinoxamine Maleate
	Ibutilide Fumarate
117–120	Etoxazene
118	Chlorotrianisene
	Tryptamine
118–119	Methylchlorophenoxyacetic Acid
118–120	Prometryne
118–122	Flutoprazepam
	Testosterone Propionate
118–128	Hydrocodone Tartrate
118.0–118.7	Pseudoephedrine
118.5–119.5	Morinamide
119	Chloramphenicol Cinnamate
	Riluzole
119–121	Mandelic Acid
119–121.5	Quinapril Hydrochloride
119–122	Terbutaline
119–123	Acebutolol
119–124	Sulfafurazole Diethanolamine
120	Clofedanol
	Methaqualone
	Metoprolol Tartrate
	Naphazoline
120–121	Rizatriptan
120–121.5	Fluvoxamine Maleate
120–122	Antazoline
	Trimetozine
120–124	Hydroxyprogesterone Caproate
120–128d	Phenoxymethylpenicillin
120–130	Quinapril Hydrochloride
121	Etilefrine Hydrochloride
	N-Benzoylmescaline
	Octamylamine Hydrochloride
121–122	Aniracetam
	Etacrynic Acid
121–123	Betanaphthol
	Sulforidazine
122–124	Succinimide
122–124d	Dextromethorphan Hydrobromide
122–125	Carbimazole
122.4	Benzoic Acid
122.5–124	Quinagolide
123d	Ethylmorphine Hydrochloride
123–124	Gestonorone Caproate
123–125	Rivastigmine Hydrogen Tartrate
123–126	Dipipanone Hydrochloride
123–127	Thiambutosine
123–129	Dihydrotachysterol
123.5–125	Bamethan
124	Picotamide
	Suprofen
	Zidovudine
124d	Cloral Betaine
124–125	Dimoxyline
	Flufenamic Acid
124–127	Butobarbital
124–136	Nadolol
124.5–126.0	Pipamperone Hydrochloride
125	Nimodipine
	Penthienate Methobromide
	Tilidate Hydrochloride
125–126	Hydroxyamfetamine
125–127	Phenglutarimide
	Sulfacarbamide
125–128	Tetrabenazine
125–130	Amygdalin
125–140d	Chloropyrilene Citrate
126	Hexethal Sodium
	Levomepromazine
126–127	Amisulpride
	Butanilicaine Phosphate
	Galantamine
	Protokylol Hydrochloride
126–128	Bemegride
	Lofexidine
	Mecloqualone
	Repaglinide
126–129	Clomethiazole Edisilate
126–130	Chlorpropamide
126–131	Etynodiol Diacetate
127	Neopine
127d	Pentobarbital Sodium
127–128	Hexestrol Dipropionate
	Tinidazole
127–128d	Atropine Oxide
	Propylhexedrine Hydrochloride
127–129	Conessine
	Tacrolimus Monohydrate
127–130	Aprindine Hydrochloride
127–131	Progesterone
127–133	Meptazinol
128	Chlorphenoxamine Hydrochloride
	Idobutal
	Mibefradil Dihydrochloride
	Prenalterol Hydrochloride
128d	Isoprenaline Sulfate
128–130	Methenamine Mandelate
128–131	Nicotinamide
128–132	Tylosin
128–133	Irgarol
128–135	Piminodine Esilate
129	Physostigmine Aminoxide
	Proguanil
	Tolbutamide
129–130	Pentobarbital
	Pyrrobutamine Phosphate
129–131	Methoxyphenamine Hydrochloride
	Paroxetine Hydrochloride Hemihydrate
130	Clonidine
130–131	Lobeline
130–131.5	Benzquinamide
130–132	Bitoscanate
	Nizatidine
	Thialbarbital Sodium
130–133	Histamine Acid Phosphate
	Tolbutamide Sodium
130–135	Chlorphenamine maleate
131	Benzfetamine Hydrochloride
	Methyl Hydroxybenzoate
131–132	Captodiame Hydrochloride
	Tirofiban Hydrochloride Monohydrate
131–133	Xylometazoline
131–135	Diazepam
131–136	Mebeverine Hydrochloride
131.5–132.5	Encainide Hydrochloride
132	Benzylmorphine
	Hydrastine
132–133	Famprofazone
	Thiamylal
132–134	Brompheniramine Maleate
	Etenzamide
132–135d	Thebacon Hydrochloride
132–137d	Cotarnine
132–143	Nicofuranose
133d	Urea
133–134	Prolintane Hydrochloride
	Ranitidine Hydrochloride
>133d	Hydroxycarbamide
134	Ambucetamide
	Chlorhexidine
	Sorbic Acid
134–135	Acetylcodeine
	Phenacetin
	Spironolactone
134–136	Alfacalcidol
	Flufenamic Acid
	Loratadine
	Practolol
134–137	Clefamide
	Muzolimine
134–138	Orphenadrine Citrate
134–145	Tiocarlide
134–147	Tetracaine Hydrochloride
135	Atropine Sulfate
	Norethandrolone
135–136	Acepromazine Maleate
	Chelidonine
	Methapyrilene Fumarate
	Proxyphylline
135–137	Levobupivacaine
135–137d	Ceftazidime Pentahydrate
135–138	Cyclopentolate Hydrochloride
	Simvastatin
135–139	Flunixin Meglumine
135–140	Alfentanil Hydrochloride
	Erythromycin
135–140d	Erythromycin Estolate
136	Fenclofenac
	Meclofenoxate Hydrochloride
136d	Sparteine Sulfate
136–137	Mephenytoin
	Sulfinpyrazone
136–138	Nicergoline
136–139	Nitroxinil
	Xylazine
136–144	Imidacloprid
137	Moclobemide
137–138	Bevantolol Hydrochloride
	Salmeterol Xinafoate
137–140	Cyclofenil
137–141	Phenoxybenzamine Hydrochloride
137.5	Quazepam
138	Bisacodyl
	Ecothiopate Iodide
	Fluoxetine Hydrochloride
	Metenolone Acetate
	Methallenestril
138–139	Butalbital
138–140	Bufotenine
	Fluconazole
	Formoterol Fumarate Dihydrate
	Phenyltoloxamine Citrate
	Zafirlukast
138–141	Dimetridazole
138–142	Pravastatin Lactone
138.5–140.5d	Verapamil Hydrochloride
139	Phenazopyridine
	Thiethylperazine Malate
139–140	Cyclopentobarbital
	Imidapril
	Pantoprazole
139–141	Zolmitriptan
140	Ajmaline Hydrochloride
	Amitriptyline Embonate
	Dichlorophenoxyacetic Acid
	Ethoheptazine Citrate
	Pentaerithrityl Tetranitrate
	Physostigmine Sulfate
	Salicylamide
	Thioproperazine

°C	Compound
140–141	Dehydroepiandrosterone
	Rabeprazole Sodium
140–141.5	Aprobarbital
140–142	Fenyramidol Hydrochloride
	Isoniazid Aminosalicylate
	Prenylamine Lactate
	Xylazine
140–144	Hyoscine Butylbromide
140–145	Phenylephrine Hydrochloride
140–146	Tylosin Tartrate
140–148	Pentapiperide Metilsulfate
140.7	Nebivolol
141	Mycophenolic Acid
141–142	Desoxycortone
	Selegiline Hydrochloride
141–143	Acebutolol Hydrochloride
	Cimetidine
	Clindamycin Hydrochloride
	Diethylcarbamazine Citrate
141–145	Benzatropine Mesilate
141–146	Ethinylestradiol
141–161	Moexipril Hydrochloride
142	Carbaryl
	Protionamide
	Trimipramine Maleate
142d	Pheniramine Aminosalicylate
142–142.5	Indeloxazine Hydrochloride
142–143	Fexofenadine
	Tramazoline
142–144	Bibenzonium Bromide
	Tuaminoheptane
142–147	Flutazolam
142–150	Colchicine
142.5	Choline Alfoscerate
143	Acetylcholine Bromide
	Mequitazine
143–144.5	Enalapril Maleate
143–148	Methoxsalen
144	Iprindole Hydrochloride
	Tetrazepam
144–145	Carbutamide
	Estradiol Valerate
144–146	Ropivacaine
144–147	Thiamazole
144–148	Quinisocaine Hydrochloride
144–149	Neostigmine Methylsulfate
144–150	Diphenadione
145	Berberine
	Butalamine Hydrochloride
	Felodipine
145–146	Caramiphen Hydrochloride
	Methandriol Diacetate
	Prazepam
	Profadol Hydrochloride
	Reboxetine Mesilate
145–146.5	Droperidol
145–147	Flecainide Acetate
	Hexobarbital
	Paraphenylenediamine
145–148	Etodolac
145–149	Bezitramide
145–150	Erythromycin Lactobionate
145–154	Azatadine Maleate
145–155	Veratrine
145–170	Moexipril Diacid Hydrochloride
145.2–146.4	Noradrenaline Hydrochloride
145.4–147.2	Pentazocine
146	Cycloguanil
146–147	Oxetacaine Hydrochloride
146–148	Atenolol
	Benserazide Hydrochloride
146–154	Mestranol
146.5–148.0	Metoclopramide
147	Papaverine
147–148	Cloricromen
	Etilefrine
	Etizolam
	Methylenedioxymethamfetamine
	Nicotinyl Tartrate
	Tofenacin Hydrochloride
147–149	Bromisoval
	Clotrimazole
	Salsalate
	Tiotixene
147–150	Cholesterol
147–152d	Adrenaline Acid Tartrate
148	Barbaloin
	Methacholine Bromide
	Tetracaine Hydrochloride
148–149	Mefruside
	Tienilic Acid
148–150	Propoxycaine Hydrochloride
	Pyrantel Tartrate
	Thialbarbital
148–151	Enalaprilat
148–152	Bromazine Hydrochloride
148.0–149.4	Haloperidol
148.5	Benazepril
149d	Distigmine Bromide
149–150	Aceclofenac
	Morazone
	Piritramide
149–151	Fentanyl Citrate
	Phenindione
149–152	Prajmalium Bitartrate
149–153	Chloramphenicol
	Estradiol Cipionate
	Fosinopril Diacid
149.1	Astemizole
149.5–152	Metenolone
150	Acetylcholine Chloride
	Heptaminol Hydrochloride
	Mifepristone
150–151	Aminosalicylic Acid
	Mepivacaine
150–153	Acemetacin
	Indinavir Sulfate
	Meprylcaine Hydrochloride
151	Aminoglutethimide
	Benzbromarone
	Salbutamol
151–152	Felbamate
	Mafenide Acetate
	Nisoldipine
151–153	Boldenone Acetate
	Ketotifen
	Nialamide
151–154	Ethyl Gallate
	Mafenide
151–155	Metharbital
152	Betahistine Hydrochloride
	Hyoscyamine Hydrobromide
	Isometheptene Mucate
152–153	Dehydroepiandrosterone
	Diethylthiambutene Hydrochloride
	Ibogaine
	Methylenedioxymethamfetamine
	Nemonapride
152–154	Hydroxyephedrine
	Lofepramine Hydrochloride
	Naproxen
	Pyridostigmine Bromide
152–157	Testosterone
152–158	Anisindione
153	Phenyl Aminosalicylate
	Trichlorophenoxyacetic Acid
153–154	Indinavir
153–155	Cabergoline Diphosphate
153–155d	Bufexamac
153–156	Entacapone
	Procaine Hydrochloride
154	Dehydroepiandrosterone sodium sulfate
	Fenbutrazate Hydrochloride
	Gestrinone
	Thebacon
154–155	Chlorhexidine Acetate
	Imolamine Hydrochloride
	Pargyline Hydrochloride
	Poldine Metilsulfate
154–156	Codeine
154–157	Cytisine
	Ethyl Biscoumacetate
154–160	Adrafinil
155	Isoprenaline
	Oxybuprocaine Hydrochloride
	Pralidoxime Mesilate
	Stanozolol
155–156	Indeloxazine Hydrochloride
155–156d	Cycloserine
155–157	Nealbarbital
155–157d	Tolmetin
155–161	Desoxycortone Acetate
155–162	Indometacin
>155d	Ceftriaxone Sodium
156	Amobarbital Sodium
	Norandrostenedione
	Omeprazole
156–157	Ketobemidone
	Moracizine
	Orphenadrine Hydrochloride
156–158	Amobarbital
	Diclofenac
156–163	Suxamethonium Chloride
157	Feprazone
	Warfarin
157d	Dihydromorphine
157–159	Celecoxib
158	Amodiaquine Hydrochloride
	Androstenedione
	Diprophylline
	Isoproturon
	Mafenide Propionate
	Mescaline Acid Sulfate
	Nitrendipine
	Suxethonium Bromide
158–159	Diuron
158–160	Amosulalol Monohydrochloride
	Lynestrenol
	Metronidazole
	Midazolam
	Thioridazine Hydrochloride
158–165	Dextropropoxyphene Napsilate
	Ethionamide
	Levopropoxyphene Napsilate
159	Aminotriazole
	Benzene Hexachloride
	Phenazocine
	Salicylic Acid
159–160	Carbocromen Hydrochloride
	Metindizate Hydrochloride
	Propantheline Bromide
	Thenium Closilate
	Warfarin
159–161	Amidefrine
	Dimetindene Maleate
	Lidoflazine
159–163	Alimemazine Tartrate
159.2–160.7	Atorvastatin Lactone
160	Amifostine
	Benzydamine Hydrochloride

°C	*Compound*
	Cefalothin
	Cilostazol
	Pempidine Tartrate
	Phenindamine Tartrate
160–161	Azacyclonol
	Ketorolac
	Metenolone
	Pipazetate Hydrochloride
	Propiomazine Maleate
160–162	Lamivudine
	Mitozantrone
	Toremifene Citrate
160–163	Didanosine
	Vinbarbital
	Zonisamide
160–165	Benzethonium Chloride
160–180	Sertraline Hydrochloride
160–190	Amantadine
161	Amiodarone Hydrochloride
	Dofetilide
161–162	Butaperazine Phosphate
161–163d	Dimethoxanate Hydrochloride
161–166	Etofylline
161–167	Hexachlorophene
161–169	Rocuronium Bromide
162	Ergometrine
	Methapyrilene Hydrochloride
162–163	Pholedrine
	Voglibose
162–165	Hexoprenaline
162–165d	Rolitetracycline
162–166	Cyclomethycaine Sulfate
	Gabapentin
	Zonisamide
162–167d	Demecarium Bromide
162–168	Isoetarine Mesilate
	Methyltestosterone
163	Atropine Methonitrate
	Candesartan Cilexetil
	Norethisterone Acetate
163–164	Clorprenaline Hydrochloride
	Famotidine
	Propranolol Hydrochloride
	Torasemide
163–164d	Amiphenazole
163–165	Spiraprilat
163–167	Methandienone
163–169	Dextropropoxyphene Hydrochloride
164	Aldosterone
	Bunitrolol Hydrochloride
164d	Econazole Nitrate
164–165	Guanoxan
	Tolrestat
	Tyramine
164–166	Boldenone
	Dicycloverine Hydrochloride
	Modafinil
164–167	Dipyridamole
	Xylazine Hydrochloride
164–168	Phenelzine Sulfate
165	Betamethasone Acetate
	Norandrostenedione
	Sulfanilamide
165d	Acetophenazine Dimaleate
165–166	Rotenone
	Stavudine
165–167	Gabapentin
	Leflunomide
165–168	Antazoline Mesilate
	Dimethyltryptamine Hydrochloride
	Secbutabarbital
	Tricyclamol Chloride
165–169	Procainamide Hydrochloride
165–170d	Edrophonium Chloride
	Isoprenaline Hydrochloride
165–171	Alfaxalone
166	Benaprizine Hydrochloride
	Lansoprazole
	Sertindole
166–168	Lorazepam
	Mannitol
	Quinaprilat (Diacid of quinapril)
166–170	Denatonium Benzoate
	Diphenhydramine Hydrochloride
	Phenazocine Hydrobromide
166–170d	Aminopromazine Fumarate
166.2	Itraconazole
167	Benziodarone
	Clemizole
	Serotonin Hydrochloride
	Sulfamethoxazole
167–168	Prilocaine Hydrochloride
167–169	Piperocaine Hydrochloride
167–170	Alfadolone
	Morantel Tartrate
167–171	Dydrogesterone
167.5–168	Indinavir
168	Naphazoline Nitrate
168d	Diethylpropion Hydrochloride
	Phenindamine Tartrate
168–169	Brallobarbital
	Chlortetracycline
	Xamoterol
168–170	Isradipine
	Naltrexone
	Rafoxanide
168–172	Fenfluramine Hydrochloride
	Phenglutarimide Hydrochloride
169	Hydroquinidine
169–170	Bunamidine Hydroxynaphthoate
	Glafenine
	Indeloxazine Hydrochloride
	Ketorolac Trometamol
169–171	Arecoline Hydrobromide
	Protriptyline Hydrochloride
169–172	Diethylstilbestrol
169.0–170.5	Paracetamol
169.0–171.2	Hydrocortisone Sodium Succinate
169.5–170	Tandospirone Citrate
170	Flunitrazepam
	Risperidone
	Thenyldiamine Hydrochloride
170d	Cloxacillin Sodium
170–171	Bephenium Hydroxynaphthoate
	Hydroquinone
	Metopimazine
	Naratriptan
	Reboxetine
170–171.8	Benperidol
170–172	Thenalidine Tartrate
170–173	Hydrocortisone Hydrogen Succinate
	Methacholine Chloride
170–174	Hexobendine Hydrochloride
	Isoniazid
170–175	Metamfetamine Hydrochloride
170–178	Triflupromazine Hydrochloride
170–179d	Betamethasone Dipropionate
>170d	Amphotericin B
171	Bacampicillin Hydrochloride
	Tramazoline Hydrochloride
171d	Methoserpidine
171–172	Trometamol
171–172d	Morazone Hydrochloride
171–173	Pindolol
171–174	Atrazine
	Cyclobarbital
171–176d	Neostigmine Bromide
171–177	Methanthelinium Bromide
172	Altretamine
	Chloropyramine Hydrochloride
	Dipyrone
	Hydroquinine
	Metomidate Hydrochloride
172d	Methylergometrine
172–173	Hydralazine
	Quetiapine Hemifumarate
172–174	Glibenclamide
	Idarubicin Hydrochloride
	Nifedipine
172–175	Mexazolam
172–176	Coumatetralyl
172–180	Oxymetholone
172–184	Potassium Hydroxyquinoline Sulfate
173	Allobarbital
	Diamorphine
	Remoxipride Hydrochloride
	Santonin
173–174	Camazepam
173–174d	Pilocarpine Nitrate
173–176	Psilocin
	Thonzylamine Hydrochloride
173–179	Estradiol
174	Carbarsone
	Etamiphylline Camsilate
	Heptabarb
	Ketorolac Trometamol
	Phenylephrine
	Stavudine
	Tolazoline Hydrochloride
174–175	Imipramine Hydrochloride
	Isotretinoin
	Lacidipine
	Normethadone Hydrochloride
	Phentolamine
	Quinidine
174–175.5	Clenbuterol Hydrochloride
174–177	Buformin Hydrochloride
	Levallorphan Tartrate
174–178	Phenobarbital
174–179	Pseudoephedrine Sulfate
174–184	Noretynodrel
174.5	Lovastatin
175	Dichlorophen
	Diloxanide
	Dimetotiazine Mesilate
	Phenobarbital Sodium
175d	Penicillamine Hydrochloride
175–176	Amoxapine
	Dyclonine Hydrochloride
175–177	Alfadolone Acetate
	Nefazodone Hydrochloride
175–178	Astemizole
	Hydroxyquinoline Sulfate
	Phenformin Hydrochloride
175–179	Floctafenine
	Syrosingopine
175–181	Dapsone
175–184	Iproniazid Phosphate
175.0–176.5	Quinidine Gluconate
175.5–176	Flupirtine Maleate
176	Fenticlor
	Methylphenobarbital
	Narceine
	Sulfadimidine
	Sulfametopyrazine
176d	Noscapine
	Troleandomycin
176–177	Dieldrin

°C	Compound
	Metaraminol Tartrate
	Methcathinone Hydrochloride
176–177d	Phenglutarimide Hydrochloride
176–178	Chloroprocaine Hydrochloride
176–181	Dithranol
176–185d	Carfenazine Maleate
177–178	Clemastine Fumarate
	Methoxymetamfetamine
177–179	Ibomal
	Terbutylazine
177–180	Naloxone
177–180d	Melphalan
177–181	Benactyzine Hydrochloride
	Dinitolmide
	Phentolamine Mesilate
177–182	Ethyl Biscoumacetate
178	Brucine
	Gelsemine
	Gliquidone
	Trifluomeprazine Maleate
	Zopiclone
178d	Mesoridazine
178–179	Amlodipine Maleate
	Pyrantel
178–179d	Clioquinol
	Zomepirac
178–180	Lobeline Hydrochloride
	Rizatriptan Benzoate
	Sulpiride
178–181	Benorilate
178.5–179.5	Ondansetron Hydrochloride Dihydrate
179	Camphor
179–180	Phenprocoumon
	Pipenzolate Bromide
179–180d	Chlorpromazine Hydrochloride
	Chlorpromazine Hydrochloride
179–181	Nomifensine
179–182	Androstenediol
	Fluoxetine Oxalate
	Nitroxoline
179–183	Sulfaphenazole
180	Fenbufen
	Labetalol Hydrochloride
	Milnacipran Hydrochloride
	Pentamidine Isetionate
	Tianeptine Sodium
	Xantinol Nicotinate
180d	Dihydralazine
	Ergotamine Tartrate
	Quinidine Polygalacturonate
180–181	Cathine Hydrochloride
	Irbesartan
	Molindone
	Pecazine Hydrochloride
	Tramadol Hydrochloride
180–182	Clobazam
	Levallorphan
	Sultiame
180–183	Tertatolol
	Tertatolol Hydrochloride
180–184	Dextromoramide
	Raltitrexed Monohydrate
180–185	Nalmefene Hydrochloride
180–192	Amantadine
>180d	Oxytetracycline Hydrochloride
181	Androstanolone
	Gliclazide
	Mescaline Hydrochloride
	Phenazocine
181d	Promazine Hydrochloride
181–182	Norpipanone Hydrochloride
181–183	Letrozole
	Oxymetazoline
	Pramocaine Hydrochloride
182	Methcathinone
	Miconazole Nitrate
	Phenmetrazine
182–183	Proxymetacaine Hydrochloride
	Sulfamethoxypyridazine
182–184	Alphachloralose
	Ethinylestradiol
	Heteronium Bromide
	Hexylcaine Hydrochloride
	Sulfacetamide
	Tolpropamine Hydrochloride
182–185	Sulindac
182–186	Etisazole Hydrochloride
182–187	Acetohexamide
182–189	Methotrexate
182.5–183.5	Pseudoephedrine Hydrochloride
182.5–184.0	Metoclopramide Hydrochloride
183	Clozapine
	Eflornithine Hydrochloride
	Eflornithine Hydrochloride Monohydrate
183–184	Etafedrine Hydrochloride
	Tacrine
183–185	Candesartan
	Idarubicin Hydrochloride
	Sirolimus
183–186	Bezafibrate
	Eucatropine Hydrochloride
	Mescaline Sulfate Dihydrate
	Trenbolone
183–187	Meptazinol Hydrochloride
183–188d	Rifampicin
183.5–184.5	Losartan
184	Clopidogrel Bisulfate
184–185	Oxedrine
184–186	Biriperone
	Diethazine Hydrochloride
	Dobutamine Hydrochloride
	Doxepin Hydrochloride
	Succinylsulfathiazole
	Troglitazone
184–190	Methdilazine Hydrochloride
185	Androsterone
	Norcodeine
	Phenothiazine
185d	Epirubicin Hydrochloride
185–186	Bamifylline Hydrochloride
	Rotenone
	Viloxazine Hydrochloride
185–186d	Pizotifen Malate
185–187	Physostigmine Salicylate
185–188	Hexestrol
185–192	Choline Theophyllinate
185–195d	Methylergometrine Maleate
	Psilocybine
186	4-Aminophenol
	Butriptyline Hydrochloride
	Citalopram Hydrobromide
	Sulfaethidole
186–187	Propyliodone
186–187d	Acetyl Sulfamethoxypyridazine
186–188	Nifuratel
186–189	Aminobenzoic Acid
	Pethidine
186–190	Dihydrocodeine Tartrate
187	Fluocortolone Pivalate
187–189	Sildenafil
187.5–190	Fluspirilene
188d	Profenamine Hibenzate
188–189	Doxepin Hydrochloride
188–190	Clostebol
	Nafarelin Monoacetate
	Nalmefene
	Trimethobenzamide Hydrochloride
188–190d	Daunorubicin Hydrochloride
	Oxedrine Tartrate
	Thiethylperazine Maleate
188–190.5	Fluocortolone
188–191	Perhexiline Maleate
188–192	Barbital
189	Moracizine Hydrochloride
	Moxonidine Hydrochloride
	Racephedrine Hydrochloride
189–189.5	DOM Hydrochloride
189–190	Benoxaprofen
189–191	Noxiptiline Hydrochloride
	Pyrazinamide
189–192	Hydroxyamfetamine Hydrobromide
189–192d	Dextromoramide Tartrate
189–193	Carbamazepine
189–195	Ethoxzolamide
190	4-Aminophenol
	Barbital Sodium
	Homatropine Methylbromide
	Oxyphenonium Bromide
	Piperazine Citrate
190d	Atropine Sulfate
	Betamethasone Valerate
	Ergotoxine
	Levomepromazine Maleate
	Ouabain
190–191	Clofedanol Hydrochloride
	Pentachlorophenol
190–192	Diprenorphine
	Phenacaine Hydrochloride Monohydrate
	Sulfapyridine
190–192d	Ascorbic Acid
190–193	Acecainide Hydrochloride
	Sulfaguanidine Monohydrate
190–194	Chlorzoxazone
	Phenylpropanolamine Hydrochloride
	Sulfadoxine
190–198	Estradiol Benzoate
	Norbormide
190–220	Flurazepam Hydrochloride
191–193	Bicalutamide
191–194	Sulfafurazole
191–197	Dexrazoxane
191.5–193	Fluquinconazole
192	Clomipramine Hydrochloride
	Fencamfamin Hydrochloride
	Tiagabine Hydrochloride
192d	Ketotifen Fumarate
192–193	Atropine Oxide Hydrochloride
	Dihydrocodeine Tartrate
	Narceine Hydrochloride
	Norpipanone Hydrobromide
	Tripelennamine Hydrochloride
192–194	Etebenecid
	Spirapril Hydrochloride
192–194d	Ambazone
192–195	Glibornuride
192–196d	Bromocriptine Mesilate
193	Acetorphine
	Fusidic Acid
	Hydroxyzine Hydrochloride
	Sulfamoxole
	Thebaine
	Zimeldine Hydrochloride
193–194	Acetyl Sulfafurazole
193–195d	Ritodrine Hydrochloride
193–196	Metaclazepam Hydrochloride
193–197	Dantron

°C	*Compound*
	Zolpidem Tartrate
193–198	Glycopyrronium Bromide
194	Apronal
	Fluvastatin Sodium
194–195	Diphemanil Metilsulfate
194–196	Methysergide
	Probenecid
194–198	Antazoline Phosphate
194–199	Hyoscine Methonitrate
195	Butaperazine Maleate
	Dimetridazole Hydrochloride
	Hyoscine Hydrobromide
	Nomifensine Maleate
195d	Ajmaline
	Aminohippuric Acid
	Apomorphine
	Benzoylecgonine
	Cocaine Hydrochloride
	Halazone
195–196	Piperidolate Hydrochloride
195–197	Bethanidine
195–197d	Propicillin Potassium
195.5–197	Clobetasol Propionate
196	Broxyquinoline
	Histapyrrodine Hydrochloride
	Morinamide Hydrochloride
	Phthalylsulfacetamide
	Zolpidem
196–197	Amitriptyline Hydrochloride
	Ethomoxane Hydrochloride
196–197d	Meticillin Sodium
196–197.5d	Carbazochrome Salicylate
196–199	Acenocoumarol
196–200d	Thiamine Mononitrate
196–202	Tridihexethyl Chloride
196–206d	Co-dergocrine Mesilate
196–208d	Isoetarine Hydrochloride
197	Hordenine Sulfate
197d	Cotarnine Chloride
197–198	Ebastine Fumarate
	Hexoprenaline Hydrochloride
	Primaquine Phosphate
197–198d	Monocrotaline
197–200d	Celiprolol Hydrochloride
198	Diperodon Hydrochloride
	Hydrocodone
	Hydroxychloroquine Sulfate
	Phentermine Hydrochloride
198d	Dimoxyline Phosphate
	Ecgonine
198–199	Dextrorphan
	Levorphanol
	Mazindol
198–200	Piroxicam
198–200d	Metallibure
198–201d	Isopropamide Iodide
198–204	Mexiletine Hydrochloride
198–206	Desoxycortone Pivalate
198.5–200.3	Ethambutol Hydrochloride
199	Norharman
199–200d	Ethylnoradrenaline Hydrochloride
199–201	Ethylmorphine
199–202	Formestane
199–203	Trimethoprim
200	Ambenonium Chloride
	Ampicillin
200d	Aconitine Nitrate
	Aminonitrothiazole
	Doxycycline Hydrochloride
	Isoxsuprine Hydrochloride
	Noscapine Hydrochloride
	Strychnine Sulfate
200–202	Phenoperidine Hydrochloride
200–202d	Sodium Fluoroacetate
200–204	Amicarbalide Isetionate
200–204d	Carbachol
200–205	Naloxone Hydrochloride
200–210	Hexocyclium Metilsulfate
200–215d	Diiodohydroxyquinoline
200–220d	Betamethasone Acetate
>200d	Lymecycline
201	Trifluperidol Hydrochloride
201–202	Diphenylpyraline Hydrobromide
	Ketobemidone Hydrochloride
	Tropisetron
201–203	Flumazenil
201–204	Cyclazocine
	Sulfadimethoxine
201–204d	Amikacin
201–208	Norethisterone
201.5–202.5	Buspirone Hydrochloride
	Timolol Maleate
202	Sulfathiazole
202–203d	Liothyronine Hydrochloride
202–205d	Etidocaine Hydrochloride
202–206	Penicillamine
203	Picrotoxin
203d	Dihydroergotamine Tartrate
	Hyoscyamine Sulfate
	Pentolonium Tartrate
203–204	Benzilonium Bromide
	Rimiterol
203–205	Mitozantrone Hydrochloride
203–205d	Carbidopa
203.5–206	Formestane
204	Acetorphine Hydrochloride
	Emepronium Bromide
	Medroxyprogesterone Acetate
	Niflumic Acid
204d	Aconitine
	Aminocaproic Acid
204–205	Cefalothin Sodium
	Pilocarpine Hydrochloride
204–205d	Doxorubicin Hydrochloride
204–209	Diphenylpyraline Hydrochloride
204–209.5	Pentostatin
205	Ecgonine
	Furaltadone
	Glipizide
	Orciprenaline Sulfate
205d	Ampicillin Sodium
	Disopyramide
	Methacycline Hydrochloride
	Prednisolone Succinate
205–206	Oxazepam
205–208	Epinastine
	Fludrocortisone Acetate
	Methylprednisolone Acetate
205–210	Chloroquine Sulfate
205–212d	Pyridoxine Hydrochloride
205–213	Tenoxicam
205.5–206.5	Methandriol
206	Guanoxan Sulfate
206d	Furosemide
	Nalorphine Hydrobromide
206–207	Epithiazide
206–207d	Sotalol Hydrochloride
206–209	Pergolide
206–210d	Thiazinamium Metilsulfate
207	Baclofen
	Cinchonidine Sulfate
	Glimepiride
	Sotalol
	Tolfenamic Acid
207d	Quinidine Sulfate
207–208	Methylephedrine Hydrochloride
207–209	Amidefrine Mesilate
	Pipoxolan Hydrochloride
207–210	Eptazocine Hydrobromide
207.5–212.0	Diltiazem Hydrochloride
208	Amodiaquine
	Guanoclor Sulfate
	Moclobemide Hydrochloride
	Nalorphine
	Sulfamethizole
208–209	Daunorubicin
208–210	Albendazole
	Endosulfan
	Moxisylyte Hydrochloride
208–212	Chlormadinone Acetate
209	Buprenorphine
	Vigabatrin
209d	Ergotoxine Esilate
209–210	Bialamicol Hydrochloride
209–211	Hydroxyephedrine Hydrochloride
	Levobunolol Hydrochloride
	Oxyclozanide
209–211d	Lormetazepam
210	Bunamidine Hydrochloride
	Mesterolone
210d	Chlortetracycline Hydrochloride
	Cinchonidine
	Opipramol Hydrochloride
210–212	Clofazimine
210–214	Levosimendan
210–215	Pyrvinium Embonate
211	Bethanechol Chloride
	Coniine Hydrobromide
211–215d	Azapetine Phosphate
211–216	Vinblastine
212	Diflunisal
	Indoprofen
	Temozolomide
212d	Adrenaline
	Beclometasone Dipropionate
	Hydrastinine Hydrochloride
	Isothipendyl Hydrochloride
212–213	Cytarabine
212–214	Brotizolam
	Lachesine Chloride
212–214d	Ergotamine
212–216	Methoxamine Hydrochloride
	Phenacemide
212–218d	Methylpiperidyl Benzilate Hydrochloride
213	Methazolamide
	Propazine
213d	Chlordiazepoxide Hydrochloride
	Dimefline Hydrochloride
213–215	Nortriptyline Hydrochloride
213–216	Cinchophen
213–218	Topotecan Hydrochloride
214d	Hexoprenaline Sulfate
	Polythiazide
	Tetracycline
214–215	Flupirtine Hydrochloride
	Loprazolam
214–216	Imidapril Monohydrochloride
	Sulfametoxydiazine
214–216d	Cyproheptadine Hydrochloride
214–217	Etorphine
214–217d	Benzylpenicillin Potassium
	Homatropine Hydrobromide
214–218	Phencyclidine Hydrobromide
	Pimozide
214–221d	Difenidol Hydrochloride
214–225d	Nifursol
215	Fazadinium Bromide
	Levacetylmethadol Hydrochloride
	Pancuronium Bromide
215d	Cinchonine Hydrochloride
215–216	Clioxanide

°C	Compound
	Desipramine Hydrochloride
	Oxcarbazepine
215–217	Butorphanol
	Trimetrexate
	Venlafaxine Hydrochloride
	Zalcitabine
215–217d	Mephentermine Sulfate
215–218d	Bromocriptine
215–219	Cyclobenzaprine Hydrochloride
216	Methyclothiazide
	Metixene Hydrochloride
216–217	Fenpiprane Hydrochloride
	Nordazepam
216–217d	Paclitaxel
216–218	Lamotrigine
216–219	Atovaquone
216.5–218d	Noradrenaline
217	Megestrol Acetate
	Mizolastine
217d	Diminazene Aceturate
217–219	Moxonidine
217–219d	Butorphanol Tartrate
217–220	Clarithromycin (chloroform and diisopropyl ether)
	Ephedrine Hydrochloride
217–221	Acetyldigitoxin
217–224	Griseofulvin
217–224d	Cortisone
	Meclozine Hydrochloride
217–225	Cyclothiazide
218	Cantharidin
218d	Sodium Ascorbate
218–219d	Solanidine
218–220	Alphaprodine Hydrochloride
	Oxycodone
	Vincristine
218–221	Dosulepin Hydrochloride
218–225	Cefixime Trihydrate
218–237	Gentamicin Sulfate
219–220	Cloricromen Hydrochloride
	Trimethoxyamfetamine
219–221	Propylthiouracil
219.3	Fasudil Hydrochloride
220	Alcuronium Chloride (brown colour)
	Amygdalin
	Cladribine
	Deslanoside
	Doxapram Hydrochloride
220d	Bendroflumethiazide
	Betamethasone Benzoate
	Chlortalidone
	Hydrocortisone Acetate
	Rimiterol Hydrobromide
220–225	Papaverine
	Pentostatin
220.5–222	Diphenoxylate Hydrochloride
221	Chlorprothixene Hydrochloride
221–223	Lofexidine Hydrochloride
	Tizanidine
221–226	Glymidine Sodium
222	Acrivastine
222d	Carbazochrome
222–223	Atropine Methobromide
	Hydroxyprogesterone
	Irinotecan
222–225	Clarithromycin (ethanol)
223	Trazodone Hydrochloride
223–225	Tirofiban
223–225d	Profenamine Hydrochloride
223–226	Buphenine Hydrochloride
223–226d	Procarbazine Hydrochloride
223–229d	Thiopropazate Hydrochloride
224	Donepezil Hydrochloride
224–226	Methylphenidate Hydrochloride
	Nitrazepam
224.4–226.8d	Danazol
225	Alfuzosin Hydrochloride
	Cetirizine Dihydrochloride
	Metformin Hydrochloride
	Pergolide Mesilate
	Suxamethonium Bromide
225d	Dexamethasone Acetate
	Hyoscine Methobromide
	Loperamide Hydrochloride
	Minoxidil
	Obidoxime Chloride
	α-Acetyldigoxin
225–226d	Pralidoxime Iodide
225–227	Levofloxacin
	Levofloxacin Hemihydrate
225–227d	Parbendazole
225–228	Trimetazidine Hydrochloride
225–230	Niclosamide
225–230d	Thioacetazone
225–236d	Apomorphine Hydrochloride
226	Dibrompropamidine Isetionate
	Ethacridine
	Phenylmethylbarbituric Acid
226–227	Chlorcyclizine Hydrochloride
	Simazine
226–227d	Procyclidine Hydrochloride
226–228	Delavirdine
	Fludrocortisone Acetate
	Flunixin
226–230	Amineptine Hydrochloride
226–232d	Prednisone Acetate
227	Metolazone
	Thioproperazine Mesilate
227d	Aztreonam
227–228d	Carbazochrome Sodium Sulfonate
227–229	Fenetylline Hydrochloride
	Tandospirone Citrate
227–231	Metildigoxin
	Metildigoxin
227–234	Dienestrol
228	Azapropazone
	Prochlorperazine Maleate
228–228.5	Alprazolam
228–229d	Ambutonium Bromide
	Mepenzolate Bromide
228–230	Acitretin
	Clostebol Acetate
	Saccharin
	Tamsulosin Hydrochloride
228–237	Methylprednisolone
228–241d	Paramethasone Acetate
229–230	Nalidixic Acid
229–231	Doxorubicin
229–233	Diamorphine Hydrochloride
230	Bumetanide
	Fluphenazine Hydrochloride
	Trioxysalen
230d	Betaine Hydrochloride
	Fenoterol Hydrobromide
230–231	Mefenamic Acid
230–232	Indoramin Hydrochloride
	Maprotiline Hydrochloride
	Vindesine
230–232d	Pheneticillin Potassium
	Promethazine Hydrochloride
230–234d	Deserpidine
230–236	Flavoxate Hydrochloride
230–240	Buclizine Hydrochloride
	Flupentixol Hydrochloride
231	Nalbuphine
231–232	Benzthiazide
	Ondansetron
	Oxyphencyclimine Hydrochloride
231–234	Cycloguanil Embonate
232	Docetaxel
232–233	Salinazid
232–235d	Droxidopa
232–247	Cetrimide
233	Diaveridine
233d	Dihydralazine Sulfate
	Fenbendazole
233–234	Bupropion Hydrochloride
	Fludrocortisone Acetate
	Pyrimethamine
233–235	Dexamethasone Sodium Phosphate
	Phencyclidine Hydrochloride
	Triazolam
233–235d	Alendronic Acid
	Prednisone
233–236	Prednisolone Pivalate
234	Chlorphentermine Hydrochloride
	Clonixin
	Yohimbine
234d	Adenosine
234–235	Colfosceril Palmitate
	Tigloidine Hydrobromide
234–236	Quinagolide Hydrochloride
234–237	Nicotinic Acid
234–238d	Sulfamerazine
234–239	Caffeine Hydrate
235	Aminoacridine Hydrochloride
	Bromhexine Hydrochloride
	Hydroxystilbamidine
	Methadone Hydrochloride
	Propamidine Isetionate
	Stanozolol
235d	Cyclopenthiazide
	Gallamine Triethiodide
	Phenazopyridine Hydrochloride
235–236d	Levothyroxine
235–238	Oxandrolone
235–238d	Cortisone Acetate
	Pralidoxime Chloride
235–255d	Emetine Hydrochloride
236	Amiphenazole Hydrochloride
236–236.5	Chlordiazepoxide
236–237d	Liothyronine
236–240d	Nitrofurazone
236–251	Etoposide
236.5–238.5	Clonazepam
237d	Quinuronium Sulfate
237–238.5d	Bromazepam
237–239	Naratriptan Hydrochloride
237–239d	Prednisolone Acetate
237–241	Antazoline Hydrochloride
238	Biperiden Hydrochloride
	Caffeine
	Dibenzepin Hydrochloride
	Harman
238d	Azathioprine
238–239	Rescinnamine
238–240	Cambendazole
238–242	Nefopam Hydrochloride
239	Dihydroergotamine
239–240	Phentolamine Hydrochloride
239–241	Fendosal
	Imidaprilat
	Morantel
240	Ametazole Hydrochloride
	Diclofenamide
	Hydroxychloroquine Sulfate
	Olsalazine Sodium
	Venlafaxine Hydrochloride
240d	Acetarsone
	Betamethasone

°C	Compound
	Digoxin
	Lysergic Acid
240–241d	Prednisolone
240–242	Amiloride
	Pyrimethamine
240–243	Diamthazole Hydrochloride
240–245d	Sulfasalazine
>240d	Lanatoside C
241	Aminoacridine
241d	Dopamine Hydrochloride
	Mannomustine
241–242d	Sodium Cromoglicate
241.5–243d	Dactinomycin
242	Clidinium Bromide
	Decoquinate
	Oxyphenisatine Acetate
	Prochlorperazine Mesilate
242d	Cycrimine Hydrochloride
	Lysergamide
242–243	Trifluoperazine Hydrochloride
242–245	Fluocortolone Hexanoate
242–245d	Loprazolam Mesilate
243	Sulfisomidine
243d	Triphenyltetrazolium Chloride
243–244	Proguanil Hydrochloride
243–245	Suxamethonium Iodide
243–250	Ropinirole
244–246	Naproxen Sodium
245d	Endrin
	Ephedrine Sulfate
	Ethacridine Lactate
	Fluclorolone Acetonide
	Histamine Hydrochloride
	Homidium Bromide
	Mecamylamine Hydrochloride
	Tocainide Hydrochloride
	Trimetaphan Camsilate
246	Clemizole Hydrochloride
	Clopamide
	Ecgonine Hydrochloride
246–247	Chlorproguanil Hydrochloride
	Galantamine Hydrobromide
246–248	Capreomycin
	Terbutaline Sulfate
247d	Amprolium Hydrochloride
247–248	Azapropazone
247–248d	Sulfaquinoxaline
247–249	Nevirapine
247–255	Fludroxycortide
248	Tryptamine Hydrochloride
248d	Barbituric Acid
	Metisazone
	Thiamine Hydrochloride
248–249d	Oxymorphone
248–250	Meclofenamic Acid
248–250d	Mepacrine Hydrochloride
248–253d	Pirenzepine Hydrochloride
249–250	Reproterol Hydrochloride
249–250d	Harmaline
249–251	Clodronic Acid
249–251d	Pyrvinium Chloride
250d	Ganciclovir
	Guanethidine Monosulfate
	Morphine Sulfate
250–252	Dexamethasone Isonicotinate
	Quinethazone
250–257	Ofloxacin
>250	Cefixime Disodium Salt
251	Salinazid
251–253	Racemorphan
252–254	Finasteride
253	Disodium Tiludronate
253–255	Capreomycin
254	Meloxicam

°C	Compound
254–256	Bufylline
	Tamsulosin
254–256d	Morphine
254.3–254.9	Inositol Nicotinate
255d	Aciclovir
	Sulfadiazine
255–256	Triclocarban
255–256.5	Deflazacort
255–257	Levobupivacaine Hydrochloride
255–257d	Ciprofloxacin
255–258d	Enoximone
255–260	Naphazoline Hydrochloride
255–265	Methaqualone Hydrochloride
255–265d	Dihydrostreptomycin Sulfate
256	Digitoxin
256–257	Galantamine Hydrochloride
	Piperazine Adipate
256–257d	Pemoline
	Tetryzoline Hydrochloride
256–262d	Protoveratrines A and B
256.5	Irinotecan Hydrochloride Trihydrate
257	Finasteride
257d	Clopenthixol Hydrochloride
257–259	Meclofenamic Acid
257–267d	Metocurine Iodide
258–260d	Pergolide Mesilate
258–262	Phenolphthalein
258–270d	Trilostane
258.5	Bupivacaine Hydrochloride
258.5d	Trihexyphenidyl Hydrochloride
259d	Furazolidone
260	Acefylline Piperazine
	Disulfamide
	Fludarabine
	Fludrocortisone
	Mafenide Hydrochloride
	Teicoplanin
260d	Acetazolamide
	Cidofovir
	Estrone
	Mebezonium Iodide
	Xipamide
260–262	Ropivacaine Hydrocloride
260–262d	Chlorhexidine Hydrochloride
260–263	Nalorphine Hydrochloride
260–264	Niridazole
261d	Harmine
261–263	Telmisartan
261–263d	Pizotifen
262–263	Ketamine Hydrochloride
262–264	Mepivacaine Hydrochloride
263	Lorcainide Hydrochloride
	Methenamine (sublimes)
264	Cinchonine
264d	Prazosin Hydrochloride
264–265	Tetramisole Hydrochloride
264–265d	Aminitrozole
	Halcinonide
	Reserpine
265d	Decamethonium Bromide
266–267	Etorphine Hydrochloride
	Hydromorphone
266–268	Clorexolone
266–269	Flugestone Acetate
267–269d	Protoveratrine A
268–270d	Protoveratrine A
268–271d	Dexamethasone
269	Tyramine Hydrochloride
269–270	Ethiazide
269–271	Thalidomide
	Triamcinolone
269.5–270.6	Ropivacaine Hydrocloride Monohydrate

°C	Compound
270	Acamprosate Calcium
	Exifone
270d	Anileridine Hydrochloride
	Cisplatin
	Fluocinolone Acetonide
	Fluoxymesterone
	Potassium Sorbate
	Trichlormethiazide
	Tubocurarine Chloride
270–272d	Oxycodone Hydrochloride
270–274	Theophylline
270–281	Azacyclonol Hydrochloride
271	Clospipramine Dihydrochloride
	Nitrofurantoin
271–273	Deferiprone
271–274	Terazosin Hydrochloride Dihydrate
272	Theophylline Hydrate
272–273	Fluticasone Propionate
	Hydroflumethiazide
272–274	Terazosin
272–275	Penciclovir
272–276	Ethisterone
272–277d	Phthalylsulfathiazole
273	Bunazosin Hydrochloride
273d	Hydralazine Hydrochloride
273–274	Hydroquinidine Hydrochloride
273–275	Epinastine Hydrochloride
	Hydrochlorothiazide
273–277	Normorphine
274	Fenoldopam Mesilate
274d	Debrisoquine Sulfate
274–276	Hexamethonium Bromide
	Naltrexone Hydrochloride
275	Arsenic Trioxide
275d	Levodopa
275–277	Penciclovir
275–285	Strychnine
276	Hydroxyprogesterone
277	Fenoldopam Hydrobromide
	Vincristine Sulfate
278	Carteolol Hydrochloride
	Dolasetron Mesilate
278–279	Terazosin Hydrochloride
278–280	Prazosin
278–282d	Riboflavin
279–280	Dantrolene
280	Bethanidine Sulfate
	Estriol
280d	Codeine Hydrochloride
	Dequalinium Acetate
	Fluorometholone
	Mebhydrolin Napadisilate
>280	Anagrelide Hydrochloride
281–282	Primidone
282	Stilbazium Iodide
282d	Fluorouracil
282–284	Mianserin Hydrochloride
283d	Neopine Hydrobromide
283–284	Tacrine Hydrochloride
283–285	Diclofenac
	Tropisetron Hydrochloride
284–286	Epinastine Hydrobromide
285d	Cyclizine Hydrochloride
	Solanine
285–288d	Amiloride Hydrochloride
286	Hydroxystilbamidine Isetionate
287–288	Methyl Benzoquate
287–292	Gemcitabine Hydrochloride
287–293	Dicoumarol
289–290	Doxazosin Hydrochloride
289–291	Meclofenamate Sodium
289–292	5-Methyltryptamine Hydrochloride

°C	Compound
290	Mebendazole
290–292	Granisetron Hydrochloride
291–294	Carbenoxolone
292–294	Triamcinolone Acetonide
295d	Phanquinone
295–296	Zomepirac Sodium
295–296d	Triamcinolone Hexacetonide
295–297d	Flucytosine
295–298	Phenytoin
296	Enoxolone
296–301	Pramipexole Dihydrochloride Monohydrate
298–300	Nedocromil
299–300d	Ibogaine Hydrochloride
300d	Allopurinol
	Fluocinonide
	Rifamycin SV
300–303d	Oxymetazoline Hydrochloride
300–305	Tiabendazole
>300	Dexamfetamine Sulfate
	Milrinone
>300d	Amfetamine Sulfate
	Xylometazoline Hydrochloride
302d	Yohimbine Hydrochloride
305	Clonidine Hydrochloride
305–315d	Hydromorphone Hydrochloride
308–309	Pipradrol Hydrochloride
>308d	Mercaptopurine
309d	Norcodeine Hydrochloride
310	Methyldopa
310d	Betaine
313	Arsenic Trioxide
315d	Dequalinium Chloride
316	Triamterene
318–320	Ciprofloxacin Hydrochloride
320–322	Benzoctamine Hydrochloride
320–323d	Pholedrine Sulfate
>320	Clopidol
326–331d	Methylthiouracil
327d	Pseudomorphine
329	Octatropine Methylbromide
330–331	Diazoxide
335	Diquat Dibromide
340d	Chlorothiazide
	Conessine Hydrobromide
>350	Alcuronium Chloride (incompletely melted)
360d	Amantadine Hydrochloride
>360	Tioguanine
373–375	Rimantadine Hydrochloride
440	Sodium Salicylate
720	Lithium Carbonate

Colour Tests

The following table was extracted from a collection of data kindly provided by Professor George Maylin, Cornell University, USA, and gives compound-specific colour reactions from a series of spray reagents applied to thin-layer chromatography systems TA, TE, TAJ, TAK, TAL and TAM.

Name	D	N	C-H	M	FES	NIN	Gibb's	H+:EtOH	ME	F	I_2
Acepromazine	orange	brown	brown	pink	pink	no rxn	–	–	–	–	–
Acetylaminobenzoic acid, 4-	no rxn	no rxn	no rxn	yellow fl	–	no rxn	–	–	red	–	wk brown
Adenylic acid, 5-	–	–	–	–	no rxn	no rxn	–	–	no rxn	no rxn	no rxn
Alphaprodine	orange	brown	brown	–	–	–	–	–	–	–	brown
Alphaprodine *N*-oxide	orange	brown	brown	–	–	–	–	–	–	–	brown
Ambroxol	wk orange	brown	brown	yellow	no rxn	pink	–	–	red	–	brown
Amcinonide	–	–	–	–	–	–	–	wk yellow	–	–	–
Amfenac	–	–	–	yellow	–	–	–	–	–	–	–
Amfetamine	wk orange	brown	brown	no rxn	no rxn	pink	–	–	–	–	–
Aminocaproic acid	–	–	–	–	–	pink	–	–	–	–	–
Aminopropiophenone, 2-	wk orange	brown	brown	–	–	pink	–	–	–	–	–
Amitriptyline	–	brown	–	–	–	–	–	–	–	–	–
Ampyrone	orange	brown	brown	–	–	wk pink	–	–	red	–	brown
Amrinone	no rxn	brown	brown	no rxn	–	no rxn	–	–	red	blue	–
Anileridine	orange	brown	brown	–	–	–	–	–	–	–	brown
Apomorphine	wk orange	brown	brown	–	–	–	–	–	–	–	green
Aspirin	–	–	–	green	–	–	–	–	–	–	–
Atropine	orange	brown	brown	–	–	–	–	–	–	–	–
Azaperol	–	brown	brown	–	–	–	–	–	–	–	–
Azaperone	–	brown	brown	–	–	–	–	–	–	–	–
Benoxaprofen	no rxn	brown	brown	fluoresce	fluoresce	no rxn	–	fluoresces	no rxn	no rxn	–
Benzoic acid	–	–	–	white	–	–	–	–	–	–	–
Benzoylecgonine	orange	brown	brown	–	–	–	–	–	–	–	brown
Benzthiazide	no rxn	wk brown	wk brown	yellow fl	brown	no rxn	no rxn	brown	no rxn	orange	–
Betamethasone	–	–	–	–	–	–	–	grey	–	–	–
Bolasterone	–	–	–	–	–	–	–	yellow	–	–	–
Boldenone	–	–	–	–	–	–	–	pink	–	–	–
Bromhexine	–	brown	brown	–	–	–	–	–	red	–	–
Bromhexine metabolite A	–	brown	brown	yellow	–	–	–	–	red	–	–
Bromhexine metabolite B	–	brown	brown	yellow	–	–	–	–	red	–	–
Bromhexine metabolite C	–	brown	brown	yellow	–	–	–	–	red	–	–
Bumetanide	–	–	–	–	–	–	–	–	orange	–	–
Bupivacaine	wk orange	brown	brown	no rxn	no rxn	–	–	–	–	–	brown
Bupivacaine, *p*-hydroxy	wk orange	brown	brown	no rxn	M yellow	–	–	–	–	–	brown
Buprenorphine	–	brown	brown	–	–	pink	–	–	–	–	–

Name	D	N	C-H	M	FES	NIN	Gibb's	H+:EtOH	ME	F	I_2
Buspirone	orange	brown	brown	no rxn	no rxn	no rxn	–	–	no rxn	no rxn	brown
Butorphanol	wk orange	brown	brown	–	no rxn	–	–	–	–	–	brown
Butylated hydroxytoluene	–	–	–	no rxn	–	–	–	–	–	–	–
Caffeine	no rxn	wk brown	dark brown	no rxn	no rxn	no rxn	no rxn	no rxn	no rxn	no rxn	wk brown
Chlorcyclizine	orange	brown	brown	–	–	–	–	–	–	–	–
(Chlorobenzoyl)benzoic acid, 2-(4-	–	brown	–	–	–	–	–	–	–	–	–
(Chlorophenyl)piperazine, 1-(M-	orange	brown	brown	pink	no rxn	wk pink	–	–	–	–	brown
Chloroprocaine, 2-	wk orange	brown	brown	–	–	pink	–	–	red	–	brown
Chlorothiazide	no rxn	no rxn	no rxn	no rxn	no rxn	no rxn	–	–	no rxn	orange	–
Chlorphenamine	orange	brown	brown	–	–	–	–	–	–	–	brown
Chlorphenesin	no rxn	brown	brown	purple/grey	–	–	–	–	red	–	brown
Chlorphenesin carbamate	–	–	–	grey/blue fl	–	–	–	–	–	–	–
Chlorpromazine	–	brown	–	–	pink	–	–	–	–	–	brown
Chlorpromazine metabolite	–	–	–	–	purple	–	–	–	–	–	–
Cholesterol	–	–	–	red/purple	–	–	–	grey	–	–	–
Cimetidine	wk orange	brown	brown	grey	yellow	–	–	–	grey/purple red	–	–
Clenbuterol	–	–	–	–	–	–	–	–		–	–
Cocaine	orange	brown	brown	no rxn	no rxn	no rxn	–	–	–	–	no rxn
Codeine	wk orange	brown	brown	–	M blue	–	–	–	–	–	brown
Corticosterone	–	–	–	–	–	–	–	grey	–	–	–
Cortisone	–	–	–	–	–	–	–	no rxn	–	–	–
Cyproheptadine	orange	brown	brown	red/yellow fl	M red	no rxn	–	–	–	–	–
Cyproheptadine epoxide	orange	brown	brown	red/yellow fl	M red	no rxn	–	–	–	–	–
Cyproheptadine *N*-oxide	orange	brown	brown	brown/ylw fl	M brown	no rxn	–	–	–	–	–
Deanol	no rxn	wk brown	brown	–	–	wk pink	–	–	no rxn	–	brown
Dehydronorketamine, 5,6-	wk orange	brown	brown	–	pink	–	–	–	orange	–	brown
Deoxycorticosterone acetate	–	–	–	–	–	–	–	brown/grey	–	–	–
Desipramine	–	–	–	–	blue	–	–	–	–	–	–
Desoximetasone	–	–	–	–	–	–	–	grey	–	–	–
Despropionyl fentanyl	orange	brown	brown	–	–	–	–	–	–	–	–
Detomidine	wk orange	brown	brown	no rxn	no rxn	–	–	–	–	no rxn	no rxn
Dexamethasone	–	–	–	–	–	–	–	grey	–	–	–
Diazepam	wk orange	brown	brown	–	–	–	–	–	–	–	wk brown
Diclofenac	wk orange	wk brown	wk brown	red/brown	–	–	–	–	no rxn	no rxn	–
Diethylpropion	wk orange	brown	brown	–	–	pink	–	–	–	–	–
Diflunisal	no rxn	no rxn	wk brown	no rxn	no rxn	no rxn	–	–	no rxn	no rxn	no rxn
Dihydrocodeine	wk orange	brown	brown	–	M blue	–	–	–	–	–	brown
Dihydrocodeine metabolite	wk orange	brown	brown	–	M blue	–	–	–	–	–	brown
Dimethoxycinnamic acid, 3,4-	orange	no rxn	no rxn	grey	grey	no rxn	–	–	no rxn	no rxn	–
Dipyrone	orange	brown	brown	–	–	wk pink	–	–	–	–	brown
Doxepin	wk orange	brown	brown	–	yellow	–	–	–	–	–	brown
Doxylamine	orange	brown	brown	–	–	–	–	–	–	–	–
Doxylamine base urine metabolite 1	orange	brown	brown	–	–	–	–	–	–	–	–
Doxylamine base urine metabolite 2	orange	brown	brown	–	–	–	–	–	–	–	–
Doxylamine enzyme hydrolysis metabolite	orange	brown	brown	–	–	–	–	–	–	–	–
Dyphylline	orange	no rxn	wk brown	–	–	–	–	–	–	–	wk brown
Ecgonine methyl ester	wk orange	brown	brown	no rxn	no rxn	no rxn	–	–	–	–	brown
Embutramide	orange	brown	brown	white	–	–	–	–	–	–	–
Ephedrine	wk orange	brown	brown	–	no rxn	pink	–	–	–	–	–

Name	D	N	C-H	M	FES	NIN	Gibb's	H+:EtOH	ME	F	I_2
Estradiol	–	–	–	–	–	–	–	pink	–	–	–
Estrone	–	–	–	–	–	–	–	pink	–	–	–
Etamiphylline	–	brown	–	–	–	–	–	–	–	–	brown
Ethacrynic acid	–	–	–	–	–	–	–	–	–	–	–
Ethinyl estradiol	–	–	–	–	–	–	–	pink	–	–	–
Ethyl aminobenzoate	wk orange	brown	brown	no rxn	no rxn	–	–	–	red	–	brown
Ethylaminopropiophenone, 2-	wk orange	brown	brown	–	–	pink	–	–	–	–	–
Ethylnicotinamide, *N*-	wk orange	brown	brown	–	–	–	–	–	–	–	–
Etidocaine	orange	brown	brown	–	–	–	–	–	–	–	–
Etodolac	–	–	–	blue	–	–	–	–	–	–	–
Fenfluramine	–	brown	brown	–	wk pink	–	–	–	–	–	–
Fenoprofen	–	–	–	green	–	–	–	–	–	–	–
Fludrocortisone	–	–	–	–	–	–	–	grey	–	–	–
Fludroxycortide	–	–	–	–	–	–	–	grey	–	–	–
Flumethasone	–	–	–	–	–	–	–	grey	–	–	–
Flunixin	wk orange	brown	brown	yellow fl	no rxn	–	–	–	no rxn	–	–
Fluocinolone acetonide	–	–	–	–	–	–	–	grey	–	–	–
Fluorometholone	–	–	–	–	–	–	–	grey	–	–	–
Fluoxymesterone	–	–	–	–	–	–	–	grey	–	–	–
Fluprednisolone	–	–	–	–	–	–	–	grey	–	–	–
Fructose	no rxn	no rxn	no rxn	no rxn	no rxn	no rxn	no rxn	no rxn	no rxn	no rxn	no rxn
Furosemide	no rxn	no rxn	no rxn	black	–	–	–	–	red	no rxn	–
Glycine xylidide	orange	brown	brown	–	–	–	–	–	–	–	no rxn
Glycopyrrolate	orange	brown	brown	–	–	–	–	–	–	–	–
Gramine	orange	brown	brown	blue	blue	no rxn	–	–	dk blue	–	–
Green 242	wk orange	brown	brown	green	M red	M black	–	–	no rxn	no rxn	–
Griseofulvin	orange	no rxn	no rxn	no rxn	no rxn	no rxn	–	–	no rxn	no rxn	–
Guaifenesin	wk orange	wk brown	–	blue	blue	–	–	–	–	–	–
Harmine	orange	–	–	–	–	–	–	–	–	–	–
Heptaminol	–	–	–	–	–	pink	–	–	–	–	–
Homatropine	–	brown	brown	–	–	–	–	–	–	–	–
Hordenine	orange	brown	brown	blue	M blue	–	–	–	–	–	brown
Hydrochlorothiazide	–	–	–	–	–	–	–	–	pink	red	–
Hydrocortisone	orange	wk brown	–	–	–	–	–	yellow/grey	–	–	–
Hydromorphone	wk orange	brown	–	–	–	–	–	–	–	–	brown
Hydroxy imipramine, 2-	–	–	–	–	yellow	–	–	–	–	–	brown
Hydroxyazaperol	–	brown	brown	–	–	–	–	–	–	–	–
Hydroxyazaperone	–	brown	brown	–	–	–	–	–	–	–	–
Hydroxybuspirone, 5-	orange	brown	brown	white	no rxn	no rxn	–	–	no rxn	no rxn	brown
Hydroxybutorphanol	wk orange	brown	brown	–	–	–	–	–	–	–	brown
Hydroxycyproheptadine	–	–	–	red	–	–	–	–	–	–	–
Hydroxydesipramine, 2-	–	–	–	–	yellow	–	–	–	–	–	brown
Hydroxydetomidine, 3-	wk orange	brown	brown	no rxn	no rxn	–	–	–	–	no rxn	no rxn
Hydroxydoxepin 1	wk orange	brown	brown	–	yellow	–	–	–	–	–	brown
Hydroxydoxepin 2	wk orange	brown	brown	–	yellow	–	–	–	–	–	brown
(Hydroxyethyl)promazine sulfoxide, 2-(1-	orange	brown	brown	purple	pink	no rxn	–	–	–	–	–
Hydroxylated mepivacaine	wk orange	brown	brown	–	–	–	–	–	–	–	brown
Hydroxylidocaine, 3-	wk orange	brown	brown	–	–	–	–	–	–	–	wk brown
Hydroxymeperidine, *p*-	–	brown	brown	–	grey	–	–	–	–	–	–

Name	D	N	C-H	M	FES	NIN	Gibb's	H+:EtOH	ME	F	I_2
Hydroxymethadone, P-	wk orange	brown	brown	–	M red	–	–	–	–	–	–
Hydroxynefopam, *p*-	wk orange	brown	brown	–	–	M blue	–	–	–	–	brown
Hydroxyprednisolone, 20-beta-	orange	brown	brown	–	–	–	–	grey	–	–	–
Hydroxyprednisone, 20-beta-	orange	brown	brown	–	–	–	–	grey	–	–	–
Hydroxypromazine, 3-	no rxn	no rxn	no rxn	red	purple	–	–	–	–	–	–
Hydroxypropranolol, 4-	wk orange	brown	brown	–	–	–	–	–	–	–	green
Hydroxytenoxicam, 5'-	orange	wk brown	wk brown	no rxn	no rxn	no rxn	–	–	no rxn	white	wk brown
Hydroxytrazodone	orange	brown	brown	blue	no rxn	no rxn	–	–	–	–	brown
Hydroxyzine	orange	brown	brown	–	–	–	–	–	–	–	–
Ibuprofen	–	–	–	grey/tan fl	–	–	–	–	–	–	–
Imipramine	–	–	–	–	blue	–	–	–	–	–	brown
Imipramine *N*-oxide	–	–	–	–	blue	–	–	–	–	–	–
Indapamide	orange	brown	brown	red	pink	pink	–	–	pink	pink	brown
Indometacin	–	–	–	grey	–	–	–	–	–	–	–
Ipratropium bromide	orange	brown	–	no rxn	no rxn	–	–	–	–	–	–
Isoetarine	orange	brown	brown	grey	M grey	pink	–	–	–	dk pink	brown
Isoetarine EH metabolite	orange	brown	brown	grey	M grey	pink	–	–	–	no rxn	brown
Isoxsuprine	orange	brown	brown	blue	M grey	–	–	–	–	–	brown
Ketamine	orange	brown	brown	–	–	–	–	–	–	–	brown
Ketoprofen	–	–	–	yellow/yellow fl	–	–	–	–	–	–	–
Ketorolac	–	brown	brown	–	–	–	–	–	red/grey	–	brown
Lenperone	orange	brown	–	–	–	–	–	–	–	–	–
Levallorphan	orange	brown	brown	no rxn	no rxn	–	–	–	–	–	brown
Levorphanol	wk orange	brown	brown	wk blue	no rxn	–	–	–	–	–	brown
Lidocaine	orange	brown	brown	–	–	–	–	–	–	–	wk brown
Maprotiline	orange	brown	brown	–	–	no rxn	–	–	–	–	–
Mazindol	–	brown	–	–	–	–	–	–	–	–	–
Meclofenamic acid	orange	no rxn	no rxn	black	–	pink	–	–	–	–	–
Medroxyprogesterone	–	–	–	–	–	–	–	green/grey	–	–	–
Medrysone	–	–	–	–	–	–	–	grey	–	–	–
Mefenamic acid	–	–	–	blue/green	–	–	–	–	–	–	–
Mephentermine	orange	brown	brown	–	–	wk pink	–	–	–	–	brown
Mepivacaine	orange	brown	brown	–	–	–	–	–	–	–	brown
Meprednisone	–	–	–	–	–	–	–	grey	–	–	–
Metamfetamine	orange	brown	brown	–	–	pink	–	–	–	–	brown
Metaproterenol	–	–	–	–	–	–	blue	–	–	–	–
Methadone	wk orange	brown	brown	–	M yellow	–	–	–	–	–	brown
Methandrostenolone	–	–	–	–	–	–	–	grey	–	–	–
Methapyrilene	orange	brown	brown	red	–	no rxn	–	–	–	–	brown
Methapyrilene BU metabolite	orange	brown	brown	red	–	pink	–	–	–	–	brown
Methapyrilene EH metabolite I	orange	brown	brown	no rxn	–	no rxn	–	–	–	–	brown
Methapyrilene EH metabolite III	orange	brown	brown	no rxn	–	no rxn	–	–	–	–	brown
Methocarbamol	orange	brown	brown	blue	blue	–	–	–	–	–	wk brown
Methoxamine	orange	brown	brown	–	M yellow	pink	–	–	–	–	–
Methyl-6-oxopipecolo-2',6' xylidide, 1-	wk orange	brown	brown	–	–	–	–	–	–	–	brown
Methylamino antipyrine, 4-	orange	brown	brown	–	–	wk pink	–	–	–	–	brown
Methylphenidate	orange	brown	brown	no rxn	no rxn	–	–	–	no rxn	–	brown
Methylprednisolone	–	–	–	–	–	–	–	red/grey	–	–	–
Methyltestosterone, 17-	–	–	–	–	–	–	–	grey	–	–	–

Name	D	N	C-H	M	FES	NIN	Gibb's	H+:EtOH	ME	F	I_2
Metolazone	orange	wk brown	–	–	–	–	–	–	–	–	–
Monoethylglycine xylidide	no rxn	brown	brown	–	–	–	–	–	–	–	no rxn
Morphine	wk orange	brown	brown	–	M blue	–	–	–	–	–	brown
Nabumetone	–	–	–	blue	–	–	–	–	–	–	–
Nabumetone metabolite M-I	–	–	–	blue	–	–	–	–	–	–	–
Nabumetone metabolite M-II	–	–	–	blue	–	–	–	–	–	–	–
Nabumetone metabolite M-III	–	–	–	blue	–	–	–	–	–	–	–
Nabumetone metabolite M-IV	–	–	–	blue	–	–	–	–	–	–	–
Nabumetone metabolite M-V	–	–	–	blue	–	–	–	–	–	–	–
Nalbuphine	wk orange	brown	brown	–	–	–	–	–	–	–	–
Naloxone	–	–	–	–	–	–	–	–	–	–	brown
Naproxen	–	–	–	green	–	–	–	orange	–	–	–
Nefopam	wk orange	brown	brown	–	M blue	–	–	–	–	–	brown
Niacinamide	wk orange	wk brown	wk brown	–	–	–	–	–	–	yellow	–
Nicotine	orange	brown	brown	–	–	–	–	–	–	–	–
Nikethamide	wk orange	brown	brown	–	–	–	–	–	–	–	–
Nikethamide *N*-oxide	wk orange	brown	brown	–	–	–	–	–	–	–	–
Nivazol	–	–	–	–	–	–	–	grey	–	–	–
Nordazepam	–	brown	brown	–	–	–	–	–	–	–	–
Nordoxepin	wk orange	brown	brown	–	yellow	–	–	–	–	–	brown
Norketamine	wk orange	brown	brown	–	–	–	–	–	–	–	brown
Norpseudoephedrine	wk orange	brown	brown	–	–	pink	–	–	–	–	–
Oxycodone	orange	brown	–	–	–	–	–	–	–	–	–
Oxymorphone	orange	brown	brown	–	–	–	–	–	–	–	brown
Oxyphenbutazone	wk orange	wk brown	wk brown	yellow	–	–	–	–	–	yellow	–
Paracetamol	no rxn	no rxn	wk brown	white/grey	no rxn	no rxn	–	–	–	blue	brown
Paramethasone	–	–	–	–	–	–	–	grey	–	–	–
Paroxetine	–	–	brown	–	blue/green	–	–	–	blue/green	–	brown
Pemoline	–	–	–	–	–	–	–	–	–	purple/pink	–
Pentachlorophenol	orange	no rxn	no rxn	no rxn	–	–	–	–	–	–	–
Pentazocine	orange	brown	brown	–	–	–	–	–	–	–	–
Pentoxifylline	–	brown	brown	–	–	–	–	–	–	–	–
Pentoxifylline, demethyl-	–	brown	brown	–	–	–	–	–	–	–	–
Perphenazine	orange	brown	brown	–	purple	–	–	–	–	–	brown
Pethidine	orange	brown	brown	no rxn	grey	–	–	–	–	–	brown
Pethidine *N*-oxide	orange	brown	brown	–	grey	–	–	–	–	–	–
Phenmetrazine	wk orange	wk brown	wk brown	–	–	–	–	–	–	–	wk brown
Phentermine	orange	fades	–	–	–	–	–	–	–	–	–
Phenylbutazone	wk orange	brown	brown	red	no rxn	no rxn	–	–	–	–	–
Phenylbutazone alchohol metabolite	–	–	–	wk red	–	–	–	–	–	–	–
Phenylpropanolamine	orange	brown	brown	–	–	pink	–	–	–	–	–
Piretanide	no rxn	no rxn	no rxn	no rxn	chars	wk pink	no rxn	wk rxn	wk red	no rxn	wk brown
Piroxicam	–	brown	–	–	–	–	–	–	–	–	–
Piroxicam metabolite	–	brown	–	–	–	–	–	–	–	–	–
Prednisolone	orange	brown	brown	–	–	–	–	grey	–	–	–
Prednisone	orange	brown	brown	–	–	–	–	yellow/grey	–	–	–
Pregnenolone	–	–	–	–	–	–	–	grey	–	–	–
Prilocaine	no rxn	brown	brown	no rxn	no rxn	no rxn	–	–	–	–	brown
Procaine	orange	brown	brown	no rxn	no rxn	no rxn	–	–	red	–	brown

Name	D	N	C-H	M	FES	NIN	Gibb's	H+:EtOH	ME	F	I_2
Progesterone	–	–	–	–	–	–	–	wk grey	–	–	–
Promazine	–	–	–	–	pink	–	–	–	–	–	brown
Propiomazine	–	–	–	–	pink	–	–	–	–	–	–
Propiomazine metabolite	–	–	–	–	pink	–	–	–	–	–	–
Propionylpromazine	–	–	–	–	pink/purple	–	–	–	–	–	–
Propoxyphene	orange	–	–	–	–	–	–	–	–	–	–
Propoxyphene metabolite I	orange	–	–	–	–	–	–	–	–	–	–
Propoxyphene metabolite II	orange	–	–	–	–	–	–	–	–	–	–
Propoxyphene metabolite III	orange	–	–	–	–	–	–	–	–	–	–
Propranolol	wk orange	brown	brown	green	grey	red	–	–	red	–	brown
Pseudoephedrine	wk orange	brown	brown	–	–	pink	–	–	–	–	–
Pyrilamine	orange	brown	brown	red	pink	no rxn	–	–	–	–	brown
Pyrilamine, acid hydrolysis metabolite	–	brown	brown	–	no rxn	–	–	–	–	–	brown
Pyrilamine, *O*-demethyl	orange	brown	brown	red	pink	no rxn	–	–	–	–	brown
Pyrilamine, *O*-demethyl *N*-demethyl	orange	brown	brown	red	pink	no rxn	–	–	–	–	brown
Ranitidine	orange	brown	brown	grey	yellow	wk pink	–	–	–	–	–
Retinal	wk orange	wk brown	wk brown	purple	yellow/green	–	–	–	–	–	–
Romifidine	orange	brown	brown	no rxn	no rxn	no rxn	–	–	no rxn	wk blue/grey	brown
Salbutamol	no rxn	brown	brown	red	no rxn	no rxn	lt blue	–	no rxn	no rxn	wk brown
Salicylic acid	–	–	–	green	–	–	–	–	–	–	–
Stanozolol	–	–	–	–	–	–	–	grey	–	–	–
Strychnine	orange	brown	brown	blue → orange	no rxn	–	–	–	–	–	–
Sulfadimethoxine	orange	brown	brown	no rxn	no rxn	no rxn	–	–	red	–	brown
Tenoxicam	orange	wk brown	wk brown	no rxn	no rxn	no rxn	–	–	no rxn	no rxn	wk brown
Testolactone	–	–	–	–	–	–	–	grey	–	–	–
Testosterone	–	–	–	–	green	no rxn	–	green	–	–	–
Tetramisole (levamisole/dexamisole)	orange	brown	brown	wk wite	no rxn	no rxn	–	–	no rxn	–	brown
Tetramisole, hydroxylated metabolite	orange	brown	brown	–	–	–	–	–	–	–	brown
Theobromine	no rxn	no rxn	brown	no rxn	no rxn	no rxn	–	–	no rxn	no rxn	–
Theophylline	no rxn	brown	brown	no rxn	no rxn	no rxn	–	–	no rxn	no rxn	–
Tiaprofenic acid	no rxn	wk brown	wk brown	no rxn	yellow	no rxn	–	lt yellow	no rxn	no rxn	wk brown
Tralonide	–	–	–	–	–	–	–	grey	–	–	–
Trazodone	orange	brown	brown	pink	no rxn	wk pink	–	–	–	–	brown
Trazodone metabolite, MW 405	orange	brown	brown	pink	no rxn	wk pink	–	–	–	–	brown
Triamcinolone	–	–	–	–	–	–	–	grey	–	–	–
Trichlormethiazide	–	–	–	–	–	–	–	–	–	red	–
Trimethoprim	orange	brown	brown	–	–	–	–	–	–	–	–
Xylazine	orange	brown	brown	–	–	–	–	–	–	–	brown
Xylazine hydroxylated metabolites	orange	brown	brown	–	–	–	–	–	–	–	brown
Zomepirac	–	–	–	–	–	–	–	–	blue	–	–

C-H, cupric chloride; D, Dragendorff spray; F, Fearon's reagent; FES, ferric chloride, ethanol, sulfuric acid; Gibb's, Gibb's reagent; H+:EtOH, conc. hydrochloric + ethanol; I_2; iodine; M, Mandelin's reagent; ME, modified Ehrlich's reagent; N, sodium nitrite; NIN, ninhydrin; no rxn, no reaction

Thin-layer Chromatographic Data

System TA (p. 405)—Rf values

Rf	*Compound*
00	Adrenaline
	Carbachol
	Cetrimide
	Decamethonium Bromide
	Decamethonium
	Demecarium Bromide
	Diminazene
	Diquat
	Distigmine Bromide
	Ethyl Nicotinate
	Gallamine Triethiodide
	Hexamethonium Bromide
	Homatropine Methylbromide
	Hydrastinine
	Mebezonium Iodide
	Neomycin
	Noradrenaline
	Paraquat
	Pentolonium Tartrate
	Quinuronium Sulfate
	Streptomycin
	Tubocurarine Chloride
01	Alcuronium Chloride
	Benserazide
	Bethanidine
	Bretylium Tosilate
	Debrisoquine
	Dibrompropamidine
	Dihydrostreptomycin
	Guanethidine
	Guanoxan
	Hexylcaine
	Homatropine
	Hydroxystilbamidine
	Kanamycin
	Mepenzolate Bromide
	Metformin
	Obidoxime Chloride
	Pancuronium Bromide
	Pentamidine
	Pentapiperide Metilsulfate
	Propamidine
	Pyritidium Bromide
	Suxamethonium Chloride
	Suxethonium Bromide
	Thiamine
02	Acetylcholine Chloride
	Ambenonium Chloride
	Amprolium Hydrochloride
	Atropine Methonitrate
	Bethanechol Chloride
	Bibenzonium Bromide
	Buformin
	Cadaverine
	Choline
	Clidinium Bromide
	Cotarnine
	Diphemanil Metilsulfate
	Ecothiopate Iodide
	Hexocyclium Metilsulfate
	Hyoscine Methonitrate
	Lachesine Chloride
	Methacholine Chloride
	Methanthelinium Bromide
	Neostigmine Bromide
	Octatropine Methylbromide
	Oxyphencyclimine
	Penthienate Methobromide
	Poldine Metilsulfate
	Thenium Closilate
	Thiazinamium Metilsulfate
	Trimetaphan Camsilate
	Valethamate Bromide
03	Ambutonium Bromide
	Benzethonium Chloride
	Benzilonium Bromide
	Chlorproguanil
	Dequalinium Chloride
	Dofamium Chloride
	Glycopyrronium Bromide
	Guanoclor
	Heteronium Bromide
	Hexoprenaline
	Oxyphenonium Bromide
	Phenformin
	Proguanil
04	Acefylline Piperazine
	Pipenzolate Bromide
	Propantheline Bromide
	Pyridostigmine Bromide
05	Amicarbalide
	Chlortetracycline
	Clomocycline
	Cytarabine
	Demeclocycline
	Domiphen Bromide
	Emepronium Bromide
	Isopropamide Iodide
	Lymecycline
	Methacycline
	Oxytetracycline Dihydrate
	Piperazine
	Pralidoxime Chloride
	Psilocybine
	Rolitetracycline
	Sparteine
	Tetracycline
06	Pyrantel
	Tramazoline
	Tricyclamol Chloride
07	Acriflavinium Chloride
07	Berberine
	Edrophonium Chloride
	Tridihexethyl Chloride
08	Desferrioxamine
	Hyoscine Butylbromide
09	Oxymetazoline
	Putrescine
10	Azacyclonol
	Betahistine
	Denatonium Benzoate
	Mequitazine
	Stilbazium Iodide
11	Δ^9-Tetrahydrocannabinol
12	Cetalkonium Chloride
	Doxorubicin
	Doxycycline
13	Benzatropine
	Deptropine
	Histamine
	Nitroxoline
	Norcodeine
	Tetryzoline
	Tolazoline
	Xylometazoline
14	Naphazoline
15	Amidefrine
	Maprotiline
	Octafonium Chloride
16	Brucine
	Mecamylamine
	Proflavine Hemisulfate
17	Ecgonine
	Normorphine
18	Atropine
	Dopamine
	Hyoscyamine
	N-Methyltryptamine
19	Halquinol
	Primaquine
	Protriptyline
20	Cetylpyridinium Chloride
	Cyclopentamine
	Mescaline
21	Atropine Oxide
	Benzoylecgonine
	Metadrenaline
22	Octamylamine
	Trimetazidine
	Vancomycin
23	Amantadine
	Betaine
	Heptaminol
	Hydromorphone
	Methoxyphenamine
	Tryptamine
24	Amiloride
	Isometheptene
	Mersalyl Acid
	Pempidine
25	Dihydromorphine
	Hydrocodone
	Mephentermine
	Oxedrine
	Serotonin
26	Ametazole
	Coniine
	Desipramine
	Dihydrocodeine
	Propylhexedrine
	Strychnine
28	Conessine
	Homochlorcyclizine

Rf	*Compound*
29	Methdilazine
	Pholedrine
30	Ephedrine
	Ethambutol
	Methenamine
31	Antazoline
	Metamfetamine
	Physostigmine Aminoxide
	Tyramine
32	Hydroxyquinoline
	Methylephedrine
	Phentolamine
33	Chlorhexidine
	Codeine
	Dextromethorphan
	Methylenedioxymethamfetamine
	Normetadrenaline
	Phenylephrine
	Pseudoephedrine
	Trimethoxyamfetamine (2,4,6-TMA)
	Tuaminoheptane
34	Nortriptyline
	Racemorphan
35	Bufotenine
	Dextrorphan
	Hydroxyamfetamine
	Hydroxyephedrine
	Levorphanol
	Neopine
36	Metindizate
	Monocrotaline
	Penicillamine
	Pholcodine
37	Morphine
	Rimantadine
38	Chloroquine
	Harmaline
	Mesoridazine
	Sulpiride
39	Azatadine
	Dimethoxanate
	Methylenedioxyamfetamine
	Psilocin
40	Cytisine
	Dimethyltryptamine
	Ethoheptazine
	Ethylmorphine
	Hordenine
	Isoprenaline
	Loprazolam
	Mexiletine
	Phenglutarimide
41	Benzylmorphine
	Etilefrine
	Perhexiline
	Xantinol Nicotinate
42	Cathine
	Dimetindene
	Ethylnoradrenaline
	Metaraminol
	Nadolol
	Profadol
	Spiramycin
	Tigloidine
	Trimethobenzamide
	Viloxazine
43	Amfetamine
	Dehydroemetine
	Furaltadone
	Mepacrine
	Tacrine
44	Acetylcodeine
	Benzydamine
	Chlorphentermine
	Cycloserine
	Etafedrine
	Furazolidone
	Hydroquinine
	Phenylpropanolamine
	Promazine
45	Atenolol
	Brompheniramine
	Chlorphenamine
	Disopyramide
	Hydroquinidine
	Hydroxychloroquine
	Oleandomycin
	Pheniramine
	Practolol
	Thebacon
	Thebaine
	Tofenacin
46	Clemastine
	Diethyltryptamine
	Diphenylpyraline
	Eucatropine
	6-Monoacetylmorphine
	Phentermine
	Pseudomorphine
	Salbutamol
	Thioproperazine
47	Acebutolol
	Diamorphine
	Hexobendine
	Iprindole
	Isoniazid
	Ketobemidone
	Metoclopramide
	Pipazetate
	Prenalterol
	Prothipendyl
	Terbutaline
	Zimeldine
48	Acepromazine
	Carbetapentane
	Carbinoxamine
	Carbocromen
	Diprophylline
	Doxylamine
	Fenfluramine
	Imipramine
	Methadone
	Orciprenaline
	Oxprenolol
	Oxymorphone
	Perazine
	Pizotifen
	Procyclidine
	Thioridazine
49	Bamipine
	Chlorpromazine
	Cinchonidine
	Cinchonine
	Gelsemine
	Mafenide
	Methyldopa
	Metoprolol
	Phanquinone
	Phenethylamine
	Pindolol
	Procainamide
	Procarbazine
	Prochlorperazine
	Tiotixene
50	Alphaprodine
	Aminopromazine
	Metixene
	Nefopam
	Oxeladin
	Oxycodone
	Phenmetrazine
	Prolintane
	Promethazine
	Propranolol
	Ranitidine
	Thenalidine
51	Amitriptyline
	Broxyquinoline
	Clomipramine
	Cyproheptadine
	DOM
	Dosulepin
	Doxepin
	Hydralazine
	Mepyramine
	Minoxidil
	Quinidine
	Quinine
	Thiethylperazine
	Tolpropamine
	Triamterene
	Triprolidine
52	Alprenolol
	Caffeine
	Chloropyramine
	Clofedanol
	Diamthazole
	Diethylcarbamazine
	Dobutamine
	Isothipendyl
	Lorazepam
	Lormetazepam
	Methapyrilene
	Moxisylyte
	Narceine
	Oxetacaine
	Pethidine
	Solanine
	Timolol
53	Acetophenazine
	Arecoline
	Azathioprine
	Butaperazine
	Cephaëline
	Chloropyrilene
	Chlorphenoxamine
	Cyclazocine
	Noxiptiline
	Pecazine
	Phenyltoloxamine
	Pilocarpine
	Sotalol
	Temazepam
	Thenyldiamine
	Theobromine
	Trifluoperazine
54	Aminoacridine
	Bromazine
	Carfenazine
	Cimetidine
	Dibenzepin
	Emetine
	Etamiphylline
	Fencamfamin
	Fenpipramide
	Morinamide
	Nicotinamide
	Nicotine
	Niridazole
	Opipramol
	Pipradrol
	Procaine

Rf	*Compound*
	Pyrrobutamine
	Tranylcypromine
	Triflupromazine
55	Ambazone
	Aminohippuric Acid
	Bamethan
	Colchicine
	Dihydralazine
	Dimenhydrinate
	Diphenhydramine
	Erythromycin
	Fenetylline
	Homidium Bromide
	Hyoscine
	Methoxamine
	Orphenadrine
	Pentifylline
	Perphenazine
	Physostigmine
	Piperocaine
	Propiomazine
	Thonzylamine
	Trimethoprim
	Tripelennamine
	Urea
56	Chlorprothixene
	Clioquinol
	Clopenthixol
	Dimetotiazine
	Imolamine
	5-Methyltryptamine
	Metopimazine
	Nicametate
	Nicotinyl Alcohol
	Nomifensine
	Normethadone
	Oxazepam
	Pipamperone
	Piperacetazine
	Zuclopenthixol
57	Chlorcyclizine
	Clorprenaline
	Clozapine
	Cyclizine
	Cyclopentolate
	Ergometrine
	Inositol Nicotinate
	Levacetylmethadol
	Levomepromazine
	Mebhydrolin
	Methylphenidate
	Nifenazone
	Nimorazole
	Phendimetrazine
	Tetracaine
	Trometamol
58	Alimemazine
	Aminobenzoic Acid
	Cyclomethycaine
	Diaveridine
	Diethazine
	Lysergic Acid
	α-Methyltryptamine
	Methyprylon
	Metronidazole
	Metyrapone
	Mianserin
	Morazone
	Nicotinic Acid
	Pericyazine
	Propoxycaine
	Proxyphylline
	Trimeperidine
59	Aletamine
	Benzoctamine
	Butriptyline
	Chloroprocaine
	Clotiapine
	Dimefline
	Isoetarine
	Nalorphine
	Nikethamide
	Phenazopyridine
	Phencyclidine
	Prajmalium Bitartrate
	Pyridoxine
	Trimipramine
	Verapamil
	Veratrine
60	Carbamazepine
	Clomifene
	Dihydroergotamine
	Dyclonine
	Ethacridine
	Ethomoxane
	Histapyrrodine
	Lysergamide
	Lysergide
	Methylpiperidyl Benzilate
	Morantel
	Pemoline
	Prazosin
	Sulfametoxydiazine
	Tocainide
	Triazolam
	Vinblastine
	Xylazine
61	Amiphenazole
	Benzonatate
	Bromazepam
	Difenidol
	Fenpiprane
	Hydrastine
	Lobeline
	Methyl Nicotinate
	Nicofuranose
	Papaverine
	Paraphenylenediamine
	Pentazocine
	Pyrimethamine
	Quinisocaine
	Thiopropazate
	Trimetozine
	Triphenyltetrazolium Chloride
62	Ajmaline
	Amodiaquine
	Chlordiazepoxide
	Clobazam
	Clonidine
	Flavoxate
	Flupentixol
	Flurazepam
	Levamisole
	Methylergometrine
	Nordazepam
	Oxybuprocaine
	Proxymetacaine
	Styramate
	Sulfadimidine
	Thiamazole
63	Benzyl Nicotinate
	Butoxyethyl Nicotinate
	Cinchocaine
	Demoxepam
	Dimetridazole
	Ergotamine
	Flunitrazepam
	Fluphenazine
	Harmine
	Ketamine
	Mazindol
	Mebeverine
	Phenindamine
	Pyrazinamide
	Trazodone
	Yohimbine
64	Adiphenine
	Benethamine
	Biperiden
	Bunamidine
	Clomethiazole
	Doxapram
	Etenzamide
	Mephenesin
	Naftidrofuryl Oxalate
	Nicergoline
	Norharman
	Noscapine
	Sulfadiazine
	Sulfisomidine
65	Bamifylline
	Beclamide
	Benzquinamide
	Bitoscanate
	Cocaine
	Dropropizine
	Ethionamide
	Etoxazene
	Ibogaine
	Mebendazole
	Mepivacaine
	Methyldopate
	Methysergide
	Metisazone
	Naloxone
	Phenazone
	Prazepam
	Protokylol
	Sulfadimethoxine
	Sulfafurazole
	Sulfaguanidine
	Sulfamerazine
	Sulfamethizole
	Sulfamethoxazole
	Sulfamethoxypyridazine
	Trifluomeprazine
	Troleandomycin
	Tropicamide
66	Alverine
	Aminophenazone
	Azaperone
	Benactyzine
	Captodiame
	Caramiphen
	Chlormezanone
	Co-dergocrine Mesilate
	Cycrimine
	Diloxanide
	Dipipanone
	Ergotoxine
	Ketazolam
	Pipobroman
	Pipotiazine
	Propanidid
	Protionamide
	Sulfasalazine
	Sulfathiazole
67	Alprazolam
	Benorilate
	Benzocaine
	Clorgiline
	Droperidol

Rf	*Compound*
	Etomidate
	Glafenine
	Haloperidol
	Levallorphan
	Lincomycin
	Medazepam
	Piminodine
	Profenamine
	Pyrvinium Embonate
	Quazepam M (3-hydroxy-*N*-dealkyl-2-oxo)
	Sulfadoxine
	Sulfaethidole
	Sulfametopyrazine
	Sulfamoxole
	Sulfanilamide
	Sulfapyridine
	Tiabendazole
68	Aconitine
	Aminotriazole
	Azapropazone
	Brotizolam M (6-hydroxy)
	Butalamine
	Crotetamide
	Dextropropoxyphene
	Dicycloverine
	Dimoxyline
	Dipyridamole
	Hydroxyzine
	Isoaminile
	Nifedipine
	Nitrazepam
	Norpipanone
	Oxypertine
	Phenazocine
	Prenylamine
	Solanidine
	Trihexyphenidyl
69	Bupivacaine
	Butetamate
	Chloramphenicol
	Clefamide
	Fenyramidol
	Fluspirilene
	Iproniazid
	Piperidolate
	Reserpine
	Sulfaphenazole
	Tetrabenazine
	Tetramisole
70	Aminosalicylic Acid
	Azapetine
	Clofazimine
	Cropropamide
	Dexpanthenol
	Diethylthiambutene
	Diperodon
	Diprenorphine
	Ethosuximide
	Fentanyl
	Harman
	Hexetidine
	Hexyl Nicotinate
	Lidocaine
	Lidoflazine
	Loperamide
	Mebanazine
	Methaqualone
	Methocarbamol
	Nialamide
	Norbormide
	Parbendazole
	Pargyline
	Piritramide
	Pramocaine
	Protoveratrine A
	Sulfacetamide
	Sulfachlorpyridazine
71	Bezitramide
	Butacaine
	Chlorquinaldol
	Disulfiram
	Flumazenil
	Isocarboxazid
	Metomidate
	Phenoperidine
	Pimozide
	Propyphenazone
	Quazepam M (3-hydroxy-2-oxo)
	Sulfaquinoxaline
72	Acetorphine
	Amiodarone
	Aniline
	Bromocriptine
	Brotizolam
	Brotizolam M (α-hydroxy)
	Carbimazole
	Chelidonine
	Chlorpropamide
	Clindamycin
	Clonazepam
	Deserpidine
	Embutramide
	Famprofazone
	Fenbutrazate
	Methazolamide
	Methoserpidine
	Midazolam
	Pentetrazol
	Tylosin
73	Ambucetamide
	Anileridine
	Benzfetamine
	Cefaloridine
	Desmetryne
	Dextromoramide
	Diethyltoluamide
	Etorphine
	Fluanisone
	Methoxyamfetamine
	Miconazole
	Nifuratel
	Phenoxybenzamine
	Rescinnamine
	Ritodrine
	Simazine
	Trifluperidol
74	Bialamicol
	Bisacodyl
	Broxaldine
	Buphenine
	Diphenoxylate
	Etisazole
	Hydroxyphenamate
	Methoprotryne
	Noxytiolin
	Quazepam
	Selegiline
75	Aminonitrothiazole
	Bromhexine
	Buclizine
	Butyl Aminobenzoate
	Cinchophen
	Diazepam
	Dinitolmide
	Glutethimide
	Meprobamate
	Padimate
	Phenprobamate
	Phensuximide
	Quazepam M (*N*-dealkyl-2-oxo)
	Quinethazone
	Sulfiram
	Theophylline
76	Ametryne
	Buprenorphine
	Butanilicaine
	Camazepam
	Cinnarizine
	Clorexolone
	Diethylpropion
	Ethinamate
	Ethoxzolamide
	Fenoterol
	Glymidine Sodium
	Meclozine
	Mesuximide
	Metaclazepam M (nor)
	Penfluridol
	Pheneturide
	Prometryne
	Sulfacarbamide
	Thiambutosine
	Tolbutamide
77	Atrazine
	Bephenium Hydroxynaphthoate
	Cyclothiazide
	Gloxazone
	Meclofenoxate
	Metaclazepam
	Oxyphenbutazone
	Phenelzine
	Pipoxolan
	Prilocaine
	Terbutryne
	Tetrazepam M (nor)
	Tybamate
78	Carbutamide
	Clemizole
	Isoxsuprine
	Quazepam M (2-oxo)
	Stanozolol
	Syrosingopine
	Tetrazepam
	Thioacetazone
79	Clioxanide
	Clopamide
	Metallibure
	Phenothiazine
	Phenylbutazone
	Rifampicin
	Triamcinolone
80	Aminitrozole
	Econazole
	Glibenclamide
	Tiocarlide
	Trichlormethiazide
81	Diamfenetide
	Propyliodone
82	Chlorphenesin
	Chlorphenesin Carbamate
	Diazoxide
	Diclofenamide
	Methoxsalen
	Oxyphenisatine
83	Apomorphine
	Crotamiton
	Nitroxinil
84	Azinphos-methyl
	Clorazepic Acid
	Dipyrone
	Indoramin

Rf	*Compound*
	Rifamycin SV
	Salinazid
85	Acetazolamide
	Chlorzoxazone
86	Hydroflumethiazide
	Methandienone
	Nifursol
	Paramethadione
87	Amygdalin
	Glipizide
	Methyclothiazide
	Methylprednisolone
	Oxyclozanide
88	Ethotoin
	Primidone
	Trilostane
89	Methyltestosterone
	Rafoxanide
90	Aspirin
	Buclosamide
	Cortisone
	Diclofenac
	Ethinylestradiol
	Fludrocortisone acetate
91	Etidocaine
	Niclosamide
	Paramethasone
92	Fenbufen
94	Cannabidiol
	Cannabinol
	Etamivan
	Indometacin
95	Fendosal
	Methyl Hydroxybenzoate
	Oxymetholone
	Paracetamol
96	Etacrynic Acid
	Fenoprofen
	Flufenamic Acid
	Flunixin
	Hydrocortisone
	Mefenamic Acid
	Methyl Salicylate
98	Anisindione

System TB (p. 405)—**Rf values**

Rf	*Compound*
00	Acebutolol
	Acenocoumarol
	Adrenaline
	Alcuronium
	Ambazone
	Amidefrine
	Amiloride
	Aminoacridine
	Apomorphine
	Astemizole M (nor)
	Atenolol
	Atropine Methonitrate
	Azacyclonol
	Bambuterol Monocarbamate
	Bamifylline
	Benorilate
	Benserazide
	Benzoylecgonine
	Bethanidine
	Bromocriptine
	Broxyquinoline
	Brucine
	Buformin
	Bufotenine
	Carbachol
	Cetrimide
	Chloramphenicol
	Chlorhexidine
	Chlorphenesin Carbamate
	Chlorproguanil
	Chlorpropamide
	Chlorzoxazone
	Cimetidine
	Cinchophen
	Clefamide
	Clenbuterol (M#2)
	Clenbuterol (M#3)
	Clidinium Bromide
	Clindamycin
	Clioquinol
	Clonazepam
	Colchicine
	Cytarabine
	Debrisoquine
	Decamethonium Bromide
	Decamethonium
	Demoxepam
	Denatonium Benzoate
	Dicoumarol
	Diminazene
	Diprophylline
	Dipyridamole
	Dipyrone
	Dobutamine
	Dopamine
	Doxazosin
	Emepronium Bromide
	Enalapril
	Epithiazide
	Ergometrine
	Ethchlorvynol
	Ethionamide
	Etofylline
	Etoxazene
	Famotidine
	Fenoterol
	Fluconazole
	Flucytosine
	Fluorometholone
	Furaltadone
	Furazolidone
	Furosemide
	Glibenclamide
	Gliclazide
	Glipizide
	Glymidine Sodium
	Guanethidine
	Guanoclor
	Guanoxan
	Harmine
	Hexachlorophene
	Hexylresorcinol
	Histamine
	Homatropine Methylbromide
	Hydrocortisone
	Hydroxystilbamidine
	Isoetarine
	Isoprenaline
	Isopropamide Iodide
	Ketoconazole
	Labetalol
	Levocabastine
	Lysergamide
	Lysergic Acid
	Mebendazole
	Mebutamate
	Meprobamate
	Mercaptopurine
	Metaclazepam M (dinor)
	Metformin
	Methanthelinium Bromide
	Methazolamide
	Methocarbamol
	Methylergometrine
	Methylprednisolone
	Metopimazine
	Minoxidil
	Morphine
	Nalbuphine
	Narceine
	Neostigmine Methylsulfate
	Niclosamide
	Nicotinamide
	Nifenazone
	Nifuratel
	Nitrazepam
	Nitrofurantoin
	Nitrofurazone
	Nizatidine
	Noradrenaline
	Norbormide
	Norcodeine
	Norharman
	Obidoxime Chloride
	Oxazepam
	Oxcarbazepine
	Oxyphenbutazone
	Oxyphenonium Bromide
	Oxytetracycline Dihydrate
	Pancuronium Bromide
	Paracetamol
	Paraquat
	Pemoline
	Pentapiperide Metilsulfate
	Pentolonium Tartrate
	Phenformin
	Pilocarpine
	Pirenzepine
	Pirenzepine M (*N*-desmethyl)
	Piroxicam M (5-hydroxy)
	Practolol
	Pralidoxime Mesilate
	Prednisolone
	Prednisone
	Proguanil
	Propantheline Bromide
	Pseudomorphine
	Psilocybine
	Pyridostigmine Bromide
	Pyridoxine
	Quazepam M (3-hydroxy-*N*-dealkyl-2-oxo)
	Remoxipride M(FLA-838)
	Remoxipride M(NCM-001)
	Remoxipride M(NCM-009)
	Resorcinol

Rf	*Compound*
	Rimiterol
	Salicylamide
	Strophanthin-K
	Sulfacarbamide
	Sulpiride
	Suxamethonium Chloride
	Tetracycline
	Thiamine
	Thiazinamium Metilsulfate
	Thiazinamium Metilsulfate M (sulfoxide)
	Tolazamide
	Trilostane
	Trimetaphan Camsilate
	Trimethoprim
	Tubocurarine Chloride
	Xamoterol
	Xipamide
01	Acefylline Piperazine
	Alprazolam
	Astemizole
	Brotizolam M (6-hydroxy)
	Butalbital
	Carbimazole
	Cephaëline
	Chlormezanone
	Clenbuterol M (hydroxy)
	Co-dergocrine Mesilate
	Cycloserine
	Cytisine
	Diazoxide
	Dihydroergotamine
	Dropropizine
	Ergotamine
	Ergotoxine
	Ethylnoradrenaline
	Glafenine
	Heptaminol
	Hexoprenaline
	Inositol Nicotinate
	Iproniazid
	Isoniazid
	Itraconazole
	Loprazolam
	Lorazepam
	Metaraminol
	Methyldopa
	Methysergide
	Metoclopramide
	Moclobemide
	Nadolol
	Nalorphine
	Nifedipine
	Nimodipine
	Niridazole
	Orciprenaline
	Oxymetazoline
	Oxyphencyclimine
	Penicillamine
	Pentamidine
	Phenazopyridine
	Phentolamine
	Phenylephrine
	Pipamperone
	Piperazine
	Piritramide
	Prazosin
	Prenalterol
	Procainamide
	Propamidine
	Protionamide
	Protokylol
	Rescinnamine
	Salbutamol
	Salinazid
	Sotalol
	Styramate
	Terbutaline
	Theobromine
	Theophylline
	Thiamazole
	Triamterene
	Triazolam
	Tryptamine
	Tuaminoheptane
	Vinblastine
02	Amiphenazole
	Bambuterol
	Brotizolam M (α-hydroxy)
	Buclosamide
	Carbamazepine
	Chlordiazepoxide
	Dihydromorphine
	Droperidol
	Etilefrine
	Felodipine
	Guaifenesin
	Harman
	Hexestrol
	Hydroquinine
	Hydroxyamfetamine
	Hydroxychloroquine
	Ketobemidone
	Mephenesin
	Metronidazole
	Nialamide
	Nitrendipine
	Pindolol
	Pipobroman
	Procarbazine
	Proxyphylline
	Pyrimethamine
	Quazepam M (3-hydroxy-2-oxo)
	Quazepam M (*N*-dealkyl-2-oxo)
	Quinine
	Reserpine
	Tocainide
	Tolazoline
	Trimethobenzamide
03	Acetophenazine
	4-Aminophenol
	Azathioprine
	Buphenine
	Caffeine
	Clorazepic Acid
	Cortisone
	Deserpidine
	Diethylstilbestrol
	Etenzamide
	Ethambutol
	Fenetylline
	Fenpipramide
	Flumazenil
	Hydromorphone
	Hydroquinidine
	Isoxsuprine
	Lysergide
	Mescaline
	Mesoridazine
	Metisazone
	Naphazoline
	Nimorazole
	Nordazepam
	Phanquinone
	Pholcodine
	Pholedrine
	Pimozide
	Pipotiazine
	Propoxycaine
	Pyrazinamide
04	Bamethan
	Carisoprodol
	Clozapine
	Ethinylestradiol
	Fluspirilene
	Hydrocodone
	Isradipine
	Methenamine
	Methoserpidine
	Nicotinyl Alcohol
	Oxedrine
	Oxypertine
	Paroxetine
	Pericyazine
	Phenazone
	Phenylpropanolamine
	Pirenzepine M (desamide)
	Quinidine
	Tizanidine
	Tramazoline
	Veratrine
	Zopiclone
05	Ambucetamide
	Atropine
	Brotizolam
	Carfenazine
	Chloroprocaine
	Ephedrine
	Ethinamate
	Ethosuximide
	Fluphenazine
	Homatropine
	Hordenine
	Neopine
	Procaine
	Psilocin
	Tacrine
	Tetrazepam M (nor-)
	Trimetazidine
06	Antazoline
	Benzocaine
	Benzylmorphine
	Bromazepam
	Butyl Aminobenzoate
	Cinchonidine
	Cinchonine
	Codeine
	Dehydroemetine
	Flecainide
	Flupentixol
	Hyoscine
	Lormetazepam
	Mequitazine
	Midazolam
	6-Monoacetylmorphine
	Opipramol
	Pentifylline
	Piperacetazine
	Propranolol
	Thiambutosine
	Timolol
	Trimethoxyamfetamine (2,4,6-TMA)
	Viloxazine
	Yohimbine
07	Ajmaline
	Benzquinamide
	Butacaine
	Clopenthixol
	Disopyramide
	Ethylmorphine
	Mazindol
	Pentetrazol
	Perphenazine

Rf	*Compound*
	Tetryzoline
	Thioproperazine
	Tiabendazole
	Tiocarlide
	Xylometazoline
	Zuclopenthixol
08	Amodiaquine
	Beclamide
	Bisoprolol
	Clobazam
	Clonidine
	Dihydrocodeine
	Etorphine
	Fenyramidol
	Metipranolol
	Morazone
	Morinamide
	Papaverine
	Profadol
	Strychnine
	Temazepam
09	Buprenorphine
	Dimethyltryptamine
	Econazole
	Estrone
	Gelsemine
	Loperamide
	Naloxone
	Nomifensine
10	Flunitrazepam
	Hexobendine
	Hydroxyzine
	Metoprolol
	Oxetacaine
	Oxymorphone
	Tiotixene
	Trazodone
11	Aconitine
	Alprenolol
	Ametazole
	Betaxolol
	Erythromycin
	Etynodiol Diacetate
	Haloperidol
	Lidoflazine
	Miconazole
	Oxprenolol
	Phenothiazine
	Trimetozine
	Triprolidine
12	Anileridine
	Camazepam
	Carbromal
	Etamiphylline
	Fluoxetine M (nor)
	Fluvoxamine
	Halofantrine (desbutyl-)
	Physostigmine
13	Clenbuterol
	Dimetotiazine
	Emetine
	Fluoxetine
	Levorphanol
	Methoxsalen
	Primaquine
	Tertatolol
	Trifluperidol
14	Butanilicaine
	Chloroquine
	Dextrorphan
	Ketazolam
	Phenmetrazine
	Racemorphan
	Remoxipride
	Testosterone
15	Bisacodyl
	Cyclazocine
	Diamorphine
	Diethyltryptamine
	Dimefline
	Diperodon
	DOM
	Hydrastine
	Mepacrine
	Nikethamide
	Tetracaine
16	Androsterone
	Diloxanide
	Dimoxyline
	Metyrapone
	Pentazocine
	Phenazocine
	Quazepam M (2-oxo)
17	Carbocromen
	Diethylcarbamazine
	Lobeline
	Methyltestosterone
	Mexiletine
	Penfluridol
	Phenglutarimide
	Pipazetate
18	Chlorphentermine
	Clorprenaline
	Dimethoxanate
	Eucatropine
	Granisetron
	Levamisole
	Maprotiline
	Methylenedioxyamfetamine
	Protriptyline
	Tetramisole
19	Amantadine
	Desipramine
	Levallorphan
20	Amfetamine
	Doxapram
	Isocarboxazid
	Loratadine
	Norethisterone
	Propanidid
	Thebacon
21	Aminophenazone
	Disulfiram
	Noscapine
22	Cholesterol
	Dibenzepin
23	Acetylcodeine
	Methoxyamfetamine
	Metomidate
	Oxybuprocaine
	Verapamil
24	Ketotifen
	Methoxamine
	Methylenedioxymethamfetamine
	Thebaine
25	Cathine
	Cinchocaine
	Mecloqualone
	Oxycodone
	Perazine
26	Acepromazine
	Benzatropine
	Carbinoxamine
	Deptropine
	Etomidate
	Meclofenoxate
	Methoxyphenamine
	Phenoperidine
	Phentermine
	Proxymetacaine
	Tofenacin
27	Diazepam
	Mebhydrolin
	Nortriptyline
	Quazepam
	Zimeldine
28	Butaperazine
	Crotetamide
	Encainide
	Ibogaine
	Metamfetamine
	Octamylamine
	Phenethylamine
29	Cropropamide
	Prilocaine
30	Alphaprodine
	Azaperone
	Diamthazole
	Flurazepam
	Methylpiperidyl Benzilate
	Thiethylperazine
31	Gestonorone Caproate
	Glutethimide
	Mepivacaine
	Moxisylyte
32	Cyclopentamine
	Cyclopentolate
	Methdilazine
	Propyphenazone
	Tetrazepam
33	Brompheniramine
	Clemizole
	Nefopam
	Trifluoperazine
34	Dihydralazine
	Ethomoxane
	Mephentermine
	Prochlorperazine
	Propiomazine
	Propylhexedrine
35	Chlorphenamine
	Etafedrine
	Lidocaine
	Methylphenidate
	Pheniramine
	Thiopropazate
36	Benzydamine
	Dimetindene
	Flavoxate
	Loxapine
	Methaqualone
	Phendimetrazine
	Piminodine
	Prazepam
	Progesterone
	Promethazine
37	Aletamine
	Cyclandelate
	Famprofazone
	Ketamine
	Methyl Nicotinate
	Pethidine
	Phenelzine
38	Cotarnine
	Hydroxyprogesterone
	Phenyltoloxamine
	Promazine
	Thenalidine
	Thonzylamine
39	Arecoline
	Coniine
	Fluanisone

Rf	*Compound*
	Mepyramine
	Mianserin
	Nicotine
	Tigloidine
	Tranylcypromine
40	Azinphos-methyl
	Bamipine
	Benactyzine
	Mebeverine
	Metaclazepam
	Normethadone
41	Bezitramide
	Chloropyramine
	Clofedanol
	Clotiapine
	Doxylamine
	Hydralazine
	Isothipendyl
	Medazepam
	Methapyrilene
	Nicametate
	Tetrabenazine
	Trimeperidine
42	Aminopromazine
	Benzyl Nicotinate
	Bupivacaine
	Chlorcyclizine
	Clorgiline
	Dextromethorphan
	Dextromoramide
	Diphenoxylate
	Diphenylpyraline
	Fenfluramine
	Nicofuranose
	Thenyldiamine
	Thioridazine
43	Fentanyl
	Noxiptiline
	Pramocaine
	Prothipendyl
44	Bromazine
	Clomethiazole
	Diphenhydramine
	Tripelennamine
45	Butoxyethyl Nicotinate
	Chlorpromazine
	Cocaine
	Cyproheptadine

Rf	*Compound*
	Dimenhydrinate
	Ethoheptazine
	Metixene
	Nisoldipine
	Phenindamine
	Pizotifen
46	Hydrastinine
	Sertraline
47	Chlorphenoxamine
	Fenbutrazate
	Levomepromazine
	Pecazine
	Triflupromazine
48	Benethamine
	Carbetapentane
	Cyclizine
	Doxepin
	Hexetidine
	Imipramine
	Lorcainide
	Mebanazine
	Orphenadrine
49	Captodiame
	Clemastine
	Conessine
	Dosulepin
	Dyclonine
	Iprindole
50	Amitriptyline
	Halofantrine
	Rimantadine
51	Chlorprothixene
	Mecamylamine
	Oxeladin
52	Broxaldine
	Naftidrofuryl Oxalate
	Tolpropamine
53	Azapropazone
	Clomipramine
	Piperocaine
	Pipoxolan
54	Alimemazine
	Cinnarizine
	Pseudoephedrine
	Pyrrobutamine
55	Cyclomethycaine
	Piperidolate
	Prenylamine

Rf	*Compound*
	Quinisocaine
56	Adiphenine
	Clomifene
	Difenidol
57	Azapetine
	Benzoctamine
	Clofazimine
	Diethazine
	Perhexiline
	Selegiline
58	Isoaminile
	Norpipanone
59	Butetamate
	Dextropropoxyphene
	Methadone
	Pipradrol
60	Dieldrin
	Diethylthiambutene
	Trifluomeprazine
61	Buclizine
	Butriptyline
	Meclozine
62	Amiodarone
	Bialamicol
	Diethylpropion
	Fencamfamin
	Levacetylmethadol
	Procyclidine
	Trimipramine
63	Aprindine
	Phenoxybenzamine
	Sulfadoxine
64	Profenamine
65	Alverine
66	Trihexyphenidyl
67	Benzfetamine
	Bromhexine
	Cycrimine
	Dicycloverine
	Dipipanone
	Prolintane
	Sparteine
68	Biperiden
	Pempidine
72	Chlordane
73	Phencyclidine
74	Heptachlor

System TC (p. 405)—Rf values

Rf	*Compound*
00	Ametazole
	Bethanidine
	Buformin
	Carbachol
	Debrisoquine
	Decamethonium Bromide
	Decamethonium
	Diminazene
	Dopamine
	Guanoclor
	Guanoxan
	Hexoprenaline
	Histamine
	Homatropine Methylbromide
	Hydrastinine
	Hydroxystilbamidine
	Isoetarine
	Lysergic Acid
	Metformin

Rf	*Compound*
	Noradrenaline
	Obidoxime Chloride
	Pancuronium Bromide
	Paraquat
	Pentamidine
	Pentolonium Tartrate
	Phenformin
	Pseudomorphine
	Suxamethonium Chloride
	Thiamine
	Thiazinamium Metilsulfate
	Tubocurarine Chloride
01	Acefylline Piperazine
	Adrenaline
	Amidefrine
	Amiloride
	Benserazide
	Benzoylecgonine
	Bufotenine

Rf	*Compound*
	Cetrimide
	Chlorproguanil
	Cotarnine
	Cycloserine
	Cytarabine
	Dipyrone
	Dobutamine
	Fenoterol
	Homatropine
	Isoprenaline
	Metaraminol
	Methyldopa
	Nadolol
	Oxedrine
	Oxymetazoline
	Oxyphenonium Bromide
	Pentapiperide Metilsulfate
	Phenylephrine
	Piperazine

Rf	*Compound*
	Practolol
	Proguanil
	Propamidine
	Salbutamol
	Sulfacarbamide
	Terbutaline
02	Atenolol
	Cinchophen
	Dihydralazine
	Ethambutol
	Ethylnoradrenaline
	Etilefrine
	Guanethidine
	Heptaminol
	Hydroxyamfetamine
	Hydroxychloroquine
	Mecamylamine
	Tetryzoline
	Tolazoline
	Tramazoline
	Tryptamine
03	Acebutolol
	Atropine
	Azacyclonol
	Conessine
	Dihydromorphine
	Minoxidil
	Narceine
	Orciprenaline
	Oxyphencyclimine
	Pempidine
	Penicillamine
	Phentolamine
	Pholedrine
	Protokylol
	Sotalol
	Sparteine
	Veratrine
04	Ambazone
	Chloroquine
	Deptropine
	Dextrorphan
	Methoxamine
	Methoxyphenamine
	Mexiletine
	Phenylpropanolamine
	Propantheline Bromide
	Pseudoephedrine
	Tacrine
	Trimetazidine
05	Azapropazone
	Cathine
	Clioquinol
	Ephedrine
	Isopropamide Iodide
	Maprotiline
	Mepacrine
	Norcodeine
	Pindolol
	Primaquine
	Procainamide
	Xylometazoline
06	Bamethan
	Benzatropine
	Broxyquinoline
	Hordenine
	Mequitazine
	Mesoridazine
	Naphazoline
	Profadol
07	Amantadine
	Antazoline
	Hydroquinine
	Levorphanol
	Metoclopramide
	Oxetacaine
	Protriptyline
	Tuaminoheptane
08	Azathioprine
	Cinchonidine
	Disopyramide
	Hydroquinidine
	Mephentermine
	Metoprolol
	Perhexiline
	Phenglutarimide
	Pyridoxine
	Triamterene
09	Amfetamine
	Cimetidine
	Dimethyltryptamine
	Etafedrine
	Hydromorphone
	Ketobemidone
	Morphine
	Prenalterol
	Psilocin
	Racemorphan
10	Cyclopentamine
	Cytisine
	Diethyltryptamine
	Doxylamine
	Mescaline
	Procarbazine
	Propranolol
11	Desipramine
	Hydralazine
	Isoniazid
	Metopimazine
	Octamylamine
	Oxprenolol
	Quinine
	Rimantadine
	Timolol
	Trimethoxyamfetamine (2,4,6-TMA)
12	Alprenolol
	Cinchonine
	Diprophylline
	Ergometrine
	Methylenedioxyamfetamine
	Neopine
	Pentazocine
	Phenelzine
	Pipamperone
	Quinidine
13	Coniine
	Cyclazocine
	Dihydrocodeine
	Dimetindene
	Eucatropine
	Mazindol
	Metamfetamine
	Methenamine
	Pheniramine
	Pipazetate
14	Buphenine
	Methylergometrine
15	Clorprenaline
	Methdilazine
16	Brompheniramine
	Fenfluramine
	Fenpipramide
	Nortriptyline
	Pericyazine
17	Brucine
	Chlorphentermine
	DOM
	Nicotinic Acid
	Nicotinyl Alcohol
18	Chlorphenamine
	Codeine
	Dextromethorphan
	Pholcodine
	Trilostane
19	Aminopromazine
	Carbinoxamine
	Cephaëline
	Ethoheptazine
	Lysergamide
	6-Monoacetylmorphine
	Piperacetazine
	Strychnine
20	Hydrocodone
	Methadone
	Salinazid
	Styramate
	Triprolidine
21	Apomorphine
	Dehydroemetine
	Methysergide
	Nicotinamide
	Tigloidine
	Tofenacin
22	Benzydamine
	Carbetapentane
	Ethylmorphine
	Harmine
	Opipramol
	Oxeladin
	Trimethoprim
23	Benzylmorphine
	Chloroprocaine
	Fluphenazine
	Imipramine
	Iproniazid
	Nalorphine
	Pemoline
	Prothipendyl
	Tocainide
	Viloxazine
24	Acepromazine
	Carbocromen
	Dimethoxanate
	Levallorphan
	Phentermine
25	Acetophenazine
	Clemastine
	Mepyramine
	Metixene
	Nialamide
	Thenyldiamine
	Zimeldine
26	Diethylcarbamazine
	Methapyrilene
27	Carfenazine
	Haloperidol
	Phenmetrazine
	Tripelennamine
28	Chloropyramine
	Diazoxide
	Dihydroergotamine
	Diphenylpyraline
	Phenethylamine
	Thonzylamine
29	Nomifensine
	Perphenazine
30	Butacaine
	Diamthazole
	Isothipendyl
	Norharman
	Promazine

Rf	Compound
	Quazepam M (3-hydroxy-*N*-dealkyl-2-oxo)
	Theophylline
	Thioridazine
	Trifluoperazine
31	Chloramphenicol
	Clonidine
	Procaine
	Procyclidine
	Pyrimethamine
	Theobromine
32	Amitriptyline
	Clopenthixol
	Isoxsuprine
	Loperamide
	Meprobamate
	Nefopam
	Pilocarpine
	Pipotiazine
	Prolintane
	Tetracaine
	Tolpropamine
	Zuclopenthixol
33	Amiphenazole
	Dimenhydrinate
	Diphenhydramine
	Dipipanone
	Flupentixol
	Mebutamate
	Orphenadrine
	Propoxycaine
	Proxyphylline
	Tranylcypromine
34	Cinchocaine
	Clomipramine
	Emetine
	Ergotamine
	Fencamfamin
	Iprindole
	Normethadone
	Pethidine
	Thebacon
	Thioproperazine
35	Alphaprodine
	Brotizolam M (6-hydroxy)
	Chlorpromazine
	Demoxepam
	Dibenzepin
	Lobeline
	Nicametate
	Nicotine
	Noxiptiline
	Phencyclidine
	Promethazine
	Triflupromazine
36	Chlorphenoxamine
	Cyclomethycaine
	Ethionamide
	Lorazepam
	Metronidazole
	Nitrazepam
	Physostigmine
37	Butaperazine
	Clofedanol
	Colchicine
	Dipyridamole
	Doxepin
	Hyoscine
	Oxymorphone
	Perazine
	Piperocaine
	Prochlorperazine
	Pyrrobutamine
	Thebaine
38	Clozapine
	Diamorphine
	Glafenine
	Levomepromazine
	Pipradrol
	Protionamide
	Yohimbine
39	Aconitine
	Alimemazine
	Alverine
	Cyclopentolate
	Etamiphylline
	Levacetylmethadol
	Lysergide
	Phenazocine
40	Aletamine
	Amodiaquine
	Dyclonine
	Furaltadone
	Harman
	Hexetidine
	Oxazepam
	Tiotixene
	Triazolam
41	Bromazepam
	Cyclizine
	Glipizide
	Methylphenidate
	Naftidrofuryl Oxalate
	Oxybuprocaine
	Proxymetacaine
	Thiethylperazine
	Trimeperidine
42	Dosulepin
	Meclofenoxate
	Propiomazine
	Pyrazinamide
43	Acetylcodeine
	Bamipine
	Bromazine
	Diethylthiambutene
	Inositol Nicotinate
	Mephenesin
44	Cyproheptadine
	Hexobendine
	Moxisylyte
	Nimorazole
	Niridazole
	Pecazine
	Thenalidine
45	Difenidol
	Fenetylline
	Mebhydrolin
	Phanquinone
	Piritramide
46	Brotizolam M (α-hydroxy)
	Chlorcyclizine
	Morazone
	Quinisocaine
47	Cocaine
	Ethomoxane
	Furazolidone
	Prazosin
	Profenamine
48	Butriptyline
	Co-dergocrine Mesilate
	Dimefline
	Dimetotiazine
	Droperidol
	Flurazepam
	Levamisole
	Loprazolam
	Phenyltoloxamine
49	Morinamide
50	Chlordiazepoxide
	Ibogaine
	Norpipanone
	Phenazopyridine
51	Benorilate
	Chlorprothixene
	Chlorzoxazone
	Diethazine
	Oxycodone
	Phendimetrazine
52	Benzoctamine
	Brotizolam
	Clomifene
	Fenyramidol
	Thiamazole
53	Benactyzine
	Clonazepam
	Mebeverine
	Thiopropazate
54	Bamifylline
	Butanilicaine
	Hydroxyzine
	Isoaminile
	Tetramisole
	Tiabendazole
	Trimipramine
55	Dextropropoxyphene
	Nordazepam
	Pramocaine
	Quazepam M (3-hydroxy-2-oxo)
56	Anileridine
	Carbamazepine
	Clefamide
	Clorazepic Acid
	Etoxazene
	Nikethamide
	Quazepam M (*N*-dealkyl-2-oxo)
57	Alprazolam
	Benzocaine
	Butetamate
	Phenindamine
58	Caffeine
	Diperodon
	Methylpiperidyl Benzilate
	Metyrapone
	Mianserin
	Pipobroman
	Tetrazepam M (nor-)
	Trazodone
	Trifluomeprazine
59	Benethamine
	Clofazimine
	Clotiapine
	Etenzamide
	Fluspirilene
	Mebendazole
	Temazepam
60	Adiphenine
	Midazolam
	Penfluridol
	Pimozide
	Vinblastine
61	Cycrimine
	Econazole
	Etorphine
	Lormetazepam
	Trihexyphenidyl
62	Ergotoxine
	Mepivacaine
	Norbormide
63	Butyl Aminobenzoate
	Chlormezanone
	Diethylpropion
	Flumazenil

Rf	Compound
	Ketamine
	Lidoflazine
64	Biperiden
	Cholesterol
	Dicycloverine
	Hydrastine
	Ketazolam
	Pentetrazol
	Phenoperidine
	Piminodine
	Prilocaine
65	Beclamide
	Glymidine Sodium
	Metomidate
	Nifedipine
	Oxypertine
	Papaverine
66	Methyl Nicotinate
	Naloxone
	Pentifylline
67	Azapetine
	Buclosamide
	Crotetamide
	Flavoxate
	Miconazole
68	Ambucetamide
	Amiodarone
	Buprenorphine
	Fluanisone
	Metaclazepam M (nor)
	Metisazone

Rf	Compound
	Pipoxolan
	Prenylamine
69	Benzquinamide
	Bromocriptine
	Butoxyethyl Nicotinate
	Clemizole
	Clomethiazole
	Cropropamide
	Mebanazine
	Selegiline
	Tetrazepam
70	Benzfetamine
	Clobazam
	Clorgiline
	Doxapram
	Nicofuranose
	Propanidid
	Verapamil
71	Benzyl Nicotinate
	Dextromoramide
	Etomidate
	Lidocaine
72	Flunitrazepam
	Trimetozine
73	Bupivacaine
	Camazepam
	Diazepam
	Metaclazepam
74	Diloxanide
	Famprofazone
	Fentanyl

Rf	Compound
	Isocarboxazid
	Medazepam
	Noscapine
	Prazepam
	Reserpine
75	Dimoxyline
	Quazepam
	Rescinnamine
76	Bisacodyl
	Phenoxybenzamine
77	Deserpidine
	Methoserpidine
	Methoxyamfetamine
	Thiambutosine
78	Cinnarizine
	Disulfiram
	Fenbutrazate
	Tetrabenazine
	Tiocarlide
79	Bezitramide
	Bromhexine
	Broxaldine
	Meclozine
	Phenothiazine
80	Bialamicol
	Methaqualone
81	Piperidolate
83	Buclizine
84	Diphenoxylate
89	Quazepam M (2-oxo)
99	Azinphos-methyl

System TD (p. 406)—**Rf values**

Rf	Compound
00	Aspirin salicyluric acid
	Barbituric Acid
	Carbazochrome
	Carbidopa
	Cinchophen
	Dipyrone
	Enalapril
	Levodopa
	Lysergic Acid
	Paramethadione
	Phthalylsulfacetamide
	Phthalylsulfathiazole
	Salicylic Acid salicyluric acid
	Sodium Cromoglicate
	Succinylsulfathiazole
	Sulfasalazine
	Valproic Acid
01	Baclofen
	Bumetanide
	Captopril
	Digoxin
	Furosemide
	Mafenide
	Nicotinic Acid
	Saccharin
	Sulfaguanidine
02	Chlorothiazide
	Nitrofurantoin
	Prenalterol
	Trifluperidol
03	Digitoxin
	Etacrynic Acid
	Flurazepam
	Loprazolam
	Lysergide
	Niflumic Acid

Rf	Compound
04	Acetazolamide
	Aloxiprin
	Chlortalidone
	Clozapine
	Dichlorophenoxyacetic Acid
	Ethyl Biscoumacetate
	Hydrochlorothiazide
	Quinethazone
	Sulfinpyrazone
05	Aminosalicylic Acid
	Brotizolam M (6-hydroxy)
	Sulfisomidine
	Triazolam
07	Alprazolam
	Aspirin salicylic acid
	Brotizolam M (α-hydroxy)
	Carbenoxolone
	Hydroflumethiazide
	Methocarbamol
	Salicylic Acid
08	Diflunisal
	Piroxicam M (5-hydroxy)
	Primidone
09	Meprobamate
	Methylchlorophenoxyacetic Acid
	Sulfathiazole
10	Chlordiazepoxide
	Mebutamate
11	Bufexamac
	Butalamine
	Chloramphenicol
	Chlorphenesin Carbamate
	Diphenadione
	Ethiazide
	Guaifenesin
12	Sulfamethizole

Rf	Compound
	Zomepirac
13	Bromazepam
	Epithiazide
	Midazolam
	Probenecid
	Styramate
	Sulfanilamide
	Tolmetin
14	Benzthiazide
	Diclofenamide
	Sulfaethidole
	Sulindac
15	Brotizolam
	Caffeine
	Demoxepam
	Paracetamol
	Quazepam M (3-hydroxy-*N*-dealkyl-2-oxo)
	Trichlormethiazide
16	Indometacin
	Sulfapyridine
17	Diiodohydroxyquinoline
	Sulfacetamide
18	Alclofenac
	Aspirin
	Cyclothiazide
	Dicoumarol
	Fenbufen
	Phenazone
19	Aminobenzoic Acid
	Clopamide
	Dantrolene
	Methyclothiazide
	Sulfamethoxypyridazine
21	4-Aminophenol
	Cyclopenthiazide

Rf	*Compound*
	Enoxolone
22	Oxazepam
	Phenacemide
	Polythiazide
	Sulfadiazine
23	Lorazepam
	Metolazone
	Sulfadimidine
	Sulfamerazine
	Sultiame
24	Sulfametoxydiazine
25	Aminophenazone
	Bendroflumethiazide
	Diclofenac
	Sulfafurazole
26	Benzoic Acid
	Sulfamethoxazole
27	Ketoprofen
29	Phenylmethylbarbituric Acid
	Sulfaphenazole
30	Flumazenil
	Flurbiprofen
	Glibenclamide
	Trilostane
31	Clorexolone
	Methyprylon
	Sulfadimethoxine
32	Aminoglutethimide
	Hexachlorophene
33	Apronal
	Chlorambucil
	Metaclazepam M (nor)
	Naproxen
	Phenytoin
34	Clorazepic Acid
	Nordazepam
	Quazepam M (*N*-dealkyl-2-oxo)
35	Alfadolone
	Clonazepam
	Nitrazepam
	Tetrazepam M (nor)
	Tybamate
36	Carisoprodol
37	Sulfadoxine
38	Chlorpropamide
	Etamivan
	Indapamide
	Phenacetin
	Pheneturide
	Phenolphthalein
	Salicylamide
	Vinylbital
	Xipamide
39	Acetohexamide
	Nalidixic Acid
40	Glibornuride
	Sulfametopyrazine
41	Barbital
	Mefenamic Acid
42	Fenoprofen
	Quazepam M (3-hydroxy-2-oxo)
43	Ethoxzolamide
45	Acetanilide
	Ketazolam
	Mefruside
46	Ibuprofen
	Lormetazepam
47	Metaclazepam
	Phenobarbital
	Phenprobamate
48	Aprobarbital
49	Acecarbromal
	Ethinamate
	Methylpentynol
50	Allobarbital
	Butobarbital
	Cyclobarbital
	Cyclopentobarbital
	Ethosuximide
	Heptabarb
	Ibomal
	Secbutabarbital
	Vinbarbital
51	Piroxicam
	Temazepam
	Tolbutamide
52	Acenocoumarol
	Amobarbital
	Bemegride
	Brallobarbital
	Griseofulvin
	Oxyphenbutazone
	Tolazamide
53	Carbromal
	Clobazam
	Ethotoin
	Hexethal
	Talbutal
54	Butalbital
	Chlorzoxazone
	Flunitrazepam
	Medazepam
55	Camazepam
	Idobutal
	Pentobarbital
	Secobarbital
56	Benzocaine
57	Tetrazepam
58	Diazepam
	Nealbarbital
59	Dichlorophen
	Quazepam M (2-oxo)
60	Triclocarban
61	Cholesterol
	Estradiol
	Propyphenazone
62	Benziodarone
	Mephenytoin
	Methyl Hydroxybenzoate
	Phenprocoumon
63	Carbimazole
	Glutethimide
	Methaqualone
64	Ethyl Hydroxybenzoate
	Prazepam
	Santonin
	Warfarin
65	Hexobarbital
	Phenindione
66	Metharbital
	Spironolactone
70	Methylphenobarbital
71	Enallylpropymal
	Glyceryl Trinitrate
	Phensuximide
73	Coumatetralyl
	Methohexital
	Thymol
74	Cyclandelate
75	Clofibrate
77	Thialbarbital
	Thiopental
78	Phenylbutazone
	Quazepam
80	Dantron
81	Ethchlorvynol
82	Clofenotane
91	Azinphos-methyl

System TE (p. 406)—Rf values

Rf	*Compound*
00	Acetylcysteine
	Alcuronium Chloride
	Amidefrine
	Aniline
	Aspirin salicyluric acid
	Atropine Methonitrate
	Baclofen
	Barbituric Acid
	Captopril
	Carbachol
	Carbenoxolone
	Carbidopa
	Cetrimide
	Decamethonium Bromide
	Decamethonium
	Doxorubicin
	Enalapril
	Enalaprilat
	Epirubicin
	Guanoxan
	Homatropine Methylbromide
	Hydroxyamfetamine
	Levodopa
	Lysergic Acid
	Mandelic Acid
	Metformin 80
	Methotrexate
	Narceine
	Nedocromil
	Neostigmine Methylsulfate
	Nicotinic Acid
	Obidoxime Chloride
	Ofloxacin
	Oxytetracycline Dihydrate
	Pancuronium Bromide
	Paraquat
	Pentolonium Tartrate
	Phthalylsulfacetamide
	Phthalylsulfathiazole
	Pralidoxime Mesilate
	Psilocybine
	Pyridostigmine Bromide
	Salicylic Acid salicyluric acid
	Sodium Cromoglicate
	Strophanthin-K
	Succinylsulfathiazole
	Sulfasalazine
	Suxamethonium Chloride
	Thiazinamium Metilsulfate
	Thiazinamium Metilsulfate M (sulfoxide)
	Trimetaphan Camsilate

Rf	*Compound*
	Trimethadione
	Tubocurarine Chloride
	Valproic Acid
01	Aminobenzoic Acid
	Clidinium Bromide
	Glycopyrronium Bromide
	Guanethidine
	Hexocyclium Metilsulfate
	Mupirocin
	Oxyphenonium Bromide
	Thiamine
02	Chlorothiazide
	Clenbuterol (M#2)
	Dipyrone
	Emepronium Bromide
	Mercaptopurine
	Methyldopa
	Nalidixic Acid
03	Acetazolamide
	Denatonium Benzoate
	Distigmine Bromide
	Isopropamide Iodide
	Penicillamine
	Penthienate Methobromide
	Perindopril (perindoprilat)
	Pirenzepine M (*N*-desmethyl)
	Piroxicam M (5-hydroxy)
04	Acitretin
	Alclofenac
	Bumetanide
	Dichlorophenoxyacetic Acid
	Fenbufen
	Fluorouracil
	Propantheline Bromide
	Sulfacetamide
	Sulfadiazine
	Sulfamethizole
	Sulindac
	Tiaprofenic Acid
	Zomepirac
05	Butaperazine
	Etacrynic Acid
	Glibornuride
	Glymidine Sodium
	Indometacin
	Methylchlorophenoxyacetic Acid
	Probenecid
	Propantheline Bromide M (xanthanoic acid)
	Sulfamethoxazole
	Sulfisomidine
	Tolmetin
06	Azathioprine
	Chlorambucil
	Clenbuterol (M#3)
	Fenoprofen
	Flurbiprofen
	Furosemide
	Ibuprofen
	Idarubicin
	Ketoprofen
	Lanatoside C
	Naproxen
	Nitrofurantoin
	Oxyphencyclimine
	Perindopril
	Rimiterol
	Sulfafurazole
07	Aminosalicylic Acid
	Benzoic Acid
	Enoxolone
	Glipizide
	Histamine
	Paramethadione

Rf	*Compound*
	Saccharin
	Tolazamide
	Trilostane
08	Azapropazone
	Cinchophen
	Sulfaethidole
	Sulfamerazine
	Sulfametopyrazine
	Sulfathiazole
09	Aloxiprin
	Aspirin
	Benzthiazide
	Dantrolene
	Flucytosine
	Gliclazide
	Oxymetholone
	Oxyphenbutazone
	Sulfamethoxypyridazine
	Sulfaphenazole
10	Aspirin salicylic acid
	Chlorpropamide
	Salicylic Acid
	Sulfadimethoxine
11	Glibenclamide
	Mefenamic Acid
	Methoxamine
	Niflumic Acid
	Theophylline
12	Acetohexamide
	Diclofenac
	Flunixin
	Levocabastine
	Meclofenamic Acid
	Phenylephrine
	Sulfametoxydiazine
	Tolbutamide
13	Adrenaline
	Chlorhexidine
	Coumatetralyl
	Sulfadimidine
	Xipamide
14	Azacyclonol
	Tenoxicam
	Tolfenamic Acid
	Trichlormethiazide
15	Anisindione
	Ethylnoradrenaline
	Pyridoxine
	Urea
	Xamoterol
16	Acenocoumarol
	Carbazochrome
	Diflunisal
	Hexobendine
	Pirenzepine
	Sulfinpyrazone
17	Piroxicam
	Pseudoephedrine
18	Bufexamac
	Dihydralazine
	Dihydromorphine
	Flufenamic Acid
	Hydromorphone
	Metaraminol
	Minoxidil
	Orciprenaline
	Proguanil
	Warfarin
19	Feprazone
	Methazolamide
	Phenprocoumon
20	Diazoxide
	Morphine
	Nadolol

Rf	*Compound*
	Salbutamol
21	Allopurinol
	Bambuterol Monocarbamate
	Isoprenaline
	Phenindione
	Terbutaline
	Xantinol Nicotinate
22	Atenolol
	Etilefrine
	Fendosal
	Heptaminol
23	Benziodarone
	Homatropine
	Niclosamide
	Remoxipride M (FLA-838)
24	Amiloride
	Atropine
	Ethyl Biscoumacetate
	Mescaline
	Phenylmethylbarbituric Acid
	Sulfapyridine
25	Diprophylline
	Ephedrine
	Famotidine
	Fenoterol
	Pholcodine
	Prenalterol
	Sulfaguanidine
	Tolazoline
26	Cotarnine
	Hyoscyamine
	Tetryzoline
	Thioproperazine M
	Tryptamine
27	Cimetidine
	Mafenide
	Mequitazine
	Naphazoline
	Pholedrine
	Remoxipride M(NCM-009)
	Triamcinolone
28	Brotizolam M (6-hydroxy)
	Clindamycin
	Diiodohydroxyquinoline
	Nizatidine
	Phenobarbital
29	Dihydrocodeine
	Isoniazid
	Labetalol
	Trimethoxyamfetamine (2,4,6-TMA)
30	Brallobarbital
	Clioquinol
	Dicoumarol
	Hexachlorophene
	Mesoridazine
	Ranitidine
	Sotalol
	Thiethylperazine M
	Tramazoline
	Triamterene
	Xylometazoline
31	Δ^9-Tetrahydrocannabinol
32	Barbital
	Ibomal
	Methoxyphenamine
	Nalorphine
	Strychnine
33	Acebutolol
	Bufotenine
	Chlorzoxazone
	Colchicine
	Diclofenamide
	Digoxin
	Ergometrine

Rf	*Compound*
	Hydrocodone
	Oxymorphone
	Phentolamine
34	Allobarbital
	Dichlorophen
	Dropropizine
	Hydrochlorothiazide
	Nalbuphine
	Oxymetazoline
	Propylhexedrine
	Sulpiride
	Theobromine
	Vinbarbital
35	Amantadine
	Codeine
	Fluconazole
	Methylephedrine
36	Carbamazepine M (OH-)
	Chloramphenicol
	Deptropine
	Digitoxin
	Ethylmorphine
	Hydroflumethiazide
	Isoetarine
	Lysergamide
	Maprotiline
	Nifenazone
	Pemoline
	Tiotixene M
	Viloxazine
37	Bambuterol
	Coniine
	Hydrastinine
	Hydroxychloroquine
	Ketobemidone
38	Acetophenazine
	Ambazone
	Etofylline
	Heptabarb
	Opipramol
	Oxetacaine
	Protriptyline
39	Carfenazine
	Cyclopentobarbital
	Dimpylate
	Guaifenesin
	Methylenedioxymethamfetamine
	Procainamide
	Vinylbital
40	Aprobarbital
	Bunitrolol
	Cyclobarbital
	Desipramine
	Hydroquinine
	Loprazolam
	Mephentermine
	Nicotinamide
	Paroxetine
	Quinethazone
	Sparteine
41	Butobarbital
	Demoxepam
	DOM
	Etamivan
	Idobutal
	Iproniazid
	Methylergometrine
	Methylphenobarbital
	Methylprednisolone
	Nitrofurazone
	Phenytoin
	Prednisolone
	Primidone
	Remoxipride M(NCM-001)
	Thiamazole
42	Carbimazole
	Chlortalidone
	Dextrorphan
	Dihydroergotamine
	Metamfetamine
	Methylenedioxyamfetamine
	Perphenazine
43	Amfetamine
	Clenbuterol M (hydroxy)
	Dantron
	Dopamine
	Ethoxzolamide
	Hydroquinidine
	Lorazepam
	Methoxyamfetamine
	Pindolol
	Pipamperone
	Tertatolol
	Thialbarbital
	Thioproperazine
44	Amobarbital
	Butalbital
	Cinchonidine
	Cinchonine
	Clopenthixol
	Dipyridamole
	Epithiazide
	Ergotamine
	Hexethal
	Methyl Hydroxybenzoate
	Metoprolol
	Nealbarbital
	Pilocarpine
	Tiotixene
	Tocainide
	Triazolam
	Zuclopenthixol
45	Brotizolam M (α-hydroxy)
	Fluphenazine
	Hydrocortisone
	Methysergide
	Nicotinyl Alcohol
	Oxazepam
	Oxprenolol
	Paracetamol
	Pentobarbital
	Phenazone
	Prednisone
	Quinine
	Secobarbital
	Thebaine
	Trimethoprim
46	Chloroquine
	Chlorphenamine
	Diphenadione
	Erythromycin
	Ethyl Hydroxybenzoate
	Flupentixol
	Fluvoxamine
	Furazolidone
	Glafenine
	Metaclazepam M (dinor)
	Metronidazole
	Pheniramine
	Phenmetrazine
	Talbutal
	Thiopropazate M
47	Alprazolam
	Antazoline
	Dextromethorphan
	Dimetindene
	Fluoxetine
	Fluoxetine M (nor)
	Methocarbamol
	Metipranolol
	Naloxone
	Perazine
	Psilocin
	Trimethobenzamide
	Zopiclone
48	Bisoprolol
	Chlorphentermine
	Fenpipramide
	Hyoscine
	Phentermine
	Pipazetate
	Secbutabarbital
	Tofenacin
	Zimeldine
49	Alprenolol
	Diamorphine
	Dimethoxanate
	Dixyrazine
	Dobutamine
	Flecainide
	Harmaline
	Propranolol
	Proxyphylline
	Quazepam M (3-hydroxy-*N*-dealkyl-2-oxo)
	Quinidine
	Thebacon
	Thiopental
50	Carbinoxamine
	Dimethyltryptamine
	Ethiazide
	Fluocortolone
	Ketoconazole
	Resorcinol
	Salicylamide
	Timolol
51	Astemizole M (nor)
	Betaxolol
	Granisetron
	Metoclopramide
	Pericyazine
	Sulfanilamide
	Tropicamide
52	Bendroflumethiazide
	Brotizolam
	Caffeine
	Chlordiazepoxide
	Chlorphenesin Carbamate
	Etizolam
	Gelsemine
	Harmine
	Hordenine
	Ketotifen
	Moclobemide
	Thenalidine
	Thiethylperazine
53	Emetine
	Hexobarbital
	Lofexidine
	Mazindol
	Methyclothiazide
	Phenolphthalein
	Pipotiazine
	Propyl Hydroxybenzoate
	Styramate
54	Acetylcodeine
	Encainide
	Fenetylline
	Hydroxyzine
	Loxapine
	Metharbital
	Oxcarbazepine

Rf	*Compound*
	Phanquinone
	Phenethylamine
	Pyrazinamide
	Remoxipride
	Sulforidazine
55	Clopamide
	Clozapine
	Dibenzepin
	Ethoheptazine
	Mexiletine
	Pentoxifylline
	Physostigmine
	Prochlorperazine
	Thiamylal
	Trifluoperazine
	Triprolidine
56	Ajmaline
	Amygdalin
	Carbamazepine
	Etafedrine
	Lysergide
	Meprobamate
	Tizanidine
57	Acecarbromal
	Aminoacridine
	Harman
	Metolazone
	Sultiame
	Vinblastine
58	Apomorphine
	Clemastine
	Clenbuterol
	Droperidol
	Enallylpropymal
	Mepyramine
	Methohexital
	Morazone
	Nimorazole
	Pyrimethamine
	Tranylcypromine
59	4-Aminophenol
	Arecoline
	Cyclothiazide
	Embutramide
	Lormetazepam
	Nefopam
	Nikethamide
	Perhexiline
	Prazosin
	Prothipendyl
60	Aminopromazine
	Clorexolone
	Disopyramide
	Doxylamine
	Eucatropine
	Hexylresorcinol
	Mebendazole
	Mebutamate
	Midazolam
	Pargyline
	Pentetrazol
	Pethidine
61	Fenfluramine
	Flumazenil
	Halofantrine M (desbutyl)
	Metixene
	Nicotine
	Piritramide
	Trichlorfon
62	Alphaprodine
	Aminophenazone
	Amiphenazole
	Buphenine
	Carbocromen

Rf	*Compound*
	Chlorphenesin
	Isoxsuprine
	Oxycodone
	Phendimetrazine
	Promazine
	Temazepam
63	Acepromazine
	Bromazepam
	Chloropyramine
	Diethyltryptamine
	Doxepin
	Isopropylaminophenazone
	Methdilazine
	Methyprylon
	Polythiazide
64	Astemizole
	Cyclopentolate
	Cyproheptadine
	Isothipendyl
	Metyrapone
	Nitrazepam
	Nomifensine
	Pizotifen
	Tetracaine
	Yohimbine
65	Aminoglutethimide
	Cyclazocine
	Diphenhydramine
	Dosulepin
	Levamisole
	Mebhydrolin
	Pecazine
	Phenacemide
	Phenylbutazone
	Promethazine
	Thenyldiamine
	Thonzylamine
	Tybamate
66	Cyclopentamine
	Cyclopenthiazide
	Ethosuximide
	Indapamide
	Mepivacaine
	Methapyrilene
	Methylphenidate
	Noxiptiline
	Pentifylline
	Tetramisole
	Trazodone
67	Apronal
	Chlorcyclizine
	Cinchocaine
	Clonazepam
	Imipramine
	Meclofenoxate
	Mefruside
	Nifuratel
	Nordazepam
	Oxeladin
	Phenyltoloxamine
	Thioridazine
68	Bemegride
	Chlormezanone
	Clorazepic Acid
	Cortisone
	Cyclizine
	Dimenhydrinate
	Diphenylpyraline
	Fluorometholone
	Flutazolam
	Mianserin
	Nicametate
	Orphenadrine
	Phenacetin

Rf	*Compound*
	Phenindamine
	Propiomazine
	Simvastatin
	Tolpropamine
	Trimetozine
	Tripelennamine
69	Amitriptyline
	Crotetamide
	Cyclobenzaprine
	Griseofulvin
	Papaverine
	Quazepam M (3-hydroxy-2-oxo)
70	Acetanilide
	Chlorphenoxamine
	Chlorpromazine
	Clonidine
	Lidoflazine
	Pentazocine
	Phenazopyridine
	Pirenzepine M (desamide)
	Testosterone
71	Alfadolone
	Ethinylestradiol
	Ethotoin
	Etynodiol Diacetate
	Flurazepam
	Fluspirilene
	Hexoprenaline
	Hydrastine
	Nifedipine
	Phenaglycodol
	Pheneturide
	Pimozide
	Procaine
	Pyrrobutamine
	Veratrine
72	Androsterone
	Azaperone
	Clomipramine
	Doxapram
	Etorphine
	Methyl Nicotinate
	Pentaerithrityl Tetranitrate
	Propanidid
	Quazepam M (*N*-dealkyl-2-oxo)
	Sertraline
73	Diethylstilbestrol
	Doxazosin
	Etomidate
	Hexestrol
	Metaclazepam M (nor)
	Methylpiperidyl Benzilate
	Methyltestosterone
	Nicergoline
	Phenprobamate
	Pramocaine
	Tetrazepam M (nor)
	Verapamil
74	Amodiaquine
	Chlorprothixene
	Cropropamide
	Etamiphylline
	Flunitrazepam
	Indoramin
	Isradipine
	Ketazolam
	Levallorphan
	Loperamide
	Mephenytoin
	Methylpentynol
	Metomidate
	Phenazocine
	Procyclidine
	Propyphenazone

Rf	*Compound*
	Thiopropazate
75	Aconitine
	Butanilicaine
	Camazepam
	Carbromal
	Carisoprodol
	Clobazam
	Econazole
	Etidocaine
	Histapyrrodine
	Isocarboxazid
	Lobeline
	Mevinphos
	Prilocaine
	Santonin
	Triclocarban
	Triflupromazine
76	Ambucetamide
	Aprindine
	Cholesterol
	Clomethiazole
	Clotrimazole
	Diazepam
	Estrone
	Etenzamide
	Ethambutol
	Ethinamate
	Fenyramidol
	Haloperidol
	Levomepromazine
	Mecloqualone
	Methanthelinium Bromide
	Methoxsalen
	Norethisterone
	Phenoperidine
	Piperocaine
77	Alimemazine
	Benzocaine
	Captodiame
	Cocaine
	Diethazine
	Felodipine
	Fencamfamin
	Fenproporex
	Flavoxate
	Methadone
	Phensuximide
	Reserpine
	Trifluperidol
78	Azapetine
	Clemizole
	Disulfiram
	Estradiol
	Etofenamate
	Fentanyl
	Loratadine
	Medazepam
	Methaqualone
	Mexazolam
	Naftidrofuryl Oxalate
	Nimodipine
	Noscapine
	Oxypertine
	Spironolactone
	Tramadol
	Xylazine
79	Anileridine
	Dextromoramide
	Hexetidine
	Itraconazole
	Ketamine
	Metaclazepam
	Progesterone
	Prolintane
	Sulfadoxine
	Tetrabenazine
	Tetrazepam
80	Bupivacaine
	Buprenorphine
	Cyclandelate
	Glutethimide
	Hexylcaine
	Hydralazine
	Lidocaine
	Lorcainide
	Methandienone
	Miconazole
	Nitrendipine
	Norpipanone
	Procarbazine
	Quazepam M (2-oxo)
	Trimipramine
81	Butetamate
	Demeton-*S*
	Deserpidine
	Diethylthiambutene
	Isoaminile
	Lacidipine
	Pipradrol
	Prazepam
	Rescinnamine
	Thymol
82	Amiodarone
	Clomifene
	Fluanisone
	Phenothiazine
	Piperidolate
83	Adiphenine
	Biperiden
	Butacaine
	Crotamiton
	Dichlorvos
	Gestonorone Caproate
	Oxybuprocaine
	Phenelzine
	Profenamine
	Quazepam
	Trihexyphenidyl
84	Clofibrate
	Dicycloverine
	Methyl Salicylate
	Penfluridol
	Phencyclidine
	Prenylamine
	Tilidate
85	Diethylpropion
	Floctafenine
	Hydroxyprogesterone
	Nisoldipine
86	Butalamine
	Cinnarizine
	Clofazimine
	Fenbutrazate
	Fludrocortisone Acetate
	Glyceryl Trinitrate
	Ibogaine
	Lindane
	Mebeverine
	Mesuximide
87	Benzfetamine
	Chlordane
	Clofenotane
	Dimoxyline
	Diphenoxylate
	Dipipanone
	Famprofazone
	Meclozine
	Metenolone
	Methoxychlor
	Phenoxybenzamine
88	Halofantrine
	Paramethasone
	Piminodine
89	Dieldrin
	Heptachlor
90	Lofepramine
91	Difenidol
94	Diquat
95	Cannabidiol
	Cannabinol
99	Azinphos-methyl
	Chlorpyrifos
	Dimethoate
	Malathion

System TF (p. 406)—**Rf values**

Rf	*Compound*
00	Acetylcysteine
	Aspirin salicyluric acid
	Baclofen
	Barbituric Acid
	Betaxolol
	Bezafibrate
	Bisoprolol
	Carbazochrome
	Cinchophen
	Clenbuterol (M#2)
	Dipyrone
	Dosulepin *S*-oxide
	Doxorubicin
	Enalapril
	Enalaprilat
	Epirubicin
	Fenoterol
	Idarubicin
	Levodopa
	Lysergic Acid
	Mandelic Acid
	Mercaptopurine
	Methotrexate
	Metipranolol
	Mupirocin
	Nedocromil
	Neostigmine Methylsulfate
	Nicotinic Acid
	Ofloxacin
	Perindoprilat
	Perindopril
	Phthalylsulfacetamide
	Phthalylsulfathiazole
	Pralidoxime Mesilate
	Pyridostigmine Bromide
	Salbutamol

Rf	*Compound*
	Salicyluric acid
	Sodium Cromoglicate
	Succinylsulfathiazole
	Sulfasalazine
	Sulforidazine
	Thiazinamium Metilsulfate M (sulfoxide)
	Trimetaphan Camsilate
	Trimethadione
	Xamoterol
	Xantinol Nicotinate
	Zopiclone
01	Alphaprodine
	Captopril
	Labetalol
	Loprazolam
	Mafenide
	Pecazine
	Saccharin
	Salicylic Acid
	Tertatolol
02	Alprazolam
	Carbidopa
	Etacrynic Acid
	Levocabastine
	Prenalterol
	Triazolam
03	Benperidol
	Flurazepam
	Glafenine
	Niflumic Acid
	Tropicamide
04	Brotizolam M (6-hydroxy)
	Sulfinpyrazone
	Theobromine
05	Clozapine
	Diflunisal
	Digoxin
	Midazolam
	Tiaprofenic Acid
	Trifluperidol
06	Dichlorophenoxyacetic Acid
	Etofylline
	Sulfaguanidine
	Tenoxicam
07	Furosemide
	Miconazole
08	xanthanoic acid
09	Metaclazepam M (dinor)
	Theophylline
10	Aloxiprin
	Aminophenazone
	Bumetanide
	Caffeine
	Digitoxin
	Sulindac
11	Chlordiazepoxide
	Itraconazole
	Methylchlorophenoxyacetic Acid
	Nitrofurazone
	Pemoline
12	Zomepirac
13	Indometacin
14	Flumazenil
	Phenazone
16	Chlorothiazide
	Sulfisomidine
17	Carbenoxolone
	Guaifenesin
18	Bromazepam
	Furazolidone
	Piroxicam M (5-hydroxy)
19	Bufexamac
	Clenbuterol (M#3)
	Diiodohydroxyquinoline
20	Fluorouracil
	Methylenedioxymethamfetamine
	Oxcarbazepine
	Sulfathiazole
	Tolmetin
21	Quinethazone
23	Fluanisone
	Methocarbamol
	Primidone
	Probenecid
	Sulfamethizole
24	Aminosalicylic Acid
	Demoxepam
	Prednisolone
25	Denatonium Benzoate
	Dinitro-orthocresol
	Ketoprofen
	Metaclazepam M (nor)
	Methyprylon
27	Diclofenac
	Methylprednisolone
28	Alclofenac
	Benzoic Acid
	Fluocortolone
	Hydrocortisone
	Prednisone
	Quazepam M (3-hydroxy-*N*-dealkyl-2-oxo)
29	Butalamine
	Loratadine
30	Aspirin
	Fenbufen
	Flurbiprofen
	Glibenclamide
	Nitrofurantoin
31	Acetazolamide
	Chloramphenicol
	Nalidixic Acid
	Tolfenamic Acid
32	Camazepam
	Dicoumarol
	Ethyl Biscoumacetate
	Paracetamol
33	Diphenadione
34	Chlorphenesin Carbamate
	Hexachlorophene
	Hydrochlorothiazide
35	Etamivan
	Mebutamate
	Metaclazepam
	Oxazepam
	Sulfaethidole
36	Dantrolene
	Meprobamate
37	Griseofulvin
	Phenacetin
38	Clopamide
	Fenoprofen
	Naproxen
	Piroxicam
39	Styramate
	Sulfadiazine
	Sulfamethoxypyridazine
40	Alfadolone
	4-Aminophenol
	Chlorambucil
	Chlortalidone
	Medazepam
	Phenacemide
41	Lorazepam
	Sulfamerazine
42	Sulfacetamide
	Sulfapyridine
43	Acetohexamide
	Acitretin
	Aminobenzoic Acid
	Chlorpropamide
	Meclofenamic Acid
	Nifuratel
	Sulfametoxydiazine
	Sultiame
44	Simvastatin
45	Acetanilide
	Clonazepam
	Isotretinoin
	Ketazolam
	Lormetazepam
	Nordazepam
	Quazepam M (*N*-dealkyl-2-oxo)
	Sulfadimidine
	Testosterone
	Tetrazepam M (nor)
	Trilostane
46	Clorazepic Acid
	Enoxolone
	Nitrazepam
	Sulfanilamide
47	Aminoglutethimide
	Carbimazole
	Clobazam
	Flunitrazepam
	Hydroflumethiazide
	Methyltestosterone
	Temazepam
48	Acecarbromal
	Acenocoumarol
	Mefenamic Acid
49	Benzbromarone
	Diazepam
	Propyphenazone
	Tetrazepam
50	Ethiazide
	Methyclothiazide
	Santonin
	Sulfametopyrazine
	Tolazamide
51	Benzthiazide
	Clorexolone
	Metolazone
	Spironolactone
	Sulfadimethoxine
	Sulfadoxine
	Sulfaphenazole
52	Androsterone
	Apronal
	Fluorometholone
	Quazepam M (3-hydroxy-2-oxo)
	Sulfafurazole
	Valproic Acid
53	Bemegride
	Carisoprodol
	Ethosuximide
	Pheneturide
54	Ethotoin
	Sulfamethoxazole
55	Carbromal
	Mexazolam
	Phenprobamate
	Phenytoin
	Prazepam
	Salicylamide
	Tolbutamide
56	Phenindione
	Progesterone
57	Etynodiol Diacetate
	Ibuprofen
	Norethisterone
	Quazepam M (2-oxo)

Rf	*Compound*
58	Benziodarone
	Estradiol
	Mefruside
	Mephenytoin
	Methoxsalen
	Phenprocoumon
59	Ethinamate
	Gestonorone Caproate
	Isradipine
	Phenolphthalein
	Phensuximide
	Triclocarban
60	Cholesterol
	Cyclothiazide
	Felodipine
	Glibornuride
	Paramethadione
	Polythiazide
	Trichlormethiazide
61	Barbital
	Chlorzoxazone
	Indapamide
	Phenylmethylbarbituric Acid
62	Benzocaine
	Cyclopenthiazide
	Epithiazide
	Glutethimide
	Metenolone
	Methylpentynol
	Oxyphenbutazone
	Warfarin
63	Hydroxyprogesterone
64	Cyclobarbital
	Diclofenamide
	Dimpylate
	Heptabarb
	Secbutabarbital
	Vinylbital
	Xipamide
65	Aprobarbital
	Butobarbital
	Cyclopentobarbital
	Ethoxzolamide
	Hexobarbital
	Hexylresorcinol
	Lacidipine
	Metharbital
	Methyl Hydroxybenzoate
	Nisoldipine
	Phenobarbital
	Vinbarbital
66	Allobarbital
	Amobarbital
	Clofibrate
	Ethyl Hydroxybenzoate
	Ibomal
	Pentobarbital
67	Butalbital
	Dichlorophen
	Hexethal
	Methylphenobarbital
	Propyl Hydroxybenzoate
	Talbutal
68	Brallobarbital
	Diethylstilbestrol
	Estrone
	Methyl Salicylate
	Nealbarbital
	Phenylbutazone
	Secobarbital
	Thymol
	Tybamate
69	Dantron
	Idobutal
70	Clidinium Bromide
	Hexestrol
71	Bendroflumethiazide
	Enallylpropymal
	Quazepam
72	Chlordane
	Glyceryl Trinitrate
	Methohexital
	Methoxychlor
	Thialbarbital
73	Benzyl Benzoate
74	Clofenotane
	Coumatetralyl
	Dieldrin
	Ethchlorvynol
	Thiopental
75	Heptachlor
	Lindane
	Thiamylal
77	Cyclandelate
93	Azinphos-methyl

System TG (p. 407)—**Rf values**

Rf	*Compound*
08	Indoprofen
09	Fenbufen
10	Tolmetin
12	Alclofenac
13	Sulindac
14	Benoxaprofen
	Ketoprofen
	Naproxen
16	Fenoprofen
	Flurbiprofen
18	Ibuprofen
19	Furosemide
20	Fenclofenac
	Indometacin
23	Phenylbutazone
	Salsalate
25	Oxyphenbutazone
28	Niflumic Acid
29	Diclofenac
30	Clonixin
32	Mefenamic Acid
33	Flunixin
	Theophylline
36	Bufexamac
37	Diflunisal
	Flufenamic Acid
38	Meclofenamic Acid
45	Feprazone
47	Theobromine

System TH (p. 410)—**Rf values**

Rf	*Compound*
03	Barbituric Acid
27	Phenylmethylbarbituric Acid
38	Phenobarbital
47	Brallobarbital
51	Barbital
53	Allobarbital
56	Vinbarbital
59	Cyclobarbital
61	Ibomal
62	Cyclopentobarbital
	Heptabarb
66	Aprobarbital
67	Butalbital
68	Butobarbital
69	Secbutabarbital
71	Idobutal
	Talbutal
72	Methylphenobarbital
74	Amobarbital
	Hexethal
75	Thialbarbital
76	Pentobarbital
78	Nealbarbital
	Secobarbital
80	Thiopental
85	Hexobarbital
86	Metharbital
87	Enallylpropymal
93	Methohexital

System TI (p. 415)—**Rf values**

Rf	*Compound*
05	Cannabidiol
30	Δ^9-Tetrahydrocannabinol
52	Cannabinol

System TJ (p. 415)—Rf values

Rf	*Compound*
20	Cannabinol
29	Δ^9-Tetrahydrocannabinol
36	Cannabidiol

System TL (p. 405)—Rf values

Rf	*Compound*
00	Adrenaline
	Bamethan
	Benzalkonium Chloride
	Berberine
	Buformin
	Carbachol
	Cetrimide
	Cetylpyridinium Chloride
	Cinchophen
	Cotarnine
	Debrisoquine
	Decamethonium Bromide
	Decamethonium
	Diminazene (aceturate)
	Diquat
	Dopamine
	Guanethidine
	Guanoclor
	Guanoxan
	Histamine
	Homatropine Methylbromide
	Hydrastinine
	Hydroxystilbamidine
	Isoetarine
	Isopropamide Iodide
	Lysergic Acid
	Mequitazine
	Metformin
	Minoxidil
	Narceine
	Obidoxime Chloride
	Oxyphencyclimine
	Oxyphenonium Bromide
	Pancuronium Bromide
	Paraquat
	Pentamidine
	Pentapiperide Metilsulfate
	Pentolonium Tartrate
	Phenformin
	Phenylephrine
	Piperazine
	Propantheline Bromide
	Pseudomorphine
	Psilocybine
	Suxamethonium Chloride
	Thiamine
	Thiazinamium Metilsulfate
	Tubocurarine Chloride
01	Acefylline Piperazine
	Atropine
	Azacyclonol
	Brucine
	Bufotenine
	Chlorproguanil
	Cytarabine
	Deptropine
	Dihydralazine
	Dihydromorphine
	Dimethoate
	Ephedrine
	Hexoprenaline
	Homatropine
	Mesoridazine
	Methyldopa
	Morphine
	Nadolol
	Oxymetazoline
	Proguanil
	Propamidine
	Trimetazidine
02	Amidefrine
	Amiloride
	Atenolol
	Benzatropine
	Chloroquine
	Chlorphenamine
	Cyclopentamine
	Cycloserine
	Cytisine
	Dehydroemetine
	Dihydrocodeine
	Dipyrone
	Ethambutol
	Hydromorphone
	Maprotiline
	Mephentermine
	Methoxyphenamine
	Phentolamine
	Pholcodine
	Protriptyline
	Racemorphan
	Strychnine
	Tetryzoline
	Tolazoline
	Tramazoline
03	Acetophenazine
	Antazoline
	Benserazide
	Broxyquinoline
	Codeine
	Conessine
	Desipramine
	Dextrorphan
	Dobutamine
	Etilefrine
	Hydroquinine
	Hydroxychloroquine
	Isoprenaline
	Methenamine
	Penicillamine
	Perazine
	Pheniramine
	Pholedrine
	Xylometazoline
04	Amantadine
	Azathioprine
	Carbinoxamine
	Diamorphine
	Ethoheptazine
	Fenoterol
	Hydrocodone
	Mecamylamine
	Neopine
	Nialamide
	Practolol
	Procarbazine
	Quinine
	Salbutamol
05	Butaperazine
	Cinchonine
	Coniine
	Diethylcarbamazine
	Glipizide
	Heptaminol
	Hordenine
	Hydroquinidine
	Loprazolam
	Metamfetamine
	Pyridoxine
	Sotalol
	Sparteine
	Terbutaline
	Thebaine
06	Acebutolol
	Brompheniramine
	Cinchonidine
	Dextromethorphan
	Dimethoxanate
	Dimethyltryptamine
	Dimetindene
	Ethylmorphine
	Hexobendine
	Ketobemidone
	Lysergamide
	Methdilazine
	Orciprenaline
	Perhexiline
	Pipazetate
	Protokylol
	Quinidine
	Thioproperazine
	Triprolidine
	Viloxazine
07	Carfenazine
	Opipramol
	Prochlorperazine
	Propranolol
	Tigloidine
	Tiotixene
	Tofenacin
08	Ambazone
	Aminopromazine
	Benzylmorphine
	Cephaëline
	Chlorphentermine
	Diphenylpyraline
	Ergometrine
	Phenglutarimide
	Pindolol
	Pipamperone
	Profadol
	Sulfacarbamide
	Thiethylperazine
	Trifluoperazine
09	Azaperone
	Benzydamine
	Clemastine
	Clioquinol
	Doxylamine
	Mepacrine
	Metoprolol
	Mexiletine

Rf	*Compound*
	Perphenazine
	Procainamide
	Prothipendyl
	Psilocin
	Timolol
10	Fluphenazine
	Pempidine
	Tacrine
11	Alphaprodine
	Alprenolol
	Clopenthixol
	Diethyltryptamine
	Fenfluramine
	Hydroxyamfetamine
	Pethidine
	Promazine
	Thebacon
	Theophylline
	Tryptamine
	Zuclopenthixol
12	Acepromazine
	Acetylcodeine
	Carbocromen
	Cimetidine
	Colchicine
	Diprophylline
	Emetine
	Eucatropine
	Mescaline
	Methylergometrine
	Metixene
	Metopimazine
	Phentermine
	Pilocarpine
	Thenalidine
	Thenyldiamine
	Trimethoprim
	Trimethoxyamfetamine (2,4,6-TMA)
13	Bamipine
	Bromazine
	Brotizolam M (6-hydroxy)
	Cyproheptadine
	Disopyramide
	Doxepin
	Imipramine
	Mazindol
	Methapyrilene
	Metoclopramide
	Nicotine
	Oxprenolol
	Thioridazine
14	Alprazolam
	Chlorcyclizine
	Dibenzepin
	Dihydroergotamine
	Fenetylline
	Isothipendyl
	Mepyramine
	Phenmetrazine
	Thonzylamine
15	Amitriptyline
	Dimenhydrinate
	Diphenhydramine
	Etafedrine
	Fenpipramide
	Methysergide
	Oxetacaine
	Phenyltoloxamine
	Primaquine
	Tolpropamine
	Tripelennamine
16	Cyclizine
	DOM
	Dosulepin
	Inositol Nicotinate
	Iprindole
	Orphenadrine
	Pecazine
	Tetracaine
	Triazolam
17	Chloropyramine
	Chlorphenoxamine
	Chlorpromazine
	Clozapine
	Etamiphylline
	Iproniazid
	Methylenedioxyamfetamine
	Nefopam
	Phanquinone
	Piperacetazine
	Promethazine
	Trimeperidine
	Veratrine
18	Amfetamine
	Clomipramine
	Hyoscine
	Pericyazine
	Physostigmine
	Pyrrobutamine
19	Hydroxyzine
	Midazolam
	Moxisylyte
	Oxeladin
20	Clorprenaline
	Hexetidine
	Isoniazid
	Mebhydrolin
	Nicametate
21	Phenindamine
	Pipotiazine
	Pyrimethamine
	Theobromine
22	Chlordiazepoxide
	Ethiazide
	Loperamide
	Meclofenoxate
	Nicotinyl Alcohol
	Triflupromazine
23	Clotiapine
	Ergotamine
	Methylphenidate
	Mianserin
	Procyclidine
24	Dimefline
	Ethylnoradrenaline
	Lysergide
	Metaraminol
	Phendimetrazine
	Tuaminoheptane
25	Caffeine
	Chlorprothixene
	Cyclazocine
	Cyclomethycaine
	Dyclonine
	Octamylamine
	Prolintane
	Salinazid
26	Cyclopentolate
	Propiomazine
27	Apomorphine
	Brotizolam
	Methadone
	Nicotinamide
	Piperocaine
28	Dimetotiazine
	Harmine
	Lorazepam
	Pentazocine
	Propoxycaine
	Quinisocaine
29	Clofedanol
	Co-dergocrine Mesilate
	Lobeline
	Nalorphine
	Nikethamide
	Proxyphylline
	Vinblastine
30	Fencamfamin
	Oxymorphone
	Procaine
31	Alimemazine
	Brotizolam M (α-hydroxy)
	Morazone
	Nomifensine
32	Benperidol
	Morinamide
33	Haloperidol
	Harman
	Methylpiperidyl Benzilate
	Nimorazole
	Norharman
34	Bamifylline
35	Cinchocaine
	Clomifene
	Naftidrofuryl Oxalate
	Proxymetacaine
	Rimantadine
36	Benzquinamide
	Droperidol
	Ethomoxane
	Lidoflazine
	Oxybuprocaine
37	Amodiaquine
	Chloroprocaine
	Miconazole
	Trazodone
	Trimipramine
38	Alverine
	Butriptyline
	Methoxamine
	Norpipanone
	Quazepam M (3-hydroxy-*N*-dealkyl-2-oxo)
39	Diethazine
	Oxycodone
	Phenethylamine
	Pipradrol
40	Flurazepam
	Furaltadone
	Glafenine
	Metronidazole
	Pemoline
	Pimozide
41	Diazoxide
	Metyrapone
	Pipobroman
	Pramocaine
42	Aletamine
	Dipyridamole
	Levamisole
	Piritramide
	Thiopropazate
	Verapamil
43	Benethamine
	Benzoctamine
	Diethylthiambutene
44	Flumazenil
45	Flavoxate
	Levallorphan
46	Levomepromazine
	Pentifylline
	Pyrazinamide

Rf	Compound
	Tetramisole
47	Butetamate
	Carbamazepine
	Chlorzoxazone
	Papaverine
48	Chloramphenicol
	Ergotoxine
	Mepivacaine
	Metomidate
	Tranylcypromine
49	Fluspirilene
	Mebendazole
	Mebeverine
	Phenazocine
	Prazosin
50	Buphenine
	Lormetazepam
51	Adiphenine
	Anileridine
	Demoxepam
	Difenidol
	Oxazepam
52	Clemizole
	Etomidate
	Hydrastine
	Trifluomeprazine
	Trimetozine
	Yohimbine
53	Benactyzine
	Bromazepam
	Clonidine
	Isoxsuprine
	Niridazole
	Phenazopyridine
	Styramate
	Temazepam
	Tiabendazole
54	Cocaine
	Dicycloverine
	Doxapram
55	Amiodarone
	Crotetamide
	Etenzamide
	Ethionamide
	Isoaminile
	Nitrazepam
	Piperidolate
	Propanidid
56	Azapetine
	Mebutamate
	Methaqualone
	Pipoxolan
	Prenylamine
57	Amiphenazole
	Chlormezanone
	Cropropamide
	Mephenesin
	Protionamide
58	Aconitine
	Clomethiazole
	Dimoxyline
	Fentanyl
	Meprobamate
	Metaclazepam M (nor)
	Oxypertine
	Phenoperidine
	Quazepam M (*N*-dealkyl-2-oxo)
59	Clorgiline
	Diazepam
	Fenyramidol
	Furazolidone
	Methyl Nicotinate
	Piminodine
	Quazepam M (3-hydroxy-2-oxo)
	Thiamazole
	Trihexyphenidyl
60	Benzyl Nicotinate
	Clorazepic Acid
	Cycrimine
	Dextromoramide
	Fluanisone
	Nordazepam
	Penfluridol
	Prilocaine
	Tetrazepam M (nor)
61	Ambucetamide
	Bromocriptine
	Butanilicaine
	Clonazepam
	Isocarboxazid
	Nicofuranose
62	Benorilate
	Butoxyethyl Nicotinate
	Clobazam
	Ibogaine
	Medazepam
	Metaclazepam
63	Etorphine
	Flunitrazepam
	Lidocaine
	Mebanazine
	Naloxone
	Pentetrazol
	Phenelzine
	Prazepam
	Pseudoephedrine
	Reserpine
64	Beclamide
	Biperiden
	Butacaine
	Diethylpropion
	Hydralazine
	Ketamine
	Methoserpidine
	Norbormide
	Noscapine
	Rescinnamine
65	Bupivacaine
	Camazepam
	Cinnarizine
66	Benzocaine
	Bisacodyl
	Deserpidine
	Diperodon
	Ketazolam
	Phencyclidine
	Profenamine
	Tetrazepam
67	Azapropazone
	Diloxanide
	Etoxazene
	Famprofazone
	Fenbutrazate
	Tetrabenazine
68	Clefamide
	Clofazimine
	Nifedipine
	Phenoxybenzamine
69	Buprenorphine
	Cholesterol
	Disulfiram
	Methoxyamfetamine
	Metisazone
	Thiambutosine
70	Benzfetamine
	Bezitramide
	Buclosamide
	Butyl Aminobenzoate
	Diphenoxylate
	Dipipanone
	Meclozine
71	Bromhexine
	Broxaldine
	Phenothiazine
	Quazepam M (2-oxo)
72	Buclizine
	Tiocarlide
73	Bialamicol
76	Quazepam
99	Azinphos-methyl

System TM (p. 418)—Rf values

Rf	Compound
00	Lysergic Acid
26	Ergometrine
27	Lysergamide
31	Methylergometrine
33	Methysergide
40	Dihydroergotamine
48	Ergotamine
64	Co-dergocrine Mesilate
67	Ergotoxine
70	Lysergide

System TN (p. 422)—Rf values

Rf	Compound
22	Paraquat
34	Gallamine Triethiodide
35	Suxamethonium Chloride
36	Hexamethonium Bromide
40	Suxethonium Bromide
56	Decamethonium Bromide
	Guanethidine
60	Choline
70	Acetylcholine Chloride

Rf	*Compound*
80	Pancuronium Bromide
85	Tubocurarine Chloride
94	Bretylium Tosilate
95	Atropine Methonitrate
100	Cetrimide

System TO (p. 422)—Rf values

Rf	*Compound*
05	Gallamine Triethiodide
10	Hexamethonium Bromide
	Paraquat
	Suxamethonium Chloride
16	Decamethonium Bromide
23	Suxethonium Bromide
35	Atropine Methonitrate
40	Bretylium Tosilate
	Tubocurarine Chloride
50	Cetrimide
	Guanethidine
60	Acetylcholine Chloride
	Choline

System TP (p. 422)—Rf values

Rf	*Compound*
00	Hydrocortisone Sodium Phosphate
08	Hydrocortisone Hydrogen Succinate
09	Triamcinolone
20	Prednisolone
23	Methylprednisolone
27	Hydrocortisone
30	Betamethasone
32	Dexamethasone
	Triamcinolone acetonide
41	Prednisone
42	Fluocinolone Acetonide
51	Fluoxymesterone
	Hydrocortisone acetate
58	Betamethasone valerate
	Fludrocortisone acetate
59	Alfadolone
60	Alfaxalone
	Testosterone
65	Diethylstilbestrol
	Methandienone
69	Oxymetholone
70	Methyltestosterone
71	Norethandrolone
	Norethisterone
72	Cortisone
	Dienestrol
	Ethinylestradiol
75	Beclometasone
77	Lynestrenol
78	Androstanolone
	Ethisterone
	Fluocortolone hexanoate
	Testosterone propionate
79	Estradiol benzoate
	Ethylestrenol
	Methallenestril
	Noretynodrel
80	Dimethisterone
	Medroxyprogesterone Acetate
	Megestrol Acetate
81	Hydroxyprogesterone Caproate
	Progesterone
83	Etynodiol Diacetate
86	Desoxycortone
	Dydrogesterone
	Mestranol
	Testosterone Phenylpropionate
87	Norethisterone Acetate
88	Chlorotrianisene
	Nandrolone

System TQ (p. 422)—Rf values

Rf	*Compound*
00	Betamethasone
	Hydrocortisone Hydrogen Succinate
	Hydrocortisone Sodium Phosphate
	Prednisolone
	Prednisone
	Triamcinolone
	Triamcinolone acetonide
02	Hydrocortisone
07	Testosterone
08	Dexamethasone
	Fluocinolone Acetonide
09	Fluoxymesterone
10	Diethylstilbestrol
	Methandienone
11	Androstanolone
	Hydrocortisone Acetate
12	Fludrocortisone Acetate
	Testosterone Propionate
16	Methyltestosterone
18	Methallenestril
20	Norethandrolone
	Progesterone
22	Alfadolone
	Alfaxalone
	Norethisterone
23	Oxymetholone
25	Dienestrol
27	Betamethasone Valerate
28	Cortisone
	Testosterone Phenylpropionate
30	Ethinylestradiol
32	Estradiol benzoate
	Noretynodrel
35	Fluocortolone Hexanoate
38	Beclometasone
39	Ethisterone
	Norethisterone Acetate
42	Dimethisterone
49	Nandrolone
50	Ethylestrenol
	Medroxyprogesterone Acetate
	Megestrol Acetate
52	Desoxycortone
	Mestranol
53	Dydrogesterone
55	Hydroxyprogesterone Caproate
	Lynestrenol
61	Etynodiol Diacetate
77	Chlorotrianisene
80	Methylprednisolone

System TR (p. 422)—Rf values

Rf	*Compound*
00	Betamethasone
	Dexamethasone
	Hydrocortisone Hydrogen Succinate
	Hydrocortisone Sodium Phosphate
	Triamcinolone
02	Prednisolone
03	Methylprednisolone
08	Hydrocortisone
10	Fluocinolone Acetonide
	Prednisone
18	Diethylstilbestrol
20	Betamethasone Valerate
	Triamcinolone Acetonide
30	Fludrocortisone Acetate
34	Dienestrol
38	Fluoxymesterone
	Hydrocortisone Acetate
40	Ethinylestradiol
55	Cortisone
70	Methallenestril
80	Alfadolone

Rf	Compound
	Ethisterone
85	Oxymetholone
87	Methandienone
	Norethisterone
89	Beclometasone
	Fluocortolone Hexanoate
90	Alfaxalone
	Androstanolone
	Mestranol
	Testosterone
91	Dimethisterone
	Methyltestosterone
	Noretynodrel
94	Ethylestrenol
95	Etynodiol Diacetate
	Norethandrolone
96	Dydrogesterone
	Estradiol Benzoate
97	Nandrolone
98	Chlorotrianisene
	Desoxycortone
	Medroxyprogesterone Acetate
	Megestrol Acetate
	Norethisterone Acetate
99	Hydroxyprogesterone caproate
	Lynestrenol
	Progesterone
	Testosterone Propionate
	Testosterone Phenylpropionate

System TS (p. 422)—**Rf values**

Rf	Compound
00	Betamethasone
	Cortisone
	Dexamethasone
	Ethisterone
	Fludrocortisone Acetate
	Hydrocortisone
	Hydrocortisone Acetate
	Hydrocortisone Hydrogen Succinate
	Hydrocortisone Sodium Phosphate
	Methylprednisolone
	Prednisolone
	Prednisone
	Triamcinolone
01	Fluocinolone Acetonide
02	Betamethasone Valerate
03	Diethylstilbestrol
05	Dienestrol
06	Triamcinolone Acetonide
16	Fluoxymesterone
40	Ethinylestradiol
42	Beclometasone
45	Alfadolone
54	Methallenestril
58	Fluocortolone Hexanoate
61	Methandienone
63	Norethisterone
	Testosterone
71	Methyltestosterone
	Noretynodrel
72	Alfaxalone
	Androstanolone
78	Norethandrolone
79	Estradiol Benzoate
82	Oxymetholone
85	Medroxyprogesterone Acetate
	Megestrol Acetate
90	Hydroxyprogesterone Caproate
	Mestranol
	Norethisterone Acetate
92	Chlorotrianisene
95	Desoxycortone
	Dimethisterone
	Nandrolone
	Progesterone
97	Lynestrenol
98	Dydrogesterone
	Testosterone Propionate
	Testosterone Phenylpropionate
99	Ethylestrenol
	Etynodiol Diacetate

System TT (p. 423)—**Rf values**

Rf	Compound
02	Phthalylsulfathiazole
	Succinylsulfathiazole
11	Sulfisomidine
21	Sulfaguanidine
24	Sulfadiazine
33	Sulfamerazine
46	Sulfamethizole
47	Sulfapyridine
50	Sulfadimidine
53	Sulfacetamide
	Sulfamethoxypyridazine
	Sulfathiazole
55	Sulfametoxydiazine
61	Sulfanilamide
74	Sulfafurazole
84	Chlorpropamide
85	Sulfadimethoxine
88	Sulfamethoxazole
89	Sulfaphenazole
90	Carbutamide
98	Tolbutamide

System TU (p. 423)—**Rf values**

Rf	Compound
01	Succinylsulfathiazole
04	Phthalylsulfathiazole
17	Sulfametoxydiazine
18	Sulfamerazine
22	Sulfadiazine
26	Sulfamethoxypyridazine
27	Carbutamide
	Sulfadimidine
33	Sulfamethoxazole
35	Tolbutamide
36	Sulfamethizole
37	Sulfacetamide
40	Sulfathiazole
43	Chlorpropamide
	Sulfapyridine
48	Sulfafurazole
49	Sulfisomidine
52	Sulfadimethoxine
70	Sulfaphenazole
90	Sulfaguanidine
96	Sulfanilamide

System TV (p. 423)—**Rf values**

Rf	Compound
01	Succinylsulfathiazole
02	Sulfamethizole
	Sulfamethoxazole
03	Chlorpropamide
	Sulfadiazine
04	Phthalylsulfathiazole
	Sulfacetamide
	Sulfafurazole
	Tolbutamide
05	Sulfathiazole
07	Carbutamide
	Sulfamerazine
13	Sulfaphenazole
15	Sulfametoxydiazine
20	Sulfisomidine
34	Sulfadimethoxine
48	Sulfaguanidine
50	Sulfamethoxypyridazine
62	Sulfadimidine
66	Sulfanilamide
73	Sulfapyridine

System TW (p. 420)—Rf values

Rf	*Compound*
19	Dimethoate
23	Mevinphos
68	Azinphos-methyl
74	Malathion
77	Parathion methyl
81	Parathion
82	Dimpylate

System TX (p. 420)—Rf values

Rf	*Compound*
00	Dichlorophenoxyacetic Acid
	Methylchlorophenoxyacetic Acid
	Omethoate
01	Methamidophos
	Monocrotophos
04	Dimethoate
	Nicotine
06	Dinitro-orthocresol
07	Trichlorfon
12	Dichlorophen
	Mevinphos
	Warfarin
14	Coumatetralyl
18	Aldicarb
	Carbaryl
	Demeton-*S*
19	Methoprotryne
20	Azinphos-methyl
	Dichlorvos
21	Desmetryne
	Triazophos
22	Linuron
	Simazine
23	Monolinuron
24	Azinphos-ethyl
26	Ametryne
27	Coumaphos
30	Parathion methyl
31	Malathion
32	Fenitrothion
	Prometryne
	Terbutryne
37	Cyfluthrin
40	Alachlor
	Deltamethrin
	Endosulfan
41	Dicamba
	Fenthion
	Parathion ethyl
43	Methoxychlor
47	Dimpylate
51	Lindane
58	Disulfoton
64	Chlorpyrifos
65	Dieldrin
71	Endrin
84	Heptachlor

System TY (p. 420)—Rf values

Rf	*Compound*
00	Methamidophos
	Methylchlorophenoxyacetic Acid
	Omethoate
01	Monocrotophos
	Nicotine
02	Dichlorophenoxyacetic Acid
	Trichlorfon
04	Dimethoate
10	Mevinphos
11	Methoprotryne
	Warfarin
12	Aldicarb
13	Demeton-*S*
16	Desmetryne
	Dichlorophen
18	Simazine
20	Dichlorvos
23	Ametryne
25	Carbaryl
30	Coumatetralyl
	Monolinuron
31	Linuron
	Prometryne
32	Terbutryne
38	Dinitro-orthocresol
	Triazophos
42	Azinphos-methyl
45	Alachlor
48	Azinphos-ethyl
50	Dimpylate
53	Malathion
61	Coumaphos
70	Dicamba
73	Parathion methyl
76	Fenitrothion
77	Endosulfan
81	Fenthion
84	Methoxychlor
	Parathion ethyl
87	Dieldrin
89	Cyfluthrin
	Disulfoton
90	Deltamethrin
	Endrin
92	Lindane
95	Chlorpyrifos
97	Heptachlor

System TZ (p. 420)—Rf values

Rf	*Compound*
15	Trichlorfon
37	Dimethoate
65	Aldicarb
68	Carbaryl
75	Dichlorvos
76	Dimpylate
77	Endosulfan
82	Fenitrothion
	Malathion
90	Fenthion
95	Deltamethrin

System TAA (p. 420)—Rf values

Rf	*Compound*
00	Tropicamide
05	Trichlorfon
08	Dimethoate
12	Aldicarb
17	Carbaryl
21	Dimpylate
33	Malathion
36	Dichlorvos
65	Fenitrothion
	Methoxychlor
68	Fenthion
72	Deltamethrin
95	Endosulfan

System TAB (p. 420)—Rf values

Rf	*Compound*
00	Dichlorvos
	Diquat
	Glyphosate (glyphosate acid)
	Paraquat
02	Dichlorophenoxyacetic Acid
	Trichlorfon
03	Dimethoate
	Mevinphos
04	Aldicarb
	Atrazine
	Dicamba
	Methylchlorophenoxyacetic Acid
	Trichlorophenoxyacetic Acid
07	Terbutryne
12	Carbaryl
24	Malathion
30	Dimpylate
50	Fenitrothion
51	Dieldrin
52	Disulfoton
55	Endrin
64	Chlordane
69	Heptachlor

System TAC (p. 420)—Rf values

Rf	*Compound*
00	Dichlorvos
	Diquat
	Glyphosate (glyphosate acid)
	Paraquat
01	Trichlorfon
02	Methylchlorophenoxyacetic Acid
	Mevinphos
	Trichlorophenoxyacetic Acid
03	Aldicarb
	Dichlorophenoxyacetic Acid
04	Carbaryl
05	Dicamba
08	Atrazine
12	Terbutryne
14	Malathion
17	Fenitrothion
20	Dimpylate
27	Dieldrin
35	Disulfoton
	Endrin
44	Chlordane
51	Heptachlor

System TAD (p. 406)—Rf values

Rf	*Compound*
00	Ambazone
	Amiloride
	Baclofen
	Barbituric Acid
	Chloropyramine
	Chloroquine
	Cytarabine
	Enalapril
	Ethambutol
	Levodopa
	Lysergic Acid
	Metformin
	Oxytetracycline Dihydrate
	Pentamidine
	Phthalylsulfacetamide
	Phthalylsulfathiazole
	Sodium Cromoglicate
	Valproic Acid
02	Dipyrone
	Mafenide
	Succinylsulfathiazole
	Sulfasalazine
04	Carbidopa
	Nicotinic Acid
	Saccharin
05	Etacrynic Acid
06	Bumetanide
	Captopril
07	Cinchophen
	Furosemide
	Sulfaguanidine
09	Benzyl Benzoate
10	Carbazochrome
11	Chlorothiazide
	Hydrochlorothiazide
13	Hydroflumethiazide
	Triamterene
14	Sulfacarbamide
15	Aminosalicylic Acid
	Methylchlorophenoxyacetic Acid
	Niflumic Acid
	Quinethazone
18	Acetazolamide
	Diflunisal
	Isoniazid
20	Trimethoprim
21	Ethyl Biscoumacetate
22	Aloxiprin
	Sulfanilamide
23	Chlortalidone
	Diclofenamide
	Trichlormethiazide
24	Aspirin salicylic acid
	Probenecid
	Salicylic Acid
25	Epithiazide
26	Cyclothiazide
	Paracetamol
	Trifluperidol
27	Cyclopenthiazide
	Methyclothiazide
	Sulfamethizole
	Sulfathiazole
	Sulfisomidine
28	Carbenoxolone
	Digoxin
	Primidone
	Sulfacetamide
29	Clozapine
30	4-Aminophenol
	Bendroflumethiazide
	Benzthiazide
	Styramate
	Sulfinpyrazone
	Tolmetin
31	Aminobenzoic Acid
	Aspirin
	Bufexamac
32	Chlorphenesin Carbamate
	Meprobamate
	Metronidazole
	Polythiazide
33	Alclofenac
	Dicoumarol
	Metolazone
	Nitrofurantoin
	Sulfafurazole
34	Chloramphenicol
	Sulfaethidole
	Sulfapyridine
	Sulindac
35	Benzoic Acid
	Mebutamate
	Quazepam M (3-hydroxy-*N*-dealkyl-2-oxo)
36	Loprazolam
	Xipamide
37	Brotizolam M (6-hydroxy)
38	Indometacin
	Methocarbamol
	Sulfadiazine
39	Clopamide
	Fenbufen
	Phenolphthalein
40	Alprazolam
	Guaifenesin
41	Brotizolam M (α-hydroxy)
	Flurazepam
	Ketoprofen
	Phenindamine
	Sulfamethoxazole
	Triazolam
42	Demoxepam
	Digitoxin
	Lorazepam
	Oxazepam
	Sulfamerazine
	Sultiame
43	Salicylamide
	Sulfamethoxypyridazine
	Sulfaphenazole
44	Hexachlorophene
	Naproxen

Rf	Compound
	Pyrazinamide
	Sulfadimidine
45	Flurbiprofen
46	Butalamine
	Indapamide
47	Bromazepam
	Clorexolone
	Diclofenac
	Enoxolone
	Sulfametoxydiazine
48	Sulfadimethoxine
49	Chlorpropamide
50	Chlorambucil
	Dantrolene
	Fenoprofen
	Phenacemide
	Phenazone
51	Ethoxzolamide
52	Acetanilide
	Phenacetin
53	Acetohexamide
	Aminoglutethimide
	Brotizolam
	Chlordiazepoxide
	Diphenadione
	Midazolam
	Nitrazepam
	Phenobarbital
	Phenytoin
54	Glibornuride
	Ibuprofen
	Mefenamic Acid
	Sulfametopyrazine
55	Caffeine
	Mefruside
	Methyl Hydroxybenzoate
	Methyprylon
	Sulfadoxine
56	Allobarbital
	Chlorzoxazone
	Clonazepam
	Ibomal
	Miconazole
	Paramethadione
	Propyl Hydroxybenzoate
	Tetrazepam M (nor)
57	Aprobarbital
	Barbital
	Brallobarbital
	Butalbital
	Clorazepic Acid
	Dichlorophen
	Ethyl Hydroxybenzoate
	Glibenclamide
	Methylpentynol
	Nordazepam
	Oxyphenbutazone
	Secbutabarbital
	Vinbarbital
58	Aminophenazone
	Amobarbital
	Butobarbital
	Cyclobarbital
	Ethinamate
	Quazepam M (3-hydroxy-2-oxo)
59	Carisoprodol
	Cyclopentobarbital
	Etamivan
	Ethosuximide
	Heptabarb
	Idobutal
	Pentobarbital
	Pheneturide
60	Acecarbromal
	Acenocoumarol
	Ethotoin
	Hexethal
	Lormetazepam
	Nealbarbital
	Phenprobamate
	Quazepam M (*N*-dealkyl-2-oxo)
	Talbutal
61	Flumazenil
	Phenprocoumon
62	Alfadolone
	Ketazolam
	Nalidixic Acid
	Secobarbital
	Tolbutamide
63	Benzocaine
	Triclocarban
64	Bemegride
	Carbromal
	Cholesterol
	Estradiol
	Warfarin
65	Benziodarone
	Metaclazepam M (nor)
	Propyphenazone
	Temazepam
	Thymol
66	Mephenytoin
	Tolazamide
	Vinylbital
67	Tetrazepam
68	Carbimazole
	Clotrimazole
	Griseofulvin
	Procarbazine
	Thiopental
69	Camazepam
	Hexobarbital
	Metharbital
	Santonin
	Thialbarbital
70	Clioquinol
	Clobazam
	Enallylpropymal
	Glutethimide
	Methylphenobarbital
	Phenindione
	Quazepam M (2-oxo)
71	Azathioprine
	Clofibrate
	Metaclazepam
	Methohexital
	Piroxicam
72	Diazepam
	Diiodohydroxyquinoline
	Flunitrazepam
	Phensuximide
	Prazepam
73	Cyclandelate
	Medazepam
75	Spironolactone
76	Phenylbutazone
78	Dantron
	Quazepam
80	Clofenotane
82	Ethchlorvynol
94	Azinphos-methyl

System TAE (p. 405)—**Rf values**

Rf	Compound
00	Alcuronium Chloride
	Amikacin
	Atropine Methonitrate
	Busulfan
	Cetrimide
	Cetylpyridinium Chloride
	Decamethonium Bromide
	Decamethonium
	Dihydralazine
	Dihydrostreptomycin
	Diquat
	Histamine
	Homatropine Methylbromide
	Kanamycin
	Neomycin
	Neostigmine Methylsulfate
	Pancuronium Bromide
	Paraquat
	Pentamidine
	Pentolonium Tartrate
	Pralidoxime Mesilate
	Pyridostigmine Bromide
	Rolitetracycline
	Streptomycin
	Suxamethonium Chloride
	Thiazinamium Metilsulfate M (sulfoxide)
	Tobramycin
	Trimetaphan Camsilate
	Trimethadione
	Tubocurarine Chloride
01	Amidefrine
	Chlorhexidine
	Cotarnine
	Denatonium Benzoate
	Deptropine
	Hydrastinine
	Piperazine
	Thiazinamium Metilsulfate
02	Distigmine Bromide
	Oxyphencyclimine
	Oxyphenonium Bromide
	Thiamine
03	Adrenaline
	Azacyclonol
	Clidinium Bromide
	Emepronium Bromide
	Glycopyrronium Bromide
	Guanethidine
	Guanoxan
	Hexocyclium Metilsulfate
	Isopropamide Iodide
	Mequitazine
	Metformin
	Methanthelinium Bromide
	Naphazoline
	Propantheline Bromide
	Tolazoline
04	Benzalkonium Chloride
	Berberine
	Carbachol

Rf	*Compound*
	Chloroquine
	Pirenzepine M (*N*-desmethyl)
	Sparteine
	Tramazoline
05	Antazoline
	Atropine
	Brucine
	Coniine
	Tetryzoline
	Xylometazoline
06	Amiloride
	Benzatropine
	Cyclopentamine
	Maprotiline
	Mephentermine
	Mescaline
	Phentolamine
	Protriptyline
	Tryptamine
07	Amantadine
	Benserazide
	Desipramine
	Ethacridine
	Homatropine
	Hydroxychloroquine
	Methoxyphenamine
	Proguanil
	Rimiterol
	Trimethoxyamfetamine (2,4,6-TMA)
08	Methylenedioxymethamfetamine
	Oxytetracycline Dihydrate
	Paroxetine
	Perhexiline
	Phenylephrine
	Prajmalium Bitartrate
	Remoxipride M(FLA-838)
	Strychnine
09	Aminoacridine
	Disopyramide
	DOM
	Metamfetamine
	Methoxyamfetamine
	Penthienate Methobromide
	Pholedrine
	Pseudoephedrine
10	Bufotenine
	Dextromethorphan
	Dextrorphan
	Dimetindene
	Ephedrine
	Methylenedioxyamfetamine
11	Dihydrocodeine
	Fluoxetine
	Fluoxetine M (nor)
	Hydrocodone
	Levodopa
	Mesoridazine
	Phentermine
12	Amfetamine
	Aminopromazine
	Brompheniramine
	Chlorphenamine
	Dihydromorphine
	Doxylamine
	Ethambutol
	Ethoheptazine
	Hexobendine
	Hexoprenaline
	Hydromorphone
	Methenamine
	Methoxamine
	Methylephedrine
	Pipazetate
	Tiotixene M
13	Acebutolol
	Carbinoxamine
	Metaraminol
	Thiethylperazine M
	Thioproperazine M
14	Atenolol
	Azapetine
	Chlorphentermine
	Diethyltryptamine
	Dimethyltryptamine
	Dopamine
	Etafedrine
	Granisetron
	Heptaminol
	Isoprenaline
	Nadolol
	Pheniramine
	Propylhexedrine
	Psilocin
	Tofenacin
15	Etilefrine
	Pholcodine
	Prothipendyl
16	Benzydamine
	Betaine
	Bunitrolol
	Encainide
	Methadone
	Salbutamol
17	Lofexidine
	Metoclopramide
	Procainamide
	Sulpiride
	Tertatolol
	Veratrine
18	Bambuterol
	Carbocromen
	Fluvoxamine
	Morphine
	Pindolol
	Pirenzepine
	Promazine
	Terbutaline
	Xamoterol
19	Bambuterol Monocarbamate
	Cinchonine
	Emetine
	Halofantrine M (desbutyl)
	Oxeladin
	Pipradrol
	Sotalol
	Triprolidine
20	Aprindine
	Benzylmorphine
	Fenfluramine
	Hydroquinidine
	Metoprolol
	Oxprenolol
	Procyclidine
	Thenalidine
	Thioridazine
	Timolol
	Zimeldine
21	Codeine
	Dimethoxanate
	Ethylmorphine
	Fencamfamin
	Hydroquinine
	Imipramine
	Methapyrilene
	Metipranolol
	Metixene
	Orciprenaline
	Perazine
	Propranolol
	Thenyldiamine
22	Ajmaline
	Alprenolol
	Betaxolol
	Bisoprolol
	Chloropyramine
	Clenbuterol
	Isothipendyl
	Mafenide
	Mepyramine
	Prolintane
	Thioproperazine
	Thonzylamine
	Tripelennamine
23	Bamethan
	Diphenylpyraline
	Lobeline
	Phencyclidine
	Thebaine
24	Bamipine
	Cinchonidine
	Cyclazocine
	Doxepin
	Erythromycin
	Ketotifen
	Piperocaine
	Thebacon
	Trimethobenzamide
25	Chlorpromazine
	Cropropamide
	Fenpipramide
	Gelsemine
	Mexiletine
	Orphenadrine
	Pyrrobutamine
	Sertraline
	Viloxazine
26	Acetylcodeine
	Butaperazine
	Clomipramine
	Diamorphine
	Ketobemidone
	Loprazolam
	Prochlorperazine
	Quinine
	Remoxipride
	Tiotixene
	Tolpropamine
	Xantinol Nicotinate
27	Amitriptyline
	Bromazine
	Diphenhydramine
	Dipipanone
	Dosulepin
	Oxymorphone
	Pecazine
	Thiethylperazine
28	Acepromazine
	Alphaprodine
	Dimenhydrinate
	Flecainide
	Pizotifen
29	Chlorphenoxamine
	Noxiptiline
	Phenelzine
30	Clenbuterol M (hydroxy)
	Clomifene
	Cyproheptadine
	Hexetidine
	Nefopam
	Oxycodone
	Promethazine
	Propiomazine

Rf	*Compound*
	Quinidine
	Tramadol
	Trifluoperazine
31	Profenamine
32	Alimemazine
	Clofedanol
	Histapyrrodine
	Labetalol
	Levomepromazine
	Mebeverine
	Phenyltoloxamine
	Triflupromazine
33	Buphenine
	Clofazimine
	Diethazine
	Pipamperone
34	Acetophenazine
	Chlorprothixene
	Narceine
	Pentazocine
	Pethidine
	Phenmetrazine
35	Chlorcyclizine
	Cocaine
	Nicametate
	Opipramol
36	Mebhydrolin
	Procaine
	Trimipramine
38	Amodiaquine
	Benzoctamine
	Dibenzepin
	Fenoterol
39	Carfenazine
	Cyclizine
	Ibogaine
	Nicotine
40	Clioquinol
	Diethylthiambutene
	Methylphenidate
	Perphenazine
	Physostigmine
	Pipotiazine
41	Arecoline
	Lorcainide
	Tranylcypromine
42	Aconitine
	Cinchocaine
	Clozapine
	Levallorphan
	Tocainide
	Zopiclone
43	Dimetotiazine
	Naftidrofuryl Oxalate
	Nicergoline
	Norpipanone
	Prenylamine
	Tetracaine
	Trihexyphenidyl
	Verapamil
44	Butacaine
	Clonidine
	Fenetylline
	Minoxidil
	Penicillamine
	Phenethylamine
45	Biperiden
	Clopenthixol
	Fluphenazine
	Isoaminile
	Nizatidine
	Trimethoprim
	Zuclopenthixol
46	Cyclopentolate

Rf	*Compound*
	Mazindol
	Meclofenoxate
	Pericyazine
	Spiramycin
	Vinblastine
47	Captodiame
	Dixyrazine
48	Butetamate
	Flavoxate
	Mianserin
	Thiopropazate M
49	Adiphenine
	Hyoscine
	Loxapine
	Phendimetrazine
50	Flupentixol
	Phenazocine
	Triamterene
51	Haloperidol
	Tetramisole
	Tizanidine
52	Benactyzine
	Flurazepam
	Loperamide
	Pilocarpine
53	Cimetidine
	Famotidine
	Levamisole
	Nomifensine
	Obidoxime Chloride
54	Amiodarone
	Apomorphine
	Oxybuprocaine
	Piperidolate
55	Astemizole M (nor)
	Dicycloverine
	Diethylpropion
	Isoniazid
	Trifluperidol
56	Astemizole
	Furazolidone
	Halofantrine
57	Flucytosine
	Hydroxyzine
	Lysergamide
	Nalorphine
58	Dihydroergotamine
	Methylpiperidyl Benzilate
	Nalbuphine
	Nifenazone
59	Caffeine
	Dropropizine
	Hydrastine
	Theobromine
60	Anileridine
	Benzfetamine
	Lysergide
	Methyldopa
	Nimorazole
61	Morazone
	Oxetacaine
	Tilidate
62	Benperidol
	Ergometrine
	Isoxsuprine
	Pramocaine
	Prilocaine
	Thiopropazate
63	Fluspirilene
	Mepivacaine
	Meprobamate
	Nalidixic Acid
	Piminodine
64	Pentoxifylline

Rf	*Compound*
	Trazodone
65	Azaperone
	Butanilicaine
	Harmine
	Moclobemide
66	Etofylline
	Metyrapone
	Phenazone
	Pyrimethamine
	Yohimbine
67	Alprazolam
	Fluanisone
	Fluconazole
68	Ergotamine
	Ketamine
	Ketoconazole
	Nialamide
	Nicotinamide
	Prazosin
	Triazolam
69	Bupivacaine
	Colchicine
	Cytarabine
	Doxapram
	Methylergometrine
	Midazolam
70	Ambazone
	Aminophenazone
	Diprophylline
	Fentanyl
	Iproniazid
	Lidoflazine
	Lysergic Acid
	Phenoperidine
71	Bamifylline
	Doxazosin
	Droperidol
	Etacrynic Acid
	Nikethamide
	Proxyphylline
	Pyrazinamide
72	Brotizolam
	Dextromoramide
	Etizolam
	Harman
	Lidocaine
	Nicotinic Acid
	Noscapine
	Penfluridol
	Pentetrazol
	Pentifylline
73	Bromazepam
	Deserpidine
	Hydralazine
	Isoetarine
	Pimozide
	Piritramide
74	Cyclophosphamide
	Methyl Nicotinate
	Naloxone
	Nicotinyl Alcohol
	Oxypertine
	Papaverine
	Theophylline
75	Allopurinol
	4-Aminophenol
	Carbimazole
	Ibuprofen
	Lincomycin
	Metronidazole
	Pyridoxine
	Sulfaguanidine
	Thiotepa
	Tiabendazole

Rf	*Compound*
76	Ambucetamide
	Brotizolam M (6-hydroxy)
	Chlordiazepoxide
	Clemizole
	Flumazenil
	Levocabastine
	Primidone
	Reserpine
77	Mercaptopurine
	Metomidate
	Miconazole
	Nifuratel
	Paracetamol
	Pargyline
	Protionamide
	Rescinnamine
78	Aspirin
	Brotizolam M (α-hydroxy)
	Broxaldine
	Disulfiram
	Econazole
	Etomidate
	Griseofulvin
	Hydrochlorothiazide
	Isopropylaminophenazone
	Methyprylon
	Nitrofurazone
	Oxcarbazepine
	Sulfadoxine
79	Carbamazepine
	Carbamazepine M (OH-)
	Cinnarizine
	Clorexolone
	Medazepam
	Methaqualone
	Nifedipine
	Sulfadimidine
	Sulfamethoxazole
	Sulfathiazole
80	Acetanilide
	Azathioprine
	Buprenorphine
	Clomethiazole
	Clotrimazole
	Dimethoate
	Etidocaine
	Fenyramidol
	Flunitrazepam
	Mebendazole
	Mecloqualone
	Meclozine
	Oxymetazoline
	Phenazopyridine
	Propanidid
	Psilocybine
	Sulfamerazine
	Sulfisomidine
	Tetrabenazine
	Thiamazole
	Trimetozine
81	Azinphos-ethyl
	Azinphos-methyl
	Clindamycin
	Clofibrate
	Demoxepam
	Dimpylate
	Glafenine
	Guaifenesin
	Metaclazepam M (dinor)
	Metaclazepam M (nor)
	Methyl Hydroxybenzoate
	Pemoline
	Pirenzepine M (desamide)
	Propyphenazone
	Strophanthin-K
	Sulfacarbamide
	Sulfadiazine
	Sulfafurazole
	Sultiame
82	Bisacodyl
	Camazepam
	Cinchophen
	Diazepam
	Dipyridamole
	Lofepramine
	Lorazepam
	Lormetazepam
	Mebutamate
	Metaclazepam
	Methoxsalen
	Naproxen
	Nordazepam
	Oxazepam
	Phenothiazine
	Phenprobamate
	Remoxipride M(NCM-001)
	Remoxipride M(NCM-009)
	Sulfametoxydiazine
	Temazepam
83	Butyl Aminobenzoate
	Clorazepic Acid
	Crotetamide
	Indometacin
	Ketazolam
	Methocarbamol
	Phenacetin
	Progesterone
	Rifampicin
	Salicylamide
	Sulfamethizole
	Sulfamethoxypyridazine
	Sulfanilamide
84	Acecarbromal
	Acetazolamide
	Barbital
	Barbituric Acid
	Benzocaine
	Bromhexine
	Bromocriptine
	Chlorambucil
	Chlormezanone
	Cholesterol
	Clobazam
	Crotamiton
	Diazoxide
	Ethosuximide
	Etorphine
	Flufenamic Acid
	Flutazolam
	Gliclazide
	Isocarboxazid
	Malathion
	Methazolamide
	Nitrofurantoin
	Phenaglycodol
	Phenoxybenzamine
	Prazepam
	Prednisone
	Spironolactone
	Tetrazepam
85	Carbromal
	Carisoprodol
	Chlorpyrifos
	Clonazepam
	Digoxin
	Dipyrone
	Enalapril
	Etamivan
	Floctafenine
	Hexobarbital
	Ketoprofen
	Methohexital
	Phenobarbital
	Sulfasalazine
	Testosterone
	Tetrazepam M (nor-)
	Tolmetin
86	Aprobarbital
	Aspirin salicylic acid
	Benorilate
	Benzyl Alcohol
	Butobarbital
	Chloramphenicol
	Demeton-*S*
	Ethinamate
	Ethinylestradiol
	Furosemide
	Glipizide
	Glutethimide
	Hydrocortisone
	Hydroxyprogesterone
	Loratadine
	Methylphenobarbital
	Methyltestosterone
	Mevinphos
	Mexazolam
	Nisoldipine
	Norethisterone
	Phanquinone
	Phenolphthalein
	Phenytoin
	Prednisolone
	Resorcinol
	Salicylic Acid
	Sulfadimethoxine
	Tiaprofenic Acid
	Tolazamide
87	Allobarbital
	Brallobarbital
	Bumetanide
	Butalbital
	Carbutamide
	Chlorphenesin Carbamate
	Chlorpropamide
	Clenbuterol (M#2)
	Clenbuterol (M#3)
	Cortisone
	Cyclandelate
	Dobutamine
	Estrone
	Etenzamide
	Ethchlorvynol
	Felodipine
	Hydroflumethiazide
	Itraconazole
	Mefenamic Acid
	Mephenesin
	Metharbital
	Methylprednisolone
	Nimodipine
	Nitrendipine
	Phenylbutazone
	Probenecid
	Propantheline Bromide M (xanthanoic acid)
	Quazepam
	Quazepam M (2-oxo)
	Saccharin
	Sulfacetamide
	Sulindac
	Tenoxicam
88	Amobarbital

Rf	*Compound*
	Azapropazone
	Chlortalidone
	Chlorzoxazone
	Clemastine
	Cyclobarbital
	Dicoumarol
	Digitoxin
	Doxycycline
	Epithiazide
	Ethyl Hydroxybenzoate
	Fenbutrazate
	Heptabarb
	Hexestrol
	Hexylresorcinol
	Isradipine
	Minocycline
	Niflumic Acid
	Piroxicam
	Piroxicam M (5-hydroxy)
	Procarbazine
	Quazepam M (3-hydroxy-2-oxo)
	Quazepam M (3-hydroxy-*N*-dealkyl-2-oxo)
	Quazepam M (*N*-dealkyl-2-oxo)
	Secbutabarbital
	Tetracycline
	Tolbutamide
	Trichlormethiazide
	Zomepirac
88.	
	Secobarbital
89	Bezafibrate
	Dieldrin
	Diflunisal
	Etofenamate
	Etynodiol Diacetate
	Indapamide
	Lanatoside C
	Sulfaphenazole
	Vinbarbital
	Vinylbital
90	Androsterone
	Beclamide
	Buclosamide
	Cyclopentobarbital
	Diclofenac
	Diphenoxylate
	Famprofazone
	Glibenclamide
	Mesuximide
	Nitrazepam
	Oxyphenbutazone
	Pentobarbital
	Propyl Hydroxybenzoate
	Trichlorfon
91	Chlordane
	Dichlorophen
	Fenticlor
	Fluorometholone
	Ibomal
92	Acenocoumarol
	Bezitramide
	Diethylstilbestrol
	Feprazone
	Glibornuride
	Metenolone
	Nealbarbital
	Pentaerithrityl Tetranitrate
	Talbutal
93	Gliquidone
	Metformin
	Niclosamide
	Phenprocoumon
	Xipamide
94	Benzbromarone
	Hexachlorophene

System TAF (p. 405)—**Rf values**

Rf	*Compound*
00	Diquat
	Paraquat
	Suxamethonium Chloride
01	Pentolonium Tartrate
	Psilocybine
02	Decamethonium Bromide
	Decamethonium
03	Histamine
04	Piperazine
07	Brucine
	Disopyramide
08	Obidoxime Chloride
10	Sparteine
11	Betaine
	Strychnine
	Tubocurarine Chloride
12	Homatropine Methylbromide
	Methenamine
13	Hydrocodone
14	Chloroquine
	Hydromorphone
	Narceine
15	Hydrastinine
	Loprazolam
	Pancuronium Bromide
16	Carbinoxamine
	Lysergic Acid
18	Oxyphencyclimine
	Thiamine
19	Dihydrocodeine
21	Chlorphenamine
22	Codeine
	Cotarnine
	Dibenzepin
	Nicotine
	Thioproperazine
23	Benzylmorphine
	Carbachol
	Morphine
	Perazine
24	Methapyrilene
	Tiotixene
25	Acetylcodeine
	Thebacon
	Thiazinamium Metilsulfate
26	Ethylmorphine
	Pheniramine
	Prochlorperazine
27	Homatropine
28	Atropine
29	Cetrimide
	Cetylpyridinium Chloride
	Prothipendyl
	Trifluoperazine
30	Cocaine
	Guanethidine
	Triprolidine
31	Propantheline Bromide
	Thonzylamine
32	Acetophenazine
	Thebaine
33	Diamorphine
	Mepyramine
	Oxycodone
	Procainamide
34	Bufotenine
	Tripelennamine
35	Isothipendyl
	Promazine
36	Oxymorphone
	Oxyphenonium Bromide
	Thenyldiamine
38	Dimethoxanate
	Physostigmine
39	Dimethyltryptamine
	Opipramol
	Tetracaine
40	Perphenazine
	Pethidine
41	Dosulepin
	Ethoheptazine
	Isopropamide Iodide
	Phendimetrazine
42	Dextromethorphan
	Procaine
44	Promethazine
45	Chlorpromazine
	Doxepin
	Flurazepam
	Phenmetrazine
	Pilocarpine
46	Alimemazine
	Mebhydrolin
47	Hyoscine
	Imipramine
48	Bromazine
	Dimenhydrinate
	Diphenhydramine
	Metformin
	Psilocin
49	Clemastine
	Dextrorphan
	Diphenylpyraline
	Fluphenazine
	Isoniazid
	Levomepromazine
	Orphenadrine
	Phenindamine
	Triflupromazine
50	Cyproheptadine
	Methylpiperidyl Benzilate
	Mianserin
51	Amitriptyline
	Chlorprothixene
	Lysergamide
52	Chlorcyclizine
	Cyclizine
	Levamisole
	Naphazoline
	Nomifensine
	Piperidolate
	Propiomazine
53	Tetramisole

Rf	*Compound*
54	Clomipramine
	Diethazine
	Theobromine
55	Caffeine
	Cimetidine
	Cinchonidine
	Profenamine
	Thioridazine
	Tolazoline
56	Berberine
	Butetamate
	Diethylpropion
	Diethyltryptamine
	Piperocaine
	Trimipramine
57	Benactyzine
	Hydrastine
59	Diprophylline
	Dipyrone
	Dopamine
	Lysergide
	Nalorphine
	Pipotiazine
	Thiopropazate
	Trimethoprim
60	Ergometrine
	Mepivacaine
	Methadone
	Pramocaine
	Tetryzoline
61	Cinchonine
	Pericyazine
	Pipamperone
	Trazodone
	Verapamil
63	Colchicine
	Indometacin
	Mescaline
	Metamfetamine
	Quinidine
64	Amiodarone
	Ephedrine
	Ergotamine
	Nialamide
	Xylometazoline
65	Hydroxyzine
	Mazindol
	Quinine
	Triamterene
	Triazolam
66	Alprazolam
	Anileridine
	Antazoline
	Benzalkonium Chloride
	Nicotinamide
	Phenazone
	Pyrrobutamine
	Theophylline
67	Nikethamide
	Phenylephrine
	Pyridoxine
	Tranylcypromine
68	Aconitine
	Aminophenazone
	Cyclopentamine
	Harmine
	Procyclidine
69	Benperidol
	Bromazepam
	Hydroquinine
	Iproniazid
	Isoprenaline
	Lidocaine
	Nicotinyl Alcohol
	Phencyclidine
	Protriptyline
70	Coniine
	Hydroquinidine
	Methylphenidate
	Metronidazole
	Midazolam
	Pyrazinamide
	Trimethoxyamfetamine (2,4,6-TMA)
	Yohimbine
71	Acebutolol
	Brotizolam
	Desipramine
	Maprotiline
72	Cinchophen
	Dipipanone
	Flumazenil
	Ibogaine
	Ketamine
	Pentazocine
73	Clemizole
	Droperidol
	Levallorphan
	Methoxamine
74	Amiloride
	Cyclazocine
	Etilefrine
	Methoxyamfetamine
	Metoprolol
	Papaverine
	Pentetrazol
	Piritramide
	Prazosin
	Salbutamol
	Tocainide
75	Amfetamine
	Carbamazepine
	Carbimazole
	Fluanisone
	Haloperidol
	Methyldopa
	Noscapine
	Timolol
	Trihexyphenidyl
76	Brotizolam M (6-hydroxy)
	Butacaine
	Clonidine
	DOM
	Guanoxan
	Harman
	Metaraminol
	Methylenedioxyamfetamine
	Trifluperidol
77	Amantadine
	Chlordiazepoxide
	Chlorphentermine
	Fentanyl
	Lidoflazine
	Methyl Nicotinate
	Orciprenaline
	Piminodine
	Terbutaline
78	Brotizolam M (α-hydroxy)
	Dextromoramide
	Fluspirilene
	Glafenine
	Mexiletine
	Oxprenolol
	Phentermine
	Pindolol
79	Bupivacaine
	Carisoprodol
	Crotetamide
	Pipradrol
	Prilocaine
	Proguanil
	Propranolol
	Rescinnamine
	Santonin
80	Chlormezanone
	Econazole
	Ketazolam
	Miconazole
	Reserpine
81	Disulfiram
	Fenoterol
	Isoxsuprine
	Loperamide
	Metomidate
	Pemoline
	Phenazocine
82	Flunitrazepam
	Lorazepam
	Lormetazepam
	Phenelzine
	Phenoperidine
	Pimozide
	Temazepam
83	Buphenine
	Camazepam
	Chlortalidone
	Cropropamide
	Demoxepam
	Medazepam
	Nordazepam
84	Acecarbromal
	Acetanilide
	Mebendazole
	Metaclazepam
	Metaclazepam M (nor)
	Methaqualone
	Salicylamide
85	Clobazam
	Clomethiazole
	Diazepam
	Etomidate
	Mebutamate
	Prenylamine
86	Clofazimine
	Fenyramidol
	Isocarboxazid
	Methyltestosterone
	Nitrazepam
87	Azinphos-methyl
	Benzocaine
	Bisacodyl
	Carbromal
	Cinnarizine
	Clonazepam
	Clorazepic Acid
	Dipyridamole
	Ethinamate
	Meprobamate
88	Ambucetamide
	Bemegride
	Bromocriptine
	Chlorpropamide
	Clioquinol
	Meclozine
	Quazepam M (*N*-dealkyl-2-oxo)
	Testosterone
	Tolbutamide
89	Glutethimide
	Mephenesin
	Penfluridol
	Phenothiazine Tf
	Prazepam
	Progesterone

Rf	*Compound*
	Quazepam M (3-hydroxy-*N*-dealkyl-2-oxo)
	Tetrazepam
90	Butyl Aminobenzoate
	Chloramphenicol
	Chlorzoxazone
	Methyl Salicylate
	Quazepam M (2-oxo)
	Quazepam M (3-hydroxy-2-oxo)
91	Hexetidine
	Oxazepam
	Resorcinol
92	Acenocoumarol
	Diethylstilbestrol
	Diphenoxylate
	Tetrazepam M (nor)
	Thymol
93	Camphor
95	Cyclandelate
96	Bezitramide
	Cholesterol
	Quazepam
97	Phenoxybenzamine
98	Hexachlorophene

System TAH (p. 418)—Rf values

Rf	*Compound*
45	Cannabinol
50	Δ^9-Tetrahydrocannabinol
60	Cannabidiol

System TAJ (p. 406)—Rf values

Rf	*Compound*
00	Acetylcysteine
	Amiloride
	Aminopromazine
	Antazoline
	Atropine
	Benzilonium Bromide
	Berberine
	Cefalothin
	Chloroquine
	Chlorphenamine
	Cimetidine
	Cinchonidine
	Debrisoquine
	Demeclocycline
	Dihydromorphine
	Dipyrone
	Dopamine
	Doxylamine
	Ephedrine
	Ethambutol
	Ethylnoradrenaline
	Guanethidine
	Harmaline
	Homatropine
	Hydroxyamfetamine
	Hydroxychloroquine
	Hyoscyamine
	Isoetarine
	Isometheptene
	Isopropamide Iodide
	Levodopa
	Mafenide
	Mecamylamine
	Mephentermine
	Metamfetamine
	Metaraminol
	Methoxamine
	Methyldopa
	Morphine
	Normorphine
	Oxymetazoline
	Oxyphencyclimine
	Perphenazine
	Phenformin
	Phentolamine
	Phenylephrine
	Phthalylsulfathiazole
	Pindolol
	Procyclidine
	Propantheline Bromide
	Propranolol
	Propylhexedrine
	Protokylol
	Pseudoephedrine
	Pseudomorphine
	Quinidine
	Saccharin
	Sparteine
	Sulfasalazine
	Terbutaline
	Δ^9-Tetrahydrocannabinol
	Trimetaphan Camsilate
	Tryptamine
01	Brompheniramine
	Hydralazine
	Nortriptyline
	Phenylpropanolamine
02	Diethyltryptamine
	Mescaline
	Mesoridazine
	Metoprolol
	Minocycline
	Narceine
	Pentazocine
	Phentermine
	Ranitidine
	Tripelennamine
03	Eucatropine
	Hordenine
	Ketobemidone
	Methylenedioxymethamfetamine
	Phenethylamine
04	Acepromazine
	Brucine
	Carbinoxamine
	Dimetindene
	Erythromycin
	Etafedrine
	Mazindol
	Methoxyamfetamine
	Nicotinic Acid
	Paroxetine
	Piperacetazine
	Protriptyline
	Strychnine
	Triamterene
05	Acetophenazine
	Etacrynic Acid
	Fendosal
	Methoxyphenamine
	Urea
06	Aconitine
	Alprenolol
	Apomorphine
	Cyclazocine
	Diflunisal
	Dihydrocodeine
	Fluphenazine
	Haloperidol
	Opipramol
	Procaine
	Promazine
07	Desipramine
	Fenfluramine
	Imipramine
08	Carfenazine
	Ethoheptazine
	Methadone
	Xylazine
09	Chloroprocaine
	Clonidine
	Emetine
	Hydrochlorothiazide
	Hydrocodone
	Hydroflumethiazide
	Isoniazid
	Nicotine
	Tetramisole
	Thioridazine
10	Butaperazine
	Codeine
	Dimethoxanate
	Furosemide
	Levallorphan
11	Azapropazone
	Chlorothiazide
	Chlorphenoxamine
	Chlorpromazine
	Lobeline
	Methylphenidate
	Phanquinone
	Propoxycaine
	Quinethazone
12	Harmine
	Methdilazine
	Pemoline
	Salicylic Acid
	Tetracaine
13	Amitriptyline
	Cocaine

Rf	*Compound*
	Ethylmorphine
	Indoramin
	Isoxsuprine
	6-Monoacetylmorphine
	Oxymorphone
14	Orphenadrine
	Pethidine
	Triamcinolone
	Trimethoprim
15	Amodiaquine
16	Butorphanol
	Metixene
17	Alclofenac
	Chlortalidone
	Ergometrine
18	Acetazolamide
	Bumetanide
	Clomipramine
	Cyproheptadine
	Nalorphine
	Physostigmine
	Prochlorperazine
19	Nalbuphine
	Normethadone
	Prednisolone
	Tiotixene
	Tranylcypromine
	Zomepirac
20	Anileridine
	Chlorprothixene
	Methapyrilene
	Phenmetrazine
	Tolmetin
21	Chlorcyclizine
22	Butriptyline
	Epithiazide
	Pilocarpine
	Profenamine
	Sulfanilamide
	Thebaine
	Thiethylperazine
23	Alphaprodine
	Cyclizine
	Cyclopentolate
	Doxepin
	Methysergide
	Nefopam
24	Difenidol
	Harman
	Molindone
	Phencyclidine
	Pyrrobutamine
	Trichlormethiazide
25	Diamorphine
	Ibogaine
	Nomifensine
	Quinisocaine
26	Hydroxyzine
	Phenazocine
27	Butacaine
	Levomepromazine
	Niflumic Acid
	Oxycodone
	Phenyltoloxamine
28	Arecoline
	Etamiphylline
	Mepivacaine
	Probenecid
29	Hexylcaine
	Primidone
30	Methyclothiazide
	Paracetamol
	Tiaprofenic Acid
31	Benzoctamine
	Benzthiazide
	Chlorphenesin Carbamate
	Methylprednisolone
32	Acetylcodeine
	Chloramphenicol
	Flurazepam
	Metronidazole
	Theobromine
33	Dextropropoxyphene
	Dihydroergotamine
	Lysergide
	Prednisone
34	Benactyzine
	Bromazepam
	Metolazone
	Nitrofurazone
	Procarbazine
	Propiomazine
	Resorcinol
	Sulfamethizole
35	Digitoxin
	Furaltadone
	Mebutamate
	Meprobamate
	Polythiazide
36	Hydrocortisone
37	Biperiden
	Diazoxide
	Droperidol
	Flunixin
	Phenindamine
38	Bendroflumethiazide
	Betamethasone
	Chlorphenesin
	Dexamethasone
	Trihexyphenidyl
39	Colchicine
	Prazosin
	Sulfafurazole
	Sulindac
40	Aspirin
	Clonixin
	Diclofenac
	Sulfadiazine
	Theophylline
	Tosylchloramide Sodium
41	Fluoxymesterone
	Methocarbamol
	Sulfachlorpyridazine
42	Demoxepam
	Dicycloverine
	Guaifenesin
	Mepenzolate Bromide
43	Fenbufen
	Stanozolol
	Sulfadimidine
44	Aminobenzoic Acid
	Carbamazepine
	Diethylpropion
	Methandienone
	Methazolamide
45	Loxapine
	Mephenesin
	Sulfamethoxazole
46	Dantrolene
	Fluorometholone
	Indometacin
	Lorazepam
	Nitrofurantoin
	Phenazopyridine
	Sulfamethoxypyridazine
	Tiabendazole
47	Flurbiprofen
	Ketamine
	Oxazepam
	Prenylamine
	Tilidate
48	Chlordiazepoxide
	Lysergic Acid
	Phenytoin
49	Naltrexone
	Pentoxifylline
	Piperidolate
50	Clonazepam
	Prilocaine
	Sulfapyridine
51	Chlorzoxazone
	Cortisone
	Diphenadione
	Ethoxzolamide
	Phenazone
	Piminodine
52	Etorphine
	Flavoxate
	Thiopropazate
53	Aminophenazone
	Benzquinamide
	Embutramide
	Nitrazepam
	Nordazepam
	Sulfadimethoxine
	Sulfadoxine
54	Amygdalin
	Azaperone
	Caffeine
	Ketoprofen
	Paramethasone
55	Benzoic Acid
	Chlormezanone
	Estradiol
	Ethinylestradiol
	Fludrocortisone
	Flufenamic Acid
	Lidocaine
	Trazodone
56	Benoxaprofen
	Benzonatate
	Hexachlorophene
	Indapamide
	Oxyphenbutazone
	Reserpine
	Vinbarbital
57	Etoxazene
58	Ethinamate
	Fenoprofen
	Mebendazole
	Naloxone
	Phenacetin
59	Azapetine
	Bupivacaine
	Fentanyl
	Ibuprofen
	Meclofenamic Acid
	Nikethamide
	Pramocaine
	Testosterone
60	Acetohexamide
	Dicoumarol
	Doxapram
	Etamivan
	Methyltestosterone
	Naproxen
61	Acecarbromal
	Diphenylpyraline
	Ethotoin
	Hyoscine
	Methyl Hydroxybenzoate
62	Buprenorphine

Rf	*Compound*
	Halcinonide
63	Estrone
64	Aniline
	Dimoxyline
	Mephenytoin
65	Chlorpropamide
	Cholesterol
	Meclozine
	Noscapine
	Phenoxybenzamine
	Temazepam
	Tolazamide
66	Cyclopentobarbital
	Etidocaine
	Papaverine
67	Diazepam
	Isocarboxazid
68	Acenocoumarol
	Griseofulvin
	Mefenamic Acid
69	Flunitrazepam
	Piroxicam
	Tolbutamide
70	Medazepam
	Oxymetholone
	Pentetrazol
71	Pargyline
73	Ethchlorvynol
	Spironolactone
	Thiopental
74	Phenelzine
75	Prazepam
76	Progesterone
77	Mecloqualone
78	Desoxycortone
81	Cyclandelate
	Phensuximide
82	Anisindione
	Methoxsalen
83	Tetrabenazine
85	Mesuximide
87	Paramethadione
88	Cannabidiol
90	Cannabinol
	Clofibrate
	Phenothiazine
	Phenylbutazone
95	Clofenotane
	Methyl Salicylate
	Triprolidine
98	Bromhexine
	Camphor
	Diquat

System TAK (p. 406)—Rf values

Rf	*Compound*
00	Acepromazine
	Acetophenazine
	Aconitine
	Amiloride
	Aminophenazone
	Aminopromazine
	Amodiaquine
	Anileridine
	Aniline
	Antazoline
	Apomorphine
	Arecoline
	Atropine
	Azaperone
	Benzilonium Bromide
	Berberine
	Brompheniramine
	Brucine
	Butaperazine
	Butorphanol
	Carbinoxamine
	Carfenazine
	Chloroprocaine
	Chloroquine
	Chlorothiazide
	Chlorphenamine
	Cimetidine
	Cinchonidine
	Cocaine
	Codeine
	Demeclocycline
	Dihydrocodeine
	Dihydromorphine
	Dimetindene
	Dipyrone
	Dopamine
	Doxylamine
	Ergometrine
	Ethambutol
	Ethylnoradrenaline
	Etorphine
	Fluphenazine
	Furaltadone
	Guanethidine
	Hordenine
	Hydrochlorothiazide
	Hydroflumethiazide
	Hydroxyamfetamine
	Hydroxychloroquine
	Hydroxyzine
	Isoetarine
	Isopropamide Iodide
	Levodopa
	Lidocaine
	Lobeline
	Mazindol
	Metaraminol
	Methadone
	Methapyrilene
	Methyldopa
	Minocycline
	Molindone
	Morphine
	Nalbuphine
	Nicotine
	Normorphine
	Oxymorphone
	Phanquinone
	Phenylephrine
	Pilocarpine
	Piperacetazine
	Prazosin
	Procaine
	Procyclidine
	Propantheline Bromide
	Propoxycaine
	Pseudomorphine
	Ranitidine
	Sparteine
	Terbutaline
	Tetracaine
	Tetramisole
	Trazodone
	Triamterene
	Tripelennamine
01	Acetazolamide
	Digitoxin
	Ephedrine
	Hydralazine
	Hyoscyamine
	Ketobemidone
	Nalorphine
	Naloxone
	Naltrexone
	Narceine
	Oxycodone
	Oxymetazoline
	Oxyphencyclimine
	Phentolamine
	Pseudoephedrine
	Δ^9-Tetrahydrocannabinol
	Trimetaphan Camsilate
02	Chlordiazepoxide
	Chlorpromazine
	Clonidine
	Cyclopentolate
	Diethylpropion
	Droperidol
	Emetine
	Erythromycin
	Etamiphylline
	Etoxazene
	Eucatropine
	Haloperidol
	Harmaline
	Homatropine
	Imipramine
	Lysergide
	Mepivacaine
	Mesoridazine
	6-Monoacetylmorphine
	Orphenadrine
	Phenindamine
	Phenylpropanolamine
	Promazine
	Protokylol
	Quinidine
	Strychnine
	Thioridazine
	Tiabendazole
03	Benactyzine
	Debrisoquine
	Diethyltryptamine
	Dihydroergotamine
	Doxapram
	Harman
	Harmine
	Hydrocodone
	Isoniazid
	Mephentermine
	Metamfetamine
	Pentazocine
	Perphenazine
	Phenformin
	Physostigmine
	Prednisolone
	Procarbazine

Rf	*Compound*
	Tilidate
	Triprolidine
04	Bromazepam
	Buprenorphine
	Dextropropoxyphene
	Diquat
	Ethylmorphine
	Isometheptene
	Ketamine
	Mepenzolate Bromide
	Methylphenidate
	Methysergide
	Paroxetine
	Phencyclidine
	Phenoxybenzamine
	Phthalylsulfathiazole
	Prednisone
05	Acetylcodeine
	Alphaprodine
	Amitriptyline
	Bupivacaine
	Butacaine
	Chlorphenoxamine
	Cyclazocine
	Diamorphine
	Epithiazide
	Hydrocortisone
	Ibogaine
	Isoxsuprine
	Opipramol
	Paracetamol
	Phentermine
	Propranolol
	Sulfanilamide
	Tiotixene
	Trichlormethiazide
	Tryptamine
06	Azapropazone
	Benzquinamide
	Benzthiazide
	Cefalothin
	Etafedrine
	Levallorphan
	Nomifensine
	Pethidine
	Pindolol
	Quinethazone
	Reserpine
	Triamcinolone
	Xylazine
07	Dexamethasone
	Lysergic Acid
08	Betamethasone
	Butriptyline
	Chloramphenicol
	Chlorprothixene
	Colchicine
	Fentanyl
	Flurazepam
	Methyclothiazide
	Metolazone
	Papaverine
	Phenmetrazine
	Polythiazide
	Theobromine
	Trimethoprim
09	Cortisone
	Loxapine
	Mescaline
	Nortriptyline
	Prochlorperazine
10	Acetylcysteine
	Chlorcyclizine
	Chlortalidone
	Dimoxyline
	Indoramin
	Nicotinic Acid
	Profenamine
11	Bendroflumethiazide
	Cyclizine
	Piperidolate
	Sulfadiazine
	Sulfafurazole
	Thebaine
	Thiethylperazine
12	Biperiden
	Ethoheptazine
	Medazepam
	Methocarbamol
	Methoxamine
	Metoprolol
	Pentoxifylline
13	Diazoxide
	Difenidol
	Methylprednisolone
	Quinisocaine
14	Benzoctamine
	Clonixin
	Doxepin
	Metronidazole
	Pemoline
	Sulfamethizole
15	Hexylcaine
	Methazolamide
	Phenyltoloxamine
	Urea
16	Clomipramine
	Cyproheptadine
	Mecamylamine
	Phenethylamine
	Propiomazine
17	Alprenolol
	Methylenedioxymethamfetamine
	Nefopam
	Sulfadimidine
	Tranylcypromine
18	Caffeine
	Chlorphenesin Carbamate
	Methoxyamfetamine
	Noscapine
	Phenazone
	Tosylchloramide Sodium
19	Etidocaine
	Levomepromazine
	Methdilazine
	Nikethamide
	Saccharin
	Sulfapyridine
20	Flunixin
	Methoxyphenamine
	Normethadone
	Pargyline
	Phenazocine
	Pramocaine
	Resorcinol
	Sulfamethoxypyridazine
21	Theophylline
22	Indapamide
	Metixene
	Prilocaine
	Trihexyphenidyl
23	Benzonatate
	Desipramine
	Sulfachlorpyridazine
24	Dantrolene
	Meclozine
	Piminodine
	Propylhexedrine
25	Dicycloverine
	Fenfluramine
	Furosemide
	Pyrrobutamine
26	Azapetine
	Fluorometholone
	Sulfamethoxazole
27	Guaifenesin
28	Bromhexine
	Protriptyline
	Sulfadimethoxine
	Sulfadoxine
29	Mephenesin
	Meprobamate
30	Sulfasalazine
32	Chlorphenesin
33	Tetrabenazine
35	Fludrocortisone
	Fluoxymesterone
36	Nitrofurazone
	Thiopropazate
38	Demoxepam
39	Paramethasone
40	Sulindac
41	Oxyphenbutazone
	Pentetrazol
	Phenacetin
42	Bumetanide
	Etacrynic Acid
	Lorazepam
44	Aminobenzoic Acid
45	Chlormezanone
	Piroxicam
46	Embutramide
47	Mebutamate
	Oxazepam
48	Diazepam
	Etamivan
	Ethoxzolamide
	Griseofulvin
49	Hyoscine
50	Diphenylpyraline
51	Acenocoumarol
52	Methyl Hydroxybenzoate
	Nitrazepam
53	Clonazepam
54	Temazepam
56	Niflumic Acid
	Phenazopyridine
	Stanozolol
57	Mebendazole
58	Acecarbromal
	Estradiol
	Ethinylestradiol
	Halcinonide
59	Flunitrazepam
	Tolmetin
60	Nordazepam
	Primidone
61	Chlorzoxazone
	Methandienone
62	Amygdalin
	Vinbarbital
63	Cyclopentobarbital
	Prenylamine
	Testosterone
64	Carbamazepine
	Diclofenac
	Spironolactone
65	Aspirin
	Methyltestosterone
	Zomepirac
66	Acetohexamide
	Estrone

Rf	*Compound*
	Ethotoin
67	Isocarboxazid
68	Fenbufen
	Fendosal
	Mecloqualone
	Methoxsalen
	Progesterone
69	Diflunisal
	Ethinamate
	Flurbiprofen
	Prazepam
70	Alclofenac
	Anisindione
	Mephenytoin
	Mesuximide
	Paramethadione
71	Cyclandelate
	Desoxycortone
	Flavoxate
	Hexachlorophene
	Phensuximide
	Probenecid
	Salicylic Acid
	Thiopental
	Tolazamide
72	Mafenide
	Nitrofurantoin
74	Diphenadione
	Oxymetholone
	Phenelzine
	Tolbutamide
75	Naproxen
76	Cannabidiol
	Ibuprofen
	Phenylbutazone
77	Cannabinol
	Ethchlorvynol
	Meclofenamic Acid
	Phenothiazine
78	Chlorpropamide
	Cholesterol
	Fenoprofen
	Flufenamic Acid
80	Benoxaprofen
	Clofibrate
	Dicoumarol
	Tiaprofenic Acid
81	Benzoic Acid
82	Ketoprofen
84	Dimethoxanate
	Phenytoin
86	Mefenamic Acid
	Methyl Salicylate
90	Indometacin
93	Clofenotane
95	Camphor

System TAL (p. 406)—Rf values

Rf	*Compound*
00	Levodopa
	Phanquinone
02	Cocaine
	Pseudomorphine
04	Chloroquine
	Demeclocycline
	Hydroxychloroquine
05	Benzilonium Bromide
	Ecgonine
06	Chlorpropamide
	Methyldopa
	Tetramisole
07	Dopamine
08	Cimetidine
	Doxylamine
	Minocycline
09	Amodiaquine
10	Ranitidine
11	Nicotine
13	Oxymorphone
14	Atropine
15	Antazoline
	Ethylnoradrenaline
	Morphine
16	Guanethidine
18	Tripelennamine
19	Hydroxyamfetamine
	Isopropamide Iodide
20	Berberine
	Butacaine
	Ethambutol
	Hordenine
	Metaraminol
	Nalbuphine
	Propantheline Bromide
	Trimetaphan Camsilate
22	Aminopromazine
	Apomorphine
	Phenylephrine
	Procaine
24	Aconitine
	Dipyrone
	Mazindol
	Oxyphencyclimine
25	Chlorphenamine
	Dihydromorphine
	Hydralazine
	Oxymetazoline
	Saccharin
	Tetracaine
26	Acetylcysteine
	Codeine
	Isoetarine
27	Carbinoxamine
	Sparteine
28	Arecoline
	Brompheniramine
	Lidocaine
	Normorphine
29	Amiloride
	Ephedrine
	Phenformin
	Phenylpropanolamine
	Terbutaline
30	Piperacetazine
	Pseudoephedrine
	Urea
31	Δ^9-Tetrahydrocannabinol
32	Chloroprocaine
33	Acetophenazine
	Eucatropine
34	Homatropine
	Hydroxyzine
	Hyoscyamine
	Phentolamine
35	Diethylpropion
	Lobeline
36	Butorphanol
	Debrisoquine
	Mephentermine
	Narceine
	Oxycodone
	Phentermine
	Procyclidine
	Tryptamine
37	Ergometrine
	Molindone
38	Dihydrocodeine
	Harmaline
	Tilidate
39	Acepromazine
	Sulfasalazine
40	Azacyclonol
	Bupivacaine
	Dimetindene
	Hydrochlorothiazide
	Ketobemidone
	Mepivacaine
	Naltrexone
	Triamterene
41	Cefalothin
	Chlorothiazide
	Diethyltryptamine
	Fluphenazine
	Promazine
42	Butaperazine
	Cyclopentolate
	Erythromycin
	Phthalylsulfathiazole
43	Hydroflumethiazide
	Isometheptene
	Ketamine
44	Etamiphylline
	Pilocarpine
	Strychnine
45	Metamfetamine
	Methadone
	Naloxone
	Propoxycaine
46	Droperidol
	Nalorphine
47	Chlorpromazine
	Isoniazid
	Orphenadrine
48	Benactyzine
	Harmine
	Methapyrilene
	Phencyclidine
	Protokylol
49	Dimethoxanate
	Etafedrine
	Propranolol
50	Harman
	Maprotiline
	Methoxamine
	Nomifensine
	Phenethylamine
	Physostigmine
	Sulfanilamide
51	Carfenazine
	Clonidine
	Dextropropoxyphene
	Mescaline
	6-Monoacetylmorphine

Rf	Compound
	Phenoxybenzamine
	Thioridazine
52	Imipramine
	Mepenzolate Bromide
	Mesoridazine
	Tranylcypromine
54	Chlorphenoxamine
	Ethylmorphine
	Hydrocodone
	Paroxetine
	Prazosin
56	Amitriptyline
	Nicotinic Acid
	Perphenazine
	Pindolol
	Quinethazone
57	Etacrynic Acid
	Methylenedioxymethamfetamine
	Pentazocine
	Profenamine
58	Emetine
	Mecamylamine
	Methoxyamfetamine
59	Lysergide
	Opipramol
	Tiabendazole
60	Acetazolamide
	Alphaprodine
	Cyclazocine
	Etorphine
	Isoxsuprine
	Pemoline
	Phenmetrazine
61	Acetylcodeine
	Azapropazone
	Butriptyline
	Haloperidol
	Trichlormethiazide
62	Furaltadone
63	Bromazepam
	Chlortalidone
	Epithiazide
	Ibogaine
64	Brucine
	Diamorphine
	Methoxyphenamine
	Piperidolate
65	Benzoctamine
	Chlorprothixene
	Ethoheptazine
	Prednisolone
	Propylhexedrine
	Theobromine
	Triamcinolone
66	Levallorphan
	Methysergide
	Quinisocaine
	Trazodone
	Trimethoprim
67	Azaperone
	Difenidol
68	Anileridine
	Fenfluramine
	Nortriptyline
	Quinidine
	Resorcinol
	Tosylchloramide Sodium
69	Diflunisal
	Methyclothiazide
	Phenyltoloxamine
	Prilocaine
	Triprolidine
70	Alprenolol
	Chlorcyclizine
	Cinchonidine
	Etoxazene
	Furosemide
	Hexylcaine
	Methylphenidate
	Metoprolol
	Polythiazide
	Salicylic Acid
	Sulfadiazine
	Sulfafurazole
	Xylazine
71	Benzthiazide
	Chloramphenicol
	Doxepin
	Nefopam
	Tiotixene
72	Bendroflumethiazide
	Cyclizine
	Desipramine
	Methdilazine
	Methocarbamol
	Pethidine
73	Biperiden
	Colchicine
	Doxapram
	Flurazepam
	Metixene
	Paracetamol
74	Guaifenesin
	Hydrocortisone
	Prednisone
	Prochlorperazine
75	Clomipramine
	Dexamethasone
	Diazoxide
	Etidocaine
	Metolazone
	Metronidazole
	Sulfamethizole
76	Aminophenazone
	Cyproheptadine
	Fenoprofen
	Protriptyline
	Thebaine
77	Buprenorphine
	Indoramin
78	Bromhexine
	Digitoxin
	Loxapine
	Mephenesin
	Meprobamate
	Methazolamide
	Methylprednisolone
	Normethadone
	Theophylline
79	Chlordiazepoxide
	Lysergic Acid
80	Betamethasone
	Bumetanide
	Chlorphenesin Carbamate
	Clonixin
	Sulfachlorpyridazine
	Trihexyphenidyl
81	Caffeine
	Levomepromazine
	Propiomazine
	Sulfamethoxazole
82	Phenindamine
83	*p*-Aminobenzoic Acid
	Cortisone
	Fendosal
	Flunixin
	Nitrofurazone
	Phenazone
	Thiethylperazine
	Tolmetin
84	Diclofenac
	Dicycloverine
	Dihydroergotamine
	Fentanyl
	Sulfamethoxypyridazine
85	Sulfapyridine
86	Chlorphenesin
	Lorazepam
	Primidone
	Pyrrobutamine
87	Mebutamate
88	Zomepirac
89	Demoxepam
	Nikethamide
	Oxazepam
	Phenacetin
90	Acecarbromal
	Alclofenac
	Aspirin
	Azapetine
	Benzonatate
	Cyclopentobarbital
	Dantrolene
	Fluorometholone
	Indometacin
	Niflumic Acid
	Pentoxifylline
	Phenazocine
	Piminodine
	Pramocaine
	Prenylamine
	Probenecid
	Procarbazine
	Sulfadoxine
91	Acetohexamide
	Benzquinamide
	Clonazepam
	Diphenadione
	Estradiol
	Estrone
	Ethinamate
	Ethinylestradiol
	Ethotoin
	Ethoxzolamide
	Fenbufen
	Fludrocortisone
	Fluoxymesterone
	Flurbiprofen
	Halcinonide
	Hexachlorophene
	Mephenytoin
	Methyl Hydroxybenzoate
	Paramethasone
	Phenazopyridine
	Stanozolol
	Thiopropazate
	Vinbarbital
92	Acenocoumarol
	Amygdalin
	Benzoic Acid
	Chlorzoxazone
	Diphenylpyraline
	Flavoxate
	Indapamide
	Isocarboxazid
	Meclofenamic Acid
	Methandienone
	Methyltestosterone
	Nitrazepam
	Nordazepam
	Oxyphenbutazone
	Reserpine

Rf	*Compound*
	Sulindac
	Temazepam
	Testosterone
	Thiopental
93	Dimoxyline
	Hyoscine
	Ibuprofen
	Mafenide
	Mebendazole
	Naproxen
	Noscapine
	Papaverine
	Pargyline
	Phenelzine
	Tolbutamide
94	Carbamazepine
	Chlormezanone
	Oxymetholone
	Paramethadione
	Piroxicam
	Prazepam
95	Anisindione
	Cyclandelate
	Flufenamic Acid
	Flunitrazepam
	Meclozine
	Medazepam
	Mefenamic Acid
	Pentetrazol
	Progesterone
	Sulfadimidine
	Tolazamide
96	Aniline
	Cholesterol
	Desoxycortone
	Diazepam
	Dicoumarol
	Etamivan
	Ethchlorvynol
	Griseofulvin
	Mecloqualone
	Methoxsalen
	Phenothiazine
	Phensuximide
	Phenytoin
	Spironolactone
97	Cannabidiol
	Cannabinol
	Clofenotane
	Clofibrate
	Phenylbutazone
	Tetrabenazine
98	Camphor
	Diquat
	Ketoprofen
	Mesuximide
	Sulfadimethoxine
	Tiaprofenic Acid
99	Benoxaprofen

System TAM (p. 422)—**Rf values**

Rf	*Compound*
09	Estradiol
13	Chlorothiazide
33	Triamcinolone
54	Prednisolone
56	Methylprednisolone
58	Hydrocortisone
60	Prednisone
64	Flumetasone
66	Dexamethasone
68	Fluocinolone Acetonide
70	Betamethasone
74	Fluoxymesterone
75	Metolazone
78	Stanozolol
86	Fluorometholone
	Oxymetholone
88	Methandienone
90	Fludrocortisone
91	Cortisone
	Desoxycortone
	Paramethasone
92	Methyltestosterone
	Testosterone
94	Ethinylestradiol
95	Estrone
96	Cholesterol
97	Progesterone

Gas Chromatographic Data

ND = not detected/not eluted

System GA (p. 444)—retention index

RI	*Compound*
0	Acemetacin
305	Dichlorodifluoromethane
361	Cryofluorane
372	Acetaldehyde
421	Ethanol
462	Enflurane
469	Acetone
484	Trichlorofluoromethane
491	Methanol
515	Ether
	Methylene Chloride
530	Isopropyl Alcohol
533	Halothane
571	Propanol
579	Methyl Ethyl Ketone
596	Ethyl Acetate
605	Chloroform
634	Trichloroethane
680	Amyl Nitrite
695t	Cloral Hydrate
701	Methoxyflurane
710	Trichloroethylene
715	Methylpentynol
756	Toluene
780	Monoethanolamine
784	Dimethyl Sulfoxide
786	Paraldehyde
789	Tetrachloroethylene
798	Ethylene Glycol
813	Piperazine
838	Urethane
857	Trichloroethanol
860	Xylene *p*-xylene
863	Xylene *m*-xylene
882	Allopurinol
884	Xylene *o*-xylene
888	Tuaminoheptane
910	Tetrachloroethane
930	Putrescine
947	Benzaldehyde
949	Chlorobutanol
981	Phenol
1000	Acefylline Piperazine
	Benzene
	Carbon Tetrachloride
1015	Ethchlorvynol
1017	Fluspirilene
1020	Metaldehyde
1035	Cadaverine
1040	Benzyl Alcohol
	o-Cresol
1052	Isometheptene
1060	*p*-Cresol
	Dimethadione
	Trimethadione M (nor)
1064	Valproic Acid
1065	Cresol *m*-cresol
1090	Trimethadione
1100	Amfetamine art (formyl)
	Methyl Nicotinate
1105	Emylcamate
1110	Cresol *p*-cresol-AC
1111	Phenethylamine
1115	Paramethadione
1120	Heptaminol
1125	Amfetamine
	Fenetylline M (amfetamine)
1133	Fenfluramine norfenfluramine
1140	Bromisoval M (OH-isovalerianic acid)
1143	Camphor
1155	Phentermine
1158	Aniline
	Phenazopyridine aniline
1160	Clomethiazole M (deschloro-2-OH-)
	Prilocaine M (OH-desacyl-)
1175	Famprofazone M (metamfetamine)
	Metamfetamine
	Propylhexedrine
1180	Benzoic Acid
	Lidocaine M (2,6-dimethylaniline)
1185	Clomethiazole M (deschloro-)
	Metamfetamine M (4-OH-, pholedrine)
1186	Naphthalene
1190	Bromisoval M (Br-isovalerianic acid)
	Methamidophos
1195	Arecoline
	Methyl Salicylate
	Salicylic acid-Me
1200	Dicamba 2,5-dichloromethoxybenzene
1205	Ethosuximide
1206	Menthol
1210	Chloroaniline 4-chloroaniline
	Hyoscine art (desacyl-)
	Methenamine
1212	Sulfafurazole
1214	Pargyline
1215	Carbromal M (carbromide)
	Nicotinyl Alcohol
1220	Paracetamol art (*p*-aminophenol)-Me_2
	Tranylcypromine
1227	Clomethiazole
1230	Cyclopentamine
	Fenfluramine
1235	Betahistine
	Chlormezanone art
	Clomethiazole M (deschloro-COOH-)
	Dimethylamfetamine
1240	Amantadine
	Hydroquinone
	Mebanazine
	Mephentermine
	Phenacetin M (hydroquinone)
1250	Pyrazinamide
1253	4-Aminophenol
	Aprindine M (*p*-aminophenol)
	Paracetamol art (*p*-aminophenol)
1258	Resorcinol
1260	Thymol
1265	Phenazopyridine 4-aminophenol
1270	Ethosuximide M (oxo)
1275	Dichlorvos
	Phenacetin M (*p*-phenetidine)
1280	Cocaine M (anhydroecgonine methylester)
1293	Aletamine
1303	Disulfoton M (sulfoxide)
	Octamylamine
1307	Salicylic Acid
1308	Salicylic Acid
1309	Aminosalicylic Acid
	Benorilate aspirin
1312	Aminotriazole
1313	Phenylpropanolamine
1320	Aldicarb
	Dichlorophenoxyacetic Acid M (2,4-dichlorophenol)
	Labetalol Art
1322	Ethosuximide M (3-OH)
1323	Linuron 3,4-dichloroaniline
1331	Apronal
1334	Phendimetrazine
1335	Nicotinic Acid
	Phenelzine
1340	Carbromal M (OH-carbromide)
1341	Nikethamide M (nicotinamide)
1344	Chlorphentermine
1350	Clonidine Art (dichlorophenyl-isocyanate)
	Mexiletine M(desamino-oxo-)
	Nicotine
	Prilocaine M (desacyl-)-AC
	Selegiline M (nor)
1353	Dimetridazole
1355	Ephedrine M (nor)-TFA_2
1360	Cathine
	Diethylpropion M (phenylpropanolamine)
	Ephedrine M (nor)
1361	Methoxyphenamine
1365	Clomethiazole M (2-OH-)
	Ephedrine
	Ethinamate
	Pseudoephedrine
1368	Acetanilide
	Eugenol
1370	Ethosuximide M (OH-ethyl)
	Tryptophan M (OH-skatole)
1373	Bemegride
1380	Acecarbromal M (desbromocarbromal)
	Carbromal M(desbromo-)

RI	*Compound*
	Clomethiazole M (deschloro-2-OH-ethyl-)
	Ephedrine M (nor-)-PFP$_2$
1388	Rimantadine
1389	Diphenyl
1390	Ametazole
	Parachlorophenol
1400	Chlormezanone M (4-chlorobenzoic acid)
	Chlorocresol
	Dimethoate M (COOH-)-Me
	Mexiletine Mexiletene
1405	Diuron 3,4-dichloroaniline
	Methylephedrine
1406	Dimethyl Phthalate
1412	Methoxyamfetamine
1413	Piroxicam
1414	Etenzamide M (desethyl)/salicylamide
	Salicylamide
1416	Fenoterol
1420	Chloroxylenol
1430	Dimethoate M (OH-)
1432	Hordenine
	Methyl Hydroxybenzoate
	Phenmetrazine
	Warfarin
1436	Nicotinamide
1438	Trichlorfon
1440	Trichlorophenoxyacetic Acid M (trichlorophenol)
1450	Hydroquinine
	Mevinphos
	Selegiline
1460	Hydroquinone M (2-OH-)
	Lidocaine M (dimethylhydroxyaniline)
1462	Butylated Hydroxyanisole
1465	Amfetamine M (OH-methoxy-)
	Hydroxyamfetamine M (methoxy-)
	Pheneturide
1470	Metharbital
1472	Cocaine M (methylecgonine)
1473	Phenacemide
1475	Propylhexedrine M (OH-)
1480	Amfetamine M (4-OH-)
	Hydroxyamfetamine
	Methyl Hydroxybenzoate M (methoxy-)
	Methylenedioxyamfetamine MDA
1486	Diethylpropion
1487	Mandelic Acid
	Protokylol
1489	Barbital
	Metharbital barbital
1490	Butylated Hydroxytoluene
	Carbaryl M (1-naphthol)
	Pholedrine
1492	Cantharidin
1497	Histamine
1500	Clonidine Art (dichlorophenylmethyl-carbamate)
	Nialamide
	Phenyltoloxamine M ((*N*-oxide)-ME$_2$ NOH)
1504	Thiotepa
1505	Propranolol M (1-naphthol-)
1510	Amfetamine M (desamino-oxo-OH-methoxy-)
	Fenfluramine norfenfluramine-AC
1513	Acecarbromal M (carbromal)
	Carbromal
1515	Pyridostigmine Bromide
1517	Mercaptopurine
1519	Etafedrine
1520	Amfetamine M (3-OH-)-PFP$_2$
	Amfetamine M (desamino-oxo-OH-)-AC
	Diphenhydramine M (nor-)
	Methylenedioxyamfetamine art (formyl)
	Phenprobamate
1525	Nikethamide
	Parathion M (*p*-nitrophenol)
1527	Methyprylon
1528	Hydralazine
1540	Bromisoval
	Deltamethrin M (COOH-)-Me
	Methyprylon M (OH-)-H$_2$O
1542	Clofibrate
1545	Aspirin
	Gliclazide Art 1-Me
1547	Acetylcysteine
	4-Aminobenzoic Acid
1550	Carbimazole thiamazole
	Pentetrazol
	Selegiline M (nor-OH-)
	Thiamazole
1555	Benzocaine
	Carbaryl M (1-naphthol)-AC
	Chlormezanone M (*N*-methyl-4-chlorobenzamide)
	Ephedrine M (nor-) -TMS$_2$
1560	Clomethiazole M (1-OH-ethyl-)
	Doxylamine M (carbinol)-H$_2$O
	Enallylpropymal
	Etenzamide
	Methylenedioxyethylamfetamine MDEA
1564	Diethyl Phthalate
1565	DOM art (formyl)
1567	Propyl Hydroxybenzoate
1568	Mephenesin
1570	Methyl Hydroxybenzoate M (OH-)-AC
	Trifluperidol M (*N*-desalkyl-oxo) 2H$_2$O
1580	Ethyl Hydroxybenzoate
	Mepyramine M (*N*-desmethoxybenzyl-)
	Selegiline M (OH-)
1583	Diethyltoluamide
1585	Methylenedioxymethamfetamine MDMA
1590	Hydrastinine
1592	Metronidazole
1593	Dichlorophenoxyacetic Acid 2,4-D-Me
	Iproniazid
1595	Omethoate
1598	Tolazoline
1600	Allobarbital
	Amfetamine M (desamino-oxo-OH-methoxy-)-AC
	Crotamiton
	Hydroxyzine M (4-chloromethylbiphenyl)
1604	Clorprenaline
1605	Methylenedioxyamfetamine MDA-PFP
	Nikethamide M (*N*-ethylnicotinamide)
1608	Nicametate
1610	Benzophenone (BPH)
	Methyprylon enol-AC
	Metipranolol M art (phenol)-AC
1615	Ibuprofen
	Methylenedioxyamfetamine MDA-TFA
1618	Aprobarbital
1620	Glibornuride art (amide)
	Gliclazide art (amide)
	Methocarbamol M (guaifenesin)
1621	Chlorproguanil
1628	Demeton-*S* demeton-*S*-methyl
1630	Ibuprofen M (3-OH-)-Me
	Vanillin
1632	Glymidine Sodium
1634	Phensuximide
	Prolintane
1640	Butoxyethyl Nicotinate
	Clofibrate M (clofibric acid)
	Dipyridamole
1645	Barbital M (barbituric acid-Me$_3$)
	Carbinoxamine M (chlorobenzoylpyridine)
	Diphenhydramine M (diphenylmethanol)
	Trometamol
1650	Guaifenesin
	Haloperidol M (*N*-desalkyl-oxo-)-2H$_2$O
	Tripelennamine M (benzylpyridylamine)
1651	Tolazamide
1655	Secbutabarbital
1660	Butobarbital
	Dinitro-orthocresol
	Etenzamide M (desethyl-)-AC
	Vinbarbital M (5-(1-ethylpropyl)-barbituric acid)
1661	Oxyphencyclimine
1665	Butalbital
	Monocrotophos
	Paracetamol
	Secobarbital M (desallyl-)
	Vinylbital M (desvinyl-)
1667	Styramate
1670	Atrazine M (desethyl-deschloro-methoxy-)
	Carbinoxamine M (carbinol)
	Gliclazide art 3
	Isoniazid
1675	Fencamfamin
	Phenacetin
1676	Dofamium Chloride
1678	Carbimazole
	Dyclonine
1680	Atrazine M (desethyl-)
	Chlorphenesin
	Mescaline
	Phenyltoloxamine M (O-desalkyl-)
1682	Hydroxyephedrine
1683	Tolbutamide
1684	Demeton
1685	Clomethiazole M (deschloro-di-OH-)
	Etilefrine
	Salol
1687	Paracetamol
	Tigloidine
1688	Crotetamide
1690	Benzene Hexachloride α-isomer
	Bisoprolol (M (phenol))
	Monolinuron M art (HOOC-)-Me
	Simazine
	Tributyl Phosphate
1699	Cetrimide
1700	Deltamethrin M (desacyl-)-HCN
	Dichlorophenoxyacetic Acid 2,4-D-isopropyl ester
	Guaifenesin M (*O*-desmethyl-)
	Idobutal
	Orphenadrine M (methylbenzophenone)
	Oxprenolol M (desamino-OH-desalkyl-)

RI	*Compound*
1703	Talbutal
1705	Mesuximide
1710	Amobarbital
	Benzene Hexachloride β-isomer
	Methylenedioxymethamfetamine MDMA-TMS
1714	Atrazine
	Tocainide
1715	Nicotine M (cotinine)
	Thiambutosine
1720	Acecarbromal
	Beclamide
	Chlorothiazide
	Clofedanol M (2-Cl-benzophenone)
	Ibomal M (desbromo-oxo-)-Me$_2$
	Methylenedioxymethamfetamine MDMA-TFA
1724	Hydroxyphenamate
1725	Dimethoate
	Methylphenidate
	Tryptophan M (tryptamine)
	Tybamate
1726	Methoxamine
1728	Chlorzoxazone
1729	Vinylbital
1730	Droperidol M (benzimidazolone)-AC$_2$
	Glibornuride Art (methylsulfonamide)
	Gliclazide art (methylsulfonamide)
	Ibomal M (desbromo-OH-)-Me$_2$
1735	Amfetamine M (desamino-oxo-di-OH-)-AC$_2$
	Pentobarbital
	Selegiline M (nor-)-AC
1738	Benzyl Benzoate
	Cropropamide
	Propazine
1740	Glibornuride art (methylsulfonamide)-Me
	Gliclazide art (methylsulfonamide)-Me
	Ketamine M (nor-OH-)-NH$_3$
	α-Methyltryptamine
	Reserpine M (trimethoxybenzoic acid)-Me
1742	Butyl Aminobenzoate
1743	Halquinol
1745	Benzene Hexachloride γ-isomer
	Lindane
	Tyramine
1748	Profadol
	Trimethoxyamfetamine
1750	Amobarbital M (3-OH-)-Me$_2$
	Buclizine M (carbinol)
	Cinnarizine M (carbinol)
	Ibuprofen M (OH-)-Me
	Mesuximide M (nor-)
	Tolpropamine M (*N*-oxide)
	Trichlorophenoxyacetic Acid methyl ester
1753	Dimethyltryptamine
	Vinbarbital
1754	Butetamate
	Nitroxinil
	Pethidine
	Phenoperidine pethidine
1755	Benzene Hexachloride δ-isomer
	Methylenedioxyethylamfetamine MDEA-PFP
1756	Ethionamide
1760	Dimpylate
	Diphenhydramine M (desamino-OH-)
	Pentachlorophenol
1765	Ibuprofen M (HOOC-)-Me$_2$
1770	Ibomal M (desbromo-OH-)
	Meclofenoxate
	Methohexital
	Methylenedioxyethylamfetamine MDEA-TFA
	N-Methyltryptamine
	Neostigmine Bromide
1780	DOM M (*O*-desmethyl-)-PFP$_2$
	Reserpine M (trimethoxybenzoic acid)
1785	Carisoprodol meprobamate
	Mephenytoin
	Meprobamate
1786	Secobarbital
1790	Lidocaine M (desethyl-)
	Vinbarbital M (5-(1-ethylpropyl)-5-hydroxybarbituric acid)
1791	Chlorpropamide
1792	Alphaprodine
1795	Brallobarbital M (desbromo-OH-)
	Dicamba
	5-Methyltryptamine
1798	Benethamine
1800	Caffeine
	Carbamazepine M (acridine)
	Desmetryne
	Dichlorophenoxyacetic Acid 2,4-D
	Ethotoin
	Haloperidol M (*N*-desalkyl-)
	Histapyrrodine M (*N*-desbenzyl-)
	Lidocaine M (monoethylglycinexylidide)
	Metharbital M (OH-)
	Naproxen M (OH-)-Me$_2$
1801	Sparteine
1802	Chlorquinaldol
1803	Nimorazole
1804	Physostigmine
1805	Dichlorophenoxyacetic Acid 2,4-D-isobutyl ester
	Ephedrine M (nor-)-AC$_2$
	Pheniramine
	Terbutylazine
1807	Dexpanthenol
	Theobromine
1808	Cotarnine
	Trimeperidine
1810	Ketamine M (nor)
	Metamfetamine M (OH-methoxy-)
	Salicylic Acid M (glycine conjugate)-Me
1811	Pipobroman
1815	Aprobarbital M (OH-)
1816	Protionamide
1819	Saccharin
1820	Alprenolol
	Lobeline
	Methyl Hydroxybenzoate M (*p*-hydroxyhippuric acid)-Me
1823	Prilocaine
1825	Methylenedioxyethylamfetamine MDEA-TMS
	Salicylic Acid M (glycine conjugate)
	Trichlorophenoxyacetic Acid isopropyl ester
1827	Tilidate bisnortilidate
1830	Carisoprodol
	Glutethimide
	Hexylresorcinol
	Isoaminile
	Methylenedioxymethamfetamine MDMA-PFP
	Morazone M(OH-phenmetrazine isomer 1)
	Phenmetrazine M (OH-) isomer 1
	Phenyltoloxamine M (desamino-OH-)
	Tilidate nortilidate
1832	Moxisylyte
1833	Tetryzoline
1835	Dichlorophenoxyacetic Acid 2,4-Dichlorophenoxybutyric acid-Me
	Phenazone
1838	Tilidate
1840	Benorilate
	Dichlorophenoxyacetic Acid 2,4-D-butyl ester
	Etomidate M (COOH-)-Me
	Ketamine
1844	Dimenhydrinate
1845	Salicylic Acid M (glycine conjugate)-Me$_2$
1850	Amfetamine M (3-OH-)-TMS$_2$
	Bromisoval M (isovalerianic acid carbamide)
	Buclizine M (chlorobenzophenone (ClBP))
	Diuron
	Hexethal
	Hydroxyzine M (4-chlorobenzophenone)
	Noxiptiline M(dibenzocycloheptanone)
	Trichlorophenoxyacetic Acid 2,4,5-T
1851	Fluoxetine (norfluoxetine)
1852	Lachesine Chloride
1853	Brallobarbital
1855	Aminophenazone M (desamino-OH-)
	Benzfetamine
	Dichloralphenazone
	Dichloralphenazone M (4-OH-phenazone)
	Hexobarbital
	Parathion methyl
	Phenazone M (4-OH-)
	Viloxazine
1857	Ethoheptazine
	Thiopental
1859	Fluoxetine (fluoxetine)
1860	Demeton-*S*-methylsulfoxide
	Methylenedioxyamfetamine MDA-AC
	Metyrapone
	Salicylamide M (OH-)-AC$_2$
	Selegiline M (OH-)-AC
1865	Carbaryl
	Cyclopentobarbital
	Glutethimide M (OH-ethyl-)
	Morazone M(OH-phenmetrazine isomer 2)
	Phenmetrazine M (OH-) isomer 2
	Secobarbital M (3′-OH-)
1866	Demeton-*S*-methylsulfone
1870	Diphenhydramine
	Etomidate
	Lidocaine
	Methyprylon M (oxo-)
1875	Ephedrine M (OH-)
	Glutethimide M (OH-phenyl-)
1876	Alachlor
1879	Ametryne
1880	Aprindine M (desindane)-AC
	Butobarbital M (3′-oxo-)
	Heptachlor
	Ibomal
	Methohexital M (OH-)
	Phenylmethylbarbituric Acid
1883	Clorgiline
1884	Primidone M (phenylethylmalondiamide (PEMA))
1885	Fluvoxamine
	Pethidine M (nor-)
	Phenoperidine norpethidine
1889	Mebutamate

RI	*Compound*
1890	Diphenhydramine M (OH-)
	Malathion M (malaoxon)
	Methylphenobarbital
	Tolmetin
1892	Parathion M (amino-)
1895	Aminophenazone
	Clenbuterol (Art (-H_2O))
	Diphenhydramine M (di-OH-)
	Parathion paraoxon
	Prolintane M (oxo-)
1899	Thiamylal
1900	Amfetamine M (4-OH-)-AC_2
	Chloropyramine M (*N*-desalkyl-)
	Clofedanol M (aldehyde)
	Etamivan
	Flurbiprofen
	Morazone M(OH-MeO-phenmetrazine)
	Orphenadrine M (nor-)
	Phencyclidine
	Phenmetrazine M (OH-methoxy-)
	Tolpropamine
	Tryptophan M (indole acetic acid)-Me
1902	Digitoxin
1903	Cyclandelate
1905	Fenitrothion
1906	Morinamide
1910	Diethyltryptamine
	Doxylamine
	Monolinuron
1913	Dibutyl Phthalate
1915	Amobarbital M (3-OH-)
	Propylhexedrine M (OH-)-AC_2
1920	Aprindine M (*N*-desalkyl-)
	Bamethan
	Butobarbital M (3′-OH-)
	Harman M (1-OH)
	Ketamine M (nor-di-OH-)-2H_2O
	Meptazinol
	Penfluridol M (*N*-desalkyl-oxo-)-2H_2O
	Propyphenazone
	Tofenacin
1923	Bibenzonium Bromide
1925	Bethanidine
	Malathion
1927	Linuron
1930	Amfetamine M (3-OH-)-AC_2
	Desipramine M (ring)
	Imipramine M (ring)
	Prometryne
	Trimipramine M (nor-ring)
	Vinbarbital M (5-(3-hydroxy-1-methylbutyl)-5-vinylbarbituric acid)
1933	Prenalterol
1935	Orphenadrine
	Primidone M (diamide)
1938	Fenthion
1939	Azapetine
1940	Butalbital M (OH-)
	Butobarbital M (3′-OH-)-AC
	Phenyltoloxamine
	Prenylamine M (desamino-OH-)-H_2O
	Terbutryne
	Tryptophan M (indole formic acid)-Me
1943	Aldrin
	Tramadol
1945	Nystatin
1948	Bunitrolol
1949	Isocarboxazid
1950	Droperidol M (benzimidazolone)
	Flufenamic Acid
	Mephenytoin M (nor)
	Parathion ethyl
	Pimozide M (benzimidazolone)
	Tetracycline
1952	Harman
1953	Phenobarbital
	Primidone M (phenobarbital)
1955	Aminophenazone M (bis-nor)
	Chlorpyrifos
	Cyclobarbital
	Dipyrone M (bis-desalkyl-)
	Glibornuride M (COOH-)-art (sulfonamide)-Me_3
	Gliclazide M (HOOC-)-art (sulfonamide)-Me_3
	Nifenazone M(desacetyl)
1960	Amobarbital M (COOH-)
	Doxylamine M (desamino-OH-)-AC
	Fenyramidol
	Ketamine M (nor-OH-)-H_2O
1964	Padimate
1965	Hexylcaine
1969	Pemoline
1970	Doxepin M (*cis-N*-oxide)
	Hexobarbital M (OH-)-H_2O
	Trifluperidol M (*N*-desalkyl-)
1971	Caramiphen
1973	Emepronium Bromide
1975	Amitriptyline M (*N*-oxide)
	Clioquinol
	Ethomoxane
1976	Tiaprofenic Acid
	Tripelennamine
1980	Aminophenazone M (nor-)
	Atropine Art (-CH_2O)
	Hexobarbital M (nor-)
	Methoxsalen
	Naproxen M (*O*-desmethyl-)-Me_2
	Piperocaine
1981	Methapyrilene
1985	Methylenedioxyethylamfetamine MDEA-AC
	Opipramol M (ring)
	Oxprenolol Art
	Psilocin
1990	Procarbazine
1995	Meptazinol M (nor-)
	Tramadol M (*O*-desmethyl-)
	Vinylbital M (OH-)-H_2O
1996	Chlorphenamine
1998	Carbamazepine M (iminostilbene)
	Tramadol M (O-desmethyl-)-AC
1999	Thenyldiamine
2005	Fencamfamin M (desethyl-)-AC
	Theophylline
	Tiocarlide
2008	Diethylthiambutene
2010	Baclofen
	Diphenhydramine M (methoxy)
	Procaine
	Triamterene
2013	Octafonium Chloride
2014	Chlorphenamine M (nor-)
	Pilocarpine
2016	Fenoprofen
2020	Alimemazine M (ring) (phenothiazine)
	Chlordane
	Dixyrazine M (phenothiazine)
	Fenamiphos
	Furosemide Art (-SO_2NH)-Me
	Hexobarbital M (oxo-)-Me
	Mequitazine M (phenothiazine)
	Promethazine M (phenothiazine)
	Vinbarbital M (OH-)-H_2O
	Xylometazoline
2021	Methadone 2-ethyl-5-methyl-3,3-diphenyl-1-pyrroline (EMDP)
2022	Cyclopentolate
	Isopropamide Iodide
2024	Gliquidone
	Tinidazole
2025	Butanilicaine
	Carbamazepine M (formyl-acridine)
	Cyclizine
	Oxcarbazepine M (formylacridine)
	Zomepirac M (-CO_2)
2026	Eucatropine
2029	Dimethoxanate
2030	Glibornuride M (OH-)-Art (sulfonamide)-Me_2
	Gliclazide M (OH-)-art (sulfonamide)-Me_2
	Quinisocaine
	Selegiline M (nor-OH-)-AC_2
2033	Isopropylaminophenazone
2035	Metoprolol
	Nefopam
2037	Pipazetate
2038	Thioacetazone
2040	Brallobarbital M (2-OH-)
	Etidocaine
	Furosemide Art (-SO_2NH)
	Ketobemidone
	Methadone 2-ethylidene-1,5-dimethyl-3,3-diphenylpyrrolidine (EDDP)
	Tiabendazole
2045	DOM M (desamino-oxo-OH-)-PFP_2
	Naproxen
	Pethidine M (OH-)
	Prothipendyl M (ring)
2046	Psilocybine
2050	Cinnarizine M (OH-methoxy-BPH) isomer 1
	Cyclobarbital M (oxo-)-Me_2
	Diphenhydramine M (OH-methoxy-BPH) isomer 1
	Diphenylpyraline M (OH-methoxy-BPH) isomer-1
	Furosemide Art (-SO_2NH)-Me_2
	Hexobarbital M (1,5-dimethyl-5-(3-oxo-1-cyclohexen-1-yl)barbituric acid)
	Methocarbamol
	Norbormide
2055	Heptabarb
	Phenindione
2057	Bufotenine
2060	Glutethimide M (OH-ethyl-)-AC
2065	Amfetamine M (OH-methoxy-)-AC_2
	Cinnarizine M (OH-BPH) isomer 1
	Cyclophosphamide
	Diphenhydramine M (OH-BPH) isomer 1
	Diphenylpyraline M (OH-BPH) isomer-1
	Mepivacaine
	Propranolol M (desamino-OH-)
2070	Berberine
	Cinnarizine M (OH-methoxy-BPH) isomer 2
	Diphenhydramine M (OH-methoxy-BPH) isomer 2
	Diphenylpyraline M (OH-methoxy-BPH) isomer-2
	Dobutamine M (*N*-desalkyl-*O*-methyl-)-AC_2
	Dopamine M (*O*-methyl-)-AC_2
	Vinbarbital M (OH-)
2072	Homatropine

RI	*Compound*
2077	Disulfoton M (sulfone)
2078	Benzoctamine
2080	Carbinoxamine
	Chlorphenoxamine
	Cinnarizine M (OH-BPH) isomer 2
	Diphenhydramine M (OH-BPH) isomer 2
	Diphenylpyraline M (OH-BPH) isomer 2
	Pheniramine M (nor-)
2085	Atropine Art (-H_2O)
	Reserpine M (trimethoxyhippuric acid)
2087	Ranitidine
2090	Clofedanol
	Clofedanol M (nor)-H_2O
	Clofenotane *op*′-DDE
	Clonidine
	Endosulfan
	Fluorouracil
2092	Brompheniramine
2093	Hexetidine
2095	Diflunisal
	Methadone M (nor-)
	Metoclopramide M (desethyl-)
	Normethadone
2098	Methoprotryne
2100	Chlorpromazine M (*N*-oxide)
	Chlorpromazine M (ring)
	Clenbuterol (clenbuterol)
	Dosulepin M (*N*-oxide)
	Histapyrrodine M (*N*-desphenyl-oxo-)-H_2O
	Lorcainide M (desacyl-)
	Naphazoline
	Perphenazine M (ring)
	Prochlorperazine M (*N*-oxide)
	Tolpropamine M (nor-)
	Verapamil M (*N*-desalkyl-)
2103	Proxyphylline
2110	Aldrin dieldrin
	Dieldrin
	Prolintane M (OH-phenyl-)-AC
2111	Dicycloverine
2114	Cycrimine
2115	Cocaine M (nor-cocaethylene)
	Primidone M (acetyl-)
	Prolintane M (OH-methoxy-phenyl-)-AC
	Xipamide art (-SO_2NH)-Me_2
2116	Thialbarbital
2120	Ascorbic Acid
	Cinnarizine M (desalkyl-) (norcyclizine)
	Cyclizine M (nor-)
	Flupentixol M (*N*-oxide)
	Fluspirilene M (desamino-OH-)
	Glycopyrronium Bromide
	Histapyrrodine M (*N*-desbenzyl-oxo-)
	Mepyramine M (*N*-desalkyl-)
	Penfluridol M (desamino-OH-)
	Perazine M (phenothiazine)
	Phenothiazine
	Pimozide M (desamino-OH-)
	Promazine M (phenothiazine)
2125	Etofylline etophylline
	Fenetylline M (etofylline)
	Lidoflazine M(desaminocarboxy-)-Me
2130	Chlorphenamine M (desamino-OH-)-AC
	Clofedanol M (OH-)-H_2O
	Dosulepin M (OH-*N*-oxide)
	Pimozide M (desamino-carboxy-)
2132	Sulfacetamide
2133	Chloropyrilene
2135	Methaqualone
	Prolintane M (OH-phenyl-)
2138	Dextromethorphan
	Pyrimethamine
	Racemorphan
2140	Atenolol Art (HOOC-)-Me
	Clofenotane *pp*′-DDE
	Dichlorophen
	Methylenedioxymethamfetamine MDMA-AC
	Phenyltoloxamine M (nor-)
2141	Disulfiram
2142	Alverine
2145	Chlortalidone
	Ephedrine M (OH-)-AC_3
	Methadone
	Pipradrol
2146	Clomipramine M (*N*-oxide)
2147	Propranolol
2150	Amfetamine M (3,4-di-OH-)-AC_3
	Atenolol Art (-H_2O)
	Carbinoxamine M (nor)
	Phenmetrazine M (OH-) isomer 1-AC_2
	Tolpropamine M (OH-)
2155	Bromazine
	Prilocaine M (OH-)
	Trioxysalen
2156	Bromocriptine
	Procyclidine
2160	Chloropyramine M (*N*-desalkyl-)-AC
	Clenbuterol (Art)
2162	Cocaine M (nor-)
2165	Tacrine
2170	Hydrochlorothiazide art (-SO_2NH)-Me
	Oxymetazoline
	Tryptophan-Me_2-AC
2173	Oxyphenonium Bromide Art
2174	Santonin
2175	Atenolol and
	Dopamine
2177	Imolamine
2180	Flurbiprofen M (OH-)-Me_2
	Rescinnamine
2181	Butriptyline
2183	Endrin
2184	Ergocryptine
2185	Sulfanilamide
2186	Adiphenine
2187	Cocaine
	Methazolamide
2188	Dextropropoxyphene
2190	Atropine
	Chloropyramine
	Cyclobarbital M (oxo-)
	Fluoxetine (noracetylfluoxetine)
	Flupentixol M (ring)
	Fluphenazine M (ring)
	Hyoscyamine
	Oxeladin
	Trifluoperazine M (ring)
	Triflupromazine M (ring)
2193	Racemorphan M (nor-)
2194	Amitriptyline
2195	Cyclobenzaprine
2199	Chlormezanone chlormezazone
2200	Etofylline-AC
	Lorcainide M (desacyl-)-AC
	Phenmetrazine M (OH-) isomer 2-AC_2
	Phenobarbital M (4-OH-)-Me_3
	Prolintane M (oxo-OH-alkyl-)
	Tolpropamine M (nor-OH-)
	Tramadol M (OH-)
2201	Mefenamic Acid
2202	Mianserin M (*N*-oxide)
2203	Thonzylamine
2205	Dropropizine
	Pethidine M (OH-)-AC
2210	Chloropyramine M (nor)
	Etamiphylline
	Mianserin
	Penfluridol M (*N*-desalkyl-)
	Phenindamine M (nor-)
2214	Norpropoxyphene
2215	Amitriptyline M (nor-)
	Nortriptyline
	Trimipramine
2218	Clofenotane *op*′-DDT
2220	Carbamazepine M (epoxide)
	Chlorcyclizine
	Chlorphenoxamine M (OH-methoxy-carbinol)-H_2O
	Clemastine M (OH-methoxy-carbinol)-H_2O
	Doxepin *cis*
	Doxepin *trans*
	Isothipendyl M(nor-)
	Mepyramine
	Mesuximide M (OH-)
	Phenyltoloxamine M (O-desalkyl-OH-)
	Tetracaine
2223	Zimeldine M (nor-)
2225	Isothipendyl
2227	Aminoglutethimide
2230	Clomipramine M (ring)
	Dextrorphan
	Fluspirilene M (desamino-carboxy-)
	Imipramine
	Isothipendyl M (bis-nor)
	Levorphanol
	Lidoflazine M(desaminocarboxy-)
	Penfluridol M (desamino-carboxy-)
	Phenindamine M (*N*-oxide)
	Triflupromazine
2232	Carbetapentane
2235	Amitriptyline M (cyclobenzaprine)
	Desipramine
	Medazepam
	Mianserin M (nor)
	Phenoxybenzamine
2240	Aminoacridine
	Carbamazepine M (OH-ring)
	Desipramine M (ring-OH-)
	Dextromethorphan dextrorphan
	Diphenhydramine M (di-nor-acetyl)
	Famprofazone M (OH-propyphenazone)-AC
	Histapyrrodine
	Imipramine M (OH-ring)
	Methaqualone M (2-formyl-)
	Metipranolol M (desamino-OH-)-AC_2
	Pentifylline
	Pethidine M (nor-)-AC
	Prolintane M (oxo-OH-methoxy-phenyl-)
2241	Chloroprocaine
	Dextrorphan M (nor-)
	Metipranolol
2243	Azacyclonol
2245	Disopyramide M (bis-desalkyl-)-NH_3
	Doxepin M (*cis*-nor-)
	Doxepin M (*trans*-nor-)
	Ketoprofen
	Phenazopyridine
	Pindolol
	Trihexyphenidyl
2250	Bamipine
	Cocaine M (cocaethylene)
	Flecainide

RI	*Compound*
	Fluoxetine (acetylfluoxetine)
	Glutethimide M (OH-phenyl-)-AC
	Mirtazapine
	Nifedipine M (dehydro-)
	Pentifylline M (di-OH-)-H_2O isomer-1
	Primidone
	Promethazine M (nor-)
	Trifluomeprazine
2253	Protriptyline
	Sulfinpyrazone
	Trimetozine
	Triprolidine
2255	Benactyzine
	Flurazepam M (desalkyl-OH-)
	Mecloqualone
	Procainamide
	Prolintane M (oxo-OH-alkyl-)-AC
	Quazepam M (2-oxo-)
2258	Triazophos
2259	Promethazine
2260	Chlorprothixene Art (Cl-thioxanthenone)
	Clopenthixol Art-(Cl-thioxanthenone)
	DOM M (OH-)-AC_2
2265	Diphenhydramine M (nor-acetyl-)
	Glibornuride M (OH-)-art (sulfonamide)-Me
	Gliclazide M (OH-)-art (sulfonamide)-Me
2266	Timolol
2269	Bupivacaine
2270	Noxiptiline Noxiptyline
	Zimeldine
2271	Diclofenac
2273	Anisindione
2275	Dimetindene
	Heptabarb 3′-hydroxyheptabarbital
	Nitrendipine M (dehydro-desethyl-) CO_2
	Prolintane M (oxo-OH-phenyl-)-AC
2276	Biperiden
2280	Diprophylline
	Doxylamine M (bis-nor-)-AC
	Medazepam M (nor-)
	Pentazocine
	Phenyltoloxamine M (OH-) isomer 1
	Trichlorophenoxyacetic Acid 2,4,5-T-isobutyl ester
2281	Pramocaine
2285	Carbamazepine
	Galantamine
	Oxcarbazepine M (carbamazepine)
	Pentifylline M (di-OH-)-H_2O isomer-2
2290	Guaifenesin M (OH-methoxy-)-AC_2
	Nifedipine M (dehydro-COOH-)
2291	Harmine
2293	Maprotiline M (nor-)
2295	Methylphenobarbital M (nor-OH-)
	Pentifylline M (OH-) isomer-1
	Phenobarbital M (4-OH-)
	Prolintane M (di-OH-phenyl-)-AC_2
	Sulpiride art (-SO_2NH)
	Tramadol M (nor-)-AC
2298	Diethylstilbestrol
2300	Aprindine M (desphenyl-)-AC
	Buclizine M (OH-ClBP)
	Doxylamine M (OH-)-AC
	Hydroxyzine M (OH-chlorobenzophenone)
	Hyoscine
	Isoxsuprine
	Mafenide M(acetyl-)-Me
	Mesuximide M (nor-OH-)
	Phenindamine M (OH-)
	Phenyltoloxamine M (OH-) isomer 2
2301	Bufylline
2302	Benzatropine
2305	Alimemazine
	Fencamfamin M (desethyl-OH-)-AC_2
2310	Chloramphenicol
	Domiphen Bromide
	Flurbiprofen M (OH-methoxy)-Me_2
	Methylphenobarbital M (OH-methoxy-)
	Tertatolol
2314	Buphenine
	Clofenotane *pp′*-DDT
	Primaquine
2315	Dihydroergotamine
2318	Antazoline
	Piperidolate
	Thenalidine
2320	Doxylamine M (OH-methoxy-)-AC
	Heptabarb 3′-oxoheptabarbitone
	Phenmetrazine M (OH-methoxy-)-AC_2
	Phenyltoloxamine M (OH-methoxy-)
	Phenyltoloxamine M (nor-OH-) isomer 1
	Phenytoin
	Trichlorophenoxyacetic Acid isooctil ester
2323	Proxymetacaine
2325	Oxazepam
	Mazindol
	Viloxazine M (di-oxo-)
2327	Mepenzolate Bromide
2330	Ambucetamide
	Disopyramide M (*N*-desalkyl-)-CHNO-AC
	Dobutamine M (*N*-desalkyl-*O*-methyl-)-AC
	Nitrendipine M (dehydro-desmethyl-) CO_2
2335	Alimemazine M (nor-)
	Iprindole
	Propoxycaine
	Tropicamide
2336	Probenecid
2337	Bromhexine
2339	Thiazinamium Metilsulfate
2340	Carbamazepine M (OH-methoxy-ring)
	Doxylamine M (nor-)-AC
	Mafenide
	Phenyltoloxamine M (nor-OH-) isomer 2
	Profenamine
2348	Amitriptyline M (*cis*-10-OH-)
	Amitriptyline M (*trans*-10-OH-)
2350	Lidocaine M (OH-)
	Reserpine (trimethoxyhippuric acid)-ME
2355	Cyproheptadine
	Levallorphan
	Oxypertine
2360	Methaqualone M (2-OH-methyl-)
	Prolintane M (oxo-OH-methoxy-phenyl-)-AC
	Viloxazine M (*O*-desethyl-)-AC_2
2365	Dextropropoxyphene M (nor-)-AC
2366	Ergotamine
2367	Phenylbutazone
2370	Betaxolol
	Diperodon
	Imipramine M (OH-methoxy-ring)-AC
	Methylphenobarbital M (OH-)
	Noxytiolin
	Phenglutarimide M (desethyl-)
2375	Codeine
	Harmaline art (dihydro-)
	Nortriptyline M (*cis*-10-OH-)
	Nortriptyline M (*trans*-10-OH-)
	Pizotifen
2376	Piperonyl Butoxide
2377	Azatadine
	Diethazine
2378	Bisoprolol (bisoprolol)
2380	Amitriptyline M (OH-)
	Benzydamine
	Dosulepin
	Feprazone
	Mephenytoin M (OH-methoxy-)
	Pentazocine M (desalkyl-)-AC_2
	Polythiazide
2384	Difenidol
2385	Atenolol
	Xipamide art (-SO_2NH)
2388	Codeine M (nor)
	Nitrazepam 2-amino-5-nitrobenzophenone
	Norcodeine
2390	Amitriptyline M (nor-OH-)
	Cannabis CBD
	Desipramine M (ring-OH-methoxy-)
	Dihydrocodeine
	Imipramine M (OH-methoxy-ring)
	Maprotiline
	Tripelennamine M (OH-)-AC
2392	Dosulepin M (sulfoxide)
2395	Dipyrone M (desalkyl-)-AC
	Nandrolone
	Neopine
	Phenprocoumon isomer 2-Me
2400	Betaxolol (Art-H_2O)
	Bisoprolol (Art(-H_2O))
	Cyproheptadine M (nor)
	Dextropropoxyphene M (nor-*N*-propionyl-)
	Dihydromorphine
	Hydrocodone M (dihydromorphine)
	Mephenytoin M (4-OH-)
	Mepivacaine M (oxo-)
	Methaqualone M (2-carboxy-)
	Tripelennamine M (OH-)
2402	Hexestrol
2405	Chlorphenamine M (OH-)-AC
	Fluspirilene M (*N*-desalkyl-oxo-)
	Morphine M (nor-) PFP_3
	Promazine M (nor-)
2406	Dibenzepin M (di-nor)
	Pentoxifylline
2410	Azatadine M (OH-alkyl-)-H_2O
	Betaxolol (Art)
	Chlorprothixene M (*N*-oxide) $(CH_3)_2NOH$
	Clopenthixol M (*N*-oxide)-$C_6H_{14}N_2O_2$
	Famprofazone M (OH-propyphenazone)
	Lorazepam
	Mepivacaine M (OH-)
	Meptazinol M (oxo-)
2413	Sotalol
2415	Benperidol M (*N*-desalkyl-)
	Clomipramine
	Pimozide M (*N*-desalkyl-)
2417	*op′*-Methoxychlor
2419	Pyrrobutamine
2420	Chlorambucil
	Chloropyramine M (bis-nor-)-AC
	Diloxanide
	Ethylmorphine
	Meclofenamic Acid

RI	*Compound*
	Tripelennamine M (nor-)
	Tripelennamine M (nor-)-AC
2421	Dosulepin M (nor)
	Dosulepin M (norsulfoxide)
2425	Clemastine
	Mafenide M(acetyl-)
2428	Diazepam
2430	Harmaline
	Tetrazepam
	Tetrazepam M (oxo)
2432	Clomipramine M (nor)
2433	Propanidid
2434	Aminopromazine
2440	Chloropyramine M (OH-)-AC
	Hydrocodone
	Morphine M (nor)-PFP_2
	Quazepam
	Tramazoline
2444	Ketazolam
2445	Etynodiol Diacetate
	Hydromorphone
	Methoxychlor
	Morphine
2449	Dibenzepin M (nor-)
2450	Acebutolol M (phenol-)
	Androstanolone dihydrotestosterone enol-TMS_2
	Cyproheptadine M (nor-OH-)-H_2O
	Dibenzepin
	Furosemide M (*N*-desalkyl-)-Me_2
	Isothipendyl M(OH-)
	Mebhydrolin
	Nomifensine M(OH-)
	Profenamine M (bis-desethyl-)-AC
	Prolintane M (oxo-di-OH-phenyl-)-AC_2
2451	Hydromorphone M (dihydromorphine)
2452	Chlordiazepoxide M (nor)
2455	Dibenzepin M (N_5-desmethyl-)
2457	Butacaine
	Clorazepic Acid
2459	Morphine M (nor)
	Normorphine
2460	Cocaine M (*m*-OH-)
	Diclofenac M (OH-)-Me_2
	Flutazolam
	Verapamil M (*N*-desalkyl-acetyl-)
2461	Azapropazone
2462	Aprindine
2464	Tramadol M (*N*,*O*-didesmethyl-)-AC_2
2465	Molindone
	Protoveratrine A protoveratrines A and B
2467	Methdilazine
2470	Astemizole M (*N*-desalkyl)
	Bromazepam M (3-OH-)
	Chloropyramine M (nor)-AC
	Chlorphenoxamine M (OH-)
	Flurazepam M (desalkyl-)
2471	Oxybuprocaine
2473	Azinphos-methyl
	Δ^9-THC
2474	Dipipanone
2475	Androsterone
	Prolintane M (oxo-di-OH-phenyl-)
2480	Chlorpromazine M (didesmethyl-)
	Chlorpromazine M (nor-)
	Fenetylline M (*N*-desalkyl-)-AC
	Imipramine M (OH-)-Me
	Metixene
	Xipamide art (-SO_2NH)-Me
2485	Dihydrotestosterone-TMS
	Perhexiline M (OH-)
	Prolintane M (oxo-di-OH-)-AC_2
2488	Norpipanone
2490	Butalamine
	Chlorprothixene Art (dihydro-)
	Nordazepam
	Lorcainide M (*N*-desalkyl-desacyl-)-AC_2
	Nordazepam
	Procyclidine M (oxo-)-H_2O
	Sulfaethidole M (acetyl-)
	Tetrabenazine
2492	Chlorprothixene
2495	Chlorpromazine
	3-Monoacetylmorphine
	Ergocristine
	Mianserin M (8-OH-)
	Tubocurarine Chloride
2500	Cannabigerol
	Dosulepin M (OH-)
	Flecainide (Art (formyl))
	Histapyrrodine M (OH-)
	Tetrabenazine M (*O*-desmethyl-OH-)
	Trihexyphenidyl M (OH-)
2502	Sulfadiazine
2503	Acetylcodeine
2505	Disopyramide
	Emetine
	Nomifensine M (isomer 1)
	Pentifylline M (OH-) isomer-2
2510	Dihydrotestosterone
	Perhexiline M (diOH-) H_2O
2514	Levomepromazine
2515	Profenamine M (desethyl-)-AC
2517	Thebaine
2520	Azatadine M (OH-alkyl-)-AC
	Buclizine M (desalkyl-) (norchlorcyclizine)
	Chlorcyclizine M (nor-)
	Hydroxyzine M (desalkyl-)
	Meclozine M (*N*-desalkyl-)
2524	Oxycodone
2525	Methaqualone M (6-OH-)
	6-Monoacetylmorphine 6-MAM
	Oxetacaine
2526	Dextropropoxyphene M (nor-amide)
2529	Chlordiazepoxide M (demoxepam)
	Demoxepam
2530	Apomorphine
	Chlorphenamine M (nor-)-AC
	Dehydroepiandrosterone DHEA
	Doxepin M (OH-dihydro-)
	Mianserin M (OH-methoxy-)
	Tetrazepam M (nor-)
2533	Thebacon
2535	Cannabinol
	Chlorphenamine M (bis-nor-)-AC
	Doxepin M (*cis*-OH-)
	Imipramine M (OH-ring)-AC
2538	Oxymorphone
2540	Azatadine M (OH-aryl-)-AC
	Doxepin M (*cis*-nor-OH-)
	Nadolol
	Pecazine
2545	Nifedipine
	Pentazocine M (OH-)
	Verapamil M (*N*-didesalkyl-acetyl-)
2550	Acecainide
	Benoxaprofen
	Harmaline M (*O*-desmethyl-)-2H
	Harmine M (*O*-desmethyl-)
	Indometacin (capillary)
	Indometacin
	N-acetylprocainamide
2551	Noretynodrel
2553	Desipramine M (2-OH-)
2555	Chloroquine M (desethyl-)
	Dextrorphan M (OH-)-AC_2
	Dimefline
	Drostanolone
	Loxapine
	Pericyazine M (ring)
	Prenylamine
2558	Clobazam
	Trimethoprim
2560	Azinphos-ethyl
	Chlorprothixene M (*N*-oxide sulfoxide) $(CH_3)_2NOH$
	DOM M (desamino-oxo-OH-)-AC_2
	Doxepin M (*trans*-OH-)
	Etamiphylline M (desethyl-)-AC
	Methaqualone M (OH-methoxy-)
	Nadolol Art
	Pentifylline M (OH-)-AC
	Prolintane M (oxo-di-OH-methoxy-)-AC_2
2565	Imipramine M (OH-)
2566	Sulfamerazine
2569	Clomipramine M (2-OH-)
2570	Benzoylecgonine
	Cocaine M (benzoylecgonine)
	Histapyrrodine M (oxo-)
	Maprotiline M (desamino-di-OH-)
	Oxycodone M (dihydro-)-AC_2
	Tetrazepam M (OH-) isomer 1
2573	Coumaphos
2574	Clomipramine M (10-OH-)
2575	Drostanolone-TMS
	Midazolam
	Trimipramine M (OH-)
2578	Ethoxzolamide
2580	Bamipine M (OH-)
	Dehydroepiandrosterone DHEA enol-TMS_2
	Promethazine M (nor-OH-)
	Tetrazepam M (OH-) isomer 2
2588	Carteolol
2590	Chlorpromazine M (OH-)-Me
	Cinchonidine
	Cinchonine
	Deltamethrin M (desacyl-)-Me
	6-Monoacetylmorphine 6-MAM-TMS
	Nifuratel
	Nomifensine M (isomer 2)
	Phenindamine M (nor-OH-)
	Promethazine M (OH-)
	Pyrazophos
	Trimipramine M (OH-methoxy-)
	Viloxazine M (OH-)-AC_2
2595	Bisoprolol (Art)
	Dehydroepiandrosterone DHEA-H_2O
	Temazepam
2600	Alimemazine M (OH-)-AC
	Androstenedione
	Desipramine M (ring-di-OH-)
	Dibenzepin M (OH-) isomer-1-AC
	Flunitrazepam
	Harmine M (*O*-desmethyl-)-AC
	Imipramine M (di-OH-ring)
	Mexazolam
	Pethidine M (nor-OH-)-AC_2
	Sulfanilamide M (acetyl-)-Me
	Sulfapyridine
2603	Flupirtine
2605	Chloroquine
	Morphine M (nor-)-TMS_3
2607	Ketotifen
2610	Celiprolol
	Imipramine M (OH-)-AC

RI	*Compound*
2612	Estrone
	Mestranol
2613	Sulfadimidine
2615	Deptropine
	Diamorphine
2617	Phenacaine
2620	Clemizole
	Enalapril
	Metoclopramide
	Metoprolol M (*O*-desmethyl-)-AC_3
	Nalorphine
	Sulfaethidole
	Testosterone
2625	Drostanolone-enol-TMS_2
	Gallamine Triethiodide
	Norethisterone
2630	Dihydrotestosterone-AC
	Prolintane M (tri-OH-)-AC_3
2635	Coumatetralyl
	Nitrendipine
2638	Amoxapine
	Loxapine M(amoxapine)
2640	Disopyramide M (*N*-desalkyl-)-AC
	Imipramine M (bis-nor-)-AC
	Metaclazepam
2645	Biperiden M (OH-)
	Methyltestosterone
2648	Prazepam
2650	Alimemazine M (OH-)
	6-Monoacetylmorphine 6-MAM-PFP
2655	Bisacodyl M (bisdesacetyl)
	Phenprocoumon M (OH-) isomer-1 Me_2
2659	Estradiol
2660	Lorcainide M (nor-)
	Lormetazepam
	Nortriptyline M (acetyl-)
	Perhexiline M (diOH-)
	Zotepine
2662	Oxymorphone M (nor-)-enol-TMS_3
2665	Alimemazine M (sulfoxide)
	Bromazepam
	Methyltestosterone enol-TMS_2
2670	Cocaine M (OH-methoxy-)
	Desipramine M (acetyl-)
	Fenbutrazate
	Temazepam M (OH-)
2672	Methandienone
2675	Flurazepam M (2-OH-ethyl-)
	Phenprocoumon isomer-2 Me_2
	Trifluperidol
2680	Benzthiazide
	Bisacodyl M (methoxybisdesacetyl)
	Dibenzepin M (ter-nor-)
	Oxycodone M (nor-)-enol-AC_3
2683	Trifluoperazine
2685	Indometacin (packed)
	Promazine M (OH-)
2686	Broxaldine
	Phenazocine
2690	Carteolol (Art)
	Fenpipramide
	Metaclazepam M(nor-)
	Nitrendipine M (dehydro-desethyl-OH-) H_2O
	Oxymorphone M (dihydro-)
	Sulfanilamide M (acetyl-)
	Tenoxicam (tenoxicam-Me_2)
	Testosterone enol-TMS_2
2694	Flurazepam M (didesethyl-)
2700	Drostanolone Propionate drostanolone-AC
	Griseofulvin
	Hydrocodone M (nor-dihydro-)-AC
	Pentifylline M (di-OH-)
2705	Azaperone
	Phenprocoumon isomer 3 Me_2
	Promazine M (sulfoxide)
2710	Dextrorphan M (nor-)-AC_2
	Promethazine M (sulfoxide)
2715	Fluanisone M (*O*-desmethyl-)
	Naloxone
2719	Ethinylestradiol
2720	Acepromazine M (dihydro-)-H_2O
	Azatadine M (nor-)-AC
	Chlorprothixene M (sulfoxide)
	Fentanyl
	Flunitrazepam M (nor)
	Phenytoin M (4-OH-)-Me_2
	Prothipendyl M (OH-)
2723	Flunitrazepam M (7-amino-)
	Oxymorphone
2727	Clomipramine M (8-OH)
	Lormetazepam decomposition product
2730	Enalapril M (enalaprilate-H_2O)-Me
	Metaclazepam M(*O*-desmethyl-)
	Metoprolol M (OH-)-AC_3
2735	Acepromazine
2738	Propiomazine
2740	Hydrocortisone
	Nitrazepam
	Phenytoin M (4-OH-methoxy-)-Me_2
2747	Clobazam M (nor-)
2748	Naftidrofuryl Oxalate
2749	Cyfluthrin
	Disulfoton
2750	Bisacodyl M (desacetyl)
	Chlorprothixene M (OH-dihydro-) isomer 1
	Dihydrocodeine M (nor)-AC_2
	Furosemide M (*N*-desalkyl-)-Me
	Prothipendyl M (sulfoxide)
2760	Hydrocodone M (nor-)-AC
2761	Butorphanol
2762	Clomipramine M (8-OH-nor)
2765	Alimemazine M (bis-nor-)-AC
	Dixyrazine M (amino-)-AC
	Fluphenazine M (amino-)-AC
2770	Dibenzepin M (OH-) isomer-2-AC
	Phenprocoumon M (OH-methoxy)-Me_2
	Phenprocoumon M (di-OH-)-Me_3
	Phenytoin M (4-OH-methoxy-)
	Pseudomorphine
2773	Oxymorphone M (nor-)-enol-TMS_4
2774	Captodiame
2775	Cannabis M (11-hydroxy-Δ^9-THC)
2780	Flurazepam
	Mequitazine
2785	Fluanisone
	Nitrazepam M (7-amino-)
2788	Oxymorphone M (nor-)-enol-TMS_2
2790	Chlorprothixene M (OH-dihydro-) isomer 2
	Dihydromorphine M (nor-)-AC_3
	Quinidine
	Temazepam M (OH-)-AC
2793	Progesterone
2795	Chlordiazepoxide
	Hexachlorophene
	Phenytoin M (OH-)
2798	Perazine
2800	Amiodarone Art (*O*-desalkyl)
	Clotrimazole
	Pholcodine phocoldine-TFA
	Prothipendyl M (OH-ring)
	Quinine
2809	Chlorpromazine M (sulfoxide)
2810	Bisacodyl M (methoxydesacetyl)
	Chlorprothixene M (OH-methoxy-dihydro-)
	Hydroquinidine
	Lorcainide
	Trichlormethiazide
	Warfarin M (OH-) isomer-1-Me_2
2811	Acebutolol
2815	Testosterone propionate
2818	Bisacodyl
2820	Bisacodyl M (bismethoxybisdesacetyl)
2823	Clonazepam
2825	Flunitrazepam M (nor-amino-)
	Papaverine
2830	Fenetylline
	Midazolam M (α-OH-)
	Warfarin M (OH-) isomer-2-Me_2
2835	Carbocromen
	Fluoxymesterone
2850	Acebutolol Art (-H_2O)
	Anileridine
	Aprindine M (OH-)-AC
	Gelsemine
2860	Prazepam M (3-OH-)
	Tripelennamine M (nor-OH-)-AC_2
2870	Warfarin M (OH-) isomer 3-Me_2
	Xantinol Nicotinate xantinol-AC_2
2872	Hydroxychloroquine
	Phenoperidine
2880	Ajmaline
	Dapsone
	Hydroxyzine
	Lorcainide M (OH-)-AC
	Naltrexone
	Profenamine M (desethyl-OH-)-AC_2
2884	Piminodine
2885	Ibogaine
2890	Bisacodyl M (bismethoxydesacetyl)
	Cinchocaine
	Clonazepam M (7-amino-)
	Sulindac
2895	Clozapine
	Dimoxyline
	Prajmalium Bitartrate M (methoxy-) Art
2896	Sulindac M (sulfide)
2900	Chlorpromazine M (norsulfoxide)
	Deltamethrin
	Metoclopramide M (desethyl-)-AC2
	Oxycodone M (nor-dihydro-)-AC_2
	Profenamine M (bis-desethyl-OH-)-AC_2
2906	Doxapram
2910	Coumatetralyl M (OH-) isomer-1-Me
2917	Chlorotrianisene
2920	Pyrrobutamine M (oxo-)
2925	Coumatetralyl M (OH-) isomer-2-Me_2
	Prajmalium Bitartrate prajmalium
	Sulfametoxydiazine sulfamethoxydiazine-Me_3
2929	Nimodipine
2930	Alimemazine M (nor-OH-)-AC_2
	Clomifene
	Ethylmorphine M (nor-)-AC_2
	Haloperidol
2931	Loxapine M(8-OH-)
2932	Pipotiazine
2934	Diphenadione
2935	Clonazepam M (amino-OH-)
	Coumatetralyl M (OH-) isomer-3-Me_2
	Oxycodone M (nor-dihydro-)-AC_3
2940	Dextromoramide
	Lorcainide M (OH-methoxy-)-AC

RI	*Compound*
2945	Camazepam
	Codeine M (nor-)-AC_2
	Quinine M (*N*-oxide)-AC
2949	Diltiazem
2950	Quinidine M (*N*-oxide)
2951	Amoxapine M (7-OH-)
	Loxapine M(7-OH-amoxapine)
2955	Estriol
	Morphine M (nor-)-AC_3
2959	Amoxapine M (8-OH)
	Loxapine M(8-OH-amoxapine)
2960	Cyproheptadine M (oxo-)
	Nalbuphine
2965	Clemizole M (oxo-)
	Miconazole
2970	Alfentanil
	Dexamethasone
	Triamcinolone
2980	Doxylamine M (OH-carbinol-)-AC
	Etizolam
	Pholcodine-PFP
2985	Acenocoumarol M(amino-)-Me_3
	Drostanolone Propionate
2988	Hydrastine
2990	Chlorpromazine M (bis-nor-)-AC
	Coumatetralyl M (OH-) isomer-4-Me_2
	Diltiazem M (desacetyl-)
	Trifluoperazine M (sulfoxide)
2995	Aprindine M (OH-methoxy-)-AC
3000	Clobazam M (OH-)
	Sultiame
	Triazolam M (α-OH-)
	Xipamide M (OH-)-Me_4
3005	Coumatetralyl M (di-OH-) isomer-1-Me_2
	Flupentixol M (dihydro-)-AC
	Oxymetholone
3010	Chloroquine M (desethyl-)-AC
	Lorcainide M (OH-dimethoxy-)-AC
	Pentamidine
3015	Benzylmorphine
3016	Encainide
3033	Etorphine
3035	Meclozine
3040	Pipamperone
3045	Alprazolam M (α-OH-)
	Mebeverine
3050	Brotizolam (M(OH) Art(-CH_2O))
	Cinnarizine
	Diltiazem M (*O*-desmethyl-)
	Fluphenazine
	Opipramol
3055	Flupentixol M (desalkyl-dihydro-)-AC
3060	Cyproheptadine M (OH-)
	Dimetotiazine
	Tiotixene
3070	Brotizolam
	Chlorpromazine M (nor-)-AC
	Coumatetralyl M (OH-methoxy-)-Me_2
	Pholcodine phocoldine
3075	Trilostane (decomposition occurs)
3078	Fenbufen
3080	Nifenazone
	Triazolam
3085	Coumatetralyl M (di-OH-) isomer-2-Me_2
	Stanozolol
3088	Cholesterol
3089	Methysergide
3095	Dextromoramide M (OH-)
3100	Alprazolam
	Bezafibrate
	Dobutamine M (*O*-methyl-)-AC_2
	Spironolactone M (canrenoic acid)
3102	Sulpiride
3105	Clozapine M (nor-)
	Coumatetralyl M (di-OH-) isomer-3-Me_3
3115	Thioridazine
3116	Strychnine
3120	Mequitazine M (sulfoxide)
3125	Etophylline clofibrate
3130	Prajmalium Bitartrate M (OH-) Art
	Spironolactone M (canrenoic acid)-ME
3132	Floctafenine
3140	Pholcodine phocoldine-TMS
3145	Fluphenazine M (desalkyl-)-AC
	Noscapine
3150	Astemizole
	Colecalciferol
	Dimetotiazine M (nor-)
	Verapamil
3152	Haloperidol M (reduced)
3155	Yohimbine
3175	Coumatetralyl M (tri-OH-)-H_2O-Me_2
	Perazine M (OH-)
3180	Sulforidazine M (ring)
	Verapamil M (nor-)
3190	Butaperazine
3194	Clorexolone
3195	Quinine M (OH-)-AC_2
	Rotenone
3200	Colchicine
	Dimetotiazine M (OH-)-AC
	Dobutamine M (*O*-methyl-)
	Prajmalium Bitartrate M (OH-methoxy-) Art
	Thioproperazine M (ring)
3205	Nitrazepam M (7-acetamido-)
3210	Dextromoramide M (OH-)-AC
3220	Dixyrazine
3225	Fluocortolone
3240	Buprenorphine art (-H_2O)
3245	Alprazolam M (OH-)
3247	Thiethylperazine
3250	Mequitazine M (sulfone)
	Pipamperone M (OH-)
	Spironolactone M (canrenone)
3255	Clobazam M (OH-MeO-)
	Sulfamethoxazole M (N^4-acetyl-)-Me
3260	Pericyazine
	Pholcodine-AC
3265	Acenocoumarol M (acetamido-)-Me_2
3269	Dextromoramide M (methoxy-)
3280	Brucine
	Spironolactone
3281	Trimethobenzamide
3287	Phytomenadione
3320	Buprenorphine art (-H_2O)-AC
3330	Trazodone
3335	Amiodarone
3340	Chlormadinone Acetate chlormadinone-H_2O
3350	Acenocoumarol M (OH-) isomer 1-Me_2
	Dixyrazine M (*O*-desalkyl-)-AC
	Dobutamine M (*O*-methyl-)-AC_3
	Testosterone dipropionate
3355	Dixyrazine M (*N*-desalkyl-)-AC
3360	Buclizine
	Buprenorphine
	Chlormadinone Acetate
	Dimetotiazine M (nor-)-AC
	Penfluridol
	Quinine M (di-OH-dihydro-)-AC_3
3380	Dimetotiazine M (bis-nor-)-AC
	Mesoridazine
	Perphenazine
	Trazodone M (OH-acetyl-)
3410	Sulfaethidole M (acetyl-)-Me_2
3415	Sulforidazine
3420	Thioridazine M (ring sulfone)
3430	Droperidol
	Lysergide M (2-oxo-3-OH-)-TMS_2
3433	Benperidol
3440	Gestonorone Caproate
3445	Lysergide LSD
3450	Clopenthixol M (desalkyl-dihydro-)-AC
3467	Thiopropazate
3490	Clopenthixol M (desalkyl-)-AC
	Clozapine M (nor-acetyl-)
3500	Acenocoumarol M(OH-) isomer 2-Me_2
	Thioridazine M (oxo-)
3514	Diphenoxylate
3515	Lysergide M (nor-)-TMS_2
	Lysergide iso-LSD-TMS
3550	Econazole
3552	Thioproperazine
3560	Piritramide
3590	Carfenazine
3595	Lysergide LSD-TMS
3620	Sulfametoxydiazine M (acetyl-)-Me
3705	Lysergide M (nor-)-TMS
3710	Sulfadiazine M (acetyl-)-Me_2
3800	Thioridazine M (side chain sulfone)
3840	Glibenclamide glibencamide-Me_2
3870	Lidoflazine
	Pimozide
ND	Acetophenazine
	Aconitine
	Alprazolam M (4-OH-)
	Amidefrine
	Aminonitrothiazole
	Amodiaquine
	Benzonatate
	Betaine
	Bezitramide
	Bunamidine
	Captopril
	Carbidopa
	Cimetidine
	Cinchophen
	Clioxanide
	Clofazimine
	Coniine
	Debrisoquine
	Decoquinate
	Diazoxide
	Dicoumarol
	Ecgonine
	Epithiazide
	Etacrynic Acid
	Etoxazene
	Flavoxate
	Furosemide
	Glafenine
	Guanethidine
	Hexamethonium Bromide
	Hexobendine
	Hydrochlorothiazide
	Hydroflumethiazide
	Lofepramine
	Loprazolam
	Metallibure
	Metformin
	Methyclothiazide
	Methyldopa
	Methylergometrine
	Metolazone
	Morantel
	Nifursol

RI	*Compound*
	Oxyclozanide
	Oxymorphone M (nor-)
	Oxyphenbutazone
	Pancuronium Bromide
	Parbendazole
	Pentapiperide Metilsulfate
	Phentolamine
	Piperacetazine
	Practolol
	Prazosin
	Propantheline Bromide
	Propyliodone
	Pyrantel
	Quinethazone
	Rafoxanide
	Reserpine
	Ritodrine
	Sulfaguanidine
	Sulfamoxole
	Sulfathiazole
	Suxamethonium Chloride
	Urea

System GB (p. 444)—**retention index**

RI	*Compound*
994	Isometheptene
1060	Ethchlorvynol
1063	Cineole
1098	Valproic Acid
1142	Amfetamine art (formyl)
1150	Amfetamine
	Amiphenazole
1157	Fenfluramine norfenfluramine
1191	Mephentermine phentermine
	Phentermine
1192	Propylhexedrine
1194	Menthol
1200	Metamfetamine
1228	Methyl Salicylate
	Salicylic acid-Me
1245	Chlormezanone art
1250	Mephentermine
1252	Fenfluramine
	Tranylcypromine
1257	Pargyline
1258	Ethosuximide
1261	Zopiclone art (aminochloropyridine)
1269	Clomethiazole
1270	Labetalol Art
1278	Phenelzine
1280	4-Aminophenol
	Paracetamol art (*p*-aminophenol)
1338	Diethylpropion M (*N*-didesethyl-)
1340	Salicylic Acid
1352	Cathine
	Diethylpropion M (phenylpropanolamine)
1353	Phenylpropanolamine
1356	Ephedrine M (nor-)
1380	Eugenol
	Nicotine
1393	Chlorphentermine
1395	Ethosuximide M (3-OH)
	Mexiletine M (desamino-oxo-)
1400	Acetanilide
1410	Ephedrine
	Methoxyamfetamine
	Pseudoephedrine
1416	Methoxyphenamine
1418	Nikethamide M (nicotinamide)
1423	Diethylpropion M (*N*-desethyl-)
1430	Cocaine M (anhydroecgonine methylester)
1431	Mexiletine
1436	Ethosuximide M (OH-ethyl)
1451	Methylephedrine
1453	Selegiline
1457	Diethylpropion M (ethylnorephedrine)
1465	Diphenhydramine M (diphenylmethane)
1472	Cocaine M (norecgonine)
1475	Felbamate
1483	Phenmetrazine
1489	Salicylamide
1504	Phendimetrazine
1510	Etafedrine
1511	Codeine
1512	Methylenedioxyamfetamine MDA
1530	Cocaine M (methylecgonine)
1532	Diethylpropion
1534	Propranolol M (1-naphthol-)
1569	Nikethamide
1572	Methylenedioxymethamfetamine MDMA
1579	Pentetrazol
1580	Phenyltoloxamine M ((*N*-oxide)-ME_2 NOH)
1581	Methyprylon
1596	Chlormezanone M (*N*-methyl-4-chlorobenzamide)
1599	Diethylpropion M (diethylnorephedrine)
1601	Methyprylon M (OH-)-H_2O
1602	Cocaine M (ethylecgonine)
1609	Iproniazid
1614	Clorprenaline
1629	Levetiracetam
1630	Methylenedioxyethylamfetamine MDEA
1632	Vanillin
1637	Ibuprofen
1645	Bupropion
	Diphenhydramine M (diphenylmethanol)
	Nicotine M (cotinine)
1648	Fenproporex
1652	DOM
1660	Glibornuride Art (methylsulfonamide)
	Gliclazide art (methylsulfonamide)
	Prolintane
1670	Doxylamine M (carbinol)-H_2O
1673	Cinnarizine M (Benzophenone)
	Cyclizine M (benzophenone)
1688	Buclizine M (4-chloromethylbiphenyl)
	Hydroxyzine M (4-chloromethylbiphenyl)
1689	Methylenedioxyamfetamine art (formyl)
1695	Glibornuride art (amide)
1698	Butalbital
1700	Orphenadrine M (methylbenzophenone)
1707	Haloperidol M (*N*-desalkyl-oxo-)-$2H_2O$
1722	Paracetamol
1724	Phenyltoloxamine M (O-desalkyl-)
1730	Phenacetin
1737	Fencamfamin
1742	Amobarbital
1751	Ethotoin
1769	Tocainide
1776	Pentobarbital
1778	Beclamide
1780	Diphenhydramine M (4-phenylmethylphenol)
1793	Methylphenidate
1804	Meclofenoxate
1806	Nefazodone *m*-chlorophenylpiperazine (*m*CPP)
	Trazodone M (mCPP)
1809	Pethidine
1827	Methohexital
	Secobarbital
1840	Ketamine M (nor-OH-)-NH_3
1842	Pethidine M (nor)
	Phenoperidine norpethidine
1854	Meprobamate
1862	Alphaprodine
	Buclizine M (4-chlorobiphenyl-methanone)
	Hydroxyzine M (4-chlorobenzophenone)
1870	Methyprylon M (oxo-)
1874	Pheniramine
1880	Carbamazepine M (acridine)
1883	Diphenhydramine M (desamino-)
1888	Norfluoxetine
1890	Pheniramine M (nor)
1895	Trimeperidine
1898	Bupropion (M (OH-))
1899	Benzfetamine
1903	Fluoxetine
1904	Caffeine
1907	Ketamine M (nor-)
1910	Glutethimide
1911	Fluvoxamine
1914	Hydralazine
1920	Theobromine
1922	Diphenhydramine M (nor-)
1923	Ethoheptazine
	Thiopental
	Viloxazine
1928	Diphenhydramine
	Phenyltoloxamine M (desamino-OH-)
1931	Ketamine M (nor-)-H_2O
1939	Ketamine
1951	Phenazone
1952	Triclofos Sodium
1958	Glutethimide M (OH-ethyl-)
1970	Doxylamine
1972	Oxprenolol
1974	Doxylamine M (nor-)
1980	Meptazinol
1981	Phencyclidine
1990	Theophylline
1992	Aminophenazone
1996	Primidone M (PEMA)
2002	Phenyltoloxamine M (nor-)
2007	Orphenadrine M (nor-)
2009	Ketamine M (nor-di-OH-)-$2H_2O$
2013	Tofenacin
2014	Desipramine M (ring)

RI	Compound
	Orphenadrine
2015	Amobarbital M (3-OH-)
2016	Butalbital M (OH-)
2019	Pentazocine M (desalkyl-)
2021	Tramadol
2029	Secobarbital M (3′-OH-)
2030	Phenyltoloxamine
	Propyphenazone
2031	Phenobarbital
2034	Thenyldiamine
2040	Glutethimide M (OH-phenyl-)
2049	Tramadol M (nor-)
2051	Amitriptyline M (*N*-oxide)
	Atropine Art (-CH_2O)
2054	Carbamazepine M (methylacridine)
	Oxcarbazepine M (methylacridine)
2056	Acebutolol M (phenol-)
2058	Ketamine M (nor-OH-)-H_2O
2062	Oxprenolol Art
2064	Carbamazepine M (iminostilbene)
2065	Chlorphenamine M (bis-nor-)
2069	Dipyrone
	Meptazinol M (nor-)
	Methadone M (EMDP)
2077	Doxepin M (*cis-N*-oxide)
2079	Chlorphenamine
2080	Psilocin
2081	Doxepin M (*trans-N*-oxide)
	Pemoline
2084	Nabumetone
2089	Acebutolol Art (desacetyl-)
2090	Atenolol Art (-H_2O)
	Metoprolol
2092	Cyclopentolate
2093	Tramadol M (*O*-desmethyl-)
2096	Ibuprofen M (2-OH-)
2104	Cyclizine
2106	Nefopam
2107	Trimipramine M (nor-ring)
2110	Heptabarb
2115	Chlorphenamine M (nor)
2116	Nefopam M (nor)
2120	Methadone M (EDDP)
	Promethazine M (phenothiazine)
2122	Tramadol M (*N*,*O*-didesmethyl-)
2128	Cinnarizine M (desalkyl-)
	Cyclizine M (nor-)
	Diphenylpyraline
2130	Mequitazine M (phenothiazine)
	Phenothiazine
	Promazine M (phenothiazine)
2134	Thiopental M (OH-)
2145	Pethidine M (OH-)
2147	Carbinoxamine
2150	Clomipramine M (*N*-oxide)
2158	Carbamazepine M (formyl-acridine)
	Oxcarbazepine M (formylacridine)
2163	Venlafaxine
2165	Clonidine
	Homatropine
2169	Verapamil M (*O*-desmethyl-didesalkyl-)
2172	Benzoctamine
2175	Dicycloverine
2184	Brompheniramine
2189	Primidone M (acetyl-)
2190	Chlorphenoxamine
2193	Verapamil M (*N*-desalkyl-)
2196	Venlafaxine M (*N*-desmethyl-)
2200	Noxiptiline M(OH-dibenzocycloheptanone)-H_2O
2203	Brompheniramine M (bis-nor)
2205	Chlorphenoxamine M (nor)
2215	Amitriptyline M (*cis*-10-OH-*N*-oxide)
2219	Brompheniramine M (nor)
2222	Methylphenobarbital
2228	Methadone
2230	Hydroxyzine M (OH-chlorobenzophenone)
	Venlafaxine M (*O*-desmethyl-)
2231	Diclofenac
2234	Propranolol
2237	Racemorphan
2239	Amitriptyline M (*trans*-10-OH-*N*-oxide)
	Diphenhydramine M (methoxy-)
	Nomifensine
2240	Diphenhydramine M (di-nor-acetyl-)
	Flecainide (Art (formyl))
2242	Pipradrol
2244	Racemorphan M (nor-)
2245	Phenindamine
2246	Verapamil M (*O*-desmethyl-desalkyl-)
2250	Atropine Art (-H_2O)
2252	Tramadol M (OH-)
2253	Topiramate
2255	Levacetylmethadol M (di-nor-)
2256	Methaqualone
	Pethidine M (nor-)-AC
2259	Cocaine M (nor-)
2261	Procyclidine
	Trazodone M (desalkylacetyl-)
2262	Levacetylmethadol M (nor-)
2264	Venlafaxine M (*N*,*O*-didesmethyl)
2266	Nefopam M (OH-)
	Oxcarbazepine oxcarbamazepine
2267	Levacetylmethadol
2268	Dextropropoxyphene
2278	Fluoxetine (noracetylfluoxetine)
2284	Amitriptyline
2286	Disopyramide M (*N*-desalkyl-)
2288	Butriptyline
2289	Cocaine
2293	Atropine
	Hyoscyamine
2300	Verapamil M (didesalkyl-)
2302	Mianserin
	Trimipramine
2304	Nortriptyline
2311	Esmolol
2314	Imipramine
2316	Chlorcyclizine
2317	Cocaine M (norcocaethylene)
2318	Triflupromazine
2319	Fluoxetine (acetylfluoxetine)
2320	Metipranolol
2322	Harmine
	Nabumetone (M (6-MNA))
2323	Dextrorphan
2328	Dextrorphan M (nor)
	Mepyramine
2329	Protriptyline
2330	Amitriptyline M (cyclobenzaprine)
	Butriptyline M (nor-)
2332	Phenoxybenzamine
	Procainamide
2333	Doxepin M (*cis*-nor)
	Moclobemide
	Promethazine M (nor-)
2335	Clomipramine M (ring)
	Desipramine M (ring-OH-)
	Pindolol
	Trimipramine M (nor-)
2337	Naproxen
2338	Desipramine
2339	Doxepin M (*trans*-nor)
2340	Medazepam
	Triprolidine
2343	Nortriptyline M (norcyclobenzaprine)
	Protriptyline M (nor-)
2345	Cocaine M (cocaethylene)
2346	Chlormezanone
2348	Mianserin M (nor-)
2350	Flurazepam M (desalkyl-)-TMS
2351	Flecainide
2354	Trihexyphenidyl
2355	Chlorcyclizine M (nor)
	Chlorpromazine M (*N*-oxide)
	Hydroxyzine M (norchlorcyclizine)
2356	Pentazocine
	Prochlorperazine M (*N*-oxide)
2360	Diphenhydramine M (nor-acetyl-)
2361	Azacyclonol
	Mirtazapine
2370	Mefenamic Acid
	Methaqualone M (2-formyl-)
	Nifedipine M (dehydro-)
	Phenazopyridine
2373	Flurazepam M (desalkyl-OH-)
	Timolol
	Venlafaxine M (*O*-desmethyl OH-) isomer 1
2376	Dimetindene
2378	Phenobarbital M (4-OH-)
2383	Promethazine
	Thiazinamium Metilsulfate (both for thiazinamium methylsulfate Art (promethazine))
2384	Primidone
2385	Nabumetone M (*O*-desmethyl)
2395	Esmolol (Art)
2396	Naproxen M (*O*-desmethyl-)
2398	Phenyltoloxamine M (nor-OH-) isomer 1
2402	Alimemazine
	Phenyltoloxamine M (nor-OH-) isomer 2
2404	Maprotiline M (nor)
2408	Venlafaxine M (*O*-desmethyl OH-) isomer 2
2420	Betaxolol
	Racemorphan M (OH-)
2421	Antazoline
2423	Benzatropine
2425	Promazine
2427	Bisoprolol
	Hyoscine
2432	Alimemazine M (nor)
2435	Carbamazepine
	Oxcarbazepine M (carbamazepine)
2437	Iprindole
	Methaqualone M (2-OH-methyl-)
2438	Oxazepam
2440	Maprotiline
	Practolol
2442	Tropicamide
2450	Venlafaxine M (nor OH-)
2452	Promazine M (nor)
2454	Amitriptyline M (*cis*-10-OH-)
2460	Cyproheptadine
	Levallorphan
2466	Amitriptyline M (*trans*-10-OH-)
2469	Atenolol
2472	Phenylbutazone
2480	Bisoprolol (Art(-H_2O))
	Cannabis CBD
	Nortriptyline M (*cis*-10-OH-)
2481	Sertraline
2486	Dosulepin
2487	Norpropoxyphene
	Procyclidine M (OH-isomer-1)
2494	Imipramine M (10-OH-)
	Nortriptyline M (*trans*-10-OH-)

RI	*Compound*
2499	Azatadine
	Citalopram
2504	Mazindol
2507	Dosulepin M (nor-)
2508	Betaxolol (Art)
2511	Clomipramine
	Dihydrocodeine
2514	Dextropropoxyphene M (nor-*N*-propionyl-)
2517	Procyclidine M (OH-isomer-2)
2519	Betaxolol (Art-H_2O)
2520	Sotalol
2521	Desipramine M (10-OH-)
2526	Norcitalopram
2527	Dihydromorphine
2528	Doxepin M (*cis*-OH-)
	Lorazepam
2533	Dosulepin M (sulfoxide)
2535	Codeine M (nor)
	Norcodeine
2540	Clomipramine M (nor)
2544	Doxepin M (*trans*-OH-)
2546	Propranolol M (4-OH-)
	Verapamil M (*N*-desalkyl-acetyl-)
2552	Ketazolam
2556	Diazepam
	Medazepam diazepam
2559	Dihydrocodeine M (nor)-TMS_2
	Flurazepam M (desalkyl-)
	Thebacon
2562	Lamotrigine
2563	Chlorphenamine M (nor)-AC
2564	Diamorphine morphine
	Morphine
2566	Dibenzepin
	Lormetazepam lorazepam-TMS_2
2569	Acebutolol Art (-H_2O)
2575	Mebhydrolin
2576	Quazepam
2578	Cannabis Δ^9-THC
2579	Tetrabenazine
	Verapamil M (*N*-didesalkyl-acetyl-)
2580	Hydrocodone
	Oxcarbazepine M (10-OH-)
2586	Dipipanone
2588	Remoxipride
2592	Metixene
2598	Hydromorphone
2599	Dihydrocodeine M (nor)
	Hydrocodone M (nor-)
2600	Meptazinol M (oxo-)
2603	Maprotiline M (desamino-di-OH-)
2608	Chlorprothixene
	Cocaine M (*m*-OH-)
	Cyproheptadine M (nor-OH-)-H_2O
	Disopyramide
2618	Chlorpromazine
	Clorazepic Acid
	Trihexyphenidyl M (OH-)
2621	Oxycodone M (nor-)-enol-TMS_2
2622	Flunitrazepam M (nor-)-TMS
2625	Diamorphine 3-monoacetylmorphine
	Nordazepam
2628	Mianserin M (8-OH-)
2631	Codeine M (nor)-TMS_2
	Trimipramine M (OH-)
2634	Nitrazepam M (7-amino-)-TMS_3
2636	Imipramine M (2-OH-)
2638	Tetrabenazine M (*O*-desmethyl-OH-)
2639	Thioridazine M (ring)
2641	Levomepromazine
2644	Cannabinol
	Doxepin M (*cis*-nor-OH-)
2645	Acetylcodeine
2646	Chlorpromazine M (didesmethyl-)
	6-Monoacetylmorphine
2649	Nefopam M (nor-di-OH)
	Pentazocine M (OH-)
2650	Bromazepam M (3-OH-)-TMS_2
	Cocaine M (*p*-OH-)
2656	Chlorpromazine M (nor)
2658	Nadolol
2662	Trimipramine M (nor-OH-)
2663	Benzoylecgonine
	Cocaine M (benzoylecgonine)
	Cocaine M (methoxycocaethylene)
2666	Oxycodone M (dihydro-)
2669	Desipramine M (2-OH-)
	Pecazine
	Procyclidine M (oxo-)-H_2O
2670	Nadolol art
2671	Doxepin M (*trans*-nor-OH-)
	Oxycodone
2673	Dextropropoxyphene M (nor-amide)
2679	Chlordiazepoxide M (nor)
2680	Bisoprolol (Art)
2683	Clobazam
2688	6-Monoacetylmorphine 6-MAM-TMS
2691	Paroxetine
2698	Clomipramine M (10-OH-)
	Methaqualone M (OH-methoxy-)
2703	Oxycodone M (nor)
2708	Nifedipine
2709	Cocaine M (OH-cocaethylene)
2715	Imipramine M (OH-methoxy-)
	Trimipramine M (OH-methoxy-)
2717	Loxapine
	Promethazine M (nor-OH-)
2722	Midazolam
2723	Oxycodone oxymorphone
2724	Acecainide
	N-Acetylprocainamide
2727	Diazepam temazepam
	Temazepam
2729	Cocaine M (OH-methoxy-)
2732	Promethazine M (norsulfoxide)
2734	Paroxetine M (desmethylenyl-3-methyl-)
2735	Clomipramine M (2-OH-)
2738	Carbamazepine M (10,11-di-OH-)
2739	Flurazepam M (bis-desethyl-)
2742	Clonazepam M (7-amino-)-TMS_2
2744	Flunitrazepam
2746	Amoxapine
	Loxapine M(amoxapine)
	Oxycodone M (nor)-enol-TMS_3
2749	Desipramine M (OH-methoxy-)
2750	Glymidine Sodium
2759	Clobazam M (nor)
2760	Bromazepam
2763	Oxycodone M (nor)-TMS_2
2769	Diamorphine
2770	Lormetazepam
2774	Nortriptyline M (acetyl-)
2775	Midazolam M (4-OH-)-TMS
2778	Flurazepam M (2-OH-ethyl-)-TMS
2779	Cocaine M (OH-methoxycocaethylene)
2781	Promazine M (OH-)
2783	Prazepam
2789	Lorcainide M (nor-)
2793	Bisacodyl M (bisdesacetyl)
	Felodipine
2797	Promazine M (nor-OH-)
	Promethazine M (sulfoxide)
2798	Trifluoperazine
2804	Flunitrazepam M (7-amino-)
2805	Alimemazine M (sulfoxide)
	Flurazepam M (2-OH-ethyl-)
2806	Chlordiazepoxide M (demoxepam)
	Demoxepam
2811	Desipramine M (acetyl-)
2816	Flunitrazepam M (nor)
2817	Alimemazine M (norsulfoxide)
2824	Acepromazine M (dihydro-)-H_2O
2829	Alimemazine M (OH-)
2832	Flupentixol M (desalkyl-)-*cis*
2833	Fentanyl
	Phenazocine
2836	Flunitrazepam M (7-amino-)-TMS
2839	Dosulepin M (norsulfoxide)
2840	Promazine M (sulfoxide)
2843	Clomipramine M (8-OH-)
2844	Acepromazine
2845	Alimemazine M (nor-OH-)
2855	Flupentixol M (desalkyl-)-*trans*
2861	Olanzapine
2866	Midazolam M (α-OH-)-TMS
2875	Promazine M (norsulfoxide)
2876	Bisacodyl M (desacetyl)
2878	Nitrazepam M (7-amino-)
2880	Clomipramine M (8-OH-nor-)
2896	Flurazepam
2900	Fenetylline
2901	Midazolam M (α-OH-)
2902	Butorphanol
2911	Olanzapine M (nor)
2915	Nitrazepam
2923	Lorcainide
2926	Acebutolol
2939	Chlorpromazine M (7-OH-)
	Mequitazine
2941	Zolpidem
2949	Nortriptyline M (norcyclobenzaprine)-AC
2956	Bisacodyl
2962	Imipramine M (di-OH-)
2973	Papaverine
2975	Cannabis M (11-hydroxy-Δ^9-THC)
2979	Quinidine
2981	Chlordiazepoxide
2982	Amlodipine
2983	Phenoperidine
2995	Desipramine M (di-OH-)
2996	Clonazepam M (7-amino-)
3000	Clonazepam
	Hydroxyzine
3003	Chlorpromazine M (sulfoxide)
3018	Doxapram M (keto-)
3024	Clozapine
3046	Chlorpromazine M (norsulfoxide)
	Doxapram
3054	Doxazosin
3068	Loxapine M (7-OH-)
3076	Diltiazem
3077	Loxapine M (8-OH-)
3086	Quinidine M (*N*-oxide)
3088	Levomepromazine M (norsulfoxide)
3092	Clozapine M (nor-)
	Diltiazem M (desacetyl-)
3094	Dextromoramide
	Haloperidol
3096	Dimetotiazine
	Nimodipine
3108	Alfentanil
	Alprazolam
3114	Diltiazem M (*N*-desmethyl-)
	Levomepromazine M (sulfoxide)
3119	Rofecoxib
3145	Trifluoperazine M (sulfoxide)
3147	Diltiazem M (*O*-desmethyl-)
3152	Haloperidol M (reduced)
3160	Acepromazine M (7-OH-)

RI	Compound
3162	Camazepam
3191	Trifluoperazine M (norsulfoxide)
3193	Meclozine
3194	Fluphenazine
3211	Etorphine
3219	Opipramol
	Triazolam
3233	Cinnarizine
3236	Loratadine
3263	Zopiclone
3275	Thioridazine M (nor-)
3292	Thioridazine
3305	Verapamil
3308	Triazolam M (α-OH-)-TMS
3310	Dextromoramide M (OH-)
3332	Lysergide (LSD)
3348	Pholcodine
3358	Noscapine
3371	Verapamil M (nor-)
3385	Diprenorphine
3400	Quetiapine
3461	Buclizine
3486	Pericyazine
3525	Amoxapine M (7-OH-)
	Loxapine M(7-OH-amoxapine)
3546	Amoxapine M (-OH-)
	Loxapine M(8-OH-amoxapine)
3562	Trazodone
3571	Prochlorperazine M (norsulfoxide)
3594	Perphenazine
3609	Clozapine M (nor-acetyl-)
3610	Buprenorphine
3626	Thioridazine M (ring sulfone)
3629	Mesoridazine
3640	Trazodone M (OH-acetyl-)
3667	Benperidol
3670	Diphenoxylate
3690	Sulforidazine
3758	Prochlorperazine M (sulfoxide)
ND	Alprazolam M (OH-)
	Benoxaprofen
	Buformin
	Captopril
	Cocaine M (ecgonine)
	Debrisoquine
	Diazoxide
	Droperidol
	Glibornuride
	Lidoflazine
	Loprazolam
	Metformin
	Nalbuphine
	Nalorphine
	Naloxone
	Naltrexone
	Pimozide
	Pipotiazine
	Triazolam M (α-OH-)
	Vigabatrin

System GC (p. 444)**—retention index**

RI	Compound
1253	Bemegride
1287	Tuaminoheptane
1383	Cathine
	Diethylpropion M (norephedrine)
	Ephedrine M (nor)
	Phenylpropanolamine
1429	Dimethylamfetamine
1440	Pargyline
1450	Phentermine
1460	Phenelzine
1467	Ephedrine
1470	Fenfluramine norfenfluramine
1480	Methylephedrine
1500	Propylhexedrine
1536	Amfetamine
1543	Pseudoephedrine
1573	Nicotine
1621	Fenfluramine
1630	Ethoheptazine
1668	Mephentermine
1670	Methoxyphenamine
1715	Diethylpropion
1722	Metamfetamine
1725	Chlorphentermine
1735	Phendimetrazine
1737	Etafedrine
1759	Tranylcypromine
1849	Prolintane
1852	Nikethamide
1873	Phenmetrazine
1880	Clorprenaline
1934	Phenylephrine
2021	Pentetrazol
2025	Pethidine
2111	Nicotine M (cotinine)
2172	Benzfetamine
2173	Dextropropoxyphene
2180	Fencamfamin
2200	Meclofenoxate
	Methylphenidate
2225	Pentazocine
2230	Doxapram
	Levorphanol
2300	Thenyldiamine
2307	Cyproheptadine
2348	Cyclizine
2370	Aminophenazone
2376	Caffeine
2378	Diphenhydramine
2409	Etamivan
2430	Carbinoxamine
2447	Diphenylpyraline
2457	Brompheniramine
	Naphazoline
2470	Methadone
2478	Pipradrol
2504	Dihydromorphine
2542	Morphine
2546	Promethazine
2563	Amiphenazole
2576	Thonzylamine
2586	Chlorphenamine
2646	Alimemazine
2669	Dimetindene
2681	Codeine
2702	Dihydrocodeine
2739	Mebhydrolin
2749	Antazoline
2894	Dipipanone
2926	Phenindamine
2954	Triprolidine
3028	Hydrocodone
3469	Anileridine
3625	Dextromoramide

System GD (p. 451)**—relative to n-$C_{16}H_{34}$**

RRT	Compound
0.4	Salsalate
0.49	Sulindac
	Indometacin
0.6	Salsalate
0.89	Ibuprofen
1.3	Flurbiprofen
1.12	Bufexamac
1.13	Alclofenac
1.18	Naproxen-Me
1.20	Diflunisal
1.26	Flufenamic Acid
	Fenclofenac
1.30	Flurbiprofen
1.31	Fenoprofen
1.36	Tolmetin
1.37	Naproxen-Me
1.38	Niflumic Acid
1.39	Flunixin
1.42	Diclofenac-Me
1.45	Ketoprofen
	Mefenamic Acid-Me
1.55	Fenclofenac
	Indometacin
1.61	Clonixin
1.62	Meclofenamic Acid
1.77	Tolmetin
1.79	Fenbufen
1.81	Feprazone
1.98	Benoxaprofen
2.05	Phenylbutazone
2.11	Oxyphenbutazone
2.27	Indoprofen
2.64	Furosemide

System GE (p. 456)—relative to phenytoin

RRT	Compound
0.04	Trimethadione
0.4	Phensuximide
0.5	*N*-desmethylmesuximide
0.06	Paramethadione
0.09	Valproic Acid
0.18	Ethosuximide
0.22	*N*-desmethylparamethadione
0.35	Mesuximide
0.55	Mephenytoin
0.57	Ethotoin
0.65	Primidone M (phenylethylmalondiamide (PEMA))
0.73	5-Ethyl-5-phenylhydantoin
0.74	Phenobarbital
	Primidone M (phenobarbital)
0.83	Carbamazepine
0.89	Primidone
1.35	Cholesterol

System GF (p. 457)—retention index

RI	Compound
1315	Amfetamine
1335	Metamfetamine
1455	Tranylcypromine
1525	Nicotine
1655	Diethylpropion
1895	Nikethamide
1935	Methylphenidate
1995	Pethidine
2050	Benzfetamine
2090	Methyprylon
2100	Benzocaine
	Pheniramine
2105	Diphenhydramine
2110	Ethoheptazine
2130	Tybamate
2150	Phencyclidine
2170	Doxylamine
2185	Orphenadrine
2195	Nicotine M (cotinine)
2230	Barbital
2240	Lidocaine
2265	Aminophenazone
	Dicycloverine
2270	Oxprenolol
2305	Methapyrilene
2310	Propyphenazone
2315	Glutethimide
2320	Cyclizine
2325	Phenacetin
2335	Chlorphenamine
2340	Allobarbital
	Caffeine
	Thenyldiamine
2345	Mepivacaine
2365	Chlorphenoxamine
2370	Dextropropoxyphene
	Methadone
2380	Hexobarbital
	Nefopam
2390	Butobarbital
2395	Butalbital
2405	Diphenylpyraline
2430	Amobarbital
2445	Benzoctamine
	Phenazone
2455	Carbetapentane
2460	Meprobamate
	Nealbarbital
2465	Butriptyline
	Pentobarbital
2470	Brompheniramine
2480	Bromazine
2485	Procyclidine
2495	Vinbarbital
2505	Trimipramine
2510	Amitriptyline
	Secobarbital
2515	Phenindamine
2540	Imipramine
2550	Cocaine
	Fluopromazine
2560	Chlorcyclizine
	Mepyramine
2570	Doxepin
2580	Methaqualone
	Procaine
2590	Protriptyline
2595	Mianserin
2600	Phenoxybenzamine
	Pramoxine
	Thiopental
	Triprolidine
2610	Carbamazepine
2620	Carbamazepine M (iminostilbene)
2640	Medazepam
2660	Atropine
	Piperidolate
2670	Nomifensine
2675	Promethazine
2710	Clemastine
	Cyproheptadine
	Dipipanone
2715	Alimemazine
	Tetracaine
2745	Promazine
	Theophylline
2765	Brallobarbital
2770	Dosulepin
2775	Profenamine
2795	Clomipramine
2800	Feprazone
	Prothipendyl
2803	Nordazepam oxazepam
2815	Pyrrobutamine
2825	Cyclobarbital
2830	Amitriptyline M (10-OH-)
2840	Dihydrocodeine
2845	Phenothiazine
2860	Codeine
	Phenylbutazone
2880	Amitriptyline (stereoisomers)
2885	Dibenzepin
	Hyoscine
2895	Metixene
2900	Oxyphencyclimine
2910	Chlorprothixene
	Disopyramide
2920	Mebhydrolin
	Methdilazine
2930	Hydrocodone
2940	Chlorpromazine
	Heptabarbital
2960	Phenobarbital
2965	Levomepromazine
	Procainamide
3010	Azapropazone
3025	Norpropoxyphene
3030	Pentazocine
3041	Nordazepam
3045	Diazepam
3050	Trifluoperazine
3210	Flurazepam
3225	Propiomazine
3230	Acepromazine
3245	Chloroquine

System GG (p. 467)—retention index

RI	Compound
2620	Medazepam
2803	Oxazepam
2910	Lorazepam
2940	Diazepam
	Ketazolam
3041	Nordazepam
3043	Demoxepam
3065	Chlordiazepoxide
3125	Clorazepic Acid
	Temazepam
3147	Clobazam
3190	Flunitrazepam
3220	Flurazepam
3280	Bromazepam
3450	Nitrazepam
3455	Clozapine
3600	Clonazepam

System GH (p. 476)—retention index

RI	*Compound*
2110	Propylcannabidiol
2170	Propyl-Δ^9-Tetrahydrocannabinol
2270	Cannabidiol
2280	Cannabicyclol
2350	Δ^9-Tetrahydrocannabinol
2430	Cannabinol
2440	Cannabigerol
2580	Cannabis M (8α-hydroxy-Δ^9-THC)
2620	Cannabis M (11-hydroxy-Δ^9-THC)
2710	Cannabis M (8α,11-dihydroxy-Δ^9-THC)
2756	Cannabis M (11-nor-Δ^9-THC-9-carboxylic acid)

System GI (p. 494)—retention time (min)

t = tailing peak

RT	*Compound*
0.7	Acetaldehyde
	Methanol
0.9	Dichlorodifluoromethane
1.9	Ethanol
	Methylene Chloride
2.0	Cryofluorane
2.5	Acetone
3.0	Trichlorofluoromethane
4.0	Isopropyl Alcohol
5.5	Propanol
5.9	Ether
6.2	Chloroform
7.3	Methyl Ethyl Ketone
8.2	Trichloroethane
8.3	Enflurane
8.5	Halothane
8.6	Carbon Tetrachloride
9.4	Ethyl Acetate
12.5t	Cloral Hydrate
14.8	Benzene
	Trichloroethylene
17.6	Methoxyflurane
17.0t	Ethylene Glycol
20.1	Methylpentynol
20.3	Amyl Nitrite
23.2	Paraldehyde
24.3	Tetrachloroethylene
24.8	Toluene
24.9	Tetrachloroethane
25.5	Trichloroethanol
29.8	Chlorobutanol
33.2	*m*-Xylene
34.2	Benzaldehyde
	p-Xylene
34.5	*o*-Xylene
35.2	Ethchlorvynol
38.2	Camphor

System GJ (p. 496)—relative to griseofulvin

RRT	*Compound*
0.16	Sulfacetamide
0.4	Sulfamoxole
0.42	Sulfafurazole
0.47	Sulfapyridine
0.49	Sulfathiazole
0.50	Sulfisomidine
0.53	Glymidine Sodium
0.71	Sulfadimidine
0.91	Sulfamethoxazole M (N^4-acetyl-)-Me
0.93	Sulfamethoxypyridazine
0.98	Sulfamethizole
1.38	Sulfametoxydiazine
1.69	N^4-acetylsulfadiazine-Me
1.71	Sulfaphenazole

System GK (p. 204)—relative to caffeine

RRT	*Compound*
	Trichlorophenoxyacetic Acid 2,4,5-T-methyl ester
0.13	Diuron (3,4-dichlorophenyl isocyanate)
	Linuron 3,4-dichlorophenyl-isocyanate
0.23	Dichlorvos
0.27	Trichlorfon
0.36	3,4-Dichloroaniline
	Paraquat (reduction product I – monoene)
0.4	Diquat monoene (reduction product I – monoene)
0.47	Carbaryl M (1-naphthol)
0.49	Dicamba
	Diquat diene
0.50	Mevinphos
0.54	Methylchlorophenoxyacetic Acid
0.58	Paraquat (reduction product II – diene)
0.65	Dichlorophenoxyacetic Acid
0.70	Demeton-*S*
0.73	Omethoate
0.74	Dinitro-orthocresol (methyl ether)
0.76	Lindane
0.78	Monolinuron
0.79	Atrazine
	Dimpylate
0.8	Simazine
0.85	Heptachlor
0.86	Dimethoate
	Disulfoton
0.88	Aldrin
0.9	Monocrotophos
0.94	Propanil
0.95	Desmetryne
0.96	Parathion methyl
0.97	Linuron
0.99	Terbutryne
1.01	Fenitrothion
1.03	Malathion
1.04	Parathion ethyl
1.06	*trans*-Chlordane
1.08	*cis*-Chlordane
1.10	Endosulfan
1.13	Dieldrin
1.18	Dichlorophenoxyacetic Acid
	Dichlorophenoxyacetic Acid (iso-octil ester)
	Tiabendazole
1.19	Endrin
1.24	Clofenotane (*op*′-DDT)
	Trichlorophenoxyacetic Acid 2,4,5-T-isooctil ester
1.27	Pyrethrin I
1.32	Clofenotane (*pp*′-DDT)
1.4	*op*′-Methoxychlor
1.46	Methoxychlor (*pp*′-methoxychlor)
1.59	pyrethrin II
1.60	Azinphos-methyl
ND	Aminotriazole

System GKA (p. 488)—retention index

RI	*Compound*
866	Aldicarb
1059	Methomyl
1102	Barban
1220	Dichlorvos
1294	Carbofuran
1394	Mevinphos

RI	*Compound*
1408	Chlorbromuron
1494	Carbaryl
1530	Methiocarb
1626	Chlorpropham
1672	MCPA
1676	Dazomet
1690	Dimethoate
1710	Atrazine
1728	Gamma-BHC
1740	Mecoprop
1756	Dichloroprop
1766	2,4-D
	2,4,5-T
1769	Diazinon
1776	Disulfoton
1802	Dinoseb
1816	Pirimicarb
1820	MCPB
1850	Phosphamidon
1866	Chlorpyrifos Methyl
1906	Terbutryne
1917	Malathion
1944	Fenitrothion
1968	Heptachlor
2008	Aldrin
2030	Captan
2092	Methidathion
2150	Iodofenphos
2170	Dieldrin
2228	Flampropisopropyl
2236	Endrin
2242	DDT (O,P)
2310	Carbophenothion
2316	Bromoxynil Octanoate
2330	DDT (P,P)
2488	Phosalone
2634	Permethrin
9999	Asulam
	Chlordane
	Dalapon
	Dicamba
	Trichlorphon

System GKB (p. 488)—retention index

RI	*Compound*
966	Aldicarb
1150	Methomyl
1174	Barban
1334	Dichlorvos
1390	Carbofuran
1510	Chlorbromuron
1532	Mevinphos
1660	Methiocarb
1706	Carbaryl
1748	Chlorpropham
1808	MCPA
1840	Gamma-BHC
1862	Mecoprop
1885	Atrazine
1888	Dimethoate
1899	Diazinon
1902	Dazomet
1906	Disulfoton
1926	Dinoseb
1954	2,4-D
1970	MCPB
1982	Dichloroprop
1984	Pirimicarb
2016	Phosphamidon
2060	Chlorpyrifos Methyl
2064	Terbutryne
2068	Heptachlor
2096	Aldrin
2107	Malathion
2110	2,4,5-T
2112	Fenitrothion
2268	Methidathion
2281	Captan
2304	Dieldrin
2342	Iodofenphos
2356	Endrin
2412	Flampropisopropyl
2428	DDT (O,P)
2472	Bromoxynil Octanoate
2494	Carbophenothion
2502	DDT (P,P)
2736	Phosalone
2836	Permethrin
9999	Asulam
	Chlordane
	Dalapon
	Dicamba
	Trichlorphon

System GKC (p. 488)—retention index

RI	*Compound*
1088	Aldicarb
1266	Methomyl
1282	Barban
1454	Dichlorvos
1498	Carbofuran
1610	Chlorbromuron
1680	Mevinphos
1780	Methiocarb
1816	Carbaryl
1888	Chlorpropham
1962	MCPA
1962	Mecoprop
2032	Diazinon
2046	2,4-D
2048	Atrazine
2055	Dichloroprop
2068	Dinoseb
2080	Disulfoton
2088	Gamma-BHC
2120	Dimethoate
2164	Pirimicarb
2188	Heptachlor
2200	Dazomet
2212	Phosphamidon
2226	Aldrin
2234	Chlorpyrifos Methyl
2246	Terbutryne
2262	MCPB
2278	Fenitrothion
2287	Malathion
2302	2,4,5-T
2475	Methidathion
2490	Captan
2528	Dieldrin
2564	Iodofenphos
2588	Flampropisopropyl
2600	Endrin
2620	Bromoxynil Octanoate
2624	DDT (O,P)
2692	DDT (P,P)
2708	Carbophenothion
2960	Phosalone
3056	Permethrin
9999	Asulam
	Chlordane
	Dalapon
	Dicamba
	Trichlorphon

System GKD (p. 488)—retention time (min)

RT	*Compound*
1.2	Methothrin
2.6	Fenpropathrin
3.2	Cyhalothrin
3.8	Permethrin
4.5	Cypermethrin
5.1	Fentalerate
5.8	Deltamethrin

System GL (p. 451)—retention index

RI	*Compound*
1210	Methyl Salicylate
1530	Salicylic Acid M (5-OH-)-Me_3
1680	Ibuprofen M (3-OH-)-Me
1800	Naproxen M (OH-)-Me_2
2115	Flufenamic Acid M (OH-)-Me_2
2120	Naproxen M (*O*-desmethyl-)-Me_2
2130	Fenoprofen M (OH-)-Me_2
2140	Niflumic Acid M(OH-) Me_2
2180	Flurbiprofen M (OH-)-Me_2
2190	Fenbufen M (acetic acid OH-)-Me_2
2225	Etodolac (etodolac-Me)
2250	Ketoprofen M(OH-)-Me_2
2460	Diclofenac M (OH-)-Me_2
2500	Phenylbutazone M (OH-alkyl)-Me
2600	Tolmetin M (COOH-)-Me_2
2880	Indometacin M (OH-)-Me_2

System GM (p. 460)—relative to iprindole

RRT	*Compound*
0.284	Fluoxetine
0.295	Fluvoxamine
0.304	Fluoxetine
0.319	Pethidine
0.357	Pethidine M (nor)
0.420	Tofenacin
0.423	Ketamine M (nor)
0.427	Ketamine
0.428	Meptazinol M (nor)
0.429	Meptazinol
0.52	Methadone M (EDDP)
0.544	Venlafaxine
0.57	Venlafaxine M (*N*-desmethyl)
0.606	Methadone
0.625	Venlafaxine M (*O*-desmethyl)
0.683	Butriptyline
0.687	Venlafaxine M (*N,O*-didesmethyl)
0.723	Amitriptyline
0.761	Butriptyline M (nor)
0.784	Imipramine
0.816	Nortriptyline
0.82	Zimeldine
0.83	Doxepin M (*cis*-nor-)
0.85	Amitriptyline M (cyclobenzaprine)
0.850	Nomifensine
0.870	Pentazocine
0.878	Protriptyline
0.879	Mianserin
0.88	Nortriptyline M (norcyclobenzaprine)
0.896	Desipramine
0.933	Doxepin M (*trans*-nor)
0.941	Zimeldine M (nor)
0.967	Moclobemide
1.000	Iprindole
1.0861	Maprotiline
1.105	Mianserin M (nor)
1.107	Maprotiline M (nor)
1.121	Citalopram
1.149	Amitriptyline M (*cis*-10-OH-)
1.168	Amitriptyline M (*trans*-10-OH-)
1.172	Clomipramine
1.22	Dextropropoxyphene
1.231	Norcitalopram
1.248	Norpropoxyphene
1.259	Dosulepin
1.261	Nortriptyline M (*cis*-10-OH-)
1.3	Dextropropoxyphene M (nor-*N*-propionyl)
1.309	Dipipanone
1.323	Nortriptyline M (*trans*-10-OH-)
1.374	Clomipramine M (nor)
1.449	Acetylcodeine
1.45	Dosulepin M (nor)
1.493	Dihydrocodeine
1.519	Codeine
1.735	Dibenzepin
1.969	Dextropropoxyphene M (nor-amide)
2.047	Paroxetine
2.831	Amoxapine
ND	Alfentanil
	Buprenorphine
	Diphenoxylate
	Diprenorphine
	Etorphine
	Morphine
	Trazodone

System GN (p. 476)—retention time (min)

See Table 28.20 for retention details.

System GO (p. 476)—Retention time (min)

See Table 28.20 for retention details.

System GP (p. 469)—retention index

RI	*Compound*
2235	Felodipine (M (dehydro-desethyl-)-Me)
2255	Nifedipine M (dehydro-)
	Nisoldipine M (dehydro-desisobutyl-)-Me
2270	Isradipine M (dehydro-deisopropyl)-Me
2280	Felodipine (M (dehydro-))
2300	Nimodipine M (dehydro-desisopropyl-desmethoxyethyl)-Me_2
	Nitrendipine M (dehydro-desethyl-)-Me
2360	Isradipine M (dehydro)
2370	Nitrendipine M (dehydro-)
2390	Nimodipine M (dehydro-desmethoxyethyl)-Me
2430	Amlodipine M (dehydro-2-$HOOC^-$)-Me
2450	Nisoldipine M (dehydro-)
2470	Perindopril M(perindoprilat)-Me_3
2560	Perindopril M(perindoprilat-H_2O)-Me_3
2615	Nisoldipine M (dehydro-OH^-)
2635	Amlodipine M (dehydro-desamino-$HOOC^-$)-Me
2645	Nimodipine M (dehydro-desisopropyl-*O*-desmethyl-HOOC)-Me
2655	Nimodipine M (dehydro-)
2665	Nimodipine M (dehydro-desisopropyl-*O*-desmethyl)-Me
2680	Enalapril M (enalaprilat)-Me_3
2695	Nifedipine M (dehydro-2-COOH-)-Me
	Nisoldipine M (dehydro-desisobutyl-2-$HOOC^-$)-Me_2
2735	Enalapril M (enalaprilat-H_2O)-Me
2740	Nimodipine M (dehydro-*O*-desmethyl-HOOC-)-Me
2865	Ramipril M (ramiprilat)-Me_3
2925	Ramipril M (ramiprilate-H_2O)-Me_3
2960	Cilazapril (M (cilazaprilate)-Me_3)
2985	Benazepril (M (benazeprilate)-Me_3)
3005	Trandolapril M perindoprilate-Me_3
3010	Cilazapril (cilazapril-Me)
3030	Benazepril (benazepril-Me)
3070	Trandolapril M perindoprilate-H_2O-Me_3
3080	Quinapril M (quinaprilate)-Me_3
3310	Quinapril M (quinaprilate-H_2O)-Me_3
3555	Losartan (losartan-2Me)
3580	Moexipril M(moexiprilate)-Me_3
3775	Moexipril M(moexiprilate-H_2O)-Me_3

System GQ (p. 497)**—retention time (min)**

RT	Compound
5.5	Lidocaine M (monoethylglycinexylidide)
5.7	Prilocaine
	Propitocaine
6.0	Lidocaine
6.8	Procaine
7.2	Mepivacaine
7.85	Cocaine
8.0	Tetracaine
10.4	Cinchocaine

System GR (p. 497)**—retention time (min)**

RT	Compound
2.8	Sevoflurane
3.4	Isoflurane
3.7	Enflurane
4.2	Halothane

System GS (p. 498)**—retention time (min)**

RT	Compound
16.1	Amitriptyline
16.3	Trimipramine
17.1	Imipramine
17.2	*cis*-Doxepin
17.5	Nortriptyline
17.6	*trans*-Doxepin
18.1	Mianserin
18.7	Desipramine
21.0	Maprotiline
21.2	Chloramitriptyline (IS)
22.0	Clomipramine
24.0	Desmethylclomipramine

System GV (p. 498)**—retention time (min)**

RT	Compound
10.4	Ketamine
11.6	Xylazine
16.6	Chlorpromazine
19.0	Azaperone
	Acetopromazine
19.7	Azaperol
20.2	Propionylpromazine
23.3	Haloperidol

System GW (p. 498)**—retention time (min)**

RT	Compound
19.3	Triflupromazine
19.8	Isothiopendyl
19.9	Promethazine
20.3	Alimemazine
20.6	Promazine
21.4	Ethopropazine
23.0	Chlorpromazine
23.6	Levomepromazine
25.6	Trifluoperazine
27.1	Perazine
28.7	Prochlorperazine
31.1	Thioridazine
32.7	Thiethylperazine
46.9	Thioproperazine

System GX (p. 476)**—retention time (min)**

See Table 28.19 for retention details.

System GY (p. 476)**—retention index**

See Table 28.19 for retention details.

System GAG (p. 495)**—relative to testosterone**

RRT	Compound
0.89	Methandriol
0.91	Nandrolone
1.2	Methandienone
1.05	Boldenone
	Methyltestosterone
1.17	Oxandrolone
1.21	Testosterone acetate
1.28	Oxymetholone
1.43	Testosterone propionate
1.5	Fluoxymesterone
1.54	Testosterone isobutyrate
1.77	Testosterone isocaproate
1.92	Testosterone enantate
2.19	Testosterone cipionate
2.36	Testosterone decanoate
2.56	Testosterone undecylate

System GAI (p. 495)**—relative to 17α-methyl-5α-androstan-3β,17β-diol**

RRT	*Compound*
0.57	Clenbuterol
0.905	Metenolone 1-methylen-5α-androstan-3α-ol-17-one
0.921	Methandienone 17α-methyl-5β-androst-1-en-3α,17β-diol
0.925	Methandienone 17α-methyl-5β,(α)-androstan-3α,17β-diol
0.943	17α-Trenbolone
0.95	5α-Dihydrotestosterone
0.96	5β-Androst-1-en-17β-ol-3-one
0.961	Boldenone
0.97	Testosterone
0.974	Drostanolone Propionate
0.993	Metenolone
1.078	17α-(2-hydroxyethyl)-5α-estran-3α,17β-diol
1.106	2-hydroxymethyl-17α-methyl-5-androstan-3,17-diol
1.111	Oxandrolone
1.117	17α-methyl-1,4-androstadien-6β,17β-diol-3-one
1.155	Fluoxymesterone
1.18	Oxymetholone 17-triol
1.31	Stanozolol
1.393	4β-Hydroxystanozolol
6.0	2-hydroxymethyl-17α-methyl-5-androstan-3

System GAJ (p. 457)**—relative to methylphenobarbital**

RRT	*Compound*
0.350	Valproic Acid
0.453	Ethosuximide
0.612	Barbital
0.689	Mesuximide mesuximide
0.732	Butobarbital
0.775	Amobarbital M (COOH-)
0.778	Butalbital
0.779	Mesuximide *N*-desmethylmesuximide
0.789	Nealbarbital
0.794	Amobarbital
0.798	Methohexital
	Vinylbital
0.803	Pentobarbital
0.865	Secobarbital
0.918	Mephenytoin
0.940	Ethotoin
	Hexobarbital
0.948	Thiopental
1.000	Methylphenobarbital
1.053	Butobarbital M (3′-OH-)
1.065	Carbamazepine M (iminostilbene)
1.074	Primidone M (PEMA)
1.087	Phenylmethylbarbituric Acid
1.138	Amobarbital M (3-OH-)
1.142	Cyclobarbital
1.150	Phenobarbital
1.188	Carbamazepine M (epoxide)
1.206	Secobarbital M (3′-OH-)
1.282	Heptabarb
1.674	Primidone
1.716	Carbamazepine
1.941	Lamotrigine
ND	Vigabatrin

Systems GAK–GAQ

For Systems GAK, GAL, GAM, GAN, GAO, GAP and GAQ see Table 2.4 (Chapter 2, p. 8).

System GAR (p. 495)**—retention time (min)**

RT	*Compound*
11.8	Dehydroepiandrosterone DHEA
11.9	Androsterone
12.3	Methandriol
12.5	Nandrolone
12.8	Boldenone
12.9	Testosterone
13.1	Methyltestosterone
13.2	Methandienone
13.5	Testosterone acetate
13.6	Boldenone acetate
13.7	Oxandrolone
	Oxymetholone
14.2	Testosterone propionate
14.6	Fluoxymesterone
15.4	Stanozolol
15.9	Testosterone isocaproate
16.7	Testosterone enantate
18.7	Boldenone benzoate
	Testosterone cipionate
19.8	Testosterone decanoate
22.4	Boldenone undecylenate

High Performance Liquid Chromatographic Data

System HA—*k* values

t = tailing peak

k	*Compound*
0.1	Acetanilide
	Acetazolamide
	Benzocaine
	Clomethiazole
	Diazepam
	Diazoxide
	Flurazepam M (desalkyl-)
	Indapamide
	Lorazepam
	Methocarbamol
	Nitrazepam
	Phenothiazine
	Phenoxybenzamine
	Proxyphylline
	Theobromine
	Theophylline
0.2	Bezitramide
	Caffeine
	Colchicine
	Diphenoxylate
	Dipyridamole
	Mebanazine
	Medazepam
	Mephenesin
	Methadone M (EMDP)
	Methaqualone
	Nicotine M (cotinine)
	Nifedipine
	Nordazepam
	Pargyline
	Pemoline
	Perhexiline
	Phenazone
0.3	Aminophenazone
	Benzquinamide
	Ergocristine
	Fenbutrazate
	Noscapine
	Papaverine
0.4	Bromhexine
	Buprenorphine
	Cimetidine
	Deserpidine
	Doxapram
	Ergocryptine
	Ergocornine
	Ergometrine
	Ergotamine
	Methylergometrine
	Methysergide
0.5	Lysergamide
	Methoserpidine
	Practolol
0.6	Dihydroergotamine
	Diprenorphine
	Droperidol
	Etorphine
	Lidocaine
	Lidoflazine
	Lofepramine
	Phentermine
	Piritramide
	Pramocaine
	Rescinnamine
	Trazodone
0.6t	Diphenoxylic acid
0.7	Buclizine
	Dextromoramide
	Fenoterol
	Lysergide
	Meclozine
	Morazone
	Narceine
	Oxypertine
	Pimozide
0.8	Cinnarizine
	Fentanyl
	Harmine
	Isoxsuprine
	Phenoperidine
	Prazosin
0.8t	Lysergic Acid
0.9	Amfetamine
	Bamethan
	Buphenine
	Bupivacaine
	Chlorphentermine
	Diethylpropion M (norephedrine)
	Ephedrine M (nor-)
	Mepivacaine
	Metaraminol
	Methoxamine
	Nomifensine
	Phendimetrazine
	Phenylpropanolamine
	Terbutaline
0.9t	Benzoylecgonine
1.0	Cathine
	Ephedrine
	Nalorphine
	Norfenfluramine
	Norpseudoephedrine
	Phenelzine
	Piminodine
	Prenylamine
	Prilocaine
	Pyrimethamine
	Salbutamol
	Thiopropazate
	Tranylcypromine
1.1	Anileridine
	Benperidol
	Clorprenaline
	Desmethylmaprotiline
	Dicycloverine
	Ecgonine
	4-Hydroxypropranolol
	Hyoscine
	Loxapine
	Nicotine
1.2	Alprenolol
	Azacyclonol
	Benzfetamine
	Butacaine
	Clonidine
	Debrisoquine
	Etamiphylline
	Flupentixol
	Fluphenazine
	Haloperidol
	2-Hydroxydesipramine
	Lidocaine M (monoethylglycinexylidide)
	Mexiletine
	Nadolol
	Phenethylamine
	Pindolol
	Pipradrol
	Pseudoephedrine
	Sotalol
	Timolol
	Tocainide
	Trifluperidol
	Trimethoprim
	Tryptamine
	Tyramine
1.2t	Nialamide
1.3	Atenolol
	Didesmethylimipramine
	Fencamfamin
	Fenfluramine
	Flurazepam
	Mescaline
	Metoprolol
	Norpropoxyphene
	Oxprenolol
	Pericyazine
	Phenazocine
	Phenylephrine
	Procainamide
	Propranolol
1.4	Diethylcarbamazine
	Hydroxyzine
	Metopimazine
	Naloxone
	Primaquine
1.5	Mephentermine
1.6	Tacrine
	Xylometazoline
1.6t	Cyclopentolate
1.7	Benactyzine
	Benzoctamine
	Butetamate
	Carfenazine

k	*Compound*
	Cyclopentamine
	Diethylpropion
	Levacetylmethadol
	Mecamylamine
	Meclofenoxate
	Methoxyphenamine
	Methylphenidate
	N-Monodesmethylorphenadrine
	Norbutriptyline
	Oxymetazoline
	Phenmetrazine
	Phentolamine
	Piperidolate
	Tofenacin
	Verapamil M (nor-)
1.7t	Labetalol
	Norpethidine
	Pethidine M (nor-)
1.8	Adiphenine
	Alverine
	Antazoline
	10-Hydroxynortriptyline
	Lorcainide
	Mazindol
	Mianserin
	Monodesethylamiodarone
	N-monodesisopropyldisopyramide
	Pentazocine
	Tramazoline
	Trihexyphenidyl
	Trimipramine M (nor-)
1.9	Acetophenazine
	Cinchocaine
	Dextropropoxyphene
	Etafedrine
	Mebeverine
	Perphenazine
	Piperacetazine
	Procaine
1.9t	Levallorphan
2.0	Diethylthiambutene
	Metamfetamine
	Monodesmethylclomipramine
	Nortriptyline
	Procyclidine
	Prolintane
	Tetracaine
	Thiamine
2.1	Cyclazocine
	Desipramine
	Dimetotiazine
	Ibogaine
	Propiomazine
	Protriptyline
	Proxymetacaine
	Quinidine
	Tolazoline
	Trimeperidine
2.2	Chlorpromazine M (nor-)
	Dipipanone
	Dosulepin M (nor-)
	Doxepin M (nor-)
	Flavoxate
	Maprotiline
	Methadone
	Norcyclizine
	Opipramol
	Quinisocaine
2.2t	Prajmalium Bitartrate
2.3	Chlorcyclizine
	Desacetylmoxisylyte
	Methylephedrine
	Ranitidine
2.4	Amiodarone
	Disopyramide
	Mianserin M(nor-)
	Naphazoline
	Profenamine
	Quinine
2.4t	Isopropamide Iodide
	Phencyclidine
2.5	Phenindamine
2.6	Physostigmine
	Verapamil
2.6t	Oxyphenonium Bromide
2.7	Bromazine
	Butriptyline
	Pirenzepine
	Triflupromazine
	Trimipramine
2.7t	Dopamine
2.8	Cocaine
	Dibenzepin
	Methadone M (EDDP)
	Oxyphencyclimine
	Pyrrobutamine
2.8t	Ajmaline
	Alphaprodine
	Ketobemidone
	Pethidine
	Pethidinic acid
2.9	Chlorphenoxamine
	Cyclizine
	10-Hydroxyamitriptyline
	Moxisylyte
	Phenglutarimide
	Tolpropamine
2.9t	Normorphine
	Zimeldine M (nor-)
3.0	*N*-Acetylprocainamide
	Chlorprothixene
	Histapyrrodine
	Nefopam
	Orphenadrine
	Oxeladin
	Trifluoperazine
3.1	Alimemazine
	Betahistine
	Bufotenine
	Cinchonidine
	2-Hydroxyimipramine
	Meptazinol
	Phenyltoloxamine
3.1t	Codeine M (nor-)
	Norcodeine
	Protokylol
	Psilocin
3.2	Cyproheptadine
	Dosulepin
	Levomepromazine
	Penthienate Methobromide
	Thonzylamine
	Triprolidine
3.2t	Glycopyrronium Bromide
	Zimeldine
3.3	Amitriptyline
	Diphenhydramine
	Ethoheptazine
3.3t	Diphenylpyraline
	Poldine Metilsulfate
3.4	Butaperazine
	Clomipramine
	Diethazine
	Pizotifen
3.5	Thenalidine
3.6	Metixene
	Tripelennamine
3.6t	6-Monoacetylmorphine
	Tigloidine
3.7	Clemastine
	Doxepin
3.7t	Apomorphine
	Benzatropine
	Ethylmorphine
	Hyoscyamine
	Thebacon
3.8	Isothipendyl
	Thiethylperazine
	Tiotixene
3.8t	Morphine
3.9	Chlorphenamine
	Mepyramine
	Pecazine
	Prochlorperazine
3.9t	Atropine
3.0t	Diamorphine
	Mebhydrolin
	Trimetazidine
4.0	Chloropyrilene
	Thenyldiamine
4.1	Acepromazine
	Brompheniramine
	Chlorpromazine
	Iprindole
	Methapyrilene
	Pheniramine
	Thioproperazine
4.1t	Mepenzolate Bromide
4.2	Chloropyramine
	Imipramine
4.2t	Homatropine
4.3t	Bretylium Tosilate
4.4	Doxylamine
	Propantheline Bromide
	Prothipendyl
4.4t	Benzylmorphine
	Levorphanol
4.6t	Dosulepin M (sulfoxide)
	Thebaine
4.7	Trimethobenzamide
4.7t	Carbinoxamine
	Dextrorphan
	Neostigmine Bromide
4.8t	Clemizole
	Codeine
5.0	Mesoridazine
	Metoclopramide
	Promethazine
5.1	Dimetindene
5.2	Emepronium Bromide
	Thioridazine
5.4	Pipazetate
5.6t	Dextromethorphan
5.7t	Dihydromorphine
5.8t	Dimethoxanate
5.9	Promazine
5.0t	Deptropine
6.0	Methdilazine
6.3t	Pyridostigmine Bromide
6.7t	Oxymorphone
6.9t	Oxycodone
6.0t	Pholcodine
7.1t	Emetine
	Hydrocodone
7.2t	Dihydrocodeine
7.7t	Cephaëline
7.9t	Hydromorphone
8.2t	Cotarnine
8.3t	Mequitazine
11.1t	Brucine
13.0t	Strychnine
15.2t	Chloroquine

System HB—*k* values

k	*Compound*
0.1	Noradrenaline
0.27	Oxedrine
0.73	Hydroxyephedrine
0.81	Tyramine
2.0	Hordenine
2.24	Hydroxyamfetamine
3.6	Phenethylamine
3.9	Phenylpropanolamine
3.87	Ephedrine M (nor-)
4.39	Cathine
5.9	Pseudoephedrine
5.68	Ephedrine
5.91	Phenelzine
8.48	Amfetamine
10.52	Metamfetamine
11.08	Dimethylamfetamine
14.95	Methoxyamfetamine
16.82	Mescaline
19.46	Phentermine
29.99	Prazepam
32.17	Methoxyphenamine

System HBA—Retention time (min)

RT	*Compound*
8.8	Erythromycin
15.7	Clarithromycin
17.1	Roxithromycin
20.7	Azithromycin

System HBB—Retention time (min)

RT	*Compound*
8.8	Erythromycin
9.6	Azithromycin
13.8	Clarithromycin
16.3	Roxithromycin

System HBC

See Table 2.5 (Chapter 2, p. 8) for retention details.

System HBD

See Table 2.5 (Chapter 2, p. 8) for retention details.

System HBE

See Table 2.5 (Chapter 2, p. 8) for retention details.

System HBF

See Table 2.5 (Chapter 2, p. 8) for retention details.

System HBG

See Table 2.5 (Chapter 2, p. 8) for retention details.

System HBH—*k* values

k	*Compound*
1.63	Bromazepam
2.92	Clonazepam
3.22	Nitrazepam
3.34	Flunitrazepam
3.35	Alprazolam
4.14	Clobazam
5.16	Lorazepam
5.18	Triazolam
5.42	Oxazepam
6.8	Temazepam
6.68	Chlordiazepoxide
7.19	Lormetazepam
8.22	Clorazepic Acid
8.97	Nordazepam
10.4	Diazepam
10.78	Ketazolam
12.98	Flurazepam
41.46	Medazepam

System HBI—*k* values

k	*Compound*
0.79	Clonazepam
0.8	Bromazepam
0.86	Flunitrazepam
0.97	Nitrazepam
1.09	Clobazam
1.13	Triazolam
1.14	Lorazepam
1.25	Oxazepam
1.28	Alprazolam
1.46	Lormetazepam
1.49	Temazepam
1.65	Chlordiazepoxide
1.84	Clorazepic Acid
1.89	Nordazepam
2.22	Ketazolam
2.29	Diazepam
3.12	Flurazepam
4.28	Prazepam
6.31	Medazepam

System HC—*k* values

k	*Compound*
0.05	Buprenorphine
0.09	Dextromoramide
0.1	Pemoline
	Phenoperidine
	Piritramide
0.15	Benzfetamine
	Noscapine
0.16	Diethylpropion
	Papaverine
0.17	Naloxone
0.19	Dextropropoxyphene
0.2	Mazindol
	Phendimetrazine
0.26	Caffeine
	Tranylcypromine
0.27	Fenetylline
0.29	Nalorphine
0.3	Phenazocine
0.35	Norpipanone
0.36	Methylphenidate
0.37	Phenelzine
0.53	Normethadone
0.55	Pethidine
0.63	Adrenaline
0.66	Diamorphine
0.67	Pentazocine
0.69	Pipradrol
0.7	Diethylpropion M (norephedrine)
	Ephedrine M (nor-)
	Phenylpropanolamine
0.72	Fencamfamin
0.78	Acetylcodeine
0.8	6-Monoacetylmorphine
0.82	Chlorphentermine
0.83	Cathine
0.85	Oxycodone
	Thebacon
0.86	Phentermine
0.88	Fenfluramine
0.9	Thebaine
0.98	Amfetamine
	Methylenedioxyamfetamine
1.03	Benzylmorphine
	Methadone
1.06	Ethylmorphine
1.08	Normetadrenaline
1.11	Etorphine
	Fentanyl
	Hydroxyamfetamine
1.13	DOM
1.21	Codeine
1.3	Morphine
	Phenethylamine
	Prolintane
1.46	Levallorphan
1.47	Tyramine
1.48	Trimethoxyamfetamine
1.55	Ethoheptazine
1.6	Phenylephrine
1.61	Dipipanone
1.63	Pholcodine
1.77	Pseudoephedrine
1.79	Ephedrine
1.83	Methylephedrine
1.89	Dimethylamfetamine
2.04	Pethidine M (nor-)
2.07	Metamfetamine
2.17	Hydrocodone
	Mescaline
2.48	Mephentermine
2.5	Dihydrocodeine
2.75	Dihydromorphine
3.2	Levorphanol
3.51	Norcodeine
3.92	Normorphine

System HD—*k* values

k	*Compound*
0.1	Dipyrone
	Nifenazone
	Paracetamol
	Phenazone
0.2	Aminophenazone
0.4	Morazone
	Salicylamide
0.5	Acetanilide
	Aspirin
0.55	Etenzamide
0.6	Phenacetin
	Piroxicam
0.7	Benorilate
	Choline Salicylate
	Salicylic Acid
1.2	Indoprofen
1.25	Sulindac
1.3	Propyphenazone
1.95	Bufexamac
	Oxyphenbutazone
2.05	Tolmetin
2.4	Ketoprofen
2.5	Famprofazone
2.6	Alclofenac
3.3	Naproxen
3.6	Salsalate
3.7	Zomepirac
4.0	Fenbufen
4.1	Diflunisal
6.5	Phenylbutazone
6.95	Indometacin
7.9	Fenoprofen
11.3	Benoxaprofen
11.5	Diclofenac
15.1	Ibuprofen
15.6	Salol
19.7	Flufenamic Acid
21.1	Mefenamic Acid

System HE—*k* values

k	*Compound*
0.91	Ethosuximide
1.35	Primidone
1.57	Sultiame
2.76	Phenobarbital
2.81	Ethotoin
6.02	Mesuximide
6.8	Pheneturide
7.97	Glutethimide
8.3	Carbamazepine
9.71	Phenytoin

System HF—*k* values

k	*Compound*
0.17	Viloxazine
0.42	Nomifensine
0.5	Dibenzepin
0.67	Naproxen
	Zimeldine
1.33	Oxypertine
1.63	Noxiptiline
	Opipramol
2.27	Doxepin
3.6	Desipramine
	Dosulepin
	Protriptyline
4.17	Imipramine
4.58	Nortriptyline
4.92	Maprotiline
5.42	Amitriptyline
6.17	Trimipramine
7.33	Butriptyline
9.92	Clomipramine
10.83	Iprindole

System HG—*k* values

k	*Compound*
1.11	Barbital
	Metharbital barbital
1.5	Phenylmethylbarbituric Acid
2.46	Allobarbital
2.69	Metharbital
3.09	Brallobarbital
	Phenobarbital
3.42	Aprobarbital
4.01	Ibomal
4.83	Vinbarbital
4.9	Secbutabarbital
5.25	Cyclobarbital
5.43	Butobarbital
6.0	Cyclopentobarbital
6.17	Butalbital
7.2	Talbutal
7.27	Methylphenobarbital
7.37	Hexobarbital
8.12	Idobutal
8.65	Enallylpropymal
9.9	Heptabarb
10.22	Nealbarbital
10.91	Amobarbital
10.96	Pentobarbital
16.28	Secobarbital
27.61	Methohexital
34.28	Hexethal

System HH—*k* values

k	*Compound*
0.63	Barbital
0.9	Phenylmethylbarbituric Acid
1.23	Phenobarbital
1.33	Allobarbital
1.72	Brallobarbital
1.99	Metharbital
2.22	Aprobarbital
2.32	Vinbarbital
2.58	Ibomal
2.61	Cyclobarbital
3.3	Secbutabarbital
3.42	Butobarbital
3.48	Butalbital
3.84	Cyclopentobarbital
	Methylphenobarbital
4.7	Talbutal
4.77	Idobutal
4.93	Heptabarb
5.67	Hexobarbital
6.19	Nealbarbital
6.96	Enallylpropymal
7.05	Amobarbital
8.07	Pentobarbital
11.47	Secobarbital
20.39	Hexethal
20.48	Methohexital

System HI—*k* values

k	*Compound*
0.46	Nitrazepam M (7-amino-)
0.68	Nitrazepam M (7-acetamido-)
1.17	Clorazepic Acid
2.32	Bromazepam
2.42	Demoxepam
2.85	Clonazepam
2.96	Nitrazepam
3.06	Clobazam M (nor-)
3.15	Flunitrazepam
3.91	Clobazam
4.27	Flurazepam M (OH-ethyl-)
4.38	Triazolam
4.47	Chlordiazepoxide M (nor-)
4.6	Lorazepam
4.62	Oxazepam
4.7	Alprazolam
5.19	Flurazepam M (desalkyl-)
5.68	Temazepam
6.32	Lormetazepam
6.41	Chlordiazepoxide
8.0	Nordazepam
9.47	Diazepam
9.75	Midazolam
12.81	Ketazolam

System HJ—*k* values

k	*Compound*
2.1	Midazolam
2.29	Diazepam
2.45	Ketazolam
3.19	Flurazepam
4.6	Prazepam
7.05	Medazepam

System HK—*k* values

k	*Compound*
0.0	Nitrazepam M (7-amino-)
0.01	Clobazam M (nor-)
0.03	Clobazam
	Demoxepam
0.04	Ketazolam
0.08	Lormetazepam
0.14	Lorazepam
0.35	Clonazepam
0.47	Flunitrazepam
0.6	Temazepam
0.73	Oxazepam
1.43	Flurazepam M (2-OH-ethyl-)

k	*Compound*
1.49	Nitrazepam
1.52	Flurazepam M (desalkyl-)
1.83	Triazolam
1.93	Nitrazepam M (7-acetamido-)
1.99	Nordazepam
2.0	Clorazepic Acid
2.19	Prazepam
2.39	Chlordiazepoxide M (nor-)
2.49	Diazepam
2.79	Alprazolam
2.87	Chlordiazepoxide
2.99	Bromazepam
4.44	Medazepam
5.9	Midazolam
6.5	Flurazepam

System HL—*k* values

k	*Compound*
7.47	Cannabis CBD
	Cannabis cannabivarin
8.18	Cannabis cannabigerol
	Cannabis tetrahydrocannabivarin
8.76	Cannabis cannabidiolic acid
11.77	Cannabis CBN
13.35	Cannabis Δ^9-THC
14.07	Cannabis Δ^8-THC
14.64	Cannabis tetrahydrocannabivaric acid
14.78	Cannabis cannabicyclol
19.09	Cannabis cannabichromene
25.83	Cannabis tetrahydrocannabinolic acid

System HM—*k* values

k	*Compound*
2.0	Digitoxigenin
2.8	Digitoxigenin Monodigitoxoside
3.7	Gitoxigenin
3.9	Digitoxigenin Bisdigitoxoside
4.5	Digoxigenin
	Gitoxigenin Monodigitoxoside
5.4	Digitoxin
5.5	Digoxigenin Monodigitoxoside
6.5	Gitoxigenin Bisdigitoxoside
6.8	Gitaloxin
8.2	Digoxigenin Bisdigitoxoside
8.6	Gitoxin
11.3	Digoxin
17.9	Lanatoside A
31.8	Lanatoside B
39.5	Lanatoside C

System HN—*k* values

k	*Compound*
0.54	Chlorothiazide
0.67	Quinethazone
0.7	Hydrochlorothiazide
1.28	Chlortalidone
1.3	Hydroflumethiazide
3.1	Trichlormethiazide
3.82	Methyclothiazide
4.01	Clopamide
4.89	Metolazone
7.26	Clorexolone
8.67	Mefruside
9.32	Benzthiazide
10.78	Cyclothiazide
15.09	Polythiazide
15.35	Bendroflumethiazide
16.45	Cyclopenthiazide

System HP—*k* values

k	*Compound*
0.0	Lysergic Acid; iso-lysegide
0.33	Lysergamide
0.5	Ergometrine
0.83	Methylergometrine
	Iso-lysergic Acid
	Lysergol
0.92	2-Oxylysergide
1.83	Lysergide
1.98	Lysergic Acid Methylpropylamide
2.33	Methysergide
7.08	Ergosine
9.58	Ergotamine
10.2	Ergocornine
11.4	Dihydroergotamine
15.2	Ergocryptine
15.9	Dihydroergocryptine
17.3	Ergocristine
17.7	Ergosinine
18.3	Dihydro-ergocristine
44.3	Bromocriptine

System HQ—*k* values

k	*Compound*
0.0	Procaine
0.24	Chloroprocaine
0.79	Lidocaine
1.09	Propoxycaine
	Mepivacaine
1.38	Prilocaine
	Proxymetacaine
2.68	Cocaine
4.42	Butanilicaine
4.59	Piperocaine
5.68	Benzoylecgonine
7.19	Bupivacaine
8.97	Butacaine
16.25	Oxybuprocaine
	Tetracaine
20.06	Benzocaine

System HR—*k* values

k	*Compound*
0.86	Bupivacaine
	Oxybuprocaine
1.33	Tetracaine
1.61	Benzocaine
2.48	Diperodon
	Pramocaine
2.78	Dyclonine
4.14	Oxetacaine
5.51	Cinchocaine
10.31	Cyclomethycaine
11.24	Quinisocaine

System HS—*k* values

k	*Compound*
0.01	Noscapine
0.04	Papaverine
0.21	Caffeine
0.35	Diamorphine
0.5	Acetylcodeine
0.8	Thebaine
1.0	6-Monoacetylmorphine
1.45	Ethylmorphine
1.9	Codeine
2.02	Quinine
2.43	Strychnine
5.16	Morphine

System HT—*k* values

k	*Compound*
2.4	Cortisone
2.5	Triamcinolone acetonide
3.4	Prednisone
4.2	Beclometasone
4.8	Dexamethasone
5.8	Hydrocortisone
7.5	Methylprednisolone
8.4	Prednisolone

System HU—*k* values

k	*Compound*
3.3	Sulfachlorpyridazine
3.8	Sulfapyridine
4.4	Sulfadoxine
4.8	Sulfamethoxazole
	Sulfaquinoxaline
4.9	Sulfamethoxazole (N^4-acetyl-)
6.0	Sulfafurazole
7.1	Sulfadimidine
7.5	Sulfamethoxypyridazine
7.7	Sulfacetamide
8.1	Sulfamerazine
8.2	Sulfametoxydiazine
8.7	Sulfadiazine
8.9	Sulfanilamide
9.6	Sulfanilamide (N^4-acetylsulfanilamide)
12.6	Sulfamoxole
13.4	Sulfathiazole
14.0	Phthalylsulfathiazole
16.8	Succinylsulfathiazole

System HV—relative to meclofenamic acid

RRT	*Compound*
0.45	Furosemide
0.52	Indoprofen
0.60	Tolmetin
0.61	Alclofenac
0.66	Ketoprofen
0.69	Oxyphenbutazone
	Salsalate
0.77	Diflunisal
0.78	Sulindac
0.81	Fenbufen
0.85	Diclofenac
0.87	Clonixin
	Indometacin
0.89	Flurbiprofen
0.91	Fenclofenac
0.92	Feprazone
0.93	Niflumic Acid
0.95	Mefenamic Acid
	Phenylbutazone
0.98	Benoxaprofen
0.99	Flunixin
	Tolmetin
1.0	Flufenamic Acid

System HW—*k* values

k	*Compound*
0.32	Aminophenazone
	Paracetamol
0.45	Dipyrone
	Nifenazone
0.95	Phenazone
2.05	Morazone
2.3	Acetanilide
2.5	Salicylamide
2.7	Aspirin
4.4	Phenacetin
4.6	Etenzamide
	Salicylic Acid
4.8	Choline Salicylate
7.7	Piroxicam
11.0	Propyphenazone
22.4	Benorilate

System HX—retention index

RI	*Compound*
0	Diquat
	Paraquat
9	Thiamine (hydrochloride)
30	Adrenaline
35	Benserazide
39	Dihydralazine
48	Pentolonium Tartrate
55	Nicotinyl Alcohol
56	Decamethonium
60	Metformin
65	Levodopa
	Pholcodine
	Pyridostigmine Bromide
	Pyridoxine
69	Methyldopa
	Nicotine
70	Fluorouracil
72	Flucytosine
79	Arecoline
	Isoprenaline
80	Phenylephrine
84	Metaraminol
118	Etilefrine
149	Acetylcysteine
150	Rimiterol
151	Orciprenaline
168	Nicotinamide
184	Phenelzine
187	Mercaptopurine
193	Hydralazine
200	Morphine
201	Enalapril
205	Pholedrine
208	Procainamide
211	Bromisoval M2
214	Coniine
215	Nicotine M (cotinine)
	Xantinol Nicotinate
217	Oxymorphone
219	Diethylcarbamazine
220	Salbutamol
221	Ephedrine
222	Isoetarine
225	Terbutaline
	Tolazoline
226	Sotalol
230	Tranylcypromine
233	Famotidine
237	Bromisoval α-(cystein-*S*-yl)isovalerylurea (M3)
	Dihydromorphine
	Pseudoephedrine
239	Ceftriaxone
	Xamoterol
240	Dropropizine
	Hydromorphone
	Psilocin
243	Atenolol
	Resorcinol
244	Amfetamine
247	Tizanidine
	Tocainide
249	Iproniazid
250	Bamethan
	Phenformin
	Prednisone
251	Cimetidine
257	Amiloride
	Metronidazole
258	Clonidine
	Phenmetrazine
259	Sulpiride
260	Nalorphine
261	Dihydrocodeine
	Tetramisole
262	Aminophenazone
	Homatropine Methylbromide
	Metamfetamine
	Theobromine
263	Phendimetrazine
264	Paracetamol
	Procaine
266	Codeine
	Methylenedioxyamfetamine
268	Acetazolamide
	Cefaclor
270	Hyoscine
271	Lisinopril
272	Homatropine
	Mescaline
274	Methoxyamfetamine
275	Diprophylline
276	Theophylline
277	Oxycodone
278	Methylenedioxymethamfetamine
280	Hydroxychloroquine
282	Chloroquine
	Fenyramidol
283	Pheniramine
286	Hydrocodone
	Trimethadione
287	Fenoterol
288	Lidocaine
	Nadolol
289	Dopexamine
	Etofylline
290	Gelsemine
	Pentetrazol
	Sulfisomidine
	Trimethoxyamfetamine (2,4,6-TMA)
291	Ethylmorphine
	Pirenzepine M (*N*-desmethyl)
	Saccharin
292	Ergometrine
	Methotrexate
293	Pirenzepine
	Proxyphylline
294	Hydrochlorothiazide
	Ketobemidone
	Mephentermine
295	Guanoxan
	Moclobemide
	Nalbuphine
296	Mepivacaine
	Physostigmine
297	Clenbuterol M(hydroxy)
	Minoxidil
298	Triamterene
299	Atropine Methonitrate
	Oxytetracycline Dihydrate
	Pipamperone
	Pyrantel
	Trimethoprim
300	Pindolol
301	Ethosuximide
302	Strychnine
303	Methoxyphenamine
304	Bambuterol Monocarbamate
	Cinchonine
	Methazolamide
	Nikethamide
305	Caffeine
306	Atropine
	Cinchonidine
307	Pemoline
308	Barbital
	Dobutamine
310	Emetine
	Nifenazone
	Sulfathiazole
311	Ketamine
	Tropicamide
312	Bromisoval M1
	Brucine
	Sulfapyridine
314	Ofloxacin
	Perindoprilat
	Tetracycline
316	Captopril
	Dipyrone
	Nitrofurazone
	Remoxipride M(FLA-838)
317	Thenyldiamine
	Timolol
318	Carbimazole
	Ciprofloxacin
	Nedocromil
319	Azaperone
	Harman
	Nitrofurantoin
320	Aminoacridine
	Methylergometrine
	Naphazoline
321	Tubocurarine Chloride
322	Primidone
	Quinidine
323	Azathioprine
324	Metoclopramide
325	Dextrorphan
	Viloxazine
326	Clenbuterol
	Metoprolol
	Thiazinamium Metilsulfate (M-sulfoxide)
327	Quinine
	Salicylamide
328	Guaifenesin
	Tramadol
329	Mexiletine
331	Zopiclone
333	Phenazone
	Sulfadimidine
	Thebacon
334	Nialamide
	Remoxipride
335	Sulfamethoxypyridazine
336	Fenetylline
	Furazolidone
	Tripelennamine
	Tyramine
338	Dimetindene
339	Harmine
	Phenacemide
340	Diamorphine
	DOM
	Fluconazole
	Thebaine
341	Remoxipride M(NCM-009)
	Tramazoline
342	Methapyrilene
344	Etorphine
	Sultiame
345	Disopyramide
	Mepacrine
	Methocarbamol
	Mexazolam

RI	*Compound*
	Pethidine
346	Allobarbital
	Clenbuterol (M#2)
347	Methyprylon
	Trimethobenzamide
348	Apomorphine
	Cocaine
	Yohimbine
349	Nomifensine
350	Aspirin
	Salicylic Acid
352	Prazosin
353	Bambuterol
	Cyclopentolate
	Isoxsuprine
	Sulfametopyrazine
354	Alcuronium Chloride
	Clindamycin
	Fencamfamin
	Oxprenolol
355	Carbamazepine M (10,11-di-OH-)
	Pentoxifylline
	Pipradrol
356	Chlorphenamine
	Levallorphan
	Strophanthin-K
357	Aprobarbital
	Mazindol
	Piperocaine
358	Bisoprolol
359	Carbinoxamine
	Ethoheptazine
	Granisetron
360	Benzoic Acid
	Narceine
361	Astemizole M(nor)
	Dibenzepin
362	Lysergide
363	Alphaprodine
	Chlordiazepoxide
	Encainide
	Papaverine
364	Mephenesin
	Remoxipride M(NCM-001)
	Sulfadoxine
365	Bromisoval
	Labetalol
366	Bupivacaine
	Crotetamide
	Tenoxicam
367	Chlortalidone
368	Busulfan
	Clozapine
	Diazoxide
	Noscapine
	Phentolamine
369	Buspirone
370	Buphenine
	Doxorubicin
	Prolintane
371	Brallobarbital
	Fenfluramine
372	Glafenine
	Pentazocine
373	Fentanyl
	Ketotifen
	Pirenzepine M (desamide)
375	Phencyclidine
377	Clopamide
	Dextrorphan
	Opipramol
	Phenacetin
	Piritramide
	Propranolol
	Secbutabarbital
378	Alfentanil
	Trazodone
379	Clidinium Bromide
	Epirubicin
	Ibomal
	Isopropamide Iodide
	Metipranolol
	Phenobarbital
	Proguanil
	Vinbarbital
380	Benzoctamine
381	Tertatolol
382	Benactyzine
	Colchicine
383	Antazoline
	Astemizole
384	Butobarbital
	Cyclobarbital
385	Droperidol
	Pipazetate
386	Betaxolol
	Trimetaphan Camsilate
387	Chlorphenesin Carbamate
	Flumazenil
388	Loprazolam
	Prothipendyl
	Triprolidine
389	Tetracaine
390	Butetamate
	Chloramphenicol
	Isothipendyl
391	Cyclopentobarbital
	Mianserin
392	Butacaine
	Isocarboxazid
393	Benperidol
	Diphenhydramine
	Dipyridamole
	Metaclazepam M(dinor)
394	Butalbital
395	Clomethiazole
396	Apronal
	Oxcarbazepine
	Phenoxybenzamine
397	Bromazepam
	Buprenorphine
	Chlorzoxazone
	Flurazepam
	Phenindamine
398	Amoxapine
	Chlorhexidine
399	Midazolam
401	Diphenylpyraline
	Prednisolone
402	Oxypertine
403	Citalopram
	Doxazosin
	Hydrocortisone
	Perazine
	Talbutal
404	Benzocaine
	Doxepin
405	Cyclizine
	Medazepam
	Oxybuprocaine
406	Procyclidine
407	Loxapine
	Promazine
409	Phenazocine
	Promethazine
410	Carbromal
	Idarubicin
	Pericyazine
411	Dihydroergotamine
	Mebhydrolin
413	Xylometazoline
415	Phenyltoloxamine
	Pramocaine
416	Demoxepam
	Ergotamine
	Heptabarb
417	Bromhexine
	Nealbarbital
418	Carbamazepine
	Methanthelinium Bromide
	Orphenadrine
	Protriptyline
419	Carfenazine
	Clenbuterol (M#3)
	Flecainide
	Hexobarbital
420	Alimemazine
	Cilazapril
	Clemizole
	Emepronium Bromide
421	Haloperidol
	Sulforidazine
422	Adiphenine
	Denatonium Benzoate
423	Fluanisone
424	Amobarbital
	Desipramine
	Metomidate
	Oxyphencyclimine
	Oxyphenonium Bromide
	Pentobarbital
	Vinylbital
425	Lorcainide
	Metaclazepam M(nor)
426	Methylprednisolone
	Paroxetine
427	Aminopromazine
	Thioproperazine
428	Amlodipine
	Dosulepin
	Perphenazine
429	Acecarbromal
	Piperidolate
	Trihexyphenidyl
430	Fluvoxamine
431	Cisapride
	Levocabastine
	Phenytoin
	Pipotiazine
	Piroxicam
432	Nifuratel
433	Aprindine
	Sulfasalazine
434	Phenoperidine
435	Furosemide
	Levomepromazine
	Metharbital
	Methylphenobarbital
	Pizotifen
436	Glutethimide
	Phenolphthalein
437	Hydroxyzine
	Imipramine
	Secobarbital
438	Maprotiline
	Mebendazole
	Triamcinolone
439	Ketoconazole
440	Amitriptyline
	Dextromoramide
	Methadone
	Propiomazine

RI	Compound
441	Oxazepam
	Propyphenazone
442	Tiotixene
443	Pecazine
444	Beclometasone
	Bromazine
	Lorazepam
	Profenamine
446	Piroxicam M (5-hydroxy)
447	Verapamil
448	Clopenthixol
	Mebeverine
	Mepyramine
	Nitrazepam
450	Chlorpropamide
	Prochlorperazine
451	Metaclazepam
	Metixene
452	Tolazamide
454	Propantheline Bromide
	Trimipramine
456	Bromocriptine
	Chlorpromazine
457	Epithiazide
	Methoxsalen
459	Chlorprothixene
	Methaqualone
	Mupirocin
	Trifluperidol
460	Sertraline
462	Clomipramine
	Fluphenazine
464	Butaperazine
465	Clonazepam
466	Norpipanone
467	Reserpine
468	Bamipine
470	Alprazolam
	Fluorometholone
	Nordazepam
	Tolmetin
471	Deptropine
472	Temazepam
473	Propyl Hydroxybenzoate
475	Clorazepic Acid
	Etomidate
	Flupentixol
476	Triazolam
477	Pyrrobutamine
	Tolbutamide
478	Glipizide
480	Methyl Salicylate

RI	Compound
	Thialbarbital
	Trifluoperazine
482	Mecloqualone
483	Flunitrazepam
	Thiopropazate
484	Brotizolam
	Tiaprofenic Acid
	Triflupromazine
485	Thiopental
487	Lormetazepam
	Thiethylperazine
488	Clobazam
	Sulindac
	Xipamide
490	Thioridazine
495	Ketoprofen
496	Rescinnamine
499	Xanthanoic Acid
500	Dipipanone
501	Clemastine
	Naproxen
	Oxyphenbutazone
503	Methohexital
504	Pimozide
508	Bendroflumethiazide
	Diflunisal
510	Loperamide
511	Tetrazepam
513	Bezafibrate
516	Thiamylal
520	Fenbufen
521	Etacrynic Acid
523	Loratadine
526	Econazole
	Probenecid
527	Nifedipine
528	Diazepam
530	Lidoflazine
531	Bisacodyl
534	Testosterone
536	Gliclazide
	Norethisterone
538	Fluspirilene
539	Ethinylestradiol
544	Estrone
546	Warfarin
549	Etynodiol Diacetate
560	Cinnarizine
561	Captodiame
563	Acenocoumarol
564	Bezitramide
574	Fenoprofen

RI	Compound
577	Ketazolam
579	Hexylresorcinol
585	Flurbiprofen
587	Meclozine
592	Diethylstilbestrol
	Spironolactone
595	Niflumic Acid
599	Dicoumarol
607	Indometacin
616	Diclofenac
	Ibuprofen
	Phenprocoumon
618	Desbutylhalofantrine
	Dimpylate
	Hexestrol
625	Nitrendipine
632	Isradipine
637	Glibenclamide
648	Prazepam
653	Meclofenamic Acid
659	Penfluridol
661	Mefenamic Acid
663	Pentaerithrityl Tetranitrate
665	Phenothiazine
668	Nimodipine
671	Flufenamic Acid
672	Phenylbutazone
	Progesterone
683	Amiodarone
690	Felodipine
	Nisoldipine
	Tolfenamic Acid
693	Stanozolol
723	Niclosamide
725	Itraconazole
741	Disulfiram
800	Halofantrine
809	Metenolone
814	Simvastatin
860	Benzbromarone
896	Estradiol
900	Lacidipine
	Methoxychlor
936	Hexachlorophene
939	Isotretinoin
990	Cannabidiol
1017	Chlordane
1054	Hydroxyprogesterone
1072	Heptachlor
1080	Cannabinol

System HY—retention index

RI	Compound
21	Noradrenaline
	Thiamine (hydrochloride)
52	Ascorbic Acid
66	*m*-Aminobenzoic Acid
77	Tyramine
79	Phenylephrine
86	Sulfanilamide
92	Pholcodine
	Sulfaguanidine
95	Suprofen
96	Fluorouracil
128	Allopurinol
131	Orciprenaline
132	Hydralazine
133	Normorphine

RI	Compound
142	Etilefrine
156	Dihydromorphine
158	Pilocarpine
160	Procainamide
166	Hydroxyamfetamine
175	Ranitidine
176	Acetylcysteine
178	Nizatidine
179	Tolazoline
181	Bufotenine
182	Dimenhydrinate
	Morphine
184	Oxymorphone
185	Psilocybine
187	Hydromorphone

RI	Compound
190	Amiloride
	Carbidopa
	Tryptamine
191	Famotidine
192	Diethylcarbamazine
194	Atenolol
	Clonidine
	Dipyrone
196	Tranylcypromine
197	Methapyrilene
201	Phenylpropanolamine
	Theobromine
203	Pargyline
204	Aminophenazone
206	Pheniramine

RI	*Compound*
208	Dihydrocodeine
	Tocainide
209	Cinchonine
211	Resorcinol
212	*p*-Aminobenzoic acid
214	Cinchonidine
216	Metamfetamine
218	Phendimetrazine
222	Tetramisole
223	Homatropine
225	Procaine
226	Acetazolamide
	Amoxicillin
	Cimetidine
	Fenproporex
	Metronidazole
	Psilocin
227	Diprophylline
	Ephedrine
228	Dimethyltryptamine
	Methoxamine
	Methoxyamfetamine
230	Diethylpropion
	Pseudoephedrine
231	Hydrocodone
232	Trimethoxyamfetamine (3,4,5-TMA)
234	Saccharin
	Sulfadiazine
	Tiabendazole
235	*o*-Aminobenzoic acid
	Norcodeine
	Sulpiride
236	Benzoylecgonine
	Lysergic Acid
237	Codeine
	Nalorphine
238	Levamisole
	Naloxone
	Salbutamol
239	Chlorothiazide
	Nikethamide
240	Minocycline
	Physostigmine
241	Paracetamol
	Phenmetrazine
	Pipamperone
	Sulfacetamide
242	Hexobarbital
	Sulfapyridine
243	Mescaline
244	Ethylmorphine
245	Debrisoquine
	Ketobemidone
	Phentermine
	Quinidine
246	Chloroquine
	Fenoterol
	Isoniazid
	Mephentermine
	Oxycodone
	Quinine
247	Sulfamerazine
248	Methylenedioxyamfetamine
249	Nadolol
	Theophylline
250	Ampicillin
	Chloroprocaine
	Lisinopril
	Timolol
251	Atropine
252	Methylenedioxymethamfetamine
253	Hyoscine
	Pindolol
254	Trimethoprim
255	Hydrochlorothiazide
256	Apomorphine
257	Mepyramine
	Strychnine
	Sulfadimidine
	Tubocurarine Chloride
258	Barbital
	Lidocaine
259	Caffeine
	Doxylamine
260	Ciprofloxacin
	Mepivacaine
	Ofloxacin
	Oxytetracycline Dihydrate
262	Guaifenesin
	Ketamine
263	Metoclopramide
	Naphazoline
	Triamterene
264	Chlorphenamine
265	Levorphanol
	Methazolamide
	Tetracycline
	Tripelennamine
266	Phenacemide
267	Brompheniramine
	Brucine
	Tramadol
269	Meptazinol
	Proxymetacaine
	Zopiclone
270	Triprolidine
	Zimeldine
271	Harmine
	Pemoline
272	Lamotrigine
	Metoprolol
273	Demeclocycline
	Viloxazine
274	Pentoxifylline
275	Bretylium Tosilate
	Sultiame
276	Diethyltryptamine
	Ergocalciferol
	Ethosuximide
	Glafenine
	Primaquine
	Thebaine
277	Ajmaline
	Fenetylline
	Methylphenidate
278	Mexiletine
279	Yohimbine
280	Butanilicaine
	Chlortetracycline
	Hydrastine
281	Acetanilide
	Disopyramide
	Pethidine
282	Clenbuterol
	Diamorphine
283	Captopril
284	Clozapine
	Oxprenolol
285	Chlordiazepoxide
	Phencyclidine
286	Astemizole
	Mazindol
287	Cyclopentolate
288	Dimetindene
	Nitrofurantoin
	Pentazocine
	Primidone
289	Cocaine
	Cyclazocine
	Dimethoate
	Fluconazole
	Noscapine
	Pyrimethamine
	Salicylamide
290	Labetalol
	Tilidate
291	Clindamycin
	Doxycycline
	Levallorphan
	Zolpidem
292	Clomethiazole
	Etorphine
294	Antazoline
	Hyoscine Butylbromide
	Morazone
295	Papaverine
296	Nomifensine
297	Methocarbamol
298	Dapsone
	Dextrorphan
	Trimethoxyamfetamine (2,4,6-TMA)
299	Diazoxide
	Fentanyl
	Mepacrine
	Phenazocine
	Phenazone
	Propranolol
300	Butorphanol
	Dibenzepin
301	Betaxolol
	Diprenorphine
	Isoxsuprine
302	Methyprylon
303	Etenzamide
305	Chlorhexidine
	Flunitrazepam
	Flurazepam
	Thioproperazine
	Trazodone
306	Midazolam
	Trifluperidol
307	Bromisoval
308	Chlortalidone
309	Fencamfamin
310	Bupivacaine
	Buspirone
	Clopamide
312	Doxapram
	Piperocaine
	Triamcinolone
313	Nefopam
314	Phenazopyridine
315	Fenfluramine
	Ketotifen
316	Doxepin
	Haloperidol
317	Alphaprodine
	Cisapride
318	Aspirin
319	Aprobarbital
320	Sulfamethoxazole
321	Carbutamide
	Ibogaine
	Tetracaine
322	Benzoctamine
	Mebendazole
	Mephenesin
323	Alprenolol
	Droperidol
	Orphenadrine
	Prochlorperazine
324	Benperidol

RI	*Compound*
	Metharbital
	Promethazine
326	Hydroxyzine
	Promazine
327	Benzoic Acid
	Berberine
	Colchicine
	Flumazenil
330	Noxiptiline
331	Bromazepam
	Butacaine
	Secbutabarbital
333	Sulfafurazole
334	Bromhexine
	Chlormezanone
	Medazepam
335	Dipyridamole
	Imipramine
	Phenacetin
	Phenobarbital
336	Brallobarbital
	Carbamazepine M (epoxide)
	Chloramphenicol
	Diphenhydramine
	Loxapine
337	Mesoridazine
	Paroxetine
338	Nortriptyline
	Profenamine
339	Buprenorphine
340	Chlorcyclizine
	Opipramol
	Prajmalium Bitartrate
	Prednisone
341	Demoxepam
	Trichlormethiazide
342	Butalbital
	Mianserin
343	Methadone
	Piritramide
344	Trifluoperazine
345	Clonixin
	Trimipramine
346	Chlorphenoxamine
347	Digoxin
	Dyclonine
	Phensuximide
348	Chlorphenesin Carbamate
	Clotiapine
349	Fluanisone
	Hydrocortisone
350	Acepromazine
	Chlorpromazine
351	Reserpine
352	Cyclobarbital
	Cyclopentobarbital
	Ibomal
	Sulfadimethoxine
353	Chlorprothixene
	Demeton-*S*
	Isocarboxazid
354	Cyproheptadine
355	Butobarbital
	Flecainide
	Salicylic Acid
	Vinblastine
356	Pericyazine
357	Idobutal
358	Benzocaine
359	Propiomazine
361	Desipramine
	Diltiazem
	Prednisolone
362	Loratadine
	Protriptyline
363	Dipipanone
	Fluvoxamine
	Vinbarbital
364	Methyclothiazide
366	Mephenytoin
	Normethadone
367	Dosulepin
368	Carbamazepine
369	Butriptyline
370	Fenbendazole
	Nitrazepam
	Propyphenazone
	Talbutal
371	Cinchocaine
	Metolazone
	Perazine
372	Cortisone
	Nordazepam
374	Acecarbromal
	Amobarbital
	Dextropropoxyphene
	Tiotixene
375	Amitriptyline
376	Benzylpenicillin
377	Carbromal
	Heptabarb
378	Cyclobenzaprine
379	Alprazolam
380	Furosemide
	Nalidixic Acid
381	Dexamethasone
	Levomepromazine
	Phenytoin
	Trihexyphenidyl
382	Nealbarbital
	Pecazine
	Piroxicam
383	Pentobarbital
385	Diphenoxylate
	Econazole
386	Verapamil
387	Mesuximide
388	Clorazepic Acid
389	Maprotiline
390	Dextromoramide
	Methylprednisolone
	Oxazepam
	Triazolam
391	Clorexolone
394	Enallylpropymal
395	Methylphenobarbital
	Perphenazine
396	Isosorbide Dinitrate
398	Meclozine
400	Fluoxetine
	Lorazepam
	Methaqualone
401	Atrazine
	Glutethimide
402	Carbaryl
403	Clonazepam
405	Clomipramine
406	Butaperazine
	Indoprofen
407	Rescinnamine
	Secobarbital
409	Naftidrofuryl Oxalate
411	Chlorpropamide
	Clopenthixol
	Monolinuron
413	Cyclomethycaine
414	Flunixin
415	Benzthiazide
417	Diuron
	Etomidate
	Mefruside
	Rifampicin
423	Glipizide
424	Tolbutamide
427	Fluoxymesterone
	Thioridazine
428	Paraoxon
429	Diazepam
430	Eugenol
431	Bisacodyl
433	Cyclothiazide
	Thiopental
434	Tolmetin
435	Flupentixol
438	Acetohexamide
	Temazepam
442	Terbutryne
445	Tolazamide
449	Methyl Salicylate
451	Hexethal
452	Tiaprofenic Acid
453	Cyclopenthiazide
454	Buclizine
	Triflupromazine
455	Chlorocresol
	Clobazam
456	Estradiol
458	Propyl Hydroxybenzoate
459	Oxyphenbutazone
461	Fenbufen
462	Sulindac
463	Lormetazepam
464	Ketoconazole
	Nifedipine
468	Digitoxin
	Naproxen
469	Flucloxacillin
471	Fluphenazine
474	Sulfinpyrazone
476	Amiodarone
	Thiamylal
483	Butyl Aminobenzoate
	Gliclazide
	Tetrazepam
484	Methohexital
488	Griseofulvin
491	Fluocinolone
495	Zomepirac
497	Etacrynic Acid
499	Glyceryl Trinitrate
500	Diloxanide
506	Camazepam
	Domiphen
	Linuron
507	Probenecid
508	Testosterone
511	Chloroxylenol
513	Azinphos-methyl
514	Warfarin
521	Estrone
522	Ketazolam
524	Fenoprofen
528	Hexylresorcinol
530	Niflumic Acid
535	Dienestrol
539	Spironolactone
544	Thymol
554	Nitrendipine
558	Naphthalene
559	Diethylstilbestrol
562	Metolachlor
570	Prazepam

RI	*Compound*
571	Glibenclamide
575	Dicycloverine
583	Diflunisal
584	Betamethasone Valerate
	Nimodipine
587	Methyltestosterone
590	Indometacin
591	Dichlorophen
592	Diclofenac
598	Coumatetralyl
	Ibuprofen
603	Dantron
628	Dimpylate
636	Clobetasol Propionate
637	Phenothiazine
643	Phenylbutazone
656	Penfluridol
667	Flufenamic Acid
	Gliquidone
676	Norethisterone
680	9-carboxy-11-nor-9-tetrahydro-cannabinol
686	Mefenamic Acid
690	Meclofenamic Acid
691	Disulfoton
698	Progesterone
703	Dithranol
711	Beclometasone Dipropionate
	Danazol
734	Disulfiram
738	Trichlorfon
766	Quazepam
824	Carbenoxolone
867	Tolnaftate
894	Testosterone Acetate
902	Cannabidiol
1003	Testosterone propionate
1028	Cannabinol

System HZ—retention time (min)

RT	*Compound*
1.4	Dipyrone
	Methyldopa
1.5	Aminosalicylic Acid
	Ascorbic Acid
	Enalapril
	Flucytosine
	Folic Acid
	Lisinopril
1.55	Allopurinol
1.6	Acetylcysteine
	Isoniazid
	Perindopril
	Theobromine
1.7	Atenolol
	Benzoylecgonine
	Cilazaprilat
	Dopamine
	Metformin
	Theophylline
1.8	*N*-Acetylprocainamide
	Cimetidine
	Ciprofloxacin
	Famotidine
	Morphine
	Olanzapine
	Pyridostigmine Bromide
	Ranitidine
	Zolmitriptan
1.9	*N*[4]-Acetylsulfapyridine
	Acetazolamide
	Caffeine
	Carbamazepine M (epoxide)
	Codeine
	Hydralazine
	Hydroxychloroquine
	Paracetamol
	Procainamide
	Sulfasalazine
2.0	Azapropazone
	Baclofen
	Dihydrocodeine
	Naloxone
	Ofloxacin
	Sotalol
	Sulpiride
	Tranylcypromine
2.1	Aminophenazone
	Captopril
	Chloroquine
	Chlorothiazide
	Colchicine
	Ephedrine
	Methylenedioxyamfetamine
	Methylergometrine
	Naratriptan
	Pentoxifylline
	Phenazone
	Primidone
	Timolol
	Tocainide
	Trandolaprilat
	Trimethoprim
2.2	Atropine
	Barbital
	O-Desmethylvenlafaxine
	Hydrochlorothiazide
	Methylenedioxymethamfetamine
	Nicorandil
	Oxcarbazepine M (10-OH-)
	Physostigmine
	Strychnine
	Sulfapyridine
	Terazosin
2.3	Chlortalidone
	Desmethylmirtazapine
	Ethosuximide
	Glafenine
	Lamotrigine
	Rivastigmine
	Sulfamethizole
	Tizanidine
	Triamterene
	Zopiclone
2.4	Alfuzosin
	Dimethyl-methyl-succinimide
	Ketamine
	Meprobamate
	Metamfetamine
	Methysergide
	Minoxidil
	Moclobemide
	Nitrofurantoin
	Phentermine
	Pindolol
2.5	Aminoglutethimide
	Celiprolol
	Clonidine
	Metoprolol
	Prazosin
	Prednisolone
2.6	Crotetamide
	Dapsone
	Flumazenil
	Lidocaine
	Mepivacaine
	Metoclopramide
	Prednisone
	Quinidine
	Quinine
	Yohimbine
2.7	Allobarbital
	Aspirin
	Pipamperone
	Prilocaine
2.8	Aprobarbital
	Diethylpropion
	Dimethoate
	Hydroquinine
	9-Hydroxy-risperidone
	Mirtazapine
	Omeprazole
2.9	Bromisoval
	Ondansetron
	Oxcarbazepine
	Sulfamethoxazole
	Tramadol
3.0	Benzoic Acid
	Brallobarbital
	Bromazepam
	Dipyridamole
	Disopyramide
	Labetalol
	Oxprenolol
	Phenobarbital
	Phentolamine
	Remoxipride
3.1	Bisoprolol
	Demoxepam
	Risperidone
	Venlafaxine
3.2	Butobarbital
	Chlordiazepoxide
	Cyclobarbital
	Cyclopentolate
	Doxapram
	Methyl Hydroxybenzoate
	Pethidine
	Zolpidem
3.3	Cocaine
	Cropropamide
	Trazodone
3.4	Butalbital
	Dexamethasone
	Dihydroergotamine
	Ergotamine
	Mesoridazine
3.5	Buspirone
	Chlorphenamine
	Droperidol
	Furosemide
	Metipranolol
3.6	Aldicarb

RT	Compound
	Benperidol
	Cetirizine
	Mazindol
3.7	Desmethylcitalopram
	Mephenytoin
	Paraoxon
	Phenytoin
	Propranolol
3.8	Betaxolol
	Oxazepam
	Pentazocine
	Proguanil
3.9	Alprenolol
	Astemizole
	Carbromal
	Clozapine
	Fenfluramine
	Heptabarb
	Opipramol
	Sulindac
4.0	Alprazolam
	Amobarbital
	Dantrolene
4.1	Bupivacaine
	Ketorolac
	Lorazepam
	Pentobarbital
	Vinylbital
4.2	Bevantolol
	Flurazepam
	Midazolam
	Nitrazepam
	Phenolphthalein
	Ramipril
	Triazolam
4.3	Benzocaine
	Hexobarbital
4.4	Desmethylcarvedilol
	Floctafenine
	Pericyazine
	Tetrabenazine
	Tetracaine
4.5	Cilazapril
	Citalopram
	Diltiazem
	Glipizide
4.6	Brotizolam
	Clonazepam
	Doxepin M (nor-)
	Methylphenobarbital
	Mianserin
4.7	Propyphenazone
	Secobarbital
	Sulfinpyrazone
4.8	Cyclizine
	Glutethimide
	Mesuximide
	Sulforidazine
4.9	Amlodipine
	Piroxicam
5.0	Buprenorphine
	Chlorpropamide
	Doxepin
5.2	Carvedilol
	Cisapride
	Flecainide
	Ketoconazole
	Methoxsalen
5.3	Mebhydrolin
	Tofenacin
5.4	Diflunisal
	Malathion
	Medazepam
	Methaqualone
	Pergolide
	Quinapril
	Tolmetin
5.5	Temazepam
5.6	Clorazepic Acid
	Flunitrazepam
	Fluvoxamine
	Paroxetine
5.7	Bromocriptine
	Dosulepin
	Hydroxyzine
	Promethazine
5.8	Diuron
	Haloperidol
	Tiaprofenic Acid
5.9	Desipramine
	Promazine
	Tolbutamide
6.0	Orphenadrine
6.1	Trandolapril
6.2	Clobazam
	Lormetazepam
	Procyclidine
6.3	Perazine
6.4	Biperiden
	Ketoprofen
	Thiazinamium Metilsulfate
6.5	Cyproheptadine
	Parathion
	Pramocaine
6.6	Lorcainide
	Maprotiline
	Nortriptyline
	Pizotifen
	Verapamil M (nor-)
6.7	Desmethylfluoxetine
	Imipramine
	Oxyphenbutazone
6.8	Meloxicam
	Naproxen
	Tiotixene
	Tolazamide
6.9	Thiopental
7.0	Desmethylsertraline
	Verapamil
7.1	Mebeverine
7.2	Nifedipine
	Perphenazine
	Sulindac
7.5	Amitriptyline
	Bromhexine
	Levomepromazine
7.6	Dextropropoxyphene
	Fluoxetine
	Trihexyphenidyl
7.7	Nefazodone
7.8	Probenecid
8.0	Valproic Acid
	Zuclopenthixol
8.2	Sertraline
8.3	Trimipramine
8.4	Diazepam
8.5	Methadone
8.8	Gliclazide
9.1	Acenocoumarol
	Chlorpromazine
9.4	Warfarin
9.5	Spironolactone
9.6	Bisacodyl
	Camazepam
9.8	Sertindole
10.1	Chlorprothixene
	Fluphenazine
10.2	Clomipramine
10.3	Deptropine
	Ketazolam
10.4	Prochlorperazine
10.7	Aceclofenac
	Flupentixol
10.9	Fenoprofen
11.8	Flurbiprofen
11.9	Pimozide
12.3	Triflupromazine
12.6	Phenprocoumon
13.2	Trifluoperazine
13.5	Thioridazine
13.6	Nabumetone
14.0	Clemastine
	Loperamide
14.2	Betamethasone
14.4	Glibenclamide
	Indometacin
14.6	Loratadine
14.8	Diclofenac
14.9	Isradipine
15.4	Thioproperazine
16.3	Thiethylperazine
16.5	Ibuprofen
17.6	Prazepam
17.7	Nimodipine
19.5	Phenylbutazone
22.0	Cinnarizine
22.5	Bezitramide
25.8	Felodipine
27.4	Diphenoxylate
33.2	Dimpylate
35.0	Propofol
35.5	Parathion
37.5	Quazepam
37.9	Tolfenamic Acid
43.4	Penfluridol
90.4	Amiodarone

System HAA—retention time (min)

RT	Compound
2.7	Adenosine
	Pholcodine
2.8	Metformin
	Noradrenaline
2.9	Pralidoxime Chloride
	Pyridoxine
3.0	Acamprosate Calcium
	Methyldopa
	Pancuronium Bromide
3.1	Aciclovir
	Amoxicillin
	Arecoline
	Flucytosine
3.2	Betahistine
	Nicotinic Acid

RT	*Compound*
	Pyridostigmine Bromide
3.3	Morphine
	Nizatidine
3.4	Enalapril
	Fluorouracil
3.5	Famotidine
3.6	Amiloride
	Atenolol
	Cimetidine
	Diprophylline
	Folic Acid
	Levodopa
3.7	Amfetamine
	Ranitidine
	Terbutaline
3.8	Ampicillin
	Cyanocobalamin
	Pyrazinamide
	Sotalol
	Sulfaguanidine
	Theobromine
3.9	Cefalexin
	Sulpiride
4.6	Pilocarpine
4.7	Dihydrocodeine
4.8	Cefixime
	Nalorphine
4.9	Theophylline
5.0	Codeine
	Coumatetralyl
5.2	Procaine
5.3	Ceftriaxone
5.4	Chloroquine
5.6	Paracetamol
5.7	Ephedrine
5.9	Bamethan
	Carteolol
	Saccharin
6.1	Clonidine
	Trimetazidine
6.7	Caffeine
6.8	Metronidazole
	Nadolol
6.9	Acetazolamide
7.0	Diaveridine
	Levamisole
	Tetramisole
7.1	Amisulpride metabolite-1
7.2	Dropropizine
7.3	6-Monoacetylmorphine
7.4	Hyoscine
8.0	Resorcinol
8.1	Methylenedioxyamfetamine
8.3	Trimethoprim
8.4	Metamfetamine
	Sulfadiazine
	Vinblastine
8.6	Ofloxacin
	Pindolol
8.7	Triamterene
8.9	Amisulpride
	Furaltadone
9.0	Apomorphine
	Sulfathiazole
9.1	Ciprofloxacin
	Methylenedioxymethamfetamine
9.2	Strychnine
9.4	Emetine
9.6	Ketamine
9.7	Benzoylecgonine
	Captopril
	Hyoscyamine
9.8	Minoxidil
9.9	Lidocaine
	Metoclopramide
	Tetracycline
10.0	Dimetridazole
10.2	Cinchonine
	Moclobemide
10.3	Bamifylline
	Timolol
10.4	Alfuzosin
	Atropine
	Barbital
10.5	Ethosuximide
10.6	Prazosin
	Tinidazole
10.7	Metoprolol
	Selegiline
10.8	Acepromazine
	Clenbuterol
	Cycloguanil
10.9	Amisulpride metabolite-2
	Pipamperone
11.0	Quinidine
	Viloxazine
11.1	Carbimazole
	Doxylamine
	Primidone
11.2	Sulfamethoxypyridazine
11.3	Quinine
11.4	Disopyramide
	Fluconazole
	Guaifenesin
11.5	Celiprolol
	Mexiletine
	Pentoxifylline
	Yohimbine
11.7	Vanillin
11.8	Pethidine
11.9	Cocaine
	Zolpidem
12.0	Clindamycin
	Lysergide
	Oxprenolol
12.1	Doxorubicin
	Papaverine
	Salicylic Acid
12.2	Furazolidone
12.3	Bisoprolol
12.5	Buspirone
	Indoramin
	Pentazocine
	Pyrimethamine
12.6	Dapsone
12.7	Nefopam
	Tenoxicam
	Trazodone
12.8	Carbinoxamine
	Noscapine
12.9	Chlorphenamine
	Melphalan
13.1	Dexamethasone
	Estriol
	Fenfluramine
	Propranolol
	Triprolidine
13.2	Astemizole
	Dipyridamole
13.3	Betamethasone
	Clidinium
	Dextrorphan
	Sulfadoxine
13.4	Betaxolol
	Loprazolam
	Phenol
	Sulfamethoxazole
	Tobramycin
13.5	Chlorhexidine
	Isothipendyl
13.6	Proguanil
	Veratrine
13.7	Perindopril
13.8	Adrafinil
	Mianserin
	Ticlopidine
	Vincristine
13.9	Brompheniramine
	Digoxin
14.0	Amineptine
	Buprenorphine
	Diltiazem
	Gentamicin
	Naloxone
	Phenobarbital
14.1	Chloramphenicol
	Doxepin
	Omeprazole
	Phenothiazine (phenothiazine ring)
	Prednisolone
	Toloxatone
14.2	Amoxapine
	Fentanyl
	Opipramol
	Prednisone
14.3	Phenothiazine (phenothiazine ring 2)
14.4	Cilazapril
	Haloperidol
14.5	Carbutamide
	Promethazine
14.6	Cisapride
	Lobeline
	Loxapine
14.7	Bacampicillin
	Bromazepam
	Pipotiazine
	Sulfadimethoxine
14.8	Biperiden
14.9	Butobarbital
	Desipramine
	Midazolam
	Tianeptine
	Trichlormethiazide
15.0	Benzydamine
	Cyproheptadine
	Nemonapride
15.1	Aldicarb
	Amlodipine
	Imipramine
15.2	Chlordiazepoxide
	Furosemide
	Pizotifen
	Thioproperazine
15.3	Fluvoxamine
	Hydroxyzine
	Paroxetine
	Trihexyphenidyl
15.4	Methyclothiazide
	Verapamil
15.5	Chlormezanone
	Maprotiline
	Nicergoline
15.6	Nortriptyline
15.7	Amphotericin B
	Cetirizine
	Ketoconazole
	Ramipril
	Simazine
15.8	Carbamazepine
	Dextromoramide
	Dextropropoxyphene
	Medazepam

RT	*Compound*
	Methadone
	Naftidrofuryl Oxalate
	Pivampicillin
	Roxithromycin
15.9	Amitriptyline
	Trimipramine
16.0	Chlorpromazine
	Clomethiazole
	Nalidixic Acid
	Perphenazine
16.1	Mebendazole
16.2	Fluoxetine
	Rifampicin
16.3	Phenytoin
	Zuclopenthixol
16.4	Clomipramine
	Reserpine
16.6	Amobarbital
	Lansoprazole
	Piroxicam
	Sulindac
16.6.	Vinylbital
16.7	Bromocriptine
16.8	Quinapril
16.9	Nitrazepam
17.0	Alprazolam
	Aprindine
	Benazepril
	Dimethyl Phthalate
	Trandolapril
17.2	Floctafenine
	Lorazepam
	Pimozide
	Thioridazine
17.4	Clonazepam
	Embutramide
	Flupentixol
	Fluphenazine
	Secobarbital
	Triazolam
17.6	Glipizide

RT	*Compound*
	Rifabutin
	Tiaprofenic Acid
17.7	Chlorpropamide
	Hydrocortisone
	Trifluoperazine
17.8	Altretamine
18.0	Carbaryl
18.1	Phenindione
18.2	Atrazine
	Estradiol
	Parbendazole
18.3	Bezafibrate
	Clofibrate
	Propyl Hydroxybenzoate
18.4	Clorazepic Acid
	Griseofulvin
18.5	Diuron
18.6	Bendroflumethiazide
	Flunitrazepam
	Temazepam
18.7	Digitoxin
18.8	Xipamide
18.9	Methylprednisolone
19.1	Bumetanide
19.2	Clobazam
	Thiopental
19.3	Cinnarizine
	Fenbufen
	Fenproporex
19.5	Benzene
	Nifedipine
19.6	Ketoprofen
20.0	Meclozine
20.1	Acenocoumarol
	Econazole
20.2	Captodiame
	Penfluridol
20.3	Diazepam
20.5	Desbutylhalofantrine
	Gliclazide
20.7	Spironolactone

RT	*Compound*
20.9	Diethylstilbestrol
	Rifamycin SV
21.2	Ciprofibrate
	Droperidol
	Fenoprofen
21.3	Flurbiprofen
	Linuron
21.5	Etodolac
21.6	Trifluperidol
21.7	Indometacin
21.9	Prometryne
	Toluene
22.0	Glibenclamide
	Niflumic Acid
22.1	Diclofenac
	Nitrendipine
22.4	Chlorambucil
	Isradipine
	Tetrazepam
22.6	Minocycline
22.9	Loratadine
23.0	Halofantrine
23.1	Pentaerithrityl
23.3	Naphthalene
23.4	Prazepam
23.8	Ibuprofen
	Progesterone
23.9	Niclosamide
24.0	Norethisterone
	Xylene
24.1	Chlormadinone
	Phenylbutazone
24.4	Felodipine
24.9	Fusidic Acid
25.1	Disulfiram
25.8	Dimpylate
26.1	Benzbromarone
26.4	Cyclandelate
27.2	Lacidipine
27.4	Methoxychlor
27.6	Piperonyl Butoxide

System HAB—retention time (min)

RT	*Compound*
1.0	Abacavir
4.0	Amprenavir
4.2	Indinavir

System HAC—retention time (min)

RT	*Compound*
2.0	Indinavir
2.5	Amprenavir
7.1	Ritonavir
8.0	Nelfinavir
8.5	Efavirenz
9.5	Saquinavir
17.3	Nelfinavir
22.2	Ritonavir
	Saquinavir

System HAD—*k* values

k	*Compound*
2.7	Lamivudine
3.2	Didanosine
3.8	Stavudine
6.6	Zidovudine
8.1	Abacavir
11.1	Nevirapine

System HAE—*k* values

k	*Compound*
6.3	Delavirdine
9.4	Amprenavir
28.6	Efavirenz

System HAF—*k* values

k	*Compound*
5.3	Clonazepam
6.6t	Bromazepam
9.1	Nitrazepam
13.7	Triazolam
15.0	Lorazepam
18.4	Etizolam
21.0	Chlordiazepoxide
29.8	Diazepam
32.2	Flutazolam

System HAK—*k* values

k	*Compound*
4.7	Carbamazepine
6.2	Clonazepam
7.6	Nordazepam
9.3	Clobazam
ND	Phenobarbital
	Phenytoin

System HAL—*k* values

k	*Compound*
1.4	Barbital
1.45	7-acetamidoclonazepam
1.55	7-aminoclonazepam
2.0	Aprobarbital
2.4	Hexobarbital
3.7	Flunitrazepam M (nor)
4.33	Clonazepam
4.4	Oxazepam
4.6	Nitrazepam
5.1	Lorazepam
6.2	Flunitrazepam
6.3	Alprazolam
6.6	Triazolam
7.7	Chlordiazepoxide
7.8	Clobazam
7.9	Nordazepam
8.1	Bromazepam
8.2	Medazepam
13.2	Diazepam

System HAM—*k* values

k	*Compound*
1.8	Theophylline
1.98	Caffeine
2.0	Paracetamol
2.2	Primidone
2.7	Sulfamethoxazole
2.8	Phenobarbital
3.1	Chlordiazepoxide
3.4	Oxazepam
3.5	Phenytoin
4.2	Lorazepam
4.3	Clonazepam
4.5	Nitrazepam
9.0	Imipramine
9.1	Desipramine
10.3	Diazepam
ND	Alprazolam
	Bromazepam
	Clobazam
	Codeine
	Ephedrine
	Levomepromazine
	Lidocaine
	Medazepam
	Nortriptyline
	Propranolol
	Thioridazine
	Triazolam

System HAO—*k* values

See Table 14.1 (Chapter 14) for retention information.

System HAP—*k* values

See Table 14.1 (Chapter 14) for retention information.

System HAR—relative to testosterone

RRT	*Compound*
0.74	Boldenone
0.78	Fluoxymesterone
0.84	Nandrolone
0.86	Methandienone
1.17	Methyltestosterone
1.25	Methandriol
1.76	Testosterone acetate
1.9	Clostebol acetate
2.01	Testosterone propionate
2.17	Testosterone isobutyrate
2.6	Testosterone enantate
2.63	Testosterone cipionate
3.18	Testosterone undecanoate

System HATa—relative to testosterone

RRT	*Compound*
1.31	Testosterone Propionate
1.48	Testosterone Phenylpropionate
1.62	Testosterone Isocaproate
1.8	Testosterone Enantate
1.94	Boldenone Undecylenate
2.05	Testosterone Cipionate
2.53	Testosterone Undecenoate
2.78	Testosterone Decanoate
3.27	Testosterone Undecylate

System HATb—relative to testosterone

RRT	*Compound*
0.7	Fluoxymesterone
0.75	Oxandrolone
0.76	Boldenone
0.84	Ethisterone
0.87	Methandienone
0.92	Nandrolone
1.13	Dehydroepiandrosterone
1.27	Methyltestosterone
1.29	Methandriol
1.52	Mesterolone
1.55	Norethandrolone
2.59	Testosterone Acetate
2.64	Oxymetholone
4.06	Testosterone Propionate

System HAV—*k* values

k	*Compound*
2.2	Celiprolol
2.3	Propranolol
3.6	Diltiazem deacetyldiltiazem
5.1	Desmethyldiltiazem
6.1	Diltiazem
6.4	Imipramine
8.2	Verapamil

System HAX—retention time (min)

RT	*Compound*
4.1	Methyldopa
4.5	Theophylline
4.7	Methotrexate
4.8	Caffeine
	Paracetamol
4.9	Guaifenesin
5.0	Methocarbamol
	Pentoxifylline
5.1	Colchicine
	Hydrochlorothiazide
5.2	Salicylic Acid
5.3	Atenolol
5.4	Phenazone
5.6	Morphine
	Nizatidine
	Phenobarbital
5.7	Fenoterol
	Metformin
5.8	Bromazepam
	Demoxepam
	Furosemide
	Hydromorphone
5.9	Diflunisal
	Pentobarbital
	Ranitidine
6.0	Chlormezanone
	Dantrolene
	Mephenytoin
	Oxazepam
6.1	Codeine
	Lorazepam
	Phenytoin
6.2	Carbamazepine
	Secobarbital
6.3	Ketorolac
	Nitrazepam
6.4	Alprazolam
	Methoxamine
	Triazolam
6.5	Clonazepam
	Hydralazine
	Oxycodone
6.6	Dobutamine
	Floctafenine
	Glutethimide
6.7	Ethylmorphine
	Nordazepam
	Triamterene
	Trimethoprim
6.8	Homatropine
	Methaqualone
6.9	Chlordiazepoxide
	Hydrocodone
	Methylenedioxyamfetamine
	Moclobemide
7.0	Atropine
	Hyoscine
	Naproxen
7.1	Metoprolol
7.2	Clobazam
7.3	Procaine
7.4	Brotizolam
	Nifedipine
7.5	Strychnine
	Zopiclone
7.7	Diazepam
	Ketazolam
	Mepivacaine
7.8	Clonidine
7.9	Diamorphine
	Metoclopramide
8.0	Fenoprofen
	Flurbiprofen
	Lidocaine
	Warfarin
8.1	Ibuprofen
8.3	Quinine
8.4	Chlorpromazine M (sulfoxide)
8.5	Glibenclamide
	Indometacin
8.6	Dipyridamole
	Droperidol
	Methylphenidate
8.7	Azacyclonol
	Diclofenac
	Doxapram
	Quinidine
8.8	Remoxipride
8.89	Cetirizine
8.9	Temazepam
9.1	Buspirone
	Naphazoline
	Risperidone
9.2	Pethidine
	Propranolol
9.3	Desacetyldiltiazem
9.4	Encainide
9.5	Pheniramine
9.6	Disopyramide
	Hydroxychloroquine
9.9	Pentazocine
10.0	Cocaine
	Fluvoxamine
10.1	Mesoridazine
	Propofol
10.2	Midazolam
	Pericyazine
10.5	Flurazepam
	Prazepam
10.7	Azatadine
10.8	Chlorphenamine
	Tetracaine
10.9	Cisapride
	Clozapine
	Loratadine
11.1	Diltiazem
	Haloperidol

RT	*Compound*
	Paroxetine
11.3	Flavoxate
11.4	Fentanyl
	Hydroxyzine
11.7	Anileridine
11.9	Quazepam
12.1	Difenidol
12.2	Diphenhydramine
	Fluoxetine
12.4	Cyclizine
12.7	Chloroquine
12.9	Doxepin
13.0	Desipramine
13.1	Mefenamic Acid
	Perphenazine
13.2	Promethazine
13.3	Verapamil
13.6	Fluphenazine
13.7	Flupentixol
	Nortriptyline
13.8	Lovastatin
14.1	Propiomazine
14.5	Sertraline
14.7	Imipramine
14.9	Alimemazine
15.1	Diethazine
15.2	Levomepromazine
	Methdilazine
15.3	Pecazine
15.5	Cyclobenzaprine
	Trimipramine
15.8	Amitriptyline
16.5	Methadone
16.6	Profenamine
17.0	Chlorpromazine
17.3	Triflupromazine
17.6	Chlorprothixene
18.3	Fluspirilene
ND	Procyclidine
	Thioridazine

System HAY—retention time (min)

RT	*Compound*
2.8	Methyldopa
2.9	Methotrexate
3.1	Atenolol
	Nizatidine
3.2	Hydroxychloroquine
	Morphine
3.3	Metformin
	Ranitidine
3.4	Codeine
	Fenoterol
	Hydromorphone
3.5	Hydralazine
	Theophylline
3.6	Chloroquine
	Ethylmorphine
	Homatropine
	Methoxamine
3.7	Hydrocodone
	Hyoscine
	Paracetamol
	Trimethoprim
3.8	Atropine
	Caffeine
	Dobutamine
	Methylenedioxyamfetamine
	Zopiclone
3.9	Guaifenesin
	Methocarbamol
	Moclobemide
	Strychnine
	Triamterene
4.0	Hydrochlorothiazide
	Procaine
4.1	Colchicine
	Diamorphine
	Metoprolol
4.2	Mepivacaine
	Pentoxifylline
4.3	Chlorpromazine M (sulfoxide)
	Clonidine
	Metoclopramide
4.4	Salicylic Acid
4.5	Azacyclonol
	Lidocaine
	Oxazepam
	Phenazone
	Pheniramine
	Quinine
4.6	Azatadine
	Desacetyldiltiazem
	Doxapram
	Quinidine
	Remoxipride
	Risperidone
4.7	Droperidol
	Methylphenidate
	Phenobarbital
	Procyclidine
4.8	Dipyridamole
	Naphazoline
	Pethidine
4.9	Disopyramide
	Encainide
	Propranolol
5.0	Buspirone
	Cocaine
	Furosemide
	Mesoridazine
5.1	Bromazepam
	Demoxepam
	Pericyazine
5.2	Clozapine
	Dantrolene
5.29	Cetirizine
5.3	Chlordiazepoxide
	Chlormezanone
	Chlorphenamine
	Phenytoin
5.4	Diltiazem
	Mephenytoin
	Tetracaine
5.5	Carbamazepine
	Flurazepam
	Pentazocine
5.6	Ketorolac
	Pentobarbital
5.8	Cisapride
	Cyclizine
	Floctafenine
	Lorazepam
	Oxycodone
	Paroxetine
5.9	Anileridine
	Fluvoxamine
	Secobarbital
6.0	Clonazepam
	Diflunisal
	Diphenhydramine
	Fentanyl
	Flavoxate
	Nitrazepam
6.1	Difenidol
	Doxepin
6.2	Glutethimide
	Haloperidol
6.3	Desipramine
	Hydroxyzine
	Midazolam
	Perphenazine
6.4	Alprazolam
	Promethazine
6.7	Methdilazine
	Temazepam
	Triazolam
6.8	Imipramine
	Nordazepam
	Nortriptyline
7.0	Pecazine
	Verapamil
7.07	Fluoxetine
7.1	Alimemazine
	Clobazam
	Cyclobenzaprine
	Propiomazine
7.2	Fluphenazine
	Levomepromazine
	Naproxen
7.3	Amitriptyline
7.4	Diethazine
	Methaqualone
7.5	Flupentixol
7.7	Sertraline
	Trimipramine
7.8	Chlorpromazine
7.9	Brotizolam
	Nifedipine
8.3	Chlorprothixene
	Profenamine
	Warfarin
8.4	Methadone
8.8	Diazepam
8.9	Fenoprofen
	Flurbiprofen
	Triflupromazine
9.2	Indometacin
	Ketazolam
9.8	Fluspirilene
	Glibenclamide
	Mefenamic Acid
	Thioridazine
10.0	Diclofenac
10.5	Ibuprofen
12.8	Prazepam
13.3	Loratadine
14.1	Diphenoxylate
14.8	Lovastatin
15.2	Propofol
17.7	Quazepam

System HAZ—*k* values

k	*Compound*
0.02	Sulpiride
0.14	Phenobarbital M (4-OH-)
0.18	Caffeine
0.19	Mianserin M (8-OH-)
0.22	Flunitrazepam M (7-amino)
0.38	Carbamazepine M (epoxide)
0.39	Desipramine M (2-OH-)
	Imipramine M (10-OH-)
	Imipramine M (2-OH-)
	Phenobarbital
0.53	Mianserin M (*N*-oxide)
0.6	Phenytoin
0.62	Chlorpromazine M (sulfoxide)
0.65	Flunitrazepam M (nor-)
0.72	Haloperidol
0.73	Flurazepam
0.79	Clonazepam
0.82	Carbamazepine
0.86	Flunitrazepam
0.88	Mianserin M (nor-)
	Nitrazepam
1.07	Triazolam
1.18	Mianserin
1.23	Oxazepam
1.43	Temazepam
1.44	Maprotiline
1.52	Desipramine
1.62	Imipramine
1.68	Chlordiazepoxide
1.71	Nortriptyline
1.76	Amitriptyline
1.82	Levomepromazine
1.85	Imipramine M (*N*-oxide)
1.88	Nordazepam
2.25	Diazepam
2.64	Chlorpromazine
3.28	Perphenazine
3.88	Thioridazine

System HBK—Retention times relative to 5-(4-Methylphenyl)-5-phenylhydantoin

RRT	*Compound*
0.000	Adenosine 5'-monophosphate
	Capreomycin
	Histamine
	Hydroxocobalamin
	Paraquat
	Vancomycin
0.003	Zanamivir
0.006	Cycloserine
	Fludarabine phosphate
	Thiamine
0.007	Dihydralazine
	Diquat
0.009	Obidoxime
0.010	Benserazide
	Hexoprenaline
	Penciclovir
	Pramipexole
0.013	Betahistine
	Cytarabine
	Ganciclovir
0.016	Amprolium
	Levodopa
	Valacyclovir
0.017	Isoniazid
0.019	Cytisine
	Gemcitabine
	Xantinol
0.020	Aciclovir
0.022	Acetarsol
	Flucytosine
	Hydroxyurea
	Nedocromil
0.023	Carbidopa
	Didanosine
	Pralidoxime
	Zalcitabine
0.024	Guanethidine
0.027	Dopamine
	Folic acid
	Mafenide
	Pyridoxine
0.028	Aztreonam
	Milrinone
	Oxedrine
0.030	Lisinopril
0.031	Famotidine
0.032	Lamivudine
	Normorphine
0.034	Amygdalin
0.035	Adrenalone
	Mitoxantrone
0.036	Diprophylline
	Metanephrine
	Riboflavin
0.038	Methotrexate
0.039	Oxymorphone
0.040	Lincomycin
	6-Mercaptopurine
	Metaraminol
	Phanquinone
0.041	Fluorouracil
0.042	Carbazochrome
	Etamiphyllin
0.044	Etilefrine
	Minocycline
	Salbutamol
	Serotonin
	Terbutaline
0.045	Arecoline
	Buformin (1-Butylbiguanide)
	Cefaclor
	Topotecan
0.046	Distigmine
	Practolol
0.049	Azatadine
0.050	Stavudine
0.051	Idoxuridine
0.053	Diethylcarbamazine
0.054	Hordenine
0.057	Ambazone
	Galantamine
	Nicametate
0.058	Omethoate
0.059	Cinchonidine
0.060	Acetylcysteine
	Procarbazine
	Pyrazinamide
0.061	Acecainide
	Aminophenazone
	Melphalan
0.063	Codeine
	Pholedrine
	Rizatriptan
0.064	Cefalexin
	Methylthiouracil
0.065	Bufotenine
0.066	Moxonidine
	Pipamperone
0.068	Cathinone
0.069	Proxyphylline
0.070	Naloxone
	Pentamidine
0.072	Dropropizine
0.073	Dopexamine
	Nifenazone
	Pilocarpine
0.074	Cefradine
	Zolmitriptan
0.075	Brucine
	Ofloxacin
0.076	Doxylamine
0.078	Fenoterol
0.079	Famciclovir
	Pseudoephedrine
0.080	Ethionamide
0.081	Homatropine
0.083	Amiphenazole
0.084	Oxytetracycline
0.087	Azathioprine
0.088	Oxycodone
	Tropicamide
0.089	Diaveridine
	Nialamide
0.091	Tubocurarine
0.093	Emetine
0.094	Bamethan
	Metyrapone
0.095	Cabergoline
	Trimethoprim
0.096	Deslanoside
0.099	Furaltadone
0.101	Methylergometrine
	Tolazoline
0.102	Tizanidine
0.103	Pentetrazol
	Physostigmine
0.104	Amphetamine
	Hydrastinine
	Lysergic acid
	Psilocin
0.105	Bacitracin
0.110	Procaine
0.111	Bamifylline
	Hyoscyamine
	Spiramycin A
0.112	Ketobemidone
	Zidovudine (AZT)
0.113	Atropine methylbromide
0.115	Rabeprazole
0.118	Thiabendazole
0.119	Aloin
	Rolitetracycline
0.122	Eucatropine
0.124	Irinotecan
0.125	Tetracycline
	Vindesine

RRT	*Compound*
0.127	Etofylline
	Phendimetrazine
0.129	Solanine
0.132	Dobutamine
0.133	Glafenine
0.136	Doxorubicin
0.138	Piritramide
0.142	Azaperone
0.143	Mandelic acid
0.146	Guaifenesin
0.147	Clindamycin
0.149	Clonidine
0.150	Aclarubicin
	Resorcinol
0.151	Methazolamide
0.152	Alfuzosin
	Propylthiouracil
0.154	Debrisoquine
	Fenetylline
0.157	Captopril
	Tetramisole
0.158	Lanatoside C
	Mepivacaine
0.159	Isosorbide mononitrate
0.160	Azapropazone
	Guanoxan
0.164	Demeclocycline
0.165	Sulfamerazine
0.168	Bunitrolol
	Formoterol
	Trimethobenzamide
0.169	Epirubicin
0.171	Mepacrine
0.173	Thenyldiamine
0.174	Dimetridazole
0.177	Rivastigmine
0.178	Mersalyl acid
	Methyl nicotinate
	Thebacon
	Tinidazole
0.181	Felbamate
	Fenproporex
0.182	Digoxin
0.185	Acriflavinium
0.186	Bunazosin
0.188	Alcuronium
	Nalmefene
0.192	Acetylcodeine
0.195	Benzquinamide
	Floctafenine
0.198	Granisetron
	4-Methylthioamphetamine (4-MTA)
	Tropisetron
0.205	Ambenonium
	Carbinoxamine
0.206	Acetyldigitoxin
	Phthalylsulfathiazole
0.209	Nevirapine
0.210	Esmolol
0.214	Dolasetron
0.215	Colchicine
	Doxycycline
0.217	Chlortetracycline
0.219	Aldosterone
0.220	Naphazoline
	Nelfinavir
0.223	Mevinphos, isomer 1
0.224	Pyrantel
0.225	Azlocillin
0.226	Ajmaline
0.227	Tripelennamine
0.228	Imolamine
	Trimetozine
0.230	Chlorphentermine
	Vanillin
0.234	Ondansetron
0.237	Yohimbine
0.238	Phthalylsulfacetamide
0.240	Hexobendine
0.241	Mizolastine
0.246	Enoximone
0.249	Docetaxel
0.253	Butanilicaine
0.255	Pantoprazole
0.256	Xylazine
0.257	Sulfamethoxypyridazine
0.259	Methapyrilene
0.260	Ambutonium
	Cyclopentolate
	Tenoxicam
0.263	Lysergide (LSD)
0.266	Atorvastatin
	Carbenicillin
0.269	Crotetamide
0.270	Benzyl alcohol
	Etamivan
0.272	Acetanilide
	Imidacloprid
	Paclitaxel
0.274	Altretamine
0.279	Narceine
0.281	Methandriol
0.282	Daunorubicin
0.283	Meclofenoxate
0.284	Proxymetacaine
	Remifentanil
0.286	Clopamide
	Finasteride
	Flumazenil
	Fluvastatin
0.288	Morazone
0.292	Thalidomide
	Vincristine
0.294	Pyrimethamine
0.296	Prednisolone
0.297	Imidapril
0.298	Natamycin
0.304	Dimethoate
	Indinavir
	Sulfadoxine
0.308	Androstenedione
0.309	Dapsone
	Loprazolam
0.312	Diclofenamide
	Perazine
	Phenazopyridine
0.314	Etoposide
	Flupirtine
0.316	Thonzylamine
	Tramazoline
0.319	Dienestrol
0.320	Ritonavir
0.323	Modafinil
0.329	Desmetryn
	Fluocinonide
	Metenolone
0.330	Ethoheptazine
0.333	Chlorphenesin
0.339	Toloxatone
0.341	Fluspirilene
	Morantel
	Prenylamine
0.343	Fludrocortisone
0.347	Buspirone
0.348	Pipradrol
0.349	Acemetacin
	Alphaprodine
	Phentolamine
0.350	Ethacridine
0.351	Benoxaprofen
0.352	Phenol
0.354	Lansoprazole
0.357	Cefalotin
0.358	Aceclofenac
0.359	Norethynodrel
0.360	Brallobarbital
0.363	Tirofiban
0.364	Benzoic acid
0.375	Chlorambucil
	Torasemide
0.376	Tamsulosin
0.378	Clemastine
	Pravastatin, diastereomer 1
0.379	Thioproperazine
0.385	Enalapril
0.389	Amsacrine
0.392	Buphenine
0.395	Fencamfamine
0.396	Liothyronine
0.401	Demecarium
0.402	Methyl 4-hydroxybenzoate
0.403	Carbocromen
	Propanidid
0.407	Benperidol
0.408	Fenpipramide
	Prothipendyl
0.409	Carbutamide
	Etidocaine
0.411	Ticlopidine
0.416	Chlorhexidine
	Norethandrolone
0.417	Dichlorophen
	Halcinonide
0.419	Droperidol
0.422	Idarubicin
0.425	Hexaconazole
	Nitrendipine
0.430	Trichloroethylene
0.432	Fenticlor
0.434	Econazole
0.442	Clofedanol
	Isradipine
0.443	Clidinium
	Tertatolol
0.444	Pipazetate
0.447	Sulfaquinoxaline
0.450	Toremifene
0.451	Dydrogesterone
	Methylprednisolone
0.454	Proguanil
0.455	Alprenolol
0.459	Benactyzine
0.460	Isoaminile
0.464	Mebendazole
	Nystatin, isomer 1
0.465	Bezitramide
0.470	Cropropamide
0.473	Donepezil
0.475	Chelidonine
0.476	Astemizole
	Clobetasol 17-propionate
	Nimodipine
0.478	Ibogaine
0.481	Aniracetam
0.482	Trichlormethiazide
0.486	Glycopyrronium
0.488	Desoxycortone acetate
0.489	Etofenamate
0.496	Cinnarizine
	Rotenone
0.499	Oxyphenisatine
0.500	Efavirenz

RRT	Compound
0.502	Malathion
	Metolachlor
0.503	Talbutal
0.507	Aldicarb
0.508	Ambucetamide
0.510	Fluticasone 17-propionate
0.512	Methoprotryne
0.513	Alachlor
	Benzylpenicillin
0.516	m-Cresol
0.521	Triazophos
0.523	Fenitrothion
0.526	Azinphos-ethyl
0.527	Nisoldipine
0.531	Captodiame
0.542	Mycophenolate mofetil
0.543	Carbromal
0.545	Diphenoxylate
	Itraconazole
	Miconazole
0.548	Buclosamide
	4-Hexylresorcinol
0.550	Oxymetazoline
0.553	Naphthalene
0.558	Bufexamac
0.560	Aprindine
0.563	Danazol
0.566	Megestrol acetate
0.568	Butetamate
	Muzolimine
0.569	Chlormadinone acetate
	Prochlorperazine
0.573	Amphotericin B
0.576	Clomifene
0.577	Progesterone
0.579	Antazoline
0.587	Fusidic acid
0.588	Chlorzoxazone
	Inositol nicotinate
0.591	Meclofenamic acid
0.592	Simazine
0.596	Felodipine
	m-Xylene
0.598	Benzaldehyde
0.599	Flumetasone
0.602	Doxazosin
0.603	Dixyrazine
0.617	Hexocyclium
0.618	Dithranol
0.621	Oxymetholone
0.622	Fluoxymesterone
	Loxapine
0.625	Medroxyprogesterone acetate
0.628	Beclometasone dipropionate
0.640	Vinylbital
0.642	Nalidixic acid
0.643	Clopenthixol
0.647	Oxybuprocaine
	Thenalidine
0.648	Acetophenone
0.649	Etomidate
0.650	Quinagolide
	Sulforidazine
0.656	Chlorquinaldol
0.663	Mibefradil
0.664	Benzyl benzoate
	Lovastatin
0.666	Difenidol
	Phenazocine
0.667	Penfluridol
0.671	Clodantoin
0.672	Bacampicillin
	Cantharidin
0.685	Phenoxymethylpenicillin (penicillin V)

RRT	Compound
0.686	Dichlorvos
	Isothipendyl
0.687	Nordazepam
0.689	Ketoconazole
0.695	Parathion (E605)
0.699	Prajmalium
0.706	Propofol
0.710	Fenthion
0.720	Clorazepate
0.726	Clorexolone
	Pyrazophos
0.732	Desonide
0.734	Enoxolone
	Triclocarban
0.735	Butaperazine
0.736	Riluzole
0.748	Nifuratel
0.751	Benzydamine
0.754	Berberine
0.761	Ketorolac
0.766	Cilazapril
0.768	Phenprobamate
0.771	Cinchophen
0.781	Bamipine
0.783	Embutramide
0.787	Dicoumarol
0.795	Carbenoxolone
	Clobetasone butyrate
	Famprofazone
	Propyliodone
0.796	Tetrazepam
0.797	Triclosan
0.802	Noxiptilin
0.804	Indoprofen
0.808	Phenyltoloxamine
0.810	Dimpylate
0.811	Diiodohydroxyquinoline
0.812	Benazepril
0.815	Propyphenazone
0.820	Moexipril
0.825	Trenbolone
0.832	Olsalazine
0.835	Pergolide
0.836	Losartan
0.837	Cyclandelate
0.842	Spirapril
0.845	Fosinopril
0.851	Diphenylpyraline
0.852	Anastrozole
0.855	Fluocortolone
0.861	Dimetotiazine
	Fluanisone
	Santonin
0.862	Oxyphenonium
0.868	Prometryn
0.869	Clemizole
0.881	Sirolimus (rapamycin)
0.886	Terbutryn
0.889	Pheneticillin
0.893	Letrozole
0.894	Simvastatin
0.910	Dequalinium
0.914	Clotiapine
0.923	Benzbromarone
0.943	Pyrethrin I
0.956	Deflazacort
0.959	Thiazinamium
0.960	Brotizolam
0.963	Disulfoton
0.965	Tolpropamine
0.966	Methanthelinium
0.968	Xylometazoline
0.981	Denatonium
0.994	Normethadone

RRT	Compound
0.997	Irbesartan
1.003	Fluorometholone
1.010	Carmustine
1.025	Nitrobenzene
1.029	Vinorelbine
1.030	Clostebol acetate
1.034	Fenbendazole
1.036	Atrazine
1.038	Benzthiazide
1.043	Telmisartan
1.044	Budipine
1.048	Cloxacillin
1.054	Rofecoxib
1.058	Adiphenine
1.059	Acitretin
1.060	Pivampicillin
1.063	Nandrolone
1.065	Bromhexine
1.067	Oxyphencyclimine
1.068	Nortriptyline
1.072	Lobeline
1.073	Methoxychlor
1.092	2,4-Dichlorophenoxyacetic acid (2,4-D)
1.096	Piperonyl butoxide
1.103	Cyclothiazide
1.109	Etisazole
1.114	Propionylpromazine
1.121	Cyclobenzaprine
1.125	Diethazine
1.128	Histapyrrodine
1.133	Pecazine
1.138	Emepronium
1.151	Metaclazepam
1.159	Levocabastine
1.174	Isosorbide dinitrate
1.176	Chlorocresol
1.177	Benzyl nicotinate
1.179	Isoproturon
1.197	Tolnaftate
1.205	Benziodarone
1.213	Menadione
1.230	Diuron
1.238	Fenpiprane
1.242	Cerivastatin
1.252	Nebivolol
1.253	Endosulfan
1.257	Butalamine
1.258	Monolinuron
1.260	Hexachlorophene
1.265	Benzene
1.269	Trandolapril
1.272	Alclofenac
1.281	Dyclonine
1.282	Griseofulvin
	Quinapril
1.290	Salmeterol
1.297	Fexofenadine
1.317	Stanozolol
1.339	Mequitazine
1.355	Atracurium
1.363	Tiagabine
1.375	Testosterone
1.380	Nicergoline
1.385	Albendazole
1.392	Propantheline
1.401	Endrin
1.418	Methyl salicylate
1.427	Chlorpyrifos
1.433	Propicillin
1.457	Ketoprofen
1.461	Digitoxin
1.482	Cyclofenil
1.484	Pipoxolan

RRT	*Compound*
1.485	Meloxicam
1.496	Chlorotrianisene
1.513	Cannabidiol
1.515	Trifluperidol
1.517	Benzethonium
1.539	Methohexital
1.570	Valethamate
1.594	Bopindolol
1.596	Norethisterone
1.614	Crotamiton
1.617	Dieldrin
1.629	4,6-Dinitro-o-cresol (DNOC)
1.643	Chlorphenoxamine
1.644	Oxeladin
1.696	Repaglinide
1.700	Clopidogrel
1.712	Tienilic acid
1.772	Propazine
1.788	Atovaquone
1.820	Chloroxylenol
1.837	Clotrimazole
1.850	Lynestrenol
1.851	17α-Methyltestosterone
1.853	Bezafibrate
	Zomepirac
1.877	Deptropine
1.901	Zotepine
1.908	Pyrethrin II
1.916	Propanil
2.041	Hexachlorobenzene
2.086	Ethisterone
2.088	Terbuthylazine
2.117	Formestane
2.123	Toluene
2.151	Probenecid
2.165	Valsartan
2.192	Heptachlor
2.214	Isotretinoin
2.241	Camazepam
2.483	Glycerol trinitrate
2.486	Padimate
2.563	Saquinavir
2.600	Diflunisal
2.689	Azinphos-methyl
2.805	Rescinnamine
2.896	Glibornuride
2.907	Fenamiphos
2.984	Cyfluthrin, isomer 1
3.041	Niflumic acid
3.114	Leflunomide
3.162	Rifabutin
3.282	Aldrin
3.339	Deltamethrin
3.353	Allylestrenol
3.471	Cetylpyridinium
4.737	Alfacalcidol
5.315	Boldenone undecylenate

Ultraviolet Absorption Maxima

In the following tables no values below 230 nm have been included although some have been recorded in the monographs in Part 2. Details of A(1%, 1 cm) values are given in the monographs in Part 2.
Table A gives the wavelengths of maximum absorption, together with the wavelengths of any subsidiary peaks in the range 230 to 360 nm, for the compounds in **acid** solution. Table B gives the wavelengths of maximum absorption in **alkaline** solution when values in acid solution are not recorded in the monographs in Part 2, or when the values in alkaline solution differ significantly from the values in acid solution. Table C gives the values in **neutral** solution for compounds for which values in acid or alkaline solution are not recorded in the monographs in Part 2, or when the values in neutral solution differ significantly from these in acid or alkaline solution.
For an unknown compound, the wavelength of maximum absorption should be compared with the tables using a tolerance of ±2 nm to give a list of possible compounds; reference may then be made to the monographs in Part 2.

A. In acid solution—wavelengths of maximum absorption from 230 nm

λ max nm	*Compound*	*Subsidiary Peaks nm*
230	Amiphenazole	261
	Amisulpride	285
	Amoxicillin	272
	Aspirin	278
	Benzoic Acid	273
	Bromazine	
	Captopril	360
	Carmustine	
	Chloroprocaine	288
	Chlorprothixene	268, 324
	Chlorpyrifos	289
	Clobazam	289
	Dehydroemetine	283
	Dichloralphenazone	
	Diprenorphine	286
	Dipyridamole	285
	Docetaxel	275, 283
	Donepezil	271, 316
	Dosulepin	303
	Emetine	282
	Ethionamide	275
	Flupentixol	
	Gliclazide	
	Methysergide	322
	Minoxidil	281
	Nabumetone	261, 270, 333
	Phenazone	
	Stanozolol	
	Vanillin	204, 278, 309
231	Aloxiprin	
	Amicarbalide	256
	Aztreonam	260
	Benperidol	249, 279
	Camazepam	313
	Celiprolol	324
	Chlortetracycline	266, 342, 371
	Clopenthixol	269, 325
	Lormetazepam	311
	Lovastatin	238, 247
	Piperocaine	274
	Pseudomorphine	
	Rifampicin	263, 336
	Ticlopidine	268, 275
	Trimetazidine	269
232	Bunitrolol	292
	Chlorcyclizine	
	Chlorpropamide	
	Cytisine	302
	Diperodon	
	Etisazole	323
	Hexylcaine	275
	Hydroxyzine	258, 263, 270
	Meprylcaine	
	Pericyazine	268
	Procarbazine	
233	Cocaine	275
	Doxorubicin	253, 290
	Floctafenine	348
	Homochlorcyclizine	258, 263, 270
	Methylenedioxyamfetamine	285
	Paroxetine	264, 270, 293
	Spiramycin	
234	Acebutolol	320
	Aconitine	275
	Aminosalicylic Acid	300
	Benzoylecgonine	274
	Etenzamide	293
	Heteronium Bromide	
	Mebendazole	288
	Methaqualone	269
	Methylenedioxymethamfetamine	285, 285
	Oxazepam	280
	Thenalidine	
	Thioproperazine	263, 312
235	Ambucetamide	
	Cambendazole	319
	Cinchonine	315
	Clomifene	292
	Dimetotiazine	262
	Disulfamide	276, 285
	Fluvastatin	305
	Furosemide	274, 342
	Hydroxychloroquine	256, 329, 343
	Nisoldipine	331
	Oxybuprocaine	298
	Propoxycaine	298
	Rotenone	292
	Salicylamide	298
	Salsalate	310
236	Cinchonidine	316
	Diltiazem	
	Flurazepam	284
	Foscarnet Sodium	
	Nitrendipine	350
	Salicylic Acid	303
	Thonzylamine	274, 316
	Toremifene	
237	Aminitrozole	345

λ max nm	Compound	Subsidiary Peaks nm
	Amodiaquine	343
	Benazepril	
	Benzbromarone	274, 281
	Chloropyrilene	312
	Clorazepic Acid	287
	Felodipine	359
	Fenyramidol	309
	Halazone	
	Methapyrilene	314
	Metolazone	271, 344
	Oxyphenbutazone	
	Phenylbutazone	
	Rifabutin	277, 326
	Risperidone	275
	Sulfinpyrazone	
	Temazepam	284, 358
238	Citalopram	237, 270
	Dropropizine	
	Halcinonide	
	Mesoridazine	262, 310
	Moclobemide	
	Nifedipine	338
	Norbormide	300
	Nordazepam	283, 361
	Penthienate Methobromide	
	Pravastatin	230, 237, 245
	Ritonavir	
	Saquinavir	292
	Thiamylal	287
	Toloxatone	271, 279
239	Acetanilide	
	Amitriptyline	
	Amlodipine	
	Bromazepam	345
	Lacidipine	282, 366
	Mepyramine	316
	Niridazole	
	Nortriptyline	
	Tetrazepam	284, 345
	Thenyldiamine	315
	Tripelennamine	314
240	Altretamine	
	Dihydralazine	274, 306
	Letrozole	273, 281
	Muzolimine	
	Prazepam	285, 360
	Propyphenazone	
	Sulfapyridine	
	Tacrine	323, 336
	Thalidomide	300
241	Amiodarone	
	Antazoline	291
	Carvedilol	285, 320, 332
	Cefaloridine	254
	Dequalinium Chloride	330
	Flavoxate	293, 320
	Mexazolam	290, 373
	Physostigmine Aminoxide	300
	Propiomazine	273, 360
242	Azaperone	312
	Butaperazine	277
	Clenbuterol	295
	Clopamide	
	Diazepam	284, 366
	Homidium Bromide	283
	Mitozantrone	276, 320
	Oleandomycin	
	Phenethylamine	247, 252, 257, 263
	Pralidoxime Chloride	292
	Prothipendyl	
	Spironolactone	
	Sulfadiazine	
	Sulfamerazine	304

λ max nm	Compound	Subsidiary Peaks nm
243	Acepromazine	279
	Acetophenazine	278
	Ascorbic Acid	
	Carfenazine	277
	Cinchophen	268, 344
	Etizolam	250, 294, 362
	Famprofazone	279
	Fluanisone	
	Isotretinoin	359
	Metallibure	
	Methacycline	524, 340
	Methotrexate	307
	Nitroxinil	350
	Piperacetazine	278
	Practolol	
	Propantheline Bromide	281
	Sulfadimidine	301
	Tiabendazole	302
244	Diamfenetide	
	Dofamium Chloride	
	Ethosuximide	
	Menadione	249, 261, 340
	Phenacetin	
245	Ajmaline	289
	Aloin	253, 300
	Bromhexine	310
	Buclosamide	297
	Chlorhexidine	
	Clozapine	297
	Haloperidol	
	Harman	300
	Isothipendyl	
	Paracetamol	
246	Amprolium Hydrochloride	262
	Chlordiazepoxide	308
	Doxazosin	331
	Famciclovir	310
	Irbesartan	
	Lisinopril	253, 258, 264, 267
	Physostigmine	302
	Prajmalium Bitartrate	290
	Terazosin	331, 250, 273
	Thiamine	
	Trazodone	274, 310
	Triphenyltetrazolium Chloride	
247	Acetohexamide	
	Cinchocaine	319
	Cyclofenil	
	Flurbiprofen	
	Gentamicin	
	Harmine	319
	Methoxsalen	304
	Norharman	300
	Phenelzine	252, 257, 263
	Phentermine	251, 257, 263
	Piminodine	253, 257, 263
	Prazosin	331
248	Aminopromazine	297
	Azapetine	
	Boldenone	
	Carbenoxolone	
	Didanosine	246, 250
	Droperidol	276
	Lobeline	
	Ondansetron	266, 310
	Oxetacaine	252, 258, 264
	Pipamperone	
	Probenecid	
	Sulfaquinoxaline	263, 348
	Valsartan	
249	Astemizole	286, 277
	Hydrastinine	306, 363
	Kanamycin	306

λ max nm	*Compound*	*Subsidiary Peaks nm*
	Nefazodone	276
	Nitroxoline	293
	Promethazine	298
	Sulfamoxole	
250	Azapropazone	
	Biriperone	286
	Chlorproguanil	
	Desipramine	
	Diethazine	298
	Histapyrrodine	295
	Hydroquinidine	316, 345
	Hydroquinine	316, 345
	Levomepromazine	302
	Noxiptiline	
	Papaverine	
	Phenmetrazine	256, 261, 263, 267
	Profenamine	299
	Quinidine	317, 345
	Quinine	317, 346
	Triamterene	360, 360
	Trimipramine	
	Zimeldine	
251	Aletamine	257, 263
	Alimemazine	300
	Alphaprodine	257, 263
	Amfetamine	257, 263
	Aminoglutethimide	257
	Bamipine	298
	Benaprizine	257, 261, 264
	Bezitramide	274
	Clomipramine	
	Cycrimine	256, 263
	Diflunisal	315
	Ephedrine	257, 263
	Etafedrine	257, 263
	Ethoheptazine	257, 263
	Exemestane	
	Felbamate	256, 262
	Fentanyl	257, 263
	Hydroxyphenamate	257, 263
	Hydroxyquinoline	308, 318, 356
	Hyoscine	257, 263
	Hyoscine Methonitrate	257, 263
	Imipramine	
	Loxapine	292
	Mandelic Acid	257, 262
	Mebanazine	257, 261, 267
	Mephentermine	257, 263
	Methcathinone	
	Methenamine	257, 263
	Methylephedrine	257, 263
	Methylphenidate	257, 264
	Methylpiperidyl Benzilate	257
	Metindizate	257
	Pargyline	256, 261, 268
	Perazine	300
	Pethidine	257, 263
	Phendimetrazine	257, 261, 267
	Phenformin	258, 264, 267
	Phenglutarimide	257, 263
	Phenylpropanolamine	257, 262
	Pipazetate	
	Procyclidine	257, 263
	Promazine	302
	Pseudoephedrine	257, 263
	Styramate	257, 263
	Thiazinamium Metilsulfate	299
	Tilidate	257, 262
	Tricyclamol Chloride	257, 263
	Tridihexethyl Chloride	257, 263
	Trimeperidine	257, 263
252	Amoxapine	297
	Anileridine	258, 264
	Atropine	258, 264
	Atropine Methonitrate	258, 264
	Bacitracin	
	Beclamide	258, 264
	Benactyzine	258, 262, 264
	Benzfetamine	258, 262, 268
	Benzilonium Bromide	258, 264
	Bethanidine	258, 264
	Biperiden	259, 264
	Caramiphen	259, 265
	Carbetapentane	258, 264
	Carteolol	288
	Cathine	258, 263
	Cyclopentolate	258, 264
	Dextropropoxyphene	257, 263
	Dicycloverine	280
	Difenidol	258
	Diphenhydramine	257
	Eucatropine	258, 264
	Fenbutrazate	257, 261, 267
	Fenproporex	257, 263
	Fenthion	
	Flunixin	327
	Gelsemine	
	Glycopyrronium Bromide	258, 264
	Hexocyclium Metilsulfate	257, 264
	Homatropine	258, 264
	Homatropine Methylbromide	258, 264
	Hyoscine Butylbromide	258, 264
	Hyoscyamine	258, 264
	Isoaminile	258, 264
	Lachesine Chloride	258, 264
	Mepenzolate Bromide	258, 261, 263
	Metaclazepam	
	Metamfetamine	257, 263
	Nelfinavir	
	Oxeladin	258, 264
	Oxyphenonium Bromide	258, 264
	Phencyclidine	258, 263, 270
	Pipenzolate Bromide	258, 262
	Piperidolate	258, 264
	Pipradrol	258
	Poldine Metilsulfate	258
	Prolintane	258, 264
	Ramipril	258
	Selegiline	258, 264
	Thiamazole	
	Trihexyphenidyl	258, 264
	Trimetaphan Camsilate	258, 264
253	Adiphenine	258, 264
	Alverine	259, 264, 268
	Ambutonium Bromide	259, 265
	Azacyclonol	259
	Benzatropine	259
	Bibenzonium Bromide	258, 264, 268
	Butetamate	258, 264
	Clidinium Bromide	259
	Cotarnine	332
	Diethylpropion	
	Diphenylpyraline	258
	Doxapram	259, 265
	Emepronium Bromide	258, 268
	Ethoxzolamide	304
	Fencamfamin	259, 265, 269
	Fenpipramide	259, 265
	Hyoscine Methobromide	258, 264
	Levacetylmethadol	258
	Medazepam	
	Methadone	259, 264, 292
	Methdilazine	302
	Normethadone	259, 265, 292
	Opipramol	338
	Pecazine	300

λ max nm	*Compound*	*Subsidiary Peaks nm*
	Pentapiperide Metilsulfate	258, 265
	Valethamate Bromide	259, 265
254	Celecoxib	
	Cinnarizine	
	Dextromoramide	259, 264
	Dimethoxanate	
	Enoxolone	
	Ethyl Hydroxybenzoate	
	Fluvoxamine	
	Irinotecan	359, 372
	Loperamide	260, 266
	Perphenazine	307
	Prochlorperazine	305
	Strychnine	
	Tropicamide	
255	Aciclovir	
	Alcuronium Chloride	291
	Aniline	261
	Chlorpromazine	239, 274, 300, 341
	Furaltadone	362
	Ganciclovir	
	Methazolamide	290
	Molindone	299
	Niflumic Acid	329
	Pentaerithrityl Tetranitrate	
	Propyl Hydroxybenzoate	
	Thiethylperazine	309
	Thiopropazate	305
	Trifluomeprazine	305
256	Fluphenazine	306
	Harmaline	
	Levobunolol	313
	Mequitazine	307
	Ofloxacin	326
	Oxcarbazepine	306
	Pemoline	262, 268
	Pivampicillin	261, 268
	Pyritidium Bromide	313
	Sulfachlorpyridazine	
	Trifluoperazine	305
	Triflupromazine	305
	Vincristine	297
257	Aminophenazone	
	Ampicillin	262, 268
	Carbarsone	
	Cefradine	
	Chloroquine	329, 343
	Clemastine	
	Cyclizine	262, 268
	Diminazene	
	Enalapril	268
	Nalidixic Acid	315
	Paraquat	
	Salinazid	327
	Tolazoline	263
258	Cefalexin	
	Cetalkonium Chloride	264, 270
	Cetirizine	
	Chlormezanone	265, 272
	Clomethiazole	
	Desmetryne	
	Dipyrone	
	Halofantrine	230, 298
	Halquinol	
	Levocabastine	263, 269
	Morazone	
	Orphenadrine	264
	Succinylsulfathiazole	281
	Tioguanine	348
	Tranylcypromine	264, 271
	Trimethobenzamide	
259	Baclofen	266, 274
	Carbenicillin	265, 327
	Ceftazidime	257, 260
	Chlorphenoxamine	
	Chlorphentermine	267, 274
	Clofedanol	265
	Demecarium Bromide	265
	Dipipanone	265, 293
	Fenpiprane	268
	Indinavir	
	Nicotine	
	Nifuratel	367
	Phenindamine	
260	Alprazolam	
	Aminoacridine	313, 326
	Aprindine	266, 272
	Dimetindene	
	Hexyl Nicotinate	
	Isopropylaminophenazone	
	Ketoprofen	
	Metyrapone	233
	Mexiletine	
	Neostigmine Bromide	266
	Nicotinyl Alcohol	
	Norpipanone	294
	Tiaprofenic Acid	305
	Tolpropamine	265, 273
261	Betahistine	
	Ceftriaxone	
	Cyclomethycaine	
	Dibrompropamidine	
	Doxylamine	
	Ethyl Nicotinate	
	Etoxazene	310
	Fluconazole	266
	Inositol Nicotinate	
	Methyl Benzoquate	
	Nicametate	
	Nicotinamide	
	Nitrofurazone	
	Pheniramine	266
	Quinisocaine	269, 331
262	Acriflavinium Chloride	
	Clorprenaline	266
	Debrisoquine	270
	Diloxanide	
	Etidocaine	271
	Mebeverine	
	Nicofuranose	
	Nifenazone	
	Pentamidine	
	Phenoxybenzamine	268, 274
	Sulfanilamide	269
	Sulfisomidine	
	Thioridazine	310, 230, 263
	Tocainide	270
	Tolmetin	315
	Veratrine	292
	Zomepirac	324
263	Benzethonium Chloride	269, 274
	Bretylium Tosilate	272, 278
	Broxyquinoline	
	Bupivacaine	271
	Carbinoxamine	
	Chlorquinaldol	330
	Denatonium Benzoate	269
	Disopyramide	269
	Itraconazole	
	Lidocaine	272
	Mepivacaine	271
	Tenoxicam	377
264	Benzoctamine	271
	Berberine	345
	Bisacodyl	
	Fenfluramine	271

λ max nm	*Compound*	*Subsidiary Peaks nm*
	Metopimazine	310
	Nikethamide	
	Pindolol	287
	Pramipexole	
	Sorbic Acid	
	Stilbazium Iodide	355
	Sulfadoxine	
	Sulfaguanidine	271
265	Acetazolamide	
	Acetone	
	Alachlor	273
	Brompheniramine	
	Brucine	300
	Butriptyline	
	Cefaclor	
	Chlorphenamine	
	Cladribine	
	Decoquinate	
	Econazole	271, 280
	Famotidine	
	Hexobendine	
	Lamotrigine	267
	Maprotiline	272
	Minocycline	354
	Phanquinone	272, 292
	Primaquine	282, 334
	Sertraline	273, 281
	Sulfafurazole	
	Sulforidazine	311
	Tetryzoline	272
	Xylometazoline	
266	Amineptine	
	Bialamicol	
	Captodiame	
	Carbutamide	
	Chlortetracycline	359
	Coniine	
	Fluorouracil	
	Gallamine Triethiodide	
	Iproniazid	
	Isoniazid	
	Milrinone	327
	Nialamide	
	Psilocin	283, 292
	Stavudine	
	Sulfacarbamide	272
	Zidovudine	
267	Butanilicaine	275
	Ethomoxane	
	Ibutilide	
	Mafenide	274
	Moracizine	
	Nefopam	275
	Penfluridol	273
	Riboflavin	
	Sirolimus	277, 288
	Topotecan	295, 316
	Tramazoline	275
	Xantinol Nicotinate	273
268	Aztreonam	281
	Clomocycline	
	Demeclocycline	
	Diethylthiambutene	288
	Ethacridine	
	Flucloxacillin	274, 344
	Mescaline	
	Metixene	
	Oxytetracycline Dihydrate	352
	Phthalylsulfacetamide	
	Psilocybine	
	Sulfamethizole	
	Thenium Closilate	275
	Vinblastine	
269	Benserazide	
	Deserpidine	
	Doxycycline	346
	Isoxsuprine	274
	Ketamine	276
	Ketoconazole	
	Lymecycline	356
	Morinamide	314
	Nadolol	276
	Octafonium Chloride	274, 281
	Pyrazinamide	312
	Sotalol	
	Trimethoxyamfetamine	
270	Alprenolol	276
	Aminobenzoic Acid	
	Clopidogrel	278, 308
	Diamthazole	293
	Distigmine Bromide	
	Etacrynic Acid	
	Etofylline	
	Mephenesin	276
	Methyclothiazide	314
	Phenol	
	Phenyltoloxamine	276
	Pyridostigmine Bromide	
	Tetracycline	356
	Theophylline	
	Warfarin	280, 303
271	4-Aminophenol	
	Ambenonium Chloride	277
	Bufylline	
	Clonidine	278
	Dinitro-orthocresol	
	Embutramide	276
	Mazindol	
	Methoxyphenamine	
	Naphazoline	281, 288, 291
	Pheneticillin	275
	Propofol	
	Sulfacetamide	
	Trimethoprim	
	Yohimbine	277, 287
272	Amidefrine	
	Amosulalol	
	Apomorphine	
	Benzocaine	278
	Bicalutamide	
	Butacaine	278
	Cyclothiazide	314
	Epithiazide	315
	Ethiazide	
	Etilefrine	
	Etodolac	
	Fenoprofen	
	Guanoclor	278
	Hydrochlorothiazide	318
	Metaraminol	
	Profadol	
	Pyrimethamine	
	Rolitetracycline	357
	Theobromine	
	Thymol	
	Tramadol	279
273	Anisindione	
	Bendroflumethiazide	325
	Bisoprolol	
	Buphenine	
	Caffeine	
	Cisapride	307
	Clonazepam	
	Coumatetralyl	283, 309
	Diclofenac	
	Diprophylline	

λ max nm	Compound	Subsidiary Peaks nm
	Edrophonium Chloride	
	Glymidine Sodium	299
	Guaifenesin	
	Hydroflumethiazide	325
	Hydroxyephedrine	
	Metoclopramide	309
	Naftidrofuryl Oxalate	283
	Oxedrine	
	Oxprenolol	
	Paclitaxel	
	Phenylephrine	
	Pimozide	280
	Proxyphylline	
	Resorcinol	
	Venlafaxine	280, 274
	Viloxazine	
274	Acefylline Piperazine	
	Atenolol	280
	Cyclopenthiazide	319
	Gemcitabine	
	Hordenine	
	Hydroxocobalamin	351
	Methoxyamfetamine	
	Methoxymetamfetamine	
	Metoprolol	280
	Pentoxifylline	
	Quinuronium Sulfate	323, 359
	Reboxetine	
	Ritodrine	
	Tyramine	
275	Bamethan	
	Clemizole	
	Esmolol	281
	Fenetylline	
	Fenoterol	
	Guanoxan	
	Hydroxyamfetamine	
	Moxisylyte	
	Pentifylline	
	Pholedrine	
	Propylthiouracil	
	Sulfadimethoxine	
276	Diaveridine	
	Dimenhydrinate	
	Glipizide	
	Insulin	
	Methylthiouracil	
	Orciprenaline	
	Salbutamol	
	Serotonin	
	Terbutaline	
277	Alclofenac	
	Ciprofloxacin	315
	Cyclazocine	
	Meclofenoxate	
	Metadrenaline	
	Metronidazole	
	Narceine	
	Omeprazole	303
	Oxymetholone	
	Tinidazole	
278	Amylmetacresol	286
	Bamifylline	
	Bufotenine	297
	Butorphanol	
	Chlorothiazide	
	Dextromethorphan	
	Diethyltryptamine	287
	Ethylnoradrenaline	
	Ibogaine	
	Isoetarine	
	Metipranolol	
	Naratriptan	284, 295

λ max nm	Compound	Subsidiary Peaks nm
	Normetadrenaline	
	Pentazocine	
	Phenazocine	
	Phentolamine	
	Procaine Benzylpenicillin	
	Teicoplanin	
	Tryptamine	287
	Tryptophan	286
	Verapamil	
279	α-Methyltryptamine	288
	Butyl Aminobenzoate	
	Chlorocresol	
	Chloroxylenol	
	Deferiprone	
	Dextrorphan	
	Diamorphine	
	Dimethyltryptamine	288
	Dobutamine	
	Isoprenaline	
	Lamivudine	
	Levallorphan	
	Levorphanol	
	Mefenamic Acid	350
	Mepacrine	343
	Methyldopa	
	Mianserin	
	Noradrenaline	
	Pergolide	280, 281
	Racemorphan	
280	Adrenaline	
	Azathioprine	
	Cetylpyridinium Chloride	
	Chlorzoxazone	
	Cytarabine	
	Dihydroergotamine	
	Dopamine	
	Etamivan	
	Hexoprenaline	
	Hydrocodone	
	Hydromorphone	
	Ketobemidone	
	Loratadine	
	Metocurine Iodide	
	Mivacurium Chloride	
	Nevirapine	
	Nitrazepam	
	Octreotide	288
	Oxycodone	
	Oxymetazoline	
	Pirenzepine	
	Rafoxanide	335
	Rimiterol	
	Sulfathiazole	
	Tamsulosin	
	Xamoterol	270, 275
	Zalcitabine	
281	Acetarsone	
	Mizolastine	288
	Naloxone	
	Naltrexone	
	Oxymorphone	
	Parbendazole	288
	Protokylol	
	Tetracaine	312
	Thebacon	
	Vancomycin	
282	Benzquinamide	
	Carbidopa	
	Clorgiline	
	Dichlorophen	
	Dolasetron	
	Dyclonine	
	Methanthelinium Bromide	

λ max nm	Compound	Subsidiary Peaks nm
	Phthalylsulfathiazole	
	Rizatriptan	
	Tetrabenazine	
283	Azatadine	
	Benzthiazide	
	Clarithromycin	
	Clofazimine	
	Dihydrocodeine	
	Dihydromorphine	
	Fazadinium Bromide	
	Formoterol	
	Pholcodine	
	Quazepam	
284	Acetorphine	
	Acetylcodeine	
	Benzylmorphine	
	Ethylmorphine	
	Etofenamate	349
	Lansoprazole	
	Nalbuphine	
	Nalmefene	298
	Norcodeine	
	Sulindac	327
	Thebaine	
285	Amiloride	361
	Cisplatin	301, 362
	Codeine	
	Dimoxyline	309, 335
	Morphine	
	Nalorphine	
	Nemonapride	314
	Neopine	
	Normorphine	
	Obidoxime Chloride	
286	Buprenorphine	
	Cyproheptadine	
	Diclofenamide	296
	Flucytosine	
	Mebhydrolin	320
	Mersalyl Acid	
	Nicergoline	
	Pramocaine	
	Remoxipride	
287	6-Monoacetylmorphine	
	Iprindole	293
	Prenalterol	
288	Dapsone	
	Idoxuridine	
	Propranolol	305, 319
289	DOM	
	Fenbendazole	302
290	Bleomycin	
	Cyclobenzaprine	
	Haloxon	312
	Methoxamine	
	Natamycin	303, 318
	Noscapine	312
	Pantoprazole	
	Pyridoxine	
	Triprolidine	
	Tylosin	
291	Carbimazole	
292	Albendazole	
	Butylated Hydroxyanisole	
	Doxepin	
	Protriptyline	
	Sulpiride	
294	Hydrastine	
	Procaine	
295	Timolol	
296	Xipamide	
297	Clotiapine	
	Ketotifen	
	Nimorazole	
298	Bunamidine	
299	Rescinnamine	
301	Oxypertine	
302	Labetalol	
	Mifepristone	
304	Zopiclone	303, 306
305	Lysergic Acid	
306	Bromocriptine	
307	Benzydamine	
308	Tiotixene	
309	Dimefline	
310	Diquat	
313	Ergometrine	
	Lysergamide	
	Methylergometrine	
	Tizanidine	319
314	Mirtazapine	252
315	Lysergide	
	Pyrantel	
316	Ergotamine	
	Sulfamethoxypyridazine	
317	Dimetridazole	
318	Indometacin	
319	Nizatidine	254
321	Carbocromen	
325	Mercaptopurine	
327	Enoximone	
329	Gloxazone	
336	Diphenadione	
340	Bumetanide	
344	Hydroxystilbamidine	
345	Glafenine	
358	Olsalazine	249

B. In alkali solution—wavelengths of maximum absorption

In this table wavelengths of maximum absorption in alkaline solution are given only for those compounds for which maxima in acid solution are not recorded in the monographs in Part 2, or for which the maxima in alkaline solution differ significantly from the maxima in acid solution.

λ max nm	Compound	Subsidiary Peaks nm
230	Buformin	
	Indometacin	279
231	Aspirin	298
	Celiprolol	324
	Flurazepam	312
	Mercaptopurine	310
	Oxybuprocaine	310
	Temazepam	313
232	Chlorhexidine	253
	Harman	284
	Thiamine	336
	Triamterene	270, 370
233	Niridazole	282
	Oxazepam	344
235	Moxisylyte	301
	Prenalterol	305
	Saccharin	268
236	Dobutamine	292

λ max nm	*Compound*	*Subsidiary Peaks nm*
	Papaverine	277, 326
237	Bromazepam	348
	Cambendazole	314
	Cyclazocine	298
	Etilefrine	290
	Ketotifen	302
	Profadol	290
	Tacrine	317
	Zopiclone	277
238	Captopril	
	Cinchocaine	325
	Clozapine	261, 297
	Fenbendazole	312
	Hexethal (pH 9.2)	253
	Hydroxyamfetamine	294
	Metaraminol	292
	Phenazocine	298
	Phenylephrine	291
	Phenylmethylbarbituric Acid	
	Pholedrine	295
	Vinbarbital (pH 9.2)	254
239	Barbital (pH 9.2)	254
	Bromocriptine	300
	Butobarbital (pH 9.2)	254
	Cresol	290
	Cyclobarbital (pH 9.2)	256
	Heptabarb (pH 9.2)	255
	Idobutal (pH 9.2)	254
	Lymecycline	267
	Pentobarbital (pH 9.2)	255
	Phenobarbital (pH 9.2)	254
	Secbutabarbital (pH 9.2)	254
	Secobarbital (pH 9.2)	254
	Talbutal (pH 9.2)	255
240	Acetazolamide	291
	Amobarbital (pH 9.2)	255
	Benzbromarone	281, 355
	Brallobarbital (pH 9.2)	256
	Butalbital (pH 9.2)	255
	Clioxanide	282, 362
	Dextrorphan	299
	Edrophonium Chloride	294
	Ibomal (pH 9.2)	257
	Levallorphan	299
	Levorphanol	299
	Nealbarbital (pH 9.2)	255
	Nordazepam	340
	Pentazocine	300
	Racemorphan	299
	Sulfadiazine	254
241	Allobarbital (pH 9.2)	256
	Aprobarbital (pH 9.2)	257
	Cyclopentobarbital (pH 9.2)	254
	Demeclocycline	276, 388
	Methapyrilene	312
	Oxedrine	291
	Salicylamide	328
242	Adrenaline	297
	Bamethan	290
	Buphenine	291
	Chloroxylenol	296
	Dichloralphenazone	256
	Hexestrol	297
	Hydroxyephedrine	290
	Iproniazid	307
	Phenazone	256
	Sulfadimidine	258
	Sulfamerazine	255
	Zolpidem	311
243	Chloropyrilene	308
	Chlorzoxazone	287
	Etizolam	
	Glymidine Sodium	317
	Harmine	275, 300
	Hexobarbital (pH 9.2&13)	
	Isoxsuprine	270, 277, 292
	Methylphenobarbital (pH 13)	
	Methysergide	320
	Minocycline	
	Propiomazine	283
244	Benoxaprofen	309
	Carbimazole	
	Chlorocresol	299
	Enallylpropymal (pH 13)	
	Metharbital (pH 9.2&13)	
	Methylphenobarbital (pH 9.2)	243
	Mexazolam	
	Morazone	263
245	Acepromazine	283
	Dichlorophen	304
	Enallylpropymal (pH 9.2)	244
	Metadrenaline	291
	Propyphenazone	265
	Salbutamol	295
	Sulfametoxydiazine	
246	Diethylpropion	
	Diprenorphine	299
	Droperidol	288
	Eugenol	296
	Labetalol	333
	Lisinopril	254, 258, 261, 267
	Methohexital (pH 9.2&13)	
	Oxytetracycline Dihydrate	269
	Thenyldiamine	310
247	Amoxicillin	291
	Antazoline	295
	Buclosamide	325
	Diminazene	
	Spironolactone	
	Sulfapyridine	
	Vinylbital	
248	Benperidol	288
	Carbarsone	
	Loxapine	298
	Mepyramine	312
	Rolitetracycline	268
	Vanillin	348
249	Acetohexamide	
	Floctafenine	359
	Pentamidine	
	Propantheline Bromide	282
	Sotalol	
	Sulfaphenazole	
	Tripelennamine	312
250	Acetarsone	299
	Allopurinol	257
	Amoxapine	299
	Clomethiazole	
	Isothipendyl	
	Prothipendyl	320
	Sulfamethoxypyridazine	
	Sulfamoxole	
	Sulfanilamide	
251	Amiodarone	
	Clomocycline	283
	Gentamicin	
	Nalorphine	298
252	Imipramine	
	Pargyline	257, 263
	Prazosin	345
	Sulfaquinoxaline	357
253	Apomorphine	
	Chlortetracycline	284, 346
	Doxorubicin	
	Hexethal (pH 13)	
	Hydroxychloroquine	330

λ max nm	*Compound*	*Subsidiary Peaks nm*
	Profenamine	302
	Sulfafurazole	
254	Barbital (pH 13)	
	Butobarbital (pH 13)	
	Chloroquine	330
	Clemizole	269, 275, 283
	Cyclopentobarbital (pH 13)	324
	Idobutal (pH 13)	
	Phenobarbital (pH 13)	
	Didanosine	
	Oxyphenbutazone	
	Parbendazole	297, 303
	Promazine	306
	Promethazine	305
	Secbutobarbital (pH 13)	
	Secobarbital (pH 13)	
	Sorbic Acid	
	Vinbarbital (pH 13)	
255	Amobarbital (pH 13)	
	Azapropazone	325
	Butalbital (pH 13)	
	Carbutamide	
	Heptabarb (pH 13)	
	Methdilazine	308
	Pentobarbital (pH 13)	
	Strychnine	278
	Sulfacarbamide	
	Talbutal (pH 13)	
256	Alimemazine	310
	Allobarbital (pH 13)	
	Brallobarbital (pH 13)	
	Cyclobarbital (pH 13)	
	Dapsone	292
	Folic Acid	283
	Methylthiouracil	
	Nikethamide	261
	Sulfacetamide	
	Sulfathiazole	
	Tropicamide	
257	Aprobarbital (pH 13)	
	Barbituric Acid (pH 9.2)	259
	Carbenoxolone	
	Ibomal (pH 13)	
	Paracetamol	
	Perphenazine	310
	Pivampicillin	311
	Succinylsulfathiazole	
	Sulfachlorpyridazine	
	Thiopropazate	
258	Methotrexate	303
	Nalidixic Acid	334
	Pheniramine	263, 268
	Trifluoperazine	308
	Zimeldine	
259	Adenosine	
	Chlormezanone	
	Cinchophen	330
	Halquinol	343
	Levomepromazine	323
	Selegiline	269
	Sulfaguanidine	
260	Cyclizine	
	Enoxolone	
	Phthalylsulfathiazole	
	Propylthiouracil	
	Sulfamethizole	
	Sulfinpyrazone	
	Tolmetin	323
	Tranylcypromine	266, 273
261	Carbinoxamine	
	Cefaloridine	
	Disopyramide	
	Nicotine	
	Zomepirac	330
262	Bromhexine	317
	Brompheniramine	269
	Chlordiazepoxide	
	Chlorphenamine	
	Coniine	268
	Cyclofenil	
	Ketoprofen	
	Minoxidil	288
	Sulfisomidine	
263	Chlorquinaldol	345
	Gliclazide	
	Nicofuranose	
	Phenindamine	
264	Aminophenazone	
	Methyclothiazide	300
	Phenylbutazone	
	Salinazid	
265	Aminobenzoic Acid	
	Aminosalicylic Acid	300
	Amprenavir	
	Cladribine	
	Diethazine	
	Dinitro-orthocresol	
	Ibuprofen	273
	Methaqualone	306
	Pecazine	
	Phthalylsulfacetamide	
266	4-Aminophenol	
	Acecainide	
	Brucine	304
	Feprazone	
	Sulforidazine	
268	Aloin	
	Dimetotiazine	
	Flucloxacillin	274, 318
	Gelsemine	
269	Mazindol	275
	Mebeverine	290
	Psilocybine	282, 292
	Sulfadimethoxine	
270	Mebendazole	355
	Mepacrine	345
	Psilocin	293
	Riboflavin	356
	Zalcitabine	
271	Furosemide	333
	Isopropylaminophenazone	
	Nitroxinil	
272	Amosulalol	
	Pericyazine	
	Sulfadoxine	
273	Amodiaquine	287
	Bendroflumethiazide	330
	Captodiame	
274	Cytarabine	
	Hydrochlorothiazide	324
	Hydroflumethiazide	333
	Isocarboxazid	
	Serotonin	323
	Theobromine	
275	Bufexamac	
	Deserpidine	
	Diclofenac	
	Meclofenamic Acid	319
	Procainamide	
	Theophylline	
	Thioridazine	313
276	Dithranol	
	Gliquidone	
277	Diflunisal	
	Ethionamide	
278	Dimenhydrinate	

λ max nm	Compound	Subsidiary Peaks nm
	Phenindione	330
279	Ambucetamide	286
	Idoxuridine	
280	Dantron	
	Diazoxide	
	Nicergoline	
	Procaine Benzylpenicillin	
	Quinidine	330
	Quinine	330
	Sulindac	327
	Tryptophan	288
	Yohimbine	
281	Ethylmorphine	
	Flunixin	
	Noscapine	315
	Trilostane	
282	Butacaine	
284	Cyproheptadine	
	Nitrofurazone	
	Nomifensine	
285	Azathioprine	
	Benzocaine	
	Butyl Aminobenzoate	
	Fenbufen	
	Mefenamic Acid	
286	Clobazam	
	Cotarnine	330
	Pyrimethamine	
287	Ketoconazole	
	Phenol	
	Trimethoprim	
288	Cinchonine	302, 315
	Methazolamide	
	Niflumic Acid	
290	Hydromorphone	
	Mersalyl Acid	
	Resorcinol	
291	Carbidopa	
	Nystatin	305, 319
	Phentolamine	
292	Chlorothiazide	
	Fendosal	
	Hydrastine	
	Oxymorphone	
	Thymol	
293	Flucytosine	
	Metallibure	
	Naltrexone	
	Warfarin	308
294	Pentaerithrityl Tetranitrate	
	Tyramine	
295	Diethylthiambutene	
	Dipyridamole	
	Ethyl Hydroxybenzoate	
	Fenoterol	
	Triclosan	
296	Noradrenaline	
	Propyl Hydroxybenzoate	
297	Benzthiazide	
	Dihydromorphine	
	Isoprenaline	
	Nalbuphine	
	Orciprenaline	
	Pirenzepine	
	Teicoplanin	
	Terbutaline	
298	Aloxiprin	
	Isoniazid	
	Morphine	
	Parachlorophenol	
	Salicylic Acid	
299	Butorphanol	
	Diamorphine	
300	Buprenorphine	
	Ketobemidone	
	Xamoterol	
302	Iprindole	
	Methyldopa	
303	Gloxazone	
	Oxymetazoline	
	Tetracaine	
	Thiopental (pH 13)	
304	Thiopental (pH 9.2)	255
305	Nimorazole	
	Tetrazepam	
	Thiamylal	
306	Rescinnamine	
	Thialbarbital (pH 13)	
307	Nialamide	
308	Lysergic Acid	
309	Albendazole	
	Lysergamide	
310	Ergometrine	
	Ergotamine	
	Hydroxystilbamidine	
	Lysergide	
	Methylergometrine	
	Phenprocoumon	
311	Coumatetralyl	
	Ethyl Biscoumacetate	
314	Dantrolene	
	Dicoumarol	
315	Oxymetholone	
317	Bumetanide	
319	Liothyronine	
	Metronidazole	
	Pentachlorophenol	
320	Tioguanine	
322	Dimetridazole	
324	Oxyclozanide	
325	Levothyroxine	
330	Harmaline	
	Xipamide	
332	Pralidoxime Chloride	280
334	Niclosamide	377
341	Salsalate	
353	Obidoxime Chloride	

C. In neutral solution—wavelengths of maximum absorption

The compounds listed below are those whose wavelengths of maximum absorption in acid or alkaline solution are not given in the monographs in Part 2, or for which the maxima in neutral solution differ significantly from those in acid or alkaline solution.

λ max nm	Compound	Subsidiary Peaks nm
230	Benzyl Benzoate	
	Bezafibrate	
	Flecainide	300
	Hexestrol	280
	Lorazepam	316
	Meclozine	266, 273
	Nalmefene	285
	Oxazepam	315

λ max nm	*Compound*	*Subsidiary Peaks nm*
	Pravastatin	237, 245
	Prilocaine	
	Temazepam	314
	Tinidazole	311
	Zuclopenthixol	268, 325
231	Atracurium	280, 281
	Camazepam	315
	Estradiol	
	Proxymetacaine	268, 310
	Simvastatin	238, 247, 237, 246
232	Celiprolol	329
	Ciprofibrate	
	Clopamide	277, 286
	Eugenol	282
	Methylenedioxymethamfetamine	285
233	4-Aminophenol	303
	Bromazepam	320
	Clioxanide	
	Doxorubicin	253, 290
	Paroxetine	264, 270, 292
	Triamterene	267
234	Bephenium Hydroxynaphthoate	263, 270, 283, 295, 352
	Cefaloridine	
	Daunorubicin	251, 288
	Quinethazone	278, 345
235	Acebutolol	328
	Androstenedione	
	Aniline	286
	Fludroxycortide	
	Gestrinone	347
236	Clobetasone Butyrate	
	Clofenotane	267
	Fluclorolone Acetonide	
	Griseofulvin	291
	Metformin	
237	Carbamazepine	285
	Cefalothin	265
	Cycloguanil	278, 289, 301
	Diltiazem	
	Risperidone	279, 285
	Trenbolone	340, 338
238	Amlodipine	
	Flugestone	
	Flumetasone	
	Methyl Salicylate	306
	Phenazopyridine	277
	Sodium Cromoglicate	326
	Triamcinolone	
239	Beclometasone	
	Clobetasol Propionate	
	Propyliodone	281
	Pyrvinium Embonate	358
	Santonin	
240	Benorilate	
	Benziodarone	275, 357
	Betamethasone	241
	Clenbuterol	295
	Cortisone	
	Dactinomycin	
	Dequalinium Chloride	326, 335
	Desoxycortone	
	Dexamethasone	
	Dimethisterone	
	Ethisterone	
	Fludrocortisone	
	Fluocinolone Acetonide	
	Fluocinonide	
	Fluoxymesterone	
	Gestonorone Caproate	
	Hydralazine	260, 304, 315
	Hydrocortisone	
	Hydroxyprogesterone	
	Methylprednisolone	
	Metomidate	
	Nizatidine	325, 313, 260, 314
	Norethandrolone	
	Norethisterone	
	Prednisolone	
	Prednisone	
	Progesterone	
	Propofol	291
	Testosterone	
241	Aldosterone	
	Altretamine	
	Benazepril	237
	Diethylstilbestrol	
	Fluorometholone	
	Medroxyprogesterone Acetate	
	Methyltestosterone	
	Metisazone	274
	Nomifensine	292
	Paramethasone	
242	Ceftriaxone	269
	Deflazacort	
	Dihydrotachysterol	251, 261
	Etomidate	
	Fluocortolone	
	Indapamide	288
	Ketazolam	
	Meclofenamic Acid	282, 331
	Salol	310
243	Buclosamide	301
	Colchicine	350
	Desonide	
	Isopropylaminophenazone	269
	Mexenone	287, 325
	Zolpidem	314, 236, 294
244	Flumazenil	
	Ketoconazole	296
	Mexazolam	
	Noxytiolin	
	Phytomenadione	249, 263, 270, 331
245	Alfuzosin	331
	Benzaldehyde	279, 289
	Clonazepam	309
	Ketorolac	312
	Methandienone	
	Terazosin	330
	Trimetozine	
246	Etebenecid	
	Felbamate	251, 256, 262
	Sultiame	
247	Azaperone	300
	Chlorotrianisene	307
	Mesuximide	252, 258, 264
	Methcathinone	
	Phensuximide	252, 258, 264
248	Bisacodyl	
	Halquinol	263, 334
	Practolol	
	Trioxysalen	296, 338
249	Aldicarb	
	Broxyquinoline	325
250	Boldenone	243
	Diuron	287
	Doxazosin	275, 282
251	Bamipine	298
	Chlorquinaldol	315
252	Atovaquone	276
	Beclamide	258, 264, 268
	Benzyl Alcohol	258, 264
	Clidinium Bromide	258, 264
	Clorexolone	
	Cyclandelate	258, 264
	Dantron	283
	Diphenoxylate	258, 264

λ max nm	*Compound*	*Subsidiary Peaks nm*
	Flunitrazepam	308
	Fluspirilene	273, 293
	Fosinopril	258, 268
	Glutethimide	258, 264
	Loratadine	
	Primidone	258, 264
	Ramipril	258, 267
	Valaciclovir	
253	Cetalkonium Chloride	258, 263, 270
	Methallenestril	264, 273, 317, 332
	Prenylamine	258, 268
	Trilostane	
254	Clostebol	
	Clotrimazole	260
	Danazol	
	Ganciclovir	264
	Phenothiazine	317
	Phenprobamate	259, 261, 265, 269
	Pyridoxine	324
255	Buclizine	260
	Clioquinol	325
	Dixyrazine	305
	Lofepramine	
	Methylthioamfetamine	254
	Nedocromil	286, 345, 378
256	Benzalkonium Chloride	262, 268
	Busulfan	
	Dithranol	288, 360
	Mifepristone	305
257	Azlocillin	320
	Benzylpenicillin	264, 325
	Ceftazidime	
	Cilostazol	
	Lorcainide	263
	Mephenytoin	264
	Methyl Hydroxybenzoate	
	Tolazamide	263, 268, 275
	Tolnaftate	
258	Alfentanil	264, 268
	Aprindine	296
	Benethamine	
	Chlorambucil	303
	Diiodohydroxyquinoline	
	Diloxanide	278
	Fosphenytoin	
	Nitrobenzene	
	Phenacemide	265
	Phenytoin	264
	Sertindole	302, 259, 302
	Syrosingopine	298
259	Ethotoin	265
	Furazolidone	367
	Isopropamide Iodide	265
	Moracizine	
	Phenaglycodol	266, 275
	Proguanil	
	Tofenacin	265, 272
260	Abacavir	285
	Aminoacridine	311, 325
	Cefalexin	
	Chloronitrotoluene	
	Chlorproguanil	
	Harmaline	344
	Melphalan	301
	Phthalylsulfathiazole	288
261	Aciclovir	
	Fluconazole	267
	Proflavine Hemisulfate	
262	Benzyl Nicotinate	
	Simazine	
263	Atrazine	
	Cerivastatin	
	Nicotinic Acid	
	Octafonium Chloride	269, 274, 282
	Tenoxicam	289
264	Bambuterol	
	Fluoxetine	268, 275
	Methyl Nicotinate	
	Miconazole	272, 280
	Pindolol	287
	Zotepine	297
265	Colecalciferol	
	Ergocalciferol	
	Pipotiazine	315
	Suprofen	291
	Triclocarban	
266	Deptropine	272
	Isradipine	278, 291, 326
	Naphthalene	275, 286
	Nitrofurantoin	367
	Zidovudine	
267	Propamidine	
	Reserpine	295
	Tienilic Acid	296
268	Domiphen Bromide	277
	Phenoxymethylpenicillin	275
	Polythiazide	317
	Vinorelbine	282, 293, 310
269	Clopidol	
	Propicillin	276
270	Fenclofenac	276
	Nadolol	278
	Thiambutosine	
	Vindesine	
272	Benzoic Acid	280
	Ciprofloxacin	322, 334
	Paradichlorobenzene	265, 282
	Sulfisomidine	
273	Fenoprofen	280
	Glimepiride	
	Indoramin	279, 289
	Methoserpidine	
274	Dibutyl Phthalate	
	Dicamba	230, 278
	Etamiphylline	
	Etodolac	
	Parathion	
	Venlafaxine	280
275	Aceclofenac	
	Chlortalidone	284
	Cisapride	308
	Cresol	279
	Dimethyl Phthalate	
	Dodecyl Gallate	
	Ecgonine	
	Ethyl Biscoumacetate	303
	Ethyl Gallate	
	Glibenclamide	300
	Methocarbamol	
	Nabilone	282
276	Mefruside	284
	Omeprazole	305
277	Bamifylline	
	Meptazinol	
	Phenolphthalein	
278	Butylated Hydroxytoluene	
	Cannabidiol	285
	Chloramphenicol	271
	Cyanocobalamin	361, 550
	Formestane	
	Mestranol	287
	Δ^9-THC	
	Δ^9-Tetrahydrocannabinolic Acid	283
279	Butoxyethyl Nicotinate	
	Carbaryl	
	Pergolide	

λ max nm	*Compound*	*Subsidiary Peaks nm*
280	Aminohippuric Acid	
	Betaxolol	
	Chlorphenesin Carbamate	288
	Clofibrate	288
	Estriol	
	Estrone	
	Methylchlorophenoxyacetic Acid	287
	Meticillin	
	Mivacurium Chloride	
	Propanidid	
	Tubocurarine Chloride	
281	Chlorphenesin	289
	Ethinylestradiol	
	Felodipine	
	Quazepam	
	Sulfiram	
282	Alclofenac	290
	Clarithromycin	
	Hexylresorcinol	
	Indoprofen	
	Milrinone	331
283	Acenocoumarol	306
	Etoposide	284, 291
	Moexipril	
	Tilmicosin	
	Triclosan	
284	Alpha Tocoferil Acetate	
	Dichlorophenoxyacetic Acid	292
	Parachlorophenol	291
285	Acetomenaphthone	322
	Chlormadinone Acetate	
	Naratriptan	296
	Phenprocoumon	310
286	Anisindione	340
	Dydrogesterone	
	Famotidine	
	Remoxipride	287
287	Megestrol Acetate	
	Mizolastine	
	Mupirocin	
	Nicergoline	

λ max nm	*Compound*	*Subsidiary Peaks nm*
288	Flufenamic Acid	339
	Ofloxacin	332
289	Aztreonam	
	Camphor	
	Clonixin	335
290	Alfadolone	
	Alfaxalone	
	Bleomycin	
	Methoxamine	
	Propranolol	306, 319
291	Protionamide	
292	Rabeprazole	
293	Benzocaine	
294	Butyl Aminobenzoate	
	Tolfenamic Acid	330
295	Hydroquinone	
	Pentachlorophenol	303
	Procaine Benzylpenicillin	
296	Bitoscanate	311
	Fenbendazole	
	Procaine	
298	Salicylic Acid	
300	Levofloxacin	
303	Clefamide	
	Oxyclozanide	
304	Famciclovir	
306	Entacapone	
307	Lamotrigine	
308	Benzonatate	
311	Gliquidone	
313	Ranitidine	
315	Rifamycin SV	
322	Morantel	
324	Nisoldipine	
327	Temozolomide	
328	Thioacetazone	
330	Loprazolam	
333	Niclosamide	
356	Carbazochrome	
386	Aminonitrothiazole	

Infra-red Peaks

The table below lists the six major absorption bands which have been selected from recorded spectra over the range 2000 to 650 cm^{-1} (5 to 15 μm). The selected peaks are the six most intense peaks, except that peaks in the region where Nujol absorbs (1490 to 1320 cm^{-1}, 6.7 to 7.6 μm) have been omitted. The peaks are arranged in descending order of amplitude. Shoulders have been chosen only if they are clearly resolved and the point of maximum absorption can be easily determined. Where there is more than one peak of the same intensity at the sixth intensity level, the choice has been arbitrary. It should be noted that, because of variations in instruments and conditions, other determinations of the spectrum may not give peaks with the same relative intensities. In particular, the order of the two most intense peaks may be reversed and this should be taken into consideration when using the index.

To identify an unknown compound, the wavenumbers of the two most intense peaks should be compared with the table, initially allowing a tolerance of $\pm 4\,cm^{-1}$, to produce a list of possible compounds. Comparison of the six most intense peaks with this list may allow a tentative identification; reference should then be made to the spectra given in the monographs in Part 2.

If a tentative identification cannot be made, it may be necessary to use a wider coverage, or to search on the third most intense peak.

Wavenumbers cm^{-1}						*Compound*
675	1262	1305	1556	1215	788	Nicotinyl Alcohol
680	665	695	778	840	950	Lindane
683	1040	1014	1053	813	1266	Lynestrenol
685	1629	776	1174	715	1205	Cetylpyridinium Chloride
688	855	704	781	917	957	Benzene Hexachloride
690	755	1235	1595	1497	811	Phenol
691	769	1529	720	1164	998	Triphenyltetrazolium Chloride
694	751	1086	1041	1010	714	Captodiame
694	1190	740	1075	1020	1694	Alverine
695	745	755	942	1146	1608	Phenethylamine
695	1723	1231	1054	1162	751	Benactyzine
696	745	1111	1022	1592	1067	Benethamine
696	1036	835	723	1255	893	Aldrin
696	1117	755	751	1030	1298	Cycrimine
697	701	749	773	1123	1219	Difenidol
697	746	714	724	1052	1515	Pargyline
697	1051	1020	1000	740	1115	Etafedrine
699	1175	760	1199	1292	1070	Mebanazine
700	720	760	940	805	1491	Meclozine
700	740	1495	1090	1605	825	Amfetamine
700	746	1030	1500	1055	1590	Phenylpropanolamine
700	747	1136	1027	1592	1075	Prenylamine
700	756	746	1128	1075	1175	Procyclidine
700	760	1298	1020	892	869	Phencyclidine
700	1040	762	1025	1605	1200	*N*-Methyltryptamine
700	1590	1123	1086	1041	751	Doxylamine
700	1664	764	1590	1315	979	Ambutonium Bromide
701	740	690	1585	1300	1065	Pipradrol
701	1230	1682	1287	973	1594	Diethylpropion
702	691	1138	964	740	1000	Cinnarizine
702	726	780	875	1618	1211	Benzalkonium Chloride
702	735	1121	997	760	1153	Biperiden
702	745	1316	1063	971	1155	Azacyclonol
702	753	858	1115	1215	1256	Moexipril
702	756	973	1206	1196	935	Trihexyphenidyl
704	765	740	1492	1092	981	Selegiline
704	1036	764	1005	1210	1595	Pseudoephedrine
704	1265	1020	1075	1612	826	Chlordane
705	920	1115	772	1045	1061	Tricyclamol Chloride
705	1095	749	759	1020	952	Bibenzonium Bromide
708	699	752	1102	742	1134	Emepronium Bromide
708	756	1042	797	738	1492	Fencamfamin
708	1250	1230	1010	765	699	Diphemanil Metilsulfate
709	1689	1296	667	935	685	Benzoic Acid
712	1022	810	1575	1310	1040	Nicotine
713	754	1103	1017	1180	991	Diphenhydramine
714	787	1205	1220	928	1515	Chloroform
716	743	851	833	1244	1618	Diethylthiambutene
716	756	701	984	1125	1496	Cyclizine
717	1492	710	769	1162	729	Tridihexethyl Chloride
720	760	775	1112	1130	1038	Nefopam
722	698	1612	1204	875	790	Cetalkonium Chloride
727	776	700	802	1515	970	Tolpropamine
728	1695	833	1086	1050	1010	Benoxaprofen
730	1285	705	1495	1610	1510	Phentermine
735	750	1310	710	1300	1590	Phenothiazine
736	1066	811	746	1245	1260	Pericyazine
737	1134	1316	695	1122	1212	Mebhydrolin
738	1650	1612	1145	1173	1040	Iprindole
740	710	1573	1175	1018	918	Diphenyl
740	747	765	1230	1110	756	Imipramine
740	1111	1063	1086	1234	724	Diethyltryptamine
740	1306	902	1095	1279	1231	Tiabendazole
742	1039	702	1052	990	1162	Methylephedrine
742	1585	1233	1035	909	1494	Tryptamine
743	1113	1235	1050	812	1010	Dimethyltryptamine
745	1510	1602	1187	1258	1035	Aprindine
745	1583	697	1019	707	1139	Fenproporex
745	1593	725	1495	690	1275	Bamipine
746	741	763	1230	1590	1104	Desipramine
747	698	1060	1491	1590	1085	Metamfetamine
747	1240	1561	1125	1095	1220	Chlorpromazine
748	765	740	833	1111	1010	Clemizole
748	918	1063	990	1111	1639	Azapetine
748	1245	1587	1282	1562	1219	Diethazine
748	1248	1260	1305	1590	1275	Alimemazine
748	1248	1590	1282	1568	1125	Profenamine
748	1279	1244	1163	1143	1570	Perazine
750	729	1052	1162	1086	1280	Metixene
750	768	1219	1250	1162	1282	Pecazine
750	1006	768	1198	1290	1219	Doxepin
751	1250	742	1220	729	1042	Mequitazine
751	1250	1234	1287	770	1162	Promazine
751	1317	1235	1504	1245	1567	Harman
752	1225	805	842	1212	1237	Clomipramine
752	1271	1124	803	984	795	Azatadine
752	1280	1569	1165	1242	1145	Prochlorperazine
753	1242	1319	1222	1277	1031	Methdilazine
754	899	1090	800	877	1587	Cinchonidine
754	1248	796	1234	1281	1211	Thioridazine
754	1653	1221	1186	1575	1316	Propiomazine
754	1656	700	1492	1590	1117	Morazone
755	1155	790	1237	1115	1126	Opipramol
756	700	1035	770	1190	735	Clofedanol
756	741	1103	1092	1046	1280	Ajmaline
756	742	768	720	775	1590	Nortriptyline
756	770	746	969	1014	1258	Amitriptyline
757	743	732	1134	1060	1020	Benzoctamine

Wavenumbers cm^{-1}						*Compound*
757	1033	1265	740	1098	1149	Butriptyline
757	1294	917	1145	1247	1155	Perphenazine
757	1295	780	1592	1162	1110	Prothipendyl
758	1229	733	1129	1259	1287	Promethazine
758	1657	1288	1210	1250	1150	Salicylic Acid
759	1140	1592	1032	1308	935	Maprotiline
759	1250	1698	699	731	1199	Cinchophen
759	1271	747	1575	1242	932	Levallorphan
760	1110	1505	1590	990	909	Cinchonine
760	1556	1645	1655	750	1612	Aminoacridine
760	1695	1169	946	–	–	Sildenafil
761	842	1618	1003	1310	827	Triazolam
763	727	747	1252	963	717	Dosulepin
763	1590	724	747	1570	1050	Dimetindene
763	1656	1063	1175	674	1093	Mazindol
764	778	800	968	988	880	Cyclobenzaprine
764	1410	1615	1380	1040	1524	Etizolam
764	1674	1708	1242	1268	829	Fenbufen
765	752	708	1075	741	1205	Clotrimazole
768	1096	1250	1288	1053	890	Pindolol
775	790	1500	1100	1022	850	Clofenotane
775	1580	825	990	1509	1146	Triprolidine
776	714	752	1501	1141	1020	Prolintane
776	1104	832	746	1030	1170	Chlorprothixene
777	756	815	786	1640	960	Cyproheptadine
790	833	1145	1186	917	980	Chlorobutanol
792	750	768	1490	730	1595	Protriptyline
793	1080	1492	1508	1385	843	Methylthioamfetamine
800	1515	1065	1130	1290	1205	Norcodeine
800	1515	1612	1587	1234	1315	5-Methyltryptamine
805	1243	1118	945	1086	833	Morphine
815	1492	699	953	1075	840	Zimeldine
817	1248	1290	1095	1160	952	Thymol
818	1493	1092	1020	848	754	Chlorphentermine
828	1590	1284	902	1148	710	Protionamide
830	1090	1051	1020	690	1300	Butylchloral Hydrate
832	1151	1673	1217	1136	1598	Haloperidol
832	1228	1066	1264	1494	1108	Bamethan
834	1507	1034	1226	1160	1601	Citalopram
835	1083	1300	970	1620	–	Cloral Hydrate
835	1510	1054	1271	1098	1611	Oxedrine
836	1261	1236	1042	1061	733	Psilocin
840	1622	1522	1084	802	1577	Histamine
840	1630	1085	1130	730	1500	Cloral Betaine
848	811	1038	700	1005	912	Dieldrin
851	750	724	1049	889	1010	Endrin
887	1538	784	823	1297	1584	Acetarsone
905	1008	999	1020	1101	985	Allylestrenol
913	970	1630	945	1063	1000	Hexamethonium Bromide
917	1126	1156	995	1030	1050	Methylpentynol
932	1255	729	718	669	815	Thiotepa
935	950	830	1010	1063	980	Ethchlorvynol
949	1089	869	1231	1000	1740	Acetylcholine Chloride
952	1123	1162	819	1111	1298	Isopropyl Alcohol
953	1198	808	784	1266	728	Clioquinol
961	888	831	1621	985	1020	Mebezonium Iodide
961	909	952	719	970	724	Cetrimide
967	1049	1226	1278	1158	1473	Fenamiphos
970	980	1185	1616	1150	1205	Hexylresorcinol
970	1080	1033	1060	1115	1495	Nalbuphine
973	1059	1079	1712	893	1000	Ergocalciferol
975	994	964	1299	1142	1165	Ethylestrenol
975	1090	1672	1110	1065	1025	Iproniazid
980	1075	1219	847	1162	1052	Cineole
980	1238	835	1157	1129	792	Hydroxyephedrine
988	725	760	706	1087	870	Chlorcyclizine
994	699	754	1049	1242	670	Ephedrine
995	1018	1087	772	1492	820	Pyrrobutamine
996	1090	1637	1600	1282	847	Obidoxime Chloride
1000	1666	833	781	1041	775	Azinphos-methyl
1002	1131	754	800	1075	694	Buclizine
1010	1065	1038	1103	1183	1126	Amphotericin B
1010	1666	819	666	1538	1176	Dimethoate

Wavenumbers cm^{-1}						*Compound*
1012	1091	817	1121	951	1000	Paradichlorobenzene
1015	1041	667	1548	1602	1190	Diamthazole
1016	1108	1050	1080	940	699	Phenelzine
1017	1030	1070	987	1090	1080	Isothipendyl
1018	1748	1174	1209	824	1250	Malathion
1019	1083	1421	1280	–	–	Mannitol
1020	925	1515	1219	1587	970	Parathion
1020	1230	1290	1210	1530	1605	Rimiterol
1020	1250	775	793	826	1190	Demeton-*S*
1020	1587	971	1562	823	1159	Dimpylate
1022	1050	990	1270	1235	1170	Dimercaprol
1023	1112	695	963	1153	743	Tranylcypromine
1023	1250	1200	970	1718	1585	Nitrofurazone
1026	1111	1312	1136	1653	990	Ascorbic Acid
1030	1143	1127	1070	1050	1630	Guanethidine
1031	952	666	798	2983	2941	Disulfoton
1031	1018	1076	975	1582	1279	Trometamol
1031	1293	907	–	–	–	Tributyl Phosphate
1033	930	805	1489	1442	1189	Methylenedioxy-methamfetamine
1033	1007	1575	1300	1078	1139	Coniine
1033	1068	1143	1123	980	1516	Kanamycin
1033	1153	1458	–	–	–	Acarbose
1035	1257	1222	1497	748	1070	Chelidonine
1040	1590	845	770	660	1260	Tobramycin
1045	695	754	704	1091	976	Cathine
1046	1026	995	1102	1078	979	Menthol
1046	1714	1278	775	2964	599	Omethoate
1047	1248	1124	1493	756	748	Mephenesin
1050	752	1239	1282	1562	1091	Mesoridazine
1050	1168	1074	1010	1108	1734	Erythromycin
1050	1630	1120	1145	1545	940	Amikacin
1052	894	901	967	862	1075	Colecalciferol
1052	1163	1122	994	1016	1730	Spiramycin
1052	1170	1108	1734	–	–	Clarithromycin
1052	1268	1500	1111	793	934	Codeine
1054	700	742	1191	1204	1075	Benzatropine
1055	830	971	1243	1359	1539	Fenitrothion
1056	967	1018	1009	870	980	Dihydrotachysterol
1058	1015	885	913	1153	966	Propylhexedrine
1059	1022	800	959	952	839	Cholesterol
1059	1040	751	760	738	1114	Deptropine
1061	1158	850	978	1320	–	Dichlorvos
1062	1002	1563	1709	1101	1258	Natamycin
1062	1618	862	1266	1653	1089	Isosorbide Dinitrate
1064	1045	1129	1499	1185	1264	Ethylmorphine
1065	1013	1298	1284	1102	1581	Mannomustine
1065	1025	695	758	1272	890	Amygdalin
1066	1690	1729	1140	1008	1242	Noretynodrel
1067	1000	1570	1175	1316	847	Nystatin
1067	1094	1007	696	1041	746	Bromazine
1070	709	1050	696	765	1101	Diphenylpyraline
1072	1058	1010	1740	1168	990	Digitoxin
1075	775	1587	1041	1030	1123	Clorprenaline
1075	1027	1145	1109	1178	1002	Cytarabine
1075	1038	1263	1228	1213	822	Salbutamol
1075	1052	1162	1111	1010	1587	Tylosin
1075	1709	1055	1020	1160	1110	Digoxin
1078	1123	772	1634	1175	1672	Sulfasalazine
1082	1130	1005	1149	1063	800	Hydroxyzine
1083	757	695	965	990	1030	Phenmetrazine
1084	1110	1584	1041	763	1010	Carbinoxamine
1085	1014	1730	1163	1130	864	Metildigoxin
1085	1319	827	1302	1038	812	Miconazole
1086	1173	1605	1010	1305	995	Orciprenaline
1086	1298	1538	1149	689	917	Sulfaethidole
1088	1490	1010	760	700	990	Chlorphenoxamine
1090	1011	700	763	1121	1210	Clemastine
1090	1061	1142	987	1050	1009	Ethambutol
1090	1230	795	1264	1247	1724	Dichlorophenoxyacetic Acid
1090	1310	805	825	1010	1040	Econazole
1092	1070	1248	1262	1582	1217	Nadolol
1092	1273	1713	1235	710	1020	Aconitine

Wavenumbers cm⁻¹						*Compound*
1093	854	1300	910	1176	1234	Hexetidine
1093	1494	1280	1011	1042	1600	Trimetazidine
1094	1113	1163	1074	975	1205	Metaldehyde
1095	1085	1015	1180	807	830	Phenaglycodol
1095	1170	946	860	846	763	Paraldehyde
1095	1605	1266	1172	1698	1527	Benzonatate
1096	950	1068	982	1175	1125	Stanozolol
1100	1120	1260	1000	780	1600	Gallamine Triethiodide
1101	1153	1270	799	1207	1316	Amidefrine
1102	704	757	1117	1042	917	Tofenacin
1102	1242	1190	1605	1517	1280	Hexoprenaline
1103	1270	772	1580	795	1240	Propranolol
1105	1045	1062	1183	1160	932	Psilocybine
1106	1702	1365	1458	–	–	Alachlor
1107	1227	926	1124	709	876	Triclofos Sodium
1109	1154	854	978	1323	–	Trichlorfon
1111	711	1162	696	763	1587	Mephentermine
1111	1052	1075	1010	1162	1190	Oleandomycin
1111	1068	1078	1592	1098	890	Mecamylamine
1111	1666	1052	1724	1250	1515	Dihydrostreptomycin
1113	1195	1205	1155	1088	1005	Etorphine
1113	1630	1495	1226	1591	1034	Ethacridine
1114	1316	1145	1081	755	1255	Trifluoperazine
1115	1176	1653	1284	1265	1600	Flufenamic Acid
1115	1495	1264	1665	1592	748	Guanoxan
1116	767	1245	1144	1084	836	Fluphenazine
1117	1316	1159	1237	1075	1030	Triflupromazine
1118	874	1288	923	1026	1036	Putrescine
1118	969	1250	1043	1500	1098	Pholcodine
1118	1070	1045	980	962	1015	Sparteine
1118	1098	1069	1044	1195	1210	Pseudomorphine
1120	1060	1625	1525	1290	880	Gentamicin
1120	1105	697	1083	752	1630	Phendimetrazine
1120	1220	1710	1088	1180	1740	Methoserpidine
1120	1225	1272	805	1584	938	Amylmetacresol
1120	1230	1680	1175	1610	1038	Vindesine
1120	1279	1594	1493	1097	1252	Ethomoxane
1121	1222	1508	1252	1205	1022	Dehydroemetine
1122	1315	1572	1237	1142	1165	Flunixin
1123	1219	1703	1585	1497	1171	Hexobendine
1123	1230	1575	1505	1616	990	Trimethobenzamide
1123	1520	1732	1337	–	–	Mivacurium Chloride
1124	1220	1087	1208	963	1618	Sulfachlorpyridazine
1125	1260	1138	1595	1650	1070	Sulfisomidine
1126	1630	1596	1235	1650	1565	Trimethoprim
1127	1242	1592	996	1513	834	Mescaline
1130	1092	1267	1247	691	1220	Glymidine Sodium
1130	1515	1587	1612	1639	1315	Ambazone
1130	1527	929	1274	1082	1592	Sulfathiazole
1130	1595	1510	1240	1000	1151	Trimethoxyamfetamine
1131	1642	1229	1110	1592	1001	Trimetozine
1135	1010	1600	1618	1630	720	Homochlorcyclizine
1138	1158	1172	1293	889	1192	Sultiame
1139	1294	1166	1495	1112	812	Diazoxide
1140	1238	1735	1175	1282	1090	Clofibrate
1141	1405	1253	–	–	–	Quazepam
1143	1585	1091	840	1529	1667	Succinylsulfathiazole
1143	1668	1565	1240	1590	1260	Furosemide
1145	1160	1599	1621	685	1306	Sulfamethoxazole
1145	1264	1552	1090	825	1600	Sulfacetamide
1145	1315	1162	1601	1642	1085	Sulfametopyrazine
1145	1595	1304	1635	682	1090	Sulfadimidine
1148	1507	1313	1592	675	1630	Sulfaphenazole
1148	1733	704	1199	735	990	Cyclopentolate
1149	1590	1560	1316	1088	1618	Sulfamerazine
1149	1603	774	962	1164	1289	Resorcinol
1149	1603	1316	1637	1099	1294	Sulfanilamide
1150	1090	757	740	1052	1123	Clopenthixol
1150	1276	1592	1107	685	1633	Dapsone
1150	1310	750	1665	1102	1248	Metopimazine
1151	1180	1125	1052	1300	1525	Hydroflumethiazide
1151	1316	1299	897	1089	1592	Mafenide
1153	1597	1140	1284	1090	925	Sulfametoxydiazine

Wavenumbers cm⁻¹						*Compound*
1155	1248	1724	761	1200	755	Methanthelinium Bromide
1156	719	765	1176	957	747	Tiotixene
1156	1042	1212	720	960	762	Thioproperazine
1157	1305	1595	1090	1123	1620	Chlorothiazide
1158	1177	1597	772	1073	1509	Trichlormethiazide
1158	1317	1590	1020	858	848	Chloroxylenol
1158	1595	715	1063	1515	1300	Methyclothiazide
1159	1045	1718	1176	700	1212	Atropine Methonitrate
1159	1599	1130	1305	1630	1088	Sulfamethoxypyridazine
1160	947	1311	1092	1078	934	Diprenorphine
1160	992	785	1512	1230	1585	Sotalol
1162	1120	1597	1071	1240	1500	Polythiazide
1162	1176	819	1041	746	909	Mefruside
1162	1176	882	702	907	1123	Diclofenamide
1163	1172	1603	1312	781	1510	Ethiazide
1163	1635	1578	1560	975	1525	Xipamide
1164	1599	1042	1508	750	700	Antazoline
1164	1730	1118	1026	1056	1195	Atropine Oxide
1165	817	1629	1200	1282	1239	Harmine
1165	1031	1681	1531	905	1264	Acetohexamide
1165	1116	1070	698	793	1202	Fenfluramine
1165	1316	1105	825	710	920	Tosylchloramide Sodium
1165	1735	710	745	1250	955	Pipotiazine
1166	1633	1598	1092	1647	690	Sulfafurazole
1167	1183	1742	1080	833	1768	Meclofenoxate
1167	1548	1316	1665	671	1115	Acetazolamide
1168	1138	1605	1309	1511	1060	Cyclopenthiazide
1169	1221	1291	1637	1083	1549	Flecainide
1170	770	1290	1620	1700	2850	Biriperone
1170	904	814	1619	1638	–	Nalmefene
1170	1155	1306	1518	1621	750	Bendroflumethiazide
1170	1490	1263	824	1224	1036	Ethoxzolamide
1170	1633	1217	1660	1715	1045	Bromocriptine
1170	1681	1527	837	1302	1592	Phthalylsulfacetamide
1170	1682	1520	1710	1050	1100	Glibornuride
1174	1638	1064	1229	1284	850	Paraquat
1175	1523	1220	840	857	1615	Hexestrol
1175	1538	1582	1510	1307	1274	Stilbazium Iodide
1175	1721	1052	874	1072	709	Hyoscine Butylbromide
1176	1314	1167	1126	1603	1269	Epithiazide
1178	934	861	980	962	773	Busulfan
1178	1605	1229	1672	1575	965	Dyclonine
1180	1160	1310	1502	1620	1590	Benzthiazide
1181	1258	1515	825	746	1119	Dimetridazole
1182	1050	1661	1730	1248	1194	Benorilate
1183	1688	1305	1755	925	1219	Aspirin
1184	1212	1761	1261	1504	931	Moxisylyte
1185	1512	1490	–	–	–	Paroxetine
1185	1620	1075	1762	1580	1290	Tienilic Acid
1187	1535	1070	1265	745	1160	Metronidazole
1188	1012	1032	1120	680	815	Bretylium Tosilate
1188	1604	1260	1028	1676	1003	Pentamidine
1188	1727	1495	1232	1162	1011	Oxyphenisatine
1190	1227	1041	1031	779	823	Clomethiazole
1190	1647	1520	1309	1764	816	Clioxanide
1190	1654	1266	1047	1600	1306	Dibrompropamidine
1190	1658	1730	1608	890	1053	Beclometasone
1192	1715	1163	1101	700	1149	Piperidolate
1195	1225	1582	1627	720	1105	Serotonin
1195	1508	1610	1580	1592	1247	Phentolamine
1195	1590	1672	1250	1562	1052	Amicarbalide
1196	1028	1667	1597	742	1053	Hydroxystilbamidine
1200	1040	770	760	1595	1090	Mexiletine
1200	1218	1168	1760	1150	1122	Acetorphine
1200	1219	1613	1048	1280	1495	Propamidine
1200	1287	1075	1114	1518	1160	Isoetarine
1200	1623	1176	1504	1515	1252	Aminonitrothiazole
1202	1220	1050	805	1185	1294	Butylated Hydroxyanisole
1203	1527	1166	1587	1155	1219	Oxyclozanide
1204	781	806	920	1265	869	Diiodohydroxyquinoline
1204	1219	1754	917	1162	1492	Cyclofenil
1205	1176	833	1250	1512	1610	Diethylstilbestrol
1205	1190	1057	1160	1220	717	Dimetotiazine

Wavenumbers cm⁻¹						Compound
1206	827	1173	1510	1248	775	Dienestrol
1208	1041	1541	1515	1634	1094	DOM
1208	1138	1744	1500	905	1194	Thebacon
1208	1182	1094	–	–	–	Amlodipine
1209	816	1515	741	1176	1105	Cresol
1209	1130	1247	1180	1770	1727	Syrosingopine
1210	1174	1042	1135	760	1010	Thenium Closilate
1210	1192	1520	760	1240	813	Hydroquinone
1210	1231	1155	1069	1610	1042	Terbutaline
1210	1248	1276	1572	1025	1525	Quinuronium Sulfate
1210	1705	1530	1600	1305	1050	Diperodon
1210	1730	1252	755	1008	1162	Pentapiperide Metilsulfate
1210	1755	1075	1105	1160	1250	Alpha Tocoferil Acetate
1210	1760	1163	1070	775	1030	Acetomenaphthone
1211	1170	1156	754	1234	810	Tolnaftate
1212	1198	1754	1162	1500	909	Bisacodyl
1212	1708	712	1112	1132	664	Etomidate
1213	1708	1305	1104	1590	1520	Proxymetacaine
1215	1170	1050	750	1520	790	α-Methyltryptamine
1215	1562	1592	1257	1087	1275	Rafoxanide
1216	1266	1132	1510	1715	1174	Mebeverine
1217	1121	1252	739	1511	1031	Viloxazine
1218	1653	695	1560	1137	1275	Pemoline
1219	1180	1112	1135	1304	696	Desflurane
1220	1120	1700	1240	1720	1265	Reserpine
1220	1611	1210	1583	1135	800	Griseofulvin
1220	1620	1192	1570	1590	1260	Ranitidine
1220	1727	1163	763	1062	1093	Mepenzolate Bromide
1222	701	1061	1008	765	1751	Poldine Metilsulfate
1222	1728	746	1265	1250	1200	Thiopropazate
1224	1005	748	1052	700	770	Hexocyclium Metilsulfate
1224	1010	1059	764	743	1036	Thiazinamium Metilsulfate
1224	1497	1241	705	1613	758	Phenazocine
1225	1044	975	1088	945	1128	Cyclophosphamide
1225	1127	1715	1100	1184	1590	Deserpidine
1225	1719	729	704	1030	1111	Oxyphenonium Bromide
1225	1745	1031	1056	1013	907	Pancuronium Bromide
1226	817	1111	1162	1245	1170	Dichlorophen
1227	1136	1111	1724	1176	1613	Vinblastine
1227	1436	1586	–	–	–	Nizatidine
1227	1739	1015	1250	1101	738	Furazolidone
1228	752	1500	1600	689	1080	Domiphen Bromide
1228	1067	917	1147	1250	1605	Estriol
1228	1499	1534	823	1163	1285	Tiocarlide
1228	1758	1710	1278	1010	1043	Alfadolone
1230	1745	1170	1685	1030	1130	Vincristine
1231	1725	1664	1466	–	–	Moracizine
1232	812	671	1010	1044	724	Methenamine
1232	824	1493	1615	792	1052	Bufotenine
1232	1043	818	1109	1490	710	Chlorphenesin
1233	768	1653	1590	858	726	Bephenium Hydroxynaphthoate
1233	1153	1205	1592	762	1003	Oxypertine
1233	1731	1272	1042	1055	1501	Acetylcodeine
1234	720	1307	1499	813	1093	Thiambutosine
1234	1605	1144	1270	1030	910	Thebaine
1235	1032	1499	925	1075	934	Hydrastinine
1235	1215	1510	1619	1030	1105	Quinine
1236	749	1047	1125	1026	1175	Methoxyphenamine
1237	1306	1580	832	1500	1531	Azathioprine
1238	1264	1609	1214	854	1054	Pentazocine
1238	1495	753	1278	1578	1608	Levorphanol
1238	1724	1646	1219	881	1597	Chlormadinone Acetate
1238	1730	1213	1050	1030	1131	6-Monoacetylmorphine
1240	750	698	1494	1598	1586	Phenoxybenzamine
1240	840	760	1515	708	1185	Octafonium Chloride
1240	1225	1507	1623	1026	1132	Hydroquinine
1240	1505	1120	826	1063	769	Benzethonium Chloride
1240	1735	702	1496	1015	1031	Levacetylmethadol
1242	746	1031	1492	1079	916	Alprenolol
1242	962	900	1786	1852	1002	Cantharidin
1242	1258	1707	1215	1100	772	Fenclofenac
1242	1280	1580	1495	1505	760	Racemorphan

Wavenumbers cm⁻¹						Compound
1242	1667	1744	1718	1203	1610	Desoxycortone
1244	1655	1513	1555	1265	836	Phenacetin
1244	1666	1510	1595	1078	880	Clefamide
1244	1728	940	1230	922	1050	Naloxone
1244	1733	1633	1204	1515	1123	Benzquinamide
1245	760	940	747	1085	1145	Dihydromorphine
1245	1054	1227	1493	1276	821	Estradiol
1245	1491	752	1030	697	1111	Phenyltoloxamine
1245	1624	1635	1600	1185	1501	Etoxazene
1245	1627	1587	1500	1560	1522	Mepacrine
1245	1764	1178	1215	911	1736	Diamorphine
1246	1293	1535	1230	1040	1607	Isoprenaline
1247	731	747	1630	813	1280	Norharman
1247	1198	1748	1499	1143	806	Methylchlorophenoxyacetic Acid
1250	752	758	1670	1626	1587	Salicylamide
1250	1510	1606	1174	813	1184	Chlorotrianisene
1250	1550	1588	1610	1090	1655	Colchicine
1250	1567	976	1098	1064	1650	Rifampicin
1251	1281	1606	1176	1674	1566	Nifursol
1252	1226	1746	1737	1012	1028	Etynodiol Diacetate
1252	1505	1298	1285	1020	1060	Ethinylestradiol
1252	1512	820	1612	1270	869	Hordenine
1253	1274	1500	945	1224	871	Adrenaline
1253	1582	1060	1090	1000	1047	Narceine
1255	761	1208	1733	745	1158	Propantheline Bromide
1255	1060	1035	1612	1291	1241	Mestranol
1255	1510	740	1230	1125	1020	Guaifenesin
1255	1647	1572	1504	757	1163	Mefenamic Acid
1258	750	1500	1120	1092	1037	Oxprenolol
1258	1508	1637	1142	1724	1220	Propanidid
1258	1513	1274	1590	1610	810	Pholedrine
1258	1514	1619	1040	860	820	Quinidine
1258	1689	1235	933	1016	1500	Alclofenac
1259	1517	1599	1102	813	1111	Hydroxyamfetamine
1260	1154	1646	750	678	1120	Saccharin
1260	1598	1637	1211	1613	920	Mexenone
1263	1249	1733	1662	1712	1630	Megestrol Acetate
1263	1304	1216	1591	1136	1063	Metaraminol
1263	1706	1106	713	698	1067	Benzyl Benzoate
1264	740	1620	1597	1152	1197	Dantron
1264	1515	1116	1229	1213	1616	Cephaëline
1265	1293	1216	1200	1066	1137	Noradrenaline
1265	1298	1204	752	985	790	Apomorphine
1266	1147	1124	1165	1233	1715	Rescinnamine
1266	1518	1595	822	1495	1612	Tyramine
1266	1600	1779	1692	1176	1120	Procaine Benzylpenicillin
1267	1193	1492	1147	966	913	Disulfiram
1267	1547	1706	1238	1020	966	Fusidic Acid
1269	825	1209	818	889	1104	Fenticlor
1269	1130	1233	1575	1249	1303	Butorphanol
1270	1085	1111	1136	1234	1035	Veratrine
1270	1490	1198	1142	968	915	Sulfiram
1270	1718	1105	710	1068	1022	Hexylcaine
1272	1734	1102	1593	1025	718	Inositol Nicotinate
1273	1595	1681	1630	1111	1163	Butyl Aminobenzoate
1274	1040	1502	1017	763	1056	Benzylmorphine
1275	1165	1598	1694	1639	1111	Butacaine
1275	1500	1118	1050	1250	782	Neopine
1275	1720	1618	717	1116	1316	Benzoylecgonine
1276	1165	1220	1317	1665	1600	Propyl Hydroxybenzoate
1276	1182	737	1139	960	1213	Hexachlorophene
1277	1212	1015	1540	870	1086	Pyridoxine
1278	1703	711	1115	1310	1040	Piperocaine
1278	1724	1108	740	699	1587	Benzyl Nicotinate
1279	1508	1263	1026	1292	1238	Papaverine
1280	1220	1160	1250	760	780	Fazadinium Bromide
1280	1250	1055	1099	801	1124	Clorgiline
1280	1650	1635	852	1090	968	Isosorbide Mononitrate
1280	1680	1598	1170	1315	1634	Benzocaine
1281	751	1718	1306	1075	1103	Nicergoline
1282	820	1709	1244	921	1493	Estrone
1282	990	1010	1587	1612	1204	Doxorubicin

Wavenumbers cm^{-1}						*Compound*
1282	1718	1111	741	1022	703	Methyl Nicotinate
1282	1724	1111	740	1020	1587	Butoxyethyl Nicotinate
1284	1601	1042	1238	1575	702	Tramadol
1285	1650	714	1587	690	1610	Phytomenadione
1286	1724	1110	740	1591	1025	Ethyl Nicotinate
1290	1673	1170	1240	1610	1590	Ethyl Hydroxybenzoate
1290	1680	1565	1270	687	772	Salinazid
1299	1256	1064	1208	1129	676	Pentolonium Tartrate
1300	744	1710	1042	694	1180	Nicotinic Acid
1301	1638	1595	1510	805	1180	Aminosalicylic Acid
1307	774	1222	711	1196	1553	Pentachlorophenol
1308	1261	1210	1136	1063	675	Pempidine
1312	790	1258	1066	1275	1030	Normorphine
1314	1176	1709	1215	818	740	Aminitrozole
1315	1063	1136	833	1204	1234	Methoxyflurane
1316	1190	930	806	1258	782	Broxyquinoline
1317	1150	1665	1170	1110	1595	Trifluperidol
1318	1180	1150	1168	1602	1060	Hydrochlorothiazide
1319	1295	622	594	–	–	Methyl Bromide
1320	1077	1503	1155	1120	947	Buprenorphine
1330	1260	1165	755	–	–	Amosulalol
1335	1240	1110	–	–	–	Fluoxetine
1353	1541	809	719	1263	1609	Chloronitrotoluene
1406	1038	850	967	1166	1271	Chlorpyrifos
1414	774	640	–	–	–	Clenbuterol
1429	1048	583	–	–	–	Androstenediol Diacetate
1449	1372	1054	942	–	–	Methandriol Dipropionate
1456	1157	1038	775	–	–	Pergolide
1457	971	717	–	–	–	Ticlopidine
1459	1621	1713	1086	–	–	Ofloxacin
1461	1202	748	–	–	–	Propofol
1470	1135	825	800	790	760	Sertraline
1477	1202	984	914	–	–	Ditiocarb
1490	762	1240	1230	741	749	Trimipramine
1490	1257	1038	1504	799	1188	Methylenedioxyamfetamine
1490	1610	697	1316	1540	827	Alprazolam
1492	1250	1271	1227	1036	1128	Protokylol
1492	1512	1598	1247	1175	1035	Mepyramine
1492	1631	1092	698	1010	1600	Fenpiprane
1494	1598	769	1562	1010	1098	Chloropyramine
1495	1271	1040	1250	1055	1149	Dihydrocodeine
1495	1592	1283	1650	1030	757	Alcuronium Chloride
1495	1637	688	750	1665	1050	Amiphenazole
1495	1694	770	1136	1562	1587	Butanilicaine
1496	1219	1022	1276	1179	1050	Methoxamine
1496	1242	1040	1300	1280	1070	Dextromethorphan
1496	1592	770	1250	955	735	Tripelennamine
1497	740	698	1028	1125	1220	Benzfetamine
1497	1527	1120	1230	1590	1620	Timolol
1499	1203	823	–	–	–	Cisapride
1500	1138	1225	1315	1157	825	Penfluridol
1500	1340	1255	1165	–	–	Tamsulosin
1500	1529	1280	1265	1052	1600	Ethylnoradrenaline
1500	1660	1280	1195	1120	1212	Brucine
1500	1665	1593	1195	1570	1265	Benserazide
1503	1287	1190	1174	813	1115	Dopamine
1503	1497	1316	1603	1089	1517	Amantadine
1504	1247	1208	1145	1225	865	Dimoxyline
1504	1277	1307	1189	1149	1565	Nitroxoline
1505	748	1600	693	1279	755	Thenalidine
1505	1121	1155	1304	805	945	Nalorphine
1505	1271	1234	1030	1587	1098	Berberine
1505	1645	1220	1155	835	775	Lidoflazine
1506	1217	738	–	–	–	Astemizole
1506	1657	1565	1263	1227	1612	Paracetamol
1507	1279	1144	680	1620	966	Fluconazole
1507	1640	1240	1258	1200	1221	Ketoconazole
1507	1729	1594	1132	1282	–	Linuron
1508	1560	1295	1587	747	1083	Clofazimine
1508	1580	1101	903	1681	1248	Carbarsone
1509	779	709	1282	1219	1190	Hydroxyquinoline
1509	1261	1620	1234	854	1030	Hydroquinidine
1510	1209	1256	1610	833	1170	Ritodrine
1510	1220	1265	1280	1125	1240	Metocurine Iodide
1510	1230	1118	1210	824	1635	Pramocaine
1510	1245	1108	1028	1175	810	Metoprolol
1510	1253	1026	1232	1149	1587	Verapamil
1510	1592	1171	1299	809	1217	Prometryne
1512	1220	750	695	1182	837	Buphenine
1512	1259	1033	808	1190	1623	Methoxyamfetamine
1512	1282	812	1200	950	785	Halquinol
1513	1243	1179	–	–	–	Venlafaxine
1513	1604	750	698	1500	732	Histapyrrodine
1513	1664	1080	1050	1302	1250	Clindamycin
1514	1240	745	1220	1043	1500	Isoxsuprine
1514	1256	1228	1110	1200	1150	Emetine
1515	1249	1091	1053	3250	830	Betaxolol
1515	1593	1550	1250	1613	1175	Thonzylamine
1515	1595	1294	1166	806	1140	Ametryne
1515	1603	1580	1661	1250	1305	Thioacetazone
1516	1228	1120	1280	1265	1165	Tubocurarine Chloride
1517	1599	1640	750	1700	692	Warfarin
1518	1242	1213	1099	840	772	Prenalterol
1520	1280	1266	1190	1200	1220	Dobutamine
1520	1562	1620	1600	1128	1290	Chlorproguanil
1520	1587	1215	806	1266	1133	Terbutryne
1522	1498	1140	1166	1097	1632	Diquat
1524	1160	1623	1718	1276	823	Glibenclamide
1524	1180	1298	1147	1573	770	Piroxicam
1524	1577	1209	1025	1147	1258	Metallibure
1526	1214	1010	1076	1041	1251	Dipyridamole
1527	835	1574	1495	1624	1095	Baclofen
1527	1387	1051	–	–	–	Altretamine
1527	1628	1575	1235	820	1080	Chlorhexidine
1527	1672	1612	738	1595	1289	Dinitolmide
1527	1726	1516	1290	1240	1215	Methyldopate
1528	1690	1650	1159	1032	900	Glipizide
1529	1162	1250	1037	1290	1123	Normetadrenaline
1529	1245	1123	730	1309	1600	Nitroxinil
1529	1537	896	1622	1153	1614	Heptaminol
1530	1300	1230	1275	1580	1715	Acetylcysteine
1530	1634	1666	1562	1587	1149	Buformin
1531	1587	1258	806	1292	1163	Desmetryne
1532	1142	1084	1710	1585	1560	Phthalylsulfathiazole
1534	1635	1492	1575	1600	1170	Proguanil
1535	1115	1250	1000	900	800	Pentetrazol
1538	811	1304	1121	1272	1175	Methoprotryne
1538	1504	753	1618	762	1095	Clopidol
1538	1600	1266	1277	1160	1117	Rimantadine
1538	1613	1098	1319	1258	1203	Aminocaproic Acid
1539	1612	1295	804	1161	1121	Atrazine
1543	898	1190	1590	1201	1506	Buclosamide
1544	1575	1641	1715	1235	1070	Riboflavin
1549	1134	699	1084	1152	1600	Sulfamethizole
1550	1005	1616	1602	1647	882	Sorbic Acid
1550	1596	1680	719	704	757	Denatonium Benzoate
1553	1621	1289	797	1103	1129	Simazine
1558	1042	1230	987	1026	1517	Noxytiolin
1559	1648	1690	1298	1270	925	Secobarbital
1562	1225	696	1211	1268	1248	Fenoprofen
1562	1642	1715	1289	1261	1210	Carbenoxolone
1563	864	1613	1212	1105	1067	Thiethylperazine
1563	1316	1647	775	928	1044	Ametazole
1565	815	1535	1255	869	847	Amodiaquine
1565	1508	1600	1120	1173	923	Cadaverine
1566	1650	863	1615	1190	740	Methysergide
1568	1537	1590	1625	1650	1500	Phenformin
1570	1255	1304	754	1227	1241	Cyclazocine
1570	1271	740	1250	765	675	Thiamazole
1571	1496	1173	1323	–	–	Propazine
1572	756	1504	775	1286	1308	Diclofenac
1572	1079	1263	1234	763	1511	Bunamidine
1572	1515	1613	1285	1650	1218	Niclosamide
1573	1538	1612	1155	800	870	Chloroquine
1574	1275	740	1246	1150	767	Carbimazole
1574	1610	1584	1536	761	822	Triamterene

Wavenumbers cm⁻¹						Compound
1575	1590	1234	752	702	1267	Profadol
1576	1631	1499	1155	1115	751	Quinisocaine
1577	756	1212	1703	1124	1274	Pizotifen
1577	1550	1526	1620	934	877	Cycloserine
1579	1608	1530	1050	1150	810	Hydroxychloroquine
1580	708	795	1225	1205	1300	Meptazinol
1580	877	741	1000	708	775	Nomifensine
1580	1030	1620	1180	1080	1260	Δ^8-Tetrahydrocannabinol
1580	1040	1620	1180	1130	1050	Δ^9-Tetrahydrocannabinol
1580	1159	1494	682	940	797	Sulfadiazine
1580	1270	1175	1030	1205	752	Levomepromazine
1580	1490	1650	1620	1065	1103	Methylergometrine
1580	1613	1660	1244	1220	1040	Doxycycline
1580	1620	1063	1075	935	740	Metformin
1582	873	990	730	1029	1081	Perhexiline
1583	1161	1596	1315	1091	1305	Sulfadoxine
1584	690	860	870	990	1010	Pheniramine
1584	745	660	1278	1190	765	Aminopromazine
1584	1298	1462	1081	–	–	Rabeprazole
1585	750	1003	1067	1565	1040	Brompheniramine
1585	1020	1050	1100	1082	115	Cyclopentamine
1585	1086	746	1010	830	1562	Chlorphenamine
1585	1264	1127	1078	1639	950	Sulfapyridine
1585	1305	1252	1131	1605	1070	Floctafenine
1585	1557	1666	1204	751	1298	Carfenazine
1585	1560	1290	762	1238	1145	Betahistine
1585	1630	1020	1210	1240	1050	Cannabidiol
1585	1656	762	685	1248	1493	Phenazopyridine
1587	1079	1228	1259	1575	1022	Gloxazone
1587	1560	760	1275	958	1493	Zomepirac
1587	1575	1197	699	1150	1248	Levamisole
1587	1669	775	1236	1222	1152	Azaperone
1587	1724	1176	1515	699	1041	Choline Salicylate
1588	808	865	1275	1140	880	Ethionamide
1588	1620	1208	1082	1160	1503	Cimetidine
1589	1742	1202	1192	1229	1245	Captopril
1590	1111	1245	1505	700	1170	Clomifene
1590	1147	1090	1314	685	1066	Sulfadimethoxine
1590	1220	1722	1050	1308	743	Suprofen
1590	1493	1277	1170	1122	1041	Pantoprazole
1590	1603	1564	1109	1188	1248	Loxapine
1590	1614	1530	1496	1254	1311	Metoclopramide
1590	1640	1500	1133	1270	1695	Azapropazone
1592	765	1558	1250	1158	1316	Methapyrilene
1592	787	758	1308	691	1015	Lysergic Acid
1592	955	870	1080	1055	1115	Piperazine
1592	1167	1141	1081	1058	–	Tilmicosin
1592	1618	1294	1188	1500	1513	Pyrvinium Embonate
1594	1273	784	696	1304	900	Phenylephrine
1594	1437	1247	–	–	–	Terazosin
1595	767	990	1562	1149	1234	Chloropyrilene
1595	1199	1285	1250	1070	765	Oxymetazoline
1595	1238	1500	760	1060	925	Dropropizine
1595	1525	1615	1550	1090	1055	Penicillamine
1595	1650	1114	914	1313	1248	Methylprednisolone
1595	1698	1240	1625	1111	1315	Chloroprocaine
1596	1153	1168	1307	1500	1075	Cyclothiazide
1596	1570	1548	1295	757	1234	Clotiapine
1597	766	1242	976	1159	1311	Thenyldiamine
1597	1068	797	1305	1279	1222	Etilefrine
1597	1168	1290	1665	1305	1625	Aminobenzoic Acid
1597	1198	1562	1220	1745	760	Aloxiprin
1597	1470	1062	843	–	–	Danazol
1597	1548	1300	702	1230	830	Clorazepic Acid
1598	1278	1615	1222	1168	1635	Dithranol
1598	1492	1238	3366	873	–	Alfuzosin
1598	1620	1765	1495	1659	771	Cloxacillin
1598	1643	1540	766	1236	1574	Cinchocaine
1600	700	830	765	964	986	Loperamide
1600	742	1293	1250	763	1500	Tetryzoline
1600	1225	1510	850	1713	1108	Dantrolene
1600	1286	1174	1688	1126	1532	Tetracaine
1600	1288	1261	1530	1123	1219	Methyldopa

Wavenumbers cm⁻¹						Compound
1600	1511	1634	1305	1200	1538	Methotrexate
1600	1512	1639	1297	1545	1570	Procainamide
1600	1560	758	1136	1101	1117	Clozapine
1600	1575	1410	765	–	–	Quetiapine
1600	1634	1501	1307	1205	1235	Clomocycline
1600	1645	1525	1225	1310	1050	Minocycline
1600	1650	1160	960	1510	1040	Quinethazone
1600	1757	1669	1224	1314	750	Propicillin
1600	1759	1409	1064	–	–	Fosinopril
1600	1764	1656	1538	715	1143	Cefaloridine
1602	1031	1074	1548	1122	857	Bromhexine
1602	1253	1298	871	1237	800	Xylometazoline
1603	1098	1381	1222	–	–	Cerivastatin
1603	1643	1293	1125	1252	1540	Prazosin
1603	1767	1622	1495	1660	794	Flucloxacillin
1604	1592	752	1181	1246	1107	Amoxapine
1605	1086	1490	1655	1505	1300	Cotarnine
1605	1232	1090	1218	1546	1156	Dinitro-orthocresol
1605	1278	1246	1670	1210	1700	Propoxycaine
1605	1493	1097	1673	1040	826	Metisazone
1605	1510	700	1160	1575	1200	Fenoterol
1605	1589	1500	749	702	–	Donepezil
1605	1625	1125	1160	1218	1263	Proflavine Hemisulfate
1605	1626	1127	1145	1276	1094	Sulfamoxole
1607	1325	1423	–	–	–	Tenoxicam
1607	1766	1673	1500	1093	1260	Meticillin
1608	820	767	1310	1210	995	Midazolam
1608	1180	1493	1250	1535	1320	Liothyronine
1608	1270	1585	1240	1300	1543	Etamivan
1608	1296	721	1580	690	775	Tolazoline
1608	1314	1292	772	706	1111	Etisazole
1608	1575	1537	1136	769	1100	Dihydralazine
1609	690	1217	1495	934	1280	Edrophonium Chloride
1610	1178	1298	700	1255	815	Medazepam
1610	1220	1570	1010	865	780	Mercaptopurine
1610	1445	1240	1095	780	–	Lofexidine
1610	1635	1588	1171	1267	1198	Diminazene
1610	1660	1165	1145	962	1012	Metolazone
1610	1778	1510	1238	1690	752	Pheneticillin
1611	1595	815	1230	1572	1170	Primaquine
1612	1204	1219	1306	1157	935	Oxymetholone
1612	1234	1515	980	1052	1176	Bufexamac
1612	1580	1660	1226	1248	1530	Tetracycline
1612	1754	1315	1123	1030	1000	Carbenicillin
1613	1524	700	768	1058	752	Fenyramidol
1613	1585	1164	1314	1085	1099	Xylazine
1613	1704	809	1250	1225	1515	Nalidixic Acid
1614	1090	1650	1583	750	715	Debrisoquine
1614	1488	1429	1404	–	–	Lamotrigine
1615	762	740	1685	1250	1570	Coumatetralyl
1615	780	1499	791	1211	800	Naphazoline
1615	1570	1450	1210	825	–	Mitoxantrone
1615	1575	1658	1224	1258	1206	Methacycline
1615	1642	1515	1250	1562	1298	Pyritidium Bromide
1616	1573	1660	1190	1298	1315	Demeclocycline
1616	1584	1665	1235	1180	1138	Oxytetracycline Dihydrate
1618	756	1577	1135	1293	1176	Benziodarone
1618	1258	1217	1712	1105	1149	Diethylcarbamazine
1618	1684	695	712	702	764	Fenpipramide
1619	1535	1215	1169	1035	–	Indinavir
1620	1050	1580	1030	1120	1228	Cannabinol
1620	1129	1230	1537	1075	1176	Sulfaguanidine
1620	1630	1540	1560	740	1317	Indoramin Hydrochloride form II
1620	1777	1500	1310	1700	703	Benzylpenicillin
1621	1513	1186	1160	1250	1205	Melphalan
1621	1757	1537	1157	3000	–	Ceftazidime
1622	1580	1666	1311	1041	1227	Chlortetracycline
1623	703	1107	717	858	1002	Dextromoramide
1624	1602	1284	1244	–	–	Nemonapride
1625	760	1260	690	1590	850	Chlordiazepoxide
1625	1121	1260	1525	1290	875	Carbidopa
1625	1520	1547	698	670	1600	Nialamide

Wavenumbers *cm^{-1}*						*Compound*
1625	1668	1257	1539	1231	971	Tioguanine
1626	1219	1003	1266	923	892	Pipobroman
1626	1307	1136	1066	1212	749	Lysergide
1626	1577	1319	1305	1148	955	Morantel
1626	1600	1274	1093	1100	1193	Parbendazole
1627	910	965	1030	1136	1063	Decamethonium Bromide
1627	1601	709	1266	761	1070	Tropicamide
1628	1195	1562	1265	1149	1041	Desferrioxamine
1628	1205	1015	–	–	–	Omeprazole
1628	1492	1260	1312	836	1077	Homidium Bromide
1628	1575	1640	1075	835	805	Pyrimethamine
1628	1585	1308	1185	1240	1148	Levothyroxine
1628	1610	1045	1182	1192	1518	Loprazolam
1629	1035	1064	1520	1282	1250	Dexpanthenol
1629	1284	794	1305	1581	1095	Diethyltoluamide
1630	748	1245	1558	1170	998	Amiodarone
1630	1111	1174	701	1192	1066	Bethanidine
1630	1610	1537	–	–	–	Entacapone
1630	1645	1598	1250	1510	1570	Diaveridine
1631	1590	1171	1181	1316	1242	Acriflavinium Chloride
1631	1712	750	1208	1136	1160	Ergotamine
1632	1555	1661	1301	861	1176	Procarbazine
1633	1121	1718	1255	759	1272	Flavoxate
1633	1245	1510	1184	805	820	Atenolol
1633	1662	1720	1705	1558	768	Co-dergocrine Mesilate
1634	754	748	1044	1212	1541	Ergometrine
1634	1233	753	1276	1114	1587	Etenzamide
1634	1587	1550	820	1089	1232	Triclocarban
1634	1602	1504	1686	1238	1538	Amiloride
1635	1260	1590	1730	1230	705	Mebendazole
1635	1305	1264	805	1069	1047	Sodium Cromoglicate
1635	1590	1291	1103	1316	712	Nikethamide
1636	1568	1225	1100	–	–	Trenbolone
1636	1620	953	1075	1040	860	Choline
1637	1278	1602	1081	699	1136	Dimefline
1637	1402	1511	1136	–	–	Zolpidem
1638	698	752	1610	1500	1070	Imolamine
1638	1522	1593	787	1562	1149	Amprolium Hydrochloride
1638	1535	1290	781	–	–	Famotidine
1639	751	1603	694	1492	1170	Butalamine
1639	775	761	1603	1250	1316	Dibenzepin
1639	1047	1534	1595	1211	971	Aminotriazole
1639	1052	1612	1086	1265	1694	Desonide
1639	1509	1527	1696	1600	1259	Acecainide
1639	1536	1460	1285	1158	1040	Nelfinavir
1639	1592	1111	1492	812	758	Hydroxycarbamide
1639	1721	758	1534	1212	1294	Ergotoxine
1640	696	736	1558	1275	1290	Beclamide
1640	1041	633	–	–	–	Aztreonam
1640	1203	896	–	–	–	Nitrendipine
1640	1535	1316	745	1575	715	Indoramin Hydrochloride form I
1640	1605	1305	1208	1132	1065	Pyrantel
1640	1610	1550	1231	1210	758	Minoxidil
1640	1685	1118	755	712	1255	Dimenhydrinate
1640	1702	1610	1232	1042	1115	Hydrocortisone
1642	1497	1234	1515	822	1019	Practolol
1645	756	707	1219	1101	1068	Oxetacaine
1645	1170	1564	1198	850	1240	Methylthiouracil
1646	1482	1590	772	735	819	Metaclazepam
1646	1490	1064	–	–	–	Zalcitabine
1646	1520	1256	1300	1046	815	Phenacaine
1647	1379	1041	–	–	–	Ganciclovir
1647	1485	1210	–	–	–	Nisoldipine
1647	1562	1117	1241	1274	1520	Levodopa
1648	1225	1702	1491	–	–	Isradipine
1648	1670	1588	1511	1302	1495	Nifenazone
1649	716	1094	1298	1153	1016	Lorcainide
1649	1068	1617	689	1272	660	Norethisterone
1650	986	1020	999	1062	1075	Aldosterone
1650	1150	1130	1315	880	1090	Chlormezanone
1650	1263	1612	1210	894	1185	Norethandrolone
1650	1280	1255	1302	1720	1180	Ketotifen

Wavenumbers *cm^{-1}*						*Compound*
1650	1520	765	1235	1272	1180	Etidocaine
1650	1523	760	1220	1123	1265	Mepivacaine
1650	1540	1565	1140	790	1311	Cytisine
1650	1576	705	769	757	1500	Isopropamide Iodide
1650	1590	765	1496	774	1176	Tacrine
1650	1618	1131	1590	1500	750	Propyphenazone
1650	1698	1538	729	1041	1205	Bamifylline
1651	1271	1714	1736	1246	1041	Fludrocortisone
1652	1248	1037	1595	1562	1063	Embutramide
1652	1700	1548	1220	760	750	Pentifylline
1653	1242	1718	816	1220	1495	Fluorouracil
1653	1508	1529	1238	1136	1597	Diamfenetide
1653	1541	1621	676	992	845	Isoniazid
1653	1548	1118	618	–	–	Bleomycin
1653	1600	768	1560	754	1730	Ethyl Biscoumacetate
1653	1610	778	795	1295	1568	Clonidine
1654	867	1036	1247	926	1282	Fluoxymesterone
1654	1400	1055	–	–	–	Boldenone Acetate
1654	1612	1708	887	1112	1085	Prednisolone
1655	1104	1075	1564	1040	1262	Lincomycin
1655	1570	1388	741	732	–	Lisinopril
1655	1600	1290	1210	1125	1075	Metenolone
1655	1617	1234	1098	1282	1123	Crotetamide
1655	1699	1755	1275	1205	815	Metharbital
1656	759	696	1613	1163	1113	Phenprocoumon
1656	767	1587	1562	1315	1298	Dichloralphenazone
1656	1513	1176	1250	1026	820	Ambucetamide
1656	1623	1235	1280	1316	1590	Crotamiton
1656	1690	750	1538	763	1282	Proxyphylline
1656	1693	1284	714	690	1226	Ketoprofen
1656	1706	748	1543	1220	1600	Etamiphylline
1656	1737	1227	705	1201	1211	Oxyphencyclimine
1656	1739	1605	758	1111	1153	Chlorquinaldol
1657	1517	1592	1378	1348	1038	Mifepristone
1658	1157	1552	668	1090	905	Tolbutamide
1658	1163	1622	1722	1176	1747	Fluocortolone
1658	1227	1600	905	1745	1034	Paramethasone
1658	1276	716	–	–	–	Boldenone Undecylenate
1658	1563	1193	1625	1166	1241	Propylthiouracil
1658	1605	1275	876	1281	1241	Dimethisterone
1658	1695	1548	763	750	1029	Xantinol Nicotinate
1658	1698	747	1548	1242	760	Caffeine
1659	1278	1370	–	–	–	Atovaquone
1660	701	1493	1263	1273	1236	Fentanyl
1660	770	1318	1305	1590	1580	Phenazone
1660	871	1615	1057	1236	1066	Testosterone
1660	1059	1630	750	699	1115	Styramate
1660	1060	1235	1612	1127	723	Ethisterone
1660	1060	1730	1080	1250	1175	Halcinonide
1660	1090	716	1618	1170	970	Phenacemide
1660	1153	1267	735	1590	1300	Vanillin
1660	1160	1239	950	1612	1090	Methyltestosterone
1660	1210	1712	1053	1140	768	Dihydroergotamine
1660	1315	1126	750	700	1620	Aminophenazone
1660	1497	1575	1070	1150	1220	Cyanocobalamin
1660	1598	752	1538	1315	1500	Acetanilide
1660	1617	1606	1710	1056	907	Betamethasone
1660	1618	1048	1237	1595	1228	Thiamine
1660	1620	886	1601	1160	1240	Methandienone
1660	1622	1697	1581	1232	1197	Dydrogesterone
1660	1685	1600	1239	1157	1212	Pipamperone
1660	1693	1085	1310	750	869	Methyprylon
1660	1700	1039	747	1562	1234	Diprophylline
1660	1700	1720	1550	762	752	Pentoxifylline
1661	1147	1599	1089	1635	1310	Carbutamide
1661	1159	1553	757	1086	909	Chlorpropamide
1661	1172	1234	1149	978	1613	Clorexolone
1661	1400	1204	1470	1300	1078	Mexazolam
1662	1159	1725	1619	1605	1285	Fluocortolone
1662	1495	762	1204	1290	1086	Lidocaine
1662	1614	1700	872	1209	1232	Progesterone
1662	1705	1496	700	765	1120	Primidone
1663	896	1622	1695	1052	1603	Dexamethasone

Wavenumbers cm⁻¹						Compound
1663	1057	1618	1609	902	1080	Triamcinolone
1663	1172	1038	1532	1285	928	Clopamide
1664	764	1050	1110	1282	775	Strychnine
1664	1585	697	1163	1562	760	Disopyramide
1664	1623	901	1733	1139	1160	Flumetasone
1664	1705	1600	1546	746	1219	Fenetylline
1665	790	1582	1000	810	1175	Hydralazine
1665	1060	1050	1320	1205	1180	Trilostane
1665	1245	1525	1495	1217	1285	Acebutolol
1665	1703	1318	1300	1278	1593	Pirenzepine
1665	1712	1636	1562	740	1180	Bufylline
1666	1086	1052	1063	1724	1639	Fluclorolone Acetonide
1666	1250	1123	724	–	–	Oxalic Acid
1666	1574	590	–	–	–	Milrinone
1666	1612	1724	884	1063	1010	Clobetasol Propionate
1667	1036	1117	1020	810	1239	Fluoroacetamide
1667	1101	1499	1125	1002	1019	Morinamide
1667	1248	1119	1215	1010	1080	Methocarbamol
1667	1259	1096	1605	1289	1070	Idoxuridine
1667	1316	740	694	1602	704	Prazepam
1667	1505	1246	1039	2932	2867	Cilostazol
1667	1522	1279	1222	787	944	Bupivacaine
1667	1626	1590	1302	797	1289	Tramazoline
1668	1541	1731	1170	1318	1291	Thiamylal
1668	1707	904	1622	1610	1246	Prednisone
1669	701	757	1087	1190	1592	Piritramide
1669	1074	1629	910	1056	1615	Fluocinolone Acetonide
1670	750	705	870	815	1595	Isocarboxazid
1670	760	783	1618	1158	1270	Lysergamide
1670	1220	1265	1587	746	1149	Acetophenazine
1670	1240	1730	1750	1070	1635	Fluocinonide
1670	1270	1590	755	1500	1575	Tolfenamic Acid
1670	1540	1300	1170	1735	1220	Thiopental
1670	1626	760	1538	1592	1298	Dofamium Chloride
1670	1658	1198	1173	–	–	Saquinavir
1670	1717	1567	745	980	1190	Theophylline
1672	1064	1179	1163	1208	1639	Dipyrone
1672	1134	1652	1050	765	1243	Guanoclor
1672	1578	1255	714	699	970	Metyrapone
1672	1613	1316	1211	1171	1100	Flurazepam
1672	1700	1093	694	1176	1615	Pheneturide
1673	1515	1628	1570	760	1224	Cycloguanil
1673	1761	1718	1237	1292	1303	Heptabarb
1674	1636	823	591	–	–	Celiprolol
1675	749	1279	1193	1163	1143	Butaperazine
1675	820	1105	1195	1308	1242	Ketazolam
1675	1084	–	–	–	–	Zidovudine
1675	1220	1265	1587	746	1562	Acepromazine
1675	1222	1269	1592	748	1560	Piperacetazine
1675	1242	1500	1615	1298	765	Fendosal
1675	1505	767	806	1136	1190	Ambenonium Chloride
1675	1540	765	1128	772	1240	Tocainide
1675	1701	1059	1045	1095	1079	Fludroxycortide
1675	1760	1317	1303	1230	853	Secbutabarbital
1675	1760	1725	1234	1282	1298	Vinbarbital
1676	1638	1548	1230	1516	1211	Flucytosine
1676	1704	1092	1620	1185	750	Apronal
1678	690	1240	1265	755	717	Demoxepam
1678	1197	1093	1290	1727	1167	Diloxanide
1678	1594	800	769	787	1298	Carbamazepine
1678	1602	825	1132	1310	800	Tetrazepam
1679	1733	1205	1178	1255	692	Nandrolone
1680	700	1602	820	738	790	Nordazepam
1680	705	1310	1220	760	1255	Methyl Salicylate
1680	1277	1730	860	1160	1145	Bemegride
1680	1510	730	1300	1220	1605	Indoprofen
1680	1643	1502	1270	820	1250	Labetalol
1680	1698	703	1618	1594	1026	Nicotinamide
1680	1709	1316	1193	1253	1040	Methohexital
1680	1718	1193	1318	1110	703	Camazepam
1680	1720	1767	1320	1245	875	Barbital
1681	727	1205	1250	1316	1110	Thalidomide
1681	847	1072	1515	816	1562	Chloramphenicol
1681	1228	1218	1706	1299	1065	Indometacin
1681	1313	705	840	1125	740	Diazepam
1682	1070	1710	1601	1140	788	Mebutamate
1682	1153	1121	1315	1610	843	Lormetazepam
1682	1512	1252	1033	–	–	Diltiazem
1682	1599	1565	770	1265	697	Methaqualone
1682	1605	768	782	1282	1583	Mecloqualone
1683	753	710	1253	696	764	Doxapram
1683	1156	1285	1307	1125	1180	Probenecid
1683	1492	1248	1220	1150	978	Diflunisal
1683	1736	1275	1512	765	1600	Oxyphenbutazone
1684	1664	704	1490	764	845	Clobazam
1685	825	750	802	1315	1230	Bromazepam
1685	1020	1600	1584	1050	1165	Pyrazinamide
1685	1033	1160	845	1190	1310	Chlortalidone
1685	1149	1317	1120	1605	826	Lorazepam
1685	1610	748	1255	1578	1532	Clonazepam
1685	1610	1300	1130	1270	1000	Thialbarbital
1685	1705	1595	1230	752	1156	Droperidol
1685	1719	1744	1315	1218	845	Pentobarbital
1686	1275	1637	1111	695	751	Phensuximide
1686	1602	1636	1191	1567	1225	Folic Acid
1686	1616	1508	1070	762	1570	Acenocoumarol
1686	1710	1200	1270	1281	704	Glutethimide
1687	700	1211	1115	1052	769	Lobeline
1687	1315	925	1219	847	1640	Allobarbital
1687	1670	1112	1603	705	1150	Temazepam
1687	1706	693	830	1136	1123	Oxazepam
1688	1069	1090	1590	1310	1140	Meprobamate
1688	1210	1200	1223	1134	1179	Ecgonine
1688	1636	1215	1588	1150	1607	Repaglinide
1689	1232	1270	857	1606	1149	Methallenestril
1689	1337	1098	–	–	–	Nimodipine
1689	1718	1550	1640	1285	672	Enallylpropymal
1690	1088	1064	700	1605	1623	Phenprobamate
1690	1205	1170	1310	1620	1270	Salsalate
1690	1225	1527	1120	1496	1310	Nifedipine
1690	1235	1497	1598	1155	750	Fluanisone
1690	1274	1605	1174	1116	772	Procaine
1690	1515	1370	1250	–	–	Formoterol
1690	1610	698	1536	745	784	Nitrazepam
1690	1610	1041	1170	1150	1010	Emylcamate
1690	1640	1602	835	665	880	Muzolimine
1690	1665	1221	1550	1595	680	Theobromine
1690	1720	1740	1310	1290	1200	Butalbital
1691	705	1245	1469	–	–	Methcathinone
1691	1113	1342	1346	1237	1458	Metolachlor
1692	1587	916	1224	1235	956	Allopurinol
1692	1730	1750	1318	1220	1630	Vinylbital
1693	1614	1082	–	–	–	Felbamate
1693	1720	1745	1316	1255	860	Aprobarbital
1693	1725	1745	1300	1210	830	Cyclobarbital
1694	660	1600	1094	1212	834	Carbromal
1694	729	1162	1282	1298	934	Etebenecid
1694	757	1587	1162	1204	1219	Benperidol
1694	1149	1587	1086	1612	684	Sulfacarbamide
1694	1176	884	819	675	1086	Tolazamide
1694	1260	1520	1155	1140	1222	Tetrabenazine
1695	1148	1220	1267	1000	1252	Alfaxalone
1695	1185	1200	1515	1623	1267	Aminoglutethimide
1695	1215	1199	1153	1587	1280	Bumetanide
1695	1250	1065	1538	1600	1140	Tybamate
1695	1505	753	1220	1230	825	Pimozide
1695	1520	1229	1610	1175	1270	Chlorambucil
1695	1527	1075	1246	1101	1319	Carisoprodol
1695	1543	766	754	1299	1258	Prilocaine
1695	1613	1497	1263	1205	1558	Decoquinate
1695	1720	1190	1200	1390	1350	Bambuterol
1695	1752	1265	833	1205	775	Nealbarbital
1696	747	1142	1120	712	1027	Ketamine
1696	1260	1020	–	–	–	Nabumetone
1696	1619	1574	1260	1100	1038	Nabilone
1696	1727	1760	1242	850	1215	Butobarbital

Wavenumbers cm⁻¹						*Compound*
1696	1728	1755	835	1290	1207	Idobutal
1697	1620	1490	1528	1107	783	Flunitrazepam
1698	1046	1277	1027	1064	1079	Androstanolone
1698	1194	1181	1250	700	1150	Phenglutarimide
1698	1496	1206	1099	–	–	Felodipine
1698	1720	1757	1316	1230	850	Hexethal
1699	1594	1242	–	–	–	Nefazodone
1700	700	766	1219	1740	1280	Phenindione
1700	1120	1179	1512	1219	1620	Anileridine
1700	1210	1601	1175	1318	753	Benzaldehyde
1700	1235	1495	1590	1100	763	Lofepramine
1700	1266	1136	1036	1156	1073	Tigloidine
1700	1283	1584	1275	1683	950	Phanquinone
1700	1610	1435	1325	830	1090	Enoximone
1700	1652	1160	1285	1295	1530	Gliquidone
1700	1660	1235	1720	1275	1750	Cortisone
1700	1660	1612	1538	1298	1219	Acefylline Piperazine
1700	1722	1210	1300	830	1622	Ibomal
1700	1755	1212	815	1319	848	Cyclopentobarbital
1700	1777	1208	1130	1303	730	Ethosuximide
1701	1220	1184	1735	1052	1672	Trimetaphan Camsilate
1702	1720	1751	1240	802	716	Phenylmethylbarbituric Acid
1703	1140	957	–	–	–	Etretinate
1703	1618	1576	1407	–	–	Daunorubicin
1703	1619	1267	–	–	–	Ciprofloxacin
1703	1728	1752	1315	1211	829	Talbutal
1704	1006	1018	1160	1270	1603	Sulindac
1704	1605	1253	775	1170	1235	Cyclomethycaine
1704	1724	1637	1600	1227	1510	Cefalothin
1704	1754	733	1052	1302	702	Mephenytoin
1705	700	1115	1492	1600	1157	Norpipanone
1705	741	1197	1160	1290	1135	Yohimbine
1705	1150	1100	1580	1020	1000	Methoxsalen
1705	1282	1030	699	1775	1086	Mesuximide
1705	1595	943	1640	742	1272	Trazodone
1705	1597	1248	777	699	1285	Ketobemidone
1706	1068	1055	1252	1238	1032	Mesterolone
1707	1162	920	667	1089	997	Gliclazide
1707	1684	1754	720	1298	1050	Methylphenobarbital
1708	698	1491	1110	1092	1030	Dipipanone
1708	701	751	1590	1190	1754	Norbormide
1708	1213	1250	1278	946	1107	Valproic Acid
1708	1218	1166	1148	688	730	Pethidine
1708	1608	1210	1755	1178	1085	Carbocromen
1709	1214	1261	1613	1294	1311	Oxybuprocaine
1709	1435	1226	997	–	–	Loratadine
1710	698	1230	1136	1175	1205	Phenoperidine
1710	1060	1245	1185	690	720	Mandelic Acid
1710	1505	1596	1220	743	1230	Fluspirilene
1710	1600	1110	880	930	1620	Trioxysalen
1710	1734	1750	1225	775	1190	Barbituric Acid
1710	1738	1275	1110	712	1037	Cocaine
1711	701	1495	1122	1032	760	Normethadone
1711	1215	1154	1176	948	690	Neostigmine Bromide
1712	1014	1300	1062	1094	946	Bethanechol Chloride
1712	1262	1135	1282	1020	1650	Arecoline
1712	1684	1670	1770	1310	1300	Phenobarbital
1713	1041	1694	1030	1052	1250	Ethinamate
1713	1075	1610	805	1010	–	Urethane
1714	1214	1136	1197	1184	1155	Dicycloverine
1714	1238	1182	1263	1167	703	Tilidate
1714	1300	1755	755	1492	1275	Phenylbutazone
1714	1618	1522	1235	–	–	Ritonavir
1715	1072	700	1603	1110	760	Hydroxyphenamate
1715	1100	1200	690	760	1020	Fenbutrazate
1715	1200	1735	1035	1087	1265	Drostanolone Propionate
1715	1300	767	1745	715	703	Feprazone
1715	1372	1463	1087	–	–	Zopiclone
1715	1540	1610	1140	1500	1220	Bezafibrate
1715	1620	1100	747	759	1237	Gelsemine
1716	700	760	820	1780	1100	Ethotoin
1716	1305	750	688	1750	1595	Sulfinpyrazone
1716	1505	1280	1639	1115	909	Naltrexone

Wavenumbers cm⁻¹						*Compound*
1717	1202	1231	1258	–	–	Oxandrolone
1717	1225	1315	1300	1095	1050	Pipazetate
1717	1632	1485	1104	–	–	Aciclovir
1718	1146	1052	–	–	–	Mupirocin
1718	1154	694	1173	1220	1060	Caramiphen
1718	1180	1174	1042	923	858	Hyoscine Methobromide
1718	1216	1108	1285	1585	1265	Orphenadrine
1718	1237	1205	1770	1513	1126	Nitrofurantoin
1718	1317	1217	1250	763	1298	Dimethoxanate
1718	1459	1389	1267	–	–	Simvastatin
1719	1501	1033	1255	934	980	Oxycodone
1720	1035	1153	1163	1063	1204	Atropine
1720	1235	1740	1295	1145	1262	Eucatropine
1720	1250	1204	1268	1495	1289	Physostigmine Aminoxide
1720	1270	1500	959	1055	800	Hydrocodone
1720	1665	1748	1200	1275	1045	Hexobarbital
1720	1700	1581	1210	1170	1300	Bromisoval
1720	1740	1774	748	698	785	Phenytoin
1721	1188	1052	–	–	–	Azithromycin
1721	1232	779	1185	1273	870	Ibuprofen
1721	1271	1107	737	1587	1022	Nicofuranose
1722	1606	1532	1772	1272	3295	Azlocillin
1722	1654	1252	1109	715	967	Alfentanil
1724	1000	1031	1062	1242	1282	Androsterone
1724	1148	1308	961	952	1612	Suxamethonium Chloride
1724	1174	1155	1223	1190	1681	Naproxen
1724	1179	1160	1195	1044	935	Homatropine Methylbromide
1724	1216	1149	1178	1124	943	Demecarium Bromide
1724	1219	1250	1111	781	1265	Carbaryl
1724	1234	1028	1692	1111	824	Chlorphenesin Carbamate
1724	1243	1200	1495	1120	1162	Physostigmine
1724	1250	1052	1020	1612	1086	Docusate Sodium
1724	1276	1111	741	1022	1590	Hexyl Nicotinate
1724	1351	1182	–	–	–	Androstenediol
1724	1652	1161	–	–	–	Flumazenil
1725	1120	1158	1176	694	1234	Carbetapentane
1725	1189	1075	–	–	–	Methandriol
1725	1231	1034	–	–	–	Boldenone Benzoate
1725	1238	1041	–	–	–	Androstenediol Dipropionate
1725	1260	1072	1460	–	–	Lovastatin
1725	1372	1062	–	–	–	Dehydroepiandrosterone
1725	1513	1189	–	–	–	Atracurium
1725	1654	1175	–	–	–	Boldenone
1725	1696	1758	1317	1240	850	Amobarbital
1726	698	1220	1160	763	1055	Pipenzolate Bromide
1726	1249	1279	1077	1586	1661	Etacrynic Acid
1727	718	1593	1198	1605	1572	Tiaprofenic Acid
1727	1193	1094	695	1248	1030	Ethoheptazine
1727	1247	1279	1034	757	1500	Hydromorphone
1727	1579	1187	–	–	–	Pravastatin
1727	1669	1258	1608	967	1188	Medroxyprogesterone Acetate
1727	1683	1251	–	–	–	Clostebol
1728	697	1183	1120	1215	1495	Diphenoxylate
1728	1156	1249	1500	1630	1010	Pyridostigmine Bromide
1728	1220	1190	1162	690	1052	Benzilonium Bromide
1728	1670	1177	1188	1716	1224	Hydroxyprogesterone
1729	1282	1590	1136	–	–	Propanil
1729	1283	1594	1130	1116	743	Nicametate
1730	853	1166	736	705	1047	Hyoscine
1730	1047	1025	1277	1095	755	Camphor
1730	1083	1056	930	1102	1200	Carbachol
1730	1158	1194	694	1265	1219	Butetamate
1730	1165	722	1280	1620	1070	Naftidrofuryl Oxalate
1730	1172	1030	735	1063	1125	Homatropine
1730	1175	725	704	776	1026	Dextropropoxyphene
1730	1200	1567	1608	751	1227	Propyliodone
1730	1230	695	726	1163	1265	Valethamate Bromide
1730	1240	769	1190	712	1011	Clidinium Bromide
1730	1240	1225	1145	941	953	Oxymorphone
1730	1616	1216	–	–	–	Famciclovir
1730	1786	730	1059	766	1309	Clodantoin
1730	1802	1098	1200	770	1295	Trimethadione
1730	1805	1100	1040	1280	1070	Paramethadione

Wavenumbers cm^{-1}						Compound
1731	1128	1221	1100	700	1080	Oxeladin
1731	1206	885	994	902	1250	Betaine
1733	755	1708	700	1286	1054	Bezitramide
1733	1287	1086	1132	744	1044	Diethyl Phthalate
1733	1667	1715	1266	1250	1618	Gestonorone Caproate
1734	1192	1212	1274	1104	1074	Cyclandelate
1734	1195	965	685	1160	720	Methylpiperidyl Benzilate
1735	1155	1178	1040	1237	1203	Octatropine Methylbromide
1735	1175	1185	1317	860	923	Hyoscine Methonitrate
1735	1175	1210	1150	705	740	Methylphenidate
1735	1219	1085	1234	1063	700	Heteronium Bromide
1735	1255	1170	1507	1135	1295	Distigmine Bromide
1736	1064	1110	1183	1242	1174	Monocrotaline
1736	1145	700	1190	1500	746	Adiphenine
1738	1010	1070	1036	1277	1605	Haloxon
1738	1160	1025	1145	1225	1050	Hyoscyamine
1738	1181	1141	1162	1195	1077	Trimeperidine
1738	1225	1164	1178	1115	1192	Glycopyrronium Bromide
1739	1227	1234	704	1064	1130	Penthienate Methobromide
1739	1238	1227	702	1058	1093	Metindizate
1739	1241	699	743	1176	1191	Lachesine Chloride
1739	1248	1066	1632	972	1128	Methacholine Chloride
1739	1674	1211	–	–	–	Benazepril
1740	1163	1638	1270	962	1012	Suxethonium Bromide
1740	1178	1134	694	1030	1055	Alphaprodine
1740	1178	1230	1265	1278	1510	Phenolphthalein
1740	1760	1815	1188	1280	1007	Dimethadione
1742	1200	1182	1240	1150	1055	Protoveratrines A and B
1743	1652	1187	756	–	–	Ramipril

Wavenumbers cm^{-1}						Compound
1744	1239	1735	1053	1004	1123	Troleandomycin
1745	1276	1038	1010	1498	1080	Noscapine
1745	1668	1590	1195	–	–	Dactinomycin
1746	1412	1034	748	–	–	Etodolac
1748	1253	1232	1520	1027	1126	Nifuratel
1750	1645	1425	1390	1187	–	Enalapril
1751	1302	1585	752	1072	693	Phenindamine
1752	1168	1104	660	1505	1020	Pilocarpine
1753	1215	700	690	1180	1020	Benaprizine
1754	1582	1678	1271	1235	1190	Cefradine
1754	1660	1181	1202	1174	1532	Phenoxymethylpenicillin
1755	1226	1250	1110	1020	1315	Furaltadone
1760	1501	1037	1260	1020	1111	Hydrastine
1760	1742	1104	1683	972	1150	Pivampicillin
1762	801	962	1149	840	1300	Chlorzoxazone
1770	1075	1788	1263	1687	1744	Bacampicillin
1773	1676	1170	1127	1115	1185	Spironolactone
1774	1046	1004	888	1609	1151	Coumaphos
1775	1610	1515	1485	1250	–	Etoposide
1775	1693	1526	1308	1497	1583	Ampicillin
1775	1693	1600	1365	1500	1560	Cefaclor
1776	1730	1183	1267	1149	1236	Acecarbromal
1777	1145	648	896	–	–	Succinimide
1778	1169	1019	1094	1402	–	Dicamba
1780	1755	1795	1123	990	1162	Picrotoxin
1786	1176	1205	1111	1149	698	Pipoxolan
1820	1163	1047	2993	2909	874	Gamma-butyrolactone
2772	1614	1329	1257	1122	–	Norfluoxetine

Mass Spectral Data of Drugs

In the following table the *m/z* values of the eight most intense ions are listed in descending order of intensity for drugs and other compounds of forensic interest. To identify an unknown compound, the *m/z* values of the two most intense ions should be compared with the table in order to produce a list of possible compounds. The eight most intense ions of the unknown can then be compared with this list. Comparison with standard spectra should then be made. Complete mass spectra for most compounds can be found in the monographs in Part 2.

Principal peaks at m/z								*Compound*
27	26	12	28	13	14	–	–	Cyanide
28	99	56	27	26	55	42	100	Succinimide
29	30	28	31	32	–	–	–	Formaldehyde
29	41	39	42	69	116	167	168	Ascorbic Acid
29	44	43	42	26	41	28	27	Acetaldehyde
29	46	45	28	44	30	47	–	Formic Acid
30	27	124	56	123	87	78	41	Hexoprenaline
30	42	43	27	44	29	31	41	Ethylenediamine Hydrate
30	43	72	102	73	42	118	99	Diminazene
30	44	41	45	86	55	43	69	Octamylamine
30	44	42	568	31	58	27	81	Pseudomorphine
30	57	82	116	99	53	55	42	Cimetidine
30	72	43	135	121	148	52	56	Guanoxan
30	86	57	41	29	39	192	42	Terbutaline
30	86	57	41	77	135	29	206	Salbutamol
30	86	57	129	74	56	41	114	Timolol
30	86	57	294	71	310	70	87	Nadolol
30	91	65	92	51	39	121	103	Phenethylamine
30	108	107	77	39	51	137	27	Tyramine
30	138	195	140	103	197	77	196	Baclofen
30	167	45	168	165	183	166	152	Didesmethyldiphenhydramine
31	32	29	30	28	33	34	27	Methanol
31	33	29	32	43	28	27	42	Ethylene Glycol
31	45	29	27	46	43	30	42	Ethanol
31	45	46	29	27	59	74	43	Phenelzine
31	49	77	29	113	51	48	115	Triclofos
31	49	77	113	115	82	51	117	Trichloroethanol
31	59	29	45	74	27	41	43	Ether
31	59	42	60	27	29	45	41	Propanol
33	131	69	79	181	51	151	101	Sevoflurane
41	43	29	55	39	57	73	81	Lanatoside C
41	43	183	167	140	184	124	109	*N*-Hydroxyaprobarbital
41	81	53	221	79	39	178	233	Methohexital
41	132	102	160	96	29	27	44	Propamidine
41	147	79	93	55	105	67	91	Trilostane
41	167	124	39	80	53	68	141	Allobarbital
41	167	168	39	124	97	141	181	Butalbital
41	173	91	135	77	55	44	69	Santonin
41	226	77	143	181	141	39	145	Alclofenac
41	229	43	329	69	344	29	283	Δ^9-THC-11-oic acid
42	28	41	29	27	86	56	39	Gamma-butyrolactone
42	31	61	43	29	27	44	41	Monoethanolamine
42	43	70	246	185	55	56	445	Thiopropazate
42	128	85	43	44	41	70	69	Barbituric Acid
42	140	112	41	85	43	71	141	Methenamine
42	248	247	32	151	45	201	69	Enoximone
42	271	258	123	56	83	240	95	Trifluperidol
42	292	56	294	109	203	201	44	Penfluridol
43	29	27	72	57	42	44	41	Methyl Ethyl Ketone
43	29	28	59	30	42	74	102	Cycloserine
43	29	39	41	45	57	68	58	Digitoxin
43	31	29	61	60	85	73	44	Isosorbide Dinitrate
43	31	57	73	60	29	55	44	Amygdalin
43	41	184	168	167	97	55	53	Thiamylal
43	44	85	86	42	129	68	30	Metformin
43	44	87	31	45	42	131	71	Paraldehyde
43	45	60	58	95	99	398	206	Rifampicin
43	45	60	120	42	92	138	44	Aloxiprin
43	55	69	81	152	210	95	180	Artesunate
43	55	299	91	147	79	253	271	Desoxycortone
43	58	42	44	30	129	36	143	Carbachol
43	58	42	143	85	171	157	102	Bethanechol Chloride
43	58	59	27	42	26	39	29	Acetone
43	58	143	42	41	40	39	128	Trimethadione
43	59	155	121	156	31	157	158	Phenaglycodol
43	61	45	70	29	27	73	42	Ethyl Acetate
43	70	29	71	27	154	41	267	Ergotoxine
43	70	55	42	41	73	61	87	Amyl Acetate
43	70	71	54	44	154	267	55	Ergocornine
43	70	71	154	41	209	69	267	Ergocryptine
43	71	55	79	91	109	123	336	Fluoxymesterone
43	91	134	92	65	39	63	135	Phenylacetone
43	91	227	268	312	79	55	77	Dydrogesterone
43	114	85	30	101	86	44	72	Buformin
43	127	195	85	44	36	152	58	Proguanil
43	129	57	56	41	72	39	58	Paramethadione
43	129	69	41	86	97	55	44	Acecarbromal
43	141	183	42	87	41	140	165	Paracetamol (mercapturic acid conjugate)
43	147	158	91	328	55	93	79	Clostebol
43	180	42	45	44	64	100	222	Acetazolamide
43	182	167	225	181	183	151	142	Trimethoxyamfetamine
43	187	42	171	229	86	144	170	Amiloride
43	221	83	236	56	223	222	55	Methazolamide
43	262	136	202	135	321	83	148	Famciclovir
43	314	121	133	91	107	57	239	Androstenediol Dipropionate
43	327	299	298	292	329	328	256	7-Acetamidoclonazepam
43	340	298	325	91	41	231	280	Norethisterone
43	398	337	72	309	95	362	217	Daunorubicin
44	30	42	41	29	27	100	55	Tuaminoheptane
44	42	124	165	163	123	93	65	Adrenaline
44	42	147	120	65	43	45	39	Amidefrine
44	42	159	43	45	184	41	109	Norfenfluramine
44	43	59	56	69	55	41	113	Heptaminol
44	43	79	93	41	135	91	81	Rimantadine
44	45	26	218	215	203	202	42	10-Hydroxynortriptyline
44	45	42	58	43	59	41	57	Topotecan
44	45	58	76	60	43	42	46	Noradrenaline
44	57	43	40	55	41	79	77	Cathine
44	59	165	166	181	179	178	43	Orphenadrine Tofenacin
44	69	41	208	210	55	71	43	Carbromal
44	70	59	277	71	191	278	203	Maprotiline
44	70	179	178	207	280	250	236	10,11-Dihydroxyprotriptyline
44	71	268	227	193	42	269	229	Monodesmethylclomipramine
44	76	77	29	45	42	95	65	Phenylephrine
44	77	76	29	95	39	58	42	Metaraminol

Principal peaks at m/z								*Compound*
44	77	79	51	45	42	107	105	Phenylpropanolamine
44	82	80	107	77	108	81	79	Hydroxyamfetamine
44	83	85	36	28	–	–	–	Trichloroacetic Acid
44	83	180	182	137	143	139	41	Bromisoval
44	91	40	42	65	45	39	43	Amfetamine
44	100	41	60	29	27	30	86	Piperazine
44	108	42	77	107	149	95	123	Oxedrine
44	121	77	120	42	106	91	39	Tocainide
44	122	78	121	65	107	91	134	Methoxyamfetamine
44	136	51	135	77	42	78	45	Methylenedioxyamfetamine
44	138	122	137	121	91	78	45	Methylthioamfetamine
44	146	147	39	41	190	42	148	Cytisine
44	166	151	57	43	91	135	209	DOM
44	167	168	165	183	105	152	77	Monodesmethyldiphenhydramine
44	180	209	227	223	77	208	179	3′-Carboxymefenamic Acid
44	194	109	67	86	238	56	85	Acefylline Piperazine
44	202	45	220	218	215	91	–	Nortriptyline
44	204	203	202	41	221	57	55	Desmethyldosulepin
44	206	162	108	51	207	201	178	Sodium Cromoglicate
44	208	117	58	193	130	57	29	Norpropoxyphene
44	209	211	250	210	224	42	251	2-Hydroxydesipramine
44	215	411	324	45	164	42	216	Etorphine
44	309	183	104	251	91	197	242	Fluoxetine
44	329	192	70	138	109	42	41	Paroxetine
45	29	43	60	42	28	44	41	Acetic Acid Glacial
45	43	27	41	39	29	59	44	Isopropyl Alcohol
45	130	44	71	42	61	115	55	2-Ethylbutyrylurea
45	156	141	69	41	43	157	55	3′-Hydroxypentobarbital
45	217	70	41	69	110	285	202	Pentazocine
46	76	57	55	56	60	47	97	Pentaerithrityl Tetranitrate
49	84	86	51	47	35	88	41	Methylene Chloride
51	29	101	149	31	69	99	32	Desflurane
55	41	42	43	70	57	29	31	Amyl Alcohol
55	44	142	141	41	61	81	82	Apronal
55	57	43	97	41	56	158	44	Carisoprodol
55	72	97	41	56	158	118	57	Tybamate
55	82	41	39	54	42	56	109	Pentetrazol
55	83	82	41	113	70	29	69	Bemegride
55	91	316	140	125	98	43	331	Betaxolol Methaneboronate
55	339	110	36	298	82	242	96	Nalmefene
55	378	43	29	57	410	379	84	Buprenorphine
56	42	83	57	77	51	97	54	Dipyrone
56	55	41	43	45	85	42	84	Cadaverine
56	84	111	69	82	54	67	45	Vigabatrin
56	100	138	110	57	237	70	41	Viloxazine
56	231	97	111	112	42	77	71	Aminophenazone
57	41	141	167	39	83	55	182	Nealbarbital
57	42	44	177	58	219	133	107	Profadol
57	58	70	42	44	188	84	43	Ethoheptazine
57	85	42	56	76	191	70	77	Phendimetrazine
57	139	351	134	121	333	313	109	Fluticasone Propionate
57	233	42	56	158	43	160	103	Norpethidine
57	328	121	145	91	105	79	239	Androstenediol Diacetate
57	328	121	146	91	105	79	159	Androstenediol
58	30	59	56	77	–	–	–	Hydroxyephedrine
58	30	59	77	29	95	65	57	Etilefrine
58	30	107	59	77	56	42	43	Pholedrine
58	30	363	44	72	29	27	364	Bialamicol
58	41	30	126	59	69	56	44	Cyclopentamine
58	41	56	30	124	65	59	93	Ethylnoradrenaline
58	42	30	51	204	146	77	44	Psilocybine
58	42	41	125	59	30	89	168	Chlorphentermine
58	42	59	30	77	107	57	51	Hordenine
58	42	69	41	30	215	202	59	10-Hydroxyamitriptyline
58	43	57	149	71	42	41	55	Acetylcholine Chloride
58	44	31	59	57	42	45	40	Dosulepin Sulfoxide
58	44	41	83	77	69	85	43	Mexiletine
58	55	41	44	43	128	59	56	Isometheptene
58	59	42	215	202	57	189	43	Cyclobenzaprine
58	59	72	45	292	218	42	–	Dimetindene
58	59	179	42	178	72	77	30	Chlorphenoxamine
58	59	202	42	203	214	217	–	Amitriptyline
58	59	221	30	42	222	255	43	Chlorprothixene
58	70	318	316	317	193	319	161	Zimeldine
58	71	26	54	167	72	42	44	Carbinoxamine
58	71	72	167	182	42	180	59	Doxylamine
58	71	72	207	42	91	59	118	Cyclopentolate
58	71	73	121	150	136	43	161	Diltiazem
58	71	91	115	129	273	–	–	Cyclopentolate H_2O
58	71	150	176	72	193	105	59	Tetracaine
58	71	208	72	59	42	89	57	Noxiptiline
58	72	29	42	71	57	59	224	Normethadone
58	72	30	77	56	44	42	73	Methylephedrine
58	72	43	78	271	57	44	77	Camazepam
58	72	59	405	–	–	–	–	Toremifene
58	72	279	234	151	192	166	165	Moxisylyte
58	73	44	45	165	42	40	181	Orphenadrine
58	73	45	43	57	167	44	165	Dimenhydrinate
58	73	45	165	59	42	166	149	Bromazine
58	73	45	167	165	166	44	152	Diphenhydramine
58	77	51	56	42	105	50	43	Methcathinone
58	77	59	56	51	42	105	91	Pseudoephedrine
58	85	86	57	84	70	43	268	8-Hydroxyclomipramine
58	85	269	268	270	271	314	242	Clomipramine
58	86	318	85	320	272	319	273	Chlorpromazine
58	91	42	41	134	65	59	40	Phentermine
58	91	59	56	30	42	121	78	Methoxyphenamine
58	91	59	134	65	56	42	57	Metamfetamine
58	91	72	71	197	185	184	92	Tripelennamine
58	97	72	71	42	191	79	78	Methapyrilene
58	97	72	71	203	191	190	42	Thenyldiamine
58	107	30	178	77	56	57	137	Dobutamine
58	111	71	42	75	59	141	113	Meclofenoxate
58	116	198	199	72	59	42	44	Dimethoxanate
58	117	208	115	193	91	179	130	Dextropropoxyphene
58	121	72	71	216	215	122	78	Thonzylamine
58	121	78	91	106	148	134	164	Methoxymetamfetamine
58	125	71	72	36	127	79	219	Chloropyramine
58	131	72	71	79	42	30	78	Chloropyrilene
58	134	91	119	179	121	42	55	Venlafaxine
58	135	77	51	55	136	105	63	Methylenedioxymethamfetamine
58	140	67	72	83	81	155	156	Propylhexedrine
58	143	115	42	156	211	128	269	Rizatriptan
58	146	56	105	77	42	106	40	Ephedrine
58	165	255	359	166	73	199	45	Captodiame
58	170	284	213	145	212	159	144	Iprindole
58	179	180	225	178	165	42	210	Nefopam
58	188	130	59	42	143	129	115	Dimethyltryptamine
58	195	59	72	388	89	315	42	Trimethobenzamide
58	204	59	42	30	146	77	44	Psilocin
58	204	146	59	42	160	43	159	Bufotenine
58	213	198	180	214	57	212	270	Promethazine
58	220	219	59	191	189	42	205	Doxepin
58	224	209	71	225	72	210	180	Dibenzepin
58	233	29	304	72	305	159	288	Entacapone
58	234	193	192	42	235	194	59	Lofepramine
58	235	85	234	236	195	193	208	Imipramine
58	236	40	202	235	203	42	44	Dosulepin
58	238	91	45	239	167	165	56	Prenylamine
58	238	208	42	324	190	–	–	Desmethylcitalopram
58	249	208	99	193	234	84	248	Trimipramine
58	251	250	211	85	42	209	296	2-Hydroxyimipramine
58	254	45	44	77	42	59	72	Clofedanol
58	254	111	227	214	45	44	71	Nizatidine
58	255	42	71	59	44	181	165	Phenyltoloxamine
58	282	30	284	355	73	283	44	Amodiaquine
58	284	86	238	198	199	85	42	Promazine
58	285	214	200	86	227	85	213	Prothipendyl
58	293	45	59	193	100	178	294	Butriptyline

Principal peaks at *m/z*								Compound
58	298	212	198	100	299	252	199	Alimemazine
58	328	100	228	185	329	242	229	Levomepromazine
58	352	86	353	85	306	42	266	Triflupromazine
58	366	59	100	266	248	84	44	Trifluomeprazine
58	427	234	59	50	42	428	91	Narceine
59	157	156	141	43	41	71	69	3′-Hydroxyamylobarbital
59	257	150	256	31	76	42	157	Dextrorphan
59	257	150	256	44	31	200	157	Levorphanol
59	271	150	270	31	214	42	171	Dextromethorphan
60	42	88	30	31	43	29	70	Benserazide
60	44	28	–	–	–	–	–	Urea
60	167	121	197	180	151	214	274	Zanamivir
63	78	45	61	46	62	48	47	Dimethyl Sulfoxide
66	120	39	65	269	205	118	77	Cyclothiazide
67	137	91	138	55	79	41	95	Dimethisterone
67	193	66	41	169	39	65	77	Cyclopentobarbital
69	43	41	44	71	167	165	55	2-Bromo-2-ethylbutyramide
69	56	71	91	261	84	119	70	Fenbutrazate
69	68	70	77	103	56	54	51	Bisnortilidate
69	83	43	79	41	81	53	80	Methylpentynol
70	41	69	75	114	42	217	68	Captopril
70	43	55	41	57	42	71	–	Amyl Nitrite
70	43	154	71	41	209	86	195	Bromocriptine
70	44	191	192	188	59	165	71	Protriptyline
70	44	207	178	279	249	–	–	10-Hydroxyprotriptyline
70	71	42	44	57	190	29	247	Ketobemidone
70	71	269	154	195	55	59	57	Dihydroergocornine
70	83	42	257	193	56	228	164	Loxapine
70	91	84	113	245	41	28	224	Lisinopril
70	96	97	71	42	43	44	169	Naratriptan
70	112	293	264	44	42	305	41	Bromhexine
70	113	141	399	43	26	72	42	Thiethylperazine
70	120	43	91	39	103	71	65	Aletamine
70	125	71	91	153	267	154	221	Ergocristine
70	125	91	153	43	41	44	244	Dihydroergotamine
70	150	151	153	77	51	118	60	Chloramphenicol
70	154	125	41	43	155	42	225	Co-dergocrine
71	42	56	43	177	77	178	105	Phenmetrazine
71	58	72	43	159	56	42	201	Quinisocaine
71	70	44	57	42	247	43	246	Pethidine
71	70	57	43	219	42	218	44	Pethidinic Acid
71	72	58	100	83	56	70	44	Diethylcarbamazine
71	91	106	177	57	72	65	30	Bethanidine
71	375	70	246	305	290	–	–	Ofloxacin
72	30	43	77	73	51	41	27	Clorprenaline
72	30	43	122	73	41	106	121	Sotalol
72	30	56	43	27	41	39	110	Prenalterol
72	30	56	73	249	98	234	102	Alprenolol
72	30	56	98	43	107	41	73	Atenolol
72	30	107	56	45	41	44	43	Metoprolol
72	30	116	56	43	160	41	158	4-Hydroxypropranolol
72	30	151	43	109	56	57	108	Practolol
72	39	42	38	94	56	51	81	Pyridostigmine Bromide
72	41	56	43	221	73	57	45	Oxprenolol
72	42	208	108	65	73	66	39	Neostigmine Bromide
72	43	30	56	151	221	41	98	Acebutolol
72	43	73	41	70	65	40	39	Orciprenaline
72	44	43	124	123	30	42	41	Isoprenaline
72	44	159	73	58	42	109	56	Fenfluramine
72	56	30	43	98	115	144	41	Propranolol
72	58	71	42	73	70	56	44	Isoaminile
72	73	43	91	224	56	71	129	Levacetylmethadol
72	73	91	293	223	165	85	71	Methadone
72	73	214	200	44	285	86	56	Isothipendyl
72	73	320	71	70	56	210	198	Dimetotiazine
72	73	340	269	197	71	70	56	Propiomazine
72	86	57	70	367	282	352	334	Bambuterol
72	91	73	44	42	56	70	65	Dimethylamfetamine
72	91	73	56	148	65	57	42	Mephentermine
72	91	114	145	75	160	117	92	Oxetacaine
72	107	56	116	43	73	41	251	Esmolol
72	116	107	100	281	73	43	325	Bisoprolol
72	133	30	116	248	134	56	41	Pindolol
72	176	91	58	177	41	42	30	Alverine
72	181	85	152	42	44	58	43	Methanthelinium Bromide
72	263	292	307	55	107	192	219	Betaxolol
73	43	84	55	69	41	44	85	Emylcamate
73	58	57	43	41	39	29	45	Digoxin
73	61	103	–	–	–	–	–	Mannitol
73	102	41	57	43	27	55	29	Valproic Acid
74	56	44	269	41	284	239	255	Mitoxantrone
75	41	57	70	43	59	56	47	Penicillamine
76	173	104	111	148	50	169	130	Thalidomide
76	239	104	240	285	241	50	75	Chlortalidone
77	51	123	50	65	93	30	78	Nitrobenzene
77	106	105	51	50	78	52	39	Benzaldehyde
77	183	308	184	105	55	51	41	Phenylbutazone
77	278	105	78	51	279	252	130	Sulfinpyrazone
78	77	52	51	50	39	79	74	Benzene
78	106	51	137	50	136	107	79	Methyl Nicotinate
78	106	135	136	51	50	79	52	*N*-Methylnicotinamide
78	350	135	176	77	97	123	110	Tenoxicam
79	77	108	101	51	50	39	40	Benzyl Alcohol
79	78	52	105	304	314	316	51	3-Hydroxybromazepam
79	96	31	113	81	70	127	78	Thioproperazine
79	105	104	51	78	52	50	77	Betahistine
81	53	330	96	82	332	64	63	Furosemide
81	83	46	110	82	112	84	117	Cloral Betaine
81	95	71	41	67	55	138	123	Menthol
81	124	54	53	125	171	45	42	Metronidazole
81	153	67	152	55	54	68	96	Gabapentin
81	223	79	41	80	157	185	77	Thialbarbital
82	30	81	54	28	55	83	41	Histamine
82	30	81	83	55	54	42	27	Ametazole
82	47	84	29	111	83	113	85	Cloral Hydrate
82	68	91	159	42	158	92	65	Pargyline
82	81	54	28	52	55	53	51	Fomepizole
82	97	42	83	96	57	94	55	Ecgonine
82	182	83	105	303	77	94	96	Cocaine
83	68	82	72	84	77	103	115	Nortilidate
83	70	261	202	217	203	82	215	Setiptiline
83	70	273	244	209	42	71	43	Clotiapine
83	84	55	56	43	71	41	62	Meprobamate
83	85	47	87	48	49	35	82	Chloroform
83	140	82	124	43	96	97	42	Deptropine
83	140	82	124	96	97	42	125	Benzatropine
84	56	85	77	105	55	30	42	Pipradrol
84	71	85	82	80	341	70	356	Conessine
84	82	80	56	43	28	30	41	Coniine
84	91	77	55	182	85	65	104	Antazoline
84	91	85	56	55	150	41	118	Methylphenidate
84	97	301	56	85	96	218	82	Flecainide
84	128	179	42	85	178	214	98	Clemastine
84	194	55	85	56	41	30	99	Perhexiline
84	204	205	85	42	55	105	77	Procyclidine
84	209	67	43	110	41	192	164	Minoxidil
85	43	42	86	44	41	75	110	Mefruside
85	56	69	55	27	44	42	109	Pipobroman
85	58	86	91	84	70	42	225	Benzydamine
85	87	101	50	103	31	66	35	Dichlorodifluoromethane
85	135	87	137	31	101	100	50	Cryofluorane
86	30	57	108	44	29	84	41	Bamethan
86	30	58	29	130	87	77	42	Diethyltryptamine
86	30	58	123	78	51	29	42	Nicametate
86	30	72	44	141	42	29	57	Butanilicaine
86	30	167	99	87	58	165	29	Adiphenine
86	30	216	87	58	100	99	56	Phenglutarimide
86	36	87	84	58	56	44	38	Amiodarone
86	36	126	30	58	38	112	99	Mepacrine
86	44	30	265	41	180	29	87	Ethomoxane
86	44	87	107	43	106	56	41	Prilocaine
86	57	41	127	190	243	90	174	Clenbuterol
86	57	277	70	292	87	114	–	Carteolol
86	57	318	259	99	112	200	333	Levobunolol

Principal peaks at m/z								*Compound*
86	58	87	42	56	77	44	43	Etafedrine
86	58	88	105	206	87	55	77	Tridihexethyl Chloride
86	58	99	56	162	132	149	205	Acecainide
86	58	250	44	57	72	291	71	Celiprolol
86	58	319	87	73	247	245	112	Chloroquine
86	71	99	58	55	56	100	87	Dicycloverine
86	87	58	30	29	84	56	42	Carbocromen
86	87	58	44	72	42	120	85	Lidocaine
86	87	58	149	111	99	57	41	Cinchocaine
86	87	99	58	84	387	315	56	Flurazepam (2-hydroxyethyl)
86	87	100	30	58	44	42	29	Clomifene
86	91	87	145	58	144	30	44	Carbetapentane
86	91	105	87	144	58	100	56	Oxeladin
86	99	29	30	100	71	87	192	Oxybuprocaine
86	99	30	87	58	71	136	100	Proxymetacaine
86	99	91	144	58	56	41	87	Caramiphen
86	99	91	191	87	119	58	248	Butetamate
86	99	100	141	87	71	44	58	Naftidrofuryl Oxalate
86	99	120	30	92	87	58	65	Procainamide
86	99	120	58	87	30	92	71	Procaine
86	99	136	30	58	178	87	71	Propoxycaine
86	99	154	30	87	58	29	156	Chloroprocaine
86	99	184	58	30	87	201	186	Metoclopramide
86	100	44	30	29	42	58	56	Diamthazole
86	105	77	87	182	99	183	58	Benactyzine
86	109	30	151	87	81	99	58	Etamiphylline
86	114	100	44	238	115	56	72	Isopropamide Iodide
86	166	251	280	57	151	70	165	Tertatolol
86	181	43	44	41	114	42	152	Propantheline Bromide
86	298	87	30	58	299	212	180	Diethazine
87	79	51	225	42	50	86	80	Furazolidone
88	42	123	124	89	77	51	44	Methyldopa
90	177	105	77	106	51	89	50	5-Phenyloxazolidine-2,4-dione
91	30	92	42	29	146	44	104	Phenformin
91	30	155	108	65	197	39	107	Tolbutamide
91	65	187	92	277	259	90	273	Trimetaphan Camsilate
91	70	208	254	117	56	160	54	Enalapril
91	79	67	201	77	105	93	120	Lynestrenol
91	79	77	55	67	93	270	105	Danazol
91	81	106	78	39	95	68	43	Ethinamate
91	92	65	39	63	93	51	89	Toluene
91	92	118	44	43	135	65	178	Phenacemide
91	106	105	77	51	39	29	92	Xylene
91	106	197	162	107	148	27	63	Beclamide
91	120	65	121	92	105	77	118	Benethamine
91	121	65	122	309	64	230	123	Benzthiazide
91	127	106	110	43	92	65	120	Isocarboxazid
91	133	176	174	44	107	92	177	Buphenine
91	146	44	119	206	41	78	77	Pheneturide
91	148	149	65	92	42	56	39	Benzfetamine
91	155	114	65	197	42	41	85	Tolazamide
91	155	197	65	84	39	95	41	Glibornuride
91	159	160	131	65	92	81	39	Tolazoline
91	177	44	106	45	78	123	51	Nialamide
91	196	198	92	197	65	77	56	Phenoxybenzamine
91	204	365	144	118	117	120	122	Benazepril
91	215	79	105	77	55	41	298	Noretynodrel
91	216	77	259	–	–	–	–	Phencyclidine
91	233	30	232	31	276	275	65	Mebhydrolin
91	269	324	55	296	295	323	297	Prazepam
92	65	108	214	156	39	109	43	Sulfaguanidine
92	91	65	103	93	39	163	77	Tropicamide
92	156	65	108	191	45	39	55	Sulfathiazole
92	156	65	191	108	55	45	174	Succinylsulfathiazole
92	156	191	65	108	76	104	50	Phthalylsulfathiazole
92	270	65	156	108	106	93	59	Sulfamethizole
92	284	156	108	65	106	93	220	Sulfaethidole
93	135	43	66	65	39	94	92	Acetanilide
94	66	39	65	40	55	38	95	Phenol
94	96	15	79	81	93	95	14	Methyl Bromide
94	138	42	108	136	41	96	97	Hyoscine
94	151	57	95	40	41	58	108	Amantadine

Principal peaks at m/z								*Compound*
95	55	41	43	59	27	39	67	Picrotoxin
95	81	41	69	55	83	67	137	Camphor
95	96	42	109	41	208	54	39	Pilocarpine
95	130	132	60	97	35	134	47	Trichloroethylene
95	327	39	329	96	122	244	67	Diloxanide
96	42	195	210	71	69	44	152	Altretamine
96	44	43	31	45	27	78	264	Hydroxystilbamidine
96	56	42	91	97	39	65	58	Selegiline
96	94	159	110	97	98	136	137	Granisetron
96	97	98	91	136	31	29	55	Pentapiperide Metilsulfate
96	105	77	97	216	42	218	51	Lobeline
96	109	97	294	95	135	121	242	Astemizole
96	293	198	211	143	183	55	115	Ondansetron
97	43	71	70	96	91	98	42	Bamipine
97	55	69	72	71	98	43	62	Mebutamate
97	56	91	68	132	173	–	–	Fenproporex
97	70	99	43	98	44	42	188	Thenalidine
97	98	296	199	55	212	96	198	Methdilazine
97	99	61	117	119	63	101	62	Trichloroethane
97	105	77	96	42	183	98	82	Mepenzolate Bromide
97	105	77	183	84	36	42	51	Methylpiperidyl Benzilate
98	41	42	55	99	77	69	44	Cycrimine
98	70	99	42	386	126	55	41	Mesoridazine
98	70	214	111	134	341	199	326	Sulpiride
98	84	71	56	41	42	99	124	Mecamylamine
98	99	44	242	70	28	111	149	Amisulpride
98	99	70	42	96	55	41	40	Mepivacaine
98	99	70	228	230	243	245	185	Remoxipride
98	99	105	77	55	41	127	111	Difenidol
98	105	55	41	99	77	218	84	Trihexyphenidyl
98	111	99	42	55	41	29	112	Norpipanone
98	111	99	147	55	41	42	96	Flavoxate
98	111	99	199	41	288	200	55	Pipazetate
98	112	99	55	42	41	211	84	Fenpipramide
98	119	91	99	124	64	41	55	Diperodon
98	135	99	70	77	97	42	112	Encainide
98	137	97	136	41	193	84	110	Sparteine
98	152	154	42	69	174	208	153	Chlormezanone
98	194	166	157	55	42	165	99	Pipoxolan
98	215	58	84	91	56	71	186	Fencamfamin
98	218	99	55	41	42	77	84	Biperiden
98	370	126	99	40	70	371	258	Thioridazine
99	56	72	165	300	228	229	242	Chlorcyclizine
99	56	167	207	194	266	195	165	Cyclizine
99	114	98	167	70	165	57	43	Diphenylpyraline
99	156	41	29	57	211	125	137	Tributyl Phosphate
99	197	44	58	112	309	41	42	Metixene
99	404	56	100	405	70	312	381	Sildenafil
100	44	72	101	77	56	42	105	Diethylpropion
100	56	42	101	55	54	41	30	Nimorazole
100	56	42	176	98	120	70	189	Molindone
100	56	101	42	185	184	41	128	Furaltadone
100	56	113	139	111	42	70	101	Moclobemide
100	56	231	132	103	115	57	70	Indeloxazine
100	58	41	101	43	56	65	30	Isoetarine
100	58	105	77	56	101	41	70	Meprylcaine
100	72	240	340	44	197	254	43	Acepromazine
100	101	44	72	198	180	42	29	Profenamine
100	113	56	101	87	378	194	91	Doxapram
100	128	70	41	42	293	56	101	Pramocaine
100	142	280	456	116	58	458	42	Halofantrine
100	265	128	266	44	98	56	101	Dextromoramide
100	286	142	56	42	239	70	185	Moracizine
101	103	105	66	47	35	31	82	Trichlorofluoromethane
102	30	72	44	116	55	173	71	Ethambutol
102	84	58	56	42	30	103	91	Bamifylline
102	245	247	304	305	306	58	126	Hydroxychloroquine
103	77	82	29	97	42	51	104	Tilidate
104	105	204	77	78	133	51	132	Ethotoin
104	132	218	51	103	77	78	52	Phenylmethylbarbituric Acid
104	189	103	78	51	77	105	52	Phensuximide

Principal peaks at *m/z*								Compound
104	189	103	117	78	91	51	146	2-Phenylglutarimide
105	77	51	122	50	39	74	76	Benzoic Acid
105	77	96	183	51	42	182	94	Clidinium Bromide
105	77	106	44	51	128	78	40	Broxaldine
105	104	77	79	244	106	108	27	Etomidate
105	111	77	96	97	183	42	51	Pipenzolate Bromide
105	129	112	77	42	313	41	55	Oxyphencyclimine
105	135	51	134	77	106	50	78	Hippuric Acid
105	177	77	209	254	210	103	181	Ketoprofen
105	210	255	77	51	78	132	91	Ketorolac
105	554	540	43	45	77	31	29	Aconitine
106	30	77	185	105	104	89	141	Mafenide
106	78	51	137	50	79	107	31	Isoniazid
106	78	177	51	178	107	149	40	Nikethamide
106	123	78	51	119	79	77	107	Salinazid
107	69	125	83	79	55	41	77	Cyclandelate
107	79	77	51	152	105	50	78	Mandelic Acid
107	108	77	79	51	39	53	50	Cresol
107	108	78	79	80	77	51	52	Fenyramidol
107	120	79	75	77	44	91	45	Styramate
107	145	268	238	121	133	159	224	Diethylstilbestrol
107	163	223	108	29	164	41	57	Bufexamac
107	165	123	95	121	–	–	–	Azaperone
107	176	90	77	70	105	42	79	Pemoline
108	81	213	54	77	136	51	43	Phenazopyridine
108	107	91	182	109	77	79	31	Mephenesin
108	109	179	137	43	81	80	110	Phenacetin
108	248	140	65	92	141	109	80	Dapsone
109	27	165	198	40	55	57	288	Mizolastine
109	76	104	92	239	65	108	43	Phthalylsulfacetamide
109	80	44	81	53	39	52	54	Aminosalicylic Acid
109	80	53	81	108	52	54	110	4-Aminophenol Aniline
109	108	80	53	51	39	91	27	Nicotinyl Alcohol
109	151	43	41	221	179	29	108	Tiocarlide
109	151	43	80	108	81	53	52	Paracetamol
109	304	231	124	258	110	83	123	Flupirtine
110	82	39	81	53	69	55	111	Resorcinol
110	263	125	262	265	264	111	89	Ticlopidine
111	96	167	112	165	71	43	42	Piperidolate
111	127	139	83	96	251	–	–	Clopamide
111	175	75	85	30	276	127	113	Chlorpropamide
112	77	105	139	55	41	96	56	Hexylcaine
112	161	85	45	163	113	114	59	Clomethiazole
112	246	105	77	55	41	44	247	Piperocaine
112	264	113	91	179	110	178	115	Dipipanone
112	344	121	41	67	55	54	345	Cyclomethycaine
113	70	42	211	351	43	71	56	Pirenzepine
113	70	55	42	41	39	85	69	Ethosuximide
113	70	114	42	221	222	56	43	Tiotixene
113	70	373	141	43	72	42	127	Prochlorperazine
113	70	407	43	141	42	127	71	Trifluoperazine
113	70	409	43	141	283	42	127	Butaperazine
113	86	116	98	117	115	58	84	Aprindine
113	100	71	43	73	81	96	376	Aclarubicin
113	339	44	70	141	43	60	340	Perazine
114	42	72	113	69	81	54	115	Thiamazole
114	44	142	365	42	223	115	205	Pericyazine
114	72	43	100	29	44	337	86	Propanidid
114	100	56	42	115	101	70	398	Pholcodine
114	115	160	72	43	86	229	42	Ropinirole
114	382	73	397	116	30	72	135	Tolterodine
115	86	79	57	56	107	100	52	Morinamide
115	117	89	53	109	51	91	39	Ethchlorvynol
115	187	139	145	157	170	259	289	Mannitol Hexaacetate
116	88	29	44	60	148	56	27	Disulfiram
117	119	47	35	121	82	84	49	Carbon Tetrachloride
117	198	196	119	129	67	127	98	Halothane
118	108	182	91	225	107	57	75	Mephenesin Carbamate
118	117	91	92	119	65	77	103	Phenprobamate
118	117	203	103	77	78	119	91	Mesuximide
120	43	138	92	121	39	64	63	Aspirin
120	92	137	65	121	39	64	53	Salicylamide
120	92	138	64	39	63	121	65	Salicylic Acid
120	92	152	121	65	64	93	63	Methyl Salicylate
120	106	78	92	51	226	41	39	Metyrapone
120	137	193	92	65	121	138	41	Butyl Aminobenzoate
120	165	92	65	137	39	121	93	Benzocaine
120	263	142	178	100	264	41	29	Butacaine
121	43	122	223	147	91	41	135	Betamethasone
121	58	72	71	214	122	215	78	Mepyramine
121	65	36	185	50	38	76	39	Halazone
121	120	69	92	195	39	93	45	Salicyluric acid
121	120	354	122	43	234	106	64	Xipamide
121	122	91	147	225	43	135	120	Prednisolone
121	122	315	43	147	223	135	41	Dexamethasone
121	152	40	93	65	–	–	–	Methyl Hydroxybenzoate
121	163	151	109	43	122	108	65	Benorilate
121	164	77	57	56	165	162	122	Ritodrine
121	318	317	173	120	362	44	31	Ethyl Biscoumacetate
121	429	280	430	389	134	122	281	Mifepristone
122	78	106	51	50	52	44	123	Nicotinamide
122	119	77	78	91	107	65	63	Formoterol
122	121	91	123	147	77	107	93	Boldenone
122	121	91	147	161	43	107	120	Ethisterone
123	31	58	106	79	43	78	51	Iproniazid
123	51	78	106	50	52	105	39	Isonicotinic Acid
123	57	42	103	44	85	124	51	Carbidopa
123	105	78	51	106	77	124	50	Nicotinic Acid
123	106	78	51	105	50	77	52	Nicofuranose
123	124	77	44	51	74	53	39	Levodopa
124	43	314	79	91	229	272	105	Progesterone
124	82	83	94	55	42	67	96	Tigloidine
124	82	94	83	42	96	103	67	Atropine
124	82	94	83	140	144	67	284	Tropisetron
124	82	168	77	105	42	94	83	Benzoylecgonine
124	107	82	83	42	77	79	94	Homatropine
124	109	198	81	77	125	52	31	Guaifenesin
124	118	198	109	43	57	125	77	Methocarbamol
124	276	58	140	56	72	125	41	Eucatropine
125	44	70	91	41	40	244	153	Ergotamine
125	70	91	153	41	244	43	71	Dihydroergocristine
125	189	230	127	191	63	232	90	Diazoxide
125	207	55	369	41	126	134	163	Cilostazol
126	44	30	42	41	55	43	58	Guanethidine
126	56	70	211	127	151	152	85	Pramipexole
126	98	41	69	58	55	127	44	Levetiracetam
126	127	84	56	–	–	–	–	Ropivacaine
126	127	174	91	70	69	55	42	Prolintane
127	43	229	44	161	231	85	186	Chlorproguanil
127	161	163	153	129	187	90	189	Triclocarban
128	96	70	39	41	27	42	29	Cantharidin
128	130	65	39	64	63	129	99	Parachlorophenol
128	130	169	87	41	129	242	171	Clofibrate
128	130	202	31	29	65	43	111	Chlorphenesin
128	130	202	43	129	111	75	204	Chlorphenesin Carbamate
128	141	268	130	270	77	143	233	Dichlorophen
129	172	128	102	101	130	76	77	Saquinavir
130	131	30	160	77	103	132	102	Tryptamine
131	167	41	103	43	132	77	289	Ciprofibrate
131	256	125	42	255	89	258	257	Clemizole
132	104	44	175	103	117	43	130	Debrisoquine
133	132	56	115	30	117	91	77	Tranylcypromine
134	93	135	144	94	116	296	136	Dolasetron
134	104	103	91	77	78	105	44	Felbamate
134	104	191	143	162	–	–	–	Norfluoxetine
135	57	91	77	43	119	105	180	Hydroxyphenamate
135	136	164	29	31	108	178	237	Adenosine
135	150	91	107	117	–	–	–	Thymol
136	43	123	148	161	113	83	414	Metenolone
136	81	137	42	41	55	130	128	Cinchonidine
136	81	322	188	55	42	41	172	Quinidine
136	123	148	83	93	107	161	–	Metenolone Acetate
136	135	52	28	137	109	29	18	Allopurinol
136	137	81	42	41	189	55	117	Quinine
136	294	81	159	55	42	41	143	Cinchonine

Principal peaks at m/z								*Compound*
136	310	135	225	149	122	155	311	Ibogaine
137	120	92	65	39	138	121	63	Aminobenzoic Acid
138	55	189	82	41	110	326	42	Hydroquinine
138	326	55	110	189	82	160	139	Hydroquinidine
138	352	215	310	214	69	321	354	Griseofulvin
139	141	357	111	359	140	113	75	Indometacin
140	84	56	41	72	69	29	39	Pempidine
140	141	84	41	29	96	56	55	Bupivacaine
141	43	183	44	140	80	108	52	Paracetamol (cysteine conjugate)
141	156	41	55	98	39	142	155	Butobarbital
141	156	41	57	39	98	157	47	Secbutabarbital
141	156	43	41	157	55	39	98	Pentobarbital
141	445	169	123	155	96	42	317	Metopimazine
142	44	140	42	198	170	41	96	Pipotiazine
142	57	42	197	185	339	240	226	Hexetidine
142	126	127	80	54	42	55	69	Zidovudine
142	143	100	155	44	112	57	29	Butalamine
142	170	44	410	42	143	43	41	Piperacetazine
143	36	70	144	38	100	–	–	Zuclopenthixol Dihydrochloride
143	70	100	144	42	98	58	56	Flupentixol
143	70	100	144	42	56	98	221	Clopenthixol
143	245	112	99	56	139	217	247	Zopiclone
145	117	122	89	105	90	63	146	Hydroxyquinoline
146	190	117	118	161	189	103	91	Primidone
146	233	103	133	91	117	115	77	4-Hydroxyglutethimide
147	43	146	42	193	118	164	44	Carbazochrome
147	73	75	117	233	148	45	149	Gamma-hydroxybutyric Acid-TMS$_2$
147	131	130	132	119	148	365	218	Indapamide
149	41	29	57	56	104	32	65	Dibutyl Phthalate
149	177	150	65	76	105	176	104	Diethyl Phthalate
150	121	56	93	39	151	66	94	Glipizide
150	152	165	41	167	43	44	130	2-Bromo-2-ethyl-3-hydroxybutyramide
150	326	163	203	251	281	41	311	Acitretin
151	72	223	123	222	152	52	29	Etamivan
151	94	122	106	51	53	149	150	Pyridoxine
151	109	136	178	177	29	207	135	Thiambutosine
151	136	121	120	180	297	77	93	Omeprazole
151	164	45	43	165	109	110	108	Aciclovir
152	119	165	163	180	60	179	153	Protionamide
152	151	81	109	51	–	–	–	Vanillin
153	93	30	65	152	154	125	110	Normetadrenaline
154	31	29	139	133	43	27	–	Deferiprone
154	70	155	167	223	225	349	153	Dihydroergocryptine
155	96	140	43	42	81	94	53	Arecoline
155	128	–	–	–	–	–	–	Trenbolone
155	140	83	98	55	41	84	69	Methyprylon
155	157	227	154	185	44	30	156	Buclosamide
155	170	112	169	55	82	41	39	Metharbital
156	92	108	65	140	253	157	43	Sulfamethoxazole
156	92	108	65	140	43	157	42	Sulfafurazole
156	141	45	157	41	29	55	27	3′-Hydroxybutobarbital
156	141	55	41	157	43	98	39	Hexethal
156	141	55	155	98	39	82	43	Barbital
156	141	157	41	55	142	98	39	Amobarbital
156	157	113	111	358	96	97	81	Tiagabine
156	158	92	77	157	314	108	65	Sulfaphenazole
158	214	57	145	124	45	70	96	Niridazole
159	157	43	198	71	172	143	105	Simvastatin
159	157	64	198	172	143	105	73	Lovastatin
159	161	81	335	333	163	337	205	Miconazole
160	103	89	131	115	76	161	104	Hydralazine
160	300	189	145	188	301	161	42	Azapropazone
162	43	63	164	30	44	98	42	Guanoclor
163	77	164	135	194	76	92	50	Dimethyl Phthalate
163	148	91	103	117	120	44	77	Phenylethylmalondiamide
163	161	119	91	206	117	107	164	Ibuprofen
163	178	91	117	41	164	77	121	Propofol
164	149	131	137	103	77	133	165	Eugenol
165	138	331	123	110	194	42	41	Pipamperone
165	234	194	235	193	196	166	179	Azapetine
166	68	95	41	53	123	–	–	3-Methylxanthine
166	68	123	53	42	41	95	–	7-Methylxanthine
166	164	129	131	168	94	133	96	Tetrachloroethylene
166	165	167	138	133	105	60	106	Ethionamide
167	41	124	168	97	39	169	45	Aprobarbital
167	41	168	124	39	97	141	67	Idobutal
167	168	41	43	97	124	39	55	Secobarbital (2,3-dihydroxypropyl)
167	168	41	97	124	39	57	53	Talbutal
167	209	43	124	39	41	53	140	Ibomal
168	137	44	139	43	152	124	167	Methoxamine
168	140	169	114	141	167	113	63	Norharman
168	167	514	548	40	166	51	–	Ceftazidime
168	227	55	212	303	140	93	42	Remifentanil
169	58	168	170	72	167	44	42	Pheniramine
169	78	171	113	115	63	51	170	Chlorzoxazone
169	92	289	65	290	39	333	184	Sulfasalazine
170	142	58	97	91	84	–	–	Fencamfamin-AC
171	43	143	41	128	55	141	159	Secobarbital
171	228	172	185	128	43	115	141	Nabumetone
172	92	156	65	108	173	39	174	Sulfanilamide
172	92	156	65	108	39	44	41	Sulfacetamide
172	98	73	367	173	56	124	55	Perindopril
172	157	173	43	41	55	69	71	Thiopental
172	187	84	57	42	188	44	43	Alphaprodine
173	117	145	78	104	94	76	147	Piroxicam
174	77	91	105	132	–	–	–	Norphenazone
174	160	104	145	117	77	91	129	Carphedon
175	56	176	91	104	86	174	85	Reboxetine
175	70	176	132	379	204	56	217	Oxypertine
175	189	190	286	173	162	271	163	Abacavir
176	59	132	150	45	193	105	29	Benzonatate
177	118	45	135	90	91	221	119	Procarbazine
178	44	135	179	77	84	107	41	Isoxsuprine
178	44	163	135	77	196	176	179	Protokylol
178	192	272	466	244	288	191	273	Cephaëline
180	55	67	109	82	42	137	70	Theobromine
180	77	181	44	179	51	209	167	*trans*-10,11-Dihydro-10,11-dihydroxy-carbamazepine
180	95	68	41	53	181	96	40	Theophylline
180	95	68	41	58	53	123	96	Bufylline
180	104	223	77	209	252	51	165	Phenytoin (4-hydroxyphenyl)
180	179	178	152	44	181	223	51	Carbamazepine-10,11-epoxide
180	209	182	152	181	30	211	138	Ketamine
180	209	252	208	152	179	181	210	Oxcarbazepine
180	223	194	254	109	95	193	166	Diprophylline
180	264	193	109	194	181	67	42	Pentifylline
181	41	182	39	124	53	138	97	Enallylpropymal
181	85	56	166	266	182	179	91	Trimetazidine
181	152	153	182	268	237	–	–	Fenbufen-Me
181	152	153	254	182	151	76	127	Fenbufen
181	263	246	182	198	154	91	65	Torasemide
181	395	198	251	397	396	199	666	Syrosingopine
182	30	181	167	211	183	151	148	Mescaline
182	57	43	55	40	69	41	181	Harman
182	288	167	156	165	243	183	157	Zolmitriptan
183	43	29	60	41	129	91	73	Ouabain
183	76	90	50	91	120	106	92	Saccharin
183	77	252	320	184	41	69	51	Feprazone
184	92	185	65	39	108	66	186	Sulfapyridine
185	36	186	98	87	43	70	221	Zuclopenthixol Acetate
185	187	255	257	123	115	157	150	Lamotrigine
185	230	141	186	184	115	170	153	Naproxen
186	42	201	56	57	187	202	71	Trimeperidine
186	114	29	72	42	113	27	109	Carbimazole
186	185	92	65	108	39	93	187	Sulfadiazine
186	218	77	295	263	105	51	158	Mebendazole
188	47	82	96	29	77	84	56	Dichloralphenazone
188	96	77	56	105	189	55	51	Phenazone
188	155	113	43	45	85	69	146	Famotidine

Principal peaks at m/z								*Compound*
188	189	159	132	53	173	131	145	Nalidixic Acid
189	104	190	77	44	105	132	103	Mephenytoin
189	105	201	285	165	166	190	134	Meclozine
189	132	117	160	91	115	103	77	Glutethimide
191	121	77	104	122	43	51	192	Amiphenazole
191	192	207	208	209	–	–	–	Amineptine
191	261	274	260	316	192	190	176	Tetrabenazine
192	193	287	176	191	286	270	285	Dehydroemetine
192	201	249	165	450	–	–	–	Losartan
192	206	272	480	288	246	205	191	Emetine
192	343	342	232	190	165	193	67	Irbesartan
193	118	140	91	56	152	–	–	Fenproporex-TFA
193	192	236	191	194	165	190	237	Carbamazepine
193	208	194	250	178	192	29	179	Mianserin
193	255	228	256	257	165	230	258	Desmethylmedazepam
194	109	55	67	82	195	42	110	Caffeine
194	180	109	193	238	95	137	81	Proxyphylline
194	195	238	193	72	178	45	196	Nomifensine
195	41	141	69	39	152	135	196	Vinbarbital
195	194	42	208	196	167	180	–	Mirtazapine
195	194	196	209	180	–	–	–	Desmethylmirtazapine
195	212	114	30	194	72	44	43	Disopyramide
195	281	196	152	280	81	77	66	Trimetozine
196	239	208	200	225	397	396	257	Amosulalol
197	241	198	77	242	104	91	103	Fenoprofen
197	256	198	257	91	103	–	–	Fenoprofen-Me
198	58	115	70	269	199	72	71	Aminopromazine
198	197	170	199	182	169	77	183	Tacrine
199	167	198	166	99	154	69	77	Phenothiazine
199	200	92	65	108	39	66	201	Sulfamerazine
199	244	200	178	179	184	183	245	Flurbiprofen
199	324	93	77	65	55	121	135	Oxyphenbutazone
200	91	243	242	84	186	166	201	Phencyclidine (1-phenylcyclohexyl)
200	185	199	171	44	84	71	131	Tetryzoline
201	81	98	175	259	176	202	242	Primaquine
201	117	167	202	251	165	118	115	Cinnarizine
201	165	203	56	187	242	299	388	Cetirizine
201	174	63	202	64	65	175	90	Tiabendazole
201	176	202	56	258	70	71	42	Morazone
201	203	165	45	299	166	202	56	Hydroxyzine
202	366	115	77	368	125	105	213	Atovaquone
203	58	44	205	54	204	72	202	Chlorphenamine
203	232	132	175	204	233	160	118	Aminoglutethimide
204	117	146	161	77	103	115	118	Phenobarbital
204	148	73	101	203	127	104	205	Levamisole
205	42	135	173	206	123	145	45	Pyrantel
205	70	231	78	135	136	42	166	Trazodone
205	77	41	39	220	130	145	131	Xylazine
205	218	123	356	219	162	95	190	Fluanisone
205	240	91	84	125	242	206	186	Pyrrobutamine
205	244	191	345	206	72	272	246	Benzquinamide
207	41	39	124	91	165	122	44	Brallobarbital
207	141	81	79	67	80	41	77	Cyclobarbital
208	193	130	115	91	165	179	207	Methadone
208	199	221	163	231	147	207	195	Zotepine
208	209	278	207	193	200	194	84	Triprolidine
209	70	224	293	115	41	156	266	Anastrozole
209	210	141	115	153	208	46	181	Naphazoline
209	257	180	208	210	77	44	194	3′-Hydroxymethylmefenamic acid
210	56	43	184	211	75	99	76	Acetohexamide
210	144	239	45	321	209	95	211	Quetiapine
210	252	371	284	312	43	178	240	Isradipine
211	143	91	283	197	70	344	97	Cilazapril
211	182	184	210	212	183	155	156	Milrinone
212	42	187	45	70	180	56	98	Dixyrazine
212	169	197	213	106	211	170	168	Harmine
212	213	122	198	44	53	91	65	Tolmetin
213	160	159	296	133	145	212	157	Ethinylestradiol
213	214	170	198	169	115	63	143	Harmaline
214	92	65	213	108	42	215	39	Sulfisomidine
214	213	92	65	215	108	39	42	Sulfadimidine
214	216	242	295	215	297	179	178	Diclofenac

Principal peaks at m/z								*Compound*
215	92	216	65	108	53	69	39	Sulfamethoxypyridazine
215	214	44	185	200	216	157	186	Tramazoline
215	230	56	77	216	96	41	39	Propyphenazone
216	215	92	65	108	54	125	39	Sulfametoxydiazine
217	159	95	43	186	143	160	218	Bicalutamide
217	190	285	215	216	284	102	218	Letrozole
218	42	219	91	165	155	193	115	Diphenoxylic Acid
218	44	191	221	219	178	42	180	Benzoctamine
218	117	118	146	103	77	91	115	Methylphenobarbital
218	174	160	161	275	219	175	162	Physostigmine
219	248	148	220	120	218	133	64	4-Hydroxyphenobarbital
220	191	204	178	192	221	233	410	Risperidone
220	221	205	147	42	193	77	118	Noscapine
221	43	78	93	80	41	141	39	Heptabarb
221	72	325	54	196	55	207	181	Ergometrine
221	81	157	80	79	155	41	77	Hexobarbital
221	199	200	186	395	251	77	214	Rescinnamine
221	314	248	261	193	236	222	315	Δ^8-THC
222	165	76	223	166	105	104	90	Phenindione
223	241	208	222	194	180	77	224	Mefenamic Acid
224	42	237	226	123	206	239	56	Haloperidol
224	82	127	55	83	141	125	113	Fluconazole
227	310	174	284	147	160	173	199	Mestranol
228	182	363	88	229	76	276	257	Clefamide
228	200	199	128	229	185	115	201	Trioxysalen
228	258	287	198	57	229	259	214	Etodolac
229	30	231	172	194	174	200	230	Clonidine
229	257	303	42	230	258	201	215	Flumazenil
230	109	82	187	243	363	42	123	Benperidol
230	187	42	217	83	82	461	96	Pimozide
230	231	58	44	42	105	173	159	Phenazocine
230	271	55	256	164	270	71	124	Cyclazocine
231	42	119	232	92	65	67	74	Azathioprine
231	147	285	232	201	132	165	166	Buclizine
231	246	314	232	121	193	74	174	Cannabidiol
232	184	233	201	186	433	95	120	Cisapride
232	250	175	204	176	233	102	78	Diflunisal
233	45	245	316	451	259	42	96	Doxazosin
233	71	316	245	43	387	234	205	Terazosin
233	383	259	245	95	56	246	234	Prazosin
234	91	74	107	70	160	55	404	Imidapril
234	146	179	206	131	91	117	118	Metisazone
235	73	250	207	161	115	128	177	Propofol-TMS
235	195	208	44	234	193	194	71	Desipramine
235	236	307	219	92	65	43	220	Zolpidem
235	250	91	233	236	65	76	132	Methaqualone
236	235	264	235	307	278	321	248	Fluvastatin
236	317	315	288	316	286	208	78	Bromazepam
238	42	239	224	240	56	72	226	Loperamide
238	210	239	287	360	150	178	67	Nitrendipine
238	210	239	354	383	338	178	310	Felodipine
239	196	268	120	197	225	77	104	Phenytoin
240	212	241	184	138	92	128	63	Dantron
241	77	242	105	44	43	195	57	2-Amino-5-nitrobenzophenone
242	43	270	269	241	103	243	76	Clorazepic Acid
242	207	244	270	243	271	269	165	Medazepam
242	229	213	42	56	43	198	312	Olanzapine
242	269	270	241	243	271	244	272	Nordazepam
243	118	190	56	91	202	–	–	Fenproporex-PFP
243	256	70	245	192	227	258	326	Clozapine
244	42	72	475	109	245	85	476	Fluspirilene
244	59	77	29	43	31	45	55	Glymidine Sodium
244	229	44	173	40	230	243	245	Xylometazoline
245	146	42	189	44	105	29	43	Fentanyl
245	257	247	193	56	246	228	259	Amoxapine
245	260	44	217	218	246	261	259	Oxymetazoline
246	42	247	91	103	165	115	56	Diphenoxylate
246	42	367	247	57	56	91	77	Phenoperidine
246	45	42	366	58	57	43	106	Piminodine
246	92	65	245	108	247	39	260	Sulfadimethoxine
246	143	403	70	404	42	248	113	Perphenazine
246	165	42	123	199	247	214	108	Droperidol

Principal peaks at m/z								*Compound*
246	243	180	315	248	245	182	167	Efavirenz
246	247	42	120	218	172	106	91	Anileridine
246	291	248	290	247	139	111	292	Zomepirac
247	189	249	191	243	55	29	245	Etacrynic Acid
247	248	249	250	219	212	106	221	Pyrimethamine
247	249	58	72	248	167	250	168	Brompheniramine
247	285	328	249	41	287	330	55	Clorexolone
248	44	249	121	136	29	164	192	Ambucetamide
248	261	219	233	247	205	318	389	Alfuzosin
250	70	207	91	251	119	148	56	Fenetylline
250	95	39	235	66	207	41	193	3′-Oxohexobarbital
251	70	253	28	41	42	139	18	Mexazolam
251	222	223	250	252	195	110	97	7-Aminonitrazepam
251	266	249	77	143	76	252	39	4′-Hydroxymethaqualone
251	280	118	91	121	119	252	189	Phenprocoumon
252	237	253	181	238	77	76	209	Anisindione
252	312	253	237	141	198	213	270	Trenbolone Acetate
253	91	213	43	105	271	79	145	Methandriol Dipropionate
253	252	43	104	254	235	77	89	Triamterene
253	288	287	289	225	259	254	41	Tetrazepam
254	143	42	70	411	113	56	157	Acetophenazine
254	256	118	255	303	305	63	45	Chlorambucil
256	121	185	43	257	65	42	214	Probenecid
256	283	284	285	257	255	258	286	Diazepam
256	284	283	285	84	257	258	255	Ketazolam
256	301	91	258	119	65	257	303	Benoxaprofen
257	55	311	77	259	313	44	312	3-Hydroxyprazepam
257	59	150	256	31	157	42	200	Racemorphan
257	77	268	239	205	267	233	259	Oxazepam
258	260	262	–	–	–	–	–	Lofexidine
260	261	42	57	184	215	217	262	Phenindamine
260	262	180	287	261	145	286	124	Quinethazone
260	302	216	215	243	189	242	188	Cambendazole
261	263	243	245	281	316	–	–	Etacrynic Acid-Me
262	264	110	138	125	152	89	77	Clopidogrel
262	308	91	124	117	223	179	160	Trandolapril
263	281	166	92	145	167	235	139	Flufenamic Acid
263	295	235	166	264	92	–	–	Flufenamic Acid-Me
264	378	192	250	320	58	165	251	Valsartan
265	251	267	133	237	135	78	211	Nevirapine
266	267	224	220	268	44	250	248	Apomorphine
266	268	264	167	165	270	202	132	Pentachlorophenol
266	268	267	255	231	102	88	176	Mazindol
267	221	207	180	223	154	196	268	Lysergamide
267	299	266	31	51	268	29	77	Fenbendazole
268	143	425	70	269	42	394	157	Carfenazine
268	224	154	180	207	223	192	179	Lysergic Acid
269	205	221	297	271	62	285	124	Hydrochlorothiazide
269	240	241	268	270	107	121	213	7-Amino-1-desmethylflunitrazepam
270	198	252	226	141	115	–	–	Trenbolone
271	43	41	311	295	312	297	91	8α-Hydroxy-Δ^9-THC
271	43	295	41	297	29	330	272	8β-Hydroxy-Δ^9-THC
271	81	150	201	148	110	272	82	Normorphine
271	273	300	272	256	77	255	257	Temazepam
272	273	41	327	145	76	42	29	Butorphanol
274	225	318	273	275	226	257	121	Phenolphthalein
274	276	159	103	262	275	278	132	Sertraline
276	111	219	42	277	97	29	100	Diethylthiambutene
277	279	165	278	241	239	242	240	Clotrimazole
279	163	323	58	277	308	280	322	Dimefline
280	105	281	501	77	183	85	147	Fexofenadine
280	143	42	70	437	406	113	56	Fluphenazine
280	253	281	206	234	252	254	264	Nitrazepam
280	314	315	286	234	288	316	240	Clonazepam
281	43	282	187	107	91	55	105	Megestrol Acetate
281	120	91	122	280	160	68	282	Phentolamine
282	236	237	281	263	145	44	93	Niflumic Acid
282	299	284	283	241	56	301	253	Chlordiazepoxide
283	44	255	282	254	284	264	256	7-Aminoflunitrazepam
283	282	256	176	157	43	41	57	Levallorphan
284	91	375	81	42	36	285	175	Benzylmorphine

Principal peaks at m/z								*Compound*
285	81	215	148	286	164	110	115	Norcodeine
285	96	229	228	70	214	115	200	Hydromorphone
285	162	42	215	286	124	44	284	Morphine
285	256	257	258	44	287	110	220	7-Aminoclonazepam
285	286	269	287	241	242	77	270	Demoxepam
285	312	313	286	266	238	294	284	Flunitrazepam
286	124	244	148	109	107	287	147	Androstenedione
286	229	91	81	287	41	77	228	Famprofazone
286	244	77	218	51	217	288	215	Desmethylclobazam
286	300	96	42	244	230	301	82	Bezitramide
287	70	44	164	42	288	59	230	Dihydromorphine
287	96	286	215	70	44	58	42	Cyproheptadine
287	245	289	331	56	29	41	57	Ciprofloxacin
288	69	178	41	287	43	289	55	Nabilone
288	91	107	105	255	79	203	93	Dehydroepiandrosterone
288	273	331	287	304	290	289	275	Flurazepam
288	290	218	146	114	63	51	148	Triclosan
288	379	91	175	172	189	378	191	Donepezil
289	245	246	210	259	211	183	291	Flutazolam
290	67	108	107	79	55	41	93	Androsterone
290	184	185	104	77	168	291	198	Sultiame
290	259	275	291	243	123	200	43	Trimethoprim
291	239	274	293	75	302	276	138	Lorazepam
291	248	43	79	91	93	107	176	Oxandrolone
293	265	264	292	43	222	223	294	7-Acetamidonitrazepam
294	248	91	110	117	209	160	297	Ramipril
295	296	238	310	119	43	251	239	Cannabinol
296	41	44	110	298	285	55	268	Cyclopenthiazide
296	195	58	297	253	196	212	84	Hexobendine
296	215	217	298	216	152	181	251	Fenclofenac
296	254	196	273	59	67	151	178	Nimodipine
296	298	205	221	64	63	41	125	Ethiazide
296	298	279	205	36	64	117	62	Trichlormethiazide
296	409	380	280	352	266	–	–	Ethylmorphine-TFA
296	459	280	266	402	430	–	–	Ethylmorphine-PFP
297	208	44	254	298	347	236	165	Amlodipine
297	298	36	98	125	143	–	–	Zuclopenthixol Decanoate
298	271	299	224	272	270	252	280	Dsmethylflunitrazepam
298	594	58	593	299	609	595	564	Tubocurarine Chloride
299	42	162	124	229	59	300	69	Codeine
299	43	41	67	300	69	231	29	11-Hydroxy-Δ^9-THC
299	162	229	123	59	42	44	300	Neopine
299	231	314	43	41	295	55	271	Δ^9-THC
299	242	59	243	42	96	70	214	Hydrocodone
300	258	77	259	283	302	231	256	Clobazam
300	302	298	299	301	193	207	264	Cisplatin
301	44	42	59	164	70	302	242	Dihydrocodeine
301	138	41	70	96	84	316	153	Carteolol Methaneboronate
301	216	44	42	70	302	203	57	Oxymorphone
302	57	85	231	91	110	79	215	Norethandrolone
302	124	43	91	79	121	105	122	Methyltestosterone
303	58	43	304	151	44	42	57	Verapamil
303	70	274	304	260	209	96	317	Nefazodone
303	262	135	175	41	55	43	95	Enoxolone
303	301	305	115	194	196	114	87	Broxyquinoline
303	331	239	255	30	158	64	159	Hydroflumethiazide
304	306	64	74	109	177	176	48	Diclofenamide
305	150	307	115	152	114	306	123	Clioquinol
305	307	306	309	308	334	102	75	Lormetazepam
308	165	309	121	55	154	98	56	Mebeverine
308	279	204	273	77	307	310	309	Alprazolam
309	96	42	58	98	70	57	44	Ketotifen
310	58	199	112	311	111	212	41	Pecazine
310	64	36	312	42	43	62	63	Methyclothiazide
310	121	353	311	43	120	92	296	Acenocoumarol
310	206	42	64	312	299	45	48	Polythiazide
310	312	311	163	325	75	39	297	Midazolam
311	255	42	44	296	310	312	174	Thebaine
311	312	41	188	80	82	81	241	Nalorphine
312	43	399	297	356	281	371	311	Colchicine
313	162	314	124	284	59	42	243	Ethylmorphine

Principal peaks at m/z								Compound
313	238	342	315	75	344	239	137	Triazolam
314	285	154	87	315	155	144	167	Pergolide
314	315	393	270	283	79	271	394	Amsacrine
315	230	316	70	44	42	258	140	Oxycodone
316	270	91	130	117	104	132	231	Quinapril
317	43	271	147	289	390	95	81	Alfadolone
317	288	359	401	43	318	289	196	Oxyphenisatine
321	278	320	292	306	191	322	304	Berberine
321	364	304	240	168	91	322	365	Bumetanide
323	221	181	222	207	72	223	324	Lysergide
327	43	369	268	310	42	215	204	Diamorphine
327	268	42	43	215	44	328	269	6-Monoacetylmorphine
327	328	41	242	286	96	229	70	Naloxone
329	284	224	268	330	285	225	270	Nifedipine
330	118	91	319	219	64	92	421	Bendroflumethiazide
331	43	71	332	121	147	131	41	Clobetasone Butyrate
332	333	304	335	176	303	334	162	Chelidonine
334	335	162	120	107	144	143	130	Strychnine
335	333	349	305	378	–	–	–	Metaclazepam
336	121	120	215	162	92	337	187	Dicoumarol
339	221	196	181	207	223	222	72	Methylergometrine
339	324	338	325	340	308	154	292	Papaverine
341	43	340	374	267	107	55	342	Spironolactone
341	44	343	342	440	70	18	344	Sertindole
341	55	36	300	342	110	243	256	Naltrexone
341	233	356	246	247	248	234	281	Sulindac
341	282	229	42	43	59	342	204	Acetylcodeine
341	298	43	44	55	284	242	–	Thebacon
342	18	28	266	313	224	239	45	Etizolam
343	70	344	109	42	113	491	56	Lidoflazine
350	91	259	352	348	65	351	107	Metolazone
351	420	73	232	233	260	405	200	Acrivastine
352	367	338	366	29	368	353	339	Dimoxyline
353	210	235	336	72	54	236	195	Methysergide
353	354	169	170	355	156	184	144	Yohimbine
355	139	113	371	341	415	–	–	Acemetacin
355	296	327	234	268	204	–	–	Ethylmorphine-AC
357	269	226	356	207	312	279	324	Tolrestat
361	277	319	276	199	318	362	43	Bisacodyl
363	206	143	42	70	207	218	113	Opipramol
371	210	270	266	284	254	268	41	Nisoldipine
372	58	110	357	272	57	373	72	Finasteride
377	43	55	246	278	59	378	41	Halcinonide
380	223	382	238	152	345	215	113	Chlorotrianisene
381	300	382	301	281	140	115	362	Celecoxib
382	266	245	280	292	384	383	294	Loratadine
385	192	146	196	234	357	–	–	Ethylmorphine-TMS
386	138	387	84	110	42	301	263	Piritramide
386	359	323	388	245	303	342	361	Quazepam
386	368	43	55	275	81	57	95	Cholesterol
388	310	215	198	173	91	–	–	Nemonapride
392	73	183	154	129	222	451	309	Carvedilol
394	245	316	210	291	176	365	313	Brotizolam
394	395	379	392	120	197	203	393	Brucine
397	115	242	398	88	143	271	62	Diiodohydroxyquinoline
409	172	452	186	245	228	130	396	Repaglinide
409	271	257	228	208	70	–	–	Tamsulosin
428	471	82	103	233	151	472	412	Nebivolol
455	457	472	474	459	456	458	473	Clofazimine
463	91	575	159	185	489	309	92	Zafirlukast
504	473	429	505	221	474	84	430	Dipyridamole
518	173	264	519	373	376	520	249	Benziodarone
578	195	577	367	351	579	366	365	Deserpidine
596	513	465	364	338	–	–	–	Indinavir
608	195	607	397	609	395	381	396	Methoserpidine
608	606	195	609	395	397	212	396	Reserpine
710	1709	769	1107	943	1133	–	–	Methadone
787	772	1138	1254	1314	742	–	–	Mianserin
1071	1035	1733	1140	1165	1640	–	–	Strophanthin-K
1119	1320	1160	1081	1253	1287	–	–	Flupentixol
1240	1495	1280	1580	756	1610	–	–	Dextrorphan
1529	740	1491	1613	1182	1141	–	–	Benzydamine
1621	1689	1250	1089	1211	1550	–	–	Methyl Benzoquate
1647	1279	843	1013	903	754	–	–	Glyceryl Trinitrate
1695	1220	707	930	773	960	–	–	Flurbiprofen
1775	1583	1684	1248	1613	1313	–	–	Amoxicillin

Mass Spectral Data of Pesticides

In the following table the m/z values of the eight most intense ions are listed in descending order of intensity; the table should be used as described under Mass Spectral Data of Drugs.

The values for m/z in this table were obtained using a quadrupole spectrometer, after gas chromatography unless otherwise stated, except for those substances marked † the data for which were obtained on a magnetic sector instrument.

			Principal peaks at m/z					*Compound*
41(100)	44(82)	45(42)	48(31)	47(29)	86(28)	87(26)	42(22)	2-Methyl-2-(methylthio)-propionaldehyde oxime (GCDP of Aldicarb)
41(100)	86(89)	58(85)	85(61)	87(50)	44(50)	55(45)	76(43)	Aldicarb (probe)
41(100)	140(85)	196(72)	74(64)	106(64)	168(53)	45(40)	227(37)	Mephosfolan
41(100)	173(83)	91(65)	135(49)	77(45)	55(43)	44(42)	69(59)	Santonin
42(100)	115(61)	61(55)	57(46)	55(43)	68(38)	161(38)	45(37)	3,3-Dimethyl-1-(methylthio)butan-2-one oxime (GCDP of Thiofanox)
43(100)	44(88)	136(80)	94(58)	47(56)	95(32)	46(30)	47(27)	Acephate (probe)
43(100)	45(99)	46(91)	94(54)	47(50)	199(49)	139(48)	68(46)	Aziprotryne
43(100)	57(98)	41(76)	55(54)	71(41)	69(27)	56(27)	42(26)	Dichlorophenoxyacetic Acid (2,4-D) (iso-octyl ester)
43(100)	57(96)	41(79)	55(47)	71(44)	69(35)	56(31)	70(28)	Trichlorophenoxyacetic Acid (2.4,5-T) (iso-octyl ester)
43(100)	57(83)	41(61)	71(48)	55(47)	162(41)	164(30)	69(29)	Dichlorprop (iso-octyl ester)
43(100)	57(94)	169(77)	41(70)	142(69)	55(52)	71(33)	56(29)	Mecoprop (iso-octyl ester)
43(100)	58(84)	44(75)	200(69)	68(43)	215(40)	41(38)	42(37)	Atrazine
43(100)	61(81)	62(67)	97(59)	45(59)	44(47)	89(47)	106(38)	Dalapon (probe)
43(100)	73(80)	59(52)	55(47)	72(46)	100(46)	44(45)	86(40)	Dodine (probe)
43(100)	86(73)	41(43)	42(31)	70(23)	44(21)	143(20)	128(19)	Tri-allate
43(100)	86(62)	41(38)	44(25)	42(24)	70(19)	128(13)	234(13)	Di-allate
43(100)	93(88)	41(42)	120(24)	65(24)	137(23)	179(21)	119(15)	Propham
43(100)	127(49)	41(35)	45(20)	44(18)	129(16)	63(12)	153(12)	Chlorpropham
43(100)	175(92)	57(84)	177(60)	4205)	258(22)	302(18)	112(15)	Oxadiazon
43(100)	211(80)	41(71)	44(57)	205(31)	163(29)	42(28)	45(25)	Dinobuton
43(100)	264(33)	306(32)	57(7)	42(6)	290(5)	145(4)	307(4)	Trifluralin
44(100)	43(60)	68(60)	212(48)	41(47)	42(34)	173(28)	172(25)	Cyanazine
44(100)	58(81)	105(69)	45(59)	42(55)	47(52)	57(36)	56(31)	Methomyl (probe)
44(100)	73(97)	159(89)	191(80)	86(72)	150(71)	72(68)	59(56)	Thiophanate-methyl (probe)
44(100)	161(44)	124(36)	187(31)	159(24)	163(23)	189(20)	216(20)	Methazole (probe)
45(100)	47(91)	58(78)	48(74)	105(71)	46(54)	42(50)	88(38)	*N*-Hydroxythioacetimidate (GCDP of Methomyl)
45(100)	188(23)	160(18)	77(7)	146(6)	224(6)	237(6)	91(5)	Alachlor
51(100)	153(76)	87(66)	222(44)	52(43)	63(43)	41(42)	69(39)	Barban
53(100)	127(20)	51(13)	164(13)	223(13)	70(10)	153(10)	50(10)	Chlorbufam
54(100)	53(93)	43(82)	124(65)	212(63)	187(61)	198(59)	285(49)	Vinclozolin
54(100)	108(89)	81(33)	190(31)	111(26)	135(25)	83(25)	80(25)	Diquat (reduction product II–diene)
56(100)	174(79)	175(31)	57(24)	176(23)	41(20)	131(16)	132(12)	Terbacil (*N*-methyl derivative)
57(100)	42(75)	68(39)	61(38)	55(34)	47(33)	115(31)	45(30)	Thiofanox
57(100)	43(94)	41(85)	196(63)	71(60)	198(59)	55(56)	223(35)	Fenoprop (iso-octyl ester)
57(100)	127(83)	43(78)	55(52)	42(25)	88(15)	128(14)	58(12)	Bromoxynil Octanoate
58	214	229	43	172	187	216	69	Propazine
61(100)	46(43)	60(15)	91(13)	258(13)	170(12)	260(11)	172(9)	Metobromuron
61(100)	46(24)	62(11)	63(10)	60(9)	124(8)	45(8)	233(6)	Chlorbromuron
61	46	126	214	99	60	63	153	Monolinuron
61	160	132	124	46	248	73	109	Linuron
66(100)	91(50)	79(47)	263(42)	65(35)	101(34)	261(25)	265(24)	Aldrin†
67(100)	81(67)	263(59)	36(58)	79(47)	82(41)	261(36)	265(33)	Endrin†
72	44	73	42	232	187	124	45	Diuron
72(100)	44(34)	73(25)	42(20)	232(19)	187(13)	124(13)	45(12)	Diuron (probe)
72(100)	44(29)	167(28)	132(25)	45(20)	77(11)	42(10)	212(10)	Chlortoluron
72	220	148	132	205	–	–	–	Isoproturon
72(100)	44(27)	183(23)	228(22)	45(21)	73(15)	168(14)	42(12)	Metoxuron (probe)
72(100)	100(81)	128(62)	44(55)	115(41)	127(36)	57(30)	55(20)	Napropamide
72(100)	164(27)	119(24)	91(22)	42(14)	44(11)	64(11)	45(10)	Fenuron
72(100)	166(85)	42(63)	44(44)	43(24)	238(23)	69(21)	167(19)	Pirimicarb
72(100)	167(86)	165(42)	239(21)	152(17)	168(14)	166(13)	73(5)	Diphenamid
72(100)	245(37)	44(31)	75(21)	45(19)	63(16)	90(14)	247(13)	Chloroxuron (probe)
73	352	454	253	144	42	212	455	Glyphosate

Principal peaks at m/z								*Compound*
75(100)	47(54)	121(43)	97(43)	65(37)	45(30)	93(27)	79(17)	Phorate
77(100)	160(77)	132(67)	44(30)	105(29)	104(27)	93(24)	76(22)	Azinphos-methyl
77	105	91	51	65	212	50	78	Benzyl Benzoate
77(100)	221(60)	88(37)	220(35)	51(26)	105(24)	223(20)	222(18)	Chloridazon
79(100)	80(61)	77(56)	44(44)	78(37)	149(34)	51(31)	117(28)	Captan
79(100)	80(42)	77(28)	78(19)	151(17)	51(13)	57(13)	92(12)	Captafol
79(100)	82(32)	81(30)	263(17)	77(17)	108(14)	265(12)	80(12)	Dieldrin†
81(100)	267(73)	109(55)	269(47)	323(26)	91(23)	170(21)	173(18)	Chlorfenvinphos
83(100)	108(73)	96(50)	54(47)	111(44)	192(44)	84(34)	55(33)	Diquat (reduction product 1-monoene)
84(100)	58(49)	43(32)	44(24)	42(10)	53(8)	55(8)	86(4)	Aminotriazole (probe)
84(100)	133(21)	42(18)	162(17)	161(15)	105(19)	77(8)	119(6)	Nicotine†
84	178	161	133	118	–	–	–	Nicotine-1′-*N*-oxide
85(100)	145(90)	93(32)	125(22)	47(21)	58(20)	63(14)	75(11)	Methidathion
87(100)	57(81)	43(62)	71(45)	41(42)	69(29)	77(19)	42(17)	MCPB (iso-octyl ester)
87(100)	58(47)	44(40)	61(29)	59(26)	60(25)	45(22)	145(20)	Vamidothion
87(100)	93(76)	125(56)	58(40)	47(39)	63(33)	79(22)	42(21)	Dimethoate
88(100)	42(25)	44(20)	208(18)	73(15)	45(10)	89(10)	76(9)	Thiram
88(100)	60(50)	109(24)	142(17)	79(14)	47(11)	111(11)	61(10)	Demeton-S-methyl
88(100)	60(63)	125(56)	61(52)	47(49)	93(47)	89(47)	63(34)	Thiometon
88	89	97	61	60	153	186	125	Disulfoton
90(100)	153(89)	125(82)	44(67)	63(40)	127(36)	155(32)	62(24)	4-Chlorophenyl isocyanate (GCDP of Monolinuron)
91	58	86	106	231	45	77	230	Norbormide
91(100)	133(70)	161(55)	117(48)	107(47)	160(43)	105(42)	115(35)	Pyrethrin II
93(100)	66(52)	94(6)	67(4)	78(3)	46(3)	54(3)	–	Aniline (GCDP of Fenuron)
93(100)	125(89)	126(68)	42(49)	47(48)	87(40)	63(31)	45(29)	Formothion
94	95	141	64	79	80	111	110	Methamidophos
96(100)	42(53)	70(50)	72(26)	150(23)	122(21)	194(14)	43(11)	Paraquat (reduction product I–monoene)
96(100)	42(64)	148(35)	192(35)	94(22)	122(22)	134(21)	44(15)	Paraquat (reduction product II–diene)
97(100)	65(35)	303(32)	125(28)	359(27)	109(27)	301(25)	357(22)	Bromophos-ethyl
97	109	362	226	65	210	125	137	Coumaphos
97(100)	109(90)	291(57)	139(47)	125(41)	137(39)	155(32)	123(24)	Parathion†
97(100)	195(59)	199(53)	65(27)	47(23)	314(21)	201(19)	125(19)	Chlorpyrifos
97(100)	279(92)	223(90)	109(67)	162(53)	251(46)	65(45)	281(42)	Dichlofenthion
98	176	42	118	41	119	51	175	Cotinine
100(100)	272(81)	274(65)	270(42)	237(33)	102(33)	65(30)	276(28)	Heptachlor†
101(100)	59(95)	41(39)	162(36)	69(28)	63(25)	42(23)	164(23)	2,4-DB (methyl ester)
101(100)	59(70)	77(40)	107(25)	41(22)	142(20)	42(15)	89(15)	MCPB (methyl ester)
104(100)	202(66)	42(42)	174(351	77(24)	103(19)	173(18)	76(16)	Metamitron
105(100)	77(47)	106(10)	292(10)	145(7)	51(7)	294(6)	172(6)	Benzoylprop-ethyl
105(100)	77(46)	276(20)	106(14)	230(12)	44(11)	156(7)	129(7)	Flamprop-methyl
105(100)	77(44)	276(21)	106(18)	278(7)	51(5)	129(4)	156(4)	Flamprop-isopropyl
106	141	77	143	140	142	52	79	Chloromethylaniline
107(100)	69(48)	77(29)	41(26)	81(21)	45(17)	78(16)	57(16)	Ethiofencarb
107(100)	91(69)	135(69)	93(67)	55(66)	121(58)	43(52)	163(48)	Jasmolin II
107(100)	93(57)	121(53)	91(50)	149(35)	105(33)	79(27)	77(26)	Cinerin II
107(100)	168(37)	77(24)	108(15)	78(15)	79(10)	45(9)	51(8)	2-Ethylthiomethylphenol (GCDP of Ethiofencarb)
107(100)	235(91)	203(85)	139(60)	123(46)	95(35)	237(32)	314(29)	Nuarimol
108(100)	219(61)	80(31)	221(22)	65(16)	53(12)	109(6)	156(5)	4-(4-Chlorophenoxy) aniline (GCDP of Chloroxuron)
109	79	110	145	139	47	15	112	Trichlorfon
109	79	185	47	145	187	83	93	Dichlorvos
109(100)	110(72)	79(69)	59(67)	58(38)	47(38)	63(37)	45(37)	Oxydemeton-methyl
109(100)	125(80)	263(56)	79(26)	63(18)	93(18)	47(13)	247(8)	Parathion-methyl
109(100)	185(18)	79(17)	187(6)	145(6)	47(5)	220(4)	110(3)	Dichlorvos†
109(100)	329(48)	331(42)	79(20)	333(14)	93(9)	240(8)	238(6)	Tetrachlorvinphos (probe)
110(100)	41(20)	43(19)	152(13)	81(11)	53(10)	64(10)	111(10)	*o*-Isopropoxyphenol (GCDP of Propoxur)
110(100)	152(47)	43(28)	58(37)	41(21)	111(20)	81(15)	64(13)	Propoxur (probe)
110(100)	156(83)	79(39)	109(32)	58(30)	47(21)	80(19)	44(17)	Omethoate
115(100)	144(78)	116(42)	89(16)	63(15)	145(8)	62(7)	50(7)	Alphanaphthol (GCDP of Carbaryl)
119(100)	72(54)	91(44)	45(38)	64(37)	74(29)	44(28)	73(24)	Carbetamide (probe)
119(100)	91(62)	64(34)	41(16)	63(16)	44(15)	43(11)	50(10)	Phenyl isocyanate (GCDP of Fenuron)
120(100)	77(66)	93(36)	43(35)	51(30)	41(27)	176(23)	104(18)	Propachlor
121(100)	122(47)	45(43)	73(39)	166(38)	165(37)	65(22)	107(21)	2-(1,3-Dioxolan-2-yl)phenol (GCDP of Dioxacarb)
121(100)	122(62)	166(46)	165(42)	73(35)	45(31)	162(21)	51(18)	Dioxacarb (probe)
121(100)	227(94)	228(15)	114(9)	152(9)	122(8)	63(5)	165(5)	Methoxychlor (*op*′)
123(100)	43(52)	55(34)	93(25)	91(24)	81(23)	164(23)	107(20)	Jasmolin I
123(100)	43(62)	91(58)	81(47)	105(45)	55(43)	133(40)	77(33)	Pyrethrin I
123(100)	43(35)	93(33)	121(27)	81(27)	150(27)	107(24)	91(24)	Cinerin I
123(100)	79(40)	43(32)	81(31)	91(29)	136(27)	107(23)	55(19)	Allethrin
123(100)	92(33)	224(29)	167(27)	63(23)	77(22)	226(22)	64(21)	Dichlofluanid
123(100)	171(67)	128(52)	143(49)	81(38)	91(28)	172(25)	45(23)	Resmethrin
125(100)	93(96)	127(75)	173(55)	158(37)	99(35)	55(23)	79(20)	Malathion†
125(100)	109(92)	79(62)	47(57)	63(44)	93(40)	51(26)	277(25)	Fenitrothion
125(100)	127(61)	44(50)	90(50)	99(33)	237(24)	63(23)	43(22)	Drazoxolon (probe)
125(100)	165(64)	75(46)	196(43)	51(43)	101(37)	127(36)	102(35)	Chlorfenprop-methyl

Principal peaks at *m/z*								Compound
125(100)	292(91)	181(90)	47(84)	153(84)	56(73)	79(61)	93(48)	Etrimfos
125(100)	377(78)	47(64)	79(59)	93(54)	109(49)	63(38)	97(37)	Iodofenphos
126(100)	151(91)	166(50)	43(39)	41(32)	51(30)	52(24)	108(16)	2,2-Dimethyl-l,3-benzodioxol-4-ol (GCDP of Bendiocarb)
127(100)	57(96)	41(34)	43(33)	55(26)	371(16)	88(13)	128(12)	Ioxynil (iso-octyl ester)
127(100)	65(48)	63(27)	129(27)	92(23)	52(20)	64(13)	128(13)	4-Chloroaniline (GCDP of Monolinuron)
127	67	58	97	109	192	79	223	Monocrotophos
127(100)	192(30)	109(27)	67(20)	43(8)	193(7)	39(6)	79(5)	Mevinphos†
128(100)	43(26)	42(18)	44(13)	129(11)	55(5)	115(4)	57(4)	Tridemorph
128(100)	43(17)	42(16)	129(10)	70(4)	117(4)	57(4)	91(4)	Fenpropiomorph
132	77	160	105	29	65	76	97	Azinphos-ethyl
133(100)	104(46)	132(45)	78(27)	105(21)	44(20)	91(17)	77(17)	*m*-Tolyl isocyanate (GCDP of Phenmedipham)
133(100)	104(52)	132(34)	91(34)	165(31)	44(27)	78(26)	77(23)	Phenmedipham
136	89	171	125	63	90	78	77	Chloronitrotoluene
137(100)	179(74)	152(65)	93(47)	153(42)	199(39)	97(38)	43(37)	Diazinon
139(100)	107(95)	111(40)	219(39)	141(33)	251(31)	75(30)	53(26)	Fenarimol
139(100)	111(39)	141(33)	75(18)	83(17)	251(16)	113(12)	253(12)	Dicofol (probe)
139(100)	111(66)	141(43)	75(40)	250(26)	44(23)	113(20)	252(17)	*pp*-Dichlorobenzophenone (GCDP of Dicofol)
141(100)	43(93)	71(74)	143(44)	41(42)	77(33)	140(25)	142(24)	Pentanochlor
141(100)	140(37)	106(68)	142(36)	143(28)	77(25)	78(10)	54(8)	3-Chloro-4-methylaniline (GCDP of Chlortoluron)
141(100)	200(51)	115(24)	142(11)	139(10)	201(7)	140(3)	116(2)	2-(1-Naphthyl)acetlc Acid (methyl ester)
141(100)	214(84)	125(68)	155(65)	46(60)	77(50)	89(47)	143(38)	Methylchlorophenoxyacetic Acid (MCPA) (methyl ester)
142(100)	114(41)	157(35)	144(32)	52(20)	116(14)	159(13)	78(13)	3-Chloro-4-methoxyaniline (GCDP of Metoxuron)
142(100)	237(96)	44(75)	214(67)	107(62)	212(61)	144(61)	249(56)	Quintozene
144(100)	115(82)	116(48)	57(31)	58(20)	63(20)	145(19)	89(14)	Carbaryl (probe)
146(100)	72(54)	44(35)	128(29)	45(28)	161(25)	42(11)	147(11)	Isoproturon
146(100)	128(34)	44(30)	161(30)	147(10)	91(4)	118(3)	117(3)	4-Isopropylphenyl isocyanate (GCDP of Propoxur)
146	148	111	75	50	150	113	147	Paradichlorobenzene
151(100)	126(58)	166(48)	51(19)	58(18)	43(17)	41(14)	223(9)	Bendiocarb (probe)
153(100)	154(20)	110(15)	109(15)	152(13)	136(10)	82(9)	80(8)	Lenacil
154(100)	55(45)	42(44)	43(35)	141(20)	128(20)	155(19)	56(16)	Dodemorph
156	50	155	52	157	51	75	102	Paraquat
159(100)	191(57)	103(38)	104(37)	52(32)	51(29)	77(22)	90(21)	Carbendazim (probe)
160(100)	161(99)	117(69)	42(45)	41(41)	162(37)	163(33)	57(31)	Terbacil
161(100)	163(66)	99(26)	90(24)	63(23)	73(13)	62(13)	126(13)	3,4-Dichloroaniline (GCDP of Diuron and Linuron)
161(100)	207(82)	83(52)	137(45)	105(41)	179(41)	133(39)	79(30)	Ethofumesate
161	57	163	217	219	63	165	90	Propanil
161	162	172	257	285	77	208	177	Triazophos
162(100)	42(87)	89(79)	44(73)	76(59)	43(53)	73(39)	45(22)	Dazomet
162(100)	164(80)	59(62)	189(56)	63(39)	191(35)	55(31)	248(27)	Dichlorprop (methyl ester)
162	238	45	146	240	163	91	77	Metolachlor
163(100)	181(79)	165(68)	91(41)	77(33)	51(29)	127(28)	115(17)	Cypermethrin
164(100)	136(84)	135(81)	108(42)	163(35)	69(30)	82(24)	96(22)	2-Methylaminobenzthiazole (GCDP of Methabenzthiazuron)
164(100)	136(73)	135(69)	163(42)	69(30)	58(25)	45(25)	57(25)	Methabenzthiazuron (probe)
164(100)	149(70)	41(27)	58(25)	131(25)	122(25)	51(23)	123(22)	Carbofuran
164(100)	149(86)	131(41)	103(36)	51(35)	122(35)	77(34)	123(33)	2,3-Dihydro-2,2-dimethylbenzofuran-7-ol (GCDP of Carbofuran)
165(100)	311(51)	77(37)	233(31)	69(26)	241(20)	239(20)	166(18)	Fluotrimazole
166(100)	209(17)	167(14)	96(12)	194(4)	55(2)	71(2)	210(2)	Ethirimol
167(100)	132(97)	169(29)	166(26)	168(16)	77(16)	76(12)	51(12)	3-Chloro-4-methylphenyl isocyanate (GCDP of Chlortoluron)
167(100)	135(93)	122(49)	43(41)	68(31)	81(31)	65(27)	149(24)	3-Methoxycarbonylaminophenol (GCDP of Phenmedipham)
167(100)	166(45)	168(12)	165(12)	124(9)	123(6)	122(5)	67(4)	Lenacil (*N*-methyl derivative)
168(100)	153(84)	45(40)	109(37)	91(31)	58(21)	57(15)	169(14)	Methiocarb (probe)
168(100)	153(70)	109(62)	45(44)	91(36)	77(18)	107(14)	65(13)	4-Methylthio-3,5-xylenol (GCDP of Methiocarb)
168(100)	183(72)	140(67)	76(40)	170(33)	112(36)	185(26)	142(25)	3-Chloro-4-methoxyphenyl isocyanate (GCDP of Metoxuron)
168(100)	318(94)	152(88)	304(79)	180(73)	42(71)	109(71)	333(69)	Pirimiphos ethyl
169(100)	143(79)	59(58)	141(57)	228(54)	107(50)	77(47)	125(35)	Mecoprop (methyl ester)
170(100)	60(61)	171(50)	172(49)	205(35)	173(29)	100(24)	207(24)	Chlorthiamid (probe)
170(100)	134(75)	198(74)	257(73)	172(40)	200(31)	108(30)	259(28)	Benazolin (methyl ester)
171(100)	44(26)	128(21)	83(20)	71(18)	98(13)	56(13)	172(11)	Hexazinone
171(100)	65(99)	173(93)	92(43)	52(12)	63(12)	141(11)	106(8)	4-Bromoaniline (GCDP of Meto-bromuron)
171(100)	173(62)	100(31)	136(24)	75(24)	50(19)	99(12)	74(11)	Dichlobenil
173	175	220	73	222	174	191	62	Dicamba
173	340	168	167	165	341	174	322	Diphenadione
176	177	149	57	119	193	41	147	Piperonyl Butoxide
180(100)	223(23)	85(14)	181(12)	55(10)	96(9)	42(8)	43(6)	Ethirimol (methyl ether)
180(100)	223(23)	181(10)	224(3)	42(2)	109(2)	150(2)	71(1)	Dimethirimol (methyl ether)
181(100)	183(97)	109(89)	219(86)	111(75)	217(68)	51(43)	221(41)	Lindane†
182(100)	121(48)	97(36)	184(32)	154(24)	111(24)	65(22)	138(20)	Phosalone†
182(100)	165(74)	89(69)	90(57)	212(48)	51(47)	65(45)	91(38)	Dinitro-orthocresol (methyl ether)
183(100)	163(29)	165(25)	44(15)	184(15)	91(13)	77(13)	127(9)	Permethrin

Principal peaks at m/z								*Compound*
187(100)	124(65)	189(64)	159(28)	126(21)	161(19)	97(10)	191(10)	3,4-Dichlorophenyl isocyanate (GCDP of Diuron and Linuron)
191(100)	193(61)	206(60)	53(57)	208(39)	141(35)	113(29)	85(16)	Chloroneb
195(100)	36(95)	237(91)	41(89)	241(79)	75(78)	239(76)	170(76)	Endosulfan†
196(100)	198(89)	59(82)	55(36)	87(34)	223(31)	200(29)	225(29)	Fenoprop (methyl ester)
198(100)	41(78)	57(54)	43(39)	47(38)	74(36)	61(34)	103(32)	Metribuzin
198(100)	196(97)	197(37)	200(34)	195(32)	170(21)	225(17)	125(16)	Picloram (methyl ester)
199(100)	45(97)	175(94)	145(70)	111(69)	109(68)	234(64)	133(62)	Dichlorophenoxyacetic Acid (2,4-D) (methyl ester)
199(100)	197(97)	90(72)	171(35)	169(31)	65(17)	62(9)	50(8)	4-Bromophenyl isocyanate (GCDP of Metobromuron)
200(100)	43(81)	186(52)	229(52)	214(50)	42(48)	68(48)	44(46)	Trietazine
201(100)	44(96)	186(72)	68(63)	173(57)	96(40)	158(38)	203(35)	Simazine†
201(100)	174(72)	63(12)	202(11)	64(11)	65(9)	175(8)	90(8)	Thiabendazole†
203(100)	201(69)	108(69)	215(60)	44(57)	213(51)	178(45)	205(41)	Tecnazene
203(100)	205(60)	234(27)	188(26)	97(21)	201(20)	190(18)	236(17)	Dicamba (methyl ester)
205(100)	207(75)	42(25)	70(16)	206(16)	162(12)	41(11)	188(11)	Bromacil
206(100)	234(67)	116(51)	174(22)	148(22)	173(19)	89(15)	88(14)	Quinomethionate
207(101)	205(89)	90(27)	63(26)	209(24)	99(24)	126(21)	62(13)	3-Chloro-4-bromoaniline (GCDP of Chlorbromuron)
208(100)	210(31)	76(20)	173(17)	209(12)	357(10)	104(9)	172(9)	Dialifos
209(100)	207(94)	211(32)	238(24)	240(23)	74(20)	109(18)	179(17)	Trichlorobenzoic Acid (2,3,6-TBA) (methyl ester)
213(100)	57(67)	58(66)	198(58)	82(44)	171(39)	43(38)	99(25)	Desmetryne
214	141	155	125	46	77	89	143	Methylchlorophenoxyacetic Acid
214	173	216	229	132	68	138	175	Terbutylazine
216(100)	127(27)	115(27)	157(20)	217(15)	129(11)	143(10)	126(6)	2-Naphthyloxyacetic Acid (methyl ester)
219(100)	221(68)	41(45)	188(41)	190(40)	56(37)	220(32)	42(31)	Bromacil (*N*-methyl derivative)
221	232	97	237	373	65	265	193	Pyrazophos
227(100)	228(15)	114(10)	152(5)	212(4)	63(3)	169(3)	115(3)	Methoxychlor (*pp*′)
233	45	42	59	179	146	109	235	Trichlorophenoxyacetic Acid (methyl ester)
233(100)	45(99)	42(86)	59(79)	179(69)	146(65)	109(65)	235(64)	Trichlorophenoxyacetic Acid (2,4,5-T) (methyl ester)
233(100)	231(82)	44(75)	124(74)	207(72)	73(30)	235(30)	205(26)	3-Chloro-4-bromophenyl isocyanate (GCDP of Chlorbromuron)
235	237	165	236	75	239	82	199	Dicophane (*pp*′-DDT)
235(100)	237(59)	165(33)	236(16)	199(12)	75(12)	239(11)	176(10)	Dicophane (*op*′-DDT)
239(100)	209(41)	43(36)	91(35)	77(33)	254(33)	51(27)	131(26)	Dinoterb (methyl ether)
242(100)	240(62)	244(48)	97(35)	62(33)	61(18)	178(16)	135(13)	2,5-Dichloro-4-bromophenol (Bromophos impurity)
245(100)	182(49)	90(46)	75(45)	63(41)	247(34)	50(32)	51(32)	4-(4-Chlorophenoxy)phenyl isocyanate (GCDP of Chloroxuron)
252(100)	43(53)	57(43)	41(41)	281(37)	253(34)	162(22)	77(22)	Pendimethalin
252(100)	254(67)	324(51)	108(49)	75(40)	322(40)	326(26)	50(22)	Tetrasul
265	308	121	43	266	187	213	251	Warfarin
273(100)	76(53)	228(35)	50(29)	229(25)	274(19)	140(13)	104(12)	Naptalam (methyl ester)
278	125	109	169	79	93	–	–	Fenthion
283(100)	285(67)	202(55)	50(55)	139(37)	63(37)	76(31)	75(28)	Nitrofen
290(100)	276(93)	125(69)	305(53)	233(44)	42(41)	109(38)	93(37)	Pirimiphos-methyl
291(100)	88(77)	276(67)	289(55)	293(53)	248(50)	274(37)	278(32)	Bromoxynil (methyl ether)
292	121	188	130	115	91	128	129	Coumatetralyl
301(100)	299(81)	303(47)	332(29)	142(26)	221(24)	330(23)	223(22)	Chlorthal Dimethyl
303	154	217	44	288	80	260	153	Fenamiphos
305(100)	43(49)	261(38)	307(37)	216(16)	306(15)	42(13)	232(13)	Dinitramine
331(100)	125(91)	329(80)	79(57)	109(53)	93(45)	47(34)	333(29)	Bromophos
373(100)	375(84)	377(46)	371(39)	44(36)	109(36)	75(35)	272(35)	*cis*-Chlordane
373(100)	375(93)	377(53)	371(47)	272(36)	237(30)	75(29)	65(28)	*trans*-Chlordane
385(100)	243(56)	370(41)	127(13)	386(10)	88(9)	228(8)	101(7)	Ioxynil (methyl ether)

Reagents

Acetate Buffer (pH 5): dissolve 13.6 g of sodium acetate and 6 mL of acetic acid in sufficient water to produce 1000 mL.

Acetic Acid: Glacial Acetic Acid: contains not less than 99% w/w of $CH_3 \cdot CO_2H$.

Acetic Acid, Dilute: contains approximately 6% w/w of $CH_3 \cdot CO_2H$.

Ammonia Buffer (pH 9.5): dissolve 10.7 g of ammonium chloride in 40 mL of 5 M ammonia and dilute with water to 1000 mL.

Ammonia Solution, Dilute: dilute 37.5 mL of strong ammonia solution to 100 mL with water. It contains about 10% w/w of NH_3.

Ammonia Solution, Strong: contains 27 to 30% w/w of NH_3.

Ammonium Polysulfide Solution: dissolve a sufficient quantity of precipitated sulfur in ammonium sulfide solution to produce a deep orange solution.

Ammonium Sulfide Solution: saturate 120 mL of 5 M ammonia with washed hydrogen sulfide and add 80 mL of 5 M ammonia. It should be recently prepared.

***p*-Anisaldehyde Reagent:** dissolve 0.5 mL of *p*-anisaldehyde in 50 mL of acetic acid and 1 mL of hydrochloric acid.

Ascorbic Acid Reagent: a 2% solution of ascorbic acid.

Barium Chloride Solution: a 10% solution of barium chloride.

Benzalkonium Chloride Solution: a solution containing 50% of a mixture of alkylbenzyldimethylammonium chlorides.

Borax Buffer 0.05 M: dissolve 19.07 g of borax in sufficient water to produce 1000 mL.

Bratton-Marshall Spray:
(a) 1% sodium nitrite (w/v) in 1% sulfuric acid (v/v). (Add 1.0 g sodium nitrite to 1.0 mL concentrated sulfuric acid in 99 mL water. Store in refrigerator)
(b) 5% ammonium sulfamate (w/v) in water. (Add 5.0 g ammonium sulfamate to 100 mL water. Store in refrigerator)
(c) 2% *N*-(1-Naphthyl)ethylenediamine dihydrochloride in ethanol (95%). (Add 2.0 g *N*-(1-naphthyl)ethylenediamine dihydrochloride to 100 mL ethanol (95%). Store in refrigerator in brown bottle)
(d) Spray in sequence a + b + c
(e) Spray with concentrated HCl
(f) Heat plate in oven at 125° for 10 min

Bromine Solution: Bromine Water: a freshly-prepared, saturated solution of bromine.

Chlorine Solution: a freshly-prepared, saturated solution of chlorine.

Chromic Acid Solution: dissolve 3 g of potassium dichromate in 10 mL of water, then carefully dilute to 100 mL with sulfuric acid with continuous stirring. The solution is stable for one month.

Cobalt Thiocyanate Solution: dissolve 6 g of cobalt nitrate and 18 g of potassium thiocyanate in 100 mL of water.

Copper Sulfate Solution: a 5% solution of copper sulfate.

Cupric Chloride: Dissolve 125 g cupric chloride in 375 mL water and 125 mL methanol.

Dimethyl Yellow Solution: a 0.2% solution of dimethyl yellow in ethanol (90%).

Dithiobisnitrobenzoic Acid Solution: dissolve 10 mg of 5,5′-dithiobis-2-nitrobenzoic acid in 100 mL of phosphate buffer (pH 7.4).

DPST Solution: dissolve 0.5 g of 2,5-diphenyl-3-(4-styrylphenyl)-tetrazolium chloride in 100 mL of ethanol; dilute 5 mL of this solution to 50 mL with 2 M sodium hydroxide immediately before use.

Dragendorff Spray: (a) mix together 2 g of bismuth subnitrate, 25 mL of acetic acid, and 100 mL of water; (b) dissolve 40 g of potassium iodide in 100 mL of water. Mix together 10 mL of (a), 10 mL of (b), 20 mL of acetic acid, and 100 mL of water. Prepare every 2 days.

Duquenois Reagent: dissolve 2 g of vanillin and 0.3 mL of acetaldehyde in 100 mL of ethanol. The reagent should be stored in the dark.

Fast Blue B Solution: a 1% solution of fast blue B salt (diazotised *o*-dianisidine). It should be freshly prepared.

Fearon's Reagent: Dissolve 0.5 g pentacyanoamine ferroate (ammonium disodium salt) in 60 mL 5% sodium hydroxide. Add 3 drops of 3% hydrogen peroxide.

Ferric Ammonium Sulfate Solution: a 10% solution of ferric ammonium sulfate.

Ferric Chloride, Ethanol, Sulfuric Acid: Dissolve 500 mg ferric chloride in 150 mL ethanol and 50 mL concentrated sulfuric acid. DANGER: exothermic reaction. Add acid to ethanol with cooling and stirring.

Ferric Chloride Solution: a 5% solution of ferric chloride.

Fluorescamine: Dissolve 50 mg fluorescamine in 100 mL methanol.

Fluorescein Solution: mix 10 mL of a saturated solution of fluorescein in acetic acid with 15 mL of acetic acid and 25 mL of strong hydrogen peroxide solution. This solution must be freshly prepared.

Formaldehyde Solution: Formalin: contains 34 to 38% w/w of formaldehyde.

Forrest Reagent: mix together equal volumes of a 0.2% solution of potassium dichromate, a 30% v/v solution of sulfuric acid, a 20% w/w solution of perchloric acid, and a 50% v/v solution of nitric acid.

FPN Reagent: mix together 5 mL of ferric chloride solution, 45 mL of a 20% w/w solution of perchloric acid, and 50 mL of a 50% v/v solution of nitric acid.

Furfuraldehyde Reagent: (a) dilute 2 mL of redistilled furfuraldehyde to 100 mL with acetone; (b) dilute 4 mL of sulfuric acid to 100 mL with acetone; prepare immediately before use. Spray with (a) first, followed by (b).

Furfuraldehyde Solution: a 10% solution of furfuraldehyde in ethanol.

Gibb's Reagent: Dissolve 500 mg 2,6-dichloroquinone-4-chloroimide in 100 mL ethanol.

Hydriodic Acid: contains about 55% w/w of HI.

Hydrochloric Acid: Concentrated: contains 35 to 39% w/w of HCl.

Hydrochloric Acid, Dilute: mix 274 g of hydrochloric acid with 726 g of water. It contains about 10% w/w of HCl.

Hydrogen Peroxide Solution, Strong: 100 volume: contains 29 to 31% w/v of H_2O_2.

Hydroxylamine Hydrochloride Solution: dissolve 3.5 g of hydroxylamine hydrochloride in 95 mL of ethanol (60%), add 0.5 mL of a 0.1% solution of bromophenol blue followed by 0.5 M potassium hydroxide in ethanol until a green tint develops in the solution, then add sufficient ethanol (60%) to produce 100 mL.

Iodine Solution: dissolve 2 g of iodine and 3 g of potassium iodide in sufficient water to produce 100 mL.

Iodobismuthous Acid Solution: mix 40 mg of bismuth subcarbonate with 0.5 mL of 0.5 M sulfuric acid and add 5 mL of a 10% solution of potassium iodide, 1 mL of 0.5 M sulfuric acid, and 25 mL of water.

Iodoplatinate Solution: dissolve 0.25 g of platinic chloride and 5 g of potassium iodide in sufficient water to produce 100 mL.

Iodoplatinate Solution, Acidified: add 5 mL of hydrochloric acid to 100 mL of iodoplatinate solution.

Lead Acetate Paper: immerse white filter paper in a mixture of 10 volumes of lead acetate solution and 1 volume of 2 M acetic acid. After drying, cut the paper into strips. Store in a well-closed container.

Lead Acetate Solution: a 10% solution of lead acetate in carbon dioxide-free water.

Ludy Tenger Reagent: dissolve 5 g of bismuth subcarbonate in 15 mL of hydrochloric acid, add 30 g of potassium iodide and then add 85 mL of water very slowly and with constant stirring. For use as a TLC spray, dilute 1 volume with 4 volumes of water.

Mandelin's Reagent: dissolve 0.5 g of ammonium vanadate in 1.5 mL of water and dilute to 100 mL with sulfuric acid. Filter the solution through glass wool.

Marquis Reagent: mix 1 mL of formaldehyde solution with 9 mL of sulfuric acid. Prepare daily.

Mercuric Chloride-Diphenylcarbazone Reagent: (a) dissolve 0.1 g of diphenylcarbazone in 50 mL of ethanol; (b) dissolve 1 g of mercuric chloride in 50 mL of ethanol; prepare the solutions daily. Mix (a) and (b) just before spraying.

Mercuric Nitrate Solution: dissolve 40 g of mercuric oxide (red or yellow) in a mixture of 32 mL of nitric acid and 15 mL of water. Store in glass containers protected from light.

Mercurous Nitrate Spray: a saturated solution of mercurous nitrate.

Mercuric Sulfate: Dissolve 4 g mercuric nitrate in 50 mL concentrated sulfuric acid:water (1:1). Make up to 250 mL with water.

Molybdate–Antimony Reagent: dissolve 10 g of ammonium molybdate in 40 mL of 2 M sulfuric acid; dissolve 0.1 g of sodium antimony tartrate in 50 mL of 2 M sulfuric acid. Mix the two solutions and dilute to 500 mL with 2 M sulfuric acid.

Naphthoquinone Sulfonate Solution: dissolve 0.3 g of sodium 1,2-naphthoquinone-4-sulfonate in 100 mL of ethanol:water (1:l).

***N*-(1-Naphthyl)ethylenediamine Solution:** a 0.5% solution of *N*-(1-naphthyl)ethylenediamine hydrochloride.

Ninhydrin Spray: add 0.5 g of ninhydrin to 10 mL of hydrochloric acid and dilute to 100 mL with acetone. Prepare daily.

Nitric Acid: Concentrated: contains 69 to 71% w/w of HNO_3.

Nitric Acid, Dilute: mix 106 mL of nitric acid with sufficient water to produce 1000 mL. It contains about 10% w/w of HNO_3.

Nitric Acid, Fuming: contains not less than 95% w/w of HNO_3.

Nitrogen Dioxide Vapour: produced by the action of nitric acid on copper turnings. For location in thin-layer chromatography the TLC plate is exposed to the nitrous fumes which are evolved.

Nitroso-naphthol Solution: a 0.2% solution of 2-nitroso-1-naphthol in ethanol.

Perchloric Acid: contains about 72% w/w of $HC1O_4$.

Perchloric Acid Solution: add 15 mL of perchloric acid to sufficient water to produce 100 mL.

Phosphate Buffer (pH 5.6): dissolve 62.4 g of sodium dihydrogen phosphate in sufficient water to produce 100 mL.

Phosphate Buffer (pH 6.88): dissolve 3.40 g (0.025 M) of potassium dihydrogen phosphate and 3.53 g (0.025 M) of anhydrous disodium hydrogen phosphate, both previously dried at 110° to 130° for 2 hours, in sufficient water to produce 1000 mL.

Phosphate Buffer (pH 7.4): (a) dissolve 9.465 g of anhydrous disodium hydrogen phosphate in water and dilute to 1000 mL; (b) dissolve 9.073 g of potassium dihydrogen phosphate in water and dilute to 1000 mL. Mix 80 mL of (a) with 20 mL of (b) to obtain a solution of pH 7.4.

Phosphoric Acid: contains 84 to 90% w/w of H_3PO_4.

Potassium Cupri-tartrate Solution: Fehling's Solution: (a) dissolve 34.64 g of copper sulfate in a mixture of 0.5 mL of sulfuric acid and sufficient water to produce 500 mL; (b) dissolve 176 g of sodium potassium tartrate and 77 g of sodium hydroxide in sufficient water to produce 500 mL. Mix equal volumes of solutions (a) and (b) immediately before use.

Potassium Cyanide Solution: a 10% solution of potassium cyanide.

Potassium Permanganate Solution, Acidified: a 1% solution of potassium permanganate in 0.25 M sulfuric acid.

Silver Nitrate Solution: a freshly-prepared 5% solution of silver nitrate.

Sodium Chloride-Potassium Chloride Solution: mix 140 mL of M sodium chloride with 50 mL of 0.1 M potassium chloride, and dilute with water to 1000 mL.

Sodium Hydroxide Solution: a 20% solution of sodium hydroxide.

Sodium Hydroxide Solution, Dilute: a 5% solution of sodium hydroxide.

Sodium Hypobromite Solution: dissolve 5 mL of bromine in 50 mL of a 40% solution of sodium hydroxide, with agitation and cooling.

Starch-iodide Paper: impregnate unglazed white paper with starch mucilage diluted with an equal volume of a 0.4% solution of potassium iodide.

Starch Mucilage: triturate 0.5 g of starch with 5 mL of water and add this, with constant stirring, to sufficient water to produce about 100 mL. Boil for a few minutes, cool, and filter. It should be freshly prepared.

Sulfuric Acid: Concentrated: contains not less than 95% w/w of H_2SO_4.

Sulfuric Acid, Dilute: mix carefully 104 g of sulfuric acid with 896 g of water and cool. It contains about 10% w/w of H_2SO_4.

Sulfuric Acid, Fuming: Oleum: prepared by the addition of sulfur trioxide to sulfuric acid and is available containing about 30% of free SO_3.

Sulfuric Acid–Ethanol Reagent: add gradually 10 mL of sulfuric acid to 90 mL of ethanol.

Tetrabutylammonium Phosphate, 0.005 M, pH 7.5: PIC Reagent A.
Marketed by Waters Associates Inc., Milford, MA 01757, USA; Waters Associates (Instruments) Ltd, Northwich, Cheshire, UK.

***p*-Toluenesulfonic Acid Solution:** dissolve 4 g of *p*-toluenesulfonic acid in 20 mL of ethanol.

Trinder's Reagent: dissolve 40 mg of mercuric chloride in 850 mL of water, add 120 mL of M hydrochloric acid and 40 g of hydrated ferric nitrate, and dilute to 1000 mL with water.

Van Urk Reagent: dissolve 1 g of *p*-dimethylaminobenzaldehyde in 100 mL of ethanol and add 10 mL of hydrochloric acid.

Vanillin: Dissolve 2 g vanillin in 100 mL concentrated sulfuric acid.

Zwikker's Reagent: mix 40 mL of a 10% solution of copper sulfate with 10 mL of pyridine and add sufficient water to produce 100 mL.

Proprietary test materials

Amberlite XAD-2: polymeric adsorbent beads for adsorbing water-soluble organic substances.
Marketed by Rohm and Haas Company, Philadelphia, PA 19105, USA: Rohm and Haas (UK) Ltd, Croydon, Surrey, UK.

Anabolic Steroid Radioimmunoassay Kits: for nandrolone and for 17α-methyl substituted anabolic steroids.
Obtainable from Prof. R. V. Brooks, Dept of Chemical Pathology, St. Thomas' Hospital Medical School, London, UK.

Carbon Monoxide in Blood: Spectrophotometric Reference Standards.
Marketed by American Hospital Supply Corporation, Evanston, IL 60201, USA: American Hospital Supply (UK) Ltd, Ashford, Middlesex, UK.

Cholinesterase Activity Assay Kit: colorimetric method for plasma or serum.
Marketed by Sigma Chemical Co., St. Louis, MO 63178, USA; Sigma London Chemical Co. Ltd, Poole, Dorset, UK.

Co-oximeter, IL 282: for the determination of carbon monoxide in blood.
Marketed by Instrumentation Laboratory Inc., Lexington, MA 02173, USA; Instrumentation Lab. UK Ltd. Warrington, Cheshire, UK.

Dextrostix: reagent strips for the approximate estimation of glucose in blood.
Marketed by Ames, Division of Miles Laboratories Inc., Elkhart, IN 46515, USA; Ames Division of Miles Laboratories Ltd, Stoke Poges, Buckinghamshire, UK.

Ethanol Assay Kit: enzymatic method for the determination of ethanol in whole blood, plasma, or serum.
Marketed by Sigma Chemical Co., St Louis, MO 63178, USA; Sigma London Chemical Co. Ltd, Poole, Dorset, UK.

Extrelut: a column containing granules of diatomaceous earth with a large pore volume.
Marketed by E. Merck, D-6100 Darmstadt, W. Germany; BDH Chemicals Ltd, Poole, Dorset, UK.

High Performance Silica Gel TLC Plates: with fluorescent indicator and concentration zone.
Marketed by E. Merck, D-6100 Darmstadt, W. Germany; BDH Chemicals Ltd, Poole, Dorset, UK.

Labstix: reagent strips for urine testing to indicate pH, and the presence of protein, glucose, ketones, and blood.
Marketed by Ames, Division of Miles Laboratories Inc., Elkhart, IN 46515, USA; Ames Division of Miles Laboratories Ltd, Stoke Poges, Buckinghamshire, UK.

Paracetamol Assay Kit: enzymatic method for the determination of paracetamol in plasma.
Marketed by Cambridge Life Sciences, Cambridge, UK.

Sephadex LH-20: a bead-formed dextran gel with hydrophilic and lipophilic properties.

Marketed by Pharmacia (Great Britain) Ltd, Milton Keynes, Buckinghamshire, UK; Pharmacia Fine Chemicals, Division of Pharmacia Inc., Piscataway, NJ 08854, USA.

Sep-Pak C-18 Cartridge: a silica cartridge for column chromatography.
Marketed by Waters Associates Inc., Milford, MA 01757, USA; Waters Associates (Instruments) Ltd, Northwich, Cheshire, UK.

Serum-Iron Assay Kit
Marketed by Travenol Laboratories Inc., Deerfield, IL 60015, USA; Lorne Laboratories Ltd, Reading, Berkshire, UK.

Subtilisin A
Marketed by Novo Enzyme Products Ltd, Windsor, Berkshire, UK.

Tox Elut: a column containing granules of diatomaceous earth with a large pore volume.
Marketed by Analytichem International Inc., Lawndale, CA 90260, USA.

Urastrat: a complete quantitative system for the determination of urea nitrogen in serum.
Marketed by General Diagnostics, Warner-Lambert (UK) Ltd, Eastleigh, Hampshire, UK.

E Numbers

E number	*Compound*
E100	Curcumin
E101	Riboflavin
E102	Tartrazine
E104	Quinoline Yellow
E110	Sunset Yellow FCF
E120	Carmine
E122	Carmoisine
E123	Amaranth
E124	Ponceau 4R
E127	Erythrosine
E129	Allura Red AC
E131	Patent Blue V
E132	Indigo Carmine
E133	Brilliant Blue FCF
E140	Chlorophylls
E141	Copper Complexes of Chlorophylls and Chlorophyllins
E142	Green S
E150	Caramel
E151	Brilliant Black BN
E153	Vegetable Carbon
E160	Alpha-, Beta-, Gamma-carotene
E160	Capsanthin
E160	Capsorubin
E160	Lycopene
E160	Beta-apo-8′ Carotenal
E160	Ethyl Ester of Beta-apo-8′ Carotenoic Acid
E161	Lutein
E161	Canthaxanthin
E162	Beetroot Red
E163	Cyanidin
E163	Delphidin
E163	Malvidin
E163	Pelargonidin
E163	Peonidin
E163	Petunidin
E170	Calcium Carbonate
E171	Titanium Dioxide
E172	Iron Oxides and Hydroxides
E173	Aluminium
E200	Sorbic Acid
E201	Sodium Sorbate
E202	Potassium Sorbate
E203	Calcium Sorbate
E210	Benzoic Acid
E211	Sodium Benzoate
E212	Potassium Benzoate
E214	Ethylparaben
E215	Ethylparaben Sodium
E216	Propylparaben
E217	Propylparaben Sodium
E218	Methylparaben
E219	Methylparaben Sodium
E221	Sodium Sulfite
E222	Sodium Bisulfite
E223	Sodium Metabisulfite
E224	Potassium Metabisulfite
E228	Potassium Bisulfite
E260	Acetic Acid, Glacial
E270	Lactic Acid
E280	Propionic Acid
E281	Sodium Propionate
E281	Anhydrous Sodium Propionate
E282	Calcium Propionate
E283	Potassium Propionate
E290	Carbon Dioxide
E296	Malic Acid
E297	Fumaric Acid
E300	Ascorbic Acid
E301	Sodium Ascorbate
E302	Calcium Ascorbate
E304	Ascorbyl Palmitate
E307	Alpha Tocopherol
E308	Gamma Tocopherol
E309	Delta Tocopherol
E310	Propyl Gallate
E311	Octyl Gallate
E312	Dodecyl Gallate
E320	Butylated Hydroxyanisole
E321	Butylated Hydroxytoluene
E322	Lecithin
E330	Anhydrous Citric Acid
E331	Sodium Citrate Dihydrate
E332	Potassium Citrate
E334	Tartaric Acid
E338	Phosphoric Acid
E339	Sodium Phosphate, Dibasic
E339	Sodium Phosphate, Monobasic
E339	Sodium Phosphate, Tribasic
E340	Dibasic Potassium Phosphate
E340	Monobasic Potassium Phosphate
E341	Calcium Phosphate, Dibasic Anhydrous
E341	Calcium Phosphate, Dibasic Dihydrate
E341	Calcium Phosphate, Tribasic
E385	Edetate Calcium Disodium
E400	Alginic Acid
E401	Sodium Alginate
E402	Potassium Alginate
E404	Calcium Alginate
E405	Propylene Glycol Alginate
E407	Carrageenan
E410	Ceratonia
E412	Guar Gum
E413	Tragacanth
E414	Acacia
E415	Xanthan Gum
E420	Sorbitol
E421	Mannitol
E431	Polyoxyl 40 Stearate
E422	Glycerin
E460	Cellulose, Microcrystalline
E460	Cellulose, Powdered
E461	Methylcellulose
E462	Ethylcellulose
E463	Hydroxypropyl Cellulose
E464	Hypromellose
E466	Carboxymethylcellulose Sodium
E471	Glyceryl Behenate
E491	Sorbitan Monostearate
E492	Sorbitan Tristearate
E493	Sorbitan Monolaurate
E494	Sorbitan Monooleate
E495	Sorbitan Monopalmitate
E500	Sodium Bicarbonate
E501	Potassium Bicarbonate
E504	Magnesium Carbonate Anhydrous
E504	Magnesium Carbonate Hydroxide
E504	Normal Magnesium Carbonate
E507	Hydrochloric Acid
E508	Potassium Chloride
E513	Sulfuric Acid
E516	Calcium Sulfate Anhydrous
E516	Calcium Sulfate Dihydrate
E516	Calcium Sulfate Hemihydrate
E524	Sodium Hydroxide
E525	Potassium Hydroxide
E530	Magnesium Oxide
E553a	Magnesium Trisilicate
E553a	Magnesium Silicate
E553b	Talc
E558	Bentonite
E559	Kaolin
E570	Stearic Acid
E621	Monosodium Glutamate
E900	Dimethicone
E901	Wax, White
E901	Wax, Yellow
E903	Wax, Carnauba
E904	Shellac
E907	Wax, Microcrystalline
E941	Nitrogen
E942	Nitrous Oxide
E943a	Butane
E943b	Isobutane
E944	Propane
E950	Acesulfame Potassium
E951	Aspartame
E952	Sodium Cyclamate
E952	Calcium Cyclamate
E952	Cyclamic Acid
E954	Saccharin
E954	Saccharin Sodium
E965	Maltitol
E965	Maltitol Solution
E966	Lactitol
E967	Xylitol
E1200	Polydextrose
E1201	Povidone
E1202	Crospovidone
E1505	Triethyl Citrate
E1518	Triacetin
E1520	Propylene Glycol

Medical Glossary

Abdominal: relating to the abdomen (the part of the body between the pelvis and the chest).

Abscess: a localised collection of pus.

Absorption rate constant: a pharmacokinetic measurement used in describing the distribution of a drug.

Acetoacetylcoenzyme A thiolase: an enzyme that catalyses the synthesis of acetoacetyl coenzyme A from two molecules of acetyl coenzyme A; it can also act as a thiolase, catalysing the reverse reaction.

Acetylation: addition of an acetyl group to a substance.

Acetylcholinesterase: a hydrolase enzyme found in red blood cells and other tissues that catalyses the cleavage of acetylcholine to choline and acetate.

α_1-Acid glycoprotein: an acute phase protein found in blood plasma that is an indication of tissue necrosis and inflammation.

Acidification of urine: administration of agents, such as ammonium chloride or ascorbic acid, to produce acidic urine.

Acidosis: disturbance of acid–base balance of the body as a result of accumulation of acid and hydrogen ions or depletion of the alkaline reserve.

Acrodynia: *see* 'Pink' disease.

Active metabolite: the pharmacologically active product of metabolism of a drug.

Acute renal failure: kidney failure of sudden onset.

Addiction: state of being physiologically and psychologically dependent on a drug.

Adenosine triphosphate: a nucleotide that occurs in all cells and acts as an energy store and is required for various metabolic reactions, including the synthesis of nucleic acids and proteins, and to produce mechanical movement.

Adipose tissue: fatty tissue.

Adrenal medulla: the inner part of the adrenal gland that synthesises catecholamines.

Adrenergic nervous system: sympathetic nerves that liberate noradrenaline at their synapses.

Adrenocortical insufficiency: reduced secretion of corticosteroids by the adrenal cortex.

Agglutination: the clumping together of red blood cells or micro-organisms that is brought about by specific antibodies called agglutinins.

Agonal: occurring at the time just before death.

Alanine aminotransferase: an enzyme found in the serum and body tissues, especially the liver, that catalyses the reversible transfer of nitrogen (as an amino group) for excretion or for incorporation into other compounds.

Albumin: the main protein in blood plasma.

Alcohol dehydrogenase: an enzyme that catalyses the oxidation of many alcohols to their corresponding aldehyde.

Aleukia: a reduced number of leukocytes (white blood cells) in the blood.

Algal: relating to or caused by algae.

Alkaline phosphatase: an enzyme that in alkaline conditions catalyses the cleavage of orthophosphate from orthophosphoric monoesters.

Alkalinisation of urine: administration of agents, such as potassium citrate or sodium bicarbonate, in order to produce alkaline urine.

Allele: any alternative form of a gene that can occupy a particular chromosomal locus.

Allergen: an agent capable of producing immediate-type hypersensitivity (allergy).

Allergic reaction: an antigen–antibody reaction that causes tissue damage and that is triggered by exposure of a sensitised individual to the particular antigen or allergen.

Alopecia: hair loss.

Alzheimer's disease: a form of dementia in which there is diffuse atrophy of the cerebral cortex.

Amanita phalloides: the 'death cap' poisonous mushroom.

Amino acid: any organic compound containing an amino and a carboxyl group.

Aminoglycoside antibiotic: a generic term used for a bactericidal antibiotic that is derived from bacteria of the *Streptomyces* and *Micromonospora* families, such as gentamicin, neomycin, and framycetin.

Aminotransferase: an enzyme that catalyses the transfer of an amino group to another molecule.

Amnesia: partial or total loss of memory.

Amylase: any enzyme that catalyses the conversion of starches into sugars.

Amyotrophic lateral sclerosis: a fatal progressive degenerative disorder that affects the upper and lower motor neurones in the brain and spinal cord.

Anabolic agent: an agent that promotes synthesis of body protein.

Anaemia: a reduction below normal of the blood-haemoglobin concentration due to lack of red blood cells and/or their haemoglobin content.

Anaerobic: occurring in the absence of molecular oxygen.

Anaesthesia: loss of sensation either by nerve or receptor damage or by the administration of an anaesthetic drug.

Anagen: the part of the hair growth cycle during which hair synthesis occurs.

Analgesic: a drug that relieves pain.

Anaphylactic shock: shock due to an allergic reaction.

Anecdotal: based on individual cases rather than on controlled studies.

Angiotensin-converting enzyme inhibitor: an antihypertensive drug that acts by inhibiting angiotensin-converting enzyme and produces vasodilatation and reduces peripheral resistance.

Anhedonia: total loss of interest or enjoyment in former pleasures or activities.

Anorexia: loss or lack of appetite for food.

Anoxia: a total lack of oxygen in the tissues.

Antagonist: an agent that blocks or reverses the effects of another drug.

Antemortem: before death.

Anti-arrhythmic: a drug that is used in the management of cardiac arrhythmias.

Antibiotic: a general term used to encompass all the different antimicrobial drugs.

Antibody: a specific substance produced in the blood as a reaction to an antigen.

Anti-cancer agent: a drug that is used to treat malignant neoplasms (cancers).

Anticoagulant: a drug, such as heparin or warfarin, that inhibits blood clotting and is used in the treatment of thromboembolic disorders.

Anticonvulsant: a drug that is used in the treatment of epilepsy or other convulsive disorders.

Antidepressant: a drug used to treat depression, includes the tricyclic antidepressants and monoamine oxidase inhibitors (MAOIs).

Antidote: a remedy that counteracts the actions of a poison.

Antiepileptic: a drug that reduces the frequency of epileptic seizures.

Antifungal: a drug, such as ketoconazole, that is used to treat fungal infections.

Antigen: a substance that is capable of initiating the production of a specific antibody (immunoglobulin) that reacts with the antigen.

Antihistamine: a drug that antagonises the actions of histamine at H_1 receptors and is used to treat type I hypersensitivity reactions and to alleviate pruritus, nausea and vomiting.

Antihypertensive: a drug that reduces blood pressure.

Anti-inflammatory: a drug that is used to reduce inflammation, includes aspirin, NSAIDs and antirheumatic drugs.

Antiparkinsonian: a drug that stimulates dopamine receptors or enhances the actions of dopamine and is used to treat Parkinson's disease.

Antipsychotic: a drug used in the treatment of psychoses (formerly called a major tranquilliser).

Antiserum: a serum, obtained from an animal that has previously been immunised against an antigen, which contains immunoglobulins against the antigen.

Anti-ulcer: an agent that prevents formation of ulcers or promotes their healing.

Antivenom: a proteinaceous material containing antitoxins that is used as an antidote to poisoning by certain snakes and arthropods.

Antiviral: a drug used in the treatment of a viral infection.

Anxiolytic: a drug that reduces anxiety.

Aorta: the artery that carries blood out of the left ventricle of the heart.

Aphonia: loss of voice.

Aphrodisiac: a drug that arouses sexual excitement.

Apnoea: cessation of breathing.

Arrhythmia: any variation from the normal rhythm of the heartbeat.

Arterial blood: oxygenated blood (bright red in colour).

Arthralgia: pain in a joint.

Aspartate aminotransferase: (aspartate transaminase, AST) an enzyme that catalyses the reversible transfer of an amino group from aspartate to alpha-ketoglutarate to form glutamate and oxaloacetate.

Asphyxia: cessation of breathing that occurs as a result of hypoxia and hypercapnia induced by breathing air lacking in oxygen.

Aspiration: removal, by suction, of excess fluid or gas from a body cavity (*see also* Gastric aspiration).

Assay: determination of the amount of a particular constituent of a mixture, or determination of the biological or pharmacological potency of a drug.

Asymptomatic: no symptoms.

Ataxia: jerky and irregular movements that are a result of defective muscular control.

Atrial flutter: a cardiac arrhythmia characterised by a rapid atrial rate.

Attention deficit disorder: a childhood mental disorder characterised by inattention and hyperactivity.

AUC: area under the plasma concentration vs time curve.

Autonomic nerves: the parasympathetic and sympathetic nervous systems that control cardiac and smooth muscle and glands.

Autopsy: postmortem examination of a body for determining the cause of death or presence of any pathological changes.

Axon: that part of a neurone that carries impulses away from the cell body.

Barbiturate: a sedative drug derived from barbituric acid.

Benzodiazepine: any of a group of compounds having a common molecular structure and acting similarly as depressants of the central nervous system.

Beta-blocker: a competitive antagonist at beta-adrenergic receptor sites.

Beta-glucuronidase: *see* Glucuronidase.

Bezoar: a deposit of foreign hard material in the gastro-intestinal or urinary tract.

Bile: a greenish-yellow fluid stored in the gall bladder and secreted by the liver into the small intestines via the bile ducts; its main constituents are bile salts, the bile pigments (bilirubin and biliverdin), and cholesterol.

Biliary excretion: excretion of a drug or metabolite into the bile.

Bilirubin: a yellow bile pigment that is mainly formed from the breakdown of haemoglobin from red blood cells in the spleen. It circulates in plasma as a complex with albumin and undergoes conjugation in the liver to form bilirubin diglucuronide, which is excreted in bile.

Bioavailability: proportion of a drug or foreign compound absorbed.

Bipolar disorder: a mood disorder in which the patient experiences alternating episodes of hypomania or mania and depression.

Blepharospasm: spasm of the muscles in the eyelid that results in the eye being almost completely closed.

Blood: the red viscid fluid that circulates through the heart and blood vessels; it consists of plasma, erythrocytes (red blood cells), leukocytes (white cells) and platelets (thrombocytes).

Blood bank: a special refrigerator used to store blood after withdrawal from donors until required for transfusion.

Blood clot: a semi-solid mass formed mainly of platelets and fibrin.

Blood urea nitrogen: the urea concentration of blood or serum stated in terms of nitrogen content; it is used as an indication of glomerular filtration rate.

Blood–brain barrier: the membranes between the circulating blood and the brain; some drugs can diffuse through these membranes into the cerebrospinal fluid, others cannot.

Bone marrow: the soft material filling the cavities of the bones.

Botulism: neurotoxicity caused by the exotoxin *Clostridium botulinum* usually as a result of eating contaminated food; symptoms include descending paralysis, gastro-intestinal disturbances, postural hypotension, dry mouth, and dilated pupils.

Bronchoconstriction: narrowing of the bronchial lumen usually as a result of bronchial smooth muscle contraction.

Buccal: relating to the cheek of the mouth.

Calcineurin phosphatase: a protein phosphatase, specific for serine and threonine, that plays an important role in activation of T lymphocytes.

Cannabinoid: any of the principles that can be extracted from cannabis, including tetrahydrocannabinol, cannabinol, and cannabidiol.

Capillary: one of the minute blood vessels that connect the arterioles and venules.

Carboxyhaemoglobin: haemoglobin in which the oxygen binding sites are occupied by carbon monoxide.

Carcinogen: any cancer-producing substance.

Carcinogenic: a substance able to cause cancer.

Carcinomatosis: a condition in which cancer is disseminated throughout the body.

Cardiac arrest: sudden cessation of the heart beat.

Cardiac arrhythmia: any abnormality in the rate or regularity of the heartbeat.

Cardiac failure: inability of the heart to pump blood at an adequate rate for tissue requirements.

Cardiac glycoside: a drug, such as digoxin, that is used to slow the heart rate in some cardiac arrhythmias and to treat heart failure.

Cardiac infarction (myocardial infarction): interruption of the blood supply to the heart muscle resulting in necrosis.

Cardiorespiratory arrest: stopping of the heart and breathing.

Cardiovascular: relating to the heart and blood vessels.

Catagen: the brief part of the hair growth cycle when anagen (growth) stops and telogen (resting) begins.

Catalepsy: term used in psychiatry to describe maintenance of a fixed body posture.

Catecholamine: any of the amines produced in the body (e.g. noradrenaline and adrenaline) that are involved in nerve transmission in the sympathetic nervous system.

Catecholmethyltransferase: a cytosolic enzyme found in the kidney, liver and central nervous system that catalyses the methylation of a catechol or catecholamine.

Catheterisation: insertion of a catheter (a tubular, flexible surgical instrument) into a body cavity to withdraw or introduce fluid.

Central nervous system (CNS): the part of the nervous system consisting of the brain and spinal cord.

Cerebral haemorrhage: bleeding into the brain.

Cerebrospinal fluid (CSF): the clear fluid filling the ventricles of the brain, the subarachnoid space, and the central canal of the spinal cord.

Cerebrovascular accident: *see* Stroke.

Charcoal haemoperfusion: the extracorporeal removal of toxic substances from the blood using charcoal as an adsorbent.

Chelating agent: an agent, such as desferrioxamine, that inhibits a toxin by reacting with it to form a less active or inactive complex.

Chelation therapy: the use of a chelating agent to manage a case of poisoning.

Cholesterol: a sterol found in the brain, nerves, liver, blood, and bile that is the precursor of bile acids and steroid hormones and is also a constituent of cell membranes.

Cholinergic: receptors that are stimulated by acetylcholine.

Cholinesterase: an enzyme found in various tissues, including plasma, that catalyses the hydrolysis of acetylcholine into choline.

Chorea: brief, involuntary muscle contractions and an inability to sustain voluntary contractions.

Chronic interstitial nephritis: chronic inflammation of the interstitial renal tissue that leads to progressive fibrosis and danger of renal failure.

Circulatory collapse: *see* Shock.

Circulatory shock: *see* Shock.

Cirrhosis: damage to cells of an organ resulting in fibrosis (usually applied to the liver).

Clearance: a pharmacokinetic term that usually refers to plasma clearance and is the rate at which plasma is cleared of a substance by processes such as excretion by the kidneys, metabolism, or dialysis.

Clot: a semi-solid mass, as in a clot of blood or lymph.

Clotting factor: one of the substances in the blood (known as factors) that are essential to the clotting process.

CNS depressant: a substance that reduces activity of the central nervous system.

Coagulated blood: blood that has clotted.

Coagulation factor: *see* Clotting factor.

Cognition: the processes in the mind that are involved in perceiving, thinking and remembering.

Colic: acute abdominal pain.

Coma: a state of complete loss of consciousness from which the patient cannot be roused even by powerful stimulation.

Competitive inhibition: reversible binding of a drug that results in inhibition of enzyme activity or antagonism at a receptor site.

Complex partial epilepsy: a seizure with impaired consciousness in which the neuronal discharges remain localised in one area of the brain.

Concretion: a deposit of hard material in a natural cavity or in tissue.

Congener: something that is closely related to another thing or shares the same functions.

Conjugation reaction: a type of metabolic reaction that involves the addition of an endogenous group to a drug molecule to produce a more polar substance that is more readily excreted by the body.

Conjunctiva: the delicate transparent membrane that lines the eyelids and covers the exposed part of the eyeball.

Convulsion: involuntary contraction of the voluntary muscles.

Corticosteroid: one of the 21-carbon steroids synthesised by the adrenal cortex which may possess either mainly glucocorticoid actions (effects on carbohydrate, fat and protein metabolism) or mineralocorticoid actions (effects on fluid and electrolyte balance).

Cotinine: the major urinary metabolite of nicotine.

Coumarin anticoagulant: any derivative of coumarin or any compound that acts like coumarin as an indirect anticoagulant, such as warfarin.

Cramp: an involuntary, painful, spasmodic muscle contraction.

Creatine: an amino acid found mainly in skeletal muscle.

Creatinine: a breakdown product of the decomposition of creatine that is excreted in the urine.

Creatinine clearance: renal clearance of endogenous creatinine (commonly used to provide an estimate of glomerular filtration rate).

Cyanosis: a bluish coloration of skin and mucous membranes caused by excessive amounts of deoxyhaemoglobin (reduced haemoglobin) in the blood.

Cyclo-oxygenase-2 inhibitor: a type of non-steroidal anti-inflammatory drug, such as celecoxib, that selectively inhibits the enzyme cyclo-oxygenase-2 and is used in the management of rheumatic disorders.

CYP3A: one of the forms of cytochrome P450.

Cysteine: a sulfur-containing non-essential amino acid produced by the hydrolysis of proteins.

Cytochrome a-a_3 complex: a complex formed in the electron transport chain that transfers electron to oxygen, reducing it to water.

Cytochrome P450: an enzyme found in the cells of most tissues that catalyses a wide range of oxygenation reactions that are responsible for the detoxification of many drugs.

Cytochrome P450 mixed function oxidase: *see* Cytochrome P450.

Cytochrome-P450 IID6: one of the forms of cytochrome P450.

Cytosolic: relating to or contained in the cytosol (liquid medium of the cytoplasm).

Deacetylation: removal of an acetyl group.

Dealkylation: removal of an alkyl group.

Deamination: removal of an amine group.

Deletion: in genetics, the loss of any part of the genetic material on a chromosome.

Delirium: an acute transient mental disturbance that may be characterised by hallucinations or illusions.

Dementia: a deterioration of cognitive processes or intellectual abilities including memory, judgement, language and abstract thinking.

Demethylation: removal of a methyl group.

Dental caries: tooth decay.

Dependency: a state in which there is a compulsive or chronic need, usually for a drug.

Depolarising substance: a substance that reduces the voltage across a biological membrane.

Depressant: a substance that reduces energy and activity by causing muscular relaxation.

Dialysis: a general term used to describe the removal of waste products and excess water from a patient by diffusion through a semi-permeable membrane, examples of specific procedures include peritoneal dialysis and haemodialysis.

Dialysis dementia: a dementia formerly seen in dialysis patients associated with high levels of aluminium in the dialysis fluid or with aluminium-containing antacids given to control phosphorus levels.

Diaphorase: any flavoprotein that catalyses the oxidation of the cofactors NAD or NADP (see below) using a non-physiological compound (such as methylene blue) as an electron acceptor.

Diaphoresis: *see* Sweating.

Diaphragm: the dome-shaped muscular membrane that separates the thorax from the abdomen.

Diarrhoea: increased frequency and liquidity of the stools.

Diffuse intravascular coagulation: *see* Disseminated intravascular coagulopathy.

Diplopia: double vision.

Disseminated intravascular coagulopathy: a bleeding disorder where there is widespread microvascular thrombosis with tissue and organ ischaemia combined with spontaneous bruising and bleeding.

Diuresis: increased production of urine.

Diuretic: an agent that promotes diuresis.

DNA: deoxyribonucleic acid, the primary genetic material of cellular organisms.

Dopamine receptor: one of several types of receptor that are stimulated by the neurotransmitter dopamine.

Drug compliance: the degree to which a patient complies with instructions for taking their prescribed medicines.

Drug conjugate: the product of a drug metabolism reaction in which the drug is combined with another moiety such as a sugar or amino acid.

Drug receptor: *see* Receptor.

Drug tolerance: the requirement for larger doses of a drug to maintain a constant response or a diminution of response to repeated constant doses of a drug.

Duodenal ulcer: a peptic ulcer (a distinct break in the gastro-intestinal mucosa) in the duodenum.

Dysarthria: impaired speech due to loss of muscular control.

Dysautonomia: dysfunction of the autonomic nervous system.

Dysphagia: difficulty in swallowing.

Dysphoria: disquiet, malaise, restlessness.

Dyspnoea: difficulty in or laboured breathing.

Eating disorder: a disorder, such as anorexia nervosa, where an abnormal feeding habit is accompanied by psychological factors.

Eczema: a term used, often synonymously with dermatitis, to refer to a variety of skin conditions characterised by redness, inflammation and itching.

EEG: *see* Electroencephalogram.

Egestion: the casting out of indigestible material.

Electrocardiogram (ECG): a graphic tracing that represents the electrical currents produced by contraction of the heart muscle.

Electroencephalogram (EEG): a recording of the electrical impulses generated by nerve cells in the brain.

Elimination: a pharmacokinetic term used to describe the removal of a drug from the body, for example by metabolism or excretion in urine or faeces.

Elimination rate constant: a pharmacokinetic definition describing the rate of clearance of a drug.

Emesis: *see* Vomiting.

Emetic: an agent that causes vomiting.

Emetic chemoreceptor: the vomiting centre in the brain, stimulation of which produces vomiting.

Emphysema: an abnormal accumulation of air in tissues or organs; often refers to pulmonary emphysema where there is distension of the alveoli of the lungs.

Encephalopathy: degenerative disease of the brain.

Endocytosis: the uptake of a substance by a cell by invagination of its membrane and formation of a vesicle.

Endogenous: arising from causes within the organism.

Endotoxin: a heat-stable toxin associated with the outer membranes of certain gram-negative bacteria that are not secreted by the cells but are only released when the cells are disrupted.

End-stage renal failure: chronic renal failure that is irreversible.

Enterohepatic recirculation: a recycling of a drug/metabolite that can occur if the compound is excreted in the bile and then undergoes metabolism by the gut flora and is reabsorbed and is subject to metabolism in the liver, excretion in the bile, etc.

Enzymatic hydrolysis: the splitting of a compound by the addition of water and facilitated by an enzyme.

Eosinophilia-myalgia syndrome: a syndrome, sometimes fatal, of eosinophilia (increased white blood cells in the blood) combined with severe generalised myalgia that has been reported in patients taking preparations containing tryptophan.

Epidermal: relating to the external layer of the skin.

Epithelium: the tissue covering internal and external surfaces of the body.

Epigastric: referring to the region of the abdomen lying over the stomach.

Epilepsy: a group of syndromes that are characterised by recurrent epileptic seizures; an epileptic seizure is a paroxysmal discharge of cerebral neurones that may manifest as various clinical signs, including impairment or loss of consciousness, abnormal motor phenomena, or sensory or autonomic disturbances.

EPO: *see* Erythropoietin.

Ergotism: poisoning from eating ergotised grain or from misuse of medicinal ergot.

Erythema: reddening of the skin.

Erythrocytes (red blood cells): non-nucleated cells in circulating blood that contain haemoglobin.

Erythropoietin (EPO): a glycoprotein hormone secreted chiefly by the kidney in the adult and by the liver in the fetus, which acts on the bone marrow cells to stimulate red blood cell production; an erythropoietin that is produced by recombinant DNA technology is available for clinical use.

Esterase: an enzyme that catalyses the breakdown of an ester to produce an alcohol and an acid.

Eumelanin: a type of melanin (black pigment) found in darkly coloured skin and hair.

Euphoria: an exaggerated feeling of well-being (physical and mental).

Exogenous: from outside the organism.

Extracellular: outside the cell.

Extrapyramidal: referring to the parts of the central nervous system that are involved in motor activities but which are outside the pyramidal tract.

Extravascular: situated or occurring outside a blood vessel.

F-actin: a polymerised form of actin, a protein that makes up muscle fibres.

Factor V: a clotting factor found in plasma but not in serum that catalyses the cleavage of prothrombin to the active thrombin.

Factor X: a clotting factor that is involved in both the intrinsic and the extrinsic pathways of blood coagulation.

Faeces: the excrement discharged from the intestines consisting of bacteria, cells exfoliated from the intestines, secretions (mainly from the liver) and a small amount of food residue.

Fatty acid: a straight chain monocarboxylic acid that occurs in fats.

Femoral: relating to the femur or thigh.

Ferrochelatase: an enzyme found in mitochondria that catalyses the insertion of ferrous iron into protoporphyrin IX to form haem.

Fetal: relating to the fetus.

Fetus: the postembryonic developing child in utero (i.e. from 9 weeks after fertilisation until birth).

Fever: elevation of the body temperature above normal.

Fibrin: the insoluble protein matrix that forms part of a blood clot and is formed from soluble fibrinogen by the enzymatic action of thrombin.

Fibrinogen: a soluble plasma protein that is converted to insoluble fibrin by the action of thrombin.

First-pass metabolism: metabolism of an orally taken drug that occurs in the gastro-intestinal tract or in the liver before the drug enters the systemic circulation.

Fit: colloquial term for an epileptic seizure.

Flaccid paralysis: a paralysis that is accompanied by loss of muscle tone and absence of tendon reflexes.

Free drug: drug in the bloodstream that is not bound to plasma proteins.

Fresh frozen plasma: a preparation prepared from centrifuged donated whole blood that is used clinically to replace clotting factors or other plasma proteins.

G-actin: a globular form of actin, a protein that makes up muscle fibres.

Gangrene: death of tissue, usually as a result of inadequate blood supply, that is followed by bacterial infection and putrefaction.

Gastric aspiration: inhalation of the stomach contents into the lungs.

Gastric lavage: irrigation of the stomach.

Gastric ulcer: a peptic ulcer (an ulceration of the mucous membrane) occurring in the stomach.

Gastroenteritis: an acute inflammation of the mucous membranes of the stomach and intestines, usually caused by bacterial infection, with symptoms including nausea, diarrhoea, abdominal pain and weakness.

Gene: a segment of a DNA molecule that contains all the information required for synthesis of a product (polypeptide chain or RNA molecule).

Genome: the complete set of hereditary factors as in chromosomes.

Genomics: the study of the structure and function of the genome.

Genotype: the complete genetic constitution of an individual.

Gilbert's syndrome: an inborn error of bilirubin metabolism where blood concentration of unconjugated bilirubin is raised but there is no blood abnormality or liver damage.

Gingival sulci: a shallow V-shaped space around the tooth.

β-Globulin: one of the globulins present in serum that constitute the majority of plasma protein.

Glomerulopathy: any disease of the glomeruli of the kidneys.

Glomerulus: a functional unit of the kidney that collects the filtrate from the blood capillaries and directs it into the kidney tubule.

Glucocorticosteroid: any of the corticosteroids that regulate carbohydrate, lipid, and protein metabolism.

Gluconeogenesis: synthesis of glucose from protein or fat that occurs when there is insufficient carbohydrate available.

Glucose-6-phosphate dehydrogenase: an enzyme that catalyses the oxidation of glucose-6-phosphate to a lactone, reducing NADP+ to NADPH, which in turn maintains levels of reduced glutathione in cells.

Glucuronidase: an enzyme that catalyses the cleavage of terminal glucuronic acid residues from a variety of β-glucuronides; it is present in the intestine where it can hydrolyse glucuronide conjugates and therefore can contribute to the recycling that is seen with some compounds (*see* Enterohepatic recirculation).

Glucuronidation: addition of glucuronic acid to form a conjugate (*see* Glucuronide conjugate).

Glucuronide conjugate: a water-soluble compound formed during metabolism of a drug that is a result of combination with α-D-glucuronic acid.

Glucuronyl transferase: an enzyme that catalyses the transfer of glucuronic acid to a substrate to form a glucuronide congugate.

Glutathione: a tripeptide, found in many tissues but especially in the liver, which acts as a cofactor for enzymes and also detoxifies harmful compounds.

Glutathione peroxidase: an enzyme found in high levels in the liver that catalyses the detoxifying reduction of peroxides (such as hydrogen peroxide or organic peroxides) via oxidation of glutathione.

Glutathione S-transferase: an enzyme that catalyses the conjugation of a wide variety of substances with glutathione.

Glycosuria: glucose in the urine.

Granuloma: an imprecise term for any small nodule formed by inflammatory cells.

Granulopenia: a reduction in the number of granulocytes (a type of white blood cell) in the blood.

Growth hormone: an anabolic hormone secreted by the pituitary gland that promotes growth of skeletal, muscular and other tissues; a growth hormone produced by recombinant DNA technology is available for clinical use.

Habituation: an older term used in describing drug dependency.

Haem: the iron protophorphyrin group that is the pigment-carrying part of haemoglobin.

Haematocrit: the proportion of the volume of a blood sample that is red blood cells.

Haematuria: blood in the urine.

Haemocyanin: a blue pigment found in the blood plasma of many molluscs and arthropods that can bind oxygen.

Haemodialysis: the removal of waste products from the blood by passing the blood through a dialysis machine.

Haemofiltration: the removal of waste products from the blood by passing the blood through filters outside the body and returning the blood to the patient.

Haemoglobin: the red oxygen-carrying pigment of red blood cells that comprises an iron-containing group called haem combined with globin; it has the ability to reversibly bind oxygen.

Haemolysis: breakdown of red blood cells causing release of haemoglobin.

Haemolytic uraemic syndrome: a syndrome (seen predominantly in children) in which intravascular platelet clumping occurs mainly in the renal vasculature causing renal impairment.

Haemorrhagic colitis: a bloody diarrhoea caused by a strain of *Escherichia coli* that is generally self-limiting but may be complicated by haemolytic uraemic syndrome.

Haemorrhagic diathesis: a predisposition to abnormal clotting and bleeding.

Haemostatic: an agent that stops bleeding.

Hair follicle: the sheath in which a hair grows.

Half life (plasma half life): the time required for the drug plasma concentration to fall to half of a certain measured concentration.

Hallucination: a false perception of an object that occurs in the absence of such an object.

Hallucinogen: an agent capable of producing hallucinations.

HCG (human chorionic gonadotrophin): a hormone produced by the placenta.

Heart block: impairment of conduction of the normal sinus node impulse through the heart.

Heparinised blood: blood that has had heparin added to it to increase the clotting time.

Hepatic clearance: removal of a drug from the blood by metabolism in the liver.

Hepatic dysfunction: impaired functioning of the liver.

Hepatic encephalopathy: a degenerative disease of the brain that usually occurs as a consequence of advanced liver disease; disturbances of consciousness occur that may progress to coma.

Hepatic failure: liver failure.

Hepatic portal system: the blood supply of the liver.

Hepatitis: inflammation of the liver.

Hepatobiliary: affecting the liver and the bile or bile ducts.

Hepatocellular carcinoma: cancer of the liver cells.

Hepatocyte: a liver cell.

Hepatolenticular degeneration: a rare autosomal disease of impaired excretion of excess copper which leads to copper accumulation in the liver, brain and other organs including the kidneys and corneas; also known as Wilson's disease.

Hepatorenal: relating to the liver and the kidneys.

Hepatotoxicity: having a destructive or harmful effect on liver cells.

Histamine: a naturally occurring substance found in all body tissues that has several functions including capillary dilatation, smooth muscle contraction, increased gastric secretion and acceleration of heart rate.

Homeostasis: the tendency to maintain a stable internal environment, such as constant body temperature or blood pressure.

Homogeneous: of the same quality or consistency throughout.

Homogenous: having a similar structure because of descent from a common ancestor.

Hormone: a chemical substance produced by an endocrine gland and circulated in the bloodstream that regulates the activity of an organ or tissues.

Human chorionic gonadotrophin: *see* HCG.

Hyaluronidase: an enzyme that catalyses the breakdown of hyaluronic acid.

Hydrolysis: the splitting of a compound by the addition of water.

Hydrophilic: a substance that has an affinity with water.

Hydroxylation: addition of a hydroxyl group.

Hyperaemia: an increase of blood in an area.

Hyperaesthesia: excessive sensitivity.

Hyperbaric oxygen: oxygen under greater than atmospheric pressure.

Hyperbilirubinaemia: excessive bilirubin in the blood, which may lead to jaundice.

Hyperimmune: having large quantities of specific antibodies in the serum.

Hyperinsulinaemia: excessively high blood insulin levels.

Hyperkalaemia: abnormally high potassium concentration in the blood.

Hyperkeratosis: thickening of the stratum corneum of the skin.

Hypermagnesaemia: abnormally high magnesium concentration in the blood.

Hypernatraemia: abnormally high sodium concentration in the blood.

Hyperpigmentation: excessive pigmentation of the skin.

Hypertension: a higher than 'normal' arterial blood pressure.

Hyperthermia: abnormally raised core body temperature (to above 37.2°).

Hyperventilation (hyperpnoea): increased breathing that results in reduced carbon dioxide tension and alkalosis.

Hypnotic: a drug used to induce sleep.

Hypocalcaemia: low blood calcium concentration.

Hypoglycaemia: decreased concentration of glucose in the blood that may produce symptoms of anxiety, cold sweat, hypothermia and delirium or coma (hypoglycaemic coma).

Hypoglycaemic agent: an agent that controls blood sugar levels and is used in the management of diabetes mellitus.

Hypoglycaemic coma: *see* Hypoglycaemia.

Hypokalaemia: low potassium concentration in the blood.

Hyponatraemia: low sodium concentration in the blood.

Hypophosphataemia: decreased amounts of phosphates in the blood; signs include haemolysis, weakness and convulsions.

Hypotension: abnormally low blood pressure.

Hypothermia: a below normal core body temperature (35° or lower).

Hypotonia: reduced tone of the skeletal muscles.

Hypotonic: displaying hypotonia; solution with a low osmotic pressure.

Hypoventilation: reduced breathing that results in increased carbon dioxide tension.

Hypoxia: low oxygen level in the tissues despite adequate perfusion by blood.

Iatrogenic: any adverse condition that is a result of treatment by a doctor.

Idiosyncrasy: an abnormal individual reaction to a drug or protein or other administered agent.

IgE: one of the immunoglobulins that act as antibodies.

Iliac: relating to the ilium, part of the hip bone.

Immune response: the response of the immune system to an antigenic stimulus.

Immunogen: a substance capable of inducing an immune response.

Immunoglobulin: one of the 5 classes of glycoproteins (IgA, IgD, IgE, IgG and IgM) that function as antibodies.

Immunostimulant: an agent capable of stimulating immune responses.

Immunosuppressant: an agent that can suppress immune responses, such as a corticosteroid or ciclosporin.

Immunotoxic: toxic to or toxicity involving the immune system.

Immunotoxin: a molecule formed by coupling a toxin to an antibody.

Impotence: failure to initiate an erection or to maintain an erection until ejaculation.

In vitro: in the test tube.

In vivo: in living tissue.

Incontinence: inability to control defaecation or urination.

Induce (metabolism): increase/enhance metabolism of a substance.

Inferior vena cava: the main trunk vein that supplies the lower limbs.

Ingestion: the taking in of food/medicines by mouth.

Inhaler: an apparatus for administering a vapour or volatilised medication by inhalation.

Insomnia: inability to sleep; abnormal wakefulness.

Insulin-like growth factor I: one of a group of polypeptide hormones believed to be responsible for many of the anabolic effects of growth hormone.

Interferon alfa: one of a large family of glycoproteins that are produced by virus-infected cells and that confer protection on uninfected cells of the same species.

Interleukin-2: a glycoprotein that stimulates the proliferation of T lymphocytes and therefore amplifies the immune response to an antigen.

International Normalised Ratio: a standardised form of the prothrombin–time ratio that allows for accurate monitoring of patients taking anti-coagulant therapy.

Interstitial nephritis: inflammation of the interstitial tissue of the kidney.

Intoxication: Poisoning.

Intracellular: within a cell.

Intramuscular: within a muscle.

Intraperitoneal: within the peritoneal cavity (abdominal and pelvic cavities).

Intravascular: within a blood vessel.

Intravenous: within a vein.

Isoform: proteins that have the same function and similar structure but are specific to different tissues.

Jaundice: a condition characterised by hyperbilirubinaemia. Mild forms are only detectable chemically; more severe forms present with yellow discoloration of sclerae, skin and mucous membranes that results from deposition of bile pigment.

Jejunum: the portion of the small intestine between the duodenum and the ileum.

Keratin: a protein that is one of the main constituents of skin, hair and nails.

Keshan disease: a fatal disease of the heart muscle caused by dietary deficiency of essential trace elements.

Ketosis: accumulation of ketone bodies in the bloodstream and body tissues due to incomplete metabolism of fatty acids.

Kidneys: the two organs in the lumbar region that filter the blood and excrete waste products in urine and regulate the concentrations of various ions in the extra-cellular fluid.

Kinin: any of a group of polypeptides found in plasma, such as bradykinin, that cause vasodilatation of most vessels but vasoconstriction of the pulmonary vessels and also alter vascular permeability.

Lacrimation: tear formation.

Lactic acidosis: a metabolic acidosis that occurs when cellular respiration is impaired (in conditions such as shock and septicaemia) producing a build up of lactic acid in the blood.

Laryngeal: relating to the larynx (voice box).

Laryngitis: inflammation of the larynx (voice box).

Laxative: an agent that promotes bowel evacuation.

Leptomeningeal: relating to the leptomeninges (the membranes that cover the brain and spinal cord).

Leptomeningeal carcinoma: cancer of the meninges (the membranes covering the brain and spinal cord), specifically the pia mater and arachnoid membranes.

Leukocyte: a white blood cell; there are several different types that are classified into two large groups, granular leukocytes (basophils, eosinophils, and neutrophils), and non-granular leukocytes (lymphocytes, and monocytes).

Leukopenia: reduction in the number of leukocytes in the blood below about $5000/mm^3$.

Lipid: a fat or fat-like substance that is characterised by being insoluble in water.

Lipid-lowering drug: a drug that reduces cholesterol and/or triglycerides in the blood and is used to treat hyperlipidaemias and to reduce cardiovascular risk.

Lipophilic: having an affinity for fat.

Loading dose: a large initial dose that is sometimes given so that therapeutic steady-state plasma concentrations are reached more quickly.

Local anaesthetic: an anaesthetic that produces reversible loss of function or sensation near to their site of application or injection by diminishing nerve impulse conduction.

Locus: in anatomy, a general term for a site in the body; in genetics, the position of a gene on a chromosome.

Lyme disease: an infectious disease, caused by *Borrelia burgdorferi* and transmitted largely by *Ixodes* ticks, that is a multi-system disease affecting the skin in the initial stages (erythema migrans), followed by variable effects on the nervous system, heart and joints.

Lymphatic: pertaining to lymph or a lymph vessel; by extension, the term is used alone to designate a lymphatic vessel or, in the plural, to designate the lymphatic system.

Lymphocyte: a type of white blood cell; there are two types, B lymphocytes that provide humoral immunity, and T lymphocytes that are responsible for cellular immunity.

Lymphocytosis: an increase in normal lymphocytes in the blood.

Lysozyme: an enzyme found in saliva and tears that acts as an antiseptic.

Macrocyte: an abnormally large red blood cell.

Malaise: a vague feeling of illness and discomfort.

Malate dehydrogenase: an enzyme found in the mitochondria and cytosol that catalyses the oxidation of L-malate to oxaloacetate.

Mania: undue elation with hyperexcitability and hyperactivity that occurs usually as a phase of bipolar disorder (manic depression).

Manic-depressive disorder: *see* Bipolar disorder.

Meconium: a dark greenish-black viscous substance that forms the first bowel movement in newborns.

Mee's lines: white lines on the fingernails that can be a sign of poisoning with trace elements and arsenic.

Melanin: a black pigment found in skin, hair and the choroid of the eye.

Meningitis: inflammation of the meninges (the membranes surrounding the spinal cord and brain) usually caused by either bacterial or viral infection.

Mercapturic acid: a cysteine conjugate excreted in the urine that is the end-product of metabolism of a glutathione conjugate.

Metabolic acidosis: disturbance of the acid–base balance due to loss of base or accumulation of (non-carbonic) acid.

Metabolism: the chemical processes that occur in the maintenance of living tissues i.e. synthesis of new tissue (anabolism) and breakdown of old tissue (catabolism); also used to describe the chemical transformation undergone by drugs in the body (biotransformation).

Metabolism inducer: a substance that can enhance the rate of metabolism by increasing the numbers of metabolising enzymes.

Metabolite: any product of metabolism.

Metallothionein: a protein that is involved in the transport of metals, such as zinc, within the body.

Methaemoglobin: a brown pigment that is a form of haemoglobin (but which is unable to transport oxygen) in which the haem portion is oxidised from the ferrous to ferric state.

Methaemoglobinaemia: the presence of methaemoglobin in the blood; symptoms depend on the amount of methaemoglobin present and can range from breathlessness on exertion through to cyanosis, fatigue, nausea and vomiting, and drowsiness which can progress to stupor and coma.

Methylation: the addition of a methyl group to a compound.

Methyltransferase: an enzyme that catalyses the transfer of a methyl group from one compound to another.

Microflora: micro-organisms present in or characteristic of a specific location.

Microsomal enzyme: a general term used for the enzymes found in the smooth endoplasmic reticulum of cells that are responsible for the metabolism of foreign compounds, the major one being the cytochrome P450 system.

Minor tranquilliser: the old term for an anxiolytic sedative, such as diazepam, used for treating anxiety disorders.

Miosis: contraction of the pupils.

Mixed-function oxidase system: cytochrome P450-dependent oxidation reactions.

Monoamine oxidase inhibitor: a drug used to treat depression that inhibits monoamine oxidase (the enzyme responsible for the metabolism of several biogenic amines).

Motility: capable of spontaneous movement.

Motor: a muscle or nerve that produces movement.

Motor paralysis: paralysis of voluntary muscles.

Mucin: a mixture of glycoproteins that are secreted by many cells and are the main constituent of mucus.

Mucosa: a mucous membrane.

Mucous membrane: a membrane or lining that contains glands that secrete mucus.

Munchausen's syndrome: a condition in which the patient repeatedly presents with an apparent acute physical illness and gives a false history.

Mutagen: a substance that causes changes in DNA.

Mutation: a permanent transmissible change in genetic material.

Mycotoxin: a fungal toxin.

Mydriasis: dilatation of the pupil of the eye.

Myocardial infarction: necrosis of heart muscle as a result of interruption of the blood supply to the area usually due to thrombosis at the site of a ruptured atheromatous plaque.

Myoglobinuria: the presence of myoglobin (the oxygen-transporting muscle protein) in the urine.

***N*-acetyltransferase:** an enzyme that catalyses the transfer of an acetyl group, often acetyl coenzyme A, to another compound.

NAD: nicotinamide adenine dinucleotide and its reduced and oxidised forms are used as co-factors in many metabolic drug reactions.

NAD+: *see* NAD.

NADH: *see* NAD.

NADP: nicotine adenine dinucleotide phosphate is used as a cofactor in many metabolic drug reactions.

Narcolepsy: repetitive, uncontrollable episodes of sleep occurring in the daytime.

Narcotic: an agent that produces deep sleep, applied especially to the opioids.

Nasal septum: the partition between the nasal cavities.

Nausea: a feeling of sickness.

***N*-dealkylation:** removal of an alkyl group from a compound where the alkyl group is attached to a nitrogen atom.

Necropsy: examination of a body after death.

Necrosis: localised death of tissue.

Neonatal: the first four weeks after birth.

Neonate: newborn infant up to four weeks old.

Neoplastic disease: generally used to refer to malignant neoplasms (cancers).

Nephrotoxicity: toxicity to kidney cells.

Neuroleptic: a drug that acts on the nervous system and is used in the treatment of psychoses (antipsychotic).

Neurological: relating to the nervous system.

Neuromuscular blocking drug: a drug that affects transmission at the neuromuscular junction and is used to produce muscle relaxation in anaesthesia.

Neuromuscular junction: the junction between the skeletal muscle fibre and the nerve that innervates it.

Neuropathy: damage to the peripheral nervous system.

Neurotoxic: toxic to the nervous system.

Neurotoxin: a toxin that is poisonous or destructive to nervous tissue.

Neurotransmitter: an endogenous substance involved in the transmission of nerve impulses, such as adrenaline.

Non-compliance: failure of the patient to comply with the dosage instructions for his/her medication.

***N*-oxidation:** formation of an *N*-oxide.

NSAID: a non-steroidal anti-inflammatory drug.

Nystagmus: repetitive involuntary and jerky movement of the eyeball.

Organophosphorous insecticide: an insecticidal compound that contains phosphorus bound to an organic compound.

Ocular: relating to the eye.

***O*-dealkylation:** metabolism of an aromatic alkyl ether to give a phenol and corresponding aldehyde.

Oedema: the presence of abnormally large amounts of fluid in the tissues of the body.

Oesophagus: the tube that extends from the pharynx to the stomach.

Oestrogens: a steroidal hormone that controls the development and maintenance of the female sex organs, secondary sex characteristics, and mammary glands as well as certain functions of the uterus.

Olfactory nerve: the nerve supplying the nose.

Opiate: an agent derived from opium.

Opioid: a narcotic with the same properties as an opiate but that is not derived from opium.

Opisthotonus: a spasm with extreme extension of the body with the head and the heels being bent backwards and the body bowed forwards.

Optic neuritis: inflammation of the optic nerve.

Oral adsorbent: a substance, such as activated charcoal, that is given by mouth to bind poisons in the gastro-intestinal tract thereby reducing their absorption.

Oral contraceptive: an oestrogen and progestogen or progestogen-only preparation that is taken by mouth for contraception.

Organic aciduria: excessive excretion of one or more organic acids in the urine.

Osteoporosis: loss of bone density.

Ototoxicity: causing damage to the ear.

Oxyhaemoglobin: oxygenated haemoglobin.

P450 enzymes: *see* Cytochrome P450.

Paediatric: relating to paediatrics; the branch of medicine that deals with the child.

Pancytopenia: reduced amounts of platelets, and red and white cells in the blood.

Papillary necrosis (renal): death of the tissue that forms the papillae in the medulla of the kidneys.

Papule: a small circumscribed elevation of the skin.

Paraesthesia: an abnormal touch sensation (often without any external stimulus), such as tingling, burning or prickling.

Paralysis: loss or impairment of motor function that may be due to damage to the nerves or muscular mechanisms.

Paranoia: behaviour characterised by delusions of persecution or of grandeur, or a combination of the two.

Parasympathetic system: a part of the autonomic nervous system.

Parent drug: the administered drug that undergoes metabolism to form an active metabolite.

Parenteral: administration of a drug (or exposure to a substance) by a route other than the gastro-intestinal tract.

Parkinson's disease: a slowly progressive neurodegenerative disease with reduced brain dopamine activity characterised by tremor, impaired voluntary movement, and loss of postural reflexes.

Parotid gland: the salivary gland.

Pathogenesis: the development and origin of disease.

Pathognomonic: a sign or a symptom that is distinctive to a particular disease and therefore allows a diagnosis to be made.

Peptide: a molecule made up of two or more amino acids.

Pericardial: relating to the pericardium, the membranous sac that surrounds the heart.

Perimortem: the time immediately before and after death.

Peripheral blood: blood in the systemic circulation.

Peripheral neuritis: inflammation of a peripheral nerve.

Peristalsis: waves of contraction and relaxation that pass along the intestines and that move the contents along.

Peritoneal dialysis: removal of waste products from the blood by irrigation of the peritoneal cavity with a dialysis solution.

Perspiration: *see* Sweating.

P-glycoprotein: a cell surface protein found in many cells, including tumour cells where it aids transport of anti-cancer drugs out of the tumour cell and is therefore responsible for drug resistance.

Pharmacodynamics: the study of the effects of drugs and the mechanisms of their actions and the correlation of these with their chemical structure.

Pharmacogenetics: the study of the relationship between genetic factors and the effects produced by drugs (often refers to side effects produced by drugs).

Pharmacokinetics: the study of the absorption, distribution and clearance (metabolism and excretion) of drugs with respect to time.

Pharmacological: relating to the properties and reactions of drugs.

Pharyngitis: inflammation of the throat.

Phase I metabolism: alteration of the foreign molecule (drug) so that a functional group is added or uncovered that can then undergo conjugation in a phase II metabolic reaction.

Phase II metabolism: a conjugation reaction (addition of another moiety) that generally increases the water solubility of the product enabling its excretion in the bile or urine.

Phenothiazine: any of a group of antipsychotic agents derived from the phenothiazine structure.

Phenotype: the physical, biochemical and physiological make-up of an individual (includes genetically and environmentally determined traits).

Pheomelanin: a sulfur-containing type of melanin found in red hair.

Phosphodiesterase: an enzyme that catalyses the hydrolysis of one of the ester linkages in a phosphodiester compound.

Phospholipase: an enzyme that catalyses the hydrolysis of an ester bond in a phospholipid.

Phospholipase A_2: an esterase that catalyses the hydrolysis of a membrane phospholipid.

Piloerection: erection of the hair.

'Pink' disease: a disease of early childhood, usually caused by mercury poisoning, and characterised by pink, swollen fingers and toes and other symptoms that include skin rashes, listlessness, irritability, failure to thrive and photophobia.

Pituitary gland: a gland located at the base of the brain attached to the hypothalamus.

Pituitary hormone: one of the hormones secreted by the pituitary gland, such as gonadotrophin or growth hormone.

Placental transfer: transfer of a substance from the mother's blood to the fetus' blood by passage through the placenta.

Plasma: the fluid fraction of blood; plasma is to be distinguished from serum (see below).

Plasma esterase: an enzyme that acts on ester bonds to produce an alcohol and an acid.

Pleural: relating to the pleura, the serous membrane that covers the surface of the lungs.

Polymerase: an enzyme that catalyses polymerisation, especially of nucleotides to polynucleotides.

Polymorphic: occurring in several or many forms.

Polypeptide: a chain of amino acids.

Polyuria: excretion of an excessive volume of urine, as in diabetes mellitus.

Portal vein: the vein that supplies blood to the liver.

Positional nystagmus: nystagmus that occurs or is altered depending on the position of the head.

Postmortem: after death.

Precursor: in biological processes, a substance that undergoes transformation/degradation to form a more active compound.

Presynaptic: situated just before the synapse (the join of two adjacent neurones).

Pre-systemic: occurring before the drug is in the systemic circulation.

Procollagen: a precursor of collagen, the protein that forms connective tissue.

Prodrug: an inactive drug that, after administration, is metabolised to produce the active pharmacological agent.

Prognosis: a forecast of the probable outcome of a disease.

Prophylaxis: an intervention that is aimed at the prevention of a disease.

Protease: an enzyme that catalyses the splitting of internal peptide bonds in a polypeptide or protein.

Protein: a nitrogenous organic compound that is composed of amino acids.

Protein binding: Non-covalent binding of a drug to a plasma protein (usually albumin).

Protein phosphatase: a hydrolase enzyme that catalyses the cleavage of phosphoryl groups from phosphoproteins.

Proteolysis: the breaking down of proteins into smaller polypeptides.

Proteolytic enzyme: an enzyme that catalyses the breakdown of proteins.

Proteomics: the study of the proteome (the complete set of proteins produced from the information encoded in a genome) under various conditions, as a means of understanding biological processes.

Prothrombin time: the time taken for a clot to form in plasma on the addition of thromboplastin and calcium.

Protozoal: relating to the Protozoa (unicellular organisms).

Provocation test: the administration of a chemical or antigen in order to assess for a response.

Proximal renal tubule: part of the nephron in the kidney.

Pruritus: Itching.

Pseudocholinesterase: a plasma enzyme that is responsible for the metabolism and inactivation of succinylcholine.

Pseudohallucination: a hallucination that the subject knows is unreal and is generated within the mind.

Psychic: relating to the mind.

Psychoactive drug: a drug that has an effect on mental state (also called a psychotropic drug).

Psychological dependence: a substance dependence in which the drug is used to obtain relief from tension or emotional discomfort rather than being associated with tolerance or withdrawal.

Psychomotor: relating to motor effects of cerebral or psychic activity.

Psychomotor skills: the motor effects of cerebral or psychic activity.

Psychosis: a severe psychiatric disorder in which there is disordered thinking and loss of contact with reality due to delusions and/or hallucinations; there may also be mood and behavioural disturbances.

Psychotropic drug: *see* Psychoactive drug.

Ptosis: drooping of the upper eyelid.

Pulmonary: relating to the lungs.

Pulmonary fibrosis: chronic inflammation and progressive fibrosis of the lungs.

Pulmonary oedema: accumulation of extravascular fluid in the lungs.

Pulse: the expansion of the arteries that is transmitted by the contraction of the left ventricle that is usually palpated at the wrist.

Pupillary dilation: dilation of the pupils of the eye.

Purgative: *see* Laxative.

Putrefaction: the process of decomposition or rotting.

Pyrogenic: causing fever.

QT-time: a measure on the electrocardiogram recording between the Q and the T points of the action potential.

Receptor: a molecular structure within a cell or on its surface that binds a specific substance or drug to elicit a specific physiologic effect.

Recombinant EPO: *see* Erythropoietin.

Recombinant growth hormone: *see* Growth hormone.

Rectal: relating to the rectum, the lower part of the large intestine that ends in the anal canal.

Red blood cells: *see* Erythrocytes.

Red cells: *see* Erythrocytes.

Reduced haemoglobin (deoxyhaemoglobin or deoxygenated haemoglobin): haemoglobin that is formed when oxyhaemoglobin releases its oxygen.

Reflux (gastric): a backward flow; usually refers to gastric reflux where the stomach contents reflux back into the oesophagus.

Regime: a regulated programme of an activity, such as exercise, diet or medication.

Regurgitation: *see* Vomiting.

Renal carcinoma: cancer of the kidney.

Renal clearance: clearance of a drug/metabolite from the blood by excretion by the kidney.

Renal dysfunction: *see* Renal impairment.

Renal failure: the progressive loss of renal function so that waste products and metabolites accumulate in the blood; it usually refers to a glomerular filtration rate of less than 10 mL/min.

Renal impairment: a reduced renal function where glomerular filtration rate is between 10 and 60 mL/min.

Renal tubule: part of the nephron in the kidney.

Respiration: the act of breathing.

Respiratory alkalosis: an increase in tissue pH that is a result of excess loss of carbon dioxide from the body, usually caused by hyperventilation.

Respiratory arrest: when breathing stops.

Respiratory failure: a condition resulting from respiratory insufficiency, in which there is persistent abnormally low arterial oxygen tension or abnormally high carbon dioxide tension.

Reticulocyte: an immature red blood cell.

Retroperitoneal: behind the peritoneum (the membrane that lines the abdominal and pelvic cavities).

Rhabdomyolysis: disintegration of muscle, associated with excretion of myoglobin in the urine.

Rhodanese: an enzyme involved in the metabolism of cyanide.

RNA: ribonucleic acid, the genetic material in RNA viruses.

Salicylate: a compound derived from salicylic acid; it is an inhibitor of prostaglandin synthesis and has analgesic, antipyretic and anti-inflammatory effects.

Saliva: the clear, alkaline secretion from the salivary glands.

Salivation: the secretion of saliva.

Sebaceous glands: the glands of the skin that secrete sebum.

Sebum: the oily secretion of the sebaceous glands.

Sedative: an agent that reduces functional activity (may also be called a tranquiliser).

Seizure: a single episode of epilepsy.

Sensory nerve: a nerve that conducts impulses from a sense organ back to the spinal cord or brain.

Serotonin: a monoamine found in the brain, blood platelets and gastro-intestinal tract that has various functions including involvement in central nervous system transmission, vascular spasm and gastro-intestinal motility.

Serous fluid: pertaining to or resembling serum.

Serum: the cell-free and fibrinogen-free fluid that remains once plasma or blood has clotted.

Shock: failure of the circulatory system to maintain adequate perfusion of vital organs.

Skeletal muscle: striated muscle that is attached to bone.

Small intestine: the proximal part of the intestine, comprising the duodenum, jejunum and ileum.

Sodium channel: a protein channel selective for the passage of sodium ions.

Somatic nerve: a nerve that supplies skeletal muscle.

Spastic paresis: a form of paralysis with associated muscle spasms and hypertonia.

Spleen: a large vascular organ in the upper part of the abdominal cavity that produces lymphocytes and plasma cells and also breaks down red blood cells.

SSRI: selective serotonin re-uptake inhibitor, such as fluoxetine, that is used for the management of depression.

Steady-state concentration: the plasma-drug concentration that is achieved with chronic dosing.

Steroid: a term used to denote a naturally occurring lipid, related to cholesterol, that has a particular ring structure, such as the adrenocortical hormones, sex hormones, bile acids and sterols.

Sterol: a steroid, such as cholesterol or ergosterol, that has a ring structure with a long side-chain at position 17 and at least one alcoholic hydroxyl group, usually at position 3.

Stimulant drug: an agent or remedy that produces stimulation.

Striated muscle: a muscle that has the appearance of fine stripes, e.g. cardiac and voluntary muscle.

Stupor: a state of marked impairment of consciousness that only responds to vigorous stimulation.

Subclavian: below the clavicle (collar-bone).

Subcutaneous: underneath the skin.

Sublingual: underneath the tongue.

Sublingual glands: salivary glands underneath the tongue.

Submandibular glands: salivary glands underneath the jaw.

Substrate: a substance upon which an enzyme acts.

Sudoresis: *see* Sweating.

Sulfhaemoglobin: (sulphaemoglobin, sulphmethaemoglobin) a sulfide oxidation product of haemoglobin that cannot transport oxygen or carbon dioxide and is formed in the body by certain drugs.

Sulfotransferase: an enzyme that catalyses the transfer of a sulfate group.

Sulfoxidation: the addition of an oxygen atom to the sulfur atom of an organic compound to form a sulfoxide.

Suppository: a solid dosage form, administered usually rectally or vaginally, in which the drug is dispersed in a base that is solid at room temperature but melts or dissolves at body temperature.

Surrogate: a substitute.

Sweat: the liquid secreted by the sweat glands.

Sweating: the secretion of sweat.

Sympathetic: a part of the autonomic nervous system.

Symptom: any subjective evidence of disease.

Synaesthesia: a sense impairment where stimulus of one part of the body may produce a sensation in a different part of the body or in a different sense, for example a sound produces a sensation of colour.

Synergism: when the effect produced by two substances together is greater than the additive effect of the two compounds.

Systemic circulation: the general circulation that carries oxygenated blood from the left side of the heart to the tissues of the body, and returns the venous blood to the heart.

Systemic lupus erythematosus: an auto-immune disease, more common in women, that is characterised by tissue damage involving the skin, joints, kidneys, central nervous system and other organs, with the most common symptom being arthralgia or arthritis.

Tachyarrhythmia: any disturbance of the heart rhythm in which the heart rate is abnormally increased.

Tachycardia: excessive rapidity in the action of the heart.

Telogen phase: the resting third phase of the hair growth cycle that follows catagen.

Teratogen: any agent or factor capable of disrupting fetal development and producing malformation.

Tetanus: uncontrolled muscle spasm that is caused by the neurotoxin produced by the bacillus *Clostridium tetani.*

Therapeutic index: the ratio of the median lethal dose to the median effective dose.

Therapeutic range: *see* Therapeutic window.

Therapeutic window: the range between the minimum and maximum doses of a drug.

Thoracic: relating to or affecting the thorax (chest).

Thrombocytopenic purpura: any form of purpura (spontaneous extravasation of blood from capillaries into the skin) in which the platelet count is decreased.

Thyroid: gland that sits on both sides of the windpipe and secretes thyroxine that controls the rate of metabolism.

Tinnitus: a sound in the ears such as buzzing, ringing, roaring or clicking.

Tissue plasminogen activator: an endogenous enzyme that converts plasminogen in blood clots to fibrinolysin that results in breakdown of the clot; several types of tissue plasminogen activator are available for clinical use for the treatment of thromboembolic disorders.

Tolerance: a decreasing response to a stimulus after prolonged exposure (*see also* Drug tolerance).

Torsade de pointes: a potentially lethal ventricular tachycardia with a characteristic ECG pattern.

Toxin: a poison.

Trachea: the windpipe that descends from the larynx to the bronchi.

Tranquilliser: a drug with a calming or soothing effect (usually refers to an anti-anxiety agent, also known as a minor tranquilliser).

Transferrin: a serum glycoprotein that binds and transports iron.

Transfusion: the introduction of blood (whole blood or blood components) directly into a blood vessel.

Transit time: a measure of the time required for faeces to pass through the colon.

Transplant: an organ or tissue that is removed from its site in the body and grafted into another site or into another individual.

Tremor: an involuntary trembling.

Tricyclic antidepressant: an antidepressant drug that possesses a three-ring molecular structure and that inhibits the neuronal re-uptake of noradrenaline in the central nervous system.

Trophic: relating to nutrition.

Trough concentration: the minimum plasma-drug concentration that occurs before administration of the following dose.

Trypsin: an enzyme present in pancreatic secretions that catalyses the breakdown of protein.

L-tryptophan: an amino acid that is an essential constituent of the diet.

Tuberculostatic drug: a drug, such as isoniazid or rifampicin, that is used in the treatment of tuberculosis.

Tubular necrosis (renal): severe damage or necrosis of the tubule cells of the kidney that causes acute renal failure.

Tyrosine hydroxylase: an enzyme found in the brain that activates molecular oxygen to catalyse the hydroxylation of tyrosine to dopa.

Uraemia: retentionin the blood of urea, creatinine and other nitrogenous products of protein metabolism.

Urea: the end-product of protein metabolism that is excreted in the urine.

Urea nitrogen: the urea concentration of blood or serum expressed in terms of nitrogen content.

Uridine diphosphate glucuronosyltransferase: one of the enzymes involved in glucuronide formation.

Urinary retention: accumulation of urine within the bladder due to inability to urinate.

Urine: the fluid excreted by the kidneys.

Urticaria: a usually transient allergic skin reaction consisting of itchy, pinkish, raised wheals.

Vaccine: a suspension or extract of attenuated or killed micro-organisms used for the prevention or treatment of infectious diseases.

Vaginal: relating to the vagina.

Vasculopathy: any disorder of the blood vessels.

Vasodilator: causing dilation of the blood vessels.

Vasospasm: a spasm of blood vessels producing vasoconstriction.

Venepuncture: insertion of a needle into a vein.

Venous blood: blood obtained from a vein.

Vertical nystagmus: an up-and-down movement of the eyes.

Vesicle: a small bladder or sac containing fluid; a skin blister.

Visual acuity: sharpness of vision.

Vitamin: a substance that is found in many foods in small amounts and is necessary in trace amounts for the normal metabolic functioning of the body.

Vitreous humour: the transparent jelly-like substance that fills the cavity inside the eye-ball between the lens and the retina.

Volume of distribution: the apparent volume of body fluids into which a drug is distributed.

Vomiting: the forcible expulsion of the stomach contents through the mouth.

Vomitus: matter that has been vomited.

Washout: irrigation or lavage of a body cavity (often the stomach).

Wheal: an itchy skin reaction, typical of urticaria, with smooth blister-type lesions that are redder or paler than the surrounding skin.

Whole blood: blood from which none of the elements have been removed.

Wilson's disease: *see* Hepatolenticular degeneration.

Withdrawal symptoms: a substance-specific mental disorder that follows the cessation of use or reduction in intake of a psychoactive substance that had been regularly used to induce a state of intoxication.

Wolff-Parkinson-White syndrome: a disturbed heart rhythm where there is atrial fibrillation in association with pre-excitation.

Xanthine: a purine derivative, such as theophylline, used for its bronchodilator properties.

Xenobiotic: a chemical foreign to a given biological system.

Subject Index

B

C

D

E

G

H

I

J

K

L

N

O

P

T